GOLDMAN-CECIL MEDICINE

GOLDMAN-CECIL MEDICINE

27TH EDITION

Volume 1

EDITED BY

LEE GOLDMAN, MD, MPH

Cournand and Richards Professor of Cardiology, Columbia University Vagelos College of Physicians and Surgeons
Professor of Epidemiology, Mailman School of Public Health
Dean Emeritus, Faculties of Health Sciences and Medicine, Columbia University Irving Medical Center
New York, New York

KATHLEEN A. COONEY, MD

George Barth Geller Distinguished Professor and Chair, Department of Medicine
Duke University School of Medicine
Durham, North Carolina

ELSEVIER

Elsevier
1600 John F. Kennedy Blvd.
Ste 1800
Philadelphia, PA 19103-2899

GOLDMAN-CECIL MEDICINE, TWENTY-SEVENTH EDITION

ISBN: 978-0-323-93038-3
Volume 1 ISBN: 978-0-323-93034-5
Volume 2 ISBN: 978-0-323-93035-2

INTERNATIONAL EDITION

ISBN: 978-0-323-93039-0
IE Volume 1 ISBN: 978-0-323-93036-9
IE Volume 2 ISBN: 978-0-323-93037-6

Notice

Practitioners and researchers must always rely on their own experience and knowledge in evaluating and using any information, methods, compounds or experiments described herein. Because of rapid advances in the medical sciences, in particular, independent verification of diagnoses and drug dosages should be made. To the fullest extent of the law, no responsibility is assumed by Elsevier, authors, editors or contributors for any injury and/or damage to persons or property as a matter of products liability, negligence or otherwise, or from any use or operation of any methods, products, instructions, or ideas contained in the material herein.

Publishing Director, Medical Reference Content: Dolores Meloni
Senior Content Development Manager: Laura Schmidt
Publishing Services Manager: Catherine Jackson
Senior Project Manager: Daniel Fitzgerald
Designer: Maggie Reid

Printed in India

Last digit is the print number: 9 8 7 6 5 4 3 2

ASSOCIATE EDITORS

Kirsten Bibbins-Domingo, PhD, MD
Lee Goldman, MD Professor of Medicine and Professor of Epidemiology and Biostatistics, University of California, San Francisco School of Medicine, San Francisco, California
Editor in Chief, Journal of the American Medical Association (JAMA) and the JAMA Network, Chicago, Illinois

Mary K. Crow, MD
Professor of Medicine, Weill Medical College of Cornell University
Mary K. Crow, MD Chair in Immunology and Inflammation Research, Hospital for Special Surgery
New York, New York

Nancy E. Davidson, MD
Professor of Medicine, Raisbeck Endowed Chair, and Chief, Division of Medical Oncology, University of Washington School of Medicine
Executive Vice President, Fred Hutchinson Cancer Center
Seattle, Washington

Jeffrey M. Drazen, MD
Distinguished Parker B. Francis Professor of Medicine, Harvard Medical School
Senior Physician, Department of Medicine, Brigham and Women's Hospital
Editor, NEJM Group
Boston, Massachusetts

Victoria J. Fraser, MD
Adolphus Busch Professor and Chair, Department of Medicine, Washington University School of Medicine in St. Louis
St. Louis, Missouri

Ali G. Gharavi, MD
Jay Meltzer Professor and Chief, Division of Nephrology, Columbia University Vagelos College of Physicians and Surgeons
New York, New York

Anthony N. Hollenberg, MD
John Wade Professor and Chair, Department of Medicine, Boston University Chobanian & Avedisian School of Medicine
Physician-in-Chief, Boston Medical Center
Boston, Massachusetts

S. Claiborne Johnston, MD, PhD
Adjunct Professor of Neurology, University of California, San Francisco School of Medicine
San Francisco, California

Anil K. Rustgi, MD
Herbert and Florence Irving Professor of Medicine and Director, Herbert Irving Comprehensive Cancer Center, Columbia University Vagelos College of Physicians and Surgeons
Chief, New York-Presbyterian Hospital/Columbia University Irving Medical Center Cancer Service
New York, New York

PREFACE

In the more than 95 years since the first edition of the *Cecil Textbook of Medicine* was published, almost everything we know about internal medicine has changed. Progress in medical science is now occurring at an ever-accelerating pace, and it is doing so within the framework of transformational changes in biomedical science, clinical practice, and the delivery of health care at individual, societal, and global levels. This textbook and its associated electronic products incorporate the latest medical knowledge in multiple formats that should appeal to students and seasoned practitioners, regardless of how they prefer to access this rapidly changing information.

Even as *Cecil's* specific information has changed, however, we have remained true to the tradition of a comprehensive textbook of medicine that carefully explains the *why* (the underlying genetics, genomics, and pathobiology of disease) and the *how* (now expected to be evidence-based from randomized controlled trials and meta-analyses). Descriptions of physiology and pathophysiology include the latest genetic advances in a practical format that strives to be useful to the nonexpert so that care can truly be as precise and personalized as possible.

Medicine has entered an era when the acuity of illness and the limited time available to evaluate a patient threaten the ability of physicians to satisfy their intellectual curiosity. As a result, the acquisition of information, quite easily achieved in this era, is often confused with knowledge. We have attempted to address this dilemma with a textbook that not only informs but also stimulates new questions and gives a glimpse of the future path to new knowledge. Grade A evidence is specifically highlighted in the text and referenced at the end of each chapter.

In addition to the information provided in the printed textbook and its electronic version, *Cecil* is commonly accessed on Elsevier's electronic Clinical Key platform. *Cecil* content and graphics are specifically organized to optimize not only its readability but also the searchability and utility of these electronic versions, which are continuously updated to incorporate new Grade A references and other evidence.

The section for each organ system begins with a chapter that summarizes an approach to patients with suspected or known dysfunction of that organ system. As summarized in E-Table 1-1, the text specifically provides clear, concise information regarding how a physician should approach more than 150 common symptoms, signs, and laboratory abnormalities, usually with a flow diagram, a table, or both for easy reference. In this way, *Cecil* remains a comprehensive text to guide diagnosis and therapy, not only for patients with suspected or known diseases, but also for patients who may have undiagnosed symptoms or signs that require an initial evaluation.

Just as each edition brings new authors, it also reminds us of our gratitude to past editors and authors. Previous senior editors of *Cecil* include a short but remarkably distinguished group of leaders of American medicine: Russell Cecil, Robert Loeb, Paul Beeson, Walsh McDermott, James Wyngaarden, Lloyd H. Smith, Jr., Fred Plum, J. Claude Bennett, Dennis Ausiello, and Andrew Schafer. As we welcome a group of outstanding new editors—Kathleen A. Cooney, Kirsten Bibbins-Domingo, Victoria J. Fraser, Ali G. Gharavi, Anthony N. Hollenberg, and S. Claiborne Johnston—we also express our appreciation to Robert C. Griggs, Donald W. Landry, Wendy Levinson, W. Michael Scheld, Allen M. Spiegel, and other associate editors from previous editions on whose foundation we continue to build. Our returning associate editors—Mary K. Crow, Nancy E. Davidson, Jeffrey M. Drazen, Anil K. Rustgi—continue to make critical contributions to the selection of authors and the review and approval of all chapters in their respective sections.

The tradition of *Cecil* is that all chapters are written by distinguished experts in each field. All told, our 409 chapters and the Appendix are written by approximately 570 individual authors. Steven A. Seifert, an author of the chapter on "Envenomation, Bites, and Stings," passed away after submitting his chapter, and we deeply mourn his passing.

The editors are most grateful for the superb editorial assistance of Maribel Lim, who expertly coordinated a team that included Caroline Davidson, Pamela Ehn, Julie Mangoff, and Joan Dupont, and without whose dedication, perseverance, and attention to detail this book never would have been possible. At Elsevier, we are most indebted to Dolores Meloni, Laura Schmidt, Daniel Fitzgerald, and Maggie Reid—dedicated professionals who have been critical to the planning and production of this edition.

This edition of *Goldman-Cecil Medicine* includes many new authors. We would also like to thank outgoing authors, who often provided figures that are included in this edition as well as tables that have been included or modified for this edition. Furthermore, because of the templated format and extensive editing that are characteristic of *Goldman-Cecil Medicine*, some new chapters incorporate principles, concepts, and organizational aspects from those prior chapters, often revised extensively prior to publication. Prior authors whose 26th edition coauthors have revised and updated their chapters include: Jeffrey L. Anderson, Gerald B. Appel, David Atkins, Richard L. Barbano, Stephen G. Baum, Hasan Bazari, George A. Beller, Paul D. Berk, Philip J. Bierman, Michael R. Bishop, William A. Blattner, William Bonnez, David M. Buchner, Edgar M. Carvalho, Troy E. Daniels, W. Lawrence Drew, George L. Drusano, David O. Freedman, John N. Galgiani, Jeffrey S. Ginsberg, Colleen Hadigan, Frederick G. Hayden, Douglas C. Heimburger, Edward W. Hook, III, Michael R. Jaff, Alain Joffe, Sian Jones, Carol A. Kauffman, Anthony E. Lang, Geoffrey S.F. Ling, Kieren A. Marr, Eric L. Matteson, William J. McKenna, Theodore E. Nash, Lindsay E. Nicolle, David L. Paterson, Srinivasa N. Raja, Daniel E. Rusyniak, George Sakoulas, Robert A. Salata, William Schaffner, W. Michael Scheld, Harry Shamoon, Richard M. Siegel, David P. Steensma, Raymond A. Strikas, and Ronald B. Turner. Special thanks also to Morton J. Kern, Gary S. Firestein, and Stephanie M. Stanford, whose excellent chapters were eliminated to save space, with their key information shortened and incorporated into other chapters. We also thank other non-returning authors from the 26th edition, many of whom had contributed to multiple editions: Grover C. Bagby, Thomas P. Bleck, Olaf A. Bodamer, Patrick J. Bosque, Lucy Breakwell, John C. Byrd, Clara Camaschella, Jane A. Cauley, William P. Cheshire, Jr., Arun Chockalingam, Steven L. Cohn, David S. Cooper, Joseph Craft, Mark R. Cullen, Stephen C. Dreskin, Thomas D. DuBose, Jr., Herbert L. DuPont, George M. Eliopoulos, Jerrold J. Ellner, Joel D. Ernst, Gregory T. Everson, Amelia Evoli, Martyn A. French, Susan I. Gerber, Dale N. Gerding, Matthew R. Golden, Richard M. Gore, Leslie C. Grammer, M. Lindsay Grayson, Lev M. Grinberg, Rajesh Gupta, H. Hunter Handsfield, David J. Hunter, Karen R. Jacobson, Stuart Johnson, Jacqueline Jonklaas, Gerald T. Keusch, Alexander Kratz, Virginia Byers Kraus, Frank A. Lederle, William M. Lee, James E. Leggett, Glenn N. Levine, Marc S. Levine, Bennett Lorber, Daniel R. Lucey, Peter Manu, Xavier Mariette, Thomas J. Marrie, Emeran A. Mayer, Stephan A. Mayer, Graeme Meintjes, Jonathan W. Mink, William E. Mitch, Bruce A. Molitoris, José G. Montoya, Daniel M. Musher, Stanley J. Naides, Anne T. Neff, Anne B. Newman, Gaetane Nocturne, James R. O'Dell, Pablo C. Okhuysen, Pankaj Jay Pasricha, Manisha Patel, Michael A. Pesce, James D. Ralston, Adam J. Ratner, Susan E. Reef, David B. Reuben, Karen Rosene-Montella, Renato M. Santos, Sam Schulman, Wun-Ju Shieh, Michael S. Simberkoff, Eric J. Small, Magdalena E. Sobieszczyk, Roland W. Sutter, Ronald G. Victor, Angela Vincent, Tonia L. Vincent, Edward H. Wagner, John T. Watson, David A. Weinstein, Anita K.M. Zaidi, Sherif Zaki, and Thomas Ziegler. We also thank Peter S. Aronson, who contributed to the chapter on "Acid-Base Disorders"; Ghada Hijazi, who contributed to the chapter on "Glycogen Storage Diseases"; Alexander Hillel, who contributed to the chapter on "Throat Disorders"; and Jason Pan, who contributed to the chapter on "Hepatic Failure and Liver Transplantation." Chapters written by public employees reflect recommendations and conclusions of the authors and do not necessarily reflect the official position of the entity for which they work.

My work on this and previous editions would not have been possible without mentors such as Robert Gifford, Eugene Braunwald, P. Roy Vagelos, and the late Lloyd H. Smith, Jr. I am also especially indebted to Jill and the entire Goldman family (Jeff, Abigail, Mira, Samuel, Daniel, Morgan, Quincy, Robyn, Tobin, Dashel, and Alden), who have not only tolerated but actually inspired the countless hours required to edit a book that attempts to sustain the *Cecil* tradition and to meet the needs of today's physicians.

LEE GOLDMAN, MD, MPH

CONTRIBUTORS

Charles S. Abrams, MD
Francis C. Wood Professor of Medicine, University of Pennsylvania Perelman School of Medicine, Philadelphia, Pennsylvania
Thrombocytopenia

Ronald S. Adler, MD, PhD
Professor of Radiology, New York University Grossman School of Medicine; NYU Langone Health, New York, New York
Imaging Studies in the Rheumatic Diseases

Anupam Agarwal, MD
Senior Vice President for Medicine and Dean, University of Alabama at Birmingham Heersink School of Medicine, Birmingham, Alabama
Acute Kidney Injury

Cem Akin, MD, PhD
Professor of Medicine, University of Michigan, Ann Arbor, Michigan
Mastocytosis

Allen J. Aksamit, Jr., MD
Professor of Neurology, Mayo Clinic College of Medicine and Science, Rochester, Minnesota
Encephalitis

Qais Al-Awqati, MB ChB
Robert F. Loeb Professor of Medicine and Professor of Physiology & Cellular Biophysics, Columbia University Vagelos College of Physicians and Surgeons, New York, New York
Structure and Function of the Kidneys; Disorders of Sodium and Water

Upton D. Allen, MBBS, MSc
Professor of Pediatrics, University of Toronto; Head, Division of Infectious Diseases, The Hospital for Sick Children, Toronto, Ontario, Canada
Epstein-Barr Virus Infection

Ban Mishu Allos, MD
Associate Professor of Medicine, Vanderbilt University School of Medicine, Nashville, Tennessee
Campylobacter *Infections*

Derek C. Angus, MD, MPH
Distinguished Professor and Mitchell P. Fink Endowed Chair, Department of Critical Care Medicine, University of Pittsburgh School of Medicine, Pittsburgh, Pennsylvania
Approach to the Patient with Shock

Frederick R. Appelbaum, MD
Professor of Medicine, University of Washington School of Medicine; Executive Senior Vice President and Deputy Director, Clinical Research Division, Fred Hutchinson Cancer Center, Seattle, Washington
The Acute Leukemias

James O. Armitage, MD
Professor of Internal Medicine, University of Nebraska Medical Center College of Medicine, Omaha, Nebraska
Non-Hodgkin Lymphomas

April W. Armstrong, MD, MPH
Professor of Dermatology and Associate Dean for Clinical Research, Keck School of Medicine of USC, Los Angeles, California
Principles of Therapy of Skin Diseases

Deborah K. Armstrong, MD
Professor of Oncology and Professor of Gynecology and Obstetrics, Johns Hopkins University School of Medicine, Baltimore, Maryland
Gynecologic Cancers

M. Amin Arnaout, MD
Professor of Medicine and Chief Emeritus, Division of Nephrology, Massachusetts General Hospital and Harvard Medical School, Boston, Massachusetts
Cystic Kidney Diseases

Robert M. Arnold, MD
Distinguished Service Professor of Medicine, University of Pittsburgh School of Medicine; Chief Medical Officer, UPMC Health System Palliative and Supportive Institute, Pittsburgh, Pennsylvania
Palliative Care

Louise Aronson, MD, MFA
Professor of Geriatrics, University of California, San Francisco School of Medicine, San Francisco, California
Epidemiology of Aging

John P. Atkinson, MD
Samuel B. Grant Professor of Medicine, Washington University School of Medicine in St. Louis, St. Louis, Missouri
Complement System in Disease

Evelyn Attia, MD
Professor of Psychiatry, Columbia University Vagelos College of Physicians and Surgeons; Director, Eating Disorders Center, Columbia University Irving Medical Center, New York, New York
Eating Disorders

Andrew D. Auerbach, MD, MPH
Professor of Medicine, University of California, San Francisco School of Medicine, San Francisco, California
Preoperative Evaluation

John Z. Ayanian, MD, MPP
Alice Hamilton Distinguished University Professor of Medicine and Healthcare Policy; Director, Institute for Healthcare Policy and Innovation, University of Michigan, Ann Arbor, Michigan
Disparities in Health and Health Care

Larry M. Baddour, MD
Professor Emeritus of Medicine, Departments of Medicine and Cardiovascular Disease, Mayo Clinic College of Medicine and Science, Rochester, Minnesota
Infective Endocarditis

Lindsey R. Baden, MD
Professor of Medicine, Harvard Medical School, Vice President of Clinical Research, Brigham and Women's Hospital, Boston, Massachusetts
Overview of Pneumonia

Thomas C. Bailey, MD
Professor of Medicine, Washington University School of Medicine in St. Louis, St. Louis, Missouri
Tuberculosis

Barbara J. Bain, MBBS
Professor of Diagnostic Haematology, St Mary's Hospital Campus of Imperial College London, London, United Kingdom
The Peripheral Blood Smear

Dean F. Bajorin, MD
Attending Physician and Member, Memorial Sloan Kettering Cancer Center; Professor of Medicine, Weill Medical College of Cornell University, New York, New York
Tumors of the Kidney, Bladder, Ureters, and Renal Pelvis

Robert W. Baloh, MD
Professor of Neurology, David Geffen School of Medicine at UCLA, Los Angeles, California
Neuro-Ophthalmology; Smell and Taste; Hearing and Equilibrium

Charles R.M. Bangham, BM, PhD, DSc
Professor and Co-Director, Institute of Infection, Imperial College London, London, United Kingdom
Retroviruses Other Than Human Immunodeficiency Virus

Jonathan Barasch, MD, PhD
Samuel W Lambert Professor of Medicine, Professor of Pathology and Cell Biology, Columbia University Vagelos College of Physicians and Surgeons, New York, New York
Structure and Function of the Kidneys; Acute Kidney Injury

Bruce Barrett, MD, PhD
Professor of Family Medicine and Community Health, University of Wisconsin School of Medicine and Public Health, Madison, Wisconsin
The Common Cold

John R. Bartholomew, MD
Professor of Medicine, Cleveland Clinic Lerner College of Medicine, Cleveland, Ohio
Other Peripheral Arterial Diseases

J.D. Bartleson, MD
Professor Emeritus of Neurology, Mayo Clinic College of Medicine and Science, Rochester, Minnesota
Mechanical and Other Lesions of the Spine, Nerve Roots, and Spinal Cord

Mary B. Barton, MD, MPP
Former Vice President, Performance Measurement, National Committee for Quality Assurance, Washington, D.C.
The Preventive Health Visit

Robert C. Basner, MD
Professor Emeritus and Special Lecturer in Medicine, Columbia University Vagelos College of Physicians and Surgeons, New York, New York
Sleep Disorders

Adam J. Bass, MD
Irving Professor of Medicine, Columbia University Vagelos College of Physicians and Surgeons, New York, New York
Neoplasms of the Esophagus and Stomach

Anne R. Bass, MD
Professor of Clinical Medicine, Weill Medical College of Cornell University; Attending Physician, Hospital for Special Surgery, New York, New York
Immunomodulatory Drugs

Julie E. Bauman, MD, MPH
Professor of Medicine, George Washington University School of Medicine and Health Sciences, Washington, D.C.
Head and Neck Cancer

Daniel G. Bausch, MD, MPH&TM
Professor of Tropical Medicine, London School of Hygiene and Tropical Medicine, London, United Kingdom; Senior Advisor for Global Health Security, FIND, Geneva, Switzerland
Viral Hemorrhagic Fevers

Arnold S. Bayer, MD
Distinguished Professor of Medicine, David Geffen School of Medicine at UCLA, Los Angeles, California; Senior Investigator, The Lundquist Institute at Harbor-UCLA, Torrance, California
Infective Endocarditis

Jeffrey J. Bazarian, MD, MPH
Professor of Emergency Medicine, University of Rochester School of Medicine & Dentistry, Rochester, New York
Traumatic Brain Injury and Spinal Cord Injury

Gonzalo M. Bearman, MD, MPH
Richard P. Wenzel Professor of Medicine and Chair, Division of Infectious Diseases, Virginia Commonwealth University School of Medicine, Richmond, Virginia
Acute Bronchitis and Tracheitis

Richard C. Becker, MD
Professor of Medicine and Physician-in-Chief, University of Cincinnati Heart, Lung and Vascular Institute, University of Cincinnati College of Medicine, Cincinnati, Ohio
Antithrombotic and Antiplatelet Therapy

J. David Beckham, MD
Professor of Medicine and Chief, Division of Infectious Diseases and Geographic Medicine, University of Texas Southwestern, Dallas, Texas
Arboviruses Causing Fever, Rash, and Neurologic Syndromes

Joshua A. Beckman, MD
Gayle and Paul Stoffel Distinguished Chair and Director, Vascular Medicine, University of Texas Southwestern, Dallas, Texas
Diseases of the Aorta

John H. Beigel, MD
Associate Director for Clinical Research, Division of Microbiology and Infectious Diseases, National Institute of Allergy and Infectious Diseases, National Institutes of Health, Bethesda, Maryland
Antiviral Therapy (Non-HIV)

Elisabeth H. Bel, MD, PhD
Professor of Respiratory Medicine, University of Amsterdam, Amsterdam, the Netherlands
Asthma

Walter Belda, Jr., MD
Professor of Dermatology, University of Sao Paulo, Sao Paulo, Brazil
Granuloma Inguinale (Donovanosis)

Eduardo E. Benarroch, MD, DSci
Professor of Neurology, Mayo Clinic College of Medicine and Science, Rochester, Minnesota
Autonomic Disorders

Joseph R. Berger, MD
Professor of Neurology, University of Pennsylvania Perelman School of Medicine, Philadelphia, Pennsylvania
Brain Abscess and Parameningeal Infections

Nancy Berliner, MD
H. Franklin Bunn Professor of Medicine, Harvard Medical School; Chief, Division of Hematology, Brigham and Women's Hospital, Boston, Massachusetts
Leukocytosis and Leukopenia; Histiocytoses

James L. Bernat, MD
Emeritus Professor of Neurology, Dartmouth Geisel School of Medicine, Hanover, New Hampshire
Coma, Disorders of Consciousness, and Brain Death

Daniel H. Bessesen, MD
Professor of Medicine, University of Colorado, School of Medicine, Aurora, Colorado
Obesity

Kirsten Bibbins-Domingo, PhD, MD
Lee Goldman, MD Professor of Medicine and Professor of Epidemiology and Biostatistics, University of California, San Francisco School of Medicine, San Francisco, California; Editor in Chief, Journal of the American Medical Association (JAMA) and the JAMA Network, Chicago, Illinois
Approach to Medicine, the Patient, and the Medical Profession: Medicine as a Learned and Humane Profession; Population Health

Leslie G. Biesecker, MD
Director, Center for Precision Health Research, National Human Genome Research Institute, National Institutes of Health, Bethesda, Maryland
Clinical Genomics—Genome Structure and Variation

Joseph J. Biundo, MD
Emeritus Professor of Medicine, Louisiana State University Medical Center, New Orleans, Louisiana
Bursitis, Tendinopathy, Other Periarticular Disorders, and Sports Medicine

Joel N. Blankson, MD, PhD
Professor of Medicine, Johns Hopkins University School of Medicine, Baltimore, Maryland
Pathobiology of Human Immunodeficiency Viruses

Karen C. Bloch, MD, MPH
Professor of Medicine (Infectious Diseases), Vanderbilt University School of Medicine, Nashville, Tennessee
Tularemia and Other Francisella *Infections*

Henk J. Blom, PhD
Professor, Department of Clinical Genetics, Erasmus University Medical Center, Rotterdam, the Netherlands
Homocystinuria and Hyperhomocysteinemia

William E. Boden, MD
Professor of Medicine, Boston University School of Medicine; Lecturer in Medicine, Harvard Medical School; Scientific Director, Clinical Trials Network, Department of Medicine, VA Boston Healthcare System, Boston, Massachusetts
Angina Pectoris and Chronic Ischemic Heart Disease

Guy Boivin, MD
Professor of Microbiology, Immunology and Infectious Diseases, Laval University and the Centre Hospitalier, Universitaire de Quebec, Quebec City, Quebec, Canada
Cytomegalovirus

Jean Bolognia, MD
Professor of Dermatology, Yale University School of Medicine, New Haven, Connecticut
Infections, Pigmentation Disorders, Regional Dermatology, and Distinctive Lesions in Black Skin

Robert A. Bonomo, MD
Professor of Medicine and Senior Associate Dean for Veterans Affairs, Case Western Reserve University School of Medicine; Associate Chief of Staff for Academic Affairs, Cleveland VA Hospital, Cleveland, Ohio
Diseases Caused by Acinetobacter *and* Stenotrophomonas *Species*

Sarah L. Booth, PhD
Professor of Biochemical & Molecular Nutrition and Director, U.S.D.A. Human Nutrition Research Center on Aging and Vitamin K Laboratory, Tufts University, Boston, Massachusetts
Vitamins, Trace Minerals, and Other Micronutrients

Ingvar G. Bosaeus, MD, PhD
Professor, University of Gothenburg; Senior Consultant, Clinical Nutrition, Sahlgrenska University Hospital, Gothenburg, Sweden
Malnutrition: Assessment and Support

David J. Brenner, PhD, DSc
Higgins Professor of Radiation Biophysics, Center for Radiological Research, Columbia University Vagelos College of Physicians and Surgeons, New York, New York
Radiation Injury

S. Louis Bridges, Jr., MD, PhD
Physician-in-Chief and Chair, Department of Medicine, Franchellie M. Cadwell Professor and Chief of Rheumatology, Hospital for Special Surgery; Chief, Division of Rheumatology, Weill Medical College of Cornell University, New York, New York
Systemic Diseases in Which Arthritis Is a Feature

Laurent Brochard, MD
Keenan Chair in Critical Care and Respiratory Medicine, Keenan Research Centre, St. Michael's Hospital, Unity Health Toronto; Professor of Medicine and Director, Interdepartmental Division for Critical Care, University of Toronto, Toronto, Ontario, Canada
Mechanical Ventilation

Robert A. Brodsky, MD
Professor of Medicine and Oncology and Director, Division of Hematology, Johns Hopkins University School of Medicine, Baltimore, Maryland
Aplastic Anemia and Related Bone Marrow Failure States

Itzhak Brook, MD
Professor of Pediatrics, Georgetown University School of Medicine, Washington, D.C.
Diseases Caused by Non–Spore-Forming Anaerobic Bacteria; Actinomycosis

Jennifer R. Brown, MD, PhD
Director, CLL Center and Institute Physician, Dana-Farber Cancer Institute; Worthington and Margaret Collette Professor of Medicine, Harvard Medical School, Boston, Massachusetts
Chronic Lymphocytic Leukemia

Enrico Brunetti, MD
Associate Professor of Infectious Diseases, Department of Clinical, Surgical, Diagnostic and Pediatric Sciences, University of Pavia; Staff Physician, Division of Infectious Diseases, San Matteo Hospital Foundation, Pavia, Italy
Cestodes

Amy E. Bryant, PhD
Affiliate Research Professor, Department of Biomedical and Pharmaceutical Sciences, Idaho State University, Meridian, Idaho
Nonpneumococcal Streptococcal Infections and Rheumatic Fever

Philip J. Budge, MD, PhD
Associate Professor of Medicine, Washington University School of Medicine in St. Louis, St. Louis, Missouri
Antiparasitic Therapy

Pierre A. Buffet, MD, PhD
Professor of Cell Biology, Faculty of Medicine, Paris University; Consultant Physician, Institut Pasteur Medical Center, Paris, France
Leishmaniasis

David A. Bushinsky, MD
John J. Kuiper Distinguished Professor Emeritus of Medicine and Professor of Pharmacology and Physiology, University of Rochester School of Medicine & Dentistry, Rochester, New York
Nephrolithiasis

Vivian P. Bykerk, MD
Professor of Medicine, Weill Medical College of Cornell University; Attending Physician, Hospital for Special Surgery, New York, New York
Approach to the Patient with Rheumatic Disease

Peter A. Calabresi, MD
Professor of Neurology, Neuroscience, and Ophthalmology, and Director of the Richard T Johnson Division of Neuroimmunology and Neurological Infections; Director of the Multiple Sclerosis Center, Johns Hopkins University School of Medicine, Baltimore, Maryland
Multiple Sclerosis and Demyelinating Conditions

Diane P. Calello, MD
Professor of Emergency Medicine; Executive and Medical Director, New Jersey Poison Information and Education System, Rutgers New Jersey Medical School, Newark, New Jersey
Acute Poisoning

David P. Calfee, MD, MS
Professor of Medicine and of Population Health Sciences, Weill Medical College of Cornell University; Chief Hospital Epidemiologist, New York-Presbyterian Hospital/Weill Medical College of Cornell University, New York, New York
Prevention and Control of Health Care–Associated Infections

S. Todd Callahan, MD, MPH
Professor of Pediatrics and Chief, Division of Adolescent and Young Health, Vanderbilt University Medical Center, Nashville, Tennessee
Adolescent Medicine

Michael Camilleri, MD, DSc
Atherton and Winifred W. Bean Professor of Medicine, Pharmacology, and Physiology, Mayo Clinic College of Medicine and Science, Rochester, Minnesota
Disorders of Gastrointestinal Motility

Juan J. Canoso, MD
Emeritus Rheumatologist, ABC Medical Center, Mexico City, Mexico; Adjunct Professor of Medicine, Tufts University School of Medicine, Boston, Massachusetts
Bursitis, Tendinopathy, Other Periarticular Disorders, and Sports Medicine

Maria Domenica Cappellini, MD
Professor of Internal Medicine, Department of Clinical Sciences and Community Health, University of Milan; and Ca'Granda Foundation-Policlinico Hospital, Milan, Italy
The Thalassemias

Blase A. Carabello, MD
Professor of Cardiovascular Sciences and Chief, Division of Cardiology, East Carolina University Brody School of Medicine, Greenville, North Carolina
Valvular Heart Disease

Laura R. Carucci, MD
Professor of Radiology, Virginia Commonwealth University School of Medicine; Section Chief of Abdominal Imaging, Director of CT and MRI Radiology, Virginia Commonwealth University Health System, Richmond, Virginia
Diagnostic Imaging Procedures in Gastroenterology

Mariana Castells, MD, PhD
Professor of Medicine, Harvard Medical School and Physician, Brigham and Women's Hospital, Boston, Massachusetts
Anaphylaxis; Drug Allergy

William H. Catherino, MD, PhD
Professor and Vice Chair-Research, Department of Gynecologic Surgery and Obstetrics, Uniformed Services University of the Health Sciences, Bethesda, Maryland
Ovaries and Pubertal Development; Reproductive Endocrinology and Infertility

Tommy E. Cederholm, MD, PhD
Professor Emeritus, Clinical Nutrition and Metabolism, Department of Public Health and Caring Sciences, Uppsala University, Uppsala, Sweden; Department of Geriatric Medicine, Theme Inflammation & Aging, Karolinska University Hospital, Stockholm, Sweden
Malnutrition: Assessment and Support

Naga P. Chalasani, MD
David W Crabb Professor, Indiana University School of Medicine; Vice President for Academic Affairs, Indiana University Health, Indianapolis, Indiana
Alcoholic and Nonalcoholic Steatohepatitis

Henry F. Chambers, MD
Professor of Medicine, University of California, San Francisco School of Medicine, San Francisco, California
Staphylococcal Infections

Larry W. Chang, MD, MPH
Professor of Medicine, Epidemiology, and International Health, Johns Hopkins University School of Medicine and Bloomberg School of Public Health, Baltimore, Maryland
Epidemiology and Diagnosis of Human Immunodeficiency Virus Infection and Acquired Immunodeficiency Syndrome; Acute Clinical Manifestations and Diagnosis of HIV

Lin Chang, MD
Professor of Medicine and Vice Chief, Vatche and Tamar Manoukian Division of Digestive Diseases, David Geffen School of Medicine at UCLA, Los Angeles, California
Irritable Bowel and Functional Upper Gastrointestinal Syndromes

Nelson J. Chao, MD, MBA
Donald D. and Elizabeth G. Cooke Professor of Medicine, Duke University School of Medicine, Durham, North Carolina
Hematopoietic Cell Transplantation

Mitali Chatterjee, MD, PhD
Professor of Pharmacology, Institute of Postgraduate Medical Education & Research, Kolkata, West Bengal, India
Leishmaniasis

Seemant Chaturvedi, MD
Stewart J Greenebaum Endowed Professor of Stroke Neurology, University of Maryland School of Medicine; Stroke Program Director, University of Maryland Medical System, Baltimore, Maryland
Hemorrhagic Cerebrovascular Disease

Lin H. Chen, MD
Associate Professor of Medicine, Harvard Medical School, Boston, Massachusetts; Director of the Travel Medicine Center, Division of Infectious Diseases and Travel Medicine, Mount Auburn Hospital, Cambridge, Massachusetts
Approach to the Patient Before and After Travel

Sharon C-A Chen, MB BS, PhD
Clinical Professor of Medicine, The University of Sydney Centre for Infectious Diseases and Microbiology, Westmead Hospital, Westmead, New South Wales, Australia
Cryptococcosis

Susan Y. Chon, MD
Professor of Dermatology, University of Texas MD Anderson Cancer Center, Houston, Texas
Urticaria, Drug Hypersensitivity Rashes, Nodules and Tumors, and Atrophic Diseases

David C. Christiani, MD
Professor of Medicine, Harvard Medical School; Physician, Pulmonary and Critical Care, Massachusetts General Hospital; Elkan Blout Professor of Environmental Genetics, Environmental Health, Harvard School of Public Health, Boston, Massachusetts
Physical and Chemical Injuries of the Lung

Edward Chu, MD, MMS
Carol and Roger Einiger Professor of Cancer Medicine; Director, Montefiore Einstein Cancer Center; Vice-President of Cancer Medicine; Albert Einstein College of Medicine and Montefiore Medicine, Bronx, New York
Neoplasms of the Small and Large Intestine

Theodore J. Cieslak, MD, MPH
Adjunct Associate Professor of Epidemiology, College of Public Health, University of Nebraska, Omaha, Nebraska
Bioterrorism

George A. Cioffi, MD
Edward S. Harkness Professor and Chair, Jean and Richard Deems Professor of Ophthalmology, Columbia University Vagelos College of Physicians and Surgeons, New York, New York
Diseases of the Visual System

Carolyn M. Clancy, MD
Assistant Undersecretary for Health, Discovery, Education and Affiliate Networks, Department of Veterans Affairs; Clinical Associate Professor of Internal Medicine, George Washington University School of Medicine and Health Sciences, Washington, D.C.
Measuring Health and Health Care

Heather Clauss, MD
Professor of Internal Medicine/Infectious Disease, Lewis Katz School of Medicine at Temple University, Philadelphia, Pennsylvania
Gram-Positive Rod Infections

Daniel J. Clauw, MD
Professor of Anesthesiology, Medicine (Rheumatology) and Psychiatry, and Director, Chronic Pain and Fatigue Research Center, University of Michigan Medical School, Ann Arbor, Michigan
Fibromyalgia

David R. Clemmons, MD
Kenan Professor of Medicine, University of North Carolina School of Medicine; Attending Physician, UNC Hospitals, Chapel Hill, North Carolina
Approach to the Patient with Endocrine Disease

Thomas M. Coffman, MD
Professor and Dean, Cardiovascular and Metabolic Disorders Program, Duke-NUS Medical School, Singapore; James R Clapp Professor of Medicine, Duke University School of Medicine, Durham, North Carolina
Vascular Disorders of the Kidney

David Cohen, MA, MD
Daniel Midler-John A. Catsimatidis Professor of Nephrology, Professor of Medicine, Columbia University Vagelos College of Physicians and Surgeons, New York, New York
Treatment of Irreversible Renal Failure

Jeffrey Cohen, MD
Chief, Laboratory of Infectious Diseases, National Institute of Allergy and Infectious Diseases, National Institutes of Health, Bethesda, Maryland
Varicella-Zoster Virus (Chickenpox, Shingles)

Myron S. Cohen, MD
Yeargan-Bate Eminent Professor of Medicine, Microbiology and Epidemiology; Associate Vice Chancellor for Global Health; Director, Institute of Global Health and Infectious Diseases, University of North Carolina School of Medicine, Chapel Hill, North Carolina
Approach to the Patient with a Sexually Transmitted Infection; COVID-19: Epidemiology, Clinical Manifestations, Diagnosis, Community Prevention, and Prognosis; Prevention of Human Immunodeficiency Virus Infection

Steven P. Cohen, MD
Professor of Anesthesiology & Critical Care Medicine, Neurology, and Physical Medicine & Rehabilitation, and Psychiatry and Behavioral Sciences and Chief, Pain Medicine Division, Johns Hopkins School of Medicine, Baltimore, Maryland; Director of Pain Research and Professor of Anesthesiology and Physical Medicine & Rehabilitation, Walter Reed National Military Medical Center, Uniformed Services University of the Health Sciences, Bethesda, Maryland
Pain

Joseph M. Connors, MD
Emeritus Professor, BC Cancer Centre for Lymphoid Cancer and the University of British Columbia, Vancouver, British Columbia, Canada
Hodgkin Lymphoma

Deborah J. Cook, MD, MSc
Professor of Medicine, Clinical Epidemiology & Biostatistics, McMaster University Michael G. DeGroote School of Medicine, Hamilton, Ontario, Canada
Approach to the Patient in a Critical Care Setting

Lucy B.M. Cook, MB BS, PhD
Consultant Hematologist, Centre for Haematology, Faculty of Medicine, Imperial College London, London, United Kingdom
Retroviruses Other Than Human Immunodeficiency Virus

Kathleen A. Cooney, MD
George Barth Geller Distinguished Professor and Chair, Department of Medicine, Duke University School of Medicine, Durham, North Carolina
Approach to Medicine, the Patient, and the Medical Profession: Medicine as a Learned and Humane Profession; Prostate Cancer

William J. Craigen, MD, PhD
Professor of Molecular and Human Genetics, Baylor College of Medicine, Houston, Texas
Approach to Inborn Errors of Metabolism

Jill P. Crandall, MD
Jacob and Jeanne Barkey Professor of Medicine and Chief, Division of Endocrinology, Albert Einstein College of Medicine, New York, New York
Diabetes Mellitus

Simon L. Croft, PhD, DSc
Emeritus Professor, Faculty of Infectious and Tropical Diseases, London School of Hygiene & Tropical Medicine, London, United Kingdom
Leishmaniasis

Mary K. Crow, MD
Professor of Medicine, Weill Medical College of Cornell University; Mary K. Crow, MD Chair in Immunology and Inflammation Research, Hospital for Special Surgery, New York, New York
Approach to Medicine, the Patient, and the Medical Profession: Medicine as a Learned and Humane Profession; The Innate and Adaptive Immune Systems; Approach to the Patient with Rheumatic Disease; Systemic Lupus Erythematosus

John A. Crump, MB ChB, MD, DTMH
Professor of Medicine, Pathology, and Global Health, Centre for International Health, University of Otago, Dunedin, Otago, New Zealand
Salmonella *Infections (Including Enteric Fever)*

Merit E. Cudkowicz, MD
Julieanne Dorn Professor of Neurology, Harvard Medical School and Chair of Neurology, Massachusetts General Hospital, Boston, Massachusetts
Amyotrophic Lateral Sclerosis and Other Motor Neuron Diseases

Charlotte Cunningham-Rundles, MD, PhD
David S Gottesman Professor of Medicine, Icahn School of Medicine at Mount Sinai, New York, New York
Primary Immunodeficiency Diseases

Kathryn M. Dahir, MD
Professor of Medicine, Director of the Program for Metabolic Bone Disorders at Vanderbilt, Vanderbilt University Medical Center, Nashville, Tennessee
Osteonecrosis, Osteosclerosis/Hyperostosis, and Other Disorders of Bone

Inger K. Damon, MD, PhD
Director, Retired, Division of High Consequence Pathogens and Pathology, Centers for Disease Control and Prevention, Atlanta, Georgia
Smallpox, Monkeypox, and Other Poxvirus Infections

Michael Daras, MD, PhD
Professor of Neurology, Columbia University Vagelos College of Physicians and Surgeons, New York, New York
Nutritional and Alcohol-Related Neurologic Disorders

Richard C. Dart, MD, PhD
Professor of Emergency Medicine, University of Colorado School of Medicine and Director, Rocky Mountain Poison and Drug Safety, Denver Health and Hospital Authority, Denver, Colorado
Envenomation, Bites, and Stings

Nancy E. Davidson, MD
Professor of Medicine, Raisbeck Endowed Chair, and Chief, Division of Medical Oncology, University of Washington School of Medicine; Executive Vice President, Fred Hutchinson Cancer Center, Seattle, Washington
Approach to Medicine, the Patient, and the Medical Profession: Medicine as a Learned and Humane Profession; Breast Cancer and Benign Breast Disorders

Kevin D. Deane, MD, PhD
Professor of Medicine, University of Colorado School of Medicine, Aurora, Colorado
Laboratory Testing in the Rheumatic Diseases

Lisa M. DeAngelis, MD
Chief Physician Executive, Memorial Sloan Kettering Cancer Center, New York, New York; Professor of Neurology, Weill Medical College of Cornell University, New York, New York
Tumors of the Central Nervous System

Malcolm M. DeCamp, MD
Professor of Surgery and Chair, Division of Cardiothoracic Surgery; K. Craig Kent Chair in Strategic Leadership, University of Wisconsin School of Medicine and Public Health, Madison, Wisconsin
Interventional and Surgical Approaches to Lung Disease

Thomas G. DeLoughery, MD
Professor of Hematology, Oregon Health & Science University, Portland, Oregon
Microcytic and Hypochromic Anemias

Carlos del Rio, MD
Leon L. Haley Jr MD Distinguished Professor of Medicine, Emory University School of Medicine; Professor of Epidemiology and Global Health, Rollins School of Public Health of Emory University, Atlanta, Georgia
COVID-19: Epidemiology, Clinical Manifestations, Diagnosis, Community Prevention, and Prognosis; Prevention of Human Immunodeficiency Virus Infection

Gabriele C. De Luca, MD, DPhil
Professor of Clinical Neurology and Experimental Neuropathology, Nuffield Department of Clinical Neurosciences, University of Oxford, Oxford, Oxfordshire, United Kingdom
Approach to the Patient with Neurologic Disease

David W. Denning, MBBS
Professor of Infectious Diseases in Global Health, The University of Manchester, Manchester, United Kingdom
Systemic Antifungal Agents

Patricia A. Deuster, PhD, MPH
Professor and Executive Director, Consortium for Health and Military Performance, Uniformed Services University, Bethesda, Maryland
Rhabdomyolysis

Amy E. DeZern, MD, MHS
Associate Professor of Oncology and Medicine, Johns Hopkins University School of Medicine, Baltimore, Maryland
Aplastic Anemia and Related Bone Marrow Failure States

Ketan K. Dhatariya, MBBS, MSc, MD, MS, PhD
Honorary Professor of Medicine, Norwich Medical School, University of East Anglia; Consultant, Elsie Bertram Diabetes Centre, Norfolk and Norwich University Hospitals NHS Foundation Trust, Norwich, Norfolk, United Kingdom
Diabetes Mellitus

Robert B. Diasio, MD
William J. and Charles H. Mayo Professor of Molecular Pharmacology and Experimental Therapeutics, Mayo Clinic College of Medicine and Science, Rochester, Minnesota
Principles of Drug Therapy

David J. Diemert, MD
Professor, Departments of Medicine and of Microbiology, Immunology and Tropical Medicine, George Washington University School of Medicine and Health Sciences, Washington, D.C.
Nematode Infections

Kathleen B. Digre, MD
Distinguished Professor of Neurology and Professor of Ophthalmology, University of Utah School of Medicine, Salt Lake City, Utah
Headaches and Other Head Pain

Vasken Dilsizian, MD
Professor of Medicine and Radiology, Department of Diagnostic Radiology and Nuclear Medicine, University of Maryland School of Medicine; Chief, Division of Nuclear Medicine, University of Maryland Medical Center, Baltimore, Maryland
Noninvasive Cardiac Imaging

Jodie A. Dionne, MD
Associate Professor of Medicine, University of Alabama at Birmingham, Birmingham, Alabama
Syphilis and Nonsyphilitic Treponematoses

Jorge Di Paola, MD
Professor of Pediatrics and Elizabeth Finney McDonnell Endowed Chair and Director, Division of Pediatric Hematology Oncology, Washington University School of Medicine in St. Louis, St. Louis, Missouri
Von Willebrand Disease and Hemorrhagic Abnormalities of Platelet and Vascular Function

Angela Dispenzieri, MD
Professor of Medicine and of Laboratory Medicine, Mayo Clinic College of Medicine and Science, Rochester, Minnesota
Amyloidosis

Sunil Dogra, MD, DNB
Professor of Dermatology, Venereology and Leprology, Postgraduate Institute of Medical Education and Research (PGIMER), Chandigarh, India
Leprosy (Hansen Disease)

James H. Doroshow, MD
Deputy Director for Clinical and Translational Research and Director, Division of Cancer Treatment and Diagnosis, National Cancer Institute, National Institutes of Health, Bethesda, Maryland
Approach to the Patient with Cancer

John M. Douglas, Jr., MD
Executive Director, Tri-County Health Department, Greenwood Village, Colorado
Papillomavirus

Jeffrey M. Drazen, MD
Distinguished Parker B. Francis Professor of Medicine, Harvard Medical School; Senior Physician, Department of Medicine, Brigham and Women's Hospital; Editor, NEJM Group, Boston, Massachusetts
Approach to Medicine, the Patient, and the Medical Profession: Medicine as a Learned and Humane Profession; Asthma

Dimitri Drekonja, MD, MS
Associate Professor of Medicine, University of Minnesota; Chief, Infectious Diseases Section, Minneapolis VA Health Care System, Minneapolis, Minnesota
Approach to the Patient with Urinary Tract Infection

Erik R. Dubberke, MD, MSPH
Professor of Medicine, Washington University School of Medicine in St. Louis, St. Louis, Missouri
Clostridial and Clostridioides *Infections*

Catherine E. DuBeau, MD
Professor of Medicine, Geisel School of Medicine at Dartmouth-Hitchcock Medical Center, Lebanon, New Hampshire
Urinary Incontinence

J. Stephen Dumler, MD
Professor and Chairperson, Joint Departments of Pathology, Uniformed Services University, Walter Reed National Military Medical Center, and Joint Pathology Center, Bethesda, Maryland
Zoonoses

Madeleine Duvic, MD
Professor and Deputy Chairman, Department of Dermatology, University of Texas MD Anderson Cancer Center, Houston, Texas
Urticaria, Drug Hypersensitivity Rashes, Nodules and Tumors, and Atrophic Diseases

Kristie Ebi, PhD, MPH
Professor of Global Health, University of Washington Center for Health and the Global Environment (CHanGE), Schools of Medicine and Public Health, University of Washington, Seattle, Washington
Effects of Climate Change on Health

Kathryn M. Edwards, MD
Sarah H. Sell and Cornelius Vanderbilt Endowed Chair and Professor of Pediatrics, Vanderbilt University School of Medicine, Nashville, Tennessee
Parainfluenza Viral Disease

N. Lawrence Edwards, MD
Professor and Vice Chairman, Department of Medicine, University of Florida; Chief, Section of Rheumatology, Malcolm Randall Veterans Administration Medical Center, Gainesville, Florida
Crystal Deposition Diseases

John W. Eikelboom, MBBS, MSc
Professor of Medicine, McMaster University Michael G. DeGroote School of Medicine, Hamilton, Ontario, Canada
Venous Thrombosis and Embolism

Lawrence H. Einhorn, MD
Distinguished Professor of Medicine, Indiana University School of Medicine, Indianapolis, Indiana
Testicular Cancer

Perry M. Elliott, MBBS, MD
Professor of Cardiovascular Medicine, Institute of Cardiovascular Science, University College London & St. Bartholomew's Hospital, London, United Kingdom
Diseases of the Myocardium and Endocardium

Ezekiel J. Emanuel, MD, PhD
Diane v.S. Levy & Robert M. Levy Professor and Vice Provost for Global Initiatives, University of Pennsylvania, Philadelphia, Pennsylvania
Bioethics in the Practice of Medicine

Matthew E. Falagas, MD, MSc, DSc
Director, Alfa Institute of Biomedical Sciences and Director, First Department of Internal Medicine, Hygeia Hospital, Athens, Greece; Adjunct Associate Professor of Medicine, Tufts University School of Medicine, Boston, Massachusetts
Pseudomonas *and* Burkholderia *Infections*

Gary W. Falk, MD, MS
Professor of Medicine, University of Pennsylvania Perelman School of Medicine, Philadelphia, Pennsylvania
Diseases of the Esophagus

James C. Fang, MD
June and John Hartman Presidential Endowed Chair, Professor, and Chief, Division of Cardiovascular Medicine, University of Utah School of Medicine; Executive Director, Cardiovascular Service Line, University of Utah Health Sciences, Salt Lake City, Utah
ST-Elevation Acute Myocardial Infarction and Complications of Myocardial Infarction

Monica M. Farley, MD
Jonas A. Shulman Professor of Medicine and Director, Division of Infectious Diseases, Emory University School of Medicine, Atlanta, Georgia
Haemophilus *and* Moraxella *Infections*

Gene Feder, MBBS, MD
Professor of Primary Care, Centre for Academic Primary Care, Population Health Sciences, Bristol Medical School, University of Bristol, Bristol, United Kingdom
Intimate Partner Violence

David J. Feller-Kopman, MD
Professor of Medicine, Geisel School of Medicine; Chief, Pulmonary and Critical Care Medicine, Dartmouth Hitchcock Medical Center, Lebanon, New Hampshire
Interventional and Surgical Approaches to Lung Disease

Thomas McDonald File, Jr., MD, MSc
Professor of Medicine and Chair, Infectious Disease Section, Northeast Ohio Medical University, Rootstown, Ohio; Chair, Infectious Disease Division, Summa Health, Akron, Ohio
Streptococcus pneumoniae *Pulmonary Infections*

Glenn I. Fishman, MD
William Goldring Professor of Medicine and Director, Leon H. Charney Division of Cardiology, New York University Grossman School of Medicine, New York, New York
Principles of Electrophysiology

John M. Flack, MD, MPH
Sergio Rabinovich Endowed Chair of Internal Medicine, Professor and Chair, Department of Medicine, Southern Illinois University, Springfield, Illinois
Arterial Hypertension

James M. Fleckenstein, MD
Professor of Medicine & Molecular Microbiology, Washington University School of Medicine in St. Louis, St. Louis, Missouri
Approach to the Patient with Suspected Enteric Infection

Lee A. Fleisher, MD
Emeritus Professor and Former Chair, Anesthesiology and Critical Care, University of Pennsylvania Perelman School of Medicine, Philadelphia, Pennsylvania
Overview of Anesthesia

Paul W. Flint, MD
Professor and Chair of Otolaryngology-Head & Neck Surgery, Oregon Health & Science University, Portland, Oregon
Throat Disorders

Evan L. Fogel, MD, MSc
Stuart Sherman Professor of Gastroenterology and Hepatology and Professor of Medicine, Indiana University School of Medicine, Indianapolis, Indiana
Diseases of the Gallbladder and Bile Ducts

Robert J. Fontana, MD
Professor of Medicine, University of Michigan Medical School, Ann Arbor, Michigan
Liver Failure and Transplantation

Chris E. Forsmark, MD
Professor of Medicine, University of Florida College of Medicine, Gainesville, Florida
Pancreatitis

Pierre-Edouard Fournier, MD, PhD
Professor of Medical Bacteriology-Virology and Hygiene, Aix-Marseille Universite and Institut Hospitalo-Universitaire Mediterranee-Infection, Marseille, France
Rickettsial Infections

Vance G. Fowler, Jr., MD, MHS
Florence McAlister Distinguished Professor of Medicine and of Molecular Genetics and Microbiology, Duke University School of Medicine, Durham, North Carolina
Infective Endocarditis

Manuel A. Franco, MD, PhD
Professor, Instituto de Genética Humana, Facultad de Medicina, Pontificia Universidad Javeriana, Bogotá, Colombia
Rotaviruses, Noroviruses, and Other Gastrointestinal Viruses

Victoria J. Fraser, MD
Adolphus Busch Professor and Chair, Department of Medicine, Washington University School of Medicine in St. Louis, St. Louis, Missouri
Approach to Medicine, the Patient, and the Medical Profession: Medicine as a Learned and Humane Profession; Introduction to Microbial Disease: Pathophysiology and Diagnostics; Legionella *Infections*

Roy Freeman, MD
Professor of Neurology, Beth Israel Deaconess Medical Center, Harvard Medical School, Boston, Massachusetts
Autonomic Disorders

Karen M. Freund, MD, MPH
Professor of Medicine and Vice Chair for Faculty Affairs and Quality Improvement, Tufts University School of Medicine, Boston, Massachusetts
Approach to Women's Health

Blake A. Froberg, MD
Associate Professor of Pediatrics and Emergency Medicine, Indiana University School of Medicine, Indianapolis, Indiana
Chronic Poisoning: Trace Metals and Others

Patrick G. Gallagher, MD
Professor of Pediatrics, Pathology and Genetics, Yale University School of Medicine, New Haven, Connecticut
Hemolytic Anemias: Red Blood Cell Membrane and Metabolic Defects

Monica Gandhi, MD
Professor of Medicine and Director of the Ward 86 HIV Clinic, University of California, San Francisco School of Medicine, San Francisco, California
COVID-19: Epidemiology, Clinical Manifestations, Diagnosis, Community Prevention, and Prognosis

Rajesh T. Gandhi, MD
Professor of Medicine, Harvard Medical School; Director of HIV Clinical Services and Education, Massachusetts General Hospital, Boston, Massachusetts
COVID-19 Treatment and Vaccination

Leonard Ganz, MD
Division Vice President, Medical Affairs and Chief Medical Officer, Cardiac Rhythm Management Division Abbott, Beaver, Pennsylvania
Electrocardiography

Hasan Garan, MD, MS
Dickinson W. Richards, Jr. Professor of Medicine, Columbia University Vagelos College of Physicians and Surgeons, New York, New York
Ventricular Arrhythmias

Guadalupe Garcia-Tsao, MD
Professor of Medicine, Yale University School of Medicine, New Haven, Connecticut and VA-CT Healthcare System, West Haven, Connecticut
Cirrhosis and Its Sequelae

William M. Geisler, MD, MPH
Professor of Medicine, University of Alabama at Birmingham Heersink School of Medicine, Birmingham, Alabama
Diseases Caused by Chlamydiae

Joel M. Gelfand, MD, MSCE
James J. Leyden Professor of Dermatology and Epidemiology and Vice Chair, Clinical Research, Departments of Dermatology and of Biostatistics, Epidemiology, and Informatics, University of Pennsylvania Perelman School of Medicine, Philadelphia, Pennsylvania
Eczemas, Photodermatoses, Papulosquamous (Including Fungal) Diseases, and Figurate Erythemas

Tony P. George, MD
Professor of Psychiatry, University of Toronto; Clinician-Scientist, Centre for Addiction and Mental Health, Toronto, Ontario, Canada
Nicotine and Tobacco

Lior Gepstein, MD, PhD
Sohnis Family Professor in Medicine, Technion - Israel Institute of Technology; Director, Cardiology Department, Rambam Health Care Campus, Haifa, Israel
Regenerative Medicine, Cell Therapy, and Gene Therapy

Morie A. Gertz, MD
Roland Seidler Jr. Professor of the Art of Medicine and Chair Emeritus, Internal Medicine, Mayo Clinic College of Medicine and Science, Rochester, Minnesota
Amyloidosis

Khalil G. Ghanem, MD, PhD
Professor of Medicine, Johns Hopkins University School of Medicine, Baltimore, Maryland
Syphilis and Nonsyphilitic Treponematoses

Ali G. Gharavi, MD
Jay Meltzer Professor and Chief, Division of Nephrology, Columbia University Vagelos College of Physicians and Surgeons, New York, New York
Approach to Medicine, the Patient, and the Medical Profession: Medicine as a Learned and Humane Profession; Approach to the Patient with Renal Disease

Cybele Ghossein, MD
Professor of Medicine and Vice Chair for Academic and Faculty Affairs, Northwestern University Feinberg School of Medicine, Chicago, Illinois
Interstitial Nephritis

Christopher J. Gill, MD, MS
Professor of Global Health, Boston University School of Public Health, Boston, Massachusetts
Whooping Cough and Other Bordetella *Infections*

Geoffrey S. Ginsburg, MD, PhD
Chief Medical and Scientific Officer, All of Us Research Program, National Institutes of Health, Bethesda, Maryland
Applications of Molecular Technologies to Clinical Medicine

Marshall J. Glesby, MD, PhD
Professor of Medicine, Weill Medical College of Cornell University, New York, New York
Systemic Manifestations of HIV/AIDS

John W. Gnann, Jr., MD
Professor of Medicine, Medical University of South Carolina, Charleston, South Carolina
Herpes Simplex Virus Infections

David L. Goldman, MD
Associate Professor of Pediatrics, Microbiology and Immunology, Children's Hospital at Montefiore/Albert Einstein College of Medicine, Bronx, New York
Mycoplasma *Infections*

Lee Goldman, MD, MPH
Cournand and Richards Professor of Cardiology, Columbia University Vagelos College of Physicians and Surgeons; Professor of Epidemiology, Mailman School of Public Health; Dean Emeritus, Faculties of Health Sciences and Medicine, Columbia University Irving Medical Center, New York, New York
Approach to Medicine, the Patient, and the Medical Profession: Medicine as a Learned and Humane Profession; Approach to the Patient with Possible Cardiovascular Disease; Bradycardias and Conduction System Delays; Supraventricular Ectopy and Tachyarrhythmias

Larry B. Goldstein, MD
Ruth L. Works Professor and Chair, Department of Neurology, and Associate Dean for Clinical Research, University of Kentucky College of Medicine; Co-Director, Kentucky Neuroscience Institute, Lexington, Kentucky
Approach to Cerebrovascular Diseases; Ischemic Cerebrovascular Disease

Anthony C. Gordon, MBBS, MD
Professor of Anesthesia & Critical Care, Imperial College London, London, United Kingdom
Shock Syndromes Related to Sepsis

Jason Gotlib, MD, MS
Professor of Medicine, Stanford University School of Medicine, Stanford Cancer Institute, Stanford, California
Polycythemia Vera, Essential Thrombocythemia, and Primary Myelofibrosis

Eduardo Gotuzzo, MD
Professor Emeritus, Alexander von Humboldt Tropical Medicine Institute, Universidad Peruana Cayetano Heredia; Principal Professor of Medicine and Tropical Diseases, National Hospital Cayetano Heredia, Lima, Peru
Cholera and Other Vibrio *Infections*

Hartmut Grasemann, MD, PhD
Professor of Pediatrics, The Hospital for Sick Children and University of Toronto, Toronto, Ontario, Canada
Cystic Fibrosis

Judith Green-McKenzie, MD, MPH
Professor, Division of Occupational & Environmental Medicine, Department of Emergency Medicine, University of Pennsylvania Perelman School of Medicine, Philadelphia, Pennsylvania
Principles of Occupational and Environmental Medicine

Harry B. Greenberg, MD
Professor of Medicine and of Microbiology and Immunology, Stanford University School of Medicine, Stanford, California
Rotaviruses, Noroviruses, and Other Gastrointestinal Viruses

Steven A. Greenberg, MD
Professor of Neurology, Brigham and Women's Hospital and Harvard Medical School, Boston, Massachusetts
Inflammatory Myopathies

David M. Greer, MD, MA
Professor and Chair of Neurology, Boston University Chobanian and Avedisian School of Medicine and Boston Medical Center, Boston, Massachusetts
Coma, Disorders of Consciousness, and Brain Death

S. Ryan Greysen, MD, MHS
Associate Professor of Medicine and Chief, Section of Hospital Medicine, University of Pennsylvania Perelman School of Medicine, Philadelphia, Pennsylvania
Medical Care of Patients with Psychiatric Diseases

Marie R. Griffin, MD, MPH
Professor Emerita of Health Policy, Vanderbilt University School of Medicine, Nashville, Tennessee
Overview of Pneumonia

Robert C. Griggs, MD
Professor of Neurology, Medicine, Pediatrics, Pathology & Laboratory Medicine, University of Rochester School of Medicine & Dentistry, Rochester, New York
Approach to the Patient with Neurologic Disease

Daniel Grossman, MD
Professor of Obstetrics, Gynecology and Reproductive Sciences, University of California, San Francisco School of Medicine, San Francisco, California
Contraception

Lisa M. Guay-Woodford, MD
McGehee Joyce Professor of Pediatrics, George Washington University School of Medicine and Health Sciences, Children's National Research Institute, Washington, D.C.
Hereditary Nephropathies and Developmental Renal/Urinary Abnormalities

Roy M. Gulick, MD, MPH
Rochelle Belfer Professor of Medicine and Chief, Division of Infectious Diseases, Weill Medical College of Cornell University; Attending Physician, New York-Presbyterian Hospital, New York, New York
Antiretroviral Treatment of Human Immunodeficiency Virus Infection

David A. Haake, MD
Health Sciences Clinical Professor of Medicine, David Geffen School of Medicine at UCLA; Staff Physician, VA Greater Los Angeles Healthcare System, Health Sciences, Los Angeles, California
Leptospirosis

Melissa M. Hagman, MD
Associate Professor of Medicine and Program Director, Internal Medicine Residency-Boise, University of Washington, Boise, Idaho
Nonpneumococcal Streptococcal Infections and Rheumatic Fever

Klaus D. Hagspiel, MD
Professor of Radiology, Medicine (Cardiology) and Pediatrics; Chief, Division of Noninvasive Cardiovascular Imaging, Department of Radiology and Medical Imaging, University of Virginia School of Medicine, Charlottesville, Virginia
Noninvasive Cardiac Imaging

Raymond C. Harris, MD
Anne and Roscoe R. Robinson Chair, Professor of Medicine, and Associate Chair, Division of Nephrology, Vanderbilt University School of Medicine, Nashville, Tennessee
Diabetes and the Kidney

Fiona P. Havers, MD, MHS
Medical Epidemiologist, National Center for Immunization and Respiratory Diseases, Centers for Disease Control and Prevention, Atlanta, Georgia
Pre-2019 Coronaviruses

Elisabeth I. Heath, MD
Professor of Oncology and Associate Director, Translational Sciences, Department of Oncology, Wayne State University School of Medicine, Karmanos Cancer Institute, Detroit, Michigan
Prostate Cancer

Frederick M. Hecht, MD
Professor of Medicine, University of California, San Francisco School of Medicine, San Francisco, California
Complementary and Integrative Medicine

Donald D. Hensrud, MD, MPH
Associate Professor of Preventive Medicine and Nutrition, Mayo Clinic College of Medicine and Science, Rochester, Minnesota
Diet and Nutrition

Jeremy Hess, MD, MPH
Professor of Emergency Medicine, University of Washington Center for Health and the Global Environment, Schools of Medicine and Public Health, University of Washington, Seattle, Washington
Effects of Climate Change on Health

Erik L. Hewlett, MD
Professor Emeritus of Medicine and of Microbiology, Immunology and Cancer Biology, University of Virginia School of Medicine, Charlottesville, Virginia
Whooping Cough and Other Bordetella *Infections*

Richard J. Hift, MMed, PhD
Professor of Medicine, University of KwaZulu-Natal, Durban, KwaZulu-Natal, South Africa
The Porphyrias

David R. Hill, MD, DTM&H
Professor of Medical Sciences and Director, Global Public Health, Quinnipiac University Frank H Netter MD School of Medicine, Hamden, Connecticut
Giardiasis

Nicholas S. Hill, MD
Professor of Medicine, Tufts University School of Medicine; Chief, Division of Pulmonary, Critical Care and Sleep Medicine, Tufts Medical Center, Boston, Massachusetts
Respiratory Monitoring in Critical Care

Christopher D. Hillyer, MD
President and Chief Executive Officer, New York Blood Center; Professor of Medicine, Weill Medical College of Cornell University, New York, New York
Transfusion Medicine

Hans H. Hirsch, MD, MSc
Professor and Senior Clinical Consultant, Transplantation & Clinical Virology, Department of Biomedicine, University of Basel; Division of Infectious Diseases & Hospital Epidemiology, Department of Acute Medicine, University Hospital Basel, Basel, Switzerland
Polyomaviruses

Marius M. Hoeper, MD
Professor of Respiratory Medicine, Hannover Medical School, Hannover, Germany
Pulmonary Hypertension

Brian D. Hoit, MD
Professor of Medicine, Physiology and Biophysics, Case Western Reserve University School of Medicine; Director of Echocardiography, Harrington Heart & Vascular Center, University Hospital Cleveland Medical Center, Cleveland, Ohio
Pericardial Diseases

V. Michael Holers, MD
Professor of Medicine and Immunology, University of Colorado School of Medicine, Aurora, Colorado
Complement System in Disease

Steven M. Holland, MD
Director, Division of Intramural Research and Chief, Immunopathogenesis Section, National Institute of Allergy and Infectious Diseases, NIH, Bethesda, Maryland
The Nontuberculous Mycobacteria

Anthony N. Hollenberg, MD
John Wade Professor and Chair, Department of Medicine, Boston University Chobanian & Avedisian School of Medicine; Physician-in-Chief, Boston Medical Center, Boston, Massachusetts
Approach to Medicine, the Patient, and the Medical Profession: Medicine as a Learned and Humane Profession; Thyroid

Steven M. Hollenberg, MD
Professor of Medicine, Emory University School of Medicine; Director, Cardiac Intensive Care, Emory Heart & Vascular Center, Atlanta, Georgia
Cardiogenic Shock

Jo Howard, MB BChir
Consultant Haematologist and Lead Clinician, Haematology, Guy's and St Thomas' National Health Service Foundation Trust; Honorary Professor, King's College London, London, United Kingdom
Sickle Cell Disease and Other Hemoglobinopathies

David J. Hunter, MBBS, MSc, M SpMed, PhD
Florance and Cope Chair of Rheumatology and Co-Director, Sydney Musculoskeletal Health Flagship, University of Sydney, Sydney, Australia
Osteoarthritis

Khalid Hussain, MB ChB, MD, MSc
Professor of Pediatrics, Weill Medical College of Cornell University-Qatar; Division Chief-Endocrinology, Department of Pediatrics, Sidra Medicine, Doha, Qatar
Hypoglycemia

Michael C. Iannuzzi, MD, MBA
Deputy Dean, Professor, and Chair of the Department of Medical Education, City University of New York School of Medicine, New York
Sarcoidosis

Robert D. Inman, MD
Professor of Medicine and Immunology, University of Toronto and Schroeder Arthritis Institute, University Health Network, Toronto, Ontario, Canada
Spondyloarthritis

Sharon K. Inouye, MD, MPH
Professor of Medicine, Harvard Medical School; Director, Aging Brain Center, Marcus Institute for Aging Research-Hebrew SeniorLife, Boston, Massachusetts
Delirium and Changes in Mental Status

Michael G. Ison, MD, MS
Chief, Respiratory Diseases Branch, Division of Microbiology and Infectious Diseases, National Institute of Allergy and Infectious Diseases, National Institutes of Health, Rockville, Maryland
Influenza; Adenovirus Diseases

Joanna C. Jen, MD, PhD
Professor of Neurology, Otolaryngology, Neurosurgery, Icahn School of Medicine at Mount Sinai, New York, New York
Neuro-Ophthalmology; Smell and Taste; Hearing and Equilibrium

Dennis M. Jensen, MD
Professor of Medicine, David Geffen School of Medicine at UCLA; Staff Physician, VA Greater Los Angeles Healthcare System; Director, Human Studies Core & GI Hemostasis Research Unit, CURE Digestive Diseases Research Center, Los Angeles, California
Gastrointestinal Hemorrhage

Michael D. Jensen, MD
Professor of Medicine, Mayo Clinic College of Medicine and Science, Rochester, Minnesota
Obesity

Robert T. Jensen, MD
Chief, Cell Biology Section, Digestive Diseases Branch, National Institute of Diabetes and Digestive and Kidney Diseases, National Institutes of Health, Bethesda, Maryland
Neuroendocrine Neoplasms

S. Claiborne Johnston, MD, PhD
Adjunct Professor of Neurology, University of California, San Francisco School of Medicine, San Francisco, California
Approach to Medicine, the Patient, and the Medical Profession: Medicine as a Learned and Humane Profession; Approach to the Patient with Neurologic Disease

Robin L. Jones, MD, BSc, MB
Professor of Medical Oncology and Head of the Sarcoma Unit, Royal Marsden Hospital and Institute of Cancer Research, London, United Kingdom
Malignant Bone Tumors, Sarcomas, and Other Soft Tissue Neoplasms

Richard C. Jordan, DDS, PhD
Professor of Pathology, Oral Pathology & Radiation Oncology, University of California, San Francisco School of Medicine, San Francisco, California
Diseases of the Mouth and Salivary Glands

Charles J. Kahi, MD, MS
Professor of Medicine, Indiana University School of Medicine, Indianapolis, Indiana
Vascular Diseases of the Gastrointestinal Tract

Laurent Kaiser, MD
Professor of Medicine and Head of the Infectious Disease Division, Geneva University Hospital (HUG), Geneva, Switzerland
Viral Hemorrhagic Fevers

Henry J. Kaminski, MD
Meta A. Neumann Professor of Neurology & Rehabilitation Medicine, George Washington University School of Medicine and Health Sciences, Washington, D.C.
Disorders of Neuromuscular Transmission

Moses R. Kamya, MBChB, MMed, MPH, PhD
Professor of Medicine, Makerere University, Kampala, Uganda; Executive Director, Infectious Diseases Research Collaboration, Kampala, Uganda
Malaria

Louise W. Kao, MD
Professor of Clinical Emergency Medicine and Director, Medical Toxicology Fellowship Program, Indiana University School of Medicine, Indianapolis, Indiana
Chronic Poisoning: Trace Metals and Others

Steven A. Kaplan, MD
Professor of Urology, Icahn School of Medicine at Mount Sinai; Director, Men's Health Program, Mount Sinai Health System, New York, New York
Benign Prostatic Hyperplasia and Prostatitis

Daniel L. Kastner, MD, PhD
NIH Distinguished Investigator and Scientific Director Emeritus, Division of Intramural Research, National Human Genome Research Institute, National Institutes of Health, Bethesda, Maryland
The Systemic Autoinflammatory Diseases

David A. Katzka, MD
Professor of Medicine, Columbia University Vagelos College of Physicians and Surgeons, New York, New York
Diseases of the Esophagus

Debra K. Katzman, MD
Professor of Pediatrics, The Hospital for Sick Children and University of Toronto; Senior Associate Scientist, Research Institute; The Hospital for Sick Children, Toronto, Ontario, Canada
Adolescent Medicine

Kenneth Kaushansky, MD
Professor of Medicine and Dean Emeritus, Renaissance School of Medicine at Stony Brook University, Stony Brook, New York
Hematopoiesis and Hematopoietic Growth Factors

Keith S. Kaye, MD, MPH
Professor of Medicine, Rutgers Robert Wood Johnson Medical School, New Brunswick, New Jersey
Diseases Caused by Acinetobacter *and* Stenotrophomonas *Species*

Armand Keating, MD
Professor of Medicine, University of Toronto, Toronto, Ontario, Canada
Hematopoietic Cell Transplantation

Robin K. Kelley, MD
Professor of Clinical Medicine, University of California, San Francisco School of Medicine, San Francisco, California
Liver and Biliary Tract Tumors

Richard B. Kennedy, PhD
Professor of Medicine and Co-Director, Vaccine Research Group, Mayo Clinic College of Medicine and Science, Rochester, Minnesota
Rubella (German Measles)

Fadlo R. Khuri, MD
President and Professor of Hematology and Medical Oncology, American University of Beirut; Adjunct Professor of Medicine, Pharmacology and Otolaryngology, Emory University School of Medicine, Atlanta, Georgia
Lung Cancer and Other Pulmonary Neoplasms

Rose Kim, MD
Associate Professor of Medicine, Cooper Medical School of Rowan University, Camden, New Jersey
Gram-Positive Rod Infections

Louis V. Kirchhoff, MD, MPH
Professor of Internal Medicine (Infectious Diseases), Psychiatry, and Epidemiology, University of Iowa Carver College of Medicine and College of Public Health, Iowa City, Iowa
Chagas Disease

Hannah Kirking, MD
Medical Epidemiologist, National Center for Immunization and Respiratory Diseases, US Centers for Disease Control and Prevention; Assistant Professor, Department of Medicine, Emory University, Atlanta, Georgia
Pre-2019 Coronaviruses

Ajay J. Kirtane, MD
Professor of Medicine, Columbia University Vagelos College of Physicians and Surgeons; Director, Cardiac Catheterization Laboratories, New York-Presbyterian/Columbia University Irving Medical Center, New York, New York
Interventional Diagnosis and Treatment of Coronary Artery Disease

Priya S. Kishnani, MD
Chen Family Distinguished Professor, Chief, Division of Medical Genetics, Department of Pediatrics, and Professor of Molecular Genetics and Microbiology, Duke University Medical Center, Durham, North Carolina
Glycogen Storage Diseases

Jeffrey D. Klausner, MD, MPH
Clinical Professor of Medicine and Population and Public Health Sciences, Keck School of Medicine of USC, Los Angeles, California
Neisseria gonorrhoeae *Infections*

Amy D. Klion, MD
Senior Clinical Investigator and Head of the Human Eosinophil Section, Deputy Chief of the Laboratory of Parasitic Diseases, National Institute of Allergy and Infectious Diseases, National Institutes of Health, Bethesda, Maryland
Eosinophilic Syndromes

Michael Klompas, MD, MPH
Professor of Medicine and Population Medicine, Department of Population Medicine, Harvard Medical School and Harvard Pilgrim Healthcare Institute; Hospital Epidemiologist, Brigham and Women's Hospital, Boston, Massachusetts
Overview of Pneumonia

David S. Knopman, MD
Robert H. and Susan M. Rewoldt Professorship in Neurology Honoring Bradley F. Boeve, M.D., Mayo Clinic College of Medicine and Science, Rochester, Minnesota
Regional Cerebral Dysfunction: Higher Mental Functions; Cognitive Impairment and Dementia

Christine J. Ko, MD
Professor of Dermatology and Pathology, Yale University School of Medicine, New Haven, Connecticut
Approach to Skin Diseases

Susheel Kodali, MD
Professor of Medicine, Columbia University Vagelos College of Physicians and Surgeons; Director, Structural Heart & Valve Center, New York-Presbyterian/Columbia University Medical Center, New York, New York
Valvular Heart Disease

Dimitrios P. Kontoyiannis, MD, ScD
Robert C. Hickey Chair in Clinical Care and Deputy Head, Division of Internal Medicine, The University of Texas MD Anderson Cancer Center, Houston, Texas
Mucormycosis; Mycetoma and Dematiaceous Fungal Infections

Barbara S. Koppel, MD
Professor of Clinical Neurology (Emeritus), New York Medical College, Valhalla, New York
Nutritional and Alcohol-Related Neurologic Disorders

Kevin M. Korenblat, MD
Professor of Medicine, Washington University School of Medicine in St. Louis, St. Louis, Missouri
Approach to the Patient with Jaundice or Abnormal Liver Tests

Bruce R. Korf, MD, PhD
Wayne H. and Sara Crews Finley Endowed Chair in Medical Genetics, Distinguished Professor of Genetics, and Associate Dean for Genomic Medicine, University of Alabama at Birmingham Heersink School of Medicine, Birmingham, Alabama
Principles of Genetics

Mark G. Kortepeter, MD, MPH
Professor of Preventive Medicine and Medicine and Vice President for Research, Uniformed Services University of the Health Sciences, Bethesda, Maryland
Bioterrorism

Anita A. Koshy, MD
Associate Professor of Neurology, University of Arizona, Tucson, Arizona
Toxoplasmosis

Shyamasundaran Kottilil, MD, PhD
Professor of Medicine and Chief of Infectious Diseases, University of Maryland School of Medicine, Baltimore, Maryland
Antiviral Therapy (Non-HIV)

Joseph A. Kovacs, MD
Senior Investigator, Critical Care Medicine Department, National Institutes of Health Clinical Center, Bethesda, Maryland
Pneumocystis *Pneumonia*

Thomas O. Kovacs, MD
Professor of Medicine, David Geffen School of Medicine at UCLA, Los Angeles, California
Gastrointestinal Hemorrhage

Kris V. Kowdley, MD
Professor of Medicine, Elson S. Floyd College of Medicine, and Director, Liver Institute Northwest, Washington State University, Seattle, Washington
Iron Overload (Hemochromatosis)

Monica Kraft, MD
Murray M. Rosenberg Professor and System Chair, Samuel Bronfman Department of Medicine, Icahn School of Medicine at Mount Sinai and Mount Sinai Health System, New York, New York
Approach to the Patient with Respiratory Disease

Christopher M. Kramer, MD
George A. Beller MD/Lantheus Medical Imaging Distinguished Professor of Cardiovascular Medicine and Chief, Cardiovascular Division, University of Virginia School of Medicine, Charlottesville, Virginia
Noninvasive Cardiac Imaging

Donna M. Krasnewich, MD, PhD
Program Director, National Institute of General Medical Sciences, National Institutes of Health, Bethesda, Maryland
Lysosomal Storage Diseases

William E. Kraus, MD
Richard and Pat Johnson Distinguished University Professor, Duke University School of Medicine, Durham, North Carolina
Physical Activity

Peter J. Krause, MD
Senior Research Scientist, Yale University School of Public Health and Yale University School of Medicine, New Haven, Connecticut
Babesiosis and Other Protozoan Diseases

Andrew T. Kroger, MD, MPH
Medical Officer, National Center for Immunization and Respiratory Diseases, Centers for Disease Control and Prevention, Atlanta, Georgia
Immunization

Daniela Kroshinsky, MD, MPH
Professor, Vice Chair of Strategic Initiatives and Faculty Development, and Director of Pediatric Dermatology, Department of Dermatology, Duke University School of Medicine, Durham, North Carolina
Macular, Papular, Purpuric, Vesiculobullous, and Pustular Diseases

John F. Kuemmerle, MD
Professor of Medicine, Virginia Commonwealth University School of Medicine, Richmond, Virginia
Inflammatory and Anatomic Diseases of the Intestine, Peritoneum, Mesentery, and Omentum

Ernst J. Kuipers, MD, PhD
Professor of Medicine, Erasmus MC University Medical Center, Rotterdam, Netherlands
Acid Peptic Disease

Jean S. Kutner, MD
Professor of Medicine, University of Colorado School of Medicine, Aurora, Colorado
Palliative Care

Daniel Laheru, MD
Ian T. MacMillan Professorship in Clinical Pancreatic Research, Johns Hopkins University School of Medicine, Baltimore, Maryland
Pancreatic Cancer

Rachel Lampert, MD
Professor of Medicine, Yale University School of Medicine, New Haven, Connecticut
Cardiac Arrest and Life-Threatening Arrhythmias

C. Seth Landefeld, MD
Professor and Chair of Medicine, University of Alabama at Birmingham Heersink School of Medicine, Birmingham, Alabama
Geriatric Assessment

Raphael J. Landovitz, MD, MSc
Professor of Medicine, Center for Clinical AIDS Research & Education, David Geffen School of Medicine at UCLA, Los Angeles, California
Prevention of Human Immunodeficiency Virus Infection

Donald W. Landry, MD, PhD
Hamilton Southworth Professor and Chair Emeritus, Department of Medicine, Columbia University Vagelos College of Physicians and Surgeons; Physician-in-Chief, Columbia University Irving Medical Center, New York, New York
Approach to the Patient with Renal Disease

Richard A. Lange, MD, MBA
Rick and Ginger Francis Endowed Professor and President, Texas Tech University Health Sciences Center El Paso; Dean, Paul L. Foster School of Medicine, El Paso, Texas
Acute Coronary Syndrome: Unstable Angina and Non–ST Elevation Myocardial Infarction

Hochang B. Lee, MD
John Romano Professor and Chair, Department of Psychiatry, University of Rochester School of Medicine & Dentistry, Rochester, New York
Psychiatric Disorders in Medical Practice

Nelson Lee, MD, MBBS
Professor, Institute for Pandemics, Dalla Lana School of Public Health, University of Toronto, Toronto, Ontario, Canada
Influenza

Andrew S. Levey, MD
Professor of Medicine and Dr. Gerald J and Dorothy R Friedman Professor Emeritus, Tufts University School of Medicine; Chief Emeritus, Division of Nephrology, Tufts Medical Center, Boston, Massachusetts
Chronic Kidney Disease

Stephanie M. Levine, MD
Professor of Medicine, University of Texas Health San Antonio, San Antonio, Texas
Alveolar Filling Disorders

Gary R. Lichtenstein, MD
Professor of Medicine, University of Pennsylvania Perelman School of Medicine; Director, Center for Inflammatory Bowel Disease, Department of Medicine, Hospital of the University of Pennsylvania, Philadelphia, Pennsylvania
Inflammatory Bowel Disease

Jeffrey M. Liebmann, MD
Shirlee and Bernard Brown Professor and Vice Chair, Department of Ophthalmology, Columbia University Vagelos College of Physicians and Surgeons, New York, New York
Diseases of the Visual System

Jane M. Liebschutz, MD, MPH
Professor of Medicine, Falk Chair in Ambulatory Medicine, and Chief, Division of General Internal Medicine, University of Pittsburgh School of Medicine, UPMC Health System, Pittsburgh, Pennsylvania
Drug Use Disorders

Henry W. Lim, MD
Former Chair, Department of Dermatology; Senior Vice President for Academic Affairs, Henry Ford Health, Detroit, Michigan
Eczemas, Photodermatoses, Papulosquamous (Including Fungal) Diseases, and Figurate Erythemas

Aldo A.M. Lima, MD, PhD
Professor, Institute of Biomedicine, Federal University of Ceara, Fortaleza, Ceará, Brazil
Cryptosporidiosis

Ajit P. Limaye, MD
Professor of Medicine and Director, Solid Organ Transplant Infectious Disease Program, Departments of Medicine and Laboratory Medicine, Division of Allergy & Infectious Diseases, University of Washington, Seattle, Washington
Cytomegalovirus

Nita A. Limdi, PharmD, PhD, MSPH
Ray L Watts Heersink Endowed Chair and Professor, Departments of Neurology and of Epidemiology; Director, Translational Pharmacogenomics Program and Associate Director, Hugh Kaul Precision Medicine Institute, University of Alabama Birmingham Heersink School of Medicine, Birmingham, Alabama
Principles of Genetics

Mark S. Link, MD
Professor of Medicine, University of Texas Southwestern Medical Center, Dallas, Texas
Electrocardiography

Catherine Liu, MD
Professor, Vaccine and Infectious Disease Division, Fred Hutchinson Cancer Center; Professor of Medicine, University of Washington, Seattle, Washington
Staphylococcal Infections

Donald M. Lloyd-Jones, MD, ScM
Eileen M. Foell Professor of Heart Research; Professor of Preventive Medicine, Medicine, and Pediatrics; Chair, Department of Preventive Medicine; Northwestern University Feinberg School of Medicine, Chicago, Illinois
Epidemiology of Cardiovascular Disease

Fred A. Lopez, MD
Richard Vial Professor and Vice Chair, Department of Medicine, Louisiana State University Health Sciences Center-New Orleans, New Orleans, Louisiana
Tularemia and Other Francisella *Infections*

Arnold Louie, MD
Professor of Medicine, Molecular Genetics and Microbiology and Associate Director, Institute for Therapeutic Innovation, University of Florida College of Medicine, Orlando, Florida
Antibacterial Chemotherapy

Jeffrey M. Lyness, MD
President and CEO, American Board of Psychiatry & Neurology, Deerfield, Illinois; Professor Emeritus of Psychiatry, University of Rochester School of Medicine & Dentistry, Rochester, New York
Psychiatric Disorders in Medical Practice

C. Ronald MacKenzie, MD
C. Ronald MacKenzie Chair in Ethics and Medicine, Hospital for Special Surgery; Professor of Clinical Medicine and Medical Ethics, Weill Medical College of Cornell University, New York, New York
Surgical Treatment of Joint Diseases

Calman A. MacLennan, BM, BCh, DPhil
Senior Program Officer—Bacterial Vaccines, Enteric and Diarrheal Diseases, Global Health, Bill & Melinda Gates Foundation, Seattle, Washington; Jenner Investigator, Jenner Institute, Nuffield Department of Medicine, University of Oxford, Oxford, Oxfordshire, United Kingdom; Professor of Vaccine Immunology and Director of BactiVac, Institute of Immunology and Immunotherapy, University of Birmingham, Birmingham, West Midlands, United Kingdom
Shigellosis

Harriet L. MacMillan, CM, MD, MSc
Chedoke Health Chair in Child Psychiatry and Distinguished University Professor of Psychiatry & Behavioural Neurosciences and of Pediatrics, Offord Centre for Child Studies, McMaster University Michael G. DeGroote School of Medicine, Hamilton, Ontario, Canada
Intimate Partner Violence

Robert D. Madoff, MD
Professor of Surgery, University of Minnesota, Minneapolis, Minnesota
Diseases of the Rectum and Anus

Jacquelyn Maher, MD
William and Mary Ann Rice Distinguished Professor of Medicine and Director of UCSF Liver Center, University of California, San Francisco School of Medicine, San Francisco, California
Alcoholic and Nonalcoholic Steatohepatitis

Lisa A. Maier, MD, MSPH
Professor of Medicine, University of Colorado, and Chief, Division of Occupational Environmental Health Sciences, National Jewish Health, Denver, Colorado
Physical and Chemical Injuries of the Lung

Frank Maldarelli, MD, PhD
Head, Clinical Retrovirology Section, HIV Dynamics and Replication Program, NCI-Frederick, Frederick, Maryland
Pathobiology of Human Immunodeficiency Viruses

Atul Malhotra, MD
Peter C Farrell Presidential Chair and Professor of Medicine, Research Chief of Pulmonary and Critical Care Medicine, and Director of Sleep Medicine, University of California, San Diego, School of Medicine, La Jolla, California
Disorders of Ventilatory Control

Mark J. Manary, MD
Helene B. Roberson Professor of Pediatrics, Washington University, St. Louis, Missouri
Severe Malnutrition

Luis A. Marcos, MD, MPH
Associate Professor of Medicine and Director of the Tick-Borne Disease Center, Division of Infectious Diseases, Department of Medicine; Department of Microbiology and Immunology, Renaissance School of Medicine at Stony Brook University, Stony Brook, New York
Trematode Infections

Ariane J. Marelli, MD, MPH
Professor of Medicine, McGill University Faculty for Medicine and Health Sciences, Director, McGill Adult Unit for Congenital Heart Disease, McGill University Health Centre, Montreal, Quebec, Canada
Congenital Heart Disease in Adults

Andrew R. Marks, MD
Wu Professor and Chair, Department of Physiology and Cellular Biophysics, Director, Helen and Clyde Wu Center for Molecular Cardiology, Columbia University Vagelos College of Physicians and Surgeons, New York, New York
Cardiac and Circulatory Function

Jonas Marschall, MD, MSc, DTM&H
Professor of Medicine, Washington University School of Medicine in St. Louis, St. Louis, Missouri
Legionella *Infections*

Paul Martin, MD
Mandel Chair in Gastroenterology and Chief, Division of Digestive Health and Liver Diseases, University of Miami Miller School of Medicine, Miami, Florida
Approach to the Patient with Liver Disease

Fernando J. Martinez, MD, MS
Bruce Webster Professor of Internal Medicine, Weill Medical College of Cornell University; Chief, Division of Pulmonary and Critical Care Medicine, Weill Medical College of Cornell University/NY Presbyterian Hospital, New York, New York
Interstitial Lung Disease

Joel B. Mason, MD
Professor of Medicine and Nutrition, Divisions of Gastroenterology and Clinical Nutrition, Tufts University; Director, Vitamins & Carcinogenesis Laboratory, U.S.D.A. Human Nutrition Research Center at Tufts University, Boston, Massachusetts
Vitamins, Trace Minerals, and Other Micronutrients

Henry Masur, MD
Chief, Critical Care Medicine Department, Clinical Center, National Institutes of Health, Bethesda, Maryland
Microbial Complications of HIV/AIDS

Amy J. Mathers, MD
Associate Professor of Medicine and Pathology, Associate Director of Clinical Microbiology, and Medical Director Antimicrobial Stewardship, University of Virginia School of Medicine, Charlottesville, Virginia
Enterobacterales: Non-Enteric Infections and Multidrug Resistance

Michael A. Matthay, MD
Professor of Medicine and Anesthesia, University of California, San Francisco School of Medicine, San Francisco, California
Acute Respiratory Failure

F. Dennis McCool, MD
Professor of Medicine, Warren Alpert Medical School of Brown University, Providence, Rhode Island
Diseases of the Diaphragm, Chest Wall, Pleura, and Mediastinum

Iain B. McInnes, PhD
Vice-Principal and Head of College of Medical, Veterinary and Life Sciences, Muirhead Chair of Medicine/Versus Arthritis Professor of Rheumatology, University of Glasgow, Glasgow, United Kingdom
Rheumatoid Arthritis

Vallerie McLaughlin, MD
Kim A. Eagle MD Endowed Professor of Cardiovascular Medicine, Professor of Medicine, and Director, Pulmonary Hypertension Program, University of Michigan Medical School, Ann Arbor, Michigan
Pulmonary Hypertension

Amy McMichael, MD
Professor of Dermatology, Wake Forest School of Medicine, Winston-Salem, North Carolina
Infections, Pigmentation Disorders, Regional Dermatology, and Distinctive Lesions in Black Skin

John J.V. McMurray, MB ChB, MD
Professor of Medical Cardiology, British Heart Foundation Cardiovascular Research Centre, University of Glasgow; Honorary Consultant Cardiologist, Queen Elizabeth University Hospital Glasgow, Glasgow, Scotland, United Kingdom
Heart Failure: Treatment and Prognosis

Kenneth R. McQuaid, MD
Professor of Clinical Medicine and Vice-Chair, Department of Medicine, University of California, San Francisco School of Medicine; Chief of the Medical Service, San Francisco Veterans Affairs Medical Center, San Francisco, California
Approach to the Patient with Gastrointestinal Disease

Paul S. Mead, MD, MPH
Chief, Bacterial Diseases Branch, Division of Vector-Borne Diseases, Centers for Disease Control and Prevention, Fort Collins, Colorado
Plague and Other Yersinia *Infections*

Robert T. Means, Jr., MD
Professor of Internal Medicine and Clinical Professor of Pathology, East Tennessee State University James H. Quillen College of Medicine, Johnson City, Tennessee
Approach to the Anemias

Michael T. Melia, MD
Associate Professor of Medicine, Johns Hopkins University School of Medicine, Baltimore, Maryland
Approach to Fever or Suspected Infection in the Normal Host

Ingo K. Mellinghoff, MD
Chair, Department of Neurology, Memorial Sloan Kettering Cancer Center; Professor of Neurology and of Neuroscience, Weill Medical College of Cornell University, New York, New York
Tumors of the Central Nervous System

Genevieve B. Melton, MD, PhD
Professor of Surgery, University of Minnesota Medical School, Minneapolis, Minnesota
Diseases of the Rectum and Anus

Samuel T. Merrick, MD
Professor of Clinical Medicine, Weill Medical College of Cornell University, New York, New York
Systemic Manifestations of HIV/AIDS

Marisa H. Miceli, MD
Clinical Professor of Infectious Diseases and Internal Medicine, University of Michigan Medical School, Ann Arbor, Michigan
Endemic Mycoses

Marc Michel, MD, MSc
Professor and Head of the Department of Internal Medicine and Clinical Immunology, Henri Mondor University Hospital, Assistance Publique Hopitaux de Paris, Université Paris-Est Créteil, Creteil, France
Autoimmune and Intravascular Hemolytic Anemias

Ali H. Mokdad, PhD
Chief Strategy Officer, Population Health, and Professor of Health Metrics Sciences, Department of Health Metrics Sciences, Institute of Health Metrics and Evaluation, University of Washington, Seattle, Washington
Global Health

Ernest Moy, MD, MPH
Executive Director, Office of Health Equity, Veterans Health Administration, Washington D.C.
Measuring Health and Health Care

Debabrata Mukherjee, MD, MS
Professor and Chairman, Department of Internal Medicine, Texas Tech University Health Sciences Center El Paso, El Paso, Texas
Acute Coronary Syndrome: Unstable Angina and Non–ST Elevation Myocardial Infarction

Andrew H. Murr, MD
Professor and Chairman, Department of Otolaryngology-Head and Neck Surgery, University of California, San Francisco School of Medicine, San Francisco, California
Approach to the Patient with Nose, Sinus, and Ear Disorders

Robert J. Myerburg, MD
Professor of Medicine, Cardiovascular Genetics, and Physiology, Department of Medicine, University of Miami Miller School of Medicine, Miami, Florida
Cardiac Arrest and Life-Threatening Arrhythmias

Kari C. Nadeau, MD, PhD
John Rock Professor of Climate and Population Studies and Chair, Department of Environmental Health, Harvard T.H. Chan School of Public Health, Boston, Massachusetts
Approach to the Patient with Allergic or Immunologic Disease

Avindra Nath, MD
Chief, Section of Infections of the Nervous System, National Institutes of Neurological Diseases and Stroke, National Institutes of Health, Bethesda, Maryland
Meningitis: Bacterial, Viral, and Other; Brain Abscess and Parameningeal Infections

Genevieve Neal-Perry, MD, PhD
Robert A. Ross Distinguished Professor and Chair, Department of Obstetrics and Gynecology, University of North Carolina School of Medicine, Chapel Hill, North Carolina
Menopause

Eric G. Neilson, MD
Vice President for Medical Affairs, Lewis Landsberg Dean, and Professor of Medicine and of Cell and Developmental Biology, Northwestern University Feinberg School of Medicine, Chicago, Illinois
Interstitial Nephritis

Christina A. Nelson, MD, MPH
Medical Officer, Bacterial Diseases Branch, Division of Vector-Borne Diseases, Centers for Disease Control and Prevention, Fort Collins, Colorado
Plague and Other Yersinia *Infections*

David B. Nelson, MD, FACOG
Gillette Professorship of Obstetrics and Gynecology, Dedman Family Scholar in Clinical Care, Associate Professor of Obstetrics and Gynecology and Chief, Division of Maternal-Fetal Medicine, University of Texas Southwestern Medical Center, Dallas, Texas
Medical Issues in Pregnancy

Lewis S. Nelson, MBA, MD
Professor and Chair, Department of Emergency Medicine; Director, Division of Medical Toxicology, Rutgers New Jersey Medical School, Newark, New Jersey
Acute Poisoning

Eric J. Nestler, MD, PhD
Nash Family Professor of Neuroscience and Director, Friedman Brain Institute, Icahn School of Medicine at Mount Sinai, New York, New York
Biology of Addiction

Kathleen M. Neuzil, MD, MPH
Myron M. Levine Professor of Medicine and Pediatrics and Director, Center for Vaccine Development and Global Health, University of Maryland School of Medicine, Baltimore, Maryland
COVID-19 Treatment and Vaccination

Lynnette K. Nieman, MD
Senior Investigator, Diabetes, Endocrinology and Obesity Branch, National Institute of Diabetes and Digestive and Kidney Diseases, National Institutes of Health, Bethesda, Maryland
Approach to the Patient with Endocrine Disease; Adrenal Cortex; Polyglandular Disorders

Alexander S. Niven, MD
Professor of Medicine, Mayo Clinic College of Medicine and Science, Rochester, Minnesota
Respiratory Testing and Function

Christopher M. O'Connor, MD
Adjunct Professor of Medicine, Duke University School of Medicine, Durham, North Carolina; CEO, Inova Heart and Vascular Institute, Fairfax, Virginia
Heart Failure: Epidemiology, Pathobiology, and Diagnosis

Francis G. O'Connor, MD, MPH
Professor of Military and Emergency Medicine and Medical Director, Consortium for Health and Military Performance, Uniformed Services University of the Health Sciences, Bethesda, Maryland
Disorders Due to Heat and Cold; Rhabdomyolysis

Patrick G. O'Connor, MD, MPH
Dan Adams and Amanda Adams Professor of Medicine and Chief, General Internal Medicine, Yale University School of Medicine, New Haven, Connecticut
Alcohol Use Disorders

Anne E. O'Donnell, MD
The Nehemiah and Naomi Cohen Chair in Pulmonary Disease Research, Georgetown University School of Medicine; Chief, Division of Pulmonary, Critical Care and Sleep Medicine, Georgetown University Medical Center, Washington, D.C.
Bronchiectasis, Atelectasis, Cavitary, or Cystic Lung Diseases

James S. O'Donnell, MD, PhD
Professor, Irish Centre for Vascular Biology, Royal College of Surgeons in Ireland, Dublin, Ireland
Von Willebrand Disease and Hemorrhagic Abnormalities of Platelet and Vascular Function

Jae K. Oh, MD
Professor of Medicine, Mayo Clinic College of Medicine and Science, Rochester, Minnesota; Director, Heart Vascular Stroke Institute, Samsung Medical Center, Seoul, Gangnam, South Korea
Pericardial Diseases

Michael S. Okun, MD
Professor and Chair of Neurology, Fixel Institute for Neurological Diseases, University of Florida College of Medicine, Gainesville, Florida
Parkinsonism; Other Movement Disorders

Sean T. O'Leary, MD, MPH
Professor of Pediatrics, University of Colorado School of Medicine, Aurora, Colorado
Papillomavirus

Jeffrey E. Olgin, MD
Gallo-Chatterjee Distinguished Professor and Chief of Cardiology, University of California, San Francisco School of Medicine, San Francisco, California
Approach to the Patient with Suspected Arrhythmia

Kenneth N. Olivier, MD, MPH
Professor of Medicine, University of North Carolina at Chapel Hill, Chapel Hill, North Carolina
The Nontuberculous Mycobacteria

Iacopo Olivotto, MD
Professor of Cardiovascular Medicine, Meyer Children's Hospital IRCCS, University of Florence, Florence, Italy
Diseases of the Myocardium and Endocardium

Nancy J. Olsen, MD
Professor of Medicine, Penn State Milton S. Hershey Medical Center, Hershey, Pennsylvania
Biologic Agents and Signaling Inhibitors

Walter A. Orenstein, MD, DSc
Professor of Medicine, Pediatrics, Epidemiology & Global Health, Emory University School of Medicine; Associate Director, Emory Vaccine Center, Atlanta, Georgia
Immunization

Thomas L. Ortel, MD, PhD
Professor of Medicine and Pathology and Chief, Division of Hematology, Duke University School of Medicine, Durham, North Carolina
Antithrombotic and Antiplatelet Therapy

John J. O'Shea, MD
Scientific Director, National Institute of Arthritis and Musculoskeletal and Skin Diseases, National Institutes of Health, Bethesda, Maryland
Biologic Agents and Signaling Inhibitors

Douglas R. Osmon, MD
Professor of Medicine, Mayo Clinic College of Medicine and Science, Rochester, Minnesota
Infections of Bursae, Joints, and Bones

Jill L. Ostrem, MD
Carlin and Ellen Wiegner Distinguished Professor of Neurology, University of California, San Francisco School of Medicine, San Francisco, California
Parkinsonism; Other Movement Disorders

Luis Ostrosky-Zeichner, MD
Professor and Division Chief, Division of Infectious Diseases, University of Texas Health Science Center at Houston; Medical Director for Epidemiology, Memorial Hermann Texas Medical Center, Houston, Texas
Mucormycosis

Catherine M. Otto, MD
J. Ward Kennedy-Hamilton Endowed Chair in Cardiology and Professor of Medicine, University of Washington School of Medicine; Director, Heart Valve Clinic, and Associate Director, Echocardiography, University of Washington Medical Center, Seattle, Washington
Echocardiography

Martin G. Ottolini, MD
Professor of Pediatrics and Director, Capstone Student Research Program, Office of the Dean, School of Medicine, Uniformed Services University of the Health Sciences, Bethesda, Maryland
Measles

Inna G. Ovsyannikova, PhD
Professor of Medicine, Mayo Clinic College of Medicine and Science, Rochester, Minnesota
Rubella (German Measles)

Peter G. Pappas, MD
Professor of Medicine, University of Alabama at Birmingham Heersink School of Medicine, Birmingham, Alabama
Candidiasis; Mycetoma and Dematiaceous Fungal Infections

Ben Ho Park, MD, PhD
Benjamin F. Byrd, Jr Chair in Oncology and Professor of Medicine, Vanderbilt University School of Medicine; Director, Vanderbilt-Ingram Cancer Center, Vanderbilt University Medical Center, Nashville, Tennessee
Cancer Biology and Genetics

Robin Patel, MD
Elizabeth P. and Robert E. Allen Professor of Individualized Medicine and Professor of Medicine and of Microbiology; Director, Infectious Diseases Research Laboratory and Vice Chair Education, Department of Laboratory Medicine and Pathology, Mayo Clinic College of Medicine and Science, Rochester, Minnesota
Introduction to Microbial Disease: Pathophysiology and Diagnostics

Thomas F. Patterson, MD
Professor of Medicine, Long School of Medicine, University of Texas Health Science Center, San Antonio; Chief, Infectious Diseases, UT Health San Antonio, San Antonio, Texas
Aspergillosis

Jean-Michel Pawlotsky, MD, PhD
Professor, Department of Virology, Henri Mondor University Hospital AP-HP, Paris-Est University & INSERM U955, Créteil, France
Acute Viral Hepatitis; Chronic Viral and Autoimmune Hepatitis

Thomas H. Payne, MD
Professor of Medicine and Professor of Biomedical Informatics and Medical Education, University of Washington School of Medicine; Adjunct Professor of Health Systems and Population Health, University of Washington School of Public Health, Seattle, Washington
Statistical Interpretation of Data for Clinical Decision Making

Elizabeth N. Pearce, MD, MSc
Professor of Medicine, Boston University Chobanian & Avedisian School of Medicine, Boston, Massachusetts
Thyroid

Richard D. Pearson, MD
Professor Emeritus of Medicine, University of Virginia School of Medicine, Charlottesville, Virginia
Antiparasitic Therapy

Trish M. Perl, MD, MSc
Professor of Medicine and H. Ben and Isabelle T. Decherd Chair in Internal Medicine in Honor of Henry M. Winans, Sr., M.D., University of Texas Southwestern Medical Center, Dallas, Texas
Enterococcal Infections

Brett W. Petersen, MD, MPH
Deputy Branch Chief, Poxvirus and Rabies Branch, Centers for Disease Control and Prevention, Atlanta, Georgia
Smallpox, Monkeypox, and Other Poxvirus Infections

William A. Petri, Jr., MD, PhD
Wade Hampton Frost Professor of Epidemiology and Vice Chair for Research, Department of Medicine, University of Virginia School of Medicine, Charlottesville, Virginia
Relapsing Fever and Other Borrelia *Infections; African Sleeping Sickness; Amebiasis*

Marc A. Pfeffer, MD, PhD
Distinguished Dzau Professor of Medicine, Harvard Medical School; Senior Physician, Brigham and Women's Hospital, Boston, Massachusetts
Heart Failure: Treatment and Prognosis

Jennifer A. Philips, MD, PhD
Theodore and Bertha Bryan Professor of Medicine and Molecular Microbiology and Co-Director, Division of Infectious Diseases, Washington University School of Medicine in St. Louis, St. Louis, Missouri
Tuberculosis

David S. Pisetsky, MD, PhD
Professor of Medicine and Immunology, Duke University School of Medicine; Medical Research Service, VA Medical Center, Durham, North Carolina
Laboratory Testing in the Rheumatic Diseases

Steven D. Pletcher, MD
Professor of Clinical Otolaryngology, University of California, San Francisco School of Medicine, San Francisco, California
Approach to the Patient with Nose, Sinus, and Ear Disorders

Ian D. Plumb, MBBS, MSc
Epidemiologist, National Center for Immunization and Respiratory Diseases, Centers for Disease Control and Prevention, Atlanta, Georgia
Pre-2019 Coronaviruses

Gregory A. Poland, MD
Lowell Leary Emeritus Mary Professor of Medicine and Director, Vaccine Research Group, Mayo Clinic College of Medicine and Science, Rochester, Minnesota
Rubella (German Measles)

Frank Powell, PhD
Professor of Medicine, University of California, San Diego School of Medicine, La Jolla, California
Disorders of Ventilatory Control

Reed E. Pyeritz, MD, PhD
William Smilow Professor of Medicine and Genetics, Emeritus, University of Pennsylvania Perelman School of Medicine, Philadelphia, Pennsylvania
Inherited Diseases of Connective Tissue

Thomas C. Quinn, MD, MSc
Professor of Medicine and Pathology and Director, Center for Global Health, Johns Hopkins University School of Medicine; Associate Director for International Research, National Institute of Allergy and Infectious Diseases, National Institutes of Health, Baltimore, Maryland
Epidemiology and Diagnosis of Human Immunodeficiency Virus Infection and Acquired Immunodeficiency Syndrome; Acute Clinical Manifestations and Diagnosis of HIV

Vincent Racaniello, PhD
Higgins Professor of Microbiology & Immunology, Columbia University Vagelos College of Physicians and Surgeons, New York, New York
COVID-19: Virology and Pathology

Jai Radhakrishnan, MD, MS
Professor of Medicine, Columbia University Vagelos College of Physicians and Surgeons; Clinical Director, Division of Nephrology, Columbia University Irving Medical Center, New York, New York
Disorders of Sodium and Water; Glomerular Disorders and Nephrotic Syndromes

Jerald Radich, MD
Professor of Medical Oncology, Clinical Research Division, Fred Hutchinson Cancer Center and University of Washington School of Medicine, Seattle, Washington
Chronic Myeloid Leukemia

Petros I. Rafailidis, MD, PhD, MSc
Associate Professor Internal Medicine-Infectious Diseases, Democritus University of Thrace; Second University Department of Internal Medicine, University General Hospital of Greece, Alexandroupolis, Greece; Senior Researcher, Alfa Institute of Biomedical Sciences, Athens, Greece
Pseudomonas *and* Burkholderia *Infections*

Ganesh Raghu, MD
Professor of Medicine and Laboratory Medicine (adjunct), University of Washington School of Medicine; Director, Center for Interstitial Lung Diseases, and Co-Director, Scleroderma Clinic, University of Washington Medical Center, Seattle, Washington
Interstitial Lung Disease

Margaret V. Ragni, MD, MPH
Professor of Medicine and Clinical Translational Science, University of Pittsburgh School of Medicine; Director, Hemophilia Center of Western Pennsylvania, Pittsburgh, Pennsylvania
Coagulation Factor Deficiencies

Proton Rahman, MD
University Research Professor of Medicine, Memorial University, St. Johns, Newfoundland, Canada
Spondyloarthritis

S. Vincent Rajkumar, MD
Edward W. and Betty Knight Scripps Professor of Medicine, Mayo Clinic College of Medicine and Science, Rochester, Minnesota
Plasma Cell Disorders

Stuart H. Ralston, MB ChB, MD
Versus Arthritis Professor of Rheumatology, University of Edinburgh, Edinburgh, United Kingdom
Paget Disease of Bone

Didier Raoult, MD, PhD
Emeritus Professor, Aix-Marseille Université and, Institut Hospitalo-Universitaire Méditerranée-Infection, Marseille, France
Bartonella *Infections; Rickettsial Infections*

Annette C. Reboli, MD
Dean and Professor of Medicine, Cooper Medical School of Rowan University, Camden, New Jersey
Gram-Positive Rod Infections

K. Rajender Reddy, MD
Founders Professor of Medicine, University of Pennsylvania Perelman School of Medicine, Philadelphia, Pennsylvania
Bacterial, Parasitic, Fungal, and Granulomatous Liver Diseases

Donald A. Redelmeier, MD
Professor of Medicine, University of Toronto; Canada Research Chair, Medical Decision Science; Senior Scientist, Evaluative Clinical Sciences, Sunnybrook Research Institute; Staff Physician, Sunnybrook Health Sciences Centre, Toronto, Ontario, Canada
Postoperative Care and Complications

Carrie A. Redlich, MD, MPH
Professor of Medicine, Pulmonary and Critical Care Medicine, Yale University School of Medicine, New Haven, Connecticut
Occupational Lung Disease

John Reilly, MD
Richard D. Krugman Endowed Chair, Dean, School of Medicine, and Vice Chancellor for Health Affairs, University of Colorado School of Medicine, Aurora, Colorado
Chronic Obstructive Pulmonary Disease

Megan E. Reller, MD, PhD, MPH
Associate Professor of Medicine, Duke University School of Medicine, Durham, North Carolina
Zoonoses

Hilary E.L. Reno, MD, PhD
Professor of Medicine, Washington University in St. Louis, St. Louis, Missouri
Diseases Caused by Chlamydiae

Neil M. Resnick, MD
Thomas Detre Professor of Medicine, University of Pittsburgh School of Medicine; Chief, Division of Geriatric Medicine and Gerontology, University of Pittsburgh Medical Center, Pittsburgh, Pennsylvania
Urinary Incontinence

Louis B. Rice, MD
Joukowsky Family Professor and Chair of Medicine, Professor of Molecular Microbiology and Immunology, Warren Alpert Medical School of Brown University, Providence, Rhode Island
Principles of Anti-Infective Therapy

E. Steve Roach, MD
Professor of Neurology, University of Texas Dell Medical School, Dell Children's Hospital, Austin, Texas
Developmental and Neurocutaneous Disorders

Jennifer G. Robinson, MD, MPH
Professor Emeritus of Epidemiology and Medicine; Director, Prevention Intervention Center, Department of Epidemiology, University of Iowa Carver College of Medicine, Iowa City, Iowa
Disorders of Lipid Metabolism

Inez Rogatsky, PhD
Professor of Microbiology and Immunology, Weill Medical College of Cornell University; Senior Scientist, Arthritis and Tissue Degeneration Program, Hospital for Special Surgery, New York, New York
Immunomodulatory Drugs

Joseph G. Rogers, MD
Adjunct Professor of Medicine, Duke University School of Medicine, Durham, North Carolina; President and CEO, Texas Heart Institute, Houston, Texas
Heart Failure: Epidemiology, Pathobiology, and Diagnosis

Jean-Marc Rolain, PharmD, PhD
Professor, Aix-Marseille Université and Institut Hospitalo-Universitaire Méditerranée Infection, Marseille, France
Bartonella *Infections*

Barrett J. Rollins, MD, PhD
Linde Family Professor of Medicine, Dana-Farber Cancer Institute, Brigham and Women's Hospital, and Harvard Medical School, Boston, Massachusetts
Histiocytoses

José R. Romero, MD
Arkansas Secretary of Health and Director of the Department of Health; Professor of Pediatrics, University of Arkansas for Medical Sciences, Little Rock, Arkansas
Enteroviruses

Jennifer B. Rosen, MD
Director, Epidemiology and Surveillance, Bureau of Immunization, New York City Department of Health and Mental Hygiene, Long Island City, New York
Mumps

Philip J. Rosenthal, MD
Professor of Medicine, University of California, San Francisco School of Medicine, San Francisco, California
Malaria

James A. Russell, MD
Professor of Medicine, University of British Columbia, Vancouver, British Columbia, Canada
Shock Syndromes Related to Sepsis

Anil K. Rustgi, MD
Herbert and Florence Irving Professor of Medicine and Director, Herbert Irving Comprehensive Cancer Center, Columbia University Vagelos College of Physicians and Surgeons; Chief, New York-Presbyterian Hospital/Columbia University Irving Medical Center Cancer Service, New York, New York
Approach to Medicine, the Patient, and the Medical Profession: Medicine as a Learned and Humane Profession; Neoplasms of the Esophagus and Stomach

Joshua D. Safer, MD
Professor of Medicine, Icahn School of Medicine at Mount Sinai, and Executive Director, Center for Transgender Medicine and Surgery, Mount Sinai Health System, New York, New York
Transgender Medicine

Sarbjit S. Saini, MD
Professor of Medicine, Johns Hopkins University School of Medicine, Baltimore, Maryland
Urticaria and Angioedema

Jane E. Salmon, MD
Collette Kean Research Chair, Hospital for Special Surgery; Professor of Medicine, Weill Medical College of Cornell University, New York, New York
Tissue Injury and Repair

Edsel Maurice T. Salvana, MD, DTM&H
Director, Institute of Molecular Biology and Biotechnology, National Institutes of Health, University of the Philippines Manila; Professor, Section of Infectious Diseases, Department of Medicine, Philippine General Hospital, Manila, Philippines
Brucellosis

Nanette Santoro, MD
Professor and E. Stewart Taylor Chair, Department of Obstetrics and Gynecology, University of Colorado School of Medicine, Aurora, Colorado
Menopause

Peter A. Santucci, MD
Professor of Medicine, Loyola University Medical Center, Maywood, Illinois
Electrophysiologic Procedures and Surgery

Mark J. Sarnak, MD, MS
Dr. Gerald J and Dorothy R Friedman Professor of Medicine and Chief, Division of Nephrology, Tufts University School of Medicine, Boston, Massachusetts
Chronic Kidney Disease

Kerry J. Savage, MD
Professor of Medicine, University of British Columbia; Medical Oncologist, British Columbia Cancer Agency, Vancouver, British Columbia, Canada
Hodgkin Lymphoma

Patrice Savard, MD, MSc
Associate Clinical Professor of Microbiology, Infectious Diseases and Immunology, Université de Montréal; Chief, Infectious Diseases Division, Centre Hospitalier de l'Université de Montréal (CHUM), Québec, Canada
Enterococcal Infections

Michael N. Sawka, PhD
Adjunct Professor, School of Biological Sciences, Georgia Institute of Technology, Atlanta, Georgia
Disorders Due to Heat and Cold

Paul D. Scanlon, MD
Professor of Medicine, Mayo Clinic College of Medicine and Science, Rochester, Minnesota
Respiratory Testing and Function

Andrew I. Schafer, MD
Professor of Medicine and Director, Richard T. Silver Center for Myeloproliferative Neoplasms, Weill Medical College of Cornell University, New York, New York
Thrombotic Disorders: Hypercoagulable States; Approach to the Patient with Bleeding or Thrombosis; Disseminated Intravascular Coagulation and Bleeding in Liver Failure

Manuel Schiff, MD, PhD
Professor of Paediatrics, Reference Center for Inborn Errors of Metabolism, Necker University Hospital, APHP and University of Paris Cité; INSERM UMRS_1163, Institut Imagine, Paris, France
Homocystinuria and Hyperhomocysteinemia

Michael L. Schilsky, MD
Professor of Medicine and Surgery, Yale University School of Medicine, New Haven, Connecticut
Wilson Disease

Thomas Rudolf Schneider, MD, PhD
Professor of Infectious Diseases, Medical Clinic 1, Department of Gastroenterology, Infectious Diseases and Rheumatology, Charite Campus Benjamin Franklin, Berlin, Germany
Whipple Disease

Robert T. Schooley, MD
Professor of Medicine, University of California, San Diego School of Medicine, San Diego, California
Epstein-Barr Virus Infection

David L. Schriger, MD, MPH
Professor Emeritus and Vice Chair of Emergency Medicine, David Geffen School of Medicine at UCLA, Los Angeles, California
Approach to the Patient with Abnormal Vital Signs

Lynn M. Schuchter, MD
Madlyn and Leonard Abramson Professor of Medicine and Director, Tara Miller Melanoma Center, University of Pennsylvania Perelman School of Medicine, Philadelphia, Pennsylvania
Melanoma and Nonmelanoma Skin Cancers

Lawrence B. Schwartz, MD, PhD
Distinguished Professor of Medicine, Virginia Commonwealth University School of Medicine, Richmond, Virginia
Anaphylaxis

Carlos Seas, MD, MSc
Associate Professor of Medicine, Universidad Peruana Cayetano Heredia; Vice Director, Alexander von Humboldt Tropical Medicine Institute, and Attending Physician, Infectious and Tropical Medicine, Hospital Nacional Cayetano Heredia, Lima, Peru
Cholera and Other Vibrio *Infections*

Steven A. Seifert, MD†
Professor of Emergency Medicine, University of New Mexico School of Medicine; Medical Director, New Mexico Poison and Drug Information Center, Albuquerque, New Mexico
Envenomation, Bites, and Stings

Julian Lawrence Seifter, MD
James G. Haidas Distinguished Chair in Medicine, Brigham and Women's Hospital and Harvard Medical School, Boston, Massachusetts
Potassium Disorders; Acid-Base Disorders

Duygu Selcen, MD
Professor of Neurology and Pediatrics, Mayo Clinic College of Medicine and Science, Rochester, Minnesota
Muscle Diseases

Magdy Selim, MD, PhD
Professor of Neurology, Harvard Medical School, and Chief, Division of Stroke and Cerebrovascular Disease, Beth Israel Hospital, Boston, Massachusetts
Hemorrhagic Cerebrovascular Disease

Carol E. Semrad, MD
Professor of Medicine, University of Chicago Pritzker School of Medicine, Chicago, Illinois
Approach to the Patient with Diarrhea and Malabsorption

Jorge Sepulveda, MD, PhD
Professor of Pathology, George Washington University School of Medicine and Health Sciences, Washington, D.C.
Reference Intervals and Laboratory Values

Pamela J. Shaw, DBE, MBBS, MD
Professor of Neurology, Sheffield Institute for Translational Neuroscience, University of Sheffield, Sheffield, United Kingdom
Amyotrophic Lateral Sclerosis and Other Motor Neuron Diseases

Beth H. Shaz, MD
Professor of Pathology and Deputy Director, Marcus Center for Cellular Cures, Duke University School of Medicine, Durham, North Carolina
Transfusion Medicine

Robert L. Sheridan, MD
Professor of Surgery, Harvard Medical School and Massachusetts General Hospital, Boston, Massachusetts
Medical Aspects of Trauma and Burns

Stuart Sherman, MD
Glen A. Lehman Professor of Gastroenterology, Professor of Medicine and of Radiology, and Director, Advanced Endoscopy, Indiana University School of Medicine, Indianapolis, Indiana
Diseases of the Gallbladder and Bile Ducts

Kaveh G. Shojania, MD
Professor and Vice Chair (Quality & Innovation), Department of Medicine, University of Toronto, Toronto, Ontario, Canada
Quality, Safety, and Value

Bo Shopsin, MD, PhD
Associate Professor, Department of Medicine and Microbiology, New York University Grossman School of Medicine, New York, New York
Staphylococcal Infections

Michael E. Shy, MD
Carver College of Medicine Chair in Inherited Neuropathies and Professor of Neurology, Pediatrics, and Molecular Physiology and Biophysics, University of Iowa Carver College of Medicine, Iowa City, Iowa
Peripheral Neuropathies

†Deceased.

Ellen Sidransky, MD
Chief, Medical Genetics Branch, National Human Genome Research Institute, National Institutes of Health, Bethesda, Maryland
Lysosomal Storage Diseases

Costi D. Sifri, MD
Professor of Medicine and Medical Director, Immunocompromised Infectious Diseases Program, University of Virginia School of Medicine, Charlottesville, Virginia
Approach to Fever and Suspected Infection in the Immunocompromised Host

Robert F. Siliciano, MD, PhD
Professor of Medicine, Johns Hopkins University School of Medicine; Investigator, Howard Hughes Medical Institute, Baltimore, Maryland
Pathobiology of Human Immunodeficiency Viruses

David L. Simel, MD, MHS
Professor of Medicine, Duke University School of Medicine; Chief, Medical Service, Durham Veterans Affairs Medical Center, Durham, North Carolina
History and Physical Examination

Karl Skorecki, MD
Professor, Azrieli Faculty of Medicine, Bar-Ilan University, Safed Gan, Israel
Regenerative Medicine, Cell Therapy, and Gene Therapy

Barbara A. Slawski, MD, MS
Professor of Medicine and Chief of Hospital Medicine, Medical College of Wisconsin, Milwaukee, Wisconsin
Principles of Medical Consultation

Arthur S. Slutsky, CM, MD
Professor of Medicine, Surgery and Biomedical Engineering, University of Toronto; St Michael's Hospital; Keenan Research Centre, Li Ka Shing Knowledge Institute, Unity Health Toronto, Toronto, Ontario, Canada
Mechanical Ventilation

Gerald W. Smetana, MD
Professor of Medicine, Harvard Medical School and Physician, Division of General Medicine, Beth Israel Deaconess Medical Center, Boston, Massachusetts
Principles of Medical Consultation

A. Gordon Smith, MD
Professor and Chair of Neurology, Virginia Commonwealth University School of Medicine, Richmond, Virginia
Peripheral Neuropathies

Stephen R. Smith, MD, MHS
Professor of Medicine, Duke University School of Medicine, Durham, North Carolina
Vascular Disorders of the Kidney

Frederick S. Southwick, MD
Professor of Medicine, University of Florida College of Medicine, Gainesville, Florida
Nocardiosis

Allen M. Spiegel, MD
Dean Emeritus and Professor of Medicine, Albert Einstein College of Medicine, Bronx, New York
Principles of Endocrinology; Polyglandular Disorders

Robert Spiera, MD
Professor of Clinical Medicine, Weill Medical College of Cornell University; Director of the Scleroderma, Vasculitis, and Myositis Center, Hospital for Special Surgery, New York, New York
Giant Cell Arteritis and Polymyalgia Rheumatica

Stanley M. Spinola, MD
Professor of Microbiology and Immunology, Medicine, and Pathology and Laboratory Medicine, Indiana University School of Medicine, Indianapolis, Indiana
Chancroid

Catherine Y. Spong, MD
Professor and Chair, Department of Obstetrics and Gynecology, Paul C. MacDonald Distinguished Chair in Obstetrics and Gynecology, University of Texas Southwestern Medical School, Dallas, Texas
Medical Issues in Pregnancy

Sally P. Stabler, MD
Professor of Medicine and Cleo Scott & Mitchell Vincent Allen Chair in Hematology Research, University of Colorado School of Medicine, Aurora, Colorado
Megaloblastic Anemias

Paul Stark, MD
Professor Emeritus of Radiology, University of California, San Diego School of Medicine; Chief, Cardiothoracic Radiology, VA San Diego Healthcare System, La Jolla, California
Imaging in Pulmonary Disease

E. William St. Clair, MD
W. Lester Brooks, Jr. Professor of Medicine, Duke University School of Medicine, Durham, North Carolina
Sjögren Syndrome

Theodore S. Steiner, MD
Professor and Head, Division of Infectious Diseases, University of British Columbia, Vancouver, British Columbia, Canada
Escherichia coli *Enteric Infections*

David S. Stephens, MD
Stephen W. Schwarzmann Distinguished Professor of Medicine and Chair, Department of Medicine, Emory University School of Medicine, Atlanta, Georgia
Neisseria meningitidis *Infections*

David A. Stevens, MD
Professor of Medicine, Stanford University Medical School, Stanford, California; President, California Institute for Medical Research, Principal Investigator, Infectious Diseases Research Laboratory, California Institute for Medical Research, San Jose, California
Systemic Antifungal Agents

Dennis L. Stevens, MD, PhD
Professor of Medicine, University of Washington School of Medicine, Seattle, Washington
Nonpneumococcal Streptococcal Infections and Rheumatic Fever

M. Barry Stokes, MB BCh
Professor of Pathology and Cell Biology, Columbia University Vagelos College of Physicians and Surgeons, New York, New York
Glomerular Disorders and Nephrotic Syndromes

James K. Stoller, MD, MS
Jean Wall Bennett Professor of Medicine, Samson Global Leadership Endowed Chair, and Chairman, Education Institute, Cleveland Clinic Lerner College of Medicine, Cleveland Clinic, Cleveland, Ohio
Respiratory Monitoring in Critical Care

John H. Stone, MD, MPH
Professor of Medicine, Harvard Medical School; Edward A. Fox Chair in Medicine, Massachusetts General Hospital, Boston, Massachusetts
The Systemic Vasculitides

Richard M. Stone, MD
Professor of Medicine, Harvard Medical School; Lunder Family Chair in Leukemia, Chief of the Medical Staff, Dana-Farber Cancer Institute, Boston, Massachusetts
Myelodysplastic Syndromes

Edwin P. Su, MD
Professor of Clinical Orthopaedics, Weill Medical College of Cornell University; Attending Orthopaedic Surgeon, Hospital for Special Surgery, New York, New York
Surgical Treatment of Joint Diseases

Ronald S. Swerdloff, MD
Professor of Medicine, David Geffen School of Medicine at UCLA, Los Angeles, California; Chief, Division of Endocrinology, Metabolism and Nutrition, Harbor-UCLA Medical Center; Senior Investigator, The Lundquist Institute, Torrance, California
The Testis and Male Hypogonadism, Infertility, and Sexual Dysfunction

Heidi Swygard, MD, MPH
Professor of Medicine, University of North Carolina at Chapel Hill, Chapel Hill, North Carolina
Approach to the Patient with a Sexually Transmitted Infection

Megan Sykes, MD
Michael J. Friedlander Professor of Medicine and Director, Columbia Center for Translational Immunology, Columbia University Vagelos College of Physicians and Surgeons, New York, New York
Transplantation Immunology

H. Keipp Talbot, MD, MPH
Associate Professor of Medicine and Health Policy, Vanderbilt University Medical Center, Nashville, Tennessee
Respiratory Syncytial Virus and Human Metapneumovirus

Rulla M. Tamimi, ScD
Professor of Population Health Sciences, Weill Medical College of Cornell University, New York, New York
Epidemiology of Cancer

Marian Tanofsky-Kraff, PhD
Professor of Medical and Clinical Psychology and of Medicine, Uniformed Services University of the Health Sciences, Bethesda, Maryland
Eating Disorders

Susan M. Tarlo, MBBS
Professor of Medicine, University of Toronto; Respiratory Physician, University Health Network, Toronto, Ontario, Canada
Occupational Lung Disease

Stephanie N. Taylor, MD
Professor of Medicine, Louisiana State University Health Sciences Center, New Orleans, Louisiana
Neisseria gonorrhoeae *Infections*

Paul S. Teirstein, MD
Chief of Cardiology and Director, Interventional Cardiology, Scripps Clinic, La Jolla, California
Interventional Diagnosis and Treatment of Coronary Artery Disease

Sam R. Telford, III, ScD
Professor of Infectious Disease and Global Health, Tufts University School of Veterinary Medicine, North Grafton, Massachusetts
Babesiosis and Other Protozoan Diseases

Rajesh V. Thakker, MD
May Professor of Medicine, Radcliffe Department of Medicine, University of Oxford, Oxford, United Kingdom
The Parathyroid Glands, Hypercalcemia, and Hypocalcemia

Judith Therrien, MD
Professor of Medicine, McGill University and Jewish General Hospital, Montreal, Quebec, Canada
Congenital Heart Disease in Adults

George R. Thompson, III, MD
Professor of Medicine, University of California–Davis School of Medicine, Sacramento, California
Endemic Mycoses

Laura Tormoehlen, MD
Associate Professor of Clinical Neurology and Emergency Medicine, Department of Neurology and Emergency Medicine, Indiana University, Indianapolis, Indiana
Chronic Poisoning: Trace Metals and Others

Antonella Tosti, MD
Fredric Brandt Endowed Professor of Dermatology, Dr. Phillip Frost Department of Dermatology and Cutaneous Surgery, University of Miami Miller School of Medicine, Miami, Florida
Diseases of Hair and Nails

Indi Trehan, MD, MPH, DTM&H
Associate Professor of Pediatrics and Adjunct Associate Professor of Global Health and of Epidemiology, University of Washington, Seattle, Washington
Severe Malnutrition

Guillermo E. Umpierrez, MD
Professor of Medicine, Emory University, Atlanta, Georgia
Diabetes Mellitus

Anthony Michael Valeri, MD
Professor of Medicine, Columbia University Vagelos College of Physicians and Surgeons; Medical Director, Hemodialysis, DaVita-Haven Dialysis Center and DaVita-Highbridge Park Dialysis Center, New York, New York
Treatment of Irreversible Renal Failure

John Varga, MD
Frederick G. Huetwell Professor and Chief, Division of Rheumatology, University of Michigan Medical School, Ann Arbor, Michigan
Systemic Sclerosis (Scleroderma)

Bradley V. Vaughn, MD
Professor of Neurology, University of North Carolina, Chapel Hill, North Carolina
Sleep Disorders

Alan P. Venook, MD
Professor of Clinical Medicine, University of California, San Francisco School of Medicine, San Francisco, California
Liver and Biliary Tract Tumors

Joseph G. Verbalis, MD
Professor of Medicine, Georgetown University; Chief, Endocrinology and Metabolism, Georgetown University Hospital, Washington, D.C.
Posterior Pituitary

Julie M. Vose, MD, MBA
Professor of Medicine and Chief, Hematology/Oncology, University of Nebraska Medical Center College of Medicine, Omaha, Nebraska
Non-Hodgkin Lymphomas

Robert M. Wachter, MD
Holly Smith Professor and Chairman, Department of Medicine, University of California, San Francisco School of Medicine, San Francisco, California
Quality, Safety, and Value

B. Timothy Walsh, MD
Ruane Professor of Psychiatry, Columbia University Vagelos College of Physicians and Surgeons and New York State Psychiatric Institute, New York, New York
Eating Disorders

Edward E. Walsh, MD
Professor of Medicine, University of Rochester School of Medicine & Dentistry, Rochester, New York
Respiratory Syncytial Virus and Human Metapneumovirus

Thomas J. Walsh, MD
Formerly Professor of Medicine, Pediatrics, and Microbiology Immunology; Director, Transplantation-Oncology Infectious Diseases, Weill Medical College of Cornell University and New York Presbyterian Hospital, New York, New York
Aspergillosis

Jeremy D. Walston, MD
Raymond and Anna Lublin Professor of Geriatric Medicine, Johns Hopkins University School of Medicine, Baltimore, Maryland
Common Clinical Sequelae of Aging

Roland B. Walter, MD, PhD, MS
Professor, Translational Science and Therapeutics Division, Fred Hutchinson Cancer Center; Professor of Medicine, University of Washington School of Medicine, Seattle, Washington
The Acute Leukemias

Christina Wang, MD
Professor of Medicine, David Geffen School of Medicine at UCLA, Los Angeles, California; Senior Associate Director, Clinical and Translational Science Institute, the Lundquist Institute and Harbor-UCLA Medical Center, Torrance, California
The Testis and Male Hypogonadism, Infertility, and Sexual Dysfunction

Kenneth K. Wang, MD
Russ and Kathy Van Cleve Professor of Gastroenterology Research, Mayo Clinic School of Medicine and Science, Rochester, Minnesota
Gastrointestinal Endoscopy

Lorraine B. Ware, MD
Professor of Medicine, Pathology, Microbiology, and Immunology, Vanderbilt University School of Medicine, Nashville, Tennessee
Acute Respiratory Failure

Cirle A. Warren, MD
Professor of Medicine, University of Virginia School of Medicine, Charlottesville, Virginia
Cryptosporidiosis

Paul B. Watkins, MD
Howard Q Ferguson Distinguished Professor, Division of Pharmacometrics and Experimental Therapeutics, Eshelman School of Pharmacy; Director, Institute for Drug Safety Sciences, University of North Carolina, Chapel Hill, North Carolina
Drug-Induced Liver Injury

Thomas J. Weber, MD
Professor of Medicine, Duke University School of Medicine, Durham, North Carolina
Approach to the Patient with Metabolic Bone Disease; Osteoporosis

Louis H. Weimer, MD
Professor of Neurology, Columbia University Vagelos College of Physicians and Surgeons, New York, New York
Nutritional and Alcohol-Related Neurologic Disorders

Geoffrey A. Weinberg, MD
Professor of Pediatrics, University of Rochester School of Medicine & Dentistry; Director, Clinical Pediatric Infectious Diseases & Pediatric HIV Program, Golisano Children's Hospital, University of Rochester Medical Center, Rochester, New York
Parainfluenza Viral Disease

Robert S. Weinstein, MD
Professor of Medicine and Director, Bone Morphometry Laboratory, University of Arkansas for Medical Sciences, Little Rock, Arkansas
Osteomalacia and Rickets

Roger D. Weiss, MD
Professor of Psychiatry, Harvard Medical School, Boston, Massachusetts; Chief, Division of Alcohol, Drugs, and Addiction, McLean Hospital, Belmont, Massachusetts
Drug Use Disorders

Roy E. Weiss, MD, PhD
Kathleen & Stanley Glaser Distinguished Chair and Chairman, Department of Medicine, University of Miami Miller School of Medicine, Miami, Florida
Neuroendocrinology and the Neuroendocrine System; Anterior Pituitary

Jeffrey I. Weitz, MD
Professor of Medicine & Biochemistry, McMaster University Michael G. DeGroote School of Medicine; Executive Director, Thrombosis & Atherosclerosis Research Institute, Hamilton, Ontario, Canada
Venous Thrombosis and Embolism

Frederick G.P. Welt, MD
Professor of Medicine, Associate Chief of Cardiovascular Medicine, and Director of the Cardiac Catheterization Laboratory, University of Utah School of Medicine, Salt Lake City, Utah
ST-Elevation Acute Myocardial Infarction and Complications of Myocardial Infarction

Richard P. Wenzel, MD, MSc
Professor and Former Chairman, Internal Medicine, Virginia Commonwealth University School of Medicine, Richmond, Virginia
Acute Bronchitis and Tracheitis

Victoria P. Werth, MD
Professor of Dermatology, University of Pennsylvania Perelman School of Medicine; Chief of Dermatology, Corporal Michael J. Crescenz VAMC, Philadelphia, Pennsylvania
Principles of Therapy of Skin Diseases

Sterling G. West, MD
Professor of Medicine, University of Colorado School of Medicine, Aurora, Colorado
Systemic Diseases in Which Arthritis Is a Feature

A. Clinton White, Jr., MD
Professor of Internal Medicine, University of Texas Medical Branch, Galveston, Texas
Cestodes

Christopher J. White, MD
Chairman and Professor of Medicine and Cardiology, Ochsner Clinical School of the University of Queensland, Ochsner Medical Institutions, New Orleans, Louisiana
Atherosclerotic Peripheral Arterial Disease

Julian White, MBBS, MD
Professor and Head, Toxinology Department, Women's and Children's Hospital, North Adelaide, South Australia, Australia
Envenomation, Bites, and Stings

Perrin C. White, MD
Audry Newman Rapoport Distinguished Chair, Pediatric Endocrinology, Professor of Pediatrics, University of Texas Southwestern Medical Center; Chief of Endocrinology, Children's Medical Center, Dallas, Texas
Sexual Development

Richard J. Whitley, MD
Distinguished Professor of Pediatrics, Loeb Eminent Scholar Chair in Pediatrics, and Professor of Microbiology, Medicine, and Neurosurgery, Pediatrics, University of Alabama at Birmingham Heersink School of Medicine, Birmingham, Alabama
Herpes Simplex Virus Infections

Michael P. Whyte, MD
Emeritus Professor of Medicine, Washington University School of Medicine in St. Louis, St. Louis, Missouri
Osteonecrosis, Osteosclerosis/Hyperostosis, and Other Disorders of Bone

Samuel Wiebe, MD, MSc
Professor of Clinical Neurosciences, Community Health Sciences, and Pediatrics; Director, Adult Epilepsy Program and Epilepsy Co-Lead, Hotchkiss Brain Institute, University of Calgary Cumming School of Medicine, Calgary, Alberta, Canada
The Epilepsies

Jeanine P. Wiener-Kronish, MD
Distinguished Henry Isaiah Dorr Professor of Research and Teaching in Anaesthesia, Harvard Medical School and Massachusetts General Hospital, Boston, Massachusetts
Overview of Anesthesia

David J. Wilber, MD
George M Eisenberg Professor of Medicine, Loyola University Chicago Stritch School of Medicine, Maywood, Illinois
Electrophysiologic Procedures and Surgery

Mark H. Wilcox, MD
Professor and Head of Medical Microbiology Research & Development, Microbiology, Leeds Teaching Hospitals & University of Leeds, Leeds, United Kingdom
Clostridial and Clostridioides *Infections*

Beverly Winikoff, MD, MPH
President, Gynuity Health Projects; Professor of Clinical Population and Family Health, Population and Family Health, Columbia University Mailman School of Public Health, New York, New York
Contraception

Jane N. Winter, MD
Professor of Medicine, Northwestern University Feinberg School of Medicine, Chicago, Illinois
Approach to the Patient with Lymphadenopathy or Splenomegaly

Marsha N. Wittink, MD, MBE
Associate Professor of Psychiatry and Family Medicine and Academic Chief, Division of Medicine in Psychiatry, University of Rochester School of Medicine & Dentistry, Rochester, New York
Medical Care of Patients with Psychiatric Diseases

Tracy A. Wolff, MD, MPH
Scientific Director, US Preventive Services Task Force Program, Center for Evidence and Practice Improvement, Agency for Healthcare Research and Quality, Rockville, Maryland
The Preventive Health Visit

Edward M. Wolin, MD
Professor of Medicine, Albert Einstein College of Medicine; Director, Neuroendocrine Tumor Program, Department of Medical Oncology, Montefiore Einstein Center for Cancer Care, Bronx, New York
Neuroendocrine Neoplasms

Gary P. Wormser, MD
Professor of Medicine and of Pathology, Microbiology and Immunology, and Pharmacology; Chief, Division of Infectious Diseases, New York Medical College, Valhalla, New York
Lyme Disease

Clyde W. Yancy, MD, MSc
Professor of Medicine, Chief of Cardiology, Professor of Medical Social Sciences, and Vice-Dean, Diversity & Inclusion, Northwestern University Feinberg School of Medicine; Associate Director, Bluhm Cardiovascular Institute, Northwestern Medicine, Chicago, Illinois
Cardiogenic Shock

Neal S. Young, MD
Chief, Hematology Branch, National Heart, Lung, and Blood Institute, National Institutes of Health, Bethesda, Maryland
Parvovirus

Vincent B. Young, MD, PhD
William Henry Fitzbutler Professor of Internal Medicine/Infectious Diseases, Professor of Microbiology and Immunology, University of Michigan Medical School, Ann Arbor, Michigan
The Human Microbiome

William F. Young, Jr., MD, MSc
Tyson Family Endocrinology Clinical Professor of Medicine, Mayo Clinic College of Medicine and Science, Rochester, Minnesota
Adrenal Medulla, Catecholamines, and Pheochromocytoma

Alan S.L. Yu, MB BChir
Harry Statland and Solon Summerfield Professor, University of Kansas Medical Center; Director, The Kidney Institute, University of Kansas Medical Center, Kansas City, Kansas
Disorders of Magnesium and Phosphorus

Peter Zimetbaum, MD
Richard and Susan Smith Professor of Cardiovascular Medicine, Harvard Medical School; Associate Chief and Director of Clinical Cardiology, Beth Israel Deaconess Medical Center, Boston, Massachusetts
Bradycardias and Conduction System Delays; Supraventricular Ectopy and Tachyarrhythmias

Jane R. Zucker, MD, MSc
Assistant Commissioner, Bureau of Immunization, New York City Department of Health and Mental Hygiene, Queens, New York
Mumps

CONTENTS

VOLUME 1

SECTION IX: VASCULAR MEDICINE

SECTION X: RESPIRATORY DISEASES

SECTION XI: CRITICAL CARE MEDICINE

SECTION XXV: RETROVIRUSES

SECTION XXVI: BEHAVIORAL MEDICINE

SECTION XXVII: NEUROLOGY

VIDEO CONTENTS

This icon appears throughout the book to indicate chapters with accompanying video available on Elsevier eBooks+.

EYE, EAR, NOSE, AND THROAT DISEASES

Cecil

I SOCIAL AND ETHICAL ISSUES IN MEDICINE

1

APPROACH TO MEDICINE, THE PATIENT, AND THE MEDICAL PROFESSION: MEDICINE AS A LEARNED AND HUMANE PROFESSION

LEE GOLDMAN, KATHLEEN A. COONEY, KIRSTEN BIBBINS-DOMINGO, MARY K. CROW, NANCY E. DAVIDSON, JEFFREY M. DRAZEN, VICTORIA J. FRASER, ALI G. GHARAVI, ANTHONY N. HOLLENBERG, S. CLAIBORNE JOHNSTON, AND ANIL K. RUSTGI

APPROACH TO MEDICINE

THE HISTORIC EVOLUTION

Medicine is a profession that incorporates science and the scientific method with the art of being a physician. The art of tending to the sick is as old as humanity itself. Even in modern times, the art of caring and comforting, guided by common sense over millennia as well as by a more recent, systematic approach to medical ethics (Chapter 2), remains the cornerstone of medicine. Without these humanistic qualities, the application of the modern science of medicine is suboptimal, ineffective, or even detrimental.

However, the essential humanistic qualities of caring and comforting can achieve full benefit only if they are coupled with an understanding of how medical science can and should be applied to all individuals regardless of their race, sex, sexual orientation, or other characteristics. Without this knowledge, comforting may be inappropriate or misleading and caring may be ineffective or counterproductive if it inhibits a sick person from obtaining appropriate, scientific medical care.

The concept of *internal medicine*, which began in 19th-century Germany, was to emphasize the underlying pathobiologic causes of disease, not just the patterns or progression of clinical manifestations. Modern medicine is based on increasingly accelerated discoveries made with this approach over the past 150 years, during which time human life expectancy has approximately doubled.[1] *Goldman-Cecil Medicine* incorporates this tradition by showing how pathobiologic abnormalities cause clinical manifestations and by emphasizing how therapies can modify this underlying pathophysiology and improve the patient's well-being.

CONTEMPORARY MEDICAL SCIENCE

The contemporary practice of medicine now includes an increasingly detailed understanding of cellular, subcellular, molecular, genetic, and epigenetic mechanisms of health and disease. For example, the understanding of microbial pathogenesis as well as that of many noninfectious (as we understand them now) inflammatory diseases (Chapter 236) is now guided by a detailed understanding of the human immune system and its response to foreign antigens (Chapters 35 to 37).

Health, disease, and an individual's interaction with the environment are also substantially determined by genetics and epigenetics. In addition to monogenic conditions, medical science increasingly understands the complex interactions that underlie multigenic traits, including diabetes mellitus, cancer, and other common health conditions (Chapter 32). The decoding of the human genome holds the promise that personalized health care increasingly can be targeted according to an individual's genetic profile, in terms of screening and presymptomatic disease management, as well as in terms of specific medications, their complex interactions, and their adjusted dosing schedules.[2]

Knowledge of the structure and physical forms of proteins helps explain abnormalities as diverse as sickle cell anemia (Chapter 149) and prion-related diseases (Chapter 371). Proteomics, which is the large-scale analysis of proteins produced by an organism, also holds extraordinary promise for developing drug targets for more specific and effective therapies. Increasingly, the effects of nurture and the environment, expressed as epigenetic modifications of DNA or chromatin, are also being deciphered, with the potential for future therapeutic interventions. A striking illustration is evolving evidence that the gut microbiome is shaped at the time of birth during vaginal delivery. Advances in our understanding of the human microbiome also raise the possibility that our complex interactions with microbes, which outnumber the cells in the human body by a factor of 10, will help explain conditions ranging from inflammatory bowel disease (Chapter 127) to obesity (Chapter 201).

EVIDENCE-BASED MEDICINE

Concurrent with these advances in fundamental human biology has been a dramatic shift in methods for evaluating the application of scientific advances to the individual patient and to populations. The randomized controlled trial, sometimes with thousands of patients at multiple institutions, has replaced anecdote as the most robust method for measuring the benefits and optimal uses of diagnostic and therapeutic interventions (Chapter 8). Yet this approach to the evaluation of therapeutics and diagnostics is being challenged. To reduce costs as well as overcome inefficiencies, redundancies, and the late failure of many clinical trials (at the phase III stage) inherent in classic randomized controlled trials, technologic advances are enabling new methods, tools, and approaches to bring clinical trials into the 21st century. These methods include disease modeling and simulation, alternative trial methods such as response-adaptive randomized designs (Chapter 8), real-world pragmatic trials, population-based studies, use of artificial intelligence and data science, implementation science, community-engaged research, novel objective outcome measures, and engagement of clinical trial "participants" (rather than "human subjects") to expand the pool of individuals willing to be involved in clinical research.

As research progresses from studies that show biologic effect, to studies that elucidate dosing schedules and toxicity, and finally to controlled trials that assess true clinical benefit, the metrics of measuring outcome has also improved from subjective impressions of physicians or patients to reliable and valid measures of morbidity, quality of life, functional status, and other patient-oriented outcomes (Chapter 9). These marked improvements in the scientific methodology of clinical investigation have expedited extraordinary changes in clinical practice, such as recanalization therapy for acute myocardial infarction (Chapter 58) and aspiration therapy for cerebrovascular clots (Chapter 377), which focus on important outcomes, including not only death but also physical function and quality of life. Just as physicians in the 21st century must understand advances in fundamental biology, similar understanding of the fundamentals of clinical study design as it applies to diagnostic and therapeutic interventions is important.

An understanding of human genomics and genetics can also help stratify and refine the approach to clinical trials by helping researchers identify fewer patients with a more homogeneous disease pattern to study the efficacy of an intervention. Such an approach has been especially relevant in cancer, in which tumors with certain genetic mutations can respond to a drug specifically designed for that target, whereas other tumors with similar histologic but different molecular characteristics will not. Germline genetic testing is now common in clinical practice, and molecular biomarkers are increasingly important for screening, surveillance, early detection, risk stratification, and therapy. Systems biology, which is the integration of all these techniques, can enable the development of new predictive, preventive, and personalized approaches to disease.

CHANGES IN MEDICAL PRACTICE

This explosion in medical knowledge and clinical research has led to increasing specialization and subspecialization, defined initially by organ system and more recently by locus of principal activity (inpatient as compared with outpatient), reliance on manual skills (proceduralist vs. nonproceduralist), or participation in research. Sophisticated computerized analyses of radiographs,[3] computed tomographic scans, magnetic resonance images, retinal images,[4] and histopathologic specimens are also poised to revolutionize the interpretation of these tests, much as computerized electrocardiographic interpretation (Chapter 42) changed clinical cardiology.

Computerized health records can avoid duplication of tests, ensure that care is coordinated among the patient's various health care providers, and increase the value of health care. Real-time electronic monitoring can be used to alert physicians about patients whose vital signs (Chapter 7) might warrant urgent evaluation to avoid more serious clinical decompensation.[5] Data derived from electronic medical records can detect patterns of drug side effects or interactions that can then guide molecular analyses that confirm new risks or even genetic diseases.[6]

Although it is too soon to know whether patients would routinely benefit from sequencing and analysis of their exome or full genome, such information is increasingly becoming affordable and more accurate, with potential usefulness for identifying Mendelian disease patterns[7] and informing reproductive planning. Despite much hope, however, genetic profiling of germline sequences has had limited positive impact on drug selection and dosing.

NEW THERAPEUTICS

Gene therapy is currently approved by the U.S. Food and Drug Administration (FDA) for only a few diseases—Leber congenital amaurosis (Chapter 391), retinal dystrophy, beta thalassemia, hemophilia (Chapter 160), and spinal muscular atrophy (Chapter 387) are examples—but many more gene therapies are in development and clinical testing. Specific DNA sequences can now be targeted with clustered regularly interspaced short palindromic repeats (CRISPR)-associated nucleases to inactivate genes or to correct a pathogenic mutation back to the reference sequence. This technique has already demonstrated durable benefits for patients with hemophilia (Chapter 160).

Cell-based therapy is now beginning to provide vehicles for the delivery of cells engineered to address a patient's particular chimeric antigen receptor (CAR).[8] CAR-T cell therapy is FDA-approved for conditions such as non-Hodgkin lymphoma (Chapter 171), acute lymphoblastic leukemia (Chapter 168), multiple myeloma (Chapter 173), melanoma (Chapter 188), and prostate cancer (Chapter 186), and it is being actively tested in other conditions. Although effective in many cases, cost and severe side effects, especially the so-called cytokine release syndrome, currently limit its widespread use.

Regenerative medicine to help heal injured or diseased organs, by the administration of cells modified to meet a patient's needs, is in its infancy. However, cultured chondrocytes are now FDA-approved to repair cartilaginous defects of the femoral condyle and the knee.

Immune checkpoint inhibitors have revolutionized the approach to treating cancer, initially melanoma (Chapter 188),[9] but now also a wide range of malignancies, with future potential efficacy for the treatment of refractory infectious diseases, autoimmune diseases, and serious allergic disorders.[10] Messenger RNA (mRNA) vaccines, which deliver antigen-encoding mRNA into immune cells, where they stimulate an adaptive immune response, have revolutionized the approach to preventing severe acute respiratory syndrome coronavirus-2 (SARS-CoV-2; Chapter 337) and are increasingly being applied to other infections.[11]

SOCIETAL IMPLICATIONS

Extraordinary advances in the science and practice of medicine have transformed the global burden of disease. For example, vaccines and other population-wide interventions, such as screening for and treating hypertension and hypercholesterolemia, have greatly reduced the burden of infectious and cardiovascular diseases. In many countries, life expectancies for men and women have been increasing, a greater proportion of deaths are occurring among people older than age 70 years, and far fewer children are dying before the age of 5 years. In the United States, however, overall life expectancy has declined in the last several years. Explanations include not only the unprecedented SARS-CoV-2 pandemic and the coronavirus-2019 (COVID-19) disease it causes, but also obesity-related diseases[12] as well as so-called deaths of despair owing to alcohol, drug overdoses, and suicide.[13] Disability from conditions such as substance abuse, mental health disorders, injuries, diabetes, musculoskeletal disease, and chronic respiratory disease have become increasingly important issues for all health systems.

Globally, but also within the United States, substantial health disparities persist based on geography, race, ethnicity, socioeconomic status, and often sexual orientation and gender identity.[14] Physicians must understand historic as well as current health disparities and the social determinants of health. They must strive to understand the benefits and needs of diverse populations and individual patients, and they must be advocates for equity, inclusion, access, and social justice in all aspects of medicine and health care.[15]

APPROACH TO THE PATIENT

Patients commonly have complaints (symptoms), but at least one third of these symptoms will not be readily explainable by any detectable abnormalities on examination (signs) or on laboratory testing. Even in the modern era of advanced diagnostic testing, the history and physical examination are estimated to contribute at least 75% of the information that informs the evaluation of symptoms, and symptoms that are not explained on initial comprehensive evaluation rarely are manifestations of a serious underlying disease. Conversely, asymptomatic patients may have signs or laboratory abnormalities, and laboratory abnormalities can occur in the absence of symptoms or signs.

Symptoms and signs commonly define *syndromes*, which may be the common final pathway of a wide range of pathophysiologic alterations. The fundamental basis of internal medicine is that diagnosis should elucidate the pathophysiologic explanation for symptoms and signs so that therapy may improve the underlying abnormality, not just attempt to suppress the abnormal symptoms or signs.

When patients seek care from physicians, they may have manifestations or exacerbations of known conditions or they may have symptoms and signs that suggest malfunction of a particular organ system. Sometimes the pattern of symptoms and signs is highly suggestive or even pathognomonic for a particular disease process. In these situations, in which the physician is focusing on a particular disease, *Goldman-Cecil Medicine* provides scholarly yet practical approaches to the epidemiology, pathobiology, clinical manifestations, diagnosis, treatment, prevention, and prognosis of entities such as acute myocardial infarction (Chapter 58), chronic obstructive lung disease (Chapter 76), inflammatory bowel disease (Chapter 127), gallstones (Chapter 141), rheumatoid arthritis (Chapter 243), hypothyroidism (Chapter 207), and tuberculosis (Chapter 299), as well as newly described disorders such as emerging zoonoses (Chapter 303), small fiber neuropathies (Chapter 388), mitochondrial diseases (Chapter 389), autoinflammatory diseases (Chapter 240), and clonal disorders of indeterminate potential (Chapter 142).

Many patients, however, have undiagnosed symptoms, signs, or laboratory abnormalities that cannot be immediately ascribed to a particular disease or cause. Whether the initial manifestation is chest pain (Chapter 39), diarrhea (Chapter 126), neck or back pain (Chapter 369), or a variety of more than 100 common symptoms, signs, or laboratory abnormalities, *Goldman-Cecil Medicine* provides tables, figures, and entire chapters to guide the approach to diagnosis and therapy (see E-Table 1-1 or the table on the inside back cover of the printed book). By virtue of this dual approach to known disease as well as to undiagnosed abnormalities, this textbook, similar to the modern practice of medicine, applies directly to patients regardless of their mode of manifestation or degree of previous evaluation.

CLINICAL REASONING AND DECISION-MAKING

The patient-physician interaction proceeds through many phases of clinical reasoning and decision making. The interaction begins with an elucidation of complaints or concerns in a respectful and socially conscious approach, followed by inquiries or evaluations to address these concerns in increasingly precise ways. The process commonly requires a careful history or physical examination (Chapter 6), ordering of diagnostic tests, integration of clinical findings with test results, understanding of the risks and benefits of the possible courses of action, and careful consultation with the patient and family to develop future plans. Physicians can increasingly call on a growing literature of evidence-based medicine to guide the process so that benefit is maximized while respecting individual variations in different patients. Throughout *Goldman-Cecil Medicine*, the best current evidence is highlighted with specific grade A references that can be accessed directly in the electronic version.

The increasing availability of evidence from randomized trials to guide the approach to diagnosis and therapy should not be equated with "cookbook" medicine. Evidence and the guidelines that are derived from it emphasize proven approaches for patients with specific characteristics. Substantial clinical judgment is required to determine whether the evidence and guidelines apply to individual patients and to recognize the occasional exceptions. Even more judgment is required in the many situations in which evidence is absent or inconclusive.[16] Evidence must be tempered by patients' preferences, although it is a physician's responsibility to avoid pre-judgment and to emphasize evidence when presenting alternative options to the patient. The adherence of a patient to a specific regimen is likely to be enhanced if the patient also understands the rationale and evidence behind the recommended option.

To optimize medical care, the physician must understand the patient as a person. This fundamental precept of doctoring includes an understanding of the patient's sexual orientation and gender identity, cultural background, social situation, family issues, financial constraints, access to health insurance, trust in the health care system, and preferences for different types of care and outcomes, ranging from maximum prolongation of life to the relief of pain and suffering (Chapters 2 and 3). If the physician does not appreciate and address these issues, the science of medicine cannot be applied appropriately, and even the most knowledgeable physician will fail to achieve the desired outcomes.

Even as physicians become increasingly aware of new discoveries, patients can obtain their own information from a variety of sources, some of which are of questionable reliability.[17] The increasing use of alternative and complementary therapies (Chapter 30) is an example of patients' frequent dissatisfaction with prescribed medical therapy. Physicians should keep an open mind regarding unproven options but must advise their patients carefully if such options may carry any degree of potential risk, including the risk that they may be relied on to substitute for proven approaches.

The principle of patient autonomy asserts that physicians make recommendations but patients make the final decisions (Chapter 2). The physician is an expert advisor who must inform and empower the patient to make decisions by integrating scientific data with their preferences and values. The physician must have an open dialogue with the patient and family regarding the full range of options and encourage shared decision-making whenever appropriate.

The rise of telemedicine, stimulated by the social distancing in response to the COVID-19 pandemic, promises to increase accessibility but at the potential detriment of the personal closeness of the patient-doctor relationship.[18] Physicians and the medical profession have the opportunity to use this indisputably convenient tool to extend health care to underserved and vulnerable populations worldwide, but they must remain vigilant to benefit from its virtues, minimize its limitations, and not exacerbate health disparities based on access to digital technology.[19]

INCORPORATING A PUBLIC HEALTH FOCUS

The physician does not exist in a vacuum, but rather as part of a complicated and extensive system of medical care and public health. In premodern times and even today in some resource-limited countries, the most important ways to promote health and reduce disease are to ensure basic hygiene, clean water, and adequate nutrition (Chapter 11). In resource-limited and high-income countries, adoption of healthy lifestyles, including better diet (Chapter 13) and appropriate exercise (Chapter 14), are the keys to reducing the epidemics of obesity (Chapter 201), coronary disease (Chapter 40), and diabetes (Chapter 210). Public health interventions to provide immunizations (Chapter 15) and to reduce injuries and the use of tobacco (Chapter 363), illicit drugs (Chapter 365), and excess alcohol (Chapter 364) can collectively produce more health benefits than nearly any other imaginable health intervention. As emphasized by the COVID-19 pandemic (Chapters 335 to 337), the public health system must play a key role in informing the populace and in promoting guidelines for individuals as well as for the health care profession.

APPROACH TO THE MEDICAL PROFESSION

Medical professionalism should emphasize three fundamental principles: the primacy of patient welfare, patient autonomy, and social justice. As modern medicine brings a plethora of diagnostic and therapeutic options, the interactions of the physician with the patient and society become more complex and potentially fraught with ethical dilemmas (Chapter 2). To help provide a moral compass that is not only grounded in tradition but also adaptable to modern times, the primacy of patient welfare emphasizes the fundamental principle of the medical profession. The physician's altruism, which begets the patient's trust, must be impervious to the social, economic, bureaucratic, and political challenges that are faced by the physician and the patient (Chapter 4).

To promote these fundamental principles, a series of professional responsibilities (Table 1-1) represents practical, daily traits that benefit the physician's own patients and society as a whole. Physicians who use these and other attributes to improve their patients' satisfaction with care are not only promoting professionalism but also reducing their own risk for liability and malpractice. Physicians have a responsibility to stay current in their field[20] and to know when a patient's best interests are served by a referral to another physician or health care clinician.

TEAMWORK, STANDARDS, AND ACCOUNTABILITY

An interesting new aspect of professionalism is the increasing reliance on team approaches to medical care, as exemplified by physicians whose roles are defined by the location of their practice—historically in the intensive care unit or emergency department and now on the inpatient general hospital floor. Quality care requires coordination and effective communication across inpatient and outpatient sites among physicians who themselves may now typically work defined hours. This transition from reliance on a single, always available physician to a team, ideally with a designated coordinator, places new challenges on physicians, the medical care system, and the medical profession. Many teams comprise health care professionals who have complementary skills, including physicians, nurses, advanced practice providers, and pharmacists. This new model emphasizes the relevance of interprofessional education that focuses on core competencies, roles, responsibilities, communication, and teamwork.[21]

The changing medical care environment is also placing increasing emphasis on standards, outcomes, and accountability. As purchasers of insurance become more cognizant of value rather than just cost (Chapter 10), outcomes ranging from patients' satisfaction to rates of screening mammography (Chapter 183) and even to mortality rates with coronary artery bypass graft surgery (Chapter 59) have become metrics by which rational choices can be made. Clinical guidelines and critical pathways derived from randomized controlled trials and evidence-based medicine can potentially lead to more cost-effective care and better outcomes.

TABLE 1-1 PROFESSIONAL RESPONSIBILITIES

Commitment to:
Professional competence
Honesty
Patient confidentiality
Maintaining appropriate relationships
Improving the quality of care
Improving access to care
Just distribution of finite resources
Scientific knowledge
Maintaining trust by managing conflicts of interest
Professional responsibilities

From Brennan T, Blank L, Cohen J, et al. Medical professionalism in the new millennium: a physician charter. *Ann Intern Med.* 2002;1136:243-246.

SOCIAL JUSTICE

The importance of social justice acknowledges that the patient-physician interaction does not exist in a vacuum. The physician has a responsibility to the individual patient and to broader society to promote equitable access to health care, to eliminate disparities in health and health care delivery, and to bring science to even the most contentious political issues. For example, research into the relationship of firearms to rates of murder and suicide[22] can be useful for preventive medicine and public policy regardless of an individual's position on background checks and licensing for gun owners. The promotion of masks and vaccines to slow the COVID-19 pandemic was an example of how science should guide behaviors, even in times of uncertainty.

Medical schools,[23] medical research,[24] the medical profession,[25] and all medical institutions must embrace the principles of diversity, equity, inclusion, and social justice in education and the workplace. These principles optimize the profession's ability to mirror the populations it serves and to maximize the ability to address disparities and inequalities in care.

These major changes in many Western health care systems bring with them many risks and concerns. If the concept of limited choice among physicians and health care providers is based on objective measures of quality and outcome, channeling of patients to better providers is one reasonable definition of better selection and enlightened competition. If the limiting of options is based overwhelmingly on cost rather than measures of quality, outcomes, and patient satisfaction, physicians and their patients can be seriously disadvantaged.

Another risk is that the same genetic information that can lead to earlier diagnosis and to more effective, personalized medicine may be used against the very people whom it is supposed to benefit—by creating a stigma, potentially raising health insurance costs, or sometimes even making someone unable to obtain life or long-term care insurance. The ethical approach to medicine (Chapter 2), genetics (Chapter 31), and genetic counseling provides means to protect against this adverse effect of scientific progress.

BALANCING PROFESSIONAL RESPONSIBILITIES

In the modern environment, the physician often has a dual responsibility: to the health care system as an expert who helps create standards, measures of outcome, clinical guidelines, and mechanisms to ensure high-quality, cost-effective care; and to individual patients who entrust their well-being to that physician to promote their best interests within the reasonable limits of the system. A health insurance system that emphasizes cost-effective, value-based care, that gives physicians and health care providers responsibility for the health of a population and the resources required to achieve these goals, that must exist in a competitive environment in which patients can choose alternatives if they are not satisfied with their care, and that places increasing emphasis on health education and prevention can have many positive effects. In this environment, however, physicians must beware of overt and subtle pressures that could entice them to underserve patients and abrogate their professional responsibilities by putting personal financial reward ahead of their patients' welfare. The physician's responsibility to represent the patient's best interests and avoid financial conflicts by doing too little in the newer systems of capitated care provides different specific challenges but an analogous moral dilemma to the historical American system in which the physician is rewarded financially for doing too much.

An ongoing challenge for a profession that values dedication, attention to detail, and selflessness is the increasing risk of suffering burnout, which is characterized by emotional exhaustion and depersonalization. For example, the medical profession's heroic response to COVID-19, despite the personal health risks and significant psychological challenges, was inspiring. Nevertheless, the longer-term effects on physicians' resiliency will be a challenge to individual physicians and the profession as a whole.[26,27] Hopefully, both individual-focused and structural or organizational modifications in the work environment can result in clinically meaningful reductions in physician burnout.[28]

In the current health care environment, all health care professionals must strive to retain and expand their scientific knowledge base, redouble their commitment to the principles of their profession, and preserve their own well-being so they can serve others. In this spirit, *Goldman-Cecil Medicine* seeks to be a comprehensive approach to the ethos, foundation, and modern practice of internal medicine.

GENERAL REFERENCES

For the General References and other additional features, please visit Elsevier eBooks+ at https://ebooks.health.elsevier.com.

2 BIOETHICS IN THE PRACTICE OF MEDICINE

EZEKIEL J. EMANUEL

It commonly is argued that the bioethical dilemmas physicians face today result primarily from modern advances in medical technology. The rise of transplantation, intensive care units, genetics, implantable devices, and other technologies have created novel bioethical concerns. In reality, however, concerns about most medical ethical issues are as old as medicine itself. The Hippocratic Oath, composed around 400 BC, attests to the need of ancient Greek physicians for advice on how to address the many bioethical dilemmas that they confronted. The Oath addresses issues of confidentiality, abortion, euthanasia, sexual relations between physicians and patients, divided loyalties, and, at least implicitly, charity care and executions. Whether we agree with its advice or not, the mere existence of the Oath reminds physicians that medical ethical conundrums are inherent to medical practice. Technology may make these issues more common and change the context in which they arise, but many, if not most, bioethical issues that physicians regularly confront are age-old.

Many physicians are taught that four main principles can be invoked to address bioethical dilemmas: autonomy, nonmaleficence, beneficence, and justice. Autonomy is the idea that people should have the right and freedom to choose, pursue, and revise their own life plans. Nonmaleficence is the idea that people should not be knowingly harmed or injured. This principle is encapsulated in the oft-repeated phrase "first, do no harm"—*primum non nocere*. Beneficence refers to the positive actions that a physician should undertake to promote the well-being of his or her patients. In clinical practice, this obligation arises from the implicit and explicit commitments and promises central to the physician-patient relationship. Finally, the principle of justice is defined by the fair distribution of benefits and burdens that result from clinical interactions.

Although helpful in providing an initial framework, these principles are too broad to have more than limited value. The principles are also frequently underdeveloped and likely to conflict with each other, thereby resulting in bioethical dilemmas. The principles themselves do not offer guidance on how they should be balanced to resolve dilemmas. Given that they are focused on physician-patient encounters, the principles are also unhelpful when addressing bioethical issues at the system or institutional level, such as the allocation of scarce vaccines. Finally, these four principles are not comprehensive and fail to encapsulate all critical values. As the severe acute respiratory syndrome coronavirus 2 (SARS-CoV-2) pandemic has made clear, other fundamental ethical principles and values include a focus on equity and priority to the worst off, duties to future generations, and professional integrity.[1]

There is no formula that can magically determine how to solve bioethical dilemmas.[2] Instead, medical professionals should follow an orderly analytic process. First, practitioners need to obtain the facts relevant to the situation. Second, they must delineate the fundamental bioethical issue. Third, they must identify all the crucial principles and values that relate to, and potentially conflict with, the case. Fourth, because many ethical dilemmas have been previously analyzed and subjected to empirical study, practitioners should examine the relevant literature so they may potentially identify new values, understand existing principles, reformulate the issue at hand, and see if there is an accepted resolution. Fifth, with this information, the practitioner must distinguish clearly unethical practices from a range of ethically permissible actions. Finally, it is important not only to come to a resolution but also to state clearly the justification for such decisions. Although unanimous decisions are ideal, the reality remains that such consensus may be elusive. Reasonable physicians must therefore take care to explain what principles they weighted highly and what interpretations they relied upon to resolve ethical dilemmas.

A multitude of bioethical dilemmas arise in medical practice each year, including issues of genetics, conscientious objection by providers, and termination of care. In clinical practice, the most common issues revolve around informed consent, termination of life-sustaining treatments, euthanasia and physician-assisted suicide, allocation of scarce resources (featured prominently during the SARS-CoV-2 pandemic and in transplantation), and conflict of interest.

PHYSICIAN-PATIENT RELATIONSHIP: INFORMED CONSENT

HISTORY

The requirement of informed consent dates as far back as Plato. The first recorded legal case on informed consent took place in England in 1767 when a patient complained that he had not given his consent for two surgeons to refracture his leg after it had healed improperly. The judge ultimately ruled that obtaining a patient's consent prior to a procedure was the "rule of the profession" and thus a legal obligation of surgeons. Failure to obtain consent, the court declared, was inexcusable. In more contemporary times, a landmark 1957 U.S. court ruling stated that physicians have a positive legal obligation to disclose information about risks, benefits, and alternative treatments to patients; this decision popularized the term *informed consent*.

DEFINITION AND JUSTIFICATION

Informed consent is a person's autonomous authorization to permit a physician—or other health professional—to undertake diagnostic or therapeutic interventions for himself or herself. The patient understands that he or she is taking responsibility for the decision while empowering someone else, the physician, to implement it. However, agreement to a course of medical treatment does not necessarily qualify as informed consent.

The four fundamental requirements for valid informed consent are: mental capacity, disclosure, understanding, and voluntariness. First, informed consent assumes that people have the mental capacity to make decisions; disease, development, or medications can compromise patients' mental capacity to provide informed consent. Adults are presumed to have the legal competence to make medical decisions, and whether an adult is incompetent to make medical decisions is a legal determination. Practically, physicians usually decide whether patients are competent based on whether they can understand the information disclosed, appreciate its significance for their own situation, and use logical and consistent thought processes in decision making. Incompetence in medical decision making does not mean a person is incompetent in all types of decision making and vice versa. Second, crucial information relevant to the decision must be disclosed, usually by the physician, to the patient. Third, the patient should understand the information and its implications for his or her interests and life goals. Finally, the patient's decision must be made voluntarily, without coercion or manipulation by the physician.

It is a mistake to view informed consent as a one-time event, such as the signing of a form. Informed consent is viewed more accurately as a process that evolves throughout the course of a patient's diagnosis and subsequent treatment.

Typically, a patient's autonomy is the value invoked to justify informed consent. Other values, such as bodily integrity and beneficence, have also been cited, especially in early legal rulings.

EMPIRICAL DATA

Extensive research on informed consent shows that physicians frequently do not communicate all the relevant information needed for patients to make an informed decision in clinical settings. The more complex the medical decisions, the more likely it is that physicians will obtain all the elements of informed consent.

Interestingly, data suggest that disclosure, both in informed consent documents and in discussion, is better in research than clinical settings, likely because of the research-specific requirement of having a written document to guide a process overseen by an independent committee, such as an institutional review board or a research ethics committee.

Patients frequently fail to recall crucial information disclosed during the process of obtaining informed consent, although they usually think they have sufficient information to make a decision. Whether patients fail to recall key information because they are overwhelmed by the information or because they find much of it not salient to their decision is unclear. The issue therefore lies more in determining what patients understand at the point of decision making, rather than what they recall later. For common medical interventions, such as elective surgery, the ideal informed consent would include the risks and benefits as quantified in randomized controlled trials, relevant data on the surgeon, the institution's clinical outcomes for the procedure, and a list of acceptable alternatives.[3]

Studies aimed at improving informed consent in clinical settings suggest that interactive media, such as interactive computer software and videos, improve patients' understanding of competing alternatives.[A1] Typically, patients who use a decision aid have greater knowledge of the evidence, feel more clear about what matters to them, have more accurate understanding of risks and benefits, and participate more in the decision-making process. Computer and web-based decision aids are now available for hundreds of common conditions and procedures.

A more modern challenge in obtaining informed consent is the introduction of electronic methods into the process, including smartphone applications in acute situations such as ischemic stroke.[A2] Digital models for informed consent often are not user-friendly for older patients, and evidence suggests that most people do not read click-through agreements on computers and mobile devices. Concern also exists that it may be challenging to obtain true voluntary choice without being able to assess the body language, tone, and emotion that can be observed during a person-to-person interaction.

One of the most important results of empirical research on informed consent is that there is a gap between the desire for information and the desire for actual decision making. Studies suggest that although most patients want information, far fewer actually want to make decisions about their own care. In one study, for example, only one third of patients desired decision-making authority, and patients' decision-making preferences were not correlated with their information-seeking preferences. Patients' preferences for decision-making authority generally increase with higher educational levels and decline with age. Most importantly, the more serious the illness, the more likely patients are to prefer that physicians make the decisions. Several studies suggest that patients who have less of a desire to make their own decisions generally are more satisfied with how the decisions are ultimately made.

PRACTICAL CONSIDERATIONS

Physicians who implement informed consent are usually concerned about the extent to which information should be disclosed and how to disclose it so it is well understood.[4] Physicians should disclose at least six fundamental elements of information to patients (Table 2-1). Because risk is usually a physician's principal concern, physicians also should disclose (1) the nature of the risks, (2) their magnitude, (3) the likelihood that the risks will occur, and (4) when the consequences might occur. Increasingly, these disclosures should include data both from clinical trials and from the institution and physician performing the test and treatments. In general, all serious risks, such as death, paralysis, stroke, infections, or chronic pain, even if rare, should be disclosed, as should common risks.

The key challenge in providing this information is doing so within reasonable time constraints and without overwhelming the patient with unnecessarily technical details. Fortunately, time constraints can be somewhat ameliorated by using interactive electronic media that allow patients to view information on their own schedules while facilitating the transfer of basic information.

TABLE 2-1 FUNDAMENTAL ELEMENTS FOR DISCLOSURE TO PATIENTS

Diagnosis and prognosis
Nature of proposed intervention
Reasonable alternative interventions
Risks associated with each alternative intervention
Benefits associated with each alternative intervention
Probable outcomes of each alternative intervention

The question of how much physicians should disclose is a state-level determination. Generally, states have adopted one of two divergent legal standards. The *physician* or *customary* standard, adapted from malpractice law, states that the physician should disclose all information "which a reasonable medical practitioner would make under the same or similar circumstances." Conversely, the *reasonable person* or *lay-oriented* standard states that physicians should disclose all information that a "reasonable person in the patient's circumstances would find material" to the medical decision. The physician standard is factual and can be determined empirically, but the patient-oriented standard, which is meant to engage physicians with patients, is hypothetical. Currently, each standard is used by about half of the United States.

The requirement of informed consent has no exceptions. In emergency situations, consent can be assumed under the belief that patients' interests are in survival and retaining maximal mental and physical functioning; as a result, reasonable persons would want treatment. In some circumstances, physicians may believe the process of informed consent could pose a serious psychological threat. In rare cases, the "therapeutic privilege" of promoting a patient's well-being trumps autonomy, but physicians should be wary of invoking this exception too readily.

If patients are deemed mentally incompetent to make medical decisions, family members—in order from spouse, children, parents, siblings, then more distant relatives—usually are selected as surrogates or proxies,[5] although there may be concerns about conflicting interests or knowledge of the patient's wishes. In the relatively rare circumstance in which a patient has formally designated a proxy, that person has decision-making authority.

The *substituted judgment* standard states that the proxy should choose what the patient would choose if he or she were competent. The *best interests* standard states that the proxy should choose what is best for the patient. However, it is often not clear what the patient would have decided, because the situation was not discussed with the patient and he or she left no advance care directive. Similarly, what is considered "best" for a patient can be controversial because of tradeoffs between quality of life and pure survival. These problems are complicated by the poor ability of many proxies to predict a patient's quality of life; proxies also tend to underestimate patients' future functional status and satisfaction. Similarly, a proxy's predictions on a mentally incapacitated patient's life-sustaining preferences are often inaccurate. In cases in which the patient is diagnosed with dementia, families tend to agree with patients on decisions regarding life-sustaining treatment two thirds of the time, better but not much better than the 50% agreement based on chance alone. Such confusion on how to decide for incapacitated patients can create conflicts among family members or between the family and medical providers. In such circumstances, an ethics consultation may be helpful.

TERMINATION OF MEDICAL INTERVENTIONS

HISTORY

Since the origins of medicine, withholding medical treatment from terminally ill patients while still providing palliative care, thereby allowing "nature to take its course," has been deemed ethical. Hippocrates argued that physicians should "refuse to treat those [patients] who are overmastered by their disease." In the 19th century, prominent American physicians advocated withholding cathartic and emetic "treatments" from the terminally ill. In 1900, the editors of *The Lancet* argued that physicians should intervene to ease the pain of death and that they did not have an obligation to prolong a clearly terminal life. The contemporary debate on terminating care began in the United States in 1976 with the *Quinlan* case, in which the New Jersey Supreme Court ruled that patients had a right to refuse life-sustaining interventions on the basis of a right to privacy, and that the family could exercise that right for a patient in a persistent vegetative state.

DEFINITION AND JUSTIFICATION

It generally is agreed that all patients have a right to refuse medical interventions. Ethically, this right is based on the patient's right to autonomy and is implied by the doctrine of informed consent. Legally, state courts have cited the right to privacy, the right to bodily integrity, and common law to justify the right to refuse medical treatment. In the 1990 *Cruzan* case, and in the subsequent physician-assisted suicide cases, the U.S. Supreme Court affirmed that there is a "constitutionally protected right to refuse lifesaving hydration and nutrition." The Court stated that "[A] liberty interest [based on the 14th Amendment] in refusing unwanted medical treatment may be inferred from our prior decisions." All patients have both a constitutional and an ethical right to refuse medical interventions. These rulings were the basis of consistent state and federal court rulings in the *Schiavo* case to permit the husband to terminate artificial nutrition and hydration for his terminally ill wife in a vegetative state (Chapter 373).

EMPIRICAL DATA

Data show that termination of medical treatments is now the norm, and the trend has shifted toward stopping medical interventions based on the preferences of patients and their surrogate decision makers. Over 85% of Americans and 90% of decedents in intensive care units do not receive cardiopulmonary resuscitation. Of decedents in intensive care units, more than 85% die after the withholding or withdrawal of medical treatments, with an average of 2.6 interventions being withheld or withdrawn per decedent.

Despite extensive public support for use of advance care directives, passage of the Patient Self-Determination Act mandating that health care institutions inform patients of their right to complete such documents, and the 2016 policy to reimburse physicians for discussing end-of-life preferences with patients, less than 40% of Americans appear to have completed any written form of end-of-life decisions. Among Americans ages 75 and older, about 20% have neither written nor talked with someone about their wishes for medical treatment at the end of life. Data suggest that although over 40% of patients required active decision making about terminating medical treatments in their final days, more than 70% lacked actual decision-making capacity, thereby highlighting the importance of completing advance directives.

Efforts to improve completion of advance care directives have generated mixed results. In La Crosse County, Wisconsin, for example, after health care organizations in the county added an "Advance Directive" section to their electronic medical records, 90% of decedents had some type of advance directive. Unfortunately, successful pilot efforts like La Crosse County's have not been widely adopted or easily scaled. A persistent problem has been that even when patients complete advance care directives, the documents frequently are not readily available, physicians do not know they exist, or they tend to be too general or vague to guide decisions. The increasing use of electronic health records should make it possible for advance directives to be available whenever and wherever the patient presents to a health care provider. Although electronic health records will help in making existing advance directives available, they will not solve the problem of actually initiating a conversation among the physician, patient, and family about advance care planning. Starting that conversation still seems to be a persistent barrier.

Just as proxies are poor at predicting patients' wishes, data show that physicians are even worse at determining patients' preferences for life-sustaining treatments. In one study, for example, 30% of family conferences between clinicians and surrogates did not discuss preferences for end-of-life decision making for patients who were at high risk of death. In many cases, life-sustaining treatments are continued even when patients or their proxies desire them to be stopped. Conversely, many physicians discontinue or never begin interventions unilaterally without the knowledge or consent of patients or their surrogate decision makers. These discrepancies emphasize the importance of engaging patients early on in their care about treatment preferences.

PRACTICAL CONSIDERATIONS

Many practical considerations are applicable to enacting the right to terminate medical treatment (Table 2-2). First, patients have a right to refuse any and all medical interventions. The question of what medical interventions can be terminated—or not started—is a recurrent topic of debate. Courts have made clear that any treatment prescribed by a physician and administered by a health care provider can be stopped if it is more harmful than beneficial. The issue is not whether the treatment is ordinary, extraordinary, or heroic, or whether it is high-technology or low-technology. Treatments that can be stopped include not only ventilators, artificial nutrition, and hydration, but also dialysis, pacemakers, ventricular assist devices, antibiotics, and any medication.[6]

Second, there is no ethical or legal difference between withholding an intervention and withdrawing it. If a respirator or other treatment is started because physicians are uncertain whether a patient would have wanted it, they always can stop it later when information clarifies the patient's wishes. Although physicians and nurses might find stopping a treatment to be more difficult psychologically, withdrawal is ethically and legally permitted—and required—when it is consonant with the patient's wishes.

Third, competent patients have the exclusive right to make decisions about terminating their own care. If there is a conflict between a competent patient and his or her family, the patient's wishes are to be followed. It is the patient's right to refuse treatment, not the family's right. For mentally incompetent patients, the situation is more complex. If the patients left clear indications of their wishes, whether as explicit oral statements or as written advance directives, these wishes should be followed. Physicians should not be overly concerned about the precise form patients use to express their wishes; because patients have a constitutional right to refuse treatment, the focus should be whether the wishes are clear and relevant to the situation. If an incompetent patient did not leave explicit indications of his or her wishes or designate a proxy, the physician should identify a surrogate decision maker and rely upon that person's judgment. Some state courts have restricted what treatments a proxy decision maker can terminate, thereby requiring the incompetent patient to have given very specific instructions about the particular treatments he or she does not want to receive and the conditions under which care should be withheld or withdrawn. This requirement severely limits the authority and power of proxy decision makers.

TABLE 2-2 PRACTICAL CONSIDERATIONS IN TERMINATION OF MEDICAL TREATMENTS

PRACTICAL QUESTION	ANSWER
Is there a legal right to refuse medical interventions?	Yes. The U.S. Supreme Court declared that competent people have a constitutionally protected right to refuse unwanted medical treatments based on the 14th Amendment.
What interventions can be legally and ethically terminated?	Any and all interventions (including respirators, antibiotics, pacemakers, ventricular assist devices, intravenous or enteral nutrition and hydration) can be legally and ethically terminated.
Is there a difference between withholding life-sustaining interventions and withdrawing them?	No. The consensus is that there is no important legal or ethical difference between withholding and withdrawing medical interventions. Stopping a treatment once begun is just as ethical as never having started it.
Whose view about terminating life-sustaining interventions prevails if there is a conflict between the patient and family?	The views of a competent adult patient prevail. It is the patient's body and life.
Who decides about terminating life-sustaining interventions if the patient is incompetent?	If the patient appointed a proxy or surrogate decision maker when competent, that person is legally empowered to make decisions about terminating care. If no proxy was appointed, there is a legally designated hierarchy, usually (1) spouse, (2) adult children, (3) parents, (4) siblings, and (5) available relatives.
Are advance care directives legally enforceable?	Yes. As a clear expression of the patient's wishes, they are a constitutionally protected method for patients to exercise their right to refuse medical treatments. In almost all states, clear and explicit oral statements are legally and ethically sufficient for decisions about withholding or withdrawing medical interventions.

Fourth, the right to refuse medical treatment does not translate into a right to demand any treatment, especially treatments that have no pathophysiologic rationale, have already failed, or are known to be harmful. Futility has become a justification to permit physicians unilaterally to withhold or withdraw treatments despite the family's requests for treatment. Some states, such as Texas, have enacted futility laws, which prescribe procedures by which physicians can invoke futility either to transfer a patient or to terminate interventions. However, the principle of futility is not easy to implement in medical practice. Initially, some commentators advocated that an intervention was futile when the probability of success was 1% or lower. This threshold seems to be based on empirical data, but it is a covert value judgment. Futility is meant to justify unilateral determinations by physicians, so it generally has been viewed as an inappropriate assertion that undermines physician-patient communication and violates the principle of shared decision making. Similar to the distinction between ordinary and extraordinary care, futility is increasingly viewed as more obfuscating than clarifying and is therefore being invoked much less often.

ASSISTED SUICIDE AND EUTHANASIA

HISTORY

Even in Hippocrates' era, euthanasia and physician-assisted suicide were controversial issues. In 1905, a bill was introduced into the Ohio legislature to legalize euthanasia; it was defeated. In the mid-1930s, similar bills were introduced and defeated in the British Parliament and the Nebraska legislature. In 1997, the U.S. Supreme Court stated that there is no constitutional right to euthanasia or physician-assisted suicide, but that there also is no constitutional prohibition against states legalizing these interventions. As of 2021, nine U.S. states and the District of Columbia have legalized physician-assisted suicide—but no state has legalized euthanasia. The Montana Supreme Court did not recognize a constitutional right to physician-assisted suicide, but it ruled that the law permitting the termination of life-sustaining treatment protected physicians from prosecution if they helped hasten the death of a consenting, rational, terminally ill patient. Importantly, the American College of Physicians does not currently support the legalization of physician-assisted suicide. Both euthanasia and physician-assisted suicide are legal in many other countries, including the Netherlands, Belgium, Luxembourg, Canada, New Zealand, and Spain, and physician-assisted suicide is legal in Switzerland and Germany. Both euthanasia and physician-assisted suicide are illegal under English law.

DEFINITION AND JUSTIFICATION

The terms *euthanasia* and *physician-assisted suicide* require careful definition (Table 2-3). So-called passive and indirect euthanasia are misnomers and not actual instances of euthanasia; rather, they are ethical and legal ways to terminate care.

Four general arguments are made against permitting euthanasia and physician-assisted suicide. First, Kant and Mill, the philosophical champions of individual autonomy, believed that autonomy itself did not allow a person voluntarily to end conditions that made them autonomous. As a result, both philosophers were against voluntary enslavement and suicide. They therefore argued that the exercise of autonomy cannot include the ending of life, which would mean ending the possibility of exercising autonomy. Second, many dying patients may experience pain and suffering as the result of not receiving appropriate care. It is therefore possible that adequate care and pain management (Chapter 26) might relieve suffering without the need for euthanasia or physician-assisted suicide (Chapter 3). Although some patients may experience uncontrolled pain despite optimal end-of-life care, relatively few give pain as the justification for seeking euthanasia or physician-assisted suicide. Third, there is a clear ethical distinction between intentionally ending a life and terminating life-sustaining treatments. Both the motivations and physical acts are different. Injecting a life-ending medication, or providing a prescription for one, is not the same as removing or refraining from introducing a bodily invasive medical intervention. Finally, permitting euthanasia and physician-assisted suicide may introduce adverse consequences. For example, disturbing reports of involuntary euthanasia and euthanasia of depressed patients have come from the Netherlands and Belgium, and many worry about coercion of expensive or burdensome patients to accept euthanasia or physician-assisted suicide. Permitting euthanasia and physician-assisted suicide is likely to lead to further intrusions of lawyers, courts, and legislatures into the physician-patient relationship.

Four parallel arguments are forwarded to permit euthanasia and physician-assisted suicide. First, it is argued that autonomy justifies euthanasia and physician-assisted suicide. To respect autonomy requires permitting individuals to decide when and how it is better to end their lives. Second, beneficence—furthering the well-being of individuals—supports permitting euthanasia and physician-assisted suicide. In some cases, living can create more pain and suffering than death; ending a painful life relieves more suffering and produces a net good for the patient. Just the reassurance of having the option of euthanasia or physician-assisted suicide, even if not used, can provide "psychological insurance" and be beneficial to people. Third, euthanasia and physician-assisted suicide are no different from termination of life-sustaining treatments that are recognized as ethically justified. In both cases, the patient consents to die; in both cases, the physician intends to end the patient's life and takes some action to end the patient's life; and in both cases, the final result is the same: the patient's death. With no difference in the patient's consent, the physician's intention, or the final result, there can be no difference in the ethical justification. Fourth, the supposed slippery slope that would result from permitting euthanasia and physician-assisted suicide is unlikely. The idea that permitting euthanasia and physician-assisted suicide would undermine the physician-patient relationship or lead to forced euthanasia is completely speculative and not borne out by the available data.

TABLE 2-3 DEFINITIONS OF ASSISTED SUICIDE AND EUTHANASIA

TERM	DEFINITION
Voluntary active euthanasia	Intentional administration of medications or other interventions to cause the patient's death with the patient's informed consent
Involuntary active euthanasia	Intentional administration of medications or other interventions to cause the patient's death when the patient was competent to consent but did not consent (e.g., the patient may not have been asked)
Nonvoluntary active euthanasia	Intentional administration of medications or other interventions to cause the patient's death when the patient was incompetent and was mentally incapable of consenting (e.g., the patient might have been in a coma)
Passive euthanasia	Withholding or withdrawal of life-sustaining medical treatments from a patient to let him or her die (termination of life-sustaining treatments)—a poor term that should not be used
Indirect euthanasia	Administration of narcotics or other medications to relieve pain with the incidental consequence of causing sufficient respiratory depression to result in the patient's death
Physician-assisted suicide	A physician provides prescription medications or other interventions to a patient with the understanding that the patient can use them to commit suicide
Physician-assisted death	Either voluntary, active euthanasia or physician-assisted suicide. This term is preferred in the United States by advocates of these practices, but the term is not used in Europe.

EMPIRICAL DATA

Attitudes and practices related to euthanasia and physician-assisted suicide have been studied extensively. Two thirds of Americans say there are some situations in which a patient should be allowed to die, but 30% say that medical professionals should always do everything possible to save a patient's life. About 60% of adults think that these interventions are moral for a person who has an incurable disease and is suffering great pain with no hope of improvement. However, public support dramatically decreases to below 40% for patients who are ready to die because living is a burden or for patients who are burdensome to their families.

Physicians and medical societies tend to be much less supportive of euthanasia and physician-assisted suicide than the public,[7] with oncologists, palliative care physicians, and geriatricians among the least supportive. Among American and British physicians, the majority opposes legalizing either practice.

Approximately 25% of American physicians have received requests for euthanasia or physician-assisted suicide, including about 50% of oncologists and a growing number of neurologists.[8] Studies also indicate that less than 5% of American physicians have performed euthanasia or physician-assisted suicide. Surveys of oncologists indicate that about 4% have performed euthanasia and about 11% have performed physician-assisted suicide during their careers.

Safeguards for euthanasia and physician-assisted suicide are frequently violated. For example, one study found that about 55% of euthanasia requests came from the family. In about 40% of euthanasia and 20% of physician-assisted suicide cases, the patient was depressed; in only half of the cases was the request repeated, irrespective of treatment.

In Oregon and Washington state, over 70% of patients receiving physician-assisted suicide had cancer. Other characteristics strongly linked to requests for physician-assisted suicide included age over 65 years,[9] White race, more formal education, and having medical insurance.

Since physician-assisted suicide was legalized in Oregon over 20 years ago, less than 0.7% of all dying patients died by physician-assisted suicide. In the Netherlands and Belgium, where both euthanasia and physician-assisted suicide are legal, less than 5% of all deaths are by these measures, with 0.4 to 1.8% of all deaths as the result of euthanasia without the patient's consent.[10]

Counterintuitively, in all jurisdictions where it has been studied, pain is not the primary motivation for requesting euthanasia or physician-assisted suicide. In Oregon, loss of autonomy, dignity, and fear of being a burden are cited by patients as the predominant motives. In addition, psychological distress, especially depression and hopelessness, seem to be more important than pain. Interviews with physicians and with patients with amyotrophic lateral sclerosis, cancer, or infection with human immunodeficiency virus show that pain is not associated with interest in euthanasia or physician-assisted suicide; instead, depression and hopelessness are the strongest predictors of interest. These findings raise important issues about the involvement of mental health experts in attempts to determine whether psychiatric treatment would change a patient's views.

Finally, data from the Netherlands and the United States suggest that there are problems in performing euthanasia and physician-assisted suicide. Dutch researchers reported that physician-assisted suicide causes complications in 7% of cases. Furthermore, the patients did not die, awoke from coma, or vomited up the medication in 15% of cases. Ultimately, in nearly 20% of physician-assisted suicide cases, the physician ended up injecting the patient with life-ending medication, converting physician-assisted suicide to euthanasia. These data raise serious questions about how to address complications of physician-assisted suicide when euthanasia is illegal or unacceptable.

PRACTICAL CONSIDERATIONS

There is widespread agreement that if euthanasia and physician-assisted suicide are used, they should be considered only after all reasonable attempts at physical and psychological palliation have failed.[11] A consensus—with slight differences—among American states and European countries has emerged on safeguards. These safeguards include: (1) the patient must be competent and must request euthanasia or physician-assisted suicide repeatedly and voluntarily; (2) in the Netherlands and other European countries, the patient must have unbearable pain or other suffering that cannot be relieved by optimal palliative interventions; by comparison, there is no requirement for unremitting suffering in the United States, but the patient must be terminally ill; (3) there should be a waiting period to ensure that the patient's desires are stable and sincere; and (4) the physician should obtain a second opinion from an independent physician. Although there have been some prosecutions in the United States, there have been no convictions—except for Dr. M. Jack Kevorkian in 1999—when physicians have participated in euthanasia and physician-assisted suicide.

ALLOCATION OF SCARCE MEDICAL RESOURCES

HISTORY

As with other medical ethical issues, decisions about the allocation of resources are not new. In 1792, Dominique Jean Larrey, Surgeon in Chief to Napoleon's Imperial Guard, devised a plan for sorting injured soldiers for emergency transport and medical treatment based on the severity of their wounds. During World War II, penicillin was finally produced in larger, but still quite limited quantities. Winston Churchill decided that priority for treatment should be given to soldiers who could be rapidly returned to active duty at the frontlines. Consequently, soldiers with sexually transmitted diseases were prioritized to receive penicillin over soldiers with severe wounds. Only a small fraction of the penicillin supply was allocated to civilians.

In the early 1960s, chronic renal dialysis was first developed in Seattle, Washington, but the number of machines was limited. To select which patients with chronic renal failure would receive dialysis, a committee used social value criteria, such as whether the person was employed, had dependents, or went to religious services. After publication of a *Life* magazine article about this so-called "God Committee," the process and criteria were roundly condemned. Eventually, Congress eliminated the allocation issue by funding all chronic renal dialysis through Medicare. Well before SARS-CoV-2 created the need to determine which patients should receive priority for ventilators and vaccines,[12] the most visible type of allocation decisions in the United States have been for solid organ transplantation, where demand for organs has regularly outstripped supply.

DEFINITION AND JUSTIFICATION

Rationing occurs in situations in which the supply of some resource (whether a medication, hospital bed, protective equipment, or operating room time) is insufficient to meet the needs of all patients who could medically benefit from the resource. Allocation or distribution is the process of determining which patients should receive priority in getting the medical resource.

Sometimes, an *absolute* scarcity of resources means that no matter how much money is spent, the supply will not be sufficient. Examples include the limited availability of organs for transplantation and, at least initially, vaccines and therapeutics for COVID. In some cases, the problem is a *relative* scarcity, where spending more money can eventually increase the supply of the resource but choices must be made in the meantime. An example was the supply of personal protective equipment or vaccines at points during the SARS-CoV-2 pandemic. Historically, many different criteria have been used for allocating scarce medical resources, including age, income, social usefulness (such as ability to fight in war), first come–first served, time on a waiting list, and medical urgency.

Fair allocation of scarce medical resources relies on four fundamental ethical values: (1) maximizing the benefits from the scarce resources, (2) treating people equally, (3) giving priority to the worst off, and (4) promoting and rewarding social value. Each of these can be interpreted and realized in at least two different ways (Table 2-4).

At least four important conclusions can be drawn about applying these ethical values and principles to allocating scarce medical resources. First, there is widespread agreement that an individual's wealth should not determine who receives scarce medical resources. Second, first come–first served should not be used because it almost invariably prioritizes people who live near medical facilities or who are wealthy and well-connected. Third, no single principle is sufficient to encapsulate all ethical values; a multi-principled allocation scheme will be required. Fourth, the combination of principles must be adopted to the particular medical situation. To save the most lives in the SARS-CoV-2 pandemic in the United States and Europe, for example, older individuals were prioritized for vaccines because they were the most likely to become severely ill and die if infected. For other illnesses, from which children are the most likely to die or transmit infections, younger people should be prioritized.

TABLE 2-4 ETHICAL VALUES FOR ALLOCATING SCARCE MEDICAL RESOURCES

VALUE	DEFINITION	PRINCIPLES OR DIFFERENT WAYS OF REALIZING THE VALUE	EXAMPLES
Maximizing benefit	Priority for resources should be given to individuals who have the best prospects of survival, as well as individuals who are likely to live for many more years if saved.	Save the most lives	Giving resources to individuals with the best chance of survival, disaster response
		Prognosis after treatment or save the most life years	Giving resources to the individuals predicted to survive the longest
Treating people equally	Nondiscrimination based irrelevant factors such as race or religion. Age can be a relevant factor if it influences prognosis or other value.	First come–first served	Time on a waiting list used in kidney transplantation
		Random selection or lottery	Selecting among otherwise equally qualified people (e.g., draft)
Giving priority to the worst off	Worst off can be defined as individuals who are sickest now or who have had the least of a critical good, such as the shortest life.	Sickest first	Severity score for liver transplantation
		Youngest first	Prioritized for influenza vaccine because they are integral to transmission
Promoting and rewarding social value	Giving resources to individuals who have helped or will help the most in the medical response.	Retrospective—reward individuals who contributed the most in the past	Prioritizes individuals who have donated organs or who have participated in prior medical research studies
		Prospective—reward individuals who are likely to contribute most in the future	Prioritize health care workers

EMPIRICAL DATA

Decisions about the allocation of medical resources are common, and different criteria are deployed in different circumstances. In the emergency department, for example, the fundamental allocation decision is which patients receive immediate attention. The primary allocation criterion used medical urgency rather than prognosis, so the sickest patient typically gets the most attention and preempts other patients. In SARS-CoV-2, priority for both personal protective equipment and vaccines was given to health care workers, who were socially useful because they could help save the lives of others, so as to follow the principle of maximizing benefit. After health care workers, the next priority for vaccines was older individuals, so as to maximize benefit by maximally reducing mortality.

The criteria for the transplantation of different organs emphasize different principles. For example, for liver transplantation (Chapter 140) the emphasis is on sickest patients, specifically those with the highest severity scores. This approach is controversial: it minimizes death on the waiting list but does not maximize lives saved with transplantation or the post-transplantation length of life saved. Conversely, in 2014, a new kidney transplant (Chapter 117) allocation scheme was introduced to emphasize the principle of prognosis or more life years by giving "higher quality" kidneys to patients with longer expected post-transplantation survival. This new approach retained the principle first come–first served but changed how "first-come" was determined. Rather than using time on the transplantation waiting list, the allocation scheme uses the time on dialysis to reduce racial and socioeconomic disparities, thereby emphasizing the principle of giving priority to the worst off. Although racial disparities have diminished, particularly for getting onto the waitlist, access disparities have persisted in part because poorer and minority patients may have barriers related to completing needed preoperative testing or receiving financial clearance.[13]

In the United States, reports on prioritizing limited SARS-CoV-2 vaccines (Chapter 337) generally invoked the principles of social usefulness and maximizing benefits by minimizing mortality. The resulting recommendations were to provide vaccines initially to health care workers and residents of long-term care facilities, with other groups prioritized by their risk of mortality (Table 2-5). Ultimately, however, the allocation was determined by individual states. For example, Florida extended the recommendations to include all persons ages 65 and older, as well as persons deemed by hospitals to be extremely vulnerable.

PRACTICAL CONSIDERATIONS

The process for implementing any allocation scheme typically has two stages. The first stage is to establish priority groups based upon the four ethical values. The second stage is to specify which priority group applies to each particular individual. For SARS-CoV-2, both stages were fulfilled. For organ transplantation, the national Organ Procurement and Transplantation Network establishes different criteria for determining priority groups, but then transplantation teams at each center determine which individual patients qualify to receive available organs based on the allocation criteria.

TABLE 2-5 ADVISORY COMMITTEE ON IMMUNIZATION POLICY'S INITIAL RECOMMENDATIONS FOR THE ALLOCATION OF COVID-19 VACCINES*

TIER OR PHASE	GROUPS RECOMMENDED	TOTAL PERSONS IN EACH GROUP (MILLIONS)
1a	Health care workers	21
	Residents of long-term care facilities	3
1b	Frontline essential workers (e.g., grocery store workers and police)	30
	Persons over age 75 years	19
1c	Persons ages 65-74 years	28
	Persons ages 16-64 years with high-risk medical conditions	81
	Essential workers not recommended for vaccination in Phase 1b (e.g., construction workers and bank tellers)	20
2	All persons over age 16 years not previously recommended	All others

*https://www.cdc.gov/mmwr/volumes/69/wr/pdfs/mm695152e2-H.pdf.

Each of these steps can be done less than ethically. The established priority groups may not adhere to the four key ethical values. For example, the decision by Florida's governor to open up initial allocation of SARS-CoV-2 vaccines for all people over age 65 years rather than for younger minority individuals with high-risk conditions was widely viewed as politically motivated. Another example is that wealthy patients often can pick organ transplant centers with shorter waiting lists or may be listed for organ transplantation at multiple centers. This ability to be listed multiple times favors the wealthy, who also can afford to be evaluated at multiple centers and fly to them when a suitable organ becomes available.

FINANCIAL CONFLICTS OF INTEREST

HISTORY

Worrying whether payment structures and fees compromise the integrity of medical decision making is not new. In 1899, a physician reported that more than 60% of surgeons in Chicago were willing to provide a 50% commission to physicians for referring cases. He subsequently argued that in some cases, this fee splitting led to unnecessary surgical procedures. A 1912 study by the American Medical Association confirmed that fee splitting was a common practice and it added to the list of physicians' financial conflicts of interest acts, which included selling patented medicines and patenting surgical instruments. In the 1990s, the ethics of pharmaceutical and biotech companies paying clinical researchers and physicians again raised the issue of financial conflicts of interest.

DEFINITION AND JUSTIFICATION

A conflict of interest occurs when a physician's secondary interests, such as making money, risks compromising or undermining a physician's primary interest, especially promoting a patient's well-being. Physicians not only have several primary interests (Table 2-6), they also have multiple secondary interests, such as earning income, raising a family, contributing to the profession, and pursuing avocational interests, such as hobbies. These secondary interests are not evil; typically, they are legitimate, even admirable. A conflict of interest occurs when one of these secondary interests could compromise pursuit of a primary interest, especially the patient's well-being.

Conflicts of interest are problematic because they can or appear to compromise the integrity of physicians' judgment, the patient's well-being, or the integrity of research. Conflicts of interest can induce a physician to do something—perform a procedure, fail to order a test, or distort data—that may not be in a patient's best interest. These conflicts can undermine the trust of both the patient and the public, not only in an individual physician but also in the medical profession at large.

Some people may believe in a distinction between actual and potential conflicts of interest, as well as claim that a conflict exists only when a physician's judgment is actually distorted or undermined. This distinction is wrong.[14] An actual conflict of interest occurs when a reasonable person could suspect that a physician's judgment could have been altered by the secondary interest. Appearances can be damaging, because it is difficult for patients and the public to determine what motives influence a physician's decision and it often is impossible to know whether judgment actually has been distorted. Financial conflicts of interest are of particular concern, not because they are worse than other types of conflicts, but because they are more pervasive, identifiable, and regulated compared with other conflicts. Since ancient times, the ethical norm has been clear: the physician's primary obligation is to the patient's well-being, and a physician's personal financial well-being comes second and should never compromise this duty.

EMPIRICAL DATA

Financial conflicts are common, and they are often underreported. The more imaging facilities and specialty referrals a practice has, the greater the utilization of medical services and the higher the health care spending—often without any benefit to the patients. In Florida, nearly 40% of physicians are owners of freestanding facilities to which they refer patients. In one study, 4 to 4.5

TABLE 2-6 PRIMARY INTERESTS OF PHYSICIANS

Promotion of the health and well-being of their patients
Advancement of biomedical knowledge through research
Education of future physicians and health care providers
Promotion of public health

times more imaging studies were ordered by self-referring physicians than by physicians who referred patients to radiologists. Similarly, urologists who had integrated radiation facilities into their practices increased their radiation use by 2.5 times compared with urologists who did not have such financial interests.

Similarly, multiple studies have shown that physicians' interaction with pharmaceutical representatives can lead to prescribing of new drugs, nonrational prescribing, and decreased use of generic drugs.[15] Industry funding for travel to continuing medical education symposia increases prescribing of the sponsor's drug. A study of 1400 FDA advisory committee members found that 13% had some financial interest in a drug company whose product was being reviewed by that committee; these members had a 63% chance of voting for its approval and an 84% chance of doing so if they sat on advisory boards for that company. A separate study found that 80% of U.S.-based hematologist-oncologists who use Twitter, often to tweet about pharmaceutical products, have at least one financial conflict of interest, with median payments of over $1000.

Regarding researcher conflicts of interest, the available data suggest that corporate funding does not appear to compromise the design and methodology of clinical research; in fact, commercially funded research may be methodologically more rigorous than government- or foundation-supported research. Conversely, data suggest that financial interests do distort researchers' interpretations and, most importantly, dissemination of research studies. Growing evidence suggests the suppression or selective publication of data unfavorable to corporate sponsors but the repeated publication of favorable results.

PRACTICAL CONSIDERATIONS

First, financial conflicts of interest are inherent in any profession in which the professional earns income from rendering a service. Second, conflicts come in many different forms, from legitimate payment for services rendered and ownership of medical laboratories and facilities, to drug company dinners, payment for attendance at pharmaceutical meetings, and consultation with companies.

Third, in considering how to manage conflicts, it is important to note that people are poor judges of their own potential conflicts. Individuals often cannot distinguish the various influences that guide their judgments, do not think of themselves as inherently bad, and do not imagine that payment shapes their judgments. Physicians tend to be defensive about charges of conflicts of interest. In addition, conflicts tend to act insidiously, subtly changing practice patterns so that they then become what appear to be justifiable norms.

Fourth, rules—whether laws, regulations, or professional standards—to regulate conflicts of interest are based on two considerations: (1) the likelihood that payment or other secondary interests would create a conflict, with greater financial interest tending to increase the risk of compromised judgment, and (2) the magnitude of the potential harm if judgment is compromised. Rules tend to be of three types: (1) disclosure of conflicts, (2) management of conflicts, and (3) outright prohibition. Federal law bans certain types of self-referral of physicians in the Medicare program. The American Medical Association and the Pharmaceutical Research and Manufacturers of America have established joint rules that permit physicians to accept gifts of minimal value but "refuse substantial gifts from drug companies, such as the costs of travel, lodging, or other personal expenses ... for attending conferences or meetings." Additionally, the Physician Payment Sunshine Act, which was passed in 2010 as part of the Affordable Care Act and went into effect in August 2013, requires that drug and device manufacturers report all payments and transfers of value given to physicians to the Centers for Medicare and Medicaid Services so that such information can be published on a searchable public website.

Fifth, there is much emphasis on disclosure of conflicts, with the implicit idea being that sunshine is the best disinfectant. Disclosure may be useful in publications for peers, but it is unclear whether this is a suitable safeguard in the clinical setting. Disclosure may instead make patients worry more. Patients may have no context in which to place the disclosure or to evaluate the physician's clinical recommendation. Furthermore, self-disclosure often is incomplete, even when required.[16] Disclosure letters revealing a physician's financial conflicts of interest can significantly improve patients' knowledge of their physicians' financial relationships with the health care industry without adversely affecting patients' trust in their physicians or leading to missed appointments.[A3] Patients who are unsure about their physician's conflicts of interest report the least amount of trust in their physician, thereby suggesting the value of transparency.

Finally, some conflicts can be avoided by a physician's own action. Physicians can refuse to engage in personal investments in medical facilities or to accept gifts from pharmaceutical companies at relatively little personal cost. In other circumstances, the conflicts may be institutionalized, and minimizing them can occur only by changing the way organizations structure reimbursement incentives. Capitation encourages physicians to limit medical services, and its potentially adverse effects are likely to be managed by institutional rules rather than by personal decisions.

FUTURE DIRECTIONS

In the near future, as genetics moves ever more into the clinical setting, practicing physicians will frequently encounter ethical issues surrounding genetic testing, counseling, and treatment. The use of genetic tests without the extensive counseling so common in research studies would alter the nature of associated bioethical issues. Because these tests have serious implications for the patient and others, scrupulous attention to informed consent is essential. The bioethical issues raised by genetic tests for somatic cell changes, such as tests that occur commonly in cancer diagnosis and risk stratification, are no different from the issues raised with the use of any laboratory or radiographic test.

In some cases, ethics consultation services may be of assistance in resolving bioethical dilemmas. However, data suggest that consultation services are used mainly for problems that arise in individual cases and are not used for more institutional or policy problems.

GENERAL REFERENCES

For the General References and other additional features, please visit Elsevier eBooks+ at https://ebooks.health.elsevier.com.

Grade A References

A1. Stacey D, Légaré F, Lewis K, et al. Decision aids for people facing health treatment or screening decisions. *Cochrane Database Syst Rev.* 2017;4:CD001431.
A2. Haussen DC, Doppelheuer S, Schindler K, et al. Utilization of a smartphone platform for electronic informed consent in acute stroke trials. *Stroke.* 2017;48:3156-3160.
A3. Rose SL, Sah S, Dweik R, et al. Patient responses to physician disclosures of industry conflicts of interest: a randomized field experiment. *Organ Behav Hum Decis Process.* 2021;166:27-38.

3

PALLIATIVE CARE

ROBERT M. ARNOLD AND JEAN S. KUTNER

By 2030, 20% of the U.S. population will be older than 65 years, and people older than 85 years constitute the fastest growing segment of the population. Owing to successes in public health and medicine, many of these people will live the last years of their lives with chronic medical conditions such as cirrhosis, end-stage kidney disease, heart failure, chronic obstructive pulmonary disease (COPD), and dementia. Even human immunodeficiency virus (HIV) and many cancers, once considered terminal, have turned into chronic diseases. More recently, palliative care has taken an important role in the care of hospitalized patients with coronavirus disease-2019 (COVID-19) infection (Chapter 337), many of whom qualify for palliative care because of underlying prior conditions, severity of acute illness, or both.[1]

The burden associated with these illnesses and their treatments is high. Chronically ill patients report multiple physical and psychological symptoms that lower their quality of life. The economic pressures associated with medical care adversely affect patients' socioeconomic status and cause family stress, especially among caregivers who spend 20 or more hours a week helping their loved ones.

Palliative care, which was developed to decrease the burden associated with chronic illness, emphasizes patient- and family-centered care that optimizes quality of life by anticipating, preventing, and treating suffering. Palliative care throughout the continuum of illness addresses physical, intellectual, emotional, social, and spiritual needs while facilitating the patient's autonomy, access to information, and choice.

Palliative care is both a subspeciality and a key component of good medicine. Specialty palliative care, delivered by an interdisciplinary team, is available concurrently with or independently of curative or life-prolonging care. Palliative and nonpalliative health care providers should collaborate and communicate about care needs while focusing on peace and dignity throughout the course of illness, during the dying process, and after death.

Given that most seriously ill patients are not seen by a palliative care subspecialist, every clinician should have basic competency in palliative care. For example, all primary care clinicians should know the basic tenets of treating pain (Chapter 26) as well as how to discuss advance directives (Chapter 2) and give "bad" news. Specialties with a high prevalence of seriously ill patients, such as critical care, cardiology, pulmonology, neurology, nephrology, and oncology, should have more advanced skills.[2–5] Interventions to promote both specialty and primary palliative care are associated with improvements in the patient's burden of symptoms and reductions in the utilization of acute care services, although its effects on quality of life and on the caregiver are less consistent.[A1-A4]

Six points deserve special emphasis. First, palliative care can be delivered at any time during the course of an illness and is often provided concomitantly with disease-focused, life-prolonging therapy. For example, most elderly patients with chronic incurable illnesses, who might benefit from palliative care, are in the last 10 years of their lives but do not consider themselves to be dying. Moreover, prognostication is an inexact science (E-Fig. 3-1). If palliative care is to have an impact on patients' lives, it should be integrated into patients' treatment plans early in the illness. The strongest data for early integration of specialty palliative care is from patients early in the course of oncologic disease.[6,A5] Second, although the specialty of palliative care has grown exponentially over the past 25 years, most patients with serious illness will never see a palliative care specialist because of shortages in the palliative care workforce. Some of the shortages may be addressed by telehealth,[7] but data on palliative care delivered this way are inconclusive.[A6] All clinicians must integrate palliative care principles if the care of seriously ill patients is to be improved. Third, palliative care primarily focuses on the burden of illness rather than treating the disease itself. Because these burdens can be physical, psychological, spiritual, or social, good palliative care requires a transdisciplinary approach. Fourth, palliative care takes the family unit (however defined by the patient) as the central focus of care. Treatment plans thus must be developed for both the patient and the family. Given data on prolonged grief disorder, treatment should continue for the family after the patient's death. Fifth, palliative care recognizes that medical treatments do not uniformly reverse the progression of disease and that patients die. At some point in a patient's illness, the treatments may be associated with more risks and cause more burden than benefit. Palliative care recognizes this reality and starts with a discussion of the patient's goals and the development of an individualized treatment plan that is consistent with these goals. Finally, disparities in palliative care mirror the inequities in health care generally.[8] Black patients have poorer symptom management, fewer discussions of goals of care, and less access to hospice.[A7] In addition, Black physicians receive less palliative care training and rate their training in palliative care as less good than their general medical education.

Many people confuse palliative care with hospice—an understandable confusion because hospice epitomizes the palliative care philosophy. The two, however, are different. In the United States, hospice services and eligibility criteria are largely driven by the Medicare Hospice Benefit. Although exceptions exist, hospice in the United States provides palliative care, primarily at home, for patients who have a life expectancy of 6 months or less and who are willing to forgo life-prolonging treatments. However, the requirement that patients must have a life expectancy of 6 months or less limits hospice's availability, as does the requirement that patients relinquish potentially life-prolonging treatments. Moreover, because doctors often are unwilling to cease these treatments until very late in the disease course, so are most patients.

PALLIATIVE CARE DOMAINS

Palliative care is a philosophy of and approach to care that addresses physical, psychological, spiritual, existential, social, and ethical domains. When caring for patients with chronic life-limiting illness, good palliative care requires that the following questions be addressed.

IS THE PATIENT PHYSICALLY COMFORTABLE?

Across many chronic conditions, patients have a large number of inadequately treated physical symptoms (Table 3-1). The reasons are multifactorial and range from inadequate education of the clinician, to societal beliefs regarding the inevitability of suffering in chronic illness, to concerns regarding opioids, to the lack of evidence-based treatments in noncancer patients.

The first step to improve symptom management is a thorough assessment. Standardized instruments such as the Brief Pain Inventory (Fig. 3-1) measure both the patient's symptoms and the effect of those symptoms on the patient's life. Use of standardized instruments (such as the Edmonton Symptom Assessment Scale [E-Fig. 3-2]) ensures that clinicians will identify overlooked or underreported symptoms and, as a result, will enhance the satisfaction of both the patient and family.

The evidence for the treatment of end-stage symptoms continues to improve. For example, palliative care can improve quality of life in patients with end-stage heart failure,[A8] who often require such help.[9] The use of nonsteroidal anti-inflammatory agents and opioids can result in effective pain management in more than 75% of patients with cancer. Advances such as intrathecal pumps and neurolytic blocks are helpful in the remaining 25% (Chapter 26). Medical marijuana, while popular, has little impact on cancer pain.[A9] The use of oxygen is not helpful for refractory dyspnea except when hypoxia has been documented, whereas use of medications for depression often can be helpful in addressing refractory dyspnea (Chapter 362). Recent data also suggest that prophylactic subcutaneous scopolamine butylbromide decreases dying patients' death rattle.[A10]

IS THE PATIENT PSYCHOLOGICALLY SUFFERING?

Patients may be physically comfortable but still suffering. Psychological symptoms and syndromes such as depression, delirium, and anxiety are common in patients with life-limiting or chronic illnesses. It may be difficult to determine whether increased morbidity and mortality are caused by the physical effects of the illness or by the psychological effects of depression and anxiety on energy, appetite, or sleep. Screening questions focusing on mood (e.g., "Have you felt down, depressed, and hopeless most of the time for the past 2 weeks?") and anhedonia (e.g., "Have you found that little brings you pleasure or joy in the past 2 weeks?") have been shown to help in diagnosing depression in this population. Increasing data show that treatment of depression in chronic illness is possible and improves both morbidity and mortality.

For patients and families facing mortality, existential and spiritual concerns are common. Progressive illness often raises questions of love, legacy, loss, and meaning. A clinician's role is not to answer these questions or to provide reassurance, but rather to understand concerns of the patient and family, how they are coping, and what resources might help. Spirituality often is a source of comfort, and clinicians can ascertain a patient's beliefs using a brief instrument such as the FICA Spiritual Assessment Tool (Table 3-2). A single screening question such as "Are you at peace?" may identify patients who are in spiritual distress and facilitate referrals to chaplains.

IS THE FAMILY SUFFERING?

Families, defined broadly as those individuals who care most for the patient, are an important source of support for most patients. Families provide informal caregiving, often at the expense of their own physical, economic, and psychological health. Good palliative care requires an understanding of how the family is coping and a search for ways to provide family members with the social or clinical resources they need to improve their well-being. Comprehensive and individually targeted interventions can reduce the burden on caregivers, although the absolute benefits are relatively small.

Because patients who are receiving palliative care often die, the treating team must address bereavement and family suffering after death. Good communication and informational brochures about receiving care in an intensive care unit can decrease family members' adverse psychological outcomes after death.[A11] A letter of condolence or a follow-up phone call to the next of kin after a patient's death is respectful and offers the opportunity to clarify questions about the patient's care. Some family members suffer from complicated grief—a recently described syndrome associated with separation and traumatic distress, with symptoms persisting for more than 6 months. Primary care clinicians, who have ongoing relationships with the loved one, and hospices, which provide bereavement services for a year after the patient's death, have the opportunity to assess whether the grief symptoms persist or worsen.

IS THE PATIENT'S CARE CONSISTENT WITH THE PATIENT'S GOALS?

The *sine qua non* for palliative care is ensuring that the treatment plan is consistent with the patient's goals and values. Some patients prefer longevity over quality of life, but a large proportion of elderly, seriously ill patients are not focused on living as long as possible. Instead, they want to maintain a sense of control, relieve their symptoms, improve their quality of life, avoid being a burden on their families, and have a closer relationship with their loved ones.

Ensuring that treatment is consistent with a patient's goals requires good communication skills (Table 3-3). The approaches to giving bad news, discussing goals of care, and talking about forgoing life-sustaining treatment have similar structures.[10] First, the patient needs to understand the basic facts about the

TABLE 3-1 APPROACHES TO THE MANAGEMENT OF PHYSICAL AND PSYCHOLOGICAL SYMPTOMS

SYMPTOM	ASSESSMENT	TREATMENT
Pain	How severe is the symptom (as assessed with the use of validated instruments) and how does it interfere with the patient's life? What is the etiology of the pain? Is the pain assumed to be neuropathic or somatic? What has the patient used in the past (calculate previous days' equal analgesic dose)?	Prescribe medications to be administered on a standing or regular basis if pain is frequent. Consider alternative medicine, concomitant analgesics, and interventional treatments for pain to minimize the use of opiates. Concomitant analgesics (e.g., corticosteroids, anticonvulsants, tricyclic antidepressants, and bisphosphonates) should be used when applicable (particularly for neuropathic pain). For mild pain: use acetaminophen or a nonsteroidal anti-inflammatory agent. For moderate pain: titrate short-acting opioids (see Table 26-6). For severe pain: rapidly titrate short-acting opioids until pain is relieved or intolerable side effects develop; start long-acting opiates once pain is controlled. Rescue doses: prescribe immediate-release opioids—10% of the 24-hour total opiate every hour (orally) or every 30 minutes (parenterally) as needed.
Constipation	Is the patient taking opioids?	Prescribe laxatives for all patients on opiates, starting with a stimulant laxative. If ineffective, add drugs from alternative classes (e.g., stimulant, osmotic laxatives, and enemas). Prescribe methylnaltrexone if still constipated.
Shortness of breath	Ask the patient to assess the severity of the shortness of breath. Does the symptom have reversible causes?	Prescribe oxygen to treat hypoxia-induced dyspnea, but *not* if the patient is not hypoxic. Cardiopulmonary rehabilitation decreases dyspnea and improves exercise tolerance. Opioids may relieve breathlessness without measurable reductions in respiratory rate or oxygen saturation; effective doses are often lower than those used to treat pain. Aerosolized opioids do not work. Fans or cool air decrease dyspnea. Use reassurance, relaxation, distraction, cognitive behavioral therapy, and massage therapy.
Fatigue	Is the patient too tired for activities of daily living? Is the fatigue secondary to depression? Is a disease process causing the symptom or is it secondary to reversible causes?	Provide cognitive education about conserving energy use. Treat underlying conditions appropriately and as consistent with patient's goals and values. Psychostimulants may help in selected diseases for limited time periods.
Nausea	Which mechanism is causing the symptom (e.g., stimulation of the chemoreceptor trigger zone, gastric stimulation, delayed gastric emptying or "squashed stomach" syndrome, bowel obstruction, intracranial processes, or vestibular vertigo)? Is the patient constipated?	Prescribe an agent directed at the underlying cause (Chapter 118). If persistent, give antiemetic around the clock. Multiple agents directed at various receptors or mechanisms may be required.
Anorexia and cachexia	Is a disease process causing the symptom, or is it secondary to other symptoms (e.g., nausea and constipation) that can be treated? Is the patient troubled by the symptom or is the family worried about what not eating means?	A nutritionist may help find foods that are more appetizing (Chapter 13). Provide counseling about the prognostic implications of anorexia (Chapter 200).
Delirium	Is the cause reversible? Is the confusion acute, over hours to days? Does consciousness wax and wane? Is there a problem of attention? Does the patient have disorganized thinking? Does the patient have an altered level of consciousness—either agitated or drowsy?	Identify underlying causes and manage symptoms (Chapter 361). Recommend behavioral therapies, including avoidance of excess stimulation, frequent reorientation, and reassurance. Ensure presence of family caregivers and explain delirium to them. Although antipsychotics are often used, the data are meager.
Depression	Over the last 2 weeks, have you been bothered (0) not at all, (1) several days, (2) more than half the days, (3) every day by: • Little interest or pleasure in doing things • Feeling down, depressed, or hopeless	Add the points for each answer. For a score >2, further evaluation is recommended, with consideration of supportive psychotherapy, cognitive approaches, behavioral techniques, pharmacologic therapies (see Table 362-5), or a combination of these interventions. Prescribe psychostimulants for rapid treatment of symptoms (within days) or selective serotonin reuptake inhibitors, which may require 3 to 4 weeks to take effect; tricyclic antidepressants are relatively contraindicated because of their side effects.
Anxiety (applicable also for family members)	Over the last 2 weeks, have you been bothered (0) not at all, (1) several days, (2) more than half the days, (3) every day by: • Feeling nervous, anxious, or on edge • Not being able to stop or control worrying	Add the points for each answer. A score of >2 should lead to a more in-depth evaluation (see Chapter 362) and consideration of supportive counseling and benzodiazepines or selective serotonin reuptake inhibitors (Table 362-9).
Spiritual distress	Are you at peace?	Inquire about spiritual support. Offer chaplain support.

Modified from Morrison RS, Meier DE. Palliative care. *N Engl J Med.* 2004;350:2582-2590.

diagnosis, possible treatments, and prognosis. The communication skill that helps clinicians communicate information is *Ask-Tell-Ask*—exploring what the patient knows or wants to know, then explaining or answering questions, and then providing an opportunity for the patient to ask more. In the hospital, where discontinuity of care is common and misunderstandings frequent, it is important to determine what the patient knows before providing information so as to keep everyone well-coordinated. When giving serious news, knowing what the patient already knows allows the clinician to anticipate the patient's reaction. Finally, information must be titrated based on the patient's preferences. Although most patients want to hear everything about their disease, a minority do not. There is no foolproof way to ascertain what any patient wants to know other than by asking.

When giving patients information, it is important to give small pieces of information, not to use jargon, and to confirm that patients understand what they have been told.[A12] Clinicians should focus on the key message the patient should hear (the headline) rather than overwhelming the patient with biomedical information. Giving information is like titrating medication dosing: one gives information, checks understanding, and then gives more information based on what the patient has heard.

After ensuring that the doctor and the patient have a shared understanding of the medical facts, clinicians should engage in an open-ended conversation about the patient's goals as the disease progresses. This strategy requires that the patient be asked about both hopes and fears. One might ask: "Given the medical situation, as you think about the future, what brings you joy and pleasure?" "If your time is limited, what are the things that are most important to achieve?" "What are your biggest fears or concerns?" "As you think about the future, what do you want to avoid or not have the doctors do?" The clinician can use an understanding of these goals to make recommendations about which treatments to provide and which treatments would not be helpful. As a result, palliative care provided early in the trajectory of illness can improve quality of life, mood, and even survival.

STUDY ID# ______ HOSPITAL ID# ______

DO NOT WRITE ABOVE THIS LINE

Brief Pain Inventory (Short Form)

Date: ___/___/___ Time: ____

Name: ______ ______ ______
Last First Middle Initial

1. Throughout our lives, most of us have had pain from time to time (such as minor headaches, sprains, and toothaches). Have you had pain other than these everyday kinds of pain today?

1. Yes 2. No

2. On the diagram, shade in the areas where you feel pain. Put an X on the area that hurts the most.

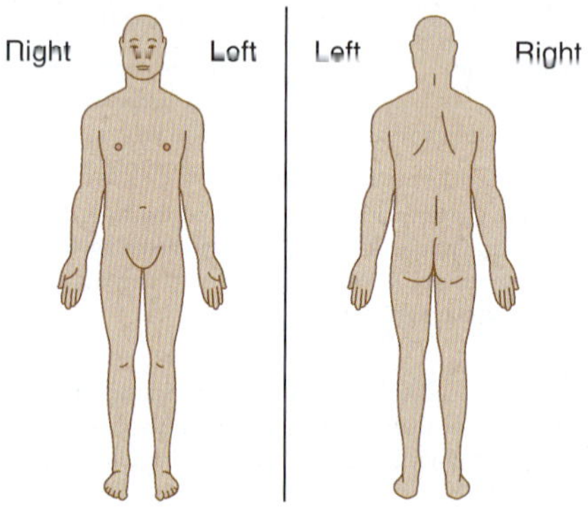

3. Please rate your pain by circling the one number that best describes your pain at its worst in the last 24 hours.

0 No pain 1 2 3 4 5 6 7 8 9 10 Pain as bad as you can imagine

4. Please rate your pain by circling the one number that best describes your pain at its least in the last 24 hours.

0 No pain 1 2 3 4 5 6 7 8 9 10 Pain as bad as you can imagine

5. Please rate your pain by circling the one number that best describes your pain on the average.

0 No pain 1 2 3 4 5 6 7 8 9 10 Pain as bad as you can imagine

6. Please rate your pain by circling the one number that tells how much pain you have right now.

0 No pain 1 2 3 4 5 6 7 8 9 10 Pain as bad as you can imagine

FIGURE 3-1. **Brief Pain Inventory (short form).** (Copyright 1991. Charles S. Cleeland, PhD, Pain Research Group. All rights reserved.)

7. What treatments or medications are you receiving for your pain?

8. In the last 24 hours, how much relief have pain treatments or medications provided? Please circle the one percentage that most shows how much relief you have received.

0% No pain	10%	20%	30%	40%	50%	60%	70%	80%	90%	100% Complete relief

9. Circle one number that describes how, during the past 24 hours, pain has interfered with your:

A. General Activity

0 Does not interfere	1	2	3	4	5	6	7	8	9	10 Completely interferes

B. Mood

0 Does not interfere	1	2	3	4	5	6	7	8	9	10 Completely interferes

C. Walking Ability

0 Does not interfere	1	2	3	4	5	6	7	8	9	10 Completely interferes

D. Normal Work (includes both work outside the home and housework)

0 Does not interfere	1	2	3	4	5	6	7	8	9	10 Completely interferes

E. Relations with Other People

0 Does not interfere	1	2	3	4	5	6	7	8	9	10 Completely interferes

F. Sleep

0 Does not interfere	1	2	3	4	5	6	7	8	9	10 Completely interferes

G. Enjoyment of Life

0 Does not interfere	1	2	3	4	5	6	7	8	9	10 Completely interferes

FIGURE 3-1, cont'd.

Clinicians often find that talking about prognosis is particularly difficult for two reasons: first, it is hard to foretell the future accurately; and second, they fear this information will "take away patients' hope." Thus, clinicians often avoid talking to patients about these issues unless specifically asked. Although some patients do not want to hear prognostic information, for many patients, this information helps them plan their lives. Patients who are told that their disease is generally terminal are more likely to spend a longer period of time enrolled in hospice and avoid aggressive treatment at the end of life, without adverse psychological consequences. Furthermore, their families usually have fewer post-death adverse psychological outcomes.

Given that one cannot guess how much information to provide, a clinician can start these conversations by asking, "Are you the kind of person who wants to hear about what might happen in the future with your illness or would you rather take it day by day?" If the patient requests the latter, the clinician can follow up by asking if there is someone else with whom he or she can talk about the prognosis. Second, before giving prognostic information, it is useful to inquire about the patient's concerns in order to provide information in the most useful manner. Finally, it is appropriate when discussing prognostic information to acknowledge uncertainty: "The course of this cancer can be quite unpredictable, and we don't have a crystal ball. I think you should be aware of the possibility that your health may deteriorate quickly, and you should plan accordingly. We probably are dealing with weeks to months, although some patients do better, and some do worse. Over time, the course may become clearer, and if you wish, I may be able to be a little more precise about what we are facing." A structured handout and conversational format, called Best Case/

TABLE 3-2 FICA SPIRITUAL ASSESSMENT TOOL

F—What is your **faith**/religion? Do you consider yourself a religious or spiritual person? What do you believe in that gives meaning/importance to life?

I—**Importance** and **influence** of faith. Is your faith/religion important to you? How do your beliefs influence how you take care of yourself? What are your most important hopes? What role do your beliefs play in regaining your health? What makes life most worth living for you? How might your disease affect this?

C—Are you part of a religious or spiritual **community**? Is this of support to you, and how? Is there a person you really love or is very important to you? How is your family handling your illness? What are their reactions/expectations?

A—How would you like me to **address** these issues in your health care? What might be left undone if you were to die today? Given the severity or chronicity of your illness, what is most important for you to achieve? Would you like me to talk to someone about religious/spiritual matters?

From Puchalski C, Romer A. Taking a spiritual history. *J Palliat Med.* 2000;3:129-137.

Worst Case, has been extensively used in surgery and nephrology,[11] both to discuss prognosis and as a way to discuss treatment alternatives (E-Fig. 3-3).

The clinician must discuss these topics in an empathic way. Palliative care conversations are as much about emotions as facts. Talking about disease progression or death may elicit negative emotions such as anxiety, sadness, or frustration. These emotions decrease a patient's quality of life and interfere with the ability to hear factual information. Empathic responses strengthen the patient-physician relationship, increase the patient's satisfaction, and make the patient more likely to disclose other concerns. The first step is recognizing when the patient is expressing emotions. Once the clinician recognizes the emotion being expressed, he or she can respond empathically.

It is also important for clinicians to recognize their own emotional reactions to these conversations. The physician's emotional reactions color impressions of the patient's prognosis, thereby making it hard to listen to the patient, and may influence the physician to hedge bad news. The clinician should become aware of her or his own emotional reactions to ensure that the conversation focuses on the patient rather than the health care provider's needs.

In addition to good communication skills, palliative care requires a basic knowledge of medical ethics and the law. For example, patients have the moral and legal right to refuse any treatment, even if refusal results in their death. There is no legal difference between withholding and withdrawing life-sustaining treatment. Differences in state laws regarding physician-assisted dying (Chapter 2), as well as use of agents such as medical marijuana or psychedelics, require clinicians to stay current regarding local legislation. When confronted with areas of ambiguity, the clinician should know how to obtain either a palliative care or ethics consultation.

During the past 50 years, a societal push has encouraged patients to designate health care proxies and to create advance care planning documents, typified by the use of living wills.[12] These documents are meant to protect patients against unwanted treatments and to ensure that as they are dying, their wishes are followed. Unfortunately, there are few empirical data showing that these documents actually change practice. Still, discussions of the documents with health professionals and family members generally provoke important conversations about end-of-life care decisions and may help families confronted with difficult situations know they are respecting their loved one's wishes.[13]

IS THE PATIENT GOING TO DIE IN THE LOCATION OF CHOICE?

Most patients say that they want to die at home. Unfortunately, most patients die in institutions—either hospitals or nursing homes. Burdensome transitions decrease quality in end-of-life care. Good palliative care requires establishing a regular system of communication to minimize transitional errors. A social worker who knows about community resources is important in the development of a dispositional plan that respects the patient's goals.

Hospice programs are an important way to allow patients to die at home. In the United States, *hospice* refers to a specific, government-regulated form of end-of-life care, available under Medicare since 1982 but subsequently adopted by Medicaid and many other third-party insurers. Hospice care typically is provided at home, a nursing home, or specialized acute care unit. Care is provided by an interdisciplinary team, which usually includes a physician, advanced practice provider, nurse, social worker, chaplain, volunteers, bereavement coordinator, and home health aides, all of whom collaborate with the primary care clinician, patient, and family. Bereavement services are offered to the family for a year after the death.

TABLE 3-3 CORE COMMUNICATION SKILLS

RECOMMENDED SKILL	EXAMPLE
A. IDENTIFYING CONCERNS AND RECOGNIZING CUES	
Elicit Concerns	
Open-ended questions	"Is there anything you wanted to talk to me about today?"
Active listening	Allowing patient to speak without interruption; allowing pauses to encourage patient to speak
Recognize Cues	
Informational concerns	Patient: "I'm not sure about the treatment options"
Emotional concerns	Patient: "I'm worried about that"
B. RESPONDING TO INFORMATIONAL CONCERNS	
"Ask-tell-ask"	Topic: communicating information about cancer stage
Ask	"Have any of the other doctors talked about what stage this cancer is?"
Tell	"That's right, this is a stage IV cancer, which is also called metastatic cancer…"
Ask	"Do you have questions about the staging?"
C. RESPONDING TO EMOTIONAL CONCERNS	
Nonverbal Empathy: S-O-L-E-R	
S	Face the patient **S**quarely
O	Adopt an **O**pen body posture
L	**L**ean toward the patient
E	Use **E**ye contact
R	Maintain a **R**elaxed body posture
Verbal Empathy: N-U-R-S-E	
N	**N**ame the emotion: "You seem worried"
U	**U**nderstand the emotion: "I see why you are concerned about this"
R	**R**espect the emotion: "You have shown a lot of strength"
S	**S**upport the patient: "I want you to know that I will still be your doctor whether you have chemotherapy or not"
E	**E**xplore the emotion: "Tell me more about what is worrying you"
D. DISCUSSING GOALS OF CARE	
R	**R**eframe that the status quo is not working: "I worry that more treatment will hurt you more than help"
E	**E**xpect emotion: "I can see this is not what you wanted to hear"
M	**M**ap the patient values: "Have you ever filled out a living will?" "Given the medical situation, what brings you joy and meaning?" "As you look at the future, what do you want to avoid?"
A	**A**lign with the patient values: "What I am hearing you say is…."
P	**P**ropose a plan

Adapted from Back AL, Arnold RM, Tulsky JA. *Discussing Prognosis.* Alexandria, VA: American Society of Clinical Oncology; 2008.

Hospices are paid on a per diem rate and are required to cover all the costs related to the patient's life-limiting illness. Because of this and the fact that the focus of hospice is on comfort rather than life prolongation, many hospices will not cover expensive treatments such as inotropic agents in heart failure or chemotherapy in cancer, even if they have a palliative effect. Not surprisingly, many hospices are experimenting with different service models that do not require patients to forgo possibly life-prolonging treatments, in an attempt to enroll patients earlier in the course of their illness and increase access to their services. The Veterans Administration and some insurance plans cover hospice services concurrently with disease-focused therapies.

Hospice care for nursing home residents is associated with less aggressive care near death but an overall increase in Medicare expenditures. By comparison, interdisciplinary palliative care for hospitalized adults with serious illness can reduce costs.[14]

GENERAL REFERENCES

For the General References and other additional features, please visit Elsevier eBooks+ at https://ebooks.health.elsevier.com.

Grade A References

A1. Kavalieratos D, Corbelli J, Zhang D, et al. Association between palliative care and patient and caregiver outcomes: a systematic review and meta-analysis. *JAMA*. 2016;316:2104-2114.
A2. Gaertner J, Siemens W, Meerpohl JJ, et al. Effect of specialist palliative care services on quality of life in adults with advanced incurable illness in hospital, hospice, or community settings: systematic review and meta-analysis. *BMJ*. 2017;357:j2925.
A3. Broese JM, de Heij AH, Janssen DJ, et al. Effectiveness and implementation of palliative care interventions for patients with chronic obstructive pulmonary disease: a systematic review. *Palliat Med*. 2021;35:486-502.
A4. Quinn KL, Shurrab M, Gitau K, et al. Association of receipt of palliative care interventions with health care use, quality of life, and symptom burden among adults with chronic noncancer illness: a systematic review and meta-analysis. *JAMA*. 2020;324:1439-1450.
A5. El-Jawahri A, LeBlanc TW, Kavanaugh A, et al. Effectiveness of integrated palliative and oncology care for patients with acute myeloid leukemia: a randomized clinical trial. *JAMA Oncol*. 2021;7:238-245.
A6. Bakitas MA, Dionne-Odom JN, Ejem DB, et al. Effect of an early palliative care telehealth intervention vs usual care on patients with heart failure: the ENABLE CHF-PC randomized clinical trial. *JAMA Intern Med*. 2020;180:1203-1213.
A7. Jones T, Luth EA, Lin SY, et al. Advance care planning, palliative care, and end-of-life care interventions for racial and ethnic underrepresented groups: a systematic review. *J Pain Symptom Manage*. 2021;62:e248-e260.
A8. Rogers JG, Patel CB, Mentz RJ, et al. Palliative care in heart failure: the PAL-HF randomized, controlled clinical trial. *J Am Coll Cardiol*. 2017;70:331-341.
A9. Boland EG, Bennett MI, Allgar V, et al. Cannabinoids for adult cancer-related pain: systematic review and meta-analysis. *BMJ Support Palliat Care*. 2020;10:14-24.
A10. van Esch HJ, van Zuylen L, Geijteman ECT, et al. Effect of prophylactic subcutaneous scopolamine butylbromide on death rattle in patients at the end of life: the SILENCE randomized clinical trial. *JAMA*. 2021;326:1268-1276.
A11. Kentish-Barnes N, Chevret S, Valade S, et al. A three-step support strategy for relatives of patients dying in the intensive care unit: a cluster randomised trial. *Lancet*. 2022;399:656-664.
A12. Gao W, Wilson R, Hepgul N, et al. Effect of short-term integrated palliative care on patient-reported outcomes among patients severely affected with long-term neurological conditions: a randomized clinical trial. *JAMA Netw Open*. 2020;3:e2015061.

4

DISPARITIES IN HEALTH AND HEALTH CARE

JOHN Z. AYANIAN

Disparities in health care and health are evident in all countries around the world. Health disparities often reflect a country's specific history, such as the legacy of conquest and colonization for American Indians and of slavery, segregation, and structural racism for Black Americans. Socioeconomic disparities in health related to poverty or lack of education occur globally and can be reduced by better educational and economic opportunities and by effective health care systems and social services.

Most efforts to understand and reduce health disparities have focused on race, ethnicity, and socioeconomic status and have sought to disentangle the relative impact of health care, health behaviors, and biologic, social, and environmental factors as contributors to these disparities. More recently, these efforts have expanded to assess a wider range of health disparities, including those faced by sexual minorities, people with disabilities, and people in disadvantaged urban or rural areas.

DEFINITIONS OF HEALTH DISPARITY AND HEALTH EQUITY

The U.S. Department of Health and Human Services defines a health disparity as a "health difference that is closely linked with economic, social, or environmental disadvantage." Conversely, health equity is defined as the "attainment of the highest level of health for all people."[1] These definitions build on U.S. National Academy of Medicine reports in which equitable health care was defined as "care that does not vary in quality due to personal characteristics, such as gender, ethnicity, geographic location, or socioeconomic status" and which identified racial and ethnic disparities in health care as an important contributor to disparities in health outcomes. Fragmented systems of care and structural racism, as well as bias and discrimination on the part of health professionals, can contribute to differential receipt of health care services, thereby leading to health disparities. However, not all differences in health care represent unacceptable disparities related to discrimination, in part because some differences in care may be related to clinical appropriateness or patients' preferences.

DEMOGRAPHIC CHANGES IN THE U.S. POPULATION

The racial and ethnic composition of the U.S. population has changed substantially in recent decades. As the population has grown from 193 million in 1965 to 332 million in 2022, almost half of this growth related to nearly 60 million new immigrants. During this time period, the non-Hispanic White proportion of the U.S. population dropped from 84 to 60% and the Black proportion rose from 11 to 13%. In contrast, the Hispanic proportion grew substantially from 4 to 18% and the Asian or Pacific Islander proportion increased from 1 to 6%. These trends are projected to continue through 2065, when the corresponding proportions of the U.S. population are projected to be 46% non-Hispanic White, 13% Black, 24% Hispanic, and 14% Asian or Pacific Islander if current immigration patterns persist.

RACIAL AND ETHNIC DISPARITIES IN HEALTH OUTCOMES

Substantial differences in life expectancy between Black and White Americans have narrowed since 1975 as life expectancy has risen.[2] Notably, as of 2018, life expectancy was about 3 years longer for Hispanic individuals relative to White individuals. In contrast, life expectancy in 2018 was 4 years shorter for Black individuals, relative to White individuals (Fig. 4-1). Overall, the all-cause mortality rate is about 25% higher in Black Americans. In 2020, coronavirus disease 2019 (COVID-19; Chapter 336) was the third leading cause of death in the United States. COVID-19 death rates have been disproportionately higher in Black and Hispanic populations, predominately because of higher infection rates rather than higher case-fatality rates.[3] As a result, during the COVID-19 pandemic in 2020, life expectancy declined from 2018 by 3.88 years for Hispanic Americans and 3.25 years for Black Americans, compared with 1.36 years for White Americans.[4] These disparities underscore the disproportionate effect that COVID-19 has had on Hispanic and Black adults.

Heart disease and cancer are the two leading causes of death for all five racial and ethnic groups officially designated by the U.S. federal government, but age-adjusted death rates for specific causes vary substantially by race and ethnicity (Table 4-1). Black Americans have the highest age-adjusted death rates, overall and due specifically to heart disease[5] and to cancer, followed by non-Hispanic White Americans. Black Americans also have the highest

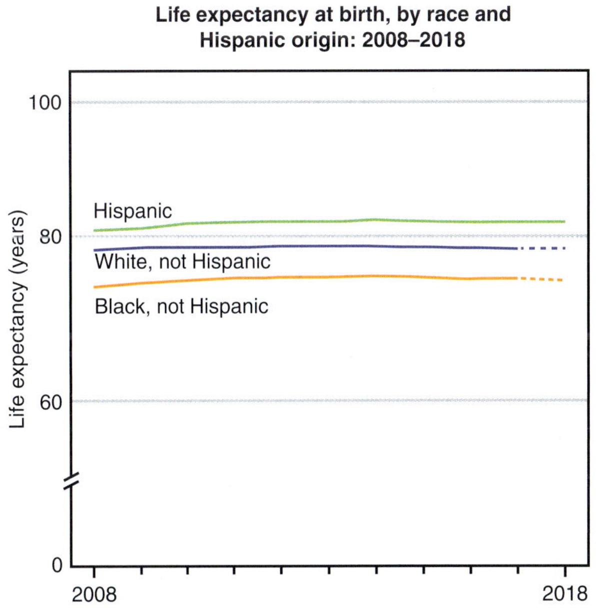

FIGURE 4-1. Life expectancy at birth. Note: Life expectancy data by Hispanic origin were available starting in 2006 and were corrected to address racial and ethnic misclassification. (Source: NCHS, *Health United States, 2019*, Figure 1 from the National Vital Statistics System [NVSS].)

TABLE 4-1 AGE-ADJUSTED DEATH RATES FOR 10 LEADING CAUSES OF DEATH BY RACE/ETHNICITY IN THE UNITED STATES, 2018*

	ALL PERSONS	WHITE, NON-HISPANIC	BLACK OR AFRICAN AMERICAN	HISPANIC OR LATINO	ASIAN OR PACIFIC ISLANDER	AMERICAN INDIAN OR ALASKA NATIVE
All causes	723.6	745.7	852.9	524.1	390.6	571.8
Heart disease	163.6	167.5	203.7	112.3	85.0	110.8
Cancer	149.1	154.4	168.7	107.4	92.6	97.2
Chronic lung disease	39.7	45.0	29.6	17.0	11.6	28.3
Cerebrovascular disease	37.1	35.9	50.8	32.0	29.4	24.2
Alzheimer disease	30.5	32.2	26.6	25.5	15.8	15.3
Diabetes mellitus	21.4	18.8	37.6	24.6	16.4	31.0
Poisoning	19.3	23.6	19.0	11.1	3.3	19.6
Influenza and pneumonia	14.9	15.0	15.8	11.7	12.8	13.7
Suicide	14.2	18.0	7.0	7.4	6.9	13.7
Kidney disease	12.9	11.6	24.8	11.6	8.3	11.4

*Per 100,000 population, from *Health, United States, 2019*. Hyattsville, MD: National Center for Health Statistics; 2020. https://www.cdc.gov/nchs/data/hus/2019/005-508.pdf.

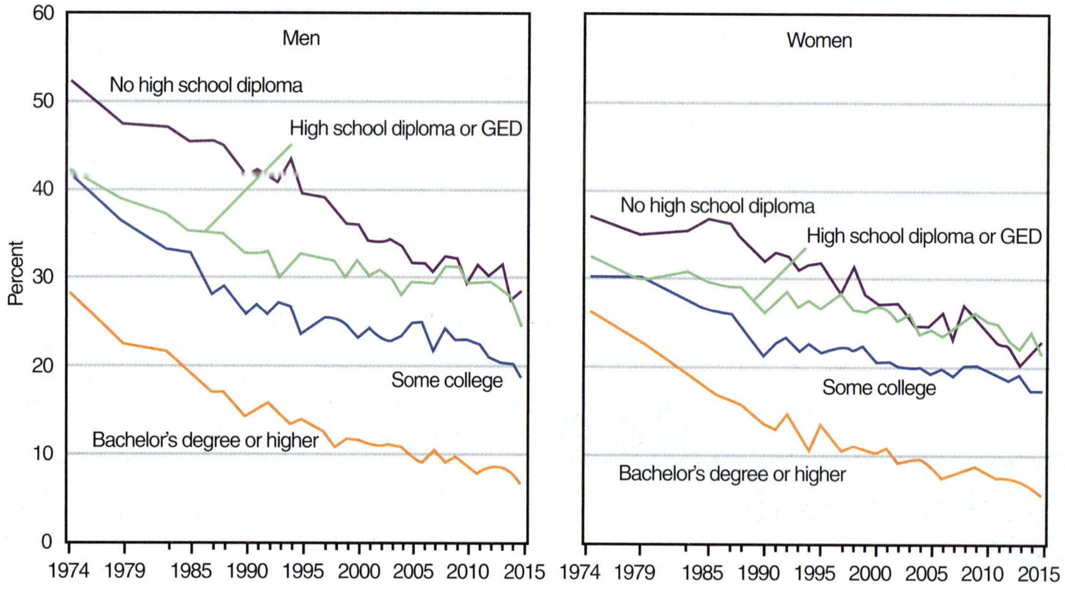

FIGURE 4-2. **Current cigarette smoking: adults aged 25+. Note: Smoked 100 cigarettes in their lifetime and now smoke every day or some days. (Source: NCHS, *Health, United States, 2016*, Figure 10 and Table 48. Data from the National Health Interview Survey [NHIS].)**

death rates from cerebrovascular disease, diabetes mellitus, and kidney disease, but lower-than-average death rates from chronic lung disease, poisoning, and suicide. Non-Hispanic White Americans, in contrast, have higher-than-average death rates from these latter three causes.

Hispanic Americans have lower-than-average death rates from all causes except diabetes mellitus (see Table 4-1). American Indians have lower-than-average death rates from most causes except diabetes mellitus and poisoning, but they also have markedly elevated death rates from chronic liver disease (27.7 deaths per 100,000 vs. 11.1 among all persons). Asian and Pacific Islander Americans together have lower-than-average death rates from each of the 10 leading causes of death, including markedly lower rates for heart disease, cancer, chronic lung disease, Alzheimer disease, poisoning, and suicide.

Major health risk factors that contribute to morbidity and mortality among adults vary substantially by race, ethnicity, and level of education.[6] Black adults have the highest age-adjusted prevalence of hypertension (43%; Chapter 64), which is a major contributor to their high rates of heart disease, cerebrovascular disease, and kidney disease, whereas the prevalence of hypertension is substantially lower among non-Hispanic White (29%), Hispanic (28%), and Asian (27%) adults. In contrast, the prevalence of diabetes mellitus is substantially higher among Black (18%), Mexican American (18%), and Asian (16%) adults than among non-Hispanic White adults (10%).[7]

Smoking rates (Chapter 363) vary widely in the United States by race/ethnicity and sex. Rates are highest among non-Hispanic White men (21%), Black men (22%), and American Indian men (28%) and women (24%). Smoking rates are intermediate among non-Hispanic White women (19%), Black women (14%), Hispanic men (16%), and Asian men (15%), and they are lowest among Hispanic women (7%) and Asian women (5%).[8]

SOCIOECONOMIC DISPARITIES IN HEALTH OUTCOMES

Socioeconomic gradients in morbidity and mortality, which are a major component of health disparities, have widened in the United States in recent years. Adults with higher educational levels and incomes have experienced substantial gains in life expectancy related to their lower smoking rates and better control of hypertension, hyperlipidemia, and other chronic health conditions and risk factors. By comparison, adults with low incomes experienced minimal gains overall prior to COVID-19.[9] For example, socioeconomic status is an independent correlate of mortality after a myocardial infarction.[10] Among middle-aged non-Hispanic White adults without postsecondary education, life expectancy has actually decreased since 1999 as a result of rising death rates from alcohol-related liver disease, drug overdoses, and suicide, and overall U.S. life expectancy has decreased since 2014.[11]

U.S. smoking rates have declined substantially since 1974, with the steepest drop among college graduates (Fig. 4-2). Higher smoking rates among less educated adults remain a major contributor to socioeconomic disparities in morbidity and mortality. The temporal improvement in smoking rates overall has been offset by marked increases in age-adjusted death rates due to drug overdoses—particularly among non-Hispanic White adults, who have had a three-fold increase in this death rate from 1999 to 2015 primarily due to opioid overdoses (Fig. 4-3).[12]

The magnitude of socioeconomic disparities in mortality vary widely by geographic region within the United States. When considering life expectancy at age 40, for example, adults with incomes in the lowest quartile can expect to survive to age 81 years in New York City and several California cities, but only to age 77 years in some cities in Ohio, Indiana, and Michigan. These disparities in life expectancy are primarily related to regional differences in the prevalence of behavioral and metabolic risk factors, including smoking, limited physical activity, obesity, hypertension, and diabetes mellitus. Among high-income counties, cancer has become the leading cause of death, whereas heart disease remains the leading cause in poorer counties.

INSURANCE COVERAGE AND ACCESS TO CARE

Health insurance coverage is an important contributor to racial, ethnic, and socioeconomic disparities in health care and health outcomes, especially for adults who are under age 65 years and do not have near-universal insurance coverage through Medicare, as do older adults.[13] Since the Affordable Care Act was enacted in 2010, 38 states have expanded Medicaid to nonelderly adults with annual incomes below 138% of the federal poverty level (<$17,775 for a single adult in 2021). In all states, adults with incomes of 100 to 400% of the federal poverty level (about $12,900 to $51,500 in 2021) have become eligible for subsidized private insurance.

With this expanded coverage, rates of uninsurance have declined substantially for poor and near-poor adults in all racial and ethnic groups since 2010 (Fig. 4-4), although they still remain substantially higher for Hispanic and Black adults (Fig. 4-5).

Health insurance is a primary determinant of access to care because it reduces financial barriers to preventive services such as smoking cessation and cancer screening and to effective care for chronic health conditions such as hypertension, diabetes, and heart disease. Uninsured adults are three to five times more likely to delay or forgo needed care or prescription medications because of cost than are adults with private insurance or Medicaid (Fig. 4-6). Gaining insurance coverage is associated with improved access to care and better health outcomes, particularly for middle-aged adults with low incomes and chronic health conditions such as hypertension and diabetes mellitus. Life expectancy is also correlated with the local availability of physicians, especially primary care doctors, but also to a lesser degree specialists as well.[14]

QUALITY OF CARE

An extensive body of research has documented substantial racial and ethnic disparities in the quality of health care provided to patients with a wide range of major conditions, including heart disease, hypertension, diabetes mellitus, kidney disease, breast cancer, and colorectal cancer. Relative to non-Hispanic

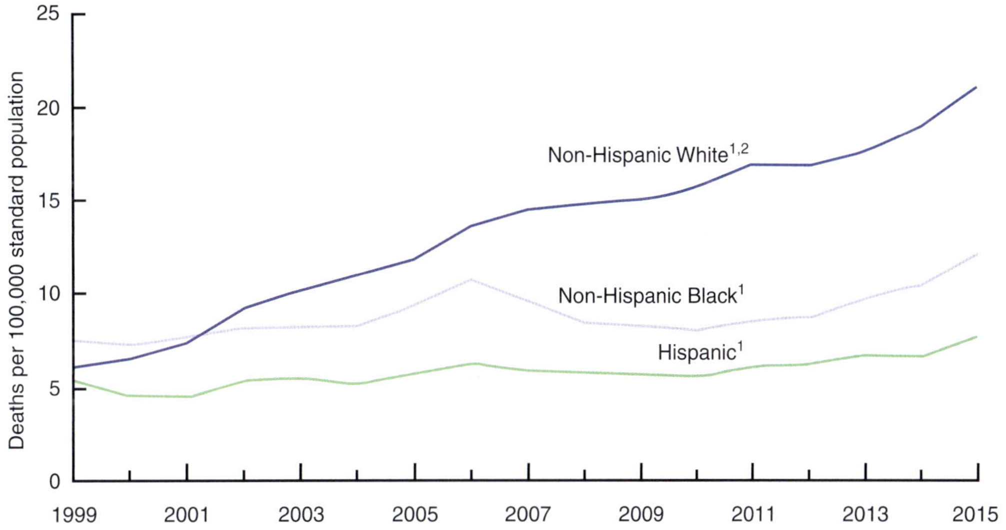

FIGURE 4-3. Age-adjusted drug overdose death rates by race and ethnicity: United States, 1999-2015. [1]Significant increasing trend, $p < 0.005$. [2]Rate for non-Hispanic White persons was significantly higher than for non-Hispanic Black and Hispanic persons, $p < 0.001$. Notes: Deaths are classified using the *International Classification of Diseases, Tenth Revision*. Drug overdose deaths are identified using underlying cause-of-death codes X40-X44, X60-X64, X85, and Y10-Y14. Deaths for Hispanic persons may be underreported by about 5%. Access data table for Figure 3 at: https://www.cdc.gov/nchs/data/databriefs/db273_table.pdf#3. (Source: Hedegaard H, Warner M, Miniño AM. *Drug overdose deaths in the United States, 1999–2015*. NCHS data brief, no 273. Hyattsville, MD: National Center for Health Statistics. 2017.)

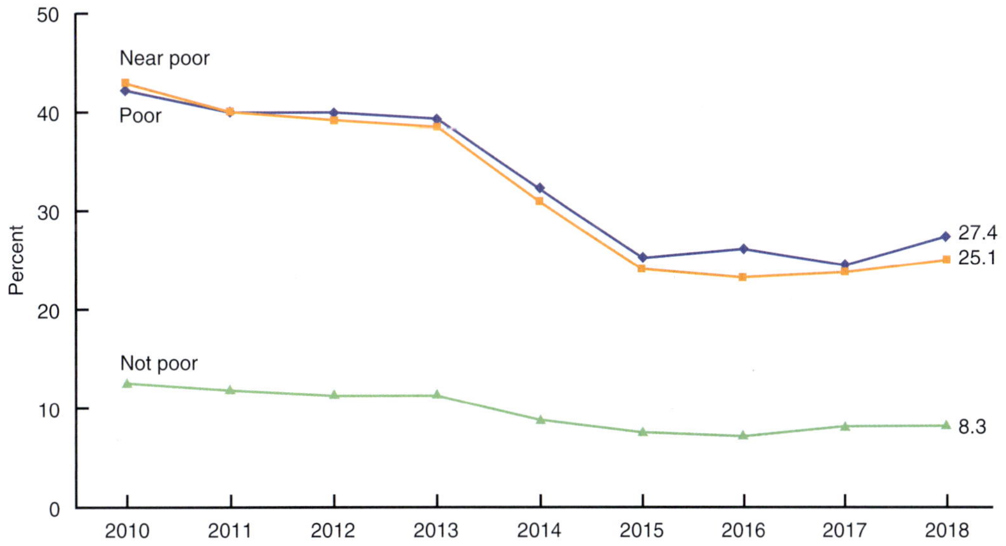

FIGURE 4-4. Percentage of adults aged 18 to 64 who were uninsured at the time of interview, by poverty status: United States, 2010-2018. Note: Data are based on household interviews of a sample of the civilian noninstitutionalized population. (Source: NCHS, National Health Interview Survey, 2010-2018, Family Core Component.)

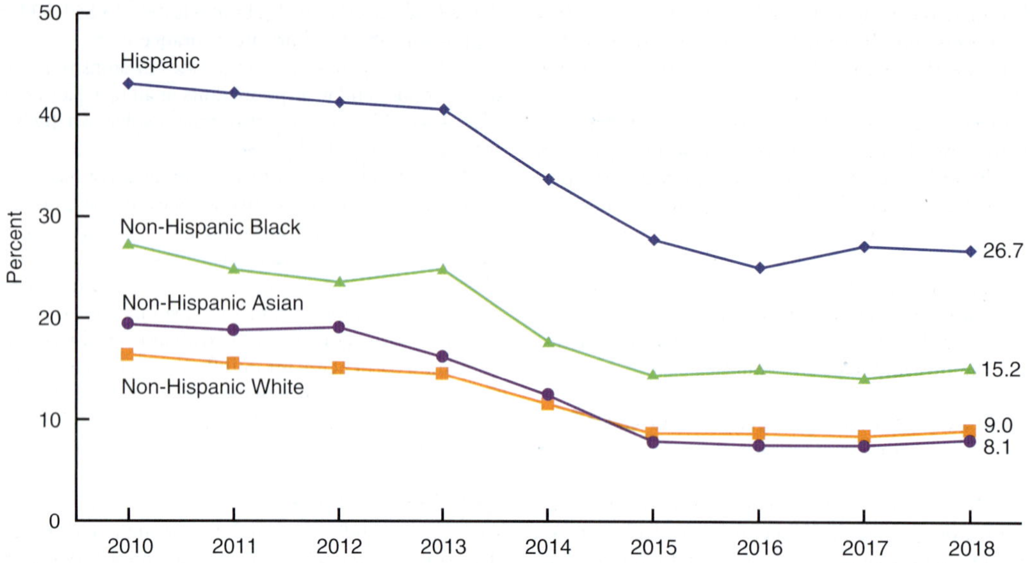

FIGURE 4-5. **Percentage of adults aged 18 to 64 who were uninsured at the time of interview, by race and ethnicity: United States, 2010-2018.** Note: Data are based on household interviews of a sample of the civilian noninstitutionalized population. (Source: NCHS, National Health Interview Survey, 2010-2018, Family Core Component.)

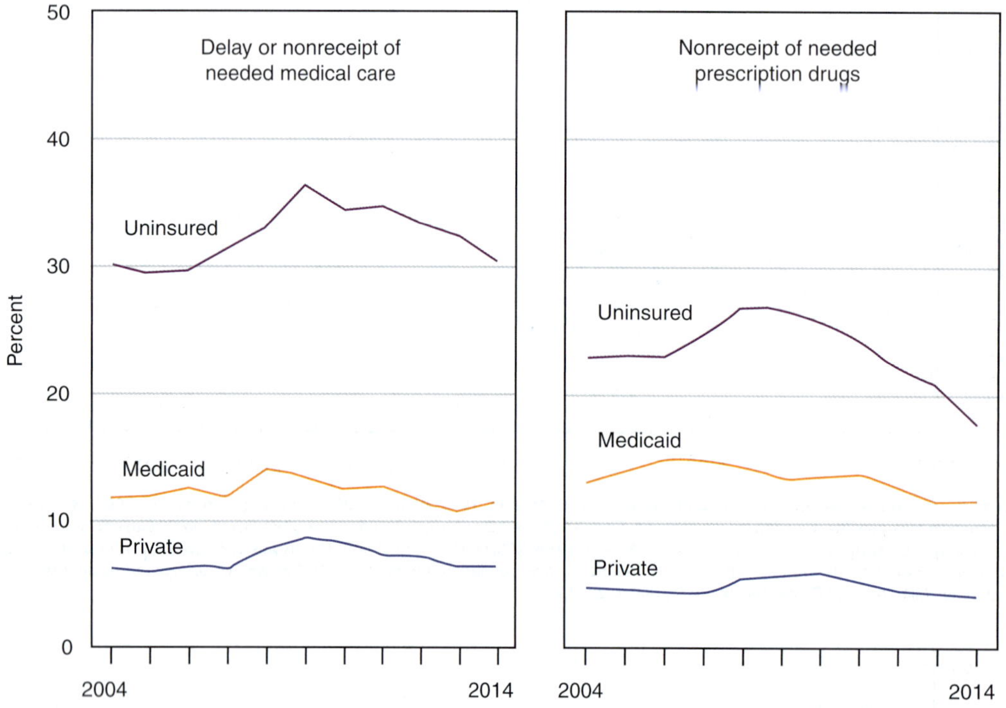

FIGURE 4-6. **Difficulty accessing care: Adults aged 18 to 64.** (Source: CDC/NCHS, Health, United States, 2015, Figure 12 and Table 63. Data from the National Health Interview Survey [NHIS].)

White adults, Black and Hispanic adults are much less likely to have good control of their hypertension or diabetes mellitus. These disparities are narrowed among Medicare enrollees nationally, and they have been eliminated in Medicare health maintenance organizations in the western United States. Over time, such improvements in the control of hypertension and diabetes mellitus may further reduce disparities in cardiovascular mortality for Black Americans relative to other racial and ethnic groups.

Similar improvements have been noted in the quality of hospital care nationally for minority patients with acute myocardial infarction, heart failure, and pneumonia, for whom the quality of hospital care is now clinically equivalent by race and ethnicity. Most notably, substantial disparities in timely percutaneous coronary interventions (Chapter 57) and in rates of influenza and pneumococcal vaccination (Chapter 15) have been eliminated for Black and Hispanic patients relative to non-Hispanic White patients.

CLINICAL APPROACHES TO REDUCE DISPARITIES

The increasing diversity of the U.S. population has created new challenges and opportunities for health care professionals and organizations to meet the needs of patients from diverse backgrounds, particularly immigrants. The federal Office of Minority Health has produced national standards for delivering culturally and linguistically appropriate health care, including the use of trained interpreters for patients with limited English proficiency. The principal standard is that health care providers should ensure quality care and services that are effective, equitable, understandable, respectful, and responsive to diverse cultural health beliefs and practices, preferred languages, health literacy, and other communication issues. Physicians and other caregivers who have undergone educational programs in cultural competencies may provide better care to diverse populations. However, this training has not clearly improved patients' outcomes, such as reducing disparities in control of glycemia, blood pressure, or cholesterol for Black adults with diabetes mellitus.

Disparities in health care often arise from fragmented systems of care, particularly for conditions that require complex services, such as cancer, cardiovascular disease, end-stage renal disease, and organ transplantation. When care requires multiple specialists or sites of care, disparities also can be reduced by emphasizing patient-centered approaches that provide better coordinated care with enhanced support for patients from disadvantaged backgrounds, such as those who are uninsured or have less education or limited English proficiency. This support may include multidisciplinary team-based care and enhanced outreach to patients and their families via care coordinators, patient navigators, and community health workers.[15]

It is also essential for clinical leaders in health care organizations to implement reporting systems (e.g., through enhanced electronic health records) to identify and monitor disparities related to race, ethnicity, language, and socioeconomic factors. These systems can be used to set measurable goals for reducing disparities in the quality and outcomes of care, motivate quality improvement programs to address clinically important disparities, and assess progress toward achieving these goals.

GENERAL REFERENCES

For the General References and other additional features, please visit Elsevier eBooks+ at https://ebooks.health.elsevier.com.

5

GLOBAL HEALTH

ALI H. MOKDAD

Efforts to improve health and reduce death and disability in populations across the world require a comprehensive understanding of what disables and kills people across countries, time, age, and sex. Before the coronavirus disease 2019 (COVID-19) pandemic, global life expectancy was increasing despite marked disparities among and often within countries. The COVID-19 pandemic is estimated to have reduced life expectancy by about 1.7 years in the United States and globally. Addressing global health requires an understanding of the leading causes of death and disability so resources can be targeted where they can be most effective.

LIFE EXPECTANCY

Life expectancy is highly variable across the globe (Fig. 5-1), ranging from 51.8 years in Lesotho to 84.8 years in Singapore.[1] Life expectancy in Africa is markedly lower than in other parts of the world. Even within a single country, however, major disparities may exist. In the United States, for example, overall life expectancy was 78.9 years in 2019, but it ranged from 74.9 years in West Virginia to 81.7 years in Hawaii. For all racial and ethnic groups, U.S. life expectancy in 2019 ranged from 64.5 years to 91.7 years.

LEADING CAUSES OF DEATHS

Cardiovascular disease and cancers have remained the leading causes of death worldwide across the last three decades (Fig. 5-2). Compared with 1990, noncommunicable disease are more prominent and infectious diseases less prominent among leading causes of death. In general, as the sociodemographic index improves over time, the burden of noncommunicable disease increases. However, such global trends mask disparities at the country level where some countries are still dealing with a heavy infectious disease burden even as they witness a rise in noncommunicable diseases.

The leading causes of death globally vary by age of death (Fig. 5-3). Before the COVID-19 pandemic, infectious diseases were responsible for more deaths in younger age groups globally, with a greater burden of noncommunicable disease in older ages. Diarrheal and lower respiratory infections are more common in younger ages, injuries and self-harm are highest in young adults, and cardiovascular disease and cancer are the main causes of death in the older age groups. The recent declines in malnutrition deaths in some countries is attributed to improved diet, water sanitation, and access to medical care. Despite this progress, however, malnutrition is still the leading cause of burden for some countries. The COVID-19 pandemic reduced life expectancy by about 1.7 years in the U.S.[2] and by about 2.3 years worldwide.

LEADING CAUSES OF DISABILITIES

Over the past three decades, cardiovascular disease has remained the leading cause of disability worldwide (as measured by lost disability-adjusted life years [DALYs], Fig. 5-4).[3] The disability burden from cancer has risen from fourth to second, primarily as a result of longer life expectancy, whereas maternal

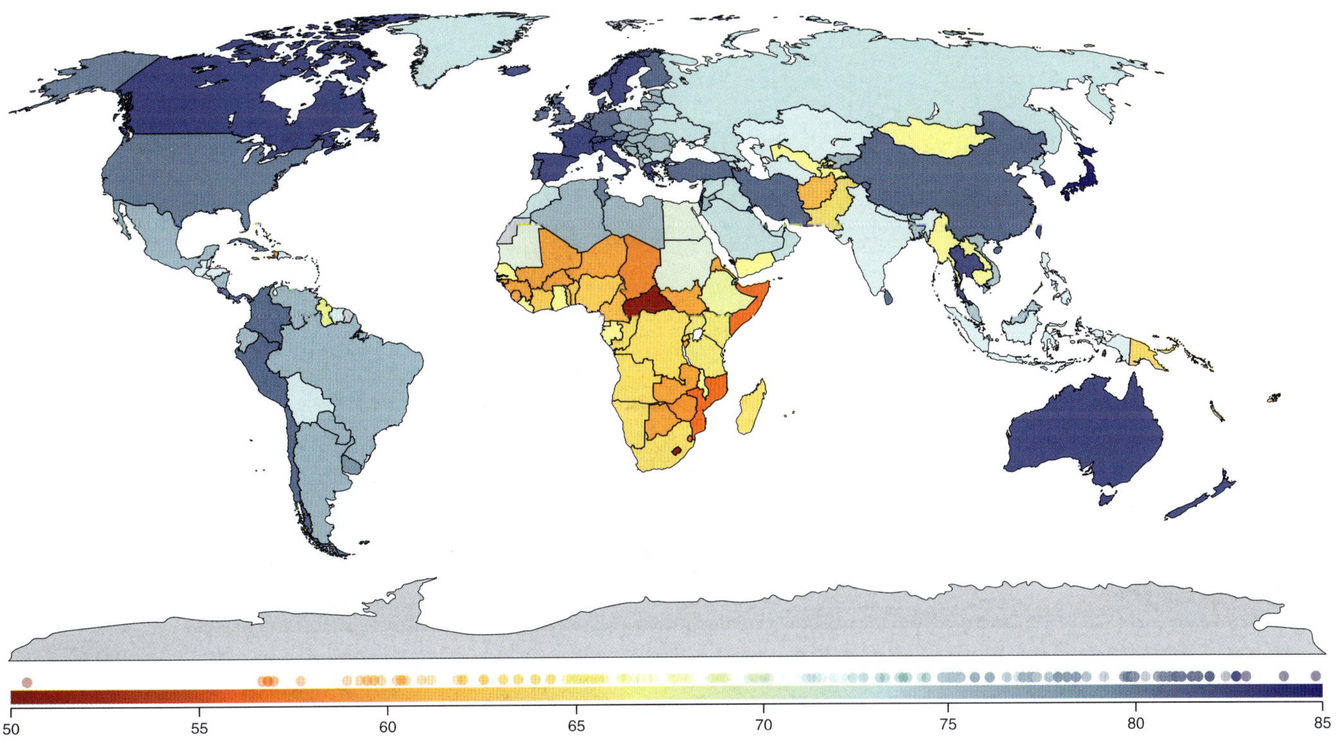

FIGURE 5-1. Life expectancy for both sexes in 2019. (Available from Global Burden of Disease 2019, Institute for Health Metrics and Evaluation. https://www.healthdata.org/data-visualization/gbd-compare. Accessed November 16, 2022.)

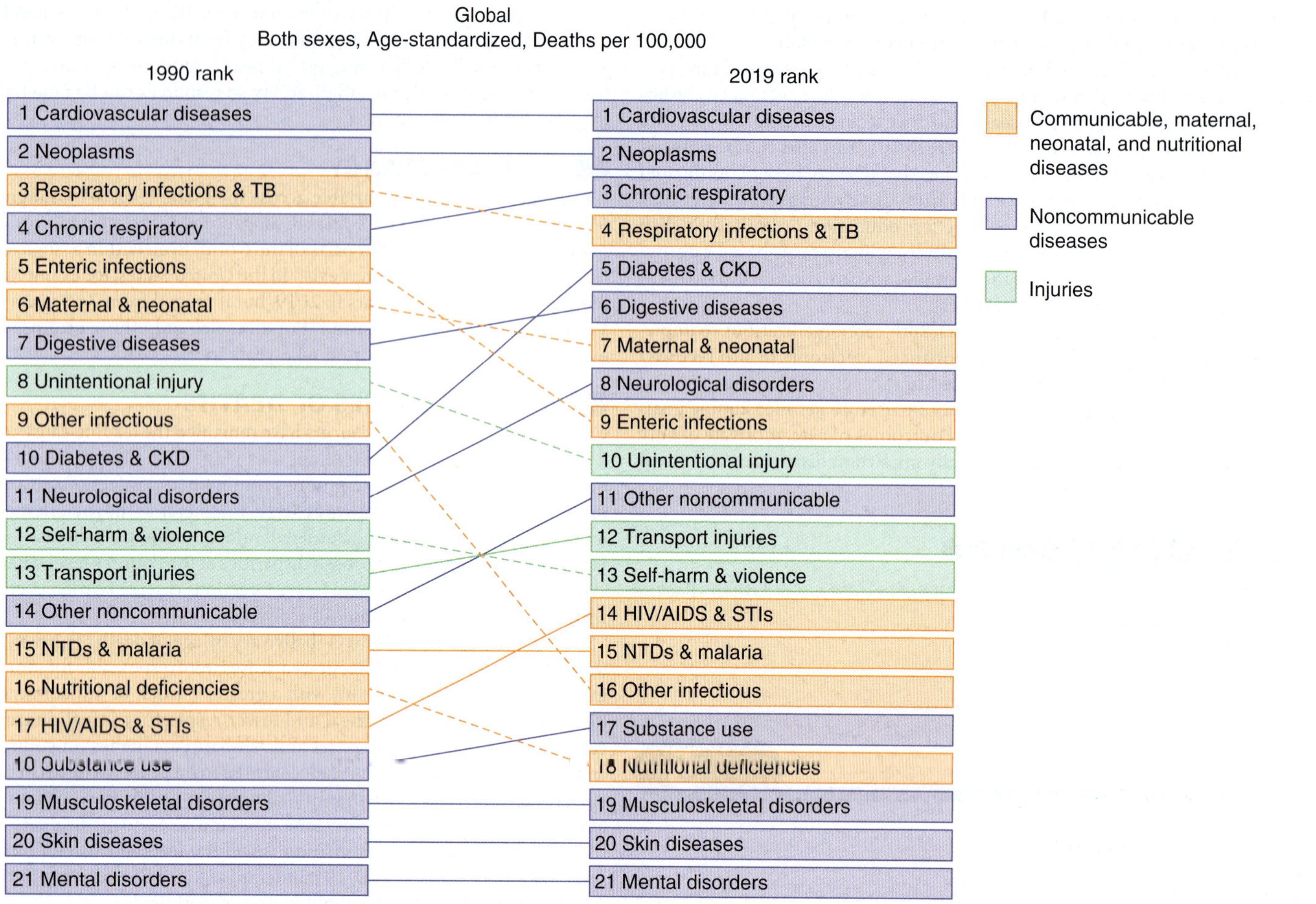

FIGURE 5-2. **Leading causes of death in 1990 and 2019 for both sexes and all ages (age standardized).** AIDS = acquired immunodeficiency syndrome; CKD = chronic kidney disease; HIV = human immunodeficiency virus; NTD = neglected tropical disease; STI = sexually transmitted infection; TB = tuberculosis. (Available from Global Burden of Disease 2019, Institute for Health Metrics and Evaluation. https://www.healthdata.org/data-visualization/gbd-compare. Accessed November 16, 2022.)

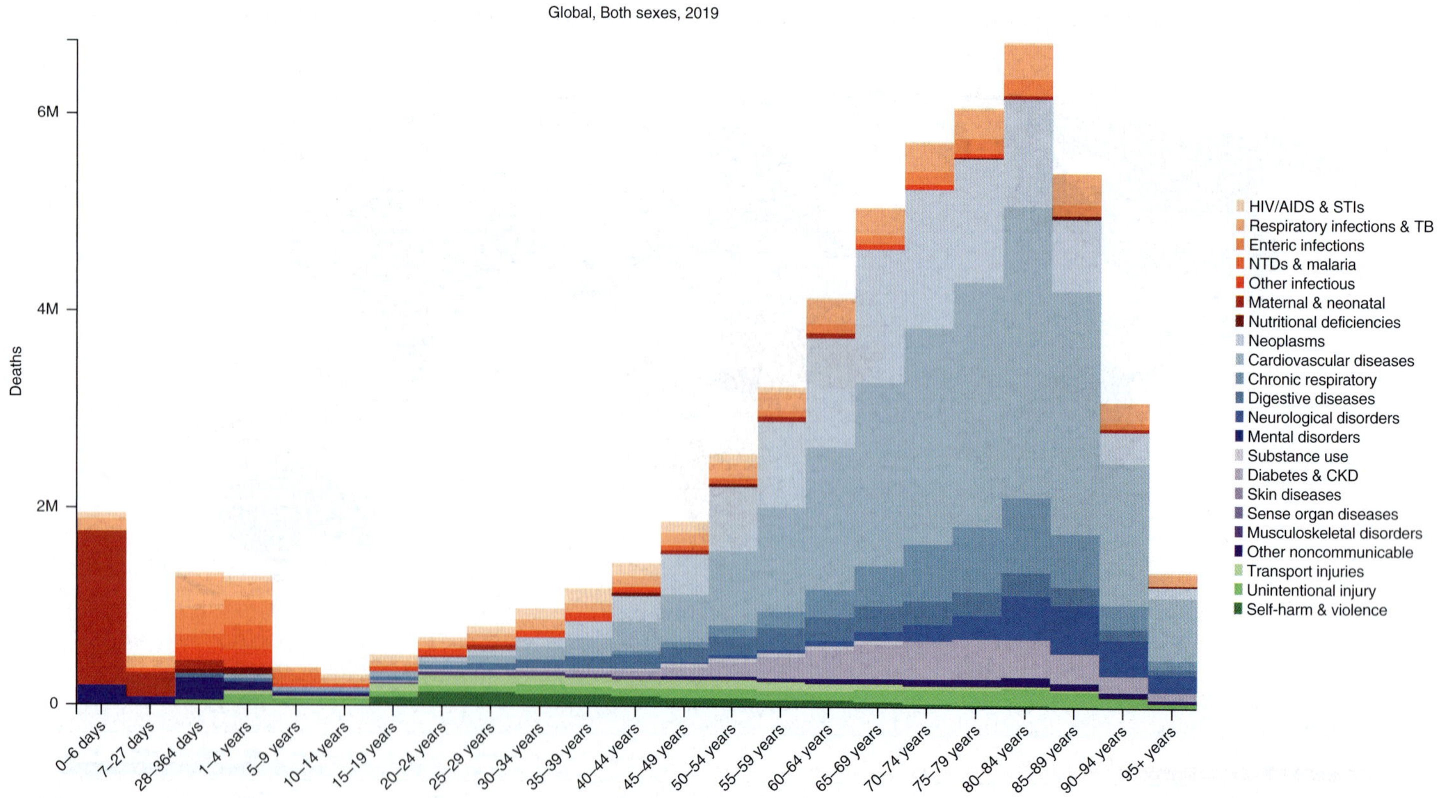

FIGURE 5-3. **Causes of death globally in 2019 by 5-year incremental age groups.** AIDS = acquired immunodeficiency syndrome; CKD = chronic kidney disease; HIV = human immunodeficiency virus; NTD = neglected tropical disease; STI = sexually transmitted infection; TB = tuberculosis. (Available from Global Burden of Disease 2019, Institute for Health Metrics and Evaluation. https://www.healthdata.org/data-visualization/gbd-compare. Accessed November 16, 2022.)

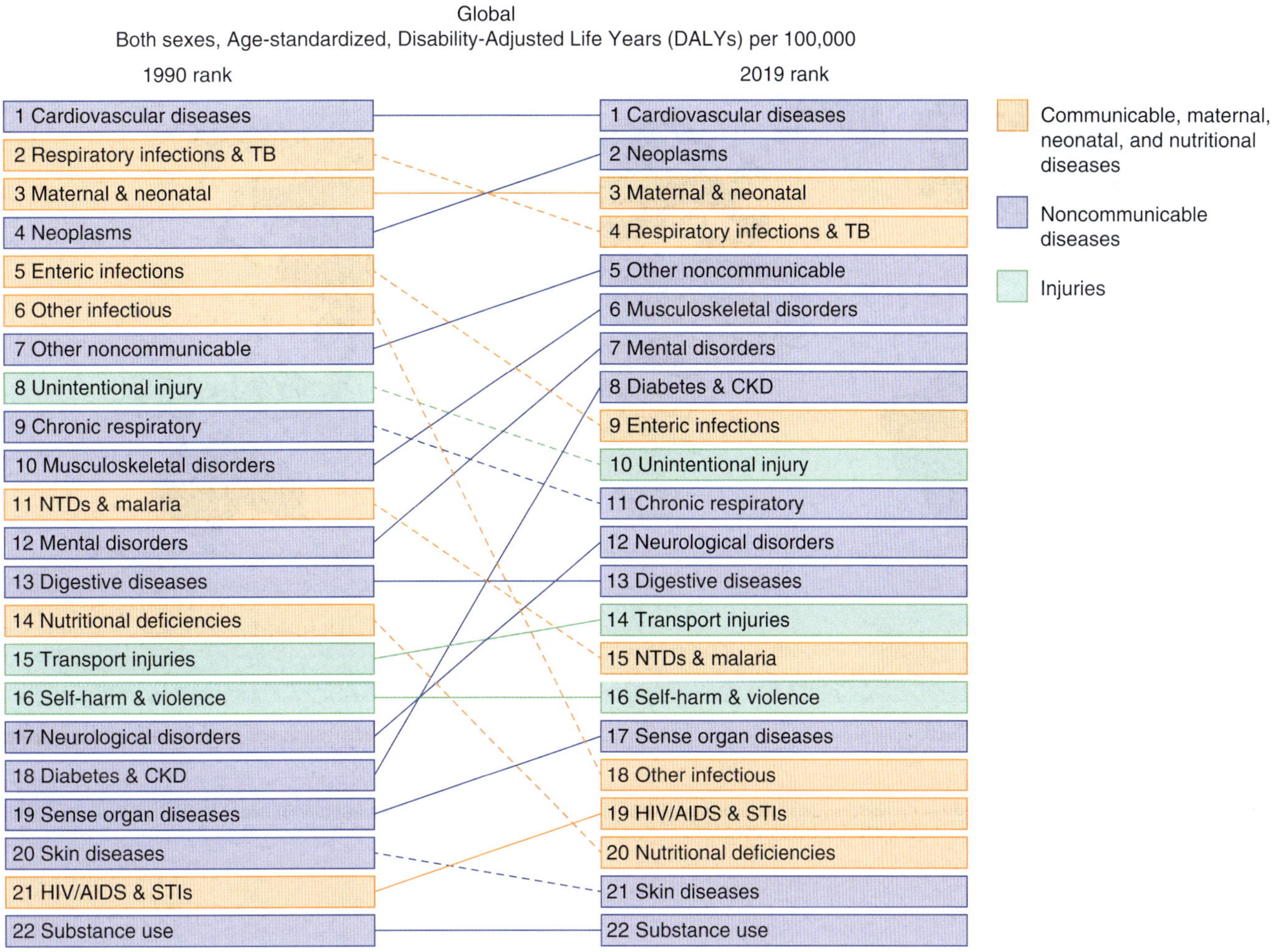

FIGURE 5-4. Leading causes of lost disability-adjusted life years 1990 and 2019 (age standardized). AIDS = acquired immunodeficiency syndrome; CKD = chronic kidney disease; HIV = human immunodeficiency virus; NTD = neglected tropical disease; STI = sexually transmitted infection; TB = tuberculosis. (Available from Global Burden of Disease 2019, Institute for Health Metrics and Evaluation. https://www.healthdata.org/data-visualization/gbd-compare. Accessed November 16, 2022.)

and neonatal diseases remained the third leading cause of lost DALYs. The burden of respiratory infections and tuberculosis has declined globally but it remains a major burden in many countries. In low-income countries, for example, respiratory infections were the second leading cause of lost DALYs.

The main contributors to increasing health loss worldwide over the past 30 years, as measured by the largest absolute increase in number of DALYs, includes six causes that largely affect older adults—ischemic heart disease (with the number of related lost DALYs increasing by 50% from 1990 to 2019), diabetes (up almost 150%), stroke (up over 30%), chronic kidney disease (up over 90%), lung cancer (up almost 70%), and age-related hearing loss (up over 80%) Additionally, four causes of disability that are common from teenage years into old age have also increased: human immunodeficiency virus (HIV; up about 130% over the past 3 decades), musculoskeletal disorders (also up about 130%), low back pain (up nearly 50%), and depressive disorders (up about 60%).

The age-standardized loss of DALYs varies substantially across the globe (Fig. 5-5).[4] In general, the burden is much higher in Africa, particularly the Central African Republic and Lesotho, compared with the remainder of the world. The burden is also high in Afghanistan. The global obesity epidemic partly explains why the number of DALYs due to ischemic heart disease rose by more than 400% in the Philippines from 1990 to 2019, and the number of lost DALYs due to diabetes rose by more than 1000% in the United Arab Emirates. In Singapore, Iceland, Norway, Ireland, Australia, New Zealand, and Qatar, more than half of all lost DALYs is now due to disability caused by noncommunicable diseases and injuries. Ethiopia, Sudan, and Bangladesh have seen 2% or greater annual reductions in age-standardized DALY rates.

LEADING UNDERLYING RISK FACTORS

Changes in mortality and morbidity reflect a variety of underlying causes.[5] Among the leading age-standardized risk factors that lead to loss of DALYs for all ages and both sexes, child and maternal malnutrition remain most prominent (Fig. 5-6). An important trend is the rise of risk factors for noncommunicable diseases, such as high systolic blood pressure, elevated fasting plasma glucose levels, and high body mass index. These risk factors vary tremendously by the sociodemographic index of countries. In countries with a low sociodemographic index, the leading risk factors for loss of DALYs are child and maternal malnutrition, air pollution, unsafe water, poor sanitation, and lack of hand-washing. By comparison, the leading risk factors in countries with high sociodemographic indexes are tobacco, high body mass index, and high fasting plasma glucose levels.

CHANGING PATTERNS OF DISEASE

Although morbidity and mortality from malnutrition and communicable diseases have declined markedly worldwide, especially in children, parts of Africa, Asia, and Latin America face not only a continued burden of persistent infectious diseases (e.g., HIV, malaria, tuberculosis, and other bacterial infections[6]) but also a rise in noncommunicable diseases (e.g., obesity, diabetes, hypertension). As the world's population ages, more and more people worldwide are now living with chronic health conditions. As a result, noncommunicable diseases, such as cardiovascular disease and diabetes, now account for nearly two-thirds of the global burden of disease, even in low- and middle-income countries.

In developing countries, malnutrition, especially in poorer and more rural areas, coexists with obesity, primarily in urban and more affluent segments of the population.[7] Rising rates of obesity (Chapter 201), diabetes (Chapter 210), smoking (Chapter 363), and often-undiagnosed hypertension (Chapter 64) in low-income countries portend a major future increase in cardiovascular diseases.[8]

THE GLOBAL HEALTH CHALLENGE

Many deaths that occur globally could have been prevented with access to high-quality health care. The Health Access and Quality of Care Index, which is

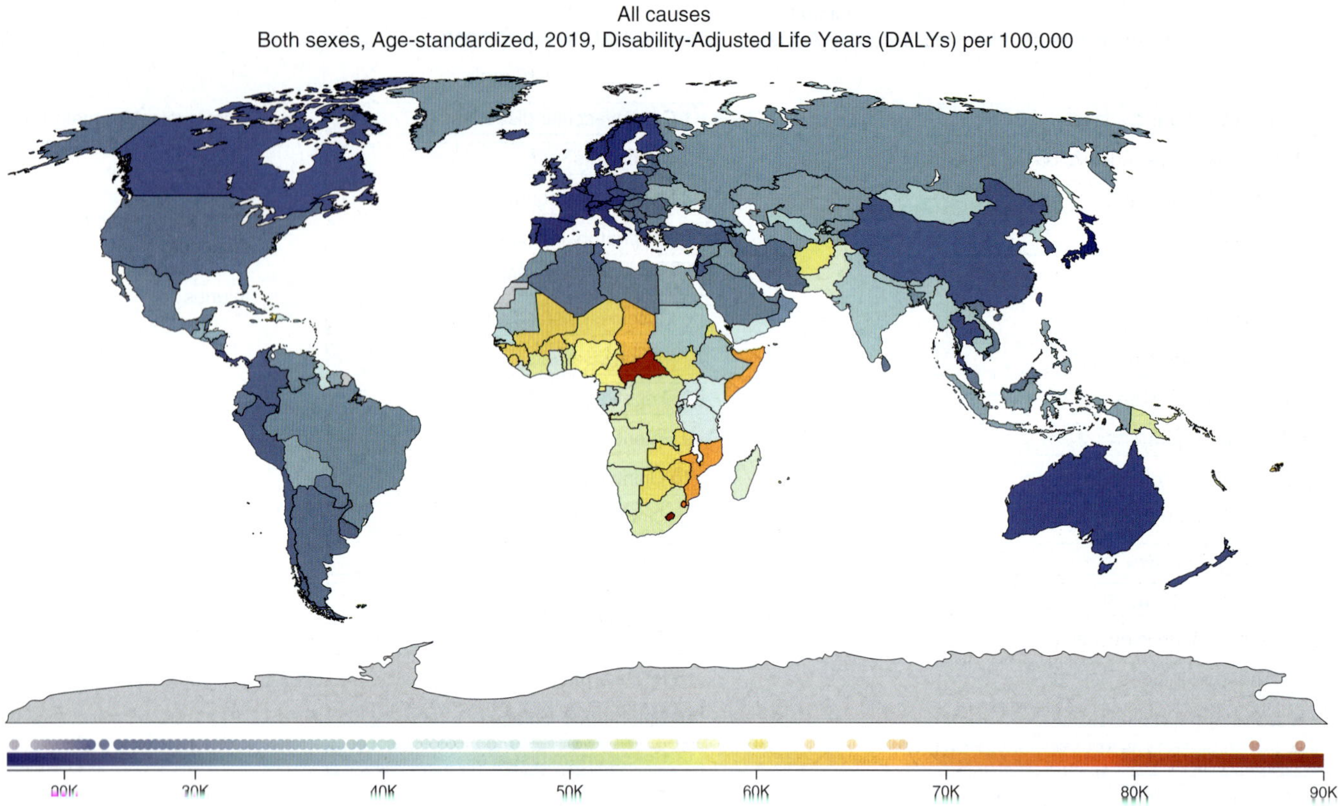

FIGURE 5-5. **Age-standardized loss of disability-adjusted life years globally.** (Available from Global Burden of Disease 2019, Institute for Health Metrics and Evaluation. https://www.healthdata.org/data-visualization/gbd-compare. Accessed November 16, 2022.)

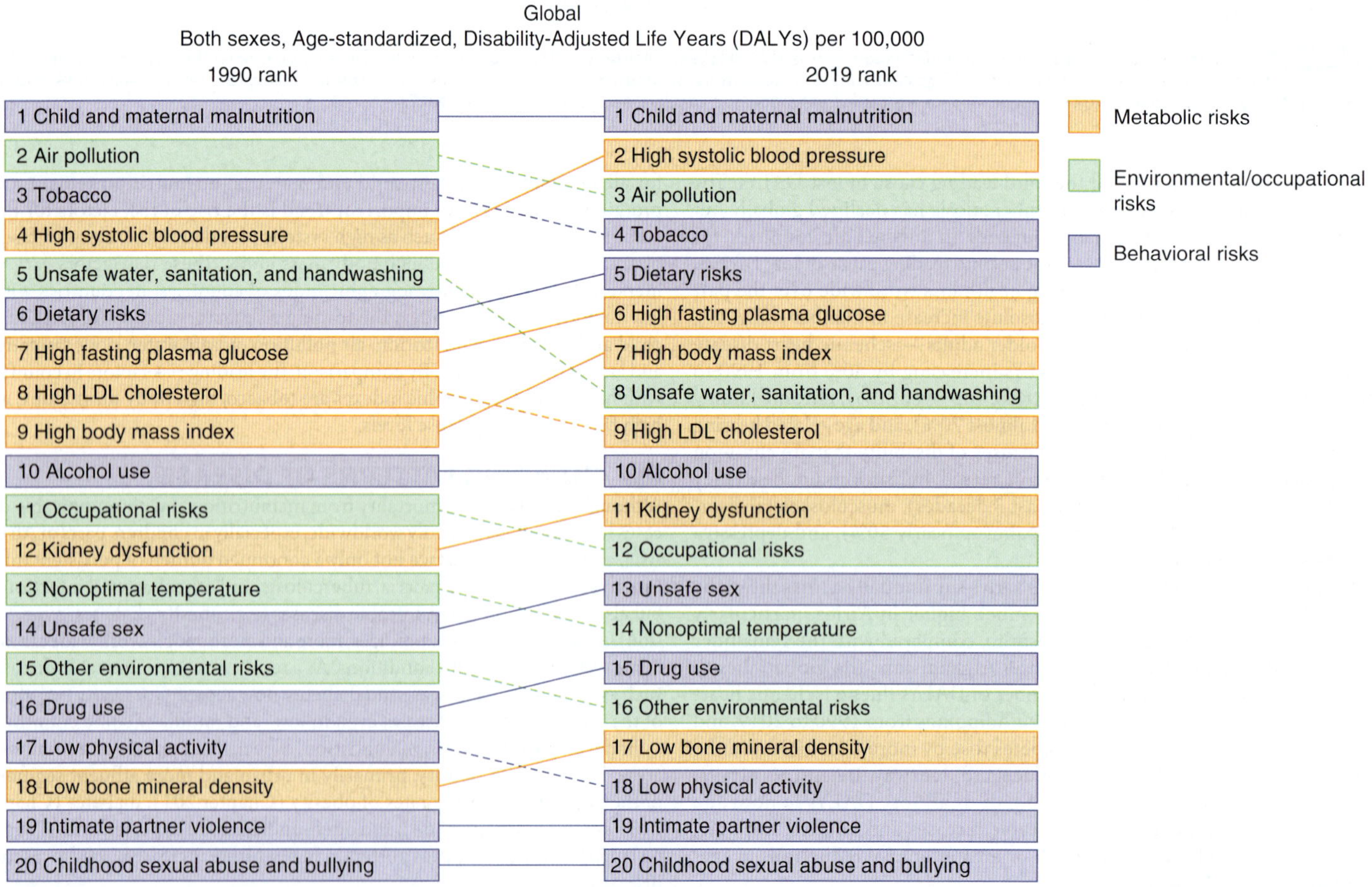

FIGURE 5-6. **Age-standardized leading risk factors for loss of disability-adjusted life years globally.** LDL = low-density lipoprotein. (Available from Global Burden of Disease 2019, Institute for Health Metrics and Evaluation. https://www.healthdata.org/data-visualization/gbd-compare. Accessed November 16, 2022.)

based on 32 causes of deaths that should not occur in the presence of effective health care,[9,10] range from a high of 97.1 (with 100 as the highest index of access and quality of care) in Iceland to a low of 18.6 in the Central African Republic. Second, health is strongly linked to economic development. Countries that made greater improvements in the human capital index (calculated as the number of years a person can be expected to work in the years of peak productivity, considering life expectancy, functional health, years of schooling, and learning)[11] had faster per capita economic growth. These findings highlight the need for countries to invest in health and education so as to improve their economies by improving the productivity of their labor forces.[12] Only by understanding the current health spending landscape can decision makers better allocate resources, technology, and innovation to improve health outcomes.

The COVID-19 pandemic has exacerbated already deep health disparities and demonstrated the weaknesses in worldwide public health systems. Vaccines and life-saving interventions have not been available in many parts of the world. Even in resource-rich countries, vaccination rates have often been disappointing. Excess global mortality from COVID-19 was about 17 million by the end of 2021,[13] with a huge impact on mental health[14] and gender equity.[15] Much of the recent gains in life expectancy have been reversed, with life expectancy falling to below what it was in 2013.

Global health efforts aimed to reduce infectious diseases and improve prenatal care have markedly improved the health of children under 10 years of age worldwide in the past few decades, with the overall burden of disease declining by approximately 55%. Unfortunately, this progress has not been matched in other age groups. For example, despite increased recognition of the importance of adolescent health to global development and future economic prosperity, the world failed to respond to health risks during adolescence and young adulthood (ages 10 to 24 years).[16]

Addressing social determinants of health could bring substantial health and economic benefits. Programs to improve diet quality (Chapter 13), increase physical activity (Chapter 14), and promote smoking cessation (Chapter 363) can yield large health benefits. Unfortunately, many low- and middle-income countries spend far less than 5% of their comparatively low gross domestic product on health care and, as a result, cannot address their domestic health needs.

As shown by the COVID-19 pandemic, infectious disease, like climate (Chapter 17), are worldwide issues regardless of the country or countries that may be initially or most responsible. The COVID-19 pandemic has demonstrated the importance of a strong public health infrastructure, as well as modern acute health care capabilities. However, global health threats will require not only country-specific resources and infrastructures but also general cooperation and responses. Affluent countries, which have provided poorer countries with low-cost or free treatments for HIV and onchocerciasis (Chapter 327), now must be encouraged to help countries with limited resources improve access to health care and public health programs. The sharing of expertise can also ensure that countries allocate resources to effective programs and wisely use limited resources.

GENERAL REFERENCES

For the General References and other additional features, please visit Elsevier eBooks+ at https://ebooks.health.elsevier.com.

II

PRINCIPLES OF EVALUATION AND MANAGEMENT

6 HISTORY AND PHYSICAL EXAMINATION

DAVID L. SIMEL

OVERVIEW

Physicians may have multiple objectives with varying degrees of importance in their encounters with patients. These goals include, but are not limited to, the translation of symptoms and signs into diagnoses, the assessment of stability or change in known conditions, the provision of information and counseling for future prevention, and the reaffirmation or alteration of therapeutic interventions. For a healthy adult with no symptoms or signs of a problem, age-specific and risk-specific screening guidelines should be followed (Chapter 12), but a comprehensive annual physical examination is not recommended.

The interaction between the patient and physician represents not only a scientific encounter but also a social ritual centered on the locus of control of patient and physician and meeting each other's expectations. Patients expect a competent assessment of their health care needs and concerns. Physicians need to feel that they have not missed something important, an occasional need to put limits on the time available for each interaction, and a need to maintain objectivity. The expertly performed rational clinical examination enhances the social ritual and the likelihood of acquiring relevant data. It also optimizes the physician's ability to understand the patient's symptoms and concerns, as well as to facilitate the healing process. The comprehensiveness of a clinical evaluation depends on the time available, whether the episode of care was prompted by specific concerns, whether the evaluation is an intake evaluation to establish a long-term relationship with the patient, or whether the setting is in acute care. The coronavirus disease 2019 (COVID-19) pandemic rapidly advanced the use of telemedicine by clinicians who were forced to learn new creative methods for the physical examination.

MEDICAL HISTORY

The history begins by asking patients to describe, in their own words, the reason for seeking medical care (Table 6-1). Although patients may have many reasons for initiating a visit to the physician, they should be encouraged to select the one or two most important concerns they have. Physicians should reassure patients with multiple worries that other concerns will not be ignored, but emphasize that it is important to understand what worries them most.

HISTORY OF THE PRESENT ILLNESS

Open-ended questions facilitate descriptions of problems in the patient's own words. Subsequently, specific questions fill in gaps and help clarify important points. However, wise clinicians realize that when they are talking, they are not listening. Nonetheless, when the patient is acutely ill, the physician should limit the amount of time spent in open-ended discussion and move promptly to the most important features that allow quick evaluation and management. In general, the history of the problem under consideration includes the following:

- Description of onset and chronology
- Location of symptoms
- Character (quality) of symptoms
- Intensity
- Precipitating, aggravating, and relieving factors
- Inquiry into whether the problem or similar problems occurred before and, if so, whether a diagnosis was established

It is often helpful to ask patients to express what they believe is the cause of the problem or what concerns them the most. This approach often uncovers other pertinent factors and helps establish that the physician is trying to meet the patient's needs.

PAST MEDICAL AND SURGICAL HISTORY

An astute clinician recognizes that patients may not report all their prior problems because they may forget, may assume that previous events are unrelated to their current problem, or simply may not want to discuss past events. Open-ended statements such as "Tell me about other medical illnesses that we did not discuss" and "Tell me about any operations you had" prompt the patient to consider other items. The physician should ask the patient about unexplained surgical or traumatic scars.

A list of current medications includes prescriptions, over-the-counter medications, vitamins, and herbal preparations. Patients who do not recall the names of medications should bring all medication bottles to the next visit. Patients may not consider topical medications (e.g., skin preparations or eye-drops) as important, so they may need prompting.

Information about allergies (Chapter 234) is particularly important, but challenging, to collect. Patients may attribute adverse reactions or intolerances to allergies, but many supposed allergic reactions are not truly drug allergies. Eliciting the patient's actual response to medications facilitates a determination of whether the response was a true allergic reaction.

SOCIAL AND OCCUPATIONAL HISTORY AND RISK FACTORS

The social history not only reveals important information but also improves understanding of the patient's unique values, support systems, and social situation. It can be helpful to ask the patient to describe what they would do during a recent typical day when they were well, and more recently if they have been affected by changes in their health or social situation. Physicians must consider whether inherent bias, especially about race, gender, and gender identity, affects their assessment of the patient.

Data that may influence risk factors for disease should be gathered, including a nonjudgmental assessment of substance abuse (Chapter 365). The tobacco history should include the use of snuff, chewing tobacco, cigar and cigarette smoking, and electronic nicotine delivery systems (Chapter 363). Alcohol use should be determined quantitatively and by the effect that it has had on the patient's life (Chapter 364). Past or present use of prescription pain medications, sedatives, or illicit substances should be assessed (Chapter 365). The sexual history should address sexual orientation and gender identity, as well as current and past sexual activity. The best way to address sexual orientation and gender identity may be to ask the patient whether they think of themselves as "lesbian, gay, or homosexual; as straight or homosexual; as bisexual; as something else; or whether they 'don't know.'"[1] The employment history should include the current and past employment history, as well as any significant hobbies. All adult patients should be asked if they served in the military. Military veterans should be asked about their combat history, years of service, and areas of deployment.[2] In patients in whom exposure to trauma has been established, screening for post-traumatic stress disorder (PTSD; Chapter 362) can be done with several simple questions (Table 6-2). Post-traumatic stress disorder is not just a consequence of military service, so all patients should be screened for prior traumatic events and their current response to them.

The physician should obtain information on socioeconomic status, insurance, the ability to afford or obtain medications, and past or current barriers to health care (Chapter 4). Marital status and the living situation (i.e., whom the patient lives with, significant stressors for that patient) are important as risk factors for disease and to determine how best to care for the patient. A patient's culture (Chapter 4) and values should be known, including any prior advance directives or desire to overrule them (Chapter 3).

FAMILY HISTORY

The family history allows risk stratification, which affects the pretest probability for an increasing number of disorders.[3] For common diseases such as heart disease, additional inquiry into the age of onset in first-degree relatives and death attributed to the disease should be obtained (Chapter 40). Patients may lack appropriate information about the absence of disease.

REVIEW OF SYSTEMS

The review of systems elicits symptoms or signs not covered or overlooked in the history of the present illness, though no evidence suggests that a complete review of symptoms is necessary at each patient evaluation (Table 6-3).[4] The review of systems is more efficient when the questions are restricted to a specific period (e.g., "a recent change in your vision" or "shortness of breath, wheezing, or coughing this past week") or by having the patient fill out a previsit questionnaire.

PHYSICAL EXAMINATION

CHAPERONES

When a guest or friend accompanies the patient, the clinician should either ask the patient if they would like their companion to stay during the examination or ask the guest to wait outside the room. Patients can be offered the option of a chaperone, especially when the clinician and patient are of different genders and a comprehensive examination is planned. Many examiners prefer a chaperone to allay their own anxieties attributable to gender differences or to

TABLE 6-1 PATIENT'S MEDICAL HISTORY

Description of the patient
Age, sexual orientation and gender identity, racial and ethnic background, language, occupation
Chief reason for seeking medical care
State the purpose of the evaluation (usually in the patient's words)
Other physicians involved in the patient's care
Include the clinician that the patient identifies as his or her primary provider or the physician who referred the patient. Record contact information for all physicians who should receive information about the visit
History of the reason for seeking medical care
In chronologic fashion, determine the evolution of the indication for the visit and then each major symptom. It is best to address the patient's reason for seeking care first rather than what the physician ultimately believes is most important
Be careful to avoid "premature closure," when a diagnosis is assumed before all the information is collected
Past medical and surgical history
List other illnesses and previous surgeries not related to the current problem
List all prescribed and over-the-counter medications with dose; remember to ask about vitamin and herbal supplements
Allergies and adverse reactions
List allergic reactions to medications and food. Record the specific reaction (e.g., hives). Distinguish allergies from adverse reactions or intolerance to medication (e.g., dyspepsia from nonsteroidal anti-inflammatory agents)
Social, occupational, and military history (see Table 6-2)
Describe the patient's current family and a typical day for patient
Risk factors/habits
- Physical activity
- Use of tobacco, alcohol, and drugs
- Risk factors for sexually transmitted disease (including human immunodeficiency virus and hepatitis)

Family history
History of any diseases in first-degree relatives and a listing of family members with any conditions that could be risk factors for the patient (e.g., cardiovascular disease at a young age, malignancy, known genetic disorders, longevity)
Review of systems (see Table 6-3)

TABLE 6-2 HISTORY OF MILITARY SERVICE AND POST-TRAUMATIC STRESS

- Tell me about your military experience.
- When and where do you/did you serve?
- What do you/did you do while in the service?
- How has military service affected you?

If the patient answers "yes" to any of the questions below, ask the patient, "Can you tell me more about that?"
- Did you see combat, enemy fire, or casualties?
- Were you or a buddy wounded, injured, or hospitalized?
- Did you ever become ill while you were in the service?
- Were you a prisoner of war?

To screen for post-traumatic stress disorder, ask, "In your life, have you ever had an experience so horrible, frightening, or upsetting that, in the past month you…"
- Have had nightmares about it or thought about it when you did not want to?
- Tried hard not to think about it or went out of your way to avoid situations that reminded you of it?
- Were constantly on guard, watchful, or easily startled?
- Felt numb or detached from others, activities, or your surroundings?

From Department of Veterans Affairs. Military Health History Pocket Card for Clinicians. https://www.va.gov/oaa/archive/Military-Health-History-Card-for-print.pdf. Accessed April 6, 2021.

achieve a perceived need for protection should the patient become concerned during the procedure.

VITAL SIGNS

Vital signs include the pulse rate and rhythm, blood pressure, respiratory rate, and body temperature. Marked abnormalities require a rapid, focused evaluation that may take precedence over the typical structural approach to the remainder of the evaluation (Chapter 7).

When the blood pressure is abnormal (Chapter 64), the measurement should be repeated, assuring that the cuff size is appropriate. Because of inherent variability in blood pressure, and the prevalence of both white coat hypertension on the one hand and masked hypertension on the other, the clinician is now advised to confirm hypertension through review of measurements obtained outside of the clinical setting.[5]

TABLE 6-3 REVIEW OF SYSTEMS*

FOCUS all questions on a specific time frame (e.g., within the past "month" or "now") and on items not already addressed during the clinical examination:
- Change in weight or appetite
- Change in vision
- Change in hearing
- New or changing skin lesions
- Chest discomfort or sensation of skipped beats
- Shortness of breath, dyspnea on exertion
- Abdominal discomfort, constipation, melena, hematochezia, diarrhea
- Difficulty with urination
- Change in menses
- Joint or muscle discomfort not already mentioned
- Problems with sleep
- Difficulty with sexual function
- Exposure to "street" drugs or medications not already mentioned
- Depression (feeling "down, depressed, or hopeless"; loss of interest or pleasure in doing things)
- A sensation of unsteadiness when walking, standing, or getting up from a chair

*Start with this basic list and adapt the items by considering factors such as age, gender, medications, and the problems identified during the examination. The process is facilitated by developing a routine personal approach to these questions, typically going through the systems from "head to toe."

Respirations should be assessed with the patient unaware that the rate is being observed. Abnormal patterns include tachypnea (rapid rate of breathing) or hypopnea (slow or shallow rate of breathing). Tachypnea is not always associated with hyperventilation, which is defined by increased alveolar ventilation resulting in a lower arterial carbon dioxide level (Chapter 89). Dyspnea is a subjective sensation claimed by the patient,[6] and patients with hypoxemia do not always complain of breathlessness. The clinician should listen for whether the patient can complete sentences without taking a breath and should observe them for increased work of breathing.

The body temperature of adults is measured with an oral electric thermometer. Tympanic thermometers vary too much in comparison with oral thermometers (−1.2° to +1.6° C vs. the oral temperature) to be reliable in hospitalized patients, but they can be useful when continuous monitoring is important.

HEAD AND NECK

Face

The examiner should note any asymmetrical facial features. Examples of asymmetry include skin lesions (Chapter 403), cranial nerve palsies (Chapter 366), parotid enlargement (Chapter 393), or the ptosis of Horner syndrome (Chapter 392). A variety of disorders may cause symmetrical, abnormal facies; examples include acromegaly (Chapter 205), Cushing syndrome (Chapter 208), and Parkinson disease (Chapter 378).

Ears

Physicians may not recognize their patient's hearing impairment (Chapter 396) unless they perform a whispered voice test. Otoscopic evaluation of the tympanic membranes should reveal a translucent membrane with an obvious cone of light reflected where the eardrum meets the malleolus (see Fig. 394-12 in Chapter 394). Cerumen impaction is an easily treated cause of diminished hearing.

Nose

Patients with nasal symptoms often incorrectly self-diagnose bacterial sinusitis (Chapter 394). The physician should inspect the nares for polyps that are obstructing, glistening, mucosal masses. Transillumination performed in a dark room is useful for diagnosing sinusitis, especially when combined with visualization of a purulent discharge, a patient's report of a poor response to decongestants or antihistamines, maxillary toothache, and the presence of discolored rhinorrhea (Chapter 394).

Mouth

The quality of the patient's dentition directly affects nutrition. Premalignant oral lesions (e.g., leukoplakia [see Fig. 393-3 in Chapter 393], nodules, ulcerations) found by generalist physicians are usually verified by dentists (Chapter 393). Patients who use smokeless tobacco products are at significantly increased risk for premalignant and malignant oral lesions (Chapter 363). Bimanual palpation of the cheeks and floor of the mouth facilitates identification of potentially malignant lesions (Chapter 393).

Eyes

The eye examination begins with simple visual inspection to look for symmetry in the lids, extraocular movements, pupil size and reaction, and the presence of redness (Chapters 391 and 392). Abnormal extraocular movements should be grouped into nonparalytic (usually chronic with onset in childhood) or paralytic causes (third, fourth, or sixth cranial nerve palsy). Pupillary abnormalities may be symmetrical or asymmetrical (anisocoria). Red eyes should be categorized by the pattern of ciliary injection, presence of pain, effect on vision, and papillary abnormalities. When the eye examination is approached systematically, the generalist physician can evaluate red eyes for conjunctivitis, episcleritis or scleritis, iritis, and acute glaucoma.

Routine determination of visual acuity can confirm a patient's report of diminished vision but does not replace the need for formal ophthalmologic evaluation in patients with visual complaints (Chapter 391). Novice examiners will find ophthalmoscopes with panoptic views easier to use than the direct ophthalmoscope, resulting in better sensitivity and specificity for optic disc abnormalities. After identifying the optic disc by ophthalmoscopy, the examiner should note the border of the disc for clarity, color, and the size of the central cup in relation to the total diameter (usually less than half the diameter of the disc). A careful observer usually can see spontaneous venous pulsations that indicate normal intracranial pressure, but about 10% of patients with normal intracranial pressure will not have spontaneous pulsations. Abnormalities of the optic disc include optic atrophy (a white disc), papilledema (see Fig. 391-25 in Chapter 391) (blurry margins with a pink, hyperemic disc), and glaucoma (a large, pale cup with retinal vessels that dive underneath and that may be displaced toward the nasal side). The generalist's examination inadequately detects early glaucomatous changes, so high-risk patients should undergo routine ophthalmologic examination for glaucoma.

After inspecting the disc, the upper and lower nasal quadrants should be examined for the appearance of vessels and the presence of any retinal hemorrhages (see Fig. 391-22 in Chapter 391) or lesions. Patients with diabetes (Chapter 210) should undergo routine examination by eye care experts because the sensitivity of a generalist's examination is not adequate to exclude diabetic retinopathy or monitor it over time.

Neck

Carotid Pulses

The carotid pulses should be palpated for contour and timing in relation to the cardiac impulse. Abnormalities in the carotid pulse contour reflect underlying cardiac abnormalities (e.g., aortic stenosis) but are generally appreciated only after detecting an abnormal cardiac impulse or murmur (Chapter 39). Many physicians listen for bruits over the carotid arteries because asymptomatic carotid bruits are associated with an increased incidence of cerebrovascular and cardiac events in older patients (Chapters 375 and 376). Unfortunately, clinical studies do not provide adequate data for judging the importance of detecting bruits in asymptomatic patients.

Jugular Veins

Inspection of the venous waveforms may facilitate the interpretation of the cardiac examination for right heart valvular lesions. The waveforms can be highlighted by shining a penlight obliquely on the vein while looking for the dynamic changes of the projected shadow on the bed linen. The examination of the neck veins is an unreliable indicator of central venous pressure or fluid responsiveness in hemodynamically unstable patients (Chapter 39). Increased respiratory collapse of the inferior vena cava seen with bedside ultrasound or increased cardiac output during passive leg raising are better examination predictors for fluid responsiveness.

Thyroid

About 4 to 7% of the general asymptomatic population will have thyroid nodules detected on physical examinations.[7] The thyroid gland is felt best when standing behind the patient and using both hands to palpate the thyroid gland gently (Chapter 207). Palpation is enhanced when the patient swallows sips of water to allow the thyroid to glide underneath the fingers. When viewed from the side, lateral prominence of the thyroid between the cricoid cartilage and the suprasternal notch indicates thyromegaly. The volume of a normal thyroid gland is no greater than the volume of the patient's distal thumb phalanx.

Lymphatic System

While palpating the thyroid, the examiner may also identify enlarged cervical lymph nodes (Chapter 154). Lymph nodes can also be palpated in the supraclavicular area, axilla, epitrochlear area, and inguinofemoral region. Simple lymph node enlargement confined to one region is common and does not usually represent an important underlying disorder. Unexpected gross lymph node enlargement in a single area or diffuse lymph node enlargement is more important. Patients with febrile illnesses, underlying malignancy, or inflammatory diseases should routinely undergo an examination of each of the aforementioned areas for lymph node enlargement.

CHEST

Inspection of the patient's posture may reveal lateral curves in the back (scoliosis) or kyphosis that may be associated with loss of vertebral height from osteoporosis (Chapter 225). When patients have back pain, the spine and paravertebral muscles should be palpated for spasm and tenderness (Chapter 369). The patient may be placed through maneuvers to assess loss of mobility associated with ankylosing spondylitis (Chapter 244), but a history of loss of lateral mobility may be just as efficient in the early stages of spondylitis.

LUNGS

The incremental value of palpation and percussion of the chest to supplement the history, auscultation, and eventual chest radiograph is unknown. Normal vesicular sounds, which approximate a 3 : 1 inspiratory : expiratory ratio with no pause between inspiration and expiration, are heard throughout most of the normal posterior chest during quiet breathing. Auscultated wheezes are continuous adventitial sounds. Crackles (formerly called rales) are discontinuous sounds heard in conditions that stiffen the lung (heart failure, pulmonary fibrosis, and obstructive lung disease[8]).

HEART

The heart examination is an important prelude to the possible ordering of further cardiac diagnostic tests.[9] The patient should be examined in the sitting and lying positions (Chapter 39). Palpation of the apical impulse in the left lateral decubitus position helps detect a displaced apical impulse and can reveal a palpable S_3 gallop. When the apical impulse is lateral to the midclavicular line, radiographic cardiomegaly and an ejection fraction of less than 50% are more likely. Most examiners auscultate in sequence the second left and right intercostal spaces, the left sternal border, and then the apex. The examiner should concentrate on the timing, intensity, and splitting of sounds with respiration. The first and second heart sounds are heard best with the diaphragm, as are pericardial rubs. Gallops (S_3 and S_4) are heard best with the stethoscope bell. High-pitched sounds are easier to hear with the diaphragm and low-pitched sounds easier to hear with the bell, while medium-pitched sounds are heard equally well with either. The location, timing, intensity, radiation patterns, and respiratory variation of murmurs should be noted. Special maneuvers during auscultation (e.g., Valsalva, auscultation during sudden squatting or standing) do not need to be performed if the results of routine precordial examination are entirely normal.

The presence of an S_3 gallop is useful for detecting left ventricular systolic dysfunction. The presence of a systolic thrill or a holosystolic murmur increases the likelihood of moderate to severe aortic stenosis or mitral regurgitation. Quiet systolic murmurs are unlikely to herald important cardiac abnormalities. A loud, early diastolic murmur or a diastolic murmur associated with an S_3 suggests severe aortic regurgitation.

BREAST

Physical breast examination by physicians is no longer recommended as a routine screening test among women at average risk. However, women may present with concerns identified through their self-examinations. The most important determinants of the accuracy of the breast examination are the duration of the examination; the patient's position; careful evaluation of the breast boundaries; the pattern of the examination; and the position, movement, and pressure of the examiner's fingers (Chapter 183). To obtain the best sensitivity, the duration of the breast examination needs to be 5 to 10 minutes' total time, but few generalist physicians perform such a lengthy examination. Clinicians should recognize that the examination may make them (or their patient) feel uncomfortable—the presence of a chaperone may give the clinician the confidence to perform an intensive examination.

The physician should palpate the breast with the pads of the fingers while the patient is supine and holding her hand first on her forehead (to flatten the lateral border of the breast) and then on her shoulder (to flatten the medial border). The examiner should make small circular motions with the fingers, moving up and down in parallel rows to span the entire breast-clavicle to the bra line. Cancerous breast lumps are difficult to distinguish from benign breast lumps, which is why breast imaging now dominates recommendations for screening and follow-up of clinical abnormalities.

ABDOMEN

When patients have an acute abdominal problem, the examination focuses initially on identifying patients who require surgical evaluation. Palpation and percussion of the abdomen of patients with no symptoms or risk factors for an abdominal disorder seldom reveal important abnormalities (Chapter 118). Palpation can reveal an asymptomatic widening of the abdominal aorta that, in older patients, suggests an abdominal aneurysm. However, palpation misses a substantial proportion of small to medium aneurysms (Chapter 63).

The presence of bowel sounds in patients with acute symptoms can be falsely reassuring because the sounds may increase early in an obstruction and then persist despite an ileus. For patients without gastrointestinal symptoms or abnormalities on palpation, auscultation for bruits is important primarily to detect renal bruits in patients with hypertension (Chapters 64 and 110). The presence of an abdominal bruit in a hypertensive patient, if heard in systole and diastole, strongly suggests renovascular hypertension.

LIVER

Detection of liver disease depends mostly on the history and laboratory evaluations (Chapter 132). By the time that signs are present on physical examination, the patient usually has advanced liver disease. The first abnormalities on physical examination associated with liver disease may be extrahepatic. The clinician should assess the patient for ascites, peripheral edema, jaundice, or splenomegaly. In patients with an enlarged liver, palpation should begin at the liver edge, but palpation of the edge below the costal margin increases the likelihood of hepatomegaly only slightly. Percussion may detect the upper border of the liver, and a span of less than 12 cm reduces the likelihood of hepatomegaly.

SPLEEN

Examination for splenomegaly in patients without findings suggestive of a disorder associated with splenomegaly almost always reveals nothing (Chapter 154). Approximately 3% of healthy teenagers may have a palpable spleen. The examination for an enlarged spleen begins first with percussion in the left upper quadrant to detect dullness. Palpation can be performed by palpating with the right hand while providing counterpressure with the left hand behind the spleen. Alternatively, the examiner can palpate with one hand without counterpressure while the patient is in the right lateral decubitus position. With the patient supine while the examiner stands cephalad to the spleen, the fingers can be hooked lightly under the left lower rib cage to feel the spleen as the patient takes a deep breath.

MUSCULOSKELETAL SYSTEM

The patient's symptoms direct the musculoskeletal examination (Chapters 236 and 242). Most patients have back pain at some point during their life (Chapter 369). The patient's history helps assess the likelihood of an underlying systemic disease (age, history of systemic malignancy, unexplained weight loss, duration of pain, responsiveness to previous therapy, intravenous drug use, urinary infection, or fever). The most important physical examination findings for lumbar disc herniation in patients with sciatica are ipsilateral straight leg raising causing pain, contralateral straight leg raising causing pain, and ankle or great toe dorsiflexion weakness. Evaluation of hip motion and pain during motion helps detect hip osteoarthritis.[10]

The generalist physician should evaluate an adult patient with knee discomfort for torn menisci or ligaments. A variety of maneuvers assess for pain, popping, or grinding along the joint line between the femur and tibia to evaluate for meniscal tears. A tear in the ligaments eliminates a discrete endpoint when the anterior, medial, or posterior ligaments are stressed. As with many musculoskeletal disorders, no single finding has the accuracy of the orthopedist's examination, which factors in the history and a variety of clinical findings.

The shoulder examination[11] is directed toward determining range of motion, maneuvers that cause discomfort, and assessment of functional disability. Hip osteoarthritis is detected by evidence of restriction of internal rotation and abduction of the affected hip. The degree of pain and disability experienced by the patient may prompt confirmation of the diagnosis and referral.

The hands and feet[12] may show evidence of osteoarthritis (local or as part of a systemic process) (Chapter 241), rheumatoid arthritis (Chapter 243), gout (Chapter 252), or other connective tissue diseases. In addition to regional musculoskeletal disorders, such as carpal tunnel syndrome, a variety of medical and neurologic conditions should prompt routine examination of the distal ends of the extremities to prevent complications (e.g., diabetes [neuropathy or ulcers] or hereditary sensorimotor neuropathy [claw toe deformity]).

SKIN

The skin should be examined under good lighting (Chapter 403). It is best to ask the patient to point out any spots on the skin of concern. Examiner agreement on some of the most important features of melanoma (asymmetry, haphazard color, border irregularity) is fair to moderate (Chapter 188). A lesion that is symmetrical, has regular borders, is only one color, is 6 mm or smaller, or has not enlarged in size is unlikely to represent a melanoma. However, an increasing number of these findings greatly enhance the likelihood of melanoma (Chapter 188).

Basal cell carcinoma and squamous cell carcinoma occur more frequently than melanoma (Chapter 188). The examiner should pay particular attention to sun-exposed areas of the nose, face, forearms, and hands.

NEUROLOGIC EXAMINATION

Full details of the neurologic examination are given in Chapter 366.

PSYCHIATRIC EVALUATION

During the general examination, much of the psychiatric assessment (including cognition) is accomplished while eliciting the routine history and performing the review of systems (Chapter 362). Observation of the patient's mannerisms, affect, facial expression, thought content, and behavior may suggest underlying psychiatric disturbances. Specific questioning for symptoms of depression (Table 362-3) is appropriate for all adult patients. Delirium (Chapter 361) is common in both medical and surgical inpatients and is recognized by fluctuating mental status. Suspect delirium when the patient has trouble carrying on a normal conversation during bedside rounds. The patient's nurse or visitors may detect delirium before the physician.

PELVIC EXAMINATION

A complete examination includes a description of the external genitalia, appearance of the vagina and cervix as seen through a speculum, and bimanual palpation of the uterus and ovaries (Chapters 184 and 219). However, current evidence is insufficient to assess whether an annual screening pelvic examination is necessary in the asymptomatic and not pregnant adult woman. In the emergency setting, all women of reproductive age with vaginal bleeding and pelvic pain should have a pregnancy test and an ultrasound to evaluate for a possible ectopic pregnancy. The diagnosis of transgender and gender incongruence should be made by clinicians with expertise in the diagnostic criteria. Likewise, the ongoing care of transgender and gender-incongruent patients is best delivered by clinicians with experience in this field (Chapter 215).[13]

MALE GENITALIA

Examination of the male genitalia should begin with a description of whether the penis is circumcised and whether there are any visible skin lesions (e.g., ulcers or warts). Palpation should confirm the presence of bilateral testes in the scrotum. The epididymis and testes should be palpated for nodules. The low incidence of testicular carcinoma means that most nodules are benign (Chapter 185).

As a screening test for prostate carcinoma, no evidence supports a digital rectal examination in the absence of an elevated serum prostate-specific antigen.[14] The generalist physician will more frequently perform a digital examination to evaluate for tenderness associated with prostatitis or enlargement causing lower urinary tract symptoms. The size of the prostate can be described by centimeters of width and height.

RECTUM

Patients can be examined while lying on their side, during a gynecologic bimanual exam, or while standing and leaning over a table. The rectal examination begins with inspection of the perianal area for skin lesions. A well-lubricated, gloved finger is placed on the anus, and while applying gentle digital pressure, the examiner asks that the patient bear down as though having a bowel movement. This maneuver facilitates entry of the finger into the rectum. A normal rectal response includes tightening of the anal sphincter around the finger. The examiner should palpate circumferentially around the length of the fully inserted finger for masses. As a screening test for colorectal carcinoma (Chapter 179), digital examination does not replace testing stool samples collected by the patient.

TELEHEALTH

The increase in telehealth visits, especially during the severe acute respiratory syndrome coronavirus 2 pandemic (Chapter 336), has made the physical examination more challenging. With the help of digital devices (for heart rate and electrocardiogram), home monitoring devices (for weight, blood pressure, and pulse oximetry), and a caregiver (if needed), a focused physical examination can be performed virtually.[15]

SUMMARIZING THE FINDINGS FOR THE PATIENT

The clinician should summarize pertinent positive and negative findings for the patient and be willing to express uncertainty, provided that uncertainty is accompanied by a plan of action (e.g., "I will reexamine you on your next visit"). The rationale for subsequent laboratory, imaging, or other tests should be explained. A plan should be established for providing further feedback and results to the patient, especially when there is a possibility that bad news may need to be delivered. Some physicians ask the patient if there is "anything else" to be covered. Patients who express additional new concerns at the end of the visit may have been fearful to address them earlier; when the problems seem non-urgent, it is acceptable to reassure the patient and offer the promise of evaluating the patient in a follow-up phone call or at the next visit.

FUTURE DIRECTIONS

The common assumption that physicians' diagnostic skills are deteriorating is not supported by evidence. There is considerable evidence that the scientific approach to understanding what is worthwhile and what is not worthwhile during the clinical examination identifies a core set of skills for clinical diagnosticians. These skills have expanded to include bedside ultrasonography,[16] which is of proven benefit in some emergency situations (Chapters 7 and 97). Because good patient outcomes at good value are driven primarily by the quality of the information obtained during the clinical examination, continued application of scientific principles to the history and physical examination should improve diagnostic skills.

GENERAL REFERENCES

For the General References and other additional features, please visit Elsevier eBooks+ at https://ebooks.health.elsevier.com.

7 APPROACH TO THE PATIENT WITH ABNORMAL VITAL SIGNS

DAVID L. SCHRIGER

Care of the patient is guided by integration of the chief complaint, history, vital signs, and findings on physical examination (Chapter 6). Physicians should be keenly aware of a patient's vital signs, because they are important markers of clinical stability. Although vital signs themselves seldom are the centerpiece of the clinical evaluation, they sometimes become the major focus of urgent care when they themselves pose a life-threatening challenge (Chapters 50, 90, 92, 95).

THE IMPORTANCE OF VITAL SIGNS

The importance of vital signs in medical care is a conundrum for proponents of an evidence-based approach to the care of patients. No experienced physician would be willing to care for patients without them, yet a formal evaluation of the utility of vital signs for making specific diagnoses would conclude that they are not particularly useful because their likelihood ratios are too close to 1 to differentiate patients who have a specific condition from those who do not (Chapter 6). For uncommon conditions, their predictive value is even worse. For example, the probability of tachycardia in a patient in thyroid storm is high, yet the probability of thyroid storm in a patient with isolated tachycardia is low. This application of Bayes theorem (Chapter 8) demonstrates why there is no justification for ordering thyroid tests for every tachycardic patient and why attempts to say "When vital sign *x* is high [low], do *y*" fail. Each vital sign can be normal or abnormal in almost every acute condition (Table 7-1), and vital signs can be transiently abnormal in healthy individuals. An algorithmic approach to testing and treatment in response to abnormal vital signs would be too vague and too complex to be of use.

TABLE 7-1 NORMAL AND PANIC RANGES FOR KEY VITAL SIGNS IN ADULTS*

	NORMAL	PANIC
Temperature	36°-38° C (96.8°-100.4° F)	40° C (104° F)
Pulse	60-100 beats/min	<45 beats/min, >130 beats/min
Respirations	12-20 breaths/min	<10 breaths/min, >26 breaths/min
Oxygen saturation	95-100%	<90%
Systolic blood pressure	90-130 mm Hg	<80 mm Hg, >200 mm Hg
Diastolic blood pressure	60-90 mm Hg	<50 mm Hg, >120 mm Hg

*Normal values are for healthy adults. Values outside these ranges are common in patients who are ill or are anxious about their health care encounter. Panic values demand the health care provider's attention in any adult patient. These values are specific (rarely present in healthy patients at rest) but not sensitive (most ill patients' vital signs will not include panic values). All vital signs must be interpreted in the context of the patient's presentation (see text).

PREDICTIVE VALUE

How can it be that vital signs are poor predictors of diagnoses but central to the practice of medicine? First, although vital signs are insufficiently predictive to be of use in rigid algorithms, these algorithms are but one of several heuristics used by physicians to diagnose and to treat patients. Pattern recognition and the hypothetical-deductive model are heuristics that are based not on average tendencies of a single factor (e.g., hypotension is present in *x*% of cases of septic shock) or a small number of factors (e.g., hypotension and tachycardia are present in *y*% of cases of septic shock) but on the complex interaction of multiple factors (e.g., because this patient is an ill-appearing elderly man with an enlarged prostate and a history of urinary tract infections, is tachycardic and hypotensive, has clear lungs and an enlarged but nontender prostate, and has an oxygen saturation of 97%, he should be treated for urosepsis [Chapter 263] while awaiting results of urinalysis and urine culture). Thus, vital signs can play an important function in medical decision making even though their likelihood ratios for specific conditions are unimpressive.

Despite their poor predictive value for any single diagnosis, abnormal vital signs help identify patients who are sicker.[1] For example, even one abnormal vital sign in the emergency department significantly increases the likelihood of adverse outcomes in elderly patients by about 50%. Abnormal vital signs on emergency department discharge increase the chance of rapid readmission, and abnormal vital signs after admission carry a 20-fold increased risk for subsequent important deterioration. Abnormal vital signs are also a key predictor of which patients are at risk of dying soon after being sent home from an emergency department or after an inpatient admission.[2]

The usefulness of vital signs is also evidenced by the finding that more severe abnormalities are associated with an even worse prognosis. For example, among hospitalized patients, one critically abnormal vital sign carries about a 1% risk for inpatient death, whereas three simultaneously abnormal vital signs carry nearly a 25% risk for inpatient death.

VITAL SIGNS AS SYMPTOMS

Abnormal vital signs are seldom the fundamental pathophysiologic problem. In shock (Chapter 92), hypotension and tachycardia are manifestations of pathophysiologic processes at cellular and molecular levels. Given the circuitous links from clinical disease to fundamental pathophysiology to abnormal vital signs, it is not surprising that the relationships between the disease states and vital signs are not strong. Until new technologies enable direct measurement of primary pathologic processes, vital signs remain an important, albeit imperfect, proxy.

The five key vital signs are temperature, pulse, blood pressure, respiratory rate, and oxygen saturation (pulse oximetry). Pulse oximetry is included because it has become widely available, is noninvasive, is relatively inexpensive, and provides information unique from the respiratory rate. Advocates have suggested that pain, smoking status, and weight be considered routine vital signs; although a case can be made for each, they are not considered here. Clinicians should never forget that the most important vital sign is what the patient looks like; general appearance is a sign that guides the intensity and urgency of the evaluation.

MEASURING VITAL SIGNS

Although obtaining vital signs is generally straightforward, the validity and reliability of measurement depend on proper technique and, for blood pressure and pulse oximetry, well-maintained equipment. In an era of increasing telehealth, in part because of the severe acute respiratory syndrome coronavirus 2 pandemic (Chapter 336), vital signs increasingly may be measured via home devices, including wearable sensors.[3]

Rectal and oral temperatures are generally accurate (Chapter 259), although oral temperatures can be falsely depressed in patients who breathe through their mouths. Axillary temperature is unreliable and should not be used. There is wide variability in the validity and reliability of measurements performed with tympanic membrane thermometers. A hypothermia thermometer is preferred in patients with suspected hypothermia, and core temperature should be measured with an esophageal, bladder, or rectal temperature sensor in patients with severe hypothermia or hyperthermia (Chapter 95).

Blood pressure must be measured with an appropriately sized cuff (Chapter 64). Automated blood pressure machines occasionally provide spurious results, and questionable values should be confirmed by manual auscultation and by checking other limbs. Pulse is best obtained by palpation because this technique provides the opportunity to assess regularity and contour; the pulse should be counted for sufficient time for an accurate rate to be obtained (at least 15 seconds). High heart rates or dysrhythmias detected on the digital readout of a cardiac monitor, whether watched near the patient, by off-site standardized cardiac telemetry, or a wearable electronic device,[4] must be confirmed by palpation because these monitors can spuriously count large P waves, T waves, or pacemaker spikes as R waves, thereby reporting a heart rate double the actual rate. Orthostatic vital signs—the comparison of blood pressure and pulse in the supine, sitting, and standing positions—are advocated by some but have proved to be insensitive and nonspecific for hypovolemia. Some degree of orthostatic hypotension is also common in patients whose hypertension (Chapter 64) is treated intensively but should not be a reason for de-escalating treatment unless required by the patient's symptoms.[5]

Because the typical respiratory rate is between 12 and 20 breaths per minute and because there is considerable breath-to-breath variation, the respiratory rate should be assessed for at least 30 seconds and preferably 1 minute. New technologies purporting to measure the respiratory rate have not proved clinically useful. Oxygen saturation is dependent on technology, so an understanding of the idiosyncrasies of the device being used is critical. Valid measurements are unlikely unless there is good correlation of the machine's pulse reading and the patient's pulse, and smartphone pulse oximetry readings are often unreliable.[6] The probe should be placed on a part of the body that is warm and well perfused. Pulse oximeters compare the absorption of light at two wavelengths, so readings may be spuriously high under conditions that change the color of oxygenated or deoxygenated hemoglobin, including carbon monoxide poisoning (Chapter 82), methemoglobinemia (Chapter 147), some of the less common hemoglobinopathies, and skin pigmentation. For example, pulse oximetry also slightly overestimates oxygen saturation in Black patients.[7]

TABLE 7-2 ABNORMALITIES REQUIRING RAPID EVALUATION IN THE ASYMPTOMATIC PATIENT

An irregularly irregular rapid pulse (if it is not known to be chronic) should trigger an evaluation of the patient's rhythm so that atrial fibrillation can be identified, evaluated, and treated (Chapter 52), thereby decreasing the patient's risk of stroke.

A heart rate above 130 beats per minute always warrants an electrocardiogram to determine the patient's rhythm and a consideration of the differential diagnosis of tachycardia (hypovolemia, anemia, and thyroid disease in particular).

A markedly elevated diastolic blood pressure (e.g., >115 mm Hg) should stimulate an evaluation for hypertensive urgencies (Chapter 64). Note that hypertension in the absence of signs of acute end-organ damage does not require acute treatment, which can reduce intracranial perfusion pressure and cause stroke. Patients with elevated blood pressure should be offered standard evaluation and treatment for chronic hypertension (Chapter 64).

Markedly low pulse or blood pressure in patients receiving cardioactive medications should lead to a confirmation that the patient is truly asymptomatic, an inquiry into the dosing of these medications, and a reconsideration of the regimen.

Markedly low pulse in elderly patients who are not receiving rate-controlling drugs should trigger an evaluation of the patient's cardiac conduction system.

Oxygen saturation below 93% in the absence of known pulmonary problems should prompt an evaluation of the patient's pulmonary status.

ROLE OF VITAL SIGNS IN MANAGEMENT OF THE PATIENT

Abnormal vital signs should be remeasured. Certain abnormalities require prompt evaluation (Table 7-2). Other vital sign abnormalities should be rechecked in the future unless they have been previously noted, in which case a work-up can be initiated, guided by the patient's past history and physical examination findings. It is critical that physicians always "treat the patient, not the vital signs."

PATIENTS WITHOUT SYSTEMIC COMPLAINTS

In patients presenting for a routine evaluation or nonsystemic complaint (e.g., knee injury), an abnormal vital sign will seldom be the harbinger of acute illness. Most commonly, an abnormal vital sign will be a false reading or a transient finding due to random variation, pain, or anxiety that requires no evaluation or treatment and can be rechecked in the future. On occasion, an abnormal vital sign will be the only or most apparent manifestation of a chronic condition or risk factor. The measurement of an elevated blood pressure leading to a diagnosis of hypertension is the classic example of the value of vital signs in such patients.

PATIENTS WHO COMPLAIN OF SYSTEMIC ILLNESS BUT DO NOT APPEAR TO BE VERY ILL

Vital signs serve two additional roles in symptomatic patients who do not appear particularly ill. First, abnormalities in vital signs provide information that may suggest or support a diagnosis. The presence of elevated temperature in a patient with productive cough, shortness of breath, and localized rales and egophony supports a diagnosis of infectious pneumonia. Vital signs may also play a role in defining therapy and triage. For example, guidelines for patients with community-acquired pneumonia (Chapter 85) formally incorporate vital signs.

The second role of vital signs in the stable symptomatic patient is to provide warning that the patient is sicker than they appear. For example, the presence of hypotension in a well-appearing patient thought to have pyelonephritis may be an indication of sepsis or hypovolemia. For vital signs to be of use, the physician must be aware of them and must incorporate them explicitly into a thought process that considers the dangerous diagnoses associated with the abnormal vital sign. The physician then must decide whether the likelihood of each potentially dangerous diagnosis is high enough to warrant specific evaluation. Unfortunately, no quick or easy rules differentiate spurious abnormalities that can be ignored from those that should trigger additional testing or treatment. What can be said is that the well-trained physician who is aware of abnormal vital signs and is willing to contemplate a change in treatment or disposition, sometimes as stimulated by automated alert systems,[8] in response to them is less likely to make mistakes.

A few specific points bear mention. First, for most vital signs, "normal" is relative. Blood pressure must be interpreted in the context of the patient. For example, a blood pressure of 88/64 mm Hg may be reasonable for an otherwise healthy, young 50-kg woman but should cause concern in a 90-kg middle-aged man. Similarly, a blood pressure of 128/80 mm Hg would be fine in a 60-year-old man but worrisome in a 34-week pregnant woman. Second, because vital signs are insensitive measures of disease, normal vital signs should not dissuade the physician from pursuing potentially critical diagnoses. For example, young, well-conditioned adults may maintain normal vital signs well into the course of shock.

USE OF VITAL SIGNS IN PATIENTS WHO APPEAR TO BE ILL

For some patients, abnormal vital signs are expected on the basis of their appearance and their symptoms. For patients in extremis, care should proceed according to established guidelines such as Advanced Cardiac Life Support (Chapter 50), Advanced Trauma Life Support, and algorithms for the treatment of shock (Chapters 93 and 94). For hospitalized patients, markedly abnormal vital signs require urgent evaluation (Table 7-3), which in some settings may trigger a rapid response team.[9] For such ill-appearing patients, two processes must occur. In one, the physician, armed with knowledge of the differential diagnosis of each abnormal vital sign and the ability to take a thorough history and to perform an appropriate physical examination, narrows the list of potential diagnoses and decides which are of sufficient probability to warrant evaluation. Simultaneously, the physician considers the list of treatment options for all diagnoses associated with the abnormal vital sign and, before establishing a diagnosis, initiates those treatments for which the potential benefit of prompt administration exceeds potential harms. For example, antibiotics for febrile patients with suspected bacterial infection, hydrocortisone for hypotensive patients at risk for hypoadrenalism (Chapter 208), and thiamine

TABLE 7-3 ABNORMAL VITAL SIGNS THAT REQUIRE URGENT EVALUATION

Heart rate
- Heart rate < 40 beats/min, especially if symptoms
- Resting heart rate > 140 beats/min

Blood pressure
- Systolic blood pressure < 90 mm Hg or > 30-40 mm Hg below patient's usual stable blood pressure
- Systolic blood pressure > 200 mm Hg for >30 min
- Diastolic blood pressure > 110 mm Hg with symptoms

Respiratory rate
- Respiratory rate < 8 breaths/min or > 35 breaths/min
- New onset of marked dyspnea, compromised airway, cyanosis

Oxygenation
- O_2 saturation < 85% for >5 min (except patients with chronic severe hypoxemia)
- Need for 100% supplemental O_2 or a nonrebreathing O_2 mask

Temperature
- Body temperature < 35° C
- Body temperature > 39° C or associated with acute decompensation

for hypothermic patients at risk for Wernicke encephalopathy (Chapter 384) may improve outcome and are unlikely to cause harm even if the patient does not have the suspected condition. Although early presumptive treatment can be life-saving in selected patients, it should not be abused; physicians must avoid knee-jerk responses that can cause harm. The current COVID-19 pandemic (Chapter 336) provides a useful example of this principle. Early in the pandemic, patients who presented with low pulse oximetry values were reflexively intubated. Only later did it become clear that this approach was not optimal, but that noninvasive ventilation and sometimes putting the patient in the prone position were better responses (Chapter 337).

DIFFERENTIAL DIAGNOSIS AND TREATMENT OPTIONS

Single Abnormal Vital Signs

Because vital signs can be abnormal in virtually any disease process, no differential diagnosis can be encyclopedic. The physician should focus initially on common diseases and diseases that require specific treatment. The thought process should begin with the chief complaint and history, and then it should incorporate information about the vital signs and the remainder of the physical examination.

Multiple Abnormal Vital Signs

Patients who are acutely ill are likely to have several abnormal vital signs. Although certain patterns of abnormal vital signs predominate in specific conditions (e.g., hypotension, tachycardia, and hypothermia in profound sepsis), no pattern can be considered pathognomonic. The physician's goal is to work toward a diagnosis while simultaneously providing treatments whose benefits outweigh potential harms.

Fever is generally accompanied by tachycardia, with the general rule of thumb that the heart rate will increase by 10 beats per minute for every 1° C increase in temperature. The absence of tachycardia with fever is known as pulse-temperature dissociation and has been reported in typhoid fever (Chapter 284), legionnaires disease (Chapter 290), babesiosis (Chapter 324), Q fever (Chapter 302), infection with *Rickettsia* spp. (Chapter 302), malaria (Chapter 316), leptospirosis (Chapter 298), pneumonia caused by *Chlamydia* spp. (Chapter 294), and viral infections such as dengue fever (Chapter 352), yellow fever (Chapter 351), and other viral hemorrhagic fevers (Chapter 351), although the predictive value of this finding is unknown.

Much can be learned by comparing the respiratory rate with pulse oximetry. Hyperventilation in the presence of high oxygen saturation suggests a central nervous system process or metabolic acidosis rather than a cardiopulmonary process. Low respiratory rates in the presence of low levels of oxygen saturation suggest central hypoventilation (Chapter 74), which may respond to narcotic antagonists.

Hypertension and bradycardia in the obtunded or comatose patient are known as the Cushing reflex, a relatively late sign of elevated intracranial pressure. Physicians should strive to diagnose and treat this condition before the Cushing reflex develops.

APPROACH TO ABNORMALITIES OF SPECIFIC VITAL SIGNS

Elevated Temperature

Normal temperature is often cited as 37° C (98.6° F), but there is considerable diurnal variation and variation among individuals.[10] Furthermore, data suggest that normal human body temperature is now closer to 36.1° C (97° F),[11] so 38° C is the most commonly cited threshold for fever. Fever thought to be due to infection should be treated with antipyretics and appropriate antimicrobials (Chapter 259). The importance of early administration of antibiotics to potentially septic patients cannot be overstated (Chapters 259 and 260). Hyperthermia (temperature above 40° C) should be treated with cooling measures such as ice packs, cool misting in front of fans, cold gastric lavage, and, for medication-related syndromes, medications such as dantrolene (Chapter 95). Most hospital anesthesia departments will have a designated kit for the treatment of malignant hyperthermia (Chapter 400).

Low Temperature

The treatment of hypothermia is guided by its cause (Chapter 95). The body's temperature decreases when heat loss exceeds heat production. Every logically possible mechanism for this phenomenon has been observed. Decreased heat production can result from endocrine hypofunction (e.g., Addison disease [Chapter 208], hypopituitarism [Chapter 205], hypothyroidism [Chapter 207]) and loss of the ability to shiver (e.g., drug-induced or neurologic paralysis or neuromuscular disorders). Malfunction of the hypothalamic regulatory system can be due to hypoglycemia (Chapter 210) and a variety of central nervous system disorders (Wernicke encephalopathy [Chapter 384], stroke [Chapter 376], tumor [Chapter 175], and trauma [Chapter 368]).[12] Resetting of the temperature set point can occur with sepsis. Increased heat loss can be due to exposure, behavioral and physical disorders that prevent the patient from sensing or responding to cold, skin disorders that decrease its ability to retain heat, and vasodilators (including ethanol). A careful history and physical examination should illuminate which of these possibilities is most likely.

Several considerations are worthy of emphasis. The spine of an obtunded hypothermic patient who is "found down" must be protected and evaluated because paralysis from a fall may have prevented the patient from seeking shelter and may have diminished the ability to produce heat. The physician should not forget to administer antibiotics to patients who may be septic (Chapter 94), thiamine to those who may have Wernicke encephalopathy (Chapter 384), hydrocortisone to those who may be hypoadrenal (Chapter 208), and thyroid hormone to those who may have myxedema coma (Chapter 207). Severely hypothermic patients (Chapter 95) should be treated gently because any stimulation may trigger ventricular dysrhythmias; even in the absence of pulses, cardiopulmonary resuscitation should be used only in patients with ventricular fibrillation or asystole.

Elevated Heart Rate

The rate, rhythm, and electrocardiogram differentiate sinus tachycardia from tachyarrhythmias (Chapters 49, 50, 52, and 53). Tachyarrhythmias can be instigated by conditions that may require specific treatment (e.g., sepsis [Chapter 94], electrolyte disorders [Chapters 102, 103, and 104], endocrine disorders [Chapter 202], and poisonings [Chapters 20 and 96]) before the arrhythmia is likely to resolve. For sinus tachycardia, treatment of the underlying cause is always paramount. Treatments may include antipyretics (for fever); anxiolytics; oral or intravenous fluids (for hypovolemia); nitrates, angiotensin-converting enzyme inhibitors, and diuretics (for heart failure and fluid overload [Chapter 46]); oxygen (for hypoxemia); α-blockers (for stimulant overdose); β-blockers (for acute coronary syndromes [Chapters 57 and 58] or thyroid storm [Chapter 207]); and lysis or anticoagulation (for pulmonary embolism [Chapter 68]). Tachycardia is often an appropriate response to a clinical condition and should not be treated routinely unless it is causing or is likely to cause secondary problems.

Low Pulse

Bradycardia (Chapter 51) can be physiologic (athletes and others with increased vagal tone), due to prescribed cardiac medications (e.g., β-blockers, calcium-channel blockers, digoxin), overdoses (e.g., cholinergics, negative chronotropic agents), disease of the cardiac conducting system, electrolyte abnormalities (severe hyperkalemia), and inferior wall myocardial infarction (Chapters 51 and 58). Asymptomatic patients do not require immediate treatment. The goal of therapy is to produce a heart rate sufficient to perfuse the tissues and alleviate the symptoms (Chapter 50). Overdoses should be treated with specific antidotes (Chapter 96). Endocrine disorders should be treated with replacement therapy. In patients with acute coronary syndrome (Chapter 57), the goal is to restore perfusion and alleviate the ischemia. Patients with profound bradycardia or hypotension may require chronotropic drugs to increase perfusion even if these agents increase myocardial oxygen demand. In normotensive patients with milder bradycardia, chronotropic agents should be used only if symptoms and ischemia cannot be resolved by other means. Atropine is the primary therapy for bradycardia; isoproterenol and cardiac pacing are reserved for those who do not respond (Chapter 51).

Elevated Blood Pressure

Elevated blood pressure does not require acute treatment in the absence of symptoms or signs of end-organ damage (Chapter 64). In patients whose blood pressure is markedly above their baseline, the history and physical examination should assess for the conditions that define "hypertensive emergency": evidence of encephalopathy, intracranial hemorrhage, ischemic stroke, heart failure, pulmonary edema, acute coronary syndrome, aortic dissection, renal failure, and preeclampsia. In the absence of these conditions, treatment should consist of restarting or adjusting the medications of patients with known hypertension and initiating a program of blood pressure checks and appropriate evaluation for those with no prior history of hypertension (Chapter 64).

The patient with a true hypertensive emergency should be treated with agents appropriate for the specific condition. Because rapid decreases in blood pressure can be as deleterious as the hypertensive state itself, intravenous agents with short half-lives, such as nitroprusside, labetalol, nitroglycerin, and esmolol, are preferred (Chapter 64).

Low Blood Pressure

Low blood pressure must be evaluated in the context of the patient's symptoms, general appearance, and physical examination findings. Treatment depends on context. The same blood pressure value may necessitate intravenous inotropic agents in one patient and no treatment in another.

In tachycardic hypotensive patients, the physician must rapidly integrate all available evidence to determine the patient's volume state, cardiac function, vascular capacitance, and the primary cause of the tachycardia (Chapter 92).[13] Not all patients with hypotension and tachycardia are in shock, and not all patients in shock will have hypotension and tachycardia. Point-of-care ultrasound (Chapter 39)[14] of the heart and inferior vena cava may be useful in differentiating the cause of shock.

Treatment of shock is based on the cause: hypovolemic, cardiogenic, or distributive (septic, neurogenic, anaphylactic) (Chapters 92 to 94). Symptomatic hypotensive patients thought to be intravascularly volume depleted should have their legs raised and receive intravenous fluid resuscitation with crystalloid or blood, depending on their hemoglobin level (Chapter 92).[15] In patients with known heart disease, patients who are frail or elderly, and patients whose volume status is uncertain, small boluses of fluid (e.g., 250 mL of normal saline), each followed by reassessment, are preferred so that iatrogenic heart failure may be avoided. Inotropic support should be reserved for patients who do not respond to fluid resuscitation. High-output heart failure should be kept in mind in patients with possible thyroid storm or stimulant overdose.

Increased Respiratory Rate

Tachypnea is a normal response to hypoxemia (see later) or acidemia (Chapter 104).[16] Treatment of tachypnea in the absence of hypoxemia is directed at the underlying cause, which often is pain (Chapter 26). Anxiolytics (e.g., diazepam, 5 to 10 mg PO or IV; lorazepam, 1 to 2 mg PO, IM, or IV) or reassurance can calm patients with behavioral causes of hyperventilation. Breathing into a paper bag has been shown to be an ineffective treatment. Pulmonary embolism (Chapter 68) does not necessarily reduce the oxygen saturation or cause a low Po_2 and should always be considered in at-risk patients with unexplained tachypnea.

Decreased Respiratory Rate

Any perturbation of the respiratory center in the central nervous system can slow the respiratory drive (Chapter 74). Narcotics and other sedatives and neurologic conditions are common causes of a decreased respiratory rate. The primary treatment of apnea is mechanical ventilation (Chapter 91), but narcotic antagonists can be tried in patients with a history or physical examination findings (miosis, track marks, opioid patch) suggestive of narcotic use or abuse (Chapter 365). In nonapneic patients, mechanical ventilation, either noninvasive or invasive (intubation), is indicated for patients who are breathing too slowly to maintain an acceptable oxygen saturation and for patients who are retaining carbon dioxide in quantities sufficient to depress mental function. Patients who are unable to protect their airway should be intubated. Oxygen should be administered to all hypopneic patients who are hypoxemic (see earlier). Patients with chronic hypoventilation (Chapter 74) may have retained HCO_3^- to compensate for an elevated Pco_2 and so may depend on hypoxia to maintain respiratory drive; in these patients, overaggressive administration of oxygen can decrease the respiratory rate, increase the Pco_2, and increase obtundation (Chapter 90).

Decreased Oxygen Saturation

In hypopneic patients, initial efforts should try to increase the respiratory rate (see earlier) and tidal volume. Regardless of etiology, oxygen, in amounts adequate to restore adequate oxygen saturation ($Po_2 > 60$ mm Hg, oxygen saturation > 90%), is the mainstay of therapy. When oxygen alone fails, noninvasive methods for improving ventilation or tracheal intubation are required (Chapter 90). Oxygen should increase the Po_2 in all patients except those who have severe right-to-left shunting (Chapter 55). Treatment of conditions that cause hypoxemia includes antibiotics (pneumonia), bronchodilators (asthma, chronic obstructive pulmonary disease), diuretics and vasodilators (pulmonary edema), anticoagulants (pulmonary embolism), hyperbaric oxygen (carbon monoxide poisoning), methylene blue (methemoglobinemia, sulfhemoglobinemia), and transfusion (anemia).

GENERAL REFERENCES

For the General References and other additional features, please visit Elsevier eBooks+ at https://ebooks.health.elsevier.com.

8 STATISTICAL INTERPRETATION OF DATA FOR CLINICAL DECISION MAKING

THOMAS H. PAYNE

Statistical techniques are core to evidence-based medicine. The scientific method is based on generating a hypothesis and designing an experiment to test that hypothesis. This powerful approach has been at the root of advances in human endeavors and particularly within medicine. A clear description of a question, a formulation of a hypothesis, a careful design of an experiment to test the hypothesis, the gathering of unbiased data, and the appropriate analysis of the results of the experiment permit the determination of whether a test or treatment is useful or not. If these steps are not conducted in a rigorous manner, statistical tests are likely to produce inaccurate or unreliable results.

INCIDENCE AND PREVALENCE

Incidence describes the number of subjects who *contract* a disease *over time* divided by the population at risk. Incidence is usually expressed as a rate (e.g., 7 per 1000 per year), but it may sometimes be a proportion, as in lifetime incidence. *Prevalence* describes the number of subjects who *have* a disease at *one point in time* divided by the population at risk; it is always a proportion. At any point in time, the prevalence of a disease is defined by the product of incidence of the disease multiplied by the average duration of the disease.

INTERPRETING DATA

Physicians are continuously confronted with data from many sources, including clinical measurements (e.g., vital signs), laboratory tests, and imaging studies. In fact, the work of the modern-day physician is in many respects one of information management. Although the physician may not conduct independent statistical analyses unaided, knowledge of the fundamentals of data analysis is critical for the ability to evaluate whether and how to integrate information into clinical practice.

This knowledge is also essential for understanding the medical literature and incorporating it into practice. Millions of research articles are published each year, and their quality varies widely. Articles published in the leading medical journals undergo rigorous statistical review, but the same is not true for most other journals. Although it generally is inadvisable to base clinical decisions upon a single study, physicians are often confronted with new information and the dilemma of how to deal with it.

Both of these goals—interpreting clinical data and understanding the medical literature—require familiarity with the laws of probability and the field of statistics.

DATA AND THEIR CHARACTERISTICS

Variability is a constant of nature. Statistical techniques represent an effort to describe data and distinguish differences that reflect random variation from those that represent true differences. First, it is necessary to define the nature of data elements being analyzed. Numeric data can vary over a wide range, with values anywhere between the extremes of that range. Blood pressure, for example, can have values of 130, 129.3, 75, and any value in between. Such data are called *continuous*. Numeric data that can only have an integer value, such as number of siblings, are called *discrete*. Other data are reasonable only if they fall into one of several categories, such as whether someone is alive or dead. These data are *categorical*. Labeling a test as positive or negative, which may depend on a somewhat judgmental threshold rather than a continuum, is another example of categorical data.

The next step in examining data is to assess how they are distributed. The distribution of values within a population (e.g., blood pressures) is often categorized as normal (i.e., Gaussian). A normal distribution is often characterized using both measures of *central tendency* (i.e., mean, median, and mode) and measures of *dispersion* around the center of the distribution (e.g., standard deviation). However, many phenomena in medicine produce distributions that are not normal (e.g., Poisson, binomial, etc.), and their analysis requires non-parametric approaches.[1]

HYPOTHESIS TESTING

In medical research, the goal is typically to discern whether two groups differ in a meaningful way, such as whether an outcome in a group that received a particular treatment differs from the outcome in a group that received no treatment or a placebo. This comparison begins with a hypothesis that is stated formally as the *null hypothesis* and is phrased in relation to an alternative hypothesis. The two hypotheses are mutually exclusive and exhaustive. So if a study compares change in blood pressure between a group that received an intervention and one that did not (controls), the null hypothesis would be that the intervention had no effect on blood pressure and the alternative hypothesis would be that it did have an effect.

A study should be designed to determine whether to accept or reject the null hypothesis. In the analysis of data collected in the study, the challenge is to determine whether differences seen in the distribution of blood pressure in people who received the treatment differed from those who did not; and if there is a difference, whether that difference is due to chance. The appropriate techniques for testing hypotheses vary depending on the nature of the data that are collected (Table 8-1).

TABLE 8-1 TYPES OF VARIABLES AND COMMONLY USED STATISTICAL METHODS

TYPE OF OUTCOME VARIABLE	EXAMPLES	ASSOCIATED STATISTICAL METHODS: BIVARIATE	ASSOCIATED STATISTICAL METHODS: MULTIVARIATE
Categorical (dichotomous)	Alive; readmission to the hospital within 30 days	2 × 2 table, chi-square analysis	Logistic regression
Categorical (nominal)	Race; cancer, tumor type	Chi-square analysis	Nominal logistic regression
Categorical (ordinal)	Glasgow Coma Scale	Mann-Whitney-Wilcoxon, Kruskal-Wallis	Ordinal logistic regression
Numerical (continuous)	Cholesterol; SF-36 scales*	*t* Test, analysis of variance	Linear regression
Numerical (count)	Number of times pregnant; number of mental health visits in a year	Mann-Whitney-Wilcoxon, Kruskal-Wallis	Poisson regression, linear models
Time to event regression	Time to breast cancer; time to viral rebound in HIV-positive subjects	Log rank	Cox proportional hazards

*Numerical scores with many values are often treated as though they were continuous.
HIV = human immunodeficiency virus; SF-36 = short-form 36-item health survey.
Courtesy of Thomas B. Newman, MD, MPH, and Charles E. McCulloch, PhD.

Since blood pressure measurements vary, any true difference between intervention subjects and control subjects may be difficult to detect if there is only a small number of study subjects; the natural, biologic dispersion of blood pressure may obscure a true difference between the two. However, if the number of subjects is increased, the ability to detect a true difference also increases, and some number should be sufficient to detect a meaningful difference if it truly exists. Below that number, the study may fail to detect a difference between blood pressure readings of the intervention and control groups even though a difference genuinely exists. This level is termed *beta* and represents the probability of a *Type II error* (i.e., failure to detect a true difference when one truly exists). When the number of subjects exceeds the minimum number, there can be greater confidence that a difference will be observed if one truly exists. The probability below which the null hypothesis can be rejected is termed the *alpha* level and represents the probability of rejecting the null hypothesis when the null hypothesis is actually true. A *Type I error* occurs when a null hypothesis is rejected although it is true. To eliminate any possibility of a Type I error would necessitate an infinite number of subjects, so by convention, a 5% or lower chance of this error is considered acceptable. Thus, at an alpha level of 0.05, a difference that is detected will be a true difference 95% of the time, but 5% of the time a random difference will be mistakenly classified as a true difference.

Because falsely concluding that a difference exists (e.g., concluding that a treatment is helpful when it is actually ineffective) is considered a more serious error than the reverse (concluding that a treatment is ineffective when, in fact, it is potentially helpful), levels for beta error typically are set much lower than those for alpha (e.g., 80%). *Power analysis* is a method for estimating the minimum sample size necessary to detect the minimum difference between groups that is defined as clinically meaningful at a specified alpha level (typically 0.05) and beta level.

P values, which are often reported in medical studies, answer the question, "If the null hypothesis were true, what would be the probability of obtaining, by chance alone, a value of the test statistic this large or larger?" For a fixed level alpha, the power of a test increases with sample size and increases with the true difference between the null hypothesis and a specified alternative.

In essence, the foundation of hypothesis testing is determining whether there is a difference and whether any difference is explained by chance. This determination hinges on probability, as well as conventions regarding tolerance for false-positive (calling a difference real when it actually is a chance effect) and false-negative (not finding a true difference) conclusions.

Study Design

When testing the hypothesis that an intervention is effective, there may be other reasons unrelated to the intervention as to why that outcome measurement might have changed. A *covariate* is another factor, different than the tested intervention, that can potentially influence the outcome under study. For example, in evaluating a medication to treat hypertension, subjects also may have been exposed to a campaign to reduce dietary salt intake. The reduction in salt intake, which could have contributed to any observed changes in blood pressure, would be considered a covariate. It is essential to adjust, or control, for these covariates. The most straightforward way is to assign the intervention to one group but also to measure the change in outcome in an otherwise similar *control* group as well. The strongest research design is the *randomized, double-blinded controlled trial* in which individuals are randomly assigned either to receive the intervention to be tested or to receive an inert or inactive substitute. Subjects in both the intervention and control groups are kept uninformed as to whether they are receiving the active intervention or substitute, and the investigator observing the outcomes is also kept unaware of who is assigned to which group. Thus, neither the subject nor the person recording results knows which arm of the intervention is being observed, and so the reporting and recording of results are insulated from belief in the power of the intervention. This approach is regarded as the most accurate way to assess the effect of an intervention, because any effect of covariates would be expected to occur nearly equally in both the intervention and control groups. Furthermore, any placebo effect is minimized by masking whether or not the subject is receiving the treatment. The advantages of randomized controlled trials make this design the accepted "gold standard" for the evaluation of new pharmacologic treatments.

However, randomized controlled trials are not always practical for many reasons, and much medical knowledge is derived from different study designs in which it is difficult to know all of the influences on the outcome. Nonrandomized studies can never guarantee adequate control for all covariates, even in very large observational data sets.[2] For example, consider whether hospital mortality rates increased or declined after a large process change, such as the installation of new computer systems to enter and communicate orders. Any changes in error rates may be due to the new computer system, but they also could be explained by heightened awareness of the risk for errors. Investigators can attempt to control for known covariates, but other covariates may not be known. For this reason, randomized trials provide the strongest evidence for causality.

A variety of other *quasi-experimental* study designs have been applied. For example, an intervention might be applied to an entire practice rather than to individual patients. Although it would be ideal to assign the intervention randomly to participating practices, such an approach may be impractical or impossible. One approach would be to introduce an intervention sequentially to individual practices in a systematic manner—which is termed a *stepped wedge* design. If this approach cannot be done in a systematic manner or if the evaluation is being conducted post hoc, the data can be retrospectively segmented into short, consecutive time periods so that the analysis can try to distinguish temporal trends from actual effects of the intervention. This design is termed an *interrupted time-series*.

When evaluating health care interventions, it is often desirable to include both a quantitative measurement of outcomes (such as mortality or hospital admissions) and observational or qualitative methods, such as surveys or structured interviews. These data are often complementary. If, for example, a study fails to show that an intervention was effective, qualitative information may reveal whether it was properly implemented and what problems prevented implementation. Qualitative methods also are important to understand the attitudes and reactions of health care personnel and patients.

Time to Event Data

A common study design is to follow a sample of patients who receive a treatment until a prespecified outcome has occurred, such as death or hospital admission. The analysis uses the time between the subject's participation in the study until the outcome. Results are often displayed graphically as a survival distribution. Some subjects may contribute data to the study but not complete it. A *Kaplan-Meier analysis* allows estimation of survival in a manner that uses data from patients who drop out of the study. A *Cox proportional hazards model* compares the survival between or among groups.[3]

Noninferiority Trials

In some research, the goal is not to find a more effective treatment but one that has other advantages, such as fewer side effects or lower cost. In these studies, called *noninferiority trials*, the purpose is to evaluate a new treatment against an existing one with the goal of demonstrating that it is at least as good. An example is comparing a new treatment with a standard treatment, in which the goal is not to find an approach that is more effective, but to find a therapy that has lower cost or fewer adverse effects with at least similar efficacy to the standard treatment.[4]

CAUSALITY

There is an important difference between association and causality. The rooster's crow is *associated* with, but does not cause, sunrise. Anoxia *causes* death. An investigator's—and the public's—belief that a treatment is beneficial is powerful, and the scientific method can help us determine the difference between belief and reality. Belief can influence biology. The placebo effect is the concept that effects can be due to belief and not to the intervention itself.

Confounding

If a covariate is related to both the outcome and to the exposure or risk factor being studied, and if it is unequally distributed between the groups being compared, it becomes a *confounder*. Since most health outcomes have many contributing causes, there often are many possible confounders. For example, in a study of the association between obesity and heart disease, age may be a confounder. Age is related to obesity and also to heart disease. If the obese subjects are older than the nonobese subjects, then differences in the outcome of heart diseases may be due to the older age of the obese subjects rather than to their obesity.

In observational studies in which randomization is not possible, steps to reduce bias due to confounding should be considered in the analysis. In an observational study of the effect of a treatment on an outcome of interest, it may be that the treatment is given to some subjects (patients) because of their characteristics, such as age or severity of illness. A variety of sophisticated statistical techniques are applied in an effort to reduce bias in observational studies. For example, a *propensity score* is the probability that a study subject would receive the exposure or treatment of interest, based on the subject's characteristics and the clinical environment.[5] Using the propensity score, it is possible to adjust for the effect of known confounding variables so that it is less likely the difference in outcome is due to confounding bias. Nevertheless, all techniques to reduce confounding depend entirely on data about relevant covariates. If such data are missing, statistical adjustment cannot produce an accurate result. A limitation of the propensity score in reducing confounding bias is that many confounders may be unknown or difficult or even impossible to measure.[6]

Machine Learning

Machine learning approaches problems by learning rules from data in contrast with expert systems. Starting with patient-level observations, algorithms sift through vast numbers of variables, looking for combinations that reliably predict outcomes.[7] This process in some ways resembles traditional regression models: there are outcomes, covariates, and statistical functions linking the two. Machine learning can handle enormous numbers of predictors and combine them in nonlinear and highly interactive ways. Optimism for machine learning should be tempered by understanding that association is not the same as causation and that vast biomedical data available to apply to these techniques may have insufficient breadth—lacking, for example, social determinants of health—or insufficient quality or biases that can make the results unreliable or even not valid.[8] Another limitation can be the difficulty in understanding and interpreting results because of the complexity and opacity of the model. Before they are of clinical use, machine learning models must be independently validated in prospective clinical trials in sites other than those in which the model was developed.[9]

STATISTICAL APPROACHES AND CHALLENGES

Multivariable Statistics

In many cases, researchers are interested in the effects of multiple predictor variables on an outcome. Particularly in observational studies, in which investigators cannot assign values of a predictor variable experimentally, it will be of interest to estimate the effects of a predictor variable of interest independent of the effects of other variables.[10] For example, in studying whether breastfeeding reduces a mother's risk for subsequent breast cancer, investigators would try to take differences in age, race, family history, and parity into account. Trying to stratify by all these variables would require a massive data set. Instead, multivariable models are used to enable the information about individual predictors to be summarized using the full data set.

Multiple Comparisons

Analyses in which multiple statistical tests are conducted can lead to a false conclusion that one of them is a positive result. The more tests conducted, the more likely it becomes that one will be positive based on chance alone even though the P value may be set to 0.05. One way to correct for this problem is to use the *Bonferroni correction*, which divides the P value for rejecting the null hypothesis by the number of hypothesis tests performed.[11]

Meta-analysis

Meta-analysis is a statistical method for drawing inferences from a sample of *studies* to derive a summary estimate and confidence interval for a parameter measured by the included studies. Meta-analysis allows for a formal combination of results while estimating and accommodating both the within-study and between-study variations.[12,13]

USING DATA FOR CLINICAL DECISIONS

An important and common element of the physician's role is to make decisions.[14] Effective decision making includes gathering information, determining whether more information is worth the additional risk and expense, and interpreting results. All of these tasks depend on a physician's skill in using data optimally. Information gathering begins with the most important data: those derived from a careful patient history and physical examination. However, the variety of available laboratory tests and diagnostic procedures greatly increases the amount of information that can be obtained and that must be ordered intelligently and interpreted correctly.[15] Appropriate use of clinical information can make important differences in patients' outcomes and in the resources required to optimize them.

TABLE 8-2 PRINCIPLES OF TEST ORDERING AND INTERPRETATION

The interpretation of test results depends on what is already known about the patient.
No test is perfect; clinicians should be familiar with its diagnostic performance and never believe that a test "forces" them to pursue a specific management strategy.
Tests should be ordered if they may provide *additional* information beyond that already available.
Tests should be ordered if there is a reasonable chance that the data will influence the patient's care.
Two tests that provide similar information should not be ordered.
In choosing between two tests that provide similar data, use the test that has lower costs or causes less discomfort and inconvenience to the patient.
Clinicians should seek all of the information provided by a test, not just an abnormal or normal result.
The cost-effectiveness of strategies using noninvasive tests should be considered in a manner similar to that of therapeutic strategies.

Courtesy of Thomas H. Lee, MD.

		Disease present: Yes	Disease present: No
Test result	Positive	a	b
	Negative	c	d

From these data, one can also calculate:

Risk ratio or relative risk (RR)	$\frac{a}{(a+b)} \div \frac{c}{c+d}$
Relative risk reduction (RRR)	$1 - RR$
Risk difference or absolute risk reduction (ARR)	$\frac{a}{(a+b)} - \frac{c}{(c+d)}$
Number needed to treat (NNT)	$\frac{1}{ARR}$
Odds ratio (OR)	$\frac{ad}{bc}$

FIGURE 8-1. **A 2×2 table evaluating use of a test to determine if a disease is present.** In this model, test sensitivity is a/(a + c), specificity is d/(b + d), and disease prevalence is (a + b)/(a + b + c + d). Positive predictive value can then be calculated as a/(a + b) and negative predictive value as d/(c + d).

Evaluating a patient who presents with new breathlessness (Chapter 71) presents an example of decision-making principles. A thorough history and physical examination set the foundation, and a spectrum of choices are considered. Is this a temporary problem or a life-threatening condition for which immediate and potentially risky testing and treatment should be recommended? (Table 8-2) The sequence in which testing is undertaken also has implications for safety and cost. Some tests are simple and fast to perform and most helpful when results are negative; others involve substantial risk and expense but can give a definitive answer.

Theories and Principles Useful in Decision Making

Much of medical practice involves risk and uncertainty. When discussing uncertainty, the concept of *probability* is useful. Probability is the likelihood that something occurs; a probability of 1.0 means it is certain to occur, and a probability of 0 means it will not occur. The term *odds* refers to a ratio of probabilities of an event (p): $Odds = p/(1 - p)$. If the probability of the event is 50% or 1 in 2, as in a coin flip, then odds of the event are 1 (or 1 : 1). If the probability is 1 in 3, or 0.33, then the odds are 0.33/0.66 or one half (1 : 2).

A simple yet instructive model of decision making is a 2 × 2 table (Fig. 8-1). A group (or *population*) of patients is divided into 4 cells. The table shows the presence or absence of a disease across the top and test results on the left. The cells in this 2 × 2 table are labeled with letters beginning with a in the upper left and d in the lower right. The *sensitivity* of a test, which is defined as the probability of positive results when the disease is known to be present, is calculated in the table as $a/(a + c)$. Test *specificity*, which is the probability of a negative test result when the disease is absent, is calculated as $d/(b + d)$. Sensitivity and specificity are referred to as *test characteristics* because they explain how a test performs in the presence or absence of disease. In clinical practice, however, tests are usually used to determine whether a disease or condition is present or absent, or at least how likely it is based on a given test result. In the 2 × 2 table, this probability, which can be calculated as $a/(a + b)$, is referred to as the *positive predictive value*. Similarly, $d/(c + d)$, which is the *negative predictive value* of the test, indicates how likely it is that the disease is absent given a negative test result.

Inspection of this 2 × 2 table shows another very important finding: how common the disease is in this population, shown as $(a + c)/(a + b + c + d)$. This calculation is analogous to the *prevalence* of the disease in the population.

A special insight from this simple 2 × 2 table is that positive and negative predictive values depend on the test characteristics, but importantly they also depend on the prevalence of the disease in this particular population of patients. Different positive and negative predictive values result when the same test is used in a population in which the disease is rare compared with when it is used in a population in which the disease is common.

This insight is the essence of *Bayes theorem*: the likelihood of the disease given a positive test result depends on both the test characteristics and on the prevalence of the disease in the population. Bayes theorem is often expressed by the formula $P(A|B) = (P(B|A) * P(A))/P(B)$, (probability of disease A given test result B is the probability of result B given disease A times the probability of disease A, divided by probability of result B), but the essence of the greatest value of Bayes theorem to physicians can be understood from the simple 2 × 2 table. Bayes theorem also implies that any new information, as from a new research result, should be interpreted in the context of prior knowledge.[16]

Another useful concept is the *likelihood ratio*, which is the prevalence of a sign (or any test result) in patients with the diagnosis of interest divided by the prevalence of the identical finding (or test result) in patients without the target diagnosis. The positive likelihood ratio is expressed by the formula $P(B|A)/P(B|\bar{A})$ (or [sensitivity] ÷ [1 − specificity]) (E-Table 8-1).

Other common measures used in decision making can be derived from these simple building blocks that come from the 2 × 2 table. *Pretest probability* in the 2 × 2 model is the same as the prevalence of disease—how common it is in that population. Before doing any test, the probability of disease is simply the prevalence in that population. After performing the test, the probability may be different—the *post-test probability*—which is why and how the test can be useful.[17]

In the 2 × 2 model, a test is defined as either positive or negative. However, it may not be clear where to draw the line (or threshold) between positive and negative. Fig. 8-2 shows three possible divisions between a positive and negative test result. The vertical line on the left excludes all patients who do not have the disease, but it classifies only half of the patients with the disease as positive. The one on the right results in all patients with the disease having a positive result but at the cost of including half of the patients who do not have the disease in the positive result. The middle line achieves a compromise—most of the patients with the disease are defined as having a positive result, and most of the patients without the disease are defined as having a negative result. Which of the three lines is chosen depends on how the test is being used. A plot of all such possible lines with the sensitivity and specificity creates a curve showing how sensitivity and specificity are related for the test: a *receiver operator characteristic (ROC)* curve. Fig. 8-3 is a common way to display this relationship. An ideal test would have a curve closer to A than to B—a high sensitivity and a high specificity. ROC curves can also be used to compare the ability of different tests to distinguish between the presence or absence of disease. Tests with higher *areas under the curve* are considered better tests.

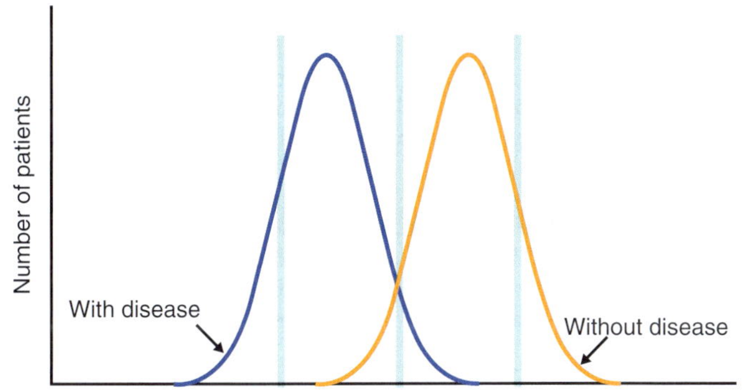

FIGURE 8-2. For each of the vertical lines, those results to the left indicate a positive result, while results on the right indicate a negative result.

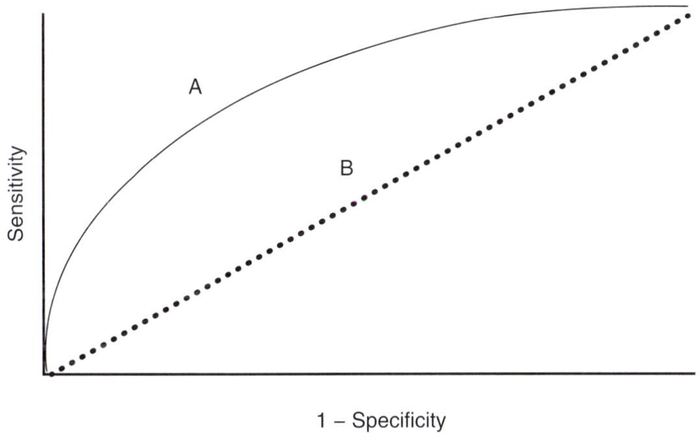

FIGURE 8-3. A receiver operator characteristic (ROC). This curve displays all the possible decision thresholds based on a test's sensitivity and specificity. The best test has very high sensitivity and specificity. In this example, A is a better test than B.

In most cases, physicians do not rely on a single test to determine whether or not a condition or disease is present. Rather, several test results and other data (which may include portions of the patient's history and findings on the physical examination), as well as findings from past records, are incorporated into that judgment. This multiplicity of information highlights one of the limitations of Bayes theorem. The results of multiple tests may not be independent of each other, but Bayes theorem assumes that they are. It is also important to be aware that it is difficult to determine the accuracy of historical and examination data—particularly if not gathered first-hand but obtained from an electronic health record, which may contain errors. Some laboratory, imaging, and pathology results may vary depending on the subjective assessment of the person who creates the report. Astute clinicians understand that data may be inaccurate or subject to differing interpretation.

When should a test be ordered? Gathering additional information—whether from history, repeated examinations, tests, or imaging—can change the likelihood of disease, as is demonstrated by the 2 × 2 table. In general terms, additional data should be obtained only if they would change the likelihood of a disease or condition at an acceptable cost and risk and if such a change in probability would affect what is recommended to the patient. "Will it change therapy?" is a common question that summarizes such thinking: Will the test lead to a diagnosis that would be treated differently? If not, then the value of the test is lower. Sometimes the most important choice is to defer further testing and to observe the patient over time—the "test of time."

Utility

The results of diagnosis and treatment vary, and the importance or value of those outcomes also varies. For example, the value of surviving may depend on quality of life and side effects endured to achieve survival. Quantifying this value can be difficult, but ultimately the most important quantification is from the patient. The term *utility* describes the value or importance of the outcome as judged by the patient or measured in some other way. In some analyses, the length of survival is adjusted by a measure of the quality of life, described as *quality-adjusted life years* or *QALYs*.[18]

DECISION-MAKING STRATEGIES

Shared Decision Making

Physicians make many decisions, some of which are simple and many of which are complex. A good physician does not make all of these decisions independently. Especially for decisions that involve risks or preferences, the wise physician involves the patient in decision making when possible. Shared decision making considers the utility of different outcomes and the patient's desires, which may vary widely from one person to the next. Shared decision making is an important element of physician-patient interaction and also has direct ties to the decision-making process.[19]

Decision Analysis

Answers to some questions involve a series of questions and probabilities that are not practical to answer with a single study or test. As a result, an approach known as *decision analysis* can be useful (E-Fig. 8-1). This analysis begins with a question, such as "should a drug be given?", which then leads to branches stemming from the yes and no answers, each of which has its own branching from what is called a chance node. Chance nodes may lead to other branches. Each chance node has several probabilities that, by definition, must add up to one. The end of each of the branches is assigned a utility. To determine, for example, if a drug should be given, the utility of each end branch is multiplied by the probability of ending on that branch, and this process is continued (or folded back) until each of the original choices is assigned a score. Using this model, the best choice is the choice with the highest score. Decision analysis can be applied to decisions in which prospective trials are impractical, such as a public health policy decision, or when a randomized controlled trial would be impractical, such as developing a strategy for screening for cervical cancer. Since probabilities assigned to some of the nodes may not be known and could plausibly be within a range, a technique known as *sensitivity analysis* can be used to determine if the key conclusions of the decision analysis model would change as the chance node probabilities change within that range. Including benefit and cost in decision analysis permits a cost-benefit (or cost-effectiveness) analysis[20] that can lead to informed decisions regarding what strategy or approach should be pursued, or whether a new technology or treatment should be adopted.

Aids to Decision Making

As the volume of text, test results, images, and genomic data rises, the limitations of human cognition often are reached. For example, most physicians are able to keep several data elements in mind when making a decision, but decision-making aids become worth considering when the number of facts to be considered rises to include a dozen or more. Some of these aids are simple *prediction rules*,[21] which can use clinical data to estimate the pretest probability of a condition. In other cases, automated systems, as simple as smartphone applications and as complex as cloud-based systems, can be helpful for diagnostic and therapeutic decision making. With progressively rising volumes of health care data and computing power, machine learning, artificial intelligence, and other analytical tools and techniques may increasingly provide additional aid to clinician decision making. Periodic modifications of decision aids and testing them using prospective (ideally randomized controlled) trials can increase their value.

To apply these concepts, consider a patient with breathlessness. Does this patient have a pulmonary embolism or some other condition? Although data derived from the history and physical examination individually have a low sensitivity, the pretest probability of pulmonary embolism (Chapter 68) can be classified as high, moderate, or low when used together to calculate a Wells score (Chapter 68). In patients so classified as having low risk, the D-dimer test has high sensitivity and therefore a high negative predictive value; as a result, a negative test reduces the risk of pulmonary embolism substantially. The D-dimer test carries a trivial risk to the patient, and its cost is low. Based on its test characteristics, a negative D-dimer result can safely exclude venous thromboembolism and limit the number of patients requiring further evaluation with imaging techniques. Conversely, in a patient with high pretest probability, a test with higher risk and expense may be warranted, such as computed tomographic pulmonary angiography, which has both a high sensitivity and a high specificity. By balancing the patient's pretest probability, as determined using a prediction rule, with a test's expenses, risks, and operating characteristics, an appropriate decision-making strategy can be developed and applied to an individual patient.

GENERAL REFERENCES

For the General References and other additional features, please visit Elsevier eBooks+ at https://ebooks.health.elsevier.com.

9 MEASURING HEALTH AND HEALTH CARE

CAROLYN M. CLANCY AND ERNEST MOY

Physicians routinely quantify a variety of health measures, including symptoms, vital signs, and findings on physical examination, to improve diagnosis, treatment, and prognostication. Similarly, measures of health care efficacy and quality of health care can and should be prioritized for several reasons.

First, the quality of care delivered is often suboptimal. Persistent variations in practice for patients with the same diagnosis reflect a combination of clinical uncertainty, individualized practice styles, patients' preferences and characteristics (age, race, ethnicity, education, income), and other factors. Both suboptimal care and varied care for the same condition undermine the historical assumption that a combination of highly trained health professionals and accredited facilities is sufficient to ensure consistent high-quality care.

Second, a major challenge in health care today, largely attributable to the successes of biomedical sciences, is the management of chronic disease for a population with an increasing life expectancy. For chronic conditions, health benefits are often and more appropriately measured in improvements in functional status or quality of life, rather than simply using mortality rates or life expectancy.

Third, increasing costs of health care are now threatening public budgets and investments in other social goals, such as education. Although the United States spends more per capita on health care than any other developed nation, the achieved outcomes lag far behind.

Finally, advances in communication and information technologies have inspired more people to play an active role in their health and health care. These innovations have accelerated demands for transparency and shared decision-making.

As health insurance and health care regulation have expanded, requirements to track and justify health care services have grown. Intensifying urgency to improve the quality of health care, reduce disparities, control costs, and enhance transparency will likely lead patients and insurers to demand more data and to link quality measures to payments for services.

Fortunately, modern technology can help to meet the demand for data. Patients can record and submit their health parameters using handheld devices connected to personal health records. Automated billing programs can track health care services, and electronic health records can assess the quality of physician care. Ultimately, fully integrated health information systems will allow patient information to be retrieved instantly and seamlessly whenever and wherever it is needed. For example, the Department of Veterans Affairs has substantial clinical and demographic data on veterans who receive care at their facilities. These data allowed rapid identification and outreach to at-risk groups early in the severe acute respiratory syndrome coronavirus 2 (SARS-CoV-2) pandemic, so that vaccines could be targeted to patients at need without ethnic, socioeconomic, or geographic disparities.[1] In addition to assessing the quality of care today, these tools offer enormous promise for learning as a byproduct of care delivery.

HOW ARE HEALTH AND HEALTH CARE MEASURED?

Three types of measures typically assess health and health care. Measures of *health* quantify the sickness or well-being of a person. Measures of *health care quality* quantify the extent to which a patient receives needed care and does not receive unnecessary care. Health care quality is assessed using measures of *structure* (e.g., education and credentialing of clinicians), *process* (adherence to professional standards and evidence-based recommendations), and *outcomes* (or end results of care, including how patients experience their care and their self-reported health and function). Measures of *health care resources* quantify the resources used (e.g., imaging, surgery, medication, intensive care) to improve the health of a patient. All measures can be summed across populations within a practice or community (Table 9-1).

Measures of health and health care often overlap (E-Fig. 9-1). Health measures that can be improved by health care, such as blood pressure or blood glucose levels, are often used as health care quality outcome measures. The delivery of quality health care requires the use of resources and the generation of direct health care costs, which may or may not improve health care at the margins of spending. Impaired health that reduces the ability to do work and earn wages but that could have been prevented by the delivery of health care contributes to the indirect costs of health care. At the intersection of health, health care quality, and health care resources are measures of health care value. These measures compare the health benefits of specific health care services with their costs.

WHY MEASURE HEALTH AND HEALTH CARE?

Measures of health and health care can be used for many purposes by different stakeholders (Table 9-2). Patients can use their own health information to track their progress, adjust their lifestyle, and plan for their future health

TABLE 9-1 MEASURES OF HEALTH AND HEALTH CARE

MEASURES OF HEALTH

- *Mortality:* rates of death typically adjusted for age and sex
- *Morbidity:* incidence and prevalence rates of diseases and their sequelae
- *Functional status:* assessments of a patient's ability to perform various actions such as activities of daily living or instrumental activities of daily living as observed by a provider or reported by the patient
- *Self-reported health status:* a patient's assessment of his or her health and well-being

MEASURES OF HEALTH CARE QUALITY

- *Health care outcomes:* the end results or health benefits derived from good health care or the health loss attributable to poor health care
- *Health care processes:* assessments of whether the right care was delivered at the right time and in the right way
- *Health care infrastructure:* the availability of resources needed to deliver high-quality health care
- *Patient perceptions of health care:* a patient's assessment of health care received, usually emphasizing patient-provider communication and shared decision making
- *Access to health care:* the ability of patients to gain entry into health care and navigate to needed resources

MEASURES OF HEALTH CARE RESOURCES

- *Health care utilization:* the quantity of health care services that are used
- *Direct costs:* the costs of providers, supplies, and equipment needed to deliver health care
- *Indirect costs:* the costs of lost wages and decreased productivity due to illness or injury that could have been prevented by appropriate health care
- *Nonmedical costs:* the costs of health care not related to the delivery of services, such as administration, advertising, research, and profits earned by health industries

TYPE OF MEASURE	EXAMPLE
HEALTH	
Mortality	Deaths due to colorectal cancer per 100,000 population
Morbidity	New AIDS cases per 100,000 population
Functional status	% of people unable to perform one or more activities of daily living
Self-reported health status	% of people reporting that their overall health is excellent
HEALTH CARE QUALITY	
Health care outcomes	Deaths per 1000 hospitalizations with pneumonia
Intermediate outcomes	% of adults with diabetes whose blood pressure is $<$140/80 mm Hg
Health care processes	% of children who were given all recommended vaccinations
Health care infrastructure	% of office-based physicians with computerized systems for recording clinical notes
Patient perceptions of health care	% of patients who always reported good communication with their regular providers
Access to health care	% of patients who were unable or delayed in receiving medical care
HEALTH CARE RESOURCES	
Health care utilization	% of people with an emergency department visit in the past year
Direct costs	Expenditures for the treatment of depression
Indirect costs	Lost wages and productivity while caring for children with asthma
Nonmedical costs	Profits earned by pharmaceutical companies

TABLE 9-2 USES OF HEALTH AND HEALTH CARE MEASURES BY USER AND UNIT OF ANALYSIS

	USES BY PROVIDERS	USES BY POLICYMAKERS	USES BY PATIENTS
Patient-level measures	Diagnosis and prognosis Monitoring treatment response and compliance	Identifying sentinel events	Tracking health and health needs Retirement and estate planning
Provider practice or health plan–level measures	Improving quality Improving efficiency Reducing disparities	Public reporting Paying for performance Provider credentialing	Selecting providers and health plans
Community-level measures	Selecting practice location	Resource allocation Policy evaluation	Selecting place to live

care needs. Patient-level measures are important to physicians, hospitals, health plans, and policymakers, whether they are used to identify sentinel events that represent quality defects (e.g., amputating the wrong leg or giving a patient the wrong medication), to initiate root cause analyses to improve health care quality, or to assess how quality output is linked to cost input (Chapter 10).

Hospitals and health plans aggregate measures over their practices to identify opportunities for raising quality, improving efficiency, and reducing care disparities. For measures for which physicians are primarily accountable, these data can be used to acknowledge and reward high-performing physicians, select physicians for inclusion on panels, and produce report cards to inform the public. Patients can use these report cards to select physicians and health plans that best match their health care needs. Regulators may examine measures to assess qualification for licensure and to identify physicians who might benefit from remedial instruction. Credentialing organizations may construct measures to demonstrate the superior performance of physicians who meet their high standards. For example, the National Committee for Quality Assurance maintains the Healthcare Effectiveness Data and Information Set that is widely used to accredit health plans, and the American Board of Internal Medicine and other specialty boards include measures of practice performance as well as measures of medical knowledge for the maintenance of certification. Measures that are aggregated to the community level can help policymakers allocate health care resources to locales with the greatest need and assess the success of any interventions.

SELECTING MEASURES BASED ON EVIDENCE

Data used to measure the structure, process, and outcomes of health care can be gathered as part of hypothesis-driven research, as a part of quality improvement, or from secondary sources of data initially collected for routine clinical care billing. The data's rigor and integrity are critical to the reliability of analyses performed on them.

In addition to the quality of the data themselves, however, the method of study design is also critical to the validity of reported findings. The most robust measures are supported by the concurrence of evidence derived from different research methodologies. In randomized controlled trials, random assignment of the intervention ensures that both patients who do and do not receive it are as similar as possible. In double-blind studies, neither the patient nor the patient's physician knows the assigned treatment. For more complex interventions, such as the use of a team to manage depression, blinding is impractical. In all settings, controls typically receive the best standard care. In some situations, patients may serve as their own controls in a time-series randomized trial. Adaptive designs incorporate strategies that assign more participants to treatment groups that are performing well, assign fewer participants to groups that are performing poorly, and investigate wide dose ranges to identify the most effective dose.[2] Pragmatic trials inform a clinical or policy decision by determining the usefulness of an intervention for real-world clinical practice. Noninferiority trials are designed to prove the equivalence of two strategies.[3]

Although the randomized trial is a rigorous way to assess treatment effects, enrollment is often limited to selected individuals who meet strict entry criteria. This approach enhances a trial's internal validity but limits its generalizability. As a result, randomized trials are ideal for establishing an intervention's efficacy, which is its potential benefit under ideal conditions, but not necessarily its *effectiveness* in the real world. *Cluster randomized trials,* which randomize the level of the provider or system, represent a practical approach to determining effectiveness.

Although randomized trials are critical for assessing efficacy and effectiveness, *observational* and *case-control* studies are also important. In a *cohort study,* persons or patients are followed to determine their outcomes as a function of whether or not they possess a particular attribute or have been exposed to a particular condition or intervention. Cohort studies can provide a direct estimate of the absolute risk for an outcome in exposed patients but cannot guarantee whether such differences are related to interventions that were not randomly allocated.[4]

In *case-control studies,* cases are defined based on having experienced an outcome not experienced by controls (Chapter 8). Information that is gleaned from existing records or interviews can determine the propor tion of case and control patients who experienced an exposure of interest. Case-control studies can achieve the same or higher statistical power as cohort studies despite enrolling fewer subjects, so they are especially attractive for investigating uncommon outcomes, such as serious adverse effects of medications when the events are too rare to study with clinical trials or cohort studies. Case-control studies are subject to misclassification bias and recall bias, and they provide estimates of relative risk but not absolute risk.

Cross-sectional studies collect data at just one point in time. They can be used to estimate the prevalence of a condition or outcome but not to make valid inferences about whether a given outcome is related to any causal attribute or event.

There are additional methodologic issues beyond the credibility and quality of the source of data for quality measures. When presented with reports suggesting less-than-perfect performance, many physicians believe that their patients are sicker or are less likely to adhere to treatment recommendations. To address these concerns, risk adjustment for severity of illness, accurate identification of patient characteristics, and assessment of outcomes over time are all critical. Case-mix adjustment methods commonly use sophisticated statistical approaches (Chapter 8) in an attempt to adjust for such potential differences and to estimate whether observed differences result from differing patient populations rather than true differences in quality of care.[5]

The precision of specific measures is also a challenge. Many stakeholders, especially payers and policymakers, are increasingly impatient and are generally more enthusiastic about the use of measures that are only "pretty good" than are providers whose care is being judged.

SELECTING MEASURES: WHICH MEASURES ARE RIGHT FOR WHAT PURPOSE?

Creating measures is different from selecting which measures are most important and meaningful. Numerous publicly available sources provide a wealth of health and health care information (E-Table 9-1). The most prominent consensus-based organization that endorses measures is the National Quality Forum, which convenes panels of experts to assess the quality of a proposed measure based on criteria that include importance, scientific acceptability, feasibility, and usability. Endorsed measures are reassessed periodically to ensure they remain up-to-date and applicable.

The National Institutes of Health Patient Reported Outcomes Measurement Information System (http://www.nihpromis.org) is a repository of standardized patient-reported health status measures and collection instruments. Domains include physical, mental, and social well-being. The Agency for Healthcare Research and Quality National Quality Measures Clearinghouse (http://www.qualitymeasures.ahrq.gov) is an inventory of evidence-based measures of health care quality. Domains include clinical quality, efficiency,

TABLE 9-3 ATTRIBUTES OF MEASURES OF HEALTH AND HEALTH CARE

MEASURE ATTRIBUTES	CRITERIA FOR PROVIDERS	CRITERIA FOR POLICYMAKERS	CRITERIA FOR PATIENTS
Measure is scientifically sound			
Based on strong evidence	Based on high-quality studies?		
Valid	Measures what is intended and includes key elements?		
Reliable	Reproducible by different measurers and providers?		
Clearly specified	Numerator, denominator, exclusions, and risk adjustment defined?		
Endorsed by independent experts	Well-accepted by scientific and medical communities?		
Condition is important Affects many people Causes high mortality or morbidity Is costly Is very unequal across populations	Important for my practice or the population I serve?	Important for population that will be affected by my policy?	Important to me?
Data collection is feasible Already available Could be collected at low cost relative to potential benefit Auditable	Available for my practice or the population I serve?	Available before and after policy implementation for affected population?	Available to me?
Findings are actionable Can be understood Can be improved Have been used successfully Have few unintended consequences	Do I know what actions I must change to improve quality? Used in practices like mine to improve quality with few unintended consequences?	Do I know what policies I must change to improve quality? Used for policies like mine to improve quality with few unintended consequences?	Do I know what actions I must take to improve my health? Used by patients like me to improve health with few unintended consequences?
When used as part of measure set, measures are: Balanced Able to be disaggregated	Represents multiple conditions, settings of care, populations, types of data (survey, administrative data, medical records), types of measures (structure, process, outcomes), and perspectives (patient, provider, system, society) as appropriate? Identifies individual measures that can be improved?		

and population health. Also related are the National Guidelines Clearinghouse (http://www.guideline.gov) and the Health Care Innovations Exchange (http://www.innovations.ahrq.gov), collections of clinical guidelines and descriptions of successful uses of measures, respectively.

Potential users should examine the attributes of specific measures to ensure that they are appropriate for their intended application (Table 9-3) and can measure change reliably and validly.[6] A number of organizations have developed scales or rating systems that summarize performance across multiple dimensions. Sometimes referred to as composite measures (e.g., a letter grade from the Leapfrog Group for hospital safety), these scales vary in comprehensiveness with little consensus regarding how components of a summary scale should be weighted. Indeed, it is not uncommon for a hospital to receive an "F" from one group and be rated a "top performer" by another. Thus, although appealing in their simplicity, the optimal use of these approaches remains unresolved.

MEASURING HEALTH AND HEALTH CARE AS PARTS OF A SYSTEM

Measuring health and health care together is also important for understanding the system as a whole. Patients, providers, and policymakers generally agree that the paramount goal of the health system is to improve health. At the population health level, however, factors other than medical care are highly influential. For example, population health is affected as much by health behaviors—such as diet, physical activity, smoking, and alcohol and drug use—as by the direct provision of medical care. Social characteristics (e.g., poverty, education, crime, and residential segregation) and physical determinants (e.g., housing and the natural and built environment) also impact population health to a greater extent than medical care (Chapter 4). Discrimination and bias have adverse effects on population health, including structural racism in social policies, such as housing and education, and algorithmic biases in clinical decision-support tools that may advantage some groups over others.[7] These issues must be addressed locally and systematically to enable all patients to derive maximal benefit from medical care and to achieve health equity. Explicitly measuring and rewarding equitable care is one component of achieving excellent care for all patients.[8,9]

Viewing medical care as a component of a system for generating and preserving population health has many implications for physicians and other health care providers. First, it emphasizes the importance of services to encourage healthy lifestyles and prevent the development of disease. For example, efforts to prevent tobacco use (Chapter 363) among adolescents (Chapter 21) may yield greater population health benefits than treating the complications of nicotine addiction later in life. Second, it serves as a reminder that patients who seek care have widely varying attributes and resources, factors that may affect their ability to comply with treatment recommendations. As a consequence, it may be important to consider medications with lower out-of-pocket costs for low-income patients and to simplify instructions to a patient's level of health literacy. Third, it recognizes how environmental factors outside of the control of physicians often have a large impact on population health. When health care measures are used to assess quality, adjustment for these factors is critical to ensure that comparisons are not biased. Fourth, it stresses the need for a culturally competent, diverse, and inclusive provider workforce. For example, in a randomized controlled trial, Black men were more likely to opt for indicated preventive services after consultation with a Black male doctor than with a non-Black male doctor.[10]

The SARS-CoV-2 pandemic has emphasized the relevance of telehealth for quality of care,[11] especially for a geographically dispersed population. However, telehealth also has the potential to worsen disparities because of differential access to and comfort with suitable devices.[12] In the Department of Veterans Affairs health care system, for example, explicit attention to the digital divide enabled rapid substitution of virtual care for in-clinic care with few disparities so that veterans with lower income, higher disability, and more chronic conditions were equally likely to receive virtual care during the pandemic.[13]

Another virtue of measuring health and health care together is to assess the value of components of the health system or the health system as a whole. U.S. national health expenditures have increased over 100 times from $27 billion (5.0% of the gross domestic product) in 1960 to $3.2 trillion in 2015 (17.8% of the gross domestic product) (Fig. 9-1). They are projected to exceed $5.5 trillion in 2025 and account for 20% of the gross domestic product. Expenditures on hospital care, physician and clinical services, prescription drugs, and the administration of health insurance account for 70% of total national health expenditures. Payers and employers can examine the cost-effectiveness of specific services and promote those that yield the largest health benefits for each dollar spent. U.S. health care processes rank much higher than health outcomes, despite the world's highest health care expenditures. In the United States the differential between the world's highest per capita expenditures but only the 46th longest life expectancy is in part because social conditions, such as poverty and lack of health insurance, may prevent even excellent medical care from achieving the best health outcomes.[14]

11

POPULATION HEALTH

KIRSTEN BIBBINS-DOMINGO

In addition to understanding the biology of health, the pathobiology of disease, and the principles of diagnosis and individual therapy, clinicians also must be familiar with the concept of population health. Population health can be defined as the health outcomes of a group of individuals, whether based on geography (Chapter 5), ethnicity or socioeconomic status (Chapter 4), age (Chapters 21 and 24), gender or gender identity (Chapter 214), or other attributes, such as employment (Chapter 16), disability, homelessness, or incarceration. The field of population health includes health outcomes, patterns of the determinants that influence health, and the policies and interventions that link these two.

Population health is also a priority for health care organizations. Improving the U.S. health care system requires simultaneous pursuit of three aims: improving the experience of care for patients, reducing per capita costs of health care, and improving the health of populations.[1] In this conceptualization, the improvement of population health is central to high-quality health care (Chapter 10), potentially augmented by changing health care financing toward rewarding value over volume and specifically incentivizing improvements in population-based outcomes. These changes in payment models have led to the creation of an infrastructure that is often referred to as "population health management."

POPULATION HEALTH MANAGEMENT

Population health management describes how a health care organization that is interested in quality, value, and improvements in population health can deploy its resources to address areas of need within a population. Population health management strategies focus not only on the care that is provided to an individual during an outpatient visit or hospitalization but also on managing the health of all patients with a particular condition as well as the entire population for which an organization has responsibility. The scope of these strategies generally includes expanded preventive services, care models that detect and intercede when early signs of health deterioration are identified, and community-based programs that address care for complex conditions outside of clinical settings, including the social issues that often complicate the management of chronic conditions.

Data suggest that population health management strategies can improve health outcomes. For example, consider the delivery of a preventive intervention such as evidence-based cancer screening to an entire population for which a health care organization has responsibility. When fecal immunochemical tests are directly mailed to all patients in a health care system, rates of screening for colon cancer increase. To be effective, however, such screening must be accompanied by rigorous plans for evaluating individuals who have a positive test result.[A1] Identifying all patients with a particular risk profile (e.g., obesity [Chapter 201] or pre-diabetes [Chapter 210]) may allow for more efficient enrollment of such patients into preventive care interventions (e.g., a diabetes prevention program). A population health management program can achieve 80 to 90% control rates for hypertension (Chapter 64) in an integrated health delivery system by focusing on structured treatment algorithms, team-based care, and an active management of hypertension registries. Online digital tools and telemedicine may allow for effective management of chronic conditions such as asthma,[A2] obesity,[A3] or diabetes.

Inherent in many population health management care models is the importance of team-based care that includes nonphysicians (e.g., nurses, nurse practitioners, pharmacists, and social workers, among others). Health care workers who work outside traditional clinical settings may be particularly important. For example, community health workers, who are trained to have basic knowledge of clinical conditions, can provide health coaching and psychosocial support, augment patient engagement by strengthening connections to outpatient care, facilitate navigation during transitions in care (e.g., from inpatient to outpatient or from primary care to specialty care), and identify relevant resources to address unmet social needs (e.g., food, housing, transportation). Outpatient models that include community health workers in the care of patients with multiple chronic conditions (e.g., diabetes, obesity, tobacco dependence, and hypertension) can improve control of these chronic conditions, improve mental health outcomes, improve quality of care, and decrease subsequent hospitalizations.[A4,A5] Similar approaches for high-risk patients at the time of hospital discharge demonstrate improvements in access to primary care and reductions in recurrent readmissions. Community health workers also have shown promise for mental health conditions such as depression (Chapter 362)[2] and geriatric conditions such as hearing loss.[A6] Economic analyses show positive returns on investment for models of care that incorporate community health workers,[3] but more widespread adoption has been limited by variability in the health care reimbursement, variability in training and licensing, and limited studies on the standardization of such interventions.[A7]

BEYOND POPULATION HEALTH MANAGEMENT TO POPULATION HEALTH

Population health management is being incorporated into traditional health systems that are seeking to improve clinical prevention, management of chronic disease, value, and quality. However, inherent in the broader concept of population health is the recognition that clinical care accounts only for about 20% of the factors responsible for health outcomes. Even after also accounting for individual behaviors that might be addressed in the health care setting, other factors (often referred to as the social determinants of health) account for far more (Fig. 11-1). These social drivers of health pose specific challenges for the delivery of health care. Patients at highest risk for poor clinical outcomes often have the highest degree of need with respect to these social drivers of health, and individual clinicians often feel ill-equipped to address these needs. The systemic nature of many social drivers of health are best addressed with broader policies and programs that are widely available to groups of individuals with similar needs rather than by simply addressing the unmet needs of an individual patient at one point in time.[4] This recognition has led to an increased interest in how physicians and health systems might move beyond targeted population health management programs to address social and structural determinants of health more directly.

Interventions focused on the social determinants of health or addressing social needs of patients in health care settings have had variable success. Increasing attention is focusing on screening all patients for social needs, with the goal of addressing any unmet needs,[A8] but interventions to address food insecurity, financial strain, and housing instability have not yet resulted in replicable approaches to guide their widespread implementation.[5] For example, a trial of providing rideshare transportation to patients with transportation needs failed to improve attendance at outpatient visits,[A9] suggesting that addressing a single determinant of health may be insufficient in patients who may also have multiple additional needs (e.g., economic, food, shelter). Providing permanent supportive housing for chronically homeless individuals who are high users of health care services can increase outpatient follow-up for mental health, decrease emergency psychiatric visits, and decrease the use of homeless shelters, but not reduce overall emergency department visits or hospitalizations.[A10] Sustainable models for addressing social needs such as housing within the context of health care delivery generally require partnerships with institutions for whom housing is their primary focus. Similarly, data on addressing food insecurity for diabetic patients in health care settings support the use of partnerships with food pantries.[A11] However, the difficulties of addressing complex social needs in high-risk patients is exemplified by the failure of an intervention based on a team of nurses, social workers, and community health workers to reduce hospital readmissions among high users of health care with medically and socially complex problems,[A12] despite high engagement of patients with the program.

Although the importance of addressing the social drivers of health is critical for improving population health, the most effective means for addressing such challenges within the context of health care delivery remains uncertain. However, data suggest five types of interventions are most likely to address social needs and thereby improve individual and population health (Fig. 11-2). All clinicians and health care organizations should be *aware* of the social determinants of health and the potential needs and assets of patients with respect to these social factors. In the context of health care delivery, clinical teams may identify and address the social needs of an individual patient by providing direct *assistance* (e.g., providing a voucher for transportation or referral to a food assistance program). *Adjustments* to clinical care may also be appropriate to minimize the burden of social need (e.g., telehealth visits for patients with transportation needs or a lower-cost diagnostic evaluation or treatment regimen for patients with limited resources). Since addressing social needs one patient at a time may not be effective or cost-effective, changes in structural factors that result in social needs for larger populations of patients are usually better addressed by *alignment* with other sectors (e.g., partnerships with housing agencies and social services to develop programs for permanent supportive housing following hospitalization) or joint *advocacy* for changes in housing policies.

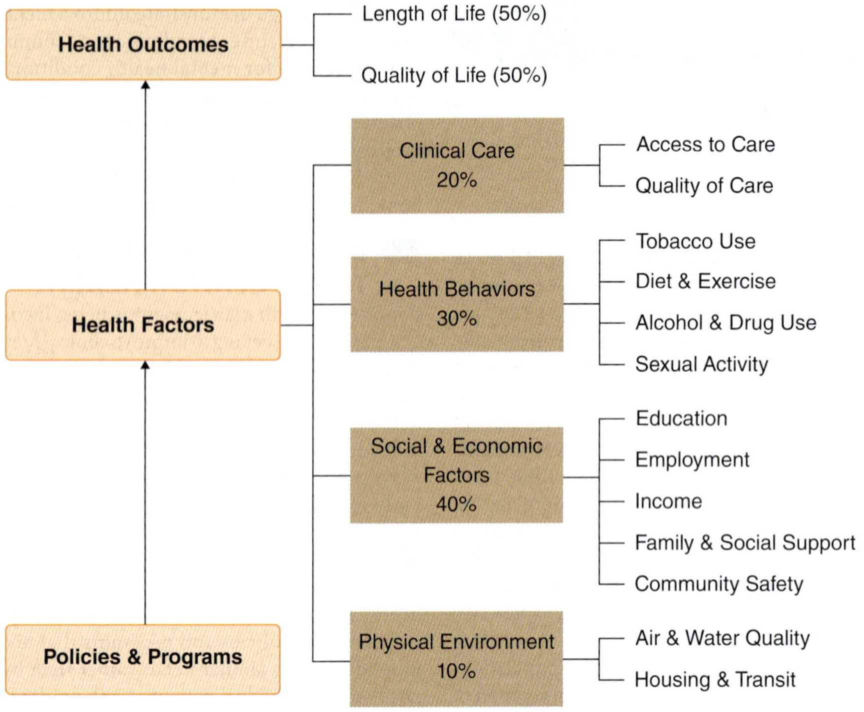

FIGURE 11-1. **Relative contribution of clinical care, individual behaviors, and social determinants of health to health outcomes.** (Adapted from National Academies of Sciences, Engineering, and Medicine Population Health Roundtable Discussion Paper.)

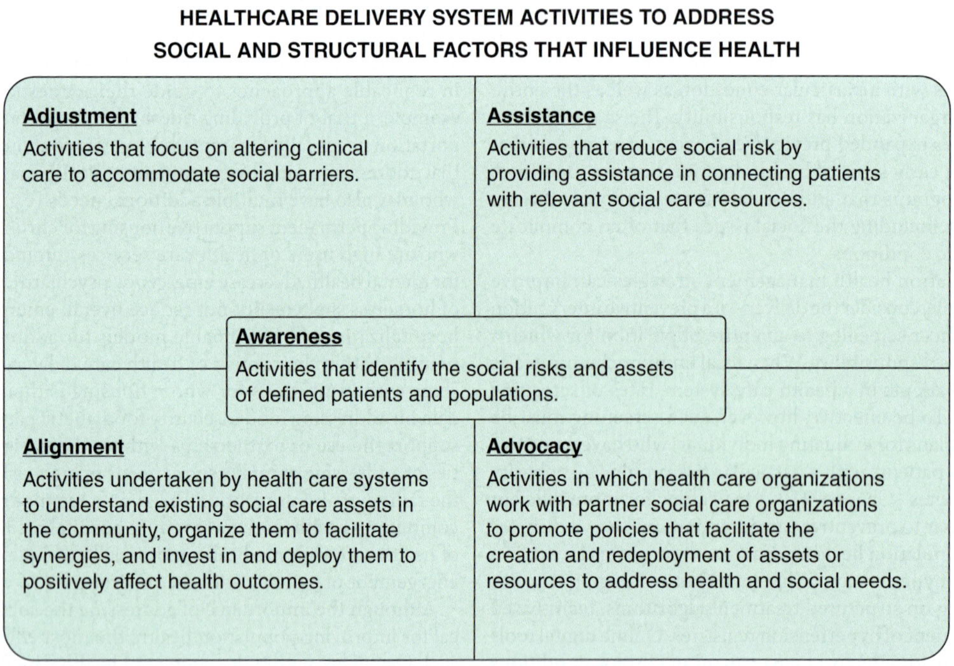

FIGURE 11-2. **The Five As: Activities of health delivery systems to address social needs and social determinants of health to improve population health.** (Adapted from the National Academies of Sciences, Engineering, and Medicine report: *Integrating Social Care into the Delivery of Health Care: Moving Upstream to Improve the Nation's Health*.)

GENERAL REFERENCES

For the General References and other additional features, please visit Elsevier eBooks+ at https://ebooks.health.elsevier.com.

Grade A References

A1. Issaka RB, Avila P, Whitaker E, et al. Population health interventions to improve colorectal cancer screening by fecal immunochemical tests: a systematic review. *Prev Med.* 2019;118:113-121.

A2. Merchant RK, Inamdar R, Quade RC. Effectiveness of population health management using the propeller health asthma platform: a randomized clinical trial. *J Allergy Clin Immunol Pract.* 2016;4:455-463.

A3. Baer HJ, Rozenblum R, De La Cruz BA, et al. Effect of an online weight management program integrated with population health management on weight change: a randomized clinical trial. *JAMA.* 2020;324:1737-1746.

A4. Kangovi S, Mitra N, Grande D, et al. Community health worker support for disadvantaged patients with multiple chronic diseases: a randomized clinical trial. *Am J Public Health.* 2017;107:1660-1667.

A5. Kangovi S, Mitra N, Norton L, et al. Effect of community health worker support on clinical outcomes of low-income patients across primary care facilities: a randomized clinical trial. *JAMA Intern Med.* 2018;178:1635-1643.

A6. Nieman CL, Betz J, Garcia M, et al. Effect of a community health worker–delivered personal sound amplification device on self-perceived communication function in older adults with hearing loss: a randomized clinical trial. *JAMA.* 2022;328:2324-2333.

A7. Vasan A, Morgan JW, Mitra N, et al. Effects of a standardized community health worker intervention on hospitalization among disadvantaged patients with multiple chronic conditions: a pooled analysis of three clinical trials. *Health Serv Res.* 2020;55:894-901.

A8. Gottlieb LM, Hessler D, Long D, et al. Effects of social needs screening and in-person service navigation on child health: a randomized clinical trial. *JAMA Pediatr.* 2016;170:e162521.

A9. Chaiyachati KH, Hubbard RA, Yeager A, et al. Association of rideshare-based transportation services and missed primary care appointments: a clinical trial. *JAMA Intern Med*. 2018;178:383-389.

A10. Raven MC, Niedzwiecki MJ, Kushel M. A randomized trial of permanent supportive housing for chronically homeless persons with high use of publicly funded services. *Health Serv Res*. 2020;55:797-806.

A11. Seligman HK, Smith M, Rosenmoss S, et al. Comprehensive diabetes self-management support from food banks: a randomized controlled trial. *Am J Public Health*. 2018;108:1227-1234.

A12. Finkelstein A, Zhou A, Taubman S, et al. Health care hotspotting—a randomized, controlled trial. *N Engl J Med*. 2020;382:152-162.

III

PREVENTIVE AND ENVIRONMENTAL ISSUES

12

THE PREVENTIVE HEALTH VISIT

MARY B. BARTON AND TRACY A. WOLFF

A general health check-up for adults has not been proven to reduce mortality, but it is associated with better recognition and treatment of chronic diseases as well as better patient-reported outcomes.[1] The value of the periodic health visit is increased by a focus on primary and secondary prevention. The appropriate preventive services, including screening and lifestyle counseling, as well as their frequency, vary with the age, sex, and individual risk factors of each patient.

The U.S. Preventive Services Task Force (USPSTF) recommendations are used by major primary care groups, many health plans, and quality organizations, and their A and B recommendations guide preventive services that are covered under the Affordable Care Act. The USPSTF bases its recommendations on two factors: an estimate of the *net benefits* (benefits minus harms) of a service and an assessment of the *certainty* of that estimate, based on the rigor of supporting studies. Grade A recommendations require high certainty of a substantial net benefit, most often from large, prospective, controlled studies that measure morbidity or mortality.[2] Grade B recommendations have at least moderate certainty of at least a moderate benefit. USPSTF recommendations are thus more conservative than those of some subspecialty organizations that may give more weight to indirect evidence, such as earlier detection of disease, and less weight to potential harms of interventions. Clinicians can draw several general conclusions from an evidence-based approach to prevention: we should be selective in our use of screening tests, especially in older patients, and involve patients in decisions about specific services for which a small chance of benefit must be balanced against possible harm.

HISTORY AND RISK ASSESSMENT

The history and risk assessment are important tools to identify individuals who may need additional screening tests or immunizations not generally recommended for their age group or who may benefit from specific counseling to promote healthy behaviors. Formal health risk appraisals should be linked to a system to provide specific feedback and targeted interventions. Risk assessment should address the following:

- Use of tobacco, alcohol, and other drugs (especially injection drugs) (Chapters 363, 364, and 365)
- Diet (Chapters 13 and 201)
- Physical activity (Chapter 14)
- Sexual behavior that may increase the risk for sexually transmitted diseases or unintended pregnancy (Chapters 264, 353, and 356)
- Family history of cancer and heart disease
- Birthplace and current residence (community risk for infectious diseases)
- Presence of chronic diseases, such as diabetes, and of other cardiovascular risk factors
- Presence of social risk factors, such as housing instability, food insecurity, financial strain

SCREENING FOR EARLY DISEASE OR ASYMPTOMATIC RISK FACTORS

Every year, new screening tests are introduced and marketed on the basis of their ability to detect unrecognized diseases or risk factors for disease. Other conditions need to be fulfilled for a screening test to be worthwhile for routine use, however (Table 12-1). Benefits of screening must be balanced against the potential harms, including false-positive results and the risks and costs of follow-up procedures or treatments. Even when tests have high specificity, the majority of positive results will be false-positive results if the test is used to screen healthy populations for uncommon conditions such as cancer (Chapter 8). There is evidence that cancer screening can lead to "overdiagnosis"—detection of slow-growing cancers that would never have caused clinical symptoms in a patient's lifetime. Overdiagnosis subjects patients to the side effects of treatment with no benefits. A relatively small number of screening tests have been proved beneficial for the general population (Table 12-2), but several screening tests are indicated for specific populations at risk (Table 12-3). Many commonly used screening tests are not recommended by the USPSTF (Table 12-4) because they provide little benefit or lack sufficient evidence to prove

TABLE 12-1 REQUIREMENTS OF AN EFFECTIVE SCREENING TEST

The disease being screened for is an important cause of morbidity and mortality.
Screening can detect disease in an early, asymptomatic phase.
Screening and treatment of patients with early disease or risk factors produce better health outcomes than does treatment of patients when they present with symptoms.
Screening test is acceptable to patients and clinicians—safe, convenient, acceptable false-positive rate, acceptable costs.
Benefits of early detection and asymptomatic treatment are sufficient to justify potential harms and costs of screening.

TABLE 12-2 PREVENTION RECOMMENDATIONS FOR THE GENERAL POPULATION: FROM THE U.S. PREVENTIVE SERVICES TASK FORCE AND OTHER SOURCES

SCREENING
Height, weight, and body mass index (BMI) calculation: periodically
Blood pressure: at least every 2 yr
Screen for alcohol misuse
Screen for unhealthy drug use
Brief screen for depression*
Total blood cholesterol, LDL, and HDL cholesterol: every 5 yr for men and women ≥20 yr with CHD risk factors and men ≥35 yr without CHD risk factors
Colorectal cancer screening: age 45-75 yr
Mammogram: at least every 2 yr for women 50-74 yr
Cervical cancer: Papanicolaou (Pap) test every 3 yr for women aged 21-29 yr; for women aged 30-65 yr, either Pap test every 3 yr or human papillomavirus (HPV) test with or without Pap every 5 yr
HIV test: at least once in all adults; repeat based on high-risk sexual activity
Hepatitis C screening at least once for persons ages 18 to 79 years, repeat based on continued risk
Chlamydia and gonorrhea: sexually active women ≤24 yr and older women at risk
Screening for bacteriuria in pregnant persons
Bone mineral density test: women ≥65 yr and high-risk women <65 yr
COUNSELING
Substance use
Tobacco cessation
Reduction of risky or harmful alcohol use
Diet and exercise
Limit saturated fat; maintain calorie balance; emphasize grains, fruits, and vegetables†
Regular physical activity
Sexual behavior
Unintended pregnancy: contraception
Interventions during pregnancy and after birth to support breastfeeding
Dental health: floss, brush with fluoride toothpaste daily
IMMUNIZATIONS
Pneumococcal vaccine (two preparations, administered 1 yr apart, age ≥65 yr)
Influenza vaccine (annual)
Tetanus-diphtheria (Td) boosters (every 10 yr)
Measles, mumps, rubella (MMR) vaccine (susceptible adults aged 19-49 yr)‡
Varicella (two doses, susceptible adults born after 1980)‡
Herpes zoster vaccine, two doses after age 50 yr
HPV vaccine (two doses, boys and girls ages 12-13 yr; three doses if given at ages 15-26 yr)
COVID-19 vaccine, with booster age >5 yr
PREVENTIVE MEDICATIONS
Multivitamin with folic acid (women planning or capable of pregnancy)

*Screening is most effective where adequate systems exist to ensure effective treatment and appropriate follow-up.
†Diet counseling is most effective when it targets at-risk groups (overweight or with CHD risk factors).
‡Immunity can be verified by serologic testing, documented history of illness, or vaccination.
CHD = coronary heart disease; COVID = coronavirus disease; HDL = high-density lipoprotein; HIV = human immunodeficiency virus; HPV = human papillomavirus; LDL = low-density lipoprotein.
USPSTF recommendations:
Sources: https://www.uspreventiveservicestaskforce.org/; other sources for Tables 12-2 and 12-3 include U.S. Department of Health and Human Services (diet, physical activity), Centers for Disease Control and Prevention (injury prevention, immunizations, dental health), and Health Resources and Services Administration (contraception).

TABLE 12-3 RECOMMENDED SCREENING AND INTERVENTIONS FOR SELECTED POPULATIONS

POTENTIAL INTERVENTION	POPULATION
SCREENING	
Diabetes screen	Adults aged 35 to 70 yr with overweight or obesity
Ultrasound examination for abdominal aortic aneurysm	Males aged 65-75 yr with current or previous smoking history
Low-dose computed tomography for lung cancer	Adults with at least 20 pack-year smoking history (current adults who smoke, and those who quit smoking within past 15 years)
Syphilis (RPR/VDRL)	High-risk sexual behavior; consider local epidemiology*
Gonorrhea screen	High-risk sexual behavior; consider local epidemiology*
Tb screening	Persons who were born in, or are former residents of, high-risk countries, congregate settings, immunosuppressed
COUNSELING	
Exercise to prevent falls	Community dwelling adults ≥65 yr at increased risk for falls
Counseling to prevent STIs	Adults at increased risk
IMMUNIZATIONS	
Hepatitis B vaccine	Exposure to blood products; IV drug use; high-risk sexual behavior; travelers to high-risk areas
Hepatitis A vaccine	Persons living in or traveling to high-risk areas; institutionalized persons and workers in these institutions; those with certain chronic medical conditions
Meningococcal vaccine	First-year college students in dormitories; military recruits; those with asplenia; travelers to high-risk areas
Varicella vaccine	Adults born after 1980 without evidence of immunity
PREVENTIVE MEDICATIONS	
Statin	Adults over 40 yr at increased risk of cardiovascular disease
Breast cancer preventive medications	Women at increased risk for breast cancer and with low risk for thromboembolic complications
HIV preexposure prophylaxis	Adults at high risk of HIV acquisition

*Routine screening may be indicated in communities or settings where infection is prevalent.
HIV = human immunodeficiency virus; IV = intravenous; RPR = rapid plasma reagin; STI = sexually transmitted infection; Tb = tuberculosis; VDRL = Venereal Disease Research Laboratory.

TABLE 12-4 INTERVENTIONS NOT RECOMMENDED FOR ROUTINE USE IN ASYMPTOMATIC AVERAGE-RISK ADULTS*

PHYSICAL EXAMINATION
Oral examination for oral cancer (I) Brief tests of mental status to detect dementia (I) Vision and hearing tests in older adults (I) Screening testicular examination (D)
BLOOD TEST
Routine blood tests for anemia Blood level of C-reactive protein to predict coronary risk (I) Blood tests for celiac disease (I) Herpes serology (D) Blood tests for ovarian cancer (D)
RADIOLOGY
Chest radiograph for lung cancer Ultrasound examination for asymptomatic carotid artery stenosis (D) Whole body computed tomographic scan Ultrasound examination for ovarian cancer Helical computed tomography for asymptomatic coronary disease (I)
OTHER
Resting or exercise electrocardiography (D) of asymptomatic coronary disease Pulmonary function tests for chronic obstructive pulmonary disease (D) Routine urine tests (for infection, cancer, or chronic kidney disease) (I) Vitamin supplements (I, D)

*These services have either insufficient evidence to support routine use (I) or at least fair evidence that they provide no benefit or that harms outweigh benefits (D).

or disprove their value. Because only about 50% of U.S. adults see a primary care physician each year,[3] the responsibility for providing preventive services may increasingly fall to other clinicians.

DEPRESSION

Depression is common and frequently undetected in primary care (Chapter 362), and screening is specifically recommended in the adult general population, including pregnant and postpartum women. The most commonly used screen, and one of the simplest, is the Patient Health Questionnaire (PHQ)-9 (Table 12-5), which has nine items, each scored from 0 to 3. The PHQ-9 takes 5 to 10 minutes to administer.[4] A total score of 10 indicates moderate depression, whereas a score of 20 generally corresponds to severe depression. To improve outcomes, however, screening for depression must be linked to an organized system with staff support to ensure follow-up diagnostic assessment and treatment.

COGNITIVE IMPAIRMENT

By comparison, routine screening for cognitive impairment is more complicated. Despite excellent screening tools (Chapters 361 and 371),[5] no specific interventions have substantial impact on progression, so the USPSTF found insufficient evidence to support screening.[A1] Nevertheless, identification of cognitive impairment is included in Medicare's wellness visits and can guide family and other caregivers in ways that are likely to benefit the patient.

HIGH BLOOD PRESSURE, ABNORMAL LIPIDS, AND OTHER CARDIOVASCULAR RISK FACTORS

Overall cardiovascular disease (CVD) risk, based on age, sex, blood pressure, lipid levels, diabetes and smoking status, should be calculated at regular intervals to guide treatment decisions to reduce cardiovascular risk. Blood pressure should be measured at least every 2 years (Chapter 64), and home measurement[6] is recommended rather than beginning treatment based on an office measurement alone.[A2] The value of blood pressure screening in adolescents (Chapter 21) is less clear.[A3]

For lipids, the most commonly used risk estimation tool relies on measures of total cholesterol and high- and low-density lipoprotein cholesterol (Chapter 190) to estimate 10-year risk of coronary heart disease (http://tools.acc.org/ASCVD-Risk-Estimator). Statins are routinely recommended for patients who already have known atherosclerotic cardiovascular disease (Chapter 190). By comparison, the USPSTF, which focuses on primary prevention for individuals at risk for developing cardiovascular disease, recommends low- to moderate-dose statins for adults ages 40 to 75 years who have at least a 10% 10-year risk of CVD and at least one CVD risk factor.[A4] Recommendations from the American Heart Association and American College of Cardiology favor treatment for those with an estimated 10-year risk as low as 7.5%, whereas the USPSTF recommends individualizing treatment decisions for adults with a 10-year CVD risk of 7.5 to 10%.[7] The USPSTF concluded evidence was insufficient to recommend for or against beginning treatment after age 75 in adults with no evidence of CVD. Although factors such as C-reactive protein, homocysteine, and coronary calcification as assessed by computed tomography (CT) are associated with an increased risk for heart disease, the USPSTF has, at least so far, found insufficient evidence to recommend their routine use in risk assessment.

ABDOMINAL AORTIC ANEURYSM

Between 5 and 9% of men older than 65 years have an abdominal aortic aneurysm (Chapter 63). The risk for aneurysm is highest in smokers and is substantially lower in women (1%). The USPSTF recommends one-time screening with ultrasound examination in men aged 65 to 75 years who are current or former smokers,[8] based on trials demonstrating as much as a 40% lower death rate from abdominal aortic aneurysm rupture in screened men, even though it does not decrease all-cause mortality.[A5]

TABLE 12-5 PATIENT HEALTH QUESTIONNAIRE-9 (PHQ-9)

Over the last 2 weeks, how often have you been bothered by any of the following problems?

USE "✔" TO INDICATE YOUR ANSWER	NOT AT ALL	SEVERAL DAYS	MORE THAN HALF THE DAYS	NEARLY EVERY DAY
1. Little interest or pleasure in doing things	0	1	2	3
2. Feeling down, depressed, or hopeless	0	1	2	3
3. Trouble falling or staying asleep, or sleeping too much	0	1	2	3
4. Feeling tired or having little energy	0	1	2	3
5. Poor appetite or overeating	0	1	2	3
6. Feeling bad about yourself—or that you are a failure or have let yourself or your family down	0	1	2	3
7. Trouble concentrating on things, such as reading the newspaper or watching television	0	1	2	3
8. Moving or speaking so slowly that other people could have noticed. Or the opposite—being so fidgety or restless that you have been moving around a lot more than usual	0	1	2	3
9. Thoughts that you would be better off dead or of hurting yourself in some way	0	1	2	3
FOR OFFICE CODING	*0*	+___	+___	+___
		=Total Score:_____		

Developed by Drs. Robert L. Spitzer, Janet B.W. Williams, Kurt Kroenke, and colleagues.

COLORECTAL CANCER

Screening can reduce both the incidence of and mortality from colorectal cancer. Options for screening men and women older than 45 years include an annual highly sensitive fecal occult blood test (FOBT) or fecal immunochemical test, a multitargeted stool DNA test every 1 to 3 years, flexible sigmoidoscopy every 5 years (or every 10 years with annual FOBT), CT colonography every 5 years, or colonoscopy every 10 years (Chapter 179).[A6]

Colonoscopy combines detection with the opportunity for biopsy and removal of lesions, so it is preferred in some guidelines. It carries higher costs and risks, however, and no single strategy has proved to be more effective or cost-effective than the alternatives. The USPSTF recommends routine screening for adults ages 45 to 75 years and selective screening in adults ages 75 to 85 years.[9]

BREAST CANCER

In large trials, mammography screening (at intervals of 1 to 2 years, with or without clinical breast examination) reduces breast cancer mortality by 15 to 30% (Chapter 183). Most trials suggest that the benefits of screening extend to women in their 40s, but the benefits are smaller and the risks for false-positive results are higher than in women aged 50 to 70 years. If a woman aged 40 to 49 years has a two-fold increased risk for breast cancer compared with the average in her age group, she will have a similar benefit-to-harm ratio for biennial screening mammography as an average-risk woman aged 50 to 74 years. No studies provide data on the benefits of screening women aged 75 and older. In a collaborative study, six independent models predicted that an average of 80% of the benefit of mammography could be achieved with biennial rather than annual mammography, whereas national mammography surveillance data indicate that false-positive results and other harms of screening would be reduced by about half if women were screened every other year instead of yearly. The USPSTF recommends biennial screening mammography for women aged 50 to 74 years, that the decision to start screening mammography in women before age 50 years should be an individual decision, and that the current evidence is insufficient to assess the balance of benefits and harms of screening mammography in women aged 75 years or older.

Although many cancers are discovered by patients, teaching women to perform breast self-examination increases the likelihood that a woman will undergo further evaluation for an unimportant finding, but it does not improve outcomes. Widespread screening for *BRCA1* or *BRCA2*, inherited mutations that increase the risk for breast cancer, is not recommended, but the USPSTF recommends that primary care providers assess risk in women who have family members with breast, ovarian, tubal, or peritoneal cancer by using one of several family history risk assessment tools designed to identify women at risk for potentially harmful mutations. Women with a positive result on risk assessment should be referred for genetic counseling.[10]

CERVICAL CANCER

Papanicolaou (Pap) screening is highly effective in preventing invasive cervical cancer, but many women in the United States are screened more often than needed. The USPSTF and a multispecialty-society collaborative endorse starting screening at age 21 years and then screening women aged 21 to 30 years every 3 years, regardless of their sexual history or HPV vaccination status (Chapter 184). In women ages 30 to 65 years, the USPSTF recommends either Pap testing every 3 years or human papillomavirus (HPV) testing with or without Pap testing every 5 years[11] (Chapters 15 and 344).[A7] Aside from its value for performing a Pap test, evidence is inadequate for recommending a pelvic examination in asymptomatic, nonpregnant women. Women who have adequate screening histories and who are not otherwise at high risk should discontinue screening after 65 years of age. Screening is not indicated in women who have undergone a total hysterectomy for benign disease. Whether women who have received the HPV vaccine (Chapter 15) need different screening strategies is not yet known.

PROSTATE CANCER

Screening with prostate-specific antigen (PSA) can increase the detection of organ-confined prostate cancer, but three large trials provided conflicting results as to whether screening lowers morbidity or mortality from prostate cancer (Chapter 186). Based on long-term follow-up of those trials and studies of early treatment of screen-detected cancer,[A8] the USPSTF concluded that PSA-based screening programs in men ages 55 to 69 years may prevent up to 1 to 2 deaths from prostate cancer and up to 3 cases of metastatic prostate cancer per 1000 men screened over 13 years.[A9] These benefits are offset by harms of screening, including an approximate 1% risk of hospitalization after biopsy. More importantly, an estimated 20 to 50% of screen-detected cancers are "overdiagnosed" (i.e., they may subject patients to risks of unnecessary treatment). Men undergoing prostatectomy have 1 in 8 chance of developing long-term urinary incontinence, and 1 in 3 men experience long-term sexual impotence. More than 1 in 7 men who have radiation therapy experience long-term erectile dysfunction, and up to 30% or so of men experience long-term bothersome bowel symptoms, including bowel urgency and fecal incontinence. Because of the small benefit of screening with the PSA and potential harms of overdiagnosis and overtreatment, the USPSTF recommends individual decision making among men aged 55 to 69 years. The USPSTF recommends against PSA screening in men aged 70 years and older due to lack of benefits and increased harms.[12]

LUNG CANCER

The USPSTF recommends annual screening with low-dose CT in adults aged 50 to 80 years who have at least a 20 pack-year smoking history and who currently smoke or have quit within the last 15 years, based on trials that reported relative reductions of death from lung cancer by 16 to 25% and of all-cause mortality by about 7%.[A10] The overall benefit of screening takes into account that individuals would have about two false positive CT scans over a lifetime of screening.[13] As many as 40% of screened persons will have another finding on CT, such as coronary artery calcification, a mass in the kidney or adrenal gland, or an aortic aneurysm.[14] These findings are of uncertain significance, but they may lead to additional procedures to evaluate them.

OSTEOPOROSIS

Tests of bone mineral density can identify men and women with a high risk for fracture as a result of osteoporosis and who may benefit from medications proved to lower the risk for fracture (Chapter 225). The USPSTF recommends screening for osteoporosis in women older than 65 years as well as in younger women who have risk factors that put them at comparable risk. The most widely used screening tool for the risk of hip fracture is bone mineral density of the hip assessed with dual-energy x-ray absorptiometry (DXA), although peripheral DXA and quantitative ultrasound are acceptable and have the advantage of portability. A tool developed by the World Health Organization (http://www.shef.ac.uk/FRAX/) incorporates bone mineral density and other risk factors, such as age and fracture history, to guide decisions.

THYROID DISEASE

Routine thyroid testing occasionally identifies patients with symptomatic but undiagnosed hypothyroidism (Chapter 207), but it more often detects subclinical hypothyroidism, which presents in 5% of women and 3% of men in the United States and is characterized by elevations in thyroid-stimulating hormone with normal levels of free thyroxine.

Because the benefits of treating subclinical hypothyroidism remain uncertain, the USPSTF does not recommend routine thyroid testing in the absence of symptoms. Clinicians should be alert to subtle signs of thyroid disease and have a low threshold for testing patients in high-risk groups, including postpartum and postmenopausal women.

DIABETES

Although the treatment of impaired fasting glucose or impaired glucose tolerance can delay progression to diabetes (Chapter 210), screening for type 2 diabetes does not improve mortality rates after 10 years of follow-up.[A11] Routine screening for diabetes beginning at age 45 years is recommended by some groups, but the USPSTF recommends screening for overweight or obese adults ages 35 to 70 years of age.[15] Clinicians should refer patients with abnormal blood glucose to intensive behavioral counseling interventions that can lower CVD risk. Although tight glucose control can reduce the incidence of microvascular disease, the benefit of early asymptomatic detection on clinically important retinopathy, neuropathy, and nephropathy is likely to be small.

HIV INFECTION

The USPSTF and Centers for Disease Control and Prevention (CDC) recommend screening for HIV infection (Chapters 356, 357, and 358) in all adolescents and adults aged 15 to 65 years,[16] including pregnant women.[17] Whether to continue screening after age 65 years depends upon risk factors such as new sexual partners. The optimal screening interval is unclear, but annual screening is reasonable in persons at very high risk, such as individuals who are actively engaged in risky sexual behaviors. Rescreening is not necessary in seronegative patients who have not been at increased risk since the last screen.

HEPATITIS B AND C INFECTIONS

Drugs for chronic hepatitis C and B infection (Chapter 135) have increased the ability to achieve viral suppression and prevent the complications of chronic liver disease in infected individuals.[A12] As a result, screening is recommended for hepatitis C in all adults ages 18 to 79 years, usually as just a one-time screen.[18] For hepatitis B, the evidence of a benefit is less clear,[A13] but screening is still recommended in adolescents and adults who are at increased risk of infection,[19] especially individuals born in countries with a high prevalence of hepatitis B or with a history of past or current injection drug use.

SEXUALLY TRANSMITTED DISEASE

Behavioral counseling is recommended to prevent sexually transmitted disease in sexually active adolescents and adults who are at increased risk.[A14,20] Screening for chlamydia and gonorrhea (Chapter 294) is recommended for all women aged 24 years and younger who are sexually active and for older women at risk.[A15,21] Nucleic acid amplification tests for chlamydia can be performed on cervical or urine specimens. Early detection of chlamydia can reduce pelvic inflammatory disease (Chapter 264), a risk factor for infertility and ectopic pregnancy. Similar benefits are likely from screening women for gonorrhea (Chapter 275). Women older than 25 years are at increased risk based on their current sexual behaviors and those of their partners. Syphilis testing is recommended in persons who are at increased risk for infection, such as persons with HIV, men who have sex with men, and people whose communities have an elevated prevalence of the disease.

VISION AND HEARING

Undetected but correctable vision (Chapter 391) and hearing (Chapter 396) problems are common in older adults and can be discovered by asking about problems and performing simple tests of visual acuity and hearing. Unfortunately, evidence is limited to show that regular screening leads to measurable benefits in function. Regular visual acuity testing is recommended for older adults by many organizations, but a large trial did not find any lasting benefits of screening, despite detecting many correctable causes of vision problems. The USPSTF concluded that evidence was insufficient[A16] to recommend routine vision or hearing screening.[22,23]

BEHAVIORAL INTERVENTIONS

Lifestyle factors contribute to a large proportion of preventable deaths in the United States. Brief interventions are effective for some behaviors such as smoking and problem drinking, but changing other behaviors usually requires more intensive approaches. The 5 As framework—ask, assess, advise, assist, and arrange—which was developed from smoking cessation research, provides a useful framework for counseling.

TOBACCO USE

Brief interventions can produce small but clinically important increases in quit rates among people who use tobacco. Effects increase with more intensive counseling and support, including the use of medication (Chapter 363).

MISUSE OF ALCOHOL AND DRUGS

The USPSTF recommends screening all adults 18 years or older for alcohol misuse (Chapter 364) with one of three tools: the 10-question AUDIT instrument, its 3-question version AUDIT-C (http://www.integration.samhsa.gov/images/res/tool_auditc.pdf), or a single question: "How many times in the past year have you had five (for men) or four (for women and adults over 65 years old) or more drinks in a day?" Brief multicontact behavioral interventions can successfully reduce alcohol consumption in at-risk adults who drink. The USPSTF also recommends screening for unhealthy drug use (Chapter 365), primarily based on the benefits of treating people with opioid use disorder.[24]

DIET AND PHYSICAL ACTIVITY

Counseling to promote a healthful diet (Chapter 13) and to promote physical activity (Chapter 14) can reduce the intake of saturated fat, increase the consumption of fruits and vegetables, and increase weekly physical activity. Studies of counseling also demonstrate small but potentially important improvements in CVD risk factors, including blood pressure, low-density lipoprotein cholesterol, and adiposity. Effects are most consistent with more intensive counseling (multiple sessions with trained counselors) and in higher-risk patients, such as those who have overweight or obesity or CVD risk factors (Chapters 14 and 13).

INJURY PREVENTION

Motor vehicle injuries are the leading cause of years of potential life lost before age 65 years. In older persons, falls are a leading cause of unintentional injury and can be reduced with exercise in community-dwelling seniors and targeted multicomponent interventions in highest-risk groups (Chapter 24). The USPSTF recommends that women of childbearing age be screened for intimate partner violence (Chapter 223)[25] but found insufficient evidence to recommend screening all elderly or other vulnerable adults for abuse and neglect.

IMMUNIZATIONS

Recommendations regarding immunization (Chapter 15) are regularly updated by the Advisory Committee on Immunization Practices of the CDC (http://www.cdc.gov/vaccines).[26]

Vaccination for COVID-19 is recommended (Chapter 337) for all adults and for children and adolescents 5 to 18 years, including a booster shot for adults. These recommendations are likely to be updated as the virus mutates or immunity wanes.

Annual influenza immunization is recommended for all adults. Pneumococcal vaccination is recommended for adults ages 65 years and older and is also indicated for younger adults with chronic heart, lung, or kidney disease; asthma; diabetes; asplenia and other immune disorders; as well as those who smoke. Two doses of varicella vaccine are recommended for all adults born in the United States after 1980 without other evidence of immunity, and two doses of zoster vaccine are recommended for all adults at age 60 years. Adults should be revaccinated once with the Tdap vaccine (tetanus, diphtheria, acellular pertussis) and every 10 years with Td; if their vaccination history is uncertain, complete primary immunization with two additional doses of Td is recommended. A series of three doses of a vaccine against HPV is recommended for young men and women ages 15 to up to age 26 years (only two doses are required for vaccination at ages 11 to 14 years) to reduce the risk for cervical cancer and genital warts, as well as to decrease transmission of the virus.

PREVENTIVE MEDICATIONS AND SUPPLEMENTS

Aspirin, postmenopausal hormone replacement therapy, breast cancer preventive medications, HIV preexposure prophylaxis (PrEP), and supplements of vitamins or minerals can carry both benefits and risks. Decisions need to consider the likely benefits (which increase with the underlying risk of the disease being prevented), the probability of harm, and the individual preferences of each patient.

ASPIRIN

In men and women without known vascular disease, aspirin reduces the risk for nonfatal myocardial infarction and ischemic stroke, but these benefits are often offset by an increased risk for serious gastrointestinal bleeding and hemorrhagic stroke.[A17] In men and women who have an elevated risk of CVD (10-year risk at least 10%), the benefits of aspirin outweigh risks by a small amount for adults ages 40 to 59 years. As a result, decisions regarding aspirin in this age range should be individualized based on additional consideration of risks and patients' values.[27] By comparison, the USPSTF found evidence that the harms outweigh the benefits in older adults[A18] and recommends against initiating aspirin therapy in adults ages 60 years or older (Chapter 70).

PREVENTIVE MEDICATIONS FOR BREAST CANCER

Tamoxifen, raloxifene, and aromatase inhibitors can reduce the incidence of invasive breast cancer in women at increased risk, but all have some harms. Tamoxifen and raloxifene increase the risk for thromboembolic events and worsen menopausal symptoms, tamoxifen also increases the risk for endometrial cancer (Chapter 184). Aromatase inhibitors worsen menopausal symptoms and are associated with gastrointestinal symptoms and musculoskeletal pain. The USPSTF recommends clinicians discuss the balance of benefits and harms of these medications with women over age 35 years who are at increased risk for breast cancer. Women most likely to benefit are those who are at low risk for the adverse effects of medications and whose 5-year risk of invasive breast cancer is 3% or higher. Online tools can be used to assess this risk (http://www.cancer.gov/bcrisktool/).

POSTMENOPAUSAL HORMONE THERAPY

Estrogen-only therapy in women over the age 50 years reduces the risk for developing diabetes and fractures in the near term, but it is also associated with a higher risk of gallbladder disease, stroke, and venous thromboembolism (Chapter 222).[A19] Combination therapy with estrogen and progestin, by comparison, reduces the risk of diabetes and fractures as well as colorectal cancer, but it increases the risk for invasive breast cancer, coronary heart disease, stroke, pulmonary embolism, gallbladder disease, urinary incontinence, and dementia.[A20] Hormone therapy is an option for younger menopausal women with persistent, troublesome menopausal symptoms (Chapter 222), but the USPSTF recommends against its routine use for preventive purposes.

HIV PREEXPOSURE PROPHYLAXIS

The use of daily tenofovir-based medications reduces the risk of HIV acquisition by about 50% in individuals who are at increased risk of HIV infection (Chapter 356).[A21] Adherence to daily use is a strong predictor of benefit. The USPSTF recommends HIV preexposure prophylaxis for persons at high risk of HIV infection, including persons with serodiscordant partners, who use condoms inconsistently with partners at high risk, or who have had a recent sexually transmitted infection. Preexposure prophylaxis is also recommended for persons who inject drugs and share needles (Chapter 365).[28]

VITAMIN AND MINERAL SUPPLEMENTATION

The USPSTF does not recommend routine use of vitamin or mineral supplements because there is no convincing evidence that multivitamins or individual or paired supplements (e.g., vitamin A, C, and D; folic acid; selenium; or calcium) reduce CVD, cancer, or all-cause mortality in community-dwelling average-risk adults. For vitamin E or beta-carotene, routine supplements are documented to be harmful. The USPSTF found insufficient evidence to support screening for vitamin D deficiency in adults[A22,29] or to suggest the routine use of calcium and vitamin D supplements for the primary prevention of fractures in ambulatory adults.

FUTURE ISSUES

Preventive care recommendations often vary based on a patient's characteristics such as age, sex, gender, and clinical risk factors, including behavior and race or ethnicity. Given well-described epidemiologic differences in the prevalence of diseases and their health impacts, prevention and treatment guidelines will likely become more specific for populations if and when sufficient evidence exists. Genomic testing has the potential for guiding personal recommendations for screening and prevention, but currently available genomic screening in average-risk individuals is limited by an incomplete understanding of the predictive value of specific genotypes in the general population, the uncertain effect of such information on clinical decisions, and concerns about the possible adverse effects of screening (e.g., anxiety, false reassurance, or discrimination). The USPSTF issues an annual report to Congress about research priorities: recent reports have focused on the need for more evidence about adult and child mental health, substance abuse and intimate partner violence, and health equity.[30]

GENERAL REFERENCES

For the General References and other additional features, please visit Elsevier eBooks+ at https://ebooks.health.elsevier.com.

Grade A References

A1. Patnode CD, Perdue LA, Rossom RC. Screening for cognitive impairment in older adults: updated evidence report and systematic review for the US Preventive Services Task Force. *JAMA.* 2020;323:764-785.

A2. Guirguis-Blake JM, Evans CV, Webber EM, et al. Screening for hypertension in adults: updated evidence report and systematic review for the US Preventive Services Task Force. *JAMA.* 2021;325:1657-1669.

A3. Gartlehner G, Vander Schaaf EB, Orr C, et al. Screening for hypertension in children and adolescents: updated evidence report and systematic review for the US Preventive Services Task Force. *JAMA.* 2020;324:1884-1895.

A4. Chou R, Cantor A, Dana T, et al. Statin use for the primary prevention of cardiovascular disease in adults: updated evidence report and systematic review for the US Preventive Services Task Force. *JAMA.* 2022;328:754-771.

A5. Guirguis-Blake JM, Beil TL, Senger CA, et al. Primary care screening for abdominal aortic aneurysm: updated evidence report and systematic review for the US Preventive Services Task Force. *JAMA.* 2019;322:2219-2238.

A6. Lin JS, Perdue LA, Henrikson NB, et al. Screening for colorectal cancer: updated evidence report and systematic review for the US Preventive Services Task Force. *JAMA.* 2021;325:1978-1997.

A7. Melnikow J, Henderson JT, Burda BU, et al. Screening for cervical cancer with high-risk human papilloma virus testing: updated evidence report and systematic review for the US Preventive Services Task Force. *JAMA.* 2018;320:687-705.

A8. Fenton JJ, Weyrich MS, Durbin S, et al. Prostate-specific antigen–based screening for prostate cancer: evidence report and systematic review for the US Preventive Services Task Force. *JAMA.* 2018;319:1914-1931.

A9. Center for Healthcare Policy and Research. Prostate-specific antigen–based screening for prostate cancer: a systematic evidence review for the U.S. Preventive Services Task Force. (Evidence syntheses, no. 154.) Rockville, MD: Agency for Healthcare Research and Quality, April 2017. AHRQ Publication No. 17-05229-EF-1.

A10. Jonas DE, Reuland DS, Reddy SM, et al. Screening for lung cancer with low-dose computed tomography: updated evidence report and systematic review for the US Preventive Services Task Force. *JAMA.* 2021;325:971-987.

A11. Jonas DE, Crotty K, Yun JDY, et al. Screening for prediabetes and type 2 diabetes: updated evidence report and systematic review for the US Preventive Services Task Force. *JAMA.* 2021;326:744-760.

A12. Chou R, Dana T, Fu R, et al. Screening for hepatitis C virus infection in adolescents and adults: updated evidence report and systematic review for the US Preventive Services Task Force. *JAMA.* 2020;323:976-991.

A13. Chou R, Blazina I, Bougatsos C, et al. Screening for hepatitis B virus infection in nonpregnant adolescents and adults: updated evidence report and systematic review for the US Preventive Services Task Force. *JAMA.* 2020;324:2423-2436.

A14. Henderson JT, Senger CA, Henninger M, et al. Behavioral counseling interventions to prevent sexually transmitted infections: updated evidence report and systematic review for the US Preventive Services Task Force. *JAMA.* 2020;324:682-699.

A15. Cantor A, Dana T, Griffin JC, et al. Screening for chlamydial and gonococcal infections updated evidence report and systematic review for the US Preventive Services Task Force. *JAMA.* 2021;326:957-966.

A16. Feltner C, Wallace IF, Kistler CE, et al. Screening for hearing loss in older adults: updated evidence report and systematic review for the US Preventive Services Task Force. *JAMA.* 2021;325:1202-1215.
A17. Zheng SL, Roddick AJ. Association of aspirin use for primary prevention with cardiovascular events and bleeding events: a systematic review and meta-analysis. *JAMA.* 2019;321:277-287.
A18. McNeil JJ, Nelson MR, Woods RL. Effect of aspirin on all-cause mortality in the healthy elderly. *N Engl J Med.* 2018;379:1519-1528.
A19. Prentice RL, Aragaki AK, Chlebowski RT, et al. Randomized trial evaluation of the benefits and risks of menopausal hormone therapy among women 50-59 years of age. *Am J Epidemiol.* 2021;190:365-375.
A20. Gartlehner G, Patel SV, Reddy S, et al. Hormone therapy for the primary prevention of chronic conditions in postmenopausal persons: updated evidence report and systematic review for the US Preventive Services Task Force. *JAMA.* 2022;328:1747-1765.
A21. Chou R, Evans C, Hoverman A, et al. Preexposure prophylaxis for the prevention of HIV infection: evidence report and systematic review for the US Preventive Services Task Force. *JAMA.* 2019;321:2214-2230.
A22. Kahwati LC, LeBlanc E, Weber RP, et al. Screening for vitamin D deficiency in adults: updated evidence report and systematic review for the US Preventive Services Task Force. *JAMA.* 2021;325:1443-1463.

TABLE 13-1 APPROXIMATE DAILY CALORIC NEEDS

		CALORIES NEEDED FOR EACH ACTIVITY LEVEL		
GENDER	AGE (YEARS)	SEDENTARY*	MODERATELY ACTIVE†	ACTIVE‡
Female	19–30	2000	2000–2200	2400
	31–50	1800	2000	2200
	51+	1600	1800	2000–2200
Male	19–30	2400	2600–2800	3000
	31–50	2200	2400–2600	2800–3000
	51+	2000	2200–2400	2400–2800

*Only light physical activity in a typical day.
†Physical activity equal to walking about 1 to 3 miles a day at 3 to 4 miles per hour, plus light physical activity.
‡Physical activity equal to walking more than 3 miles per day at 3 to 4 miles per hour, plus light physical activity.

13

DIET AND NUTRITION

DONALD D. HENSRUD

DIETARY REQUIREMENTS

The recommended dietary allowances for essential nutrients are the average daily level of intake shown to be sufficient to meet the nutrient requirements of nearly all (97 to 98%) healthy people. By comparison, the dietary reference intakes take into consideration the accumulating evidence on the relationships of diet and nutritional status to chronic diseases, such as coronary heart disease, cancer, diabetes, and the other leading causes of death. Dietary reference intakes recommend intake levels that not only prevent deficiencies but also may promote long-term health and disease prevention.

In this way, dietary guidelines have expanded from focusing on preventing deficiencies of isolated nutrients to preventing chronic disease, a goal that is especially important now that about 50% of all adult Americans have one or more preventable chronic diseases and over 70% of adults are overweight or obese. The 2020-2025 Dietary Guidelines for Americans translates average caloric requirements (Table 13-1) into specific recommendations that can reduce the likelihood of becoming overweight or obese.

NUTRITION'S INFLUENCE ON MORTALITY AND MORBIDITY

EVIDENCE OF CONNECTIONS BETWEEN DIET AND DISEASE

Deficiency conditions of specific nutrients have been well documented, but establishing conclusive relationships between diet and chronic diseases often relies on epidemiologic studies that are susceptible to unrecognized confounding and cannot infer causality. Nevertheless, the totality of consistent evidence from large population studies and randomized trials in at-risk individuals have brought clarity to the characteristics of dietary patterns that promote optimal health.

Diet should not be considered in isolation because other lifestyle factors also influence the risk of chronic diseases. The greatest nutritional public health problems in the United States and in many other parts of the world are overweight and obesity, with their associated comorbidities. Body weight is ultimately determined by the balance between energy intake through diet and energy expenditure through physical activity (Chapter 14). Recommendations for health promotion and disease prevention must include diet and physical activity, as well as other lifestyle factors.

DISEASES INFLUENCED BY NUTRITION

Of the 10 leading causes of death in the United States (Table 13-2),[1] 6 are related to diet, 4 to excess alcohol use (Chapter 364), and 6 to obesity (Chapter 201). Major causes of morbidity that often underlie causes of death (e.g., obesity, chronic liver disease, and hypertension) are also directly related to diet and nutrition.

TABLE 13-2 MAJOR CAUSES OF DEATH (2019) AND MORBIDITY IN THE UNITED STATES RELATED TO DIETARY FACTORS

CAUSE OF DEATH	NUMBER	%
1. Heart disease*,†	659,000	23
2. Cancer*,†,‡	600,000	21
3. Accidents‡	173,000	6
4. Chronic lower respiratory diseases†	157,000	6
5. Cerebrovascular diseases*,†,‡	150,000	5
6. Alzheimer disease*,†	121,000	4
7. Diabetes mellitus*,†	88,000	3
8. Kidney disease*	52,000	2
9. Pneumonia/influenza	50,000	2
10. Suicide‡	48,000	2
MORBIDITY		
1. Obesity*		
2. Chronic liver disease and cirrhosis†,‡		
3. Hypertension*,†		
4. Diverticular disease and constipation*		
5. Osteoporosis*		

*Related to diet and nutrition.
†Related to obesity.
‡Related to excess alcohol use.

The 2020-2025 Dietary Guidelines for Americans (Table 13-3)[2] outline critical ways for health professionals to help Americans make healthy choices. Although dietary recommendations promulgated by major professional societies for risk reduction and/or management of the major chronic diseases vary somewhat in their details (E-Table 13-1),[3–6] the close agreement among these recommendations enhances their credibility.

Cardiovascular Disease

Of the seven major risk factors for coronary heart disease, four are related to diet: hypercholesterolemia (Chapter 190), hypertension (Chapter 64), obesity (Chapter 201), and diabetes (Chapter 210). Elevated plasma low-density lipoprotein (LDL) cholesterol is a strong risk factor for coronary heart disease and is raised by increasing consumption of dietary saturated fat and *trans* fat. *Trans* fat also lowers high-density lipoprotein (HDL) cholesterol. Saturated fat is found in meat, full-fat dairy products, and tropical oils. *Trans* fat, which comes almost entirely from partially hydrogenated oils and has no health benefits, was removed from processed foods in 2018 by the U.S. Food and Drug Administration. Less emphasis is placed on limiting dietary cholesterol in recent guidelines because dietary cholesterol has a lesser effect on LDL cholesterol than saturated fat and is often found in the same foods. Limiting foods that contain saturated fat also limits dietary cholesterol. LDL cholesterol levels can be lowered by substituting healthier unsaturated fats (polyunsaturated or monounsaturated oils) or carbohydrates (preferably whole grains) for saturated fat. LDL cholesterol can also be lowered modestly by increasing the intake of soluble fiber and phytosterols from legumes, fruits, vegetables, and flax seed, as well as by consuming proteins and isoflavones from soy foods.

TABLE 13-3 DIETARY GUIDELINES FOR AMERICANS, 2020-2025: KEY RECOMMENDATIONS

1. Follow a healthy dietary pattern at every life stage.
   - For about the first 6 months of life, exclusively feed infants human milk.
   - At about 6 months, introduce infants to nutrient-dense complementary foods.
   - From 12 months through older adulthood, follow a healthy dietary pattern.
2. Customize and enjoy nutrient-dense food and beverage choices to reflect personal preferences, cultural traditions, and budgetary considerations.
3. Focus on meeting food group needs with nutrient-dense foods and beverages, and stay within calorie limits.
   - The core elements that make up a healthy dietary pattern include:
     - Vegetables of all types—dark green; red and orange; beans, peas, and lentils; starchy; and other vegetables
     - Fruits, especially whole fruit
     - Grains, at least half of which are whole grain
     - Dairy, including fat-free or low-fat milk, yogurt, and cheese, and/or lactose-free versions and fortified soy beverages and yogurt as alternatives
     - Protein foods, including lean meats, poultry, and eggs; seafood; beans, peas, and lentils; and nuts, seeds, and soy products
     - Oils, including vegetable oils and oils in food, such as seafood and nuts
4. Limit foods and beverages higher in added sugars, saturated fat, and sodium, and limit alcoholic beverages.
   - Added sugars—Less than 10% of calories per day starting at age 2. Avoid foods and beverages with added sugars for those less than 2 years of age
   - Saturated fat—Less than 10% of calories per day starting at age 2
   - Sodium—Less than 2300 milligrams per day, and even less for children younger than age 14
   - Alcoholic beverages—Adults of legal drinking age can choose not to drink or to drink in moderation by limiting intake to 2 drinks or less in a day for men and 1 drink or less in a day for women

Adapted from the *Dietary Guidelines for Americans, 2020-2025*. 9th ed. U.S. Department of Agriculture and U.S. Department of Health and Human Services. December 2020. https://www.dietaryguidelines.gov/. Accessed January 24, 2022.

Diet also can influence the risk of coronary heart disease in ways independent of LDL cholesterol and traditional risk factors, such as inflammation, oxidative stress, endothelial function, insulin sensitivity, and others. Consistent evidence from meta-analyses of large cohort studies has shown decreased cardiovascular and total mortality with increasing consumption of fruits and vegetables, whole grains, and nuts, as well as decreased incident coronary heart disease and total mortality from fish and olive oil.[7,8] Randomized trials are generally consistent with cohort studies, and a Mediterranean dietary pattern (Fig. 13-1) composed of many of these food groups can favorably affect cardiovascular risk factors and outcomes.[A1–A3] Diets such as the Dietary Approaches to Stop Hypertension (DASH) diet (Table 13-4) can reduce the incidence of cardiovascular disease by 30%.[A4] Higher-carbohydrate diets also can lower the risk of coronary heart disease in men by 20%, whereas the higher–unsaturated fat and higher-protein diets can reduce the risk by 30%.

Sodium intake clearly influences blood pressure, but much controversy has surrounded whether reducing sodium intake would truly be beneficial. In a cluster randomized trial in China, providing a salt substitute that was 75% sodium chloride and 25% potassium chloride to persons over age 60 years or with a history of stroke reduced cardiovascular events and death by 12 to 13% over a mean follow-up of 4.75 years.[A5] These data support the salt recommendations in Table 13-3.[9]

Moderate consumption of alcohol, defined as no more than one drink daily for women and two for men, has been associated with reduced risk of coronary heart disease, primarily by raising HDL cholesterol, inhibiting platelet aggregation, and stimulating fibrinolytic activity. National dietary data indicate that added sugar is associated with increased cardiovascular mortality. In addition, consumption of red and particularly processed meat has been associated with increased cardiovascular and total mortality.[10]

Cancer

About one third of cancers are due to suboptimal habits in diet,[11] physical activity, and weight management. Because cancer consists of many different conditions that share a common feature of uncontrolled abnormal cell division, risk factors, including diet, vary among different types of cancer. Nutrients, non-nutritive dietary constituents, and nutritional status can influence the risk for cancer through many different mechanisms, such as free radical scavenging

The Mediterranean Diet

Food/Food Group	Recommended Intake*	Tips
Vegetables	4 or more servings each day (one portion each day should be raw vegetables)	Eat a variety of colors and textures; a serving is 1 cup raw or ½ cup cooked vegetables.
Fruits	3 or more servings each day	Make fruit your dessert
Grains	4 or more servings each day	Choose mostly whole grains. 1 serving = 1 slice bread or ½ cup cooked oatmeal
Fats/Oils	Olive oil: 4 Tablespoons or more each day	Choose extra virgin olive oil and use in salad dressings and cooking; choose avocado or natural peanut butter instead of butter or margarine
Dried Beans/Nuts/Seeds	Nuts/Seeds: 3 or more servings each week Beans/Legumes: 3 or more servings each week	1 ounce or 1 serving = 23 almonds or 14 walnut halves; 1 serving of beans = ½ cup
Fish and Seafood	2-3 times each week	Choose salmon, sardines, and tuna, which are rich in omega-3 fatty acids
Herbs and Spices	Use daily	Season foods with herbs, garlic, onions, and spices instead of salt
Yogurt/Cheese/Egg and Poultry	Choose daily to weekly	Choose low-fat yogurt and cheeses; choose skinless chicken or turkey instead of red meat
Alcohol/Wine	Men: 1-2 glasses each day Women: 1 glass each day	Always ask your clinician if alcohol is ok for you to consume.

FIGURE 13-1. Mediterranean Diet. Choosing a diet similar to one eaten by people living around the Mediterranean Sea may lower the risk of cardiovascular disease and have additional health benefits. The diet is mostly plant-based with high amounts of fresh vegetables, fruits, nuts, dried beans, olive oil, and fish. *Serving sizes should be individualized to meet energy and nutrient needs. Red meats, processed meats, and sweets should be limited. (Adapted from Mediterranean Diet. https://www.nutrition.va.gov/docs/UpdatedPatientEd/Mediterraneandiet.pdf. U.S. Department of Veterans Affairs. Accessed January 24, 2022.)

TABLE 13-4 DIETARY APPROACHES TO STOP HYPERTENSION (DASH)

FOOD GROUP	SERVINGS PER DAY 1600 CALORIES	2000 CALORIES	2600 CALORIES	SERVING SIZES	EXAMPLES AND NOTES	SIGNIFICANCE OF EACH FOOD GROUP TO THE DASH EATING PLAN
Grains*	6	6–8	10–11	1 slice bread 1 oz dry cereal† ½ cup cooked rice, pasta, or cereal	Whole wheat bread and rolls, whole wheat pasta, English muffin, pita bread, bagel, cereals, grits, oatmeal, brown rice, unsalted pretzels, and popcorn	Major sources of energy and fiber
Vegetables	3–4	4–5	5–6	1 cup raw leafy vegetable ½ cup cut-up raw or cooked vegetable ½ cup vegetable juice	Broccoli, carrots, collards, green beans, green peas, kale, lima beans, potatoes, spinach, squash, sweet potatoes, tomatoes	Rich sources of potassium, magnesium, and fiber
Fruits	4	4–5	5–6	1 medium fruit ¼ cup dried fruit ½ cup fresh, frozen, or canned fruit ½ cup fruit juice	Apples, apricots, bananas, dates, grapes, oranges, grapefruit, grapefruit juice, mangoes, melons, peaches, pineapples, raisins, strawberries, tangerines	Important sources of potassium, magnesium, and fiber
Fat-free or low-fat milk and milk products	2–3	2–3	3	1 cup milk or yogurt 1½ oz cheese	Fat-free (skim) or low-fat (1%) milk or buttermilk; fat-free, low-fat, or reduced-fat cheese; fat-free or low-fat regular or frozen yogurt	Major sources of calcium and protein
Lean meats, poultry, and fish	3–6	6 or less	6	1 oz cooked meats, poultry, or fish 1 egg‡	Select only lean meats; trim away visible fat; broil, roast, or poach; remove skin from poultry	Rich sources of protein and magnesium
Nuts, seeds, and legumes	3 per week	4–5 per week	1	⅓ cup or 1½ oz nuts 2 Tbsp peanut butter 2 Tbsp or ½ oz seeds ½ cup cooked legumes (dry beans and peas)	Almonds, hazelnuts, mixed nuts, peanuts, walnuts, sunflower seeds, peanut butter, kidney beans, lentils, split peas	Rich sources of energy, magnesium, protein, and fiber
Fats and oils§	2	2–3	3	1 tsp soft margarine 1 tsp vegetable oil 1 Tbsp mayonnaise 2 Tbsp salad dressing	Soft margarine, vegetable oil (such as canola, corn, olive, or safflower), low-fat mayonnaise, light salad dressing	The DASH study had 27% of calories as fat, including fat in or added to foods
Sweets and added sugars	0	5 or less per week	<2	1 Tbsp sugar 1 Tbsp jelly or jam ½ cup sorbet, gelatin 1 cup lemonade	Fruit-flavored gelatin, fruit punch, hard candy, jelly, maple syrup, sorbet and ices, sugar	Sweets should be low in fat

*Whole grains are recommended for most grain servings as a good source of fiber and nutrients.
†Serving sizes vary between ½ cup and 1¼ cups, depending on cereal type. Check the product's Nutrition Facts label.
‡Because eggs are high in cholesterol, limit egg yolk intake to no more than four per week; two egg whites have the same protein content as 1 oz of meat.
§Fat content changes serving amount for fats and oils. For example, 1 Tbsp of regular salad dressing equals one serving; 1 Tbsp of a low-fat dressing equals one-half serving; 1 Tbsp of a fat-free dressing equals zero servings.
oz = ounce; Tbsp = tablespoon; tsp = teaspoon.
Adapted from National Heart, Lung and Blood Institute. In brief: your guide to lowering your blood pressure with DASH. NIH Publication No. 06-5834. https://www.nhlbi.nih.gov/files/docs/public/heart/dash_brief.pdf. Accessed January 24, 2022.

and DNA repair. Supplementation with individual nutrients has had limited success in preventing and treating cancer. Therefore, as with heart disease, a focus on foods and dietary patterns provides the best nutritional approach to preventing cancer.

Obesity (Chapter 201) is now recognized as a major risk factor for at least 12 cancers, perhaps by elevating serum levels of insulin and leptin, inducing insulin resistance, and creating a chronic inflammatory state (Chapter 164). Excess alcohol intake (Chapter 364) also increases the risk for many cancers, including liver, breast, and the entire gastrointestinal tract.

Lung Cancer

Although the most important causal factor in the number-one cancer killer, lung cancer (Chapter 177), is cigarette smoking, consumption of fruit is inversely associated with the risk of lung cancer in both smokers and nonsmokers. Two large, randomized trials of supplementation with β-carotene reported increased mortality from lung cancer and all causes, primarily in smokers and former smokers, so β-carotene supplementation should be avoided.

Breast Cancer

The number-two cause of cancer deaths in women is breast cancer (Chapter 183). Postmenopausal breast cancer is positively associated with obesity, especially when excess adiposity is located predominantly in the abdomen. Paradoxically, the risk of premenopausal breast cancer is decreased with obesity. Alcohol increases and lactation probably decreases the risk of both types of breast cancer.

Colorectal Cancer

Colorectal cancer (Chapter 179) is the third leading cause of cancer mortality in men and women. The risk for colorectal cancer correlates positively with the intake of red and processed meats, obesity, and alcohol. The World Health Organization has classified processed meat as a carcinogen and red meat as a probable carcinogen. Foods that contain dietary fiber (as opposed to fiber per se), dairy products, and calcium appear to decrease risk.[12,13]

Prostate Cancer

Although studies have evaluated different dietary factors on the risk of prostate cancer, the clearest risk factor is obesity.

Liver Cancer

The strongest risk factor for liver cancer is alcohol, but obesity also increases risk in part via nonalcoholic fatty liver disease (Chapter 138). Aflatoxins are a strong risk factor, primarily outside the United States where they are more prevalent in the food supply. Coffee appears to be protective against liver cancer.

Pancreas Cancer

Associations exist between pancreas cancer and various dietary factors, but causality is not clear except for obesity, which increases risk.

Recommendations

Although there are differences among dietary risks for different cancers, the American Cancer Society Guidelines for Cancer Prevention are generally similar to other major dietary guidelines: consuming a plant-based diet, regular physical activity, and maintenance of a healthy body weight. Alcohol intake is the primary difference between guidelines to prevent heart disease, for which moderate consumption may be beneficial, and guidelines to prevent cancer, for which consumption increases risk even at low levels for some cancers, such as breast cancer and head and neck cancer. Randomized trials with isolated nutrients including carotenoids, vitamins C and E, folic acid, selenium, and even dietary fiber have not shown a benefit for reducing the risk of cancer. Whole plant foods contain hundreds of different vitamins, nutrients, and other phytochemicals that may collectively reduce the risk of cancer more than specific nutrients.

Hypertension

Elevated blood pressure (Chapter 64) is a major risk factor for stroke (Chapters 376 and 377), coronary heart disease (Chapter 40), heart failure (Chapter 45), peripheral vascular disease (Chapter 65), and renal disease (Chapter 116). Five lifestyle factors can reduce blood pressure: weight loss if overweight or obese, the DASH diet, increased physical activity, sodium restriction, and alcohol restriction. Obesity, especially abdominal obesity, is associated with hypertension, and weight reduction is the strongest lifestyle change that decreases blood pressure. The DASH diet (see Table 13-4) can lower blood pressure as much as drug treatment (11.6/5.3 mm Hg) in individuals with hypertension.

Diabetes Mellitus

Type 2 diabetes mellitus (Chapter 210) is strongly associated with obesity, especially abdominal obesity, so maintenance of a desirable body weight throughout life is of major importance in both preventing and treating type 2 diabetes. Sugar consumption does not have a large impact on developing diabetes, except to the extent that it may promote weight gain. However, sugar-sweetened beverages contribute to weight gain and an increased risk of type 2 diabetes. A high–glycemic index (a measure of the amount a food increases blood glucose) diet also increases risk. Red and particularly processed meats increase the risk of type 2 diabetes. Coffee intake decreases the risk of diabetes in a dose-dependent fashion. A Mediterranean dietary pattern (see Fig. 13-1) higher in healthy fat can lead to slightly better glucose control than a high-carbohydrate diet. However, a higher-carbohydrate diet can still be utilized, provided that calories are controlled and preferably whole grains are emphasized. An overall healthy eating pattern helps also reduce the risk for cardiovascular disease, which is the main cause of death in patients with diabetes.

Osteoporosis

Adequate intake of calcium, vitamin D, and protein in childhood is important for achieving optimal peak bone mass in adulthood and preventing osteoporosis (Chapter 225) later in life. Dairy products are the primary source of calcium for most children. Adults should try to achieve the recommended dietary allowance for calcium (1000 mg/day until age 50 for women and age 70 for men, then 1200 mg/day), primarily through dietary calcium with supplemental calcium as necessary. The optimum intake and blood level of vitamin D are controversial. Adults should try to achieve an intake of vitamin D at the level of the recommended dietary allowance (600 IU/day until age 70, then 800 IU/day). Fruit and vegetable intake is associated with increased bone density through various mechanisms. Vitamin K, magnesium, and zinc are involved in bone metabolism, but supplementation has not been demonstrated to be beneficial to bone health. Excessive supplementation with vitamin A increases the risk of fracture, as does excess alcohol consumption.

Other Conditions

Obesity

Obesity is the most prevalent nutritional disorder in the United States (see Chapter 201). The metabolic syndrome (a constellation that includes obesity with a large waist circumference, increased levels of serum glucose and triglycerides, high blood pressure, and a reduced HDL cholesterol level) is strikingly prevalent in the United States and is a major risk factor for coronary heart disease, cancer, type 2 diabetes, and hypertension (Chapter 64). Globally, and even in some locales in the United States, malnutrition (Chapter 198) may exist in close proximity to overweight and obesity.[14,15]

Intestinal Diverticular Disease

Low dietary fiber intake causes constipation (Chapter 118), and it is thought to be a cause of intestinal diverticular disease (Chapter 128).

Dementia

Although physical activity is the strongest lifestyle factor that is associated with the avoidance of cognitive decline, dietary factors also play a role. Observational studies suggest that Mediterranean and DASH diets may help preserve cognitive function, in part by reducing the risk of cerebrovascular disease. Limited data raise the probability that even more emphasis on increasing the intake of green leafy vegetables, berries, fish, nuts, and olive oil, as well as limiting the intake of red meats, pastries, and sweets, may be even more beneficial.

Congenital Neural Tube Defects

Inadequate maternal folic acid intake (Chapter 199) has been definitively proven to be a major risk factor for congenital neural tube defects, such as spina bifida and myelomeningocele. For this reason, cereal and grain products have been fortified with folic acid in the United States since 1998, and supplementation with folic acid is recommended in all women capable of becoming pregnant (Chapter 219).

Dietary Supplements

Relatively few dietary supplements have demonstrated benefit in preventing disease. Although higher blood concentrations of vitamin C, carotenoids, and vitamin E are associated with lower mortality, this finding appears to be because they are markers of a better diet.[16] Meta-analyses of randomized, controlled trials of antioxidants have reported increased total mortality from vitamin A, vitamin E, and β-carotene. Vitamin D and calcium are necessary for adequate bone health, and vitamin D may have other health benefits, but the evidence is inconclusive. For example, vitamin D supplementation does not improve musculoskeletal health,[A6] reduce the risk of depression,[A7] or reduce the risk of cancer, cardiovascular disease, or mortality in adults.[A8] Although multivitamins are one of the most widely used dietary supplements, with over one third of Americans taking them, there is little evidence that they prevent cardiovascular disease or cancer. Fish consumption is associated with decreased cardiovascular disease, yet randomized trials have found no benefit from omega-3 supplementation,[A9] with the exception of icosapent ethyl (a highly purified eicosapentaenoic acid ethyl ester at 4 g daily), which can reduce future cardiovascular events by 25% in patients who already have very high-risk cardiovascular disease and have elevated serum triglyceride levels (135 to 499 mg/dL).[A10] By comparison, dietary supplements with vitamins C and E, zinc, copper, lutein, and zeaxanthin may benefit patients with early macular degeneration.[A11]

TRANSLATING EVIDENCE INTO DIETARY CHANGE

The evidence is strong that dietary habits can influence the incidence and severity of many incapacitating or lethal diseases.[17–19] No justification exists for the belief that modification of the "usual" American diet is unnecessary or futile. The following statement from the Scientific Report of the 2020 Dietary Guidelines Advisory Committee concisely outlines the optimal dietary pattern based on current evidence: "Common characteristics of dietary patterns associated with positive health outcomes include higher intake of vegetables, fruits, legumes, whole grains, low- or non-fat dairy, lean meat and poultry, seafood, nuts, and unsaturated vegetable oils and low consumption of red and processed meats, sugar-sweetened foods and drinks, and refined grains."[20] Various organizations have provided dietary recommendations generally consistent with this statement (see E-Table 13-1). The U.S. Departments of Agriculture and of Health and Human Services have developed and periodically revised the Dietary Guidelines for Americans (see Table 13-3). The Dietary Guidelines list three dietary patterns of eating that are consistent with the guidelines and people can use as a practical template to follow: the Healthy U.S., Healthy Vegetarian, and Healthy Mediterranean. A food guidance system, now called MyPlate (Fig. 13-2), is part of a larger communications initiative to help consumers make better food choices. Physicians can influence their patients' health by encouraging them to optimize their dietary habits and providing them with instructional materials, assistance from dietitians, or behavioral counseling,[A12] particularly in patients who are overweight, obese, or have other cardiovascular risk factors.[21]

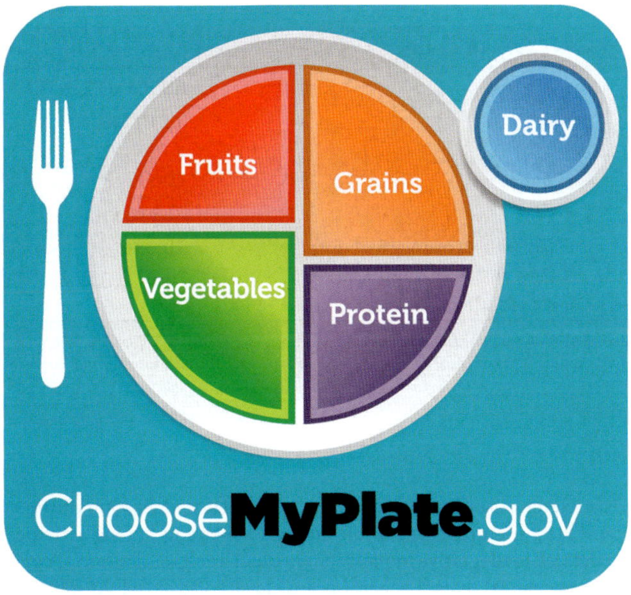

FIGURE 13-2. **U.S. Department of Agriculture's MyPlate.** MyPlate illustrates that a substantial proportion of dietary intake should be derived from vegetables, fruits, and grains, as contrasted with many Americans' expectation that protein sources should dominate. For more information, see www.ChooseMyPlate.gov.

GENERAL REFERENCES

For the General References and other additional features, please visit Elsevier eBooks+ at https://ebooks.health.elsevier.com.

Grade A References

A1. Rees K, Takeda A, Martin N, et al. Mediterranean-style diet for the primary and secondary prevention of cardiovascular disease. *Cochrane Database Syst Rev*. 2019;3:CD009825.

A2. Estruch R, Ros E, Salas-Salvadó J, et al. Primary prevention of cardiovascular disease with a Mediterranean diet. *N Engl J Med*. 2018;378:e34.1-e34.14.

A3. Delgado-Lista J, Alcala-Diaz JF, Torres-Peña JD, et al. Long-term secondary prevention of cardiovascular disease with a Mediterranean diet and a low-fat diet (CORDIOPREV): a randomised controlled trial. *Lancet*. 2022;399:1876-1885.

A4. Filippou CD, Tsioufis CP, Thomopoulos CG, et al. Dietary Approaches to Stop Hypertension (DASH) diet and blood pressure reduction in adults with and without hypertension: a systematic review and meta-analysis of randomized controlled trials. *Adv Nutr*. 2020;11:1150-1160.

A5. Neal B, Wu Y, Feng X, et al. Effect of salt substitution on cardiovascular events and death. *N Engl J Med*. 2021;385:1067-1077.

A6. Bolland MJ, Grey A, Avenell A. Effects of vitamin D supplementation on musculoskeletal health: a systematic review, meta-analysis, and trial sequential analysis. *Lancet Diabetes Endocrinol*. 2018;6:847-858.

A7. Okereke OI, Reynolds CF 3rd, Mischoulon D, et al. Effect of long-term vitamin D3 supplementation vs placebo on risk of depression or clinically relevant depressive symptoms and on change in mood scores: a randomized clinical trial. *JAMA*. 2020;324:471-480.

A8. Manson JE, Cook NR, Lee IM, et al. Vitamin D supplements and prevention of cancer and cardiovascular disease. *N Engl J Med*. 2019;380:33-44.

A9. Manson JE, Cook NR, Lee IM, et al. Marine n-3 fatty acids and prevention of cardiovascular disease and cancer. *N Engl J Med*. 2019;380:23-32.

A10. Bhatt DL, Steg PG, Miller M, et al. Cardiovascular risk reduction with icosapent ethyl for hypertriglyceridemia. *N Engl J Med*. 2019;380:11-22.

A11. Evans JR, Lawrenson JG. Antioxidant vitamin and mineral supplements for slowing the progression of age-related macular degeneration. *Cochrane Database Syst Rev*. 2017;7:CD000254.

A12. Patnode CD, Redmond N, Iacocca MO, et al. Behavioral counseling interventions to promote a healthy diet and physical activity for cardiovascular disease prevention in adults without known cardiovascular disease risk factors: updated evidence report and systematic review for the US Preventive Services Task Force. *JAMA*. 2022;328:375-388.

14

PHYSICAL ACTIVITY

WILLIAM E. KRAUS

DEFINITIONS

Physical activity can be broadly defined as bodily movement produced by skeletal muscles. *Exercise* refers to the subset of physical activity involving a structured program to improve physical fitness. *Health-enhancing physical activity* refers to the subset of physical activities that result in health benefits—generally activity involving large muscle groups of the body and substantial expenditures of energy. The two most important types of health-enhancing physical activity are moderate- to vigorous-intensity aerobic physical activity and moderate- to vigorous-intensity muscle strengthening activity.

Regular physical activity improves *health-related physical fitness*—the physiologic components of fitness that influence the risk of disease, functional limitations, disability, and premature mortality. These components include cardiorespiratory endurance (aerobic capacity); skeletal muscle strength, power, and endurance; body composition and bone strength; balance, flexibility, and reaction time.

The primary attributes of physical activity are *type* (mode), *frequency*, *duration*, and *intensity*. Types of physical activity (e.g., walking, swimming, lifting, stretching) are grouped according to their main physiologic effects into well-known categories: *aerobic* (or "cardio"), *muscle strengthening*, *flexibility*, and *balance*. Intensity is the effort level during activity. For aerobic activity, the *absolute intensity* is measured in metabolic equivalents (METs). One MET is the resting metabolic rate, which is commonly taken to be 3.5 mL O_2/kg/minute in adults. The *relative intensity* is measured as the percentage of oxygen uptake reserve (aerobic capacity) required to perform an activity (Table 14-1). In practice, the generally linear relationship between heart rate and oxygen uptake makes it reasonable to use the heart rate to monitor the relative intensity of exercise. When the heart rate is not monitored, options for estimating relative intensity (Table 14-2) include the "talk test" and Rating of Perceived Exertion scale, where 6 equals no exertion and 20 equals maximal exertion.

The *volume* (or amount) of activity is the product of frequency, duration, and intensity. Volume can be measured (e.g., by questionnaires) as MET-minutes per week (a sum of the MET intensity of all activities multiplied by the minutes each activity is performed). Volume can also be assessed using wearable devices, such as accelerometers, which are calibrated to translate body movement into measures of volume.

TABLE 14-1 EXAMPLES OF MET LEVEL REQUIREMENTS

PHYSICAL ACTIVITY	MET	ACTIVITIES OF DAILY LIVING
LIGHT-INTENSITY ACTIVITIES	**<3**	**LIGHT ACTIVITIES**
Sleeping	0.9	Bathing in tub/eating
Watching television	1.0	Writing, desk work, typing
Walking, 1.7 mph (2.7 km/h), level ground, strolling, very slow	2.3	Light housework Warm shower - sitting
Walking, 2.5 mph (4 km/h)	2.9	Fixing meals
MODERATE-INTENSITY ACTIVITIES	**3 TO 6**	**MODERATE ACTIVITIES**
Bicycling, stationary, 50 watts, very light effort	3.0	Washing floors
Walking 3.0 mph (4.8 km/h)	3.3	Warm shower - standing
Calisthenics, home exercise, light or moderate effort general	3.5	Grocery shopping/vacuuming
Walking 3.4 mph (5.5 km/h)	3.6	Mowing lawn - riding
Bicycling, <10 mph (km/h), leisure, to work or for pleasure	4.0	Gardening - weeding and raking Gardening - digging
Bicycling, stationary, 100 watts, light effort	5.5	Snow shoveling
VIGOROUS-INTENSITY ACTIVITIES	**>6**	**VIGOROUS ACTIVITIES**
Jogging, general	7.0	Mowing lawn - walking
Calisthenics (e.g., push-ups, sit-ups, pull-ups, jumping jacks), heavy, vigorous effort	8.0	Chopping wood
Running jogging, in place	8.0	Carpentry work
Rope jumping	10.0	

MET = metabolic equivalents.
Data from St. Mary's General Hospital.

TABLE 14-2 CRITERIA FOR ASSESSING RELATIVE AND ABSOLUTE INTENSITY OF AEROBIC ACTIVITY

	RELATIVE INTENSITY			ABSOLUTE INTENSITY
Intensity	Percentage of heart rate reserve or oxygen uptake reserve	Rating of Perceived Exertion	Talk Test	MET Level
Sedentary behavior	<20*	<9	Can sing	1.0-≤1.5
Light	20-39*	9-11	Can sing	>1.5-<3.0
Moderate	40-<60	12-14	Can talk without pausing for breath, but cannot sing	3.0-<6.0
Vigorous	>60	14-17	Cannot talk without pausing for breath	≥6.0

*Information in table adapted from multiple sources, including guidelines by the American College of Sports Medicine (ACSM) (*ACSM's Guidelines for Exercise Testing and Prescription*. Eleventh Edition. Lippincott Williams & Wilkins: 2022). Note ACSM classifies >90%-100% of heart rate reserve and rating of perceived exertion levels of 18-20 as "near maximal to maximal." The table provides guidelines for individuals to characterize the intensity of physical activity.
MET = metabolic equivalents (see text for details).

TABLE 14-3 KEY PHYSICAL ACTIVITY GUIDELINES FOR ADULTS

All adults should avoid inactivity. Some physical activity is better than none, and adults who participate in any amount of physical activity gain some health benefits.

For substantial health benefits, adults should do at least 150 min (2.5 hr)/wk of moderate-intensity aerobic activity or 75 min (1.25 hr)/wk of vigorous-intensity aerobic activity, or an equivalent combination of moderate- and vigorous-intensity aerobic activity. However, recent evidence shows that bouts of exercise lasting less than 10 minutes also have health benefits.

For additional and more extensive health benefits, adults should increase their aerobic physical activity to 300 min (5 hr)/wk of moderate-intensity or 150 min (2.5 hr)/wk of vigorous-intensity aerobic physical activity, or an equivalent combination of moderate- and vigorous-intensity activity. Additional health benefits are gained by engaging in physical activity beyond this amount.

Adults should also do muscle-strengthening activities that are moderate or high intensity and involve all major muscle groups on 2 or more days/wk, as these activities provide additional health benefits.

Adapted from U.S. Department of Health and Human Services. 2018 Physical Activity Guidelines for Americans. https://health.gov/paguidelines/pdf/paguide.pdf. Washington, DC: U.S. Accessed January 4, 2022.

EPIDEMIOLOGY

Physical Activity Levels

About 50% of U.S. adults report that they meet public health guidelines (Table 14-3) for moderate-to-vigorous physical activity, about 25% report that they meet guidelines for muscle-strengthening activity, and about 25% of adults report that they meet both guidelines.[1] Among U.S. men and women ages 17 to 42 years, about 70% report adequate physical activity for military service, but only about one third are both adequately active and eligible based on their body mass index.[2] In the United States, men, White individuals, younger people, and people with greater incomes and education on average report more physical activity. Furthermore, although recreational physical activity is either stable or slightly improving, Americans have experienced a steady decline in occupational physical activity over the past five decades, and it is likely that levels of physical activity around the home have also declined.

Preventive Health Benefits in Adults

There is strong evidence that health-enhancing physical activity (Table 14-2) reduces the risk for premature mortality and coronary artery disease (Chapter 59), stroke (Chapter 376), high blood pressure (Chapter 64), adverse lipid profile (Chapter 190), type 2 diabetes mellitus (Chapter 210), metabolic syndrome, osteoporosis (Chapter 225), colon cancer (Chapter 179), breast cancer (Chapter 183), obesity (Chapter 201), and depression (Chapter 362).[3,4] The reduction in risk is substantial: for example, when active and inactive adults are compared, the risk reduction is greater than or equal to 30% for all-cause mortality, cardiovascular disease,[5] stroke, hypertension, colon cancer, and type 2 diabetes. Randomized trials show that multicomponent exercise programs, most commonly focused on balance training and muscle-strengthening activity, reduce the risk of falls and fall-related fractures by as much as 40%,[A1] and balance training likely improves physical function in older adults.[A2] Randomized trials show that exercise in older adults reduces the risk of hospitalization and mortality by 30%.[A3] Health-enhancing aerobic and muscle-strengthening activities also reduce the risk for cognitive impairment in older adults and improve cognition in adults over age 50 years,[A4] in part because levels of glycosylphosphatidylinositol, which is produced in the liver, increase with exercise and mitigate aging in the brain.[6] However, exercise does not slow cognitive decline in patients with mild to moderate dementia (Chapter 371).[A5] Some evidence also suggests that physical activity reduces the risk for anxiety disorders, osteoarthritis, sleep disorders, and back pain, as well as many types of cancer.

By some estimates, 10% or more of aggregate U.S. health care expenditures are related to inadequate physical activity. The benefits of physical activity are independent of other risk factors. For example, a sedentary obese smoker achieves health benefits from exercise, even if they continue to smoke and remain obese. When a healthy diet, regular activity, and abstinence from smoking occur together, the lifestyle effects are dramatic.

Mechanisms of Effect and Dose Response

The health benefits of physical activity are due to multiple incompletely understood physiologic effects. For example, physical activity reduces blood pressure in people with hypertension (Chapter 64).[A6] Possible mechanisms include reducing sympathetic activity and increasing vagal tone, reducing norepinephrine levels, releasing vasodilators such as endorphins, reducing insulin resistance, reducing plasma renin levels, and preventing overweight and obesity. In adults with type 2 diabetes, the effects of physical activity on skeletal muscle include changes in contractile protein isoforms, mitochondrial volume and functional capacity, metabolic regulation, intracellular signaling, and neuromuscular function.[A7]

Rather than its intensity or frequency, the dominant determinant of the health benefits of physical activity is likely the total weekly volume (amount) of moderate-to-vigorous physical activity. Substantial health benefits begin to accrue with a volume of 500 to 1000 MET-minutes/week. An adult can accumulate 500 MET-minutes by walking at 3.0 miles per hour (a 3.3-MET activity) on 3 days a week for 50 minutes (3.3 METs × 3 × 50 minutes = ≈500 MET-minutes). When measured by caloric expenditure, this volume of walking in a 75-kg (165-lb) adult expends an extra 430 kcal in addition to the 190 kcal that would have been expended at rest.

The dose-response relationship between moderate-to-vigorous physical activity volume and health benefits is curvilinear. The marginal benefit of activity at even low amounts is substantial, and the marginal benefit decreases with greater amounts of activity. Mortality risks fall by 20% with minimal activity, by 30% in people who meet the minimum recommendation of 7.5 MET hours of activity per week, and by about 40% in people who perform more than twice that amount.

The dose of moderate-to-vigorous physical activity reflects both energy expenditure (amount) and intensity. Thus, some health benefits should occur at low energy expenditure (i.e., low doses of moderate-to-vigorous physical activity) and at low intensity (i.e., light intensity). For example, 15 minutes per day (90 minutes per week) of moderate-intensity activity is associated with about a 15% decrease in mortality. Even at lower levels of moderate-to-vigorous physical activity, more energy expenditure from light-intensity activity, as indicated by less sitting time, is associated with lower mortality. However, greater amounts of moderate-to-vigorous physical activity (e.g., about 60 to 75 minutes per day) may be sufficient to eliminate the adverse effects of sitting. Muscle-strengthening activity also appears to be associated with lower risk of all-cause mortality, independent of the

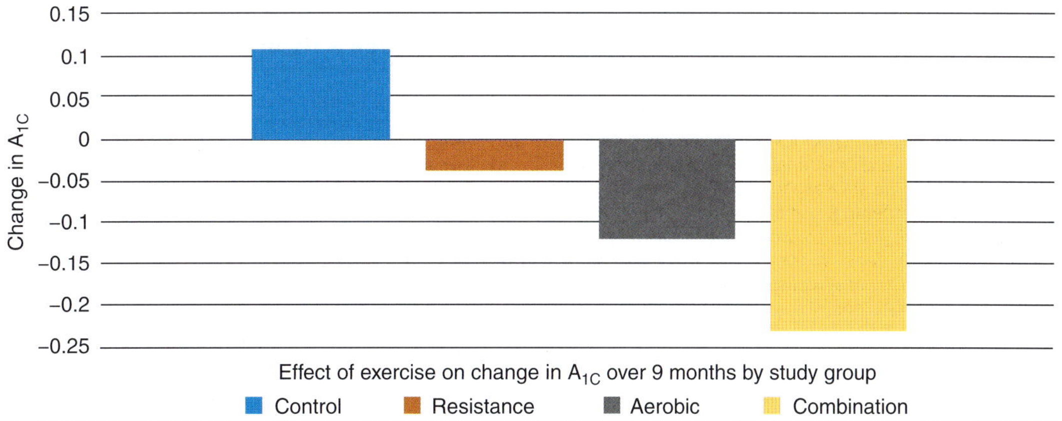

FIGURE 14-1. Changes in hemoglobin A_{1c} levels in a 9-month randomized trial comparing three exercise interventions to a control in adults with type 2 diabetes (total N = 262). The largest improvement in A_{1c} occurred with combined aerobic exercise and resistance training (muscle-strengthening activity). (Data from Church TS, Blair SN, Cocreham S, et al. Effects of aerobic and resistance training on hemoglobin A_{1c} levels in patients with type 2 diabetes: a randomized controlled trial. *JAMA*. 2010;304:2253-2262.)

amount of aerobic activity. Additionally, a combination of strength training and aerobic training produces greater health benefits than either alone to promote physical function in older adults, to lower hemoglobin A_{1c} levels in people with diabetes (Fig. 14-1), and to improve insulin sensitivity in adults with metabolic syndrome.

TREATMENT

Therapeutic Health Benefits in Adults

Clinical practice guidelines assign a substantial therapeutic role to physical activity in patients with coronary heart disease, high blood pressure (Chapter 64), type 2 diabetes (Chapter 210), obesity (Chapter 201), osteoporosis (Chapter 225), osteoarthritis (Chapter 241), claudication (Chapter 65), and chronic obstructive pulmonary disease (Chapter 76). Physical activity also plays a role in the management of depression and anxiety disorders (Chapter 362), elevated cholesterol levels (Chapter 190), pain (Chapter 26), heart failure (Chapter 46),[A8] syncope (Chapter 50), stroke (Chapter 375), back pain (Chapter 369), dementia (Chapter 371), and constipation (Chapter 123), as well as in the prophylaxis of venous thromboembolism (Chapter 68). Although there is more evidence for the therapeutic effects of aerobic exercise, muscle strengthening exercise also can have therapeutic effects, which can be additive or synergistic to those of aerobic exercise alone.

Health Risks of Physical Activity

Physical activity and exercise have some risks. Musculoskeletal injuries are by far the most common type of activity-related adverse event. The risk of injury depends on the type and volume of activity. The weekly volume of activity is directly related to the risk of musculoskeletal injuries, but when following public health guidelines of about 500 to 1000 MET-minutes/week, the risk of injury is low. The risk of injury is directly related to the rate of increase in the dose of activity, with more rapid increases having greater risk. Previous musculoskeletal injuries, excess weight, and low physical fitness also increase the risk of injury.

Relatively vigorous physical activity acutely increases the risk for sudden cardiac death (Chapter 50) and acute myocardial infarction (Chapter 58). However, the risk of sudden death and nonfatal events during and immediately after physical activity is extremely low—well below 1 event per 1,000,000 person-hours of activity. Importantly, physically active adults are protected from fatal and nonfatal cardiac events, with about 70% reduction in their risk of sudden death. This protection occurs because the time spent in vigorous activity per day is relatively small, so the risk of sudden cardiac death secondary to vigorous activity is far outweighed by the protective effect on cardiac events during the remainder of the day.

Recommended Amounts of Aerobic Activity for Prevention

To obtain substantial health benefits from physical activity, adults should partake in at least 150 minutes/week of moderate-intensity aerobic activity or 75 minutes/week of vigorous-intensity activity. Adults can do a combination of both moderate- and vigorous-intensity activity, using the rule of thumb that 1 vigorous-intensity minute of activity is equivalent to 2 moderate-intensity minutes.[7,8] Although previous recommendations were for bouts of aerobic activity of at least 10 minutes, bouts less than 10 minutes also appear to provide health benefits.

Recommended Amounts of Muscle-Strengthening Activity for Prevention

Adults should perform activities that strengthen the major muscle groups of the body at least 2 days each week. The major muscle groups are the legs, hips, back, chest, abdomen, shoulders, and arms.

Flexibility Activity

Flexibility activities are an important part of a complete physical activity regimen, but there is insufficient evidence that flexibility activities provide any health benefits, even for preventing injuries. Flexibility training may facilitate the types of physical activity that have health benefits. If so, flexibility training may be more important for people with reduced flexibility, such as older adults with age- and disease-related changes in range of motion.

Balance Activity

Balance training is recommended for adults at increased risk for falls, such as those older than 65 years with impaired gait or balance or frequent falls. Examples of balance exercises include sideways walking, backward walking, heel walking, and standing using a narrow base of support. Tai chi is an evidence-based approach to prevent falls. Preferably, adults at risk for falls should do balance training at least 3 days/week in the context of an evidence-based fall prevention program.

Sedentary Behavior

Increasing light-intensity activities by decreasing sedentary behavior is helpful for achieving and maintaining a healthy weight and reducing adverse health events. For example, more sedentary time is associated with greater risk of all-cause mortality, cardiovascular disease, some cancers, and type 2 diabetes.

Guidelines for Weight Management

The amount of activity required to maintain a healthy body weight varies widely among adults. For some adults, the amount of physical activity recommended in the guidelines will result in a stable, healthy body weight. Many adults, however, need greater amounts of activity to achieve a healthy weight.[9] These individuals should restrict their caloric intake and gradually increase their weekly physical activity to the point that is effective in achieving and maintaining a healthy body weight for them.

Additional Guidelines for Older Adults

In addition to balance training, older adults should be encouraged to be as active as feasible.[A9] For example, older adults who cannot do 150 minutes/week of moderate-intensity activity should be as active as their abilities and conditions allow. Resistance training and tai chi may be especially beneficial.[A10] Older adults should determine their level of physical activity using relative intensity, not absolute intensity. This latter guideline seeks to avoid inappropriately high levels of effort in older adults who have low fitness.

Recommending Physical Activity in Clinical Settings

Promoting physical activity in clinical settings involves essentially the same steps as the "5 A's" of smoking cessation (Chapter 363): ask, advise, assess, assist, arrange. Consistent with this approach, physicians should be knowledgeable in four domains: how to assess physical activity; how to make safe recommendations/prescriptions for physical activity in both healthy people and people with chronic conditions[10]; how to use effective behavioral interventions; and how to engage in their own active lifestyle for professional balance and as role models for patients.

Health care providers should ask and advise patients about physical activity regularly.[A11,11] One quality-of-care measure assesses whether asking and advising are done at least once a year in older adults. Some recommend that physical activity should be a "vital sign" that is assessed at every visit. Adults—especially older adults—identify their health care providers as an important source of advice on physical activity. Behavioral counseling is recommended for adults even if they have no cardiovascular risk factors. Intensive behavioral counseling is recommended for adults who are overweight or obese and have additional risk factors for cardiovascular disease. Such counseling should be a component of community programs that promote physical activity in people at increased risk for type 2 diabetes.

Lifestyle Prescription

A lifestyle prescription refers to approaches that integrate physical activity into daily life. For example, rather than walking specifically for exercise, a person walks to work or walks for pleasure as a recreational activity. Common ways to integrate physical activity into daily life are walking and biking for transportation, performing yard work, and gardening. Use of wearable devices such as pedometers to track physical activity can increase steps per day by about 2000 above baseline and increase adherence to lifestyle prescriptions. More total steps per day are associated with lower all-cause mortality, whereas step intensity is not, after controlling for total steps.[12]

Tailoring the Recommendation

Recommendations should be tailored to individual abilities, individual preferences, medical conditions, and behavior techniques that improve adherence. Interventions are more likely to be successful if they include mutual goal setting, regular feedback, graded tasks, and use of equipment, such as a step monitor.[A12] Most people prefer home-based programs, which can provide health benefits that are similar to those of programs conducted elsewhere.[A13]

A target level of physical activity below that of preventive recommendations is appropriate for adults who have very low physical fitness, a large burden of chronic disease (e.g., severe chronic obstructive lung disease), or major functional limitations. An assessment of the nature of the activity limitation and the individual's capabilities and preferences can determine the target activity level and other details of the activity recommendation. Often, promoting physical activity in such adults relies on health care and community resources designed for people with preexisting limitations, such as cardiac rehabilitation, pulmonary rehabilitation, and exercise classes for adults with arthritis.

Risk Management

Strategies to reduce injury during physical activity include increasing physical activity gradually over time, selecting activities in which collision or contact with people or objects is unusual, increasing physical fitness, using appropriate gear and sports equipment (e.g., bike helmets), engaging in activities in safe environments, and following basic safety rules and policies. Popular activities such as walking, biking, swimming, and gardening have a low risk of injury. When individuals are increasing their level of physical activity, they should start with relatively moderate-intensity activity, increase the duration and frequency first, and then the intensity later. In general, adding 5 to 15 minutes of moderate-intensity activity per session, two to three times a week, to a person's usual activities carries a low risk of musculoskeletal injury and no known risk of sudden cardiac death.

There is no evidence of any protective value for medical consultation or of supervised exercise in healthy people of any age who seek to increase their level of physical activity. The U.S. Preventive Services Task Force recommends against routine screening for coronary disease in adults at low risk. Even in adults who are at high risk for coronary disease, there is insufficient evidence to recommend for or against screening with resting electrocardiography, exercise treadmill testing, electron-beam computed tomography, or C-reactive protein concentrations.

Coordination between Medical Care and the Community

Many factors that affect physical activity levels in Americans, such as the characteristics of the communal environment (e.g., parks and recreational facilities) and the social environment (e.g., crime and social support), are difficult to influence in medical care settings. Community-level interventions that address such characteristics are essential to promoting physical activity. Effective community-based interventions include school physical education, social support interventions, community-wide campaigns, and enhancement of access to places where physical activity is possible. Medical care and community efforts should be synergistic and mutually supportive. For example, health plans should advocate for evidence-based community interventions. Community programs should serve as resources for evidence-based therapeutic activity for selected chronically ill adults, such as exercise classes designed to reduce the risk of falls.

GENERAL REFERENCES

For the General References and other additional features, please visit Elsevier eBooks+ at https://ebooks.health.elsevier.com.

Grade A References

A1. Guirguis-Blake JM, Michael YL, Perdue LA, et al. Interventions to prevent falls in older adults: updated evidence report and systematic review for the US Preventive Services Task Force. *JAMA.* 2018;319:1705-1716.

A2. Sherrington C, Fairhall NJ, Wallbank GK, et al. Exercise for preventing falls in older people living in the community. *Cochrane Database Syst Rev.* 2019;1:CD012424.

A3. de Souto Barreto P, Rolland Y, Vellas B, et al. Association of long-term exercise training with risk of falls, fractures, hospitalizations, and mortality in older adults: a systematic review and meta-analysis. *JAMA Intern Med.* 2019;179:394-405.

A4. Northey JM, Cherbuin N, Pumpa KL, et al. Exercise interventions for cognitive function in adults older than 50: a systematic review with meta-analysis. *Br J Sports Med.* 2018;52:154-160.

A5. Lamb SE, Sheehan B, Atherton N, et al. Dementia and physical activity (DAPA) trial of moderate to high intensity exercise training for people with dementia: randomised controlled trial. *BMJ.* 2018;361:1-11.

A6. Naci H, Salcher-Konrad M, Dias S, et al. How does exercise treatment compare with antihypertensive medications? A network meta-analysis of 391 randomised controlled trials assessing exercise and medication effects on systolic blood pressure. *Br J Sports Med.* 2019;53:859-869.

A7. Sampath Kumar A, Maiya AG, Shastry BA, et al. Exercise and insulin resistance in type 2 diabetes mellitus: a systematic review and meta-analysis. *Ann Phys Rehabil Med.* 2019;62:98-103.

A8. Taylor RS, Long L, Mordi IR, et al. Exercise-based rehabilitation for heart failure: Cochrane systematic review, meta-analysis, and trial sequential analysis. *JACC Heart Fail.* 2019;7:691-705.

A9. Lamb SE, Bruce J, Hossain A, et al. Screening and intervention to prevent falls and fractures in older people. *N Engl J Med.* 2020;383:1848-1859.

A10. Di Lorito C, Long A, Byrne A, et al. Exercise interventions for older adults: a systematic review of meta-analyses. *J Sport Health Sci.* 2021;10:29-47.

A11. Patnode CD, Redmond N, Iacocca MO, Henninger M. Behavioral counseling interventions to promote a healthy diet and physical activity for cardiovascular disease prevention in adults without known cardiovascular disease risk factors: updated evidence report and systematic review for the US Preventive Services Task Force. *JAMA.* 2022;328:375-388.

A12. Samdal GB, Eide GE, Barth T, et al. Effective behaviour change techniques for physical activity and healthy eating in overweight and obese adults; systematic review and meta-regression analyses. *Int J Behav Nutr Phys Act.* 2017;14:1-14.

A13. Buckingham SA, Taylor RS, Jolly K, et al. Home-based versus centre-based cardiac rehabilitation: abridged Cochrane systematic review and meta-analysis. *Open Heart.* 2016;3:1-15.

15

IMMUNIZATION

ANDREW T. KROGER AND WALTER A. ORENSTEIN

GENERAL CHARACTERISTICS OF IMMUNIZATIONS

Immunization protects against disease or the sequelae of disease through the administration of an immunobiologic—a vaccine, toxoid, immune globulin preparation, or antitoxin. Protection induced by immunization can be active or passive (Tables 15-1 and 15-2).

ACTIVE IMMUNIZATION

Administration of a vaccine or toxoid causes the body to produce an immune response against the infectious agent or its toxins. Active immunization generally results in long-term immunity, although the onset of protection may be delayed because it takes time for the body to respond. Vaccines consist of suspensions of live (usually attenuated) microbes, nonlive microbes, or proteins of microbes. Nonlive recombinant vaccines[1] are genetically engineered, so they cannot be considered inactivated because they never consisted of whole microbes. By comparison, nonlive vaccines that are not produced via genetic engineering retain the characterization "inactivated." Toxoids are modified bacterial toxins that retain immunogenic properties but lack toxicity. With live attenuated vaccines, small quantities of living organisms multiply within the recipient until an immune response cuts off replication. In most recipients, a single dose of most live vaccines generally induces a long-term immune response that closely parallels natural infection. Additional doses are recommended to ensure high rates of population immunity.

PASSIVE IMMUNIZATION

Passive immunization using immune globulins or antitoxins delivers preformed antibodies to provide rapid temporary immunity. Immune globulins obtained from human blood may contain antibodies to a variety of agents, depending on the pool of human plasma from which they are prepared. Specific immune globulins are made from the plasma of donors with high levels of antibodies to

TABLE 15-1 PASSIVE IMMUNIZATIONS FOR ADULTS

DISEASE	NAME OF MATERIAL*†§	COMMENTS AND USE
Acquired immunodeficiency syndrome (AIDS)	Immune globulin intravenous (IGIV)	To prevent bacterial infection
Botulism	For non-infant botulism: in the United States, equine botulism antitoxin (BAT) against toxin types A, B, C, D, E, F, G For infant botulism: in the United States, botulism immune globulin types A and B; BabyBIG	Equine heptavalent antitoxin for treatment of non-infant botulism; available from CDC through state or local health department—contact emergency number of local or state health department. Human immune globulin for treatment of infant botulism available from the California Department of Health, Infant Botulism Treatment and Prevention Program, (510)231-7600
Chronic immune demyelinating polyneuropathy (CIDP)	Immune globulin intravenous (IGIV)	To improve neuromuscular ability
Chronic lymphocytic leukemia (CLL)	Immune globulin intravenous (IGIV)	To prevent bacterial infection
Cytomegalovirus	Cytomegalovirus immune globulin intravenous	Prophylaxis for bone marrow and kidney transplant recipients
Digoxin intoxication	Digoxin immune Fab, ovine	
Diphtheria	Diphtheria antitoxin, equine	Treatment of established disease; allergic reactions possible to serum of equine origin, available only from CDC
Erythroblastosis fetalis	Rho (D) immune globulin, intramuscular Rho (D) immune globulin, intravenous	Rh-negative women who are pregnant with Rh-positive infants
Hepatitis A	Immune globulin, intramuscular (IGIM)	Preexposure and postexposure prophylaxis for travelers and others who need protection before immunity can be achieved with hepatitis A vaccination
Hepatitis B	Hepatitis B immune globulin	Prophylaxis for needle stick or mucous membrane contact with HBsAg-positive persons, for sexual partners with acute hepatitis B or carriers of hepatitis B, for infants born to mothers who are carriers of HBsAg, for infants whose mother or primary caregiver has acute hepatitis B
Hypogammaglobulinemia	Immune globulin, intravenous, subcutaneous, intramuscular	Maintenance therapy
Idiopathic thrombocytopenic purpura	Immune globulin, intravenous (IGIV)	Therapy for acute episodes
Measles	Immune globulin, intramuscular (IGIM) Immune globulin, intravenous (IGIV)	Prevention or modification of disease in exposed persons, not for control of outbreaks; particularly indicated for unvaccinated infants aged <6 months, pregnant persons without evidence of measles immunity, and severely immunocompromised persons
Multifocal motor neuropathy	Immune globulin intravenous (IGIV)	To improve muscle strength
Rabies	Rabies immune globulin	Postexposure prophylaxis of animal bites
Scorpion sting	Centruroides (scorpion) immune F(ab')2, equine	Specific for *Centruroides* genus scorpions (e.g., Arizona bark scorpion)
Snakebite, coral snake	Antivenin (*Micrurus fulvius*), equine; North American coral snake antivenin	Specific for North American coral snake, *Micrurus fulvius*
Snakebite, crotalidae	Antivenin (Crotalidae) polyvalent, equine Crotalidae immune F(ab')2, equine	Effective for viper and pit viper bites, including rattlesnakes, copperheads, moccasins
Spider bite, black widow	Antivenin (*Lactrodectus mactans*), equine	Specific for black widow spider, *Latrodectus mactans*, and other members of the genus
Tetanus	Tetanus immune globulin	Management of tetanus-prone wounds in persons without adequate prior active immunization and treatment of tetanus
Vaccinia	Vaccinia immune globulin, intravenous (IGIV)	Treatment of eczema vaccinatum, vaccinia necrosum, and severe inadvertent inoculations such as ocular vaccinia after vaccinia (smallpox) vaccination; available only from CDC
Varicella	Varicella-zoster immune globulin	Prevention or modification of disease in exposed persons. Indicated for persons who are at high risk for complications from varicella, who have not had varicella or varicella vaccine, and who are exposed to varicella or herpes zoster: immunocompromised persons, newborn infants whose mothers have varicella around the time of delivery (i.e., 5 days before to 2 days after), hospitalized premature infants born at ≥28 weeks of gestation whose mothers do not have evidence of immunity to varicella, hospitalized premature infants born at <28 weeks of gestation or who weigh ≤1,000 g at birth, regardless of their mothers' evidence of immunity to varicella, pregnant persons; should be given as soon as possible after exposure and within 10 days

*All products to be administered intramuscularly, unless otherwise indicated.
†All products derived from humans unless otherwise specified.
§Table revisions provided by John Grabenstein.
CDC = Centers for Disease Control and Prevention; HBsAg = hepatitis B surface antigen.

TABLE 15-2 SELECTED IMMUNIZING AGENTS INDICATED FOR ADULTS*

DISEASE	IMMUNIZING AGENT	INDICATIONS	SCHEDULE	MAJOR CONTRAINDICATIONS (C) AND PRECAUTIONS (P)	COMMENTS
Adenovirus	Adenovirus type 4 and type 7 live oral vaccine	Military: for prevention of febrile acute respiratory disease caused by type 4 and type 7 adenovirus	One oral dose (two tablets)	C: Pregnancy C: Severe allergic reaction (e.g., anaphylaxis) to a vaccine component C: Inability to swallow whole tablets without chewing P: Altered immunocompetence P: Moderate or severe acute illness	Avoid pregnancy for 6 weeks after vaccination Virus may be shed in stool: exercise caution for 28 days after vaccination in contact with children younger than 7 years, pregnant persons, or immunosuppressed persons
Anthrax	Anthrax vaccine, adsorbed, inactivated vaccine	Preexposure prophylaxis of persons at high risk of exposure (e.g., military, certain laboratory workers) Consider with antibiotics for postexposure prophylaxis	0.5-mL dose IM at 0, 4, and 6 weeks and boosters at 12 and 18 months, then booster every 3 years thereafter If used after exposure, three doses at 0, 2, and 4 weeks with 60 days of antimicrobial therapy; antibiotics should be continued for 14 days after third dose	C: Severe allergic reaction to a vaccine component or after a prior dose P: Moderate or severe acute illness	Effectiveness against aerosol exposure inferred primarily from animal data A dose-sparing schedule of two doses with 2-4 week interval exists if there is a supply shortage
Cholera	Cholera vaccine, live attenuated oral cholera vaccine		One 100-mL oral dose before travel; booster doses are not presently recommended	C: Severe allergic reaction to a vaccine component or after a prior dose P: Moderate or severe acute illness Limited or lack of data on use of vaccine in: • Pregnant persons • Immunocompromised persons • Children <18 yr and adults 65 yr and older	All travelers to cholera-affected areas should follow safe food and water precautions and proper sanitation and personal hygiene measures as primary strategies to prevent cholera
COVID-19 (three types of vaccines)	1. mRNA vaccine (non-live messenger RNA encoding the novel SARS-2 coronavirus [NCoV2] spike protein)	Pfizer-BioNTech COVID-19 vaccine: authorized for ages 6 months through 11 years and approved for ages 12 years and older Moderna COVID-19 vaccine approved for ages 18 years and older	The information in this row/column is current for ADULTS only: Two brands (no preference) BNT162b2 two 0.3-mL doses separated by 3-8 weeks mRNA-1273 two 0.5-mL doses separated by 4-8 weeks A third dose of mRNA vaccine is recommended 28 days after the primary series for persons ages 5 years and older who are immunosuppressed. A booster dose of mRNA vaccine is recommended at least 2 months after the primary series for persons ages 12 years or older. The dose must be Pfizer-BioNTech for persons 12 years through 17 years of age. A booster dose is also recommended for persons ages 12 years old and older who were immunosuppressed upon receipt of the primary series and received an additional dose. The booster dose should be administered at least 2 months after the additional dose	C: History of severe allergic reaction to a prior dose of vaccine C: History of a known allergy to a component of the COVID-19 vaccine P: History of an immediate allergic reaction to any vaccine other than COVID-19 vaccine or to any injectable therapy (i.e., intramuscular, intravenous, or subcutaneous vaccines or therapies [excluding subcutaneous immunotherapy for allergies, i.e., "allergy shots"]) P: A history of a nonsevere, immediate (onset less than 4 hours) allergic reaction after a dose of one type of COVID-19 vaccine (i.e., mRNA or Janssen) is a precaution only to like-type vaccine (i.e., if the history is to an mRNA vaccine, this precaution is to any mRNA vaccine; if the history is to a COVID-19 vector vaccine, this precaution is to any COVID-19 vector vaccine) P: An allergy-related contraindication to one type of a COVID-19 vaccine is a precaution to other-type COVID-19 vaccine (i.e., if the contraindication is to mRNA vaccine, the precaution is to any COVID-19 vector vaccine; if the contraindication is to COVID-19 vector vaccine, the precaution is to any mRNA vaccine) P: History of myocarditis or pericarditis after a dose of an mRNA or Novavax COVID-19 vaccine P: Moderate or severe acute illness P: History of multisystem inflammatory syndrome	If a precaution on the basis of allergy, observe patient for 30 minutes instead of just 15 minutes Increased risk (3.5 cases per 1 million doses) of myocarditis and pericarditis. The highest risk is in males ages 12 years to 29 years

TABLE 15-2 SELECTED IMMUNIZING AGENTS INDICATED FOR ADULTS*—cont'd

DISEASE	IMMUNIZING AGENT	INDICATIONS	SCHEDULE	MAJOR CONTRAINDICATIONS (C) AND PRECAUTIONS (P)	COMMENTS
	2. Non-replicating adenovirus vector vaccine	Not licensed: Emergency Use Authorization Only: 18 years of age and older	One 0.5-mL dose	C: History of severe allergic reaction to a prior dose of vaccine C: History of a diagnosed allergy to a component of the COVID-19 vaccine C: Thrombosis with thrombocytopenia following receipt of a previous Janssen COVID-19 vaccine (or other COVID-19 vaccines not currently authorized in the United States that are based on adenovirus vectors, e.g., AstraZeneca) is a contraindication for Janssen COVID-19 only P: History of an immediate allergic reaction to any vaccine other than COVID-19 vaccine or to any injectable therapy (i.e., intramuscular, intravenous, or subcutaneous vaccines or therapies [excluding subcutaneous immunotherapy for allergies, i.e., "allergy shots"]) P: A history of a nonsevere, immediate (onset less than 4 hours) allergic reaction after a dose of one type of COVID-19 vaccine (i.e., mRNA or Janssen) is a precaution only to like-type vaccine (i.e. if the history is to an mRNA vaccine the precaution is to any mRNA vaccine; if the history is to a COVID-19 vector vaccine, the precaution is to any COVID-19 vector vaccine) P: An allergy-related contraindication to one type of a COVID-19 vaccine is a precaution to other-type COVID-19 vaccine (i.e., if the contraindication is to mRNA vaccine, the precaution is to any COVID-19 vector vaccine; if the contraindication is to COVID-19 vector vaccine, the precaution is to any mRNA vaccine) P: History of Guillain-Barré syndrome within 6 weeks of Janssen COVID-19 vaccine P: Moderate or severe acute illness	If a precaution on the basis of allergy, observe patient for 30 minutes instead of just 15 minutes Increased risk (7 cases in 1 million doses in persons ages 18 years to 49 years, and 1 case per million doses in persons age 50 years and older) of thrombosis with thrombocytopenia. An increased risk is in females age 18 to 49 years Increased risk (7.8 cases per million doses) of Guillain-Barré syndrome, especially in males ages 50 to 64 years

TABLE 15-2 SELECTED IMMUNIZING AGENTS INDICATED FOR ADULTS*—cont'd

DISEASE	IMMUNIZING AGENT	INDICATIONS	SCHEDULE	MAJOR CONTRAINDICATIONS (C) AND PRECAUTIONS (P)	COMMENTS
	3. Protein subunit vaccine	Novavax COVID-19 vaccine authorized for 12 years and older	NVX-CoV2373 two 0.5-mL doses separated by 3-8 weeks. A booster is recommended at least 2 months after the primary series (preferentially the booster dose should be an mRNA vaccine)	C: History of severe allergic reaction to a prior dose of vaccine C: History of a known allergy to a component of the COVID-19 vaccine P: History of an immediate allergic reaction to any vaccine other than COVID-19 vaccine or to any injectable therapy (i.e., intramuscular, intravenous, or subcutaneous vaccines or therapies [excluding subcutaneous immunotherapy for allergies, i.e., "allergy shots"]) P: A history of a nonsevere, immediate (onset less than 4 hours) allergic reaction after a dose of one type of COVID-19 vaccine (i.e., mRNA or Janssen) is a precaution only to like-type vaccine (i.e., if the history is to an mRNA vaccine, this precaution is to any mRNA vaccine; if the history is to a COVID-19 vector vaccine, this precaution is to any COVID-19 vector vaccine). Note that Janssen and Novavax vaccines contain polysorbate. mRNA vaccines do not contain polysorbate P: An allergy-related contraindication to one type of a COVID-19 vaccine is a precaution to other-type COVID-19 vaccine (i.e., if the contraindication is to mRNA vaccine, the precaution is to any COVID-19 vector vaccine; if the contraindication is to COVID-19 vector vaccine, the precaution is to any mRNA vaccine). Note that Janssen and Novavax vaccines contain polysorbate. mRNA vaccines do not contain polysorbate P: History of myocarditis or pericarditis after a dose of an mRNA or Novavax COVID-19 vaccine P: Moderate or severe acute illness P: History of multisystem inflammatory syndrome	

TABLE 15-2 SELECTED IMMUNIZING AGENTS INDICATED FOR ADULTS*—cont'd

DISEASE	IMMUNIZING AGENT	INDICATIONS	SCHEDULE	MAJOR CONTRAINDICATIONS (C) AND PRECAUTIONS (P)	COMMENTS
Diphtheria	Tetanus and diphtheria toxoids combined Adult preparation of pertussis antigens combined with tetanus and diphtheria toxoids (Tdap)	All adults	For incompletely immunized adults, three total 0.5-mL doses IM needed for primary series: two doses IM 4 weeks apart, third dose 6-12 months after second dose; it is preferable that the first dose is Tdap, subsequent doses can be Tdap or Td Booster (Tdap or Td) every 10 years No need to repeat if schedule is interrupted	C: History of neurologic reaction after a previous dose (Tdap only) C: Severe allergic reaction to a vaccine component or after a prior dose P: Moderate or severe acute illness	Tetanus and diphtheria toxoids combined with acellular pertussis vaccine (Tdap) preferred as one-time booster for all persons who have not previously received Tdap
Ebola	Live, recombinant viral vector vaccine: backbone: vesicular stomatitis virus (VSV), with gene encoding for envelope glycoprotein of *Z. ebolavirus*	Responders to an outbreak of Ebola In United States, health care workers in federally designated Ebola Treatment Centers or other staff working in biosafety level 4 facilities	One 1-mL dose	C: Hypersensitivity or allergy to a vaccine component P: Moderate or severe acute illness	Avoid kissing or sharing razors, eating utensils, toothbrushes, drinking cups, or needles for 2 weeks Avoid donating blood or contact with high-risk persons, or exposure of livestock to blood or body fluids for 6 weeks Use barrier methods for sexual interaction for 2 months
Haemophilus influenzae type b	Hib conjugate vaccines	Adults who have anatomic or functional asplenia and who are vaccine naïve or hematopoietic cell transplant recipients	Adults who have functional and anatomic asplenia and who are vaccine naïve: 1 dose Adults who have received a hematopoietic cell transplant: 3 doses at 1-month intervals	C: Severe allergic reaction to a vaccine component or after a prior dose P: Moderate or severe acute illness	
Hepatitis A	Inactivated hepatitis A vaccine	Travelers to highly or intermediately endemic countries Men who have sex with men Persons who use illegal drugs (injection and noninjection) Persons who work with hepatitis A virus–infected primates or who do research with the virus Persons with chronic liver disease Homeless persons HIV-infected persons	Two 0.5-mL doses at least 6 months apart for persons aged ≥1 year	C: Severe allergic reaction to a vaccine component or after a prior dose P: Moderate or severe acute illness	Should be considered for outbreak control Should be administered to all adults in settings where patients with indications are seen Adults with HIV can be tested at least 1 month after receipt of HepA vaccine to confirm immunity. If negative, a revaccination dose can be considered.

TABLE 15-2 SELECTED IMMUNIZING AGENTS INDICATED FOR ADULTS*—cont'd

DISEASE	IMMUNIZING AGENT	INDICATIONS	SCHEDULE	MAJOR CONTRAINDICATIONS (C) AND PRECAUTIONS (P)	COMMENTS
Hepatitis B	Three inactivated hepatitis B virus subunit vaccines containing HBsAg; one vaccine containing HBsAg and a CpG 1018 adjuvant	All adults ages 18 through 59 years Adults ages 60 years and older with any of the following health conditions: 1. Health care and public safety workers potentially exposed to blood 2. Clients and staff of institutions for the developmentally disabled 3. Hemodialysis patients 4. Men who have sex with men 5. Users of illicit injectable drugs 6. Recipients of clotting factors 7. Household and sexual contacts of HBV carriers 8. Inmates of long-term correctional facilities 9. Persons treated for sexually transmitted diseases or with multiple sexual partners 10. Travelers with close contact for ≥6 months with populations with high prevalence of HBV carriage 11. Persons with chronic liver disease 12. HIV-infected persons 13. Persons with diabetes mellitus 14. Incarcerated persons	Vaccine without CpG adjuvant: three doses IM at 0, 1, and 6 months volume of dose (Recombivax-HB and Engerix-B, 18- to 19-year-olds: 0.5 mL; 20-year-olds and older: 1 mL; PreHevbrio: 18-year-olds and older: 1 mL) Vaccine with CpG adjuvant: two 0.5-mL doses 1 month apart	C: Severe allergic reaction to a vaccine component or after a prior dose C: Hypersensitivity to yeast P: Moderate or severe acute illness	Pregnancy is not a contraindication Health care workers who have contact with patients or blood, sexual contacts of persons with chronic HBV infection, hemodialysis patients, and other immunosuppressed persons should be tested 1-2 months after vaccination to determine serologic response Consider vaccination in any adult age 60 years and older
Herpes zoster	Recombinant zoster vaccine (RZV), a subunit vaccine containing varicella-zoster virus glycoprotein E	All adults age 50 years and older Immunocompromised adults ages 19 through 49 years of age	Two 0.5-mL doses IM 2-6 months apart	C: Allergy to vaccine components P: Moderate or severe acute illness P: Active zoster disease	
Human papillomavirus (HPV)	Noninfectious recombinant vaccine prepared from purified virus-like particles of L1 capsid proteins of HPV types 6, 11, 16, 18, 31, 33, 45, 52, and 58 (nine-valent; bivalent and quadrivalent vaccines, while licensed, are no longer available in the United States)	Routine vaccination of adolescents with catch-up vaccination for adults through age 26 years. Shared clinical decision-making regarding HPV vaccination is recommended for some adults ages 27 through 45 years	Two 0.5-mL doses IM at 0 and 6-12 months if the first dose was administered before the 15th birthday Three 0.5-mL doses IM at 0, 1 to 2, and 6 months if first dose was administered at age 15 years or older Three 0.5-mL doses IM at 0, 1 to 2, and 6 months for persons who are immunocompromised, have an autoimmune disease, or have a malignant neoplasm, regardless of age at first dose	C: Severe allergic reaction to a vaccine component or to a prior dose P: Moderate or severe acute illness	The vaccine will not protect against existing infections Because vaccines do not protect against all HPV types, screening for cervical cancer among vaccinated persons should occur as for unvaccinated persons

TABLE 15-2 SELECTED IMMUNIZING AGENTS INDICATED FOR ADULTS*—cont'd

DISEASE	IMMUNIZING AGENT	INDICATIONS	SCHEDULE	MAJOR CONTRAINDICATIONS (C) AND PRECAUTIONS (P)	COMMENTS
Influenza (three types of vaccines: inactivated virus vaccine [IIV] exists as high-dose influenza vaccine, adjuvanted influenza vaccine, and standard-dose influenza vaccine)	Inactivated virus vaccine (IIV)	All adults, with greatest priority for those at higher risk for influenza complications (e.g., ≥50 years old, persons with underlying medical conditions, pregnant persons) or in contact with those at higher risk (e.g., health care workers, and persons with close contact with children <5 years)	Annual vaccination; see annual ACIP recommendation The volume of the dose varies by brand and age: 0.5 mL or 0.7 mL	C: Severe allergic reaction to an influenza vaccine component (except eggs) or after a prior dose P: Moderate or severe acute illness P: Guillain-Barré syndrome within 6 weeks of prior dose of influenza vaccine	Optimum timing of vaccination for most people is by the end of October. However, vaccination can occur throughout the influenza season, particularly for persons at high risk for complications and their contacts who were not vaccinated earlier. Only one dose of influenza vaccine per season is recommended for adults
	Live attenuated influenza virus (LAIV)	Adults through 49 years of age	Administered intranasally (0.2 mL) See annual ACIP recommendations	C: Persons <2 years or ≥50 years C: Pregnant persons C: Hypersensitivity to components of vaccine (except eggs) C: Anatomic or functional asplenia (including sickle cell disease) C: Cochlear implant C: Cerebrospinal fluid (CSF) leak C: Use of influenza antivirals C: Use of high-dose aspirin or high-dose aspirin-containing therapy C: Close contacts or a caregiver of someone with severe immunocompromise (requiring a protective environment) P: Persons with underlying disorders that place them at high risk of influenza complications (including asthma) P: Have history of Guillain-Barré syndrome within 6 weeks of prior dose of influenza vaccine P: Moderate or severe acute illness	Can be used for household contacts and health care workers caring for immunocompromised patients if the patient does not require a protected environment
	Recombinant influenza vaccine (RIV)	Adults	Annual vaccination (one 0.5-mL dose)	C: Severe allergic reaction to any component of the vaccine P: Moderate or severe acute illness P: Guillain-Barré syndrome within 6 weeks of prior dose of influenza vaccine	
Japanese encephalitis	Inactivated Japanese encephalitis virus vaccine	Travelers to Asia spending at least 1 month in endemic areas during transmission season	Two 0.5-mL doses IM on days 0 and 28. The FDA approved an alternate 0- and 7-day schedule	C: Pregnancy P: Moderate or severe acute illness	
Measles	Live virus vaccine (with mumps and rubella [MMR])	All adults born after 1956 without history of live vaccine on or after first birthday, laboratory confirmation of disease, or detectable measles antibody Persons born before 1957 generally can be considered immune	One 0.5-mL dose sufficient for most adults; two doses at least 1 month apart indicated for persons entering college or medical facility employment, traveling abroad, or at risk of measles during outbreaks	C: Altered immunity (e.g., leukemia, lymphoma, generalized malignant disease, congenital immunodeficiency, immunosuppressive therapy) C: Anaphylactic hypersensitivity to neomycin or gelatin C: Pregnancy P: Thrombocytopenia P: Immune globulin or other blood products within prior 3-11 months P: Untreated tuberculosis P: Moderate or severe acute illness	Persons with anaphylactic allergies to eggs may be vaccinated (see text) Vaccine should be administered to persons with asymptomatic HIV infection and should be considered for other patients with HIV infection except those with severe immunocompromise

TABLE 15-2 SELECTED IMMUNIZING AGENTS INDICATED FOR ADULTS*—cont'd

DISEASE	IMMUNIZING AGENT	INDICATIONS	SCHEDULE	MAJOR CONTRAINDICATIONS (C) AND PRECAUTIONS (P)	COMMENTS
Meningococcal disease (two types of vaccines)	1. Meningococcal conjugate vaccines containing polysaccharide of serogroups A, C, W, and Y	All persons with persistent complement component deficiencies or complement inhibitor use, HIV infection, or anatomic or functional asplenia Persons who will travel to areas where meningococcal infection is hyperendemic or epidemic Microbiologists routinely exposed to *Neisseria meningitidis* People at increased risk during an outbreak (e.g., unvaccinated or undervaccinated first-year college students living in residence halls, military recruits) Other persons at risk during an outbreak	A two-dose primary series recommended for individuals with complement component deficiency or complement inhibitor use, HIV infection, or anatomic or functional asplenia; others should receive a single dose Individuals at ongoing increased risk of meningococcal disease should receive a booster dose every 5 years	C: Allergic reactions to a component of the vaccine, including diphtheria or tetanus toxoid, or to other diphtheria toxoid-, CRM197-, or tetanus-toxoid-containing vaccines (depending on vaccine) P: Moderate or severe acute illness	
	2. Recombinant meningococcal B protein vaccines containing either two alleles of one protein (MenB-FHbp) or three proteins as well as one protein-containing outer membrane vesicle (MenB-4 C) (ages 10 years and older)	All persons with persistent complement component deficiencies or complement inhibitor use or anatomic or functional asplenia Certain laboratory workers May be useful during localized outbreaks May be administered to young adults before age 24 years to provide short-term protection against most strains of serogroup B meningococcal disease	For healthy persons who are not at increased risk for meningococcal disease, either a 2-dose series of MenB-4C at 0 and 1 mo, or a 2-dose series of MenB-FHbp at 0 and 6 months (each dose 0.5 mL). For persons at increased risk for meningococcal disease, including during serogroup B outbreaks, MenB-FHbp should be given as a 3-dose series at 0, 1-2, and 6 months. For persons at increased risk, the 2-dose series of MenB-4C at 0 and 1 month remains in effect. The same vaccine product should be used for all doses Booster dose is recommended 1 year after the primary series and every 2-3 years thereafter for those who continue to be at increased risk Booster dose is indicated in an outbreak of serogroup B disease if 6 months or more have passed since completion of the primary series	C: Severe allergic reaction to a vaccine component or after a prior dose P: Latex sensitivity (MenB-4C only) P: Moderate or severe acute illness P: Pregnancy	Evidence supports use of MenB vaccines in all persons at increased risk for serogroup B meningococcal disease Shared clinical decision making for young adults not at increased risk
Mumps	Live virus vaccine (measles and rubella [MMR])	All adults born after 1956 without history of live vaccine on or after first birthday, laboratory confirmation of disease, or detectable mumps antibody Persons born before 1957 generally can be considered immune	One 0.5-mL dose sufficient for most adults Two doses at least 1 month apart indicated for persons entering college or medical facility employment or traveling abroad, or at risk of mumps during outbreaks	C: Altered immunity (e.g., leukemia, lymphoma, generalized malignant disease, congenital immunodeficiency, immunosuppressive therapy) C: Anaphylactic hypersensitivity to neomycin or gelatin C: Pregnancy P: Immune globulin or other blood products within prior 3 to 11 months P: Thrombocytopenia if administered with measles vaccine P: Moderate or severe acute illness	Persons with anaphylactic allergies to eggs may be vaccinated Persons previously vaccinated with two doses of a mumps-containing vaccine who are identified by public health as at increased risk for mumps because of a mumps outbreak should receive a third dose of a mumps-containing vaccine to improve protection against mumps disease and related complications

TABLE 15-2 SELECTED IMMUNIZING AGENTS INDICATED FOR ADULTS*—cont'd

DISEASE	IMMUNIZING AGENT	INDICATIONS	SCHEDULE	MAJOR CONTRAINDICATIONS (C) AND PRECAUTIONS (P)	COMMENTS
Pertussis	Adult preparation of pertussis antigens combined with tetanus and diphtheria toxoids (Tdap)	Catch-up vaccination for all persons ≥13 years May be given whenever tetanus-toxoid–containing vaccine is indicated One dose per pregnancy	One 0.5-mL dose Pregnant persons: one dose during each pregnancy preferably early in the period between 27 and 36 weeks of gestation	C: History of neurologic reaction after a previous dose (Tdap only) C: Severe allergic reaction to a vaccine component or after a prior dose P: Moderate or severe acute illness	Two preparations are available, one licensed for all persons ≥10 yr, one for 10 to 64 yr olds
Pneumococcal disease (three vaccines)	15-valent pneumococcal conjugate vaccine (PCV15) 23-valent pneumococcal polysaccharide vaccine (PPSV23) 20-valent pneumococcal conjugate vaccine (PCV20)	All adults age 65 years or older and adults ages 19 to 64 years at risk for invasive pneumococcal disease (including asthma), diabetes mellitus, alcohol use disorder, cirrhosis, cerebrospinal fluid leaks, splenic dysfunction or anatomic asplenia, Hodgkin disease, lymphoma, multiple myeloma, chronic renal failure, nephrotic syndrome, immunosuppression, HIV infection, cigarette smokers ages 19 years and older), who previously have not received PCV13 or whose pneumococcal vaccination history is unknown	Choose either: PCV20 or PCV15 followed by PPSV23 1 year later (can consider an 8-week interval between PCV15 and PPSV23)	C: Severe allergic reaction to a vaccine component or after a prior dose P: Moderate or severe acute illness	Persons who have previously received PCV13 should receive PPSV23. If PPSV23 is unavailable, they may receive PCV20
Poliomyelitis	Inactivated poliovirus vaccine (IPV)	Certain adults who are at greater risk of exposure to wild-type or vaccine-derived poliovirus than the general population, including laboratory workers, health care workers, and travelers to countries where poliomyelitis is epidemic or endemic or specific populations with disease caused by poliovirus	For unvaccinated adults, two 0.5-mL doses IM or SQ 4 weeks apart and a third dose 6-12 months after the second; if <4 weeks available before protection is needed, a single dose of IPV and ensure that the series is complete after travel For incompletely immunized adults, complete primary series of three doses of IPV or prior oral poliovirus vaccine (OPV); no need to restart interrupted series; a mixed series can be considered complete A single dose of IPV can be given to adults who previously received a primary series but now are at high risk, such as those traveling to an endemic area	C: Severe allergic reaction to a vaccine component or after a prior dose P: On theoretical grounds, pregnant persons should not receive IPV, but if immediate protection is needed, IPV can be used P: Moderate or severe acute illness	
Rabies	Inactivated vaccine, HDCV or PCECV	High-risk persons, including animal handlers, selected laboratory and field workers, and persons traveling for ≥1 month to areas with high risk of rabies	Preexposure prophylaxis: for persons 18 years old and older, two doses of 1 mL IM on days 0 and 7 Confirmation of immunity recommended for laboratory workers, bat handlers, and animal handlers	C: History of severe hypersensitivity reaction P: Moderate or severe acute illness	Further doses needed after exposure Persons traveling to high-risk areas should receive booster dose at 1 to 3 years

TABLE 15-2 SELECTED IMMUNIZING AGENTS INDICATED FOR ADULTS*—cont'd

DISEASE	IMMUNIZING AGENT	INDICATIONS	SCHEDULE	MAJOR CONTRAINDICATIONS (C) AND PRECAUTIONS (P)	COMMENTS
Rubella	Live virus vaccine (with mumps and measles [MMR])	Adults, particularly persons of childbearing age, who lack history of rubella vaccine, laboratory confirmation of disease, and detectable rubella-specific antibodies in serum Persons in institutions where rubella outbreaks may occur, such as hospitals, the military, and colleges Persons born before 1957, except those who can become pregnant, generally can be considered immune	One 0.5-mL SQ dose	C: Pregnancy, altered immunity (e.g., leukemia, lymphoma, generalized malignant disease, congenital immunodeficiency, immunosuppressive therapy) C: Anaphylactic hypersensitivity to neomycin C: Administration of blood products should not contraindicate postpartum vaccination P: Thrombocytopenia if administered with measles vaccine P: Immune globulin or other blood products within prior 3 to 11 months P: Moderate or severe acute illness	People who can become pregnant should be counseled to avoid pregnancy for 1 month after vaccination
Smallpox (two types of vaccines)	Live vaccinia virus	Persons working with orthopox viruses	One 0.0025-mL dose intracutaneously with a bifurcated needle Boosters every 10 years and perhaps every 3 years for persons working with virulent orthopox viruses	C: History or presence of eczema or other acute, chronic, or exfoliative skin condition in patient or a close household or personal contact C: Immunosuppression or pregnancy in patient or a close household or personal contact C: Breast-feeding C: Allergy to a vaccine component P: History of heart disease P: Moderate or severe acute illness No contraindications if exposed to smallpox	Some complications of vaccination are treatable with vaccinia immune globulin Vaccine is effective 3-4 days after exposure to variola and perhaps longer to prevent or to modify the illness Serious adverse events are rare but significant, including eczema vaccinatum, progressive vaccinia, myopericarditis, autoinoculation, and encephalitis Vaccinia is transmissible
	Live, nonreplicating vaccinia vector vaccine	Adults at risk for smallpox or monkeypox infection	Two 0.5-mL doses SQ, 4 weeks apart	P: Allergy to a vaccine component (based on FDA package insert) P: Altered immunocompetence	
Tetanus	Tetanus and diphtheria toxoids combined (Td) Adult preparation of pertussis antigens combined with tetanus and diphtheria toxoids (Tdap)	All adults	For incompletely immunized adults, three total 0.5-mL doses IM needed for primary series: two doses IM 4 weeks apart, third dose 6-12 month after second dose; preferable that first dose is Tdap, subsequent doses can be Tdap or Td Booster (Tdap or Td) every 10 years No need to repeat if schedule is interrupted	C: History of neurologic or severe allergic reaction after a prior dose C: History of neurologic reaction after a previous dose (Tdap only) P: Moderate or severe acute illness P: Guillain-Barré syndrome <6 weeks after previous dose of tetanus-toxoid–containing vaccine	Special recommendations for wound treatment (see text) Persons with Guillain-Barré syndrome within the first 6 weeks after immunization, particularly adults who received a prior primary series, probably should not be revaccinated in most circumstances One-time booster of Tdap for all adults
Typhoid fever	Vi capsular polysaccharide vaccine Live attenuated Ty21a oral vaccine	Travelers to areas where the risk of prolonged exposure to contaminated food and water is high May be considered for family and intimate contacts of carriers and laboratory workers who work with *Salmonella* Typhi	Vi polysaccharide vaccine: one dose IM 0.5 mL; boosters every 2 years Oral vaccine: four doses on alternate days; repeat series every 5 years if risk continues	C: Severe local or systemic reaction to a prior dose C: Ty21a vaccine should not be administered to persons with altered immunity or those receiving antimicrobial agents P: Moderate or severe acute illness	Cumulative efficacy at 2.5 to 3.0 years: Vi capsular polysaccharide: 55%, Ty21a: 48% Food and water precautions essential

Indications

H. influenzae type b vaccine is recommended for adults who have anatomic and functional asplenia (e.g., sickle cell disease) who are vaccine naïve and adults who have received a haematopoietic cell transplant (HCT; Chapter 163). For naïve adults with functional and anatomic asplenia, one dose of Hib is recommended. For all adults post-HCT, regardless of previous vaccination, three doses of Hib are recommended with intervals of 1 month.

Adverse Reactions

The contraindication to Hib vaccine is a severe allergic reaction (e.g., anaphylaxis) following a prior dose or to a vaccine component. The precaution to Hib vaccine is severe or moderate acute illness.

HEPATITIS A

Two inactivated hepatitis A (Chapter 134) vaccines are available in the United States. Seroconversion rates after a single dose of either vaccine in persons older than 1 year exceed 95%, and protection is expected to persist for at least 25 years.

Indications

For adults, the vaccine is indicated primarily for persons traveling to countries (generally those in the developing world) with high or intermediate endemicity for hepatitis A, but it is also recommended for other groups at high risk for infection or for development of severe hepatitis. In addition, vaccine is routinely recommended for children 12 to 23 months of age, with catch-up through 18 years of age. Vaccination also is recommended for unvaccinated persons 1 year of age and older for postexposure prophylaxis after close contact with an infected person or exposure to a contaminated food or water source. For postexposure prophylaxis, persons 40 years of age and older who have altered immunocompetence or chronic liver disease should receive immune globulin in addition to hepatitis A vaccine. Health care workers have not been shown to be at higher risk than the general population for hepatitis A and do not need routine immunization. Although food handlers are not at increased risk for hepatitis A compared with the general population, the consequences of infection or suspected infection in this group, which can lead to extensive public health investigations, may make vaccination cost-effective in some settings. Doses vary by age and product. All schedules call for a second dose at least 6 months after the first dose.

Adverse Reactions

The most common adverse reaction after hepatitis A vaccination is tenderness and soreness at the injection site. Although rare and more serious adverse events have been reported in temporal association with vaccination, no causal relationships have been established.

HEPATITIS B

Hepatitis B (Chapter 134) vaccine was the first vaccine known to prevent cancer. It also can prevent acute and chronic complications of hepatitis B, including an estimated 1800 deaths annually in the United States from liver cancer, cirrhosis, and fulminant hepatic disease. Currently produced vaccines contain HBsAg derived from insertion of the gene for HBsAg into *Saccharomyces cerevisiae*. When it is administered in a three-dose series, hepatitis B vaccine produces adequate antibody responses (anti-HBs ≥10 mIU/mL) in more than 90% of healthy adults younger than 40 years and in more than 95% of healthy infants, children, and adolescents. By age 60 years, protective levels of antibody develop in only 75% of vaccinated persons. A new adjuvanted hepatitis B vaccine was licensed in 2017. It consists of recombinant HBsAg, produced in yeast cells (*Hansenula polymorpha*) combined with a novel cytosine phosphoguanine (CpG)–enriched oligodeoxynucleotide (ODN) phosphorothioate immunostimulatory adjuvant (CpG 1018 adjuvant). It is administered in a two-dose series, 1 month apart. The duration of vaccine-conferred immunity is not known, although follow-up of vaccinees for more than 20 years indicates persistence of protection against clinically significant infections (i.e., detectable viremia and clinical disease). Booster doses are not currently recommended. Vaccine must be injected intramuscularly in the deltoid.

Indications

Hepatitis B vaccine is indicated for all adults ages 18 through 59 years and for adults ages 60 years of age and older who are at increased risk of infection or increased risk of complications from hepatitis B infection (see Fig. 15-1 and E-Table 15-1), including all persons ages 19 through 59 years with diabetes. Vaccination of persons who are below age 60 years and without risk factors is based on shared clinical decision making. Universal screening for HBsAg is recommended for all pregnant persons; three doses of vaccine and one dose of hepatitis B immune globulin are recommended for infants of acutely or chronically infected mothers.

Postvaccination serologic testing is recommended for health care workers, immunosuppressed persons, and sexual contacts of persons with chronic hepatitis B infection. If the test is negative, one additional dose of vaccine should be given and the individual should be retested. If this second test is negative, the remaining doses of the series should be given. If the individual still has a negative serology, they are considered a nonresponder. Postvaccination serologic testing is recommended for patients on dialysis 1 year after the final dose in the series. If the test is negative, one booster dose should be given, with follow-up testing 1 year later and then annually.

Adverse Reactions

The most common adverse reaction is soreness at the injection site. Rare instances of Guillain-Barré syndrome, leukoencephalitis, optic neuritis, transverse myelitis, rheumatoid arthritis, type 1 diabetes, and autoimmune disease have been reported, but causal associations have not been confirmed with any systemic immune complications.

HUMAN PAPILLOMAVIRUS

Three licensed HPV vaccines (Chapter 344) contain virus-like particles of the L1 capsid protein of HPV types 16 and 18, which account for about 66% of cases of cervical cancer in the United States. HPV vaccines are prophylactic (i.e., they prevent new infections). These vaccines have reduced the incidence of vaccine-type HPV infection,[A8] as well as the risk of cervical intraepithelial neoplasia.[10] Two of these vaccines, bivalent and quadrivalent, remain licensed but are no longer available in the United States. The nine-valent vaccine (9vHPV) also contains virus-like particles of the L1 capsid protein of HPV types 6 and 11, which are the most common causes of anogenital warts. This vaccine also contains L1 capsid proteins of types 31, 33, 45, 52, and 58, which cause an additional 15% of cervical cancers. HPV type 16 accounts for most of the other cancers caused by HPV infection. Overall, 9vHPV can prevent over 90% of cancers that are caused by HPV.

Indications

Routine vaccination of 11- to 12-year-old girls and boys is recommended in a two-dose schedule at 0 and 6 to 12 months for persons initiating vaccination before age 15 years and a three-dose schedule at 0, 1 to 2, and 6 months for persons initiating vaccination at age 15 years or older or who are immunosuppressed. Vaccine can be given to persons starting at age 9 years. Catch-up vaccination is recommended for all persons through 26 years. Shared clinical decision making is recommended for adults who are age 27 through 45 years and who are not adequately vaccinated.

Adverse Reactions

The most commonly reported local symptoms are injection site pain, redness, and swelling. The most common generalized symptoms are dizziness, syncope, nausea, vomiting, fatigue, headache, fever, and urticaria.

INFLUENZA

Influenza vaccines for seasonal influenza include intramuscular inactivated influenza vaccine, recombinant influenza vaccine, containing the same four virus types as the inactivated vaccine, and intranasal live attenuated influenza vaccine. Live attenuated vaccine (LAIV), which consists of four cold-adapted, temperature-sensitive attenuated viruses, one for each of the expected circulating strains, uses viruses that have been reassorted with circulating strains to contain six internal genes from the parent virus and genes for the surface hemagglutinin and neuraminidase of an A(H3N2), A(H1N1), and two B strains.

Indications

Annual influenza (Chapter 332) vaccination is indicated for all adults, but especially persons at high risk of complications from the disease: all persons aged 50 years and older; adults who have chronic pulmonary, cardiovascular, renal, hepatic, neurologic, hematologic, or metabolic disorders; persons who are immunosuppressed; women who are or will be pregnant during the influenza season; residents of long-term care facilities; American Indians or Alaska Natives; and persons who are morbidly obese. To reduce transmission of influenza to high-risk patients, health care personnel and household contacts of high-risk patients, including contacts of children younger than 5 years, also should be vaccinated annually. Providers should offer vaccination by the end of October, if possible. Pregnant persons in the third trimester should be vaccinated as soon as vaccine becomes available. Vaccination levels are still low in most adult populations in the United States and require more aggressive vaccination efforts.

The efficacy of inactivated influenza vaccine varies with the host's condition and the degree to which antigens in the vaccine match viruses that circulate during the following season. A high-dose inactivated vaccine consists of four times the hemagglutinin for each of the four strains compared with standard-dose vaccine. An inactivated adjuvanted vaccine contains standard doses of each of the four hemagglutinins but also contains MF59 as an adjuvant. Both the high-dose and adjuvanted vaccine are produced in eggs.

In recent years, the effectiveness of the vaccine has averaged about 30% for preventing laboratory-confirmed outpatient illness in persons 50 years and older and about 45% for preventing influenza-like illness in residents of long-term care facilities.[11] Protection often varies depending upon the type of influenza, and protection is higher with higher vaccine doses.[12] Live attenuated vaccine is licensed only for nonpregnant persons aged 2 through 49 years without underlying conditions that place them at high risk of complications from influenza. LAIV may be used for appropriately aged contacts of high-risk persons but is generally not recommended for contacts of severely immunosuppressed patients, such as patients with bone marrow transplants.

The high-dose and adjuvanted vaccines are recommended only for adults over age 65 years. Aside from LAIV, which is recommended only for persons ages 2 to 49 years, there is no preference for one vaccine over another for the general population. All influenza vaccines can be used in all adults provided they have no contraindications.

Influenza vaccination also reduces cardiovascular events. Vaccination efforts should begin as soon as the vaccine becomes available and should continue throughout the season. Peak influenza activity usually recurs in January or February, and influenza season continues through March.

Adverse Reactions

The most common side effect of inactivated vaccine is soreness at the injection site. Fever, malaise, and myalgia may begin 6 to 12 hours after vaccination and persist for 1 or 2 days, although such reactions are most common in children exposed to vaccine for the first time. The most common adverse events after live attenuated influenza vaccine in adults are runny nose, headache, and sore throat. Guillain-Barré syndrome may occur at a rate of about one case per 1 million doses.

MEASLES

Indications

Measles (Chapter 338) immunization is recommended for all persons born in or after 1957 without laboratory evidence of immunity, laboratory confirmation of prior disease, or documentation of prior appropriate vaccination. Most adults are considered to have been appropriately vaccinated if they received one dose of vaccine on or after their first birthday. However, adults who are at increased risk of exposure to measles or transmission of it (e.g., health care personnel, college students, international travelers) should receive a second dose if they did not get a second dose as children, unless they have serologically documented immunity, have laboratory confirmation of disease, or were born before 1957. Persons embarking on foreign travel should have received two doses of MMR vaccine or have other evidence of measles immunity as defined before. Persons born before 1957 are usually immune as a result of natural infection and do not require vaccination, although vaccination is not contraindicated if they are believed to be susceptible.

During educational institutional outbreaks of measles, all persons who have not received two doses or who lack other evidence of measles immunity should be vaccinated. Although measles vaccine can be administered only with mumps and rubella as MMR, individuals already immune to one or more of the components may receive MMR without harm.

Measles vaccine is contraindicated for pregnant persons on theoretical grounds, for persons with altered immunocompetence (except those with HIV infection who are not severely immunocompromised), and for persons with a history of severe allergic reaction (e.g., anaphylaxis) to a prior dose or to a vaccine component. Patients with anaphylactic reactions to eggs can be vaccinated without prior skin testing.

Adverse Reactions

MMR vaccine can cause fever (<15%), rash (5%), transient lymphadenopathy (20%), or parotitis (<1%). Febrile reactions, which usually are otherwise asymptomatic, generally occur 7 to 12 days after vaccination and persist for 1 or 2 days. MMR vaccination can rarely cause anaphylaxis, febrile seizures in children, thrombocytopenic purpura, transient arthralgia, and measles inclusion body encephalitis in persons with demonstrated immunodeficiencies.

MENINGOCOCCAL DISEASE

Three quadrivalent meningococcal vaccines are available against disease caused by serogroups A, C, W, and Y of *Neisseria meningitidis* (Chapter 274). One conjugate vaccine consists of each serogroup-specific polysaccharide covalently linked to 48 μg of diphtheria toxoid and is licensed for persons 9 months to 55 years of age. The second conjugate vaccine consists of the polysaccharides linked to CRM_{197} and is licensed for persons 2 months to 55 years of age. The third conjugate vaccine consists of the polysaccharides linked to tetanus toxoid and is licensed for persons 2 years old and older. The four serogroups in each vaccine account for approximately half of meningococcal disease cases in the United States, including in persons 11 years of age or older (Chapter 274). Conjugate vaccines induce immunologic memory and result in higher and more durable levels of high-avidity antibodies. The duration of immunity for MenACWY is estimated at between 3 and 5 years.

Two recombinant meningococcal serogroup B vaccines are licensed in the United States for persons 10 through 25 years of age. One vaccine (MenB-4C) contains three outer membrane proteins as well as protein-containing outer membrane vesicles, and the other (MenB-FHbp) contains two different alleles of the outer membrane protein (FHbp). Because of the low incidence of serogroup B meningococcal disease, evidence of vaccine effectiveness was inferred based on demonstration of immune response, as measured by serum bactericidal activity using human complement, against a small number of serogroup B strains.

Indications

Routine vaccination with MenACWY is recommended for all adolescents at 11 through 18 years of age, with a first dose administered at age 11 or 12 years and revaccination at age 16 years. For adolescents who receive a first dose between ages 13 and 15 years, a booster dose is recommended at age 16 to 18 years. Meningococcal vaccination is also recommended for unvaccinated and undervaccinated college freshmen who will live in dormitories, for military recruits, for persons at risk during a community outbreak attributable to a vaccine serogroup, and for persons who travel to or live in areas with hyperendemic or epidemic disease (e.g., the "meningitis belt" of sub-Saharan Africa, stretching from Mauritania to Ethiopia). For persons at ongoing increased risk of meningococcal disease (i.e., microbiologists with frequent exposure to *N. meningitidis* in culture and persons with persistent complement component deficiencies, splenic dysfunction, asplenia, or HIV infection), MenACWY vaccination is also recommended, with revaccination every 5 years.

MenB vaccines are recommended for a narrower group of persons at increased meningococcal disease risk compared with MenACWY: persons with persistent complement component deficiencies (including inherited or chronic deficiencies in C3, C5 to C9, properdin, factor D, factor H, or who are taking eculizumab or ravulizumab); anatomic or functional asplenia; microbiologists routinely exposed to isolates of *N. meningitidis;* and those at increased risk because of a serogroup B meningococcal disease outbreak. MenB vaccines are not recommended routinely for first-year college students in residence halls, military recruits, or international travelers. A MenB vaccine series may be administered on the basis of shared vaccine decision making to adolescents and young adults aged 16 to 23 years to provide short-term protection against most strains of serogroup B meningococcal disease. The preferred age for MenB vaccination is 16 to 18 years.

Both MenB-4C and MenB-FHbp are administered in a two-dose series for healthy individuals. For individuals at increased risk of serogroup B meningococcal disease, one of the MenB vaccines (MenB-FHbp) is recommended in a three-dose series. For individuals at continued increased risk, a booster dose is recommended 1 year after completion of the primary series and then every 2 to 3 years thereafter based on continuing risk. For persons at risk in an outbreak who may have received previous doses of MenB vaccine, a booster dose may be given 1 year after the primary series or as little as 6 months after the primary series if recommended by public health officials. MenB vaccines are not interchangeable, and the same brand of MenB vaccine should be used for all primary series doses and the booster doses. The current low prevalence of disease, coupled with lack of data for making policy recommendations for MenB vaccines, resulted in ACIP's determining insufficient evidence exists to make a routine public health recommendation that all adolescents be vaccinated with MenB vaccine. Given the seriousness of meningococcal disease and the availability of licensed vaccines, ACIP agreed sufficient evidence exists to encourage shared clinical decision making about MenB vaccination for adolescents and young adults who are not otherwise at increased risk for serogroup B meningococcal disease.

Adverse Reactions

The most common adverse reactions to MenACWY are injection site reactions and systemic symptoms, such as headache and malaise, which generally persist for 1 or 2 days. An excess risk of Guillain-Barré syndrome was initially reported after vaccination with one of the three MenACWY vaccines but has not been confirmed in subsequent studies.

Injection site reactions are common with MenB vaccines. The most common systemic adverse reactions observed within the 7 days after receipt of MenB vaccines are fatigue, headache, and myalgia.

MUMPS

Indications

Mumps (Chapter 340) vaccine is indicated for all persons without evidence of immunity. For most adults, such evidence consists of a prior history of vaccination on or after the first birthday, laboratory evidence of immunity, or laboratory confirmation of disease. For adults at high risk, including health care personnel, international travelers, and students at post–high school educational institutions, two doses of mumps vaccine constitute acceptable evidence of immunity. Most persons born before 1957 can be considered immune as a result of natural infection, although vaccination is not contraindicated if such persons are thought to be susceptible. Persons who were previously vaccinated with two doses of a mumps-containing vaccine and who are identified by public health officials as at increased risk for mumps because of a mumps outbreak should receive a third dose of a mumps-containing vaccine to improve protection against mumps disease and related complications.

Mumps vaccine is contraindicated for pregnant persons on theoretical grounds, for persons with moderate to severe acute febrile illnesses, and for persons with altered immunocompetence. When it is combined with measles vaccine, it may be given to persons with asymptomatic HIV infection and considered for persons with symptomatic infection if they are not severely immunocompromised. Patients with anaphylactic reactions to eggs can be vaccinated without skin testing.

Adverse Reactions

Adverse events after the vaccine strain used in the United States are uncommon but include fever, parotitis, and allergic reactions. Thrombocytopenic purpura has been reported rarely after MMR (see also, Measles, Adverse Reactions).

PERTUSSIS

Each of the two vaccines licensed for boosting immunity to pertussis (Chapter 289) in adults is combined with tetanus and diphtheria toxoids as Tdap, which has a lower content of pertussis antigens compared with the childhood pertussis-containing vaccines (DTaP). Boostrix (GlaxoSmithKline), which is licensed for adolescents and adults 10 years of age and older, contains three pertussis antigens—toxoid (PT), filamentous hemagglutinin (FHA), and pertactin (PRN). Adacel (Sanofi Pasteur), which is licensed for 10 through 64 years of age, contains five pertussis antigens: PT, FHA, PRN, and two fimbriae. Both vaccines, when they are administered to previously vaccinated adolescents and adults, induce serologic responses that are comparable to those induced with effective childhood vaccination.

Indications

A single dose of Tdap is indicated for all adolescents at 11 to 12 years of age. All adults who have not received Tdap should receive it regardless of the interval since their last tetanus or diphtheria toxoid–containing vaccine. Tdap can be given at any interval after a prior Td. All pregnant persons should receive one dose of Tdap vaccine during each pregnancy, optimally early in the period between 27 and 36 weeks of gestation to maximize maternal antibody response and passive antibody transfer to the infant. Persons not vaccinated during pregnancy should receive Tdap postpartum if they have never previously been vaccinated with it. With the exception of pregnant persons, booster doses of Tdap are not recommended. However, in any circumstance in which a tetanus-toxoid vaccine is indicated generally, Tdap may substitute for Td, unless there is a contraindication to the pertussis component.

Adverse Reactions

Adverse events, usually local reactions, are similar to the adult preparation of Td alone compared with Tdap vaccine (see the section on tetanus and diphtheria later).

PNEUMOCOCCAL DISEASE

Pneumococcal polysaccharide vaccine (PPSV23) consists of purified polysaccharide capsular antigens from 23 types of *Streptococcus pneumoniae* (Chapter 268). Most adults, including elderly patients and those with alcoholic cirrhosis and diabetes mellitus, have a two-fold or greater rise in type-specific antibodies within 2 to 3 weeks of vaccination. Vaccination is approximately 60% effective against invasive pneumococcal disease, but its efficacy against pneumonia in high-risk populations, such as patients with alcoholic cirrhosis or Hodgkin disease, is not clear.[A9]

Pneumococcal conjugate vaccines (PCV15) contains conjugated capsular antigen from the serotypes for which the previously recommended PCV13 is protective, plus serotypes 22F and 33F. PCV20 contains conjugated capsular antigen from the serotypes for which the previously recommended PCV13 is protective, plus serotypes 8, 10A, 11A, 12F, 15B, 22F, and 33F.

Three pneumococcal vaccines are currently recommended for all adults ages 65 years and older. For patients who are PCV13-naïve, clinicians may choose PCV20 or choose PCV15 followed by PPSV23 a year later. Adults ages 19 through 64 years who have a high-risk condition for invasive pneumococcal disease (asthma, diabetes mellitus, cirrhosis, cerebrospinal fluid leaks, splenic dysfunction or anatomic asplenia, Hodgkin disease, lymphoma, multiple myeloma, chronic renal failure, nephrotic syndrome, immunosuppression, HIV infection, cigarette smoking) and who previously have not received PCV13 should receive either a dose of PCV20 or PCV15 followed by PPSV23 8 weeks to a year later.

Indications

The preponderance of information supports the use of pneumococcal vaccines in high-risk populations, including all persons 65 years and older and persons 19 years or older with conditions (Table 15-2). Special efforts should target hospitalized patients. Approximately two thirds of patients who are admitted later with pneumococcal disease had been hospitalized for other reasons within the preceding 5 years.

Because immunity may decrease 5 years or more after initial vaccination with PPSV23, a single booster dose of PPSV23 should be considered at that time for adults at highest risk of disease (such as asplenic patients) and for adults who lose antibody rapidly (such as patients with nephrotic syndrome or renal failure). Persons 65 years or older who received a dose more than 5 years earlier when they were younger than 65 years also should be revaccinated. Because of the rarity of severe reactions in revaccinated patients, persons with indications for vaccination but with unknown histories of prior vaccination should be vaccinated.

Adverse Reactions

Local reactions to PPSV23 are frequent, but less than 3% of vaccinees experience severe local reactions or systemic symptoms such as fever and malaise. Severe events, such as anaphylaxis or Arthus-like reactions at the site of injection, are rare. PCV13 reactions include pain, redness, and swelling at the injection site; limitation of movement of the injected arm; fatigue; and headache.

POLIOMYELITIS

Since 2000, inactivated poliovirus vaccine (IPV) has replaced the live attenuated oral poliovirus vaccine (OPV) in the United States because OPV vaccine caused about eight to nine polio cases per year in the United States among recipients or their contacts (Chapter 349). Trivalent OPV containing types 1, 2, and 3 has been replaced by bivalent OPV containing types 1 and 3 in all countries using OPV. In addition, there is a recommendation that all countries should include at least one dose of IPV in their immunization schedules.

Indications

Routine vaccination of persons 18 years of age or older is not recommended. If adults who are unvaccinated, are incompletely vaccinated, or have unknown vaccination status travel to areas where wild poliovirus is endemic or epidemic, they should receive a series of three doses: two doses of IPV administered at an interval of 4 to 8 weeks, with a third dose administered 6 to 12 months after the second. If three doses of IPV cannot be administered, alternatives include the following: three doses of IPV administered 4 weeks or more apart; two doses of IPV administered 4 weeks or more apart if less than 8 weeks remain before protection is needed; and, if less than 4 weeks remain before protection is needed, a single dose of IPV. If fewer than three doses are administered, the remaining doses needed to complete a three-dose series should be administered when feasible, at the intervals recommended, especially if the person remains at increased risk for poliovirus exposure.

As a precaution, adults (≥18 years of age) who are traveling to areas where poliomyelitis cases are occurring and who have received a routine series with either IPV or OPV in childhood should receive another dose of IPV before departure. For adults, available data do not indicate the need for more than a single lifetime booster dose with IPV.

Adverse Reactions

Minor local reactions (pain, redness) commonly occur after IPV. Because IPV contains trace amounts of streptomycin, polymyxin B, and neomycin, allergic reactions may occur in persons allergic to these antibiotics.

RABIES

Two inactivated rabies vaccines are licensed in the United States. Human diploid cell vaccine (HDCV), which is prepared from the Pitman-Moore strain of rabies virus, also contains small amounts of neomycin sulfate, albumin, and phenol red indicator. The purified chick embryo cell vaccine (PCECV), which is prepared from the Flury LEP rabies virus strain, also contains small amounts of polygeline, human serum albumin, potassium glutamate, and sodium ethylenediamine tetra-acetic acid (EDTA). Both vaccines are given intramuscularly.

Indications

Rabies (Chapter 383) vaccine is indicated for preexposure prophylaxis of high-risk persons, including animal handlers, selected laboratory and field workers, and persons traveling for more than 1 month to areas where rabies is a constant threat. For both rabies vaccines, the preexposure regimen consists of two 1-mL intramuscular injections on days 0 and 7, followed by a titer at regular intervals depending on risk. If the titer is negative, a booster dose should be administered. Adults at intermediate risk (veterinarians, travelers) may receive a third dose of vaccine instead of a titer, provided that it is administered between 21 days through 3 years following the first dose.[13] Postexposure treatment depends on prior exposure to vaccine (Chapter 383). Persons being treated for the first time should be given human rabies immune globulin as well as four doses of vaccine at days 0, 3, 7, and 14.

Adverse Reactions

Local reactions (e.g., pain at the injection site, redness, swelling, and induration) are common after both rabies vaccine preparations. Hypersensitivity reactions have been reported in up to 6% of persons after booster doses of HDCV.

RUBELLA

Indications

One dose of rubella vaccine (Chapter 339) is indicated for adults born in 1957 or later without evidence of immunity and for women of any age who lack evidence of immunity and who are considering becoming pregnant. Persons without a prior history of vaccination on or after the first birthday, laboratory evidence of immunity, or laboratory confirmation of disease should be considered as lacking evidence of immunity. A single dose of vaccine is 95% or more effective. Many persons receive two doses of rubella vaccine by the two-dose schedule of MMR.

Rubella vaccine is contraindicated for persons with moderate to severe acute illnesses and persons with reduced immunocompetence. When it is given with measles vaccine, it may be administered to persons with asymptomatic HIV infection and considered for symptomatic persons who are not severely immunocompromised. Rubella vaccine is grown in human diploid cells and can be administered without problems to persons with egg allergies.

Adverse Reactions

Follow-up of pregnant persons who had no evidence of immunity and who received rubella vaccines within 3 months of the estimated date of conception showed no evidence of defects compatible with congenital rubella syndrome in their offspring. Nevertheless, vaccine is contraindicated in pregnant persons on theoretical grounds, and conception should be delayed for 1 month after rubella vaccination.

Arthralgia develops among about 25% of nonimmune postpubertal females after vaccination with rubella vaccine. Symptoms generally begin 1 to 3 weeks after vaccination, usually are mild, persist for about 2 days, and rarely recur. These symptoms are less common in postpubertal males compared with females. Other infrequent adverse events include transient peripheral neuritis and pain in the arms and legs. Thrombocytopenic purpura is rare when rubella vaccine is administered as MMR.

TETANUS AND DIPHTHERIA

Tetanus (Chapter 271) toxoid is one of the most effective immunizations, with more than 95% protection after a primary series of three doses. In persons aged 7 years or older, it should always be used in combination with diphtheria (Chapter 272) toxoid (Td), which is more than 85% effective in preventing disease. Combinations that also include pertussis antigens (Tdap) are preferred to Td for routine immunization of adolescents and adults who have yet to receive Tdap as well as for pregnant persons (for whom Tdap is recommended during every pregnancy). Doses need not be repeated if the schedule is interrupted. A booster dose of Tdap or Td is recommended every 10 years.

Indications

After a wound, persons of unknown immunization status or persons who have received fewer than three doses of tetanus toxoid should receive a dose of Tdap or Td regardless of the severity of the wound. Td also is indicated for persons who have previously received three or more doses if more than 10 years has elapsed since the last dose, in the case of clean and minor wounds, and if more than 5 years has elapsed for all other wounds. However, the benefit of an adult tetanus or diphtheria booster is probably very, very small.[14] Persons who have never received a dose of Tdap should receive it instead of Td for wound management. Tetanus immune globulin should be administered simultaneously at a separate site to persons who have wounds that are not clean and minor if they have not previously received at least three doses of toxoid.

Adverse Reactions

Most reactions to Td consist of local inflammation and low-grade fever. Exaggerated local (Arthus-like) reactions, with extensive painful swelling, often from shoulder to elbow, are occasionally reported 2 to 8 hours after receipt of a diphtheria- or tetanus-containing vaccine, particularly in persons who have received frequent doses of diphtheria or tetanus toxoid. Severe systemic reactions, such as generalized urticaria, anaphylaxis, Guillain-Barré syndrome, and other neurologic complications, rarely have been reported after receipt of tetanus toxoid.

VARICELLA: CHICKENPOX

A single dose of live attenuated varicella vaccine (Oka strain), which can be combined with MMR vaccine, protects 70 to 90% of recipients against any disease and more than 95% of recipients against severe disease, but a two-dose schedule is recommended. Whether immunity wanes with increasing time after vaccination is unclear. Use of vaccine has been associated with dramatic decreases in the incidence of varicella.

Indications

Persons 13 years or older without evidence of immunity to varicella should receive two doses at least 4 weeks apart. Evidence of immunity to varicella for adults includes documentation of two doses of varicella-containing vaccine (varicella or MMRV) at least 28 days apart, laboratory evidence of immunity or laboratory confirmation of disease, birth in the United States before 1980, or diagnosis or verification of a history of varicella or herpes zoster disease by a health care provider. Serologic screening of adults in some situations may be cost-effective, provided that identified susceptible adults are vaccinated. Serologic testing is not indicated after vaccination. The vaccine is contraindicated in persons who are immunocompromised, persons with anaphylactic allergies to vaccine components, and pregnant persons. Postexposure vaccination within 3 days of exposure can reduce the likelihood of symptomatic infection by about two-thirds. The varicella vaccine formulation marketed in the United States is temperature sensitive, so it must be stored at −50°C to −15°C to retain potency.

Adverse Reactions

The most common side effect is soreness at the injection site, which is reported in 25 to 35% of recipients 13 years or older. Varicella-like rashes at the injection site (median of two lesions) have been reported in 3% of recipients in this age group after the first dose and in 1% after the second dose. Nonlocalized rashes with a median of five lesions have been reported in 5.5% of recipients after the first dose and in 0.9% after the second dose. Although the vaccine virus can cause herpes zoster (shingles), especially in children, the incidence is substantially lower than would be expected after natural varicella (Chapter 346). More severe events in temporal relation to the vaccine have been reported rarely, but a causal relationship has not been established. Transmission of vaccine virus to a contact is extremely rare and probably occurs only from vaccinees in whom a varicella-like rash developed.

VARICELLA-ZOSTER

Recombinant zoster vaccine (RZV), a subunit vaccine containing varicella-zoster virus glycoprotein E with the $ASO1_B$ adjuvant system, is about 97% effective for the prevention of herpes zoster in persons ages 50 to 69 years and about 91% effective in persons aged 70 years and older.[15] This is the only zoster vaccine available in the United States.

Indications

Recombinant zoster subunit vaccine (RZV) is recommended for all adults ages 50 years and older and for adults ages 18 through 49 years who are immunosuppressed. The vaccine is recommended even in adults who previously received live zoster vaccine or had herpes zoster, and it is not necessary to elicit a history of varicella or to test for varicella immunity before administering RZV. The vaccine is administered intramuscularly as two doses separated by 2 to 6 months.[16]

Adverse Reactions

Local reactions (erythema, pain or tenderness, and swelling at the injection site) are common. Moderate or severe local reactions occur in about 10% of RZV vaccine recipients, and moderate or severe systemic reactions also occur in about 10%. If an individual has a reaction to the first dose, it does not affect their likelihood of a reaction to the second dose.

VACCINES INTENDED PRIMARILY FOR INTERNATIONAL TRAVELERS

Evaluation of people before travel should include a review and provision of routine vaccines recommended on the basis of age and other individual characteristics. Recommendations for specific vaccines related to travel will depend on itinerary, duration of travel, and host factors. Detailed recommendations are available at www.cdc.gov/travel.[17]

CHOLERA

Indications

Cholera (Chapter 278) vaccine is indicated for adult travelers (aged 18 to 64 years) from the United States to areas of the world with endemic or epidemic cholera caused by toxigenic *Vibrio cholerae* O1 within the past year (https://wwwnc.cdc.gov/travel/). Lyophilized CVD 103-HgR (Vaxchora, PaxVax) is a single-dose, live attenuated oral cholera vaccine. Its efficacy against severe diarrhea (defined as fecal output >3 L/24 hours) after oral toxigenic *V. cholerae* O1 challenge is estimated to be 90% at 10 days after vaccination and 80% at 3 months after vaccination.[18] There is no recommendation for use of booster doses at this time.

Adverse Reactions

Available safety data indicate no harms except for a slightly elevated risk for mild diarrhea among vaccine recipients.

JAPANESE ENCEPHALITIS

Indications

Japanese encephalitis (Chapter 352) vaccine is indicated primarily for travelers to Asia who will spend a month or longer in endemic areas during the transmission season, especially if travel will include rural areas. In all instances, travelers should be advised to take personal precautions to reduce exposure to mosquito bites. An older vaccine was reported to be 80 to 91% effective in preventing clinical disease, and the current whole virus inactivated vaccine (Ixiaro, Intercell Biomedical) was licensed on the basis of comparable immunogenicity. The primary series consists of two 0.5-mL doses given intramuscularly on days 0 and 28, for patients 2 months and older, with the second dose administered at least 1 week before travel. If the primary series was administered more than 1 year previously, a booster dose may be given before the next potential exposure to the virus. The FDA has approved an alternate 0- and 7-day schedule for persons 18 years old and older.

Adverse Reactions

Headache, myalgia, and local reactions (pain and tenderness) occur in more than 10% of vaccinees. However, the incidence rates of these events were similar to those in a comparison group that received a placebo with aluminum hydroxide.

TYPHOID

Indications

The cumulative efficacy at 2.5 to 3.0 years for the live attenuated Ty21a oral vaccine is about 50%, whereas the cumulative efficacy at 2.5 to 3.0 years for the capsular polysaccharide vaccine is about 55%. Typhoid (Chapter 284) vaccine is indicated primarily for travelers to areas where the risk of prolonged exposure to contaminated food and water is high. Because the vaccine is not always effective, food and water precautions are still essential. The vaccine also may be considered for family or other intimate contacts of typhoid carriers and laboratory workers who work with *Salmonella* Typhi. The capsular polysaccharide vaccine is approved for persons 2 years old and older. The live attenuated Ty21a oral vaccine is approved for persons ages 6 years and older. For adults and children 6 years and older, either of the vaccines may be used. For Ty21a, one enteric-coated capsule is taken every other day for four doses. Alternatively, a single dose of the ViCPS vaccine may be given. The duration of protection with Ty21a is not known; repetition of the primary series is recommended every 5 years for persons at risk. Boosters are recommended every 2 years for the ViCPS vaccine if persons continue to be at risk. The ViCPS vaccine can be given to children as young as 2 years.

Adverse Reactions

Fever and headache may occur after receipt of typhoid vaccines. Stomach pain, nausea, and rash are rarely observed.

YELLOW FEVER

Indications

Yellow fever (Chapter 351) occurs only in areas of South America and Africa. Vaccination with a single dose of the live attenuated 17D strain of virus confers protection to almost all recipients for at least 10 years. For most persons only a single dose is recommended. However, a booster dose is recommended every 10 years for at-risk laboratory personnel and certain previously vaccinated travelers (pregnant persons before travel to at-risk areas; hematopoietic stem cell transplant recipients vaccinated before transplant; HIV-infected persons; and travelers who will be in a higher-risk setting based on season, location, activities, and duration of their travel, such as travelers who plan to spend a prolonged period in endemic areas or those traveling to highly endemic areas such as rural West Africa during peak transmission season or an area with an ongoing outbreak).

Yellow fever vaccine should not be given to immunocompromised persons or persons with anaphylactic allergies to eggs. The vaccine is contraindicated in pregnant persons on theoretical grounds, although pregnant persons who must travel to a high-risk area may be vaccinated.

Adverse Reactions

Adverse reactions (fever, aches, and soreness, redness, or swelling where the injection was given) occur in up to 25% of vaccinees. Anaphylaxis has been reported in 0.8 to 1.8 persons per 100,000 doses of vaccine distributed. A rare syndrome (0.25 case per 100,000 doses distributed) of multiple organ system failure with high rates of mortality called viscerotropic disease has been reported, primarily among older adults and persons who have undergone thymectomy or have severe thymic dysfunction. Meningoencephalitis, Guillain-Barré syndrome, acute disseminated encephalomyelitis, and bulbar palsy have been reported in 1 per 125,000 doses and are more common in older vaccinees. In patients 60 years and older who are going to spend time in yellow fever–endemic zones, yellow fever vaccine should be administered with caution and only after careful counseling.

VACCINES FOR POSSIBLE BIOTERRORISM AGENTS

ANTHRAX

Anthrax (Chapter 272) vaccine adsorbed (AVA) is prepared from a cell-free filtrate of a nonencapsulated strain of anthrax and contains many cell products, including protective antigen. Protective antigen is responsible for binding to cells, allowing transport of lethal factor and edema factor into host cells. A recombinant protective antigen (rPA) vaccine is in clinical trials.

Indications

Preexposure prophylaxis consists of a three-dose primary intramuscular schedule at 0 and 4 weeks and at 6 months, with booster doses at 12 and 18 months, followed by boosters every 3 years thereafter. Protective efficacy of an earlier form of the vaccine against cutaneous anthrax was 92.5%. Animal models suggest efficacy against inhalation anthrax. Preexposure vaccination is recommended for persons engaged in work involving exposure to high concentrations of *Bacillus anthracis* or in activities with high potential for aerosol production. Vaccine is recommended in conjunction with antibiotics for postexposure prophylaxis after exposure to aerosolized *B. anthracis* spores. The recommended regimen is three doses of AVA administered at 0, 2, and 4 weeks, combined with 60 days of antibiotics, which should be continued for at least 14 days after the third dose of vaccine (Chapter 272).

Adverse Reactions

The most common adverse events are local reactions, including subcutaneous nodules, which are thought to be due to the deposition of the aluminum-containing adjuvant in subcutaneous tissue. These adverse events are less common with intramuscular injections than with subcutaneous injections.

SMALLPOX

Two licensed vaccines are available for prevention of smallpox. ACAM 2000 vaccine uses live vaccinia virus, an orthopox virus that is distinct from variola and cowpox viruses and that provides cross-protection from smallpox. Smallpox vaccine is close to 100% effective when it is administered properly with a bifurcated needle. The skin usually does not need any special preparation. If alcohol is used for cleaning, the skin should be allowed to dry before vaccination to avoid inactivation of the vaccine. The needle is held perpendicular to the skin with 15 punctures for all vaccinees, made rapidly with enough vigor to ensure that a trace of blood appears within 15 to 20 seconds. With a primary take, the vaccination site should become reddened and pruritic within 3 or 4 days after vaccination; a large vesicle with a red areola forms and becomes pustular by 7 to 11 days. The lesion scabs by the third week.

Jynneos vaccine is a live, nonreplicating vaccinia vector vaccine, which uses the modified vaccinia Ankara strain. It is approved for persons ages 18 years and older for prevention of smallpox and/or monkeypox infection. Its efficacy is inferred through comparison of immunogenicity with ACAM 2000. It is administered as a subcutaneous injection in two doses 4 weeks apart.

Indications

The vaccine is indicated for persons who work with orthopox viruses. To increase preparedness for a smallpox attack, vaccination is often recommended for persons who will serve on public health or health care response teams. The duration of immunity is unclear. Revaccination is recommended at least every 10 years for persons who continue to be at risk. Contraindications for both vaccines include a history of severe allergic reactions (e.g., anaphylaxis) to a previous dose of vaccine or to a component. Immunosuppression is a contraindication to the ACAM 2000 live virus vaccine. Other contraindications to ACAM 2000 include history or presence of eczema, other chronic or exfoliative skin conditions, and pregnancy in the patient or a close household or other contact. Persons who are younger than 1 year, are breast-feeding, or have allergies to vaccine components should not be vaccinated. Because of reports of postvaccination cardiac events, vaccination should be deferred in persons with ischemia or other severe heart diseases or persons at high risk for ischemic heart disease events (https://www.cdc.gov/smallpox/clinicians/vaccination.htm). In the event of exposure to variola, the risk of disease outweighs any contraindications. Should variola be introduced into a community, vaccination would be indicated for all exposed persons and their close contacts to prevent further spread, and recommendations for more widespread vaccination would have to be evaluated on a case-by-case basis.

Adverse Reactions

For ACAM 2000, fever is the most common adverse event. Other more serious complications include eczema vaccinatum, which is a local or disseminated vaccinia infection in persons with a history of eczema or other exfoliative dermatitis; vaccinia necrosum, which occurs in immunocompromised persons; autoinoculation, especially of the eye, which can cause keratitis and scarring; generalized vaccinia; myopericarditis; and encephalitis. The risk for death from vaccinia is about one case per 1 million primary vaccinations. The most common adverse events to Jynneos include local reactions, myalgia, and headache.

EBOLA

Ervebo is a live attenuated vector vaccine with vesicular stomatitis virus as the vector with the gene encoding the glycoprotein of Ebola strain Zaire ebolavirus (Chapter 351). It is administered as a single intramuscular (IM) dose.

Indications

Ervebo is recommended for persons 18 years old and older who are responders to an outbreak of Ebola or who work in federally designated Ebola treatment centers in the United States. Additionally, vaccine is recommended for persons who work in biosafety level 4 facilities in the United States.

Adverse Reactions

The most common adverse reactions include local reactions, headache, and fever. Arthralgia and arthritis also occur, particularly in women and persons with a past history of arthritis. History of severe allergic reaction (e.g., anaphylaxis) to a previous dose of or to a component of the vaccine is a contraindication. After receiving a dose of vaccine, recipients should avoid kissing or sharing razors, eating utensils, toothbrushes, drinking cups, or needles for 2 weeks. Vaccine recipients should avoid donating blood, contact with high-risk persons, or exposure of livestock to blood or body fluids for 6 weeks. Barrier methods for sexual interaction should be used for 2 months.

OTHER AGENTS

Other organisms or products that have been considered potential bioterrorism threats include plague (Chapter 288) and botulinum toxin (Chapter 271). Poisoning with botulinum toxin can be treated with a trivalent antitoxin available from the Centers for Disease Control and Prevention (see https://www.cdc.gov/laboratory/drugservice/formulary.html). An experimental heptavalent botulinum toxoid can be obtained from the Centers for Disease Control and Prevention for laboratory workers at high risk for exposure to toxin. Preexposure vaccination is not warranted or feasible for the general population.

GENERAL REFERENCES

For the General References and other additional features, please visit Elsevier eBooks+ at https://ebooks.health.elsevier.com.

Grade A References

A1. Koufoglou E, Kourlaba G, Michos A. Effect of prophylactic administration of antipyretics on the immune response to pneumococcal conjugate vaccines in children: a systematic review. *Pneumonia (Nathan)*. 2021;13:7.

A2. Wysocki J, Center KJ, Brzostek J, et al. A randomized study of fever prophylaxis and the immunogenicity of routine pediatric vaccinations. *Vaccine*. 2017;35:1926-1935.

A3. El Sahly HM, Baden LR, Essink B, et al. Efficacy and safety of the mRNA-1273 SARS-CoV-2 vaccine. *N Engl J Med*. 2021;384:403-416.

A4. Thompson MG, Stenehjem E, Grannis S, et al. Effectiveness of Covid-19 vaccines in ambulatory and inpatient care settings. *N Engl J Med*. 2021;385:1355-1371.

A5. Lopez Bernal J, Andrews N, Gower C, et al. Effectiveness of Covid-19 vaccines against the B.1.617.2 (delta) variant. *N Engl J Med*. 2021;385:585-594.

A6. Thompson MG, Burgess JL, Naleway AL, et al. Prevention and attenuation of Covid-19 with the BNT162b2 and mRNA-1273 vaccines. *N Engl J Med*. 2021;385:320-329.

A7. Bar-On YM, Goldberg Y, Mandel M, et al. Protection of BNT162b2 vaccine booster against Covid-19 in Israel. *N Engl J Med*. 2021;385:1393-1400.

A8. D'Addario M, Redmond S, Scott P, et al. Two-dose schedules for human papillomavirus vaccine: systematic review and meta-analysis. *Vaccine*. 2017;35:2892-2901.

A9. Kraicer-Melamed H, O'Donnell S, Quach C. The effectiveness of pneumococcal polysaccharide vaccine 23 (PPV23) in the general population of 50 years of age and older: a systematic review and meta-analysis. *Vaccine*. 2016;34:1540-1550.

16

PRINCIPLES OF OCCUPATIONAL AND ENVIRONMENTAL MEDICINE

JUDITH GREEN-MCKENZIE

Occupational and environmental medicine is a multidisciplinary field that focuses on how to recognize, diagnose, treat, and prevent injuries and illnesses that arise from exposures at work and in the environment, as well as to improve the health, well-being, and safety of employees, their families, and their communities, locally and globally.[1] Physicians in occupational and environmental medicine collaborate with employers, safety personnel, industrial hygienists, occupational health nurses, ergonomists, human resources specialists, labor union leaders, and others. They must also be conversant with how environmental exposures can lead to illness.

Physicians who specialize in occupational and environmental medicine may have a responsibility to the employer as well as the worker.[2] All physicians who assess the possibility of work-related injury or illness also must be cognizant of the regulatory environment affecting their work.

OCCUPATIONAL AND ENVIRONMENTAL MEDICINE REGULATORY ENVIRONMENT

Occupational and environmental medicine grew out of a necessity to provide protections for workers in the context of the heightened awareness about industrial accidents and exposures as well as the liability of employers for workplace injuries and illnesses. Its development has been embedded in an evolving regulatory environment, and the two together have led to improved occupational health outcomes.[3]

WORKERS' COMPENSATION

Workers' compensation is a "no-fault" system in which monetary compensation is provided to workers for medical and rehabilitation costs as well as lost wages related to illnesses or injuries that arose out of or during the course of employment, regardless of cause. Employers are held responsible for compensation, and the injured worker accepts the standard amount of permitted compensation. Workers' compensation is now the third largest source of support for disabled workers after Social Security and Medicare.

WORK-RELATED DISABILITY

Physicians and other providers may be asked to determine the extent of their patient's disability under the workers' compensation system. In general, disability is an inability or limitation in performing activities, roles, and tasks within a social or physical environment. Disability differs from impairment, which refers to an anatomic or functional abnormality or loss. Individuals with the same impairment may have different degrees of disability, which may vary depending on factors such as economic demand, educational factors, job description, and age. Workers' compensation defines four types of disability:

- *Temporary total disability:* Inability to work for a period, but recovery is expected. Lost wage (indemnity) benefits are paid to the worker while on disability.
- *Permanent total disability:* Inability to undertake gainful employment, and further treatment will not lead to recovery. Indemnity benefits are paid to the worker.
- *Temporary partial disability:* The worker can perform some work duties (modified duty) and can return to work if a suitable placement can be found.
- *Permanent partial disability:* Permanent loss of one or several functions. Work is possible but in a modified duty capacity or at a different job.

Maximal medical improvement or *permanency* is said to have occurred when an injured worker has recovered as much as they are likely to recover and have likely reached a stage of permanent disability. Although the condition may improve over time, the best decision must be made with the information at hand at the time.

If an employer provides modified duty that the employee can perform, then this option can reduce payment for lost wages (indemnity costs) and thus reduce the overall cost of workers' compensation. This approach also keeps the employee in the work culture, thereby easing the way to return to full-duty work, if and when achievable. In fact, most injured workers return to full-duty work.

APPROACH TO THE PATIENT

SALIENT FEATURES OF THE OCCUPATIONAL AND ENVIRONMENTAL MEDICINE HISTORY

Two simple initial questions during the history taking—"What is your job? and "Where do you work?"—can help clinicians ascertain whether work may play a role in the patient's present illness and past medical history. If the condition is work related, a directed occupational and environmental history is essential to document any relationship to work so as to establish the background for any future workers' compensation claim. Otherwise the worker may be denied workers' compensation if the case is not clearly presented, or may at least experience a delay in receiving such benefits.

When a workers' compensation claim is filed, the adjuster who reviews the case relies greatly on the provider's initial medical note to determine whether to accept the claim. The physician and document must query about the mechanism of the injury or the nature of the exposure to assess any potential work-relatedness. In addition to usual questions to explore an injury, additional information should be elicited for a work-related claim:

- Reason for visit: chief complaint, which will guide future questions
- Mechanism of injury: helps ascertain work-relatedness
- Age: can help estimate time to recovery
- Handedness (right/left): may affect modified duty assigned by the provider
- Place of work: to appraise type of work potentially available (e.g., options that the worker may be able to perform)
- Job title: may help determine if modified duty is necessary
- Description of job duties: helps determine how to design modified duty work
- Prior injuries: can help the clinician determine longevity at work (e.g., if the employee had similar prior surgery, the clinician can explore potential preventive measures with the employee and the employer)
- Whether others are injured similarly: may suggest population level prevention
- Comorbid conditions: can influence current and future injuries and return-to-work arrangements
- Social history: determine living arrangements and whether help at home or duties at home may affect recovery
- Is the employee currently working: may help infer severity of injury or illness, thereby informing return to work status (modified or full duty)

In addition to detailed questions exploring an exposure, the clinician should elicit information about:

- The nature of exposure: agent and place of exposure (work, home, community)
- A standard exposure history: such as with the Exposure Survey created by the Agency for Toxic Substance and Disease Registry (E-Fig. 16-1)
- A safety data sheet (SDS): contains physical data, potential hazards, and handling and safety precautions data on all the potential toxins at work
- Symptom temporality: to determine if symptoms improve away from work or in a different environment, as in occupational asthma compared with asthma that has environmental triggers (Chapter 75)
- Time of peak symptoms: helps with temporality if during work hours
- Duration of symptoms: recent or remote onset
- Organ system involved (e.g., skin manifestations may suggest an agent with direct contact)
- Type of personal protective equipment used: determine adequacy
- Current work duties: help assess degree of potential exposure
- Occupational history using a standard survey (see E-Fig. 16-1): to determine exposures from prior jobs (e.g., sensitizers such as diisocyanate or beryllium)
- Length of employment: potential for sustained exposure
- Similar symptoms in other employees: ascertain if presentation is unique
- Smoking history: may be synergistic for a respiratory agent
- Family history of allergy: to determine atopy

CLINICAL IMPLICATIONS

ACUTE INJURIES

In the United States, approximately three million nonfatal workplace injuries and illnesses are reported annually. Over 50% of these injuries require modified duty, job transfer, or time away from work. The most commonly reported injuries are sprains, strains, and tears; soreness or pain; cuts, lacerations, and punctures; bruises and contusions; and fractures (Table 16-1).[4] Fractures result in the most lost work days. Initial management is basic first aid followed by referral, as necessary, to emergency care or an appropriate specialist.

Eye injuries are common and may be prevented with the use of appropriate personal protective equipment, such as eye protection for healthcare personnel conducting a procedure where a splash from a body fluid is possible or the use of welding goggles to prevent photokeratoconjunctivitis in a welder.

CLINICAL SYNDROMES

Environmental and occupational hazards especially affect individuals who have underlying diseases, chronic health conditions, or habits that increase their risk. For example, individuals who smoke have a higher risk of developing more severe lung disease from occupational exposures (Chapter 81).

Occupational or environmental diseases may be difficult to distinguish from other diseases that cause similar symptoms or signs. For acute syndromes, proximal exposure to toxins, often with similar symptoms in others, is a helpful clue. For more recurrent symptoms, a cyclic pattern in which symptoms worsen on workdays and improve on days off, is helpful. For chronic symptoms, such as hepatic dysfunction or neurologic findings, a more long-standing work or environmental exposure or toxin should be considered, and such a link is more likely if multiple individuals are affected.

For potential exposure to heavy metals (Chapter 20), blood levels can be diagnostic. For other exposures, a trial of withdrawal followed by re-challenge can be very helpful when it can be safely implemented.

TABLE 16-1 COMMON OCCUPATIONAL MUSCULOSKELETAL INJURIES

ANATOMICAL LOCATION	INJURY
Neck and Back Injury	Acute back or neck pain Disk herniation
Shoulder	Acromioclavicular joint separation Adhesive capsulitis Brachial plexus neuropathy Impingement syndrome Labral tear Rotator cuff tear Rotator cuff tendinosis Shoulder dislocation Subacromial bursitis Supraspinatus tendinitis
Elbow	Anterior interosseous syndrome Elbow dislocation Elbow fracture Lateral and medial epicondylitis Olecranon bursitis Pronator syndrome Radial tunnel entrapment Ulnar collateral ligament injury Ulnar nerve entrapment at elbow
Hand	Carpal tunnel syndrome De Quervain tenosynovitis Dupytren contracture Mallet finger Radius fracture Scaphoid fracture Trigger finger Ulnar fracture Wrist sprain
Hip	Bursitis Labral tear Tendonitis
Knee	Anterior cruciate ligament injury Collateral ligament injury Knee pain Medial and lateral meniscal injury Patellofemoral pain Posterior cruciate ligament injury
Ankle	Fracture Inversion or inversion injury
Eye Injury	Cataract Chemical or thermal burn Corneal abrasion Foreign body Splash to eye of infectious fluid Trauma
Ear Injury	Hearing loss due to acoustic or physical trauma Ototoxic hearing loss Sensorineural noise induced hearing loss
Occupational Infections	Bloodborne pathogen exposures Hepatitis B and C Herpes B virus Human immunodeficiency virus Influenza virus Severe acute respiratory syndrome coronavirus 2 Tuberculosis
Occupational Skin Manifestations	Allergic dermatitis from allergens such as latex and chromate Bedbugs Infectious agents such as herpes simplex Irritant contact dermatitis from cleansers and solvents Scabies Skin cancer from arsenic or polycyclic aromatic hydrocarbons

Common Clinical Syndromes

Although environmental and occupational exposures can cause or exacerbate many clinical syndromes, certain syndromes are especially common or problematic (Table 16-2).

TABLE 16-2 COMMON OCCUPATIONAL AND ENVIRONMENTAL HEALTH CONDITIONS IN GENERAL PRACTICE

CONDITION	EXPOSURE SETTINGS	COMMENT
Asthma	Virtually any indoor or outdoor workplace	New-onset, recrudescent, or exacerbated asthma
Interstitial, parenchymal, and inflammatory lung disorders	Dusts, metals, and organic materials	All parenchymal disorders have one or more environmental causes
Cancers of the respiratory tract	Asbestos, radon, silica, combustion fumes, tars, and some metals	Smokers are more likely to be affected
Sensorineural hearing loss	Noise, metals, and solvents	High-frequency loss, especially in younger workers
Musculoskeletal disorders of trunk and limbs	Heavy or repetitive activities or postures	Cold, vibration, and work stress contribute
Upper airway irritation	Dust and fumes	More common in smokers and atopic persons
Nonspecific building-related illness	Office work	Must exclude *specific* causes
Dermatitis, allergic or irritant	Repeated exposure to unprotected skin	Work and environmental exposures should be considered in every case
Multiple chemical sensitivities	Any	Complication of adverse environmental exposure

From Cullen MR. Principles of occupational and environmental medicine. In: Goldman L, Schafer AI, eds. *Goldman-Cecil Medicine*, 26th ed. Philadelphia: Elsevier; 2020: Chapter 16.

Asthma

Numerous workplace antigens ranging from animal dander, to latex, to small molecules are responsible for as much as 20% of adult-onset asthma (Chapter 75). The temporal relationship of symptoms to work may be the only clue, and resolution after removal from the toxic environment is the only way to establish the diagnosis.

Chronic Lung Diseases

Coal workers' pneumoconiosis (Chapter 81), silicosis (Chapter 81), and chronic berylliosis can all resemble sarcoidosis (Chapter 83) on a chest radiograph, and all may exacerbate any underlying chronic obstructive pulmonary disease (Chapter 76).[5,6] Asbestosis (Chapter 81) resembles idiopathic pulmonary fibrosis (Chapter 80) except for its pleural involvement. Hypersensitivity pneumonitis (Chapters 80 and 81) occurs in agricultural settings or wherever microbes contaminate work materials. Bronchiolitis obliterans is seen in workers in facilities that produce microwave popcorn or coffee as a result of exposure to diacetyl or 2,3-pentanedione. Inorganic chemicals can cause allergic alveolitis.

Respiratory Cancers

Occupational exposure to coal dust, asbestos, silica, polyaromatic hydrocarbons, diesel exhaust, pitch, asphalt, radon, chromium, and formaldehyde have been implicated in lung cancer (Chapter 177), and their risks are synergistic with cigarette smoking. Asbestos is also the major risk factor for malignant mesothelioma (Chapters 86 and 177).

Sensorineural Hearing Loss

Noise is second only to aging as a cause of high-frequency sensorineural hearing loss (Chapter 394).[7] Hearing protection can mitigate or prevent hearing loss and is required for major occupational noise exposure. Exposure to ototoxic workplace chemicals, such as aniline dyes used commercially to dye fabric, also may lead to hearing loss.

Musculoskeletal Disorders

Low back pain (Chapter 369) is the most common work-related musculoskeletal complaint. In addition to usual care, workplace preventive measures are key.

Other chronic musculoskeletal injuries include carpal tunnel syndrome (Chapter 388), epicondylitis, and De Quervain tenosynovitis. Physical therapy and medications are often helpful, but modifying the causal work and leisure activities is a key intervention.

Skin Conditions

Erythematous rashes commonly are caused by workplace or other exposures to latex, plastics, irritating chemicals, heat pressure, or friction. Identification and elimination of the precipitant is critical. Allergy testing (Chapter 230) by a consultant is helpful in difficult cases.

Common Exposures

Thousands of toxins (Table 16-3) and other hazards can potentially cause or exacerbate a wide range of conditions, but certain basic principles and clinical approaches can guide the assessment of their role in causing signs or symptoms in individual workers. The major determinants of the risk for clinical disease are exposure and absorption, which together determine the dose of the toxin.

Sick Building Syndrome

The inability to provide safe heating, air-conditioning, and air exchange in indoor spaces can result in nonspecific symptoms such as headache, fatigue, cough, and even skin rashes in multiple occupants in the affected building.[8] Molds and other microbial materials may be the cause, but a specific irritant may not be discovered despite extensive testing. Remediation of identifiable sources usually alleviates the problem, but sometimes empirical cleaning or replacement of systems may be required.

Metals

Exposures to lead and arsenic (Chapter 20) are now uncommon in the workplace but have been associated with contamination of drinking water in the United States and globally. Mercury (Chapter 20) is found in large ocean fish. Manganese (Chapter 20) in welding fumes and various alloys can cause extrapyramidal Parkinson-like symptoms and autonomic dysfunction. Blood or urine levels are generally the best way to make the diagnosis.

Solvents, Organohalides, Herbicides, and Pesticides

Petroleum derivatives, which are commonly components of workplace and household products, are irritating and sometimes neurotoxic or hepatotoxic (Chapter 96). Dioxin, which is produced by the combustion of chlorine-containing materials, can cause soft tissue sarcomas (Chapter 187) and perhaps other cancers. Glyphosate, which had been a common herbicide, is associated with about a 40% increased risk of non-Hodgkin lymphoma (Chapter 171). Exposure to pyrethroid insecticides is associated with increased mortality.[9]

Particulate Matter

Ambient air pollution is a major contribution not only to lung disease but also to cardiovascular disease[10,11] and all-cause mortality.[12] Some estimates suggest that indoor and outdoor air pollution cause 6 to 7 million annual deaths worldwide, about two-thirds of which are attributable to outdoor pollution. Respiratory irritants include sulfur dioxide, and small particulate matter that may be laden with proinflammatory polyaromatic hydrocarbons, which especially result from burning wood, coal, or diesel fuel.

Water

In addition to toxins such as lead and arsenic, more than 800 million people worldwide consume unclean drinking water that can be contaminated with bacteria, nontuberculous mycobacteria, and protozoa. Such contaminated water causes about 3.75 million deaths worldwide each year.

Disease outbreaks attributable to water can result in serious acute, chronic illness as well as result in a fatality, especially if one is immunocompromised. Water contamination is not distributed evenly. It may depend on seasonality, for example, where enteric infection and water-related illnesses occur more commonly during the periods of rain abundance, as in areas where bimodal rainfall patterns are experienced. Besides climatic events, the degree of contamination can also depend on the number of pathogens present in the water source, how old and well maintained the system is, and whether the water quality is inspected regularly.

Molds and Dusts

Molds, with or without a detectable odor, often stimulate an allergic airway response[13] (Chapter 230), sometimes as part of a broader contamination of indoor air handling systems. Mineral dusts include silica,[14] fibrous glass, mineral wool, and other synthetic fibers.

Radiation

Radiation exposure is discussed in Chapter 18.

Global Warming and Climate Change

Please see Chapter 17.

OCCUPATIONAL SAFETY STANDARDS

The Occupational Safety and Health Administration (OSHA) issues, promulgates, and enforces standards for workplace safety and health. The National Institute of Occupational Safety and Health (NIOSH), which is part of the Centers for Disease Control and Prevention, does not have authority to set standards, but its reviews regarding chemicals, toxicology, and other hazards provide evidence to help inform the process of setting standards to protect workers' health and safety. These evidence-based standards were created to protect workers and are enforced through workplace inspections and penalties that are assessed for noncompliance. Even for hazards for which clear standards do not exist, the employer is required to protect employees from potentially dangerous exposures.

MEDICAL SURVEILLANCE

Medical surveillance is the systematic, ongoing monitoring of workers who have exposure or potential exposure to occupational hazards. This measurement and assessment then inform secondary prevention measures and the ability to evaluate the effectiveness of prevention strategies.

HIERARCHY OF CONTROLS

The hierarchy of hazard controls, developed through the National Institute of Occupational Safety and Health, is a 5-tiered system that describes the most to least robust ways by which workers can be protected from a hazard. First is elimination, such as banning dichlorodiphenyltrichloroethane (DDT) use in agriculture. Next is substitution, such as using sesquisulfide in lieu of white phosphorus in matches, thereby successfully eliminating jawbone necrosis in workers. Third is the use of engineering controls to eliminate the hazard, as in using safety devices to reduce needlestick exposures in health care personnel. Fourth are administrative controls, such as social distancing to reduce the spread of coronavirus-19 (COVID-19) infection. Finally is the use of personal protective equipment, such as hearing protection to reduce noise exposure, when the hazard itself cannot be eliminated.

ENVIRONMENTAL MEDICINE

Physicians and other providers may be called upon to understand and manage medical concerns that arise from environmental exposures.[15] Tasks may include conducting a risk assessment, managing and communicating risk, making recommendations about possible human health effects, and assessing, understanding, and interpreting regulatory issues. The severity and urgency of environmental issues, such the adverse ramifications of a changing climate (Chapter 17) or environmental justice (e.g., neighborhoods being differentially affected by toxic waste), may vary geographically but remain major challenges. Being able to elicit a detailed environmental history may help reveal presenting diagnoses. Examples include a cardiac event precipitated by exposure to particulate matter 2.5 ($PM_{2.5}$) air pollution, heat-related illness from working in a hot environment without acclimatization or with inadequate access to shade and/or hydration, or a vector-borne disease (e.g., Lyme disease) in an area where the organism was not previously found but has emerged because of climate change.

ENVIRONMENTAL STANDARDS

Key statutes to address these environmental hazards include:

- The Resource Conservation and Recovery Act, which created the framework for the proper management of hazardous and nonhazardous solid waste.
- The Comprehensive Environmental Response, Compensation, and Liability Act, which established the federal Superfund program in 1980 to clean up uncontrolled or abandoned hazardous waste sites as well as accidents, spills, and other emergency releases of pollutants and contaminants into the environment.
- The Emergency Planning and Community Right-to-Know Act of 1986, which addressed the environmental and safety hazards posed by the storage and handling of toxic chemicals.

WELLNESS AND RESILIENCY

Workplaces must not only treat and prevent illness and injury but also promote health and well-being. Wellness, resiliency, and prevention of burnout have

TABLE 16-3 SELECT OCCUPATIONAL AND ENVIRONMENTAL HAZARDS

GROUP	HAZARD	EFFECT/SYMPTOMS	OCCUPATION/POTENTIAL SOURCE
Noxious Gases	Argon	Simple asphyxiant	Welder
	Ammonia	Pulmonary irritant, acute respiratory distress syndrome	Refrigeration; ammonia injection into soil as nitrogen-containing plant nutrient
	Carbon monoxide	Chemical asphyxiant	Mechanic, firefighter, blast furnace
	Helium	Simple asphyxiant	Electronics, aircraft manufacture
	Hydrogen cyanide	Chemical asphyxiant	Agricultural workers, plastics industry
	Hydrogen fluoride	Pulmonary irritant, ARDS	Glass etching
	Nitrogen	Simple asphyxiant, silo-fillers' disease	Welder, firefighter
Industrial Dusts Pneumonoconioses	Asbestos	Asbestosis, mesothelioma, lung cancer, pleural plaques, colon, renal and stomach cancer	Mining
	Coal	Emphysema, coal workers' pneumoconiosis	Coal mining, welders, diesel exhaust
	Silica	Silicosis	Sand blasting, granite countertop manufacture
Other Inorganic Dusts	Iron	Siderosis	Welding
	Tin	Stannosis	Tin
Vegetable Dusts	Cotton, flax, hemp	Byssinosis	Yarn and cotton manufacturer
	Flour dust	Occupational asthma	Baker
	Fungi in moldy hay	Farmer lung	Farming, agriculture
	Organic dusts or aerosols	Hypersensitivity pneumonitis	Mushroom farming, composting installations, vegetable storage
	Plicatic acid from western red cedar	Occupational asthma	Logging, house construction
	Sugar cane (fungus)	Bagassois	Sugar cane farming
Metals	Beryllium	Beryllium disease	Foundries, metal fabricators
	Cadmium	Pulmonary edema	Battery manufacturing, silver soldering
	Chromium	Lung cancer, nasal sinus cancer, sensitization	Welding on stainless steel, spray painting, operating chrome plating baths
	Cobalt	Asthma, allergic contact dermatitis, cardiomyopathy	Knee/hip replacement degradation
	Copper	Metal fume fever	Welding
	Lead	Lead toxicity, lethargy, wrist drop, lead line, anemia	Environmental lead, Ayurveda medication, battery production, glazes
	Magnesium	Metal fume fever	Welding, brazing
	Manganese	Parkinsonian syndrome	Welding, ore crushing, metallurgy
	Mercury—inorganic	Erethism, tremor, proteinuria	Amalgam workers, battery maker, fluorescent lamp maker
	Mercury—organic	Paresthesias, cognitive changes, cerebral palsy	Food chain: biomethylation of inorganic mercury by aquatic organisms
	Nickel	Sensitizer, dermatitis, asthma, nasal cancer	Welding alloys, stainless steel, plating
	Vanadium pentoxide	Pneumonitis, bronchitis, eye irritation	Cleaning fireboxes under boilers
	Zinc	Metal fume fever	Welding
Organic Compounds	Aliphatic hydrocarbon-n-hexane	Neuropathy, lipoid pneumonia	Solvent use, industrial cleaner and degreaser, mineral oil lubricants use
	Aromatic hydrocarbons—benzene	Aplastic anemia, leukemia	Shoe cements use, printing, fuel component
	Chlorinated hydrocarbons (e.g., trichloroethylene)	Headache, irritability, CNS depression, beverage/alcohol intolerance	Dry cleaning, chemical synthesis
	Chlorinated aromatics (e.g., dioxin)	Chloracne	Pulping and pesticide manufacturing
	Fluorinated hydrocarbons (e.g., perfluorochemicals)	Possibly carcinogen	Stain-resistant textiles and carpeting, water-repellent clothes, ski wax, Teflon manufacture
	Halogenated hydrocarbons (e.g., chloroform)	Nephrotoxicity, respiratory depression	Building, paper and board industries
Plastics	Acrylates/methacrylates	Irritant, contact allergen	Plexiglass manufacture, caulk use
	Fluoropolymers (e.g., Teflon)	Polymer fume fever	Teflon manufacture
	Vinyl chloride	Hepatic angiosarcoma	Vinyl chloride monomer, polymerization operations
Pesticides	Carbamates (e.g., carbaryl [Sevin])	Acetylcholine esterase inhibition	Pesticide manufacturing and application, forestry, pest management
	Fumigants (e.g., dibromochloropropane)	Oligospermia	Soil fumigant
	Fungicides (e.g., pentachlorophenol)	Aplastic anemia, chloracne	Wood preservative (telephone poles), dock, pier, and wharf structures
	Herbicides (e.g., paraquat)	Pulmonary fibrosis	Agriculture, forestry
	Organophosphates (e.g., parathion)	Acetylcholine esterase inhibition, paresthesias	Pesticide, agriculture, forestry
	Pyrethrins (e.g., permethrin)	Paresthesias with skin contact, dermatitis	Forestry, agriculture
Physical Hazards	Cold	Hypothermia, frostbite	Construction worker, outdoor trades
	Dysbarism	Fatigue, mottled skin, eardrum rupture	Commercial and sport divers
	Heat	Heat-related illness	Outdoor worker, athlete, farm worker
	Infrared radiation	Lens, cornea, retinal damage, skin burns	Glass blowing, smelting, foundry and forge operations
	Ionizing radiation	Cancer	Nuclear medicine, x-ray technician
	Lasers	Mild burns, cataracts	Welding, cosmetic surgery
	Noise	Hearing loss	Construction, mining, animal worker
	Radiofrequency radiation (radio waves and microwaves)	Burns	Telecommunications, electrosurgery
	Ultraviolet radiation	Photokeratoconjunctivitis or welders flash, cataracts	Plumbers, welders, machinery fitters, assemblers, toolmaker
	Vibration	Vibration white finger	Jackhammering, chainsawing

ARDS = acute respiratory distress syndrome; CNS = central nervous system.

become key issues throughout the workforce, and especially among health care workers, exacerbated by the COVID-19 pandemic.[16] For example, the provision of physical relaxation options can reduce stress among health care workers.[A1] Building collective and individual wellness and resiliency is a valuable skill to prevent burnout, which is an important occupational hazard that affects the personal and professional lives of employees and can have a substantial negative impact on patients, clients, and the financial well-being of institutions. The organization of work is a significant factor in causing and propagating burnout, and addressing such issues requires surveillance to identify the magnitude of the problem, careful consideration of key potential explanations, and a coordinated effort among front-line workers, mental health services, institutional leadership, and relevant stakeholders.[17,18]

EMERGENCY PREPAREDNESS AND DISASTER MANAGEMENT

The key roles for occupational and environmental medicine, as highlighted during the early months of the COVID-19 pandemic, include skills in emergency preparedness, emergency management, assessment of exposures, identification of hazards, disease prevention, surveillance, and population health. Knowledge of specific threats (including chemical, biologic, radiologic, and physical hazards) and bioterrorism agents (Chapter 19) can help protect employees, families, and the population at large. Emergency management planning includes resource mobilization, communication, procurement of medical products, financing, and contingency planning, often with the collaboration with local, state, or federal agencies. Addressing the mental health and safety needs of employees and responders is also critical.

ROLE OF THE INDIVIDUAL CLINICIAN

Clinicians must be agile to meet the challenges presented by the changing nature of work and our environment. They must recognize that care extends beyond merely attending to the clinical ailment in one worker to consider workplace risks that might affect other workers. Clinicians must consider both work-related and nonoccupational causes of illnesses, with the understanding, for example, that orthopedic or neurologic conditions may predispose to workplace injuries, and vice versa, that underlying lung disease may predispose to environmental pulmonary disease, and that preexisting anxiety or depression can exacerbate burnout. Referral to an occupational and environmental medicine specialist, who is trained in preventing, mitigating, and controlling hazards and managing workforces on a population level, is indicated when the degree of complexity rises above the scope of the general clinician.

GENERAL REFERENCES

For the General References and other additional features, please visit Elsevier eBooks+ at https://ebooks.health.elsevier.com.

Grade A Reference

A1. Zhang M, Murphy B, Cabanilla A, et al. Physical relaxation for occupational stress in healthcare workers: a systematic review and network meta-analysis of randomized controlled trials. *J Occup Health*. 2021;63:e12243.

17

EFFECTS OF CLIMATE CHANGE ON HEALTH

JEREMY HESS AND KRISTIE EBI

Climate is an important contextual element for human health and well-being. Anthropogenic climate change has demonstrated that long-held assumptions about the climate's stationarity are no longer valid, and our health systems and activities urgently need to be adjusted, in some cases fundamentally, to accommodate the ongoing shift in weather patterns. Health care education and practice must change, as well. To reduce harm, the health sector as a whole has an obligation to reduce its greenhouse gas emissions aggressively, and individual clinicians should acquire basic familiarity with the drivers and impacts of climate change, as well as priority strategies to reduce and manage risk.[1] Clinicians should understand how climate change will affect their patients and the communities in which they practice, and they should become proactive in improving the sustainability of health systems and services.

HOW CLIMATE CHANGE AFFECTS HEALTH

Climate, which is the multi-decade average of weather patterns in a given location, is the basis for long-term expectations, whereas weather is more variable and shapes day-to-day experiences. However, the implicit assumption that past climate is predictive of future weather patterns is no longer true. Anthropogenic climate change, driven by human emissions of greenhouse gases into the atmosphere, is undermining the assumption of stationarity.

Climate, which is a fundamental driver of health and disease,[2] determines the ecology of life in a particular place, including the social ecology of human settlement. Despite usual climatic variability, such as the recurring El Niño southern oscillation, the earth's climate has been quite stable within a relatively narrow range for millennia.[3]

Because of human emissions of greenhouse gases into the atmosphere, climatic expectations are no longer based on historical experience, with potentially profound implications for human health and, therefore, for public health and medical practice. Climate change affects health security, health determinants, risks for specific diseases, and how the health system's infrastructure and capacity will be able to respond to the challenges of the 21st century.

Anthropogenic climate change operates through simple physical principles. As a result of increased emissions of greenhouse gases (principally carbon dioxide but also methane, hydrofluorocarbons, and a host of other short-lived species), the earth's atmosphere is retaining a larger fraction of the sun's energy. This energy is transferred into land, water, and the atmosphere. For example, with more energy from warmer oceans, storms are stronger, contain more precipitation, and create more floods. Increased atmospheric heat dries out soils more quickly, and heat waves are stronger and persist for longer. Warming melts land-based ice and snow, thereby raising sea levels. Warming also speeds the photochemical reactions that are responsible for the formation of ground-level ozone, which is an air pollutant. Carbon dioxide levels in the oceans equilibrate with levels in the atmosphere, thereby increasing the concentration of carbonic acid; this weak acid dissolves calcium carbonate, thereby threatening collapse of marine ecosystems built on animals with shells. These impacts are already discernible with global average surface warming of 1.2° C above preindustrial temperatures. High-emission scenarios for the duration of the 21st century would result in 5.7° C of warming by the end of the century. Widespread, catastrophic impacts become increasingly likely with each additional unit of warming. For example, up to 90% of warm water corals are projected to die at 1.5° C of warming.

The implications for human health and well-being are significant. Health impacts result from a combination of underlying population-level vulnerability based on socio-demographics and health status, climate sensitivity of relevant disease pathways, and lack of investments in protective measures that could reduce exposure and promote prompt recovery in the event of expected adverse impacts.

The environmental impacts from climate change (Fig. 17-1) affect a wide range of pathways. Some pathways are relatively direct, such as heat exposure, which causes heat exhaustion and heat stroke (Chapter 95), as well as exacerbating stress on the cardiovascular, respiratory, and renal systems. Heat also affects determinants of health by reducing economic productivity and increasing the likelihood of violent crime. Extreme weather, including heat waves, storms, floods, wildfire, and climatic events such as droughts have significant health impacts by increasing injuries, exacerbations of chronic disease, anxiety, and depression.

Climate change also affects a wide range of other, less direct pathways that are important to human health, from air pollution (heat and sunlight affect the development of ground-level ozone and wildfires release particulate air pollution) to aeroallergens (the onset and intensity of pollen season are correlated with temperature).[4] Infectious diseases are particularly sensitive to climatic shifts as a result of changes in the reproductive rates and geographic distribution of pathogens (Chapter 303) including vectors that can transmit waterborne and foodborne diseases, such as the tick that can carry Lyme

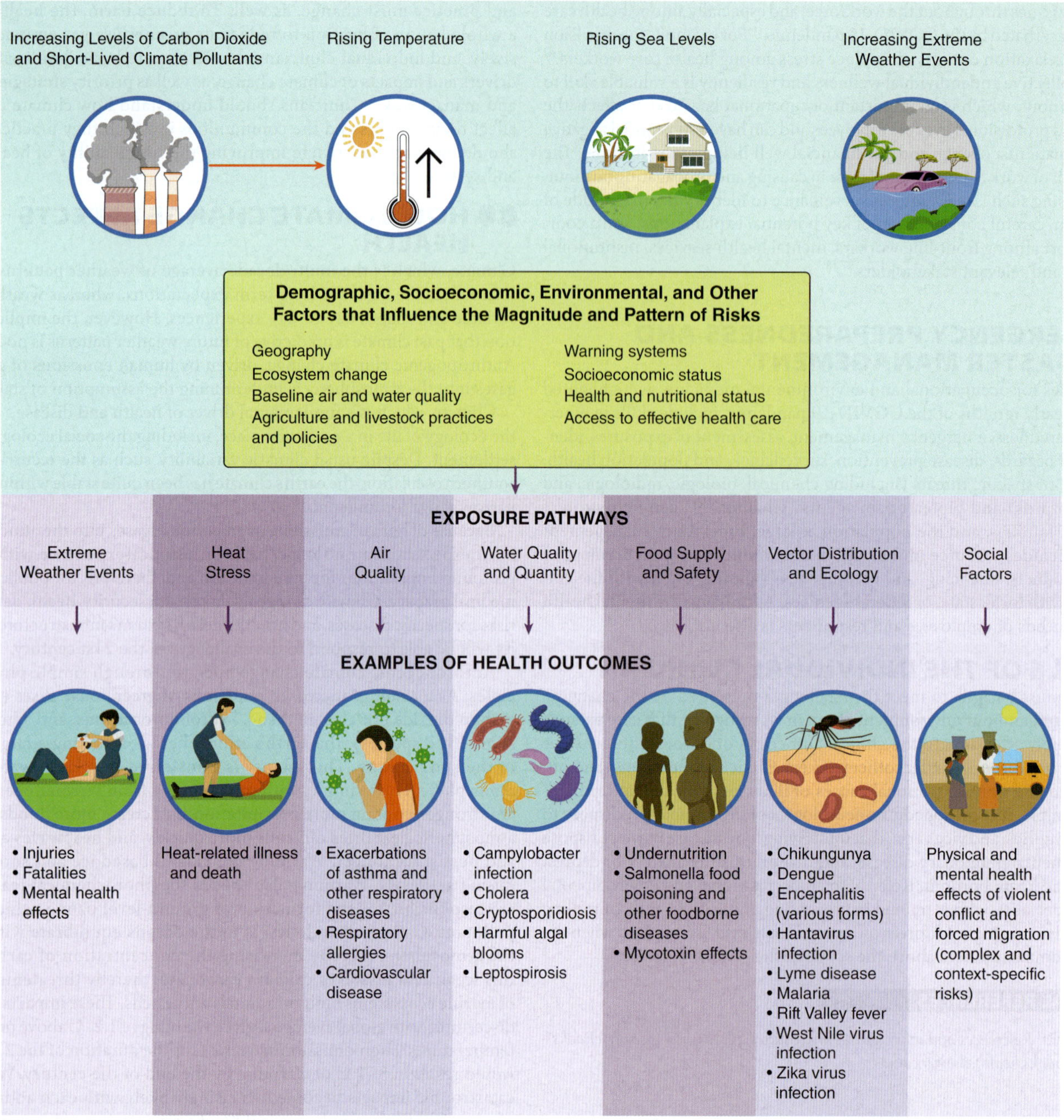

FIGURE 17-1. Major health risks associated with climate change. (From Haines A, Ebi K. The imperative for climate action to protect health. *N Engl J Med.* 2019;380:263-273. Reproduced with permission.)

disease (Chapter 296) and the mosquitoes that can carry dengue fever, Zika virus, chikungunya, and yellow fever (Chapters 351 and 352), and skin and soft tissue infections.[5] Nutritional impacts derive from several different pathways, including disruption of food production from extreme weather, decreased protein and micronutrient content of staple crops, and collapse of productive ecosystems that are key for subsistence.[6] On a macro level, rising sea levels and ecologic stressors are expected to lead to widespread and challenging migration and displacement.

RECENT EVIDENCE AND PROJECTED IMPACTS OF CLIMATE CHANGE ON HEALTH

Health impacts of climate change are already apparent. Patterns of emergence include sentinel events and outbreaks (Table 17-1), shifts in endemicity, introduction and establishment of new diseases, and changing patterns of underlying risks and stressors that affect determinants of health. For instance, heat-related mortality rates are increasing globally, and 37% of heat-related mortality can now be attributed to climate change.[7]

An outbreak of *Vibrio parahaemolyticus* (Chapter 278) in Alaska in 2004 shifted the range of that pathogen over 1000 km to the north; Lyme disease (Chapter 296) is moving steadily northward on the North American continent[8]; ragweed allergy (Chapter 230), historically rare in Europe, is becoming increasingly prevalent[9]; and rising sea levels are requiring relocation from a wide range of coastal communities (see Fig. 17-1).[10] Other shifts, such as changes in the range of *Aedes albopictus,* which transmits Zika, dengue, and chikungunya (Chapters 351 and 352), and *Phlebotomus,* which transmits leishmaniasis (Chapter 319), are driven by climate change and increase risk of these infectious diseases.[11]

The timing and magnitude of the most severe impacts will depend on multiple choices made at the societal level in coming decades. Substantial future warming is inevitable based on greenhouse gas emissions to date. Through roughly mid-century, choices regarding health and social protections, including the degree to which societies invest in basic physical and mental health care, health systems, education, economic protection, and climate-resilient infrastructure, will be the primary determinant of climate impacts. The extent to which climatic hazards and associated stresses could cause severe impacts after mid-century, overwhelming protections in many locations, is a function of preparedness and of how successfully the world is able to reduce greenhouse gas emissions in the next two decades.

HEALTH CARE PROFESSIONALS AND CLIMATE CHANGE

Clinicians should have a basic understanding of what constitutes a climate-resilient health system and how climate change may affect the populations for which they care. Practitioners should advocate for reducing the health sector's substantial greenhouse gas emissions and participate in building climate-resilient health systems (E-Fig. 17-1).

Although this framework is primarily designed for public health officials and leaders of health systems, it has clear relevance to clinicians across the health sector. An emphasis on leadership, for example, highlights the need for clinicians to speak publicly about preparing for climate change and its impacts so as to prioritize planning and public-facing policies, measures, and engagements.[12] The emphasis on ensuring climate-smart risk monitoring and early warning encompasses a wide range of activities, from surveillance of indicators of climate change (e.g., extreme heat events and heat-related illness; pollen season parameters and allergic respiratory disease) to an understanding of how shifts in climate may affect individual and community health. Other important aspects of adapting to climate change in the health sector include engagement in disaster planning and preparedness exercises (in anticipation of more frequent and severe extreme heat events, storms, wildfires, and power failures), as well as the development and implementation of early warning systems[13] for extreme events, and promoting disaster risk reduction to prevent and limit adverse health impacts from disasters.

Reducing greenhouse gas emissions from the health sector is also an important priority.[14] The health sector's emission of greenhouse gases constitutes approximately 4% of the global total,[15] larger than global emissions from air travel. In the United States, the percentage is even higher—the health sector is responsible for nearly 10% of emissions.[16] These emissions are clearly associated with health harms from co-emitted air pollution. In the United States, for example, air pollution from health care causes the loss of nearly 400,000 disability-adjusted years of life[17] and approximately 4.2 million premature deaths globally each year. The harms from air pollution associated with the health care sector in the United States are of the same order of magnitude as harms associated with medical errors.

RESEARCH PRIORITIES FOR CLIMATE CHANGE AND HEALTH

The health sector also must develop additional evidence to support the practice innovations that will be needed to respond to the challenges that climate change presents.[18,19] Areas of emphasis include understanding how climate change harms health; how to diagnose these harms in individuals and across populations; how to devise, implement, and evaluate interventions to reduce these harms; and how to make more accurate prognostic estimates about how current trends and potential interventions could affect the future.

TABLE 17-1 EXAMPLES OF CLIMATE-RELATED HAZARDS, UNDERLYING VULNERABILITIES, AND INFECTIOUS DISEASE OUTCOME

HAZARD	VULNERABILITY	INFECTIOUS DISEASE OUTBREAKS
U.S. hurricane Katrina	Lack of water, sanitation, and hygiene in large shelters for evacuees	Norovirus gastroenteritis
Mozambique cyclones Idai and Kenneth	Lack of water, sanitation, and hygiene and overcrowding in camps for displaced	Diarrheal diseases, malaria
128 flooding, storm, and drought events	Displacement	Measles, cholera, cutaneous leishmaniasis, dengue
Yemen heavy rainfall and elevated temperature	Contamination of surface water	Cholera
Pakistan monsoon flooding	Record-breaking floods	Acute diarrhea, leptospirosis, malaria, leishmaniasis
European heavy rain	Overwhelmed water treatment and distribution systems	Waterborne diseases, such as cryptosporidium
African drought	Water scarcity and hygiene	Cholera

Source: Modified from Semenza JC, Rocklov J, Ebi KL. Climate change and cascading risks from infectious diseases. *Infect Dis Ther*. 2022;11:1371-1390; https://doi.org/10.1007/s40121-022-00647-3.

GENERAL REFERENCES

For the General References and other additional features, please visit Elsevier eBooks+ at https://ebooks.health.elsevier.com.

18

RADIATION INJURY

DAVID J. BRENNER

IONIZING RADIATION

DEFINITIONS

The ionizing radiations are x- and gamma rays, alpha and beta particles, and (indirectly) neutrons. Unlike non-ionizing radiations such as radio waves, microwaves, infrared light, visible light, and ultraviolet (UV) radiation, ionizing radiations have enough energy to knock electrons out of atomic or molecular orbits, thereby potentially breaking chemical bonds in key biomolecules such as DNA.

A key difference among the various ionizing radiations is their ability to penetrate matter (Fig. 18-1). For example, alpha particles have very limited range, measured in micrometers. Because alpha particles cannot penetrate skin, their health significance is entirely in the context of internal exposure by inhalation or ingestion of alpha-emitting radioactive materials. Beta particles, which have intermediate ranges, can typically be stopped by a piece of paper. By contrast, x-rays, gamma rays, and neutrons are highly penetrating and are hard to shield.

Ionizing radiations are emitted by radioactive materials, which can either be naturally occurring or can be man-made, using machines such as nuclear reactors. The amount of ionizing radiation emitted by a radioactive material is determined by its activity, measured in becquerels (1 Bq = 1 radioactive disintegration/second) or Curies (Ci).

Radioactivity should be distinguished from absorbed dose, which is a measure of how much ionizing energy is actually absorbed by a structure of interest, such as a person or an organ. The basic measurement unit of absorbed dose, which is the energy deposited per unit mass, is the Gray (1 Gy = 1 J/kg). *Equivalent dose* takes into account the fact that not all types of radiation are equally effective, *effective dose* takes into account the fact that not all organs in the body are equally sensitive to ionizing radiation, and *collective dose* is a measure of the effective dose delivered summed over a whole exposed population (Table 18-1).

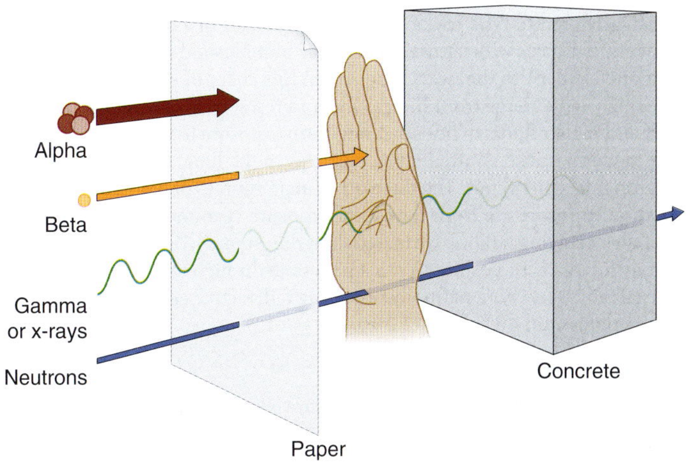

FIGURE 18-1. Schematic illustration of the relative ranges of alpha particles, beta rays, x- or gamma rays, and neutrons as they penetrate through matter.

TABLE 18-1 STANDARD QUANTITIES AND UNITS ASSOCIATED WITH EXPOSURE TO IONIZING RADIATION

QUANTITY	DEFINITION	UNITS
Absorbed dose	Energy per unit mass	Gray (Gy)
Equivalent dose	Average dose × radiation-type-specific radiation weighting factor	Sievert (Sv)
Effective dose	Sum of equivalent doses to all exposed organs, each multiplied by an appropriate organ-relative sensitivity factor	Sievert (Sv)
Collective dose	Sum of effective doses to a population of exposed individuals	Person-Sv

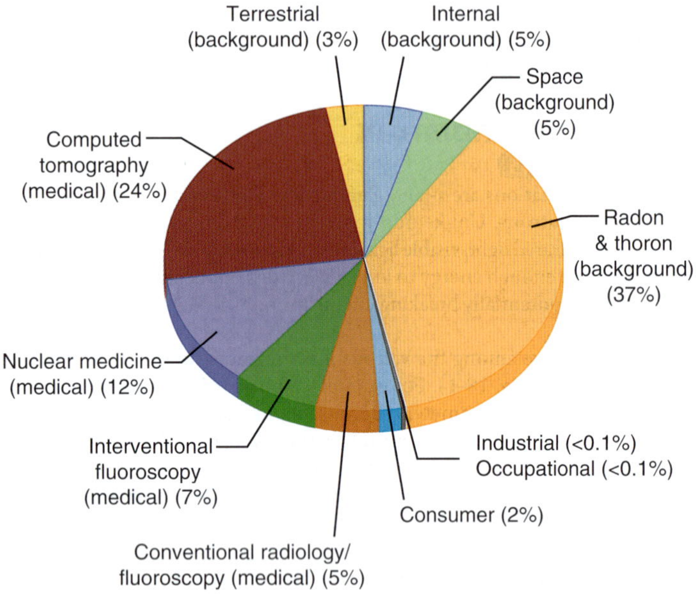

FIGURE 18-2. **The major sources of radiation exposure to an average individual in the United States.** (From Hall EJ, Giaccia AJ. *Radiobiology for the Radiologist*. 7th ed. Philadelphia: Lippincott Williams & Wilkins; 2012.)

EPIDEMIOLOGY

Radiation exposure can come from natural sources, therapeutic or diagnostic medical exposures, or accidental exposures to individuals or to large populations. Natural sources and radiologic examinations are the major (and about equal) contributors to the overall collective radiation dose to the U.S. population (Fig. 18-2).

Natural Sources of Ionizing Radiation

The largest naturally occurring source of radiation is from radon gas, which is an alpha-particle emitter. Radon is a constituent component of all rocks, particularly granite-type rocks. Radon is a member of a chain of radioactive elements that starts with naturally occurring uranium and radioactively decays from one element to the next; uniquely in this chain of elements, radon is a gas, which can emerge from the ground and result in high levels in the basement and higher floors of houses. Long-term exposure to radon gas can cause lung cancer because emitted alpha particles in the lung can damage cells in the bronchial epithelium. The three other main sources of naturally occurring radiation exposure are from terrestrial exposure (gamma rays emitted from naturally occurring radioactive materials in the ground), from space radiations (mainly intergalactic cosmic rays that penetrate through the atmosphere), and internal radiation (from naturally occurring radioactive elements in the body, such as potassium-40).

Medical Exposures

The single largest source of medical exposure is computed tomography (CT), which on average contributes about 25% of the collective dose to the U.S. population. This source of exposure is recent because CT has been commonly used only since the 1980s. Now, however, about 70 million CT scans are performed annually in the United States. In addition to CT, nuclear medicine, interventional fluoroscopy, and conventional radiography together constitute about 25% of the overall collective dose to the U.S. population.

TABLE 18-2 ESTIMATED RELEASES OF RADIOACTIVE IODINE AND RADIOACTIVE CESIUM FROM THE FOUR HISTORICALLY BIGGEST NUCLEAR POWER PLANT ACCIDENTS

	^{131}I (TBq)	$^{137/134}$Cs (TBq)
Windscale, 1957	750	20
Three Mile Island, 1979	1	0.000001
Chernobyl, 1986	1,800,000	110,000
Fukushima, 2011	~500,000	~20,000

Radiologic Accidents

Since the widespread introduction of nuclear power plants, major radiologic accidents have become an intermittent, although rare, source of radiation exposure. The accidents at Chernobyl in 1986 and at Fukushima in 2011 released far more radioactivity than any other accidents (Table 18-2). For those individuals exposed to low radiation doses, many common symptoms reported in the immediate aftermath were not necessarily physical health problems directly attributable to radiation exposure but rather psychological and psycho-social effects.[1]

Radiologic Terrorism

In the broadest of terms, two different types of such threats exist, one from an improvised nuclear device and the other from a radiologic dispersal device, sometimes called a *dirty bomb*.[2,3] The two are very different in terms of their potential consequences and also their likelihood of occurrence.

The consequences of exploding an improvised nuclear device, perhaps similar to those detonated at Hiroshima or Nagasaki, although more likely exploded at ground level, would be devastating in terms of loss of life and major injuries. For example, a 20-kT daytime surface improvised nuclear device explosion in midtown Manhattan might involve 2.2 million people exposed to high radiation doses, of whom perhaps only 1.6 million might survive.

By contrast, the consequences of exploding a radiologic dispersal device or dirty bomb, dispersing what could be very small or very large amounts of radioactive material, would likely involve a relatively small spatial area in which individuals are significantly exposed, as well as a much larger area in which individuals are exposed to very low levels of radioactivity. The significance of a dirty bomb depends on the amount of radioactivity in the device and the efficiency with which the explosion aerosolizes and disperses the radioactive material. Of course, the consequences of a radiologic dispersal device extend beyond health effects and could potentially involve large-scale social and economic disruption.

PATHOBIOLOGY

Ionizing radiation can both mutate cells and cause cell death. The key initial damage site is a DNA double-strand break, although other types of damage are possible. This double-strand break is generally repaired by a variety of mechanisms, the most important of which for ionizing radiation damage is nonhomologous end rejoining. Imprecise nonhomologous end rejoining can lead to small mutations, whereas double-strand break misrepair (i.e., the wrong ends of breaks being rejoined to each other) can lead to chromosomal translocations, inversions, telomere fusions, and other large-scale chromosomal structural alterations.

Although chromosomal translocations, inversions, and point mutations are typically nonlethal lesions, such radiation-induced chromosomal aberrations can be the initial lesions associated with carcinogenesis. For example, the initial event in many hematopoietic cancers (Chapters 168 and 170) is often a recurrent translocation, which in turn results in the fusion of genes located at the translocation breakpoints. Radiation-induced point mutations and deletions also are often associated with loss of heterozygosity in tumor suppressor genes.

Misrepair of double-strand breaks can also result in dicentric chromosome aberrations and centric rings (Chapter 166), which are generally lethal lesions that cause reproductive cell death in which a cell loses its ability to divide. A second, quite different mechanism of radiation-induced cell death is apoptosis, or programmed cell death, that, for example, is important after radiation exposure of hematopoietic cells and jejunal crypt cells.

CLINICAL MANIFESTATIONS

The consequences of radiation exposure are dose dependent and are also dependent on whether the exposure is to the whole body or only part of the body. After high doses of whole-body exposure, the major consequences are acute radiation syndromes, which may be fatal. After high doses of partial-body exposure, such as after radiotherapy, the consequences are highly organ specific. These high-dose tissue reactions are deterministic, meaning that there typically is a threshold below which the effects are not seen, with the severity of the effect increasing with increasing dose. By contrast, the major concern at lower doses is with stochastic effects, in which there is no dose threshold, and it is the probability of the effect that increases with increasing dose. The most important example here is radiation-induced cancer.

Acute Radiation Syndromes

The radiation dose needed to mitotically kill active dividing cells is far less than the dose needed to remove the functioning ability of differentiated cells. As a result, acute radiation syndromes generally relate to the failure of precursor cells to provide replacements for functional cells within an organ, when the latter need replacement. Acute radiation syndromes typically progress through four stages: prodromal, clinical latency, manifest illness, and recovery or death.

Prodromal Stage

Prodromal (early) symptoms occur shortly after irradiation, with the radiation dose determining the severity, duration, and onset. Typical prodromal symptoms include nausea, vomiting, anorexia, fatigue, diarrhea, abdominal cramping, and dehydration. At very high doses, these symptoms can appear within a few minutes of exposure; but at somewhat lower doses, they may not appear for many hours, if at all.

Latency Period

After the prodromal stage, a latency period typically precedes manifest illness. This delay occurs because the subsequent syndromes (hematopoietic or gastrointestinal) involve the failure of relevant tissues to self-renew, and manifest illness does not occur until after the typical cellular turnover times in these tissues.

Manifest Illness

The *hematopoietic syndrome* results from whole-body or significant partial-body exposure to 3 to 9 Gy. At these doses, radiation kills mitotically active hematopoietic precursor cells. Symptoms then result from lack of circulating blood elements some 4 to 8 weeks later as circulating cells die and are not replaced. The hematopoietic syndrome may manifest as infections and possible hemorrhage, impairment of immune mechanisms, and potentially multiple-organ failure.

The *gastrointestinal syndrome* usually occurs after whole-body or significant partial-body exposure of about 8 Gy and above. These doses lead to death of intestinal stem cells in the regenerating crypts. Symptoms then result when differentiated cells of the villi are naturally sloughed off, but stem cells are unable to produce new cells, thereby leading to depopulation of the epithelial lining of the gastrointestinal tract. After a latency period of about 7 days, loss or significant shortening of the villi on the intestinal epithelium leads to bacterial growth and increased risk for sepsis. Common symptoms include anorexia, nausea, vomiting, prolonged bloody diarrhea, abdominal cramps, dehydration, and weight loss. Should death occur, it is typically 7 to 10 days later.

At extremely high radiation doses, death is typically from the *cerebrovascular syndrome* within a few days after exposure. The cause of death is believed to be because changes in permeability of small blood vessels in the brain lead to cerebral edema.

Organ-Specific Late Effects after Radiotherapy

Iatrogenic organ-specific late effects follow quite predictably after targeted radiation therapy in which the organ in question is irradiated, although the severity of the response is less predictable.[4] These tissue effects can be divided into global organ responses and focal responses, in which a particular part of the organ is differentially irradiated (Table 18-3).

As one example, significant radiation exposure to the heart increases the risk for subsequent major heart disease.[5,6] These risks have been most notable in women who have had radiotherapy for left-sided breast cancer (Chapter 183), patients treated with mantle radiation for Hodgkin lymphoma (Chapter 172), and some patients treated for lung tumors adjacent to the heart. Radiation effects to the heart can be wide ranging, including to the coronary arteries, the myocardium, the heart valves, and the pericardial sac. The increased risk, which is proportional to the cardiac dose, begins a few years after exposure and continues throughout life. These radiation risks appear to be multiplicative of the natural background cardiac risks, so patients with preexisting cardiac risk factors are likely to have greater absolute increases in their risk for radiation-induced cardiac disease. Radiation damage to the lungs (Chapter 82)[7] and colorectal area (Chapter 128)[8] also can cause significant morbidity.

TABLE 18-3 TYPICAL ORGAN-SPECIFIC DETERMINISTIC LATE EFFECTS AFTER HIGH-DOSE RADIOTHERAPY

ORGAN	LOCAL END POINT	GLOBAL END POINT
Brain, cranial nerves	Focal weakness, vision loss	Neurocognitive deficit
Lung	Bronchial stricture	Shortness of breath
Heart	Coronary stenosis	Pericarditis, cardiomyopathy
Bladder	Bleeding	Urinary frequency, diarrhea
Bowel	Ischemia, bleeding	Enteritis

Adapted with changes from Rubin P, Constine LS, Marks LB, eds. *ALERT—Adverse Late Effects of Cancer Treatment*. Vol. 1: General Concepts and Specific Precepts. Heidelberg: Springer; 2014.

Stochastic Effects of Radiation

In contrast to the deterministic organ-based effects of radiation, ionizing radiation also produces stochastic effects, whereby the severity of the disease is not dose dependent, but the probability of an effect increases with increasing dose. These effects are largely due to radiation-induced mutations of target cells, as opposed to cell killing, with by far the most important effect being radiation carcinogenesis. Other potential radiation-induced stochastic health effects include deleterious radiation-induced genetic effects to subsequent generations.

Radiation Carcinogenesis

In general, radiation acts as a multiplier of natural background cancer rates, although there are exceptions, such as radiation-induced breast cancer, in which the radiation risks are largely independent of the natural background rates, and prostate cancer, which generally is not a radiogenic tumor. Most radiation-induced cancers occur many years after radiation exposure, typically in the same "cancer-prone" years (about 55 to 75 years of age), as do naturally occurring cancers. Exceptions include radiation-induced hematopoietic cancers and radiation-induced thyroid cancers, both of which typically occur within a few years of radiation exposure. Sensitivity to radiation-induced cancer is age dependent, with people exposed at younger ages having higher lifetime cancer risks.

Most of what is known quantitatively about the radiation-induced risks for cancer comes from studies of atomic bomb survivors, who had measurable increased subsequent risks for cancer: at a 1 Gy dose at follow-up more than 50 years later, atomic bomb survivors showed a 64% increased risk of solid cancer in females and a 20% increase in males. Despite much study, hereditary effects in the children of atomic bomb survivors was not detected.

Long-term survivors of radiation therapy also have a small but significantly increased risk of radiation-associated second cancers.[9] At low radiation doses, for example, below 0.1 Gy, epidemiologic studies are difficult to perform and interpret because of the difficulty in quantifying a small excess cancer risk above the natural human lifetime cancer risk of about 40%. However large-scale epidemiologic studies in children who have received CT scans or had small radioactive iodine exposures at Chernobyl showed an increased risk of radiation-induced cancer.

Radiation Cataractogenesis

Ionizing radiation induces ocular cataracts (Chapter 391) with a probability, severity, and latency related to the radiation dose.[10] Studies of atomic bomb survivors, Chernobyl cleanup workers, astronauts, and radiologic technicians have all shown increased incidence of cataracts, even at radiation doses below 1 Gy. Radiation cataractogenesis is a result of radiation damage to dividing cells in the lens. Because there are essentially no mechanisms in the lens for removal of damaged cells, the resulting nontranslucent lens fibers migrate toward the posterior pole of the lens, where they represent the first stage of a cataract. Posterior subcapsular cataracts are less common than nuclear or cortical cataracts in the general population but are the type most commonly associated with ionizing radiation.

DIAGNOSIS

The diagnosis of radiation injury can be considered in two different contexts. The first context is when the radiation dose is not known, and the goal is to estimate the dose that was delivered in order to optimize treatment. Examples include accidents and radiologic terrorism scenarios. The second context is when the radiation dose is known, in particular after radiotherapy. Here the sequelae (see Table 18-3) are predictable, but the timing and the severity of the injury are less predictable.

Radiation Biodosimetry

For an individual exposed to a large whole-body radiation dose, the first critical task is to estimate the radiation dose that the individual received, because different syndromes (hematopoietic, gastrointestinal, cerebrovascular) are associated with different radiation dose ranges. The technique for estimating exposures to individuals is known as *radiation biodosimetry*. In this diagnostic process, a small amount of a body tissue, such as blood or urine, is analyzed, and dose-dependent end points in the sample are measured to provide an estimated dose. The most common end point of DNA damage, such as micronuclei, in blood samples, can now be assessed by commonly available high-throughput technologies. Other practical endpoints include gene expression in blood or induction of metabolites in urine.

Post-Radiotherapy Sequelae

Deterministic radiation-induced organ syndromes are seen at reasonably predictable intervals after radiation therapy. For example, radiation pericarditis (Chapter 62) can develop during treatment or months to years later, initially with an effusion and progressing to pericardial constriction. Radiation enterocolitis (Chapter 126) can develop 6 to 12 months after radiation doses of 40 to 60 Gy for prostate cancer or gynecologic malignancies. Radiation-induced pulmonary injury can be detected in up to 50% of patients who receive thoracic radiation therapy, but only a minority of them will develop clinical symptoms (Chapter 82). In addition, the majority of all radiotherapy patients experience acute skin or mucosal toxicity, in particular radiation dermatitis, oral mucositis, and xerostomia.

TREATMENT

Whole-Body Exposure Syndromes

For exposures below 2 Gy, no immediate treatment is needed (Fig. 18-3). For patients with potential hematopoietic syndrome (doses between 2 and 10 Gy), the two primary treatment approaches are: first, antibiotics and barrier nursing, which can raise the human LD_{50} (the dose at which 50% of exposed individuals die) from about 4 Gy to 8 Gy; and second, granulocyte colony-stimulating factor (G-CSF).[11] Subcutaneous G-CSF, filgrastim (10 μg/kg daily for up to 2 weeks), or pegfilgrastim (two 6-mg doses one week apart) are approved by the U.S. Food and Drug Administration (FDA) for the treatment of patients with radiation-induced myelosuppression following a radiologic/nuclear incident. A placenta-derived adherent stromal cell has been approved by the FDA for emergency treatment of acute radiation exposure in a possible nuclear event.[12]

The role of bone marrow transplantation in treating individuals with the hematopoietic syndrome is probably quite limited at doses less than about 9 Gy. In the aftermath of the Chernobyl accident, for example, 13 individuals underwent bone marrow transplantation, and three deaths were directly attributed to the sequelae of the procedure in patients in whom the transplantation was not indicated based on their exposure. Conservative treatment regimens, including antibiotics, cytokine therapy, transfusions, and nursing, are clearly effective, but current treatment options are very limited at doses above about 10 Gy, when the gastrointestinal syndrome becomes the dominant cause of death.

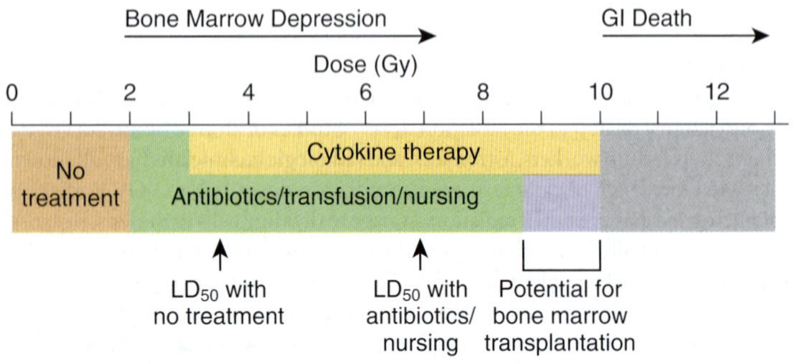

FIGURE 18-3. Schematic recommended treatment for acute radiation syndromes, as a function of the estimated dose that the individual received. Note the very narrow dose window for which bone marrow transplantations are potentially useful. GI = gastrointestinal; Gy = Gray units; LD_{50} = dose of radiation expected to kill 50% of exposed cells within 30 days. (Adapted with changes from Hall EJ. *Radiobiology for the Radiologist*. 7th ed. Philadelphia: Lippincott Williams & Wilkins; 2012.)

Radiotherapy Sequelae

Proton beam therapy may have the potential to reduce side effects compared with other modern versions of radiation therapy.[A1] However, these benefits appear to be limited to specific situations, especially locally advanced esophageal cancer and pediatric brain tumors,[13] and the cost-benefit ratio of proton beam therapy is uncertain. Comparatively few drugs have been approved by the FDA for minimizing radiotherapy-associated sequelae. Amifostine (200 mg/m^2 given intravenously daily before each fraction of radiation therapy)[14] is FDA-approved for minimizing radiotherapy-associated xerostomia, but its use has been limited by significant toxicity, and data on its efficacy are conflicting.[15] Several drugs have been designed to mitigate or treat the damage caused by radiation therapy, particularly to the mucosal barrier. Palifermin, which is a recombinant human keratinocyte growth factor, is FDA-approved (60μg/kg/day administered as an IV bolus injection for 3 consecutive days before therapy and 3 consecutive days after therapy for leukemia or lymphoma) to decrease the incidence or duration of severe oral mucositis.[A2] Avasopasem (a superoxide dismutase mimetic at 90mg given before each therapy) can reduce mucositis in patients who receive radiation therapy for head and neck cancer.[A3] Oral glutamine[A4] and zinc[A5] have shown some benefit for reducing the severity of radiation-induced oral mucositis. However, no medications have been consistently effective for reducing the gastrointestinal side effects of pelvic radiotherapy.[A6]

For radiotherapy-induced dermatitis, mucositis, and xerostomia, treatments include topical agents for dermatitis (Chapter 405), analgesics for mucositis, and saliva substitutes for xerostomia. Beyond dermatitis, mucositis, and xerostomia, radiation-induced deterministic tissue effects are typically treated in the same way as their non-radiation-induced counterparts. For example, the treatment of radiation-induced coronary artery disease is no different than the approach to coronary diseases in general (Chapters 56 to 59). However, the management of acute and chronic gastrointestinal symptoms after radiotherapy requires a more specialized approach because of the risk for local stricture (Chapter 128).

PREVENTION

Countermeasures after Radiologic Accidents or Terrorism

Three FDA-approved pharmaceuticals can limit the radiation dose caused by exposures to specific radioisotopes: potassium iodide for radioactive iodine; Prussian blue for radioactive cesium or thallium; and diethylenetriamine pentaacetate (DTPA) for plutonium, americium, or curium. Although these pharmaceutical countermeasures can limit the organ doses and therefore the health consequences produced by these specific radioisotopes, they cannot be used to treat any of the adverse clinical effects caused by them.

The administration of potassium iodide (KI), which contains nonradioactive iodine, saturates the thyroid with nonradioactive iodine and thereby prevents radioactive iodine from being absorbed into the thyroid, where it can cause thyroid cancer (Chapter 207). The protective effects of KI last about 24 hours, so it should be taken daily (130 mg for adults, 65 mg for children >3 years of age, 32 mg for children 1 to 3 years of age, 16 mg for infants) while there is a likelihood of exposure.

Prussian blue (Radiogardase: ferric hexacyanoferrate [II]) binds cesium in the gastrointestinal tract and limits its reabsorption into the blood stream, thereby reducing the biologic half-life of cesium in the body from about 110 days to about 30 days and limiting the organ toxicities that it produces. The recommended dose of Prussian blue is 3 g orally three times daily for adults and 1 g orally three times daily for children 2 to 12 years of age, for a minimum of 30 days.

DTPA is a chelating agent that binds to radioactive plutonium, americium, and curium, thereby decreasing their persistence in the body. DTPA comes in two forms, Ca-DTPA and Zn-DTPA, with the calcium form considered more effective over the first 24 hours of exposure, and the zinc form preferable at later times, although both are effective over several weeks. They are administered intravenously (or with a nebulizer), with a daily intravenous dose of 1 g for adults and 14 mg/kg for children younger than 12 years.

Several radiation countermeasure drugs have been developed to counteract the symptoms of acute radiation syndromes, have been demonstrated effective in animal models, and are undergoing trials prior to FDA approval.

Medical Imaging

CT is a superb diagnostic tool, and individual CT radiation–associated risks are small; as a result, a great majority of the approximately 90 million CT scans performed annually in the United States generally provide far more benefits than risks. However, organ doses from CT are typically far larger than those from conventional radiographic examinations, so CT should operate under the dual principles of optimization and justification. Optimization involves reducing the radiation dose per CT, using improved protocols and technology.

In terms of justification—making sure that all CT scans are clinically justified, a substantial proportion of CT scans could potentially be replaced by other modalities, such as magnetic resonance imaging for some head examinations and selective use of ultrasound for diagnosing appendicitis. For example, CT scans performed in patients who undergo appendectomy are associated with about a 25% higher risk of subsequent hematologic malignancy.[16] In addition, many CT scans could be avoided entirely by following usage appropriateness criteria.

NON-IONIZING RADIATION INJURY

Ionizing radiations uniquely have sufficient energy to cause DNA strand breaks, which in turn can lead to cell killing and mutations. By contrast, non-ionizing radiations, such as radio waves, microwaves, infrared radiation, and visible light, do not have sufficient energy to break DNA strands, and none of these radiations have been associated with health hazards. One exception is ultraviolet (UV) radiation, which is generally a mutagen and a carcinogen. A second possible exception is radiofrequency radiation, although in this case the epidemiologic evidence and mechanistic considerations do not provide strong evidence of health risks.

ULTRAVIOLET RADIATION

UV radiations, which are part of the non-ionizing electromagnetic spectrum, cover a wavelength from about 150 to 400 nm (intermediate between visible light and x-rays). In turn, these UV wavelengths are subcategorized as UVA (400 to 320 nm), UVB (315 to 280 nm), and UVC (280 to 150 nm).

Sunlight is by far the largest source of UV radiation to humans. Because of filtering in the atmosphere, about 95% of the UV spectrum that reaches the earth's surface is UVA, the remainder is nearly all UVB, and almost no UVC penetrates the ozone layer to reach the earth. Other sources of UV exposures include tanning beds and booths. Industrial exposures include welding arcs, plasma torches, germicidal and blacklight lamps, electric arc furnaces, hot-metal operations, mercury-vapor lamps, and some lasers.

PATHOBIOLOGY

UV radiations do not penetrate deeply into human tissues, so the injuries they cause are principally to the skin and eyes. The biologic effects of UV radiation are primarily attributable to its absorption in DNA, where pyrimidine dimers and their products are produced. These products are generally very efficiently removed, primarily through nucleotide excision repair but also through base excision repair, but errors in these repair processes ultimately can result in mutations. Although most UV radiation in sunlight is UVA, UVB is much more efficiently absorbed by nucleic acids, and most of the biologic effects of sunlight are associated with UVB.

The damaging effects of UV radiation are exacerbated in patients who have underlying defects in nucleotide excision repair. For example, studies of patients with xeroderma pigmentosum have provided key evidence of the link between UV light and skin cancer. In addition, the effects of UV are often enhanced in patients who are taking medications that contain photodynamic agents, such as tetracyclines, fluoroquinolones, nonsteroidal anti-inflammatory drugs, diuretics, statins, phenothiazines, thioxanthenes, and antifungals. Such drug-related phototoxic reactions typically resolve after the drug is discontinued.

CLINICAL MANIFESTATIONS

The major acute effects of UVB exposure are sunburn and erythema, whereas UVA exposure is rarely the direct cause of sunburn. All UV radiations are well-established skin carcinogens (Chapter 188). Squamous cell carcinomas and basal carcinomas are typically associated with multiple or chronic exposures to sunlight, whereas melanoma is linked primarily to episodes of acute sunburn. Lighter-skinned individuals, whose skin and eyes contain less melanin, are more prone to all UV effects because melanin acts as a photoprotector. Acute exposures of the eye to UVB (Chapter 391) can cause "welder flash" (photokeratitis), and chronic exposures are associated with cataracts as well as pterygium.

PREVENTION

Excessive exposure to sunlight or other sources of UV radiation should be avoided, especially in fair-skinned individuals. UV radiation–screening lotions or creams and UV radiation–blocking sunglasses should be used when appropriate.

During significant exposure to sunlight, it is important to use a broad-spectrum sunscreen that provides protection from UVB as well as UVA. Standard recommendations are use of sunscreen with a sun protection factor (SPF) of 30, with reapplication at least every 2 hours. Likewise, sunglasses should be rated to block 99% or 100% of UVB and UVA radiation.

FAR-UVC RADIATION

A particular UV wavelength, far UVC (207 to 222 nm), is an effective antibactericidal and antiviral agent, including against severe acute respiratory syndrome coronavirus 2 (Chapter 336).[17] Because of its very limited penetration, it may be safe for human exposure, unlike typical UVC radiation.

RADIOFREQUENCY RADIATIONS

Radiofrequency radiations are also part of the non-ionizing electromagnetic spectrum (E-Fig. 18-1). Examples are radiation emitted from mobile phones (800 to 2000 MHz),[18] electric power lines (50/60 Hz),[19] low-frequency magnetic fields,[20] and airport whole-body scanners (24 to 30 GHz). Biologic studies of these low-level radiofrequency exposures have generally not shown measurable genotoxicity.

Numerous epidemiologic studies have focused on the effects of electric power line proximity and of cell phone usage. Although some early studies showed positive associations between exposure and health detriment, these studies have generally not proved consistent or repeatable. Further studies are, however, warranted, and an ongoing prospective European study is following 290,000 adult cell phone users over a 20-year period.

GENERAL REFERENCES

For the General References and other additional features, please visit Elsevier eBooks+ at https://ebooks.health.elsevier.com.

Grade A References

A1. Lin SH, Hobbs BP, Verma V, et al. Randomized phase IIB trial of proton beam therapy versus intensity-modulated radiation therapy for locally advanced esophageal cancer. *J Clin Oncol.* 2020;38:1569-1579.

A2. Mazhari F, Shirazi AS, Shabzendehdar M. Management of oral mucositis in pediatric patients receiving cancer therapy: a systematic review and meta-analysis. *Pediatr Blood Cancer.* 2019;68:1-9.

A3. Anderson CM, Lee CM, Saunders DP, et al. Phase IIb, randomized, double-blind trial of GC4419 versus placebo to reduce severe oral mucositis due to concurrent radiotherapy and cisplatin for head and neck cancer. *J Clin Oncol.* 2019;37:3256-3265.

A4. Peng T-R, Lin H-H, Yang L-J, et al. Effectiveness of glutamine in the management of oral mucositis in cancer patients: a meta-analysis of randomized controlled trials. *Support Care Cancer.* 2021;29:4885-4892.

A5. de Menêses AG, Normando AGC, Porto de Toledo I, et al. Effects of oral supplementation in the management of oral mucositis in cancer patients: a meta-analysis of randomized clinical trials. *J Oral Pathol Med.* 2020;49:117-125.

A6. Lawrie TA, Green JT, Beresford M, et al. Interventions to reduce acute and late adverse gastrointestinal effects of pelvic radiotherapy for primary pelvic cancers. *Cochrane Database Syst Rev.* 2018;1:CD012529.

19 BIOTERRORISM

MARK G. KORTEPETER AND THEODORE J. CIESLAK

Physicians play critical roles at the point of entry into the medical system and as consultants for emergency services, so they should be familiar with potential epidemiologic clues that an attack has occurred, general clinical aspects of agents considered to be the greatest threats, and the means by which to alert the appropriate public health authorities if they suspect intentional use.

EPIDEMIOLOGIC CLUES

As with any other outbreak, the response to a potential act of bioterrorism relies on public health fundamentals.[1,2] Except for direct evidence of a release, no other single feature can be considered definitive proof of bioterrorism, but multiple simultaneous features should raise the suspicion of an unnatural event (Table 19-1).

Victims of a chemical or conventional weapon attack would likely become ill shortly after a release or explosion, whereas victims of a silent biologic weapon attack would likely present for care in a delayed fashion to different care providers, dispersed in space and time due to the pathogen's incubation period. One way in which a bioterror attack might differ from a natural outbreak is in the unusual presentation of illness. For example, a disease that typically occurs on the skin or causes gastrointestinal illness might instead exhibit respiratory features (e.g., anthrax, plague). Another clue could be illnesses that are unresponsive to standard therapies because of an unusual antibiotic sensitivity profile. Suspicion should also be raised by finding a disease outside the location or season in which it typically occurs.

AGENTS OF CONCERN

Among the myriad human infectious pathogens, a relatively small number possess the requisite properties to be considered potential weapons that could cause widespread disease, so-called weapons of mass destruction. The U.S. Centers for Disease Control and Prevention (CDC) has designated six as category A due to their ability to cause large-scale disruption, the need for preparedness, and fear their release might engender (Table 19-2).[3] These agents can be formulated to remain stable in aerosol, which allows their potential efficient spread via the air over a large population.

TABLE 19-1 EPIDEMIOLOGIC CLUES OF A BIOWEAPON ATTACK

A large outbreak, especially in a discrete population
Many cases of unexplained illness or deaths
More severe disease than expected for a specific pathogen or failure to respond to standard therapy
Unusual manifestation of illness, such as inhalational disease from agents not typically causing clinical illness
An unusual disease for a given geographic area or transmission season, especially in the absence of a competent vector
Multiple simultaneous or serial epidemics
A single case of a rare disease (smallpox, some viral hemorrhagic fevers, inhalational anthrax, pneumonic plague)
Unusual strains or variants of organisms, or antimicrobial resistance patterns different from those known to be circulating
Higher attack rates among those outside a protected area or lower rates among those inside a protected area or shelter
Outbreaks of the same disease occurring simultaneously in noncontiguous areas
A zoonotic disease occurring in humans but not in animals
Direct evidence or intelligence of a release (equipment, munitions, tampering) or other identified vehicle of spread (spray device, contaminated letter)
A downwind pattern of casualty location

Modified from Stanek SA, Saunders D, Alves DA, et al. *USAMRIID's Medical Management of Biological Casualties Handbook*, 9th ed. September 2020. Found at www.usamriid.army.mil under reference materials tab. Accessed October 30, 2021.

ANTHRAX

EPIDEMIOLOGY

Anthrax, caused by infection with the gram-positive bacillus *Bacillus anthracis* (Chapter 272), is a worldwide scourge of herbivores. Most human cases have had direct occupational contact with infected animals or their hides, hair, or bone, although a recent outbreak occurred among injection drug users in the United Kingdom. Endemic areas include underdeveloped parts of sub-Saharan Africa and Southeast Asia, where humans interact closely with animals that have not been vaccinated. Sporadic cases occur in the United States, typically along the trails of the historic cattle drives in the central plains. Animals are typically infected while grazing in areas contaminated with anthrax spores, which can survive in the soil for decades and can be formulated as a stable desiccated powder. Although most cases worldwide are cutaneous, the spore form of the organism can be milled into the ideal particle size (2 to 6 μm) for infecting the lungs and causing inhalational disease.

PATHOBIOLOGY AND CLINICAL MANIFESTATIONS

Exposure to spores can occur through a break in the skin, through the gastrointestinal tract, or by inhalation. Spores are taken up by macrophages and replicate in the local skin, or are transported to the regional lymph nodes in the gastrointestinal tract or lungs. While replicating, the bacilli secrete lethal toxin, which causes local necrosis, and edema toxin, which causes significant local edema. Untreated or unrecognized infection can result in bacteremia, systemic toxemia, and death.

Cutaneous anthrax can be readily recognized by the astute clinician based on two clinical manifestations caused by its toxins: a black eschar, from which anthrax gets its name (from the Greek *anthrakis*, for coal), and surrounding edema that is out of proportion to the size of the lesion. The lesion starts as a papule that becomes a vesicle and eventually develops a central, black, necrotic area. Although this form of disease is readily treatable, it can lead to a 20% case-fatality rate if it is not recognized and treated appropriately. Gastrointestinal anthrax, which occurs after ingestion of infected, undercooked meat, is much more difficult to recognize and can have a case-fatality rate

TABLE 19-2 CENTERS FOR DISEASE CONTROL AND PREVENTION CATEGORY A BIOTERROR AGENTS

DISEASE (AND AGENT)	DIAGNOSTIC ASSOCIATIONS	WEAPONIZATION RATIONALE	TREATMENT* (SEE TEXT FOR DETAIL)
Anthrax (*Bacillus anthracis;* Chapter 272)	Hemorrhagic mediastinitis	Highly lethal inhalational disease; stable spores survive desiccation; can be formulated as aerosol	**Ciprofloxacin** (400 mg q8h) or (a) levofloxacin (750 mg q24h) or moxifloxacin (400 mg q24h) plus either (b) **meropenem** (2 g q8h) or imipenem (1 g q6h) or doripenem (500 mg q8h) plus (c) **linezolid** (600 mg q12h) or clindamycin (900 mg q8h) or rifampin (600 mg q12h) or chloramphenicol (1 g q6-8h)[†]
Smallpox (variola virus; Chapter 343)	Synchronous exanthem	Virions stable in environment; population immunologically naïve	Supportive care; brincidofovir and tecovirimat are now licensed treatments
Plague (*Yersinia pestis;* Chapter 288)	Hemoptysis	Contagious through respiratory droplets; "Black Death" conjures fear	Gentamicin (5 mg/kg qd) or ciprofloxacin (400 mg q12h), doxycycline (200 mg × 1, then 100 mg q12h), or levofloxacin 500 mg q24h or moxifloxacin 400 mg q24h
Tularemia (*Francisella tularensis;* Chapter 287)	Plague-like illness	Bacteria stable in environment; very low infectious dose	Same as for plague[‡]
Botulism (botulinum toxins; Chapter 271)	Descending, flaccid paralysis	Highly potent toxin; lends itself to food and water use; cases consume vast resources	Supportive care; ventilator support; botulinum antitoxin may halt (but will not reverse) symptom progression
Viral hemorrhagic fevers (Chapter 351; see E-Table 19-1)	Hemorrhagic diatheses	Fear factor is paramount; few countermeasures exist	Supportive care; ribavirin may be beneficial in select cases (e.g., Lassa fever, New World arenaviruses, Crimean-Congo hemorrhagic fever virus, hemorrhagic fever renal syndrome) when it is given under an experimental protocol: 30 mg/kg load, then 16 mg/kg q6h for 4 days, then 8 mg/kg q8h for 6 days; for Ebola virus (Zaire), two approved therapies are either REGN-EB3 or mAb114

*All therapeutic agents listed in this table should be administered intravenously.
[†]Preferred treatments are in **bold**.
[‡]Note that levofloxacin and moxifloxacin are now licensed by the U.S. Food and Drug Administration for the treatment of plague, but not for tularemia.
qd = once daily.

of 50% or more. Reported in the United States for the first time after an animal-hide drum circle event in 2009, the disease causes fever, abdominal pain, diarrhea, hematochezia, hematemesis, and ascites. Paracentesis may yield hemorrhagic ascites.

Inhalational anthrax is of greatest concern after an aerosolized bioweapon attack. After an incubation period that averages 1 to 6 days but can be up to 43 days, patients present with fever, profound drenching sweats, nausea, vomiting, diarrhea, shortness of breath, cough, and chest pain. Without prompt recognition and appropriate therapy, individuals can deteriorate rapidly with increasing dyspnea, stridor, cyanosis, and respiratory failure. Engorgement and hemorrhage of mediastinal lymph nodes with accompanying mediastinitis lead to the clinical hallmark of a widened mediastinum on the chest radiograph in about 60% of cases. Patients may also develop large hemorrhagic pleural effusions and infiltrates. Bacteremic dissemination can lead to widely metastatic infection in the gastrointestinal tract and meninges.

DIAGNOSIS

B. anthracis can be identified by Gram stain or culture of tissue or body fluids, including skin biopsy for cutaneous disease, peripheral blood, pleural effusions, and cerebrospinal fluid but not sputum. A chest radiograph may provide initial clues to inhalational disease with manifestations such as hilar or paratracheal fullness and pleural effusions. A chest computed tomography scan can confirm mediastinal adenopathy. Other techniques, such as fluorescent antibody staining or polymerase chain reaction (PCR), may provide more rapid diagnosis.

TREATMENT

The approach to the management of patients[4] infected with or exposed to anthrax differ among patients with meningitis and patients in whom meningitis has been excluded. For patients in whom meningitis is present or cannot be excluded, three antibiotics are administered intravenously (preferred drugs are in bold):

- **Ciprofloxacin** (400 mg q8h) or levofloxacin (750 mg q24h) or moxifloxacin (400 mg q24h) plus
- **Meropenem** (2 g q8h) or imipenem (1 g q6h) or doripenem (500 mg q8h) plus
- **Linezolid** (600 mg q12h) or clindamycin (900 mg q8h) or rifampin (600 mg q12h) or chloramphenicol (1 g q6-8h).

If meningitis has been excluded, a two-drug regimen can be used:

- **Ciprofloxacin** or levofloxacin or moxifloxacin or meropenem or imipenem or doripenem or vancomycin (penicillin G or amoxicillin can also be used if the infecting strain is known to be susceptible) plus
- **Clindamycin or linezolid** or doxycycline or rifampin

A monoclonal antibody, raxibacumab (single dose of 40 mg/kg IV during 2 hours and 15 minutes after premedicating with diphenhydramine 25 to 50 mg IV), is approved for additional therapy of inhalational anthrax along with antibiotics on the basis of animal efficacy data. Intravenous anthrax immune globulin, which has been given as adjunctive therapy to a small number of patients, is approved in the United States for use in addition to antibiotics for inhalational anthrax. Another antibody, obiltoxaximab (16 mg/kg IV), is also approved by the Food and Drug Administration (FDA) to treat inhalational anthrax in combination with appropriate antibacterial drugs or to prevent inhalational anthrax based on its efficacy in animals and safety in healthy human volunteers.[5]

PREVENTION

The anthrax vaccine,[6] which is effective at preventing all forms of disease, has been reserved primarily for at-risk ranchers or veterinarians who have regular contact with herbivores, as well as for laboratory research personnel and military personnel. The vaccine is given as five doses intramuscularly over 18 months (day 0, followed by 1, 6, 12, and 18 months), with annual boosters if continued risk exists.

After a known exposure, chemoprophylaxis is recommended with ciprofloxacin (500 mg orally twice daily) or doxycycline (100 mg orally twice daily) for 60 days, although shorter durations are likely to be effective, especially if combined with vaccination. If the vaccine is available, three doses may be given concomitantly with antibiotics, but it is not licensed for this purpose and must be administered under an investigational protocol. Raxibacumab (dosed as before) is also approved for prophylaxis if antibiotics are not available.[7]

PROGNOSIS

Factors associated with survival from anthrax include administration of a multiple-drug antibiotic regimen or anthrax antiserum given during the prodromal phase, as well as pleural fluid drainage. Case-fatality rates in untreated patients approach 100%, although 55% of the victims of inhalation anthrax survived in a 2001 outbreak, likely owing to the use of multiple antibiotics and modern intensive care.

SMALLPOX

EPIDEMIOLOGY

Although smallpox was declared eradicated in 1980, concerns exist about undeclared stores outside approved repositories in the United States and Russia. The recent discoveries of unaccounted for vials of variola in the United States provide some credence to this concern. In addition to near-universal susceptibility, the environmental stability of smallpox viral particles makes it a formidable potential weapon.[8]

Smallpox is caused by variola virus, an orthopoxvirus (Chapter 343) that is closely related to cowpox, vaccinia, monkeypox, and Alaskapox. Variola generally spreads to household and other close contacts, but it can spread via aerosolized droplet nuclei as well as by direct contact with patient secretions or fomites. Health care providers who are caring for patients or unsuspecting individuals who have contact with contaminated objects are also at risk.

PATHOBIOLOGY AND CLINICAL MANIFESTATIONS

Infection initially occurs in the respiratory mucosa, is followed by replication in the regional lymph nodes, and leads to an asymptomatic primary viremia that seeds the reticuloendothelial system. Approximately 1 week after infection (range, about 1 to 2 weeks), a secondary viremia seeds the skin. At this time, the sudden onset of illness includes fever, headache, backache, and vomiting. Within 2 or 3 days of this prodrome, and often as the temperature falls, the characteristic rash begins with small papules in a centrifugal pattern (more on the face and extremities than on the trunk) that progress in synchronous fashion during the next week to vesicles, umbilicated pustules, and finally scabs. Lesions are deep seated and can be intensely painful. Individuals are contagious at the onset of the rash and are considered free of contagion only after the scabs have separated.

DIAGNOSIS

Chickenpox (varicella; Chapter 346), which might be confused with early or mild smallpox, occurs predominantly on the trunk rather than on the extremities (a centripetal pattern), and the lesions occur in successive crops, so macules, papules, pustules, and scabs can be seen simultaneously. In addition, varicella is transmissible before onset of the rash, but contagiousness abates when all the lesions are scabbed. Other diseases in the differential diagnosis of smallpox include monkeypox (Chapter 343), Alaskapox, other poxviruses, disseminated vaccinia in a vaccine recipient or contact, disseminated herpes zoster (Chapter 346) or herpes simplex (Chapter 345), impetigo (Chapter 408), drug eruptions (Chapter 407), contact dermatitis (Chapter 405), erythema multiforme (Chapter 406), and rickettsialpox (Chapter 302).

Clinical recognition of the characteristic rash (Fig. 19-1) should raise suspicion of smallpox. Diagnosis would likely come from PCR or viral culture of skin or blood samples or from acute and convalescent serologies.

TREATMENT

The primary therapy for smallpox remains supportive care, although tecovirimat (600 mg orally every 12 hours for 14 days) is approved by the U.S. FDA to treat all poxvirus infections and is included in the strategic national stockpile.[9] Brincidofovir (4 mg/kg, once weekly for two doses, maximum 200 mg), which is an oral analog of cidofovir, is also an approved treatment.

PREVENTION

Vaccination uses vaccinia, an orthopoxvirus related to variola. In the event of an outbreak, postexposure vaccination within 4 days can prevent or ameliorate disease and might be applied in a method of surveillance and containment, as was used during global eradication. The U.S. government has stockpiled enough doses for the entire U.S. population of a live replicating cell-culture-derived product (ACAM2000) for use in a national emergency. The surveillance and containment, or ring, vaccination method combines active case finding with vaccination of potential contacts within a certain radius around the cases. Health care providers would need to be vaccinated, and airborne

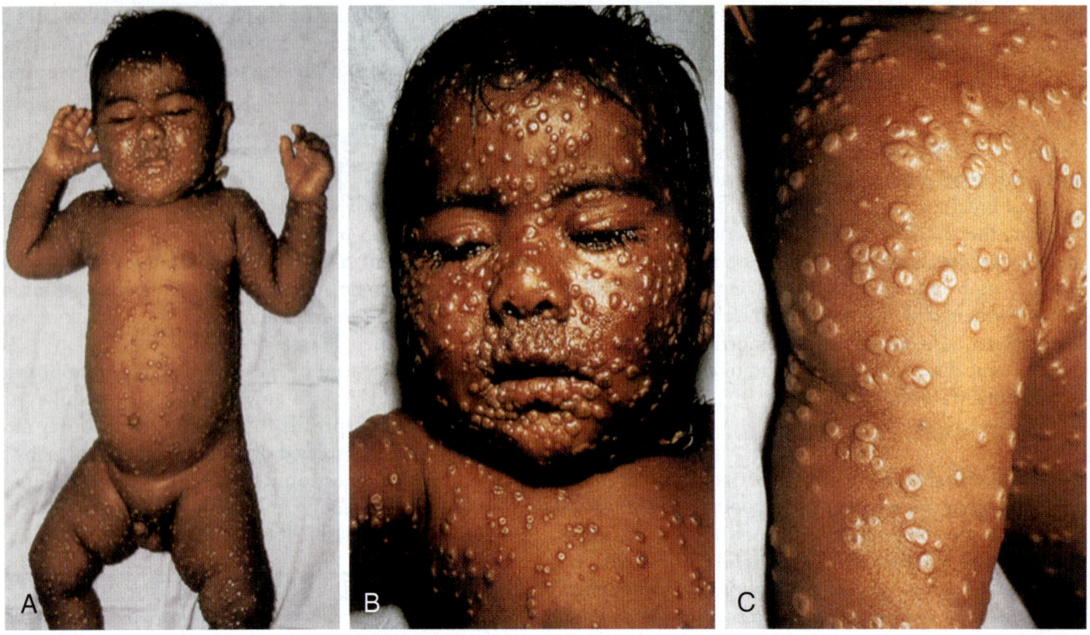

FIGURE 19-1. **Smallpox. A, Demonstrates centrifugal nature of the rash. B, Demonstrates coalescences of some pustules. C, Demonstrates umbilicated pustules.** (From Fenner F, Henderson DA, Arita A, et al. *Smallpox and its Eradication*. Geneva: World Health Organization; 1988.)

and contact precautions (HEPA filter masks, negative-pressure rooms, gowns, gloves, eye protection) would be recommended in the hospital environment. Because the vaccine is a live agent, it is contraindicated in individuals who are immunocompromised and in individuals who have eczema or significant exfoliative skin conditions. Even in normal hosts, the vaccine can be associated with inoculation of other locations on the body, spread to close contacts, disseminated disease, postvaccine encephalitis, progressive vaccinia in individuals with defective cell-mediated immunity, eczema vaccinatum in people with prior eczema, and pericarditis or myocarditis.[10] In the postexposure setting, risks and benefits must be weighed regarding which individuals at risk for complications might receive vaccine and whether vaccinia immune globulin might be administered concomitantly. First-line therapy for significant vaccine reactions is vaccinia immune globulin. A novel live, but nonreplicating, vaccinia-based vaccine, Jynneos, was recently approved by the FDA for the prevention of smallpox as well as monkeypox. Although this product is expected to alleviate some of the concerns associated with the replicating vaccine, its requirement for two doses would complicate its use in a postexposure setting.[A1]

PROGNOSIS

The case-fatality rate for the typical form of smallpox, variola major, is approximately 30%, but wide variations exist. In the minority of individuals who develop hemorrhagic smallpox or flat-type smallpox, the case-fatality rate approaches 100%. A different viral strain, variola minor, has case-fatality rates of only about 1%. Survivors of smallpox are often left with lifelong scarring from the lesions. Blindness and bone deformities, especially in children, are also known complications.

PLAGUE

EPIDEMIOLOGY

Plague, which is caused by the gram-negative coccobacillus *Yersinia pestis* (Chapter 288), was responsible for hundreds of millions of deaths during three historic pandemics. Plague was used as a weapon by the Japanese before World War II when they released infected fleas in Chinese cities, and it was included in the former Soviet Union's biologic weapon arsenal. Plague is transmissible through the respiratory route, so an aerosol release could have devastating effects.

Each year in the United States, several human cases are reported, usually in the Southwest. Most of these cases are bubonic, although occasional pneumonic plague has been linked to infections in domestic cats.

PATHOBIOLOGY AND CLINICAL MANIFESTATIONS

Plague is manifested in three ways.[11] Bubonic plague, which is the most common form, occurs after the bite of an infected flea. The organism spreads through the local lymphatics to the regional lymph nodes. As replication occurs, the lymph node or group of lymph nodes becomes swollen and extremely tender. Because most flea bites occur on the lower extremities, the inguinal and femoral lymph nodes are most often affected. Untreated bubonic plague can progress to septicemic plague after organisms gain entry to the blood stream. In addition, patients can develop necrosis of cooler areas of the body, such as the tip of the nose, ears, or digits, due to a temperature-dependent coagulase produced by the organism.

Septicemic plague may also occur in the absence of an antecedent bubo. Meningitis may occur from seeding through the blood stream.

In pneumonic plague, the lungs are seeded secondarily by bacteremia from septicemic plague or primarily when a person inhales infectious droplets. Although naturally occurring pneumonic plague is rare, this form of disease is the major concern after intentional release of aerosol. In patients with pneumonic plague, the disease can be spread to others. One of the hallmarks of the disease is the potential for purulent sputum to become hemorrhagic. Although hemoptysis can certainly be seen with other diseases (Chapter 71), the presentation of clusters of multiple patients with hemoptysis should prompt the clinician to consider plague.

DIAGNOSIS

Plague bacilli are readily identified by their bipolar appearance or Gram, Wright-Giemsa, or Wayson stains, and they can be cultured from sputum or other infected body fluid, such as blood, fluid from a bubo, or cerebrospinal fluid. Other diagnostic methods include PCR for the F1 antigen, direct fluorescent antibody staining of body fluids, and serology by enzyme-linked immunosorbent assay or passive hemagglutination. However, serology is primarily useful in retrospect, because patients must be treated empirically before a serologic response occurs.

TREATMENT

Drug options include streptomycin (if available, 1 g IM twice daily for 7 to 10 days or for 3 days after the fever remits) or gentamicin (5 mg/kg IM or IV daily or a 2-mg/kg load followed by 1.7 mg IM or IV three times daily also for 7 to 10 days). Alternative choices (all for 7 to 10 days or for 3 days after fever and symptoms have resolved) include doxycycline (200-mg IV load, then 100 mg IV every 12 hours), ciprofloxacin (400 mg IV every 12 hours), levofloxacin (500 to 750 mg IV once daily), and moxifloxacin (400 mg IV once daily) (Table 19-2).[12] The drug of choice for plague meningitis is chloramphenicol (25- to 30-mg/kg IV load, followed by 50 to 60 mg/kg/day every 6 hours; on favorable clinical response, the dose can be reduced to 25 to 30 mg/kg/day every 6 hours). CDC now recommends the addition of either levofloxacin (750 mg once daily) or moxifloxacin (400 mg once daily) to chloramphenicol, when feasible.

PREVENTION

Use of standard precautions is appropriate for bubonic plague. Droplet precautions should be applied for patients with pneumonic plague, including a private room where caregivers wear masks, gowns, gloves, and eye protection within 3 to 6 feet of the patients. These precautions should be continued until the patient demonstrates improvement and has been receiving effective antibiotics for 72 hours. Oral ciprofloxacin (500 to 750 mg twice daily), levofloxacin (500 to 750 mg once daily), doxycycline (100 mg twice daily), or moxifloxacin (400 mg once daily) is recommended for postexposure prophylaxis for 7 days beyond the period of exposure in household contacts or individuals suspected of exposure in either the endemic or bioterrorism setting.[13]

No licensed vaccine for plague currently exists in the United States, and a previously licensed whole-cell killed vaccine is no longer available. New vaccines are being studied.

PROGNOSIS

Case-fatality rates are 50% or more for untreated bubonic plague and nearly 100% for untreated septicemic and pneumonic plague. These fatality rates can be significantly reduced with prompt recognition and appropriate therapy.

TULAREMIA

Tularemia (Chapter 287) is caused by infection with the gram-negative, aerobic nonmotile coccobacillary organism *Francisella tularensis*.[14] A zoonotic disease of rabbits, ground squirrels, and other small mammals, tularemia can infect humans by skin or mucous membrane contact with body fluids or tissues of infected animals or from the bite of infected deerflies, mosquitoes, or ticks. Disease rarely occurs by inhalation of contaminated dusts or ingestion of contaminated food or water. One outbreak was associated with groundskeepers in Martha's Vineyard. Fewer than 150 cases of naturally occurring human tularemia are typically reported each year. However, the environmental stability of *F. tularensis* as well as its very low infectious dose (as few as 10 organisms) makes it a potential weaponization threat.

CLINICAL MANIFESTATIONS AND DIAGNOSIS

Clinical manifestations of tularemia depend on the route of exposure. Although six different forms have been described, tularemia is perhaps more simplistically compared with plague, with glandular forms analogous to bubonic plague, as well as pneumonic and typhoidal forms that present a clinical picture similar to what is seen in pneumonic and septicemic plague. A preponderance of these latter forms would be expected after an intentional release by aerosol. After an incubation period of 2 to 10 days, symptoms begin with fever and proceed to include severe exhaustion, substernal chest pain, nonproductive cough, and weight loss.

A diagnosis can be made by isolating the organism from blood, sputum, skin, or mucus membrane lesions, but culture may be difficult because of unusual growth requirements and overgrowth of commensal organisms. Molecular technologies are available in specialized laboratories, but serology is the most common method of diagnosis, often in retrospect. Because of the risk of spread to microbiology laboratory personnel, it is important to notify the laboratory if infection with this organism is suspected.

TREATMENT AND PROGNOSIS

Treatment of tularemia is similar to that of plague, with aminoglycosides for 7 to 10 days; streptomycin and gentamicin are considered the drugs of choice, although ciprofloxacin is a newer potential alternative (Table 19-2). Doxycycline/tetracycline and chloramphenicol are second-line choices because their use has been associated with relapses, and the recommended duration of therapy is 14 to 21 days.

Person-to-person spread is unusual, and standard precautions are adequate in caring for ill individuals. For known exposures, consensus recommendations in a bioterrorism setting call for doxycycline (100 mg) or ciprofloxacin (500 mg) orally twice a day for 14 days as postexposure prophylaxis. A live attenuated vaccine has proven efficacy in preventing disease due to laboratory exposures and aerosol challenge in human volunteers, but it is not readily available to the public.

The case-fatality rate for untreated pneumonic and typhoidal tularemia is 35%, but this rate can be reduced to less than 5% with appropriate treatment.

BOTULISM

Botulism is caused by exposure to one of eight related neurotoxins (A to H) produced by strains of *Clostridium botulinum* (Chapter 271), a ubiquitous, anaerobic, spore-forming, gram-positive bacillus. Botulinum toxins, which are among the most toxic substances known, can be lethal in doses as low as 0.001 μg/kg. These toxins block release of acetylcholine from presynaptic nerve terminals, thereby resulting in a generalized flaccid paralysis with autonomic dysfunction. Although most toxins are unstable in the environment and thus constitute dubious weaponization threats, the potent nature of botulinum toxin, coupled with the ease with which it might be used to contaminate food and water, makes it a concern. Naturally occurring human botulism is limited to types A, B, and E, although other toxin serotypes can produce an identical clinical syndrome. For this reason, a heptavalent antitoxin with activity against serotypes A to G was licensed in 2013.

CLINICAL MANIFESTATIONS AND DIAGNOSIS

Botulism typically develops after a latent period ranging from hours to several days. Initial manifestations involve bulbar palsies, ptosis, photophobia, blurred vision, and other signs of cranial nerve dysfunction.[15] Symptoms progress craniocaudally, thereby leading to dysphonia, dysphagia, and, ultimately, a descending symmetrical paralysis. In fatal cases, death typically results from respiratory muscle failure.

Although botulism may mimic other neurologic disorders, such as myasthenia gravis (Chapter 390) and Guillain-Barré syndrome (Chapter 388), the occurrence of an outbreak involving multiple cases of descending, symmetrical, flaccid paralysis should make diagnosis of botulism relatively straightforward.

TREATMENT AND PROGNOSIS

Supportive care measures, including meticulous attention to ventilatory support, are the mainstay of botulism management. Patients may require such support for several months, so the management of a large-scale botulism outbreak would be resource intensive. Antitoxin should be administered as soon as possible to prevent progressive disease. Botulism is not contagious, so standard precautions are appropriate. The first victims of an outbreak may have higher case-fatality rates because of delays in recognition. Patients who recover can have long-term sequelae, such as dyspnea on exertion, fatigue, and weakness.

VIRAL HEMORRHAGIC FEVERS

EPIDEMIOLOGY

Viral hemorrhagic fever (Chapter 351) describes a clinical syndrome caused by four families of RNA viruses: filoviruses (Ebola and Marburg), arenaviruses ("Old World" Lassa fever and "New World" South American viruses, Machupo, Junin, and others), bunyaviruses (hantaviruses, Crimean-Congo hemorrhagic fever, and Rift Valley fever), and flaviviruses (yellow fever and dengue) (E-Table 19-1). Agents of greatest concern from a bioterrorism perspective include the filoviruses and arenaviruses, which are infectious by the aerosol route, can replicate well in cell culture for large-scale production, and have a clinical syndrome of hemorrhage and fever that engenders fear. The massive outbreak of Ebola virus disease in West Africa in 2013-2016 and a subsequent outbreak in eastern Democratic Republic of the Congo in 2018-2020 demonstrated the devastation that a hemorrhagic fever virus can have on a population, even in the absence of an intentional release, in an environment conducive to spread, including limited medical infrastructure, mobile populations, mistrust of government, and close contact during burial practices, among other factors.[16]

PATHOBIOLOGY AND CLINICAL MANIFESTATIONS

Once virus gains entry through the skin, mucous membranes, or respiratory tract, replication occurs in macrophages and dendritic cells. Organisms are then transported to regional lymph nodes and eventually through the lymphatics and blood stream to target organs, such as the liver and spleen, where local necrosis occurs. The body responds with activation of cytokines and chemokines, and massive depletion of lymphocytes disables the host's adaptive immune response. A sepsis-like picture ensues, with declining mean arterial pressure, increased vascular permeability, and a bleeding diathesis.

Clinical features of the hemorrhagic fevers include the acute onset of malaise, sore throat, fever, skin flushing, conjunctival injection, prostration, myalgias, and nonbloody diarrhea. These viruses have significant differences in the prominence of individual clinical findings. For example, dengue, the filoviruses, and Lassa more commonly cause a maculopapular rash in the first week. The filoviruses and South American viruses more typically cause obtundation and encephalitis. Although all of these viruses produce modest elevations of aminotransferase levels, yellow fever and Rift Valley fever are known for causing significant hepatic dysfunction, thereby resulting in icterus and jaundice. Depending on a number of factors, including virulence, route of exposure, inoculum, and other host factors, illness can progress in the second week to overt signs of bleeding, including petechiae, purpura, ecchymoses, and oozing from venipuncture sites. Electrolyte abnormalities and large-volume gastrointestinal losses were reported during the 2013-2016 West Africa Ebola outbreak. Massive bleeding occurs uncommonly; but if it does, the source is usually the gastrointestinal tract. Severe cases will demonstrate a combination of neurologic and hematologic abnormalities.

DIAGNOSIS

Numerous common diseases should be considered in the differential diagnosis of a viral hemorrhagic fever, including rickettsial infections (Rocky Mountain spotted fever, ehrlichia, anaplasma, and African tick typhus; Chapter 302), leptospirosis (Chapter 298), meningococcemia (Chapter 274), typhoid (Chapter 284), and falciparum malaria (Chapter 316). However, a viral hemorrhagic fever should be considered in patients who present with a clinically compatible syndrome, especially if a cluster of cases is seen.

Laboratory features may include thrombocytopenia, elevated aminotransferase levels, leukopenia, anemia (although an elevated hematocrit may be seen in patients with significant vascular leakage, as is sometimes seen with dengue and hantaviruses), hematuria, and proteinuria.

PCR, viral culture, immunoglobulin M–specific enzyme-linked immunosorbent assay, acute and convalescent serology, or immunohistochemistry on autopsy specimens can establish the diagnosis. Routine clinical specimens and any attempt at viral isolation require a biosafety level 3 or 4 laboratory with expert consultation from the CDC or the U.S. Army Medical Research Institute of Infectious Diseases.

TREATMENT

Two licensed therapies now exist for Ebola virus: Inmazeb (a cocktail of three monoclonal antibodies) and Ebanga (a single monoclonal antibody). Both showed significantly decreased fatality rates in the 2018-2020 outbreak in eastern Democratic Republic of Congo.[A2] Even with this success, however, supportive care remains a primary means of management for all viral hemorrhagic fevers, with close attention to fluid status, electrolytes, avoidance of procedures that cause bleeding and medications that impair platelet function, use of blood products as necessary, use of vasopressors for hypotension, and dialysis for renal failure. Close attention to fluid status has significantly reduced mortality from dengue, and aggressive fluid repletion has been needed to address significant loss of fluid volume due to diarrhea, electrolyte abnormalities, and protein/nutritional depletion in Ebola infections.[17] Oral ribavirin or intravenous ribavirin (see Table 19-2) under an approved experimental protocol can reduce mortality in Lassa hemorrhagic fever and also appears to be beneficial against Argentine hemorrhagic fever (Junin virus) and hantaviruses that cause hemorrhagic fever with renal syndrome. Ribavirin has no apparent efficacy against filoviruses (Ebola or Marburg) or flaviviruses (dengue, yellow fever).

PREVENTION

Vaccines licensed by the U.S. FDA are available against only two specific agents, yellow fever and Ebola.[A3] Experimental vaccines exist against Junin virus and Rift Valley fever virus, but these vaccines have been used primarily to protect laboratory workers.

Certain viral hemorrhagic fevers (primarily Ebola, Marburg, Lassa, and Crimean-Congo hemorrhagic fever) produce high-level viremia during the period of greatest bleeding risk and body fluid production, thereby making them notorious for causing nosocomial outbreaks. In general, these outbreaks occur in environments, such as sub-Saharan Africa, where basic infection control practices are inadequate because of limited resources (e.g., lack of gowns, gloves, and eye protection as well as reuse of unsterilized needles and syringes). Spread of these viruses in the nosocomial environment can be significantly reduced with standard precautions that limit contact with blood and body fluids. In caring for patients who may spread disease, the use of masks, gowns, gloves, and eye protection is recommended. Many cases in the United States and Europe are cared for in biocontainment units specifically designed to reduce nosocomial spread to caregivers.[18]

PROGNOSIS

Hemorrhagic viruses exhibit a wide range of mortality rates, ranging from less than 1% with Rift Valley fever to 80 to 90% with untreated Ebola Zaire (E-Table 19-1). Despite the notoriety of these viruses for causing hemorrhage, the majority of individuals do not die of blood loss. Rather, death results from a sepsis-like picture (Chapter 94), including a loss of vascular hemostasis, disseminated intravascular coagulation, hypotension, renal failure, shock, and death. Provision of intensive care appears to have benefit.

RESPONSE TO A BIOTERRORISM ATTACK

Even a relatively small bioterror event can have profound consequences. After the 2001 anthrax mailings, thousands of people were prescribed antibiotic prophylaxis, and government buildings were closed for decontamination. Since that event, significant improvements in future responses to a bioterrorism event include the licensure, manufacture, and storage of enough smallpox vaccine for everyone in the United States; production of anthrax and botulinum antitoxins for the strategic national stockpile; and development of protocols and authority for response.

The early detection of the release of a pathogen remains a significant challenge. The 2013-2016 Ebola outbreak also identified shortcomings in preparedness, which may be mitigated, in part, by establishing a network of biocontainment units.

A framework for pandemic preparedness, which applies to bioterrorism preparedness as well,[19] includes four main features: ensuring the global community commits appropriate financial resources and monitors progress; reinforcing national public health capabilities and infrastructure; strengthening the leadership role of the World Health Organization; and enhancing the scientific armory against infectious diseases.

Unfortunately, the response to the coronavirus-2019 (COVID-19) pandemic demonstrated that, despite lessons learned from both the 2001 anthrax attacks and the 2013-2016 Ebola outbreak, significant challenges remain in public health preparedness. There is a critical need to reassess our response capability and capacity for the next public health emergency.[20]

In any future bioterror attack,[21] early warning signs might include clusters of patients with mediastinal adenopathy or widened mediastinum on the chest radiograph, a centrifugal pustular rash (smallpox), pneumonia and hemoptysis (plague), descending flaccid paralysis (botulism), or hemorrhagic manifestations and impaired clotting (viral hemorrhagic fever). Should such a cluster be identified or suspected, physicians should contact the local county or city health department, the state health department, and potentially the CDC. Unlike a natural outbreak, a potential bioterror outbreak also requires a rapid dialogue between public health and law enforcement authorities, because patient and environmental samples constitute evidence against a perpetrator and must be handled under chain of custody. Physicians also must be prepared not only to protect themselves and their patients but also to serve as community resources, regardless of whether an outbreak is natural or terrorist in origin.

GENERAL REFERENCES

For the General References and other additional features, please visit Elsevier eBooks+ at https://ebooks.health.elsevier.com.

Grade A References

A1. Pittman PR, Hahn M, Lee HS, et al. Phase 3 trial of modified vaccinia Ankara as a vaccine against smallpox. *N Engl J Med.* 2019;381:1897-1908.

A2. Mulangu S, Dodd LE, Davey RT , Jr, et al. A randomized, controlled trial of Ebola virus disease therapeutics. *N Engl J Med.* 2019;381:2293-2303.

A3. Henao-Restrepo AM, Camacho A, Longini IM, et al. Efficacy and effectiveness of an rVSV-vectored vaccine in preventing Ebola virus disease: final results from the Guinea ring vaccination, open-label, cluster-randomised trial (Ebola Ça Suffit!). *Lancet.* 2017;389:505-518.

20 CHRONIC POISONING: TRACE METALS AND OTHERS

LOUISE W. KAO, LAURA TORMOEHLEN, AND BLAKE A. FROBERG

About 80% of the elements in the periodic table are metals or metalloids, and various metals are in contact with humans in the home, workplace, and environment. Metals are part of a number of normal physiologic processes, such as iron in hemoglobin, but also can cause a number of toxic adverse effects.[1–3]

LEAD TOXICITY

EPIDEMIOLOGY

Lead (Pb) is a silver-gray, malleable metal that is resistant to corrosion. It has no known physiologic use, so any lead in the human body should be considered contamination.

The most common sources of lead poisoning are lead-based paints, lead-contaminated dust, and lead-contaminated soil. Other sources include plumbing, solder, batteries, retained bullets, toys, curtain weights, necklace charms, food containers, and cosmetics, including Nigerian eyeliners. Adults in occupations such as battery manufacturing, welding, construction, mining, glass blowing, rifle ranges, and shipbuilding have the highest lead exposures. Other less common but important routes of exposure include lead-contaminated moonshine and lead-containing ethnic folk remedies (e.g., greta and azarcon in Mexico).

Children in lower socioeconomic areas have the highest exposures to lead,[4] and the majority of the scientific literature is biased toward pediatric studies. Much of what we have learned, however, is applicable to adults.

PATHOBIOLOGY

Lead's most devastating effects are on the central nervous system (CNS) of children. By disrupting the intracellular junction of capillary endothelium, lead impairs the blood-brain barrier and further increases its CNS absorption. Lead also increases capillary leak, which in severe cases can result in cerebral edema.

Lead inhibits several enzymes involved in heme synthesis: aminolevulinic acid synthetase, δ-aminolevulinic acid dehydratase, coproporphyrinogen decarboxylase, and ferrochelatase. Lead also inhibits the enzyme erythrocyte pyrimidine-5-nucleotidase and, as a result, impairs RNA degradation and contributes to red cell hemolysis. Collectively, the inhibition of these enzymes results in decreased concentrations of hemoglobin and a shorter lifespan of red blood cells.

By depositing lead-protein complexes in renal proximal tubular cells, lead interferes with normal mitochondrial function, thereby resulting in decreased reabsorption of glucose, amino acids, and phosphate. Chronically exposed persons can develop renal failure from tubular atrophy, interstitial fibrosis, and glomerular sclerosis.

Although lead has not been associated with specific bone-related disorders, the skeletal system serves as the main reservoir for lead; with chronic exposure, lead stores in bone can have a half-life of 5 to 19 years. As a result, tissues may be subjected to increased lead exposure during times of accelerated bone turnover, such as during childhood growth, after fracture of a long bone, or during pregnancy.

CLINICAL MANIFESTATIONS

Lead poisoning can be subtle and difficult to diagnose because many of its historical clinical associations (e.g., neuropathy, gout, abdominal colic) are rarely seen today. In children, the most concerning long-term complications of environmental lead exposure are developmental cognitive deficits, especially when lead concentrations in young children exceed 100 μg/dL. Subacute neurologic problems include ataxia, lethargy, seizures, and coma. Adults can also experience severe neurologic symptoms (e.g., seizures and cerebral edema) with plumbism, but typically only when whole blood lead levels are higher than 150 μg/dL. More commonly, the neurologic problems caused by lead in adults are manifested as memory problems,[5] insomnia, depression, personality changes, and an increased risk of cardiovascular disease. Higher childhood blood levels are also associated with changes on measures of brain structure seen on magnetic resonance imaging (MRI).[6]

Other clinical effects of lead poisoning, in both children and adults, include a normocytic or microcytic anemia, abdominal pain, hepatotoxicity, and pancreatitis. The classic finding of peripheral neuropathy with footdrop and wristdrop is well described in adults but only occasionally seen in children. Nephrotoxicity most commonly is manifested as Fanconi syndrome (Chapter 113) with aminoaciduria, glycosuria, and phosphaturia. A consequence of this toxicity is impaired uric acid clearance and gout (Chapter 252). High lead levels may increase the risk of hypertension.

DIAGNOSIS

Existing evidence is insufficient to recommend screening for elevated blood lead levels in asymptomatic individuals,[7] so the diagnosis of lead intoxication involves a high level of clinical suspicion. The best initial test is a whole blood lead level collected in a certified lead-free tube (Table 20-1). The blood lead level can be falsely elevated in individuals who have received chelation therapy in the prior 7 days. Capillary lead levels can be falsely elevated by skin contaminated with lead.

Radiographic imaging can support the diagnosis of lead poisoning and sometimes detect a lead-containing object or a retained bullet. Bone x-ray fluorescence technology can estimate bone lead levels, which can reflect chronic lead exposure, but this test is not commonly available.

TREATMENT

The first step in the management of patients with elevated lead levels is prompt removal of the source, although the effectiveness of household environmental clean-up and educational initiatives is disappointing.[A1,A2] If lead comes from a work-related source, the Occupational Safety and Health Administration should be contacted. Chelation increases excretion of lead in a 24-hour urine sample and thereby decreases blood concentrations, but studies to date with the chelating agent succimer (2,3-dimercaptosuccinic acid, DMSA) in children have not shown improved neuropsychological function despite success in reducing blood lead levels. The current recommendation is that asymptomatic adults with blood lead levels of less than 70 μg/dL do not require chelation, patients with mild symptoms or blood lead levels between 70 and 100 μg/dL should receive oral chelation, and patients with lead-induced encephalopathy or blood lead levels above 100 μg/dL should receive parenteral chelation. Although DMSA is approved by the Food and Drug Administration only for children, it also is commonly used in adults (Table 20-2).

Whole bowel irrigation with a polyethylene glycol–electrolyte solution should be considered if a patient has retained a gastrointestinal lead object. Patients who have lead-containing bullet fragments lodged in soft tissues or joint spaces may need to have them surgically removed.

PROGNOSIS

Despite controversy about long-term recovery from lead-associated cognitive deficits in children, adults with neurologic symptoms improve with removal of the exposure. The hematologic and nephrotoxic effects of lead also are reversible.

TABLE 20-1 DIAGNOSTIC TESTING FOR METALS: REFERENCE RANGES

METAL	SERUM LEVEL	WHOLE BLOOD LEVEL	SPOT URINE	24-HOUR URINE
Lead		<5 μg/dL		
Mercury		<10 μg/L	<20 μg/L	<5 μg/L creatinine
Arsenic		<5 μg/L		<50 μg/L or <100 μg/g creatinine
Cadmium		<5 μg/L		<3 μg/g creatinine
Aluminum	<2 μg/L	<12 μg/L		<4-12 μg/g creatinine
Bismuth	<1 μg/dL	<5 μg/dL	<20 μg/L	
Cobalt	0.1-1.2 μg/L		0.1-2.2 μg/L	
Manganese	0.4-0.85 μg/L	4-15 μg/L		<10 μg/L
Silver	<0.5 μg/L			<1 μg/L
Thallium		<2 μg/L		<5 μg/L
Zinc	109-130 μg/dL	600-1000 μg/dL		<500 μg/day

Modified from Nelson L, Howland M, et al., eds. *Goldfrank's Toxicologic Emergencies*. 11th ed. New York: McGraw-Hill Medical; 2019.

TABLE 20-2 CHELATORS FOR ADULT HEAVY METAL POISONING

SYMPTOMS	CHELATOR	RECOMMENDED DOSE†	ADVERSE EFFECTS
LEAD			
Asymptomatic, BLL* < 70 µg/dL	None		
Mild-moderate, BLL 70-100 µg/dL	DMSA	10 mg/kg tid PO × 5 days, then bid for 14 days	Nausea, vomiting, diarrhea, rash, elevations in aminotransferase levels, neutropenia
Encephalopathy, BLL > 100 µg/dL	BAL +	4 mg/kg deep IM q4h × 5 days	Local injection site (pain, redness, sterile abscess); nausea, vomiting, diarrhea; anxiety, hypertension, tachycardia, fever; contraindicated in peanut allergy
	$CaNa_2EDTA$‡	1500 mg/m²/day (approximately 50-75 mg/kg/day, maximum 3 g) either continuous infusion or in 2-4 divided IV doses for 5 days, adjusted for renal insufficiency	Renal toxicity (from metal chelate), constitutional symptoms, transient hypotension
MERCURY			
Acute (elemental or inorganic, but not organic) with moderate/severe symptoms	BAL	5 mg/kg deep IM q4h for 2 days, then 2.5 mg/kg q6h for 2 days, then 2.5 mg/kg bid for 7 days or until symptoms improve and the patient is able to take oral medication, at which point DMSA should be considered	Local injection site (pain, redness, sterile abscess); nausea, vomiting, diarrhea; anxiety, hypertension, tachycardia, fever; contraindicated in peanut allergy
Chronic (elemental or inorganic) or organic with symptoms	DMSA	10 mg/kg tid PO × 5 days, then bid for 14 days	Nausea, vomiting, diarrhea; mild elevations in aminotransferase levels
ARSENIC			
Acute exposure with moderate to severe symptoms	BAL	3 mg/kg deep IM q4h × 2 days, then bid for 7 to 10 days	Local injection site (pain, redness, sterile abscess); nausea, vomiting, diarrhea; anxiety, hypertension, tachycardia, fever; contraindicated in peanut allergy
Chronic exposure with moderate symptoms§	DMSA	10 mg/kg tid PO × 5 days, then bid for 14 days	Nausea, vomiting, diarrhea; mild elevations in aminotransferase levels
ALUMINUM			
Acute or chronic exposure in dialysis patient with encephalopathy	Deferoxamine	See *http://kidneyfoundation.cachefly.net/professionals/KDOQI/guidelines_bone/guide12.htm*	Hypotension, increased risk of sepsis, acute lung injury
THALLIUM			
Acute thallium poisoning with moderate to severe symptoms	Prussian Blue	3 g tid PO until the urinary thallium excretion is less than 0.5 mg/day	Constipation, blue stool

*Adult recommendations.

†Chelation doses in general are not well studied or validated, with the exception of lead in children. Optimal dosing is not well established, particularly for BAL. Doses listed are author's suggestions.

‡Start 4 hours after first dose of BAL is administered.

§Benefit in this setting is not established.

BAL = British anti-Lewisite, dimercaprol; bid = twice daily; BLL = blood lead level; DMSA = 2,3-dimercaptosuccinic acid, succimer; EDTA = ethylenediaminetetraacetic acid; h = hour; IM = intramuscularly; IV = intravenously; PO = orally; qd = daily; tid = three times daily.

MERCURY TOXICITY

EPIDEMIOLOGY

Mercury (Hg) is a naturally occurring metal with three distinct forms. Although all forms are neurotoxic, elemental mercury (Hg^0) also causes pulmonary toxicity, inorganic mercury (Hg^+ or Hg^{++}) causes gastrointestinal and renal toxicity, and organic mercury (ethyl, methyl, alkyl, or phenyl) is a teratogen.

Elemental mercury is found in dental amalgams, thermometers, fluorescent lamps, batteries, and some paints. Occupational exposures may occur in dentists and dental hygienists, painters, gold extractors, bronzers, electroplaters, metallurgists, paper pulp manufacturers, miners, ceramic workers, and other workers who use mercury in processing. Mercury thermometers are becoming increasingly rare, and many countries have banned them because of potential mercury toxicity. Toxicity from elemental mercury is caused primarily from breathing its volatilized vapor.

Inorganic mercury has been used historically as a medicinal, cosmetic, and topical antiseptic in the forms of HgCl (calomel) and $HgCl_2$ (mercuric chloride). It is also used in the tanning industry, in taxidermy, in manufacturing of fireworks, and in dye manufacturing. Inorganic mercury may also be found in patent medicines, folk remedies (such as empacho among Mexican Americans), skin lightening creams, and Asian herbal remedies. Toxicity may occur from ingestion, inhalation, or dermal absorption.[8]

Organic mercury compounds can be classified as short-chain alkyl (such as methyl mercury), long-chain alkyl, and aryl compounds. The aryl compounds, such as thimerosal, behave like inorganic mercurial compounds. Methyl mercury has caused several large-scale human poisoning epidemics.

Soil and marine organisms methylate inorganic mercury from the air and industrial waste. Through a process known as bioamplification, methyl mercury concentrates in the tissues of marine life, reaching highest concentrations in large predatory fish such as tuna and swordfish. Fish consumption is now the largest route of organic mercury exposure in the general population, and organic mercury levels have been increasing in the United States even as levels of inorganic mercury have been declining.[9] Organic mercury is also used as a fungicide, pesticide, wood preservative, and medicinal antiseptic or preservative (Mercurochrome and thimerosal). Toxicity is typically by ingestion.

PATHOBIOLOGY

The pathophysiology of mercury poisoning is related to its disruption of cell physiology by binding to sulfhydryl, phosphoryl, carboxyl, and amide groups, thereby causing widespread dysfunction of normal cellular mechanisms. Each type of mercury causes differential effects depending on its route of exposure, solubility, and lipophilicity.

Elemental mercury is poorly absorbed by ingestion. If gastrointestinal motility or mucosal integrity is compromised, however, elemental mercury may ionize into more readily absorbed forms. Elemental mercury toxicity occurs primarily by inhalation of the vapor into the alveoli, where it is well absorbed in the pulmonary circulation and readily crosses the blood-brain barrier. In the brain, it interferes with multiple cellular processes, including protein and nucleic acid synthesis. Mercury also inhibits catechol-*O*-methyltransferase, thereby elevating circulating catecholamine levels.

Inorganic mercury is absorbed after ingestion, initially binds the gastrointestinal mucosa, and accumulates in the kidneys, where it exerts direct oxidative damage. Although it does not readily cross the blood-brain barrier, CNS toxicity can be seen with chronic exposures because of the prolonged elimination rate. Mercuric ions do not appear to cross the placental barrier.

Organic mercury compounds are readily absorbed after ingestion and inhalation and are moderately absorbed after dermal exposure, particularly if skin is not intact. Owing to its high lipid solubility, organic mercury crosses the blood-brain barrier and concentrates in the CNS. It can also cross the placental barrier and concentrate in the fetus. Organic mercury concentrates in red blood cells, distributes throughout the body, and is primarily eliminated in the feces. Some forms of organic mercury are metabolized in the body to inorganic mercury compounds. Toxicity results from its inhibition of enzyme systems and interference with cellular maturity, microtubule function, and neurotransmitter synthesis and uptake.

CLINICAL MANIFESTATIONS

Elemental Mercury

The manifestations of elemental mercury toxicity vary depending on the dose and chronicity of the exposure. Inhalation of high concentrations of mercury vapor, as may occur in an industrial setting, may result in cough, chills, fever, and shortness of breath. Nausea, vomiting, and weakness may result. This syndrome may progress to a severe acute lung injury and respiratory as well as renal failure. Chronic exposure to lower concentrations of mercury vapor produces a classic triad of tremor, gingivostomatitis, and neuropsychiatric disturbances. The mercurial tremor may be both static and intentional. Sudden episodic bursts of tremor, also called tetanus mercurialis, have been described. Neuropsychiatric manifestations of mercury poisoning, also known as erethism, include fatigue, insomnia, memory dysfunction, social withdrawal, shyness, and depression. Acrodynia, or pink disease, has been described after elemental or inorganic mercury exposure, most notably in children after exposure to mercurial teething powder and diaper ointment. This syndrome is manifested as an erythematous, hyperkeratotic, often desquamating rash on the palms, soles, and face in conjunction with a papular rash. Acrodynia is also associated with an idiosyncratic hypersensitivity to mercury ions and mercury poisoning, which itself can increase circulating catecholamines and mimic pheochromocytoma (Chapter 209). Common findings include tremor, diaphoresis, tachycardia, and hypertension.

Inorganic Mercury

Inorganic mercury poisoning can occur after dermal or mucosal absorption of mercury-containing cosmetics and teething powders as well as after accidental or intentional ingestion of mercuric chloride antiseptics. After acute ingestion, a hemorrhagic gastroenteritis is typically followed by renal failure from acute tubular necrosis. Chronic exposure is associated with erethism, renal dysfunction, and neurologic manifestations such as sensorimotor neuropathy, constriction of visual fields, tremor, and delirium.

Organic Mercury

Human toxicity from organic mercury was first recognized when the dumping of mercury-containing waste into Minamata Bay in Japan led to a large-scale poisoning of the population, whose primary dietary staple was fish from the bay. In what is now called Minamata disease, patients presented with paresthesia, ataxia, dysarthria, tremor, and constriction of visual fields or "tunnel vision."[10] These symptoms can be progressive and sometimes fatal. Children born to these exposed mothers (congenital Minamata disease) suffered mental retardation, limb deformities, chorea, seizures, and microcephaly. In a large Korean study, higher mercury levels were associated with depression in women but not men, and even then only in women with low fish consumption.[11] In the United States, organic mercury exposure from seafood has not been significantly associated with cardiovascular or all-cause mortality.[12] Nevertheless, higher circulatory levels of mercury (along with aluminum and cadmium) are found in patients with Alzheimer disease than in controls.

With organic mercury toxicity, symptoms are typically delayed for weeks to months. Other symptoms that follow organic mercury poisoning include mucous membrane irritation after ingestion and dermatitis after cutaneous exposure. However, no cardiovascular toxicities have been reported with up to moderate elevation in blood mercury levels.

DIAGNOSIS

The diagnosis of mercury poisoning should be considered on recognition of the characteristic signs and symptoms coupled with a known or suspected exposure. Whole blood and urine mercury levels can confirm the exposure, but the correlation between levels and symptoms is inconsistent. In the setting of elemental mercury ingestion or injection, radiographs may also be useful. In a nonoccupationally exposed patient, whole blood mercury concentration should not exceed 10 μg/L, and a 24-hour urine mercury concentration should not exceed 20 μg/L (Table 20-1); urine must be collected in an acid-washed container. In general, urine concentrations are more reliable for monitoring of exposure and the response to therapy, but whole blood concentration is the preferred monitoring test for methyl mercury poisoning.

The ratio of red blood cells to plasma mercury can differentiate organic mercury toxicity from inorganic mercury toxicity because organic mercury concentrates significantly in red blood cells. Hair analysis is unreliable because of the potential for external contamination. The practice of obtaining urine mercury levels after a chelation challenge is not recommended because levels obtained in this way are difficult to interpret.

TREATMENT

Treatment is primarily symptomatic and supportive, with removal from the source of exposure. In cases of acute exposure, decontamination may be required. In cases of occupational or environmental exposure, environmental decontamination and surveillance by local or federal agencies may be necessary. After inhalation of elemental mercury vapor, support of respiratory function is crucial. After ingestion of inorganic mercury salts, fluid resuscitation, usually with normal saline, is needed to correct intravascular depletion, and renal replacement therapy may be required in cases of oliguric renal failure. Mercury compounds are poorly cleared by extracorporeal elimination measures, such as hemodialysis or peritoneal dialysis.

If dietary fish is the likely cause of an elevated mercury level, affected individuals should avoid eating any fish or shellfish for 1 month, after which blood or urine mercury levels should be reanalyzed. If mercury levels have declined into the normal range, as is usually the case, low-mercury fish (shrimp, canned light tuna, salmon, pollock, catfish) can be reintroduced into the diet at a frequency of no more than two meals per week.

Chelation therapy will increase urinary elimination of mercury (Table 20-2), and limited clinical data support its use early after acute poisonings. Oral DMSA, which is the chelator of choice, is generally well tolerated. If oral administration is not possible, dimercaprol (British anti-Lewisite, BAL) can be used except after methyl mercury exposure, in which it is contraindicated because it may shift mercury into the brain.

PROGNOSIS

The neurotoxicity that follows significant poisoning from all types of mercury may be irreversible, particularly in the setting of organic mercury poisoning, in which the diagnosis is often delayed. Nevertheless, 33 of 40 symptomatic children affected in the contaminated grain outbreak of 1971 in Iraq improved during a 2-year observation period. Acute renal failure after elemental or inorganic mercury poisoning can sometimes resolve. Patients with acrodynia have been reported to recover completely after chelation therapy and removal of the exposure.

ARSENIC TOXICITY

EPIDEMIOLOGY

Arsenic (As), which is found in soil, minerals, rocks, and metal ores, is present in all living organisms. It exists in several forms: elemental, inorganic (As^{3+} trivalent arsenite and As^{5+} pentavalent arsenate), gaseous (arsine, AsH^3), and organic. Elemental and organic arsenic have low toxicity, whereas gaseous arsine and inorganic arsenic are highly toxic. Arsenic's medicinal properties were recognized as early as 400 BC, and it has been used throughout history as a medicinal as well as a component of pigments, cosmetics, and famously as a poison.

Human exposure to arsenic may occur through contaminated air, groundwater, soil, and food, particularly seafood, rice, and produce.[13] Marine organisms, especially shellfish, contain organic arsenicals arsenobetaine and arsenocholine, which are commonly reported in laboratory assays as elevated arsenic level but exert no known toxic effects.

In Bangladesh, ongoing epidemic arsenic poisoning from contaminated groundwater has affected millions of persons. Taiwan, Chile, the Cordoba province in Argentina, West Bengal, and other regions in the Ganga plain also have elevated levels of naturally occurring arsenic and cases of arsenic poisoning.

Occupational exposure to arsenic occurs in the microelectronics industry, where arsenide crystals are used to etch circuits on microchips. Arsine gas is liberated when inorganic arsenic contacts acid, as may occur in occupations such as metal smelting, galvanizing, and semiconductor manufacturing. Arsenic compounds are also used in the production of paint, fungicide, insecticide, pesticide, herbicide, wood preservatives, ceramics, and glass, and employees in these industries may also be potentially exposed.

Arsenic compounds may still be found in folk remedies and patent medicines. Modern medicinal uses of arsenic include arsenic trioxide (Trisenox) for the treatment of acute promyelocytic leukemia and other hematologic malignancies (Chapter 168), and melarsoprol (which is not commercially available in the United States), for the treatment of African trypanosomiasis (Chapter 317).

PATHOBIOLOGY

The toxicologically significant arsenic compounds are inorganic (trivalent and pentavalent). Arsine gas, which is also toxic, causes acute hemolysis. After absorption, inorganic arsenic binds to hemoglobin and is distributed to the liver, kidney, heart, and lungs. In the liver, arsenic is methylated to form monomethylarsonic and dimethylarsinic acid, both of which are less toxic. Arsenic concentrates in keratin-rich tissues, such as hair, skin, and nails. Much of an ingested dose of arsenic is eliminated in the urine. The mechanism of toxicity is by binding sulfhydryl groups of critical enzymes, including those of the Krebs cycle, thereby resulting in impaired gluconeogenesis, impaired oxidative phosphorylation, and ultimately depletion of cellular energy stores. DNA damage and an impaired DNA repair mechanism contribute to carcinogenic effects. Pentavalent arsenate may substitute for phosphate in biochemical reactions and disrupt normal oxidative phosphorylation. Arsenic also affects cardiac conduction by blocking cardiac potassium channels. Arsenic can alter gene expression through induction, downregulation, and upregulation of various genes involved in apoptosis, cell signaling, and growth factor response.

Arsine is a colorless, nonirritating gas. After inhalation, it is absorbed rapidly and binds to erythrocytes, where it exerts oxidative stress and causes severe Coombs-negative intravascular hemolysis. Renal failure is due to hemoglobin pigment deposition as well as to the direct toxic effects of arsine on renal tubular cells.

CLINICAL MANIFESTATIONS

The initial clinical features after acute ingestion of inorganic arsenic are nausea, vomiting, bloody diarrhea, and abdominal pain. Severe manifestations such as seizures, delirium, and coma are seen after large exposures. Within several days, hematologic findings such as pancytopenia can be seen. QT prolongation, which can develop acutely or chronically, can lead to dysrhythmias such as torsades de pointes. After gastrointestinal symptoms improve, distal symmetrical peripheral neuropathy develops, potentially accompanied by weakness or encephalopathy.

Chronic exposures affect the bone marrow, skin, and peripheral nervous system.[14] Dermatologic effects include patchy or diffuse alopecia, hyperpigmentation, and melanosis as well as hyperkeratosis on the palms and soles. The pigmentation of chronic poisoning commonly appears in a finely freckled, "raindrop" pattern of symmetrical pigmentation or depigmentation that is particularly pronounced on the trunk and extremities. Nails may exhibit transverse white bands, which are known as Mees lines (Chapter 409) and reflect growth interruption during poisoning. Anemia, pancytopenia, neutropenia, thrombocytopenia, and eosinophilia can be seen. Neuropathy, which is a hallmark of arsenic poisoning, is a diffuse, symmetrical, ascending, painful sensorimotor neuropathy, most prominent in a stocking-glove distribution. In severe poisoning, ascending weakness and paralysis may result in respiratory failure that mimics Guillain-Barré syndrome (Chapter 388). Arsenic exposure also causes a dose-dependent decline in lung function.[15] Peripheral vascular disease, including peripheral vascular gangrene (black foot disease), can develop in chronically exposed patients. Even low to moderate chronic arsenic exposure increases the long-term risk of cardiovascular disease. Arsenic is a human carcinogen, and exposed populations have an increased risk of developing malignant neoplasms in the lung, skin, and bladder.[16]

Arsine gas produces a clinical triad of abdominal pain, hemolysis, and hematuria, typically occurring hours after exposure. Patients may initially have headache, weakness, nausea, and vomiting. Several weeks after an acute exposure, peripheral neuropathy may develop.

DIAGNOSIS

Blood arsenic, urine arsenic, and urine arsenic metabolites can be used to confirm recent or ongoing exposure. In the unexposed individual, blood arsenic should be below 1 μg/L; hair and nail levels should be less than 1 ppm.[17]

However, arsenic clears from the blood quickly, so urine levels are most helpful to diagnose chronic or past exposure. Arsenic levels above 50 μg in a spot urine test warrant a 24-hour test. Urine is collected in a metal-free polyethylene container, and levels exceeding 50 μg or 100 μg/g creatinine in a 24-hour collection require further scrutiny (Table 20-1). Patients who have recently ingested seafood may have urine arsenic levels exceeding 1500 μg/L exclusively from organic arsenic, so differentiating inorganic from nontoxic organic arsenic is often critical. Total arsenic levels in hair or nails, where arsenic accumulates, are useful indicators of past exposures.

In patients with chronic arsenic exposure, a complete blood count may show anemia (normocytic, normochromic, or megaloblastic), leukopenia, and thrombocytopenia. A peripheral smear may show basophilic stippling (see Fig. 143-14) or karyorrhexis. Renal dysfunction, hepatic enzyme elevation, and hyperbilirubinemia may be seen as well. The electrocardiogram may show QT prolongation and nonspecific ST-T wave changes. Nerve conduction studies typically show evidence of a distal symmetrical sensorimotor axonopathy. Conduction slowing may be seen in severe poisoning.

TREATMENT

Initial treatment of arsenic toxicity includes supportive care, fluid repletion, decontamination if needed, and removal of the source of exposure. Hemodialysis may be required in patients who have significant renal dysfunction.

In cases of severe acute poisoning from inorganic arsenic, chelation is beneficial if it is instituted early. Dimercaprol (BAL; see Table 20-2), which is the traditional chelating agent for arsenic, is effective in decreasing morbidity and mortality if it is administered within minutes to hours of acute exposure. The oral analogue of BAL, dimercaptosuccinic acid (DMSA, succimer) is also useful for subacute or chronic arsenic poisoning. 2,3-dimercapto-1-propanesulfonic acid (DMPS) has also been used successfully but is neither approved by the Food and Drug Administration nor commercially available in the United States. In chronic inorganic arsenic intoxication, however, a clear benefit of chelation therapy has not been demonstrated.

Hemolysis caused by arsine gas poisoning should be treated with prompt exchange transfusion. Exchange transfusion can restore functional erythrocytes, remove hemoglobin pigments, remove arsenic itself, and remove toxic products formed in the arsine-hemoglobin reaction.

PROGNOSIS

Outcomes after arsenic poisoning are influenced by the dose, type of arsenic compound, and route and chronicity of exposure. Acute high-dose arsine gas inhalation with severe and rapid systemic toxicity can be fatal. With appropriate treatment, however, recovery has been reported. After acute inorganic arsenic ingestion, rapid diagnosis and treatment, including chelation, can significantly reduce mortality. After acute or chronic arsenic poisoning, electrocardiographic abnormalities and bone marrow suppression are generally reversible after exposure ceases, but encephalopathy and neuropathy may be permanent. Skin changes, such as hyperpigmentation and hyperkeratoses, can progress to cancer but also can improve with mitigation of exposure.

CADMIUM TOXICITY

EPIDEMIOLOGY

Cadmium (Cd) is primarily found in zinc ores as cadmium sulfide. Serious human exposures usually come from industrial use, including the production of nickel-cadmium batteries, electroplating, soldering, and welding. Workplace exposures occur through inhalation of dust containing oxides of cadmium or fumes from welding or smelting of metals containing cadmium.[18] Depending on the particle size, more than 50% of cadmium can be absorbed through the lungs, but little cadmium is absorbed through the gastrointestinal tract. Many plants take up cadmium from the environment, but poor oral bioavailability and relatively low food concentrations make ingestion of food an unlikely source of significant cadmium. An exception is when cadmium-containing industrial waste is dumped in agricultural regions, such as happened in Japan in the 1950s, when cadmium-containing mining waste in waterways that irrigated rice fields caused a large outbreak of osteomalacia, painful fractures, and renal disease ("itai-itai", or ouch-ouch syndrome). Today, a common source of environmental cadmium exposure is through smoking, because tobacco concentrates cadmium from the soil. Compared with nonsmokers, an average smoker has twice the concentration of total body cadmium.

PATHOBIOLOGY

Cadmium commonly exists as a divalent ion (Cd^{2+}) in salts such as cadmium sulfide and cadmium oxide. As with other divalent metals, it binds to and inhibits sulfhydryl-containing proteins and enzymes, thereby resulting in oxidative stress, cellular apoptosis, or necrosis. To survive in an environment where metals are ubiquitous, mammals have developed numerous antioxidant systems for protection. The one best studied in cadmium is the protein metallothionein, which is an intracellular, cysteine-rich protein especially found in the liver and kidney, where it is a potent protective antioxidant that binds to ionized cadmium.[19] Slow release of cadmium from the cadmium-metallothionein complex results in a long biologic half-life of over 20 years.

CLINICAL MANIFESTATIONS

The most life-threatening manifestation of cadmium toxicity is acute chemical pneumonitis (Chapters 81 and 82). In persons who are exposed to high concentrations of cadmium fumes (e.g., smelter or welders), cadmium pneumonitis is manifested like metal fume fever with fever, malaise, myalgias, and elevated white blood cell counts that develop within 12 hours of exposure. Unlike metal fume fever, which typically resolves within a few days, cadmium pneumonitis can progress, with symptoms of dyspnea, hemoptysis, pulmonary edema, and respiratory distress, as well as diffuse bilateral alveolar infiltrates on the chest radiograph.

The most problematic manifestation of chronic cadmium exposure is renal failure. As with lead, cadmium can damage the proximal tubules of the kidney and result in Fanconi syndrome (Chapter 113). Cadmium, bound to metallothionein, accumulates in the kidney; once metallothionein binding is saturated, toxicity can develop. Unlike the acute pulmonary manifestations, renal symptoms of cadmium toxicity may have a latency of decades. Clinically, the signs of renal disease from cadmium are not different from those of other causes of proximal tubular disease, with proteinuria being the most common finding. Patients will often manifest secondary symptoms of renal dysfunction, such as osteoporosis, osteomalacia, or ureteral stones owing to impaired calcium metabolism. Hypertension and anemia from cadmium exposure are also likely secondary to its renal toxicity.

DIAGNOSIS

No laboratory tests can aid in the diagnosis of cadmium pneumonitis, so physicians must rely on their clinical suspicion or on alveolar infiltrates on a chest radiograph in a cadmium-exposed worker who presents with influenza-like symptoms. Patients may present with an initially benign clinical picture and progress to respiratory failure.

Diagnosis of renal toxicity from chronic cadmium exposure relies predominantly on a 24-hour urine cadmium level standardized to grams of creatinine in a certified laboratory experienced in heavy metal testing (Table 20-1). In nonexposed nonsmokers, cadmium values should average about 0.08 μg/g creatinine. For patients with levels above 3 μg cadmium/g creatinine, a medical evaluation and renal testing are indicated. Levels at or above 7 μg cadmium/g creatinine require removal from the workplace. Urinary β_2-microglobulin levels increase as proximal tubular function worsens and can serve as a useful early marker of toxicity; levels above 300 μg/g creatinine should raise concern for early kidney disease.

TREATMENT

Because of the progression of potentially life-threatening pulmonary symptoms in cadmium pneumonitis, any patient presenting with influenza-like symptoms after working with heated cadmium should be admitted for observation. If the metal a patient was welding or cutting is not known, any clinical or radiographic signs of noncardiogenic pulmonary edema would also warrant hospital admission for supplemental oxygen and pulmonary support.

There are no effective specific treatments for acute or chronic cadmium toxicity. Chelation therapy is not recommended. Cessation of exposure is recommended but is not likely to reverse renal or pulmonary damage.

PROGNOSIS

Patients with cadmium pneumonitis can survive with aggressive supportive treatment, but severe cases can result in death, and survivors can have persistent restrictive lung disease. Because of its long half-life in the kidney, cadmium-induced renal damage is largely irreversible unless it is detected early when body burden is low (urinary cadmium < 10 μg/g creatinine).

SYNDROMES SPECIFIC TO OTHER TOXIC METALS

ALUMINUM (DIALYSIS DEMENTIA)

In the 1970s, patients who had renal failure and who were exposed to aluminum-containing phosphate binders or aluminum-contaminated dialysis fluid developed progressive neurologic impairment and seizures. Also known as dialysis dementia, this syndrome developed during weeks to years and was often fatal if undetected. Aluminum-containing phosphate binders and dialysis fluids are no longer used in patients with renal failure, and at-risk dialysis patients are screened for aluminum toxicity. As a result, this phenomenon has decreased over time,[20] but occasional outbreaks continue to be reported, typically owing to contamination of dialysis fluid with aluminum from electric pumps or drums.

Aluminum is found in air, soil, and water and is a component of metal alloys used in the home, such as cookware. Aluminum is also found in some antacids (sucralfate) and as aluminum potassium sulfate (Alum), which is used to treat hemorrhagic cystitis. Additional iatrogenic sources of aluminum include total parenteral nutrition solutions and vaccines. Ingested aluminum is not metabolized by the body and is excreted unchanged by the kidney. In patients who have impaired renal function, aluminum is bound to transferrin and concentrates primarily in bone. Smaller amounts, however, are distributed to the heart, liver, kidney, and brain. Ingested aluminum is thought to affect several biochemical functions, including neurotransmitter manufacture, uptake, and release. Aluminum also affects erythropoiesis and the normal function of bone, likely partially by interference with parathyroid function.

CLINICAL MANIFESTATIONS AND DIAGNOSIS

Clinical effects in patients with chronic exposures include anemia, osteomalacia, and neurologic effects including memory loss, tremor, dyspraxia, encephalopathy, and seizures.[21] A relationship between aluminum and Alzheimer dementia has been proposed, but the complex characteristics of aluminum bioavailability make it difficult to produce conclusive evidence.

Serum and urine aluminum levels can be obtained to estimate exposure. A serum aluminum concentration should not exceed 2 μg/L, and a 24-hour urine concentration is expected to be 4 to 12 μg per gram of creatinine in a patient with typical background aluminum exposure (Table 20-1).

TREATMENT AND PROGNOSIS

Management of aluminum toxicity centers on removal of the source of exposure. The only chelator with proven benefit is deferoxamine (Table 20-2), which has a high affinity for aluminum and forms a dialyzable aluminum-deferoxamine complex. If neurologic dysfunction is detected early, successful treatment and full recovery have been reported with deferoxamine.

BISMUTH (BISMUTH ENCEPHALOPATHY)

Bismuth salts used to treat gastrointestinal disorders include bismuth subgallate, bismuth citrate, bismuth subnitrate, and bismuth subsalicylate (the active ingredient in Pepto-Bismol). Bismuth (Bi) is poorly absorbed from the gastrointestinal tract and is still used today to treat peptic ulcer disease and diarrhea. It also is used as an oral deodorant for patients with colostomies. Idiopathic bismuth toxicity is almost always associated with the chronic ingestion of over-the-counter preparations.

CLINICAL MANIFESTATIONS AND DIAGNOSIS

Bismuth toxicity is manifested primarily as a subacute encephalopathy with ataxia and incoordination followed by progressive memory loss, behavioral changes, insomnia, and muscle cramps. As symptoms progress, a common feature is limb myoclonus when patients are startled or as they fall asleep. As symptoms worsen, myoclonus can progress to involve the entire body, including the tongue, and can occur without stimulus. Seizures can also develop.

The diagnosis of bismuth encephalopathy can be difficult. Blood and urine levels can indicate exposure to bismuth (Table 20-1) but do not correlate with symptoms. Furthermore, electroencephalographic findings, laboratory tests, and imaging studies are not specific. Because of its similarity in onset and symptoms, bismuth encephalopathy is often misdiagnosed as Creutzfeldt-Jakob disease (Chapter 371) or other progressive encephalopathies. Therefore, any patient in whom these diagnoses are being entertained should be screened for the use of bismuth products. Because bismuth causes black stools, the finding of heme-negative black stool in a patient with a rapidly progressing encephalopathy warrants an investigation for bismuth toxicity.

TREATMENT AND PROGNOSIS

The treatment of bismuth encephalopathy is to stop the use of the offending agent. Although case reports have reported benefits with metal chelators (e.g., DMSA, BAL, and 2,3-dimercapto-1-propanesulfonic acid; see Table 20-2), the rarity of the disorder makes a clinical trial impossible. Ethylenediaminetetraacetic acid (EDTA) may increase brain bismuth concentrations, so it should not be used. Although deaths have occurred from bismuth encephalopathy, full recovery is possible if the offending drug is stopped and if the patient receives modern supportive care.

COBALT (THYROID AND CARDIAC TOXICITY)

Cobalt (Co) is an essential trace element that serves as the catalytic center of vitamin B_{12}. Toxicity is associated with chronic ingestion of cobalt salts and more recently from cobalt-containing metal prostheses. One of the side effects of chronic ingestion is polycythemia (Chapter 152). By stabilizing hypoxia-inducible transcription factors that normally respond to low concentrations of oxygen, cobalt mimics hypoxia and stimulates erythropoietin production. In the 1950s, cobalt chloride was used to treat iron deficiency anemia. Some of these patients developed hypothyroidism and goiter because of cobalt's ability to inhibit tyrosine iodinase. In addition, cobalt has caused dilated cardiomyopathy with pericardial effusions in adults who consumed large amounts of beer in which cobalt salts had been added as a foam stabilizer. Cobalt can cause neurotoxicity with symptoms of hearing loss, visual impairment, and polyneuropathy.

Current concern for cobalt toxicity is predominately for patients who have cobalt-chromium prosthetic joints. Cobalt liberated from a prosthesis has been linked to hypothyroidism (Chapter 207), dilated cardiomyopathy (Chapter 47), and neurotoxicity with metal-on-ceramics arthroplasty and metal-on-metal prosthetics.

DIAGNOSIS AND TREATMENT

The diagnosis in a patient with a cobalt-containing joint replacement requires symptoms of polycythemia, hypothyroidism, cardiomyopathy, and neurotoxicity. In these patients, a blood chromium level above 7 μg/L should stimulate a referral for a possible joint revision.

There is little evidence that chelation improves outcomes in cobalt-poisoned patients.

SILVER (ARGYRIA)

Silver (Ag) is a precious metal long used in coinage and for its antibacterial properties. Silver is a broad-spectrum antimicrobial and commonly used as a topical antimicrobial in bandages, catheters, and medical devices. The ingestion of colloidal silver preparations as a "natural" supplement accounts for the majority of recent cases of significant toxicity.

When it is ingested continually, silver will be deposited in the skin and the liver.[22] The primary chronic toxicity of silver is argyria, which is a permanent blue-gray discoloration of the skin owing to silver deposition over time (Fig. 20-1). Argyria can result from inhalation, ingestion, mucosal absorption, or dermal application or exposure. Argyria may be localized to the site of exposure, such as with corneal argyria, which was seen in the past from the use of colloidal silver–containing eye drops, or at the site of silver earrings and rings. Rarely, argyria has been reported after the implantation of silver-containing medical devices.

DIAGNOSIS AND TREATMENT

The diagnosis of argyria is primarily based on history and physical examination. Localized skin biopsy, typically to differentiate argyria from malignant lesions, will show characteristic black-brown globules that are adherent to the dermal elastic fibers, blood vessels, basement membranes, hair follicles, and sweat glands on light microscopy; refractile particles on darkfield microscopy; and the presence of silver on scanning electron microscopy with energy dispersive radiography.

Chelation therapy is not effective for argyria, but successful laser treatment has been reported.[23]

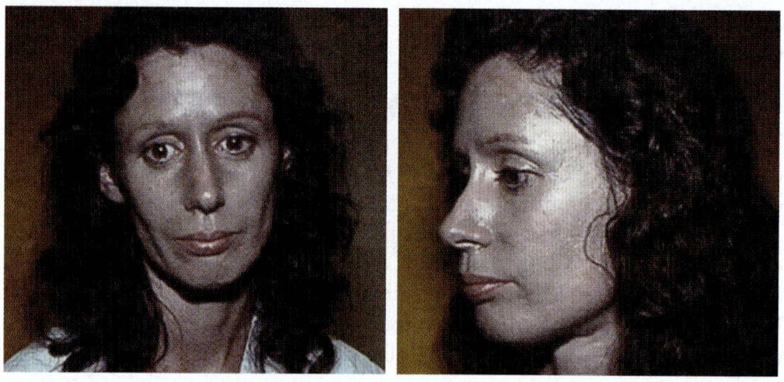

FIGURE 20-1. Frontal and side views of a 36-year-old woman with argyria show the gray discoloration of her face and neck. (From Jacobs R. "Argyria: my life story," *Clin Dermatol*. Elsevier, 2006;24:66-69. Figure 3.)

THALLIUM (NEUROPATHY AND ALOPECIA)

Thallium (Tl) has no beneficial role in the human body. Its salts are odorless, tasteless, well absorbed in the gastrointestinal tract, and very toxic. These characteristics make it a potential homicidal agent, and patients with thallium poisoning should always be considered potential victims of a crime. By interfering with potassium and sulfhydryl-containing enzymes, thallium interrupts normal energy production. Although it is toxic to all organs, the peripheral nervous system and integumentary system are the most sensitive.

The earliest clinical sign of thallium poisoning is a rapidly progressive, painful sensory polyneuropathy. Within 2 or 3 days of exposure, patients will describe painful burning paresthesias in their feet. These paresthesias can progress up the legs and, over time, can involve the hands. Motor nerves can also be affected, and profound weakness, including in respiratory muscles, can be misdiagnosed as Guillain-Barré syndrome (Chapter 388). Cranial neuropathies have also been reported. Thallium toxicity causes painless hair loss, typically beginning 5 to 14 days after exposure and sometimes progressing to total body alopecia. Skin and nails can also be affected, with scaling of palms, acne-like lesions of the face, and Mees lines in the nails. Other neurologic symptoms of thallium poisoning include hallucinations, altered mental status, insomnia, psychosis, ataxia, and coma. Constipation, myalgias, pleuritic chest pain, arrhythmias, and hypotension can also occur.

Systemic toxicities often develop before hair loss and because not all patients lose their hair, clinicians should consider thallium as a possible cause of any rapidly progressive painful neuropathy. In patients with thallium poisoning, a pulled hair will often have darkening of the hair root when visualized under a low-power light microscope.

DIAGNOSIS AND TREATMENT

The diagnosis of thallium poisoning requires the identification of elevated concentrations of thallium in a 24-hour urine sample (normal, <20 μg/specimen). Because thallium undergoes enterohepatic circulation and is eliminated in the feces, treatment requires binding of thallium in the gut. The most effective antidote is Prussian blue (a complex of potassium hexacyanoferrate), with recommended doses ranging from 3 g orally three times a day up to 250 mg/kg three times a day. Patients with thallium toxicity have received plasma exchange and continuous renal replacement therapy, but the benefit of these therapies is unknown.[24]

ZINC (MYELOPATHY)

Zinc (Zn) is an essential mineral that is necessary for normal cellular functioning. It is involved in the catalytic activity of more than 200 enzymes and plays an important role in olfaction, taste, immune function, protein synthesis, and DNA synthesis. It is found naturally in a wide variety of foods and is absorbed in the jejunum, where it binds to metallothioneins. Patients at risk for zinc deficiency include those with intestinal bypass, Crohn disease, and patients receiving total parenteral nutrition without adequate zinc supplementation. Zinc deficiency is manifested as a triad of dermatitis, diarrhea, and alopecia, which is reversible after zinc repletion.

In the setting of zinc overload, metallothioneins are upregulated; because copper has a higher affinity for metallothioneins, the result is increased copper binding and subsequent elimination of copper. Zinc-induced copper deficiency has been reported after overuse of zinc-containing supplements, with the improper use of zinc-containing denture adhesives, and from the presence of retained zinc-containing coins such as pennies.

The hematologic manifestations of zinc-induced copper deficiency include sideroblastic anemia, leukopenia, neutropenia, and myelodysplastic syndrome, all of which are reversible with zinc cessation alone. In addition, a syndrome of myeloneuropathy,[25] characterized by a spastic gait and sensory ataxia, is also associated with zinc overload/copper deficiency and may improve with copper supplementation and zinc cessation.[26]

Diagnostic testing in patients suspected of zinc overload should include serum or urine zinc concentrations (Table 20-1), serum copper levels, and ceruloplasmin levels. In patients with myeloneuropathy, nerve conduction studies may show a sensory neuropathy, and MRI may show increased T2 signal in the dorsal columns of the cervical spinal cord.

TREATMENT

Treatment of zinc overload–induced copper deficiency is primarily by cessation of zinc exposure and repletion of copper. Although there is no standard dosing regimen, a common recommendation is 2 to 8 mg/day of oral elemental copper. Various chelation regimens have been reported, but data are insufficient to support their routine use in the setting of chronic toxicity.

MANGANESE (PARKINSONISM)

Manganese (Mn) is an essential element necessary for the function of several enzymes, including superoxide dismutase and glutamine synthetase. Although there is no clear syndrome associated with manganese deficiency, a well-described constellation of symptoms and findings is associated with manganese toxicity. Dose-dependent manganese toxicity, primarily with chronic occupational exposure, results from inhalation of high concentrations of either manganese dust (e.g., in miners) or manganese fumes (e.g., smelting, grinding, and rarely welding). Toxicity has also been reported with overuse of supplements or use of illicit methcathinone synthesized with potassium permanganate.

The mechanism of neurotoxicity from manganese exposure is likely multifactorial, including neuroinflammation, dysregulation of mitochondrial function and cell signaling, oxidative stress, altered metabolism of neurotransmitters, and alterations in manganese transporters and homeostasis.[27] Manganese causes selective toxicity in the globus pallidus, striatum, and substantia nigra pars reticulata.

CLINICAL MANIFESTATIONS

The symptoms of manganism develop insidiously after years of exposure. Patients first develop changes in appetite, muscle weakness, and apathy. On occasion, patients will develop signs of central excitation and can have what is termed manganese psychosis. Symptoms often progress to difficulties with gait, speech, and facial expression.[28] The gait abnormalities involve a slow and clumsy gait with the inability to walk backward. Patients often freeze while turning and frequently fall. Symptoms can progress to muscle hypertonia in extension and a peculiar gait in which patients walk on the balls of the feet with their ankles extended. Patients also develop stuttering speech, masked facies, sleep disturbances, and myalgias. Unlike with idiopathic Parkinson disease (Chapter 378), patients with manganism do not typically develop a resting tremor or resting dementia, and their symptoms do not typically respond to levodopa therapy.[29]

DIAGNOSIS

Although there is no definitive test of manganese toxicity, a history of exposure, confirmatory laboratory testing (Table 20-1), radiographic studies, and clinical symptoms can support the diagnosis. The best laboratory test is a whole blood manganese level (normal, $<15\ \mu g/L$), with elevated levels indicative of exposure but not necessarily correlating directly with symptoms. Because manganese can concentrate in the globus pallidus, MRI often will show an intense T1-weighted signal in the globus pallidus bilaterally. However, MRI is indicative of manganese exposure but does not correlate with clinical symptoms. Because of the differences in the affected brain regions between manganese toxicity and Parkinson disease, fluorodopa positron emission tomography (PET) scanning can help differentiate between these disorders: patients with manganese toxicity will typically have normal PET scans, whereas patients with Parkinson disease have abnormal scans.

TREATMENT

Manganism is not typically responsive to treatment, but removal from exposure is important. Although chelation with $CaNa_2EDTA$ has been associated with increased urinary elimination of manganese, patient outcomes would not be expected to improve with chelation.

GENERAL REFERENCES

For the General References and other additional features, please visit Elsevier eBooks+ at https://ebooks.health.elsevier.com.

Grade A References

A1. Nussbaumer-Streit B, Mayr V, Dobrescu AI, et al. Household interventions for secondary prevention of domestic lead exposure in children. *Cochrane Database Syst Rev.* 2020;10:CD006047.

A2. Braun JM, Hornung R, Chen A, et al. Effect of residential lead-hazard interventions on childhood blood lead concentrations and neurobehavioral outcomes: a randomized clinical trial. *JAMA Pediatr.* 2018;172:934-942.

IV

AGE-SPECIFIC AND GERIATRIC MEDICINE

21

ADOLESCENT MEDICINE

DEBRA K. KATZMAN AND S. TODD CALLAHAN

Adolescence, a period of transition between childhood and adulthood, is marked by critical biologic, psychological, social, and cognitive changes. During this unique developmental period, patterns of behaviors and lifestyle choices are established that can influence current and future health, and unique medical and psychological problems can emerge. Adult-oriented health care providers play a pivotal role in engaging youth in their health and in providing health care to adolescents.

NORMAL PHYSICAL GROWTH AND DEVELOPMENT

Biologic growth and development in adolescents are signified by the onset of puberty (Chapter 217), which varies temporally among adolescents and explains why adolescents of the same chronologic age can vary greatly in physical appearance. The first visible sign of puberty among girls is usually thelarche, or the development of breast buds, which occurs on average at 10 years in White girls and 1 year earlier in African American girls (Chapter 217).

Menarche occurs 2 to 4 years after the initial appearance of breast buds and pubic hair. The average age of menarche is 12.9 years for White American girls and 12.2 years for African American girls. Menstrual periods are not always regular during the first 2 years after menarche. At menarche, only 20% of cycles are ovulatory; it may take up to another 4 years for 80% of cycles to be ovulatory. The average time for completion of puberty in girls is 4 years (range, 1.5 to 8.0 years).

Puberty begins about 1 year later in boys than in girls. The first physical signs of puberty in boys, testicular enlargement and thinning of the scrotum, occur at 10 years. Adrenarche usually begins about 6 months later (Chapter 216), and facial hair appears about 3 years after the appearance of pubic hair. The completion of puberty in boys averages 3 years (range, 2 to 5 years).

Pubertal weight gain accounts for about half of a person's ideal adult body weight. Peak weight gain follows the linear growth spurt by 3 to 6 months in adolescent girls and by about 3 months in adolescent boys. The average weight gain during puberty among adolescent girls is 15 to 55 lb or 7 to 25 kg (mean gain, 38.5 lb or 17.5 kg). Overall, adolescent boys gain 15 to 65 lb or 7 to 30 kg during puberty (mean gain, 52.2 lb or 23.7 kg).

Boys' body fat levels decrease during adolescence, dropping to 12% body fat by the end of puberty. On average, adolescent girls' lean body mass falls from 80 to 75%, whereas their average body fat levels increase from 16 to 27% by the end of adolescence. By the time adolescent girls are 16 years of age and adolescent boys are 18 years of age, they have accrued more than 90% of their adult skeletal mass.

Sexual maturity ratings (SMRs), also known as Tanner stages, are used to describe the progression of secondary sexual characteristics that occur in adolescents, irrespective of chronologic age. SMR is based on the development of breasts and the appearance of pubic hair among girls (E-Fig. 21-1) and on testicular and penile development and the appearance of pubic hair among boys (E-Fig. 21-2). SMR 1 corresponds to the prepubertal stage: puberty has not begun and no sexual development has occurred. SMR 2 to SMR 5 indicates the progression of puberty to adulthood. Once young people reach SMR 5, they have fully developed secondary sexual characteristics. Sexual maturation correlates with linear growth, changes in weight and body composition, and hormonal changes.[1] Sexual maturation provides important assurance of the normal progression of puberty or identification of abnormal pubertal development.

NORMAL PSYCHOSOCIAL DEVELOPMENT

Adolescence is often divided into three psychosocial developmental phases: early adolescence (11 to 13 years), middle adolescence (14 to 16 years), and late adolescence (17 to 21 years). In early adolescence, adolescents begin to separate from their parents and establish an individual identity. As adolescents pull away from parents in search of their own identity, their peer group begins to take on increasing salience.

At the beginning of adolescence, cognitive abilities are dominated by concrete thinking. Young adolescents lack abstract reasoning capabilities, problem-solving skills needed to overcome barriers to behavioral changes, and the ability to appreciate how current behaviors can affect future health status.

Middle adolescence is characterized by growth in emotional autonomy and increasing separation from family. The adolescents' peer groups play a powerful role, and adolescents are increasingly involved in partnering relationships that include dating, sexual experimentation, and adverse health behaviors such as smoking cigarettes, drinking alcohol, using street drugs, and being truant. Abstract reasoning skills emerge but often regress to concrete thinking when adolescents are faced with stressful situations. These adolescents begin to understand the relationship between health behaviors and future health status, but peer pressure may make it challenging for them to make appropriate health-related choices.

During late adolescence, young people become increasingly more emotionally independent. Peer group values become less important, and young people spend more time in a relationship with one person. This late stage of adolescence is characterized by the development of a strong personal identity. Abstract reasoning skills expand, and older adolescents have problem-solving skills that help them overcome challenges to behavioral change.

VITAL STATISTICS

Morbidity and mortality among 10- to 19-year-olds are often the result of risky behaviors and environmental factors (Table 21-1).[2] Unintentional injury is the leading cause of death in this age group. Malignant neoplasms, suicide, and homicide are the next three leading causes. Most deaths due to intentional injury (i.e., suicide and homicide) are theoretically preventable.

UNINTENTIONAL AND INTENTIONAL INJURIES

Unintentional injuries account for 25 to 35% of all deaths among 10- to 19-year-olds. Major causes of unintentional injuries include motor vehicle accidents, drowning, fire, poisoning, and falls. Factors that contribute to adolescent injuries include socioeconomic factors (adolescents from low-income families are at greatest risk for injury), environmental factors (hazards such as all-terrain vehicles, backyard swimming pools, firearms, kerosene heaters, and gang activity), school environment, and developmental factors.

Suicide (Chapter 362) rates have been increasing among 10- to 19-year-olds since 1999, and suicide is now the second leading cause of death among youth 10- to 14-year-olds and 15- to 19-year-olds. In both age groups, Native Americans have the highest rates, followed by White American youth; African American and Asian American youth have substantially lower rates. The rate of attempted suicide is almost five times greater among gay, lesbian, and transgender (sexual minority) students (29%) compared with heterosexual students (6.4%).[3] The estimated ratio of attempted-to-completed suicides among adolescents ranges between 50:1 and 100:1. The most common methods used in suicide attempts are drugs and alcohol, whereas suffocation, hanging, or use of firearms is associated with completed suicides. Suicide death rates caused by firearms are almost seven times higher in 15- to 19-year-old boys than in comparably aged girls.

Homicide is the third leading cause of death among 15- to 19-year-olds and the fourth leading cause among younger adolescents. Among African American males, however, it is the leading cause of death among 15- to 19-year-olds

TABLE 21-1 LEADING CAUSES OF DEATH AMONG 10- TO 19-YEAR-OLDS, U.S., 2019

AGES 10-14		AGES 15-19	
CAUSE	**NUMBER (%)**	**CAUSE**	**NUMBER (%)**
All causes	3,164 (100)	All causes	10,258 (100)
Unintentional injury	778 (24.6)	Unintentional injury	3,537 (34.5)
Suicide	534 (16.9)	Suicide	2,210 (21.5)
Malignant neoplasms	404 (12.8)	Homicide	1,877 (18.3)
Homicide	191 (6.0)	Malignant neoplasms	589 (5.7)
Congenital anomalies	189 (6.0)	Heart disease	288 (2.8)
Heart disease	87 (2.7)	Congenital anomalies	188 (1.8)
Chronic lower respiratory disease	81 (2.6)	Influenza and pneumonia	71 (0.7)
All others	900 (28.4)	All others	1,498 (14.6)

Data from the Centers for Disease Control and Prevention's Web-based Statistics Query and Reporting System (WISQARS™). Available at https://wisqars.cdc.gov/data/lcd/home. Accessed March 13, 2023.

(97% involving firearms) and the second leading cause among those 10 to 14 years old (92% firearm-related).

Approximately 1 in 8 9th- to 12th-grade students who dated or "went out with someone" report being the victim of physical or sexual dating violence in the prior 12 months.[4] For both physical and dating violence, the prevalence is higher among females than males (9 versus 7% and 13 versus 4%, respectively). Among 9th- to 12th-grade students, almost 16% report being electronically bullied and 20% report being bullied on school property. Being the victim of bullying is associated with a wide variety of mental health problems. When adolescent bullies become adults, they are more likely than their peers to become violent or abusive towards partners, spouses, and children.

OTHER DISEASES

Excluding intentional and unintentional injuries, cancer is the leading cause of death in adolescents. Cancers of major importance in adolescents include Hodgkin lymphoma (Chapter 172), germ cell tumors (Chapter 185), central nervous system tumors (Chapter 175), non-Hodgkin lymphoma (Chapter 171), thyroid cancer (Chapter 207), malignant melanoma (Chapter 188), and acute lymphoblastic leukemia (Chapter 168).

In adolescents, the course of severe acute respiratory syndrome coronavirus 2 (SARS-CoV-2) infection tends to be much milder than in adults, but severe illness, death, and long-term adverse effects can occur.[5] Vaccines against SARS-CoV-2 are at least as effective in adolescents as in young adults.[6]

APPROACH TO THE ADOLESCENT PATIENT

When interviewing adolescent patients, the clinician should consider their physical, cognitive, and psychosocial developmental stage; their growing autonomy and increasing role in taking responsibility for managing their own health and well-being; and their individual progression from childhood to adulthood. Chronologic age is not a guarantee that all adolescents will be at the same stage of development. The clinician should offer adolescent health care in a sensitive, flexible, and developmentally and culturally appropriate manner.

The clinician can meet with the adolescent alone at first to give the message that the adolescent is the patient and the clinician is most eager to hear what the adolescent has to say. This is also an opportunity to assess the adolescent's capacity for autonomous decision making. Conversely, the clinician can meet with the adolescent and their parents or guardians together for the initial part of the interview and then meet with the adolescent alone; this approach permits the clinician to develop an understanding of the reason for the visit from the perspective of the adolescent and the adolescent's parents or guardians and to communicate that input from both the adolescent and the parents or guardians is highly valued. This approach also provides an opportunity for the clinician to observe the interaction between the adolescent and parents or guardians. The final approach to the interview is to greet the adolescent and family and request a meeting with the parents or guardians alone. This approach allows the parents or guardians to discuss concerns about the adolescent that they may not feel comfortable raising in the presence of the adolescent. Having this information may improve the focus of the visit. In this approach, the encounter with the parents or guardians is then followed by the clinician's meeting with the adolescent alone. With this interview structure, it is important that the adolescent be present from the time the adolescent meets with the clinician until the end of the visit, so that the adolescent does not perceive a breach of confidentiality.

CONFIDENTIALITY

Issues of consent and confidentiality are central in the clinician-adolescent interaction. When confidentiality is guaranteed, adolescents are more likely to seek necessary medical care, to disclose sensitive information, and to trust their clinician. Under these circumstances, most adolescents will involve their parents in their care at some point. Parents appreciate education about the concept of confidentiality and recognize the importance of allowing the adolescent the opportunity to speak alone with the clinician. Confidentiality is also important for clinicians to make an accurate diagnosis and to provide treatment.

Confidentiality and defining the limits of confidentiality should be discussed with the adolescent and their parents or guardians at the beginning of the interview. The adolescent and family need to know that the clinician will intervene if the clinician believes that the adolescent's actions may cause the adolescent, or another person, significant harm or that the adolescent is in imminent danger. Examples of situations in which the clinician would not maintain confidentiality when dealing with young people include disclosure of current suicidal or homicidal intent. The legal definition of confidentiality varies, depending on geographic location, and clinicians should be familiar with local laws.

Another goal of the interview is to build rapport with the adolescent and their parents or guardians. Clinicians can establish rapport at the start of the interview by creating an environment that is nonjudgmental, unintimidating, and supportive. It is helpful to encourage the adolescent to talk about themself—friends, hobbies, school. The clinician should listen carefully to the adolescent's statements and feelings. Sensitivity to and understanding of the adolescent's developmental stage, sexual orientation, gender identity, and cultural background are important in interviewing and interpreting answers accurately. The clinician should be respectful of the adolescent's growing need to be independent and desire to be treated as an individual person. Taking the time to build rapport is key to engaging the adolescent in a discussion of their personal health concerns with the clinician.

PREVENTIVE HEALTH CARE

Preventive health care for adolescents (Chapters 12 and 15) should promote physical and mental health and healthy physical, psychological, and social growth and development. Positive behaviors such as exercise (Chapter 14) and nutritious eating (Chapter 13) should be encouraged, and health risk behaviors such as unsafe driving, high-risk sexual behaviors, and use of tobacco (Chapter 363), drugs, and alcohol (Chapter 364) should be discouraged. Because lifelong health habits are established during adolescence, it is an important time to invest in health promotion and preventive services.

The U.S. Preventive Services Task Force recommends screening and counseling of all adolescents about depression[7] and obesity and ensuring that all adolescents are up-to-date on their immunizations for tetanus, diphtheria, pertussis, varicella, measles, mumps, rubella, hepatitis A and B, meningococcus (A, C, Y, W-135), influenza, polio, and human papillomavirus (HPV; Chapter 15). In addition, at-risk adolescents should be counseled about sexually transmitted infections (e.g., human immunodeficiency virus [HIV], chlamydia, gonorrhea, and syphilis) and advised about immunizations for pneumococcus and meningococcal serotype B.

COMPONENTS OF THE ADOLESCENT CARE HEALTH VISIT

History

Open-ended, nonjudgmental, developmentally appropriate, and gender-neutral questions help put the adolescent at ease and produce informative answers (Chapter 12). In addition to a standard medical history, the assessment should include a psychosocial history from the adolescent, either through a screening questionnaire or during the interview with the adolescent alone. The HEEADSSS assessment, a valuable screening tool for obtaining a comprehensive psychosocial history, covers the following topics:

- **H**ome: family members, living arrangements, and relationships
- **E**ducation/**E**mployment: academic or vocational success and future plans
- **E**ating: concerns about weight or body image or disordered eating attitudes and behaviors; dietary intake
- **A**ctivities: recreational activities, dating, and relationships
- **D**rugs: use of tobacco or e-cigarettes, alcohol, illicit drugs, anabolic steroids, nonmedical use of prescription medications, and driving while intoxicated or after using drugs
- **S**exuality: sexual orientation, sexual behaviors (including abstinence), and sexual abuse
- **S**uicide (mental health): feelings of sadness, loneliness, depression; or suicidal ideation, attempts, and nonsuicidal self-injury
- **S**afety: risk of unintentional injury or violence, fighting; or weapon carrying; seat belts when driving motor vehicles; bicycle helmets, and sports-related protective gear.

Physical Examination

In general, the adolescent physical examination should occur without a parent or guardian present. In some situations, the adolescent is asked whether they would prefer to have a chaperone in the room during the physical examination. A male clinician should request that a female chaperone be present during the physical examination of a female patient, especially during the breast and genital examination. In theory, a female clinician should request a male chaperone be present during the genital examination of a male patient.

Care should be taken to ensure the adolescent's privacy. Providing an examination gown that covers the trunk and genital area is important. Talking with the adolescent during the examination also tends to increase comfort; explaining the procedures and commenting on the results are helpful. A comprehensive physical examination (Chapter 12) should include measuring the adolescent's weight and height, calculating their body mass index, plotting these measurements on standardized growth charts, and determining the adolescent's SMR.

Adolescent cardiovascular risk factors are associated with adult cardiovascular events.[8] However, the U.S. Preventive Services Task Force currently states that it cannot make recommendations for or against screening adolescents for high blood pressure.[9]

A thorough sexual history must be obtained to determine which anatomic sites (oral, anal, vaginal, urethral) should be screened for sexually transmitted infections. Annual screening for *Chlamydia trachomatis* and *Neisseria gonorrhoeae* is recommended for sexually active adolescents. A self-collected vaginal swab is the preferred specimen for testing women, whereas a first-catch urine specimen is preferred for men to screen for urethral infection (and is acceptable for women as well). Adolescents 13 years and older should be screened at least once for HIV infection. Screening intervals for all sexually transmitted infections should be based on the patient's sexual behaviors.

Routine cervical cancer screening is not recommended in adolescents.[10] However, screening is appropriate in young women with HIV infection, human papillomavirus infection, immune deficiency, or a prior abnormal cervical screening result. Indications for a pelvic examination in an adolescent include symptoms of vaginal or uterine infection, menstrual irregularities (e.g., amenorrhea, dysfunctional uterine bleeding, menorrhagia, and severe dysmenorrhea), undiagnosed abdominal or pelvic pain, tenderness, mass, trauma, sexual abuse, or assault.

Conclusion of the Health Visit

At the conclusion of the adolescent health visit, the clinician should review the findings with the adolescent and talk about what happens next. The adolescent should have the opportunity to ask questions, get clarification, make comments, and respond to suggestions. The clinician should discuss with the adolescent what information will remain confidential. The clinician should then meet with the adolescent and the parents or guardians (if they have accompanied the adolescent to the health visit) to review the outcomes and to discuss the nonconfidential issues.

SEXUAL AND REPRODUCTIVE HEALTH

Care related to sexual and reproductive health includes issues of adolescent sexual development, sexual orientation, sexual behaviors, gender identity (Chapter 214), pregnancy, and, if indicated, contraception. When obtaining a sexual history, it is important that clinicians avoid assumptions about a teen's gender identity, gender expression, or sexual attraction; doing so will likely preclude receiving correct information.

In the United States, the percentage of teens having sex before the age of 13 is 3.4%: 2.0% of girls and 4.8% of boys.[11] The proportion of young people who have had sexual intercourse increases as they age through adolescence: one in five 15-year-olds and two-thirds of 18-year-olds report having had sex.[12] About 40% of adolescents aged 15 to 19 years reported ever having had penile-vaginal intercourse, 45% ever having had oral sex with a different-sex partner, and 9% ever having had anal sex with a different-sex partner. Among adolescents aged 15 to 19 years who had had penile-vaginal sex, 75% of females and 48% of males reported that their first intercourse was with a steady partner.[13] About 10% of adolescents have had four or more sex partners during their lives, and over 50% of sexually active high-school students report condom use during their last sexual encounter. Nearly 12% of adolescent females between 9th and 12th grade report having been forced to have intercourse. Adolescents are more likely to report engaging in oral than in vaginal sex because they perceive oral sex as significantly less risky (fewer health, social, and emotional consequences) than vaginal sex, but adolescents who engage in oral sex also are more likely to engage in vaginal sex.

In 2019, about 170,000 babies were born to women aged 15 to 19 years in the United States. This birth rate of 16.7/1,000 women in this age group represented an historic low for the United States.[14] Even so, the United States has the highest adolescent birth rate of any developed country. Adolescent pregnancy is more common among American Indian/Alaska Native, Black, and Hispanic girls, as well as among girls from low-income families. Abortion rates in this age group have decreased by almost 50% since 1990, mostly attributable to decreased sexual activity and increased use of effective contraception.

CONTRACEPTION

The use of effective contraceptive methods is a cornerstone of preventing adolescent pregnancy. Sexually active teens require ready access to confidential care that offers effective, safe, and affordable types of birth control. The most commonly used contraceptive method in adolescents is the condom, followed by withdrawal and oral contraceptive pills.[15] Hormonal delivery systems, such as transdermal patches, vaginal rings, and long-acting reversible contraceptives, are convenient and effective (Chapter 220). Long-acting reversible contraceptive methods (intrauterine devices and contraceptive implants) are now recommended as the contraceptive method of choice for young women because of their high effectiveness. In choosing a method of contraception, dual protection against HIV and other sexually transmitted infections should be recommended. Routine counseling about and advance provision of emergency contraception is an important part of the public health strategy to reduce teen pregnancy rates (Chapter 220).

SEXUALLY TRANSMITTED INFECTIONS

Young people ages 15 to 24 account for over half (55%) of all new sexually transmitted infections in the United States (Chapter 264). In 2019, adolescents 15 to 19 years of age accounted for 25% of the reported cases of chlamydia (Chapter 294) and 15% of the cases of gonorrhea (Chapter 275) in the United States. The overall prevalence of *Chlamydia trachomatis* infections among 14- to 19-year-olds is approximately 2%, but the prevalence varies and is higher among young women than men. In adolescents, HIV infection (Chapter 353) is contracted primarily as a sexually transmitted infection, and youth 13 to 24 years of age represent over 20% of all new diagnoses of HIV infection in the United States. HPV (Chapter 344), which is the most prevalent of all sexually transmitted infections in 15- to 24-year-olds, has a prevalence of about 20% in adolescent girls 14 to 17 years of age. HIV and syphilis are of particular concern among African American and Hispanic male adolescents with same-sex partners.

Adolescents are at increased risk for acquiring sexually transmitted infections for several reasons, including elevated rates among sex partners and inconsistent or incorrect condom use. Sexual minority youth may have particular difficulty accessing appropriate sexual health services. Adolescent girls may have persistent cervical columnar epithelium that is more susceptible than squamous epithelium to infection with *Neisseria gonorrhoeae, Chlamydia trachomatis*, and HPV as well as lower levels of immunoglobulin A in their cervical mucus. For many adolescents, treatment may be delayed owing to an inability to access confidential health care services, lack of health insurance, stigma, shame, poverty, and drug use.

Chlamydial infections (Chapter 294) are overwhelmingly asymptomatic. When symptoms are present, they may be so mild or short-lived that they are easily ignored. Otherwise, clinical presentations and treatments of sexually transmitted infections (Chapter 264) in adolescents are similar to those in adults.

To maximize the likelihood of successful treatment of these infections, an observed single-dose therapy is preferred, when available. In addition, whenever possible, expedited partner therapy, which is the treatment of sexual partners without requiring a prior clinical evaluation or prevention counseling, reduces the risk of recurrent sexually transmitted infections better than standard management and should be used within 60 days wherever state law permits. Clinicians should consider the use of expedited partner therapy for partners exposed to heterosexual males and females with chlamydia or gonorrhea infections, especially when in-person evaluation and treatment are unlikely (Chapter 264).[16] For prevention, the U.S. Preventive Services Task Force recommends behavioral counseling for sexually active adolescents.[17]

OBESITY

The prevalence of obesity among adolescents between ages 16 and 19 years is 20%.[18] Obese adolescents are significantly more likely to become severely obese in adulthood. The health consequences of adolescent obesity include sleep apnea, diabetes and its complications,[19] and cardiovascular diseases. Interventions should focus on changing behavior, modifying diet,[A1] increasing physical activity, reducing screen time, assessing for obesity-related physical and mental health issues, and improving sleep patterns. Pharmacotherapy can be considered after a formal program of intensive lifestyle modifications has failed to limit weight gain or to ameliorate comorbidities.[A2] Bariatric surgery may be considered as an option for adolescents with severe obesity (Chapter 201).

MENTAL HEALTH

About 25% of female adolescents and about 10% of male adolescents in the United States have depression.[20] Approximately 75% of lifetime cases of depression[21] and anxiety (Chapter 362) start by age 24 years. The most common mental disorders in adolescents (age 13 to 18 years) in the United States by lifetime prevalence are anxiety (32%), behavior (19%), and mood disorders (14%). About 10% of adolescents have attention-deficit/hyperactivity disorder,[22] about half of whom are on medications.[23] Adolescents diagnosed with one of these mental health problems often have other comorbid disorders.

Screening for anxiety[24] and depression[25] is recommended in adolescents. Left undiagnosed or untreated, these disorders can influence development, education, social relationships, and participation in the workforce.

EATING DISORDERS

Eating disorders (Chapter 200) commonly begin during adolescence. For adolescent-onset eating disorders, early recognition and aggressive treatment are critical to a successful outcome. The medical complications of eating disorders in adolescents include faltering growth, pubertal delay, low bone mineral density, and changes in brain structure and cognitive function. These complications, which occur early in the disease process, may not be completely reversible.

The goals of treatment are to restore physical health, normal eating behavior patterns, and mental health and to reduce the impact of the eating disorder on the quality of life. Adolescents should be treated at a facility where the health professionals understand eating disorders and have experience in treating adolescents. Successful management strategies for adolescents with eating disorders include early restoration of a normal nutritional and physiologic state, involvement of the family in the treatment, and incorporation of an interdisciplinary team in the treatment. Family-based therapy is an effective first-line, outpatient treatment for adolescents with eating disorders and helps protect against relapse.

SUBSTANCE USE AND SUBSTANCE USE DISORDERS

Nearly half of adolescents try an illicit drug (Chapter 365) by the time they finish high school. Just over 60% of adolescents consume alcohol (Chapter 364) by the end of high school, and about 40% report having been drunk at least once in their life. Adolescents who begin using alcohol or drugs before 15 years of age are more than five times more likely to develop an addiction later in life compared with those who first use alcohol at 21 years of age.

Nearly 30% of 12th-grade students report vaping in the last 30 days, with 25% vaping nicotine and 12% vaping marijuana. About 25% of U.S. adolescents have used marijuana in the past year, a percentage that has remained relatively stable over the last decade with an increasing proportion using e-cigarettes or vaping systems as the delivery device. Similarly, adolescents are now more likely to use e-cigarettes than to smoke conventional cigarettes (Chapter 363); however, those who use e-cigarettes are more likely than nonusers to initiate conventional cigarette use as well.[26] In 2004, almost 10% of 12th-graders reported nonmedical use of prescription opioids (Chapter 365), but that number dropped to 2% in 2020.[27]

Adolescent drug use is the result of a complex interaction among genetic, social, environmental, and personal risk factors. Boys tend to initiate drug and alcohol use at younger ages than girls do, but once girls begin to experiment, they are just as likely as boys to use drugs. Boys are more likely to consume marijuana, steroids, and smokeless tobacco, whereas girls are more likely to use amphetamines and methamphetamine.

Adolescents with poor self-esteem and low motivation, as well as those without an attachment to school and/or with poor academic achievement, have a greater propensity for alcohol and drug use compared with those without these characteristics. Adolescents with a family history of alcohol or other drug use are also at greater risk. Adolescents are less likely to succumb to external pressures toward drug use if they have a strong sense of attachment to parents who clearly communicate their disapproval of drug use.

Signs and symptoms suggestive of substance use or substance use disorders include changes in physical appearance, poor hygiene or dress, wearing long-sleeved shirts to hide scarring at injection sites, persistent cough or bronchitis, difficulty sleeping, sudden weight loss or weight gain, sudden changes in personality, aggressive behavior, irritability, nervousness, giddiness, changes in peer group, increased isolation from peers or family, depression, loss of interest in once-favorite activities, decline in performance or attendance at school or work, forgetfulness, increased secretiveness, money or objects disappearing from the household, and prescription drugs that seem to be used up too quickly.

A validated screening tool for alcohol and substance use (Table 21-2) should be used in adolescents.[28] Those answering yes to one question should receive feedback regarding the adverse effects of substance use. Those who answer yes to two or more questions are at high risk for substance use problems and require further assessment or referral (Chapters 364 and 365).[A3] Urine drug testing has low sensitivity for detection of drug use, and there is no consensus about its role for screening of adolescents.

Alcohol and drug use contributes to more than 40% of adolescent deaths from motor vehicle crashes, to suicide attempts, and to an increased risk for subsequent use and dependence and related problems in adulthood. Historically, treatment for substance use disorders in adolescents and young adults has been based on abstinence. More recently, however, a harm-reduction approach has gained acceptance. Adolescents discontinue drug and alcohol use mainly because of concern about their negative effects, and community-based interventions can be effective. Individual interventions appear to have a larger effect size than family-based interventions[A4] in reducing alcohol abuse, with the effect size decreasing over time.

TABLE 21-2 CRAFFT SCREENING TOOL FOR DRUG AND ALCOHOL USE IN ADOLESCENTS

The adolescent is instructed, "Please answer these next questions honestly. Your answers will be kept confidential. During the past 12 months, did you . . ."
- Drink any alcohol (more than a few sips)?
- Smoke any marijuana or hashish?
- Use anything else to get high?

If the adolescent answers no to the three opening questions, the provider only needs to ask the adolescent the first question—the CAR question. If the adolescent answers yes to any one or more of the three opening questions, the provider asks all six CRAFFT questions.
- **C**—Have you ever ridden in a CAR driven by someone (including yourself) who was "high" or had been using alcohol or drugs?
- **R**—Do you ever use alcohol or drugs to RELAX, feel better about yourself, or fit in?
- **A**—Do you ever use alcohol/drugs while you are by yourself, ALONE?
- **F**—Do you ever FORGET things you did while using alcohol or drugs?
- **F**—Do your family or FRIENDS ever tell you that you should cut down on your drinking or drug use?
- **T**—Have you gotten into TROUBLE while you were using alcohol or drugs?

CRAFFT is a mnemonic acronym of the first letters of key words in the six screening questions. The questions should be asked exactly as written.

CHRONIC ILLNESS AND TRANSITION

The prevalence of chronic diseases in adolescents has increased significantly because advances in medical technology and treatments have increased the survival of young people with childhood diseases formerly considered lethal. About 18% of adolescents in the United States live with a chronic illness. Chronic illness may affect the adolescent's development, or the adolescent's development may affect the illness. For example, cystic fibrosis (Chapter 77) may delay puberty and hinder normal peer development. Puberty can exacerbate diabetes mellitus (Chapter 210). Increased risk-taking by adolescents with diabetes, asthma, or chronic renal failure can hinder their compliance with their medication regimen.

Adolescents in general, and those with special health care needs in particular, require a smooth, seamless, coordinated, and developmentally appropriate transition to support their engagement in the adult health care system.[29] The patient, family, and pediatric and adult health care systems should view the transition as a natural part of the developmental process of care for all adolescents. The recommended elements of a transition plan include early individualized planning and preparation of patient, family, and health care teams; tailored written transition plans; coordination by both the transferring and receiving physicians; introductory meetings for young adults with their new providers before transfer; transfer at a time of disease stability rather than during a period of instability; and the introduction of transition coordinators who act as liaisons between the pediatric and adult health care system.

GENERAL REFERENCES

For the General References and other additional features, please visit Elsevier eBooks+ at https://ebooks.health.elsevier.com.

Grade A References

A1. Boff RM, Liboni RPA, Batista IPA, et al. Weight loss interventions for overweight and obese adolescents: a systematic review. *Eat Weight Disord.* 2017;22:211-229.

A2. Weghuber D, Barrett T, Barrientos-Pérez M, et al. Once-weekly semaglutide in adolescents with obesity. *N Engl J Med.* 2022;387:2245-2257.

A3. U.S. Preventative Services Task Force. Screening and behavioral counseling interventions to reduce unhealthy alcohol use in adolescents and adults: updated evidence report and systematic review for the U.S. Preventive Services Task Force. *JAMA.* 2018;320:1910-1928.

A4. Tanner-Smith EE, Lipsey MW. Brief alcohol interventions for adolescents and young adults: a systematic review and meta-analysis. *J Subst Abuse Treat.* 2015;51:1-18.

22

EPIDEMIOLOGY OF AGING

LOUISE ARONSON

DEMOGRAPHY

For decades, the world's population has aged at an unprecedented rate. Both proportions and absolute numbers of people living into old age have increased. As of 2020, 1 billion people were age 60 years or older, and by 2050 people over age 65 years are projected to account for 1 in 6 people worldwide. Between 1990 and 2019, people over age 80 nearly tripled, a number expected to triple again by 2050, thereby reaching 426 million. As a result of these marked shifts, the World Health Organization declared 2020 to 2030 the Decade of Healthy Ageing, and the United Nations has recognized aging as one of four global population "mega-trends."[1]

In 2021 in the United States, people ages 65 years and older accounted for 16% of the population, and people over age 80 years comprised 4% of the population, with those numbers expected to double and triple, respectively, by 2050.[2] So-called baby boomers (i.e., people born between 1946 and 1964 and one of the largest generations in American history) play a key role in shaping national demographic trends. By the 2030s, when all baby boomers are over age 65 years, older Americans will constitute 21% of the population, and the country will have more elderly people than children. Since millennials (people born between 1981 and 1995) outnumber baby boomers, these trends are projected to continue for generations.

Three demographic factors within this larger transformation have important implications for health. First, marked inequalities in life expectancies persist across ethnic and racial groups (Chapter 4), among sexual minorities, and in geographic location within the United States.[3] Second, a somewhat smaller but still significant gender gap exists in longevity. In 2019, for example, average life expectancy at age 65 years was 18.2 years for males and 20.8 years for females. Third, the longevity curve has flattened since 2010 as a result of a leveling of the decline in mortality from cardiovascular disease (Chapter 40) despite increases in deaths from drug overdose (Chapter 365), suicide (Chapter 362), obesity (Chapter 201), and Alzheimer disease (Chapter 371), as well as the emergence of severe acute respiratory syndrome coronavirus 2 (SARS-CoV-2; Chapter 336).[4] Improvements in life expectancy will therefore require attention to social determinants of health across the life span.

DISEASE AND DISABILITY IN OLDER ADULTS

MORBIDITY AND MULTIMORBIDITY

Over 85% of older adults have one or more chronic health conditions (Table 22-1), the most common of which are hypertension (Chapter 64), hyperlipidemia (Chapter 190), arthritis (Chapter 236), heart disease (Chapter 40), and diabetes (Chapter 210). The prevalence of individual diseases varies by sex, race, and ethnicity. For example, more older Black adults than White adults report hypertension (about 70% vs. about 55%), and more women have arthritis than men (about 60% vs. about 45%). Nevertheless, over 82% of adults ages 65 to 74 years and 73% of adults ages 75 years and older describe their overall health as good to excellent. Self-reported health worsens not only with advanced age but also by race; 12 to 14% of Native, Black, and Latino Americans report fair to poor health compared with just over 8% of White or Asian Americans. Over age 70 years, nearly 14% of Americans have dementia (Chapter 371) and a majority have sensory impairments, including problems with balance (75%), hearing (26%), and vision (15%). The lifetime risk of dementia increases with age, is higher in women than in men (for reasons that include greater longevity as well as hormonal and environmental factors), and is nearly two times higher in Black adults than White adults.

Multimorbidity, which is the state of having multiple comorbid conditions, is the norm with advancing age. About 65% of adults over age 65 years have two or more chronic health conditions, nearly a quarter have four or more such conditions, and the prevalence of multiple chronic conditions is increasing. After adjustment for other factors, Black adults have earliest onset and highest prevalence of multimorbidity, whereas Latino adults develop multimorbidity most rapidly with aging. Quality care of older adults requires consideration of sociodemographic risk, the impact of the treatment of one condition on others, the masking of diseases by symptoms of other diseases, and burden of the treatment.

The degree of multimorbidity predicts future disability. The proportion of older adults with self-reported difficulty in activities of daily living increases stepwise as their number of medical conditions increases. Multimorbidity is also associated with poorer lower extremity strength and balance, which are predictors of disability, and slower gait speed, which is a powerful predictor of mortality in old age. Multiple chronic diseases have more than an additive effect on physical functioning and hence disability.

GERIATRIC SYNDROMES

Geriatric syndromes (Chapter 24), which are common and highly morbid conditions in older adults, are not linked to a single disease or pathologic process but rather occur when accumulated impairments across multiple domains result in a single, recognizable phenomenon. For example, falls (Chapter 24) occur in people with a wide range of risk factors: poor vision, foot problems, cognitive impairment, disorders of gait and balance, fear of falling, sarcopenia, neurologic diseases, polypharmacy, and medications that can cause orthostatic hypotension. Other geriatric syndromes include urinary incontinence (Chapter 115), frailty (Chapter 24), impaired sleep (Chapter 374), delirium (Chapter 361), pressure ulcers (Chapter 24), cognitive impairment (Chapter 371), and malnutrition (Chapter 197). Geriatric syndromes adversely affect health outcomes and may be caused or exacerbated by medical treatments.

SUBCLINICAL DISEASE

The risks of disability and mortality among older adults are elevated by asymptomatic or unrecognized disease. Nonspecific symptoms may be inaccurately attributed to aging or a comorbid condition. For example, magnetic resonance imaging reveals subclinical vascular changes consistent with a prior stroke in about one third of older adults without a history of stroke. Although subclinical cardiovascular disease doubles the risk of falls, frailty, dementia, and death, when and how to intervene to prevent these outcomes remains unclear. Noninvasive testing also yields higher rates of conditions such as hypothyroidism (Chapter 207), peripheral arterial disease (Chapter 65), chronic obstructive pulmonary disease (Chapter 76), and osteoarthritis (Chapter 241) than are documented clinically, perhaps in part because other limitations mask their subclinical impact.

OBESITY

Obesity (Chapter 201) is a major cause of preventable life-years lost, and its impact on morbidity (e.g., physical limitations, diabetes) and mortality (e.g., cardiovascular disease, cancer) increases with age. Over age 60 years, about one third of White adults, 40% of Latino adults, and 50% of Black adults are obese. Obesity disproportionately affects older women, especially Black women and low-income women, in whom it increases the risk of disability, low quality of life, nursing home placement, and death. However, the prevalence of obesity declines after age 75 years, in part because of selective survivorship and in part because of the increasing prevalence of serious comorbid diseases that result from the pro-inflammatory state of obesity.

TABLE 22-1 U.S. ADULTS WITH CHRONIC CONDITIONS, MULTIMORBIDITY, 2018

	NO CHRONIC CONDITIONS		*1 CHRONIC CONDITION*		*≥2 CHRONIC CONDITIONS*	
AGE	**% POPULATION**	**N**	**% POPULATION**	**N**	**% POPULATION**	**N**
18 to 44 years	73%	83,444	21%	23,841	7%	7,723
45 to 64 years	37%	30,404	30%	25,250	33%	27,383
≥65 years	12%	6,382	24%	12,280	64%	32,748

Source: National Center for Chronic Disease Prevention and Health Promotion. https://www.cdc.gov/pcd/issues/2020/20_0130.htm.

DISABILITY

Disability in older adults can be slowly progressive and chronic (e.g., arthritis), subacute and potentially reversible (e.g., post-hospitalization), or sudden and catastrophic (e.g., after a stroke). Levels of disability range from challenges in work, social, or recreational activities, thereby requiring adaptation or substitution, to an inability to be independent in household tasks, to the loss of basic self-care capabilities and the need for long-term personal care (see Chapter 23).

Fortunately, most older adults are not disabled. Although some degree of loss in physical function with advancing age is inevitable, the effects of age are highly variable, both between and within individuals. For example, self-reported physical limitations are about 6.5% through age 45 years, but they increase to 17% between ages 46 to 64 years, to 27% at age 65 years, and to 45% at age 75 years and beyond. After age 65 years, the prevalence of physical disability is higher among women in each age subgroup, as well as in American Indians, Alaska Natives, Latinos, people below the federal poverty level, and people living in the South U.S. Census region. Between the ages of 65 to 74 years, just 4% of Americans need personal care, but that number rises to 21% in Americans over age 85 years.

Noncatastrophic disability has a preclinical phase, during which people limit or modify their function but are not yet disabled. The onset of disability occurs with frequent transitions between independent and dependent states, thereby often offering multiple opportunities for intervention.[5] Major disabling conditions include arthritis, cardiovascular disease, chronic back pain, and dementia. However, joint and cardiac disease do not always cause limitations in the elderly, whereas sensory impairment and falls have substantial impact on disability.

FRAILTY

Frailty (Chapter 24) is defined as an age-related syndrome of decreased physiologic reserve, increased vulnerability to stress, and adverse health outcomes. Its phenotype has been described as including at least three of the following: weakness, fatigue, low activity, slow movement, and weight loss.[6] Frailty is also characterized by poor physical function, accumulation of physical deficits, and the cumulative burden of disease. Loss of muscle mass, which is termed sarcopenia, is also a key component of frailty.[7] Experimental data suggest that sestrins, which are stress-induced regulators that affect cell metabolism, may be critical for maintaining muscle mass and strength.

The prevalence of frailty, which increases with age, is under 5% below age 70 years but rises steeply thereafter to over 30% above age 80 years. In all older age groups, frailty is more common in women than men, and it is more prevalent in populations with high rates of chronic disease and socio-demographic disadvantage.[8] Importantly, frailty is not a steady state; both progression and reversion are common, although it eventually usually becomes a pre-death condition.

In clinical settings, frailty can be assessed using a validated instrument (see Table 24-1). Weakness can be assessed in an office setting by measuring grip strength (<30 kg in men and <20 kg in women). Although frailty itself is a risk factor for poorer outcomes and high health care costs, it also is associated with falls, fractures, cognitive decline, depression, low quality of life, loneliness, disability, nursing home admission, and hospitalization.

MORTALITY

Mortality rises with age. U.S. death rates are 1.7% per year between the ages of 65 to 74 years, increasing to 4.3% per year between the ages of 75 to 84 years, and to 13.2% per year in Americans age 85 years and older.[9] Before the coronavirus-2019 (COVID-19) pandemic, the top five causes of death for Americans ages 65 and older were cardiovascular disease (37%), cancer (about 27%), chronic lower respiratory disease (about 8%), cerebrovascular disease (about 8%), and Alzheimer disease (about 8%). Since 1980, cardiovascular disease and cancer have remained the top causes of death, whereas death rates for Alzheimer disease, diabetes, and unintentional injuries have increased (Table 22-1). Cancer was the leading cause of death and diabetes the fifth most common among the young-old ages 65 to 74 years, whereas Alzheimer disease and stroke are more common in the old-old ages 85 years and older. In 2020, however, COVID-19 became the third leading cause of death among all older age subgroups (Fig. 22-1),[10] and especially in frail elderly.[11]

HEALTHY AGING

LONGEVITY AND HEALTHY AGING

About 15 to 25% of longevity is estimated to be heritable. Other key determinants include a mother's health during pregnancy, lifetime exposures to infectious diseases and environmental hazards, psychosocial stress, nutrition (Chapter 13), physical activity (Chapter 14), and avoidance of smoking

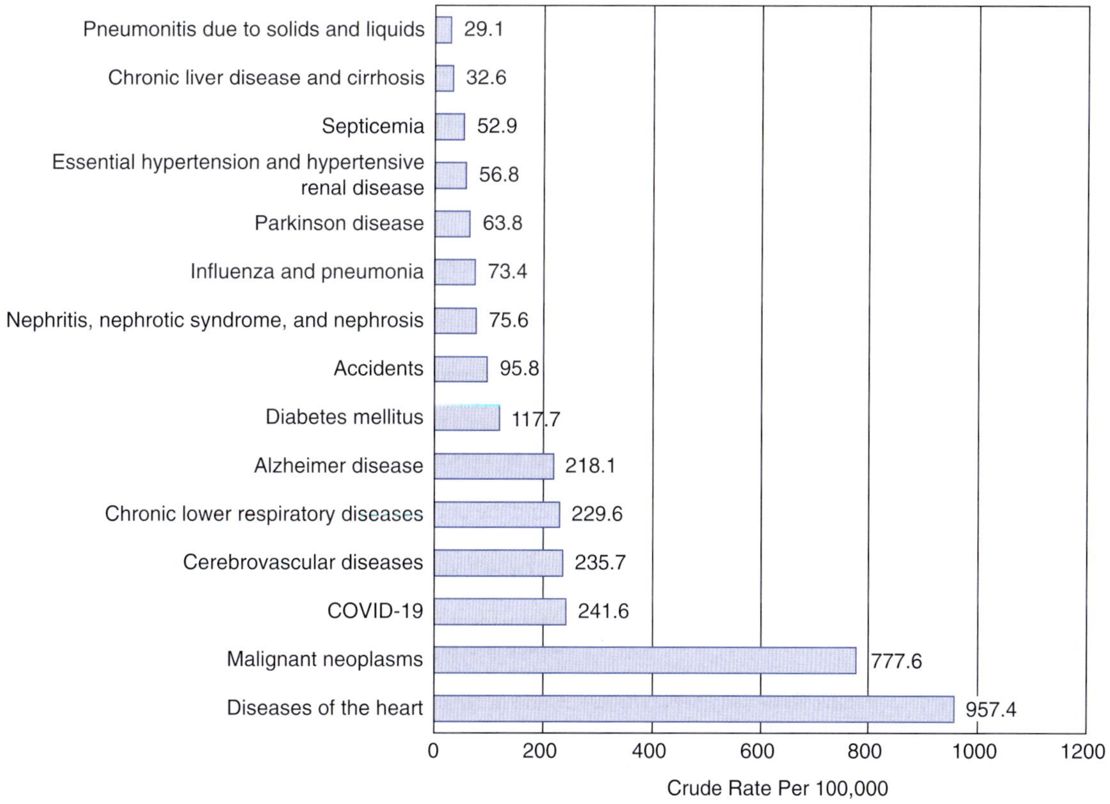

FIGURE 22-1. Underlying causes of death in Americans over age 65 years. (Centers for Disease Control and Prevention, National Center for Health Statistics. Provisional Multiple Cause of Death on CDC WONDER Online Database, released 2021. Data are from the final Multiple Cause of Death Files, 2018-2019, and from provisional data for years 2020-2021, as compiled from data provided by the 57 vital statistics jurisdictions through the Vital Statistics Cooperative Program. Accessed at http://wonder.cdc.gov/mcd-icd10-provisional.html on Dec 20, 2021 2:16:53 PM.)

TABLE 22-2 LIFE EXPECTANCY AND HEALTH EXPECTANCY AT AGE 60 BY GENDER AND GEOGRAPHY

	LIFE EXPECTANCY (IN YEARS)		*HEALTH LIFE EXPECTANCY (IN YEARS)*	
REGION	**MALE**	**FEMALE**	**MALE**	**FEMALE**
Global	**18.3**	**21.0**	**14.1**	**16.1**
Africa	16.0	17.6	12.1	13.3
Americas	19.8	22.9	15.5	17.7
Eastern Mediterranean	18.0	19.7	13.4	14.4
Europe	19.7	23.6	15.5	18.3
Southwest Asia	17.7	20.1	13.2	14.8
Western Pacific	18.5	21.6	14.4	16.6

Source: World Health Organization and United States Census Bureau. https://www.census.gov/library/stories/2021/05/long-life-does-not-always-mean-a-healthy-life-in-old-age.html.

(Chapter 363) and drugs of abuse (Chapter 365). Primary molecular pathways involved in aging include insulin and insulin growth factor-1, sirtuins, mechanistic target of rapamycin (mTOR), and AMP-activating protein kinase (AMPK). Each of these mechanisms affects autophagy, the catabolic process that enables cells to recycle dysfunctional material and maintain energy homeostasis. Metabolism, proteostasis, inflammation, epigenetics, macromolecular damage, and stem cells are among the critical, interrelated factors affecting healthy aging.

Emerging geroscience suggests the possibility that biological rate of aging may be slowed by nutritional, behavioral, genetic, and pharmacological interventions. Senolytics are compounds, such as flavonoids, that are being evaluated as potential supplements to slow the progression of aging.[12] Although many hormone levels decline with aging, hormone replacement with estrogen (Chapter 222), growth hormone (Chapter 205), testosterone (Chapter 216), and adrenal androgens (Chapter 208) have not been proven beneficial for longevity and have known harms.

Critical to consideration of longevity is the concept of "health span," defined by the World Health Organization as the average number of years lived in full health. Worldwide, life expectancy at age 60 years is 18.3 years in men and 21 years in women, but health life expectancy is only about 14 years in men and 16 years in women (Table 22-2).

Between 1991 and 2018, the health span of older Americans increased, with fewer elderly individuals reporting fair or poor health. Despite these overall gains, however, considerable disparities persist based on economic status, with fair or poor health reported by 21% of Americans age 65 years and older below the poverty level compared with just 4% of Americans in that age range with incomes at 400% of the poverty level or higher.

PREVENTION

Intensive blood pressure control to systolic blood pressure to less than 130 mm Hg lowers cardiovascular events in adults ages 60 to 80 years.[A1] Statins effectively reduce cardiovascular and all-cause mortality when used for primary prevention, even in individuals up to at least age 75 years.[A2] In healthy elderly, low-dose aspirin not only does not improve disability-free survival but also actually increases all-cause mortality.[A3] Antiresorptive and anabolic agents can slow the progression of osteoporosis and reduce the risk of fractures in women.[A4] Multifactorial interventions to prevent falls, fractures, and serious fall injuries do not appear to be helpful as currently designed.[A5,A6] Exercise reduces functional decline in community-dwelling elderly persons.[A7] Tai Chi continues to be the most effective exercise for preventing falls in community-dwelling older adults, whereas resistance training is useful to reduce the risk of disability.[A8] Biobehavioral approaches can decrease disability in low-income elders.[A9] Hearing aids significantly improve hearing-related function, but their long-term benefit to prevent disability or dementia is not yet known.[A10]

GENERAL REFERENCES

For the General References and other additional features, please visit Elsevier eBooks+ at https://ebooks.health.elsevier.com.

Grade A References

A1. Zhang W, Zhang S, Deng Y, et al. Trial of intensive blood-pressure control in older patients with hypertension. *N Engl J Med*. 2021;385:1268-1279.

A2. Gencer B, Marston NA, Im K, et al. Efficacy and safety of lowering LDL cholesterol in older patients: a systematic review and meta-analysis of randomised controlled trials. *Lancet*. 2020;396:1637-1643.

A3. McNeil JJ, Woods RL, Nelson MR, et al. Effect of aspirin on disability-free survival in the healthy elderly. *N Engl J Med*. 2018;379:1499-1508.

A4. Wang QY, Ding N, Dong YH, et al. Pharmacological treatment of osteoporosis in elderly people: a systematic review and meta-analysis. *Gerontology*. 2021;67:639-649.

A5. Lamb SE, Bruce J, Hossain A, et al. Screening and intervention to prevent falls and fractures in older people. *N Engl J Med*. 2020;383:1848-1859.

A6. Bhasin S, Gill TM, Reuben DB, et al. A randomized trial of a multifactorial strategy to prevent serious fall injuries. *N Engl J Med*. 2020;383:129-140.

A7. Li P-S, Hsieh C-J, Tallutondok EB, Peng H-J. The dose-response efficacy of physical training on frailty status and physical performance in community-dwelling elderly: a systematic review and meta-analysis of randomized controlled trials. *Healthcare (Basel)*. 2022;10:586.

A8. Li F, Harmer P, Fitzgerald K, et al. Effectiveness of a therapeutic tai ji quan intervention vs a multimodal exercise intervention to prevent falls among older adults at high risk of falling: a randomized clinical trial. *JAMA Intern Med*. 2018;178:1301-1310.

A9. Szanton SL, Leff B, Li Q, et al. CAPABLE program improves disability in multiple randomized trials. *J Am Geriatr Soc*. 2021;69:3631-3640.

A10. Feltner C, Wallace IF, Kistler CE, et al. Screening for hearing loss in older adults: updated evidence report and systematic review for the US Preventive Services Task Force. *JAMA*. 2021;325:1202-1215.

23 GERIATRIC ASSESSMENT

C. SETH LANDEFELD

The goal of geriatric assessment is to improve quality of life, independence, and longevity by identifying conditions that may be ameliorated and by informing patients' decisions. Geriatric assessment evaluates specific domains that are often impaired in older people and that reduce quality of life, ability to live independently, and life expectancy; and the personal and social context of the older person.

RATIONALE

The premise of geriatric assessment is that older individuals desire "life, liberty, and the pursuit of happiness." Fulfillment of these desires depends on the older person's abilities, their environment, and the person-environment fit, all of which should be assessed and managed to achieve the older person's goals.

Geriatric assessment and management by a clinician or multidisciplinary team identifies conditions that are often undetected but can be ameliorated; they also provide information about prognosis, patients' values, and preferences.[1] Geriatric assessment improves outcomes in hospitalized older adults and in older adults with advanced cancer, and possibly in others.[A1–A5]

FUNCTION

Decline in the function of every organ system occurs at a rate of about 1% per year after age 30 years. Geriatric assessment evaluates functions that directly affect how older people live in the world each day. These functions generally depend on the central or peripheral nervous system, although they can be affected by dysfunction in other organ systems.

INITIAL OBSERVATION

Geriatric assessment begins with observation of the patient and companions, looking for signs of geriatric syndromes such as dementia (Chapter 371), depression (Chapter 362), impaired mobility (Chapter 24), or elder abuse. Is the patient alone or accompanied? Bright or dulled? Well groomed? Conversant? At ease with a companion? Does the patient stand briskly and without assistance? Is the gait normal?

FUNCTIONAL STATUS

Functional status refers to the ability of an individual to perform activities that are needed to fulfill social and community roles. These activities, which are acquired during childhood, are often lost in reverse order with progressive failure of the brain or another organ. For example, children learn first to feed themselves, later to dress, and later to work, whereas a person with dementia may first lose the ability to work, later to dress, and later to feed.

Activities of daily living (ADLs) are performed daily: feeding, maintaining continence, toileting, transferring, bathing, grooming, and dressing. People with an impairment, such as difficulty standing, may maintain independence in ADLs by using an appliance, such as a raised toilet seat and support stand. ADL dependency—needing the help of another person to perform an activity—can be caused by an acute illness but often results from a neurologic condition such as neurodegenerative disease or stroke.

Instrumental ADLs are performed to live at home: preparing meals, housework, laundry, shopping, driving or using public transportation, using the telephone, and handling medications and finances. Dependency in instrumental ADLs can be caused by physical limitations from chronic disease or by dementia (Chapter 371), and it is often an early sign of undiagnosed dementia. Dependency in instrumental ADLs often can be ameliorated by a variety of public and private services (e.g., taxis or rideshare, laundry and cleaning services, and Meals on Wheels).

Dependency in ADLs and instrumental ADLs are present in about 10% and 20%, respectively, of people ages 75 years or older living in the community and are very frequent in hospitalized elders. These dependencies are strong predictors of long-term institutionalization and death.

Advanced ADLs are the ability to fulfill societal, community, and family roles. They can be assessed by asking the person whether they perform an activity, such as playing a musical instrument, or performed it previously. Loss of advanced ADLs may indicate mild cognitive impairment, dementia, or physical limitations.

COGNITION AND COMPETENCY

Mild cognitive impairment does not interfere with independent ADLs. By comparison, dementia (Chapter 371), which is cognitive decline in one or more domains not explained by delirium (Chapter 361) or another mental disorder (Chapter 362, interferes with independence in instrumental ADLs.

The incidence of dementia increases from less than 1% per year at age 65 years to 5% per year at age 85 years. Treating hypertension with a target of 120 mm Hg systolic (Chapter 64) is the only intervention demonstrated to reduce the incidence of dementia and mild cognitive impairment.

Although screening for cognitive impairment is not recommended, detection can lead to identification of treatable conditions (e.g., medication side effects, depression, or hearing impairment). Symptoms of cognitive decline, such as forgetfulness, disorientation, and changes in personality, require cog nitive testing. Disorientation to year is about 85% sensitive and 95% specific for cognitive impairment. The Mini-Cog test (Table 361-5), also has high sensitivity and specificity.

Decision-making capacity is specific to each decision. Patients are competent when they can do all of the following:

- Make and express personal preferences.
- Comprehend the risks and benefits of the intervention.
- Comprehend the implications of the decision.
- Give rational reasons for the decision.

If the patient is not competent, the decision should be made by a surrogate or, if a surrogate is not available, by the physician, as specified by state law (Chapter 2).

MOOD AND AFFECT

Universal screening is recommended to assess mood and affect.[2] A positive answer to either of these two questions has a 95% sensitivity and 65% specificity for a major depressive disorder:

1. During the past month, have you often been bothered by feeling down, depressed, or hopeless?
2. During the past month, have you often been bothered by little interest or pleasure in doing things?

All patients should be screened once and also after major life events, such as retirement or a serious illness, and whenever the clinician senses sadness or aversion on seeing a patient.

VISION

Impaired visual acuity is associated with worse functional status, worse quality of life, falls, depression, and social isolation. The prevalence of impaired visual acuity with refractive correction increases from 1% at age 65 years to nearly 20% in persons aged 80 years or older.

Although screening has not been recommended for older adults,[A6] it is useful for the clinician to ask a simple question: whether the patient has difficulty driving, watching television or reading, or doing any of their daily activities because of their eyesight, even while wearing eyeglasses. Impaired visual acuity is determined using the Snellen eye chart (E-Fig. 391-1) as worse than 20/40; 20/200 is the legal threshold for blindness.

HEARING

Hearing loss (Chapter 396) is common, often unrecognized and untreated, and associated with social isolation, functional decline, depressive symptoms, and cognitive impairment. Presbycusis initially affects high frequencies and often-associated central auditory processing disorders can further decrease the ability to understand words over background noise. Routine screening for hearing loss is not recommended,[3] but hearing tests are warranted when the patient, the caregiver, or the physician visit reveals a potential loss of hearing because amplification with a hearing aid, cochlear implant, or assisted listening device can be very helpful.[4]

To detect hearing loss, the clinician can ask, "Do you feel you have hearing loss or have any difficulty hearing?" The whisper test has high sensitivity and specificity: the clinician stands 2 feet behind the patient, occludes one ear, rubs the tragus, whispers a combination of 6 numbers and letters, and then asks the patient to repeat the sequence. The whisper test is positive if fewer than 3 numbers and letters are repeated correctly. Hearing loss also can be detected by a handheld otoscope with a built-in audiometer and by tests on personal computers and smartphones.

When hearing loss is detected, the patient's companion can be asked about its severity and effects on functioning. When hearing is diminished, it is important to examine the ear. If substantial cerumen is found, it must be removed, sometimes by a specialist, and then the hearing evaluation can be performed again.

NUTRITION

The patient should be asked whether a change in weight has occurred over the last year and whether any change was intentional. Weight should be measured and the body mass index (BMI) calculated in kg/m^2 (Chapter 201): BMI of less than 18.5 is underweight, 18.5 to 24.9 is normal, 25 to 29.9 is overweight, 30 to 39.9 is obese, and 40.0+ is severely obese.

Obesity (Chapter 201) affects more than 40% of older Americans and is associated with poorer function and mobility, many chronic diseases, and decreased life expectancy. Obesity and its adverse effects are ameliorated by intensive, multicomponent interventions that may include bariatric surgery.

Unintentional weight loss (Chapter 118) of 5% or more is associated with increased mortality and should prompt evaluation for an underlying cause of malnutrition (Chapter 198), including depression, dementia, dental disease, cancer, malabsorption, poverty, and neglect. Protein and energy supplementation (Chapter 198) increase survival in hospitalized patients who are undernourished on admission. Screening for deficiency of vitamin D or B_{12} is not recommended because of insufficient evidence.[5]

MOBILITY AND LIFE SPACE

Mobility without the assistance of another person depends on the environment and assistive devices. For example, a person may walk the aisles of a grocery store with a shopping cart but be unable to walk across a parking lot without assistance. Life-space mobility, which is the distance through which a person moves over a month, varies from being restricted to a room to traveling outside the region.

Gait speed predicts survival, although less in the very old: for example, 65 year-old men with gait speeds of 1.6 meter (m) per second (s) and 0.8 m/second have median survivals of 32 years and 15 years, respectively; 90-year-old men with gait speeds of 1.6 m/second and 0.8 m/second have median survivals of 8 years and 6 years, respectively. Gait speed also predicts survival in women, and survival in women is generally 20% or more longer than in men of the same age and gait speed.

Mobility can be assessed with two questions:

1. For health or physical reasons, do you have difficulty climbing up 10 steps? Walking ¼ mile?
2. Because of underlying health or physical reasons, have you modified how you climb 10 steps or how frequently? Walk ¼ mile?

The clinician should then evaluate risk factors for impaired mobility, including low physical activity, obesity, symptoms that limit mobility, and chronic diseases that cause organ failure. By observing how the patient arises from a chair, the patient's gait, and the strength of major muscle groups, the clinician can assess the likely causes of poor mobility and whether they may be amenable to physical therapy or other interventions.

RISK OF FALLS

Poor balance is associated with high all-cause mortality,[6] and falls (Chapter 24), which are the 11th most frequent cause of death among people ages 75 years or older, kill almost as many people as prostate cancer and breast cancer combined. One third of community-dwelling persons older than age 65 years fall each year, and the risk increases with age.

On an annual basis, patients should be asked: "Have you fallen in the last year?, Are you afraid of falling?" If the answer to either question is yes, the clinician could measure orthostatic blood pressure, determine nutritional status, assess visual acuity, and examine the feet and knees (for causes of mobility impairment), the strength of the legs and arms, sensation and proprioception of the feet, balance, gait, and cognition. The Timed Up and Go approach measures how long it takes a person to stand up from a chair, walk 10 feet, turn, return, and sit down again; if the sequence requires more than 12 seconds or reveals any gait abnormalities, the patient is at increased risk for falls.[7]

When possible, any medications that affect balance, alertness, or judgement should be discontinued. Older people at increased risk for falls benefit from exercise programs.[A7]

CONTINENCE

Incontinence of urine (Chapter 115) or stool (Chapter 131) and urinary tract symptoms decrease quality of life, limit social function and life space, and can lead to falls and admission to long-term care facilities. Urinary incontinence, which occurs in one third of older women, usually improves with specific interventions, often without medication or surgery.[A8-A9] Three quarters of older men experience urinary frequency, nocturia, or urgency, almost always related to prostate conditions (Chapter 115). Fecal incontinence with at least monthly loss of stool occurs in 8% of men and women aged 50 years and older.

Every elderly patient should be asked: "Have you had urinary incontinence to the extent that it is bothersome?" Further questions determine the frequency and severity of the symptoms and often the pattern (overflow, urge, stress, or mixed incontinence; Chapter 115).

FRAILTY

Frailty (Table 24-1) is global decline in physical function associated with unintentional weight loss of 10 pounds in the last year, self-reported exhaustion, low physical activity, weak grip strength, and slow walking speed.[8] The presence of three or more of these characteristics predicts a five-fold increase in mortality as well as hip fractures, cognitive decline, and adverse outcomes of surgery and hospital care.

SEXUALITY

Among older people in excellent or very good health, nearly 80% of individuals ages 66 to 75 years old and nearly 40% of individuals ages 76 to 85 years old are sexually active. Sexual activity is associated with better cardiovascular health, greater self-esteem, and higher life enjoyment.[9] Nonetheless, sexual problems are common, and sexually transmitted infections have increased in older adults.

Each elderly patient should be asked: "Do you have sex?" The risk for sexually transmitted infections should be assessed (Chapter 264), with behavioral counseling for patients who are at risk.

SELF-NEGLECT AND ABUSE

More than 10% of older people suffer mistreatment, which includes emotional, financial, physical, and sexual abuse, as well as self-neglect and neglect by others. Self-neglect is most common, especially among persons ages 75 years or older and individuals with lower socioeconomic status, cognitive impairment, or physical disability.

To identify difficulties that can lead to self-neglect, patients should be asked how they manage their daily lives: "Are you afraid of anyone?, Has anybody hurt you?, Is anyone taking or using your money without your permission?" Family caregivers should be asked: "Are your elder's needs more than you are able to handle? Are you worried that you might hit your elder? Have you hit your elder?"

Most states have laws that require clinicians to report a reasonable suspicion of abuse or self-neglect to adult protective services.

MEDICATION REVIEW

Polypharmacy is common and can cause drug-drug interactions as well as other adverse effects such as nonadherence. The patient and caregiver should be asked to bring all prescribed and over-the-counter medicines to each visit. The physician should record all the medications and determine which may lead to drug-drug interactions or potentially have harms that exceed their benefits; commercially available drug interaction programs are useful (e.g., Drug Interactions Checker for Drugs, Food and Alcohol: https://www.drugs.com/drug_interactions.html). Drug safety can be improved by goal-directed programs and by explicit deprescribing, which is the process of withdrawing medications, usually one at a time under the supervision of a health professional, with the goal of improving outcomes and minimizing potential harms of polypharmacy.[10,11]

THE BUILT AND SOCIAL ENVIRONMENTS

BUILT ENVIRONMENT

The ability of an older person to live safely as they wish depends on how their home environment and community fit their abilities and needs. Inability to access needed services can lead to self-neglect. Decisions about the appropriateness of the home environment often involve a tension between safety and autonomy. This determination can be based on two questions:

1. Is the home safe, given the patient's cognitive and functional abilities?
2. Can the patient access needed community services, such as stores and a bank?

Home safety to reduce risk for falls can be assessed by a home health agency or by the patient using a brochure from the Centers for Disease Control and Prevention (CDC). (Check for Safety: A Home Fall Prevention Checklist for Older Adults: https://www.cdc.gov/steadi/pdf/check_for_safety_brochure-a.pdf).

SOCIAL SUPPORT

Older persons with loss of independence of ADLs or instrumental ADLs usually require help with important decisions and with daily activities. Informal (i.e., unpaid) support from family and friends is an important source of help,[12] but the clinician should also determine who is available to help the patient and who has durable power of attorney for health care and finances.

FINANCIAL ASSESSMENT

Insufficient money to pay for food, housing, and medical care increases the risk for functional decline and death. If financial security is in doubt, the patient should be asked: "Do you have enough money to pay for groceries? Bills? Medication? Medical/dental bills? A small emergency? A major emergency?" The answers can guide further questions as to whether the patient is a beneficiary of Medicare or Medicaid, is a veteran, or has private health or long-term care insurance. For example, insurance or veterans' benefits can pay for home assistance and daycare.

PROGNOSIS

Prediction of functional status, ability to live independently, and survival inform planning and decisions by older persons and their families. Life expectancy, which is the median length of survival for a group of people, varies according to age, gender, and race (E-Table 23-1 and https://www.cdc.gov/nchs/data/nvsr/nvsr69/nvsr69-12-508.pdf). Life expectancy can be estimated more precisely by incorporating clinical characteristics with online calculators (e.g., see https://eprognosis.ucsf.edu/calculators/). For example, just a few criteria such as male sex (1 point), dependent ADL (2 points for 1 to 4 ADLs and 5 points for 5 dependent ADLs), and 4 clinical characteristics (heart failure, 2 points; serum creatinine >3 mg/dL, 2 points; albumin level 3.0 to 3.4 g/dL or <3.0 g/dL, 1 or 2 points, respectively; nonmetastatic or metastatic cancer, 3 or 8 points, respectively) can classify hospitalized older adults into groups with median 1-year mortality rates of 4% (0 or 1 point), 19% (2 or 3 points), 34% (4 to 6 points), and 64% (>6 points), respectively.

For treatments and screening tests, it is important to determine whether the "time to benefit" (how long it will take for the long-term benefit to exceed the short-term risk) exceeds the life expectancy.[13] For example, an intervention for which benefit exceeds harm after 5 to 10 years (e.g., cancer screening) is unlikely to benefit a person with a life expectancy of 3 years.

GOALS AND PREFERENCES

Life goals often change over time, and advance care planning unfortunately does not necessarily improve end-of-life care.[14] Each year and after major

TABLE 23-1 FUNCTIONAL ASSESSMENT ELDERLY INDIVIDUALS

ASPECT BEING ASSESSED	PREVISIT QUESTIONNAIRE: LENGTH OF SCREEN IN MINUTES	PREVISIT QUESTIONNAIRE: INSTRUMENTS	ADMINISTERED BY INTERVIEW: LENGTH OF SCREEN IN MINUTES*	ADMINISTERED BY INTERVIEW: INSTRUMENTS
Functional status	<2	Activities of daily living* Instrumental activities of daily living*		
Advance directives	<2	Single question about having advance directives		
MEDICAL ASSESSMENT				
Visual impairment	<2	Single question*	<2	Snellen eye chart (see E-Fig. 391-1)
Hearing impairment	<2	Single question*	<2 (if needed)	Whisper test*
Cognitive problems	<2		≥5	Mini-cog (see Table 361-5)
Mind, affective problems	≥5	PHQ-2* and 9 (see Table 12-5)	<2	
Falls, mobility, balance	<2	Simple questions	<2	Timed Up and Go test*
Medication review	≥5	Inspection of medication bottles		
Malnutrition	<2	Single question*	<2	Weight
Urinary incontinence	<2	Single question*	<2	International Consultation on Incontinence Modular Questionnaire short form if single question is positive (see Chapter 115)
Frailty	<2	Questions (see Table 24-1)	<2	Gait speed, grip strength
Preventive services	≥5	Specific questions		
OTHER DIMENSIONS				
Environment	≥5	Home safety checklist		
Social support	<2	Single question		
Financial status			<2	Insurance status

*See text.
PHQ = Patient Health Questionnaire (see text).
Modified from Reuben DB. Geriatric Assessment. In: Goldman L, Schafer A, eds. *Goldman-Cecil Medicine*. 26th ed. Philadelphia: Elsevier; 2020.

life events, a patient should be asked questions such as: "As you look to the future, what is important to you?," and "What can I do for you today and over the coming months?" Goals may include long-term survival, survival to an event in the foreseeable future, living at home, maintenance of a role, or control of symptoms (e.g., pain or dyspnea). Clinicians can suggest what goals are achievable, what actions can achieve specific goals, and the risks of actions and their possible consequences. Symptom-focused management can improve survival.[A10]

PREVENTIVE SERVICES

Preventive services that benefit older people include vaccinations, screening tests for selected asymptomatic diseases, and behavioral counseling. Vaccinations recommended by the CDC for older adults (Chapter 15) are annual inactivated or recombinant influenza vaccination, two one-time pneumococcal vaccinations (PCV13 and PPSV23 administered 1 year apart), herpes zoster recombinant vaccination (two doses of RZV), and tetanus-diphtheria (Td) or tetanus-diphtheria-pertussis (Tdap) vaccination every 10 years.

Preventive services for which current evidence demonstrates net benefit are recommended by U.S. Preventive Services Task Force for older adults (Chapter 12; http://epss.ahrq.gov/ePSS/search.jsp). Screening is recommended for colorectal cancer and breast cancer to age 75 years and for lung cancer in past or current smokers up to age 80 years. Other recommendations (E-Table 23-2) pertain to screening for hypertension (Chapter 64), abdominal aortic aneurysm (Chapter 63), prediabetes or diabetes (Chapter 210), osteoporosis (Chapter 225), depression (Chapter 362), unhealthy use of alcohol or drugs (Chapters 364 and 365), and certain infections (e.g., human immunodeficiency virus, syphilis, gonorrhea and chlamydia, hepatitis B, hepatitis C, and latent tuberculosis). Aspirin for primary prevention is not recommended in adults ages 60 years or older.[A11]

GERIATRIC ASSESSMENT IN PRACTICE

Geriatric assessment asks questions that can be completed by the patient, caregiver, or office staff, as well as by clinicians (a physician, advanced practice nurse, social worker, and/or physical therapist). Tests can be completed by office staff or a clinician (Table 23-1). Geriatric assessment identifies syndromes, impairments, and disabilities that require a targeted plan to guide management by the principal physician or other clinician over time.

Geriatric assessment is especially useful in hospitalized older adults, but it is reasonable to perform it annually in individuals over age 75 years, patients with multiple chronic diseases, and patients who have survived after major illnesses. Many elements of geriatric assessment are included in Medicare's Initial Preventive Physical Exam and the Annual Wellness Visit (see Medicare Wellness Visits – ICN MLN6775421 February 2021 [https://www.cms.gov] for covered services).

GENERAL REFERENCES

For the General References and other additional features, please visit Elsevier eBooks+ at https://ebooks.health.elsevier.com.

Grade A References

A1. Ellis G, Gardner M, Tsiachristas A, et al. Comprehensive geriatric assessment for older adults admitted to hospital. *Cochrane Database Syst Rev*. 2017;9:CD006211.
A2. Eamer G, Taheri A, Chen SS, et al. Comprehensive geriatric assessment for older people admitted to a surgical service. *Cochrane Database Syst Rev*. 2018;1:CD012485.
A3. Shields L, Henderson V, Caslake R. Comprehensive geriatric assessment for prevention of delirium after hip fracture: a systematic review of randomized controlled trials. *J Am Geriatr Soc*. 2017;65:1559-1567.
A4. Mohile SG, Mohamed MR, Xu H, et al. Evaluation of geriatric assessment and management on the toxic effects of cancer treatment (GAP70+): a cluster-randomised study. *Lancet*. 2021;398:1894-1904.
A5. Shepperd S, Butler C, Cradduck-Bamford A, et al. Is comprehensive geriatric assessment admission avoidance hospital at home an alternative to hospital admission for older persons? A randomized trial. *Ann Intern Med*. 2021;174:889-898.
A6. Chou R, Dana T, Bougatsos C, et al. Screening for impaired visual acuity in older adults: updated evidence report and systematic review for the US Preventive Services Task Force. *JAMA*. 2016;315:915-933.
A7. US Preventive Services Task Force. Interventions to prevent falls in community-dwelling older adults. *JAMA*. 2018;319:1696-1704.
A8. Burgio KL, Kraus SR, Johnson TM, 2nd, et al. Effectiveness of combined behavioral and drug therapy for overactive bladder symptoms in men: a randomized clinical trial. *JAMA Intern Med*. 2020;180:411-419.
A9. Diokno AC, Newman DK, Low LK, et al. Effect of group-administered behavioral treatment on urinary incontinence in older women: a randomized clinical trial. *JAMA Intern Med*. 2018;178:1333-1341.
A10. Denis F, Basch E, Septans AL, et al. Two-year survival comparing web-based symptom monitoring vs routine surveillance following treatment for lung cancer. *JAMA*. 2019;321:306-307.
A11. Davidson KW, Barry MJ, Mangione CM, et al. Aspirin use to prevent cardiovascular disease: US Preventive Services Task Force recommendation statement. *JAMA*. 2022;327:1577-1584.

24

COMMON CLINICAL SEQUELAE OF AGING

JEREMY D. WALSTON

EPIDEMIOLOGY

Older adults make up the majority of patients actively treated in the health care system, in large part owing to their increased burden of chronic diseases but also because of their marked vulnerability to adverse health outcomes, such as functional and cognitive decline (Chapter 361), falls, delirium (Chapter 361), and frailty. This age-related vulnerability is thought to have its basis in altered biology that results in tissue and physiologic system changes, which in turn may contribute to many of these conditions and to the chronic disease states commonly seen in older adults. Importantly, these biologic changes are likely to be heterogeneous and to occur at different chronologic ages and in different organs at different rates (Fig. 24-1). These complex age-related biologic changes represent a source of vulnerability that sets the stage for the marked increase in clinical sequelae observed in older adults.

PATHOBIOLOGY

Age-Related Cellular and Molecular Changes

The multiple biologic changes of aging affect important homeostatic functions and can lead to altered cellular function, declines in tissue resiliency, and cellular dropout. Although the exact contributions of each of these biologic changes are not yet known, improvements in precision medicine approaches may facilitate future targeted prevention and treatment strategies. For example, autophagy, an intracellular process responsible for the recycling of damaged or redundant organelles or proteins, becomes less effective with aging.[1] The result is an intracellular accumulation of dysfunctional mitochondria and proteins, which in turn can trigger cellular dysregulation through increased levels of free radicals, lower mitochondrial energy production, and programmed cell death or apoptosis. Senescent cell populations arise with increasing age and lead to alterations in tissue and immune system function.[2] For example, some fibroblasts and fat cells evolve toward a senescent cell phenotype whereby reproduction and cell death are less likely to take place and survival persists in an altered, less functional state. These senescent cells secrete inflammatory cytokines and other bioactive molecules that pathologically alter surrounding tissues. Senescent T-cell populations also evolve with increasing age, perhaps related to early-life viral infections. Senescent T cells are less able to respond appropriately to immunogenic signals, thereby increasing vulnerability to infections. Another biologic age-related change is an increasing tendency for apoptosis, or programmed cell death. Although apoptosis is a normal cellular program that kills and disassembles damaged or redundant cells in all tissues, it accelerates with age and likely contributes to the vulnerability to chronic disease states, such as Parkinson disease (Chapter 378), heart failure (Chapter 45), and the generalized loss of cell number in many tissues. Finally, evidence suggests that increased activity in transforming growth factor-β signaling may play an important role in the fibrotic changes that are observed in the heart, skeletal muscle, and lung tissue and that result in functional decrements with increasing age. Importantly, these aging-related molecular and cellular changes are heterogeneous and may affect individuals at different ages and in different tissues. However, the end results are increased susceptibility to chronic disease states, frailty, declines in function and cognition, and ultimately mortality.

Physiologic System Dysregulation and Its Consequences

Dysfunction in multiple physiologic stress response systems also plays a role in late-life vulnerability. Chronic diseases such as diabetes, vascular disease, chronic obstructive pulmonary disease, depression, and heart failure activate the innate immune system, the sympathetic nervous system, and the hypothalamic-pituitary-adrenal axis, which in turn increases the production of cortisol and the inflammatory cytokine interleukin-6 (IL-6). These responses further exacerbate aging-related clinical conditions, such as osteoporosis and hypertension, and increase vulnerability to frailty, functional decline, accidental injury, and worsening chronic disease states (E-Fig. 24-1).

CLINICAL MANIFESTATIONS

Some clinical manifestations are related not to physiologic aging but rather to cumulative exposures, such as with sun-related skin cancer (Chapter 188), or the delayed expression of genetic abnormalities, such as Huntington disease (Chapter 379) or polycystic kidney disease (Chapter 112). However, many organs and systems become less functional with age. For example, a healthy 70-year-old will have only about 50% of the lung function (Chapter 71) and renal function (Chapter 101) of a young adult. The resultant lack of physiologic reserve capacity does not affect day-to-day function but can greatly affect the ability to recover from a severe illness that exhausts the body's reserve capacity.

Despite normal baseline temperatures, older adults are more susceptible to hypothermia or hyperthermia (Chapter 95) after environmental exposure, even though they are less likely to develop fever with infections. For example, patients with pneumonia (Chapter 85) may present with confusion and dehydration rather than with fever and cough. Among older persons with critical illness, more than half die within 1 month or experience significant functional decline over the following year.

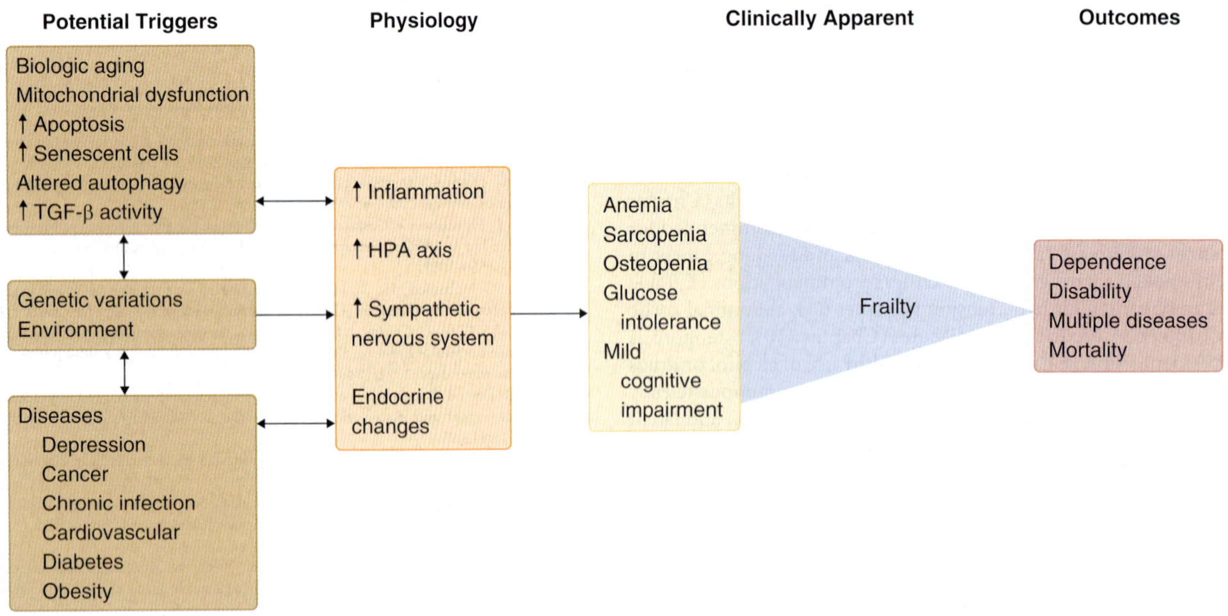

FIGURE 24-1. **Comprehensive model pathway for biologic vulnerability to adverse outcomes in aging.** HPA = hypothalamic-pituitary-adrenal; TGF-β = transforming growth factor-β.

EFFECTS OF AGING ON SPECIFIC ORGANS AND SYSTEMS

CARDIOVASCULAR SYSTEM

Between the ages of 20 and 80 years, left ventricular systolic function does not change, but the left ventricle gradually thickens. The result is that left ventricular filling in early diastole declines by 50%, and ventricular filling becomes more dependent on atrial contraction (Chapter 41).[3] Although atherosclerosis is the most important cause of symptomatic cardiac disease in elderly people, the age-associated vascular stiffness results in an age-related increase in heart failure despite normal systolic function (Chapter 45). With the gradual loss of up to 90% of sinus node pacemaker cells by the age of 80 years, both the resting heart rate and the maximal heart rate with exercise decline. Conduction system dysfunction contributes to an increase in the prevalence of atrial fibrillation, which is seen in about 4% of community-dwelling older individuals (Chapter 52) and can develop in up to one third of the elderly after surgery (Chapter 401). Heart valves thicken and stiffen, and the prevalence of aortic stenosis and mitral annular calcifications rises (Chapter 60), often causing heart murmurs.

Stiffening of the aorta causes an increase in systolic blood pressure, whereas diastolic blood pressure often stays stable or even declines (Chapter 64). Hypertensive patients age 80 years and older should generally be treated according to current recommendations for people older than 65 years, with a systolic blood pressure goal of less than 120 mm Hg likely associated with lower cardiovascular and all-cause mortality for otherwise healthy older adults.[A1-A2] However, some older adults, especially frail elders, may not tolerate systolic blood pressures this low without side effects, so treatment must be individualized. For some patients over age 80 years, a modest reduction in their multidrug regimen may sustain target blood pressure levels with fewer side effects.[A3] Blood pressure control reduces the incidence of cognitive impairment and dementia (Chapter 371) in older persons with mild cognitive deficits,[A4] and discontinuation of antihypertensive treatment does not improve cognitive, psychological, or general daily functioning.[A5] There is little evidence, however, of the impact of maintaining a lower blood pressure on those who are over age 90 years.

The combination of impaired ventricular filling and the inability to increase the heart rate with stress contributes to the postural hypotension that is seen in 20% of older individuals (Chapter 49), as well as their predisposition to falls and syncope with stresses that younger individuals would tolerate. The reduced ability of the elderly to tolerate cardiovascular stress must be recognized and anticipated whenever they experience a major illness. In addition, coronary artery disease can limit cardiac reserve and increase the risk that hypotension will cause a secondary myocardial infarction.

Hyperlipidemia is common in older adults, and statins are effective in this age group for reducing coronary heart disease events.[A6-A7] However, their favorable cost-effectiveness for primary prevention in persons over age 75 years can be offset by even minor geriatric-specific side effects, and these drugs can be discontinued safely in the setting of advanced, life-limiting illness.[A8] Low-dose aspirin is not beneficial in healthy elderly people because its side effects outweigh its benefits.[A9-A10] However, low-dose edoxaban (15 mg daily) may be a safe and effective option to prevent systemic embolization in elderly patients who otherwise seem not to be safe candidates for anticoagulation.[A11]

All adult cardiac conditions become more common with aging. Exercise training can improve endurance and decrease age-related cardiac stiffness.[A12] Treatment recommendations for specific cardiac abnormalities must balance the potential benefit of targeted interventions against the common multimorbidities seen with aging.[4]

RESPIRATORY SYSTEM

The chest wall stiffens with advancing age, and the lungs lose elastic recoil (Chapter 73).[5] Maximal vital capacity declines by about 40%, but oxygen exchange declines by about 50% because of the additive effect of progressive ventilation-perfusion mismatching (Chapter 73). As a result, the arterial Po_2 of many 80-year-olds is about 70 to 75 mm Hg. The clinical manifestations are often progressive shortness of breath with exercise (Chapter 71) and an increased susceptibility to community-acquired pneumonia (Chapter 85) and even to aspiration pneumonia.

GASTROINTESTINAL SYSTEM

Taste and smell (Chapter 395) decline with advancing age. Food tends to taste less sweet and more bitter.

The esophageal sphincter can become lax (Chapter 124), thereby increasing reflux and even aspiration. Atrophic gastritis reduces the risk of duodenal ulcer but also the absorption of iron (Chapter 145) and vitamin B_{12} (Chapter 150). Delayed gastric emptying can lead to a sense of early satiety and decreased appetite.

A gradual decline in the number of hepatocytes decreases the weight of the liver by about one third by the age of 90 years and decreases the liver's ability to metabolize drugs (Chapter 25). Distal colonic motility from the rectosigmoid to the anal canal declines, and more than 60% of elderly individuals develop constipation (Chapter 122). Diverticula (Chapter 128) become more common with age and are seen in up to 50% of people older than age 80 years.

URINARY SYSTEM

Glomerular filtration declines by about 1% per year, and kidney size declines by about one third in older adults (Chapter 101). Maximal concentrating capacity declines, and it becomes more difficult to excrete a salt load or to conserve water in the face of dehydration.

The bladder becomes more irritable with advancing age and may generate less power, which is especially a problem in men with prostatic hypertrophy (Chapter 114). By comparison, urinary incontinence (Chapter 115) is more prevalent in women. Residual bladder urine volume increases, and nocturia is common. Vaginal and urethral atrophy predispose women to urinary tract infections (Chapter 263).

The kidney is more susceptible to the effects of medications, particularly nonsteroidal anti-inflammatory drugs, which can result in sodium and fluid retention and subsequent hypertension. In elderly individuals, a slight acidemia results from impaired acid excretion and may contribute to the development of osteoporosis.

ENDOCRINE SYSTEM

Growth hormone levels fall with advancing age (Chapter 205), thereby resulting in decreased muscle strength, thinning of bones and skin, and increased central fat. However, growth hormone replacement does not appear to result in improved muscle strength. Levels of thyroid hormones do not decline with age (Chapter 207). Parathyroid hormone levels, however, commonly increase, especially in women, probably in response to the kidney's declining ability to maintain normal serum levels of phosphorus and calcium (Chapters 184 and 227).

The ability of the pancreas to release insulin is blunted with advancing age (Chapter 210), but the kidney's clearance of insulin also decreases. The net result is maintained plasma insulin levels in the fasting state but an increased likelihood of postprandial or stress-induced hyperglycemia. Dramatic declines in estrogen and progesterone production precipitate menopause at an average age of 51 years (Chapter 222). Testosterone levels begin to decrease in men by about 50 years of age, often with resulting declines in sexual function but not in the potency of semen (Chapter 216). Testosterone supplements reverse the muscle loss and sexual implications of declining testosterone levels, but their safety and effect on the risk of cardiovascular complications are uncertain.[6,7]

IMMUNE SYSTEM

Declines in the responsiveness of the immune system explain why the incidence of autoimmune conditions, such as systemic lupus erythematosus (Chapter 245) and multiple sclerosis (Chapter 380), declines in the elderly. However, this same decline explains increased morbidity and mortality with infectious diseases and the increased risk of reactivating infections such as tuberculosis (Chapter 299) and herpes zoster (Chapter 346). These risks emphasize the importance of vaccination against herpes zoster, influenza, pneumococcal pneumonia, and tetanus in the elderly (Chapter 15).

HEMATOPOIETIC SYSTEM

Hematopoiesis (Chapter 142) is generally sustained with aging, except in response to marked stress and inflammatory pathway activation. The one exception is that the hematocrit declines somewhat in older men, presumably owing to their lower testosterone levels. Clonal hematopoiesis, which is the proliferation of a single cell, is more common with aging and increases the risk of cancer, cardiovascular disease, and all-cause mortality.[8]

INTEGUMENTARY SYSTEM

With aging, the epidermis and dermis adhere less tightly and the subcutaneous tissue thins, thereby making the skin feel looser and more likely to wrinkle and ulcerate. Clinical sequelae include senile purpura (Fig. 24-2) as tears in small venules after bumps or abrasions (Chapter 407). Ultraviolet light exposure also predisposes to skin cancer (Chapter 188), rosacea (Chapter 406), xerosis, and hair loss (Chapter 409). Wound healing is also compromised, and complete skin healing can take 5.5 weeks instead of 3.5 weeks in individuals older than age 65 years.

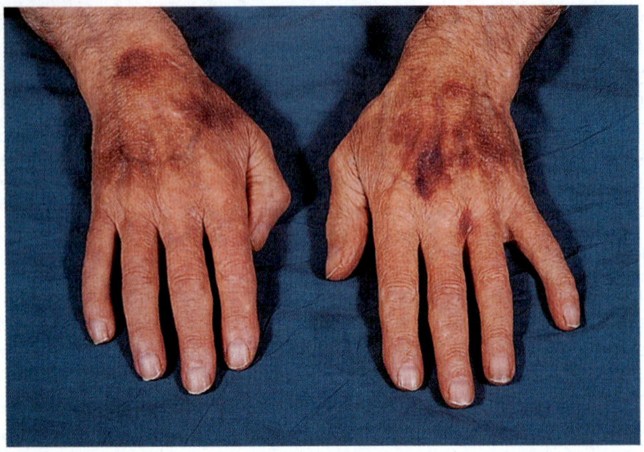

FIGURE 24-2. **Senile purpura is a common and benign condition that results from impaired collagen production and capillary fragility in some older adults.** In the absence of other signs of disease, no investigation is necessary. (From Forbes CD, Jackson WF. *Color Atlas and Text of Clinical Medicine*. 3rd ed. London: Mosby; 2003.)

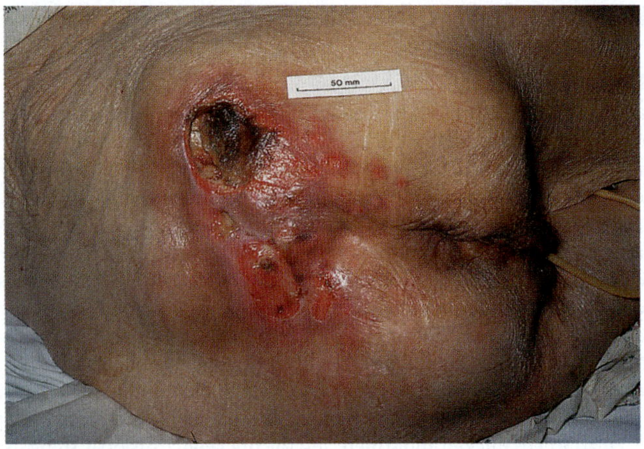

FIGURE 24-3. **Severe sacral pressure sore, one of the serious but preventable complications of immobility.** (From Forbes CD, Jackson WF. *Color Atlas and Text of Clinical Medicine*. 3rd ed. London: Mosby; 2003.)

Pressure Sores

Older adults are more prone to pressure sores when they are bedridden. Pressure sores, which are necrotic areas of muscle, subcutaneous fat, and skin, usually occur between underlying bone and a hard surface (or a soft surface during a prolonged time) as a result of compression and subsequent ischemia (Fig. 24-3). A continuous-pressure threshold of only 30 to 35 mm Hg is needed to cause pressure sores, and a standard mattress can generate pressures five times as high. In addition to pressure injury, other contributing factors include shear injury from rubbing constantly against underlying surfaces, burning injury from friction of the superficial skin layers, and moisture that softens the skin, makes it stick to underlying surfaces, and provides easy access for infection.

TREATMENT AND PREVENTION

Safe positioning, regular turning, avoidance of direct pressure, pressure-reducing beds, and advanced static mattresses or advanced static overlays can reduce the incidence of pressure sores. Alternating air mattresses or overlays are not recommended.[9] Pressure sores should be photographed to establish a baseline. The wound should be freed of any pressure to prevent additional pressure ulcers. Wet-to-dry dressings are a mainstay, and semiocclusive and occlusive dressings also can be helpful. Protein or amino acid supplementation enriched with zinc and antioxidants,[A13] hydrocolloid or foam dressings, and adjunctive electrical stimulation may be useful. Surgical or chemical débridement is often required. Topical or systemic antibiotics (Chapter 261) may be needed. Pressure ulcers usually heal within 6 months, but surgical repair is sometimes required.

MUSCULOSKELETAL SYSTEM

Bone mass and density decrease by about 1% per year but by up to 2 to 3% per year in the first 5 to 10 years after menopause in women (Chapters 222 and 225). In older women with osteopenia, bisphosphonate therapy (e.g., zoledronate, four 5-mg infusions at 18-month intervals)[A14] significantly reduces the risk of nonvertebral or vertebral fractures within 1 year[A15] and therefore is useful in women with a life expectancy longer than 1 year. Tendons and ligaments become less elastic, thereby contributing to a higher incidence of rupture, especially of the Achilles tendon. Sarcopenia is common in older adults.[10] For example, muscle mass declines by about 25% by the age of 70 years and by 30 to 40% by the age of 80 years unless it is offset by exercise.

CLINICAL PHARMACOLOGY

Older adults take a disproportionate share of all prescription (Chapter 25) and nonprescription (Chapter 30) medications, and they are at increased risk of drug-drug interactions. Because older adults have less muscle mass and more fat as a proportion of total body weight, they are more sensitive to the effects of water-soluble drugs and have prolonged effects from lipophilic drugs. Declines in renal and hepatic function reduce the clearance of most drugs, although drugs that are conjugated and glucuronidated are cleared relatively normally. Older people also are more likely to be nonadherent to prescribed regimens owing to the number of medications and their cost, mental impairment, and medication side effects.

SENSORY AND SLEEP

In addition to age-related cognitive decline (Chapters 361 and 361), hearing loss develops in about 25% of individuals older than 65 years (Chapter 396), with decreased neural transmission leading to difficulty in discriminating important sounds from background noise. Presbycusis diminishes the ability to hear high-frequency sounds.

The thickening and stiffening of the lens diminish the ability to focus on nearby objects and increase glare (Chapter 391). Transmission of light through the lens may decline by 50% or more, so elderly individuals require more ambient light. Vitreal detachment causes floaters that also can interfere with vision. Decreased tear production causes dryness of the eyes. All of these conditions contribute to a decline in visual acuity to the extent that 40% of men and 60% of women older than 65 years have a visual acuity of 20/70 or worse.

Older adults tend to have difficulty in sleeping (Chapter 374) yet spend much more time in bed. Sleep apnea also becomes more common with advancing age (Chapter 374).

FRAILTY

EPIDEMIOLOGY

Frailty in older adults is a geriatric syndrome of weakness, slowness, and weight loss, owing to an aggregate of comorbid conditions. Frailty serves as a clinical indicator of which older adults are at high risk for adverse outcomes, including delirium (Chapter 361), falls, and mortality.[11,12] Measures of frailty are also increasingly utilized to identify older adults who are at highest risk for adverse health outcomes related to procedures or medical treatments, including intensive care,[13] general surgery,[14] hip fracture surgery,[15] or coronavirus disease 2019 (COVID-19) infection.[16]

PATHOBIOLOGY

The biology that differentiates vulnerable or frail older adults from resilient or robust older adults is complex and multisystemic in nature. For example, diminished heart rate variability, which is a marker of dysregulated sympathetic nervous system activity, is associated with aging, frailty, and cardiac arrhythmias. Frail older adults have significantly higher levels of salivary cortisol during the afternoon nadir period, thereby suggesting chronically increased activity of the hypothalamic-pituitary-adrenal axis. Elevated levels of inflammatory cytokines, especially IL-6, tumor necrosis factor-α receptor 1 (TNFR1), and C-reactive protein, are strongly related to functional decline, frailty, chronic disease, and mortality in older adults, probably owing to increased fat, more senescent cells, and free radical production from altered mitochondria. IL-6 is likely to have a negative impact on stem cells and satellite cells, which in turn may contribute to the chronic anemia and age-related declines in skeletal muscle (sarcopenia) and bone mass (osteopenia) commonly observed in frail, older adults. TNFR1 stimulates apoptosis and necroptosis, which are cell programs that lead to cell death and possibly tissue depletion and vulnerability later in life. In addition to stress response systems, endocrine factors that normally maintain muscle mass play a role in frailty. For example, the adrenal androgen dehydroepiandrosterone sulfate and insulin-like growth factor 1 are significantly lower in frail adults. Future preventive or treatment strategies to reduce frailty and improve resiliency may target some of these stress responses or endocrinologic changes.

CLINICAL MANIFESTATION AND DIAGNOSIS

Validated frailty screening tools (Table 24-1) enable physicians to identify patients at highest risk of side effects, adverse outcomes, and mortality and to develop preventive interventions that will decrease risk and improve quality of life. One approach is to measure physiologic parameters such as grip strength, walking speed, and weight loss, as well as to gather information about activity and fatigue levels. With use of this approach, the prevalence of frailty rises with increasing age; approximately 10% of community-dwelling adults older than 65 years meet these frailty criteria and subsequently are at increased risk of functional decline, falling, hospitalization, and death, even after adjustment for age, socioeconomic and smoking status, and multiple common disease states.

TREATMENT AND PREVENTION

Interventions should be targeted to the specific characteristics of a patient's frailty. Increasing physical exercise is the mainstay of most programs.[A16] Focused prevention of iatrogenic injuries or recurrent hospitalizations and remediation of symptoms are often warranted for frail vulnerable older adults (Fig. 24-4). Physical activity, exercise interventions, and nutritional supplementation can reduce disability and symptoms and improve quality of life across the spectrum of robust to frail older adults. In addition, exercise and weight loss together improve function in obese and frail older adults. Other options include a team-based approach that engages the patient, family members, caregivers, health care providers, and social workers. Classic palliative care (Chapter 3), with appropriate pain management, less invasive treatment plans, limited hospital visits, and organized home care plans, can greatly improve quality of life. If the patient has frequently been admitted to an inpatient setting, a program for all-inclusive care or a medical daycare setting may help prevent recurrent admissions and improve quality of life. Once admitted to the hospital, frail older adults may benefit from being congregated in a unit that specializes in their care and can provide attention to their functionality, continence, sleep disturbances, delirium, and palliative care issues.

TABLE 24-1 FOUR COMMONLY USED INSTRUMENTS TO MEASURE FRAILTY IN OLDER ADULTS, WITH RELEVANT MEASUREMENT DOMAINS AND SCORING CRITERIA

INSTRUMENT	DOMAINS	SCORING
Physical frailty (biologic syndrome model)*	Physical function (slowness, low activity, weakness), nutritive (weight loss), and exhaustion	Score range: 0-5 Frail = ≥3 criteria present Intermediate/pre-frail = 1-2 criteria present Robust = 0 criteria present
Cumulative Deficit Frailty Model (comorbidity model)†	Diseases, ability in ADL, health attitudes/values, and symptoms/signs from the clinical and neurologic examinations	Number of deficits present and divided by the number of deficits taken into consideration Higher proportion equates to a higher level of frailty
Vulnerable Elders Survey (VES-13)‡	Physical function and ADL/IADL disability	Score range: 0-10 Frail = score ≥3
1994 Frailty measure (functional domains model)§	Physical function, nutritive function, cognitive function, sensory problems	Subject scoring a 3 or higher on at least one item in any domain is considered to have a problem or difficulty in that domain Frail = problems/difficulties in ≥2 domains

*Fried LP, Tangen CM, Walston J, et al. Frailty in older adults: evidence for a phenotype. *J Gerontol A Biol Sci Med Sci*. 2001;56:M146-M156.
†Rockwood K, Andrew M, Mitnitski A. A comparison of two approaches to measuring frailty in elderly people. *J Gerontol A Biol Sci Med Sci*. 2007;62:738-743.
‡Saliba D, Elliott M, Rubenstein LZ, et al. The Vulnerable Elders Survey: a tool for identifying vulnerable older people in the community. *J Am Geriatr Soc*. 2001;49:1691-1699.
§Strawbridge WJ, Shema SJ, Balfour JL, et al. Antecedents of frailty over three decades in an older cohort. *J Gerontol B Psychol Sci Soc Sci*. 1998;53:S9-S16.
Details on the use and implementation of these tools can be found in the referenced articles.
ADL = activities of daily living; IADL = instrumental activities of daily living.

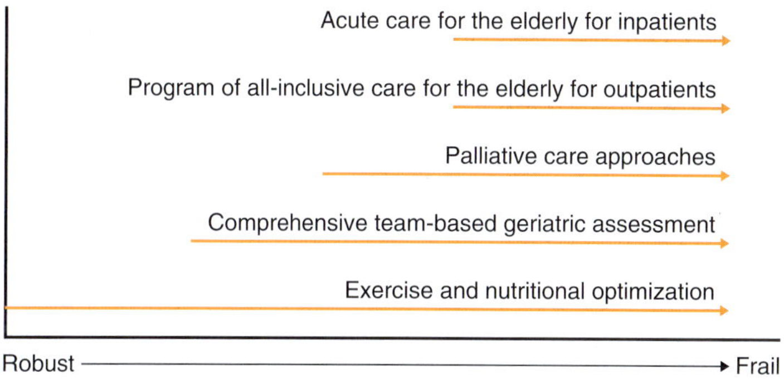

FIGURE 24-4. Assessment and treatments in frail and vulnerable older adults.

PROGNOSIS

Frailty increases the likelihood for development of influenza or influenza-like illness in the 6 months after vaccination; the likelihood of requiring care in a skilled nursing or long-term care facility after hospitalization for general surgery; the likelihood of poor outcomes in patients with cardiovascular disease; poor renal transplant graft function and early hospital readmission after transplantation; falls, hospitalization, and mortality in patients on hemodialysis for chronic renal failure; and the risk of death in aging intravenous drug users. Biologic differences between frail and non-frail older adults (see Fig. 24-1) drive the marked vulnerability to adverse outcomes observed in the frail subjects.

FALLS

Falls are a common manifestation of frailty. Contributing factors include cardiopulmonary disease, poor eyesight, hearing loss, balance disturbances, weakness, movement disorders, neuropathies, poor judgment, depression, osteoporosis, arthritis, and foot disorders.[17] The risk of falling also increases in patients who take more prescription medications, especially hypnotics, muscle relaxants, antihypertensive agents, diuretics, and antidepressant medications. Environmental risks include stairs, loose objects, rugs, poor lighting, poorly fitting shoes, uneven pavements, and slippery surfaces.

Patients who have fallen or have a fear of falling should have a falls assessment, including measuring orthostatic blood pressure, assessing vision, reviewing medications, and testing balance, gait, and lower extremity strength.[18,19] Exercise alone and exercise combined with other interventions (e.g., vision assessment and treatment; environmental modification) lower the risk compared with usual care,[A17–A19] but intensive, nurse-led, individualized plans may not provide incremental benefit over good baseline care.[A20,A21] Data on vitamin D supplementation to reduce falls have been inconclusive, but recent trials indicate no benefit.[A22,A23]

GENERAL REFERENCES

For the General References and other additional features, please visit Elsevier eBooks+ at https://ebooks.health.elsevier.com.

Grade A References

A1. Zhang W, Zhang S, Deng Y, et al. Trial of intensive blood-pressure control in older patients with hypertension. *N Engl J Med*. 2021;385:1268-1279.
A2. Williamson JD, Supiano MA, Applegate WB, et al. Intensive vs standard blood pressure control and cardiovascular disease outcomes in adults aged ≥75 years: a randomized clinical trial. *JAMA*. 2016;315:2673–82.
A3. Sheppard JP, Burt J, Lown M, et al. Effect of antihypertensive medication reduction vs usual care on short-term blood pressure control in patients with hypertension aged 80 years and older: the OPTIMISE randomized clinical trial. *JAMA*. 2020;323:2039-2051.
A4. Hughes D, Judge C, Murphy R, et al. Association of blood pressure lowering with incident dementia or cognitive impairment: a systematic review and meta-analysis. *JAMA*. 2020;323:1934-1944.
A5. Moonen JE, Foster-Dingley JC, de Ruijter W, et al. Effect of discontinuation of antihypertensive treatment in elderly people on cognitive functioning—the DANTE study Leiden: a randomized clinical trial. *JAMA Intern Med*. 2015;175:1622-1630.
A6. Cholesterol Treatment Trialists' Collaboration. Efficacy and safety of statin therapy in older people: a meta-analysis of individual participant data from 28 randomised controlled trials. *Lancet*. 2019;393:407-415.
A7. Gencer B, Marston NA, Im K, et al. Efficacy and safety of lowering LDL cholesterol in older patients: a systematic review and meta-analysis of randomised controlled trials. *Lancet*. 2020;396:1637-1643.
A8. Kutner JS, Blatchford PJ, Taylor DH Jr, et al. Safety and benefit of discontinuing statin therapy in the setting of advanced, life-limiting illness: a randomized clinical trial. *JAMA Intern Med*. 2015;175:691-700.

A9. McNeil JJ, Nelson MR, Woods RL, et al. Effect of aspirin on all-cause mortality in the healthy elderly. *N Engl J Med*. 2018;379:1519-1528.
A10. McNeil JJ, Woods RL, Nelson MR, et al. Effect of aspirin on disability-free survival in the healthy elderly. *N Engl J Med*. 2018;379:1499-1508.
A11. Okumura K, Akao M, Yoshida T, et al. Low-dose edoxaban in very elderly patients with atrial fibrillation. *N Engl J Med*. 2020;383:1735-1745.
A12. Howden EJ, Sarma S, Lawley JS, et al. Reversing the cardiac effects of sedentary aging in middle age—a randomized controlled trial: implications for heart failure prevention. *Circulation*. 2018;137:1549-1560.
A13. Cereda E, Klersy C, Serioli M, et al. A nutritional formula enriched with arginine, zinc, and antioxidants for the healing of pressure ulcers: a randomized trial. *Ann Intern Med*. 2015;162:167-174.
A14. Reid IR, Horne AM, Mihov B, et al. Fracture prevention with zoledronate in older women with osteopenia. *N Engl J Med*. 2018;379:2407-2416.
A15. Deardorff WJ, Cenzer I, Nguyen B, et al. Time to benefit of bisphosphonate therapy for the prevention of fractures among postmenopausal women with osteoporosis: a meta-analysis of randomized clinical trials. *JAMA Intern Med*. 2022;182:33-41.
A16. Martínez-Velilla N, Casas-Herrero A, Zambom-Ferraresi F, et al. Effect of exercise intervention on functional decline in very elderly patients during acute hospitalization: a randomized clinical trial. *JAMA Intern Med*. 2019;179:28-36.
A17. Guirguis-Blake JM, Michael YL, Perdue LA, et al. Interventions to prevent falls in older adults: updated evidence report and systematic review for the US Preventive Services Task Force. *JAMA*. 2018;319:1705-1716.
A18. Liu-Ambrose T, Davis JC, Best JR, et al. Effect of a home-based exercise program on subsequent falls among community-dwelling high-risk older adults after a fall: a randomized clinical trial. *JAMA*. 2019;321:2092-2100.
A19. de Souto Barreto P, Rolland Y, Vellas B, et al. Association of long-term exercise training with risk of falls, fractures, hospitalizations, and mortality in older adults: a systematic review and meta-analysis. *JAMA Intern Med*. 2019;179:394-405.
A20. Bhasin S, Gill TM, Reuben DB, et al. A randomized trial of a multifactorial strategy to prevent serious fall injuries. *N Engl J Med*. 2020;383:129-140.
A21. Lamb SE, Bruce J, Hossain A, et al. Screening and intervention to prevent falls and fractures in older people. *N Engl J Med*. 2020;383:1848-1859.
A22. Bischoff-Ferrari HA, Vellas B, Rizzoli R, et al. Effect of vitamin D supplementation, omega-3 fatty acid supplementation, or a strength-training exercise program on clinical outcomes in older adults: the DO-HEALTH randomized clinical trial. *JAMA*. 2020;324:1855-1868.
A23. Appel LJ, Michos ED, Mitchell CM, et al. The effects of four doses of vitamin D supplements on falls in older adults: a response-adaptive, randomized clinical trial. *Ann Intern Med*. 2021;174:145-156.

V CLINICAL PHARMACOLOGY

25

PRINCIPLES OF DRUG THERAPY

ROBERT B. DIASIO

Depending on the conditions, a drug may produce different effects ranging from no effect to a desirable effect to an undesirable toxic effect. Clinicians must learn how to choose the correct drug dosage for different conditions to ensure effective and safe therapy. To do so, clinicians must understand pharmacokinetics—the movement of a drug over time through the body—and pharmacodynamics—the relationship between drug concentration and drug effect (Fig. 25-1), as well as drug interactions and adverse drug responses. Genomics is increasingly helpful both for individualizing therapy as well as in the design of new drugs.[1]

PHARMACOKINETIC PRINCIPLES

Administration

The most efficient and straightforward means of administering a drug into the systemic circulation is by intravenous injection of a bolus. With this route, the full amount of a drug is delivered into the systemic circulation almost immediately. The same dose also may be administered as an intravenous infusion over a longer period, thereby resulting in a decrease in the peak plasma concentration and an accompanying increase in the time the drug is present in the circulation. Many other routes of administration can be used, including sublingual, oral, transdermal, rectal, inhalational, subcutaneous, and intramuscular; each of these routes carries not only a potential delay in the time it takes the drug to enter the circulation but also the possibility that a large fraction of it will never reach the circulation.

Absorption

Absorption refers to the transfer of a drug from the site of administration to the systemic circulation. Many drugs cross a membrane barrier by passive diffusion and enter the systemic circulation. Because passive diffusion in this setting depends on the concentration of the solute at the membrane surface, the rate of drug absorption is affected by the concentration of free drug at the absorbing surface. Factors that influence the availability of free drug thus affect drug absorption from the administration site; this effect can be exploited to design medications that release a drug slowly into the circulation by prolonging drug absorption. With certain sustained-released oral preparations, the rate of dissolution of the drug in the gastrointestinal tract determines the rate at which the drug is absorbed (e.g., timed-release antihistamines). Similarly, a prolonged drug effect can be obtained by the use of transdermal medications (e.g., nitroglycerin) or intramuscular depot preparations (e.g., benzathine penicillin G).

First-Pass Effect

Some drugs that are administered orally are absorbed relatively efficiently into the portal circulation but are metabolized by the liver before they reach the systemic circulation. Because of this "first-pass" or "presystemic" effect, the oral route may be less suitable than other routes of administration for such drugs. A good example is nitroglycerin, which is well absorbed but efficiently metabolized during the first pass through the liver. However, the same drug can achieve adequate systemic levels when it is given sublingually or transdermally.

Bioavailability

The extent of absorption of a drug into the systemic circulation may be incomplete. The bioavailability of a particular drug is the fraction (F) of the total drug dose that ultimately reaches the systemic circulation from the site of administration. This fraction is calculated by dividing the amount of the drug dose that reaches the circulation from the administration site by the amount of the drug dose that would enter the systemic circulation after direct intravenous injection into the circulation (essentially the total dose). Bioavailability can range from 0, in which no drug reaches the systemic circulation, to 1.0, in which essentially all of the drug is absorbed. The bioavailability of a drug may vary in different formulations because the overall absorption differs. This variability is a concern with the increasing use of generic preparations.

Distribution

After delivery of a drug into the systemic circulation, either directly by intravenous injection or after absorption, the drug is transported throughout the body, initially to well-perfused tissues and later to areas that are less perfused. This distribution phase can be assessed best by plotting the drug's plasma concentration on a log scale versus time on a linear scale (Fig. 25-2). For an intravenously administered drug, for which absorption is not a factor, the initial phase—from immediately after administration through the rapid fall in concentration—represents the distribution phase, during which a drug rapidly disappears from the circulation and enters the tissues. This phase is followed by the elimination phase (see later), when drug in the plasma equilibrates with drug in the tissues. During this latter phase, the drug's plasma concentration is thought to be related to drug effect.

Volume of Distribution

The volume of distribution relates the amount of drug in the body to the concentration of drug in the plasma. It is calculated by dividing the dose that ultimately gets into the systemic circulation by the plasma concentration at time zero (C_{p0}):

$$\text{volume of distribution} = \text{dose}/C_{p0} \quad (1)$$

The C_{p0} can be calculated by extrapolating the elimination phase back to time zero (see Fig. 25-2). The volume of distribution is best considered the "apparent volume of distribution" because it represents the apparent volume

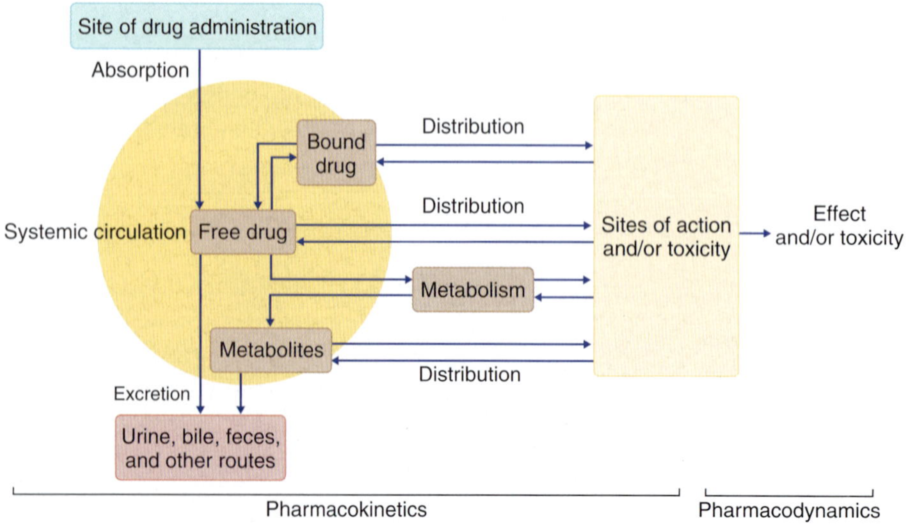

FIGURE 25-1. **Schematic of a drug's movement through the body, from the site of administration to production of a drug effect.** The relationship between pharmacokinetics and pharmacodynamics is shown.

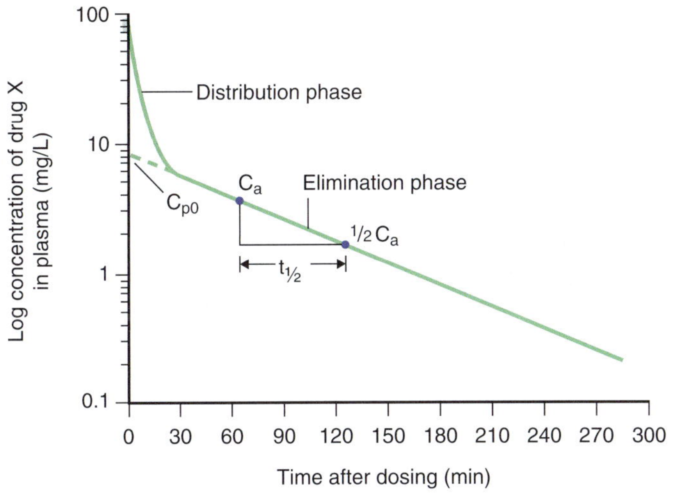

FIGURE 25-2. Representative drug concentration versus time plot used in pharmacokinetic studies. Concentration of drug is plotted with a logarithmic scale on the ordinate, and time is plotted with a linear scale on the abscissa. The resultant curve has two phases: the distribution phase, which is the initial portion of the plotted line when the concentration of drug decreases rapidly; and the later elimination phase, during which there is an exponential disappearance of drug from the plasma over time. The *dotted line* extrapolated from the elimination phase back to time zero is used to calculate plasma concentration at time zero (C_{p0}). During the elimination phase, the half-life ($t_{1/2}$) can be calculated as the time it takes to decrease the concentration by half (shown here as the time needed to decrease from concentration C_a to ½ C_a).

needed to contain the entire amount of the drug, assuming it is distributed throughout the body at the same concentration as in the plasma. Volume of distribution can vary widely for commonly used drugs (E-Table 25-1). Volume of distribution is useful for calculating a loading dose and appreciating how various changes can affect a drug's half-life.

Elimination

Drugs are removed from the body by two major mechanisms: hepatic elimination, in which drugs are metabolized in the liver and excreted through the biliary tract; and renal elimination, in which drugs are removed from the circulation by either glomerular filtration or tubular secretion. For most drugs, the rates of hepatic and renal elimination are proportional to its plasma concentration, a relationship that is often described as a "first-order" process. Two measurements, clearance and half-life, are used to evaluate elimination.

Clearance

The efficiency of elimination can be assessed by quantifying how fast the drug is cleared from the circulation. Drug clearance is a measure of the volume of plasma cleared of drug per unit of time. It is similar to the clinical measurement used to assess renal function—creatinine clearance, which is the volume of plasma from which creatinine is removed per minute. Total drug clearance (Cl_{tot}) is the rate of elimination by all processes (El_{tot}) divided by the plasma concentration of the drug (C_p):

$$Cl_{tot} = El_{tot}/C_p \tag{2}$$

Drugs may be cleared by several organs, but renal clearance and hepatic clearance are the two major mechanisms, so total drug clearance (Cl_{tot}) for most drugs is essentially the sum of renal clearance and hepatic clearance:

$$Cl_{tot} = Cl_{Ren} + Cl_{Hep} \tag{3}$$

Some drugs have clearances as low as <3 mL/minute, whereas aspirin is cleared at greater than 500 mL/minute. Aminoglycosides are cleared almost entirely by the kidneys, whereas aspirin, carbamazepine, and phenytoin are cleared less than 5% by the kidneys.

Drug clearance is affected by several factors, including blood flow through the organ of clearance, protein binding to the drug, and activity of the clearance processes in the organs of elimination (e.g., glomerular filtration rate and tubular secretion in the kidney, enzyme activity in the liver). Drug clearance is not affected by the volume of distribution of drug throughout the body because clearance mechanisms act only on drug in the circulation.

Half-Life

The amount of time needed to eliminate a drug from the body depends on the clearance and the volume of distribution. The first-order elimination constant (K_e) represents the proportion of the apparent volume of distribution that is cleared of drug per unit of time during the drug's exponential disappearance from the plasma over time (elimination phase):

$$K_e = Cl/\text{volume of distribution} \tag{4}$$

The value of this constant for a particular drug can be determined by plotting drug concentration versus time on a log-linear plot (see Fig. 25-2) and measuring the slope of the straight line obtained during the exponential (elimination) phase.

The time needed to eliminate the drug is best described by its half-life ($t_{1/2}$), which is the time required during the elimination phase (see Fig. 25-2) for the plasma concentration of the drug to be decreased by half. Mathematically, the half-life is equal to the natural logarithm of 2 (representing a reduction of drug concentration to half) divided by K_e. Substituting for K_e from Equation 4 and calculating the natural logarithm of 2, the half-life can be represented by the following equation:

$$t_{1/2} = 0.693\ \text{volume of distribution}/Cl \tag{5}$$

From this equation, one can predict that at any given clearance, as the volume of distribution increases, the half-life increases. Similarly, at a given volume of distribution, the half-life decreases as the clearance increases. Because a disease may affect volume of distribution and clearance differently, the half-life may increase, decrease, or not change much at all.

The half-life is useful to predict how long it takes for a drug to be eliminated from the body. For any drug that has a first-order elimination, one would expect that by the end of the first half-life, the drug would be reduced to 50%; by the end of the second half-life, to 25%; by the end of the third half-life, to 12.5%; by the end of the fourth half-life, to 6.25%; and by the end of the fifth half-life, to 3.125%. In general, a drug can be considered essentially eliminated after five half-lives, when less than 5% of the effective concentration remains.

CLINICAL APPLICATION OF PHARMACOKINETIC PRINCIPLES

Using a Loading Dose

To attain a desired therapeutic concentration rapidly, a loading dose is often used. In determining the amount of drug to be given, the clinician must consider the volume of distribution within the body into which the drug will be distributed.

$$\text{Loading dose} = \text{desired concentration} \times \text{volume of distribution} \tag{6}$$

Rapid administration of an entire loading dose may produce an initially high peak concentration that results in toxicity. This problem can be avoided either by administering the loading dose as a divided dose, by administering the drug as an infusion (with an intravenous drug), or by taking advantage of the slower access to the circulation from various other routes (e.g., oral dosing). For example, phenytoin may require a loading dose to achieve a therapeutic level (10 to 20 mg/L) rapidly. Because the volume of distribution for phenytoin is approximately 0.6 L/kg, the loading dose (see Equation 6) is 420 mg/L to attain a minimally therapeutic level of 10 to 20 mg/L in a 70-kg adult. However, administration of 420 mg of phenytoin by intravenous bolus carries the risk for cardiac arrest and death. By taking advantage of the reduced bioavailability (F = 0.8) and slow absorption of oral phenytoin, the loading dose can be administered safely as an oral dose of 500 mg.

The equation for the loading dose can also be used to calculate the dose needed to "boost" an inadequate blood level of drug to a desired therapeutic range. If therapeutic monitoring (see later under Drug Monitoring as a Guide to Therapy) shows that the phenytoin level is 5 mg/L and the desired level is 15 mg/L, it is necessary to multiply the difference needed to achieve the desired concentration (15 mg/L) by the volume of distribution (0.6 L/kg) to determine the dose (in mg/kg) necessary to achieve this drug level. In a 70-kg individual, 0.6 mg/kg is multiplied by 70 kg to obtain the calculated loading dose (420 mg) that can be administered safely. A 500-mg oral dose with a bioavailability of less than 1 (e.g., F = 0.8) would deliver to the systemic circulation the approximate amount needed and avoid the risks associated with rapid intravenous administration.

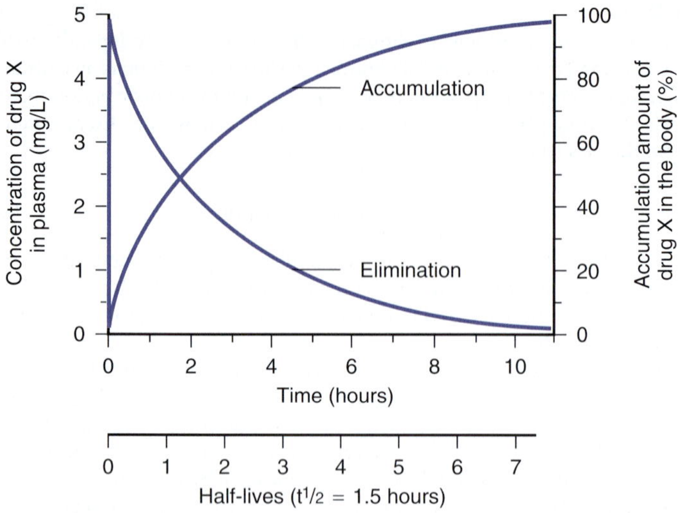

FIGURE 25-3. Representative plot of the mirror-image relationship between the elimination of drug (after drug is discontinued) and the accumulation of drug (during infusion). The plot shows the concentration on the left *y*-axis and time on the upper *x*-axis. The lower *x*-axis shows the time in half-lives, and the *y*-axis on the right shows the percentage of drug in the body. After five half-lives, elimination is essentially complete, and accumulation is essentially at a steady state.

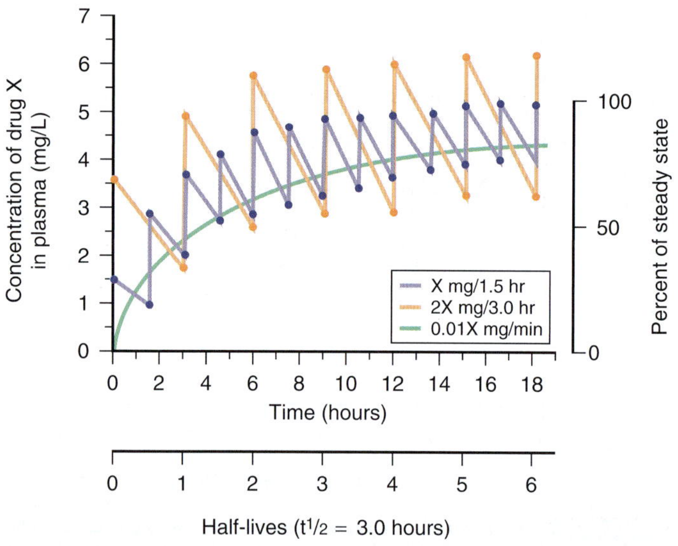

FIGURE 25-4. Accumulation of drug over time, approaching a steady state. Time is depicted in hours (upper *x*-axis) and half-lives (lower *x*-axis, showing that steady state is reached in approximately five half-lives). The *green line* depicts the pattern produced by an infusion of a hypothetical drug at a dose of 0.01X. The *orange line* shows the pattern resulting from oral administration of a 2X dose every 3 hours, and the *blue line* represents the pattern produced by oral administration of dose X every 1.5 hours.

Determining Drug Accumulation

Continuing to administer a drug, either as a prolonged infusion or as repeated doses, results in accumulation until the drug level reaches a steady state at which plasma and tissue levels remain constant because the amount of drug being administered equals the amount being eliminated. The elimination half-life determines not only the time course of drug elimination but also the time course of drug accumulation (Fig. 25-3). As with drug elimination, five half-lives is the approximate time needed to reach steady state during drug accumulation. Whereas drugs with short half-lives accumulate rapidly, drugs with long half-lives require a longer time to accumulate, thereby potentially delaying the achievement of therapeutic levels. For drugs with long half-lives, a loading dose may be needed to obtain rapid drug accumulation and a more rapid therapeutic effect.

With each change in drug dose or rate of infusion, a change in steady state occurs. Although it is not obvious for drugs with short half-lives, the effects of dose adjustments for drugs with longer half-lives are delayed, and the time varies directly with the drug's half-life.

Using a Maintenance Dose

After steady state is reached in approximately five half-lives, with either a continuous infusion or intermittent doses, the rate of drug administered equals the rate of drug eliminated. For an intravenous drug, the administration rate is the infusion rate (I); for a drug administered by another route (e.g., orally), the administration rate is the dose per unit of time (D/t). Equation 7 shows that the rate of elimination (total) equals $Cl_{tot} \times C_p$. With an intravenously administered drug, because the infusion rate equals the elimination rate at steady state, it follows that

$$I = Cl_{tot} \times C_p \quad (7)$$

Similarly, with an orally administered drug, the dose administered per unit of time equals the elimination rate at steady state, with the result that

$$D/t = Cl_{tot} \times C_p \quad (8)$$

These equations show the direct relationship between the dose and the resultant plasma concentration at steady state. This relationship is independent of the distribution of the drug. By use of these equations, it is possible to determine the infusion rate or the interval and dose needed to achieve and maintain a specified drug concentration in the plasma.

When a drug is administered intermittently, it approaches steady-state concentration over time, with a pattern similar to that observed with continuous infusion (Fig. 25-4). With intermittent drug administration, such as with an oral dose, the drug concentration fluctuates; the magnitude of fluctuation between the peak and trough concentrations depends on the interval of administration, drug half-life, absorption characteristics, and site of administration. As the intervals decrease below the half-life, the fluctuation decreases and approaches the curve produced by an intravenous infusion. With timed-release formulations, orally administered drugs reach peak concentration more slowly but persist longer in the plasma.

Decreasing the Drug Level

At times, it may be necessary to decrease the plasma drug level while maintaining therapy (e.g., when signs of toxicity become apparent or a potentially dangerously high concentration of drug is noted; see later). The most effective and rapid response is to discontinue the drug; the length of time for which the drug is discontinued is determined by the estimated half-life of the drug in the specific patient. After discontinuation of the drug for a time based on its half-life, the total clearance (Cl_{tot}) of the drug can be used to determine what infusion rate (I, Equation 7) or dose and interval (D/t, Equation 8) must be used to achieve the new desired concentration (C_p).

Effect of Dose Increases on Elimination Kinetics

Not all drugs behave the same when the dose is increased. For most drugs, elimination follows first-order or linear kinetics; the amount of drug eliminated is directly proportional to the concentration of drug in the plasma (Fig. 25-5A). However, a few drugs have a different pattern of elimination. For example, ethanol, phenytoin, and aspirin have dose-dependent, nonlinear saturation kinetics. As the dose of drug increases and the concentration of drug in the plasma rises, the relative amount of drug being eliminated falls (i.e., the clearance decreases) until the rate of drug metabolism is at its maximum. At this point, drug elimination is said to be zero order, and the drug concentration in plasma starts to increase much more (no longer linearly) with each subsequent increase in dose (Fig. 25-5B).

DRUG MONITORING AS A GUIDE TO THERAPY

Although published pharmacokinetic data (usually population averages) are useful to determine initial drug dosing, modification of the dose may be needed in an individual patient. For some drugs (e.g., certain antihypertensive agents or anticoagulants), the therapeutic effects (e.g., blood pressure or coagulation) can be quantified easily over a range of concentrations, thereby permitting adequate drug adjustment. For many other drugs (e.g., some antiarrhythmic or antiseizure medications), therapeutic effects over a range of concentrations are not readily detectable. With these drugs, the plasma concentration may provide further guidance in optimizing therapy if the plasma concentration of the drug is a reflection of its concentration at the site of action and the drug effects are reversible. A third, much smaller group of drugs produces irreversible effects (e.g., aspirin inhibition of platelet aggregation). With these drugs, plasma drug concentration does not correlate with drug effect, and drug monitoring is not useful.

To use drug concentration as a guide to therapy, the range of effective but safe concentrations, or the *therapeutic window*, is usually determined from a dose-response curve generated from a population of patients who have been examined closely for therapeutic and toxic effects (Fig. 25-6). The *therapeutic*

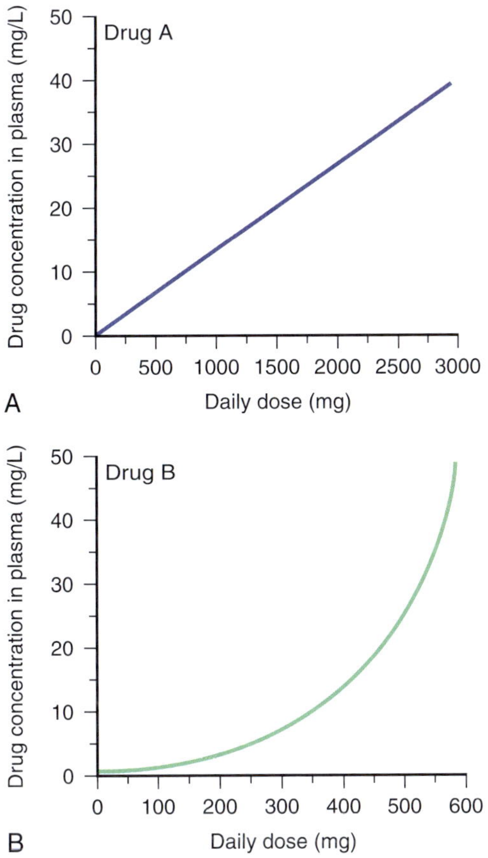

FIGURE 25-5. **Effect of increasing the dose of a drug on its serum concentration. A, Drug A follows first-order or linear kinetics. B, Drug B follows zero-order or nonlinear (or saturable) kinetics.**

index, which is a useful measure of drug toxicity, is calculated by dividing the 50% value from the toxicity curve by the 50% value from the efficacy curve. Because these curves are generated from population data, the values may not be applicable to all individuals.

Drug monitoring is especially useful when a drug is used to treat a serious or life-threatening disease and it is essential to avoid inadequate doses (because a therapeutic effect is often critical) as well as excessive doses (because of the risk for toxicity). In contrast, it is not necessary to assay levels of drugs used to treat noncritical diseases (when inadequate treatment is not a serious problem) or for which the therapeutic index is large (when relative overtreatment is not likely to produce toxicity).

Problems with Interpreting Drug Concentration

The time of blood collection, perhaps more than any other factor, contributes to the misinterpretation of drug levels. If sampling is performed too early, while the drug is still in the distribution phase, the drug level may be high and not reflect drug concentration at the site of action. It is therefore important to sample after the distribution phase.

For many drugs administered intermittently, such as intravenous antibiotics (e.g., vancomycin), a trough level, which is obtained immediately before the next dose is administered, is most useful for making decisions about dose adjustments. For drugs administered by infusion or intermittently at short intervals, the best time to draw blood is during steady state.

Protein binding is another major factor that contributes to the misinterpretation of drug levels. Free drug (not bound to protein and able to equilibrate with tissues and to interact with the site of action) is the critical drug concentration when therapeutic decisions are being made. Many drugs are tightly bound to plasma protein, however. Many commonly used drugs (e.g., aspirin, carbamazepine, and phenytoin), have protein binding of more than 75%, so assessment of the total drug level may not be helpful. Unfortunately, assessment of the "true" free drug concentration also may be inaccurate, particularly if the fraction of drug bound to protein varies. In addition, the drug's binding may be decreased by disease or by other drugs, thereby leading to increased unbound drug levels that alter the interpretation of the measured drug concentrations. Kidney and liver disease can change the binding of certain drugs

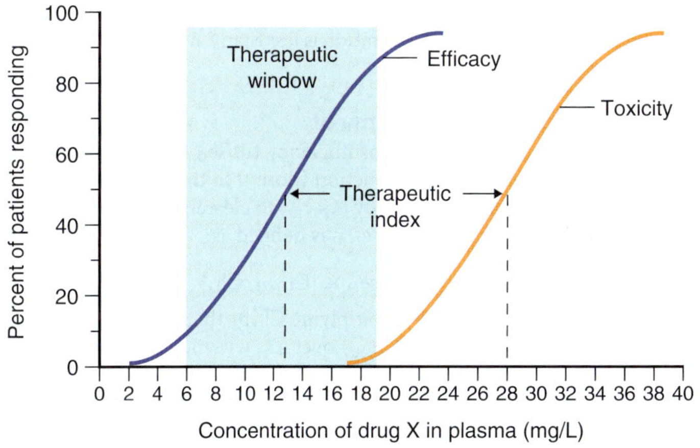

FIGURE 25-6. **Pattern produced in a dose-response population study in which both effect and toxicity are measured. The therapeutic window is shown as the range of therapeutically effective concentrations, which includes most of the efficacy curve and less than 10% of the toxicity curve. The therapeutic index is calculated by dividing the 50% value on the toxicity curve by the 50% value on the efficacy curve.**

(e.g., phenytoin) to protein because of a decrease in protein (e.g., decreased albumin, as in nephrotic syndrome or liver disease) or as a result of competition for protein binding by endogenously produced substances (e.g., uremia in kidney disease, hyperbilirubinemia in liver disease). Similarly, other drugs being administered may compete for binding to protein. A major problem secondary to these changes in protein binding is that free drug is not typically measured in many of the common drug assays used by clinical laboratories. Lastly, changes in drug binding to protein can affect the pharmacokinetics of the drug; the volume of distribution increases as protein binding decreases.

The usefulness of a drug assay is also limited by physiologic changes that may alter the response at a particular drug concentration. An example is the response produced by increasing levels of phenytoin in the presence of reduced protein binding (e.g., with hypoalbuminemia or renal impairment), where changes in phenytoin's blood concentration will be exaggerated.

Tolerance, which is a reduced response to a given concentration of drug with continued use, is commonly observed with the continued use of opioids (e.g., in terminal cancer patients). After long-term administration, the same drug concentration is no longer associated with the same pain relief. Positive (placebo) or negative (nocebo) effects may also be associated with many drugs and may mimic their known benefits or toxicities.[2]

ADJUSTMENTS OF DRUG DOSE WITH DISEASE

Kidney Disease

The major questions to be answered when determining whether a drug dosage needs to be adjusted in the setting of kidney disease are: is the drug primarily excreted through the kidneys, and are increased drug levels likely to be associated with toxicity? If the answer to both questions is yes, a drug is likely to accumulate and become toxic as renal clearance decreases unless the drug dose is reduced.

To obtain the desired concentration over time in the presence of decreased clearance, adjustments can be made by decreasing the dose while maintaining the dose interval, maintaining the dose but increasing the interval between doses, or a combination of both (E-Table 25-2). With these adjustments, it may be possible to achieve an average concentration similar to that obtained with normal renal function, but there may be concomitant marked changes in the magnitude of peak and trough values. In choosing the type of drug adjustment, the clinician should consider not only the therapeutic index of the drug but also whether an effective concentration must be achieved quickly and maintained within a narrow range (i.e., maintaining an average drug concentration and avoiding trough levels at which the drug is ineffective); and whether toxicity is associated with elevated (i.e., peak) drug concentrations.

Renal drug clearance correlates with creatinine clearance (whether the drug uses glomerular filtration or tubular secretion), so any adjustment of drug dose in kidney disease can use the creatinine clearance to estimate the dose needed. The creatinine clearance (Cl_{cr}), which is used as an estimate of glomerular filtration rate, may be calculated directly from the serum creatinine concentration by the following equation:

$$Cl_{cr} = [(140 - \text{age}) \times \text{weight (kg)}] / [72 \times \text{serumcreatinine (mg/dL)}] \qquad (9)$$

The calculated creatinine clearance should be multiplied by 0.85 for females when the serum creatinine concentration is less than 5 mg/dL and renal function is not rapidly changing.

Using Clearance for Dose Adjustment

The dose of a drug used in renal insufficiency ($dose_{D\text{-}RI}$) is proportional to the dose used with normal renal function ($dose_D$) in the same ratio as clearance of the drug in renal insufficiency ($Cl_{D\text{-}RI}$) to clearance with normal renal function (Cl_D). By rearranging, $dose_{D\text{-}RI}$ is defined as:

$$Dose_{D\text{-}RI} = dose_D \times [Cl_{D\text{-}RI}/Cl_D] \quad (10)$$

The $Cl_{D\text{-}RI}$ can be estimated by multiplying Cl_D by the ratio of the creatinine clearance in renal insufficiency ($Cl_{cr\text{-}RI}$) over Cl_{cr} with normal renal function:

$$Cl_{D\text{-}RI} = Cl_D \times [Cl_{cr\text{-}RI}/Cl_{cr}] \quad (11)$$

As shown in Equation 3, total clearance is the sum of clearance by renal and nonrenal (typically hepatic) mechanisms. Any nonrenal clearance is assumed to remain normal, and only the renal clearance is adjusted, with total clearance being reduced only to the extent that renal clearance is reduced. The dose may be calculated from the total (adjusted) clearance and the desired plasma concentration by either Equation 7 or Equation 8.

However, the calculated dose is only an initial guide to the needed dose. By monitoring the drug response or the plasma drug concentration at various times after initial dosing, further dose adjustments can be made as necessary. From a practical perspective, most clinical dose adjustments in the presence of renal dysfunction can be guided by published tables based on changes in glomerular filtration rate and the effectiveness of dialysis in removing the drug. Computerized decision support systems are particularly effective in guiding medication dosing for inpatients with renal insufficiency.

Loading Dose in Renal Insufficiency

For drugs that are typically administered with a loading dose in patients with normal renal function, the same approach can be used in patients with renal insufficiency to ensure that the desired concentration is achieved rapidly. For drugs typically administered without a loading dose, the prolonged half-life that results from renal insufficiency may delay the time required to reach a steady state. In this setting, a loading dose (equal to the amount needed to reach steady state with normal renal function) should be followed by lower or less frequent maintenance doses.

Liver Disease

Although many drugs are biotransformed in the liver, no useful laboratory test can guide dose adjustments. If the liver's capacity to produce protein (reflected by a low albumin concentration and prolonged prothrombin time) is reduced significantly, the clearance of drugs metabolized by the cytochrome P-450 enzymes is probably reduced as well.

One special situation that can develop with chronic liver disease and may require dose adjustment is portal hypertension with a portacaval shunt (Chapter 139). In this situation, hepatic blood flow decreases and hepatic clearance also decreases, thereby reducing the first-pass effect and resulting in higher concentrations of drug reaching the systemic circulation. Drugs with a large hepatic extraction that are typically administered orally (e.g., propranolol to lower portal vein pressure) may appear in the systemic circulation at higher, potentially toxic concentrations.

Hemodynamic Diseases

Decreased cardiac output and hypotensive conditions lead to decreased perfusion of the organs, including those responsible for eliminating drugs. The drug dose can be adjusted for decreased renal perfusion by the use of creatinine clearance. The effect of decreased hepatic blood flow on pharmacokinetics is more difficult to assess. For drugs that have a high hepatic extraction (e.g., lidocaine), decreased hepatic blood flow suggests a need for dose reduction.

Altered hemodynamics also may affect the distribution of selected drugs. Drugs that have a relatively large volume of distribution (e.g., lidocaine) may be affected by conditions leading to hypotension, such as shock, thereby resulting in a decrease in the apparent volume of distribution and a need to reduce the loading dose to avoid potentially toxic drug levels.

In general, in the setting of severely compromised hemodynamics, it is advisable to be conservative and to avoid potentially toxic loading and maintenance doses. Drug levels and the clinical status should be monitored closely, and drug doses should be adjusted as necessary.

TABLE 25-1 GENERAL RECOMMENDATIONS FOR DRUG USE IN ELDERLY PATIENTS

- Clearance of drugs eliminated by the kidneys may be reduced by 50%.
- Drugs eliminated primarily by the liver typically do not require dose adjustments for age, except for drugs with high hepatic clearances, which may be affected by the age-related decrease in hepatic blood flow.
- Because of the potential for increased target organ sensitivity in elderly people, only the lowest effective dose should be used.
- Frequent reviews of the patient's drug history should be conducted, including both prescription and over-the-counter medications, keeping in mind the increased potential risk for drug interactions and adverse drug responses.

APPROACH TO DRUG OVERDOSE

The pharmacokinetic principles discussed earlier can be used to determine the best approach for drug removal in the setting of a drug overdose (Chapter 96), particularly if hemodialysis or hemoperfusion remove a substantial fraction of the total body load of drug. For drugs with a large volume of distribution (e.g., warfarin), only a small amount can be removed because clearance affects only the amount of drug present in the plasma, and a large portion of the drug is outside the plasma compartment. Similarly, for a drug with high clearance value (e.g., metformin), hemoperfusion may increase the overall clearance only minimally and is not indicated.

DRUG USE IN ELDERLY PATIENTS

Administering drugs to elderly patients (Chapter 24) is perhaps the most challenging area of adult therapeutics because of several factors: the increasing likelihood of multiple illnesses, often with multisystemic involvement; the need for these patients to take multiple drugs (often prescribed by different physicians); and the increasing probability of altered pharmacokinetics and pharmacodynamics. These factors together contribute to a significantly increased frequency of drug interactions and adverse drug responses in this group of patients (Table 25-1).

Pharmacokinetic Changes with Age

Pharmacokinetic changes can be secondary to the general physiologic effects of aging, such as alteration in body composition, or to specific changes in pharmacokinetically important organs (e.g., kidneys, liver). The distribution of drugs tends to change dramatically with age, mainly because of changes in body composition. Most typical is the increase in total body fat, with the accompanying decrease in lean body mass and total body water. The concentration of plasma proteins may also change; in particular, the albumin level may decrease as the liver ages. For water-soluble drugs that are not bound to plasma proteins, the apparent volume of distribution is reduced; in contrast, for lipid-soluble drugs, the volume of distribution is increased. Changes in metabolism also accompany aging, but these changes alone do not typically account for altered pharmacokinetics.

The clearance of many drugs is decreased in the elderly because cardiac output and blood flow to the kidneys and liver may be decreased. Glomerular filtration rate may be reduced by 50%. Hepatic elimination of drugs is less affected, except for drugs with a high hepatic clearance (e.g., lidocaine). The elimination half-life of many drugs is increased with aging as a consequence of a larger apparent volume of distribution and a decreased hepatic or renal clearance (see Equation 5).

Pharmacodynamic Changes with Age

Pharmacodynamic changes are a result of changes in the responsiveness of the target organ. Elderly individuals typically require lower drug doses, even if the pharmacokinetics are little changed. For example, antianxiety drugs and drugs from the sedative-hypnotic class may produce increased central nervous system depression in elderly patients at concentrations that are well tolerated in younger adults.

INTERACTIONS AMONG DRUGS

Because patients are typically treated with multiple agents, even for a single disease, the possibilities for drug interactions are great. Many clinically important drug interactions typically involve a drug with a low therapeutic index (e.g., warfarin) and an easily detectable pharmacologic effect (e.g., bleeding), such that a small increase in the amount of drug produces a significant effect (toxicity).

It is difficult to assess the prevalence of drug interactions in either the inpatient or the ambulatory setting, particularly because no formal and comprehensive surveillance mechanism is available. However, the risk for drug interactions seems to be increasing, particularly for critically ill, hospitalized patients who are frequently taking more than 10 medications.[3]

There are basically two types of drug interaction: pharmacokinetic drug interactions, caused by a change in the amount of drug or active metabolite at the site of action; and pharmacodynamic drug interactions (without a change in pharmacokinetics), caused by a change in drug effect.

Pharmacokinetic Drug Interactions

Less Drug at the Site of Action

Decreased Absorption

The gastrointestinal lumen is perhaps the best example of an area where drug interactions can result in decreased drug absorption. Some commonly used drugs can illustrate this type of interaction. For many drugs, a physicochemical interaction prevents the drug from being absorbed. For example, metal ions (e.g., aluminum, calcium, and magnesium in antacids and iron in supplements to treat iron deficiency) form insoluble complexes with tetracyclines and can act as chelating agents. Other commonly used medications that decrease absorption include kaolin-pectin suspensions, which are used to treat diarrhea and can significantly inhibit the absorption of coadministered drugs.

Drugs that are particularly susceptible to changes in pH may have decreased absorption when they are administered with other drugs that either affect gastric acidity or alter the extent of exposure to low pH. Proton pump inhibitors or histamine-2 receptor antagonists may elevate gastric pH, which can inhibit the dissolution and subsequent absorption of drugs that are weak bases (e.g., ketoconazole). Medications that delay gastric emptying (e.g., belladonna alkaloids) can increase the degradation of a coadministered acid-labile drug (e.g., levodopa), thereby resulting in decreased absorption.

Altered Distribution

Drugs that use the same active transport process to reach their site of action can compete at the level of transport, thereby resulting in lower levels of drug reaching that site. Examples of this type of interaction include the interaction of phenothiazines (e.g., chlorpromazine) with tricyclic antidepressants (e.g., amitriptyline).

Increased Metabolism

Many drugs (e.g., phenytoin, ethanol, griseofulvin, rifampin) and toxic compounds (e.g., cigarette smoke, certain chlorinated hydrocarbons) can increase the hepatic metabolism of other drugs (e.g., corticosteroids, cyclophosphamide, cyclosporine, certain β-adrenergic blockers, theophylline, warfarin) by inducing the activity of the cytochrome P-450 super family of monooxygenase enzyme (see medicine.iupui.edu/clinpharm/ddis/ for more information).

More Drug at the Site of Action

Increased Absorption

Any drug that increases the rate of gastric emptying (e.g., metoclopramide) can potentially increase the absorption of acid-unstable drugs. Also, drugs that decrease intestinal motility (e.g., anticholinergics) may increase the absorption of drugs that are relatively poorly absorbed (e.g., metformin) by increasing the drug's contact time with the absorbing surface.

Altered Distribution

Drugs bound to protein are limited in their distribution (particularly at the site of action) and are not available for metabolism or excretion. Drugs can compete with each other for binding to plasma proteins, resulting in drug interactions. Phenytoin and warfarin are both greater than 90% bound to protein. When both are coadministered, phenytoin can displace warfarin, thereby leading to an increased anticoagulant effect and possible bleeding.

Decreased Metabolism

One of the most impressive drug interactions is produced when one drug inhibits the metabolism of another, thereby leading to the second drug's accumulation and a significant risk for toxicity. An example of this type of interaction occurs when 6-mercaptopurine, an antileukemic drug with a low therapeutic index, is used with allopurinol, often administered to control hyperuricemia. The interaction may result in potentially life-threatening toxicity.

Some drugs can inhibit the metabolism of many other drugs because many drugs share the same metabolic pathway. This consideration is particularly relevant for drugs that share CYP-450 pathways. It is estimated that CYP2D6 accounts for the metabolism of approximately 25% of all currently prescribed drugs, including antidepressants, neuroleptics, β-blockers, opioids, antiemetics, antiarrhythmics, and even some cancer chemotherapy drugs. Some commonly used drugs such as cimetidine can inhibit the metabolism of drugs from several different classes, such as diazepam, imipramine, lidocaine, propranolol, theophylline, and warfarin. Agents such as amiodarone inhibit the metabolism of calcium-channel blockers, phenytoin, and warfarin. Of particular importance with amiodarone is its half-life of 1 to 2 months; it continues to inhibit drug metabolism for several months after it has been discontinued.

Other drugs are notable because their metabolism is inhibited by a variety of different drugs. The metabolism of warfarin is inhibited not only by cimetidine and amiodarone but also by many other drugs, including alcohol, allopurinol, disulfiram, metronidazole, phenylbutazone, sulfinpyrazone, and trimethoprim-sulfamethoxazole. Similarly, the metabolism of phenytoin is inhibited by chloramphenicol, clofibrate, disulfiram, isoniazid (slow acetylators; see Table 25-3), phenylbutazone, and valproic acid.

Although most of these examples involve enzymes that metabolize the drug within the liver, drug-metabolizing enzymes outside the liver also may be affected by certain drugs. Perhaps the best-known example is monoamine oxidase, which can be affected by nonspecific monoamine oxidase inhibitors, thereby resulting in the accumulation of catecholamines at multiple sites after their release in response to the eating of tyramine-containing foods such as aged cheese, aged or cured meats, and any spoiled meat, poultry, or fish.

Decreased Excretion

Drugs can compete for the active transporters present in the kidney. Most of these interactions involve the acid transporters. The best-known interaction is probenecid's inhibition of penicillin transport, thereby leading to decreased penicillin clearance and thus higher plasma levels, an interaction that was helpful when penicillin was in short supply. A similar inhibitory effect on the renal excretion of methotrexate can be produced by salicylates, phenylbutazone, and probenecid. The active transport of basic drugs (e.g., metformin and dofetilide) can also be inhibited by other drugs (e.g., cimetidine).

Pharmacodynamic Drug Interactions

With pharmacodynamic interactions, drugs interact at the level of the receptor (target) or may produce additive effects by acting at separate sites on cells. An example of the first is the interaction of a β-blocker with epinephrine, which blocks β-adrenergic receptors; as a result, the α-adrenergic effects of epinephrine are unopposed. This undesirable interaction can result in severe hypertension. The additive effects of drugs are exemplified by aspirin, which can increase the bleeding time by acting on platelets, and direct-acting oral anticoagulants, which affect clotting (Chapter 70). The result is an increased risk for hemorrhage. Similarly, β-adrenergic blockers and calcium-channel blockers have additive negative inotropic effects when they are coadministered.

DIAGNOSIS AND PREVENTION OF DRUG INTERACTIONS

For a drug interaction to be recognized, the index of suspicion must be high, particularly whenever multiple drugs are used together. Several clinical settings should raise concern about the possibility of drug interactions and alert the clinician as to how to avoid them (Table 25-2). Because of the ever-increasing list of known and suspected drug interactions, it is impossible for a clinician to remember all or even many of the possible interactions, so it is best to consult one of a number of websites (e.g., www.drugs.com/drug_interactions.html and reference.medscape.com/drug-interactionchecker) that maintain current information on drug interactions.

Another type of drug interaction is between components of food (e.g., grapefruit juice) or natural products (e.g., herbs) and drugs. By inhibiting the intestinal CYP-450 3A4 enzyme system, grapefruit juice can raise levels of drugs metabolized by this pathway (e.g., saquinavir, cyclosporine, verapamil) and result in toxicity or adverse drug effects. It is now recognized that a number of foods and herbs can affect drug-metabolizing enzymes, such as the CYP-450s (see medicine.iupui.edu/clinpharm/ddis/).

ADVERSE REACTIONS TO DRUGS

An adverse drug response is an undesired effect produced by a drug at standard doses, which typically necessitates reducing or stopping the suspected agent and may require treatment of the noxious effect produced. Further harm may occur with continued or future therapy with the drug.

EPIDEMIOLOGY

The financial impact of adverse drug responses is estimated to be more than $100 billion per year. The actual incidence of adverse drug responses is difficult to quantify because many cases are either not recognized or not

TABLE 25-2 HIGH-RISK SITUATIONS THAT RAISE CONCERNS ABOUT POSSIBLE DRUG INTERACTIONS AND HOW TO PREVENT THEM

HIGH-RISK SITUATIONS

- The use of any drug with a low therapeutic index (e.g., anticoagulant agents, antiarrhythmic agents, anticonvulsant agents, lithium carbonate, oral hypoglycemic agents).
- As the number of drugs being used concurrently increases, the risk for drug interactions disproportionately increases, particularly with more than 10 drugs.
- Critically ill patients who have multisystemic disease with compromised renal, hepatic, cardiac, or pulmonary function.
- Patients who have the acquired immunodeficiency syndrome or an immunocompromised state.
- Patients with various behavioral and psychiatric disorders (e.g., patients who take many prescription drugs as well as illicit drugs and alcohol).

STEPS CAN BE TAKEN TO PREVENT DRUG INTERACTIONS

- When taking the medical history, document all drugs the patient is taking (and has recently taken), including prescription, over-the-counter, and other addictive drugs.
- Minimize the number of drugs being taken by frequently reviewing the patient's drug list to ensure that each drug continues to be needed.
- Have a high degree of suspicion when medications that have a low therapeutic index and are known to have a high risk for drug interactions are used.
- Be especially alert in high-risk clinical settings, such as occur with critically ill patients.
- Consider adverse drug interactions in the differential diagnosis whenever any change occurs in a patient's course.

reported. The incidence may approach 20% for outpatients (even higher for patients taking more than 15 drugs) and 2 to 7% for inpatients. The incidence of adverse drug responses increases exponentially with more than four drugs. Meta-analyses of several prospective studies suggest that adverse drug responses are now the fourth leading cause of death in hospitalized patients. Each year, adverse drug events cause an estimated four emergency department visits per 1000 individuals in the United States, with an estimated 100,000 drug-related emergency hospitalizations just in patients older than age 65 years. The most common drug classes implicated are anticoagulants, antibiotics, diabetes drugs, and opioid analgesics.[4] The incidence of adverse drug responses is likely to increase because of more prescribed and over-the-counter medications being used. Electronic medical records have the potential to predict adverse drug events and hopefully to prevent them.[5,6]

PATHOBIOLOGY

Most adverse drug responses are caused by an exaggerated (but predictable) pharmacologic effect of the drug or by a toxic or immunologic effect of the drug or a metabolite (not typically expected).

Predictable Toxic Responses to Drugs

Exaggerated drug responses that cause adverse drug effects may be due to any condition, including genetic factors,[7] that alter pharmacokinetics or pharmacodynamics. Molecular changes in the genes coding for drug-metabolizing enzymes include autosomal recessive polymorphisms associated with the debrisoquine-sparteine, *N*-acetylation, and mephenytoin types or classes of drugs (Table 25-3). Individuals with autosomal recessive genes are typically "poor metabolizers," with potentially altered pharmacokinetics that result in elevated plasma drug concentrations and can lead to toxicity. For example, the variability of response to warfarin (Chapter 70) is now understood to be due to single-nucleotide polymorphisms in the cytochrome P-450 2C9 (*CYP2C9*) and vitamin K epoxide reductase (*VKOR*) genes.

A particularly impressive example occurs with certain cancer chemotherapeutic agents that have a relatively narrow therapeutic window and the potential to produce severe cytotoxicity (e.g., deficiency in dihydropyrimidine dehydrogenase activity can result in life-threatening toxicity after the administration of 5-fluorouracil). These defects typically are not recognized until the patient is given the drug. They are often described as "pharmacogenetic" syndromes.

Other genetic alterations do not affect metabolism specifically and do not produce a range of quantitative changes. These defects can produce "qualitative" defects and are often associated with structural defects. The classic example is glucose-6-phosphate dehydrogenase. Individuals who are deficient in this enzyme cannot tolerate the oxidative stress produced by some drugs, thereby leading to hemolysis (Chapter 147). Drugs that can produce this clinical picture include aspirin, nitrofurantoin, primaquine, probenecid, quinine, sulfonamides, sulfones, and vitamin K. Another similar defect is deficiency of methemoglobin reductase, which results in an inability to maintain iron in hemoglobin in the ferrous state, causing methemoglobinemia (Chapter 144) after exposure to oxidizing drugs such as nitrites, sulfonamides, and sulfones.

Unpredictable Toxic Responses to Drugs

Other toxic or immunologic adverse drug responses are not predictable and are not obviously due to an increase in drug concentration (pharmacokinetic) or drug effect (pharmacodynamic). Unpredictable toxic responses include direct reactions between a drug and a specific organ (e.g., platinum-containing drugs, such as cisplatin, can produce direct toxicity in the kidney and the eighth cranial nerve, and a wide range of drugs can cause liver injury [Chapter 136]). With other drugs, metabolism to an active intermediate must occur first. With a standard dose of acetaminophen, no untoward effects occur because the relatively small amount of reactive metabolite formed by oxidative metabolism is detoxified rapidly by reduced glutathione. In the presence of an overdose (Chapter 96), the glutathione is depleted, and the remaining reactive metabolite can damage the liver.

Immunologic reactions to drugs are generally not produced by the drug alone. Similar to other low-molecular-weight compounds (<1000 D), they are typically not antigenic themselves. When a drug or reactive metabolite combines with a protein to form a drug-protein complex, it can become antigenic, capable of eliciting an immune response.

Perhaps the most impressive form of drug allergy (Chapter 234) is anaphylaxis (Chapter 233), which is due to an immunoglobulin E–mediated hypersensitivity. Many drugs from different classes have been shown to produce this type of drug allergy. The best-known example is the anaphylactic response produced by penicillin, which can occur after its administration by any route. Skin testing with penicillin G, penicilloic acid, or penicilloyl polylysine can identify patients at risk and should be performed in those with a suspected penicillin allergy who need treatment with penicillin. If the skin test result is

TABLE 25-3 GENETIC POLYMORPHISMS OF DRUG-METABOLIZING ENZYMES

TYPE	PRIMARY DRUG EXAMPLES	OTHER DRUGS THAT ARE SUBSTRATES	INCIDENCE OF "POOR METABOLIZERS" (%)	ENZYME INVOLVED
Debrisoquine-sparteine polymorphism	Amitriptyline, codeine, tamoxifen	Antidepressants, antiarrhythmics, β-adrenergic receptor–blocking drugs, codeine, dextromethorphan, neuroleptics	5-10 (Whites)	Cytochrome P-450 IID6 (CYP2D6)
Mephenytoin polymorphism	Mephenytoin	Mephobarbital, hexobarbital, diazepam, omeprazole	4 (Japanese, Chinese, 15-20)	Cytochrome P-450 IIC (CYP2C)
N-acetylation polymorphism	Isoniazid, sulfadiazine	Hydralazine, phenelzine, procainamide, dapsone, sulfamethazine, sulfapyridine, aminoglutethimide, aminosalicylic acid, sulfasalazine	40-70 (Japanese, 10-20)	*N*-acetyltransferase (NAT2)
Methyl conjugation polymorphism	Catecholamines	L-Dopa, methyldopa	25-30 (Whites)	Catechol-*O* methyltransferase (COMT)

positive, the patient must undergo desensitization before receiving penicillin. If the skin test result is negative, penicillin can be administered with caution.

DIAGNOSIS AND PREVENTION OF ADVERSE DRUG RESPONSES

Although many of the well-known adverse drug effects are due to a relatively small group of drugs, every drug has the potential to cause an adverse reaction. A physician should always consider the possibility of an adverse drug reaction in the differential diagnosis even if none has been previously reported to an updated website (e.g., www.fdable.com) for the particular drug. Health care professionals are encouraged to report any adverse events or product problems on a one-page form that can be sent by mail, fax, or electronically to the U.S. Food and Drug Administration (https://www.fda.gov/safety/medical-product-safety-information/medwatch-forms-fda-safety-reporting).

In many instances, it is readily apparent that a specific drug has produced an adverse reaction, such as the appearance of a rash in an otherwise healthy patient who was recently prescribed a single drug (e.g., penicillin).[8] In other cases, the effect produced by the drug may be difficult to discern from other disease states. In still other cases, the adverse effect may mimic the illness being treated (e.g., development of an arrhythmia in a patient being treated with an antiarrhythmic drug).

A patient's list of prescription drugs should be reviewed at each visit, and potential interactions with any nonprescription drugs should also be assessed. Screening tools[9] that can identify potentially inappropriate or unnecessary drug prescriptions can also reduce the risks of adverse drug reactions.[A1,A2]

The recent severe acute respiratory syndrome coronavirus 2 pandemic (Chapters 335 to 337) has resulted in external pressures to bring new drugs to market quickly. However, this public health crisis has also emphasized the need for the careful application of basic principles of clinical pharmacology in drug development.[10]

USEFULNESS OF GENOMIC DATA

In addition to being useful for avoiding adverse drug effects (see earlier), genomic data (e.g., the presence of a specific genetic variant) can also help inform the clinician of the optimal drug or dose for a specific patient. With oncologic drugs, genomic data from the tumor of an individual patient often can be useful in making a specific therapeutic decision (see www.fda.gov/drugs/science-and-research-drugs/table-pharmacogenomic-biomarkers-drug-labeling) (Chapter 164). An example is vemurafenib, which is an orally bioavailable, adenosine triphosphate (ATP)-competitive, small-molecule inhibitor of BRAF(V600E) kinase and which is effective against melanoma and potentially other malignancies[A3] that have a specific mutation in their *BRAF* gene—a valine-to-glutamic acid mutation at residue 600 (V600E) that results in the oncogene protein product, BRAF(V600E) kinase and markedly elevates activity in the MAPK signaling pathway.

Knowledge about tumor genetics also can guide new drug development. For example, the observation that the overall survival of patients with advanced non-small-cell lung cancer or colorectal cancer is approximately 1 to 2 years in patients who have a p.G12C mutation in their *KRAS* gene led to a search for a *KRAS*-targeted drug. Sotorasib, which is a covalent small-molecule inhibitor that irreversibly targets the cysteine residue at codon 12 of *KRAS*, thereby locking the protein into an inactive state, has shown potential activity in the treatment of several cancers that carry this mutation.[11] In contrast, genotype-guided selection of an oral P2Y12 inhibitor compared with conventional clopidogrel therapy without point-of-care genotyping did not reduce a composite end point of cardiovascular death, myocardial infarction, stroke, stent thrombosis, or severe recurrent ischemia.[A4,12]

GENERAL REFERENCES

For the General References and other additional features, please visit Elsevier eBooks+ at https://ebooks.health.elsevier.com.

Grade A References

A1. Hill-Taylor B, Walsh KA, Stewart S, et al. Effectiveness of the STOPP/START (screening tool of older persons' potentially inappropriate prescriptions/screening tool to alert doctors to the right treatment) criteria: systematic review and meta-analysis of randomized controlled studies. *J Clin Pharm Ther.* 2016;41:158-169.

A2. O'Connor MN, O'Sullivan D, Gallagher PF, et al. Prevention of hospital-acquired adverse drug reactions in older people using screening tool of older persons' prescriptions and screening tool to alert to right treatment criteria: a cluster randomized controlled trial. *J Am Geriatr Soc.* 2016;64:1558-1566.

A3. Chapman PB, Robert C, Larkin J, et al. Vemurafenib in patients with BRAFV600 mutation-positive metastatic melanoma: final overall survival results of the randomized BRIM-3 study. *Ann Oncol.* 2017;28:2581-2587.

A4. Pereira NL, Farkouh ME, So D, et al. Effect of genotype-guided oral P2Y12 inhibitor selection vs conventional clopidogrel therapy on ischemic outcomes after percutaneous coronary intervention: the TAILOR-PCI randomized clinical trial. *JAMA.* 2020;324:761-771.

26

PAIN

STEVEN P. COHEN

DEFINITION

In 2020, the International Association for the Study of Pain redefined pain as "an unpleasant sensory and emotional experience associated with, or resembling that associated with, actual or potential tissue damage."[1] This definition removes the connection between the perception of pain and its stimulus, and it also acknowledges that pain may occur in the absence of ongoing tissue damage, such as with fibromyalgia or phantom limb pain.[2] One implication of this construct is that pain is always subjective. Hence, a patient's report of pain should be accepted at face value in the absence of evidence to the contrary, even though some treatments may be tailored to objective evidence.

EPIDEMIOLOGY

Pain is ubiquitous in life, usually serving as a warning sign of impending or actual injury to the organism. It is older than mankind has existed, dating back to our most primitive ancestors. Pain is also a vital diagnostic clue for physicians. Pain is the most common symptom for which patients seek medical attention, with three of the top 10 reasons being osteoarthritis (Chapter 241), back pain (Chapter 369), and headaches (Chapter 367).

Recent data in the United States estimate a pain point prevalence of 20%, including 8% of people reporting high-impact chronic pain.[3] In the United Kingdom, the prevalence of chronic pain has been estimated to be 40 to 45%, with moderate-to-severe disabling pain affecting between 10.4% and 14.3% of people.

Populations at high risk for chronic pain include the elderly, people residing in rural areas, minority individuals, service members and veterans, and individuals with physical and psychological morbidities. Reasons for these disparities may include cultural issues, access to care, and differential treatment. Many chronic pain conditions including headaches, abdominal pain, and widespread pain disorders are more common in females.

PATHOBIOLOGY

The biopsychosocial model posits that biological, psychological, and social factors play a role in chronic pain (Fig. 26-1). The relationship between psychopathology in pain is bidirectional, with many conditions strongly associated with the persistence of pain after acute injury. Social factors that can negatively affect treatment include low job satisfaction, smoking, sedentary lifestyle, and secondary gain. Functional imaging has demonstrated that the brains of chronic pain patients are different than normal individuals, and that they undergo morphologic alterations such as general and disease-specific diminutions in gray matter as a consequence of chronic pain.

Nociception is the physiologic activation of specialized peripheral receptors (*nociceptors*) by stimuli that are potentially damaging to tissue (e.g., mechanical [tumor growth, incision], thermal, or chemical [ischemia or infection]). In addition to nociceptors that respond to specific stimuli, polymodal nociceptors respond to multiple modalities.

In contrast, pain is a conscious experience that results not only from activation of nociceptive pathways (sensory-discriminative component) but is also influenced by alterations in somatosensory processing following tissue injury, psychosocial factors (affective-motivational component), past experience, and expectations (cognitive-evaluative component). Once a stimulus is detected, it is converted into an electrical nerve signal through activation of transduction channels (e.g., transient receptor potential channels) expressed on the axonal membrane (*transduction*). These action potentials are conveyed along the axons of unmyelinated (C) or thinly myelinated (A-delta) nerve fibers through specific pathways (*transmission*). Modulation refers to the attenuation

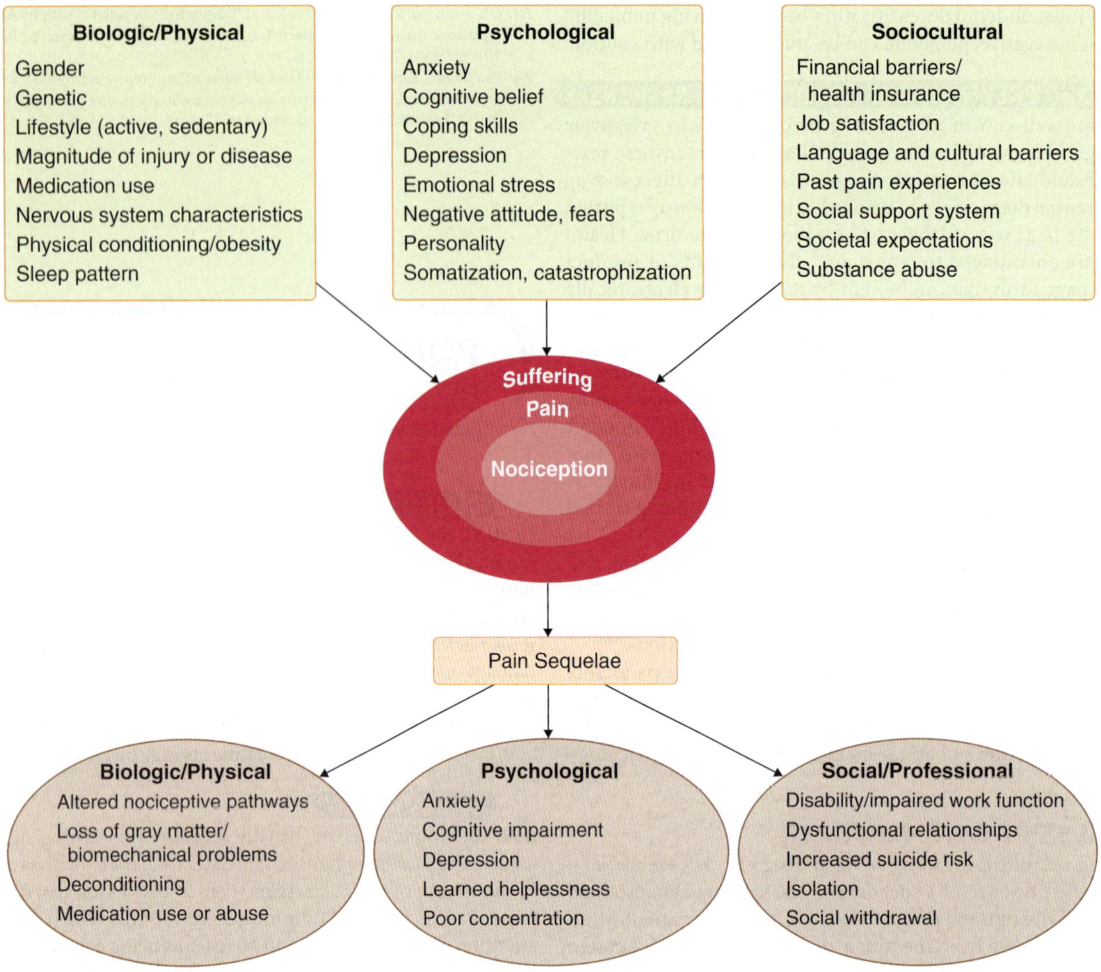

FIGURE 26-1. **Biopsychosocial model of pain.**

(or amplification) of pain signals through intrinsic inhibitory activity within the peripheral and central nervous systems (e.g., intrinsic brain and spinal neurons that release a plethora of neurotransmitters) before being perceived as unpleasant *(perception)*, though in some cases pain signals may be enhanced during this process (e.g., wind-up). Pathologic pain results when injury- or disease-induced changes in the peripheral and/or central nervous systems lead to enhanced pain signaling. One example is *peripheral sensitization*, which is characterized by spontaneous ectopic activity in injured nerves and dorsal root ganglion cells, as well as enhanced sensitivity to stimuli.

Prolonged and repeated activation of nociceptive afferent fibers produces *central sensitization*, a state of hyperexcitability of central pain-signaling neurons with activation of *N*-methyl-D-aspartate (NMDA) receptors by glutamate. Loss of inhibitory interneurons and altered balance between descending inhibitory and excitatory modulatory mechanisms play a key role in the maintenance of pain. Other central neuroplastic changes that contribute to neuropathic pain include deafferentation hyperactivity following spinal cord or avulsion injuries, loss of large fiber inhibition, and reorganization of central connections of primary afferent fibers. Central and peripheral sensitization are considered to be the prime culprits responsible for pain induced by innocuous stimuli (allodynia) and increased pain to normally noxious stimuli (hyperalgesia), both of which are commonly observed in neuropathic pain. In some patients, this nociplastic process serves as the primary mechanism (e.g., fibromyalgia).

Nature versus Nurture

Chronic pain is a prototypical example of the interplay between genes and environment. Heritability is estimated to account for between 30% and 60% of the variance in pain response and plays a role in both the perception of acute pain and the transition to chronic pain.

A pain syndrome can result from a single gene mutation with high penetrance (e.g., primary erythromelalgia; Chapter 66), but multiple gene abnormalities usually promote a predisposition to pain, which requires a subsequent inciting event. For example, back pain, despite the large influence of environmental and psychosocial factors, is estimated to have a heritability of between 21% and 67%. Chronic pain in parents and a parent's pain-related cognitions are associated with pain in early adolescence, before degenerative processes typically manifest, and may have a genetic as well as environmental explanation.

Neuropathic, Nociceptive, Nociplastic, and Mixed Pain

Pain can be etiologically classified as nociceptive, neuropathic, nociplastic, or mixed (Tables 26-1 and 26-2). This distinction is important because it affects decision making at all levels of care (e.g., whether to obtain magnetic resonance imaging [MRI] for subacute spinal pain, what type of medications to prescribe, and prognosis).

Nociceptive pain, which is the most common type of pain, results from an injury or disease affecting somatic structures and includes conditions such as arthritis and mechanical spine pain.[4] Nociceptive pain can be subdivided into somatic pain involving injury to skin, muscles, and joints, and visceral pain, which results from pathology affecting internal organs (e.g., pancreatitis, angina, renal stones). In contrast to somatic pain, visceral pain is usually poorly localized, referred to somatic regions (e.g., myocardial ischemia radiating into the arm), and tends to be associated with a greater affective-motivational component than somatic pain. Reasons for these differences include a lower density and different types of nociceptors, and convergence with afferent pathways in the spinal cord.

Neuropathic pain,[5] which accounts for between 15% and 25% of chronic pain, is caused by a lesion or disease that affects the somatosensory system. Neuropathic pain may be associated with a greater decrement in quality of life than comparable degrees of nociceptive pain. One subtype of neuropathic pain is central pain, which manifests as a constellation of sensory, motor, and sometimes autonomic symptoms following a lesion or disease affecting the central nervous system.

Nociplastic pain[6] arises from altered nociception despite no clear evidence of actual or threatened tissue damage, no biomarkers, and no evidence of a disease or lesions affecting the somatosensory system. Formerly known as

TABLE 26-1 CLASSIFICATION AND PREVALENCE OF COMMON PAIN CONDITIONS

NEUROPATHIC		*NOCICEPTIVE*		*NOCIPLASTIC*[1]	*MIXED*
PERIPHERAL[2]	**CENTRAL**	**SOMATIC**	**VISCERAL**		
Peripheral neuropathy (1-3%)	Central post-stroke pain (8%)	Arthritis (25-40% in people >40 yr)	Endometriosis (10% in women of reproductive age)	Irritable bowel syndrome[1] (5-15%)	Headache[1] (15% for migraine, 20-30% for tension-type)
Postherpetic neuralgia (annual incidence 0.1-0.2%), lower with varicella zoster vaccine	Spinal cord injury (30-50%)	Myofascial pain (5%-10%)	Interstitial cystitis[1,4] (0.2-1% of women)	Fibromyalgia[1] (3-6%), generalized diffuse pain 7-13%	Cancer[5] (lifetime prevalence 30-40%)
Chronic postsurgical pain (2-10% after surgery)	Multiple sclerosis (25%)	Connective tissue disorders (0.2-0.5%)	Ulcers/gastritis/esophagitis (3-9%)	Complex regional pain syndrome type I[1] (0.006-0.05%, 3-20% after orthopedic surgery)	Low back pain[6] (annual prevalence rate 15-45%)
Phantom limb pain (30-60%)	Parkinson disease (10%)	Burn pain[3] (annual incidence of burns requiring hospitalization 0.01%)	Cholecystitis/appendicitis (10-20% of people have gallstones and up to one third develop cholecystitis)	Temporomandibular disorder (5-12%)[1]	Neck pain[6] (annual prevalence rate 15-40%)
Trigeminal neuralgia (0.01%)	Seizure disorder (1-3%)				Ischemic pain[7] (5-10% prevalence for peripheral vascular disease)
Radiculopathy/spinal stenosis (3-10%)					
Nerve entrapment syndromes (e.g., carpal tunnel, thoracic outlet, meralgia paresthetica; 5-10% collectively)					

[1]Strong female predominance.
[2]Prevalence rates represent the proportion of the population who suffers from the condition except for phantom limb pain in which the prevalence is based on those with limb amputation.
[3]Third-degree burns may be associated with neuropathic pain.
[4]Also sometimes considered nociplastic pain (bladder pain syndrome).
[5]Neuropathic pain occurs in 20-50% of cases and may occur secondary to tumor invasion, surgery, chemotherapy, and radiation treatment.
[6]Neuropathic pain may predominate or accompany nociceptive pain in 20-50% of cases.
[7]Typically nociceptive, but long-standing pain may result in ischemic neuropathy.

TABLE 26-2 CATEGORIZATION OF PAIN STATES

CLINICAL CHARACTERISTIC	NEUROPATHIC PAIN	NOCICEPTIVE PAIN	NOCIPLASTIC PAIN
Etiology	Disease or injury affecting the nervous system	Tissue or potential tissue damage	Maladaptive changes that affect nociceptive processing
Descriptors	Lancinating, shooting, electrical-like	Throbbing, aching, pressure-like	Similar to neuropathic pain; visceral pain (irritable bowel syndrome, bladder pain syndrome) may be diffuse, aching, gnawing, or sharp
Sensory deficits	Frequent (e.g., numbness, tingling, pricking)	Infrequent and in nondermatomal or non-nerve distribution	Common, in nondermatomal or non-nerve distribution
Motor deficits	Neurologic weakness may be present	May have pain-induced weakness	Generalized fatigue common; weakness due to deconditioning
Hypersensitivity	Pain frequently evoked with nonpainful (allodynia) stimuli	Uncommon except for hypersensitivity in the immediate area of an acute injury	Very common and diffuse
Pain pattern	Distal radiation common	Distal radiation less common; proximal nondermatomal radiation frequent around anatomic structure	Diffuse spread not following anatomic referral pattern; patients often have multiple nociplastic conditions
Paroxysms	Exacerbations common and unpredictable	Exacerbations less common and associated with activity	Common, often related to psychosocial stressors
Autonomic signs	Can occur in ⅓ to ½ of patients	Uncommon	Sympathetic nervous system hyperactivity common

"functional pain syndromes," these conditions include fibromyalgia (Chapter 253), irritable bowel syndrome (Chapter 123), and some forms of chronic headache. Coexisting conditions may include augmented sensory processing (e.g., photophobia), diminished inhibitory pathways, and a higher co-prevalence of mood and sleep disorders. For example, over 50% of patients with chronic pain exhibit some form of sleep disturbance (Chapter 374), with the prevalence being even higher in nociplastic pain states.

Mixed pain disorders[7] contain components of neuropathic, nociceptive, and sometimes nociplastic pain (e.g., nonspecific low back pain). An example is cancer-related pain, which can result from tissue invasion or as a consequence of therapy (e.g., surgery, chemotherapy, and radiation therapy), can involve sensory nerves, and can be exacerbated by anxiety and sleep disorders. In some studies, mixed pain conditions account for more than 50% of chronic pain.

CLINICAL MANIFESTATIONS AND DIAGNOSIS

Multiple classification systems describe pain based on duration, anatomic source, and mechanisms. Acute pain results from injury or inflammation, has survival value, and plays a role in healing by preventing reinjury. In contrast, chronic pain is perhaps best construed as a "disease" that serves no useful purpose. Although no clear threshold defines when acute pain becomes pathologic, it is generally accepted that pain persisting beyond the expected healing period, or lasting over 3 months, constitutes chronic pain.

History

The evaluation of pain begins with a thorough history. Since no test or biomarker can reliably identify pain, a patient's pain complaints should always be taken seriously in the absence of objective evidence to the contrary.

A comprehensive history should include the location of pain, its quality, inciting event(s), exacerbating and relieving factors, associated symptoms and signs (e.g., numbness), magnitude, interference with activities, and response to prior treatments. The severity of pain should be assessed, usually on a 0 to 10 visual analogue scale, as mild (1-3), moderate (4-7), or severe (>7 on a 0-10 scale). Because there are subtle differences among pain scales, repeat assessments or response to therapy are ideally gauged using the same instrument. For mentally incapacitated patients, age-appropriate substitute scales or facial expressions can be used. In assessing response to therapy, a 30% or greater reduction in pain constitutes meaningful improvement. However, pain also must be considered in the context of functional capacity, psychologic and emotional well-being, sleep status, and ability to work.

Neuropathic pain is characterized by positive and negative symptoms. Positive symptoms reflect abnormal excitability of the nervous system, whereas negative symptoms, such as a loss of sensation, are usually the result of loss of axons/neurons. Paresthesias and other symptoms suggestive of sensory dysfunction are indicative of neuropathic pain, especially when they occur in a dermatomal or nerve distribution. Descriptors such as "shooting" and "electrical" are more apt to be associated with neuropathic pain. Other positive symptoms observed in neuropathic pain states include pain evoked by normally innocuous stimuli (allodynia) and an exaggerated or prolonged pain response to noxious stimuli (hyperalgesia/hyperpathia).

Nociceptive pain is classically exacerbated by movements that stress the anatomic structure (e.g., walking for arthritis, head movements for neck pain). "Throbbing" and "aching" tend to be identified with nociceptive pain states such as arthritis.

Nociplastic pain is typically characterized by diffuse symptoms (e.g., widespread pain, coexisting nociplastic conditions, or multiple pain locations). It is often accompanied by concomitant symptoms such as fatigue, insomnia, multiple chemical sensitivities, mild cognitive impairment (e.g., memory difficulties), and sensitivity to light and/or sound. *Mixed pain syndromes* in conditions such as cancer are characterized by more than one type of pain.

The evaluation of a patient in pain also must include a psychosocial history. Between half and two thirds of patients with chronic pain have depression (Chapter 362), anxiety disorders, somatoform disorders, or substance abuse disorders (Chapters 364 and 365).

Physical Examination

Since pain is a frequent manifestation of systemic disease, examination of the patient in pain should encompass all bodily systems. Although a finding on examination is almost never pathognomonic, it frequently helps guide diagnostic testing or treatment. Unlike acute pain, chronic pain is usually not associated with autonomic activation and altered vital signs. Numbness in the distribution of a nerve or nerve root suggests neuropathic pain, but nondermatomal sensory changes can accompany nociplastic and nociceptive pain as well. Focal allodynia and hyperalgesia are hallmarks of neuropathic pain. The most common forms of neuropathy are associated with sensory deficits in a glove-stocking distribution, but other patterns occur as well (Chapter 388).

When evaluating muscle strength, a distinction should be made between pain-induced and neurologic weakness (Chapter 366), with the latter often occurring in conjunction with muscle atrophy or asymmetric reflexes. Widespread physical findings such as diffuse tenderness or nonanatomic pain patterns may indicate central sensitization, opioid-induced hyperalgesia, a somatic symptom disorder, or another psychiatric illness (e.g., new-onset depression).

Psychologic Assessment

The lifetime prevalence of coexisting psychiatric illness in patients with chronic pain ranges from 50% to over 80%, and 30% to 60% of chronic pain sufferers experience symptoms of depression, anxiety, or posttraumatic stress (Chapter 362). These psychiatric conditions are strong predictors for the development of chronic pain after an episode of acute pain and are associated with poorer treatment outcomes. The clinician must screen all pain patients for psychological conditions that can adversely affect treatment (Table 26-3), including maladaptive behaviors and secondary diagnoses such as somatic symptom disorders and poor coping skills.

Diagnostic Tests

Imaging can be helpful in diagnosing the cause of pain, but it lacks specificity. For example, the correlation between findings on MRI and the intensity of spinal pain is modest at best, with more than 50% of asymptomatic individuals having abnormalities on lumbar, thoracic, and cervical films (Chapter 369). Musculoskeletal imaging should be reserved for patients who have serious or progressive deficits or "red flags," such as suspected malignancy, infection, or fractures.[8] For chronic pain disorders such as primary headaches, abdominal pain, or pelvic pain, imaging should be reserved for the evaluation of new-onset symptoms or a significant change in symptoms.

Electromyography and nerve conduction studies (Chapter 366) can diagnose injury to large nerve fibers. However, these studies are associated with both false-negative and false-positive results and are not sensitive for detecting impairment of small nerve fibers. For small-fiber neuropathies, a skin biopsy demonstrating decreased nerve fiber density can be valuable.

TABLE 26-3 PSYCHOSOCIAL FACTORS ASSOCIATED WITH CHRONIC PAIN

Multiple pain complaints
Poor job satisfaction/low pay
Inadequate coping skills, catastrophization
Fear-avoidance behavior
Manual labor/physically stressful job
Obesity
Somatization
Smoking
Low resiliency
Low baseline activity levels
Secondary gain (e.g., worker's compensation, ongoing litigation)
Older age
Low education level
High disease burden (e.g., pain intensity/disability, opioid use)
Substance misuse, including opioids
Neurologic symptoms
Anxiety
Depressed mood
Emotional distress

TREATMENT

In managing pain, realistic goals must be established, and individually tailored treatment regimens should be developed to achieve these ends. A key goal is to alleviate suffering, which can be the consequence of loss of physical function, social isolation, familial distress, and a sense of inadequacy.

Interdisciplinary pain programs can be more effective than unidimensional approaches and cost-effective when properly administered. The stepped care model recommends starting therapy with the least resource-intensive services and progressing to specialty care within a biopsychosocial framework. Within this paradigm, self-care can include weight loss if appropriate; a healthy lifestyle, including exercise[A1] and proper sleep hygiene; smoking cessation; and ergonomic modifications when indicated (Fig. 26-2). Whenever possible, nonopioid options are preferred.[9]

Pharmacologic Therapies

Antipyretic Analgesics

Acetaminophen, aspirin, and other nonsteroidal anti-inflammatory drugs (NSAIDs) form a cornerstone of pain pharmacotherapy (Table 26-4). These antipyretic analgesics exert their antinociceptive effects by inhibiting cyclooxygenase, the rate-limiting enzyme in the production of prostaglandins, which sensitize nociceptors and regulate inflammation. Whereas aspirin and NSAIDs act both centrally and peripherally, thereby making them effective topical agents for inflammatory conditions, acetaminophen is a weaker analgesic that acts primarily in the central nervous system (and possibly also via cannabinoid 1 and transient receptor potential cation channel subfamily V member 1 receptors) and is largely devoid of anti-inflammatory effects.

The main drawback of these nonopioid analgesics is their relatively limited therapeutic efficacy. Acetaminophen is often ineffective for spinal pain and usually provides only minimal, short-term benefit for knee or hip osteoarthritis.[A2] NSAIDs generally provide limited benefit for spinal pain and osteoarthritis compared with placebo.[A3]

A major concern for antipyretic agents is their side effects. For NSAIDs, these include bleeding, gastrointestinal ulceration, renal toxicity, and an increased risk of cardiovascular events. Cyclooxygenase-2 selective inhibitors such as celecoxib or the addition of a protein pump inhibitor (Table 124-1) may attenuate the risk of gastrointestinal bleeding, but the incidence of adverse renal or cardiovascular events remains increased, especially in patients who are elderly, have multiple comorbid conditions, and take many medications. In these and other situations, topical NSAIDs (e.g., diclofenac) can be useful for focal rheumatologic disorders, with fewer side effects.[A4]

Adjuvant Analgesics

For the treatment of neuropathic pain (Table 26-5), antidepressants and anticonvulsants (gabapentin and pregabalin) should be the two first-line classes of medications.[A5] Depending on the drug and condition, these medications can provide significant pain relief beyond that observed with placebo in 15% to 30% of patients with neuropathic pain, and may provide preemptive effects before surgery. In terms of efficacy, tricyclic antidepressants are superior to serotonin and norepinephrine reuptake inhibitors, which in turn are more efficacious

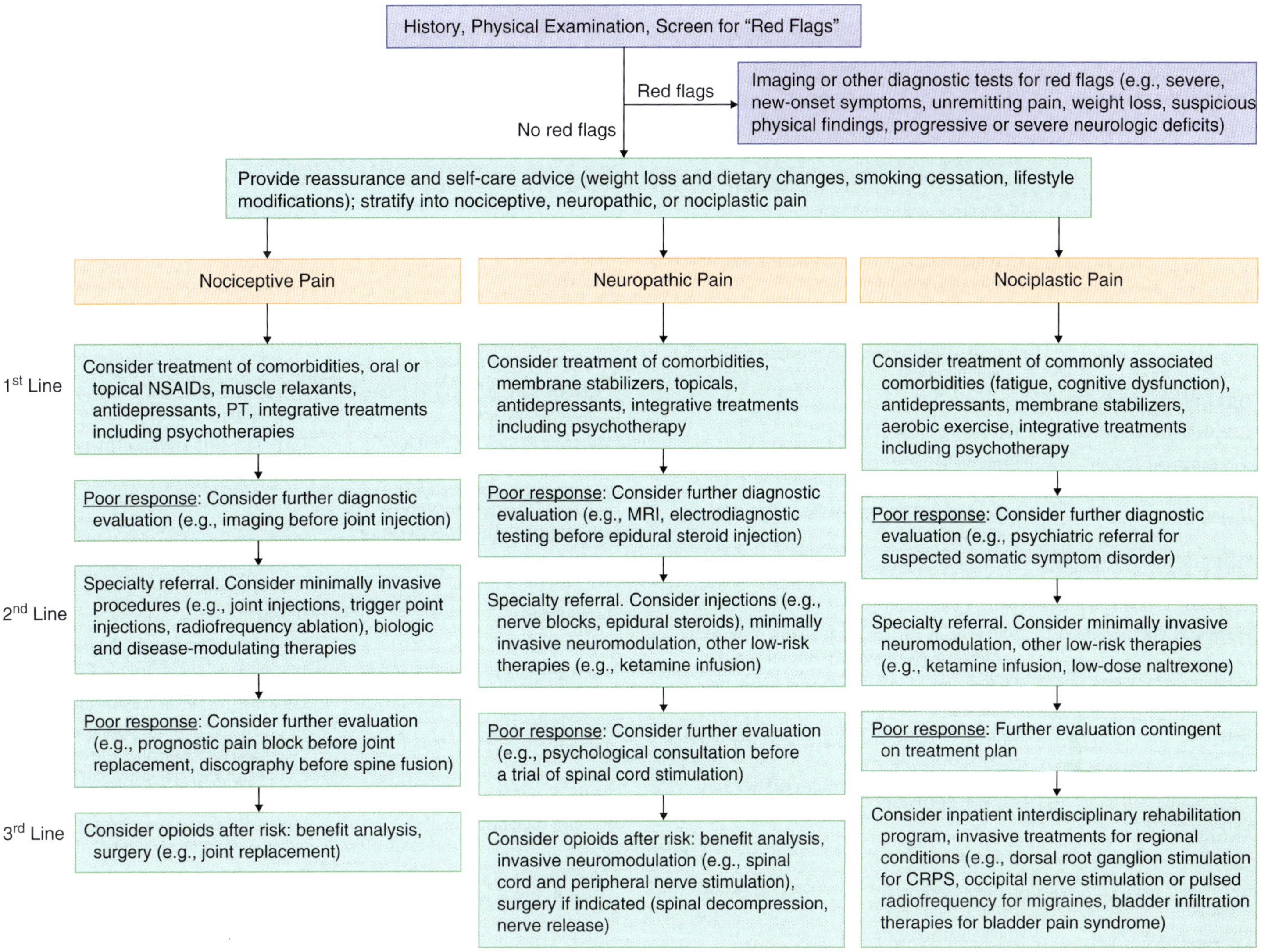

FIGURE 26-2. Approach to patient with chronic pain. CRPS = complex regional pain syndrome; MRI = magnetic resonance imaging; NSAIDs = nonsteroidal anti-inflammatory drugs; PT = physical therapy.

than serotonin specific reuptake inhibitors. Nortriptyline and imipramine have fewer side effects than amitriptyline and are preferable first-choice agents for neuropathic pain. Antidepressants are also effective for headaches (Chapter 367), nociplastic pain, and musculoskeletal disorders.

Although antidepressants are more versatile in that they have proven benefit in myriad pain conditions, gabapentin and pregabalin may be better than antidepressants for prototypical "lancinating-type" neuropathic pain. Gabapentin and pregabalin also act additively with antidepressants and opioids.[10]

When gabapentin and pregabalin are ineffective or intolerable, alternative anticonvulsants that act via different mechanisms may be tried. For trigeminal neuralgia (Chapter 367), carbamazepine remains the treatment of choice, though adverse effects such as agranulocytosis limit its utility. Other adjuvants that may be effective in certain contexts include topical agents such as lidocaine and capsaicin,[A6] NMDA antagonists (e.g., ketamine), and skeletal muscle relaxants/antispasticity drugs (e.g., baclofen).

Cannabinoids can treat chronic pain by binding to two receptors: CB1, which is expressed in high concentrations in the central nervous system (and is responsible for most of their euphoric effects) and along pain pathways, and CB2, which is found mainly on immune cells in peripheral tissue and contains anti-inflammatory properties.[11] FDA-approved cannabinoids are dronabinol, nabilone, and cannabidiol, none of which is currently approved for pain. Unfortunately, controlled trials have found that cannabinoids have limited benefit for chronic pain and a high rate of adverse effects.[A7] Nevertheless, some patients may benefit from their antiemetic and appetite-stimulating properties, as well as improved sleep and decreased anxiety. Serious side effects of cannabinoids may include cognitive and motivational impairment and psychological effects such as delusions, hallucinations, panic disorders, depression, and addiction.

Opioid Analgesics

Opioid analgesics (Table 26-6) are a mainstay of treatment for cancer pain but are no longer considered first-line treatment for any noncancer pain because of limited evidence that they improve quality of life compared with nonopioid analgesics despite their abuse potential.[A8] For nociplastic pain, opioids may be less effective than for other pain categories, and some evidence actually supports the efficacy of opioid antagonists (e.g., low-dose naltrexone) for nociplastic pain.

Optimizing therapy with opioid analgesics requires carefully balancing the beneficial and undesirable effects (Table 26-7), including not only addiction but also nausea, constipation, sedation, itch, respiratory depression, and endocrine deficiency that leads to sexual dysfunction and accelerated osteoporosis.[12] Opioids that are predominantly eliminated by the kidneys, such as morphine, must be used with caution in patients with renal dysfunction; in this situation, alternatives include fentanyl and methadone.

The increasing use of prescription opioids for chronic pain has been associated with a dramatic increase in opioid-related deaths, a trend that has been amplified by the coronavirus disease 2019 (COVID-19) pandemic (Chapter 365). The long-term use of opioids can be associated with tolerance, hyperalgesia, physical dependence, and addiction. The rates of abuse and addiction, which vary substantially across studies, are heavily dependent on the population selected, surveillance, and differences in applying definitions. Rates of misuse are estimated at between 20% and 30%, and the incidence of addiction is less than 8% in carefully selected populations (E-Fig. 26-1). Sometimes the only way to distinguish between tolerance and opioid-induced hyperalgesia is with a long-term drug holiday. Cross-tolerance among opioids is incomplete, and a strategy often used to combat tolerance is opioid rotation, which may result in a 30% to 50% reduction in the equi-analgesic dose.

Tramadol and tapentadol represent a class of analgesic drugs that have dual mechanisms of action. Tramadol is a weak agonist that inhibits the reuptake of norepinephrine and serotonin. Along with the typical opioid-related side effects, seizures have been reported. Tapentadol, which is about twice as strong as tramadol, functions as a mu opioid agonist with a ceiling effect and as a norepinephrine reuptake inhibitor.

TABLE 26-4 COMMONLY USED NONSTEROIDAL ANTI-INFLAMMATORY DRUGS (NSAIDS)

DRUG SUBSTANCE	USUAL DOSE
OVER-THE-COUNTER	
Acetaminophen	325-650 mg orally q4-6h 650 mg q4h PRN IV or up to 1000 mg q6h PRN IV
Acetylsalicylic acid	325-650 mg orally q4-6h
Ibuprofen	200-800 orally q6-8h (200 mg available over-the-counter) 400-800 mg q6h IV PRN
Naproxen	220-550 mg orally q12h (220 mg available over-the-counter); extended release: 750-1000 mg orally q24h; 1500 mg orally may be given if well-tolerated
ORAL PRESCRIPTION	
Celecoxib (COX-2 selective)	100-200 mg orally q12-24h
Diclofenac	50 mg orally q8h 75 mg q24h IM
Diflunisal	Initial dose 500-1000 mg orally then 250-500 mg orally q8-12h
Etoricoxib (COX-2 selective; not available in United States)	30-90 mg orally daily
Etodolac (COX-2 selective)	300 mg orally q8-12h or 400-500 mg orally q12h; extended release 400-1000 mg orally q24h
Ketoprofen	25-50 mg orally q6-12h; extended release 100-200 mg orally daily
Ketorolac	Initial dose 20 mg orally, then 10 mg orally q4-6h 10-30 mg q4-6h IM or IV
Indomethacin	25-50 mg orally q6-8h; extended release 75 mg orally q12-24h
Mefenamic acid	Initial dose 500 mg orally, then 250 mg orally q6h, for up to 1 wk
Meloxicam (COX-2 selective)	5-15 mg orally in once or twice per day dosing 30 mg daily IV
Nabumetone (COX-2 selective)	1000-2000 mg orally daily
Oxaprozin	600-1200 mg orally daily
Piroxicam	Initial dose 40 mg orally, then 20 mg orally daily
Sulindac	150-200 mg orally q12h
TOPICAL CREAM	
Diclofenac	Apply up to 4 g q6h as needed; available over-the-counter in United States
Ketoprofen	Apply 2-4 g q6-12h as needed; not available in United States

h = hour; IM = intramuscular; IV = intravenous.

TABLE 26-5 RECOMMENDATIONS FOR THE PHARMACOLOGIC TREATMENT OF CHRONIC NEUROPATHIC PAIN

FIRST-LINE DRUGS/DRUG CLASSES	TYPICAL TOTAL DAILY DOSE AND REGIMEN
Gabapentin	1200–3600 mg, in three divided doses
Gabapentin extended release	1200–3600 mg, in one or two divided doses
Pregabalin	300–600 mg, in two divided doses
Duloxetine	60–120 mg, in one or two divided doses
Tricyclic antidepressants (e.g., nortriptyline, amitriptyline)	25–150 mg, usually once per day
SECOND-LINE DRUGS	
Capsaicin 8% patches (for peripheral neuropathic pain)	1-4 patches to the painful area for 30-60 min once every 3 mo
Lidocaine patches (for peripheral neuropathic pain)	1-3 patches to the region of pain once per day for up to 12 h
THIRD-LINE DRUGS AND THOSE RECOMMENDED IN SELECTIVE CIRCUMSTANCES	
Botulinum toxin A (subcutaneously)	50–200 units to the painful area once every 3 mo
Lamotrigine	200-400 mg in two divided doses
Carbamazepine	400-1200 mg in two divided doses
Oxcarbazepine	1200-2400 mg in two divided doses
Venlafaxine	150-225 mg in two or three divided doses
Ketamine (infusion)	No standard therapy for chronic pain in terms of rate or number of treatments, though higher cumulative doses (e.g., >400 mg) appear more effective
Baclofen (intrathecal, oral)	15-80 mg in three or four divided doses. Oral to intrathecal ratio 100 : 1
Tramadol, tapentadol, and pure mu-agonist opioids	See Table 26-6

All medications are oral unless otherwise indicated.

Recommendations based on Schlereth T. Guideline "diagnosis and non interventional therapy of neuropathic pain" of the German Society of Neurology (Deutsche Gesellschaft für Neurologie). *Neurol Res Pract*. 2020;2:16.

Butorphanol, nalbuphine, and pentazocine are opioid agonist-antagonist drugs. These drugs should be used with caution, particularly in patients who are receiving other opioid agonists, because they may precipitate withdrawal or reduce the effectiveness of pure opioid agonists. Buprenorphine, which is a long-acting partial agonist at the mu opioid receptor and an antagonist at other opioid receptors, is available in various formulations as a stand-alone analgesic and in combination with naloxone for treatment of opioid addiction.

Combination Pharmacotherapies
Guidelines suggest that when monotherapy is ineffective, multiple agents that act at different sites and ideally have antagonistic adverse effects may be combined (E-Fig. 26-2). Controlled trials have found that gabapentin plus nortriptyline, gabapentin plus morphine, nortriptyline plus morphine, and mirtazapine plus pregabalin provide superior benefit than either drug alone for neuropathic pain.[A9]

Psychologic Treatment
Relaxation techniques such as biofeedback and guided imagery are effective for a wide array of acute and chronic pain conditions but may be especially useful in individuals with high levels of anxiety. Cognitive-behavioral therapy, which is a structured form of psychotherapy predicated on the replacement of negative thought patterns and behaviors with more constructive ones, enhances inhibitory pain signals and also can be effective for associated symptoms such as fatigue and insomnia.[A10,A11] Ideal candidates include motivated patients in whom distorted thinking (e.g., catastrophization) and counterproductive behaviors (e.g., fear-avoidance) amplify pain. In patients with personality disorders and ingrained maladaptive behaviors, which may also predispose to pain and pain-related disability, long-term psychotherapy may be necessary.

Physical Treatments
The use of physical therapies to provide pain relief and enhance function is a cornerstone of integrative treatment. Physical therapists evaluate, educate, and provide minimally invasive procedural interventions to help prevent and alleviate pain and dysfunction. These interventions include addressing causes of pain (e.g., correcting gait abnormalities) and providing treatments (e.g., hot and cold packs, joint manipulation).

Exercise is an effective treatment for many forms of chronic pain, and it also is a means to prevent injury. Exercise reduces the sensitivity to pain but is more beneficial for improving function than for relieving pain and more beneficial for musculoskeletal and diffuse pain than for neuropathic pain.[A12]

Interventional therapies
Local Injections and Nerve Blocks
Local injections of lidocaine may be tried for diagnostic, therapeutic, and prognostic purposes. In appropriate patients (especially trigger point injections for myofascial pain, intra-articular injections for osteoarthritis, and nerve blocks with corticosteroids for nerve entrapment syndromes), injections can provide intermediate-term pain relief, facilitate rehabilitation, and improve quality of life. For radicular leg pain, spinal injections can provide limited benefit.[A13] Patients

TABLE 26-6 FORMULATIONS, DOSAGES, AND PHARMACOLOGIC INFORMATION ON COMMONLY PRESCRIBED OPIOIDS

PURE OPIOID AGONISTS				
DRUG	**EQUIANALGESIC DOSAGE (ORAL UNLESS SPECIFIED)**	**READILY AVAILABLE ROUTES OF ADMINISTRATION**	**DURATION OF ACTION**	**COMMENTS**
Morphine	30 mg	IV, IM, PO, PR; SR formulation	3-6 h for short-acting, 8-12 h for SR	Reference standard for all opioids. Renally excreted active metabolite
Oxycodone	20 mg	PO, PR; SR formulation	3-6 h for short-acting, 8-12 h for SR	Widely available in combination form with nonopioid analgesics. Greater euphoric effects than morphine. Popular among recreational users
Hydromorphone	3-6 mg	PO, PR, IV, IM, SR formulation	3-6 h, 18-24 h for SR	Higher PO: IV conversion ratio than other opioids. SR form reserved for opioid-tolerant patients, and contraindicated in patients with recent monoamine oxidase inhibitor use
Hydrocodone	30-60 mg	PO, SR formulation	3-6 h, 12-24 h for SR	Wide variation in morphine equivalent dose. Most commonly prescribed opioid in United States. Typically used in combination form with nonopioid analgesic acetaminophen. IR products containing <15 mg hydrocodone are Schedule III in the United States. SR form available without acetaminophen
Oxymorphone	10 mg	PO, IV, IM, PR; SR formulation	4-8 h, 8-12 h for SR	Coingestion of alcohol with SR formulation can lead to rapid increase in plasma levels and overdose. Very low (10%) oral bioavailability
Methadone	2-10 mg (see comments)	PO, PR, IV	6-12 h for pain	Morphine: methadone conversion varies according to dose and length of opioid use, ranging from 3 : 1 to > 20 : 1 in patients on very high doses. Any physician with a Schedule II DEA license may prescribe for pain. May take 5-7 days to reach steady state due to long half-life. ECG monitoring recommended with higher doses. Other properties such as NMDA receptor antagonism and reuptake inhibition of serotonin and norepinephrine may slow tolerance and increase efficacy for neuropathic pain
Levorphanol	3 mg	PO, IM, IV	4-10 h	2 : 1 oral to IV conversion ratio. Agonist at mu, kappa, and delta receptors. Multiple mechanisms of action, including inhibition of serotonin and norepinephrine reuptake, NDMA receptor antagonism and sigma receptor agonism. Long half-life exceeded only by methadone
Fentanyl	12.5 μg/h (TD) = 30 morphine milliequivalents/day Dosing 100-1200 μg for TM Potency for TM formulations varies from 1/8 that of morphine for buccal or sublingual tablets or lozenges to 1/5 for films or oral sprays	TD, TM	72 h for TD; 1.5-3 h for TM	TD and TM formulations may be useful in patients with poor bowel function. Rapid onset (<10 min) iontophoretic TD system available for postoperative pain TD: Wide variation in conversion ratios and doses depending on route. Delivery system may be associated with fewer gastrointestinal side effects, and include buccal, sublingual, and intranasal routes TM delivery associated with more rapid (10 min) onset than immediate-release oral opioids. FDA approved for breakthrough cancer pain in opioid-tolerant patients
Sufentanil	15-30 μg (~7.5 times as potent as fentanyl)	TM	1-3 h	Rapid onset, wide variation in conversion ratio. For use only in health care and battlefield settings. 15 and 30 μg dosages approved in Europe and United States. Not approved for home use or for longer than 72 h
Propoxyphene	200 mg	PO, PR	3-6 h	Removed from market in United States. Wide variation in morphine equivalent dose. Often used in combination form with nonopioid analgesics. Toxic metabolite may accumulate with excessive use, especially in elderly. Weak antagonist at NMDA receptor
Meperidine	300 mg	PO, PR, IM, IV	2-4 h	Toxic metabolite may accumulate with excessive use, especially in patients with renal insufficiency. Associated with tachycardia and hypertension. Concurrent use with monoamine oxidase inhibitors may result in fatal reactions. May cause more "euphoria" than other opioids. IM absorption erratic

TABLE 26-6 FORMULATIONS, DOSAGES, AND PHARMACOLOGIC INFORMATION ON COMMONLY PRESCRIBED OPIOIDS—cont'd

DRUG	TYPICAL DOSING/ ANALGESIC POTENCY	READILY AVAILABLE ROUTES OF ADMINISTRATION	DURATION OF ACTION	COMMENTS
AGONIST-ANTAGONISTS, PARTIAL AGONISTS				
Buprenorphine Buprenorphine/ Naloxone (4 : 1 ratio for opioid addiction)	0.3-24 mg SL 5-70 μg/h (TD) 2-24 mg/day (tablets and films about 30 times as potent as morphine; TD patch 10-15 times as potent)	TM, PR, IV, TD	8-12 h for TM, 7 days for SR, once daily for stable buprenorphine/ naloxone combination	Partial mu agonist and kappa antagonist that may precipitate withdrawal in opioid-dependent patients on high doses. Lower abuse potential and fewer side effects than pure agonists. Not readily reversed by naloxone. Schedule III drug in United States. Primarily used in combination with naloxone as sublingual or buccal tablets and films for opioid dependence. May prolong QT interval
Butorphanol	1 mg/spray, repeat after 60-90 min (IN) 1-2 mg (IV/IM) (~7 times as potent as morphine)	IN, IM, IV, PO	3-5 h	Mixed agonist-antagonist at mu receptor and antagonist at kappa receptor. Commonly used as nasal spray to treat migraine headache, and less commonly for labor pain. Significant abuse potential
Nalbuphine	1 : 1 parenteral analgesic potency ratio to morphine (~0.8 : 1.0 [equianalgesic] times as potent as morphine)	SQ, IM, IV	3-6 h	Mixed agonist-antagonist, often used for labor and delivery. Sometimes used to treat refractory opioid-induced pruritus
Pentazocine Pentazocine/ Naloxone (Talwin) (100 : 1 ratio of pentazocine to naloxone)	90 mg (~3 times as potent as morphine)	PO, SQ, IM, IV	3-4 h parenteral, 3-8 h PO	Mixed agonist-antagonist. (−) enantiomer is kappa agonist. Naloxone added in 1970s (Talwin) to prevent abuse. Commonly prescribed in preparation with acetaminophen
WEAK, DUAL-ACTION OPIOID AGONISTS				
Tramadol	50-100 mg, up to 400 mg/day (1/10th as potent as morphine)	PO	4-6 h, 24 h for SR	Dual action involves inhibition of serotonin and norepinephrine reuptake. Affinity for mu opioid receptor 6000× less than morphine. Analogue of codeine with active metabolite in which differences in metabolism may influence drug effects. Available in combination form with acetaminophen. Maximum recommended dose of 400 mg/day. Avoid concurrent use of monoamine oxidase inhibitors. Recently moved to FDA category Schedule IV in United States
Tapentadol	50-100 mg, up to 600 mg/day (⅓ to ⅔ as potent as morphine)	PO	4-6 h, 12 h for SR	Dual action involves inhibition of norepinephrine reuptake. May have fewer of certain side effects than morphine, such as gastrointestinal and respiratory depression. Maximum dose 600 mg/day. Avoid concurrent use of monoamine oxidase inhibitors. Schedule II in United States. Approved for diabetic neuropathy

DEA = Drug Enforcement Administration; ECG = electrocardiogram; FDA = U.S. Food and Drug Administration; IM = intramuscular; IN = intranasal; IR = immediate release; IV = intravenous; NMDA = N-methyl-D-aspartate; PO = oral; PR = rectal; SL = sublingual; SR = sustained release; TD = transdermal; TM = transmucosal.

who have concomitant psychosocial issues (e.g., secondary gain, untreated depression) or a greater burden of disease, are taking opioids, and have a discordance between their symptoms and the findings on physical examination or imaging are unlikely to benefit. Although the theoretical benefits of adding a corticosteroid to lidocaine include blocking the inflammatory cascade (thereby suppressing ectopic discharges from injured nerves and inhibiting the synthesis of prostaglandins), the incremental benefit of adding corticosteroids to a local anesthetic for nerve blocks or to epidural or joint injections is small.[A14] In patients who benefit from local injections, translating the temporary relief into long-term improvement necessitates addressing the underlying cause, which often requires rehabilitation and psychotherapy.

Biologic therapies such as bone marrow concentrate and platelet-rich plasma have shown inconsistent results in the treatment of musculoskeletal disorders and peripheral nerve injuries.[A15] In patients with lumbar facet joint pain, sacroiliac joint pain, or knee osteoarthritis, evidence supporting radiofrequency denervation is mixed.[13] In patients with cancer pain, neurolytic procedures targeting the celiac plexus for upper abdominal pain and the superior hypogastric plexus for pelvic pain may provide significant benefit lasting several months.

Electrical Stimulation

The most common form of electrical stimulation[14] is transcutaneous electrical nerve stimulation. The evidence supporting transcutaneous electrical nerve stimulation to treat chronic pain is mixed, with evidence of limited, short-term benefit for neuropathic pain[A16] but not for back pain. Spinal cord stimulation is a neuromodulatory technique in which an electrode is inserted epidurally to stimulate the dorsal column. Conventional, high-frequency, and burst stimulation have all been shown to be effective for chronic pain, with mixed evidence supporting one modality over another. The strongest evidence for spinal cord stimulation is to treat complex regional pain syndrome, ischemic pain, and back pain with predominantly radicular pain after unsuccessful back surgery.

Peripheral nerve stimulation is used for patients with neuropathic pain in the distribution of one or two nerves and for headaches (Chapter 367), with relief sometimes persisting for more than 1 year for neuropathic pain but mixed evidence for efficacy in migraine headaches.[15] In patients with intractable chronic pain unresponsive to conservative measures, deep brain and motor cortex stimulation may be considered, with the strongest evidence for neuropathic pain.

Surgery

Surgical interventions are often advocated in patients who have failed conservative measures. A traumatic neuroma is an inexorable consequence of cutting or burning a nerve, formed as a result of unregulated and disorganized nerve regeneration. Neuromas have been shown to fire ectopic pain signals and are often quite painful. Hence, neurolytic procedures are rarely successful in the

TABLE 26-7 GUIDELINES FOR OPIOID THERAPY

1. Nonpharmacologic and nonopioid pharmacologic therapy are preferred for subacute and chronic pain and should be used before initiating opioid therapy. For acute pain, consider opioid therapy only if the benefits are anticipated to outweigh the risks.
2. Establish realistic goals before starting opioid therapy and discuss how therapy will be discontinued.
3. Before starting opioids and during treatment, risk factors for harm should be evaluated, and strategies to mitigate risk (e.g., offering naloxone) should be incorporated in patients who are at risk of overdose.
4. Initiate therapy with immediate-release opioids.
5. Start with the lowest effective dose; carefully reassess benefits and risks when dosage is increased. Avoid increasing doses to levels likely to yield diminishing benefits relative to risks.
6. For patients who are already receiving higher opioid dosages, clinicians should carefully weigh benefits and risks and exercise care when reducing or continuing the opioid dosage. If risks outweigh benefits of continued opioid therapy, clinicians should optimize other therapies and work closely with patients to taper to lower dosages gradually or, if warranted, appropriately taper and discontinue opioids. In the absence of life-threatening or extenuating circumstances, opioid therapy should not be discontinued abruptly, and clinicians should not abruptly or rapidly reduce opioid dosages.
7. For the treatment of acute pain, clinicians should prescribe no greater quantity than needed for the expected duration of pain severe enough to require opioids.
8. Evaluate the patient within 1 to 4 weeks after starting opioids, and reevaluate the benefits and harms within 3 months or more frequently as indicated.
9. When prescribing opioids for acute, subacute, or chronic pain, review the patient's history of use of controlled substance with a prescription drug monitoring program.
10. When prescribing opioids for subacute or chronic pain, consider toxicology testing to assess for prescribed medications as well as other prescribed and nonprescribed controlled substances.
11. Clinicians should use extreme caution when prescribing opioids and benzodiazepines concurrently and consider whether the benefits outweigh risks when concurrently prescribing opioids and other central nervous system depressants.
12. For patients with opioid use disorder (Chapter 365), offer or arrange treatment with medications (e.g., buprenorphine or methadone).

Adapted from Dowell D, Ragan KR, Jones CM, Baldwin GT, Chou R. CDC guideline for prescribing opioids—United States, 2022. Available at https://www.cdc.gov/mmwr/volumes/71/rr/pdfs/rr7103a1-H.pdf.

long-term treatment of neuropathic pain. Total joint replacement (Chapter 255) is an increasingly common treatment for osteoarthritis of the knee or hip, but up to 40% of patients will experience significant pain following arthroplasty. Surgery done solely to remove a painful body part (e.g., orchiectomy, limb amputation) rarely results in long-term benefit.

Complementary and Alternative Therapies

Pain is the most common indication for complementary and alternative medical treatments (Chapter 30), with utilization rates approaching 40%. Some of the most popular modalities are acupuncture, chiropractic, nutraceuticals, Tai Chi, and yoga, all of which are beneficial in certain contexts. However, the magnitude of benefit tends to be modest, and little evidence supports one modality over another or against conventional medical treatments. Other supplements that have been used to treat chronic pain include omega-3 polyunsaturated fatty acids, natural eggshell membrane, turmeric, ginger, magnesium, and vitamin B_{12}.

Back Pain

In many populations, back pain is the leading cause of pain worldwide. Careful diagnostic assessment is required. For pain that has a clear anatomic cause and does not respond to medications, physical therapy, injections, and surgery may all be considered (Chapter 369).[A17]

Pain Management in Vulnerable Populations

Persons at particularly high risk for chronic pain include individuals with intellectual disabilities, older adults, indigent people, and torture survivors.[16] For these vulnerable populations, focus should be on the utilization of tools to assess pain and monitor treatment compatible with cognitive abilities, adapting therapy to individual circumstances, understanding age-related differences in drug pharmacokinetics, and ensuring autonomy and dignity.

Older adults have higher pain thresholds and lower pain tolerance; they are more likely to report pain, often with multiple comorbid conditions, than are younger adults. The increased risk for drug-related adverse effects in this population is the basis for the popular recommendation, "start low and go slow" in the titration of drugs. Age-related physiologic factors that can decrease the therapeutic dose of opioid and nonopioid analgesics include changes in volume of distribution and protein binding, decreased metabolism, decreased excretion, and increased pharmacologic sensitivity. Thus, nonpharmacologic interventions such as ergonomic modifications, tailored physical therapy and exercise programs, nutritional consultation, psychobehavioral approaches, and injections should be considered in appropriate patients.[17]

FUTURE DEVELOPMENTS

Research is addressing the genotyping and phenotyping of chronic pain patients both to identify individuals at high risk for chronification of pain and to guide treatment. Neuroimaging and molecular biomarkers may, in the future, help to measure nociception and pain, and also function as objective indicators of treatment response.

Regenerative therapies (Chapter 34) seek to facilitate the body's ability to repair, replace, restore, and/or regenerate diseased or damaged tissue. Some treatments, such as platelet-rich plasma, are commonly used to treat musculoskeletal conditions with mixed results. Others, such as stem cell therapy, are also being investigated for nerve injury and degenerative conditions. The approach to managing pain must consider the reality of spiraling health care costs and opioid addiction (Chapter 365).

GENERAL REFERENCES

For the General References and other additional features, please visit Elsevier eBooks+ at https://ebooks.health.elsevier.com.

Grade A References

A1. Ferro Moura Franco K, Lenoir D, Dos Santos Franco YR, et al. Prescription of exercises for the treatment of chronic pain along the continuum of nociplastic pain: a systematic review with meta-analysis. *Eur J Pain*. 2021;25:51-70.
A2. Machado GC, Maher CG, Ferreira PH, et al. Efficacy and safety of paracetamol for spinal pain and osteoarthritis: systematic review and meta-analysis of randomised placebo controlled trials. *BMJ*. 2015;350:h1225.
A3. Machado GC, Abdel-Shaheed C, Underwood M, et al. Non-steroidal anti-inflammatory drugs (NSAIDs) for musculoskeletal pain. *BMJ*. 2021;372:n104.
A4. Maloney J, Pew S, Wie C, et al. Comprehensive review of topical analgesics for chronic pain. *Curr Pain Headache Rep*. 2021;25:7.
A5. Mathieson S, Maher CG, McLachlan AJ, et al. Trial of pregabalin for acute and chronic sciatica. *N Engl J Med*. 2017;376:1111-1120.
A6. Derry S, Rice AS, Cole P, et al. Topical capsaicin (high concentration) for chronic neuropathic pain in adults. *Cochrane Database Syst Rev*. 2017;1:CD007393.
A7. Stockings E, Campbell G, Hall WD, et al. Cannabis and cannabinoids for the treatment of people with chronic noncancer pain conditions: a systematic review and meta-analysis of controlled and observational studies. *Pain*. 2018;159:1932-1954.
A8. Thornton JD, Goyat R, Dwibedi N, et al. Health-related quality of life in patients receiving long-term opioid therapy: a systematic review with meta-analysis. *Qual Life Res*. 2017;26:1955-1967.
A9. Gilron I, Tu D, Holden RR, et al. Combination of morphine with nortriptyline for neuropathic pain. *Pain*. 2015;156:1440-1448.
A10. Cherkin DC, Anderson ML, Sherman KJ, et al. Two-year follow-up of a randomized clinical trial of mindfulness-based stress reduction vs cognitive behavioral therapy or usual care for chronic low back pain. *JAMA*. 2017;317:642-643.
A11. Pei JH, Ma T, Nan RL, et al. Mindfulness-based cognitive therapy for treating chronic pain a systematic review and meta-analysis. *Psychol Health Med*. 2021;26:333-346.
A12. Geneen LJ, Moore RA, Clarke C, et al. Physical activity and exercise for chronic pain in adults: an overview of Cochrane Reviews. *Cochrane Database Syst Rev*. 2017;4:CD011279.
A13. Oliveira CB, Maher CG, Ferreira ML, et al. Epidural corticosteroid injections for lumbosacral radicular pain. *Cochrane Database Syst Rev*. 2020;4:CD013577.
A14. Shanthanna H, Busse J, Wang L, et al. Addition of corticosteroids to local anaesthetics for chronic non-cancer pain injections: a systematic review and meta-analysis of randomised controlled trials. *Br J Anaesth*. 2020;125:779-801.
A15. Belk JW, Kraeutler MJ, Houck DA, et al. Platelet-rich plasma versus hyaluronic acid for knee osteoarthritis: a systematic review and meta-analysis of randomized controlled trials. *Am J Sports Med*. 2021;49:249-260.
A16. Johnson MI, Paley CA, Jones G, et al. Efficacy and safety of transcutaneous electrical nerve stimulation (TENS) for acute and chronic pain in adults: a systematic review and meta-analysis of 381 studies (the meta-TENS study). *BMJ Open*. 2022;12:e051073.
A17. Zaina F, Tomkins-Lane C, Carragee E, et al. Surgical versus non-surgical treatment for lumbar spinal stenosis. *Cochrane Database Syst Rev*. 2016;2016:CD010264.

27

BIOLOGY OF ADDICTION

ERIC J. NESTLER

DEFINITION

Drug addiction involves compulsive substance use despite serious negative consequences. Harmful drug use and addiction are significant contributors to medical morbidity and mortality both directly as a result of the toxic effects of abused drugs and indirectly through accidents, violence, nonsterile needle use, smoking, and other health hazards. By far the greatest contributors to illness and death are the widely used legal drugs, tobacco (Chapter 363) and alcohol (Chapter 364), although illegal addictive drugs and abused prescription drugs also exact a significant toll. An increasing impact of cannabinoids is expected as legal restrictions against such drugs are eased and their use increases. In addition, addiction creates enormous burdens on society by impairing the function of the addicted person in multiple life roles, disrupting families and neighborhoods, and motivating crime.

Compulsive use, the cardinal feature of addiction, means that the affected person cannot control substance use for a significant period of time despite powerful reasons to do so, such as drug-related health problems, drug-associated arrests, or the threat of losing one's job or spouse.[1] In the outpatient setting, addiction can be remarkably frustrating to treat: drug seeking and administration are apparently voluntary behaviors that an otherwise sentient person seems unwilling to control. Even after significant efforts have been exerted to get an addicted patient into drug treatment, relapse is common, even long after the last withdrawal symptom has cleared. Relapses are often precipitated by stress or by reminders of drug use (cues) that may range from familiar drug use contexts (such as smoking after a meal) to interactions with drug-using friends, the smell of marijuana or tobacco smoke, and body feelings previously associated with drug seeking (so-called interoceptive cues).

Drug users may repeatedly take drugs to gain pleasure or to escape from negative feelings, including the aversive feelings that may occur when drugs wear off.[2,3] As a result of repeated drug administration over time, initial protein targets for the drugs and their downstream signaling pathways (Table 27-1) are excessively stimulated and may thus undergo homeostatic adaptations. These adaptations can produce tolerance (the need for increasing drug doses to achieve desired affects) or dependence (revealed by withdrawal symptoms between drug doses or with drug cessation). Both tolerance and dependence can contribute to ongoing drug use and to dosage increases; however, neither tolerance nor dependence alone explains compulsive use. First, tolerance and dependence occur not only with repeated use of many addictive drugs (e.g., heroin, alcohol) but also with many nonaddictive drugs (e.g., β-adrenergic antagonists, α_2-adrenergic agonist antihypertensive agents, nitrates, selective serotonin reuptake inhibitor antidepressants). Second, some highly addictive drugs, such as cocaine, may produce little physical dependence and withdrawal in some individuals who nonetheless exhibit compulsive use. Finally, if dependence and withdrawal were necessary factors in addiction, the phenomenon of late, post-detoxification relapse would not be the major clinical problem that it is. Although these forms of homeostatic adaptation play a role in addiction, other types of plasticity within the nervous system are more significant.

RISK FACTORS FOR ADDICTION

Only a minority of individuals who use drugs go on to become addicted. The best-established risk factors for addiction are male sex and family history. Across countries and cultures, males have a greater risk for both heavy drug use and addiction, with risk ratios in the range of 1.4:1 to 2:1, but the sex ratios have narrowed in many countries, especially for tobacco use and alcohol. Moreover, females who succumb to addiction tend to do so more quickly after initial drug exposures, and drug use during pregnancy can have enormously deleterious effects on the fetus.[4]

Genes play a major role in familial risk as evidenced by twin and adoption studies. Twin studies consistently show higher rates of concordance for heavy drug use and addiction within monozygotic twin pairs than within dizygotic twin pairs. Adoption studies demonstrate that individuals adopted early in life tend to resemble their biologic rather than their adoptive parents with respect to patterns of alcohol use. Large population genetic studies suggest that the heritable risk for addiction to any of several substances, including opioids, stimulants, nicotine, alcohol, and marijuana, is roughly the same and varies between 30 and 60%, depending on the study. Adverse life events (e.g., stress, trauma) are important noninherited factors that also determine an individual's risk for addiction.

Although genes clearly play a significant role in vulnerability to addiction, only a small portion (<10%) of the specific genetic variants that confer risk have been identified with certainty. Like all common neuropsychiatric disorders, addiction risk is highly genetically complex; there is evidence from linkage and association studies for contributions by many hundreds of genetic variants, each with a very small effect.[5–7] The strongest genetic risk factors identified to date are variations in genes that encode acute drug targets, such as nicotinic cholinergic receptor subunits, although each contributes only a very small portion of the overall heritable risk. However, the task of gene identification is complicated by the challenges of phenotype definition. There are no objective medical tests with which to make the diagnosis, and there may be independent genetic and nongenetic risk factors for different stages of substance use disorders, such as drug experimentation, addiction, and treatment responsiveness. Moreover, twin and family studies suggest that there may be both shared and unshared genetic risk factors as well as epigenetic changes[8] underlying addictions to different drugs. As in other genetically complex disorders, it is hoped that with the identification of numerous risk-conferring variants, it will be possible to identify key biochemical pathways involved in addiction pathogenesis, which will then suggest potential targets for new and more effective treatments.

REWARD CIRCUITRY: THE NEURAL SUBSTRATE OF ADDICTION

The survival and perpetuation of species require that animals, including humans, learn to predict threats and also learn the circumstances under which they can

TABLE 27-1 PROPERTIES OF ADDICTIVE DRUGS

DRUG	NEUROTRANSMITTER	DRUG TARGET	EFFECT AFTER BINDING
Opioids (morphine, heroin, oxycodone, fentanyl)	Endorphins; enkephalins	μ and δ opioid receptor (agonist)	Activate G_i/G_o; activate K^+ channels
Psychostimulants (cocaine, amphetamines)	Dopamine (DA)	Dopamine transporter (DAT)* (antagonist)	Increase synaptic DA; stimulate presynaptic and postsynaptic DA receptors
Nicotine	Acetylcholine	Nicotinic acetylcholine receptor (nAChR) (agonist)	Stimulate cation channel (may desensitize)
Alcohol[†]	γ-Aminobutyric acid (GABA) Glutamate	$GABA_A$ receptor (agonist) *N*-methyl-D-aspartate (NMDA) receptor (antagonist)	Activate Cl^- channel Inhibit Na^+/Ca^{2+} entry
Marijuana (Δ^9-tetrahydrocannabinol)	Anandamide; 2-arachidonoylglycerol	Cannabinoid CB_1 (agonist)	Activate G_i/G_o; activate K^+ channels
Phencyclidine, ketamine	Glutamate	NMDA receptor (antagonist)	Inhibit Na^+/Ca^{2+} entry

*The psychostimulants also interact with the norepinephrine and serotonin transporters, but under normal conditions, it is the DAT that is critical for rewarding and addictive properties. Unlike cocaine, amphetamines enter dopamine nerve terminals through the DAT and interact with a second target, the vesicular monoamine transporter (VMAT), to release DA into the cytoplasm and thence, through the DAT, to release it into the synapse.

[†]Alcohol binds to and affects many other protein targets (e.g., several types of ion channels) that also contribute to its overall actions.

Modified from Hyman SE, Malenka RC, Nestler EJ. Neural mechanisms of addiction: the role of reward-related learning and memory. *Annu Rev Neurosci*. 2006;29:565-598.

obtain "rewards," such as food, water, shelter, and opportunities for mating. A simple operational definition of reward is a stimulus that elicits approach and consummatory behaviors. Several interconnected neural circuits, highly conserved in evolution, control an individual's responses to rewarding and aversive stimuli (E-Fig. 27-1). Dopamine-releasing neurons in the ventral tegmental area of the midbrain and their major target neurons in the nucleus accumbens in the ventral striatum serve as a rheostat that detects and drives responses to rewards and threats. The amygdala and hippocampus are crucial for forming reward- and fear-related memories. The dorsal striatum (caudate and putamen) mediates well-learned behaviors and habits. Finally, several regions of the prefrontal cortex exert executive control over these subcortical systems. Addiction involves abnormal functioning of this entire circuit.[9,10]

The neurotransmitter dopamine, released from ventral tegmental area nerve terminals in the nucleus accumbens, plays the key (albeit not the only) role in binding rewards and reward-associated cues to adaptive reward-seeking responses. In animals, implanted electrodes can record firing of dopamine neurons; microdialysis catheters and electrochemical methods can be used to detect dopamine that has been released from presynaptic terminals. In humans, positron emission tomography (PET) permits indirect measures of dopamine release by observing the displacement of a positron-emitting D_2 dopamine receptor ligand previously bound to receptors after a stimulus or pharmacologic challenge. Such methods show that natural rewards cause firing of neurons in the ventral tegmental area and release of dopamine in the nucleus accumbens and other forebrain regions. When dopamine action does not occur because of lesions in dopamine neurons, blockade of postsynaptic dopamine receptors, or inhibition of dopamine synthesis, rewards no longer motivate the behaviors necessary to obtain them.

The role of dopamine has been elucidated in patients with Parkinson disease (Chapter 378), which results from the death of midbrain dopamine neurons; however, neurons within the substantia nigra, which project to the dorsal striatum, are more severely affected than neurons within the ventral tegmental area. Patients are generally treated with l-dopa, a dopamine precursor, but as the disease progresses, other drugs may be needed, including selective D_2 dopamine receptor agonists. A minority of patients treated with these D_2 dopamine receptor agonists develop new risky, goal-directed behaviors, such as compulsive gambling or shopping. These behaviors generally cease when the D_2 dopamine receptor agonist is withdrawn, presumably because these agents can combine with endogenous dopamine from preserved neurons in the ventral tegmental area to overstimulate the nucleus accumbens and other components of the reward circuitry. These observations not only underscore the role of dopamine in motivation and reward seeking but also suggest that behavioral addictions share neural substrates with drug addiction.[11,12]

The precise pattern of firing of dopamine neurons and the resulting synaptic release of dopamine in forebrain circuits shape behavior so as to maximize future reward. In a basal state, dopamine neurons have a slow tonic pattern of firing. When a new, unexpected, or greater-than-expected reward is encountered, a phasic burst of firing of dopamine neurons causes a transient increase in synaptic dopamine. When a reward is predicted from known cues and is exactly as expected, there is little change from the tonic pattern of firing, that is, only small additional dopamine release. When a predicted reward is omitted or less than expected, dopamine neurons pause their firing to levels below their tonic rate. Phasic increases in synaptic dopamine signify that the world is better than expected, facilitate learning of new predictive information, and bind the newly learned predictive cues to action.

Dopamine is not the only neurotransmitter that signals reward. Other neurotransmitters, including acetylcholine, endogenous opioid peptides (e.g., enkephalin and endorphin), and endogenous lipid substances called endocannabinoids (because cannabinoid drugs like marijuana are agonists at their receptors), are also released in the reward circuitry in response to natural rewards.

PROPERTIES OF ADDICTIVE DRUGS

Addictive drugs are chemically diverse, and these interact with different molecular targets in the nervous system (Table 27-1). They also exhibit significant differences from each other in many of their physiologic and behavioral effects.[13–15] For example, cocaine and amphetamines are stimulants that increase arousal, may cause anxiety, and at lower doses enhance cognitive performance. Alcohol, which is a depressant, is anxiolytic at low doses and degrades cognitive performance. Heroin and other opioids, which are analgesic, cause drowsiness, constipation, and pupillary constriction. The shared behavioral effect of all addictive drugs is the liability, in vulnerable individuals, of causing compulsive use. The shared pharmacologic property that is a major mediator of addiction is the ability to increase levels of synaptic dopamine in the nucleus accumbens and other regions of the forebrain. For example, cocaine blocks the dopamine uptake transporter that normally clears dopamine from synapses. Amphetamines cause reverse transport of dopamine into synapses through the dopamine uptake transporter. Opioids, nicotine, cannabinoids, and alcohol cause dopamine release, and they act by different initial mechanisms to stimulate dopamine neurons in the ventral tegmental area or to release them from resting inhibitory control. The first three of these drugs also induce reward through nondopamine mechanisms (i.e., by activating cholinergic, opioid, or cannabinoid receptors). By comparison, alcohol directly affects γ-aminobutyric acid and glutamate receptors within the reward circuitry (Table 27-1).

Natural rewards, such as food or sexual opportunities, regulate the firing of dopamine neurons through highly processed sensory information, both external and interoceptive. Addictive drugs short-circuit this kind of information processing by acting directly on proteins that control dopamine and other signals in the reward circuitry. Acting by such direct pharmacologic mechanisms, addictive drugs typically produce greater quantities of synaptic dopamine and other reward-related neurotransmitters over longer times compared with natural rewards. In addition, addictive drugs provide a grossly pathologic learning signal by occluding pauses in dopamine and other neuron firing, even when drug use proves less pleasurable than expected or even aversive. For example, when the inhalation of smoke causes painful coughing, it might seem that the brain would signal an experience that is worse than expected with a resulting decrement in the firing rate of neurons in the ventral tegmental area. However, because nicotine causes dopamine release pharmacologically, independent of the smoker's actual experience, reward circuits, unavailable to conscious introspection, still receive a positive message that reinforces nicotine-seeking and nicotine use. In short, addictive drugs, by virtue of their effects on dopamine and related neurotransmitters, always signal "better than expected."

DRUG-INDUCED NEURAL PLASTICITY RELEVANT TO ADDICTION

Neurobiologic research on addiction has focused intensely on compulsive aspects of drug use, the ability of specific cues to activate drug seeking and craving, and the long persistence of stress- and cue-dependent relapse risk. As described previously, compulsive drug use and the power of drug-associated cues reflect the usurpation of the brain's reward circuitry by drugs of abuse. The persistence of addiction reflects long-term changes in neurons and synapses, as well as their interacting circuits. These long-lived alterations in gene expression can be attributed to drug-induced epigenetic mechanisms, such as modifications of chromatin.[16]

Long-term changes in gene expression may render the addicted person susceptible to stress and may also create persistent changes in hedonic state and mood regulation that may motivate drug taking. By themselves, however, changes in gene expression do not explain the ability of exquisitely specific cues to activate drug seeking or, if seeking is impeded, intense subjective drug craving. The ability of specific cues to activate drug seeking and wanting is based on long-term associative memories consolidated under the influence of dopamine and other reward signals, in part via changes in gene expression.[17,18] Long-term memory formation represents perhaps the most persistent changes in brain function that may occur in adult life. The neural substrates of memory are likely to include alterations in synaptic weights, such as long-term potentiation or long-term depression, and physical remodeling of dendritic spines.

Cues that can reinitiate drug use include environmental stimuli (e.g., persons with whom drugs have been used, drug paraphernalia) and body feelings. Because addictive drugs reliably increase synaptic dopamine and other reward-related neurotransmitters as a result of their direct pharmacologic actions—indeed, they produce excessive and grossly distorted reward signals—the brain receives a powerful impetus to connect the circumstances in which the drugs have been used with the motivation to take drugs again. Addictive drugs also activate transcription factors, such as the cyclic adenosine monophosphate response element binding protein, and alter the composition of activator protein 1 complexes in brain reward circuits.[19] Cocaine, opioids, and other addictive drugs regulate many genes downstream of these and other transcription factors. Even if the drug is no longer pleasurable, these signals continue to reinforce drug wanting and seeking. Moreover, the certainty and magnitude of these signals give drugs a marked advantage over natural rewards and other learned goals, including prosocial activities.

GENERAL REFERENCES

For the General References and other additional features, please visit Elsevier eBooks+ at https://ebooks.health.elsevier.com.

28

IMMUNOMODULATORY DRUGS

ANNE R. BASS AND INEZ ROGATSKY

Even with the availability of targeted biologic treatments (Chapter 29), synthetic immunomodulatory drugs remain the cornerstone of therapy for many autoimmune conditions, including rheumatoid arthritis, juvenile inflammatory arthritis, psoriatic arthritis, and systemic lupus erythematosus (Table 28-1). When used for rheumatic diseases, these agents are often referred to as disease-modifying antirheumatic drugs (DMARDs). Orally bioavailable and relatively inexpensive, these agents target intracellular processes important for the survival and/or function of immune cells. Many, although not all, of these agents are immunosuppressive; that is, they predispose patients to infection. With the exception of glucocorticoids, synthetic immunomodulatory agents are slow acting, generally taking 2 to 3 months to have their therapeutic effect. Some synthetic immunomodulatory drugs are U.S. Food and Drug Administration (FDA)–approved for a narrow group of conditions but are used more widely in clinical practice. For example, mycophenolate mofetil is FDA-approved for the prevention of transplant rejection but is often used to treat systemic lupus erythematosus.

GLUCOCORTICOIDS

First introduced into clinical practice in the early 1950s, glucocorticoids remain among the most commonly prescribed class of medications worldwide, primarily due to their extremely potent immunosuppressive and anti-inflammatory properties and very low cost. Despite their efficacy, serious side effects associated with glucocorticoid use prompted the race for "selective," less toxic, glucocorticoid-like compounds; however, no such new-generation glucocorticoids have yet become available. A fundamental difference setting glucocorticoids apart from other anti-inflammatory medications is that they are modeled after endogenously produced steroid hormones with numerous functions in normal mammalian physiology. Hence, "adverse effects" of their administration are not "off-target" but rather reflect expected responses of biologic systems receiving these hormones in excess of their physiologic levels and irrespective of the normal circadian cycle of glucocorticoid secretion. Endogenous glucocorticoids are produced from cholesterol by the adrenal cortex along with structurally similar mineralocorticoids (the unifying term *corticosteroids* refers to both types of molecules). These hormones signal through the glucocorticoid and mineralocorticoid receptors, respectively; however, the main endogenous glucocorticoid, cortisol, can bind both receptors. Most synthetic clinically used glucocorticoids have much higher affinity for the glucocorticoid receptors.[1]

GLUCOCORTICOID RECEPTOR

The human glucocorticoid receptor gene (*NR3C1*) encodes the main 795–amino acid GRα protein that is responsible for the majority of glucocorticoid activities and a GRβ splice variant that differs from GRα in its unique C-terminus beyond amino acid 728 and does not bind hormone. The physiologic significance of the β-isoform has been debated and likely differs between cell types depending on how much β-isoform is expressed; it has been reported to function as a dominant-negative inhibitor of GRα in certain contexts. In addition, the alternate translation start sites of GRα may give rise to different isoform combinations present in different tissues. GRα protein is a member of the nuclear receptor family—the largest family of mammalian transcription factors. Upon activation by its endogenous or synthetic hormonal ligand, cytoplasmic heat-shock protein-bound GRα undergoes structural changes and translocates to the cell nucleus, where it either binds DNA directly—typically, a specific palindromic sequence known as a glucocorticoid response element—or is tethered to DNA through protein:protein interactions with other DNA-bound regulators, particularly those of the activator protein-1 (AP1) and nuclear factor-κB (NF-κB) families (Fig. 28-1). In each case, GRα can activate or repress transcription. Commonly, however, GRα binding to palindromic glucocorticoid response elements leads to activation of associated genes, whereas binding to AP1/NF-κB represses transcription of their target genes (Fig. 28-1). Anti-inflammatory and immunosuppressive properties of glucocorticoids result both from direct activation of anti-inflammatory (interleukin [IL]-10, dual specificity phosphatase-1 [Dusp1], glucocorticoid-inducible leucine-zipper [Gilz], TNFAIP3/A20, and others) and repression of AP1- and/or NF-κB–driven pro-inflammatory genes.

The extremely broad consequences of glucocorticoid actions stem from the fact that the GRα protein is expressed essentially in every cell in the body. In each cell type, the glucocorticoid receptor activates and represses hundreds of genes, thereby leading to specific physiologic effects. Recent genome-wide analyses of GRα binding and glucocorticoid-regulated transcriptomes revealed a striking level of specificity in the glucocorticoid receptor's actions, whereby even in closely related cell types (e.g., different types of white blood cells), glucocorticoid receptor–regulated genes display a mere 15% overlap. This finding indicates that cell-specific variables (e.g., chromatin packaging and accessibility to transcription factor binding), the composition of GRα interacting accessory proteins (e.g., coactivators and corepressors that associate with GRα in a cell- and binding site–specific manner), and the physiologic state of the cell play major roles in specifying glucocorticoid function (Fig. 28-1).

PHYSIOLOGIC AND PHARMACOLOGIC EFFECTS OF GLUCOCORTICOIDS IN DIFFERENT TISSUES

Glucocorticoids and Inflammation

One of the most well-known effects underlying the widespread use of glucocorticoids is suppression of inflammation. This effect stems from dramatic reduction

TABLE 28-1 RECOMMENDED GLUCOCORTICOID DOSE TAPERING SCHEDULES, SUBJECT TO INDIVIDUAL VARIABILITY AND REQUIRING MONITORING OF PATIENT'S CLINICAL RESPONSE*

STARTING DOSE OF PREDNISONE (OR EQUIVALENT)	PROGRESSIVE DECREASE OF DAILY DOSE
>40 mg daily	5-10 mg daily every 1-2 weeks
20-40 mg daily	5 mg daily every 1-2 weeks
10-19 mg daily	2.5 mg daily every 2-3 weeks
5-9 mg daily	1 mg daily every 2-4 weeks
<5 mg daily	0.5 mg daily every 2-4 weeks

*Recommended schedules can be modified for individual patients, depending on the disease and the duration of glucocorticoid treatment.

Adapted from Guerrero Pérez F, Marengo AP, Villabona Artero CV. The unresolved riddle of glucocorticoid withdrawal. *J Endocrinol Invest.* 2017;40:1175-1181.

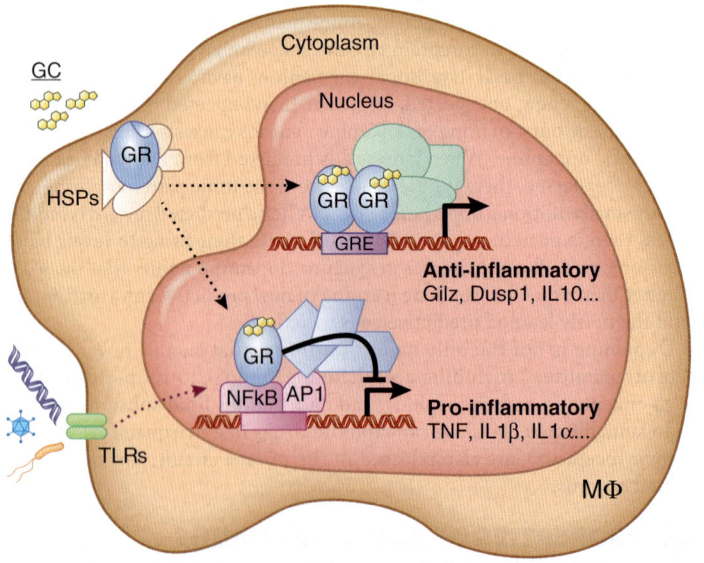

FIGURE 28-1. **Glucocorticoid receptor (GR) signaling pathway.** Unliganded GR is cytoplasmic and bound by heat-shock proteins (HSPs) that maintain its competence for glucocorticoid (GC) ligand binding. When GC-bound, GR undergoes structural change, translocates to the nucleus, and associates with specific genomic glucocorticoid response elements (GREs) (two hexameric head-to-tail [inverted] half-sites separated by three base pairs) or tethers to DNA through protein:protein interactions with AP1 and NF-κB, the effector pro-inflammatory transcription factors downstream of toll-like receptors (TLRs). In each case, a number of coactivator and corepressor proteins associate with GR in a binding site–specific manner. Some proteins encoded by genes activated and repressed by GR in a macrophage (MΦ) through direct DNA binding and tethering, respectively, are listed. AP1 = activator protein 1; IL = interleukin; NFκB = nuclear factor kappa light chain enhancer of activated B cells; TNF = tumor necrosis factor.

in the transcription of genes encoding inflammatory cytokines (tumor necrosis factor [TNF], IL-1α, IL-1β, IL-12p40, IL-6), chemokines (Cxcl10, Ccl2, Ccl3, Ccl4, Ccl5), and cell adhesion molecules (ICAM, ELAM), along with other mediators of inflammation (such as those produced through the activity of cyclooxygenase-2 and phospholipase A2: prostaglandins, leukotrienes, and arachidonic acid metabolites) produced by macrophages, endothelial cells, fibroblasts, and other cell types. These changes yield a less inflammatory environment, reducing leukocyte and lymphocyte trafficking, as well as their numbers, due to both a decrease in proliferation and an increase in apoptosis for certain cell subsets. It should be noted that glucocorticoid receptor–mediated apoptosis, specifically of immature and transformed lymphocytes, makes glucocorticoids the drug of choice for numerous hematologic malignancies.

Physiologically, glucocorticoid production in inflammatory conditions is triggered through the activation of the hypothalamic-pituitary-adrenal (HPA) axis by inflammatory cytokine signaling when the local mechanisms to control inflammation fail. This effect is transient and self-limited due to a negative feedback loop back to the hypothalamus that suppresses excessive HPA activity.[2] Pharmacologically, prolonged or high-dose glucocorticoid administration is not susceptible to HPA-mediated inhibition and may lead to immunosuppression and increased susceptibility to infections. It is important to note that the effect of glucocorticoids on immune cell types is not indiscriminately suppressive but modulatory and generally favors Th2-type T-cell responses while suppressing Th1; similarly, glucocorticoids inhibit the function of inflammatory macrophages while promoting macrophage commitment to the homeostatic anti-inflammatory phenotype.

Glucocorticoids and Metabolism in the Liver, Adipose Tissue, and Muscle

As the name suggests, endogenous glucocorticoids are critical mediators of glucose, as well as lipid and protein metabolism. In the liver, glucocorticoids are essential for maintaining normal blood glucose levels during fasting, awakening, and periods of stress, partly by increasing the hepatic responsiveness to glucagon. This occurs through stimulation of gluconeogenesis (indeed, GR activates genes encoding rate-limiting enzymes of gluconeogenesis such as *PEPCK*). Glucocorticoids have also been implicated in the regulation of fatty acid metabolism in the liver. In the adipose tissue, glucocorticoids both increase adipocyte differentiation and decrease lipolysis upon chronic exposure; the result is to promote visceral fat accumulation. Finally, in the skeletal muscle, glucocorticoids inhibit protein synthesis while promoting proteolysis to provide amino acids for gluconeogenesis.

The compound systemic effects of glucocorticoid excess on the key metabolic tissues—the liver, adipose tissue, and muscle—are perhaps best highlighted in patients with Cushing syndrome (Chapter 208) resulting from pituitary or adrenocortical adenomas or long-term administration of glucocorticoid medications. These include glucose intolerance due to increased gluconeogenesis in the liver and antagonism of the effects of insulin on peripheral glucose utilization, fasting and postprandial hyperglycemia, and reduced insulin sensitivity[3]—typical signs of type 2 diabetes and metabolic syndrome (Chapter 210). Patients with Cushing syndrome often present with dyslipidemia due to both an increase in triglyceride and total cholesterol levels and adipocyte differentiation in the visceral adipose tissue, ultimately leading to centripetal adiposity. Finally, catabolic effects of high circulating glucocorticoids in the muscle result in skeletal muscle atrophy and weakness.

Glucocorticoids and the Cardiovascular System

Glucocorticoids are required to maintain blood volume and pressure, as well as normal arteriolar tone and cardiac output. Consequently, sustained exposure to high-dose glucocorticoids results in elevated blood pressure—an effect observed both in patients with Cushing syndrome and in individuals treated with glucocorticoids. Of note, in Cushing syndrome, a part of this effect is a consequence of increased retention of water and sodium by the kidneys—an activity of mineralocorticoid receptors, rather than glucocorticoid receptors, activated by endogenous cortisol. However, synthetic glucocorticoids lacking any mineralocorticoid receptor–binding activity have an independent glucocorticoid receptor–mediated effect on blood pressure by suppressing the production of vasodilators (e.g., prostaglandins and endothelial nitric oxide) while stimulating the responsiveness to vasoconstrictors (e.g., vasopressin and catecholamines) and augmenting the expression of angiotensin II receptors, ultimately increasing peripheral vascular resistance (Chapter 64).

Glucocorticoids and the Bones

Two of the most debilitating adverse effects of glucocorticoid treatment are osteoporosis (Chapter 225)[4] and osteonecrosis (Chapter 229). Glucocorticoids have a spectrum of functions in normal bone physiology by acting upon both key cell types: osteoblasts and osteoclasts (Chapter 225). Glucocorticoids are required for normal bone growth and remodeling; they stimulate osteoclastogenesis, in part, by activating the expression of RANK ligand—a critical growth factor for osteoclast maturation—while inhibiting the expression of its decoy receptor osteoprotegerin in surrounding osteoblasts and stromal cells, ultimately leading to bone resorption. At the same time, glucocorticoids inhibit osteoblast proliferation and differentiation (by shifting stromal cell differentiation from osteoblasts to adipocytes) and promote their apoptosis. Clinically, these activities may result in significant bone loss and an increased risk of fractures, especially with prolonged use (>3 months) of oral corticosteroids or high cumulative doses of potent topical corticosteroids.[5] Fortunately, however, these effects can be lessened by co-administration of bisphosphonates, denosumab (a RANK ligand inhibitor at 60 mg subcutaneously every 6 months), or teriparatide (a recombinant parathyroid hormone at 20 μg subcutaneously daily).[A1]

Glucocorticoids and the Central Nervous System

At normal levels, glucocorticoids have long been known to be critical in the hippocampus, where they facilitate memory and learning. There is also extensive evidence that excessive glucocorticoids (including endogenous glucocorticoids during a sustained period of stress) are associated with decreased hippocampal cellularity, impaired memory, and changes in mood, cognition, and reasoning. Similarly, although adequate levels of glucocorticoids are protective against acute traumatic stress, repeated high-dose glucocorticoid treatment mimics chronic stress and induces dendritic lengthening in the basolateral amygdala—a region responsible for developing fear, anxiety, and aggression. Notably, experimental evidence also shows that exposure of the brain to increased amounts of glucocorticoids early in life or even in utero may have long-lasting consequences for the HPA axis and glucocorticoid-regulated processes such as metabolism and cardiovascular function.

Overall, while physiologic, diurnal, or acute stress-induced secretion of glucocorticoids is essential for normal brain functions and protection from stress-induced damage, sustained elevated levels of glucocorticoids cause a spectrum of central nervous system pathologies whose severity depends on the dose, duration, and time of exposure, as well as genetic, epigenomic, and environmental factors at play.

Clinical Use

Glucocorticoids are approved for use in a wide variety of inflammatory conditions at a range of doses and durations. Glucocorticoids can be used for short-term management of disease flares, such as in patients with asthma, gout, rheumatoid arthritis, juvenile inflammatory arthritis, or psoriatic arthritis, and for patients experiencing acute allergic reactions. A short course of corticosteroids also improves outcomes in ventilated patients with coronavirus 2019 diseases (Chapter 337). Other conditions require sustained glucocorticoid use to maintain disease remission, such as sarcoidosis, ulcerative colitis, eczema, minimal change glomerulonephritis, systemic lupus erythematosus, dermatomyositis, temporal arteritis, and polymyalgia rheumatica. Low doses (≤10 mg) are often adequate for rheumatoid arthritis and polymyalgia rheumatica, whereas high doses (e.g., prednisone 1 mg/kg) are required for the acute management of giant cell arteritis, lupus nephritis, and dermatomyositis. Inhaled glucocorticoids can be used for the management of asthma and chronic obstructive pulmonary disease, whereas intra-articular glucocorticoids are used to control localized joint symptoms in patients with inflammatory arthritis and osteoarthritis. Repeated intra-articular glucocorticoid injections can be associated with more rapid cartilage loss in osteoarthritis patients, however. Finally, glucocorticoids can be administered topically for the treatment of psoriasis, eczema, and other skin conditions.

Management of glucocorticoids in the perioperative period for patients on chronic steroid therapy has been traditionally based on an assumption that supraphysiologic dose increases are always required to avoid the development of adrenal insufficiency. Based on the negative results of a small number of randomized trials to test this assumption and more recent clinical experience, along with the risks of hypertension, fluid retention, hyperglycemia, and infection with the routine use of high-dose glucocorticoid supplementation, this practice should be reserved for special situations. With (1) major surgical procedures, (2) the presence of volume-refractory hypotension, or (3) in patients requiring chronic physiologic replacement therapy for adrenal insufficiency, it has been recommended that patients should receive their steroid dose right up to the time of surgery, followed by hydrocortisone 50 to 100 mg intravenously started prior to surgery, followed by a 200-mg continuous infusion over 24 hours or by 50 to 100 mg repeated every 8 hours for at most 48 to 72 hours postoperatively (based on the known normal secretory rate of cortisol of 75 to 150 mg daily during anesthesia and major surgery).[6] Either of these regimens should be immediately followed by replacement with the patient's oral glucocorticoid therapy. Conversely, perioperative supplemental glucocorticoids are not indicated for minor or intermediate-intensity surgical procedures, for patients who are chronically taking prednisone (or equivalent) at doses of 10 mg or less daily, for patients who are on every-other-day steroids, or for patients who are using only topically administered steroids. In all these cases, treating physicians should be promptly reactive, with exogenous glucocorticoids administered in case of unexpected postoperative hypotension or other manifestations of adrenocortical insufficiency. The recommendations for withholding supraphysiologic steroid therapy perioperatively in the settings described earlier do not apply to individuals taking chronic glucocorticoid replacement for adrenal failure or to generally any surgery in children chronically treated with glucocorticoids.

Toxicity and Monitoring

Glucocorticoid toxicity is dose and duration dependent. Even inhaled glucocorticoids for asthma (Chapter 75) have metabolomic side effects,[7] and just a short burst of high-dose oral glucocorticoid therapy increases the short-term risk of gastrointestinal bleeding, heart failure, and sepsis by about three-fold.[8] Common toxicities include weight gain, Cushing syndrome, osteoporosis, osteonecrosis, diabetes, hypertension, hyperlipidemia, posterior subcapsular cataracts, increased intraocular pressure, skin fragility, poor wound healing, gastrointestinal tract bleeding and perforation, mood changes, myopathy, and predisposition to infection, including opportunistic ones. Glucocorticoids administered to children can also result in growth retardation. Patients starting glucocorticoids should be counseled to take supplemental calcium and vitamin D; additional treatments to prevent osteoporosis depend on the anticipated dose and duration of glucocorticoid treatment, the patient's age, and baseline osteoporosis risk.

Because patients on exogenous glucocorticoids can develop secondary adrenal insufficiency, the dose of glucocorticoids should be tapered gradually to accommodate a slow return of adrenal function (Table 28-1). Different tapering regimens for glucocorticoids in different diseases are based on a very low quality of evidence. Considering the sizable individual variation in response to tapering, it is unlikely that a secure, uniform glucocorticoid tapering schedule applicable to all patients will be determined in the foreseeable future, as recently summarized. A systematic, broadly based review estimated the risk of clinical or subclinical adrenal insufficiency after glucocorticoid withdrawal to be approximately 30% after use of a variety of types of glucocorticoids in several underlying diseases. The problem of this apparently high rate of adrenal insufficiency is compounded by its difficulty in recognition, because symptoms and signs are usually nonspecific (e.g., nausea, vomiting, abdominal cramps, fatigue) and insidious in onset. Dosage, duration of treatment, administration route, age, fragility, underlying disease, and even laboratory testing of serum cortisol level are not completely useful in predicting adrenal insufficiency. Some generalizations can be made regarding glucocorticoid withdrawal[9]:

1. Hypothalamic-pituitary-adrenal (HPA) axis suppression mostly occurs after oral or parenteral glucocorticoid treatment that leads to higher systemic levels of glucocorticoids, but it may also appear with cutaneous, ototopical, or ophthalmic administration.
2. HPA suppression is improbable in patients who have received glucocorticoid treatment for less than 3 weeks.
3. HPA suppression is improbable in patients who have received daily prednisone at a dose of less than 5 mg (or equivalent) or alternate-day prednisone at doses of less than 10 mg (or equivalent).
4. Repeated biochemical monitoring for adrenal insufficiency with glucocorticoid withdrawal is impractical. If needed, a first assessment that measures morning serum cortisol level (between 8:00 and 9:00 AM) may be helpful but not conclusive in most cases. Among classical stimulatory tests to diagnose adrenal insufficiency, the insulin tolerance test is considered the gold standard, but it requires medical supervision because of its risk and is contraindicated in several populations. A standard-dose corticotropin analog test may be more reliable and accurate than the morning cortisol level, but it is cumbersome.
5. Patients who have adrenal insufficiency upon glucocorticoid withdrawal usually respond symptomatically to reinstitution of glucocorticoid therapy.
6. During the year after discontinuing glucocorticoids, patients should be well educated on the risks of adrenal insufficiency[10] and know that they may require glucocorticoids in situations of stress (such as surgery or significant medical illness) to compensate for reduced adrenal glucocorticoid production.

Notwithstanding the complex variables that determine the effectiveness and safety of glucocorticoid tapering, which may also include genetic determinants, an example of a general tapering scheme might be a stable reduction of 10 to 20% with monitoring of clinical response of the patient (see Table 28-1).

Glucocorticoid use in pregnancy can be associated with low-birthweight babies and may slightly increase the risk of cleft palate, but glucocorticoids are commonly used in pregnancy when needed by the mother (Chapter 221). Prednisone and prednisolone are metabolized to an inactive form by placental 11β-hydroxysteroid dehydrogenase and do not reach the fetus. In contrast, fluorinated glucocorticoids such as dexamethasone and betamethasone do cross the placenta and are used predelivery to treat the fetus and induce fetal lung maturation.

IMMUNOMODULATORY AGENTS

Hydroxychloroquine

Mechanism of Action

The mechanism of action of hydroxychloroquine is not fully understood, but the drug is known to reduce lysosomal activity and autophagy (the process in which organelles and proteins are sequestered into vesicles that fuse with lysosomes to be broken down and used as fuel for other cellular needs). Hydroxychloroquine also reduces the presentation of class II major histocompatibility complex autoantigens, as well as signaling through toll-like receptors 7 and 9. Hydroxychloroquine is given as a once- or twice-daily oral dose; it is readily absorbed and has a long half-life due to extensive tissue uptake.

Clinical Use

Hydroxychloroquine was developed to treat malaria but is also approved for the treatment of systemic lupus erythematosus (Chapter 245) and rheumatoid arthritis (Chapter 243). Hydroxychloroquine can help to control lupus skin disease, arthritis, serositis, and mild hematologic abnormalities, and discontinuing hydroxychloroquine increases the risk of a lupus flare. Hydroxychloroquine is not used as primary treatment for lupus nephritis, but the drug can help reduce the risk of end-stage renal disease in these patients. Hydroxychloroquine also reduces the risk of type 2 diabetes and venous thromboembolism, lowers cholesterol levels, and improves overall lupus survival. In patients with rheumatoid arthritis, hydroxychloroquine is a component of "triple therapy" (along with sulfasalazine and methotrexate), which is as effective as methotrexate plus a TNF inhibitor. Hydroxychloroquine is also used in some inflammatory and rheumatic skin diseases, mainly as a steroid-sparing agent.

Toxicity and Monitoring

Hydroxychloroquine can cause retinopathy, which is treatment dose and duration related. Retinopathy risk can be minimized by using a dose less than or equal to 5 mg/kg and by referring the patient for ophthalmologic screening. Hydroxychloroquine can also be associated with pruritus, areas of blue-gray "bruiselike" skin pigmentation, particularly on the lower extremities, cardiomyopathy, prolongation of the QT interval, proximal myopathy, and peripheral neuropathy. Hydroxychloroquine is not associated with fetal malformations and is generally continued during pregnancy in lupus patients in order to prevent a disease flare.

Sulfasalazine

Mechanism of Action

Sulfasalazine is metabolized by intestinal bacteria to sulfapyridine and 5-aminosalicylic acid (5-ASA). Sulfapyridine is well absorbed, whereas most of the 5-ASA remains in the intestine. 5-ASA appears to be responsible for the therapeutic effect of sulfasalazine in ulcerative colitis (Chapter 127) through an unknown mechanism. It should be noted that 5-ASA is a weak cyclooxygenase 1 and 2 inhibitor, and traditional nonsteroidal anti-inflammatory agents, which strongly inhibit cyclooxygenase, actually worsen colitis. How sulfasalazine ameliorates rheumatoid arthritis is unknown. Sulfasalazine is given in split daily doses ranging from 2 to 4 g/day.

Clinical Use

Sulfasalazine is approved for the treatment of ulcerative colitis (Chapter 127), as well as polyarticular juvenile inflammatory arthritis and rheumatoid arthritis. In rheumatoid arthritis, sulfasalazine is a component of "triple therapy" (along with hydroxychloroquine and methotrexate), which has been shown to be as effective as methotrexate plus a TNF inhibitor. Sulfasalazine is also used in the treatment of psoriatic arthritis.

Toxicity and Monitoring

Sulfasalazine can be associated with severe hypersensitivity reactions and should never be given to individuals with sulfa or aspirin allergy. Sulfasalazine can also cause agranulocytosis (Chapter 153) and aplastic anemia (Chapter 151). More common side effects of sulfasalazine include gastrointestinal upset, headache, and liver dysfunction.

Sulfasalazine has not been associated with fetal abnormalities; however, because sulfasalazine can inhibit folate absorption, folic acid supplementation is especially important in pregnant women taking the drug. Sulfasalazine can cause reversible oligospermia, and alternative treatments should be considered in male patients attempting to conceive a child.

IMMUNOSUPPRESSIVE AGENTS

Methotrexate

Mechanism of Action

Methotrexate inhibits dihydrofolic acid reductase, which results in antiproliferative effects via reduced synthesis of purines, pyrimidines, and polyamines. Methotrexate polyglutamates (metabolites) also inhibit aminoimidazole carboxamide ribonucleotide transformylase, an inhibitor of adenosine deaminase. This results in high intracellular levels of adenosine, which, when released, can have anti-inflammatory effects on neutrophils, macrophages, and lymphocytes. Oral absorption of methotrexate is dose dependent and varies among individuals. Subcutaneous dosing can be used to ensure bioavailability and helps to reduce gastrointestinal side effects. Methotrexate is excreted largely through glomerular filtration and active tubular secretion, and dose reduction is important in individuals with renal insufficiency, such as the elderly. Methotrexate is administered weekly as either a single dose or in three divided doses 12 hours apart over a 24-hour period. Although high-dose methotrexate (20 to 25 mg per week) is associated with greater efficacy than lower doses (5 to 15 mg per week), dosages are generally "ramped up" while monitoring for dose-dependent toxicities.

Clinical Use

Along with cyclosporine and acitretin, methotrexate is approved as one of the conventional systemic immunomodulatory treatments of psoriasis (Chapter 405). Several biologic agents have since emerged for the treatment of moderate to severe psoriasis. Methotrexate is FDA-approved for the treatment of rheumatoid arthritis,[11] polyarticular juvenile inflammatory arthritis, and psoriatic arthritis. Methotrexate monotherapy is recommended as the first-line treatment in patients with early rheumatoid arthritis, with or without glucocorticoid therapy (Chapter 243). If disease activity remains high, then methotrexate can be combined with hydroxychloroquine and/or sulfasalazine or combined with a biologic DMARD, generally a TNF inhibitor or a Janus kinase inhibitor. In patients with psoriatic arthritis (Chapter 244), methotrexate is effective in treating peripheral arthritis and psoriasis but is not effective in treating enthesitis, dactylitis, or nail or spine involvement.

Toxicity and Monitoring

In addition to predisposing patients to infection, methotrexate can cause liver toxicity and bone marrow suppression.[12] Complete blood counts and liver function testing should be performed monthly for 3 months at the initiation of therapy (and after changes in dose) and every 3 to 4 months thereafter. Renal function should also be monitored because a fall in glomerular filtration rate reduces methotrexate clearance. Alcohol should be avoided in patients on methotrexate, and methotrexate should not be prescribed to individuals with underlying liver disease. Patients with psoriasis (Chapter 405), particularly patients who have diabetes or who are obese, appear to be at higher risk of liver toxicity than patients with rheumatoid arthritis. Liver biopsy may be recommended in psoriatic patients who have received a cumulative methotrexate dose between 1.5 and 4 grams, depending on their level of risk. Non-Hodgkin lymphoma (Chapter 171) has been reported in patients treated with methotrexate, including some cases that regressed without additional treatment upon withdrawal of methotrexate. Methotrexate can be associated with acute pneumonitis or pulmonary fibrosis, and smokers are at increased risk for pulmonary toxicity. In patients with rheumatoid arthritis, methotrexate-induced lung injury can sometimes be difficult to distinguish from rheumatoid lung disease. Stomatitis, nausea, malaise, and fatigue are other relatively common side effects of methotrexate. Toxicity can be lessened by administration of folic acid 1 mg daily or folinic acid 5 mg weekly 12 to 24 hours after each methotrexate dose.

Methotrexate is teratogenic and can also cause fetal death. It is contraindicated in pregnant women and nursing mothers, and it should not be used for at least 3 months before planned conception in either men or women.

PURINE AND PYRIMIDINE INHIBITORS

Leflunomide

Mechanism of Action

Leflunomide inhibits dihydro-orotate dehydrogenase and thereby results in decreased pyrimidine synthesis and antiproliferative effects. Leflunomide is given as a daily 20-mg dose. It has a long half-life (≈2 weeks) due to biliary recycling, and using a loading dose (100 mg daily × 3 days) at treatment initiation leads to a more rapid clinical response. Leflunomide has both renal (early) and fecal (late) elimination, and in cases of severe leflunomide toxicity, a cholestyramine washout (cholestyramine 8 g three times daily × 11 days) causes rapid drug elimination. Without a washout, leflunomide metabolites remain detectable in the blood for up to 2 years.

Clinical Use

Leflunomide is FDA-approved for the treatment of rheumatoid arthritis (Chapter 243), where it improves signs and symptoms of the disease and prevents structural damage. Leflunomide is also used in the management of peripheral arthritis in patients with psoriatic arthritis.

Toxicity and Monitoring

Leflunomide can cause severe liver injury, including fatal liver failure. Leflunomide can also cause marrow suppression and predispose patients to infection. Liver function testing and complete blood counts should be performed monthly for 3 to 6 months at the initiation of therapy and every 2 to 3 months thereafter. If there is a three-fold rise in aminotransferase levels, then leflunomide should be discontinued and a cholestyramine washout used. As with methotrexate, there are reports of leflunomide-associated interstitial lung disease. Leflunomide commonly causes diarrhea and mild alopecia. Minor side effects may resolve with leflunomide dose reduction. Although there are no data specifically linking leflunomide to the development of malignancy, the risk of lymphoma may be increased in any patient on immunosuppressive therapy.

Leflunomide is teratogenic and can also cause fetal death; it is contraindicated in pregnant women and nursing mothers, and it should not be used in women of childbearing age who are not using contraception. Women planning pregnancy should stop leflunomide and use a cholestyramine washout. Pregnancy should not be attempted until the blood leflunomide M1 metabolite level is less than 0.02 mg/L on two separate tests at least 2 weeks apart.

Mycophenolate Mofetil

Mechanism of Action

Mycophenolate mofetil is rapidly metabolized to mycophenolic acid, the active metabolite.[13] Mycophenolic acid blocks the function of inosine monophosphate dehydrogenase and thereby inhibits the de novo pathway of guanosine synthesis. Because T and B lymphocytes lack salvage pathways to synthesize purines, mycophenolate mofetil acts preferentially on lymphocytes. In addition to these antiproliferative effects, mycophenolate mofetil reduces antibody formation by B cells. Mycophenolate mofetil is given orally twice daily, with dose reduction in patients with severe renal impairment.

Clinical Use

Mycophenolate mofetil is approved for use in kidney, liver, and heart transplant (Chapter 38) recipients in combination with cyclosporine and glucocorticoids. Mycophenolate mofetil has also been shown to be as effective as cyclophosphamide in inducing remission of lupus nephritis and superior to azathioprine in maintaining remission of lupus nephritis (Chapter 245). Mycophenolate mofetil is as effective as cyclophosphamide in the management of scleroderma-related interstitial lung disease.

Toxicity and Monitoring

Mycophenolate mofetil can cause neutropenia and other cytopenias. Nausea and diarrhea are common with the drug. Mycophenolate mofetil increases the risk of infection and may also increase the risk of lymphoma.

Mycophenolate mofetil is a pregnancy category D drug that has been associated with congenital malformations and miscarriages and is contraindicated in pregnancy. Reliable contraception should be used in women of childbearing age on mycophenolate mofetil, and contraception should be continued for at least 6 weeks after discontinuing the drug. Breast-feeding should also be avoided in mothers on mycophenolate mofetil.

Azathioprine and 6-Mercaptopurine

Mechanism of Action

Azathioprine is a derivative of 6-mercaptopurine (6-MP), and their effects are similar. Both drugs are activated by hypoxanthine-guanine phosphoribosyltransferase (HGPRT) to form 6-thioguanine nucleotides that can be incorporated into DNA, causing cytotoxicity. Other drug metabolites inhibit the enzyme glutamine-5-phosphoribosylpyrophosphate amidotransferase, required for de novo purine synthesis. Both drugs result in dose-dependent suppression of delayed-type hypersensitivity and cytotoxicity. Azathioprine and 6-MP are metabolized in the liver and in erythrocytes via two pathways, one using thiopurine S-methyltransferase (TPMT) and the other using xanthine oxidase. Ten percent of the population is heterozygous for a nonfunctioning TPMT allele and 0.3% are homozygous for this allele, resulting in intermediate or low to absent TPMT levels, respectively. Patients with low or absent TPMT can experience life-threatening myelosuppression when given azathioprine or 6-MP, while those with intermediate levels benefit from lower drug dosages. TPMT testing (level or genotype) can help identify individuals at increased risk of myelotoxicity, but because myelotoxicity can occur even in the presence of normal TPMT levels, all patients require close monitoring of complete blood counts, particularly at the initiation of therapy and with any dose change. The second route of azathioprine and 6-MP inactivation, via xanthine oxidase, can be inhibited by xanthine oxidase inhibitors, such as allopurinol or febuxostat, used in the treatment of gout. The dose of azathioprine or 6-MP must be reduced when one of these drugs is used. Azathioprine and 6-MP are given as a single or split daily dose. The daily dose of azathioprine in patients with autoimmune diseases and as maintenance to prevent transplant rejection is 1 to 3 mg/kg.

Clinical Use

Azathioprine is approved for the treatment of rheumatoid arthritis, though rarely used for this indication, and as adjunctive therapy in the prevention of renal transplant rejection (Chapter 117). 6-MP is approved for the treatment of acute lymphatic leukemia as part of a combination regimen. Azathioprine and 6-MP can help to maintain remission in ulcerative colitis[14] and are sometimes used as steroid-sparing agents in Crohn disease (Chapter 127). Azathioprine is most commonly used as a steroid-sparing agent in systemic lupus erythematosus (Chapter 245).

Toxicity and Monitoring

Bone marrow suppression is common and dose-related in patients receiving azathioprine or 6-MP, and it can result in leukopenia, anemia, and thrombocytopenia. Gastrointestinal side effects, including nausea, vomiting, diarrhea, and elevated liver enzymes, are common, and azathioprine can also cause pancreatitis. Complete blood counts and measurement of liver enzymes should be performed every 1 to 2 weeks during the first month of treatment and with every change in dose, every 2 weeks for an additional 2 months, and then every 3 months thereafter. Azathioprine and 6-MP are associated with an increased risk of infections, lymphoma, and skin cancer. Rare cases of hepatosplenic T-cell lymphoma have been reported in inflammatory bowel disease patients receiving azathioprine.

Azathioprine and 6-MP are categorized as pregnancy category D drugs because they can be associated with prematurity, low birthweight, neonatal leukopenia, thymic hypoplasia, and hypogammaglobulinemia. However, immunologic effects on the fetus generally normalize within 1 year, and azathioprine is not associated with fetal malformations. For this reason, azathioprine is often continued in pregnant lupus patients, especially if they have a recent history of nephritis.

IMMUNOPHILIN-BINDING AGENTS, INCLUDING CALCINEURIN INHIBITORS

Cyclosporine

Mechanism of Action

Cyclosporine binds to cyclophilin A, the predominant immunophilin in T cells, and this binding enhances cyclophilin's inhibition of calcineurin. Calcineurin is stimulated during T-cell activation to activate nuclear factor of activated T cells (NFAT), which in turn leads to the production of IL-2 and other cytokines important in the immune response. Calcineurin also indirectly enhances activation of NFκB, which is critical for T-cell function and survival. Cyclosporine also has calcineurin-independent inhibitory effects on the mitogen-activated protein kinase (MAPK) pathway. Cyclosporine is metabolized by cytochrome P-450 3A (CYP3A) in the liver, and 95% of excretion is biliary. Drug clearance is also strongly stimulated by P-glycoprotein expression on intestinal enterocytes. Cyclosporine is given twice daily as a divided oral dose. Daily dosages for patients with rheumatic diseases are lower than maintenance doses used to prevent transplant rejection (2 to 4 mg/kg vs. 7 to 9 mg/kg, respectively). Trough drug levels should be measured to determine the optimal therapeutic dose, especially in transplant patients. Therapeutic drug concentrations differ with the measurement technique, institution, indication, and protocol. Drug interactions occur when cyclosporine is co-administered with inhibitors or inducers of CYP3A or P-glycoprotein. Azole antifungal agents, macrolide antibiotics, and calcium-channel blockers increase cyclosporine levels, whereas many anticonvulsants and St. John's wort decrease cyclosporine levels.

Clinical Use

Cyclosporine is FDA-approved for the treatment of severe plaque psoriasis (Chapter 405) and to prevent allogeneic kidney, heart, and liver transplant rejection (Chapter 38). It is also approved for the treatment of active rheumatoid arthritis but is not commonly used for this indication. In patients with psoriasis, cyclosporine is generally used intermittently and for less than 12 weeks to avoid cumulative toxicity. Cyclosporine is also a first-line treatment for pure red cell aplasia (Chapter 151). Voclosporin, a cyclosporine analogue, is approved for the treatment of active lupus nephritis in patients who are on background therapy with mycophenolate mofetil.

Toxicity and Monitoring

Cyclosporine can cause hypertension, renal insufficiency, hyperkalemia, and hyperuricemia. In patients with rheumatoid arthritis and psoriasis, blood pressure and creatinine levels should be monitored every 2 weeks during initiation of treatment and every 1 to 3 months during long-term use. If the creatinine level rises 25% above baseline, then testing should be repeated and the dosage reduced 25 to 50% if there is no improvement. Nonsteroidal anti-inflammatory drugs (NSAIDs) should be avoided in patients taking cyclosporine. Psoriasis patients treated with cyclosporine who have been previously treated with PUVA or methotrexate are at increased risk of skin cancer. Cyclosporine also increases the risk of lymphoma and predisposes patients to infection. More common side effects of cyclosporine include hypertrichosis, gum hyperplasia, and tremor.

Cyclosporine is a pregnancy category C drug. Limited experience in pregnant transplant recipients suggests that cyclosporine is not associated with fetal malformations but is associated with low-birthweight babies. Breast-feeding should be avoided in mothers on cyclosporine.

Tacrolimus

Mechanism of Action

Tacrolimus binds to the T-cell immunophilin FK-binding protein 12 (FKBP-12), and this complex inhibits activation of calcineurin (see Cyclosporine, Mechanism of Action). As with cyclosporine, tacrolimus also has calcineurin-independent inhibitory effects on the MAPK pathway. Tacrolimus is metabolized by CYP3A in the liver and is more than 90% excreted in feces. Drug interactions occur when tacrolimus is co-administered with inhibitors or inducers of CYP3A. Tacrolimus is given twice daily as a divided oral dose, with dose adjustments made based on trough levels.

Clinical Use

Tacrolimus is approved for the prevention of allogeneic kidney, heart, and liver transplant rejection, and graft survival is similar to that achieved with cyclosporine-based regimens. Tacrolimus should be used in combination with azathioprine or mycophenolate mofetil in heart and kidney transplant recipients.

Toxicity and Monitoring

Tacrolimus, particularly at high doses, can cause nephrotoxicity and hypertension and should not be used in combination with cyclosporine. Like cyclosporine, tacrolimus can also cause hyperkalemia, headache, and tremor, and it is associated with an increased risk of infections, lymphoma, and skin cancers. Tacrolimus is associated with new-onset type 2 diabetes in approximately 20% of transplant recipients, but it reverses in about one third of them by 1 year post-transplant. Tacrolimus has been associated with cardiac hypertrophy, which is reversible upon dose reduction or drug discontinuation. Tacrolimus given by injection can be associated with anaphylaxis, likely due to castor oil derivatives contained in the IV formulation, and should be avoided unless oral administration is impossible.

Tacrolimus has not been associated with fetal malformations, but it has been associated with preterm birth, as well as hyperkalemia and renal impairment during pregnancy. Breast-feeding should be avoided in mothers taking tacrolimus.

Sirolimus

Mechanism of Action

Sirolimus, like tacrolimus, binds to the immunophilin FKBP-12. However, unlike tacrolimus, the sirolimus/FKBP-12 complex inhibits activation of the mammalian target of rapamycin (mTOR) and has no effect on calcineurin. mTOR inhibition blocks antigen- and cytokine-driven T-cell proliferation and also inhibits antibody production. mTOR is also an important modulator for aging and age-related diseases. mTOR inhibitors may have anticancer activity for many types of malignancies. Sirolimus is given once daily as an oral dose, and excretion is over 90% in feces. Sirolimus has a long half-life, and dose adjustments should not be more frequent than every 7 to 14 days, guided by trough levels. A loading dose more rapidly achieves therapeutic levels, both when sirolimus treatment is initiated and when dose adjustments are made. Like cyclosporine, sirolimus is a substrate for CYP3A4 and P-glycoprotein, and concomitant use of strong inducers or inhibitors of CYP3A4 or P-glycoprotein should be avoided when possible. When given concomitantly with cyclosporine, sirolimus should be administered 4 hours after cyclosporine to minimize their interaction. The dose of sirolimus often needs to be increased after cyclosporine is withdrawn.

Clinical Use

Sirolimus is approved for the prevention of allogeneic renal transplant rejection and is used in combination with cyclosporine and glucocorticoids starting at the time of transplant (Chapter 117). Cyclosporine can be withdrawn 3 to 12 months after transplant, depending on the patient's risk of rejection. Sirolumus is also approved for the treatment of patients with lympangioleiomyomatosis (Chapter 80).

Toxicity and Monitoring

Patients taking sirolimus are at increased risk of lymphoma and infection. Sirolimus can be associated with angioedema (particularly when used together with ACE inhibitors), fluid accumulation, and delayed wound healing. Sirolimus can be associated with renal insufficiency, particularly when used with cyclosporine, and the new onset of proteinuria. Patients on sirolimus can develop hyperlipidemia and are at risk for rhabdomyolysis when given HMG-CoA reductase inhibitors, particularly if they are receiving concomitant cyclosporine.

Sirolimus is contraindicated in pregnancy, given its antiproliferative effects. Breast-feeding should also be avoided in mothers taking sirolimus.

ALKYLATING AGENTS

Cyclophosphamide

Mechanism of Action

Cyclophosphamide is a prodrug that is metabolized in the liver by CYP-450 enzymes to alkylating molecules that cause DNA cross-linking. This occurs preferentially in rapidly proliferating cells, such as tumor and hematopoietic cells.

Clinical Use

Cyclophosphamide is approved for the treatment of a variety of malignancies, as well as minimal change nephrotic syndrome, but is also used in the treatment of lupus nephritis and antineutrophil cytoplasmic antibodies (ANCA)–associated vasculitis. The use of cyclophosphamide for these conditions has declined, however, as less toxic therapies, such as mycophenolate mofetil for lupus nephritis and rituximab for ANCA-associated vasculitis, have been shown to be equally efficacious.

Toxicity and Monitoring

Cyclophosphamide causes myelosuppression and predisposes patients to infections (including opportunistic ones), and cyclophosphamide metabolites can cause hemorrhagic cystitis. Cardiac toxicity is also seen. Cyclophosphamide increases the risk of secondary malignancies and increases the risk of bladder cancer even in patients who do not experience hemorrhagic cystitis during treatment. Cyclophosphamide commonly causes nausea and hair loss. Cyclophosphamide should not be used together with a TNF inhibitor because of an increased risk of solid tumors with this combination.

Cyclophosphamide can cause infertility, and the risk is higher the older the patient and the greater the cumulative cyclophosphamide dose. Treatment with a GnRH agonist prior to each dose of cyclophosphamide can help to protect gonadal function. Cyclophosphamide causes fetal malformations and miscarriages and should not be used in pregnancy or during lactation.

GENERAL REFERENCES

For the General References and other additional features, please visit Elsevier eBooks+ at https://ebooks.health.elsevier.com.

Grade A Reference

A1. Ding L, Hu J, Wang D, et al. Efficacy and safety of first- and second-line drugs to prevent glucocorticoid-induced fractures. *J Clin Endocrinol Metab*. 2020;105:600-613.

29 BIOLOGIC AGENTS AND SIGNALING INHIBITORS

NANCY J. OLSEN AND JOHN J. O'SHEA

Many of the drugs used by clinicians, even if effective and safe, were discovered empirically, meaning their molecular target was not necessarily known in advance. By comparison, therapeutic agents derived from biologic molecules and other targeted therapies have transformed many areas of medicine over the past two decades. A significant advantage of this new type of drug is the possibility of acting on specific molecules directly involved in disease pathogenesis. The concept of targeted agents carried with it the promise of reduced toxicity compared to empirically generated agents. Although this promise may not have been universally fulfilled, most targeted drugs have relatively good margins of safety and their usage in many areas of medicine has steadily increased. The efficacy (or lack thereof) of targeted therapies has also contributed to understanding of disease mechanisms.

Targeted therapeutics can be broadly classified as "biologics," meaning that they are produced from natural sources or living organisms. In this chapter though, we will be focusing on products engineered to be produced by cells using biotechnology methods. In general, these are large molecules administered by intravenous or subcutaneous routes. Newer additions to this class are small molecules synthesized and designed for specific targets. The targeting of specific signaling pathways was challenging given the similarities of some of these molecules, such as kinases, which may contribute to many intracellular processes. Nevertheless, many of these obstacles have been successfully overcome, resulting in a class of novel therapeutics.

Targeted therapies such as biologic agents and signaling inhibitors have applications in many areas of medicine, including cancer as well as immune-mediated dermatologic, rheumatologic, infectious, neurologic, hematologic, and cardiovascular disease. The range of possible and approved indications is almost endless and will continue to be an area of intense research and development.

BIOLOGIC AGENTS

Several types of biologics have been used as targeted therapies (Table 29-1; Fig. 29-1). One widely used class of drugs is recombinant proteins, including cytokines, interferons, growth factors, and colony-stimulating factors. Examples include granulocyte colony-stimulating factor (G-CSF; filgrastim, lenograstim), used to treat neutropenia, and interleukin (IL)-2 (aldesleukin), approved for treatment of melanoma and renal cell carcinoma. Classic endocrine mediators that engage receptors and activate intracellular signaling pathways, such as growth hormone, can be considered in this category as well (Chapter 205).

In addition to cytokines, humans produce endogenous cytokine antagonists. An example is anakinra, which is a recombinant version of a naturally occurring protein, the IL-1 receptor antagonist. The drug, like the natural protein, blocks binding of IL-1 to its receptor, thereby preventing signaling. It differs from the native human protein by the addition of one terminal amino acid. It is approved to treat rheumatoid arthritis (Chapter 243) and some childhood inflammatory syndromes.

Many of the commonly used biologics are monoclonal antibodies, which were initially derived from mice using hybridoma technology. By comparison, chimeric immunoglobulins are engineered to have murine variable regions of the component heavy and light chains attached to human constant regions. An example is infliximab, which targets the cytokine tumor necrosis factor-α (TNF-α). However, antichimeric antibodies develop in some treated patients and have the potential to block their efficacy. Further refinements using phage display techniques led to development of completely humanized monoclonal immunoglobulin Gs (IgGs); the TNF-α–targeting product adalimumab was an early example. More than 100 monoclonal antibodies have now been approved for diverse indications.[1]

A variation on monoclonal antibody therapy is the creation of antibody drug conjugates, meaning that other moieties, including small molecules, are chemically linked to the antibodies; examples include brentuximab vedotin and trastuzumab emtansine. The former is used in Hodgkin's lymphoma (Chapter 172) and targets CD30 with an antibody coupled to monomethyl auristatin E to effect cell killing. The latter targets *HER2* on cancer cells by the antibody and kills the cells with its "warhead."

Another approach to designing biologic therapeutics is with fusion proteins. Most of these agents are receptors that are fused to other human proteins like the Fc portion of immunoglobulins. These agents may target soluble or cell-bound molecules such as cytokines by functioning as decoy receptors that prevent binding of the mediator to its receptor. The first major therapeutic application of this technology was etanercept, which combines the human TNF-α receptor with a human Fc portion of the IgG molecule. An alternative strategy is to graft biologically active peptides onto the Fc domain of IgG, as in romiplostim, a thrombopoietin receptor agonist, approved for treatment of immune thrombocytopenia (Chapter 158). Cytokine fusion molecules also can be created. An example is IL-2 linked to a peptide of diphtheria toxin that was

TABLE 29-1 CLASSES OF BIOTHERAPEUTICS

CLASS	TYPES	EXAMPLES
Recombinant proteins	Cytokines Growth factors IL-1 receptor antagonist	Aldesleukin (IL-2) Filgrastim Anakinra
Monoclonal antibodies	Murine Chimeric Humanized	OKT3 Infliximab Adalimumab
Antibody-drug conjugates	Tumor cytotoxics	Brentuximab vedotin
Fusion proteins	Decoy receptors Immunotoxins	Etanercept Denileukin diftitox
Engineered cells	CAR-T cells	Tisagenlecleucel

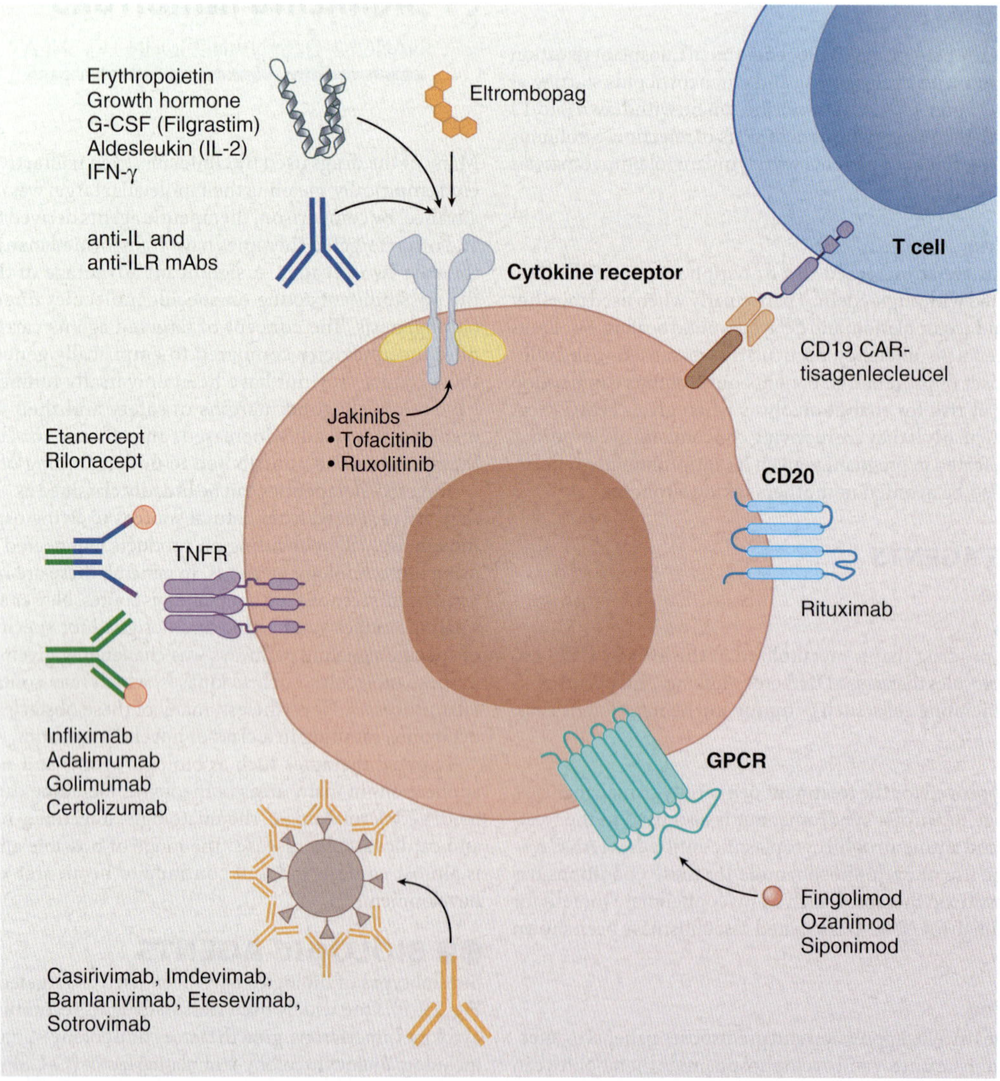

FIGURE 29-1. **Biologics and signaling inhibitors that have clinical applications as targeted therapeutics take many forms.** Recombinant cytokines and growth factors, monoclonal antibodies, and fusion proteins may target small molecules or cells. Newer approaches include cells that are engineered to target tumors and small molecular weight kinase inhibitors that block intracellular signaling pathways. The clinical applications of these therapies are numerous, ranging from malignancies to autoimmune diseases. CAR = chimeric T cell antigen receptor; G-CSF = granulocyte colony-stimulating factor; GPCR = G protein–coupled receptor; IFN = interferon; IL = interleukin; ILR = interleukin receptor; TNFR = tumor necrosis factor receptor.

approved for treatment of cutaneous T-cell lymphoma but was subsequently removed from the market because of toxicities, especially visual loss.

A more recently developed class of biologics is engineered cells. Perhaps the most exciting example of this therapy is chimeric antigen receptor (CAR)-T cells.[2,3] Such cells are a remarkable example of gene therapy in which T cells are directed to tumor cells by transduction with engineered antigen receptors. Approved CAR-T cells include tisagenlecleucel, axicabtagene ciloleucel, and lisocabtagene maraleucel, all of which target malignant B cells and represent the first examples of engineered living cells being approved.

SPECIFIC TYPES OF BIOLOGIC AGENTS

Biologic agents also can be considered in groups defined by their corresponding targets. Examples include soluble mediators (e.g., cytokines, complement proteins, antibodies, and growth factors), viruses,[4] and cells (including malignant cells and normal cells, especially T and B lymphocytes).

BIOLOGICS THAT TARGET SOLUBLE PROTEINS

Cytokines

The cytokine TNF-α binds to two receptors (TNFR55 and TNFR75), where it contributes to host responses against infection. When TNF-α production is uncontrolled, chronic inflammation can cause subsequent tissue damage in diseases such as rheumatoid arthritis (Chapter 243). Both monoclonal antibodies and soluble TNF-α receptor molecules are efficacious in inhibiting the activity of TNF-α (Table 29-2). These biologics all neutralize soluble TNF-α, but the monoclonal antibodies are more effective at also binding and preventing signaling of transmembrane forms of the cytokine. Efficacy of these approved biologics in rheumatoid arthritis and other conditions was shown in large, randomized, placebo-controlled trials in combination with methotrexate or as monotherapy.[A1,A2] However, these agents are not completely interchangeable,[5] as shown by the lack of utility of etanercept in treatment of granulomatous diseases such as Crohn disease (Chapter 127), for which infliximab is efficacious.[A3] Adverse effects of TNF blockade include an increased risk of infection, especially reactivation of latent tuberculosis, and therefore screening tests to exclude tuberculosis are required before its use.

RANKL, which is another member of the TNF superfamily, promotes osteoclast differentiation and bone resorption. Denosumab is a recombinant human monoclonal antibody that targets RANKL, which interferes with differentiation, activation, and survival of osteoclasts. It is indicated for treatment of postmenopausal osteoporosis (Chapter 225) and in men and women at high risk of bone loss after treatment with androgen deprivation therapy or aromatase inhibitors, respectively. Conversely, sclerostin, which is a product of osteocytes, inhibits bone formation; romosozumab targets sclerostin and is approved for the treatment of postmenopausal osteoporosis.

B cell activating factor (BAFF, aka Blys, CD257) is also in the TNF family. Belimumab is an anti-BAFF monoclonal antibody approved to treat adults with active systemic lupus erythematosus (Chapter 245). A fusion protein targeting CD257, blisibimod, is being investigated as a treatment for IgA nephropathy (Chapter 107).

IL-1 is an important driver of fever and induction of acute phase protein synthesis. Three approved therapeutics for IL-1 blockade are available at this time (Table 29-2): recombinant human IL-1 receptor antagonist (anakinra), a receptor fusion molecule (rilonacept) displaying both the IL-1 receptor and the IL-1 receptor accessory protein, and a fully human monoclonal antibody against IL-1β (canakinumab). Efficacy of anakinra in adult rheumatoid arthritis was somewhat disappointing, but subsequent studies in children with inflammatory arthritis showed significant therapeutic effects. It has become clear that IL-1β is the key inflammatory mediator of the autoinflammatory syndromes (Chapter 240), and IL-1 blockade using these agents has been approved for treatment of these conditions. An advantage of IL-1 blockade is a lower risk of infections than with TNF-α inhibitors. Canakinumab also has been shown to prevent recurrent cardiovascular events in patients who have suffered a myocardial infarction and who have elevated C-reactive protein (CRP) levels (Chapter 58).

Daclizumab, a humanized monoclonal IgG1 that targets the high-affinity IL-2 receptor by binding IL-2R alpha chain is approved for the prevention of acute renal transplant rejection but was discontinued in 2009. In 2016 it was approved for relapsing forms of multiple sclerosis (Chapter 380).

Dupilumab binds to the alpha chain subunit that is shared by the IL-4 and IL-13 receptors and inhibits signaling of both of these type 2 cytokines. It is approved for treatment of atopic dermatitis, asthma, and rhinosinusitis with polyps.

TABLE 29-2 APPROVED BIOTHERAPEUTICS TARGETING TNF-α, INTERLEUKIN-1, AND INTERLEUKIN-6

TARGET	THERAPEUTIC	DESCRIPTION	APPROVED INDICATIONS
TNF-α	Infliximab	Chimeric mAb	Rheumatoid arthritis, psoriatic arthritis, psoriasis, ankylosing spondylitis, Crohn disease
	Etanercept	Receptor fusion molecule	Rheumatoid arthritis, psoriatic arthritis, psoriasis, ankylosing spondylitis, polyarticular juvenile idiopathic arthritis
	Adalimumab	Humanized mAb	Rheumatoid arthritis, psoriasis, hidradenitis suppurativa, adult and pediatric Crohn disease, ankylosing spondylitis, polyarticular juvenile idiopathic arthritis
	Golimumab	Human IgG1 mAb	Rheumatoid arthritis, psoriatic arthritis, ankylosing spondylitis, ulcerative colitis
	Certolizumab pegol	Pegylated Fab′ fragment of a mAb	Rheumatoid arthritis, psoriatic arthritis, Crohn disease
IL-1	Anakinra	Recombinant human IL-1 receptor antagonist	Rheumatoid arthritis, cryopyrin-associated periodic syndromes
	Rilonacept	Recombinant receptor fusion molecule	Cryopyrin-associated periodic syndromes
	Canakinumab	Human IgG1 mAb	Systemic juvenile idiopathic arthritis, adult and pediatric familial Mediterranean fever, TNF receptor-associated periodic syndrome, hyper IgD syndrome
IL-6	Tocilizumab	Recombinant humanized mAb	Rheumatoid arthritis, giant cell arteritis, systemic juvenile idiopathic arthritis, polyarticular juvenile idiopathic arthritis
	Sarilumab	Human IgG1 mAb	Rheumatoid arthritis

IgD = immunoglobulin D; IgG = immunoglobulin G; IL = interleukin; mAb = monoclonal antibody; TNF = tumor necrosis factor.

IL-5 is important for eosinophil maturation and activation. Three anti-IL-5 monoclonal antibodies, mepolizumab, reslizumab, and benralizumab are approved for the treatment of asthma (Chapter 75) and eosinophilia (Chapter 156).

Similar to IL-1, IL-6 is a prototypic inflammatory cytokine, which drives production of TNF-α, IL-1, and IL-17.[6] Therapeutic blockade of IL-6R with tocilizumab and sarilumab is approved for treatment of inflammatory joint conditions in adults and children (Table 29-2). Subcutaneous tocilizumab is approved for the treatment of giant cell arteritis (Chapter 250). Tocilizumab use is associated with increased risk of varicella zoster virus infection as well as liver and cholesterol abnormalities. Satralizumab is an IL-6R monoclonal antibody approved for neuromyelitis optica (Chapter 392). Siltuximab is an IL-6 antibody approved for multicentric Castleman disease (Chapter 171).

IL-12 and IL-23 are dimeric cytokines that share a subunit (p40). Ustekinumab targets this common p40 chain, preventing binding of both cytokines to their corresponding receptors, which are expressed primarily on activated T cells. Ustekinumab is an approved treatment for psoriasis (Chapter 405), psoriatic arthritis (Chapter 244), and Crohn disease (Chapter 127). Agents that target the p19 subunit of IL-23, including guselkumab, tildrakizumab, and risankizumab are approved for the treatment of psoriasis and psoriatic arthritis.

The IL-17 family includes 6 members, with IL-17A and IL-17F sharing sequence similarities and having the greatest role in development of autoimmunity. Neutralizing antibodies to IL-17A (secukinumab and ixekizumab) and IL-17R (brodalumab) are approved by the U.S. Food and Drug Administration to treat ankylosing spondylitis, psoriasis, and psoriatic arthritis.[A4,7]

Interferons are important for host defense, especially against viruses but are overexpressed in autoimmune disease, particularly systemic lupus erythematosus. Anifrolumab binds to IFN-alpha receptor 1 (IFNAR1) and thereby blocks IFN-α and IFN-β. In phase III trials, anifrolumab reduced lupus disease activity, improved skin rash and arthritis, and reduced corticosteroid use. It is now approved for treatment of moderate or severe systemic lupus erythematosus.[A5] Emapalumab targets IFN-γ and is approved for hematophagocytic lymphohistiocytosis (Chapter 155).[8]

Thymic stromal lymphopoietin (TSLP) is an epithelial-derived cytokine that has a role in allergic disease, upregulates other cytokines and is elevated in the airways of patients with asthma. A recent phase II trial showed efficacy of an anti-TSLP monoclonal antibody, tezepelumab, in patients with non-eosinophilic asthma.

Antibodies

IgE antibodies mediate allergic diseases by binding through the Fc portion of the molecule to specific receptors, FcεRI and CD23/FcεRII. Omalizumab is an approved humanized IgG1 monoclonal antibody that binds free IgE and prevents receptor binding and signaling. Indications for treatment with omalizumab include allergic asthma that has failed other therapies and chronic spontaneous urticaria (Chapter 232). Because of the elevated risk of allergic reactions, subcutaneous injections of this drug must be administered in a medical office rather than in the home.

Complement

Tissue damage in allergic and immune disorders is often mediated by complement proteins, so targeting these molecules is a useful therapeutic approach. Eculizumab and ravulizumab are anti-C5 monoclonal antibodies that prevent the formation of the membrane attack complex and block chemotactic activity of C5a. They are approved to treat paroxysmal nocturnal hemoglobinuria (Chapter 146) and are available in some countries for the treatment of atypical hemolytic uremic syndrome. Investigational applications include age-related macular degeneration. An inhibitor of C5a, avacopan, is being investigated for treatment of antineutrophil cytoplasm antibody (ANCA)-associated vasculitis.[A6]

BIOLOGIC AGENTS THAT TARGET CELLS

B Lymphocytes

The humoral arm of the immune response mediates many autoimmune disorders through production of autoantibodies. Therefore, blockade or targeted elimination of B lymphocytes and inhibition of B cell–derived cytokines has been used therapeutically in diseases such as systemic lupus erythematosus (Chapter 245) and rheumatoid arthritis.[9] Rituximab is a chimeric monoclonal antibody that targets CD20 B cells for deletion. It was first used for treatment of B-cell lymphomas (Chapter 171) and is now also approved for treatment of rheumatoid arthritis. Consensus documents also suggest that rituximab may be useful as treatment for organ-damaging systemic lupus erythematosus that has failed other therapies. Ocrelizumab is a humanized monoclonal antibody that targets an overlapping epitope of CD20 and is an FDA-approved treatment for multiple sclerosis (Chapter 380). Obinutuzumab and ofatumumab are anti-CD20 monoclonal antibody approved for lymphoma and being studied for autoimmune disease. Targeting CD19 rather than CD20 is of interest as an alternative approach because of the potential for depleting long-lived plasma cells and early B cells that are not CD20-positive, while at the same time sparing regulatory B cells. Anti-CD19 antibodies are currently in trials for autoimmune diseases and malignancies. Blinatumomab is a bispecific agent that targets CD3 on T cells and CD19 on B cells and is approved for acute lymphoblastic leukemia (Chapter 168).

T Lymphocytes

The central role of T lymphocytes in the immune response makes this cell subset an attractive target for treatments of autoimmune disease and graft rejection as well as cancer immunotherapy. Therapies targeting the T-cell surface marker CD3 have been available for several decades and are still in limited use for the treatment of transplant rejection. The first humanized therapeutic monoclonal antibody was alemtuzumab, which targeted the CD52 molecule on T and B lymphocytes. An unexpected and as yet unexplained consequence of this treatment was long-standing lymphopenia, limiting its use. Ibalizumab is anti-CD4 monoclonal antibody for treatment of human immunodeficiency virus (HIV).

Costimulatory and Checkpoint Molecules

Another approach is inhibition of costimulatory signals required for full T-cell activation. The best example is the fusion protein abatacept, in which the extracellular portion of cytotoxic T lymphocyte antigen-4 (CTLA-4) is coupled to the extracellular portion of human IgG1. This molecule, which inhibits costimulatory signals between CD28 and CD80/86, is FDA approved for the treatment of rheumatoid arthritis (Chapter 243). Addition of abatacept to cyclophosphamide, however, did not improve the outcome of lupus nephritis in a trial. In general, infectious complications associated with abatacept are lower than with drugs that block TNF-α. Physiologically, CTLA4 binds CD80/CD86 and delivers a signal that inhibits T-cell activation. Antibodies that target CTLA4 and other negative regulators of T-cell activation (PD1, PDL1) represent a new class of drugs, checkpoint inhibitors, that are currently in use to treat various cancers (Chapter 164).[10] Examples include ipilimumab, nivolumab, atezolizumab, pembrolizumab, cemiplimab, avelumab, and durvalumab. Checkpoint inhibitors may induce immune-related adverse effects and can exacerbate autoimmune diseases.[11]

Adhesion Molecules

Another way to manipulate T cells in the immune response is to block migration to sites of inflammation. Natalizumab, which is a human monoclonal antibody against α_4-integrin, achieves this effect and is approved to treat relapsing/remitting forms of multiple sclerosis. A safety concern with natalizumab is the risk of progressive multifocal leukoencephalopathy (Chapter 341), a fatal condition associated with reactivation of the JC virus in immunosuppressed individuals. Vedolizumab is a monoclonal antibody that targets α4β7 integrin and is approved for ulcerative colitis and Crohn disease.[A7]

Growth Factor Receptors

Growth factor receptors, also known as receptor tyrosine kinases, are key regulators of normal cellular function but can also have major roles in cancer. Multiple monoclonal antibodies that target epidermal growth factor receptors (EGFRs) are approved, including trastuzumab and pertuzumab (breast cancer; Chapter 183); cetuximab and panitumumab (colorectal cancer; Chapter 179); and necitumumab (small cell lung cancer).

The vascular endothelial growth factor (VEGF) family of growth factors is involved in angiogenesis and has been implicated in pathogenesis of malignant disease, the development of metastases, and in forms of retinopathy. Bevacizumab and ramucirumab are biologics that target VEGF to treat malignancies including metastatic colon cancer (Chapter 179). VEGF inhibitors ramucirumab, brolucizumab, and ranibizumab are approved for treatment of macular degeneration (Chapter 391). Another approach to targeting VEGF is with the recombinant fusion protein aflibercept, which is composed of binding domains of the two human receptors for VEGF fused to human IgG1 Fc.

Other Therapeutic Targets Engaged By Monoclonal Antibodies

Aside from cancer, autoimmunity, and allergic disease, biologics are used in the treatment of a wide variety of additional disorders. For instance, the proprotein convertase subtilisin/kexin type 9 (PCSK9) binds to low-density lipoprotein (LDL) receptors and facilitates their degradation. The PSCK9 monoclonal antibodies alirocumab and evolocumab promote recycling LDL receptors and are approved for treatment of hypercholesterolemia (Chapter 190). Caplacizumab is a monoclonal antibody that targets von Willebrand factor and is used for the treatment of acquired thrombocytopenic purpura (Chapter 158). Crizanlizumab targets P-selectin approved for vaso-occlusive crisis in sickle cell disease, and lanadelumab targets kallikrein for treatment of hereditary angioedema (Chapter 232). Litifilimab, a monoclonal antibody to blood dendritic cell antigen 2 (BDCA2), has shown potential for the treatment of cutaneous lupus erythematosus.[A8]

Calcitonin gene–related peptide (CGRP) is a potent vasodilator involved in the pathophysiology of migraine (Chapter 367). Galcanezumab and fremanezumab target CGRP and erenumab targets CGRP receptor for migraine prevention. Aducanumab binds aggregated amyloid β and is approved for the treatment of Alzheimer disease, although controversy remains regarding its efficacy and cost-effectiveness (Chapter 371).

Biologics are also used in the treatment of infectious disease. Raxibacumab is a monoclonal antibody directed against the protective antigen component of lethal toxin of *Bacillus anthracis* (Chapter 272). Palivizumab is a monoclonal antibody that binds the F protein of respiratory syncytial virus (Chapter 330) and is used to prevent severe disease. For severe acute respiratory syndrome coronavirus 2, antispike monoclonal antibodies, including casirivimab, imdevimab, bamlanivimab, etesevimab, and sotrovimab, have been used for prevention and treatment (Chapter 337).

SMALL MOLECULE TARGETED THERAPIES

In addition to recombinant cytokines, small molecule agonists of cytokine receptors have been generated. Eltrombopag is a small molecule thrombopoietin receptor agonist that is approved for treatment of cases of immune thrombocytopenia (ITP) that are resistant to other therapies. It has the advantage of oral dosing (Chapter 158). The original approval for ITP was subsequently expanded with addition of severe aplastic anemia (Chapter 151), in which efficacy is due to actions on stem cells that result in production of other cell lines. This interesting precedent suggests that many other small molecule cytokine receptor agonists and antagonists might be useful therapeutics.

Seven-transmembrane receptors, including chemokine receptors, are very "druggable" targets. Two examples of drugs that target chemokine receptors include maraviroc, a small, orally available molecule that targets the chemokine receptor CCR5. This receptor is an essential cofactor for HIV entry into the cell, which is the mechanism of its antiretroviral effects. Fingolimod, ozanimod, and siponimod are small molecule receptor modulators that target sphingosine-1-phosphate receptor (S1PR1), which is critical for trafficking of T cells and vascular integrity. These agents are approved for multiple sclerosis, and ozanimod is also approved for treatment of ulcerative colitis.[12]

SIGNALING INHIBITORS

An alternative to targeting cytokines extracellularly is to use small molecules that block intracellular signaling pathways activated by binding of cytokines to their specific receptors. An advantage of this approach is that the drugs are administered orally. Because of the ultimately similar downstream cytokine targets, a basic safety principle is that biologics and signaling inhibitors are generally not recommended for use in combination. Janus kinases (JAKs) are critical for signaling by a large family of cytokines, presenting an especially attractive therapeutic target.[13,14] First-generation JAK inhibitors, or jakinibs, inhibit multiple JAKs and thus a large number of cytokines (Table 29-3). Jakinibs are approved for the treatment of rheumatoid arthritis, psoriatic arthritis, juvenile arthritis, and ulcerative colitis and are being investigated for the treatment of a number of other autoimmune and dermatologic conditions.[15,16] Polycythemia vera and related myeloproliferative neoplasms are due to gain-of-function *JAK2* mutations. Ruxolitinib inhibits JAK1 and JAK2 and is approved for the treatment of myeloproliferative neoplasms (Chapter 152) and acute graft-versus-host disease. First-generation jakinibs inhibit JAK2, which mediates signaling of many cytokines, including growth hormone, erythropoietin, thrombopoietin, IL-11, granulocyte colony-stimulating factor (G-CSF), and granulocyte macrophage (GM)-CSF; as a result, treated patients may develop anemia and other cytopenias. Although these effects are not usually severe enough to lead to discontinuation of treatment, newer selective jakinibs are being developed that spare JAK2.

Bruton tyrosine kinase has a critical role in B-cell function.[17] The Bruton tyrosine kinase inhibitors ibrutinib, acalabrutinib, and zanubrutinib are FDA approved to treat chronic lymphocytic leukemia (Chapter 169), Waldenström macroglobulinemia, and lymphoma. In all, more than 35 kinase inhibitors have been approved for multiple indications, including many cancers.

CONCLUSION

The use of biologic agents and signaling inhibitors has led to major improvements in the treatment of a wide variety of diseases, ranging from autoimmunity to malignancies. These targeted therapies have also provided insights into basic pathogenetic mechanisms in many of these disorders. Future directions are likely to focus on improved targeting, with greater selectivity for disease processes while sparing normal pathways, thereby reducing off-target effects. Expansion into other areas of medicine is also likely, with borrowed, modified, or completely new agents.

TABLE 29-3 APPROVED JANUS KINASE INHIBITORS

DRUG	TARGET	INDICATION
Ruxolitinib	JAK1/JAK2	MPN, acute GvHD
Tofacitinib	JAK1/JAK2/JAK3	RA, PsA, UC, polyarticular JIA
Baricitinib	JAK1/JAK2	RA, COVID-19 (EU)
Upadacitinib	JAK1	RA
Filgotinib	JAK1	RA (approved in EU, Japan)
Peficitinib	Multiple JAKs	RA (approved in Japan, Korea)
Fedratinib	JAK2/FLT3/RET/BRD4	MPN

COVID = coronavirus disease; EU = European Union; GvHD = graft versus host disease; JIA = juvenile idiopathic arthritis; MPN = myeloproliferative neoplasms; PsA = psoriatic arthritis; RA = rheumatoid arthritis; UC = ulcerative colitis.

GENERAL REFERENCES

For the General References and other additional features, please visit Elsevier eBooks+ at https://ebooks.health.elsevier.com.

Grade A References

A1. Donahue KE, Gartlehner G, Schulman ER, et al. AHRQ comparative effectiveness reviews. *Drug therapy for early rheumatoid arthritis: a systematic review update.* Rockville (MD): Agency for Healthcare Research and Quality (US); 2018.

A2. Emery P, Pope JE, Kruger K, et al. Efficacy of monotherapy with biologics and JAK inhibitors for the treatment of rheumatoid arthritis: a systematic review. *Adv Ther.* 2018;35:1535-1563.

A3. Fukushima K, Sugita A, Futami K, et al. Postoperative therapy with infliximab for Crohn's disease: a 2-year prospective randomized multicenter study in Japan. *Surg Today.* 2018;48:584-590.

A4. Deodhar A, Blanco R, Dokoupilová E, et al. Improvement of signs and symptoms of nonradiographic axial spondyloarthritis in patients treated with secukinumab: primary results of a randomized, placebo-controlled phase III study. *Arthritis Rheumatol.* 2021;73:110-120.

A5. Morand EF, Furie R, Tanaka Y, et al. Trial of anifrolumab in active systemic lupus erythematosus. *N Engl J Med.* 2020;382:211-221.

A6. Jayne DRW, Merkel PA, Schall TJ, et al. Avacopan for the treatment of ANCA-associated vasculitis. *N Engl J Med.* 2021;384:599-609.

A7. Sandborn WJ, Baert F, Danese S, et al. Efficacy and safety of vedolizumab subcutaneous formulation in a randomized trial of patients with ulcerative colitis. *Gastroenterology.* 2020;158:562-572.

A8. Werth VP, Furie RA, Romero-Diaz J, et al. Trial of anti-BDCA2 antibody litifilimab for cutaneous lupus erythematosus. *N Engl J Med.* 2022;387:321-331.

30 COMPLEMENTARY AND INTEGRATIVE MEDICINE

FREDERICK M. HECHT

In addition to the pharmaceutical and surgical therapies that have been central to advances in medical care, a large proportion of people across the globe also use health care treatments that fall outside of conventional medical care. The United States' National Center for Complementary and Integrative Health of the National Institutes of Health has defined complementary health care as "health care approaches developed outside of mainstream Western, or conventional, medicine" when they are used together with conventional medicine, and as alternative medicine when they are used in place of conventional medicine. Integrative medicine is an approach to medical practice that includes conventional medical therapies as well as nonpharmaceutical and nonsurgical therapies that have not always been incorporated or emphasized in conventional medicine but for which some evidence base now exists. This approach typically includes the use of lifestyle, mind-body practices, or natural products. Because these therapies typically receive little or no attention during medical education and because of conflicting claims and limitations in the quality of existing evidence, counseling patients about these therapies can be challenging.

USE OF INTEGRATIVE AND COMPLEMENTARY TREATMENTS

An estimated one third of Americans over 18 years of age have used some form of integrative health approach in the past 12 months, and the percentage appears to be increasing. The most commonly used practices included natural products, yoga and tai chi, deep breathing, meditation, chiropractic and osteopathic manipulation, and massage. Integrative medicine techniques have also become a common component of pain management in patients with cancer.[1]

MIND AND BODY PRACTICES

MEDITATION

Meditation and related contemplative practices involve various techniques to self-regulate attention. Often derived from different spiritual traditions, meditation has been used for centuries to achieve states of mental and emotional calm, increased awareness of physical sensations and emotional states, and improved attention. More recently, meditation practices are often used in the secular arena, increasingly within health care settings, to help manage stress, improve emotional regulation skills, and address other mental and physical health issues.

Among the different approaches to meditation, the two general types that have received the most study are *mindfulness-based* meditation and *concentration-mantra* meditation. Mindfulness meditation involves practices aimed at "paying attention in a particular way, on purpose, in the present moment, and nonjudgmentally." For example, the Mindfulness-based Stress Reduction program and related programs in health care settings aim to improve the ability of patients to cope with chronic pain. This approach is at least as effective as approaches such as cognitive-behavioral therapy for treating chronic low back pain (Chapter 369), and both approaches are more effective than usual medical care alone.[A1] In patients treated with opiates for chronic pain, mind-body therapies can reduce the intensity of pain and reduce opioid doses, with the largest effect sizes from meditation approaches.[A2]

Another important application of mindfulness-based approaches has been to address mood regulation, particularly in conditions such as depression (Chapter 362). In patients who have experienced at least one prior episode of significant depression, mindfulness-based cognitive therapy, which combines some elements of cognitive-behavioral therapy with mindfulness practices, can reduce relapse rates by about 20% compared with continuing antidepressant medication alone,[A3] without increasing costs. As a result, mindfulness-based cognitive therapy is now recommended as one of the standard-of-care approaches to prevent relapse of depression in the United Kingdom. Mindfulness-based interventions are also increasingly integrated into the workplace in a variety of ways, including web-based programs and classes on yoga or meditation.

A common form of mantra-based meditation is transcendental meditation. A more generic form is mantra meditation, which may evoke a relaxation response. Limited evidence suggests that this approach can lower blood pressure and improve depressive symptoms.

YOGA AND TAI CHI

Although yoga, tai chi, and qigong are practiced for different purposes and with a variety of styles, their goal is to achieve health benefits that go beyond general physical fitness. The focused attention during movement practices can be viewed as a form of moving meditation.

Tai chi can improve balance and reduce the risk of falls by about 50% in the elderly.[A4] In addition, regular tai chi can significantly improve psychological outcomes, including reductions in stress[A5] and depression. Yoga also is effective for low back pain and has been incorporated into guidelines for managing chronic low back pain.[A6] In patients with hypertension, yoga has been reported to decrease systolic blood pressure by up to 10 mm Hg,[A7] although the quality of data is low.

Yoga can be practiced in a variety of ways, and the actual yoga practices are important when suggesting yoga to patients. For example, yoga that is effective for low back pain has been specifically tailored to low back pain—a gentle yoga style to avoid postures that might exacerbate back pain, while focusing on postures and methods that are thought to be useful. Yoga programs designed for conditions such as low back pain are available at some medical centers and yoga studios. If specifically tailored classes are not available, many yoga studios offer restorative yoga classes, which are less likely to include postures and movements that may exacerbate low back pain and are more likely to include a focus on mindful movement and body awareness that may be helpful for low back pain.

MANUAL THERAPIES

Manual therapies include a broad range of physical treatments commonly used by physical therapists, massage therapists, chiropractors, and osteopaths. These therapies typically include massage and manipulation of muscles, as well as techniques to mobilize joints.

Massage therapy is effective for conditions such as neck and shoulder pain,[2] and massage is commonly used for sports injuries, delayed-onset muscle soreness after strenuous exercise, and other causes of muscle pain. The mechanisms though which massage therapy works are not fully understood. However, studies using muscle biopsies after exercise-induced muscle injury have found that massage decreases the production of inflammatory cytokines and increases indicators of cell repair such as mitochondrial biogenesis. Massage therapy has also been shown to reduce anxiety and blood pressure. One important issue for clinicians to understand is the wide range of massage techniques and different types of expertise among massage therapists. Some forms, such as Swedish massage, are aimed largely at relaxation. Other forms of massage, such as sports massage and deep tissue massage, tend to use greater pressure and techniques specifically aimed at enhancing recovery from muscle injury. When referring a patient for massage for issues such as sports injury, it may be helpful to make sure the massage therapist has specific training and experience in working with sports injuries.

Spinal manipulation, which involves applying a controlled force to a joint of the spine, is typically performed by chiropractors or osteopathic physicians but also can be performed by physical therapists and some physicians. Although spinal manipulation has sometimes been viewed with suspicion in conventional medicine, a growing body of evidence supports its use in specific conditions.[3] For example, spinal manipulative therapy is somewhat effective for reducing acute low back pain,[A8,A9] and is now included in the American College of Physicians recommendations for treatment of acute low back pain. Although serious adverse events after spinal manipulation, such as vertebral artery dissection, appear to be very rare, they emphasize the need for skilled practitioners who are properly trained to perform it.[4]

ACUPUNCTURE AND TRADITIONAL CHINESE MEDICINE

Acupuncture,[5] which has been practiced in China for thousands of years, involves placing thin needles in specific sites, or acupuncture points, which are often stimulated in a variety of ways, such as by spinning the needle. Controversy exists as to whether the benefits of acupuncture are due to a placebo effect versus actual effects of the needle insertion. Data from meta-analysis suggest that about 50% of its benefits are consistent with a placebo effect, but it still improves pain compared with sham treatment, such as stimulation of an acupuncture point without a needle penetrating the skin.[A10,A11] Substantial evidence also indicates that acupuncture can decrease the duration of postoperative ileus,[A12] as well as nausea and vomiting after chemotherapy or surgery.[6]

Other components of traditional Chinese medicine include an assessment of potential imbalances or blockages in the circulation of *qi*, or vital energy, through the body; the use of herbal medicine; and recommendations for diet and exercise (including qigong). Evidence for these broader elements of traditional Chinese medicine is still limited. Data are also limited for the true benefit of Ayurveda (traditional medicine from the Indian subcontinent), which includes some elements of yoga along with components parallel to traditional Chinese medicine.

NATURAL PRODUCTS

Natural products encompass vitamins, minerals, herbs (also known as botanicals), and probiotics, all of which are often sold as dietary supplements. Although many of these products have anecdotal support, evidence of efficacy is limited for most of them.[7] Under the 1994 Dietary Supplement Health and Education Act, dietary supplements are considered to be food, so manufacturers are not required to obtain Food and Drug Administration (FDA) approval before marketing any supplement that was already available before 1994 ("grandfathered status"). By comparison, new dietary ingredients introduced after 1994 require reasonable evidence of safety, which must be reviewed before marketing.

Some dietary supplements can cause severe adverse effects, in part due to impurities or excessive levels of certain active ingredients,[8] and in aggregate they represent the second most common cause of drug-induced liver disease (Chapter 136). The Dietary Supplement and Nonprescription Drug Consumer Protection Act of 2006 requires that physicians in hospitals report any serious adverse event associated with a dietary supplement (using a form available on the FDA website: MedWatch Form 3500A). The updated status of different natural products is available on the National Center for Complementary and Integrative Health website (https://nccih.nih.gov/health/herbsataglance.htm), and the National Institutes of Health Office of Dietary Supplements has additional information on the current status of different dietary supplements (https://ods.od.nih.gov/factsheets/list-all/).

Although rigorous research has not found evidence that clearly supports the use of many nutritional supplements, intriguing exceptions exist. An example is turmeric (a traditional medicine from the Indian subcontinent), which is high in curcumin, a curcuminoid that has substantial anti-inflammatory and antioxidant properties. Data suggest that a curcuminoid preparation may be more effective than placebo for decreasing pain and improving postexercise recovery.[9]

Potential Interactions with Drug Therapies

One reason for medical providers to be aware of dietary supplements their patients are taking is that some supplements may have potential interactions with other medications. An example is St. John's wort, which may improve depression, although well-designed studies have failed to show that it is more effective than placebo. St. John's wort induces several cytochrome P-450 isoenzymes, and it has significant interactions with a variety of medications that are metabolized through this system, including warfarin, cyclosporine, oral contraceptives, certain antiretrovirals, and selective serotonin reuptake inhibitors. Other herbal supplements with significant potential for drug interactions include goldenseal and ginseng.

VITAMIN AND MINERAL SUPPLEMENTS

Vitamin and mineral supplements are popular and widely used. Observational studies have linked consumption of various micronutrients, or measurements of these micronutrients in blood, to a reduced risk of certain diseases. However, supplementation of vitamins and minerals for the general population has been disappointing, and a number of randomized trials of nutrient supplementation have not only failed to find evidence of benefit but have actually demonstrated harm (Chapter 199).

Together, these considerations suggest that clinicians should focus on having patients follow an overall healthy eating pattern (Chapter 13) that is low in processed foods and high in nutrient-rich foods, rather than relying on dietary supplements. A Mediterranean diet pattern (Fig. 13-1), for example, can reduce cardiovascular risk, and this type of diet should provide adequate micronutrients for most patients. Special conditions in which evidence suggests benefit from micronutrient supplementation include pregnancy (Chapter 221) and conditions such as chronic pancreatitis with pancreatic insufficiency (Chapter 130).

Probiotics and Prebiotics

Growing evidence shows that the human gut microbiome (Chapter 257) has a variety of important influences on health. Probiotics, which are live microorganisms that are thought to be beneficial in the human gut, are available naturally in yogurt and other fermented foods or as dietary supplements. Prebiotics, which are nondigestible food ingredients that promote the growth of beneficial microorganisms, are another potential approach to improving the gut microbiome.

The most impressive evidence for how changing the gut microbiome can treat a medical condition comes from the studies in which fecal transplants from healthy individuals have been used to treat recurrent *Clostridioides difficile*–associated colitis (Chapters 261 and 271).[A13] Probiotics also can reduce the incidence of antibiotic-induced diarrhea.[A14] For irritable bowel syndrome, data have found probiotics may improve global symptoms by about 20%[10] but overall are mixed, and so are the recommendations of professional societies. In trials showing benefit, the most frequently included strains have been *Lactobacillus acidophilus*, followed by *Streptococcus thermophilus*, *Bifidobacterium breve*, and *Bifidobacterium longum*.

OVERVIEW

Although more evidence is needed on many fronts, evidence-based integrative health therapies are increasingly being included in medical practice. When used appropriately, these approaches may expand the tools available to health care practitioners and the options that can be recommended to patients. Many patients may appreciate choices other than drugs in different conditions. For some conditions, such as pain, the use of nonpharmacologic treatments may reduce the risk of harm from conventional treatments, such as overuse of narcotics. Yoga, tai chi, mindfulness-based meditation, self-massage, and acupressure also can be incorporated into telemedicine.[11]

GENERAL REFERENCES

For the General References and other additional features, please visit Elsevier eBooks+ at https://ebooks.health.elsevier.com.

Grade A References

A1. Cherkin DC, Sherman KJ, Balderson BH, et al. Effect of mindfulness-based stress reduction vs cognitive behavioral therapy or usual care on back pain and functional limitations in adults with chronic low back pain: a randomized clinical trial. *JAMA*. 2016;315:1240-1249.

A2. Garland EL, Brintz CE, Hanley AW, et al. Mind-body therapies for opioid-treated pain: a systematic review and meta-analysis. *JAMA Intern Med*. 2020;180:91-105.

A3. Kuyken W, Warren FC, Taylor RS, et al. Efficacy of mindfulness-based cognitive therapy in prevention of depressive relapse: an individual patient data meta-analysis from randomized trials. *JAMA Psychiatry*. 2016;73:565-574.

A4. Huang ZG, Feng YH, Li YH, et al. Systematic review and meta-analysis: Tai Chi for preventing falls in older adults. *BMJ Open*. 2017;7:1-8.

A5. Zou L, Sasaki JE, Wei GX, et al. Effects of mind-body exercises (Tai Chi/yoga) on heart rate variability parameters and perceived stress: a systematic review with meta-analysis of randomized controlled trials. *J Clin Med*. 2018;7:404.

A6. Zhu F, Zhang M, Wang D, et al. Yoga compared to non-exercise or physical therapy exercise on pain, disability, and quality of life for patients with chronic low back pain: a systematic review and meta-analysis of randomized controlled trials. *PLoS One*. 2020;15:e0238544.

A7. Park SH, Han KS. Blood pressure response to meditation and yoga: a systematic review and meta-analysis. *J Altern Complement Med*. 2017;23:685-695.

A8. Paige NM, Miake-Lye IM, Booth MS, et al. association of spinal manipulative therapy with clinical benefit and harm for acute low back pain: systematic review and meta-analysis. *JAMA*. 2017;317:1451-1460.

A9. Nguyen C, Boutron I, Zegarra-Parodi R, et al. Effect of osteopathic manipulative treatment vs sham treatment on activity limitations in patients with nonspecific subacute and chronic low back pain: a randomized clinical trial. *JAMA Intern Med*. 2021;181:620-630.

A10. Nielsen A, Dusek JA, Taylor-Swanson L, et al. Acupuncture therapy as an evidence-based nonpharmacologic strategy for comprehensive acute pain care: the academic consortium pain task force white paper update. *Pain Med*. 2022;23:1582-1612.

A11. Vickers AJ, Vertosick EA, Lewith G, et al. Acupuncture for chronic pain: update of an individual patient data meta-analysis. *J Pain*. 2018;19:455-474.

A12. Wang Y, Yang J-W, Yan S-Y, et al. Electroacupuncture vs sham electroacupuncture in the treatment of postoperative ileus after laparoscopic surgery for colorectal cancer: a multicenter, randomized clinical trial. *JAMA Surg*. 2023;158:20-27.

A13. Hui W, Li T, Liu W, et al. Fecal microbiota transplantation for treatment of recurrent *C. difficile* infection: an updated randomized controlled trial meta-analysis. *PLoS One*. 2019;14:e0210016.

A14. Liao W, Chen C, Wen T, et al. Probiotics for the prevention of antibiotic-associated diarrhea in adults: a meta-analysis of randomized placebo-controlled trials. *J Clin Gastroenterol*. 2021;55:469-480.

VI

GENETICS

31

PRINCIPLES OF GENETICS

BRUCE R. KORF AND NITA A. LIMDI

The elucidation of the structure and function of the genome is one of the great triumphs of modern science. The relevance of inheritance to health and disease probably has been recognized throughout history, but now the rules governing inheritance and the mechanisms whereby genetic information is stored and used are coming to light. Application of this knowledge to medical practice had long been focused on rare monogenic and chromosomal disorders. Major contributions have been made in these areas in genetic testing, genetic counseling, prenatal diagnosis, newborn screening, carrier screening, and, to an increasing extent, treatment. The era of genomic medicine[1] provides powerful new approaches to the management of both rare and common disorders.

GENETIC ARCHITECTURE OF DISEASE

It may be argued that no disorder is completely determined either by genetic or nongenetic factors. Even monogenic conditions, such as phenylketonuria, are modified by the environment, in this case by dietary intake of phenylalanine. Genetically determined host factors are known to modify susceptibility to infection or other environmental agents. Even individuals who are victims of trauma may find themselves at risk in part because of genetic traits that affect behavior or ability to perceive, escape, or recover from danger.

The number of genetic variants that contribute to a disease phenotype, the degree to which each contributes, and the frequency of these variants in the population is referred to as the genetic architecture of disease (Fig. 31-1).[2] Conditions may be largely determined by a single gene, with other genes playing a smaller role in modifying the phenotype, or may result from the accumulation of small effects of many genes. From a medical perspective, it is helpful to divide the genetic contribution to disease into three categories: (1) high-penetrance monogenic or chromosomal disorders; (2) monogenic versions of common disorders; and (3) complex, multifactorial disorders. Each of these affects medical practice in distinctive ways.

HIGH-PENETRANCE MONOGENIC OR CHROMOSOMAL DISORDERS

High-penetrance monogenic or chromosomal disorders are what most clinicians think of as "genetic conditions." They include rare but familiar single-gene disorders, such as neurofibromatosis, Marfan syndrome, and cystic fibrosis, and chromosomal abnormalities, such as trisomy 21 (Down syndrome). Several thousand distinct human genetic disorders have been described and catalogued in Mendelian Inheritance in Man (available at www.omim.org). These disorders include dominant, recessive, and sex-linked disorders, as well as conditions due to variants within the 16.6-kilobase mitochondrial genome. These disorders also include chromosomal syndromes that are associated with duplication or deletion of small regions

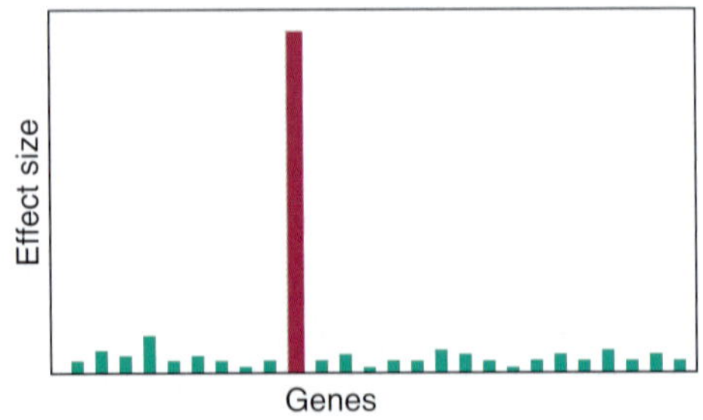

FIGURE 31-1. Diagram illustrating concept of genetic architecture. Different genes are indicated on the x-axis, and their effect size (the degree to which a particular gene contributes to the phenotype) is shown on the y-axis. A disorder associated with variants in a single gene shows a large effect size from that single gene (shown in red). Many other genes (shown in blue) with smaller effect sizes may modify the phenotype, but the major gene is alone sufficient to cause the phenotype.

of the genome and that may result in specific syndromes, such as Williams syndrome (deletion of contiguous loci from a region of chromosome 7), intellectual disability, or autism spectrum disorder.

ROLE OF THE NONSPECIALIST IN MANAGEMENT OF RARE GENETIC DISORDERS

Most clinicians have limited experience with specific rare genetic disorders and are likely to need to refer such patients to a specialist for assistance with diagnosis and management. Nevertheless, the nonspecialist has an important role in the care of these patients. This role begins with realization that the patient may have such a disorder and arrangement for diagnostic evaluation. Many genetic disorders produce obvious signs or symptoms that should prompt referral even if they are not immediately suggestive of a diagnosis. Others can be more subtle, with nevertheless significant consequences if the diagnosis is missed. An example is Marfan syndrome (Chapter 239). The physician needs to be alert to the physical characteristics of patients with Marfan syndrome because life-threatening aortic dissection can be avoided with appropriate monitoring and treatment.

The management of patients with rare genetic disorders may require the assistance of a specialist, but the nonspecialist is likely to be the first contact when an affected individual is ill. The primary care physician should be familiar with the disorder and major potential complications. For example, patients who have neurofibromatosis type 1 (Chapter 385) and who experience chronic back pain require more aggressive evaluation than would be typical for an unaffected individual with back pain because they may be presenting with a malignant peripheral nerve sheath tumor. A good working relationship between the specialist and nonspecialist is crucial to effective care.

The nonspecialist also has an important role in supporting the patient and helping to explain the choices that may be offered for management. This role includes providing support for patients who have disorders that cannot be treated and for the emotional impact that accompanies knowledge that a disorder may be transmitted to one's offspring or shared with other relatives. Most patients have little understanding of the mechanisms of genetics and genetic disease. Although the responsibility to explain these issues may reside with specialists and counselors, the primary care physician has an important supportive role.

GENOMIC APPROACHES TO RARE DISORDERS

Identification of genes that underlie rare disorders enables molecular diagnostic tests to detect pathogenic variants. A database of testing laboratories can be found at www.ncbi.nlm.nih.gov/gtr/. Cytogenomic microarray analysis can reveal small deletions or duplications in individuals with conditions such as autism spectrum disorder, for whom standard chromosomal analysis is unrevealing. Sequencing the entire coding region of the genome (exome sequencing) or the entire genome (genome sequencing) is now being applied clinically.[3] Screening for carrier status for autosomal recessive disorders has been offered for many years, with specific ancestry groups being offered testing for conditions of high prevalence in their group. Genomic approaches are now making it possible to increase the number of conditions tested, thereby enabling a comprehensive screen of dozens or even hundreds of genes regardless of ancestry.[4] Prenatal screening for trisomy and some pathologic copy number changes can be offered noninvasively by analysis of fetal DNA in maternal blood.[5] Newborn screening is being expanded beyond inborn errors of metabolism such as phenylketonuria and galactosemia, with the advent of tandem mass spectrometry and the availability of a standardized panel of tests.[6] Genome sequencing is also effective for identifying genetic disorders in newborns in intensive care nurseries, thereby providing information that can guide management.[7] Genome sequencing has also been evaluated as an approach to newborn screening,[8,A1] though challenges include the inability to detect all pathologic variants associated with treatable newborn diseases, as well as concerns about identification of currently untreatable or later-onset disorders.

Finally, treatment of some monogenic disorders is becoming feasible. Therapies that use either pharmaceuticals or gene or enzyme replacement strategies are in use or being tested for many conditions. The principles of management of genetic disorders are evolving rapidly, and care of patients increasingly requires active partnership among specialists, primary care physicians, and patient advocates. Moreover, individuals with congenital disorders such as Down syndrome are routinely surviving to adulthood and require primary care physicians who are familiar with their special needs.

MONOGENIC VERSIONS OF COMMON DISORDERS

Not all monogenic disorders produce rare phenotypes, and not all common disorders have complex multifactorial causes. Some common disorders occur in families as single-gene traits, mostly with an autosomal dominant inheritance. Age of onset can be variable, and penetrance is usually incomplete (i.e., not all individuals who carry a pathogenic variant become symptomatic). Examples include several cancer predisposition syndromes (e.g., hereditary breast and ovarian cancer, Lynch syndrome, familial adenomatous polyposis, Li-Fraumeni syndrome, and various multiple endocrine neoplasia syndromes), inherited forms of cardiomyopathy, long QT syndrome, and maturity-onset diabetes of the young.[9]

GENETIC TESTING FOR MONOGENIC COMMON DISORDERS

Genetic tests for disorders associated with inherited forms of common disorders are now available, usually as panels that test for variants in multiple genes known to be associated with specific disorders. As with any medical test, the physician must consider the clinical utility of testing before a test is ordered. For example, compelling evidence supports the value of making an early diagnosis of hemochromatosis because the complications can be prevented, but not reversed, by phlebotomy and subsequent monitoring of iron stores. Individuals at risk for colon cancer can be offered surveillance with colonoscopy or surgical resection of the colon to reduce the risk for cancer. Individuals at risk for breast and ovarian cancer likewise can be offered surveillance, chemoprevention, or surgery.

Potential risks of genetic testing, such as guilt or stigmatization, also must be considered. The Genetic Information Nondiscrimination Act of 2008 (GINA)[10] protects individuals in the United States from the use of genetic information as a basis for determining eligibility for employment or health insurance in most instances. Protection does not, however, extend to life insurance or disability insurance. Some states have genetic nondiscrimination laws that exceed the protections of GINA.

ROLE OF THE NONSPECIALIST IN MANAGEMENT

The role of the physician in dealing with monogenic disorders includes recognition of individuals at risk and participation in the creation of a plan of care.[11] The most valuable screening tool is the family history. Directed questioning about a family history of monogenic disorders (especially breast, ovarian, and colon cancer, as well as hypercholesterolemia, hypertension, cardiomyopathy, arrhythmia, deep vein thrombosis, cirrhosis, kidney disease, and diabetes) can help identify the occasional patient with Mendelian segregation of these conditions. Even if the information is of uncertain reliability, eliciting a family history can prompt referral for further evaluation, documentation of the family history, and consideration for genetic testing.

The advent of exome or genome sequencing for diagnosis of rare disorders has opened the possibility of identification of individuals at risk based on secondary findings. The American College of Medical Genetics and Genomics has recommended that testing laboratories evaluate a list of genes for which identification of a pathogenic variant can lead to management to reduce risk, if the patient or parent opts into receiving this information.[12] This information would be shared even if the individual being sequenced is a child, because the condition may have relevance to the eventual health of the child, as well as parents and other relatives.

COMPLEX, MULTIFACTORIAL DISORDERS

Understanding the genetics of common disorders is one of the great challenges of modern medicine, with the promise of major returns in terms of prevention, diagnosis, and treatment. The etiology of these disorders is complex in that they result from an interplay of genes, environment, and individual lifestyles.

GENOME-WIDE ASSOCIATION STUDIES

Dissection of the genetic contribution to common disease cannot be accomplished by study of rare variants or family-based linkage studies. Most efforts have focused on study of large patient cohorts, comparing the association of genetic variants in affected cases as compared with control subjects. The ability to test millions of genetic variants rapidly across the genome has enabled genome-wide association studies (GWAS) to identify variants associated with common disorders. Hundreds of such associations have been found, either because genetic variants themselves contribute to risk or are closely linked with other variants that are involved in the disorder (linkage disequilibrium).

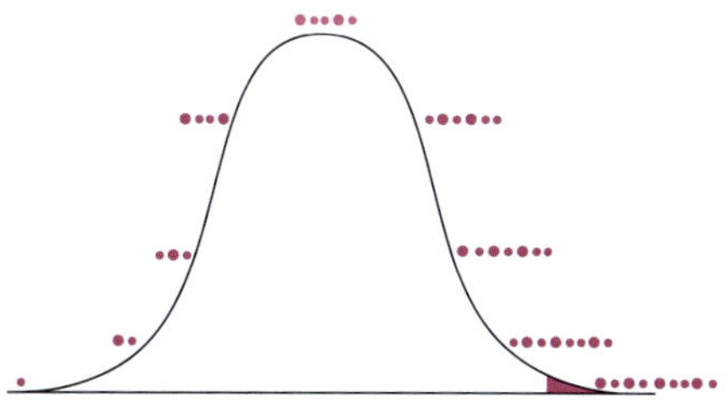

FIGURE 31-2. **Concept of polygenic risk score. Individual variants are indicated by red dots, with the effect size depicted by the size of the dot. The phenotype is indicated as showing a normal distribution in the population, with the least affected individuals to the left and the most affected to the right. There is a gradient of numbers of genomic variants along the distribution, with the most severely affected, indicated by the red area under the curve to the right, having the highest polygenic risk score (i.e., the sum of all associated genetic variants weighted by their effect size). In reality, the number of variants incorporated into a polygenic risk score is far larger than shown here.**

GENETIC RISK ASSESSMENT

The goal of genetic risk assessment is the identification of individuals at risk for disease before the onset of signs or symptoms. In principle, the genetic factors could be identified at any time in life by testing a DNA sample. Persons found to be at risk can be offered treatment in advance of onset of the disease to avoid complications or might be advised to modify their lifestyle to avoid exposure to dietary or environmental factors that might increase risk of disease.

Polygenic Risk Scores

The contribution to multifactorial disease risk of any one genetic variant is too small to be clinically useful, but risk is additive across multiple variants. Summing the number of risk-associated variants, each weighted by effect size (i.e., the odds ratio of disease in carriers of a specific allele compared with noncarriers) results in a polygenic risk score (Fig. 31-2).[13] Individuals at the upper end of the distribution of a polygenic risk score for a particular trait may have a risk comparable to persons with a single gene Mendelian trait, and they likewise can be offered management to mitigate that risk. Studies are underway to test the clinical utility of polygenic risk scores and determine how they can be integrated into clinical care.[14,15] Specific risk alleles and effect sizes may differ in populations of different ancestry, thereby limiting the portability of polygenic scores across populations. To date most GWAS studies have been performed on populations of European ancestry, so a major effort is required to engage populations historically under-represented in genetics research to enable application of polygenic scores across diverse populations and to avoid exacerbating health disparities.[16]

POPULATION SCREENING

The possibility of early identification of individuals at risk of disease raises the question of the utility of population screening. Some research-based population screening programs have been instituted, based on lists of actionable genomic variants (i.e., variants that are highly predictive of disease for which treatment is beneficial prior to onset of symptoms). The Centers for Disease Control and Prevention have identified a list of "Tier 1 conditions" (specifically hereditary breast and ovarian cancer, Lynch syndrome, and hypercholesterolemia) for which population screening may be beneficial. Low-cost genotyping has also spawned an industry of direct-to-consumer genomic testing for a limited repertoire of tests subject to approval by the Food and Drug Administration.

PHARMACOGENETIC TESTING

Response to medications, the principal treatment modality for acute and chronic diseases, is highly variable, ranging from inadequate efficacy to adverse drug reactions. Variations in genes associated with drug pharmacodynamics and pharmacokinetics (absorption, distribution, metabolism, and excretion) has a significant effect on response and dose requirements (Table 31-1). The Clinical Pharmacogenetic Implementation Consortium (https://cpicpgx.org/guidelines/) and the Food and Drug Administration (https://www.fda.gov/medical-devices/precision-medicine/table-pharmacogenetic-associations) provide clinical guidance on the use of genotypic information to optimize medication regimens. With approximately 15 to 30% of response variability explained by genetic variants, pharmacogenetics has become a valuable tool for optimizing the selection and dosing of medications, and it is poised to

TABLE 31-1 GENES IN WHICH COMMON POLYMORPHISMS AFFECT RATES OF DRUG METABOLISM OR ACTION

GENE	EXAMPLES OF AFFECTED DRUG(S)
CYP2B6	efavirenz
CYP2C19	amitriptyline, clopidogrel, citalopram, escitalopram
	omeprazole, rabeprazole, lansoprazole, pantoprazole
	voriconazole
CYP2C9	lornoxicam, meloxicam, phenytoin, piroxicam, tenoxicam
	fosphenytoin, phenytoin
	warfarin
CYP2D6	doxepin, clomipramine, amitriptyline, nortriptyline, desipramine, metoprolol, imipramine
	atomoxetine, codeine, fluvoxamine, ondansetron, oxycodone, paroxetine, tamoxifen, tramadol, tropisetron
CYP3A5	tacrolimus
CYP4F2	warfarin
DPYD	capecitabine, fluorouracil
G6PD	rasburicase, tafenoquine
HLA-A	carbamazepine, oxcarbazepine
HLA-B	abacavir
	allopurinol
	phenytoin, carbamazepine, oxcarbazepine
IFNL3	peginterferon-alpha-2a/2b
NUDT15	azathioprine, thioguanine, mercaptopurine
SLCO1B1	simvastatin
TPMT	azathioprine, thioguanine, mercaptopurine
UGT1A1	atazanavir, irinotecan
VKORC1	warfarin

play an increasing role in clinical care.[17] Benefits include customizing drug selection and dosing, increasing the likelihood of therapeutic benefit without a prolonged trial and error period, and improving safety and cost-effectiveness.

GENERAL REFERENCES

For the General References and other additional features, please visit Elsevier eBooks+ at https://ebooks.health.elsevier.com.

Grade A Reference

A1. Pereira S, Smith HS, Frankel LA, et al. Psychosocial effect of newborn genomic sequencing on families in the babyseq project: a randomized clinical trial. *JAMA Pediatr*. 2021;175:1132-1141.

32 CLINICAL GENOMICS—GENOME STRUCTURE AND VARIATION

LESLIE G. BIESECKER

CLINICAL GENOMICS

Genomics is a biomedical discipline that addresses the structure, function, evolution, mapping, and editing of all of the DNA of an organism. Genomics also encompasses a broad and rapidly changing suite of technologies that use high-throughput assays to assess the molecular basis of heritable disease.[1]

The growth of genomic medicine is exemplified by the more than 3 million individuals who already have been evaluated using genome sequencing and many others using exome sequencing. At least 1 of every 25 of patients has a mendelian genetic disorder, and many more have polygenic disorders. This simple arithmetic indicates that practicing clinicians are likely to have sequenced patients in their practices and must learn to recognize and manage individuals with inherited diseases.

A genome is the nuclear DNA included in 23 pairs of chromosomes: 22 autosomes plus two sex chromosomes (XX in females and XY in males). The diploid genome (2n) comprises two haploid copies, each of about 3 billion base pairs (bp). Two haploid genomes are reconstituted in the fertilized embryo as a diploid genome, for a total of 6 billion nucleotides. The protein coding genetic sequences include about 23,000 genes and comprise a minority (about 2%) of the human genome. The many other biologically relevant sequences include noncoding RNAs and conserved regulatory elements. In spite of this biologic complexity, clinicians can focus on the 2% of the genome that encode genes, because those genes harbor the variations that are currently best understood as being important for diagnosing and managing patients.

GENE

Genes, which are the units of heredity, are the biologic basic of the transmission of genetic traits and diseases. Genes comprise segments of DNA that encode the information carried by the gene. Precisely mapping the gene onto the nucleotides of the genome can be challenging, because it can be difficult to appreciate all of the disparate DNA elements, such as enhancers and promoters, that contribute to gene regulation and function.

Genomic DNA is configured in a two-stranded, double-helical macromolecule. A DNA strand comprises millions of one of four nucleotides: two purine bases, adenine (A) and guanine (G), and two pyrimidine bases, thymine (T) and cytosine (C). Two such strands, in opposite orientation and with an elegant twist, compose the double helix. Three consecutive nucleotides (triplet codon) of coding DNA specify an amino acid. The 64 possible different codons code for only 20 amino acids, so more than one codon triplet can code for a single amino acid. The information that codes for proteins in most protein-coding genes is broken up into several segments, referred to as exons, which are separated by noncoding introns (Fig. 32-1). The entire gene (exons and introns) is transcribed into messenger RNA (mRNA) by RNA polymerase. In the subsequent splicing process, the intervening introns are deleted; then the spliced, mature mRNA is translated into a polypeptide. At the end of the open reading frame of the gene, the polypeptides are terminated by one of three termination codons.

PATTERNS OF INHERITANCE

MENDELIAN INHERITANCE

Many heritable traits in humans can be attributed to variation of a single gene (monogenic) and segregate in a mendelian inheritance pattern[2]: autosomal dominant, autosomal recessive, or sex-linked. An understanding of inheritance begins with understanding the genotype, which is the status (normal or variant) of a given pair of alleles of genes in an individual. For females, inheritance is straightforward because they have 23 pairs of homologous chromosomes (22 pairs of autosomes and one pair of X chromosomes), whereas males have 22 pairs of autosomes, but only one X and one Y chromosome. Thus, in females, the status of all genes is either homozygous normal (both normal), homozygous variant (both variant), heterozygous (one of each), or compound heterozygous (two different, but both variant). By comparison, genes on the X chromosome of males can be either hemizygous normal or hemizygous variant, to denote the fact that they only have one X chromosome. Only a few genes have alleles on the X and the Y chromosome.

Autosomal dominant inheritance is the pattern that results from a disorder in which the gene is located on an autosome (i.e., not a sex chromosome) and harbors just one copy of an abnormal allele (heterozygote) that is sufficient to cause the phenotype (Fig. 32-2A). The phenotype of an individual who harbors two identical abnormal alleles (homozygote) or two different abnormal alleles (compound heterozygote) is also abnormal. The heterozygous genotype is much more common than the homozygous or compound heterozygous genotype. If a parent is heterozygous, the variant is present in only one of their two alleles, and there is a 50% chance of transmission to each offspring. In pedigree analysis, autosomal dominant inheritance is recognized as a vertical transmission of the trait—from parent to child. However, there is a nuance in dominant inheritance. A trait is formally called autosomal dominant only when the phenotype of the heterozygote is the same as the homozygous variant (see Fig. 32-2A). In reality, this relationship is true for very few human disorders, Huntington

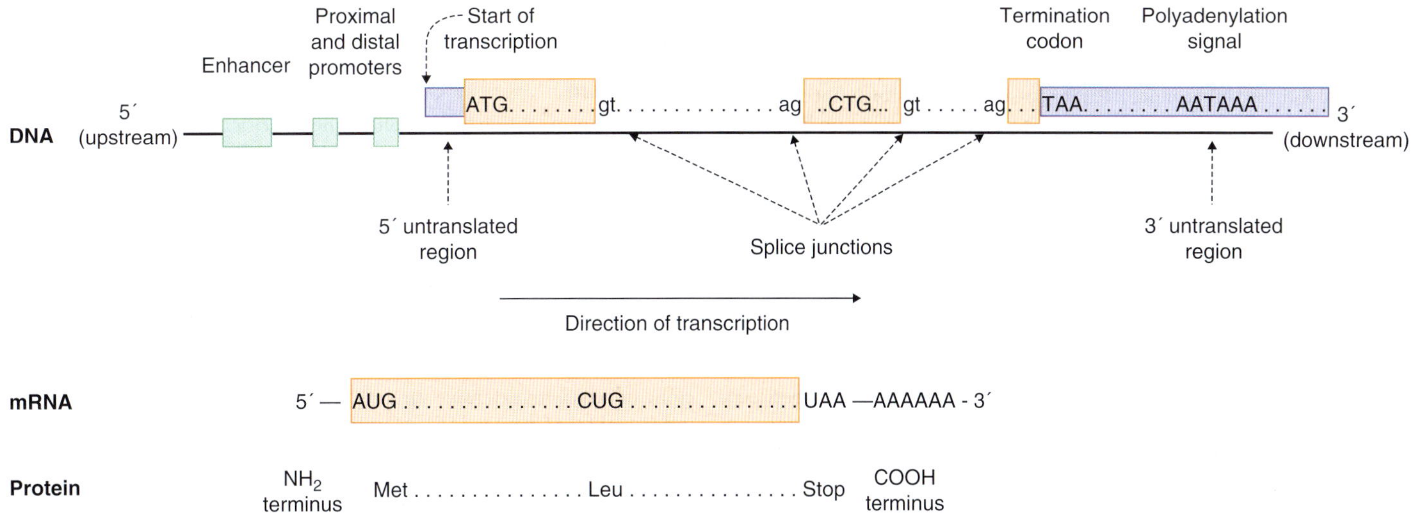

FIGURE 32-1. Gene structure. Illustration of the general structure of a gene. Three exons are depicted as rectangles, comprising sequences that code for proteins *(orange)* or are noncoding *(blue)*. Note that the translation typically starts with an ATG triplet, which encodes the amino acid methionine. The upstream portion of a gene corresponds to the NH_2 terminus, and the downstream portion encodes the COOH terminus of the encoded protein. Enhancers and promoters are shown as *green* rectangles. A = adenine; C = cytosine; G = guanine; T = thymine; u = uracil.

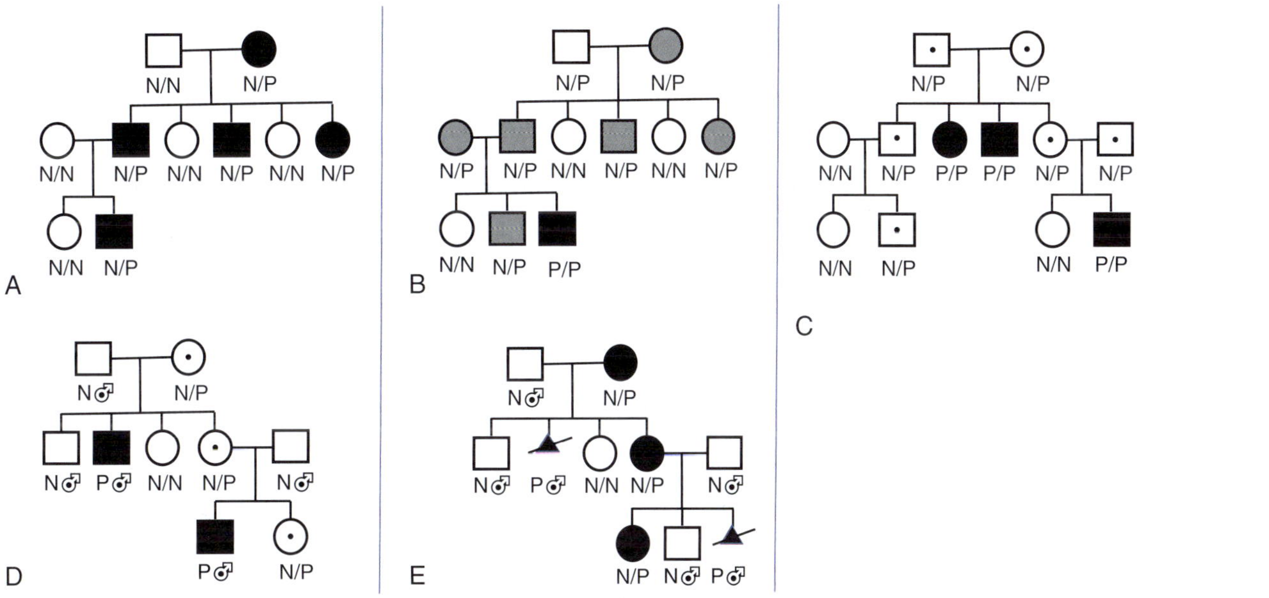

FIGURE 32-2. Modes of inheritance. In the classic mendelian modes of inheritance, the inheritance pattern that is observed in families is determined by the biologic effects of the variants in the gene. In autosomal dominant inheritance (**A**), the pattern reflects the fact that the abnormal variant allele causes a phenotype when only one copy is present and it overrides the normal allele. Two copies of the variant can cause the same severity as one, or it may be more severe (see **B**). In semidominant inheritance (**B**), the effects of the abnormal variants are additive—so two copies of the variant are more severe than one. In autosomal recessive inheritance, (**C**) one copy of the abnormal variant causes little or no abnormality, and so only individuals with two variant alleles have the disorder. The sex-linked inheritance patterns (**D, E**) parallel the same ideas as for the autosomal patterns, with the caveat that males only have one copy of the gene, and thus have fewer combinations of alleles. Squares = male; circles = female; black symbols = affected individuals; symbols with a dot in center = carriers; white symbols = unaffected individuals; gray symbols = individuals affected with phenotype of intermediate severity; black triangle crossed out = terminated pregnancy.

disease being one. For most disorders that are described as having autosomal dominant inheritance, the phenotype of the heterozygote is intermediate in severity between that of the two homozygous states (normal and variant) (see Fig. 32-2B). The classic example is familial hypercholesterolemia, in which the heterozygote phenotype has moderate hypercholesterolemia (low-density cholesterol levels of 190 to 500 mg/dL), whereas the homozygous (or compound heterozygous) variant phenotype is much more severe (levels >500 mg/dL). The formal term for this characteristic is semidominant (or incompletely dominant) inheritance. In humans, most pathogenic variants of this type are sufficiently rare that there are very few matings in which both parents are heterozygous for pathogenic variants in the same gene, so homozygosity is not commonly observed in their offspring. In common usage, all human traits that follow either the "true" autosomal dominant or the semidominant patterns are called autosomal dominant. One final type of dominant inheritance is codominant, best known as the inheritance pattern of the ABO blood type system, in which both alleles are expressed independently, and neither dominates the other.

Autosomal recessive inheritance is the pattern that results from variants in which the phenotype of the heterozygote (termed a "carrier") is unaffected (Fig. 32-2C). This characteristic is the main distinction between autosomal recessive inheritance as compared with autosomal dominant inheritance. In autosomal recessive inheritance, the affected individuals have two pathogenic variants at a single locus, one on each chromosome. These variants can either be the same (homozygous) or distinct (compound heterozygous). Typically, both pathogenic variants are inherited, one each, from an unaffected carrier parent. Because there is a 1 in 2 chance of transmission of the pathogenic variant from each parent, there is a 1 in 4 chance that an offspring will inherit the pathogenic variants from both parents (½×½). Autosomal recessive inheritance is observed as horizontal occurrence of the trait—that is, multiple affected siblings, but no parent-to-child transmission because the carrier parents are unaffected. Occasionally heterozygotes may manifest a mild phenotype, which is indeed the same situation described above for what was termed semidominant inheritance. However, if the heterozygous phenotype is very mild or only detectable with sophisticated and sensitive phenotyping, the trait is considered to have an autosomal recessive inheritance pattern.

In sex-linked inheritance, the gene is on the X chromosome (it is sometimes called X-linked inheritance). Father-to-son transmission is not observed because if a father is affected, he harbors the pathogenic variant on his sole X chromosome; he can either transmit his X chromosome with the pathogenic variant (in which case the offspring must be female) or he can transmit his Y chromosome, which cannot have the pathogenic variant (in which case the offspring is male). Males only have one X chromosome, so when they harbor an abnormal allele, their genotype is said to be hemizygous. All daughters of affected fathers are therefore heterozygotes for the pathogenic variant. The clinical manifestations of sex-linked inherited disorders is complicated by X-inactivation. This X-inactivation process provides a degree of similarity in gene expression between the sexes—males only have one X chromosome, so gene dosage is 1.0. The X-inactivation process balances expression between males and females by randomly silencing the expression of most genes on X on one of the two chromosomes in females, leading to a functional gene dosage of 1.0.

Taking X-inactivation into account and the various combinations of genotype and phenotype that can manifest in sex-linked disorders, there are two classic patterns. The sex-linked recessive inheritance pattern (see Fig. 32-2D) is typically associated with a partial loss of function allele, which reduces, but does not abrogate gene function and is not cell-lethal. This inheritance pattern typically only manifests in affected males. Female heterozygotes, having one normal allele of the gene, are unaffected because 50% dosage is sufficient for normal function. This principle assumes random X-chromosome inactivation. However, females with incomplete X-inactivation can manifest the phenotype of what is typically a sex-linked recessive inheritance pattern disorder. In sex-linked recessive inheritance, heterozygous (carrier) females have a 1 in 2 probability that each male offspring is affected and a 1 in 2 probability that each female offspring is a heterozygous carrier. If the disorder is such that affected males can reproduce, all of their male offspring are unaffected, and all their female offspring are heterozygous carriers. The classic description of sex-linked dominant inheritance (see Fig. 32-2E) is typically associated with more severe alleles, which are cell-lethal. This lethality leads to nonviability of the male embryos, so the pathogenic variant is not observed in males. Female heterozygotes are affected and have a 1 in 2 chance that each female offspring will also be affected; there is also a 1 in 2 chance a male will receive the variant, but all affected males die early in development.

Formally, the terms autosomal dominant, autosomal recessive, and sex-linked describe inheritance patterns, not genes, diseases, alleles, or variants. Although this distinction may seem arcane, it is important because the inheritance pattern descriptor can be confused with the descriptor for the cellular basis of the disease. This is most obvious for cancer susceptibility traits caused by variants in tumor suppressor genes (see Chapter 166). The inheritance pattern of the clinical trait, which is increased susceptibility to cancer, is autosomal dominant. Biologically, however, such disorders are often described as cellular recessives, because the phenotype of cancer only manifests following a secondary, somatic variant in the gene, thereby causing the cells to be homozygous or compound heterozygous for variants in the gene. As well, it is best to associate disease or abnormal phenotypes to pathogenic variants in the gene, not to the gene itself. In this respect, one should describe a patient as "having a pathogenic variant in a Lynch syndrome gene," instead of saying the person "has the Lynch syndrome gene." It is also nonsensical to say that a patient "has the Lynch syndrome gene" because in fact essentially all humans have two copies of such genes. As well, it is incorrect to say that colon cancer is "caused by the Lynch syndrome gene." Genes do not cause disease—they "cause" normal and abnormal physiology.

NONMENDELIAN INHERITANCE

Genetic disorders can present with multiple occurrences in a family (multiplex) or as a single occurrence (simplex). Simplex occurrence of disease can be explained by a classic mendelian autosomal recessive, X-linked recessive, or autosomal dominant inheritance pattern. For the autosomal recessive pattern, it may be simply by chance in the family; for the X-linked recessive pattern, it may have been inherited silently through females in prior generations; and in either, it may develop through a de novo (new) mutation. However, simplex occurrence disease also might be due to nonmendelian inheritance such as genomic imprinting, uniparental disomy, digenic inheritance, mosaicism, and mitochondrial DNA variants. For these reasons, the clinician should be alert for families in which only a single individual is apparently affected. Other atypical modes of inheritance not further considered here include mitochondrial inheritance, imprinting, digenic inheritance, and uniparental disomy.

Mosaicism

An important exception to mendelian inheritance is the concept of mosaicism.[3] Mosaicism is defined as the presence of two or more cell lines that originated from the same zygote but have distinct chromosomal or gene variant complements. A chimera is when the cells originated from different zygotes, as is the case in an individual who receives transplanted tissue. Some mosaic disorders can manifest patchy pigmentary abnormalities that follow the lines of Blaschko. Mosaicism is common in a number of well-recognized disorders, such as seborrheic keratoses of the skin, which are caused by somatic variants in *PIK3CA* or *FGFR3*, and paroxysmal nocturnal hemoglobinuria, which is associated with somatic variants in *PIGA*. Mosaicism is also the genomic basis of cancer—a clone of cells with extensive variants that originated from a normal cell in an individual (see Chapter 166). Mosaicism can also arise in the hematopoietic lineage with age. This phenomenon has become important in internal medicine in the phenomenon of clonal hematopoiesis of indeterminant potential (CHIP). This condition causes an elevated risk of myelodysplastic conditions, vascular disease, and other disorders, most commonly in older individuals.[4,5]

Mosaicism can also affect the risk of recurrence for genetic diseases. A parent can harbor two or more cell lines in the gonads (germline mosaicism) or in somatic cells. The level of mosaicism in the somatic cells may be low enough or limited to non-critical tissues or organs such that the parent appears unaffected, or they may be affected in a patchy pattern (Fig. 32-3). Mosaicism should be suspected when two or more children of healthy parents develop a disease that is typically inherited in an autosomal dominant pattern.

GENOMIC VARIATION IN HUMANS

Variation in the genome is the fundamental biologic basis of all heritable traits and diseases.[6] This spectrum of genomic variation runs the gamut from one base pair (a single nucleotide variant [SNV]) to 3×10^9 base pairs (triploidy, which is three copies of a genome, rather than the normal two), and everything in between. The categories of genomic variation that are described later represent slices of that spectrum of variation, and are handy categorical clusters of this variation (much as red, orange, yellow, green, cyan, blue, and violet are useful but arbitrary slices of the continuous, visible electromagnetic spectrum). Another dimension of the broad and continuous spectrum of genomic variation is the relationship of this variation to health and disease. A given single nucleotide variant can be so devastating that it is 100% lethal early in embryonic development. On the other extreme, each of us has over a million single nucleotide variants that have no known biologic consequences.

MUTATION AND VARIANTS

The process of changing a genome from one state to another is termed a mutation. Mutation is a process, not a state. Mutation is defined as the process of a change in nucleotide sequence owing to errors of DNA replication, recombination, or repair, radiation, chemical mutagens, or transposons. A variant is a state of the genome such that one or more nucleotides differ from the reference sequence. At first this may seem arbitrary and unsatisfying—it seems to be dodging the issue of whether a variant is normal or abnormal, disease-associated, or benign. But there is utility and merit to this approach because it is not so simple that at a given position an adenine is normal whereas a cytosine, guanine, or thymine is abnormal. Genetic variation can be complex and subtle, so the new formulation is simply to define a reference sequence, but not necessarily call it normal or abnormal. Because the reference is based on sequences from actual human beings, it is a mix of both. Then a variant is simply described as being different from, or the same as, the reference. Genomic variants can be inherited from a parent (hereditary, constitutional, or germline variants; see Fig. 32-2A–D) and thus be present in every cell, or variants can be acquired in only some tissues during development or any time during life (somatic or mosaic variants) (see Fig. 32-3).

SINGLE NUCLEOTIDE VARIANTS AND OTHER SMALL VARIANTS

Single nucleotide variants are defined as a change of one nucleotide at a given position. Nonsynonymous variants are gene changes that can either lead to a single amino acid change (missense); alter the reading frame and thereby lead to alteration in the downstream protein structure (frameshift) or introduce a stop codon (premature termination codon) that truncates the protein prematurely (nonsense); or abolish the specific site at which splicing of an intron takes place during the processing of precursor mRNA into mature mRNA (splice site). Most mRNAs with nonsense variants are inactivated and

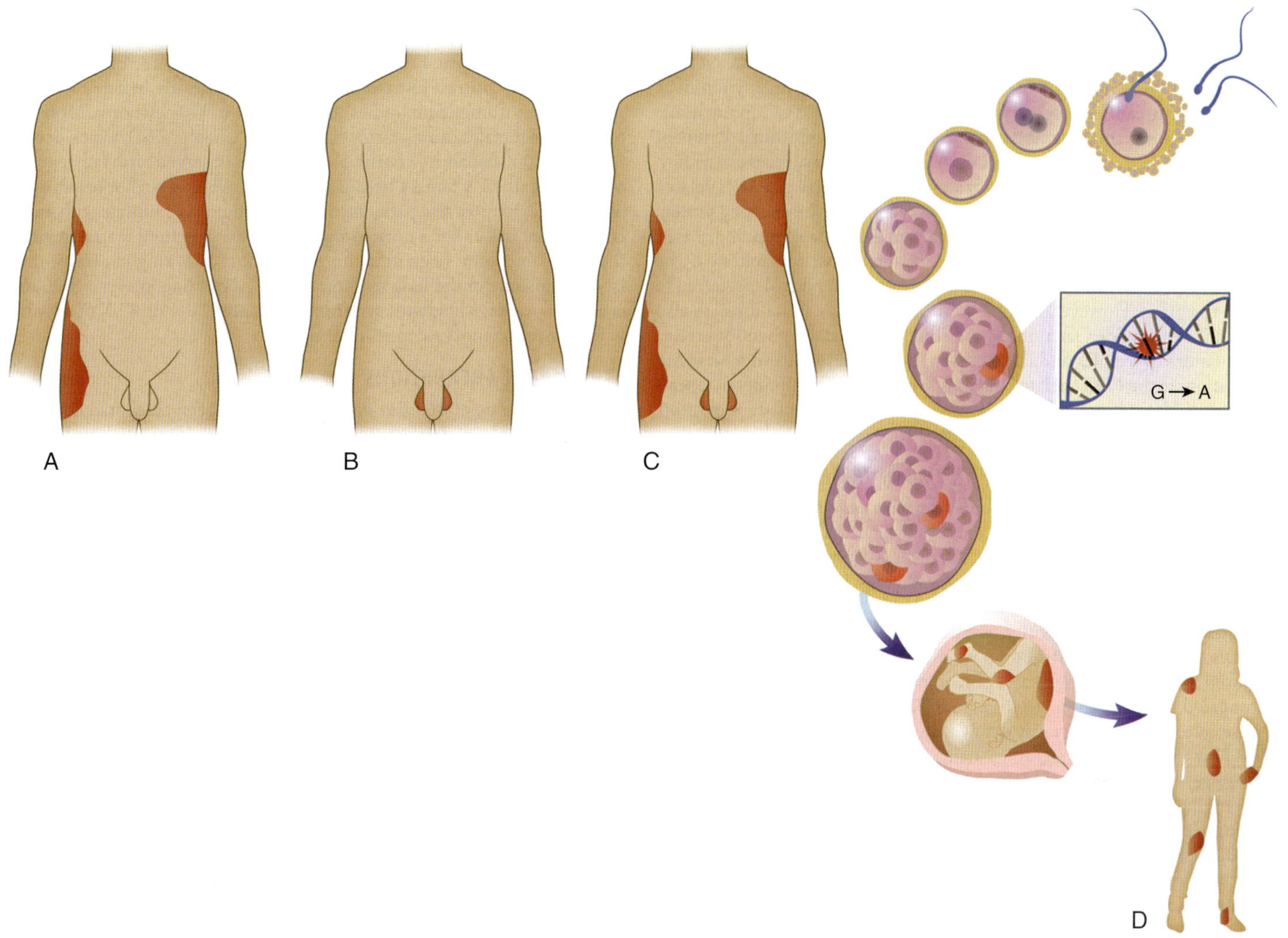

FIGURE 32-3. **Types of mosaicism.** Mosaicism is categorized into germline and somatic. A given individual can harbor a mosaic variant in one of two general categories of cells: germline or nongermline (somatic) cells. Thus, an individual can harbor in either (**A** or **B**) or both (**C**) of these compartments. How mosaicism is generated is illustrated in **D**. After fertilization, in a multicellular embryo, one cell undergoes a mutation and all of the cells that derive from that cell harbor the variant. (From Spinner N, Biesecker LG. Mosaicism in human disease. *Nat Rev Genet*. 2013;14:307-320.)

removed from cells by a surveillance mechanism called nonsense mediated decay. The most common mutation, cytosine to thymine, is about 10-fold more common than other base changes and occurs in the methylated CpG dinucleotide (a cytosine-guanine sequence) because methylated cytosine can be deaminated and converted to thymine.

Any two unrelated humans differ on average by about 3.5 million single nucleotide variants (≈0.1% of the 3 billion bp reference haploid genome). Whereas most of these single nucleotide variants lie outside of the exons, on average about 20,000 single nucleotide variants occur in coding regions; among these variants, about 7000 to 10,000 are nonsynonymous (i.e., change the encoded amino acid). Single nucleotide variants located outside of the protein-coding regions can still have phenotypic effects, such as by modifying gene regulatory elements, altering the binding sites for transcription factors, generating splicing variants, or affecting noncoding RNAs. The former term, single nucleotide polymorphism (SNP), was initially defined as a DNA variation that is present in greater than 1% of the population, but this term is now discouraged because "polymorphism" carried with it connotations of being "benign," which is clearly false for a substantial number of single nucleotide polymorphisms.

Variants are divided into substitutions, insertions, and deletions. Variants in protein-coding sequence that change the protein structure are termed nonsynonymous, whereas those that do not lead to protein changes are termed synonymous. Synonymous variants can still have functional consequences, such as by generating a new (abnormal) splice site or an exon splice enhancer, or by affecting regulatory elements. A set of consecutive single nucleotide variants (or other variants) that lie on a single chromosome is defined as a haplotype. A nonrandom association of markers in a population not interrupted by meiotic recombination (crossing over) is described as linkage disequilibrium. More than 100,000 single nucleotide variants have been shown to cause mendelian disorders. Many of these disorders are cataloged in locus-specific databases (http://www.hgvs.org/locus-specific-mutation-databases), the Human Gene Mutation Database (http://www.hgmd.cf.ac.uk/ac/index.php), and ClinVar (https://www.ncbi.nlm.nih.gov/clinvar/).

DELETIONS, INSERTIONS, AND INDELS

These variations are less common than single nucleotide variants. They comprise small nucleotide alterations, including deletions of one to a moderate number of nucleotides, insertions of one or a moderate number of nucleotides (which may be a duplication of adjacent DNA or nucleotides from elsewhere in the genome), and variants that comprise both a deletion of one or more nucleotides and an insertion of one or more nucleotides. Many of these variants are cataloged in the same databases as described earlier for single nucleotide variants.

TANDEM REPEATS

The genome contains a large number of repetitive elements, the most clinically important of which are the short tandem repeats (e.g., dinucleotides, trinucleotides, and tetranucleotides—$[GT]_n$, $[CAA]_n$, or $GATA]_n$—called microsatellites). These highly polymorphic repeats can have a wide range of copy numbers of their repeating subunits.[7] A number of these markers can be used to derive a nearly unique pattern of genotypes for each individual, as is used in identification for criminal forensic and paternity analysis (https://www.fbi.gov/services/laboratory/biometric-analysis/codis).

The instability of these repeats leads them to be unstable (dynamic) within individuals; humans can be complex mosaics of a range of repeat lengths among their cells. Pathogenic dynamic expansion of trinucleotide, tetranucleotide, and pentanucleotide repeat sequences can cause disease whether located in coding regions (e.g., $[CAG]_n$ triplet in *HTT*-related Huntington disease), noncoding introns (e.g., $[GAA]_n$ in *FXN*-related Friedreich ataxia), in the upstream noncoding part of the gene (e.g., $[CGG]_n$ in *FMR1*-related fragile X syndrome), or in the downstream noncoding part of the gene (e.g., $[CTG]_n$ in myotonic dystrophy) regions. These variants can cause disease in an autosomal dominant pattern (e.g., *DMPK*-related myotonic dystrophy), autosomal recessive pattern (e.g., *FXN*-related Friedreich ataxia), or sex-linked pattern (e.g., *FMR1*-related fragile X syndrome) owing to a gain or loss of function of the encoded protein that is altered by the repeat mutation. For each of the unstable repeat diseases, a repeat number threshold exists, above which the disease is manifested. The number of repeats below that threshold but greater than normal is referred to as a pre-mutation. However, in some of these genes, pre-mutations are also associated with a milder, later onset, and sometimes distinct phenotype (e.g., ovarian failure in females and late-onset neurologic disorders in males with premutations in the *FMR1*-related fragile X syndrome). The number of repeats tends to expand in subsequent generations—a phenomenon called anticipation, which typically occurs in a sex-specific manner.

STRUCTURAL VARIANTS AND COPY NUMBER VARIANTS

It has long been recognized that genomes can have large-scale variation in the amount of DNA or the arrangement of DNA, as delineated by microscopic chromosomal analysis. Recent technologic advances (Chapter 33) have improved the ability to identify and characterize these variations. High-resolution analysis of human genome sequences has identified both moderate scale and higher order architectural features, with a potential to cause genomic instability and extensive submicroscopic structural variations. Copy number variant is the term used to describe a larger scale gain or loss of DNA from a chromosome, as compared to an insertion, deletion, or indel, as described above. Again, all of these categories are arbitrarily defined, and some of these categories more reflect how they are detected rather than a biologically based categorization. On average, each individual harbors about 1000 copy number variants, with sizes ranging from 500 bp to 1.2 Mb (million base pairs). These structural variations consist of copy number gains or losses, including deletions, insertions, duplications, and triplications, as well as balanced rearrangements such as genomic inversions and balanced translocations. The frequency of smaller copy number variants (<1 kb, kilobase pair) and indels (insertion or deletion of bases <100 bp) is higher than the larger rearrangements, because they are biologically better tolerated. The number of copy number variants is far smaller than the number of single nucleotide variants, but if one counts the base pairs that are abnormal, more base pairs are in copy number variants than in single nucleotide variants in any given individual.

Copy number variants are associated with mendelian diseases, nonmendelian traits (e.g., complex diseases), and common traits (including neurobehavioral traits),[8] but they also can be benign. Copy number variants can cause disorders by disrupting the gene structure or by changing the copy number of dosage-sensitive genes. However, copy number variants that involve nongenic sequences and leave a gene intact also can have long-range effects by changing the expression of neighboring genes. The Toronto Database of Genomic Variants (http://projects.tcag.ca/variation) summarizes copy number variants, and many clinically relevant copy number variants are also included in the Database of Chromosomal Imbalance and Phenotype in Humans using Ensembl Resources (DECIPHER) (https://www.deciphergenomics.org/).

CHROMOSOMAL ABERRATIONS

Chromosomal aberrations are the class of genomic variation that causes the greatest perturbation of DNA. Chromosomal aberrations, which can be divided into numerical and structural aberrations, occur in about 1 in 160 live births. Although many of the associated phenotypes are rare, the general clinician is likely to have individuals with the more common disorders in their practice.

Most numerical chromosome aberrations result in prenatal lethality. Numerical aberrations are classified as either polyploidy (number of chromosomes are in multiples of the haploid set of 23 chromosomes) or aneuploidy (with extra or missing chromosomes not in multiples of the haploid set). A normal female chromosome complement is 46,XX and male is 46,XY. Polyploidies such as triploidies (69,XXX, 69,XXY, and 69,XYY) are caused by abnormal fertilization of the egg by two sperms, whereas tetraploidies (92,XXYY or 92,XXXX) are caused by a failure in zygote division. Among *viable* chromosomal aneuploidies, the most common trisomies and monosomies involve chromosomes X, Y, 21, 18, and 13 and arise as a result of meiotic nondisjunctions. These aneuploidies are the most common because these four chromosomes have the smallest number of biallelically transcribed genes. The only autosomal trisomies compatible with life are Down syndrome (trisomy 21, 1 in every 670 newborns) (E-Fig. 32-1A),[9,10] Edwards syndrome (trisomy 18, 1 in 7500 newborns), and Patau syndrome (trisomy 13, 1 in every 22,700 newborns). In contrast to trisomies, all monosomies are lethal.

Sex chromosome aneuploidies are found in 1 in 440 newborns. Monosomy X (45,X) in females causes Turner syndrome (Chapter 214), which occurs in 1 in every 4000 female newborns. However, this observed birth rate represents only 1% of all 45,X fetuses because more than 99% of such fetuses result in miscarriage. In most live patients, the 45,X cell line is a mosaic with another cell line that has either a normal karyotype or a structural rearrangement of the X chromosome (e.g., deletion of the short arm, ring chromosome, or isochromosome of the long or short arms). About one in every 1000 males is either 47,XXY Klinefelter syndrome (Chapter 214) or 47,XYY (typically with at most phenotypic manifestations).

STRUCTURAL ABERRATIONS

Chromosomal deletions and duplications have been categorized as microscopically visible or submicroscopic, as terminal or interstitial, and as recurrent or nonrecurrent. Balanced reciprocal translocations, which result from an exchange of the DNA material between two chromosomes, are found in about 1 in 600 individuals. During meiosis, the translocation chromosomes segregate and lead to the transmission of either balanced or unbalanced products being transmitted to progeny. The unbalanced products often lead to either spontaneous miscarriage or birth of a child with typically serious clinical consequences. When a fragment of one chromosome is translocated internally into another chromosome's arm, the aberration is termed an insertion or insertional translocation. Insertional translocations occur more than 100 times more frequently than originally recognized. The carrier of a balanced translocation has up to a 50% chance of abnormal progeny. Other less common structural chromosomal abnormalities include inversions, ring chromosomes, isochromosomes, complex chromosome rearrangements, and heterochromatin variants.

ASSAYING GENETIC VARIATION

Genomic assays vary based upon the size of the aberration that is being targeted. Chromosomal aberrations longer than about 5 Mb can be detected by light microscopy (cytogenetics) after specific staining that generates a characteristic banding pattern (e.g., G-banded karyotype analysis). Submicroscopic rearrangements, such as microdeletions or microduplications (30 kb to 5 Mb), can be analyzed using fluorescence in situ hybridization (FISH).[11] Overall, light microscopic techniques are declining in favor of molecular assays but are still necessary to detect balanced rearrangements.

The development of array-based comparative genomic hybridization (array CGH) or single nucleotide polymorphism chip-based testing allows determination of chromosome imbalances and copy number variants, with the level of resolution depending only on the number, size, and distance between the arrayed interrogating probes. Millions of these oligonucleotide probes can be synthesized on one glass slide. Oligonucleotide probes are also used on single nucleotide polymorphism arrays, which, unlike microarray-based CGH, can generate association studies or detect uniparental disomies. The widespread diagnostic use of array CGH and single nucleotide polymorphism chips has not only increased the sensitivity for detecting diseases associated with copy number variants but also has led to the discovery of many additional copy number variant–associated disorders. To detect genomic imbalances, an alternative is a quantitative polymerase chain reaction–based technique called multiplex ligation-dependent probe amplification (MLPA). MLPA provides a simple, rapid, and sensitive method to detect dosage alterations in selected genomic regions.

Most recently, several next-generation sequencing technologies enabled simultaneous and massively parallel DNA sequencing (Chapter 33). These technologies facilitate panel testing (simultaneous assay of multiple genes implicated in a particular phenotype), exome sequencing (the coding regions of the genome), and genome sequencing. Next-generation sequencing methods generate far larger quantities of data at less expense; however, the raw sequence data that are generated from individual amplified DNA template sequences have shorter read lengths, which can be difficult to map uniquely to the genome. Thus, neither exome sequencing nor genome sequencing is truly "whole exome" or "whole genome." Nevertheless, next-generation sequencing of a patient's genome (e.g., 30-fold coverage with respect to the haploid human reference genome sequence) can generate robust and accurate individual genomic evaluation. These next-generation sequencing technologies have led to an explosion in gene discovery and an increasing understanding of the mechanistic bases of genetic disorders. Exome sequencing alone currently has about a 25% yield for clinical diagnosis in patients with phenotypic syndromes of unknown cause—a significant improvement over previously available testing modalities.

Recent advances and the relatively widespread use of array CGH, single nucleotide polymorphism-chips, and next-generation sequencing technologies have transformed the understanding and diagnosis of human disease (Chapter 33). As sequencing becomes less expensive and more available, the understanding of human evolution, disease, and treatment is advancing rapidly.

GENETIC TEST REPORTS

Whereas gene changes formerly were termed "polymorphism" if they are benign and "mutation" if they are disease- or trait-associated, these terms have been replaced. Instead, a gene state different from reference is termed a variant, and the term variant is modified by an adjective such as "benign," "likely benign," of "unknown significance," "likely pathogenic," or "pathogenic."[12] Clinicians will increasingly encounter genetic test reports with descriptors such as "likely pathogenic variant" or "benign variant," or "variant of unknown significance." The involvement of genetic counselors can greatly improve the transmission of genetic information to patients and their families.[13]

As with all forms of medical testing, genetic test results are probabilistic. Some, such as the finding of nonmosaic trisomy 21, confer an extremely high likelihood (for all practical purposes, 100%) of phenotypic abnormality in the patient. Others, such as a novel nonsense variant in a patient with suspected *BRCA1*-related hereditary breast and ovarian cancer susceptibility, may be reported as likely pathogenic.

Distinct variants in a gene can cause the same phenotype (allelic heterogeneity) or distinct phenotypes (phenotypic heterogeneity). By contrast, the same abnormal clinical phenotype can be caused by variants in different genes (genetic or locus heterogeneity). This complexity has led to a proposal to designate human single gene diseases by the dyad of gene and phenotype. For example, *MSH2*-related Lynch syndrome.

Based on the functional consequences, variants are also categorized by their consequences into loss-of-function or gain-of-function variants. The former—also known as hypomorphic (partial loss) or amorphic (null) loss of function (complete loss)—affect the dosage-sensitive or haploinsufficient genes, in which decreased production of a protein is not sufficient for normal function. Gain-of-function variants increase the function or add a new function for the protein (neomorphic), whereas dominant negative variants encode a protein that interacts antagonistically with the normal product from the other allele (antimorphic).

Adult medicine practitioners are increasingly likely to encounter genetic testing results in their practices, whether in a diagnostic setting (e.g., an individual with early onset cancer), a secondary findings setting (e.g., a parent of a child sequenced for autism found to have malignant hyperthermia), or in a direct-to-consumer testing setting (e.g., an unanticipated breast and ovarian cancer susceptibility result from ancestry testing). Familiarity with genetic and genomic test results will allow clinicians to integrate these results seamlessly into their practices and use them to improve the care of their patients.

GENOMICS AND GENETICS AS A NORMAL PART OF MEDICINE

Nongeneticists are sometimes intimidated or concerned about using genetic diagnostics in their practices, and there is some historical basis for this concern. Clinical genetics is associated with a tragic legacy of eugenics, the thoroughly discredited concept that our species should be "improved" by preventing the reproduction of individuals deemed to be genetically undesirable or unfit. The modern clinical practice of genetics seeks to improve the health and lifespan of individuals with genetic disorders, theoretically increasing the frequency of pathogenic variants in the population because successfully treated individuals can live longer and reproduce.[14] The theoretical qualifier is important because, in the larger picture, this effect on the population is much smaller than that of the natural mutation rate. Nevertheless, reproductive genetics can still elicit concerns of eugenic tendencies. Although no overtly eugenic laws or medical practices persist, concerns linger that the very availability of prenatal testing and selective termination, coupled with social and economic pressures against disease and disability, comprise a subtle eugenic bias in reproductive medicine.

The important takeaway from this history and sociology of genetics is that adult medicine clinicians seeking to improve the health of their patients should not hesitate to use genetic and genomic diagnosis and targeted therapeutics because of any lingering fears of the eugenic history of the field. In this respect, genetics is just like any other technologically advanced component of modern medicine. It can have bioethical conundrums (Chapter 2), which may be different from those in other specialties, but these issues are not overall greater or more worrisome than those in other disciplines. Clinicians should ignore protestations that genetics and genomics is somehow exceptional from all other aspects of medicine, or something to be avoided or discouraged. A genetic or genomic test used to diagnose and treat an adult with cardiac disease is no different than a catheter, an ultrasound, or a troponin level—another arrow in the modern biomedical quiver that has great potential to improve health and extend longevity.

GENERAL REFERENCES

For the General References and other additional features, please visit Elsevier eBooks+ at https://ebooks.health.elsevier.com.

33

APPLICATIONS OF MOLECULAR TECHNOLOGIES TO CLINICAL MEDICINE

GEOFFREY S. GINSBURG

The Human Genome Project, an enabler of the systematic exploration of the molecular underpinnings of disease, has led to the expectation that these insights would lead to a transformation of medical practice. However, most diseases are still defined by their anatomic location and clinical symptoms and are treated with one-size-fits-all therapies that fail to account for the unique biologic background of the individual and of the diseased tissues. Genome-based technologies can probe the molecular architecture of disease and the genetic backgrounds of the individuals who harbor them to improve the potential for more precise diagnostics and therapeutic strategies.[1] The Human Genome Project (https://www.genome.gov/human-genome-project) provided the foundation for precision medicine along with advances in genotyping and sequencing technologies, bioinformatics, systems biology, and computational biology. Today, precision medicine aims to build on this foundation, translating these discoveries into clinical practice, with the ultimate goal of improved health and health care for individuals and for populations.

MOLECULAR TECHNOLOGIES ALONG THE CONTINUUM FROM HEALTH TO DISEASE

In 2015, the United States embarked on a Precision Medicine Initiative to enroll over 1 million people in what is now called the "*All of Us*" research program (https://allofus.nih.gov/). The shared data from sequencing, electronic medical records (EMRs), personal reported information, and digital health technologies provide a platform for assessing the biology of disease as well as a paradigm that will allow for more informed decisions along the continuum from health to disease (Fig. 33-1). Precision health care is now being used in clinical practice across the lifespan (Table 33-1). DNA testing is used for reproductive counseling for couples who are planning a pregnancy and for prenatal testing with sequencing assays of fetal DNA in the maternal circulation to assess for mendelian and developmental disorders. Sequencing in the neonatal intensive care unit (ICU) is becoming more common for diagnoses and determination of treatment options for gravely ill infants. Sequencing is also being used to end the diagnostic odyssey for many children (and some adults) with rare and undiagnosed diseases. For the early assessment of disease risk, family history still may be the most powerful tool. However, genomic risk scores are being defined to complement family history for certain chronic diseases. Although lagging the dramatic decline in cost and increase in throughput of DNA sequencing, technology platforms that measure the "expressed genome" (RNA, proteins, metabolites) are increasingly being used to define physiologic states in response to the environment, to classify disease states, to diagnose current disease, and to predict future clinical outcomes. These approaches, which form the basis for a new molecular classification and taxonomy of disease and diagnosis, can provide more precise ways to screen for and to detect disease at its earliest molecular manifestations, often preclinically. In addition, the selection of certain drugs increasingly can be guided by a patient's underlying genetic makeup as well as by the molecular makeup of the disease. Given that a disease's evolution from baseline risk often occurs over many years (see Fig. 33-1), periodic molecular and digital profiling defines a novel form of health care that focuses on health assessments and disease prevention with proactive management rather than the current paradigm of acute intervention and crisis management.

GENOMES, DISEASE, AND TREATMENT

A key question in medicine is to what extent genetic variation influences the likelihood of disease onset, affects the natural history of disease in combination with the environment and social factors, or provides clues relevant to the management of disease. Genome sequencing is providing new approaches for the diagnosis, study, and treatment of disease.

NEWBORN SCREENING, PRENATAL DIAGNOSIS, AND PRE-CONCEPTION CARRIER TESTING

A natural outcome of identifying genes for rare mendelian disorders (Chapter 32) is the application of these findings to earlier detection, at birth (newborn screening), in utero (prenatal diagnosis), or pre-conception (carrier testing).

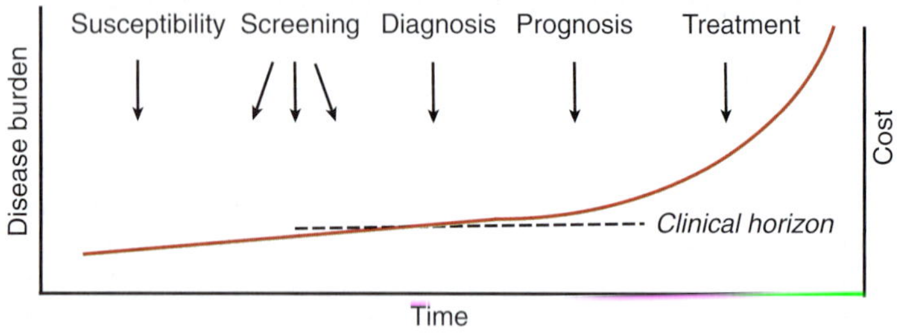

FIGURE 33-1. Use of molecular technologies across the continuum from health to disease. Various molecular technologies may now be used to complement the traditional approach to evaluating health and disease across the lifespan. The *red curve* indicates the course of a chronic disease over time. The *dashed line* indicates when clinical symptoms are manifest. Overall, the goal is to shift the detection and treatment paradigm to the left. (Adapted from Ginsburg GS, Willard H. eds. *Genomic and Personalized Medicine*. 3rd ed. Academic Press; 2016.)

Newborn screening—mandatory, state-supported public health programs meant to protect newborn children by screening them for rare, treatable (and thus preventable) disorders at birth—has been steadily increasing from an average of five conditions in 1995 to a panel of 35 core disorders currently recommended by the U.S. Department of Health and Human Services.[2] Rapid genome sequencing (about 19.5 hours from test to result) has been used to treat patients with undiagnosed and potentially fatal disorders in the neonatal ICU.[3] As the number of conditions considered for newborn screening will undoubtedly grow, rapid sequencing can potentially broaden and foreshorten differential diagnosis, thereby resulting in fewer empirical treatments as well as faster progression to genetic and prognostic counseling.[4,5]

Cell-free fetal DNA circulating in maternal blood can be analyzed by next-generation sequencing technologies to identify fetal aneuploidy from cell-free fetal DNA in maternal plasma. Noninvasive prenatal testing of trisomy 21 eliminates the need for invasive procedures, while also greatly expanding the number of genetic variants that have traditionally been detected in utero.

Before conception, carrier screening enables couples to assess their risk of having a child with a recessive mendelian disorder (Chapter 32) and use this information to guide their reproductive decisions. There are over 1000 rare, *recessive* mendelian disorders for which the underlying genetic mutation is known. Though individually rare, these mutations can have a sizable public health impact considering that each person is estimated to carry on average 2.8 mutations[6] for known severe recessive disorders.

SEQUENCING: A DRIVER OF PRECISION MEDICINE

Genome-wide association studies (GWASs) have identified over 275,000 unique single nucleotide variant trait associations from large cohorts of patients and controls across numerous diseases (https://www.ebi.ac.uk/gwas/). GWAS has been a transformative approach to identifying common genetic variation across the entire human genome in an unbiased fashion, thereby offering an unprecedented opportunity to uncover new biologic pathways of disease. Gene editing technologies using Clustered Regularly Interspaced Short Palindromic Repeats (CRISPR) and Transcription Activator-Like Effector Nucleases (TALEN) are changing the approach to defining the biology of genetic variants discovered by GWAS and sequencing.[7,8]

Since 2001, the cost of sequencing a human genome has dropped from more than $3 billion per genome to $500. Using next-generation sequencing technology, a sequencing laboratory can sequence more than 60 genomes

TABLE 33-1 APPLICATION OF MOLECULAR DIAGNOSTICS ALONG THE CONTINUUM FROM HEALTH TO DISEASE

TIME POINT IN CLINICAL DECISION MAKING	*CANCER*		*CARDIOVASCULAR DISEASE*	
	TEST	**INDICATION**	**TEST**	**INDICATION**
Risk/susceptibility	*BRCA1, BRCA2* *HNPCC* *TP53, PTEN*	Breast, ovarian Colon Sarcomas	*9p21*, GeneSeq, various polygenic risk scores LongQTNext/RhythmNext	CAD LQTS
Screening	HPV genotypes	Cervical	*APOB, LDLR, LDLRAP1, PCSK9*	Familial hypercholesterolemia
Diagnosis	Cancer origin OVA1	Cancer of unknown primary Ovarian mass malignancy	*ABCC9, AKAP9, ANK2, CACNA1C, CACNA2D1, CACNB2, CALM1, CALM2, CALM3, CASQ2, CAV3, DES, DSC2, DSG2, DSP, GPD1L, HCN4, JUP, KCND3, KCNE1, KCNE1L, KCNE2, KCNE3, KCNH2, KCNJ2, KCNJ5, KCNJ8, KCNQ1, LMNA, NKX2-5, PKP2, PLN, RANGRF, RYR2, SCN10A, SCN1B, SCN2B, SCN3B, SCN4B, SCN5A, SNTA1, TGFB3, TMEM43, TRDN, TRPM4, TTN* TnI, BNP, CRP	Long QT syndrome ACS
Prognosis	Oncotype DX (21-gene assay) MammaPrint (70-gene assay) HER2/neu, ER, PR	Breast	Under development	
Drug response*	*BCR-ABL* *EML4-ALK*	Imatinib (CML) Crizotinib (NSCL)	*CYP2C19* *CYP2C9, VKORC1*	Clopidogrel Warfarin
Monitoring	CTCs	Tumor recurrence or progression	AlloMap	Transplant rejection

*Additional drug-gene pairs can be found in E-Table 33-1.

ACS = acute coronary syndromes; BNP = brain natriuretic peptide; CAD = coronary artery disease; CRP = C-reactive protein; CTCs = circulating tumor cells; ER = estrogen receptor; HPV = human papillomavirus; LQTS = long QT syndrome; PR = progesterone receptor; TnI = troponin I.

Data from Ginsburg GS, Willard H. eds. *Genomic and Personalized Medicine*. 3rd ed. Academic Press; 2016.

per day, thereby allowing direct measurement not just of common variants, but also theoretically of all variation in a genome. It is estimated that the population frequency of germline variants is approximately 1 in every 1000 of the 3.2 billion nucleotide positions, thereby giving rise to approximately 3 million variants in a given human genome. The challenge lies in determining the meaning of variants, many of which occur in noncoding regions of the genome whose function is largely unknown, and their potential for causing disease. The significance of the noncoding variants remains poorly understood. As a result, the focus clinically has been on exome sequencing (which examines variation in the coding sequences that constitute 1 to 2% of the genome), in which mutations may have predictable effects on downstream protein structure. Genome interpretation is a key bottleneck in the ubiquitous application of sequencing to clinical medicine.[9] With increasing efforts to encourage data sharing and the creation of interoperable data stores, definitive diagnoses from genomic data should become more common.[10] Of note, the American Colleges of Medical Genetics and Genomics currently defines 73 actionable variants in the human genome (https://www.ncbi.nlm.nih.gov/clinvar/docs/acmg/) that, when found, should be discussed with the patients who harbor them.

RISK PREDICTION FOR COMMON COMPLEX DISEASES

Despite strong statistical associations linking genetic variants with complex diseases in GWAS, the low relative risk of the disease allele (generally <2) limits their use for risk assessment. Notable exceptions include the genetic variations underlying inherited breast cancer syndromes, Lynch syndrome, and familial hypercholesterolemia, for which some variants have enabled preventive treatment or screening of family members as well as their consideration as part of population screening programs.

Despite the advancements in genetic testing, a simple family history continues to be among the best tools to identify risks for common diseases.[11] In fact, for conditions with high heritability, such as cardiovascular disease, family history is a much stronger predictor of disease than any single or combination of genetic/genomic markers. One model suggests that neither family history nor genetic testing should be used as a standalone but that the real power for disease prediction, risk assessment, and differential diagnosis comes from their combined use. Recently, polygenic risk scores have been derived from GWAS and sequencing data to enhance the prediction of genetic susceptibility of individuals to disease. Polygenic risk scores for an individual are calculated as weighted counts of thousands of risk variants that they carry, where the risk variants and their weights have been identified in GWASs. Whether polygenic risk scores are ready for clinical use is a matter of debate because many of them have been derived on data from individuals of European ancestry and may not apply to other ancestral groups. In addition, the utility of polygenic risk scores has not always been compared with more traditional risk calculators or family history, so it is not clear whether polygenic risk scores are superior to other risk assessment tools that are already available clinically.

CLINICAL SEQUENCING FOR RARE DISEASES AND DIAGNOSTIC DILEMMAS

Nearly 7000 mendelian disorders have a known molecular basis (http://omim.org/). However, there are nearly as many suspected mendelian traits for which the molecular basis remains to be identified. The potential for clinical sequencing to find the underlying cause and identify treatment options for these rare, sometimes debilitating diseases has led to the formation of various large national and international rare disease consortia. In some specialized clinical centers and through programs such as the National Human Genome Research Institute's Undiagnosed Diseases Program (http://www.genome.gov/27544402), clinical sequencing is being offered to patients with suspected genetic diseases, the so-called "diagnostic dilemmas." To date, about 30% of the more than 1500 participants have received a diagnosis based on their genome sequencing data.[12,13]

PHARMACOGENOMICS: GERMLINE GENETIC VARIANTS AND DRUG RESPONSE

Over the past decade a plethora of genomic markers of efficacy, adverse events, and dosing of therapeutics have been discovered and recommended for clinical use (see E-Table 33-1), but their uptake into clinical practice has been variable, despite their clear actionability. In some cases, such as with the *HLA-B**5701 genotype for the drug abacavir for the treatment of human immunodeficiency virus (HIV) and *HLA-B**1502 for the antiseizure drug carbamazepine, carriers of these genotypes should avoid the drug entirely to eliminate a specific serious adverse event. In other cases, such as *TPMT* for mercaptopurine or *CYP2C9/VKORC1* for warfarin, adjusting the dose of drug based on genotype can help to avoid toxicity and improve efficacy. *Actionability* is not enough to ensure uptake of pharmacogenomics testing as exemplified with the anti-platelet drug clopidogrel, for which despite having an FDA "black box warning" for efficacy in individuals carrying the *CYP2C19* genetic variant, there is often no clear consensus among physicians on its use. Genetic markers that predict reduced therapeutic efficacy may face a high hurdle for established drugs, unless there is strong evidence of the test's clinical validity and utility.

One barrier to implementation of pharmacogenetic testing in clinical practice is the difficulty in translating genetic laboratory test results into actionable prescribing decisions for affected drugs. The Clinical Pharmacogenomics Implementation Consortium was formed to address this barrier to clinical implementation of pharmacogenetic tests by creating, curating, and posting freely available, peer-reviewed, evidence-based, updatable, and detailed gene/drug clinical practice guidelines (https://cpicpgx.org/). These guidelines follow standardized formats, include systematic grading of evidence and clinical recommendations, use standardized terminology, and are peer-reviewed.

CANCER PHARMACOGENOMICS: SOMATIC SEQUENCING OF TUMOR DNA FOR TARGETING DRUG THERAPIES

Cancer arises as a result of somatic DNA mutations that confer a growth advantage upon the cells in which they have occurred, thereby giving rise to tumors (Chapter 166). Comparison of the genetic profiles of tumors and the surrounding normal tissue can reveal the acquired DNA variations that drive growth and that may reveal targets for treatment. The idea of pairing medicines with specific tumor markers in a targeted fashion was first demonstrated when detailed molecular studies of breast tumors led to the discovery of human epidermal growth factor receptor 2 (HER-2), a biomarker overexpressed in approximately 30% of breast tumors and associated with adverse outcomes. Subsequently, trastuzumab (Herceptin), a humanized monoclonal antibody targeting HER-2, was developed and shown to have increased efficacy in patients whose tumors tested positive. HER-2 testing is now part of the standard evaluation and management of breast cancer (Chapter 183). In the past decade, other examples of cancer therapies with companion diagnostics emerged (https://www.mycancergenome.org/). For example, *EGFR* mutation testing has markedly improved the efficacy of gefitinib and erlotinib, small molecule drugs for the treatment of non–small cell lung cancer (Chapter 177) that target *EGFR*. In metastatic colorectal cancer (Chapter 179), tumors with mutated *KRAS* are usually resistant to treatment with cetuximab and panitumumab, thereby leading the American Society of Clinical Oncologists and the U.S. Food and Drug Administration (FDA) to recommend withholding the drugs in these patients. Next-generation sequencing now allows a comprehensive assessment of actionable tumor markers that indicate the potential for a specific therapeutic to have efficacy in a given tumor (https://www.mycancergenome.org/). In 2011, two cancer drugs received accelerated approval by the FDA for use with a companion diagnostic test: crizotinib for the treatment of patients with locally advanced or metastatic non–small cell lung cancer (Chapter 177) with its companion diagnostic designed to detect the *EML4-ALK* fusion gene, and vemurafenib for the treatment of patients with metastatic or unresectable melanoma positive for *BRAF* V600E mutations (Chapter 188). The International Cancer Genome Consortium (https://www.icgc.org/) and the Cancer Genome Atlas (http://cancergenome.nih.gov/) represent international collaborative efforts to define the spectrum of mutations found in tumors, mapping the genomic landscape of cancer. These efforts provide a foundation from which to develop additional therapeutic strategies against new targets; however, even when successful, the results may be short-lived as therapeutic resistance evolves. Despite the promise of next-generation sequencing, an integrated interdisciplinary approach is needed to select the best therapeutic option for any given patient. Molecular tumor boards have become a powerful platform to foster debate, discussions, and overall communication and decision making for the use of next-generation sequencing data to select therapy.[14]

MICROBIAL SEQUENCING FOR INFECTIOUS DISEASE DIAGNOSIS

In infectious disease, diagnosis of pathogens by next-generation sequencing may supplant the need to first grow microorganisms in culture, previously a major impediment to pathogen identification. For example, in 2003, sequencing of samples from infected patients with the severe acute respiratory syndrome (SARS) identified the causative agent as a coronavirus. Comparison of sequences of multiple isolates of an organism from a single epidemic gives a picture of the organism's evolution, thereby allowing inference as to where the outbreak began and how the infection spread.[15] Sequencing has been a key for diagnosis, rapid vaccine development, and population health surveillance during the SARS-coronavirus-2 (SARS-CoV-2) pandemic.[16] The clinical application of next-generation sequencing to infectious disease also has been highlighted when the source of a carbapenem-resistant *Klebsiella pneumoniae* outbreak at the National Institutes of Health Clinical Center was identified by sequencing isolates of the bacteria in real time and tracing the source to a single individual who had been discharged 3 weeks earlier.

THE EXPRESSED GENOME

COMPLEX MULTIMARKER GENOMIC TESTS FOR DISEASE DIAGNOSIS AND PROGNOSIS

Beyond DNA sequence, measures of gene expression, proteins, metabolites, and epigenetic changes are being used to generate comprehensive profiles of biologic systems in health and disease. Many of the computational challenges of analyzing these large, complex datasets are being addressed to yield next-generation biomarkers that are multianalyte, diagnostic, prognostic, and predictive. A growing number of marketed tests now typically measure protein or RNA levels, often with complex algorithms, thereby enabling diagnosis and prognosis. One example examines expression of 21 genes in tumor tissue to determine the likelihood of disease recurrence in women with early-stage hormone estrogen receptor–positive breast cancer. The test analyzes expression levels and converts them to a recurrence risk score, which has been shown to help guide treatment in patients, reduce overall health care costs, and improve outcomes and is currently covered by many major insurance companies. Other examples include MammaPrint (Agendia, Inc.), which analyzes the expression of 70 genes to determine whether patients are at high or low risk of breast cancer recurrence; and AlloMap (CareDx, Inc.), an 11 blood gene RNA signature for monitoring rejection following cardiac transplant.

Some, but not all, of the marketed in vitro diagnostic multianalyte index assays have demonstrated analytical and clinical validity, but evidence of clinical utility is usually lagging. Moreover, the very nature of these tests presents challenges to insurers, who grapple not only with limited data on clinical utility, but also how to reimburse such tests that are composed of both a laboratory component and an associated algorithm used to score risk, the latter part being integral to realizing the test's value.

METABOLIC AND PROTEIN PROFILING

Endophenotypes are the various molecular domains that exist at intermediate levels of organization between the genotype and the phenotype, including metabolomics and proteomics.[17] A metabolic profile is very similar to some of the traditional targeted profiles, such as a lipid profile, although it is more comprehensive. Metabolomics measures changes in the metabolic or chemical milieu that are downstream of genomic and proteomic alterations. Humans contain an estimated 5000 or so discrete small molecule metabolites, and the identification of metabolic fingerprints for specific diseases may have particular practical utility for the development of therapies because metabolic changes immediately suggest enzymatic drug targets. Similar to genomics and proteomics, metabolomics may be useful in disease diagnosis, prognosis, and drug development. In particular, metabolomics likely will be a valuable tool in assessing drug toxicity. These tools are being applied to diverse areas such as diabetes, obesity, cardiovascular disease, cancer, and mental disorders.

The large-scale study of proteins, termed proteomics, allows for the identification of proteins and of their differential expression between two physiologic states (e.g., health and a specific disease). Quantitative proteomics, in which global differences in protein abundances are measured, continues to be a priority area for biomarker discovery and molecular medicine. This area has been dominated by stable isotope approaches, but recent label-free quantitative methods rely on the measured intensity of a peptide ion and compare this intensity to intensity in other samples. Label-free methods have the advantage of higher throughput and fewer sample manipulation steps. Multiple- or selected-reaction monitoring of specific peptides within biofluids allows quantitation of absolute abundance of proteins in clinical samples. Although this technology is relatively immature in its applications to human health and disease compared with RNA and metabolic profiling, it is anticipated that these methods, combined with the development of mass spectroscopy technology, will advance proteomics to more routine use in diagnosis, prognosis, and pharmacogenomics within the coming years.[18]

IMPLEMENTING PRECISION MEDICINE IN CLINICAL PRACTICE

Despite progress and momentum in the discovery of genomic information with great potential to affect health care, significant challenges and barriers have limited the broad use of genomics in clinical practice (Table 33-2).[19]

EVIDENCE GENERATION

The adoption of genomic medicine is significantly hampered by gaps in the evidence of its clinical utility or impact on health and economic outcomes. Evidence is needed to demonstrate that genomic approaches deliver improved health outcomes in a cost-effective and affordable manner. As genome-based technologies mature scientifically, mechanisms must be put into place to ensure ongoing assessment and evidence generation of their value to patients, providers, and health systems. The pace of discovery far outweighs the ability to assess the value of each technology using traditional approaches such as randomized controlled clinical trials. Advancing the field likely will be best served by drawing upon a range of evidence sources, including randomized trials, pragmatic clinical trials, observational studies, and mining of data from EMRs.[20]

One strategy for developing the evidence base is to use continuous data collection among diverse populations after a drug or diagnostic test has entered the marketplace. A framework that guides implementation and ensures ongoing evidence generation, either after these products have been approved by regulators and entered the market or across a dedicated genomic medicine implementation network, could ultimately enhance the pace of adoption. Ongoing post-market data capture and evidence development is a paradigm that has been broadly underutilized but could be used to assess the economic impact of genomic medicine approaches.

IMPLEMENTATION OF PRECISION MEDICINE IN HEALTH CARE SYSTEMS

Generating the evidence base for precision medicine requires overcoming many practical and logistic challenges such as the absence of supporting information

TABLE 33-2 CHALLENGES AND SOLUTIONS TO ENABLE PRECISION MEDICINE IN PRACTICE

CHALLENGE	POTENTIAL SOLUTIONS
Evidence generation	• Balance the use of evidence generated from randomized controlled trials, the analysis from large datasets, and observational studies • A framework that ensures ongoing evidence generation once products have been approved by regulators and entered the market • Final regulatory and payer approval contingent on the inclusion of a health economic analysis
Implementation and education	• Standardized structured data and common data elements in EMRs • A centralized global genomic medicine toolbox to include optimized decision support tools • Increased investment in implementation science and diffusion research, as well as the outcomes and public health impact • Incentives to encourage adoption of precision medicine best practices by clinicians and health care delivery systems • Modular genomic medicine education programs for clinicians • Integration of genomics into core curricula in professional training • Educational programs, beginning at early educational stages, to emphasize precision and related concepts
Data ownership, privacy, and sharing	• Incentives among the public, private industry, academics, and government • Data governance and ownership frameworks • Privacy measures and risks associated with data breaches
Participant diversity, engagement, and trust	• A research agenda to understand participant preferences, beliefs, literacy, and values in precision medicine research and clinical care • Programs should reach out and engage underserved populations • Community advisors and ambassadors

Adapted from Ginsburg GS, Finkelman E, Balatbat C, et al. *Precision Medicine: A Global Action Plan for Impact.* Doha, Qatar: World Innovation Summit for Health; 2016.

technology (IT) infrastructure, data standards and interoperability, decision support technology, and funding for implementation and translational research. EMRs can enable linkage between genetic information and other health information to produce new understandings of health and disease. EMRs have been suggested as a possible solution for delivering actionable genomic information to providers. However, even where EMRs are available, they are largely unprepared to handle genomic information. Compounding this problem is a lack of standards for how such data should be stored. This challenge is referred to as interoperability, or the ability of IT programs to communicate with other systems both in terms of the data and codes they contain and the operating systems they use. In addition, standards for structured data, or common data elements, to be captured in EMRs must be developed. Having these structured data will allow datasets to be aggregated across health systems and research cohorts to be created across institutions. An example of work being done to enable the integration of genomic information is the DIGITizE Action Collaborative of the National Academies of Science, Medicine and Engineering (http://www.nationalacademies.org/hmd/Activities/Research/GenomicBasedResearch/Innovation-Collaboratives/EHR.aspx).

Clinical decision support is becoming more relevant as the sheer volume of information providers need to have "just in time" increases and also as clinical conditions continue to be subdivided and treated differently. Clinical decision support has the power to use genetic information to guide decision making, reduce cognitive load, and potentially limit medication errors. Clinical decision support, empowered by a robust IT infrastructure, represents an important approach for ensuring adherence to evidence-based precision medicine in clinical practice as well as a platform from which to share clinical success and cost-savings information.

Education of key stakeholder groups is a critical need for implementation and adoption of genomic medicine technologies. Most health professional educational programs are devoid of the practical information for understanding the use of genomic medicine testing, interpretation of the results, and how to counsel patients. These gaps must be filled for both the workforce currently in practice and for the workforce of the future.

DATA OWNERSHIP, PRIVACY, AND SHARING

Data sharing among health care systems, industry, researchers, clinicians, and patients is integral to evidence generation and to advancing the understanding of health and disease. Prototypes for sharing genomic and clinical data on a centralized platform are being developed (E-Table 33-2), but the IT costs prohibit some health care systems from participating in data sharing. As a result, underserved populations may be underrepresented in or completely absent from the shared datasets. Amassing larger and more diverse datasets and sharing these data with smaller or resource-limited health settings will be critical for their inclusion in precision medicine strategies in the future.

Policy and regulatory frameworks must address participants' concerns related to data ownership and privacy. Given the intrinsic identifiable nature of genomic data, patients have concerns about their privacy and rights.[21] Because obtaining participant consent is a necessary first step to gathering research data, the informed consent process could be made more standardized and streamlined globally, including implementing and standardizing nontraditional electronic consent tools to make it easier on patients and researchers.

Legislation prohibiting discrimination based on genetic information, such as the Genetic Information Nondiscrimination Act of 2008[22] in the United States, is an important step toward allaying the public's fears of how their (genomic) data might be used. The informed consent process might be further enabled by a framework that (1) addresses the risks to and concerns of patients and the general public, (2) provides information on what privacy protections are currently in place, and (3) provides information on how data sharing promotes the public good.

PARTICIPANT ENGAGEMENT AND TRUST

Participants are truly the key enablers of precision medicine. Their genomic and personal information contributes to research and eventually to evidence generation. Their appetite for data sharing will encourage implementation of genomics into health care. Their trust that personal data will be used effectively and ethically will enable data sharing. Initiatives that pursue deeper engagement between participants and the clinical care and research components of their various health care systems will enable the field to progress. Engagement is being enhanced through several channels, including traditional education approaches (for providers, patients, and the general public) and with patient and health advocacy organizations.

Due to the longitudinal nature of evidence generation in precision medicine, continuous efforts should be made to engage and update participants on the existing and/or potential risks and benefits of participating in precision medicine research to help secure an ongoing research partnership with participants and their families. Engagement strategies with the participant should pay attention to the diversity of health literacy and numeracy (such that risk information, for example, can be understood) of the population. The degree to which individuals engage with research and clinical care depends on their ability to access and understand their health care information, relevant consent documents, and the potential impact of testing and treatment on their clinical outcomes. Efforts could be made to not only ensure that information is provided to participants (perhaps through patient portals connected to precision medicine–enabled EMRs), but also to ensure that such materials are context sensitive and culturally appropriate. Genomic and precision medicine may exacerbate existing health disparities; therefore, additional efforts will be required to ensure that diverse ethnic and cultural groups are informed, engaged, and represented to ensure maximum impact of precision medicine to improve health outcomes.[23] A recent framework for a social contract between genomic medicine researchers and participants in the United Kingdom may be a useful model for both researchers and clinicians.[24]

GENERAL REFERENCES

For the General References and other additional features, please visit Elsevier eBooks+ at https://ebooks.health.elsevier.com.

34 REGENERATIVE MEDICINE, CELL THERAPY, AND GENE THERAPY

LIOR GEPSTEIN AND KARL SKORECKI

CELL THERAPY

DEFINITION

A remarkable clinical need exists for the development of methods to facilitate the regeneration of injured or diseased tissues and organs. This need stems from the unrelenting prevalence of trauma, congenital disorders, ischemia, and degenerative processes, which becomes increasingly urgent as the global population expands and ages. Cancer also is tied to this field, both directly (replacement of lost vital organ function as a result of cancer invasion or treatment modalities, cell-based delivery of cancer immune and gene therapies) and indirectly (e.g., role of stem cells in cancer pathogenesis and risk of tumorigenesis in stem cell–based therapies). Recent developments in stem cell biology, molecular interventions, biopolymers, and other related biological and engineering disciplines have paved the way to the emerging research and clinical discipline of regenerative medicine.

REGENERATIVE MEDICINE

Regenerative medicine seeks to harness methods for the replacement or repair of dysfunctional cells, tissue, or organs in an attempt to restore normal function. It therefore draws upon therapies from the three conventional pillars of medical therapeutics (pharmaceuticals, biologics, and medical devices) as well as from the newest technology platforms, namely, cell therapy, tissue engineering, and molecular therapies. The long-term goal of regenerative medicine is to replace the lost functions of tissues and organs, and, consequently, to develop curative strategies for unmet clinical needs such as diabetes, heart failure, chronic kidney disease, traumatic and ischemic tissue loss, and neurodegenerative disorders, among others.

Cell Therapies

Cell therapies involve the application of cells to achieve a therapeutic benefit. Although achieving tissue and organ regeneration through cell replacement represents an important goal of cell therapy, additional therapeutic benefits could be obtained by immunomodulatory effects (e.g., for prevention of graft-versus-host disease), by acting as a vehicle for the delivery of genes or gene

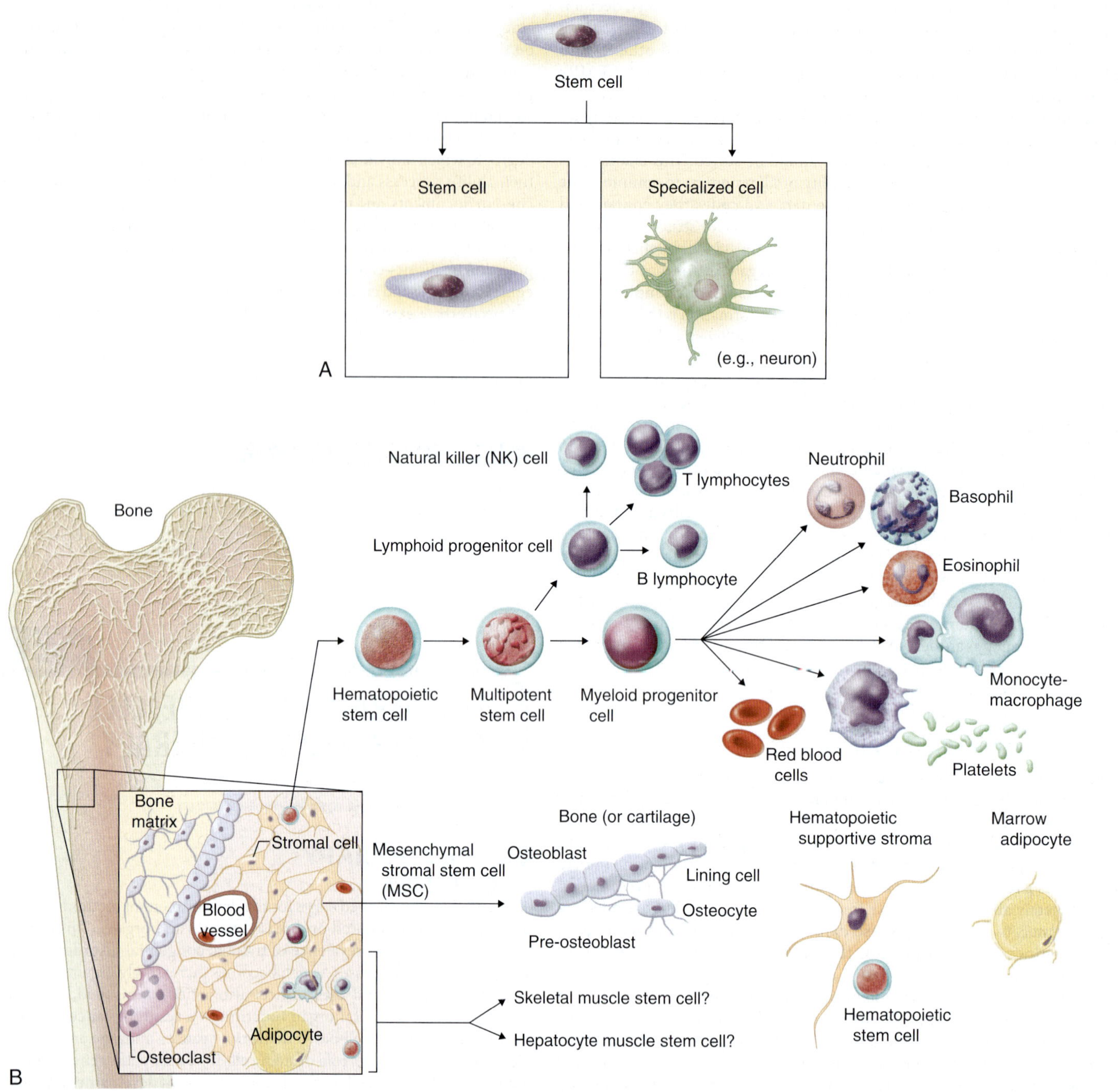

FIGURE 34-1. **A, Asymmetrical cell division. Although this property was considered a required characteristic for stem cells based on their original description in the adult hematopoietic system, not all cell types currently named as stem cells necessarily display this property. For instance, human embryonic stem cells divide by symmetrical cell division. B, Adult stem cells. Adult stem cells can be multipotent and have the capacity to differentiate into a limited number of different cell types, often restricted to a given tissue or organ system, as in the case of adult hematopoietic or epidermal stem cells. Two stem cell types have been isolated from adult bone marrow: the hematopoietic stem cell (HSC) that can give rise to all blood cell types and the supporting mesenchymal stromal cell (MSC). MSCs have immunomodulatory effects and can give rise to some differentiated cell types.**

products, and by the genetic engineering of immune cells (e.g., in chimeric antigen receptor [CAR] T-cell–based therapies).

Stem Cells

Stem cells possess two defining properties: (1) the capacity for self-renewal and (2) the ability to differentiate into cell types with specialized cellular functions (Fig. 34-1A). Their effects may occur through the process of asymmetrical cell division at the individual stem cell level or at the cell population level wherein a subset of cells differentiates and the remaining stem cells remain dormant or replicate themselves as stem cells. After asymmetrical cell division, non–stem cell derivatives may either generate a pool of organ system–restricted, transit-amplifying cells with enhanced proliferative capacity or continue to differentiate by epigenetic and gene expression profile changes until reaching the terminally differentiated state. For example, bone marrow cells are capable of reconstituting the adult hematopoietic system (Fig. 34-1B). These hematopoietic stem cells constitute the basis for hematopoietic stem cell transplantation, the only form of stem cell therapy performed routinely in clinical practice (Chapter 163).

The different stem cell types can be classified based on the protein or transcription factors they express, but also according to their replicative capacity (limited versus unlimited), the scope or potency of differentiation (e.g., pluripotent, multipotent, oligopotent, unipotent), and their place in the life history of the organism (developmental or post-developmental).

ADULT (POSTNATAL) STEM CELLS. After birth, many tissues are thought to contain a subpopulation of cells with the capacity for extended self-renewal, combined with the ability to differentiate into more mature cell types with specialized functions (Fig. 34-1). Adult stem cells, thought to represent less than 0.01% of the total number of cells, are located in specialized supportive

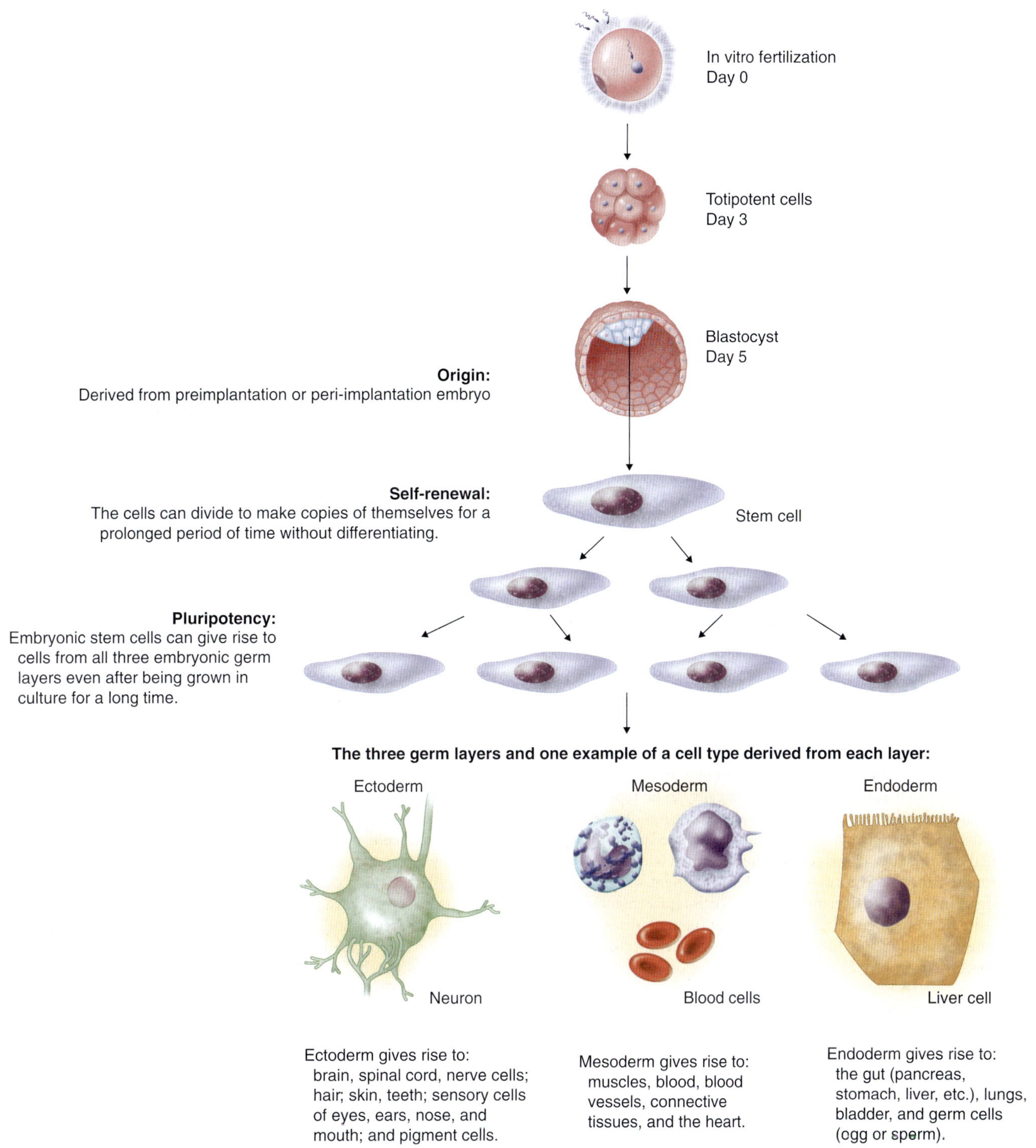

FIGURE 34-2. Embryonic stem cells. Totipotency refers to the capacity to differentiate into all cell types in an organism, including extraembryonic tissues, placenta, and umbilical cord, a property confined to the fertilized egg itself, including the cells derived from the first few cell divisions after fertilization. Pluripotency refers to the capacity to differentiate into all the specialized cell types derived from the three germ layers (ectoderm, mesoderm, endoderm) of the developing embryo and is a hallmark feature of embryonic stem cells, derived from the inner cell mass of the preimplantation blastocyst.

niche compartments and respond to cues in their local microenvironment. Adult tissues reported to contain putative stem cells include bone marrow (hematopoietic and mesenchymal compartments), blood vessel endothelium, dental pulp, epithelia of the skin, adipose tissue, digestive system, cornea, retina, testis, and liver. Similar stem/progenitor cells were also reported in organs historically not thought to contain such cells, such as the central nervous system. Whether adult stem cells represent remnants of developmental stem cells that persist into adulthood for the purposes of organ maintenance and repair or represent a distinct cell type dedicated for this latter purpose is not clear. Importantly, in many organs, despite the presence of such tissue-specific stem cells, their regenerative capacity is still inadequate to deal with massive cell loss, such as occurs following ischemic brain injury.

EMBRYONIC AND INDUCED PLURIPOTENT STEM CELLS. In contrast to adult stem cells that have relatively limited differentiation potency, cells in the developing preimplantation embryo retain the capacity to differentiate into all tissues in the body. Consequently, human embryonic stem cells, which can be isolated from the inner cell mass of human blastocysts generated for in vitro fertilization, can be propagated indefinitely in the undifferentiated state using special culture conditions, while retaining the capacity to differentiate into cell derivatives of all three germ layers (ectoderm, mesoderm, and endoderm) (Fig. 34-2). Using combinations of different growth factors, human embryonic stem cells can be induced to differentiate into several cell types, including neurons and glia, cardiomyocytes, vascular endothelial and smooth muscle cells, pancreatic β-cells, hepatocytes, and blood cells (e.g., platelets, red blood cells).

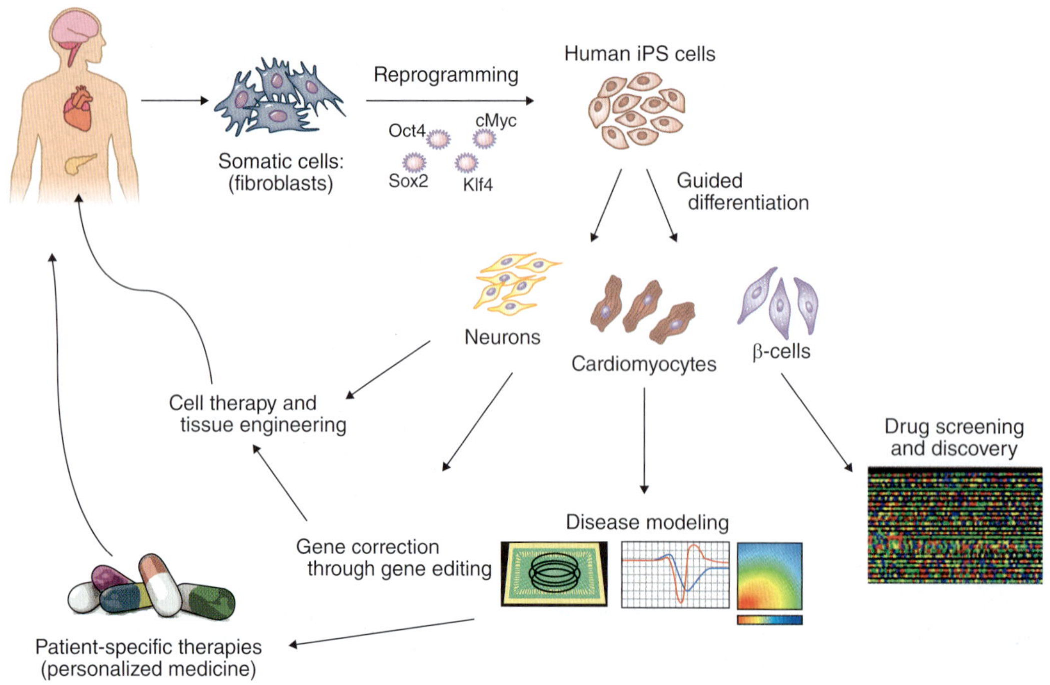

FIGURE 34-3. Potential applications of human induced pluripotent stem cells (hiPSCs). Patient-specific hiPSCs can be generated by reprogramming adult-somatic cells (e.g., fibroblasts) with a set of transcription factors and then coaxing them to differentiate into a variety of cell lineages. The patient-specific hiPSC cell derivatives can then be transplanted back into the patient in an autologous manner for regenerative medicine applications. In a similar manner, disease/patient-specific hiPSC-based models of inherited disorders can be generated ("disease-in-a-dish models") and used to improve the understanding of genetic disorders, to develop drugs, and to optimize patient-specific therapies. Gene editing techniques can be used to correct mutations and for transplantation of healthy cells.

One of the limitations in using human embryonic stem cells is the inability to derive such cells from adult individuals, thereby preventing their utilization in a patient-specific manner. This limitation was overcome with the introduction of the human induced pluripotent stem cell technology. This approach allows adult somatic cells (such as fibroblasts or blood cells) to be reprogrammed into pluripotent stem cells through the transient expression of a set of transcription factors linked to pluripotency. The human induced pluripotent stem cells generated can then be coaxed to differentiate into a wide variety of cell types. Importantly, since hiPSCs can be generated in a patient-specific manner, the technology can be used to develop autologous cell-replacement strategies that can preempt immunologic rejection, to generate patient/disease-specific models of genetic disorders, and to establish screens for drug testing and drug discovery (Fig. 34-3).

Conceptual Cell Therapy Approaches for Regenerative Medicine

Historically, the field of cell therapy can be traced to the transfusion of blood and blood products, solid organ transplantation, in vitro fertilization, and bone marrow transplantation. Nevertheless, beyond the aforementioned therapies and the recent emergence of CAR T-cell therapy for hematologic malignancies, additional cell therapy approaches are considered experimental and are still at different stages of preclinical and clinical development (Fig. 34-4).[1]

BONE MARROW–DERIVED STEM/PROGENITOR CELLS AND MESENCHYMAL STROMAL CELLS. Studies of bone marrow–derived hematopoietic or mesenchymal stem cells were based initially on the assumption that these adult stem cells may display some degree of plasticity, thereby allowing them to transdifferentiate into the relevant cell types (such as heart cells, nerve cells, and liver cells) following engraftment into the appropriate tissue environment. Although mounting evidence suggests that such transdifferentiation probably does not occur to a significant extent, many of these studies reported varying degrees of functional improvement in different organs. It now seems that the clinical benefit relates to growth factors that are secreted by the engrafted cells ("paracrine hypothesis") and augment endogenous tissue repair, improve tissue vascularization, modulate inflammation, and protect tissues at risk. Nevertheless, despite numerous trials for several indications, no mesenchymal stromal cell therapies are currently FDA approved in the United States.

DELIVERY OF EXTRACELLULAR VESICLES. Extracellular vesicles are intrinsic mediators of intercellular communication and allow functional transfer of biomolecules (lipids, proteins, DNA, mRNA, and microRNAs) between diverse locations.[2] Extracellular vesicles represent a collective term for vesicles that are secreted or shed by cells and can be categorized into groups, either by their size or mechanisms of formation and release. Examples include apoptotic bodies (1 to 5 μm), microparticles (100 to 1000 nm), and exosomes (<100 nm). Extracellular vesicles have attracted considerable interest both as potential biomarkers for disease and as therapeutic agents.

Many stem cells may exert their beneficial effect in tissue repair/regeneration by a paracrine effect, potentially acting by transferring biologically active molecules via extracellular vesicles. Delivery of extracellular vesicles may possess several advantages over stem cell therapy, such as reduced cost, easier manufacturing and delivery, and limited immunogenicity. Extracellular vesicles can also be used as a novel drug delivery approach by engineering the cells from which they are created to confer unique properties tailored for specific applications.

DELIVERY OR ACTIVATION OF TISSUE-SPECIFIC STEM CELLS OR INDUCTION OF CELL PROLIFERATION. In contrast to the conventional dogma, recent evidence suggests that several organs believed to lack regenerative capacity (such as the brain, pancreas, and kidney) do possess such ability, albeit at a limited capacity. Whether this capability is due to the presence of tissue-specific stem/progenitor cells or due to the replication capability of terminally differentiated cells is still a matter of debate.

Significant efforts have been made in recent years to isolate such putative tissue-specific stem/progenitor cells based on the expression of general or specific stem cell markers or unique culturing properties. Current efforts to utilize these findings for regenerative medicine are focused either on the isolation, ex vivo expansion, and transplantation of such putative stem/progenitor cells back to their respective native organs or on the augmentation of their endogenous reparative potential in vivo.

The final strategy aims to boost endogenous organ repair through the replication of terminally differentiated tissue-specific cells. Such strategies can either augment the inherent physiologic capability of a given organ (for example, insulin secretagogues for pancreatic β-cells) or attempt to induce replication in cells that have already withdrawn from the cell cycle, such as in the case of cardiomyocytes. Such regeneration strategies in the heart, for example, focus on attempting to replicate molecular and cellular pathways involved in the transient regeneration capacity reported in the neonatal mammalian heart[3] or by genetic approaches promoting adult cardiomyocytes to reenter the cell cycle.

ENGRAFTMENT OF HUMAN FETAL TISSUES OR XENOTRANSPLANTATION USING GENETICALLY MODIFIED ANIMALS. The most straightforward

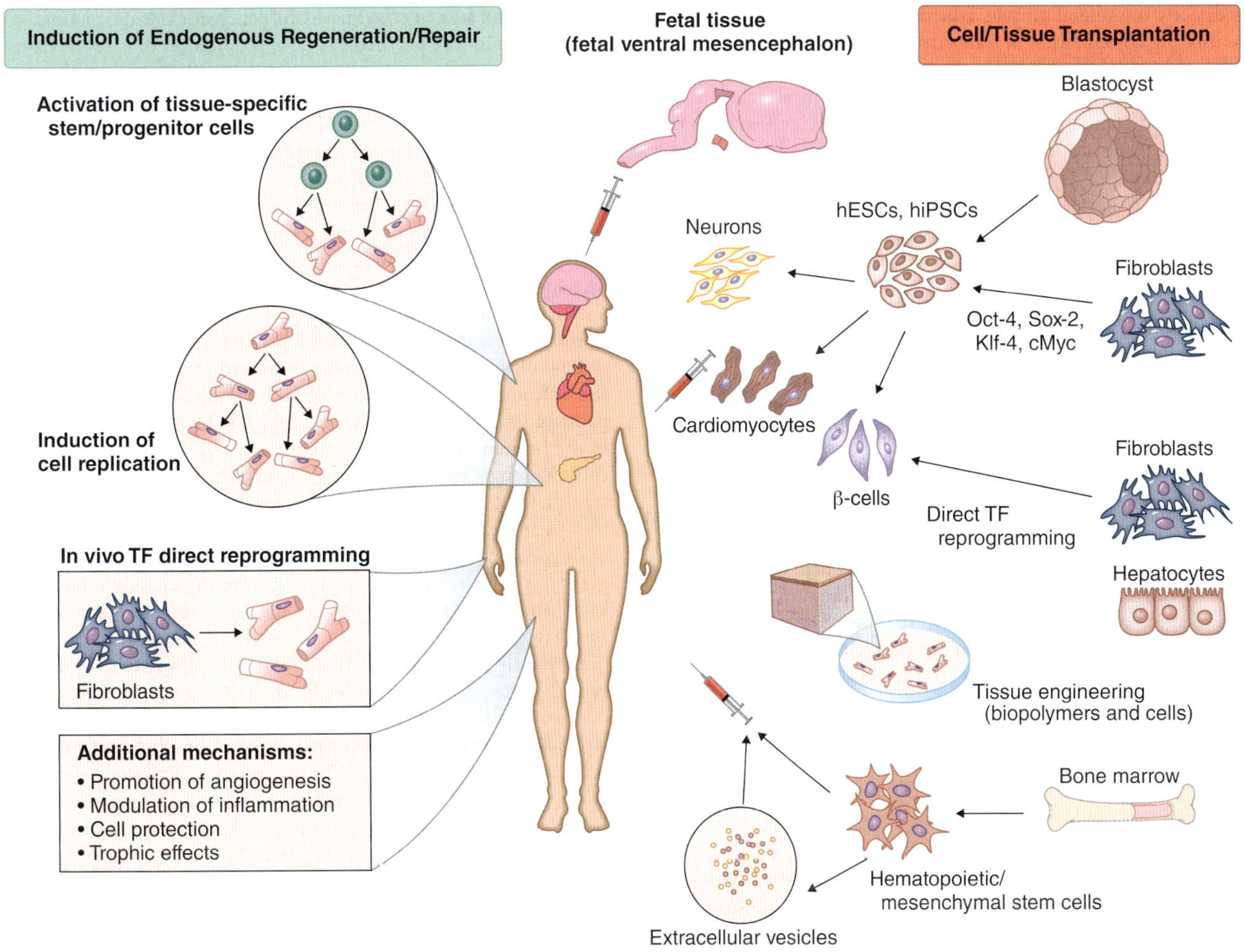

FIGURE 34-4. Conceptual framework for regenerative medicine approaches. These strategies can be divided into those attempting to augment endogenous regeneration or those focusing on transplantation of cells. The former could be achieved through the activation of putative tissue-specific stem/progenitor cells, through induction of cell replication, by in vivo transcription factor (TF)–based direct reprogramming (directly converting one somatic cell type such as fibroblasts into another), and by several other indirect means (e.g., modulation of inflammation, induction of angiogenesis, trophic effect, protection of tissue at risk). Cell sources that can be used for cell transplantation include fetal tissues (e.g., dopaminergic-rich fetal ventral mesencephalon for Parkinson disease), pluripotent stem cell (hESCs and hiPSCs)–derived cell lineages, and somatic cells that can be generated ex vivo by direct transcription factor–based reprogramming of fibroblasts. More recently, delivery of extracellular vesicles (EVs) derived from such cell sources were suggested as a potential alternative to cell therapy. Finally, the aforementioned cell sources can be combined with biopolymers as a tissue-engineering strategy. hESC = human embryonic stem cell; hiPSC = human induced pluripotent stem cell.

approach for organ repair would be to replace the missing cells/tissues/organs with identical counterparts. During prenatal human development, cells of fetal origin often show enhanced proliferative capacity as well as the ability to differentiate into more than one type of mature or specialized cell. Moreover, animal studies have demonstrated that transplantation of tissues harvested from developing organs may give rise to entire functioning organs such as kidneys, lungs, and pancreas. Nevertheless, to date, the only fetal-derived cells that have been used in human clinical applications are the dopaminergic cells derived from the developing fetal nervous system for the treatment of Parkinson disease, with conflicting evidence for success (Chapter 378).

An alternative to the use of human tissue/organ donors may be xenotransplantation, focusing on the use of transgenic pigs as sources for organ transplantation. Several genetically modified pig lines have been generated (most recently using the CRISPR/Cas9 genome editing system), aiming to overcome the main obstacles of immune rejection of the xenografts, physiologic incompatibilities, and transmission of zoonotic pathogens. These advancements have allowed proof-of-concept implantation of kidneys derived from such genetically modified pigs into two legally dead people with no discernible brain function.[4] More recently, a heart from a genetically modified pig was implanted in a patient who had terminal heart failure and was not a candidate for conventional heart transplantation.[5] The pigs were genetically modified to knock out three endogenous swine genes and to knock in six human genes, thereby reducing the immune rejection of the xenografts and particularly the hyperacute rejection associated with the presence of highly immunogenic glycoprotein derivatives in the vasculature of the pig's organs.

TRANSPLANTATION OF EX VIVO DIFFERENTIATED HUMAN PLURIPOTENT STEM CELLS. Numerous preclinical studies have demonstrated the ability of human embryonic stem cell derivatives to engraft, survive, and improve organ performance in a wide spectrum of relevant animal disease models (including, for example, heart failure, Parkinson disease, and diabetes). Nevertheless, the inability to create patient-specific human embryonic stem cells from adult individuals, the ethical issues arising from destructive use of human embryos, and the anticipated immune rejection associated with such allogeneic cell transplantation may hinder their clinical utilization. The human induced pluripotent stem cell technology may provide a potential solution to these challenges, since it generates patient-specific cells that could be coaxed to differentiate into a variety of lineages and subsequently transplanted in an autologous or allogeneic manner.

A flurry of clinical trials using human embryonic stem cells or human induced pluripotent stem cell lineages[6] have focused on the retina (transplantation of retinal pigmented epithelial cells for the treatment of macular degeneration) and other ophthalmologic disorders (retinitis pigmentosa and corneal disorders),[7] on spinal cord injury (using oligodendrocyte progenitors), and on neurodegenerative disorders such as Parkinson disease (using dopaminergic neurons) and amyotrophic lateral sclerosis. Additional targeted disorders include heart failure, pancreatic type 1 diabetes, cartilage defects, and cancer. Early clinical trials indicate that these procedures are safe and well tolerated, but many technical, regulatory, and conceptual challenges remain.

DIRECT REPROGRAMMING. In contrast to approaches involving human induced pluripotent stem cells, which seek to initially reprogram somatic cells into a pluripotent state followed by differentiation into specific cell lineages, direct reprogramming aims to convert the phenotype of one mature cell type directly into another. The prototype for such a strategy was the demonstration that *MyoD*, a master regulator of skeletal muscle formation, can convert fibroblasts directly to skeletal muscle. Based on the experimental approach used to identify the combination of transcription factors that can reprogram somatic cells into human induced pluripotent stem cells, researchers identified a combination of lineage-specific developmental transcription factors that can convert terminally differentiated fibroblasts or other somatic cells into neuronal cells, β-cells, different hematopoietic cell lineages, and cardiomyocyte-like cells. Despite the unique potential of such strategies, direct reprogramming has not yet reached clinical trials, and in many cases the transdifferentiated cells cannot recapitulate the full extent of the phenotypic properties of the native cells.

Tissue Engineering

Tissue engineering is an interdisciplinary technology that combines principles from life sciences and engineering with the goal of developing functional substitutes for damaged tissues and organs. Regardless of the specific clinical application, tissue-engineering strategies usually involve the utilization of combinations of biomaterials (to generate supporting three-dimensional scaffolds), cells, and biologically active factors. The scaffold serves many purposes, including the control of the shape and size of the engrafted tissue, the delivery of biologic signals and adequate biomechanical support to the cells, the induction of vascularization of the graft, and the protection of the cells from physical damage. Scaffolds used in tissue engineering approaches are commonly divided into two general categories: cellular scaffolds that are seeded ex vivo with cells prior to the in vivo transplantation and acellular scaffolds that depend on cells in the recipient to repopulate the scaffold with subsequent reconstitution. Efforts have mainly concentrated on the musculoskeletal system (bone and cartilage repair) but have also targeted other organs such as the heart and even complex organ structures such as the esophagus, trachea, and urinary bladder. More recently, advances in organ decellularization/recellularization methodologies and three-dimensional bioprinting have allowed the generation of clinically relevant, anatomically accurate engineered tissues and organs.

Specific Disease Applications in Cell Therapy

Although a growing number of experimental cell therapies have reached various stages of clinical trials, as yet none have become established or approved treatments, with the aforementioned exception of hematopoietic stem cells, CAR T cells, and solid organ transplantation. Nonetheless, significant advances may be on the horizon.

NEURODEGENERATIVE DISORDERS. The central nervous system has limited capacity for regenerating lost tissue in both slowly progressive degenerative neurologic conditions (e.g., Parkinson disease, Alzheimer disease, or amyotrophic lateral sclerosis) and in acute injuries that lead to rapid cell loss (e.g., ischemic stroke or traumatic spinal cord injury). Stem cell–based therapies are being explored as potential novel therapeutic paradigms for both acute and chronic neurodegenerative disorders. These procedures could potentially act through the following mechanisms: (1) cell replacement, whereby cells (precommitted to a specific neuronal or glial lineages) are transplanted to replace the specific subtypes of cells that were lost (i.e., dopaminergic neurons in Parkinson disease, motor neurons in amyotrophic lateral sclerosis, or a mixture of different neuronal and glial subtypes in other disorders); (2) trophic support, whereby the engrafted cells are used to promote the survival of affected neurons or glia or stimulate endogenous repair of the diseased brain through the secretion of neurotrophic factors; and (3) modulation of the inflammatory process thought to contribute to the pathogenesis of many neurodegenerative processes.

In Parkinson disease (Chapter 378) cell-replacement therapy suggested significant improvement in motor function after intrastriatal implantation of fetal mesencephalic dopamine-rich tissue obtained from aborted human fetuses aged 6 to 9 weeks. Further progress, however, has been limited by lack of sufficient tissue to treat a large number of affected patients, the variability in functional outcome, reports of serious dyskinesias in a subset of treated patients, and ethical considerations.

Given these limitations, stem cell derivatives could offer a viable alternative by either replacing the dopaminergic neurons or by slowing the degeneration process and restoring the integrity of the nigrostriatal pathway through the release of trophic factors. Preclinical engraftment studies demonstrate that such cells can survive in animal models of Parkinson disease and exert beneficial functional effects following cell maturation. Initial clinical trials using human pluripotent stem cells have begun. The program that has advanced the most has been the transplantation of retinal pigment epithelium derived from human embryonic stem cells and human induced pluripotent stem cells for the treatment of macular degeneration (Chapter 391).

DIABETES MELLITUS. Successful pancreatic transplantation and improved glucocorticoid-free protocols for transplantation of islets of Langerhans can not only restore glucose control in patients with diabetes mellitus but can also prevent or even reverse some of the disease's complications (Chapter 210).[8] However, whole organ or islet-based transplantation approaches are limited both by immunologic rejection and an available source of transplantable tissues. These challenges have motivated the search for cell types that can replace or augment deficient β-cell function.

The differentiation of human embryonic stem cells and human induced pluripotent stem cells into precursor or early-stage β-cells is a potential option. The engraftment of either β-cell progenitors (which are expected to develop and mature in vivo) or more mature β-cells/islet-like tissues can sometimes normalize glucose levels in treated patients.

One of the problems in using β-cells for cell-replacement therapy is that the autoimmune destruction of endogenous β-cells, which underlies the pathogenesis of type 1 diabetes, will probably also result in the destruction of the human induced pluripotent stem cell–derived β-cells. To overcome this challenge, efforts are being made either to genetically manipulate the transplanted cells or to develop encapsulation biotechnologies to deliver the cells in an immunoprotective environment.

Beyond the derivation of new β-cells from pluripotent stem cells, progress has also been made in reprogramming closely related cell types to β-cells by overexpressing master regulatory transcription factors. An additional regenerative strategy focuses on increasing pancreatic β-cell mass by inducing their replication. This therapeutic approach would mainly target type 2 patients with diabetes by decreasing the burden on existing but overworked β-cells.

Finally, several clinical trials have explored the efficacy of mesenchymal stem cells, both as supporting cells to protect existing β-cells and as a source for newly generated β-cells. There is some evidence to suggest that transplantation of mesenchymal stem cells can be effective to a certain degree in type 2 diabetes, but its efficacy in type 1 diabetes is controversial.

STEM CELL–DERIVED PLATFORMS FOR DISEASE MODELING, PERSONALIZED MEDICINE, AND DRUG DISCOVERY. In addition to the generation of cells for regenerative applications, the ability to grow a wide variety of different specialized cell types of human origin in culture (in combination with advances in organ-on-a-chip, tissue engineering, and three-dimensional bioprinting technologies) provides unparalleled opportunities for disease modeling, gene and drug discovery, and drug testing. The advent of human induced pluripotent stem cell technology has further revolutionized this field. Different types of patient-specific human induced pluripotent stem cell–derived neurons, cardiomyocytes, skeletal muscle, blood cells, hepatocytes, and other cell types propagated in cell culture recapitulate disease-relevant phenotypes of a wide array of genetic disorders. Mechanistic insights derived using this approach have enabled predictive testing of existing therapies in a patient-specific manner (personalized medicine) as well as development and preclinical testing of evolving therapies.

GENE THERAPY

Gene therapy can be broadly defined as the transfer of genetic material into cells to restore or correct a cellular dysfunction or to provide a new cellular function in an attempt to cure a disease or to improve the clinical status of a patient. Recent clinical successes include entirely novel initiatives in treating primary immunodeficiency syndromes,[9] blood disorders,[10,11] and leukodystrophies; the improvement of vision in patients with retinal disease[12]; innovative approaches targeting chronic and acute viral infections; and highly encouraging outcomes in treating cancer.[13]

Clinically approved gene therapy agents include fomivirsen for the treatment of cytomegalovirus retinitis, the viral delivery of the lipoprotein lipase (*LPL*) gene for the treatment of LPL deficiency, voretigene neparvovec-rzyl for the treatment of Leber retinal dystrophy, and onasemnogene abeparvovec for the treatment of spinal muscular atrophy. An alternative to the direct in vivo gene delivery approach is the ex vivo genetic engineering of cells that are then engrafted to the patient.[14] The first clinical approval of this strategy involved the ex vivo genetic modification of harvested hematopoietic stem cells to express a functional product of the adenosine deaminases gene for the treatment of severe combined immunodeficiency. A turning point in the field was the development of CAR T cells,[15] which are a genetically modified cellular immunotherapy that can rescue patients who have hematologic malignancies (and recently also certain solid tumors) and who have failed prior conventional therapies.

Classifications and Mechanisms of Action

In general, somatic gene therapy applications can be divided into those aiming to correct or treat genetic disorders and those targeting nongenetic diseases by altering cell, tissue, and organ function. Traditional gene therapy efforts for inherited disorders have mainly focused on the exogenous expression of genes encoding the missing or abnormal proteins. Current and future efforts are expected to shift the focus from uncontrolled overexpression of the missing protein to correcting the mutation at the DNA level (gene editing strategies). For nongenetic disorders, efforts are aimed at overexpressing various proteins in an attempt to alter cellular function (e.g., to increase contractility in heart failure by expressing proteins related to calcium handling), to protect tissue at risk (e.g., in acute kidney injury), to exert paracrine effects through local secretion of specific proteins by the engineered cells (e.g., to promote angiogenesis in ischemic tissues or to induce neurotrophic effects in neurodegenerative disorders), and even to secrete certain proteins and hormones (e.g., to correct bleeding disorders by secreting coagulation factors or to treat anemia by secreting erythropoietin). Finally, major efforts have focused on using gene therapy tools for cancer immunotherapies.

Gene therapy efforts can be divided into ex vivo strategies and direct in vivo strategies. The former involve initial harvesting of cells from a patient, followed by their genetic modification, selection, and amplification in the laboratory, and eventually delivery of the modified cells back to the patient to achieve the desired therapeutic effect. This strategy is attractive for the genetic modification of stem cells or other cell types that could reconstitute relevant tissues and organs following transplantation. Prominent examples include the genetic modification of hematopoietic stem cells for treatment of hematopoietic disorders and various CAR T-cell strategies. Finally, next-generation therapeutic strategies are expected to use genetically engineered cells also to carry drugs and oncolytic viruses to treat intractable tumors and to modulate several tissue processes through the secretion of angiogenic, neurotrophic, and anti-inflammatory molecules.

The in vivo gene therapy approach involves the delivery of the relevant transgene (via different vectors) directly to the targeted tissue. The stable or transient expression of the transgene only in the relevant cells/tissues can be achieved by combining localized delivery, tropism of the vector used to the tissue of interest, and expression of the transgene under the control of a cell/tissue-specific promoter.

Gene Therapy Delivery Methods

Gene therapy agents are often composed of two elements: the genetic material itself (i.e., the DNA expression cassette, short interfering RNA, or an antisense molecule) and the vector delivery system. The latter is often the more complex and limiting component. It is therefore important to tailor the specific vector type for each gene therapy application to allow the most efficient delivery with minimal adverse effects. Vectors used for gene therapy can be classified into nonviral or viral vectors.

Gene therapy mediated by nonviral vectors is referred to as transfection and consists of the direct delivery of naked DNA by injection or in combination with liposomes (cationic lipids mixed with nucleic acids), nanoparticles, and other means. Although nonviral vectors are less toxic and immunogenic and can be produced in large amounts, their efficacy may be transient and insufficient. The efficiency of nonviral vector delivery could be enhanced by different physical methods, such as electroporation (for muscle, skin, and tumors), gene gun (for DNA vaccination), and ultrasound-assisted delivery (for cardiovascular and tumor-related applications).

Gene therapy mediated by viral vectors is referred to as transduction and has become the dominant clinical delivery approach. The idea is to harness the innate ability of viruses to deliver genetic material into the infected cell. Viruses used in gene therapy have been modified to enhance safety, increase specific uptake, and improve efficiency. Viral vectors are derived from viruses with either RNA (retroviruses and lentiviruses) or DNA (adenovirus, adeno-associated virus [AAV], herpes simplex virus [HSV], and poxvirus [vaccine virus]) genomes. Viral vectors can also be integrating, by inserting themselves into the recipient's genome, or nonintegrating, by forming an extrachromosomal genetic element. Integrating vectors, such as gamma-retroviral vectors and lentiviral vectors, are generally used to transfect actively dividing cells. Integrating vectors, however, may carry the risk of insertional mutagenesis, with clinical oncogenic transformations reported for retroviruses. Nonintegrating vectors, such as adenoviral vectors and adeno-associated virus vectors, can be used to transduce quiescent or slowly dividing cells, but they are quickly (in the case of adenoviral vectors) lost from cells that divide rapidly.

Adenoviral vectors and retroviral vectors featured prominently in early gene therapy trials. There has been a movement away from both, however, because of a death that was linked to the toxicity of the adenoviral vector and the leukemic transformation associated with the retroviral vector. These vectors have been replaced with adeno-associated virus and lentiviral vectors. Other viral vectors may be tailored for specific settings. For example, in gene therapies for pain management a replication-defective herpes simplex virus vector is used due to its tropism for nerves, whereas different oncolytic viruses are used in oncology because of their tropism to cancer cells.

Diseases Treated by Gene Therapy

HUMAN STEM CELL–BASED GENE THERAPY. Human stem cells are the preferred target for ex vivo gene therapy since their genetic modification would ensure a steady supply of their gene-corrected progeny in the body. Consequently, such approaches have the potential to treat conditions in which mature hematopoietic lineages fail to develop or to function correctly. The process of hematopoietic stem cell–based gene therapy involves the initial isolation of these progenitors from the bone marrow or peripheral blood using antibodies targeting the CD34 surface marker, followed by ex vivo genetic modification (using lentiviral vectors or gene editing techniques) for expression of the corrective transgene. Before the modified cells are administered back to the patient, the recipient is usually treated with a preconditioning chemotherapy regimen to deplete endogenous progenitors and to favor engraftment of the gene-corrected cells.

Despite the convincing clinical improvement observed in the first-generation human stem cell–based gene therapies for immunodeficiency, the adverse consequences resulting from the random integration of retroviruses have stalled progress in this field for many years. The recent shift to the use of lentiviral vectors and gene editing tools with improved efficacy and safety has renewed interest in the approach. Consequently, human stem cell–based gene therapies have been successfully tested in severe inherited diseases of the immune system (Wiskott-Aldrich syndrome and X-linked severe combined immunodeficiency) and in diseases of the blood (β-thalassemia) and nervous system (adrenoleukodystrophy and metachromatic leukodystrophy).

LIVER. A striking gene therapy success has been to induce the liver to produce coagulation factors for the treatment of coagulopathies, such as hemophilia B (Chapter 160), in which raising circulating coagulation factor levels from <1% (in affected individuals) into the range of 5% may be sufficient for effective treatment.

Cardiovascular disease. The cardiovascular system is emerging as an attractive target for nucleic acid–based therapies.[16] These efforts have focused on novel lipid-lowering approaches, on achieving therapeutic angiogenesis for chronic ischemic heart disease and critical limb ischemia, on improving cardiac function in heart failure, and on correcting monogenic cardiovascular diseases.

The use of traditional gene therapy strategies and emerging RNA and genome editing therapies have led to the development of clinical programs for the prevention and management of atherosclerotic cardiovascular diseases by targeting lipid metabolism. These include early-stage clinical trials employing recombinant adeno-associated virus (rAAV)–based liver-directed human LDL receptor (LDLR) gene delivery for the treatment of homozygous familial hypercholesterolemia. The emerging role of RNA-based therapies resulted in development of antisense oligonucleotides or short interfering RNA strategies for lowering apolipoprotein (a), proprotein convertase subtilisin/kexin type 9, *apoCIII*, and *ANGPTL3*. These highly successful lipid-altering strategies have either reached advanced clinical trials or were already approved clinically (i.e., inclisiran, a siRNA-based therapy targeting PCSK9 (Chapter 190).[A1]

The use of genes to promote angiogenesis to augment perfusion of the ischemic myocardium or to treat critical limb ischemia has been the focus of two decades of preclinical research using a variety of angiogenic mediators. Overall, these gene therapy approaches were very successful in various animal models, but human trials provided inconsistent results. Another important gene therapy target has been heart failure and various cardiomyopathies. One effort that reached advanced clinical trials was the expression of the sarcoplasmic reticulum calcium ATPase (SERCA2a), which led to the restoration of abnormal calcium transients and improved cardiac contractility in animal models with heart failure. However, human trials failed to demonstrate clinical benefits, most probably due to inefficient myocardial transgene expression. Nevertheless, efforts focusing on additional targets are ongoing.

CANCER (SEE ALSO CHAPTER 164). One of the most exciting opportunities for gene therapy lies in the cancer arena. Gene therapy strategies targeting cancer include the use of naturally occurring or modified viruses to induce cytotoxic or growth inhibitory effects in cancer cells, gene therapies to boost the immune response to tumor antigens, and mRNA antitumor vaccines.

Antitumor cytotoxicity and growth inhibition. Oncolytic viruses are therapeutically useful anticancer viruses that preferentially infect and damage malignant tissues without causing harm to normal tissues. Cancer selectivity takes advantage of deficiencies characterizing many tumor types, such as deficient innate antiviral response mechanisms, susceptibility to cell injury pathways (e.g., reactive oxygen species), deficient tumor suppressors, and restoration of defective cell death pathways such as apoptosis. Several viruses such as the Newcastle disease virus (which activates the innate or adaptive immune response), reovirus (which activates host protein kinases to shut down protein production), and mumps virus preferentially target cancer cells, thereby causing cell death and tumor regression. Other oncolytic viruses include modified versions of Coxsackie, herpes, vaccinia, adeno, rhabdo, and measles viruses.

Although the foregoing approaches have inherent anticancer activity, viruses such as vesicular stomatitis poliovirus can be genetically engineered to engender oncolytic activity. Beyond the direct viral cytopathic effect, viral vectors can be engineered to deliver genes to cancer cells that will result in tumor cell death. Tumor cell selectivity for activation of such genes can be achieved using promoters that are activated only in cancer cells (e.g., human telomerase or survivin) or in specific types of tumors (e.g., probasin in prostate cancer, ceruloplasmin in ovarian cancer, or HER2 in breast cancer). Suicide gene therapy involves delivery of a pro-drug activating enzyme (suicide gene) that converts nontoxic pro-drugs to cytotoxic metabolites.

Oncorine, which is a recombinant oncolytic virus that selectively replicates in p53-deficient tumors, is used in China for patients with squamous head and neck or esophageal cancer. Talimogene laherparepvec is a recombinant human herpes simplex virus modified to optimize local spread and elaboration of human granulocyte-macrophage colony stimulating factor. This agent is an oncolytic virus approved by the FDA for the treatment of locally advanced or metastatic cutaneous melanoma and is under study for the treatment of hepatocellular, pancreatic, and other solid tumors.

Gene therapies aiming to boost the immune response to tumor antigens. Immunotherapeutic approaches are rapidly emerging as the "fifth pillar" (along with surgery, radiation, chemotherapy, and growth factor pathway–targeted therapies) in the treatment of cancer. Among these approaches, CAR T-cell anticancer therapy can be considered a form of combined gene and cell therapy. The approach is based upon ex vivo genetic engineering of T cells from the cancer patient (Fig. 34-5). CAR T-cell therapy requires drawing blood from the patient, separating the T cells, and genetically engineering the T cells ex vivo to express surface CARs and then expanding them in vitro. CARs are synthetic molecules which enable the engineered T cells to recognize and attach to a specific protein, or antigen, on tumor cells. Following a prior chemotherapy immunodepletion step, the CAR T cells are infused into the patient. Infused CAR T cells multiply in the patient, where they target, attack, and kill cells expressing the surface antigen corresponding to the genetically engineered CAR. This process may elicit an extensive massive cytokine release response, which is an "on-target" adverse effect, whose clinical management using corticosteroids and anti–interleukin-6 drugs, along with the treatment of other adverse effects (e.g., neurotoxicity), is a *sine qua non* for the overall success of this novel anticancer therapy approach.

The CAR T-cell therapies, which have been extensively studied and approved for clinical use, target the CD19 surface antigen on B cells and are effective for B-cell malignancies, including childhood acute lymphocytic leukemia and diffuse B-cell lymphomas. The remarkable success of CAR T-cell therapy to achieve durable remissions, even in relapsed or poor prognosis disease, has now led to the successful extension of CAR T-cell therapy targeting the CD22 and CD123 antigens in leukemias and the BCMA protein in myeloma.[A2]

RNA-Based Therapeutics

Recent advances in the generation, purification, and cellular delivery of RNA have allowed the development of several types of RNA-based therapeutics.[17] These diverse RNA-based therapies include approaches that (1) inhibit protein generation by promoting RNA degradation and/or inhibition of protein translation (antisense oligonucleotides, small interfering RNAs, or microRNAs); (2) bind receptors and inhibit signal transduction (aptamers); or (3) induce protein expression (mRNA therapeutics) (Fig. 34-6).

Antisense Oligonucleotide, Small Interfering RNAs, and microRNAs

ANTISENSE OLIGONUCLEOTIDES. Antisense oligonucleotides are short, single-stranded oligonucleotides that can pair with complementary sequences in endogenous messenger RNA (mRNA) transcripts, thereby altering their processing and eventually affecting specific protein translation (Fig. 34-6).[18] By binding to their targets, antisense oligonucleotides can modulate the splicing of pre-mRNAs (allowing skipping or inclusion of a targeted exon), induce the degradation of target mRNAs (by the RNase H-mediated degradation process), or block the translation of mRNAs into proteins (by steric hindrance of ribosomal activity).

Several antisense oligonucleotide drugs have already received clinical approval, and several others are in advanced clinical trials, Eteplirsen is a representative of a group of morpholino-oligos approved to treat Duchenne muscular dystrophy (Chapter 389), which is caused by mutations that produce a premature stop codon and a nonfunctional dystrophin protein (most commonly in exon 51 of the *DMD* gene). Eteplirsen recognizes and hybridizes to exon 51 of the dystrophin gene, thereby modulating the pre–messenger RNA splicing process to exclude exon 51 from the mature mRNA. This process restores the reading frame and leads to translation of a shortened, but functional, dystrophin protein. Similarly, nusinersen is used to treat spinal muscular atrophy (Chapter 387) by binding to the *SMN2* gene pre-mRNA, thereby inducing the inclusion of exon 7 and, consequently, the stability of the translated protein as an alternative to the mutated SMN1 protein.[A3] Mipomersen induces the degradation of apolipoprotein B mRNAs to treat familial hypercholesterolemia (Chapter 190), whereas inotersen is used to treat familial amyloid polyneuropathy (Chapter 174) caused by the mutations in the transthyretin (*TTR*) gene.[A4]

SMALL INTERFERING RNA (SIRNA). RNA interference (RNAi) regulates gene expression through a highly precise mechanism of sequence-directed gene silencing by specific mRNA degradation. Whereas the antisense oligonucleotide techniques are based on single-stranded RNA, the molecule utilized in the RNAi pathway is small interfering RNA (siRNA), a short-sized,

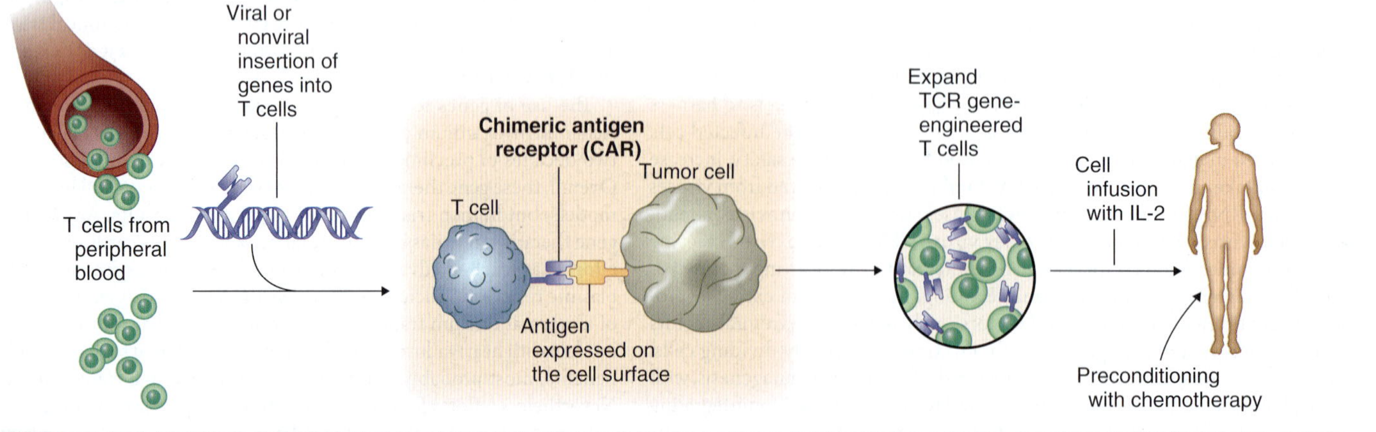

FIGURE 34-5. **CAR T-cell anticancer therapy.** CAR T cells are genetically engineered ex vivo to produce chimeric antigen receptors (CARs) on their surfaces. They are then expanded in the laboratory and reinfused into the patient. IL = interleukin; TCR = T-cell receptor. (Adapted from National Cancer Institute publication at https://www.cancer.gov/about-cancer/treatment/research/car-t-cells. Credit: National Cancer Institute.)

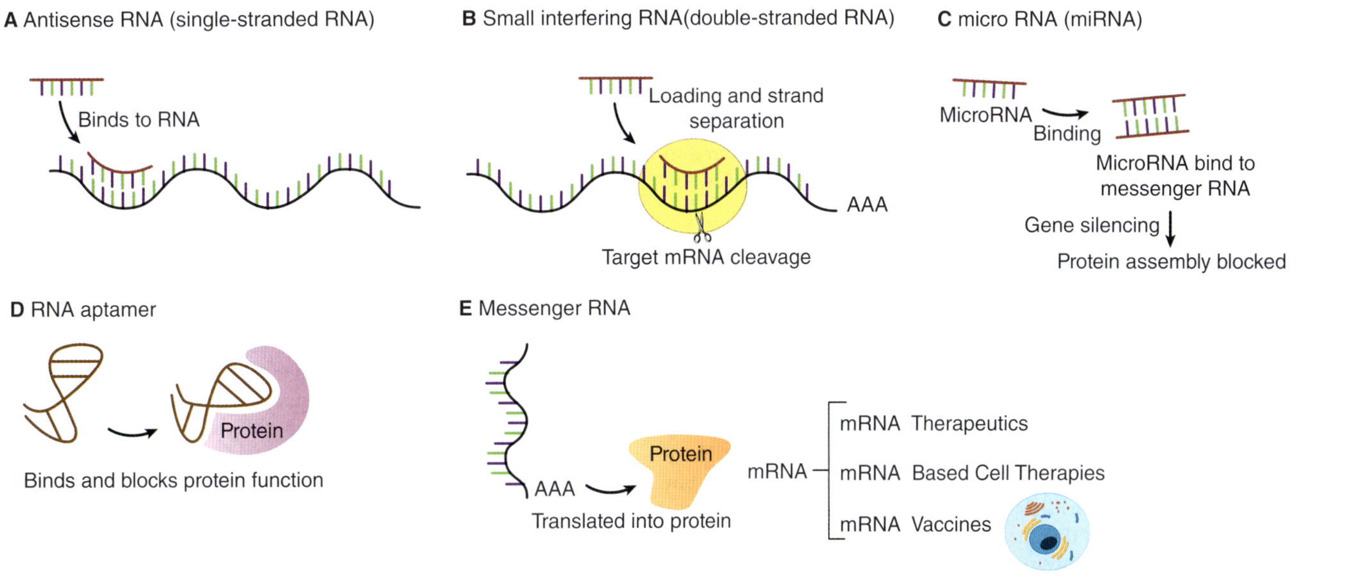

FIGURE 34-6. **RNA therapies. A, Antisense RNA. The single-stranded antisense RNA hybridizes to the target mRNA. After binding, it modulates the splicing of pre-mRNA and/or induces the degradation of mRNA and/or inhibits the translation of mRNA into protein. B, Small interfering RNA (siRNA). siRNAs are short (20 to 25 nucleotides), double-stranded RNA molecules that use the RNAi pathway to degrade a target mRNA in a sequence-specific manner. After loading into the RNA-induced silencing complex (RISC), one strand is removed after strand separation. The guide strand then guides the RISC to the target mRNA, which is recognized and cleaved. C, microRNA (miRNA). miRNAs are small, noncoding RNA molecules that regulate the expression of multiple mRNAs by blocking translation or promoting degradation of the target mRNAs. D, RNA aptamers. The RNA aptamer can bind to a specific protein and block its function. E, Synthetic messenger RNA. After the messenger RNA (mRNA) is introduced into the cells, cellular machinery, including the ribosome, translates its information into a protein, the final product that can work as an enzyme or antigen. The mRNA-based therapies can be divided into three conceptual groups: (1) replacement therapy (mRNA therapeutics), (2) mRNA-based vaccines, and (3) mRNA-based cell therapy. mRNA = messenger RNA.**

double-stranded RNA (Fig. 34-6). After being loaded into the cell's RNA-induced silencing complex (RISC), the double strands of siRNA are separated and one strand is discarded. The remaining RNA strand binds to the target mRNA sequence specifically, and the RISC machinery induces its degradation.

The use of RNAi for therapeutic applications is based on repressing the function of proteins implicated in several disease states such as cancer, age-related macular degeneration, and amyloidosis. In addition, siRNA-based, allele-specific silencing (resulting in reduced expression of the mutated "toxic" allele) can be used to target a variety of dominant-negative genetic disorders, such as Huntington disease (Chapter 379).

Currently, several siRNA-based therapeutics received FDA approval. The first approved siRNA drug, patisiran, exerts its effect by targeting the 3' untranslated region of transthyretin mRNA in the liver. By suppressing the expression of TTR, patisiran can prevent the systemic deposition of amyloid aggregates and is indicated to treat adult patients with polyneuropathy due to hereditary TTR amyloidosis (Chapter 174).[A5] Givosiran, which is intended to treat acute hepatic porphyria (Chapter 194),[A6] targets aminolevulinate synthase 1 mRNA in the liver and reduces the levels of the disease-causing neurotoxic intermediate proteins. Inclisiran binds to and cleaves the mRNA sequence of proprotein convertase subtilisin/kexin type 9 (PCSK9), thereby interfering with LDL receptor recycling in the liver and reducing LDL levels for more than 6 months (Chapter 190). Similarly, olpasiran was shown to reduce the levels of lipoprotein(a), another cardiovascular risk factor.[A7] Lumasiran, which targets glycolate oxidase,[19] reduces hepatic oxalate production for the treatment of primary hyperoxaluria type 1 (Chapter 189).

MICRORNA (MIRNA) MIMICS AND INHIBITORS. MicroRNAs are small, noncoding RNA molecules that regulate the expression of multiple mRNAs by blocking their translation or inducing their degradation. The miRNA-based therapeutics can be categorized into miRNA mimics and miRNA inhibitors (Fig. 34-6). The former are double-stranded RNA molecules that mimic the function of endogenous miRNAs, whereas the latter are single-stranded RNA oligos designed to interfere with specific endogenous miRNAs. Although no miRNA-based drugs are currently approved, promising candidates in clinical trials include miRNA inhibitors targeting specific miRNAs thought to play a role in hematologic malignancies, in solid tumors such as glioblastoma multiforme, in chronic hepatitis C, and in tissue repair. Potential therapeutic targets of miRNA mimics include keloid and pathologic fibrosis as well as modulation of the tumor microenvironment of different solid cancers.

APTAMERS. Aptamers are short, single-stranded nucleic acids that can bind to a variety of proteins, peptides, carbohydrates, and other molecules by virtue of their tertiary structure (Fig. 34-6). Consequently, aptamers can serve as agonists, antagonists, bispecific activity, and even carriers for other drugs. In this regard, aptamers have the potential to replace monoclonal antibody–based therapies. Pegaptanib, the first RNA aptamer drug, was developed to treat the wet type of age-related macular degeneration (Chapter 391). It acts by binding to vascular endothelial growth factor (VEGF), thereby preventing the formation of abnormal and leaky blood vessels. Other aptamers are currently in clinical trials for indications ranging from diabetic nephropathy, to multiple type of cancers (lung, pancreatic, and glioblastoma), to coagulation disorders.

MESSENGER RNA-BASED THERAPEUTICS. mRNAs serve as the intermediates between the coding genomic DNA and the encoded proteins. Synthetic mRNA is engineered to mimic naturally occurring mRNA, so as to prevent it from being recognized as foreign biologic material and being destroyed by the immune system. One of the most advanced approaches is to encase the mRNA in lipid nanoparticles. However, the activity of synthetic mRNAs is still transient, ranging from days to weeks.

Replacement therapy. In replacement therapy, modified RNA is administered to replace or compensate for a defective gene or protein or to supply therapeutic proteins. Many rare genetic diseases can be targeted using this approach. In cystic fibrosis (Chapter 77), for example, the mRNA encoding CFTR, a chloride channel that is defective in this disease, is delivered to lung epithelial cells by nebulization. Other mRNA-based therapeutic applications are being developed for different metabolic, infectious, and cardiac diseases. The largest number of mRNA-based applications are in the cancer arena, focusing mainly on immuno-oncology applications.

mRNA-based vaccines. Synthetic mRNAs encoding specific antigens can be used for vaccination to induce immunity against infections (prophylactic vaccines) or to harness the immune system to fight specific cancer types (therapeutic vaccines). For the former, the SARS-CoV-2 pandemic revealed the potential of the modified RNA technology for prophylactic vaccination (Chapter 337).[A8,A9]

MRNA ANTI-TUMOR VACCINES. Once in the body, the delivered mRNA directs cells that take up the mRNA (such as dendritic cells) to produce proteins that may stimulate an immune response against targeted proteins present in tumor cells. After taking up and translating the mRNA, dendritic cells present the resulting proteins, or antigens, to immune cells such as T cells, thereby starting the immune response. As in the case of CAR T-cell therapy, personalizing the vaccine for the antigens relevant to a given patient tumor, or developing banks for vaccines relevant to characterized tumor neo-antigens, are likely to be the future manner in which antitumor mRNA vaccines join in the repertoire of gene and cell therapy for malignant disease.

Cell therapy. Cell therapy may be enhanced by the mRNA approach by generation of engineered cells with unique properties tailored for specific applications. The cells may be obtained in an autologous manner, from pluripotent stem cells, or from a cell bank. Subsequently, candidate cells are therapeutically modified ex vivo with mRNA encoding the desired proteins (such as CARs or reprogramming or transdifferentiation factors) and delivered to the patient. In contrast to genetically modified cells with DNA plasmids, the effects achieved by mRNA expression are temporary.

GENOME EDITING

The center of gravity for gene therapy may be shifting from the addition of a therapeutic gene by conventional gene therapy strategies to genome editing, whereby a pathogenic mutation can be corrected at its natural location in the genome using programmable nucleases. Such programmable nucleases include zinc-finger nucleases (ZFNs), transcription activator-like effector nucleases (TALENs), and the more recently described clustered regulatory interspaced short palindromic repeat associated nuclease Cas9 (CRISPR-Cas9).[20] These genome-editing methodologies can be used not only to correct mutations but also to inactivate (or knock out) deleterious mutations in diseased cells, to disrupt viral DNA, and to add therapeutic transgenes. Such genome-editing therapies have already entered advanced preclinical and clinical testing for a variety of indications.[21]

Genome Editing Mechanisms of Action

Programmable nucleases act as highly specific molecular scissors engineered to target a specific sequence in the genome and introduce a double-strand break in the DNA just proximal to the targeted site (Fig. 34-7). The predominant cellular pathway to repair double-stranded DNA breaks is nonhomologous end-joining, which joins two double-stranded break ends by direct ligation with no or little homology between the joined ends. As a result, nonhomologous end-joining is associated with a high probability for error by resulting in the insertion or deletion of a few nucleotides at the break site. The resulting insertion-deletion (*indel*) mutations can therefore be exploited to selectively inactivate genes (Fig. 34-7A) and specifically genes that are responsible for the abnormal clinical phenotype.

The same logic can also be extended to protect against infectious or genetic diseases by inactivating wild-type genes that favor the pathologic processes. Examples include inducing loss-of-function mutations in the CCR5 T-cell receptor to treat HIV infection, in the *PCSK9* gene to treat hypercholesterolemia, and in the *TTR* gene to treat ATTR amyloidosis-related polyneuropathy.[22] The first approved gene editing clinical trial involved the use of zinc finger nucleases to target the *CCR5* locus in autologous CD4+ T cells ex vivo by adenoviral vectors for the treatment of HIV infection. Clinical follow-up revealed that the transfer of the gene-edited T cells into patients was well tolerated and that the *CCR5*-knockout cells were protected to a certain extent from infection with CCR5-tropic HIV. Similarly, programmable nucleases may also be used to target foreign DNA, such as viral genomes, thereby specifically targeting and inactivating viral-specific genes without affecting host human-specific DNA. Such an approach is in clinical trials targeting human papilloma virus (HPV). Finally, targeting of two nucleases to make two double-stranded breaks around an insertion (Fig. 34-7B) may be useful for treatment of nucleotide expansion disorders such as spino-cerebellar ataxia and Huntington disease.

An alternative mechanism to resolve the DNA cleavage is by homology directed repair between the endogenous DNA and an exogenously introduced donor fragment containing the normal nucleotide sequence (Fig. 34-7C). In this fashion, the pathogenic mutation is permanently corrected back to the normal sequence. This mutation correction approach preserves the architecture of the genome and maintains gene control under the normal cellular regulatory elements and could therefore be used to target a wide array of genetic disorders.

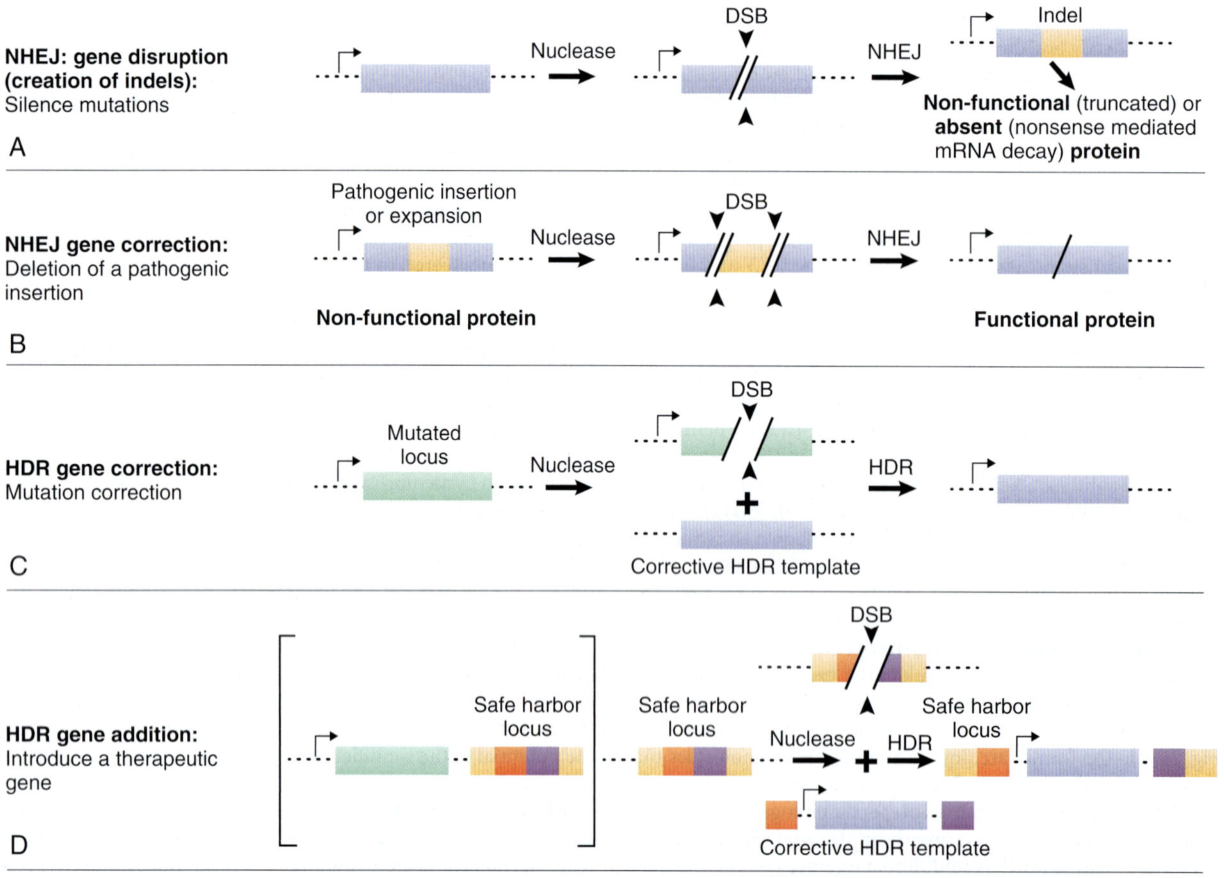

FIGURE 34-7. Conceptual therapeutic genome-editing modifications. The specific type of genome-editing therapeutic strategy depends on the nature of the mutation/disease. **A,** Nonhomologous end-joining (NHEJ) gene disruption. For gene disruption, expression of the pathologic protein is suppressed by introducing a double-stranded break (DSB) at the desired gene locus. The ineffective endogenous NHEJ repair mechanism leads to formation of indels in the gene of interest, often resulting in frameshift mutations that create premature stop codons and a nonfunctional protein product (truncated protein) or nonsense mediated decay of transcripts (no protein). **B,** NHEJ gene correction. Two DSBs targeted to both sides of a pathogenic expansion or insertion may be resolved by NHEJ, causing a deletion of the intervening sequences to mediate therapy. **C,** Homology directed repair (HDR) gene correction. For mutation correction, the HDR gene correction mechanism is used. A DSB is induced near the mutation site. HDR repair of the break site is achieved with an exogenous template, correcting the mutation and restoring normal gene function. **D,** Gene editing. This approach introduces a therapeutic transgene into either the native or a non-native (safe harbor site) locus in the genome. A DSB is induced at the desired locus, and an HDR template containing the relevant transgene and associated transcription control elements is introduced to the nucleus. mRNA = messenger RNA.

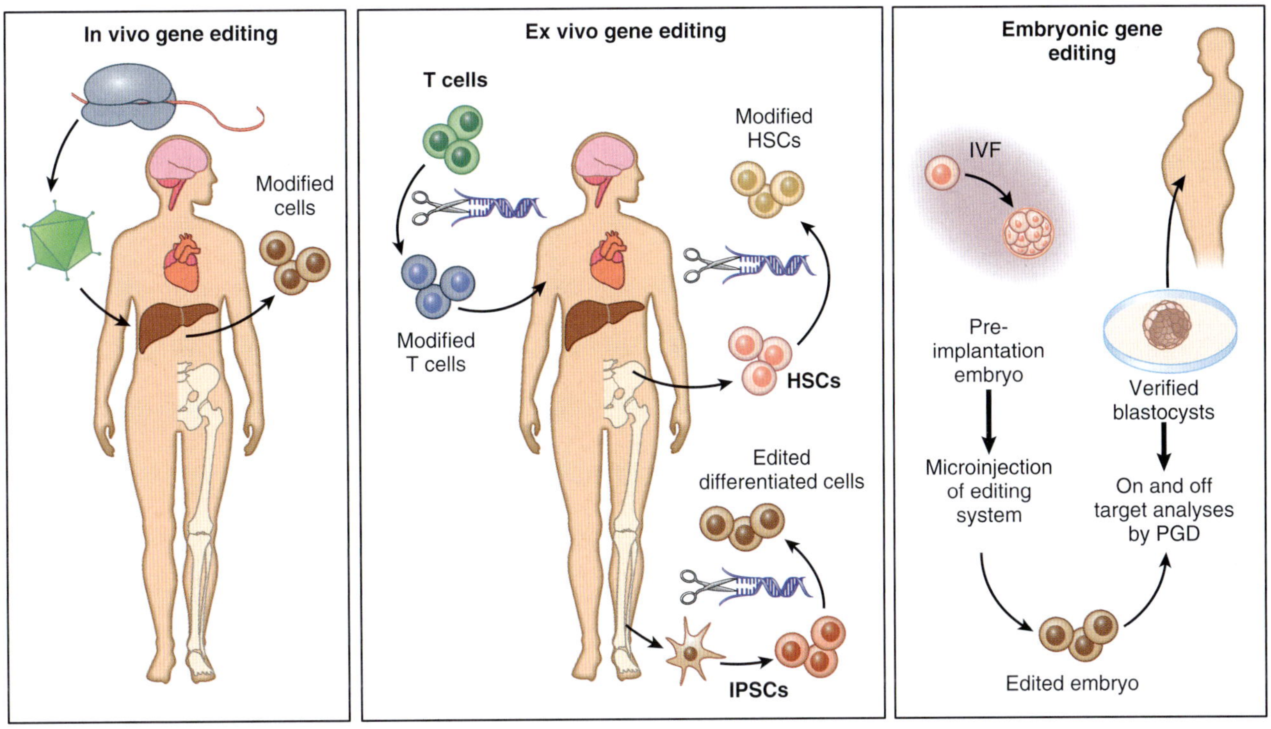

FIGURE 34-8. Ex vivo versus in vivo therapeutic genome therapy strategies. In ex vivo editing therapy, cells are removed from a patient, undergo genome editing, are expanded, and are then engrafted back to the patient to repopulate the diseased organ/tissues with healthy cells. Unique candidates for such an approach are HSCs, which can then be reintroduced by bone marrow transplantation. Alternative candidates are patient-specific iPSCs, which can be generated from a diseased individual, genetically modified, coaxed to differentiate into the desired cell lineage (e.g., heart cell, nerve cells, liver cells) and then transplanted back to the same patients. In vivo therapy involves genome editing of cells in situ. Delivery could be systemic or localized, with the preferred candidate organs being the liver, muscle, brain, and eye. For embryonic correction, the early-stage embryo formed during in vitro fertilization can undergo gene editing, and the corrected blastocyst can then be returned to the mother. HSCs = hematopoietic stem cells; iPSCs = induced pluripotent stem cells; IVF = in vitro fertilization; PGD = preimplantation diagnosis.

Finally, site-specific nucleases may also bring a unique value by enabling insertion of therapeutic transgenes (Fig. 34-7D) into specific safe harbor locations in the human genome, thereby ensuring long-term expression of the transgene, achieving better control over transgene copy number and expression levels, and reducing the potential for random insertional mutagenesis. Gene insertion may be used to secrete certain factors or to favorably alter the phenotype of the genetically modified cell.

The aforementioned strategies for gene modifications can be utilized either via a direct in vivo approach to modify existing cells (e.g., targeting liver cells) or alternatively by an initial ex vivo cell modification step followed by in vivo transplantation of genetically modified cells (Fig. 34-8).

The first clinical trials involving CRISPR/Cas9 in China and later in the United States involved the ex vivo disruption of the programmed death 1 (PD-1) gene in extracted T cells, which were then reinjected into the patients to generate more efficacious cancer immunotherapies to treat multiple myeloma, pancreatic and lung cancer, or glioblastoma. More than 100 ongoing clinical trials of CRISPR/Cas gene editing and other gene editing technologies in different disease types have confirmed the safety and feasibility of the technique for human gene therapy. These trials focus primarily on five clinical fields: blood disorders, cancer, ophthalmologic disorders, chronic infections, and protein-folding disorders.

Efforts in treating blood disorders have focused on development of CRISPR-based treatments of sickle cell anemia (Chapter 149) and β-thalassemia (Chapter 148).[23] Both hemoglobinopathies could theoretically be cured by isolating hematopoietic stem cells from the patients and using genome editing to either correct the disease-causing mutation in β-globin or to activate the expression of γ-globin, a fetal form of hemoglobin that could substitute for defective β-globin. The edited stem cells are then transplanted back into the patient. All patients treated so far showed normal or near-normal hemoglobin levels. The challenge for these approaches will be to achieve efficient, robust, and specific gene modification of the ex vivo hematopoietic stem cells since they cannot undergo effective clonal expansion. CRISPR/Cas9 may also be used to improve cell-based immunotherapies such as next-generation CAR T cells, which are safer, more controllable, and more efficacious.

In cases in which somatic approaches do not look promising, researchers are considering a third approach by making permanent changes to the genomes of human embryos. From a medical perspective, this approach has the advantage that gene correction will be permanent, so neither the treated person nor any of their descendants will carry the disease allele. In principle, the procedure would involve manipulating embryos at a very early stage, in conjunction with in vitro fertilization (Fig. 34-8). In a proof-of-concept study, a genetic mutation in the *MYBPC3* gene (causing hypertrophic cardiomyopathy) was corrected in viable preimplantation human embryos. In this and other studies, the embryos were never implanted, but the feasibility of this controversial approach was demonstrated.

GENERAL REFERENCES

For the General References and other additional features, please visit Elsevier eBooks+ at https://ebooks.health.elsevier.com.

Grade A References

A1. Wright RS, Ray KK, Raal FJ, et al. Pooled patient-level analysis of inclisiran trials in patients with familial hypercholesterolemia or atherosclerosis. *J Am Coll Cardiol.* 2021;77:1182-1193.

A2. Rodriguez-Otero P, Ailawadhi S, Arnulf B, et al. Ide-cel or standard regimens in relapsed and refractory multiple myeloma. *N Engl J Med.* 2023;388:1002-1014.

A3. Mercuri E, Darras BT, Chiriboga CA, et al. Nusinersen versus sham control in later-onset spinal muscular atrophy. *N Engl J Med.* 2018;378:625-635.

A4. Benson MD, Waddington-Cruz M, Berk JL, et al. Inotersen treatment for patients with hereditary transthyretin amyloidosis. *N Engl J Med.* 2018;379:22-31.

A5. Adams D, Gonzalez-Duarte A, O'Riordan WD, et al. Patisiran, an RNAi therapeutic, for hereditary transthyretin amyloidosis. *N Engl J Med.* 2018;379:11-21.

A6. Balwani M, Sardh E, Ventura P, et al. Phase 3 trial of RNAi therapeutic givosiran for acute intermittent porphyria. *N Engl J Med.* 2020;382:2289-2301.

A7. O'Donoghue ML, Rosenson RS, Gencer B, et al. Small interfering RNA to reduce lipoprotein(a) in cardiovascular disease. *N Engl J Med.* 2022;387:1855-1864.

A8. Jackson LA, Anderson EJ, Rouphael NG, et al. An mRNA vaccine against SARS-CoV-2—preliminary report. *N Engl J Med.* 2020;383:1920-1931.

A9. Walsh EE, Frenck RW Jr, Falsey AR, et al. Safety and immunogenicity of two RNA-based Covid-19 vaccine candidates. *N Engl J Med.* 2020;383:2439-2450.

VII

PRINCIPLES OF IMMUNOLOGY AND INFLAMMATION

35

THE INNATE AND ADAPTIVE IMMUNE SYSTEMS

MARY K. CROW

THE IMMUNE SYSTEM IN HOST DEFENSE

The immune system, comprising cells, the molecules they produce, and the organs that organize those components, evolved over millions of years in response to infections with pathogenic microorganisms. Its essential role in maintaining health is based on recognition and elimination or control of those foreign microbes. Central to its efficacy is its capacity to distinguish foreign and dangerous invaders from self-components.[1] In addition to host defense, the immune system is involved in the prevention of malignancy by surveying and recognizing self-cells that express novel antigens,[2] as well as in resolution and repair of tissue damage.

The immune system is described as including an *innate immune system* and an *adaptive immune system*. The former provides the first and rapid line of defense to a foreign stimulus.[3] The latter, dependent on activation by cells of the innate immune system, develops a more specific response targeted to the offending organism and generates memory for that stimulus that can be elicited rapidly should that organism be encountered on a later occasion.[4]

Immune system cells derive from precursor cells of the hematopoietic lineage in the bone marrow (Chapter 142) and populate discrete lymphoid organs, including lymph nodes, spleen, and thymus, as well as skin and intestine. Cells of the innate immune system serve as sentinels at locations that are likely to encounter foreign organisms, and after activation they often travel to a local lymphoid organ. The induction of the adaptive immune response occurs in the context of structured aggregates of innate and adaptive immune cells in the lymphoid organs. Once activated and differentiated to produce effector molecules, immune system cells can be sampled in blood as they travel to sites of infection or tissue damage. There they interact directly with target cells to mediate cell death. Alternatively, they provide activating signals to expand or regulate a response or secrete high local levels of immunomodulatory proteins called cytokines. Cytokines communicate among cells within the immune system or between immune system cells and cells in other tissues.[5]

Important advances in characterization of the cell surface and intracellular pattern recognition receptors, particularly the Toll-like receptor (TLR) family and signaling pathways used by innate immune cells to implement a defensive response, are now understood to have relative specificity for pathogen-associated molecular patterns that are characteristic of categories of microbes.[6] In contrast to those receptor systems that initiate an innate immune response, the protein products that implement the response, whether to expand the reaction, promote cell trafficking to the most relevant location, or shape the differentiation programs of adaptive immune system cells, do not show specificity based on the initial triggering stimulus. The products of the innate immune system can be highly effective at ablating or limiting the extent of infection and can generate a tissue repair program that establishes a satisfactory resolution of the episode of infection.

In contrast to recognition of structural patterns common in the microbial world by cells of the innate immune system, the adaptive immune system is designed to respond to the entire continuum of antigens.[7] This goal is achieved through two principal types of antigen recognition receptors: T-cell receptors and antibodies. α/β T-cell receptors, which are the most abundant class of T-cell receptors, interact specifically with epitopes formed by a small linear peptide embedded in major histocompatibility complex (MHC) molecules on the surface of antigen-presenting cells. Antibodies, or immunoglobulins, are expressed as cell surface receptors on B cells or are secreted, with both having the same specificity for antigen by recognizing conformational structures formed by the tertiary configuration of proteins.

The cells and products of the immune system function as an exquisitely regulated complex system. Inherited variations in hundreds of genes have evolved, under pressure of microbial challenge, to ensure adequate defense against pathogenic organisms across the human population. However, in any one individual, the composite genetic profile can generate vulnerability to infection or, alternatively, autoimmune or inflammatory disease.

CELLULAR ELEMENTS OF THE INNATE IMMUNE SYSTEM

Monocytes and Macrophages

Monocytes circulate in the peripheral blood with a half-life of 1 to 3 days. Macrophages arise from circulating patrolling monocytes that have migrated out of the circulation and have proliferated and differentiated in tissue. Tissue-resident macrophages may represent a separate yolk sac–derived cell lineage, with their differentiation influenced by tissue-specific factors, and include alveolar macrophages in the lung, Kupffer cells in the liver, osteoclasts in bone, microglia in the central nervous system, and type A synoviocytes in the synovial membrane.[8] Macrophages secrete myriad products, including hydrolytic enzymes, reactive oxygen species, cytokines, and chemokines. Macrophages engulf microorganisms and foreign particles directly and can be activated by protein complexes containing antibodies that bind to cell surface receptors for the Fc portion of immunoglobulin molecules (Fc receptors, or FcRs). These encounters activate intracellular signaling pathways that induce transcription of target genes, primarily those encoding mediators that promote inflammation or enzyme-mediated death of the microbe. Cytokines from other immune system cells, including interferon (IFN)-γ or interleukin (IL)-4, can drive macrophage differentiation toward the production of mediators that are primarily pro-inflammatory or to a wound healing functional profile. Researchers have characterized those functional phenotypes as M1 or M2, although it is recognized that the context of an innate immune response will determine the functional response, with composite profiles common. In addition to responding to foreign microbes,[9] macrophages contribute to the elimination of senescent or apoptotic cells through a process called efferocytosis and in a manner that avoids induction of an inflammatory response.[10] Macrophages also interact with other cell types through complementary cell surface adhesion or costimulatory receptors. After capturing antigen, they can function as antigen-presenting cells for T lymphocytes, and they can interact with non–immune system cells such as endothelial cells or fibroblasts.

Dendritic Cells

Dendritic cells comprise a complex family of cells that perform essential functions in the innate immune response and serve as a bridge to activation of an adaptive immune response. Myeloid dendritic cells incorporate antigens derived from invading microbes, travel to nearby lymph nodes, and present processed antigenic peptides to T cells in the form of peptide–MHC molecule complexes. They are the most effective antigen-presenting cells[11] based on expression of cell surface costimulatory molecules, and they produce cytokines, including IL-12 and IL-23, after interaction with pathogen-associated molecular patterns (PAMPs). They thereby contribute to the shaping of the T-cell differentiation program to generate effector cell functions. Plasmacytoid dendritic cells are highly efficient producers of type I IFN, a key mediator of host defense against viral infections, after interaction of nucleic acids with their endosomal Toll-like receptors.

Natural Killer Cells

Natural killer (NK) and NK T cells provide early defense against viral infections and other intracellular pathogens while adaptive responses are developing. NK cells are sensitized by cytokines, including type I IFNs, released from plasmacytoid dendritic cells and macrophages, and secrete abundant IFN-γ, which activates macrophages and other cells. They also are poised to kill virus-infected cells by injecting pore-forming enzymes and granzymes. Activation of NK cells is inhibited by interaction with self-MHC class I molecules on target cells. When those self-histocompatibility antigens are not present, NK cell–mediated killing is implemented. NK cells are important in tumor surveillance because they are able to kill MHC class I–deficient tumor cells that are no longer susceptible to adaptive immune responses. In addition to NK cells, innate lymphoid cells, a type of lymphocyte that participates early in innate immune responses but does not express rearranged receptors, are a focus of current study and are particularly important in immune responses in the gut.[12]

Neutrophils

Neutrophils are the most abundant circulating white blood cells. They are recruited rapidly to inflammatory sites and can phagocytose and digest microbes (Chapter 153). Activation of neutrophils and phagocytosis is facilitated through the triggering of FcRs or complement receptors. Microbe-containing phagosomes fuse with lysosomes, which contain enzymes, proteins, and peptides that inactivate and digest microbes. Beyond their phagocytic capability, neutrophils produce a variety of toxic products in the respiratory burst, which is a process accompanied by an increase in oxygen consumption. During the respiratory burst, oxygen radicals are generated by nicotinamide adenine dinucleotide phosphate (NADPH) oxidases. Neutrophils also contribute to host defense through extrusion of DNA and associated proteins in the form of neutrophil extracellular traps to which bacteria can stick, facilitating their clearance. Despite their effective contributions to the innate immune response and microbial host defense, neutrophils can generate considerable collateral damage. Neutrophil extracellular traps have the capacity to induce production of cytokines by plasmacytoid dendritic cells and may damage vascular endothelial cells.[13] Secretion of neutrophil granule contents, particularly their enzymes (myeloperoxidase, elastase, collagenase, and lysozyme), causes direct cellular injury and damages macromolecules at inflamed sites.

Eosinophils

In contrast to macrophages and neutrophils, eosinophils are only weakly phagocytic but are potent cytotoxic effector cells against parasites. Their major effector mechanism is the secretion of cationic proteins (major basic protein, eosinophil cationic protein, and eosinophil-derived neurotoxin). These proteins are released into the extracellular space, where they directly destroy the invading microorganism but can also damage host tissue (Chapter 156).

Basophils and Mast Cells

Basophils and tissue mast cells secrete inflammatory mediators such as histamine, prostaglandins, leukotrienes, and some cytokines. Release of these substances is triggered when cell surface immunoglobulin E (IgE) receptors encounter monomeric IgE. They play a role in atopic allergies, in which allergens bind immunoglobulin (IgE) and cross-link FcεRs. Mast cells have been observed in rheumatoid arthritis synovial tissue and have been implicated in local inflammatory responses (Chapter 235). Like plasmacytoid dendritic cells and macrophages, mast cells express Toll-like receptors and FcRs and produce cytokines after encountering immune complexes composed of Toll-like receptor ligands.

PRINCIPLES OF INNATE IMMUNE SYSTEM ACTIVATION: RECOGNITION OF IMMUNE STIMULI AND GENERATION OF EFFECTOR FUNCTION

Recognition Receptors and Triggers of an Innate Immune Response

Toll-like Receptors

The innate immune system uses both cell surface and intracellular pattern recognition receptors to recognize conserved structures on microbes (PAMPs). Examples of PAMPs are bacterial lipopolysaccharides, peptidoglycans, mannans, bacterial DNA, double-stranded RNA, and glucans. The discovery and characterization of the Toll-like receptor (TLR) family of receptors and their relevant ligands have focused attention on the mechanisms that allow an innate immune response to shape the nature of the resulting inflammatory or repair programs, as well as the T-cell effector functions that follow recognition of antigens from the relevant pathogen. The Toll-like receptors have in common leucine-rich domains and bind PAMPs common to classes of pathogenic organisms. For example, TLR-4, a cell surface–expressed pattern recognition receptor, binds lipopolysaccharide of gram-negative bacteria, and TLR-2 recognizes bacterial peptidoglycans and lipoproteins, often based on dimerization with other Toll-like receptor family members. Important advances in understanding systemic autoimmune diseases have followed the characterization of endosomal Toll-like receptors with relative specificity for single-stranded RNA (TLR-7 and TLR-8), demethylated 5′-cytosine-phosphate-guanine-3′ (CpG)-enriched DNA (TLR-9), and double-stranded RNA (TLR-3, which has both cell surface and endosomal forms). The distribution of particular Toll-like receptors among cells of the innate immune system varies, contributing to the distinct roles played by those cells in immune responses. The Toll-like receptors alert the immune system that a microbe, typically a bacterium in the case of TLR-2 and TLR-4 or a virus in the case of TLR-3, TLR-7, TLR-8, and TLR-9, is threatening the host. But in some cases, when an immune complex with self-nucleic acid gains access to an endosomal Toll-like receptor, a self-directed innate immune response can be initiated or amplified.[14]

Cytoplasmic Nucleic Acid Sensors

Following the description of the Toll-like receptor family and their capacity to recognize microbial and self-nucleic acids, a second category of intracellular innate immune system receptors was defined that recognize RNA or DNA from microbes, primarily viruses, that gain access to the cell cytoplasm. The DExD/H-box family of helicases include retinoic acid–inducible gene I (RIG-I) and melanoma differentiation–associated protein 5 (MDA5), described as members of the RIG-I–like receptor (RLR) family that recognizes viral RNAs with particular structural characteristics that distinguish them from most host RNAs (Fig. 35-1). Cytoplasmic DNA receptors also have been defined, with cyclic guanosine monophosphate–adenosine monophosphate synthase (cGAS) identified as an important sensor of cytoplasmic DNA that triggers an innate immune response after interacting with the stimulator of IFN genes (STING). Whether RNA or DNA triggers these cytoplasmic sensors, the results are transcription and production of IFN-β and other pro-inflammatory cytokines that orchestrate the early phase of an antiviral immune response. The aryl hydrocarbon receptor represents an additional cytosolic receptor that can be triggered by various ligands and demonstrates crosstalk with other intracellular pathways.[15]

NOD Receptors

The nucleotide-binding oligomerization domain (NOD)–like receptor (NLR) family comprises components of an intracellular structure called the inflammasome, a signaling platform that organizes innate immune system activation in response to some stimuli.[16] The inflammasome can activate caspase 1, an enzyme important for maturation of the pro-inflammatory cytokines IL-1β and IL-18. The NLRP3-containing inflammasome has been best studied and implicated in the inflammatory response to monosodium urate crystals, the triggers of gout attacks (Chapter 252). Mutations in the *NLRP3* gene are the basis of chronic autoinflammatory syndromes that are associated with exaggerated production of IL-1 (reviewed in Chapter 240).

C-Type Lectin Receptors

Members of the C-type lectin receptor family have a carbohydrate recognition domain and a calcium-binding domain that promotes signaling after interaction with carbohydrate-expressing microbes as well as self-molecules. Dendritic cell–specific intracellular adhesion molecule-3 grabbing non-integrin (dendritic cell-SIGN) is an example of a family member that recognizes high–mannose-containing structures on foreign antigens and supports dendritic cell activation. Mannose receptors on macrophages, dendritic cells, and other cell types, such as renal mesangial cells, participate in clearance of microbes as well as antigen trapping for presentation to adaptive immune system cells. The selectin family of proteins has a lectin domain, binds to carbohydrate ligands, and mediates the first steps of leukocyte migration. L-selectin is present on virtually all leukocytes; P-selectin and E-selectin are expressed on activated endothelial cells, and P-selectin is also stored in platelets. Selectins capture floating leukocytes and initiate their attachment and rolling on activated endothelial cells.

Scavenger Receptors

Scavenger receptors comprise a diverse family of receptors with the common functional role of binding various ligands and transporting or removing nonself or altered-self targets. They can participate in clearance of microorganisms and cholesterol transport but also contribute to disease pathology. For example, among the scavenger receptors is the receptor for oxidized low-density lipoproteins, which can promote generation of lipid-laden macrophages and atherosclerosis when accumulated in excess, and receptors for relatively inert substances such as silicon, which drive an inflammatory response once taken into phagocytic cells. Scavenger receptors also participate in activation of the inflammasome, as can occur after binding serum amyloid A protein.

Immunoglobulin-like Domain-Containing Receptors

The immunoglobulin-like killer inhibitory receptor (KIR) family of receptors participates in distinguishing self-cells from cells of foreign origin or tumor cells expressing modified self-molecules. NK cells are ready to produce their toxic mediators, but they are held in check by inhibitory receptors that recognize MHC class I or MHC class I–like molecules. The observation that NK cells kill target cells lacking MHC class I molecules recognized as self led to the missing-self hypothesis. By screening cell surfaces for the expression of MHC class I molecules, the innate immune system collects information about the intactness of tissues, emphasizing the crucial role of MHC class I molecules as markers of tissue integrity. The Triggering Receptors Expressed by Myeloid cells (TREM) family of cell surface receptors has emerged as important regulators of inflammation.[17] TREM-1 synergizes with other pathogen-recognizing receptors in anti-viral responses, and TREM-2 participates in innate immunity in Alzheimer disease.[18]

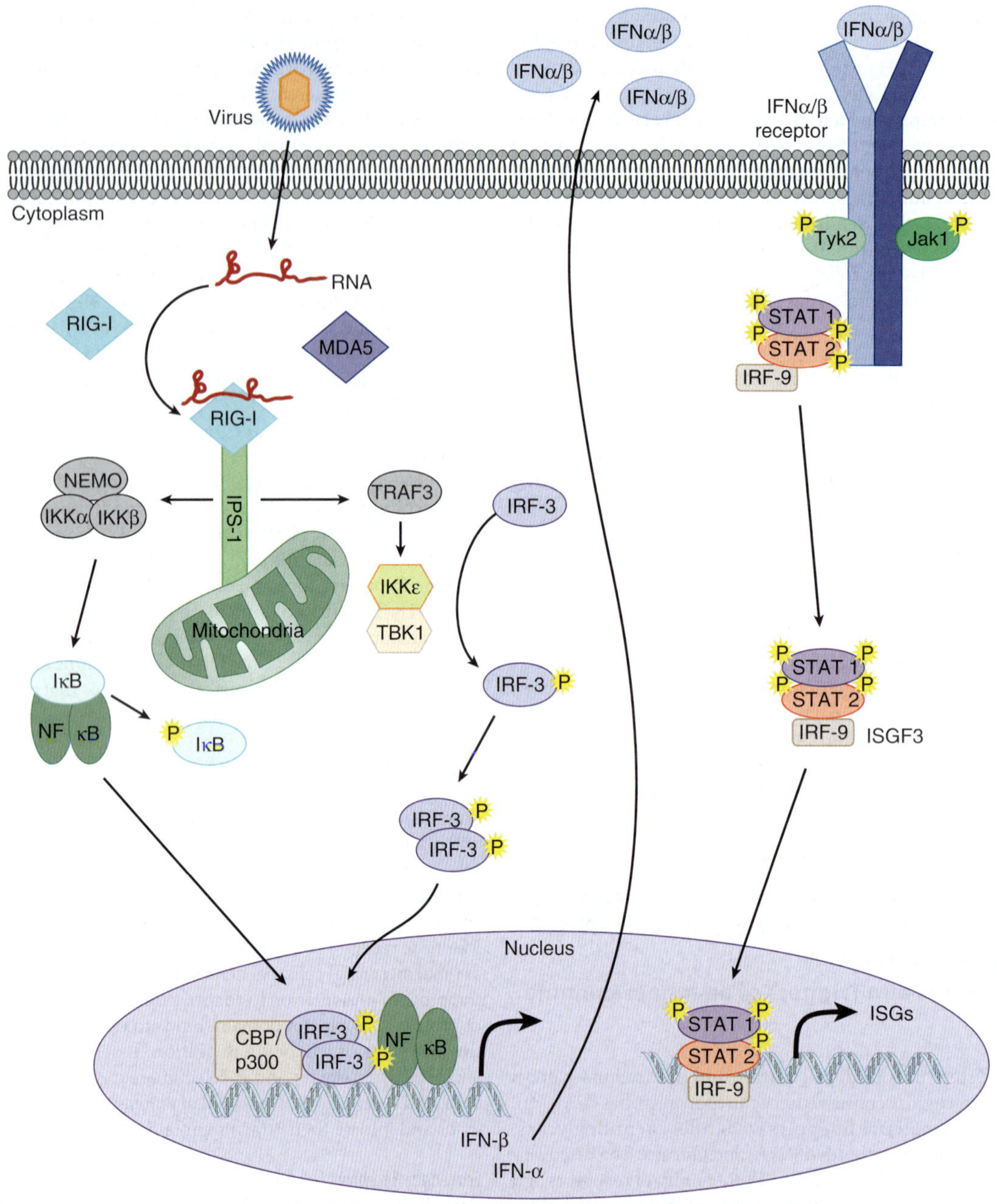

FIGURE 35-1. **Induction of an antiviral type I interferon (IFN) response.** Cytoplasmic sensors of RNA, including retinoic acid–inducible gene 1 (RIG-I) and melanoma differentiation-associated protein 5 (MDA5), trigger a signaling cascade that results in translocation of interferon regulatory factor 3 (IRF-3) to the nucleus and transcription of interferons. Those cytokines promote an antiviral immune response after binding to their receptor and activating the Janus kinase (JAK)–signal transducer and activator of transcription (STAT) pathway. CBP/p300 = CREB binding protein; IFN = interferon; IκB = inhibitor of κB; IKK = inhibitor of nuclear factor κB kinase subunit; IPS-1 = interferon-β promoter stimulator-1; IRF = interferon regulatory factor; ISG = interferon-stimulated gene; ISGF3 = interferon-stimulated gene factor 3; NEMO = nuclear factor-κB essential modulator; NF-κB = nuclear factor κB; P = phosphate; RIG-1 = retinoic acid-inducible gene 1; RNA = ribonucleic acid; STAT = signal transducer and activator of transcription; TBK1 = TANK-binding kinase 1; TRAF3 = TNF (tumor necrosis factor) receptor–associated factor; Tyk = tyrosine kinase. (From Wilkins C, Gale M Jr. Recognition of viruses by cytoplasmic sensors. *Curr Opin Immunol*. 2010;22:41-47.)

Fc and Complement Receptors

Most cells of the innate immune system possess FcRs that specifically interact with the constant region (Fc portion) of immunoglobulins and can bind antibodies attached to antigens. The isotype of the antibody determines which cell type is activated in a given response. Triggering of most FcRs transmits activating signals; however, inhibitory FcRs on B cells and macrophages can limit responses. Ligation of an FcγR on macrophages or neutrophils triggers phagocytosis of the antigen, activation of the respiratory burst, and induction of cytotoxicity. On NK cells, FcγRs initiate antibody-dependent cell-mediated cytotoxicity. FcRs on plasmacytoid dendritic cells are important for bringing immune complexes into endosomes containing Toll-like receptors. FcRs on mast cells, basophils, and activated eosinophils bind monomeric IgE with extremely high affinity. Cross-linking of the constitutively cell surface–bound IgE induces cell activation and the release of cytoplasmic granules. Some immunoglobulin isotypes fix complement, and complement receptors on monocytes amplify cell activation induced by antigen-antibody-complement immune complexes (Chapter 37). Complement receptor 1 (CR1) binds C3b and C4b, initial degradation products of complement activation, and when activated promotes phagocytosis of a complement-bearing immune complex. CR3 and CR4 are β_2-integrins and bind the degradation product iC3b.

Cytokine and Chemokine Receptors

Cells of the innate immune system express receptors for many cytokines, soluble low-molecular-weight glycoproteins that derive from many cellular sources. Binding of IFN-γ, produced by NK or type 1 helper T cells (T_H1 cells), by its receptor on monocytes activates a differentiation program that expands an inflammatory response. Receptors for IL-4 on monocytes induce a gene transcription program that is more supportive of a wound healing and repair program. Tumor necrosis factor-α (TNF-α) is a product of activated macrophages but also binds to those same cells through its specific receptor, expanding an inflammatory response. Innate immune cells also express receptors for IL-6, which induces acute phase reactants, and type I IFN. These

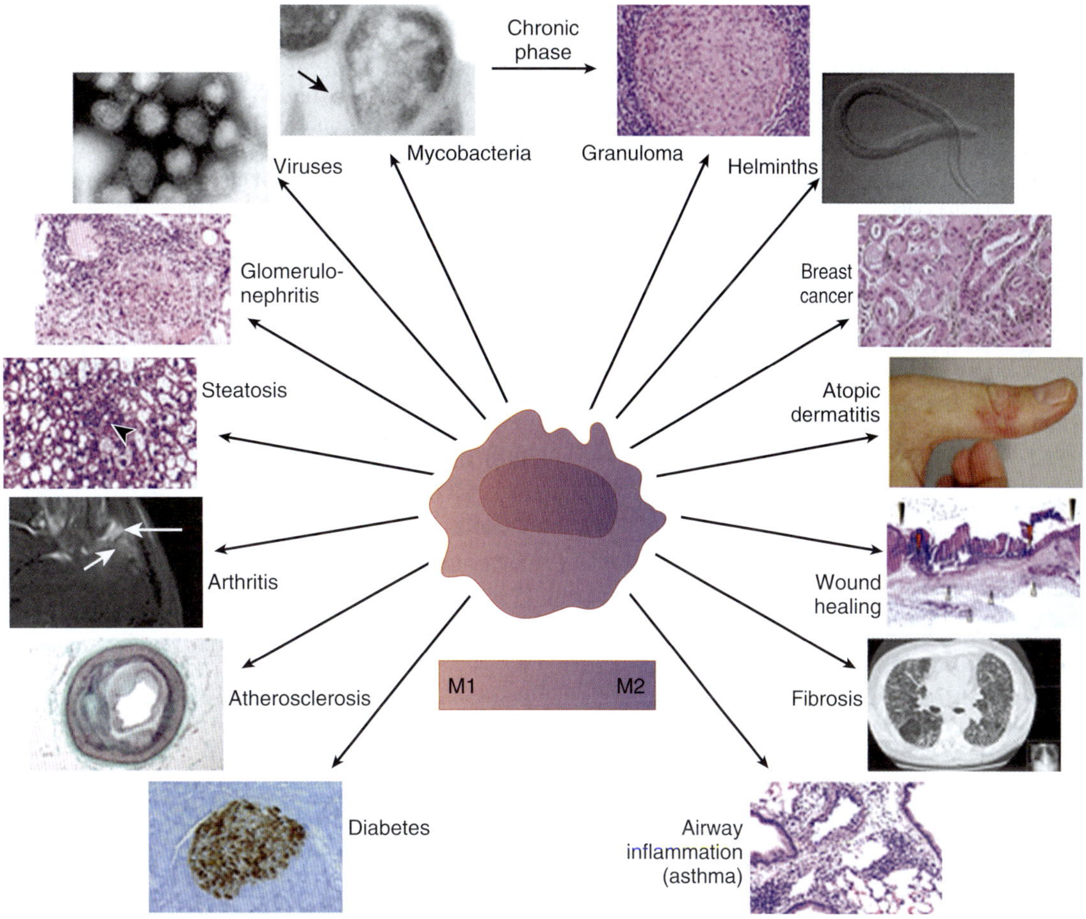

FIGURE 35-2. **Schematic representation of macrophage plasticity and polarization in pathology.** Dynamic changes occur over time with evolution of pathology: a switch from M1 (pro-inflammatory/classically activated) to M2 (anti-inflammatory/alternatively activated) macrophage polarization characterizes the transition from early to chronic phases of infection. Moreover, mixed phenotypes or populations with different phenotypes can coexist. (From Sica A, Mantovani A. Macrophage plasticity and polarization: in vivo veritas. *J Clin Invest*. 2012;122:787-795.)

mediators orchestrate a broad host defense program in response to virus infection (Fig. 35-2). Chemokine receptors include many family members that are differentially distributed among immune system cells and sense the gradient generated by soluble chemokines, resulting in attraction of cells to sites where they are needed to implement inflammatory or immune functions.

Signaling Pathways, Cell Differentiation, and Effector Mediators of the Innate Immune System

Each family of innate immune system receptors uses a complex network of molecules to transmit information from the cell surface or its cytoplasm to the nucleus, resulting in induction of a broad gene transcription and protein synthesis program that implements the next phase of the response. The contributions of each of the signal transduction pathways to the overall innate immune response will depend on the proteins produced and will determine whether the resulting cell products focus on ablating the damaging effects of virus infection on the host, limiting the inflammation and tissue damage that follow a bacterial or fungal infection, or healing a tissue wound through the production of scar tissue.

Receptor-Mediated Signaling Pathways

Certain common cell signaling systems are used by many cells and receptor systems. Arguably the most important is the nuclear factor κ light chain enhancer of activated B cells (NF-κB) pathway. NF-κB is a rapid-acting transcription factor because it preforms in cells of the innate immune system and does not require new protein synthesis to take action. Its activity is induced by ligation of Toll-like receptors and many cytokine receptors. Its component transcription factors translocate to the cell nucleus after degradation of an inhibitory component, inhibitor of κB (IκB), and bind to promoter regions of genes encoding mediators of inflammation and cell proliferation. Other important pathways are mediated by the IFN regulatory factor (IRF) family, including transcription factors that are activated by endosomal Toll-like receptors or by cytoplasmic nucleic acid sensors in response to ligation by DNA or RNA, usually from viral sources. IRF-3 is particularly important for promoting transcription of IFN-β, typically produced early in an antivirus innate immune response. IRF-7 is particularly supportive of IFN-α production induced by endosomal Toll-like receptors and is constitutively present in plasmacytoid dendritic cells, the most active producers of IFN-α.

The Janus kinase (JAK)–signal transducer and activator of transcription (STAT) pathway is used by many cytokine receptors and involves sequential enzymatic reactions by kinases that eventuate in translocation of STAT proteins to the nucleus, where they bind to gene promoters and induce transcription and synthesis of products important in implementing immunoregulation and inflammation.[19]

TNF receptor family members activate a complex signaling pathway that involves proteins called TNF receptor–associated death domain (TRADD) proteins and TNF receptor–associated factors (TRAFs), ultimately activating the NF-κB and the mitogen-activated protein (MAP) kinase pathways.

The TGF-β receptor is a serine/threonine receptor kinase that phosphorylates cytoplasmic proteins of the SMAD family, which act as transcription factors after receptor engagement by TGF-β. TGF-β signaling can play an important role in terminating an innate immune response and initiating a wound healing or tissue repair program.

It is apparent that common intracellular signaling strategies are used by many of the receptor systems that activate and regulate the innate immune system, with ligand-receptor engagement triggering the activation of kinases that phosphorylate downstream pathway proteins, and result in translocation of important transcription factors from cytoplasm to nucleus where new gene transcription takes place.

Soluble Products of the Innate Immune Response

Cells of the innate immune system are the principal producers of many pro-inflammatory and regulatory cytokines already mentioned and are also their targets. In addition to the cytokines described, cells of the innate immune system produce chemokines that attract immune system cells to sites of tissue damage or infection, and they produce cell survival and differentiation factors that help to develop an adaptive immune response. Macrophages and dendritic cells produce IL-12 and IL-23 to support the development of effector T-cell programs, and they produce B-cell–activating factor (BAFF), a soluble member of the TNF family.[20] BAFF supports B-cell survival and can provide costimulatory signals to B cells that have received antigen-specific activation signals through their surface B-cell antigen receptors, promoting differentiation to antibody-producing plasma cells.

Components of the complement system, a group of plasma enzymes and regulatory proteins that are converted from inactive pro-enzymes to active enzymes in a controlled and systematic cascade, are crucial in linking microbial recognition to cellular effector function (Chapter 37). Mannose-binding lectin circulates in the plasma, functioning as an opsonin, and is involved in activation of the complement pathway. C-reactive protein, an acute phase protein, participates in opsonization by binding to bacterial phospholipids. Macrophages and neutrophils are important in the initiation phase of an innate immune response through their production of antimicrobial defensins, cysteine-rich cationic proteins, and cathelicidin peptides, such as LL37. Both categories of mediators can assist in killing of microbes in phagosomes. Neutrophils extrude stimulatory DNA in the form of neutrophil extracellular traps or release mitochondrial DNA, along with DNA-associated proteins like high-mobility group box 1 (HMGB1) that amplifies Toll-like receptor responses in plasmacytoid dendritic cells or macrophages.

Role of the Innate Immune System in Localization, Expansion, and Resolution of the Immune Response

Localization of Innate Immune System Cells

Most cells of the innate immune response are free agents, moving through blood or lymph in transit from one site to another. Mobility of those cells is required for effective initiation of a response to invading microbes. Cells use a multistep process of adherence and activation. Initially, leukocytes roll on activated endothelial cells, activate chemokine receptors, increase adhesiveness, and eventually migrate through the endothelial layer across a chemokine gradient. The selectin family of proteins mediates the first steps of leukocyte migration. P-selectin and E-selectin are expressed on activated endothelial cells, and P-selectin is also stored in platelets. Selectins capture floating leukocytes and initiate their attachment and rolling on activated endothelial cells. To transform attachment and rolling into firm adhesion, the concerted action of chemokines, chemokine receptors, and integrins is necessary. Integrins are heterodimers formed of many different α chains and β chains; different α/β combinations are expressed on different cell subsets. Only after activation can integrins interact with ligands on endothelial cells. Activation involves modification of the cytoplasmic domain of the β chain, which leads to a structural change of the extracellular domains. This process is termed *inside-out signaling*. The last step of homing is transendothelial migration. Here, the firmly attached leukocytes migrate through the endothelial cell monolayer and the basement membrane of the vessel wall.

Transition to an Adaptive Immune Response

Movement of innate immune system cells is also required to transition a host response from primarily one depending on cells of the innate immune system to one that engages T and B lymphocytes. Dendritic cells resident in the skin and gut serve as sentinels and a first line of defense against invading organisms. When those cells are activated following sensing of PAMPs by pattern recognition receptors and following uptake of microbial components by those cells, the dendritic cells migrate to local lymph nodes where their contents can be sampled by T cells. As noted, activated macrophages, dendritic cells, and plasmacytoid dendritic cells produce cytokines that shape the differentiation program of T cells. In addition, cell surface costimulatory molecules induced after Toll-like receptor-mediated activation, such as CD80 and CD86, provide essential accessory activation signals to T cells to ensure their effective activation. Macrophages and dendritic cells also support the development of an adaptive immune response through their production of survival and differentiation factors.

Role of Innate Immune System Cells in Resolution of an Immune Response and Wound Repair

Macrophages are particularly important in resolving an immune response and organizing the repair of damaged tissue. A classic paradigm describing pro-inflammatory/classically activated (M1) and anti-inflammatory/alternatively activated (M2) macrophages (see earlier under Monocytes and Macrophages) is likely to be overly simplistic. Yet it is clear that in the course of a chronic infection, macrophages can shift their functional profile from M1 to M2, in some cases promoted by the T-cell cytokines IL-4 and IL-13, to develop a gene expression program that includes production of TGF-β, supportive of a fibrotic response, and IL-10, a cytokine that inhibits antigen-presenting cell function. Although an M1-like profile driven by IFN-γ is highly productive in achieving initial control over a pathogenic invading microbe, and M2-derived mediators promote wound healing, it should be recognized that either macrophage phenotype, and complex in-between profiles, also can be associated with pathologic states (see Fig. 35-2). A family of polyunsaturated fatty acid (PUFA)-derived innate immune system mediators, termed specialized pro-resolving mediators, includes lipoxins, resolvins, protectins, and maresins.[21] These mediators stimulate clean up of inflammatory sites, limit further inflammation, and help to restore homeostasis following an episode of immune system activation. Current research is investigating the innate immune mechanisms that account for such diverse diseases as atherosclerosis (Chapter 65), viewed as associated with M1 macrophages, and idiopathic pulmonary fibrosis (Chapter 80), possibly involving M2-like macrophages, as well as the role of resolvins at sites of chronic inflammation such as rheumatoid synovial tissue.

CELLULAR ELEMENTS OF THE ADAPTIVE IMMUNE SYSTEM

T Cells

T precursor cells are derived from hematopoietic progenitors that migrate to the thymus, a primary lymphoid tissue, where all the subsequent stages of T-cell maturation occur (Fig. 35-3). Pre-T cells express two enzymes, RAG recombinase and terminal deoxynucleotidyl transferase, enabling them to recombine T-cell receptor genes. The β chain of the T-cell receptor is rearranged first and is expressed together with a pre-T-cell receptor α chain. Signals from the immature T-cell receptor complex induce thymocyte proliferation

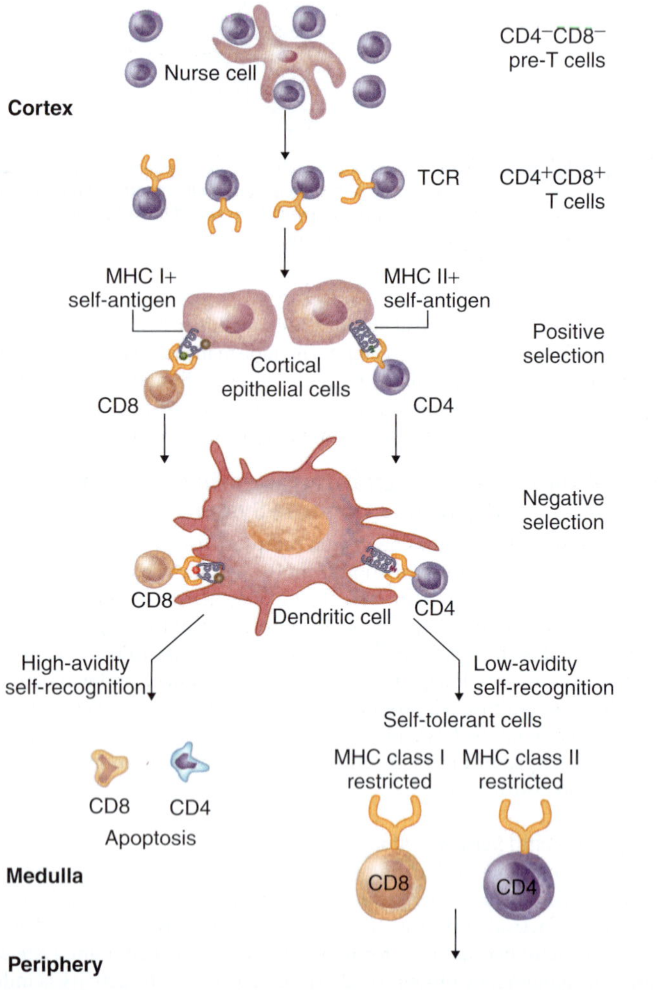

FIGURE 35-3. Maturation of T cells in the thymus. Precursors committed to the T-cell lineage arrive in the thymus and begin to rearrange their T-cell receptor (TCR) genes. Immature T cells with receptors binding to self–major histocompatibility complex (MHC) on cortical epithelial cells receive signals for survival (positive selection). At the corticomedullary junction, surviving T cells probe self-antigens presented by dendritic cells and macrophages. T cells reacting strongly to self-antigens are deleted by apoptosis (negative selection). T cells released into the periphery are tolerant toward self and recognize foreign antigens in the context of self-MHC.

and expression of both CD4 and CD8 molecules, so-called double-positive thymocytes. Subsequently, the T-cell receptor α chain is recombined, with formation of a mature T-cell receptor. From here, the thymocyte undergoes differentiation and selection steps modulated by the thymic microenvironment, thereby resulting in formation of a T cell that can migrate to secondary lymphoid tissues and is poised to recognize antigenic peptides.

Early-stage thymocytes reside in the thymic cortex, where they mostly interact with epithelial cells. They then migrate toward the medulla, encountering dendritic cells and macrophages at the corticomedullary junction. Thymic stromal cells regulate T-cell proliferation by secreting lymphopoietic growth factors, such as IL-7. Interactions of the T-cell receptor with MHC molecules expressed on epithelial cells and on dendritic cells or macrophages determine the fate of the thymocyte. Low-avidity recognition of peptide-MHC complexes on thymic cortical cells by the T-cell receptor results in positive selection, thereby rescuing cells from apoptotic cell death. Following positive selection, thymocytes migrate toward thymic medullary epithelial cells, which selectively express and present peripheral tissue antigens in order to mediate negative selection of autoreactive T cells. Thymocytes that express a receptor not fitting any MHC antigen complex die by neglect. High-affinity interaction between the T-cell receptor and peptide-MHC complex induces apoptotic death of the recognizing T cell. This process of negative selection eliminates T cells with specificity for self-antigens and is responsible for central tolerance to many autoantigens. While undergoing selection, T cells continue to differentiate. Double-positive thymocytes expressing both CD4 and CD8 engage either MHC-I or MHC-II with low-moderate affinity T-cell receptors, thereby resulting in differentiation to CD8 or CD4 single-positive T cells, respectively. These single-positive cells are now mature and ready for exit and migration to secondary lymphoid organs, including the spleen, lymph nodes, and mucosal lymphoid tissues, following chemokine cues and using adhesion molecules to enter. They exist in these tissues as quiescent naïve cells until receiving the appropriate antigenic signal for activation and development of subsequent effector function.

B Lymphocytes

Lymphoid stem cells differentiate into B-lineage cells in the bone marrow, supported by a specialized microenvironment of nonlymphoid stromal cells that supply necessary chemokines, including stromal cell–derived factor 1 (CXCL12) and cytokines (IL-7). Precursor B cells undergo sequential rearrangements of heavy chain and light chain immunoglobulin genes. On pre-B cells, the membrane μ chain is associated with a surrogate light chain to form a pre-B-cell receptor. Signals provided through this receptor induce proliferation of progeny that subsequently rearrange different light chain gene segments.

Immature B cells that express receptors directed against self-antigens are lost through negative selection and clonal deletion. Cross-linking of surface IgM by multivalent self-antigens causes immature B cells to die. Such self-reactive B cells can be rescued from death by replacing the light chain with a newly rearranged light chain that is no longer self-reactive, a process named *receptor editing*. On maturation, B cells begin additionally to express surface IgD. B cells positive for IgD and IgM are exported from the bone marrow and migrate to peripheral lymphoid tissues following a chemokine gradient (Fig. 35-4). Colocalization of T and B cells in secondary lymphoid tissues facilitates their interaction following a pathogen challenge. This response enables B cells to receive T-cell help for the former's activation and differentiation to generate memory cells and allows the antibody secretion that is required for responses to protein antigens.

PRINCIPLES OF ADAPTIVE IMMUNE SYSTEM ACTIVATION: RECOGNITION OF ANTIGEN AND GENERATION OF EFFECTOR FUNCTION

Lymphocytes and Lymphoid Tissue

The immune system uses specialized lymphoid microstructures to bring antigens to the site of lymphocyte traffic and accumulation. Secondary lymphoid organs include the spleen for blood-borne antigens, the lymph nodes for antigens encountered in peripheral tissues, and the mucosa-associated, bronchial-associated, and gut-associated lymphoid tissues, where antigens from epithelial surfaces are collected. Lymphocytes circulate through secondary lymphoid organs, constantly searching for their antigen.[22] Their homing to lymph nodes is facilitated by specialized microvessels, called high endothelial venules, which provide the proper structure for them to leave the circulation and enter the tissue. Secondary lymphoid tissues have developed several

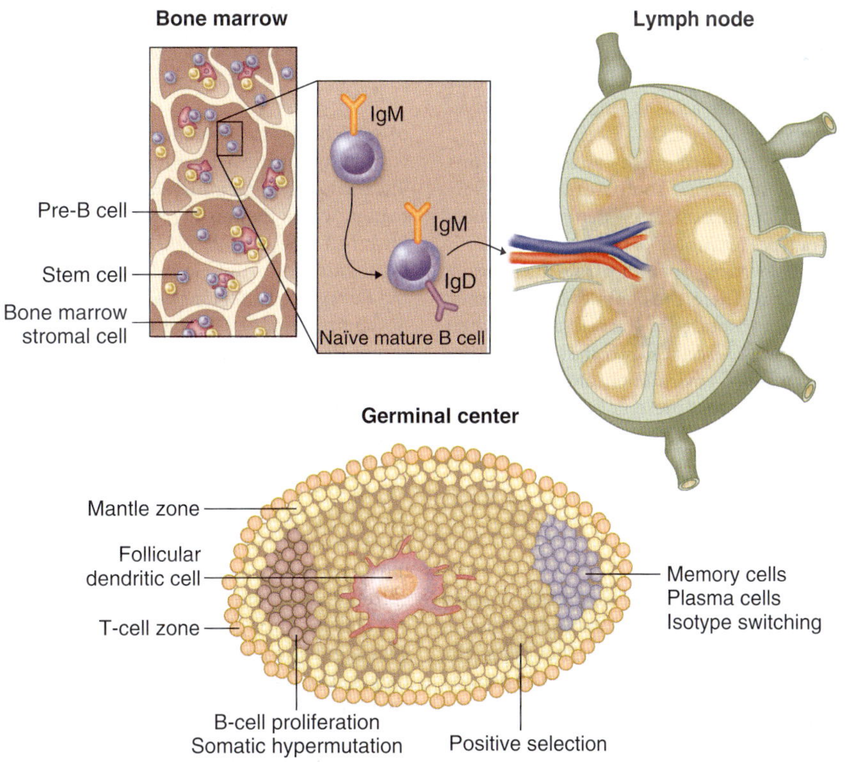

FIGURE 35-4. B-cell development and differentiation. The early stages of B-cell development occur in the bone marrow, with cells progressing through a developmental program determined by the rearrangement and expression of immunoglobulin (Ig) genes. Immature B cells with receptors for multivalent self-antigens die in the bone marrow. Surviving B cells coexpress IgD and IgM surface receptors. They are seeded into peripheral lymphoid organs, where they receive signals to survive. Antigen-binding B cells and antigen-presenting B cells that receive help from antigen-specific T cells are activated through membrane-bound and secreted molecules. Activated B cells migrate into the follicles, forming germinal centers, and undergo somatic hypermutation of immunoglobulin genes. Cells with high affinity for antigens presented on the surface of follicular dendritic cells are selected to differentiate into long-lived antibody-secreting plasma cells that migrate to the bone marrow. Cells differentiating into long-lived memory B cells have a range of antigen affinities, enabling more diverse responses upon reinfection by pathogens.

strategies to sequester the relevant antigen. Antigens in peripheral tissue are encountered first by dendritic cells that, after activation, are mobilized to transport antigens into the local lymph nodes by the draining lymph. These antigen-bearing dendritic cells enter the lymph nodes through the afferent lymphatic vessel and settle in the T-cell–rich zones to present processed antigens to T cells. The net result of this process is an accumulation and concentration of the antigen in an environment that can be readily screened by infrequent antigen-specific T cells.

B cells are segregated from T cells in the lymph nodes and are localized in follicles. Naïve B cells may engage antigen as they circulate through secondary lymphoid tissues, for example as presented to them by migratory dendritic cells or macrophages in the subcapsular region of lymph nodes. If, on antigen engagement, B cells find their cooperating (cognate) T cells at the borders of the T-cell–rich areas and the follicle, they both receive cues to enter germinal centers and send similar signals back to their cognate follicular helper T cells. Germinal centers contain a network of follicular dendritic cells that capture particulate antigen or immune complexes on the cell surface. This unprocessed antigen is taken up by antigen-specific B cells, processed and presented, and recognized by antigen-specific T_{FH} cells. Germinal centers are essential for generating long-lived antibody-secreting plasma cells and memory B cells.

Antigen Processing and Presentation

T cells bearing α/β T-cell receptors recognize peptide fragments that are displayed in the context of MHC class I and class II molecules through a process termed antigen presentation. The two classes of MHC molecules are used as restriction elements by two different subsets of T cells. $CD4^+$ T cells recognize antigenic peptides embedded into MHC class II molecules, whereas $CD8^+$ T cells bind peptides complexed with MHC class I molecules. Generally, MHC class II molecules are expressed only on specialized, so-called professional, antigen-presenting cells, such as dendritic cells, monocytes, macrophages, and B cells, whereas class I proteins are displayed by virtually all nucleated cells, facilitating recognition by $CD8^+$ T cells of peptides from viruses that often have a broad range of target tissues. Peptides bound to MHC class II molecules typically derive from extracellular antigens that are captured and internalized into endosomes to be digested by proteinases, notably cathepsin. Occasionally, however, intracellular proteins or membrane proteins are also funneled into this pathway. MHC class II molecules are assembled in the endoplasmic reticulum in association with a protein called the invariant chain (Fig. 35-5). The molecules are transported to the endosome, where the invariant chain is removed from the peptide-binding cleft, making the cleft accessible to peptides derived from extracellular proteins. MHC class II molecules, stabilized by peptides of 10 to 30 amino acids in length, are displayed on the cell surface, where they are recognized by $CD4^+$ T cells.

MHC class I–associated peptides are generated in the cytosol by the proteasome, a large cytoplasmic multiprotein enzyme complex (see Fig. 35-5), thereby allowing killer $CD8^+$ T cells to recognize microbial peptides produced within infected cells. Specialized transporter proteins, called transporter in antigen processing (TAP), facilitate translocation of peptides from the cytosolic proteasome to the endoplasmic reticulum. There, the peptides bind to newly formed MHC class I molecules and are transported to the cell surface, where they are recognized by antigen-specific $CD8^+$ T cells. MHC class I–associated peptides may also originate in the extracellular environment and be presented to T cells through the appropriately named cross-presentation pathway. This pathway enables $CD8^+$ T cells to recognize foreign peptides (e.g., from viruses) that are derived from infected and dying cells that are ingested by myeloid cells and then presented by MHC class I molecules.

Structure of Antigen-Specific Receptors

T-Cell Receptors

T-cell receptors are dimers of α chains and β chains or of γ chains and δ chains, each of which contains three complementarity-determining binding sites in the N-terminal domain. These complementarity-determining sites define the specificity of the T-cell receptor. Most α/β T-cell receptors recognize peptide fragments in the context of MHC molecules, although certain ones bind glycolipid antigens, for example, from mycobacteria, displayed by molecules with structural similarity to MHC. γ/δ T-cell receptors are more variable and can recognize peptides or certain glycolipid antigens in the context of MHC-like molecules, or even unprocessed antigens.

Antibodies

Antibodies consist of two identical heavy chains and two identical light chains, which are covalently linked by disulfide bonds. The amino (N)-terminal domain of each chain is variable and represents the recognition structure that interacts with the antigen. Each antibody has two binding arms of identical specificity. The carboxy (C)-terminal ends of the heavy and light chains form the constant region, which defines the subclass of the antibody (κ or λ for light chains; IgM, IgA, IgD, IgE, or IgG for heavy chains). Additional subclasses can be distinguished for IgG and IgA. The constant region of antibodies includes the Fc region. Fc regions can polymerize (IgA) or pentamerize (IgM), both in the presence of a J (joining) chain. Fc regions are also the ligand for Fc receptors (FcRs) on cells of the innate immune system.

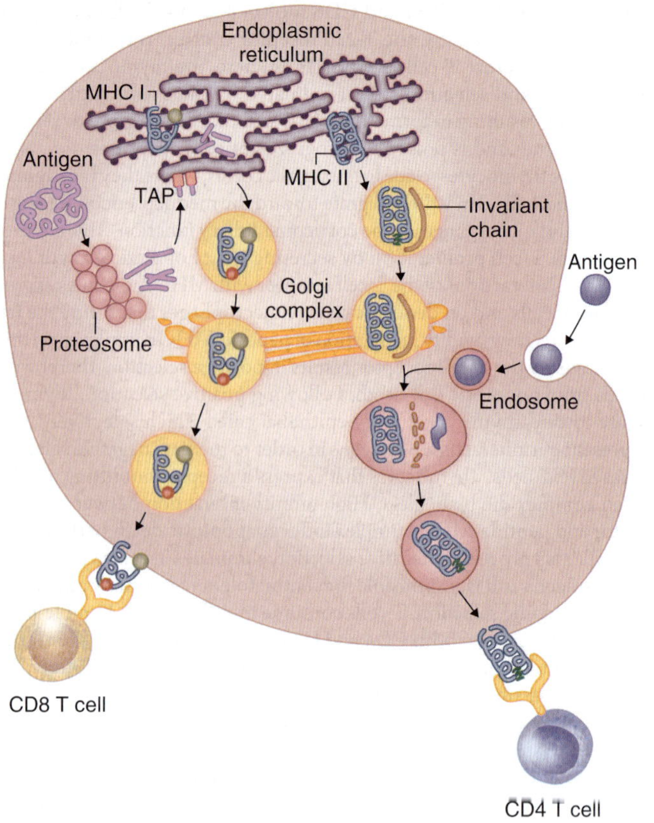

FIGURE 35-5. Pathways of antigen processing and delivery to major histocompatibility complex (MHC) molecules. Cytosolic proteins are broken down by the proteosome to generate peptide fragments, which are transported into the endoplasmic reticulum by specialized peptide transporters (TAP). After peptides are bound to MHC class I molecules, MHC-peptide complexes are released from the endoplasmic reticulum and travel to the cell surface, where they are ligands for $CD8^+$ T-cell receptors (TCRs). Extracellular foreign antigens are taken into intracellular vesicles, called *endosomes,* and proteases are activated that digest antigens into peptide fragments. After fusing with vesicles that contain MHC class II molecules, antigenic peptides are placed in the antigen-binding groove. Loaded MHC class II–peptide complexes are transported to the cell surface, where they are recognized by the TCRs of $CD4^+$ T cells.

Specificities of T-Cell Receptors and Antibodies

The repertoires, or total number of specificities, of T-cell receptors and antibodies are extremely diverse and have been estimated in the human to account for up to 10^{18} or higher and 10^{11} combinations, respectively. This enormous diversity reflects the anticipatory nature of adaptive immune receptors and must be acquired; it cannot be genetically encoded in contrast to that of innate receptors. T-cell receptor β chains and δ chains are assembled by the recombination of variable, diversity, joining, and constant region segments of T-cell receptor genes. Immunoglobulin heavy chains are formed from four gene segments—the variable, diversity, joining, and constant region gene segments. Also, immunoglobulin light chains and T-cell receptor α chains and γ chains lack the diversity segment and are composed of three gene segments. During T-cell receptor or antibody rearrangement, gene segments are cut out by nucleases and recombined at the DNA level to form linear coding units for each receptor gene. An enormous diversity of receptors is generated as each receptor or antibody uses a different combination of gene segments; the recombination and repair process is imprecise, introducing nucleotide variations at the variable-diversity, diversity-joining, and variable-joining junctions; and random nucleotides can be inserted at the junctional region by an enzyme, terminal deoxyribonucleotidyl transferase.

Once generated, T-cell receptor sequences remain unchanged. This rule does not apply to immunoglobulins, which undergo modification, including replacement of an entire variable region, or receptor editing, to modify those receptors that inadvertently bind self-antigens; class switching, in which the variable-diversity-joining unit combines with different constant region genes; or somatic hypermutation, in which the antigen-contact areas of the antibody undergo mutations to improve the affinity. The latter two events occur in secondary lymphoid tissues, such as the spleen, lymph nodes, and mucosal lymphoid tissue, where immune responses to antigens are initiated.

T-Cell Stimulation and Accessory Molecules

MHC-peptide recognition by the T-cell receptor, the first signal for T-cell activation, leads to receptor clustering and phosphorylation of the intracellular portion of the CD3 protein complex, the signaling component of the receptor, by receptor-associated tyrosine kinases. These events transmit signals to the nucleus and initiate activation of the T cell. The coreceptors CD4 and CD8, through their interaction with MHC class II and class I molecules, respectively, support CD3-mediated signals. This first activation signal delivered by the T-cell receptor and coreceptors needs to be complemented by the interaction of accessory molecules on the T cell and their ligands on the antigen-presenting cell. A spectrum of accessory molecules has been identified, of which the best known is CD28, which are engaged by CD80 and CD86 on antigen-presenting cells. Engagement of CD28 provides to the T cells a second, or costimulatory, signal that ensures T-cell survival and expansion. CD28-mediated signals are mandatory for the expression of many activation markers on the responding T cells and, in particular, for the secretion of IL-2. In the absence of such a second signal, T cells are rendered nonresponsive and anergic or undergo apoptosis. Additionally, adhesion molecules (integrins) stabilize the interactions between T cells and antigen-presenting cells. Signals from the T-cell receptor result in the activation of many genes and entry of the T cell into the cell cycle.

Three major variables determine the outcome of T-cell receptor stimulation: the duration and affinity of the T-cell receptor-antigen interaction, the maturation stage of the responding T cell, and the nature of the antigen-presenting cell. Antigen-presenting cells are gatekeepers in the initiation of T-cell responses. They can upregulate the expression of accessory molecules that provide costimulatory signals. MHC-peptide complexes are particularly dense on dendritic cells, enabling them to activate naïve T cells. In contrast, memory and effector cells have a lower threshold for activation and can react to antigens presented on peripheral tissue cells.

Another set of accessory molecules can limit the activation of T cells and have been identified as therapeutic targets, with inhibitors promoting activation and expansion of T cells with potential to inhibit or eliminate tumor cells.[23] CTLA-4 and PD-1 are expressed on T cells after cell activation and limit their expansion when ligated by CD80 or CD86 or PD-L1, respectively, but the so-called immune checkpoint inhibitors block those accessory molecules, with the goal of reversing peripheral tolerance to tumor antigens.

B-Cell Stimulation and Accessory Molecules

Mature, but naïve, B cells in secondary lymphoid organs are activated by soluble and cell-bound antigens to develop into antibody-secreting effector cells. B cells respond to a large variety of antigens, including proteins, polysaccharides, and lipids. Binding of antigen to cell surface IgM molecules induces B-cell receptor clustering, the initial step in B-cell activation. In addition to the antigen-binding immunoglobulin, the B-cell receptor comprises two proteins, Ig-α and Ig-β. The Ig-α/Ig-β heterodimer functions to transduce a signal and initiates the intracellular signaling cascade, analogous to the CD3 molecule of the T-cell receptor. Thus, the composition of the B-cell receptor, with ligand-binding and signal-transducing units, and the signaling events that lead to gene induction, are similar to those of the T-cell receptor. Both receptors are enhanced by coreceptors. The B-cell receptor-coreceptor complex is composed of CD81, CD19, and CD21, analogous to the T-cell receptor coreceptors CD4 and CD8. CD21 binds to complement fragments on opsonized antigens that are bound by the B-cell receptor, thereby resulting in phosphorylation of the intracellular tail of CD19 by tyrosine kinases and augmentation of the B-cell receptor–mediated signal.

Like naïve T cells, naïve B cells require accessory signals in addition to triggering of their antigen-binding receptor. They receive second signals either from follicular helper T cells or from thymus-independent antigens such as bacterial polysaccharides that can induce antibody production in the absence of helper T cells.[24] In contrast, in the case of protein antigens, which are thymus- or T-dependent, the initial B-cell receptor stimulation prepares the cell for subsequent interaction with follicular helper T cells. These activated B cells start to enter the cell cycle; upregulate cell surface molecules, such as CD80 and CD86, which provide costimulatory signals to T cells; and upregulate certain cytokine receptors. As such, these B cells are prepared to activate helper T cells and to respond to cytokines secreted by those T cells, but they cannot differentiate into antibody-producing cells in the absence of T-cell help. Survival and differentiation factors produced by myeloid cells, such as B-cell–activating factor, also stimulate B cells and help to maintain the B-cell pool.

Signaling Pathways, Cell Differentiation, and Effector Mediators of the Adaptive Immune System

T-Cell Differentiation

T-cell activation induces T-cell proliferation, with the goal of clonally selecting and expanding antigen-specific T cells. Antigen-specific $CD8^+$ T cells expand several thousand–fold; $CD4^+$ T cells expand somewhat less. During the phase of rapid growth, T cells differentiate from naïve T cells that are essentially devoid of effector functions into effector T cells that are needed for clearance of infectious organisms, or pathogens. The transition into effector cells is associated with a fundamental shift in functional profiles. First, effector T cells do not require costimulation to function and can scan tissues that lack professional antigen-presenting cells. Second, they switch the expression of chemokine receptors and adhesion molecules to gain access to peripheral tissues. Finally, they gain effector functions.

The principal effector function of $CD8^+$ T cells is to lyse infected, antigen-bearing target cells. On activation, $CD8^+$ T cells acquire cytotoxic functions and, using a variety of receptors and adhesion molecules, can emigrate from secondary lymphoid organs to peripheral tissue sites seeking cells infected by viruses or intracellular bacteria displaying pathogen-derived peptides on MHC class I molecules. On recognizing the appropriate MHC class I–peptide complex, $CD8^+$ T cells induce apoptosis of target cells using specialized lytic granules. A pore-forming protein, perforin, is released from the lytic granules and inserted into the target cell membrane. Proteases (granzymes) are injected into the target cells to initiate the apoptotic process by activating enzyme cascades. $CD4^+$ T cells can also induce apoptosis but by a different mechanism. On activation, they express cell surface molecules such as Fas ligand (CD178) and TRAIL, which initiate the apoptotic cascade selectively in cells expressing the respective ligands Fas (CD95) or the death receptors DR4 and DR5.

Compared with $CD8^+$ T cells, the spectrum of options for $CD4^+$ T cells is larger. They are generally characterized as helper T, or T_H, cells because they produce cytokines and express cell surface molecules that promote the effector function of other lymphocytes and phagocytes. On activation, different subsets of $CD4^+$ effector T cells can be distinguished based on the preferential production of certain cytokines (see E-Table 35-1). T_H1 T cells predominantly produce IFN-γ and tumor necrosis factor-α (TNF-α) and are involved in cell-mediated immunity, such as delayed-type hypersensitivity reactions. These cytokines, among other actions, promote macrophage activation that is critical for protective responses against intracellular pathogens such as mycobacteria and listeria. T_H2 T cells preferentially produce IL-4, IL-5, and IL-13, cytokines that promote eosinophil maintenance, expansion, and tissue accumulation, as well as macrophage function; these are all important for host protection following infection with helminths, such as schistosomes and other worms. T_H17 T cells produce IL-17, critical for neutrophil expansion and function, with killing of extracellular bacteria, such as streptococci, and pathogenic fungi. These cells may also produce IL-22 that promotes host-protective function at barrier surfaces, such as the skin and gut. Follicular helper T (T_{FH}) cells home to lymphoid follicles, where B cells congregate, where they express CD40 ligand (CD154) and other surface proteins along with cytokines, including IL-21, IL-4, and IFN-γ, that are critical for B-cell maturation to plasma cells and memory B cells. The decision as to which differentiation pathway to take is made during the early stages of naïve T-cell activation by antigen-presenting cells in secondary lymphoid organs. Pathway differentiation depends on several factors, including (1) the cytokines produced by the activating antigen-presenting cell and other innate cells in the microenvironment, (2) the nature of costimulatory signals, and (3) the avidity of the T-cell receptor-MHC antigen interaction. $CD4^+$ T-cell subset, or lineage, development is generally correlated with the expression of specific transcription factors (T-bet for T_H1, GATA3 for T_H2, RORγt for

T_H17, and Bcl6 for T_{FH} cells). However, lineage commitment among differentiated $CD4^+$ T cells is not absolute, and transition between different effector types is possible.

Regulatory T Cells

Depending on their cytokine profile, $CD4^+$ T cells have the ability to cross-regulate each other, influence T-cell differentiation, and suppress T-cell effector activity. T cells with regulatory activity generated during the normal immune response are IL-10– and transforming growth factor-β (TGF-β)–producing cells. In addition, specialized subsets of regulatory T (Treg) cells are characterized by expression of the transcription factor forkhead box P3 (Foxp3).[25] Naturally occurring $Foxp3^+$ Treg cells are generated during T-cell development in the thymus and recognize self-antigens. $Foxp3^+$ Treg cells can also arise from conventional $CD4^+$ T cells in the periphery. Treg cells are important in peripheral tolerance, controlling the expansion of autoreactive T cells. They also play a role in immune responses to pathogens by virtue of their ability to suppress T-cell effector function and consequently downmodulate the inflammatory response incited by the former, a natural consequence of pathogen elimination. Treg cells may also specialize according to their tissue environment, for example, selectively to regulate inflammation promoted by T_H1, T_H2, and T_H17 cells, respectively, and to regulate T_{FH} cells that drive production of autoantibodies by B cells in autoimmune diseases. A principal difference between natural and induced Treg cells is that the latter largely survey mucosal and other environmentally exposed surfaces.

In addition to secretion of IL-10 and TGF-β, which can dampen inflammatory responses, and functioning as a sink for pro-inflammatory cytokines such as IL-2, Tregs may also express the T-cell molecule cytotoxic T-lymphocyte antigen (CTLA)-4 (CD152) that, like CD28, engages CD80 and CD86 on antigen-presenting cells. In contrast to CD28, which receives a positive signal from CD80 and CD86, engagement of these molecules on antigen-presenting cells by CTLA-4 on Tregs suppresses the ability of antigen-presenting cells to activate naïve T cells.

T-Cell Homeostasis

Effective immunity depends on the ability of the immune system to generate large numbers of antigen-specific T cells rapidly, yet the space in the T-cell compartment is limited. To avoid competition for space and resources and to prevent perturbation of T-cell diversity by lifelong exposure to antigens, the adaptive immune system employs several counterbalancing mechanisms. In the later stages of the activation process, a strong negative signal derives from interaction of CTLA-4 with CD80/CD86 on antigen-presenting cells. In addition, T cells undergo activation-induced cell death. Activated $CD4^+$ T cells begin to secrete Fas ligand and acquire sensitivity to Fas-mediated death, inducing apoptotic suicide and fratricide in neighboring T cells. These mechanisms impose constraints in the early stages of the T-cell antigen response. Other mechanisms control the rapid decline of expanded antigen-specific T cells when elimination of the antigen has been achieved. Removal of the driving antigen causes a deprivation of cytokines and costimulatory molecules, and growth factor–deprived T cells die from apoptosis. It has been estimated that only 5% of the antigen-expanded population survives after antigen clearance, becoming memory cells that are poised to respond if the host is again challenged by the same offending pathogen.

B-Cell Differentiation

Differentiation of B cells activated by protein antigens depends on interaction with helper T cells. B cells use their antigen receptor not only to recognize antigens but also to internalize them. After processing endocytosed antigens, MHC class II–peptide complexes appear on the cell surface, where antigen-specific $CD4^+$ T cells detect them. Also, B cells express costimulatory molecules and provide optimal conditions for T-cell activation. On activation, $CD4^+$ T cells express CD154, also known as CD40 ligand, on their surface and are able to stimulate the CD40 molecule on their B-cell partner. CD40-CD154 interaction is essential for subsequent B-cell proliferation and differentiation. Cytokines secreted by the helper T cells act in concert with CD154 to amplify B-cell differentiation and to determine the antibody type by controlling isotype switching. Cytokines drive isotype switching by stimulating the transcriptional activation switch regions upstream of heavy chain constant region genes and ultimately facilitating excision of the IgM heavy chain gene and recombination of the VDJ segments with one of the downstream constant regions, IgG, IgA, or IgE. A population of B cells that is prominent in aging, in autoimmune disease and after virus infection or vaccination, called age-associated B cells (ABCs), appears to require signals through endosomal TLR-7, along with B-cell receptor and cytokine signals, for differentiation to autoantibody-secreting cells.[26]

T-cell–dependent B-cell differentiation and maturation take place in germinal centers, specialized areas in secondary lymphoid tissues where B cells rapidly proliferate and mutate the variable, or antigen-binding portion, of their immunoglobulin surface receptors. Those B cells bearing receptors with mutations that confer the highest affinity for antigen are selected for survival with the help of specific signals delivered by follicular helper T cells, whereas those with mutations conferring lesser affinity die by apoptosis. This process enables affinity maturation of B cells that most efficiently bind antigen and thereby facilitate antigen removal and pathogen clearance.

Generating Memory and Tolerance

Memory

An important consequence of adaptive immunity is the generation of immunologic memory, the basis for long-lived protection after a primary infection. Memory induction by vaccination is one of the landmark successes in medicine. Immunologic memory is defined as the ability to respond more rapidly and effectively to pathogens that have been encountered previously. As a direct result of clonal expansion and selection in antigen-driven responses, the frequencies of antigen-specific memory B cells and memory T cells are increased 10-fold to 1000-fold compared with the naïve repertoires. In addition to increased frequencies, memory T cells and B cells are functionally different from their naïve counterparts. Memory cells are long-lived and survive in the presence of certain cytokines without the need for continuous antigenic stimulation, guaranteeing immunologic memory for the life expectancy of the individual cell. Memory B cells produce predominantly IgG and IgA antibodies with evidence of somatic hypermutation and high affinity for the antigen. High-affinity IgE antibodies are also produced upon challenge with certain pathogens, such as helminths, and upon allergen exposure. Cell surface expression of high-affinity antibodies allows more efficient antigen uptake, thereby enhancing the crucial interaction with T cells. On antigen encounter, memory B cells change to antibody-secreting plasma cells, or re-enter the germinal center, where the high affinity of their immunoglobulin receptor gives them a competitive advantage over naïve B cells in antigen binding, leading to affinity maturation of somatically mutated antibody molecules.

Because the T-cell receptor does not undergo isotype switching or affinity maturation, memory T cells are more difficult to distinguish from naïve or effector T cells. Memory T cells lack activation markers and need antigen stimulation to resume effector functions. In contrast to naïve T cells, memory T cells have a lower activation threshold and are less dependent on costimulatory signals. In essence, their requirements for antigen stimulation are fewer, and their clonal size is larger, permitting fast, efficient responses to secondary antigen encounters.

Tolerance

Unresponsiveness to self is a fundamental property of the immune system and is required to maintain tissue integrity of the host. Because of the extraordinary complexity and variability of the repertoires of T- and B-cell antigen receptors, mechanisms of self/nonself discrimination are particularly applicable to the adaptive immune system. For T and B cells, antigen-specific receptors are generated randomly, and the entire spectrum of antigens can be recognized. Several different mechanisms are used, collectively called *tolerance*.[27] Tolerance in the adaptive immune system is antigen specific, and failure of self-tolerance results in immune responses against self-antigens. In central tolerance, self-reactive lymphocytes are deleted during development. In the bone marrow, B cells that express receptors directed against self-antigens are eliminated through clonal deletion. The process of negative selection is particularly important for T cells, and mutations in a gene called *AIRE* are associated with failure to delete self-reactive cells effectively in the thymus.[28] Even in the healthy setting, not all self-reactive T cells are centrally purged from the repertoire, and all T cells have some degree of self-reactivity, which is necessary for positive selection in the thymus and peripheral survival. Mechanisms of peripheral T-cell tolerance include (1) anergy, (2) peripheral deletion, (3) clonal ignorance, and (4) suppression of immune responses by regulatory T cells. T-cell anergy is transient and is actively maintained. MHC-peptide presentation to T cells by immature or inactivated, resting antigen-presenting cells or on cells other than peripheral antigen-presenting cells results in anergy because of the lack of expression of costimulatory molecules. Peripheral deletion is induced as a consequence of hyperstimulation.

Hyperstimulation of T cells (e.g., by high doses of antigen and high concentrations of IL-2) preferentially activates pro-apoptotic pathways and causes elimination of the responding T-cell specificity. Clonal ignorance is defined as the presence of self-reactive lymphocytes that fail to recognize or respond to peripheral antigens. These cells remain responsive to antigenic challenge if given in the right setting. An example of clonal ignorance is nonresponsiveness to sequestered antigens that are not accessible to the immune system. Treg cells play a pivotal role in maintaining peripheral tolerance. Harnessing the frequencies and function of Foxp3 $CD4^+$ T cells may offer a promising approach to restoring peripheral tolerance in treating autoimmune diseases or facilitating transplantation tolerance.

A critically important mechanism of peripheral B tolerance is maintained through the absence of T-cell help. B lymphocytes that recognize self-antigens in the periphery in the absence of T-cell help are rendered anergic or are unable to enter lymphoid follicles, where they could receive T-cell help, effectively excluding them from immune responses.

CONTRIBUTION OF THE INNATE AND ADAPTIVE IMMUNE RESPONSES TO PATHOGENESIS OF DISEASE

Immunodeficiency and Autoimmunity

Characterization of genetic polymorphisms and mutations in immune system genes that are associated either with apparent vulnerability to infection or inappropriate self-reactivity and autoimmunity has provided important insights into immune mechanisms that are essential for host defense and maintenance of immune tolerance. Mutations in components of innate and adaptive immune system pathways that recognize, respond to, or regulate the response to viruses or bacteria characterize immunodeficiencies that can be life-threatening (see Chapter 231).[29] In some cases, those vulnerabilities are revealed only in the setting of an infection with an agent not previously encountered. For example, recent reports describe previously healthy men who developed severe disease in the setting of severe acute respiratory syndrome coronavirus-2 (SARS-CoV-2) infection and were found to have mutations in the *TLR7* gene, thereby impairing the type I IFN response.[30]

Autoimmune and inflammatory diseases occur in about 5% of the general population. The mechanisms that account for the generation of autoreactive T cells, responses directed to modified self-antigens, and the well-established associations of certain MHC alleles with autoimmune diseases are areas of active investigation.[31] Although many autoimmune diseases may result from failure of tolerance mechanisms or dysfunction of the regulatory pathways that control adaptive immune responses, excessive activation of an innate immune response can set the stage for a self-reactive T- or B-cell response. Polymorphisms in genes encoding components of innate immune signaling pathways can amplify an immune response, thereby resulting in increased and sustained production of type I IFN, IL-1, or TNF-α. Endogenous ligands with potential to activate Toll-like receptors can act as effective immune stimuli in the setting of a pro-inflammatory environment associated with oxidative or apoptotic cell damage. Alterations in degradation of endogenous RNA and DNA based on single-gene mutations can result in activation of cytosolic nucleic acid sensors, sustained type I IFN production, skin lesions, and central nervous system involvement in diseases termed type I interferonopathies.[32] The inflammasome and its component proteins, including the NOD-like receptors, are recognized as mediators of inflammatory responses induced in some autoinflammatory syndromes (Chapter 240).

Many models of autoimmunity rely on the hypothesis that peripheral anergy is broken. Microbial infection or bacterial components in the gut microbiome (Chapter 257) may trigger an immune response that primes the immune system for an exaggerated and self-directed response to a subsequent trigger through epigenetic modifications.[33] Autoreactive B cells that recognize self-antigen complexed with foreign antigen may result in activation of T cells specific for the foreign antigen that then provide help to B cells specific for the self-antigen. Tolerance mechanisms of anergy or clonal ignorance can fail if a foreign antigen is sufficiently different from a self-antigen to initiate an immune response but sufficiently similar for activated T cells to elicit T-cell and B-cell effector functions (molecular mimicry).

GENERAL REFERENCES

For the General References and other additional features, please visit Elsevier eBooks+ at https://ebooks.health.elsevier.com.

36 TISSUE INJURY AND REPAIR

JANE E. SALMON

THE INFLAMMATORY RESPONSE: INNATE IMMUNE MECHANISMS

Inflammation is a vital physiologic response triggered by noxious agents that challenge homeostasis of the body. The innate immune system provides the first level of defense against signals of danger, including pathogenic microorganisms and sterile incursions such as trauma, cancer, ischemia, and metabolic perturbations. Host defense mechanisms generate a rapid protective response, render pathogens harmless, and repair damaged tissue. These highly controlled responses normally protect against further injury, but pathologic inflammation can be inappropriately triggered or inadequately controlled and, in some cases, lead to marked destruction of the extracellular matrix as well as to organ dysfunction.

Invading pathogens or environmental stresses stimulate tissue resident cells by engaging receptors that activate innate immunity. Innate immune responses are also required to initiate specific adaptive immune responses. Designed for rapid responses (minutes to hours), innate immunity relies on the body's ability to recognize conserved features that are present in pathogens but not in the uninfected host. Common motifs trigger innate immune responses, in contrast to the exquisite antigen specificity and precision of adaptive responses, which are slow to develop (days to weeks; Chapter 35).

An adaptive immune response is essential for host protection when innate mechanisms fail to contain the pathogen or injury.

INITIATORS AND EFFECTORS

Triggers of an innate inflammatory response can be classified as pathogen-associated molecular patterns (PAMPs), conserved molecular motifs of infectious agents, and damage-associated molecular patterns (DAMPs), which are signals of host cellular distress. A variety of pattern recognition receptors and cells of innate and adaptive immunity sense PAMPs and DAMPs. PAMP receptors, such as toll-like receptor (TLR) proteins, that are expressed on the cell surface or the inner leaflet of cytoplasmic vesicles, serve as sentinels that rapidly activate innate immune responses, thereby protecting the host from infection. DAMP recognition receptors within the cytoplasm sense "danger" signals that originate from stress, whether toxic environmental (e.g., urate) or cellular (e.g., adenosine triphosphate [ATP]), and respond to microenvironmental damage. Tissue injury induced by trauma or noxious stimuli triggers DAMP receptors to initiate inflammatory responses, thereby leading to microvascular damage, extravasation of leukocytes, and leakage of plasma proteins into the tissue (Fig. 36-1).

Upon encountering a pathogenic agent or tissue injury, the innate immune system is challenged to integrate multiple signals to initiate a proper protective response. Inflammasomes are cytoplasmic multiprotein complexes that comprise a sensor protein, inflammatory caspases, and, in some cases, an adapter protein that connects the two. Inflammasomes (Chapter 35) constitute fundamental processing units that contribute to PAMP and DAMP sensing and coordinate downstream signaling. Inflammasomes are activated by a range of endogenous and exogenous stimuli, thereby leading to enzymatic activation of a caspase and resulting in secretion of interleukin-1β (IL-1β) and IL-18, as well as apoptotic and pyroptotic cell death.

Resident tissue cells, mainly macrophages, dendritic cells, eosinophils, and mast cells that are activated by pattern recognition receptors, are the initiators of acute inflammation. These cells express surface or cytoplasmic pattern recognition receptors and, at the onset of an infection or other injury, they are activated and release inflammatory mediators that are responsible for the clinical signs of inflammation and tissue damage (see Fig. 36-1). Chemical factors produced during inflammation, including histamine, bradykinin, serotonin, leukotrienes, and prostaglandins, sensitize pain receptors, cause local vasodilation, and attract phagocytes, especially neutrophils. Neutrophils help to eliminate microbes but also can damage tissues owing to phagocytosis, the generation of reactive oxygen species, and degranulation, which releases proteases. Neutrophils also extrude chromatin fibers that contain antimicrobial peptides and enzymes, called neutrophil extracellular traps (NETs),[1] and that immobilize and kill invading

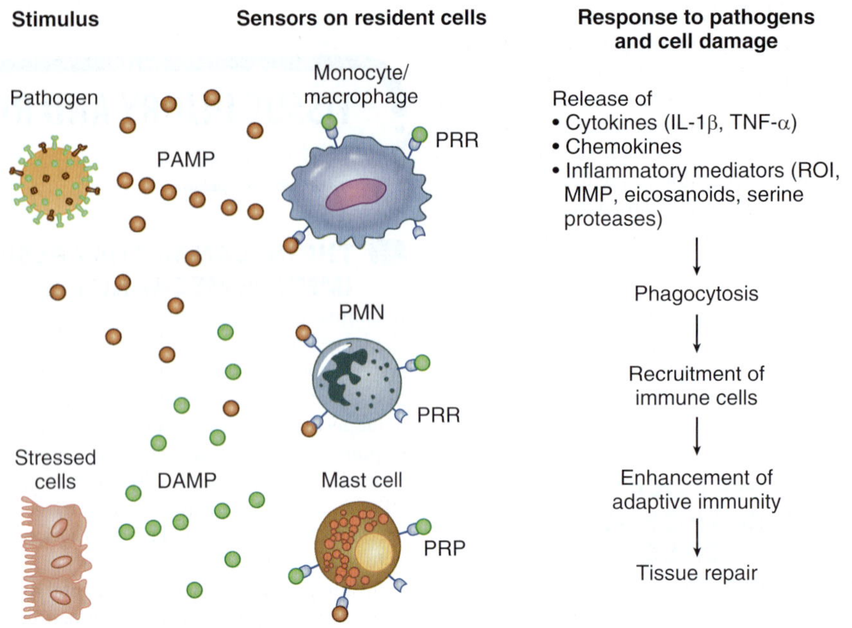

FIGURE 36-1. **Pathogens release PAMPs and stressed, injured cells release DAMPS, both of which bind to pattern recognition receptor on immune cells and stimulate an innate immune response that is accompanied by inflammation, activation of adaptive immunity, and eventually processes to resolve the infection injury and allow for tissue repair.** DAMP = damage-associated molecular pattern; IL-1β = interleukin-1beta; MMP = matrix metalloproteinase; PAMP = pathogen-associated molecular pattern; PMN = polymorphonuclear leukocytes; PRR = pattern recognition receptor; ROI = reactive oxygen intermediate; TNF-α = tumor necrosis factor-alpha.

microorganisms. NETs also may contribute to autoimmunity by binding to and presenting extracellular autoantigens or by stimulating thrombus formation. Neutrophils trigger other parts of the immune system by releasing factors that summon additional leukocytes and lymphocytes.

Local activation of the innate immune response quickly triggers a variety of signals that recruit other inflammatory cells (see Fig. 36-1). Resident vascular endothelial cells, mast cells, dendritic cells, and interstitial fibroblasts also release soluble mediators, including eicosanoids, chemokines, and pro-inflammatory cytokines. Pro-inflammatory members of the IL-1 family (IL-1α, IL-1β, IL-18, and IL-33) and tumor necrosis factor-α (TNF-α) have pleiotropic activities; they enhance adhesion molecule expression on endothelial cells, induce proliferation of endogenous cells, stimulate antigen presentation, and amplify the inflammatory response. Newly arrived inflammatory cells and locally stimulated cells also produce reactive toxic intermediates plus a variety of proteases (e.g., matrix metalloproteinases, serine proteases, and cysteine proteases). Enzymes that degrade the extracellular matrix regulate inflammatory tissue turnover, thereby damaging tissue, releasing matrix-bound growth factors and cytokines, and promoting the retention of newly recruited cells. In most situations, the normal physiologic response is an exquisitely coordinated program that uses proteolytic enzymes to remodel the extracellular matrix and promote a supportive environment for wound healing rather than tissue damage.

THE INFLAMMATORY RESPONSE: ADAPTIVE IMMUNE MECHANISMS

The adaptive immune response is a crucial component of host defense against infection, but unlike the innate response, it is learned rather than intrinsic. Its distinguishing and unique feature is the ability to recognize pathogens specifically, based on clonal selection of lymphocytes bearing antigen-specific receptors. Effector mechanisms that eliminate pathogens in adaptive immune responses are essentially identical to those of innate immunity. The specific antigen recognition feature of the adaptive immune response seems to have been appended to the preexisting innate defense system. As a result, the inflammatory cells and molecules of the innate immune system are essential for the effector functions of B and T lymphocytes.

In addition to initiating protective responses, antigens unassociated with infectious agents also may elicit adaptive immune responses. Many clinically important diseases are characterized by normal immune responses directed against an inappropriate antigen, typically in the absence of infection. Immune responses directed at noninfectious antigens occur in allergy and hypersensitivity, in which the antigen is an innocuous foreign substance, and in autoimmunity, in which the response is to a self-antigen. Adaptive immune responses mediate tissue injury in allergy, hypersensitivity, and autoimmunity.

INITIATORS AND EFFECTORS

Effector actions of antibodies depend on recruiting cells and molecules of the innate immune system. Antibodies are adapters that bind antigens to nonspecific inflammatory cells and direct their destructive effector responses. Antibodies also activate the complement system (Chapter 37), which enhances opsonization of antigens, recruits phagocytic cells, and amplifies (or "complements") antibody-triggered damage. The isotype or class of antibodies produced determines which effector mechanisms are engaged.

Cell-bound receptors for immunoglobulin (Ig) constitute the link between humoral and cellular aspects of the immune cascade and play an integral part in the process by which foreign and endogenous opsonized material is identified and destroyed. These cell-based binding sites for antibodies, termed *Fc receptors*, interact with the constant region (Fc portion) of the immunoglobulin heavy chain of a particular antibody class regardless of its antigen specificity. Accessory cells that lack intrinsic specificity, such as neutrophils, macrophages, and mast cells, are recruited to participate in inflammatory responses through the interaction of their Fc receptors with antigen-specific antibodies. Distinct receptors for different immunoglobulin isotypes are expressed on different effector cells.

Receptors for IgG (FcγRs) are a diverse group of receptors expressed as hematopoietic cell surface molecules on phagocytes (macrophages, monocytes, neutrophils), platelets, mast cells, eosinophils, and natural killer (NK) cells.[2] FcγRs often are expressed as stimulatory and inhibitory pairs. Triggering of stimulatory FcγRs initiates a series of events, including phagocytosis; antibody-dependent, cell-mediated cytotoxicity; secretion of granules; and release of inflammatory mediators, such as cytokines, reactive oxidants, and proteases. Extensive structural diversity among FcγR family members leads to differences in binding capacity, signal transduction pathways, and cell type–specific expression patterns. The structure of the Fc domain of IgG dictates interactions with FcγRs and can lead to pro- or anti-inflammatory responses. The strength of interactions between immune complexes and various FcγRs is determined by structural diversity within IgG subclasses (IgG1, IgG2, IgG3, IgG4) and post-translational modifications of their Fc domains.[3] This diversity allows IgG complexes to activate a broad program of cell functions relevant to inflammation, host defense, and autoimmunity. Phagocyte activation is triggered by stimulatory FcγRs, facilitating the recognition, uptake, and destruction of antibody-coated targets, whereas multivalent IgG binding to FcγRs on platelets leads to platelet aggregation and thrombosis, and binding to FcγRs on NK cells mediates cytotoxicity of antibody-coated targets.

IgE binds to high-affinity FcεRs on mast cells, basophils, and activated eosinophils.[4] In contrast to FcγRs, which are low affinity and bind to multivalent IgG rather than circulating individual IgG molecules, FcεRs can bind monomeric IgE. A single mast cell may be armed with IgE molecules specific for different antigens, all bound to surface FcεRs. Mast cells, localized beneath the mucosa of the gastrointestinal and respiratory tracts and the dermis of the skin, await exposure to multivalent antigens, which cross-link surface IgE bound to FcεRs and cause release of histamine-containing granules and generation of cytokines and other inflammatory mediators (Chapter 235). IgE-mediated activation of eosinophils, which are normally present in the connective tissue of underlying respiratory, urogenital, and gut epithelium, leads to the release of highly toxic granule proteins, free radicals, and chemical mediators such as prostaglandins, cytokines, and chemokines (Chapter 156). These mediators amplify local inflammatory responses by activating endothelial cells and recruiting and activating more eosinophils and leukocytes. Prepackaged granules and high-affinity FcεRs that bind to free monomeric IgE enable an immediate response to pathogens or allergens at the first site of entry, a location where FcεR-bearing cells reside.

Inhibitory FcγRs, which modulate activation thresholds and terminate stimulating signals, are key elements in the regulation of effector function. Given that inhibitory and stimulatory Fc receptors are often coexpressed on the same cells, the effector response to a specific stimulus in a particular cell represents the balance between stimulatory and inhibitory signals. Inhibitory FcγRs can dampen responses triggered by FcεRs on mast cells and FcγR-mediated inflammation at sites of immune complex deposition.

Effector activities targeted by IgG and IgM also may be mediated by components of the complement system (Chapter 37). Antigen-bound multimeric immunoglobulin can initiate activation of the classic pathway of complement, causing enhanced phagocytosis of antigen-antibody complexes, increased local vascular permeability, and recruitment and activation of inflammatory cells. The target of injury is specified by the antibody, and the extent of damage is determined by the synergistic activities of immunoglobulin and complement.

Antigen-specific effector T cells also may initiate tissue injury. On exposure to an appropriate antigen, memory T cells are stimulated to release cytokines and chemokines that activate local endothelial cells and recruit and activate macrophages and other inflammatory cells. The effector cells directed by T-cell-derived cytokines, or cytolytic T cells themselves, mediate tissue damage. T helper 1 (T_H1) cells produce interferon-γ (IFN-γ) and activate macrophages to cause injury, whereas T_H2 cells produce IL-4, IL-5, and eotaxin (an eosinophil-specific chemokine) and trigger inflammatory responses in which eosinophils predominate. T_H17 cells secrete several effector molecules, including IL-17, which act on both immune and nonimmune cells to trigger differentiation; release of antimicrobial molecules, cytokines, and chemokines; and recruitment to sites of inflammation.[5] T_H effector subsets, more recently identified, include follicular T helper cells (T_{FH}), which provide help to B cells in germinal centers and thus are key regulators of humoral responses and antibody production.

HYPERSENSITIVITY REACTIONS

In predisposed individuals, innocuous environmental antigens may stimulate an adaptive immune response, immunologic memory, and, on subsequent exposure to the antigen, inflammation. Damage to epithelial surfaces lies at the origin of various manifestations of allergic disease. The epithelium of the lungs, gut, and skin are sensors of environmental stimuli, and alterations to their epithelial surfaces drives a type 2 immune response that underlies atopic diseases.[6] These "overreactions" of the immune system to harmless environmental antigens (allergens), called *hypersensitivity* or *allergic reactions* (Chapter 230), produce tissue injury and can cause serious disease. Hypersensitivity reactions are grouped into four types according to the effector mechanisms by which they are produced (Table 36-1). The effectors for types I, II, and III hypersensitivity reactions are antibody molecules, whereas type IV reactions are mediated by antigen-specific effector T cells.

Autoimmune disease is characterized by the presence of antibodies and T cells specific for self-antigens expressed on target tissues. The mechanisms of antigen recognition and effector function that lead to tissue damage in autoimmune disease are similar to the mechanisms elicited in response to pathogens and environmental antigens. These mechanisms resemble certain hypersensitivity reactions and may be classified accordingly. Autoimmune disease caused by antibodies directed against cell surface or extracellular matrix antigens corresponds to type II hypersensitivity reactions; disease caused by formation of soluble immune complexes that subsequently are deposited in tissue corresponds to type III hypersensitivity; and disease caused by effector T cells corresponds to type IV hypersensitivity. Typically, several of these pathogenic mechanisms are operative in autoimmune disease. However, IgE responses are not associated with damage in autoimmunity.

Type I Hypersensitivity Reactions

Type I hypersensitivity reactions (Fig. 36-2) are triggered by the interaction of antigen with antigen-specific IgE bound to FcεRs on mast cells, which causes mast cell activation. Proteolytic enzymes and toxic mediators, such as histamine, are released immediately from preformed granules, and chemokines, cytokines, and leukotrienes are synthesized after activation. Together, these mediators increase vascular permeability, break down tissue matrix proteins, promote eosinophil production and activation (IL-3, IL-5, and granulocyte-macrophage colony-stimulating factor [GM-CSF]), and cause influx of effector leukocytes (TNF-α, platelet-activating factor, and macrophage inflammatory protein [MIP-1]), constriction of smooth muscle, stimulation of mucus secretion, and amplification of T_H2 cell responses (IL-4 and IL-13). Eosinophils and basophils, which are activated through cell surface FcεRs, rapidly release highly toxic granular proteins (major basic protein, eosinophil peroxidase, and collagenase) and, over a longer period, produce cytokines (IL-3, IL-5, and GM-CSF), chemokines (IL-8), prostaglandins, and leukotrienes that activate epithelial cells, leukocytes, and eosinophils to augment local inflammation and tissue damage.

FcεR-bearing effectors act in a coordinated fashion. The immediate allergic inflammatory reaction initiated by mast cell products is followed by a late-phase response that involves recruitment and activation of eosinophils, basophils, and T_H2 lymphocytes. The manifestations of IgE-mediated reactions depend on

TABLE 36-1 FOUR MAJOR TYPES OF IMMUNOLOGICALLY MEDIATED HYPERSENSITIVITY REACTIONS*

IMMUNOLOGIC SPECIFICITY	TYPE I (IgE ANTIBODY)	TYPE II (IgG ANTIBODY)	TYPE III (IgG ANTIBODY)	TYPE IV (T CELLS): T_H1 CELLS	TYPE IV (T CELLS): T_H2 CELLS	TYPE IV (T CELLS): T_H17 CELLS	TYPE IV (T CELLS): T CELLS
Antigen	Soluble antigen allergen	Cell- or matrix-associated antigen	Soluble antigen	Soluble antigen	Soluble antigen	Soluble antigen	Cell-associated antigen
Effector mechanism	FcεRI- or FcγRIII-dependent mast cell activation, with release of mediators/cytokines	FcγR⁺ cells (phagocytes, NK cells), complement	FcγR⁺ cells, complement	Macrophage activation	Eosinophil activation	Macrophage activation, neutrophil activation	Direct cytotoxicity
Examples	Systemic anaphylaxis, asthma, allergic rhinitis, urticaria, angioedema	Certain drug reactions and reactions to incompatible blood transfusions	Arthus reaction and other immune complex–mediated reactions (e.g., serum sickness, subacute bacterial endocarditis)	Contact dermatitis, tuberculin reaction	Chronic allergic inflammation (e.g., chronic asthma, chronic allergic rhinitis)	Contact dermatitis, atopic dermatitis, asthma, rheumatoid arthritis	Contact dermatitis (e.g., poison ivy), reactions to certain virus-infected cells, some instances of graft rejection

*Hypersensitivity reactions were classified into four types by Coombs and Gell (1963) and modified by Janeway and colleagues (2001).

FcγR = Fc receptor for immunoglobulin G; FcεR = Fc receptor for immunoglobulin E; Ig = immunoglobulin; NK = natural killer.

From Coombs RRA, Gell PGH. Classification of allergic reactions responsible for clinical hypersensitivity and disease. In: Gell PGH, Coombs RA, eds. *Clinical Aspects of Immunology*. Oxford, UK: Blackwell; 1963; and Janeway C, Travers P, Walport M, Shlomchick M. *Immunobiology: The Immune System in Health and Disease*. 5th ed. New York: Garland Publishing; 2001.

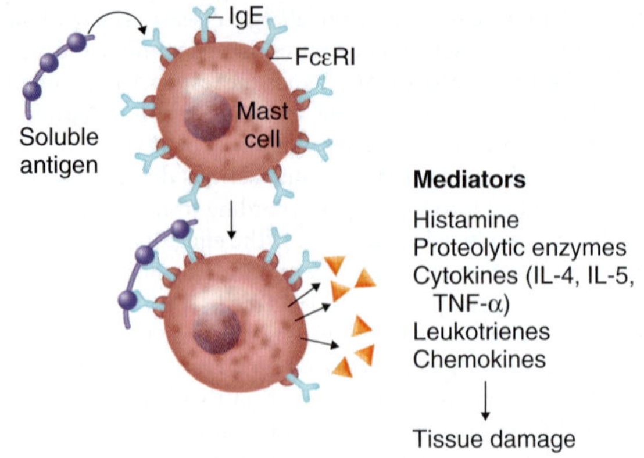

FIGURE 36-2. Type I hypersensitivity. Type I responses are mediated by immunoglobulin E (IgE), which induces mast cell activation. Cross-linking of the Fc receptor for IgE (FcεR) on mast cells, triggered by the interaction of multivalent antigen with antigen-specific IgE bound to FcεR, causes the release of preformed granules containing histamine and proteases. Cytokines, chemokines, and lipid mediators are synthesized after cell activation. IL = interleukin; TNF = tumor necrosis factor.

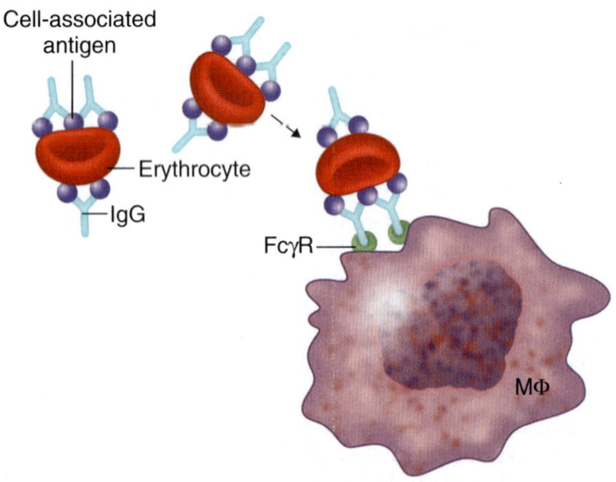

FIGURE 36-3. Type II hypersensitivity. Type II responses are mediated by immunoglobulin G (IgG) directed against cell surface or matrix antigens, which initiates effector responses through the Fc receptor for IgG (FcγR) and complement. The relative contributions of these pathways vary with the IgG subclass and the nature of the antigen. Only FcγR-mediated phagocytosis by macrophages (MΦ) is depicted in this figure. Activation of complement components would result in binding of C3b to the red blood cell membrane, rendering red blood cells susceptible to phagocytosis and leading to formation of the membrane attack complex and cell lysis.

the site of mast cell activation. Mast cells reside in vascular and epithelial tissue throughout the body. In a sensitized host (an individual with IgE responses to antigens), re-exposure to antigen leads to type I hypersensitivity responses only in the mast cells exposed to the antigen. Inhalation of antigens produces bronchoconstriction and increased mucus secretion (asthma and allergic rhinitis); ingestion of antigens causes increased peristalsis and secretion (diarrhea and vomiting); and the presence of subcutaneous antigens initiates increased vascular permeability and swelling (urticaria and angioedema). Blood-borne antigens cause systemic mast cell activation, increased capillary permeability, hypotension, tissue swelling, and smooth muscle contraction—the characteristics of systemic anaphylaxis.[7]

Type II Hypersensitivity Reactions

Type II hypersensitivity reactions (Fig. 36-3) are caused by chemical modification of cell surface or matrix-associated antigens that generates "foreign" epitopes to which the immune system is not tolerant. B cells respond to this antigenic challenge by producing IgG, which binds to these modified cells and renders them susceptible to destruction through complement activation, phagocytosis, and antibody-dependent cytotoxicity This phenomenon is seen clinically when drugs interact with blood constituents and alter their cellular antigens. Hemolytic anemia caused by immune-mediated destruction of erythrocytes (Chapter 146) and thrombocytopenia caused by destruction of platelets (Chapter 158), both type II hypersensitivity reactions, are adverse effects of certain drugs. Chemically reactive drug molecules bind covalently to the surface of red cells or platelets creating new epitopes that in a small subset of individuals are recognized as foreign antigens by the immune system and stimulate production of IgM and IgG antibodies reactive with the conjugate of drug and cell surface protein. Penicillin-specific IgG binds to penicillin-modified proteins on red blood cells and triggers activation of the complement cascade. Activation of complement components C1 through C3 results in covalent binding of C3b to the red cell membrane and renders circulating red cells susceptible to phagocytosis by FcγR and complement receptor–bearing macrophages in the spleen or liver. Activation of complement components C1 through C9 and formation of the membrane attack complex cause intravascular lysis of red cells. The factors that predispose only some people to drug-induced type II hypersensitivity reactions are unknown. Penicillin, quinidine, and methyldopa have been associated with hemolytic anemia and thrombocytopenia through this mechanism. Another example is heparin-induced thrombocytopenia or thrombosis, a severe, life-threatening complication that occurs in 1 to 3% of patients exposed to heparin (Chapter 158). Interactions among heparin, human platelet factor 4, antibodies to the human platelet factor 4–heparin complex, platelet FcγRIIA, and splenic FcγRs (which remove opsonized platelets) are involved in the pathogenesis of this disease.

Autoantibodies directed at antigens on the cell surface or extracellular matrix cause tissue damage by mechanisms similar to type II hypersensitivity reactions. IgG or IgM antibodies against erythrocytes lead to cell destruction in autoimmune hemolytic anemia because opsonized cells (coated with IgG or IgM and complement) are removed from the circulation by phagocytes in the liver and spleen or are lysed by formation of the membrane attack complex. Platelet destruction in autoimmune thrombocytopenic purpura occurs through a similar process. Because nucleated cells express membrane bound complement regulatory proteins, they are less sensitive to lysis through the membrane attack complex, but when coated with antibody, they become targets for phagocytosis or antibody-dependent cytotoxicity. This mechanism is responsible for autoimmune and alloimmune neutropenia (Chapter 153).

IgM and IgG antibodies recognizing antigens within tissue or binding to extracellular antigens cause local inflammatory damage through FcγR and complement mechanisms.[8] Pemphigus vulgaris (Chapter 406) is a serious blistering disease that results from a loss of adhesion between keratinocytes caused by autoantibodies against the extracellular portions of desmoglein 3, an intercellular adhesion structure of epidermal keratinocytes. Another example of a type II hypersensitivity reaction is Goodpasture disease (Chapter 79), in which antibodies against the α_3-chain of type IV collagen (the collagen in basement membranes) are deposited in glomerular and lung basement membrane. Tissue-bound autoantibodies activate monocytes, neutrophils, and basophils through FcγRs, initiating release of proteases, reactive oxidants, cytokines, and prostaglandins. Local activation of complement, particularly C5a, recruits and activates inflammatory cells and amplifies tissue injury. Neighboring cells are lysed by assembly of the membrane attack complex or by FcγR-initiated, antibody-dependent cytotoxicity.

Autoantibodies against cell surface receptors produce disease by stimulating or blocking receptor function. In myasthenia gravis (Chapter 390), autoantibodies against the acetylcholine receptors on skeletal muscle cells bind the receptor and induce its internalization and degradation in lysosomes, thereby reducing the efficiency of neuromuscular transmission and causing progressive muscle weakness. In contrast, Graves disease (Chapter 207) is characterized by autoantibodies that act as agonists. Autoantibodies to thyroid-stimulating hormone receptors bind the receptor, mimicking the natural ligand, inducing thyroid hormone overproduction, disrupting feedback regulation, and causing hyperthyroidism.

Type III Hypersensitivity Reactions

Type III hypersensitivity reactions (Fig. 36-4) are caused by tissue deposition of small soluble immune complexes that contain antigens and high-affinity IgG antibodies directed at these antigens. Localized deposition of immune complexes activates FcγR-bearing mast cells and phagocytes and initiates the complement cascade, all effectors of tissue damage.

Immune complexes are generated in all antibody responses. The formation and the fate of immune complexes depend on the biophysical and immunologic properties of the antigen and the antibody. Larger aggregates fix complement more efficiently, present a broader multivalent array of ligands for complement and FcγRs to bind, and are taken up more readily by mononuclear phagocytes in the liver and spleen and thereby removed from the circulation. Smaller immune complexes, which form in antigen excess—as occurs early in an immune response—circulate in the blood and are deposited in blood

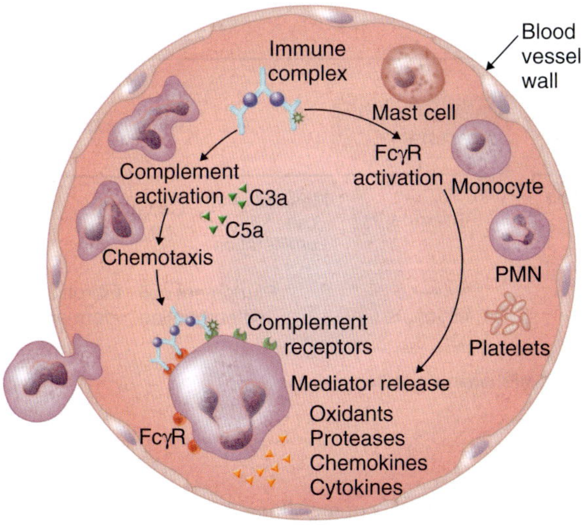

FIGURE 36-4. **Type III hypersensitivity. Type III responses are mediated by immunoglobulin G (IgG) directed against soluble antigens. Localized deposition of immune complexes activates mast cells, monocytes, neutrophils, and platelets bearing the Fc receptor for IgG (FcγR), and initiates the complement cascade, all effectors of tissue damage. Generation of complement activation products C3a and C5a recruits and stimulates inflammatory cells and amplifies effector functions. PMN = polymorphonuclear leukocyte (also called *neutrophil*).**

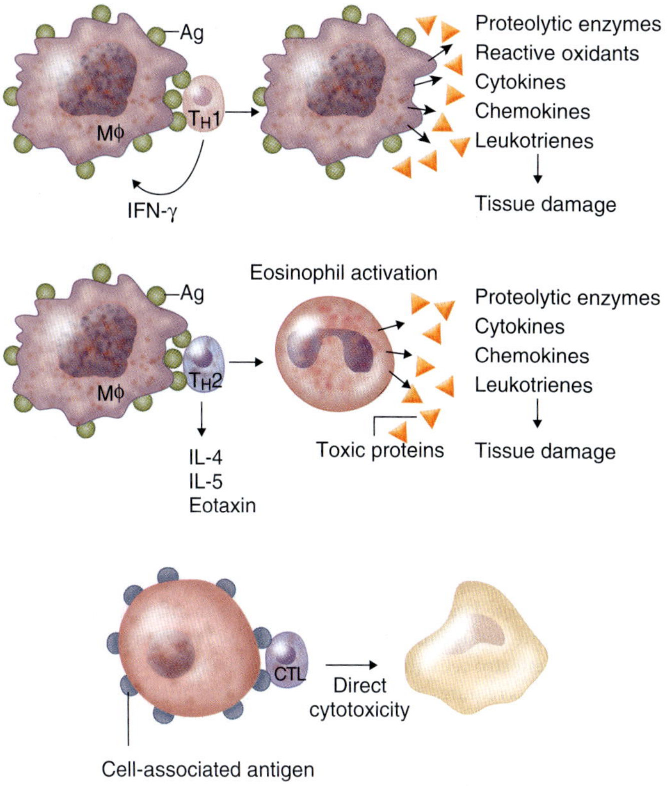

FIGURE 36-5. **Type IV hypersensitivity. Type IV responses are mediated by T cells through three different pathways. In the first, type 1 helper T (T_H1) cells recognize soluble antigens (Ag) and release interferon-γ (IFN-γ) to activate effector cells, in this case macrophages (MΦ), and cause tissue injury. In T_H2-mediated responses, eosinophils predominate. T_H2 cells produce cytokines to recruit and activate eosinophils, leading to their degranulation and tissue injury. In the third pathway, damage is caused directly by cytolytic T lymphocytes (CTL). IL = interleukin.**

vessels, where they initiate inflammatory reactions and tissue damage through interactions with FcγRs and complement receptors.

Serum sickness (Chapter 230)[9] is a systemic type III hypersensitivity reaction, historically described in patients injected with therapeutic horse antiserum for the treatment of bacterial infections. In general, serum sickness occurs after the injection of large quantities of a soluble antigen. Clinical features include chills, fever, rash, urticaria, arthritis, and glomerulonephritis. Disease manifestations become evident 7 to 10 days after exposure to the antigen, when antibodies are generated against the foreign protein and form immune complexes with these circulating antigens. Immune complexes are deposited in blood vessels, where they activate phagocytes and complement, producing widespread tissue injury and clinical symptoms. The effects are transient, however, and resolve after the antigen is cleared.

A syndrome similar to serum sickness occurs in chronic infections in which pathogens persist in the face of continued immune response. In subacute bacterial endocarditis (Chapter 61), antibody production continues but fails to eliminate the infecting microbes. As the pathogens multiply, generating new antigens, immune complexes form in the circulation and are deposited in small blood vessels, where they lead to inflammatory damage of skin, kidney, and nerve. Hepatitis B virus infection (Chapters 134 and 135) may be associated with immune complex deposition early in its course, during a period of antigen excess, because antibody production in response to hepatitis B surface antigen is as yet relatively insufficient; some anicteric patients may present with acute arthritis. Mixed essential cryoglobulinemia, which may be associated with hepatitis C viral infection (Chapters 134 and 135), is an immune complex–mediated vasculitis in which deposition of complexes containing IgG, IgM, and hepatitis C antigens causes inflammation in peripheral nerves, kidneys, and skin. Serum sickness also can develop in transplant recipients who are treated with mouse monoclonal antibodies specific for human T cells to prevent rejection, and in patients with myocardial infarction who are treated with the bacterial enzyme streptokinase to effect thrombolysis.

Systemic lupus erythematosus (Chapter 245), the prototypical immune complex–mediated autoimmune disease, is characterized by circulating IgG directed against common cellular constituents, typically DNA and DNA-binding proteins. Small immune complexes are deposited in skin, joints, and glomeruli and initiate local tissue damage.

Type IV Hypersensitivity Reactions

Type IV hypersensitivity reactions (Fig. 36-5), also known as *delayed-type hypersensitivity reactions*, are mediated by antigen-specific effector T cells.[10] These reactions are distinguished from other hypersensitivity reactions by the lag time from exposure to the antigen until the response is evident (1 to 3 days). Antigen is taken up, processed, and presented by macrophages or dendritic cells. T_H1 effector cells that recognize the specific antigen (these are scarce and take time to arrive) are stimulated to release chemokines, which recruit macrophages to the site, release cytokines that mediate tissue injury and growth factors that stimulate monocyte production. IFN-γ activates macrophages and enhances their release of inflammatory mediators, whereas TNF-α and TNF-β activate endothelial cells, enhance vascular permeability, and damage local tissue. The prototypical type IV hypersensitivity reaction is the tuberculin test, but similar reactions can occur after contact with sensitizing antigens (e.g., poison ivy, certain metals) and lead to epidermal reactions characterized by erythema, cellular infiltration, and vesicles. $CD8^+$ T cells also may mediate damage by direct toxicity.

In contrast to T_H1-mediated hypersensitivity reactions, in which the effectors are macrophages, eosinophils predominate in T_H2-mediated responses. T_H2 effector T cells are associated with tissue damage in chronic asthma (Chapter 75). T_H2 cells produce cytokines to recruit and activate eosinophils (IL-5 and eotaxin), leading to degranulation, further tissue injury, and chronic, irreversible airway damage.

Additional T_H effector cells, such as T_H17 cells, mediate tissue damage. T_H17 cells produce IL-17 family cytokines, as well as IL-21, IL-22, and GM-CSF, that regulate innate effectors and orchestrate local inflammation by inducing release of pro-inflammatory cytokines and chemokines, proliferation and activation of effector cells and other target cells, recruitment of neutrophils, and enhanced T_H2-mediated inflammation, all of which amplify allergic and autoimmune responses. T_H17 cells have been implicated in allergic disorders (atopic dermatitis, asthma) and autoimmune and inflammatory diseases (psoriasis, inflammatory bowel disease, rheumatoid arthritis, systemic lupus erythematosus, multiple sclerosis), and chronic transplant rejection.

In some autoimmune diseases, effector T cells specifically recognize self-antigens to cause tissue damage, either by direct cytotoxicity or by inflammatory responses mediated by activated macrophages. In type 1 insulin-dependent diabetes mellitus, T cells mediate destruction of β cells of the pancreatic islets. IFN-γ–producing T cells specific for myelin basic proteins have been implicated in multiple sclerosis. Rheumatoid arthritis (Chapter 243) is another autoimmune disease caused, at least in part, by activated T_H1 cells.

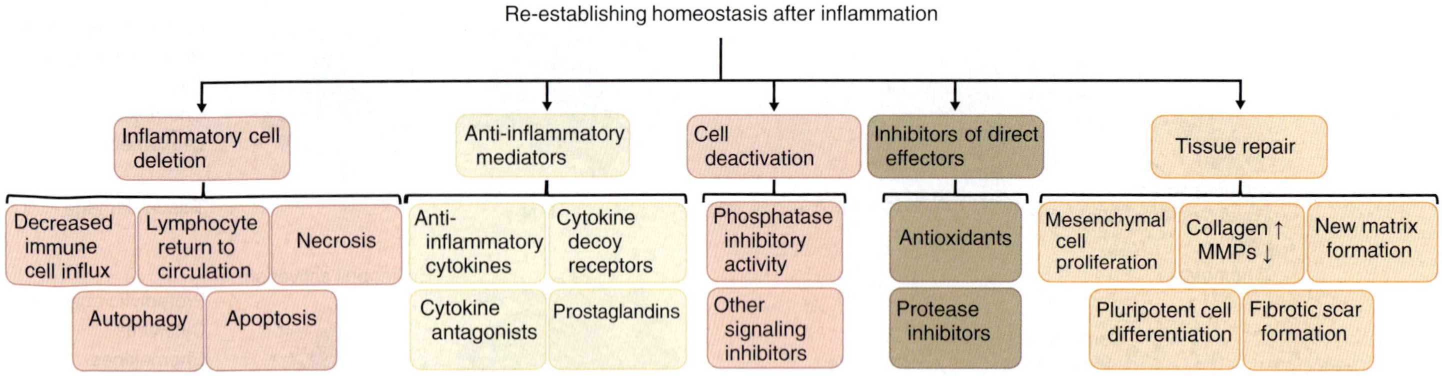

FIGURE 36-6. **Mechanisms that resolve inflammation and lead to repair of the extracellular matrix. MMPs = matrix metalloproteinases.**

TISSUE REPAIR AND RESOLUTION OF INFLAMMATION

Transient inflammation is a normal physiologic response, but serious injury results when unabated inflammation persists. After an inflammatory response is initiated, homeostasis must be reestablished by removing or deactivating mediators and effector cells, thereby permitting damaged tissues to repair. This resolution process requires cellular responses such as apoptosis and necrosis, the generation of anti-inflammatory cytokines and antioxidants, and the production of protease inhibitors (Fig. 36-6).

CELLULAR RESPONSES

Removal of inflammatory cells is accomplished by suppressing the production of chemotactic factor and the expression of vascular adhesion molecules, thereby releasing cells (particularly lymphocytes) from tissues so they can return to the circulation through the lymphatic system or by directly causing cell death via necrosis, apoptosis, or autophagy. However, the release of cellular contents by dying cells may be deleterious, and defective apoptosis or the persistence of apoptotic cells can contribute to chronic inflammation and to autoimmune diseases.

Some immune cells disappear during the resolution phase, whereas other cells expand.[11] For example, mesenchymal cells, such as fibroblasts, typically proliferate to produce new matrix, which in turn contracts to form fibrotic scar tissue. DNA synthesis in these stromal cells is induced by locally produced growth factors, such as platelet-derived growth factor. TGF-β stimulates fibroblasts to proliferate and changes their phenotype to healing by driving matrix formation through increased production of collagen and suppressed expression of matrix metalloproteinases. Mesenchymal stem cells also can differentiate into organ-specific lineages and, in the appropriate milieu, become bone cells, chondrocytes, adipocytes, or other terminally differentiated stromal cells.

SOLUBLE MEDIATORS AND INHIBITORS OF DAMAGING EFFECTORS

Resident and infiltrating cells release anti-inflammatory cytokines. TGF-β and IL-10 are produced by macrophages, interstitial fibroblasts, or T cells. T-cell cytokines (e.g., IL-4, IL-10, and IL-13) suppress the expression of matrix metalloproteinases by IL-1- or TNF-stimulated cells. TGF-β suppresses the production of collagenase, increases the deposition of collagen, and induces the tissue production of metalloproteinase inhibitors, thereby decreasing the activity of matrix metalloproteinases.

In addition, intracellular safety mechanisms regulate inflammatory signaling pathways to ensure that the process is self-limited. For example, kinases in growth factor receptors and other intracellular pathways activated by pro-inflammatory cytokines require phosphorylation to amplify enzyme activity, but phosphatases remove these phosphates so that kinases return to their resting inactive form.

Catalase and superoxide dismutase, which are antioxidant enzymes, inactivate toxic reactive oxygen intermediates released by phagocytes. The removal of toxic metabolites is facilitated by glutathione peroxidases and glutathione reductase.

Protease inhibitors are produced to regulate endogenous proteases and thereby to reduce the likelihood that collateral tissue damage will occur. For example, serine protease inhibitors (e.g., antithrombin III, plasminogen activator inhibitors 1 and 2, and α_1-antitrypsin) attenuate inflammation and resolve blood clots. Tissue inhibitors of metalloproteinases bind to activated matrix metalloproteinases and irreversibly block their catalytic sites to inhibit enzyme function. Examples of disease states characterized by an unfavorable balance between tissue inhibitors of metalloproteinases and matrix metalloproteinases include loss of cartilage in arthritis and progression of tumor metastases. Inhibition of pro-inflammatory cytokines and growth factors is associated with increased production of matrix protein and decreased activity of matrix metalloproteinases.

GENERAL REFERENCES

For the General References and other additional features, please visit Elsevier eBooks+ at https://ebooks.health.elsevier.com.

37

COMPLEMENT SYSTEM IN DISEASE

JOHN P. ATKINSON AND V. MICHAEL HOLERS

The complement system consists of plasma and membrane proteins that participate in host defense against infections and in clearance of cellular and extracellular debris, as well as in a wide variety of autoimmune and inflammatory states (Fig. 37-1).[1–3] Complement is essential in innate immunity and a potent effector arm of adaptive (humoral) immunity. It is a *first* responder, especially in blood, to bacterial and viral invasion (Table 37-1). It helps to maintain sterility ("guardian of the intravascular space") by depositing within seconds its opsonic and membrane-perturbing fragments on a pathogen's surface. A second major activity of complement is to promote the inflammatory response via the release of soluble fragments *(anaphylatoxins)* that act in both extracellular and intracellular sites. These fragments bind to their receptors, thereby leading to cellular activation, including chemokinesis and chemotaxis by phagocytic cells, and enhancing protection against infections. Furthermore, the deposition of complement fragments on immune complexes keeps them from precipitating and promotes their adherence to red blood cells (RBCs) for a hand-off to monocytes and dendritic cells in the liver and spleen.

Through these interactions, complement also instructs the adaptive immune response. Antigens decorated by complement proteins are more efficiently taken up by, or held in place for presentation to, monocytes, follicular-dendritic cells, B lymphocytes, and other antigen-presenting cells, thereby resulting in an adaptive immune response (Chapter 35). For example, complement activation is required for an optimal antibody response to most foreign antigens. In this way, the complement system is often called "nature's adjuvant." Individuals lacking a functional complement system are predisposed to bacterial infections, predominantly by encapsulated organisms, including streptococcus, staphylococcus, *Haemophilus* spp, and *Neisseria* spp. Surprisingly, a complete deficiency of C1q, which is an early component of the classical complement pathway, strongly predisposes to autoimmune diseases, particularly systemic lupus erythematosus (SLE).[4] This association suggests that complement is required not only for host defense against foreign agents but also to identify and safely clear self-materials (debris removal), particularly RNA and DNA species[5] in conditions such as rhabdomyolysis.[6]

A remarkable feature of the complement system is that it reacts within seconds (Table 37-2). In less than 2 minutes, it can coat an encapsulated gram-positive bacterium with several million C3b opsonic fragments and lyse gram-negative bacteria by insertion of its terminal components (the membrane attack complex). It works faster if driven by immunoglobulin M (IgM) or IgG binding to an antigen on a microbial membrane to activate and focus the cascade. Antibodies and lectins direct the activation process to the pathogen's surface. Overall, the complement cascade is designed to become engaged on the surface of a pathogen, particularly bacteria. Plasma and membrane *regulators of complement activation* inhibit formation on normal "self" cells.

Much of complement-mediated pathology revolves around the alternative pathway's amplification loop. This loop is key in triggering activation early in an immune response; however, it must be rigorously regulated to prevent activation on normal self and excessive activation on injured self.[7] Approximately half of the proteins associated with the complement system are dedicated to the control of its activation and effector functions, especially to maintain homeostasis of the alternative pathway's amplification loop.

In clinical medicine, the complement system participates in three pathologic processes: (1) an inherited decrease in functional activity leading to increased susceptibility to bacterial infections and to autoimmunity, (2) undesirable tissue damage upon activation by autoantibodies and immune complexes, and (3) excessive activation at sites of tissue injury in individuals carrying genetic variants in regulators (Tables 37-3 and 37-4).

Knowledge of how complement is activated and how it can be controlled points to opportunities for the development of therapeutic agents such as anti-C5 monoclonal antibody therapy, which has been approved to treat complement-dependent hemolytic and autoimmune disorders.

ACTIVATION OF COMPLEMENT

CLASSICAL PATHWAY

The binding of IgM or IgG to a target antigen activates this exceptionally powerful and quick-acting pathway to destroy microbes (Figs. 37-2 and 37-3). The classical pathway reaction cascade is designed to opsonize and perturb the surface membrane of microorganisms. Of course, autoantibodies also trigger this highly efficient classical pathway. Complement action mediated by immune complexes may then lead to cellular and tissue damage. Instructive examples of autoantibodies and complement-mediated diseases are immune hemolytic anemias, myasthenia gravis, and bullous pemphigoid. The basic problem or pathologic defect in this type of human disease is the formation of the autoantibody. A misidentification of self has occurred because of a breaking of tolerance. In this pathologic situation, the complement system is working at the behest of the autoantibody.

TABLE 37-1 COMPLEMENT SYSTEM IN HOST DEFENSE AGAINST BACTERIA AND VIRUSES

THE ACTIVITY	THE PLAYERS
Opsonization	(C3b > C4b, C1q, MBL)*
Membrane perturbation including lysis (the membrane attack complex)	(C5b-C9)
Pro-inflammatory via cellular activation (the anaphylatoxins and their receptors)	(C3a, C4a, C5a)

*C3b is the major opsonin of the complement system. C1q and MBL (mannose- or mannan-binding lectin) both participate in classical and lectin pathway activation, respectively, but also bind to their specific receptors upon attachment to a target.

TABLE 37-2 SALIENT FEATURES OF THE COMPLEMENT SYSTEM

Ancient innate system of immunity predominantly found in blood (the "guardian of the intravascular space")
Capable of rapidly opsonizing and lysing bacteria and viruses (millions of active fragments can be deposited on a target)
Works in seconds!
Most proteins are synthesized by the liver, but local production is also important to outcomes
Constantly turning over (AP protein C3 "ticks over" at a rate of 1 to 2%/hr)
The AP also features a feedback or amplification loop, which requires tight control
Effector arm of the humoral immune system (IgM, IgG, and IgA)
Critical for clearance of self-debris (garbage removal)
After immunoglobulins and albumin, complement proteins are among the most abundant in blood
Nature's adjuvant (almost all foreign antigens are coated with complement fragments); instructs the adaptive immune response
A deficiency of an activator leads to bacterial infections or autoimmunity (SLE)
A deficiency of a regulator leads to undesirable cellular and tissue damage at sites of injury or degeneration (excessive activation): atypical hemolytic uremic syndrome, age-related macular degeneration

aHUS = atypical hemolytic uremic syndrome; AMD = age-related macular degeneration; AP = alternative pathway; Ig = immunoglobulin; SLE = systemic lupus erythematosus.

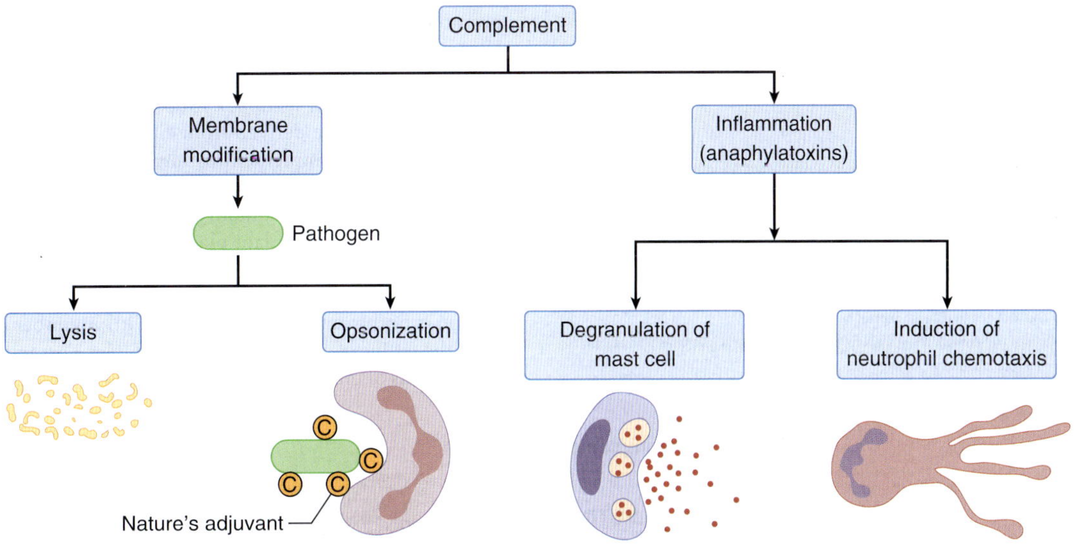

FIGURE 37-1. Function of the complement system. The most important function of the complement system is to alter the membrane of the pathogen by coating its surface with clusters of activation fragments. In one case, they facilitate the key process of opsonization in which C4b and C3b interact with complement receptors. In the other case, as with certain gram-negative bacteria and viruses, the membrane attack complex lyses the organism. The second critical function of complement is to activate cells and thus promote inflammatory and immune responses. The complement fragments C3a and C5a (known as anaphylatoxins) stimulate many cell types such as mast cells to release their contents and stimulate phagocytic cells to migrate to sites of inflammation (chemotaxis) and T cells to modulate metabolism and promote polarization. Through these phenomena of opsonization and cell activation, complement serves as nature's adjuvant to prepare, facilitate, and instruct the host's adaptive immune response. Because extracellular complement activation occurs in a few seconds, this innate immune system initially engages most pathogens, especially those that try to enter the vascular space. As will be illustrated, these basic functions are also required to handle immune complexes and prevent autoimmunity. (Modified from Arthritis Foundation. *Primer on the Rheumatic Diseases*, 12th ed. Atlanta, GA: Arthritis Foundation; 2001.)

The classical pathway is also activated by means other than the formation of IgM- and IgG-bearing immune complexes. β-Amyloid in the neuritic plaques of patients with Alzheimer disease directly engages the classical pathway via an interaction with C1q (Table 37-5). Likewise, C-reactive protein (CRP) and serum amyloid protein bind to chromatin and other ribonucleoprotein complexes released from apoptotic cells, and these types of complexes activate the classical pathway. The classical pathway also plays a key role in the opsonization and removal of nuclear debris. Approximately 80% of patients with hereditary absence of C1q or C4 develop SLE. Deposits of CRP and activated C1 have been demonstrated in ischemic tissue such as infarcted human myocardium. These observations indicate that classical pathway activation via these antibody-independent means is critical in protecting against autoimmune responses by facilitating debris clearance.

Regulation of classical pathway activation occurs at two levels. First, the *ser*ine *p*rotease *in*hibitor (serpin) known as the C1-inhibitor (C1-INH) blocks the activity of many proteases, including factor XIIa, kallikrein, and factor XIa of the clotting system as well as C1r, C1s, and MASP2 of the complement system. The importance of C1-INH is exemplified by its role in hereditary angioedema (Table 37-6). In this dominantly inherited disease, a deficiency of C1-INH allows uncontrolled proteolysis of C4 and C2 and generation of bradykinin, leading to recurrent swelling episodes. This serpin prevents chronic activation of the classical pathway cascade and, after a few minutes, helps to shut down the system. Classical pathway activation is also regulated by multiple inhibitors at the key step of C3 activation. These plasma and membrane proteins inhibit C3 convertase formation on healthy self. Membrane regulators are highly expressed on most cell types, where they prevent activation on normal self and overexuberant activation on altered self.

TABLE 37-3 PARTICIPATION OF THE COMPLEMENT SYSTEM IN HUMAN DISEASE

Activation by autoantibody (formation of immune complexes)
Engagement with modified self (clearance of debris or garbage) • Degenerative processes (diseases of aging such as age-related macular degeneration) • Cell and tissue damage (ischemia-reperfusion injury; atypical hemolytic uremic syndrome)

TABLE 37-4 PATHOLOGIC CONDITIONS ASSOCIATED WITH COMPLEMENT ACTIVATION

Examples of diseases in which complement activation contributes to the immunopathology:
Atypical hemolytic uremic syndrome*†
Paroxysmal nocturnal hemoglobinuria†
Age-related macular degeneration*†
Membranoproliferative glomerulonephritis (types 1, 2, and 3)†‡
Myasthenia gravis‡
Neuromyelitis optica spectrum disorder
Bullous pemphigoid‡
Systemic lupus erythematosus/antiphospholipid syndrome‡
Rheumatoid arthritis‡
Immune hemolytic anemias‡
Immune vasculitis (ANCA-positive syndromes)‡
Ischemia reperfusion injury*†
Allotransplantation‡
Amyotrophic lateral sclerosis‡
Transplantation rejection‡
Serum sickness‡
Exposures to foreign materials (e.g., membranes, nanoparticles, gene therapy viruses)*

*Injury, ischemia, trauma, degeneration, or foreign body is the trigger (innate immune activation).
†Lack of adequate regulation contributes to disease pathogenesis.
‡Antibody-dependent activation of the complement system (adaptive humoral immune activation).
ANCA = antineutrophil cytoplasmic antibody.

LECTIN PATHWAY

The protein mannose-binding lectin (MBL) is a member of the collectin family that also includes pulmonary surfactants A and D. MBL has a structure similar to C1q in that it consists of several subunits; namely, a globular recognition head domain for carbohydrates and a collagen-like tail that interacts with serine proteases. In the case of MBL, the globular domain is a lectin (protein) that binds to repeating mannose and *N*-acetylglucosamine residues on the surface of pathogens (see Figs. 37-2 and 37-3). Many microorganisms are recognized by MBL, including gram-positive and gram-negative bacteria, mycobacteria, fungi, parasites, and viruses (including human immunodeficiency virus 1 [HIV-1]). In general, as would be expected, mammalian glycoproteins and glycolipids are not readily recognized by MBL and the related lectins (ficolins and collectins) that activate the lectin pathway.

Three serine proteases, MASP-1, MASP-2, and MASP-3, associate with MBL (and the ficolins and collectins) through their collagen-like domain. This is analogous to the association of C1r and C1s with C1q. Activation of MASP-2, with some help from MASP-1, results in cleavage of C2 and C4, leading to formation of the classical/lectin pathway C3 convertase (C4b2a).

Genetic variations in the structural and regulatory portions of the MBL gene lead to wide differences in serum levels. A low level of MBL is associated with recurrent infections in children and adults and is a risk factor for the development of SLE. More striking is the association of low levels of MBL with infections in the setting of the treatment of SLE. For example, heterozygous MBL deficiency has been associated with a four-fold increase in the risk of bacterial pneumonia and homozygous deficiency with a more than 100-fold increase.[8]

ALTERNATIVE PATHWAY

The alternative pathway takes advantage of the fact that C3 undergoes spontaneous, chronic, low-grade activation (Fig. 37-4; see also Figs. 37-2 and 37-3). This C3b may covalently attach to any cell; however, on normal self, amplification of the cascade is blocked by inhibitors. In contrast, deposition on polysaccharides of bacterial membranes and to other targets, such as endotoxin and virally infected cells, leads to a rapid engagement of this pathway. These sites, similar to immune complexes and almost any type of biomaterial (cardiopulmonary bypass and hemodialysis membranes, nanoparticles, and so on), lack regulators, so rapid, massive activation may occur. IgA also has the capacity to promote activation of the alternative pathway.

During spontaneous activation, called *tickover*, small amounts of activated C3 are continuously generated (C3 turns over in blood at 1 to 2%/hour). It can initiate a feedback loop and cleave more C3 to C3b. Also, the initial C3b may be derived from either the classical or lectin pathway. Thus, activation of complement by any one of the three pathways has the potential to be rapidly magnified. The alternative pathway C3 convertase is negatively controlled (to maintain homeostasis), both in the fluid phase and on host cells, by two abundant plasma proteins and two widely expressed membrane proteins.[9]

The central role of the alternative pathway as an amplifier of complement activation is borne out by its association with a number of clinicopathologic states in the setting of deficient regulation (Tables 37-6 and 37-7). For example, multiple forms of membranoproliferative glomerulonephritis (Chapter 107)

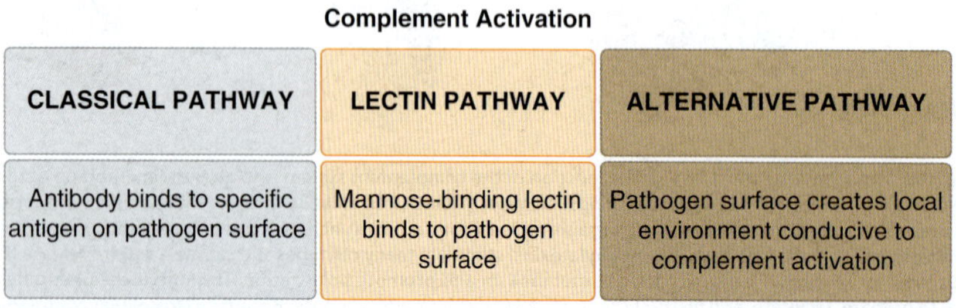

FIGURE 37-2. The three pathways of complement activation. The system is designed to be most efficient on a membrane surface. However, complement activation in the fluid phase, as, for example, in serum sickness, also occurs. In addition, the alternative pathway is continuously at a low level turning over (tickover) in the fluid phase (see Fig. 37-3).

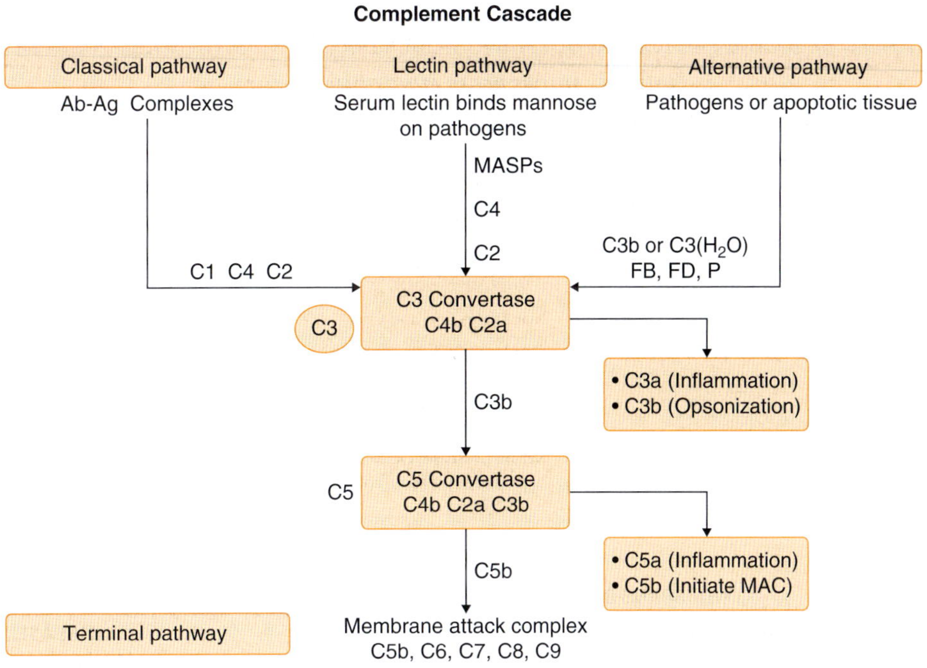

FIGURE 37-3. **Classical and lectin pathway activation.** Ab = antibody; Ag = antigen; FB = pro-enzyme factor B; FD = protease factor D; MAC = membrane attack complex; MASP = mannan-associated serine protease; P = complement factor P.

TABLE 37-5 TISSUE INJURY OR DEGENERATION AND COMPLEMENT ACTIVATION*

Age-related macular degeneration
Osteoarthritis (degenerative joint disease)
Ischemic stroke
Myocardial infarction
Traumatic injury (e.g., brain, liver, kidney, gut)
Ischemia-reperfusion injury
Burns
Acute respiratory distress syndrome
Septic shock
Multiorgan failure syndromes
Alzheimer disease

*In these conditions, complement activation leads to deposition of fragments at the site of injury; however, how much of the tissue injury is attributable to complement system is unknown. In many cases, animal models support a pathologic role for the complement system. Only in age-related macular degeneration is there also powerful genetic evidence in humans to indicate a key role for the complement system.

are associated with excessive deposition of C3 fragments in the kidney because of either the presence of autoantibodies (C3 or C4 nephritic factors) that stabilize C3 convertases or a genetic deficiency in complement regulatory protein (factor H or factor I). Likewise, atypical hemolytic uremic syndrome[10] (i.e., not associated with a preceding enteropathic infection featuring a Shiga-like toxin) occurs (Chapter 158) in individuals who harbor heterozygous missense mutations in factor H, membrane cofactor protein (MCP), or factor I or have gain-in-function mutations in factor B or C3. Genome-wide association and targeted deep sequencing studies have also linked age-related macular degeneration and diabetic retinopathy[11] (Chapter 391) to functional coding mutations in factor H and factor I and, more uncommonly, in factor B and C3. Finally, rodent models of rheumatoid arthritis, SLE, and antineutrophil cytoplasmic antibody (ANCA)–positive vasculitic syndromes[12] are ameliorated if the alternative pathway is disrupted.

C3 AND C5 CONVERTASES

The three activation pathways converge at C3. A remarkable feature of C3 is the presence of a thioester bond. Buried within the three-dimensional structure of the C3 protein lies a γ-carboxy group of a reactive glutamic acid residue linked to a cysteine in an "internal thioester." Upon its cleavage, for a few microseconds, a covalent attachment can occur via an ester or amide linkage to any nearby hydroxyl or amino group. Most of the cleaved thioester bonds are hydrolyzed by water to produce a form of C3 (known as C3 [H_2O]); however, a substantial percentage forms an amide or ester bond to amino groups or carbohydrates, thereby covalently attaching C3b to a target's surface. Also, the addition of a C3b to C4b2a (classical/lectin pathway C3 convertase) or to C3bBb (alternative pathway C3 convertase) then forms a convertase for C5 (C3bBbC3b for the alternative pathway and C4bC2aC3b for the classical/lectin pathway).

REGULATORS OF COMPLEMENT ACTIVATION AT THE C3 AND C5 STEPS

The regulators of complement activation (see Table 37-6) limit the production of C3b, primarily by the alternative pathway C3 convertases. Because the addition of C3b to a C3 convertase makes it a C5 convertase, regulation of the two enzyme complexes is linked. Modulation of their activity on host cells limits tissue destruction and the production of inflammatory mediators.

The complement activation regulatory proteins control complement activation by two processes. *Decay-accelerating activity* refers to when the inhibitor transiently binds to C3b or C4b in the convertase and thereby dissociates the other members of the complex, rendering it enzymatically inactive (as the component released is the catalytic domain of the protease). The second is cofactor activity, which requires recognition of C3b or C4b by a plasma cofactor protein. Upon this interaction, the protease, factor I, cleaves C3b or C4b. Cleavage of C3b by factor I renders the convertase irreversibly inactive (generates iC3b, which cannot participate in convertase formation).

MEMBRANE ATTACK COMPLEX

The cleavage of C5 generates C5a, the most potent of the complement anaphylatoxins, and C5b. C5b associates with C6 and C7 to create a lipophilic trimer as the initial part of the membrane attack complex (see E-Fig. 37-1). The C5b67 trimer inserts into the lipid bilayer and serves as a binding site for C8 and C9. C9 self-polymerizes, leading to 12 to 18 C9 molecules that form a ring structure, completing the membrane attack complex. The membrane attack complex resembles a doughnut with a 10-nm pore running through the center. This pore allows water and ions to enter the cells, ultimately leading to osmotic lysis. Many pathogens such as gram-positive bacteria possess a capsule that makes them resistant to lysis. Opsonization leading to phagocytosis is thus the major means of eliminating such organisms.

The membrane attack complex appears to be essential only for elimination of *Neisseria* spp. Individuals completely deficient in C5, C6, C7, C8, or C9 are at an increased risk only for meningococcal and gonococcal infections (Chapters 274 and 275). C9 deficiency is a common immunodeficiency in Japan, with a heterozygote frequency of 3 to 5%. Thus, heterozygous deficiency seems to not be deleterious to the population in general but may have a selective advantage.

TABLE 37-6 SOLUBLE AND MEMBRANE FACTORS REGULATING COMPLEMENT

SOLUBLE FACTORS REGULATING COMPLEMENT			
NAME	**LIGAND OR BINDING FACTOR**	**FUNCTIONAL ACTIVITY**	**PATHOLOGY, IF DEFICIENT**
C1-INH	C1r, C1s, mannan-binding lectin-associated serine protease (MASP-2)	Binds to and displaces C1r and C1s from C1q and mannan-binding lectin-associated serine protease (MASP-2) from mannan or mannose binding lectin (MBL)	Hereditary angioedema
C4bp* (C4 binding protein)	C4b, glycosaminoglycans	Displaces C2a (decay-accelerating activity); cofactor for C4b cleavage by factor I (cofactor activity)	No clinical syndrome clearly defined
CPN-1 (carboxypeptidase-N)	C3a, C5a	Inactivates C3a and C5a	Urticaria and angioedema
Factor H*†	C3b, C3d, glycosaminoglycans	Displaces Bb from alternative pathway C3 and C5 convertases (decay-accelerating activity) and is a cofactor for factor I to cleave C3b (cofactor activity)	Age-related macular degeneration, atypical hemolytic uremic syndrome, C3 glomerulopathies, bacterial infections secondary to low C3
Factor I†	C3b, C4b	Serine protease; cleaves C3b and C4b, requires a cofactor protein (cofactor activity)	Age-related macular degeneration, atypical hemolytic uremic syndrome, bacterial infections secondary to low C3
Protein S (vitronectin)	C5b67	Inhibits membrane attachment by C5b67	None defined
MEMBRANE-BOUND FACTORS REGULATING COMPLEMENT			
NAME	**LIGAND OR BINDING FACTOR**	**FUNCTIONAL ACTIVITY**	**DISEASE, IF DEFICIENT**
Decay-accelerating factor (CD55)	C3 and C5 convertases	Prevents binding and displaces Bb from alternative pathway convertase and C2a from CP or LP convertases, respectively	Paroxysmal nocturnal hemoglobinuria Polyneuropathy syndromes CD55 deficiency with hyperactivation of complement, angiopathic thrombosis, and protein-losing enteropathy (CHAPLE syndrome)
Membrane cofactor protein (MCP, CD46)	C3b, C4b	Cofactor for factor I (cofactor activity)	Atypical hemolytic uremic syndrome, immune deficiency
Protectin (CD59)	C8, C9	Inhibits MAC formation and insertion	Paroxysmal nocturnal hemoglobinuria
Complement receptor type 1 (CD35) (immune adherence or C4b/C3b receptor)	C3b, C4b, C3, and C5 convertases	Cofactor for factor I to cleave C4b and C3b (cofactor activity); displaces Bb from C3b and C2a from C4b to inhibit convertases (decay-accelerating activity)	No complete deficiency described; decreased levels in immune complex–mediated diseases such as lupus
Complement receptor of the immunoglobulin superfamily (CRIg)	C3b, iC3b, C3c	Inhibits activation of alternative pathway	None defined

*Factors H and C4bp also bind to surfaces, particularly at sites of tissue and cellular injury, where they carry out regulatory activity.

†If heterozygous deficient, the individual is predisposed to age-related macular degeneration and atypical hemolytic uremic syndrome. If homozygous deficient, the AP turns over excessively, resulting in kidney disease (C3 glomerulopathies) and bacterial infections (secondary to the very low C3).

$(C3b)_2$ Bb = alternative pathway C5 convertase; C3bC4bC2a = classical and lectin pathway C5 convertase; C4bC2a = classical and lectin pathway C3 convertase; MAC = membrane attack complex.

Extensive complement activation during an inflammatory response can result in sufficient membrane attack complex deposition to produce host cell lysis. Host cells, however, have mechanisms in place to resist the osmotic changes caused by the membrane attack complex and to block assembly of the membrane attack complex as it is formed (the protein is known as protectin or CD59). Rather, the nonlethal effects of sublytic membrane attack complex deposition are more likely to contribute to pathology. In most cells, this occurs through a general activation of multiple cell signaling pathways.

The response to membrane attack complex deposition at sites of complement activation depends on the cell type (Table 37-8). In phagocytic cells, such as neutrophils or macrophages, sublytic membrane attack complex insertion leads to the production of reactive oxygen species (e.g., superoxide, hydrogen peroxide) as well as release of prostaglandins and leukotrienes. Platelets undergoing a "membrane attack complex insertion" expose phosphatidylserine on their outer membrane, facilitating assembly of blood coagulation enzyme complexes on their surfaces with a potentially procoagulant effect. On endothelial cells, membrane attack complex deposition induces the synthesis of interleukin-1α (IL-1α), which leads to further autocrine and paracrine endothelial cell activation. It stimulates a procoagulant state by (1) altering the phospholipid composition of the endothelial membrane; (2) inducing the synthesis of tissue factor and upregulating the synthesis of plasminogen activator inhibitor; (3) upregulating the expression of adhesion molecules, including intercellular adhesion molecule 1 (ICAM-1) and E-selectin; and (4) stimulating endothelial cells to proliferate through growth factor production. In summary, although cell death does not usually occur, deposition of the sublytic levels of membrane attack complex leads to a potentially dangerous situation, with increased inflammation, a procoagulant state, and cellular proliferation. Of course, part of this response is necessary at sites of injury to eliminate pathogens and debris and to facilitate wound repair. The short duration of complement activation and the presence of inhibitors help to maintain homeostasis.

Regulation of membrane attack complex formation is important clinically (Fig. 37-5). Two plasma proteins, S-protein (vitronectin) and possibly clusterin, bind the C5b-7 complex and prevent its association with the lipid membrane. C8 and multiple C9 molecules adhere to this soluble complex, termed *soluble C5b-9*, which is lytically inactive. CD59 (protectin) is a membrane-bound inhibitor of membrane attack complex formation. This small glycoprotein is attached to the cell membrane through a glycosyl phosphatidylinositol tail (GPI anchor). It binds to C5b-8, inserted in the cell membrane, to prevent binding to and polymerization of C9. The expression of CD59 is defective in patients with paroxysmal nocturnal hemoglobinuria (Chapter 146), owing to the failure to synthesize the GPI anchor used by this and many other membrane proteins (including decay-accelerating factor [DAF]) to insert on the cell. The clinical features of paroxysmal nocturnal hemoglobinuria are primarily chronic hemolysis and intermittent thrombosis. Hemolysis is caused by complement activation on red cells because of a lack of DAF and particularly CD59. Thrombosis (Chapter 67) is likely secondary to intravascular complement activation, leading to endothelial cell activation. The primary defect is an acquired somatic hematopoietic stem cell mutation of a gene on the X chromosome responsible for encoding the first enzyme in the pathway to synthesize a GPI anchor.

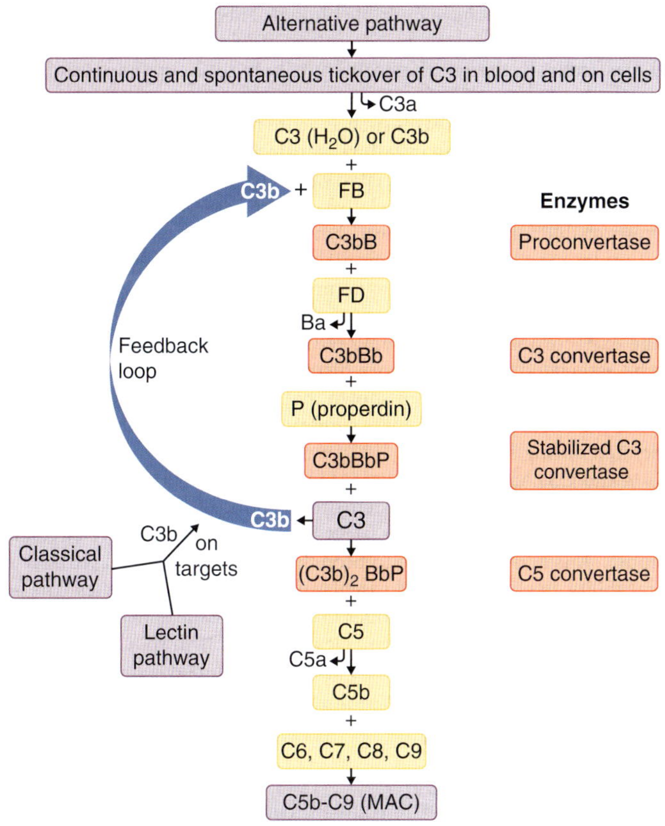

FIGURE 37-4. Complement activation pathways. In the reaction cascade shown, C3b or C3 (H_2O) binds the pro-enzyme factor B (FB), and the C3bB or C3 (H_2O)B complex then is cleaved by the protease factor D (FD). FD is generated by the cleavage of inactive pro-FD to active FD by the protease MASP-3. The addition of properdin (P) to the enzyme complex increases the half-life of the enzyme complex approximately 10-fold. Although the source of the C3b can be from spontaneous turnover or via lectin pathway (LP) and classical pathway (CP) activation, the alternative pathway (AP) feedback loop commonly takes over to generate much of C3b that binds to a target. The alternative pathway is continuously turning over. If activated C3b or C3 (H_2O) remains in the fluid phase, it is rapidly inhibited by the plasma regulators factor H and factor I. If activated C3b binds to normal or healthy self, it is prevented from forming a convertase by the ubiquitously expressed membrane cofactor protein (MCP [CD46]) and decay-accelerating factor (DAF [CD55]) (not shown). DAF both prevents B from binding to C3b and "kicks out" the catalytic Bb domain (a temporary stop), but MCP is a permanent stop because, upon its binding, the C3b is proteolytically cleaved to inactive C3b (iC3b) by the serine protease factor I. The feedback loop is a powerful amplification system. A single *Escherichia coli* organism in blood can be coated with several million C3bs in a couple of minutes!

ANAPHYLATOXINS

The anaphylatoxins serve a key early role in initiating a local inflammatory response as they trigger pathways to prepare a cell to face a pathogen or injury (Table 37-9). Similar to the membrane attack complex, anaphylatoxins are another major source of potential pathologic damage to self that results from complement activation. These peptides, C3a and C5a, are cleaved from their respective proteins during complement activation. They are 77 (C3a) or 74 (C5a) amino acids long and contain a key carboxy (C)-terminal arginine. They interact with the anaphylatoxin receptors. In plasma, the C-terminal arginine is removed by carboxypeptidase-N from anaphylatoxins not bound to their receptors. Depending on the response studied, this removal totally inactivates the anaphylatoxin or reduces its potency by about 1000-fold.

TABLE 37-8 RESPONSES TO SUBLYTIC MEMBRANE ATTACK COMPLEX ACTIVATION

CELL TYPE	EFFECTS
Most cells	Increased intracellular calcium flux Activation of G proteins Activation of protein kinases Activation of transcription factors Proliferation
Neutrophils and macrophages	Release of reactive oxygen species Activation of phospholipase A_2 Release of prostaglandins, thromboxane, and leukotrienes
Platelets	Release of adenosine triphosphate Increased P-selectin expression Procoagulant membrane changes
Endothelial cells	Increased synthesis of IL-1α Increased release of tissue factor Increased release of von Willebrand factor Increased synthesis of basic fibroblast and platelet-derived growth factors
Synoviocytes	Increased synthesis of prostaglandins Increased synthesis of interleukin-6 Increased production of matrix metalloproteinase
Glomerular epithelium	Activation of phospholipase A_2 Synthesis of prostaglandin Increased synthesis of collagen and fibronectin
Oligodendrocytes	Increased synthesis of myelin basic protein and proteolipids Increased proliferation

TABLE 37-7 COMPLEMENT SYSTEM MEDIATES THE DISEASE PROCESS AND ITS INHIBITION TREATS THE CONDITION

DISEASE	PATHOPHYSIOLOGY	ETIOLOGY	TREATMENT	FDA APPROVED
Paroxysmal nocturnal hemoglobinuria (Chapter 146)	Lyse red blood cells	Acquired hematopoietic somatic stem cell mutation in gene required for synthesis of glycosylphosphatidylinositol (GPI) anchor	Monoclonal antibody to C5 Peptide C3 convertase inhibitor	Yes Yes
Atypical hemolytic uremic syndrome (Chapter 158)	Damage to endothelial cells	Inherited loss-of-function variants in alternative pathway regulators or gain of function variants in alternative pathway activators	Monoclonal antibody to C5	Yes
Hereditary angioedema (Chapter 232)	Bradykinin generation	Autosomal dominant variants in the C1-inhibitor gene	C1 inhibitor replacement Bradykinin receptor blockage Kallikrein inhibitors	Yes Yes Yes
Age-related macular degeneration (Chapter 391)	Degeneration of the retina	Inherited variants in a regulator (factor H or factor I) or gain-in-function in an alternative pathway component (C3 or factor B)	Clinical trials in progress	No
Neuromyelitis optica spectrum disorder (Chapter 392)	Damage to spinal cord and optic nerve	Complement-fixing autoantibodies to aquaporin-4 typically found	Monoclonal antibody to C5	Yes
Myasthenia gravis (Chapter 390)	Degeneration of neuromuscular junction	Complement-fixing autoantibodies to acetylcholine receptor	Monoclonal antibody to C5	Yes

FDA = Food and Drug Administration.

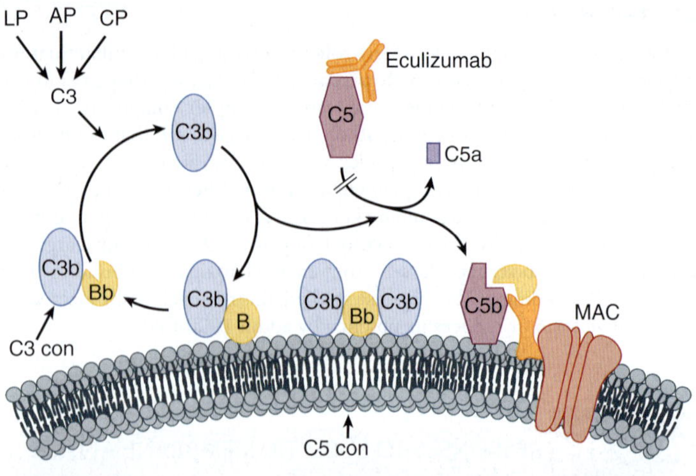

FIGURE 37-5. **Complement activation and the mechanism of action of eculizumab (monoclonal antibody [mAb] to C5).** The alternative pathway (AP) constantly undergoes "tickover" but can also be primed by the classical pathway (CP) and lectin pathway (LP). The C3b that is formed interacts with factor B (B), which is then cleaved by factor D to form a C3 convertase (C3Bb). As more C3b is generated, a fraction binds to the C3 convertase to form a C5 convertase. Monoclonal antibody to C5 (eculizumab) prevents the cleavage of C5 by the C5 convertase. Not shown is that properdin binds to both the C3 and C5 convertases to increase their half-lives approximately five- to 10-fold (from ≈30 seconds to several minutes). (Modified from Wong EK, Goodship TH, Kavanagh D. Complement therapy in atypical haemolytic uraemic syndrome [aHUS]. *Mol Immunol*. 2013;56:199-212.)

TABLE 37-9 DISTRIBUTION OF ANAPHYLATOXIN RECEPTORS AND THEIR CELLULAR RESPONSES

CELL TYPE	RESPONSES
C5aR (CD88)	
Neutrophils	Chemotaxis
Eosinophils	Enzyme release
Basophils	Generation of reactive oxygen species
Mast cells	Upregulation of adhesion molecules
Monocytes	Increased synthesis of interleukin-1, interleukin-6, and interleukin-8
	Prostaglandin and leukotriene synthesis
Hepatocytes	Increased synthesis of acute phase reactants
Pulmonary epithelium	Increased interleukin-8
Neuronal cells	Cellular activation
Endothelial cells	Increased expression of P-selectin
Renal epithelial/mesangial cells	Proliferation and synthesis of growth factors
C3aR	
Eosinophils	Chemotaxis
Mast cells	Enzyme release
Platelets	Generation of reactive oxygen species
	Upregulation of adhesion molecules
Epithelial, endothelial, etc.	Cellular activation

IL = interleukin.

The C5a receptor (C5aR [CD88]) is a seven-transmembrane-spanning protein that couples ligand binding to G-protein signaling. Expressed on myeloid cells, particularly neutrophils and eosinophils, it mediates the potent chemoattractant property of C5a for both of these cell types. Signaling through CD88 leads to rapid secretion of all granule contents. These contents include lipases and proteases as well as lactoferrin from neutrophils and peroxidase, major basic protein, and cationic protein from eosinophils. C5a also induces the release of cytokines, such as tumor necrosis factor (TNF), IL-1, IL-6, IL-8, and adhesion molecules, promoting the inflammatory response. The C5aR is expressed by numerous other tissues, including hepatocytes, bronchial and alveolar epithelium, vascular endothelium, renal mesangial and tubular epithelial cells, and brain neuronal cells. These cells are activated by receptor engagement, leading to production and release of cytokines, chemokines, and prostaglandins and to cellular proliferation.

The C3a receptor is also a seven-transmembrane-domain protein. It is expressed on almost all myeloid cells, including mast cells, where it mediates the release of allergic mediators. The C3aR also has been detected on many tissues, including in the brain and lung.

The anaphylatoxins have multiple biologic effects. In general, they cause smooth muscle contraction and recruitment of granulocytes, monocytes, and mast cells. In theory, they can contribute to the pathophysiology of any inflammatory condition. In disease models, C3a and C5a have been shown to play a role in diseases such as acute respiratory distress syndrome (ARDS), multisystem organ failure, septic shock, myocardial ischemia-reperfusion injury, ANCA-associated vasculitis, asthma, rheumatoid arthritis, SLE, and inflammatory bowel disease. The anaphylatoxin peptides also are responsible for the "postpump" syndrome seen in patients undergoing cardiopulmonary bypass or hemodialysis. Exposure of blood to dialysis or perfusion membranes leads to complement activation. Within minutes of starting bypass, there is a sharp increase in the levels of C3a and C5a in the extracorporeal circuit being returned to the patient. This increase can be associated with respiratory distress, pulmonary hypertension, and pulmonary edema. It has been shown that the length of time that patients stay on the ventilator after bypass surgery correlates with the level of C3a generated during reperfusion.

C3a and C5a have been implicated in the initiation and prolongation of ARDS (Chapter 90) and multisystem organ failure. After severe trauma, levels of C3a have been measured that suggest activation of the entire circulating C3 pool. This activation leads to bronchoconstriction, increased vascular permeability, hypotension, and vascular plugging with leukocytes. The activation of white blood cells continues the cycle of tissue damage with further complement activation. Continued elevation of C3a in shock or ARDS is a poor prognostic sign. C3a and C5a also appear to play a major role in the pathogenesis of asthma (Chapter 75).

COMPLEMENT RECEPTORS

Opsonization of target by C4b and C3b is effective in preventing infections because these two complement fragments (and the further cleavage products in the case of C3b) are ligands for complement receptors (E-Fig. 37-2). After covalent attachment of C4b and C3b, immune adherence occurs between the opsonized microbe and immune cells, predominantly neutrophils, monocytes, and macrophages. Complement opsonins are highly effective mediators of immune adherence. On phagocytic cells, this is the prelude to the ingestion and destruction of the target antigen. On red cells, immune adherence is followed by transfer of the C4b/C3b-coated cargo to monocytes and macrophages in the liver and spleen. CR1 is particularly efficient at immune adherence. Proteolytic modification of C3b leads to iC3b, which is a ligand for the highly phagocytic CR3 and CR4. A further degradation of iC3b to C3d leads to an interaction with CR2 to lower the threshold of B-cell activation. Overall, the process is designed with two goals in mind: (1) destruction by phagocytosis of the microbe and (2) coating of microbial antigens for an adaptive immune response. For example, follicular dendritic cells and B lymphocytes express CR1, CR2, CR3, and CR4 that facilitate complement-coated antigens to be bound, internalized, and presented to other immune cells. CR3 and CR4 facilitate phagocytosis, and CR2 on follicular dendritic cells facilitates immunologic memory generation.

COMPLEMENT INHIBITORS

Given the many disease states in which complement is one of the central mediators of pathology, it is no surprise that complement inhibitors are in preclinical or clinical development for treatment of human diseases (see Table 37-2 and E-Fig. 37-2). These inhibitors take several different forms. Whereas some are variations of physiologic inhibitors, others are the products of molecular biologic searches for novel compounds.[13,14]

It is important to consider where in the complement pathway to design an inhibitor to act. Inhibition of the activation pathways limits the production of biologically active peptides. Inhibiting the activation of C3 not only prevents the generation of the C3a anaphylatoxin but also may leave the patient susceptible to infection by limiting the deposition of C3b on targets as an opsonin. Inhibition of C3b deposition would decrease the patient's ability to clear immune complexes, potentially resulting in renal, pulmonary, and vascular damage. It also might promote the development of antibodies to self-antigens.

Inhibition of the C5 convertases is an attractive goal because it would prevent the generation of the C5a anaphylatoxin and the membrane attack complex (see Fig. 37-5). This strategy would inhibit complement activation without limiting C3b deposition. Inhibitors based on this concept have been successful; the monoclonal antibody to C5 is approved by the U.S. Food and Drug Administration (FDA) to treat paroxysmal nocturnal hemoglobinuria and atypical hemolytic-uremic syndrome (Chapter 158) as well as neuromyelitis optica spectrum disorder (Chapter 392) and myasthenia gravis (Chapter 390).

Other concerns about complement inhibition include whether it is short or long term and whether it is systemic or local. Long-term inhibition of complement, particularly at one of the early steps, is likely to predispose to infection and possibly autoimmunity. Short-term (hours to days) inhibition at any step is unlikely to cause problems. Given that inflammation is usually a local phenomenon, several mechanisms are being tested to target complement inhibitors to these sites. In this way, higher levels of inhibition can be achieved when needed and with lower doses of inhibitor.

NATURAL COMPLEMENT INHIBITORS

Naturally occurring compounds that control complement activation include products or extracts of plants, fungi, insects, bacteria, viruses, and venoms. The mechanism of complement inhibition by some of these natural products is known and is of clinical and experimental importance. In particular, to protect themselves from the host's complement system, poxviruses, herpesviruses, and flaviviruses produce either mimics of the human regulators that they at one time hijacked from their hosts or proteins that bind the hosts' regulators such as the plasma protein factor H. Bacteria also express a wide variety of inhibitors of the human complement system. *Staphylococcus aureus*, for example, synthesizes up to 10 distinct proteins that inhibit at almost every key step of the complement cascade. Cobra venom factor (CVF) is a modified form of cobra C3b secreted by venom glands in the oral cavity. It is a 144,000-dalton glycoprotein that forms an alternative pathway convertase in association with host factor B. Upon injection, CVF leads to massive activation of the alternative pathway, resulting in shock and pulmonary microvascular injury in experimental animals. It is resistant to the host's inhibitors because the site for that interaction is altered on CVF. Perhaps the most widely used natural inhibitor of complement activation is heparin. It decreases activation of the classical pathway and alternative pathway. In clinical practice, the anticomplementary effect of heparin has been used to prevent complement activation during cardiopulmonary bypass. Measurement of complement activation products such as C3a or soluble C5b-9 after bypass showed decreases of 35 to 70% for adult and pediatric patients when heparin-coated extracorporeal circuits were used. Although numerous studies have looked at the decrease in complement activation by heparin-coated bypass circuits, there have been few attempts to correlate this with clinical outcome.

ANTI-C5

The complement inhibitor that has achieved the widest attention as a therapeutic agent to stop complement activation is a monoclonal antibody that targets C5 and prevents its cleavage to C5a (potent anaphylatoxin) and C5b (initiator of the membrane attack complex) (see Fig. 37-5). The generation of the C3b and C4b still occurs, allowing opsonization of pathogens and formation of immune complexes. Because activation of early complement components is also important for the maintenance of tolerance to self-antigens, inhibition of C5 activation is less worrisome than inhibition of C3 activation. The one consequence of C5 deficiency in humans is an increased risk of *Neisseria* infections (Chapters 274 and 275) that can largely be mitigated through vaccination. The anti-C5 monoclonal antibody eculizumab has been approved for use in patients with paroxysmal nocturnal hemoglobinuria, atypical hemolytic uremic syndrome, neuromyelitis optica, and myasthenia gravis. Additional inhibitors targeting the C3 convertase, specific complement receptors, and early pathway-specific activation mechanisms are all under active development and clinical trials.

The complement system is undergoing a renaissance. There are several reasons but probably the foremost is the discovery of mutations in complement regulators leading to atypical hemolytic uremic syndrome and age-related macular degeneration. Second is the therapeutic success of a monoclonal antibody to C5 in the treatment of atypical hemolytic uremic syndrome and paroxysmal nocturnal hemoglobinuria. Third is the introduction of purified C1-INH, kallikrein inhibitors, and a bradykinin receptor antagonist to prevent and treat swelling attacks in hereditary angioedema. Last, intriguing recent data implicate the complement system in the pathophysiology of multiple disorders, including age-related macular degeneration, ischemia/reperfusion injury, organ regeneration, brain development (pruning of undesirable synapses), intracellular metabolomics and polarization processes, obesity, asthma, T-cell activation phenomena associated with allergic and rheumatic diseases,[15,16] and more.

GENERAL REFERENCES

For the General References and other additional features, please visit Elsevier eBooks+ at https://ebooks.health.elsevier.com.

38 TRANSPLANTATION IMMUNOLOGY

MEGAN SYKES

DEFINITION

Clinical transplantation encompasses transplantation of organs and islets of Langerhans containing insulin-producing β cells, in which it is necessary to overcome the host-versus-graft (HVG) immune response to avoid rejection, as well as hematopoietic cell transplantation (Chapter 163), in which it is necessary to contend with not only the HVG but also the graft-versus-host (GVH) immune response. Because preparations of bone marrow or mobilized peripheral blood stem cells contain mature T cells, their administration to conditioned and consequently immunoincompetent recipients is associated with the risk for GVH disease (GVHD). Transplanted organs and tissues include corneas, kidneys, livers, hearts, lungs, small intestines, pancreases, hands, and faces. Uterine, penile, and laryngeal transplantation are composite tissue transplants that have only recently become possible, and the numbers performed are consequently quite low.

Transplants originating from a member of the same species are referred to as *allotransplants*. However, transplants from other species, termed *xenografts*, provide a promising solution to the severely inadequate supply of allogeneic organs and tissues, and may be used in the future. Transplants of tissues or cells originating from the recipient, either by processing of cells from the recipient's own organ (e.g., islets of Langerhans following pancreatectomy for chronic pancreatitis) or cell populations (e.g., $CD34^+$ hematopoietic progenitor and stem cells collected from leukapheresis products following mobilization from the bone marrow before high-dose radiation or chemotherapy to treat cancer) are referred to as *autologous*. In the future, these transplants may include stem cell–derived autologous cells used for therapeutic purposes.

ANTIGENS IN TRANSPLANTATION

The major antigens recognized during graft rejection and the cell types targeting them are summarized in Table 38-1.

MAJOR HISTOCOMPATIBILITY ANTIGENS

The major histocompatibility complex (MHC; human leukocyte antigens [HLAs] in the human) controls adaptive and some innate immune responses and is of central importance in many immune-mediated diseases. The MHC also presents the strongest immunologic obstacle to all types of allografts. The HLA molecules include two major isoforms, termed class I and class II, and are all encoded in the MHC complex of chromosome 6. Although all HLA molecules have a similar general structure, class I and class II molecules show different expression patterns, with class I MHC expressed on most cells of the body, whereas class II antigens are expressed mainly on antigen-presenting cell populations, such as dendritic cells, macrophages, and B cells, as well as thymic epithelial cells involved in T-cell selection. Class II MHC can also be expressed on human vascular endothelial cells and activated T cells.

The function of both classes of MHC molecules is to present peptide antigens to T-cell receptors, allowing adaptive immune responses to occur (Chapter 35). Class I molecules typically present eight- to nine-amino acid peptides derived from cytosolic proteins (e.g., viral proteins) that are transported into the endoplasmic reticulum, where they are processed and loaded onto class I molecules. CD8 molecules interact with the α_3 domain of the class I heavy chain, thereby strengthening the interaction of $CD8^+$ T cells that recognize class I–peptide complexes. Peptides presented by class II MHC molecules, on the other hand, are mostly 10- to 20-mers derived from exogenous proteins (e.g., phagocytosed bacteria) that are processed through the endosomal processing pathway, and these are recognized by receptors of T cells whose CD4 molecules strengthen the overall T cell–antigen-presenting cell interaction. The class I presentation pathway is of particular importance in allowing destruction of virally infected cells, consistent with the expression of class I MHC on almost all cell types in the body. An exception occurs when class I molecules present peptides from exogenous antigens, thereby resulting in cross-presentation and cross-priming of T cells. Class II MHC presentation of exogenous antigens takes place primarily on professional antigen-presenting cells and B cells, consistent with the role of $CD4^+$ T cells in initiating immune responses by activating antigen-presenting cells, providing direct and indirect

TABLE 38-1 LYMPHOCYTES INVOLVED IN GRAFT REJECTION

CELL TYPE	ANTIGENS RECOGNIZED	FUNCTION	RELEVANCE
$CD4^+$ T cells	Allogeneic class II MHC (+ peptide) Self class II MHC + donor peptide	Antigen-presenting cell activation Help (cytokines and costimulation) Proinflammatory cytokine production Cytotoxicity Regulatory function	Organ allografts Cellular allografts Xenografts GVHD
$CD8^+$ T cells	Allogeneic class I MHC (+ peptide) Self class I MHC + donor peptide	Cytotoxicity Cytokine production Regulatory function	Organ allografts Cellular allografts Xenografts GVHD
NK cells	Class I MHC (activates or inhibits NK cell function) Other activating ligands	Cytotoxicity Cytokine production	Organ allografts Cellular allografts Xenografts
B cells	Class I and class II MHC Blood group antigens Xenogeneic carbohydrates	Antibody-mediated rejection (hyperacute, acute humoral, and chronic rejection)	Organ and hematopoietic cell allografts Cellular allografts Xenografts GVHD

CTL = cytotoxic T lymphocyte; GVHD = graft-versus-host disease; MHC = major histocompatibility complex; NK = natural killer.

(through activated antigen-presenting cells that also present peptides on class I molecules) "help" for $CD8^+$ cytotoxic T lymphocytes, and providing help for antibody-producing B cells. B cells are able to focus the antigens recognized by their specific surface immunoglobulin receptors by binding and internalizing these antigens, which enter the endosomal antigen-processing pathway and become presented by class II molecules on that B cell. This ability of B cells preferentially to present peptides derived from their cognate antigens to CD4 T cells recognizing those alloantigens is very important in driving alloantibody production.

A number of MHC molecules have been crystallized, both alone and with T-cell receptors that recognize them. The structure of class I and II MHC molecules is similar overall and includes both the peptide-binding cleft formed by a β-pleated sheet and two α-helices forming the sides of the cleft (E-Fig. 38-1). However, class I and II MHC molecules also have significant structural differences, as summarized in E-Table 38-1. T-cell receptors interact physically with both the α-helices of the MHC molecules and side chains of the peptide that is bound in the groove, thereby representing a trimolecular MHC-peptide–T-cell receptor interaction (see E-Fig. 38-1). The most variable ("hypervariable") portion of the T-cell receptor, which is produced by V-D (for TCRβ)-J somatic rearrangements and N insertions in the T-cell receptor α and β chains, known as complementarity-determining region 3 (CDR3), recognizes specific MHC-peptide complexes.

The HLA molecules are all encoded within a 3.6-million base-pair region that encodes more than 200 genes, including complement and tumor necrosis factor (TNF) genes and many others in addition to MHC that have immunologic functions. The organization of the HLA region is illustrated in E-Figure 38-2. The class II region contains two α- and β-chain genes, only one of which is functional, for each of HLA-DQ and DP. However, the DR locus contains different numbers of β-chains for different HLA alleles. Some of these DR β-chains are pseudogenes, but various HLA-DR alleles contain either one or two functional β-chain genes.

One of the striking features of HLA molecules (and the MHC of most mammalian species) is their extensive polymorphism.[1] The class I and class II regions contain thousands of defined HLA alleles. Because the primary function of antigen presentation to T cells is to permit responsiveness to and clearance of pathogenic microorganisms, this polymorphism may have evolved to maintain the diversity of immune responsiveness to various pathogens within a population, thereby avoiding annihilation of that population by a single microorganism that might not be presented well by a particular MHC. According to the most recently accepted nomenclature, HLA alleles are identified by the locus (e.g., HLA-A), followed by an asterisk, and then a unique number with up to four sets of digits separated by colons.[2] The first set describes the allele group (e.g., HLA-A*02), which usually corresponds to a serologically defined antigen, and the second set indicates the specific allele (e.g., HLA-A*02:101). The third and fourth sets of digits are of less practical importance because they identify silent nucleotide substitutions in different alleles and variations in the nontranslated regions of the gene, respectively.

Within certain populations, however, the level of diversity within allele groups may be quite limited because of the common genetic origin of the allele. For example, for the originally serologically defined HLA-DR3 allele group, there is little diversity among Northern Europeans, such that most carry the DRB1*0301 allele. Thus, for this population, it is reasonable to refer to the serologic HLA-DR3 type as defining this allele. Certain alleles predominate within racial groups. For example, as few as five DRB1 alleles predominate among Northern Europeans, with each allele represented in 10 to 30% of this population (E-Table 38-2).

Most organ transplantations are performed across HLA disparities, and the strong immunosuppressive regimens used in transplant recipients are designed to prevent rejection by this exceptionally strong immune response. In contrast to T-cell responses to peptide antigens derived from foreign proteins, which are recognized by a very small fraction of naïve T cells (in the range of 1 in 10^5), a very high proportion, estimated at 1 to 10% of the T-cell repertoire, recognizes MHC alloantigens. The application of high-throughput sequencing of the hypervariable regions of T-cell receptors of those T cells that proliferate to allogeneic MHC has directly demonstrated the large number of T-cell clones contributing to this response.[3] The strong immunogenicity of allogeneic MHC molecules relates to the manner in which T cells are selected in the thymus; developing thymocytes do not survive unless they can weakly recognize a self MHC/peptide complex on a thymic stromal cell. This process is termed *positive selection*. Thymocytes whose receptors have high affinity for self/MHC complexes are deleted, however, so strongly autoreactive T cells rarely make it into the peripheral T-cell pool. Allogeneic antigens are not part of this *negative selection* process. The net result of these two selection steps and the inherent cross-reactivity of T-cell receptors is that the T-cell "repertoire" recognizes allogeneic MHC molecules, providing a barrier to organ and hematopoietic cell transplantation. In the case of organ transplantation, in which long-term pharmacotherapy with powerful immunosuppressive drugs is used in an effort to prevent graft rejection, this can translate into improved results with HLA-matched organs. Despite the disadvantage of prolonged cold ischemia associated with transportation of a deceased donor graft, a pediatric kidney transplant study has shown superior outcomes with well-matched deceased donor kidneys compared with poorly matched living donor transplants.[4] Because of the high rates of late graft loss associated with de novo anti-HLA antibody formation, efforts have aimed to reduce this outcome by identifying HLA mismatches that are less likely to induce these alloantibodies.

For hematopoietic cell transplantation (Chapter 163), the risks for GVHD and marrow graft failure are so greatly amplified in the presence of extensive HLA mismatches that such transplantations have been largely avoided in the past. Disparities in the highly polymorphic class I and class II molecules predispose to GVHD. The risk of GVHD is increased by HLA-DPB1 mismatching, despite its lower polymorphism, especially when the regulatory region variant rs9277534 is a high-expression allele in recipients but low-expression in donors. If a sufficiently matched, related donor is unavailable, a search has typically been conducted through large registries containing millions of volunteer unrelated donors. Because of its extensive polymorphism, truly MHC-identical, unrelated donors can be difficult to find in the human population at large. For individuals with common HLA genotypes, the likelihood of finding a matched unrelated donor is markedly greater than that for individuals with rare genotypes. This situation relates in part to the phenomenon of *linkage disequilibrium*, wherein alleles at nearby loci are found together on the same chromosomal segment, or *haplotype*, more frequently than would be predicted by chance. The pattern of linkage disequilibrium is different in different racial groups, so the chance of finding a truly genotypically identical haplotype is greatest within the same population.

Advances in the ability to perform transplants from alternative donors have increased the availability of hematopoietic cell transplantation in individuals who lack an HLA-identical related donor (Chapter 163). Advances in avoiding GVHD in haploidentical related donor hematopoietic cell transplantation have increased the safety of HLA-mismatched hematopoietic cell transplantation, thereby yielding outcomes that may be superior to those using matched unrelated donors in some cases and comparable to results using matched sibling donors.

MINOR HISTOCOMPATIBILITY ANTIGENS

"Minor" histocompatibility antigens are peptides derived from polymorphic proteins presented by an MHC molecule. Even genotypically HLA-identical siblings have many different minor histocompatibility antigens that are sufficient to induce graft rejection if immunosuppressive pharmacotherapy is not used. Additionally, significant GVHD frequently (about 30 to 50% of the time) complicates hematopoietic cell transplantation between HLA-identical siblings, even with the use of pharmacologic immunoprophylaxis. Minor histocompatibility antigens, which can result from genetic polymorphisms in protein-coding regions or from homozygous loss-of-function variants in hematopoietic cell transplant donors or organ transplant recipients, render recipient and donor organs more susceptible to GVHD and rejection, respectively. An example of the latter is the *LIMS1* locus, which encodes a cell surface protein for which a homozygous loss-of-function variant is associated with anti-LIMS1 IgG2 and IgG3 antibodies and an increased risk of kidney allograft rejection. Another example is Y chromosome-encoded genes, which result in significantly increased graft rejection rates and GVHD in male-to-female and female-to-male organ and hematopoietic cell transplants, respectively.

OTHER ANTIGENS

The major blood group (ABO) antigens can be the targets of a dramatic "hyperacute" rejection process that occurs when mismatched vascularized grafts are transplanted. Recognition of blood group antigens on the endothelial surface of the graft vessels by recipient "natural" antibodies (antibodies that are present without known sensitization to the antigens) activates the complement and coagulation cascades, resulting in rapid graft thrombosis and ischemia. A similar outcome can occur after transplantation to an individual with preformed antidonor HLA antibodies resulting from presensitization by prior transplantations, transfusions, or pregnancies. Antibodies against other polymorphic antigens, such as MHC class I–related chain A (MICA), have been associated with graft rejection. In the past, transplantation could not be successfully performed in the presence of a positive antidonor crossmatch. However, considerable success has been achieved in the transplantation of ABO-mismatched kidneys, livers, and hearts (the latter in the neonatal period only) and in transplantation of kidneys to highly presensitized patients. In the case of kidney and liver transplantation, initial removal of the antibody and sometimes depletion of B cells, as well as the infusion of intravenous immunoglobulin (IVIG), has led to these successes.[5] Additional agents under investigation include proteosome inhibitors, interleukin-6 blockers, complement inhibitors, and IgG-degrading enzymes.[6] ABO-mismatched neonatal heart transplantation has succeeded because the transplantations are performed before the recipient has developed high levels of anti–blood group antigen antibodies, and the B cells seem to be rendered tolerant to the donor blood group antigen by the grafting process. Recognition of blood group antigens can also be of significance in hematopoietic cell transplantation, in which ABO barriers are routinely crossed in both directions. This can cause hemolysis of recipient erythrocytes if the mismatch is in the GVH direction, but this complication can be avoided by washing the cellular product before infusion. Mismatches in the HVG direction can cause more persistent problems due to ongoing destruction of donor erythropoietic cells, resulting in pure red cell aplasia. More often, however, donor erythropoiesis is successfully established, and antidonor isohemagglutinins disappear from the circulation. With the increasing application of HLA-mismatched donor hematopoietic cell transplantation, the importance of HLA alloantibodies in causing graft failure has recently been recognized and may require similar desensitization procedures to those used in sensitized organ allograft recipients.[7]

A and B blood group antigens are the consequence of the presence or absence of specific glycosylation enzymes in different individuals. Likewise, an antigenic specificity of the utmost importance in xenotransplantation is a carbohydrate epitope, Galα1–3Galβ1–4GlcNAc (αGal), which is produced by a specific galactosyl transferase. Humans and Old World monkeys lack a functional αGal transferase and produce high levels of natural antibodies against the ubiquitous αGal epitope. Because animals of interest as xenograft sources (e.g., pigs) express αGal at high levels on their vascular endothelium, transplantation of vascularized organs from pigs results in hyperacute rejection. The development of αGal-knockout pigs, therefore, was an important milestone that advanced the field of xenotransplantation. The more recent recognition of non-Gal carbohydrate natural antibody targets on cells of αGal-knockout pigs has led to further genetic modifications of these potential source animals, a procedure that has been greatly facilitated by current gene editing techniques.

In another type of transplant reaction, recognition as foreign results not from the presence of an antigen, but paradoxically from the absence of a self MHC molecule. Natural killer (NK) cells express a series of surface inhibitory and activating receptors that, collectively, determine whether the NK cell does or does not kill a potential target cell. The ligands for the inhibitory receptors are MHC class I molecules, and the receptors recognize specific groups of alleles. An NK cell may kill an allogeneic target that lacks a self MHC inhibitory ligand. This phenomenon can result in rapid bone marrow rejection in animal models and may be of significance in HLA-mismatched hematopoietic cell transplantation. The possible role of NK cells in organ allograft rejection is controversial, but they are thought to be of importance in organ xenotransplantation. NK cells clearly play a strong role in the rejection of xenogeneic hematopoietic cells, an observation that is relevant in one approach to inducing tolerance (see later discussion).

MECHANISMS OF REJECTION AND GRAFT-VERSUS-HOST DISEASE

CELLULAR MEDIATORS

Many different cell types participate in rejection responses, and considerable redundancy exists. T cells are key players in most forms of rejection, with the exception of rejection induced by antibodies in the absence of T-cell help, such as hyperacute and acute vascular rejection induced by natural antibodies. Several studies have suggested a dominant role for memory T cells in causing rejection, but it is difficult to distinguish whether "memory" T cells detected after a transplant converted from naïve T cells before or after the transplant.

DIRECT, SEMIDIRECT, AND INDIRECT ALLORECOGNITION

T-cell responses are induced by antigen-presenting cells that present alloantigens. Alloantigen recognition may be categorized as *direct*, *semidirect*, and *indirect* (Fig. 38-1). Direct allorecognition denotes recognition of donor antigens on donor antigen-presenting cells provided by the graft. The extraordinarily high frequency of T cells with alloreactivity is caused by direct recognition of allogeneic MHC. However, T cells with these specificities may also detect their ligands on recipient antigen-presenting cells, as these may pick up intact donor MHC-peptide complexes transferred in exosomes. This "semidirect" pathway may be important in maintaining strong direct alloresponses long after donor antigen-presenting cells in a grafted organ have been replaced by those of the recipient. Indirect recognition is the recognition of donor antigens

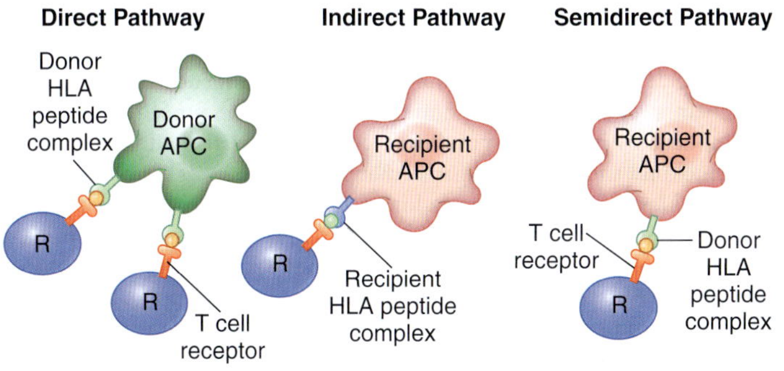

FIGURE 38-1. **Direct and indirect allorecognition.** Direct allorecognition involves the recognition by a T-cell receptor of major histocompatibility complex (MHC) molecules (with or without a peptide) on a donor antigen-presenting cell. Indirect allorecognition involves recognition by the T-cell receptor of a donor peptide presented on a recipient antigen-presenting cell that has picked up and processed donor antigens.

that are picked up, processed, and presented on recipient MHC molecules on recipient antigen-presenting cells. The indirect response is more similar to "normal" T-cell responses, in which professional antigen-presenting cells present peptide antigens to T cells that are present at relatively low frequency in the naïve repertoire. The indirect response, like the semidirect response, can be maintained by the constantly renewed pool of recipient antigen-presenting cells. The indirect response is of particular importance in inducing antibody responses.

EFFECTOR MECHANISMS OF REJECTION

T cells can promote graft rejection through several effector mechanisms. One is the antibody-dependent processes that have already been discussed. CD4 T cells provide cognate help to B cells when their T-cell receptors (TCRs) recognize complexes of self MHC with donor MHC–derived peptide antigens produced by B cells whose surface Ig receptors recognize and pick up the donor MHC antigen. Antidonor antibody can lead to the pathologic picture of acute humoral rejection and may also participate in a slower process of chronic rejection. Chronic rejection of kidney and heart allografts is characterized by unique vascular lesions with intimal thickening and loss of the vessel space. Chronic rejection of lung allografts is termed obliterative bronchiolitis. The mechanisms underlying these chronic rejection lesions are not well understood, and several different immune processes may in fact lead to similar lesions. Induced responses to autoantigens exposed by injured graft tissue have been implicated in several forms of chronic rejection.

Another major effector pathway leading to graft rejection involves cytotoxic T lymphocytes, which are predominantly CD8$^+$ but also include CD4$^+$ T cells. Several effector mechanisms lead to killing of target cells by cytotoxic T lymphocytes, including granzyme/perforin-mediated and Fas/Fas ligand (FasL) pathways and other members of the TNF/TNF-receptor families. Because CD8$^+$ cells recognize class I MHC molecules, which are widely expressed, it is not difficult to envision graft destruction by CD8$^+$ cytotoxic T lymphocytes. CD8$^+$ cytotoxic T lymphocytes may be activated through an antigen-presenting cell that is stimulated initially through contact with an alloreactive CD4$^+$ cell. This is one form of CD4 "help" for CD8$^+$ cells. In addition, CD8$^+$ cells may be dependent on cytokines such as interleukin-2 (IL-2) produced by CD4$^+$ cells for their expansion and cytotoxic differentiation. However, there are also many examples of CD8$^+$ cell–mediated rejection that is independent of "help" from CD4$^+$ cells. Class II MHC, which is recognized by CD4$^+$ T cells, is less widely expressed on graft tissues than is class I MHC, although it may be induced on endothelial cells and graft parenchymal cells in the presence of inflammatory cytokines such as interferon-γ (IFN-γ).

In addition to cytotoxic mechanisms resulting from direct allorecognition, CD4$^+$ and CD8$^+$ T cells with indirect specificity seem also to be capable of causing graft destruction under some circumstances. Cytokines such as IFN-γ and TNF-α, as well as innate cellular mediators, have been implicated in some instances, but in general, the pathways of indirect graft destruction are not well understood.

THE ROLE OF T-CELL TRAFFICKING

Rejection processes require trafficking of T cells into the graft, which occurs after the initial activation of naïve T cells in the lymphoid tissues. Naïve T cells can migrate into lymph nodes because of their expression of the CCR7 chemokine receptor and the adhesion molecule L-selectin. These T cells are activated by migratory graft antigen-presenting cells that also enter the lymph nodes. T-cell activation is associated with loss of CCR7 and L-selectin expression and acquisition of a new set of chemokine receptors and adhesion molecules that allow rolling and adhesion on the graft endothelium and entry into the graft parenchyma. Inflammation in the graft, such as that induced by ischemia-reperfusion injury and the transplantation procedure, as well as that induced by initially responding T cells, is associated with upregulation of chemokines and adhesion ligands that promote entry of lymphocytes into the graft. Nevertheless, well-healed-in grafts can be slowly rejected by adoptively transferred memory T cells, demonstrating that acute graft injury and inflammation are not essential for rejection in the presence of an established memory T-cell response. Rejection of hematopoietic cell grafts may involve many of the same mechanisms as those discussed for solid organs, although less detailed work has been done in this area.

MECHANISMS OF GRAFT-VERSUS-HOST DISEASE

Initiation of GVHD (Chapter 163) requires that donor T cells recognize host alloantigens. Donor T cells infiltrate a variety of recipient epithelial tissues, namely skin, the intestine, and liver. Animal models have demonstrated clear roles for both CD4$^+$ and CD8$^+$ cells in initiating GVHD, and each subset is able to do so independently of the other. The mechanisms of GVHD include activation of alloreactive donor T cells by recipient antigen-presenting cells within the recipient lymphoid tissues, leading to the differentiation of effector cells with direct cytotoxic activity and cytokine production in response to host antigens. A prominent role is played by TNF-α, whose production is induced in part by the translocation of bacteria across the intestinal wall, promoting innate immune system activation through toll-like receptors (Chapter 35). An intensely pro-inflammatory environment is produced by the combination of conditioning-induced tissue injury and disruption of mucosal barriers, bacterial activation of the innate immune system, and the GVH alloresponse. An important role is now appreciated for the inflamed microenvironment in target tissues in promoting the trafficking of GVH-reactive T cells into these tissues.

STRATEGIES TO PREVENT GRAFT-VERSUS-HOST DISEASE

In view of the critical role of donor T cells in inducing GVHD, an obvious strategy for preventing this complication is to remove mature T cells from the marrow graft. This approach has indeed been shown in both animal models and clinical studies to prevent GVHD effectively. However, there are several disadvantages to this approach. One is that adult humans, particularly those who have undergone prior chemotherapy and radiotherapy, have little remaining thymic tissue and therefore demonstrate sluggish T-cell recovery, leading to serious opportunistic infections. For example, the inclusion of antihuman T-lymphocyte immune globulin in a myeloablative conditioning regimen for patients with acute leukemia significantly lowers the rate of chronic GVHD but does not significantly improve survival.[A1]

T-cell depletion of hematopoietic cell grafts used to treat hematologic malignancies may be associated with an increased relapse rate due to loss of a graft-versus-tumor (GVT) effect, which is in large part mediated by GVH alloreactivity. Separation of GVHD from GVT effects is a major goal of research in hematopoietic cell transplantation, and some promising strategies are being explored (E-Table 38-3).[8] For example, Janus kinase inhibitors show promise for prevention of GVHD[9] and for the treatment of steroid-refractory GVHD after hematopoietic cell transplantation (Chapter 163).[A2,A3] Trials of low-dose IL-2 have shown efficacy in preventing chronic GVHD, apparently by expanding regulatory T cells. Infusion of expanded regulatory T cells has also entered clinical trials,[10] and infusion of mesenchymal stromal cells has shown benefit in treating refractory GVHD.[11] Preventing T-cell trafficking into epithelial target tissues of GVHD is a particularly promising approach because of the theoretical preservation of graft-versus-tumor effects in lymphohematopoietic tissues. Chemokine receptor blockade is a promising approach to achieving this goal.

A third disadvantage of T-cell depletion is that it eliminates the engraftment-promoting effect conferred by alloreactive T cells, resulting in increased rates of allograft failure, especially in the setting of HLA-mismatched transplantation. NK-cell recognition in the GVH direction resulting from the absence in the recipient of a class I MHC ligand (E-Fig. 38-3) that can trigger a donor NK-cell inhibitory receptor (KIR) may promote donor hematopoietic cell engraftment and antitumor effects against acute myeloid leukemias in the setting of T-cell–depleted, HLA-mismatched hematopoietic cell transplantation. The role of donor-recipient KIR mismatch and of polymorphisms in KIR genotype and expression in antitumor effects, GVHD, and infectious immunity in hematopoietic cell transplantation is complex and may vary with different diseases and types of transplant conditioning, in addition to different types of donor-recipient mismatch.

Clinically, pharmacologic immunosuppressive prophylaxis is usually used in at least the first 6 months after hematopoietic cell transplantation to minimize the complication of GVHD. Posttransplant cyclophosphamide significantly reduces the risk of GVHD although it does not increase overall survival.[A4] Additionally, HLA-matched or closely matched donors are chosen whenever possible because GVHD increases in frequency and severity as increased HLA barriers are transgressed. These measures, nevertheless, are insufficient, and GVHD remains a major complication of hematopoietic cell transplantation. Therefore, many of the new strategies being explored in organ transplantation and other fields are also being examined for the prevention of GVHD in experimental models. It should be borne in mind, however, that tolerance of donor T cells to recipient alloantigens (see later discussion) might not be entirely beneficial in the hematopoietic cell transplantation setting for the treatment of malignant disease because loss of GVH alloreactivity is likely to come with loss of antitumor effects.

STRATEGIES TO PREVENT ALLOGRAFT REJECTION

NONSPECIFIC IMMUNOSUPPRESSION

Immunosuppressive drugs are the mainstay of clinical organ transplantation, and improvements in these drugs following the discovery of cyclosporine have extended organ transplantation to include hearts, lungs, pancreases, livers, and other organs and tissues in the past 40 years. The mechanisms of action of these agents, which typically include a calcineurin inhibitor, an anti-proliferative drug, and corticosteroids, are discussed in Chapter 28. However, it is noteworthy that, despite these improvements and their enormous impact on early graft survival, pharmacologic agents have been less effective in attenuating late graft loss. Because chronic immunologic rejection processes and side effects of the immunosuppressive drugs themselves are responsible for much of this late graft loss, improved immunosuppressive agents and induction of immune tolerance (see later discussion) are major research goals in transplantation.

COSTIMULATORY BLOCKADE

As understanding of immune responses has increased, recent years have seen the exploration of numerous biologic agents, including antibodies and small molecules targeting receptors of the immune system, as well as cell-based therapies,[12] in efforts to improve allograft survival. Because of the central role played by T cells in the immune response, considerable attention has been focused on blockers of T-cell costimulation. When a naïve T cell recognizes antigen through its unique TCR, additional "costimulatory" signals are required to allow full activation, expansion, and differentiation to occur. These signals are provided by antigen-presenting cells in the form of ligands (e.g., B7-1, B7-2) for costimulatory receptors (e.g., CD28) on the T cell. Cross-talk between the T cell and the antigen-presenting cell (e.g., due to CD40 activation by CD154 upregulation on the activated T cell) further amplifies the costimulatory activity of the antigen-presenting cell, allowing it to effectively activate other T cells as well. The CD154 (T cell)–CD40 (B cell) interaction also promotes Ig class switching and functioning of B cells as antigen-presenting cells. Blockade of these processes (e.g., by CTLA4Ig and anti-CD154 or CD40 monoclonal antibodies [mAbs]) has led to marked prolongation of allograft survival in stringent rodent and large-animal models. Robust, systemic tolerance to donor antigens has been achieved in rodents receiving bone marrow transplantation with costimulatory blockade and little or no additional conditioning. Some of these agents have joined the armamentarium of immunosuppressive agents in clinical trials in transplantation and autoimmune diseases. Although the optimal protocol for its use is still in development, CTLA4Ig has permitted sparing of nephrotoxic calcineurin inhibitors, with improved long-term patient and renal allograft survival.[13] Although anti-CD154 antibodies have been associated with thromboembolic complications, precluding further evaluation in transplantation trials, recently developed nonthrombogenic anti-CD154 and anti-CD40 antibodies have shown promise in preclinical studies and have entered clinical trials.[14] Numerous additional costimulatory and inhibitory pathways that affect T cell responses have been described, and these all are potential targets for further manipulation of the alloresponse.

IMMUNE TOLERANCE

Immune tolerance denotes a state in which the immune system is specifically unreactive to the donor graft (or recipient in the case of GVH reactivity) while remaining normally responsive to other antigens.[15] Tolerance is distinct from the state produced by nonspecific immunosuppressive agents, which increase risks for infection and malignancy. Numerous approaches to tolerance induction have been described in rodent models, largely owing to the strong tolerogenicity of primarily vascularized heart, liver, and kidney grafts in these animals. Such grafts are less tolerogenic in humans, and few of these strategies have been effectively applied clinically to date. Since the test for tolerance is graft acceptance without continuous immunosuppressive therapy (i.e., without the standard of care), tolerance protocols being evaluated clinically should first demonstrate efficacy in stringent animal models, including highly immunogenic grafts such as MHC-mismatched skin in rodents and vascularized organ graft models in large animals.

The three major mechanisms of T-cell tolerance are deletion, anergy, and suppression (often referred to as "regulation"). *Deletion* denotes the destruction of T cells with receptors that recognize donor antigens; it can be achieved during T-cell development in the thymus, for example, by induction of mixed chimerism in T-cell–depleted hosts. Deletion can also be applied to mature T cells in the periphery, for example, by transplantation of a tolerogenic organ or marrow graft in combination with blockade of costimulatory molecules. *Anergy* denotes the inability of T cells to respond fully to antigens they recognize, and it can be induced by antigen presentation without costimulation. *Suppression* has attracted considerable interest since the discovery that constitutively $CD25^+$ T cells of the $CD4^+$ subset have suppressive activity that is dependent on expression of the transcription factor Forkhead Box Protein 3 (FoxP3). These and other types of suppressive T cells (e.g., NKT cells, regulatory $CD8^+$ cells and B cells, myeloid-derived suppressor cells, regulatory monocytes, and dendritic cells) have been implicated in rodent transplantation tolerance models and in prevention of autoimmunity. The use of expanded regulatory cells has recently entered clinical trials in both transplantation and autoimmune disease, including both antigen-specific and nonspecific ("polyclonal") regulatory cell therapy,[16] as well as chimeric antigen receptor (CAR) Tregs.[17] Other regulatory cell types, including tolerogenic monocytes and dendritic cells, have demonstrated safety in early clinical trials.[18] However, in the absence of large animal studies demonstrating the efficacy of these cellular therapies in achieving tolerance and without validated biomarkers for tolerance, rapid immunosuppression withdrawal to test tolerance induction is not the goal of these studies. There is also interest in strategies for activating or expanding regulatory T cells in vivo, thereby favoring the suppressive immune response over destructive alloimmunity.

The developments in animal models and understanding of immune mechanisms described here have provided impetus for efforts to achieve immune tolerance in clinical transplantation. Every transplantation center has anecdotal cases of patients who have removed themselves from chronic immunosuppression without experiencing graft rejection. However, for every such patient, there are dozens more who have experienced rejection on dose reduction or removal of immunosuppressive drugs. Trials of slow withdrawal of nonspecific immunosuppressive therapy have had very little success in renal allograft recipients and higher success rates in a very highly selected group of liver allograft recipients, especially children with long-term rejection-free graft survival.[19] Application of this approach to a larger subset of patients will depend on future advances in the ability to identify biomarkers that are predictive of success. "Tolerance signatures" with sufficient predictive value to allow such withdrawal to be safely undertaken have not yet been identified.

One approach developed in animal models has been successfully applied to the induction of immune tolerance in a small group of patients receiving renal allografts. This approach, involving bone marrow transplantation after nonmyeloablative conditioning, which is less toxic than standard hematopoietic cell transplantation conditioning, was shown to be effective in the most stringent rodent and large-animal models before being evaluated clinically. Initial success using combined kidney and bone marrow transplantation in patients with renal failure due to multiple myeloma led to pilot studies in patients with renal failure without malignant disease, with encouraging results. This protocol involved induction of transient chimerism in combination with a kidney allograft from HLA-mismatched related donors and was free of the complication of GVHD. Mechanistic studies, including a high-throughput sequencing-based approach to identifying and tracking donor-reactive T-cell clones, implicated an early role for regulatory T cells followed by gradual clonal deletion in the long-term tolerance.[20] Another nonmyeloablative approach has succeeded in achieving more durable chimerism and tolerance, but only in the HLA-identical sibling transplant setting,[21] and a third approach has led to full donor chimerism across extensive HLA barriers, but with significant toxicity, including GVHD.[22] With further refinements of this approach and proof of efficacy in large animal models, it is hoped that transplantation of all organ types might ultimately be routinely performed without the need for chronic immunosuppressive therapy, with its attendant complications and limited ability to control chronic rejection. Because autoimmune diseases are major contributors to end-stage renal disease, β-cell loss in type 1 diabetes, and other types of organ failure, the potential for tolerance strategies to reverse autoimmunity while inducing allograft tolerance is also a source of hope. All these approaches must, however, be undertaken with the caution that successful regimens could also lead to immune tolerance to active infectious organisms.

GENERAL REFERENCES

For the General References and other additional features, please visit Elsevier eBooks+ at https://ebooks.health.elsevier.com.

Grade A References

A1. Kroger N, Solano C, Wolschke C, et al. Antilymphocyte globulin for prevention of chronic graft-versus-host disease. *N Engl J Med.* 2016;374:43-53.

A2. Zeiser R, Polverelli N, Ram R, et al. Ruxolitinib for glucocorticoid-refractory chronic graft-versus-host disease. *N Engl J Med.* 2021;385:228-238.

A3. Jagasia M, Perales MA, Schroeder MA, et al. Ruxolitinib for the treatment of steroid-refractory acute GVHD (REACH1): a multicenter, open-label phase 2 trial. *Blood.* 2020;135:1739-1749.

A4. Broers AEC, de Jong CN, Bakunina K, et al. Posttransplant cyclophosphamide for prevention of graft-versus-host disease: results of the prospective randomized HOVON-96 trial. *Blood Adv.* 2022;6:3378-3385.

A5. Shaked A, DesMarais MR, Kopetskie H, et al. Outcomes of immunosuppression minimization and withdrawal early after liver transplantation. *Am J Transplant.* 2019;19:1397-1409.

VIII

HEART DISEASES

39 APPROACH TO THE PATIENT WITH POSSIBLE CARDIOVASCULAR DISEASE

LEE GOLDMAN

Patients with cardiovascular disease may present with a wide range of symptoms and signs, each of which may be caused by noncardiovascular conditions. Conversely, patients with substantial cardiovascular disease may be asymptomatic. Because cardiovascular disease is a leading cause of death in the United States and other developed countries, it is crucial that patients be evaluated carefully to detect early cardiovascular disease, that symptoms or signs of cardiovascular disease be evaluated in detail, and that appropriate therapy be instituted.

In evaluating a patient with known or suspected heart disease, the physician must determine quickly whether a potentially life-threatening condition exists. In these situations, the evaluation must focus on the specific issue at hand and be accompanied by the rapid performance of appropriately directed additional tests. Examples of potentially life-threatening conditions include acute myocardial infarction (MI) (Chapter 58), unstable angina (Chapter 57), suspected aortic dissection (Chapter 63), pulmonary edema (Chapter 46), and pulmonary embolism (Chapter 68).

USING THE HISTORY TO DETECT CARDIOVASCULAR SYMPTOMS

Patients may complain spontaneously of a variety of cardiovascular symptoms (Table 39-1), but sometimes these symptoms are elicited only by obtaining a careful, complete medical history. In patients with known or suspected cardiovascular disease, questions about cardiovascular symptoms are key components of the history of present illness; in other patients, these issues are a fundamental part of the review of systems.

CHEST PAIN

Chest discomfort or pain is the cardinal manifestation of myocardial ischemia resulting from coronary artery disease or any condition that causes myocardial ischemia by an imbalance of myocardial oxygen demand compared with myocardial oxygen supply (Chapter 56). Women[1] and older individuals may be less likely to complain of classic anginal pain despite equivalent or even more advanced coronary disease.

New, acute, often ongoing pain may indicate an acute myocardial infarction, unstable angina, or aortic dissection; a pulmonary cause, such as acute pulmonary embolism or pleural irritation; a musculoskeletal condition of the chest wall, thorax, or shoulder; or a gastrointestinal abnormality, such as esophageal reflux or spasm, peptic ulcer disease, or cholecystitis (Table 39-2). The chest discomfort of an acute coronary syndrome (Chapter 57) or a myocardial infarction commonly occurs without an immediate or obvious precipitating clinical cause and builds in intensity for at least several minutes; the sensation can range from annoying discomfort to severe pain (Chapter 58).[2,3] Although a variety of adjectives may be used by patients to describe the sensation, physicians must be suspicious of any discomfort, especially if it radiates to the neck, shoulder, or arms.

The chest discomfort of unstable angina is clinically indistinguishable from that of an acute myocardial infarction except that the former may be precipitated more clearly by activity and may be more rapidly responsive to antianginal therapy (Chapter 57). Aortic dissection (Chapter 63) classically presents with the sudden onset of severe pain in the chest and radiating to the back; the location of the pain often provides clues to the location of the dissection. Ascending aortic dissections commonly present with chest discomfort radiating to the back, whereas dissections of the descending aorta commonly present with back pain radiating to the abdomen. The presence of back pain or a history of hypertension or other predisposing factors, such as Marfan syndrome, should prompt a careful assessment of peripheral pulses to determine whether the great vessels are affected by the dissection and of the chest radiograph to evaluate the size of the aorta. If this initial evaluation is suggestive, further testing with transesophageal echocardiography, computed tomography (CT), or magnetic resonance imaging (MRI) is indicated. The pain of pericarditis (Chapter 62) may simulate the pain of an acute myocardial infarction, may be primarily pleuritic, or may be continuous; a key physical finding is a pericardial rub. The pain of pulmonary embolism (Chapter 68) is commonly pleuritic in nature and is associated with dyspnea; hemoptysis also may be present. Pulmonary hypertension (Chapter 69) of any cause may be associated with chest discomfort with exertion; it commonly is associated with severe dyspnea and often is associated with cyanosis.

Recurrent, episodic chest discomfort may be noted with angina pectoris and with many cardiac and noncardiac causes (Chapter 56). A variety of stress tests (Table 39-3) can be used to provoke reversible myocardial ischemia in susceptible individuals and to help determine whether ischemia is the pathophysiologic explanation for the chest discomfort (Chapter 56).

TABLE 39-1 CARDINAL SYMPTOMS OF CARDIOVASCULAR DISEASE

Chest pain or discomfort
Dyspnea, orthopnea, paroxysmal nocturnal dyspnea, wheezing
Palpitations, dizziness, syncope
Cough, hemoptysis
Fatigue, weakness
Pain in extremities with exertion (claudication)

DYSPNEA

Dyspnea, which is an uncomfortable awareness of breathing, is commonly caused by cardiovascular or pulmonary disease. A systematic approach (see Fig. 71-2) with selected tests nearly always reveals the cause.[4] Acute dyspnea can be caused by myocardial ischemia, heart failure, severe hypertension, pericardial tamponade, pulmonary embolism, pneumothorax, upper airway obstruction, acute bronchitis or pneumonia, or some drug overdoses (e.g., salicylates). Subacute or chronic dyspnea is also a common presenting or accompanying symptom in patients with pulmonary disease (Chapter 71). Dyspnea also can be caused by severe anemia (Chapter 144) and can be confused with the fatigue that often is noted in patients with systemic and neurologic diseases (Chapters 236 and 366).

In heart failure, dyspnea typically is noted as a hunger for air and a need or an urge to breathe. The feeling that breathing requires increased work or effort is more typical of airway obstruction or neuromuscular disease. A feeling of chest tightness or constriction during breathing is typical of bronchoconstriction, which is commonly caused by obstructive airway disease (Chapters 75 and 76) but also may be seen in pulmonary edema. A feeling of heavy breathing, a feeling of rapid breathing, or a need to breathe more is classically associated with deconditioning.

In cardiovascular conditions, chronic dyspnea usually is caused by increases in pulmonary venous pressure as a result of left ventricular failure (Chapters 45 and 46) or valvular heart disease (Chapter 60). Orthopnea, which is an exacerbation of dyspnea when the patient is recumbent, is caused by increased work of breathing because of either increased venous return to the pulmonary vasculature or loss of gravitational assistance in diaphragmatic effort. Paroxysmal nocturnal dyspnea is severe dyspnea that awakens a patient at night and forces the assumption of a sitting or standing position to achieve gravitational redistribution of fluid. Of note is that acute diuresis relieves the dyspnea of severe heart failure, but the degree of relief is not always directly related to the amount of diuresis.

PALPITATIONS

Palpitations (Chapter 49) describe a subjective sensation of an irregular or abnormal heartbeat. Palpitations may be caused by any arrhythmia (Chapters 52 and 53) with or without important underlying structural heart disease. Palpitations should be defined in terms of the duration and frequency of the episodes; the precipitating and related factors; and any associated symptoms of chest pain, dyspnea, lightheadedness, or syncope. The history can determine whether the palpitations are caused by an irregular or a regular heartbeat. The feeling associated with a premature atrial or ventricular contraction, often described as a "skipped beat" or a "flip-flopping of the heart," must be distinguished from the irregularly irregular rhythm of atrial fibrillation or the rapid but regular rhythm of supraventricular tachycardia. Associated symptoms of chest pain, dyspnea, lightheadedness, dizziness, or diaphoresis suggest an important effect on cardiac output and mandate further evaluation. In general, evaluation begins with ambulatory electrocardiography (ECG; Table 39-4), which is always indicated in patients who have palpitations in

TABLE 39-2 CAUSES OF CHEST PAIN

CONDITION	LOCATION	QUALITY	DURATION	AGGRAVATING OR RELIEVING FACTORS	ASSOCIATED SYMPTOMS OR SIGNS
CARDIOVASCULAR CAUSES					
Angina	Retrosternal region; radiates to or occasionally isolated to neck, jaw, epigastrium, shoulder, or arms (left common)	Pressure, burning, squeezing, heaviness, indigestion	<2-10 min	Precipitated by exercise, cold weather, or emotional stress; relieved by rest or nitroglycerin; atypical (Prinzmetal) angina may be unrelated to activity, often early morning	S_3 or murmur of papillary muscle dysfunction during pain
Rest or unstable angina	Same as angina	Same as angina but may be more severe	Usually <20 min	Same as angina, with decreasing tolerance for exertion or at rest	Similar to stable angina but may be pronounced; transient heart failure can occur
Myocardial infarction	Substernal and may radiate like angina	Heaviness, pressure, burning, constriction	≥30 min but variable	Unrelieved by rest or nitroglycerin	Shortness of breath, sweating, weakness, nausea, vomiting
Pericarditis	Usually begins over sternum or toward cardiac apex and may radiate to neck or left shoulder; often more localized than the pain of myocardial ischemia	Sharp, stabbing, knifelike	Lasts many hours to days; may wax and wane	Aggravated by deep breathing, rotating chest, or supine position; relieved by sitting up and leaning forward	Pericardial friction rub
Aortic dissection	Anterior chest; may radiate to back	Excruciating, tearing, knifelike	Sudden onset, unrelenting	Usually occurs in setting of hypertension or predisposition, such as Marfan syndrome	Murmur of aortic insufficiency, pulse or blood pressure asymmetry; neurologic deficit
Pulmonary embolism (chest pain often not present)	Substernal or over region of pulmonary infarction	Pleuritic (with pulmonary infarction) or angina-like	Sudden onset; minutes to <1 hr	May be aggravated by breathing	Dyspnea, tachypnea, tachycardia; hypotension, signs of acute right ventricular failure, and pulmonary hypertension with large emboli; rales, pleural friction rub, hemoptysis with pulmonary infarction
Pulmonary hypertension	Substernal	Pressure; oppressive	Similar to angina	Aggravated by effort	Pain usually associated with dyspnea; signs of pulmonary hypertension
NONCARDIAC CAUSES					
Pneumonia with pleurisy	Localized over involved area	Pleuritic, localized	Brief or prolonged	Painful breathing	Dyspnea, cough, fever, dull to percussion, bronchial breath sounds, rales, occasional pleural friction rub
Spontaneous pneumothorax	Unilateral	Sharp, well localized	Sudden onset, lasts many hours	Painful breathing	Dyspnea; hyperresonance and decreased breath and voice sounds over involved lung
Musculoskeletal disorders	Variable	Aching	Short or long duration	Aggravated by movement; history of muscle exertion or injury	Tender to pressure or movement
Herpes zoster	Dermatomal in distribution	Burning, itching	Prolonged	None	Vesicular rash appears in area of discomfort
Esophageal reflux	Substernal, epigastric	Burning, visceral discomfort	10-60 min	Aggravated by large meal, postprandial recumbency; relief with antacid	Water brash
Peptic ulcer	Epigastric, substernal	Visceral burning, aching	Prolonged	Relief with food, antacid	
Gallbladder disease	Epigastric, right upper quadrant	Visceral	Prolonged	May be unprovoked or follow meals	Right upper quadrant tenderness may be present
Anxiety states	Often localized over precordium	Variable; location often moves from place to place	Varies; often fleeting	Situational	Sighing respirations, often chest wall tenderness

Modified from Andreoli TE, Carpenter CCJ, Griggs RC, et al. Evaluation of the patient with cardiovascular disease. In: *Cecil Essentials of Medicine*, 6th ed. Philadelphia: WB Saunders; 2004:34-35.

the presence of coronary artery disease, structural heart disease, or substantial accompanying symptoms.[5] In such patients, more detailed evaluation is also warranted (see Fig. 49-3).

Lightheadedness or *syncope* (Chapter 49) can be caused by any condition that decreases cardiac output (e.g., bradyarrhythmia, tachyarrhythmia, obstruction of the left ventricular or right ventricular inflow or outflow, cardiac tamponade, aortic dissection, or severe pump failure), by reflex-mediated vasomotor instability (e.g., vasovagal, situational, or carotid sinus syncope), or by orthostatic hypotension (see Table 49-1). Neurologic diseases (e.g., migraine headaches, transient ischemic attacks, or seizures) also can cause transient loss of consciousness. The history, physical examination, and ECG can often diagnose the cause of syncope (see Table 49-2). Syncope caused by a cardiac arrhythmia usually occurs with little warning. Syncope with exertion or just after conclusion of exertion is typical of aortic stenosis and hypertrophic obstructive cardiomyopathy. In many patients, additional testing is required to document central nervous system disease, the cause of reduced cardiac output, or carotid sinus syncope. When the history, physical examination, and ECG do not provide helpful diagnostic information that points toward a specific cause of syncope, it is imperative that patients with heart disease or an abnormal ECG be tested with continuous ambulatory ECG monitoring to diagnose a

TABLE 39-3 COMMON EXERCISE TEST PROTOCOLS*

PROTOCOL	STAGE	DURATION (min)	GRADE (%)	RATE (mph)	METABOLIC EQUIVALENTS AT COMPLETION	FUNCTIONAL CLASS
Modified Bruce protocol†	1	3	0	1.7	2.5	III
	2	3	10	1.7	5	II
	3	3	12	2.5	7	I
	4	3	14	3.4	10	I
	5	3	16	4.2	13	I
Naughton protocol‡	0	2	0	2	2	III
	1	2	3.5	2	3	III
	2	2	7	2	4	III
	3	2	10.5	2	5	II
	4	2	14	2	6	II
	5	2	17.5	2	7	I

*Ramp protocols in which the workload is gradually increased on the basis of the patient's estimated functional capacity to achieve maximal effort in approximately 10 minutes are also useful.
†Commonly used in ambulatory patients.
‡Commonly used in patients with recent myocardial infarction, unstable angina, or other conditions that are expected to limit exercise.
Modified from Braunwald E, Goldman L, eds. *Primary Cardiology*. 2nd ed. Philadelphia: WB Saunders; 2003.

TABLE 39-4 INDICATIONS FOR AMBULATORY ELECTROCARDIOGRAPHIC MONITORING

History, physical examination, or 12-lead electrocardiogram suggests a possible arrhythmia
Known coronary or structural heart disease or a family history of genetic arrhythmia or sudden cardiac death
Symptoms warrant targeted therapy that depends on diagnosing the specific arrhythmia
Patient requires reassurance or a specific diagnosis because of anxiety or other concerns

possible arrhythmia; in selected patients, formal electrophysiologic testing may be indicated (Chapter 49). In patients with no evident heart disease, tilt testing (Chapter 49) can help detect reflex-mediated vasomotor instability.

OTHER SYMPTOMS

Nonproductive *cough* (Chapter 71), especially a persistent cough (see Fig. 71-1), can be an early manifestation of elevated pulmonary venous pressure and otherwise unsuspected heart failure. *Fatigue* and *weakness* are common accompaniments of advanced cardiac disease and reflect an inability to perform normal activities. A variety of approaches have been used to classify the severity of cardiac limitations, ranging from class I (little or no limitation) to class IV (severe limitation) (Table 39-5). *Hemoptysis* (Chapter 71) is a classic presenting finding in patients with pulmonary embolism, but it is also common in patients who have mitral stenosis, pulmonary edema, pulmonary infections, and malignant neoplasms (see Table 71-6). *Claudication*, which is pain in the extremities with exertion, should alert the physician to possible peripheral arterial disease (Chapters 65 and 66).

COMPLETE MEDICAL HISTORY

The complete medical history should include a thorough review of systems, family history, social history, and past medical history (Chapter 12). The review of systems may reveal other symptoms that suggest a systemic disease as the cause of any cardiovascular problems. The family history should focus on premature atherosclerosis or evidence of familial abnormalities, such as may be found with various causes of the long QT syndrome (Chapter 53) or hypertrophic cardiomyopathy (Chapter 47).

The social history should include specific questioning about cigarette smoking, alcohol intake, and use of illicit drugs. The past medical history may reveal prior conditions or medications that suggest systemic diseases, ranging from chronic obstructive pulmonary disease, which may explain a complaint of dyspnea, to hemochromatosis, which may be a cause of restrictive cardiomyopathy. A careful history to inquire about recent dental work or other procedures is crucial if bacterial endocarditis is part of the differential diagnosis.

PHYSICAL EXAMINATION FOR DETECTION OF SIGNS OF CARDIOVASCULAR DISEASE

The cardiovascular physical examination, which is a subset of the complete physical examination (Chapter 6), provides important clues to the diagnosis of asymptomatic and symptomatic cardiac disease and may reveal cardiovascular manifestations of noncardiovascular diseases. The cardiovascular physical examination begins with careful measurement of the pulse and blood pressure (Chapter 7). If aortic dissection (Chapter 63) is a consideration, blood pressure should be measured in both arms and, preferably, in at least one leg. When coarctation of the aorta is suspected (Chapter 55), blood pressure must be measured in at least one leg and in the arms. Discrepancies in blood pressure between the two arms also can be caused by atherosclerotic disease of the great vessels. Pulsus paradoxus, which is more than the usual 10-mm Hg drop in systolic blood pressure during inspiration, is typical of pericardial tamponade (Chapter 62).

GENERAL APPEARANCE

The respiratory rate may be increased in patients with heart failure. Patients with pulmonary edema are usually markedly tachypneic and may have labored breathing. Patients with advanced heart failure may have Cheyne-Stokes respirations.

Systemic diseases, such as hyperthyroidism (Chapter 207), hypothyroidism (Chapter 207), rheumatoid arthritis (Chapter 243), scleroderma (Chapter 246), and hemochromatosis (Chapter 196), may be suspected from the patient's general appearance. Marfan syndrome (Chapter 239), Turner syndrome (Chapter 217), Down syndrome (Chapter 32), and a variety of congenital anomalies also may be readily apparent.

OPHTHALMOLOGIC EXAMINATION

Examination of the fundi may show diabetic (see Fig. 391-22) or hypertensive retinopathy (see Fig. 391-24) or Roth spots (see Fig. 391-26) typical of infectious endocarditis. Beading of the retinal arteries is typical of severe hypercholesterolemia. Osteogenesis imperfecta, which is associated with blue sclerae, also is associated with aortic dilation and mitral valve prolapse. Retinal artery occlusion (see Fig. 391-27) may be caused by an embolus from clot in the left atrium or left ventricle, a left atrial myxoma, or atherosclerotic debris from the great vessels. Hyperthyroidism may present with exophthalmos and typical stare (see Fig. 391-5), whereas myotonic dystrophy, which is associated with atrioventricular block and arrhythmia, often is associated with ptosis and an expressionless face (see Fig. 389-2).

JUGULAR VEINS

The external jugular veins help in assessment of mean right atrial pressure, which normally varies between 5 and 10 cm H_2O; the height (in centimeters) of the central venous pressure is measured by adding 5 cm to the height of the observed jugular venous distention above the sternal angle of Louis (Fig. 39-1). The normal jugular venous pulse, best seen in the internal jugular vein (and not seen in the external jugular vein unless insufficiency of the jugular venous valves is present), includes an *a* wave, caused by right atrial contraction; a *c* wave, reflecting carotid artery pulsation; an *x* descent; a *v* wave, which corresponds to isovolumetric right ventricular contraction and is more marked in the presence of tricuspid insufficiency; and a *y* descent, which occurs as the tricuspid valve opens and ventricular filling begins (Fig. 39-2). Abnormalities of the jugular venous pressure (Fig. 39-3) as detected on physical examination or point-of-care ultrasonography[6] are useful in detecting heart failure, and they

TABLE 39-5 A COMPARISON OF THREE METHODS OF ASSESSING CARDIOVASCULAR DISABILITY

CLASS	NEW YORK HEART ASSOCIATION FUNCTIONAL CLASSIFICATION	CANADIAN CARDIOVASCULAR SOCIETY FUNCTIONAL CLASSIFICATION	SPECIFIC ACTIVITY SCALE
I	Patients with cardiac disease but without resulting limitations of physical activity Ordinary physical activity does not cause undue fatigue, palpitation, dyspnea, or anginal pain	Ordinary physical activity, such as walking and climbing stairs, does not cause angina Angina with strenuous or rapid or prolonged exertion at work or recreation	Patients can perform to completion any activity requiring ≥7 metabolic equivalents, for example, can carry 24 lb up 8 steps; carry objects that weigh 80 lb; do outdoor work (shovel snow, spade soil); do recreational activities (skiing, basketball, squash, handball, jog or walk 5 mph)
II	Patients with cardiac disease resulting in slight limitation of physical activity They are comfortable at rest Ordinary physical activity results in fatigue, palpitations, dyspnea, or anginal pain	Slight limitation of ordinary activity Walking or climbing stairs rapidly, walking uphill, walking or stair climbing after meals, in cold, in wind, or when under emotional stress, or only during the few hours after awakening Walking >2 blocks on the level and climbing >1 flight of ordinary stairs at a normal pace and in normal conditions	Patient can perform to completion any activity requiring ≥5 metabolic equivalents but cannot and does not perform to completion activities requiring ≥7 metabolic equivalents, e.g., have sexual intercourse without stopping, garden, rake, weed, roller skate, dance foxtrot, walk at 4 mph on level ground
III	Patients with cardiac disease resulting in marked limitation of physical activity They are comfortable at rest Less than ordinary physical activity causes fatigue, palpitations, dyspnea, or anginal pain	Marked limitation of ordinary physical activity Walking 1 or 2 blocks on the level and climbing >1 flight in normal conditions	Patient can perform to completion any activity requiring ≥2 metabolic equivalents but cannot and does not perform to completion any activities requiring ≥5 metabolic equivalents, for example, shower without stopping, strip and make bed, clean windows, walk 2.5 mph, bowl, play golf, dress without stopping
IV	Patients with cardiac disease resulting in inability to carry on any physical activity without discomfort Symptoms of cardiac insufficiency or of the anginal syndrome may be present even at rest If any physical activity is undertaken, discomfort is increased	Inability to carry on any physical activity without discomfort—anginal syndrome may be present at rest	Patient cannot or does not perform to completion activities requiring ≥2 metabolic equivalents; cannot carry out activities listed above (Specific Activity Scale, class III)

From Goldman L, Hashimoto B, Cook EF, et al. Comparative reproducibility and validity of systems for assessing cardiovascular functional class: advantages of a new specific activity scale. *Circulation.* 1981;64:1227-1234. Reproduced by permission of the American Heart Association.

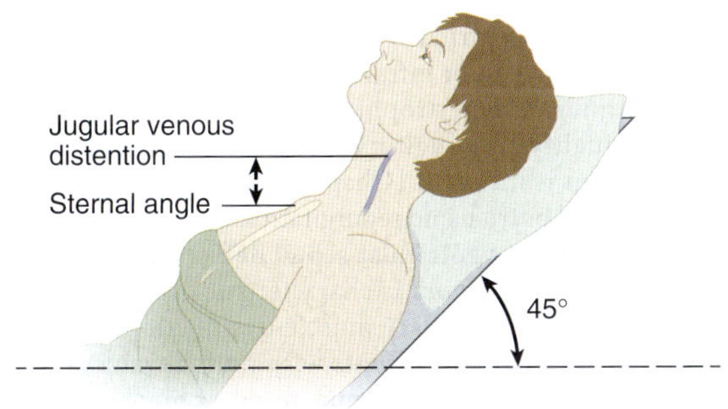

FIGURE 39-1. **Jugular venous distention is defined by engorgement of the internal jugular vein more than 5 cm above the sternal angle at 45 degrees.** The central venous pressure is the observed venous distention above the sternal angle plus 5 cm.

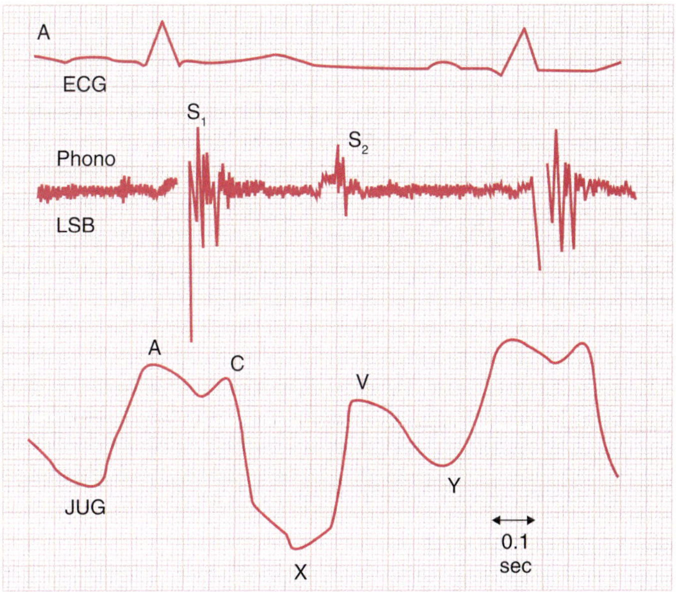

FIGURE 39-2. **Normal jugular venous pulse.** ECG = electrocardiogram; JUG = jugular vein; LSB = left sternal border; phono = phonocardiogram; S_1 = first heart sound; S_2 = second heart sound.

correlate well with brain natriuretic peptide levels (Chapter 45) and echocardiographic evidence of an elevated pulmonary artery pressure (Chapter 43). The jugular venous pressure also helps in the diagnosis of pericardial disease, tricuspid valve disease, and pulmonary hypertension (Table 39-6).

CAROTID PULSE

The carotid pulse should be examined in terms of its volume and contour. The carotid pulse (Fig. 39-4) may be increased in frequency and may be more intense than normal in patients with a higher stroke volume secondary to aortic regurgitation, arteriovenous fistula, hyperthyroidism, fever, or anemia. In aortic regurgitation or arteriovenous fistula, the pulse may have a bisferious quality. The carotid upstroke is delayed in patients with valvular aortic stenosis (Chapter 60) and has a normal contour but diminished amplitude in any cause of reduced stroke volume.

CARDIAC INSPECTION AND PALPATION

Inspection of the precordium may reveal the hyperinflation of obstructive lung disease or unilateral asymmetry of the left side of the chest because of right ventricular hypertrophy before puberty. Palpation may be performed with the patient either supine or in the left lateral decubitus position; the latter position moves the left ventricular apex closer to the chest wall and increases the ability to palpate the point of maximal impulse and other phenomena. Low-frequency phenomena, such as systolic heaves or lifts from the left ventricle (at the cardiac apex) or right ventricle (parasternal in the third or fourth intercostal space), are felt best with the heel of the palm. With the patient in the left lateral decubitus position, this technique also may allow palpation of an S_3 gallop in cases of advanced heart failure or an S_4 gallop in cases of poor left ventricular distensibility during diastole. The left ventricular apex is more diffuse and sometimes may be frankly dyskinetic in patients

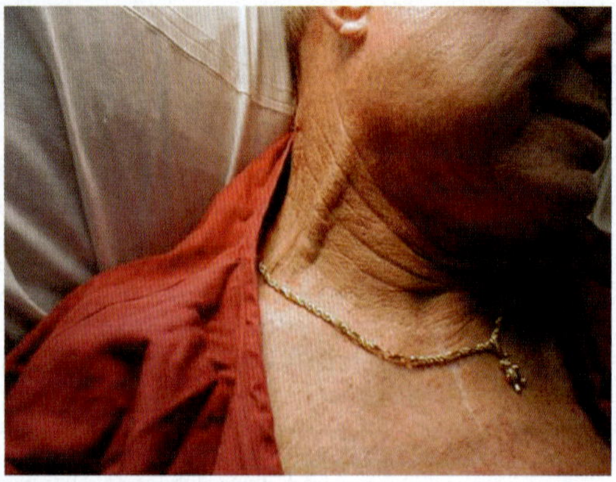

FIGURE 39-3. **Typical distention of the internal jugular vein.** (From http://courses.cvcc.vccs.edu/WisemanD/jugular_vein_distention.htm.)

TABLE 39-6 ABNORMALITIES OF VENOUS PRESSURE AND PULSE AND THEIR CLINICAL SIGNIFICANCE

Positive hepatojugular reflux	Suspect heart failure, particularly left ventricular systolic dysfunction (echocardiography recommended)
Elevated systemic venous pressure without obvious *x* or *y* descent, quiet precordium, and pulsus paradoxus	Suspect cardiac tamponade (echocardiography recommended)
Elevated systemic venous pressure with sharp *y* descent, Kussmaul sign, and quiet precordium	Suspect constrictive pericarditis (cardiac catheterization and MRI or CT recommended)
Elevated systemic venous pressure with a sharp brief *y* descent, Kussmaul sign, and evidence of pulmonary hypertension and tricuspid regurgitation	Suspect restrictive cardiomyopathy (cardiac catheterization and MRI or CT recommended)
A prominent *a* wave with or without elevation of mean systemic venous pressure	Exclude tricuspid stenosis, right ventricular hypertrophy caused by pulmonary stenosis, and pulmonary hypertension (echo-Doppler study recommended)
A prominent *v* wave with a sharp *y* descent	Suspect tricuspid regurgitation (echo-Doppler or cardiac catheterization to determine etiology)

CT = computed tomography; MRI = magnetic resonance imaging.
From Braunwald E, ed. *Heart Disease: A Textbook of Cardiovascular Medicine.* 5th ed. Philadelphia: WB Saunders; 1997.

with advanced heart disease. The distal palm is best for feeling thrills, which are the tactile equivalent of cardiac murmurs. By definition, a thrill denotes a murmur of grade 4/6 or louder. Higher-frequency events may be felt best with the fingertips; examples include the opening snap of mitral stenosis or the loud pulmonic second sound of pulmonary hypertension.

AUSCULTATION

The first heart sound (Fig. 39-5), which is largely produced by closure of the mitral and—to a lesser extent—the tricuspid valves, may be louder in patients with mitral valve stenosis and intact valve leaflet movement and less audible in patients with poor closure caused by mitral regurgitation (Chapter 60). The second heart sound is caused primarily by closure of the aortic valve, but closure of the pulmonic valve is also commonly audible. In normal individuals, the louder aortic closure sound occurs first, followed by pulmonic closure. With expiration, the two sounds are virtually superimposed. With inspiration, by comparison, the increased stroke volume of the right ventricle commonly leads to a discernible splitting of the second sound. This splitting may be fixed in patients with an atrial septal defect (Chapter 55) or a right bundle branch block. The split may be paradoxical in patients with left bundle branch block or other causes of delayed left ventricular emptying. The aortic component of the second sound is increased in intensity in the presence of systemic hypertension and decreased in intensity in patients with aortic stenosis. The pulmonic second sound is increased in the presence of pulmonary hypertension.

Early systolic ejection sounds are related to forceful opening of the aortic or pulmonic valve. These sounds are common in congenital aortic stenosis, with a mobile valve; in hypertension, with forceful opening of the aortic valve; and in healthy young individuals, especially when cardiac output is increased. Midsystolic or late systolic clicks are caused most commonly by mitral valve prolapse (Chapter 60). Clicks are relatively high-frequency sounds that are heard best with the diaphragm of the stethoscope.

An S_3 corresponds to rapid ventricular filling during early diastole. It may occur in normal children and young adults, especially if stroke volume is increased. After about 40 years of age, however, an S_3 should be considered abnormal; it is caused by conditions that increase the volume of ventricular filling during early diastole (e.g., mitral regurgitation) or that increase pressure in early diastole (e.g., advanced heart failure).[7] A left ventricular S_3 gallop is heard best at the apex, whereas the right ventricular S_3 gallop is heard best at the fourth intercostal space at the left parasternal border; both are heard best with the bell of the stethoscope. An S_4 is heard rarely in young individuals but is common in adults older than 40 or 50 years because of reduced ventricular compliance during atrial contraction; it is a nearly ubiquitous finding in patients with hypertension, heart failure, or ischemic heart disease.

The opening snap of mitral and, less commonly, tricuspid stenosis (Chapter 60) occurs at the beginning of mechanical diastole, before the onset of the rapid phase of ventricular filling. An opening snap is high pitched and is heard best with the diaphragm; this differential frequency should help distinguish an opening snap from an S_3 on physical examination. An opening snap commonly can be distinguished from a loud pulmonic component of the second heart sound by the differential location (mitral opening snap at the apex, tricuspid opening snap at the left third or fourth intercostal space, pulmonic second sound at the left second intercostal space) and by the longer interval between S_2 and the opening snap.

Heart murmurs may be classified as systolic, diastolic, or continuous (Table 39-7).[8] Murmurs are graded by intensity on a scale of 1 to 6. Grade 1 is faint and appreciated only by careful auscultation; grade 2, readily audible; grade 3, moderately loud; grade 4, loud and associated with a palpable thrill; grade 5, loud and audible with the stethoscope only partially placed on the chest; and grade 6, loud enough to be heard without the stethoscope on the chest. Systolic ejection murmurs usually peak in early to mid-systole when left ventricular ejection is maximal; examples include fixed valvular, supravalvular, or infravalvular aortic stenosis and pulmonic stenosis. The murmur of hypertrophic obstructive cardiomyopathy has a similar ejection quality, although its peak may be later in systole when dynamic obstruction is maximal (Chapter 47). Pansystolic murmurs are characteristic of mitral or tricuspid regurgitation or with a left-to-right shunt from conditions such as a ventricular septal defect (left ventricle to right ventricle). A late systolic murmur is characteristic of mitral valve prolapse (Chapter 60) or ischemic papillary muscle dysfunction. Ejection quality murmurs also may be heard in patients with normal valves but increased flow, such as occurs with marked anemia, fever, or bradycardia secondary to congenital complete heart block; they also may be heard across a valve that is downstream from increased flow because of an intracardiac shunt. Maneuvers such as inspiration, expiration, standing, squatting, and hand gripping can be especially useful in the differential diagnosis of a murmur; however, echocardiography commonly is required to make a definitive diagnosis of cause and severity (Table 39-8).

High-frequency, early diastolic murmurs are typical of aortic regurgitation and pulmonic regurgitation from a variety of causes. The murmurs of mitral and tricuspid stenosis begin in early to mid-diastole and tend to diminish in intensity later in diastole in the absence of effective atrial contraction, but they tend to increase in intensity in later diastole if effective atrial contraction is present.

Continuous murmurs may be caused by any abnormality that is associated with a pressure gradient in systole and diastole. Examples include a patent ductus arteriosus, ruptured sinus of Valsalva aneurysm, arteriovenous fistula (of the coronary artery, pulmonary artery, or thoracic artery), and a mammary souffle. In some situations, murmurs of two coexistent conditions (e.g., aortic stenosis and regurgitation, atrial septal defect with a large shunt and resulting flow murmurs of relative mitral and pulmonic stenosis) may mimic a continuous murmur.

Although experienced examiners may still be able to diagnose meaningful valvular heart disease accurately by auscultation, most general physicians are not nearly so accurate, even after training. As a result, echocardiography (Chapter 43) is critical to the evaluation of patients with suspected structural heart disease.

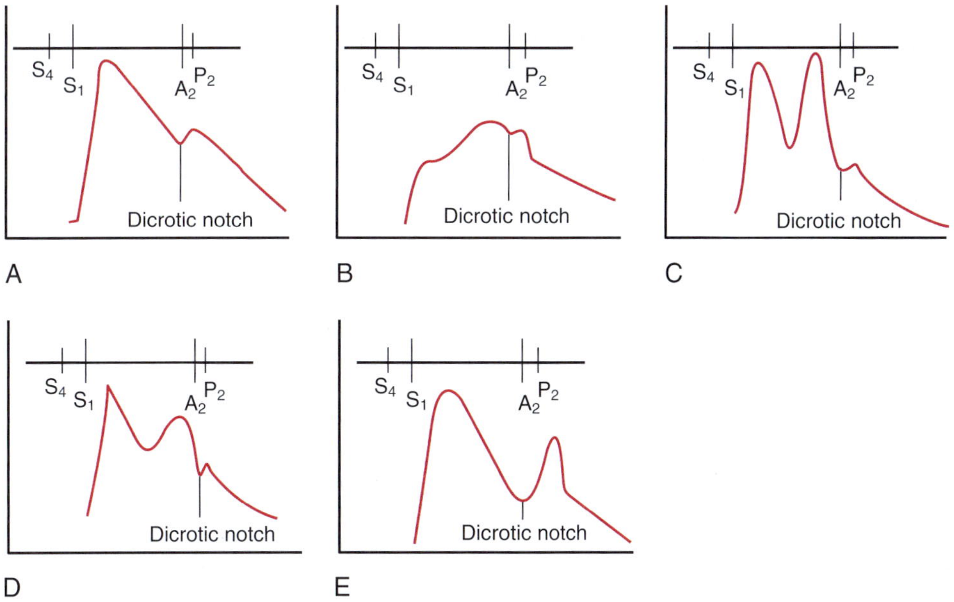

FIGURE 39-4. **Schematic diagrams of the configurational changes in the carotid pulse and their differential diagnosis.** Heart sounds also are illustrated. **A,** Normal. **B,** Anacrotic pulse with slow initial upstroke. The peak is close to the second heart sound. These features suggest fixed left ventricular outflow obstruction, such as valvular aortic stenosis. **C,** Pulsus bisferiens, with percussion and tidal waves occurring during systole. This type of carotid pulse contour is observed most frequently in patients with hemodynamically significant aortic regurgitation or combined aortic stenosis and regurgitation with dominant regurgitation. It rarely is observed in patients with mitral valve prolapse or in normal individuals. **D,** Pulsus bisferiens in hypertrophic obstructive cardiomyopathy. This finding rarely is appreciated at the bedside by palpation. **E,** Dicrotic pulse results from an accentuated dicrotic wave and tends to occur in sepsis, severe heart failure, hypovolemic shock, and cardiac tamponade and after aortic valve replacement. A_2 = aortic component of the second heart sound; P_2 = pulmonary component of the second heart sound); S_1 = first heart sound; S_4 = atrial sounds. (From Chatterjee K. Bedside evaluation of the heart: the physical examination. In: Chatterjee K, Chetlin MD, Karliner J, et al, eds. *Cardiology: An Illustrated Text/Reference.* Philadelphia: JB Lippincott; 1991:3.11-3.51.)

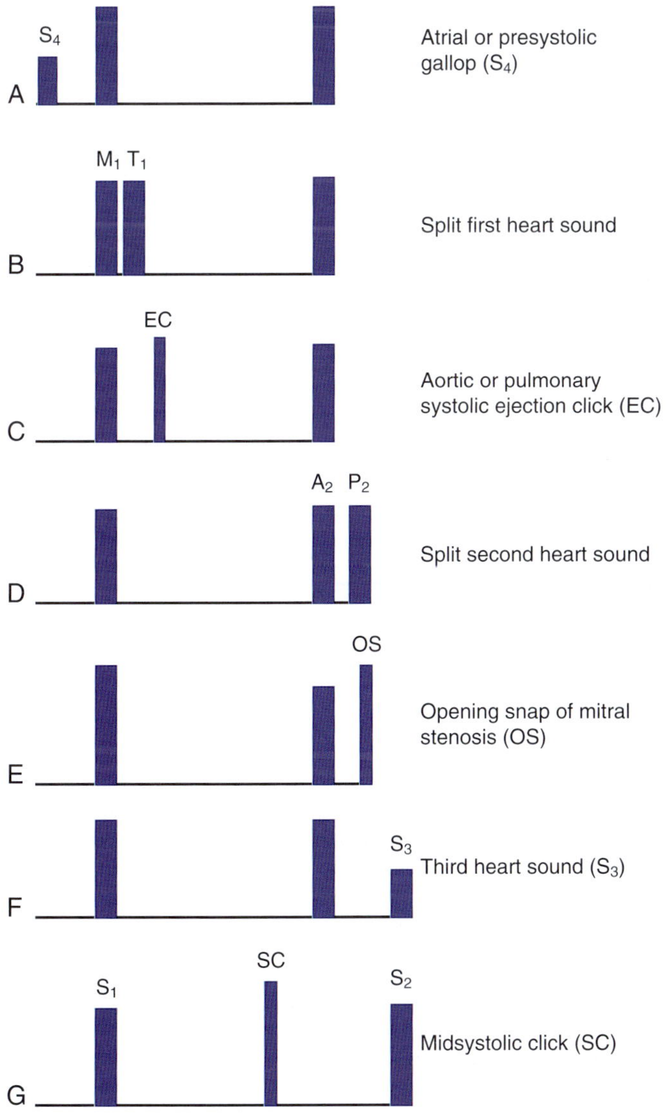

FIGURE 39-5. **Timing of the different heart sounds and added sounds.** (Modified from Wood P. *Diseases of the Heart and Circulation.* 3rd ed. Philadelphia: JB Lippincott; 1968.)

ABDOMEN

The most common cause of hepatomegaly in patients with heart disease is hepatic engorgement from elevated right-sided pressures associated with right ventricular failure of any cause. Hepatojugular reflux is elicited by pressing on the liver and showing an increase in the jugular venous pressure; it indicates advanced right ventricular failure or obstruction to right ventricular filling. Evaluation of the abdomen also may reveal an enlarged liver caused by a systemic disease, such as hemochromatosis (Chapter 196) or sarcoidosis (Chapter 83), which also may affect the heart. In more severe cases, splenomegaly and ascites also may be noted. Large, palpable, polycystic kidneys (Chapter 112) commonly are associated with hypertension. A systolic bruit suggestive of renal artery stenosis (Chapter 110) or an enlarged abdominal aorta (Chapter 63) is a clue of atherosclerosis.

EXTREMITIES

Extremities should be evaluated for peripheral pulses, edema, cyanosis, and clubbing. Diminished peripheral pulses suggest peripheral arterial disease (Chapters 65 and 66). Delayed pulses in the legs are consistent with coarctation of the aorta and are seen after aortic dissection.

Edema (Fig. 39-6) is a cardinal manifestation of right-sided heart failure. When it is caused by heart failure, pericardial disease, or pulmonary hypertension, the edema is usually symmetrical and progresses upward from the ankles; each of these causes of cardiac edema commonly is associated with jugular venous distention and often with hepatic congestion.[9] Unilateral edema suggests thrombophlebitis or proximal venous or lymphatic obstruction (Fig. 39-7).[10] Edema in the absence of evidence of right-sided or left-sided heart failure suggests renal disease, hypoalbuminemia, myxedema, or other noncardiac causes. Among unselected patients with bilateral edema, about 40% have an underlying cardiac disease, about 40% have an elevated pulmonary blood pressure, about 20% have bilateral venous disease, about 20% have renal disease, and about 25% have idiopathic edema. In patients who have chronic leg edema with recurrent cellulitis, leg compression therapy can reduce the risk of subsequent cellulitis.[A1]

Cyanosis (Fig. 39-8) is a bluish discoloration caused by reduced hemoglobin exceeding about 5 g/dL in the capillary bed. Central cyanosis is seen in patients with poor oxygen saturation resulting from a reduced inspired oxygen concentration or inability to oxygenate the blood in the lungs (e.g., as a result of advanced pulmonary disease, pulmonary edema, pulmonary arteriovenous fistula, or right-to-left shunting); it also may be seen in patients with marked erythrocytosis. Methemoglobinemia (Chapter 144) also can present with cyanosis. Peripheral cyanosis may be caused by reduced blood flow to the extremities secondary to vasoconstriction, heart failure, or shock.

TABLE 39-7 SOME COMMON CAUSES OF HEART MURMURS*

	USUAL LOCATION	COMMON ASSOCIATED FINDINGS
SYSTOLIC		
Holosystolic		
Mitral regurgitation	Apex → axilla	↑ with handgrip; S_3 if marked mitral regurgitation; left ventricular dilation common
Tricuspid regurgitation	LLSB	↑ with inspiration; right ventricular dilation common
Ventricular septal defect	LLSB → RLSB	Often with thrill
Early to midsystolic		
Aortic valvular stenosis	RUSB	Ejection click if mobile valve; soft or absent A_2 if valve immobile; later peak associated with more severe stenosis
Fixed supravalvular or subvalvular	RUSB	
Dynamic infravalvular	LLSB → apex + axilla	Hypertrophic obstructive cardiomyopathy; murmur louder if left ventricular volume lower or contractility increased, softer if left ventricular volume increased†; can be later in systole if obstruction delayed
Pulmonic valvular stenosis	LUSB	↑ with inspiration
Infravalvular (infundibular)	LUSB	↑ with inspiration
Supravalvular	LUSB	↑ with inspiration
"Flow murmurs"	LUSB	Anemia, fever, increased flow of any cause‡
Mid to late systolic		
Mitral valve prolapse	LLSB or apex → axilla	Preceded by click; murmur lengthens with maneuvers that decrease left ventricular volume†
Papillary muscle dysfunction	Apex → axilla	Ischemic heart disease
DIASTOLIC		
Early diastolic		
Aortic regurgitation	RUSB, LUSB	High-pitched, blowing quality; endocarditis, diseases of the aorta, associated aortic valvular stenosis; signs of low peripheral vascular resistance
Pulmonic valve regurgitation	LUSB	Pulmonary hypertension as a causative factor
Mid to late diastolic		
Mitral stenosis, tricuspid stenosis	Apex, LLSB	Low pitched; in rheumatic heart disease, opening snap commonly precedes murmur; can be caused by increased flow across normal valve‡
Atrial myxomas	Apex (L), LLSB (R)	"Tumor plop"
Continuous		
Venous hum	Over jugular or hepatic vein or breast	
Patent ductus arteriosus	LUSB	
Arteriovenous fistula		
Coronary	LUSB	
Pulmonary, bronchial, chest wall	Over fistula	
Ruptured sinus of Valsalva aneurysm	RUSB	Sudden onset

*See also Chapters 55 and 60.

†Left ventricular volume is decreased by standing or during prolonged, forced expiration against a closed glottis (Valsalva maneuver); it is increased by squatting or by elevation of the legs; contractility is increased by adrenergic stimulation or in the beat after an extrasystolic beat.

‡Including a left-to-right shunt through an atrial septal defect for tricuspid or pulmonic flow murmurs and a ventricular septal defect for pulmonic or mitral flow murmurs.

LLSB = left lower sternal border (fourth intercostal space); LUSB = left upper sternal border (second and third intercostal spaces); RLSB = right lower sternal border (fourth intercostal space); RUSB = right upper sternal border (second and third intercostal spaces).

TABLE 39-8 SENSITIVITY AND SPECIFICITY OF BEDSIDE MANEUVERS IN THE IDENTIFICATION OF SYSTOLIC MURMURS

MANEUVER	RESPONSE	MURMUR	SENSITIVITY (%)	SPECIFICITY (%)
Inspiration	↑	RS	100	88
Expiration	↓	RS	100	88
Valsalva maneuver	↑	HC	65	96
Squat to stand	↑	HC	95	84
Stand to squat	↓	HC	95	85
Leg elevation	↓	HC	85	91
Handgrip	↓	HC	85	75
Handgrip	↑	MR and VSD	68	92
Transient arterial occlusion	↑	MR and VSD	78	100

HC = hypertrophic cardiomyopathy; MR = mitral regurgitation; RS = right sided; VSD = ventricular septal defect.

Modified with permission from Lembo NJ, Dell'Italia IJ, Crawford MH, et al. Bedside diagnosis of systolic murmurs. *N Engl J Med.* 1988;318:1572-1578.

Clubbing (Fig. 39-9), which is loss of the normal concave configuration of the nail as it emerges from the distal phalanx, is seen in patients with cyanotic congenital heart disease (Chapter 55), but in adults it is usually related to pulmonary abnormalities such as lung cancer (Chapter 177).[11]

EXAMINATION OF THE SKIN

Examination of the skin may reveal bronze pigmentation typical of hemochromatosis (Chapter 196); jaundice (see Fig. 132-1) characteristic of severe right-sided heart failure or hemochromatosis; or capillary hemangiomas typical of hereditary hemorrhagic telangiectasia (see Fig. 159-3), which also is associated with pulmonary arteriovenous fistulas and cyanosis. Infectious endocarditis may be associated with splinter hemorrhages (Fig. 39-10),[12] Osler nodes (see Fig. 61-2), or Janeway lesions (Chapter 61). Xanthomas (E-Fig. 39-1) are subcutaneous deposits of cholesterol seen on the extensor surfaces of the extremities or on the palms and digital creases; they are found in patients with severe hypercholesterolemia.

LABORATORY STUDIES

All patients with known or suspected cardiac disease should have an ECG. The ECG (Chapter 42) helps identify rate, rhythm, conduction abnormalities, and possible myocardial ischemia or myocardial infarction. Blood testing in patients with known or suspected cardiac disease should be targeted to the conditions in question. In general, a complete blood cell count, thyroid indices, and lipid levels are part of the standard evaluation. Genetic screening has become increasingly useful in individuals who have a family history of cardiomyopathy, arrhythmias, or sudden death.[13]

The chest radiograph (Chapter 44) yields important information on chamber enlargement, pulmonary vasculature, and the great vessels. Point-of-care ultrasonography is increasingly being used in acute care settings to distinguish heart failure from pulmonary causes of dyspnea,[14] to diagnose severe valvular heart disease, and to evaluate suspected pericardial tamponade.[15]

For patients who have acute chest pain or other symptoms that suggest acute myocardial ischemia, the probability of an acute myocardial infarction can be estimated by integrating information from the history, physical examination, and ECG. If the ECG shows evidence of ST-segment or T-wave changes that are consistent with myocardial ischemia and that are not known to be old, admission is mandatory, and acute interventions are often required (Chapters 57 and 58). In other patients who have suggestive symptoms but a nondiagnostic ECG, rapid testing with a high-sensitivity troponin assay is very helpful for guiding triage decisions (Chapter 57). An undetectable high-sensitivity troponin level at presentation reduces the probability of acute MI or an acute coronary event to less than 1%.[16] A protocol in which the ECG and troponin level are repeated in 2 hours is as good as longer observation periods for evaluating patients with acute chest pain and suspected myocardial infarction. However, the advent of high-sensitivity troponin assays has also greatly increased the risk for a false-positive diagnosis of myocardial infarction, especially because of chronic troponin elevations in many cardiac conditions and in some elderly patients (Chapter 57). In this acute setting, early CT angiography does not improve clinical outcomes compared with invasive coronary angiography (Chapter 57).[A2]

In patients who have dyspnea or other symptoms or signs of potential heart failure, a pro–B-type natriuretic peptide level (Chapter 45) is very useful for their emergency evaluation. A level <300 pg/mL nearly excludes the diagnosis of heart failure.[17]

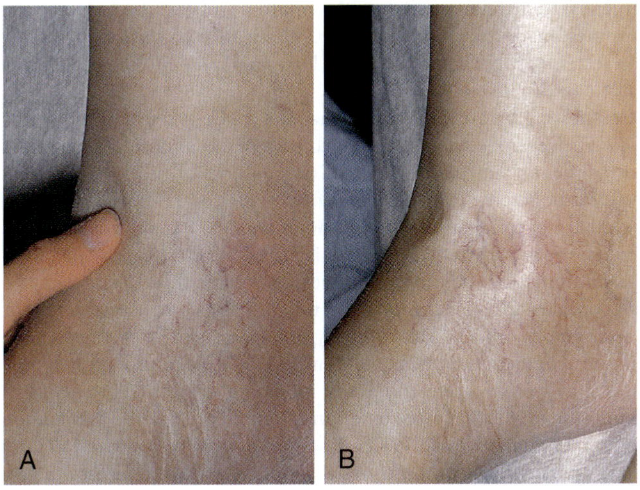

FIGURE 39-6. A and B, Pitting edema in a patient with cardiac failure. A depression ("pit") remains in the edema for some minutes after firm fingertip pressure is applied. (From Forbes CD, Jackson WD. *Color Atlas and Text of Clinical Medicine*. 3rd ed. London: Mosby; 2003.)

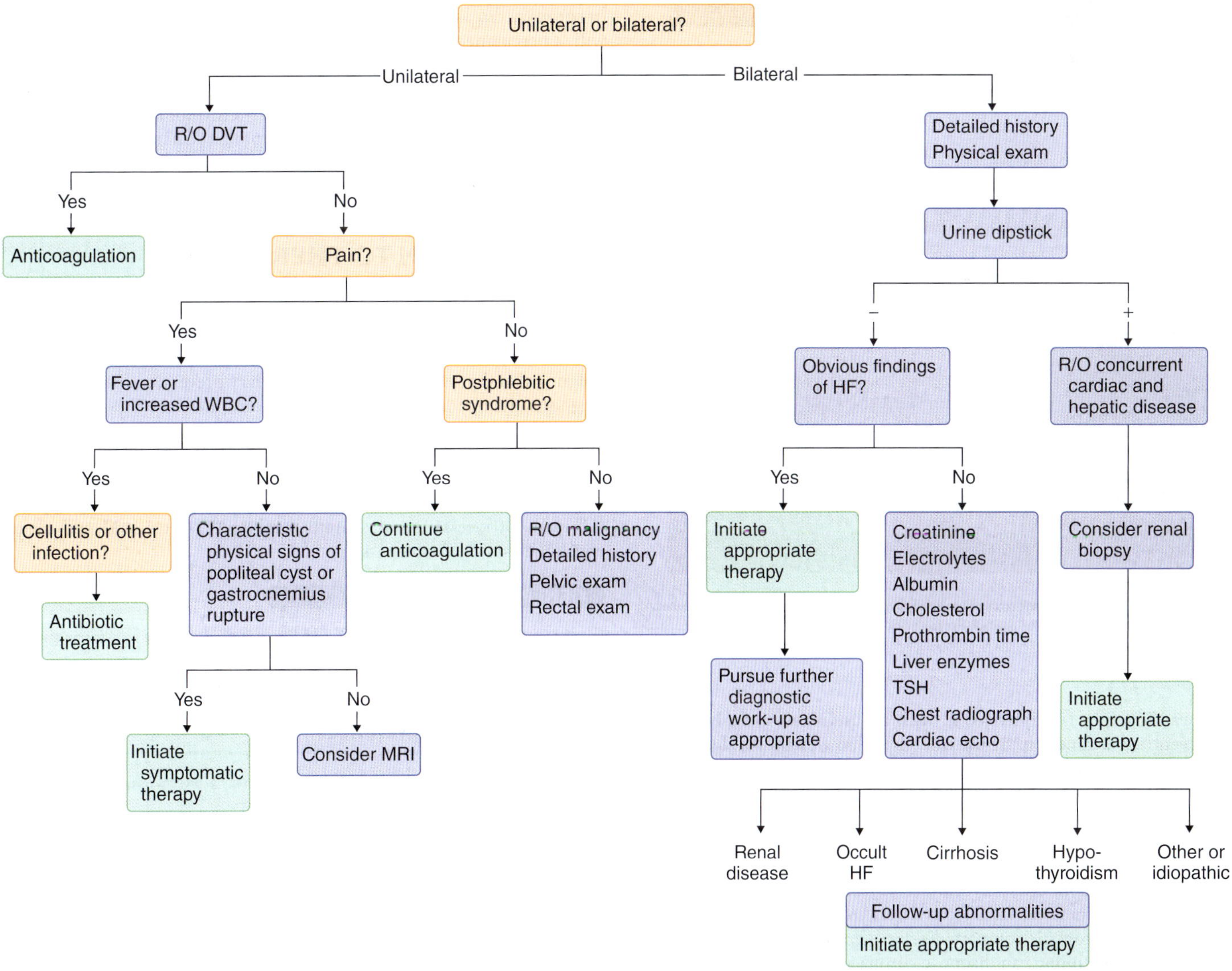

FIGURE 39-7. Diagnostic approach to patients with edema. DVT = deep vein thrombosis; HF = heart failure; MRI = magnetic resonance imaging; R/O = rule out; TSH = thyroid-stimulating hormone; WBC = white blood cell count. (From Chertow G. Approach to the patient with edema. In: Braunwald E, Goldman L, eds. *Primary Cardiology*. 2nd ed. Philadelphia: WB Saunders; 2003.)

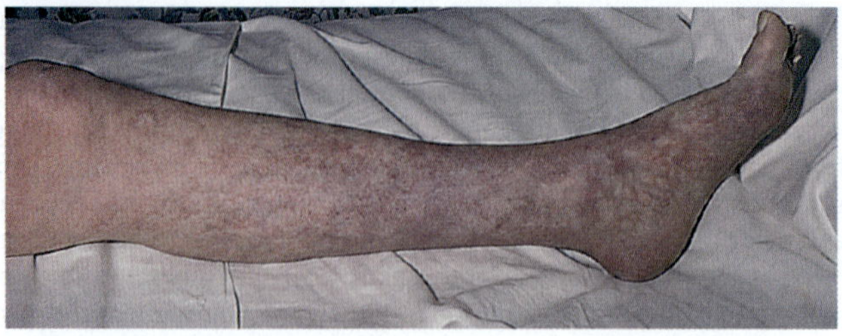

FIGURE 39-8. Arterial embolism causing acute ischemia and cyanosis of the leg. Initial pallor of the leg and foot was followed by cyanosis. (From Forbes CD, Jackson WD. *Color Atlas and Text of Clinical Medicine*. 3rd ed. London: Mosby; 2003.)

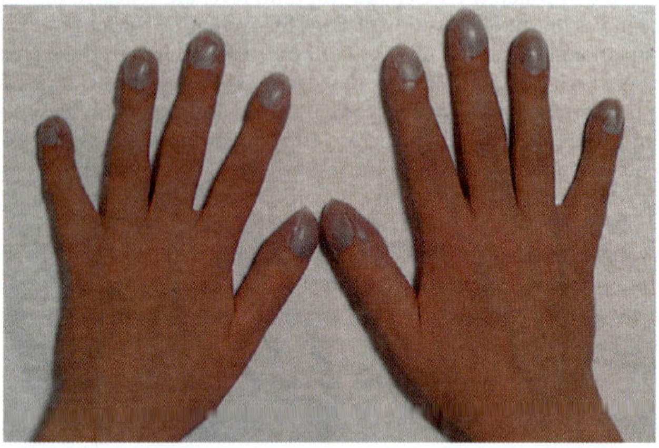

FIGURE 39-9. Severe finger clubbing in a patient with cyanotic congenital heart disease. (From Forbes CD, Jackson WD. *Color Atlas and Text of Clinical Medicine*. 3rd ed. London: Mosby; 2003.)

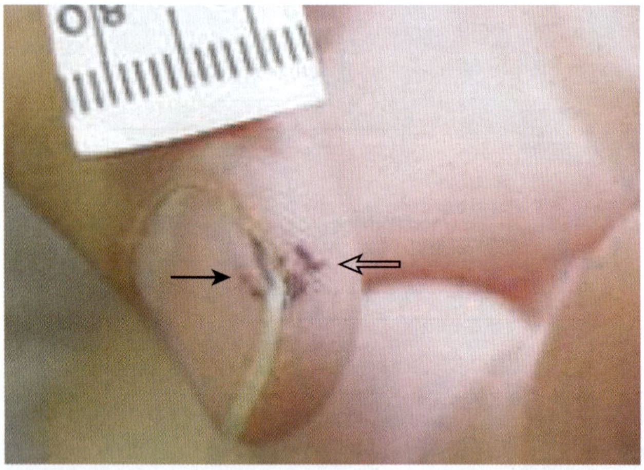

FIGURE 39-10. Splinter hemorrhage (*solid arrow*) and Janeway lesions (*open arrow*). These findings should stimulate a work-up for endocarditis. (Courtesy of Daniel L. Stulberg, MD.)

Echocardiography (Chapter 43) is the most useful test to analyze valvular and ventricular function. By use of Doppler flow methods, stenotic and regurgitant lesions can be quantified. Handheld ultrasonography performed by generalists can improve the assessment of left ventricular function, cardiomegaly, and pericardial effusion. Transesophageal echocardiography is the preferred method to evaluate possible aortic dissection and to identify clots in the cardiac chambers. Radionuclide studies (Chapter 44) can measure left ventricular function, assess myocardial ischemia, and determine whether ischemic myocardium is viable. CT can detect coronary calcium, which is a risk factor for symptomatic coronary disease (Chapter 44).[18]

Multislice CT scanning can diagnose coronary disease. In a randomized trial of emergency department patients at low to intermediate risk for a possible acute coronary syndrome, coronary CT angiography resulted in a higher rate of discharge from the emergency department (50% vs. 23%), a shorter length of stay (median, 18 vs. 24.8 hours), and a higher rate of detection of coronary disease (9% vs. 3.5%) without any change in the rate of serious adverse events. However, in a subsequent randomized trial of emergency department patients with symptoms suggestive of acute coronary syndromes but without ischemic ECG changes or an initially positive troponin test, incorporating coronary CT angiography into the triage strategy did not decrease overall costs of care.

Stress testing by exercise or pharmacologic stress is useful to precipitate myocardial ischemia that may be detected by ECG abnormalities, perfusion abnormalities on radionuclide studies, or transient wall motion abnormalities on echocardiography. These tests are often crucial for the diagnosis of possible myocardial ischemia (see Figs. 56-1, 56-2, and 56-3) and for understanding the prognosis in patients with known ischemic heart disease.

In symptomatic patients with suspected coronary disease, the strategies of initial coronary CT angiography and functional testing using exercise electrocardiography, nuclear stress testing, or stress echocardiography provide equivalent clinical outcomes over a median follow-up of 2 years,[A3] but CT angiography may be preferable when follow-up is extended to 5 years.[A4] In patients whose chest pain portends an intermediate risk for stable underlying coronary artery disease, CT coronary angiography is as good as invasive coronary angiography in terms of guiding therapy over at least 3.5 years.[A5] However, none of these tests are currently recommended in asymptomatic individuals, either routinely or prior to participation in sports or other physical activities.

Cardiac catheterization (Chapter 59) can measure precise gradients across stenotic cardiac valves, judge the severity of intracardiac shunts, and determine intracardiac pressures. Coronary angiography provides a definitive diagnosis of coronary disease and is a necessary prelude to coronary revascularization with a percutaneous coronary intervention or coronary artery bypass graft surgery (Chapter 59).

Continuous ambulatory ECG monitoring can help diagnose arrhythmias. A variety of newer technologies allow longer-term monitoring in patients with important but infrequently occurring symptoms (Chapter 49). Formal invasive electrophysiologic testing can be useful in the diagnosis of ventricular or supraventricular wide-complex tachycardia, and it is crucial for guiding a wide array of new invasive electrophysiologic therapies (Chapter 54).

APPROACH TO THERAPY

The history, physical examination, and laboratory evaluation should help the physician establish the cause of any cardiovascular problem; identify and quantify any anatomic abnormalities; determine the physiologic status of the valves, myocardium, and conduction system; determine functional capacity; estimate prognosis; and provide primary or secondary prevention. Improvements in diagnosis, therapy, and prevention have contributed to a 70% or so decline in age-adjusted cardiovascular death rates in the United States since the 1960s. Key preventive strategies that should be part of the approach to every patient, with or without heart disease, include dietary modification (Chapter 13), recognition and treatment of hypertension (Chapter 64) and hyperlipidemia (Chapter 190), cessation of cigarette smoking (Chapter 363), and adequate physical exercise (Chapter 14).

GENERAL REFERENCES

For the General References and other additional features, please visit Elsevier eBooks+ at https://ebooks.health.elsevier.com.

Grade A References

A1. Webb E, Neeman T, Bowden FJ, et al. Compression therapy to prevent recurrent cellulitis of the leg. *N Engl J Med*. 2020;383:630-639.

A2. Gray AJ, Roobottom C, Smith JE, et al. Early computed tomography coronary angiography in patients with suspected acute coronary syndrome: randomised controlled trial. *BMJ*. 2021;374:n2106.

A3. Foy AJ, Dhruva SS, Peterson B, et al. Coronary computed tomography angiography vs functional stress testing for patients with suspected coronary artery disease: a systematic review and meta-analysis. *JAMA Intern Med*. 2017;177:1623-1631.

A4. Singh T, Bing R, Dweck MR, et al. Exercise electrocardiography and computed tomography coronary angiography for patients with suspected stable angina pectoris: a post hoc analysis of the randomized SCOT-HEART trial. *JAMA Cardiol*. 2020;5:920-928.

A5. DISCHARGE Trial Group, Maurovich-Horvat P, Bosserdt M, et al. CT or invasive coronary angiography in stable chest pain. *N Engl J Med*. 2022;386:1591-1602.

40

EPIDEMIOLOGY OF CARDIOVASCULAR DISEASE

DONALD M. LLOYD-JONES

Cardiovascular diseases remain the leading causes of death, disability, and medical costs in the world, and they are expected to remain so for the foreseeable future. Cardiovascular disease manifests in a number of different ways, including: congenital heart and vascular malformations (Chapter 55); coronary heart disease (Chapters 56, 57, 58, and 59); heart failure (Chapter 46); cardiomyopathies (Chapter 47); valvular heart disease (Chapter 60); dysrhythmias (Chapters 49, 50, 51, 52, and 53); pericardial diseases (Chapter 62); aortic (Chapter 63), peripheral (Chapter 65), and cerebrovascular diseases (Chapter 375); systemic hypertension (Chapter 64); vasculitides (Chapter 249); venous thromboembolic disease (Chapter 68); and pulmonary vascular hypertension (Chapter 69). Of these, coronary heart disease, stroke, and heart failure, which share many common underlying risk factors, have by far the largest impact on the population in terms of incidence, prevalence, quality of life, and medical costs.

BURDEN IN THE UNITED STATES

Cardiovascular diseases have been the leading cause of death in the United States in every year of the 20th and 21st centuries except for 1918, when the influenza epidemic surpassed them. Even during the severe acute respiratory disease coronavirus 2 (SARS-CoV-2) pandemic (Chapter 336), cardiovascular disease remained the leading cause of death. Cardiovascular diseases account for 1 in 3 deaths in the United States annually, or more than 850,000 deaths, including about 420,000 women and slightly more men. The overall age-adjusted annual rate of death due to cardiovascular disease in the United States is about 219 per 100,000 persons, with higher rates in men than in women and in Black than in White, Hispanic, or Asian Americans.[1] Because of secular trends in risk factors and the development of effective treatments over the last 50 years, cardiovascular disease mortality rates declined by approximately 70% from their peak in the 1960s, but rates have been constant since 2011.[2]

Cardiovascular diseases also are the leading cause of hospitalizations and medical costs in the United States. Each year about 5 million Americans are hospitalized for cardiovascular disease, over 1 million of which are due to coronary heart disease and approximately 1 million more each are due to heart failure and stroke. The United States currently spends approximately $360 billion annually on direct costs for cardiovascular diseases, and total costs are projected to exceed $800 billion annually by 2030.

In the United States, about 20.1 million adults (7.2%) have coronary heart disease, 45% of whom have had a myocardial infarction. Each year, Americans suffer over 1 million new and recurrent myocardial infarctions, with about 365,000 deaths due to coronary heart disease, a large percentage of which are sudden cardiac deaths. There are 7.6 million stroke survivors (2.7%) in the United States, with the proportion twice as high in Black than in White Americans, and 795,000 new or recurrent strokes occur every year. Stroke rates are especially high in the so-called "stroke belt" in the southeastern United States. At present, 6 million Americans (2.1%) have chronic heart failure, with prevalence 50% higher in men than women and in individuals who identify as Black. With aging, the risks for stroke and heart failure tend to increase at younger ages in women and Black Americans than in White men, whose coronary risk increases earlier.

GLOBAL BURDEN

Cardiovascular diseases, including coronary heart disease and stroke, became the leading cause of death and disability globally in the early 21st century (E-Fig. 40-1). About 80% of cardiovascular deaths and events now occur in low- and middle-income countries, and the onset of cardiovascular disease tends to be at an earlier age in these countries.[3] For example, about 50% of coronary deaths occur before age 70 years in India, whereas only 25% occur by that age in high-income countries.[4] Unfavorable global trends in eating patterns, high rates of smoking, and increasing burdens of obesity, diabetes, and hypertension are driving the burden of cardiovascular disease. Although stroke was the dominant cause of death and disability in East Asian countries for decades owing to high sodium intake and resulting hypertension, recent changes in diet, activity levels, and smoking have made coronary heart disease an equivalent or greater health burden in this area of the world.

RISK FACTORS FOR CARDIOVASCULAR DISEASE

ESTABLISHED RISK FACTORS

A number of causal factors have been established for cardiovascular disease based on their strength and consistency of associations, specificity, temporality, and biologic plausibility. Furthermore, these established risk factors explain the vast majority of risk for incident myocardial infarction. Longitudinal cohort studies demonstrate that 90% of individuals who suffer a myocardial infarction have at least one established clinical risk factor prior to their first event, and adverse levels of nine risk factors and behaviors collectively account for 90% or more of the risk for myocardial infarction in men and women, in older and younger individuals, and in all regions of the world. These nine risk factors and behaviors include smoking (Chapter 363), elevated apolipoprotein B/apolipoprotein A1 ratio (Chapter 190), hypertension (Chapter 64), diabetes (Chapter 210), abdominal obesity (Chapter 201), psychosocial factors, lower consumption of fruits and vegetables (Chapter 13), alcohol intake (Chapter 364), and physical inactivity (Chapter 14). Many of the established risk factors tend to cluster in a *metabolic syndrome*, which is characterized by abdominal adiposity, insulin resistance, hyperglycemia, elevated blood pressure, elevated triglyceride levels, and lower high-density lipoprotein (HDL)-cholesterol levels. This clustering of cardiovascular risk factors can lead to synergistic increases in the risk for events.

Age is the most powerful risk factor for the development of most cardiovascular diseases, especially stroke (Chapter 376), heart failure (Chapters 45 and 46), and atrial fibrillation (Chapter 52). Chronologic age integrates a person's aggregate exposure to multiple physiologic and environmental factors on the cardiovascular system. The incidence of cardiovascular disease at least doubles with each additional decade of age in adulthood until the oldest ages, when the heavy burden of competing causes of mortality (Chapter 22) limits further progression. Newer methods of assessing biologic age, as compared with chronologic age, may lead to improved assessment of cardiovascular risk.[5]

The impact of a person's *sex* on cardiovascular disease is important. Women tend to develop risk factors later in life than do men, and women's cardiovascular disease incidence rates lag men's by approximately 10 years. The precise contributions of sex hormones to these age trends are uncertain, but many women develop worsening risk factor levels, particularly with regard to lipids, blood pressure, weight, and insulin resistance, during and after the menopausal transition (Chapter 222). Pregnancy is a cardiovascular stress test, and adverse outcomes of pregnancy are markers of risk for future cardiometabolic disease.[6]

Large disparities in cardiovascular disease are noted by *self-identified race* or ethnicity, but the established causal risk factors have broadly similar effects in all racial and ethnic groups. Hypertension tends to be more prevalent in individuals of African ancestry, especially in environments with higher sodium intake, and to have a somewhat stronger association with cardiovascular events, especially heart failure and stroke. Compared with Whites, individuals of East Asian and South Asian descent have a greater risk for developing metabolic syndrome, insulin resistance, and diabetes at a lower overall body mass index. A substantial proportion of the differences in cardiovascular risks and outcomes observed across race and ethnic groups can be attributed to differences in social determinants of health (education, socioeconomic position, health care access; Chapter 4),[7] but racial differences still exist after considering these factors.[8]

Blood lipid levels (Chapter 190), including the total serum cholesterol level and its subfractions, particularly low-density lipoprotein (LDL) cholesterol, have significant, continuous, and graded associations with the risk of coronary heart disease. Cumulative exposure is more predictive than any single measurement, elevated levels earlier in life are associated with greater risk,[9] and earlier reduction in lipid levels will have greater absolute benefit.[10] By comparison, independent, direct associations of blood lipids with stroke and heart failure events are much weaker. Apolipoprotein B–containing particles comprise the subpopulation of circulating cholesterol-containing particles that represent the atherogenic lipoprotein fractions. These particles are considered to be the central actors in the initiation and promotion of atherogenesis on the basis of a substantial body of epidemiologic, clinical, and basic science evidence. Among U.S. adults aged 20 years and older, 38.1% (or about 94 million) have total cholesterol levels above the desirable range of less than 200 mg/dL, and 11.5% (28 million) have elevated levels at or over 240 mg/dL. Mean total cholesterol levels have been falling sharply in recent decades, because of changes in dietary composition but also because of more widespread use of lipid-lowering medications. In the 1970s, mean total cholesterol concentrations were approximately 220 mg/dL, whereas currently they are just under 200 mg/dL. These improvements have been a major contributor to the decline in coronary death rates over the same time period. Randomized clinical trials have unequivocally established LDL cholesterol (and the particles that carry it) as a causal agent for coronary heart disease, and LDL cholesterol-lowering therapies (Chapter 190) are effective at reducing rates of both coronary heart disease and stroke significantly and substantially.[A1,11]

Blood pressure (Chapter 64) has a strong, continuous, and independent association with incident coronary heart disease, stroke, and heart failure events. In worldwide studies of nearly one million individuals, the risk at every age for all types of cardiovascular disease death doubled with each 20 mm Hg higher systolic blood pressure and each 10 mm Hg higher diastolic blood pressure, beginning at a blood pressure of 115/75 mm Hg. In 2017, U.S. blood pressure guidelines lowered the definition of hypertension to 130 mm Hg systolic or higher or 80 mm Hg diastolic or higher; under this definition nearly half of U.S. adults have hypertension, and its prevalence has been increasing owing to the obesity epidemic. In the United States, rates of treatment and control were gradually increasing prior to the SARS-CoV-2 pandemic, which caused a significant decline.[12] Hypertension has stronger relative associations with stroke and heart failure than with coronary heart disease, in part because of its effects on myocardial and cerebrovascular remodeling. The effective treatment of hypertension reduces the risk of stroke, heart failure, and coronary heart disease events. Current data suggest that a treatment goal of lower than 120 mm Hg systolic (with an average achieved systolic pressure of 120 to 124 mm Hg) reduces cardiovascular events and all-cause mortality compared with a goal of lower than 140 mm Hg systolic in patients without preexisting heart failure or diabetes.[13] For patients with diabetes, a goal of lower than 130 mm Hg is reasonable.[14]

Cigarette smoking (Chapter 363) is one of the strongest risk factors for cardiovascular disease events. After adjustment for other risk factors, smoking confers two- to three-fold higher risk for all manifestations of cardiovascular disease, especially coronary heart disease and peripheral arterial disease. Fortunately, consistent public health efforts have reduced the prevalence of smoking in the United States from about 45% in the 1960s to just under 15% currently. The prevalence of smoking remains higher in many European and Asian countries, and its continued increase in some parts of the world drives unfavorable trends in cardiovascular morbidity and mortality. A large body of evidence indicates that environmental exposure to tobacco smoke in nonsmokers ("second hand" or "passive" smoking) also increases risk for cardiovascular events substantially (Chapter 363) and contributes to the population burden of disease. Substantial data also support the benefits of smoking cessation for reducing the risks of a subsequent coronary event and death.[15,16]

Overweight and obesity have been increasing in the United States and worldwide. Prior to 1985, fewer than 10% of Americans were obese, defined as having a body mass index of 30 kg/m^2 or higher. Now, however, approximately 70% (170 million) of U.S. adults are overweight or obese, with 40% being obese (Chapter 201). Thirty-five percent (26 million) of U.S. children ages 2 to 19 years are overweight or obese (Chapter 201), with roughly half in each stratum. Major societal changes in the availability of food and in dietary content, coupled with reductions in physical activity, have produced this unprecedented epidemic. Although overweight and obesity themselves tend to be weak independent predictors of cardiovascular events in the short term, they are major drivers of elevated blood pressure, elevated blood glucose levels, and adverse lipid profiles that are themselves major contributors to the incidence of cardiovascular disease in the short and long term. The existence of an "obesity paradox," in which individuals diagnosed with cardiovascular disease who are overweight or obese appear to live longer than normal weight individuals, appears to represent earlier onset of cardiovascular disease owing to overweight, with shorter total longevity and more time spent with cardiovascular disease.[17]

Blood glucose (Chapter 210) and its surrogate marker for chronic levels, hemoglobin A_{1c}, have a continuous and independent association with cardiovascular events.[18] People with diabetes, whether diagnosed or undiagnosed, have two- to three-fold higher adjusted risk for cardiovascular events compared with persons without diabetes, and they also have substantially higher risks for developing chronic kidney disease (Chapter 116). Whereas diabetes was relatively uncommon before the 1980s, the obesity epidemic has led to a dramatic increase in the prevalence of type 2 diabetes and of impaired fasting glucose levels, termed *prediabetes*, with worsening of glycemic control in the United States over the past 20 or so years.[19] At present in the United States, 26 million people, representing 9.8% of all adults, have diagnosed diabetes, and another 9.4 million (about 3.7% of adults) have undiagnosed diabetes. Fully 92 million more adults, or about 38% of adults, currently have prediabetes. Diabetes disproportionately affects non-White racial and ethnic groups, such as American Indians, Black Americans, South Asians, East Asians, and Latinos, who appear to have greater probability of insulin resistance at lower body mass index, in much greater proportions than Whites. Unfortunately, tight control of glucose levels in persons with diabetes has not been associated consistently with significant reductions in risk for macrovascular cardiovascular disease (Chapter 210). However, treatment of type 2 diabetes with sodium-glucose cotransporter-2 inhibitors or glucagon-like peptide-1 receptor agonists can reduce the risk of cardiovascular events (Chapter 210).[A2,20]

Adverse diet (Chapter 13) is a major contributor to obesity, diabetes, hypertension, and dyslipidemia. Healthy eating patterns emphasize a lower caloric intake and focus on fruits and vegetables, healthy fats from nuts and olive oil, lean sources of protein such as fish, whole grains, a reduced sodium intake, and limiting the intake of processed foods, unhealthy fats, and simple sugars.[21] This eating pattern is typical of the Mediterranean diet (Fig. 13-1), which has been shown to be associated with lower cardiovascular disease incidence,[A3,A4] and the similar DASH (Dietary Approaches to Stop Hypertension) eating pattern (Table 13-4). The consumption of more sodium and less potassium is associated with a higher risk of cardiovascular disease,[22] and using a salt substitute (75% sodium chloride, 25% potassium chloride) in patients who have a history of stroke or who are over age 60 years and have hypertension can reduce cardiovascular events and all-cause death.[A5] By comparison, supplemental vitamins, minerals, and n-3 fatty acids, independent of eating pattern, have not been shown conclusively to reduce cardiovascular risk,[A6,A7] even in patients with diabetes or preexisting heart disease.[A8-A10]

Alcohol (Chapter 364) has a complex association with cardiovascular events. Moderate intake of one serving of alcohol per day is associated with a modestly lower risk for cardiovascular disease, but it is unlikely that this association is causal.[23] At higher levels of intake, however, risks for total mortality, hypertension, stroke, and heart failure clearly increase. Whereas heavy alcohol use and patterns of binge use are associated with heart failure and atrial fibrillation, alcohol's association with atherosclerotic cardiovascular disease is less clear.

Physical inactivity (Chapter 14) *and a sedentary lifestyle* are significant risk factors for cardiovascular disease.[24] Individuals who participate in no physical activity are at highest risk for events. The risk is significantly lower for people who participate in even minimal physical activity, and risks decrease further with greater activity levels, particularly to the extent they contribute to higher objective physical fitness. The biology and risks of sedentary time may be more than just the absence of physical activity, since sedentary lifestyle, as measured best by the hours of time spent in front of a television or computer screen, seems to have an adverse effect independent of time spent doing physical activity.

Family history is clearly an important cardiovascular risk factor, independent of other measurable risk factors. Genetic variants that influence cardiovascular risk factors over the lifespan, such as blood pressure and lipid levels, affect lifetime risk even more than would be estimated by adult epidemiologic or intervention studies. However, ideal levels of cardiovascular health do not appear to be genetically programmed. The heritability of ideal cardiovascular health is less than 20%, thereby suggesting strong environmental and behavioral influences on the development of cardiovascular disease.

NOVEL RISK MARKERS

Blood markers of inflammation and *target organ damage* such as C-reactive protein, high-sensitivity troponin, or natriuretic peptide levels have demonstrated significant associations with incident and recurrent cardiovascular events, independent of established risk factors. However, inflammatory markers have contributed very little additional utility for the identification of patients at risk for cardiovascular disease. Measures of myocardial damage in apparently healthy individuals appear to have more potential clinical utility.

Noninvasive cardiac testing and imaging have demonstrated ability to detect preclinical disease and guide appropriate preventive pharmacotherapeutic decisions for higher risk individuals, or avoidance of drug therapy in individuals who are thought to be at risk but do not have evidence of preclinical disease. For example, electrocardiographic evidence of left ventricular hypertrophy confers significant excess risk for coronary heart disease over and above the presence of hypertension and other risk factors. Higher levels of coronary calcification on computed tomographic (CT) imaging of the heart (Chapter 44) or greater carotid intima-media thickness measured by B-mode ultrasound of the carotid arteries portend a higher risk of future cardiovascular events. Because these imaging markers detect evidence of the actual underlying diseases of interest (i.e., left ventricular hypertrophy or atherosclerosis), rather than nonspecific risk factors, they are more effective at identifying individuals at high risk for incident clinical events, such as heart failure, stroke, and myocardial infarction. Of the available modalities, CT screening for coronary artery calcification is the preferred and widely available means for detecting individuals at near-term risk. For example, asymptomatic individuals with coronary artery calcium scores of more than 100 Agatston units have relative hazards for a coronary event that are 7- to 10-fold higher than in individuals without any coronary calcification, even after adjustment for major established risk factors. Coronary calcium scoring is the most effective and reliable means for reclassifying risk after a quantitative risk assessment using established risk factors,[25] with the ability to more correctly classify lower-risk individuals who nonetheless will have a cardiovascular event as well as higher-risk individuals who will not.

Polygenic risk scores, which can quantify genetic variation across the entire genome, have been examined for their ability to predict risk above and beyond the traditional, routinely measured clinical risk factors. To date, such scores have demonstrated statistically significant but clinically modest ability to add value to cardiovascular risk stratification in middle-aged and older individuals.[26,27]

ASSESSMENT OF RISK FOR CARDIOVASCULAR DISEASE

Estimation of Short-Term Risk

Adverse levels of any single risk factor or risk marker are associated with elevated risk for incident cardiovascular events. However, combinations of adverse risk factors are additive and sometimes synergistic for increasing risk. To improve the prediction of cardiovascular events and provide quantitative risk assessment, a number of multivariable risk equations or scores, such as the Pooled Cohort Equations,[28] have been developed. The vast majority of risk scores available have focused on predicting 10-year absolute risk, and essentially all include age, sex, smoking status, cholesterol, and blood pressure, with some also including diabetes, family history, body mass index, socioeconomic status, or novel biomarkers. The end points of interest for diverse risk equations have varied widely, from the prediction of cardiovascular death alone to the prediction of fatal and nonfatal major coronary events, major atherosclerotic events (coronary disease and stroke), or a broader range of cardiovascular events (including heart failure, coronary revascularization, angina, or claudication). As an example, the 10-year risk for incident atherosclerotic cardiovascular disease can be predicted in 50-year-old men and women according to sex, race, and different levels of risk factors (E-Fig. 40-2), and the risks are dramatically higher with a greater risk factor burden.

Lifetime Risk Estimation

Despite the widespread use of 10-year risk estimates to guide prevention strategies, this approach has important limitations. For example, one consequence of the substantial weighting of age in 10-year risk equations is that younger men and women, even those with substantial risk factor burden, do not tend to have a high short-term risk. When treatment thresholds are applied to quantitative risk estimates for clinical guidelines, men younger than 50 years of age and women under 60 years of age will infrequently exceed those thresholds. Therefore, recent guidelines have considered longer risk horizons, such as 30 years or the remaining lifespan. The established risk factors are all associated with lifetime risks for cardiovascular disease, but the nature of the relationships sometimes differs from short-term associations because of competing risks. For example, smoking is a strong risk factor for near-term cardiovascular events but a weaker discriminator of lifetime risk for cardiovascular events because of the simultaneous and substantial risk for cancer death, which limits the lifetime risk for cardiovascular disease among smokers. As a result, lifetime risk estimates may enhance communication for individual patients, but how they should be used in decision making regarding the institution of preventive drug therapy in younger individuals is less certain.

PREVENTION OF CARDIOVASCULAR DISEASE

Because patients with prevalent cardiovascular disease are at the highest risk, preventive interventions such as lifestyle modifications and drug therapy to reduce risk are most effective and cost-effective when used as therapy for secondary prevention of recurrent events, or complications such as heart failure. Examples of intensive lifestyle modification and of proven therapies include cardiac rehabilitation, antiplatelet therapy, LDL cholesterol–lowering therapy, antihypertensive medications, mineralocorticoid receptor antagonists, and certain classes of diabetes medications, as well as implantable devices that may prevent complications such as fatal ventricular dysrhythmias (Chapter 54).

For primary prevention, asymptomatic individuals may be at risk because of a heritable family history of premature cardiovascular disease, one or more markedly elevated risk factors, or multiple modestly elevated risk factors. Aspirin has no net benefit over placebo in healthy elderly individuals, in whom it actually reduces disability-free survival and overall survival,[A11,A12,29] without significantly reducing the risk of cardiovascular disease.[A13] Even in patients with diabetes or patients at moderate risk of cardiovascular disease, any benefits for preventing future cardiovascular events are offset by aspirin's side effects.[A14-A16]

The current primary prevention paradigm is to match the intensity of prevention efforts to the absolute risk of the patient.[A17] Appropriate lifestyle interventions (e.g., smoking cessation, weight loss, dietary modification) are recommended for all individuals, whereas drug therapy is recommended only for individuals in whom the absolute benefits can be expected to outweigh any potential adverse drug effects and to be cost-effective in doing so. In underserved or resource-limited settings, polypill formulations containing a statin plus several blood pressure–lowering medications in one pill, with or without aspirin, have been effective in reducing lipid levels, blood pressure,[A18] and even major cardiovascular events[A19-A21] compared with placebo or usual care. Treatment that restores optimal risk factor levels, however, does not imply that the treated individual will now have the very low incidence rates observed in people who have maintained optimal risk factor levels throughout young adulthood and into middle age. As a result, a concept gaining in importance is *primordial prevention*, which is the prevention of the development of risk factors in the first place. Primordial prevention requires a focus on health behaviors that may prevent the development of dyslipidemia, diabetes, and hypertension, as well as population-level strategies that attempt to create an environment conducive to favorable health behaviors. Mobile applications may help with the self-management that is likely critical for such efforts.[29]

CARDIOVASCULAR HEALTH: A NEW PARADIGM

In addition to resuming declines in mortality rates from cardiovascular diseases and stroke in the United States, a newer goal is to promote cardiovascular health in individuals and the population, monitor it over time, and improve it by concerted action. Central to the concept of cardiovascular health is the observation that optimal levels of seven health behaviors and health factors (Table 40-1) are associated with ideal cardiovascular health. Although about 40% of American adults believe they are in ideal cardiovascular health, fewer than 1% have all seven metrics at ideal levels, principally because of a poor-quality diet. Persons who maintain high levels of cardiovascular health from young age to middle age have extremely favorable outcomes from middle to older ages,[30] including: a markedly increased longevity; a better quality of life; a substantially lower incidence of fatal and nonfatal cardiovascular disease events; a lower incidence of other chronic diseases of aging, including cancer, dementia, and venous thromboembolism; a lower burden of subclinical atherosclerosis (e.g., carotid intima-media thickness, coronary artery calcification); higher levels of cognitive function in middle and older ages; and reduced medical care costs. These outcomes are observed in all segments of the population, as well as across all ages and both sexes.

People who pursue healthy lifestyles from young adulthood to middle age are far more likely to preserve ideal cardiovascular health than those who pursue none: 60% of the former group compared with only 3% of the latter group maintained ideal cardiovascular health factors into middle age. Cardiovascular health promotion thus represents a major paradigm shift and opportunity in public health efforts. If even 50% of U.S. adults could preserve ideal cardiovascular health into mid-life, an estimated 900,000 events would be prevented annually.[31]

FUTURE OF CARDIOVASCULAR EPIDEMIOLOGY

Decades of success in observational epidemiology research continue to provide novel insights into trends and risk markers for cardiovascular disease, as well as the influence of in utero and early life exposures on the life course of cardiovascular diseases. New techniques to characterize environmental and behavioral exposures, physiology, health status, and precursors of disease include epigenetics, proteomics, metabolomics, and high-resolution imaging. With these tools, epidemiologic research has advanced to improve the characterization of the life course of cardiovascular diseases in living individuals and populations and to understand the complex interplay of genes and environment. For example, studies of the genotypes of individuals at the extremes of the distribution of LDL cholesterol levels led to the discovery of polymorphisms in the proprotein convertase subtilisin/kexin type 9 (*PCSK9*) gene. Although such polymorphisms are uncommon, specific missense and nonsense mutations in White and Black men and women are associated with significantly lower lifelong levels of LDL cholesterol and substantially lower lifetime risks for coronary heart disease. *PCSK9* has since become an established therapeutic target for reducing atherosclerotic cardiovascular risk. Other genes discovered

TABLE 40-1 DEFINITIONS OF POOR, INTERMEDIATE, AND IDEAL CARDIOVASCULAR HEALTH FOR EACH OF SEVEN METRICS IN ADULTS AND CHILDREN

METRIC	POOR	INTERMEDIATE	IDEAL
CURRENT SMOKING			
Adults	Yes	Former, ≤12 mo	Never or quit >12 mo
Children	Tried in last 30 days	—	Never tried; never smoked whole cigarette
BODY MASS INDEX			
Adults	30 kg/m²	25-29.9 kg/m²	<25 kg/m²
Children	>95th percentile	85th-95th percentile	<85th percentile
PHYSICAL ACTIVITY			
Adults	None	1-149 min moderate or 1-74 min vigorous activity per week	≥150 min moderate or ≥75 min vigorous activity per week
Children	None	1-59 mins moderate or vigorous activity daily	≥60 mins moderate or vigorous activity daily
HEALTHY DIET SCORE*			
Adults	Meets 0-1 components	Meets 2-3 components	Meets 4-5 components
Children	Meets 0-1 components	Meets 2-3 components	Meets 4-5 components
TOTAL CHOLESTEROL			
Adults	≥240 mg/dL	200-239 mg/dL or treated to goal	<200 mg/dL untreated
Children	≥200 mg/dL	170-199 mg/dL	<170 mg/dL untreated
BLOOD PRESSURE			
Adults	SBP ≥140 mm Hg or DBP ≥90 mm Hg	SBP 120-139 mmHg or DBP 80-89 mm Hg or treated to goal	<120/<80 untreated
Children	>95th percentile	90th-95th percentile or SBP ≥120 mm Hg or DBP ≥80 mm Hg	<90th percentile untreated
FASTING GLUCOSE			
Adults	≥126 mg/dL	100-125 mg/dL or treated to goal	<100 mg/dL untreated
Children	≥126 mg/dL	100-125 mg/dL or treated to goal	<100 mg/dL untreated

*Healthy diet score consists of five components, including low sodium intake, low sugar-sweetened beverage consumption, and higher consumption of fruits/vegetables, fish, and whole grains.

DBP = diastolic blood pressure; SBP = systolic blood pressure.

Adapted from Coorey GM, Neubeck L, Mulley J, et al. Effectiveness, acceptability and usefulness of mobile applications for cardiovascular disease self-management: systematic review with meta-synthesis of quantitative and qualitative data. *Eur J Prev Cardiol.* 2018;25:505-521.

through genetic epidemiology investigations, such as the angiopoietin-like 3 gene (*ANGPTL3*), are also rapidly becoming therapeutic targets.[A22]

A second emerging focus in cardiovascular epidemiologic research has been the study of effects of interventions in populations through public health and social policies. For example, studies have demonstrated marked reductions in hospitalizations for acute myocardial infarction occurring rapidly after the initiation of indoor smoking bans in diverse settings. Modeling studies have synthesized data from numerous epidemiologic sources to show that approximately 50 to 75% of the reductions in coronary death rates in Western countries may be attributable to population changes in risk factor levels, despite being offset by a recent worsening in obesity and diabetes prevalence, with the remainder likely attributable to advances in medical and surgical therapies. The widespread availability of electronic health records and wearable device technologies offer substantial promise for future cardiovascular epidemiology studies in ever-larger and well-defined segments of the population.

GENERAL REFERENCES

For the General References and other additional features, please visit Elsevier eBooks+ at https://ebooks.health.elsevier.com.

Grade A References

A1. Sabatine MS, Wiviott SD, Kyung AI, et al. Efficacy and safety of further lowering of low-density lipoprotein cholesterol in patients starting with very low levels: a meta-analysis. *JAMA Cardiology.* 2018;3:823-828.

A2. Palmer SC, Tendal B, Mustafa RA, et al. Sodium-glucose cotransporter protein-2 (SGLT-2) inhibitors and glucagon-like peptide-1 (GLP-1) receptor agonists for type 2 diabetes: systematic review and network meta-analysis of randomised controlled trials. *BMJ.* 2021;372:m4573.

A3. Estruch R, Ros E, Salas-Salvado J, et al. Primary prevention of cardiovascular disease with a Mediterranean diet supplemented with extra-virgin olive oil or nuts. *N Engl J Med.* 2018;378:e1-e14.

A4. Delgado-Lista J, Alcala-Diaz JF, Torres-Peña JD, et al. Long-term secondary prevention of cardiovascular disease with a Mediterranean diet and a low-fat diet (CORDIOPREV): a randomised controlled trial. *Lancet.* 2022;399:1876-1885.

A5. Neal B, Wu Y, Feng X, et al. Effect of salt substitution on cardiovascular events and death. *N Engl J Med.* 2021;385:1067-1077.

A6. Manson JE, Cook NR, Lee IM, et al. Vitamin D supplements and prevention of cancer and cardiovascular disease. *N Engl J Med.* 2019;380:33-44.

A7. Manson JE, Cook NR, Lee IM, et al. Marine n-3 fatty acids and prevention of cardiovascular disease and cancer. *N Engl J Med.* 2019;380:23-32.

A8. Aung T, Halsey J, Kromhout D, et al. Associations of omega-3 fatty acid supplement use with cardiovascular disease risks: meta-analysis of 10 trials involving 77917 individuals. *JAMA Cardiol.* 2018;3:225-234.

A9. Kalstad AA, Myhre PL, Laake K, et al. Effects of n-3 fatty acid supplements in elderly patients after myocardial infarction: a randomized, controlled trial. *Circulation.* 2021;143:528-539.

A10. Nicholls SJ, Lincoff AM, Garcia M, et al. Effect of high-dose omega-3 fatty acids vs corn oil on major adverse cardiovascular events in patients at high cardiovascular risk: the STRENGTH randomized clinical trial. *JAMA.* 2020;324:2268-2280.

A11. McNeil JJ, Woods RL, Nelson MR, et al. Effect of aspirin on disability-free survival in the healthy elderly. *N Engl J Med.* 2018;379:1499-1508.

A12. McNeil JJ, Nelson MR, Woods RL, et al. Effect of aspirin on all-cause mortality in the healthy elderly. *N Engl J Med.* 2018;379:1519-1528.

A13. McNeil JJ, Wolfe R, Woods RL, et al. Effect of aspirin on cardiovascular events and bleeding in the healthy elderly. *N Engl J Med.* 2018;379:1509-1518.

A14. Guirguis-Blake JM, Evans CV, Perdue LA, et al. Aspirin use to prevent cardiovascular disease and colorectal cancer: updated evidence report and systematic review for the US Preventive Services Task Force. *JAMA.* 2022;327:1585-1597.

A15. Bowman L, Mafham M, Wallendszus K, et al. Effects of aspirin for primary prevention in persons with diabetes mellitus. *N Engl J Med.* 2018;379:1529-1539.

A16. Gaziano JM, Brotons C, Coppolecchia R, et al. Use of aspirin to reduce risk of initial vascular events in patients at moderate risk of cardiovascular disease (ARRIVE): a randomised, double-blind, placebo-controlled trial. *Lancet.* 2018;392:1036-1046.

A17. O'Connor EA, Evans CV, Rushkin MC, et al. Behavioral counseling to promote a healthy diet and physical activity for cardiovascular disease prevention in adults with cardiovascular risk factors: updated evidence report and systematic review for the US Preventive Services Task Force. *JAMA.* 2020;324:2076-2094.

A18. Muñoz D, Uzoije P, Reynolds C, et al. Polypill for cardiovascular disease prevention in an underserved population. *N Engl J Med.* 2019;381:1114-1123.

A19. Roshandel G, Khoshnia M, Poustchi H, et al. Effectiveness of polypill for primary and secondary prevention of cardiovascular diseases (PolyIran): a pragmatic, cluster-randomised trial. *Lancet.* 2019;394:672-683.

A20. Yusuf S, Joseph P, Dans A, et al. Polypill with or without aspirin in persons without cardiovascular disease. *N Engl J Med.* 2021;384:216-228.

A21. Joseph P, Roshandel G, Gao P, et al. Fixed-dose combination therapies with and without aspirin for primary prevention of cardiovascular disease: an individual participant data meta-analysis. *Lancet.* 2021;398:1133-1146.

A22. Raal FJ, Rosenson RS, Reeskamp LF, et al. Evinacumab for homozygous familial hypercholesterolemia. *N Engl J Med.* 2020;383:711-720.

41

CARDIAC AND CIRCULATORY FUNCTION

ANDREW R. MARKS

The heart has the daunting task of pumping sufficient amounts of blood to meet both its own metabolic demands and those of the other organs. Unique among all the organs, the heart's failure to perform its task for even a few minutes causes death. The heart continuously fulfills this physiologic role with a variety of electrical, contractile, and structural functions that control the flow of blood to the organs.

STRUCTURE OF THE HEART

CARDIAC DEVELOPMENT

In humans, the formation of a linear heart tube from the primary cardiac crescent occurs between days 21 and 23 of gestation. Looping of the heart tube and trabecular formation of the ventricle occur at 26 days of gestation (E-Fig. 41-1). At 6 weeks, the embryonic interventricular communication closes, followed by thickening and remodeling of the ventricular walls in the first trimester. By the end of week 7, heart development is essentially finished, although the heart continues to enlarge throughout gestation.

ELECTRICAL CELLS

The heart is a muscular pump controlled by regular electrical discharges from specialized muscle cells in the conduction system (Chapter 48). The molecular basis for the electrical activity of the heart is the activation of specific ion-conducting channels (Fig. 41-1). Coordinated activation and inactivation of cardiac ion channels regulate the membrane potential of the cardiac cells, thereby resulting in a rapid sequence of depolarization followed by repolarization. This electrical activity, which is manifested on the body surface as the electrocardiogram (ECG), is known as the action potential, and it is responsible for activating the contraction of the cardiac muscle. At a typical heart rate of 70 beats per minute, the heart beats about 100,000 times per day, or 37 million beats a year, corresponding to 3 billion beats during a lifespan of 80 years. Failure to propagate the signal throughout the heart (e.g., heart block) or abnormal rhythms (arrhythmias) that are either too slow (bradycardia) or too fast (tachycardia) can result in death (Chapter 49). Studies indicate that cardiac arrhythmias may be triggered by leak of calcium inside the cardiomyocytes, thereby suggesting a possible novel therapeutic target for a new generation of antiarrhythmic agents.

ION CHANNELS

Sodium, potassium, and calcium channels determine the electrical activity of the heart by opening and closing in a highly choreographed pattern that determines the action potential of the heart. The electrical regulation of the heart, which is reflected in the relative concentrations of ions inside and outside the heart muscle cells, determines the five phases of the action potential (Chapter 48). The action potential is initiated when the opening of sodium channels results in a rapid influx of sodium (phase 0) down its concentration gradient (≈145 mmol outside the heart muscle cell, ≈10 mmol inside). After a brief early repolarization due to activation of potassium channels (phase 1), the rapid sodium influx depolarizes the cell, thereby activating calcium channels that allow calcium influx (phase 2) down its concentration gradient (≈3 mmol outside, ≈100 nmol inside). This calcium influx triggers excitation-contraction coupling that results in pumping by the heart. Potassium channels then open and cause repolarization (phase 3) as potassium fluxes out of the cell down its concentration gradient (≈4 mmol outside, ≈135 mmol inside). The membrane potential returns to the resting level of about −90 mV (phase 4). Genetic mutations in the genes encoding ion channels have been linked to inherited forms of ventricular and atrial arrhythmias (Chapters 52 and 53).

CONDUCTION SYSTEM

Specialized pacemaker cells in the sinoatrial node (Fig. 41-2) have slightly higher (less negative) resting potentials and gradually depolarize during phase 5 owing to the activity of the potassium and calcium channels and the hyperpolarization-activated cyclic nucleotide–gated channels that are responsible for a small inward (depolarizing) current. In the normal heart, pacemaker cells are the first cells to depolarize, and they trigger the subsequent depolarization of the cells in specialized conducting fibers that propagate the electrical signal throughout the heart muscle in a highly regular and integrated fashion. Electrical activation (depolarization) spreading through the atria to the atrioventricular (AV) node is reflected as the P wave on the ECG (Chapter 42). The slowing of conduction in the AV node accounts for the PR interval on the ECG. After passing through the AV node, the depolarizing signal enters the bundle of His,

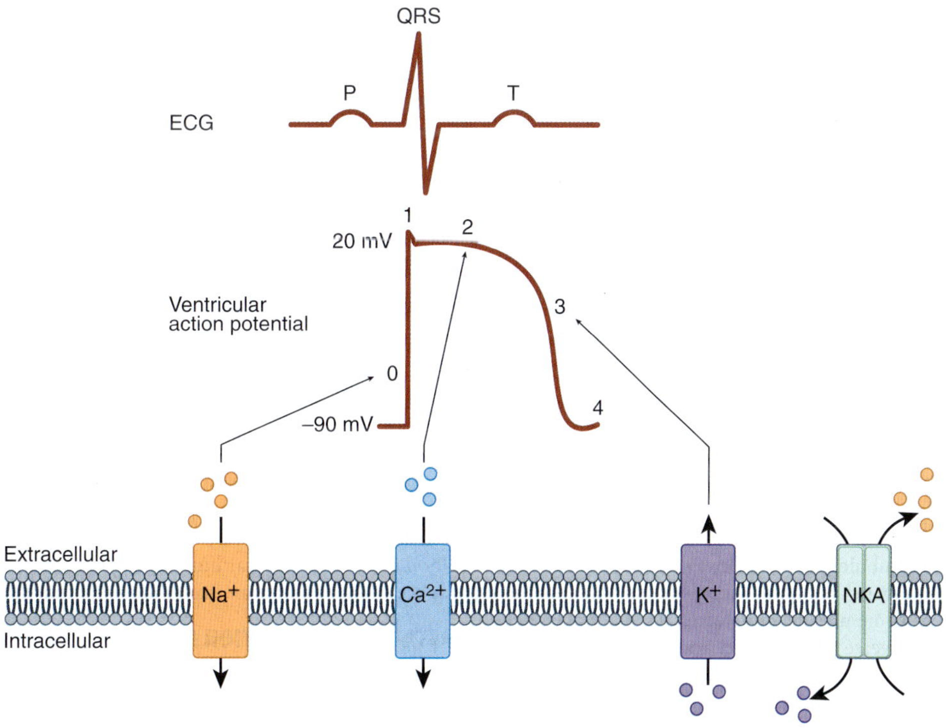

FIGURE 41-1. Cardiac action potential and ion channels. Myocardial contraction begins when sodium channels open and positively charged sodium ions flow into the cell and cause membrane depolarization (phase 0). During phases 1, 2, and 3, calcium ions flow into the cell through L-type calcium channels, while potassium flows out of the cell through voltage-gated potassium channels. These three phases correspond to myocardial contraction, which corresponds to the QRS complex on the surface electrocardiogram (ECG). The sodium-potassium adenosine triphosphatase (NKA) helps return the system to its resting state.

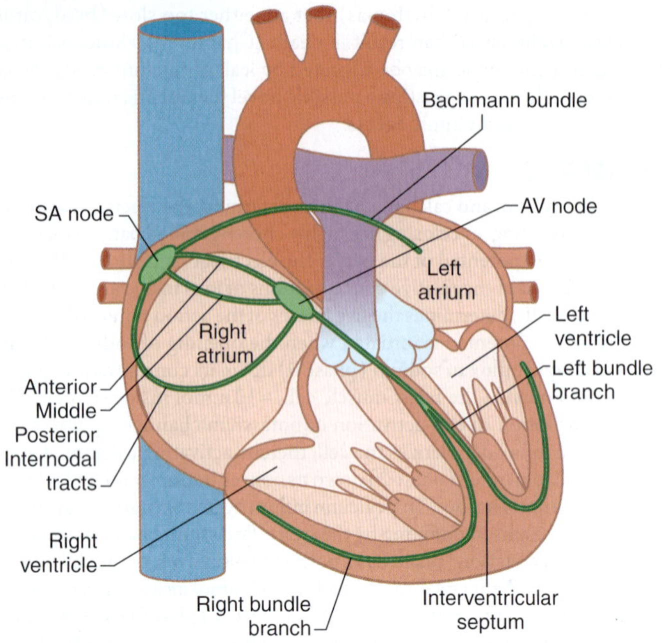

FIGURE 41-2. Cardiac anatomy. Cardiac anatomy comprises electrical and structural components. The electrical impulse that directs cardiac contraction originates in the sinoatrial (SA) node and is rapidly conducted through the atria by specialized conduction tracts. The impulses merge at the atrioventricular (AV) node, where, after a brief pause, they are rapidly conducted into the ventricles through the bundle of His, which is composed of specialized Purkinje cells. Blood moves from the atria into the ventricles through the tricuspid and mitral valves, respectively, during diastole. During systole, blood from the ventricles is pumped into the pulmonary artery and aorta through the pulmonic and aortic valves, respectively.

where conduction is rapid. The bundle of His divides into the right and left bundle branches, which conduct the depolarizing signals into the ventricles and account for the QRS complex on the ECG. Repolarization is represented by the ST segment and the T and U waves of the ECG.

CONTRACTILE CELLS

Heart muscle is composed of billions of individual cells known as cardiomyocytes, which contain an elaborate machinery required for coordinated contraction that pumps blood. Each cardiomyocyte is connected to its neighbors through specialized junctions that enable them to work as a single contractile unit.

The cardiomyocytes are filled with specialized contractile proteins arranged in highly regulated units, called sarcomeres, that give the muscles characteristic patterns known as striations (E-Fig. 41-2). Hence, like skeletal muscle, cardiac muscle is termed striated, as opposed to smooth muscles that form the vasculature and other organs such as the bladder, uterus, and stomach. Cardiomyocytes are also loaded with mitochondria that provide the energy (adenosine triphosphate [ATP]) required to fuel the heart's lifelong contractions (systole) and relaxations (diastole).

ULTRASTRUCTURE

The basic unit of the contractile system is the sarcomere, which is defined anatomically as the distance between two Z lines that anchor thin filaments composed of actin, tropomyosin, and troponin. Thin filaments slide past thick filaments (composed of myosin and titin) in a calcium-dependent manner to shorten the sarcomere length. Mutations in the genes encoding contractile proteins have been linked to dilated and hypertrophic cardiomyopathies (Chapter 47).[1,2] The contractile proteins are surrounded by a calcium-filled membrane called the sarcoplasmic reticulum. The sarcoplasmic reticulum forms specialized associations with the transverse tubules, which are invaginations of the plasma membrane and contain voltage-gated calcium channels. When the muscle is activated by depolarization of its membrane, this electrical signal travels deep into the muscle through the transverse tubules. Inside the muscle, the electrical depolarizing signal activates the voltage-gated channels, which open to allow a small amount of calcium to enter the muscle cells. This influx of calcium in turn activates the type 2 ryanodine receptor (RyR2), calcium-release channels on the sarcoplasmic reticulum. The RyR2 channels open and release enough calcium from the sarcoplasmic reticulum to raise the calcium concentration in the myoplasm about 10-fold. As a result, calcium binds to troponin C in the thin filaments and causes a conformational change that enables cross-bridging between actin and myosin, thereby leading to sliding of the filaments, shortening of the sarcomere, and muscle contraction. Hydrolysis of ATP provides the energy required for the generation of force by the actin-myosin interaction. The conversion of electrical energy (depolarization of the cell membrane) to mechanical energy is known as excitation-contraction coupling. Relaxation of the heart muscle occurs when calcium is pumped back into the sarcoplasmic reticulum through the sarcoendoplasmic reticulum ATPase.

Signals That Regulate Contraction

Contractile force can be enhanced during stress by activation of the β-adrenergic pathway, which increases both the amount of calcium released and the rate of calcium uptake in the sarcoplasmic reticulum (E-Fig. 41-3). β-Agonists (e.g., epinephrine or norepinephrine) bind to β-adrenergic receptors to activate adenylyl cyclase, which generates cyclic adenosine monophosphate and activates protein kinase A. Protein kinase A phosphorylates phospholamban, the voltage-gated calcium channel, the ryanodine receptor/calcium release channel, and sarcomeric regulatory proteins, thereby resulting in increased release of calcium from the sarcoplasmic reticulum and enhanced contractility of the heart.

Nonmuscle Cells

Although the heart is a muscular pump, 60 to 70% of its cells are cardiac fibroblasts, not muscle cells. These fibroblasts provide critical components of the extracellular matrix that determine the structure of the heart. Collagen, which is produced by the cardiac fibroblasts, is a major component of the extracellular matrix, where it forms a network that surrounds the cardiomyocytes and creates tissue that is able to withstand the stress of constant pumping. In certain pathologic conditions, including hypertension, myocardial infarction, and heart failure, the cardiac fibroblasts respond to stress by generating excess extracellular matrix, resulting in fibrosis, which can impair cardiac function.[3] Indeed, a number of commonly used therapies for heart disease, including lipid lowering with statins or fibrates and antihypertensive treatments with angiotensin-converting enzyme inhibitors, β-blockers, and angiotensin receptor blockers, exert part of their beneficial effects on cardiac fibroblasts by reducing fibrosis, thereby resulting in favorable "reverse" remodeling of the heart. Resident fibroblast lineages mediate pressure overload–induced cardiac fibrosis.

ANATOMY OF THE HEART

The primary pumping chamber of the heart is the thick-walled left ventricle, which is composed of billions of cardiomyocytes connected end to end through gap junctions. The right ventricle is a thinner-walled chamber, divided from the left ventricle by the *interventricular septum*. Above the ventricles are the right and left atria, which are thin-walled chambers that receive low-pressure venous blood; they are separated from the ventricles by the *tricuspid valve* on the right side and the *mitral valve* on the left side. These valves are attached to *papillary muscles* that emerge from the ventricular walls through *chordae tendineae*. The pressure gradient between the ventricles and the atria opens the AV valves. The papillary muscles help establish the positions of the valve leaflets and prevent regurgitant flow during contraction. The *aortic and pulmonary valves* separate the left and right ventricles from their arterial connections and enable blood flow out of the ventricles.

CORONARY BLOOD FLOW

The coronary arteries receive blood from the aorta, directly above the aortic valve, and travel through the epicardium that surrounds the heart to supply blood to the heart muscle (see Fig. 59-1 in Chapter 59). The diastolic blood pressure in the ascending aorta just above the aortic valve determines most of the flow of blood into the normal (nonstenosed) coronary arteries while the heart is relaxed. During systole, coronary flow is determined by the left ventricular intracavitary pressure, which equals the pressure within the inner myocardial wall, where coronary arteries are compressed during systole. Coronary blood flows to the epicardium during both systole and diastole but flows to the endocardium predominantly during diastole.

METABOLIC REGULATION OF THE CARDIOVASCULAR SYSTEM

Cardiac muscle requires constant coronary perfusion to supply oxygen and other metabolites. Increased energy consumption due to enhanced contractility necessitated by increased pressures or higher heart rates (e.g., during exercise) can be met only by increased coronary blood flow. Signals that augment coronary blood flow (by up to six-fold) include nitric oxide, adenosine, bradykinins, prostaglandins, and carbon dioxide. The breakdown of ATP is the source of adenosine, whereas nitric oxide is produced by the action of nitric oxide synthases that metabolize the amino acid L-arginine. Autoregulatory mechanisms, including constriction in response to increased luminal pressures and dilation in response to reduced pressure, also play a role in determining coronary artery blood flow. Other metabolic factors that cause vasoconstriction include endothelin peptides, serotonin, 5-hydroxytryptamine, thromboxane, angiotensin II, and β_1-adrenergic stimulation.

Sympathetic and parasympathetic pathways of the autonomic nervous system and the renin-angiotensin system exert potent regulatory effects on cardiovascular function. The sympathetic nervous system plays the key role in the response to stress (e.g., the fight-or-flight response) by increasing heart rate and myocardial contractility and decreasing vascular tone. Regulation of cardiovascular function by the sympathetic nervous system is mediated by norepinephrine that is released at the nerve endings and by epinephrine from the adrenal gland. β-Adrenergic signaling is mediated by epinephrine, which increases the heart rate and vasodilates the central arterial bed, thereby resulting in reduced afterload, which in turn helps augment cardiac output.

The sinoatrial and AV nodes are regulated by parasympathetic innervation that slows the pacemaker's rate of firing and conduction through the AV node by the release of acetylcholine. Vasoconstriction of the venous system is mediated by the sympathetic nervous system, which limits fluid and blood loss after trauma.

The renin-angiotensin system also regulates blood pressure, peripheral vasoconstriction, and contractility in coordination with the sympathetic nervous system. Both the sympathetic nervous system and the renin-angiotensin system are chronically activated in heart failure (Chapter 45), in which the resulting maladaptive remodeling of the cardiovascular system promotes the progression of heart failure. Decreased perfusion to the kidney, decreased delivery of sodium to the macula densa, or increased sympathetic activity results in the release of the hormone renin from the macula densa cells within the juxtaglomerular apparatus of the kidney. Renin results in the production of angiotensin II, a potent constrictor of peripheral and coronary arteries. In turn, angiotensin II causes the release of the sodium-retaining hormone aldosterone from the adrenal gland (Chapter 208). Together, these signals result in sodium retention and increased arterial blood pressure.

PHYSIOLOGY OF THE HEART AND CIRCULATORY CONTROL

CARDIAC ENERGETICS

The major immediate source of energy in the heart is the oxidation of fatty acids and glucose. When oxygen supply is limited, glucose metabolism is favored because it generates more ATP per oxygen consumed. The heart has virtually no ability to conduct anaerobic metabolism (i.e., glycolysis) and therefore is dependent on oxygen for its function. For example, heart function deteriorates immediately under conditions of hypoxia, ischemia, and carbon monoxide poisoning.

Basal metabolism, total mechanical work performed by the heart, contractility, and heart rate determine the oxygen and energy consumption of the heart. During excitation-contraction coupling, two key steps require energy consumption (ATP hydrolysis): release of the myosin head–actin interaction and reuptake of calcium into the sarcoplasmic reticulum.

The mechanical work of the heart is determined by the total *pressure-volume area*, which is related to the number of actin-myosin cross-bridges formed during the contraction. It is the sum of the external work performed by the heart in pumping blood from the ventricle to the aorta (represented by the area inside the pressure-volume loop) plus energy stored in the myocardium at the end of contraction. Enhanced contractility requires increased oxygen consumption because an increased amount of calcium released from the sarcoplasmic reticulum requires increased ATP and oxygen consumption to pump the released calcium back into the sarcoplasmic reticulum through the sarcoplasmic reticular ATPase. On the basis of these principles, increasing the heart rate requires increased oxygen consumption. If the heart rate increases from 70 to 140 beats per minute during exercise or stress, oxygen consumption increases almost two-fold above the basal value.

CONTRACTILITY AND RELAXATION

The Cardiac Cycle

In resting humans, the heart beats approximately once per second. With each beat, the heart cycles through a series of four hemodynamic events represented by changes in pressures and volumes (E-Fig. 41-4) as well as electrical activity as represented by the ECG. When the heart muscle is relaxed at end diastole, the ventricular pressure is at its resting level (*end-diastolic pressure*) and the ventricular volumes are at their maximal value (*end-diastolic volume*). Aortic pressure declines as the blood ejected into the aorta during the previous ventricular contraction flows to the peripheral circulation. Atrial contraction provides a final boost to ventricular volume immediately before ventricular systole. Ventricular contraction increases the pressure in the ventricle; when this pressure exceeds the pressure in the atrium, the mitral valve closes. However, because ventricular pressure remains less than aortic pressure, the aortic valve remains closed, and no blood enters or leaves the ventricle during this first phase of the cardiac cycle, the *isovolumic contraction* phase. During systole, ventricular pressure eventually exceeds aortic pressure, at which time the aortic valve opens, blood is ejected into the aorta, and ventricular volume decreases during the *ejection* phase of the cycle. At the end of systole when contraction is maximum, ejection ends, and the ventricular volumes are at their lowest (*end-systolic volume*). The volume of the ejected blood, which is termed the stroke volume (SV), is defined as the difference between the end-diastolic and end-systolic volumes. The ejection fraction (EF), defined as the percentage of end-diastolic volume (EDV) ejected during a contraction ($EF = 100 \times SV/EDV$), is an index of heart function. The next phase in the cycle occurs when the heart muscle relaxes, ventricular pressures are less than the aorta pressure, and the aortic valve closes. During this *isovolumic relaxation* phase, ventricular volumes remain constant because, once again, both the mitral and aortic valves are closed. When ventricular pressures fall below atrial pressures, the mitral and tricuspid valves open, and blood flows from the atria into the ventricles during the *filling* phase.

These four phases of the cardiac cycle can be represented by a *pressure-volume diagram* (E-Fig. 41-5), which plots the instantaneous ventricular pressure versus volume to calculate the *pressure-volume loop*. Similar effects occur on the left and right sides of the heart, but with higher pressures on the left side (Table 41-1).

Pressure-Volume Relationships

The volume of a ventricular chamber correlates with length of its muscles and sarcomeres. In the left ventricle, with its circular cross section, Laplace's law defines the relationship among pressure in the chamber (P), muscle tension (T, force/unit cross-sectional area of the muscle), chamber wall thickness (h), and internal radius of the chamber (R): $P \approx 2 \cdot T \cdot h/R$. Both calcium and the length of the heart muscle determine force (Fig. 41-3). Each muscle is composed of a linear array of sarcomere bundles. Maximal force is achieved at a sarcomere length of about 2.2 to 2.3 µm, which results in the optimal overlap of thick and thin filaments. When the sarcomere length is less than 2.0 µm, the ends of the thin filaments contact each other, thereby resulting in a reduction in force. Conversely, when sarcomeres are stretched beyond 2.3 µm, force decreases owing to reduced overlap between myosin heads and actin.

Force-length relationships, which are determined by measuring the force developed at different muscle lengths while preventing the muscle from shortening (isometric contractions), characterize the systolic and diastolic contractile properties of cardiac muscle. With increasing muscle length, end-systolic force increases to a greater degree than does end-diastolic force. The

TABLE 41-1 RANGE OF NORMAL RESTING HEMODYNAMIC VALUES

PRESSURE
Central venous (mean): 0-5 mm Hg
Right atrial (mean): 0-5 mm Hg
Right ventricular (systolic/diastolic): 20-30/0-5 mm Hg
Pulmonary artery (systolic/diastolic): 20-30/8-12 mm Hg
Left atrial (mean): 8-12 mm Hg
Left ventricular (systolic/diastolic): 100-150/8-12 mm Hg
Aortic (systolic/diastolic): 100-150/70-90 mm Hg
VOLUME-RELATED MEASURES
Right ventricular end-diastolic volume: 70-100 mL
Left ventricular end-diastolic volume: 70-100 mL
Stroke volume: 40-70 mL
Cardiac index: 2.5-4 L/min/m^2
Ejection fraction: 55-70%
ARTERIAL RESISTANCE
Systemic vascular resistance: 10-20 mm Hg · min/L
Pulmonary vascular resistance: 0.5-1.5 mm Hg · min/L

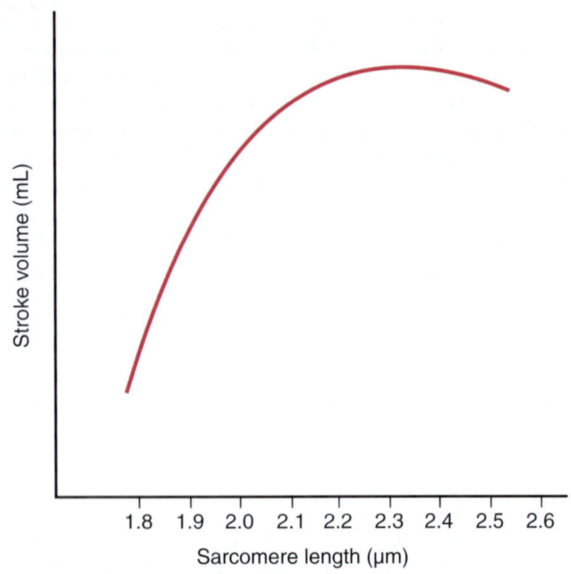

FIGURE 41-3. Frank-Starling law. Cardiac output, represented as stroke volume (end-systolic volume minus end-diastolic volume), as a function of initial sarcomere stretch. The greater the initial stretch on the fibers during diastole, referred to as preload, the more force is generated during systole.

difference in force at end diastole versus end systole increases as muscle length increases as a result of the greater developed force of the stretched muscle. This relationship of force to length is referred to as the Frank-Starling law of the heart.

Work of the Heart

Cardiovascular performance is reflected in the arterial blood pressure and cardiac output (mean arterial blood flow), which in turn are dependent on four factors: preload, afterload, ventricular contractility, and heart rate.

Preload, which refers to the degree to which sarcomeres are stretched just before systole, is defined as the end-diastolic pressure or volume. The Frank-Starling law of the heart dictates that ventricular pressure and output vary with preload, so a decrease in preload decreases end-diastolic volume and pressure, peak pressure, and stroke volume. Conversely, increased preload increases ventricular pressure and output, subject to the limits to which preload pressures can be increased. Left ventricular end-diastolic pressures of 20 to 25 mm Hg and greater cause exudation of fluid into the alveoli and pulmonary edema (Chapter 45).

Afterload refers to the stress that the ventricle must overcome to eject blood. Peak arterial pressure reflects the peak stress imposed on cardiomyocytes according to Laplace's law (described previously as $P \approx 2 \cdot T \cdot h/R$). As long as there is no left ventricular outflow obstruction, arterial pressure reflects myocyte afterload, as does *total peripheral resistance* (TPR), which corresponds to the tone of the resistance vessels. TPR is the ratio between the mean pressure decrease across the arterial system (mean arterial pressure [MAP] minus mean central venous pressure [CVP]) and cardiac output (CO): $TPR = (MAP - CVP)/CO$. When TPR is increased, the pressure-volume relationship shifts such that peak pressure is increased, whereas stroke volume and ejection fraction are decreased.

Contractility of cardiac muscle (*myocardial contractility*) or a ventricle (*ventricular contractility*) is the intrinsic ability to generate force independent of preload or afterload. When ventricular contractility is increased, the pressure-volume relationship shifts so that pressure, stroke volume, and ejection fraction are increased at constant preload volume and arterial resistance. By comparison, ventricular contractility is decreased in dilated cardiomyopathy (Chapter 47), and atrial contractility is decreased by the atrial myopathy that may precede and commonly follow atrial fibrillation.[3]

Cardiac output is measured in liters per minute and is equal to the amount of blood ejected at each heartbeat (stroke volume in liters per beat) multiplied by the number of beats per minute. As a result, *heart rate* is a powerful determinant of cardiac performance. Cardiac output and mean arterial pressure can be related to preload, afterload, contractility, and heart rate through the Frank-Starling curves, which plot end-diastolic pressure versus cardiac output or mean arterial pressure, to yield an overall picture of left ventricular function.

CARDIOVASCULAR RESPONSES TO STRESSORS

EXERCISE

Exercise requires dramatic increases in cardiac function combined with remodeling of the peripheral circulation to meet the enhanced metabolic demands of critical organs and to redirect blood flow to those organs. Indeed, the oxygen consumption during exercise can increase as much as 18-fold. About one third of the requirement for increased oxygen consumption is met by improved extraction of oxygen from the blood in the muscles (reducing venous saturation from about 75% to about 25%) and the remainder by increasing cardiac output as much as six-fold. Increased cardiac function is achieved largely through sympathetic stimulation and reduction in vagal tone, which combine to increase the heart rate, contractility, ejection fraction, filling rates, and systolic blood pressure and to decrease aortic impedance. In young healthy individuals, heart rate can increase from a baseline of 60 to 70 beats per minute at rest to as much as 170 to 200 beats per minute with exercise. To increase rather than to decrease cardiac output at these high heart rates, which can limit ventricular filling and stroke volume, contractility must also increase through a phenomenon known as the positive force frequency relationship, or Bowditch phenomenon. Along with increased cardiac contractility, arterial vasodilation in the aorta and other major arteries reduces the resistance to cardiac outflow. Both enhanced cardiac contractility and arterial vasodilation are triggered by the same sympathetic nervous system signals. With increased cardiac outflow, venous return also must increase so that preload can be maintained as well as possible to enhance cardiac function by the Frank-Starling mechanism. In response to the stress of repeated exercise (e.g., in trained athletes), the heart may undergo physiologic hypertrophy, which should be distinguished from the pathologic hypertrophy that is triggered by hypertension, myocardial infarction, and chronic activation of neurohormonal pathways (e.g., the renin-angiotensin system) (E-Fig. 41-6).

HEART FAILURE

Heart failure can be defined as the inability of the heart to provide sufficient blood flow to meet the metabolic demands of the organs (Chapter 45). Heart failure can be due to systolic dysfunction with volume overload, most often as the consequence of ischemic heart disease (myocardial infarction) or as the end-stage consequence of hypertension. Systolic heart failure is characterized by increases in the size of the various cardiac chambers (rightward shift of the end-diastolic pressure-volume relationship). In another form of heart failure, known as *diastolic heart failure*, the heart is not necessarily increased in size, and systolic function is preserved.[4] Emerging data implicate altered regulation of calcium inside the cardiomyocyte in the pathogenesis of both the cardiac and skeletal muscle weakness that is seen in heart failure, as well as in atrial fibrillation,[5] which is the most common arrhythmia associated with heart failure.

AGING

Prolongation of contraction and relaxation times, which are common abnormalities in older individuals, may be related to cardiac hypertrophy as a consequence of the high prevalence of hypertension with advancing age (Chapter 64). A progressive "stiffening" of the large arteries with advancing age increases resistance, although the mechanism underlying this change is not understood. The heart rate and contractile responses to sympathetic signals are reduced and lead to a diminished ability to respond to conditions of acute overload, such as increased blood pressure or an acute myocardial infarction.

CARDIAC REGENERATION

Some animals, such as zebrafish, can regenerate substantial portions of their hearts after injury, sometimes by recruiting atrial myocytes to replace damaged ventricular myocytes. In mammals, however, cardiomyocytes stop proliferating right after birth. Any subsequent enlargement of the heart in response to stress (e.g., hypertension) or loss of myocardium (e.g., myocardial infarction) is limited to hypertrophy of existing cardiomyocytes. Studies, however, have shown that micro-RNAs (miRNAs) can activate cardiomyocyte proliferation and repair by enabling the terminally differentiated cardiomyocytes to re-enter the cell cycle and proliferate. These miRNAs are short, noncoding RNAs that downregulate target messenger RNAs by binding to partially complementary sequences and reducing the expression of the encoded proteins. In mice, miRNAs can induce cardiac regeneration and prevent loss of heart function after myocardial infarction, thereby raising the possibility for a better understanding and potential treatment of cardiac diseases. To date, however, stem cell therapy has been disappointing for heart failure[A1] and for acute myocardial infarction.[6]

IMPAIRED CIRCULATORY FUNCTION: ATHEROSCLEROSIS

Atherosclerosis, which is an age-dependent process of progressive damage to arterial vessels, can impair coronary blood flow and result in myocardial ischemia (Chapter 56) and infarction (Chapters 57 and 58). Atherosclerosis is linked to cardiac risk factors including elevated cholesterol levels, hypertension, cigarette smoking, obesity, genetics (positive family history), and diabetes. Atherosclerosis can lead to partial or complete blockages of arteries due to formation of atherosclerotic plaques comprised of lipoproteins, inflammatory cells, and connective tissue. Atherosclerotic plaques may rupture, thereby leading to thromboses and arterial occlusions that result in myocardial infarction (Chapters 57 and 58), ischemic stroke (Chapter 376), and peripheral arterial disease (Chapter 65). Repeated atherosclerotic-induced ischemic attacks can result in dilated cardiomyopathy and heart failure (Chapter 45). An estimated 90% of cases of myocardial infarction (Chapter 58), 60% of strokes (Chapter 376), most cases of heart failure (Chapter 45), and up to one third of all cases of dementia (Chapter 371) are due to atherosclerosis.

RISK FACTORS FOR ATHEROSCLEROSIS

The major risk factors that promote the development of atherosclerosis are an elevated low-density lipoprotein (LDL) cholesterol level (Chapter 190); cigarette smoking (Chapter 363); diabetes (Chapter 210); hypertension (Chapter 64); and a family history of coronary heart disease, ischemic stroke, or peripheral arterial disease. Other conditions that increase the risk of atherosclerotic disease or events include a low high-density lipoprotein (HDL) level (Chapter 190), obesity, hyper-triglyceridemia, high plasma levels of lipoprotein (a), hyperfibrinogenemia, homocystinuria, and physical inactivity (Chapter 40).

An atherogenic lipoprotein phenotype (characterized by the predominance of small, dense LDL particles, hypertriglyceridemia, and low plasma HDL cholesterol concentration) with the metabolic syndrome is associated with atherogenic and thrombotic factors, including raised levels of plasma fibrinogen, plasminogen activator inhibitor-1, and coagulation factor VII, as well as platelet hyperactivity. The inflammatory biomarker C-reactive protein does not cause atherosclerosis but reflects ongoing inflammation that may accelerate the atherosclerotic process.[7]

PATHOPHYSIOLOGY OF ATHEROSCLEROSIS

When LDL accumulates in the inner wall of arteries (intima), it becomes oxidized, thereby resulting in the release of chemokines and adhesion molecules that promote inflammation, chiefly marked by the recruitment of monocytes, which become macrophages (E-Fig. 41-7). Macrophages accumulate cholesterol and become cholesterol-laden foam cells. Other macrophages produce proinflammatory mediators, including tumor necrosis factor (TNF), interleukin-1, proinflammatory eicosanoids, oxygen and nitrogen free radicals, and prothrombotic factors.

PLAQUE ACTIVATION, THROMBOSIS, AND INFARCTION

The atherosclerotic process typically is silent for months, years, and even decades, and it may never result in clinical manifestations.[8] However, if the plaque ruptures thrombotic occlusion of the artery may ensue (Fig. 41-4). Platelet aggregates that form on these exposed surfaces are stabilized by a fibrin network. Tissue factor, expressed in the vascular smooth muscle cells and macrophages of the atherosclerotic plaque, is the primary cellular initiator of the blood coagulation cascade that leads to fibrin formation. Atherothrombi expand rapidly and can fill the lumen within minutes, thereby leading to ischemia and infarction.

Matrix metalloproteinases and cysteine proteinases, which are produced by macrophages, are found at sites of plaque rupture and have been implicated in rupture, but their effects on the composition and size of lesions are complex. Cell death may be an important trigger of plaque rupture. Apoptotic cells contained in the plaque are usually removed by efferocytosis. If this process fails, secondary necrosis ensues, thereby leading to reduced mechanical integrity and accumulation of prothrombotic material from dead cells.

ANTIATHEROSCLEROTIC THERAPY

Current treatment of atherosclerosis focuses on reduction of risk factors, including smoking cessation, dietary and pharmacologic reduction of LDL cholesterol (Chapter 190), management of blood pressure (Chapter 64), treatment of hyperglycemia (Chapter 210), hypertriglyceridemia (Chapter 190), obesity (Chapter 201), and physical inactivity (Chapter 14).

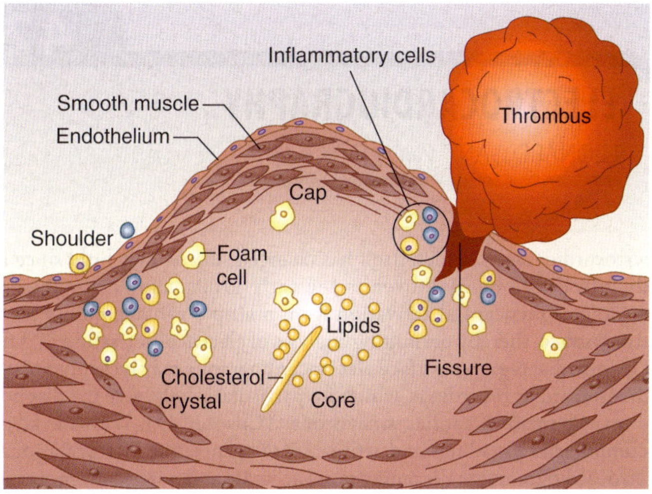

FIGURE 41-4. Plaque rupture and atherothrombosis. The advanced atherosclerotic plaque has a central core with lipids (especially cholesterol), live and dead cells, necrotic material from dead foam cells, and calcium salts. The plaque is overlaid by a fibrous cap that consists of smooth muscle cells and collagen (produced by the muscle cells) and covered by an intact layer of endothelial cells. Inflammatory cells (macrophages, T cells, mast cells, dendritic cells, and occasional B cells) are interspersed with these components and are particularly abundant in the shoulder regions of plaques, where fissures (also called ruptures) may expose thrombogenic core material (e.g., lipids, collagen, tissue factor) to blood components. This event triggers platelet aggregation and humoral coagulation, thereby leading to thrombus formation at the site of fissuring. Thrombi may expand locally to obstruct blood flow or they may detach to cause embolization.

Cholesterol-lowering with statins,[A2] ezetimibe,[A3] and proprotein convertase subtilisin kexin type 9 (PCSK9) antibodies[A4] can reduce atherosclerotic lesions, inhibit their progression, and lower the rate of subsequent coronary events and all-cause mortality. More recently, inhibition of the hepatic synthesis of PCSK9 using a single subcutaneous injection of inclisiran has resulted in LDL cholesterol reductions of 50% or so for 18 months.[A5,A6]

Aspirin[A7] and other inhibitors of platelet aggregation,[9] β-adrenergic receptor blockers, and angiotensin-converting enzyme inhibitors or angiotensin II antagonists are also part of the routine secondary prevention of coronary heart disease (Chapters 56, 57, and 58). Inhibitors of platelet aggregation are widely used for secondary prevention of atherosclerotic cardiovascular disease. Aspirin inhibits formation of proaggregatory prostaglandins, whereas other inhibitors of platelet aggregation modulate expression of platelet adhesion molecules. In addition to medical therapies, interventional therapies such as stenting and coronary artery bypass surgery (Chapter 59) also have greatly impacted the health burden of atherosclerosis.

GENERAL REFERENCES

For the General References and other additional features, please visit Elsevier eBooks+ at https://ebooks.health.elsevier.com.

Grade A References

A1. Tripathi A, Khan MS, Khan AR, et al. Cell therapy for nonischemic dilated cardiomyopathy: a systematic review and meta-analysis of randomized controlled trials. *Stem Cells Transl Med.* 2021;10:1394-1405.
A2. Chou R, Dana T, Blazina I, et al. Statins for prevention of cardiovascular disease in adults: evidence report and systematic review for the US Preventive Services Task Force. *JAMA.* 2016;316:2008-2024.
A3. Zhan S, Tang M, Liu F. Ezetimibe for the prevention of cardiovascular disease and all-cause mortality events. *Cochrane Database Syst Rev.* 2018;11:CD012502.
A4. Schmidt AF, Carter JL, Pearce LS, et al. PCSK9 monoclonal antibodies for the primary and secondary prevention of cardiovascular disease. *Cochrane Database Syst Rev.* 2020;10:CD011748.
A5. Ray KK, Wright RS, Kallend D, et al. Two phase 3 trials of inclisiran in patients with elevated LDL cholesterol. *N Engl J Med.* 2020;382:1507-1519.
A6. Raal FJ, Kallend D, Ray KK, et al. Inclisiran for the treatment of heterozygous familial hypercholesterolemia. *N Engl J Med.* 2020;382:1520-1530.
A7. Guirguis-Blake JM, Evans CV, Senger CA, et al. Aspirin for the primary prevention of cardiovascular events: a systematic evidence review for the U.S. Preventive Services Task Force. *Ann Intern Med.* 2016;164:804-813.

42

ELECTROCARDIOGRAPHY

LEONARD GANZ AND MARK S. LINK

Electrocardiography, which itself has changed surprisingly little since initially introduced by Einthoven in the early 1900s, allows simultaneous recording of myocardial activation from multiple vantage points on the body's surface, thereby permitting analysis of electrical activation in different myocardial regions. Surface electrocardiography may be supplemented with intracardiac recordings, which are particularly helpful in the diagnosis and management of cardiac arrhythmias (Chapter 49). With the advent of computerized readings and artificial intelligence, the interpretations of electrocardiograms are becoming more accurate and potentially more diagnostic of certain disease conditions.

NORMAL FUNCTION AND ELECTROCARDIOGRAM

NORMAL CARDIAC ACTIVATION

Electrical activation of the heart depends on the spread of a depolarizing wave front from pacemaker cells through cardiac muscle, as well as via specialized conducting tissues (Fig. 42-1). Under normal circumstances, cells in the sinoatrial (SA) nodal complex in the high lateral epicardial right atrium near the superior vena cava spontaneously depolarize at the highest rate and therefore constitute the dominant cardiac pacemaker (Chapter 48). This electrical wave front spreads throughout the right and left atria; specialized conducting tracts called the Bachmann bundle speed the depolarizing wave front to the left atrium. Electrical atrial activation triggers atrial muscular contraction, thereby propelling blood through the tricuspid and mitral valves into the right and left ventricles. Normally, the atrioventricular (AV) node, where conduction delay is physiologic, serves as the only electrical connection linking the atria and ventricles; the AV valve rings are insulated. The depolarizing wave front exits the AV node into the bundle of His, a specialized conducting tissue capable of rapid conduction. The bundle of His bifurcates into right and left bundle branches; the left bundle branch divides into the left anterior and left posterior fascicles. The bundle branches and their more distal ramifications of specialized conducting tissue are called the Purkinje system. From these specialized conducting tissues, the depolarizing wave front enters into and then moves through ventricular muscle. As in the atria, ventricular electrical depolarization initiates muscular contraction, which pumps blood through the semilunar valves into the pulmonary and systemic circulations. After electrical depolarization, a period of electrical recovery, or repolarization, is necessary before repeated depolarization.

At the cellular level, a complex orchestration of ion channels opening and closing determines the membrane potential throughout this process. The flow of ions into and out of the myocardial cells inscribes an action potential, which reflects depolarization and repolarization, as well as the spontaneous depolarization of pacemaker cells (Chapter 48).

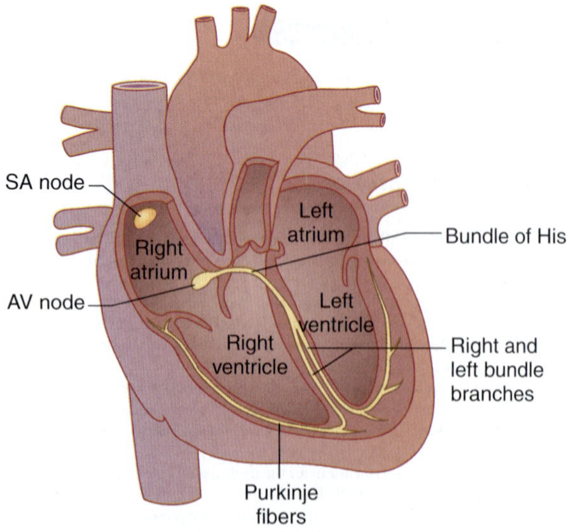

FIGURE 42-1. Cardiac conduction system. The normal conducting system consists of pacemaker cells in the sinoatrial (SA) nodal complex, specialized intra-atrial conducting tracts (including Bachmann bundle), the atrioventricular (AV) node, the His-Purkinje system, and working atrial and ventricular myocardium.

THE ELECTROCARDIOGRAPHIC WAVES

Labeled alphabetically, beginning with the P wave, the basic waves of the electrocardiogram (ECG) correspond to these electrical events (Fig. 42-2). The P wave represents atrial muscular depolarization. The morphology of the P wave is reflective of atrial structure. Under normal circumstances, the PR interval, which is the segment from the onset of the P wave to the onset of the QRS complex, represents the delay between atrial and ventricular depolarization. The QRS complex represents ventricular muscular depolarization; the disparity between ventricular and atrial muscle mass typically yields a QRS complex much larger in voltage amplitude than the P wave. Recorded from multiple vantage points, the QRS complex harbors tremendous information about the structure and function of ventricular tissue. The ST segment and T wave (and occasionally the U wave) reflect ventricular repolarization, a process of electrical recovery that must take place before the ventricle can be depolarized again. The J (junction) point denotes the end of the QRS complex and beginning of the ST segment. Atrial muscle also requires repolarization before the next depolarizing wave front. Because ventricular mass far exceeds atrial muscular mass, the low-amplitude atrial repolarization wave is buried underneath the QRS complex and therefore not manifested on the ECG.

One rarely seen ECG finding, the J wave (of Osborn), breaks with the alphabetic convention of the other electrocardiographic waves. Defined as a positive deflection on the QRS downstroke or at the J point, the J wave is seen most commonly in hypothermia (see Fig. 42-3). It also has been described in hypercalcemia and brain injury, and it may connote risk of idiopathic ventricular fibrillation (see later).

ELECTROCARDIOGRAPHY STANDARDS

A standard ECG is recorded on paper (and frequently digitally) with 1-mm ("small" boxes) as well as 5-mm ("big" boxes) gridlines (see Fig. 42-2). Voltage amplitude is measured on the vertical axis (typically 10 mm equaling 1 mV) and time on the horizontal axis. Because the usual ECG recording speed is 25 mm/sec, each 1-mm gridline (small box) represents 0.04 second

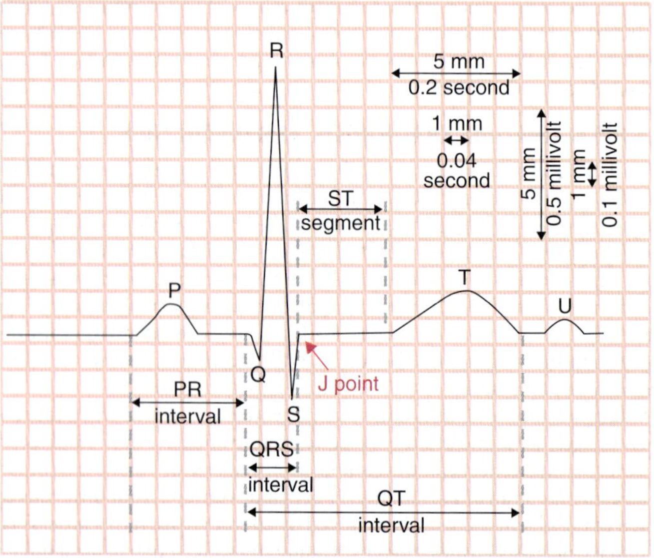

FIGURE 42-2. Inscription of a normal electrocardiogram (ECG). Sinoatrial nodal depolarization is not visible on the surface ECG; the P wave corresponds to atrial muscular depolarization. The PR interval denotes conduction through the atrial muscle, atrioventricular node, and His-Purkinje system. The QRS complex reflects ventricular muscle depolarization. The ST segment and T wave correspond to ventricular repolarization. The J point lies at the junction of the end of the QRS complex and beginning of the ST segment. The QT interval is measured from QRS onset to T wave offset. Note the gridlines. On the horizontal axis, each 1-mm line ("small" box) denotes 0.04 second (40 msec); a "big" box denotes 0.2 second (200 msec). On the vertical axis, 1 mm (small box) corresponds to 0.1 mV; 10 mm (two big boxes) therefore denotes 1 mV.

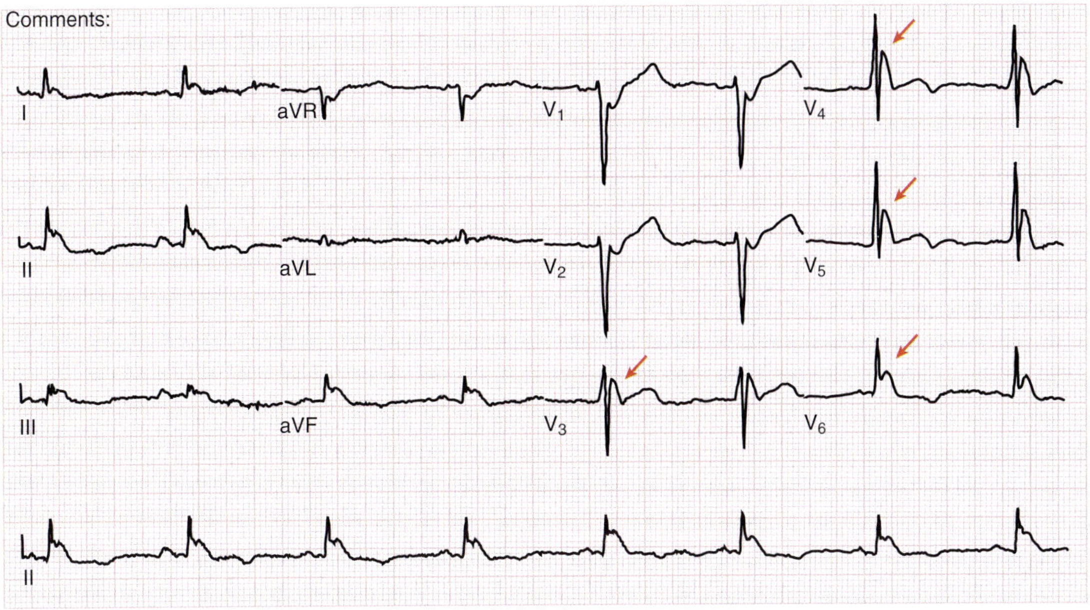

FIGURE 42-3. **J wave (of Osborn). This ECG was recorded in a 40-year-old diabetic woman with profound hypothermia (26.6° C), diabetic ketoacidosis, and hypokalemia. Note the massive J waves in leads V_3-V_6, and smaller J waves in leads I, II, III, and aVF. Other notable findings include sinus bradycardia and QT prolongation.**

(40 msec), and each 5-mm gridline (big box) equals 0.2 second (200 msec). These parameters, which are typically printed on the ECG to aid in proper interpretation, are the usual calibration or standardization, but they can be modified in unusual circumstances.

A standard ECG is recorded over a 10-second period, although a rhythm or monitor strip can be recorded for substantially longer if necessary. Multiple leads are typically recorded simultaneously from the top to the bottom of the page. The usual groupings of leads include I, II, and III; aVR, aVL, and aVF; V_1, V_2, and V_3; and V_4, V_5, and V_6 (see later). Each group of leads is recorded for 2.5 seconds. A single lead (or multilead) rhythm strip is recorded below for the entire 10 seconds. Thus, as the ECG is scanned from left to right, one sees 10 seconds of cardiac activity, with each complex recorded simultaneously in multiple leads.

NORMAL INTERVALS

Each of the various ECG waves and intervals has normal ranges, defined from large numbers of electrocardiographic recordings in (presumably) healthy subjects (Table 42-1; see Fig. 42-2).

The RR interval (identical to the PP interval in sinus rhythm), which is the measurement from R wave to R wave (or P wave to P wave), allows calculation of the heart rate. Because there are 60,000 msec in a minute, the heart rate (HR) in beats per minute can be easily calculated from the RR or PP interval in milliseconds:

$$HR = \frac{60{,}000}{RR}$$

Although traditionally the normal resting adult heart rate range has been defined as 60 to 100 beats per minute, a range of 50 to 90 at rest may actually be more reflective of normal physiology. Various stressors (exercise, pain, fever, anemia, etc.) increase the heart rate; a lower heart rate is noted after eating and during sleep. Resting heart rates tend to decrease with age. When the heart rate is grossly irregular, as in atrial fibrillation (Chapter 52), the RR interval can be averaged over a number of cardiac cycles to estimate the heart rate. Because a standard ECG records 10 seconds in time, the heart rate (beats per minute) will equal the number of beats recorded on a standard ECG multiplied by 6. Alternatively, in a regular rhythm, the heart rate can be estimated by counting the number of big boxes between consecutive QRS complexes or P waves (i.e., 2 large boxes = 150 beats per minute, 3 large boxes = 100 beats per minute, 4 large boxes = 75 beats per minute, 5 large boxes = 60 beats per minute, and so on.).

TABLE 42-1 NORMAL ELECTROCARDIOGRAPHIC INTERVALS

Heart rate	50-100 beats per minute
P wave duration	<0.12 sec (120 msec)
PR interval	0.09-0.20 sec (90-200 msec)
QRS duration	0.075-0.11 sec (75-110 msec)
QTc	males: 0.39-0.45 sec (390-450 msec); females: 0.39-0.46 sec (390-460 msec)
QRS axis	−30 to +90 degrees

P Wave Duration

The P wave duration, from the beginning to the end of a P wave, is typically less than 0.12 second (120 msec, three small boxes) in length. A broader P wave reflects an intra-atrial and/or interatrial conduction delay. Abnormalities in P wave amplitude, morphology, and axis may reflect atrial enlargement.

PR Interval

The PR interval, measured from the onset of the P wave to the onset of the QRS complex, normally lasts between 0.09 and 0.2 second (90 to 200 msec). One-to-one AV conduction with a PR interval greater than 0.2 second has traditionally been called *first-degree AV block*, but *delayed AV conduction* may be a more appropriate term. Conduction through the atrial tissue, the AV node, and the His-Purkinje system all contribute to the PR interval. When the PR interval is prolonged, delay is usually present in the AV node, although other sites of delay are possible. A short PR interval may reflect ventricular preexcitation (Wolff-Parkinson-White syndrome), a junctional rhythm, or enhanced AV nodal conduction (Chapters 49 and 52).

QRS Complex

The QRS complex, which reflects ventricular muscular electrical activation, carries important information in patients with coronary artery disease, cardiomyopathy, metabolic abnormalities, and other conditions. Capital letters (Q, R, S) denote large-amplitude deflections (≥5 mm or 0.5 mV), whereas lowercase letters (q, r, s) signify low-amplitude deflections (<5 mm or 0.5 mV). Q, q, S, and s waves are negative excursions from the isoelectric baseline, whereas R and r waves are positive deflections. Q and q waves are initial negative deflections, and S and s waves are negative deflections that follow a positive deflection (R or r wave); a QS complex is an entirely negative deflection. Q waves may reflect prior infarction (Chapters 56-58). An R′ or r′ wave refers to a second positive deflection after an S (or s) wave. The duration of the QRS complex reflects the time required for ventricular depolarization. Ventricular activation usually requires at least 0.075 second (75 msec, nearly two small boxes). There is some debate regarding the upper limit of the normal range for QRS duration; a recent consensus document specified 0.11 second (110 msec, nearly three small boxes). If the QRS duration is prolonged, an intraventricular and/or interventricular conduction delay is present. Particular patterns of interventricular conduction delay have been termed bundle branch block (see later).

QT Interval

The QT interval is measured from the onset of the QRS complex to the end of the T wave. Although the QT interval is generally felt to reflect ventricular repolarization, it also includes the time required for ventricular depolarization (QRS duration). The QT interval is generally measured in leads II, V_5, and V_6 (see later) and reported as the longest interval among the three, averaged over three to five cycles. If the QT interval cannot be accurately measured in these leads, other leads may be used. The QT interval must be corrected to allow comparison of this interval at differing heart rates. The most commonly used approach, Bazett's formula, defines a corrected QT interval (QTc):

$$QTc = \frac{QT}{\sqrt{RR}}$$

Bazett's formula works reasonably well at heart rates in the normal range but overcorrects at high rates and undercorrects at low rates. Irregular rhythms (notably atrial fibrillation) complicate calculation of the QTc. Some investigators recommend measuring at least three QT intervals to get an average, and then using an RR interval averaged over 10 cycles. More complex regression formulas have been developed to correct the QT interval at different heart rates. For example, the Fridericia formula

$$QTc = \frac{QT}{\sqrt[3]{RR}}$$

may be more accurate than Bazett's formula in atrial fibrillation and better at predicting adverse outcomes, but it has not achieved widespread clinical use.

The presence of a U wave complicates measurement of the QT (and therefore QTc) interval; it may be unclear where the T wave ends and where the U wave begins. In general the U wave should not be included as part of the QT interval; instead, the slope of the T wave to the baseline (before the P wave) should be extrapolated to determine the true QT interval. The QTc in a given patient may vary somewhat during the course of the day and is slightly longer in young and middle-aged women than in men. The upper limit of a normal QTc is somewhat debatable, but a cutoff of 0.45 second (450 msec) in men and 0.46 second (460 msec) in women is generally used. Repolarization and thus the QT interval are sensitive to drug effects as well as to abnormal electrolytes, coronary ischemia, and central nervous system events. Patients with widened QRS complexes frequently have prolonged QT and QTc intervals. In these patients, the JT interval (from J point to the end of T wave) may be a more accurate index of repolarization, but normal standards have not been established. However, a reasonable correction factor is to subtract the excess QRS interval (i.e., measured QRS − 80) from the QT interval. Patients with a prolonged QTc, whether congenital or acquired, may be at risk for torsades de pointes ventricular tachycardia (Chapter 53). A very short QTc interval (<320 to 340 msec) is unusual, and the very rare patient with the short QT syndrome is also at risk for malignant ventricular arrhythmias.

ELECTROCARDIOGRAPHIC LEADS

Recording a single ECG lead allows calculation of the heart rate and, frequently, accurate diagnosis of the heart rhythm. When the ECG is recorded from multiple skin leads simultaneously, the direction (or vector) of activation as the electrical wave front moves through the heart can be inferred. Although a number of different lead systems are possible (and some are actually used in research settings), standard electrocardiography uses 12 vantage points (i.e., leads), derived from 10 electrodes, 6 on the chest wall and 4 on the limbs. In reality, only three limb leads are actually used to generate recordings; the right leg lead serves as an electrical ground. The limb leads, called the frontal plane leads, generate bipolar and augmented unipolar lead recordings. The chest or precordial electrodes record unipolar recordings. Bipolar leads record the potential difference between two skin electrodes. In unipolar recordings, the lead of interest, the exploring electrode, is compared with a reference electrode. By convention, a positive deflection is recorded if the electrical wave front is moving toward the positive electrode in a bipolar pair or toward the exploring electrode in a unipolar lead.

The bipolar limb leads measure potential differences between electrodes on pairs of limb electrodes and closely resemble Einthoven's original string galvanometer recordings. Lead I compares the right arm (negative) and left arm (positive), lead II the right arm (negative) and left leg (positive), and lead III the left arm (negative) and left leg (positive) (E-Fig. 42-1). Because the direction of both atrial and ventricular depolarization is away from the right arm and toward the left arm, a positive P wave and QRS complex are generally recorded in lead I. Similarly, the P wave and QRS complexes are positive in leads II and III in normal sinus rhythm because atrial and ventricular activation proceeds in a craniocaudal direction.

Leads aVR, aVL, and aVF are augmented unipolar leads in which the potential in each limb is compared with a reference electrode. For lead aVR, the potential of the right arm is compared with a reference composed of the left arm and left leg electrodes. Lead aVL compares the left arm potential with a reference combining the right arm and left leg; aVF compares the left leg with a right and left arm reference. Because atrial and ventricular activation normally moves from right to left and in a craniocaudal direction, the P wave and QRS complex are negative in lead aVR but positive in lead aVF. In lead aVL, P waves and QRS complexes are generally upright, although an rS complex may be recorded, particularly in young patients.

The precordial electrodes are positioned at specific points on the chest wall (E-Fig. 42-2A). These unipolar leads compare electrical potential between the chest electrode and a reference electrode called the Wilson central terminal. The Wilson central terminal combines the right arm, left arm, and left leg potentials through 5000-Ω resistors. The six precordial leads define atrial and ventricular activation with respect to a somewhat transverse plane through the chest wall (E-Fig. 42-2B). In this plane, atrial activation moves from right to left. Initial ventricular activation involving the septum is directed from left to right; left ventricular depolarization, which dominates right ventricular depolarization because of the differential in myocardial mass, then moves apically and laterally. In lead V_1, to the right of the sternum, the P wave is biphasic (reflecting right and then left atrial activation). Initial ventricular activation of the septum inscribes an r wave, whereas subsequent activation away from lead V_1 records a dominant S wave. In lead V_6, the P wave is positive, and initial ventricular septal depolarization inscribes a tiny "septal" q wave (usually ≤0.02 second). Subsequent ventricular depolarization records a dominant R wave.

Right-sided chest leads should be recorded when right ventricular abnormalities are suspected. RV_3, the reflection of lead V_3 in the right chest, is routinely recorded in pediatric patients because of the possibility of congenital heart disease. In adults, ST elevation in lead RV_3 is quite specific for acute right ventricular infarction in patients who are being evaluated for an acute inferior wall myocardial infarction.

AXIS

An axis of electrical activation can be defined in the frontal plane axis by combining the bipolar and augmented unipolar limb leads (E-Fig. 42-3A). By convention, the axis parallel to lead I, toward the left, is called 0 degrees. A frontal plane axis between −30 and +90 degrees is normal; other axes are abnormal (E-Fig. 42-4). Mild right axis deviation beyond +90 degrees is a normal variant in children and adolescents. The frontal plane axis can be estimated by identifying the limb lead in which the QRS complex is most nearly isoelectric (a similar amplitude of positive and negative deflections); the axis is perpendicular to this lead (see E-Fig. 42-3B). Because two lines pointing 180 degrees apart can be drawn perpendicular to any given line, examination of the other limb leads defines the direction in which the axis points. If the QRS complex is positive in any given limb lead, the axis will be oriented toward that limb lead, not away from it. Alternatively, the axis is in the normal range if the QRS complexes are primarily positive in both leads I and II.

An axis per se is not defined in the precordial leads. Rather, because the typical progression from leads V_1 to V_6 is from a predominantly negative to a positive QRS complex, the transition point is usually defined as the point at which the amplitude of the R wave first exceeds the amplitude of the S wave. Clockwise rotation (transition zone at V_4 or later) may portend a higher risk of future coronary events, and counterclockwise rotation (transition zone at V_3 or earlier) a lower risk of events.

APPROACH TO INTERPRETING THE ELECTROCARDIOGRAM

Physicians' deficiencies in ECG interpretation[1] can be reduced by using a stepwise approach to ensure that no features of the tracing will be overlooked (Table 42-2).[2]

TABLE 42-2 STEPWISE APPROACH TO INTERPRETING THE ELECTROCARDIOGRAM

Estimate the heart rate
Define the heart rhythm as regular vs. irregular
- Note the relationship of P waves to QRS complexes
- Identify any pauses or premature beats
- If an unsustained arrhythmia is present, note its rate, onset (gradual vs. acute), and termination

Measure intervals (PR, QRS duration, QT)
Calculate/estimate QTc
Estimate QRS axis
Examine P wave morphology, duration, and axis
Examine QRS progression and transition in precordial leads
Examine QRS complexes in regional groupings (septal leads [V_1, V_2], anterior leads [V_2, V_3, V_4], lateral leads [I, aVL, V_5, V_6], inferior and posterior leads [II, III, aVF, V_1, V_2])
Examine ST segments in regional groupings
Examine T waves in regional groupings

NORMAL ELECTROCARDIOGRAM

Figure 42-4 is an example of a normal ECG. Sinus rhythm occurs at about 78 beats per minute, with minor variations in the RR intervals (sinus arrhythmia). The PR interval, QRS duration, and QTc are all normal. The QRS complex is most nearly isoelectric in lead aVL, so the QRS axis will be perpendicular to lead aVL. Because aVL points to −30 degrees, the QRS axis must be approximately −120 or +60 degrees. Because the QRS complex is positive in leads I and II (large R waves), the QRS axis is approximately +60 degrees. The transition in the precordial leads is typically at lead V_3 or V_4. The P wave is biphasic in lead V_1 and then positive in the other precordial leads. Septal q waves, reflecting not lateral infarction but rather normal early septal depolarization, are present in leads V_5 and V_6. Small q waves in the inferior leads are a normal variant.

ABNORMAL ELECTROCARDIOGRAM

Electrocardiography in patients with coronary artery disease is reviewed in Chapters 56 to 58 and in patients with arrhythmias in Chapters 48 to 54.

Conduction Abnormalities and Axis Deviation

Abnormalities of the specialized conduction system (i.e., His-Purkinje system) reflect slow or absent conduction in a particular structure (Table 42-3 and Fig. 42-5). Left anterior or posterior fascicular block does not prolong QRS duration beyond 120 msec. Incomplete bundle branch refers to QRS patterns that are morphologically similar to left or right bundle branch block, but with a duration of less than 0.12 second (120 msec). An interventricular conduction delay is generally defined as a QRS duration of more than 0.11 second (110 msec). When the QRS has a duration of at least 0.12 second (120 msec), it often has the configuration of a specific bundle branch block. An isolated left bundle branch block in an otherwise healthy person is associated with a two-fold higher risk for development of a cardiovascular event or dying of a cardiovascular cause. As a result, this finding should trigger an evaluation for possible cardiac disease. By comparison, a complete right bundle branch block generally has not traditionally been associated with an increased risk, although one study suggested up to a 30% increased risk in cardiovascular mortality.

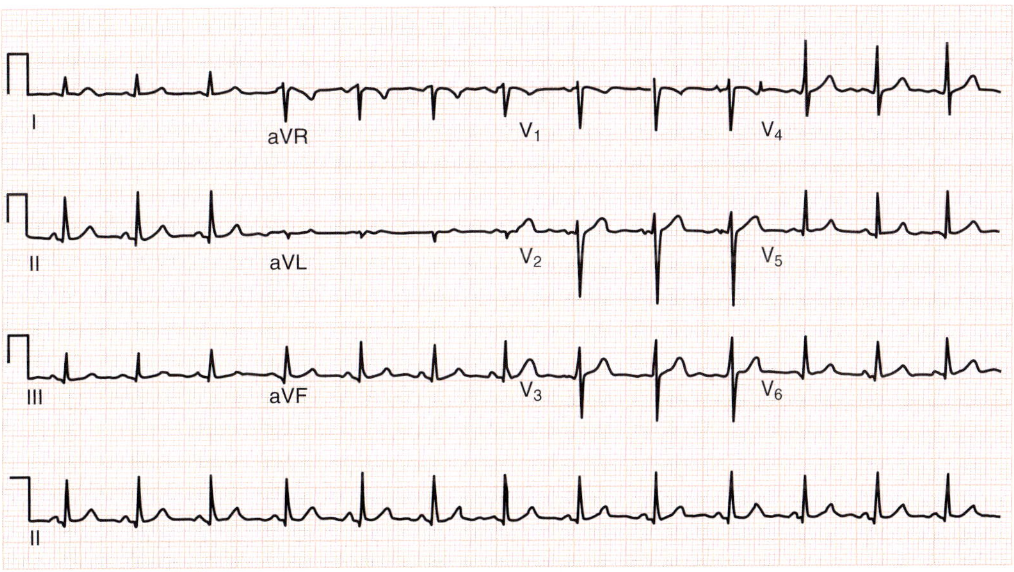

FIGURE 42-4. Normal electrocardiogram. The heart rate is approximately 78 beats per minute, with minor irregularity. Sinus arrhythmia is present. The axis is approximately +60 degrees. The PR, QRS, and QT intervals are approximately 140, 90, and 360 msec, respectively. P wave morphology, duration, and axis are normal. The transition is at lead V_4. No abnormal Q waves are present. ST segments are isoelectric, and T waves are concordant with QRS complexes.

TABLE 42-3 FASCICULAR AND BUNDLE BRANCH BLOCKS

	QRS DURATION	AXIS	QRS MORPHOLOGY	ST SEGMENTS AND T WAVES
LAFB	<0.12 sec (120 msec)	−45 to −90 degrees	Delayed transition across the precordium qR aVL	Normal
LPFB	<0.12 sec (120 msec)	+90 to +180 degrees	Delayed transition across the precordium rS I, aVL qR in III, aVF	Normal
RBBB	≥0.12 sec (120 msec)	Normal	rsr′, rsR′, rSR′ in V_1 (and usually V_2); wide S in V_6 and I	Discordant in V_1 and V_2
RBBB with LAFB	≥0.12 sec (120 msec)	−45 to −90 degrees	rsr′, rsR′, rSR′ in V_1 (and usually V_2); wide S in V_6 and I	Discordant in V_1 and V_2
RBBB with LPFB	≥0.12 sec (120 msec)	+90 to +180 degrees	rsr′, rsR′, rSR′ in V_1 (and usually V_2); wide S in V_6 and I	Discordant in V_1 and V_2
LBBB	≥0.12 sec (120 msec)	Variable	rS or QS in V_1 (S wide and notched); wide notched R without q in V_5, V_6, and I Wide notched R with or without small q in aVL	Discordant in V_1 to V_6

LAD = left axis deviation; LAFB = left anterior fascicular block; LBBB = left bundle branch block; LPFB = left posterior fascicular block; RBBB = right bundle branch block.

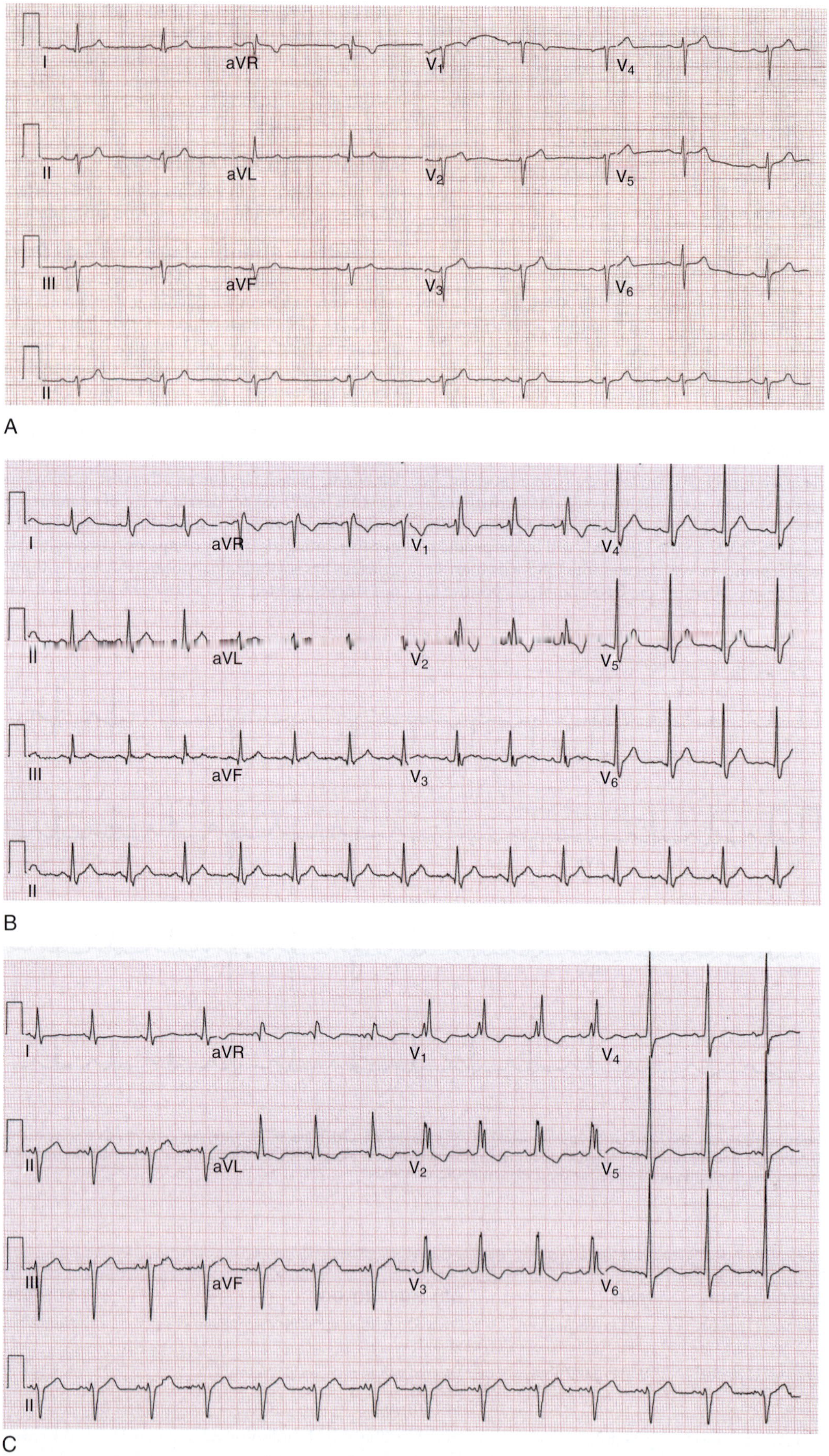

FIGURE 42-5. **Fascicular and bundle branch blocks. A,** Left anterior fascicular block (LAFB). Left axis deviation is present; the axis is approximately –60 degrees. The QRS duration is normal, and there is a delay in R wave progression across the precordial leads (late transition). Small q waves are present in leads I and aVL and small r waves in leads II, III, and aVF. **B,** Right bundle branch block (RBBB). The QRS is widened, with an rsR′ pattern in lead V_1 and a wide terminal S wave in lead V_6. ST segments are downsloping, and T waves are discordant with the QRS complex in the right precordial leads. The axis is normal, and signs of normal septal activation (q waves in lead V_6) are present. **C,** RBBB and LAFB. In addition to features diagnostic of RBBB, an axis of –60 degrees is present.

Continued

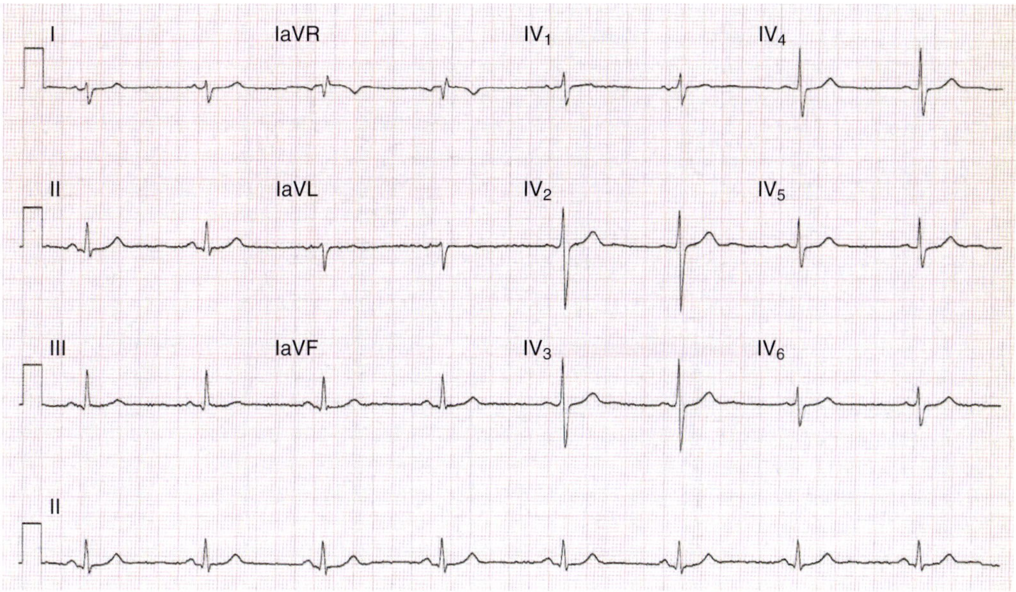

D

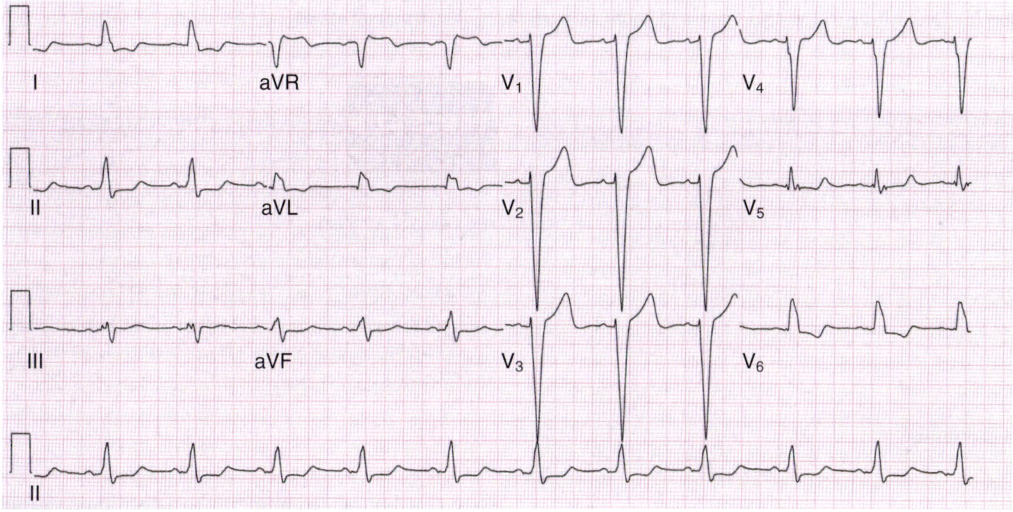

E

FIGURE 42-5, cont'd. **D, Left posterior fascicular block (LPFB). Right axis deviation (+120 degrees) is present. QRS duration is normal, and R wave progression across the precordial leads is delayed. Leads I and AVL have rS complexes, and the inferior leads have insignificant q waves. E, Left bundle branch block (LBBB). The QRS is widened, with a broad, notched complex in leads I, aVL, and the left precordial leads. Small r waves and broad, deep S waves are present in the right precordial leads. With LBBB, the axis is usually normal or deviated to the left. ST segments and T waves are discordant with the QRS complex throughout the precordium.**

Chamber Hypertrophy

A number of criteria for defining left ventricular hypertrophy (LVH; Fig. 42-6) and right ventricular hypertrophy (RVH) have been proposed. All of the LVH criteria suffer from poor sensitivity (ranging from 30 to 50%), although the specificity is reasonable (85 to 95%). The Cornell voltage criterion, developed with an echocardiographic standard for LVH, simply adds the S wave amplitude in V_3 and the R wave amplitude in aVL; a total greater than 2.0 mV in women and 2.8 mV in men implies LVH. In many clinical settings, the Cornell criterion has replaced the more complicated Romhilt-Estes criteria, which assign points for QRS amplitude, repolarization abnormalities ("strain" pattern), left axis deviation, and other electrocardiographic features. These criteria adjusted for body weight also appear to be the preferred method for detecting LVH in obese individuals. RVH is much less common than LVH. Electrocardiographic criteria for diagnosing RVH have even lower sensitivity (10 to 20%) than for LVH, although the specificity is similar. The Sokolow-Lyon criterion for RVH adds the R wave amplitude in V_1 to the S wave amplitude in lead V_5 or V_6; a sum of 1.05 mV or greater implies RVH.

Low QRS Voltage

Low QRS voltage is defined as limb lead voltage less than 5 mm (0.5 mV) in all leads or precordial voltage less than 10 mm (1 mV) in all leads. The differential diagnosis is broad (Table 42-4), and many patients will not have a clinically apparent underlying explanation.

Repolarization Abnormalities

Abnormalities of the ST segment or T waves, or both, are extremely common (Table 42-5). T waves may be in the same direction (concordant) with the QRS complex or discordant. Electrolyte and other metabolic abnormalities, drug effects (particularly digoxin and antiarrhythmic drugs), and secondary effects caused by LVH, bundle branch block, or pacing are all commonly encountered. Abnormal depolarization patterns frequently beget abnormal repolarization.

Early repolarization, which is a relatively common pattern of ST segment elevation and which was previously thought to be benign, occurs more commonly in patients who have idiopathic ventricular fibrillation compared with controls and also has been associated with an increased relative risk of cardiac mortality. The absolute risk of sudden death in apparently healthy patients with the early repolarization pattern remains quite low, however. Whether the "early repolarization syndrome" is a distinct arrhythmic syndrome or a predisposing factor in patients with other arrhythmic substrate(s) is unclear.

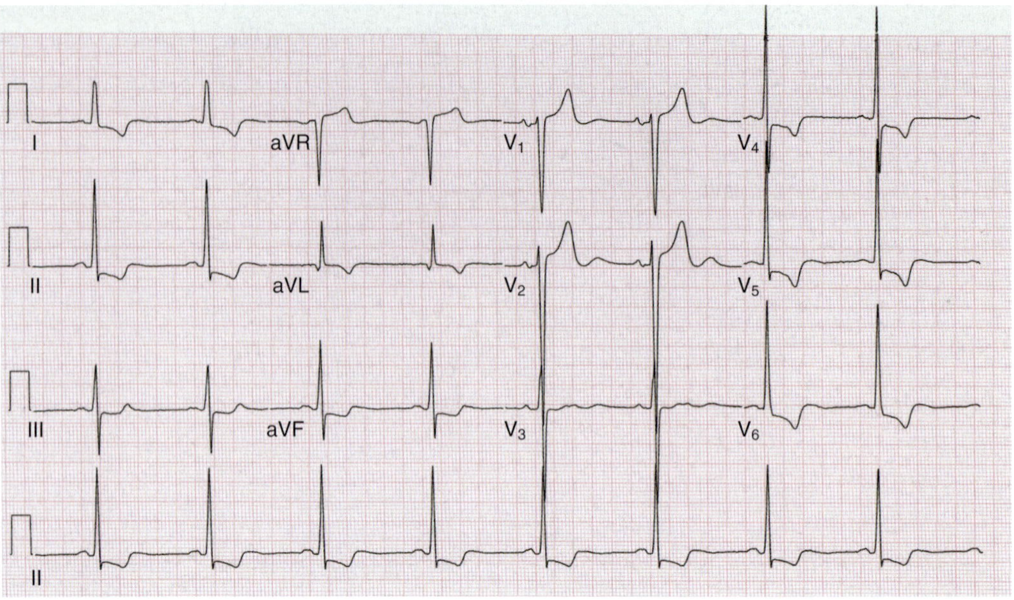

FIGURE 42-6. **Left ventricular hypertrophy.** Note the striking S wave amplitude in the right precordial leads and R wave amplitude in the left precordial leads. Repolarization abnormalities are present in the left precordial leads, as well as the limb leads. The S wave amplitude in V_3 (2.4 mV) plus the R wave amplitude in aVL (1.0 mV) total 3.4 mV, easily satisfying the Cornell voltage criteria in this 76-year-old hypertensive man. Sinus bradycardia (50 beats per minute) is present as well.

TABLE 42-4 CAUSES OF LOW QRS VOLTAGE
Normal variant
Pericardial effusion
Myocardial infarction
Cardiomyopathy
Hypothyroidism
Obesity
Sarcoidosis
Amyloidosis
Chronic obstructive pulmonary disease
Anasarca

TABLE 42-5 CAUSES OF REPOLARIZATION ABNORMALITIES
Athlete's heart
Early repolarization (normal variant)
Myocardial ischemia/injury
Pericarditis
Electrolyte abnormalities
Left ventricular hypertrophy
Intraventricular conduction delay/bundle branch block
Drug effects (digitalis, antiarrhythmic drugs, etc.)
Long QT syndrome
Stroke/neurologic catastrophe

COMPUTERIZED ELECTROCARDIOGRAPHIC READINGS

Automatic computerized ECG interpretations are generally accurate for calculating heart rates, axes, and intervals, but most if not all such systems require over-reading by a physician who will also compare the current ECG to older ECGs. In one large study of patients who received a prehospital ECG, automated interpretation for ST elevation MI (STEMI) had sensitivity and specificity of about 93% and 99%, respectively. False-positive interpretations were due primarily to artifact and nonischemic causes of ST elevation; false-negatives were rare, but related primarily to algorithmic shortcomings. Another study comparing three automated algorithms, however, reported much lower sensitivities and specificities. However, computerized readings are not reliable for diagnosis of rhythm disturbances,[3] and an over-reading by a physician remains mandatory to confirm the cardiac rhythm.

Despite these current limitations, emerging artificial intelligence systems are more accurate than cardiologists with regard to a number of ECG characteristics, such as timing intervals, P-wave morphology, QRS morphology, and left ventricular hypertrophy.[4,5] For example, artificial intelligence ECG analysis can diagnose left ventricular systolic dysfunction in patients who present with dyspnea,[6] predict which patients are at risk for developing atrial fibrillation or ischemic stroke,[7,8] and diagnose hypertrophic cardiomyopathy. These and other enhancements are likely to revolutionize ECG reading in the future.

TABLE 42-6 GENERALLY BENIGN FINDINGS IN ATHLETES' ECGS
Sinus arrhythmia, sinus bradycardia, wandering atrial rhythm, junctional rhythm
First-degree AV block
Mobitz I (Wenckebach) second-degree AV block
Incomplete RBBB
Isolated voltage criteria for LVH (without repolarization abnormalities, left axis deviation, left atrial abnormality, pathologic Q waves, etc.)
Early repolarization pattern

ELECTROCARDIOGRAMS IN ATHLETES

Extensive physical training leads to structural, electrophysiologic, and autonomic adaptations that can appear abnormal on an uninformed ECG reading.[9] Among the most important are rhythms suggesting hypervagotonia, early repolarization, and increased chamber size (Table 42-6 and Fig. 42-7). Differentiation between physiologic adaptations to exercise and potentially life-threatening abnormalities can be difficult and often requires expert consultation. The early repolarization pattern is seen frequently in athletes and may not necessarily imply significant risk in this setting.

ELECTROCARDIOGRAM IN CORONAVIRUS-19 DISEASE

Patients with coronavirus-19 disease (COVID-19; Chapter 336) may have a variety of tachyarrhythmias related to fever, hypoxia, and myocardial

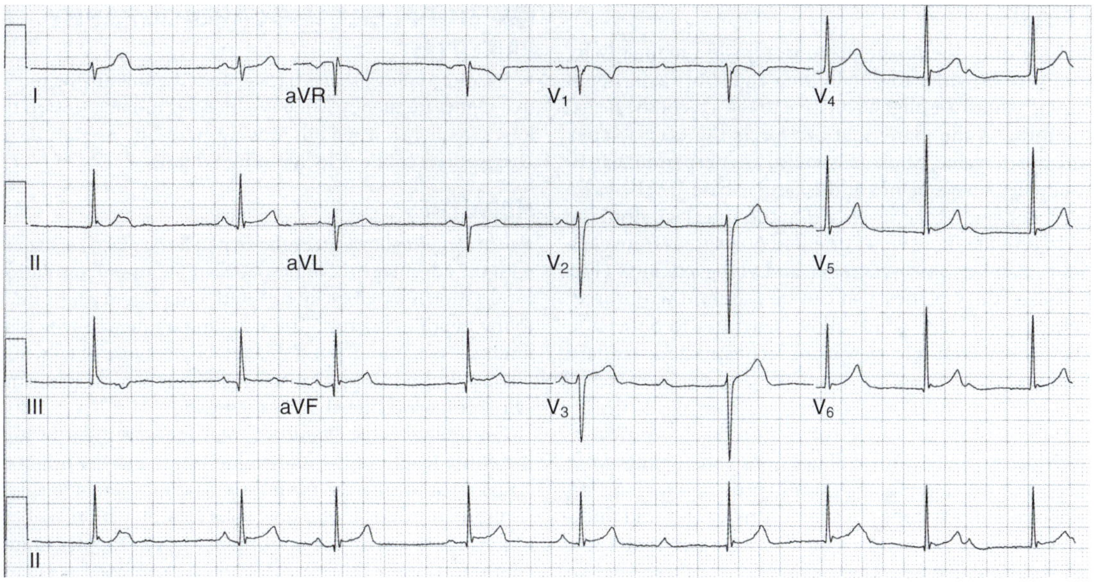

FIGURE 42-7. **Athlete's heart.** Bradycardia, variable P wave morphology, Mobitz I (Wenckebach) second-degree AV block, and junctional escape beats all reflect hypervagotonia in this thin, 18-year-old athlete. Mild right axis deviation is present, not uncommon in adolescents and young adults. Prominent S waves are present in leads V_2 and V_3, though formal voltage criteria for LVH are absent. Note sinus P waves following junctional beats that are blocked; this is not abnormal physiology.

involvement. New-onset atrial fibrillation (Chapter 52), QT-interval prolongation, ST-segment and T-wave changes, and ventricular arrhythmias (Chapter 53) are associated with a poorer prognosis, although they likely are markers of a poor prognosis rather than mediators.[10,11]

SCREENING ELECTROCARDIOGRAMS

Though frequently recommended by cardiologists and primary care physicians, screening ECGs and exercise ECGs (i.e., exercise stress test) have not been shown to improve outcomes in asymptomatic adults. The U.S. Preventive Services Task Force recommends against obtaining a screening resting or exercise ECG in asymptomatic adults who are at low risk of coronary heart disease events (Chapter 12). [A1,12] For asymptomatic adults at intermediate or high risk, evidence is insufficient to make a recommendation. The American College of Cardiology specifically recommends against performing pre-procedure ECG screening in low-risk, asymptomatic patients (Chapter 399).[13] Electrocardiographic screening of competitive athletes prior to participation remains controversial,[14] as does whether improved ECG interpretation should lead to reconsidering a screening ECG in the military.[15]

AMBULATORY ELECTROCARDIOGRAPHY

Ambulatory electrocardiography (Chapter 49) is used primarily to correlate symptoms, such as palpitations and light-headedness, with intermittent cardiac arrhythmias. Wearable devices such as smartwatches to screen for arrhythmias, especially atrial fibrillation, can increase the ability to detect asymptomatic events by about 10-fold and can guide the institution of prophylactic anticoagulant treatment, with about a 1% net absolute benefit in persons age 75 years after 7 years of follow-up.[A2] The reliability and validity of wearable devices to detect myocardial ischemia is less proven.[16]

GENERAL REFERENCES

For the General References and other additional features, please visit Elsevier eBooks+ at https://ebooks.health.elsevier.com.

Grade A References

A1. Jonas DE, Reddy S, Middleton JC, et al. Screening for cardiovascular disease risk with resting or exercise electrocardiography: evidence report and systematic review for the US Preventive Services Task Force. *JAMA*. 2018;319:2315-2328.

A2. Svennberg E, Friberg L, Frykman V, et al. Clinical outcomes in systematic screening for atrial fibrillation (STROKESTOP): a multicentre, parallel group, unmasked, randomised controlled trial. *Lancet*. 2021;398:1498-1506.

43 ECHOCARDIOGRAPHY

CATHERINE M. OTTO

Echocardiography is the clinical standard for evaluation of cardiac function in patients with known or suspected heart disease.[1] This chapter reviews the basic principles of echocardiography, standard imaging approaches, quantitative measurements, and clinical indications.[2,3] The specific indications for echocardiography and additional echocardiographic images are presented in other chapters on individual types of cardiovascular diseases.

ECHOCARDIOGRAPHIC IMAGING

PRINCIPLES

Echocardiography is based on the use of a piezoelectric crystal that converts electrical to mechanical energy, and vice versa, allowing both transmission and reception of an ultrasound signal. The frequency of ultrasound waves used for diagnostic imaging ranges from 2 to 10 MHz, with lower frequencies having greater tissue penetration and higher frequencies providing better image resolution. Each transducer consists of a complex array of piezoelectric crystals arranged to provide images in a fanlike two- or three-dimensional image, with the narrow top of this sector scan indicating the origin of the ultrasound signal. Transducers also include an acoustic lens that determines the focal depth, height, and width of the ultrasound beam.

Images are generated on the basis of the reflection of ultrasound from acoustic interfaces, for example, the boundary between the blood in the left ventricle and the myocardium. The time delay between transmission and reception is used to determine the depth of origin of the ultrasound reflection. The depths of the reflected signals from multiple ultrasound beams are combined to generate an image. The speed of signal analysis allows acquisition of two-dimensional images at slower frame rates. Ultrasound is strongly attenuated by bone and air, so echocardiography relies on acoustic "windows," where ultrasound can penetrate to the heart while avoiding the ribs and lungs. With transthoracic imaging, the patient is positioned to bring the cardiac structures close to the chest wall, usually in a left lateral decubitus position, and the transducer is placed on the chest, with use of gel to provide acoustic coupling between the transducer and skin. Standard transthoracic acoustic windows are parasternal, apical, subcostal, and suprasternal notch.

STANDARD IMAGE PLANES

From the parasternal window, the image plane is adjusted manually by an experienced health care provider to obtain long and short axis views. Standard cardiac imaging planes are aligned relative to the axis of the heart, with the long axis defined as the plane that intersects the cardiac apex and the middle of the aortic valve. Short axis views are perpendicular to this long axis, with standard image planes at the cardiac base (aortic valve level), mitral valve, and midventricular levels. From the apical window, the transducer is rotated to provide three views oriented 60 degrees from each other, producing a four-chamber, a two-chamber, and a long axis view (Fig. 43-1; Video 43-1). These image planes also can be acquired with three-dimensional ultrasound transducers, which allow structures to be seen in a cutaway three-dimensional anatomic view or in reconstructed standard two-dimensional planes.

MEASUREMENTS

Echocardiography provides accurate cardiac dimensions and volumes from 3D and 2D recordings. The measurements typically provided include left ventricular end-diastolic and end-systolic chamber diameter and wall thickness, left atrial diameter or volume, and aortic sinus diameter. Left ventricular ejection fraction (EF) is determined from three-dimensional data sets or two orthogonal two-dimensional views (Figs. 43-2 and 43-3; Video 43-2). End-diastolic and end-systolic ventricular volumes (EDV and ESV, respectively) are calculated by validated formulas, and the EF is calculated as:

$$EF = (EDV - ESV)/EDV$$

LIMITATIONS

Echocardiography is an accurate, widely available imaging approach. In some patients, image quality may be suboptimal because of poor tissue penetration (e.g., excessive adipose tissue, position of the lungs relative to the heart), but images are nondiagnostic in less than 5% of patients. Reflections are stronger when the interface is perpendicular to the ultrasound beam, so structures that are parallel to the beam may not be visible, an artifact called *echo dropout*. This potential limitation is avoided by using multiple transducer positions and imaging planes. Ultrasound artifacts, such as beam width, shadowing, and reverberations, may be misinterpreted by inexperienced observers.

DOPPLER ECHOCARDIOGRAPHY

PRINCIPLES

Ultrasound energy that is backscattered from moving red blood cells is shifted to a higher frequency when the blood is moving toward the transducer and a lower frequency when it is moving away. The magnitude of this Doppler shift corresponds to the velocity of blood flow.

MODALITIES

Pulsed Doppler allows measurement of flow velocity at a specific intracardiac site with the advantages of high spatial and temporal resolution. However, spatial localization is based on intermittent sampling at a time interval corresponding to the depth of interest. The sampling frequency, which is depth dependent, limits the maximum detectable velocity because of a phenomenon called *signal aliasing*. Pulsed Doppler usually allows recording of normal intracardiac flow velocities, which are about 1 m/second.

Continuous-wave Doppler allows measurement of high velocities along the entire length of the ultrasound beam, but the origin of the high-velocity signal must be inferred from the two-dimensional images. With stenotic and regurgitant valves, blood flow velocities may be as high as 5 to 6 m/second, requiring the use of the continuous-wave Doppler mode. Both pulsed and continuous-wave Doppler velocities are displayed as a graph of velocity versus time, with the density of the spectral display corresponding to signal strength.

Color Doppler flow imaging is a modification of pulsed Doppler in which the flow velocity is displayed across a two-dimensional or three-dimensional image with a color scale to indicate direction and velocity. The advantage is a visually appealing display of intracardiac flow patterns. Disadvantages are low temporal resolution (frame rates of 10 to 30 per second) and poor velocity resolution due to signal aliasing.

Tissue Doppler uses the Doppler principle to record the velocity of motion of the myocardial wall. Tissue Doppler recordings of the myocardium adjacent to the mitral annulus are used to evaluate diastolic ventricular function. Speckle tracking strain imaging allows direct evaluation of myocardial mechanics (E-Fig. 43-1).

MEASUREMENTS

A standard echocardiographic study includes pulsed Doppler measurement of antegrade flow velocities (transmitral and transaortic), evaluation for valve regurgitation by continuous-wave and color Doppler modalities, and estimation

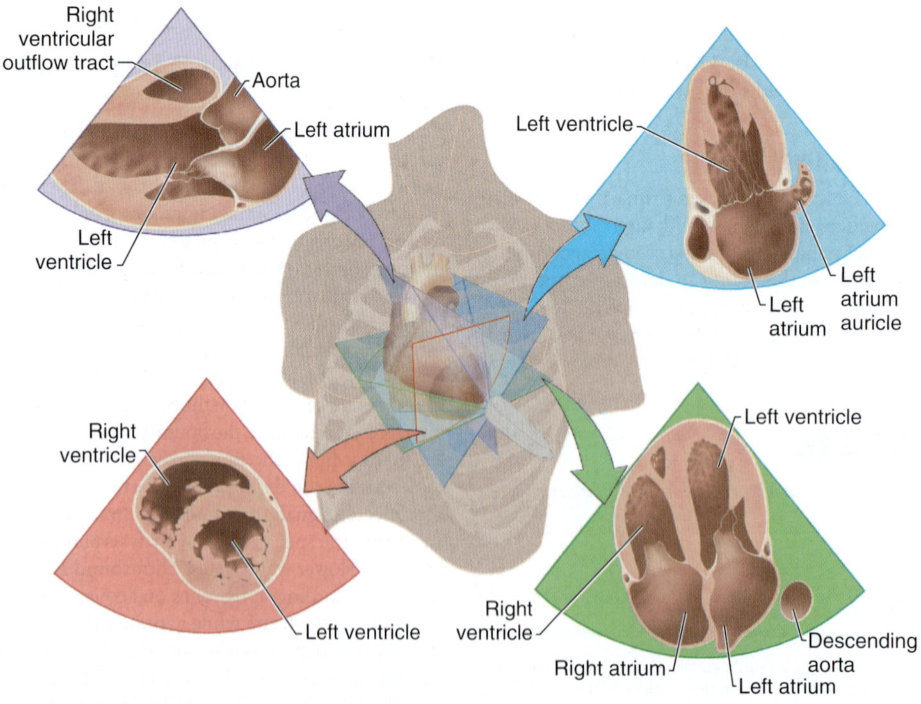

FIGURE 43-1. The four basic image planes used in transthoracic echocardiography. A parasternal transducer position, or "window," is used to obtain long and short axis views. The long axis view (*purple outline*) extends from the left ventricular apex through the aortic valve plane. The short axis view is perpendicular to the long axis view, resulting in a circular view of the left ventricle (*red outline*). The transducer is placed at the ventricular apex to obtain the two-chamber (*blue outline*) and four-chamber (*green outline*) views, each of which is about a 60-degree rotation from the long axis view and perpendicular to the short axis view. The four-chamber view includes both ventricles and both atria. The two-chamber view includes the left ventricle and left atrium; sometimes the atrial appendage is visualized. See Video 43-1. (From Otto CM. *Textbook of Clinical Echocardiography*. 6th ed. Philadelphia: Elsevier; 2018.)

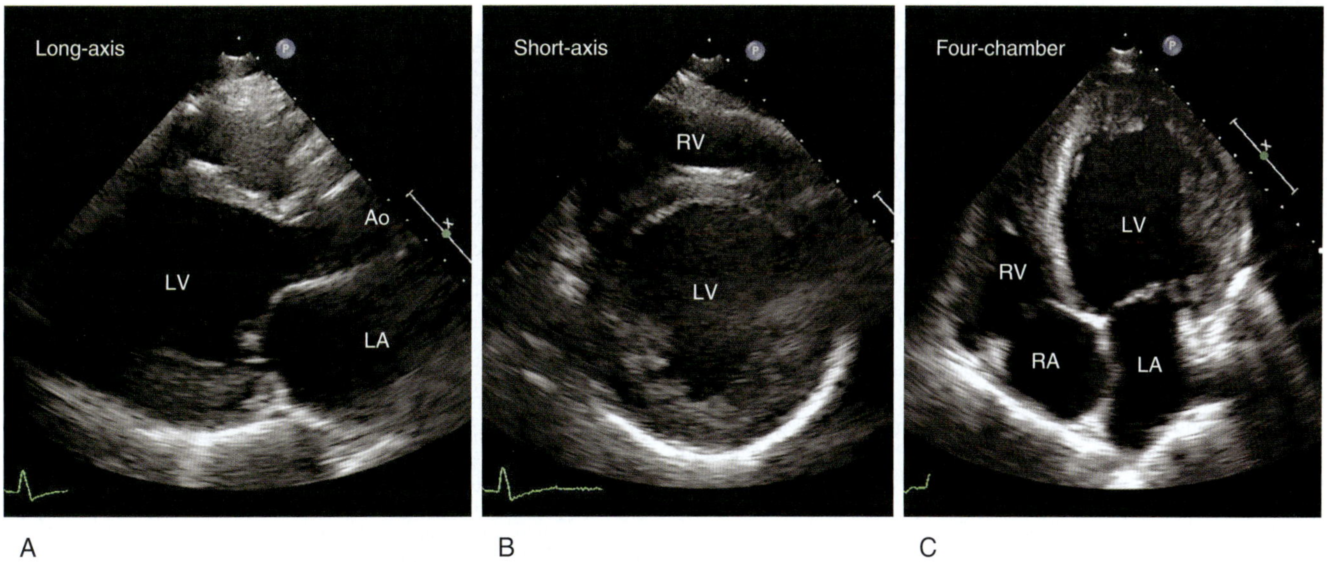

FIGURE 43-2. **Dilated cardiomyopathy on echocardiography.** This example shows severe left ventricular dilation and systolic dysfunction in standard image planes of the **(A)** parasternal long axis (*left*), **(B)** parasternal short axis (*center*), and **(C)** apical four chamber (*right*). Ao = aorta; LA = left atrium; LV = left ventricle; RA = right atrium; RV = right ventricle. See Video 43-2.

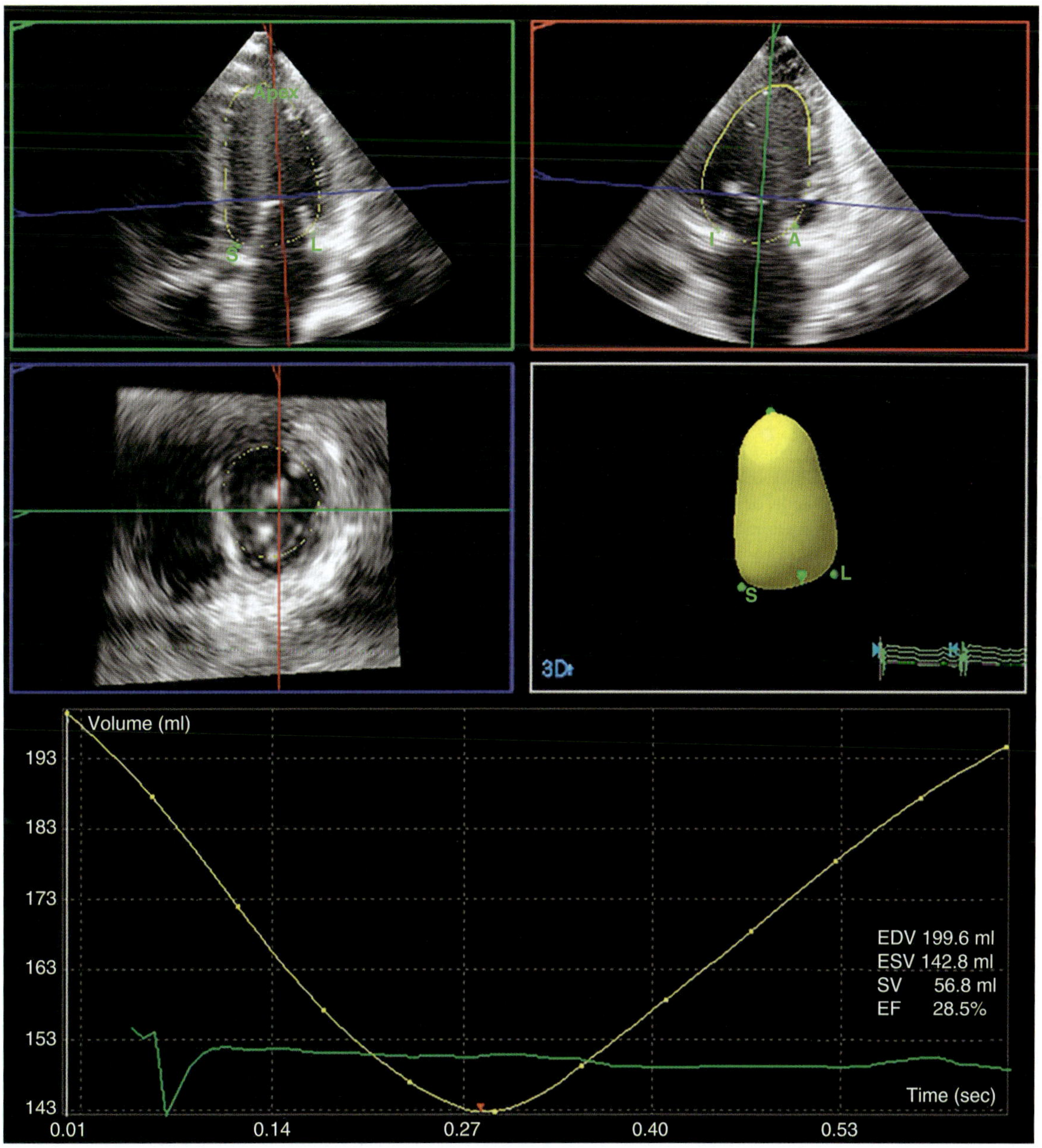

FIGURE 43-3. **Three-dimensional echocardiographic measurement of left ventricular volumes and ejection fraction.** Three-dimensional imaging shows the ventricle in four-chamber (*upper left*), two-chamber (*upper right*), and short axis (*lower left*) views derived from the three-dimensional image acquisition. The left ventricular chamber is reconstructed in the lower right. The ejection fraction is 28.5%.

of pulmonary systolic pressure based on the velocity of tricuspid regurgitation. Other Doppler measurements depend on the specific clinical indication.

Quantitative measurements using Doppler data are derived from two basic concepts: volume flow rate and the pressure-velocity relationship. Stroke volume (SV, in cubic centimeters) is calculated as the volume of a cylinder, where the base is the spatial cross-sectional area (CSA, in square centimeters) of flow, determined as the area of a circle from a two-dimensional diameter measurement. The height of the cylinder is the distance the average blood cell travels in one cardiac cycle, which is the velocity-time integral (VTI, in centimeters) of flow. Therefore,

$$SV\left(cm^3\right) = CSA\left(cm^2\right) \times VTI\,(cm)$$

This approach has been validated to measure transaortic, transmitral, and transpulmonic flow. Measurement of volume flow rate at two different intracardiac sites allows quantitation of intracardiac shunts and valvular regurgitation.

The relationship between the pressure gradient (ΔP) across a narrowing and the velocity (v) of blood flow is described by the simplified Bernoulli equation:

$$\Delta P = 4v^2$$

This equation calculates the maximum and mean gradients across stenotic valves, estimates pulmonary systolic pressure, and evaluates intracardiac hemodynamics with regurgitant valves.

ECHOCARDIOGRAPHIC APPROACHES

Transthoracic echocardiography is the standard clinical approach in most patients with suspected or known cardiac disease (Table 43-1). Advantages are that it is noninvasive, has no known adverse effects, and provides detailed data on cardiac anatomy and physiology. Limitations include poor image quality in some patients, limited visualization of structures distant from the transducer (e.g., atrial septum, left atrial appendage), and inability to visualize structures distal to prosthetic heart valves due to acoustic shadowing.

Transesophageal echocardiography offers superior image quality because of a shorter distance between the transducer and the heart, the absence of interposed bone or lung, and the use of a higher-frequency transducer (Table 43-2). Transesophageal echocardiography usually is well tolerated, but it entails some risk, because most clinicians do this procedure with the patient under moderate sedation. Transesophageal echocardiography is much more sensitive than transthoracic echocardiography for detection of left atrial thrombus (95% vs. 50%), valvular vegetations (99% vs. 60%), and prosthetic mitral valve regurgitation (Fig. 43-4).

Point-of-care ultrasound refers to the use of smaller, less expensive ultrasound systems carried by the physician to perform quick, limited examinations in the emergency department, at the inpatient bedside, or in the outpatient setting (Table 43-3).[4] Point-of-care echocardiography units range from pocket sized to laptop sized. Some are very simple, with only two-dimensional imaging and limited controls; other systems provide high-quality imaging and all Doppler modalities. Point-of-care imaging does not replace a complete echocardiogram but instead serves as an adjunct to the physical examination, particularly in the acute care setting, such as to distinguish ventricular dilation from a pericardial effusion, to estimate ventricular systolic performance, or to screen for aortic stenosis.

Contrast echocardiography may be performed with intravenous injection of agitated saline to opacify the heart chambers. These microbubbles are relatively large and do not pass through pulmonary capillaries. Therefore, appearance of contrast material in the left atrium within one or two beats after right heart opacification is consistent with an intracardiac shunt. Although blood flow occurs predominately from the left to right atrium for most atrial-level shunts, a small amount of right-to-left shunting, which is the basis of this approach, also occurs.

Contrast echocardiography also may be performed with commercially available microbubbles in the range of 1 to 5 μm. Because these microbubbles are smaller than the pulmonary capillaries, opacification of the right heart chambers is followed by opacification of the left ventricle, which can enhance the evaluation of systolic function when image quality is suboptimal, especially during stress echocardiography (Fig. 43-5).

Three-dimensional echocardiography is recommended to quantify left ventricular function and to evaluate complex structural heart disease. It also is essential to guide complex transcatheter interventions (Fig. 43-6; Video 43-3).

Stress echocardiography is a standard approach for evaluating patients with known or suspected coronary artery disease with a high sensitivity (85 to 95%) and specificity (80 to 90%).[5] Although myocardial infarction results in thinning and akinesis of the affected wall, resting myocardial function is normal in the absence of infarction, even when severe epicardial coronary disease is present. The increased myocardial demand associated with exercise or pharmacologic stress leads to myocardial ischemia, which results in a regional wall motion abnormality, often before the onset of chest pain or electrocardiographic changes (Fig. 43-7; Video 43-4).

In patients who can exercise, standard views of the left ventricle are recorded at baseline and immediately after maximal treadmill or bicycle exercise, with the rest and exercise images compared in a side-by-side format. Myocardial ischemia is present if resting wall motion is normal but hypokinesis or akinesis is seen after exercise. The pattern of regional wall motion accurately identifies the area of myocardium at risk and is reasonably reliable for identification of the affected coronary artery. With three-vessel coronary disease, rather than a regional wall motion abnormality, the only clue on imaging may be an absence of the expected decrease in chamber size at peak exercise, caused by diffuse ischemia. Interpretation of an exercise echocardiogram includes exercise duration, hemodynamic response, symptoms, and electrocardiographic changes in addition to the echocardiographic images.

TABLE 43-1 INDICATIONS FOR TRANSTHORACIC ECHOCARDIOGRAPHY IN PATIENTS WITH CARDIAC SIGNS OR SYMPTOMS AND IN THE ACUTE CARE SETTING

CARDIAC SIGNS AND SYMPTOMS

- Cardiac symptoms including chest pain, shortness of breath, palpitations, syncope/presyncope, TIA, stroke, or peripheral embolic event
- Abnormal cardiac murmur (any diastolic murmur or systolic murmur grade 3 or louder)
- Atrial fibrillation, SVT, VT, frequent or exercise-induced VPCs
- Evaluation of pulmonary hypertension
- Suspected infective endocarditis (native or prosthetic valve) with positive blood cultures or a new murmur

ACUTE CARE SETTING

- Hypotension or hemodynamic instability of suspected cardiac etiology
- Acute chest pain with suspected MI but nondiagnostic ECG
- Elevated cardiac biomarkers without other features of ACS
- Suspected complications of acute MI
- Evaluation of ventricular function after ACS
- Respiratory failure of uncertain etiology
- Guidance of therapy with acute pulmonary embolism

ACS = acute coronary syndrome; ECG = electrocardiogram; MI = myocardial infarction; SVT = supraventricular tachycardia; TIA = transient ischemic attack; VPCs = ventricular premature contractions; VT = ventricular tachycardia.
Modified from Otto CM. *Textbook of Clinical Echocardiography*. 6th ed. Philadelphia: Elsevier; 2018.

TABLE 43-2 INDICATIONS FOR TRANSESOPHAGEAL ECHOCARDIOGRAPHY AS THE INITIAL OR SUPPLEMENTAL TEST

- Suspected endocarditis with a moderate or high pretest probability (e.g., staphylococcal bacteremia, fungemia, prosthetic heart valve, or intracardiac device)
- Suspected complications of endocarditis (e.g., abscess, fistula)
- Suspected prosthetic mitral valve dysfunction
- Evaluation of posterior structure (e.g., atrial baffles) in patients with congenital heart disease
- Evaluation of patients with atrial fibrillation or flutter to facilitate clinical decision making with regard to anticoagulation, cardioversion, or radio frequency ablation
- Evaluation for cardiac source of embolus with no identified source on TTE
- Evaluation of valve structure and function to evaluate suitability for surgical or transcatheter valve interventions
- Suspected acute aortic disease, including dissection and transection (although CT preferred for this indication)
- Guidance for transcatheter interventions for structural heart disease, such as closure of a patent foramen ovale or atrial septal defect, or transcatheter edge-to-edge repair for valve regurgitation
- Reevaluation for interval changes compared with prior TEE when a change in therapy is anticipated

CT = computed tomography; PFO/ASD = patent foramen ovale/atrial septal defect; TEE = transesophageal echocardiography; TTE = transthoracic echocardiography.
Modified from Otto CM. *Textbook of Clinical Echocardiography*. 6th ed. Philadelphia: Elsevier; 2018.

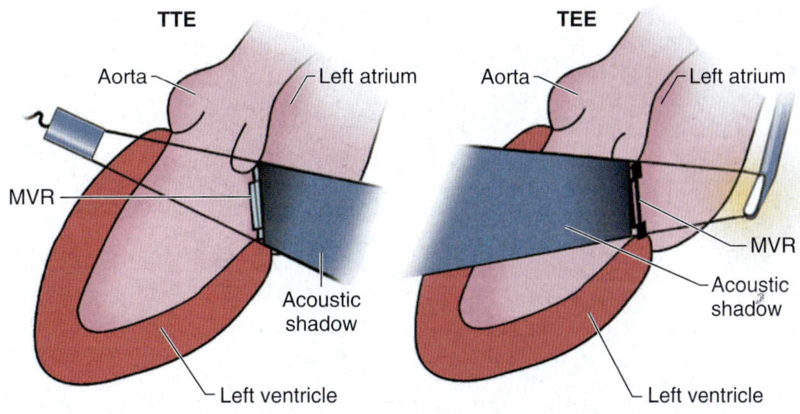

FIGURE 43-4. The problem of acoustic shadowing from a prosthetic mitral valve replacement (MVR). *Left,* With transthoracic echocardiography (TTE), the acoustic shadow distal to the prosthetic valve obscures the left atrium, limiting assessment of valve regurgitation by Doppler techniques. *Right,* With transesophageal echocardiography (TEE), the left atrium now can be evaluated for valvular regurgitation. However, the acoustic shadow now obscures the left ventricle. (From Otto CM. *Textbook of Clinical Echocardiography*. 5th ed. Philadelphia: Elsevier; 2018.)

TABLE 43-3 INDICATIONS FOR POINT-OF-CARE ECHOCARDIOGRAPHY

Urgent clinical evaluation (emergency department or intensive care unit)
• Left ventricular size (volume status) and systolic function
• Right ventricular size and systolic function
• Pericardial effusion/tamponade
Screening at-risk populations (athletes, rheumatic heart disease, etc.)
Frequent serial exams for known abnormality (e.g., response to heart failure therapy)

In patients who are unable to exercise, stress testing can be performed with a graded intravenous infusion of dobutamine, beginning at 5 to 10 μg/kg/minute and gradually increasing to a maximum dose of 40 μg/kg/minute. If needed, atropine is used to achieve 85% of the maximum predicted heart rate. In addition to evaluation for myocardial ischemia, myocardial viability is evidenced by an improvement in endocardial motion from baseline to low-dose dobutamine, with subsequent worsening of function at higher doses—the "biphasic" response.

Intracardiac echocardiography is performed with an ultrasound probe on a catheter that is inserted into the right side of the heart through the femoral vein. Intracardiac echocardiography is used in the cardiac catheterization laboratory to guide percutaneous closure of a patent foramen ovale (PFO) and other procedures. In the electrophysiology laboratory, intracardiac echocardiography can help guide catheter positioning and identify complications.

CARDIAC FUNCTION MEASUREMENTS

In addition to qualitative descriptions of cardiac anatomy and physiology, echocardiography provides precise and accurate quantification of cardiac function (including ventricular systolic and diastolic function), the severity of valve stenosis and regurgitation, and a noninvasive estimate of pulmonary pressures.[6]

SYSTOLIC VENTRICULAR FUNCTION

Left ventricular volumes and ejection fractions are routinely measured by two-dimensional biplane or three-dimensional imaging approaches. When actual measurements are not possible, overall left ventricular systolic function is graded by visual estimation, with an approximate correspondence to EF as follows: normal (EF > 55%), mildly reduced (EF, 40 to 55%), moderately reduced (EF, 20 to 40%), and severely reduced (EF < 20%). Cardiac output calculations are not routine but may be helpful for noninvasive monitoring of therapy in patients with heart failure. Because EF measurements are affected by preload and afterload, measures that are less dependent on loading conditions, including the end-systolic dimension or volume, are generally preferred for clinical decision making in situations such as the timing of surgery for chronic valvular regurgitation.

Speckle tracking strain imaging is less load-dependent than standard imaging and allows evaluation of global and regional ventricular function. A reduction in global longitudinal strain may be seen before a detectable reduction in the ejection fraction in patients with inherited cardiomyopathies or after treatment with cardiotoxic chemotherapy.[7]

Quantitative evaluation of right ventricular function by echocardiography is difficult because of the complex shape of the chamber. Useful measurements include the basal diameter, the tricuspid annular plane systolic excursion, and the systolic Doppler tissue velocity at the annulus. Cardiac magnetic resonance imaging provides more accurate quantitation of right ventricular volumes and function when it is clinically needed.

DIASTOLIC VENTRICULAR FUNCTION

Evaluation of diastolic ventricular function is challenging because the patterns of ventricular filling are affected by preload, heart rate, and coexisting valvular regurgitation in addition to the diastolic properties of the ventricle. However, echocardiography can classify diastolic function on the basis of the combination of left ventricular inflow, pulmonary vein flow, tissue Doppler velocities, and isovolumic relaxation time. An estimate of left ventricular filling pressure (e.g., left ventricular end-diastolic pressure) also can be inferred by these approaches.

VALVULAR STENOSIS

Echocardiography is the clinical standard for evaluating patients with known or suspected valvular heart disease and is far more accurate than cardiac auscultation for diagnosis.[8] When significant valvular stenosis is a concern but echocardiography is not diagnostic or seems discordant with other clinical information, measurement of valve calcification by computed tomography (Chapter 44) or of a serum brain natriuretic protein level may be helpful. In current practice, cardiac catheterization is rarely performed to diagnose the severity of valve stenosis, although coronary arteriography may be indicated before valve surgery to evaluate the coronary anatomy and to determine whether concomitant myocardial revascularization may be indicated (Chapter 56).

In patients with aortic stenosis, the most direct measure of stenosis severity is the antegrade velocity across the valve, indicating mild (<3 m/second), moderate (3 to 3.9 m/second), or severe (≥4 m/second) valve obstruction. The maximum and mean transaortic pressure gradients also can be calculated by the Bernoulli equation. Accurate evaluation depends on a careful examination by an experienced echocardiographer.

Aortic valve area (AVA) is calculated by the continuity equation, based on the concept that volume flow rates proximal to and within the narrowed orifice are equal:

$$AVA \times VTI_{AS} = CSA_{LVOT} \times VTI_{LVOT}$$

or

$$AVA = (CSA_{LVOT} \times VTI_{LVOT}) / VTI_{AS}$$

where LVOT is left ventricular outflow tract, VTI is velocity-time integral, CSA is cross-sectional area, and AS is aortic stenosis (Fig. 43-8). It is especially important to calculate the AVA when left ventricular systolic dysfunction accompanies aortic valve disease. In some patients, low-dose dobutamine stress echocardiography is helpful in distinguishing ventricular dysfunction caused by severe aortic stenosis from primary myocardial disease with concurrent moderate stenosis.

The evaluation of mitral stenosis (see Fig. 60-4) focuses on the calculation of valve area, both from direct planimetry of the area of the orifice on three-dimensional or two-dimensional images and from the deceleration slope of the

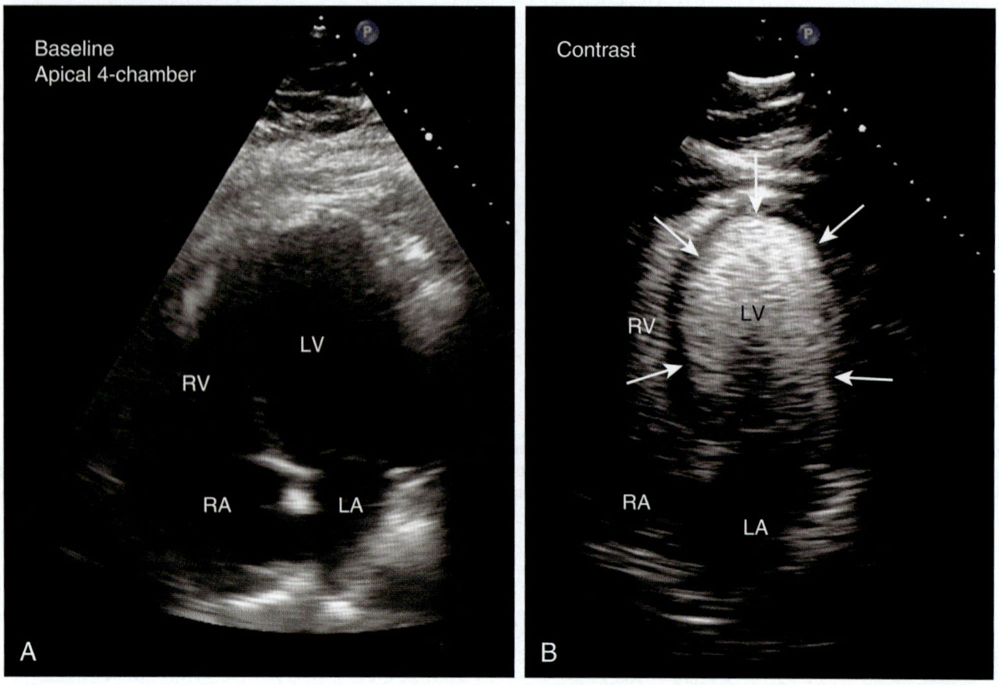

FIGURE 43-5. **Poor-quality apical view (A) with marked improvement in definition of the left ventricular cavity after opacification by contrast echocardiography (B). The arrows indicate improved identification of the left ventricular endocardial border for calculation of ejection fraction. LA = left atrium; LV = left ventricle; RA = right atrium; RV = right ventricle.**

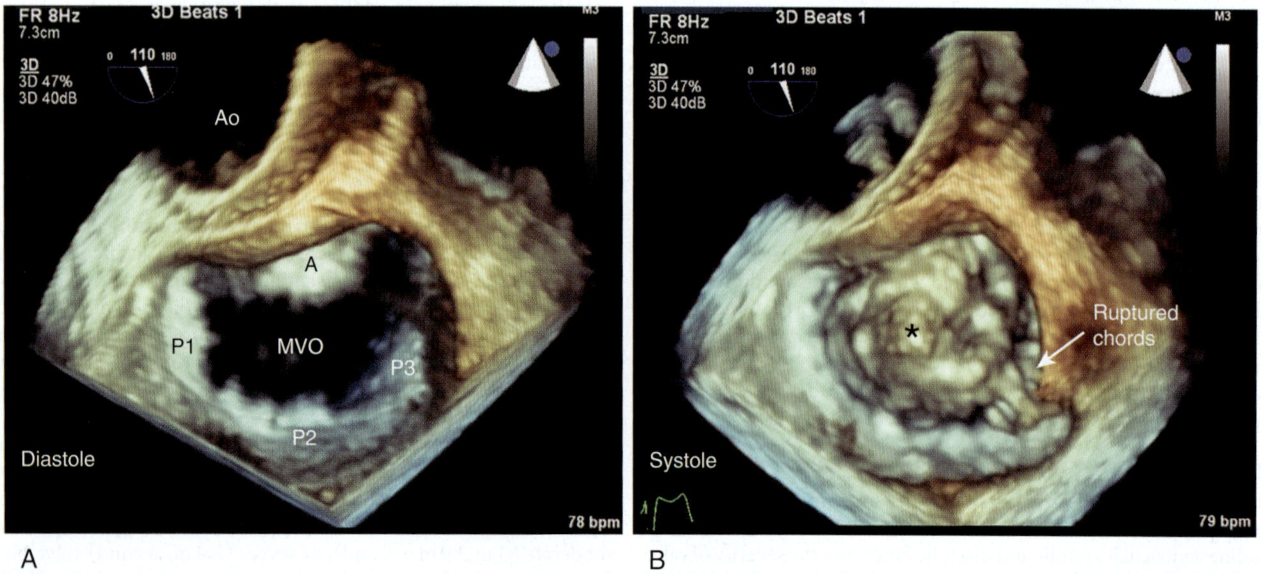

FIGURE 43-6. **The surgeon's three-dimensional view of the mitral valve from the left atrial side of the valve with the aortic valve at the top of the image.** In diastole, the anterior (A) leaflet and posterior leaflet (with P1, P2, and P3 scallops) are seen in the open position, with the normal mitral valve orifice (MVO). In systole (B), severe prolapse of the anterior leaflet is seen, particularly one bulging section (*asterisk*), and a flail segment with two small ruptured chords (*arrow*) is well visualized. These abnormalities cause severe, posteriorly directed mitral regurgitation. Ao = aorta. See Video 43-3. (From Otto CM. *Textbook of Clinical Echocardiography*. 6th ed. Philadelphia: Elsevier; 2018.)

Doppler curve (pressure half-time method). The mean transmitral gradient, which is dependent on the heart rate and volume flow rate as well as the severity of the stenosis, is not recommended to define the severity of mitral stenosis.

VALVULAR REGURGITATION

The current approach to evaluating valvular regurgitation (see Figs. 60-5 and 60-8) is based on the proximal geometry of the regurgitant jet, with measurement of the narrowest jet width (vena contracta). When further quantification is needed, regurgitant volume, regurgitant fraction, and regurgitant orifice area are calculated. Although color flow visualization of the flow disturbance may be helpful for detecting regurgitation and for understanding the mechanism of valve dysfunction, this approach should no longer be used to evaluate severity.

For aortic regurgitation, a narrow vena contracta (<3 mm) indicates mild regurgitation, whereas a wide vena contracta (>6 mm) indicates severe regurgitation. Additional evaluation of the severity of aortic regurgitation is based on the presence of holodiastolic flow reversal in the abdominal aorta and the density and slope of the continuous-wave Doppler velocity curve. The approach to evaluating mitral regurgitation (see Fig. 60-5) is similar, beginning with measurement of the vena contracta. In addition to calculation based on transmitral versus transaortic volume flow rates, the proximal acceleration of flow into the regurgitant orifice allows evaluation with central regurgitant jets based on the proximal isovelocity surface area method.

PULMONARY PRESSURES

Estimation of pulmonary artery systolic pressure (PAP) is a standard component of any echocardiographic study. The systolic pressure difference between the right ventricle and right atrium is calculated from the peak velocity in the tricuspid regurgitant (V_{TR}) jet, with use of the Bernoulli equation. Then, the right atrial pressure (RAP) is estimated from the size and appearance of the inferior vena cava. Because right ventricular and pulmonary artery systolic pressures are equal (in the absence of pulmonic stenosis),

$$PAP = 4(V_{TR})^2 + RAP$$

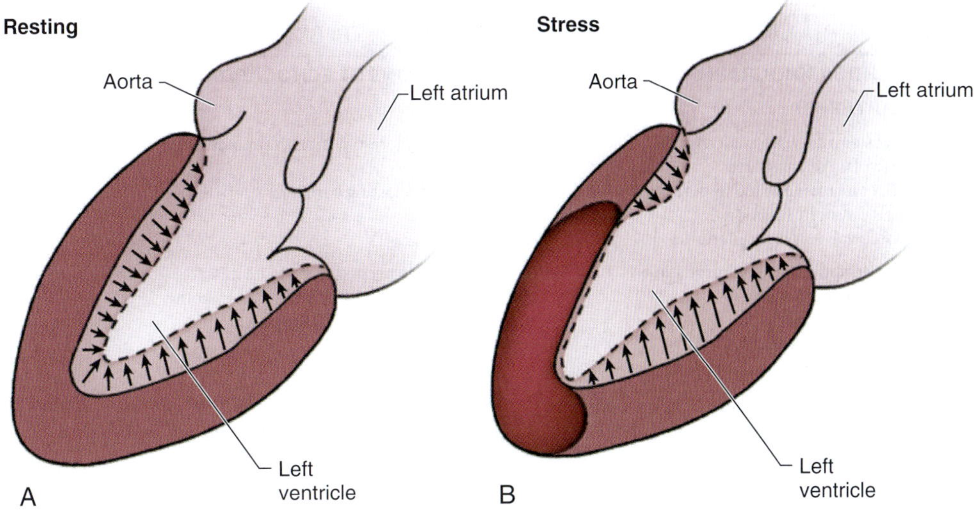

FIGURE 43-7. The concept of stress echocardiography in a patient with 70% stenosis in the proximal third of the left anterior descending coronary artery. At rest (A), endocardial motion and wall thickening are normal. After stress (B), either exercise or pharmacologic, the middle and apical segments of the anterior wall become ischemic, showing reduced endocardial wall motion and wall thickening. If the left anterior descending coronary artery extends around the apex, the apical segment of the posterior wall also will be affected, as shown here. The normal segment of the posterior wall shows compensatory hyperkinesis. See Video 43-4. (From Otto CM. *Textbook of Clinical Echocardiography*. 6th ed. Philadelphia: Elsevier; 2018.)

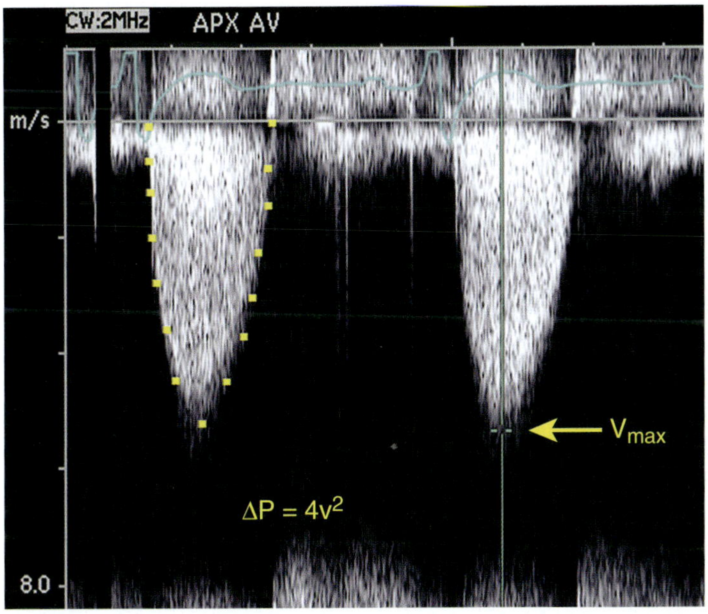

FIGURE 43-8. In a patient with aortic stenosis, the aortic jet velocity is recorded with continuous-wave Doppler from the window that yields the highest-velocity signal. Maximum velocity (V_{max}) is used to calculate the maximum systolic gradient. The Doppler curve is traced, as shown, to calculate the mean systolic gradient with the Bernoulli equation, by which the pressure gradient (ΔP) equals four times the square of the velocity.

A small amount of tricuspid regurgitation is present in most patients, so pulmonary pressures can be estimated with this approach in more than 90% of patients. Because this approach measures only pulmonary systolic pressure, not pulmonary vascular resistance, invasive evaluation may still be needed in some clinical situations (Chapter 69).

THE ECHOCARDIOGRAPHIC EXAMINATION

CLINICAL INDICATIONS

Currently, echocardiography is not recommended for screening of the general population in developed countries, but it is an effective approach to the initial evaluation of many cardiac signs and symptoms (Table 43-4),[9] with a better sensitivity than the clinical evaluation for detecting left ventricular dysfunction and valvular heart disease. Screening can also be effective in low-resource settings with a high prevalence of rheumatic heart disease.[10] A transthoracic examination is appropriate initially in most patients, although transesophageal imaging is needed for some specific diagnoses, such as concern for para-valvular abscess in patients with infected endocarditis and to exclude left atrial thrombosis before cardioversion (Chapter 52). Resting echocardiography is not helpful for diagnosis of coronary artery disease; stress imaging is needed if this diagnosis is suspected (Chapter 56). In patients with known cardiac disease, echocardiography is used to evaluate severity, to assess the results of medical and surgical interventions, and to guide procedures. Point-of-care ultrasound is useful for rapid screening to evaluate overall left ventricular function and to detect pericardial effusion (Fig. 43-9; Video 43-5).[11–13]

NORMAL FINDINGS

Trace to mild valve regurgitation is considered "physiologic" and is seen with 70 to 80% of mitral valves, 80 to 90% of tricuspid valves, and 70 to 80% of pulmonic valves in normal individuals. The prevalence of aortic regurgitation increases with age, but it is found in only 5% of young normal adults; the presence of aortic regurgitation raises the possibility of subtle aortic valve or root abnormalities.

A patent foramen ovale (Chapter 55) is present in 25 to 35% of normal individuals and may be identified by color Doppler or by contrast echocardiography. Use of the Valsalva maneuver enhances identification of a patent foramen ovale because the slight elevation in right atrial pressure may lead to a brief right-to-left shunt. The significance of a patent foramen ovale in patients without clinical events is unclear. Other common anatomic variants seen on echocardiography include aberrant chords (or "webs") in the left ventricle; small, linear, mobile echoes associated with the valves (Lambl's excrescences); and normal ridges in the left and right atria.

Unexpected abnormal findings also may be found on studies requested for other indications. A bicuspid aortic valve is present in 1 to 2% of the population; most of these patients are asymptomatic until late in life, so many cases are diagnosed "incidentally" by echocardiography. Aortic valve sclerosis, which is a frequent unexpected echocardiographic diagnosis, is a marker of cardiovascular disease and an increased risk of myocardial infarction even if valve function is normal.

INTEGRATING THE ECHOCARDIOGRAPHIC AND CLINICAL FINDINGS

The echocardiographic request should indicate the specific reason for the study and any relevant symptoms or signs. The echocardiographic examination then can be tailored to answer the clinical question.

The echocardiographic results should be interpreted in conjunction with other clinical data. If the echocardiographic data seem discrepant with the clinical data, the requesting physician should review the images with the echocardiographer to identify areas of uncertainty and to determine the next best diagnostic step.

TABLE 43-4 INDICATIONS FOR TRANSTHORACIC ECHOCARDIOGRAPHY (TTE) BY KNOWN DIAGNOSIS

CLINICAL DIAGNOSIS	KEY ECHOCARDIOGRAPHIC FINDINGS	LIMITATIONS OF ECHOCARDIOGRAPHY	ALTERNATIVE APPROACHES
VALVULAR HEART DISEASE (CHAPTER 60)			
Valve stenosis	Cause of stenosis, valve anatomy Transvalvular ΔP, valve area Chamber enlargement and hypertrophy LV and RV systolic function Associated valvular regurgitation	Possible underestimation of the stenosis severity Possible coexisting coronary artery disease	Cardiac catheterization; CMR
Valve regurgitation	Mechanism and cause of regurgitation Severity of regurgitation Chamber enlargement LV and RV systolic function PA pressure estimate	TEE may be needed to evaluate mitral regurgitant severity and valve anatomy (especially before MV repair)	Cardiac catheterization; CMR
Prosthetic valve function	Evidence for stenosis Detection of regurgitation Chamber enlargement Ventricular function PA pressure estimate	TTE is limited by shadowing and reverberations TEE is needed for suspected prosthetic MR due to "masking" of the LA on TTE	Cardiac catheterization; fluoroscopy
Endocarditis (Chapter 61)	Detection of vegetations (TTE sensitivity, 70-85%) Presence and degree of valve dysfunction Chamber enlargement and function Detection of abscess Possible prognostic implications	TEE more sensitive for detection of vegetations (>90%) A definite diagnosis of endocarditis also depends on bacteriologic criteria TEE more sensitive for detection abscess	Blood cultures and clinical findings also are diagnostic criteria for endocarditis
CORONARY ARTERY DISEASE			
Acute myocardial infarction (Chapters 57 and 58)	Segmental wall motion abnormality reflects "myocardium at risk" Global LV function (EF) Complications: Acute MR vs. VSD Pericarditis LV thrombus, aneurysm, or rupture RV infarct	Coronary artery anatomy itself is not directly visualized	Coronary angiography (by catheterization or CT) Radionuclide or PET imaging for myocardial perfusion
Angina (Chapter 56)	Global and segmental LV systolic function Exclude other causes of angina (e.g., AS, HCM)	Resting wall motion may be normal despite significant CAD Stress echocardiography is needed to induce ischemia and wall motion abnormality	Coronary angiography Radionuclide or PET imaging ETT
Pre-revascularization/ post-revascularization (Chapter 59)	Assess wall thickening and endocardial motion at baseline Improvement in segmental function after procedure	Dobutamine stress or contrast echocardiography is needed to detect viable but nonfunctioning myocardium	CMR Coronary angiography Radionuclide or PET imaging Contrast echocardiography
End-stage ischemic disease	Overall LV systolic function (EF) PA pressures Associated MR LV thrombus RV systolic function	—	Coronary angiography (by catheterization or CT) Radionuclide or PET imaging CMR for myocardial viability
CARDIOMYOPATHY (CHAPTERS 45-47)			
Dilated	Chamber dilation (all four) LV and RV systolic function (qualitative and EF) Coexisting atrioventricular valve regurgitation PA systolic pressure LV thrombus	Indirect measures of LVEDP Accurate EF may be difficult if image quality is poor	CMR for LV size, function, and myocardial fibrosis LV angiography with left and right heart hemodynamics
Restrictive	LV wall thickness LV systolic function LV diastolic function PA systolic pressure	Must be distinguished from constrictive pericarditis	Cardiac catheterization with direct, simultaneous RV and LV pressure measurement after volume loading CMR
Hypertrophic	Pattern and extent of LV hypertrophy Dynamic LVOT obstruction (imaging and Doppler) Coexisting MR Diastolic LV dysfunction	Exercise echo to detect inducible LV outflow tract obstruction	CMR Strain and strain rate imaging
HYPERTENSION (CHAPTER 64)			
	LV wall thickness and chamber dimensions LV hypertrophy LV diastolic dysfunction LV systolic function Aortic valve sclerosis Mitral annular calcification	Diastolic dysfunction precedes systolic dysfunction, but detection is challenging because of age and other factors	Speckle tracking; strain and strain rate imaging LV twist and torsion
PERICARDIAL DISEASE (CHAPTER 62)			
	Pericardial thickening Detection, size, and location of PE Two-dimensional signs of tamponade physiology Doppler signs of tamponade physiology	Diagnosis of tamponade is a hemodynamic and clinical diagnosis Constrictive pericarditis is a difficult diagnosis Not all patients with pericarditis have an effusion	Intracardiac pressure measurements for tamponade or constriction CMR or CT to detect pericardial thickening

TABLE 43-4 INDICATIONS FOR TRANSTHORACIC ECHOCARDIOGRAPHY (TTE) BY KNOWN DIAGNOSIS—cont'd

CLINICAL DIAGNOSIS	KEY ECHOCARDIOGRAPHIC FINDINGS	LIMITATIONS OF ECHOCARDIOGRAPHY	ALTERNATIVE APPROACHES
DISEASES OF THE AORTA (CHAPTER 63)			
Aortic root dilation	Cause of aortic dilation Accurate aortic root diameter measurements Anatomy of sinuses of Valsalva (especially Marfan syndrome) Associated aortic regurgitation	The ascending aorta is only partially visualized on TTE in most patients	CT CMR TEE
Aortic dissection	Two-dimensional images of ascending aorta, aortic arch, descending thoracic and proximal abdominal aorta Imaging of dissection "flap" Associated aortic regurgitation Ventricular function	TEE more sensitive (97%) and more specific (100%) Cannot assess distal vascular beds	Aortography CT CMR TEE
CARDIAC MASSES (CHAPTER 47)			
LV thrombus	High sensitivity and specificity for diagnosis of LV thrombus Suspect with apical wall motion abnormality or diffuse LV systolic dysfunction	Technical artifacts can be misleading 5-MHz or higher frequency transducer and angulated apical views needed	LV thrombus may not be recognized on radionuclide or contrast angiography
LA thrombus	Low sensitivity for detection of LA thrombus, although specificity is high Suspect with LA enlargement, MV disease	TEE needed to detect LA thrombus reliably	TEE
Cardiac tumors	Size, location, and physiologic consequences of tumor mass	Extracardiac involvement is not well seen Cannot distinguish benign from malignant tumor or tumor from thrombus	TEE CT CMR (with cardiac gating) Intracardiac echocardiography
PULMONARY HYPERTENSION (CHAPTER 69)			
	PA pressure estimate Evidence of left-sided heart disease to account for increased PA pressures RV size and systolic function (cor pulmonale) Associated TR	Indirect PA pressure measurement Difficult to determine pulmonary vascular resistance accurately	Cardiac catheterization
CONGENITAL HEART DISEASE (CHAPTER 55)			
	Detection and assessment of anatomic abnormalities Quantitation of physiologic abnormalities Chamber enlargement Ventricular function	No direct intracardiac pressure measurements Complicated anatomy may be difficult to evaluate if image quality is poor (TEE is helpful)	CMR with three-dimensional reconstruction Cardiac catheterization TEE Three-dimensional echocardiography

AS = aortic stenosis; CAD = coronary artery disease; CMR = cardiac magnetic resonance; CT = computed tomography; EF = ejection fraction; ETT = exercise treadmill test; HCM = hypertrophic cardiomyopathy; LA = left atrium; LV = left ventricle; LVEDP = left ventricular end-diastolic pressure; LVOT = left ventricular outflow tract; MR = mitral regurgitation; MV = mitral valve; ΔP = pressure gradient; PA = pulmonary artery; PE = pericardial effusion; PET = positron emission tomography; RV = right ventricle; TEE = transesophageal echocardiography; TR = tricuspid regurgitation; TTE = transthoracic echocardiography; VSD = ventricular septal defect.

From Otto CM. *Textbook of Clinical Echocardiography*. 6th ed. Philadelphia: Elsevier; 2018.

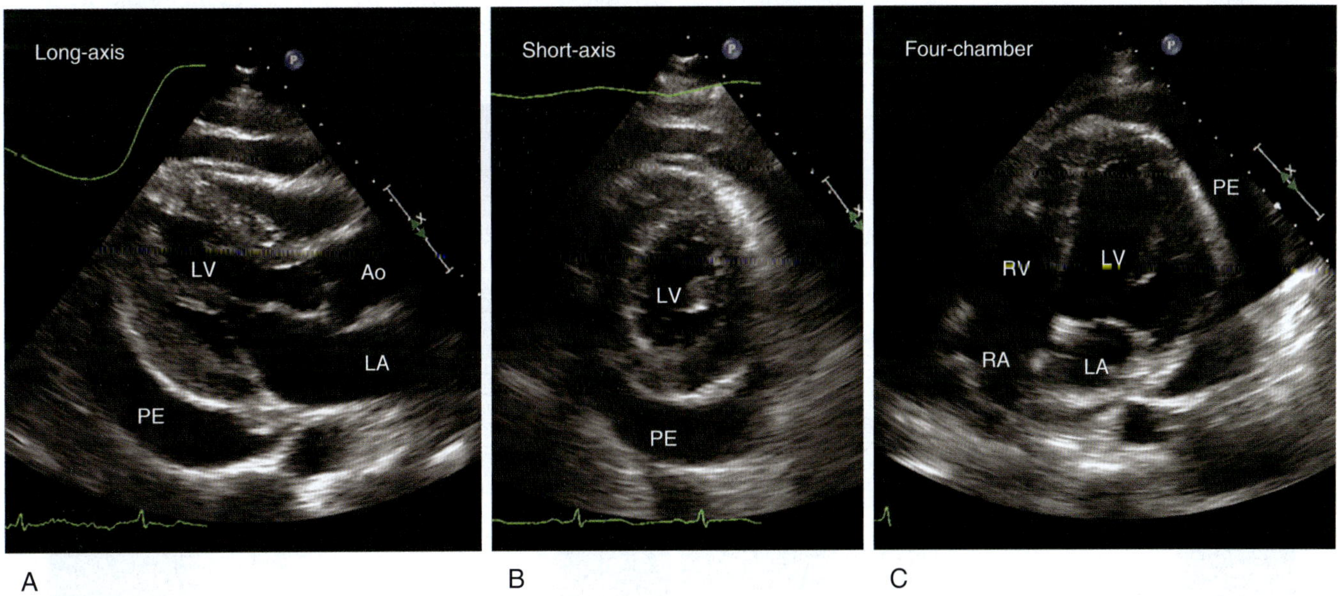

FIGURE 43-9. Pericardial effusion. A large echo-free space is seen anterior and posterior to the cardiac structure in the **(A)** parasternal long axis view (*left*), **(B)** short axis view (*center*), and **(C)** apical four-chamber view (*right*) consistent with a pericardial effusion (PE). Ao = aorta; LA = left atrium; LV = left ventricle; RA = right atrium; RV = right ventricle. See Video 43-5.

GENERAL REFERENCES

For the General References and other additional features, please visit Elsevier eBooks+ at https://ebooks.health.elsevier.com.

44

NONINVASIVE CARDIAC IMAGING

CHRISTOPHER M. KRAMER, VASKEN DILSIZIAN, AND KLAUS D. HAGSPIEL

RADIOGRAPHY OF THE HEART

Chest radiography is a widely available, relatively inexpensive, and rapid imaging modality, with an average effective radiation dose of 0.03 to 0.1 mSv. The heart is best evaluated on posteroanterior (PA) and lateral radiographs, with the heart closest to the image detector.

On the chest radiograph, the heart appears as a homogeneous shadow surrounded by lungs, so diagnostic assessment of the heart and great vessels is based on the size and shape of the cardiac silhouette, rather than on direct visualization of the heart's internal anatomy. Nevertheless, the size and shape of the heart and their changes over time, together with the appearance of the pulmonary vasculature, aid in the diagnosis of cardiac diseases. The radiographic appearance of the heart is also influenced by the radiographic technique, projection, body habitus, degree of inspiration, and whether the patient is supine or erect during the examination.

On the PA projection, the normal heart is located in the middle mediastinum, with approximately two thirds projecting to the left of the midsternum (Fig. 44-1). The superior segment of the right heart border is a more or less straight line formed by the superior vena cava and right innominate vein. The inferior segment is convex and formed by the right atrium. The left heart border consists of three segments: the aortic arch superiorly, the main pulmonary artery in the middle, and the left ventricle inferiorly. The left atrial appendage is situated in the junction between the lower and middle segments; if enlarged, it can appear as a separate, prominent segment. The inferior border of the heart sometimes is not well differentiated from the diaphragm (see Fig. 44-1).

On lateral chest images, the right ventricle and its outflow tract form the anterior heart border, with the right ventricle in contact with the lower third of the sternum. Lung between the sternum and the posteriorly curving right ventricle and its outflow tract forms the retrosternal clear space. The posterior heart border, which is seen between the carina and the diaphragm on lateral images, consists of the left atrium superiorly and the left ventricle inferiorly. The inferior vena cava courses obliquely upward before it joins the right atrium. The ascending aorta, aortic arch, and proximal descending thoracic aorta are usually well seen on lateral images (see Fig. 44-1).

Alterations of the contour of the heart are generally caused by dilation of the atria, ventricles, or blood vessels. Chest images are not sensitive for detecting cardiac hypertrophy unless it is severe.

Comprehensive cardiovascular analysis of chest radiographs requires evaluation of the size and morphology of the heart and the great vessels, the pulmonary vasculature, and the presence and positioning of any calcifications or implanted devices such as valves, pacemakers, and defibrillators.

RADIOGRAPHIC ASSESSMENT OF HEART SIZE

The cardiothoracic ratio (see Fig. 44-1) estimates the size of the heart. A value of less than 0.5 is considered normal on a radiograph taken during

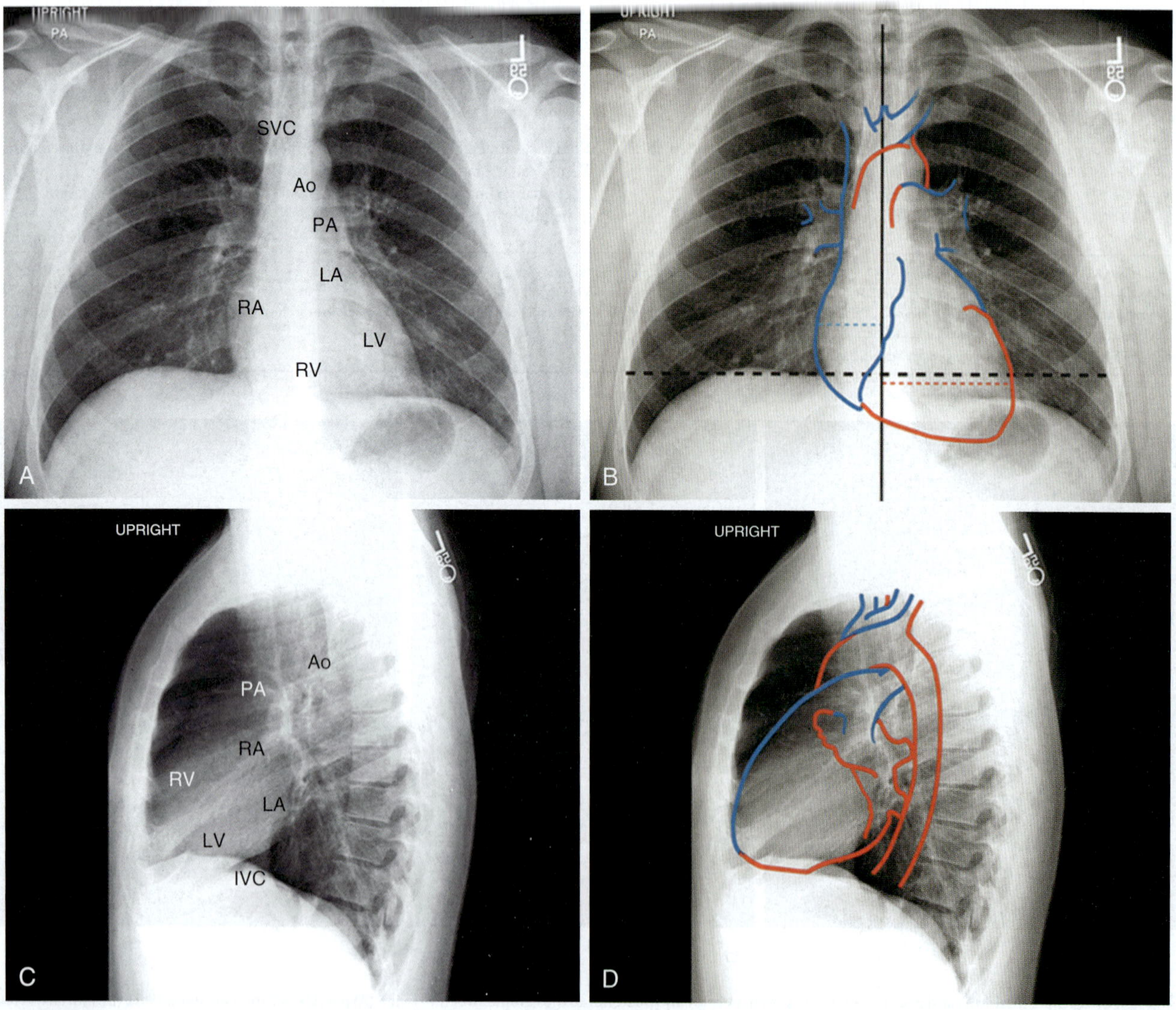

FIGURE 44-1. Normal anatomy. Posteroanterior (A) and lateral (B) chest radiograph projections in a healthy 28-year-old man. The cardiac chambers and the great vessels are marked on the corresponding drawings (B, D). The cardiothoracic ratio (C) is calculated by dividing the maximum transverse diameter of the cardiac silhouette (*blue line:* widest distance of the right heart border from the midpoint of the spine; *red line:* widest distance from the left heart border to the midpoint of the spine) through the distance between the internal margin of the ribs at the top of the right diaphragm (*black line*). Ao = aorta; IVC = inferior vena cava; LA = left atrium; LV = left ventricle; PA = pulmonary artery; RA = right atrium; RV = right ventricle; SVC = superior vena cava.

deep inspiration. Pectus excavatum deformities (Chapter 86) and epicardial fat pads can result in an abnormally large cardiothoracic ratio despite a normal-sized heart. Dilation of the left ventricle, which increases the cardiothoracic ratio, appears as a concave mid-left heart border and lengthening of the entire left heart border, with a downward pointing apex projecting below the diaphragm on PA views (Fig. 44-2). Extension of the posterior margin of the left ventricle more than 2 cm posterior to the inferior vena cava on the lateral film is considered a sign of left ventricular enlargement. Localized rather than global left ventricular enlargement usually indicates the presence of ventricular aneurysms (Chapter 58). Left ventricular hypertrophy without dilation usually is not detectable on chest radiographs.

The most common cause of left atrial enlargement is secondary to left ventricular dysfunction, especially left ventricular dilation. Isolated enlargement of the left atrium is usually a sequela of mitral valve abnormalities or atrial fibrillation. Enlargement of the left atrium can also occur with left ventricular hypertrophy without dilation in patients with aortic stenosis (Chapter 60) or hypertrophic cardiomyopathy (Chapter 47). Straightening of the left heart border between the main pulmonary artery and the left ventricle just below the left main bronchus owing to enlargement of the left atrial appendage is one of the earliest signs of left atrial enlargement; with increasing size, this segment becomes convex. A double contour within the right cardiac border (double density sign), splaying of the carina, and elevation of the right main bronchus are less frequent signs (Fig. 44-3).

The right ventricle normally does not form part of the heart's border on PA radiographs, but significant right ventricular enlargement can lead to an abnormal convexity of the left heart border, with elevation and leftward displacement of the cardiac apex. The best radiographic indication of right ventricular enlargement is obliteration of the retrosternal clear space in the lateral view owing to dilation of the right ventricular outflow tract (Fig. 44-4).

Dilation of the right atrium causes the lower segment of the right heart border to become more prominent and increasingly round. In more severe cases, the entire right heart border is enlarged, and in extreme cases, the right atrium can become border-forming on the lateral view (see Fig. 44-3).

PERICARDIAL EFFUSION

Large pericardial effusions cause significant enlargement of the cardiac silhouette despite a normal superior mediastinum—the so-called water-bottle sign. The fluid in the pericardial sac will obscure the hilar vessels on a PA chest film (Fig. 44-5), unlike cardiomegaly without effusion, in which the hilar structures often are relatively conspicuous. Posterior displacement of the pericardial fat line on lateral images is also a valuable finding for the detection of pericardial effusions.

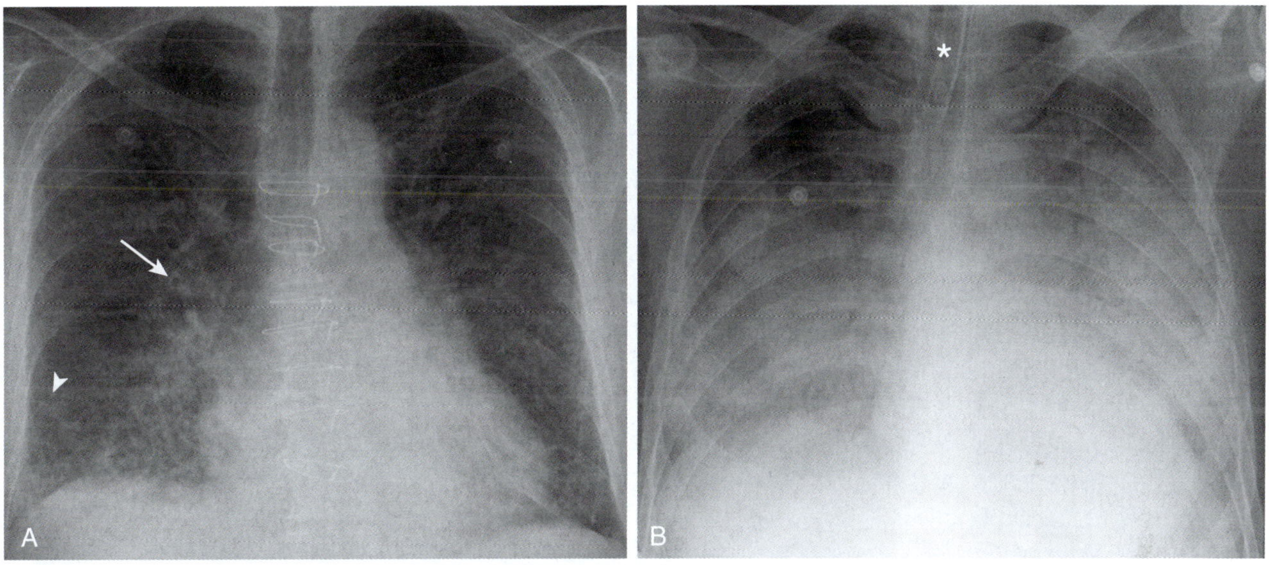

FIGURE 44-2. Left ventricular enlargement and pulmonary edema in two different patients. The image on the left (**A**) was obtained in a patient who had acute myocardial infarction and who had previously undergone aortic bypass grafting (sternotomy wires and bypass clips are seen). Interstitial edema is evidenced by the presence of vascular redistribution, Kerley B lines (*arrowhead*), and peribronchial cuffing (*arrow*). The image on the right (**B**) was obtained in a patient with cardiogenic alveolar edema. The left ventricle is significantly enlarged, and there is extensive bilateral air space consolidation with air bronchogram. Note normal position of an endotracheal tube (*asterisk*) and a nasogastric tube.

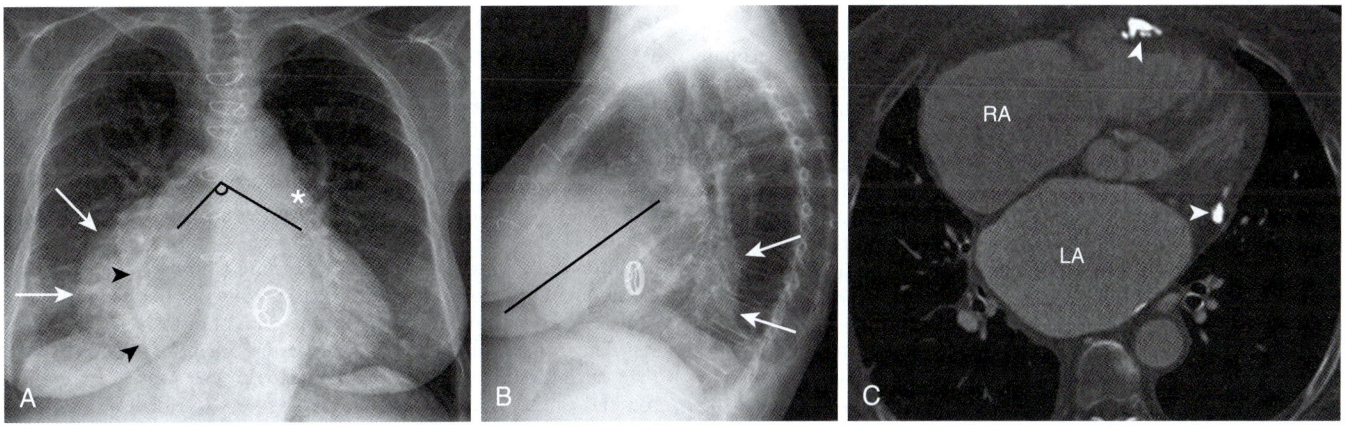

FIGURE 44-3. Biatrial enlargement in a patient who has undergone mitral valve repair. The posteroanterior (**A**) chest radiograph shows a prominent left atrial appendage (*asterisk*), the double density sign (*arrowheads*), and splaying of the carina. There is also enlargement of the right atrium, as evidenced by prominence and round shape of the right side border on the posteroanterior view (*arrows*). Posterior bulging of the heart (*arrows*) owing to biatrial enlargement is seen on the lateral view (**B**). Interstitial pulmonary edema is present. The location of the cardiac valves is best assessed on a lateral view (**B**) by drawing a line from the carina to the anterior costophrenic recess (*black line*). The pulmonic and aortic valves usually are positioned superior to this line, and the tricuspid and mitral valves are inferior to it. A computed tomographic image (**C**) also demonstrates biatrial enlargement as well as pericardial calcifications (*arrowheads*). LA = left atrium; RA = right atrium.

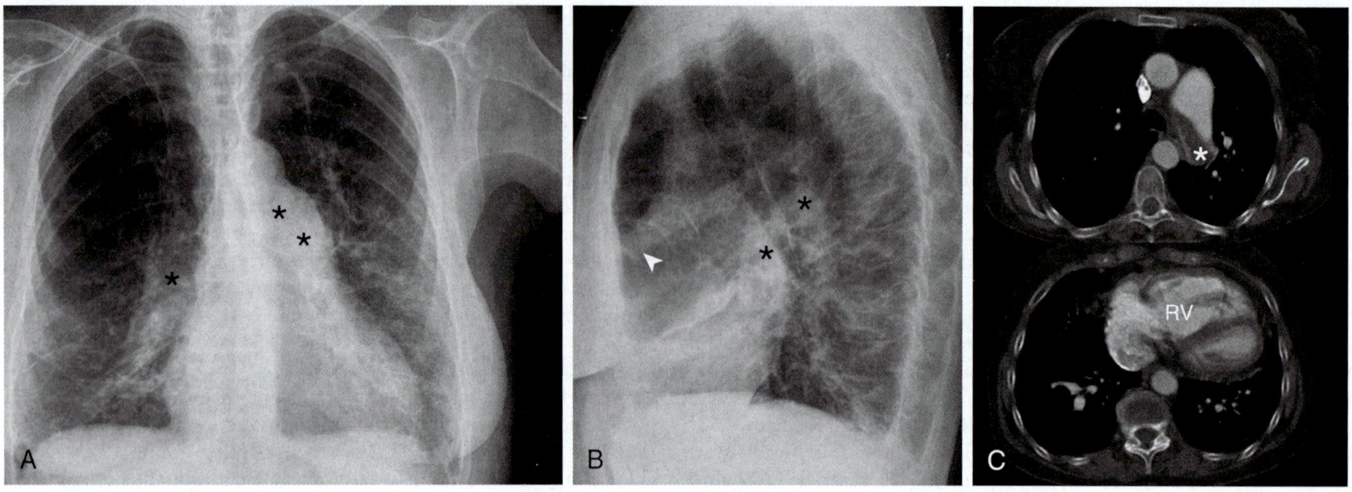

FIGURE 44-4. Pulmonary arterial hypertension in a patient with severe pulmonary emphysema and chronic pulmonary embolism. Enlarged central pulmonary arteries (*asterisks*) and the pruned-tree sign can be seen on the posteroanterior (**A**) and lateral (**B**) projections. Hyperlucency in both upper lobes is present owing to extensive pulmonary emphysema. Right ventricular enlargement has obliterated the retrosternal clear space on the lateral view (*arrowhead*) (**B**). The computed tomographic scan demonstrates dilated central pulmonary arteries with wall-adherent chronic pulmonary embolus (*asterisk*) (**C**) as well as right ventricle (RV) dilation and hypertrophy.

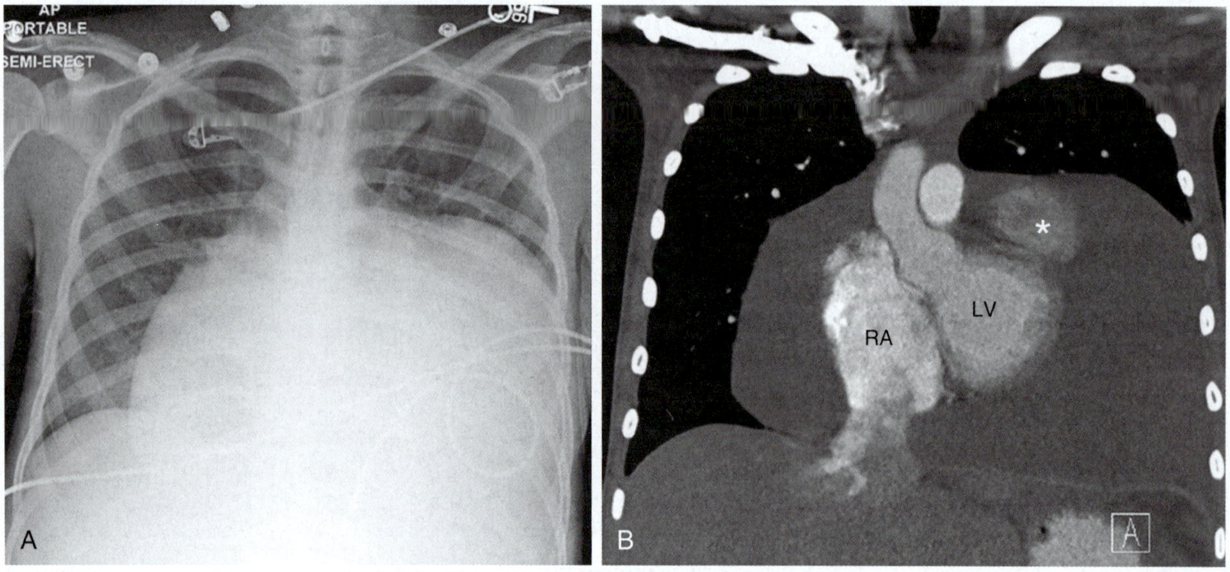

FIGURE 44-5. A 17-year-old girl presenting with massive pericardial effusion. The posteroanterior radiograph (**A**) shows the water-bottle sign; the hilar vessels are obscured. A coronal reformatted computed tomographic scan (**B**) shows the fluid in the pericardial sac as well as dilation of the right atrium and the left atrial appendage (*asterisk*). LV = left ventricle; RA = right atrium.

PULMONARY VASCULATURE

The large and medium-sized pulmonary arteries and veins can be seen on the radiograph as linear shadows, and their size and appearance correlate with pulmonary blood flow and pulmonary venous pressure. The vessels in the lower lung zones are normally larger than in the upper zones as a result of the normal distribution of pulmonary blood flow (see Fig. 44-1). In patients with right-to-left shunts (Chapter 55), the pulmonary vasculature is decreased in caliber. In left-to-right shunts, the vascularity is increased, and the vessels are sharply outlined if the patient does not have heart failure (Fig. 44-6). With increasing pulmonary venous pressure, as is seen in heart failure (Chapters 45 and 46), the vessels in the upper zone enlarge on the chest radiograph. With further increases in pulmonary venous pressures, fluid extravasates into the pulmonary interstitium, and the pulmonary vessels lose their sharp demarcation. Horizontal lines in the periphery of the lungs (Kerley B) and vertical lines in the upper lobes (Kerley A) represent thickened interlobular septae. Fluid in the interstitium of the bronchial walls causes peribronchial thickening or cuffing (see Fig. 44-2). In more advanced cases, the lungs show a diffuse ground-glass appearance that masks the vascular structures, and pulmonary edema ultimately develops (see Fig. 44-2). Long-standing pulmonary arterial hypertension leads to dilation of the central pulmonary arteries with abrupt change in caliber instead of the normal tapering. The size and number of the peripheral arterial branches diminish, resulting in a pruned-tree appearance (see Fig. 44-4).

CALCIFICATIONS

Calcifications can often be seen on chest radiographs. In the heart, calcifications most frequently involve the valves and the mitral annulus (Chapter 60). Most aortic valvular calcifications are degenerative in nature and occur in otherwise normal valves, but their incidence is increased in bicuspid valves or in patients who have had rheumatic fever. Calcification of the mitral annulus is common and usually an asymptomatic finding. Coronary artery calcifications are frequent but are rarely seen on chest radiographs. Calcifications of the ventricles are most often seen in patients with prior myocardial infarction or ventricular aneurysms (Fig. 44-7). Pericardial calcifications tend to be thicker than calcifications in the myocardium and, in severe cases, can entirely surround the heart (see Fig. 44-3).

IMPLANTED DEVICES

A great number of devices can be seen on a chest radiograph, and it is important to be familiar with their appearance to assess their correct position and integrity. The accurate assessment of device position can occasionally require cross-sectional imaging (see Figs. 44-2, 44-3, and 44-7).

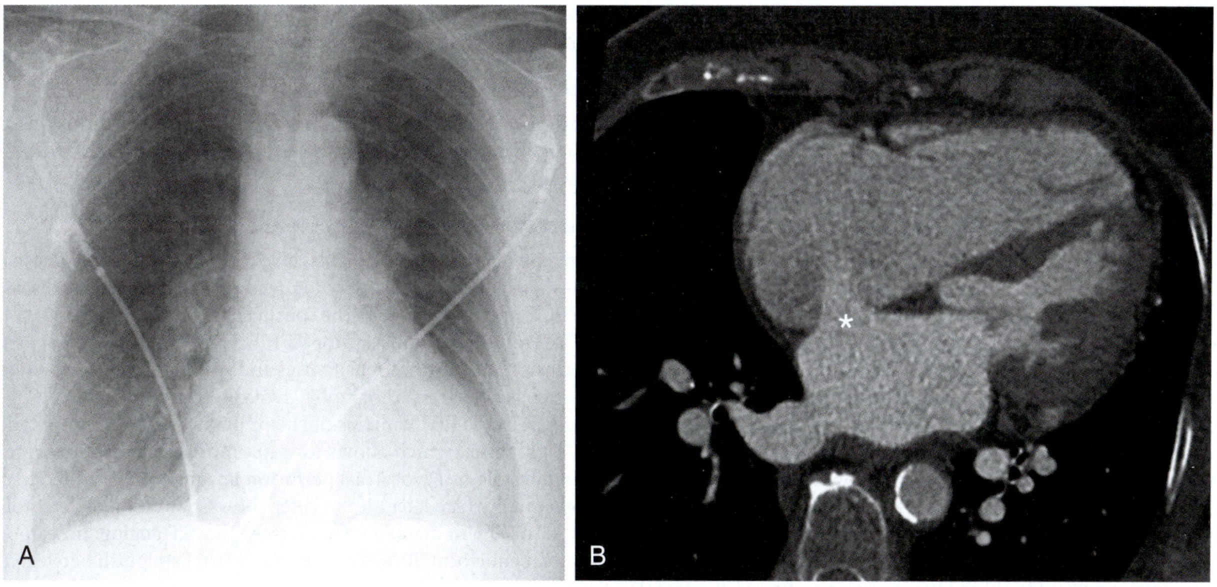

FIGURE 44-6. Female patient with known secundum type atrial septal defect. The posteroanterior radiograph (**A**) shows enlargement of the pulmonary arteries, shunt vascularity, and enlargement of the right heart border. A computed tomographic scan (**B**) shows the septal defect (*asterisk*) with left-to-right shunt. Enlargement of the right heart is also seen.

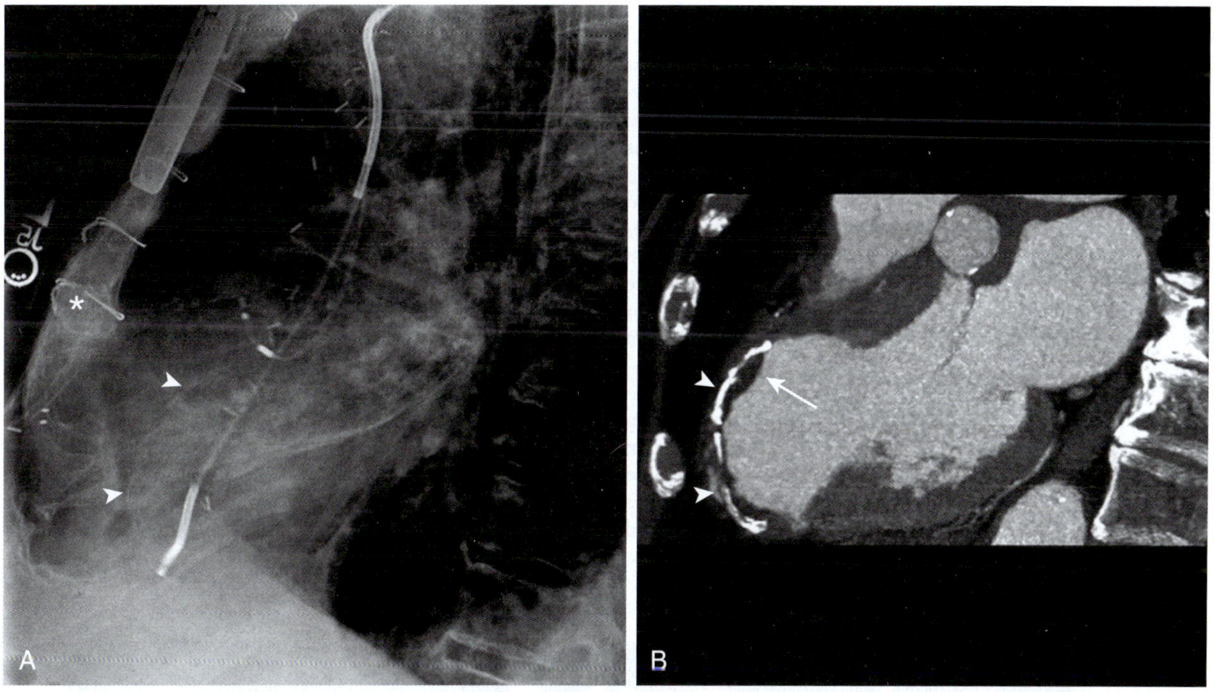

FIGURE 44-7. Calcified chronic myocardial infarction. Lateral radiograph (**A**) demonstrates thin curvilinear calcifications (*arrowheads*) in the region of the left ventricular apex. A reformatted cardiac computed tomographic scan (**B**) shows aneurysmal dilation and thinning of the apex, curvilinear calcifications, and thrombus (*arrow*). Dual-chamber pacer leads, aortocoronary bypass clips, and fracture of the most inferior sternotomy wire (*asterisk*) are also seen on the lateral radiograph (**A**).

CHARACTERISTIC APPEARANCE OF CARDIAC SILHOUETTE

Certain constellations of findings on chest radiographs can be characteristic of specific disorders. For example, in mitral stenosis, left atrial enlargement, pulmonary venous hypertension, a small aortic knob, and enlargement of the main pulmonary artery are typical findings. In aortic stenosis, left ventricular enlargement, calcifications of the aortic valve, and dilation of the ascending aorta are often present. In pulmonic valve stenosis, enlargement of the pulmonary trunk is the most common radiographic sign, with or without signs of right ventricular enlargement. In atrial septal defects, the heart is usually normal in size, with prominent pulmonary vasculature (shunt vascularity). In ventricular septal defects, the left atrium and left ventricle are prominent, and shunt vascularity is present. A number of classic chest radiographic signs have been described for patients with more complex congenital heart disease (Chapter 55). These findings include the egg-on-a-string sign in transposition of the great arteries, the gooseneck sign in endocardial cushion defects, the boot-shaped heart in tetralogy of Fallot (E-Fig. 44-1), the figure-of-3 and reversed figure-of-3 signs in coarctation of the aorta, the box-shaped heart in Ebstein anomaly, the snowman sign in total anomalous pulmonary venous return, and the scimitar sign in partial anomalous pulmonary venous return. Due to earlier diagnosis and treatment of congenital heart disease, the diagnostic role of chest radiography for these conditions is limited today, but it remains a useful technique for monitoring the progression of disease and its response to treatment.

NUCLEAR CARDIOLOGY

The techniques of nuclear cardiology permit the noninvasive imaging of myocardial perfusion, function, metabolism, and innervation by use of radionuclide imaging agents and gamma or positron cameras with associated computer processing.[1,2] All these techniques are based on acquiring images of radioactivity emanating from tracers localized in heart muscle or in the blood pools of the left and right ventricles. Myocardial perfusion imaging is the most commonly performed nuclear cardiology technique, most often in conjunction with either exercise or pharmacologic stress intended to produce flow heterogeneity between relatively hypoperfused and normally perfused myocardial regions.

MYOCARDIAL PERFUSION IMAGING

AGENTS AND TECHNIQUES

For the assessment of myocardial perfusion using single-photon emission computed tomography (SPECT) technology, ^{99m}Tc-labeled perfusion agents or thallium-201 (^{201}Tl) are used for exercise or pharmacologic stress perfusion imaging to evaluate patients with suspected or known coronary heart disease (CHD). Of the various ^{99m}Tc-labeled agents, ^{99m}Tc-sestamibi and ^{99m}Tc-tetrofosmin are the most common. These ^{99m}Tc agents permit simultaneous assessment of regional and global left ventricular function and volumes with ECG-gated SPECT technology. Advantages of positron emission tomography (PET) myocardial perfusion imaging compared with SPECT include higher sensitivity and specificity for the detection of coronary artery disease at a lower radiation dose, reduced image acquisition time (less likelihood of patient motion), higher resolution images, and better soft tissue attenuation (such as for the breast and diaphragm), with added information regarding absolute quantitative hyperemic myocardial blood flow and reserve flow (Chapter 59).

In patients with chest pain or shortness of breath, myocardial perfusion imaging is commonly performed with exercise so as to induce coronary hyperemia and link the symptoms during exercise to the location, extent, and severity of abnormal perfusion patterns. In patients who are unable or incapable of exercising to greater than 85% of the maximum predicted heart rate for their age, pharmacologic stress testing with a vasodilator can be used to induce coronary hyperemia. Vasodilator stress typically causes a modest increase in heart rate and decline in arterial pressure. Options include dipyridamole, adenosine, the selective A_{2A} adenosine receptor agonist regadenoson, or the inotropic/chronotropic agent dobutamine. Dobutamine stress is preferred in patients who have bronchospasm or a history of asthma, or who have consumed caffeine, which is an adenosine receptor antagonist, within 12 hours before testing. Patients who experience side effects such as hypotension and chest pain during vasodilator infusion should be treated with intravenous aminophylline, which is an adenosine antagonist. Unlike exercise stress, however, the perfusion defect induced with pharmacologic vasodilator stress may merely represent the heterogeneity in coronary flow rather than true myocardial ischemia.

Exercise or pharmacologic stress myocardial perfusion images are compared with images acquired at rest. Stress-induced perfusion abnormalities in regions that exhibit normal perfusion at rest are termed reversible perfusion defects, and such regions represent viable, ischemic myocardium with blunted coronary blood flow reserve (Fig. 44-8). Conversely, perfusion abnormalities that are seen both on stress and rest myocardial perfusion images are termed fixed or irreversible defects and most often suggest an area of prior myocardial infarction, particularly if the defect is severe.

CLINICAL APPLICATIONS

The major indications for stress and rest myocardial perfusion imaging are to diagnose coronary heart disease, to assess prognosis, and to detect myocardial viability.

Detection of Coronary Heart Disease

Exercise or pharmacologic stress myocardial perfusion imaging in patients with chest pain yields a sensitivity for detecting coronary heart disease of 88% for SPECT and 93% for PET. The specificity for excluding coronary heart disease is 76% for SPECT and 81% for PET. Exercise or pharmacologic stress SPECT perfusion imaging has sensitivities and specificities that are superior to those of exercise electrocardiography (ECG) testing alone.

SPECT and PET cameras can help combined with a computed tomography (CT) scanner, which allows for multimodality hybrid imaging of anatomy and physiology. Myocardial perfusion imaging can be added to coronary CT angiography (see later) if the latter shows an intermediate coronary stenosis of 50 to 70% in diameter. Conversely, the CT angiogram can be performed after an equivocal SPECT or PET study to distinguish between true-positive and false-positive perfusion defects. Hybrid imaging also permits combined coronary artery calcium scoring with myocardial perfusion.

Assessment of Prognosis

Stress myocardial perfusion imaging does not appear to add any useful prognostic information over exercise ECG testing alone in patients who achieve 10 metabolic equivalents or more of workload (Chapter 39) without ischemic ST segment depression on the exercise ECG or in low-risk women with good physical capacity. In other situations, however, the extent of fixed and reversible defects on SPECT and PET perfusion image can provide important incremental prognostic information when added to clinical characteristics, the resting left ventricular ejection fraction, and exercise ECG stress test variables. For example, nondiabetic patients with chest pain and a normal stress myocardial perfusion scan have a less than 1% per year rate of subsequent cardiac death or myocardial infarction and are generally appropriate candidates for medical therapy (Chapter 56) or even further diagnostic evaluation to search for a noncardiac cause of chest pain (Chapters 39 and 123). Conversely, patients with high-risk stress imaging results, such as transient ischemic left ventricular cavity dilation on stress images (E-Fig. 44-2), may benefit from early referral for coronary angiography and possible coronary revascularization (Chapter 59), even if symptoms are mild.

One significant limitation of SPECT myocardial perfusion imaging is its inability to identify multivessel and left main coronary artery disease in some patients who have balanced ischemia, in which uptake of the imaging agent at peak stress is homogeneously diminished throughout the left ventricular

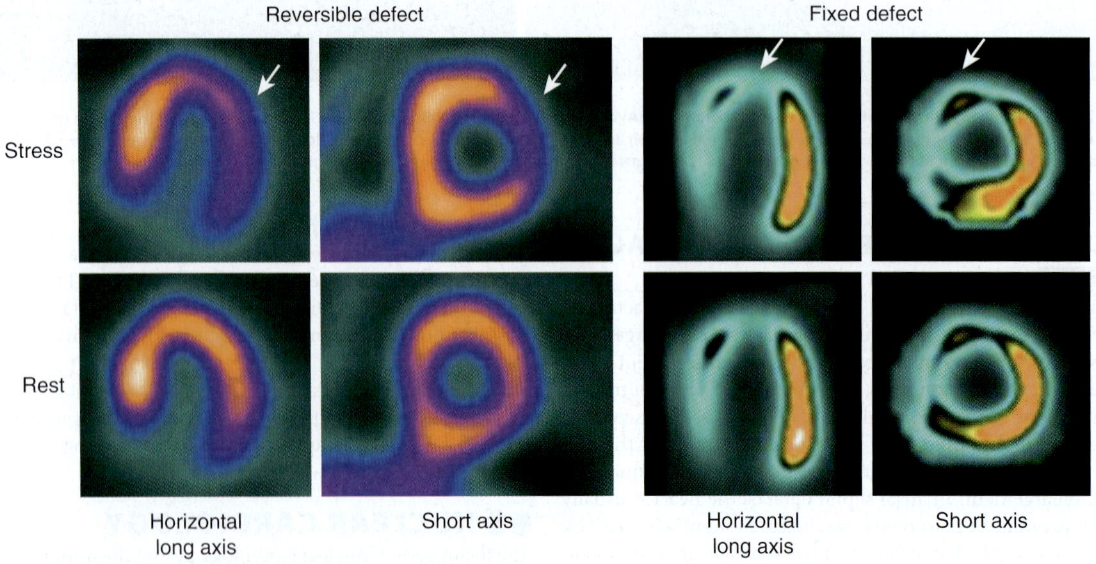

FIGURE 44-8. **Examples of reversible and fixed myocardial perfusion defects. A,** Paired stress and rest images show a reversible defect in the lateral region, thereby indicating myocardial ischemia related to the left circumflex coronary artery territory. **B,** Fixed defects in the anterior, apical, and interventricular septum, representing prior transmural myocardial infarction related to the left anterior descending coronary artery.

myocardium because of diffusely reduced flow in regions supplied by all three major coronary arteries. Quantitative PET myocardial perfusion imaging will identify these patients by demonstrating regional and/or global reduction in absolute hyperemic myocardial blood flow and an abnormal coronary flow reserve.[3]

Determination of Myocardial Viability

In some patients, fixed perfusion defects may not represent permanently infarcted myocardium but rather represent stunned or hibernating viable myocardium that has the potential to recover function after coronary revascularization. Myocardial viability usually is assessed using PET technology, with fluorine-18-labeled 2-deoxyglucose (FDG) to assess regional myocardial metabolism, and either nitrogen-13 (^{13}N) ammonia or rubidium-82 (^{82}Rb) to assess regional myocardial perfusion. FDG is a glucose analogue that is taken up initially in myocardial cells and is trapped by conversion to FDG-6-phosphate. In dysfunctional myocardial regions, increased FDG activity on clinical PET images in areas of diminished regional blood flow (termed mismatch defect) is indicative of hibernating but viable myocardium. After coronary revascularization, the left ventricular ejection fraction can improve by about 10 percentage points in such patients. However, this postintervention improvement in ejection fraction does not predict which patients with ischemic cardiomyopathy will have better survival after coronary revascularization.[A1-A2] Conversely, decreased (or absent) glucose utilization in dysfunctional myocardial regions with concomitant reduction of blood flow (termed match defect) is indicative of permanently scarred, infarcted myocardium.

INFILTRATIVE CARDIOMYOPATHIES

CARDIAC SARCOIDOSIS

The combination of PET perfusion imaging with FDG can diagnose the inflammation of cardiac sarcoidosis (E-Fig. 44-3) and monitor its response to therapy (Chapters 47 and 83).[4] The high cellular uptake of FDG in sarcoidosis is related to the inflammatory cell infiltrates that have high glycolytic activity to satisfy their large energy demands.

CARDIAC AMYLOIDOSIS

Transthyretin cardiac amyloidosis (Chapters 47 and 174) can be diagnosed with Tc-99m-pyrophosphate (^{99m}Tc-PYP) scintigraphy. In a patient with typical features of cardiac amyloid on echocardiography or cardiac magnetic resonance (MR), Grade 2 or 3 ^{99m}Tc-PYP uptake in the absence of a clonal plasma cell process (Chapter 173) is diagnostic of transthyretin cardiac amyloidosis (E-Fig. 44-4).[5]

IMAGING OF VENTRICULAR FUNCTION

Although echocardiography (Chapter 43) is the dominant noninvasive tool for measuring ventricular function, it can also be measured with radionuclide angiography using technetium-99m (^{99m}Tc)-labeled red blood cells or other ^{99m}Tc-labeled agents that are injected intravenously. Because ^{99m}Tc remains within the blood pool, serial imaging studies can be acquired during several hours. Acquisition of the images is synchronized with the QRS complex on the ECG through a multigated approach by which each cardiac cycle is divided into multiple frames. A uniform diminution of left ventricular systolic function without regional wall motion abnormalities suggests nonischemic dilated cardiomyopathy (Chapter 47), whereas depressed global function associated with regional wall motion abnormalities suggests ischemic heart disease. Left ventricular function can also be assessed by gated SPECT myocardial perfusion imaging.

CARDIAC COMPUTED TOMOGRAPHY

For CT, imaging with high spatial and temporal resolution and ECG gating during a breath-hold yields snapshots of the heart reconstructed from the same phase of the cardiac cycle.[6] Coronary CT angiography can capture a three-dimensional image of the heart in one to two heartbeats on the latest generation scanners as well as provide coronary artery calcium scoring without the use of contrast and with little radiation. Coronary CT angiography requires 60 to 80 mL of iodinated contrast. With latest generation scanners, radiation doses of 1 to 2 mSv are achievable although radiation can still be on the order of 5 to 20 mSv on older 64-detector scanners. β-Blockade is often used to achieve a heart rate of 60 beats per minute or less to optimize imaging, and irregular rhythms such as atrial fibrillation may diminish image quality.

CORONARY ARTERY CALCIUM SCORING

Coronary calcium is an indicator of the burden of atherosclerotic plaque, although there is no correlation of the amount of local coronary calcium with the physiologic or anatomic significance of an underlying coronary stenosis. Calcium scores are generally calculated as an Agatston score, which corresponds to each coronary lesion's calcium area multiplied by the maximal CT attenuation value of that lesion, and then summed for the entire coronary tree (Fig. 44-9). High scores confer an increased risk for future cardiac events and death, with overall 15-year mortality rates in asymptomatic patients ranging from 3 to 28% with coronary artery calcification scores from 0 to 1000 or greater.[7] Calcium scores are age, gender, and race dependent, but they predict coronary heart disease events independently of standard risk factors. The utility of calcium scoring is highest in patients who are at intermediate risk for coronary heart disease, based on Framingham risk data (Chapter 40). By comparison, a calcium score in otherwise low- or high-risk patients will rarely change management, although very high calcium scores may sometimes encourage cardiac stress testing.

CORONARY COMPUTED TOMOGRAPHIC ANGIOGRAPHY

Coronary CT angiography is an excellent technique to diagnose anomalous coronary arterial anatomy in adults (E-Fig. 44-5). For detection of coronary artery disease, positive-predictive values are in the range of 64 to 91%, and negative-predictive values approach 99%. Thus, the technique is an excellent

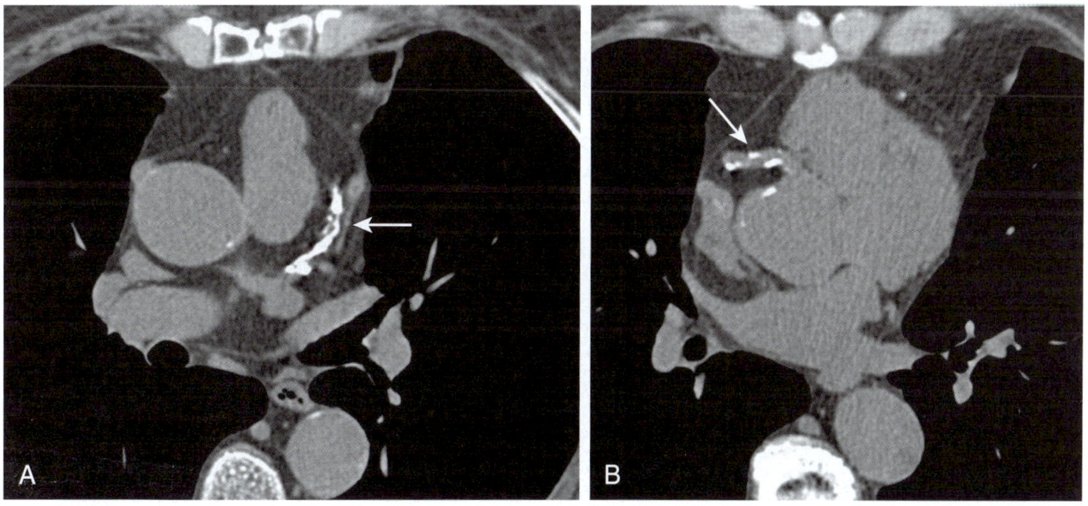

FIGURE 44-9. Non-contrast-enhanced computed tomography axial slices through the heart at two locations for coronary calcium scoring as risk assessment in an asymptomatic patient. A, The slice includes the left anterior descending artery with extensive calcification in its proximal portion (*arrow*). **B,** The slice includes the right coronary artery with proximal spotty calcification (*arrow*). This patient's calcium score was 457, putting him in a higher risk group regardless of his Framingham risk score.

way to exclude (Fig. 44-10) or detect significant coronary artery disease in the three major coronary vessels (Fig. 44-11). A limitation of the technique, however, is its lower specificity in heavily calcified vessels, which are more common in elderly patients. The accuracy for detecting stenoses in bypass grafts is quite high, although evaluation of native vessel coronary artery disease is limited in these patients owing to extensive calcification and smaller size vessels. Imaging within most coronary stents has proved difficult. Measurement of coronary artery-specific fractional flow reserve using computational flow dynamics can improve upon the accuracy (especially specificity) of angiography (E-Fig. 44-6).

Coronary CT angiography is not recommended as a routine screening test in asymptomatic patients, even those with diabetes. However, it is especially useful in selected situations, such as in low- or low-intermediate-risk patients with chest pain, patients who present to the emergency department with chest pain but without ECG changes or elevations of cardiac biomarkers (Chapters 39 and 57), or patients with equivocal or nondiagnostic stress testing. Some guidelines recommend CT angiography as the initial test for diagnosing coronary diseases in symptomatic patients.[8,9] In patients who have acute non-ST elevation MI, CT angiography has a high positive and negative predictive value as compared with invasive angiography and may be an alternative in lower risk patients with this clinical presentation.[10]

In symptomatic patients with suspected coronary disease, the strategies of initial coronary CT angiography and functional testing using exercise electrocardiography, nuclear stress testing, or stress echocardiography provide equivalent clinical outcomes at an equivalent cost over a median follow-up of 2 years.[A3,A4] CT angiography is associated with similar outcomes and fewer complications or revascularizations compared with invasive angiography in patients who have intermediate-risk chest pain.[A5] However, CT angiography can improve outcomes compared with standard care in patients with stable chest pain by stimulating the use of more aggressive medical therapies without increasing rates of coronary angiography or coronary revascularization.[A6] The extent and severity of coronary disease found at CT angiography correlate with subsequent all-cause mortality in a similar fashion to catheter-based coronary angiography. Low-attenuation, noncalcified plaque is the most potent predictor of subsequent myocardial infarction,[11] whereas progression of calcification is associated with a mildly increased risk of subsequent events after adjusting for other risk factors.[12] In asymptomatic patients, however, CT angiography does not improve risk stratification over calcium scoring.

OTHER CARDIAC APPLICATIONS

The same data acquired by coronary CT angiography can be reformatted and used for functional cardiac imaging, including measurement of left ventricular volumes, ejection fraction, wall thickness, and global and segmental wall motion. CT angiography can complement echocardiography to evaluate cardiac anatomy in patients with congenital heart disease. CT can evaluate pericardial thickness and calcification in patients with suspected constrictive pericarditis (see Fig. 62-9) and can evaluate native and prosthetic valvular structures (E-Fig. 44-7) and cardiac masses when imaging with other modalities is inadequate.

CT angiography is often used to image the left atrium and pulmonary venous anatomy and to exclude left atrial thrombus prior to electrical cardioversion or pulmonary vein ablation for atrial fibrillation (Chapter 54). CT is an important

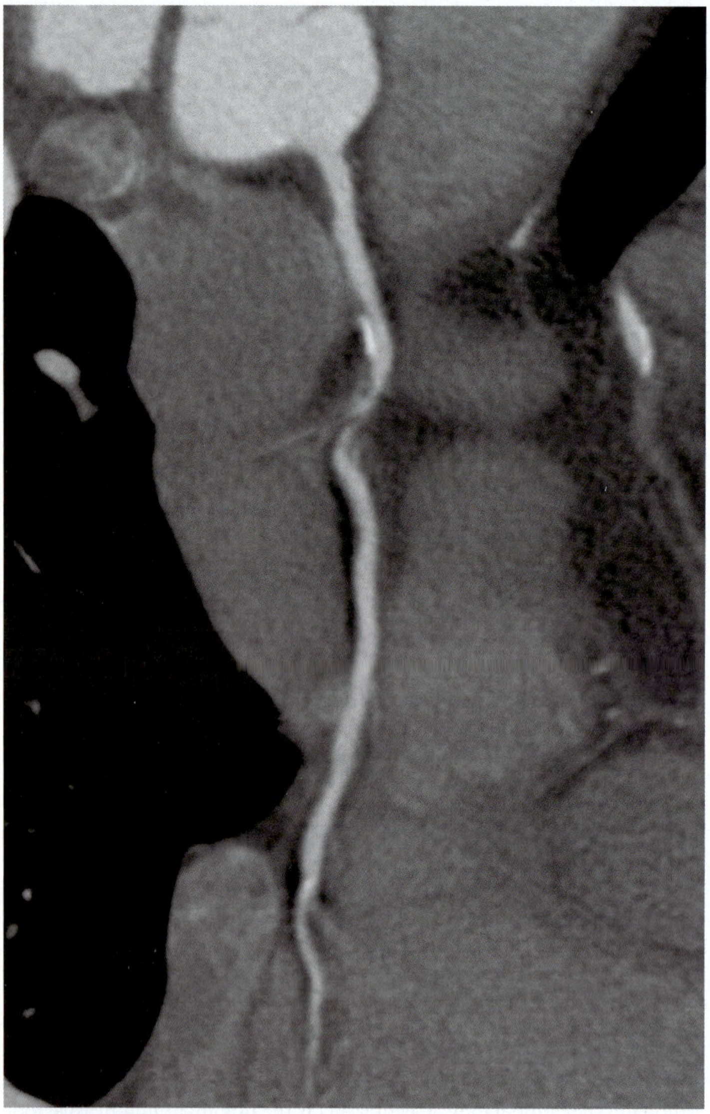

FIGURE 44-11. Contrast-enhanced computed tomographic coronary angiogram of the left anterior descending artery (LAD) in a 54-year-old man who presented to an emergency department with risk factors but atypical chest pain. The mid LAD demonstrates mixed obstructive plaque with calcified and noncalcified components.

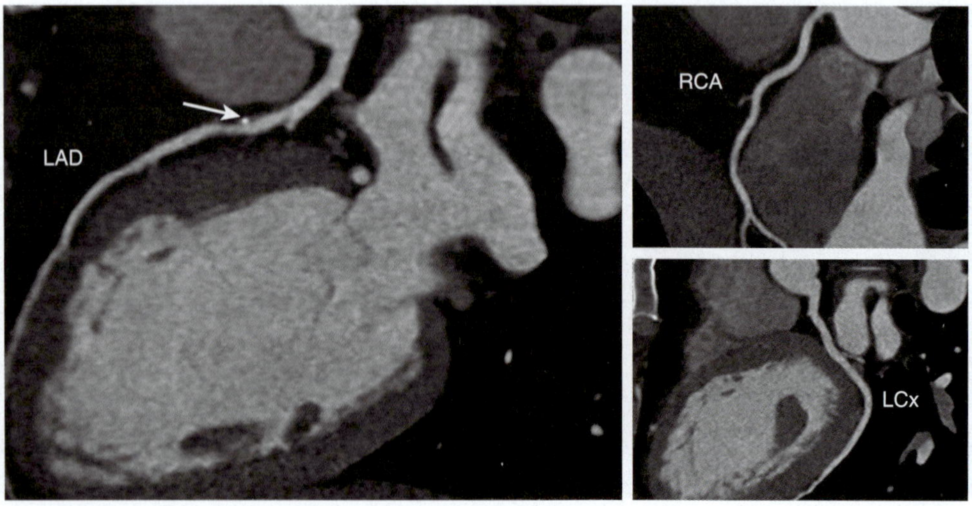

FIGURE 44-10. Contrast-enhanced computed tomographic coronary angiogram obtained on a dual-source 64-detector scanner in a patient with atypical chest pain. The left anterior descending (LAD) artery has a nonobstructive lesion (*arrow*) containing both noncalcified (soft) plaque, which appears dark, and a focal area of calcification. The right coronary artery (RCA) and left circumflex coronary artery (LCx) are normal.

tool for peri-preprocedural planning in patients being considered for transcatheter valve replacement (Chapter 60).

CARDIOVASCULAR MAGNETIC RESONANCE IMAGING

INDICATIONS, CONTRAINDICATIONS, AND PULSE SEQUENCES

Cardiac MR is a versatile and flexible imaging modality that can be applied in diverse cardiovascular conditions using either 1.5- or 3-Tesla (T) scanners. Advantages of cardiac MR include the lack of ionizing radiation, the variety of tissues that can be characterized, and the ability to image the heart in any arbitrary plane. Images typically are obtained using ECG gating and breath-hold techniques.

Although some metallic devices are contraindications to cardiac MR, patients with newer pacemaker and defibrillator systems can be imaged by carefully following the manufacturer's instructions. In addition, some non-pacemaker-dependent patients with older pacemaker and defibrillator models can be scanned safely with close monitoring and testing, as well as reprogramming of the device after the procedure. Cardiac MR is safe for all prosthetic heart valves and intracoronary stents. Gadolinium-based contrast agents can be associated with nephrogenic systemic fibrosis in patients with a glomerular filtration rate of less than 30 mL/minute/1.83 m^2 (Chapter 246), but this risk is very low with current cyclic contrast agents.

A comprehensive cardiac MR study includes evaluation of cardiac structure, function, tissue characteristics (T1, T2, T2*, and extracellular volume [ECV]) mapping, perfusion, and scarring or fibrosis. Cardiac MR is highly accurate for the noninvasive quantitative assessment of ventricular volumes and ejection fraction. The components of the examination are tailored to the particular diagnostic question at hand.

SPECIFIC CLINICAL APPLICATIONS

CORONARY ARTERY DISEASE

For detection of myocardial ischemia, first-pass gadolinium perfusion imaging during vasodilator stress with adenosine or regadenoson shows defects, generally in the subendocardium, that persist for at least five heartbeats during the first pass of contrast in patients with CHD (Fig. 44-12). Imaging is often repeated at rest after approximately 10 minutes to be sure any defect seen with stress was not either artifactual or caused by an infarct (the latter is excluded in combination with late gadolinium enhancement). Cardiac MR stress testing is more accurate than SPECT, is a strong predictor of cardiac events and survival, and is cost-effective in the evaluation of patients with chest pain.[13] In patients with suspected angina, cardiac MR can reduce unnecessary angiography within 12 months compared with routine clinical care but not compared with myocardial perfusion scintigraphy.[A7] Cardiac MR perfusion can be used to assess coronary flow. In patients with stable angina, cardiac MR perfusion is as good as the measurement of fractional flow reserve by invasive angiography for predicting future coronary events and may reduce referral for coronary revascularization.[A8] Coronary CT angiography has superior spatial resolution and accuracy compared with cardiac MR for imaging of the coronary arteries, but cardiac MR coronary imaging is useful for the diagnosis of anomalous coronary arteries.

Cardiac MR with late gadolinium enhancement is the gold standard technique for assessment of myocardial scar caused by myocardial infarction, with a better accuracy than nuclear imaging approaches, especially for smaller non–Q wave infarctions (Fig. 44-13). In acute myocardial infarction, cardiac MR T2-weighted techniques can assess the myocardium at risk and estimate the amount of salvaged myocardium owing to reperfusion. Areas of low signal in the subendocardial core of the infarction represent regions of microvascular obstruction with severe capillary destruction and are a marker of subsequent adverse left ventricular remodeling and poorer outcome. To assess myocardial viability in patients with chronic coronary heart disease, cardiac MR with late gadolinium enhancement has the best sensitivity for recovery of function with revascularization, but low-dose dobutamine contractile reserve has better specificity.

CARDIOMYOPATHIES

Cardiac MR should not be routinely performed in all patients with new onset heart failure,[A9] but it is very helpful in identifying patterns of scar or fibrosis that typify specific causes of cardiomyopathy (Chapter 57). Cardiac MR measurements of left ventricular mass and left atrial volume can be used to estimate left ventricular filling pressures and to predict survival in patients who have heart failure.[14] In nonischemic dilated cardiomyopathy, late gadolinium enhancement is associated with an adverse prognosis,[15] regardless of the left ventricular ejection fraction. In patients who have chest pain, elevated

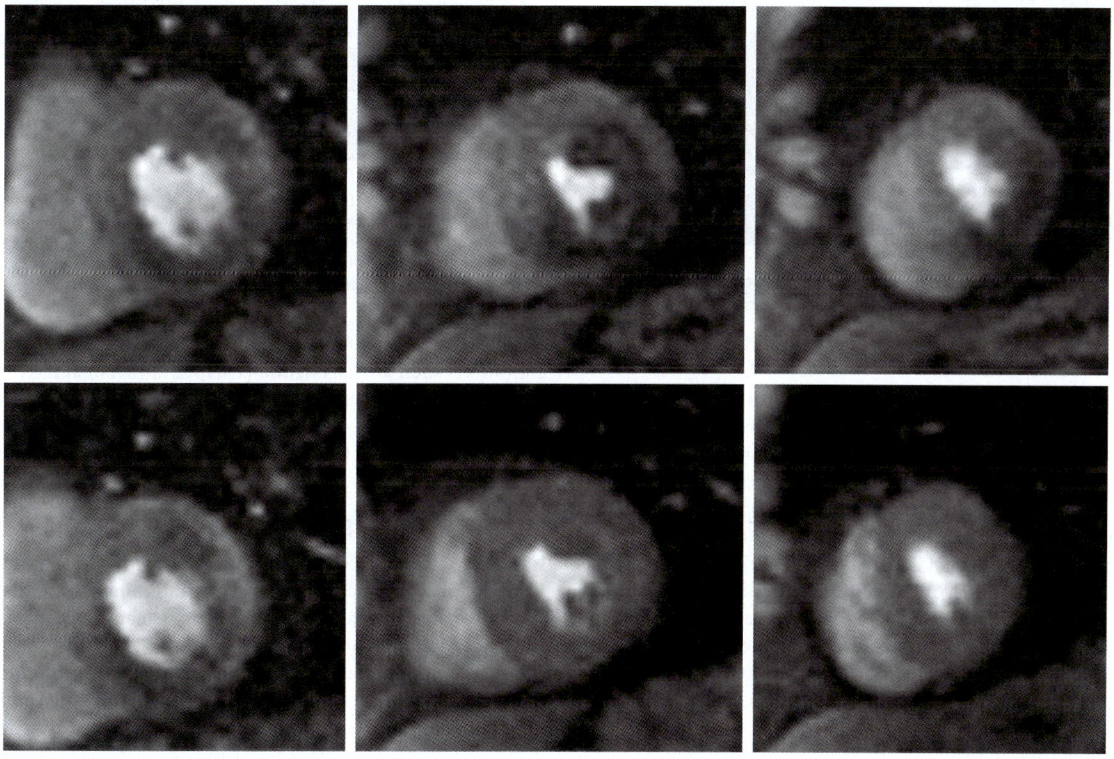

FIGURE 44-12. Set of first-pass gadolinium-enhanced magnetic resonance perfusion images during adenosine stress (*top row*) and at rest (*bottom row*) at the base (*left*), mid-ventricle (*center*), and apex (*right*). The stress images demonstrate a large perfusion deficit in the anterolateral and inferolateral walls (from 1 o'clock to 7 o'clock), especially in the mid-ventricle and apex, whereas the same regions appear normal at rest.

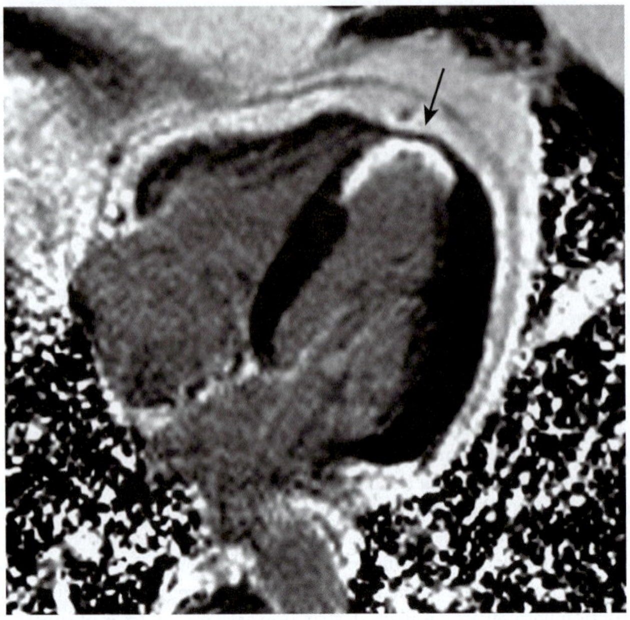

FIGURE 44-13. Late gadolinium-enhanced four-chamber long axis image in a patient with a scar (*arrow*) from a prior anterior myocardial infarction.

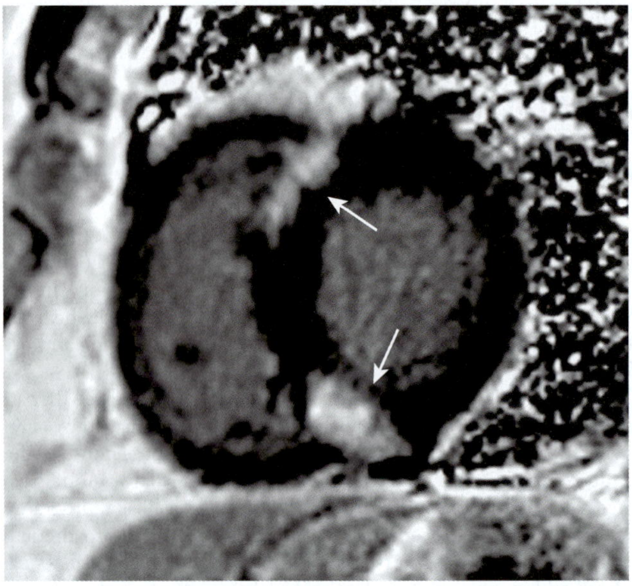

FIGURE 44-15. Late gadolinium-enhanced magnetic resonance short axis image of a 35-year-old man with hypertrophic cardiomyopathy demonstrates a classic pattern of enhancement, which identifies fibrosis (*arrows*) in the right ventricular insertion sites.

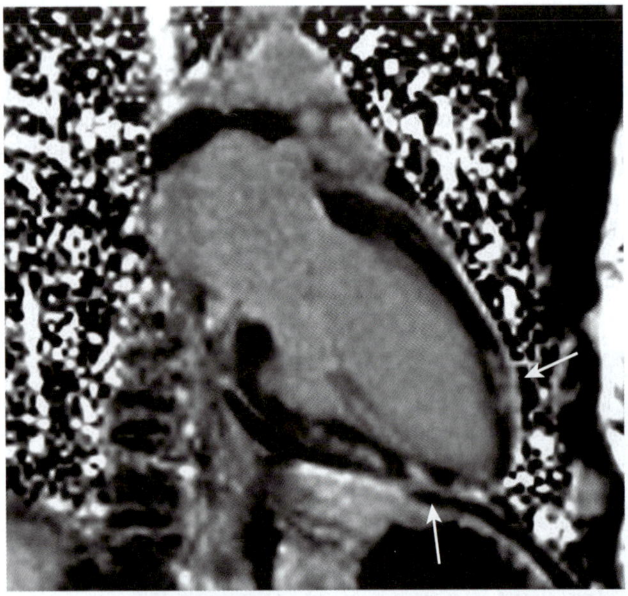

FIGURE 44-14. Gadolinium-enhanced image in a 22-year-old man shows patchy subepicardial enhancement (*arrows*) characteristic of acute myocarditis.

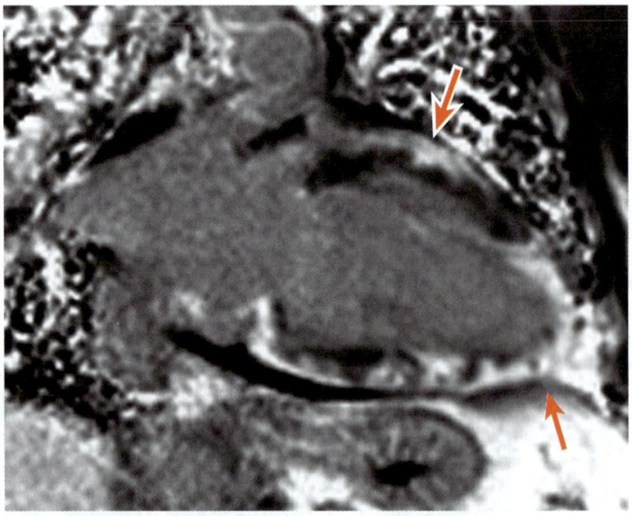

FIGURE 44-16. Late gadolinium-enhanced magnetic resonance image in a 47-year-old man with heart failure, heart block, and hilar lymphadenopathy shows patchy late gadolinium enhancement in a noncoronary distribution, including subepicardial anterior wall enhancement (*upper arrow*) and near transmural apical enhancement (*lower arrow*) consistent with myocardial sarcoidosis.

troponin levels, but a negative coronary arteriogram, cardiac MR is ideally suited to identify myocarditis or unusual causes of myocardial infarction,[16] (Fig. 44-14) (Chapter 47). In patients with hypertrophic cardiomyopathy (Chapter 47), cardiac MR is more sensitive than echocardiography for identifying increased regional wall thickness and can demonstrate late gadolinium enhancement (Fig. 44-15), the extent of which correlates with the risk of sudden death. Cardiac amyloidosis (Chapters 47 and 174) can be seen as diffuse subendocardial, transmural, or patchy late gadolinium enhancement. In cardiac sarcoidosis (Chapters 47 and 83; Fig. 44-16), patchy midwall and/or subepicardial fibrosis is readily identified, is complementary to PET (see earlier), and is more sensitive than endomyocardial biopsy. Cardiac MR is also useful for diagnosing the myocarditis associated with coronavirus disease 2019 (Chapter 336).[17]

Cardiac MR is often used to diagnose arrhythmogenic ventricular cardiomyopathy (Fig. 44-17; Chapters 47 and 53), which is characterized by global right ventricular dilation and regional akinesis or dyskinesis. In iron overload conditions such as thalassemia (Chapter 148), imaging of T2* can identify the extent of iron overload and can be used to follow the effects of chelation therapy. Rarer causes of cardiomyopathy, such as ventricular noncompaction and Chagas disease (Chapters 47 and 318), also have characteristic cardiac MR findings.

AORTIC DISEASE, PERICARDIAL DISEASE, AND MASSES

Cardiac MR is an excellent test to image aneurysms but is a second-line test to detect acute aortic dissection or intraluminal aortic hematoma (see Fig. 63-5) in stable patients. Cardiac MR is also an excellent test for the evaluation of chronic pericardial disease (Fig. 44-18) because it accurately identifies pericardial thickness as well as adherence of the pericardium to the epicardium in constrictive pericarditis. Real-time imaging can demonstrate ventricular interdependence, a hallmark of this disease. Cardiac MR is also an ideal tool to diagnose intracardiac (Fig. 44-19) and extracardiac masses such as myxomas, thrombus, and tumors (Chapter 47), owing to its high spatial resolution and ability to perform tissue characterization.

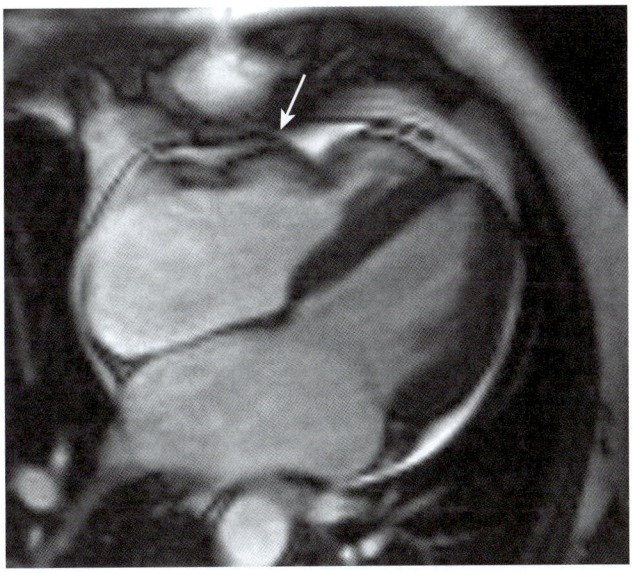

FIGURE 44-17. Magnetic resonance image in a 27-year-old woman with arrhythmogenic ventricular cardiomyopathy demonstrates regional right ventricular (RV) systolic dysfunction, which is the hallmark of the disease. The *arrow* points to a region of RV dyskinesis at end systole, and the RV appears like an accordion at end systole.

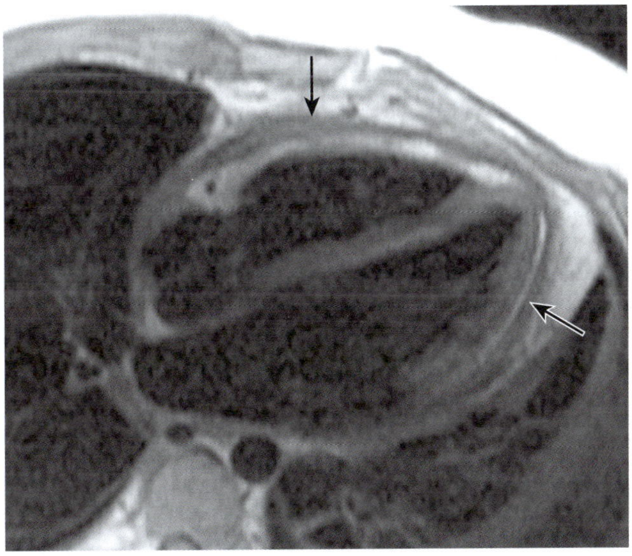

FIGURE 44-18. Magnetic resonance image of a 35-year-old man with dyspnea many years after mantle radiation for Hodgkin lymphoma shows a thickened pericardium (*arrows*) circumferentially around the left and right ventricles.

CONGENITAL HEART DISEASE

Cardiac MR is useful for the assessment of both simple and complex congenital heart disease and is often used as an adjunct to echocardiography (Chapter 55). For example, phase velocity cardiac MR readily quantifies blood flow through the major blood vessels, thereby facilitating accurate assessment of the ratio of pulmonary to systemic blood flow in the presence of shunts. Cardiovascular MR is particularly valuable for assessing abnormalities of the great vessels, such as aortic coarctation (Fig. 44-20), extracardiac anatomy, or anomalous pulmonary venous drainage, and in patients with complex congenital heart disease who have undergone prior corrective or palliative shunt surgery, such as in tetralogy of Fallot or hypoplastic left heart syndrome. Cardiac MR is uniquely able to measure right ventricular volumes accurately, an often important determination in this setting.

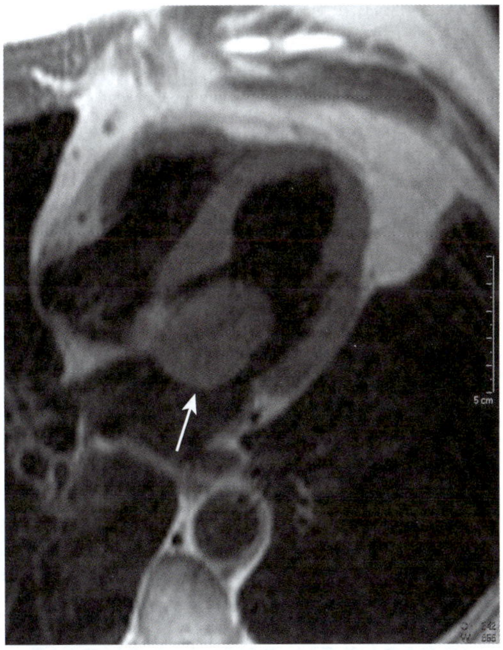

FIGURE 44-19. Diastolic magnetic resonance image of a large left atrial myxoma (*arrow*) showing that it is attached to the atrial septum and is prolapsing across the mitral valve.

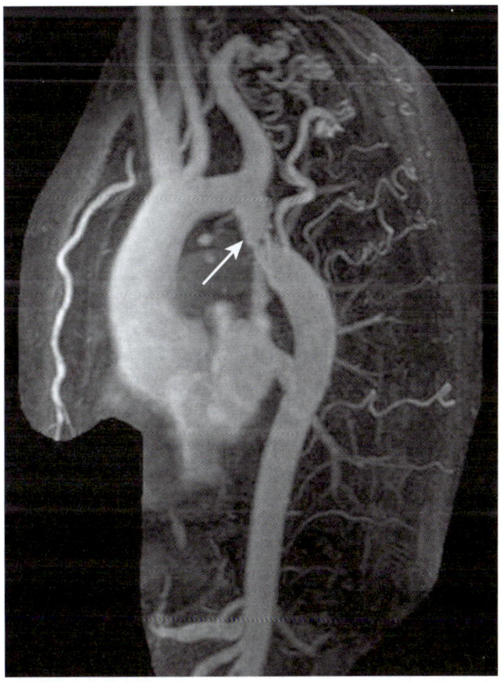

FIGURE 44-20. Three-dimensional contrast-enhanced magnetic resonance angiogram in a patient with an aortic coarctation (*arrow*).

GENERAL REFERENCES

For the General References and other additional features, please visit Elsevier eBooks+ at https://ebooks.health.elsevier.com.

Grade A References

A1. Velazquez EJ, Lee KL, Jones RH, et al. Coronary artery bypass surgery in patients with ischemic cardiomyopathy. *N Engl J Med*. 2016;374:1511-1520.

A2. Panza JA, Ellis AM, Al-Khalidi HR, et al. Myocardial viability and long-term outcomes in ischemic cardiomyopathy. *N Engl J Med.* 2019;381:739-748.
A3. Douglas PS, Hoffmann U, Patel MR, et al. Outcomes of anatomical versus functional testing for coronary artery disease. *N Engl J Med.* 2015;372:1291-1300.
A4. Foy AJ, Dhruva SS, Peterson B, et al. Coronary computed tomography angiography vs functional stress testing for patients with suspected coronary artery disease: a systematic review and meta-analysis. *JAMA Intern Med.* 2017;177:1623-1631.
A5. DISCHARGE Trial Group, Maurovich-Horvat P, Bosserdt M, et al. CT or invasive coronary angiography in stable chest pain. *N Engl J Med.* 2022;386:1591-1602.
A6. Newby DE, Adamson PD, Berry C, et al. Coronary CT angiography and 5-year risk of myocardial infarction. *N Engl J Med.* 2018;379:924-933.
A7. Greenwood JP, Ripley DP, Berry C, et al. Effect of care guided by cardiovascular magnetic resonance, myocardial perfusion scintigraphy, or NICE guidelines on subsequent unnecessary angiography rates: the CE-MARC 2 randomized clinical trial. *JAMA.* 2016;316:1051-1060.
A8. Nagel E, Greenwood JP, McCann GP, et al. Magnetic resonance perfusion or fractional flow reserve in coronary disease. *N Engl J Med.* 2019;380:2418-2428.
A9. Paterson DI, Wells G, Erthal F, et al. OUTSMART HF: a randomized controlled trial of routine versus selective cardiac magnetic resonance for patients with nonischemic heart failure (IMAGE-HF 1B). *Circulation.* 2020;141:818-827.

45

HEART FAILURE: EPIDEMIOLOGY, PATHOBIOLOGY, AND DIAGNOSIS

JOSEPH G. ROGERS AND CHRISTOPHER M. O'CONNOR

DEFINITION

Heart failure is a clinical syndrome that results when abnormalities in myocardial structure and function impair cardiac output or decrease filling of the ventricles. Clinical characteristics of the heart failure syndrome include dyspnea, fatigue, impaired exercise performance, and edema. Congestion is a common but not universal feature, so the term *congestive heart failure* is no longer used.

EPIDEMIOLOGY

Current estimates are that more than 64 million people worldwide have heart failure.[1] Most studies estimate the prevalence of heart failure to be 1 to 2% of the total adult population, with a lifetime risk that ranges between 20 to 45% depending upon age, race, and geography. Although the overall prevalence of the disease appears to be stabilized or decreasing, it is increasing in younger and older individuals as well as individuals with a preserved ejection fraction. Heart failure is the leading cause of hospitalization in patients older than age 65 years, and once a patient is hospitalized for heart failure, the 30-day risk of rehospitalization is 25%, with a 10% risk of 30-day postdischarge mortality. Although survival has improved, the absolute mortality rates for heart failure remain approximately 50% within 5 years of diagnosis.

Nearly half of patients with heart failure have a preserved ejection fraction. Compared with patients who have heart failure with reduced ejection fraction, heart failure patients with a preserved ejection fraction tend to be older and are more likely to be women with a prior history of hypertension and diabetes. The mortality rate of patients who have heart failure with a preserved ejection fraction is similar to the rate for patients with reduced ejection fraction.[2] Hospitalization and rehospitalization rates are comparable for heart failure patients regardless of their ejection fractions.

Disparities

Black Americans are at increased risk for incident heart failure compared with White Americans and also have more frequent hospitalizations. Black patients with heart failure also have a higher mortality rate than White populations. The reasons for these disparities include racial differences in risk factors, the causes of heart failure, access to care, and response to therapies. However, there is a growing literature to support systemic racial inequities and even racism as an important underlying explanation.[3] Hispanics represent a growing population of heart failure patients in the United States with an incidence rate between those of Black and White Americans.

Classification

The classification of heart failure considers the disease state and progression, degree of exercise intolerance (Chapter 39), measurement of the left ventricular ejection fraction, and its underlying cause.[4] In the first approach, heart failure is classified by its progression through four stages from pre-disease to advanced symptoms (Fig. 45-1). The second approach evaluates functional states by standardized classification systems such as the New York Heart Association classification, the Canadian Cardiovascular Society system, or other validated measures of exercise tolerance (see Table 39-5). Functional status is the most appropriate way to understand a patient's limitations and the impact of heart failure on quality of life. It also correlates with prognosis and is commonly used as a secondary end point in clinical trials. A third approach is to describe heart failure based upon ejection fraction. This method stratifies patients into those with reduced (<40%), midrange (40 to 50%), and preserved (>50%) ejection fraction. This approach also helps in understanding the patient's underlying pathophysiologic process and in guiding therapeutic decisions. Classification based on etiology, usually ischemic versus nonischemic (Chapter 47), is useful in guiding the diagnostic evaluation and in tailoring treatment.

Causes of Heart Failure

Heart failure has numerous causes (Table 45-1). In developed countries, coronary artery disease, usually with a prior myocardial infarction, accounts for nearly 70% of heart failure cases (Chapter 58). Comorbid conditions such as hypertension (Chapter 64),[5] diabetes (Chapter 210),[6] and obesity (Chapter 201)[7] are commonly associated with heart failure. Diseases of the myocardium

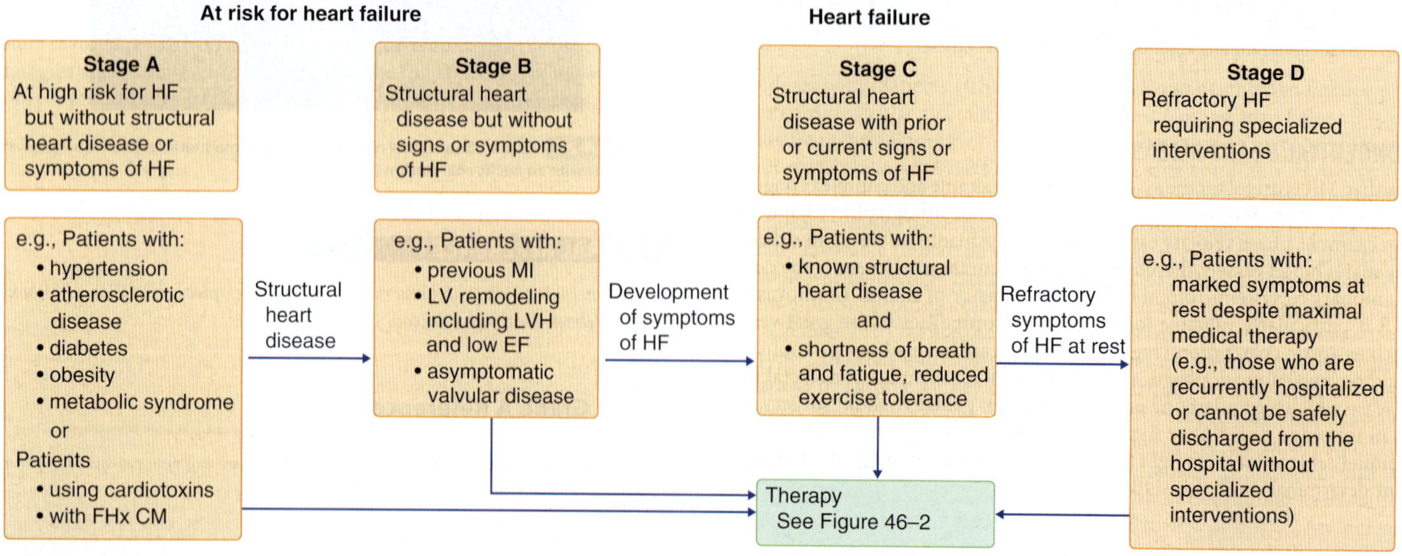

FIGURE 45-1. **Stages of heart failure.** EF = ejection fraction; FHx CM = family history of cardiomyopathy; HF = heart failure; LV = left ventricle; LVH = left ventricular hypertrophy; MI = myocardial infarction. (Modified from Heidenreich PA. 2022 AHA/ACC/HFSA guideline for the management of heart failure: a report of the American College of Cardiology/American Heart Association Joint Committee on Clinical Practice Guidelines. *Circulation.* 2022;145:e895-e1032.)

TABLE 45-1 CAUSES OF HEART FAILURE

Coronary artery disease or prior myocardial infarction or ischemic injury
Hypertension
Familial and genetic disorders, including dilated cardiomyopathies, hypertrophic cardiomyopathies, storage diseases, and muscular dystrophies
Valvular disease: valvular stenosis or regurgitation
Toxic/drug-induced damage, including prior chemotherapy
Infiltrative processes, such as sarcoid, amyloid, and hemochromatosis (i.e., restrictive cardiomyopathy)
Arrhythmia-related dysfunction, including premature ventricular contraction–induced cardiomyopathy and atrial tachyarrhythmia–related dysfunction
Arrhythmogenic right ventricular cardiomyopathy
Pulmonary heart disease, including cor pulmonale
Infectious agents, including viral infections and Chagas disease
Immunologically mediated myocardial injury
Intra- and extra-cardiac shunts
Constrictive pericarditis (i.e., nonmyocardial processes)
Nutritional disorders, such as beriberi
Inflammatory heart disease such as systemic lupus erythematosus
High-output states, such as chronic anemia, thyrotoxicosis

TABLE 45-2 FACTORS THAT MAY PRECIPITATE ACUTE DECOMPENSATION OF CHRONIC HEART FAILURE

Myocardial ischemia or infarction
Arrhythmias
Worsening hypertension
Worsening mitral or tricuspid regurgitation
Initiation of medications that worsen heart failure (calcium antagonists, β-blockers, nonsteroidal anti-inflammatory drugs, antiarrhythmic agents, chemotherapeutic drugs, antidiabetic drugs)
Failure to adhere to guideline-directed management
Dietary indiscretion
Iatrogenic volume overload (transfusion, fluid administration)
Alcohol consumption
Fever or infection
Anemia
Thyroid abnormalities
Exposure to environmental toxins
Exposure to high altitude
Pregnancy

(Chapter 47), valves (Chapter 60), and pericardium (Chapter 62), as well as endocrinopathies, metabolic abnormalities, and genetic conditions,[8] may cause heart failure. Chemotherapy (e.g., anthracyclines and trastuzumab; Chapter 164) and chest radiation (Chapter 18) may damage the myocardium. Reversible myocardial dysfunction from toxin exposure (e.g., cocaine [Chapter 365] and excessive alcohol intake [Chapter 364]), persistent tachycardia (Chapters 52 and 53), and severe mental/emotional stress (e.g., takotsubo cardiomyopathy [Chapter 47]) may cause ventricular dysfunction that typically resolves following withdrawal of the inciting etiology. Right-sided heart failure is most commonly caused by left-sided heart failure, but it also can result from pulmonary thromboembolic disease (Chapter 68), chronic lung disease (Chapters 76 and 80), and pulmonary arterial hypertension (Chapter 69).[9]

The underlying causes of heart failure vary by region. For instance, Chagas cardiomyopathy (Chapter 47) is prevalent in Central and South America. Rheumatic valvular disease is a common cause of heart failure in developing countries but is infrequent in developed countries.

Acute decompensation of heart failure may be related to worsening of the primary cause, a new cardiac or pulmonary condition, the influence of other disease states that require increased cardiac output, poor adherence to medical therapies, or the addition of medications used to treat other conditions (Table 45-2). As a result, a systematic approach to the clinical evaluation is critical. Some patients will have decompensated heart failure that requires hospitalization, whereas others will have heart failure as a comorbidity during hospitalization for another problem.

PATHOBIOLOGY

A number of factors contribute to the development and progression of heart failure (Table 45-3). The relative contribution of these mechanisms to the overall pathophysiologic manifestations of heart failure (E-Fig. 45-1) varies in individual patients.

TABLE 45-3 PATHOBIOLOGIC MECHANISMS OF HEART FAILURE

Hemodynamics
Neurohormones
Cardiorenal interactions
Abnormal calcium cycling
Cell death
Myocardial genetics

Heart Failure with a Reduced Ejection Fraction

A central tenet of heart failure is that myocardial dysfunction limits the heart's ability to pump blood at a rate commensurate with the requirements of metabolizing tissues or that it can do so only in the setting of elevated cardiac filling pressures. The pathobiology of the failing heart results in maladaptive regulation of multiple neurohormonal pathways that reduce intrinsic cardiac contractility and cause prototypical ventricular remodeling (Chapter 41). Alterations in cardiac extracellular matrix and replacement fibrosis increase the connective tissue content and further impair systolic and diastolic function (Chapter 41). Several neurohormonal pathways regulate myocardial fibrosis, including aldosterone, matrix metalloproteinases, tissue inhibitors of metalloproteinases (TIMPS), TNF-alpha, and ST2.

Adrenergic nervous system activation plays a pivotal role in the development and progression of left ventricular dysfunction. Reduced pulse pressure activates arterial baroreceptors and stimulates sympathetic nervous system activity, elevated levels of circulating norepinephrine, and increased release of norepinephrine by several organs, including the heart. Exposure of cardiac myocytes to chronically elevated levels of norepinephrine reduces the density of their β-adrenergic receptors, downregulates signaling pathways, and is directly toxic to the cells. The renin-angiotensin-aldosterone system, which is also activated relatively early in heart failure, causes vasoconstriction and sodium retention. The presumptive mechanisms of induction include renal hypoperfusion, β-adrenergic system stimulation, and hyponatremia. Adrenergic and renin-angiotensin-aldosterone system activation stimulate the failing heart and support the circulation in the short term. Over time, however, the prolonged activation of these systems causes maladaptive remodeling and further ventricular dysfunction. In addition, the sympathetic nervous system and renin-angiotensin-aldosterone system are co-regulated, such that increased activity of each pathway stimulates a simultaneous increase in the other.

Natriuretic peptides counterbalance the vasoconstricting and sodium-retaining properties of the renin-angiotensin-aldosterone system and sympathetic nervous systems by causing both arterial and venous vasodilation, natriuresis, and diuresis. The extent of natriuretic pathway activation is a marker of the severity of heart failure and is associated with adverse outcomes, including the risk for hospitalization and death.

Many patients with heart failure have elevated levels of endothelin and arginine vasopressin. Arginine vasopressin induces vasoconstriction through a vascular (V_1) receptor and reduces free water clearance through a renal tubular (V_2) receptor. Endothelin causes prolonged vasoconstriction, reductions in glomerular filtration, and pulmonary arteriolar constriction.

Cardiorenal interactions highlight the integral role of kidney dysfunction in the worsening of heart failure, with both organs contributing to the retention of sodium and water. In most patients with chronic heart failure, the kidneys are anatomically and structurally normal, but passive venous congestion and reduced renal perfusion lead to worsening renal function and a vicious cycle of progressive dysfunction of both organ systems. Renal failure may limit the ability to use inhibitors of the renin-angiotensin-aldosterone system to treat heart failure.

Abnormal calcium cycling reduces the calcium content in the cardiac sarcoplasmic reticulum owing to diastolic leak through altered ryanodine receptors. The reduced calcium content of the sarcoplasmic reticulum alters the contraction interactions between cardiac myosin and actin myofilaments. In addition, a loss of function of cardiac SERCA2a (sarcoendoplasmic reticulum calcium transport ATPase 2a) pumps, which are responsible for removal of cytoplasmic calcium, affects ventricular relaxation and causes diastolic dysfunction.

In all forms of heart failure, a variety of stimuli (e.g., elevated neurohormone levels, adrenergic activation, inflammatory mechanisms, and toxin exposure) accelerate cell death. Elevated serum levels of proinflammatory cytokines (including tumor necrosis factor-α, interleukin-1β, and interleukin-6) induce contractile dysfunction, myocardial fibrosis, and myocyte necrosis, perhaps by mediating some of the deleterious responses to catecholamines and angiotensin II.

Persistent tachycardia (e.g., atrial fibrillation with rapid ventricular response) also can result in heart failure, presumably related to chronic hyperadrenergic stimulation.[10] In some patients, the tachycardic response to heart failure may itself contribute to worsening heart failure. These forms of heart failure may be reversible, depending on the relative contribution of the tachycardia to the underlying myocardial dysfunction.

Genetic mutations are increasingly identified as important mediators of the cardiac structural and functional abnormalities linked to symptomatic heart failure (see E-Table 47-1). The majority of familial cardiomyopathies (Chapter 47), most of which are inherited in an autosomal dominant fashion, are related to defects in cytoskeletal or nuclear proteins. Inherited cardiomyopathies are also associated with muscular dystrophies, infiltrative diseases such as hemochromatosis, and mitochondrial disorders. A low plasma transthyretin concentration is a marker of transthyretin tetramer instability associated with a higher risk of heart failure in the general population even in the absence of amyloidosis.[11]

Heart Failure with a Preserved Ejection Fraction

The pathophysiologic mechanism of heart failure with a preserved ejection fraction is complex and includes alterations in cardiac structure and function, vascular abnormalities, end-organ dysfunction, and interrelated comorbidities (Table 45-4).[12] In principle, diastolic dysfunction in heart failure with a preserved ejection fraction can result from increased ventricular stiffness due to hypertrophy and interstitial fibrosis as well as from abnormal ventricular relaxation due to dysfunctional calcium cycling. Although there are many potential causes of heart failure with preserved ejection fraction, most patients have current or prior hypertension; the resulting left ventricular hypertrophy and fibrosis are responsible for increased chamber stiffness. Ischemic heart disease also may contribute to heart failure with a preserved ejection fraction by virtue of subendocardial fibrosis or as a result of intermittent ischemic dysfunction. Age itself is a crucial predisposing factor because it causes loss of myocytes (apoptosis), increased fibrosis with shifts to more rigid forms of collagen, and loss of vascular compliance.

Myocardial relaxation is an energy-dependent process. Processes that interfere with myocardial energy metabolism, such as ischemia, compromise myocardial relaxation. These changes reduce ventricular compliance and increase filling pressures. Elevated filling pressures raise the pulmonary capillary wedge pressure and contribute to the sensation of dyspnea. Diastolic dysfunction may remain asymptomatic for years, but increasing age, renal dysfunction, hypertension, and progressive left ventricular dysfunction are associated with the development of symptomatic heart failure. The resting hemodynamic profile in heart failure with preserved ejection fraction is frequently normal, but physiologic perturbations such as tachycardia or exercise result in exaggerated increases in filling pressures. This phenomenon accounts for the exertional limitations seen in this syndrome.[13] Furthermore, because atrial contraction is responsible for a disproportionately large proportion of ventricular diastolic filling into a noncompliant ventricle, atrial fibrillation can exacerbate symptoms. Abnormalities in ventricular relaxation and myocardial stiffness limit ventricular filling, so patients may have a narrow window for optimal fluid volume. Modest volume overload can substantially exacerbate symptoms of dyspnea, and diuresis may precipitate symptomatic hypotension owing to ventricular underfilling. Although isolated diastolic dysfunction can occur, the majority of patients with ventricular dysfunction have both systolic and diastolic components. As a result, it is preferable to characterize patients as having heart failure with a preserved ejection fraction or heart failure with a reduced ejection fraction rather than as having systolic or diastolic heart failure.

High-output heart failure is seen in severe anemia and hyperthyroidism (Chapter 207). It is also seen in patients with vasodilative states such as obesity (Chapter 201), late-stage liver disease (Chapter 140), arteriovenous shunts, hypoxic-hypercapnic lung disease, and myeloproliferative/myelofibrotic disorders with extramedullary hematopoiesis (Chapter 152).

TABLE 45-4 CONTRIBUTIONS TO HEART FAILURE WITH PRESERVED EJECTION FRACTION

Left ventricular hypertrophy
Hypertension
Myocardial fibrosis
Subendocardial fibrosis (from intermittent ischemia, especially with diabetes)
Arterial stiffness
Endothelial dysfunction
Inflammation

CLINICAL MANIFESTATIONS

The diagnosis of heart failure may be apparent when patients present with classic symptoms of shortness of breath in combination with a clinical examination consistent with volume overload. A previous history of a myocardial infarction or poorly controlled hypertension should increase the clinician's suspicion for the diagnosis. In contrast, the diagnosis may be missed or delayed in patients who experience a more insidious course with vague symptoms, such as fatigue and exercise intolerance. The use of biomarkers such as natriuretic peptides has significantly improved diagnostic accuracy in recent years.

The evaluation of a patient with suspected heart failure should proceed in an organized and focused manner (Fig. 45-2 and Table 45-5).

Symptoms

Shortness of Breath

Dyspnea (Chapter 71) is the most common but nonspecific symptom of heart failure, and patients with predominant lung disease or anemia may have similar symptoms. In most heart failure patients, dyspnea is present only with activity. It is the most common reason that patients seek care for heart failure, both during the chronic state and with acutely decompensated heart failure. The most important cause of dyspnea is pulmonary congestion that increases the accumulation of interstitial or intra-alveolar fluid, reduces lung compliance, and increases the work of breathing (E-Fig. 45-2). The relief of dyspnea is a primary treatment goal because of its effect on quality of life and its association with worse in-hospital and postdischarge outcomes.

When dyspnea occurs in the recumbent position, it is called *orthopnea.* Orthopnea results from the increase in venous return from the extremities and splanchnic circulation to the central circulation with changes in posture. The increase in ventricular preload raises pulmonary venous and pulmonary capillary hydrostatic pressures. Orthopnea is clinically characterized by the number of pillows a patient requires to sleep comfortably without shortness of breath. Patients with orthopnea may report an inability to sleep in a bed and instead may sleep sitting upright. Orthopnea is a specific symptom of heart failure, and it correlates well with the severity of pulmonary congestion.

Bendopnea is defined as dyspnea that occurs while bending over. The mechanism of bendopnea is poorly defined but appears to be related to increases in left ventricular filling pressures during bending in patients with a baseline elevation in pulmonary capillary wedge pressure. There appears to be an association between bendopnea and baseline mismatch of left- and right-sided filling pressures (i.e., elevated wedge pressure out of proportion to right atrial pressure). The clinical spectrum of this symptom and its relationship to outcomes are not well understood, but recent data suggest that this symptom may be more common than has previously been recognized.

Paroxysmal nocturnal dyspnea is acute, severe shortness of breath that awakens the patient from sleep. Paroxysmal nocturnal dyspnea usually occurs about 1 hour after the patient lies in a recumbent position and subsides with sitting or standing. Paroxysmal nocturnal dyspnea results from increased venous return and the mobilization of interstitial fluid from the splanchnic circulation and lower extremities, with accumulation of alveolar edema. Paroxysmal nocturnal dyspnea is relatively uncommon but almost always represents severe heart failure, and it appears to be associated with increased mortality.

Fatigue

Fatigue occurs in more than 90% of patients with heart failure. Although nonspecific and difficult to quantify, it can be an occult and troublesome manifestation of heart failure.

Chest Pain

Chest pain (Chapter 39) may be mediated by myocardial ischemia related to underlying coronary artery disease or increased wall stress that is proportional

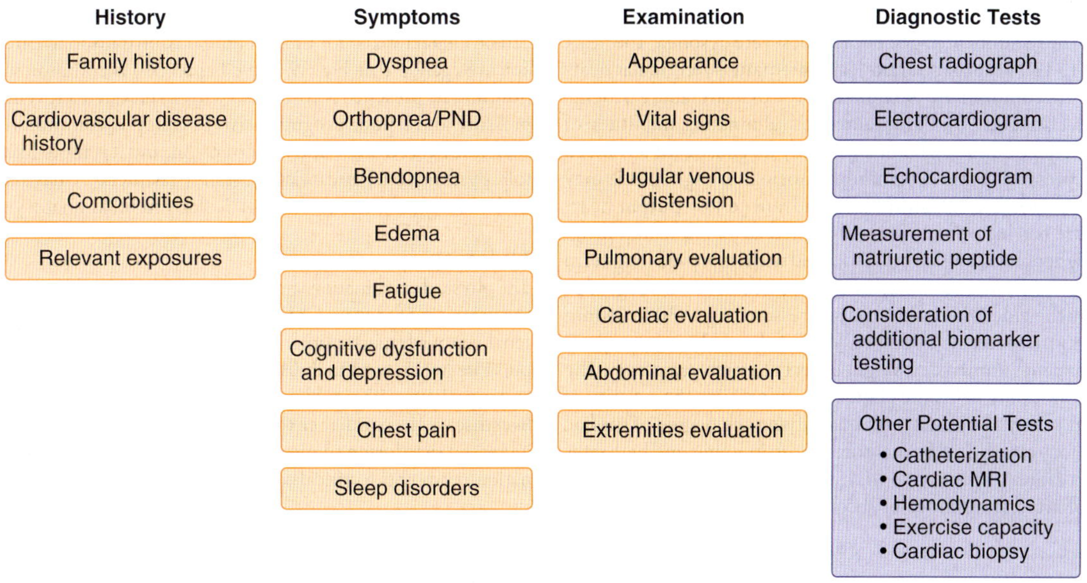

FIGURE 45-2. **Diagnostic evaluation of heart failure. The various components of the diagnostic evaluation of heart failure patients are presented from the history, symptoms, and examination to diagnostic testing. MRI = magnetic resonance imaging; PND = paroxysmal nocturnal dyspnea.**

TABLE 45-5 APPROACH TO THE DIAGNOSIS OF HEART FAILURE

Obtain a history and physical examination to identify disorders or behaviors that might cause or exacerbate heart failure.
Obtain a family history to aid in diagnosis of heritable causes of heart failure.
Assess volume status and vital signs at each encounter.
Patients with suspected new-onset or acute heart failure should undergo chest radiography to assess heart size and pulmonary congestion and to detect other diseases that may cause or contribute to the patient's symptoms.
A 12-lead electrocardiogram should be obtained for all patients presenting with heart failure.
Echocardiography should be performed during the initial evaluation of patients with heart failure to assess ventricular function and valve function.
Measurement of natriuretic peptides is recommended for the following indications: To support the diagnosis of heart failure in ambulatory patients with dyspnea as well as in those with possible acute heart failure, especially in the setting of an uncertain diagnosis. To establish prognosis or disease severity in heart failure.
The initial evaluation of patients presenting with heart failure should include a complete blood count, urinalysis and renal function, serum electrolytes, glucose and lipid profile, liver function tests, and thyroid-stimulating hormone.
Hemodynamic monitoring is recommended to guide therapy in patients who have respiratory distress or clinical evidence of impaired perfusion in whom the adequacy or excess of intracardiac filling pressures cannot be determined from clinical assessment.

Modified from Yancy CW, Jessup M, Bozkurt B, et al. 2013 ACCF/AHA guideline for the management of heart failure: a report of the American College of Cardiology Foundation/American Heart Association Task Force on Practice Guidelines. *J Am Coll Cardiol.* 2013;62:e147-e239.

to the degree of left ventricular dilation. Left ventricular hypertrophy may cause chest pain from a mismatch between oxygen supply and demand. Patients with amyloid heart disease can have chest pain owing to transient ischemia caused by deposition of amyloid protein in the medial layer of myocardial arterioles.

Cardiac Cachexia

As heart failure progresses, patients may develop constitutional symptoms, including nausea, vomiting, anorexia, abdominal pain, and muscle wasting. The development of cardiac cachexia is associated with a poor prognosis.[14] In many patients, these symptoms arise from right-sided heart failure, with or without concomitant tricuspid regurgitation, and resulting passive venous congestion in the abdominal vasculature or liver. Patients with significant hepatic congestion may develop right upper quadrant abdominal pain and jaundice that can be difficult to distinguish clinically from gallbladder disease or other abdominal conditions (Chapter 141). In patients with advanced cardiogenic shock (Chapter 93), severe abdominal pain can be a particularly ominous sign of abdominal ischemia (Chapter 129).

Cognitive Dysfunction and Mood Disorders

Cognitive dysfunction (Chapter 371) is common, particularly in elderly heart failure patients. Confusion can be a manifestation of worsening heart failure related to relative hypotension or precipitated by medications used to treat heart failure. Although intrinsic brain function itself is not affected in most patients with heart failure, cerebral hypoperfusion in advanced heart failure can cause memory impairment, limited attention span, and altered mentation.

Depressive symptoms (Chapter 362) occur in up to 25% of patients with heart failure. Depressive symptoms can be detected by simple questions such as the Patient Health Questionnaire depression module (see Chapter 23), which has an 80% predictive value for depression and is associated with worse outcomes in heart failure patients.

Sleep Disorders

Sleep-disordered breathing is observed in upward of 70% of heart failure patients and is associated with increased morbidity and mortality. Patterns of sleep-disordered breathing include obstructive sleep apnea and central sleep apnea/Cheyne-Stokes respiration (Chapter 74). Patients may have both types, and the relative proportion of each type varies with the severity of heart failure and its treatment. Nocturnal rostral fluid movement from the lower extremities of heart failure patients may worsen obstructive sleep apnea. Central sleep apnea is due in part to the instability of the ventilatory control systems in heart failure.

Chronic sleep-disordered breathing also causes a series of derangements that may precipitate or exacerbate heart failure. Sleep-disordered breathing increases blood pressure and the risk of arrhythmias.

Symptoms of sleep-disordered breathing (Chapter 374) include hypersomnolence, choking or gasping during sleep, recurrent awakenings, unrefreshing sleep, daytime fatigue, and impaired concentration or memory. The symptoms may be difficult to distinguish from other symptoms of heart failure, including unrefreshing sleep due to orthopnea and paroxysmal nocturnal dyspnea. Treatment of sleep-disordered breathing with continuous positive airway pressure ventilation improves quality of life and left ventricular ejection fraction, but these effects are attenuated after 3 months.[A1] The use of adaptive servo-ventilation increases mortality and should be avoided in this patient population.[A2]

Physical Examination

A carefully performed physical examination is critical to make an accurate diagnosis, assess comorbid conditions, understand the patient's underlying hemodynamic state, and estimate prognosis.[15]

Global Observation and Vital Signs

The patient's general appearance may provide details related to the acuity and severity of the heart failure. Patients with severe symptoms may be pale or diaphoretic and unable to speak in complete sentences. In extreme circumstances, they may be unable to lie recumbent in bed because of severe dyspnea. The heart rate may be elevated (>100 beats per minute), and premature ventricular beats or atrial arrhythmias are common. Approximately 30% of heart failure patients have atrial fibrillation (Chapter 52). Pulsus alternans (alternating amplitude of successive beats) is an uncommon sign but is virtually diagnostic for advanced heart failure. Blood pressure is most commonly normal or high, but it may be low (systolic blood pressure <90 mm Hg) in advanced low-output heart failure. Blood pressure has historically been identified as an important prognostic marker (i.e., higher blood pressure is associated with improved long-term outcomes), but these associated data may not be applicable to all subgroups of patients, especially the elderly. A narrow pulse pressure (e.g., <30 to 35 mm Hg) is indicative of more severe heart failure. Weight should be assessed and compared with the patient's known dry weight or recent weight trajectory. The assessment of weight not only helps the clinician to appreciate the severity of volume overload, but it may also assist with quantifying the degree of cardiac cachexia. The respiratory rate should be measured. Both low rates and high rates may be seen in heart failure. Likewise, both hypothermia and hyperthermia can be informative of impending shock or secondary causes of heart failure.

Jugular Veins

Examination of the jugular veins assesses right atrial pressure (see Fig. 39-2). Right atrial pressure can be estimated by measuring the height of the jugular pulse in centimeters above the sternal angle and adding 5 cm H_2O (normal = 8 cm H_2O; see Fig. 39-3). An alternative is to assess the height of the veins in relationship to the clavicle. Jugular pulsations can be distinguished from carotid pulsations by their more lateral location, lack of palpability, and a visible double waveform. It may also be useful to compare the timing to the contralateral carotid or radial pulse. If the jugular pulsation is not seen in the neck, the right atrial pressure may be either very high or low. The presence of abdominal-jugular reflux, which is a sign of abnormally elevated right-sided filling pressures, should be assessed by putting sustained pressure on the right upper quadrant of the abdomen for 30 seconds; a positive finding is at least a 1-cm rise in the jugular pressure, which then slowly declines when abdominal pressure is removed. Either an elevated jugular venous pressure or an abnormal abdominal jugular reflux has been reported in 80% of patients with advanced heart failure.

An additional important finding in the neck is evidence of tricuspid regurgitation, which is visualized as a large *cv* wave (see Fig. 39-3). This finding is often corroborated by hepatic pulsations, which can be detected during the abdominal examination. Difficulty palpating the carotid pulses may suggest low cardiac output from heart failure, aortic stenosis, or carotid artery disease (see Fig. 39-4).

Pulmonary Examination

Despite elevated left ventricular filling pressures that are transmitted back into the left atrium and pulmonary circulation, most patients with heart failure do not have evidence of pulmonary congestion on physical examination. The lungs of chronic heart failure patients undergo adaptive changes and have robust lymphatic drainage to compensate for elevated filling pressures. However, a subset of patients may develop alveolar fluid accumulation, which is appreciated as rales (Chapter 71) and which are an independent predictor of prognosis among patients with heart failure and a reduced ejection fraction.[16] These findings are more common in patients with acute pulmonary edema due to sudden decompensation from an inciting event.

Fluid may also accumulate in the pleural space related to the increased transudation of fluid and impaired lymphatic drainage in the setting of elevated systemic venous pressures (Chapter 86). The clinician should listen and percuss for the possible presence of pleural effusions (Chapter 86), which tend to lateralize to the right side owing to the greater surface area of the lungs and the position of the diaphragm.[17] The diagnosis of a moderate or large pleural effusion is critical because draining the effusion may improve dyspnea.

Cardiac Examination

The cardiac examination is the cornerstone of the evaluation of the patient with heart failure. Visual inspection and palpation may reveal a right ventricular heave, suggestive of right ventricular dysfunction and underlying pulmonary hypertension. The location, size, and duration of the point of maximal impulse against the chest wall may provide details related to the degree of left ventricular dilation; the impulse is typically laterally displaced in the setting of left ventricular enlargement and may be sustained in the setting of left ventricular hypertrophy.

Auscultation of the heart sounds provides important information related to the underlying rhythm and frequency of ectopic beats. Auscultation of a loud P2 or the ability to hear a P2 beyond the pulmonic listening area suggests pulmonary hypertension. The presence (or worsening) of valvular disorders (Chapter 60) can be characterized for their potential contribution to cardiac dysfunction. An apical S_3 gallop (see Fig. 39-5 in Chapter 39) is common in severe LV dysfunction, and its presence is correlated with an elevated left ventricular end-diastolic pressure and a poor prognosis. An S_4 gallop is common in patients who have ischemic heart disease and hypertension, and it is more likely indicative of diastolic dysfunction. Pericardial effusions (Chapter 62) may also occasionally occur in the setting of heart failure, particularly in inflammatory cardiomyopathies.

Abdomen

The physical examination should estimate the size of the liver and spleen and elicit the presence of ascites (Chapter 132). Abdominal venous congestion may cause renal venous hypertension and subsequent renal dysfunction. An enlarged and pulsatile liver is seen in individuals with markedly elevated right heart pressures and in patients with significant tricuspid insufficiency. In the setting of irreversible liver disease (i.e., cardiac cirrhosis), patients with heart failure are at a substantially increased risk during surgical interventions. Thus, a thorough abdominal examination represents a critical component of the evaluation of heart failure patients.

Extremities

Edema (Chapter 39) results from the retention of sodium due to low cardiac output and reduced renal perfusion pressures, which ultimately result in elevated right-sided filling pressures, increased hydrostatic pressures in the venous circulation, and transudation of fluid into dependent interstitial spaces, especially in the ankles or lower extremities. Edema is commonly measured on a scale of 0 to 3+, but this system has marked interobserver variation. Peripheral edema is a nonspecific finding, and edema due to heart failure must be distinguished from edema related to medication use (e.g., calcium-channel blockers, thiazolidinediones, or nonsteroidal anti-inflammatory drugs), venous insufficiency, or hypoproteinemia.

The temperature of the extremities should also be assessed. Cool extremities suggest low cardiac output or concomitant peripheral arterial disease (Chapter 65).

DIAGNOSIS

Patterns of Presentation

The initial presentation ranges from subtle outpatient findings to acute decompensation that requires hospitalization (see Figs. 45-3 and 45-4). In critically ill patients with respiratory compromise, the distinction between cardiac pulmonary edema compared with acute respiratory distress syndrome (Chapter 90) can be challenging.[18]

An initial presentation of heart failure may represent the gradual progression of known but previously asymptomatic (stage A or B) heart failure or be the first indication of altered cardiac function. In patients without an antecedent history of heart failure, precipitating factors, such as acute myocardial infarction (Chapter 58), tachyarrhythmias (Chapters 52 and 53), previously unrecognized or new valvular abnormalities (Chapter 60), toxic injury (including alcohol excess), or acute myocarditis (Chapter 47), should be considered.

When patients with stage C or D heart failure present with worsening symptoms, precipitating factors may also include myocardial ischemia, arrhythmias, or worsening of valvular function (see Table 45-2). Other conditions can include anemia, infection, thyroid abnormalities, and any disease process that may accompany or require a higher cardiac output. In many patients, however, the worsening may be gradual, augured by subtle signs and symptoms (Fig. 45-5).

Electrocardiography

A 12-lead electrocardiogram (Chapter 42) should be obtained for all patients who present with possible heart failure to evaluate the cardiac rhythm, identify current ischemia or prior myocardial infarction, and detect evidence of left ventricular hypertrophy. Rhythm abnormalities may be responsible for the development or exacerbation of underlying cardiac dysfunction. For example, an underlying tachyarrhythmia can lead to the development of left ventricular systolic dysfunction that is reversible with appropriate intervention. Q waves suggest coronary artery disease as a likely contributor to ventricular dysfunction. Voltage criteria for left ventricular hypertrophy support a diagnosis of hypertensive heart disease, including heart failure with a preserved ejection fraction. Underlying conduction abnormalities, such as delayed ventricular conduction (i.e., bundle branch morphology), determine eligibility criteria for cardiac resynchronization therapy in appropriate patients (Chapters 46 and 54) and have important prognostic implications. Holter monitoring sometimes may be helpful to determine the burden of ventricular arrhythmias or ectopic beats because tachycardia-mediated cardiomyopathies may be reversible with medical or ablation therapy.

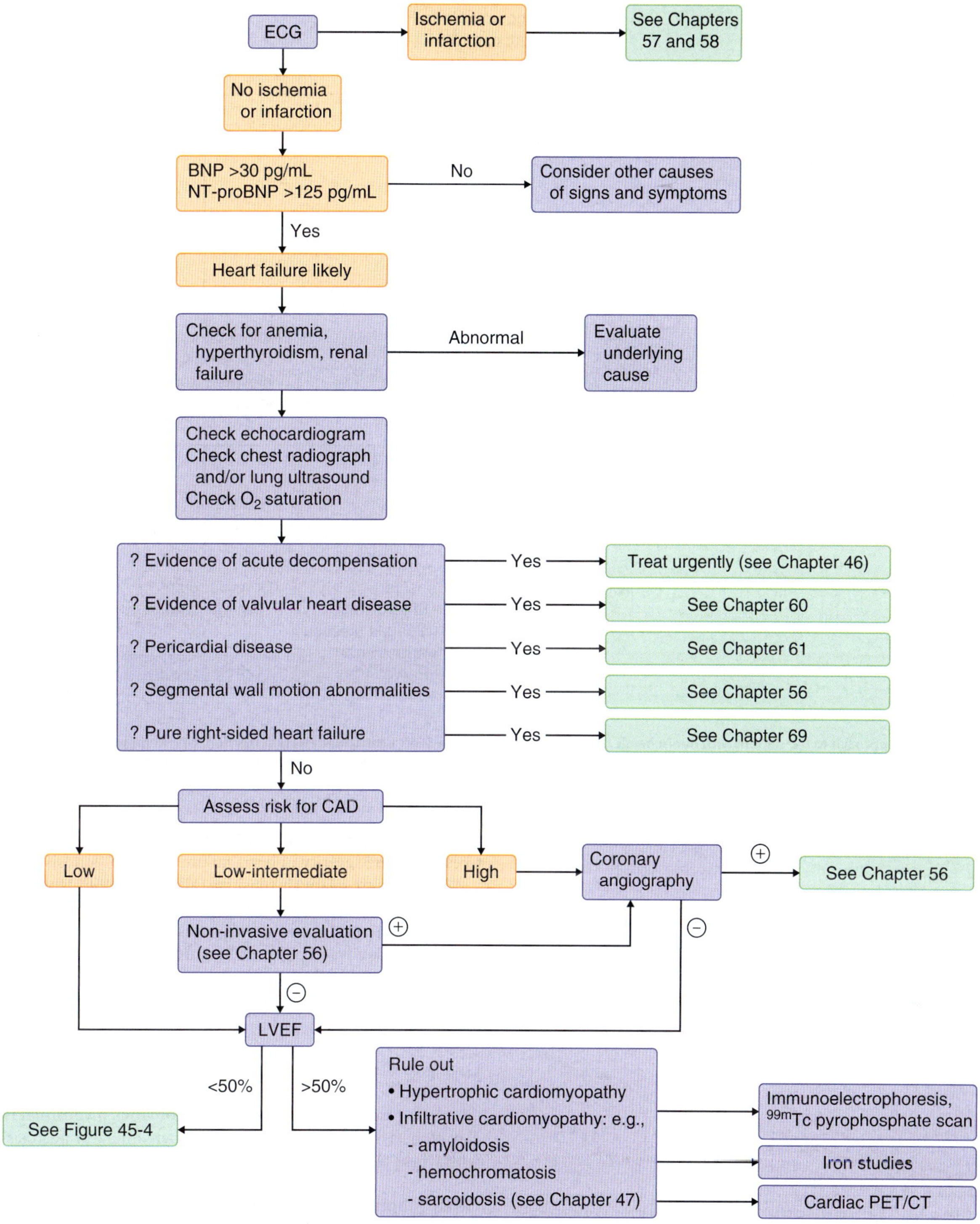

FIGURE 45-3. **Diagnostic approach to the patient with suspected heart failure.** BNP = brain natriuretic peptide; CAD = coronary artery disease; CT = computed tomographic scan; ECG = electrocardiogram; LVEF = left ventricular ejection fraction; NT-proBNP = N-terminal pro-B-type natriuretic peptide; PET = positron emission tomography.

Chest Radiography

Patients with suspected new-onset or worsening heart failure should undergo chest radiography to assess heart size and pulmonary congestion as well as to detect other diseases that may cause or contribute to the patient's symptoms. Many patients with acute heart failure but only a minority of those with chronic heart failure have clear evidence of pulmonary venous hypertension (upper lobe vascular redistribution, enlarged pulmonary veins) or pulmonary edema (perihilar or patchy peripheral infiltrates; see Fig. 44-2). Pleural effusions, usually on the right if unilateral but often bilateral, are also identified on the chest radiograph (see Fig. 86-3). Chest radiography may also play a role in identifying the location of the lead placement of intracardiac devices, such as biventricular pacemakers. Inappropriate lead placement may be observed in patients with worsening heart failure symptoms.

Laboratory Testing

The initial evaluation of patients presenting with heart failure should include a complete blood count to detect anemia and systemic diseases with hematologic manifestations; urinalysis and tests of renal function to assess underlying renal disease; serum electrolyte values to identify abnormalities needing treatment and to provide a baseline for subsequent therapy; glucose level and lipid profile to diagnose diabetes and dyslipidemia, which should be carefully managed in patients with heart failure; and thyroid-stimulating hormone level. Markers of hepatic congestion, such as elevated serum aminotransferase and bilirubin levels (Chapter 133), also should be measured because they have prognostic importance. Screening for hemochromatosis (Chapter 196) or human immunodeficiency virus (HIV) infection is reasonable in selected patients with heart failure. Diagnostic tests for rheumatologic diseases (Chapter 236), amyloidosis (Chapter 174), or pheochromocytoma (Chapter 209) are

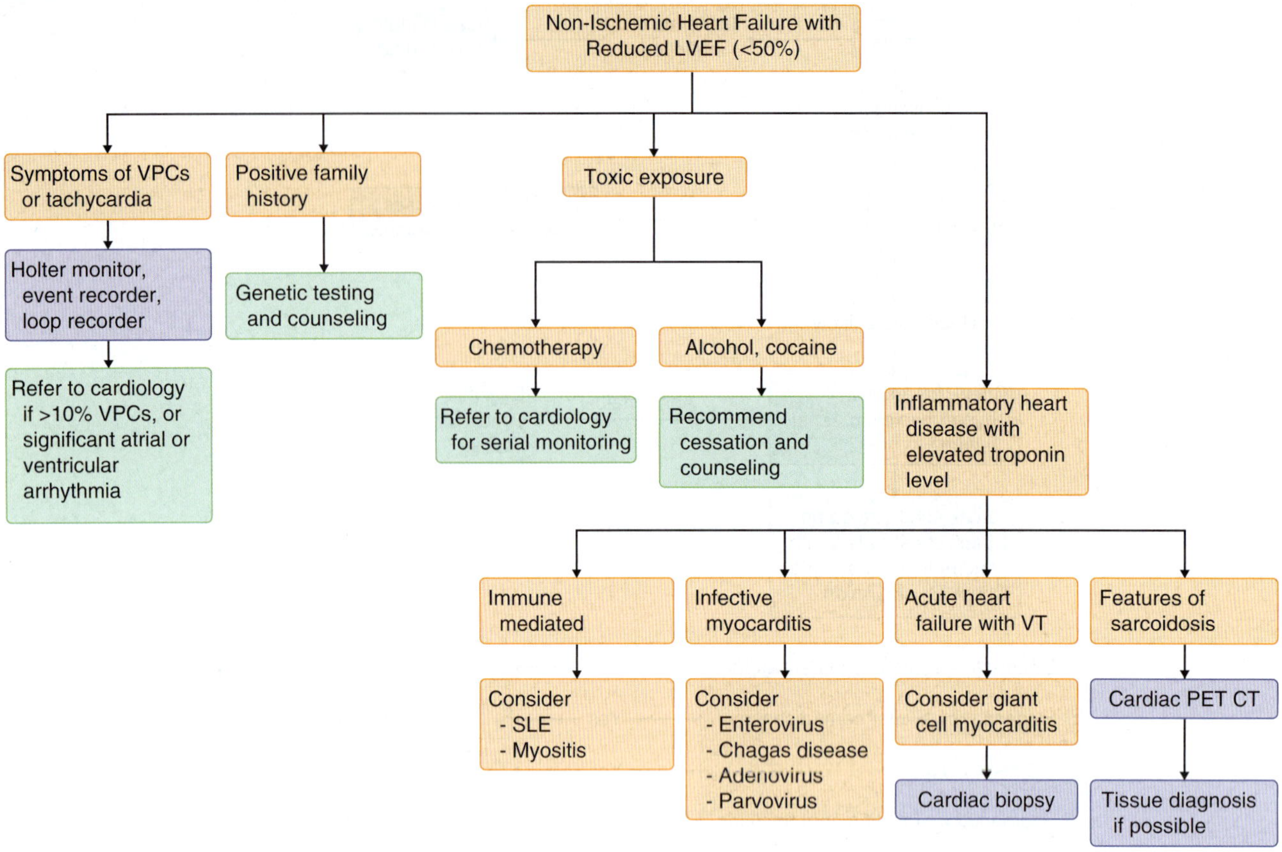

FIGURE 45-4. Diagnostic approach to the patient with nonischemic heart failure and a reduced left ventricular ejection fraction. CT = computed tomographic scan; LVEF = left ventricular ejection fraction; PET = positron emission tomography; SLE = systemic lupus erythematosus; VPC = ventricular premature contraction; VT = ventricular tachycardia.

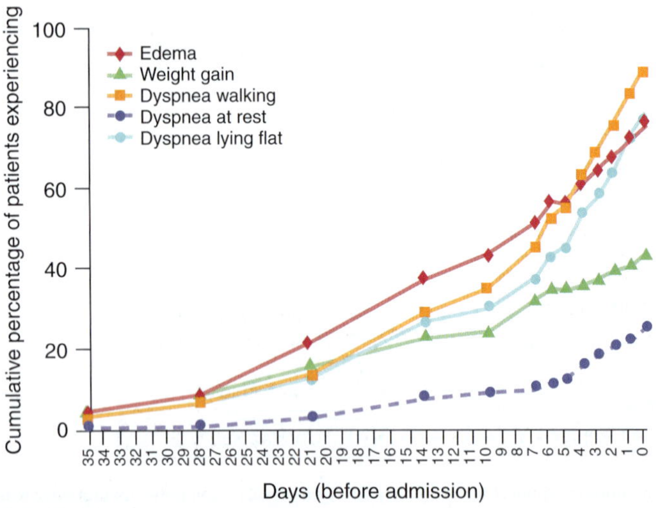

FIGURE 45-5. Number of days from onset of worsening of selected symptoms of heart failure to admission to the hospital: cumulative percentage of patients. (From Schiff GD, Fung S, Speroff T, et al. Decompensated heart failure: symptoms, patterns of onset, and contributing factors. *Am J Med.* 2003;114:625-630.)

not routinely indicated but rather should be targeted to patients with other ancillary findings suggestive of these conditions. Viral antibody titers yield relatively little incremental information and are rarely indicated in the evaluation of heart failure.

Natriuretic Peptides

Brain natriuretic peptide (BNP) and its amino-terminal fragment (NT-proBNP) provide incremental diagnostic and prognostic information above and beyond the history and physical examination in patients with heart failure. A natriuretic peptide level should be measured to support the diagnosis of heart failure in ambulatory patients with dyspnea, as well as in patients with possible acute heart failure, especially in the setting of an uncertain diagnosis. It also is useful to estimate the severity of heart failure and its prognosis.

BNP levels are relatively sensitive (about 95 to 99%) but less specific (about 50 to 60%) markers for diagnosing clinically confirmed heart failure. Circulating levels are influenced by comorbid processes. For example, obesity reduces BNP levels, whereas advancing age and renal dysfunction are associated with higher levels. Most heart failure therapies reduce BNP levels, but the usefulness of BNP-guided heart failure therapy is not well established.[A3,A4]

Troponin

Owing to the increased sensitivity of currently available troponin assays, the majority of patients admitted with acute heart failure have elevations in circulating troponin even without any obvious myocardial ischemia. These elevations, which suggest ongoing myocyte injury or necrosis, are associated with worse clinical outcomes and mortality.[19]

Other Biomarkers: Galectin-3 and ST2

A number of additional biomarkers characterize inflammation, myocyte injury, neurohormonal upregulation, and extracellular matrix turnover in patients with heart failure (E-Table 45-1). In the future, strategies that combine multiple biomarkers into a risk stratification model may prove additive to clinical judgment.

Echocardiography

An echocardiogram should be obtained during the initial evaluation of patients with heart failure to assess ventricular and valvular function. Repeated echocardiograms are also indicated when patients have a significant change in their clinical status or receive treatment that may have had a significant effect on cardiac function. In contrast, routine repeated measurements of left ventricular function in the absence of a change in clinical status or treatment should not be performed.

Echocardiography (Chapter 43) allows the assessment of systolic and diastolic ventricular function (see Figs. 43-2 and 43-3). Wall thickness, chamber size, and regional wall motion abnormalities provide evidence of the underlying etiology of heart failure with a diminished or preserved ejection fraction.[20] Echocardiography also evaluates valvular dysfunction (Chapter 60), which may be the result of or cause worsening ventricular function or symptoms. Quantitative measurements of pulmonary artery pressure and central venous pressure help characterize the degree of pulmonary hypertension and may guide diuretic therapies in circumstances in which the jugular veins are difficult to visualize. Detection of atrial or ventricular thrombi requires anticoagulation. Novel methods using ventricular strain analysis and three-dimensional echocardiography can provide additional insights about myocardial performance.

Point-of-Care Ultrasound

Point-of-care ultrasonography has gained increasing acceptance as a noninvasive tool for the detection and quantification of jugular venous distention[21] and pulmonary congestion[22] in both ambulatory and hospitalized patients with potential heart failure. However, adding ultrasound to the standard clinical evaluation has not been shown to reduce admission rates or mortality, although it may reduce future urgent visits for worsening symptoms.[A5]

Nuclear Cardiology and Coronary Angiography

Significant coronary artery disease is common in adults with heart failure and should prompt careful evaluation for ischemia, which is common not only in patients who have heart failure with a reduced ejection fraction but is also found (either as epicardial stenosis or microvascular dysfunction) in about 90% of patients who have heart failure with a preserved ejection fraction[23] (Chapters 39, 43, 44, and 56). When myocardial ischemia may be contributing to heart failure, coronary arteriography (Chapter 59) is reasonable to assess eligibility for revascularization.

The most powerful predictors of prognosis for patients with ischemic cardiomyopathy are a history of prior myocardial infarction, stenosis of 75% or greater of the left main or proximal left anterior descending artery, stenosis of 75% or greater of two or more epicardial vessels, and the severity of ventricular dysfunction. Coronary computed tomographic angiography (Chapter 44) may represent a noninvasive modality for assessing coronary disease in appropriately selected patients.

Noninvasive imaging (Chapter 44) to detect myocardial ischemia and viability is reasonable in patients who present with de novo heart failure and in patients who have known coronary artery disease and no angina, unless they are not eligible for revascularization. Viability assessment is reasonable in select situations in planning revascularization for patients who have heart failure and coronary artery disease.[24] However, stress testing to assess myocardial viability so far has not been able to identify patients who will benefit from revascularization compared with medical therapy alone.

For suspected cardiac transthyretin amyloidosis (Chapters 47 and 174), which is responsible for about 6% of cases of heart failure with a preserved ejection fraction,[25] a ^{99m}Tc-pyrophosphate scan is highly sensitive and specific. Typical findings avoid the need for a confirmatory biopsy.[26]

The single-photon emission computed tomography tracer *m*-iodobenzylguanidine (mIBG) has been widely used for studying causes and effects of cardiac sympathetic hyperactivity. Cardiac sympathetic imaging with mIBG is a noninvasive tool that may assist with the risk stratification of patients with heart failure. With mIBG imaging, the myocardial uptake and distribution can be visually assessed and quantified by calculating a heart-to-mediastinum ratio. This approach provides a highly reproducible index of cardiac sympathetic activity. Further study is required to determine the role of this imaging modality in heart failure risk stratification and clinical care.

Cardiac Magnetic Resonance Imaging

Cardiac magnetic resonance imaging (Chapter 44) provides accurate measurements of left ventricular volume and ejection fraction, and it is useful when echocardiography is inadequate. It is also helpful to assess for potential infiltrative cardiomyopathies when the cause of heart failure, especially heart failure with a preserved ejection fraction, is unclear. Late gadolinium enhancement (see Fig. 44-16) adds important prognostic information related to the risks of ventricular arrhythmias and mortality.

Myocardial Biopsy

Guidelines indicate that endomyocardial biopsy should not be performed in the routine evaluation of patients with heart failure. However, endomyocardial biopsy may be useful in patients who present with heart failure when a specific suspected diagnosis would influence therapy. For example, in patients with acute myocarditis or giant cell myocarditis and in patients with sarcoid or amyloid cardiomyopathy (Chapter 47), the appropriate pathologic diagnosis may inform treatment recommendations and prognosis. In certain circumstances, biopsy may be performed along with genetic testing (e.g., transthyretin gene mutation) to inform decisions on management and counseling of family members.

Assessment of Exercise Capacity

A heart failure patient's exercise capacity can be quantified by several testing modalities, including 6-minute walk distance and cardiopulmonary exercise testing (Chapter 73). Although these tests are not routinely recommended, they are helpful for determining the relative contribution of cardiac compared with pulmonary causes of functional limitation. The results of cardiopulmonary exercise testing are critical to determine candidacy for heart transplantation or placement of a ventricular assist device (Chapter 46). A maximal oxygen consumption of less than 14 mL/kg/minute is associated with a sufficiently poor prognosis that transplantation or implantation of a left ventricular assist device is warranted. Serial cardiopulmonary exercise testing, the 6-minute walk test, or the 60-foot walk test also can be useful to follow the disease course of specific patients objectively.

Invasive Diagnostics and Hemodynamic Monitoring

Invasive monitoring may be useful in selected patients who have acute heart failure, who have persistent symptoms despite adjustment of standard therapies, and whose fluid status or perfusion is uncertain. However, the routine use of pulmonary artery catheters should be discouraged.

Up to 30% of patients with heart failure with a reduced ejection fraction have an implantable device that detects arrhythmias and can provide hemodynamic assessment. Indirect measures, such as changes in impedance or heart rate variability, are precursors to worsening heart failure symptoms. Chronic hemodynamic monitors (i.e., direct measures of pulmonary pressures and right ventricular pressures) have been approved by the U.S. Food and Drug Administration and are now available for the serial measurement of left ventricular filling pressure surrogates. Interrogation of these devices may become part of the routine diagnostic follow-up to guide therapy[27] in patients who have respiratory distress or clinical evidence of impaired perfusion in whom the adequacy or excess of intracardiac filling pressures cannot be determined by clinical assessment.

CONSEQUENCES OF MISDIAGNOSIS

The diagnosis of heart failure may be straightforward in a patient with dyspnea, signs of congestion, and an elevated BNP level. Conversely, many patients have multiple comorbid conditions that make the assessment of shortness of breath a diagnostic dilemma. Pulmonary conditions such as chronic obstructive pulmonary disease (Chapter 76) represent the most common reason for misdiagnosis. The BNP level and echocardiogram provide useful information to make this distinction. Other potential causes of edema or volume overload include renal failure (Chapter 117), venous thrombosis (Chapter 68), and venous insufficiency. If left ventricular systolic function is normal, it may be difficult to make a conclusive determination of the relative role of heart failure with preserved ejection fraction compared with other concomitant conditions, such as pericardial constriction, severe obesity, deconditioning, chronic anemia, or other systemic illnesses. BNP levels may be helpful in some circumstances. In other situations, exercise testing or invasive hemodynamic testing may be necessary to establish the appropriate diagnosis. Misdiagnosis can result in excessive and unnecessary diagnostic testing, higher costs, and increased morbidity and mortality because of the inappropriate use or nonuse of heart failure therapies.

GENERAL REFERENCES

For the General References and other additional features, please visit Elsevier eBooks+ at https://ebooks.health.elsevier.com.

Grade A References

A1. Voigt J, Emani S, Gupta S, et al. Meta-analysis comparing outcomes of therapies for patients with central sleep apnea and heart failure with reduced ejection fraction. *Am J Cardiol.* 2020;127:73-83.

A2. Cowie MR, Woehrle H, Wegscheider K, et al. Adaptive servo-ventilation for central sleep apnea in systolic heart failure. *N Engl J Med.* 2015;373:1095-1105.

A3. McLellan J, Bankhead CR, Oke JL, et al. Natriuretic peptide-guided treatment for heart failure: a systematic review and meta-analysis. *BMJ Evid Based Med.* 2020;25:33-37.

A4. Stienen S, Salah K, Moons AH, et al. NT-proBNP (N-terminal pro-B-type natriuretic peptide)-guided therapy in acute decompensated heart failure: PRIMA II randomized controlled trial (can NT-proBNP-guided therapy during hospital admission for acute decompensated heart failure reduce mortality and readmissions?). *Circulation.* 2018;137:1671-1683.

A5. Mhanna M, Beran A, Nazir S, et al. Lung ultrasound-guided management to reduce hospitalization in chronic heart failure: a systematic review and meta-analysis. *Heart Fail Rev.* 2022;27:821-826.

46

HEART FAILURE: TREATMENT AND PROGNOSIS

JOHN J.V. MCMURRAY AND MARC A. PFEFFER

EVALUATION AND MANAGEMENT OF HEART FAILURE

Heart failure is an overarching term for a syndrome (i.e., a constellation of signs and symptoms) that encompasses a vast spectrum of cardiovascular disorders and is associated with a greatly heightened risk for death and nonfatal adverse cardiovascular events (Chapter 45). Treatment is initially directed toward prevention of cardiac injury (e.g., due to hypertension or myocardial infarction) or toward limiting structural progression if cardiac damage has already occurred (e.g., left ventricular remodeling with declining left ventricular ejection fraction) and delaying the development of symptomatic heart failure. When symptoms develop, treatments are also directed at improving functional status as well as prognosis.

At least one in five adults will develop heart failure. In the United States, 6.5 million people have heart failure, and 1.25 million patients are discharged from U.S. hospitals annually with a primary diagnosis of heart failure.[1] The estimated cost of heart failure in the United States exceeds $30 billion per year. Randomized controlled clinical trials (RCTs) supply the framework for quantifying what different therapeutic approaches can offer. Even when they are definitive, RCTs generate data only about average risks and benefits of the tested therapeutic option in a selected cohort. Because an individual patient's responses can only be inferred from the overall estimated group responses, RCTs cannot definitively direct the approach of every patient or answer the myriad questions that confront the practitioner regarding the specific circumstances of the patient. Another major limitation of RCTs is the relatively narrow time frame of observation, generally only months to several years, compared with epidemiologic experiences during decades. Despite these limitations, RCTs are the premier tool of evidence-based medicine, and the field of heart failure has fortunately been the focus of relatively high-quality RCTs that have provided robust evidence to improve clinical care and prognosis (Table 46-1). Indeed, the implementation of evidence from RCTs into clinical practice has resulted in impressive temporal improvements in survival after discharge from a first hospital admission for heart failure. Moreover, the age at which symptomatic heart failure first becomes evident has increased. Despite these tangible advances, heart failure continues to be a leading cause of morbidity and mortality in elderly people.

STAGES OF HEART FAILURE

Guidelines for the evaluation and management of chronic heart failure use a staging classification to underscore the evolution and progression of heart failure severity (Fig. 46-1).[2,3] This classification emphasizes the use of different strategies and therapeutic options across the full spectrum of the syndrome, from prevention of heart failure to palliation of patients with end-stage disease.

TABLE 46-1 THERAPIES OF PROVEN BENEFIT IN HEART FAILURE

Angiotensin-converting enzyme inhibitors
Angiotensin receptor blockers
β-Blockers
Mineralocorticoid receptor antagonists
Sacubitril-valsartan
Sodium-glucose cotransporter 2 inhibitors
Hydralazine-isosorbide dinitrate
Ivabradine
Digitalis
Vericiguat
Cardiac resynchronization therapy
Cardioverter-defibrillator
Ventricular assist device
Heart transplantation
Exercise training

INDIVIDUALS AT RISK FOR DEVELOPMENT OF HEART FAILURE (STAGE A)

Stage A designates patients at risk for development of heart failure based on concomitant cardiovascular diseases such as hypertension, coronary artery disease, and diabetes mellitus. Also included in stage A are individuals with prior exposure to cardiotoxic agents such as doxorubicin (Chapter 164) and those with a family history of a cardiomyopathy (Chapter 47). Although these predisposing factors do not by themselves technically constitute the syndrome of heart failure, the guidelines stress the importance of identifying individuals with modifiable factors because this represents an important opportunity to reduce the reservoir of patients at risk.

Population-based preventive approaches can reduce the incidence of heart failure. For example, public health programs targeting the eradication of the insect vector for *Trypanosoma cruzi* (Chapter 318) have reduced the incidence of Chagas cardiomyopathy (Chapter 47) in endemic regions of South and Central America.

Other population-based approaches to reduce the incidence of heart failure require specific screening efforts to identify individuals with modifiable risk factors. The most important, although unfortunately nonmodifiable, risk factor for the development of heart failure is advanced age; the incidence of heart failure rises sharply per decade after the age of 45 years (Chapter 45). For each decade of age after 45 years, the incidence of heart failure doubles, and heart failure is the leading hospital diagnosis for patients older than 65 years in the United States.

HYPERTENSION

Of the modifiable factors, hypertension (Chapter 64) undoubtedly contributes the greatest population-attributable risk for heart failure. In other words, even though the increased risk for heart failure in an individual with hypertension is modest, the high prevalence of hypertension in the general population means that at a population level, hypertension is the major cause of heart failure.

The contribution of hypertension to the risk for heart failure was a consistent finding from all major cardiovascular epidemiologic studies, and the earliest RCTs of antihypertensive therapy showed unambiguous reductions in the risk for heart failure. Of the components of blood pressure, elevated systolic pressure has a greater influence on the incidence of heart failure than does diastolic pressure. In fact, aging is associated with a progressive rise in systolic blood pressure and fall in diastolic pressure as the compliance of the arterial tree diminishes (Chapter 64). In community-based studies, isolated systolic hypertension and elevated pulse pressure have been the most predictive blood pressure measurements for development of heart failure. Antihypertensive treatment to a systolic blood pressure goal of 130 mm Hg appears to reduce the risk of developing heart failure.[A1] Reduction to lower than 120 mm Hg systolic provides additional benefit for reducing nonfatal cardiovascular events and all-cause mortality in patients without diabetes or prior heart failure,[A2] but at the cost of more hypotension, electrolyte abnormalities, and renal impairment. The current blood pressure goal is lower than 120 mm Hg for selected patients at high cardiovascular risk without diabetes or prior heart failure and lower than 130 mm Hg otherwise (Chapter 64).

DIABETES

Individuals with diabetes (Chapter 210) are also at heightened risk for premature cardiovascular mortality and morbidity, including heart failure. Type 2 diabetes frequently clusters with hypertension, obesity, and a sedentary lifestyle, thereby exacerbating the risks associated with each condition. However, the glucose level is an independent risk factor for cardiovascular events, including heart failure. Unlike hypertension, where pharmacologic therapy has had a generally favorable impact on reducing the risk of heart failure, historically, glucose-lowering therapy has not been shown to reduce this risk. However, sodium-glucose cotransporter 2 (SGLT2) inhibitors (e.g., dapagliflozin 10 mg daily; Chapter 210) reduce the risk of heart failure hospitalization in patients with type 2 diabetes and cardiovascular risk factors, preexisting cardiovascular disease, or chronic kidney disease (Chapter 116) with or without type 2 diabetes.[A3] The glucagon-like peptide-1 (GLP-1) receptor agonists may also reduce the risk of developing heart failure,[A4] but not to the extent seen with SGLT2 inhibitors.[A5] The α-glucosidase inhibitor acarbose, insulin, and the meglitinide nateglinide do not increase the risk of developing heart failure in patients with impaired glucose tolerance, diabetes, or both.[A6] An increase in risk of heart failure was reported with saxagliptin, although this increased risk has not been seen with other dipeptidyl peptidase-4 (DPP-4) inhibitors.[4]

By comparison, thiazolidinediones cause retention of sodium and water and should not be used in patients at risk for developing heart failure.

Trials

Therapy	Stage A	Stage B	Stage C	Stage D
Antihypertensive agents	✓	✓	✓	
Statins	✓	✓	(✓)	(✓)
β-blockers		✓	✓	✓
ACE inhibitors	✓	✓	✓	✓
Angiotensin II receptor blockers (ARBs)		✓	✓	✓
Sodium glucose cotransporter 2 inhibitors (SGLT2i)	✓	✓	✓	
Hydralazine/ nitrates			✓	✓
ARNI			✓	✓
Digoxin			✓	✓
Ivabradine			✓	✓
Mineralocorticoid antagonists			✓	✓
Implantable cardioverter-defibrillator (ICD)		✓	✓	(✓)
Cardiac resynchronization therapy (CRT)			✓	✓
Left ventricle assist device (LVAD)				✓

Stage A	Stage B	Stage C	Stage D
High risk for HF without structural heart disease or symptoms of HF	Structural heart disease but without signs or symptoms of HF	Structural heart disease with prior or current symptoms of HF	Refractory HF requiring specialized interventions
Patients with • Hypertension • Atherosclerotic disease • Diabetes • Obesity • Metabolic syndrome or • Patients using cardiotoxins with family history of cardiomyopathy (FHx CM)	Patients with • Previous MI • LV remodeling including LVH and low EF • Asymptomatic valvular disease	Patients with • Known structural heart disease • Shortness of breath and fatigue, reduced exercise tolerance	Patients with marked symptoms at rest despite maximal medical therapy (e.g., those who are recurrently hospitalized or cannot be safely discharged from the hospital without specialized interventions)

THERAPY
Goals
• Treat hypertension
• Encourage smoking cessation
• Treat lipid disorders
• Encourage regular exercise
• Discourage alcohol intake, illicit drug use
• Control metabolic syndrome
Drugs
• ACE inhibitor or ARB as appropriate for patients with vascular disease or diabetes
• SGLT2i in patients with type 2 diabetes
	THERAPY
	Goals
	• Treat hypertension
	• Encourage smoking cessation
	• Treat lipid disorders
	• Encourage regular exercise
	• Discourage alcohol intake, illicit drug use
	• Control metabolic syndrome
	Drugs
	• ACE inhibitor or ARB as appropriate for patients with vascular disease or diabetes
	• β-blockers in appropriate patients
	• SGLT2i in patients with type 2 diabetes
	Devices in selected patients
	• Implantable defibrillators
		THERAPY
		Goals
		• Treat hypertension
		• Encourage smoking cessation
		• Treat lipid disorders
		• Encourage regular exercise
		• Discourage alcohol intake, illicit drug use
		• Control metabolic syndrome
		• Dietary salt restriction
		Drugs for routine use
		• Diuretics for fluid retention
		• ACE inhibitor or ARNI
		• β-blockers
		• Mineralocorticoid antagonists
		• SGLT2i
		Drugs in selected patients
		• ARBs
		• Digitalis
		• Hydralazine/nitrates
		• Ivabradine
		Device in selected patients
		• Biventricular pacing (CRT)
		• Implantable defibrillators
			THERAPY
			Goals
			• Appropriate measures under stages A,B,C
			• Decision re: appropriate level of care
			Options
			• Compassionate end-of-life care/hospice
			• Extraordinary measures
			  • Heart transplantation
			  • Chronic inotropes
			  • Permanent mechanical support
			  • Experimental surgery or drugs

FIGURE 46-1. **Stages of heart failure and therapies at various stages of heart failure (HF). Check marks indicate therapies proved by randomized trials to be beneficial; check marks in brackets indicate benefits uncertain.** ACEI = angiotensin converting enzyme inhibitor; ARB = angiotensin receptor blocker; ARNI = angiotensin receptor/neprilysin inhibitor; CRT = cardiac resynchronization therapy; EF = ejection fraction; FHx CM = family history of cardiomyopathy; HF = heart failure; LV = left ventricle; LVH = left ventricular hypertrophy; MI = myocardial infarction; SGLT2i = sodium glucose cotransporter 2 inhibitors.

OTHER RISK FACTORS

Treatment of atherosclerotic risk factors, such as hypercholesterolemia (Chapter 190), and promotion of measures that encourage healthier lifestyles, such as smoking cessation (Chapter 363), weight control (Chapter 201), adoption of a Mediterranean diet (Chapter 13), and aerobic exercise (Chapter 14), should also reduce the number of individuals who progress from stage A to stage B (structural heart disease but without symptoms of heart failure). ACE inhibitors and SGLT2 inhibitors protect against the development of heart failure in patients with diabetes mellitus or with evidence of atherosclerosis. Elevated natriuretic peptide levels and elevated troponin levels may help identify patients with an elevated risk of developing heart failure.

Many anticancer drugs can cause myocardial damage and heart failure, as can mediastinal radiotherapy. Pericardial constriction can be a result of previous radiotherapy, and malignant pericardial involvement can cause effusion and tamponade (Chapter 62).

PRE–HEART FAILURE (STAGE B): ASYMPTOMATIC STRUCTURAL OR FUNCTIONAL HEART DISEASE

Stage B identifies asymptomatic (New York Heart Association or Canadian Cardiovascular Society class I; Chapter 45) patients who have a structural or functional cardiac disorder (e.g., left ventricular hypertrophy, enlargement, or dysfunction and valvar abnormalities) but do not have the signs and symptoms, such as dyspnea and fatigue, of the heart failure syndrome. In addition to history, physical examination, and electrocardiography (Chapter 42), more extensive screening with echocardiography (Chapter 43) or other imaging modalities (Chapter 44) is often required to detect patients with asymptomatic cardiac structural abnormalities.

A patient who has an acute myocardial infarction not complicated by early heart failure is an obvious example of someone who transitions from stage A to stage B. Rapid mechanical or pharmacologic coronary reperfusion is one of the immediate goals of therapy, with the aim of limiting the extent of myocardial injury and reducing the risk for death and future development of heart failure (Chapters 57 and 58). Survivors of the acute phase of myocardial infarction, a well-studied stage B cohort, are at particularly high risk for the future development of heart failure, with an overall annual incidence of 2% per year—but higher in patients who are older, have a lower left ventricular ejection fraction, do not routinely perform at least moderate exercise, or have concomitant hypertension or diabetes mellitus. For example, a clinically stable asymptomatic patient who has recovered from a myocardial infarction but who is older than 60 years with a left ventricular ejection fraction of less than 50% and a history of diabetes and hypertension has an estimated 30% 5-year likelihood of experiencing death or heart failure; without diabetes or hypertension, the 5-year estimated rate becomes 12%. By comparison, a younger myocardial infarction survivor who has a left ventricular ejection fraction over 50% and does not have hypertension or diabetes would be anticipated to have a 5-year rate for heart failure or death of only 3%. Measures of right ventricular function and biomarkers such as natriuretic peptides and troponin provide further independent incremental prediction for the risk for developing heart failure. With the continued improvements in care of patients with acute myocardial infarction (Chapters 57 and 58) and the use of implantable cardioverter-defibrillators (ICDs) after myocardial infarction in patients with reduced left ventricular ejection fraction, this pool of stage B patients, who represent a reservoir for new-onset heart failure, has been expanding. An ICD is recommended in patients who have a left ventricular ejection fraction of 30% or less and who survive at least 40 days after an acute myocardial infarction to reduce the risk for death (Chapter 58).

The impaired left ventricle, often due to a prior myocardial infarction, can undergo progressive chamber enlargement. This process, also termed left ventricular remodeling, describes the time-dependent and often insidious structural alterations of the impaired left ventricle, whereby the relationship of the left ventricular cavity volume increases out of proportion to mass, so the overall ventricular geometry becomes more distorted, usually more spherical. This distortion of left ventricular geometry often leads to mitral regurgitation. These structural changes produce regional and global increases in myocardial wall stress, which can promote further remodeling and contribute to the progressive deterioration of cardiac function and structure often associated with the later stages of symptomatic heart failure.

TREATMENT

The treatment of heart failure is guided by the stage of symptoms and signs (see Fig. 46-1) as well as a robust literature on therapies proved to be beneficial by randomized trials (Fig. 46-2).[5]

Angiotensin-Converting Enzyme Inhibitors and Angiotensin Receptor Blockers

Mechanistic studies confirm that ACE inhibitors inhibit progressive left ventricular enlargement by reducing wall stress during the entire cardiac cycle as well as by more direct inhibition of the intracellular signaling pathways involved in myocardial hypertrophy and interstitial fibrosis. This attenuation of ventricular remodeling by ACE inhibitors reduces the development of symptomatic heart failure or death, including sudden and unexpected deaths, in stage B asymptomatic patients with left ventricular dysfunction by about 20%.

Several ACE inhibitors are effective as prophylactic therapy for high-risk stage B patients, and the target dose of each agent is established (Table 46-2). Therefore, patients with left ventricular systolic dysfunction, heart failure, or both complicating acute myocardial infarction should receive an ACE inhibitor to reduce the risk for chronic heart failure, reinfarction, stroke, and death. The angiotensin receptor blocker (ARB) valsartan is as effective as captopril in reducing risk for cardiovascular death and other nonfatal cardiovascular outcomes, thereby providing an alternative pharmacologic class of agents for patients who cannot tolerate an ACE inhibitor because of cough or angioedema. Importantly, in patients with left ventricular dysfunction or acute heart failure in the context of a myocardial infarction, the combination of an ACE inhibitor and ARB is not better than either alone, so combination therapy is not recommended in this setting. Unlike in stage C heart failure, sacubitril/valsartan is not clearly superior to an ACE inhibitor.[A7]

β-Blockers

β-Adrenergic receptor blockers (β-blockers) have long been known to reduce death and recurrent myocardial infarction when they are administered during the acute phase of myocardial infarction in patients without pulmonary congestion (Chapter 58). However, carvedilol (Table 46-3) also improves survival, reduces subsequent nonfatal myocardial infarctions, and has a favorable trend for reduced hospitalizations for heart failure in patients with a recent myocardial infarction and reduced left ventricular ejection fraction (≤40%) when it is added to an ACE inhibitor and should be considered in such patients. For stage B patients whose left ventricular dysfunction does not have an ischemic etiology, the evidence for β-blockers is less firm.

Treatment of Arrhythmias

Functional as well as structural problems may lead to the development of heart failure. For example, a persistently rapid ventricular rate in patients with atrial fibrillation can cause a rate-related (tachycardia-induced) cardiomyopathy (Chapter 52). Adequate pharmacologic control of the ventricular rate or interventions to restore sinus rhythm or to ablate re-entry pathways (Chapter 54) may reduce the risk for heart failure.

Other Therapies

Any treatments that control hypertension or reduce the risk for myocardial infarction will benefit stage B patients. Examples include statins, antiplatelet agents, and smoking cessation. Sodium glucose cotransporter 2 (SGLT2) inhibitors also reduce the risk that patients with type 2 diabetes, established cardiovascular disease, or chronic kidney disease will develop heart failure.

SYMPTOMATIC HEART FAILURE (STAGES C AND D)

The development of symptoms and signs of the heart failure syndrome defines the transition from patients in the asymptomatic "at-risk" stages (A and B) to those who fulfill the clinical diagnosis of symptomatic heart failure (Chapter 45). This transition to the symptomatic phase underscores the progressive nature of heart failure and heralds a marked decline in prognosis. In one study, for example, the 2-year mortality rate was 27% in symptomatic patients compared with 10% in asymptomatic patients despite similarly reduced left ventricular ejection fractions and comorbidities.

HEART FAILURE PHENOTYPES BASED ON LEFT VENTRICULAR EJECTION FRACTION

Patients with heart failure are divided into three main categories defined by their left ventricular ejection fraction: heart failure with a reduced ejection fraction (HFrEF, ≤40%),[6] mildly reduced ejection fraction (HFmrEF, 41% to 49%),[7] or preserved ejection fraction (HFpEF, ≥50%).[8] Some patients with an ejection fraction ≤40% have a follow-up measurement >40%, often as a result of treatment. This fourth group of patients are said to have heart failure with improved ejection fraction (HFimpEF). Strong evidence helps guide the treatment of patients who have heart failure with a reduced ejection fraction, but less robust evidence is available for the other subtypes of heart failure.

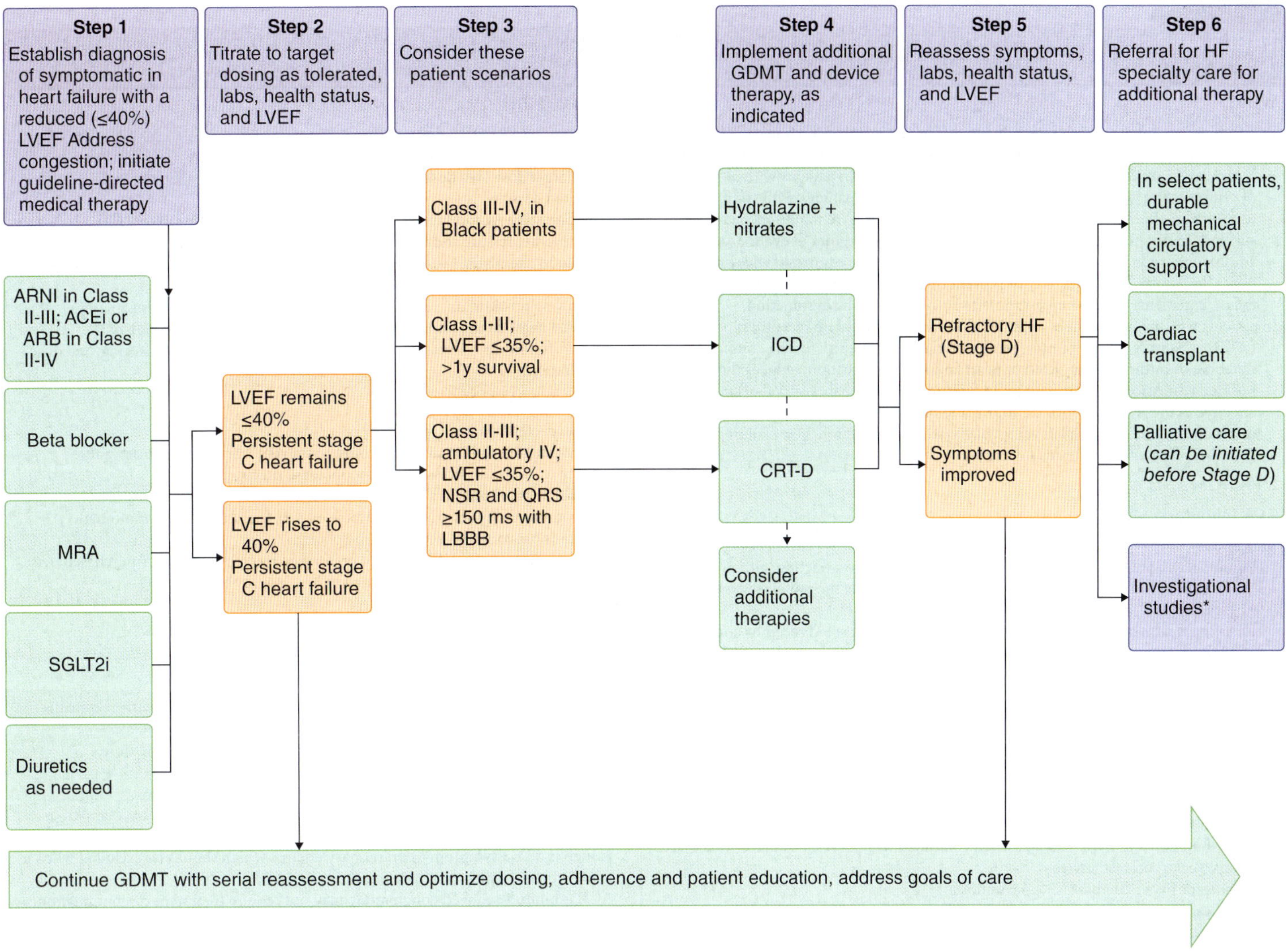

FIGURE 46-2. **General approach to stage C heart failure with a reduced ejection fraction.** *Participation in investigational studies is appropriate for stage C, NYHA class II and III heart failure (HF). ACEI = angiotensin-converting enzyme inhibitor; ARB = angiotensin-receptor blocker; ARNI = angiotensin receptor-neprilysin inhibitor; CRT-D = cardiac resynchronization therapy with defibrillator; eGFR = estimated glomerular filtration rate; GDMT = guideline-directed medical therapy; HR = heart rate; ICD = implantable cardiovascular-defibrillator; LBBB = left bundle branch block; LVEF = left ventricular ejection fraction; MRA = mineralocorticoid receptor antagonist; NSR = normal sinus rhythm; SGLT2i = sodium glucose cotransporter 2 inhibitor. (From Heidenreich PA, Bozkurt B, Aguilar D, et al. 2022 AHA/ACC/HFSA guideline for the management of heart failure: a report of the American College of Cardiology/American Heart Association Joint Committee on Clinical Practice Guidelines. *Circulation*. 2022;145:e895-e1032.)

TREATMENT

The goals of treatment for patients with stage C and stage D heart failure are relief of symptoms, avoidance of hospital admission or other manifestations of worsening heart failure, and prevention of premature death. In general, the preventive measures that are of value during stages A and B should be sustained in patients with stages C and D heart failure.

Heart Failure with Reduced Left Ventricular Ejection Fraction

Pharmacologic Treatment

Drugs are the mainstay of the treatment of patients with symptomatic heart failure on the basis of the cumulative experiences from RCTs, particularly for patients with reduced left ventricular ejection fraction.[9] However, devices and surgery have an important and increasing role in patients with advanced symptomatic heart failure (stages C and D; see Fig. 46-1). Exercise clearly improves well-being and clinical outcomes, but the evidence base for other lifestyle interventions is less robust. The organization and delivery of care can also have a substantial impact on outcomes.

Although diuretics are required to control fluid retention in most patients who have symptomatic heart failure with a reduced ejection fraction, four other life-saving foundational therapies should be prescribed in any order for all patients, wherever possible: an angiotensin receptor neprilysin inhibitor, a β-blocker, a mineralocorticoid receptor antagonist, and a sodium-glucose cotransporter 2 (SGLT2) inhibitor. The key principles guiding the use of these therapies are that all should be initiated as quickly as possible, usually starting at low doses, and up-titrated to the evidence-based target (see later).

Diuretics

MECHANISM OF ACTION. Conventional diuretics (see Table 102-4 in Chapter 102) act by blocking sodium reabsorption in the loop of Henle and distal renal tubule, thereby enhancing urinary excretion of sodium and water.

CLINICAL BENEFITS. Although not proven to improve mortality and morbidity in large trials, diuretics are required in nearly all patients with symptomatic heart failure (stages C and D) to relieve dyspnea and the signs of sodium and water retention ("congestion"), that is, peripheral and pulmonary edema.[10] No other treatment relieves symptoms and the signs of sodium and water overload as rapidly and effectively. Once a patient needs a diuretic, treatment is usually necessary for the rest of the patient's life, although the dose and type of diuretic may vary.

PRACTICAL USE. The key principle is to prescribe the minimum dose of diuretic needed to maintain an edema-free state ("dry weight"). Excessive use can lead to electrolyte imbalances, such as hyponatremia, hypokalemia (and risk for digitalis toxicity), hyperuricemia (and risk for gout), and uremia. The risk for renal dysfunction is increased by concomitant use of nonsteroidal anti-inflammatory drugs (NSAIDs). Diuretic-induced hypovolemia may also cause symptomatic hypotension and prerenal azotemia. Restriction of dietary sodium intake may help reduce, but does not eliminate, the requirement for diuretics. Diuretic dosing should be flexible, with temporary increases for evidence of fluid retention (e.g., increasing symptoms, weight gain, edema) and decreases for evidence of hypovolemia (e.g., as a consequence of increased electrolyte loss due to gastroenteritis, decreased fluid intake, or both).

In some patients with milder symptoms of heart failure and preserved renal function (stage C), a thiazide diuretic such as chlorthalidone may suffice. In

TABLE 46-2 PRACTICAL GUIDANCE ON THE USE OF ANGIOTENSIN-CONVERTING ENZYME INHIBITORS AND ANGIOTENSIN RECEPTOR BLOCKERS IN PATIENTS WITH HEART FAILURE DUE TO LEFT VENTRICULAR SYSTOLIC DYSFUNCTION

WHY?

Randomized trials have conclusively shown that angiotensin-converting enzyme (ACE) inhibitors increase survival, reduce hospital admissions, and improve New York Heart Association (NYHA) class and quality of life in patients with *all* grades of symptomatic heart failure. Other randomized trials in patients with systolic dysfunction after acute myocardial infarction show that ACE inhibitors increase survival. In patients with heart failure, the composite end point of death or hospital admission is reduced by higher doses of an ACE inhibitor compared with lower doses. ACE inhibitors also delay or prevent the development of symptomatic heart failure in patients with *asymptomatic* left ventricular systolic dysfunction.

In patients who are intolerant of an ACE inhibitor, an angiotensin receptor blocker (ARB) is indicated. For example, candesartan reduces the risk for the composite outcome of cardiovascular death or heart failure hospitalization, reduces the risk of hospital admission for heart failure, and improves functional class. Valsartan is as effective as the ACE inhibitor captopril in reducing mortality and cardiovascular morbidity in patients with left ventricular systolic dysfunction, heart failure, or both complicating acute myocardial infarction.

IN WHOM AND WHEN?

ACE Inhibitors/ARBs

Indications
- Potentially all patients with heart failure and a low ejection fraction, although usually an angiotensin receptor-neprilysin inhibitor (ARNI) is the preferred treatment (see later).
- First-line treatment (along with a β-blocker, mineralocorticoid receptor antagonist [MRA], and sodium glucose cotransporter 2 [SGLT2] inhibitor) in patients with NYHA class II to IV heart failure; start as early as possible in course of disease.
- ACE inhibitors (and probably ARBs) are also of benefit in patients with asymptomatic left ventricular systolic dysfunction (NYHA class I).

Contraindications
- ACE inhibitors only—history of angioedema
- Known bilateral renal artery stenosis
- Combination with an angiotensin receptor blocker-neprilysin inhibitor (valsartan/sacubitril)—risk of angioedema if combined with an ACE inhibitor (and renal dysfunction and hyperkalemia when combined with an ACE inhibitor or an ARB)

Cautions/seek specialist advice
- Significant hyperkalemia ($K^+ > 5.0$ mmol/L)
- Significant renal dysfunction (creatinine 221 μmol/L or >2.5 mg/dL)
- Symptomatic or severe asymptomatic hypotension (systolic blood pressure <90 mm Hg)

Potential drug interactions of particular concern
- K^+ supplements/K^+-sparing diuretics (e.g., amiloride and triamterene [beware combination preparations with furosemide])
- Mineralocorticoid receptor antagonists (spironolactone, eplerenone), ARBs, NSAIDs*
- "Low-salt" substitutes with a high K^+ content
- Angiotensin receptor blocker-neprilysin inhibitor (sacubitril/valsartan)—see earlier (contraindicated)

WHERE?

In the community for most patients

Exceptions—see Cautions/seek specialist advice

WHICH ACE INHIBITOR AND WHAT ORAL DOSE?

	STARTING DOSE	TARGET DOSE
Captopril	6.25 mg three times daily	50 mg three times daily
Enalapril	2.5 mg twice daily	10-20 mg twice daily
Lisinopril	2.5-5.0 mg once daily	20-35 mg once daily
Ramipril	2.5 mg once daily	5 mg twice daily or 10 mg once daily
Trandolapril	0.5 mg once daily	4 mg once daily

WHICH ARB AND WHAT ORAL DOSE?

	STARTING DOSE	TARGET DOSE
Candesartan	4 or 8 mg once daily	32 mg once daily
Valsartan	40 mg twice daily	160 mg twice daily
Losartan	50 mg once daily	150 mg daily

HOW TO USE?

Start with a low dose (see doses in previous column).

Double dose typically at 2-week intervals.

Aim for target dose (see doses in previous column) or, failing that, the highest tolerated dose.

Remember: *some* ACE inhibitor/ARB is better than *no* ACE inhibitor/ARB.

Monitor blood pressure and blood chemistry (urea/blood urea nitrogen, creatinine, K^+).

Check blood chemistry 1 to 2 weeks after initiation and 1 to 2 weeks after final dose titration.

When to stop up-titration, reduce dose, stop treatment—see Problem Solving.

A specialist heart failure nurse or pharmacist may assist with education of the patient, follow-up (in person or by telephone), biochemical monitoring, and dose up-titration.

ADVICE TO PATIENT

Explain expected benefits (see Why?).

Treatment is given to improve symptoms, to prevent worsening of heart failure leading to hospital admission, and to increase survival.

Symptoms improve within a few weeks to a few months of starting treatment.

Advise patients to report principal adverse effects, (i.e., dizziness/symptomatic hypotension, cough)—see Problem Solving.

Advise patients to avoid NSAIDs* not prescribed by a physician (self-purchased over-the-counter) and salt substitutes high in K^+—see Problem Solving.

PROBLEM SOLVING

Asymptomatic low blood pressure
- Does not usually require any change in therapy

Symptomatic hypotension
- If dizziness, lightheadedness, or confusion and a low blood pressure, reconsider need for nitrates, calcium-channel blockers,† and other vasodilators.
- If no signs or symptoms of congestion, consider reducing diuretic dose.
- If these measures do not solve problem, seek specialist advice.

Cough
- Cough is common in patients with heart failure, many of whom have smoking-related lung disease.
- Cough is also a symptom of pulmonary edema, which should be excluded when a new or worsening cough develops.
- ACE inhibitor–induced cough rarely may not require treatment discontinuation.
- When a troublesome cough does develop (e.g., one stopping the patient from sleeping) and can be proved to be due to ACE inhibition (i.e., recurs after ACE inhibitor withdrawal and rechallenge), substitution of an ARB should be considered.

Worsening renal function
- Some rise in urea (blood urea nitrogen), creatinine, and potassium is to be expected after initiation of an ACE inhibitor/ARB; if an increase is small and asymptomatic, no action is necessary.
- An increase in creatinine of up to 50% above baseline, or 266 μmol/L (3 mg/dL), whichever is the smaller, is acceptable.
- An increase in potassium to ≤5.5 mmol/L is acceptable but must be rechecked.
- If urea, creatinine, or potassium does rise excessively, consider stopping concomitant nephrotoxic drugs (e.g., NSAIDs*) and other potassium supplements or retaining agents (triamterene, amiloride, spironolactone-eplerenone) and, if no signs of congestion, reducing the dose of diuretic.
- If greater rises in creatinine or potassium than those outlined earlier persist despite adjustment of concomitant medications, the dose of the ACE inhibitor should be halved and blood chemistry rechecked within 1 to 2 weeks; if there is still an unsatisfactory response, specialist advice should be sought.
- If potassium rises to >5.5 mmol/L or creatinine increases by >100% or to above 310 μmol/L (3.5 mg/dL), the ACE inhibitor/ARB should be stopped and specialist advice sought. Concomitant use of a K^+ binder (e.g., patiromer; see Chapter 103) may allow an ACE inhibitor/ARB (or ARNI) to be continued in patients developing hyperkalemia.
- Blood chemistry should be monitored frequently and serially until potassium and creatinine have plateaued.

*Avoid nonsteroidal anti-inflammatory drugs (NSAIDs) unless essential.

†Calcium-channel blockers should be discontinued unless absolutely essential (e.g., for angina or hypertension).

Note: It is rarely necessary to stop an ACE inhibitor/ARB, and clinical deterioration is likely if treatment is withdrawn. Ideally, specialist advice should be sought before treatment discontinuation.

Modified from McMurray J, Cohen-Solal A, Dietz R, et al. Practical recommendations for the use of ACE inhibitors, β-blockers, mineralocorticoid receptor antagonists and angiotensin receptor blockers in heart failure: putting guidelines into practice. *Eur J Heart Fail.* 2005;7:710-721.

TABLE 46-3 PRACTICAL GUIDANCE ON THE USE OF Β-BLOCKERS IN PATIENTS WITH HEART FAILURE DUE TO LEFT VENTRICULAR SYSTOLIC DYSFUNCTION

WHY?

Several major randomized controlled trials have shown conclusively that certain β-blockers increase survival, reduce hospital admissions, and improve New York Heart Association (NYHA) class and quality of life when added to standard therapy (diuretics, digoxin, and angiotensin-converting enzyme [ACE] inhibitors) in patients with heart failure. Carvedilol is substantially more effective than a low dose of short-acting metoprolol.*

IN WHOM AND WHEN?

Indications
- Potentially *all* patients with *euvolemic* heart failure with mild to moderate symptoms; patients with severe heart failure should be referred for specialist advice.
- First-line treatment (along with an angiotensin receptor-neprilysin inhibitor [ARNI] or ACE inhibitor or angiotensin receptor blocker [ARB], mineralocorticoid receptor antagonists [MRA], and sodium-glucose cotransporter 2 [SGLT2] inhibitor) in patients with *euvolemic* NYHA class II to III heart failure; start as early as possible in course of disease.

Contraindications
- Asthma
- Second- or third-degree atrioventricular block

Cautions/seek specialist advice
- Severe (NYHA class IV) heart failure
- Current or recent (<4 weeks) exacerbation of heart failure (e.g., hospital admission with worsening heart failure, heart block, or heart rate <60 beats/minute).
- Persisting signs of congestion, hypotension/low blood pressure (systolic < 90 mm Hg), raised jugular venous pressure, ascites, marked peripheral edema

Potential drug interactions of particular concern
- Verapamil, diltiazem (should be discontinued)†
- Digoxin, amiodarone

WHERE?

- In the community in stable patients (NYHA class IV/severe heart failure patients should be referred for specialist advice)
- Not in unstable patients hospitalized with worsening heart failure
- Other exceptions—see Cautions/seek specialist advice

WHICH β-BLOCKER AND WHAT ORAL DOSE?

	STARTING DOSE	TARGET DOSE
Bisoprolol	1.25 mg once daily	10 mg once daily
Carvedilol	3.125 mg twice daily	25-50 mg twice daily
Metoprolol CR/XL	12.5-25 mg once daily	200 mg once daily*
Nebivolol	1.25 mg once daily	10 mg once daily

HOW TO USE?

- Start with a low dose (see dose shown in previous column).
- Double dose at *not less than* 2-week intervals.
- Aim for target dose (see dose shown in previous column) or, failing that, the highest tolerated dose.
- Remember: *some* β-blocker is better than *no* β-blocker.
- Monitor heart rate, blood pressure, and clinical status (symptoms, signs—especially signs of congestion, increased body weight).
- Check blood chemistry 1 to 2 weeks after initiation and 1 to 2 weeks after final dose titration.
- When to stop up-titration, reduce dose, stop treatment—see Problem Solving.
- A specialist heart failure nurse may assist with education of the patient, follow-up (in person or by telephone), and dose up-titration.

ADVICE TO PATIENT

- Explain expected benefits (see Why?).
- Treatment is given to improve symptoms, to prevent worsening of heart failure leading to hospital admission, and to increase survival.
- Symptomatic improvement may develop slowly after starting treatment, and treatment for 3 to 6 months or longer may be required before the full effects on left ventricular size and function are observed.
- *Temporary* symptomatic deterioration *may* occur during initiation or up-titration phase; in the long term, β-blockers improve well-being.
- Advise patient to report deterioration (see Problem Solving) and that deterioration (tiredness, fatigue, breathlessness) can usually be easily managed by adjustment of other medication; patients should be advised not to stop β-blocker therapy without consulting the physician.
- To detect and to treat deterioration early, patients should be encouraged to weigh themselves daily (after waking, before dressing, after voiding, before eating) and to increase their diuretic dose should their weight increase persistently (>2 days) by >1.5-2.0 kg.‡

PROBLEM SOLVING

Worsening symptoms or signs (e.g., increasing dyspnea, fatigue, edema, weight gain)
- If increasing congestion, increase dose of diuretic or halve dose of β-blocker (if increasing diuretic does not work).
- If marked fatigue (or bradycardia—see later), halve dose of β-blocker (rarely necessary); review patient in 1 to 2 weeks; if not improved, seek specialist advice.
- If serious deterioration, halve dose of β-blocker or stop this treatment (rarely necessary); seek specialist advice.

Low heart rate
- If <50 beats/minute and worsening symptoms, halve dose of β-blocker or, if severe deterioration, stop β-blocker (rarely necessary).
- Review need for other heart rate–slowing drugs (e.g., digoxin, amiodarone, diltiazem, or verapamil†).
- Arrange electrocardiogram to exclude heart block.
- Seek specialist advice.

Asymptomatic low blood pressure
- Does not usually require any change in therapy.

Symptomatic hypotension
- If dizziness, lightheadedness, or confusion and a low blood pressure, reconsider need for nitrates, calcium-channel blockers,† and other vasodilators.
- If no signs or symptoms of congestion, consider reducing diuretic dose.
- If these measures do not solve problem, seek specialist advice.

*Metoprolol tartrate should not be used in preference to an evidence-based β-blocker in heart failure.

†Calcium-channel blockers should be discontinued unless absolutely necessary, and diltiazem and verapamil are generally contraindicated in heart failure.

‡This is generally good advice for all patients with heart failure.

Note: β-Blockers should not be stopped suddenly unless absolutely necessary (there is a risk for a "rebound" increase in myocardial ischemia or infarction and arrhythmias). Ideally, specialist advice should be sought before treatment discontinuation.

Modified from McMurray J, Cohen-Solal A, Dietz R, et al. Practical recommendations for the use of ACE inhibitors, β-blockers, mineralocorticoid receptor antagonists and angiotensin receptor blockers in heart failure: putting guidelines into practice. *Eur J Heart Fail.* 2005;7:710-721.

more advanced heart failure (stage D) or in patients with concomitant renal dysfunction, a loop diuretic such as furosemide is often needed. Loop diuretics cause a rapid onset of an intense but relatively short-lived diuresis compared with the longer lasting but gentler effect of a thiazide diuretic. The timing of administration of a loop diuretic, which need not be taken first thing every morning, can be adjusted according to the patient's social activities. The dose may be postponed or even temporarily omitted if the patient has to travel or has another activity that might be compromised by the prompt action of the diuretic. In severe heart failure (stage D), the effects of long-term administration of a loop diuretic may be diminished by increased sodium reabsorption at the distal tubule. This problem can be offset by use of the combination of a loop diuretic and a thiazide or thiazide-like diuretic (e.g., hydrochlorothiazide or metolazone), which act in synergy with a loop diuretic by blocking sodium reabsorption in different segments of the nephron.[A8] This combination requires more frequent monitoring of electrolytes and renal function for diuretic-induced hyponatremia, abnormalities of the serum potassium level, and prerenal azotemia. The combination of a loop diuretic with the proximally acting carbonic anhydrase inhibitor acetazolamide can augment decongestion in the acute setting.[A9]

A period of intravenous loop diuretic, given either as bolus injections or by continuous infusion, may be required either in the ambulatory setting or as an in-patient in patients who become resistant to the action of oral diuretics. Why this resistance develops is uncertain, but factors thought to be important include impaired absorption of oral diuretics due to gut edema, hypotension, reduced renal blood flow, renal venous congestion, and adaptive changes in the nephron. In cases of severe resistant volume overload, mechanical removal of fluid by ultrafiltration may be considered.

Patients receiving a combination of diuretics require careful monitoring of blood chemistry and clinical status.

Although they are highly effective in relieving symptoms and signs, diuretics alone are not sufficient for treatment of heart failure. The addition of other disease-modifying treatments will slow structural progression, better maintain clinical stability, and reduce the risk for hospital admission and premature death.

ACE Inhibitors and Angiotensin Receptor Blockers (ARBs)

MECHANISM OF ACTION. ACE inhibitors inhibit the enzyme that converts the inactive decapeptide angiotensin I to the active octapeptide angiotensin II (and that also breaks down bradykinin). In patients with heart failure, excessive angiotensin II is thought to exert myriad harmful actions mediated through stimulation of the angiotensin II type 1 receptor subtype (AT1R), including vasoconstriction (which increases ventricular afterload), excessive growth of myocytes and the extracellular matrix (contributing to maladaptive left ventricular remodeling), activation of the sympathetic nervous system, prothrombotic actions, and augmentation of the release of arginine vasopressin and the retention of sodium (both directly and through stimulation of secretion of aldosterone, which activates the mineralocorticoid receptor). ARBs selectively block the action of angiotensin II at the AT1 receptor. Although pharmacologically distinct from ACE inhibitors, their clinical effects are similar.

ACE inhibitors also reduce the breakdown of bradykinin, and the resultant accumulation of bradykinin is directly or indirectly responsible for two of the specific adverse effects of ACE inhibitors: cough and angioedema. ARBs do not inhibit kininase II or the breakdown of bradykinin, so they do not cause cough and are associated with lower rates of angioedema than are ACE inhibitors. This difference between ARBs and ACE inhibitors explains why the combination of neprilysin (which also breaks down bradykinin and may itself cause angioedema) and an ARB is safe (and why the combination of an ACE inhibitor and a neprilysin inhibitor poses a significant risk of angioedema and is not recommended).

CLINICAL BENEFITS. Clinical trials have shown that treatment with an ACE inhibitor, when it is used alone or added to diuretics and digoxin, decreases left ventricular size, improves ejection fraction, reduces symptoms and hospital admissions, and prolongs survival. These agents also reduce the risk of developing myocardial infarction and possibly diabetes and atrial fibrillation. Consequently, treatment with an ACE inhibitor is recommended for all patients with left ventricular systolic dysfunction, irrespective of symptoms or etiology. ACE inhibitors are not a substitute for a diuretic but mitigate diuretic-induced hypokalemia.

When used as the sole agent in heart failure, ARBs produce benefits similar to those of ACE inhibitors. An ARB may be used as a substitute in patients who have cough or angioedema with an ACE inhibitor. When they are used in clinically effective doses, other adverse effects such as hypotension, renal dysfunction, and hyperkalemia are encountered as frequently as with an ACE inhibitor.

PRACTICAL USE. As early as possible in a patient's treatment, the combination of an ARB with a neprilysin inhibitor (i.e., sacubitril/valsartan) is preferred because of the additional benefit of neprilysin inhibition. If the combination is not tolerated, an ACE inhibitor or an ARB can be used. The only contraindications are a history of angioedema (for an ACE inhibitor), current symptomatic hypotension, and bilateral renal artery stenosis (Chapter 110); the latter is often associated with a prompt and marked increase in serum levels of blood urea nitrogen and creatinine when renal perfusion is reduced precipitously by inhibiting the production and actions of angiotensin II. Combined use of an ACE inhibitor and an ARB is contraindicated because it results in increased side effects without an increase in efficacy.

Treatment should be started in a low dose (see Table 46-2), with the dose gradually increased toward a target dose of proven benefit in a clinical trial. The patient should be evaluated for symptomatic hypotension, uremia, and hyperkalemia after each dose increment; these adverse effects are uncommon and can usually be resolved by reduction in the dose of diuretic (if the patient is edema free) or concomitant hypotensive or nephrotoxic medications (e.g., nitrates, calcium-channel blockers, or NSAIDs). A dry, nonproductive cough occurs in approximately 5% of patients treated with an ACE inhibitor, and if it is troublesome, substitution of an ARB is recommended. In the rare cases of angioedema (Chapter 232), the ACE inhibitor should be stopped and not used again; an ARB can be cautiously substituted (see later).

Neprilysin Inhibition

Neprilysin is an enzyme that breaks down natriuretic peptides and other vasoactive substances, including adrenomedullin and bradykinin. Inhibiting neprilysin augments the concentrations of these substances, which have vasodilator and natriuretic actions, and also inhibits pathologic growth, including hypertrophy and fibrosis. Because neprilysin also degrades angiotensin II, a neprilysin inhibitor must be combined with an agent that blocks the renin-angiotensin system. Because ACE and neprilysin each degrade bradykinin, inhibiting both enzymes leads to a significant increase in the risk of angioedema. Consequently, an ARB (valsartan) combined with a neprilysin inhibitor (sacubitril), termed an angiotensin receptor neprilysin inhibitor (ARNI), is preferred. When added to a β-blocker and a mineralocorticoid receptor antagonist, sacubitril/valsartan (97/103 mg twice daily) reduces heart failure hospitalization, cardiovascular mortality, death from all causes, and other measures of progressive worsening of heart failure compared with adding enalapril (10 mg twice daily).[A10] Compared with enalapril, sacubitril/valsartan causes more hypotension and slightly more angioedema but less renal dysfunction and hyperkalemia. Neprilysin inhibition increases levels of B-type natriuretic peptide but not NT pro-B-type natriuretic peptide.

PRACTICAL USE. Sacubitril/valsartan, which is recommended as first-line starting therapy instead of an ACE inhibitor or an ARB, can be initiated in patients hospitalized with decompensated heart failure.[A11] Switching to sacubitril/valsartan should be considered in patients who have persisting symptoms despite tolerating treatment with an ACE inhibitor or ARB (Table 46-4). Because neprilysin inhibition with sacubitril increases bradykinin, a history of angioedema is a contraindication to sacubitril/valsartan. Sacubitril/valsartan should never be combined with an ACE inhibitor, and a "wash-out" period of 36 hours is required between stopping an ACE inhibitor and starting the ARNI. Because neprilysin inhibition increases a number of vasodilator peptides, hypotension is more common with sacubitril/valsartan than with an ACE inhibitor or ARB, and switching is not recommended in a patient with a systolic blood pressure lower than 95 mm Hg.

β-Blockers

MECHANISM OF ACTION. Heart failure is characterized by excessive activation of the sympathetic nervous system, which causes vasoconstriction and sodium retention, thereby increasing cardiac preload and afterload and often inducing myocardial ischemia or arrhythmias. In addition, norepinephrine can cause hypertrophy of myocytes and augment their apoptosis. β-Blockers counteract many of these harmful effects of the hyperactivity of the sympathetic nervous system. A rapid heart rate is an important prognostic factor in heart failure among patients in sinus rhythm, and β-blockers reduce heart rate.

CLINICAL BENEFITS. The long-term addition of a β-blocker to an ARNI, an SGLT2 inhibitor, a diuretic, and a mineralocorticoid receptor antagonist further improves left ventricular systolic function and symptoms, reduces hospital admissions, and strikingly improves survival. Consequently, a β-blocker is recommended for all patients with symptomatic systolic dysfunction, irrespective of etiology and severity, and the combination of a β-blocker with an ARNI (or an ACE inhibitor or ARB) is a cornerstone of the treatment of symptomatic heart failure (see Fig. 46-1). Treatment with a β-blocker, added to an ARNI (or ACE inhibitor or ARB), a mineralocorticoid receptor antagonist, and an SGLT2 inhibitor is generally recommended for all patients with symptoms (functional classes II to IV) and left ventricular systolic dysfunction, irrespective of etiology.

In a retrospective analysis of pooled data from 11 randomized trials in patients with heart failure, β-blockers improved the left ventricular ejection fraction but did not appear to reduce all-cause mortality in patients with atrial fibrillation, whereas they reduced mortality by 27% in patients who were in sinus rhythm.[A12] Although the interpretation of these results is controversial, β-blockers remain the preferred treatment for control of the ventricular rate in patients who have both atrial fibrillation and heart failure with a reduced ejection fraction because of their excellent safety profile.

PRACTICAL USE. The major contraindications to use of a β-blocker are asthma (although it is important to note that the dyspnea caused by pulmonary congestion can be confused with reactive airway disease) and second- or third-degree atrioventricular block. Initiation of treatment during an episode of acute decompensated heart failure should also be avoided until the patient is stabilized. In addition, caution is advised in patients with a heart rate below 60 beats per minute or a systolic blood pressure below 90 mm Hg. It is recommended that a β-blocker shown to produce benefits in a randomized trial be used.

As with an ARNI (or an ACE inhibitor or ARB), mineralocorticoid receptor antagonist, and SGLT2 inhibitor, β-blockers should be introduced as early as possible in a patient's treatment, started in a low dose (see Table 46-3), and increased gradually toward a target dose used in a clinical trial (the "start low–go slow" approach). The patient should be checked for symptomatic hypotension and excessive bradycardia after each dose increment, but both of these side effects are uncommon, and hypotension can often be resolved by reduction in the dose of other nonessential blood pressure–lowering medications (e.g., nitrates and calcium-channel blockers). Bradycardia is more likely in patients who are also taking digoxin or amiodarone, and the simultaneous use of these agents should be reviewed if excessive bradycardia occurs. On occasion, symptomatic worsening and fluid retention (e.g., weight gain or edema) may occur after initiation of a β-blocker or during dose up-titration; these side effects usually can be resolved by a temporary increase in the diuretic dose without necessitating discontinuation of the β-blocker.

Treatment with a β-blocker should be given for life, although the dose may need to be decreased (or, rarely, treatment discontinued) temporarily during

TABLE 46-4 PRACTICAL GUIDANCE ON THE USE OF A COMBINED ANGIOTENSIN RECEPTOR BLOCKER-NEPRILYSIN INHIBITOR (SACUBITRIL/VALSARTAN) IN PATIENTS WITH HEART FAILURE DUE TO LEFT VENTRICULAR SYSTOLIC DYSFUNCTION

WHY?

In one major randomized trial, patients who had symptomatic heart failure and who were previously treated with an angiotensin-converting enzyme (ACE) inhibitor or angiotensin receptor blocker (ARB) were randomized to an ARB plus a neprilysin inhibitor (ARNI) sacubitril/valsartan or the ACE inhibitor enalapril, added to standard pharmacologic therapy (diuretics, β-blockers, mineralocorticoid receptor antagonists [MRAs], and digoxin). Patients treated with sacubitril/valsartan had a better survival, fewer hospital admissions, and improved New York Heart Association (NYHA) class and quality of life compared with patients who were treated with enalapril.

IN WHOM AND WHEN?

Indications
- Potentially all patients with heart failure and a low ejection fraction
- First-line treatment (along with a β-blocker, MRA, and SGLT2 inhibitor) in patients with functional class II to IV heart failure as the preferred alternative to an ACE inhibitor or ARB.

Contraindications
- History of angioedema
- Known bilateral renal artery stenosis
- Combination with an ACE inhibitor or ARB—risk of angioedema if combined with an ACE inhibitor (and renal dysfunction and hyperkalemia when combined with ACE inhibitor or an ARB)

Cautions/seek specialist advice
- Significant hyperkalemia ($K^+ > 5.0$ mmol/L)
- Significant renal dysfunction (creatinine 221 μmol/L or >2.5 mg/dL)
- Symptomatic or asymptomatic hypotension (systolic blood pressure < 95 mm Hg)

Potential drug interactions of particular concern
- K+ supplements/K+-sparing diuretics (e.g., amiloride and triamterene [beware combination preparations with furosemide])
- Mineralocorticoid receptor antagonists (spironolactone, eplerenone), NSAIDs*
- "Low-salt" substitutes with a high K+ content
- ACE inhibitor/ARB—see earlier (contraindicated)

WHERE?

In the community for most patients
Exceptions—see Cautions/seek specialist advice

WHAT ORAL DOSE?

STARTING DOSE usually sacubitril/valsartan 49 mg/51 mg twice daily if switching from ACE inhibitor/ARB (24 mg/26 mg twice daily if starting de novo)
TARGET DOSE sacubitril/valsartan 97/103 mg twice daily

HOW TO USE?

As for ACE inhibitors/ARBs
ACE inhibitor treatment must be stopped for 36 hours before starting sacubitril/valsartan (to minimize risk of angioedema)

ADVICE TO PATIENT

As for ACE inhibitors/ARBs

PROBLEM SOLVING

As for ACE inhibitors/ARBs (manage cough related to neprilysin inhibition in same way as ACE inhibitor–induced cough)

*Avoid nonsteroidal anti-inflammatory drugs (NSAIDs) unless essential.
SGLT2 = sodium glucose cotransporter 2.

episodes of acute decompensation if the patient shows signs of circulatory underperfusion or refractory congestion.

Mineralocorticoid Receptor (Aldosterone) Antagonists (MRAs)

MECHANISM OF ACTION. Aldosterone, which is the second effector hormone in the renin-angiotensin-aldosterone cascade, has detrimental vascular, renal, autonomic, and cardiac actions when it is produced in excess in patients with heart failure. Excessive aldosterone promotes sodium retention and hypokalemia, and it is believed to contribute to myocardial fibrosis, all of which predispose to arrhythmias. Aldosterone mediates its effects by activating the mineralocorticoid receptor, which is also stimulated by other endogenous corticosteroids. Mineralocorticoid receptor antagonists block these undesirable actions and, at high doses, also act as potassium-sparing diuretics.

CLINICAL BENEFITS. The mineralocorticoid receptor antagonist spironolactone improves symptoms, reduces hospital admissions, and increases survival when it is added to an ACE inhibitor (and diuretics and digoxin) in patients with a reduced left ventricular ejection fraction and severely symptomatic heart failure. Eplerenone, another mineralocorticoid receptor antagonist, reduces mortality and morbidity when it is added to both an ACE inhibitor and β-blocker in patients with a reduced left ventricular ejection fraction and heart failure with mild symptoms (NYHA class II). Consequently, a mineralocorticoid receptor antagonist should be considered in all patients with symptomatic (class II to IV) heart failure and reduced ejection fraction in addition to an ARNI (or ACE inhibitor or ARB), β-blocker, and an SGLT2 inhibitor.[A13] When begun, a mineralocorticoid receptor antagonist should be given indefinitely.

PRACTICAL USE. Treatment with a mineralocorticoid receptor antagonist should be initiated with a low dose (Table 46-5) with careful monitoring of serum electrolytes and renal function. Hyperkalemia and uremia are the adverse effects of greatest concern (as with ACE inhibitors, ARBs, or an ARNI), and a mineralocorticoid receptor antagonist should not be given to patients with a serum potassium concentration of more than 5.0 mmol/L, serum creatinine concentration above 2.5 mg/dL (>221 μmol/L), or other evidence of markedly impaired renal function. The importance of selection of patients and dose is underscored by reports of a worrisome incidence of serious hyperkalemia in community practice settings. Spironolactone can have antiandrogenic effects, especially painful gynecomastia, in men; because eplerenone has less of an action on the androgen receptor, it is a reasonable substitute in patients who experience this adverse effect.

Sodium Glucose Cotransporter 2 (SGLT2) Inhibitors

MECHANISM OF ACTION. The SGLT2 is found in the renal proximal tubule, where it is responsible for the reabsorption of glucose filtered at the glomerulus. Inhibition of SGLT2 results in increased urinary excretion of glucose and sodium, along with an osmotic diuresis. Whether this action completely or partly explains the benefit of these drugs in patients with heart failure (and chronic kidney disease) is unknown. In addition to increased glycosuria and a resultant reduction in blood glucose, the other consistent effects of SGLT2 inhibitors are an increase in hematocrit, reduced rate of long-term decline in glomerular filtration rate (after an initial dip in this measure), and a modest decrease in blood pressure.[11] Many other actions of SGLT2 have been speculated, but not confirmed, in humans.

CLINICAL BENEFITS. Clinical trials have shown that adding an SGLT2 inhibitor to a renin-angiotensin system blocker (or ARNI), β-blocker, and a mineralocorticoid receptor antagonist decreases left ventricular size, improves ejection fraction, reduces symptoms and hospital admissions, and prolongs survival in men and women, regardless of whether or not they have type 2 diabetes, chronic renal disease, or a recent worsening of their heart failure.[A14–A17] These agents also reduce the risk of worsening kidney function[A18] and possibly of developing diabetes. Consequently, treatment with an SGLT2 inhibitor is recommended for all patients with symptomatic heart failure and a reduced ejection fraction, irrespective of diabetes status. SGLT2 inhibitors mitigate MRA-induced hyperkalemia.

PRACTICAL USE. As with an ARNI (or an ACE inhibitor or ARB), β-blocker, and mineralocorticoid receptor antagonist, an SGLT2 inhibitor should be introduced as early as possible in a patient's treatment. The only contraindications are type 1 diabetes, a history of diabetic ketoacidosis, and severe renal dysfunction (estimated glomerular filtration rate <20 mL/min/1.73 m^2). In patients with type 2 diabetes (Chapter 210), other glucose-lowering therapy may need to be adjusted, especially if there is a recent history of hypoglycemia. The dose of Insulin should not be decreased by more than 25%, and it is prudent to discuss changes in insulin dosage with an endocrinologist before commencing an SGLT2 inhibitor.

Unlike other treatments for heart failure, SGLT2 inhibitors are prescribed as a single dose, and no up-titration is required (Table 46-6). Treatment may lead to a modest initial, but short-lived, diuresis and small decline in estimated glomerular filtration rate, although neither of these is usually a clinical problem. It is advisable to check kidney function within a month of starting treatment, especially in patients with a very low baseline estimated glomerular filtration rate. A clinically meaningful change in blood pressure is rare. Genital skin fungal infections may occur in 5 to 10% of patients, are rarely troublesome, and can usually be treated with an antifungal cream. In the rare cases of ketoacidosis (Chapter 210), the SGLT2 inhibitor should be discontinued immediately. Patients at greatest risk of ketoacidosis are those who are concurrently taking insulin or who may be insulin-deficient (e.g., as a result of previous pancreatitis). SGLT2 inhibitors should be temporary withheld in situations that might trigger ketoacidosis (i.e., illness leading to decreased food and fluid intake or stopping or reducing the dose of insulin), including elective surgery, for which SGLT2 inhibitors should be discontinued 3 days preoperatively.

Second-Line Treatments for Heart Failure with Reduced Left Ventricular Ejection Fraction

Several secondary agents are available for selected patients with heart failure (Fig. 46-3).

TABLE 46-5 PRACTICAL GUIDANCE ON THE USE OF MINERALOCORTICOID RECEPTOR ANTAGONISTS (MRAS) IN PATIENTS WITH HEART FAILURE DUE TO LEFT VENTRICULAR SYSTOLIC DYSFUNCTION

WHY?

Treatment with an MRA (spironolactone or eplerenone) increases survival, reduces hospital admissions, and improves New York Heart Association (NYHA) class when added to standard therapy (diuretic, digoxin, ACE inhibitor/ARB, and β-blocker) in patients with symptomatic (NYHA class II to IV) heart failure.
Eplerenone also increases survival and reduces hospital admission for cardiac causes in patients with left ventricular systolic dysfunction and heart failure (or diabetes) complicating *acute* myocardial infarction.

IN WHOM AND WHEN?

Indications
- Potentially all patients with symptomatic heart failure (NYHA class II to IV)
- First-line therapy (along with an angiotensin receptor-neprilysin inhibitor [ARNI], an ACE inhibitor, or an ARB], plus a β-blocker and an SGLT2 inhibitor) in patients with symptomatic heart failure (NYHA class II to IV) and an LVEF ≤40%

Cautions/seek specialist advice
- Significant hyperkalemia ($K^+ > 5.0$ mmol/L)†
- Significant renal dysfunction (creatinine >221 μmol/L or 2.5 mg/dL)†

Potential drug interactions of particular concern
- K^+ supplements/K^+-sparing diuretics (e.g., amiloride and triamterene; beware combination preparations with furosemide)
- ACE inhibitor, ARBs, ARNIs, NSAIDs‡
- "Low-salt" substitutes with a high K^+ content

WHERE?

In the community or in the hospital
Exceptions—see Cautions/seek specialist advice

WHICH ORAL DOSE?†

	STARTING DOSE	TARGET DOSE
Spironolactone	25 mg once daily or on alternate days	25-50 mg once daily
Eplerenone	25 mg once daily	50 mg once daily

HOW TO USE?

Start with a low dose (see dose shown in previous column).
Check blood chemistry at 1, 4, 8, and 12 weeks; 6, 9, and 12 months; 6-monthly thereafter.
If K^+ rises above 5.5 mmol/L or creatinine rises to 221 μmol/L (2.5 mg/dL), reduce dose to 25 mg on alternate days and monitor blood chemistry closely.
If K^+ rises to >6.0 mmol/L or creatinine to >310 μmol/L (3.5 mg/dL), stop MRA immediately and seek specialist advice.
A specialist heart failure nurse may assist with education of the patient, follow-up (in person or by telephone), biochemical monitoring, and dose up-titration.

ADVICE TO PATIENT

Explain expected benefits (see Why?).
Treatment is given to improve symptoms, to prevent worsening of heart failure leading to hospital admission, and to increase survival.
Symptom improvement occurs within a few weeks to a few months of starting treatment.
Avoid NSAIDs‡ not prescribed by a physician (self-purchased over-the-counter agent) and salt substitutes high in K^+.
If diarrhea or vomiting occurs, patients should stop the MRA and contact the physician.

PROBLEM SOLVING

Worsening renal function/hyperkalemia
- See How to Use? section.
- Major concern is hyperkalemia (>6.0 mmol/L)
- Conversely, a high-normal potassium level may be desirable in patients with heart failure, especially if they are taking digoxin.
- It is important to avoid other K^+-retaining drugs (e.g., K^+-sparing diuretics such as amiloride and triamterene) and nephrotoxic agents (e.g., NSAIDs‡)

Concomitant use of a K^+ binder (e.g., patiromer [Chapter 103] may allow an MRA to be continued in patients who develop hyperkalemia with an MRA.
Some "low-salt" substitutes have a high K^+ content.
Male patients treated with spironolactone may develop breast discomfort or gynecomastia (these problems are significantly less common with eplerenone).

†It is extremely important to adhere to these cautions and doses in light of recent evidence of serious hyperkalemia with spironolactone in usual clinical practice in Ontario.
‡Avoid nonsteroidal anti-inflammatory drugs (NSAIDs) unless essential.
ACE = angiotensin converting enzyme; ARB = angiotensin receptor blocker; ARNI = angiotensin receptor/neprilysin inhibitor; MRA = mineralocorticoid receptor antagonist; NSAID = nonsteroidal anti-inflammatory drug; SGLT2 = sodium-glucose cotransporter 2.
Modified from McMurray J, Cohen-Solal A, Dietz R, et al. Practical recommendations for the use of ACE inhibitors, β-blockers, aldosterone antagonists and angiotensin receptor blockers in heart failure: putting guidelines into practice. *Eur J Heart Fail.* 2005;7:710-721.

Sinus Node Inhibitors: Ivabradine

MECHANISM OF ACTION. Ivabradine is the first of a new class of drugs developed to inhibit the mixed sodium-potassium channel or current (also known as the funny channel, abbreviated as I_f or I_{kf}) in the sinoatrial node and, in so doing, reduce heart rate. Reduction in heart rate is the only known cardiac action of ivabradine, which has this effect only in patients in sinus rhythm.

CLINICAL BENEFITS. In patients with symptomatic heart failure (NYHA class II to IV), a reduced ejection fraction (≤35%), and sinus rhythm with a rate of 70 beats per minute or higher, ivabradine improves symptoms and ejection fraction and reduces the risk for hospitalization for heart failure (but not mortality) when added to an ACE inhibitor (or ARB or, presumably, ARNI), a β-blocker, and a mineralocorticoid receptor antagonist.[A19]

PRACTICAL USE. Ivabradine should be considered in patients who have persistent symptoms (NYHA class II to IV) despite treatment with a diuretic and other disease-modifying therapies (i.e., an ARNI [or ACE inhibitor or ARB], β-blocker, and a mineralocorticoid receptor antagonist) and who are in sinus rhythm with a heart rate of 70 beats per minute or greater. Ivabradine is not a substitute for a β-blocker and is not effective in atrial fibrillation. Treatment should be started at 5 mg twice daily, increased to 7.5 mg twice daily after 14 days unless the heart rate is 60 beats per minute or less, and reduced usually to 2.5 mg twice daily if the rate is less than 50 beats per minute. Symptomatic bradycardia and visual disturbance (phosphenes) are uncommon but require the dose be reduced or ivabradine be discontinued. Ivabradine also may increase the risk of developing atrial fibrillation, which should prompt discontinuation of the drug. Ivabradine should not be used in combination with agents that prolong the QT interval (e.g., amiodarone) and must be used cautiously with inhibitors (including grapefruit juice) or inducers of CYP3A4.

Soluble Guanylate Cyclase Stimulator: Vericiguat

MECHANISM OF ACTION. Vericiguat stimulates soluble guanylate cyclase, thereby converting guanosine triphosphate to cyclic guanosine monophosphate and increasing phosphokinase G levels. Phosphokinase G levels cause relaxation of vascular and cardiac muscle. Stimulation of this pathway may also prevent pathologic fibrosis and muscle hypertrophy, which contribute to adverse vascular and cardiac remodeling.

CLINICAL BENEFITS. In patients with symptomatic heart failure, a reduced ejection fraction (<45%), and a recent hospital admission (or intravenous diuretic) for worsening heart failure, vericiguat reduces the risk for hospitalization for heart failure (but not mortality) when added to an ACE inhibitor (or ARB or ARNI), a β-blocker, and a mineralocorticoid receptor antagonist.[A20]

PRACTICAL USE. Vericiguat may be considered in patients who have persistent symptoms (functional class II to IV) despite treatment with a diuretic and other disease-modifying therapies (i.e., an ARNI [or ACE inhibitor or ARB], β-blocker, a mineralocorticoid receptor antagonist and an SGLT2 inhibitor) following a hospitalization for heart failure or need for outpatient intravenous diuretics. Treatment should be started at 2.5 mg orally once daily with food, and the dose should be doubled approximately every 2 weeks as tolerated to reach the target maintenance dose of 10 mg once daily. Hypotension is the most common side effect. Vericiguat also increases the risk of anemia. Concomitant use of vericiguat with a phosphodiesterase type 5 inhibitor is not recommended because of the potential for hypotension.

Digoxin

MECHANISM OF ACTION. Digitalis glycosides inhibit the cell membrane Na^+, K^+-ATPase pump, thereby increasing intracellular calcium and myocardial contractility. In addition, digoxin is thought to enhance parasympathetic and reduce sympathetic nervous activity as well as to inhibit renin release.

CLINICAL BENEFITS. In the only large RCT that examined the effects of starting (as opposed to withdrawing) digoxin, digoxin did not reduce mortality but did decrease the risk for admission to hospital for worsening heart failure and improve quality of life when it was added to a diuretic and an ACE inhibitor. In patients in sinus rhythm, the addition of digoxin can be considered if heart failure remains symptomatic despite standard treatment with a diuretic

TABLE 46-6 PRACTICAL GUIDANCE ON THE USE OF SODIUM GLUCOSE COTRANSPORTER 2 (SGLT2) INHIBITORS IN PATIENTS WITH HEART FAILURE DUE TO LEFT VENTRICULAR SYSTOLIC DYSFUNCTION

WHY?

Treatment with SGLT2 inhibitors (dapagliflozin or empagliflozin) increases survival, reduces hospital admissions, and improves symptoms/quality of life class when added to standard therapy (diuretic, an angiotensin receptor blocker-neprilysin inhibitor [ARNI] or ACE inhibitor/ARB], a β-blocker, and an MRA) in patients with symptomatic (NYHA class II to IV) heart failure. SGLT2 inhibitors also slow the rate of decline in estimated glomerular filtration rate over time.

IN WHOM AND WHEN?

Indications
- Potentially all patients with symptomatic heart failure (NYHA class II to IV)
- First-line therapy (along with ARNI [or ACE inhibitor/ARB], β-blocker and MRA) in patients with symptomatic heart failure (NYHA class II to IV) and an LVEF ≤40%

Contraindications
- Previous diabetic ketoacidosis
- Estimated glomerular filtration rate <20 mL/min/1.73 m^2

Cautions/seek specialist advice
- Significant renal dysfunction (estimated glomerular filtration rate <30 mL/min/1.73 m^2)
- Recurrent hypoglycemia
- Insulin treatment if hypoglycemia or if "tight" glycemic control (i.e., glycated hemoglobin <7%)
- Possible pancreatic insufficiency (e.g., due to previous pancreatitis)
- History of genital fungal infection
- Possibility that excessive alcohol consumption and ketogenic low-carbohydrate diets may increase the risk of ketoacidosis (or cause diagnostic confusion)

Potential drug interactions of particular concern
- Glucose-lowering therapy, especially insulin or insulin secretagogues (such as sulfonylureas) because of small risk of hypoglycemia if "tight" glycemic control (i.e., glycated hemoglobin <7%)

WHERE?

In the community or in the hospital
Exceptions—see Cautions/seek specialist advice

WHICH ORAL DOSE?

	STARTING DOSE	TARGET DOSE
Dapagliflozin	10 mg once daily	10 mg once daily
Empagliflozin	10 mg once daily	10 mg once daily

HOW TO USE?

Start with dose shown earlier
Check kidney function at 4-8 weeks; earlier if baseline estimated glomerular filtration rate <30 mL/min/1.73 m^2. Regular monitoring not needed unless concerning initial decline in kidney function (rare).
A specialist heart failure nurse may assist with education of the patient, follow-up (in person or by telephone), and biochemical monitoring.

ADVICE TO PATIENT

Explain expected benefits (see Why?).
Treatment is given to improve symptoms, to prevent worsening of heart failure leading to hospital admission, and to increase survival.
Symptomatic improvement occurs within a few weeks to a few months after starting treatment.
Advise of small (5-10%) risk of genital fungal skin infection—more common in women and in noncircumcised men. Probably less common in people without diabetes. Genital skin hygiene important.
Advise of small (<5%) risk of hypoglycemia—only in patients with type 2 diabetes and probably only in those treated with insulin or insulin secretagogues. More likely in individuals with "tight" glycemic control (i.e., glycated hemoglobin <7%).
Advise temporary withholding of SGLT2 inhibitor and/or stopping/reducing insulin dose in situations that might trigger diabetic ketoacidosis (e.g., illness leading to decreased food and fluid intake). For example, stop SGLT2 inhibitors 3 days preoperatively. Ketoacidosis has not been observed in patients without type 2 diabetes, and the greatest risk is in patients treated with insulin or insulin secretagogues.

PROBLEM SOLVING

Most common problem is genital fungal skin infection
- Can usually be treated with an antifungal cream and does not usually require treatment interruption; oral antifungal therapy is an alternative.

Major concern is ketoacidosis, which is rare but serious
- Diagnosis may be delayed because blood glucose may not be elevated (or greatly elevated).
- Symptoms and signs that should raise concern are abdominal pain, vomiting, confusion, "pear drop/fruity" breath
- Other typical problems (e.g., breathlessness, thirst) are not helpful in patients with heart failure
- Some increase in ketones with SGLT inhibitors is common (up to 1 mmol/L)

ACE = angiotensin converting enzyme; ARB = angiotensin receptor blocker; ARNI = angiotensin receptor/neprilysin inhibitor; LVEF = left ventricular ejection fraction; MRA = mineralocorticoid receptor antagonist; SGLT2 = sodium glucose cotransporter 2.

and key disease-modifying drugs (i.e., an ARNI [or ACE inhibitor or ARB], a β-blocker, a mineralocorticoid receptor antagonist, and an SGLT2 inhibitor). However, digoxin has not been as well studied and may not be as safe as ivabradine when used in conjunction with contemporary therapies. In patients with atrial fibrillation, digoxin may be used at an earlier stage if a β-blocker fails to control the ventricular rate during exercise (Chapter 52). Digoxin can also be used to control the ventricular rate when β-blocker treatment is being initiated or up-titrated.

If the effect of digoxin is needed urgently, loading with 10 to 15 μg/kg lean body weight, given in three divided doses 6 hours apart, may be used. The maintenance dose should be one third of the loading dose. Smaller maintenance doses (e.g., one fourth of the loading dose and not more than 62.5 μg/day) should be used in elderly patients and in patients with reduced renal function as well as in patients with a low body mass. Monitoring of the serum digoxin concentration is recommended because of the narrow therapeutic window. A steady state is reached 7 to 10 days after treatment is started; blood should be collected at least 6 hours (and ideally 8 to 24 hours) after the last dose. The currently recommended therapeutic range is 0.5 to 1.0 ng/mL.

Digoxin can cause anorexia, nausea, arrhythmias, confusion, and visual disturbances, especially if the serum concentration is above 2.0 ng/mL. Hypokalemia increases susceptibility to the adverse effects. The dose of digoxin should be reduced in elderly patients and in patients with renal dysfunction. Certain drugs increase serum digoxin concentration, including amiodarone.

Hydralazine and Isosorbide Dinitrate

MECHANISM OF ACTION. Hydralazine is a powerful direct-acting arterial vasodilator. Its mechanism of action is not understood, although it may inhibit enzymatic production of superoxide, which neutralizes nitric oxide and may induce nitrate tolerance. Nitrates dilate both veins and arteries, thereby reducing preload and afterload by stimulating the nitric oxide pathway and increasing cyclic guanosine monophosphate in vascular smooth muscle. Neither drug on its own, nor any other direct-acting vasodilator, has been demonstrated to be beneficial in heart failure.

CLINICAL BENEFITS. The addition of hydralazine and isosorbide dinitrate reduces mortality, hospital admissions for heart failure, and heart failure symptoms when added to standard disease-modifying drugs (i.e., an ACE inhibitor [or presumably an ARB or ARNI, a β-blocker, mineralocorticoid receptor antagonist, and an SGLT2 inhibitor) in Black patients with functional class III or IV symptoms and an ejection fraction of 45% or less. The dose is a fixed combination of 37.5 mg of hydralazine and 20 mg of isosorbide dinitrate; if one tablet is tolerated, a second is given 12 hours later. Then the tablet is given three times daily for 3 to 5 days, at which point the dose is increased to the target maintenance of two tablets three times daily (i.e., a daily dose of 225 mg hydralazine and 120 mg isosorbide dinitrate). It is uncertain whether hydralazine/isosorbide dinitrate is an effective addition to standard therapy in non–African American patients.

PRACTICAL USE. Other than for Black patients, the main indication for hydralazine and isosorbide dinitrate is as a substitute in patients who are intolerant to an ARNI (or ACE inhibitor or ARB), primarily because of renal dysfunction. However, many patients who cannot tolerate these three drugs because of hypotension also do not tolerate hydralazine and isosorbide dinitrate. Hydralazine and isosorbide dinitrate can also be used as additional treatment in non–African Americans who remain symptomatic with other proven therapies. The main dose-limiting adverse effects of hydralazine and isosorbide dinitrate are headache and dizziness. A rare adverse effect of higher doses of hydralazine, especially in slow acetylators, is a systemic lupus erythematosus–like syndrome (Chapter 245).

Omega-3 Polyunsaturated Fatty Acids

In one trial, 1 gram of n-3 PUFA (850 to 852 mg eicosapentaenoic acid and docosahexaenoic acid as ethyl esters in the average ratio of 1 : 1.2) per day led to a

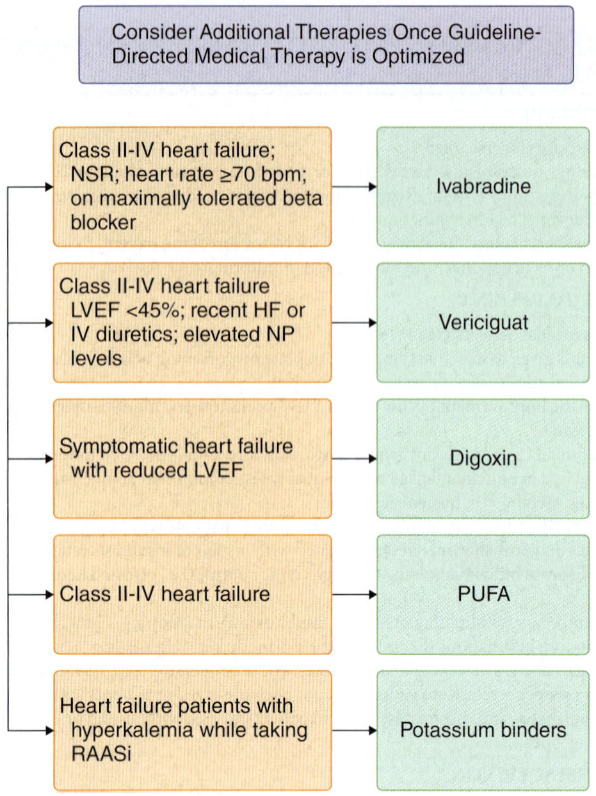

FIGURE 46-3. Second-line treatments for heart failure with reduced left ventricular ejection fraction. bpm = beats per minute; HR = heart rate; IV = intravenous; LVEF = left ventricular ejection fraction; NP = natriuretic peptide; NSR = normal sinus rhythm; PUFA = polyunsaturated fatty acids; RAASi = renin-angiotensin-aldosterone system inhibitor. (Reprinted with permission *Circulation*. 2022;145:e895-e1032 ©2022 American Heart Association, Inc.)

TABLE 46-7 SOME COMMON PRECIPITATING CAUSES OF HEART FAILURE

Myocardial ischemia or infarction
Atrial fibrillation or other supraventricular tachycardias
Uncontrolled hypertension
Valvular disease
Ventricular tachycardia
Pulmonary embolism
Pericardial disease
Sepsis
Anemia
Poor dietary or medical adherence
Adverse drug effects
Hyperthyroidism or hypothyroidism
Unknown/unexplained*

*Commonly, no clear precipitant is identified.

Adapted from Kimmelstiel CD, DeNofrio D, Konstam MA. Heart failure. In: Wachter RM, Goldman L, Hollander H, eds. *Hospital Medicine*, 2nd ed. Philadelphia: Lippincott Williams & Wilkins; 2005:360.

small reduction in cardiovascular morbidity and mortality in patients with heart failure. Although this agent may have beneficial anti-inflammatory and antiarrhythmic effects, its current role in the treatment of heart failure is uncertain, especially because trials in survivors of acute myocardial infarction have not shown benefit (Chapter 58).

Other Agents

The selective cardiac myosin activator omecamtiv mecarbil has shown inconsistent effects and is not approved by the U.S. Food and Drug Administration to treat heart failure. Other treatments have been tested in randomized trials and have been shown to have a neutral (e.g., amlodipine) or uncertain (e.g., bosentan and etanercept) effect on mortality and morbidity or to increase mortality (e.g., dronedarone, milrinone, flosequinan, vesnarinone, and moxonidine). The direct renin inhibitor aliskiren is inferior to an ACE inhibitor and is not recommended as an alternative to an ACE inhibitor (or ARB or ARNI) in patients with heart failure and a reduced ejection fraction. The potential role of cardiac stem cell therapy remains uncertain.[12]

Other Pharmacologic Issues

Some therapies that are of proven value for cardiovascular conditions that underlie or are associated with heart failure are of uncertain benefit (antiplatelet treatment, Chapter 70) or do not improve outcomes (statins, Chapter 190) in patients with persistent, symptomatic heart failure. Newer direct-acting oral anticoagulants or warfarin is indicated in patients with atrial fibrillation to reduce the risk for thromboembolism, unless patients have contraindications to their use (Chapter 52). Anticoagulants may also be used in patients with evidence of intracardiac thrombus (e.g., detected during echocardiographic examination) or systemic thromboembolism but otherwise are not indicated in patients who are not in atrial fibrillation.[A21] The many interactions of warfarin with other drugs, including some statins and amiodarone (Chapter 70), must always be considered. Heparin prophylaxis (Chapter 70) against deep vein thrombosis is indicated when patients with heart failure are bed bound, such as during hospital admission. Vaccination against influenza,[A22] pneumococcal infection, and severe acute respiratory syndrome coronavirus 2 (SARS-CoV-2) is advised (Chapter 15) in all patients with heart failure because these infections can lead to severe clinical deterioration.

Refractory Heart Failure and Pulmonary Edema

Patients presenting with acute heart failure include those who develop heart failure de novo as a consequence of another cardiac event, usually a myocardial infarction,[13] and those who present for the first time with decompensation of previously asymptomatic and often unrecognized cardiac dysfunction (patients previously with pre–heart failure [stage B], a transition with profound prognostic implications). However, because of frequent recurrences, most episodes of decompensation occur in patients with established, chronic heart failure that has worsened as a result of the unavoidable natural progression of the syndrome, with an intercurrent cardiac (e.g., arrhythmia) or noncardiac (e.g., pneumonia) event, or as a consequence of an avoidable reason, such as nonadherence with treatment or use of an agent that can alter renal function. Although it is not always identified, searching for a reversible precipitant is an important aspect of the initial therapy plan (Table 46-7). Many patients with decompensated heart failure experience worsening over a period of days or weeks before presenting to their doctor, during which time rising pulmonary artery pressure may be detected by an implantable pressure sensor.

Most patients with decompensated heart failure require admission to the hospital, especially if pulmonary edema is present. In contrast to the ambulatory setting, data from RCTs generally are not available to guide effective therapy for worsening of chronic heart failure or new-onset acute heart failure.[14] The principal goals of management of this heterogeneous group of patients are to relieve symptoms, the most important of which is extreme dyspnea, and to maintain or to restore vital organ perfusion. Importantly, using the acute admission period as an opportunity to commence evidence-based therapy and to titrate it rapidly after discharge results in a significant reduction in the risk of readmission and death.[A23]

The early administration of an intravenous bolus or infusion of a loop diuretic and, in hypoxemic patients, oxygen are the key first-line treatments. A small RCT suggested that high-dose diuretic (more than 2.5 times the previous oral dose) resulted in greater relief of dyspnea and congestion compared with low-dose diuretic (same intravenous dose as prior oral dose), but at the expense of more, albeit transient, renal dysfunction. Torsemide and furosemide are equally effective.[A24] A continuous infusion of furosemide may increase urine output compared with intermittent boluses but has not been shown to reduce mortality. An intravenous opiate may also be used cautiously in selected patients to relieve anxiety and distress, but at the risk of reducing ventilatory drive.

Noninvasive ventilation using a tight-fitting mask to provide positive-pressure ventilation reduces respiratory distress and metabolic disturbances more rapidly than standard oxygen therapy but has not reduced short-term mortality. Intravenous infusion of a nitrate (e.g., continuous intravenous infusion of 20 to 200 μg/mm of nitroglycerin, titrated according to the symptomatic response and hemodynamic measurements, particularly arterial blood pressure) may also be valuable in patients with hypertension or myocardial ischemia (Fig. 46-4).

Intravenous nesiritide can reduce the pulmonary capillary wedge pressure more promptly than intravenous nitroglycerin but has minimal effect on dyspnea and does not improve other clinical outcomes, and early intensive ventilator therapy is no better than usual care. In volume-overloaded patients with severe heart failure unresponsive to diuretics, ultrafiltration is an option at specialized centers, although it was not superior to intensified pharmacologic therapy in a recent trial.

In patients with marked hypotension or other evidence of organ hypoperfusion, an inotropic agent such as dobutamine (continuous intravenous infusion of 2.5 to 25 μg/kg/min, titrated according to hemodynamic and heart rate response and induction of arrhythmias or myocardial ischemia) or a phosphodiesterase inhibitor (e.g., milrinone) should be considered, although neither treatment has ever been shown to reduce in-hospital deaths. In some countries, the calcium sensitizer levosimendan is also available for use in these patients. In general, potent inotropic agents should be used in a cardiac-monitored setting at the lowest clinically effective dose and for the shortest duration possible (Chapter 93). Although low-dose dopamine (intravenous infusion of 2.5 μg/kg/mm) is often administered in an attempt to improve diuresis and renal function, such benefits have not been confirmed in RCTs.

Devices and Surgery

In critically ill patients (Chapter 93), temporary percutaneous mechanical circulatory support guided by invasive hemodynamic measurements may also be considered. The aim of treatment is to support the patient's circulation and vital organ function until either the patient's own heart recovers or a definitive operative procedure can be performed (e.g., percutaneous coronary intervention, implantation of a ventricular assist device, or cardiac transplantation).

Implantable Cardioverter-Defibrillators

About half of patients with heart failure die suddenly, mainly as the result of a ventricular arrhythmia. The relative risk for sudden death, as opposed to death from progressive heart failure, is greatest in patients with milder symptoms. In patients with more advanced heart failure, progressive pump failure deaths are relatively more common. Antiarrhythmic drugs do not improve survival in heart failure. ICDs (Chapter 54), however, reduce the risk for death in selected patients after myocardial infarction (Chapter 58) and, in one large RCT, improved survival in patients with class II to III heart failure and systolic dysfunction who were otherwise treated with what was considered optimal medical therapy at the time. However, a large RCT with longer follow-up found no reduction in all-cause mortality when an ICD was added to excellent contemporary pharmacologic and device therapy in older patients with nonischemic heart failure.[A25] Currently, in addition to their role in patients with an ischemic etiology, the balance of evidence also favors use of an ICD in patients who have nonischemic heart failure,[A26] limited comorbidity (i.e., a low risk of noncardiovascular death), an anticipated survival of at least a year, and a left ventricular ejection fraction remaining at 35% or less despite at least 3 months of treatment with disease-modifying therapy (i.e., an ARNI [or ACE inhibitor or ARB], β-blocker, mineralocorticoid receptor antagonist, and an SGLT2 inhibitor).

Cardiac Resynchronization Therapy

About 30% of patients with heart failure and a reduced ejection fraction have substantial prolongation of the QRS duration on the surface electrocardiogram, which is a marker of abnormal electrical activation of the left ventricle

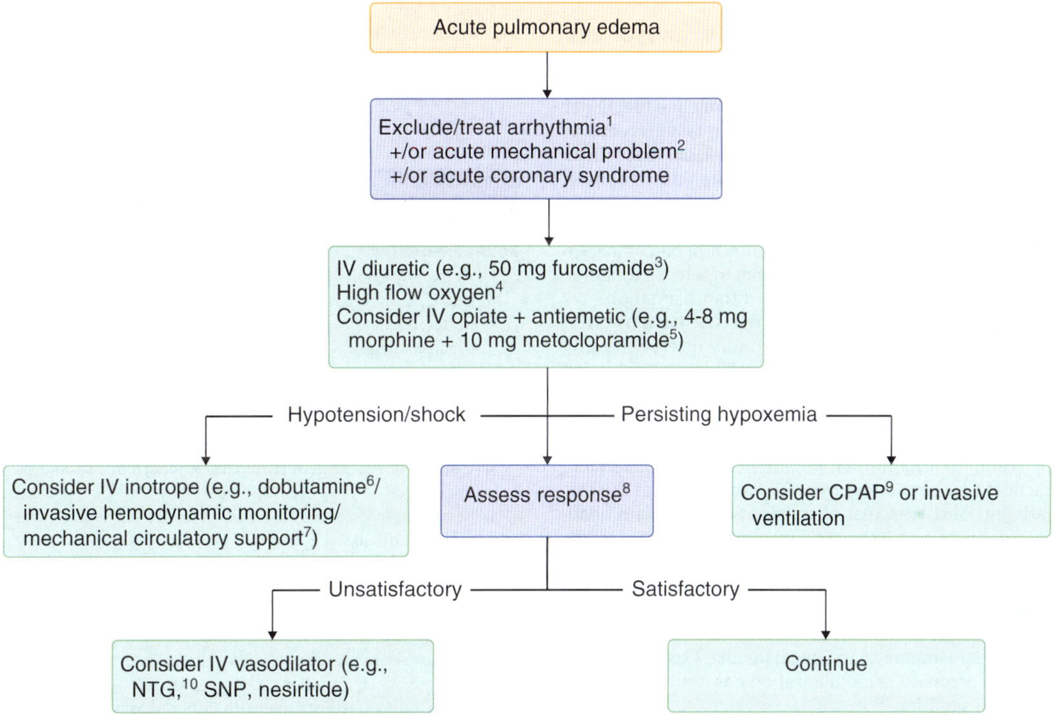

1 Casual arrhythmia (e.g., ventricular tachycardia). It can be difficult to determine whether atrial fibrillation is a primary cause of acute pulmonary edema or secondary to it. An ECG is an essential investigation.
2 Acute mechanical problems include ventricular septal rupture and mitral valve papillary muscle rupture. Mechanical support (e.g., an intra-aortic balloon pump) and urgent surgery should be considered. An echocardiogram should be performed as soon as possible, especially in a patient without a prior diagnosis of heart failure/other relevant heart disease (e.g., prior myocardial infarction or valve disease).
3 Dose of diuretic depends on prior diuretic use and renal function—a lower dose may suffice if preserved renal function and no prior diuretic use.
4 Oxygen causes an increase in systemic vascular resistance and a reduction in heart rate and cardiac output and should only be administered to patients with hypoxemia.
5 Consider if patient is agitated/distressed/in pain; may cause respiratory depression and dose should be reduced in very elderly.
6 An intravenous infusion of dobutamine may be started at a dose of 2.5 μg/kg/min, doubling every 15 minutes according to response and tolerability (dose titration usually limited by excessive tachycardia, arrhythmias, or ischemia). A dose above 20 μg/kg/min is rarely needed.
7 For example, an intra-aortic balloon pump
8 Improvement in symptoms and peripheral perfusion and adequate urine output—patient should be monitored closely, and usually a response will occur within 30 minutes. Bladder catheterization may help in monitoring urine output.
9 Continuous positive airways pressure (CPAP) is valuable in severe pulmonary edema, especially if associated with hypoxemia. Endotracheal intubation and invasive mechanical ventilation should be considered in patients with persisting hypoxemia and physical ventilatory exhaustion.
10 If systolic blood pressure is adequate (>100 mm Hg), an intravenous infusion of nitroglycerin (NTG) can be considered. Start at a dose of 10 μg/min and double every 10 minutes according to response and tolerability (usually dose up-titration is limited by hypotension). A dose of more than 100 μg/min is rarely needed.

FIGURE 46-4. **Approach to the patient with acute pulmonary edema.** IV = intravenous; NTG = nitroglycerin; SNP = sodium nitroprusside.

causing dyssynchronous contraction, less efficient ventricular emptying, and, often, mitral regurgitation. Atrioventricular coupling may also be abnormal, as reflected by a prolonged PR interval, as may interventricular synchrony. Cardiac resynchronization therapy (CRT) with atrial-biventricular or multisite pacing optimizes atrioventricular timing and improves synchronization of cardiac contraction. In symptomatic patients (NYHA class II to IV) who are in sinus rhythm, have marked systolic dysfunction (left ventricular ejection fraction ≤35%), and have a wide QRS, the addition of CRT to optimal medical therapy and an ICD improves pump function, reduces mitral regurgitation, relieves symptoms, and significantly prolongs exercise capacity. CRT also substantially reduces the risk for death and for hospital admission for worsening heart failure in such patients.[15] Many other outcome measures, including quality of life, are also improved. Whether CRT is beneficial in patients in atrial fibrillation or with non–left bundle branch block (LBBB) QRS widening is uncertain. All patients in sinus rhythm with persistent symptoms (NYHA class II to IV) and an ejection fraction of 35% or less despite optimal disease-modifying medical therapy (ARNI [or ACE inhibitor or ARB], β-blocker, mineralocorticoid receptor antagonist, and an SGLT2 inhibitor) should be considered for CRT if they have a QRS duration 130 msec or longer, especially if they have LBBB morphology, with the greatest benefit seen in patients with a QRS duration 150 msec or longer. Conversely, patients with a QRS duration less than 130 msec may be harmed by CRT. The value of new pacing modes, such as left bundle branch or[A27] His-bundle pacing,[A28] is also being explored in heart failure.

Surgery

With the exception of cardiac transplantation and ventricular assist devices, there are no generally accepted criteria for surgical intervention. Use of operative procedures is variable among centers and greatly dependent on local experience and expertise. Expert imaging and detailed hemodynamic and functional assessments are usually required when any patient with heart failure is considered for surgery, and close liaison between the relevant experts in these fields is essential. The collective expertise in surgical centers is often used to make highly individualized decisions about whether to operate and what procedures will be attempted. "Established" operative treatments for patients with heart failure include coronary artery bypass grafting, surgery, surgical or percutaneous interventions for aortic valve stenosis and mitral valve incompetence (Chapter 60), implantation of ventricular assist devices,[16] and heart transplantation.

PERCUTANEOUS CORONARY INTERVENTION OR CORONARY ARTERY BYPASS GRAFTING. Percutaneous coronary intervention or coronary artery bypass grafting (Chapter 59), as appropriate, is indicated for relief of angina. The extent of ischemia and residual myocardial viability can be determined by noninvasive assessments such as dobutamine echocardiography (Chapter 43), magnetic resonance imaging (Chapter 44), and positron emission tomographic scanning (Chapter 44) in patients with impaired left ventricular ejection fraction. Coronary artery bypass grafting reduces the risk for cardiovascular death and cardiovascular hospitalization (including heart failure hospitalization) in patients with ischemic cardiomyopathy, an ejection fraction of 35% or less, and coronary artery disease amenable to coronary-artery bypass grafting.[A29] The net benefit is not apparent until approximately 2 years after randomization because of the perioperative mortality related to surgery. Coronary artery bypass grafting is therefore recommended in such patients who are otherwise fit for surgery and have an anticipated life expectancy of 2 years or more. Percutaneous coronary revascularization has not been proven to have similar benefits in this situation.[A30]

CARDIAC TRANSPLANTATION. Cardiac transplantation remains the most accepted (Table 46-8) surgical intervention in end-stage heart failure.[17] Selection criteria usually focus on patients with refractory heart failure, that is, those with severe symptoms and functional limitations (peak oxygen consumption of less than 12 mL/kg per minute), as well as a particularly worrisome clinical course and prognosis attributed to their cardiac condition. These patients are often dependent on intravenous inotropic agents and mechanical support.

Over 3800 heart transplants are performed annually in the United States. The major limitation is the scarcity of donor organs, although increasing acceptance of heart donation after circulatory death has helped ease this problem. Cardiac xenotransplantation is experimental but a potentially promising additional way to address this shortage.[18] Absolute and relative exclusion criteria for heart transplantation (Table 46-9) include advanced age, serious comorbid conditions, and nonreversible pulmonary vascular resistance of more than 6 Wood units.

To diagnose allograft rejection, which can be antibody-mediated or cell-mediated, transjugular endomyocardial biopsies are usually performed weekly for 1 month, every other week for 2 months, and then every 1 to 2 months for the first year. In patients who are asymptomatic on low doses of corticosteroids, a gene expression profile of peripheral blood[19] can provide equivalent clinical outcomes despite fewer biopsies.[A31] Cellular rejection is usually easily treated with high-dose corticosteroids, but humoral rejection may require more aggressive immunosuppression (Chapter 38).

Another form of chronic rejection is transplant vasculopathy, which occurs at an annual rate of 5 to 10%. Patients are more likely to present with fatigue, heart failure, myocardial infarction, ventricular arrhythmia, or sudden death than with

TABLE 46-8 INDICATIONS FOR HEART TRANSPLANTATION

Indications for referral of ambulatory patients with chronic heart failure

1. Patients who have limiting symptoms on exertion despite optimal medical therapy
2. Patients who require frequent hospital admission (two or more in 12 months) despite adequate therapy and adherence
3. Deteriorating renal function or inability to clear congestion without adversely affecting renal function
4. The need to decrease the dose or discontinue prognostically beneficial medication due to symptoms (often hypotension) or side effects such as renal dysfunction
5. Worsening right ventricular function or rising pulmonary artery pressure
6. High or rising natriuretic peptide levels despite optimal therapy
7. Frequent episodes of ventricular arrhythmias despite optimal drug and electrophysiologic therapy
8. Anemia, weight loss, hyponatraemia, or liver dysfunction attributable to heart failure

Indications for urgent inpatient referral

1. Inability to wean intravenous inotropic therapy
2. Need for percutaneous mechanical circulatory support to treat a patient in cardiogenic shock
3. Ventilatory support with use of positive airway pressure for intractable pulmonary edema
4. Refractory ventricular arrhythmias

From Bhagra SK, Pettit S, Parameshwar J. Cardiac transplantation: indications, eligibility and current outcomes. *Heart*. 2019;105:252-260.

TABLE 46-9 CARDIAC TRANSPLANTATION CONTRAINDICATION CRITERIA

1. Active infection (patients with chronic viral infection such as hepatitis B, hepatitis C, and human immunodeficiency virus may be considered if viral titres are undetectable on treatment or following treatment without evidence of other organ damage).
2. Symptomatic cerebral or peripheral vascular disease.
3. Diabetes mellitus with end-organ damage (e.g., nephropathy, neuropathy, proliferative retinopathy). Poorly controlled diabetes with glycosylated hemoglobin persistently >7.5% or 58 mmol/mL is a relative contraindication.
4. Current or recent neoplasm: risk of recurrence should be discussed with the oncologist.
5. Severe lung disease: FEV1 and FVC <50% predicted or evidence of parenchymal lung disease.
6. Irreversible renal dysfunction with estimated glomerular filtration rate <30 mL/min/1.73 m^2.
7. Irreversible liver dysfunction (e.g., cirrhosis).
8. Recent pulmonary thromboembolism (generally in the last 3 months).
9. Pulmonary hypertension with pulmonary artery systolic pressure >60 mm Hg, transpulmonary gradient ≥15 mm Hg and/or pulmonary vascular resistance >5 Wood units. If irreversible with either pharmacologic manipulation or mechanical unloading of the left ventricle, this is an absolute contraindication to isolated heart transplantation.
10. Psychosocial factors including history of non-compliance with medication, inadequate social support, ongoing or recent drug or alcohol use disorder, current smoker.
11. Obesity (body mass index >35 kg/m^2 or weight >140% of ideal body weight).
12. Other multisystem disease with poor long-term survival.

FEV1 = forced expiratory volume in one second; FVC = forced vital capacity.

From Bhagra SK, Pettit S, Parameshwar J. Cardiac transplantation: indication, eligibility and current outcomes. *Heart*. 2019;105:252-260.

exertional angina. Patients are typically screened with annual coronary angiography, stress echocardiography, or positron emission tomography. Treatment emphasizes high-dose statins (see Table 190-2 in Chapter 190) and mTOR inhibitors (e.g., sirolimus or everolimus), but repeat transplantation may be required.

The survival rate after heart transplantation is currently about 85 to 90% at 1 year, 70 to 75% at 5 years, and 20% at 20 years. Transplant vasculopathy and malignancies account for about one third of deaths among patients who survive for 10 or more years.

MECHANICAL CIRCULATORY SUPPORT. Given the scarcity of organ donors, durable mechanical circulatory support using a left ventricular (or biventricular) assist device (LVAD) may be used as a "bridge to transplantation" or, in some centers, as a permanent and definitive alternative to transplantation ("destination therapy").[20] Mechanical circulatory support may also be used as a "bridge to candidacy" (i.e., to try to improve a patient's clinical status sufficiently to become eligible for transplantation). A continuous axial-flow device can provide a 65% 2-year survival free of repeat device surgery or disabling stroke. A newer ventricular magnetically levitated centrifugal-flow pump may provide better short-term and 2-year outcomes than the axial-flow pump.[A32]

Because not every hospital could or should be expected to offer all these levels of support for patients with advanced heart failure, there is a general recognition that such services should be concentrated in a limited number of tertiary centers. Centers implanting these devices use criteria such as persistent (>2 months) severe symptoms despite optimal drug and device therapy and other features placing patients at high risk for death (e.g., left ventricular ejection fraction <25%, three or more heart failure hospitalizations in the prior 12 months, peak oxygen consumption <12 mL/kg per minute, dependence on intravenous inotropic therapy, progressive end-organ dysfunction, and deteriorating right ventricular function) to decide who should be considered for mechanical circulatory support.

Organization of Care and Remote Monitoring

Several studies have shown that organized, nurse-led, multidisciplinary care can improve outcomes in patients with heart failure, particularly by reducing recurrent hospital admissions. Thus it is recommended that all patients with heart failure be enrolled in a disease management program. The most successful disease management approach seems to involve education of the patients, their families, and caregivers about heart failure and its treatment (including flexible diuretic dosing and reinforcing the importance of adherence), recognizing (and acting on) early deterioration (dyspnea, sudden weight gain, edema), and optimizing proven pharmacologic treatments. Both home-based and office-based approaches are effective. Even telephone follow-up is of value. New technology enabling noninvasive home telemonitoring of physiologic measures (e.g., heart rate and rhythm, blood pressure, temperature, respiratory rate, weight, and estimated body water content) and implanted devices, which collect similar data and may be interrogated remotely, are also being tested as aids to monitoring and management, but studies to date have not given consistent results. An alert embedded into the electronic health record can provide outpatients with personalized recommendations for increasing the use of guideline-directed medical therapies.[A33] Despite the usefulness of brain-type natriuretic peptide (BNP) in the diagnosis of heart failure and as a prognostic measure, treatment guided by BNP levels has not been shown in randomized trials to be consistently better than standard, evidence-based care.[A34] Conversely, treatment based on hemodynamic data transmitted from an implantable pulmonary artery pressure sensor may reduce heart failure hospitalizations over a 6- to 12-month period.[A35]

Education

Education of the patient, family, and caregivers is valuable (Table 46-10). Self-detection of early signs and symptoms of deterioration provides for earlier intervention. Counseling on the proper use of therapies, with an emphasis on adherence, is critical.

Useful patient-oriented material is available from several reliable sources: the Heart Failure Society of America (https://hfsa.org/patient-hub/heart-failure-facts-information), American Heart Association (http://www.heart.org/HEARTORG/Conditions/HeartFailure/Heart-Failure_UCM_002019_SubHomePage.jsp), National Heart, Lung and Blood Institute (http://www.nhlbi.nih.gov/health/dci/Diseases/Hf/HF_WhatIs.html), the Heart Failure Association of the European Society of Cardiology (https://www.heartfailurematters.org/), and other organizations.

Medication Use Counseling

When appropriate, a patient should be taught how to adjust the dose of diuretic within individualized limits. The dose should be increased (or a supplementary diuretic added) if there is evidence of fluid retention (symptoms of congestion) and decreased if there is evidence of hypovolemia (e.g., increased thirst associated with weight loss or postural dizziness, especially during hot weather or an illness causing decreased fluid intake or sodium and water loss). If hypovolemia is more marked, the doses of other medications also will have to be reduced.

The expected effects, beneficial and adverse, of other drugs should also be explained in detail (e.g., possible association of cough with ACE inhibitor). It is useful to inform patients that improvement with many drugs is gradual and may become fully apparent only after several weeks or even months of treatment. It is also important to explain the need for up-titration of the dose of an ARNI (or ACE inhibitor or ARB), a β-blocker, a mineralocorticoid receptor antagonist, and an SGLT2 inhibitor to the evidence-based target level, a goal that again may require weeks or even months to achieve. Patients should be advised not to use NSAIDs without consultation and to be cautious about using herbal or other nonproprietary preparations (Chapter 30).

Adherence

Education and counseling of the patient, caregiver, and family promote adherence, which is associated with better outcomes. Drug adherence can also be helped by home visits, specialized follow-up programs, and certain pharmacy aids, such as dose allocation (pill-organizing) boxes.

TABLE 46-10 TOPICS THAT SHOULD BE DISCUSSED WITH A PATIENT WITH HEART FAILURE AND WITH HIS OR HER FAMILY AND CAREGIVERS

GENERAL ADVICE
Explain what heart failure is and why symptoms occur
Causes of heart failure
How to recognize symptoms
What to do if symptoms occur
Self-weighing (to identify fluid retention)
RATIONALE FOR TREATMENTS
Importance of adhering to pharmacologic and nonpharmacologic (e.g., dietary) treatments
Smoking advice
Prognosis
DRUG COUNSELING
Rationale (i.e., benefits of individual drugs)
Dose and time of administration
Potential adverse effects (and what, if any, action to take)
What to do in case of missed or skipped doses
Self-management (e.g., flexible diuretic dosing)
REST AND EXERCISE
Rest
Exercise and activities related to work
Daily physical activity
Sexual activity
Rehabilitation
PSYCHOSOCIAL ASPECTS
Depression
Cognitive function
Social support
VACCINATIONS AND IMMUNIZATIONS
Influenza
Pneumococcal
OTHER
Travel
Driving
Dietary and social habits
Control sodium intake when necessary (e.g., some patients with severe heart failure)
Avoid excessive fluids in severe heart failure
Avoid excessive alcohol intake and illicit drugs

Modified from McMurray JJ, Adamopoulos S, Anker SD, et al. ESC Guidelines for the diagnosis and treatment of acute and chronic heart failure 2012: the Task Force for the Diagnosis and Treatment of Acute and Chronic Heart Failure 2012 of the European Society of Cardiology. Developed in collaboration with the Heart Failure Association (HFA) of the ESC. *Eur Heart J.* 2012;33:1787-1847.

Lifestyle Modification

Exercise

Tailored, structured, supervised aerobic exercise is safe and improves functional capacity and quality of life in patients with heart failure.[A36] An appropriate exercise prescription may also reduce hospitalizations and mortality in patients with heart failure. Regular physical activity or exercise training, if available, is recommended for all patients with heart failure who are able to participate.

Diet, Nutrition, and Alcohol

Most guidelines advocate avoidance of foods containing relatively high salt content in the belief that doing so may reduce the need for diuretic therapy, although the benefits of severe sodium restriction to less than 1 gram of sodium per day are unproven.[A37] This recommendation is based on clinical experience, which suggests that excess sodium intake can be a precipitant of clinical decompensation. Some salt substitutes have a high potassium content, which can lead to hyperkalemia.

Restriction of fluid intake is indicated only during episodes of decompensation associated with peripheral edema or hyponatremia. In these situations, daily intake should be restricted to 1.5 to 2.0 L to help facilitate reduction in extracellular fluid volume and to avoid hyponatremia.

Reducing excessive weight will reduce the work of the heart and may lower blood pressure (Chapter 64). Conversely, malnutrition is common in severe heart failure, and the development of cardiac cachexia is an ominous sign. Reduced food intake is sometimes caused by nausea (e.g., related to digoxin use or hepatosplenic congestion) or abdominal bloating (e.g., due to ascites). In these cases, small frequent meals and high-protein and high-calorie liquids may be helpful.

In severe decompensated heart failure, eating and bending may be difficult because of dyspnea—so called "bendopnea."

Moderate alcohol intake is not thought to be harmful in heart failure, although excessive intake can cause cardiomyopathy and atrial arrhythmias in susceptible individuals. In patients with suspected alcoholic cardiomyopathy, abstinence from alcohol may improve cardiac function.

Smoking

Smoking causes peripheral vasoconstriction, which is detrimental in heart failure. Nicotine replacement therapy (Chapter 363) is believed to be safe in heart failure. The safety of bupropion in heart failure is uncertain, especially because it is known to increase blood pressure, and varenicline may increase cardiovascular risk.

Sexual Activity

Sexual activity need not be restricted in patients with compensated heart failure, although dyspnea may be limiting. In men with erectile dysfunction (Chapter 216), treatment with a cyclic guanine monophosphate phosphodiesterase type 5 inhibitor can be useful, but these drugs must not be taken within 24 hours of prior nitrate use, and nitrates must not be restarted for at least 24 hours afterward. Caution should be exercised when sildenafil or another type-5 phosphodiesterase inhibitor is used in addition to sacubitril/valsartan and vericiguat because of the risk of hypotension.

Driving

Patients with heart failure can continue to drive, provided their condition does not induce undue dyspnea, fatigue, or other incapacitating symptoms. Patients with recent syncope, cardiac surgery, percutaneous coronary intervention, or device placement may be restricted from driving, at least temporarily, according to local regulations. Patients holding an occupational or commercial license may also be subject to additional restrictions.

Traveling

Short flights are unlikely to cause problems for a patient with compensated heart failure. For patients with an LVAD, travel should be planned in advance and in conjunction with the heart failure team.[21] Cabin pressure is generally maintained to provide an oxygen level no lower than equivalent to 6000 feet above sea level, which should be well tolerated in patients without severe pulmonary disease or pulmonary hypertension. Longer journeys may cause limb edema and dehydration, owing to insensible fluid loss, aggravated by caffeinated drinks and alcohol, thereby predisposing to venous thrombosis. Avoidance of dehydration is especially important in patients with an LVAD because the function of these devices is sensitive to blood volume. Adjustment of the dose of diuretics and other treatments should be discussed with the patient wishing to travel to a warm climate or a country where the risk for gastroenteritis is high. It is also advisable for heart failure patients to carry a list of medications and contact information for their health care provider and device cards for airport security. In those with an LVAD, contact with a health care provider at the patient's destination may be advisable.

Comorbidity

Comorbid conditions, which are common and important in patients with heart failure, may be due to the underlying cardiovascular disease that caused or contributed to heart failure (e.g., hypertension, coronary artery disease, diabetes mellitus), may arise as a complication of heart failure (e.g., arrhythmias), or can result from an adverse effect of treatment given for heart failure (e.g., gout). The exact causes of other comorbidities in heart failure, such as diabetes (Chapter 210), depression (Chapter 362), sleep apnea (Chapter 374), renal dysfunction (Chapter 116), and anemia (Chapter 144), are complex and uncertain. These and other comorbid conditions, such as chronic obstructive pulmonary disease and asthma, are important because they are a major determinant of prognosis and may limit the use of certain treatments for heart failure (e.g., renal dysfunction limiting use of ACE inhibitors or asthma limiting β-blockers) and because treatment of comorbidities may affect the stability of heart failure (e.g., NSAIDs needed for rheumatic conditions can cause salt and water retention and renal dysfunction). Both prevention (e.g., diabetes mellitus) and treatment (e.g., anemia) of comorbidities are being evaluated as a potential new therapeutic goal in heart failure.

Angina and Ischemia

β-Blockers are of benefit in both angina (Chapter 56) and heart failure. Similarly, ivabradine, which reduces heart rate by inhibiting the I_f current in the sinus node, is also beneficial in both angina and heart failure. Nitrates relieve angina but on their own are not of proven value in chronic heart failure. Calcium-channel blockers should generally be avoided in heart failure because they have a negative inotropic action and cause peripheral edema; only amlodipine has been shown to have no adverse effect on survival, but it may increase the risk for pulmonary edema. Trimetazidine, ranolazine, and nicorandil are antianginal drugs that are available in certain countries; their safety in patients with heart failure is uncertain. Percutaneous and surgical (Chapter 59) revascularization is also of value in relieving angina in selected patients with heart failure (see later). Coronary artery bypass grafting may reduce the risk for death from cardiovascular causes and cardiovascular hospitalization (including heart failure hospitalization) in selected heart failure patients with angina and a reduced ejection fraction.

Atrial Fibrillation

Atrial fibrillation (Chapter 52) may be the cause of or a consequence of heart failure in a patient presenting with atrial fibrillation and a rapid ventricular rate, and the distinction can be difficult, especially because prolonged atrial fibrillation may lead to a rate-related cardiomyopathy. Thyrotoxicosis (Chapter 207) and mitral valve disease (Chapter 60), especially stenosis, must be excluded. Alcohol abuse should also be considered. β-Blockers and digoxin are given to control the ventricular rate. The patient should be supervised closely after the initiation of these treatments because underlying sinus node dysfunction may raise the risk for bradycardia. If the patient presents emergently with severe heart failure, shock, or myocardial ischemia, urgent electrical or pharmacologic cardioversion may be considered (Chapter 54). Catheter ablation (Chapter 52) can reduce hospitalizations and mortality in selected patients with heart failure and atrial fibrillation,[A38] even if the left ventricular ejection fraction is normal,[A39] whereas a strategy of maintaining sinus rhythm with antiarrhythmic drug therapy alone is not superior to controlling the ventricular rate in patients with atrial fibrillation and heart failure. If pharmacologic therapy fails to control the ventricular rate and catheter ablation is contraindicated or unsuccessful, atrioventricular node ablation and pacing may be required (Chapter 54).[22] There is a strong indication for thromboembolism prophylaxis with a direct-acting anticoagulant or warfarin in patients who have heart failure with paroxysmal, persistent, or permanent atrial fibrillation (Chapter 52).

Asthma and Reversible Airway Obstruction

Asthma is a contraindication for use of a β-blocker, but most patients with chronic obstructive pulmonary disease (Chapter 76) can tolerate a β-blocker. Pulmonary congestion can mimic chronic obstructive pulmonary disease. Systemic administration of a corticosteroid to treat reversible airway obstruction may cause sodium and water retention and exacerbate heart failure, whereas inhalation therapy is better tolerated.

Diabetes Mellitus

The prevalence and incidence of diabetes mellitus are high in heart failure. β-Blocker treatment is not contraindicated and is of benefit in patients with diabetes and heart failure. In patients who have heart failure and type 2 diabetes, the SGLT2 inhibitors are the preferred antidiabetic agents.[23] Using sacubitril/valsartan reduces the glycated hemoglobin level and the need to institute insulin treatment compared with using an ACE inhibitor.

Neither insulin nor glucagon-like peptide-1 (GLP-1) receptor agonists (GP-1 Ras) increase the risk of developing heart failure, and both are considered to be safe in patients with heart failure. By comparison, several agents are not recommended in patients with severe heart failure. Thiazolidinediones cause sodium and water retention, metformin may cause lactic acidosis in patients with severe heart failure, and saxagliptin, which increases the risk for developing heart failure, should be avoided. Although there is no evidence of a similar risk with other dipeptidyl peptidase-4 inhibitors, these medications also are not recommended.

Abnormal Thyroid Function

Both thyrotoxicosis and hypothyroidism can cause heart failure (and thyrotoxicosis can cause atrial fibrillation, which may precipitate heart failure). Amiodarone can also induce both hypothyroidism and hyperthyroidism, the latter being particularly difficult to diagnose. The risk for thyroid dysfunction may be less with the related antiarrhythmic agent dronedarone, but dronedarone increases mortality in severe heart failure and should be avoided in patients with stage C or D heart failure or recently decompensated heart failure.

Gout and Hyperuricemia

Hyperuricemia and gout (Chapter 252) are common in heart failure and can be caused or aggravated by diuretic treatment. Sacubitril/valsartan and SGLT2 inhibitors reduce serum uric acid levels. Acute gout attacks are better treated with colchicine, oral steroids, or intra-articular steroids rather than with an NSAID. Allopurinol can prevent gouty attacks more safely than febuxostat.[A40]

Renal Dysfunction

Most patients with heart failure have a reduced glomerular filtration rate. ACE inhibitors, ARBs, sacubitril/valsartan, mineralocorticoid receptor antagonists, and SGLT2 inhibitors often cause an early, but small, further reduction in glomerular filtration rate and rise in serum blood urea nitrogen and creatinine levels, which, if limited, should not lead to discontinuation of treatment. Marked increases in blood urea nitrogen and creatinine, however, should prompt consideration of underlying renal artery stenosis (Chapter 110). Renal dysfunction may also be caused by sodium and water depletion (e.g., due to excessive diuresis, diarrhea, and vomiting) that leads to relative hypovolemia and hypotension. Conversely, renal venous congestion can contribute to renal impairment in patients who are markedly volume-overloaded. Nephrotoxic agents such as NSAIDs are also a common cause of renal dysfunction in heart failure.

Prostatic Obstruction

For prostatic disease (Chapter 114), a 5α-reductase inhibitor may be preferable to an α-adrenoceptor antagonist, which can cause hypotension and salt and water retention.

Iron Deficiency and Anemia

Iron deficiency is very common in heart failure, for reasons that are uncertain, and may be present without concomitant anemia. Several trials have shown that intravenous ferric carboxymaltose or ferric derisomaltose (Chapter 145) improves symptoms, quality of life, and functional capacity when administered to patients who have a serum ferritin level <100 ng/mL or serum ferritin 100 to 299 ng/mL with a transferrin saturation <20%. In patients with heart failure, this treatment can substantially reduce the risk of hospital readmission for heart failure.[A41,A42]

A normocytic, normochromic anemia (Chapter 144) is also common in heart failure, in part because of the high prevalence of renal dysfunction. Malnutrition, blood loss, and underlying iron deficiency may be contributing factors. SGLT2 inhibitors increase the hematocrit and hemoglobin and often correct anemia, possibly by reducing plasma volume and increasing erythropoiesis. The erythropoiesis-stimulating agent darbepoetin is not of benefit in heart failure patients with anemia.

Depression

Depression (Chapter 362) is common in patients with heart failure, perhaps partly owing to disturbance of the hypothalamic-pituitary axis and other neurochemical pathways but also as a result of social isolation and the adjustment to chronic disease. Depression is associated with worse functional status, reduced adherence to treatment, and poor clinical outcomes. Both psychosocial interventions and pharmacologic treatment are helpful. Selective serotonin reuptake inhibitors are believed to be the best-tolerated pharmacologic agents, whereas tricyclic antidepressants should be avoided because of their anticholinergic actions and potential to cause arrhythmias.

Sleep Apnea

Sleep-disordered breathing, including both obstructive and central sleep apnea (Chapter 374), is common in patients with heart failure. Continuous positive airway pressure can improve the symptoms of obstructive sleep apnea in selected patients (Chapter 374), but adaptive servo-ventilation increases the risk of death in patients with heart failure and central sleep apnea.

Drugs to Use with Caution in Heart Failure

Patients with heart failure, especially if it is severe, often have renal and hepatic dysfunction, so any drug excreted predominantly by the kidneys or metabolized by the liver may accumulate (Chapter 25). Similarly, because of their extensive comorbidity, patients with heart failure are inevitably treated with multiple drugs, thereby increasing the risk for drug interactions.

Drugs that should be avoided, if possible, in heart failure include most antiarrhythmic drugs (including dronedarone, although amiodarone and dofetilide may be used), most calcium-channel blockers (with the possible exception of amlodipine, although this drug may increase the risk for pulmonary edema), corticosteroids, NSAIDs, cyclooxygenase-2 inhibitors, thiazolidinediones, saxagliptin, metformin, many antipsychotics (e.g., clozapine), and antihistamines. The U.S. Food and Drug Administration recently raised the concern that the dopamine agonist pramipexole used to treat Parkinson disease (Chapter 378) also might increase the risk for developing heart failure. Some salt substitutes contain substantial amounts of potassium and must be used cautiously. Other dietary constituents (e.g., grapefruit and cranberry juice) and supplements such as St. John's wort can interact with drugs taken by patients with heart failure, especially warfarin and digoxin. α-Adrenoceptor antagonists, commonly given for prostatic symptoms (Chapter 114), may cause hypotension and fluid retention. A variety of anticancer drugs, including trastuzumab, may aggravate heart failure (see Table 164-2).

Other Subtypes of Heart Failure

Heart Failure with Mildly Reduced Left Ventricular Ejection Fraction

In patients with heart failure and a left ventricular ejection fraction >40%, the SGLT2 inhibitors dapagliflozin and empagliflozin (each 10 mg once daily)[24] reduce the risk of heart failure hospitalization substantially and also improve symptoms and health-related quality of life.[A43,A44] In addition, retrospective analyses of several trials suggest that patients with a left ventricular ejection fraction in the range of 41 to 49% respond favorably to other treatments (e.g., an ARNI [or ACE inhibitor or ARB], a β-blocker, and a mineralocorticoid receptor antagonist) shown to be effective in patients with heart failure and a reduced ejection fraction. These therapies can be used to treat patients with heart failure and mildly reduced ejection fraction, along with diuretics as needed to control fluid retention (Fig. 46-5).

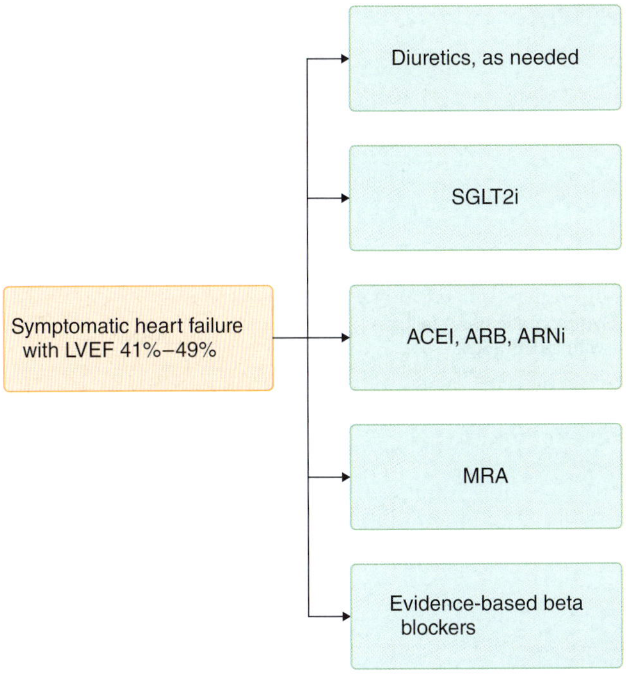

FIGURE 46-5. Treatments for heart failure with mildly reduced left ventricular ejection fraction. ACEI = angiotensin-converting enzyme inhibitor; ARB = angiotensin-receptor blocker; ARNI = angiotensin receptor-neprilysin inhibitor; LVEF = left ventricular ejection fraction; MRA = mineralocorticoid receptor antagonist; SGLT2i = sodium glucose cotransporter 2 inhibitor. (Reprinted with permission *Circulation*. 2022;145:e895-e1032 ©2022 American Heart Association, Inc.)

Heart Failure with Preserved Left Ventricular Ejection Fraction

For patients with heart failure and a left ventricular ejection fraction ≥50%, SGLT2 inhibitors (e.g., dapagliflozin 10 mg once daily or empagliflozin 10 mg once daily) reduce the risk of hospitalization for heart failure and improve symptoms and health-related quality of life. Diuretics, as needed to control fluid retention, are also valuable. However, no international consensus exists regarding other pharmacologic therapy (Fig. 46-6). Treatment of the underlying cardiovascular and other disorders that contribute to symptomatic stage C and stage D of heart failure with preserved left ventricular ejection fraction, such as hypertension, myocardial ischemia, and diabetes, is critical and is as for stages A and B (see earlier). In patients with atrial fibrillation, restoration of sinus rhythm or control of the ventricular rate with a β-blocker or a rate-limiting calcium-channel blocker can help control symptoms, although excessive rate control of atrial fibrillation or sinus rhythm may make these patients worse rather than better (Chapter 52). In patients with heart failure and preserved ejection fraction, ivabradine has no benefit on exercise capacity, and isosorbide mononitrate treatment tends to worsen activity levels. Infiltrative cardiomyopathies such as amyloidosis respond to disease-specific therapies (Chapter 47).

Heart Failure Due to Valvular Heart Disease

Heart failure also can arise as a result of regurgitant and stenotic valve disease (Chapter 60). It can sometimes be difficult to determine whether mitral regurgitation is primary or secondary in a patient with heart failure and left ventricular dilation, although a prior history of known valve disease or rheumatic fever may suggest a primary valve problem. The objective of treatment of primary valve disease is the prevention of heart failure by surgical repair or replacement of the diseased valve or valves (Chapter 60). The development of overt heart failure is an ominous sign, sometimes requiring emergent valve replacement (e.g., aortic stenosis) but sometimes indicating that valve replacement may not be possible (e.g., because of severe pulmonary hypertension).

Aortic Stenosis

Evaluation of the aortic valve (Chapter 60) can be difficult in patients with poor left ventricular systolic function. Such patients may have insufficient cardiac output to generate a high gradient across even a severely stenotic valve. Conversely, a calcified and degenerate but nonstenotic aortic valve may appear stenosed simply because it does not open normally in patients with very low cardiac output. A calculated valve area provides a better assessment of the severity of aortic stenosis in these patients. Stress echocardiography (Chapter 43) may help assess the potential for ventricular recovery after relief of aortic stenosis. Transcatheter valve replacement is a valuable technique for patients who have aortic stenosis but are at very high risk for open valve replacement.

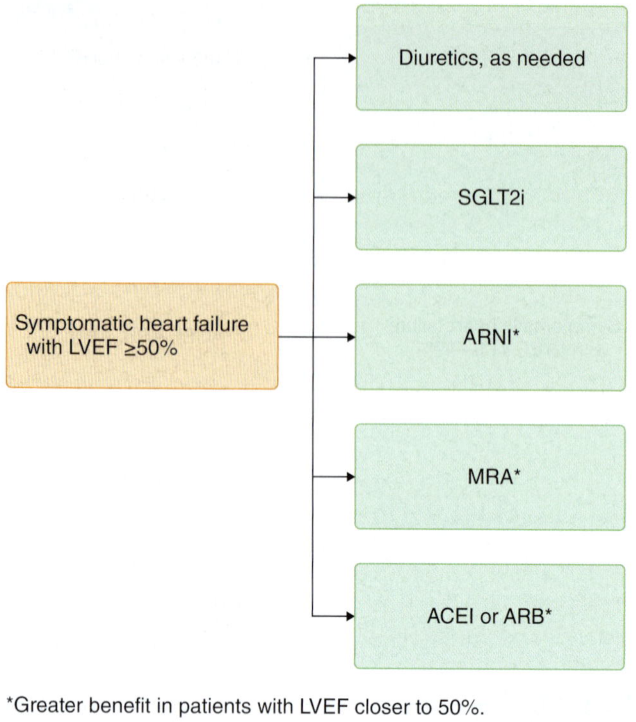

FIGURE 46-6. Treatments for heart failure with preserved left ventricular ejection fraction. ACEI = angiotensin-converting enzyme inhibitor; ARB = angiotensin-receptor blocker; ARNI = angiotensin receptor-neprilysin inhibitor; LVEF = left ventricular ejection fraction; MRA = mineralocorticoid receptor antagonist; SGLT2i = sodium glucose cotransporter 2 inhibitor. (Reprinted with permission *Circulation*. 2022;145:e895-e1032 ©2022 American Heart Association, Inc.)

Mitral and Tricuspid Regurgitation

Mitral regurgitation can be a primary cause (organic) or a secondary manifestation (functional) in a patient with heart failure and left ventricular dilation (Chapter 60). In primary mitral regurgitation, surgery sometimes will result in clinical improvement, but some patients with advanced left ventricular dysfunction will not achieve substantial benefit (e.g., mitral valve surgery in a patient with long-standing severe mitral regurgitation). Valve repair is preferable to valve replacement, although neither procedure is proven to improve survival. Generally, medical and device therapy (e.g., CRT) is preferred to isolated valve surgery for secondary regurgitation. The role of transcatheter mitral valve repair is still evolving. Two recent trials have reported conflicting findings, but one suggested that this approach could provide a durable reduction in the risk of death and hospitalization for heart failure in carefully selected patients.[A45] Concomitant tricuspid valve repair may also provide some benefit in patients who have heart failure with both mitral and tricuspid valve regurgitation,[A46] but more data will be required before it can be routinely recommended.

Heart Failure Due to Nonischemic Dilated Cardiomyopathy

Patients with heart failure and normal coronary arteries should be evaluated for possible reversible causes. Untreated hypertension is now an unusual cause of dilated cardiomyopathy in the United States, but hypertension was once a leading cause in the United States and remains a major consideration in many parts of the world. Infiltrative cardiomyopathies (e.g., hemochromatosis, amyloid, sarcoid) and arteritides sometimes have specific recommended therapies (Chapters 47, 83, 174, and 196). Chagas disease (Chapter 318) must be considered in patients from endemic areas. Alcohol and other toxins (e.g., chemotherapeutic agents) are other recognized causes of dilated cardiomyopathy. Dilated cardiomyopathy can also develop in the peripartum period. Most cases of nonischemic dilated cardiomyopathy are usually labeled "idiopathic" (i.e., no specific etiology can be determined), although many may have a genetic origin, especially if there is a positive family history. In many centers routine genetic testing is undertaken in younger patients with unexplained dilated cardiomyopathy, especially in individuals with a family history of heart failure or sudden death and in those with conduction disease (e.g., bundle branch block). First-degree relatives of patients with genetic cardiomyopathies should be counseled and screened. Irrespective of etiology, nonischemic dilated cardiomyopathy should be treated in the same way as dilated ischemic cardiomyopathy.

Heart Failure Due to Hypertrophic Cardiomyopathy

Heart failure can arise in patients with hypertrophic cardiomyopathy because of predominant diastolic dysfunction, associated mitral incompetence, or the development of systolic dysfunction. The management of hypertrophic cardiomyopathy and its complications is often very different from the management of dilated cardiomyopathy (Chapter 47), thereby underscoring the value of echocardiography in the evaluation of the patient with heart failure.

Outpatient Follow-Up

In patients being sent home from the hospital, discharge planning and subsequent management to reduce the risk for readmission are important. Ideally, an effective oral diuretic regimen should have been identified, and fluid-volume and biochemical stability should have been achieved. This optimization of volume status and development of a stable oral regimen before discharge is thought to reduce the risk for early readmission. Treatment with an ARNI (or ACE inhibitor or ARB), a β-blocker, a mineralocorticoid receptor antagonist, and SGLT2 inhibitor should be started in the stabilized patient before discharge. Outpatient follow-up should be arranged to ensure that any of those treatments that have not been started before discharge are initiated after discharge and that the dose of each drug is increased, as tolerated, to the appropriate target.

The key to successful follow-up is the careful tracking of clinical symptoms and the patient's weight, which often involves interviewing not only the patient but also family members, who may be more aware of changes in status than the patient is. Treatment of established heart failure based on natriuretic peptide levels does not appear to improve outcomes compared with best standard care. Continuity of care and seamless transitions from the inpatient to the outpatient setting are crucial aspects of optimal management. Patients with advanced heart failure and patients requiring frequent hospitalization require special attention. Programs that provide telephone-based tracking of daily weights and symptoms can detect deterioration in time to intervene before the need for hospitalization, and an implanted pulmonary artery pressure monitor may be valuable in selected patients. Although these programs may be costly, several evaluations have found them to be cost-effective. Because the care of these patients requires considerable experience and expertise, specialized disease management programs and clinics have been developed and may provide additional benefit compared with traditional care.

PROGNOSIS

The prognosis of patients with heart failure has improved with advances in therapy. Although it is difficult to predict prognosis in individual patients, until recently patients with symptoms at rest (NYHA class IV) have a 30 to 50% annual mortality rate, patients who are symptomatic with mild activity (class III) have mortality rates of 10 to 20% annually, and patients with symptoms only with moderate activity (class II) have a 5 to 10% annual mortality rate. Mortality rates are higher in older patients, men, patients with a reduced left ventricular ejection fraction[25] or underlying coronary heart disease, and patients with higher serum levels of certain biomarkers (e.g., natriuretic peptides and high-sensitivity troponin).[26]

End-of-Life Considerations

Although predicting the trajectory of illness in patients with advanced heart failure is notoriously difficult, it is often apparent when a patient has progressed to end-stage heart failure, commonly associated with concomitant renal failure. In these circumstances, the expertise of the palliative care team may be especially helpful (Chapter 3).[27] Useful websites providing information on palliative care relevant to heart failure are available (https://getpalliativecare.org/whatis/disease-types/congestive-heart-failure-palliative-care/, http://www.goldstandardsframework.org.uk/, and http://www.palliativecarescotland.org.uk/content/links, https://www.hospiceuk.org/what-we-offer/clinical-and-care-support/heart-failure-and-hospice-care). Medications such as parenteral opiates (with an antiemetic) and benzodiazepines may be particularly helpful in relieving dyspnea, anxiety, and pain that arises from ascites, hepatic congestion, lower limb edema, and pressure points. At this stage in the patient's illness, it may be appropriate to discuss withdrawal of conventional treatment, deactivation of an ICD to avoid undesired and unpleasant electrical discharges, and a do-not-resuscitate order if the patient and others involved in the patient's care agree that comfort care is appropriate. Hospice care may be chosen by some at this point.

GENERAL REFERENCES

For the General References and other additional features, please visit Elsevier eBooks+ at https://ebooks.health.elsevier.com.

Grade A References

A1. The Blood Pressure Lowering Treatment Trialists' Collaboration. Pharmacological blood pressure lowering for primary and secondary prevention of cardiovascular disease across different levels of blood pressure: an individual participant-level data meta-analysis. *Lancet*. 2021;397:1625-1636.
A2. The Blood Pressure Lowering Treatment Trialists' Collaboration. Age-stratified and blood-pressure-stratified effects of blood-pressure-lowering pharmacotherapy for the prevention of cardiovascular disease and death: an individual participant-level data meta-analysis. *Lancet*. 2021;398:1053-1064.
A3. Zou X, Shi Q, Vandvik PO, et al. Sodium-glucose cotransporter-2 inhibitors in patients with heart failure: a systematic review and meta-analysis. *Ann Intern Med*. 2022;175:851-861.
A4. Sattar N, Lee MMY, Kristensen SL, et al. Cardiovascular, mortality, and kidney outcomes with GLP-1 receptor agonists in patients with type 2 diabetes: a systematic review and meta-analysis of randomised trials. *Lancet Diabetes Endocrinol*. 2021;9:653-662.
A5. Zelniker TA, Wiviott SD, Raz I, et al. Comparison of the effects of glucagon-like peptide receptor agonists and sodium-glucose cotransporter 2 inhibitors for prevention of major adverse cardiovascular and renal outcomes in type 2 diabetes mellitus. *Circulation*. 2019;139:2022-2031.
A6. Holman RR, Coleman RL, Chan JCN, et al. Effects of acarbose on cardiovascular and diabetes outcomes in patients with coronary heart disease and impaired glucose tolerance (ACE): a randomised, double-blind, placebo-controlled trial. *Lancet Diabetes Endocrinol*. 2017;5:877-886.
A7. Pfeffer MA, Claggett B, Lewis EF, et al. Angiotensin receptor-neprilysin inhibition in acute myocardial infarction. *N Engl J Med*. 2021;385:1845-1855.
A8. Trulls JC, Morales-Rull JL, Casado J, et al. Combining loop with thiazide diuretics for decompensated heart failure: the CLOROTIC trial. *Eur Heart J*. 2023;44:411-421.
A9. Mullens W, Dauw J, Martens P, et al. Acetazolamide in acute decompensated heart failure with volume overload. *N Engl J Med*. 2022;387:1185-1195.
A10. Charuel E, Menini T, Bedhomme S, et al. Benefits and adverse effects of sacubitril/valsartan in patients with chronic heart failure: a systematic review and meta-analysis. *Pharmacol Res Perspect*. 2021;9:e00844.
A11. Velazquez EJ, Morrow DA, DeVore AD, et al. Angiotensin-neprilysin inhibition in acute decompensated heart failure. *N Engl J Med*. 2019;380:539-548.
A12. Cleland JGF, Bunting KV, Flather MD, et al. Beta-blockers for heart failure with reduced, mid-range, and preserved ejection fraction: an individual patient-level analysis of double-blind randomized trials. *Eur Heart J*. 2018;39:26-35.
A13. Burnett H, Earley A, Voors AA, et al. Thirty years of evidence on the efficacy of drug treatments for chronic heart failure with reduced ejection fraction: a network meta-analysis. *Circ Heart Fail*. 2017;10:1-12.
A14. Vaduganathan M, Docherty KF, Claggett BL, et al. SGLT-2 inhibitors in patients with heart failure: a comprehensive meta-analysis of five randomised controlled trials. *Lancet*. 2022;400:757-767.
A15. McMurray JJV, Solomon SD, Inzucchi SE, et al. Dapagliflozin in patients with heart failure and reduced ejection fraction. *N Engl J Med*. 2019;381:1995-2008.
A16. Bhatt DL, Szarek M, Steg PG, et al. Sotagliflozin in patients with diabetes and recent worsening heart failure. *N Engl J Med*. 2021;384:117-128.
A17. Voors AA, Angermann CE, Teerlink JR, et al. The SGLT2 inhibitor empagliflozin in patients hospitalized for acute heart failure: a multinational randomized trial. *Nat Med*. 2022;28:568-574.
A18. Nuffield Department of Population Health Renal Studies Group; SGLT2 inhibitor Meta-Analysis Cardio-Renal Trialists' Consortium. Impact of diabetes on the effects of sodium glucose co-transporter-2 inhibitors on kidney outcomes: collaborative meta-analysis of large placebo-controlled trials. *Lancet*. 2022;400:1788-1801.
A19. Bryan Richard S, Huang B, Liu G, et al. Impact of ivabradine on the cardiac function of chronic heart failure reduced ejection fraction: meta-analysis of randomized controlled trials. *Clin Cardiol*. 2021;44:463-471.
A20. Armstrong PW, Pieske B, Anstrom KJ, et al. Vericiguat in patients with heart failure and reduced ejection fraction. *N Engl J Med*. 2020;382:1883-1893.
A21. Zannad F, Anker SD, Byra WM, et al. Rivaroxaban in patients with heart failure, sinus rhythm, and coronary disease. *N Engl J Med*. 2018;379:1332-1342.
A22. Loeb M, Roy A, Dokainish H, et al. Influenza vaccine to reduce adverse vascular events in patients with heart failure: a multinational randomised, double blind, placebo controlled trial. *Lancet Glob Health*. 2022;10:e1835-e1844.
A23. Mebazaa A, Davison B, Chioncel O, et al. Safety, tolerability and efficacy of up-titration of guide-line-directed medical therapies for acute heart failure (STRONG-HF): a multinational, open-label, randomised, trial. *Lancet*. 2022;400:1938-1952.
A24. Mentz RJ, Anstrom KJ, Eisenstein EL, et al. Effect of torsemide vs furosemide after discharge on all-cause mortality in patients hospitalized with heart failure: the TRANSFORM-HF randomized clinical trial. *JAMA*. 2023;329:214-223.
A25. Butt JH, Yafasova A, Elming MB, et al. NT-proBNP and ICD in nonischemic systolic heart failure: extended follow-up of the DANISH trial. *JACC Heart Fail*. 2022;10:161-171.
A26. Beggs SAS, Jhund PS, Jackson CE, et al. Non-ischaemic cardiomyopathy, sudden death and implantable defibrillators: a review and meta-analysis. *Heart*. 2018;104:144-150.
A27. Wang Y, Zhu H, Hou X, et al. Randomized trial of left bundle branch vs biventricular pacing for cardiac resynchronization therapy. *J Am Coll Cardiol*. 2022;80:1205-1216.
A28. Whinnett ZI, Shun-Shin MJ, Tanner M, et al. Effects of haemodynamically atrio-ventricular optimized His bundle pacing on heart failure symptoms and exercise capacity: the His Optimized Pacing Evaluated for Heart Failure (HOPE-HF) randomized, double-blind, cross-over trial. *Eur J Heart Fail*. 2023;25:274-283.
A29. Velazquez EJ, Lee KL, Jones RH, et al. Coronary-artery bypass surgery in patients with ischemic cardiomyopathy. *N Engl J Med*. 2016;374:1511-1520.
A30. Perera D, Clayton T, O'Kane PD, et al. Percutaneous revascularization for ischemic left ventricular dysfunction. *N Engl J Med*. 2022;387:1351-1360.
A31. Kobashigawa J, Patel J, Azarbal B, et al. Randomized pilot trial of gene expression profiling versus heart biopsy in the first year after heart transplant: early invasive monitoring attenuation through gene expression trial. *Circ Heart Fail*. 2015;8:557-564.
A32. Mehra MR, Goldstein DJ, Cleveland JC, et al. Five-year outcomes in patients with fully magnetically levitated vs axial-flow left ventricular assist devices in the MOMENTUM 3 randomized trial. *JAMA*. 2022;328:1233-1242.
A33. Ghazi L, Yamamoto Y, Riello RJ, et al. Electronic alerts to improve heart failure therapy in outpatient practice: a cluster randomized trial. *J Am Coll Cardiol*. 2022;79:2203-2213.
A34. Pufulete M, Maishman R, Dabner L, et al. B-type natriuretic peptide-guided therapy for heart failure (HF): a systematic review and meta-analysis of individual participant data (IPD) and aggregate data. *Syst Rev*. 2018;7:112.
A35. Lindenfeld J, Zile MR, Desai AS, et al. Haemodynamic-guided management of heart failure (GUIDE-HF): a randomised controlled trial. *Lancet*. 2021;398:991-1001.
A36. Kitzman DW, Whellan DJ, Duncan P, et al. Physical rehabilitation for older patients hospitalized for heart failure. *N Engl J Med*. 2021;385:203-216.
A37. Ezekowitz JA, Colin-Ramirez E, Ross H, et al. Reduction of dietary sodium to less than 100 mmol in heart failure (SODIUM-HF): an international, open-label, randomised, controlled trial. *Lancet*. 2022;399:1391-1400.
A38. Parkash R, Wells GA, Rouleau J, et al. Randomized ablation-based rhythm-control versus rate-control trial in patients with heart failure and atrial fibrillation: results from the RAFT-AF trial. *Circulation*. 2022;145:1693-1704.
A39. Gu G, Wu J, Gao X, et al. Catheter ablation of atrial fibrillation in patients with heart failure and preserved ejection fraction: a meta-analysis. *Clin Cardiol*. 2022;45:786-793.
A40. White WB, Saag KG, Becker MA, et al. Cardiovascular safety of febuxostat or allopurinol in patients with gout. *N Engl J Med*. 2018;378:1200-1210.
A41. Graham FJ, Pellicori P, Kalra PR, et al. Intravenous iron in patients with heart failure and iron deficiency: an updated meta-analysis. *Eur J Heart Fail*. 2023. [Epub ahead of print.]
A42. Kalra PR, Cleland JGF, Petrie MC, et al. Intravenous ferric derisomaltose in patients with heart failure and iron deficiency in the UK (IRONMAN): an investigator-initiated, prospective, randomised, open-label, blinded-endpoint trial. *Lancet*. 2022;400:2199-2209.
A43. Packer M, Butler J, Zannad F, et al. Effect of empagliflozin on worsening heart failure events in patients with heart failure and preserved ejection fraction: EMPEROR-preserved trial. *Circulation*. 2021;144:1284-1294.
A44. Solomon SD, McMurray JJV, Claggett B, et al. Dapagliflozin in heart failure with mildly reduced or preserved ejection fraction. *N Engl J Med*. 2022;387:1089-1098.
A45. Sorajja P, Whisenant B, Hamid N, et al. Transcatheter repair for patients with tricuspid regurgitation. *N Engl J Med*. 2023. [Epub ahead of print.]
A46. Gammie JS, Chu MWA, Falk V, et al. Concomitant tricuspid repair in patients with degenerative mitral regurgitation. *N Engl J Med*. 2022;386:327-339.

47

DISEASES OF THE MYOCARDIUM AND ENDOCARDIUM

PERRY M. ELLIOTT AND IACOPO OLIVOTTO

MYOCARDIAL DISEASE

A substantial minority of cases of heart failure result from familial (genetic) or nonfamilial (acquired) disorders, which can be confined to the heart or be multisystem disorders. The term *cardiomyopathy* refers to myocardial disorders in which the heart muscle is structurally and functionally abnormal in the absence of coronary artery disease (Chapter 58), hypertension (Chapter 64), valvular disease (Chapter 60), or congenital heart disease (Chapter 55) sufficient to cause the observed myocardial abnormality. Cardiomyopathies are classified according to ventricular morphology and pathophysiology into four major types: dilated cardiomyopathy, hypertrophic cardiomyopathy, restrictive cardiomyopathy, and arrhythmogenic cardiomyopathy (Table 47-1 and Fig. 47-1). Diseases that do not fit into these groups (such as endocardial fibroelastosis and left ventricular noncompaction) are termed unclassified cardiomyopathies. Mixed phenotypes can exist; for example, patients with hypertrophic and dilated cardiomyopathies frequently have a restrictive left ventricular physiology or develop ventricular dilation.

HYPERTROPHIC CARDIOMYOPATHY

DEFINITION AND EPIDEMIOLOGY

Hypertrophic cardiomyopathy is defined as unexplained left ventricular hypertrophy in the absence of abnormal loading conditions (valve disease, hypertension, congenital heart defects) sufficient to explain the degree of hypertrophy. The disease occurs worldwide and in all racial groups, with a prevalence of between 0.2 and 0.5%.

PATHOBIOLOGY

Hypertrophic cardiomyopathy is usually familial with autosomal dominant inheritance. Mutations in sarcomeric contractile protein genes (E-Table 47-1) account for approximately 50 to 60% of cases.[1] More than 1400 different mutations have been identified, with marked variation in disease penetrance and clinical expression. The most common involved genes are *MYH7*, which

TABLE 47-1 PROFILES OF MYOCARDIAL DISEASE

	HYPERTROPHIC	DILATED	RESTRICTIVE	ARRHYTHMOGENIC
Causes	Genetic (see E-Table 47-1) Infiltrative or storage disease	Myocarditis (see Table 47-3) Metabolic/endocrine Genetic (see E-Table 47-1)	Infiltrative or storage diseases (see Table 47-7) Endomyocardial (e.g., Löffler, carcinoid) Genetic (see E-Table 47-1)	Genetic (see E-Table 47-1)
LV ejection fraction	Increased or normal	Reduced	Normal or reduced	LV and RV normal or mildly reduced until end stage
LV end-diastolic dimension	Usually decreased	Increased	Normal	LV and RV normal or mildly increased until end stage
LV wall thickness	Increased	Normal	Normal or mildly increased	Normal
Atrial size	Increased	Increased	Increased; may be massive	Atria normal until end stage
Valvular disease	Mitral regurgitation (SAM)	Mitral (functional); tricuspid regurgitation in late stages	Mitral and tricuspid regurgitation, rarely severe	
Common symptoms	Dyspnea; chest pain, syncope, palpitation, fatigue Late: orthopnea, PND	Dyspnea, fatigue Late: orthopnea, PND	Dyspnea Late: orthopnea, PND, right-sided heart failure	Palpitations, syncope End stage: right and/or left heart failure
Arrhythmia	Atrial fibrillation, ventricular tachycardia; conduction block in *PRKAG2*, mitochondrial; Fabry disease	Ventricular tachyarrhythmias; heart block in Chagas disease, giant cell myocarditis, laminopathies	Atrial fibrillation; conduction block in sarcoidosis, amyloidosis, desminopathy	Biventricular ectopy and tachycardia

LV = left ventricle; PND = paroxysmal nocturnal dyspnea; PRKAG2 = protein kinase, AMP-activated, gamma 2 noncatalytic subunit mutation; RV = right ventricle; SAM = systolic anterior motion of mitral valve.

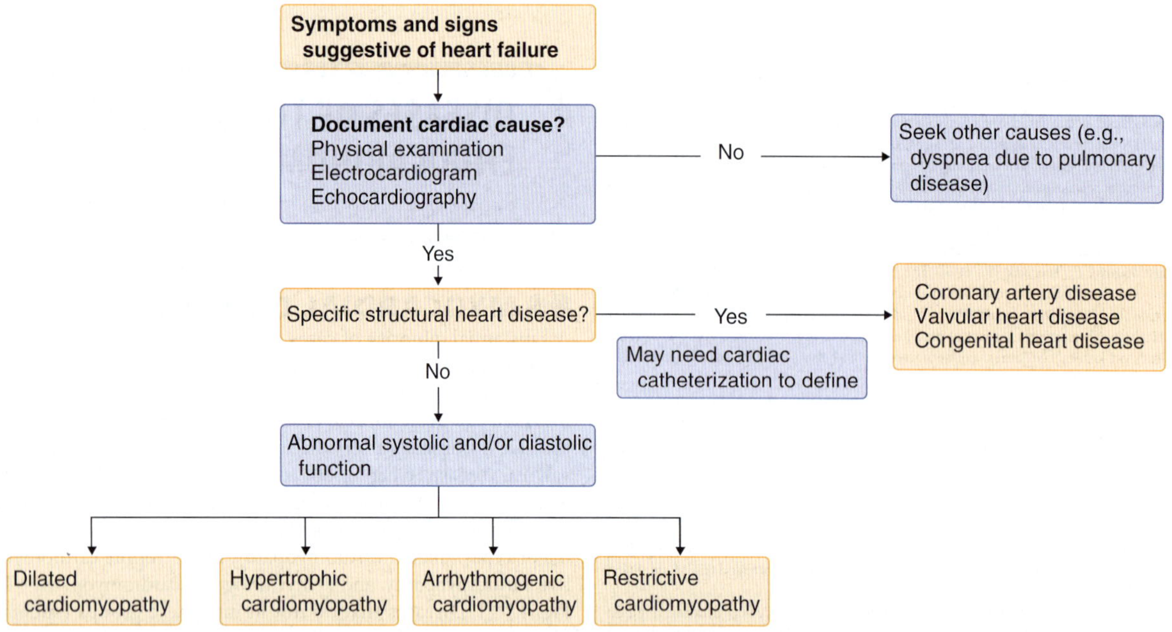

FIGURE 47-1. Initial approach to classification of cardiomyopathy. The evaluation of symptoms or signs consistent with heart failure first includes confirmation that they can be attributed to a cardiac cause. Although this conclusion is often apparent from routine physical examination and electrocardiography, echocardiography serves to confirm cardiac disease and provides clues to the presence of other cardiac diseases, such as valve disease or congenital heart disease. Having excluded these conditions, cardiomyopathy is generally considered to be dilated, restrictive, or hypertrophic, as shown in Table 47-1. Patients with apparently normal cardiac structure and contraction are occasionally found to demonstrate abnormal intracardiac flow patterns consistent with diastolic dysfunction but should also be evaluated carefully for other causes of their symptoms. Most patients with so-called diastolic dysfunction also demonstrate at least borderline criteria for left ventricular hypertrophy, frequently in the setting of chronic hypertension and diabetes. A moderately decreased ejection fraction without marked dilation or a pattern of restrictive cardiomyopathy may represent either a distinct entity or a transition between acute and chronic disease.

codes for the cardiac β-myosin heavy chain, and *MYBPC3*, which codes for myosin binding protein C. A similar clinical phenotype is seen in association with other uncommon genetic disorders, including Noonan syndrome (Chapter 55), Friedreich ataxia (Chapter 389), neurofibromatosis (Chapter 385), hereditary spherocytosis (Chapter 147), respiratory chain disorders, glycogen storage diseases (Chapter 191), and lysosomal storage disorders (Chapter 192), especially Fabry and Danon disease.

Pathology

In its original classical form, hypertrophic cardiomyopathy causes asymmetric myocardial hypertrophy preferentially involving the anteroseptal wall. However, a wide spectrum of patterns is now recognized, including concentric, midventricular, and apical. Older individuals often have hypertrophy that is limited to the basal portion of the sigmoid-shaped septum, frequently in the context of sporadic, genotype-negative disease. The right ventricular free wall and papillary muscles are often involved. The papillary muscles are often hypertrophied, are displaced anteriorly, may be bifid, and occasionally are implanted directly into the mitral leaflet, with poorly developed or absent chordae. The mitral leaflets are consistently elongated, irrespective of the degree of hypertrophy, and are prone to developing systolic anterior motion and dynamic outflow obstruction. Myocardial crypts, apical hypertrabeculation, and apical-septal myocardial bundles constitute ancillary phenotypic traits, which can be found also in genotype-positive individuals who lack myocardial hypertrophy. Apical aneurysms may develop, particularly in patients with mid-apical hypertrophy and mid-ventricular obstruction.

At the histologic level, hypertrophic cardiomyopathy is characterized by hypertrophy of cardiomyocytes, areas of myocytic disarray, and interstitial fibrosis. Myocyte disarray refers to architectural disorganization of the myocardium, with adjacent myocytes aligned obliquely or perpendicular to each other in association with increased interstitial collagen. The myofibrillar architecture within the myocyte is also disorganized. The coronary microcirculation is affected, with medial and intimal hyperplasia that can obliterate the vessel's lumen and impair vasodilatation.

Pathophysiology

Genetic mutations associated with hypertrophic cardiomyopathy can result in an overall gain of function of the sarcomere, thereby leading to abnormal cellular metabolism and an inefficient utilization of energy. Myocardial hypertrophy, which is a compensatory mechanism to this altered metabolic state, contributes to diastolic dysfunction. Myocardial fibrosis is common and contributes to progressive systolic dysfunction.

About 50% of patients develop left ventricular outflow tract obstruction at rest or with exercise owing to systolic anterior movement of the mitral valve leaflets. Obstruction may also occur at the mid-ventricular level in patients who have distal hypertrophy because of systolic obliteration of the ventricular cavity with the interposition of an abnormally positioned papillary muscle; this type of obstruction is associated with the development of apical aneurysms. The occurrence and severity of obstruction typically vary over time in individual patients and are exacerbated by dehydration, standing, increased adrenergic states, vasodilators, and ingestion of food and alcohol.

CLINICAL MANIFESTATIONS

Most patients are asymptomatic or have only mild or intermittent symptoms, and the diagnosis is often made as a result of family screening or the incidental detection of a heart murmur or an electrocardiographic (ECG) abnormality. However, a lack of symptoms may reflect the patient's long-term adaptation to diminished exercise. Symptoms can develop at any age, even many years after the appearance of ECG or echocardiographic manifestations of left ventricular hypertrophy. On occasion, sudden death or syncope may be the initial presentation.

Symptomatic progression is usually slow and associated with a gradual deterioration in left ventricular function over decades, often associated with the development of atrial fibrillation. Less than 5% of patients have rapid, symptomatic deterioration and often develop refractory heart failure owing to hypokinetic and/or restrictive evolution.

Approximately 20 to 30% of adults develop chest pain (Chapters 39 and 56), which may occur on exertion, at rest, or nocturnally. Postprandial angina associated with mild exertion is typical. Mild to moderate dyspnea on exertion is relatively common. Occasionally, patients may develop paroxysmal nocturnal dyspnea, often due to paroxysmal arrhythmias such as atrial fibrillation. Approximately 20% of patients experience syncope (Chapters 39 and 49),[2] and a similar proportion complain of presyncope. Angina and syncope are most frequent in patients who have dynamic left ventricular outflow obstruction. Palpitations (Chapter 49) are frequent and are usually attributable to supraventricular or ventricular ectopy.

DIAGNOSIS

The initial diagnostic evaluation must include a comprehensive medical history focusing on cardiovascular symptoms, a family history focusing on premature cardiac disease or death, a careful physical examination, a 12-lead ECG, and a two-dimensional echocardiogram.[3] A three- to four-generation family history, which should be obtained in all patients with a new diagnosis of cardiomyopathy, helps determine the probability of familial disease and its mode of inheritance.

Clinical examination of the cardiovascular system is often normal. In the presence of left ventricular outflow tract obstruction, the arterial pulse has a rapid upstroke and downstroke (sometimes with a bisferiens character), the apex beat is sustained or double (reflecting a palpable atrial impulse followed by left ventricular contraction), and auscultation will demonstrate a systolic ejection murmur that is heard loudest at the left sternal edge and that radiates to the right upper sternal edge and apex (Chapter 39). Most patients with left ventricular outflow tract obstruction also have the murmur of functional mitral regurgitation, which results from failure of the mitral valve leaflets to coapt due to the systolic anterior motion of the mitral valve. Physiologic and pharmacologic maneuvers that decrease afterload or venous return (e.g., standing, Valsalva maneuver, inhalation of amyl nitrite) or increase contractility (e.g., a post-extrasystole beat) will increase the intensity of the murmur, whereas interventions that increase afterload and venous return (e.g., squatting or handgrip) will reduce it (see Table 39-8). In contrast, physical signs in most patients who do not have left ventricular outflow tract obstruction are subtle and are limited to features that reflect the hyperdynamic contraction (rapid upstroke pulse) and poorly compliant right (prominent *a* wave in jugular venous pressure) and left (S_4 gallop, double-apex beat) ventricles (Chapter 39).

The general evaluation must always include an overview of potential extracardiac manifestation, which may help distinguish classic disease from rare genotypes that have radically different pathobiology, clinical course, and therapeutic strategies. These diseases include lysosomal storage diseases such Fabry, Danon, and Pompe diseases (Chapter 191); syndromes such as Noonan and LEOPARD; and mitochondrial diseases. Noonan syndrome is characterized by short stature, developmental delay, cutaneous abnormalities, hypertelorism, ptosis, low-set posteriorly rotated ears, and webbed neck. These features are shared with the less common LEOPARD syndrome (Noonan syndrome with multiple lentigines [NSML]). Angiokeratomas, anhidrosis, Raynaud-like symptoms with neuropathy, cornea verticillata, retinal vascular dilation, tinnitus, diarrhea, and proteinuria are typical features of Fabry disease (Chapter 192). Patients with mitochondrial diseases such as mitochondrial encephalomyopathy, lactic acidosis, and strokelike episodes (MELAS) have a matrilinear pattern of inheritance and present with short stature, lactic acidosis, severe exercise intolerance, neurosensory deafness, juvenile-onset diabetes, and strokelike episodes.

Diagnostic Testing

More than 95% of patients have abnormal ECG findings, but no changes are disease specific. The most common abnormalities are increased QRS voltage consistent with left ventricular hypertrophy, left axis deviation (15 to 20%), abnormal Q waves (25 to 30%, most commonly in inferolateral leads), and ST segment or T wave changes (>50%). An isolated increase in the QRS voltage without ST segment changes or T wave inversion is rare in hypertrophic cardiomyopathy. The presence of predominantly distal or apical thickening is associated with giant negative T wave inversion, which is maximal in leads V_3 and V_4.

Two-dimensional echocardiography (Chapter 43), which is the mainstay of diagnostic imaging, may be complemented by magnetic resonance imaging (MRI; Chapter 44) and computed tomography (CT; Chapter 44) for more precise definition of the extent and distribution of the hypertrophy and other relevant phenotypic features. The hypertrophy is often asymmetric and involves the anterior and posterior intraventricular septum (Fig. 47-2). The hypertrophy, however, may be more generalized and involve the free wall of the left ventricle, or it may be localized and confined to areas other than the septum, such as the apex (E-Fig. 47-1), lateral wall, or posterior wall of the left ventricle. Hypertrophy can completely obliterate the left ventricular outflow tract (E-Fig. 47-2). Systolic anterior motion of the mitral valve prevents normal coaptation of the mitral leaflets and results in mitral regurgitation (E-Fig. 47-3).

The echocardiogram also can measure left ventricular outflow tract obstruction, both at rest and after provocative maneuvers. Patients with an outflow tract gradient of 30 mm Hg or more are considered to have obstructive disease, with severe obstruction defined as a gradient ≥50 mm Hg. Exercise echocardiography is essential to assess the severity of dynamic obstruction on effort, particularly in physically active individuals, because resting values may be falsely reassuring.

Most patients with hypertrophic cardiomyopathy have left atrial enlargement as well as echocardiographic evidence of diastolic dysfunction. Magnetic resonance imaging provides accurate characterization of tissue and allows the identification of edema and replacement fibrosis (E-Fig. 47-4), while also aiding in the exclusion of rare mimics of hypertrophic cardiomyopathy such as amyloidosis (Chapter 174). Late in the disease, patients often develop left ventricular dilation (E-Fig. 47-5.)

When it is available, cardiopulmonary exercise testing with metabolic gas exchange measurements provides an accurate and reproducible assessment of exercise capacity, which can be followed serially, and it is most useful in patients who have evidence of myocardial fibrosis and progressive heart failure. Cardiac catheterization is rarely required for diagnosis or management, but it may be indicated when measurement of intracardiac pressures is required to guide therapeutic decisions (e.g., in patients with severe mitral regurgitation) and for the exclusion of coexistent coronary artery disease in patients with chest pain.

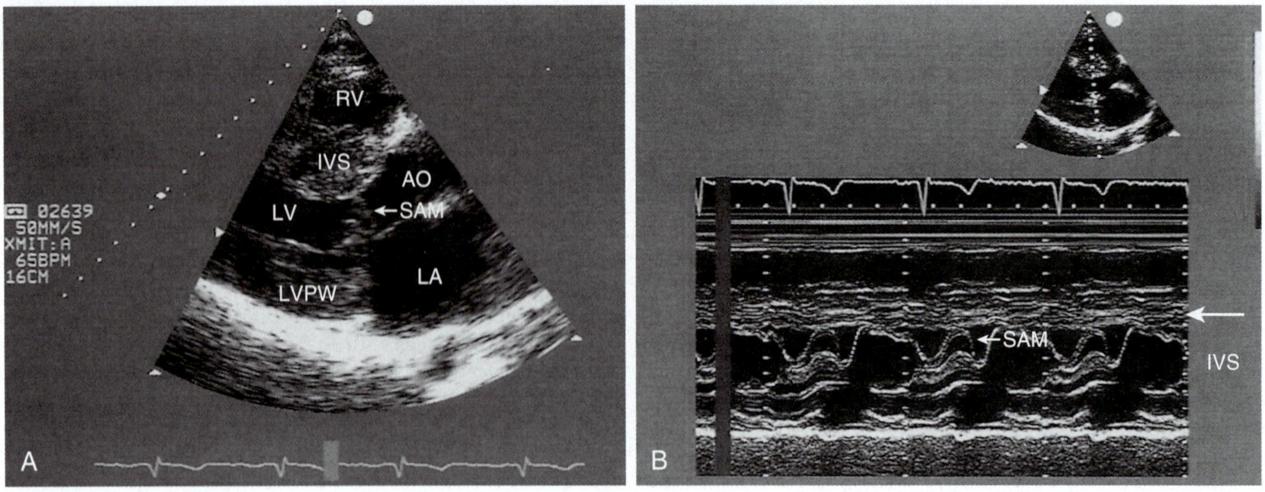

FIGURE 47-2. **Hypertrophic obstructive cardiomyopathy. A, The two-dimensional long axis parasternal view shows the chambers of the heart. The left ventricle posterior wall (LVPW) is thickened, and the most striking abnormality is the hypertrophy of the interventricular septum (IVS). In 25% of patients, systolic anterior motion of the mitral valve (SAM) causes dynamic obstruction to left ventricular outflow. B, This phenomenon is more clearly shown in the parasternal long axis M-mode echocardiogram. The massive thickening of the septum is also obvious in the M-mode image (IVS). AO = aorta; LA = left atrium; LV = left ventricle; RV = right ventricle. (From Forbes CD, Jackson WF. *Color Atlas and Text of Clinical Medicine,* 3rd ed. London: Mosby; 2003.)**

Diagnostic Criteria

Hypertrophic cardiomyopathy is defined by a maximal left ventricular wall thickness value of 15 mm or more. A value of 13 mm is considered diagnostic in relatives of probands with an unequivocal diagnosis, particularly if they have a defined genotype. In children, a wall thickness of more than 2 standard deviations above the mean, corrected for age and body size, is generally accepted as diagnostic. In the presence of other causes of left ventricular hypertrophy, such as long-standing systemic hypertension or aortic stenosis, the diagnosis of hypertrophic cardiomyopathy may be problematic. However, secondary hypertrophy rarely exceeds 15 mm, tends to be concentric, and usually lacks the typical valvular and subvalvular mitral abnormalities of hypertrophic cardiomyopathy. Hypertrophy in the highly trained athlete is mild, is rare in women, and typically occurs in association with increased left ventricular dimensions and stroke volume. An ECG tracing showing Q waves or inferolateral repolarization changes in an athlete favors the diagnosis of hypertrophic cardiomyopathy.

TREATMENT

No medical treatments have proven benefit to modify the underlying pathobiology of hypertrophic cardiomyopathy or to slow the long-term progression of the disease. As a result, medical therapy is directed at the control of symptoms, outflow obstruction, and arrhythmias (Fig. 47-3).[4,5] Exceptions include specific therapies for lysosomal storage diseases, such as Pompe disease (Chapter 191) and Fabry disease (E-Fig. 47-6; Chapter 192), and for Friedreich ataxia (Chapter 389). The treatment of the remaining patients with hypertrophic cardiomyopathy focuses on the counseling of family members, the management of symptoms, lifestyle advice related to exercise,[A1] and the prevention of disease-related complications.

Genetic Testing and Familial Screening

Genetic counseling should be offered to all newly diagnosed patients with hypertrophic cardiomyopathy. Genetic testing using next-generation sequencing panels or whole-exome sequencing can exclude rare genotypes and guide cascade screening in families in whom a pathogenic or likely pathogenic variant is identified. However, such variants are found in less than 50% of probands, and a negative test does not exclude the diagnosis of hypertrophic cardiomyopathy. When a pathogenic or likely pathogenic variant is identified, family members may be tested. However, genetic testing remains controversial in minors in the absence of clinical abnormalities, and the pros and cons of early genotyping (versus clinical follow-up) should be carefully considered on an individual basis. Individuals who test positive should be followed at regular intervals, even when the clinical evaluation is negative, because late onset of the disease has been described. Healthy family members in whom the genetic variant is excluded can be reassured and avoid such follow-up evaluations.

Screening with a 12-lead electrocardiogram and echocardiogram takes place at intervals of 12 to 18 months, usually starting at the age of 12 years (unless there is a family history of premature sudden death, the child is symptomatic or a competitive athlete, or there is a clinical suspicion of left ventricular hypertrophy), until full growth and maturation are achieved (usually by the age of 18 to 21 years). Thereafter, if there are no signs of disease expression, screening approximately every few years is advised because the onset of left ventricular hypertrophy may be delayed until well into adulthood in some families. Modified diagnostic criteria (see Table 47-2) consider the high probability that otherwise unexplained ECG and echocardiographic findings in first-degree relatives reflect incomplete disease expression.

Symptomatic Management

Medical Therapy

In patients who have nonobstructive cardiomyopathy, β-blockade may improve chest pain and dyspnea. The dose (starting at a dose equivalent to metoprolol 150 mg/day or propranolol 120 mg/day) should be titrated to achieve a target heart rate of 50 to 70 beats per minute at rest and 130 to 140 beats per minute at peak exercise. Non-dihydropyridine calcium antagonists such as verapamil (starting at a dose of 120 mg/day) and diltiazem (starting at a dose of 180 mg/day) are useful alternatives, particularly in patients with refractory chest pain, but high doses (e.g., verapamil >480 mg/day, diltiazem >360 mg/day) may be required.

In patients with symptoms caused by left ventricular outflow tract obstruction, the main aim of treatment is to reduce intraventricular gradients. Approximately 60 to 70% of patients improve with β-blockers,[A2] although high doses (equivalent to propranolol at 480 mg/day) are frequently required, and side effects are often limiting. When β-blockade alone is ineffective, disopyramide (a negative-inotropic antiarrhythmic agent), titrated to the maximal tolerated dose (usually between 400 and 600 mg/day), may be effective in up to two thirds of patients, but side effects related to the anticholinergic effects (e.g., dry eyes and mouth, urinary retention) limit its use. Disopyramide should be given concomitantly with a β-blocker (e.g., propranolol 120 to 240 mg/day), which will slow the heart rate and also blunt rapid atrioventricular nodal conduction should supraventricular arrhythmias develop. In patients who have left ventricular outflow tract obstruction and are taking a β-blocker and disopyramide, other QT-prolonging drugs (e.g., sotalol or amiodarone) must be avoided because of the potential proarrhythmic effect. In patients with outflow tract gradients, verapamil can be effective, but caution is required in patients with severe obstruction or elevated pulmonary pressures.

Allosteric inhibitors of cardiac myosin, such as mavacamten (at doses as low as 5 mg orally daily), can reduce obstruction and improve both exercise capacity and quality of life.[A3-A5] Data suggest a benefit in patients with nonobstructive hypertrophic cardiomyopathy as well.[6]

Diuretics (e.g., furosemide, 20 to 40 mg orally, followed by 20 mg/day) are seldom required; if needed in patients who have pulmonary congestion caused by elevated pulmonary pressures due to left ventricular dysfunction, the dose and duration of diuretic therapy should be minimized because injudicious use of these drugs can be dangerous, particularly in patients who have severe diastolic impairment or labile obstruction.

Losartan (100 mg/day) and valsartan (320 mg/day) are safe and may somewhat improve cardiac structure and function, but they have no benefit in terms of slowing the progression of disease.[A6,A7] Similarly, ranolazine (1000 mg twice daily) is safe for reducing ventricular ectopy, but it does not change exercise performance, plasma prohormone brain natriuretic peptide levels, diastolic function, or quality of life.[A8]

Interventional Therapy

Surgical myectomy or percutaneous alcohol septal ablation is indicated in patients who have refractory, symptomatic outflow obstruction (gradient

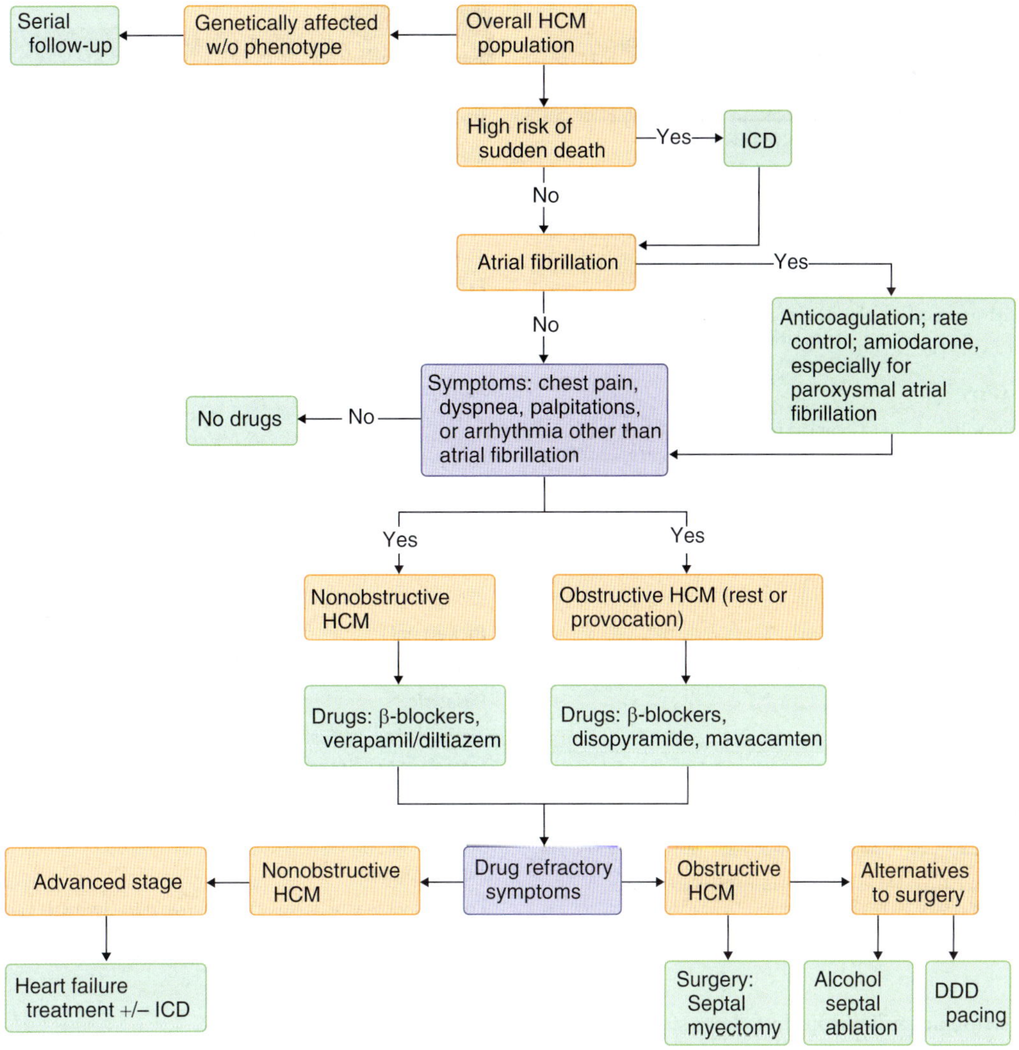

FIGURE 47-3. Approach to the management of hypertrophic cardiomyopathy (HCM). DDD = dual chamber; ICD = implantable cardioverter-defibrillator. (Modified from Maron BJ, McKenna WJ, Danielson GK, et al. American College of Cardiology/European Society of Cardiology clinical expert consensus document on hypertrophic cardiomyopathy. *J Am Coll Cardiol*. 2003;42:1687-1713.)

>50 mm Hg) despite optimized medical therapy or who are intolerant to it, with data suggesting that alcohol septal ablation may be preferred.[7] Both procedures are safe and effective in expert hands, although surgery is more effective for relieving gradients. Multidisciplinary evaluation by an expert team is advisable to determine the most appropriate therapeutic strategy for an individual patient.

The most commonly performed surgical procedure, which is extended ventricular septal myectomy, either abolishes or substantially reduces the gradient in 95% of cases, reduces mitral regurgitation, and improves exercise capacity and symptoms. Surgery should be performed in an experienced center, where mortality rates should be less than 1% for isolated myectomy. The main complications (atrioventricular block, ventricular septal defects) are uncommon (2 to 5%). When concomitant procedures (e.g., mitral valve repair or replacement, coronary artery bypass grafting) are required or when other significant comorbidities are present, perioperative mortality rates are higher (4 to 5%).

In experienced centers, the selective injection of alcohol into a septal perforator branch of the left anterior descending coronary artery to create a localized septal scar has benefits and risks that are comparable to surgery. The main nonfatal complication is atrioventricular block requiring a pacemaker in 5 to 20% of patients.

In the presence of end-stage disease with extensive myocardial fibrosis and refractory symptoms, heart transplantation is the only therapeutic option. Conversely, a left ventricular assist device is technically challenging to implant and is rarely used because of the small size of the left ventricle.

Atrial Fibrillation

Atrial fibrillation, which is one of the most common complications of hypertrophic cardiomyopathy, occurs in about 25% of patients. In general, the principles of managing atrial fibrillation in patients with hypertrophic cardiomyopathy are similar to those in other conditions (Chapter 52), including the use of anticoagulation because of the significant risk of systemic embolization. Treatment with low-dose amiodarone, 1000 to 1400 mg/week, is effective in maintaining sinus rhythm and in controlling the ventricular response during breakthrough episodes, but it is usually avoided in young patients because of its toxicity. Disopyramide, dofetilide, or sotalol (see Table 52-2) are safe but less effective. In patients who have permanent atrial fibrillation, a ß-blocker, verapamil, or diltiazem are usually required for rate control (see Chapter 52). Transcatheter ablation may be considered in selected patients, but its long-term efficacy is less than 50%, and repeated procedures are often necessary. Marked left atrial dilatation, older age, and worse symptomatic status predict failure to maintain sinus rhythm following ablation.

Prevention of Sudden Death

The overall risk for sudden death in children and adults with hypertrophic cardiomyopathy is approximately 0.5 to 1% per year, but a minority of individuals have a much greater risk for life-threatening ventricular arrhythmia. All patients with hypertrophic cardiomyopathy should be advised to avoid competitive sports and intense physical exertion, which are typical precipitants of sudden death.

The most powerful predictor of sudden cardiac death in hypertrophic cardiomyopathy is a history of previous cardiac arrest. Such patients should receive an implantable cardioverter-defibrillator (ICD; Chapter 54).

In patients without such a history, the identification of high-risk patients can be challenging. The most useful predictors of the risk for sudden death (https://doc2do.com/hcm/webHCM.html) are a family history of premature (<40 years of age) sudden cardiac death, unexplained syncope (unrelated to neurocardiogenic mechanisms), flat or hypotensive blood pressure response to upright exercise, nonsustained ventricular tachycardia on ambulatory ECG monitoring or during exercise, and severe left ventricular hypertrophy on echocardiography (defined as a maximal left ventricular wall thickness of 30 mm or more). Patients without any risk factors do not warrant an ICD. For patients with one risk factor, decisions about an ICD should be individualized on the basis of the patient's age and severity of disease and level of risk that is acceptable to the patient.

TABLE 47-2 DIAGNOSTIC CRITERIA FOR HYPERTROPHIC CARDIOMYOPATHY IN FIRST-DEGREE RELATIVES OF AFFECTED PATIENTS*

MAJOR CRITERIA	MINOR CRITERIA
ECHOCARDIOGRAPHY	
Left ventricular wall thickness ≥13 mm in the anterior septum or posterior wall or ≥15 mm in the posterior septum or free wall	Left ventricular wall thickness of 12 mm in the anterior septum or posterior wall or of 14 mm in the posterior septum or free wall
Severe SAM of the mitral valve (septal-leaflet contact)	Moderate SAM of the mitral valve (no mitral leaflet–septal contact) Redundant mitral valve leaflets
ELECTROCARDIOGRAPHY	
Left ventricular hypertrophy with repolarization changes (Romhilt and Estes)	Complete bundle branch block or (minor) interventricular conduction defects (in left ventricular leads)
T wave inversion in leads I and aVL (≥3 mm with QRS-T wave axis difference ≥30 degrees), V_3-V_6 (≥3 mm), or II and III and aVF (≥5 mm)	Minor repolarization changes in left ventricular leads Deep S wave in lead V_2 (>25 mm)
Abnormal Q waves (>40 msec or >25% R wave) in at least two leads from II, III, aVF (in absence of left anterior hemiblock), and V_1-V_4; or I, aVL, V_5-V_6	Unexplained chest pain, dyspnea, or syncope

*The diagnosis of hypertrophic cardiomyopathy in first-degree relatives of patients with the disease is based on the presence of one major criterion, two minor echocardiographic criteria, or one minor echocardiographic criterion and two minor electrocardiographic criteria.

aVF = augmented voltage unipolar left foot lead; aVL = augmented voltage unipolar left arm lead; SAM = systolic anterior motion.

Modified from McKenna WJ, Spirito P, Desnos M, et al. Experience in clinical genetics in hypertrophic cardiomyopathy. *Heart*. 1997;77:130-132.

PROGNOSIS

Most patients with hypertrophic cardiomyopathy follow a stable and benign course with a low risk for adverse events and a survival similar to that of age- and gender-matched normal populations, but many experience progressive symptoms caused by atrial arrhythmia and gradual deterioration in left ventricular systolic and diastolic function (E-Fig. 47-7). With modern therapy, heart failure–related deaths have become more common than sudden deaths. The mortality rate related specifically to hypertrophic cardiomyopathy is 0.53% per year, with 5- and 10-year cardiomyopathy-related survival rates of 98% and 94%, respectively. The annual incidence of stroke varies from 0.56 to 0.8% per year, rising to 1.9% in patients older than 60 years, and 23% of strokes are fatal. The development of severe systolic heart failure is associated with a poor prognosis, with an overall mortality rate of up to 11% per year. The incidence of infective endocarditis is 1.4 per 1000 person-years overall but 3.8 per 1000 person-years in patients with obstruction.

MYOCARDITIS

DEFINITION AND EPIDEMIOLOGY

Myocarditis, which is an inflammatory process involving the myocardium, can be caused by infections, immune-mediated damage, or toxins (Table 47-3).[8] The incidence and prevalence of myocarditis are difficult to estimate because the clinical presentation varies from asymptomatic ECG abnormalities to hemodynamic collapse and sudden death. Population estimates of the prevalence of myocarditis range from 1 in 100,000 to 1 in 10,000, whereas postmortem studies report myocarditis in up to 12% of young victims of sudden cardiac death. Myocarditis may also be the clinical presentation of the inflammatory phase of an arrhythmogenic cardiomyopathy.

Worldwide, the most common infective myocarditis is Chagas disease, caused by *Trypanosoma cruzi*, a protozoan organism endemic in rural areas of South and Central America (Chapter 318).[9] In the Western world, viral myocarditis is the most common cause of inflammatory heart disease. Human immunodeficiency virus (HIV) infection (Chapter 353) is associated with lymphocytic myocarditis and is a strong predictor of poor prognosis. Smallpox vaccination (Chapter 15) causes myopericarditis with a reported incidence of 7.8 cases per 100,000 vaccine administrations. Other rare myocarditides include giant cell myocarditis, myocarditis complicating autoimmune disorders such as systemic lupus erythematosus (Chapter 245), cocaine abuse (Chapter 365), and as a complication of combination immune checkpoint inhibitor therapy (Chapter 164).

TABLE 47-3 CAUSES OF MYOCARDITIS

INFECTION
Viral
Coxsackievirus, human immunodeficiency virus, echovirus, severe acute respiratory syndrome coronavirus-2, adenovirus, influenza, measles, mumps, parvovirus, poliovirus, rubella, varicella-zoster virus, herpes simplex virus, cytomegalovirus, hepatitis C virus, rabies virus, respiratory syncytial virus, vaccine virus, dengue virus, yellow fever virus
Protozoal
Trypanosoma cruzi, Toxoplasma gondii
Bacterial
Brucella, Corynebacterium diphtheriae, Salmonella, Haemophilus influenzae, Mycoplasma pneumoniae, Neisseria meningitidis (meningococcus), *Streptococcus pneumoniae, Staphylococcus, Mycobacterium, Neisseria gonorrhoeae* (gonococcus), *Vibrio cholerae*
Spirochetal
Treponema pallidum, Borrelia, Leptospira
Fungal
Aspergillus, Candida, Cryptococcus, Actinomyces, Blastomyces, Histoplasma, Coccidioides
Rickettsial
Coxiella burnetii, Rickettsia rickettsii, Rickettsia tsutsugamushi
Parasitic
Trichinella spiralis, Echinococcus granulosus, Taenia solium
IMMUNE-MEDIATED DISORDERS
Alloantigens
Heart transplant rejection
Autoantigens
Eosinophilic granulomatosis with polyangiitis (formerly Churg-Strauss syndrome), celiac disease, Whipple disease, giant cell myocarditis, Kawasaki disease, systemic lupus erythematosus, systemic sclerosis, sarcoidosis, scleroderma, polymyositis, thrombocytopenic purpura
Allergens (Drugs)
Penicillin, sulfonamides, tetracycline, methyldopa, streptomycin, tricyclic antidepressants, thiazide diuretics, dobutamine, indomethacin
TOXIC CAUSES
Drugs
Anthracyclines, catecholamines, amphetamines, cocaine, cyclophosphamide, 5-fluorouracil, trastuzumab, interferon, interleukin-2, checkpoint inhibitors, clozapine
Physical Agents
Electric shock, radiation, hyperpyrexia
Heavy Metals
Copper, iron, lead
Others
Arsenic, snake bite, scorpion bite, wasp and spider stings, phosphorus, carbon monoxide
GENETIC DISORDERS
Inherited cardiomyopathies with immune-mediated pathogenesis (dilated and right ventricular cardiomyopathy)

PATHOBIOLOGY

Myocarditis is defined histologically by the presence of myocyte injury, with degeneration or necrosis, and an inflammatory infiltrate not due to ischemia. Four patterns are recognized: *active myocarditis*, with myocyte degeneration or necrosis and definite cellular infiltrate with or without fibrosis; *borderline myocarditis*, with a definite cellular infiltrate without evidence of myocardial cellular injury; *persistent myocarditis*, with continued active myocarditis on repeated biopsy; and *resolving or resolved myocarditis*, characterized by a diminished or absent infiltrate with evidence of connective tissue healing on repeated biopsy. Despite their widespread use, the so-called Dallas criteria have low specificity and sensitivity, with a diagnostic yield as low as 10 to 20% in some series. Therefore, newer virology techniques used in conjunction with conventional light microscopy include nested polymerase chain reaction or reverse transcription polymerase chain reaction on RNA and DNA extracted from endomyocardial biopsy specimens and immunohistochemical staining for subtypes of infiltrating lymphocytes and abnormal expression of cellular adhesion molecules on interstitial or endothelial cells.

VIRAL MYOCARDITIS

Most data on the pathology of viral myocarditis come from murine models. Initially, there is direct invasion of the myocardium by cardiotropic viruses, which enter the cardiomyocyte through receptor-mediated endocytosis. The viral genome, which is translated intracellularly to produce viral protein or is incorporated into the host cell genome, may contribute to myocyte dysfunction by cleaving dystrophin. In the second phase, activation of the host immune system, including recruitment of natural killer cells and macrophages, increases the expression of proinflammatory cytokines such as interleukin-1 and tumor necrosis factor. Activation of $CD4^+$ T lymphocytes promotes clonal expansion of B lymphocytes, thereby resulting in further myocardial cell damage, inflammation, and the production of circulating antiheart antibodies directed against contractile, structural, and mitochondrial proteins. This autoimmune response may result in long-term ventricular remodeling by direct effects on myocardial structural components or alterations in the extracellular matrix.

CLINICAL MANIFESTATIONS

Some patients report prodromal symptoms of viremia, including fever, myalgia, coryzal symptoms, and gastroenteritis, but many individuals with myocarditis are asymptomatic and manifest only transient ECG abnormalities, such as nonspecific ST segment and T wave abnormalities, pathologic Q waves, and low QRS voltages. Less common presentations include acute myocardial infarction with angiographically normal coronary arteries (Chapter 58), atrioventricular block (Chapter 52), and ventricular arrhythmias (Chapter 53). Patients with impairment of left ventricular function may present with symptoms and signs of fulminant cardiogenic shock (Chapter 93) with acute cardiovascular collapse. In some cases, sudden cardiac death is the first presentation.

DIAGNOSIS

The diagnosis of myocarditis requires a high index of suspicion because it may mimic other common conditions.[10] There are no typical features on echocardiography, but impaired left or right ventricular systolic performance (with or without ventricular dilation), regional wall motion abnormalities, left (or right) ventricular thrombus, diastolic impairment, and pericardial effusions may be present. Cardiac magnetic resonance imaging can detect myocardial inflammation and myocyte injury, with pericellular and cellular edema.

Routine blood tests, such as full blood count and erythrocyte sedimentation rate, are usually unhelpful. Serum markers of myocardial injury, such as troponins T and I, may be elevated, but myocarditis may be proven by biopsy even in the absence of elevated serum troponin levels. Increased levels of autoantibodies against myocardial proteins (such as myosin and the adenine nucleotide translocator protein) are biomarkers of autoimmune myocarditis and correlate with progressive worsening of ventricular function. A microRNA designated as has-miR-Chr8:96 is seen in myocarditis but rarely in myocardial infarction.[11]

Cardiac magnetic resonance imaging with gadolinium enhancement can show evidence of myocarditis (Fig. 47-4), but cardiac catheterization with right ventricular endomyocardial biopsy remains the "gold standard" diagnostic test. In the United States, biopsy has generally been reserved for patients with heart failure refractory to standard management, features suggestive of systemic disease (e.g., connective tissue disease [Chapter 239], amyloidosis [Chapter 174], hemochromatosis [Chapter 196], sarcoidosis [Chapter 83]), or suspicion of giant cell myocarditis because of new-onset heart failure associated with tachyarrhythmias or conduction disease. By comparison, a European consensus statement recommends endomyocardial biopsy to achieve an etiologic diagnosis and to guide potential novel treatment options in patients with "clinically suspected myocarditis."

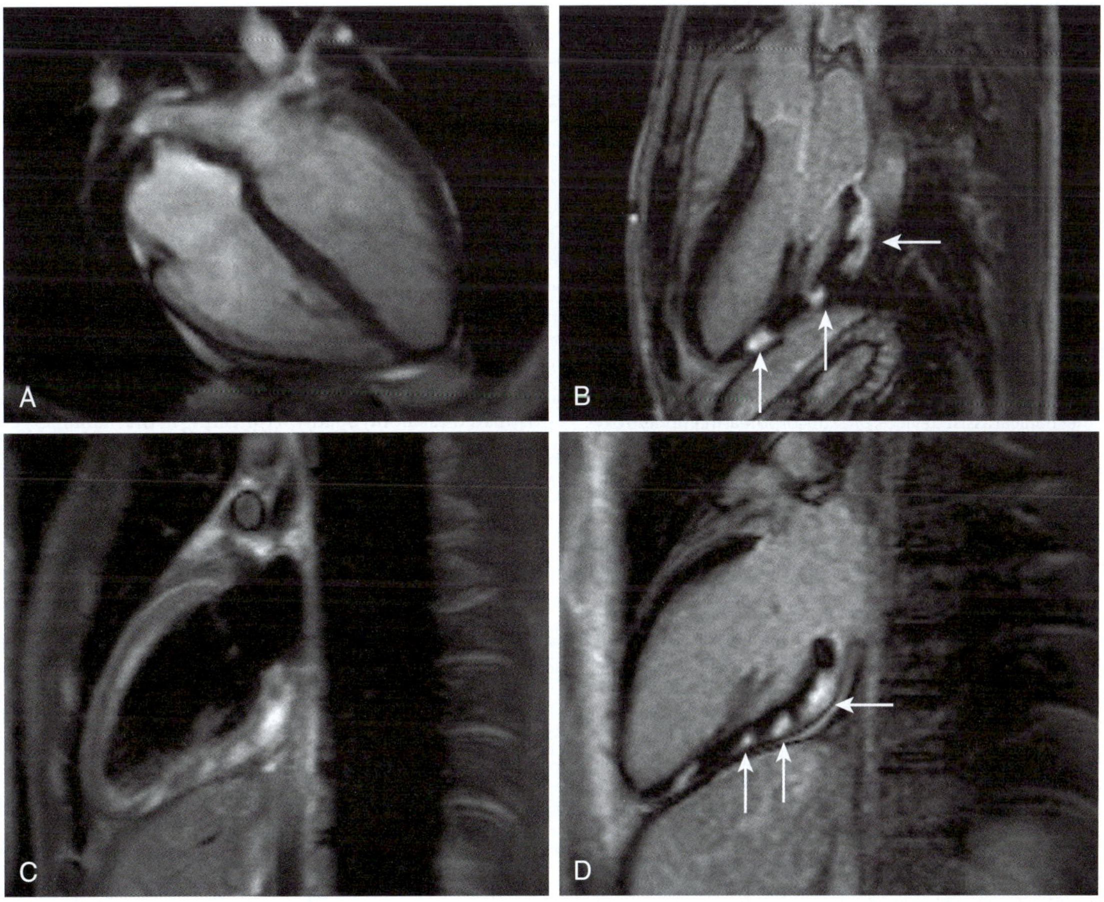

FIGURE 47-4. **A 17-year-old man presenting with apparent acute myopericarditis.** The four-chamber end-diastolic view (A) presents a mildly dilated left ventricle. There is patchy late gadolinium enhancement involving the inferior and lateral walls (B, D, *arrows*). Edema is seen on T1 imaging (C), and there is extensive late enhancement. The differential diagnosis of this appearance also includes sarcoid and giant cell myocarditis.

Specific Causes

Viral myocarditis may be suspected from the clinical picture of recent febrile illness, often with prominent myalgias, followed by angina-like chest pain, dyspnea, or arrhythmias. Elevated troponin levels support the diagnosis, and increasing viral titers (to coxsackievirus, echovirus, adenovirus, or influenza virus) are consistent with recent infection. The correlation with biopsy-proven myocarditis is strongest with HIV and Lyme disease. Clinical cardiomyopathy occurs in 10 to 40% of patients infected with HIV due to the HIV infection itself or to coinfection with cytomegalovirus.

Giant Cell Myocarditis

Giant cell myocarditis, which accounts for 10 to 20% of biopsy-positive cases of myocarditis, is manifested with the rapid onset of chest pain, fever, and hemodynamic compromise, often with ventricular tachycardia or atrioventricular block. When ventricular tachyarrhythmias or progressive heart failure are major features of clinically suspected myocarditis, particularly in a young person, endomyocardial biopsy is recommended to determine whether giant cell myocarditis is present.

Lyme Disease and Toxoplasmosis

Lyme carditis (Chapter 296)[12] is classically manifested with conduction system abnormalities resulting from infection with *Borrelia burgdorferi*, which is diagnosed serologically. Toxoplasmosis (Chapter 320) myocarditis, due to intermittent rupture of cysts in the myocardium, can cause atypical chest pain, arrhythmias, pericarditis, and symptomatic heart failure. Diagnosis is made from antibody titers.

Severe Acute Respiratory Syndrome Coronavirus-2

Myocarditis is a rare complication of SARS-CoV-2 infection (Chapter 336), with an apparent excess incidence rate of 40 extra events per million persons.[13] The risk of myocarditis also appears to be increased (1 to 10 per million persons) within a week of receiving the first dose of both adenovirus and mRNA vaccines, with a higher increased risk after the second dose of mRNA vaccines (Chapter 337). The risk of vaccine-associated myocarditis after vaccination seems to be higher in people under age 40 years.

Immune-Mediated Myocarditis

Many systemic immune-mediated diseases may present as myocarditis with lymphocytic, eosinophilic, and granulomatous myocardial infiltrates.[14] Specific disorders include sarcoidosis (Chapter 83), systemic lupus erythematosus (Chapter 245), systemic sclerosis (Chapter 246), the antiphospholipid syndrome (Chapter 160), dermato-polymyositis (Chapter 248), eosinophilic granulomatosis with polyangiitis, and other vasculitis syndromes (Chapter 249). Myocarditis can also occur in some organ-specific immune-mediated diseases such as chronic inflammatory bowel diseases (Chapter 127). Hypersensitivity reactions, especially to drugs (Chapter 234), can cause myocarditis that is often associated with peripheral eosinophilia and can be confirmed by endomyocardial biopsy.

TREATMENT

The first-line treatment of myocarditis is supportive with afterload reduction and diuresis (Chapter 46). Patients with fulminant acute myocarditis may require inotropic support, mechanical assist devices, or extracorporeal membrane oxygenation (Chapter 93). After initial stabilization, patients with symptoms and signs of heart failure should receive angiotensin-converting enzyme inhibitors, diuretics, β-blockers, and anticoagulants in accordance with standard guidelines (Chapter 46). Patients with intractable and deteriorating heart failure may require cardiac transplantation (Chapter 46).

The role of immunosuppression is uncertain. In one randomized, placebo-controlled trial of 111 adults with biopsy-proven myocarditis, there was no difference in mortality or improvement in left ventricular function in patients treated with prednisolone plus either cyclosporine or azathioprine. Conversely, in a randomized trial of patients who had major histocompatibility complex expression on endomyocardial biopsy samples and who were randomized to prednisolone (1 mg/kg/day tapering to a maintenance dose of 0.2 mg/kg/day for a total of 90 days) and azathioprine (1 mg/kg/day for a total of 100 days) versus placebo, left ventricular ejection fraction improved in the immunosuppressed group, but no difference was observed in mortality or rates of transplantation or rehospitalization during a 2-year follow-up period. Immunosuppression appears to be beneficial for patients with giant cell myocarditis, and current recommendations extend immunosuppression to other biopsy-proven, infection-negative immune-mediated forms of myocarditis including eosinophilic myocarditis, cardiac sarcoidosis, and lymphocytic myocarditis that is refractory to conventional heart failure therapy.[A9] The optimal regimens remain to be determined, and intravenous immune globulin therapy is not helpful.

PROGNOSIS

Patients with acute myocarditis with mild heart failure or symptoms suggestive of myocardial ischemia or infarction typically improve within weeks without sequelae. An acute presentation of myocarditis with advanced heart failure (ejection fraction <35%) may resolve but can lead to chronic left ventricular dysfunction (dilated cardiomyopathy) or progress to death or cardiac transplantation. Patients who present with acute fulminant myocarditis, however, may have an excellent prognosis, with survival rates of more than 90%. Overall, however, biopsy-proven viral myocarditis is associated with a long-term mortality of almost 20% at 4.7 years, and the presence of biventricular dysfunction at presentation is the best predictor of all-cause mortality. Giant cell myocarditis is usually fatal without heart transplantation, but it can be stabilized by early diagnosis and prompt introduction of immunosuppression.[15]

DILATED CARDIOMYOPATHY

DEFINITION AND EPIDEMIOLOGY

Dilated cardiomyopathy is a heart muscle disorder defined by dilation and impaired systolic function of the left ventricle or both ventricles, in the absence of coronary artery disease, valvular abnormalities, or pericardial disease. In adults, the estimated prevalence is 1 in 250.[16] In children, dilated cardiomyopathy is the most common cardiomyopathy, accounting for up to 58% of cases. Overall, males and females are approximately equally affected, except for dilated cardiomyopathy associated with neuromuscular disorders or inborn errors of metabolism, for which there is male predominance because some of these conditions have an X-linked inheritance.

PATHOBIOLOGY

A number of conditions are associated with dilated cardiomyopathy, including neuromuscular disorders, inborn errors of metabolism, and malformation syndromes. When no identifiable cause is found, the disease is termed idiopathic dilated cardiomyopathy.

Genetic Dilated Cardiomyopathy

Between 20 and 50% of individuals with dilated cardiomyopathy have evidence of familial disease (see E-Table 47-1).[17] Autosomal dominant inheritance, which accounts for the majority of familial cases, has two major forms: isolated dilated cardiomyopathy, which is manifested with a clinical picture of heart failure, and dilated cardiomyopathy, in which an associated arrhythmia (i.e., atrial fibrillation, conduction system disease, ventricular tachycardia, or fibrillation) is usually the initial manifestation. The latter cardiomyopathy may also result in heart failure or be associated with a skeletal myopathy. Genes implicated in nonsyndromic dilated cardiomyopathy include cytoskeletal and sarcomeric protein genes. Truncating mutations in *TTN*, the gene encoding the sarcomere protein titin, occur in approximately 25% of familial cases of dilated cardiomyopathy and in 18% of sporadic cases. Genes implicated in arrhythmogenic forms of dilated cardiomyopathy include desmosomal, intermediate filament, nuclear envelope, and ion channel genes. Mutations in the lamin A/C gene, which encodes a nuclear envelope protein, cause atrial and ventricular arrhythmia and progressive atrioventricular conduction disease, which may precede the development of dilated cardiomyopathy. Truncating in the filamin C gene, which encodes an important intermediate filament protein, causes a mixed arrhythmogenic and dilated cardiomyopathy phenotype, typically with lethal ventricular arrhythmias in adolescents and young adults and with subsequent heart failure in survivors.

X-linked inheritance accounts for between 2 and 5% of familial cases of dilated cardiomyopathy. Neuromuscular disorders account for 26% of cases, 90% of which are Duchenne, Becker, and Emery-Dreifuss muscular dystrophies (Chapter 389). Isolated X-linked dilated cardiomyopathy, also caused by mutations in the dystrophin gene, is characterized by raised serum creatine kinase muscle isoforms but does not result in clinical signs or symptoms of skeletal muscular dystrophy.

Acquired Dilated Cardiomyopathy

Common acquired causes of dilated cardiomyopathy include infectious myocarditis, chemotherapy (Chapter 164), radiation therapy (Chapter 18), alcohol (Chapter 364), cocaine (Chapter 365), nutritional deficiencies (Chapter 197), iron overload (Chapter 196), inflammatory and autoimmune disorders (Chapters 245 and 249), endocrinopathies (Chapter 207), and pregnancy (Chapter 221). Tachycardia-mediated cardiomyopathy (tachycardiomyopathy) is rare and usually reverses once the tachycardia is controlled.

CLINICAL MANIFESTATIONS

The symptoms and signs associated with dilated cardiomyopathy depend on the age of the patient and the degree of left ventricular dysfunction. Although the first presentation may be with sudden death or a thromboembolic event, most patients present with symptoms of high pulmonary venous pressure or low cardiac output (Chapter 45), which can be acute, sometimes precipitated by intercurrent illness or arrhythmia, or chronic. Increasingly, dilated cardiomyopathy is diagnosed incidentally in asymptomatic individuals during family screening.

Adults initially present with reduced exercise tolerance and dyspnea on exertion. With worsening left ventricular function, patients may develop dyspnea at rest, orthopnea, paroxysmal nocturnal dyspnea, peripheral edema, and ascites. Symptoms related to mesenteric ischemia, such as abdominal pain after meals, nausea, vomiting, and anorexia, may dominate, especially in children. Arrhythmia symptoms, such as palpitations, presyncope, and syncope, can occur at any age.

In advanced disease, features of low cardiac output include sinus tachycardia, weak peripheral pulses, and hypotension. The jugular venous pressure may be elevated, and the apical impulse is displaced. Peripheral edema, hepatomegaly, and ascites are common in patients with heart failure. Auscultation of the chest typically reveals basal crackles. Auscultation of the heart may reveal the presence of a third (and sometimes also a fourth) heart sound. In patients with functional mitral regurgitation, a pansystolic murmur may be heard at the apex and radiate to the axilla, but frequently no murmurs are heard, even in the presence of mitral incompetence, especially if cardiac output is very low.

DIAGNOSIS

The electrocardiogram may be normal but more typically shows sinus tachycardia, nonspecific ST segment and T wave changes (most commonly in the inferior and lateral leads), atrial enlargement, and voltage criteria for ventricular hypertrophy. Atrioventricular block raises the possibility of mutations in the lamin A/C or desmin gene. Supraventricular and ventricular arrhythmias are common, particularly in patients who have pathogenic variants in *TTN, DSP, RBM20, LMNA,* and *FLNC.* The chest radiograph is usually abnormal, with an increased cardiothoracic ratio (>0.5) reflecting left ventricular and left atrial dilation. Patients with pulmonary edema have increased pulmonary vascular markings and pleural effusion.

On echocardiography, the presence of ventricular end-diastolic dimensions greater than 2 standard deviations above body surface area–corrected means (or greater than 112% of predicted dimension) and fractional shortening less than 25% are sufficient to make the diagnosis. Other common features include functional mitral and tricuspid regurgitation and abnormalities of diastolic left ventricular function. Cardiac magnetic resonance imaging may show areas of myocardial fibrosis (E-Fig. 47-8).

Other recommended tests (Table 47-4) include a complete blood count and tests of renal, thyroid, and hepatic function. Levels of serum creatine kinase should be measured in all patients with dilated cardiomyopathy because this may provide important clues to the etiology. For example, dystrophin-linked dilated cardiomyopathy has been diagnosed in up to 8% of men with dilated cardiomyopathy and should be considered in men with increased serum creatine kinase levels and an X-linked family history. Other cardiac biomarkers, such as troponin I and troponin T, can be elevated. Plasma B-type natriuretic peptide levels predict survival, hospitalization rates, and listing for cardiac transplantation. Symptom-limited exercise testing, combined with respiratory gas analysis, is a useful technique to assess functional limitation and disease progression in patients with stable dilated cardiomyopathy.

Cardiac catheterization is rarely needed except perhaps to exclude severe coronary artery disease or to provide more precise information about possible valvular heart disease. Endomyocardial biopsy may be diagnostic for myocarditis and for some metabolic or mitochondrial disorders but is rarely advised. Hemodynamic assessment of left ventricular end-diastolic and pulmonary artery pressures may be necessary before transplantation.

TABLE 47-4 LABORATORY EVALUATION OF CARDIOMYOPATHY

CLINICAL EVALUATION
History and physical examination to identify cardiac and noncardiac disorders*
Assessment of ability to perform routine and desired activities*
Assessment of volume status*
LABORATORY EVALUATION
Electrocardiogram*
Chest radiograph*
Ambulatory electrocardiographic monitoring
Two-dimensional and Doppler echocardiogram*
Chemistry
Serum sodium,* potassium,* glucose, creatinine,* blood urea nitrogen,* calcium,* magnesium*
Albumin,* total protein,* liver function tests,* serum iron, ferritin, creatine kinase, thyroid-stimulating hormone,* brain natriuretic peptide, troponin level
Urinalysis
Hematology
Hemoglobin/hematocrit*
White blood cell count with differential,* including eosinophils
Erythrocyte sedimentation rate
INITIAL EVALUATION IN SELECTED PATIENTS ONLY
Titers for suspected infection
Acute viral titers
Human immunodeficiency virus, Epstein-Barr virus
Lyme disease, toxoplasmosis
Chagas disease
Catheterization with coronary angiography in patients with angina who are candidates for intervention*
Serologic studies for active rheumatologic disease
Endomyocardial biopsy

*Level I recommendations.

Adapted from Hunt SA, Abraham WT, Chin MH, et al. ACC/AHA 2005 guideline update for the diagnosis and management of chronic heart failure in the adult. *Circulation.* 2005;112:e154-e235.

TREATMENT

Supportive therapy includes sodium and fluid restriction, avoidance of alcohol and other toxins, and use of established heart failure medications (Chapter 46). Rest and avoidance of exercise should be recommended only for patients who have myocarditis, peripartum cardiomyopathy, or desmosomal or lamin AC mutations. For other patients, a submaximal exercise regimen is desirable to sustain mobility, to avoid deconditioning, and to maintain physical and psychological health. Patients with atrial fibrillation or with echocardiographic evidence of a left atrial or left ventricular mural thrombosis should be anticoagulated, preferably with a direct-acting anticoagulant (Table 70-6), or with warfarin to an international normalized rate of 2.0 to 3.0 (Table 70-4). An ICD is preferred to medication for primary prevention against sudden cardiac death from ventricular arrhythmia,[A10] and some patients require management for advanced heart failure (Chapter 46) with cardiac resynchronization therapy, inotropic medications, ventricular assist devices, and cardiac transplantation (Chapter 46).

Family Screening

When a pathogenic gene variant has been identified in a proband, cascade genetic testing should be considered in first-degree relatives.[18] The detection of early disease in a family member offers an opportunity to initiate treatment, usually with an angiotensin-converting enzyme inhibitor (e.g., ramipril or perindopril 5 mg daily) or ß-blocker (e.g., bisoprolol 5 mg daily or carvedilol 12.5 or 25 mg twice daily), although the efficacy of such therapy remains to be proven. Precise algorithms to guide the interval of serial evaluation remain to be determined. Even in the absence of a positive genetic test, evaluation of first-degree relatives by history, physical examination, a 12-lead ECG, and a two-dimensional echocardiogram should be considered.

PROGNOSIS

The prognosis of idiopathic and genetically determined dilated cardiomyopathy is related to the etiology, the severity of disease at the time of presentation, and the response to treatment. Most patients improve with treatment, but the 5-year survival is less than 50% in patients who present with severe disease (e.g., ejection fraction <25%, left ventricular end-diastolic dimension >65 mm, peak oxygen consumption <12 mL/kg/minute).

Specific Causes of Dilated Cardiomyopathy

Alcoholic Cardiomyopathy

In the United States, excess alcohol consumption (Chapter 364) contributes to more than 10% of cases of heart failure.[19] Alcohol and its metabolite, acetaldehyde, are cardiotoxins. Myocardial depression is initially reversible but, if alcohol consumption is sustained, can lead to myocyte vacuolization, mitochondrial abnormalities, and myocardial fibrosis. Even in chronic stages, however, the heart failure represents a sum of both reversible and irreversible myocardial dysfunction. The amount of alcohol necessary to produce symptomatic cardiomyopathy in susceptible individuals is not known but has been estimated to be six drinks (~4 oz of pure ethanol) a day for 5 to 10 years. Frequent binging without heavy daily consumption may also be sufficient. Alcoholic cardiomyopathy can develop in patients without social evidence of an alcohol problem. Abstinence leads to improvement in at least 50% of patients with severe symptoms, some of whom normalize their left ventricular ejection fractions. Patients with other causes of heart failure also should limit alcohol consumption.

Chemotherapy

Anthracycline (doxorubicin, daunorubicin, epirubicin) cardiotoxicity (Chapter 164) causes characteristic histologic changes on endomyocardial biopsy with overt heart failure in 5 to 10% of patients who receive doses of 450 mg/m^2 of body surface area or more. Most cardiotoxicity occurs within the first year and is associated with a higher anthracycline dose and a lower left ventricular ejection fraction. Patients who have received anthracyclines in the prepubertal period without apparent cardiotoxicity may develop cardiac failure in young adulthood. The risk is higher in patients who have lower baseline ejection fractions, concomitant radiation therapy, or higher doses of anthracycline. Cyclophosphamide and ifosfamide can cause acute severe heart failure and malignant ventricular arrhythmias. Some tyrosine kinase inhibitors (e.g., sunitinib) cause a reduction in systolic function, especially in the presence of coronary artery disease, but there is good response to withdrawal and conventional medical therapy (Chapter 164). 5-Fluorouracil can cause coronary artery spasm and depressed left ventricular contractility. Up to 11% of patients who receive trastuzumab (Chapter 183), a recombinant monoclonal antibody that binds to human epidermal growth factor type 2, develop dilated cardiomyopathy, which is reversible after withdrawal and conventional drug treatment. The risk for cardiotoxicity increases with previous anthracycline and radiation treatment. Interferon alfa may be associated with hypotension and arrhythmias in up to 10% of patients, and interleukin-2 rarely has been associated with cardiotoxicity. Immune checkpoint inhibitors, which activate antitumor T lymphocytes that then attack cancer cells, can lead to off-target effects, including myocarditis, heart failure, and cardiogenic shock.

The use of ß-blockers (e.g., carvedilol, starting at 6.25 mg twice daily and increasing to 25 mg twice daily in the absence of heart failure, bradycardia, or atrioventricular block)[A11] or renin–angiotensin system blockers (e.g., enalapril, starting at 1.25 mg or 2.5 mg twice daily, increasing to 10 mg twice daily as tolerated with systolic blood pressure >90 mm Hg) with chemotherapy has been associated with better subsequent left ventricular function. However, small sample sizes and potential publication bias limit the clinical interpretability of these findings.

Metabolic and Endocrine Disease

Excess catecholamines, as in pheochromocytoma (Chapter 209), may injure the heart by compromising the coronary microcirculation or by direct toxic effects on myocytes. *Cocaine* (Chapter 365) increases synaptic concentrations of catecholamines by inhibiting reuptake at nerve terminals; the result may be an acute coronary syndrome or chronic cardiomyopathy.

Thiamine deficiency from poor nutrition or alcoholism (Chapter 199) can cause beriberi heart disease, with vasodilation and high cardiac output followed by low output. Calcium deficiency (Chapter 227) resulting from hypoparathyroidism, gastrointestinal abnormalities, or chelation directly compromises myocardial contractility.

Hypophosphatemia (Chapter 105), which may occur in alcoholism, during recovery from malnutrition, and in hyperalimentation, also reduces myocardial contractility. Patients with magnesium depletion (Chapter 105) due to impaired absorption or increased renal excretion (Chapter 105) also may present with left ventricular dysfunction.

Hypothyroidism (Chapter 207) depresses contractility and conduction and may cause pericardial effusions, whereas *hyperthyroidism* increases cardiac output, can worsen underlying heart failure, and may rarely be the sole cause of heart failure. The presenting sign of diabetes (Chapter 210) can be cardiomyopathy, especially with diastolic dysfunction, independent of epicardial coronary atherosclerosis, for which it is a major risk factor. Obesity (Chapter 201) can cause cardiomyopathy with increased ventricular mass and decreased contractility, which improve after weight loss, or it can aggravate underlying heart failure from other causes.

Peripartum Cardiomyopathy

Peripartum cardiomyopathy appears in the last month of pregnancy or in the first 5 months after delivery in the absence of preexisting cardiac disease (Chapter 221).[20] The incidence is between 1 in 3000 and 1 in 15,000 deliveries, with increased risk in older mothers or in the setting of twins, malnutrition, tocolytic therapy, toxemia, or hypertension. Lymphocytic myocarditis, which is found in 30 to 50% of biopsy specimens, suggests an immune component, perhaps cross-reactivity between uterine and cardiac myocyte proteins or an enhanced susceptibility to viral myocarditis. Enhanced oxidative stress triggers activation of cathepsin D, which is a ubiquitous lysosomal enzyme that cleaves serum prolactin in its antiangiogenic and proapoptotic 16-kD form, and that appears to promote endothelial inflammation and impair metabolism and contraction of cardiomyocytes. About 15% of patients have truncating mutations in the same genes that have been implicated in dilated cardiomyopathy, especially the *TTN* gene. Presentation is usually with orthopnea and dyspnea on minimal exertion, most often within the first weeks after delivery when the excess volume of pregnancy would normally be mobilized. Preexisting cardiac disease must be excluded.

TREATMENT

Diuretics facilitate postpartum diuresis, and angiotensin-converting enzyme inhibitors improve symptoms (Chapter 46).[21] Oral bromocriptine (2.5 mg twice daily for 2 weeks, then daily for 6 weeks) can significantly improve the recovery of left ventricular function and may reduce deaths.[A12] The prognosis is improvement to normal or near-normal ejection fraction during the next 6 months in more than 50% of patients. About 4% require heart transplantation, and about 9% die suddenly or from complications of heart transplantation.

Overlap with Restrictive Cardiomyopathy

Diseases causing primarily restrictive cardiomyopathies can occasionally overlap to cause a picture consistent with dilated cardiomyopathy. For example, hemochromatosis (Chapter 196) and sarcoidosis (Chapter 83) should be considered in evaluating any patient with a cardiomyopathy. Amyloidosis (Chapter 174) is less commonly confused with dilated than with hypertrophic cardiomyopathy but should be considered in a patient who has a thick-walled ventricle with depressed contractile function.

ARRHYTHMOGENIC RIGHT VENTRICULAR CARDIOMYOPATHY

DEFINITION AND EPIDEMIOLOGY

Arrhythmogenic right ventricular cardiomyopathy (ARVC; Chapter 53) is a genetically determined type of cardiomyopathy that is characterized histologically by loss of cardiomyocytes with replacement by fibrous or fibrofatty tissue in the right ventricular myocardium; clinically by ventricular arrhythmias, heart failure, and sudden cardiac death; and histologically by cardiomyocyte loss and replacement. The disease is seen in patients of European, African, and Asian descent, with an estimated prevalence between 1 in 1000 and 1 in 5000 adults.

PATHOBIOLOGY

Arrhythmogenic right ventricular cardiomyopathy is inherited as an autosomal dominant disease with incomplete penetrance, although recessive forms with cutaneous manifestations are recognized (see E-Table 47-1). Most cases are caused by heterozygous mutations in genes encoding components of the desmosomal junction of cardiomyocytes. The most common occur in plakophilin 2, desmocollin 2, desmoplakin, and desmoglein 2. Homozygous mutations in plakoglobin and desmoplakin are responsible for the rare autosomal recessive forms (Naxos disease and Carvajal syndrome, respectively). A highly penetrant and lethal mutation in the transmembrane cytoplasmic protein 43 (TMEM43) has been described in families from Newfoundland. Other genes that rarely cause arrhythmogenic right ventricular cardiomyopathy include desmin (*DES*), phospholamban (*PLN*), and lamin (*LMNA*).

Pathology

The main pathologic feature is progressive loss of right ventricular myocardium, which is replaced by adipose and fibrous tissue. These changes begin in the inflow, outflow, and apical regions of the right ventricle. Aneurysm formation in these areas is typical. Progressive myocardial involvement may lead to global right ventricular dilation. Right ventricular disease is often associated with fibrofatty substitution of the left ventricular myocardium, with the posterolateral wall preferentially affected.

Mutations in desmosomal protein genes may increase the susceptibility of the myocardium to the damaging effects of mechanical stress. The acute phase of myocardial injury may be accompanied by inflammation. The predilection for the right ventricle has been explained by its thin wall and greater distensibility. As desmosomal proteins interact with many other proteins, including components of the cellular cytoskeleton and intermediate filaments, it is possible that ventricular dysfunction occurs as the result of reduced cytoskeletal integrity and impaired force transduction. Some desmosomal proteins, in particular plakoglobin, are also important signaling molecules that regulate the transcription of many other genes.

Inflammatory infiltrates are present in about 70% of patients in autopsy series. People with arrhythmogenic right ventricular cardiomyopathy also have raised levels of cytokines and anti-DSG2 (desmoglein) antibodies.

CLINICAL MANIFESTATIONS

By convention, the natural history of arrhythmogenic right ventricular cardiomyopathy is divided into phases, but it is not inevitable that patients will progress through all phases. In the early phase, patients are usually asymptomatic, but resuscitated cardiac arrest and sudden death may be the initial manifestations, particularly in adolescents and young adults. The overt arrhythmic phase usually begins in adolescents and young adults, when patients note palpitations or syncope. Symptomatic sustained arrhythmias are usually accompanied by ECG, morphologic, and functional abnormalities of the right ventricle sufficient to fulfill diagnostic criteria for arrhythmogenic right ventricular cardiomyopathy. A small proportion of patients progress to a more advanced phase, which is characterized by diffuse right or left ventricular impairment that requires conventional treatment for heart failure (Chapter 46). Cardiac sarcoidosis (Chapter 83; see later) has many similarities with arrhythmogenic right ventricular cardiomyopathy in terms of presentation and clinical features, and it is sometimes clinically indistinguishable.

DIAGNOSIS

Clinical evaluation includes inquiry for symptoms of arrhythmia (syncope, presyncope, sustained palpitation); a family history of premature cardiac symptoms or sudden death; 12-lead, 24-hour, and maximal exercise ECG testing; and two-dimensional echocardiography with specific right ventricular views. Contrast echocardiography may be required to obtain better endocardial definition of the right ventricular myocardium and apex of the left ventricle. Magnetic resonance imaging (Chapter 44) provides accurate assessment of ventricular volumes as well as noninvasive characterization of the characteristic fibrous tissue and fat that establish the diagnosis and provide prognostic information (Figs. 44-17 and 47-5).[22]

Ventricular arrhythmias with a left bundle branch block morphology, consistent with a right ventricular origin, are characteristic. However, the ECG and arrhythmic manifestations are not specific to arrhythmogenic right ventricular cardiomyopathy and overlap with many other disease states, so standard criteria are recommended for diagnosis (Table 47-5). Because these criteria are highly specific but lack sensitivity for detection of early disease, more sensitive criteria are recommended for first-degree relatives of known cases (Table 47-6). The diagnosis in a proband also raises the possibility of mutation analysis in the family to identify those at risk and in need of serial evaluation as well as those who need no specific follow-up.

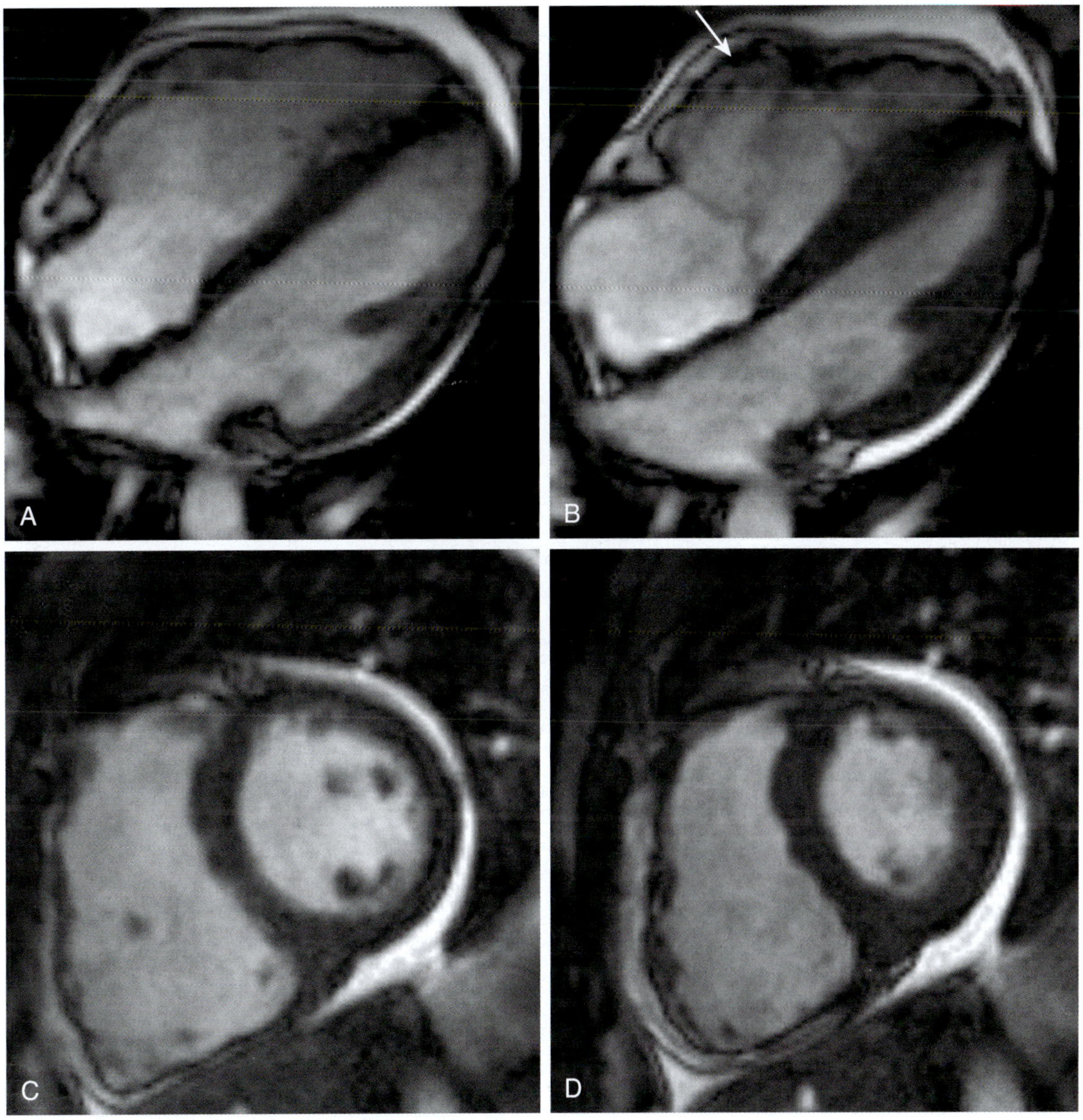

FIGURE 47-5. A 21-year-old man with arrhythmogenic right ventricular cardiomyopathy. End-diastolic (A) and end-systolic (B) frames from a four-chamber view, with a dilated and impaired right ventricle with a basal wall motion abnormality (*arrow*), confirmed on end-diastolic (C) and end-systolic (D) short axis views. This individual had no scar in the left ventricle with well-preserved systolic function; scar imaging in the thin right ventricle (with adjacent fat and small effusion) was equivocal.

TABLE 47-5 REVISED TASK FORCE CRITERIA FOR ARRHYTHMOGENIC RIGHT VENTRICULAR CARDIOMYOPATHY IN PROBANDS*

CRITERIA	
MAJOR	**MINOR**
I. GLOBAL OR REGIONAL DYSFUNCTION AND STRUCTURAL ALTERATIONS*	
By Two-Dimensional Echo • Regional RV akinesia, dyskinesia, or aneurysm • *and* 1 of the following (end diastole): PLAX RVOT ≥32 mm (corrected for body size [PLAX/BSA] ≥19 mm/m^2) PSAX RVOT ≥36 mm (corrected for body size [PLAX/BSA] ≥21 mm/m^2) *or* fractional area change ≤33%	**By Two-Dimensional Echo** • Regional RV akinesia or dyskinesia • *and* 1 of the following (end diastole): PLAX RVOT ≥29 to <32 mm (corrected for body size [PLAX/BSA] ≥16 to <19 mm/m^2) PSAX RVOT ≥32 to <36 mm (corrected for body size [PSAX/BSA] ≥18 to <21 mm/m^2) *or* fractional area change >33% to ≤40%
By MRI • Regional RV akinesia or dyskinesia or dyssynchronous RV contraction • *and* 1 of the following: RV end-diastolic volume indexed to BSA ≥110 mL/m^2 (male) or ≥100 mL/m^2 (female) *or* RV ejection fraction ≤40%	**By MRI** • Regional RV akinesia or dyskinesia or dyssynchronous RV contraction • *and* 1 of the following: RV end-diastolic volume indexed to BSA ≥100 to <110 mL/m^2 (male) or ≥90 to <100 mL/m^2 (female) *or* RV ejection fraction >40% to ≤45%
By RV angiography • Regional RV akinesia, dyskinesia, or aneurysm	
II. TISSUE CHARACTERIZATION OF WALL	
• Residual myocytes <60% by morphometric analysis (or <50% if estimated), with fibrous replacement of the RV free wall myocardium in ≥1 sample, with or without fatty replacement of tissue on endomyocardial biopsy	• Residual myocytes 60% to 75% by morphometric analysis (or 50% to 65% if estimated), with fibrous replacement of the RV free wall myocardium in ≥1 sample, with or without fatty replacement of tissue on endomyocardial biopsy
III. REPOLARIZATION ABNORMALITIES	
• Inverted T waves in right precordial leads (V_1,V_2, and V_3) or beyond in individuals >14 years of age (in the absence of complete right bundle branch block QRS ≥120 msec)	• Inverted T waves in leads V_1 and V_2 in individuals > 14 years of age (in the absence of complete right bundle branch block) or in V_4, V_5, or V_6 • Inverted T waves in leads V_1, V_2, V_3, and V_4 in individuals >14 years
IV. DEPOLARIZATION/CONDUCTION ABNORMALITIES	
• Epsilon wave (reproducible low-amplitude signals between end of QRS complex to onset of the T wave) in the right precordial leads (V_1 to V_3)	• Late potentials by SAECG in ≥1 of 3 parameters in the absence of a QRS duration ≥110 msec on the standard ECG • Filtered QRS duration (fQRS) ≥114 msec • Duration of terminal QRS <40 μV (low-amplitude signal duration) ≥38 msec • Root-mean-square voltage of terminal 40 msec ≥20 μV • Terminal activation duration of QRS ≥55 msec measured to the end of the QRS, including R′, in V_1, V_2, or V_3, in the absence of complete right bundle branch block
V. ARRHYTHMIAS	
• Nonsustained or sustained ventricular tachycardia of left bundle branch morphology with superior axis (negative or indeterminate QRS in leads II, III, and aVF and positive in lead aVL)	• Nonsustained or sustained ventricular tachycardia of RV outflow configuration, left bundle branch block morphology with inferior axis (positive QRS in leads II, III, and aVF and negative in lead aVL) or of unknown axis • >500 ventricular extrasystoles per 24 hours (Holter)
VI. FAMILY HISTORY	
• ARVC confirmed in a first-degree relative who meets current Task Force criteria • ARVC confirmed pathologically at autopsy or surgery in a first-degree relative • Identification of a pathogenic mutation† categorized as associated or probably associated with ARVC in the patient under evaluation	• History of ARVC in a first-degree relative in whom it is not possible or practical to determine whether the family member meets current Task Force criteria • Premature sudden death (<35 years of age) due to suspected ARVC in a first-degree relative

*Hypokinesis is not included in this or subsequent definitions of right ventricular (RV) regional wall motion abnormalities for the proposed modified criteria.

†A pathogenic mutation is a DNA alteration associated with ARVC that alters or is expected to alter the encoded protein, is unobserved or rare in a large non-ARVC control population, and either alters or is predicted to alter the structure or function of the protein or has demonstrated linkage to the disease phenotype in a conclusive pedigree.

ARVC = arrhythmogenic right ventricular cardiomyopathy; aVF = augmented voltage unipolar left foot lead; aVL = augmented voltage unipolar left arm lead; BSA = body surface area; ECG = electrocardiogram; MRI = magnetic resonance imaging; PLAX = parasternal long axis view; PSAX = parasternal short axis view; RVOT = right ventricular outflow tract; SAECG = signal-averaged electrocardiogram. Diagnostic terminology for original criteria: this diagnosis is fulfilled by the presence of 2 major, 1 major plus 2 minor, or 4 minor criteria from different groups. Diagnostic terminology for revised criteria: definite diagnosis: 2 major, 1 major and 2 minor, or 4 minor criteria from different categories; borderline: 1 major and 1 minor or 3 minor criteria from different categories; possible: 1 major or 2 minor criteria from different categories.

From Marcus FI, McKenna WJ, Sherrill D, et al. Diagnosis of arrhythmogenic right ventricular cardiomyopathy/dysplasia: proposed modification of the task force criteria. *Circulation.* 2010;121:1533-1541.

Differential Diagnosis

The differential diagnosis includes other inherited cardiomyopathies, the inherited arrhythmia syndromes (long QT syndrome, Brugada syndrome, and catecholaminergic polymorphic ventricular tachycardia; Chapter 53), cardiac sarcoidosis, myocarditis, and causes of right ventricular dilation such as intracardiac or extracardiac shunts (Chapter 55). The differentiation from so-called benign right ventricular outflow tract tachycardia may be problematic, although the 12-lead ECG and right ventricular imaging studies are typically normal, and no familial disease is present. Some patients with desmosomal protein gene mutations demonstrate left ventricular involvement early in the disease (e.g., truncating variants in desmoplakin), whereas survivors may develop a predominant left ventricular dilated cardiomyopathy phenotype with a risk of lethal arrhythmias.

TREATMENT

Pharmacologic treatment is the first-line therapy for patients with well-tolerated, non–life-threatening ventricular arrhythmias, such as frequent ventricular extrasystoles. Treatment of patients with symptomatic ventricular arrhythmias is with an ICD,[23] with supplemental sotalol (160 to 240 mg/day) or even amiodarone (maintenance dose of 200 mg/day). Catheter ablation (Chapter 54) may be required in patients with drug-refractory incessant ventricular arrhythmia

TABLE 47-6 ARRHYTHMOGENIC RIGHT VENTRICULAR CARDIOMYOPATHY: CRITERIA FOR DIAGNOSIS OF FIRST-DEGREE RELATIVES WHO DO NOT FULFILL CRITERIA AS PROBANDS*

ARVC in a first-degree relative plus one of the following:	
ECG	T wave inversion in right precordial leads (V_2 and V_3)
Signal-averaged ECG	Late potentials seen on signal-averaged ECG
Arrhythmia	Left bundle branch block–type ventricular tachycardia on ECG, on Holter monitoring, or during exercise testing; >200 extrasystoles during a 24-hour period
Structural or functional abnormality of the right ventricle	Mild global right ventricular dilation or reduction in ejection fraction with normal left ventricle; mild segmental dilation of the right ventricle; regional right ventricular hypokinesia

*Any one criterion is adequate for the diagnosis.
ARVC = arrhythmogenic right ventricular cardiomyopathy; ECG = electrocardiogram.
From Hamid MS, Norman M, Quraishi A, et al: Prospective evaluation of relatives for familial arrhythmogenic right ventricular cardiomyopathy reveals a need to broaden diagnostic criteria. *J Am Coll Cardiol.* 2002;40:1445-1450.

TABLE 47-7 CAUSES OF RESTRICTIVE CARDIOMYOPATHIES

INFILTRATIVE DISORDERS
Amyloidosis Sarcoidosis
STORAGE DISORDERS
Hemochromatosis Fabry disease Glycogen storage diseases
FIBROTIC DISORDERS
Radiation Scleroderma Drugs (e.g., doxorubicin, serotonin, ergotamine)
METABOLIC DISORDERS
Carnitine deficiency Defects in fatty acid metabolism
ENDOMYOCARDIAL DISORDERS
Endomyocardial fibrosis Hypereosinophilic syndrome (Löffler endocarditis)
MISCELLANEOUS CAUSES
Carcinoid syndrome

or frequent recurrences of ventricular tachycardia after implantation of an ICD, although recurrence is common.

Retrospective analyses of clinical and pathologic series have identified a number of possible predictors of adverse outcome in probands, including an early age at onset of symptoms, competitive sporting activity, severe right ventricular dilation, left ventricular involvement, syncope, episodes of complex ventricular arrhythmias or VT, and increased QRS dispersion on the 12-lead electrocardiogram. ICD implantation is recommended for the prevention of sudden cardiac death in patients with documented sustained ventricular tachycardia or ventricular fibrillation and a reasonable expectation of survival with a good functional status for longer than 1 year. ICD implantation may also be appropriate in patients with extensive disease, including those with left ventricular involvement, or undiagnosed syncope when ventricular tachycardia or ventricular fibrillation has not been excluded as the cause.

Standard heart failure therapy, including diuretics, angiotensin-converting enzyme inhibitors, and β-blockers, is indicated in patients in whom arrhythmogenic right ventricular cardiomyopathy has progressed to severe heart failure or biventricular systolic dysfunction (Chapter 46). Anticoagulation should be considered in the presence of atrial fibrillation (Chapter 52), marked ventricular dilation, or ventricular aneurysms. In patients in whom heart failure is refractory, cardiac transplantation (Chapter 46) should be considered.

PROGNOSIS

Most data on prognosis are derived from small, high-risk populations. By the age of 40 years, event-free survival is 50 to 60% in patients with Naxos disease and some autosomal dominant forms. In patients who have syncope or sustained ventricular arrhythmias and are treated with an ICD, freedom from appropriate shock therapy is about 75% at 48 months after implantation, with 96% of patients alive. Risk factors for sudden cardiac death include genotype,[24] severe right ventricular disease, left ventricular involvement, and a history of unexplained syncope.

RESTRICTIVE CARDIOMYOPATHY

DEFINITION AND EPIDEMIOLOGY

Restrictive cardiomyopathies (Table 47-7) are characterized by stiffness, impaired filling, elevated left ventricular diastolic pressures, and reduced diastolic volume of the left or right ventricle despite normal or near-normal systolic function and wall thickness.[25] Primary (idiopathic) forms are very uncommon, whereas secondary forms, in which the heart is affected as part of a multisystem disorder, usually present at the advanced stage of an infiltrative disease (e.g., amyloidosis or sarcoidosis) or a systemic storage disease (e.g., hemochromatosis). Idiopathic restrictive cardiomyopathy affects both male and female patients and may be manifested in children and young adults.

PATHOBIOLOGY

Approximately 30% of patients with idiopathic restrictive cardiomyopathy have familial disease, and most of these patients will have mutations in the cardiac sarcomere protein genes, particularly *TNNI3* and *MYH7*. These individuals may present with phenotypes that overlap with hypertrophic cardiomyopathy (Fig. 47-6). Mutations in the gene (*DES*) that encodes desmin, which is an intermediate filament, cause restrictive cardiomyopathy associated with skeletal myopathy and cardiac conduction system abnormalities. Wild-type, transthyretin-related cardiac amyloidosis (Chapter 174) is the most prevalent form of restrictive cardiomyopathy, and it increases in frequency in older patients. However, restriction is present only in the late stages of disease, when patients have extensive amyloid infiltration of the myocardial interstitium.

Restrictive cardiomyopathy is seen in hemochromatosis (Chapter 196) and sarcoidosis (Chapter 83), and it also is increasingly seen in cancer survivors as a consequence of diffuse biventricular fibrosis, most often with a nonischemic pattern, caused by chemotherapy (especially high-dose anthracyclines) and chest radiotherapy (Chapter 18).

The macroscopic features of restrictive cardiomyopathy include biatrial dilation and small ventricular cavities. In many hearts, there is thrombus in the atrial appendages and patchy endocardial fibrosis. The histologic features of restrictive cardiomyopathy vary, depending on the cause, but patchy interstitial fibrosis and myocyte disarray can be seen in patients with pure restrictive cardiomyopathy. Amyloidosis, hemochromatosis, and sarcoidosis are among the systemic diseases that cause restrictive cardiomyopathy (see later).

CLINICAL MANIFESTATIONS

Most patients present with symptoms and signs of heart failure and supraventricular arrhythmias, including atrial fibrillation (Chapter 52) and heart block (Chapter 51). Common symptoms include dyspnea on exertion, recurrent respiratory tract infections, general fatigue, and weakness. Symptoms may progress rapidly to dyspnea at rest, orthopnea, paroxysmal nocturnal dyspnea, and abdominal discomfort due to hepatic engorgement. Many patients complain of chest pain and palpitation. Rarely, sudden death is the initial manifestation of the disease.

Physical examination typically reveals an elevated jugular venous pressure, which has a prominent *y* descent and fails to fall (or rises) during inspiration (Kussmaul sign). On cardiac auscultation, the pulmonary component of the second heart sound may be loud if pulmonary vascular resistance is high. A third heart sound and occasionally a fourth heart sound commonly produce a gallop rhythm. Peripheral edema, ascites, and hepatomegaly are common.

DIAGNOSIS

No ECG findings are diagnostic, but the most frequent ECG abnormalities include P mitrale and P pulmonale, nonspecific ST segment and T wave abnormalities, ST segment depression, and T wave inversion, usually in the inferolateral leads. Voltage criteria for left and right ventricular hypertrophy may be present. Some patients with amyloidosis have low-voltage QRS complexes. Conduction abnormalities include intraventricular conduction delay and abnormal Q waves.

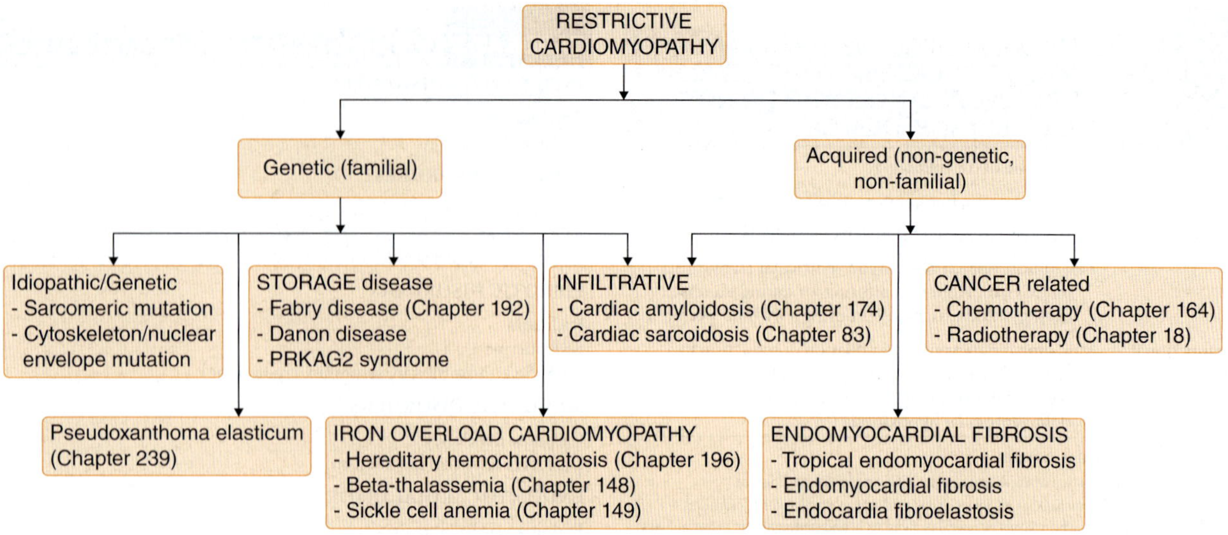

FIGURE 47-6. **Classification of restrictive cardiomyopathies.** (Adapted from Ditaranto R, Caponetti AG, Ferrara V, et al. Pediatric restrictive cardiomyopathies. *Front Pediatr.* 2022;9:745365.)

On cardiac imaging, both atria are markedly dilated and can dwarf the size of the ventricles in patients with normal global systolic function and a nonhypertrophied, nondilated left ventricle. Pulsed-wave Doppler velocities typically show increased early diastolic filling velocity, decreased atrial filling velocity, increased ratio of early diastolic filling to atrial filling, decreased E wave deceleration time, and decreased isovolumic relaxation time. Pulmonary vein and hepatic vein pulsed-wave Doppler velocities demonstrate higher diastolic than systolic velocities, increased atrial reversal velocities, and atrial reversal duration greater than mitral atrial filling duration. Tissue Doppler imaging usually shows reduced diastolic annular velocities and an increased ratio of early diastolic tissue Doppler annular velocity to mitral early diastolic filling velocity, reflecting elevated left ventricular end-diastolic pressures.

The characteristic hemodynamic feature on cardiac catheterization is a deep and rapid early decline in ventricular pressure at the onset of diastole (Table 62-6 and E-Fig 47-9), with a rapid rise to a plateau in early diastole ("dip-and-plateau" or "square root sign") (Fig. 47-7). Left ventricular end-diastolic, left atrial, and pulmonary capillary wedge pressures are markedly elevated, usually 5 mm Hg or more above right atrial and right ventricular end-diastolic pressures. Volume loading and exercise accentuate the difference between left-sided and right-sided pressures.

The diagnostic evaluation aims to exclude potentially reversible conditions and to distinguish restrictive cardiomyopathy from constrictive pericarditis (Chapter 62). Definitive etiologic diagnosis relies on the demonstration of disease-specific features, such as amyloid protein in amyloidosis (Chapter 174), noncaseating granulomas in sarcoidosis (Chapter 83), abnormal iron studies in hemochromatosis (Chapter 196), or reduced α-galactosidase A levels in Fabry disease (Chapter 192). Endomyocardial biopsy is rarely required to make these diagnoses.

TREATMENT

Diuretics are the main therapy for heart failure symptoms (Chapter 46), but they must be carefully administered so as not to reduce left ventricular filling pressures to the point of hypotension. Angiotensin-converting enzyme inhibitors and β-blockers are commonly recommended despite few data on their benefit. However, all atrioventricular blocking agents, including β-blockers, must be used with caution, because an increase in heart rate is the only mechanism to increase cardiac output in the face of augmented oxygen requirements (e.g., during physical activity). In patients with secondary restrictive cardiomyopathies, specific treatment of the underlying systemic disease is indicated whenever possible (see later). Referral for assessment for possible heart transplantation should be considered early before refractory pulmonary hypertension may develop.

PROGNOSIS

In adults with restrictive cardiomyopathy, the clinical course is usually slow and protracted. Survival from the time of diagnosis is often 10 years or more, except for AL amyloidosis, which progresses much more rapidly. Symptoms of heart failure are generally progressive and respond poorly to treatments for heart failure.

SPECIFIC CLINICAL SYNDROMES

SARCOIDOSIS

The frequency of myocardial involvement in patients with sarcoidosis (Chapter 83) is difficult to determine because it is frequently subclinical and patchy in nature. Postmortem studies suggest that the heart is involved in at least 25% of patients, but clinical cardiac involvement occurs in less than 10% of patients. Clinical manifestations of ventricular dysfunction include heart failure, conduction abnormalities, atrial and ventricular arrhythmias, pericardial effusion, valvular dysfunction, and, rarely, sudden cardiac death. Right-sided heart failure secondary to pulmonary hypertension may occur in patients with extensive fibrotic lung disease. Myocardial infiltration by sarcoid granulomas results in restrictive or dilated cardiomyopathy. The most common site is in the lateral wall of the left ventricle. Papillary muscle involvement is responsible for the most common valvulopathy, mitral regurgitation. Granuloma formation in the basal interventricular septum may cause conduction abnormalities. Ventricular arrhythmias, usually monomorphic ventricular tachycardia, are frequent and may be life-threatening.

DIAGNOSIS

The diagnosis of cardiac sarcoidosis can be challenging given its patchy involvement of the heart.[26] Magnetic resonance imaging identifies areas of edema and fibrosis (the latter evident as patchy areas of late gadolinium enhancement [Fig. 44-16]), whereas ^{18}F-Fluorodeoxyglucose positron emission tomography/computed tomography may demonstrate cardiac inflammation in the active phase of disease (E-Fig. 44-3). In patients with such noninvasive findings, histologic confirmation then may be obtained by a biopsy of other affected organs, such as mediastinal lymph nodes or the liver.

TREATMENT AND PROGNOSIS

Corticosteroid therapy (Chapter 83) may improve arrhythmias. However, heart failure may worsen despite such therapy, so immunosuppressants such as mycophenolate mofetil, methotrexate, or azathioprine may be required. An ICD is generally indicated for ventricular arrhythmias. Estimates for 1-, 5-, and 10-year transplantation-free cardiac survival are 97%, 90%, and 83%, respectively, but heart failure at presentation predicts a poor outcome, with a 10-year transplantation-free cardiac survival of only 53%.

AMYLOIDOSIS

EPIDEMIOLOGY AND PATHOBIOLOGY

Amyloidosis can result in deposition of amyloid protein in the atria, ventricles, coronary vessels, conduction system, and valves. The degree of cardiac involvement varies among subtypes. Hematologic disorders (Chapter 173) associated with excessive light chain (AL) immunoglobulin production are a common cause of cardiac amyloid. Familial forms caused by the accumulation of mutant proteins (transthyretin or apolipoprotein A) (Chapter 174)

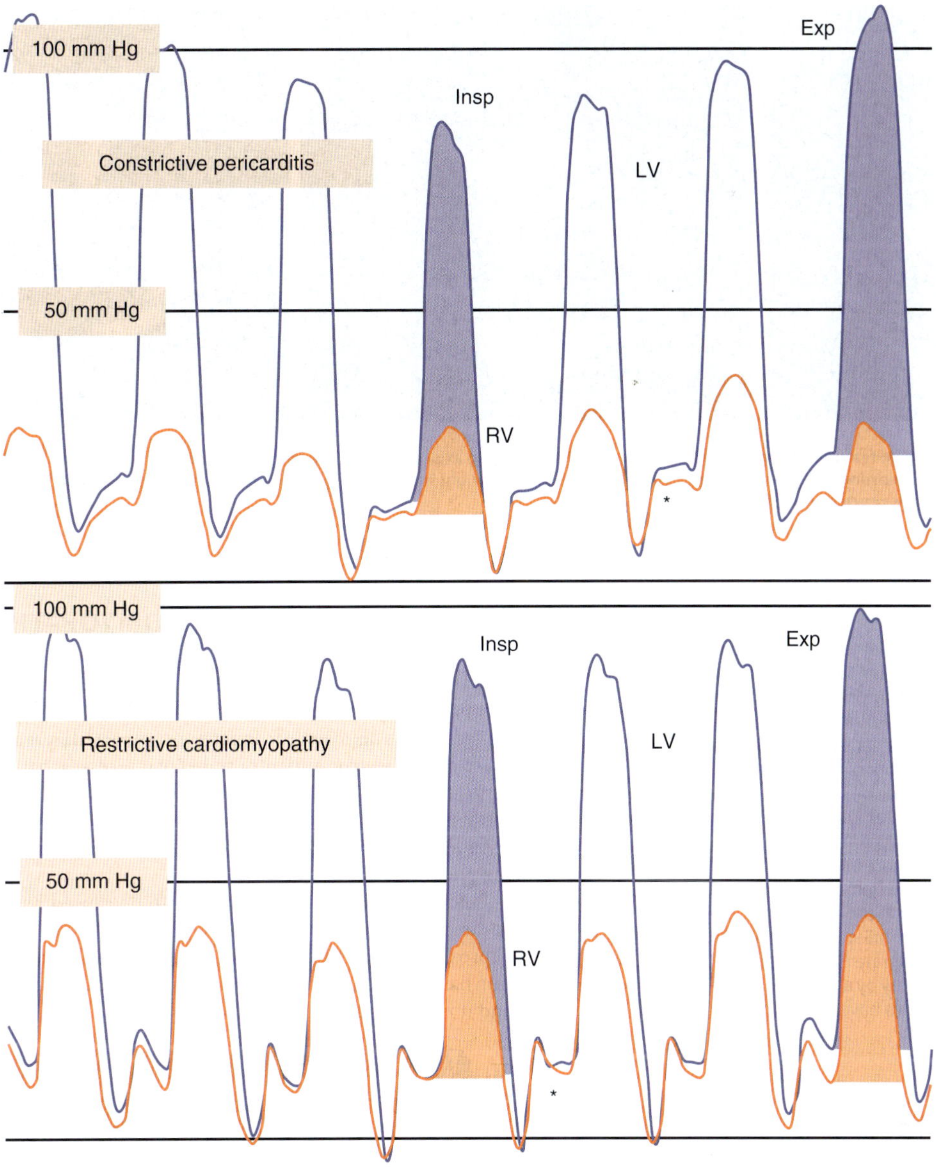

FIGURE 47-7. **Simultaneous RV and LV hemodynamic assessment in constrictive pericarditis and restrictive cardiomyopathy.** *Top*, Left ventricular (LV) (blue) and right ventricular (RV) (orange) hemodynamic pressure tracings in constrictive pericarditis. End-diastolic filling pressures are elevated and a "square root" sign is present on both pressure tracings (*). Enhanced ventricular interdependence is present, demonstrated by visualization of the systolic area index; RV (gray) and LV (dark gray) areas under the curve are shown for both inspiration (Insp) and expiration (Exp). During inspiration, there is an increase in the area of the RV pressure curve and decrease in the area of the LV pressure curve. *Bottom*, LV and RV pressure tracings in restrictive cardiomyopathy. Although end-diastolic filling pressures are elevated and a square root sign (*) is present, there is no evidence of enhanced ventricular interdependence, with parallel changes in LV and RV pressure curve areas. (Adapted from Geske JB, Anavekar NS, Nishimura RA, et al. Differentiation of constriction and restriction: complex cardiovascular hemodynamics. *J Am Coll Cardiol*. 2016;68:2329-2347.)

have variable cardiac involvement. Secondary amyloidosis, due to deposition of serum amyloid A protein in chronic inflammatory diseases, rarely affects the heart. In late-onset systemic amyloidosis, cardiomyopathy is caused by deposition of normal wild-type transthyretin (TTR); this disease nearly always affects elderly persons (>70 years), with a clinical course that is considerably slower than with other types of amyloid.

DIAGNOSIS

If cardiac amyloidosis is suspected, blood and urine should be analyzed for evidence of a plasma cell dyscrasia (Chapters 173 and 174). The ECG tracing in most forms of cardiac amyloid characteristically shows decreased voltage despite increased wall thickness on echocardiography. Characteristic two-dimensional echocardiographic findings in advanced cardiac amyloidosis are biventricular hypertrophy, thickened valves and interatrial septum, dilated atria, and a small pericardial effusion. The myocardium has a hyperreflective granular texture (Fig. 47-8), best seen on digital image analysis.[27] Echo Doppler in advanced disease demonstrates a restrictive left ventricular filling pattern. Cardiac magnetic resonance imaging may show subendocardial late gadolinium enhancement with abnormal gadolinium kinetics, but it has a 10 to 20% false-negative and false-positive rate.

Transthyretin-related cardiac amyloidosis is particularly avid for 99mTc-phosphate bone tracers (see E-Fig. 44-4). In the setting of a positive 99mTc-phosphate scan without evidence for a plasma clone on blood and urine testing, a diagnosis of transthyretin cardiomyopathy can be made without a biopsy. If both the phosphate scan and blood tests are negative, cardiac amyloidosis is very unlikely. For patients with evidence for a plasma cell dyscrasia, a histologic diagnosis is still required because the presence of uptake on a 99mTc-phosphate scan is not 100% specific for amyloid transthyretin cardiomyopathy.

A definitive diagnosis of amyloidosis requires a tissue biopsy specimen, which can be obtained from other sites. For example, fine-needle aspiration of abdominal fat is positive for amyloid deposits in more than 80% of patients with AL amyloidosis, but is less sensitive for diagnosing other forms of amyloid. If the result is negative, endomyocardial biopsy has a very high sensitivity.

TREATMENT AND PROGNOSIS

Specific therapies to impede precursor protein production and fibril formation should be implemented whenever possible (Chapter 174).[28] Tafamidis (20 to 80 mg daily) can reduce the rate of functional decline and all-cause mortality in transthyretin amyloid cardiomyopathy, but the survival benefit may not be

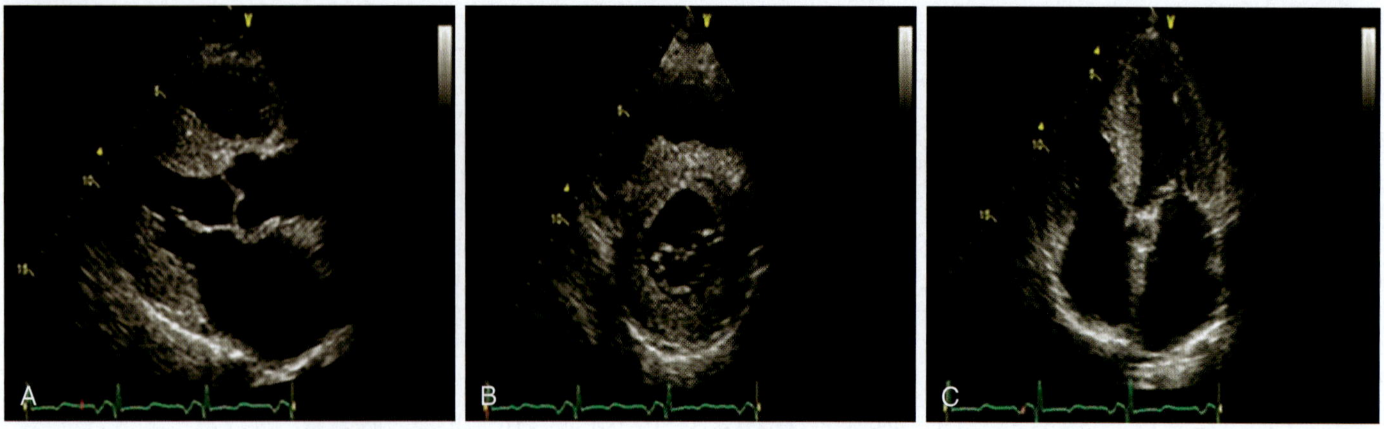

FIGURE 47-8. Typical echocardiographic features of cardiac amyloidosis. **A,** Parasternal long axis showing concentric left ventricular hypertrophy, bright myocardium, and left atrial dilatation. **B,** Parasternal short axis showing concentric left ventricular hypertrophy and bright myocardium. **C,** Apical four-chamber view showing concentric left ventricular hypertrophy and biatrial dilatation. (Images courtesy of Professor Elliott.)

evident until after 2 years of treatment.[A13,A14] Patisiran (0.3 mg/kg intravenously every 3 weeks) may reduce functional decline and adverse cardiac outcomes.[A15] All patients with atrial fibrillation (Chapter 52) should receive anticoagulation (Chapter 70) because of the high intrinsic risk of thromboembolism.

For heart failure (Chapter 46), diuretics, often in high doses (e.g., furosemide, 40 to 80 mg daily), are the mainstay of the palliative heart failure regimen. ß-blockers, angiotensin-converting enzyme inhibitors, and angiotensin II receptor blockers should be used cautiously because they are often poorly tolerated and of unproven efficacy in cardiac amyloidosis. Aldosterone inhibitors might be helpful in advanced cases. Patients may be hypersensitive to digoxin because of enhanced drug binding with amyloid fibrils. Cardiac transplantation remains controversial, but heart transplantation (Chapter 46) with high-dose chemotherapy and with stem cell transplantation (Chapter 163) has been used in patients with AL amyloidosis.

Patients with amyloidosis with heart failure have had a median survival time of less than 1 year and a 5-year survival rate of less than 5%, but new therapies such as tafamidis have reduced mortality by about 30%. Most deaths occur suddenly. Patients with familial amyloidosis have a slower course than do patients with a monoclonal gammopathy.

HEREDITARY HEMOCHROMATOSIS

Hereditary hemochromatosis (Chapter 196) is an autosomal recessive disorder caused by excessive iron deposition in various organs, including the liver, spleen, pancreas, endocrine glands, and heart. In Whites, its prevalence is between 1 in 200 and 1 in 500, with an even higher prevalence in the Irish population. The most common form is caused by mutations in the *HFE* gene, with two missense mutations (*C282Y* and *H63D*) accounting for most cases.

Most patients with classic disease present between the ages of 40 and 60 years with hyperpigmentation, diabetes mellitus, and hepatomegaly. Up to 35% of patients with hemochromatosis experience heart failure, and 36% develop arrhythmias.[29] Restrictive physiologic features dominate early in the disease, followed by ventricular dilation.

DIAGNOSIS

The diagnosis is generally made from the clinical picture, an elevated serum iron level, and a high transferrin saturation. Because paramagnetic ferritin and hemosiderin interact with nearby hydrogen nuclei in tissue water, appropriate MRI sequences evaluating the relaxation time T_2^* is highly sensitive for detecting myocardial iron deposition. Genetic testing is essential, and the diagnosis can be confirmed by endomyocardial biopsy.

TREATMENT

Phlebotomy and iron chelation therapy with deferoxamine (Chapter 196) may improve cardiac function before cell injury becomes irreversible. Standard heart failure treatment (Chapter 46) is generally recommended. Death from hemochromatosis results more often from cirrhosis and liver carcinoma than from cardiac disease.

UNCLASSIFIED CARDIOMYOPATHIES

LEFT VENTRICULAR NONCOMPACTION

Left ventricular noncompaction (LVNC) refers to an abnormal ventricular morphology that is characterized by a thin outer layer of normal or compacted myocardium with an inner noncompacted layer consisting of prominent muscular trabeculae and intra-trabecular recesses that communicate with the ventricular cavity. Current evidence suggests that the compact wall grows by intrinsic proliferation rather than by compaction of the preexisting trabecular layer. For this reason, the term excessive trabeculation is being used to describe the phenomenon.

Left ventricular noncompaction can be caused by genetic variants, most commonly in cardiac sarcomeric proteins *MYH7, MYBPC,* and *TTN,*[30] in approximately one-third of patients. However, left ventricular noncompaction has also been reported in athletes, healthy controls, and pregnant women, and it is more frequent in Black individuals.

CLINICAL MANIFESTATIONS AND DIAGNOSIS

When extensive areas are involved, ventricular systolic performance may be impaired and lead to an increased risk of ventricular arrhythmias and systemic emboli. Various diagnostic imaging criteria have been proposed, with MRI (Fig. 47-9) being more sensitive than echocardiography, Excessive trabeculation can be seen in isolation or in association with congenital heart anomalies, cardiomyopathies, and even in physiologic conditions such as pregnancy and highly trained athletes. As a result, extreme caution is needed when diagnosing left ventricular noncompaction, particularly in situations in which physiologic remodeling of the ventricle results in prominent ventricular trabeculae.

TREATMENT AND PROGNOSIS

Treatment, when necessary, is for associated heart failure (Chapter 46), arrhythmias (Chapters 50 and 53), and the risk of emboli (Chapter 70). Natural history and prognosis are not well-established.

TAKOTSUBO SYNDROME

Takotsubo syndrome causes transient left ventricular apical dysfunction that mimics myocardial infarction (Chapter 58).[31] About 90% of affected patients are women, especially postmenopausal women.

Catecholamines play a central role in the pathobiology, with acute episodes often triggered by sudden, unexpected stress or major physical illness or trauma. Many patients have abnormalities in both the structure and activity of brain areas that are related to both emotions and the sympathetic nervous system. Microvascular dysfunction and abnormal vasomotor reactivity are common findings, but it is not clear if these findings are the cause or consequence of an acute episode. Myocardial inflammation, which occurs during the acute phase, may persist in the chronic phase and may contribute to long-term morbidity.

CLINICAL PRESENTATION AND DIAGNOSIS

About 35% of events are triggered by emotional events and about 30% of events are triggered by physical events, with no obvious triggers in the remainder of

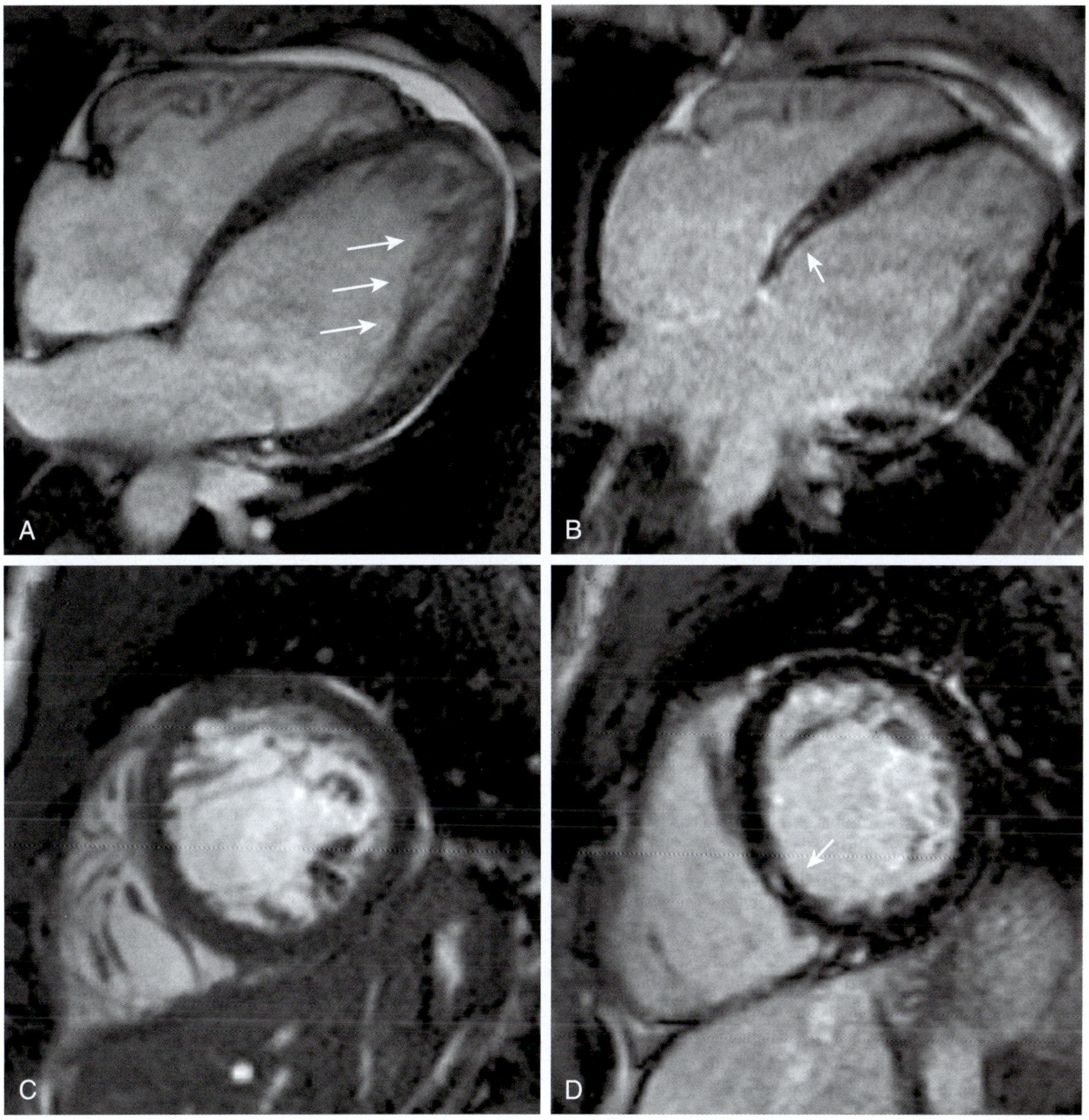

FIGURE 47-9. **A 23-year-old White man with left ventricular noncompaction.** Four-chamber end-diastolic (**A**) and short axis (**C**) views show left ventricular dilation, prominent trabeculae (*long arrows*), and poorly formed papillary muscles. The ejection fraction was 55%. There is limited mid-myocardial septal late gadolinium enhancement (**B, D,** *short arrows*).

patients. The clinical presentation is usually similar to acute myocardial infarction (Chapter 58), with chest pain, dyspnea, ST-segment elevation or depression, and T-wave inversion on the resting ECG, as well as elevation of serum cardiac troponin levels. Coronary arteriography, which reveals normal epicardial vessels, differentiates Takotsubo syndrome from acute myocardial infarction.

TREATMENT

Conservative treatment with rehydration and removal of the determinants of stress usually results in resolution of the symptoms, ECG changes, and wall motion abnormalities within hours.[32] Patients with left ventricular systolic dysfunction (ejection fraction <40%) should be treated with angiotensin-converting enzyme inhibitors and β-blockers, as in patients who have had an ST elevation myocardial infarction (Chapter 58). Patients may be weaned from both medications once left ventricular function has recovered if patients have no other complications such as tachyarrhythmias or hypertension.

PROGNOSIS

Takotsubo syndrome has a 4 to 5% in-hospital mortality related to cardiogenic shock and cardiac arrest. Survivors may experience long-term cardiac and noncardiac health problems, with an increased long-term mortality.

DISEASES OF THE ENDOCARDIUM

Endocardial fibrosis, fibroelastosis, and thrombosis are subclassified into endomyocardial diseases with hypereosinophilia (hypereosinophilic syndromes) and endomyocardial disease without hypereosinophilia (e.g., endomyocardial fibrosis) (see Table 47-7).

HYPEREOSINOPHILIC SYNDROME

Hypereosinophilic syndromes are a rare and heterogeneous group of disorders defined as persistent blood eosinophilia ($>1.5 \times 10^9$/L) for more than 6 consecutive months, associated with evidence of eosinophil-induced organ damage in the absence of causes of hypereosinophilia, such as allergic drug reactions, parasitic, and malignant disorders (Chapter 156). Pathogenic mechanisms include stem cell mutations that lead to expression of PDGFRA-containing fusion genes, mainly the *FIP1L1-PDGFRA* fusion gene, with constitutive tyrosine kinase activity and sustained overproduction of interleukin-5 by activated T-cell subsets. Clinically, hypereosinophilic syndrome can be classified into chronic eosinophilic leukemia, lymphocytic hypereosinophilic syndrome, myeloproliferative hypereosinophilic syndrome, and idiopathic hypereosinophilic syndrome. The term organ-restricted eosinophilic disease, such as eosinophilic gastroenteritis, dermatitis, or pneumonia, is used when a specific organ or tissue is the exclusive target of eosinophilic infiltration and damage. The term Löffler fibroplastic endocarditis with eosinophilia has been used to describe cardiac damage caused by direct toxicity of circulating eosinophils in patients with persistent hypereosinophilia, but its use is now discouraged.

CLINICAL MANIFESTATIONS AND DIAGNOSIS

Hypereosinophilic syndrome is a rare disorder that tends to occur in patients 20 to 50 years of age, but all age groups are affected. Cardiac involvement generally evolves in three phases: an early necrotic stage that involves the endomyocardium, which is usually asymptomatic but can be manifested as acute heart failure; a thrombotic stage, in which thrombi develop on the ventricular endocardium, sometimes causing peripheral emboli; and the final fibrotic stage, endomyocardial fibrosis, which causes restrictive cardiomyopathy and damage to atrioventricular valves.[33] Chest pain, cough, dyspnea or orthopnea, and edema of the lower extremities are typical symptoms. Some patients may develop arrhythmias.

The characteristic two-dimensional echocardiographic findings include endocardial thickening, apical obliteration of one or both ventricles by an echogenic material, hyperdynamic contraction of the spared ventricular walls with bilateral atrial enlargement, and a restrictive pattern on echo Doppler. Endomyocardial biopsy, which should be considered when myocardial involvement is suspected and which remains the gold standard for diagnosis, shows eosinophils and/or their granular products in cardiac tissue.

TREATMENT

Patients should be treated as for the hypereosinophilic syndrome (Chapter 156). Heart failure (Chapter 46) and cardiac arrhythmias (Chapter 52 and 53) should be managed in accordance with consensus guidelines. Chronic oral anticoagulation (Chapter 70) is indicated in patients who have an intracavitary thrombus and/or recurrent thromboembolic events.

TROPICAL ENDOMYOCARDIAL FIBROSIS

Tropical endomyocardial fibrosis is probably the most common type of restrictive cardiomyopathy worldwide.[34] The disease occurs predominantly within the tropics and affects mostly children and adolescents, usually from low socioeconomic backgrounds. Its cause is unknown, but potential contributors include infection, autoimmunity, genetic predisposition, ethnicity, diet, climate, and poverty.

Severe hypereosinophilia is found in some patients early in the initial stage of the illness; it is characterized by febrile illness, pancarditis, facial and periorbital swelling, pruritus, urticaria, and neurologic symptoms. This phase is followed by ventricular thrombosis that affects the apices and the subvalvular apparatus and then evolves to endocardial fibrosis. The final stage is characterized by restrictive physiology, atrioventricular valve regurgitation, and marked atrial dilation. Death results from complications of chronic heart failure but can occur suddenly from thromboembolism or arrhythmia.

Atrial fibrillation is common at presentation. In advanced disease, the electrocardiogram shows low-voltage QRS complexes, nonspecific ST-T wave changes, and conduction abnormalities. Echocardiography demonstrates apical obliteration, reduction of ventricular cavity size, and tethering or retraction of mitral or tricuspid leaflets or both. There is no specific laboratory test, and hypereosinophilia is present only early in the disease.

There is no specific treatment for endomyocardial fibrosis. Medical treatment is used to control the heart failure (Chapter 46) and arrhythmias (Chapters 52 and 53). Surgical endocardial resection, combined with valve repair or replacement, has an early postoperative mortality between 15 and 30%. The overall prognosis is poor, with about a 45% mortality rate at 1 year, increasing to nearly 90% at 3 years.

CARCINOID SYNDROME

EPIDEMIOLOGY AND PATHOBIOLOGY

Carcinoid tumors are rare (1 in 100,000) neuroendocrine malignant neoplasms originating mostly from enterochromaffin cells in the gastrointestinal tract (Chapter 213). Carcinoid syndrome, with flushing, diarrhea, and bronchospasm, occurs after tumor cells metastasize to the liver and the vasoactive substances produced by the tumors enter the systemic circulation through the hepatic vein. Carcinoid heart disease occurs in up to 70% of cases of carcinoid syndrome.

The typical cardiac lesion is the carcinoid plaque, which is composed of smooth muscle cells, myofibroblasts, and elastic tissue that forms a fibrous layer on the endocardial surface of the right ventricle and atrium, the valve leaflets, and the subvalvular apparatus, including the chordae and papillary muscles. The tricuspid valve plaques tend to develop on the ventricular side of the leaflets, where they adhere to the mural endocardium and cause valvular regurgitation. On the pulmonary valve, the predominant lesion is stenosis. In patients with a patent foramen ovale, left-sided valvular involvement can occur. Occasional patients may have concomitant myocardial metastases and pericardial effusions from direct tumor invasion.

The most common presentation is dyspnea with signs and symptoms of right-sided heart failure. The electrocardiogram and radiograph are nonspecific. Echocardiography shows thickening of the tricuspid valve, the subvalvular apparatus, and the pulmonary valve. In severe disease, the tricuspid leaflets are retracted and fixed, with loss of normal coaptation. Similar findings can be seen on cardiac magnetic resonance imaging.

TREATMENT AND PROGNOSIS

Treatment of the underlying carcinoid with a somatostatin analogue can improve systemic symptoms (Chapter 213).[35] Valve replacement now has an operative mortality of less than 10% (Chapter 213). Without treatment, patients with carcinoid heart disease have a mean life expectancy of 1.6 years, but cardiac surgery for valve disease is associated with a better outcome.[36]

NONBACTERIAL THROMBOTIC (MARANTIC) ENDOCARDITIS

EPIDEMIOLOGY AND PATHOBIOLOGY

Platelet-fiber masses that are adherent to the mitral or aortic valves are seen in about 20% of patients with malignant tumors, especially mucin-producing adenocarcinomas, melanomas, leukemias, and lymphomas. The lesions are sterile, commonly verruciform, and without accompanying inflammation.

CLINICAL MANIFESTATIONS AND DIAGNOSIS

Nonbacterial thrombotic endocarditis is virtually always asymptomatic but occasionally is a source of systemic emboli. Because of the small size of many of the emboli, the first presentation is often with cerebral symptoms. Larger lesions are detectable by echocardiography, but even transesophageal echocardiography is not sufficiently sensitive to identify lesions that may be found at autopsy and that may have been the source of systemic emboli.

TREATMENT

No treatment has been proved efficacious. However, systemic anticoagulation similar to that used in patients with tumor-associated deep venous thrombosis is often tried (Chapters 68 and 157).

CARDIAC TUMORS

Cardiac tumors can involve any part of the heart (Fig. 47-10).

MYOCARDIAL TUMORS

Most primary cardiac tumors (Table 47-8) are benign. However, all tumors that extend from other tissues into the heart are malignant, as are metastatic lesions.[37]

EPIDEMIOLOGY AND PATHOBIOLOGY

Primary tumors of the heart are unusual, with a prevalence of 1 in 2000 to 1 in 4000 in autopsy series. Nearly all these primary tumors are benign myxomas, although fibromas, lipomas, and fibroelastomas also occur. Rhabdomyomas are seen in children, especially with tuberous sclerosis (Chapter 385). The rare primary malignant tumors include sarcomas, especially angiosarcomas (see Table 47-8). Rarely, a primary mesothelioma or lymphoma may originate in the heart.

Up to 20% of advanced cancers may involve the pericardium, epicardium, or cardiac chambers either by direct extension of the primary tumor or by metastatic disease. Direct extension occurs principally from cancers of the lung, breast, esophagus, and mediastinum. Extension through the inferior vena cava to the right atrium and even to the right ventricle occurs with cancers of the kidney, adrenal gland, and liver. Metastatic spread is most common with melanomas or lymphomas.

PERICARDIAL TUMORS

CLINICAL MANIFESTATIONS

Pericardial tumors almost always result from direct extension of tumors, principally lung and breast, which produce a pericardial effusion that can progress to cardiac tamponade (Chapter 62). Patients typically are asymptomatic or minimally symptomatic in terms of the cardiac involvement until the effusion is large, although they often may be very ill because of progressive tumor elsewhere.

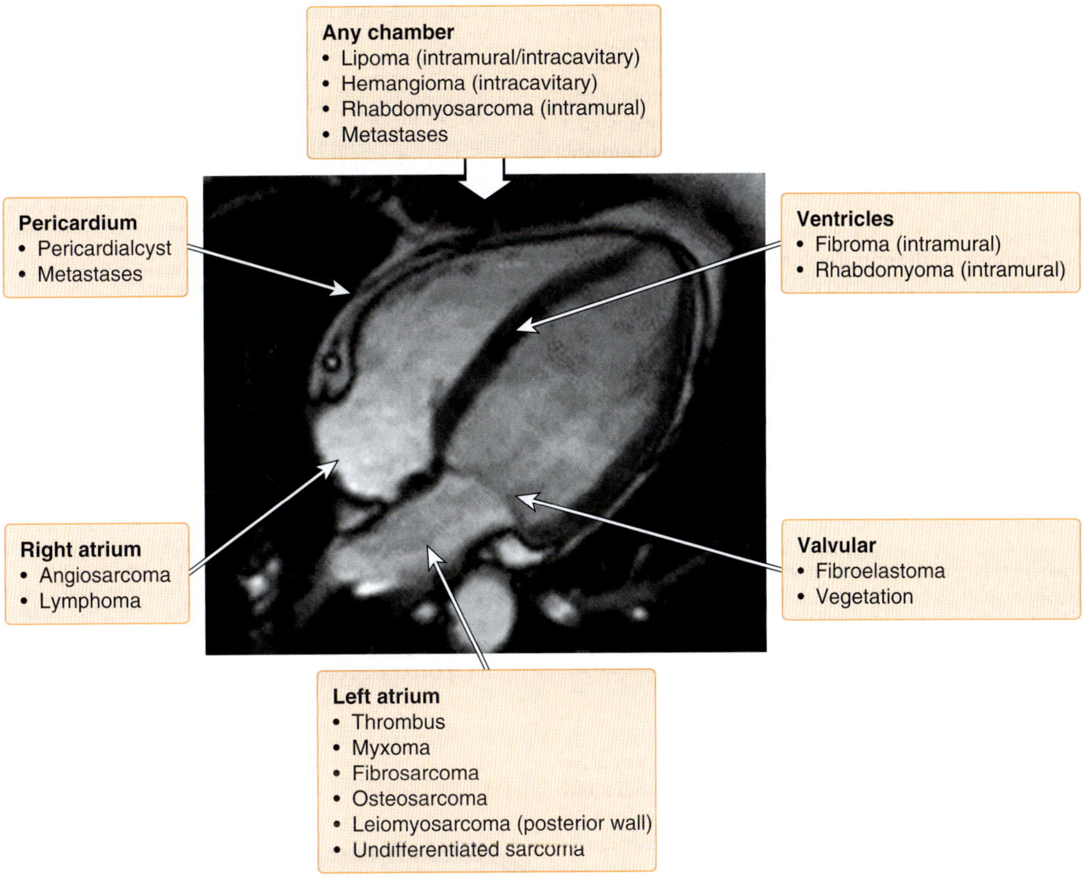

FIGURE 47-10. **The typical locations of the most common cardiac tumors.** Note, however, that the location of the various conditions can vary, and many cardiac tumors can occur in any chamber. (From Motwani M, Kidambi A, Herzog BA, et al. MR imaging of cardiac tumors and masses: a review of methods and clinical applications. *Radiology*. 2013;268:26-43.)

TABLE 47-8 CARDIAC TUMORS

PRIMARY
Benign
Myxoma
Lipoma
Fibroma
Rhabdomyoma
Fibroelastoma
Malignant
Sarcoma
Mesothelioma
Lymphoma
SECONDARY
Direct Extension
Lung cancer
Breast cancer
Mediastinal tumors
Metastatic Tumors
Malignant melanoma
Leukemia
Lymphoma
Venous Extension
Renal cell cancer
Adrenal cancer
Liver cancer

DIAGNOSIS

The diagnosis is often suspected in a patient with advanced malignant disease on the basis of evidence of heart failure, hypertension, or arrhythmia and is confirmed by echocardiography. The differentiation between pericardial involvement by tumor and postradiation pericarditis depends on pericardiocentesis, often guided by echocardiography, and cytologic examination.

TREATMENT

Cardiac tamponade must be treated with urgent pericardiocentesis, preferably under echocardiographic or radiologic guidance (Chapter 62). Although such a procedure can be life-saving and provide short-term to intermediate-term palliation, control of the effusion often requires prolonged drainage, administration of intrapericardial chemotherapeutic agents, or limited or full pericardiectomy (Chapter 62). Some patients with pericardial tumors may respond to aggressive systemic chemotherapy, but recurrent accumulation of fluid is sufficiently likely that creation of a pericardial window should be considered before hospital discharge.

PROGNOSIS

In many cases, a tumor that is causing pericarditis has extended or will eventually extend through the pericardial space and into the myocardium, so no therapy is likely to be successful. The prognosis is very poor, except in unusual cases in which the tumor responds dramatically to systemic therapy.

INTRACAVITARY TUMORS

MYXOMA

DEFINITION AND EPIDEMIOLOGY

A myxoma is a benign polypoid neoplasm that originates from endocardial cells and is attached to the interatrial septum, usually protruding into the left atrium but occasionally into the right atrium and rarely into the ventricles. Myxomas are more common in women, especially between the ages of 30 and 60 years, than in men. These tumors can be familial and are rarely associated with other systemic abnormalities.

CLINICAL MANIFESTATIONS

Myxomas are slow growing and usually do not produce symptoms or signs until they enlarge. The typical presentation is with a tumor embolus, whereby usually small portions of the myxoma break loose and cause a single embolism or a shower of emboli. However, a large embolism from a myxoma can be of sufficient size to obstruct a medium-sized artery. Some patients have systemic symptoms, including fever, malaise, and arthralgias, as part of a clinical syndrome that may be confused with bacterial endocarditis (Chapter 61) or a collagen vascular disease. Large myxomas can prolapse into the mitral valve orifice during diastole, or they may obstruct blood flow from the left atrium to the left ventricle and mimic rheumatic mitral stenosis.

DIAGNOSIS

A myxoma large enough to obstruct the mitral orifice can produce an audible "tumor plop" when the myxoma prolapses and obstructs blood flow during diastole, at the same time that the opening snap of mitral stenosis would typically be heard. If obstruction is incomplete, the tumor plop may be followed by a diastolic rumble. As obstruction becomes more severe, cardiac output may fall precipitously. Echocardiography (Chapter 43) is usually definitive; transesophageal echocardiography provides a higher sensitivity than does transthoracic echocardiography, and magnetic resonance imaging can be helpful.

TREATMENT

Surgical removal is generally curative, although myxomas can be multiple or recur in about 5% of cases. Follow-up postoperative echocardiography is generally recommended. However, the optimal frequency and duration for follow-up screening are uncertain.

OTHER PRIMARY INTRACAVITARY TUMORS

Papillary fibroelastomas are rare, typically frondlike tumors that may arise from a cardiac valve, often the mitral valve, and are generally detected incidentally by echocardiography. However, like myxomas, they can be manifested with systemic or even coronary emboli. Surgical excision is usually successful.

Angiosarcomas, which are more frequent in men than in women, typically involve the pericardium and right atrium. They cause obstruction with clinical signs and symptoms of right-sided heart failure. These sarcomas are generally not amenable to therapy.

EXTENSION OF TUMOR INTO THE CARDIAC CAVITIES

Direct extension of tumor up the inferior vena cava into the right atrium can be seen with renal cell carcinomas and less commonly with liver and adrenal cancers. In some cases, tumor extension is accompanied by adherent clot, and either the tumor or the clot may cause obstruction or pulmonary emboli (Chapter 68). No treatments are generally successful, and the prognosis is grim.

INTRAMYOCARDIAL TUMORS

Primary malignant intracardiac tumors are rare, with an incidence rate of about 35 per 100 million. The most common tumors are sarcomas (Chapter 187), lymphomas (Chapters 171 and 172), and mesotheliomas (Chapters 86 and 177). Current overall survival rates for these tumors at 5 years are about 10%, 35%, and 25%, respectively.

Benign tumors in the myocardium include lipomas, fibromas, and rhabdomyomas. Primary malignant tumors include sarcomas, lymphomas, and mesotheliomas. Metastatic tumors include melanomas, lymphomas, and leukemias. The tumors may be clinically silent, or they may produce arrhythmias or even impinge on coronary arteries, thereby causing ischemic syndromes. Large tumors may protrude into the cardiac chamber and cause obstruction. Therapies are not successful, except for occasional patients whose metastatic tumors may respond to systemic chemotherapy or whose primary tumors have been cured by heart transplantation.

GENERAL REFERENCES

For the General References and other additional features, please visit Elsevier eBooks+ at https://ebooks.health.elsevier.com.

Grade A References

A1. Saberi S, Wheeler M, Bragg-Gresham J, et al. Effect of moderate-intensity exercise training on peak oxygen consumption in patients with hypertrophic cardiomyopathy: a randomized clinical trial. *JAMA.* 2017;317:1349-1357.

A2. Dybro AM, Rasmussen TB, Nielsen RR, et al. Randomized trial of metoprolol in patients with obstructive hypertrophic cardiomyopathy. *J Am Coll Cardiol.* 2021;78:2505-2517.

A3. Olivotto I, Oreziak A, Barriales-Villa R, et al. Mavacamten for treatment of symptomatic obstructive hypertrophic cardiomyopathy (EXPLORER-HCM): a randomised, double-blind, placebo-controlled, phase 3 trial. *Lancet.* 2020;396:759-769.

A4. Ismayl M, Abbasi MA, Marar R, et al. Mavacamten treatment for hypertrophic cardiomyopathy: a systematic review and meta-analysis of randomized controlled trials. *Curr Probl Cardiol.* 2023;48:101429.

A5. Spertus JA, Fine JT, Elliott P, et al. Mavacamten for treatment of symptomatic obstructive hypertrophic cardiomyopathy (EXPLORER-HCM): health status analysis of a randomized, double-blind, placebo-controlled, phase 3 trial. *Lancet.* 2021;397:2467-2475.

A6. Ismayl M, Abbasi MA, Marar R, et al. Mavacamten treatment for hypertrophic cardiomyopathy: a systematic review and meta-analysis of randomized controlled trials. *Curr Probl Cardiol.* 2023;48:101429.

A7. Ho CY, Day SM, Axelsson A, et al. Valsartan in early-stage hypertrophic cardiomyopathy: a randomized phase 2 trial. *Nat Med.* 2021;27:1818-1824.

A8. Olivotto I, Camici PG, Merlini PA, et al. Efficacy of ranolazine in patients with symptomatic hypertrophic cardiomyopathy: the RESTYLE-HCM randomized, double-blind, placebo-controlled study. *Circ Heart Fail.* 2018;11:e004124.

A9. Lu C, Qin F, Yan Y, et al. Immunosuppressive treatment for myocarditis: a meta-analysis of randomized controlled trials. *J Cardiovasc Med (Hagerstown).* 2016;17:631-637.

A10. Alba AC, Foroutan F, Duero Posada J, et al. Implantable cardiac defibrillator and mortality in non-ischaemic cardiomyopathy: an updated meta-analysis. *Heart.* 2018;104:230-236.

A11. Avila MS, Ayub-Ferreira SM, de Barros Wanderley MR Jr, et al. Carvedilol for prevention of chemotherapy-related cardiotoxicity: the CECCY trial. *J Am Coll Cardiol.* 2018;71:2281-2290.

A12. Hilfiker-Kleiner D, Haghikia A, Berliner D, et al. Bromocriptine for the treatment of peripartum cardiomyopathy: a multicentre randomized study. *Eur Heart J.* 2017;38:2671-2679.

A13. Maurer MS, Schwartz JH, Gundapaneni B, et al. Tafamidis treatment for patients with transthyretin amyloid cardiomyopathy. *N Engl J Med.* 2018;379:1007-1016.

A14. Elliot P, Drachman BM, Gottlieb SS, et al. Long-term survival with tafamidis in patients with transthyretin amyloid cardiomyopathy. *Circ Heart Fail.* 2022;15:e008193.

A15. Solomon SD, Adams D, Kristen A, et al. Effects of patisiran, an RNA interference therapeutic, on cardiac parameters in patients with hereditary transthyretin-mediated amyloidosis: an analysis of the APOLLO study. *Circulation.* 2019;139:431-443.

48 PRINCIPLES OF ELECTROPHYSIOLOGY

GLENN I. FISHMAN

The rhythmic beating of the heart reflects the tightly regulated and exquisitely integrated activity of numerous protein complexes that control the flow of ions across cell membranes, including channels, transporters, exchangers, and gap junction channels.[1] The human heart beats almost 3 billion times during a normal lifespan, and even brief periods of dysfunction may lead to life-threatening consequences. Thus, the failure rate of cardiac rhythmicity is exceptionally low. Nonetheless, inherited syndromes, as well as acquired heart disease, may affect cardiac rhythmicity, and these disorders lead to substantial morbidity and mortality, including sudden cardiac death (Chapter 50). This chapter reviews the molecular, cellular, and organ-level determinants of cardiac rhythmicity and relates these principles to fundamental mechanisms responsible for clinically important arrhythmias.

BASIC CONCEPTS

The function of the heart as a highly dynamic pump is intricately entwined with the tightly regulated electrical activation of its constituent cardiomyocytes. During each cardiac cycle, an electrical impulse known as an *action potential* is spontaneously generated by a relatively small number of pacemaker cells in the sinoatrial node, which is located at the junction of the right atrium and the superior vena cava. The impulse then propagates through the right and left atrium, which is represented by the P wave on the electrocardiogram (ECG; Chapter 42). After depolarizing the atria, the impulse enters the atrioventricular (AV) node, which is located in the inferior septal region of the right atrium, where a delay occurs. This delay allows time for the atria to contract and fill the ventricles. The delay in the AV node represents most of the isoelectric portion of the PR interval on the ECG (Fig. 42-2). The usual duration of atrial activation, including delay in the AV node, is up to 140 msec and can be measured directly as the atrial-His interval. The impulse then travels into the specialized infranodal conducting system, which is composed of the His bundle, right and left bundle branches, and Purkinje network. The Purkinje network, which extends throughout the ventricular endocardium, rapidly conducts impulses, thereby allowing nearly simultaneous activation of the ventricles. Once out of the Purkinje network, the impulse proceeds relatively slowly from the endocardial to epicardial surface of the ventricles.

The QRS complex on ECG represents depolarization of the bundle branches and ventricular myocardium.

Subpopulations of myocytes within the heart have unique electrical properties that reflect regional specialization. Myocytes within the sinoatrial and AV nodes produce spontaneous action potentials that reflect their pacemaking function. Cells within the His-Purkinje network are optimized to rapidly deliver excitatory current to the large mass of ventricular myocardium, whereas ventricular myocytes display action potentials optimized to facilitate excitation-contraction coupling, that is, to trigger the release of calcium ions from the sarcoplasmic reticulum and to promote the actomyosin cross-bridge formation that underlies cardiac contraction (Chapter 41). Abnormalities in cardiac electrophysiology, whether the result of mendelian disorders, oligogenic syndromes, or environmental stressors that evoke acquired heart disease, can lead to disturbances in the initiation, propagation, or conduction of electrical impulses and, as a result, to a wide variety of arrhythmic syndromes.

IONIC BASIS OF CARDIAC ELECTROPHYSIOLOGY

THE CARDIAC ACTION POTENTIAL

The cardiac action potential (Fig. 48-1) is a recording of a cell's membrane potential, V_m, versus time. During each cardiac cycle, ions move back and forth across the cardiomyocyte cell membrane, thereby changing V_m. The cardiac action potential, which reflects the integrated behavior of numerous individual ionic currents, is largely dominated by the movement of Na^+, Ca^{2+}, and K^+ ions. These ions traverse the cell membrane through ion-selective pores formed by assemblies of integral membrane-spanning proteins and accessory proteins. The behavior of these ionic pathways is highly regulated, and permeation of specific ions is influenced by multiple factors, the most prominent of which are changes in membrane potential (i.e., voltage gating), ligand binding, second messengers such as cyclic adenosine monophosphate, and post-translational modification. Channel function and, by extension, action potential behavior are dynamically tuned in response to normal physiologic factors, especially heart rate. However, a number of pathologic stressors influence channel activity, including acquired syndromes that are associated with cardiac hypertrophy and failure, as well as an ever-growing number of congenital diseases. Regardless of the underlying pathology, the effects on action potential behavior may trigger arrhythmic activity.

The cardiac action potential is divided into phases, each reflecting the major ionic movements that take place. In working cardiomyocytes, such as ventricular or atrial myocytes, the *resting membrane potential* during diastole, or phase 4 of the cardiac action potential, is determined by the baseline ionic and charge gradients that exist across the sarcolemmal membrane. These gradients are generated by pumps and transporters, the most important of which is the Na^+, K^+-ATPase. This energy-requiring electrogenic pump, which is the major target of ouabain-like compounds such as digoxin, extrudes three Na^+ ions from the intracellular compartment in exchange for two K^+ ions, thereby resulting in directionally opposite gradients of Na^+ ions (outside > inside) and K^+ ions (inside > outside). Under resting conditions, a subset of membrane channels highly permeable to K^+ is open, but those that allow for the passage of other ions such as Na^+ or Ca^{2+} are only minimally permeable. As a consequence, the concentration gradient promotes the movement of potassium ions from inside to outside of the cell, until the resulting excess of negative charge within the cell balances the diffusional forces and an electrochemical equilibrium is established. The equilibrium potential for a given ion is calculated by the *Nernst equation*, where E_{eq} is the equilibrium potential, R is the universal gas constant, T is the absolute temperature, z is the valence of the ionic species, and F is Faraday constant:

$$E_{eq} = \frac{RT}{zF} ln\left(\frac{[X]_{out}}{[X]_{in}}\right)$$

If the cell membrane were *only* permeable to K^+ ions, at the measured concentrations of intracellular and extracellular K^+, the resting membrane potential would be approximately −100 mV. However, because of the slight but measurable permeability to other ionic species, which have Nernst potentials that are less negative than that for K^+, the actual resting membrane potential in a typical ventricular cardiac myocyte is closer to −85 mV.

When the cardiac cell is depolarized to its excitatory threshold, an action potential is triggered through a series of highly regulated time-dependent changes in ionic conductances (see Fig. 48-1B). The fast sodium current is activated and very rapidly depolarizes the membrane during phase 0 of the

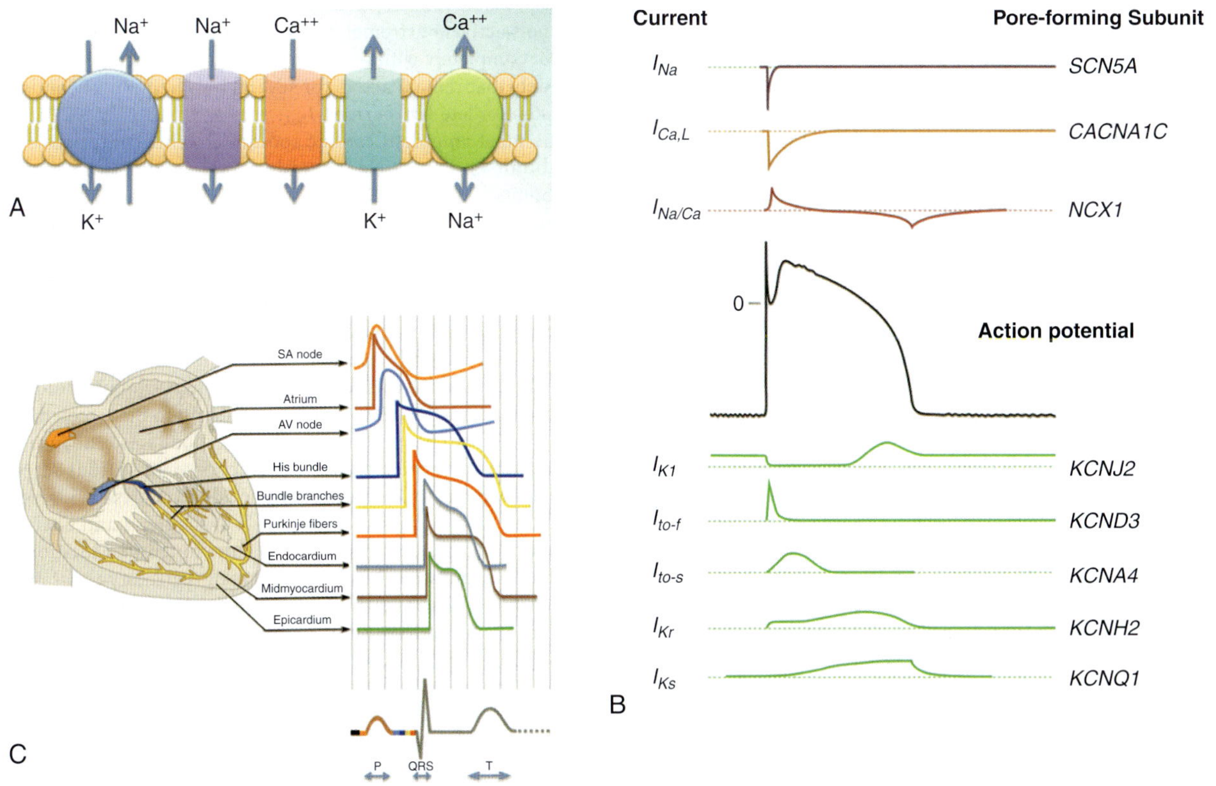

FIGURE 48-1. Ion channels and the cardiac action potential. A, Key channels involved in cardiac excitability and generation of the cardiac action potential. Inward currents are carried by Na^+ channels *(purple)* and Ca^{2+} channels *(red)*. Repolarizing currents are primarily carried by K^+ channels *(blue)*. The Na^+/K^+ ATPase is an energy-requiring exchanger that pumps Na^+ out of the cell in exchange for K^+ and is essential for establishing resting ionic gradients and the resting membrane potential. **B,** Time course and relative magnitude of ionic currents active during the cardiac action potential. Inward currents are represented by downward deflections and outward currents by upward deflections. **C,** Action potentials from different regions of the heart and their relationship to the surface electrocardiogram are indicated. (Adapted from Marbán E. Cardiac channelopathies. *Nature*. 2002;415:213-218.)

action potential. The sodium current is inactivated at the peak of depolarization, which is approximately +40 mV. The increase in V_m during phase 0 activates several additional voltage-gated currents. A transient outward potassium current, or I_{to}, partially *re*polarizes the cell, thereby producing a small notch in the action potential, denoted as phase 1. The increase in V_m during phase 0 also activates, albeit more slowly, the inward L-type calcium current, $I_{Ca\text{-}L}$. It is this trigger for Ca^{2+} that is responsible for Ca^{2+}-induced release from the sarcoplasmic reticulum and is integral to the process of excitation-contraction coupling (Chapter 41). The inward Ca^{2+} current is balanced by several outward repolarizing currents, including the rapid component of the delayed rectifier potassium current I_{Kr}, the slow component of the delayed rectifier potassium current I_{Ks}, and the electrogenic Na^+-Ca^{2+} exchanger, thereby resulting in a plateau in the action potential known as phase 2. When the outward potassium currents increase and the calcium current decreases at the end of phase 2, the action potential progresses to phase 3, which is the phase of rapid repolarization. The inward rectifier potassium current I_{K1} contributes significantly to this final phase of repolarization and brings the action potential back to its resting membrane potential, or phase 4, at which point the cell is primed for another action potential.

Action potential recordings from atrial cardiomyocytes and from cells of the His-Purkinje system are qualitatively similar to those described previously, but with some notable differences that primarily reflect the differential expression of repolarizing potassium currents that tend to abbreviate (in the case of atrial cells) or lengthen (for Purkinje cells) the action potential duration (see Fig. 48-1C).

The relatively small populations of cells in the sinoatrial node (SAN) and atrioventricular node (AVN) express unique complements of ionic currents that are responsible for spontaneous depolarization during phase 4 and the triggering of action potentials. Pacemaker cells express substantially less I_{K1} compared with ventricular myocytes, and as a consequence, their minimum V_m is −65 mV, and they do not repolarize to the same extent as working ventricular cardiomyocytes. In addition, pacemaker cells display what is known as the funny current, I_f, which is activated by *hyper*polarization and carried by sodium. Activation of I_f during phase 4 slowly depolarizes the cell membrane. In addition, a subsarcolemmal calcium clock contributes to diastolic depolarization through the spontaneous, rhythmic release of Ca^{2+} from the sarcoplasmic reticulum, a process that is linked to the voltage clock through the activity of the sodium-calcium exchange current, I_{NCX}. Inasmuch as there is minimal fast inward I_{Na} expressed in nodal cells, the action potential triggered by this spontaneous phase 4 depolarization is due to activation of calcium currents carried by $I_{Ca,L}$ and $I_{Ca,T}$. The magnitude of I_f and I_{Ca}, and hence the slope of phase 4 depolarization as well as the upstroke velocity of the action potential in pacemaker cells, is augmented by adrenergic stimulation, which produces a chronotropic response.

Owing to considerable regional heterogeneity in the density of individual ionic currents, even within distinct compartments of the heart such as the ventricular myocardium, not all ventricular action potentials are identical (see Fig. 48-1C). Much of this heterogeneity is due to differences in the magnitude of various repolarizing K^+ currents. For example, although electrotonic coupling through gap junction channels mitigates this intrinsic heterogeneity, action potentials recorded from epicardial, mid-myocardial, and endocardial cells show substantial differences in morphology, both at rest and especially in response to provocative stimuli such as changes in rate or pharmacologic agents. Moreover, action potential morphology is not static; it varies in response to changes in physiologic state. *Action potential duration adaptation*, which reflects the normal shortening of the action potential observed during increased heart rate, provides a mechanism to preserve adequate time for ventricular filling during diastole. Action potential duration shortening in this setting is due to a net increase in repolarizing currents, primarily from increased I_{Ks} and reverse-mode I_{NaCa}. This adaptation is regulated, at least in part, by the kinetics of activation and inactivation of the channels that are responsible for these currents, as well as their modulation by various signaling cascades, such as those regulated by the autonomic nervous system. However, maladaptive regulation of ionic currents is a frequent manifestation of acquired forms of heart disease, and this pathologic electrical remodeling may amplify intrinsic heterogeneities in cardiac electrophysiology and form a substrate that promotes arrhythmic behavior.

IMPULSE PROPAGATION

In the intact heart, action potentials not only must be generated but also must propagate from cell to cell as a wave of excitation throughout the atrial and ventricular myocardium. For successful propagation, the upstream excited cell must provide sufficient charge to bring the membrane potential, V_m, of downstream cells up to their excitation threshold potential. Gap junctions, which comprise arrays of intercellular channels, provide the structural basis for this electrotonic flow of current from cell to cell. For propagation to be successful, the ratio of the charge generated to charge consumed during the excitation cycle, known as the safety factor, must be greater than 1.

Unlike nerves, the action potential duration of human cardiomyocytes is quite long, on the order of 200 msec. This longer action potential duration is required so that each myocyte has sufficient time for contraction and relaxation before the next heartbeat. Impulses that arrive too early in the cardiac cycle will not produce normal action potentials. If the impulse occurs during the upstroke or plateau phase (phases 0 to 2), the sodium channels will not have had sufficient time to recover from fast inactivation, and the cell displays *absolute refractoriness*. If the impulse occurs somewhat later, during phase 3 of the action potential, a supranormal stimulus is required to overcome the potassium currents that remain active during the terminal portion of the action potential, a phenomenon known as *relative refractoriness*. Moreover, because not all of the sodium channels will have recovered from inactivation, the rate of rise of voltage during phase 0 of the premature beat may be diminished.

MOLECULAR BASIS OF CARDIAC ELECTROPHYSIOLOGY

The individual currents that are responsible for cardiac excitability reflect the integrated behavior of various protein complexes that are assembled into ion-specific channels, transporters, and exchangers.[2,3] At the molecular level, ion channels comprise multi-subunit glycoproteins, including a pore-forming major, or α-subunit, and one or several accessory proteins (E-Fig. 48-1). The latter influence a range of channel properties, including trafficking of the major subunit to the sarcolemmal membrane, as well as regulation of channel biophysical properties, that is, the opening and closing of the channel in response to various factors such as membrane voltage, ligands, mechanical stimuli, second messengers, or post-translational modification.

SODIUM CHANNELS

Voltage-gated sodium channels are responsible for the activation and propagation of the cardiac action potential. Not surprisingly, acquired and inherited syndromes that affect the function of voltage-gated sodium channels in the heart are responsible for a broad range of arrhythmic phenotypes. Cardiac sodium channels activate extremely rapidly, within 1 msec, and begin to inactivate almost completely within several milliseconds. The very small proportion of channels that remain active for several hundred milliseconds results in the persistent or late Na^+ current, I_{NaL}.

The most abundant cardiac sodium channel comprises a pore-forming α-subunit known as $Na_v1.5$ and several smaller accessory subunits, or β-subunits, designated $Na_v\beta1$ to 4. The α-subunit is an approximately 260-kD protein that consists of four homologous domains, each comprising six transmembrane segments.[4] Substantial experimental work has identified the key regions of the protein that regulate channel properties, including voltage dependence, activation, and inactivation, as well as the binding sites for pharmacologic agents such as local anesthetics, antiarrhythmic drugs, and neurotoxins. The β-subunits are single-membrane-spanning proteins that associate with $Na_v1.5$ through their extracellular immunoglobulin-fold domains. They serve to increase the delivery of the α-subunit to the sarcolemmal membrane and to influence channel function. The β-subunits also enhance the subcellular localization of the channel and its interactions with various adaptors, signaling molecules, and cytoskeletal proteins. In addition to $Na_v1.5$, several "neuronal" α-subunits are expressed at low levels in the heart and likely contribute to regional heterogeneity in sodium channel function. Mutations in $Na_v1.5$, in specific β-subunits, and in several interacting regulatory and scaffolding proteins all may influence the behavior of the sodium current in the heart and thereby produce a range of arrhythmic syndromes, including long QT syndrome type 3 (LQT3) and Brugada syndrome (Chapter 53).[5]

The I_f current contributes to phase 4 depolarization in pacemaker cells and is a reflection of the activity of hyperpolarization-activated cyclic nucleotide gated, or *HCN* channels. The full channels are composed of dimers of *HCN* proteins, each of which has six transmembrane domains. *HCN4* and *HCN1* are the predominant isoforms found in the nodes, whereas *HCN2* is found throughout the conduction system. Binding of cyclic adenosine monophosphate, a key second messenger in the adrenergic signaling cascade, to the carboxy terminus of the channel shifts activation positively, thereby increasing the slope of phase 4 depolarization and linking autonomic tone to heart rate.

CALCIUM CHANNELS

Voltage-gated calcium channels are important for generating the action potential in the sinoatrial and atrioventricular nodes and for excitation-contraction coupling in virtually all contractile cardiomyocytes.[6] The dominant forms expressed in the heart are the L-type (large and long-lasting) and the T-type (tiny and transient) calcium channels, both of which include pore-forming α-subunits, similar in overall structure to that of voltage-gated sodium channels.

L-type Ca^{2+} channels comprise an α_1 subunit, a noncovalently bound β accessory subunit ($Ca_v\beta1$-4), and an alternatively spliced α_2-δ-subunit that is post-translationally processed through cleavage and disulfide bond formation. The dominant α_1-subunit in the heart is $Ca_v1.2$, whereas $Ca_v1.3$ is restricted primarily to nodal and atrial cells. Both α_1-subunits are alternatively spliced to produce variants that are uniquely regulated.

The related T-type calcium channels are also found in the heart but display distinct biophysical properties compared with L-type Ca^{2+} channels; they activate at more negative voltages (−70 mV) and inactivate more rapidly. The major isoform expressed in the heart is $Ca_v3.1$ and, to a lesser extent, $Ca_v3.2$. These channels are normally restricted to the nodes, Purkinje cells, and atrial myocytes. In pacemaking cells, the T-type currents contribute to phase 4 depolarization. Mutations in Ca^{2+} channel subunits are also responsible for a number of arrhythmic syndromes, including Timothy syndrome (LQT8) and a subset of individuals with Brugada syndrome.

POTASSIUM CHANNELS

Numerous classes of potassium channels are expressed in the heart, where they contribute to repolarization and maintenance of the resting membrane potential.[7] The heterogeneous expression of potassium channels in different regions and cell types is largely responsible for the variable action potential morphologies that are observed. As with sodium and calcium channels, potassium channels are formed from the assembly of pore-forming subunits along with various accessory β-subunits. However, α-subunits of potassium channels include between two and six transmembrane domains, and the full channel is formed as a dimer or tetramer, depending on the specific subfamily. Dysregulation of expression and function of potassium channels is quite common in many acquired forms of heart disease. The resulting loss of repolarizing currents leads to action potential duration prolongation and acquired long QT syndrome. In addition, heritable mutations that diminish potassium currents are responsible for several forms of inherited long QT syndrome, whereas gain of function mutations may produce the short QT syndrome.

Voltage-gated potassium channels, or *Kv* channels, are activated by membrane depolarization. Numerous classes of *Kv* channels have been identified in the heart. The α-subunits are six transmembrane domain proteins. Unlike sodium and calcium channels, functional potassium channels are formed by the assembly of four such subunits and various β-subunits. The transient outward current is composed of two components, $I_{to,fast}$ and $I_{to,slow}$; both are rapidly activated and contribute to phase 1 of the cardiac action potential, but their recovery kinetics differ. $I_{to,fast}$ is particularly prominent in the epicardial layer of the ventricles, especially in the right ventricle. This differential expression is thought to contribute to the pathology of J wave syndromes, including Brugada syndrome.

The other major class of voltage-gated potassium channels in the heart is responsible for the delayed rectifier currents, broadly classified as I_K currents.[8] These channels include the ultra-rapidly activating I_{Kur}, which is restricted to atrial myocytes, and the delayed rectifier currents, I_{Kr} and I_{Ks}, both of which contribute to phase 3 repolarization of the cardiac action potential. I_{Kr} activates and inactivates rapidly and shows strong inward rectification; that is, current moves more easily (but not exclusively) in the inward direction than in the outward direction, although it is the outward current that is physiologically relevant. I_{Ks} activates slowly and does not display inward rectification. Both currents also show marked regional heterogeneity. Numerous cardiac and noncardiac medications, as well as heritable syndromes that reduce the magnitude of these currents (particularly I_{Kr}), result in action potential duration prolongation and acquired or heritable long QT syndrome.

The second major class of potassium currents in the heart are the *Kir* currents carried by inwardly rectifying potassium channels. I_{K1} is observed in both atrial and ventricular cardiomyocytes. Conductance through these channels is high at negative membrane potentials, so this current is critical for terminal repolarization (phase 3) and for setting the resting membrane potential (phase 4). Another inwardly rectifying potassium current is carried by I_{KATP} channels. The full channels include not only the pore-forming subunit but also auxiliary *SUR* subunits, which are targets for channel inhibition by the sulfonylurea class of drugs. Because I_{KATP} currents are inhibited by intracellular adenosine triphosphate, they are activated in the setting of ischemia. The augmented outward current shortens action potential duration and abbreviates systole, thereby diminishing energetic requirements. Thus I_{KATP} channels provide a link between metabolic state and membrane excitability. Importantly, the resulting action potential duration shortening diminishes refractoriness, which may enhance the risk for re-entrant arrhythmias. The last major class of inward rectifiers includes the acetylcholine- and adenosine-activated potassium channels, which are encoded by $K_{ir}3.1$ and $K_{ir}3.4$. These channels, which are enriched in nodal and atrial cardiac myocytes, are activated when ligands bind to muscarinic or purinergic G protein–coupled receptors, which facilitate the uncoupling of $G_{\beta\gamma}$ from G_α and the activation of the K_{ir} channels by the released $G_{\beta\gamma}$.

GAP JUNCTION CHANNELS

Gap junction channels, which are responsible for the electrotonic coupling of cardiac myocytes, are essential for normal impulse propagation throughout the myocardium. The channels are formed by the hexameric assembly of connexin monomers, each of which is a tetramembrane spanning protein. Connexin 43[9] is the dominant isoform expressed in ventricular and atrial myocardium, whereas connexin 40 is also abundantly expressed in the atrium. The nodes express variable amounts of connexin 45 and connexin 30.2, and the bundle branches and Purkinje fibers express significant levels of connexin 40. Gap junctions in the node integrate the intrinsic beating rate of each nodal cell into a single functional unit. Abnormalities in connexin expression and function, a process known as pathologic gap junction remodeling, are observed in atrial and ventricular myocardium in many acquired forms of heart disease. The remodeling contributes to aberrant impulse propagation and predisposes to arrhythmic behavior. In addition, germline or somatic mutations in cardiac connexin genes are associated with arrhythmic syndromes, especially atrial fibrillation.

MECHANISMS OF ARRHYTHMOGENESIS

Cardiac arrhythmias, which are disturbances in the rate or rhythm of the heartbeat, are a reflection of abnormal impulse formation or conduction. Inasmuch as cardiac myocytes reside within a complex multicellular environment and are electrotonically coupled by gap junction channels, arrhythmic syndromes almost always reflect a complex interplay of individual, or *cell autonomous*, properties within a multicellular network. Most clinically important arrhythmias arise in the setting of acquired heart disease, in which pathologic *electrical remodeling*, resulting from dysregulation of ion channel expression or function, accompanies *structural remodeling*. However, many arrhythmic syndromes, including those that are drug-induced, result from, or are exacerbated by, genetic variations, including disease-causing alterations in coding regions that directly affect the function of proteins, which regulate cardiac electrophysiology, as well as sequence variants in regulatory or other noncoding genome regions, which appear to regulate transcriptional and post-transcriptional behavior.

DISORDERS OF IMPULSE FORMATION

In the healthy heart, the sinus node, which is located at the junction of the right atrium and the superior vena cava, is the predominant pacemaker. Secondary pacemakers with intrinsically slower pacing rates are found further downstream in the specialized conduction system within the atrioventricular node and the His-Purkinje system. The firing rate of pacemaker cells is regulated primarily by autonomic tone: sympathetic stimulation increases the slope of phase 4 depolarization, whereas parasympathetic stimulation decreases the slope by augmenting repolarizing currents. Nodal suppression may result from pharmacologic agents, such as β-adrenergic blockers, calcium channel blockers, or digitalis, as well as from fibrotic diseases. Moreover, mutations in several genes that affect the voltage clock (*SCN5A* and *HCN4*), the calcium clock (*RYR2* and *CASQ2*), or both (*ANKB*) may cause familial sinus node dysfunction.

Conversely, under pathologic conditions, myocardial cells outside the specialized conduction system may exhibit spontaneous activity, a phenomenon termed *abnormal automaticity*. Abnormal automaticity is

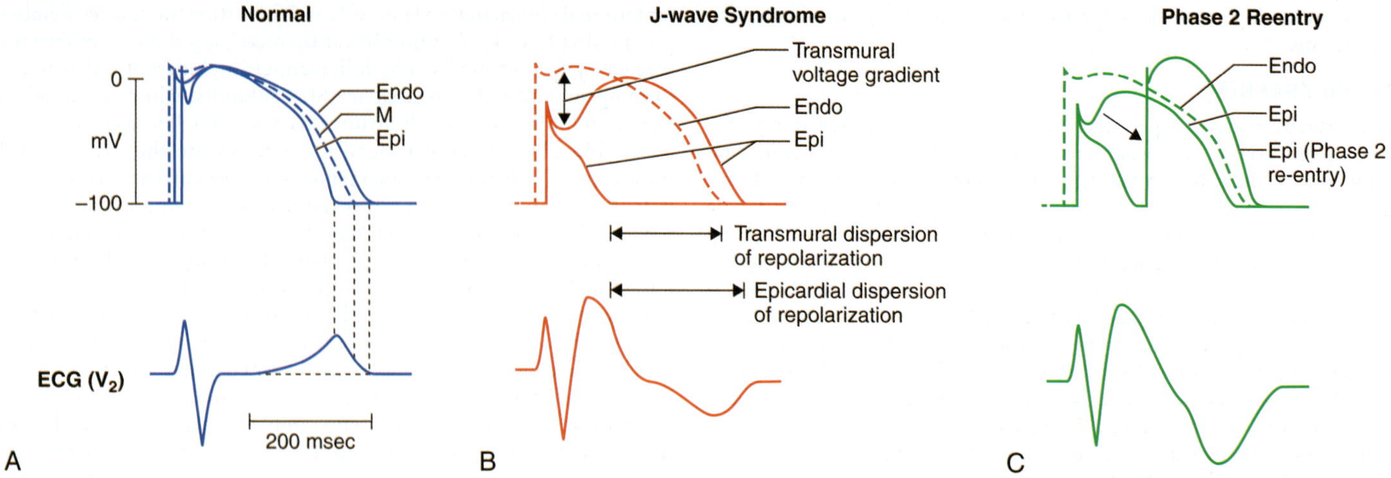

FIGURE 48-2. **Cellular basis for J-wave syndromes and phase 2 re-entry. Under normal conditions, the ST segment is isoelectric because of the absence of transmural voltage gradients at the level of the action potential plateau. Accentuation of the phase I notch under pathophysiologic conditions, such as loss-of-function of I_{Na} or gain-of-function of I_{to} leads to loss of the action potential dome at some epicardial sites but not others, producing ST and T wave changes typically observed in Brugada syndrome. Loss of the action potential dome in epicardium but not endocardium results in the development of a marked transmural dispersion of repolarization and conduction of the action potential dome, from sites at which it is maintained to sites at which it is lost, thereby causing local reexcitation via a phase 2 re-entry mechanism. (Modified from Antzelevitch C, Brugada P, Brugada J, et al. Brugada syndrome: from cell to bedside. *Curr Probl Cardiol.* 2005;30:9-54.)**

most often seen with ischemia or reperfusion, in which maximum diastolic potentials are reduced to approximately −60 mV to −50 mV, a level at which Na^+ or Ca^{2+} channels may reach their activation threshold and trigger action potentials.

AFTERDEPOLARIZATIONS AND TRIGGERED ACTIVITY

During cardiac repolarization, a number of inward and outward currents are active, and small changes in conductance of individual channels can markedly affect the trajectory of repolarization. *Afterdepolarizations,* which are abnormal oscillations in membrane potential, occur either during (early afterdepolarizations) or after (delayed afterdepolarizations) an action potential.[10] Afterdepolarizations of sufficient magnitude to evoke an action potential produce triggered activity. Early afterdepolarizations are almost always observed in the setting of abnormal action potential duration prolongation, which provides sufficient time for *re*-activation of L-type Ca^{2+} channels during the plateau phase of the action potential. Thus, congenital syndromes, as well as bradycardia, hypokalemia, hypomagnesemia, antiarrhythmic medications, and many noncardiac drugs, are associated with QT prolongation and promote early afterdepolarizations. Conversely, rapid pacing and drugs that shorten the action potential duration tend to suppress early afterdepolarizations. Early afterdepolarizations in the setting of action potential duration prolongation often trigger *torsades de pointes* (Chapter 53), a polymorphic ventricular tachycardia, especially when there is increased dispersion of repolarization. Delayed afterdepolarizations, in contrast, are usually the result of intracellular Ca^{2+} overload and are typically seen in the setting of catecholamine excess, ischemia, toxic concentrations of digitalis-like agents, and some congenital syndromes, including catecholaminergic polymorphic ventricular tachycardia. The excessive Ca^{2+} load activates the electrogenic Na^+-Ca^{2+} exchanger, producing a depolarizing transient inward current, I_{TI}.

DISORDERS OF IMPULSE CONDUCTION

During each cardiac cycle, impulses must be generated in pacemaker cells within the sinus node, and a wave of excitation must propagate throughout the atria, travel down the specialized conduction system (including the atrioventricular node and His-Purkinje network), and then activate the ventricular myocardium. Processes that diminish intercellular coupling, such as fibrosis or calcification of the specialized conduction system, can diminish the safety factor for conduction and produce varying degrees of heart block. Inherited defects in conduction have been observed with mutations in sodium channel subunits *SCN5A* and *SCN1B*, which affect phase 0 of the cardiac action potential; in *KCNJ2*, which affects terminal repolarization and the resting membrane potential; and in a number of developmental disorders that affect the cardiac conduction system, such as Holt-Oram syndrome, Emery-Dreifuss muscular dystrophy, and myotonic dystrophy type 1. Conduction block may also be seen with the secondary electrical remodeling that is associated with structural heart disease and with many cardioactive drugs.

RE-ENTRY

Re-entry is considered the most common mechanism responsible for clinically significant cardiac arrhythmias, including both supraventricular and ventricular disorders. Fundamentally, re-entry involves self-perpetuating waves of excitation that circulate around an inexcitable obstacle. Depending on the number of re-entrant waves within a tissue (one or multiple), their size, and their spatial stability, the surface ECG may reveal a relatively organized rhythm, such as atrial flutter or monomorphic ventricular tachycardia, or a seemingly disorganized rhythm, such as atrial fibrillation or polymorphic ventricular tachycardia. Re-entry normally requires the presence of unidirectional block within a "fast" conducting pathway around an obstacle, combined with recirculation of the impulse from a second "slow" pathway in the retrograde direction, as might be the case at a bifurcating Purkinje-ventricular junction or around scar tissue of a healed myocardial infarction (E-Fig. 48-2). However, the "obstacle" may also be viable myocardium that is inexcitable owing to its intrinsic electrophysiologic properties, such as cellular uncoupling or refractoriness, a phenomenon referred to as *functional block.* Because refractoriness is critically dependent on the action potential duration, areas of myocardium with prolongation of the action potential duration may form a suitable substrate for functional re-entry.

Heterogeneity in action potential duration and the concomitant *dispersion of refractoriness* also play critical roles in the maintenance of arrhythmic behavior, especially through a phenomenon known as *phase 2 re-entry.* This term refers to the flow of current during phase 2 of the cardiac action potential from a depolarized cell to neighboring cells that are more fully repolarized and not refractory to reexcitation. This principle is best characterized in the J wave syndromes,[11] especially Brugada syndrome, in which loss of function of inward currents (I_{Na} or I_{Ca}) or gain of function of outward currents (I_{to}, $I_{K\text{-}ATP}$) causes loss of the action potential dome during phase 2 and an abbreviated action potential duration in a subset of cardiac myocytes. Current can then flow into these cells from neighboring cells in which the action potential dome is maintained, thereby causing local reexcitation, a closely coupled extrasystole, and the initiation of re-entry. In Brugada syndrome, this process is thought to arise in the right ventricular outflow tract, where the transient outward current density is significantly greater in the epicardium compared with the endocardium (Fig. 48-2).

GENERAL REFERENCES

For the General References and other additional features, please visit Elsevier eBooks+ at https://ebooks.health.elsevier.com.

49

APPROACH TO THE PATIENT WITH SUSPECTED ARRHYTHMIA

JEFFREY E. OLGIN

CLINICAL MANIFESTATIONS

Patients with suspected arrhythmias can present in a variety of ways. Typical symptoms include palpitations, syncope, and presyncope (dizziness). On occasion, arrhythmias can manifest more subtly as exercise intolerance, lethargy, and vague complaints of malaise or without any symptoms at all. Conversely, arrhythmias occasionally manifest as aborted sudden cardiac death (cardiac arrest; Chapter 50). The specific differential diagnosis, prognosis, and treatment of these symptoms are determined by the severity of the symptom (i.e., whether it results in syncope) and whether the patient has underlying structural heart disease. In general, the likelihood of a life-threatening arrhythmia, such as ventricular tachycardia or ventricular fibrillation, in a patient with symptoms of palpitations or syncope is significantly greater in a patient who has structural heart disease. Therefore, the determination of whether structural heart disease is present is a key step in the diagnosis and prognosis of patients with suspected arrhythmias. The exception to this general rule is in patients with a significant family history suggestive of an inherited arrhythmia syndrome (e.g., long QT syndrome, Brugada syndrome), for whom a family history of syncope and/or sudden death should prompt referral to a cardiac electrophysiologist.

Palpitations

Palpitations, defined as an awareness of an irregular or rapid heartbeat, are most commonly due to ectopic beats—namely, premature atrial contractions (PACs; Chapter 52) and premature ventricular contractions (PVCs; Chapter 53)—or to tachyarrhythmias. A careful history can often distinguish benign palpitations from those that need further evaluation. It can be useful to have the patient tap out with a finger what the palpitations feel like. An irregularly irregular pattern suggests atrial fibrillation, whereas a more regular, rapid pattern suggests a sustained tachycardia. A reliable symptom suggesting that palpitations are caused by a tachyarrhythmia, particularly a supraventricular tachycardia, is the sensation of a regular, rapid-pounding sensation in the neck. Conversely, most patients who complain of symptoms from PACs or PVCs are often more aware of the post-extrasystolic pause or the accentuated output of the post-extrasystolic beat than of the actual premature beat itself. Most patients who have symptoms suggestive of premature beats but not of sustained tachycardia do not require further evaluation if they have no other symptoms and no evidence of structural heart disease—that is, an otherwise normal cardiac history, physical examination, and electrocardiogram (ECG; see Table 39-4). If, however, the symptoms are not due to a single occasional extrasystole or are accompanied by presyncope or syncope, further evaluation is required (Fig. 49-1). Antiarrhythmic therapy is usually not necessary to treat PACs or PVCs unless the symptoms are frequent or severe. β-Blockers (e.g., metoprolol 25 mg/day or atenolol 25 mg/day) are first-line therapy in highly symptomatic patients with documented PACs or PVCs. Recent data suggest that patients in whom PVCs exceed 24% of beats during 24-hour monitoring may have a higher risk of developing PVC-induced cardiomyopathy.[1]

Palpitations are the most common presentation of tachyarrhythmias, whereas bradyarrhythmias rarely manifest as palpitations. Most tachyarrhythmias in patients without structural heart disease are due to supraventricular tachycardias (Chapter 52) that resolve spontaneously within several seconds. When the tachyarrhythmia is more prolonged, it often resolves with simple interventions that increase vagal (parasympathetic nervous system) influence on the heart (generally the atrioventricular [AV] node). Patients themselves can cough several times, perform the Valsalva maneuver, exhale forcefully against a closed glottis for several seconds, immerse their face in ice water, or even rub gently on their eyeballs. A physician can use carotid sinus massage (Chapter 52), performed by pressing and rubbing the carotid pulse just below the angle of the mandible for 5 to 15 seconds. This maneuver should be avoided in elderly patients and in patients with a history of cerebrovascular accident, known carotid artery stenosis, or carotid bruit on auscultation. In patients with structural heart disease, palpitations may signify ventricular tachycardia (Chapter 53), particularly if they occur with syncope or presyncope. An occasional patient without structural heart disease may have idiopathic ventricular

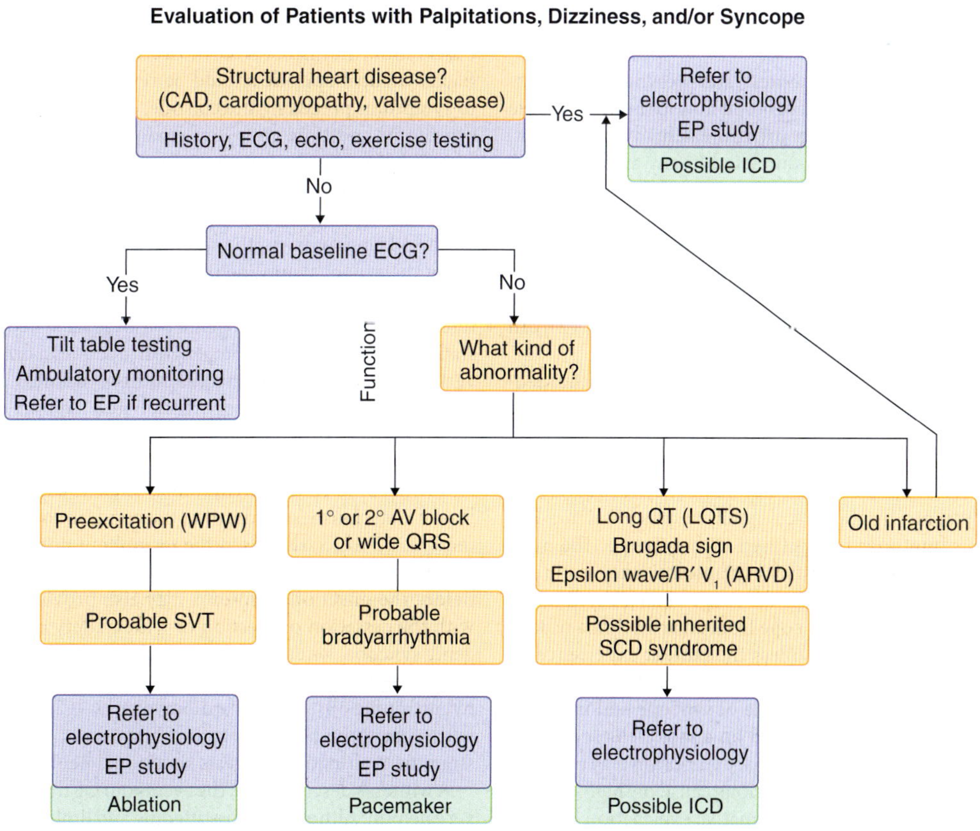

FIGURE 49-1. Algorithm for evaluating patients with symptoms of palpitation, dizziness, or syncope. ARVD = arrhythmogenic right ventricular dysplasia; AV = atrioventricular; CAD = coronary artery disease; ECG = electrocardiogram; echo = echocardiogram; EP = electrophysiology; ICD = implantable cardioverter-defibrillator; LQTS = long QT syndrome; SCD = sudden cardiac death; SVT = supraventricular tachycardia; WPW = Wolff-Parkinson-White syndrome.

TABLE 49-1 CAUSES OF SYNCOPE AND THEIR PREVALENCE

NEUROCARDIOGENIC CAUSES
Vasovagal (8-41% of patients)
Situational (1-8% of patients)
Micturition
Defecation
Swallow
Cough
Carotid sinus syncope (0.4% of patients)
Neuralgias
Psychiatric disorders
Medications, exercise
ORTHOSTATIC HYPOTENSION (4-10% OF PATIENTS)
DECREASED CARDIAC OUTPUT
Obstruction to flow (1-8% of patients)
Obstruction to left ventricular outflow or inflow: aortic stenosis, hypertrophic obstructive cardiomyopathy, mitral stenosis, myxoma
Obstruction to right ventricular outflow or inflow: pulmonic stenosis, pulmonary embolism, pulmonary hypertension, myxoma
Other heart disease
Pump failure, myocardial infarction, coronary artery disease, coronary spasm, tamponade, aortic dissection
ARRHYTHMIAS (4-38% OF PATIENTS)
Bradyarrhythmias: sinus node disease, second- and third-degree atrioventricular block, pacemaker malfunction, drug-induced bradyarrhythmias
Tachyarrhythmias: ventricular tachycardia, torsades de pointes (e.g., associated with congenital long QT syndrome or acquired QT prolongation), supraventricular tachycardia
NEUROLOGIC AND PSYCHIATRIC DISEASES (3-32% OF PATIENTS)
Migraine
Transient ischemic attacks
UNKNOWN (13-41% OF PATIENTS)

Adapted from Kapoor W. Approach to the patient with syncope. In: Braunwald E, Goldman L, eds. *Primary Cardiology*, 2nd ed. Philadelphia: Saunders; 2003.

TABLE 49-2 CLINICAL FEATURES SUGGESTING SPECIFIC CAUSES

DIAGNOSTIC CONSIDERATION
Neurocardiogenic
Symptoms after prolonged motionless standing; sudden unexpected pain; fear; or unpleasant sight, sound, or smell
Syncope in a well-trained athlete after abrupt cessation of exertion (without heart disease)
Situational syncope during or immediately after micturition, cough, swallowing, or defecation
Syncope with throat or facial pain (glossopharyngeal or trigeminal neuralgia)
Organic Heart Disease (e.g., coronary artery disease, aortic stenosis, primary arrhythmia, obstructive hypertrophic cardiomyopathy, pulmonary hypertension)
Brief loss of consciousness, no prodrome, history of heart disease
Syncope during exertion
Family history of sudden death
Neurologic
Seizures: confusion for >5 min after regaining consciousness
Transient ischemic attack, subclavian steal, basilar migraine: syncope associated with vertigo, dysarthria, diplopia, arm exercise
Migraine: syncope associated with antecedent headaches
Other Vascular
Carotid sinus: syncope with head rotation or pressure on the carotid sinus (as in tumors, shaving, tight collars)
Orthostatic hypotension: syncope immediately on standing
Subclavian steal or aortic dissection: differences in blood pressure or pulse between the two arms
Drug-Induced
Patient is taking a medication that may lead to long QT syndrome, orthostasis, or bradycardia
Psychiatric Illness
Frequent syncope, somatic complaints, no heart disease, inconstant circumstances of events

Adapted from Kapoor WN. Syncope. *N Engl J Med*. 2000;343:1856-1862.

tachycardia (typically arising from the ventricular outflow tracts; Chapter 53), but such patients generally have a more benign course than patients with structural heart disease and are readily curable with ablation (Chapter 54).

Presyncope and Syncope

Syncope, defined as a sudden loss of consciousness, and presyncope, or lightheadedness, are caused by global impairment of blood flow to the brain (Table 49-1). Syncope can be a manifestation of tachyarrhythmias, bradyarrhythmias, or neurocardiogenic syncope, or it can be unrelated to any arrhythmia. A careful history and physical examination are necessary to exclude other cardiac causes (e.g., acute ischemia, aortic stenosis) or neurologic causes. Important historical features that suggest an arrhythmic cause are an association with palpitations and the lack of any neurologic deficits preceding or following the event. Left ventricular outflow obstruction, due either to aortic stenosis (Chapter 60) or hypertrophic obstructive cardiomyopathy (Chapter 47), can present as syncope, often during or just after exertion.

Important differential diagnoses include conditions other than lightheadedness that may be termed dizziness by the patient. Vertigo (Chapter 396), a sense of imbalance or of the "room spinning," and ataxia (Chapter 379) can usually be distinguished by the history and physical examination. The possibility of seizures (Chapter 372) must also be evaluated; syncope from an arrhythmia or neurocardiogenic syncope occasionally results in seizure-like activity, and seizures can sometimes be confused with syncope. The most important distinguishing feature is that postictal symptoms, a key feature of seizure disorders, are absent when syncope is the result of an arrhythmia or a neurocardiogenic event. Patients with syncope from an arrhythmia usually awaken without any neurologic residual, unless the patient experienced a cardiac arrest with prolonged hypoxia and required resuscitation. Among patients who are hospitalized with a first episode of syncope and in whom pulmonary embolism cannot be excluded based on a low Wells score (see Table 68-3) and a negative D-dimer assay, pulmonary embolism may be found in 25% of patients who do not have another obvious cause of their syncope and in about 13% of patients who do have an alternative explanation for their syncope. By comparison, among all patients who present to an emergency department with syncope, only about 1.5% of patients appear to have pulmonary emboli.[2]

Because most spells of episodic loss of consciousness occur outside medical observation, the history is the most critical part of the evaluation (Table 49-2).[3] Each syncopal episode should be reviewed in detail, with special attention to symptoms preceding the episode, events during unconsciousness, and the symptoms and time course of regaining orientation after consciousness is restored. Information from a witness can be essential to the evaluation. About 20% of syncopal events are associated with an injury, but recurrent neurocardiogenic events are less likely to result in injury.[4]

The patient's presymptomatic activity and positioning, as well as symptoms when the syncopal episode began, are important clues to diagnosis. Seizures or cardiac arrhythmias can occur in any body position, but recumbent patients rarely develop neurocardiogenic (vasovagal) syncope and never have orthostatic hypotension. Prodromal lightheadedness, dizziness (but uncommonly vertigo), bilateral tinnitus, nausea, diffuse weakness, and dimming of vision are symptoms of cerebral hypoperfusion and support the diagnosis of syncope, which may be from a cardiac, orthostatic, or neurocardiogenic cause. Loss of consciousness so rapid that a prodrome is absent may occur with seizures and with some cardiac arrhythmias such as asystole, which typically causes loss of consciousness within 4 to 8 seconds in the upright position but usually requires 12 to 15 seconds in the recumbent position. Palpitations during the prodrome suggest a tachyarrhythmia. The activity of the patient immediately before the onset of symptoms may also provide clues. Syncope associated with the cessation of exertion or with anxiety or pain suggests neurocardiogenic syncope, whereas symptoms during exertion suggest an arrhythmia or left ventricular outflow obstruction due to aortic stenosis (Chapter 60) or hypertrophic obstructive cardiomyopathy (Chapter 47). Syncope associated with a change in posture suggests orthostatic causes, whereas syncope while straining at urination suggests situational neurocardiogenic syncope.

A witness's description of the events during the episode of unconsciousness is very helpful. Although body stiffening and limb jerking occur with generalized seizures, similar movements can result from cerebral hypoperfusion, especially if perfusion is not restored rapidly. Such muscle jerking is often multifocal and can be synchronous or asynchronous. In contrast to epileptic seizures, which generally produce tonic-clonic activity for at least 1 to 2 minutes, muscle jerking in syncope rarely persists for longer than 30 seconds. If an arrhythmia continues or the patient is physically maintained upright, tonic stiffening of the body followed by jerking movements of the limbs can occur. Occasionally, motor movements identical to a tonic-clonic seizure occur, and a mistaken diagnosis of epilepsy can be made. Urinary incontinence during the spell is frequently used to support or refute a diagnosis of epilepsy; however, fainting with a full bladder can result in incontinence, whereas seizures with an empty bladder will not. Tongue biting favors seizures.

The time frame over which consciousness and orientation are regained is perhaps the most important clue in differentiating seizures from syncope. Recovery of orientation after neurocardiogenic syncope occurs within seconds of regaining consciousness. Recovery of orientation after self-reversible arrhythmia-associated syncope is usually proportional to the duration of the unconsciousness and is usually rapid (0 to 10 seconds). Life-threatening arrhythmias (e.g., prolonged asystole or ventricular fibrillation) usually do not resolve without resuscitation, and the confusion after regaining consciousness may be permanent owing to ischemic brain injury (Chapter 50). By comparison, the period of confusion after seizures, often accompanied by agitation, continues for 2 to 20 minutes after recovery of consciousness.

DIAGNOSIS

The likelihood of an arrhythmic cause of syncope is higher in patients with underlying heart disease, a systolic blood pressure below 90 or above 180 mm Hg, a QRS duration >130 msec, or a QTc interval >480 msec. Arrhythmias are generally categorized as bradyarrhythmias (slow heart rates; see Chapter 51), tachyarrhythmias (fast heart rates; see Chapters 52 and 53), or premature beats (single extrasystoles from the atrium or the ventricle—PACs [see Fig. 52-1 or PVCs [see Fig. 53-1], respectively) (see Table 49-1). Although not a primary arrhythmia, neurocardiogenic syncope is a related diagnostic and management issue because its symptoms are frequently similar to those of arrhythmias and because neurocardiogenic syncope secondarily results in bradycardia (see later). A systematic approach can optimize the likelihood of identifying the cause of transient loss of consciousness (Table 49-3).[5]

TABLE 49-3 SUMMARY OF CLINICAL RECOMMENDATIONS FOR TRANSIENT LOSS OF CONSCIOUSNESS

TOPIC	RECOMMENDATIONS
Initial assessment	Detailed history, especially from witnesses Full clinical examination 12-lead ECG
Uncomplicated faints	Suggestive features include: Posture: occurrence during prolonged standing or similar previous episodes avoided by lying down Provoking factors, such as pain or a medical procedure Prodromal symptoms, such as sweating or feeling warm or hot before TLoC Further investigation and specialist referral are not needed.
Epilepsy	Suggestive features are a bitten tongue; head turning to one side during TLoC; no memory of abnormal behavior that occurred before, during, or after TLoC; unusual posturing; prolonged limb jerking (brief seizure-like activity often occurs during syncope, including uncomplicated faints); confusion after the event; or prodromal déjà vu or jamais vu. If features of epilepsy are present, arrange for early review by an epilepsy specialist. Do not arrange for EEG before neurologic assessment. Note that brief seizure-like activity often occurs during syncope, including uncomplicated faints. Do not suspect epilepsy unless suggestive features are present. Arrange for cardiovascular assessment if the cause of TLoC is unclear.
Urgent specialist referral	Give immediate treatment for clinically urgent problems (such as complete AV block or severe bleeding). Arrange for urgent specialist cardiovascular assessment for patients at risk for a severe adverse event (such as those with long QT interval, cardiac arrhythmia, or structural heart disease).
Further cardiovascular assessment	Focus on specific disorders that may cause TLoC, such as orthostatic hypotension, the carotid sinus syndrome, structural heart disease, or cardiac arrhythmia. Assessment should include repeated history, clinical examination, and 12-lead ECG. For suspected cardiac arrhythmia or unexplained TLoC, use ambulatory ECG for further assessment: Very frequent episodes: use 24- to 48-hour Holter monitoring. Moderately frequent episodes: use external event monitoring. Infrequent episodes: use an implantable event recorder. In patients who are sick or worrisome enough for hospital admission and do not have both a low Wells score (see Chapter 68) and a negative D-dimer assay, evaluate for possible pulmonary embolism (computed tomographic pulmonary angiography or ventilation-perfusion lung scanning).

AV = atrioventricular; ECG = electrocardiography; EEG = electroencephalogram; TLoC = transient loss of consciousness.

Adapted from Cooper PN, et al. Synopsis of the National Institute for Health and Clinical Excellence Guideline for management of transient loss of consciousness. *Ann Intern Med.* 2011;155:543-549.

Bradyarrhythmias

Bradyarrhythmias (Chapter 51) can be due to dysfunction in the sinoatrial node, AV node, or His-Purkinje system (below the AV node). Sinus bradycardia manifests as a slow atrial (sinus) rate and can occur at rest or as an inappropriately slow rate during exercise (chronotropic incompetence). Sinus arrest can be intermittent, when transient loss of sinus activity (loss of the P wave on the ECG) causes brief sinus pauses, or persistent, with prolonged loss of atrial activation. The sinus rate and even the presence of sinus pauses are influenced by autonomic tone. Therefore, healthy individuals—particularly younger patients and well-trained athletes (with high vagal tone)—have occasional sinus slowing, often during sleep. A sinus pause of more than 3 seconds is considered pathologic if it is associated with symptoms while a patient is awake. Sinus bradycardia and sinus arrest can also be the result of medications, typically β-blockers and calcium-channel blockers. When not "physiologic" or due to medications, sinus bradycardia and sinus arrest are the result of intrinsic conduction system disease. Sinus bradycardia, especially if it is intermittent, can also signify disease of the right coronary artery.

Bradyarrhythmias from AV nodal disease result from the failure of impulse conduction from the atrium to the ventricle. Like the sinus node, the AV node is dramatically affected by autonomic tone. Mobitz type I second-degree AV block (Wenckebach block; see Fig. 51-6) can be seen during periods of high vagal tone (such as while sleeping) and is not necessarily pathologic; for example, it does not progress to complete heart block and is not associated with a widened QRS. Many drugs, such as β-blockers and calcium-channel blockers, commonly cause first-degree AV block and should be considered a potential cause of any degree of AV block. Mobitz type II block (see Fig. 51-7) signifies that the level of AV block is below the AV node in the His-Purkinje system, which is not sensitive to autonomic tone; the resulting QRS is widened, and there is a high likelihood of progression to complete heart block (third-degree AV block; see Figs. 51-8 and 51-9). Idiopathic paroxysmal AV block, detected by continuous ECG monitoring, can also cause syncope. Intermittent complete heart block, which can result in drop attacks or Stokes-Adams attacks, is usually preceded by abnormal baseline findings on the ECG, such as a bundle branch block or second-degree AV block.

Tachyarrhythmias

Tachyarrhythmias can arise from the atrium or AV node (supraventricular tachycardias) or from the ventricle (ventricular tachycardias). Supraventricular tachyarrhythmias that may be associated with palpitations, presyncope, or syncope include atrial tachycardia (see Fig. 52-11), AV nodal re-entrant tachycardia (see Fig. 52-8), AV junctional tachycardia (see Fig. 52-9), atrial flutter (see Fig. 52-12), atrial fibrillation (see Fig. 52-13), or sometimes in association with accessory conduction pathways that facilitate the re-entry needed to sustain the arrhythmia (AV reciprocating tachycardia). Ventricular tachyarrhythmias include the various forms of ventricular tachycardia (see Figs. 53-1 through 53-6).

Neurocardiogenic Syncope and Related Syndromes

Neurocardiogenic syncope is the sudden onset of lightheadedness or loss of consciousness as a result of autonomic reflexes and is more common in younger patients (teenage to third decade of life). It is sometimes called a vasovagal episode, a common faint, or situational syncope if it is clearly induced by a particular activity (e.g., micturition syncope). Some families have autosomal dominant vasovagal syncope, which is genetically heterogeneous but seems to be linked to chromosome 15q26.

In neurocardiogenic syncope, heightened parasympathetic output, either due to direct stimulation (e.g., micturition, defecation, abdominal pain, or other gastrointestinal conditions) or as a reflex in response to sympathetic stimulation (e.g., seeing blood, abrupt cessation of exercise), results in arterial dilation (called the vasodilatory response) and an inhibition of sinus and

AV node activity (the cardioinhibitory response). The result is a transient decrease in blood pressure, often manifested as lightheadedness or syncope. Because they are associated with parasympathetic (vagal) output, episodes are frequently accompanied by nausea, diaphoresis, and salivation. Twin analyses provide strong evidence for genetic factors in vasovagal syncope.

Rarely, situational syncope is associated with swallowing or coughing. Swallowing can trigger brain stem reflexes that lead to vagally induced bradyarrhythmias, with resultant syncope. This phenomenon may or may not be associated with severe pain in the tonsillar pillar, which may radiate to the ear (i.e., glossopharyngeal neuralgia; Chapter 367). Cough-related syncope can occur with severe, repeated coughing, which may increase thoracic pressure and result in increased vagal tone or a transient reduction in outflow from the intracranial veins, followed by a transient increase in intracranial pressure and impaired blood flow.

A related cause of syncope is carotid body hypersensitivity, in which vagal tone is increased by direct stimulation of the carotid body. This condition is frequently seen in older patients (particularly men older than 60 years), in whom episodes are associated with mechanical stimulation of the neck (e.g., turning the head, shaving, wearing a tight collar or necktie). Use of β-blockers, calcium-channel blockers, and digitalis can exacerbate or predispose to this condition. This form of syncope is diagnosed by documenting pauses longer than 3 seconds in response to carotid sinus massage.

Postural or orthostatic hypotension can result in recurrent syncope. The history confirms that the patient is in the upright posture during spells, that the prodromal symptoms are those of cerebral hypoperfusion, and that the symptoms are relieved with recumbency. The diagnosis is supported by detecting a decrease of 30 mm Hg or greater in systolic blood pressure or a decrease of 10 mm Hg or greater in diastolic blood pressure between recumbent and upright postures. The many causes include drugs, polyneuropathies (Chapter 388), postural orthostatic tachycardia syndrome (a ≥30 beat per minute increase in heart rate when standing),[6] and neurodegenerative disorders (Chapter 378).

Cerebrovascular syncope results from cerebral hypoperfusion due to vascular phenomena, as opposed to generalized hypotension caused by arrhythmias or neurocardiogenic reflexes. Loss of consciousness can be a component of a basilar artery transient ischemic attack, but other brain stem symptoms nearly always precede or accompany the unconsciousness. Vertigo is most frequent, but diplopia or visual field disturbances, hemifacial or perioral numbness, and dysarthria or ataxia are also common. Recovery of consciousness may require 30 to 60 minutes. Although the diagnosis is suggested by the history and clinical presentation, imaging studies can be useful to confirm the diagnosis. Carotid Doppler studies may show various degrees of stenosis, especially in older patients. However, unconsciousness requires bihemispheric dysfunction; thus, unilateral carotid stenosis alone does not cause syncope. Transcranial Doppler studies or magnetic resonance angiography of the basilar artery is indicated only if brain stem ischemic symptoms are present in addition to loss of consciousness; false-positive tests are common, especially with increasing age.

Other syndromes that can cause syncope include subclavian artery stenosis, which may result in retrograde blood flow from the vertebral artery to one arm, with resultant brain stem hypoperfusion (i.e., subclavian steal syndrome). Asymmetry in upper extremity systolic blood pressure, typically averaging 45 mm Hg, is nearly always present. Brain stem symptoms are similar to those in basilar transient ischemic attacks, including loss of consciousness, but a subsequent stroke from subclavian steal is rare. Syncope may also occur in up to 10% of patients with basilar artery migraine (Chapter 367). It can have a postural (orthostatic) manifestation or be associated with other basilar artery symptoms.

Neuropsychiatric syncope is a diagnosis of exclusion but is suggested by young age, frequent spells, multiple symptoms (e.g., dizziness, vertigo, lightheadedness, numbness), and duplication of the patient's symptoms by hyperventilation with the mouth open for 2 to 3 minutes. Whereas syncope and seizures occur with the eyes open, often with gaze deviation, psychogenic events frequently begin with eye closing.

Seizures (Chapter 372) can cause loss of consciousness and occasionally present clinically as syncope. However, seizures usually have a characteristic presentation and include a postictal phase, whereas most patients experiencing a syncopal episode quickly regain consciousness, except when cerebral perfusion is so compromised as to cause a secondary seizure or persistent anoxia and brain damage.

Diagnostic Tests

Electrocardiography

The baseline ECG is critical in the evaluation of a patient with palpitations or syncope. The presence of ventricular preexcitation, as manifested by a short PR interval and a delta wave (see Fig. 52-10), establishes the likely diagnosis of Wolff-Parkinson-White syndrome in a patient with palpitations and AV reciprocating tachycardia (Chapter 52); a 12-lead ECG can also be used to determine the location of the responsible accessory pathway. The baseline ECG provides useful predictive information about the likelihood of conduction system abnormalities being responsible for bradyarrhythmias (e.g., sinus bradycardia suggests sinus node dysfunction, a prolonged PR interval suggests AV nodal disease, and a widened QRS suggests disease below the AV node). The ECG is also useful in diagnosing prior myocardial infarction (i.e., pathologic Q waves), which raises the likelihood of ventricular tachycardia as a potential cause of syncope or palpitations. Abnormalities such as a prolonged QT interval in a patient with syncope and a family history of syncope or sudden death suggest one of the congenital long QT syndromes (Chapter 50). An incomplete right bundle branch block with coved ST segment elevation in ECG lead V_1 or V_2 in a patient with syncope or palpitations suggests Brugada syndrome, whereas an epsilon wave, incomplete right bundle branch block, and inverted T waves in V_1 are suggestive of right ventricular dysplasia (Chapter 47). All these syndromes carry an increased risk for recurrent syncope and sudden death if untreated (Chapters 50 and 53). The short QT syndrome (QTc ≤330 msec or QTc ≤360 plus a family history of sudden death) also predisposes to ventricular arrhythmias. Since some of these ECG findings (especially those suggestive of Brugada syndrome and even long QT syndrome) may be transient or episodic, lack of these findings does not exclude these syndromes in patients with syncope and a strong family history.

In one study, electrocardiographic screening for 14 days increased the detection of atrial fibrillation in older adults and led to a small reduction in adverse events.[A1] However the U.S. Preventive Services Task Force found evidence to be insufficient to recommend such screening.[7]

Performing an ECG during an episode of palpitations is extremely useful in making a definitive diagnosis. For narrow–QRS complex tachycardias, the specific supraventricular tachycardia can often be surmised from the 12-lead ECG obtained during symptoms (Fig. 49-2). Moreover, for wide–QRS complex tachycardias, the 12-lead ECG is useful in distinguishing a supraventricular tachycardia (with aberrancy) from a ventricular tachycardia (Fig. 49-3). The presence of fusion beats or AV dissociation during a wide–QRS complex tachycardia leads to the diagnosis of ventricular tachycardia. For ventricular tachycardias, the morphology of the QRS complex is useful in determining the location of the ventricular tachycardia focus and in identifying idiopathic ventricular tachycardia (right ventricular outflow tract or fascicular), which has a much more benign course than ventricular tachycardia in the setting of coronary disease (Chapter 53).

The effect of carotid sinus massage, vagal maneuvers, or adenosine (given as a rapid intravenous bolus of 6 mg and repeated at a dose of 12 mg if the initial dose is ineffective) is also useful in narrowing the differential diagnosis of a tachycardia. These maneuvers slow conduction through the AV node. Therefore, tachycardias that terminate with either maneuver are likely to involve the AV node as a critical component of the re-entrant circuit (AV nodal re-entrant tachycardia or AV re-entrant tachycardia). If the maneuver induces AV block but does not immediately terminate the arrhythmia, likely causes are atrial fibrillation, atrial flutter, and atrial tachycardias (or occasionally ventricular tachycardia if the QRS is wide). On rare occasions, atrial tachycardias and some idiopathic ventricular tachycardias terminate in response to adenosine (but usually not at precisely the same time as AV block). Important clues to the specific mechanism can be obtained at the onset or termination of tachycardia, so obtaining a continuous 12-lead ECG during carotid sinus massage or the administration of adenosine is very useful.

During bradycardias, the ECG is useful in determining the level of the conduction system (sinus node, AV node, or His bundle) responsible for the bradycardia. Sinus bradycardia is diagnosed when a slow (<50/minute at rest) atrial rate (P wave) conducts to the ventricle. Sinus arrest or sinus pauses are diagnosed by absent or dropped P waves. First-degree AV block (see Fig. 51-5) is defined as a prolonged PR interval (>200 msec), and second-degree AV block is defined by P waves that occasionally do not conduct to the ventricle (P wave without an ensuing QRS); Mobitz type I second-degree AV block (also known as Wenckebach block; see Fig. 51-6) is characterized by progressive lengthening of the PR interval until one P wave does not conduct to the ventricle. This form of AV block is often seen in younger patients, is usually benign, and rarely progresses to complete AV (third-degree) block. Mobitz type II second-degree AV block (see Fig. 51-7), which is characterized by the sudden, unexpected loss of conduction of a P wave to the ventricle (dropped QRS), signifies disease of the His-Purkinje system and often progresses to complete heart block. Complete heart block or third-degree AV block (see Figs. 51-8 and 51-9) is diagnosed by the dissociation of P waves from QRS complexes, with an atrial rate faster than the ventricular rate.

Ambulatory Monitoring

For intermittent symptoms such as palpitations, dizziness, or syncope, it is often difficult to obtain a 12-lead ECG while the symptoms are occurring.

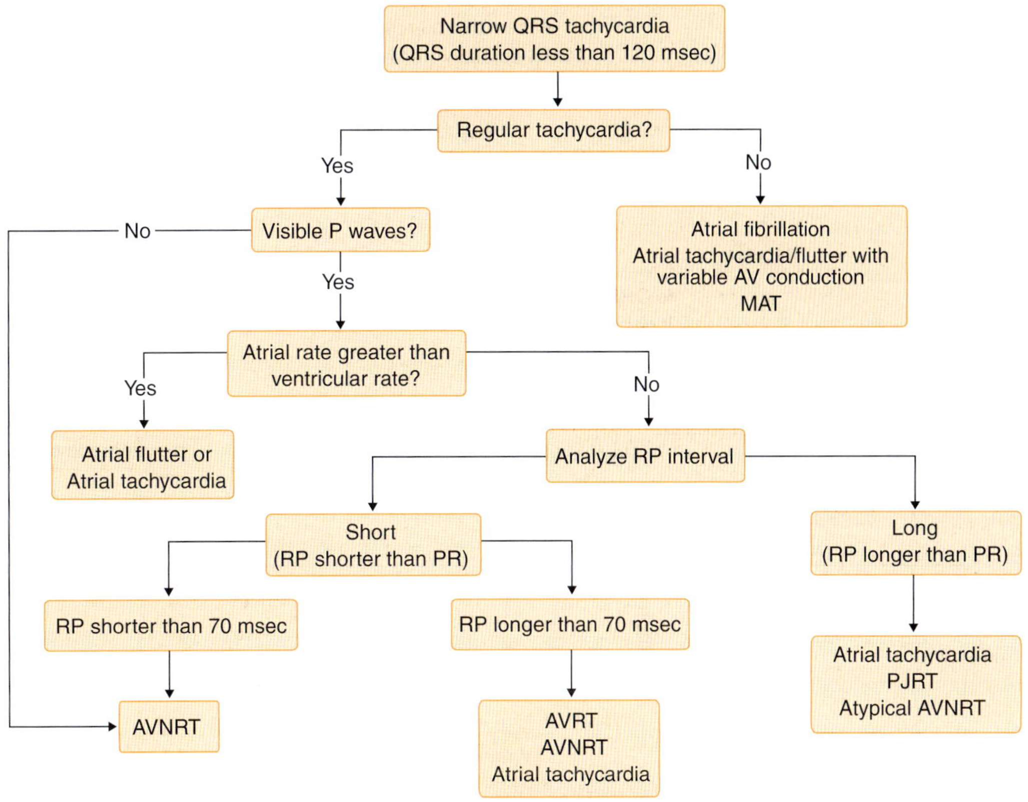

FIGURE 49-2. ECG algorithm for diagnosis of narrow-complex tachycardias. AVNRT = atrioventricular nodal reciprocating tachycardia; AVRT = atrioventricular reciprocating tachycardia; MAT = multifocal atrial tachycardia; PJRT = permanent form of junctional reciprocating tachycardia. (From Blomstrom-Lundqvist C, Scheinman MM, Aliot EM, et al. ACC/AHA/ESC guidelines for the management of patients with supraventricular arrhythmias—executive summary. *Circulation*. 2003;108:1871-1909.)

Therefore, ambulatory monitoring, which allows ECG monitoring over long periods, is a vital diagnostic tool. There are currently four general types of ambulatory monitors: Holter monitors, which continuously record the ECG for 24 to 48 hours (or extended monitors that can record continuously for longer); event recorders, which are wearable loop recorders that record only during specific events (when the patient activates the recorder because of symptoms or the recorder detects a heart rate above or below a specified threshold) and can be worn for 1 month or more; mobile cardiac outpatient telemetry that functions similarly to external event recorders but transmits data in real time through a wireless network to a central monitoring center and can be worn for up to 1 month; and implantable loop recorders, which function similarly to event recorders but can be used for up to 3 years. More recently, consumer-directed smartphone ECGs attach to a smartphone and can record an on-demand single-lead ECG rhythm strip or can use light-sensing photoplethysmography to detect irregular heart rhythms (such as atrial fibrillation) and heart rates. The choice among ambulatory monitoring methods is largely determined by the frequency and severity of the symptoms and the likelihood of capturing an episode during a given monitoring period.

Ambulatory monitoring is diagnostic only if abnormalities occur during symptoms or if the patient has typical symptoms without any concurrent abnormalities. A "normal" monitoring record is nondiagnostic if the patient does not have symptoms during the period.

Holter Monitors

Holter monitors use either a tape (in older devices) or digital media (in newer devices) to record a 3-, 5-, or 12-lead surface ECG continuously, usually for 24 to 48 hours but for 3 weeks or more when indicated. Processing, printing, and analysis of the recordings are performed offline with commercial systems. In addition to recording the rhythm, analyses of heart rate variability and ST segment changes and accurate counts of PACs and PVCs can be automated. Some systems allow extrapolation to produce a "virtual" 12-lead recording at any time during the monitoring period. Holter monitoring is useful for detecting symptoms that are frequent (multiple times daily) and for diagnosing sinus node dysfunction (sinus node arrest, sick sinus syndrome) or intermittent AV block. It can also be useful to assess the adequacy of ventricular rate control in a patient with atrial fibrillation or burden of PVCs. New form factors have enabled longer, more comfortable monitors (such as a self-contained patch) that can record for several weeks.

Traditional Holter monitors have largely been replaced by the more convenient and longer-lasting extended monitors using a single-lead patch. Traditional Holters remain useful, however, for situations in which having more than one simultaneous lead is helpful, for example, in differentiating supraventricular tachycardia (SVT) with aberrancy from ventricular tachycardia (VT) or localizing the source of a PVC or VT.

Event Monitors

Event monitors, also known as loop recorders, are designed to record intermittent episodes during long periods (weeks to months) and are thus useful for patients with less frequent symptoms. The system records the ECG into a loop buffer that is continuously updated and overwritten. The duration of memory varies from a few seconds to a few minutes and is usually programmable. When activated, the information is "locked" into memory and continues to record forward for a preprogrammed amount of time. Newer systems allow both patient-activated (when symptoms occur) and event-triggered (when the heart rate is above or below a preset threshold) recording.[8] Some recorders have algorithms to detect and record atrial fibrillation automatically, regardless of the heart rate. After episodes have been recorded, the patient transmits the recording over the telephone to centralized receivers. Some event monitors require leads similar to Holter monitors, whereas others are worn on the wrist or are put into small credit card–sized devices that are placed on the chest during symptoms. The latter type is useful only in patients whose symptoms last for several minutes and who do not have syncope.

Mobile Cardiac Outpatient Telemetry

Mobile cardiac outpatient telemetry units are similar to external event monitors, except that data are transmitted wirelessly in real time to a monitoring center. These devices are useful for patients in whom intermittent symptoms are severe or the differential diagnosis includes potentially dangerous arrhythmias that should be diagnosed expeditiously. For example, a wearable ECG sensor patch can expedite the diagnosis of atrial fibrillation in patients at high risk for it.[A2] The monitoring center also has the ability to dispatch emergency medical services if necessary.

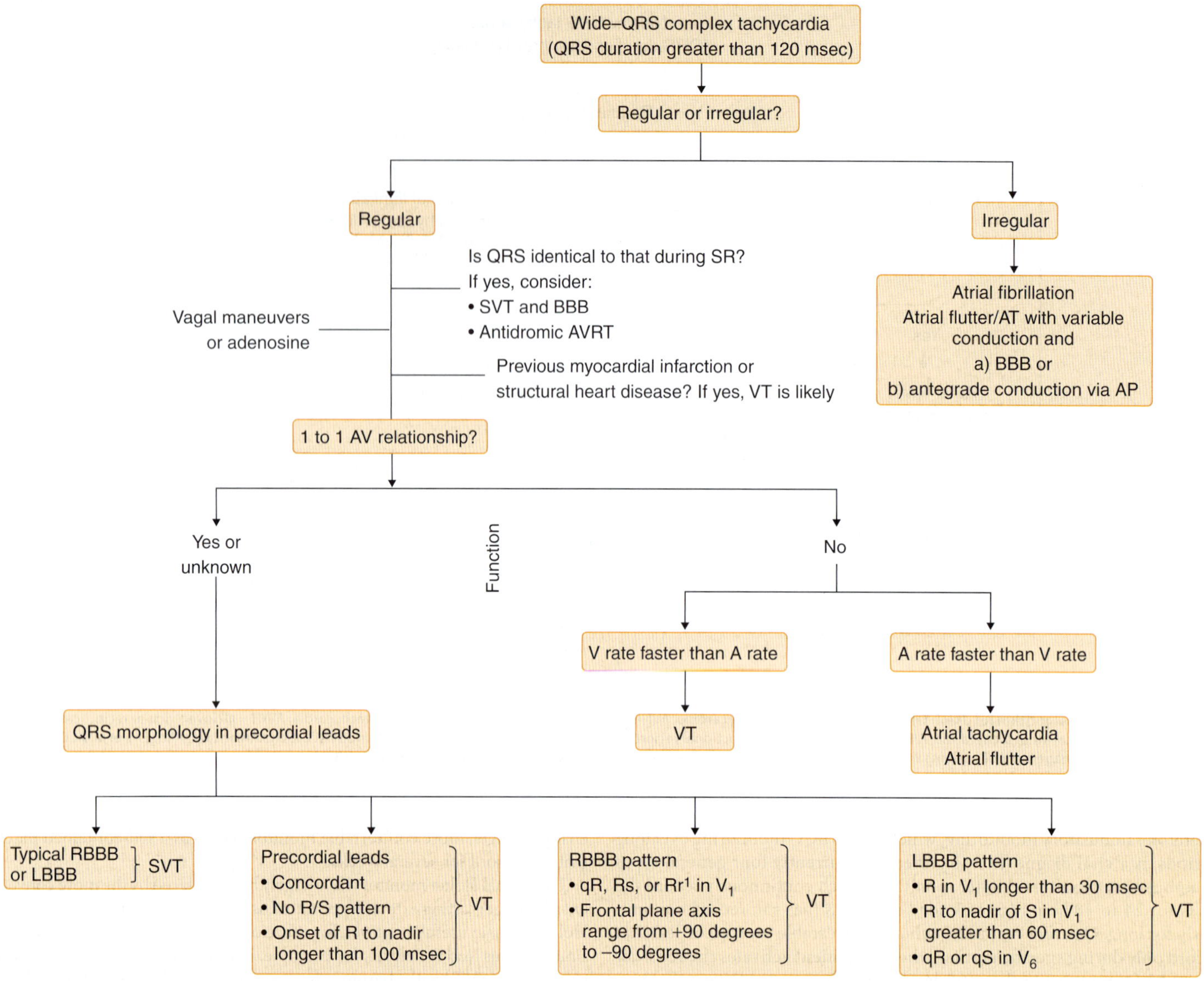

FIGURE 49-3. **ECG algorithm for diagnosis of wide-complex tachycardias. A = atrial; AP = accessory pathway; AT = atrial tachycardia; AV = atrioventricular; AVRT = atrioventricular reciprocating tachycardia; BBB = bundle branch block; LBBB = left bundle branch block; RBBB = right bundle branch block; SR = sinus rhythm; SVT = supraventricular tachycardia; V = ventricular; VT = ventricular tachycardia. (From Blomstrom-Lundqvist C, Scheinman MM, Aliot EM, et al. ACC/AHA/ESC guidelines for the management of patients with supraventricular arrhythmias—executive summary. *Circulation*. 2003;108:1871-1909.)**

Implantable Loop Recorders

Implantable loop recorders are small devices with integrated leads that are placed in a small subcutaneous pocket during a simple surgery, usually performed in the electrophysiology laboratory. They function similarly to event recorders in terms of recording ECGs. Patients can activate the device with a small transmitter, or the device can be autotriggered on the basis of preprogrammed heart rates. The device can be interrogated by a computer, similar to the way pacemakers are interrogated to program the device's parameters and to retrieve ECGs that have been recorded. Newer devices can wirelessly communicate with a telephone-connected base station in the home to upload data after an event. In patients with recurrent, difficult-to-diagnose syncope, an implantable loop recorder is better than the combination of tilt testing, an external loop recorder, and electrophysiologic testing for establishing an arrhythmic diagnosis. In patients ages 70 to 79 years or with a history of ischemic stroke, implantable loop recorders are significantly more likely than prolonged external monitoring to detect paroxysmal atrial fibrillation,[A3-A5] but the clinical benefits of better diagnosis appear to be negligible.

Consumer-Based Rhythm Monitors

With the growth of smartphones and wearable devices, patients can purchase consumer-grade devices to monitor their heart rate and heart rhythm. These devices use one of two general approaches[9,10]: use of the light sensor on the back of a smartwatch to measure *pulse* rate and rhythm using photoplethysmography or single-lead ECG devices that connect to a smartphone or are integrated into a smartwatch. Both of these devices use internal algorithms to provide automated simple interpretations of the heart rhythm (e.g., normal, possible atrial fibrillation or undetermined) and heart rate to the user. The ECG devices also record a single-lead ECG, which may be useful for a physician to interpret for possible arrhythmias. Currently, these devices are designed and approved to screen for atrial fibrillation but not other abnormal rhythms. These devices should not generally substitute for other, more established types of ambulatory monitoring to diagnose patients with suspected arrhythmias, with the possible exception of screening for atrial fibrillation.

Tilt Table Testing

Tilt table testing is used to confirm the diagnosis of neurocardiogenic syncope.[11] The test involves continuous heart rate and blood pressure monitoring during head-up tilting. After baseline measurements in the supine position, the patient is tilted head-up at 60 to 80 degrees for 60 minutes. Some laboratories use isoproterenol or nitroglycerin as additional provocation. A positive result is a sudden and precipitous fall in blood pressure and heart rate, with concurrent reproducibility of symptoms (syncope). Because there is an appreciable false-positive rate, the test is best used as a confirmatory test in patients with a history suggestive of neurocardiogenic syncope or in patients with syncope in whom structural heart disease and other causes of syncope have been excluded.

Electrophysiologic Studies

Electrophysiologic studies involve the placement of several transvenous catheters in the heart to make temporary measurements of intracardiac electrograms and to perform pacing. Electrophysiologic studies are useful to identify the precise mechanism of tachyarrhythmias and are a necessary prelude to curative ablation (Chapter 54). Most arrhythmias, especially those with re-entrant mechanisms, can be readily induced during electrophysiologic studies. In addition, the existence and characteristics of accessory AV pathways (i.e., those responsible for Wolff-Parkinson-White syndrome or other re-entrant tachyarrhythmias) can be readily assessed by an electrophysiologic study. In patients with previous myocardial infarction, electrophysiologic studies are useful in determining the existence of a substrate for ventricular arrhythmias (Chapter 53), which may be treated with ablation or implantable defibrillators (Chapter 54). Electrophysiologic studies are also useful to determine the integrity of the conduction system and the precise mechanism of bradyarrhythmias that may be causing syncope. Therefore, electrophysiologic studies may be indicated in patients with documented or suspected tachyarrhythmias as a prelude to curative ablation in patients with documented or suspected supraventricular tachycardia or idiopathic ventricular tachycardia; in patients with a previous myocardial infarction (but left ventricular ejection fraction >30 to 35%) and syncope, presyncope, or palpitations to exclude ventricular tachycardia; and in patients with severe or prolonged symptoms and no apparent diagnosis by history or ambulatory monitoring in the setting of an abnormal ECG. However, with the advent of implantable loop recorders capable of prolonged electrocardiographic monitoring and the known benefit of implantable cardioverter-defibrillator therapy in many patients with depressed left ventricular function, the role of invasive diagnostic cardiac electrophysiologic studies has been substantially reduced in patients with unexplained syncope in patients with reduced left ventricular function.

Other Tests

Echocardiography

Echocardiography (Chapter 43) can be useful to ensure that a patient does not have underlying structural heart disease, which can be an important prognostic factor in patients with ventricular tachycardia or syncope. Echocardiography should be performed in patients who present with near-syncope or syncope that is not obviously neurocardiogenic to ensure that there is no valvular or myocardial cause.

Exercise Testing

Exercise testing (Chapters 39 and 56) can be useful to assess arrhythmias, particularly in patients whose symptoms are exercise related. Exercise testing can also be useful in the evaluation of patients with bradyarrhythmias to diagnose chronotropic incompetence, and it can differentiate AV block due to autonomic tone (improves with exercise) from intrinsic conduction disease (generally worsens with an increasing rate).

Neurologic Testing

Routine electroencephalography (Chapter 366) is not helpful because a single study may be normal, even in epileptic patients. Structural brain diseases rarely cause episodic loss of consciousness, and routine brain imaging studies are indicated only in patients with focal neurologic findings. Carotid Doppler (Chapter 376) studies can document stenosis, but unconsciousness requires bihemispheric dysfunction. Transcranial Doppler or magnetic resonance angiography of the basilar artery is indicated only in patients with symptoms suggestive of brain stem ischemia.

TREATMENT

Treatment of syncope depends on the underlying cause (Chapters 52 and 53),[12,13] as well as the risk of recurrence. One approach to risk stratification is the Canadian Syncope Risk Score (Tables 49-4 and 49-5).[14] Immediate hospital admission (e.g., observation in a chest pain unit, syncope unit, or the equivalent) is recommended when the patient has a Canadian Syncope Risk Score of greater than 3 or high-risk characteristics (see Table 49-6); the cause of syncope is unclear (especially in elderly patients, otherwise fragile, or worrisome patients); the syncope resulted in significant injury; the patient is suspected of having a cardiac or cerebrovascular cause of syncope; or the patient meets criteria established by professional societies (Table 49-7). Patients at highest risk have a systolic blood pressure below 90 mm Hg, a history of myocardial infarction or heart failure, a complaint of shortness of breath, an abnormal initial ECG, or a hematocrit less than 30%.

Until the cause of the syncope is determined and treated, patients should be instructed to avoid situations that may cause injury as a result of the syncope, especially if there is no prodrome and episodes are frequent. Careful consideration should be given to driving restrictions, which may be mandatory depending on local laws, and restrictions on dangerous work-related activity (e.g., for pilots, heavy machine operators, bus drivers) until definitive therapy is given.

TABLE 49-4 THE CANADIAN SYNCOPE RISK SCORE

	POINTS
History and physical examination	
Vasovagal characteristics*	−1
History of heart disease†	1
Systolic blood pressure < 90 mm Hg or > 180 mm Hg‡	2
Laboratory data	
Troponin level elevated	2
QRS axis < −30° or > 100°	1
QRS duration > 130 ms	1
Corrected QT interval > 480 ms	2
Emergency department clinical diagnosis	
Vasovagal syncope	−2
Cardiac syncope	2
Total score (−3 to 11)	

*Triggered by prolonged standing, fear, emotion, pain, or being in a warm crowded place.
†Coronary or valvular heart disease, heart failure, cardiomyopathy, history of ventricular or atrial arrhythmias, or cardiac rhythm device.
‡At any time from presentation until emergency department discharge.
Thiruganasambandamoorthy V, Kwong K, Wells GA, et al. Development of the Canadian Syncope Risk Score to predict serious adverse events after emergency department assessment of syncope. *CMAJ*. 2016;188:E289-E298.

TABLE 49-5 SERIOUS 30-DAY OUTCOMES BASED ON THE CANADIAN SYNCOPE RISK SCORE

RISK	# OF POINTS	SERIOUS OUTCOMES*	DEATHS
Very low	−3 to −2	0.2%	0
Low	−1 to 0	0.7%	0
Medium	1 to 3	8%	0.1%
High	4 to 5	19%	3%
Very High	6 to 11	51%	9%

*Serious arrhythmia (e.g., pacemaker/defibrillator, cardioversion to treat an arrhythmia) or nonarrhythmic serious conditions such as myocardial infarction, new serious structural heart disease, aortic dissection, pulmonary embolism, severe pulmonary hypertension, significant hemorrhage, subarachnoid hemorrhage, any other serious condition causing syncope, or death.
Thiruganasambandamoorthy V, Kwong K, Wells GA, et al. Development of the Canadian Syncope Risk Score to predict serious adverse events after emergency department assessment of syncope. *CMAJ*. 2016;188:E289-E298.

Cardiac Syncope

In patients with a cardiac cause of syncope, targeted treatments include valve replacement for aortic stenosis (Chapter 60); medications for hypertrophic cardiomyopathy (Chapter 47); a pacemaker for bradyarrhythmias (Chapters 52 and 54) and for carotid body hypersensitivity; cardioversion, an implantable cardioverter-defibrillator, ablation, or medications for tachyarrhythmias (Table 49-8; Chapters 50 through 53); and fluid repletion for orthostatic hypotension. Even when a pacemaker is implanted in a patient with syncope attributed to bradycardia, the 5-year incidence of recurrent syncope approaches 20%.[15]

Neurocardiogenic Syncope

In patients with neurocardiogenic syncope, the most effective therapies are behavioral: avoidance of triggers, wearing of compression stockings, and maintenance of adequate hydration and salt intake. Lying down with the feet elevated and performing isometric hand exercises may abort an acute episode. Patients should specifically be taught how to tense their arms and legs and grip their hands during prodromal symptoms to increase peripheral resistance and systemic blood pressure.

If neurocardiogenic syncope recurs despite education and lifestyle changes, fludrocortisone (0.1 mg/day, starting dose, increasing to 0.2 mg daily if tolerated or decreasing to 0.05 mg daily if not) can expand intravascular volume and reduce syncopal episodes[A6] but has not been definitively proven to prevent syncope. Midodrine (usually 5 to 10 mg three times daily), an α_1-receptor agonist and vasoconstrictor, has shown benefit,[A7] but other α-agonists have not. Fluoxetine (10 to 40 mg daily) may be useful in patients with recurrent neurocardiogenic syncope triggered by anxiety.[A8] β-blockers (e.g., pindolol 5 to 15 mg twice daily) can be of limited benefit. High dietary sodium intake is useful for reducing the change in heart rate in the postural tachycardia syndrome.[A9]

Pacemakers reduce recurrent neurocardiogenic syncope in selected patients with primarily a cardioinhibitory component or with severely asystolic neurally mediated syncope. For example, in patients older than 40 years with frequent syncopal episodes (at least three episodes in 2 years) and either (a) demonstrated bradycardia (asystole or AV block) during an event (≥3 seconds during a

TABLE 49-6 CHARACTERISTICS OF HIGH-RISK SYNCOPE, GENERALLY REQUIRING MONITORING, ADMISSION, AND/OR SPECIALIST CONSULTATION

HISTORY
During exertion In supine position New onset of chest discomfort Palpitations before syncope Family history of sudden death Heart failure or left ventricular ejection fraction <35% Aortic stenosis or left ventricular outflow obstruction Cardiomyopathy (dilated or hypertrophic) Arrhythmogenic right ventricular cardiomyopathy Previously documented ventricular arrhythmia Coronary artery disease Congenital heart disease Pulmonary hypertension Previous ICD implantation
PHYSICAL EXAMINATION
Lowest systolic blood pressure <90 mm Hg Sinus bradycardia (<40 bpm) Suspected valvular heart disease
LABORATORY EVALUATION
Anemia (hemoglobin <9 g/dL) Hypoxia
ELECTROCARDIOGRAM
New (or previously unknown) ischemic changes, left bundle branch block, or nonsinus rhythm Bifascicular block Prolonged QTc (>450 ms) Brugada pattern

Adapted from Costantino G, Sun BC, Barbic F, et al. Syncope clinical management in the emergency department: a consensus from the first international workshop on syncope risk stratification in the emergency department. *Eur Heart J*. 2016;37:1493-1498.

TABLE 49-7 INDICATIONS FOR INITIAL OBSERVATION AND RAPID EVALUATION OF SYNCOPE

EUROPEAN SOCIETY OF CARDIOLOGY*	CANADIAN CARDIOVASCULAR SOCIETY†
Known coronary or structural heart disease, heart failure, or prior arrhythmia	Heart failure or history of ischemic, arrhythmic, obstructive, or valvular heart disease
ECG showing nonsustained ventricular tachycardia, bifascicular block, sinus bradycardia <50 beats/min, sinoatrial block, preexcitation, or evidence of an inherited disease	Abnormal ECG: arrhythmia, conduction disease, new ischemia, or evidence of prior myocardial infarction
Syncope during exertion or when supine, palpitations preceding syncope, family history of sudden cardiac death	Systolic blood pressure <90 mm Hg
Important comorbidities (e.g., severe anemia, electrolyte disturbance)	Comorbid conditions: age >60 years, dyspnea, hematocrit <30%, hypertension, cerebrovascular disease, family history of sudden death before age 50 years, syncope while supine, syncope during exercise, syncope with no prodromal symptoms

*Moya A, Sutton R, Ammirati F, et al. Guidelines for the diagnosis and management of syncope (version 2009): the Task Force for the Diagnosis and Management of Syncope of the European Society of Cardiology (ESC). *Eur Heart J*. 2009;30:2631-2671.

†Sanatani S, Chau V, Fournier A, et al. Canadian Cardiovascular Society and Canadian Pediatric Cardiology Association Position Statement on the Approach to Syncope in the Pediatric Patient. *Can J Cardiol*. 2017;33:189-198.

ECG = electrocardiogram.

TABLE 49-8 ARRHYTHMIC CAUSES OF PALPITATIONS AND SYNCOPE

		SYMPTOMS				
ETIOLOGY	**SPECIFIC ARRHYTHMIA**	**PALPITATIONS**	**DIZZINESS**	**SYNCOPE**	**TREATMENT**	**COMMENTS**
BRADYARRHYTHMIAS						
Sinus node dysfunction	Sinus bradycardia	No	Occasional	Rare	Pacemaker if symptoms	Can be seen in association with neurocardiogenic syncope
	Sinus arrest	Occasional	Yes	Occasional	Pacemaker	Pause >3 sec
	Sick sinus syndrome	Occasional	Yes	Occasional	Pacemaker	
AV nodal disease	First-degree AV block	No	No	No	None	
	Type I second-degree AV block	Occasional	No	No	None	Can be seen in association with neurocardiogenic syncope
	Type II second-degree AV block	Occasional	Rare	No	Pacemaker if severe	Can progress to complete heart block
	Third-degree AV block	Yes	Yes	Yes	Pacemaker	
Tachy-brady syndrome		Yes	Yes	Occasional	Treat tachycardia if possible Pacemaker	Can also be manifestation of sick sinus syndrome

TABLE 49-8 ARRHYTHMIC CAUSES OF PALPITATIONS AND SYNCOPE—cont'd

ETIOLOGY	SPECIFIC ARRHYTHMIA	SYMPTOMS: PALPITATIONS	SYMPTOMS: DIZZINESS	SYMPTOMS: SYNCOPE	TREATMENT	COMMENTS
TACHYARRHYTHMIAS						
SVT	Atrial tachycardia	Yes	Occasional	Rare	Ablation β-Blockers (e.g., metoprolol, atenolol)* Calcium-channel blockers (e.g., diltiazem)*	
	Atrial flutter	Yes	Occasional	Rare	Ablation Antiarrhythmic drugs (e.g., amiodarone)* Cardioversion (acute episode)	Often difficult to control rate
	Atrial fibrillation	Yes	Occasional	Rare	Ventricular rate control Warfarin Antiarrhythmic drugs (e.g., amiodarone)* Cardioversion (acute episode) Ablation	
	AV nodal re-entrant tachycardia	Yes	Yes	Rare	Ablation β-Blockers (e.g., metoprolol, atenolol)* Calcium-channel blockers (e.g., diltiazem)*	
	AV re-entrant tachycardia (WPW)	Yes	Yes	Rare	Ablation Antiarrhythmic drugs*	
VT	Idiopathic (RV outflow tract, fascicular)	Yes	Yes	Occasional	Ablation	Absence of structural heart disease Low risk for sudden death
	VT secondary to CAD, cardiomyopathy	Yes	Yes	Yes	ICD Amiodarone (400 mg qd)* Ablation	Increased incidence of sudden death
	Bundle branch re-entry	Yes	Yes	Yes	Ablation	Usually in the setting of LV dysfunction and baseline intraventricular conduction delay
	Genetic syndromes (e.g., long QT syndrome, Brugada, arrhythmic right ventricular dysplasia)	Occasional	Yes	Yes	ICD	Not always a clear family history Increased incidence of sudden death
Ectopy	PACs	Occasional	No	No	None β-Blockers (e.g., atenolol, metoprolol) if symptomatic*	
	PVCs	Occasional	No	No	None β-Blockers (e.g., atenolol, metoprolol) if symptomatic*	Benign in absence of structural heart disease
NEUROCARDIOGENIC SYNCOPE		No	Yes	Yes	Behavioral (hydration, avoid triggers, abort episodes) Midodrine (10 mg tid)	

*See Table 52-2 for drug doses.

AV = atrioventricular; CAD = coronary artery disease; ICD = implantable cardioverter-defibrillator; LV = left ventricle; PACs = premature atrial contractions; PVCs = premature ventricular contractions; RV = right ventricle; SVT = supraventricular tachycardia; VT = ventricular tachycardia; WPW = Wolff-Parkinson-White syndrome.

syncopal episode or ≥6 seconds during a presyncopal episode) or (b) a positive tilt test, dual-chamber pacing reduces subsequent syncope significantly.[A10, A11]

In syncope related to glossopharyngeal neuralgia (Chapter 367), the pain can usually be prevented by carbamazepine (400 to 1000 mg/day total in divided doses of 2 to 3 times per day orally). In refractory cases, 300 mg/day in divided doses of 1 to 4 times per day of phenytoin can be added.

Neurological Syncope

Patients who are at risk for basilar artery stroke should be treated with aspirin and should be considered for other treatments (e.g., surgery, stent placement) appropriate for their symptoms and anatomy (Chapter 376). For subclavian stenosis, repair of the stenosis is the treatment of choice. For other patients with cerebrovascular disease, the potential value of antithrombotic therapy and cerebral revascularization procedures must be considered according to standard criteria (Chapter 376). Seizures require anti-epileptic medications (Chapter 372). Basilar artery migraine requires careful medical therapy (Chapter 367).

PROGNOSIS

One syncopal event predicts a substantial risk for recurrent syncope. Although a history of syncope itself does not appear to increase the risk for a motor vehicle crash,[16] patients with cardiac or cerebrovascular causes have higher mortality rates than patients with definable noncardiac causes or those without a definable cause. For otherwise healthy individuals discharged with a primary diagnosis of syncope, the subsequent risk for all-cause mortality is increased by 6%, with stroke increased by 35%, and a cardiovascular hospitalization by 75%. Among patients who come to an emergency department, the overall death rate is about 7.5% at 1 year. In patients with inherited arrhythmias, such as long QT syndrome (Chapter 53), syncope worsens prognosis. Compared with other patients with supraventricular tachycardia, syncope per se does not increase mortality but does increase the likelihood of needing medical or ablation therapy (Chapter 54).

TABLE 49-9 DRIVING IN PATIENTS WITH ARRHYTHMIAS

CARDIOVASCULAR DISORDER	DRIVING RESTRICTION
SVT: atrial fibrillation, atrial flutter, narrow-complex SVT, wide-complex SVT	No driving if symptomatic Can drive if asymptomatic for 1 month (3-6 months for wide-complex SVT)
VT, VF	No driving for 6 months
Bradyarrhythmias	No restriction if asymptomatic; no driving if syncope occurs
After successful catheter ablation	Can drive after recovery from procedure
After pacemaker implantation	No driving for 1 week (4 weeks for commercial drivers)
After ICD implantation	No driving for 6 months (barred from commercial driving)

ICD = implantable cardioverter-defibrillator; SVT = supraventricular tachycardia; VF = ventricular fibrillator; VT = ventricular tachycardia.

Adapted from Banning AS, Ng GA. Driving and arrhythmia: a review of scientific basis for international guidelines. *Eur Heart J.* 2013;34:236-244.

In patients with arrhythmias, a key issue is whether they should be allowed to drive a motor vehicle. Consensus recommendations vary depending on the arrhythmia and its treatment (Table 49-9).

GENERAL REFERENCES

For the General References and other additional features, please visit Elsevier eBooks+ at https://ebooks.health.elsevier.com.

Grade A References

A1. Kahwati LC, Asher GN, Kadro ZO, et al. Screening for atrial fibrillation: updated evidence report and systematic review for the US Preventive Services Task Force. *JAMA.* 2022;327:368-383.

A2. Steinhubl SR, Waalen J, Edwards AM, et al. Effect of a home-based wearable continuous ECG monitoring patch on detection of undiagnosed atrial fibrillation: the mSToPS randomized clinical trial. *JAMA.* 2018;320:146-155.

A3. Bernstein RA, Kamel H, Granger CB, et al. Effect of long-term continuous cardiac monitoring vs usual care on detection of atrial fibrillation in patients with stroke attributed to large- or small-vessel disease: the STROKE-AF randomized clinical trial. *JAMA.* 2021;325:2169-2177.

A4. Buck BH, Hill MD, Quinn FR, et al. Effect of implantable vs prolonged external electrocardiographic monitoring on atrial fibrillation detection in patients with ischemic stroke: the PER DIEM randomized clinical trial. *JAMA.* 2021;325:2160-2168.

A5. Svendsen JH, Diederichsen SZ, Højberg S, et al. Implantable loop recorder detection of atrial fibrillation to prevent stroke (The LOOP Study): a randomised controlled trial. *Lancet.* 2021;398:1507-1516.

A6. Sheldon R, Raj SR, Rose MS, et al. Fludrocortisone for the prevention of vasovagal syncope: a randomized, placebo-controlled trial. *J Am Coll Cardiol.* 2016;68:1-9.

A7. Lei LY, Raj SR, Sheldon RS. Midodrine for the prevention of vasovagal syncope: a systematic review and meta-analysis. *Europace.* 2022;24:1171-1178.

A8. Flevari P, Leftheriotis D, Repasos E, et al. Fluoxetine vs. placebo for the treatment of recurrent vasovagal syncope with anxiety sensitivity. *Europace.* 2017;19:127-131.

A9. Garland EM, Gamboa A, Nwazue VC, et al. Effect of high dietary sodium intake in patients with postural tachycardia syndrome. *J Am Coll Cardiol.* 2021;77:2174-2184.

A10. Baron-Esquivias G, Morillo CA, Moya-Mitjans A, et al. Dual-chamber pacing with closed loop stimulation in recurrent reflex vasovagal syncope: the SPAIN Study. *J Am Coll Cardiol.* 2017;70:1720-1728.

A11. Bignole M, Russo V, Arabia F, et al. Cardiac pacing in severe recurrent reflect syncope and tilt-induced asystole. *Eur Heart J.* 2021;42:508-516.

50 CARDIAC ARREST AND LIFE-THREATENING ARRHYTHMIAS

ROBERT J. MYERBURG AND RACHEL LAMPERT

Sudden cardiac arrest is characterized by an abrupt loss of consciousness because of absence of cerebral blood flow owing to loss of cardiac pumping action. If not treated promptly, it will lead to central nervous system injury within minutes and a progressively increasing risk of death. Sudden cardiac arrest is often forewarned by a change in cardiovascular status, as indicated by the onset or worsening of symptoms related to transient arrhythmias, such as palpitations, lightheadedness, or near-syncope or syncope (Chapter 49). Other forewarnings may include new or worsening chest pain, dyspnea, or weakness. In individual patients, however, these warning symptoms have limited sensitivity and predictive power for sudden cardiac arrest because they also predict acute coronary syndromes (Chapter 57) and acute myocardial infarction (MI) (Chapter 58) in the absence of expressed arrhythmia. Further, sudden cardiac arrest is often the first manifestation of cardiac disease.

EPIDEMIOLOGY

The population burden of sudden cardiac arrest leading to sudden cardiac death is described by the rule of 50 s—specifically, sudden cardiac death accounts for about 50% of all cardiovascular deaths, about 50% of which are first cardiac events in apparently healthy individuals with unrecognized disease, and resulting in 50% of the loss of years of productivity owing to cardiovascular diseases.[1] The incidence in the general population over the age of 35 years is 1 to 2 per 1000 per year. Among adolescents and young adults, it is 1 per 100,000 per year. Most sudden cardiac arrests occur out of hospital (>375,000/year in the United States, with an average survival rate of 10%), and an additional 200,000 or so occur in hospital, with about a 25% survival rate.

Coronary artery disease is the most common cause of sudden cardiac arrest, either during acute events or as a consequence of chronic disease. Patients with advanced ischemic and nonischemic cardiomyopathies (Chapter 47) and with heart failure (Chapters 45 and 46) are at higher risk, although the incidence in heart failure appears to be decreasing as a result of improved long-term therapies. Patients with either common or rare acquired and inherited arrhythmia syndromes (Chapters 52 and 53) are also at increased risk for sudden cardiac arrest. In addition, both competitive athletes and individuals participating in high-intensity recreational athletic activities have a low but finite increase in risk for sudden cardiac arrest. Risk is higher in males and in association with specific sports, such as basketball and football in the United States and cycling, jogging, and soccer in Europe. In adolescents and young adults in the United States, hypertrophic cardiomyopathy (Chapter 47) is the most commonly identified structural cause in competitive athletes.[2] In individuals under 35 years, 40% of patients have no structural cardiac abnormalities at autopsy ("sudden unexplained death"), among whom about 25% have a clinically relevant variant in postmortem genetic testing.[3] Beyond the age of 30 to 35 years, coronary artery disease is more common (Chapter 58). Offspring in families in which sudden cardiac arrest was the initial manifestation of heart disease are themselves at increased risk for arrest as the initial manifestation of heart disease, thereby emphasizing the importance of a careful family history for assessing risk.[4]

PATHOBIOLOGY

In the past, ventricular fibrillation (VF) and pulseless ventricular tachycardia (VT) were the most common initially identified electrical mechanisms of sudden cardiac arrest (Chapter 53), largely in association with acute MI. However, asystole and pulseless electrical activity are now the first recorded rhythm in the majority of both in-hospital and out-of-hospital cases. Asystole may be primary or may follow deterioration or active termination of VF by electrical cardioversion. Pulseless electrical activity is defined as primary when it is the initial rhythm noted in patients with predisposing cardiac disorders and as secondary when it occurs in the setting of noncardiac predisposing factors, such as hypoxemia, metabolic disorders, massive pulmonary embolism, or blood loss.

Premature ventricular contractions (PVCs) and short runs of nonsustained VT may forewarn a long-term risk for sudden cardiac arrest, primarily when associated with advanced structural heart disease, but there is no evidence that suppression of chronic PVCs is protective. In contrast, sustained wide-QRS tachycardias are of greater concern and should be considered of ventricular origin, because of their potentially high immediate risk, until determined otherwise (Chapter 49).

It is important to recognize that not all out-of-hospital sudden deaths are cardiac in origin. Other causes include pulmonary embolism (Chapter 68), ruptured aortic aneurysm (Chapter 63), aortic dissection (Chapter 63), and acute neurologic events such as intracerebral or subarachnoid hemorrhage (Chapter 377).[5,6]

CLINICAL MANIFESTATIONS AND DIAGNOSIS

Pulselessness, in conjunction with the absence of respiratory efforts or only gasping or agonal respirations and absence of responsiveness, is diagnostic of cardiac arrest. Although the absence of a carotid or femoral pulse is a primary diagnostic criterion for health care professionals, palpation for a pulse is no longer recommended for lay responders. The absence of respiratory efforts or severe stridor with persistence of a pulse suggests a primary respiratory arrest that may lead to cardiac arrest in a short time.

In the out-of-hospital setting, the rhythm can be diagnosed by an automatic external defibrillator, when available. In the inpatient setting, electrocardiographic monitoring should be started immediately. The underlying arrhythmia can be VF, VT, supraventricular tachycardia, bradycardia, asystole, or pulseless electrical activity, with the latter implying electrical activity during which no pulse is generated (Fig. 50-1). VF is recognized by the disorganized electrical activity with no recognizable QRS. If the electrocardiogram (ECG) reveals pulseless electrical activity, potentially treatable causes include hypovolemia (Chapter 102), hypoxia (Chapter 90), cardiac tamponade (Chapter 62), tension pneumothorax (Chapter 86), drug overdose (Chapter 96), hypothermia (Chapter 95), and hyperkalemia (Chapter 103). For a wide-complex tachycardia, differentiating VT from a supraventricular tachycardia can be more challenging (see Fig. 49-3 and Table 53-2).

For at least 50% of survivors of a cardiac arrest, the arrest represents the first manifestation of cardiac disease, and diagnosing the underlying cause is critical for treatment to and prevent recurrence. The leading causes of out-of-hospital cardiac arrest are ischemic heart disease, structural heart disease, and primary arrhythmias (Table 50-1), but a variety of severe noncardiac conditions can also be responsible and are more frequent when a patient arrests in a hospital.

Systematic clinical testing should start with an ECG, blood testing for electrolytes and toxicology, echocardiography, and imaging for coronary artery disease or coronary artery anomalies. Cardiac magnetic resonance imaging (Chapter 44) is more sensitive than echocardiography and should also be performed if the diagnosis remains elusive. If the underlying diagnosis remains unclear after initial testing, provocative stress testing may reveal arrhythmic syndromes such as catecholaminergic ventricular tachycardia (Chapter 53) or a subclinical arrhythmogenic cardiomyopathy, and pharmacologic testing may unmask other rare arrhythmic syndromes. Genetic testing can reveal an underlying abnormality in about 10 to 30% of patients whose other tests have been unrevealing.[6]

TREATMENT

The management of a patient during cardiac arrest emphasizes actions to maintain blood flow to preserve the viability of the central nervous system, heart, and other vital organs, while striving to restore spontaneous circulation as quickly as possible. These goals are accomplished by assessing the patient and contacting an emergency response system (EMS), followed quickly by initiating basic life support (BLS), early defibrillation for patients with VF or pulseless VT, advanced life support (ACLS) as needed, and post–cardiac arrest care.

Cardiopulmonary resuscitation (CPR) performed by bystanders in the community or at sporting events before EMS arrival is associated with a 30-day

TABLE 50-1 CAUSES OF OUT-OF-HOSPITAL CARDIAC ARREST

CARDIAC CAUSES
- Ischemic heart disease with or without acute myocardial infarction
- Cardiomyopathy (e.g., myocarditis, hypertrophic, infiltrative, dilated), arrhythmogenic right ventricular cardiomyopathy
- Valvular heart disease
- Pericardial tamponade
- Congenital heart disease, including coronary artery anomalies
- Arrhythmia without ischemic or structural heart disease (e.g., Wolff-Parkinson-White syndrome, long QT syndrome, Brugada syndrome, catecholaminergic polymorphic ventricular tachycardia)

NONCARDIAC CAUSES
- Traumatic or nontraumatic bleeding
- Cerebrovascular accident
- Aortic dissection or rupture
- Hypoxia (e.g., pulmonary embolism, pneumonia, carbon monoxide poisoning, asthma, or chronic obstructive pulmonary disease)
- Drug overdose
- Hypoglycemia
- Hypothermia or hyperthermia
- Epilepsy
- Tension pneumothorax
- Septic shock
- Electrolyte abnormalities
- Severe dehydration

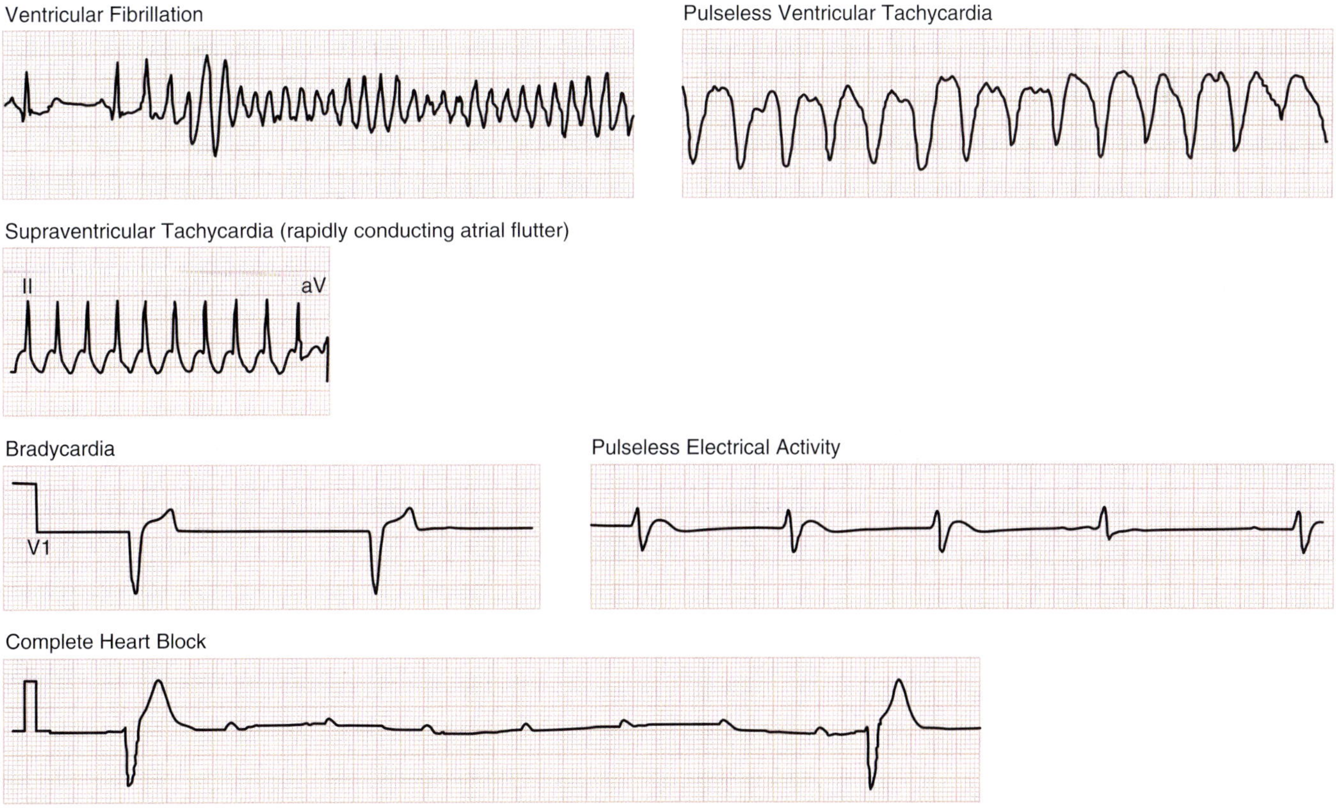

FIGURE 50-1. Electrical mechanisms associated with cardiac arrest. Shockable mechanisms include ventricular fibrillation and pulseless ventricular tachycardia. Pulseless electrical activity (as distinct from pulseless ventricular tachycardia) is a mechanical rather than an electrical disorder, and shocks are not indicated.

survival rate that is more than twice as high as that associated with no CPR before the arrival of EMS.[7,8] A mobile-phone system dispatch of lay volunteers trained in CPR and located within about one third of a mile of the victim can increase the rate of lay response by about 40%.[A1] In the United States, however, Black and Hispanic persons are 20 to 35% less likely to receive bystander CPR regardless of the location of their arrest.[9]

Basic Life Support

After an initial evaluation for response to voice or tactile stimulation, observation for respiratory movements and skin color, and simultaneous palpation of major arteries for the presence of a pulse, the determination that a life-threatening incident is in progress should prompt immediate contact with EMS (911).

When a cardiac arrest is confirmed, the goal of BLS is to establish perfusion as quickly as possible using CPR or the concept of cardiocerebral resuscitation (see later). The algorithm of BLS is compression-airway-breathing, based on the recognition that compression alone is the primary maneuver because the patient is better perfused by minimizing interruptions between compressions and can be harmed by excessive ventilation.

A precordial thump may be attempted by a trained rescuer as part of an initial response, although its added benefit is questionable. The technique involves one or two blows delivered firmly to the junction of the middle and lower thirds of the sternum from a height of 8 to 10 inches. It should not be used in an unmonitored patient with a perceptible rapid tachycardia or without complete loss of consciousness because of concern about converting organized electrical activity into VF.

Prompt initiation of CPR, which can be performed by professional and paraprofessional personnel, by emergency medical technicians, and by trained laypersons, is the key element for successful resuscitation. The delay between diagnosis and starting CPR should be minimal. If only one witness is present, the only activity that should precede BLS is telephone contact (911) of EMS. The untrained lay bystander can be prompted on how to perform CPR by the EMS telecommunicator.

Clearing the airway includes tilting the head backward and lifting the chin, in addition to exploring the airway for foreign bodies—including dentures—and removing them. The Heimlich maneuver, which entails wrapping the arms around the victim from the back and delivering a sharp thrust to the upper part of the abdomen with a closed fist, should be performed if there is reason to suspect a foreign body lodged in the oropharynx, as suggested by severe respiratory stridor, in contrast to slow agonal respirations or apnea, especially in a patient who is eating at the time of the arrest. When the person at the scene has insufficient physical strength to perform the maneuver, mechanical dislodgment of a foreign body can sometimes be achieved by abdominal thrusts with the unconscious patient in a supine position. If there is suspicion that respiratory arrest precipitated the cardiac arrest, particularly in the presence of a mechanical airway obstruction, a second precordial thump should be delivered after the airway has been cleared.

With the head properly positioned and the oropharynx clear, mouth-to-mouth respiration can be initiated. With the exception of Heimlich maneuvers, however, mechanical ventilation strategies are now reserved for EMS responders and medical professionals, rather than bystanders. Devices for establishing ventilation include plastic oropharyngeal airways, esophageal obturators for establishing ventilation, a masked Ambu bag, and endotracheal tubes. Intubation is the preferred procedure, but time should not be sacrificed, even in the in-hospital setting, while awaiting an endotracheal tube or a person trained to insert it. Temporary support with Ambu bag ventilation is the usual method in the hospital until endotracheal intubation can be accomplished. When ventilatory support is provided by EMS responders in the out-of-hospital setting, the lungs should be inflated twice in succession after every 30 chest compressions.

Circulatory support, which is the primary element of BLS, is intended to maintain blood flow until definitive steps can be taken to restore effective cardiac contractions. The rationale is based on the hypothesis that chest compression maintains an externally driven pump function by sequential emptying and filling of its chambers, with competent valves favoring forward flow. The palm of one hand is placed over the lower sternum while the heel of the other rests on the dorsum of the lower hand. The sternum is then depressed with the resuscitator's arms straight at the elbows to provide a less tiring and more forceful fulcrum at the junction of the shoulders and back. A force sufficient to depress the sternum at least 2 inches (>5cm) should be applied, with abrupt relaxation. The cycle is carried out at a rate of about 100 compressions per minute. Compression-only CPR is as good as, if not perhaps slightly better than, compression plus rescue breathing, in part because it may be more effective than compression-ventilation sequences, encourages more bystander CPR by untrained or remotely trained bystanders who lack confidence, and also allays concerns about mouth-to-mouth ventilation of unknown victims in the absence of mechanical airway devices.[A2,A3] An alternative is a compression-ventilation ratio of 30:2 for single responders to victims through adulthood and for two responders to adult victims. For two-rescuer CPR for infants and children, the recommended compression-ventilation ratio is 15 : 2. Another recently suggested modification is the "hands-only" (cardiac-only, compression-only) technique, which uses 200 successive compressions without interruption. In the prehospital setting, therapeutic hypothermia is not beneficial.[A4]

Intermediate Life Support: Automated External Defibrillators

Despite the benefit of BLS, time to defibrillation is the major determinant of survival for victims in VF or pulseless VT. Because ACLS strategies are generally implemented by in-hospital personnel or out-of-hospital EMS responders, an intermediate strategy is for nonconventional first responders to use automated external defibrillators. These devices prompt the user to deliver a defibrillation shock when deemed appropriate by a computerized rhythm detection system integrated into the device. The operators can be trained police officers, security guards, airline personnel, or trained or untrained lay bystanders (Table 50-2). A number of studies have suggested improved survival rates when such strategies are deployed in public sites,[A5] but an initial study of a home deployment strategy was disappointing. Further study is warranted because 70 to 80% of out-of-hospital cardiac arrests occur at home, with survival rates less than 6%. Automated external defibrillators, which serve as an intermediate supplement to the BLS-ACLS sequence, are intended to attempt earlier defibrillation while awaiting the arrival of ACLS-trained emergency personnel.

Advanced Cardiac Life Support

ACLS methods, other than those directly related to control of tachyarrhythmias, are guided by comprehensive protocols to aid responders over a broad expanse of clinical circumstances and mechanisms of cardiac arrest, ranging from transient clinical events to end-stage multisystem disease. The primary goals of ACLS are to restore a hemodynamically effective cardiac rhythm, optimize ventilation, and maintain and support the restored circulation. During ACLS, the first priority is prompt cardioversion or defibrillation of persisting pulseless VT or VF, if appropriate equipment is immediately available. If cardiac arrest has occurred for 4 to 5 minutes before the availability of a defibrillator, a short period of cardiac compressions immediately before defibrillation increases the probability of survival. The administration of epinephrine in this setting to all patients can increase 30-day overall survival but not survival with a favorable neurologic outcome.[A6] In the in-hospital setting, vasopressin (20 IU) plus methylprednisolone (40 mg) similarly can increase the likelihood of a return to spontaneous circulation but not of a favorable neurologic outcome.[A7] If the initial attempt to restore circulation is

TABLE 50-2 AUTOMATED EXTERNAL DEFIBRILLATOR STRATEGIES FOR RAPID RESPONSE TO CARDIAC ARRESTS CAUSED BY VENTRICULAR FIBRILLATION

DEPLOYMENT	EXAMPLES	RESCUERS	ADVANTAGES	LIMITATIONS
Emergency vehicles	Police cars Fire engines Ambulances	Trained emergency personnel	Experienced users Broad deployment Objectivity	Deployment time Arrival delays Community variations
Public access sites	Public buildings Stadiums, malls Airports Airliners	Security personnel Designated rescuers Random laypersons	Population density Shorter delays Lay and emergency personnel access	Low event rates Inexperienced users Panic and confusion
Multifamily dwellings	Apartments Condominiums Hotels	Security personnel Designated rescuers Family members	Familiar locations Defined personnel Shorter delays	Infrequent use Low event rates Geographic factors
Single-family dwellings	Private homes Apartments Neighborhood "heart watch"	Family members	Immediate access Familiar setting	Acceptance Victim may be alone One-time user; panic

unsuccessful, continued on-scene resuscitation may be preferred to immediate transfer to a hospital.[10] In patients who do not respond to standard defibrillation, either rapid sequential shocks from two defibrillators or switching the pads to an anterior-posterior position is preferable to repeated standard shocks.[A8]

After the initial attempt to restore a hemodynamically effective rhythm, the patient is intubated and oxygenated, if needed. Electrical pacing of the heart should be attempted if a severe bradyarrhythmia or asystole is present (Chapter 54). An intravenous line is established to deliver medications. After intubation, the goal of ventilation is to reverse hypoxemia and not merely to achieve a high alveolar P_{O_2}. When available, oxygen rather than room air should be used to ventilate the patient, and arterial O_2 saturation should be monitored, when possible. In the out-of-hospital setting, a face mask or an Ambu bag by means of an endotracheal tube is generally used.

Approach to Specific Arrhythmias

Tachyarrhythmic Cardiac Arrest

Slow, well-tolerated monomorphic VTs, especially in the absence of structural heart disease, can usually be treated with antiarrhythmic drugs or β-adrenergic blocking agents in some circumstances (see Tables 52-2 and 52-3 in Chapter 52). In contrast, when rapid VT or VF is identified on a monitor or by telemetry, immediate cardioversion or defibrillation should be performed (Fig. 50-2). When a reversible cause, such as an acute ischemic syndrome or electrolyte disturbance,

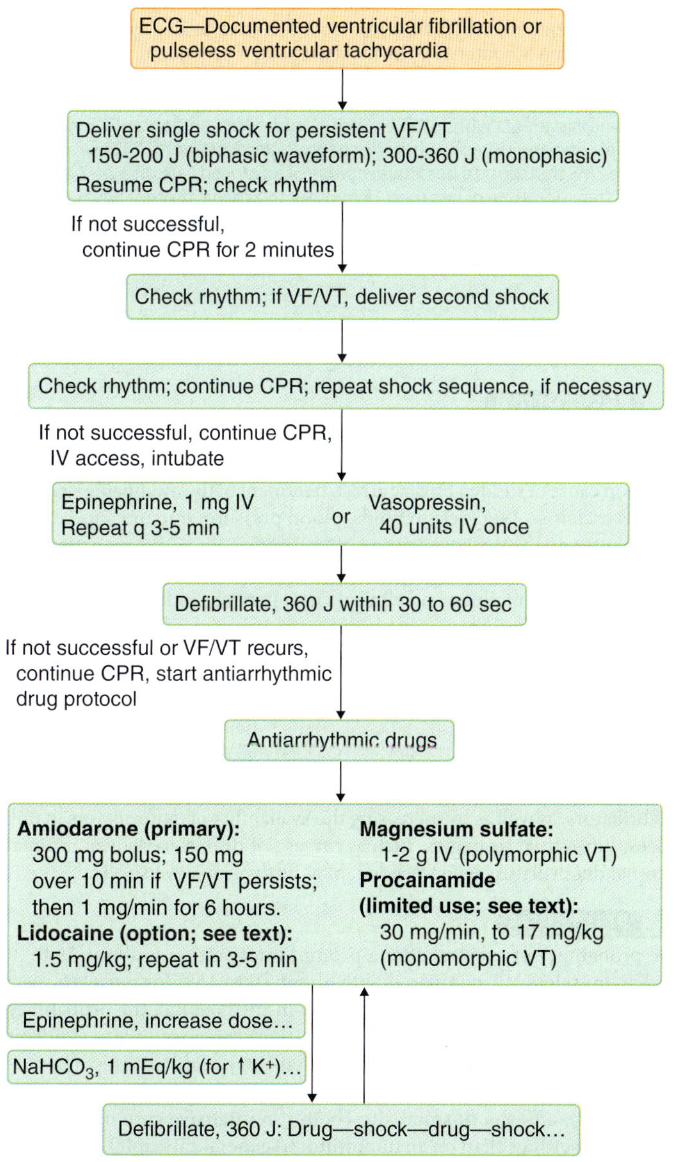

FIGURE 50-2. General algorithm for advanced cardiac life support (ACLS) response to ventricular fibrillation (VF) or pulseless ventricular tachycardia (VT). For more detail, see the ACLS guidelines in the Grade A References. *Note:* In a 2008 advisory, 200 compression-only sequences were suggested as an alternative to standard cardiopulmonary resuscitation (CPR) cycles between shocks, and this approach is under consideration for future guidelines. ECG = electrocardiogram; IV = intravenous; K^+ = potassium; $NaHCO_3$ = sodium bicarbonate.

is the apparent mechanism, normal rhythm can be successfully restored in up to 90% of VF victims weighing up to 90 kg with a direct current (DC) biphasic shock of up to 200 joules delivered within 2 to 3 minutes, or if such equipment is not available, a monophasic shock of up to 360 joules. Failure of the initial shock to restore an effective rhythm is a poor prognostic sign.

After a single shock, the patient should be checked immediately for restoration of a spontaneous pulse; CPR should be continued for five cycles if a pulse remains absent. Subsequently, a second shock should be delivered, followed by epinephrine 1 mg intravenously (IV). If a pulse is still absent, CPR is repeated for five cycles before the next shock. Epinephrine may be repeated at 3- to 5-minute intervals with defibrillator shocks in between, but high-dose epinephrine does not appear to provide added benefit. Vasopressin (40 U given IV once) is an equally good alternative to epinephrine,[A8] but the combination does not appear to be better than either alone.

SVTs can precipitate cardiac arrest in two circumstances. One is in patients with high-grade coronary artery disease, in whom rapid heart rates can cause myocardial ischemia because of the dependence of coronary blood flow on the diastolic interval. In this setting, the arrhythmia should be treated urgently by restoring sinus rhythm or slowing the heart rate, either by medical therapy (e.g., intravenous adenosine, β-blockers, or calcium channel blockers) (Chapter 52) or by electrical DC cardioversion (Chapter 54). The second mechanism of concern is atrial fibrillation in patients with Wolff-Parkinson-White syndrome, who may have ventricular rates greater than 240 beats per minute when the accessory pathway has a short refractory period (see Fig. 52-10 in Chapter 52). This abnormality, which can trigger VF or cause hypotensive VT, requires prompt slowing or termination of the SVT (Chapter 52).

Pharmacotherapy for Resistant Arrhythmias

For a patient who continues in VF or pulseless VT despite multiple attempts at DC cardioversion after epinephrine, or who has recurrent episodes of VF or VT after cardioversion, the likelihood of return of spontaneous circulation and survival to hospitalization may be increased by administering intravenous antiarrhythmic agents while continuing resuscitative efforts (see Fig. 50-2). Amiodarone and lidocaine are equivalent to each other and better than placebo when the cardiac arrest is witnessed by bystanders or EMS, but neither is better than placebo for patients who suffer unwitnessed arrests.[A9]

Amiodarone is given as a 150-mg intravenous bolus over a 10-minute period, followed by 1 mg/minute for up to 6 hours and 0.5 mg/minute thereafter. Additional bolus dosing, to a maximum of 500 mg, can be tried if the initial bolus is unsuccessful. The lidocaine dose is a 1.0- to 1.5-mg/kg intravenous bolus, with the dose repeated in 2 minutes. Neither drug needs to be given as a routine to individuals who respond to initial defibrillation with a persistently stable rhythm. For patients who remain electrically unstable or have recurrent episodes of VT or VF after initial defibrillation and oxygenation, continued antiarrhythmic therapy is indicated.

If there is sufficient clinical evidence that the cardiac arrest was associated with an acute coronary syndrome or that recurrent arrhythmias are precipitated by ischemia, lidocaine may be used in preference to amiodarone. Under other circumstances, intravenous amiodarone may be the preferred initial drug. Under all circumstances, the alternative drug may be tried if the initial choice fails. Intravenous procainamide (loading infusion of 100 mg/5 minutes to a total dose of 500 to 800 mg, followed by a continuous infusion at 2 to 5 mg/minute) is now rarely used but may be tried in those with persisting, hemodynamically unstable arrhythmias.

In patients with acute hyperkalemia as the triggering event for resistant VF, hypocalcemia, or arrest potentially caused by excess doses of calcium-blocking drugs, 10% calcium gluconate (5 to 20 mL infused at a rate of 2 to 4 mL/minute) may be helpful. Otherwise, calcium should not be used routinely during resuscitation, even though ionized Ca^{2+} levels may be low during resuscitation from cardiac arrest.

Resistant forms of polymorphic VT (*torsades de pointes*), rapid monomorphic VT, ventricular flutter (rate >260/minute), or resistant VF may respond to magnesium sulfate ($MgSO_4$) (1 to 2 g given IV over a 1- to 2-minute period) or to β-blocker therapy (propranolol, 1-mg boluses IV to a total dose of up to 15 to 20 mg or metoprolol 5 mg IV, up to 20 mg). $MgSO_4$ is specifically indicated for polymorphic VTs due to inherited or acquired (drug-induced) long QT patterns (Chapter 53). This VT pattern also occurs with marked hypokalemia. Potassium chloride (20 mEq/hour intravenously) should be included in the treatment of patients with these arrhythmias if their serum potassium level is less than 3 mEq/L. However, hypokalemia also may follow the acid-base and electrolyte shifts associated with prolonged arrests and should not be considered a primary cause of the cardiac arrest in that circumstance.

Asystole, Bradyarrhythmias, and Pulseless Electrical Activity

The approach to a patient with symptomatic bradyarrhythmia, asystolic arrest, or pulseless electrical activity differs from the approach to patients with tachyarrhythmic events (pulseless VT or VF). Effective CPR is critical because no electrical strategies are effective for restoring circulation. As soon as this mechanism of cardiac arrest is recognized, efforts should focus on continuous CPR, intubation, and establishing intravenous access. Possible reversible causes, including hypovolemia, hypoxia, cardiac tamponade, tension pneumothorax, preexisting

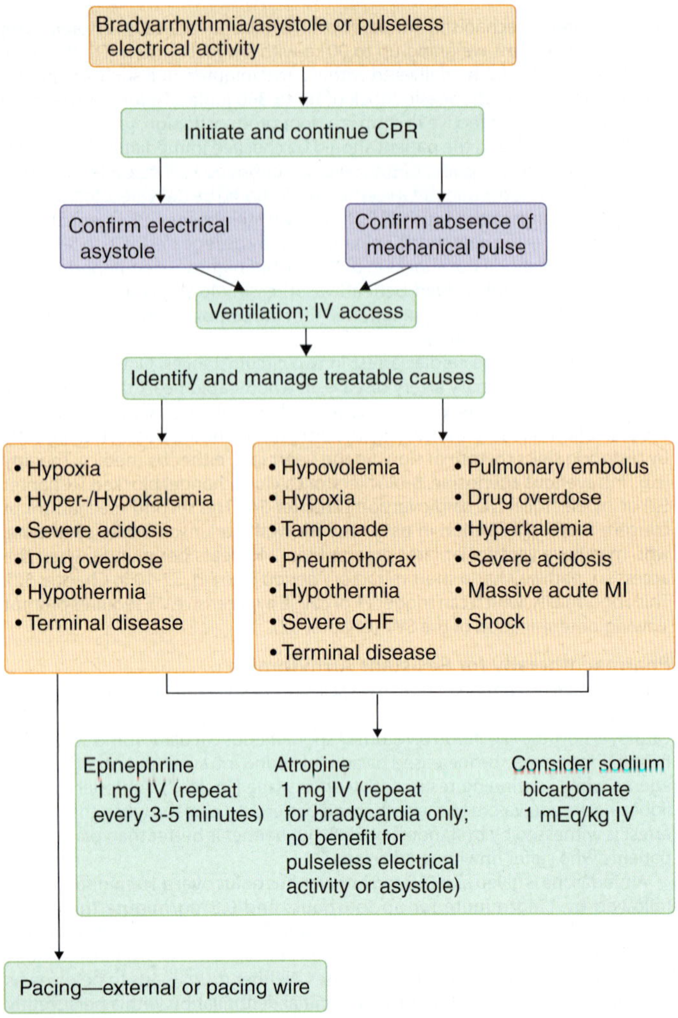

FIGURE 50-3. General algorithm for advanced cardiac life support response to bradycardic or asystolic cardiac arrest or pulseless electrical activity. For more detail, see the Grade A References. CHF = congestive heart failure; CPR = cardiopulmonary resuscitation; IV = intravenous; MI = myocardial infarction.

acidosis, drug overdose, hypothermia, and hyperkalemia, must be identified and treated immediately (Fig. 50-3). Respiratory causes of pulseless electrical activity or asystole may respond promptly to appropriate interventions, as do tamponade and hypovolemic causes. Epinephrine (1.0 mg IV every 3 to 5 minutes) or isoproterenol (up to 15 to 20 μg/minute IV), which are commonly used in an attempt to elicit spontaneous electrical activity or increase the rate of a bradycardia, have only limited success. However, one randomized trial of patients with cardiac arrest requiring vasopressors showed that combined vasopressin-epinephrine plus methylprednisolone during CPR and stress-dose hydrocortisone in postresuscitation shock improved survival to hospital discharge with favorable neurologic status compared with epinephrine-saline placebo. In the absence of an intravenous line, epinephrine (1 mg, i.e., 10 mL of a 1 : 10,000 solution) may be given by the intracardiac route, despite the danger of coronary artery or myocardial laceration. Sodium bicarbonate (1 mEq/kg) may be tried for known or strongly suspected preexisting hyperkalemia or bicarbonate-responsive acidosis but is no longer recommended for routine use. Atropine is no longer recommended for management of bradyarrhythmic cardiac arrests because of lack of efficacy.

External pacing (Chapter 54) should be tried for out-of-hospital bradycardic or asystolic cardiac arrests, although existing data suggest little effect on outcome. In-hospital, external pacing is generally used during the initial response to a bradycardic or asystolic arrest, but it should be superseded by transvenous pacing if the arrest is prolonged, if continuous pacing is needed, or if the external device fails to pace. Unfortunately, an *asystolic* patient continues to have a very poor prognosis.

Postresuscitation Care

After return of spontaneous circulation, particularly following a prolonged resuscitation, attention shifts to the elements of injury caused by cardiac arrest. The four components of the post–cardiac arrest syndrome include brain injury,[11] myocardial dysfunction, systemic ischemia-reperfusion responses, and control of persistent precipitating factors. The therapeutic goal is to maintain a stable electrical, hemodynamic, and central nervous system status. Specific therapy is determined by the clinical circumstances. The most pressing issue is the presence of anoxic encephalopathy, which is a strong predictor of in-hospital death and postarrest disability. To prevent postarrest encephalopathy, therapeutic cooling to prevent hyperthermia improves neurologic outcomes, but a target of 36°C appears to be as good as targeted hypothermia.[A10,A11] After 24 to 48 hours of cooling, patients should be gradually rewarmed to 37°C. For patients who suffer in-hospital cardiac arrest, therapeutic hypothermia does not appear to be beneficial.

During or after therapy targeted to restoration of an electrically stable cardiac rhythm, the patient's general metabolic state should be addressed by improving oxygenation and reversing acidosis. Intravenous sodium bicarbonate (1 mEq/kg), with up to 50% of this dose repeated every 10 to 15 minutes during the course of CPR, is recommended for patients with known or suspected preexisting bicarbonate-responsive causes of acidosis, for certain drug overdoses (Chapter 96), and after prolonged and unsuccessful attempts at resuscitation. Caution must be exercised, however, because excessive quantities of sodium bicarbonate can be deleterious by causing alkalosis, hypernatremia, and hyperosmolality. Furthermore, goal-directed optimization of oxygenation does not improve neurologic outcomes.[A12] When possible, arterial pH, P_{O_2}, and P_{CO_2} should be monitored during the resuscitation. Myocardial injury (Chapter 58) and hemodynamic dysfunction (Chapter 93) are managed by standard techniques, and a mean arterial blood pressure target of 63 mm Hg is as good as a target of 77 mg Hg.[A13]

In parallel with postarrest therapeutic support, diagnostic actions are also indicated, especially when the arrest is suspected to be due to an acute coronary syndrome (Chapter 57). The most pressing is cardiac catheterization followed by coronary interventions (Chapter 59) to help control unstable rhythms associated with persisting ischemia and to preserve myocardium in survivors.[12] However, in patients without ST elevation, immediate angiography is no better than delaying angiography until after neurologic recovery.[A14,A15] These activities require EMS transport to hospitals capable of advanced care on a 24-7 basis. An added transport time of less than 15 minutes to achieve prompt advanced care has been suggested as an appropriate tradeoff. A 2-day course of amoxicillin-clavulanate (1 g, 200 mg) can reduce the risk of ventilator-associated pneumonia but not mortality at 28 days.[A16]

PREVENTION

Prevention of sudden cardiac arrest should focus on preventing the underlying diseases whenever possible. Since coronary artery disease is the most common cause of sudden cardiac arrest, treatment of the modifiable risk factors of atherosclerosis (e.g., serum lipids, blood pressure, smoking, and exercise; see Chapter 40) is the cornerstone of prevention. In addition, patients who have known cardiac diseases, such as patients with a history of myocardial infarction or heart failure, and clinical characteristics indicative of a high risk of ventricular arrhythmias, can benefit from insertion of an implantable cardioverter defibrillator (Chapters 46 and 53). Screening of highly competitive and professional athletes with a history and physical examination is recommended to detect undiagnosed cardiac disease, and an ECG adds further diagnostic sensitivity.[13]

Public health initiatives can improve survival after cardiac arrest by increasing the number of people trained in CPR and in how to use automated external defibrillators, as well as by increasing the availability of defibrillators in public places. Innovative strategies, such as the use of drones to deliver automated external defibrillators when needed, may further improve survival.

PROGNOSIS

The probability of survival after a prompt intervention is about 25 to 30% for VF/pulseless VT compared with about 10 to 15% for pulseless electrical activity and less than 5% for asystole. In the hospital, the probability of survival is determined by the specific patient category (acute syndromes better than end-stage diseases), the mechanism of cardiac arrest (better for tachyarrhythmias than for bradyarrhythmias, asystole, or pulseless electrical activity), and the hospital site (better in intensive care units or other monitored settings than on an unmonitored general care unit).[14] Immediate defibrillation in highly protected settings, such as a cardiac catheterization laboratory where response times of less than 60 seconds are the norm, is associated with greater than a 90% survival rate for VF in the absence of pathophysiologic conditions that tend to perpetuate the potentially fatal arrhythmia. In many acute care settings, including patients with acute coronary syndromes (Chapters 57 and 58), outcomes also can be excellent. For other in-hospital settings and most out-of-hospital settings, the absolute number and proportion of survivors remain low.

The most important determinant of survival from sudden cardiac arrest is time to CPR and defibrillation. Some public locations amenable to very rapid response times achieve survival rates of 50% or higher. If, however, 3 to 4 minutes elapse from the onset of sudden cardiac arrest to attempted defibrillation, the survival rate falls below 50% in most in-hospital and out-of-hospital circumstances. Survival rates continue to fall rapidly thereafter, decreasing to 25% or less by 4 to 6 minutes and to less than 10% by 10 minutes. Although immediate defibrillation is preferred within the first few minutes after the onset, a brief period of CPR improves survivability when the time to defibrillation exceeds 4 to 5 minutes.

The 10-year survival among patients who are discharged alive is about 60%.[15] Long-term prognosis after discharge is determined by a number of factors, including pre-event ventricular function, history of heart failure, and the severity of residual neurologic injury. Bystander resuscitation and defibrillation not only improve survival but also reduce the rate of brain damage and nursing home admission.

Overall, about 40% of patients who survive out-of-hospital cardiac arrest have good quality of life and functional status. Patients whose sudden cardiac arrests are due to a transient arrythmia, who have preserved left ventricular function, and who have minimal, if any, neurologic defects, have a good prognosis. In contrast, patients with advanced heart disease have annual mortality rates that range from 10 to 50%. Most patients who survive but who do not have a predictably reversible cause will receive an implantable cardioverter defibrillator for secondary prevention (Chapter 54). Survivors who receive an implantable defibrillator after a sudden cardiac arrest not due to transient factors (Chapter 54) achieve a relative risk reduction of 25 to 30%, with absolute risk decreasing from 21 to 25% to 15 to 18% over a 2-year follow-up.[A17]

GENERAL REFERENCES

For the General References and other additional features, please visit Elsevier eBooks+ at https://ebooks.health.elsevier.com.

Grade A References

A1. Ringh M, Rosenqvist M, Hollenberg J, et al. Mobile-phone dispatch of laypersons for CPR in out-of-hospital cardiac arrest. *N Engl J Med.* 2015;372:2316-2325.
A2. Nichol G, Leroux B, Wang H, et al. Trial of continuous or interrupted chest compressions during CPR. *N Engl J Med.* 2015;373:2203-2214.
A3. Zhan L, Yang LJ, Huang Y, et al. Continuous chest compression versus interrupted chest compression for cardiopulmonary resuscitation of non-asphyxial out-of-hospital cardiac arrest. *Cochrane Database Syst Rev.* 2017;3:CD010134.
A4. Szarpak L, Filipiak KJ, Mosteller L, et al. Survival, neurological and safety outcomes after out of hospital cardiac arrests treated by using prehospital therapeutic hypothermia: a systematic review and meta-analysis. *Am J Emerg Med.* 2021;42:168-177.
A5. Holmberg MJ, Vognsen M, Andersen MS, et al. Bystander automated external defibrillator use and clinical outcomes after out-of-hospital cardiac arrest: a systematic review and meta-analysis. *Resuscitation.* 2017;120:77-87.
A6. Perkins GD, Ji C, Deakin CD, et al. A randomized trial of epinephrine in out-of-hospital cardiac arrest. *N Engl J Med.* 2018;379:711-721.
A7. Andersen LW, Isbye D, Kjærgaard J, et al. Effect of vasopressin and methylprednisolone vs placebo on return of spontaneous circulation in patients with in-hospital cardiac arrest: a randomized clinical trial. *JAMA.* 2021;326:1586-1594.
A8. Cheskes S, Verbeek PR, Drennan IR, et al. Defibrillation strategies for refractory ventricular fibrillation. *N Engl J Med.* 2022;387:1947-1956.
A9. Kudenchuk PJ, Brown SP, Daya M, et al. Amiodarone, lidocaine, or placebo in out-of-hospital cardiac arrest. *N Engl J Med.* 2016;374:1711-1722.
A10. Holgersson J, Meyer MAS, Dankiewicz J, et al. Hypothermic versus normothermic temperature control after cardiac arrest. *NEJM Evidence.* 2022;1.
A11. Dankiewicz J, Cronberg T, Lilja G, et al. Hypothermia versus normothermia after out-of-hospital cardiac arrest. *N Engl J Med.* 2021;384:2283-2294.
A12. Schmidt H, Kjaergaard J, Hassager C, et al. Oxygen targets in comatose survivors of cardiac arrest. *N Engl J Med.* 2022;387:1467-1476.
A13. Kjaergaard J, Møller JE, Schmidt H, et al. Blood-pressure targets in comatose survivors of cardiac arrest. *N Engl J Med.* 2022;387:1456-1466.
A14. Desch S, Freund A, Akin I, et al. Angiography after out-of-hospital cardiac arrest without ST-segment elevation. *N Engl J Med.* 2021;385:2544-2553.
A15. Nikolaou NI, Netherton S, Welsford M, et al. A systematic review and meta-analysis of the effect of routine early angiography in patients with return of spontaneous circulation after out-of-hospital cardiac arrest. *Resuscitation.* 2021;163:28-48.
A16. François B, Cariou A, Clere-Jehl R, et al. Prevention of early ventilator-associated pneumonia after cardiac arrest. *N Engl J Med.* 2019;381:1831-1842.
A17. Kolodziejczak M, Andreotti F, Kowalewski M, et al. Implantable cardioverter-defibrillators for primary prevention in patients with ischemic or nonischemic cardiomyopathy: a systematic review and meta-analysis. *Ann Intern Med.* 2017;167:103-111.

51 BRADYCARDIAS AND CONDUCTION SYSTEM DELAYS

PETER ZIMETBAUM AND LEE GOLDMAN

BRADYCARDIAS

DEFINITION

The normal human heart rate is typically defined as 60 to 100 beats per minute, and rates below 60 per minute are defined as bradycardia. Bradycardias can be a result of sinus node dysfunction or of atrioventricular (AV) block (Table 51-1). However, many individuals have heart rates below 60 per minute at rest and especially during sleep without any symptoms or signs of hypoperfusion. A bradyarrhythmia is best defined as a heart rate below 60 per minute associated with signs or symptoms, or an awake non–sinus rhythm rate below 60 per minute even in the absence of symptoms.

EPIDEMIOLOGY

Bradycardia (heart rate below 60 beats per minute) is very common, with an estimated prevalence of about 15% in adult males and 7% in adult females.[1] It is even more common (50 to 80% prevalence) in endurance athletes.[2] The prevalence of bradycardia actually diminishes with age, presumably because of age-related declines in parasympathetic activity. During sleep, bradycardia is even more common, with studies of healthy adults showing sinus bradycardia below 40 beats per minute in 20 to 25% of individuals, sinus pauses of two seconds or more in 5 to 10%, first-degree AV block in 8 to 12%, and second-degree Wenckebach block in about 5 to 10%.

However, an overwhelming majority of bradycardias are asymptomatic in individuals who can raise their heart rates to meet increased cardiac demands when needed. As a result, only an estimated 0.26% of U.S. adults have a cardiac pacemaker implanted for any indication, including bradycardia.

PATHOBIOLOGY

The normal cardiac impulse begins in the sinus node complex, which is located at the junction of the right atrium and the superior vena cava. It then travels through the right atrium and primarily activates the left atrium through the coronary sinus. The time it takes to activate the atria is represented by the P wave on the electrocardiogram (ECG). After depolarizing the atria, the impulse enters the AV node, which is located in the inferior septal region of the right atrium, where a delay occurs. This delay allows time for the atria to contract and fill the ventricles. In most individuals, the impulse travels through the AV node over a uniform functional pathway or route. Some people have two or more functional pathways called dual AV nodal pathways (fast and slow pathways). The delay in the AV node represents most of the isoelectric portion of the PR interval on the ECG (E-Fig. 51-1). The usual duration

TABLE 51-1 BRADYCARDIAS

SINUS NODE DYSFUNCTION
Sinus bradycardia <45 beats/min
Sinoatrial exit block
First-degree
Second-degree
Third-degree
Sinus arrest
Bradycardia-tachycardia syndrome
ATRIOVENTRICULAR BLOCK
First-degree
Second-degree
Mobitz type I (Wenckebach phenomenon)
Mobitz type II
Higher degree (e.g., 2 : 1, 3 : 1)
Third-degree
Atrioventricular node
His-Purkinje system

of atrial activation including delay in the AV node is up to 140 msec and can be measured directly as the atrial-His interval. The impulse then travels into the specialized infranodal conducting system, that is, through the His bundle, then right and left bundle branches, and into the Purkinje network. The Purkinje network extends or fans out throughout the ventricular endocardium. Impulses conduct rapidly through the Purkinje network, thereby allowing nearly simultaneous activation of the ventricles. A small portion of the isoelectric segment of the PR interval represents infranodal conduction. This infranodal conduction through the His-Purkinje system (HPS) also can be measured directly (His-ventricle interval) and should take between 40 and 60 msec. Once out of the Purkinje network, the impulse proceeds relatively slowly from the endocardial to epicardial surface of the ventricles. The QRS complex on ECG represents depolarization of the bundle branches and ventricular myocardium.

The normal heart rate is generated by tissues or pacemaker cells with intrinsic automaticity. The sinus node cells produce the greatest rate (60 to 100 beats per minute) of automaticity and suppress other potentially automatic (AV junctional, 40 to 55 beats per minute; His-Purkinje cells, 15 to 40 beats per minute) tissues with slower rates of depolarization. The sinus node and AV node are heavily influenced by the parasympathetic (vagal) and sympathetic (adrenergic) nervous systems. At rest, the parasympathetic system controls sinus node automaticity. With exertion or emotional or physical stress, a withdrawal of parasympathetic tone and an increase in heart rate, which is then perpetuated by sympathetic tone, further increase heart rate. Sinus arrhythmia refers to the normal variation in heart rate with inspiration and expiration. With inspiration, a withdrawal of vagal tone increases heart rate; by comparison, expiration is associated with a drop in heart rate (Fig. 51-1). During sleep, a dominance of vagal tone slows heart rate.

Most bradyarrhythmias are caused by intrinsic idiopathic fibrocalcific degeneration of the cardiac conduction system (Table 51-2). Some patients have congenital heart block,[3] and familial bradycardia can occur. The conduction system also can be damaged by ischemia and myocardial infarction, especially below the AV node. Infiltrative diseases, such as amyloidosis (Chapter 174). Sarcoidosis (Chapter 83)[4] and collagen vascular diseases, such as scleroderma (Chapter 246) or advanced rheumatoid arthritis (Chapter 243), can affect any part of the conduction system. Hypothyroidism (Chapter 207) is also commonly associated with sinus bradycardia.

Systemic infections such as Lyme disease (Chapter 296) can affect the cardiac conduction system. A myocardial abscess in bacterial endocarditis (Chapter 61) can present with acute conduction delays. Iatrogenic causes include medications (Table 51-3),[5] valve replacement surgery (whether open or catheter-based), and intracardiac procedures.[6] Even percutaneous placement of a pulmonary artery catheter can precipitate transient heart block.

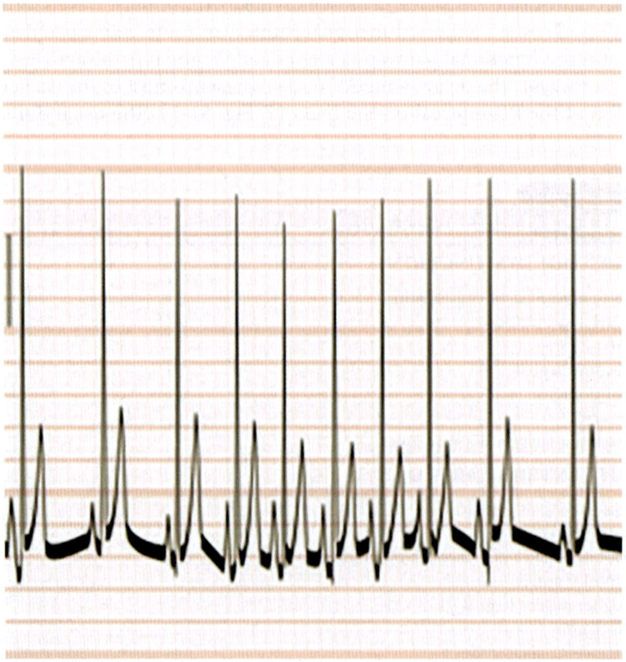

FIGURE 51-1. Sinus arrhythmia. Note the variation in sinus rates, which fluctuate with normal variations in autonomic tone.

BRADYARRHYTHMIAS

Bradyarrhythmias may be caused by dysfunction of the sinus node, AV node, or His-Purkinje system (see Table 51-1).

CLINICAL MANIFESTATIONS

Sinus bradycardia and various degrees of AV nodal blocks can occur asymptomatically during sleep in healthy individuals. Asymptomatic first- and second-degree AV block, particularly when partially or completely reversed by exercise, is usually benign. Persistent second-degree and third-degree AV nodal block is abnormal and is often associated with dizziness, fatigue, exertional dyspnea, worsening of heart failure, near-syncope, or syncope. Third-degree AV block with a good junctional escape mechanism that accelerates during exercise, as often noted in patients with congenital AV block, may remain asymptomatic. Patients with congenital heart block may not appreciate their potential for a more active lifestyle because of the lack of a reference point but often feel much better when an appropriate heart rate acceleration can be achieved after pacemaker therapy.

DIAGNOSIS

Bradycardias are typically diagnosed by the ECG. In symptomatic patients with symptoms suggestive of bradyarrhythmia, 24-hour Holter monitoring or prolonged loop monitoring usually can make the diagnosis, but some patients may require formal electrophysiologic testing (Chapter 49). Any bradycardias,

TABLE 51-2 CONDITIONS ASSOCIATED WITH BRADYCARDIA AND CONDUCTION DISORDERS

DEGENERATIVE FIBROSIS
ISCHEMIA/INFARCTION
CARDIOMYOPATHY/MYOCARDITIS
INFILTRATIVE DISORDERS
Amyloidosis Hemochromatosis Lymphoma Sarcoidosis
INFECTION
Chagas disease Diphtheria Infectious endocarditis Lyme disease Toxoplasmosis
RHEUMATOLOGIC CONDITIONS
Rheumatoid arthritis Scleroderma Systemic lupus erythematosus
NEUROMUSCULAR CONDITIONS
Myotonic dystrophy Emery Dreifuss syndrome
CARDIAC PROCEDURES
Valve surgery (open or percutaneous) Passage of a pulmonary artery catheter
CONGENITAL
Congenital anatomic lesions Arrhythmic mutations*
NEUROCARDIOGENIC EPISODES
Increased vagal tone Carotid sinus hypersensitivity Physical conditioning
ENDOCRINE/METABOLIC
Hypothyroidism Acidosis Hyperkalemia or hypokalemia Hypothermia Hypoxia

*For example, *HCN4, KCNQ1, SCN5A*.
Source: American Heart Association, Inc.

TABLE 51-3 COMMONLY USED MEDICATIONS THAT CAN PRECIPITATE OR UNMASK SINUS BRADYCARDIA OR ATRIOVENTRICULAR NODE ABNORMALITIES

CARDIAC DRUGS
β-blockers (including β-blocker eye drops for glaucoma) Non-dihydropyridine calcium channel blockers (e.g., diltiazem, verapamil)
ANTIARRHYTHMIC DRUGS
Sotalol Propafenone Amiodarone Dronedarone Flecainide
PSYCHOACTIVE DRUGS
Opioid analgesics Selective serotonin reuptake inhibitors Tricyclic antidepressants Lithium Phenothiazine Phenytoin Cannabis Cholinesterase inhibitors (e.g., donepezil)
OTHER
Uncommonly used agents, including clonidine, digoxin, ivabradine, methyldopa, propofol, reserpine, remdesivir

Source: American Heart Association, Inc.

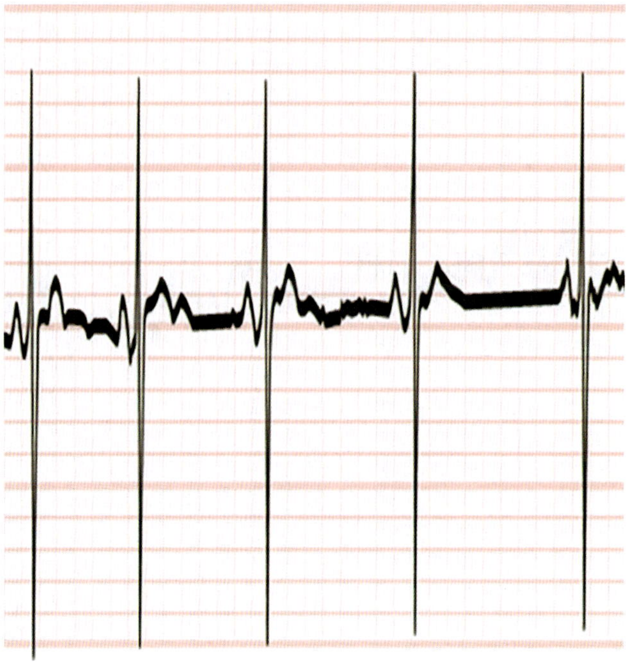

FIGURE 51-2. Sinus bradycardia. Progressive sinus bradycardia, in this case related to heightened vagal tone while sleeping.

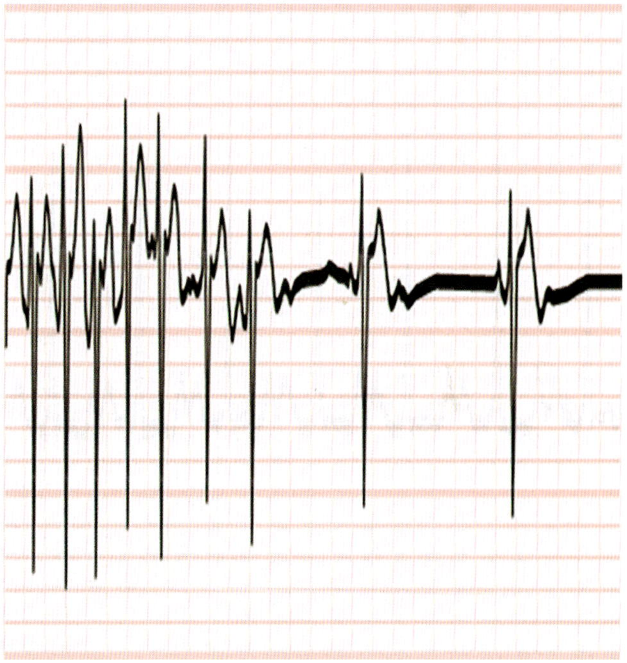

FIGURE 51-3. Electrocardiographic evidence of tachy-brady syndrome. Atrial fibrillation with a tachycardic ventricular response followed by conversion to sinus bradycardia.

including sinus node dysfunction and AV nodal block, can be caused at least in part by vagal influences, such as vasovagal episodes, vomiting, abdominal surgery, and upper and lower gastrointestinal invasive procedures. Syncope, sometimes caused by the bradycardia and sometimes by vasodepression with hypotension, may result (Chapters 39 and 49). Medications, infiltrative diseases, fibrocalcific degeneration, and a variety of other causes must be considered. Lyme disease also is a common cause of reversible complete heart block, usually localized to the AV node.

The evaluation should also include echocardiography (Chapter 43) to evaluate for structural heart disease and cardiac function. If myocardial ischemia is suspected, exercise testing (Chapters 44 and 56) should be performed. If an underlying endocarditis (Chapter 61), an infiltrative or inflammatory cardiomyopathy (Chapter 47), or adult congenital heart disease (Chapter 55) is suspected, either cardiac computed tomography or cardiac magnetic imaging should be performed (Chapter 44).

SPECIFIC BRADYARRHYTHMIAS

SINUS BRADYCARDIA AND SINUS NODE DYSFUNCTION

Sinus bradycardia (Fig. 51-2) is generally defined as a sinus rate of less than 60 beats per minute. It should be noted, however, that sinus rates as low as 45 to 50 beats per minute, particularly at rest, can be physiologically normal. Sinus node dysfunction[7] encompasses a group of disorders including sinus bradycardia, sinoatrial exit block, sinus arrest (pause of >2 to 3 seconds) during sinus rhythm, chronotropic incompetence, and tachycardia-bradycardia (tachy-brady) syndrome.[8] Sinus node dysfunction in combination with symptoms such as fatigue, dizziness, near or complete syncope (Chapters 39 and 49), or worsening of heart failure (Chapter 45) is called sick sinus syndrome. The tachy-brady syndrome is often identified by a prolonged delay in sinus node recovery following the termination of atrial fibrillation (AF) (Fig. 51-3). Sinoatrial exit block refers to the electrophysiologic phenomenon of sinus node firing with delay or block of the impulse as it travels from the sinus node to the surrounding atrial tissue (Fig. 51-4). Sinoatrial exit block can be first degree, second degree (type 1 or 2), and third degree. First-degree sinoatrial block is difficult to diagnose from the surface ECG. Second-degree sinoatrial exit block type 1 is manifest by progressive PP shortening preceding the sinus pause. The PP interval following the pause must be greater than twice the PP interval that preceded the pause. Second-degree sinoatrial exit block type 2 is characterized by a pause equaling an exact multiple of the sinus rate (i.e., constant PP interval before and after the pause). High-degree sinoatrial exit block refers to the absence of multiple P waves with a pause still corresponding to an absolute multiple of the underlying PP intervals, and third-degree AV block results in a complete absence of sinus P waves.

Chronotropic incompetence refers to the inability to increase the sinus rate appropriately in response to exercise or other physiologic demand. In most patients, chronotropic incompetence is manifest by a maximal heart rate of less than 100 beats per minute.

ATRIOVENTRICULAR CONDUCTION DISTURBANCES

AV conduction disturbances refer to abnormal conduction in the AV node or in the HPS below the AV node. Electrical transmission through the AV conduction system is primarily limited by the AV node, which conducts in a decremental fashion to prevent excessively rapid conduction to the ventricles. The normal AV node rarely conducts faster than 200 beats per minute and

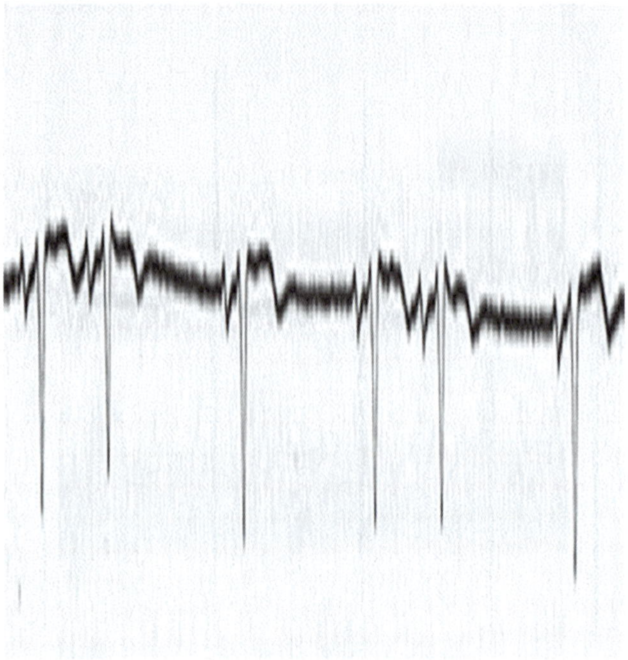

FIGURE 51-4. **Sinoatrial block.** Sinoatrial exit block, probably type 2, is characterized by a pause equaling an exact multiple of the sinus rate.

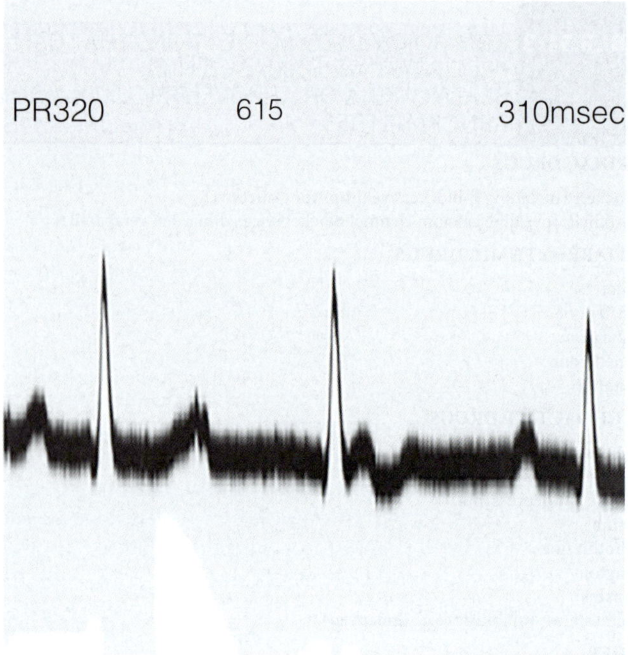

FIGURE 51-6. **Mobitz I block.** Progressive PR prolongation from 320 to 615 msec, followed by a blocked P wave. The subsequent conducted PR interval is less than the PR interval before the dropped P wave.

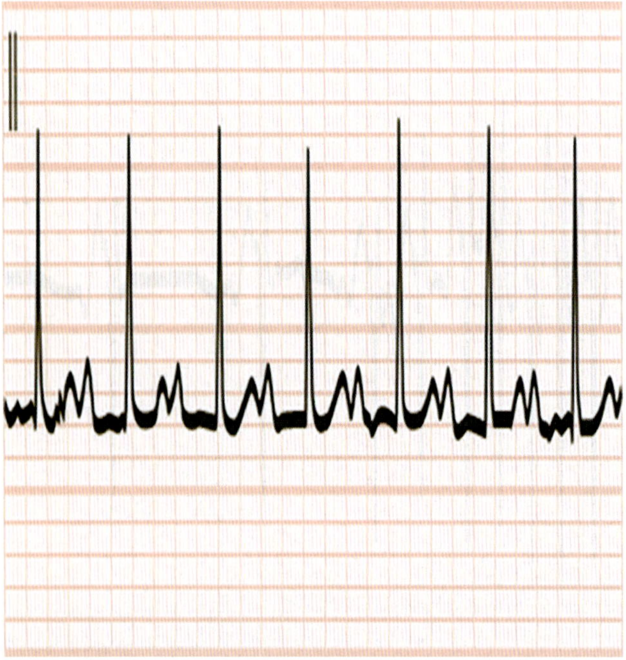

FIGURE 51-5. **First-degree atrioventricular (AV) block.** Note the prolonged (>200 msec) AV conduction.

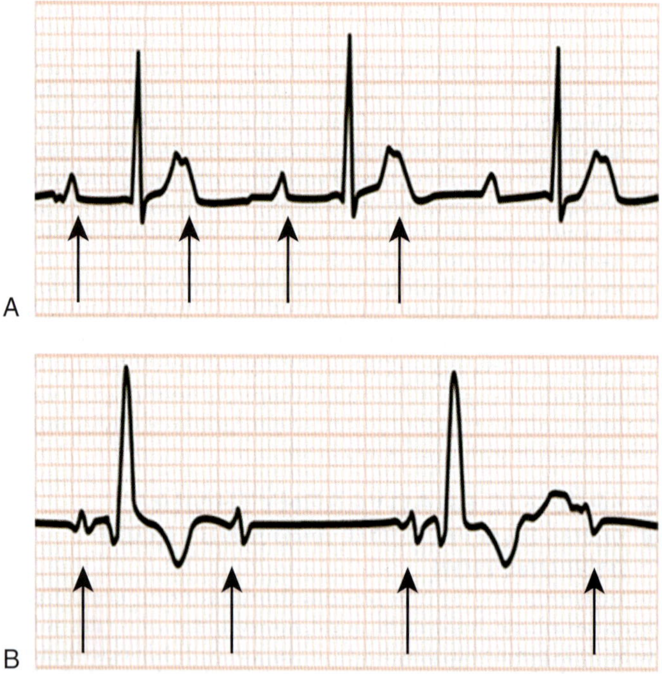

FIGURE 51-7. **Two-to-one conduction in the atrioventricular (AV) node and below the AV node. A,** Two-to-one conduction, with the conducted beats demonstrating a prolonged PR interval (>300 msec) and a narrow QRS, indicating Mobitz I block in the AV node. **B,** Normal-duration conducted PR interval and a wide QRS duration favoring Mobitz II block into an infranodal site of block.

slows with aging. The AV node is heavily influenced by autonomic tone and may conduct more than 200 beats per minute in the presence of heightened sympathetic and withdrawal of parasympathetic tone. Conduction through the HPS is faster and nondecremental.

The AV blocks are classified as first, second, high, and third degree.[9] First-degree AV block is a misnomer because nothing is actually blocked; rather, there is delay, usually in the AV node, manifest by a prolonged PR interval (Fig. 51-5). However, 50% or more of patients who have first-degree AV block either have detectable higher-degree AV block on prolonged monitoring or develop higher-grade block within about a year after the detection of asymptomatic first-degree AV block.[10] Second-degree AV block is divided into Mobitz type I (Wenckebach) or Mobitz type II. Mobitz type I is defined by progressive PR prolongation with eventual block after a P wave (Fig. 51-6). The initial PR prolongation is longest, the subsequent RR intervals shorten, and the PR interval following the blocked P wave is shorter than the last conducted PR interval before the blocked P wave. Mobitz type I usually occurs in the AV node. Mobitz type II, which is characterized by the abrupt failure of conduction after a P wave without preceding PR prolongation, usually represents conduction disease below the AV node. In patients with 2 : 1 block (two P waves for every QRS), it can be difficult to determine whether the block is Mobitz I in the AV node or Mobitz II below the AV node. Clues to conduction disease in the AV node include a prolonged PR interval (i.e., >300 msec) and a narrow QRS duration. Clues to conduction disease below the node include a normal PR interval but with bundle branch block (Fig. 51-7).

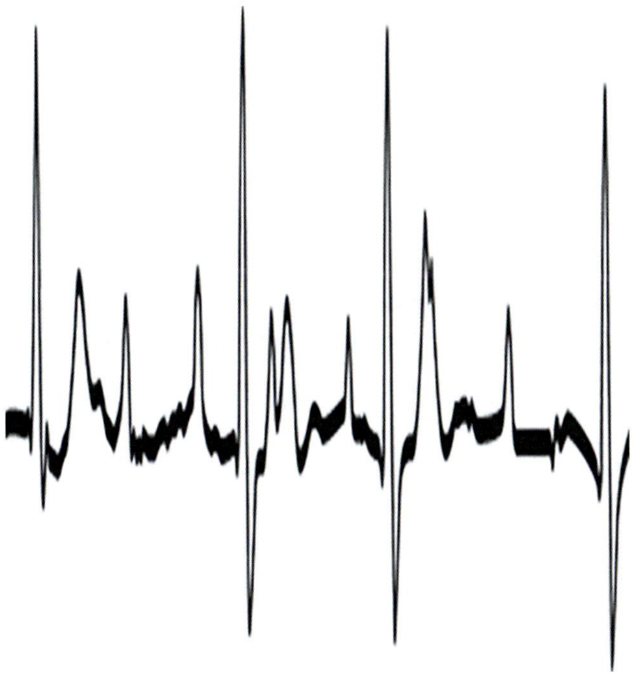

FIGURE 51-8. **High-degree atrioventricular block.** Periods of complete heart block with three nonconducted P waves (the first of which is buried in the first QRS complex) followed by two P waves, the second of which is conducted to the ventricle with a long PR interval. The subsequent three P waves are once again nonconducted, with the last P wave buried in the last QRS complex.

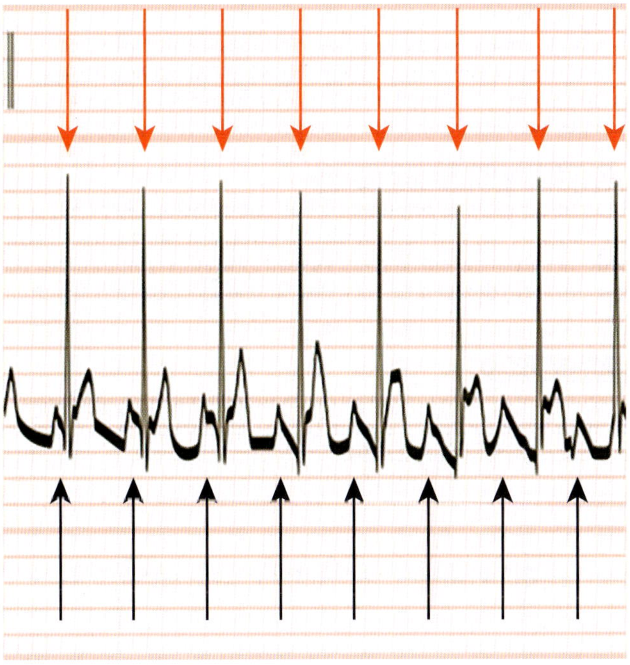

FIGURE 51-9. **Complete heart block with the atrial beats *(black arrows)* dissociated from the ventricular beats *(red arrows)*.** Note the ST elevation in leads III and aVF indicating acute inferior myocardial infarction as the cause of complete heart block.

High-degree or advanced AV block, which is a form of second-degree block with multiple or successive nonconducted P waves, or both (Fig. 51-8), frequently recurs or persists. Third-degree block (or complete heart block) refers to a rhythm in which the atrial and ventricular activity occurs independently, and the atrial rate usually exceeds the ventricular rate.[11] Third-degree heart block can be seen with sinus rhythm or any atrial tachyarrhythmia with a regular escape rhythm in the AV junction or below (Fig. 51-9). Sometimes there is no escape rhythm, and heart block results in asystole. Complete heart block, particularly when it is acute and accompanied by an escape rhythm, can be associated with marked QT prolongation, which signifies a risk for torsades de pointes (Chapter 53). For this reason, patients who undergo AV node ablation have their pacemakers set at 80 beats per minute for at least 6 weeks after the procedure to prevent QT prolongation and torsades de pointes. Eventually, the pacing rate can be reduced to more physiologic levels without the ongoing risk for ventricular arrhythmia. Complete heart block and other types of severe bradyarrhythmia may present with syncope if there is a prolonged pause before an escape rhythm develops. More often, these rhythms present with fatigue and dyspnea. The blood pressure is often elevated owing to peripheral vasoconstriction, and there may be renal insufficiency secondary to reduced cardiac output.

The term AV dissociation refers to any rhythm in which the atria and ventricles beat independently of one another. If the atrial rate is faster than the ventricular rate, it is called complete heart block or third-degree AV block. AV dissociation with an atrial rate slower than the subsidiary pacemaker is usually seen with junctional or ventricular tachycardias.

TREATMENT

The treatment of sinus node dysfunction and AV blocks consists of first removing any medications that may precipitate dysfunction (see Table 51-3).[12] Although some patients will recover normal conduction, the susceptibility to medications usually indicates an underlying conduction abnormality that may worsen over time. For example, asymptomatic sinus bradycardia (<50 per minute) in middle-aged or older adults does not appear to be associated with incident cardiovascular disease or mortality except in patients who take heart rate–modifying drugs.

Asymptomatic sinus node dysfunction requires no therapy. Asymptomatic AV nodal block, particularly if the QRS escape complex is narrow, also can be managed without intervention unless the QT interval is markedly prolonged, in which case a pacemaker should be considered.

For acutely symptomatic sinus node dysfunction and second- and third-degree AV block, urgent management includes intravenous atropine (1 mg) or isoproterenol (usually 1 to 2 μg/minute infusion) to increase the heart rate. Temporary cardiac pacing (Chapter 54) may be required. If sinus node dysfunction or AV block is due to transient abnormalities, such as drug-induced or acute ischemic syndromes, temporary pacing is usually sufficient; however, when intra-His or infra-His block is suspected (e.g., exercise-induced AV block or asymptomatic Mobitz type II block) and the site can be documented with His bundle recording, permanent pacing (see Tables 54-1 and 54-2) is the only effective long-term therapy, and consensus recommendations for pacemaker implantation should guide its use (Chapter 54).

For all forms of persistent symptomatic sinus node dysfunction or second- or third-degree AV block, permanent pacing is the therapy of choice (Chapter 54). However, recurrent syncope occurs despite a pacemaker in about 20% of patients over the subsequent 5 years.[13] In patients who have the tachy-brady syndrome, permanent pacing is usually required to prevent symptomatic bradycardia if medications are required to treat the tachycardia (Chapter 52).[14] In patients with AV block and systolic dysfunction, biventricular pacing is preferred. The only exception is Lyme disease, in which most cases of heart block resolve within a week of antibiotic therapy (Chapter 296). A newer form of physiologic pacing paces the His or left bundle branch region of the right ventricle (Chapter 54). This type of pacing stimulates the native conduction system and results in more synchronous contraction of the left and right ventricles than occurs with placement of a pacemaker into the apex or wall of the right ventricle. Cardiac neural ablation attempts to improve sinus node and AV node conduction by ablating the parasympathetic ganglia that innervate the sinus and AV nodes. This therapy has been used to treat neurocardiogenic syncope (Chapter 49) and is also being investigated for patients with sinus node dysfunction and varying degrees of AV nodal block.

INTRAVENTRICULAR BLOCKS

Given the anatomy of the intraventricular cardiac conduction system, patients can have conduction blocks or delays in either of the two fascicles (anterior or posterior) of the left bundle branch, a block or delay in the right bundle branch, or any combination of these three. As long as any one of the three conducts adequately, the patient's ECG will show the delays in the other(s): left anterior block (see Fig. 42-5A), with an axis of −45° or more negative; left posterior fascicular block (see Fig. 42-5D), with an axis of +120° or more positive; complete left bundle branch block (see Fig. 42-5E); or right bundle branch block (see Fig. 42-5B). Right bundle branch block also can occur in combination with either left anterior or left posterior fascicular block (see Fig. 42-5C). If all are delayed but at least one conducts, the patient will also have Mobitz type II block as described earlier. If all three are blocked, the patient has complete heart block (as described earlier). These intraventricular conduction delays or blocks can be caused by any of the structural (non-neurogenic, nonmedication) causes of AV block. However, by far the most common causes are ischemic heart disease, especially for the left bundle, and intrinsic degenerative changes.

In aggregate, about 1% of individuals have a bundle branch block at age 50 years, but the prevalence increases to about 17% by age 80 years. Left posterior fascicular block[15] is unusual and nearly always associated with right bundle branch block; it must be distinguished from much more common causes of right axis deviation, such as right ventricular hypertrophy, pulmonary embolism, and lateral wall myocardial infarction. Left anterior fascicular block, defined as an axis of −45° to −90°, is found in about 1% of otherwise healthy adults. However, it can be associated with degenerative disease of the conduction system, myocardial fibrosis, coronary artery disease, and structural heart diseases.

Complete left bundle branch block[16] is seen in fewer than 0.1 to 0.5% of healthy individuals but up to 25% of patients with heart failure. About 50 to 60% of patients have underlying coronary or structural heart disease.

Right bundle branch block is present in about 0.5 to 1% of the normal adult population.[17] Potential underlying causes include degenerative or infiltrative or inflammatory heart diseases, prior myocardial infarction, or severe lung disease. Transient right bundle branch block can be precipitated by the passage of pulmonary artery catheter.

CLINICAL MANIFESTATIONS AND DIAGNOSIS

Intraventricular conduction delays themselves are typically asymptomatic. However, left bundle branch block causes ventricular dyssynchrony, whereby the right ventricle contracts before the left ventricle. In some patients, this dyssynchrony also leads to mitral regurgitation. The result can be the precipitation or worsening of heart failure.

The evaluation centers on determining the risk for progression to complete heart block and determining cause, especially otherwise undiagnosed ischemic heart disease. When an intraventricular conduction delay is found on an ECG, the first task is to seek any prior ECGs to determine if the abnormality is new, whether the abnormality is or is not associated with hitherto undiagnosed underlying heart disease.[18] In patients who are presenting with suspected myocardial ischemia, a new left bundle branch block is the equivalent of ischemic ECG changes and warrants appropriate evaluation for a possible acute myocardial infarction (Chapters 57 and 58). In the setting of a possible pulmonary embolism (Chapter 68), a new right bundle branch block suggests right ventricular strain and severe pulmonary hypertension. Symptoms of syncope or presyncope suggest that the intraventricular blocks may be associated with high-degree heart block.

The routine evaluation should include echocardiography and a stress test (using echocardiography or radionuclides). Cardiac magnetic resonance imaging is recommended if there is any suspicion of an infiltrative cardiomyopathy. Rhythm monitoring (Chapter 49) is indicated if the intraventricular conduction abnormality is associated with prolongation of the PR interval, evidence of alternating right and left intraventricular blocks, or any symptoms of light-headedness or presyncope.

TREATMENT

Treatment for intraventricular conduction delays is targeted at any underlying cause. However, rhythm-specific treatments are sometimes indicated. In patients with heart failure (Chapter 46), for example, left bundle branch block is often an indication for biventricular pacing (Chapter 54). For patients with bifascicular block and syncope, pacemaker implantation is preferable to an implantable cardiac monitor,[A1] regardless of the morphology of the block or the PR interval.[19] For patients with new bifascicular block (either left bundle branch block alone or right branch block plus a left fascicular block) in combination with PR prolongation, a pacemaker is often placed prophylactically because of the high risk for progression to complete heart block, especially in the setting of an acute myocardial infarction (Chapter 47).

PROGNOSIS

The risk of all-cause mortality is increased by about two- to three-fold in individuals with left bundle branch block, about six-fold higher in the presence of underlying heart disease, and probably only minimally if exercise testing and cardiac magnetic resonance imaging show no evidence of underlying heart disease.[20] For right bundle branch block, mortality is increased in the presence of underlying heart disease; for idiopathic cases, the risk of mortality is not increased, but the long-term risk of requiring a cardiac pacemaker may be higher. The combination of right bundle branch block with either left anterior or left posterior fascicular block portends a high risk for needing a pacemaker, but prophylactic pacing is not indicated in the absence of symptoms such as syncope.

GENERAL REFERENCES

For the General References and other additional features, please visit Elsevier eBooks+ at https://ebooks.health.elsevier.com.

Grade A Reference

A1. Sheldon R, Talajic M, Tang A, et al. Randomized pragmatic trial of pacemaker versus implantable cardiac monitor in syncope and bifascicular block. *JACC Clin Electrophysiol.* 2022;8:239-248.

52

SUPRAVENTRICULAR ECTOPY AND TACHYARRHYTHMIAS

PETER ZIMETBAUM AND LEE GOLDMAN

SUPRAVENTRICULAR ARRHYTHMIAS WITH A NORMAL RATE

Atrial premature beats (APBs) can arise from the right or left atrium or the pulmonary veins. The P wave, which differs from the P wave of sinus rhythm unless the APB originates near the sinus node, always precedes the QRS complex (Fig. 52-1). If the P wave is blocked, however, it is not followed by a QRS complex. A blocked premature atrial contraction may be confused with second-degree atrioventricular (AV) block, unless its prematurity is recognized, or with sinus node dysfunction, if it is inconspicuous. Altered appearance of the ST-T segment is often a clue to the presence of a P wave. A premature QRS complex with the morphology of the underlying sinus rhythm in the absence of a premature P wave represents an AV junctional beat (Fig. 52-2).

An ectopic atrial rhythm refers to a nonsinus atrial rhythm from a single focus with a single P wave morphology (Fig. 52-3). Wandering atrial pacemaker refers to an ectopic atrial rhythm with at least three distinct P wave morphologies at rates between 50 and 100 beats per minute (Fig. 52-4).

CLINICAL MANIFESTATIONS

APBs are most often asymptomatic but can occasionally be experienced as palpitations (Chapter 49). Similarly, ectopic atrial rhythms, including a wandering atrial pacemaker, are virtually always asymptomatic. Rarely, ectopic atrial rhythm can be very slow and associated with symptoms of fatigue.

DIAGNOSIS

The diagnoses of APBs, ectopic atrial rhythms, and wandering atrial pacemakers are all made by an electrocardiogram (ECG), an ambulatory Holter monitor, or an event recorder (Chapter 49).

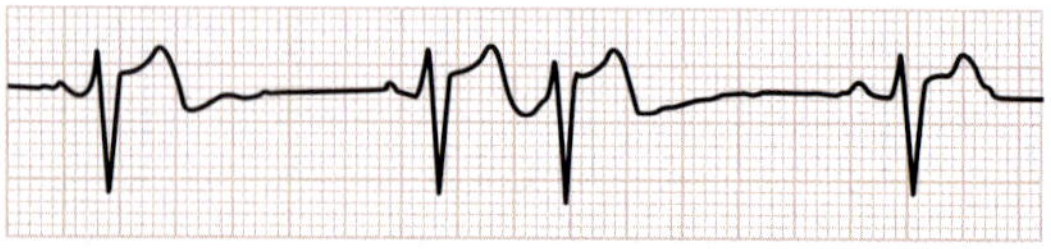

FIGURE 52-1. Atrial premature beat. Sinus rhythm with an atrial premature beat as the third complex in the rhythm strip. The P wave is buried in the preceding T wave.

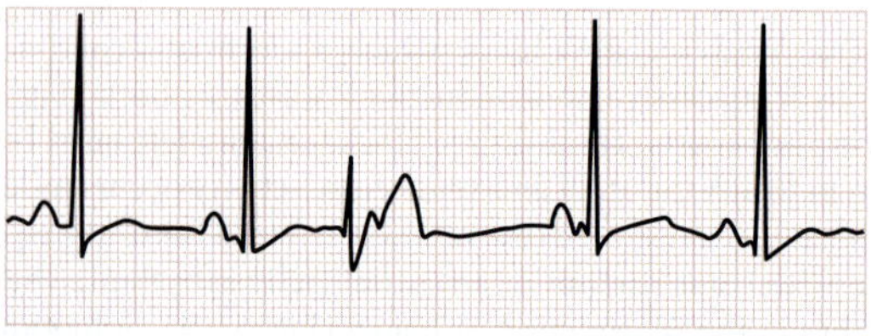

FIGURE 52-2. Junctional premature beat. The premature beat is narrow but slightly different in morphology compared with the surrounding sinus beats. This premature beat is from the atrioventricular junction or slightly more distal in the fascicles. The inverted P wave following the QRS represents retrograde activation of the atria.

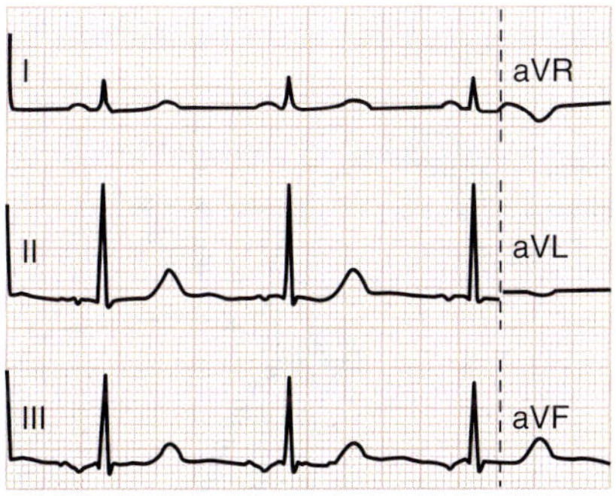

FIGURE 52-3. **Ectopic atrial rhythm.** The inverted P waves in leads II, III, and aVF indicate a nonsinus P wave originating in the low right atrium.

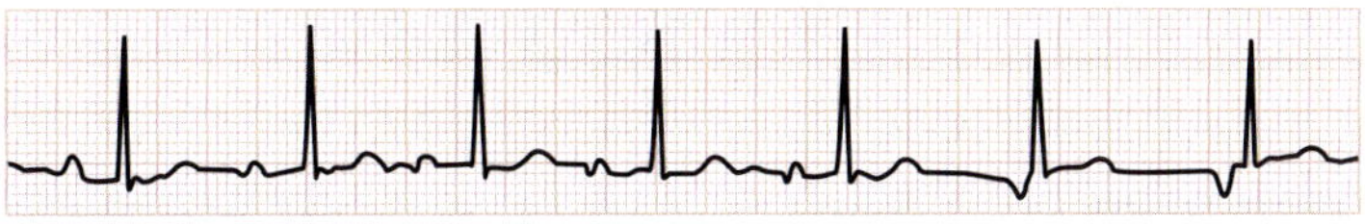

FIGURE 52-4. **Wandering atrial pacemaker.** Rhythm with three distinct P wave morphologies.

TREATMENT AND PROGNOSIS

Premature atrial contractions do not generally require treatment unless they are associated with significant symptoms. Treatment consists primarily of β-blockers (e.g., metoprolol XL, 25 to 100 mg daily) or calcium-channel blockers (e.g., long-acting diltiazem, 180 to 300 mg daily). Ectopic atrial rhythms and wandering atrial pacemakers are rarely symptomatic and are not treated with medications. Rarely, a slow ectopic rhythm associated with fatigue can be treated with atrial pacing at a rate faster than the ectopic atrial rhythm. Very frequent premature atrial contractions may portend a higher risk of atrial fibrillation (AF)[1] and other serious atrial arrhythmia, and they are associated with an increased long-term risk of stroke and clinical cardiovascular disease.

SUPRAVENTRICULAR TACHYARRHYTHMIAS

The supraventricular tachycardias (SVTs) are defined as arrhythmias with three or more beats at a rate of greater than 100 beats per minute (Table 52-1). In the United States, the incidence and prevalence of paroxysmal supraventricular tachycardias are estimated to be about 93 per 100,000 people and 480 per 100,000 people, respectively.[2]

The beats, which can be regular or irregular, are usually narrow complex but can be wide complex when associated with bundle branch block (aberration) or conduction over an accessory pathway. Atrial dilation, acute or chronic heart failure, pulmonary embolism, acute or chronic inflammatory states, or scars from prior surgery involving atrial myocardium or pericardium are among the causes of atrial tachyarrhythmias.

The most important clues for diagnosing the type of SVT include the ventricular response rate, regularity, and, if known, the suddenness of the onset of tachycardia. The QRS is regular during sinus tachycardia, atrial flutter, AV nodal re-entrant tachycardia, AV re-entrant tachycardia, and atrial tachycardia; it is irregular with AF, atrial flutter with variable AV block, multiple atrial premature contractions, and multifocal atrial tachycardia. Sudden onset and termination suggest acute AF, atrial flutter, AV nodal re-entrant tachycardia, AV reciprocating tachycardia, and atrial tachycardia. Gradual onset and recession are more suggestive of sinus tachycardia, nonparoxysmal junctional tachycardia and some forms of atrial tachycardia. The QRS complex during SVT is usually narrow but can be wide in the setting of aberrant conduction through the ventricles because of its very fast rate in the presence of coexisting disease in the bundle branches.[3]

SVTs can produce symptoms specifically related to the rhythm itself (Chapter 49), including fatigue, palpitations, dizziness, shortness of breath, chest discomfort, presyncope, and syncope. These symptoms are mostly related to the rapidity of the ventricular response and are most prevalent at the onset of the arrhythmia. In contrast to other forms of SVT, asymptomatic episodes of AF are common in patients who also have symptomatic AF.

TABLE 52-1 SUPRAVENTRICULAR TACHYCARDIAS

	R-R REGULARITY	P WAVE MORPHOLOGY
ATRIAL TACHYCARDIAS		
Sinus tachycardia	Regular	Positive in II, III, aVF; negative in aVR
Sinus node re-entry	Regular	Positive in II, III, aVF; negative in aVR
Atrial tachycardia, unifocal	Regular	P different from sinus
Atrial tachycardia, multifocal	Irregular	Three or more different P wave morphologies
Atrial flutter, common: Counterclockwise	Regular; irregular if variable AV block	Sawtooth flutter waves; regular waveform; negative in II, III, aVF, positive in V_1, negative in V_6
Clockwise		Positive in II, III, aVF; negative in V_1; positive in V_6
Atrial flutter: uncommon	Regular; irregular if variable AV block	Pattern different than common atrial flutter (counterclockwise or clockwise)
Atrial fibrillation	Irregularly irregular	Irregular fibrillation waves
AV JUNCTIONAL TACHYCARDIAS		
AV re-entry (using accessory pathways)		
Orthodromic	Regular	Retrograde P in ST-T wave
Antidromic	Regular preexcited, except in irregular preexcited atrial fibrillation	Retrograde P, short RP
Slow conducting	Regular	Retrograde P at end of T wave or later (long RP)
Atriofascicular (antidromic)	Regular preexcited	Retrograde P, short RP
AV nodal re-entry		
Common (slow-fast)	Regular	Retrograde P obscured by QRS or alters the end of QRS (short RP)
Uncommon (fast-slow)	Regular	Retrograde P at end of T wave or later (long RP)
Others (slow-slow)	Regular	PR-RP approximately equal
Nonparoxysmal junctional tachycardia*	Regular, slow rate	AV dissociation
Automatic junctional tachycardia*	Regular	AV dissociation

*Site of origin is usually infranodal.
AV = atrioventricular.

Incessant SVT and uncontrolled ventricular rates can cause tachycardia-related cardiomyopathy (Chapter 45), which is reversible with control of these arrhythmias. In some situations, however, the clinical presentation may be dominated by the underlying condition that precipitates the arrhythmia, such as fever, physical stress, hypovolemia, heart failure (Chapter 45), hypoxia, sympathomimetic or parasympatholytic medications, thyrotoxicosis (Chapter 207), and pheochromocytoma (Chapter 209).

The fundamental principle for the diagnosis of a supraventricular tachycardia is the identification of the rhythm on a 12-lead ECG, on a continuous ECG monitor, or on a wearable device such as a smart watch with ECG capability (Chapter 49). The latter two methods will also determine any correlation between an identified arrhythmia and a patient's symptoms. Chronically implanted devices such as pacemakers and an implantable cardioverter-defibrillator (ICD) also allow identification of SVTs.

SINUS TACHYCARDIA

Sinus tachycardia (Fig. 52-5) is an arrhythmia that is almost always a physiologic response to an emotional or physical stress such as anxiety, exercise, anemia, hypotension, hypoxemia, fever, thyrotoxicosis, or heart failure. It is

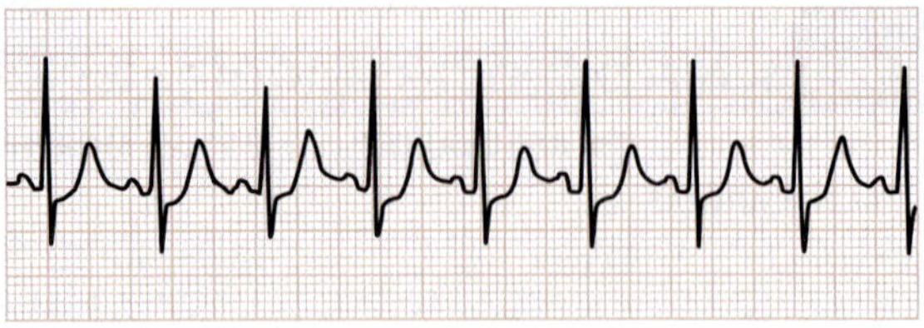

FIGURE 52-5. Sinus tachycardia at 120 beats/minute.

characterized by a gradual increase and decrease in heart rate and rarely exceeds 180 beats per minute. In rare cases, it may be a nonphysiologic condition called inappropriate sinus tachycardia, which is characterized by sinus tachycardia that develops in response to minimal stress and that continues beyond the time when the normal response would have slowed.

Sinus node re-entry is a rare form of SVT caused by re-entry in the sinus node. As opposed to physiologic sinus tachycardia, sinus node re-entry begins abruptly, is often triggered by a premature atrial beat, and ends abruptly. The P wave morphology is identical to sinus rhythm.

TREATMENT AND PROGNOSIS

Sinus tachycardia rarely should be treated directly. Instead, treatment should focus on identifying and treating any precipitating underlying conditions, especially heart failure (Chapter 46), pulmonary disease (Chapters 75 and 76), fever, anemia, thyroid disease (Chapter 207), or pheochromocytoma (Chapter 209). In the occasional patients who require treatment for symptoms that are associated with inappropriate sinus tachycardia, β-blockers (e.g., metoprolol succinate starting at 25 mg daily and titrating upward as needed) are generally chosen as first-line therapy. Alternatively, ivabradine (5 mg twice daily) provides significant improvement and can completely eliminate symptoms in approximately 50% of patients.[4] Rarely, catheter-based sinus node modification can be performed when medications are ineffective and symptoms are intractable. The prognosis is poorly understood and likely highly variable.

ATRIAL TACHYCARDIA

The term atrial tachycardia refers to a group of SVTs that originate from focal anatomic locations in the atria and propagate in a centrifugal pattern (Fig. 52-6). These locations include the pulmonary veins, crista terminalis in the right atrium, tricuspid or mitral annulus, coronary sinus, atrial septa, left atrial appendage, aortomitral continuity, or regions of scar tissue from previous cardiac surgery. Atrial tachycardias, which are usually regular rhythms that rarely exceed 200 beats per minute, may present in young age but more often develop later in life. Atrial tachycardias can be re-entrant, triggered, or automatic in mechanism.

TREATMENT AND PROGNOSIS

Some forms of atrial tachycardia are paroxysmal and may remit spontaneously without treatment. When they do not, electrical mapping and ablation (Chapter 54) of atrial tachycardia are highly effective and are increasingly offered as first-line therapy.[5] Alternatively, atrial tachycardias can be managed with medications such as β-blockers (e.g., metoprolol starting at 25 mg twice daily), calcium-channel blockers (e.g., diltiazem starting at 180 mg long-acting daily), or other antiarrhythmic drugs (see Table 52-2). Some forms of atrial tachycardia are incessant and can predispose to a tachycardia-related cardiomyopathy (Chapter 47).

MULTIFOCAL ATRIAL TACHYCARDIA

Multifocal atrial tachycardia (Fig. 52-7), which is a unique form of atrial tachycardia characterized by three or more P wave morphologies, is distinguished from wandering atrial pacemaker when the rate is 100 beats per minute or more, rather than less than 100 beats per minute. It is an irregular rhythm and occurs almost exclusively in patients with advanced pulmonary disease.

TREATMENT AND PROGNOSIS

Multifocal atrial tachycardia is relatively unresponsive to medical therapy, is very difficult to ablate, and is best treated by management of the underlying pulmonary or cardiac disorder. If absolutely required for acute symptoms, options include intravenous diltiazem, verapamil, or metoprolol (see Table 52-2). Cardioversion can restore normal sinus rhythm, but multifocal atrial tachycardia generally recurs quickly. Prognosis is largely determined by the underlying pulmonary disease.

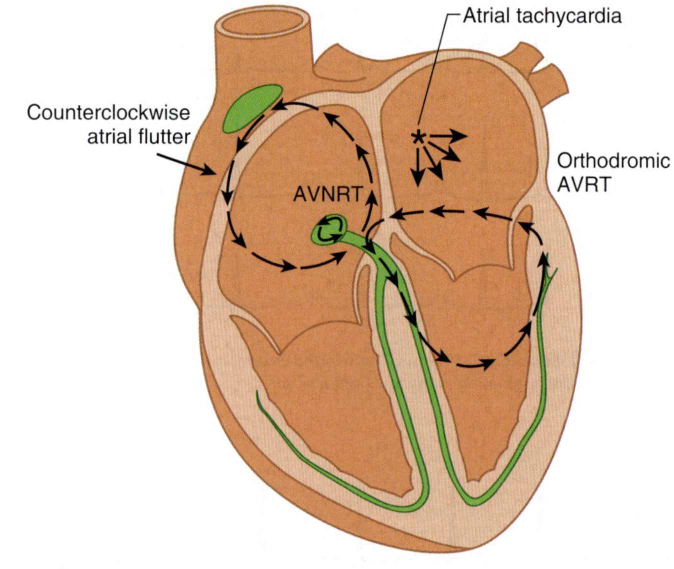

FIGURE 52-6. Diagram of the site and mechanism of common forms of supraventricular tachycardia. AVNRT = atrioventricular nodal re-entrant tachycardia; AVRT = atrioventricular re-entrant tachycardia.

ATRIOVENTRICULAR NODAL RE-ENTRANT TACHYCARDIA

AV nodal re-entrant tachycardia (also called AVNRT) is a common form of SVT in all age groups, but it presents most often in young adulthood and frequently occurs after a change in position. It is more common in women than men and may develop or be exacerbated by pregnancy or certain phases of the menstrual cycle. Patients with AV nodal re-entrant tachycardia have two functional AV nodal pathways (dual pathways). Typically, an APB blocks in one pathway (fast pathway) and conducts slowly over the other pathway (slow pathway). If this beat conducts back up the fast pathway and then re-enters the slow pathway, AV nodal re-entry occurs (Fig. 52-8). This re-entrant circuit is confined to the AV node, and the result is that both the atria and ventricles are activated nearly simultaneously. P waves may not be visible on the ECG because they are buried in the QRS complex. When P waves are present, they usually are seen just after the QRS and have a negative or superior axis (negative in leads II, III, and aVF; short RP tachycardia) (see Fig. 52-6). Atypical AV nodal re-entrant tachycardia is rare and occurs with conduction down the fast pathway and up the slow pathway, with a long interval between the preceding R wave and subsequent negative P wave (e.g., long RP tachycardia).

Symptoms associated with AV nodal re-entrant tachycardia most often include palpitations, occasionally include a sense of fullness in the neck, and may include a beat-to-beat distention of the neck veins, known as a "frog sign" and associated with contraction of the atria while the tricuspid and mitral valves are closed (cannon a waves; see Chapter 39).

TREATMENT AND PROGNOSIS

Carotid sinus massage, which has a vagal effect on the AV node, can terminate SVTs such as AV nodal re-entrant tachycardia that depend on the AV node as part of the circuit. For documented intermittent episodes of atrial tachycardia, the patient also can be instructed to try a Valsalva maneuver to terminate the arrhythmia, with higher response rates if performed in a semi-recumbent position and combined with supine repositioning and straight leg raising immediately afterward.[A1] Longer-term preventive pharmacologic management typically includes daily β-blocker or calcium channel blocker therapy (see Table 52-2). Unfortunately, use of these agents once the arrhythmia has started is usually unsuccessful. Radiofrequency ablation is the definitive approach to manage AV nodal re-entrant tachycardia and can cure more than 95% of cases, but with about a 0.5 to 1% risk of causing complete heart block that will require a pacemaker.

JUNCTIONAL TACHYCARDIA

Primary junctional tachycardia refers to a focal (non-re-entrant) tachycardia originating in the AV junction (Fig. 52-9). A number of different forms of junctional tachycardia have differing clinical patterns. Digitalis toxicity was a leading cause when it was a commonly prescribed drug.

TABLE 52-2 ANTIARRHYTHMIC DRUGS: DOSES AND SIDE EFFECTS

ANTIARRHYTHMIC DRUG AND COMMON USE	DOSE/METABOLISM	SIDE EFFECTS AND REQUIRED MONITORING	SELECTED DRUG INTERACTIONS
RATE CONTROL			
β-Blockers (selected)	Hepatic, renal Only renal (atenolol, nadolol) IV: esmolol, 250-500 μg over 1 min, then 50-300 μg/kg/min over 4 min; metoprolol, 2.5- to 5-mg bolus over 2 min, up to 3 doses 10 min apart Oral: acebutolol, 200-600 mg bid; atenolol, 25-100 mg qd; carvedilol, 3.125-50 mg bid; metoprolol, 25-150 mg bid; nadolol, 20-120 mg qd; nebivolol, 5-40 mg qd; propranolol, 10-120 mg bid	Fatigue, depression, bronchospasm, impotence	Minimal, except for carvedilol and metoprolol, whose levels may be increased by amiodarone, propafenone, quinidine, fluoxetine, haloperidol, paroxetine, and cimetidine
Calcium-channel blocker (nondihydropyridine)	Hepatic Inhibit CYP 3A4 IV: diltiazem, 20-mg bolus over 2 min, then 5-15 mg per hour maintenance infusion; verapamil, 5- to 10-mg bolus over 2 min (if no response, an additional 10 mg after 30 min and then a 0.005-mg/kg/min infusion) Oral: verapamil long-acting 120-480 mg qd Diltiazem long-acting 180-300 mg qd	Constipation, rash, peripheral edema	Inhibits CYP 3A4—will increase levels of alprazolam, carbamazepine, dihydropyridine, cyclosporine, HMG-CoA inhibitors. Verapamil (but not diltiazem) increases digoxin levels
Digoxin	Renal, hepatic, gastrointestinal, 0.125-375 mg/day orally	Anorexia, nausea, fatigue, confusion, altered vision with green-yellow halos	Levels of or sensitivity to digoxin increased by hypokalemia, quinidine, verapamil, amiodarone, propafenone, renal failure, hypoxia, decreased muscle mass Levels of or sensitivity to digoxin decreased by malabsorption, hyperkalemia, hypocalcemia
RHYTHM CONTROL			
Adenosine	Erythrocyte, endothelial cell 6-mg IV push, followed if necessary by 12 mg after 1-2 min	Nausea, headache, flushing, chest pain, bronchospasm (contraindicated if asthma)	Methylxanthines compete for adenosine receptors with adenosine Dipyridamole decreases the metabolism of adenosine
Amiodarone	Hepatic half-life 50 days PO load 10 g over 7-10 days, then 400 mg for 3 wk, then 200 mg/day for atrial fibrillation Maintenance dose of 400 mg/day for VT Dose reduce load for bradycardia or QT prolongation IV: 150- to 300-mg bolus, then 1 mg/min infusion for 6 hr, followed by 0.5 mg/min thereafter	Pulmonary (acute hypersensitivity pneumonitis, chronic interstitial infiltrates), hepatitis Thyroid (hypothyroidism or hyperthyroidism) Photosensitivity, blue-gray discoloration with chronic high dose, nausea, ataxia, tremor, alopecia Avoid if identified thyroid nodule LFTs two to three times a year, TFTs twice yearly, PFTs and CXR at initiation and CXR yearly thereafter QT prolongation expected; reduce dose if exceeds 500 msec	Inhibits CYP 450 enzymes—increases concentrations of warfarin, digoxin, cyclosporine, alprazolam, carbamazepine, HMG-CoA inhibitors, phenytoin, and quinidine
Sotalol	Renal: 80-120 mg bid orally Max dose, 240 mg bid orally	Bronchospasm QT prolongation/torsades de pointes	No significant interactions
Ibutilide	Hepatic CYP 3A4 1 mg IV over 10 min, repeat after 10 min if necessary	Nausea QT prolongation and torsades de pointes Must monitor for 4 hr after drug initiation	None
Propafenone	Hepatic 150-300 mg q8h or sustained release 225-425 mg bid orally	Metallic taste, dizziness, SIADH Atrial flutter, ventricular tachycardia	May decrease the metabolism of warfarin Increase digoxin levels
Flecainide	Renal, hepatic CYP 2D6 50-100 mg bid orally; max dose, 300-400 mg/day	Dizziness, headache, visual blurring Atrial flutter, ventricular tachycardia	May increase digoxin levels Flecainide levels increased by amiodarone, haloperidol, quinidine, cimetidine, and fluoxetine
Disopyramide	Renal, hepatic (CYP 3A4) Dose: 100-400 mg q8-12h orally; max dose, 800 mg/24 hr Reduce dose for renal or hepatic dysfunction	Anticholinergic (contraindicated for narrow-angle glaucoma): dry mouth, urinary retention, constipation, blurry vision QT prolongation/torsades de pointes	None
Procainamide	Mostly hepatic—rapid acetylators produce more NAPA; NAPA renally cleared PO dose: 50 mg/kg/24 hr IV dose: 1 g over 25 min, then 20-60 μg/kg/min infusion Reduce dose for renal dysfunction or low cardiac output	Rash, fever, arthralgias, drug-induced lupus, particularly in slow acetylators Agranulocytosis QT prolongation/torsades de pointes	Procainamide clearance reduced by trimethoprim, cimetidine, and ranitidine

TABLE 52-2 ANTIARRHYTHMIC DRUGS: DOSES AND SIDE EFFECTS—cont'd

ANTIARRHYTHMIC DRUG AND COMMON USE	DOSE/METABOLISM	SIDE EFFECTS AND REQUIRED MONITORING	SELECTED DRUG INTERACTIONS
Quinidine	Hepatic CYP 3A4 (70%), renal (30%) Dose: sulfate—600 mg tid orally, gluconate—324 to 648 mg q8h orally Dose reduced for renal failure	Thrombocytopenia, cinchonism Pruritus, rash QT prolongation/torsades de pointes	↑ Digoxin and amiodarone concentrations Quinidine inhibits CYP 2D6 and may increase drugs metabolized by this enzyme (e.g., ↑ effect of tricyclic antidepressants, haloperidol, some β-blockers, fluoxetine, opioids) Quinidine metabolism inhibited by cimetidine Quinidine metabolism increased by phenobarbital, phenytoin, and rifampicin
Dofetilide	Renal, hepatic CYP 3A4 CrCl >60 mL/min (500 µg bid orally), CrCl 40-60 (250 µg bid orally), CrCl 20-39 mL/min (125 µg bid orally)	QT prolongation and torsades de pointes Three days of in-hospital monitoring is required during drug initiation	Contraindicated with verapamil, ketoconazole, cimetidine, megestrol, prochlorperazine, and trimethoprim Hydrochlorothiazide increases dofetilide levels Must discontinue amiodarone at least 3 mo before dofetilide initiation
Ivabradine	2.5 mg starting dose, 5 mg bid orally for 1 mo followed by increase to 7.5 bid if needed	Sinus bradycardia Headaches Visual brightness	Azole antifungals, macrolide antibiotics, nefazodone, nelfinavir, ritonavir
Dronedarone	Hepatic CYP 3A4 half-life 30 hr PO 400 mg bid orally Improved absorption with food	Reduces the secretion of creatinine without a reduction in GFR Hepatic failure Avoid in heart failure	Increases digoxin levels (dose reduce digoxin by half) May increase myositis with simvastatin Avoid grapefruit

bid = twice daily; CrCl = creatinine clearance; CXR = chest radiograph; CYP = cytochrome P-450; GFR = glomerular filtration rate; HMG-CoA = 3-hydroxy-3-methylglutaryl coenzyme A; IV = intravenous administration; LFT = liver function test; max = maximum; NAPA = *N*-acetyl procainamide; PFT = pulmonary function test; PO = oral administration; qd = daily; SIADH = syndrome of inappropriate diuretic hormone; TFT = thyroid function test; VT = ventricular tachycardia.

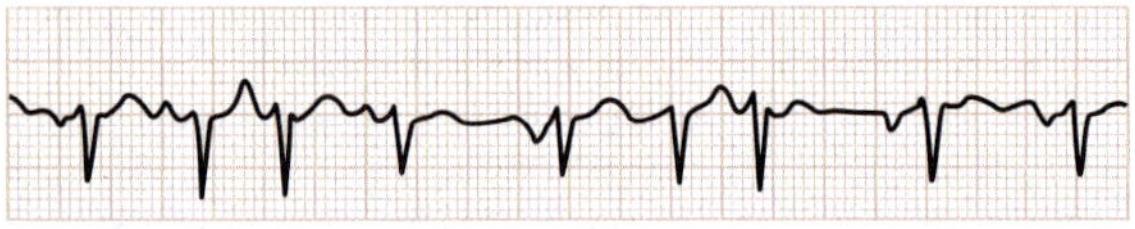

FIGURE 52-7. Multifocal atrial tachycardia. An atrial tachycardia with three different P wave morphologies.

Nonparoxysmal junctional tachycardia is a benign arrhythmia that rarely exceeds 120 beats per minute and typically exhibits a "warm-up" and "cool-down" pattern. A more rapid paroxysmal form of junctional tachycardia occurs in young adults and is often associated with exercise. Congenital junctional ectopic tachycardia, which occurs in the pediatric population, is associated with very rapid rates and a risk for tachycardia-related cardiomyopathy.

TREATMENT AND PROGNOSIS

When junctional tachycardia is not a re-entrant arrhythmia, treatment is either medically, with amiodarone or ivabradine (see Table 52-2),[A2] or with radiofrequency catheter ablation. Reported efficacies are in the 90% range.

ACCESSORY PATHWAY TACHYCARDIAS

Tachycardias associated with an accessory pathway or bypass tract are called AV re-entrant tachycardia (also called AVRT). These tachycardias most often conduct down the normal AV conducting system and back up the accessory pathway (orthodromic AV re-entrant tachycardia) (see Fig. 52-6). Antidromic tachycardia is rare and represents conduction down the accessory pathway and back up the normal conducting system or, less commonly, a second accessory pathway. Wolff-Parkinson-White syndrome is defined by the presence of delta waves or preexcitation on the ECG in sinus rhythm (Fig. 52-10), in combination with a history of AV re-entrant tachycardia. It is important to recognize, however, that many patients with ventricular preexcitation never get AV re-entrant tachycardia. In addition, up to 40% of patients with accessory pathways have AF. Because accessory pathway tissue, unlike the AV node, is usually nondecremental, a rapidly conducting accessory pathway may allow AF to conduct to the ventricles at excessive rates and precipitate ventricular fibrillation. Drugs such as digoxin, which accelerate accessory pathway conduction, should be avoided in these patients.

The ECG during orthodromic AV re-entrant tachycardia can have a narrow complex, but a wide QRS complex will be seen if there is aberration from a bundle branch block, especially at more rapid rates. The retrograde P wave is negative in leads I and aVL if it conducts over a left lateral accessory pathway and negative in leads II, III, and aVF if it conducts over a septal or posteroseptal accessory pathway (Fig. 52-11). The P wave occurs later (after the preceding R wave) compared with AV nodal re-entrant tachycardia because in AV re-entrant tachycardia, the impulse must conduct beyond the AV node and into the ventricle before returning to the atria over an accessory pathway. In antidromic AV re-entrant tachycardia, the QRS complex is wide with a slurred upstroke and resembles that seen with ventricular tachycardia as opposed to a bundle branch block. Antidromic conduction with AF is often fast, broad, and irregular (see Fig. 52-10).

Palpitations are the most common symptoms. If AF with rapid conduction occurs over the accessory pathway (preexcited AF), more significant symptoms such as light-headedness, syncope, or even cardiac arrest may occur.

TREATMENT

The acute management of AV re-entrant tachycardia, particularly if there is evidence of preexcitation, is intravenous adenosine (6 mg intravenous push, followed by another 12 mg after 1 to 2 minutes if needed). Intravenous procainamide (1 g over 25 minutes is an alternative, but direct electrical cardioversion is a safe, effective, and generally preferred option if adenosine is unsuccessful. Intravenous calcium channel blockers and β-blockers can potentially be used (see Table 52-2), but the risk of associated vasodilation and hypotension with a resultant reflex adrenergic response can cause a dangerous acceleration in conduction over the accessory pathway, so they require great caution and should be used only under expert supervision.

The longer term management of AV re-entrant tachycardia is best accomplished with an electrophysiologic study and ablation of the accessory pathway (Chapter 54). If an invasive approach is not available or preferred by the patient or if the accessory pathway is in a location that is difficult to access or associated with high risk of damage to the conduction system (i.e., risk of complete heart block), oral medications, including β-blockers (e.g., metoprolol 25 to 50 mg daily) or antiarrhythmic drugs (e.g., flecainide 100 to 150 mg twice daily) can be considered.

ATRIAL FLUTTER

Atrial flutter is an arrhythmia with an atrial rate of approximately 300 beats per minute and a ventricular response of 150 (2 : 1), 100 (3 : 1), or slower multiples. Typical atrial flutter is a macro-re-entrant circuit that circulates in the

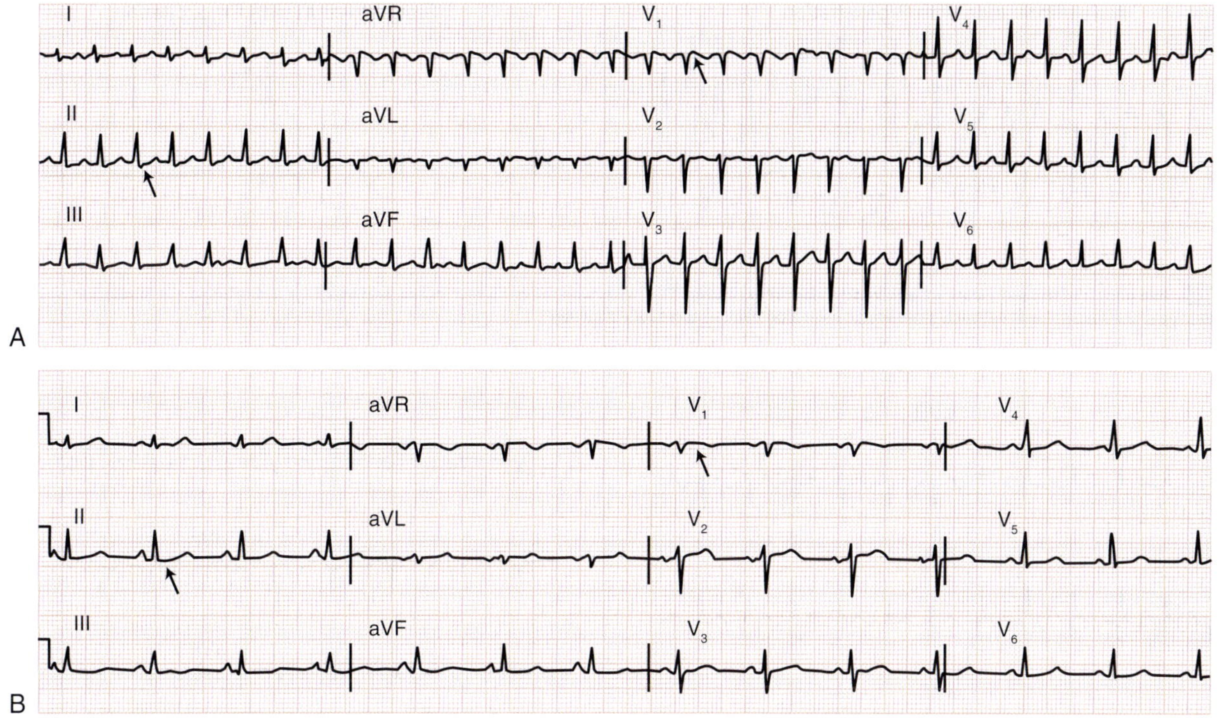

FIGURE 52-8. **Electrocardiograms demonstrating different rhythms in the same patient. A,** Atrioventricular nodal re-entrant tachycardia, with *arrows* indicating retrograde P waves (negative in lead II, positive in V_1). **B,** Same patient in sinus rhythm. The absence of a negative deflection at the end of the QRS in lead II and positive deflection in V_1 confirms that those findings in panel A were retrograde P waves.

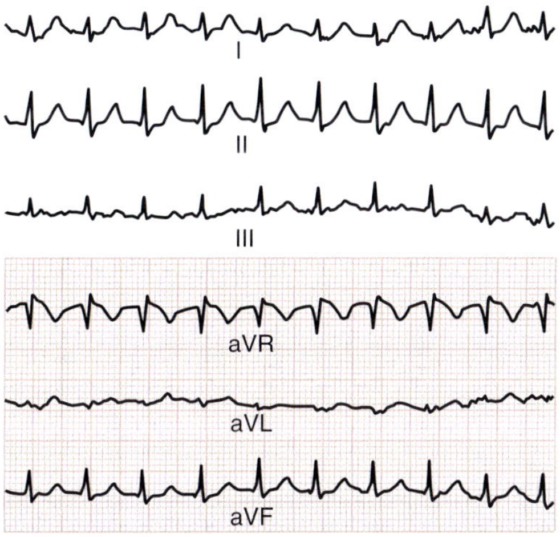

FIGURE 52-9. **Junctional tachycardia.** A tachycardia without evident P waves. The negative deflections at the end of leads II, III, and aVF represent retrograde P waves. This rhythm is impossible to distinguish from atrioventricular nodal re-entrant tachycardia on the surface electrocardiogram.

right atrium in a clockwise or counterclockwise loop (Fig. 52-12). The inferior portion of typical flutter uses the narrow region between the inferior vena cava and tricuspid annulus as a critical isthmus of conduction. Typical atrial flutter almost always occurs in patients with underlying cardiovascular or pulmonary disease. It can also develop in patients who receive antiarrhythmic drugs (e.g., sodium-channel blocking drugs) for AF. Atypical atrial flutter refers to macro-re-entrant atrial circuits that do not use this critical cavotricuspid isthmus of tissue. These atypical forms of atrial flutter often occur in the left atrium after mitral valve surgery or catheter ablation of AF. Typical atrial flutter can be recognized by a "sawtooth" P wave morphology, which is predominantly negative in leads II, III, and aVF and positive in V_1 (counterclockwise atrial flutter) or positive in leads II, III, and aVF and negative in V_1 (clockwise atrial flutter).

If the rate of atrial flutter is well controlled by effective atrioventricular block, patients may be asymptomatic. More rapid ventricular rates are associated with palpitations, light-headedness, syncope, or shortness of breath. Atrial flutter also can precipitate heart failure or myocardial ischemia in patients with underlying heart disease. If high-grade atrioventricular block develops, light-headedness and even syncope can be seen as with other bradycardias (see Chapter 51).

TREATMENT AND PROGNOSIS

It can be very difficult to control the ventricular rate of acute atrial flutter, which generally must be treated by restoring sinus rhythm. In some cases, successful treatment of precipitating problems such as hypoxia, fever, and electrolyte abnormalities will lead to spontaneous conversion, and such treatment is often required to sustain sinus rhythm once it is achieved.

Intravenous ibutilide (1 g over 10 minutes, repeated after 10 minutes if needed) is approximately 60% effective for converting atrial flutter to sinus rhythm, but direct current electrical cardioversion (Chapter 54) is the preferred approach and is highly (>95%) effective for restoring sinus rhythm. As is true of AF (see later), electrical or pharmacologic cardioversion should not be performed unless the episode of atrial flutter is believed to be less than 48 hours in duration, a transesophageal echocardiogram has excluded clot in the left atrial appendage, or the risk for stroke has been minimized by achieving a therapeutic level of anticoagulation, preferably with a direct-acting oral anticoagulant (e.g., dabigatran, rivaroxaban, apixaban, or edoxaban; see Table 70-6) or with a therapeutic international normalized ratio (INR) of 2 to 3 with warfarin (see Table 70-4), for the prior 4 weeks. Since the effective ventricular rate in atrial flutter depends on the degree of atrioventricular block, a titrated β-blocker (e.g., metoprolol starting at 25 to 50 mg daily) or calcium channel blocker (e.g., diltiazem starting at 180 to 240 mg daily) can provide temporary rate control while awaiting cardioversion. However, very careful follow-up is critical because of the challenge of balancing the degree of atrioventricular block.

As with AF, atrial flutter is rarely an isolated occurrence and can be expected to recur. Even if patients are minimally symptomatic because atrioventricular block results in a physiologic heart rate, patients are likely to have variable block, and hence an unstable heart rate, over time. For these reasons, radiofrequency ablation of the cavotricuspid isthmus is 95% curative for the typical form of atrial flutter and is the preferred choice for most patients (Chapter 54). The first-line therapy for atypical atrial flutter is also often catheter ablation, but the likelihood of success is lower,[6] so either antiarrhythmic drug therapy or simply recurrent cardioversion for infrequent recurrences are also reasonable approaches. Because patients with atrial flutter have a 3% per year risk for thromboembolism, patients at risk for recurrence should also receive long-term anticoagulation similar to what is recommended for AF (see later). If atrial flutter ablation is successful, however, the risk for recurrence is very small, and long-term anticoagulation is not necessary. Prognosis is generally related to any underlying comorbid conditions that may have precipitated the atrial flutter.

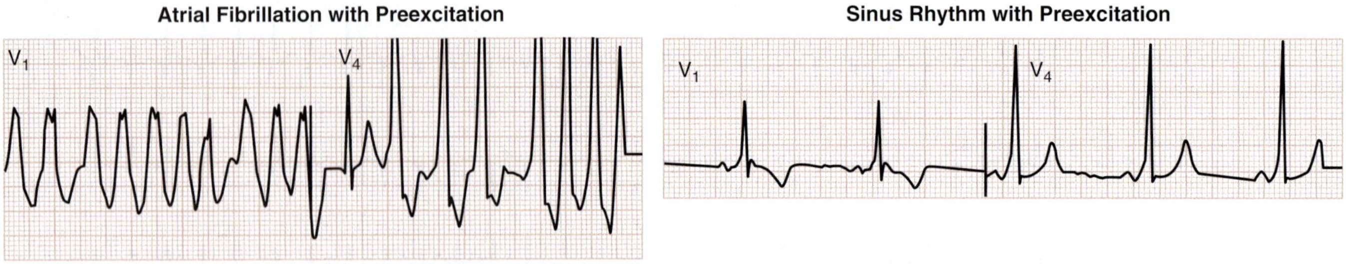

FIGURE 52-10. **Two panels of the same patient with ventricular preexcitation.** The rhythm on the left is fast, broad, and irregular, indicating atrial fibrillation with conduction over an accessory pathway. The rhythm on the right is sinus with conduction over an accessory pathway.

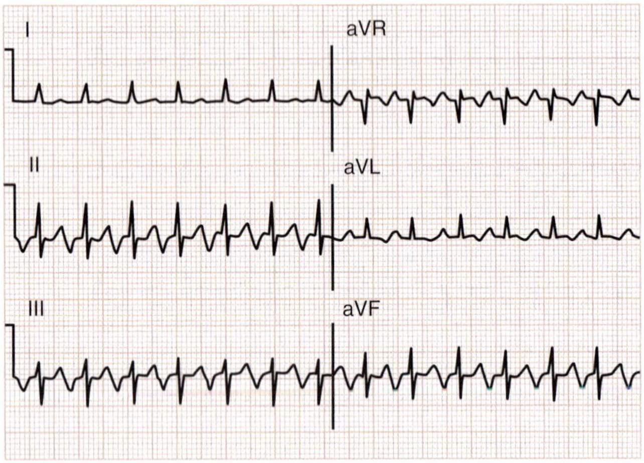

FIGURE 52-11. **Atrioventricular re-entrant tachycardia.** Negative P waves are seen in leads II, III, and aVF indicative of retrograde conduction to the atria over a septal accessory pathway.

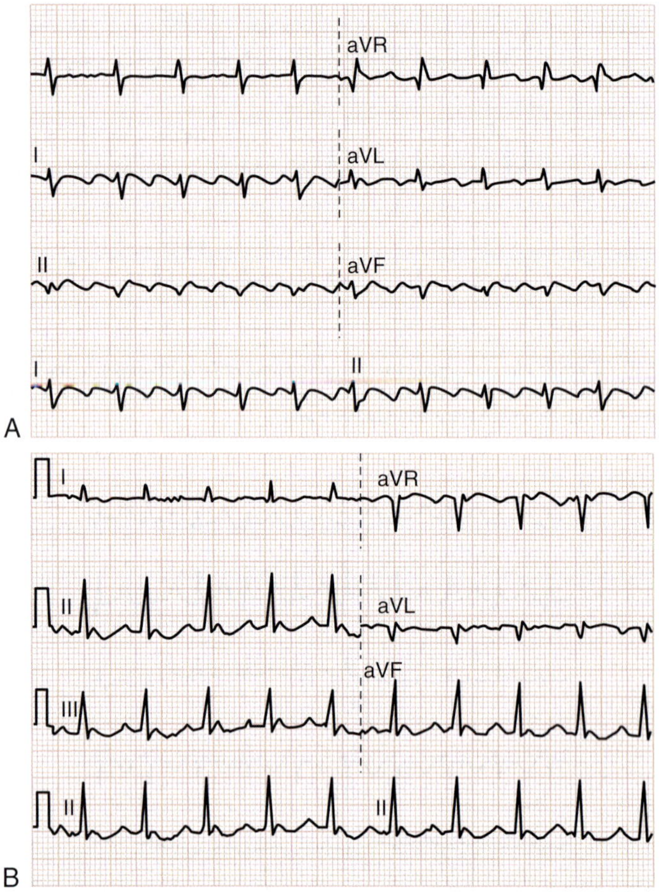

FIGURE 52-12. **Two examples of atrial flutter. A,** Typical counterclockwise right atrial flutter with classic sawtooth flutter waves seen in leads II, III, and aVF. **B,** Clockwise right atrial flutter.

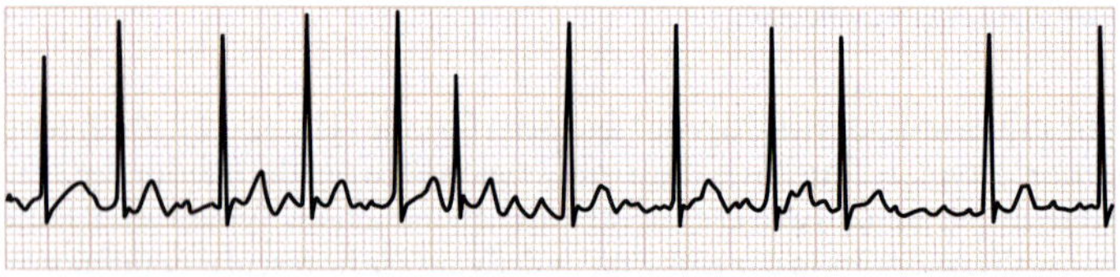

FIGURE 52-13. **Coarse atrial fibrillation.** The wavy baseline is suggestive of atrial activity and can be misinterpreted as P waves or flutter waves. The irregularity of the QRS complexes indicates that this is atrial fibrillation.

ATRIAL FIBRILLATION

AF is identified by the absence of P waves and the presence of an irregularly irregular ventricular rate. Coarse AF, which describes the presence of residual atrial activity on the ECG, is generally best seen in lead V_1 with the absence of P wave–like activity in other leads (Fig. 52-13). AF can be present with a regular ventricular rate when there is concomitant AV dissociation (e.g., complete heart block or ventricular tachycardia).

AF, which is the most common arrhythmia in clinical practice,[7] afflicts more than 2 million Americans. The likelihood of developing AF increases with aging, with an anticipated three-fold increase in prevalence as the U.S. population ages in the next 20 years. AF is almost always a recurrent disorder, with the possible exception of AF that develops in association with hyperthyroidism (Chapter 207) and surgery (Chapter 401). AF can be paroxysmal (terminates spontaneously) or persistent (persists for at least 7 days or until cardioverted).

In addition to its association with aging, AF frequently occurs in association with hypertension (Chapter 64) or other comorbid conditions such as diabetes mellitus (Chapter 210), thyrotoxicosis (Chapter 207), heart failure (Chapter 45), coronary artery disease (Chapter 56), valvular heart disease (Chapter 60), or lung disease such as chronic obstructive pulmonary disease (Chapter 76)[8] or obstructive sleep apnea (Chapter 374). About 20% of patients have no associated comorbidity. Some patients develop AF after binges of alcohol use ("holiday heart")[9] or after parasympathetic surges, such as occur after vigorous exercise or a large meal (vagally induced AF). Long-term significant alcohol use can also result in an increased risk of AF. Excessive caffeine intake is an often cited but very rare cause of AF.

AF requires a trigger in the form of atrial premature depolarizations, which often originate in the pulmonary veins and which, in the susceptible individual, result in AF. The susceptibility to AF may relate to changes in the electrical function of the left atrium. Prolonged periods of AF can lead to electrical and structural remodeling of the atria and promote the further perpetuation of AF.

AF results in the loss of the atrial contribution to ventricular filling. This so-called loss of atrial kick is generally well tolerated in normal individuals, in whom only about 15% of ventricular filling is the result of atrial contraction. In patients who have stiff, noncompliant ventricles (e.g., patients with aortic stenosis, hypertrophic or restrictive cardiomyopathy, or long-standing hypertension), however, up to 40% of ventricular filling may be related to atrial contraction, so stroke volume may fall noticeably in such patients.

Silent or asymptomatic AF may be identified on a permanently placed device such as a pacemaker or implantable defibrillator or on a wearable device.[A3] By convention, at least 2 minutes of a sustained arrhythmia consistent with AF must be present to make the diagnosis of AF. Currently, the U.S. Preventive Services Task Force concludes that evidence is insufficient to determine whether screening for AF should be recommended.[10]

CLINICAL MANIFESTATIONS AND DIAGNOSIS

The most common symptoms associated with AF include palpitations, dyspnea, chest pain, and fatigue.[11] Most patients have symptoms with the new onset of AF, but it is common for these symptoms to dissipate over time with recurrent or persistent AF, especially if the heart rate is in the physiologic range. Syncope (Chapter 49) can occasionally occur and is usually a consequence of a conversion pause that occurs when AF terminates and a delay ensues before the resumption of sinus rhythm.

The primary morbidity associated with AF is thromboembolism. Thromboembolism in patients with nonvalvular AF typically results from thrombus that forms in the left atrial appendage and later dislodges from it. The risk for thromboembolism is related to the presence of underlying vascular disease but not to the pattern of AF (paroxysmal or persistent). For example, even subclinical ("silent") AF is associated with a 2.5-fold increased risk for ischemic stroke or systemic embolism. However, the risk for embolization is further increased in the first 3 to 4 weeks after cardioversion, when the gradual return of atrial mechanical function can result in a particularly high risk for thromboembolism. The risk for thromboembolism in AF increases with age, diabetes mellitus, hypertension, previous embolic episodes, vascular disease, and heart failure. The lowest incidence (<1% annually) is in patients younger than 65 years with lone AF. AF is associated with about a 1.4-fold higher risk for cognitive impairment and dementia, with or without a history of clinical stroke. About 12% of clinical embolic events are extracranial, about 70% of which affect the extremities, with most of the remainder affecting the visceral mesenteric circulation.

AF with a rapid ventricular response can also result in biventricular dysfunction, termed tachycardia-induced cardiomyopathy (Chapter 45). This complication is generally associated with ventricular rates over 120 beats per minute for at least a few weeks. In many instances, patients with this complication are relatively asymptomatic while in AF and, as such, do not seek medical attention until evidence of heart failure develops.

The initial diagnostic evaluation of AF should include blood work (hematocrit and blood levels of potassium, creatinine, and thyroid-stimulating hormone at a minimum), as well as an echocardiogram to evaluate for possible underlying ventricular dysfunction or valvular disease. A stress test to exclude ischemia is not required as a routine part of the evaluation unless the patient otherwise has clinical evidence of atherosclerosis or coronary artery disease from the history, physical examination, ECG, or echocardiogram.

TREATMENT

Recent-Onset Atrial Fibrillation

In the presence of hypotension, acute myocardial ischemia, or new or worsening heart failure, prompt cardioversion is generally indicated. However, precipitating conditions such as hypoxia, fever, and electrolyte abnormalities also should be addressed to increase the likelihood that cardioversion will be successful and the patient will remain in sinus rhythm.

For acute AF without hypotension, hemodynamic compromise, or acute ischemia, at least one attempt to restore normal sinus rhythm is almost always warranted. However, a short period of rate control is appropriate because about 50% of patients with acute-onset AF will spontaneously revert to sinus rhythm within the first 48 to 96 hours. Therefore, even in patients with mildly symptomatic recent-onset AF, a "wait-and-see" approach with delayed cardioversion if the AF does not resolve within 48hours is as good as early cardioversion in achieving a return to sinus rhythm at 1 month.[A4] Rate control is crucial and can be accomplished with esmolol, metoprolol, verapamil, or diltiazem (see Table 52-2); digoxin is usually a third-line agent (Fig. 52-14).

Before cardioversion, either pharmacologic or electrical (Chapter 54), however, the risk for clot formation must be mitigated in all patients who have AF of more than 48 hours' duration.[12] The first step generally is to perform transesophageal echocardiography (Chapter 43). If the transesophageal echocardiogram shows no evidence of a left atrial clot, cardioversion can be undertaken without systemic anticoagulation. If the patient has risk factors for stroke in association with AF, however, most clinicians administer anticoagulation during the cardioversion and for the subsequent 4 weeks. If the transesophageal echocardiogram shows evidence of clot, 4 consecutive weeks of pre-cardioversion anticoagulation is required, preferentially with therapeutic doses of dabigatran, rivaroxaban, apixaban, or edoxaban (see Table 70-6), rather than with heparin and warfarin. If warfarin is used (see Table 70-4), an international normalized ratio (INR) of at least 2.0 is required.

For a first episode of acute AF (<48 hours' duration), cardioversion can be attempted using electrical cardioversion (Chapter 54) or medications. Electrical cardioversion, which is performed with a minimum of 200 joules, is successful in more than 90% of cases.[A5] Medical options include procainamide (15mg/kg intravenously over 30min), ibutilide (1 mg intravenously over 10minutes, repeated after 10minutes if necessary), or a single dose of propafenone (600mg) or flecainide (300mg). For recent-onset AF of less than 48hours' duration, the success rate is approximately 50%. Approximately 3 hours of postadministration monitoring is required when these antiarrhythmic agents are used owing to a risk of proarrhythmia, including but not limited to QT prolongation and torsades de pointes. This limitation often makes this option impractical compared with treatment with immediate cardioversion.

Atrial Fibrillation of Uncertain Duration

Since the duration of AF may be hard to identify definitively, it is prudent to assume that the duration of AF has been greater than 48 hours when contemplating a cardioversion strategy (see Fig. 52-14) unless there is absolute certainty of the timing of onset. In this setting, a transesophageal echocardiogram should be performed to assess for possible clot in the left atrium. If negative, cardioversion (either medical or electrical) is as for recent-onset AF. If, however, clot is seen, then the patient must be anticoagulated for 1 month unless symptoms truly warrant urgent cardioversion. Anticoagulation also must be maintained for at least 3 to 4 weeks after successful cardioversion. Even in the absence of clot, long-term anticoagulation is commonly recommended for patients with paroxysmal or recurrent AF.

Chronic Rhythm and Rate Therapy

Catheter Ablation

After the treatment and hopefully resolution of a first episode of AF and the mandatory 1 month of anticoagulation, the strategy of rhythm control within the first year with catheter ablation to isolate the pulmonary veins electrically from the remainder of the atrium (see Chapter 54) and/or with an antiarrhythmic drug confers about a one-third lower rate of death (1.0 vs. 1.3 deaths/100 person years),[A6] due to the safety and efficacy of catheter ablation,[13] which is significantly superior to anti-arrhythmia medications,[A7–A10] and the widespread use of direct-acting oral anticoagulants. Early rhythm control with catheter ablation is especially beneficial in patients who have heart failure.[A11–A13]

Medical Rhythm Control

Rhythm control with medication alone is not superior to rate control in terms of major adverse events but may be chosen for bothersome symptoms. If catheter ablation is not selected, repeat electrical or pharmacologic cardioversion can be attempted with the same medications used for an initial episode or with oral amiodarone (typically a 10-g loading dose given in equal daily amounts over 1 to 2 weeks, followed by 400 to 600mg a day for the remainder of a month).

To prevent recurrent AF, the pharmacologic options work by blocking sodium channels, potassium channels, or a combination of ion channels, thereby slowing cardiac conduction (sodium channels) and/or prolonging cardiac repolarization (potassium channels), as well as modulating the autonomic nervous system. The choice of antiarrhythmic drug is based on the patient's underlying clinical condition (Table 52-3).[14]

Amiodarone (usually 200mg daily), which is the most widely used medication for the prevention of recurrent AF, has an efficacy of 60 to 70% at 1 year and is significantly more effective than propafenone, flecainide, dofetilide, or sotalol, which are the recommended alternatives. It is associated with a number of drug interactions, most notably with warfarin and digoxin. Its associated risk for thyroid, liver, and lung toxicities, related in part to the iodine moieties on this compound, necessitate careful monitoring. Dronedarone (400mg twice daily), which is related to amiodarone but has no iodine and a shorter 15-hour half-life, is well tolerated in terms of non-cardiovascular side effects but carries an increased risk for heart failure, stroke, and death in patients with permanent AF. As a result, it should be discontinued in patients in whom sinus rhythm is not well maintained.

Quinidine, procainamide, and disopyramide are predominantly sodium-channel blocking drugs that also block potassium channels at slow heart rates. Each of these drugs is moderately successful in AF, with about 50% of treated patients in sinus rhythm at 1 year, but each also has idiosyncratic non-cardiovascular toxicities that can significantly limit their utility (see Table 52-2). Propafenone and flecainide are sodium-channel blockers that are also used for the maintenance of sinus rhythm. These drugs are moderately effective, with a 50% rate of sinus rhythm at 1 year, and are generally well tolerated, but they must be avoided in patients with structural heart disease, particularly with a history of prior myocardial infarction and impaired left ventricular function, because of a risk for drug-induced ventricular arrhythmia. Dofetilide is a potassium-channel blocking medication that is moderately effective for suppressing AF but carries a dose-dependent risk for QT prolongation and torsades de pointes.

Rate Control

If a strategy of rate control is chosen, it is important to confirm a heart rate of 70 to 100 beats per minute at rest and less than 140 beats per minute with exercise, preferably by monitoring the heart rate during exercise on an exercise treadmill test or with an ambulatory monitor. More strict rate control is not beneficial. Failure to confirm rate control can result in the development of tachycardia-induced cardiomyopathy. First-line therapy for rate control includes β-blockers (e.g., metoprolol 25 to 50mg daily) or non-dihydropyridone calcium-channel

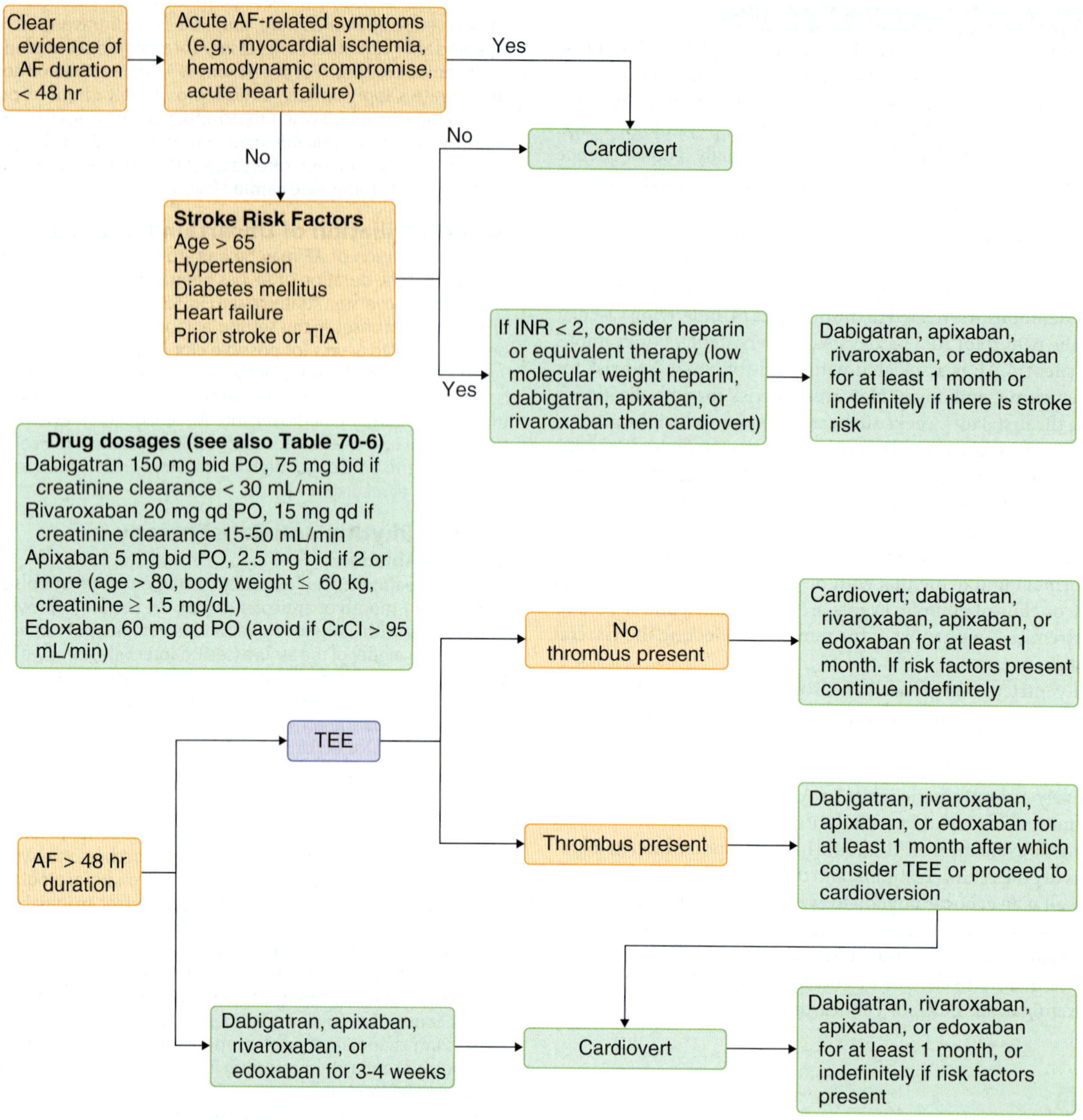

FIGURE 52-14. **Management of recent-onset atrial fibrillation (AF). bid = twice daily; CrCl = creatinine clearance; INR = international normalized ratio; qd = daily; TEE = transesophageal echocardiography; TIA = transient ischemic attack.**

TABLE 52-3 SELECTION OF ANTIARRHYTHMIC DRUGS

PATIENT'S CHARACTERISTICS	ANTIARRHYTHMIC DRUG CHOICES
No structural heart disease	*First line:* flecainide, propafenone, dronedarone, sotalol *Second line:* amiodarone, dofetilide
Depressed left ventricular ejection fraction with heart failure	*First line:* amiodarone, dofetilide *Avoid:* dronedarone, flecainide, propafenone
Coronary artery disease without heart failure	*First line:* sotalol, dronedarone, dofetilide, amiodarone *Avoid:* flecainide, propafenone
Hypertrophic cardiomyopathy	*First line:* amiodarone, sotalol *Second line:* disopyramide

blockers (e.g., diltiazem 180 to 240 mg daily); digoxin (usually 0.125 to 0.25 mg daily) can also be used but is generally less well tolerated.[A14] Interestingly, β-blockers do not appear to reduce all-cause mortality when used in patients whose AF is complicated by heart failure, but it is not clear whether digoxin is preferred in this setting. From a practical perspective, patients commonly require a combination of medications (e.g., metoprolol plus diltiazem) to achieve goal heart rates. In some patients, rate control is difficult to achieve because of inefficacy of or intolerance to medical therapy. In these patients, ablation of the AV junction can be performed with placement of a single chamber or biventricular pacemaker.[A15]

Chronic Persistent AF

In patients with chronic existing AF, catheter ablation is now recommended first-line therapy because of its efficacy of about 70% for preventing recurrent AF with an excellent safety profile.[A16] When available, the benefits of catheter ablation over medical therapy are even more striking in patients who have heart failure, in whom it provides a very clear survival advantage (Chapter 46). A second procedure typically is offered to patients who have recurrent AF following a first catheter-based procedure. Interestingly, continuing previously ineffective antiarrhythmic therapy after ablation can further reduce the risk of recurrent AF.[A17]

The surgical maze procedure is nearly always reserved for patients who have a concomitant reason for open heart surgery (e.g., coronary artery bypass grafting and/or a valve operation). The maze procedure is performed from an endocardial or epicardial approach with the same fundamental goal of electrical isolation of the pulmonary veins. In addition, a surgical maze procedure includes the clipping or resection of the left atrial appendage. The success rate for the procedure is comparable to or slightly better than that of catheter-based pulmonary vein isolation.

Paroxysmal AF

Paroxysmal AF refers to recurrent episodes of AF that resolve either spontaneously or with medical treatment. Paroxysmal AF may manifest as a breakthrough arrhythmia in patients who are on chronic medical therapy to suppress AF or in patients who are on no treatment or may be taking a medication (such as a β-blocker or diltiazem) to slow the rate of any future episode of AF. Unfortunately, most behavioral efforts to limit the recurrence of AF have largely proven ineffective. One exception is in regular alcohol drinkers, for whom abstinence from alcohol can reduce the likelihood of recurrent paroxysmal AF by about one third.[A18] Prophylactic rhythm control can be tried, but outcomes are not as good as with ablation,[A19] and medication side effects often are limiting.

For paroxysmal AF, catheter ablation is preferred because it significantly reduces the risk of recurrent atrial arrhythmias and hospitalizations, significantly improves quality of life,[A20] and also results in about a one-third reduction in the risk of major adverse events.[A21] The success rate is improved if it is performed before patients with paroxysmal AF develop persistent AF.

The other option is prophylactic rate control, typically with low-dose metoprolol (25 to 50 mg daily, with the option for an additional dose at the onset of AF and again 6 hours later if rapid AF develops) or diltiazem (180 to 240 mg daily). Another option is so-called pill-in-the-pocket therapy with a single dose of propafenone (600 mg) or flecainide (300 mg) when the paroxysmal AF episode occurs (see Fig. 52-14).

Thromboembolic Prophylaxis

Long-term anticoagulation therapy (Fig. 52-15) is generally recommended in all patients who have persistent or paroxysmal AF and a CHADS VASC score of 2 or more (Table 52-4). When paroxysmal AF is detected by screening in asymptomatic individuals by intermittent electrocardiograms or an implantable loop recorder, prophylactic anticoagulation is of little or limited value in preventing major complications.[A22,A23]

For patients with a single risk factor for stroke in association with AF, the decision to anticoagulate can be at the preference of the patient and physician.[15,16] For thromboembolic prophylaxis in patients who have AF with a mechanical prosthetic valve or rheumatic heart disease, warfarin anticoagulation (Table 70-4) is the approach of choice.[A24] For other patients, however, direct-acting oral anticoagulant medications (Table 70-6 in Chapter 70) have replaced warfarin because of their ease of use, superior or equivalent efficacy, and excellent safety profile.[A25] Options include rivaroxaban (an oral factor Xa inhibitor at 20 mg per day), apixaban (an oral factor Xa inhibitor at 5 mg twice daily), dabigatran (a direct thrombin inhibitor at 150 mg twice daily), and edoxaban (30 or 60 mg once daily). All four drugs are eliminated by the kidney (apixaban 25%, edoxaban 50%, rivaroxaban 65%, and dabigatran 85%), so they are not recommended in patients with substantial renal dysfunction, and their doses should be reduced in patients with moderate renal dysfunction (see Chapter 70).[17] Even in patients older than 75 years, these agents appear to be at least as effective as warfarin with a lower risk of life-threatening bleeding.[18] In very elderly patients who are not considered candidates for full-dose anticoagulation, low-dose edoxaban (15 mg daily) is safe and efficacious.[A26] In patients who cannot take these agents because of renal failure, warfarin titrated to an INR of 2.0 (Chapter 70) is indicated.

Idarucizumab (4 to 5 g intravenously) can rapidly reverse dabigatran,[19] and andexanet alfa (400- to 800-mg bolus over 15 to 30 minutes followed by a 400- to 960-mg infusion) can reverse rivaroxaban or apixaban and achieve good to excellent hemostasis in about 75% of bleeding patients within 12 hours (Chapter 70).[20]

In patients with AF and stable coronary disease (Chapter 59), rivaroxaban (10 mg once daily for patients with a creatinine clearance of 15 to 49 mL/minute or 15 mg once daily for patients with a creatinine clearance of ≥50 mL/minute) alone is safer and as efficacious as combining it with an anti-platelet agent.[A27] In patients with AF after an acute coronary syndrome (Chapter 57) or a coronary stent, standard-dose apixaban (5 mg twice daily or 2.5 mg twice daily for patients who meet two or more of the following dose-reduction criteria: are at least 80

TABLE 52-4 CURRENT RECOMMENDATIONS FOR THROMBOEMBOLIC PROPHYLAXIS FOR PATIENTS WITH ATRIAL FIBRILLATION BASED ON RISK FACTORS FOR STROKE

RISK FACTORS*	RECOMMENDATIONS
Heart failure (1 point) Hypertension (1 point) Age ≥65 (1 point), ≥75 (2 points) Diabetes (1 point) Stroke/TIA (2 points) Vascular disease (1 point) Female sex (1 point)	2 or more points: anticoagulation with warfarin or a direct oral anticoagulant 1 point: anticoagulation or no therapy depending on the preference of the patient and treating physician 0 points: no therapy

*Based on the CHA_2DS_2-VASc risk stratification scoring system.

TIA = transient ischemic attack.

Data from January CT, Wann S, Alpert JS, et al. 2014 AHA/ACC/HRS guideline for the management of patients with atrial fibrillation: a report of the American College of Cardiology/American Heart Association Task Force on Practice Guidelines and the Heart Rhythm Society. *J Am Coll Cardiol.* 2014;64:e1-e76.

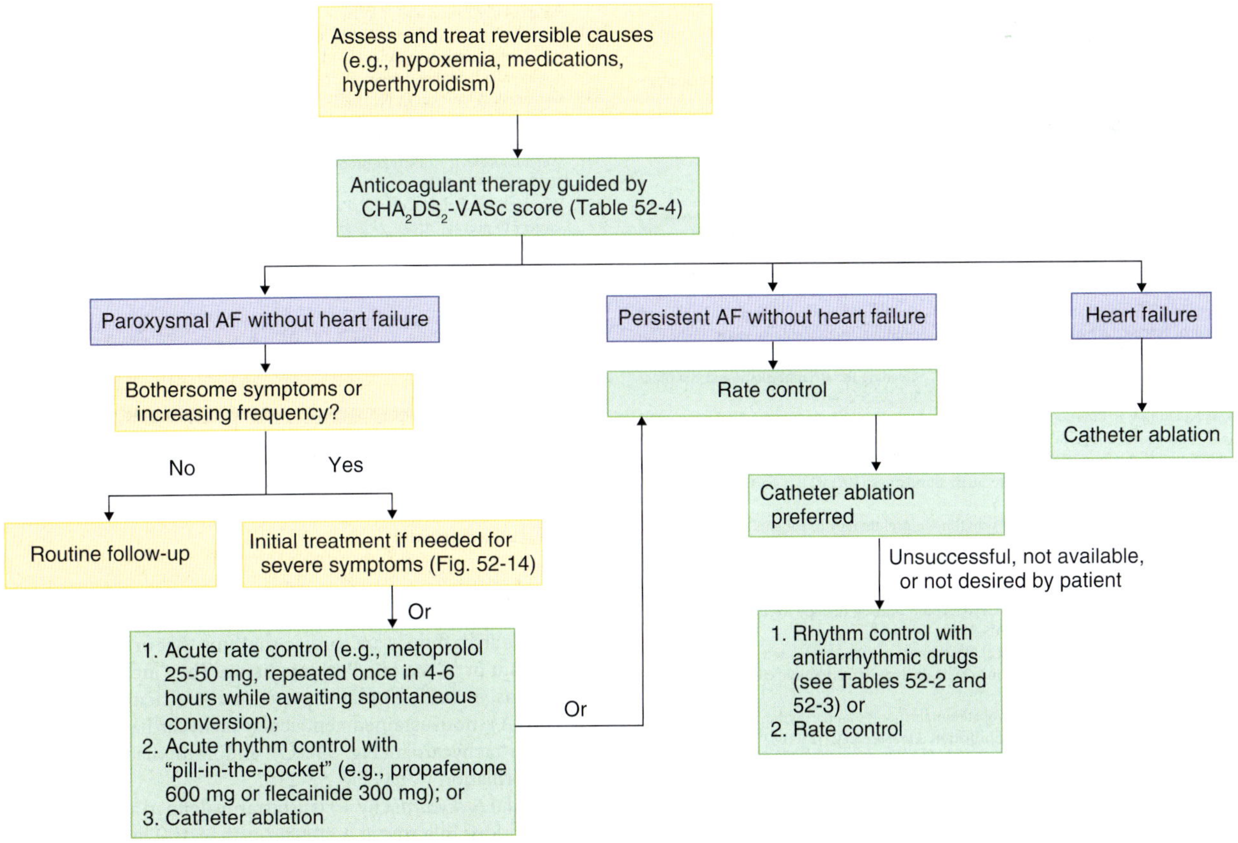

FIGURE 52-15. Treatment of recurrent paroxysmal or chronic persistent fibrillation (AF). Direct oral anticoagulants are strongly preferred over warfarin. If warfarin is used, the goal international normalized ratio is generally 2 to 3. (Adapted from Prystowsky EN, Padanilam BJ, Fogal RI. Treatment of atrial fibrillation. *JAMA.* 2015;314;278-288.)

years of age, weigh no more than 60 kg, or have a serum creatinine level of 1.5 mg/dL or higher) plus a P2Y_{12} inhibitor such as clopidogrel (75 mg once daily) is safer and as efficacious as the two drugs plus aspirin.[A28] Another efficacious option for stented patients is dual therapy with dabigatran (110 or 150 mg twice daily) plus clopidogrel (75 mg once daily) or ticagrelor 180 mg once daily.[A29] The addition of dabigatran, rivaroxaban, or apixaban to aspirin under expert supervision is preferable to adding warfarin.[A30] At the time of an invasive procedure (Chapter 399), bridging anticoagulation is no better than interrupting anticoagulation[A31] except perhaps for the very highest risk patients.[21]

For patients with mechanical valves, warfarin must be used. However, rivaroxaban (20 mg daily) is safer and more effective for patients with AF and a bioprosthetic valve.[A32] Edoxaban is non-inferior to warfarin in patients who are in atrial fibrillation after transcatheter aortic valve replacement.[A33] Oral inhibition of factor XIa is a promising alternative to factor X inhibition.[A34]

For patients at very high risk of bleeding or with serious bleeding on anticoagulation, surgical removal of the left atrial appendage or exclusion of the left atrial appendage with an implanted device is a non-inferior alternative to anticoagulation.[A35,A36] Surgical exclusion of the left atrial appendage is increasingly performed when patients with AF undergo coronary artery bypass graft surgery, and in this situation it is associated with a reduction in the risk of subsequent stroke and bleeding.[A37] With this procedure, serious complications occur in about 2% of patients, and the net benefits from reduced bleeding may increase over time.[22]

PROGNOSIS

Paroxysmal AF can occur as a self-remitting arrhythmia for decades or can progress to permanent AF. Patients with persistent AF generally progress to permanent AF unless sinus rhythm is restored.

The major long-term risks of AF are stroke, which occurs at a rate of about 4% per year in the absence of anticoagulation but only about 0.5% per year with anticoagulation, with individual risks influenced by the presence of specific risk factors (see Table 52-4). The risk is about half as high with paroxysmal AF compared with persistent AF, but even a single paroxysmal AF event is clearly linked to an increased risk of stroke.[23] Persistent AF also increases the likelihood of new or worsening heart failure, especially in patients who have a poorly compliant left ventricle, because of the absence of atrial contraction. Poor rate control can result in tachyarrhythmia-induced left ventricular dysfunction. Prognosis is also linked to any underlying comorbid conditions that may precipitate AF or contribute to a rapid ventricular response.

GENERAL REFERENCES

For the General References and other additional features, please visit Elsevier eBooks+ at https://ebooks.health.elsevier.com.

Grade A References

A1. Appelboam A, Reuben A, Mann C, et al. Postural modification to the standard Valsalva manoeuvre for emergency treatment of supraventricular tachycardias (REVERT): a randomised controlled trial. *Lancet.* 2015;386:1747-1753.
A2. Arvind B, Kothari SS, Juneja R, et al. Ivabradine versus amiodarone in the management of postoperative junctional ectopic tachycardia: a randomized, open-label, noninferiority study. *JACC Clin Electrophysiol.* 2021;7:1052-1060.
A3. Gladstone DJ, Wachter R, Schmalstieg-Bahr K, et al. Screening for atrial fibrillation in the older population: a randomized clinical trial. *JAMA Cardiol.* 2021;6:558-567.
A4. Pluymaekers N, Dudink E, Luermans J, et al. Early or delayed cardioversion in recent-onset atrial fibrillation. *N Engl J Med.* 2019;380:1499-1508.
A5. Stiell IG, Sivilotti MLA, Taljaard M, et al. Electrical versus pharmacological cardioversion for emergency department patients with acute atrial fibrillation (RAFF2): a partial factorial randomised trial. *Lancet.* 2020;395:339-349.
A6. Kirchhof P, Camm AJ, Goette A, et al. Early rhythm-control therapy in patients with atrial fibrillation. *N Engl J Med.* 2020;383:1305-1316.
A7. Wazni OM, Dandamudi G, Sood N, et al. Cryoballoon ablation as initial therapy for atrial fibrillation. *N Engl J Med.* 2021;384:316-324.
A8. Andrade JG, Wells GA, Deyell MW, et al. Cryoablation or drug therapy for initial treatment of atrial fibrillation. *N Engl J Med.* 2021;384:305-315.
A9. Turagam MK, Musikantow D, Whang W, et al. Assessment of catheter ablation or antiarrhythmic drugs for first-line therapy of atrial fibrillation: a meta-analysis of randomized clinical trials. *JAMA Cardiol.* 2021;6:697-705.
A10. Kuniss M, Pavlovic N, Velagic V, et al. Cryoballoon ablation vs. antiarrhythmic drugs: first-line therapy for patients with paroxysmal atrial fibrillation. *Europace.* 2021;23:1033-1041.
A11. Rillig A, Magnussen C, Ozga AK, et al. Early rhythm control therapy in patients with atrial fibrillation and heart failure. *Circulation.* 2021;144:845-858.
A12. Parkash R, Wells GA, Rouleau J, et al. Randomized ablation-based rhythm-control versus rate-control trial in patients with heart failure and atrial fibrillation: results from the RAFT-AF trial. *Circulation.* 2022;145:1693-1704.
A13. Packer DL, Piccini JP, Monahan KH, et al. Ablation versus drug therapy for atrial fibrillation in heart failure: results from the CABANA trial. *Circulation.* 2021;143:1377-1390.
A14. Kotecha D, Bunting KV, Gill SK, et al. Effect of digoxin vs bisoprolol for heart rate control in atrial fibrillation on patient-reported quality of life: the RATE-AF randomized clinical trial. *JAMA.* 2020;324:2497-2508.
A15. Brignole M, Pentimalli F, Palmisano P, et al. AV junction ablation and cardiac resynchronization for patients with permanent atrial fibrillation and narrow QRS: the APAF-CRT mortality trial. *Eur Heart J.* 2021;42:4731-4739.
A16. Chen C, Zhou X, Zhu M, et al. Catheter ablation versus medical therapy for patients with persistent atrial fibrillation: a systematic review and meta-analysis of evidence from randomized controlled trials. *J Interv Card Electrophysiol.* 2018;52:9-18.
A17. Duytschaever M, Demolder A, Phlips T, et al. Pulmonary vein isolation with vs. without continued antiarrhythmic drug treatment in subjects with recurrent atrial fibrillation (POWDER AF): results from a multicentre randomized trial. *Eur Heart J.* 2018;39:1429-1437.
A18. Voskoboinik A, Kalman JM, De Silva A, et al. Alcohol abstinence in drinkers with atrial fibrillation. *N Engl J Med.* 2020;382:20-28.
A19. Andrade JG, Deyell MW, Macle L, et al. Progression of atrial fibrillation after cryoablation or drug therapy. *N Engl J Med.* 2023;388:105-116.
A20. Blomström-Lundqvist C, Gizurarson S, Schwieler J, et al. Effect of catheter ablation vs antiarrhythmic medication on quality of life in patients with atrial fibrillation: the CAPTAF randomized clinical trial. *JAMA.* 2019;321:1059-1068.
A21. Packer DL, Mark DB, Robb RA, et al. Effect of catheter ablation vs antiarrhythmic drug therapy on mortality, stroke, bleeding, and cardiac arrest among patients with atrial fibrillation: the CABANA randomized clinical trial. *JAMA.* 2019;321:1261-1274.
A22. Svendsen JH, Diederichsen SZ, Højberg S, et al. Implantable loop recorder detection of atrial fibrillation to prevent stroke (the LOOP study): a randomised controlled trial. *Lancet.* 2021;398:1507-1516.
A23. Svennberg E, Friberg L, Frykman V, et al. Clinical outcomes in systematic screening for atrial fibrillation (STROKESTOP): a multicentre, parallel group, unmasked, randomised controlled trial. *Lancet.* 2021;398:1498-1506.
A24. Connolly SJ, Karthikeyan G, Ntsekhe M, et al. Rivaroxaban in rheumatic heart disease–associated atrial fibrillation. *N Engl J Med.* 2022;387:978-988.
A25. Carnicelli AP, Hong H, Connolly SJ, et al. Direct oral anticoagulants versus warfarin in patients with atrial fibrillation: patient-level network meta-analyses of randomized clinical trials with interaction testing by age and sex. *Circulation.* 2022;145:242-255.
A26. Okumura K, Akao M, Yoshida T, et al. Low-dose edoxaban in very elderly patients with atrial fibrillation. *N Engl J Med.* 2020;383:1735-1745.
A27. Yasuda S, Kaikita K, Akao M, et al. Antithrombotic therapy for atrial fibrillation with stable coronary disease. *N Engl J Med.* 2019;381:1103-1113.
A28. Khan SU, Osman M, Khan MU, et al. Dual versus triple therapy for atrial fibrillation after percutaneous coronary intervention: a systematic review and meta-analysis. *Ann Intern Med.* 2020;172:474-483.
A29. Harskamp RE, Fanaroff AC, Lopes RD, et al. Antithrombotic therapy in patients with atrial fibrillation after acute coronary syndromes or percutaneous intervention. *J Am Coll Cardiol.* 2022;79:417-427.
A30. Bennaghmouch N, de Veer A, Bode K, et al. Efficacy and safety of the use of non-vitamin K antagonist oral anticoagulants in patients with nonvalvular atrial fibrillation and concomitant aspirin therapy: a meta-analysis of randomized trials. *Circulation.* 2018;137:1117-1129.
A31. Douketis JD, Spyropoulos AC, Kaatz S, et al. Perioperative bridging anticoagulation in patients with atrial fibrillation. *N Engl J Med.* 2015;373:823-833.
A32. Guimarães HP, Lopes RD, de Barros E, et al. Rivaroxaban in patients with atrial fibrillation and a bioprosthetic mitral valve. *N Engl J Med.* 2020;383:2117-2126.
A33. Van Mieghem NM, Unverdorben M, Hengstenberg C, et al. Edoxaban versus vitamin K antagonist for atrial fibrillation after TAVR. *N Engl J Med.* 2021;385:2150-2160.
A34. Piccini JP, Caso V, Connolly SJ, et al. Safety of the oral factor XIa inhibitor asundexian compared with apixaban in patients with atrial fibrillation (PACIFIC-AF): a multicentre, randomised, double-blind, double-dummy, dose-finding phase 2 study. *Lancet.* 2022;399:1383-1390.
A35. Osmancik P, Herman D, Neuzil P, et al. 4-Year outcomes after left atrial appendage closure versus nonwarfarin oral anticoagulation for atrial fibrillation. *J Am Coll Cardiol.* 2022;79:1-14.
A36. Lakkireddy D, Thaler D, Ellis CR, et al. Amplatzer Amulet left atrial appendage occluder versus Watchman Device for stroke prophylaxis (Amulet IDE): a randomized, controlled trial. *Circulation.* 2021;144:1543-1552.
A37. Whitlock RP, Belley-Cote EP, Paparella D, et al. Left atrial appendage occlusion during cardiac surgery to prevent stroke. *N Engl J Med.* 2021;384:2081-2091.

53 VENTRICULAR ARRHYTHMIAS

HASAN GARAN

DEFINITIONS

Ventricular arrhythmias are cardiac rhythms that originate in the ventricular myocardium or in the His-Purkinje tissue. They include a wide spectrum of arrhythmias, including isolated premature ventricular contractions (PVCs) (Fig. 53-1A), nonsustained ventricular tachycardia (Fig. 53-1B), sustained ventricular tachycardia (Fig. 53-1C), and immediately life-threatening ventricular fibrillation (VF) (Fig. 53-2).

Ventricular tachycardia (VT) is arbitrarily defined as three or more ventricular contractions in a row at a rate faster than 100 beats per minute (see Fig. 53-1B). The definition of *sustained* VT—a continuous ventricular rhythm, at a rate faster than 100 beats per minute, with no interruption for 30 seconds

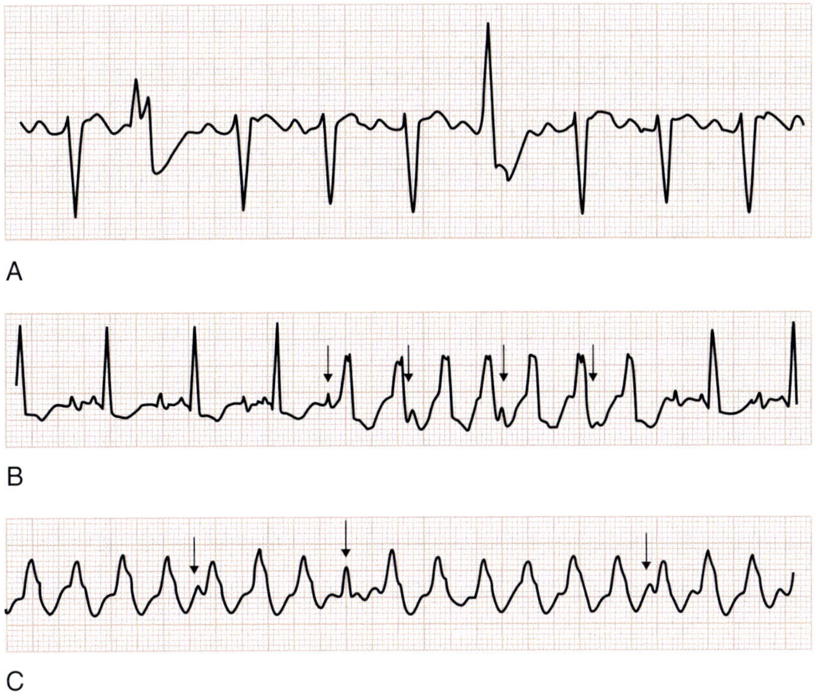

FIGURE 53-1. Ventricular arrhythmias. A, Multifocal premature ventricular beats. B, Nonsustained monomorphic ventricular tachycardia (VT). Note dissociated P waves indicated by *arrows*. C, Sustained monomorphic VT. Dissociated P waves are indicated by *arrows*, and the eighth beat in the tracing is a fusion beat.

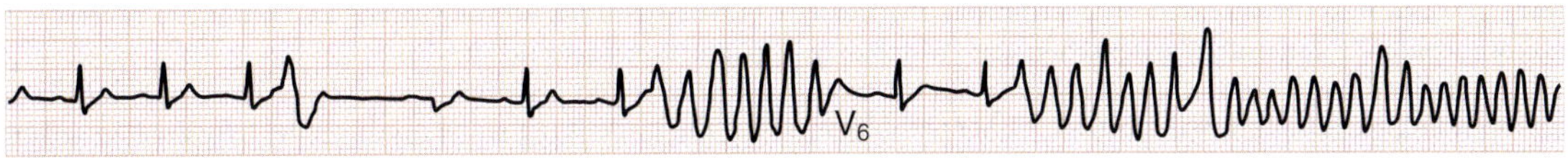

FIGURE 53-2. This electrocardiogram in a patient with idiopathic ventricular fibrillation (VF) shows recurrent, closely coupled premature ventricular contractions (PVCs) and the initiation of VF by one of these closely coupled PVCs.

or longer—is equally arbitrary. However, most sustained VTs are much faster than 100 beats per minute (see Fig. 53-1C), persist for more than 30 seconds, and cause a substantial decrease in ventricular function and cardiac output, especially in patients with underlying organic heart disease, thereby resulting in acute heart failure, hypotension, syncope, or even circulatory collapse.

Monomorphic VT is electrocardiographically defined as a wide-complex tachycardia with no change in QRS configuration, frontal axis, or horizontal axis from one beat to the next (Fig. 53-3A). Polymorphic VT is characterized by beat-to-beat changes in the QRS morphology and axis, and very fast polymorphic VT may be difficult to distinguish from *ventricular fibrillation* (VF) (Fig. 53-3B). VF, which is a grossly irregular ventricular rhythm usually at a rate faster than 300 beats per minute, appears as low-amplitude continuous electrical activity on the surface electrocardiogram (ECG) and generates no cardiac output. Torsades de pointes and bidirectional polymorphic VT are two distinct subtypes of polymorphic VT. *Pleomorphic* VT describes the phenomenon of multiple clinical monomorphic VTs, each with distinct QRS configurations and axis observed at different times in the same patient.

EPIDEMIOLOGY

The prevalence of PVCs is a function of sampling method and duration, and PVCs may be seen in 50% of apparently healthy individuals if the monitoring time is 24 hours or longer. Asymptomatic PVCs may, however, be a marker of more serious underlying heart disease.

Nonsustained VT may be recorded in up to 3% of apparently healthy individuals with no identifiable heart disease. The prevalence of PVCs and nonsustained VT not only increases with age but also with the presence and severity of an underlying heart disease. Therefore, the finding of nonsustained VT often leads to a cardiac evaluation to exclude organic heart disease, even if it is incidentally discovered in an asymptomatic patient. The prevalence of nonsustained VT rises to 7 to 12% in the late phase of myocardial infarction (MI) and may be as high as 80% in patients with advanced heart failure owing to dilated cardiomyopathy (Chapter 47).

Approximately 10% of patients with documented sustained VT have no identifiable heart disease, in which case idiopathic VT is diagnosed. The prevalence of idiopathic VT is estimated to be only 15.5 in 100,000 in men and 12.3 in 100,000 in women.

VT or VF in patients with advanced organic heart disease accounts for an estimated 50% of all annual cardiovascular deaths in the United States. The nature of the underlying heart disease in patients dying of VT or VF is age dependent. Before 30 years of age, the heart diseases most commonly associated with VT and VF are genetically inherited cardiomyopathies or channelopathies (Chapter 47), whereas acute MI and cardiomyopathy (either ischemic or dilated nonischemic) are the most common underlying heart diseases in individuals older than 40 years. In about 15% of cases of sudden cardiac death without obvious underlying organic heart disease identifiable at autopsy, postmortem genetic analysis may identify a clinically actionable pathologic mutation in an ion channel that predisposes to VT and VF.

PATHOBIOLOGY

Based on their underlying mechanisms, ventricular arrhythmias are classified as re-entrant, triggered, or automatic (Chapter 48). Re-entry, commonly the result of activation in adjacent circuits sharing a common pathway referred to as the isthmus, is initiated by the simultaneous presence of conduction block in one pathway and abnormally slow conduction in an adjacent pathway, thereby allowing recovery of excitability in the former (E-Fig. 53-1A). One type of triggered activity results from early afterdepolarizations, which are rapidly repetitive depolarizations occurring during the late phase of the action potential in the setting of an abnormally delayed repolarization process (E-Fig. 53-1B). Another type of triggered activity results from delayed afterdepolarizations, which reach depolarization threshold and cause repetitive action potentials in the setting of elevated intracellular calcium concentrations (see E-Fig. 53-1B). Automatic arrhythmias arise from accelerated pacemaker activity (E-Fig. 53-1C).

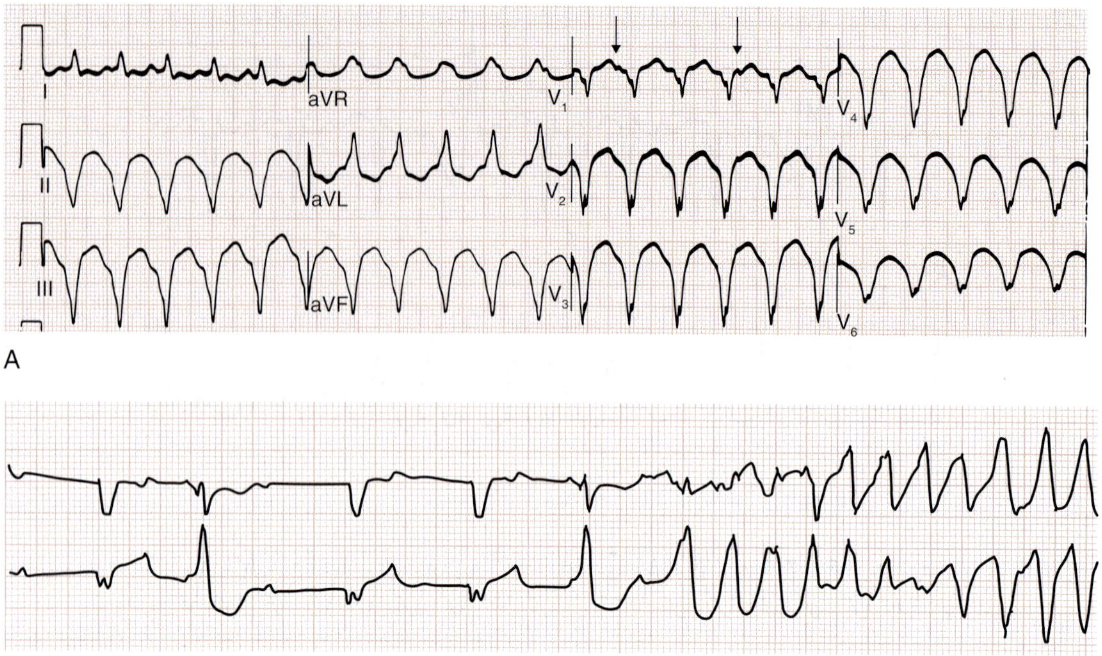

FIGURE 53-3. A, Monomorphic ventricular tachycardia (VT) in a patient with a prior myocardial infarction. The *arrows* identify P waves in lead V_1, showing atrioventricular dissociation. No R wave is recorded in any of the precordial leads V_1 to V_6 during VT. B, Polymorphic VT in a patient with chronic ischemic cardiomyopathy and marked first-degree atrioventricular block. There is no QT prolongation before the onset of the polymorphic VT.

Sustained re-entrant activation in the diseased myocardium is the most common cause of monomorphic VT and usually arises when scar (which may be subendocardial, transmural, or subepicardial), resulting from prior ischemic injury, creates an electrophysiologically abnormal substrate. Other pathologic conditions capable of creating a substrate for re-entry include inflammation (e.g., myocarditis), granuloma (e.g., cardiac sarcoidosis), fibrofatty infiltration (e.g., arrhythmogenic right ventricular cardiomyopathy), genetically caused sarcomeric disarray (e.g., hypertrophic cardiomyopathy), infiltration (e.g., amyloidosis, hemochromatosis), and iatrogenic scar (e.g., surgical repair of tetralogy of Fallot). These substrates may also result in polymorphic VT and VF by a similar re-entrant mechanism.

Triggered activity resulting from delayed afterdepolarizations is thought to be the underlying mechanism for most idiopathic monomorphic VT that has a focal site of origin in the right or left ventricular outflow tract, in one of the sinuses of Valsalva, the area of aortomitral continuity, or in the myocardial segment termed the left ventricular summit. Idiopathic VT from re-entry in the fascicles of the left bundle branch has a relatively narrow QRS complex that mimics right bundle branch block (RBBB) and anterior or posterior fascicular block. Idiopathic fascicular VTs may be electrocardiographically difficult to distinguish from idiopathic papillary muscle VTs. In Brugada syndrome, the primary cause is genetically acquired abnormal conduction in the epicardium of the right ventricular outflow tract.

Torsades de pointes, which is a specific type of polymorphic VT that derives its name from the rotating of the QRS axis, is caused by early afterdepolarizations that arise during a delayed repolarization process in the setting of genetic long QT syndromes or acquired long QT during therapy with QT-prolonging drugs. The cause may be either diminished outflowing repolarizing potassium currents, enhanced inflowing sodium currents due to incomplete inactivation of the sodium channel, or increased inflowing calcium currents. Although many episodes terminate spontaneously, the rates are usually very fast, and episodes of torsade can transform into sustained VF.

Bundle branch re-entry, which incorporates the right and the left bundle branches distally joined by the slowly conducting septal myocardium, may cause one or two nonsustained ventricular beats in a normal heart. However, sustained bundle branch re-entry occurs when myocardial disease causes chamber enlargement and bundle branch elongation and/or disease in the conduction system causes abnormally slow conduction, thereby creating the scenario for sustained bundle branch re-entry. The common type of bundle branch re-entry has anterograde activation over the right bundle and uses the left bundle retrogradely, thereby resulting in a left bunch branch block (LBBB) pattern on the surface ECG, but the reverse direction with RBBB pattern may also occur.

Accelerated pacemaker activity in an ectopic location, with rates exceeding the underlying sinus rhythm rate, may arise in settings such as transient inflammation, excess digoxin levels, intracellular calcium loading, electrolyte imbalance, and coronary reperfusion following occlusion. Bidirectional VT is thought to result from calcium overload of the myocytes owing to congenitally acquired, abnormal ryanodine receptor or calsequestrin function, or from digitalis toxicity, and it may transform to more malignant polymorphic VT and VF.

Finally, there is no consensus regarding the mechanisms underlying VF. Theoretically, VF may be initiated when a premature contraction falls in the vulnerable period of the action potential, thereby precipitating a re-entrant wave that breaks into sister wavelets and results in high-frequency electrical activity. In fact, VF may be regarded as an end stage for a variety of severe electrophysiologic abnormalities that result in chaotic activation.

CLINICAL MANIFESTATIONS

Ventricular arrhythmias can present in a variety of clinical settings (Table 53-1). They may be asymptomatic and detected only by an irregular pulse on a physical examination, on a routine ECG, or on an exercise test. Symptomatic ventricular arrhythmias can present as palpitations, dizziness, syncope (Chapters 39 and 49), shortness of breath, or sudden cardiac arrest (Chapter 50). The diagnosis may be confirmed by ambulatory ECG monitoring (Chapter 49), but more extended monitoring by a loop recorder may be needed to detect arrhythmias that may be rare and intermittent. Ambulatory monitoring can also help correlate arrhythmias with any symptoms they may cause. In some patients, exercise testing can be helpful for diagnosis.

Acute Myocardial Infarction

VT and VF may arise as early as minutes to hours after the onset of symptoms during coronary thrombosis, and prehospital VT and VF during acute MI are responsible for a large proportion of out-of-hospital sudden cardiac deaths (Chapter 50). The incidence of peri-infarction VF has declined over the past two decades, perhaps related to the widespread application of successful early coronary revascularization (Chapter 59) during acute MI. Among patients with ST elevation MI who now reach the hospital, about 3 to 4% develop VT, mostly during the acute phase. The incidence of VT in patients with non–ST elevation MI (Chapter 57) is lower, about 1%. Accelerated idioventricular rhythm (AIVR) is an automatic ventricular rhythm that is faster than the sinus rate but usually less than 120 beats per minute. It may occur

TABLE 53-1 VENTRICULAR TACHYCARDIA AND CARDIAC DIAGNOSIS

STRUCTURAL HEART DISEASE
Acquired heart disease
Acute myocardial infarction
Prior myocardial infarction, ischemic heart disease
Nonischemic dilated cardiomyopathy
Hypertensive heart disease
Valvular heart disease
Cardiac sarcoidosis
Cardiac amyloidosis
Other infiltrative diseases (e.g., Chagas disease)
Cardiac tumors
Congenital heart disease
Arrhythmogenic right ventricular cardiomyopathy
Hypertrophic cardiomyopathy
Genetic dilated cardiomyopathies
Iatrogenic
Surgically repaired congenital heart disease
Left ventricular assist devices
NO STRUCTURAL HEART DISEASE
Idiopathic ventricular tachycardia
Right and left ventricular outflow tract tachycardias
Left intrafascicular reentry
Papillary muscle tachycardias
Ion channel/ryanodine receptor mutations
Long QT syndromes
Catecholaminergic polymorphic ventricular tachycardia
Short QT syndrome
Mixed etiology
Brugada syndrome
Idiopathic ventricular fibrillation

TABLE 53-2 DISTINGUISHING VENTRICULAR TACHYCARDIA FROM SUPRAVENTRICULAR TACHYCARDIA WITH ABERRANT CONDUCTION

VENTRICULAR TACHYCARDIA	SUPRAVENTRICULAR TACHYCARDIA
AV dissociation	Same QRS morphology as preexisting bundle branch block in sinus rhythm
aVR: initial R > S or initial R or Q >40 msec	V_1: rsR′
Absence of any R waves in V_1 to V_6	
V_1 to V_6: onset of R to S >100 msec in any lead	
QRS duration >160 msec	
Initial R wave in aVR	

AV = atrioventricular.

immediately following coronary reperfusion after an acute MI, and it typically terminates spontaneously.

DIAGNOSIS

Not every wide-complex tachycardia is VT (Fig. 49-3). The diagnosis is straightforward when a His bundle electrogram is recorded during a wide-complex tachycardia in the cardiac electrophysiology laboratory, but diagnosis on a standard 12-lead ECG may be challenging (Table 53-2). The differential diagnosis of a sustained regular-rate wide-complex tachycardia includes any type of supraventricular tachycardia with aberrant conduction (Chapter 52), supraventricular tachycardia with ventricular preexcitation, bundle branch re-entry, and myocardial VT. The clinical setting and the patient's background (e.g., history of previous MI or cardiomyopathy) play a major role in making an accurate diagnosis. A wide-complex tachycardia in a young and otherwise healthy individual with no structural heart disease is more likely to be a supraventricular tachycardia (SVT) conducted with aberration or with preexcitation, but it also may be idiopathic VT. Establishing a definitive diagnosis is critically important.

The most reliable electrocardiographic observation in favor of VT is evidence of atrioventricular (AV) dissociation, that is, the absence of any relationship between the atrial and ventricular rate, with the ventricular rate faster than the atrial rate (see Fig. 53-1C), or a regular wide-complex tachycardia with the atria fibrillating. Such findings immediately exclude SVT with aberration or preexcitation except for extremely rare cases of junctional tachycardia with aberrant conduction or nodo-fascicular/nodo-ventricular reentrant tachycardia. However, the absence of AV dissociation does not exclude VT because 1:1 ventriculoatrial conduction is present in about 50% of VTs and can be seen on the 12-lead ECG in 25% of cases. Fusion beats (which occur when an occasional sinus beat conducts through the AV node and reaches the His-Purkinje system at the same time as the VT source activates the myocardium, thereby resulting in a beat with a morphology that is the hybrid of a conducted QRS complex and the VT complex; Fig. 53-1C) also confirm AV dissociation but are observed only when VT rates are relatively slow.

Another approach is to rely on ECG lead aVR, where the presence of an initial R wave, notching on the initial downstroke of a predominantly negative QRS complex, and the width of an initial r-wave or q-wave > 40 ms strongly suggest VT. Other findings that favor VT include a QRS duration longer than 160 msec, or longer than 140 msec with an RBBB pattern. The absence of an RS complex in all precordial ECG leads or an interval of more than 100 msec from the onset of R to the nadir of S wave favors VT (Fig. 53-4; and see Fig. 53-3A). The absence of any R waves in the QRS complexes recorded from all six precordial leads (see Fig. 53-3A), described as *negative concordance*, strongly suggests VT, but is not a common finding. Prominent R waves observed in all six precordial ECG leads, termed *positive concordance*, may be seen in SVT with left ventricular preexcitation in patients without structural heart disease but otherwise also suggests VT with a basal site of origin. A wide-complex tachycardia with a QRS morphology identical to that of aberrantly conducted sinus rhythm manifesting bundle branch block (BBB) on a previously recorded ECG in the same patient should raise suspicion of bundle branch re-entry VT if the ECG shows AV dissociation, which excludes 1 : 1 aberrantly conducted supraventricular tachycardia.

If AV dissociation is not present, the differential diagnosis includes SVT with aberrant conduction, but the rare condition of preexcitation with an atriofascicular accessory pathway should also be considered in a patient with LBBB pattern and 1 : 1 AV ratio. A monomorphic wide-complex tachycardia with an irregular rate, manifested by more than 60-msec difference in cycle length from one beat to the next, is likely to be atrial fibrillation (AF) or atrial flutter, with variable AV block and aberrant conduction or with preexcitation. It is important to emphasize that severe electrolyte imbalances or the use of antiarrhythmic drugs diminishes the predictive accuracy of all of these diagnostic clues.

Sustained polymorphic wide-complex tachycardia with marked beat-to-beat changes in the QRS morphology is either atrial fibrillation with varying degrees of preexcitation from one beat to the next or ventricular tachycardia that either terminates spontaneously or transforms into VF. Torsades de pointes is frequently pause dependent—typically starting when a premature beat falls on the T wave of the beat following a long RR interval (Fig. 53-5). Finally, bidirectional VT manifesting a unique feature of beat-by-beat axis alternans may occur with digitalis toxicity or in congenital catecholaminergic polymorphic VT syndrome.

Several different algorithms based on the configurations of the QRS complexes have high sensitivity, high specificity, and acceptable predictive accuracy for distinguishing epicardial VT from endocardial VT (Table 53-3). If the site of origin is epicardial, the rapidly conducting His-Purkinje system is not available immediately, and the intramyocardial conduction delay produces a slurred initial component of the QRS complex, often called a *pseudo-delta wave*, which is manifested as a slow rate of rise of voltage before it reaches the intrinsicoid deflection (Fig. 53-6). Early recognition of ECG findings suggesting an epicardial origin of VT is important in planning and preparing a patient before a catheter ablation procedure (Chapter 54) because the epicardial approach requires a special technique in the cardiac electrophysiology laboratory.

Diagnostic cardiac electrophysiology testing (Chapter 49) may be indicated in patients who have organic heart disease and recurrent syncope but in whom the history, physical examination, ECG, echocardiogram, and ambulatory cardiac rhythm monitoring fail to clarify the cause, especially if the patient has a history of MI or cardiomyopathy, either of which increases the probability that VT may be the cause of syncope.

Identifying the Underlying Cause of Ventricular Arrhythmias

In patients with ventricular arrhythmia, the first step is to conduct a careful evaluation to exclude any underlying structural heart disease. This evaluation must include a comprehensive history and physical examination (Chapter 39),

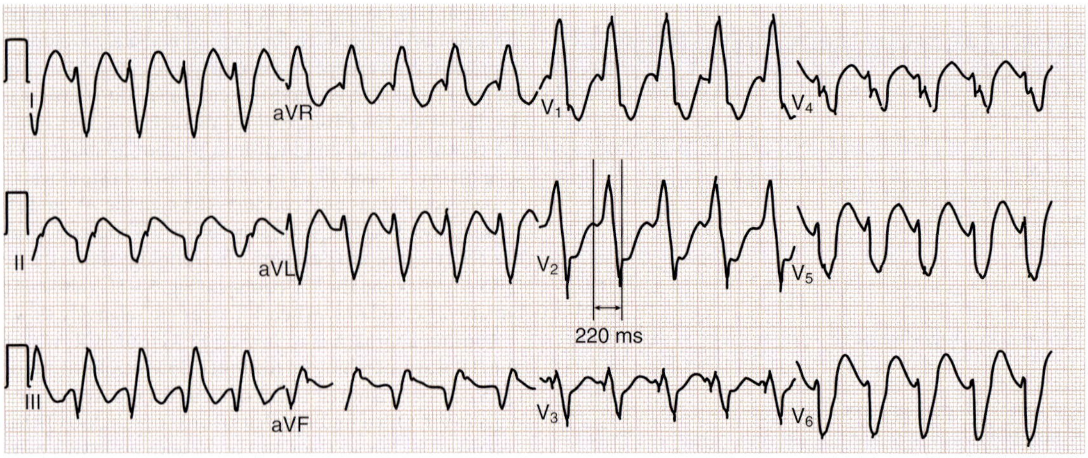

FIGURE 53-4. Monomorphic ventricular tachycardia in a patient with chronic ischemic cardiomyopathy. In lead V_2, the duration from the onset of the R wave to the nadir of the S wave is 220 msec. See text for further explanation.

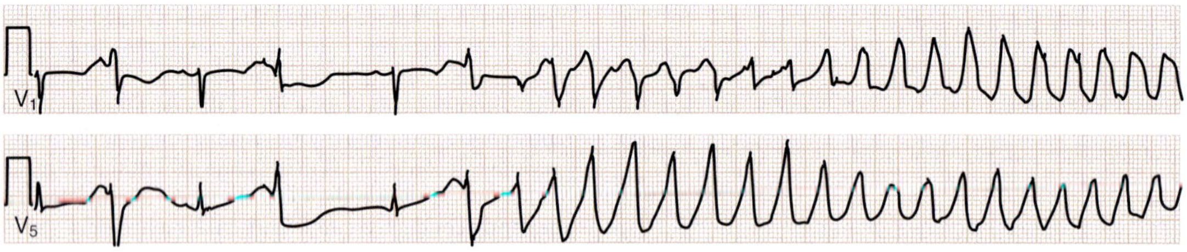

FIGURE 53-5. Torsades de pointes (TdP) in a patient with a markedly prolonged QT interval. A premature ventricular beat just after the peak of the T wave initiates TdP. As the tachycardia progresses, the rotation or the "twist" in the QRS axis is clearly observed in lead V_1, with the polarity of the signal changing gradually from negative to positive.

TABLE 53-3 ELECTROCARDIOGRAPHIC PARAMETERS TO HELP PREDICT AN EPICARDIAL ORIGIN OF VENTRICULAR TACHYCARDIA

PARAMETER	CRITERIA
Pseudo-delta wave	>75 msec favors epicardial site
Intrinsicoid deflection time	>85 msec favors epicardial site
Onset of R to nadir of S in precordial leads	>120 msec favors epicardial site
QRS duration	Epicardial longer
Q waves during VT in lead I	Favors epicardial site
Q waves during VT in II, III, aVF	Favors endocardial site
aVR/aVL amplitude ratio	Epicardial higher

VT = ventricular tachycardia.

electrocardiography, echocardiography (Chapter 43), extended cardiac rhythm monitoring (Chapter 49), and stress testing (Chapter 56). The family history may provide clues for the presence of an inherited cardiomyopathy (Chapter 47) or channelopathy. Cardiac magnetic resonance imaging (Chapter 44) is indicated in patients who are suspected of having sarcoidosis or arrhythmogenic right ventricular cardiomyopathy, and for risk stratification in patients with cardiomyopathy. Other tests to consider include 99 m technetium-pyrophosphate scan in patients suspected to have transthyretin cardiac amyloidosis (Chapters 47 and 174) and positron emission tomography to detect active myocardial inflammation (Chapter 44), conditions which predispose to ventricular tachyarrhythmias.

Despite a comprehensive evaluation, about 10 to 15% of patients will have VT with no identifiable structural or genetically identifiable cause. Most of the idiopathic monomorphic VTs are in one of two categories, distinguishable by ECG morphology. VTs that arise in the right or left ventricular outflow tract typically manifest an inferiorly directed frontal axis (E-Fig. 53-2); the QRS configurations and polarity observed in the right precordial leads (V_1 and V_2) may further discriminate the sites of origin as the right or the left ventricular outflow tract or one of the sinuses of Valsalva. VT originating in the right sinus of Valsalva closely resembles VT originating in the right ventricular outflow tract. In VT originating in the left sinus of Valsalva, the R wave duration and R/S wave amplitude ratio in leads V_1 and V_2 are significantly increased compared with VT from the right ventricular outflow tract. By comparison, idiopathic left ventricular tachycardia resulting from intrafascicular re-entry usually manifests RBBB and left axis deviation, but there may also be right axis deviation. The QRS complexes typically are not very wide because the involved region is His-Purkinje tissue adjacent to the interventricular septum. Idiopathic VT arising in one of the left ventricular papillary muscles has QRS complexes similar to those of intrafascicular re-entry (E-Fig. 53-3). Either of these typical patterns in a patient with no structural heart disease suggests idiopathic VT. Conversely, sustained VT that does not fall into either of these two broad categories should always raise a high index of suspicion that organic heart disease may be present.

Chronic Ischemic Heart Disease and Post–Myocardial Infarction Ventricular Tachycardia

In survivors of ST elevation MI (Chapter 58), the risk of sudden cardiac death is 10 times higher during the first month than later during recovery. The prevalence of sustained VT by 6 weeks is about 1%, and VT may occur as late as 15 to 20 years after the acute MI without any intervening event. VT commonly, but not invariably, reflects poor left ventricular function. The electrophysiologic substrate is the surviving but electrophysiologically abnormal tissue embedded in the infarcted zone, which creates the conditions responsible for re-entry. The areas that harbor pathways underlying re-entry may be identified by low-amplitude fractionated endocardial electrograms recorded in late systole during sinus rhythm or in mid-diastole during VT in the cardiac electrophysiology laboratory. Up to 16% of the VTs in ischemic heart disease are of epicardial origin. The same pathologic substrate may cause polymorphic VT and VF that, unlike torsades de pointes, do not depend on a long QT interval.

Nonischemic Dilated Cardiomyopathy

The most common cause of sustained monomorphic VT in nonischemic cardiomyopathy (Chapter 47) is also re-entry within the myocardium, but it differs from the post-infarction VT of chronic ischemic heart disease. The pathologic substrates tend to be located in basal, lateral, and often perivalvular

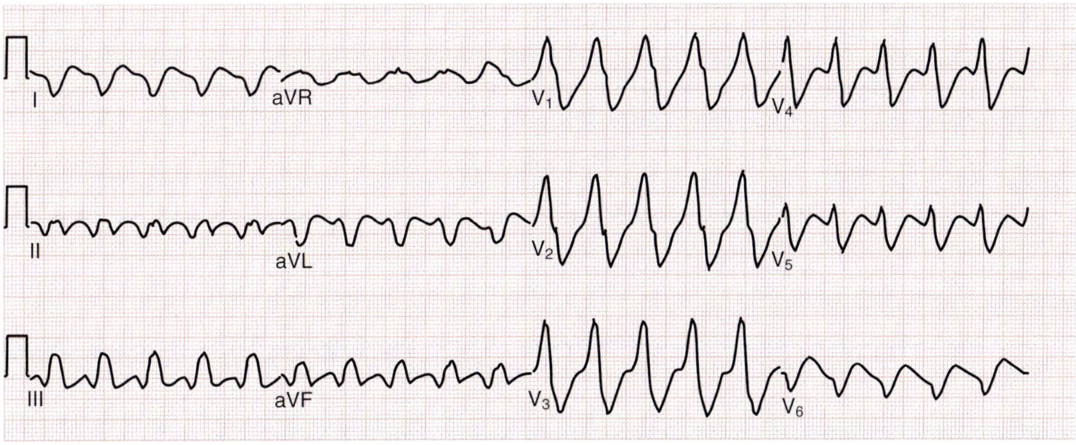

FIGURE 53-6. **Monomorphic epicardial ventricular tachycardia in a patient with nonischemic dilated cardiomyopathy.** The positive polarity pseudo-delta wave is prominent in the right precordial leads, and the negative polarity pseudo-delta wave is prominent in the inferior limb leads.

left ventricular areas, which may correlate with the location of intramyocardial or subepicardial scarring identified by imaging studies. The proportion of monomorphic VTs due to bundle branch re-entry is higher in nonischemic dilated cardiomyopathy compared with chronic ischemic heart disease.[1] Also, VT in nonischemic dilated cardiomyopathy is more likely to have an epicardial origin—as high as 35% overall and reaching 70% in Chagas disease.

Rapidly Reversing Cardiomyopathy

Patients with stress-induced cardiomyopathy (Chapter 47) will recover over several days to weeks, and patients with viral myocarditis may also recover relatively rapidly. Despite recovery of their ventricular systolic function, subgroups of patients with a history of myocarditis have a higher incidence of subsequent VT and mortality than the healthy controls over long-term follow-up.

Heart Failure

The failing heart from any underlying cause (Chapter 45) is highly vulnerable to ventricular arrhythmias. The proportion of sudden arrhythmic death depends on heart failure class and may be as high as 60% in class II to III heart failure. In patients with class IV heart failure, however, the fatal arrhythmia is more often an agonal bradyarrhythmia. Re-entrant VT is common, especially in patients whose heart failure is due to advanced ischemic heart disease, but triggered activity resulting from derangements of calcium homeostasis may also play a prominent role. In addition, hormonal factors, electrolyte abnormalities, and changes in autonomic nervous system activity also increase the vulnerability of the failing heart to ventricular arrhythmias.

Inflammatory and Infiltrative Disease

Among patients with sarcoidosis (Chapter 83), about 40 to 50% have cardiac involvement, which may first manifest as progressive AV block, VT, or both. Although the true prevalence of VT in sarcoidosis is not known, in the selected patients who have received implantable cardiac defibrillators (ICDs) for cardiac sarcoidosis diagnosed by endomyocardial biopsy, cardiac magnetic resonance imaging, or cardiac positron emission tomographic scans, about 15% per year have appropriate ICD discharges for sustained VT. Patients with other infiltrative heart diseases such as amyloidosis (Chapter 174), Fabry disease (Chapter 192), and hemochromatosis (Chapter 196) also have an elevated risk for VT and life-threatening ventricular arrhythmias.

Adult Congenital Heart Disease

VT may occur in the setting of any adult congenital heart disease with a ventricular surgical scar or patch, as is seen after repair of tetralogy of Fallot or a ventricular septal defect closure. It may also occur in a failing systemic right ventricle (Chapter 55). In patients with surgically repaired tetralogy of Fallot, the right ventricular outflow tract, with its scarring and artificial material, serves as an ideal milieu for re-entry and VT. In these patients, the prevalence of VT is about 5 to 10%, and about 2% have sudden cardiac death.

Genetically Inherited Cardiomyopathies

Hypertrophic cardiomyopathy (Chapter 47) is responsible for more than one third of sudden cardiac deaths in patients younger than age 25 years (Chapter 50), and mortality in young hypertrophic cardiomyopathy patients is almost exclusively due to VT and VF. Neither genetic testing nor a cardiac electrophysiology study can definitively identify patients at high risk for VT and VF, and the estimation of risk is based on findings such as a history of syncope, documented nonsustained VT especially in a young patient, a markedly thickened (>3 cm) interventricular septum, and a paradoxical decrease in blood pressure during exercise. Recent studies suggest that the extent of late gadolinium enhancement on cardiac magnetic resonance imaging may be a reliable predictor of serious ventricular arrhythmias in patients with hypertrophic cardiomyopathy.

Arrhythmogenic right ventricular cardiomyopathy[2] is a congenital cardiomyopathy (Chapter 47), usually with an autosomal dominant inheritance. The fibrofatty infiltration of the right ventricular myocardium, which may also involve the interventricular septum and the left ventricle, results in progressive electrophysiologic abnormalities, which may be manifest on the surface ECG as an epsilon wave (Fig. 53-7). The markedly altered conduction characteristics are conducive to re-entry. The incidence of VT in arrhythmic right ventricular cardiomyopathy is related to the severity of the pathologic myocardial changes and ranges from 25 to 100%, depending on the penetrance and the expressivity of the disease. VT typically is initiated by exercise and mimics LBBB in the precordial ECG leads. However, unlike idiopathic right ventricular outflow tract VT, the frontal axis may not be inferiorly directed, and multiple endocardial and epicardial sites of origin exist in about 60% of cases. Vigorous exercise may accelerate the progression of cardiomyopathy and increase the incidence of ventricular arrhythmia.

Genetically Inherited Ventricular Arrhythmias

Several genetically acquired syndromes, including the long QT syndromes, Brugada syndrome, and catecholaminergic polymorphic VT, increase the risk for sudden cardiac death due to ventricular tachyarrhythmias. Despite the remarkable genetic heterogeneity of long QT syndrome, most cases are LQT1, LQT2, and LQT3, which result from loss-of-function mutations in genes *KCNQ1* and *KCNH2* that code for two different potassium channels or gain-in-function mutations in the *SCN5A* gene that codes for the sodium channel.[3] The other genetic mutations are extremely rare. The VT of long QT syndrome is torsades de pointes, and both bradycardia and pauses increase its probability in patients who are predisposed. The incidence of torsades de pointes is influenced by multiple factors, including age, gender, the particular genetic mutation, and the magnitude of QT prolongation (Fig. 53-8A).

The electrocardiographic hallmark of Brugada syndrome, which also predisposes to ventricular tachyarrhythmias and sudden cardiac death, is coved ST segment elevations in the right precordial leads (Fig. 53-8B). In some cases, this pattern may not be present except when the patient is febrile. The inheritance is autosomal dominant, but the genetics are complex. A pathogenic variant of the *SCN5A* gene is present in less than 20% of the cases. Catecholaminergic polymorphic VT is a rare genetic condition resulting from abnormal calcium homeostasis. It is characterized by exercise-induced, wide-complex tachycardia manifesting alternating ECG axes from one beat to

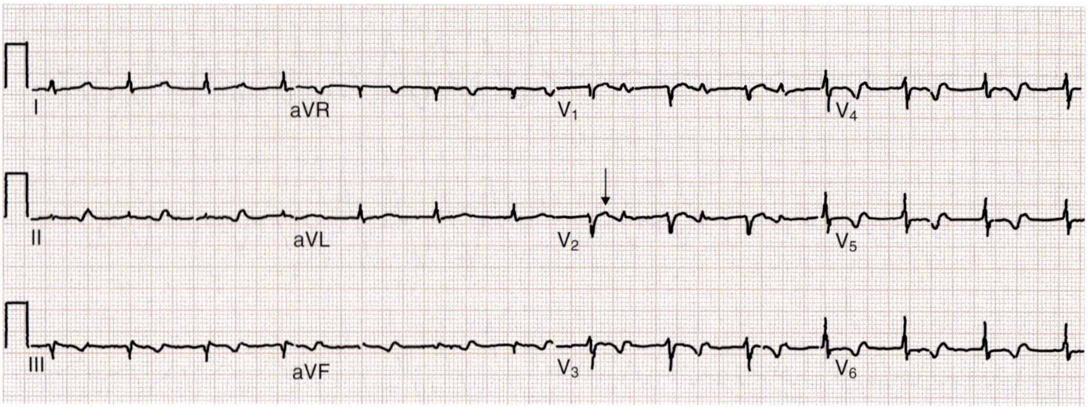

FIGURE 53-7. This electrocardiogram was recorded in a patient with arrhythmogenic right ventricular cardiomyopathy, marked first-degree heart block, and recurrent ventricular tachycardia. Epsilon waves, marked by the *arrow*, are visible in the right precordial leads.

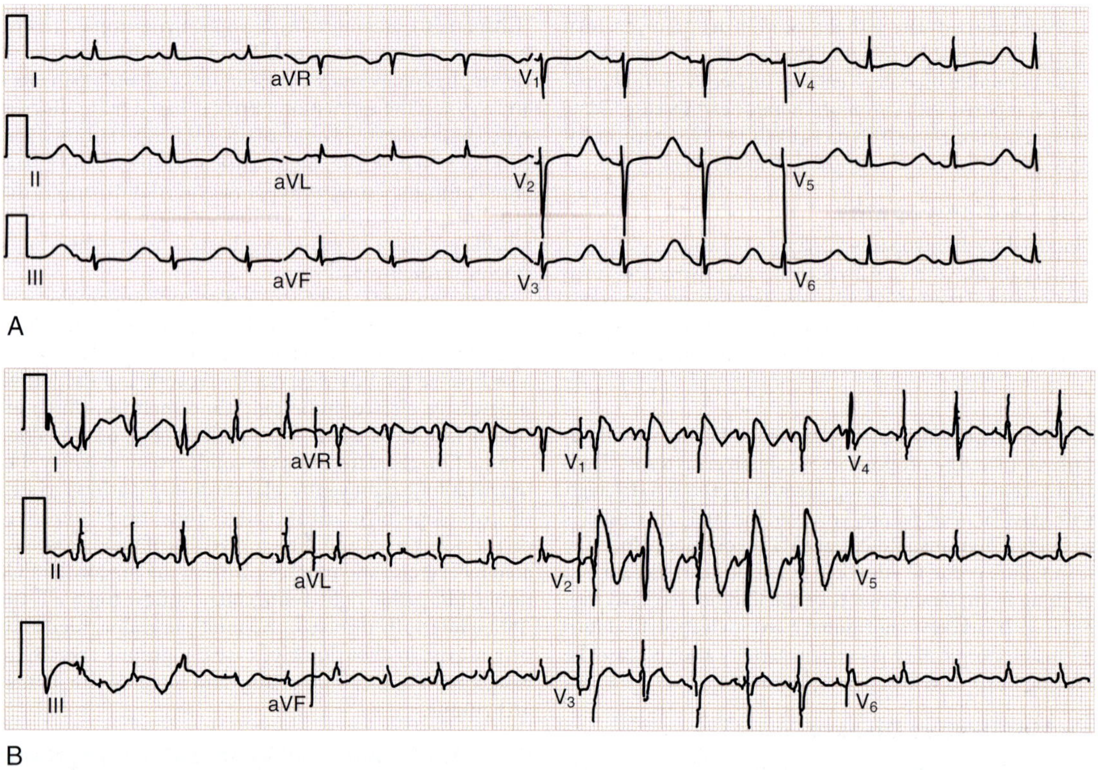

FIGURE 53-8. A, Electrocardiogram showing a QT interval of 640 msec in a woman with LQT1 syndrome, with the terminal portion of the Q wave merging with the P wave. B, Electrocardiogram of a man with Brugada syndrome, showing the typical "coved" elevation in lead V_1.

the next. This condition also predisposes the patient to exercise-induced VF. In addition, a chromosomal haplotype causing overexpression of dipeptidyl peptidase-like protein-6 has been described in one type of familial idiopathic VF,[4] which is a rare but challenging subset of inheritable arrhythmia syndromes causing sudden cardiac death.

Iatrogenic Ventricular Tachycardia and Ventricular Fibrillation

QT-prolonging drugs, including class III antiarrhythmic drugs (see www.torsades.org), may precipitate torsades de pointes and VF in genetically predisposed individuals even if the baseline QTc is normal or borderline.[5] Class IC antiarrhythmic drugs may cause life-threatening VT in patients with ischemic or any other organic heart disease and in patients with Brugada syndrome. Ventricular scarring owing to aneurysmectomy, tetralogy of Fallot repair, ventricular septal defect repair, alcohol ablation of the interventricular septum to relieve dynamic outflow tract obstruction in hypertrophic cardiomyopathy, or implantation of a left ventricular assist device may create a substrate for re-entry and VT.

TREATMENT

Acute Management of Ventricular Tachycardia and Ventricular Fibrillation

The management of hemodynamically unstable VT and VF should conform to the guidelines for advanced cardiac life support (Chapter 50), with an emphasis on prompt defibrillation. For patients who have sustained VT with modest hypotension and normal mental status, intravenous drug therapy with lidocaine (given as a 50-mg bolus), procainamide (10 mg/kg or a total of 1000 mg over 20 minutes), or amiodarone (150 mg infused intravenously over 10 minutes) may be tried. In one randomized trial, procainamide was superior to amiodarone for promptly terminating wide-complex tachycardia with fewer adverse effects.[A1] Lidocaine, which is more efficacious at faster heart rates, is effective for terminating VT, but not for preventing recurrences, except in the setting of acute ischemia. By comparison, amiodarone is more effective at slower heart rates and therefore is better for preventing recurrent VT after sinus rhythm is restored. Intravenous calcium-channel blocker therapy should not be given unless the mechanism is known with certainty to be verapamil-sensitive idiopathic left ventricular tachycardia in a patient who does not have organic heart disease.

The most important factors in preventing early recurrence are the prompt identification and reversal of any precipitating causes. Examples include hypokalemia and other electrolyte imbalances, low oxygen saturation, intravenous β-agonist agents or milrinone, acute heart failure (Chapter 46), or myocardial ischemia (Chapters 57 and 58). Heart failure should be rigorously treated (Chapter 46) and the presence of residual myocardial ischemia suspected if VF is recurrent.

Treatment of Electrical Storm

Electrical storm describes frequently recurrent VT or VF requiring repeated shocks from an implanted cardioverter-defibrillator (ICD) or external defibrillations. Electrical storm rarely occurs in nonischemic cardiomyopathy or in genetically acquired ventricular arrhythmias. When this condition is encountered in the setting of ischemic heart disease, relief of ischemia is of paramount importance. If the electrical storm continues even after coronary reperfusion, insertion of an intra-aortic balloon pump and use of an intravenous β-blocker therapy, preferably with a short half-life drug (e.g., esmolol 500 μg/kg load over 1 minute, then 50 to 200 μg/kg per minute by intravenous infusion) should be considered. Intravenous lidocaine (2 to 4 mg per minute) or intravenous amiodarone (0.5 to 1.0 mg per minute) may also be used. Catheter ablation, if possible, may reduce the recurrence rate and potentially improve survival.[6] For recurrent ventricular arrhythmias refractory to traditional therapies, noninvasive radioablation (see later) or left-sided or bilateral cardiac sympathetic denervation may be effective. Another potential option is renal denervation.[7]

Treatment of PVCs and Idiopathic Ventricular Tachycardia

In the absence of structural heart disease, there is no convincing evidence that ventricular ectopic activity influences survival. Therefore PVCs do not need treatment in asymptomatic patients.[8] If ventricular ectopy results in symptoms that substantially decrease quality of life, a cardioselective β-blocker (e.g., metoprolol 50 mg twice daily or atenolol 50 mg once daily) is a safe but not a very effective first-choice therapy. If the frequency of PVCs and nonsustained VT reaches a critical level, however, the arrhythmia itself may result in decreased systolic ventricular function even in the absence of any other cause for cardiomyopathy. These patients should be treated aggressively, including catheter mapping and ablation (Chapter 54), to avoid progressive cardiomyopathy and heart failure without subjecting the patient to the potential adverse effects of antiarrhythmic drugs.

Although cardiac arrest resulting from transformation of idiopathic VT to VF is exceedingly rare, sustained VT at a rate faster than 200 beats per minute commonly causes cardiopulmonary symptoms and may cause syncope (Chapter 49), even in the absence of structural heart disease. Idiopathic VTs of outflow tract origin may respond to β-blocker therapy (e.g., metoprolol 50 mg every 12 hours or atenolol 50 mg daily), and a few may respond to an empirical trial of calcium-channel blockers (e.g., sustained-release diltiazem 120 to 240 mg daily or sustained-release verapamil 120 to 240 mg daily). However success rates are low, ranging from 25 to 50%. The so-called idiopathic left ventricular tachycardia resulting from left fascicular re-entry frequently responds to verapamil (e.g., sustained-release 180 to 360 mg daily), but papillary muscle VT may not.

Catheter ablation therapy (Chapter 54) can cure 80 to 90% of cases of idiopathic ventricular arrhythmia with a low risk (<1%) and should be considered as a preferred alternative to long-term antiarrhythmic drug therapy.[9] If careful catheter mapping in the right ventricular outflow tract does not yield a suitable target, the left ventricular outflow tract, right or left sinus of Valsalva, or the aortomitral continuity may be the site of origin. Failures are usually due to an inability to induce the arrhythmia reliably with electrophysiologic testing or VT that originates in epicardial sites beyond safe access for an ablation catheter (e.g., close proximity to a coronary artery).

By comparison to the relatively benign prognosis of idiopathic sustained VT, idiopathic VF accounts for 5 to 10% of all cases of sudden cardiac death (Chapter 50) in patients without organic heart disease. The appropriate treatment for survivors of idiopathic VF is no different than for any other survivor of VF (i.e., ICD therapy), but some patients may have findings on electrophysiologic testing that are amenable to catheter ablation—which may decrease the risk for recurrence but still does not obviate the need for ICD protection.

Therapy for Ventricular Tachycardia and Ventricular Fibrillation in Structural Heart Disease

Implantable Cardiac Defibrillator Therapy and Antiarrhythmic Drugs

Sustained VT or VF in patients with organic heart disease is a primary indication for ICD therapy.[10,11,A2] A subcutaneous ICD is as safe and effective as a transvenous ICD for patients who do not have an indication for pacing.[A3]

After an acute MI, an ICD implanted as primary prevention therapy reduces mortality in patients who have survived more than 40 days and have a left ventricular ejection fraction of 30% or less.[A4] For patients who have class II or III heart failure regardless of the etiology of their organic heart disease and who have a left ventricular ejection fraction of less than 35%, an ICD also significantly reduces sudden cardiac death, although it may not prolong life in patients with nonischemic heart failure because of the high burden of death from other causes.[A5] By comparison, ICDs do not reduce mortality when routinely implanted soon after MI or in patients after recent coronary artery revascularization.

In patients with ischemic heart disease and a chronically depressed ejection fraction of less than 30%, insertion of an ICD reduces the mortality rate by 20%, from 36 to 29%, over the next 5 years. By comparison, amiodarone (Table 52-3) reduces the risk of sudden arrhythmic death but does not improve survival. In patients with advanced organic heart disease, the presence of frequent PVCs and nonsustained VT portend a poor prognosis, but suppression of ventricular ectopic activity with antiarrhythmic drugs does not improve prognosis; in fact, suppression of PVCs with class IC antiarrhythmic drugs in patients with prior MI increases mortality. Therefore, antiarrhythmic drugs currently serve as palliative treatment to modify the course of VT in patients with an ICD, rather than as definitive therapy. Amiodarone (100 to 400 mg daily) is more successful than β-blockers or sotalol for this palliative therapy of VT.[A6]

In patients who are clinically unstable because of incessant VT, reversible precipitating factors should be sought and, if present, corrected promptly. Intravenous β-blockers (e.g., esmolol 50 to 200 μg/kg per minute) and amiodarone (0.5 to 1.0 mg per minute) constitute first-line therapy. Intravenous lidocaine (e.g., 2 to 4 mg per minute) can be added, especially if myocardial ischemia is present, and emergent catheter ablation may be considered.

Catheter Ablation

Catheter ablation is usually also palliative rather than definitive treatment for VT in patients with structural heart disease, but it can significantly reduce the frequency of recurrent VT, ICD discharge, and adverse cardiac events.[A7,A8] Catheter ablation is most successful when clinical VT can be reproduced in the cardiac electrophysiology laboratory and tolerated for a long enough period to allow detailed catheter mapping and to validate the underlying mechanism and site of origin. Catheter ablation can be performed safely in patients with advanced heart failure. However, preventive catheter ablation before ICD implantation is not clearly better than reserving ablation for patients who need it as supplemental therapy.[A9]

Radioablation

Application of stereotactic body radiation is an investigational noninvasive method of treatment for recurrent VT,[12] especially VT storm.[13] The precise location of the target requires a synthesis of anatomic and electrophysiologic data using cardiac magnetic resonance imaging (MRI), cardiac single photon emission computed tomography (SPECT), a 12-lead ECG recorded during VT, and electrophysiologic imaging information. A single fraction of 25 Gy is delivered to the VT substrate while avoiding healthy tissue. Late postprocedure complications include exacerbation of heart failure and pericarditis.

Torsades de Pointes and Catecholinergic Polymorphic VT

In an acute setting with frequently recurrent torsades de pointes, magnesium sulfate (1 to 2 g intravenous infusion over 10 to 30 minutes) may be effective. Temporary pacing should be considered if the patient exhibits excessive bradycardia or prolonged pauses.

An ICD is recommended for patients who present with aborted cardiac arrest. Otherwise, the first line of preventive therapy for torsades de pointes in patients with long QT syndrome is β-blocker therapy (e.g., metoprolol 50 to 100 mg daily, atenolol 50 mg daily, or nadolol 40 mg daily and titrated as tolerated), but its success is influenced by gender and the magnitude of QT prolongation, as well as by the specific genotype. However, about 25% of patients continue to experience ventricular arrhythmias on full doses of β-blocker therapy and require an ICD. Left cardiac sympathetic denervation can substantially reduce the incidence of torsades de pointes and syncope in high-risk patients, as well as decrease the frequency of shocks in patients with an ICD.

β-Blockers (Table 52-3) are also the drugs of choice for catecholaminergic polymorphic VT, with ICD therapy recommended for patients with recurrent syncope or documented VT while on β-blocker therapy. Oral flecainide (Table 52-3) may be an effective adjunct in such patients.

Treatment of Genetically Acquired Ventricular Tachycardia and Ventricular Fibrillation

Most of the VTs observed in patients with arrhythmogenic right ventricular cardiomyopathy may be reproducibly induced by programmed cardiac stimulation and are amenable to catheter ablation. Nearly half of these VTs have an epicardial site of origin, and simultaneous endocardial and epicardial catheter mapping and ablation may be the most effective method of treatment. However, catheter ablation cannot substitute for concomitant ICD therapy. In patients with hypertrophic cardiomyopathy, ICD therapy is routinely recommended, especially in young high-risk patients (Chapter 47), and amiodarone may sometimes be useful.

For Brugada syndrome, catheter ablation of the electrophysiologically abnormal substrate in the right ventricular outflow tract epicardium can lead to eventual disappearance of the pathognomonic ST elevation on the ECG. Quinidine (600 to 900 mg daily in three or four divided doses) is the only antiarrhythmic drug that appears to be useful to treat this syndrome. However, follow-up periods are not long enough to know whether catheter ablation or quinidine can obviate the need for an ICD in high-risk patients who have unprovoked Brugada pattern in their resting ECG and have a history of syncope.

Iatrogenic Ventricular Tachycardia

For sustained monomorphic VT in patients with surgically repaired congenital heart disease, catheter mapping and ablation are recommended. The techniques are similar to those used for catheter ablation of ischemic VT. Although sustained VT or VF during the course of left ventricular assist device therapy is usually well tolerated acutely, recurrent intractable VT or VF can result in right heart failure and in frequent ICD shocks, both of which may carry significant morbidity. Amiodarone (200 to 400 mg daily) and β-blocker therapy (e.g., metoprolol 100 to 200 mg daily) may be effective in at least rendering VT no longer incessant, and catheter ablation therapy has occasionally been tried in refractory VT with modest success.

PROGNOSIS

VT or VF in the early minutes or hours of acute MI has not been shown to affect the long-term prognosis in patients who survive to hospital discharge. Sustained monomorphic VT occurring after the hyperacute phase but within the next few days of an anterior wall MI portends poor prognosis, with about a seven-fold increase in subsequent mortality, because it usually occurs after the necrosis of a large amount of myocardium.

The modern natural course of untreated VT and VF perhaps can best be assessed from prospective studies of patients receiving ICD therapy. Among patients who have had documented sustained VT, appropriate ICD therapy for VT or VF occurs in about 70% of patients within 2 years and 85% of patients within 3 years. For patients who have survived cardiac arrest, the rate is about 70% at 3 years. These figures underscore the high rate of recurrence of VT and VF in patients with organic heart disease presenting with sustained ventricular arrhythmias.

The prognosis of patients with PVCs or nonsustained VT is less well known but is critically dependent on the underlying heart disease. No study to date has shown any survival benefit of treating PVCs or nonsustained VT in patients who do not have underlying organic heart disease and who do not develop a cardiomyopathy as a result of their ventricular ectopic activity. In high-risk patients who have ischemic heart disease, a left ventricular ejection fraction of less than 40%, and electrically induced sustained VT, the 2-year rate of cardiac arrest or death from ventricular arrhythmia is more than 30%.

GENERAL REFERENCES

For the General References and other additional features, please visit Elsevier eBooks+ at https://ebooks.health.elsevier.com.

Grade A References

A1. Ortiz M, Martin A, Arribas F, et al. Randomized comparison of intravenous procainamide vs. intravenous amiodarone for the acute treatment of tolerated wide QRS tachycardia: the PROCAMIO study. *Eur Heart J.* 2017;38:1329-1335.

A2. Alba AC, Foroutan F, Duero Posada J, et al. Implantable cardiac defibrillator and mortality in non-ischaemic cardiomyopathy: an updated meta-analysis. *Heart.* 2018;104:230-236.

A3. Knops RE, Olde Nordkamp LRA, Delnoy PHM, et al. Subcutaneous or transvenous defibrillator therapy. *N Engl J Med.* 2020;383:526-536.

A4. Kolodziejczak M, Andreotti F, Kowalewski M, et al. Implantable cardioverter-defibrillators for primary prevention in patients with ischemic or nonischemic cardiomyopathy: a systematic review and meta-analysis. *Ann Intern Med.* 2017;167:103-111.

A5. Kober L, Thune JJ, Nielsen JC, et al. Defibrillator implantation in patients with nonischemic systolic heart failure. *N Engl J Med.* 2016;375:1221-1230.

A6. Claro JC, Candia R, Rada G, et al. Amiodarone versus other pharmacological interventions for prevention of sudden cardiac death. *Cochrane Database Syst Rev.* 2015;12.

A7. Arenal Á, Ávila P, Jiménez-Candil J, et al. Substrate ablation vs antiarrhythmic drug therapy for symptomatic ventricular tachycardia. *J Am Coll Cardiol.* 2022;79:1441-1453.

A8. Tung R, Xue Y, Chen M, et al. First-line catheter ablation of monomorphic ventricular tachycardia in cardiomyopathy concurrent with defibrillator implantation: the PAUSE-SCD randomized trial. *Circulation.* 2022;145:1839-1849.

A9. Willems S, Tilz RR, Steven D, et al. Preventive or deferred ablation of ventricular tachycardia in patients with ischemic cardiomyopathy and implantable defibrillator (BERLIN VT): a multicenter randomized trial. *Circulation.* 2020;141:1057-1067.

54 ELECTROPHYSIOLOGIC PROCEDURES AND SURGERY

PETER A. SANTUCCI AND DAVID J. WILBER

TRANSTHORACIC CARDIOVERSION AND DEFIBRILLATION

Transthoracic defibrillation, which rapidly delivers a stored charge to the heart across two surface pads or paddle electrodes, is used emergently for life-threatening tachycardias (Chapter 50). Cardioversion, which refers to shock delivery synchronized with the QRS complex, is advised in patients with either supraventricular arrhythmias (Chapter 52) or ventricular tachycardia (VT; Chapter 53) because a nonsynchronized shock coincident with the vulnerable period of the T wave may precipitate ventricular fibrillation (VF). The shock extinguishes tachyarrhythmias by simultaneously depolarizing large portions of the atria and/or ventricles. Defibrillation is used for disorganized rhythms in which synchronization to the QRS complex is not appropriate, such as VF or rapid polymorphic VT. In these emergent situations, attempts to synchronize may delay delivery of the shock.

The success of cardioversion or defibrillation is affected by the shock waveform and shock strength. Biphasic shock waveforms are recommended because they are significantly more effective than monophasic waveforms at equivalent energies. Shock energies vary by indication and between defibrillator units but are generally from 50 to 360 J. Other technique-dependent variables that maximize the energy delivered to the heart include increasing paddle pressure, delivery of the shock during expiration, and repetitive shocks. Patient-related factors that may decrease the probability of successful cardioversion and defibrillation include metabolic disturbances, a longer duration of arrhythmia, cardiac enlargement, chronic obstructive pulmonary disease, barrel-chested habitus, and higher body weight. Elective cardioversion is performed with the patient in the fasting state, usually with a short-acting anesthetic agent.

PRECAUTIONS AND COMPLICATIONS

Cardioversion of atrial fibrillation (AF) and atrial flutter (Chapter 52) may be complicated by thromboembolism, but this risk can be minimized by excluding the presence of an atrial thrombus on a transesophageal echocardiogram or by therapeutic anticoagulation with a direct-acting anticoagulant for at least 3 weeks before elective cardioversion (see Fig. 52-14, and Chapters 52 and 70). All patients should be anticoagulated for 1 month after cardioversion if AF or atrial flutter has been present for longer than 48 hours.

VF may rarely occur even when shocks are synchronized to the QRS complex. The risk is increased with electrolyte disturbances and digitalis toxicity, so elective cardioversion should be delayed in such patients. Although patients may develop mild elevations of serum troponin levels after cardioversion, sometimes with transient ST segment elevation, clinical myocardial dysfunction is rare. Post-shock bradycardia or asystole sometimes can require atropine (0.5 to 3.0 mg intravenously) or emergency transcutaneous pacing. If a patient has a pacemaker or an implantable cardioverter-defibrillator (ICD), the shocking electrodes should be placed as far away from the generator as possible and at a right angle from the pacemaker leads if feasible. Both the generator and pacing threshold should be checked after the procedure.

CARDIAC IMPLANTABLE ELECTRONIC DEVICES

Pacemakers are implanted to eliminate bradycardia, and ICDs offer highly effective protection for life-threatening ventricular tachyarrhythmias (Chapter 53). Cardiac resynchronization pacing is an essential tool for managing heart failure (Chapter 46) and is available in devices with or without the capacity for defibrillation. Implantable loop recorders, which are the preferred approach for detecting occult, infrequent, and short-lived paroxysmal arrhythmias (Chapter 49), are especially useful for patients who have syncope or may have occult AF as the cause of a stroke.

Modern devices are highly programmable and provide a wealth of diagnostic information that the clinician can use to diagnose abnormalities and to tailor therapy. The diagnostic data regarding the device's performance and the presence of arrhythmias can be routinely transmitted directly from home to the appropriate health care provider.

An important issue is the use of magnetic resonance imaging (MRI) in patients with an implanted cardiac device. Historically, such devices were considered a contraindication to MRI, but most newer devices and leads are now engineered to be classified as "MRI conditional." These patients can safely undergo MRI with appropriate management. Even patients with more modern MRI nonconditional devices often can safely undergo MRI for both thoracic and nonthoracic indications,[1] provided that the patients are appropriately screened and that their devices are reprogrammed according to standard protocols.[A1]

TEMPORARY PACING

Temporary pacing is used in patients who may not require long-term pacing as well as in emergencies, such as asystolic cardiac arrest (Chapter 50). Transcutaneous pacing with electrode pads applied to the chest wall may be the quickest option and can be life-saving, but it is uncomfortable and should be used sparingly. Usually, however, time allows for temporary pacemaker leads to be inserted percutaneously, typically through an internal jugular or subclavian vein, and to be positioned gently in the right ventricular apex, ideally under fluoroscopic guidance. Another indication for temporary pacing is to maintain a higher heart rate (typically 85 to 100 beats per minute) in order to suppress torsades de pointes (Chapter 53) until the causative factor, such as an offending drug, has been eliminated. Prophylactic temporary pacing is used in patients who have high-degree atrioventricular (AV) block in the setting of an acute myocardial infarction (Chapter 58) and for patients who are at a high risk for developing symptomatic bradycardia during an interventional or surgical cardiac procedure (e.g., during transcatheter aortic valve replacement; Chapter 60).

The most common complication of temporary pacing is infection. The risk can be minimized by proper sterile technique, limiting temporary pacing to 48 hours, or replacing the lead at that time under optimal sterile conditions.

PERMANENT PACING

Indications for Permanent Pacemaking for Bradycardias

Pacemakers are implanted either to alleviate symptoms caused by bradycardia or to prevent severe symptoms in patients in whom symptomatic bradycardia is likely to develop (Tables 54-1 and 54-2).[2] The most common bradycardia-induced symptoms are dizziness or lightheadedness, syncope or near-syncope (Chapters 39 and 49), fatigue, and heart failure. Exercise intolerance caused by a poor heart rate response to exertion (chronotropic incompetence) is another common indication. Because these symptoms can be nonspecific, documentation of an association between symptoms and bradycardia should be obtained whenever possible before a pacemaker is recommended.[3] In some patients, a simple electrocardiogram (ECG) may be sufficient to document the need for a pacemaker. If the bradycardia is intermittent, other diagnostic testing, such as 24-hour ambulatory monitoring, a continuous external or implantable loop recorder, an implantable event monitor, or an electrophysiology test (Chapter 49), may be needed to document a relationship between symptoms and bradycardia.

Correctable causes of bradycardia (Chapter 51) should be excluded. Examples include hypothyroidism (Chapter 207), electrolyte disturbances, and medications such as β-adrenergic blocking agents, calcium-channel blocking agents, digitalis, and antiarrhythmic medications (Chapters 51 and 52). Other temporary causes of bradycardia that may not require a permanent pacemaker include acute ischemia or infarction, perioperative bradycardia following cardiac surgery, and neurocardiogenic causes. Patients with sleep-related bradycardia or transient pauses do not generally warrant permanent pacing. At times, a pacemaker is necessary to allow continued treatment with a medication that is responsible for the bradycardia, such as an antiarrhythmic medication or an AV nodal blocking agent needed for AF with a rapid ventricular response.

Pacing Systems

Permanent pacing systems most commonly consist of a pulse generator connected with one to three leads implanted into the heart to sense intrinsic activity and to deliver pacing pulses as needed. Pacemaker leads are inserted percutaneously via the axillary or subclavian vein, or by cephalic vein cutdown. Less often, leads are placed epicardially during cardiac surgery. Atrial leads are often placed in the right atrial appendage, but they may be placed in a variety of locations, in part based on local electrical threshold measurements. Ventricular leads are typically positioned in the right ventricular apex, right ventricular septum, or outflow tract, and they are commonly secured in place with a helical screw, known as "active fixation," for biventricular pacing (Fig. 54-1).

TABLE 54-1 CLASS I INDICATIONS* FOR IMPLANTATION OF A PERMANENT PACEMAKER

SINUS NODE DYSFUNCTION
Symptomatic sinus bradycardia
Symptomatic chronotropic incompetence
Symptomatic sinus bradycardia resulting from required drug therapy
ATRIOVENTRICULAR BLOCK
Third-degree and advanced second-degree AV block associated with symptomatic bradycardia
Third-degree and advanced second-degree AV block in an awake patient with asystole of >3 seconds or an escape rate of <40 beats per minute or with an infranodal escape rhythm
Atrial fibrillation with a pause of ≥5 sec
Third-degree and advanced second-degree AV block due to postoperative AV block that is not expected to resolve
Third-degree and advanced second-degree AV block with neuromuscular diseases such as myotonic muscular dystrophy, Kearns-Sayre syndrome, and Erb dystrophy
Asymptomatic third-degree AV block if cardiomegaly or left ventricular dysfunction is present, or if the block is below the AV node
CHRONIC BIFASCICULAR BLOCK
Advanced second-degree or intermittent third-degree AV block
Type II second-degree AV block
Alternating bundle branch block
AFTER ACUTE PHASE OF MYOCARDIAL INFARCTION
Second-degree infranodal AV block with alternating bundle branch block
Third-degree infranodal AV block
Transient advanced second-degree or third-degree infranodal AV block and associated bundle branch block
Persistent symptomatic second-degree or third-degree AV block
CAROTID SINUS SYNDROME
Recurrent syncope caused by spontaneous carotid sinus stimulation or carotid sinus pressure that induces asystole of >3 sec in duration

*Class I indications are conditions for which a pacemaker is indicated.

AV = atrioventricular.

Adapted from Gillis AM, Russo AM, Ellenbogen KA, et al. HRS/ACCF expert consensus statement on pacemaker device and mode selection. *J Am Coll Cardiol*. 2012;60:682-703.

TABLE 54-2 CLASS IIA INDICATIONS* FOR IMPLANTATION OF A PERMANENT PACEMAKER

SINUS NODE DYSFUNCTION
Heart rate of <40 beats per minute when a clear association between symptoms consistent with bradycardia and the actual presence of bradycardia has not been demonstrated
Syncope of unclear etiology when sinus node dysfunction is demonstrated by electrophysiologic testing
ATRIOVENTRICULAR BLOCK
Persistent third-degree AV block with an escape rate of >40 beats per minute in an asymptomatic adult without cardiomegaly
Asymptomatic second-degree infranodal AV block
First-degree or second-degree AV block associated with symptoms similar to pacemaker syndrome
Asymptomatic type II second-degree AV block with a narrow QRS
CHRONIC BIFASCICULAR BLOCK
Syncope, when other potential causes of syncope have been excluded
An HV interval of ≥100 msec
Pathologic pacing-induced infranodal AV block during electrophysiologic testing
CAROTID SINUS SYNDROME
Syncope without clear provocative events and with asystole of >3 sec during carotid sinus pressure

*Class IIA indications are conditions for which a pacemaker is reasonable.

AV = atrioventricular; HV = His-ventricle.

Adapted from Tracy CM, Epstein AE, Darbar D, et al. 2012 ACCF/AHA/HRS focused update of the 2008 guidelines for device-based therapy of cardiac rhythm abnormalities: a report of the American College of Cardiology Foundation/American Heart Association Task Force on Practice Guidelines. *J Am Coll Cardiol*. 2012;60:1297-1313.

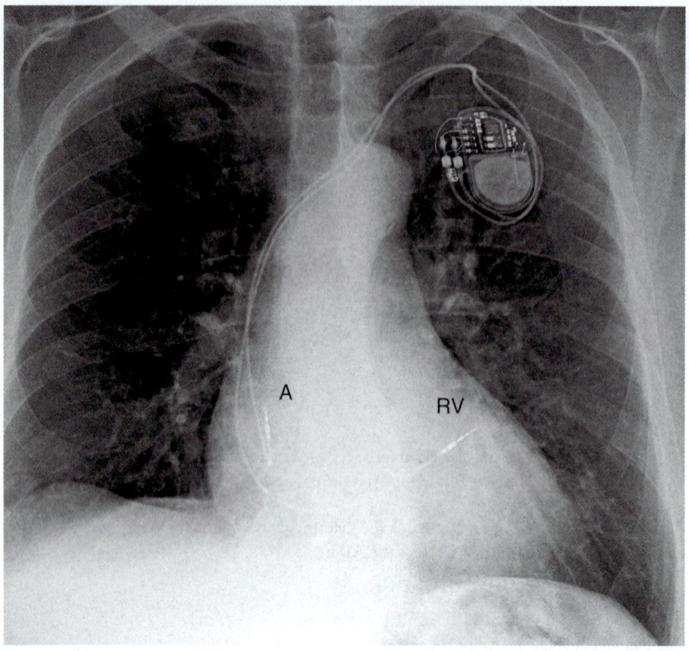

FIGURE 54-1. Chest radiograph of a patient with a dual-chamber (atrial and right ventricular) pacemaker.

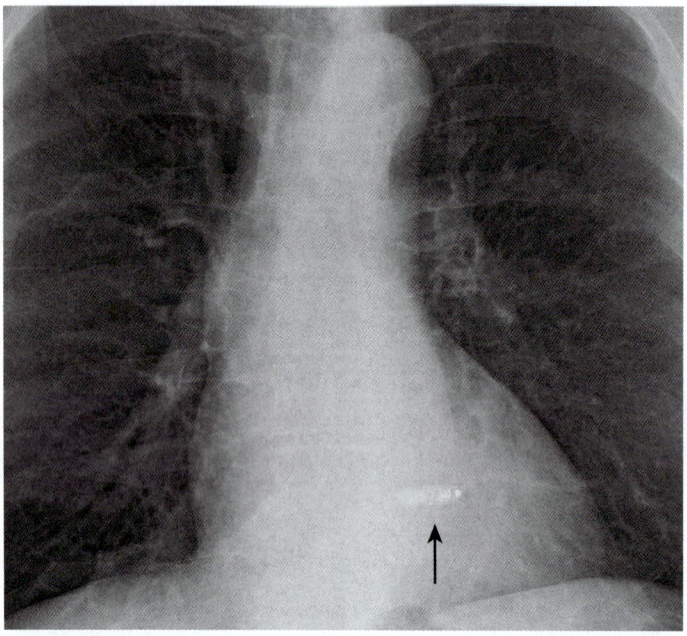

FIGURE 54-2. Chest radiograph of a leadless pacemaker (arrow) positioned in the right ventricle.

A leadless pacing system,[4] with a miniaturized generator and delivery system combined into a single unit, can be implanted, typically in the right ventricle (Fig. 54-2). These leadless pacemakers are commonly used in patients who have permanent AF and AV block. However, they also can frequently sense and track atrial mechanical activity to pace the ventricle while maintaining AV synchrony in patients with AV block and sometimes are used in patients who are in sinus rhythm with AV block.

With traditional systems, pulse generators are powered by lithium-based pacemaker batteries, which have an 8- to 12-year (or more) lifespan and can weigh less than 30 g. These generators typically are implanted subcutaneously in the infraclavicular region. The programmability of many different parameters has become standard, as has the ability of the pacemaker to provide diagnostic and telemetric data.

Synchronous biventricular pacing can preserve the ventricular synchrony that is lost when only one ventricle is paced and the other's activation is delayed. The usual option is biventricular pacing with one lead in the right ventricle

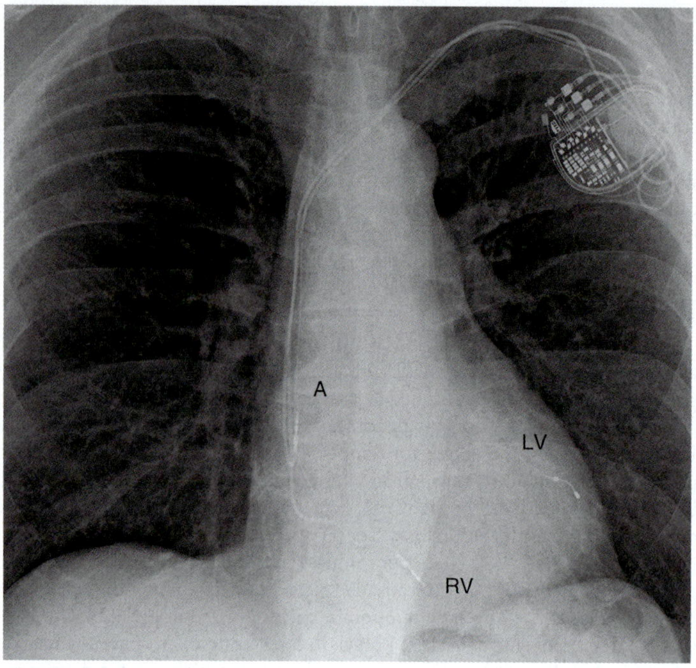

FIGURE 54-3. Chest radiograph of a patient with an atrial and biventricular pacemaker.

and one in the coronary venous system to pace the lateral left ventricle (Fig. 54-3), typically with an atrial lead in patients who are not in permanent atrial fibrillation. Permanent His-bundle pacing is also increasingly being used to maintain the patient's intrinsic conduction system, thereby avoiding ventricular dyssynchrony.[5] Yet another emerging option for physiologic pacing is left bundle branch area pacing, which may produce lower and more stable pacing thresholds in some patients.[A2] Each paced beat will have a configuration that depends on the site of the pacing lead (Fig. 54-3).

Pacing Modes and Programming

Pacing modes are described by a simple code. The first letter represents the chamber being paced (A for atrium, V for ventricle, D for dual chamber). The second letter identifies the chamber whose depolarizations are being sensed by the pacemaker (A, V, D, or O for no sensing). The third letter indicates whether the pacemaker is functioning in an inhibited (I) mode, a tracking (T) mode, in both modes (D), or asynchronously (O). The fourth letter designates whether the pacemaker can modulate the pacing rate, usually by increasing pacing rates with physical activity (R).

The most appropriate pacing mode must be determined for each individual and may change with the patient's status. By far the most common permanent pacing modes now used in the United States are DDD and DDDR. VVI and VVIR modes are used mainly in patients who have chronic AF with symptomatic pauses or bradycardia. Mode-switching pacemakers can pace in the DDD mode during sinus rhythm and automatically switch to rate-responsive (VVIR) ventricular pacing during paroxysmal AF or other supraventricular arrhythmias. Automatic mode switching from AAI(R) to DDD(R) is also available for patients with sinus node dysfunction and intermittent AV block.

Many patients' devices are programmed at settings chosen to minimize the right ventricular pacing burden, not only to conserve the battery, but also to reduce pacing-induced ventricular dyssynchrony, which sometimes can lead to impaired ventricular function. This potential side effect is particularly a concern in patients who have a normal intrinsic QRS duration and then undergo single-chamber right ventricular pacing. However, in patients who require resynchronization therapy, a very high percentage of ventricular pacing is the goal.

In patients with sinus node dysfunction, atrial or dual-chamber pacing significantly reduces the risk for AF and improves quality of life compared with ventricular pacing. Because such patients are at substantial risk of symptomatic AV block, initial dual-chamber pacing is commonly used, although atrial pacing alone is an option for selected patients with normal AV conduction. Because chronotropic incompetence is frequent in this patient population, a rate-responsive mode (AAIR or DDDR) is usually recommended. In patients with AV block, dual-chamber pacing improves quality of life, reduces the risk for developing AF, and avoids the 7 to 25% risk for developing the pacemaker syndrome, which consists of symptoms of weakness, lightheadedness, exercise intolerance, or palpitations owing to the absence of AV synchrony during single-chamber ventricular pacing. For these reasons, current consensus guidelines recommend dual-chamber pacing for most patients with sinus node dysfunction or AV block.

Synchronous biventricular pacing or His-bundle pacing is preferred in bradycardic patients who have a left ventricular ejection fraction of 50% or below and who are expected to need pacing for more than 40% of their heartbeats. With atrial pacing, this synchrony can simulate normal cardiac function. In patients who require permanent pacing, the risk of future ventricular arrhythmias guides the need for simultaneous insertion of an implantable cardioverter defibrillator.

The electrocardiogram of paced patients depends on the site and frequency of pacing (Fig. 54-4)

COMPLICATIONS OF PACEMAKERS

Complications can be either acute or late. About 1 to 2% of patients develop acute complications from the implantation procedure itself, including infection,[6] pneumothorax, cardiac tamponade owing to pericarditis or perforation of the atrium or ventricle, lead dislodgement, subclavian vein thrombosis, and pocket complications. The subcutaneous pocket may develop a hematoma, seroma, dehiscence, or local infection. Pocket hematomas can be painful and increase the risk of infection. Their occurrence can be minimized by meticulous operative technique and postoperative care, as well as by interrupting anticoagulation when feasible. In patients who require uninterrupted anticoagulation, a strategy of continued oral anticoagulant treatment at the time of implantation of a pacemaker or an ICD markedly reduces the incidence of clinically significant device-pocket hematoma compared with bridging therapy with heparin.

Late complications include venous thrombosis or obstruction (including the superior vena cava syndrome; Fig. 86-8), the pacemaker syndrome, pacing-induced ventricular dyssynchrony that can cause heart failure, infection, and various forms of pacemaker malfunction. The latter include failure to pace, failure to capture, and sensing abnormalities, most often resulting

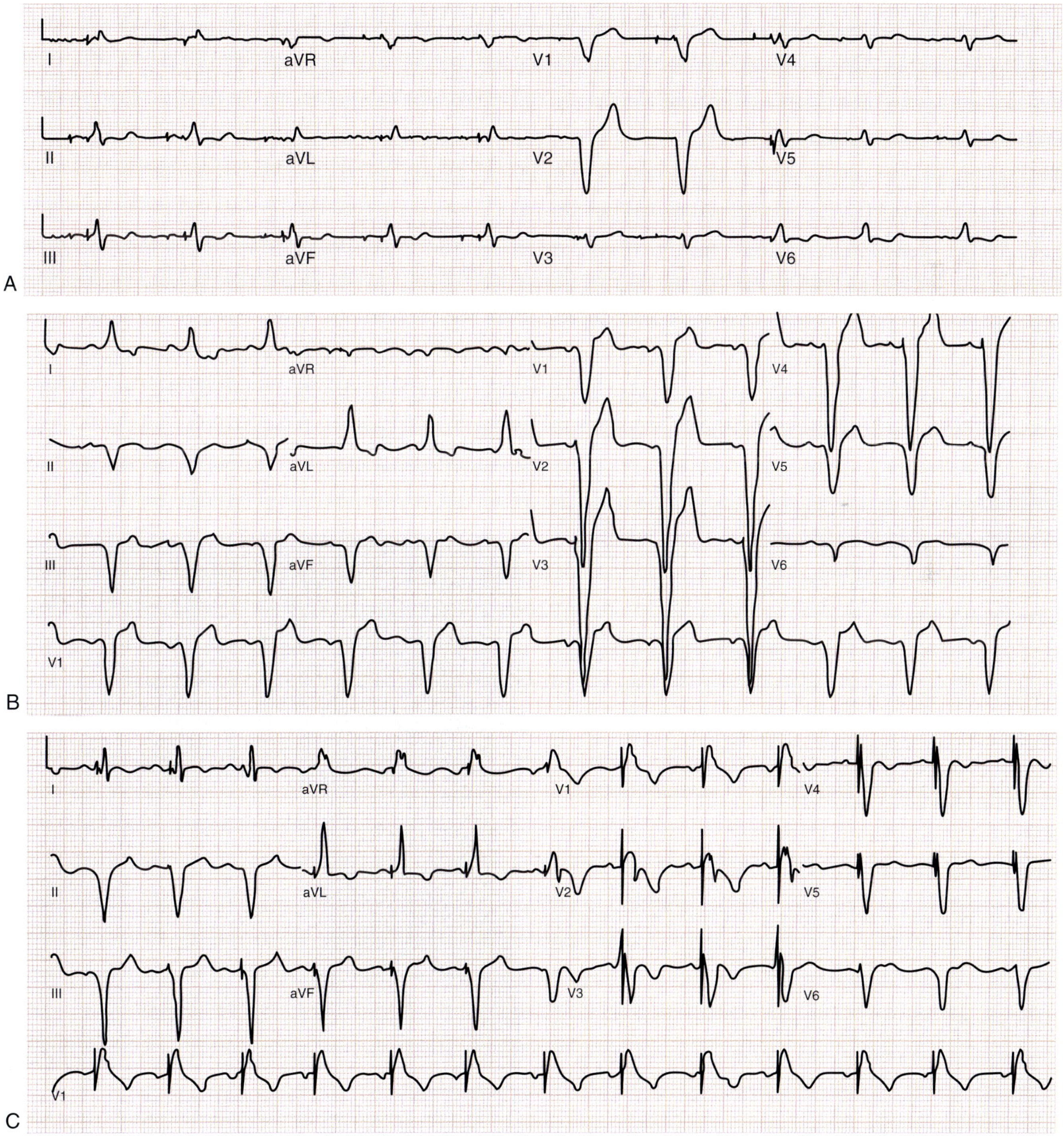

FIGURE 54-4. Electrocardiogram of patients with pacemakers. **A,** Dual-chamber atrial and right ventricular pacing. **B,** Right ventricular pacing. In this tracing, pacing is tracking the sinus P waves that are sensed with an atrial lead (with a single-chamber ventricular pacemaker, the P waves would be dissociated). **C,** Same patient after being upgraded to a biventricular pacemaker. Note the changes in lead V_1 and V_2 and the partial narrowing of the QRS that are often seen by adding simultaneous pacing of the left ventricle.

from lead abnormalities (conductor fractures, insulation breaks or changes at the lead-tissue interface). Pacemaker infections typically involve primarily the subcutaneous pacemaker pocket, but long-term resolution of infection generally requires removal of both the pulse generator and leads as well as extended antibiotic therapy (Chapter 61). Nearly 40% of patients have coexisting valve involvement, predominantly tricuspid valve infection (Chapter 61), with mortality rates as high as 15% in the hospital and 20 to 25% at 1 year. Less commonly, pulse generator malfunctions, including premature battery depletion, may occur. Long-term problems may also result from inappropriate programming. The emerging use of leadless pacing eliminates many of the risks of conventional pacing systems and is becoming increasingly common as experience grows and the technology advances.

IMPLANTABLE CARDIOVERTER-DEFIBRILLATORS AND CARDIAC RESYNCHRONIZATION THERAPY

Abnormal and prolonged ventricular activation, indicated by a QRS duration greater than 120 msec, may cause dyssynchronous activation of the left ventricle and, as a result, diminished systolic function. Right ventricular pacing, particularly from the apex, also is associated with a delayed activation sequence and, as a result, interventricular and intraventricular mechanical dyssynchrony. Cardiac resynchronization therapy requires synchronized pacing of both ventricles or physiologic pacing by means of His-bundle pacing or left bundle branch pacing.[7]

Implantable Cardioverter-Defibrillators

Indications

ICDs are a highly effective method for detecting and terminating life-threatening ventricular arrhythmias (Chapter 53). They are used both for secondary prevention following an episode of sustained VT or VF and for primary prevention in individuals at high risk for sudden cardiac death (Table 54-3). Examples include patients with ischemic or nonischemic dilated cardiomyopathy with a left ventricle ejection fraction of 35% or less and class II or III heart failure,[A3] as well as selected patients with conditions such as hypertrophic cardiomyopathy, Brugada syndrome, and long QT syndrome (Chapters 47, 53, and 58).[8]

ICD Pulse Generators and Leads

Procedures for implanting transvenous ICDs are analogous to those used for permanent pacemakers. The pulse generators, although still somewhat larger than pacemakers (with some models now <1 cm in thickness, <28 mL in volume, and around 60 g), deliver biphasic shocks at programmable energies while recording the electrogram during the arrhythmia and its treatment (E-Fig. 54-1). They also can provide anti-tachycardia pacing, as well as dual-chamber bradycardia pacing or cardiac resynchronization pacing therapy.

ICD implantation and lead configuration (Figure 54-5) are designed to deliver sufficient energy to the ventricular myocardium to ensure reliable defibrillation. The most common pathway for this energy is from the implanted pectoral pulse generator to a coil electrode on the distal portion of the transvenous lead that is positioned in the right ventricle (E-Fig. 54-2). The majority of transvenous ICD pulse generators can deliver up to 30 to 40 J, which exceeds the typical defibrillation energy threshold of 10 to 15 J, thereby allowing a substantial margin of safety for defibrillation.

An alternative to a transvenous ICD is the subcutaneous ICD.[9] However, subcutaneous systems currently have a larger pulse generator, somewhat shorter battery longevity, and do not provide usual bradycardic, anti-tachycardic, or resynchronization pacing therapy. The pulse generator must deliver higher stored energy (80 J) compared with transvenous defibrillation to ensure an adequate margin of safety for defibrillation, but data show that the device's effectiveness for sensing and terminating VF is comparable to that of transvenous systems.[A4] It is an attractive option for patients who have had prior complications from transvenous systems (e.g., vein thrombosis, infection) or issues with intravenous access, as well as for primary prevention in patients in whom frequent shocks or the need for pacing are not anticipated. However, the choice of an ICD system must be individualized to a patient's overall needs.

Programming of ICDs

The goals of ICD programming are to provide the appropriate detection of all arrhythmias, the discrimination of ventricular from supraventricular rhythms, and appropriate anti-tachycardia pacing and shocks only when needed for sustained arrhythmias. The shocks are programmed to provide an adequate margin of safety for reliable cardioversion and defibrillation. In addition, bradycardic pacing therapy should be optimized to provide an appropriate heart rate response to exertion while minimizing right ventricular pacing. Conversely, the ventricles are ideally paced for all beats in patients in whom cardiac resynchronization (see later) is needed.

ICD recipients may have sustained monomorphic VT that can be painlessly terminated by appropriately timed, overdrive anti-tachycardia pacing. ICD shocks

TABLE 54-3 INDICATIONS FOR IMPLANTABLE CARDIOVERTER-DEFIBRILLATOR IMPLANTATION

CLASS I*: SECONDARY PREVENTION
Cardiac arrest survivor (VF or unstable sustained VT not associated with a completely reversible cause)
Spontaneous sustained VT (irrespective of stability) and structural heart disease
Syncope of unknown origin associated with clinically relevant and hemodynamically significant sustained VT or VT induced at electrophysiologic testing
CLASS I*: PRIMARY PREVENTION
Prior myocardial infarction (≥40 days), LVEF <35%, NYHA class II or III
Prior myocardial infarction (≥40 days), LVEF <30%, NYHA class I
Nonischemic dilated cardiomyopathy, LVEF ≤35%, NYHA class II or III
Prior myocardial infarction, LVEF <40%, spontaneous NSVT, inducible sustained VT or VF at electrophysiologic testing
CLASS IIA†
Nonischemic dilated cardiomyopathy, significant LV dysfunction, and syncope
Sustained VT and normal or near-normal ventricular function
Hypertrophic cardiomyopathy and one or more risk factors for sudden death
Arrhythmogenic right ventricular cardiomyopathy and one or more risk factors for sudden death
Long QT syndrome with syncope or VT despite β-blocker therapy
Nonhospitalized patients awaiting cardiac transplantation
Brugada syndrome and syncope or VT
Catecholaminergic polymorphic VT and syncope or VT on β-blocker therapy
Cardiac sarcoidosis, giant cell myocarditis, or Chagas disease

*Class I indications are conditions for which an implantable cardioverter-defibrillator is indicated.
†Class IIA indications are conditions for which an implantable cardioverter-defibrillator is reasonable.
LVEF = left ventricular ejection fraction; NSVT = nonsustained ventricular tachycardia; NYHA = New York Heart Association; VF = ventricular fibrillation; VT = ventricular tachycardia.
Adapted from Tracy CM, Epstein AE, Darbar D, et al. 2012 ACCF/AHA/HRS focused update of the 2008 guidelines for device-based therapy of cardiac rhythm abnormalities: a report of the American College of Cardiology Foundation/American Heart Association Task Force on Practice Guidelines. *J Am Coll Cardiol*. 2012;60:1297-1313.

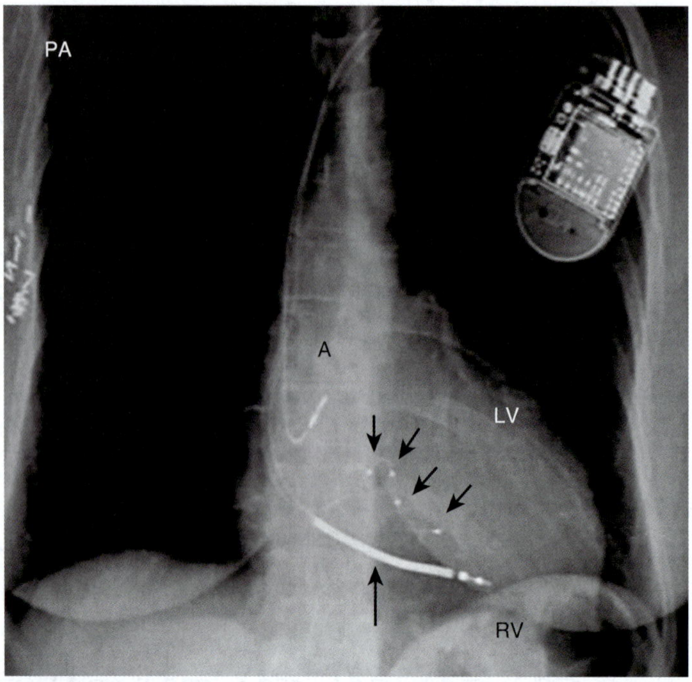

FIGURE 54-5. **Typical position of the left ventricular (LV) pacing lead *(short arrows)* with four poles, in a posterolateral branch of the coronary sinus in a patient with a cardiac resynchronization device. Atrial (A) and right ventricular (RV) implantable cardioverter-defibrillator leads are also present in typical locations. Note the presence of a defibrillator coil on the distal right ventricular lead *(long arrow),* indicating that the device is also capable of defibrillation. PA = posteroanterior.**

are uncomfortable and are not intended for routine conversion of more benign tachycardias. Optimal anti-tachycardia pacing can successfully terminate VT without a shock while also minimizing the risk that it will accelerate into VF.

ICDs incorporate a variety of programmable discrimination algorithms designed to withhold unnecessary therapies for brief episodes of rapid supraventricular arrhythmias, especially sinus tachycardia or AF. In addition, many ventricular arrhythmias will self-terminate within seconds, so algorithms designed to delay therapy for a short time can reduce unnecessary shocks. Optimal programming reduces the patient's discomfort, maximizes the life of the pulse generator battery, and reduces the potential adverse effects of unneeded shocks. Incorporating higher rate cutoffs, detection delay, rhythm discriminators, and anti-tachycardia pacing can reduce inappropriate device shocks by 50% and mortality by 30% compared with standard ICD programming, without significantly increasing the risk for syncope. Many athletes with ICDs can engage in vigorous and competitive sports without physical injury or failure to terminate the arrhythmia.

Indications for Cardiac Resynchronization Therapy

Resynchronization therapy promotes more synchronous ventricular contraction and results in "reverse remodeling" with a reduction in ventricular volumes, improved systolic function, and clinical improvement in heart failure (Chapter 46). In clinical trials of patients with reduced systolic function, QRS duration longer than 120 msec, and class III or ambulatory class IV heart failure, the addition of cardiac resynchronization therapy to guideline-directed medical therapy is associated with an approximately 30% reduction in hospitalizations and a 24 to 36% reduction in total mortality. Functional improvement in heart failure symptoms and quality of life is seen in a majority of patients, but 30 to 40% of patients may not improve symptomatically. Superior outcomes are associated with longer QRS durations (>150 msec) and a left bundle branch block QRS configuration, whereas patients with imaging-identified mechanical dyssynchrony alone, in the absence of QRS prolongation, do not improve.

Clinical trials have also established that the benefit of cardiac resynchronization therapy extends to patients with less severe heart failure symptoms (class I or II), in whom it appears to delay the onset of symptomatic heart failure and significantly reduce heart failure events over the next 1 to 7 years if the ejection fraction is 30% or less and the QRS duration is more than 130 msec, especially in patients with left bundle branch block. As noted previously, cardiac resynchronization therapy is also recommended for the treatment of bradycardia in patients who have a left ventricular ejection fraction of 50% or less and who likely will have more than 40% paced beats. The role of physiologic His-bundle and left bundle branch pacing continues to evolve. Evidence suggests the clinical results match or exceed those of biventricular pacing.[10] Current accepted usage largely follows indications for cardiac resynchronization therapy (Table 54-4).

TABLE 54-4 INDICATIONS FOR IMPLANTATION OF A CARDIAC RESYNCHRONIZATION THERAPY (CRT) DEVICE

CLASS I INDICATIONS*
LVEF ≤35%, sinus rhythm, LBBB (≥150 msec), NYHA class II, III, or ambulatory class IV on guideline-directed medical therapy
CLASS IIA INDICATIONS†
LVEF ≤35%, sinus rhythm, LBBB (120-149 msec), NYHA class II, III, or ambulatory class IV on guideline-directed medical therapy
LVEF <35%, sinus rhythm, non-LBBB (≥150 msec), NYHA class III or ambulatory class IV on guideline-directed medical therapy
LVEF ≤35%, atrial fibrillation, on guideline-directed medical therapy, and both: • Requires ventricular pacing or otherwise meets CRT criteria • Near 100% pacing with CRT can be achieved by either atrioventricular node ablation or pharmacologic rate control
LVEF ≤35% on guideline-directed medical therapy and are undergoing new or replacement device implantation with anticipated requirement for significant (>40%) ventricular pacing
In patients who have atrioventricular block, an indication for permanent pacing, a left ventricular ejection fraction between 36 and 50%, and are expected to require ventricular pacing more than 40% of the time, it is reasonable to choose pacing methods that maintain physiologic ventricular activation (e.g., cardiac resynchronization therapy or His bundle pacing) rather than right ventricular pacing.

*Class I indications are conditions for which CRT is indicated.
†Class IIA indications are conditions for which CRT is reasonable.
LBBB = left bundle branch block; LVEF = left ventricular ejection fraction; NYHA = New York Heart Association (functional class).
Adapted from Brignole M, Auricchio A, Baron-Esquivias G, et al. 2013 ESC Guidelines on cardiac pacing and cardiac resynchronization therapy: the Task Force on cardiac pacing and resynchronization therapy of the European Society of Cardiology (ESC). Developed in collaboration with the European Heart Rhythm Association (EHRA). *Eur Heart J*. 2013;34:2281-2329; Tracy CM, Epstein AE, Darbar D, et al. 2012 ACCF/AHA/HRS focused update of the 2008 guidelines for device-based therapy of cardiac rhythm abnormalities: a report of the American College of Cardiology Foundation/American Heart Association Task Force on Practice Guidelines. *J Am Coll Cardiol*. 2012;60:1297-1313; Kusumoto FM, Schoenfeld MH, Barrett C, et al. 2018 ACC/AHA/HRS guideline on the evaluation and management of patients with bradycardia and cardiac conduction delay: executive summary: a report of the American College of Cardiology/American Heart Association task force on clinical practice guidelines, and the Heart Rhythm Society. *J Am Coll Cardiol*. 2019;74:932-987.

Combined Resynchronization and Cardioverter Defibrillator Therapy

In patients who meet criteria for both cardiac resynchronization therapy and an ICD, implantation of a device with both functions (CRT-D) may provide additional mortality benefit. The burden of comorbidity does not appear to compromise the clinical benefits of cardiac resynchronization therapy plus an ICD compared with an ICD alone.[A5] However, cardiac resynchronization therapy alone may be appropriate for some patients with more advanced heart failure, extensive comorbidity, and limited life expectancy when the primary objective is symptomatic improvement, and the added value of defibrillation is not desired or less clear.[A6]

Complications

Many of the complications related to ICDs and cardiac resynchronization therapy are similar to those associated with pacemakers. Overall, major complications occur in 2 to 3% of new ICD implants and are more common during pulse generator replacement (5 to 6%). Use of an absorbable antibiotic-eluting envelope can significantly reduce the risk of major infection and should be considered in patients at high risk.[A7]

Long-term complications are primarily related to late infection and lead failure. Given their larger size and complexity, ICD leads are more likely to fail (1 to 4% annually) than are pacemaker leads (<0.5% annually). Lead failure is most often due to insulation failure or fracture of the conductor wires. Cardiac resynchronization therapy devices have the highest likelihood of procedure-related complications or lead dislodgement, predominantly owing to dislodgement of the coronary sinus lead. Phrenic nerve stimulation, which may occur with left ventricular pacing, manifests as a left-sided thumping sensation that is generally palpable; it can often be corrected with programming adjustments. In underserved countries, a resterilized pacemaker or defibrillator can be implanted with infection and failure rates similar to new devices.[11]

Although an occasional therapeutic ICD discharge is common, flurries of discharges require urgent evaluation to determine the cause. Such causes can range from flurries of VT or VF, which may have a correctable precipitant (e.g., an electrolyte imbalance, drug toxicity), to AF or another supraventricular tachycardia (SVT) with a rapid ventricular response, lead fracture, or insulation failure. An important consideration is the potential psychological impact of ICD shocks, and some patients may require psychiatric help in managing anxiety after receiving one or more shocks. In some cases, antiarrhythmic drug therapy (see Tables 52-2 and 52-3), catheter ablation, or both may reduce or eliminate the arrhythmias associated with frequent shocks (Chapter 53).

CATHETER ABLATION

Catheter ablation is a common and often preferred method for treating various forms of tachycardia. For appropriate arrhythmias, ablation often has higher success rates and is more definitive when compared with medical therapy. In addition, the treatment can be curative for some arrhythmias and avoid the need for chronic medication or future urgent intervention. Ablation is used for arrhythmias that depend upon a critical anatomic site, region, or regions of myocardial tissue that can be selectively necrosed to eliminate the arrhythmia. Depending on the arrhythmia, the target sites for ablation may be selected based on location, by substrate, by a local electrogram during a diagnostic electrophysiologic study (Chapter 49), by various mapping techniques, or by the response to maneuvers during an episode of sustained tachycardia. For some arrhythmias, reproduction of the clinical arrhythmia during diagnostic electrophysiologic testing (Chapter 49) is critical and can be facilitated by judicious use of sedation and intravenous infusion of catecholamines or other agents. Electroanatomic mapping has facilitated the ablation of many forms of tachyarrhythmias, allowed for substantial reductions in the need for fluoroscopy, and enabled ablation of complex arrhythmias with good success rates (E-Fig. 54-3).

TISSUE EFFECTS OF APPLIED ENERGY

Catheter ablation is performed by several means, including radio frequency energy, cryoablation, and laser ablation. The most common form uses radio frequency energy, typically in the range of 300 to 750 kHz, applied in a unipolar fashion between a small catheter-tip electrode in contact with the targeted myocardium and a large dispersive cutaneous patch electrode. Irreversible myocyte injury occurs with a tissue temperature higher than 50° C, with visually apparent tissue destruction at higher than 60° C. Saline irrigation of the electrode reduces heating at the tissue-electrode interface, allows for higher energy delivery when needed, moves the zone of maximal heating deeper into the tissue, and thus can allow for larger and deeper lesions with less risk of surface char and coagulum. Among other energy sources, cryoablation is the most widely used, whereas laser, microwave, and ultrasound have limited applications at present. Pulsed field ablation, which is still investigational, utilizes non-thermal electrical fields that are rapid and tissue-selective, thereby potentially reducing the risk of collateral injury.[12]

The most common serious complication of ablation is cardiac tamponade, owing to mechanical perforation of the heart by an electrode catheter. Rarely, high-degree AV block can occur when the target is near the AV node. Pulmonary vein stenosis is a rare complication of AF ablation. Also, depending on the type of ablation, collateral injury may occur to a phrenic nerve, the esophagus, or other nearby tissues. When epicardial ablation is performed, usually via percutaneous subxiphoid pericardial access, the coronary arteries could potentially be injured if ablation is delivered too nearby.

CATHETER ABLATION OF SUPRAVENTRICULAR TACHYCARDIAS

Catheter ablation is the recommended first-line treatment for paroxysmal SVT, Wolff-Parkinson-White (WPW) syndrome, or typical atrial flutter that is symptomatic enough to warrant therapy (Chapter 52). For atypical atrial flutters, ablation is becoming more common as success rates now approach those for typical atrial flutter. Ablation is rarely recommended for inappropriate sinus tachycardia because outcomes are less predictable, often partial, and may result in undesired sinus node dysfunction.

AV nodal re-entrant tachycardia (Chapter 52), which is the most common type of paroxysmal SVT, is successfully eliminated in 98% of cases (with a <1% risk for high-degree AV block), usually by radio frequency ablation of the "slow" limb of the re-entry circuit, most often at the posteroseptal aspect of the right atrium.

Accessory pathways are the next most common cause of paroxysmal SVT and can be due to manifest accessory pathways showing preexcitation (WPW syndrome) or concealed pathways that conduct only in retrograde fashion (no preexcitation on an ECG). Left-sided accessory pathways are ablated by using either a retrograde aortic or a transseptal approach, whereas right-sided and septal lesions are ablated with a venous approach. Detailed mapping is essential to identify the optimal site to ablate the accessory pathway, usually on either the atrial or the ventricular aspect of the mitral or tricuspid annulus. For the ablation of an accessory pathway, the success rate is 90 to 98%, with an overall complication rate of 2 to 3% and a less than 0.1% risk for a fatal complication.

Atrial tachycardias often arise in the right atrium and are mapped using a venous approach, but left atrial tachycardias require a transseptal approach. Approximately 10 to 20% of patients with atrial tachycardia have more than one focus and may be associated with other forms of SVT, particularly AV nodal re-entrant tachycardia. If the atrial tachycardia originates from a single site, ablation has about a 90% success rate, and complications are rare. For patients with multiple sources of atrial tachycardia, long-term success rates are lower.

Typical atrial flutter (Chapter 52), which arises in the right atrium, can be eliminated by ablation directed at a critical isthmus located in the low right atrium, between the tricuspid annulus and the inferior vena cava. The long-term success rate is more than 90%, with a less than 1% risk for serious complications.

ABLATION FOR ATRIAL FIBRILLATION

The primary aim of ablation for AF currently is to reduce the burden of recurrent episodes of AF in patients with symptoms and thereby to improve quality of life. Catheter ablation of AF has been effective in treating paroxysmal, persistent, and long-standing persistent (>1 year) AF. The optimal approach for the ablation of AF (Chapter 52) is an area of active investigation, but pulmonary vein isolation remains the cornerstone of most AF ablation procedures. For patients with recurrent paroxysmal AF, a primary driver of the arrhythmia is from focal sources in the regions surrounding the proximal portions of the pulmonary vein and sometimes other thoracic veins as they insert into atrial myocardium. Focally triggered arrhythmias may arise from other right and left atrial sites in 10 to 20% of patients.

For patients with recurrent symptomatic paroxysmal AF despite at least one antiarrhythmic drug trial, catheter ablation significantly reduces the risk for recurrent atrial arrhythmias by 50 to 70% and significantly improves quality of life compared with continued attempts to control the arrhythmia with alternative drug therapy.[13,14] The strategy of early intervention to maintain sinus rhythm (including ablation and/or antiarrhythmic drugs) may reduce mortality and stroke compared with standard medical care[A8] (see Chapter 52). First-line ablation therapy, without the requirement for prior antiarrhythmic drug failure, results in similar improvements and may lead to lower rates of recurrences.[A9–A11] For patients with symptomatic heart failure, and especially for patients who require an ICD or cardiac resynchronization therapy, catheter ablation is clearly the preferred initial therapy because it reduces all-cause mortality.[A12–A14]

Because AF is a progressive disease, however, the window of opportunity for intervention to prevent progression from paroxysmal to permanent AF or to prevent stroke, heart failure, or death may be limited. In patients with persistent AF, pulmonary vein isolation is also commonly performed early after diagnosis because it is less successful in patients with persistent AF of longer than 1 year's duration.[15]

Due to limited responses with pulmonary vein isolation alone, a variety of additional ablation targets have been tried, with mixed and often disappointing results. However, low-voltage myocardium-guided ablation can be helpful in selected patients.[A15]

Overall, the 1-year success rate of catheter ablation is 75 to 85% for paroxysmal AF and 60 to 75% for persistent AF. The most serious complications of AF ablation are atrial perforation, thromboembolism, and atrioesophageal fistula, with an overall risk of about 2%. Other complications are phrenic nerve injury, pulmonary vein stenosis, or vascular access issues. Left atrial macro-re-entrant arrhythmias, which can be a sequela of AF ablation, may require additional ablation.

In patients with refractory AF associated with an uncontrolled ventricular rate despite pharmacologic AV node blockade, ablation of the AV node can improve symptoms, functional capacity, and left ventricular function. In AV node ablation, third-degree AV block is intentionally induced with a success rate that approaches 100%. When the ablation lesions are placed sufficiently proximal in the AV junction, a junctional escape rhythm usually can be preserved. All patients require a permanent pacemaker to provide adequate rate response to physical activity.

ABLATION OF VENTRICULAR ARRHYTHMIAS

Ablation to manage ventricular arrhythmias is most commonly used for sustained VT, idiopathic monomorphic VT, and VT associated with structural heart disease, including ischemic cardiomyopathy, nonischemic dilated cardiomyopathy, arrhythmogenic right ventricular cardiomyopathy, sarcoidosis, congenital heart disease, and the Brugada syndrome.[16] However, it also may be used in selected patients with ventricular fibrillation or frequent premature ventricular contractions.

Ablation for the treatment of idiopathic VT carries a high (85% to 100%) success rate (Chapter 53), whether it arises in the outflow tract of the right ventricle or arises from other sites, including the AV valve annuli, the sinuses of Valsalva, the left ventricular septum, or the papillary muscles. Given these outcomes, ablation is recommended in symptomatic patients, either after failure of initial drug therapy or as first-line therapy, depending in part on the patient's preference. Complications are rare, and patients can usually avoid medications or an ICD.

By comparison, VT in patients with coronary artery disease and other forms of structural heart disease usually arises in diseased tissue in either ventricle. In patients with a prior myocardial infarction, ablation is often performed endocardially adjacent to or within an area of previous infarction in the left ventricle (E-Fig. 54-3). In patients with recurrent VT despite antiarrhythmic medications, VT ablation is more effective than an escalation of drug therapy.[A16]

In other forms of structural disease, percutaneous epicardial ablation may be needed. Ablation may not always be curative, but it may markedly diminish the frequency of VT episodes and reduce discharges of an ICD. Success rates range from 65 to 95%, with serious complications in about 5% of patients.

Although radio frequency catheter ablation is the most common method, other forms of ablation are sometimes used. An emerging noninvasive option is ablation via electrophysiology-guided stereotactic body radiotherapy.[17]

ARRHYTHMIA SURGERY

ATRIAL FIBRILLATION

Surgical ablation of AF can involve isolation of the pulmonary vein or a full biatrial Maze procedure, in which a series of incisions or linear lesions created by cryoablation or radio frequency ablation subdivides the atria into smaller segments unlikely to sustain AF. The most common current indication for the Maze procedure is the treatment of symptomatic AF in patients undergoing other cardiac surgical procedures, such as coronary revascularization or valve replacement or repair. AF surgery added to mitral valve surgery significantly reduces the recurrence of AF in patients with persistent or long-standing persistent AF. A variety of simpler and even minimally invasive operative procedures have been developed for AF, but their long-term efficacy and role in the treatment of AF are still being defined.

VENTRICULAR TACHYCARDIA

Surgical treatment by subendocardial resection or cryoablation of scar tissue (Chapter 53) in patients with a prior myocardial infarction can eliminate VT in selected patients (E-Fig. 54-4), with a success rate of 85 to 90%, but it carries an operative mortality rate of 5 to 15% even in experienced centers. Because of this high mortality and the development of catheter-based techniques, this procedure is generally limited to patients who have refractory VT or who have recurrent VT and other indications for cardiac surgery, such as large aneurysms associated with heart failure or the need to implant a left ventricular assist device.

CLOSURE OF THE LEFT ATRIAL APPENDAGE

The left atrial appendage, where blood tends to stagnate, is by far the most common site of origin for thromboembolism in patients with AF. Occlusion, removal, or isolation of the left atrial appendage can protect patients from stroke and thromboembolic events. In patients who are not suitable candidates for long-term anticoagulation (typically due to a propensity for bleeding or to poor adherence), occlusion of the left atrial appendage is at least as efficacious and safe as persisting with anticoagulation.[A17] The most widely used technique deploys an endocardial occlusion device, inserted percutaneously via transeptal puncture to the ostium of the left atrial appendage. After endothelialization of the luminal surface, these devices generally do not require long-term anticoagulation. Risks include dislodgement, residual leaks, and device-related thrombus. In patients who have AF and are undergoing cardiac surgery for another indication, epicardial closure of the left atrial appendage (amputation, stapling, or clip) can significantly reduce the risk of ischemic stroke or systemic embolism compared with anticoagulation alone during a mean follow-up of nearly 4 years.[A18]

GENERAL REFERENCES

For the General References and other additional features, please visit Elsevier eBooks+ at https://ebooks.health.elsevier.com.

Grade A References

A1. Nazarian S, Hansford R, Rahsepar AA, et al. Safety of magnetic resonance imaging in patients with cardiac devices. *N Engl J Med.* 2017;377:2555-2564.
A2. Wang Y, Zhu H Jr, Hou X, et al. Randomized trial of left bundle branch vs biventricular pacing for cardiac resynchronization therapy. *J Am Coll Cardiol.* 2022;80:1205-1216.
A3. Kolodziejczak M, Andreotti F, Kowalewski M, et al. Implantable cardioverter-defibrillators for primary prevention in patients with ischemic or nonischemic cardiomyopathy: a systematic review and meta-analysis. *Ann Intern Med.* 2017;167:103-111.
A4. Knops RE, Olde Nordkamp LRA, Delnoy PHM, et al. Subcutaneous or transvenous defibrillator therapy. *N Engl J Med.* 2020;383:526-536.
A5. Zeitler EP, Friedman DJ, Daubert JP, et al. Multiple comorbidities and response to cardiac resynchronization therapy: MADIT-CRT long-term follow-up. *J Am Coll Cardiol.* 2017;69:2369-2379.
A6. Kober L, Thune JJ, Nielsen JC, et al. Defibrillator implantation in patients with nonischemic systolic heart failure. *N Engl J Med.* 2016;375:1221-1230.
A7. Tarakji KG, Mittal S, Kennergren C, et al. Antibacterial envelope to prevent cardiac implantable device infection. *N Engl J Med.* 2019;380:1895-1905.
A8. Kirchhof P, Camm AJ, Goette A, et al. Early rhythm-control therapy in patients with atrial fibrillation. *N Engl J Med.* 2020;283:1305-1316.
A9. Andrade JG, Wells GA, Deyell MW, et al. Cryoablation or drug therapy for initial treatment of atrial fibrillation. *N Engl J Med.* 2021;384:305-315.
A10. Wazni OM, Dandamudi G, Sood N, et al. Cryoballoon ablation as initial therapy for atrial fibrillation. *N Engl J Med.* 2021;384:316-324.
A11. Andrade JG, Deyell MW, Macle L, et al. Progression of atrial fibrillation after cryoablation or drug therapy. *N Engl J Med.* 2023;388:105-116.
A12. Marrouche NF, Brachmann J, Andresen D, et al. Catheter ablation for atrial fibrillation with heart failure. *N Engl J Med.* 2018;378:417-427.
A13. Packer DL, Piccini JP, Monahan KH, et al. Ablation versus drug therapy for atrial fibrillation in heart failure: results from the CABANA trial. *Circulation.* 2021;143:1377-1390.
A14. Turagam MK, Garg J, Whang W, et al. Catheter ablation of atrial fibrillation in patients with heart failure: a meta-analysis of randomized controlled trials. *Ann Intern Med.* 2019;170:41-50.
A15. Huo Y, Gaspar T, Schönbauer R, et al. Low-voltage myocardium-guided ablation trial of persistent atrial fibrillation. *NEJM Evid.* 2022;1:EVIDoa2200141.
A16. Sapp JL, Wells GA, Parkash R, et al. Ventricular tachycardia ablation versus escalation of antiarrhythmic drugs. *N Engl J Med.* 2016;375:111-121.
A17. Brouwer TF, Whang W, Kuroki K, et al. Net clinical benefit of left atrial appendage closure versus warfarin in patients with atrial fibrillation: a pooled analysis of the randomized PROTECT-AF and PREVAIL studies. *J Am Heart Assoc.* 2019;8:e013525.
A18. Whitlock RP, Belley-Cote EP, Paparella D, et al. Left atrial appendage occlusion during cardiac surgery to prevent stroke. *New Engl J Med.* 2021;384:2081-2091.

55 CONGENITAL HEART DISEASE IN ADULTS

JUDITH THERRIEN AND ARIANE J. MARELLI

The convergence of major progress in medicine, pediatrics, and cardiovascular surgery has resulted in the survival of an increasingly large number of adult patients with congenital heart disease. An estimated 2.4 million people are currently living with congenital heart disease in the United States, two thirds of whom are adults. Adult care providers are becoming increasingly responsible for these patients, commonly in concert with a cardiologist and a tertiary care facility.

EPIDEMIOLOGY

Congenital heart defects are diagnosed in approximately 1% of births in the United States. An overall prevalence of 3 to 4 per 1000 adults has been documented. The median age of patients with *severe* lesions has increased from childhood to late adolescence. Advances in medical and surgical therapy have increased the survival of patients with congenital heart defects. Nearly 300,000 people in the United States are estimated to have severe congenital heart disease, defined as a combination of at least two or more abnormalities, typically associated with cyanosis at birth.

Bicuspid aortic valve occurs in about 2% of the general population, is the most common congenital cardiac anomaly encountered in adult populations, and accounts for up to half of surgical cases of aortic stenosis in adults (Chapter 60). Atrial septal defects (ASDs) constitute 30 to 40% of cases of congenital heart disease in adults, with ostium secundum ASD accounting for 7% of all congenital lesions. A solitary ventricular septal defect (VSD) represents 15 to 20% of all congenital lesions and is the most common lesion observed in children; its high spontaneous closure rates explain the lesser prevalence in adults. Patent ductus arteriosus (PDA) accounts for 5 to 10% of all congenital cardiac lesions in infants with a normal birthweight. Pulmonary stenosis and coarctation of the aorta represent 3 to 10% of all congenital lesions.

Tetralogy of Fallot is the most common cyanotic congenital anomaly observed in adults. Together with complete transposition of the great arteries, these lesions account for 5 to 12% of congenital heart disease in infants. More complex lesions, such as tricuspid atresia, univentricular heart, congenitally corrected transposition of the great arteries, Ebstein anomaly, and double-outlet right ventricle, account for 2.5% or less of all congenital heart disease.

PATHOBIOLOGY

Genetic Determinants

About 20% of congenital heart defects are associated with a syndrome or chromosomal anomaly, and the most common such chromosomal anomaly is Down syndrome (trisomy 21), in which about 50% of patients have defects of the endocardial cushions and the ventricular septum. VSDs also occur in 90% of patients with trisomy 13 and trisomy 18. The most frequently observed defects in patients with Turner syndrome (45,X) are aortic coarctation, aortic stenosis, and atrial septal defect. About 15% of patients with tetralogy of Fallot have a deletion on chromosome 22q11; prevalence is higher in those with a right aortic arch. Abnormalities involving the chromosomal band 22q11 can also result in a group of syndromes, the most common of which is DiGeorge syndrome. The shared phenotypic features are designated CATCH-22 syndromes, that is, a combination of cardiac defects, abnormal facies, thymic hypoplasia, cleft palate, and *h*ypocalcemia. For families with a child who carries a congenital cardiac malformation due to a chromosomal anomaly, the risk of the cardiac malformation in future children is related to the risk of recurrence of the chromosomal anomaly itself.

Typically, single mutant genes are also associated with syndromes of cardiovascular malformations, although not every patient with the syndrome has the characteristic cardiac anomaly. Examples include osteogenesis imperfecta (autosomal recessive; Chapter 239), associated with aortic valve disease; Jervell and Lange-Nielsen syndrome (autosomal recessive) and Romano-Ward syndrome (autosomal dominant), associated with a prolonged QT interval and sudden death; and Holt-Oram syndrome (autosomal dominant), in which an ASD occurs with a range of other skeletal anomalies. Osler-Weber-Rendu telangiectasias (Chapter 159) are associated with pulmonary arteriovenous fistulas. Williams syndrome (Chapters 31 and 32) occurs with supravalvular aortic stenosis in most cases. Noonan syndrome is associated with pulmonary stenosis, ASD, and hypertrophic cardiomyopathy. Although autosomal dominant inheritance has been implicated for both, most cases are sporadic. Deletion at chromosome 7q11.23 has been identified in patients with Williams syndrome, and a gene defect has been mapped to 12q22-qter in patients with Noonan syndrome (Chapter 47).

The risk for recurrence when the mother carries a sporadically occurring congenital lesion varies from 2.5 to 18%, depending on the lesion. Obstructive lesions of the left ventricular outflow tract have the highest recurrence rates in offspring. When the father carries the lesion, 1.5 to 3% of the offspring are affected. When a sibling has a congenital cardiac anomaly, the risk for recurrence in another sibling varies from 1 to 3%.

Genetic screening for the 22q11.2 microdeletion should be considered if patients with tetralogy of Fallot plan to have children. Without the 22q11 deletion, the risk of congenital heart disease in the fetus is 4 to 6%.

CLINICAL MANIFESTATIONS

History

Congenital heart disease is a lifelong condition during which the patient and the lesion evolve concurrently. The differential diagnosis of native and surgical anatomy in the adult with an unknown diagnosis depends on whether the patient is cyanotic or acyanotic. On completion of the evaluation, the following questions should be answered (Fig. 55-1): What is the native anatomy? Has this patient undergone surgery for the condition? What, if any, are the residual hemodynamic sequela?

Physical Examination

Physical examination of the heart and circulation includes the general physical appearance, the arterial pulse, the jugular venous pulse, the chest inspection, precordial percussion and palpation, and auscultation (Chapter 39).

Laboratory Investigations

A 12-lead electrocardiogram (ECG), chest radiograph, and baseline oxygen saturation should be part of every initial assessment. Two-dimensional transthoracic echocardiography (Chapter 43) and Doppler and color flow imaging are used to establish the diagnosis and to monitor the evolution of documented hemodynamic complications. Transesophageal echocardiographic examination is particularly useful in adults and is increasingly important during interventional catheter-guided therapy and surgery. Magnetic resonance imaging (Chapter 44) and computed tomography (Chapter 44) are useful adjuncts. Cardiac catheterization for congenital heart disease has shifted from pure diagnosis to include intervention. Coronary arteriography is recommended for adults older than 40 years in whom surgical intervention is contemplated.

SIMPLE LESIONS

ISOLATED SHUNT LESIONS

Hemodynamic complications of significant shunts relate to volume overload and chamber dilation of the primary chamber receiving the excess left-to-right shunt and to damage to the pulmonary vascular bed. The size and duration of the shunt determine the clinical course and therefore the indications for closure. The degree of shunting is a function of both the size of the communication and, depending on its location, biventricular compliance or pulmonary and systemic vascular resistance. Clinically apparent hemodynamic sequelae of shunts are typically apparent or can be expected to occur when pulmonary to systemic flow ratios, as inferred by Doppler echocardiography or measured by cardiac catheterization, exceed 1.5 : 1. Secondary enlargement of the cardiac chambers receiving excess shunt flow in diastole occurs if the shunt size is hemodynamically significant; in addition, the pulmonary artery becomes enlarged as pulmonary pressure rises.

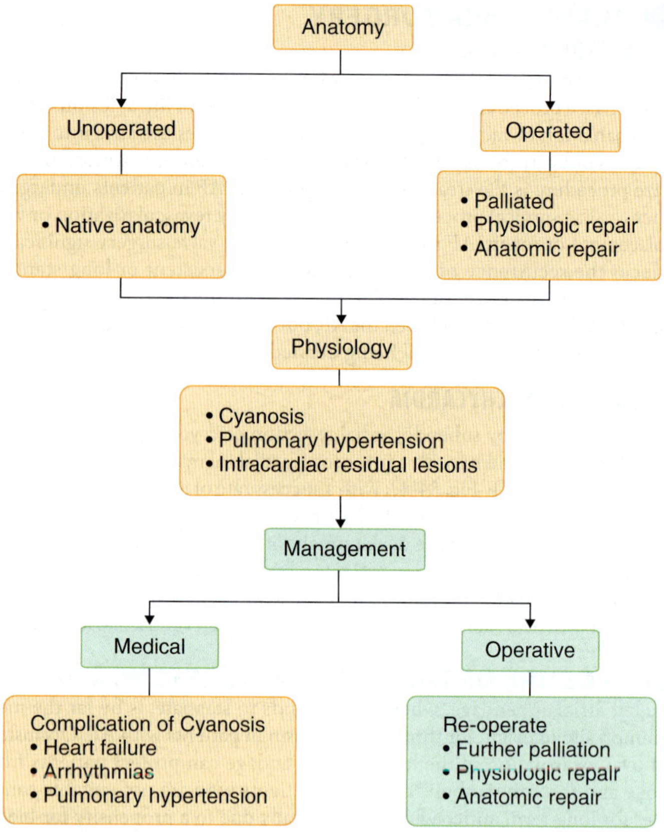

FIGURE 55-1. **The goals of complete clinical assessment in congenital heart disease are to define the anatomy and residual sequela to determine appropriate management and follow-up.**

PATENT FORAMEN OVALE AND ATRIAL SEPTAL DEFECT

Classification of ASDs is based on anatomic location. Most commonly, an ostium secundum ASD occurs in the central portion of the interatrial septum as a result of an enlarged foramen ovale or excessive resorption of the septum primum (Video 55-1). The combination of a secundum ASD and acquired mitral stenosis is known as *Lutembacher syndrome*, the pathophysiology of which is determined by the relative severity of each. Abnormal development of the embryologic endocardial cushions results in a variety of atrioventricular canal defects, the most common of which consists of a defect in the lower part of the atrial septum in the ostium primum location, typically accompanied by a cleft mitral valve and mitral regurgitation. The sinus venosus defect, which accounts for 2 to 3% of all interatrial communications, is located superiorly at the junction of the superior vena cava and right atrium and is generally associated with anomalous drainage of the right-sided pulmonary veins into the superior vena cava or right atrium. Less commonly, interatrial communications can be seen at the site of the coronary sinus, typically associated with an anomalous left superior vena cava.

The pathophysiology is determined by the effects of the shunt on the heart and pulmonary circulation. Right atrial and right ventricular dilation occurs as shunt size increases with pulmonary to systemic flow ratios greater than 1.5 : 1. Superimposed systemic hypertension and coronary artery disease modify left ventricular compliance and favor left-to-right shunting. Mitral valve disease can occur in up to 15% of patients older than 50 years. Right-sided heart failure, atrial fibrillation, or atrial flutter can occur as a result of chronic right-sided volume overload and progressive ventricular and atrial dilation. Stroke can result from paradoxical emboli, atrial arrhythmias, or both. A rise in pulmonary pressure occurs because of the increased pulmonary blood flow. Pulmonary hypertension is unusual before 20 years of age but is seen in 50% of patients older than 40 years. The overall incidence of pulmonary vascular obstructive disease is 15 to 20% in patients with ASD. Eisenmenger complex (see later) with reverse shunting, a late and rare complication of isolated secundum ASD, is reported in 5 to 10% of patients.

Up to 30% of adults have evidence of a pink-patent foramen ovale without hemodynamic evidence of shunt at rest. Clinical studies have demonstrated that the prevalence of patent foramen ovale is three times higher in patients with cryptogenic stroke (Chapter 376), particularly before the age of 55 years, because of right-to-left shunting and paradoxical embolization of material from the venous circulation.

DIAGNOSIS

Atrial Septal Defect

Although most ASDs are minimally symptomatic in the first three decades, more than 70% become impaired by the fifth decade.[1] Initial symptoms include exercise intolerance, dyspnea on exertion, and fatigue caused most commonly by right-sided heart failure and pulmonary hypertension. Palpitations, syncope, and stroke can occur with the development of atrial arrhythmias.

Precordial palpation typically discloses a normal left ventricular impulse unless the patient also has mitral valve disease. If the patient has a significant left-to-right shunt, the right ventricular impulse usually can be felt in the left parasternal area in end expiration or in the subxiphoid area in end inspiration. A dilated pulmonary artery can sometimes be felt in the second left intercostal space. On auscultation, the hallmark of an ASD is the wide and fixed splitting of the second heart sound, because the increase in venous return elevates the right atrial pressure during inspiration, thereby decreasing the degree of left-to-right shunting and offsetting the usual phasic respiratory changes. Pulmonary valve closure, as reflected by P_2, is delayed because of right ventricular overload and the increased capacitance of the pulmonary vascular bed. A soft midsystolic murmur generated by the increased flow across the pulmonary valve is usually heard in the second left interspace. In the presence of a high left-to-right shunt volume, increased flow across the tricuspid valve is heard as a mid-diastolic murmur at the lower left sternal border. With advanced right-sided heart failure, evidence of systemic venous congestion is present.

The ECG characteristically shows an incomplete right bundle branch block pattern (Fig. 55-2). Right axis deviation and atrial abnormalities, including a prolonged PR interval, atrial fibrillation, and flutter, are also seen. Typically, the chest radiograph shows pulmonary vascular plethora with increased markings in both lung fields consistent with increased pulmonary blood flow (see Fig. 44-6). The main pulmonary artery and both its branches are dilated. Right atrial and right ventricular dilation can be seen. Echocardiography is diagnostic and provides important prognostic information (E-Fig. 55-1). Ostium primum and secundum ASDs are easily identifiable with transthoracic imaging, but a sinus venosus ASD can be missed unless it is specifically sought. With Doppler study, pulmonary artery pressures can be quantified, and the interatrial shunt ratio can be estimated.

Patent Foramen Ovale

A patent foramen ovale without a resting shunt is not detectable on physical examination and is not associated with ECG abnormalities. The diagnosis is established by transesophageal Doppler echocardiography accompanied by injections of agitated saline to detect a right-to-left shunt during the Valsalva maneuver (Chapter 39).

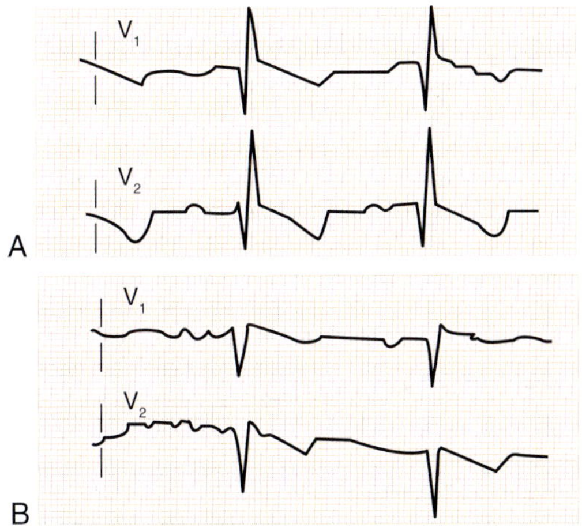

FIGURE 55-2. Electrocardiographic hallmark in atrial septal defect. Right precordial leads V_1 and V_2 illustrate two variants of an incomplete right bundle branch block pattern, the rSrT pattern (A) and the rsR′ pattern (B).

TREATMENT AND PROGNOSIS

Closure of an ASD, either percutaneously or surgically, is indicated in the presence of right-sided heart enlargement, with or without symptoms. In patients older than 40 years with symptoms and significant shunts, closure improves functional status and survival. A centrally located ASD or patent foramen ovale measuring up to 3.5 cm can be occluded by transcatheter techniques in a cardiac catheterization laboratory.[1,2] Advantages of this approach include the avoidance of sternotomy and cardiopulmonary bypass.[A1] Surgical closure is usually reserved for patients in whom concomitant repair of associated valvular anomalies is required, anomalous pulmonary veins are present, or device closure is not technically feasible.

In the presence of a significant shunt, closure of an ASD before 25 years of age without evidence of pulmonary hypertension results in a long-term outcome that is similar to that of age- and sex-matched controls. Advanced age (60 years) is not a contraindication to ASD closure in the presence of a significant shunt because a significant number of patients will show evidence of symptomatic improvement, although such late closure may not improve longevity.[3] Preoperative pulmonary artery pressure and the presence or absence of pulmonary vascular disease are important predictors of successful interventional outcome.

In patients who have had a cryptogenic stroke,[4] the presence of an atrial septal aneurysm may be more predictive of recurrent stroke than the size of the shunt.[5] Percutaneous closure of a patent foramen reduces the risk of recurrent stroke and chronic anticoagulations at the expense of a higher rate of periprocedure complications,[A2-A5] and closure is commonly recommended if the infarct appears to be embolic and no other cause can be identified.[6] A residual shunt after closure portends a higher risk of future stroke, with the risk generally proportional to the magnitude of the residual shunt.[7] By comparison, closure of a patent foramen ovale is not recommended as a treatment for migraine headache (Chapter 367).[8]

VENTRICULAR SEPTAL DEFECT

For anatomic classification of VSDs, the interventricular septum can be divided into four regions. Defects of the membranous septum, or infracristal VSDs, are located in a small translucent area beneath the aortic valve and account for up to 80% of VSDs. These VSDs typically show a variable degree of extension into the inlet or outlet septum, hence their designation as perimembranous (Video 55-2). Infundibular defects or supracristal outlet VSDs occur in the conal septum above the crista supraventricularis and below the pulmonary valve. Inlet defects are identified at the crux of the heart between the tricuspid and mitral valves and are usually associated with other anomalies of the atrioventricular canal. Defects of the trabecular or muscular septum can be multiple and occur distal to the septal attachment of the tricuspid valve and toward the apex.

Approximately half of all native VSDs are small, and more than half of them close spontaneously; moderate or even large VSDs may also close in 10% or less of cases. The highest closure rates are observed in the first decade of life; spontaneous closure in adult life is unusual.

Patients who have a small defect with trivial or mild shunts are defined as those with a shunt of less than 1.5 and normal pulmonary artery pressure and vascular resistance. Minimal or mild defects usually cause no significant hemodynamic or physiologic abnormality.

Patients with moderate defects have a shunt ratio of greater than 1.2, with elevated pulmonary artery pressure but not elevated pulmonary vascular resistance. Patients with a large and severe defect have an elevated left-to-right shunt (1.5 : 1 or higher) with high pulmonary pressure and elevated pulmonary vascular resistance. A moderate or severe defect causes left atrial and ventricular dilation consistent with the degree of left-to-right shunting. Shunting across the ventricular septum occurs predominantly during systole when left ventricular pressure exceeds that on the right; diastolic filling abnormalities occur in the left atrium. With moderate or severe defects, the right side of the heart becomes affected as a function of the rise in pulmonary artery pressure and pulmonary blood flow.

Eisenmenger complex develops in about 10% of patients with VSDs, usually when there is no resistance to flow at the level of the defect, which can be as large as the aorta. When a systolic pressure gradient is present between the ventricles, the physiologic severity may be trivial or mild but can also be moderate or severe.

DIAGNOSIS

An adult with a VSD most commonly has a small restrictive lesion that either was small at birth or has undergone some degree of spontaneous closure. Patients with a trivial or mild shunt across a small, restrictive VSD are usually asymptomatic. Physical examination discloses no evidence of systemic or pulmonary venous congestion, and jugular venous pressure is normal. A thrill may be palpable at the left sternal border. Auscultation reveals normal S_1 and S_2 without gallops. A grade 4 or louder, widely radiating, high-frequency, pansystolic murmur is heard maximally in the third or fourth intercostal space and reflects the high-pressure gradient between the left and right ventricles throughout systole. The striking contrast between a loud murmur and otherwise normal findings on cardiac examination is an important diagnostic clue. The ECG and chest radiograph are also normal in patients with small VSDs.

Patients with moderately sized VSDs typically are symptomatic as children and are therefore more likely to have repair at a young age. Adults with large, nonrestrictive VSDs that have not been operated on typically have had Eisenmenger complex for most of their lives. If not, they usually have a combination of pulmonary hypertension and left-sided volume overload resulting from a significant left-to-right shunt. Such patients are rarely seen today in developed countries but may still be encountered in the developing world.

In adults, shortness of breath on exertion can be the result of both pulmonary venous congestion and elevated pulmonary pressure. On physical examination, a diffuse palpable left ventricular impulse occurs with a variable degree of right ventricular hypertrophy and an accentuated second heart sound. A systolic murmur persists as long as pulmonary vascular resistance is below systemic resistance. The ECG commonly shows left atrial enlargement and left ventricular hypertrophy. The chest radiograph shows shunt vascularity with an enlarged left atrium and ventricle. The degree of pulmonary hypertension determines the size of the pulmonary artery trunk.

Echocardiography can identify the defect and determine the significance of the shunt by assessing left atrial and ventricular size, pulmonary artery pressure, and presence or absence of right ventricular hypertrophy. Cardiac catheterization is reserved for those in whom surgery is considered. Adults with a small defect of no physiologic significance need not be studied invasively. Those with Eisenmenger complex have severe pulmonary vascular disease and are not surgical candidates. Patients who have a moderately sized shunt that appears hemodynamically significant and in whom pulmonary pressures are elevated are most likely to benefit from direct measurements of pulmonary vascular resistance and reactivity.

TREATMENT AND PROGNOSIS

Patients with Eisenmenger complex have pulmonary vascular resistance that is prohibitive to surgery. For this group of patients, management centers on the medical complications of cyanosis (see later). In a few patients with small defects, complications can relate to progressive tricuspid insufficiency caused by septal aneurysm formation or to acquired aortic insufficiency when an aortic cusp becomes engaged in the high-velocity jet flow generated by the defect. The intermediate group of patients with a defect of moderate physiologic significance should have their VSDs closed unless closure is contraindicated by high pulmonary vascular resistance. For a perimembranous VSD, transcatheter closure is as effective as open surgical closure and has a lower rate of minor adverse events.[9]

Cumulative survival, which is about 85% at 40 years, is slightly lower than in the general population. Cumulative event-free survival after surgery is about 70% at 40 years, and a concomitant cardiac lesion (e.g., patent ductus arteriosus) and aortic cross-clamp time are determinants of late events. Late results after operative closure of isolated VSDs include residual patency in up to 20% of patients, only about 5% of whom need a reoperation. Rhythm disturbances after surgical closure of VSDs include tachyarrhythmias and conduction disturbances. Right bundle branch block occurs in one third to two thirds of patients, whereas first-degree atrioventricular block and complete heart block occur in less than 10%. Sudden cardiac death after surgical repair of VSD occurs in 2% of patients.

PATENT DUCTUS ARTERIOSUS

The ductus arteriosus connects the descending aorta to the main pulmonary trunk near the origin of the left subclavian artery (E-Fig. 55-2). Normal postnatal closure results in fibrosis and degenerative changes in the ductal lumen, leaving in its place the residual ligamentum arteriosum, which rarely can become part of an abnormal vascular ring.

The physiologic consequences of a PDA are determined by its size and length as well as by the ratio of pressure and resistance of the pulmonary and aortic circulations on either end of the duct. If systolic and diastolic pressure in the aorta exceeds that in the pulmonary artery, aortic blood flows continuously down a pressure gradient into the pulmonary artery and then returns to the left atrium. The left atrium and subsequently the left ventricle dilate, whereas the right side of the heart becomes progressively affected as pulmonary hypertension develops.

A small PDA has continuous flow throughout the entire cardiac cycle without left-sided heart dilation, pulmonary hypertension, or symptoms. However, patients with a small PDA develop infectious endarteritis at a rate of about 0.45% per year after the second decade, and closure should be considered.

A PDA is of moderate or large size but still restrictive when a left-to-right shunt occurs throughout systole and diastole is of variable duration. Left atrial or ventricular dilation and pulmonary hypertension will vary with the quantity of left-to-right shunting, as well as with the secondary effects on the pulmonary vascular bed. Symptoms generally increase by the second and third decades and include dyspnea, palpitations, and exercise intolerance. As heart failure, pulmonary hypertension, or endarteritis develops, mortality rises to 3 to 4% per year by the fourth decade, and two thirds of patients die by 60 years of age. Eisenmenger complex with systemic or suprasystemic pulmonary pressure and a right-to-left shunt develops in 5% of patients with an isolated PDA.

DIAGNOSIS

In patients with Eisenmenger physiology, a right-to-left shunt from the pulmonary artery to the descending aorta results in decreased oxygen saturation in the lower extremities compared with the upper extremities. This difference in cyanosis and clubbing is most prominent in the toes. With a large left-to-right shunt, the pulse pressure widens as diastolic flow into the pulmonary artery lowers systemic diastolic pressure. The arterial pulse becomes bounding as a result of increased stroke volume. Precordial palpation discloses variable left and right ventricular impulses as determined by the relative degree of left-sided volume overload and pulmonary hypertension. In the presence of a continuous aortopulmonary gradient, the classic "machinery" murmur of a PDA can be heard at the first or second left intercostal space below the left clavicle. As the pulmonary pressure rises, the diastolic component of the murmur becomes progressively shorter. With the development of Eisenmenger physiology and equalization of aortic and pulmonary pressure, the entire murmur may disappear, and the clinical findings are dominated by pulmonary hypertension.

In older patients, the chest radiograph shows calcification at the location of the PDA. Characteristically, the ascending aorta and pulmonary artery are dilated, and the left-sided chambers are enlarged. Echocardiography may not directly visualize the PDA but can accurately identify it by a Doppler signal that often parallels the length of the murmur. Cardiac catheterization to assess pulmonary vascular resistance is commonly indicated before closure.

TREATMENT AND PROGNOSIS

Ibuprofen can accelerate the closure of PDA in premature infants but may not reduce the need for an interventional procedure to eliminate the shunt.[A6] After ligation of a PDA in infancy or early childhood, cardiac function is commonly normal, and no special follow-up is required. If pulmonary artery pressure and pulmonary vascular resistance are substantially elevated, preoperative evaluation should assess the degree of reversibility. With Eisenmenger complex, closure is contraindicated. Closure of a PDA either percutaneously or surgically is indicated in the presence of left-sided heart enlargement or if prior endarteritis has occurred. Reported operative mortality rates vary from less than 1 to 8%, depending on the presence of calcification and the degree of pulmonary hypertension. Transcatheter or coil occlusion is an accepted procedure in adults. Residual shunt rates vary from 0.5 to 8%, depending on the device used.

PULMONARY ARTERIOVENOUS FISTULAS

Pulmonary arteriovenous fistulas can occur as isolated congenital disorders or as part of generalized hereditary hemorrhagic telangiectasia (Osler-Weber-Rendu syndrome; Chapter 159). These fistulas typically occur in the lower lobes or the right middle lobe and can be small or large, single or multiple. The arterial supply usually comes from a dilated, tortuous branch of the pulmonary artery.

The most common finding is that of abnormal opacity on a chest radiograph in a patient with buccal ruby patches or in an otherwise healthy adult who has mild cyanosis. Shunting between deoxygenated pulmonary arterial blood and the oxygenated pulmonary venous blood results in a physiologic right-to-left shunt. The degree of shunting is typically small and not significant enough to result in dilation of the left atrium and ventricle. Heart failure is unusual. Hemoptysis can result if a fistula ruptures into a bronchus. In patients with hereditary hemorrhagic telangiectasia, angiomas occur on the lips and mouth as well as in the gastrointestinal tract and on pleural, liver, and vaginal surfaces. Epistaxis is most common, but cerebrovascular accidents can also occur. Patients with hereditary hemorrhagic telangiectasia can have symptoms that resemble those of a transient ischemic attack even in the absence of right-to-left shunting. On physical examination, cyanosis and clubbing can be notable or barely detectable. Auscultation can disclose soft systolic or continuous noncardiac murmurs on the chest wall adjacent to the fistula. The murmur typically increases with inspiration. The ECG is usually normal. The chest radiograph shows one or more densities, typically in the lower lobes or in the right middle lobe. An echocardiogram can confirm the presence of the fistula by showing early opacification of the left atrium in the absence of any other intracardiac communication when saline is injected into a peripheral vein. The absence of a hemodynamically significant shunt can be confirmed by documenting normal cardiac chamber size.

If the hypoxemia is progressive or if a neurologic complication is documented to have occurred because of paradoxical emboli, fistula closure should be considered.[10] Options include percutaneous catheter techniques (e.g., embolization) if the fistula is small and accessible or a pulmonary wedge resection or lobectomy if the fistula is large. Multiple or recurrent fistulas create a major therapeutic challenge.

ISOLATED OBSTRUCTIVE LESIONS OF THE RIGHT AND LEFT VENTRICULAR OUTFLOW TRACT

Complications of obstructive lesions of the outflow tract relate to the secondary effects of exposure to pressure overload in the chamber proximal to the obstruction. The inability to increase systemic or pulmonary blood flow in the face of a fixed obstruction can cause exercise intolerance, inadequate myocardial perfusion, ventricular arrhythmias, and sudden death.

RIGHT VENTRICULAR OUTFLOW TRACT OBSTRUCTION

Obstruction of the right ventricular outflow tract can occur at the level of the pulmonary valve (see later), above it in the main pulmonary artery or its branches, or below it in the right ventricle itself. Supravalvular and branch pulmonary artery stenoses are important and common complications in patients with tetralogy of Fallot (see later). Residual supravalvular pulmonary stenosis is sometimes seen after palliative pulmonary artery banding to decrease pulmonary blood flow in patients with large left-to-right shunts. Congenital branch pulmonary artery stenosis can occur in isolation or with valvular pulmonary stenosis, shunt lesions, or a variety of syndromes.

VALVULAR PULMONARY STENOSIS

Isolated congenital valvular pulmonary stenosis (Chapter 60) is a common lesion due to a bicuspid valve in 20% of cases, a dysplastic valve caused by myxomatous changes and severe thickening in 10% of cases, and an abnormal trileaflet valve in most of the remaining cases. Fusion of the leaflets results in a variable degree of thickening and calcification in older patients.

DIAGNOSIS

A patient with moderate or even severe pulmonary stenosis may be asymptomatic. With severe stenosis, exercise intolerance can be associated with presyncope and ventricular arrhythmias. Progressive right-sided heart failure is the most common cause of death. On physical examination of patients with significant pulmonary stenosis, jugular venous pressure has a dominant *a* wave, reflecting a noncompliant right ventricle. Palpation discloses a sustained parasternal lift of right ventricular hypertrophy. An expiratory systolic ejection click is characteristic if the leaflets are still mobile. In moderate or severe stenosis, a grade 3 or louder systolic murmur can be heard and felt in the second left interspace. The length of the murmur increases as it peaks progressively later in systole with an increasing degree of obstruction. If right-sided heart failure occurs, tricuspid insufficiency and systemic venous congestion develop. The ECG can show right axis deviation and tall, peaked right atrial P waves in lead II. With more than mild stenosis, the R wave exceeds the S wave in lead V_1. On chest radiography, the main pulmonary artery can be dilated even if the stenosis is mild. Characteristically, the left pulmonary artery is more dilated than the right because of the leftward direction of the high-velocity jet. A variable degree of right ventricular hypertrophy is manifested as right-sided chamber enlargement. Echocardiography can establish the diagnosis and determine the severity by Doppler ultrasound examination, so cardiac catheterization is not required.

TREATMENT AND PROGNOSIS

The 25-year survival of patients with valvular pulmonary stenosis is greater than 95%. For patients with mild (<50 mm Hg gradients) and moderate (50 to 80 mm Hg gradients) pulmonary stenosis, bacterial endocarditis, complex ventricular arrhythmias, and progression of the stenosis are uncommon.

Depending on symptoms, percutaneous balloon valvotomy should be considered for patients with isolated valvular pulmonary stenosis and mean Doppler gradients of 30 mm Hg or greater unless there is moderate or severe pulmonary regurgitation. In the presence of a doming valve, pulmonary valvuloplasty is the procedure of choice for adults,[11] who achieve persistently good results at 10-year follow-up. When valvuloplasty cannot be performed or is unsuccessful, transcatheter pulmonary valve replacement provides good hemodynamic and clinical outcomes for at least 7 years after implantation. For patients with hypoplastic pulmonary arteries or subvalvular stenosis (double-chambered right ventricle), surgical resection of right ventricular muscle bands can be performed.

LEFT VENTRICULAR OUTFLOW TRACT OBSTRUCTION

Stenosis of the left ventricular outflow tract can occur at, below, or above the aortic valve. Discrete subaortic stenosis, most commonly caused by a fibromuscular ring just below the valve, accounts for 15 to 20% of all cases of congenital obstruction of the left ventricular outflow tract. Concomitant aortic insufficiency occurs in 50% of cases. Supravalvular aortic stenosis results from thickened media and intima above the aortic sinuses; early coronary atherosclerosis or even ostial coronary obstruction can occur.

CONGENITAL VALVULAR AORTIC STENOSIS

The normal aortic valve has three cusps and commissures. A unicuspid aortic valve accounts for most cases of severe aortic stenosis in infants (Chapter 60). A bicuspid aortic valve, which occurs in about 0.8% of infants[12] and is the most common congenital cardiac malformation, functions normally at birth but often becomes gradually obstructed as calcific and fibrous changes occur.

DIAGNOSIS

Symptoms include angina, exertional dyspnea, presyncope, and syncope and may progress to heart failure. The auscultatory hallmark of a bicuspid aortic valve in an adolescent or young adult is an audible systolic ejection click that is typically of a higher pitch than the first heart sound and is best heard not at the cardiac base but at the apex. The sound is caused by sudden movement of the stenotic valve as it moves superiorly in systole and is followed by the typical aortic stenosis murmur (Chapter 60). When significant calcification of the valve results in reduced mobility, the ejection sound is no longer heard. The diagnosis is easily confirmed by two-dimensional echocardiography, with which the number and orientation of aortic cusps can readily be identified.

TREATMENT AND PROGNOSIS

Conservative management is generally indicated for mild stenosis with a peak gradient of less than 25 mm Hg, but close supervision is required because 20% of these patients require an intervention during long-term follow-up. Unlimited athletic participation is allowed only for asymptomatic patients with peak gradients of less than 20 to 25 mm Hg, a normal ECG, and a normal exercise test result. Aortic valvuloplasty can be considered in young adults, but calcification limits its success, and valve replacement is usually required (Chapter 60). For adults, treatment decisions are similar to those for aortic stenosis from other causes. For patients with subvalvular aortic stenosis, surgical intervention is indicated in the presence of peak gradients above 50 mm Hg, symptoms, or progressive significant aortic insufficiency.

The estimated overall 25-year survival rate for patients with congenital valvular aortic stenosis diagnosed in childhood is 85%. Children with initial peak cardiac catheterization gradients of less than 50 mm Hg have long-term survival rates of higher than 90%, as opposed to survival rates of 80% in those with gradients of 50 mm Hg or greater.

COARCTATION OF THE AORTA

Aortic coarctation typically occurs just distal to the left subclavian artery at the site of the aortic ductal attachment or its residual ligamentum arteriosum. Less commonly, the coarctation ridge lies proximal to the left subclavian. A bicuspid aortic valve is the most common coexisting anomaly, but VSDs and PDAs are also seen.

The most common complications of aortic coarctation are systemic hypertension (Chapter 64) and secondary left ventricular hypertrophy with heart failure. Heart failure occurs most commonly in infants and then after 40 years of age. The high pressure proximal to the obstruction stimulates the growth of collateral vessels from the internal mammary, scapular, and superior intercostal arteries to the intercostals of the descending aorta. Collateral circulation increases with age and contributes to perfusion of the lower extremities and the spinal cord. Aneurysms occur most notably in the ascending aorta and in the circle of Willis. Premature coronary disease is thought to be related to the resulting hypertension. Complications, including bacterial endarteritis at the coarctation site or, more commonly, endocarditis at the site of a bicuspid aortic valve, cerebrovascular complications, myocardial infarction, heart failure, and aortic dissection, occur in 2 to 6% of patients, more frequently in those with advancing age who have not undergone surgery.

DIAGNOSIS

Young adults may be asymptomatic with incidental systemic hypertension and decreased lower extremity pulses. Coarctation should always be considered in adolescents and young adult men with unexplained upper extremity hypertension. The pressure differential can cause epistaxis, headaches, leg fatigue, or claudication. Older patients have angina, symptoms of heart failure, and vascular complications.

On physical examination, the lower half of the body is typically slightly less developed than the upper half. Blood pressure measurements should be obtained in each arm and one leg; an abnormal measurement is an increase of less than 10 mm Hg in popliteal systolic blood pressure compared with arm systolic blood pressure. The diastolic pressure should be the same in the upper and lower extremities. A pressure differential of more than 30 mm Hg between the right and the left arms is consistent with compromised flow in the left subclavian artery. Right brachial palpation characteristically reveals a strong or even bounding pulse compared with a slowly rising or absent femoral, popliteal, or pedal pulse. Examination of the eyegrounds can reveal tortuous or corkscrew retinal arteries. Precordial palpation is consistent with left ventricular pressure overload. On auscultation, a systolic ejection sound reflecting the presence of a bicuspid aortic valve should be sought. The coarctation itself generates a systolic murmur heard posteriorly, in the midthoracic region, the length of which correlates with the severity of the coarctation. Over the anterior of the chest, systolic murmurs reflecting increased collateral flow can be heard in the infraclavicular areas and the sternal edge or in the axillae.

In adult coarctation, the most common finding on the ECG is left ventricular hypertrophy. On the chest radiograph, the location of the coarctation segment between the dilated left subclavian artery above and the leftward convexity of the descending aorta below results in the "3 sign" (Fig. 55-3). Bilateral rib notching as a result of dilation of the posterior intercostal arteries is seen on the posterior of the third to eighth ribs when the coarctation is below the left subclavian artery. Unilateral rib notching sparing the left ribs is observed when the coarctation occurs proximal to the left subclavian artery. Transthoracic echocardiography documents the gradient in the descending aorta and determines the presence of left ventricular hypertrophy. Magnetic resonance imaging (Chapter 44) is the best modality for visualizing the anatomy of the descending aorta. Cardiac catheterization should measure pressures and assess collaterals when surgery is contemplated.

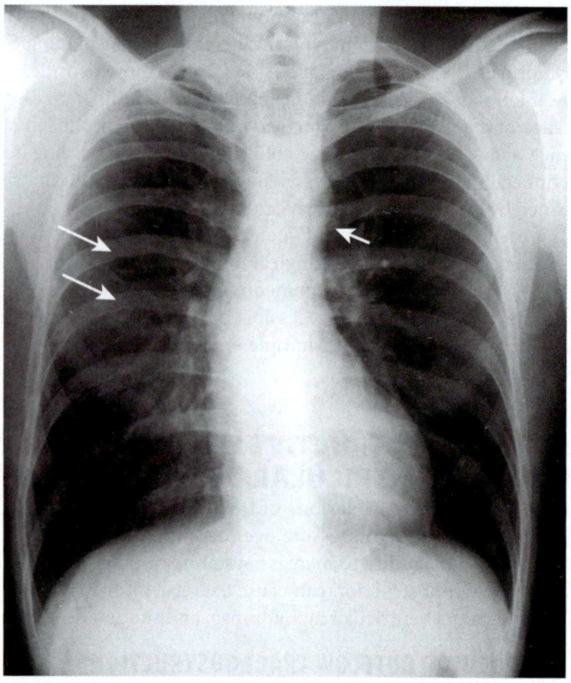

FIGURE 55-3. Chest radiograph of a patient with coarctation of the aorta. The radiographic "3 sign" formed by the dilated subclavian artery above and the dilated aorta below (*short arrow*) is shown. Note the notching, best seen at the level of the seventh and eighth ribs (*long arrows*). The dilated ascending aortic segment can also be seen.

TREATMENT AND PROGNOSIS

Intervention, typically catheter-based in adults,[13] is recommended in patients who have systemic hypertension with a peak gradient of 20 mm Hg or more on cardiac catheterization or who have evidence of significant collateral flow on imaging studies. Fifty percent of patients repaired when they are older than 40 years have residual hypertension, whereas those who have undergone surgery between the ages of 1 and 5 years have a less than 10% prevalence of hypertension on long-term follow-up.

ANOMALIES OF THE SINUSES OF VALSALVA AND CORONARY ARTERIES

SINUS OF VALSALVA ANEURYSMS

At the base of the aortic root, the aortic valve cusps are attached to the aortic wall, above which three small pouches, or sinuses, are seated. The right coronary artery originates from one sinus and the left main coronary artery from a second; the third is called the *noncoronary sinus*. A weakness in the wall of the sinus can result in aneurysm formation with or without rupture. In more than 90% of cases, the aneurysm involves the right or noncoronary cusp. Rupture typically occurs into the right side of the heart at the right atrial or ventricular level with a resulting large left-to-right shunt driven by the high aortic pressure.

A previously asymptomatic young man typically has chest pain and rapidly progressing shortness of breath sometimes after physical strain. The physical examination is consistent with significant heart failure. Even if the communication is between the aorta and the right side of the heart, biventricular failure is not unusual. The classic murmur is loud and continuous, often with a thrill. A murmur of aortic insufficiency secondary to damage to the adjacent aortic valve may be superimposed. The chest radiograph shows volume overload of both ventricles with evidence of shunt vascularity and pulmonary venous congestion. The echocardiogram is diagnostic. Cardiac catheterization can verify the integrity of the coronary artery adjacent to the ruptured aneurysm.

Even though symptoms may abate as the heart dilates, progressive cardiac decompensation typically results in death within 1 year of the rupture. A ruptured sinus of Valsalva aneurysm therefore requires urgent surgical repair.

CORONARY ARTERY FISTULAS

Fistulas arise from the right or left coronary arteries and in 90% of cases drain into the right ventricle, the right atrium, or the pulmonary artery in order of decreasing frequency. Typically, young patients are asymptomatic, but supraventricular arrhythmias are seen with progressive dilation of the intracardiac chambers. Angina can occur as the fistula creates a coronary steal by diverting blood away from the myocardium. Heart failure is seen with large fistulas. A continuous murmur heard in a young, otherwise normal acyanotic, asymptomatic patient should suggest the diagnosis. Most fistulas are associated with a small shunt, and hence the murmur is often less than grade 3 and is heard in the precordial area. Unless the shunt is large, the ECG is normal, as is the chest radiograph. The echocardiogram, especially the transesophageal echocardiogram, is diagnostic. Percutaneous transcatheter closure with coil embolization is preferred, but surgical ligation is also an alternative.

ANOMALOUS ORIGIN OF THE CORONARY ARTERIES

The left main coronary artery normally arises from the left sinus of Valsalva and courses leftward, posterior to the right ventricular outflow tract. The right coronary artery arises from the right sinus of Valsalva and courses rightward to the right ventricle. Isolated ectopic or anomalous origins of the coronary arteries (see Fig. 55-4) are seen in 0.6 to 1.5% of patients undergoing coronary angiography.[14]

The most common anomaly is ectopic origin of the left circumflex artery from the right sinus of Valsalva, followed by anomalous origin of the right coronary artery from the left sinus and anomalous origin of the left main coronary artery from the right sinus. If the anomalous coronary artery does not course between the pulmonary artery and aorta, the prognosis is favorable.

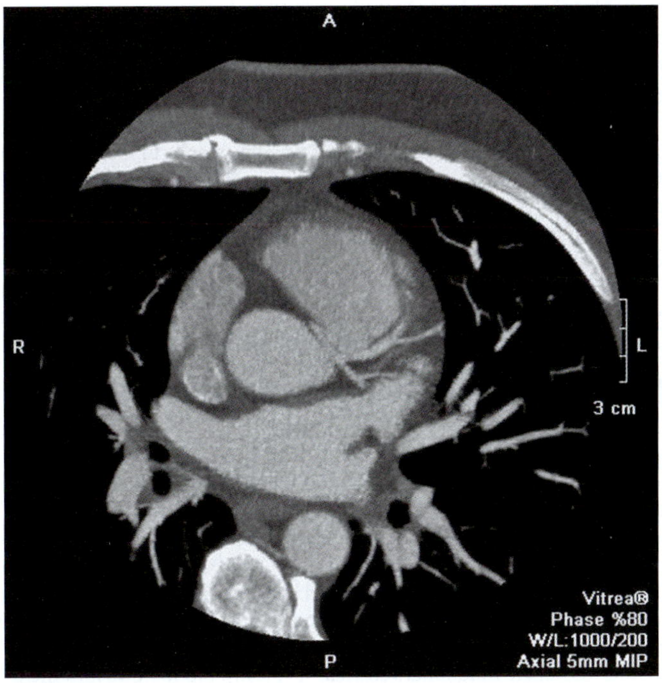

FIGURE 55-4. Frame from a computed tomographic angiographic study showing the origin of the left main coronary artery arising from the right sinus of Valsalva and coursing anteriorly between the aorta and pulmonary artery. (From Kern MJ, Kirtane AJ. Catheterization and angiography. In: Goldman L, Schafer AI, eds. *Goldman-Cecil Medicine*. 26th ed. Philadelphia: Elsevier; 2020.)

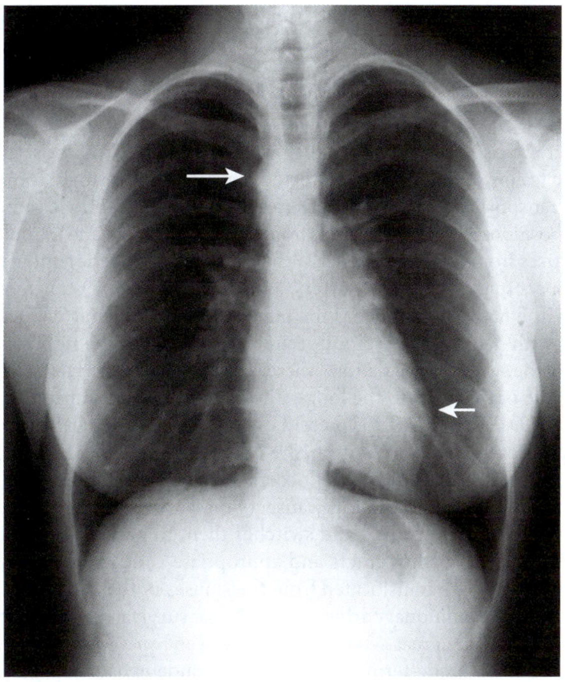

FIGURE 55-5. Chest radiograph of an adult after tetralogy of Fallot repair. A right aortic arch with rightward indentation of the trachea (*long arrow*) can be seen. The right ventricular apex remains upturned (*short arrow*). Note the sternal wires consistent with intracardiac repair, clarifying the fullness of the pulmonary artery segment often seen after extensive enlargement of the right ventricular outflow tract.

Risks of ischemia, myocardial infarction, and death are greatest when the left main coronary artery courses between both great vessels.

Coronary arteries can also originate from the pulmonary trunk. If both the right and left arteries originate from the pulmonary trunk, death usually occurs in the neonatal period. If only the left anterior descending coronary artery originates from the pulmonary trunk, the rate of survival to adulthood is approximately 10%, depending on the development of collateral retrograde flow to the anomalous artery from a normal coronary artery. This collateral flow may cause a continuous murmur along the left sternal border, congestive heart failure from the large shunt, and a coronary steal syndrome as blood is diverted away from the normal artery.

A single coronary ostium can provide a single coronary artery that branches into right and left coronary arteries, the left then giving rise to the circumflex and the anterior descending arteries. The ostium can originate from the right or left aortic sinus. The coronary circulation is functionally normal unless one of the branches passes between the aorta and the pulmonary artery.

Diagnostic procedures include angiography, magnetic resonance imaging, and transesophageal echocardiography. For an anomalous coronary artery that originates from the pulmonary artery, surgical reimplantation into the aorta is preferred. For an anomalous artery that courses between the pulmonary artery and aorta, a bypass graft to the distal vessel is preferred.

SPECIFIC COMPLEX LESIONS

TETRALOGY OF FALLOT

Tetralogy of Fallot, the most common cyanotic malformation, is characterized by superior and anterior displacement of the subpulmonary infundibular septum, which causes the tetrad of pulmonary stenosis, VSD, aortic override, and right ventricular hypertrophy. The VSD is perimembranous in 80% of cases. Additional cardiac anomalies include a right-sided aortic arch in up to 25% of patients. An anomalous left anterior descending artery originating from the right coronary cusp and crossing over the right ventricular outflow tract is seen in 10% of cases. Other associated anomalies include ASD, left superior vena cava, defects of the atrioventricular canal, and aortic insufficiency. With pulmonary atresia, pulmonary blood flow occurs through aortic to pulmonary collaterals.

Complete surgical repair in childhood consists of patch closure of the VSD and relief of the right ventricular outflow tract obstruction. Adequate pulmonary blood flow is ensured by reconstruction of the distal pulmonary artery bed. Previous palliative shunts are usually taken down. Complete repair in childhood yields a 90 to 95% 10-year survival rate with good functional results, and 30-year survival rates may be as high as 85%.

After repair, residual pulmonary stenosis, proximal or distal, can be seen. Some degree of pulmonary insufficiency is common, particularly if a patch has been inserted at the level of the pulmonary valve or if a pulmonary valvotomy has been performed. Residual VSDs can be found in up to 20% of patients. Patients may be asymptomatic or may have symptoms related to long-term complications after surgical repair. Symptoms can reflect residual right ventricular pressure or volume overload or arrhythmias at rest or with exercise. Angina can occur in a young patient if surgical repair has damaged an anomalous left anterior descending artery as it courses across the right ventricular outflow tract. In acyanotic adults, clubbing commonly regresses.

On physical examination, a right ventricular impulse is often felt as a result of residual pulmonary insufficiency or stenosis. A systolic murmur can represent residual pulmonary stenosis, residual VSD, or tricuspid insufficiency. A diastolic murmur can reflect aortic or pulmonary insufficiency. Ventricular arrhythmias are common after repair, with an incidence of sudden death as high as 5%.

The ECG in unrepaired tetralogy of Fallot shows right axis deviation, right atrial enlargement, and dominant right ventricular forces over the precordial leads. The most common finding after repair is complete right bundle branch block, which is seen in 80 to 90% of patients. The chest radiograph typically shows an upturned apex with a concave pulmonary artery segment giving the classic appearance of a boot-shaped heart. Figure 55-5 demonstrates the findings in an adult after repair. The apex is persistently upturned, although the pulmonary artery segment is no longer concave. Echocardiography can confirm the diagnosis and document intracardiac complications in repaired and unrepaired patients. Shunt patency can be determined by Doppler examination. Magnetic resonance imaging can accurately document stenosis in the distal pulmonary artery bed. Cardiac catheterization is reserved for patients in whom operative or reoperative treatment is contemplated or in whom the integrity of the coronary circulation needs to be verified.

Patients with a change in exercise tolerance, angina, or evidence of right-sided heart failure and those with symptomatic arrhythmias or syncope should be referred for complete evaluation. Surgical reintervention is generally considered when right ventricular pressure is more than two thirds the systemic pressure because of residual right ventricular outflow tract obstruction, free pulmonary regurgitation with right ventricular dysfunction, sustained arrhythmias, or a residual VSD causes a significant shunt.

Patients should be seen yearly by an adult congenital heart specialist for assessment of right ventricular function, pulmonary valve dysfunction, and arrhythmia. Surveillance should include a history, physical examination, and

12-lead ECG. Sudden cardiac death can occur in 3 to 6% of patients observed between 20 and 30 years, sometimes despite favorable hemodynamics.[15]

COMPLETE TRANSPOSITION OF THE GREAT ARTERIES

Complete transposition of the great arteries is the second most common cyanotic lesion, and surgically corrected adults are increasingly common. In simple transposition of the great arteries, the atria and ventricles are in their normal positions, but the aorta arises from the right ventricle, and the pulmonary artery arises from the left ventricle. When the aorta is anterior and rightward with respect to the pulmonary artery, as is most common, D-transposition is present. The native anatomy has the pulmonary and systemic circulations in parallel, with deoxygenated blood recirculating between the right side of the heart and the systemic circulation, whereas oxygenated blood recirculates from the left side of the heart to the lungs. The condition is incompatible with life unless a VSD, PDA, or ASD is present or an ASD is created; a hemodynamically significant VSD is present in 15% of cases. Subpulmonary obstruction of the left ventricular outflow tract occurs in 10 to 25% of cases.

The arterial switch operation transects the aorta and pulmonary artery above their respective valves and switches them to become realigned with their physiologic outflow tracts and appropriate ventricles. The proximal coronary arteries are translocated from the sinuses of the native aorta to the neoaorta (native pulmonary artery). The 22-year survival rate of patients with transposition of the great arteries who underwent operation between 1990 and 2009 is 93%. Long-term complications include neoaortic regurgitation, supravalvular stenosis, and coronary artery complications.

CONGENITALLY CORRECTED TRANSPOSITION OF THE GREAT ARTERIES

In congenitally corrected transposition of the great arteries, the great arteries are transposed, the ventricles are inverted, but the atria remain in their normal position. The systemic circulation (left atrium, morphologic right ventricle, and aorta) and pulmonary circulation (right atrium, morphologic left ventricle, and pulmonary artery) are in series. The patient is therefore acyanotic unless an intracardiac shunt is also present. The right ventricle is aligned with the aorta and performs lifelong systemic work, which accounts in part for its eventual failure. Patients with congenitally corrected transposition of the great arteries and no other associated defects can remain free of symptoms until the sixth decade, at which time significant atrioventricular valve regurgitation, failure of the right (systemic) ventricle, supraventricular arrhythmias, and heart block occur.

EBSTEIN ANOMALY

In Ebstein anomaly of the tricuspid valve, the right side of the heart consists of three anatomic components: the right atrium proper, the true right ventricle, and the atrialized portion of the right ventricle between the two. The displaced septal and posterior tricuspid leaflets lie between the atrialized right ventricle and the true right ventricle. Functionally, the valve is regurgitant because it is unable to appose its three leaflets during ventricular contraction. Valvular regurgitation and asynchronous, abnormal right ventricular function cause the dilation and right-sided heart failure observed in the more severe forms of the lesion. The wide spectrum of severity of the anomaly is based on the degree of tricuspid leaflet tethering and the relative proportion of atrialized and true right ventricle. The most common associated cardiac defect, a secundum ASD or patent foramen ovale, is reported in more than 50% of patients. On physical examination, a clicking "sail sound" is heard as the second component of S_1 when tricuspid valve closure becomes loud and delayed.

The 12-lead ECG typically shows highly peaked P waves with a wide, often bizarre-looking QRS complex. Preexcitation (Chapter 52) occurs in 20% of patients, whereas supraventricular tachyarrhythmias, atrial fibrillation, and atrial flutter occur in 30 to 40% of patients.

When patients of all ages are taken together, the predicted mortality is approximately 50% by the fourth or fifth decade. Complications include atrial arrhythmias, cyanosis, and, if there is an intra-atrial communication, stroke.

Intervention is considered when functional status or cyanosis worsens, significant atrial arrhythmias are documented, or a cerebrovascular accident occurs. Surgical options include replacement or repair of the tricuspid valve and closure of the ASD.

ATRIOVENTRICULAR CANAL DEFECT

A partial atrioventricular canal defect refers to an ostium primum ASD with a cleft mitral valve. The anomaly is manifested as a hemodynamic combination of an ASD with a variable degree of mitral regurgitation. The 12-lead ECG shows the typical findings of left axis deviation with a Q wave in leads I and aVL and a prolonged PR interval. The echocardiogram shows a defect in the inferior portion of the interatrial septum and a cleft mitral valve.

A complete atrioventricular canal defect is an uncommon defect consisting of a primum ASD, an inlet VSD that usually extends to the membranous interventricular septum, and a common atrioventricular valve. Adults who have not been operated on usually have Eisenmenger syndrome.

Surgical repair consists of closing the interatrial or interventricular communication with reconstruction of the common atrioventricular valve or closure of the cleft in the mitral valve. An adult who has undergone repair may have significant residual regurgitation of the mitral or tricuspid valve. Even after surgery, acquired subaortic obstruction can occur.

UNIVENTRICULAR HEART AND TRICUSPID ATRESIA

The terms *single ventricle, common ventricle*, and *univentricular heart* have been used interchangeably to describe the double-inlet ventricle, in which one ventricular chamber receives flow from both the tricuspid and mitral valves. In 75 to 90% of cases, the single ventricle is a morphologic left ventricle. Obstruction of one of the great arteries is common.

In tricuspid atresia, no orifice is found between the right atrium and right ventricle, and an underdeveloped or hypoplastic right ventricle is present. The morphologic left ventricle is consistently normally developed and therefore becomes the single functional ventricle. Typically, blood flows into the right atrium, then through an obligatory ASD and to the left atrium, where it then proceeds to the left ventricle. Variable features include a VSD, the abnormal position of the great arteries, and the relative degree of pulmonary stenosis, all of which are used to classify tricuspid atresia.

Adult patients rarely have not been operated on. They may be acyanotic after the Fontan operation. At 5-year follow-up, 80% or more of Fontan survivors are in New York Heart Association functional class I or II, with successful pregnancy reported in a small number of patients. When patients of all ages are considered together, 10-year survival rates vary from 60 to 70%. Late deaths are due to reoperation, arrhythmia, ventricular failure, protein-losing enteropathy, and liver dysfunction. Yearly follow-up with specialized imaging is recommended.

Anomalies of Pulmonary Venous Return

In partial anomalous pulmonary venous return, one or more, but not all four, pulmonary veins are not connected to the left atrium. The most common pattern has the right pulmonary veins connected to the superior vena cava, usually with a sinus venosus ASD.

In total anomalous pulmonary venous return, all the pulmonary veins connect abnormally to either the right atrium or one of the systemic veins above or below the diaphragm. Concurrent obstruction of the pulmonary veins is present when drainage occurs below the diaphragm and variable when drainage occurs above it. An ASD is essential to sustain life. One third of cases occur with major complex cardiac malformations. Surgical treatment is indicated.

In cor triatriatum, the pulmonary veins drain into an accessory chamber that is usually connected to the left atrium through an opening of variable size. The hemodynamic consequences are determined by the size of this opening and are similar to those of mitral stenosis.

Dextrocardia and Mesocardia

In dextrocardia, the heart is on the right side of the thorax with or without situs inversus. When the heart is right sided with inverted atria, the stomach is right sided, and the liver is left sided, the combination is dextrocardia with situs inversus. The heart usually functions normally, and the diagnosis is often fortuitous. The heart sounds are louder on the right side of the chest, and the liver is palpable on the left. The chest radiograph shows a right-sided cardiac apex with a lower left hemidiaphragm and a right-sided stomach bubble. The ECG shows an inverted P and T wave in lead I with a negative QRS deflection and a reverse pattern between aVR and aVL. A mirror-image progression is seen from V_1 to a right-sided V_6 lead. An echocardiogram should be performed to ensure that intracardiac anatomy is normal.

When dextrocardia with situs solitus occurs, the ventricles are inverted, but not the viscera and therefore not the atria. Associated severe cardiac malformations are typical. In mesocardia, the heart is centrally located in the chest with normal atrial and visceral anatomy. The apex is central or rightward displaced on the chest radiograph. Typically, no associated cardiac malformations are present.

SPECIALIZED ISSUES

Pulmonary Hypertension and Its Complications

Pulmonary hypertension (Chapter 69) secondary to structural disease of the heart or circulation can occur with or without an increase in pulmonary vascular resistance. Pulmonary vascular obstructive disease occurs when pulmonary vascular resistance rises and becomes fixed and irreversible. *Eisenmenger physiology* designates the physiologic response of shunt lesions in which a right-to-left shunt occurs in response to an elevation in pulmonary vascular resistance.

In the most common congenital anomalies, pulmonary hypertension is a result of increased pulmonary blood flow because of a native left-to-right shunt. Examples include ASD, a large-sized VSD, PDA, and a variety of complex lesions. The rate at which pulmonary hypertension progresses to become pulmonary vascular obstructive disease varies from one lesion to another and depends at least in part on the source of pulmonary blood flow. Pulmonary hypertension typically develops in patients with an ASD after the fourth decade; Eisenmenger syndrome is a late complication seen in only 5 to 10% of cases. In contrast, in patients with a large VSD or persistent PDA, progressive elevation in pulmonary vascular resistance occurs rapidly because the pulmonary vascular bed is exposed not only to the excess volume of the left-to-right shunt but also to systemic arterial pressures. As a result, Eisenmenger complex develops in approximately 10% of patients with a large VSD during the first decade.

The term *Eisenmenger syndrome*[16] should be reserved for patients in whom pulmonary vascular obstructive disease is present and pulmonary vascular resistance is fixed and irreversible. These findings, in combination with the absence of left-to-right shunting, render the patient inoperable.

The clinical manifestations of Eisenmenger syndrome include dyspnea on exertion, syncope, chest pain, congestive heart failure, and symptoms related to erythrocytosis and hyperviscosity. On physical examination, central cyanosis and digital clubbing are hallmark findings. Systemic oxygen saturations typically vary between 75 and 85%. The pulse pressure narrows as the cardiac output falls. Examination of jugular venous pressure can reveal a dominant *a* wave reflecting a noncompliant right ventricle until tricuspid insufficiency is severe enough to generate a large *v* wave. A prominent right ventricular impulse is felt in the left parasternal border in end expiration or in the subcostal area in end inspiration. A palpable pulmonary artery is commonly felt. The pulmonary component of the second heart sound is increased and can be felt in most cases. Pulmonary ejection sounds are common when the pulmonary artery is dilated with a structurally normal valve. Right atrial gallop is heard more frequently when the *a* wave is dominant. A murmur of tricuspid insufficiency is common, but the inspiratory increase in the murmur (Carvallo sign) disappears when right ventricular failure occurs. In diastole, a pulmonary insufficiency murmur is often heard. The 12-lead ECG shows evidence of right atrial enlargement, right ventricular hypertrophy, and right axis deviation. Chest radiographic findings include a dilated pulmonary artery segment, cardiac enlargement, and diminished pulmonary vascular markings. Echocardiography confirms the right-sided pressure overload and pulmonary artery enlargement as well as the tricuspid and pulmonary insufficiency. Cardiac catheterization is indicated if doubt exists about the potential reversibility of the elevated pulmonary vascular resistance in a patient who might otherwise benefit from surgery.

Cyanosis occurs when persistent venous-to-arterial mixing results in hypoxemia. Adaptive mechanisms to increase oxygen delivery include an increase in oxygen content, a rightward shift in the oxyhemoglobin dissociation curve, a higher hematocrit, and an increase in cardiac output. When cyanosis is not relieved, chronic hypoxemia and erythrocytosis result in hematologic, neurologic, renal, and rheumatic complications.

TREATMENT AND PROGNOSIS

In patients with Eisenmenger syndrome, pulmonary vasodilator therapy (e.g., bosentan 62.5 mg twice daily for 4 weeks, then 125 mg twice daily) may improve hemodynamics and exercise capacity after 4 months of use. Chronic oxygen therapy is unlikely to benefit hypoxemia caused by right-to-left shunting in the setting of a fixed pulmonary vascular resistance. Oxygen therapy may be considered for cyanotic patients during long-distance flights.

Indications for phlebotomy are symptomatic hyperviscosity in an iron-replete patient and prevention of excessive bleeding perioperatively. In the iron-replete state, moderate to severe hyperviscosity symptoms typically occur when hematocrit levels exceed 65%. If no evidence of dehydration is present, removal of 500 mL of blood during a 30- to 45-minute period should be followed by quantitative volume replacement with normal saline or dextran (E-Fig. 55-3). The procedure may be repeated every 24 hours until symptomatic improvement occurs.

Treatment of spontaneous bleeding is dictated by its severity and the abnormal hemostatic parameters (E-Fig. 55-4). For severe bleeding, platelet transfusions, fresh-frozen plasma, vitamin K, cryoprecipitate, and desmopressin have been used. Reduction in erythrocyte mass also improves hemostasis, so cyanotic patients undergoing surgery should have prophylactic phlebotomy if the hematocrit is greater than 65%.

Symptomatic hyperuricemia and gouty arthritis (Chapter 252) can be treated as necessary with colchicine, probenecid, or allopurinol. Nonsteroidal anti-inflammatory drugs are best avoided, given the baseline hemostatic anomalies in these patients.

Endocarditis Prophylaxis

Prolonged survival of patients with complex congenital heart disease has resulted in a population at increased risk for infective endocarditis (Chapter 61), which usually involves left-sided heart valves.[17] Adults with congenital heart disease should be informed about the risks of endocarditis. Any unexplained fever requires blood cultures to be drawn before antibiotics are initiated. Thorough transthoracic and transesophageal echocardiograms should be performed to assess the presence of vegetations. If infection of prosthetic material is suspected, early consultation with a specialist who has access to a congenital heart surgeon should be initiated because of the potential for rapid deterioration. The risk of endocarditis is highest in patients with cyanotic congenital heart disease and prosthetic material.

Antibiotic prophylaxis before dental procedures that involve manipulation of the gingiva, periapical regions of the teeth, or mucosal tissue is indicated in patients with previous infective endocarditis, unrepaired cyanotic lesions, palliative shunts or conduits, prosthetic valves or prosthetic materials used for valve repair, repaired congenital heart disease with prosthetic material or transcatheter device within 6 months of intervention, and repaired congenital heart disease with residual lesions at or adjacent to the site of a prosthetic patch or device (Chapter 61). It is also reasonable to consider prophylaxis against endocarditis before vaginal delivery at the time of membrane rupture in such patients. Prophylaxis is not indicated for nondental procedures in the absence of active infection.

Exercise

The goal of exercise evaluation is to assess the functional results of therapeutic interventions and to provide guidelines for exercise prescriptions. Patients with residual hemodynamic lesions or unrepaired congenital cardiac anomalies should be evaluated on an annual basis with a physical examination, an ECG, and a cardiac ultrasonographic examination if indicated. Pertinent additional tests may include Holter monitoring and exercise testing. Attention should be directed to the detection of pulmonary hypertension; arrhythmias; myocardial dysfunction; and symptoms such as exercise-induced dizziness, syncope, dyspnea, or chest pain.

Patients beyond 6 months after repair of a single shunt lesion without pulmonary hypertension, arrhythmias, or evidence of myocardial dysfunction can participate in all sports (E-Table 55-1).[18] With residual shunts, if the peak pulmonary artery pressure is less than 40 mm Hg in the absence of ventricular dysfunction or significant arrhythmias, patients can enjoy a free range of activity. Patients with elevated pulmonary vascular resistance are at risk of sudden death during intense exercise; although most self-limit their activity, participation in competitive sports is contraindicated. Patients with aortic and pulmonary stenosis should be counseled as recommended earlier, according to gradient severity. For patients with uncomplicated aortic coarctation, athletic participation is permitted if the arm-leg blood pressure gradient is 20 mm Hg or less at rest and the peak systolic blood pressure during exercise is normal. For patients after tetralogy of Fallot repair, repair of transposition of the great arteries, and the Fontan operation, exercise recommendations vary according to residual ventricular function and the presence or absence of arrhythmias.

Older Patients

Overall survival is similar to the general population in patients without cyanosis, univentricular physiology, genetic disorders, ventricular dysfunction, residual hemodynamic lesions, or acquired late complications. However, median survival is only 56 years in patients with one or more of these risk factors. Among women who become pregnant, fetal growth retardation is about 30% more common if the congenital heart condition is simple, but complex congenital lesions are associated with a 60% increased risk of fetal growth retardation and an 80-fold increased risk of maternal death.

The increasing number of older adults are surgical survivors who are subject to developing the full range of age-related cardiac conditions as well as late complications from their surgically repaired congenital anomaly.[19] Careful attention to blood pressure (Chapter 64), lipid levels (Chapter 190), and other preventive approaches (Chapter 40), including physical activity (Chapter 14), diet (Chapter 13), and smoking cessation (Chapter 363), is critically important. Neurodevelopmental problems in childhood and adolescence also may contribute to detectable cognitive decline (Chapter 371) and dementia in adulthood.

GENERAL REFERENCES

For the General References and other additional features, please visit Elsevier eBooks+ at https://ebooks.health.elsevier.com.

Grade A References

A1. Villablanca PA, Briston DA, Rodes-Cabau J, et al. Treatment options for the closure of secundum atrial septal defects: a systematic review and meta-analysis. *Int J Cardiol.* 2017;241:149-155.
A2. Søndergaard L, Kasner SE, Rhodes JF, et al. Patent foramen ovale closure or antiplatelet therapy for cryptogenic stroke. *N Engl J Med.* 2017;377:1033-1042.
A3. Saver JL, Carroll JD, Thaler DE, et al. Long-term outcomes of patent foramen ovale closure or medical therapy after stroke. *N Engl J Med.* 2017;377:1022-1032.
A4. Mas JL, Derumeaux G, Guillon B, et al. Patent foramen ovale closure or anticoagulation vs. antiplatelets after stroke. *N Engl J Med.* 2017;377:1011-1021.
A5. Ahmad Y, Howard JP, Arnold A, et al. Patent foramen ovale closure vs. medical therapy for cryptogenic stroke: a meta-analysis of randomized controlled trials. *Eur Heart J.* 2018;39:1638-1649.
A6. Sung SI, Lee MH, Ahn SY, et al. Effect of nonintervention vs oral ibuprofen in patent ductus arteriosus in preterm infants: a randomized clinical trial. *JAMA Pediatr.* 2020;174:755-763.

56

ANGINA PECTORIS AND CHRONIC ISCHEMIC HEART DISEASE

WILLIAM E. BODEN

DEFINITION

Angina pectoris and myocardial ischemia most commonly result from an obstruction or stenosis of one or more of the epicardial coronary arteries by atheromatous plaque, but it is increasingly recognized that both angina and ischemia can occur in the absence of epicardial coronary artery obstruction—particularly in women, who may exhibit microvascular angina and ischemia. Both coronary stenosis and obstruction can result when a plaque ruptures acutely to cause severe myocardial ischemia, thereby culminating in a myocardial infarction or an acute coronary syndrome (Chapters 57 and 58) with associated symptoms of angina, dyspnea, heart failure (Chapters 45 and 46), and arrhythmic complications (Chapters 50, 52 and 53) that may result in sudden cardiac death.

Angina pectoris results from an imbalance in myocardial oxygen supply and demand when an increase in activity or emotional stress increases cardiac workload, or "demand," with a concomitant increase in heart rate, blood pressure, and contractility, which, in turn, leads to an increase in left ventricular (LV) wall tension. However, stenotic coronary arteries are unable to augment antegrade flow, or "supply," adequately in response to this increase in demand. Such an imbalance classically results in chest discomfort (Chapter 39) of varying intensity and duration. Angina pectoris is generally defined as a discomfort in the chest or adjacent areas that occurs predictably and reproducibly at a certain level of exertion and is relieved with rest or nitroglycerin.

Chronic angina may result from epicardial coronary obstruction, vasospasm of the epicardial coronary arteries or microcirculation, or a noncoronary or nonvascular process, such as myocardial energy derangements, blood rheology abnormalities, or extravascular microcirculatory compression. Stable angina and chronic myocardial ischemia have been variably termed "chronic coronary syndromes," "stable ischemic heart disease," or "chronic coronary disease." Given the multiplicity of causes and precipitants of angina and ischemia in the nonacute setting, the term "chronic ischemic heart disease" is favored as being more accurately descriptive and inclusive of these multiple pathogenetic processes and triggers.

Grading of Angina Pectoris

The Canadian Cardiovascular Society (CCS) angina grading scale is a widely used four-point ordinal scale that classifies angina pectoris from mild (class I: angina occurring only during strenuous or prolonged physical activity) to severe (class IV: inability to perform any activity without angina, or angina at rest) and includes the full spectrum of angina from chronic stable to unstable (see Table 39-5). Operationally, the CCS angina scale permits clinicians to categorize patients as mild or stable (generally CCS classes I and II) versus severe or unstable (typically CCS classes III and IV). For classification purposes, subjects with stable ischemic heart disease generally exhibit CCS class I to II symptoms, which are typically provoked by exertion. Other grading systems include a specific activity scale, which is based on the metabolic cost of specific activities, and an anginal score, which integrates the clinical features and tempo of angina with electrocardiographic changes and offers independent prognostic information beyond that provided by age, sex, ventricular function, and coronary anatomy.

EPIDEMIOLOGY

More than 85 million American adults (more than 1 in 3) have at least one type of cardiovascular disease, which includes more than 17 million persons with coronary heart disease (Chapter 40), including 7.6 million who have survived a myocardial infarction (MI), nearly 10 million with angina pectoris, 5.7 million with heart failure, and 6.6 million with stroke (of all types). Among adults aged 60 to 79 years, approximately 25% of men and 16% of women have coronary heart disease, and among persons older than age 80 years, the percentages increase to 37% and 23%, respectively.[1] The Global Burden of Disease Study estimates that cardiovascular diseases are the leading cause of death globally. An estimated 18 million people died from cardiovascular disease in 2019, representing 32% of all global deaths.[2]

In 2019, before the severe acute respiratory syndrome coronavirus 2 pandemic, coronary heart disease accounted for 365,000 of the 650,000 or so U.S. deaths due to heart disease, or about 55%. The number of coronary heart disease deaths is expected to rise in the coming decade as a consequence of the aging of the U.S. population as well as the epidemic rise in obesity (Chapter 201), type 2 diabetes (Chapter 210), and metabolic syndrome, which may give rise to an increasing risk for premature coronary artery disease in younger generations.

PATHOBIOLOGY

Angina is the most frequent clinical expression of myocardial ischemia. Ischemia, which rapidly develops when a mismatch arises between myocardial oxygen needs and myocardial oxygen supply, can be manifested clinically in many ways besides angina, from no symptoms (e.g., silent myocardial ischemia) to unstable angina, MI, or sudden cardiac death. It may remain stable for many years in selected patients or may be rapidly progressive with an abrupt change in frequency and tempo during days to weeks. Conversely, atherosclerosis, which is the most common cause of myocardial ischemia, may evolve for years without any manifestations of ischemia.

Chronic angina and ischemia may be due to a variety of pathogenetic mechanisms, the most common of which is an obstructed or stenotic coronary artery. Alternative mechanisms include microvascular dysfunction, vasoconstriction at the site of a dynamic stenosis, or mural thrombosis, as well as noncoronary or nonvascular processes, such as derangements in myocardial energy supply or demand, abnormalities in blood rheology, and extravascular microcirculatory compression.[3,4]

Two major pathogenetic mechanisms may result in myocardial ischemia and angina in the chronic setting: so-called *demand angina*, which is caused by an increase in myocardial oxygen requirements and workload, and *supply angina*, which is caused by diminished oxygen delivery to myocardial tissue. Demand angina is a consequence of the increased myocardial oxygen requirements that occur with increased physical activity, emotion, or stress. In a patient with decreased myocardial perfusion owing to chronic atherosclerotic narrowing of a coronary artery, this increased demand may precipitate angina. Other extracardiac precipitants of angina include the excessive metabolic demands imposed by fever, thyrotoxicosis (Chapter 207), severe anemia (Chapter 144) from blood loss, tachycardia from any cause (Chapters 50, 52, 53), hypoglycemia (Chapter 211), and pain (Chapter 26).

By contrast, supply angina may occur in patients with either acute coronary syndrome (Chapter 57) or chronic ischemic heart disease by transient reductions in myocardial oxygen delivery as a consequence of coronary vasoconstriction with resulting dynamic coronary stenosis. In the presence of coronary luminal narrowing due to atherosclerosis, superimposed platelet thrombi and leukocytes may elaborate vasoconstrictor substances, such as serotonin and thromboxane A_2, whereas endothelial damage in diseased coronary arteries may decrease production of vasodilator substances such as nitric oxide and adenosine. The result is an abnormal physiologic vasoconstrictor response to exercise and other stimuli, such as exogenously administered adenosine, or the paradoxical vasoconstrictor response to the typical flow-mediated reactive hyperemia associated with brachial artery compression. Some patients with normal coronary angiograms or non–flow-limiting stenoses may exhibit dynamic obstruction alone, which can cause myocardial ischemia and result in angina at rest (Prinzmetal [variant] angina). Conversely, in patients with flow-limiting coronary stenoses, only a minor increase in dynamic obstruction can reduce blood flow sufficiently to cause myocardial ischemia.

The pathophysiologic basis for angina and myocardial ischemia has important implications for the selection of anti-ischemic agents. In patients with *demand angina*—in which increases in myocardial oxygen requirements are triggered by increases in heart rate, blood pressure, and contractility—therapeutic agents that reduce heart rate and wall tension, such as β-blockers or non-dihydropyridine calcium antagonists, will often provide the most clinical benefit. By comparison, nitrates and calcium antagonists with more potent vasodilatory properties (particularly the dihydropyridines) will be more beneficial to alleviate angina and ischemia mediated by coronary vasoconstriction and reductions in myocardial oxygen delivery.

Although the most common cause of chronic ischemic heart disease is atherosclerotic coronary artery narrowing and flow-limiting obstruction to epicardial blood flow, obstructive coronary artery disease may also have nonatherosclerotic causes, including congenital abnormalities of the coronary arteries (Chapter 55), coronary artery dissection, myocardial bridging, coronary arteritis in association with systemic vasculitides (Chapter 249), and radiation-induced coronary disease (Chapter 18). Importantly, myocardial ischemia and angina pectoris may occur commonly in the absence of obstructive coronary artery disease, a syndrome that is termed ischemia with nonobstructive coronary arteries (INOCA).[5] Angina and ischemia may also be associated with aortic valve disease, principally aortic stenosis (Chapter 60), hypertrophic cardiomyopathy (Chapter 47), and dilated cardiomyopathy.

CLINICAL MANIFESTATIONS

History

It is important to recognize that there are many causes of chest discomfort (see Table 39-2), that angina-like chest pain may not represent ischemic heart disease (Fig. 56-1), that ischemic heart disease causes symptoms other than anginal pain (Table 56-1), and that nonatherosclerotic coronary artery abnormalities may cause ischemic chest pain (Table 56-2).

Angina pectoris has four cardinal clinical features: the character of the discomfort, its site and distribution, its provocation, and its duration. The character of anginal discomfort is typically described as a pressure sensation that conveys a feeling of strangling and anxiety (Chapter 39), but patients may also use descriptors such as heaviness, squeezing, constricting, viselike, suffocating, and crushing. In some patients, especially women and the elderly, the quality of the sensation is more vague and atypical. Some patients may describe the discomfort as a burning sensation in the mid-epigastrium or as an uncomfortable, numb sensation. *Anginal equivalents* (i.e., symptoms of myocardial ischemia other than angina), such as dyspnea, fatigue, lightheadedness or dizziness, and gastric eructations, also may be manifestations of ischemic heart disease.

The site and distribution of anginal discomfort are predominantly midsternal or retrosternal but can be precordial. Radiation is common, usually to the left side of the neck and shoulder and down the ulnar surface of the left arm; radiation to the right arm is less common. Throat tightness or discomfort is a very important angina equivalent and should be a warning of coronary obstruction. Discomfort radiating to the jaw is common and must be distinguished from dental pain. Epigastric discomfort alone or in association with chest pressure may occur. Provocation of angina is classically caused by physical exertion or activity, emotional stress, exposure to the cold, sexual intercourse, or eating a large meal. Angina that occurs at rest or nocturnally often heralds a change in the pattern from stable to unstable and may indicate that there is an incipient plaque rupture leading to an acute coronary syndrome (ACS). Vasospastic (or Prinzmetal) angina may occur spontaneously at rest or nocturnally without provocation.

The typical duration of an episode of angina pectoris is brief. An episode usually begins gradually and reaches its maximal intensity during a period of

TABLE 56-1 NON–CHEST PAIN SYMPTOMS OF CHRONIC ISCHEMIC HEART DISEASE

DYSPNEA
Dyspnea on exertion Dyspnea at rest Paroxysmal nocturnal dyspnea Temporal change of increasing exertional dyspnea with declining effort tolerance
NON–CHEST LOCATIONS OF DISCOMFORT (EITHER EXERTIONAL OR AT REST)
Neck or mandibular discomfort or pain Throat tightness Shoulder discomfort Upper arm or forearm discomfort (more often left-sided) Interscapular or infrascapular discomfort
MID-EPIGASTRIC OR ABDOMINAL
Mid-epigastric burning, often postprandially Sharp abdominal pain (atypical, but more common in women) Right upper quadrant discomfort (may mimic gallbladder disease or pancreatitis) Nausea or vomiting (often associated with increased vagal tone secondary to inferior myocardial ischemia or infarction)
DIAPHORESIS
EXCESSIVE FATIGUE AND WEAKNESS
Often a discernible prodrome of increasing fatigue with declining effort tolerance
DIZZINESS AND SYNCOPE
Uncommon, unless precipitated or exacerbated by alterations in heart rate or rhythm (e.g., bradyarrhythmia, tachyarrhythmia, heart block), blood pressure (e.g., hypotension), or cardiac output (e.g., decreased cerebral perfusion)

	Typical/Definite Anginal Pain		Atypical/Probable Anginal Pain		Non-anginal Chest Pain		Dyspnea	
Age	Men	Women	Men	Women	Men	Women	Men	Women
30–39	3%	5%	4%	3%	1%	1%	0%	3%
40–49	22%	10%	10%	6%	3%	2%	12%	3%
50–59	32%	13%	17%	6%	11%	3%	20%	9%
60–69	44%	16%	26%	11%	22%	6%	27%	14%
70+	52%	27%	34%	19%	24%	10%	32%	12%

FIGURE 56-1. Pretest probabilities of coronary artery disease by age, sex, and symptoms. The regions shaded yellow denote the groups in which noninvasive testing is most beneficial. The regions shaded pink denote the groups with pretest probabilities of coronary artery disease between 5 and 15%, in which testing for diagnosis may be considered after assessing the overall clinical likelihood. (Adapted from Knuuti J, Wijns W, Saraste A, et al. 2019 ESC Guidelines for the diagnosis and management of chronic coronary syndromes. *Eur Heart J.* 2020;41:407-477.)

TABLE 56-2 NONATHEROSCLEROTIC CAUSES OF ISCHEMIC CHEST PAIN

PRIMARY CARDIAC CAUSES
Coronary artery abnormalities
Coronary spasm
Coronary arteritis
Coronary dissection
Coronary artery anomalies
Radiation-induced coronary disease
Myocardial bridging
Aortic stenosis
Hypertrophic cardiomyopathy
Dilated cardiomyopathy
Tachycardia
PRIMARY NONCARDIAC CAUSES
Anemia
Sickle cell disease
Hypoxemia
Carbon monoxide poisoning
Hyperviscosity (e.g., polycythemia)
Hyperthyroidism
Pheochromocytoma

minutes before abating. It is unusual for angina pectoris to peak and trough in less than a minute, and it is common that patients with exertional angina usually prefer to rest, to sit, or to stop walking during episodes that may be precipitated by the offending activity. Chest discomfort that persists for more than 15 to 20 minutes, especially at rest or nocturnally, is likely to represent ACS or MI. By contrast, features that suggest a noncardiac etiology of angina pectoris include pleuritic pain, pain reproduced by movement or palpation of the chest wall, sharp or constant pain lasting for many hours, pain or discomfort that a patient can localize to the chest wall with the tip of one finger, and very brief episodes of pain lasting seconds (Chapter 39). Typical angina pectoris is generally relieved within minutes by rest or the use of sublingual, oral, or cutaneous nitroglycerin. The response to sublingual nitroglycerin is often a helpful diagnostic tool, although some noncardiac pain (e.g., esophageal spasm) may also respond to nitroglycerin.

Although chest discomfort is usually the predominant symptom of ischemia, it is not invariably seen in all patients with chronic ischemic heart disease. Many individuals may complain predominantly or exclusively of dyspnea, diminishing exercise tolerance, fatigue, or weakness. Others will first present with an abnormal exercise test result or other evidence of myocardial ischemia without any symptoms (so-called *silent myocardial ischemia*). Some patients may present with cardiac arrhythmias or even sudden cardiac death.

Physical Examination

Many patients with chronic ischemic heart disease present with normal physical findings (Chapter 39), but a diligent physical examination may reveal findings that represent either the consequences of myocardial ischemia or evidence of risk factors for coronary heart disease. Inspection of the eyes may reveal a corneal arcus, and examination of the skin may show xanthomas (see E-Fig. 39-1). Retinal arteriolar changes are common in patients with coronary heart disease who have hypertension or diabetes mellitus (see Figs. 391-22 and 391-24).

The cardiac examination is generally of limited benefit in evaluating patients with chest discomfort or establishing a diagnosis of stable ischemic heart disease. During an episode of chest discomfort, myocardial ischemia may produce either a third or fourth heart sound.

Myocardial ischemia also can cause a transient holosystolic or mid-late systolic apical murmur due to reversible papillary muscle dysfunction that results in mitral regurgitation. These murmurs are more prevalent in patients with extensive coronary artery disease, especially with inferior or inferoposterior ischemia due to right coronary artery disease. It is important to distinguish such a murmur from the murmur of aortic stenosis or obstructive hypertrophic cardiomyopathy (see Tables 39-7 and 39-8). A displaced LV apical impulse, particularly if dyskinetic, is a sign of significant LV systolic dysfunction.

If patients have coexisting heart failure, an elevated jugular venous pressure, pulmonary rales, an S_3 gallop, and peripheral edema may be present (Chapter 45). The physical examination may reveal other implicating or contributing conditions, such as thyroid enlargement (Chapter 207) or severe anemia (Chapter 144).

DIAGNOSIS

In addition to a careful history and physical examination, assessment of patients with chronic ischemic heart disease includes the 12-lead electrocardiogram (ECG), measurement of biochemical and inflammatory markers, and noninvasive diagnostic testing (Chapter 44). The first goal is to assess the patient's probability of ischemia so that an appropriate evaluation can expedite effective therapy (Fig. 56-2). An acute syndrome with discomfort on minimal exertion or at rest requires urgent evaluation and treatment (Chapters 39 and 57), whereas a chronic syndrome with effort-related symptoms can be evaluated on an outpatient basis if an ECG does not show evidence of an acute myocardial infarction (Chapter 58), an acute coronary syndrome (Chapter 57), pericarditis (Chapter 62), or a worrisome arrhythmia (Chapters 51 to 53; Fig. 56-3).[6]

Resting Electrocardiogram

Although there may be focal, diagnostic findings of ST segment depression or T wave inversions (Fig. 56-4) on the resting ECG in patients with chronic ischemic heart disease, even those with extensive anatomic coronary artery disease may have a normal tracing at rest. In addition to myocardial ischemia, other conditions that can produce ST-T wave abnormalities include LV hypertrophy and dilation due to long-standing hypertension and valvular heart disease (e.g., aortic stenosis, hypertrophic cardiomyopathy), electrolyte abnormalities, neurogenic effects, and antiarrhythmic drugs. The presence of new ST-T wave abnormalities on the resting ECG, however, can be helpful in the diagnosis of coronary artery disease and may correlate with the severity of the underlying heart disease.

In addition to focal ST-T wave abnormalities, the ECG may reveal various conduction disturbances, most frequently left bundle branch block and left anterior fascicular block (Chapter 42). The finding of abnormal Q waves is relatively specific for the presence of previous MI but may not help determine when such an event occurred. Arrhythmias, especially ventricular premature beats (Chapter 53), may be present on the ECG but have a low sensitivity and specificity for coronary artery disease.

During a spontaneous episode of angina pectoris or during exertion or stress, the ECG becomes abnormal in 50% or more of patients with normal resting ECGs. The most common abnormality observed is focal ST segment depression, usually in one or more ECG lead groups, which signifies the presence of subendocardial ischemia. On occasion, transient but diminutive ST segment elevation and normalization of previous resting ST-T wave depression or inversion (pseudonormalization) may develop during chronic angina and ischemia, although ST segment elevation is far more commonly observed in ACS patients with plaque rupture.

Chest Radiography

Unless there is a history of prior MI, heart failure, or structural heart disease, the chest radiograph (Chapter 44) is usually normal in patients with stable angina and chronic ischemic heart disease. If an enlarged cardiac silhouette is present, it is generally indicative of a previous MI with LV dilation and cardiac remodeling. Other causes of cardiomegaly include long-standing hypertension (Chapter 64), concomitant valvular heart disease (Chapter 60), pericardial effusion (Chapter 62), and nonischemic cardiomyopathy (Chapter 47).

Laboratory Testing

In patients with new-onset or worsening symptoms, serial troponin measurements can distinguish MI and ACS from chronic ischemic heart disease (Chapters 57 and 58). The plasma levels of brain natriuretic peptide (BNP) and N-terminal pro-BNP, which increase in response to spontaneous or provoked ischemia, do not reliably distinguish stable from acute coronary syndromes but are associated with the risk of future cardiovascular events in patients who are at risk for coronary disease.

All patients with chronic angina should have biochemical evaluation of total cholesterol, low-density lipoprotein (LDL) cholesterol, high-density lipoprotein (HDL) cholesterol, triglycerides, serum creatinine (estimated glomerular filtration), and fasting blood glucose levels. In patients with known or suspected diabetes, a hemoglobin A_{1C} level should be obtained (Table 56-3). Other biochemical markers that are not routinely recommended but are associated with higher risk of future cardiovascular events include lipoprotein (a), apolipoprotein B, small dense LDL cholesterol, and lipoprotein-associated

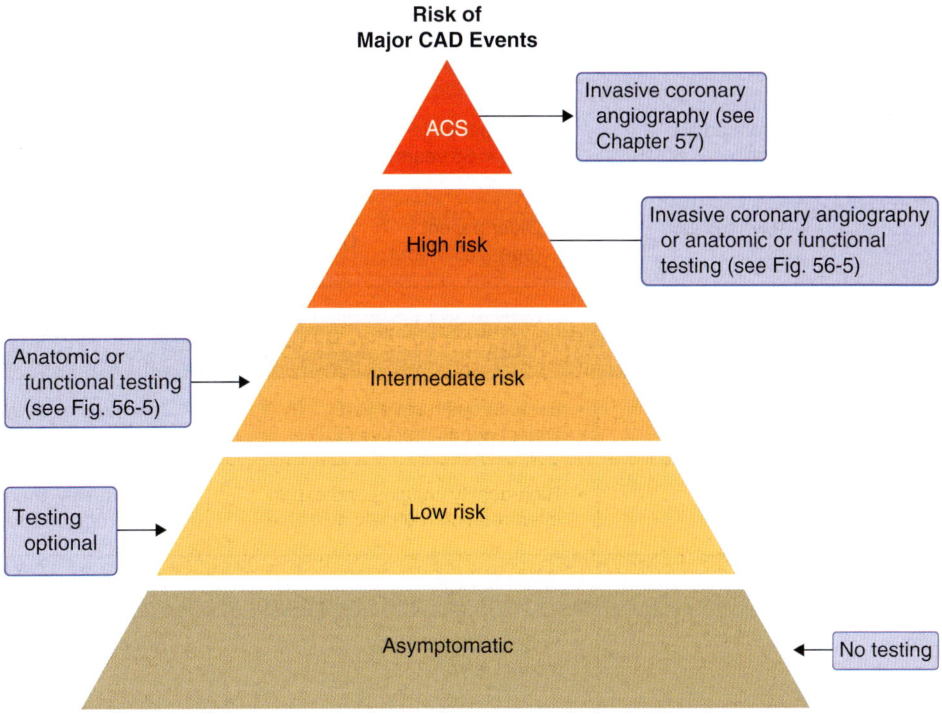

FIGURE 56-2. **Guide to when to consider noninvasive and invasive tests.** ACS = acute coronary syndrome (see Chapter 57). (From Gulati M, Levy PD, Mukherjee D, et al. 2021 AHA/ACC/ASE/CHEST/SAEM/SCCT/SCMR guideline for the evaluation and diagnosis of chest pain: a report of the American College of Cardiology/American Heart Association joint committee on clinical practice guidelines. *Circulation*. 2021;144:e368-e454.)

phospholipase A_2. Homocysteine levels correlate with the risk for development of coronary heart disease, but randomized trials have failed to demonstrate a reduction of clinical events when elevated homocysteine levels are reduced; as a result, routine screening for an elevated homocysteine level is not recommended.

High-sensitivity C-reactive protein, which is an acute-phase reactant of inflammation, has a strong and consistent relationship to the risk of future cardiovascular events, and an elevated level may warrant more aggressive diagnostic evaluation and therapy. Similarly, elevated levels of N-terminal pro-B-type natriuretic peptide can predict worse outcomes in patients with stable ischemic heart disease.

Differential Diagnosis of Angina

Many common noncardiac disorders may be manifested with clinical features that can be confused with angina pectoris (see Table 39-2). In some instances, symptoms may be indistinguishable from ischemic heart disease. For example, many patients with angina have coexisting esophageal disorders (Chapter 124), and both angina and esophageal discomfort may be relieved by nitroglycerin (Chapter 39). A distinguishing feature from angina is that esophageal discomfort is often relieved by antacids, proton pump inhibitors, or food.

Costochondritis can mimic angina but can typically be distinguished by the presence of well-localized pain on palpation. However, pressure, if it is applied too firmly to the anterior chest wall during examination of a patient with suspected angina pectoris, may elicit symptoms of discomfort even in normal subjects. Cervical radiculopathy may cause pain radiating to the shoulders, neck, or upper arms and can be confused with angina. However, this condition typically causes a constant ache that is often exacerbated by neck movement or rotation and may be accompanied by a focal sensory deficit or radiculopathy.

Pulmonary hypertension (Chapter 69) can cause exertional chest discomfort that may share many of the characteristics of angina pectoris. It is believed that right ventricular ischemia during physical exertion may cause this discomfort along with associated symptoms of exertional dyspnea, dizziness, and syncope. Findings on physical examination typically include a parasternal lift, a loud (and sometimes palpable) pulmonary component of the second heart sound, and findings of right ventricular hypertrophy on electrocardiography.

Chest discomfort may also be an important presenting clinical feature of pulmonary embolism (Chapter 68). Physical findings typically include tachycardia and tachypnea, an accentuated pulmonic component of the second heart sound, and occasionally a right-sided S_4 gallop. Pleuritic discomfort suggests pulmonary infarction, whereas a history of pain exacerbated by inspiration or deep breathing, along with a pleural friction rub, usually helps distinguish it from angina pectoris.

Acute pericarditis (Chapter 62) may be confused with the discomfort of angina pectoris, but pericarditis tends to cause chest pain that is generally sharp, is not relieved by rest or nitroglycerin, is exacerbated by movement or deep breathing, and is associated with a pericardial friction rub that may be evanescent. Aortic dissection (Chapter 63), which may be manifested with acute, severe chest pain, may be confused with an acute MI but generally not with angina.

Pretest Probability in Patients with Angina or Ischemic Equivalents

When symptoms of angina or exertional dyspnea prompt consideration of coronary heart disease and the need for additional cardiac evaluation, the clinician should first make a probability estimate of the likelihood that obstructive coronary disease is present. A number of validated risk assessment models exist that, in general, are useful in calculating this probability as follows:

- Low Pretest Probability: less than 10% pretest probability of coronary heart disease;
- Intermediate Pretest Probability: between 10% and 90% pretest probability of coronary heart disease;
- High Pretest Probability: greater than 90% pretest probability of coronary heart disease.

Recent evidence suggests that the pretest probability of detecting obstructive coronary disease among middle-aged men and women with typical angina has declined appreciably, to 32% and 44% in men aged 50 to 59 and 60 to 69 years, respectively, and to just 13% and 16% in women aged 50 to 59 and 60 to 69 years, respectively (see Fig. 56-1). These data reinforce the observation that epicardial coronary obstruction may be less common than previously believed and that other causes of chronic myocardial ischemia, such as coronary vasospasm, microvascular angina, and ischemia with nonobstructive coronary arteries, may be as frequent, if not more frequent.

Noninvasive Testing

Noninvasive stress testing with a standard electrocardiographic treadmill or bicycle exercise, radionuclide imaging (Chapter 44), stress echocardiography (Chapter 43), or newer diagnostic modalities such as cardiac magnetic resonance (CMR; Chapter 44) and positron emission tomography (PET; Chapter 44)

Pretest likelihood of CAD	Low →	No testing necessary →		Option for CAC for ASCVD risk stratification	(see Chapter 44)
	Intermediate-high →	Younger patient (age < 65 years)	**OR**	Less obstructive CAD suspected →	CCTA favored (see Chapter 44)
	Intermediate-high →	Older patient (age ≥ 65 years)	**OR**	More obstructive CAD suspected →	Stress testing favored

	Favors use of CCTA	Favors use of stress imaging
Goal	• Exclude obstructive CAD • Detect nonobstructive CAD	• Ischemia-guided management
Availability and expertise	• High-quality imaging and expert interpretation routinely available	• High-quality imaging and expert interpretation routinely available
Likelihood of obstructive CAD	• Age <65 years	• Age ≥65 years
Prior test results	• Prior functional study inconclusive	• Prior CCTA inconclusive
Other compelling indications	• Patient unable to exercise • Anomalous coronary arteries • Require evaluation of aorta or pulmonary arteries	• Suspect scar (especially if PET or stress CMR available) • Suspect coronary microvascular dysfunction (when PET or CMR available)

Stress testing information

	ETT	Stress echocardiography	SPECT MPI	PET MPI	Stress CMR MPI
Patient capable of exercise	✓	✓	✓		
Pharmacologic stress indicated		✓	✓	✓	✓
Quantitative flow				✓	✓
LV dysfunction/scar		✓	✓	✓	✓

FIGURE 56-3. Approach to choosing diagnostic testing in suspected angina pectoris or chronic ischemic heart disease. ASCVD = atherosclerotic cardiovascular disease; CAC = coronary artery calcium; CAD = coronary artery disease; CCTA = coronary computed tomography angiography; CMR = cardiovascular magnetic resonance; ETT = exercise tolerance test; LV = left ventricular; MPI = myocardial perfusion imaging; PET = positron emission tomography; SPECT = single-photon emission computed tomography. (From Gulati M, Levy PD, Mukherjee D, et al. 2021 AHA/ACC/ASE/CHEST/SAEM/SCCT/SCMR guideline for the evaluation and diagnosis of chest pain: a report of the American College of Cardiology/American Heart Association joint committee on clinical practice guidelines. *Circulation*. 2021;144:e368-e454.)

are useful and clinically important options for establishing the diagnosis and prognosis in patients with chronic ischemic heart disease (Fig. 56-5). The predictive accuracy of these tests is defined not only by their sensitivity and specificity but also by the prevalence of disease (or pretest probability) in the population under study. Noninvasive testing should be performed only if the incremental information is likely to alter the planned management strategy. Thus, the value of noninvasive stress testing is limited in patients with a very low likelihood of ischemic heart disease (Chapter 44) and is greatest when the pretest likelihood is intermediate because the test result is likely to have the greatest effect on the post-test probability of coronary artery disease and, hence, on clinical decision making.[7]

Each noninvasive test has a sensitivity and specificity (Table 56-4) that, when combined with a patient's pretest probability (see Table 56-1), can yield a post-test probability that may essentially rule in or rule out significant for coronary artery disease (Fig. 56-6).[8] The choice among tests depends on the patient's characteristics (see Figs 56-3 and 56-5). Stress testing can be performed carefully in patients with mild aortic valve stenosis or hypertrophic cardiomyopathy but generally should be avoided in patients with severe disease.

Cardiac Computed Tomographic Angiography

Cardiac computed tomographic angiography (CCTA; Chapter 44) is a highly sensitive method to detect coronary calcification (see Fig. 44-9), which is strongly associated with coronary atherosclerosis, and can also provide noninvasive angiography of the proximal coronary arteries. Although coronary calcification is a highly sensitive (approximately 90%) finding in patients with coronary artery disease, the specificity for identifying patients with obstructive coronary artery disease is much lower (approximately 50%). Because of the potential unnecessary testing from false-positive results, CCTA is currently not recommended as a routine screening approach for suspected obstructive coronary artery disease in individuals who are asymptomatic or are at low risk (<10% 10-year estimated risk of coronary events).

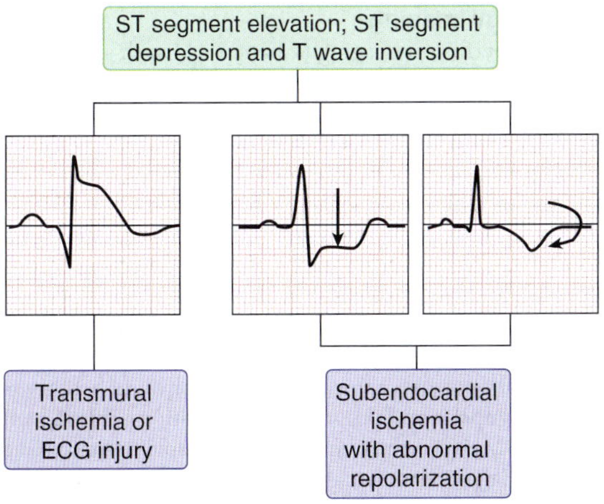

FIGURE 56-4. Ischemic ST segment shifts and repolarization changes on electrocardiogram (ECG).

TABLE 56-3 BLOOD TESTS TO OBTAIN ROUTINELY (OR SELECTIVELY*) IN PATIENTS WITH CHRONIC STABLE ISCHEMIC HEART DISEASE

LIPID LEVELS
Low-density lipoprotein (LDL) and high-density lipoprotein (HDL) cholesterol
Triglyceride level
*LDL electrophoresis (especially apolipoprotein B and small dense LDL)
*Lipoprotein (a)
*Lipoprotein-associated phospholipase A_2
METABOLIC EVALUATION
Fasting plasma glucose concentration
Serum creatinine level
Thyroxine level
*Hemoglobin A_{1c} in patients with known or suspected diabetes
MARKERS OF INFLAMMATION OR CARDIAC FUNCTION
*High-sensitivity C-reactive protein
*Brain natriuretic peptide
PROTHROMBOTIC ASSESSMENT
Plasma fibrinogen
Platelet count
*Factor V Leiden
*D-dimer
*Plasminogen activator inhibitor type 1
TO ASSESS OTHER POTENTIAL CARDIAC RISK FACTORS
*Serum homocysteine level

By contrast, selective screening of intermediate-risk patients may be reasonable because a high calcium score may reclassify such individuals as higher risk and thereby lead to more intensive risk factor modification and treatment.[9] In symptomatic patients who have an intermediate pretest probability of obstructive coronary artery disease, stress myocardial perfusion imaging and CCTA are equivalent in predicting the composite end point of death, MI, or hospitalization for ACS.[A1,A2] A negative CCTA portends a very favorable prognosis. Since CCTA identifies both obstructive and nonobstructive coronary artery disease, however, it appears to provide better overall prognostic information[A3,A4] and has replaced functional testing in some recent guidelines. CCTA is also a diagnostic alternative to invasive coronary angiography for patients who have stable chest pain and an intermediate probability of obstructive coronary disease.[A5]

Exercise Electrocardiography

An exercise ECG is the preferred test in patients who have suspected angina pectoris and are considered to have a moderate probability of coronary artery disease if the resting ECG is interpretable (i.e., ST segments are not obscured by structural heart disease or medication), provided subjects are capable of achieving an adequate workload. Interpretation of the exercise ECG should include the exercise capacity achieved (duration and metabolic

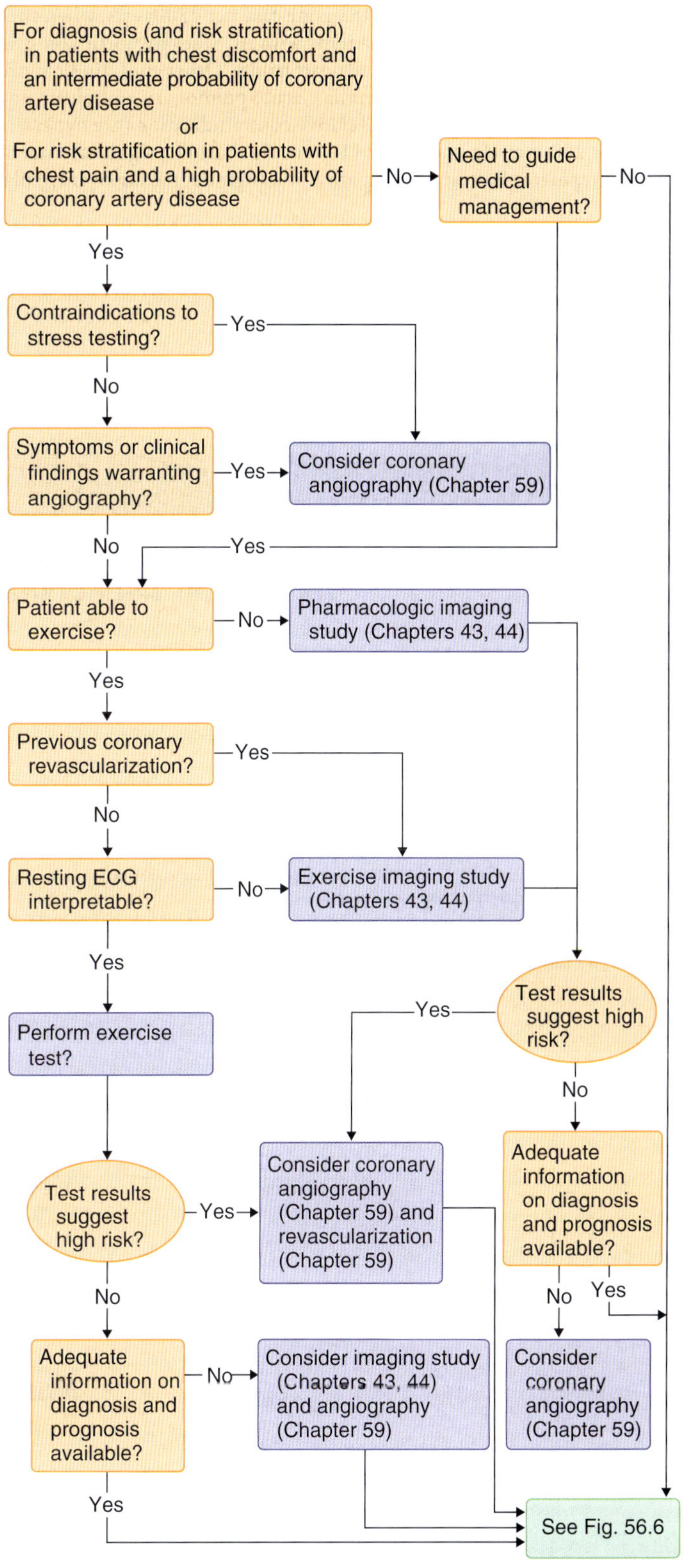

FIGURE 56-5. Approach to the use of stress testing and angiography for the evaluation of chronic stable angina. ECG = electrocardiogram. (Modified from American College of Cardiology/American Heart Association Task Force on Practice Guidelines. Management of patients with chronic stable angina. *ACC/AHA/ACP-ASIM Pocket Guidelines*. Philadelphia: Elsevier Science; 2000.)

equivalents of the external workload), the magnitude and extent of ST segment deviation, the clinical and hemodynamic responses to exercise, and the rapidity with which the heart rate returns to normal after exercise (recovery phase).

The exercise test protocol is usually adjusted to a patient's tolerance, aiming for 6 to 12 minutes of exercise time (i.e., Bruce protocol stages II to IV) to achieve maximal oxygen consumption and to elicit objective evidence of inducible ischemia, if present. Exercise stress testing is generally safe, with death or MI occurring in less than one case per 2500 tests, when such provocative testing is avoided in patients with ACS, severe aortic stenosis, severe hypertension, or uncontrolled heart failure. Other contraindications are acute MI, symptomatic arrhythmias, acute pulmonary embolism, and suspected acute aortic dissection. Relative contraindications are hypertension above 200 mm Hg systolic or 110 mm Hg diastolic, significant aortic stenosis, hypertrophic cardiomyopathy, and high-degree atrioventricular block.

Concomitant antianginal therapy (notably the use of β-blockers) reduces the sensitivity of exercise testing as a screening tool. If the purpose of the exercise test is to diagnose ischemia, it should be performed, whenever possible, before β-blockers are initiated or 2 to 3 days after their discontinuation.

TABLE 56-4 APPROXIMATE SENSITIVITIES AND SPECIFICITIES OF COMMON NONINVASIVE TESTS TO DIAGNOSE CORONARY ARTERY DISEASE

TEST	SENSITIVITY (%)	SPECIFICITY (%)
Stress ECG	58	62
Stress echocardiography	85	82
CCTA	97	78
SPECT	87	70
PET	90	85
Stress CMR	90	80

CCTA = coronary computed tomography angiography; CMR = stress cardiac magnetic resonance; ECG = electrocardiogram; PET = positron emission tomography; SPECT = single-photon emission computed tomography (exercise stress SPECT with or without dipyridamole or adenosine); stress echocardiography = exercise stress echocardiography.

Adapted from Knuuti J, Ballo H, Juarez-Orozco LE, et al. The performance of non-invasive tests to rule-in and rule-out significant coronary artery stenosis in patients with stable angina: a meta-analysis focused on post-test disease probability. *Eur Heart J*. 2018;39:3322-3330.

Nuclear Cardiology Imaging

Stress myocardial perfusion imaging (Chapter 44) with single-photon emission computed tomography (SPECT) with simultaneous electrocardiographic testing (see Fig. 44-8) is particularly helpful in the diagnosis of coronary artery disease in patients with abnormal resting ECGs and among those in whom ST segment responses cannot be interpreted accurately, such as patients with repolarization abnormalities caused by LV hypertrophy, those with left bundle branch block, and those receiving digitalis. Its sensitivity and specificity are superior to exercise electrocardiography alone in detecting coronary artery disease (especially multivessel disease), in identifying regional perfusion defects that may localize to and correlate with diseased vessels, and in delineating the magnitude and extent of ischemic and infarcted myocardium. Treadmill testing is preferred for patients who can perform such physical activity because of the additional diagnostic and prognostic information achieved with graded exercise. In the 40 to 50% of patients who are unable to exercise adequately, however, myocardial perfusion imaging with pharmacologic vasodilator stress with dipyridamole, adenosine, or regadenoson may be the preferred approach to noninvasive testing.

Stress Echocardiography (Chapter 43)

Stress two-dimensional echocardiography with exercise or pharmacologic stress can detect regional ischemia by identifying new wall motion abnormalities (see Fig. 43-7). Additional clinical information about associated structural heart disease, chamber dimensions, and valve function can be readily obtained. Exercise echocardiography can detect the presence of coronary artery disease with an accuracy similar to that achieved with stress myocardial perfusion imaging and is useful for localizing and quantifying ischemic myocardial segments. Pharmacologic stress is usually performed with dobutamine in patients who are unable to exercise and in those unable to achieve adequate heart rates with exercise.

Stress Cardiac Magnetic Resonance Imaging (Chapter 44)

Pharmacologic stress perfusion with CMR imaging is becoming increasingly available in many centers and may provide additional diagnostic capability in detecting the presence of structural heart disease, in addition to suspected coronary artery disease. CMR with gadolinium enhancement is the most accurate way to diagnose a scar from a prior MI (see Fig. 44-13). Preliminary

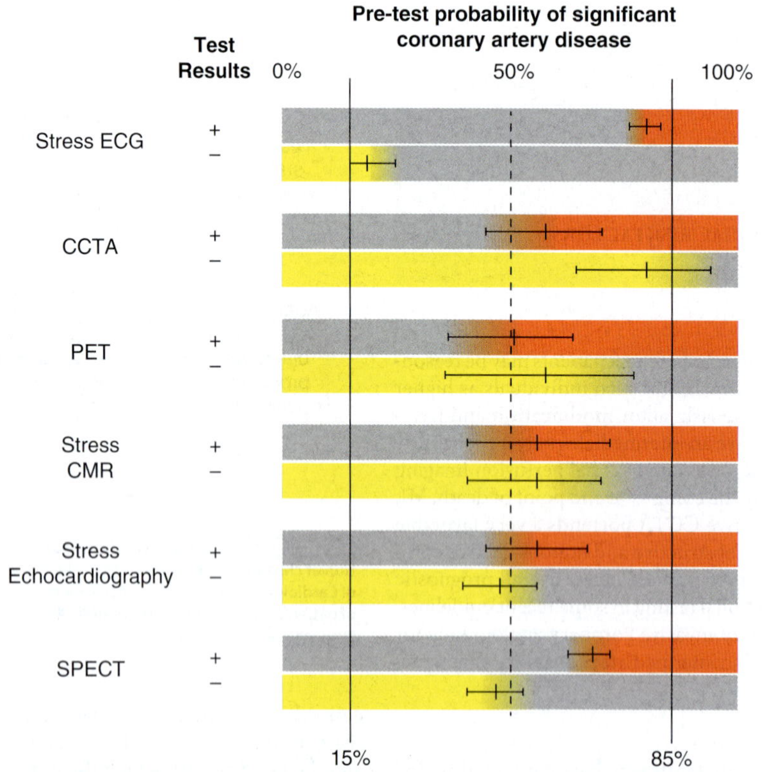

FIGURE 56-6. Ability of noninvasive tests to rule in or rule out significant coronary artery disease. Yellow = range where a negative test can rule out coronary artery disease to a threshold below 15%; red = range where a positive test can rule in coronary artery disease at a threshold above 85%. CCTA = coronary computed tomography angiography; CMR = stress cardiac magnetic resonance; ECG = electrocardiogram; PET = positron emission tomography; SPECT = single-photon emission computed tomography (exercise stress SPECT with or without dipyridamole or adenosine); stress echocardiography = exercise stress echocardiography. (From Knuuti J, Ballo H, Juarez-Orozco LE, et al. The performance of non-invasive tests to rule-in and rule-out significant coronary artery stenosis in patients with stable angina: a meta-analysis focused on post-test disease probability. *Eur Heart J*. 2018;39:3322-3330.)

TABLE 56-5 CORONARY ANGIOGRAPHY FOR DIAGNOSIS AND RISK STRATIFICATION IN PATIENTS WITH CHRONIC ANGINA AND STABLE ISCHEMIC HEART DISEASE

FOR INITIAL DIAGNOSTIC INDICATION
Recommended on the Basis of Evidence or General Consensus
Patients with suspected angina and evidence of intermediate-high risk, moderate-severe ischemia on noninvasive testing, or a changing angina pattern who have survived sudden cardiac death or serious ventricular arrhythmia
Weight of Evidence or Opinion Is in Favor
Uncertain diagnosis after noninvasive testing, and the benefit of a more certain diagnosis outweighs the risk and cost of coronary angiography
Inability to undergo noninvasive testing because of disability, illness, or morbid obesity
Occupational requirement for a definitive diagnosis
Suspected nonatherosclerotic cause of myocardial ischemia
Suspicion of a coronary spasm
High pretest probability of left main or three-vessel disease
Recurrent hospitalization for chest pain in the absence of definitive diagnosis
Overriding desire for a definitive diagnosis and a greater than low probability of CAD
Not Recommended
Significant comorbidity in patients in whom the risk of coronary arteriography outweighs the benefit of the procedure
Overriding personal desire for a definitive diagnosis and a low probability of CAD
FOR INITIAL RISK STRATIFICATION OR TREATMENT INDICATION
Recommended on the Basis of Evidence or General Consensus
With disabling (CCS class III and class IV) chronic stable angina despite medical therapy
With high-risk criteria on noninvasive testing regardless of anginal severity
Patients with angina who have survived sudden cardiac death or serious ventricular arrhythmia
Angina and symptoms and signs of congestive heart failure
Clinical characteristics that indicate a high likelihood of severe CAD
Weight of Evidence or Opinion Is in Favor
Significant left ventricular dysfunction (EF < 45%), CCS class I or class II angina, and demonstrable ischemia but less than high-risk criteria on noninvasive testing
High-risk criteria suggesting ischemia on noninvasive testing
Inadequate prognostic information after noninvasive testing
Clinical characteristics that indicate a high likelihood of severe CAD
CCS class I or class II angina, preserved left ventricular function (EF > 45%), and less than high-risk criteria on noninvasive testing
CCS class III or class IV angina that improves to class I or class II with medical therapy
CCS class I or class II angina but intolerance (unacceptable side effects) to adequate medical therapy
Not Recommended
CCS class I or class II angina in patients who respond to medical therapy and who have no evidence of ischemia on noninvasive testing
Patients who prefer to avoid revascularization after adequate explanation

CAD = coronary artery disease; CCS = Canadian Cardiovascular Society; EF = ejection fraction.
Modified from Gibbons RJ, Abrams J, Chatterjee K, et al. ACC/AHA 2002 guideline update for the management of patients with chronic stable angina—summary article: a report of the American College of Cardiology/American Heart Association Task Force on Practice Guidelines (Committee on Management of Patients with Chronic Stable Angina). *Circulation.* 2003;107:149-158.

data suggest that cardiovascular magnetic resonance imaging may be equally sensitive but more specific than fractional flow reserve (see "Diagnostic Coronary Angiography") for determining which patients will benefit from revascularization.[A6]

Diagnostic Coronary Angiography

Despite the continued evolution of noninvasive diagnostic testing, invasive coronary angiography (Chapter 59) remains the "gold standard" for anatomic definition of obstructive coronary artery disease. Among patients who have a clinical diagnosis of stable angina and chronic myocardial ischemia and who are referred for coronary angiography, a 70% or more luminal diameter narrowing is found in one (about 25%), two (about 25%), or all three (about 25%) epicardial coronary arteries in about 75% of cases; another 5 to 10% of patients have obstruction of the left main coronary artery; and the remaining 15 to 20% have no flow-limiting coronary obstructions. These data emphasize the persisting role of coronary angiography for diagnostic purposes (Table 56-5), but angiography is also helpful for risk stratification in patients with clear-cut angina and chronic ischemic heart disease. In patients with less severe coronary stenoses (i.e., 50 to 70% on angiography), coronary

TABLE 56-6 USING THE RESULTS OF NONINVASIVE RISK STRATIFICATION TO GUIDE CLINICAL DECISION MAKING

HIGH RISK (>3% ANNUAL MORTALITY RATE)
Severe resting left ventricular dysfunction (LVEF < 35%)
High-risk treadmill score (≤−11)*
Severe exercise left ventricular dysfunction (exercise LVEF <35%)
Stress-induced large perfusion defect (particularly if anterior)
Stress-induced multiple perfusion defects of moderate size
Large, fixed perfusion defect with left ventricular dilation or increased lung uptake (^{201}Tl)
Stress-induced moderate perfusion defect with left ventricular dilation or increased lung uptake (^{201}Tl)
Echocardiographic wall motion abnormality (involving more than two segments) developing at a low dose of dobutamine or at a low heart rate (<120 beats/min)
Stress echocardiographic evidence of extensive ischemia
INTERMEDIATE RISK (1-3% ANNUAL MORTALITY RATE)
Mild to moderate resting left ventricular dysfunction (LVEF = 35-49%)
Intermediate-risk treadmill score (−11 < score < 5)*
Stress-induced moderate perfusion defect without left ventricular dilation or increased lung intake (^{201}Tl)
Limited stress echocardiographic ischemia with a wall motion abnormality only at higher doses of dobutamine involving two segments or less
LOW RISK (<1% ANNUAL MORTALITY RATE)
Low-risk treadmill score (≥5)*
Normal or small myocardial perfusion defect at rest or with stress†
Normal stress echocardiographic wall motion or no change of limited resting wall motion abnormalities during stress†

*Score = (duration of exercise in minutes) − (5 × mm of ST segment depression) − (4 × angina score), where 0 = no angina, 1 = nonlimiting angina, and 2 = angina that causes discontinuation of the test.

†Although the published data are limited, patients with these findings will probably not be at low risk in the presence of either a high-risk treadmill score or severe resting left ventricular dysfunction (LVEF < 35%).

LVEF = left ventricular ejection fraction; Tl = thallium.

From Gibbons RJ, Abrams J, Chatterjee K, et al. ACC/AHA 2002 guideline update for the management of patients with chronic stable angina—summary article: a report of the American College of Cardiology/American Heart Association Task Force on practice guidelines (Committee on the Management of Patients with Chronic Stable Angina). *J Am Coll Cardiol.* 2003;41:159-168.

intravascular ultrasonography can substantially enhance the quantification of obstruction and vulnerability of the coronary atheroma to future instability. Alternatively, an invasive physiologic approach with use of a pressure wire positioned proximal and distal to a coronary stenosis can measure the severity of the stenosis and determine whether functionally significant flow reduction (i.e., a decreased fractional flow reserve [FFR] <0.8) is present. This technique may be useful when there is a borderline (50 to 60%) visual coronary stenosis at angiography, particularly if such a stenosis subtends an ischemic myocardial segment observed on noninvasive testing. An FFR below 0.8 is generally considered to represent a sufficiently important reduction in coronary flow to justify proceeding to percutaneous coronary intervention (Chapter 59) to reduce symptoms and the subsequent need for urgent revascularization.[A7] By contrast, an FFR of 0.8 or higher would indicate that myocardial revascularization of the stenotic coronary artery would be of little benefit clinically.

Risk Stratification

Clinical and noninvasive criteria can be used in a complementary fashion to refine the estimate of risk for the individual patient with chronic ischemic heart disease (Table 56-6). Clinical characteristics that include age, male sex, diabetes mellitus, previous MI, and symptoms typical of angina are predictive of the presence of coronary artery disease. Heart failure and LV dysfunction (generally defined by an ejection fraction <50%), the severity and extent of angina, and associated symptoms such as dyspnea are also important predictors of outcome in patients with chronic ischemic heart disease.

The simple classification of disease into single-, double-, or triple-vessel or left main coronary artery disease remains the most widely used approach (Table 56-8). Additional prognostic information is provided by the severity and extent of coronary luminal narrowing and its location. For example, high-grade lesions of the left main coronary artery or its equivalent, as defined by severe proximal left anterior descending and proximal left circumflex coronary artery disease, are particularly life-threatening. The SYNTAX trial has permitted the

TABLE 56-7 TREATMENT OF PATIENTS WITH STABLE ANGINA

GENERAL MEASURES

Rule out and control aggravating conditions
- Associated noncardiac diseases
- Associated cardiac disease
- Use of drugs aggravating angina

Smoking cessation
Dietary counseling for body weight and lipid control
Exercise prescription
Treat to targets
- Hypertension
- Blood lipids
- Diabetes

PHARMACOLOGIC THERAPY: RECOMMENDATIONS FOR PHARMACOTHERAPY TO PREVENT MI AND DEATH AND TO REDUCE SYMPTOMS

Recommended on the Basis of Evidence or General Consensus

Aspirin in the absence of contraindications
β-Blockers as initial therapy in the absence of contraindications in patients with prior MI or without prior MI
Angiotensin-converting enzyme inhibitor in all patients with CAD who also have diabetes or left ventricular systolic dysfunction
Low-density lipoprotein–lowering therapy in patients with documented or suspected CAD, with a target <55 mg/dL using high-potency statins, ezetimibe, and PCSK9 inhibitors
Sublingual nitroglycerin or nitroglycerin spray for the immediate relief of angina
Calcium-channel antagonists or long-acting nitrates as initial therapy for reduction of symptoms when β-blockers are contraindicated
Calcium-channel antagonists or long-acting nitrates in combination with β-blockers when initial treatment with β-blockers is not successful
Calcium-channel antagonists and long-acting nitrates as a substitute for β-blockers if initial treatment with β-blockers leads to unacceptable side effects

Weight of Evidence or Opinion Is in Favor

Rivaroxaban 2.5 mg twice daily added to low-dose (81-100 mg daily) aspirin
Clopidogrel when aspirin is contraindicated
Long-acting non-dihydropyridine calcium-channel antagonists instead of β-blockers as initial therapy
Weight reduction and increased physical activity in persons with metabolic syndrome
Consider fibric acid derivatives for high-risk patients with elevated triglycerides if LDL-cholesterol is at target on statin therapy
Angiotensin-converting enzyme inhibitor in patients with CAD or other vascular disease

Not Recommended

Dipyridamole
Chelation therapy

CAD = coronary artery disease; HDL = high-density lipoprotein; LDL = low-density lipoprotein; MI = myocardial infarction; PCSK9 = proprotein convertase subtilisin/kexin type 9.
From Fihn SD, Blankenship JC, Alexander KP, et al. 2014 ACC/AHA/AATS/PCNA/SCAI/STS focused update of the guideline for the diagnosis and management of patients with stable ischemic heart disease: a report of the American College of Cardiology/American Heart Association Task Force on Practice Guidelines, and the American Association for Thoracic Surgery, Preventive Cardiovascular Nurses Association, Society for Cardiovascular Angiography and Interventions, and Society of Thoracic Surgeons. *J Am Coll Cardiol.* 2014;64:1929-1949.

TABLE 56-8 CURRENT RECOMMENDATIONS FOR MYOCARDIAL REVASCULARIZATION IN PATIENTS WITH CHRONIC STABLE ANGINA

CABG SURGERY VERSUS MEDICAL THERAPY

Among patients with medically refractory angina pectoris, CABG surgery is indicated for symptom improvement.

Among patients with medically stable angina pectoris, CABG surgery is indicated to prolong life in left main coronary artery disease or three-vessel disease (regardless of left ventricular function) and, possibly, to help symptoms.

CABG surgery may be indicated for prolongation of life if the proximal left anterior descending coronary artery is involved (regardless of the number of diseased vessels).

CABG surgery may reduce the composite end point of death, myocardial infarction, or stroke in diabetic patients with extensive multivessel (two- to three-vessel) coronary artery disease compared with medical therapy.
CABG surgery can reduce symptoms, cardiovascular events, and death in diabetic patients with stable angina.

PCI VERSUS MEDICAL THERAPY

For the initial management of patients with stable ischemic heart disease, PCI does not reduce the risk of death, myocardial infarction, or other major cardiovascular events when it is added to optimal medical therapy.

Among patients with symptomatic angina pectoris, PCI is indicated to improve symptoms.

PCI may be indicated in the presence of severe myocardial ischemia, regardless of symptoms. PCI does not appear to improve survival compared with medical treatment among patients with one- or two-vessel disease.

In the absence of symptoms of myocardial ischemia, PCI is not indicated (merely for the presence of an anatomic stenosis).

PCI VERSUS CABG SURGERY

For single-vessel disease, PCI and CABG surgery provide excellent symptom relief, but repeated revascularization procedures are required more frequently after PCI. Intracoronary stenting is preferred to regular PCI, but direct comparison with CABG surgery is limited.

For treating diabetic patients with two- or three-vessel disease, CABG surgery is the treatment of choice.

For nondiabetic patients, multivessel PCI and CABG surgery are acceptable alternatives. The choice of PCI or CABG surgery for initial treatment depends primarily on local expertise and the patient's and physician's preferences.

In general, PCI is preferred for patients at low risk and CABG surgery for patients at high risk.

CABG = coronary artery bypass graft; PCI = percutaneous coronary intervention.

identification of subsets of coronary artery disease patients into three tertiles of low-, moderate-, and high-risk anatomic findings based on multiple lesional characteristics (see Table 56-7). Although the plaque that is causing the most severe chronic stenosis is not necessarily the one that will subsequently rupture to cause an acute coronary syndrome or acute MI, the underlying extent and severity of the coronary stenoses are nevertheless potent predictors of the likelihood of a critical plaque rupture somewhere in the epicardial coronary arterial circulation.

TREATMENT

Comprehensive management of angina and chronic ischemic heart disease (Fig. 56-7) entails multiple therapeutic approaches to the identification and treatment of associated diseases that can precipitate or worsen angina and ischemia (Table 56-8): cardiac risk factor identification and intervention; application of pharmacologic and nonpharmacologic interventions for secondary prevention; pharmacologic and symptomatic management of angina and ischemia; and myocardial revascularization with percutaneous coronary intervention (PCI) or coronary artery bypass graft (CABG) surgery, when indicated (Table 56-8).[10,11] A multidimensional management approach integrates all of these considerations, often simultaneously, in each patient. Among pharmacotherapies, three drug classes are classified as being "disease modifying" in that they have been demonstrated to reduce mortality and morbidity in patients with chronic ischemic heart disease and preserved LV function: antiplatelet agents such as aspirin; inhibitors of the renin-angiotensin-aldosterone system, especially angiotensin-converting enzyme (ACE) inhibitors; and effective lipid-lowering agents, principally statins (Chapter 40). In patients who have type 2 diabetes, the use of either a sodium-glucose cotransporter-2 inhibitor or a glucose-like peptide-1 agonist can reduce cardiac events (Chapter 210). Other therapies, such as nitrates, β-blockers, calcium antagonists, and ranolazine, can reduce symptomatic myocardial ischemia, ameliorate or prevent angina, and improve exercise performance, but they have not been shown to reduce mortality in patients with chronic ischemic heart disease.

Medical Therapy

Careful attention to lifestyle and the management of coronary risk factors is essential (Fig. 56-8). Such secondary prevention strategies can reduce the risk of progressive coronary disease, morbidity, and mortality.

Drugs That Alter Lipid Metabolism

Each 1% increase in the LDL cholesterol level results in a 2 to 3% increase in the risk for coronary events (Chapter 40). Large, randomized clinical trials in patients with ischemic heart disease have shown a consistent and significant reduction in mortality and cardiac events with statin therapy (Chapter 190). Patients with stable angina and documented ischemic heart disease should routinely be treated with statins[A8] (see Table 190-2). Current U.S. guidelines

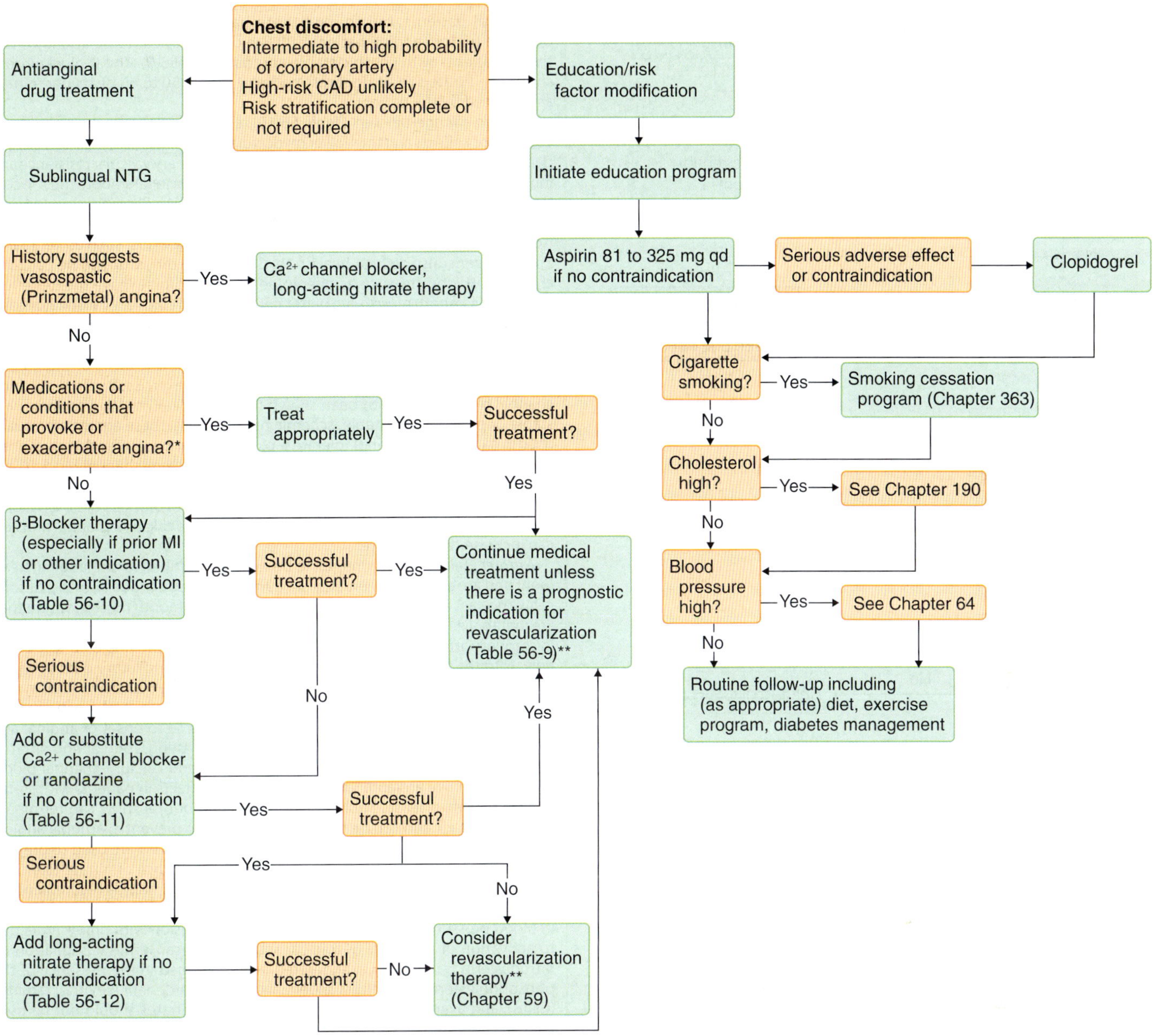

FIGURE 56-7. Algorithm for the oral treatment of stable angina. Both pathways (Antianginal Drug Treatment and Education/Risk Factor Modification) must be completed. *Conditions that exacerbate or provoke angina: medications: vasodilators, excessive thyroid replacement, vasoconstrictors; other medical problems: profound anemia, uncontrolled hypertension, hyperthyroidism, hypoxemia; other cardiac problems: tachyarrhythmias, bradyarrhythmias, valvular heart disease (especially AS), hypertrophic cardiomyopathy. **At any point in this process, based on coronary anatomy, severity of anginal symptoms, and patient preferences, it is reasonable to consider evaluation for coronary revascularization. Unless a patient is documented to have left main, three-vessel, or two-vessel CAD with significant stenosis of the proximal left anterior descending coronary artery, there is no demonstrated survival advantage associated with revascularization in low-risk patients with chronic stable angina; thus, medical therapy should be attempted in most patients before considering PTCA or CABG. AS = aortic stenosis; CABG = coronary artery bypass graft; CAD = coronary artery disease; MI = myocardial infarction; NTG = nitroglycerin; PTCA = percutaneous transluminal coronary angioplasty; qd = once daily. (Modified from American College of Cardiology/American Heart Association Task Force on Practice Guidelines. Management of Patients with Chronic Stable Angina. *ACC/AHA/ACP-ASIM Pocket Guidelines*. Philadelphia: Elsevier Science; 2000.)

recommend high-potency statin therapy (e.g., atorvastatin up to 80 mg per day or rosuvastatin up to 40 mg per day) with periodic monitoring of LDL levels to a target of less than 70 mg/dL, whereas European guidelines recommend a more stringent LDL target of less than 55 mg/dL. With the documentation of additional benefit from ezetimibe and PCSK9 antagonists, most U.S. cardiologists have also adopted these more intensive targeted levels.[12]

Ezetimibe added to statins lowers LDL and reduces subsequent cardiovascular events in patients who have survived an acute coronary syndrome,[A9] even when statins have reduced LDL levels to 50 to 100 mg/dL. PCSK9 inhibitors, which can reduce LDL levels by 60% and LDL levels to less than 30 mg/dL in most patients, are an effective option for patients with elevated LDL levels despite statins, with or without ezetimibe, and further reduce dyslipidemic residual risk, especially in high-risk patients (Chapter 190).[A10]

A pure eicosapentaenoic acid derivative (an icosapent ethyl ester) can significantly reduce cardiovascular death, MI, and stroke as well as all-cause mortality when added to statins in patients who have ischemic heart disease, well-controlled LDL levels (40 to 100 mg/dL), and elevated baseline triglyceride levels (135 to 500 mg/dL).[A11] However, bile acid sequestrants, fibrates, and various fish oil preparations (Chapters 190) targeted to reduce the triglyceride level or raise the HDL cholesterol level have failed to reduce clinical events when added to statins.[A12] Drug therapies directed specifically at raising low levels of HDL with either niacin or cholesteryl ester transfer protein inhibitors have been uniformly disappointing and are not recommended.

Angiotensin-Converting Enzyme Inhibitors

ACE inhibitors and angiotensin receptor blockers (see Table 64-7) reduce cardiac events, cardiovascular mortality, and all-cause mortality in patients with risk factors for or with previously diagnosed coronary artery disease, including high-risk patients with vascular disease or diabetes and patients with chronic ischemic heart disease and no clinical evidence of heart failure. However, the incremental benefit of such agents in otherwise well-treated patients without high-risk features remains less clear.[A13]

Antiplatelet Agents and Anticoagulants

Aspirin reduces the risk of adverse cardiovascular events in patients with angina and chronic ischemic heart disease, and in the absence of contraindications,

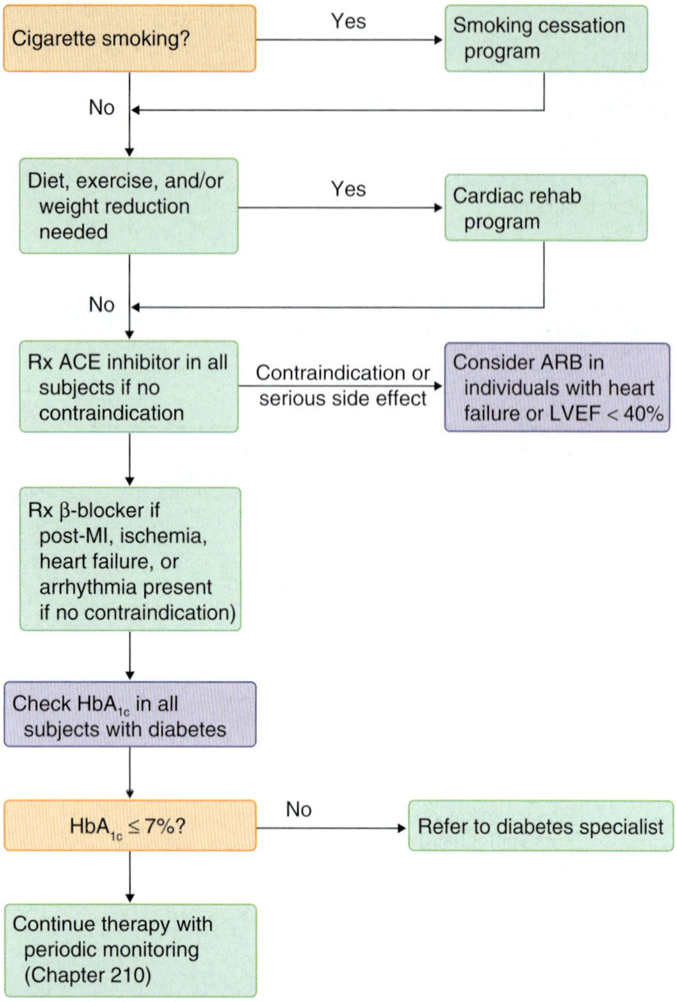

FIGURE 56-8. Approach to lifestyle interventions and pharmacotherapy. ACE = angiotensin-converting enzyme; ARB = angiotensin receptor blocker; HbA_{1c} = hemoglobin A_{1c}; LVEF = left ventricular ejection fraction; MI = myocardial infarction; Rx = prescribe.

should be administered routinely. In such patients, low-dose aspirin (81 mg daily) is as effective as 325 mg daily, with a similar bleeding risk but overall better adherence.[A14]

Although dual antiplatelet therapy with clopidogrel, prasugrel, or ticagrelor (Chapter 70) is of proven benefit when combined with aspirin to reduce the composite end point of death, MI, or stroke in ACS patients and in patients who undergo PCI,[13] especially with drug-eluting stents (Chapters 57, 58, and 59), these agents have not been shown to be superior to low-dose (75 to 162 mg/day) aspirin alone in patients who have stable angina and chronic ischemic heart disease, because any reduction in cardiovascular events is at least offset by an increase in major bleeding events.[A15] For patients who cannot tolerate aspirin or have aspirin insensitivity, clopidogrel (75 mg once daily), prasugrel (10 mg once daily), and ticagrelor (60 mg twice daily) are indicated. A direct-acting anticoagulant (see Table 70-6) is required in patients who have atrial fibrillation (Chapter 52).

Low-dose rivaroxaban (2.5 mg twice daily) combined with low-dose aspirin (81 to 100 mg daily) is superior to aspirin alone for reducing the composite primary endpoint of cardiovascular death, MI, or stroke,[A16] including a 23% reduction in death in patients with stable coronary artery disease,[A17] although it causes more bleeding. Warfarin is generally as effective as aspirin for preventing coronary events in patients with angina and is preferred to aspirin for patients with concomitant atrial fibrillation (Chapter 52), but has it been superseded by direct-acting anticoagulants, except in patients with prosthetic heart valves.

Therapeutic Agents to Reduce Angina and Ischemia

The goal of antianginal therapy is to reduce symptoms of cardiac ischemia and to improve quality of life.[14] β-Blockers, which prevent the binding of catecholamines to the β-adrenergic receptor, lower heart rate and myocardial contractility, thereby reducing myocardial workload, myocardial oxygen demand, and ischemia and anginal symptoms. β-Blockers raise the ischemic threshold and delay or prevent the onset of angina with exercise. β-Blockers also reduce the rate of secondary cardiac events and sudden cardiac death in post-MI patients, but to date there have been no placebo-controlled outcome trials in angina patients. All β-blockers appear to be equally effective in patients with chronic stable angina (Table 56-9). The β-blocker dose should be titrated to a target resting heart rate of 50 to 60 beats per minute as tolerated by the patient.

Calcium-channel blockers (Table 56-10) reduce afterload by their peripheral vasodilatory effects and thus lower myocardial workload and myocardial oxygen demand. Calcium-channel blockers also reduce coronary vascular resistance and inhibit coronary vasospasm by preventing coronary arterial smooth muscle contraction. This favorable reduction in myocardial oxygen demand, coupled with an increase in myocardial oxygen supply, results in a reduction in angina and ischemia. Non-dihydropyridine calcium-channel blockers, such as verapamil and diltiazem, also reduce heart rate. Conversely, dihydropyridine calcium-channel antagonists, such as nifedipine and amlodipine, have greater effect on vascular smooth muscle, are better peripheral and coronary vasodilators, and hence may have advantages for use in the hypertensive patient with angina. In randomized clinical trials, calcium-channel blockers and β-blockers are generally equally effective in relieving angina, improving time to onset of angina, and improving time to ischemic ST depression during exercise. Because calcium-channel blockers have not been shown to reduce death or MI in patients with stable or previously unstable ischemic heart disease, these agents are usually used in patients who cannot tolerate β-blockers or who require additional pharmacotherapy to control their symptoms. When calcium-channel blockers are used with β-blockers, care must be taken not to cause symptomatic bradycardia with verapamil and diltiazem. When calcium-channel blockers are used alone, diltiazem is often preferred because dihydropyridine calcium-channel blockers can increase the heart rate.

Nitrates (Table 56-11) continue to be widely prescribed for antianginal treatment and are effective when they are administered sublingually, orally, or topically. They act as vasodilators by entering vascular smooth muscle, where they are metabolized to nitric oxide, which relaxes vascular smooth muscle, including in coronary arteries. These effects reduce angina by improving coronary blood flow. Nitrates also lower preload because of their venodilatory effects, with a resulting reduction in LV end-diastolic pressure and wall tension, which in turn lowers subendocardial oxygen demand. When nitrates are used in patients with stable angina, they improve exercise tolerance, time to onset of angina, and ST segment depression during treadmill exercise testing. Long-acting nitrates, which are frequently combined with β-blockers and calcium-channel blockers, have additive antianginal and anti-ischemic effects in patients with stable ischemic heart disease. Sublingual nitroglycerin or oral spray can terminate an angina attack and can be used as prophylaxis to prevent exertional angina. Long-acting nitrates administered orally or transdermally are used to prevent angina and to improve exercise tolerance. For avoidance of nitrate tolerance or tachyphylaxis, an 8- to 12-hour nitrate-free interval daily is recommended. Nitroglycerin and nitrates can cause vasodilation-induced headache, a decrease in blood pressure, and, more rarely, severe hypotension with bradycardia due to activation of the vagal Bezold-Jarisch reflex. Because the vasodilation by nitroglycerin is markedly exaggerated and prolonged in the presence of the phosphodiesterase inhibitors sildenafil (Viagra), vardenafil (Levitra), tadalafil (Cialis), and avanafil (Stendra), these agents and nitrates should not be used concurrently.

Ranolazine (initiated at a dose of 500 mg twice daily and titrated up to a maximal dose of 1000 mg twice daily) acts by reducing intracellular calcium overload in ischemic myocytes by inhibiting late inward sodium current entry. The net effect of reduced late inward sodium current is a reduction in LV wall tension and myocardial oxygen demand, thereby reducing angina and ischemia. Ranolazine increases exercise tolerance in patients with stable angina, reduces episodes of recurrent ischemia, and provides additional antianginal benefit in patients who are already receiving intensive antianginal therapy with β-blockers and calcium-channel blockers, but it has not been documented to reduce the composite primary end point of cardiac death, MI, or recurrent ischemia in a trial of patients after an acute coronary syndrome.[A18]

Treating Inflammation

Low-dose colchicine (0.5 mg daily) can reduce the composite primary outcome of cardiac death, MI, stroke, and ischemia-driven revascularization by about 30% compared with placebo, but the reduction in cardiac deaths has been at least counterbalanced by an increase in noncardiovascular death.[A19,A20] Injections of a monoclonal antibody (canakinumab) targeting interleukin-1beta (IL-1β), administered in combination with standard of care (including lipid-lowering therapy) in patients with a prior MI and an hsCRP greater than or equal to 2 mg/L, reduces the primary composite end point of nonfatal MI, stroke, and cardiovascular death by 15% during a median 3.7 years of follow-up.[A21] Whether the treatment of inflammatory pathways will become a part of standard secondary prevention care remains uncertain.

Myocardial Revascularization

Coronary revascularization with CABG surgery (but not PCI) (Chapter 59) prolongs life, reduces major cardiovascular events, and improves health status, quality of life, and functional capacity in selected patients with chronic, stable ischemic heart disease who meet certain anatomic criteria: the presence of

TABLE 56-9 CLINICAL USE OF B-BLOCKERS

COMPOUND BY RECEPTOR ACTIVITY	INTRINSIC SYMPATHOMIMETIC ACTIVITY*	MEMBRANE STABILITY EFFECT	HALF-LIFE (hr)	EXCRETION	ORAL DOSE
β_1 AND β_2					
Propranolol	–	++	1-6	Hepatic	20-80 mg bid-tid
Propranolol long-acting	–	++	8-11	Hepatic	80-360 mg/day
Nadolol	–	–	40-80	Renal	40-80 mg/day
Pindolol	+	+	3-4	Renal	2.5-7.5 mg tid
Sotalol	–	–	7-18	Renal	40-160 mg bid
Timolol	–	–	4-5	Hepatic-renal	10-15 mg bid
β_1 SELECTIVE					
Acebutolol	+	+	3-4	Hepatic	200-600 mg bid
Atenolol	–	–	6-9	Renal	50-200 mg/day†
Bisoprolol	–	–	9-12	50% renal	5-20 mg/day
Metoprolol	–	–	3-7	Hepatic	50-200 mg bid
Metoprolol long-acting	–	–	14-25	Hepatic	25-400 mg
Esmolol	–	–	4.5 min	Esterases in red cells	Bolus 500 μg/kg 50-300 μg/kg/min IV
β_1, β_2, α_2					
Labetalol	+	–	6	Hepatic	200-600 mg bid
Carvedilol	–	+	6-10	Hepatic	25-50 mg bid

*Presence commonly associated with maintenance of or increase in heart rate; absence associated with decrease in heart rate.
†Atenolol may be used in older individuals at a lower dose of 25 mg once daily.
bid = twice daily; IV = intravenous; tid = three times daily.
From Théroux P. Angina pectoris. In: Goldman L, Ausiello DA, eds. *Cecil Textbook of Medicine*. 23rd ed. Philadelphia: Saunders Elsevier; 2008.

TABLE 56-10 PROPERTIES OF ORAL CALCIUM-CHANNEL BLOCKING DRUGS IN CLINICAL USE

DRUGS	USUAL DOSE	ELIMINATION HALF-LIFE (HR)	*HEMODYNAMIC EFFECT* HR	PVR	SIDE EFFECTS
DIHYDROPYRIDINES					
Nifedipine PA*	10-40 mg bid	10	↑↑	↓↓↓	Hypotension, dizziness, flushing, edema, constipation
Nifedipine XL*	30-120 mg/day	24	↑	↓↓	
Amlodipine	2.5-10 mg/day	30-50	=	↓↓↓	Headache, edema
Felodipine	2.5-10 mg/day	11-16	↑	↓↓↓	Headache, dizziness
Isradipine	2.5-10 mg bid	8	=	↓↓↓	Headache, fatigue
Nicardipine	20-40 mg tid	2-4	↑	↓↓↓	
Nicardipine SR*	30-60 mg bid	8-10	↑	↓↓	Headache, dizziness, flushing, edema
Nisoldipine	10-40 mg/day	7-12	=	↓↓↓	Same as for nifedipine
Nitrendipine	20 mg/day or bid	5-12	↑	↓↓↓	Same as for nifedipine
OTHERS					
Bepridil	200-400 mg/day	24-40	↓	↓	Arrhythmias, dizziness, nausea
Diltiazem	30-90 mg tid	4-6	↓	↓	Hypotension, dizziness, bradycardia, edema
Diltiazem CD*	120-540 mg/day	—	↓	↓	
Verapamil	80-160 mg tid	3-8	↓	↓↓	
Verapamil SR*	120-480 mg/day	—	↓	↓↓	Hypotension, heart failure, edema, bradycardia

*PA, XL, SR, CD: long acting.
bid = twice daily; HR = heart rate; PVR = peripheral vascular resistance; tid = three times daily.
From Théroux P. Angina pectoris. In: Goldman L, Ausiello DA, eds. *Cecil Textbook of Medicine*. 23rd ed. Philadelphia: Saunders Elsevier; 2008.

TABLE 56-11 CLINICAL USE OF NITROGLYCERIN AND NITRATES

	DOSE	DURATION OF ACTION	INDICATION
NITROGLYCERIN			
Sublingual or buccal spray	0.15-1.5 mg	Relief of angina	Before or at onset of pain
Ointment	7.5-40 mg	8-12 hr	Prophylaxis of angina
Transdermal	0.1-0.8 mg/hr	8-16 hr	Prophylaxis of angina
Intravenous	5-400 μg/hr	Ongoing; increasing doses as needed	Recurrent chest pain, systemic hypertension, left-sided heart failure
ISOSORBIDE DINITRATE			
Oral	5-40 mg tid	6-8 hr	Prophylaxis of angina
ISOSORBIDE-5-MONONITRATE			
Oral	20 mg bid	8-12 hr	Prophylaxis of angina
Oral, slow release	30-240 mg/day	12-20 hr	Prophylaxis of angina

bid = twice daily; tid = three times daily.
From Théroux P. Angina pectoris. In: Goldman L, Ausiello DA, eds. *Cecil Textbook of Medicine*. 23rd ed. Philadelphia: Saunders Elsevier; 2008.

significant left main coronary artery disease, three-vessel coronary artery disease, or multivessel coronary artery disease in patients who have an LV ejection fraction below 50% or have diabetes.[15]

Comparisons of PCI with Optimal Medical Therapy

Numerous randomized clinical trials have compared PCI with medical therapy in stable angina patients. PCI improves angina symptoms but does not reduce the risk of death, MI, or other major cardiovascular events when it is added to optimal medical therapy as an initial management strategy in patients with chronic ischemic heart disease,[A22-A26] including patients with a chronic total occlusion of a major coronary artery.[A27] As a result, optimal medical therapy to control symptoms is a justifiable and more cost-effective initial management strategy for patients with chronic ischemic heart disease, even if they have diabetes,[16] with revascularization reserved only for patients in whom medical therapy is ineffective in controlling anginal symptoms.[17]

For patients who have stable angina and coronary lesions with reduced fractional flow reserve below 0.8 in one or more visually stenotic arteries (≥50% stenosis), initial PCI significantly reduces the need for hospitalization for urgent revascularization but has not been shown to reduce the composite end point of MI or death.[A28] Thus, intensive secondary prevention with proven pharmacotherapies combined with lifestyle modification is of paramount importance in reducing major cardiovascular events in such patients and must be considered the foundation of treatment.

Comparisons of CABG with Medical Therapy

Randomized trials comparing CABG with medical therapy indicate that a greater severity of ischemia, a greater extent of anatomic coronary disease, and the presence of LV systolic dysfunction favor a greater magnitude of survival benefit of CABG over medical therapy. CABG prolongs survival in patients with significant left main coronary artery disease irrespective of symptoms, in patients with multivessel coronary artery disease and impaired LV function (ejection fraction < 50%), and in patients with two- or three-vessel coronary artery disease that includes the proximal left anterior descending coronary artery. Patients with extensive multivessel coronary artery disease appear to derive a survival benefit from CABG surgery, particularly if they also have diabetes, whereas PCI may be considered appropriate for symptom relief, particularly in patients with one- or two-vessel coronary artery disease. It is also worth emphasizing, however, that the randomized trials of CABG surgery compared with medical therapy were conducted more than 40 years ago, and subsequent improvements in both medical therapy and CABG surgery make it increasingly difficult to extrapolate these earlier findings to contemporary clinical practice.

Comparisons of PCI with CABG Surgery for Multivessel Coronary Artery Disease

In patients with isolated left main disease, PCI appears to be approximately equivalent to CABG for the combined end point of death, stroke, or myocardial infarction, but there may be a survival advantage with CABG.[A29] In patients with severe three-vessel disease or left main disease with additional stenoses, however, CABG is superior to PCI, especially in patients with diabetes.[A30] In terms of death and MI, as well as the composite of death, MI, and stroke, CABG surgery is superior to both PCI and optimal medical therapy in reducing the composite outcome of death or MI in stable ischemic heart disease patients who have diabetes and two- and three-vessel coronary disease during a 5-year follow-up,[A31] but not at 10 years.[A32]

These data emphasize that, among patients who remain symptomatic despite intensive treatment or who have substantial ischemia or extensive coronary artery disease, revascularization with either PCI or CABG is appropriate. If, however, the goal of revascularization is to improve survival or reduce clinical events, CABG surgery is generally superior to PCI in symptomatic patients who have stable ischemic heart disease and who have more anatomically complex disease, including three-vessel or left main coronary artery disease and in diabetic patients with multivessel coronary disease for at least 5 years (see Table 56-8; Chapter 58).[18,19] Although PCI appears to provide equivalent survival outcomes in lower-risk patients (principally in patients with one- or two-vessel coronary disease), repeated procedures are more often needed during follow-up.

Refractory Angina

Occasional patients may have refractory angina despite medications and revascularization.[20] One alternative is enhanced external counterpulsation (EECP), which is generally administered as 35 sequential treatments (1 hour daily; 5 days/week) during 7 weeks. EECP does not reduce ischemia on myocardial perfusion imaging, and the mechanisms underlying its effects are poorly understood. Possible mechanisms include durable hemodynamic changes that reduce myocardial oxygen demand, improvement in myocardial perfusion by diastolic augmentation of retrograde coronary flow, and improved endothelial function. Although EECP increased the time to ST segment depression during exercise testing, reduced angina, and improved health-related quality of life for at least 1 year in one randomized, double-blind study of patients with chronic stable angina, its role in the treatment of angina remains unclear. In patients who have refractory angina despite medical therapy and are not candidates for revascularization, reduction of coronary venous return via the coronary sinus can potentially redistribute flow to areas of ischemic myocardium and is an experimental approach to reducing symptoms and improving quality of life.

OTHER ANGINAL SYNDROMES

VARIANT ANGINA OR PRINZMETAL ANGINA

The diagnosis of variant or Prinzmetal angina is based on the documentation of transient ST segment elevation during an episode of chest pain in the absence of a severe, fixed coronary stenosis.[21] Prinzmetal variant angina typically is caused by an occlusive spasm superimposed on a coronary artery stenosis that otherwise does not limit blood flow significantly. In some patients, however, no underlying stenoses are seen. Associated Raynaud phenomenon and migraine headache have been described in some patients, suggesting that the syndrome may be part of a more generalized vasospastic disorder.

The chest discomfort occurs predominantly at rest, although approximately one third of patients may also experience pain during exercise. There is a predilection for the pain to wake the patient in the early morning hours when sympathetic activity is increasing. The syndrome is often cyclical; periods of exacerbation with repetitive episodes of chest pain may persist only for seconds or be more prolonged and severe, alternating with periods with few or no symptoms. The symptoms are typically relieved by nitroglycerin. The ST segment elevation accompanying the pain signifies transmural ischemia due to total abrupt occlusion of a nonsignificant epicardial coronary stenosis in the absence of adequate collateral circulation. The subsequent rapid reperfusion may explain the high prevalence of severe life-threatening arrhythmias.

Coronary angiography, with a provocative test for spasm, such as injection of acetylcholine into the affected coronary artery, usually precipitates the syndrome. Such testing is useful to establish the diagnosis and to assess the response to therapy, especially in patients with normal or nearly normal coronary angiograms, in whom the diagnosis is otherwise unclear. Dihydropyridine calcium-channel blockers (e.g., amlodipine, 5 to 10 mg orally per day) are preferred in patients with Prinzmetal angina.

MICROVASCULAR ANGINA WITH NORMAL CORONARY ANGIOGRAPHY

Angina can occur despite normal coronary arteries, even after an acetylcholine challenge.[22] The majority of patients who have angina or ischemia with nonobstructive coronary arteries on angiography have occult coronary abnormalities that can be detected by cardiac MR imaging[23] (Chapter 44) or by a detailed coronary catheterization. Such detailed testing may reveal increased coronary resistance and an inability to increase coronary resistance and to increase coronary flow in response to stimuli such as exercise, adenosine, dipyridamole, and atrial pacing.

Symptoms occur most frequently at rest and often in relation to emotional stress. Periods of exacerbation commonly alternate with symptom-free periods. The syndrome is more frequent in women, and some patients have an altered perception of pain or hypersensitivity to certain stimuli.

The diagnosis requires objective documentation of ischemia based on ST-T segment changes, a metabolic abnormality, a transient regional perfusion defect or new wall motion abnormality on echocardiography, or endothelial dysfunction that limits blood flow reserve. Abnormal endothelium-dependent vasoreactivity can be associated with regional myocardial perfusion defects on SPECT and PET imaging.

β-Blockers or heart rate–lowering calcium-channel blockers may be useful, particularly when a relative tachycardia, hypertension, or decreased heart rate variability on Holter monitoring is present. Nitroglycerin can relieve symptoms in approximately 50% of patients, and long-acting nitrates are also sometimes helpful.

The prognosis is generally favorable and not different from that of a general age-matched population in the absence of coronary artery disease.[24,25] However, some studies have indicated that an ischemic response to exercise is associated with increased mortality.

SILENT MYOCARDIAL ISCHEMIA

Up to 20% of patients with ischemic heart disease may not present with angina and are often described as having silent myocardial ischemia. Some patients are totally asymptomatic despite obstructive coronary artery disease, which may be severe. Others have silent ischemia after a prior documented MI. The third and most common form occurs in patients who may also exhibit the usual forms of chronic stable angina, unstable angina, and Prinzmetal angina. When monitored, these patients, who typically have silent ischemia episodes in addition to symptomatic ischemia, are sometimes referred to as having *mixed angina*. This mixed angina is estimated to be present in approximately one third of all treated patients with angina, although an even higher prevalence has been reported in diabetic patients. In these patients, about 85% of ambulant ischemic episodes occur without chest pain, and 66% of angina episodes are not accompanied by ST segment depression, suggesting that overt angina pectoris is merely the "tip of the ischemic iceberg." Pharmacologic agents that reduce or abolish episodes of symptomatic ischemia also reduce or abolish episodes of silent ischemia.

PROGNOSIS

Modern treatments have improved the prognosis of patients with chronic ischemic heart disease to an annual mortality rate of 1 to 3% and a 1 to 2% rate of major ischemic events. The 1-year rate of cardiovascular death is now 1.9% (95% confidence interval [CI], 1.7 to 2.1), with a 2.9% (95% CI, 2.6 to 3.2) rate of all-cause mortality and a 4.5% (95% CI, 4.2 to 4.8) rate of the combined outcome of cardiovascular death, MI, or stroke. Even in patients who have refractory angina and are not candidates for revascularization, modern medical treatment is associated with a 1-year mortality of only 4% and a 9-year mortality of 30%.

In a large majority of patients, anginal symptoms greatly improve or even resolve, often without any change in medical therapy.[26] Recurrent angina is a common subsequent complaint in many patients with chronic ischemic heart disease, even those who were initially treated successfully with PCI. About 30% of patients continue to experience angina one or more times per week, with associated greater physical limitation and worse quality of life, and almost 80% of patients who underwent initially successful PCI for chronic angina still take one or more antianginal agents at 1 year. Exercise rehabilitation may slightly increase exercise capacity but otherwise does not have any clear prognostic implications.[A33]

Patients with chronic stable angina require follow-up on a regular basis (in general, at least every 6 to 12 months). At each visit, a detailed history and physical examination should be performed to discern any important developments such as:

- A change in physical activity
- Any change in the frequency, severity, or pattern of angina
- Tolerance of and adherence to the prescribed medical regimen
- Modification of cardiac risk factors
- The development of new or worsened comorbid illnesses

In addition to a lipid profile and blood glucose level, an ECG should be obtained if medications have changed, and echocardiography as well as electrocardiography is indicated if there are new findings on the history or physical examination. However, routine noninvasive surveillance is not needed in stable patients.

Selection of optimal treatment requires a full understanding of the potential risks and benefits of each treatment approach. In patients who have stable symptoms and who have not had an adequate trial of medical therapy, there is no need to proceed to an invasive evaluation before multifaceted medical therapy and lifestyle intervention are implemented for at least 3 to 6 months.[27] Such an initial approach of aggressive medical therapy and lifestyle intervention is strongly recommended and supported by professional guidelines. Finally, it is important to emphasize that the results of randomized trials involving both pharmacotherapy and revascularization must be individualized for specific patients, while a multidisciplinary approach to clinical decision making can ensure that all therapeutic options are fully and transparently discussed so that patients are offered the most appropriate evidence-based treatment recommendations that are tailored to the level of ischemic risk and coronary anatomic findings.

GENERAL REFERENCES

For the General References and other additional features, please visit Elsevier eBooks+ at https://ebooks.health.elsevier.com.

Grade A References

A1. Douglas PS, Hoffmann U, Patel MR, et al. Outcomes of anatomical versus functional testing for coronary artery disease. *N Engl J Med.* 2015;372:1291-1300.

A2. Mark DB, Anstrom KJ, Sheng S, et al. Quality-of-life outcomes with anatomic versus functional diagnostic testing strategies in symptomatic patients with suspected coronary artery disease: results from the PROMISE randomized trial. *Circulation.* 2016;133:1995-2007.

A3. Budoff MJ, Mayrhofer T, Ferencik M, et al. Prognostic value of coronary artery calcium in the PROMISE study (prospective multicenter imaging study for evaluation of chest pain). *Circulation.* 2017;136:1993-2005.

A4. Singh T, Bing R, Dweck MR, et al. Exercise electrocardiography and computed tomography coronary angiography for patients with suspected stable angina pectoris: a post hoc analysis of the randomized SCOT-HEART trial. *JAMA Cardiol.* 2020;5:920-928.

A5. Maurovich-Horvat P, Bosserdt M, Kofoed KF, et al. CT or invasive coronary angiography in stable chest pain. *N Engl J Med.* 2022;386:1591-1602.

A6. Nagel E, Greenwood JP, McCann GP, et al. Magnetic resonance perfusion or fractional flow reserve in coronary disease. *N Engl J Med.* 2019;380:2418-2428.

A7. Zimmermann FM, Omerovic E, Fournier S, et al. Fractional flow reserve-guided percutaneous coronary intervention vs. medical therapy for patients with stable coronary lesions: meta-analysis of individual patient data. *Eur Heart J.* 2019;40:180-186.

A8. Koskinas KC, Siontis GCM, Piccolo R, et al. Effect of statins and non-statin LDL-lowering medications on cardiovascular outcomes in secondary prevention: a meta-analysis of randomized trials. *Eur Heart J.* 2018;39:1172-1180.

A9. Zhan S, Tang M, Liu F, et al. Ezetimibe for the prevention of cardiovascular disease and all-cause mortality events. *Cochrane Database Syst Rev.* 2018;11:CD012502.

A10. Schmidt AF, Carter JL, Pearce LS, et al. PCSK9 monoclonal antibodies for the primary and secondary prevention of cardiovascular disease. *Cochrane Database Syst Rev.* 2020;10:CD011748.

A11. Bhatt DL, Steg PG, Miller M, et al. Cardiovascular risk reduction with icosapent ethyl for hypertriglyceridemia. *N Engl J Med.* 2019;380:11-22.

A12. Khan SU, Lone AN, Khan MS, et al. Effect of omega-3 fatty acids on cardiovascular outcomes: a systematic review and meta-analysis. *EClinicalMedicine.* 2021;38:100997.

A13. Bangalore S, Fakheri R, Wandel S, et al. Renin angiotensin system inhibitors for patients with stable coronary artery disease without heart failure: systematic review and meta-analysis of randomized trials. *BMJ.* 2017;356:1-10.

A14. Jones WS, Mulder H, Wruck LM, et al. Comparative effectiveness of aspirin dosing in cardiovascular disease. *N Engl J Med.* 2021;384:1981-1990.

A15. Steg PG, Bhatt DL, Simon T, et al. Ticagrelor in patients with stable coronary disease and diabetes. *N Engl J Med.* 2019;381:1309-1320.

A16. Connolly SJ, Eikelboom JW, Bosch J, et al. Rivaroxaban with or without aspirin in patients with stable coronary artery disease: an international, randomised, double-blind, placebo-controlled trial. *Lancet.* 2018;391:205-218.

A17. Eikelboom JW, Connolly SJ, Bosch J, et al. Rivaroxaban with or without aspirin in stable cardiovascular disease. *N Engl J Med.* 2017;377:1319-1330.

A18. Salazar CA, Basilio Flores JE, Veramendi Espinoza LE, et al. Ranolazine for stable angina pectoris. *Cochrane Database Syst Rev*. 2017;2:CD011747.
A19. Nidorf SM, Fiolet ATL, Mosterd A, et al. Colchicine in patients with chronic coronary disease. *N Engl J Med*. 2020;383:1838-1847.
A20. Fiolet ATL, Opstal TSJ, Mosterd A, et al. Efficacy and safety of low-dose colchicine in patients with coronary disease: a systematic review and meta-analysis of randomized trials. *Eur Heart J*. 2021;42:2765-2775.
A21. Ridker PM, Everett BM, Thuren T, et al. Antiinflammatory therapy with canakinumab for atherosclerotic disease. *N Engl J Med*. 2017;377:1119-1131.
A22. Maron DJ, Hochman JS, Reynolds HR, et al. Initial invasive or conservative strategy for stable coronary disease. *N Engl J Med*. 2020;382:1395-1407.
A23. Mark DB, Spertus JA, Bigelow R, et al. Comprehensive quality-of-life outcomes with invasive versus conservative management of chronic coronary disease in ISCHEMIA. *Circulation*. 2022;145:1294-1307.
A24. Spertus JA, Jones PG, Maron DJ, et al. Health-status outcomes with invasive or conservative care in coronary disease. *N Engl J Med*. 2020;382:1408-1419.
A25. Bangalore S, Maron DJ, Stone GW, et al. Routine revascularization versus initial medical therapy for stable ischemic heart disease: a systematic review and meta-analysis of randomized trials. *Circulation*. 2020;142:841-857.
A26. Hochman JS, Anthopolos R, Reynolds HR, et al. Survival after invasive or conservative management of stable coronary disease. *Circulation*. 2023;147:8-19.
A27. Werner GS, Martin-Yuste V, Hildick-Smith D, et al. A randomized multicentre trial to compare revascularization with optimal medical therapy for the treatment of chronic total coronary occlusions. *Eur Heart J*. 2018;39:2484-2493.
A28. Fearon WF, Zimmermann FM, De Bruyne B, et al. Fractional flow reserve-guided PCI as compared with coronary bypass surgery. *N Engl J Med*. 2022;386:128-137.
A29. Stone GW, Kappetein AP, Sabik JF, et al. Five-year outcomes after PCI or CABG for left main coronary disease. *N Engl J Med*. 2019;381:1820-1830.
A30. Gaudino M, Hameed I, Farkouh ME, et al. Overall and cause-specific mortality in randomized clinical trials comparing percutaneous interventions with coronary bypass surgery: a meta-analysis. *JAMA Intern Med*. 2020;180:1638-1646.
A31. Mancini GBJ, Boden WE, Brooks MM, et al. Impact of treatment strategies on outcomes in patients with stable coronary artery disease and type 2 diabetes mellitus according to presenting angina severity: a pooled analysis of three federally-funded randomized trials. *Atherosclerosis*. 2018;277:186-194.
A32. Wang R, Serruys PW, Gao C, et al. Ten-year all-cause death after percutaneous or surgical revascularization in diabetic patients with complex coronary artery disease. *Eur Heart J*. 2021;43:56-67.
A33. Long L, Anderson L, Dewhirst AM, et al. Exercise-based cardiac rehabilitation for adults with stable angina. *Cochrane Database Syst Rev*. 2018;2:CD012786.

57

ACUTE CORONARY SYNDROME: UNSTABLE ANGINA AND NON–ST ELEVATION MYOCARDIAL INFARCTION

RICHARD A. LANGE AND DEBABRATA MUKHERJEE

DEFINITION

The term *acute coronary syndrome* is used to describe the continuum of myocardial ischemia (unstable angina pectoris) or infarction (with or without concomitant ST segment elevation). The patient with *unstable angina* has cardiac chest pain that is new, worsening (i.e., more severe, prolonged, or frequent than previous episodes of angina), or occurring at rest, *without* serologic evidence of myocyte necrosis—that is, no elevation of serum concentrations of troponin. The patient with cardiac chest pain *with* serologic evidence of myonecrosis and without ST elevation is said to have a *non–ST elevation myocardial infarction* (MI). Because unstable angina and non–ST elevation MI are characterized by the absence of ST elevation, they are collectively termed *non–ST elevation acute coronary syndrome* (Fig. 57-1). The patient with acute-onset cardiac chest pain, serologic evidence of myonecrosis, and persistent (>20 minutes) ST segment elevation is said to have an *ST elevation MI* (Chapter 58).

EPIDEMIOLOGY

Almost 1.2 million individuals in the United States are hospitalized annually with acute coronary syndrome, of whom approximately two thirds have non–ST elevation acute coronary syndrome. More than half of patients with non–ST elevation acute coronary syndrome are older than 65 years, and almost half are women. Non–ST elevation acute coronary syndrome is more common in individuals with one or more risk factors for atherosclerosis (Chapter 40), peripheral vascular disease, or a chronic inflammatory disorder, such as rheumatoid arthritis, psoriasis, or infection.

Most patients with non–ST elevation acute coronary syndrome have so-called type 1 MI, which is precipitated by rupture of a coronary arterial atherosclerotic plaque, with subsequent platelet aggregation and thrombus formation, leading in turn to diminished blood flow in the involved artery. Type 2 MI is myocardial injury in the milieu of a mismatch between oxygen supply and demand. Substantial reductions in oxygen supply, for example, can be caused by severe systemic arterial hypotension, anemia, or hypoxemia; dramatic increases in oxygen demand can be caused by tachycardia, severe systemic arterial hypertension, or thyrotoxicosis. In patients thought to have type 2 MI, therapy should be directed at the underlying cause.

PATHOBIOLOGY

The precipitating event in almost all patients with non–ST elevation acute coronary syndrome is coronary arterial atherosclerotic plaque rupture or erosion, with subsequent platelet aggregation and thrombus formation, leading to subtotal occlusion of the involved artery (type 1 MI). In an occasional patient, total thrombotic occlusion of the artery leads to non–ST elevation acute coronary syndrome rather than to ST elevation MI when extensive collateral blood supply perfuses the region of myocardium that is distal to the occluded artery.

Some patients have a mismatch between myocardial oxygen supply and demand caused by a secondary process other than coronary artery disease (type 2 MI). For example, intense vasospasm of a segment of an epicardial coronary artery, due to focal endothelial dysfunction (i.e., Prinzmetal angina) or drug ingestion (caused, for example, by cocaine, chemotherapeutic agents, or one of the serotonin receptor agonist "triptans"), causes a transient or sustained compromise of coronary arterial blood flow, with resultant non–ST elevation acute coronary syndrome. Spontaneous coronary arterial dissection, which occurs most often in peripartum women and patients with vasculitis, also may result in non–ST elevation acute coronary syndrome.

Plaque Rupture

Coronary arterial atherosclerotic plaque rupture (Chapter 41) or erosion is the initiating event in most patients with non–ST elevation acute coronary syndrome. Several factors may play a role in the deterioration of the protective fibrous cap that separates the atheroma in the vessel wall from the coronary arterial lumen. Local and systemic inflammation, mechanical features, and anatomic changes contribute to the transformation of a stable atherosclerotic plaque to a so-called vulnerable plaque, the rupture of which triggers platelet adherence, activation, and aggregation, with subsequent thrombus formation.

The deposition of oxidized low-density lipoprotein in the coronary arterial wall stimulates an inflammatory response, which results in the accumulation of macrophages and T lymphocytes at the plaque border. These inflammatory cells secrete cytokines (e.g., tissue necrosis factor, interleukin-1, interferon-γ), which inhibit collagen synthesis and deposition, as well as enzymes (e.g., matrix metalloproteinases and cathepsins), which promote collagen and elastin degradation, thereby rendering the overlying fibrous cap vulnerable to rupture.

Systemic inflammation may play a role in plaque rupture, as evidenced by the predisposition of individuals with chronic gingivitis, psoriasis, systemic lupus erythematosus, rheumatoid arthritis, and chronic or acute infection to develop acute coronary syndrome. Angiographic and angioscopic studies of the coronary arteries of acute coronary syndrome patients often demonstrate plaque ulceration and thrombosis at more than one site, thereby suggesting that a systemic and diffuse inflammatory process is present.

The mechanical characteristics and location of coronary arterial plaques appear to influence their stability. For example, thin fibrous caps are more likely to erode or to rupture than are thick ones. Sites of low shear stress, such as vessel bifurcations, have reduced production of endothelial vasodilator substances (i.e., nitric oxide and prostacyclin), accelerated accumulation of lipids and inflammatory cells, increased degradation of the extracellular matrix, and thinning of the fibrous cap, all of which contribute to plaque instability.

Detailed histologic examination of evolving atherosclerotic plaques reveals a rich neovascularization that is the result of angiogenic peptides, such as fibroblast growth factors, vascular endothelial growth factor, placental growth factor, oncostatin M, and hypoxia-inducible factor, which are secreted by smooth muscle cells, inflammatory cells, and platelets. This neovascularization

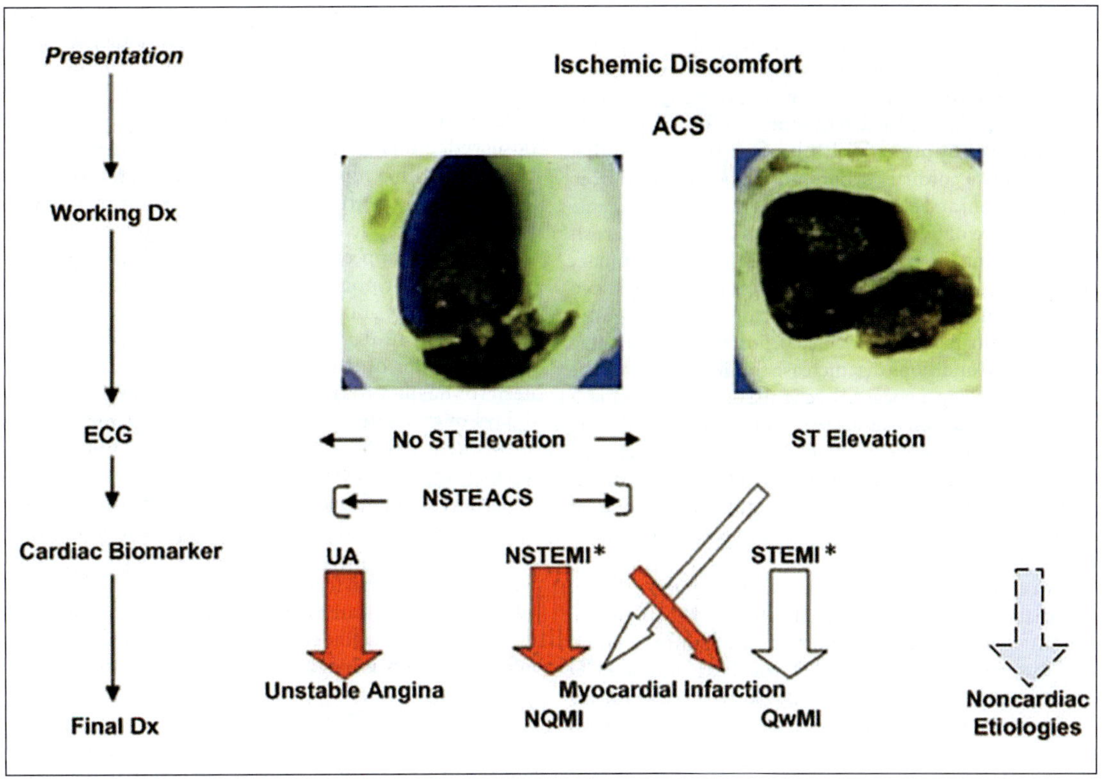

FIGURE 57-1. Acute coronary syndrome (ACS). Symptomatic, morphologic, electrocardiographic, and serologic findings in patients with various kinds of ACS. Patients with ACS usually complain of chest pain. If the involved coronary artery is totally occluded by a fresh thrombus (shown on the *right*), the patient's electrocardiogram (ECG) reveals ST segment elevation, cardiac biomarkers subsequently are elevated, and the patient is diagnosed with an ST elevation myocardial infarction (STEMI). In some cases, initial ST elevation can lead to non-Q wave myocardial infarction. If the involved coronary artery is partially occluded by fresh thrombus (shown on the *left*), the patient's ECG does not show ST segment elevation. If cardiac biomarkers are not elevated, the patient is diagnosed with unstable angina (UA). If cardiac biomarkers remain negative or are not elevated during hospitalization, the final diagnosis remains unstable angina. If cardiac biomarkers are elevated, the patient is diagnosed with a non–ST elevation MI (NSTEMI). Most patients presenting with NSTEMI develop NQMI, but a few may develop QwMI. Dx = diagnosis; NQMI = non–Q wave myocardial infarction; NSTEACS = non-ST elevation acute coronary syndrome; QwMI = Q wave myocardial infarction; UA = unstable angina.

contributes to the growth of atheroma and to leukocyte trafficking, plaque hemorrhage, and destabilization.

Thrombus Formation

Platelets play a pivotal role in the pathobiology of the acute coronary syndrome. After erosion or rupture of a vulnerable plaque, circulating platelets *adhere* to the exposed subendothelial proteins, after which they are *activated*. With activation, the platelets change shape from discoid to stellate, thereby increasing the surface area on which thrombin formation can occur. The platelets then release the contents of their intracellular granules (i.e., thromboxane, serotonin, adenosine diphosphate [ADP], von Willebrand factor, fibrinogen) into the immediate environment and promote focal vasoconstriction of the adjacent arterial segment and activation of nearby platelets. Platelets also increase the number of glycoprotein IIb/IIIa receptors on their surface and the affinity of these receptors to bind circulating fibrinogen. The result is platelet *aggregation*, which occurs as fibrinogen binds to the glycoprotein IIb/IIIa receptors of adjacent platelets, thereby creating a "platelet plug."

With formation of the platelet plug, the coagulation system activates and generates thrombin, which is a powerful stimulator of further platelet activation and aggregation. Thrombin also converts fibrinogen to fibrin, which is incorporated into the thrombus. Subtotal coronary arterial occlusion by this platelet-rich thrombus compromises blood flow in the involved artery, thereby resulting in an imbalance of oxygen supply and demand of the myocytes perfused by the artery. Distal embolization of platelet-rich thrombi from the site of a ruptured plaque may contribute to the compromise in blood flow. If the supply-demand imbalance is transient, the involved myocytes become ischemic but do not die because the ischemia is of insufficient duration to cause necrosis. The patient typically complains of cardiac chest pain at rest, but serologic evidence of myonecrosis, as evidenced by elevated serum concentrations of troponin, is absent; a diagnosis of *unstable angina* is made. In contrast, if the supply-demand imbalance is sustained, ischemic myocytes begin to die, and infarction occurs. The patient typically complains of cardiac chest pain at rest, and serologic evidence of myonecrosis confirms the diagnosis of *non–ST elevation MI*.

CLINICAL MANIFESTATIONS

Symptoms

The patient with non–ST elevation acute coronary syndrome typically complains of retrosternal pressure, squeezing, or heaviness that may be intermittent and recurrent or persistent (Chapter 39). If the episodes are intermittent and recurrent, the duration of each episode may range from only a few minutes to several hours. The chest pain may radiate to the left arm, neck, or jaw, and it may be accompanied by diaphoresis, nausea, abdominal pain, dyspnea, or syncope.

Atypical presentations are not uncommon and may include aching or vague chest discomfort, epigastric pain, acute-onset indigestion, unexplained fatigue, or dyspnea. Such atypical complaints are often observed in younger (25 to 40 years of age) and older (>75 years of age) patients; women; and patients with diabetes mellitus, chronic renal insufficiency, or dementia.

Physical Examination

The patient with non–ST elevation acute coronary syndrome often has normal findings on physical examination. On occasion, evidence of left ventricular dysfunction (Chapter 45), such as basilar rales or a ventricular gallop, hypotension, or peripheral hypoperfusion, may accompany an acute episode or appear shortly thereafter. An important goal of the physical examination is to exclude other potential causes of the patient's symptoms, including both noncardiac causes (i.e., costochondritis, pneumothorax, pulmonary embolism, pneumonia) and other cardiac disorders not attributable to myocardial ischemia (i.e., aortic dissection, pericarditis, severe systemic arterial hypertension, arrhythmias; Chapter 49). Accordingly, differences in blood pressure between the upper and lower limbs, decreased lung sounds, friction rubs, and pain on sternal palpation suggest a diagnosis other than non–ST elevation acute coronary syndrome. Other findings on physical examination—such as an elevated blood pressure, tachycardia, pallor, or increased sweating or tremor—point toward precipitating conditions, such as uncontrolled hypertension (Chapter 64), arrhythmias (Chapters 52 and 53), anemia (Chapter 144), or thyrotoxicosis (Chapter 207).

DIAGNOSIS

The patient with suspected acute coronary syndrome should be evaluated promptly because an expedient and accurate diagnosis permits the timely initiation of appropriate therapy, which can reduce the rate of complications.[1] The initial assessment should be directed at determining whether the patient's symptoms are likely to be caused by myocardial ischemia, MI, or some other disorder. The likelihood of acute coronary syndrome can be estimated from the history, physical examination, and electrocardiogram (ECG). In the acute setting, the presence or absence of traditional risk factors for atherosclerosis is less important for determining the presence or absence of acute coronary syndrome than are the patient's symptoms, ECG findings, and serologic evidence of myonecrosis. As a result, these long-term risk factors are not integral in determining whether an individual should be evaluated, hospitalized, or treated for acute coronary syndrome. Conditions that increase the likelihood that the symptomatic patient is experiencing myocardial ischemia or MI include older age, diabetes mellitus, extracardiac vascular disease, and chest pain radiating to the left arm, neck, or jaw as the presenting symptom. Myocardial ischemia is highly likely if anginal symptoms are accompanied by ECG abnormalities (i.e., Q waves, ST segment depression or elevation ≥1 mm in magnitude, or T wave inversion in multiple precordial leads) or elevated serum concentrations of troponin.

In a patient with known coronary artery disease, typical symptoms are likely to be caused by myocardial ischemia or MI rather than by another condition, particularly if the patient confirms that the symptoms are similar to previous anginal episodes. Conversely, a young individual who has a normal ECG and no risk factors for atherosclerosis is unlikely to be having acute coronary syndrome even when complaining of chest pain with features consistent with ischemia or infarction.

It is important to inquire about the use of cocaine and methamphetamines in the patient with suspected acute coronary syndrome, especially in those who are younger than 40 years or have few traditional risk factors for atherosclerosis. These drugs can increase myocardial oxygen demand and concomitantly decrease oxygen supply by causing vasospasm and thrombosis. A urine toxicologic analysis should be considered when substance abuse is suspected as a cause of acute coronary syndrome.

Electrocardiogram

An ECG, which should be performed and interpreted within 10 minutes or less of the patient's arrival at a facility, is particularly valuable if it is obtained during a symptomatic episode. If the patient has persistent (>20 minutes) ST segment elevation, prompt reperfusion therapy should be initiated (Chapter 58). Transient ST segment abnormalities that develop during a symptomatic episode at rest and resolve when the patient is asymptomatic strongly suggest non–ST elevation acute coronary syndrome. ST segment depression (or transient ST segment elevation) and T wave abnormalities occur in up to 50% of patients.

A completely normal ECG does not exclude the possibility of non–ST elevation acute coronary syndrome; in fact, about 5% of patients who are discharged from the emergency department and ultimately diagnosed with acute coronary syndrome have a normal ECG. Ischemia or infarction in the territory of the left circumflex coronary artery often escapes detection with a standard 12-lead ECG, but it may be detected with right-sided leads (V_4R and V_3R) or posterior leads (V_7 to V_9). In the patient whose initial ECG is normal, serial ECGs (e.g., 15- to 30-minute intervals during the first hour) should be performed routinely and during symptomatic episodes, and they should be compared with previous tracings to identify new ST segment or T wave abnormalities. Deep (>2 mm), symmetrical T wave inversion in the anterior chest leads is often associated with a hemodynamically significant stenosis of the left main or proximal left anterior descending coronary artery.

Serum Biomarkers

Unfortunately, the initial history, physical examination, and ECG alone cannot confirm or exclude an acute coronary syndrome. By comparison, modern high-sensitivity assays can detect troponin (Chapter 58) in the blood within 2 hours of the onset of symptoms in patients with non–ST elevation MI.

Risk Assessment and Triage

The greatest safety comes from continued observation or admission of patients who have a positive troponin level on presentation or at serial testing, have evidence of ischemia on their ECG, or have symptoms indicative of an acute exacerbation of prior coronary disease.[2,3] Because a single normal serum troponin measurement is insufficient to exclude MI in a patient with a very recent onset of symptoms, patients with suspected MI based on the clinical presentation or with ischemic ECG changes may be observed, either in the emergency department or in a chest pain evaluation unit, with a repeated troponin measurement (and a repeated ECG) at 3 or so hours after the onset of symptoms or whenever chest pain recurs.[4] A negative high-sensitivity troponin level at 2 to 3 hours after the onset of symptoms is sufficient to identify patients who do not have ST elevation or non–ST elevation MI (Fig. 57-2),[A1,A2] and patients with negative results and no ECG findings of ischemia have a sufficiently low risk (a 0.4% 30-day risk of MI or death) that they can safely complete the remainder of their evaluation as outpatients if they have no other need for hospitalization.[5–8] Noninvasive cardiac testing performed within 3 days of the initial presentation is associated with a modestly reduced subsequent risk of serious cardiac events, but its value in patients with normal troponin levels is likely small.[9]

Serum troponin concentrations can be measured with point-of-care instruments at the patient's bedside by desktop devices or handheld rapid qualitative assays.[10] The advantage of point-of-care systems for avoiding delays must be weighed against their higher costs and the need for stringent quality control. In addition, point-of-care assays are qualitative or semiquantitative and observer dependent, whereas the central laboratory provides more accurate quantitative information concerning biomarker concentrations.

Noninvasive Testing

A chest radiograph may identify pulmonary causes of chest pain and may show a widened mediastinum in aortic dissection (Chapter 63). The patient considered to have a low likelihood for acute coronary syndrome (on the basis of the history, physical examination, ECG, and serum biomarkers) should undergo timely stress testing (Chapter 39). Although stress testing does not absolutely establish or exclude the presence of coronary artery disease, it has the advantage of also defining a patient's exercise tolerance, which helps tailor therapeutic decisions. Alternatively, multidetector coronary computed tomographic angiography, which has a high (>98%) negative predictive value to exclude coronary artery disease when it is performed and interpreted at experienced centers, can help reduce the length of hospital stay when the findings are normal in emergency department patients at low to intermediate risk of possible acute coronary syndrome. However, coronary computed tomographic angiography does not have incremental value in patients with a negative troponin assay and a nonischemic ECG.[A3] Conversely, the patient who is believed to be at higher risk or who continues to have typical ischemic chest pain with ECG abnormalities or elevated cardiac biomarkers should not undergo stress testing or coronary computed tomographic angiography but rather should either undergo coronary angiography or be rendered symptom free with medical therapy before stress testing.

An echocardiogram may be helpful in the patient with chest pain if the ECG is nondiagnostic (i.e., minimal ST segment or T wave abnormalities). If left ventricular hypokinesis or akinesis is observed during an episode of chest pain and then improves when symptoms resolve, myocardial ischemia is likely. In the patient with anterior T wave inversion of uncertain etiology, hypokinesis of the left ventricular anterior wall suggests that the observed T wave abnormality is due to a severe stenosis of the left anterior descending coronary artery. Because echocardiography can help evaluate and identify alternative causes for the patient's chest pain (i.e., myocarditis [Chapter 47], aortic dissection [Chapter 63], or pulmonary embolism [Chapter 68]), it is recommended in patients whose diagnosis is uncertain.

Coronary Angiography

Coronary angiography (Chapter 59) should be performed in patients who are thought to be at high risk for death, MI, or recurrent ischemia in the ensuing days, weeks, and months (see later); in patients who have spontaneous or inducible myocardial ischemia despite appropriate medical therapy; and in patients who have a confusing or difficult clinical presentation and a subsequent inconclusive noninvasive evaluation. The results of angiography help determine whether revascularization is appropriate and, if so, whether it should be attempted by coronary artery bypass grafting or percutaneous coronary intervention (PCI) (Chapter 59).

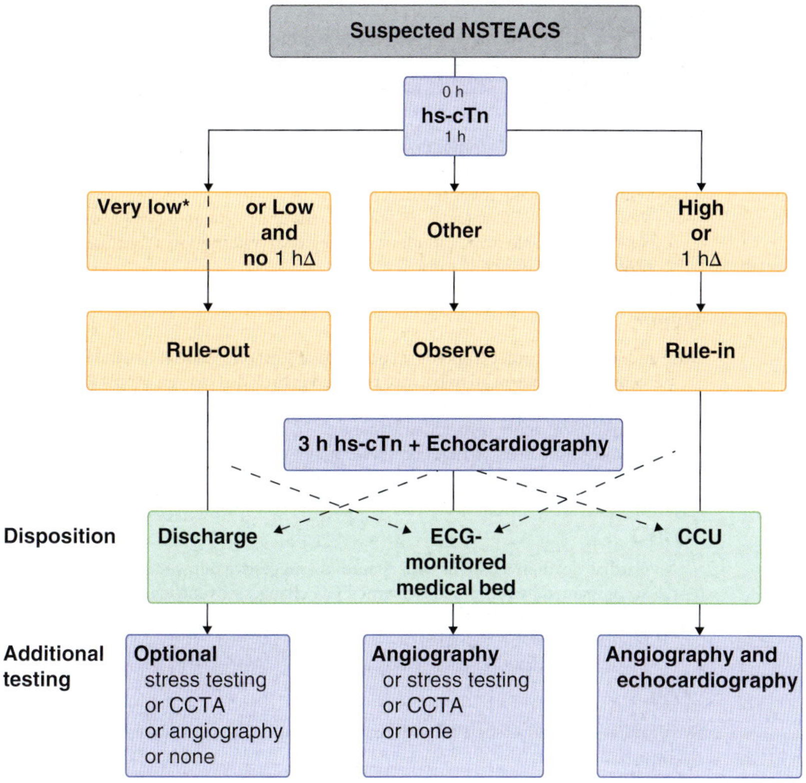

FIGURE 57-2. **Initial triage for patients with symptoms suggestive of a non-ST elevation acute coronary syndrome (NSTEACS) using high-sensitivity cardiac troponin assays.** 0 h/1 h rule-out and rule-in algorithm using high-sensitivity cardiac troponin assays in hemodynamically stable patients presenting with suspected NSTEACS to the emergency department. 0 h and 1 h refer to the time from the first blood test. NSTEMI can be ruled out at presentation if the hs-cTn concentration is very low. NSTEMI can also be ruled out by the combination of low baseline levels and the lack of a relevant increase within 1 h (no 1hΔ). Patients have a high likelihood of NSTEMI if the hs-cTn concentration at presentation is at least moderately elevated or hs-cTn concentrations show a clear rise within the first hour (1hΔ). CCTA = coronary computed tomography angiography; CCU = coronary care unit; hs-cTn = high-sensitivity cardiac troponin; NSTEACS = non-ST elevation acute coronary syndrome; NSTEMI = non-ST elevation myocardial infarction. *Only applicable if chest pain onset >3 h. (Adapted from Collet JP, Thiele H, Barbato E, et al. 2020 ESC guidelines for the management of acute coronary syndromes in patients presenting without persistent ST-segment elevation. *Eur Heart J.* 2021;42:1289-1367.)

In patients with non–ST elevation acute coronary syndrome, coronary angiography demonstrates significant stenosis of the left main coronary artery in about 15% of patients, of all three major epicardial coronary arteries in about 30 to 35% of patients, of two of the three epicardial arteries in about 20 to 30% of patients, and of one major epicardial artery in 20 to 30% of patients. About 15% of patients have no coronary arterial narrowing of hemodynamic significance. Women with non–ST elevation acute coronary syndrome are likely to have less extensive coronary artery disease than men have, and patients with non–ST elevation MI usually have more extensive disease than those with unstable angina.

On angiography, the coronary arterial lesion responsible for signs and symptoms (the so-called culprit lesion) typically is asymmetrical or eccentric, with scalloped or overhanging edges and a narrow base or neck, features that reflect underlying plaque disruption and thrombus formation. Although obvious thrombus is visible by angiography in only one third of patients, coronary angioscopy shows plaque rupture with overlying thrombus in the majority. Interestingly, the culprit lesion often is not severely stenotic when it is assessed on recently performed angiograms; in fact, two thirds of culprit lesions previously had less than 50% luminal diameter narrowing (and therefore would not have been considered appropriate for revascularization).

After the initial triage decision is made, therapeutic interventions are based on the risk of adverse events in the ensuing hours, days, weeks, and months—estimated by either the Thrombolysis in Myocardial Infarction (TIMI) or Global Registry of Acute Coronary Events (GRACE) risk algorithm—balanced against the risk of a bleeding complication from intensive medical therapy (Table 57-1) or an adverse event from an invasive cardiac procedure. On the basis of this initial assessment, the patient's therapy should be tailored to minimize the likelihood of adverse events.

Although serum markers of myonecrosis represent only one of the TIMI or GRACE risk variables, the presence of this variable alone identifies the patient as being at high risk. However, although elevated serum markers indicate myonecrosis, they provide no insight into its cause because myonecrosis can occur with disease entities other than coronary artery disease (e.g., pulmonary embolism, decompensated heart failure, severe hypertension or tachycardia, anemia, sepsis). Thus, in evaluation of the patient with possible acute coronary syndrome, the presence of elevated serum markers should be assessed in conjunction with other variables.

Increasing age is associated with a higher incidence of both ischemic events and of complications from intensive medical therapy and invasive cardiac procedures. Even though elderly individuals are at increased risk of treatment-related complications, they nonetheless derive a greater absolute and relative benefit from such intensive therapy compared with younger individuals. Apart from this initial risk assessment, the patient's general medical and cognitive status, anticipated life expectancy, and, most important, personal preferences should be evaluated and considered.

Differential Diagnosis

The current universal definition of MI recognizes five different types (Table 57-2),[11] including ST elevation (Chapter 58) MI or non–ST elevation MI related to an acute coronary thrombosis (type 1); MI caused by a mismatch between myocardial supply and demand (type 2); MI associated with sudden cardiac arrest but not documented antemortem (type 3, Chapter 50); and MI associated with a percutaneous coronary intervention (type 4) or coronary artery bypass graft surgery (type 5, Chapter 59). The use of high-sensitivity troponin assays increases the detection of all five types.

Cardiac injury with troponin elevation but without other evidence of ischemia can also occur after cardiac and noncardiac procedures (Chapter 401). Several cardiac and noncardiac conditions, some of which are potentially life-threatening, may mimic non–ST elevation acute coronary syndrome. The patient with a pulmonary embolism (Chapter 68) will often complain of chest pain and dyspnea and may have ECG abnormalities and an elevated serum troponin concentration. Aortic dissection (Chapter 63) should be considered and excluded because the therapies for non–ST elevation acute coronary syndrome are contraindicated in patients with this condition. Stroke (Chapter 376) and subarachnoid hemorrhage (Chapter 377) may be accompanied by ECG abnormalities, left ventricular segmental wall motion abnormalities, and elevated serum biomarker concentrations. Underlying chronic cardiac conditions, such as valvular heart disease (i.e., aortic stenosis, aortic regurgitation) and hypertrophic cardiomyopathy (Chapter 47), may be associated with symptoms similar to those of non–ST elevation acute coronary syndrome, elevated serum biomarker concentrations, and ECG abnormalities. Myocarditis (Chapter 47), pericarditis (Chapter 62), and myopericarditis often cause chest pain that resembles angina, ECG abnormalities, and elevated serum biomarker concentrations; an influenza-like or upper respiratory tract infection (including severe acute respiratory syndrome coronavirus 2) often precedes or accompanies these conditions. Patients with "stress cardiomyopathy" (takotsubo syndrome) typically have chest pain, ST segment abnormalities and deeply inverted T waves, and mildly elevated serum biomarker concentrations (Chapter 47). In rural areas without emergency medicine specialists or cardiologists, diagnostic support from a tertiary center can improve diagnostic accuracy.[A4]

TABLE 57-1 RISK VARIABLES FOR ISCHEMIC EVENTS AND BLEEDING COMPLICATIONS

RISK VARIABLES PREDICTIVE OF DEATH, MYOCARDIAL INFARCTION, OR RECURRENT ISCHEMIA

Thrombolysis in Myocardial Infarction (TIMI) Score*

Age >65 yr
Three or more risk factors for atherosclerosis
Known coronary artery disease (previous coronary arteriography or myocardial infarction)
Two or more episodes of anginal chest pain at rest in the 24 hr before hospitalization
Use of aspirin in the 7 days before hospitalization
ST segment deviation ≥0.5 mV
Elevated serum concentrations of troponin or CK-MB

Global Registry of Acute Coronary Events (GRACE)†

Age
Heart failure (Killip) class
Heart rate
Systolic blood pressure
ST segment deviation
Cardiac arrest during presentation
Serum creatinine concentration
Elevated serum markers of myonecrosis

RISK FACTORS FOR BLEEDING COMPLICATIONS WITH INTENSIVE THERAPY‡

Female gender
Older age
Renal insufficiency
Low body weight
Tachycardia
Systolic arterial pressure (high or low)
Anemia
Diabetes mellitus

*Individuals with three or more of these variables are considered to be at high risk, whereas those with none, one, or two are considered to be at low risk.
†Each variable is assigned a numerical score on the basis of its specific value, and the eight scores are summed to yield a total score, which is applied to a reference nomogram to determine the patient's risk. The GRACE application tool is available online at www.outcomes-umassmed.org/grace. (From Brieger D, Fox KA, Fitzgerald G, et al. Predicting freedom from clinical events in non-ST-elevation acute coronary syndromes: the Global Registry of Acute Coronary Events. *Heart.* 2009;95:888-894.)
‡The patient's bleeding risk can be estimated with the tool available at https://reference.medscape.com/calculator/53/crusade-score-for-post-mi-bleeding-risk. (From Subherwal S, Bach RG, Chen AY, et al. Baseline risk of major bleeding in non-ST-segment-elevation myocardial infarction: the CRUSADE [Can Rapid risk stratification of Unstable angina patients Suppress ADverse outcomes with Early implementation of the ACC/AHA Guidelines] Bleeding Score. *Circulation.* 2009;119:1873-1882.)
From Diez JG, Cohen M. Balancing myocardial ischemic and bleeding risks in patients with non-ST-segment elevation myocardial infarction. *Am J Cardiol.* 2009;103:1396-1402.

TABLE 57-2 UNIVERSAL DEFINITION OF MYOCARDIAL INFARCTION

TYPE 1

Rise and/or fall of cardiac troponin values, with at least one value above the 99th percentile and at least one of the following:
- Symptoms of acute myocardial ischemia
- New ischemic ECG changes or development of new pathologic Q waves
- New loss of viable myocardium or new regional wall motion abnormality consistent with an ischemic cause on imaging
- Coronary thrombus on angiography, intracoronary imaging, or autopsy

TYPE 2

Rise and/or fall of cardiac troponin values, with at least one value above the 99th percentile, evidence of an imbalance between myocardial oxygen supply and demand unrelated to acute coronary thrombosis, and at least one of the following:
- Symptoms of acute myocardial ischemia
- New ischemic ECG changes or development of new pathologic Q waves
- New loss of viable myocardium or new regional wall motion abnormality consistent with an ischemic cause on imaging

TYPE 3

- Cardiac death in a patient with symptoms suggestive of myocardial ischemia accompanied by presumed ischemic ECG changes or ventricular fibrillation, before blood samples for biomarkers can be obtained or increases in cardiac biomarkers can be identified
- Myocardial infarction detected on autopsy

TYPE 4

Myocardial infarction associated with a percutaneous coronary intervention

TYPE 5

Myocardial infarction related to coronary artery bypass graft surgery

ECG = electrocardiogram.
Thygesen K, Alpert JS, Jaffe AS, et al. Fourth universal definition of myocardial infarction (2018). *Circulation.* 2018;138:e618-e651.

TREATMENT

The goals of treatment of the patient with non–ST elevation acute coronary syndrome are to prevent recurrent ischemia (by correcting the imbalance between myocardial oxygen supply and demand), to prevent thrombus propagation, and to stabilize the vulnerable plaque.[12,13] Antianginal medications, such as nitroglycerin (see Table 56-11), β-adrenergic blockers (see Table 56-9), and calcium-channel blockers (see Table 56-10), favorably affect myocardial oxygen supply and demand, thereby preventing recurrent ischemia. Antiplatelet and antithrombotic agents retard thrombus propagation, and statins promote plaque stabilization.

Once the patient's risk status is established, therapy is initiated and tailored to the patient's risk of sustaining a subsequent ischemic cardiac event or a treatment-related complication (Table 57-3). For example, the patient considered to be at low risk of a subsequent ischemic event does not benefit from intensive antithrombotic therapy or routine coronary angiography and revascularization. Conversely, in patients considered to be at high risk of sustaining an ischemic event, optimal therapy—including coronary angiography and revascularization (if appropriate)—results in a 20 to 40% decrease in the risk of recurrent ischemia and MI and an approximately 10% reduction in mortality, with about an 18-month postponement of recurrent MI or death.[A5] An invasive approach also appears to be preferable in patients over age 75 years.[A6]

Every patient with non–ST elevation acute coronary syndrome, regardless of their level of risk, should promptly receive antianginal medications, antiplatelet therapy, and a statin, unless contraindicated. A patient considered to be at low risk may receive unfractionated heparin, but more intensive anticoagulant therapy is not necessary because such therapy increases the risk of bleeding without further reducing the risk of an ischemic cardiac event. Routine coronary angiography and revascularization are not beneficial and should be reserved for the patient with recurrent ischemia despite intensive medical therapy.

Conversely, the high-risk patient should receive antianginal medications, antiplatelet therapy, a statin, intensive anticoagulant therapy, and coronary angiography followed by revascularization (if indicated). In the patient whose coronary anatomy is suitable, revascularization reduces the incidence of ischemia and recurrent MI, and it also improves survival in certain patients (see later).

Antianginal Therapy

Nitroglycerin

Nitroglycerin (see Table 56-11), which is a venodilator at low doses and an arteriolar dilator at higher doses, may prevent recurrent ischemia in patients with unstable angina, but no studies of sufficient statistical power have determined whether it reduces the risk of MI in this population of patients. In patients who complain of recurrent symptoms, nitroglycerin should be given sublingually or by buccal spray (0.3 to 0.6 mg). Patients with ongoing or recurrent chest pain should receive intravenous nitroglycerin (5 to 10 μg/minute with use of nonabsorbable tubing), with escalation of the dose in increments of 10 μg/minute until symptoms resolve or adverse effects develop. Nitroglycerin's most common adverse effects are headache, nausea, dizziness, hypotension, and reflex tachycardia.

Nitrate tolerance can be avoided by periodically providing the patient with a nitrate-free period (i.e., a brief cessation of drug administration). Nitroglycerin should not be given to patients who have received a phosphodiesterase-5 inhibitor (i.e., sildenafil, tadalafil, or vardenafil) within the previous 24 to 48 hours, because severe hypotension may ensue.

β-Adrenergic Blockers

β-Adrenergic blockers diminish symptoms and the risk of MI in patients with acute coronary syndrome who are not already taking a β-blocker at the time of hospitalization. In the normotensive patient without ongoing chest pain or tachycardia and without contraindications to β-blockers, metoprolol should be initiated at 25 to 50 mg orally every 6 to 8 hours, with the dose increased (to 100 mg twice daily) as necessary to control heart rate, blood pressure, and symptoms. In high-risk patients and in patients with tachycardia or elevated systemic arterial pressure, metoprolol should be administered intravenously

TABLE 57-3 MANAGEMENT STRATEGIES FOR PATIENTS WITH ACUTE CORONARY SYNDROME

THERAPY	INITIATION	DURATION	DOSE, ROUTE, AND DURATION	BENEFIT VS. PLACEBO (REDUCED INCIDENCE OF ...)
LOW-RISK PATIENT				
Antianginal				
β-Blocker*	Within 24 hr	Hospitalization ± indefinitely	Metoprolol, 25-50 mg orally twice daily, titrated up to 100 mg twice daily; or atenolol, 50-100 mg orally daily	Recurrent ischemia
Nitroglycerin	Immediately	Hospitalization ± indefinitely	0.3-0.6 mg sublingually or 5-10 μg/min IV initially and increased by 10 μg/min every 5 min	Not studied
Diltiazem or verapamil[†]	Immediately	Hospitalization ± indefinitely	30-90 mg orally four times daily or up to 360 mg of long-acting preparation orally daily	MI, recurrent ischemia
Lipid Lowering				
Statins (with other lipid-lowering medications as needed; see Chapter 190)	Immediately	Indefinitely	Atorvastatin, 40-80 mg; or rosuvastatin, 20-40 mg orally daily	Recurrent ischemia
Antiplatelet				
Aspirin	Immediately	Indefinitely	162-325 mg orally initial dose, then 81 mg orally daily	Death, MI
Clopidogrel	Immediately	1-12 mo	300 mg orally initial dose, then 75 mg orally daily	MI, recurrent ischemia
Anticoagulant				
Unfractionated heparin	Immediately	2-5 days	IV bolus of 60 U/kg, then 12 U/kg/hr IV adjusted to achieve an aPTT of 50 to 70 sec	Death or MI (combined)
HIGH-RISK PATIENT				
Antianginal				
β-Blocker*	Within 24 hr	Hospitalization ± indefinitely	Metoprolol, 25-50 mg orally twice daily, titrated up to 100 mg twice daily; or atenolol, 50-100 mg orally daily	Death, MI, recurrent ischemia
Nitroglycerin	Immediately	Hospitalization ± indefinitely	0.3-0.6 mg sublingually or 5-10 μg/min IV initially and increased by 10 μg/min every 5 min	Not studied
Diltiazem or verapamil[†]	Immediately	Hospitalization ± indefinitely	30-90 mg orally four times daily or up to 360 mg of long-acting preparation orally daily	MI, recurrent ischemia
Lipid Lowering				
Statin	Before hospital discharge	Indefinitely	Atorvastatin, 40-80 mg; or rosuvastatin, 20-40 mg orally daily	Recurrent ischemia
Antiplatelet				
Aspirin *and*	Immediately	Indefinitely	162-325 mg orally initial dose, then 81 mg orally	Death, MI
Clopidogrel *or*	Immediately	12 mo	300-600 mg orally initial dose, then 75 mg orally daily	MI, recurrent ischemia
Prasugrel *or*	At time of PCI	12 mo	60 mg orally initial dose, then 10 mg orally daily	Cardiovascular death, MI or stroke (combined)[‡]
Ticagrelor	Immediately	12 mo	180 mg orally initially, then 90 mg twice daily	Vascular death, MI or stroke (combined)[‡]
Glycoprotein IIb/IIIa inhibitor (eptifibatide, tirofiban, or abciximab)	At time of PCI	12-24 hr after PCI	Abciximab, IV bolus of 0.25 mg/kg, then 0.125 μg/kg/min IV (max. 10 μg/min) for 12 hr; or eptifibatide, IV bolus of 180 μg/kg, then 2.0 μg/kg/min IV for 18-24 hr; or tirofiban, 0.4 μg/kg/min IV for 30 min, then 0.1 μg/kg/min IV for 12 to 24 hr	MI
Anticoagulants				
Enoxaparin *or*	Immediately	Duration of hospitalization (up to 8 days); discontinue after successful PCI	1 mg/kg subcutaneously twice daily	MI, recurrent ischemia[§]
Unfractionated heparin *or*	Immediately	2 to 5 days; discontinue after successful PCI	IV bolus of 60 U/kg, then 12 U/kg/hr IV adjusted to achieve an aPTT of 50 to 70 sec	Death or MI (combined)
Bivalirudin *or*	Immediately (only in patients managed with an early invasive strategy)	Up to 72 hr; discontinue 4 hr after PCI	0.10 mg/kg loading dose followed by 0.25 mg/kg/hr	Bleeding[#]

TABLE 57-3 MANAGEMENT STRATEGIES FOR PATIENTS WITH ACUTE CORONARY SYNDROME—cont'd

THERAPY	INITIATION	DURATION	DOSE, ROUTE, AND DURATION	BENEFIT VS. PLACEBO (REDUCED INCIDENCE OF ...)
Fondaparinux	Immediately	Duration of hospitalization (up to 8 days); if used during PCI, it must be coadministered with another anticoagulant with factor IIa activity	2.5-mg subcutaneous injection once daily	Bleeding[¶]
Invasive Management				
Coronary angiography followed by revascularization (if appropriate)	Up to 36-80 hr after hospitalization; within 24 hr in "very high risk" patients			MI, recurrent ischemia

*Avoid in the patient with signs of decompensated heart failure, evidence of low-output state, increased risk for cardiogenic shock, or other contraindications to β-blockade (e.g., PR interval >0.24 sec, second- or third-degree atrioventricular block without a cardiac pacemaker, active asthma, or reactive airway disease).
†Avoid in patients with clinically significant left ventricular dysfunction, increased risk for cardiogenic shock, PR interval >0.24 sec, or second- or third-degree atrioventricular block without a cardiac pacemaker.
‡Compared with clopidogrel.
§Compared with unfractionated heparin.
‖As monotherapy compared with heparin and glycoprotein IIb/IIIa inhibitor combination.
¶Compared with enoxaparin.
aPTT = activated partial thromboplastin time; IV = intravenous; MI = myocardial infarction; PCI = percutaneous coronary intervention.
Modified from Lange RA, Hillis LD. Optimal management of acute coronary syndromes. *N Engl J Med*. 2009;260:2237-2240.

(three boluses of 5 mg each given 5 minutes apart) initially, after which an oral dose should be initiated. A reasonable target heart rate is 50 to 60 beats per minute at rest.

β-Blockers should not be administered to patients with decompensated heart failure, hypotension, hemodynamic instability, or advanced atrioventricular block. Because most patients with chronic obstructive pulmonary disease or peripheral vascular disease tolerate β-blockers without difficulty, these conditions should not automatically preclude their use.

Calcium-Channel Blockers

Calcium-channel blockers, which cause arterial vasodilation, increase coronary arterial blood flow and lower systemic arterial pressure. The non-dihydropyridine calcium-channel blockers diltiazem and verapamil slow heart rate and are recommended for the patient with a contraindication to a β-adrenergic blocker or persistent or recurrent symptoms despite treatment with nitroglycerin or a β-blocker. Oral diltiazem (30 to 90 mg four times daily of the short-acting preparation or up to 360 mg once daily of the long-acting preparation) is the preferred calcium-channel blocker because it reduces the incidence of myocardial ischemia and recurrent MI in patients with non–ST elevation acute coronary syndrome. Diltiazem is contraindicated in patients with left ventricular systolic dysfunction or pulmonary vascular congestion. Caution should be exercised when combining a β-blocker with diltiazem because the two drugs may act synergistically to depress left ventricular systolic function as well as sinus and atrioventricular nodal conduction. Patients with acute coronary syndrome should not be prescribed short-acting nifedipine unless they are already receiving a β-blocker because it may increase the risk of death. By comparison, the risks and benefits of long-acting dihydropyridines are not well defined.

Antiplatelet Agents

Patients with acute coronary syndrome should receive dual antiplatelet therapy (aspirin and a $P2Y_{12}$ ADP receptor inhibitor) acutely and for up to 1 year unless they have an aspirin allergy, active bleeding, or are at high risk of bleeding.[14] Aspirin (162 to 325 mg initially, then 81 mg daily, continued indefinitely; Chapter 70) reduces the risk of death or MI by about 50%. The choice of which ADP receptor antagonist to use in combination with aspirin is determined by each patient's characteristics (i.e., risk of bleeding), medication costs, and pharmacologic properties of the agent (see the following details). The patient who is allergic to or intolerant of aspirin should be treated with a $P2Y_{12}$ ADP receptor inhibitor (clopidogrel, ticagrelor, or prasugrel [if PCI treated]) alone. Patients who are treated with drug-eluting coronary stenting (see later) and who are at high risk of bleeding may discontinue $P2Y_{12}$ ADP receptor inhibitor therapy after 3 to 6 months.[A7] Among these three options, prasugrel and ticagrelor decrease ischemic events but increase bleeding compared with clopidogrel.[A8] De-escalation to clopidogrel or low-dose prasugrel (e.g., 5 mg rather than 10 mg daily) at 3 to 6 months can provide equivalent benefits with lower bleeding risks.[A9]

$P2Y_{12}$ ADP Receptor Inhibitors

Clopidogrel (Chapter 70) has antiplatelet activity that is synergistic with aspirin because the two agents inhibit different platelet-activating pathways. Clopidogrel is a prodrug that must be metabolized by the cytochrome P-450 system to the active form. Polymorphisms in the cytochrome P-450 isoform CYP2C19, which are present in 15 to 20% of individuals, slow metabolism of the prodrug to the active form, thereby reducing the magnitude of platelet inhibition. Drugs that are potent inhibitors of the CYP2C19 enzyme (e.g., omeprazole, esomeprazole, cimetidine, fluconazole, ketoconazole, voriconazole, etravirine, felbamate, fluoxetine, and fluvoxamine) should not be administered with clopidogrel because they affect the metabolism to its active form and reduce its antiplatelet effects. In patients with non–ST elevation acute coronary syndrome, the addition of clopidogrel (a loading dose of 300 to 600 mg, then 75 mg daily for up to 1 year) to aspirin reduces the composite end point of cardiovascular death, nonfatal MI, or stroke by 20% (2.1% reduction in absolute risk) compared with treatment with aspirin alone. The benefit of an aspirin-clopidogrel combination was seen as early as 24 hours after drug initiation and persisted for the 12 months of the study, despite an increase in minor bleeding.

Prasugrel (Chapter 70) has a greater antiplatelet effect and a more rapid onset of action than clopidogrel. In patients with acute coronary syndrome who are referred for PCI, prasugrel in combination with aspirin reduces ischemic events (i.e., a combination of cardiovascular death, nonfatal MI, and stroke) by 20% compared with concomitant clopidogrel and aspirin (2.2% absolute risk reduction) therapy. However, this benefit is obtained at a 0.5% increased risk of life-threatening bleeding and a 0.3% increased risk of fatal bleeding. Compared with ticagrelor, prasugrel can significantly reduce the 1-year risk of death, myocardial infarction, or stroke, with a slightly lower risk of bleeding.[A10] In combination with aspirin, it is administered as a 60-mg oral loading dose followed by a 10-mg daily maintenance dose. Diminishing the dose from 10 mg daily to 5 mg daily at 1 month may sustain its anti-ischemic benefits but reduce bleeding, thereby improving its net clinical benefit.[A11] Because prasugrel-associated bleeding complications are highest in patients with a previous stroke or transient ischemic attack, age older than 75 years, or a body weight of less than 60 kg, it should not be used in patients with any of these features.

Ticagrelor (Chapter 70) does not require hepatic activation, and it has more rapid onset and more pronounced platelet inhibition than clopidogrel. It is a reversible inhibitor of the $P2Y_{12}$ receptor, so platelet function returns more rapidly after discontinuation than with clopidogrel. In a randomized trial in non–ST elevation acute coronary syndrome patients, the addition of ticagrelor to aspirin reduced the composite end point of vascular death, nonfatal MI, or stroke by about 15% compared with treatment with clopidogrel and aspirin but increased non–procedure-related bleeding by an absolute 0.7%. In combination with aspirin, ticagrelor is administered as a 180-mg oral loading dose, followed by a 90-mg twice-daily maintenance dose. In patients who receive ticagrelor, the daily aspirin maintenance dose should be 100 mg or less, and ticagrelor should not be used in patients with a history of intracranial hemorrhage. Even in patients more than 1 year after a non–ST elevation MI, treatment with ticagrelor at 60 or 90 mg twice daily in addition to aspirin significantly reduces the risk of cardiovascular death, MI, or stroke but not of overall death because of an increased risk of major bleeding.

Cangrelor, which is the only intravenous $P2Y_{12}$ receptor antagonist, is administered as a bolus (30 μg/kg before the PCI procedure), followed by an infusion (4 μg/kg per minute for at least 2 hours or through the duration of the intervention, whichever is longer), as an adjunct during PCI to reduce the risk of periprocedural MI, repeated coronary revascularization, and subacute thrombosis in patients who are not being treated with an oral $P2Y_{12}$ inhibitor and are not planned to receive a glycoprotein IIb/III inhibitor. To maintain platelet inhibition after discontinuation of the cangrelor infusion, oral options include clopidogrel (600 mg immediately after discontinuing cangrelor), prasugrel (60 mg immediately after discontinuing cangrelor), or ticagrelor (180 mg at any time during the cangrelor infusion or immediately after it).

Glycoprotein IIb/IIIa Inhibitors

Glycoprotein IIb/IIIa inhibitors (Chapter 70) block platelet aggregation in response to all potential agonists, so they are the most potent antiplatelet agents available. Three glycoprotein IIb/IIIa inhibitors, each of which must be administered parenterally, are available: abciximab is the Fab fragment of a monoclonal antibody to the receptor, eptifibatide is a peptide, and tirofiban is a peptidomimetic molecule.

Glycoprotein IIb/IIIa inhibitors reduce the incidence of recurrent ischemic events in patients with non–ST elevation acute coronary syndrome who undergo PCI but not in patients who are managed with medical therapy alone. When a glycoprotein IIb/IIIa inhibitor is administered to PCI patients, it should be initiated at the time of angiography because its routine administration beforehand carries an increased bleeding risk and no improvement in outcomes. The glycoprotein IIb/IIIa inhibitor infusion (see Table 57-3) typically is continued for 12 to 24 hours after PCI.

Anticoagulants

Anticoagulant therapy should be administered to all patients with acute coronary syndrome unless a contraindication, such as active bleeding, is present. For the patient in whom a noninvasive, ischemia-guided management strategy is selected, treatment with unfractionated heparin, low-molecular-weight heparin (LMWH), or fondaparinux is appropriate, with fondaparinux recommended for the patient at increased risk of bleeding. For the patient in whom an invasive management strategy is selected, unfractionated heparin and LMWH are the agents of choice. Although bivalirudin may be preferred in patients undergoing PCI, it is not used in the initial management of the patient with acute coronary syndrome.

Low-Molecular-Weight Heparin

LMWHs (Chapter 70), which are fragments of unfractionated heparin, exert a more predictable anticoagulant effect, have a longer half-life, and are less likely to cause thrombocytopenia compared with unfractionated heparin. Because they provide predictable and sustained anticoagulation with once- or twice-daily subcutaneous administration, monitoring of their anticoagulant effect is not required.

LMWH is superior to unfractionated heparin in preventing MI or death during hospitalization in non–ST elevation acute coronary syndrome patients who have elevated serum cardiac biomarkers, as well as in those considered to be at high risk for recurrent ischemia (see Table 57-1). In the low-risk patient, unfractionated heparin and LMWH have similar efficacy.

Two LMWHs, enoxaparin and dalteparin, are approved for the treatment of the patient with non–ST elevation acute coronary syndrome. The dose of enoxaparin is 1 mg/kg subcutaneously twice daily, and the dose of dalteparin is 120 IU/kg (maximum, 10,000 IU) subcutaneously twice daily. Therapy should be continued for the duration of the hospitalization, up to 8 days, or until revascularization is performed (whichever occurs first). In obese (>120 kg), thin (<60 kg), or renally impaired (creatinine clearance <30 mL/minute) patients, the LMWH dose should be adjusted to achieve an anti–factor Xa concentration of 0.5 to 1.5 IU/mL 4 to 6 hours after drug administration. LMWH should be avoided in the patient with a history of heparin-induced thrombocytopenia. In the patient with renal failure, treatment with LMWH has been associated with the development of hyperkalemia.

Heparin

Unfractionated heparin (Chapter 70) exerts its anticoagulant effect by accelerating the action of circulating antithrombin; it prevents thrombus propagation but does not lyse existing thrombi. In the patient with non–ST elevation acute coronary syndrome, the addition of heparin to aspirin reduces the rate of in-hospital ischemic events (i.e., death or MI) by 33%.

Unfractionated heparin should be initiated with an intravenous bolus of 60 U/kg, followed by a continuous infusion of approximately 12 U/kg/hour (maximum, 1000 U/hour), adjusted to maintain the activated partial thromboplastin time (aPTT) at 1.5 to 2.5 times control (i.e., 50 to 70 seconds) or a heparin concentration at 0.3 to 0.7 U/mL (by anti–factor Xa determinations). The infusion should be continued for 48 hours or until revascularization is performed, whichever occurs sooner. Frequent monitoring of the aPTT or heparin concentration is necessary because the anticoagulant response to a standard dose of unfractionated heparin varies widely among individuals; even when a weight-based nomogram (see Table 68-6) is followed, the aPTT is outside the therapeutic range more than one third of the time.

Mild thrombocytopenia occurs in 10 to 20% of patients treated with unfractionated heparin. In 1 to 5% of patients, a more severe form of thrombocytopenia develops. This antibody-mediated response usually occurs 4 to 14 days after the initiation of treatment (although it may appear more quickly in patients who received heparin within the preceding 6 months) and is associated with thromboembolic sequelae in 30 to 80% of patients (Chapter 158).

Fondaparinux

Fondaparinux (Chapter 70), which is a selective factor Xa inhibitor, does not require dose adjustment and monitoring. Fondaparinux does not cause thrombocytopenia. Fondaparinux is as effective as enoxaparin in preventing ischemic cardiac events but with 50% fewer major bleeding episodes (2.2% vs 4.1%). Because an increased incidence of catheter-related thrombosis has been reported after fondaparinux treatment, it is not recommended for patients who are likely to undergo coronary angiography. Fondaparinux is a desirable anticoagulant for the acute coronary syndrome patients who are managed in an ischemia-guided fashion, especially patients at higher risk of a bleeding complication with anticoagulant therapy, but not for other patients.

For the patient with acute coronary syndrome, fondaparinux is administered as a 2.5-mg subcutaneous injection once daily for up to 5 days or until hospital discharge. Its use is contraindicated in patients with severe renal impairment and in those who weigh 50 kg or less, and it should not be used as the sole anticoagulant during a PCI.

Bivalirudin

Bivalirudin, a direct thrombin inhibitor, is currently recommended as an alternative anticoagulant for patients undergoing PCI. In patients whose acute coronary syndrome is managed with an ischemia-guided strategy, its administration in a setting other than the cardiac catheterization laboratory is not recommended. In the patient undergoing PCI, bivalirudin (0.75 mg/kg intravenous bolus followed by an infusion of 1.75 mg/kg/hour for up to 4 hours after the PCI) is as effective as unfractionated heparin[A12] and as combination heparin and glycoprotein IIb/IIIa inhibitor therapy in preventing ischemic events, but it causes fewer major bleeding episodes. Bivalirudin is the anticoagulant of choice for the patient with acute coronary syndrome who has heparin-induced thrombocytopenia.

Direct-Acting Oral Anticoagulants

Adding a direct-acting oral anticoagulant (e.g., apixaban, rivaroxaban, and dabigatran) to a single antiplatelet agent appears to have little effect on bleeding or cardiovascular complications in patients with acute coronary syndrome. By comparison, adding one to dual antiplatelet therapy appears to increase significant bleeding about 2.2-fold with only a modest 14% reduction in adverse cardiac events.[A13] Factor Xa inhibition with low-dose rivaroxaban (2.5 mg twice daily) plus aspirin may be considered as a treatment option for maintenance treatment beyond 12 months after PCI for acute coronary syndrome inpatients at high thrombotic risk but without an increased risk for major or life-threatening bleeding.

Cholesterol Reduction

Prompt initiation of statin therapy is recommended in all patients with non–ST elevation acute coronary syndrome to promote plaque stabilization and to restore endothelial function. Moreover, when statin therapy is initiated during the patient's hospitalization (rather than at hospital discharge), long-term medical compliance is substantially improved. In the absence of contraindications, high-dose atorvastatin (40 to 80 mg daily) or rosuvastatin (20 to 40 mg daily) should be given orally regardless of the baseline serum low-density lipoprotein (LDL) cholesterol concentration. A lower dose is not as effective in reducing ischemic events, and the goal for LDL reduction is to 70 mg/dL or lower. If a statin alone does not achieve this goal, ezetimibe (10 mg daily) and/or an inhibitor of proprotein convertase subtilisin/kexin type 9 (e.g., alirocumab 300 mg or evolocumab 320 mg subcutaneously every 4 weeks; Chapter 190) should be added to achieve it. The addition of ezetimibe provides incremental benefit even in patients who have achieved an average LDL level of 70 mg/dL, especially if they have other high-risk characteristics such as diabetes or age over 70 years.[A14,A15]

Recurrent or Refractory Unstable Angina

In most patients hospitalized with non–ST elevation acute coronary syndrome, symptoms do not recur after the institution of appropriate antianginal therapy. The occasional patient with continued or recurrent chest pain despite optimal medical therapy is at high risk for an MI. For the patient with refractory myocardial ischemia or hemodynamic instability despite optimal medical therapy, intra-aortic balloon counterpulsation can reduce the incidence of ischemic episodes until revascularization can be performed. Intra-aortic balloon function is synchronized with the patient's ECG so that it inflates during diastole and deflates during systole, thereby augmenting coronary arterial blood flow and reducing myocardial oxygen demand by decreasing afterload. Intra-aortic balloon counterpulsation causes lower limb ischemia in approximately 3% of patients in whom the device is placed, but this complication usually resolves with its removal.

Coronary Revascularization

Coronary revascularization is performed to relieve angina that is persistent or recurrent despite optimal medical therapy, to prevent recurrent ischemia or MI in patients at high risk for a subsequent ischemic event, and to improve survival in patients with suitable coronary arterial anatomy.

Coronary revascularization is successful in relieving symptoms in 90% of the patients with angina refractory to medical therapy. Whether coronary bypass surgery or PCI is the more appropriate method of revascularization is determined by the location and severity of coronary arterial stenoses and the presence of comorbid medical conditions that may affect the performance or safety of the revascularization procedure (Chapter 59).

The patient who has been rendered symptom free with optimal medical therapy should undergo an assessment to determine whether he or she is at high risk or relatively low risk of sustaining a cardiac ischemic event (death, MI, or recurrent ischemia) in the ensuing days, weeks, and months and a bleeding complication from intensive medical therapy or an invasive cardiac procedure. Patients who are at low risk of having a subsequent ischemic event (those with a normal serum troponin concentration; age younger than 75 years; and zero, one, or two TIMI risk variables) should be evaluated noninvasively for inducible ischemia before hospital discharge. If the patient has spontaneous or provocable ischemia, coronary angiography and, if appropriate, revascularization should be performed.

The acute coronary syndrome patient with a detectable serum troponin concentration, age older than 75 years, or three or more TIMI risk variables is considered to be at high risk for a subsequent event and should be referred for routine coronary angiography and revascularization (if appropriate) during the hospitalization because this management strategy reduces the incidence of subsequent ischemic cardiac events.[A16] In most patients, early (within 24 hours of hospitalization) invasive therapy is no better at preventing death, MI, or stroke than somewhat delayed (median, 60 hours) invasive management,[A17] although it is associated with a modest decrease in the occurrence of recurrent ischemia. In contrast, in the one third of patients considered to be at very high risk (GRACE risk score of >140, corresponding to an incidence of in-hospital death or MI of >20%), an early invasive management strategy is superior to a delayed strategy in reducing the incidence of death, MI, or stroke. The benefit of an invasive strategy appears to extend even to patients over age 80 years.[15]

The patient with clinical features or noninvasive test results suggestive of severe coronary artery disease (i.e., left ventricular dysfunction, hemodynamic instability, life-threatening ventricular arrhythmias, or extensive inducible ischemia) should be referred for coronary angiography (Table 57-4) to determine if left main or three-vessel coronary arterial disease is present because patients with these coronary anatomic findings derive a survival benefit with coronary revascularization compared with medical therapy (Chapter 59). In patients who are taking a $P2Y_{12}$ ADP receptor inhibitor and in whom coronary artery bypass grafting can be delayed, the drug should be discontinued (5 days for clopidogrel or ticagrelor and at least 7 days for prasugrel) to allow dissipation of the antiplatelet effect. The timing of coronary bypass surgery in patients treated with a $P2Y_{12}$ ADP inhibitor should balance a potential increased risk of bleeding against the risks of delaying surgery.

For PCI, a single-stage complete revascularization is probably preferred compared with staged revascularization of the culprit artery immediately followed by other significant stenoses later (Chapter 59).[A18] Stenting can be performed safely at centers without on-site cardiac surgery.

Complications

Patients with non–ST elevation acute coronary syndrome can develop recurrent ischemic events or any of the complications associated with ST elevation MI, including arrhythmias, heart failure, and mechanical complications (Chapter 58). However, the acute complications other than recurrent ischemia occur less often in patients with non–ST elevation acute coronary syndrome because the amount of myocardial damage usually is less.

Because intensive medical therapy in conjunction with invasive management can lead to life-threatening bleeding complications, the patient's risk of such should be assessed before these therapies are instituted. Female gender, older age, renal insufficiency, low body weight, tachycardia, high or low systolic arterial pressure, anemia, and diabetes mellitus predict an increased risk of major bleeding, often due to excessive dosing of antiplatelet or anticoagulant agents. The bleeding risk can be estimated with the tool available at https://www.mdcalc.com/calc/1784/crusade-score-post-mi-bleeding-risk.

TABLE 57-4 SELECTION OF INITIAL TREATMENT STRATEGY: INVASIVE VERSUS CONSERVATIVE

GENERALLY PREFERRED STRATEGY	PATIENT CHARACTERISTICS
Invasive	Recurrent angina or ischemia at rest or with low-level activities despite intensive medical therapy Elevated troponin level New or presumably new ST segment depression Signs or symptoms of heart failure or new or worsening mitral regurgitation High-risk findings from noninvasive testing Hemodynamic instability Sustained ventricular tachycardia PCI within 6 months Previous CABG High-risk score (e.g., TIMI, GRACE) Mild to moderate renal dysfunction Diabetes mellitus Reduced left ventricular systolic function (EF <40%)
Conservative	Low-risk score (e.g., TIMI [0 or 1] or GRACE [<109]) Low-risk, troponin-negative female patients Patient or physician preference in the absence of high-risk features

CABG = coronary artery bypass grafting; EF = ejection fraction; GRACE = Global Registry of Acute Coronary Events; PCI = percutaneous coronary intervention; TIMI = Thrombolysis in Myocardial Infarction.

Integrated Approach to Treatment

Although the treatment of the patient with non–ST elevation acute coronary syndrome should be individualized, taking into account the specific features of the disease and the particular circumstances of the patient, algorithms nonetheless provide a useful framework (Fig. 57-3). Smoking cessation (Chapter 363), cholesterol lowering (Chapter 190), and control of blood pressure (Chapter 64), obesity, and diabetes mellitus (Chapter 210) are important long-term prevention strategies. A polypill strategy with aspirin (100 mg daily), ramipril (2.5 to 10 mg daily), and atorvastatin (20 to 40 mg daily) is preferred to usual care for preventing recurrent myocardial ischemic events.[A19] Maintaining adherence long term with medical therapy appears to reduce the risk of a future ischemic event by up to 80%.

PROGNOSIS

Because the number of ECG leads demonstrating ST segment depression and the magnitude of such depression are indicative of the extent and severity of myocardial ischemia and MI, it is not surprising that ST segment depression correlates with the patient's prognosis. Compared with patients without ST segment depression, the patient with non–ST elevation acute coronary syndrome who has ST segment depression of 1 mm or greater in two or more leads is almost four times as likely to die within 1 year, and the patient with ST segment depression of 2 mm or greater in magnitude is almost six times as likely to die within 1 year. If ST segment depression of 2 mm or greater is present in more than one region of the ECG, the mortality is increased 10-fold. Even the 20% of patients with acute coronary syndrome who have only 0.5 to 1 mm of ST segment depression have an adverse prognosis. Patients with ST segment depression also have a higher risk for subsequent cardiac events compared with patients with only T wave inversions (>1 mm).

The magnitude of the serum troponin concentration predicts short-term (30 days) and long-term (1 year) risks of recurrent MI and death, independent of ECG abnormalities or markers of inflammatory activity. Patients with a high-sensitivity troponin level <5 ng/L are at low risk for an event in the next 30 days, but risks increase progressively into higher levels even if the levels are stable and therefore not indicative of acute coronary syndrome.

C-reactive protein measured with a highly sensitive assay, which is a widely used marker of inflammation, has no role in the diagnosis of acute coronary syndrome but is predictive of long-term (6 months) mortality among patients with troponin-negative non–ST elevation acute coronary syndrome. Elevated serum concentrations of natriuretic peptides (B-type natriuretic peptide [BNP] or its N-terminal prohormone [NT-pro-BNP]) are associated with

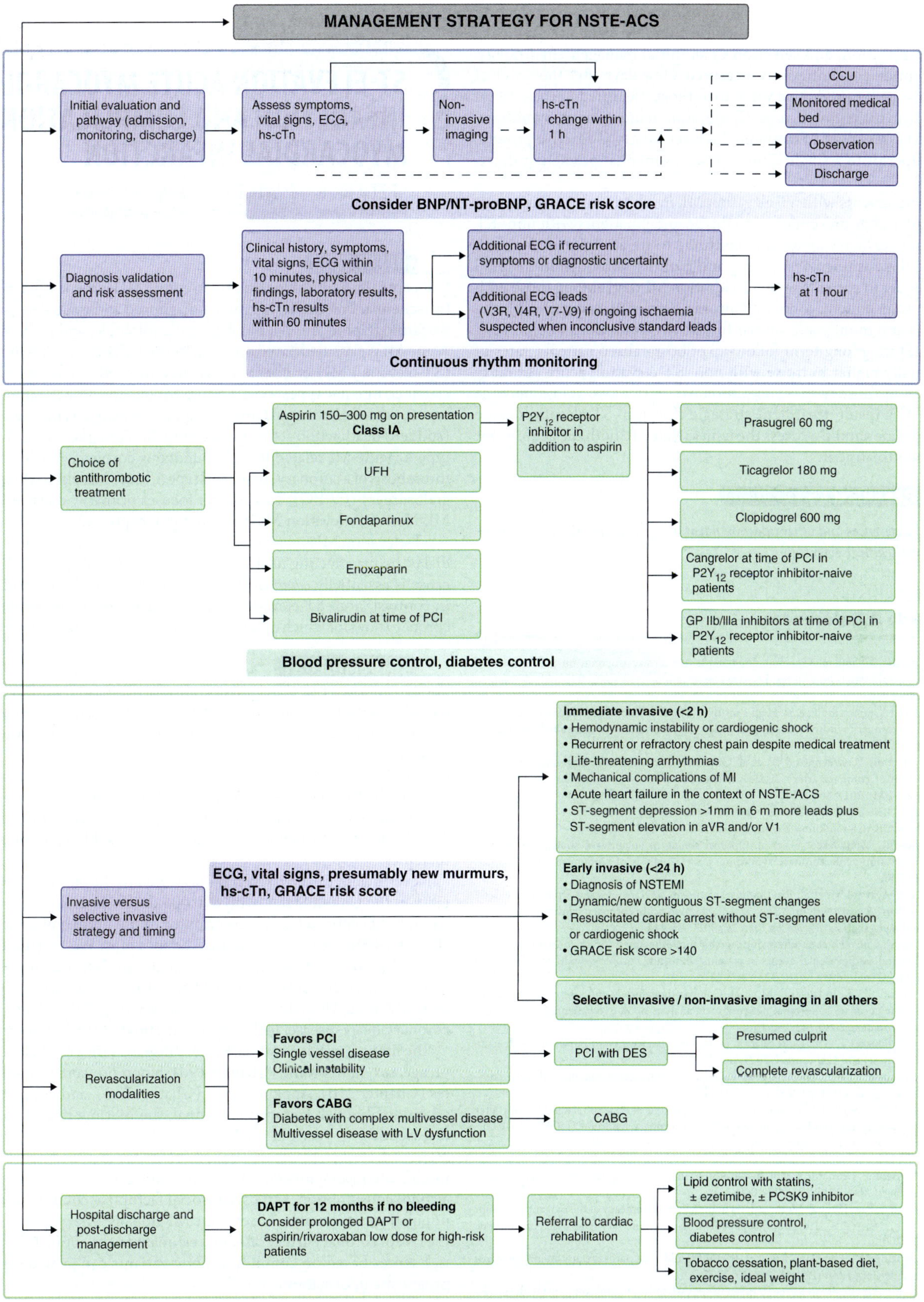

FIGURE 57-3. **Approach to the patient with non–ST elevation acute coronary syndrome (NSTE-ACS).** BNP = B-type natriuretic peptide; CABG = coronary artery bypass grafting; CCU = coronary care unit; DAPT = dual antiplatelet therapy; DES = drug-eluting stent; ECG = electrocardiogram/electrocardiography; GP = glycoprotein; GRACE = Global Registry of Acute Coronary Events; hs-cTn = high-sensitivity cardiac troponin; LV = left ventricular; MI = myocardial infarction; NSTE-ACS = non-ST elevation acute coronary syndrome; NSTEMI = non-ST elevation myocardial infarction; NT-proBNP = N-terminal pro-B-type natriuretic peptide; PCI = percutaneous coronary intervention; PCSK9 = proprotein convertase subtilisin kexin 9; UFH = unfractionated heparin. (Adapted from Collet JP, Thiele H, Barbato E, et al. ESC guidelines for the management of acute coronary syndromes in patients presenting without persistent ST-segment elevation. *Eur Heart J.* 2021;42:1289-1367.)

a three- to five-fold increased mortality in patients with non–ST elevation acute coronary syndrome, although they have limited value for diagnosis, initial risk stratification, and selection of an initial management strategy. Natriuretic peptide concentrations measured a few days after the onset of symptoms have better predictive value than those measured at the time of hospitalization. In patients with non–ST elevation acute coronary syndrome, a simultaneous assessment of troponin, high-sensitivity C-reactive protein, and BNP is superior to a single biomarker assessment at predicting short-term outcome.

In contrast to patients with ST elevation MI, in whom most events occur before or shortly after presentation to the hospital, patients with non–ST elevation acute coronary syndrome continue to be at high risk for such events during the ensuing days, weeks, and months. Although in-hospital mortality is higher in patients with ST elevation MI than among those with non–ST elevation acute coronary syndrome (7 vs. 5%, respectively), the mortality rates at 6 months are similar for the two conditions (12 vs. 13%, respectively). During long-term follow-up of hospitalized patients, rates of death are actually higher in those with non–ST elevation acute coronary syndrome than in those with ST elevation MI, with a two-fold difference after 4 years. As a result, treatment strategies for non–ST elevation acute coronary syndrome should address the issues related to both the acute event and longer-term treatment.

GENERAL REFERENCES

For the General References and other additional features, please visit Elsevier eBooks+ at https://ebooks.health.elsevier.com.

Grade A References

A1. Anand A, Lee KK, Chapman AR, et al. High-sensitivity cardiac troponin on presentation to rule out myocardial infarction: a stepped-wedge cluster randomized controlled trial. *Circulation.* 2021;143:2214-2224.

A2. Shah ASV, Anand A, Strachan FE, et al. High-sensitivity troponin in the evaluation of patients with suspected acute coronary syndrome: a stepped-wedge, cluster-randomised controlled trial. *Lancet.* 2018;392:919-928.

A3. Siontis GC, Mavridis D, Greenwood JP, et al. Outcomes of non-invasive diagnostic modalities for the detection of coronary artery disease: network meta-analysis of diagnostic randomised controlled trials. *BMJ.* 2018;360:1-14.

A4. Dee F, Savage L, Leitch JW, et al. Management of acute coronary syndromes in patients in rural Australia: The MORACS randomized clinical trial. *JAMA Cardiol.* 2022;7:690.

A5. Jobs A, Mehta SR, Montalescot G, et al. Optimal timing of an invasive strategy in patients with non-ST-elevation acute coronary syndrome: a meta-analysis of randomised trials. *Lancet.* 2017;390:737-746.

A6. Garg A, Garg L, Agarwal M, et al. Routine invasive versus selective invasive strategy in elderly patients older than 75 years with non-ST-segment elevation acute coronary syndrome: a systematic review and meta-analysis. *Mayo Clin Proc.* 2018;93:436-444.

A7. Kim BK, Hong SJ, Cho YH, et al. Effect of ticagrelor monotherapy vs ticagrelor with aspirin on major bleeding and cardiovascular events in patients with acute coronary syndrome: the TICO randomized clinical trial. *JAMA.* 2020;323:2407-2416.

A8. Navarese EP, Khan SU, Kołodziejczak M, et al. Comparative efficacy and safety of oral P2Y12 inhibitors in acute coronary syndrome: network meta-analysis of 52 816 patients from 12 randomized trials. *Circulation.* 2020;142:150-160.

A9. Shoji S, Kuno T, Fujisaki T, et al. De-escalation of dual antiplatelet therapy in patients with acute coronary syndromes. *J Am Coll Cardiol.* 2021;78:763-777.

A10. Schüpke S, Neumann F-J, Menichelli M, et al. Ticagrelor or prasugrel in patients with acute coronary syndromes. *N Engl J Med.* 2019;381:1524-1534.

A11. Kim HS, Kang J, Hwang D, et al. Prasugrel-based de-escalation of dual antiplatelet therapy after percutaneous coronary intervention in patients with acute coronary syndrome (HOST-REDUCE-POLYTECH-ACS): an open-label, multicentre, non-inferiority randomised trial. *Lancet.* 2020;396:1079-1089.

A12. Valgimigli M, Frigoli E, Leonardi S, et al. Bivalirudin or unfractionated heparin in acute coronary syndromes. *N Engl J Med.* 2015;373:997-1009.

A13. Khan SU, Arshad A, Riaz IB, et al. Meta-analysis of the safety and efficacy of the oral anticoagulant agents (apixaban, rivaroxaban, dabigatran) in patients with acute coronary syndrome. *Am J Cardiol.* 2018;121:301-307.

A14. Cannon CP, Blazing MA, Giugliano RP, et al. Ezetimibe added to statin therapy after acute coronary syndromes. *N Engl J Med.* 2015;372:2387-2397.

A15. Bach RG, Cannon CP, Giugliano RP, et al. Effect of simvastatin-ezetimibe compared with simvastatin monotherapy after acute coronary syndrome among patients 75 years or older: a secondary analysis of a randomized clinical trial. *JAMA Cardiol.* 2019;4:846-854.

A16. Tegn N, Abdelnoor M, Aaberge L, et al. Invasive versus conservative strategy in patients aged 80 years or older with non-ST-elevation myocardial infarction or unstable angina pectoris (after eighty study): an open-label randomised controlled trial. *Lancet.* 2016;387:1057-1065.

A17. Kofoed KF, Kelbaek H, Hansen PR, et al. Early versus standard care invasive examination and treatment of patients with non-ST-segment elevation acute coronary syndrome. *Circulation.* 2018;138:2741-2750.

A18. Gaffar R, Habib B, Filion KB, et al. Optimal timing of complete revascularization in acute coronary syndrome: a systematic review and meta-analysis. *J Am Heart Assoc.* 2017;6:1-11.

A19. Castellano JM, Pocock SJ, Bhatt DL, et al. Polypill strategy in secondary cardiovascular prevention. *N Engl J Med.* 2022;387:967-977.

58

ST-ELEVATION ACUTE MYOCARDIAL INFARCTION AND COMPLICATIONS OF MYOCARDIAL INFARCTION

FREDERICK G.P. WELT AND JAMES C. FANG

DEFINITION

Conceptually, acute myocardial infarction (MI) is myocardial necrosis caused by ischemia. Practically, MI can be diagnosed and evaluated by clinical, electrocardiographic (ECG), biochemical, radiologic, and pathologic methods. Acute MI is classified based on whether the ECG shows ST-segment elevation (ST-elevation MI) or not (non–ST-elevation MI). Acute MI can be further classified into five types: type 1, acute MI due to coronary atherothrombosis; type 2, acute MI due to a demand/supply mismatch; type 3, acute MI causing (sudden) death without the opportunity for biomarker or ECG confirmation; type 4, acute MI related to a percutaneous coronary intervention (PCI) or thrombosis of a coronary stent[1]; and type 5, acute MI related to coronary bypass graft surgery (CABG). This chapter focuses primarily on type 1 ST-elevation MI. Non–ST-elevation MI is covered in Chapter 57.

ST-elevation MI is characterized by profound ("transmural") acute myocardial ischemia affecting relatively larger areas of myocardium. The underlying cause is essentially *complete* interruption of regional myocardial blood flow. In contrast, non–ST-elevation MI is characterized by *incomplete* blockage of coronary flow, for which different acute therapies are appropriate (Chapter 57).

EPIDEMIOLOGY

The age-adjusted risk of hospitalization and death from cardiovascular disease and MI has declined since the 1960s. Data from Medicare beneficiaries show a continued reduction in rates of hospitalization for MI in patients over age 65 years.[2]

The declines in cardiovascular disease and MI have been particularly noteworthy for ST-elevation MI, with rates falling by two-thirds since 2008. ST-elevation MI currently comprises 25% or less of acute coronary syndromes. This decline is attributable to changing demographics, lifestyles, and medical therapies.

Nevertheless, cardiovascular disease remains the number one cause of mortality in the United States, with 690,000 deaths in 2020 (21% of all deaths), and it has become a leading contributor to the burden of disease worldwide (Chapter 40) as developing countries adopt a more Western lifestyle. Coronary artery disease is the leading cardiovascular disease, causing about 600,000 first acute MIs, 200,000 recurrent MIs, and an estimated 170,000 "silent" MIs annually in the United States. Each year, about 365,000 Americans die from coronary heart disease, including about 100,000 attributable to acute MI.

The lifetime risk for coronary artery disease varies dramatically depending on age, sex, lipid profile (Chapter 190), blood pressure (Chapter 64), diabetes (Chapter 210), smoking status (Chapter 363), and family history. When all modifiable risk factors are optimal, the lifetime risk of coronary artery disease for a 45-year-old is estimated to be less than 5%; with two or more major risk factors, by comparison, it is 50% for men and 31% for women. All modifiable risk factors combined (including obesity, diet, physical activity, alcohol consumption, and psychosocial factors) account for over 90% of the population-attributable risk of acute MI globally. The genetic contribution to the risk of coronary artery disease is estimated to be about 40%, and polygenic risk scores based on common genetic variants can provide supplementary prognostic information.

Pathobiology

The usual initiating mechanism of acute MI is fissure or rupture of a vulnerable, lipid-laden atherosclerotic coronary plaque, thereby resulting in exposure of circulating blood to highly thrombogenic plaque core and matrix materials (Chapter 41). Based on both postmortem pathologic techniques and in vivo optical coherence tomography, up to one third of acute MIs may be due to superficial erosion of fibrous caps both in lesions with necrotic cores and in lesions that are predominantly fibrocellular (Chapter 41). A minority of lesions responsible for MI are characterized as a calcified nodule that fractures.[3] Regardless of the initiating insult, platelets adhere, are activated, and aggregate at the site of injury. Thrombin is generated, thereby accelerating platelet activation, and the resulting fibrin traps red blood cells and leads to the formation of thrombus. A totally occluding thrombus typically leads to ST-elevation MI. By comparison, partial occlusion, or occlusion in the presence of collateral circulation, results in a non–ST-segment elevation acute coronary syndrome, often with ST depression or T-wave inversion (Chapter 57). Ischemia resulting from reduced coronary flow leads to myocardial cell injury or death, ventricular dysfunction, and cardiac arrhythmias. Myocardial necrosis begins after as little as 15 to 20 minutes of coronary occlusion and proceeds rapidly in a wave front from endocardium to epicardium. Partial myocardial salvage can be achieved by reperfusion within 3 to 6 hours, the degree of salvage being inversely proportional to the duration and extent of ischemia. The extent of myocardial necrosis also depends on metabolic demand and collateral blood supply.

About 10% of acute MIs are caused by conditions other than critical epicardial coronary atherosclerosis.[4] These other mechanisms include microvascular disease, endothelial dysfunction, coronary artery dissection,[5,6] coronary emboli, in situ thrombosis, vasculitis, primary vasospasm, infiltrative or degenerative disease, diseases of the aorta, congenital anomalies of a coronary artery, or trauma (Table 58-1).

CLINICAL MANIFESTATIONS

History

Acute MI may present with typical ischemic-type chest discomfort or atypically with dyspnea, nausea, epigastric discomfort, malaise, and/or unexplained weakness. Ischemic-type chest discomfort, usually the most prominent clinical symptom in acute MI, is perceived as a persistent (>10-20 minutes), diffuse, deep, and heavy retrosternal pressure or burning sensation; it rarely is perceived as sharp pain and generally not as stabbing pain (see Table 39-2 in Chapter 39). The discomfort associated with acute MI is qualitatively similar to that of angina pectoris but more severe and persistent (Chapters 39 and 56).

The primary location of typical ischemic pain is most consistently retrosternal, but it also can present left parasternal, left precordial, or across the anterior chest (Chapter 39). On occasion, discomfort is predominantly perceived in the anterior neck, jaw, arms, or epigastrium. It generally is somewhat diffuse; highly localized pain (finger point) is rarely angina or acute MI. The most characteristic pattern of radiation is to the left arm, but the right arm or both arms can be involved. The shoulders, neck, jaw, teeth, epigastrium, and interscapular areas also are sites of radiation. Discomfort above the jaws or below the umbilicus is not typical of acute MI. Associated symptoms often include nausea, vomiting, diaphoresis, weakness, dyspnea, restlessness, and apprehension.

The discomfort of acute MI is not reliably relieved by rest or nitroglycerin. The onset of acute MI usually is unrelated to exercise or other apparent precipitating factors. Nevertheless, acute MI may begin during or within a few hours following physical or emotional stress and is more common in this situation than is explained by chance.

It is estimated that at least 20% of acute MIs are painless ("silent") or atypical (unrecognized). Elderly patients, especially women, and patients with diabetes are particularly prone to painless or atypical MI, which is the presentation of MI in as many as one third to one half of such patients. Because the prognosis is worse in elderly and diabetic patients, diagnostic vigilance is required. In these patients, acute MI can be manifested as sudden dyspnea (which can progress to pulmonary edema), weakness, lightheadedness, nausea, and vomiting. Confusional states, sudden loss of consciousness, a new rhythm disorder, and an unexplained fall in blood pressure are other uncommon presentations. The differential diagnosis of ischemic chest discomfort also should include gastrointestinal disorders (e.g., reflux esophagitis; Chapter 124), musculoskeletal pain (e.g., costochondritis), anxiety or panic attacks, pleurisy or pulmonary embolism (Chapter 68), and acute aortic dissection (see Table 39-2 in Chapter 39 and Chapter 63).

Physical Examination

No physical findings are diagnostic or pathognomonic of acute MI. The physical examination often is entirely normal or may reveal only nonspecific abnormalities. An S_4 gallop frequently is found if it is carefully sought. Blood pressure often is initially elevated, but it may be normal or low. Signs of sympathetic hyperactivity (tachycardia, hypertension, diaphoresis, or any combination of these three) often accompany anterior wall MI, whereas parasympathetic hyperactivity (bradycardia, hypotension, or both) is more common with inferior wall MI.

The examination is best focused on an overall assessment of cardiac function. Adequacy of vital signs and peripheral perfusion should be noted. Signs of cardiac failure, both left and right sided (e.g., S_3 gallop, pulmonary congestion, elevated neck veins), should be sought, and observation for arrhythmias and mechanical complications (e.g., new murmurs) is essential. If hypoperfusion is present, determination of its primary cause (e.g., hypovolemia, right-sided heart failure, left-sided heart failure) is critical to management.

DIAGNOSIS

The diagnosis of acute MI has traditionally rested on the triad of ischemic-type chest discomfort, electrocardiographic abnormalities, and elevated serum cardiac biomarkers of necrosis. Acute MI was considered present when at least two of the three were present. With their increasing sensitivity and specificity, serum cardiac troponin levels (i.e., troponin I [TnI] and troponin T [TnT])

TABLE 58-1 CONDITIONS OTHER THAN CORONARY ATHEROSCLEROSIS THAT CAN CAUSE ACUTE MYOCARDIAL INFARCTION

Coronary emboli	Causes include aortic or mitral valve lesions, left atrial or ventricular thrombi, prosthetic valves, fat emboli, intracardiac neoplasms, infective endocarditis, and paradoxical emboli
Thrombotic coronary artery disease	Can occur with oral contraceptive use, sickle cell anemia and other hemoglobinopathies, polycythemia vera, thrombocytosis, thrombotic thrombocytopenic purpura, disseminated intravascular coagulation, antithrombin III deficiency and other hypercoagulable states, macroglobulinemia and other hyperviscosity states, multiple myeloma, leukemia, malaria, and fibrinolytic system shutdown secondary to impaired plasminogen activation or excessive inhibition
Coronary vasculitis	Seen with Takayasu disease, Kawasaki disease, polyarteritis nodosa, lupus erythematosus, scleroderma, rheumatoid arthritis, and immune-mediated vascular degeneration in cardiac allografts
Coronary vasospasm	Can be associated with variant angina, nitrate withdrawal, cocaine or amphetamine abuse, and angina with "normal" coronary arteries
Infiltrative and degenerative coronary vascular disease	Can result from amyloidosis, connective tissue disorders (e.g., pseudoxanthoma elasticum), lipid storage disorders and mucopolysaccharidoses, homocystinuria, diabetes mellitus, collagen vascular disease, muscular dystrophies, and Friedreich ataxia
Spontaneous coronary dissection	Over 90% of cases occur in younger women. The dominant predisposing cause is fibromuscular dysplasia (Chapter 63); other causes include various arteriopathies and pregnancy-related conditions. Precipitating factors include extreme physical and emotional stressors, intense hormonal therapy, and labor, delivery, and postpartum status. About 50% of cases present as an ST-elevation myocardial infarction, and the estimated 10-year rate of subsequent major adverse cardiac events is about 50%.
Coronary ostial occlusion	Associated with aortic dissection, luetic aortitis, aortic stenosis, and ankylosing spondylitis syndromes
Congenital coronary anomalies	Including Bland-White-Garland syndrome of anomalous origin of the left coronary artery from the pulmonary artery, left coronary artery origin from the anterior sinus of Valsalva, coronary arteriovenous fistula or aneurysms, and myocardial bridging with secondary vascular degeneration
Trauma	Associated with and responsible for coronary dissection, laceration, or thrombosis (with endothelial damage secondary to trauma such as angioplasty) and direct myocardial injury with radiation and cardiac contusion
Augmented myocardial oxygen requirements exceeding oxygen delivery	Encountered with aortic stenosis, aortic insufficiency, hypertension with severe left ventricular hypertrophy, pheochromocytoma, thyrotoxicosis, methemoglobinemia, carbon monoxide poisoning, shock, and hyperviscosity syndromes

have assumed a dominant role in confirming the diagnosis of acute MI in patients with suggestive clinical or electrocardiographic features.

Electrocardiography

In patients with a possible acute MI, a 12-lead ECG should be obtained immediately, with a goal of less than 10 minutes after arrival at a health care facility. Although the initial ECG is neither perfectly sensitive nor specific in patients who develop acute ST-elevation MI, it plays a critical role in initial stratification, triage, and management (Chapter 39).[7] In an appropriate clinical setting, a pattern of ST-segment elevation of 2 mm (0.2 mV) or more at the J point in V_2 to V_3 in men or 1.5 mm (0.15 mV) or more in women in the absence of left ventricular (LV) hypertrophy or 1 mm (0.1 mV) or more in two or more other contiguous chest or limb leads suggests coronary occlusion causing marked myocardial ischemia. In such patients, emergency reperfusion (primary angioplasty or fibrinolysis) should be performed unless it is contraindicated. Hyperacute T-wave changes may suggest the diagnosis in the early phase of ST-elevation MI before the onset of ST elevation. A new or presumably new left bundle branch block, which may obscure ST elevation analysis, may suggest an ST-elevation MI equivalent in the appropriate clinical setting. ST depression in two or more precordial leads V_1 to V_4 may indicate transmural posterior injury due to occlusion of the left circumflex coronary artery; extending ECG analysis to leads V_7 to V_9 (i.e., over the left posterior chest) can help confirm this diagnosis. Other ECG patterns (ST-segment depression, T-wave inversion, nonspecific changes, normal ECG) in association with ischemic chest discomfort are consistent with a non–ST-segment elevation acute coronary syndrome and are treated with different triage and initial management strategies (Chapter 57).

Electrocardiographic Evolution

Serial ECG tracings improve the sensitivity and specificity of the ECG for the diagnosis of acute MI and assist in assessing the outcomes of therapy. When typical ST-segment elevation persists for hours and is followed within hours to days by T-wave inversions and Q waves, the diagnosis of acute MI can be made with virtual certainty. The ECG changes in acute ST-elevation MI evolve through three overlapping phases: hyperacute or early acute, evolved acute, and chronic (stabilized).

Early Acute Phase

This earliest phase begins within minutes, persists, and evolves during hours. T waves increase in amplitude and widen over the area of injury (hyperacute pattern). ST segments evolve from concave to straightened to convex upward patterns (acute pattern). When prominent, the acute injury pattern of blended ST-T waves can take on a tombstone appearance (Figs. 58-1 and 58-2). ST-segment depressions that occur in leads opposite those with ST-segment elevation are known as reciprocal changes and are associated with larger areas of injury and a worse prognosis but also with greater potential for benefit from reperfusion therapy.

Other causes of ST-segment elevation must be considered and excluded (Table 58-2). These conditions include pericarditis (Chapter 62), left ventricular hypertrophy with J point elevation, and normal variant early repolarization (Chapter 42). Pericarditis (or perimyocarditis) is of particular concern because it can mimic acute MI clinically, but fibrinolytic therapy is *not* indicated and can be hazardous.

Evolved Acute Phase

During the second phase, ST-segment elevation begins to regress, T waves in leads with ST-segment elevation become inverted, and pathologic Q or QS

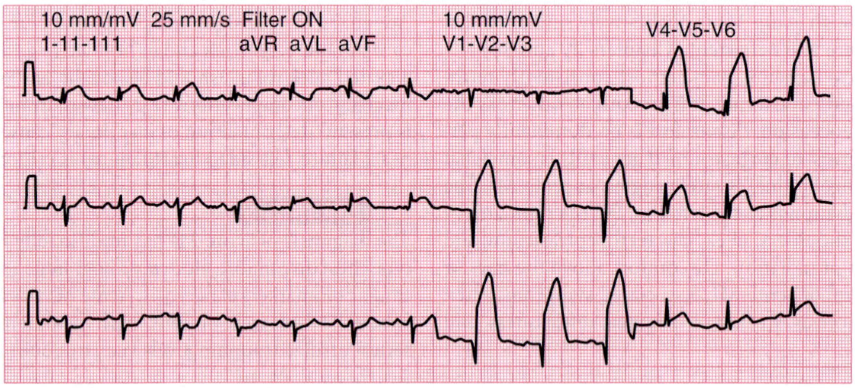

FIGURE 58-1. **Electrocardiographic tracing shows an acute anterolateral myocardial infarction.** Note ST-segment elevation in leads I, aVL, and V_1 to V_6 with Q waves in V_1 to V_4.

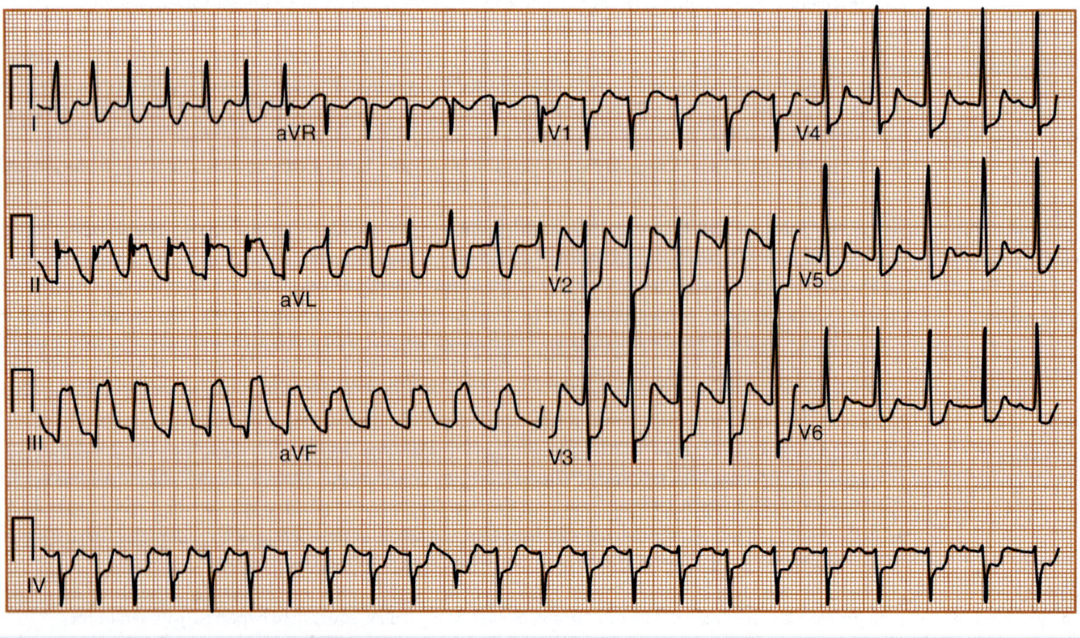

FIGURE 58-2. **Electrocardiographic tracing shows an acute inferoposterior myocardial infarction.**

TABLE 58-2 CONDITIONS THAT CAN MIMIC ST-SEGMENT ELEVATION MYOCARDIAL INFARCTION

Early repolarization with noncoronary chest pain
Myocarditis
Pericarditis
Takotsubo syndrome (stress cardiomyopathy)
Hyperkalemia
Brugada syndrome

waves become fully developed (>0.03-second duration or depth >30% of R wave amplitude or both).

Chronic Phase

Resolution of ST-segment elevation is variable. Resolution is usually complete within 2 weeks of inferior MI, but it can be delayed further after anterior MI. Persistent ST-segment elevation, often seen with a large anterior MI, is indicative of a large area of akinesis, dyskinesis, or ventricular aneurysm. Symmetrical T-wave inversions can resolve during weeks to months or can persist for an indefinite period; hence, the age of an MI in the presence of T-wave inversions is often termed indeterminate. Q waves usually do not resolve after anterior MI but often disappear after inferior wall MI.

Early reperfusion therapy accelerates the time course of ECG changes to minutes or hours instead of days to weeks. ST segments recede rapidly, T-wave inversions and loss of R waves occur earlier, and Q waves may not develop or progress and occasionally may regress. Indeed, failure of ST-segment elevation to resolve by more than 50 to 70% within 1 to 2 hours suggests failure of fibrinolysis and should prompt referral for urgent angiography and consideration of "rescue angioplasty."

True Posterior Myocardial Infarction and Left Circumflex Myocardial Infarction Patterns

True posterior MI presents a mirror-image pattern of ECG injury in leads V_1 to V_2 to V_4 (Fig. 58-2). The location of injury of an isolated true posterior MI by magnetic resonance imaging actually involves portions of the lateral left ventricular wall and is typically caused by occlusion of a nondominant left circumflex artery. In the precordial leads, the acute phase is characterized by ST-segment depression rather than by ST-segment elevation. The evolved and chronic phases show increased R wave amplitude and widening instead of Q waves. Recognition of an isolated true posterior acute MI pattern is challenging but important because the diagnosis should lead to an immediate reperfusion strategy. Extending the ECG to measure left posterior leads V_7 to V_9 increases sensitivity for detection of acute left circumflex–related injury patterns (i.e., ST-segment elevation) with excellent specificity (Chapter 42). Other causes of prominent upright anteroseptal forces include right ventricular hypertrophy, ventricular preexcitation variants (Wolff-Parkinson-White syndrome; Chapter 52), cardiomyopathies, right bundle branch block, and normal variants with early R wave progression. New appearance of these changes or the association with an acute or evolving inferior MI usually allows the diagnosis to be made.

Right Ventricular Infarction

Proximal occlusion of the right coronary artery before the acute marginal branch can cause right ventricular infarction as well as acute inferior MI in about 30% of cases. Because the prognosis and treatment of acute inferior MI differ in the presence of right ventricular infarction, it is important to make this diagnosis. The diagnosis is assisted by obtaining right precordial ECG leads, which are routinely indicated for inferior acute MI (Chapter 42). Acute ST-segment elevation of at least 1 mm (0.1 mV) in one or more leads V_4R to V_6R is both sensitive and specific (>90%) for identifying acute right ventricular injury, and Q or QS waves effectively identify right ventricular infarction.

Diagnosis in the Presence of Bundle Branch Block

The presence of left bundle branch block often obscures ST-segment analysis in patients with suspected acute MI. The presence of a new (or presumed new) left bundle branch block in association with clinical (and laboratory) findings suggesting acute MI is associated with high mortality; patients with new-onset left bundle branch block benefit substantially from reperfusion therapy and should undergo triage and treatment in the same way as patients with ST-elevation MI do. Certain ECG patterns, although relatively insensitive, suggest acute MI if they are present in the setting of left bundle branch block: Q waves in two of leads I, aVL, V_5, and V_6; R wave regression from V_1 to V_4; ST-segment elevation of 1 mm or more in leads with a positive QRS complex; ST-segment depression of 1 mm or more in leads V_1, V_2, or V_3; and ST-segment elevation of 5 mm or more associated with a negative QRS complex. The presence of right bundle branch block usually does not mask typical ST-T wave or Q wave changes except in rare cases of isolated true posterior acute MI, which are characterized by tall right precordial R waves and ST-segment depressions.

TABLE 58-3 NON–MYOCARDIAL INFARCTION CAUSES OF AN ELEVATED TROPONIN LEVEL

OTHER CARDIAC CAUSES
Myocardial injury: cardiac contusion, surgery, ablation, shocks
Myocardial inflammation: myocarditis, pericarditis
Heart failure
Cardiomyopathies: infiltrative, stress, hypertensive, hypertrophic
Aortic dissection
Severe aortic stenosis
Tachycardias
PULMONARY CAUSES
Pulmonary embolism
Pulmonary hypertension
Respiratory failure
NEUROLOGIC CAUSES
Stroke
Intracranial hemorrhage
OTHER
Shock: septic, hypovolemic, cardiogenic
Renal failure

Modified from Thygesen K, Alpert JS, Jaffe AS, et al. Fourth universal definition of myocardial infarction. *Circulation*. 2018;138:e618-e651.

Differential Diagnosis

Although ST-elevation MI is often an easy diagnosis to make on the basis of the presentation and test results (see later), other considerations include acute pericarditis (Chapter 62), acute myocarditis (Chapter 47), stress-induced cardiomyopathy (takotsubo syndrome) (Chapter 47), hyperkalemia, and early repolarization (see Table 58-2). All but early repolarization can be associated with abnormal biomarkers, but none are associated with a coronary occlusion. Early coronary angiography is advised when the cause of ST-segment elevation is unclear (see Table 58-1).

Serum Cardiac Biomarkers of Necrosis

Cardiac-derived troponin-I and troponin-T are proteins specific to sarcomeres. Serial measurement of cardiac troponins is the preferred biomarker approach for differentiating acute MI from unstable angina and non-acute coronary syndromes. In the appropriate clinical setting, acute MI is indicated by a rising and/or falling pattern of troponin, with one or more value(s) above the 99th percentile upper reference limit. High-sensitivity troponin assays can greatly reduce the likelihood of acute MI after a single negative sample and effectively exclude MI in 1 to 2 hours.[8] Such testing has increased the ability to diagnose type 1 MIs (attributable to atherothrombotic events) as well as type 2 MIs (attributable to acute imbalances in myocardial oxygen supply and demand). However, high-sensitivity assays also can lead to an increasing number of false-positive diagnoses of acute MI, because they sometimes can detect increased troponin levels in a number of non-MI settings: myocarditis (Chapter 47); other causes of cardiac injury, such as cardiac, renal, and respiratory failure (Chapter 90); stroke (Chapter 376) and intracranial hemorrhage (Chapter 377); septic shock (Chapter 94); and chronic structural heart diseases (Chapter 56; Table 58-3).[9] As a result, the clinician always must consider the clinical context as well as the finding of a temporal rise and fall of troponin levels.

High-sensitivity troponin assays measure troponin-T, which can be elevated in patients with renal failure (Chapter 117); in this situation, a troponin-I measurement, if available, is preferred. Troponin levels are maximally sensitive at 8 to 12 hours, peak at 10 to 24 hours, and persist for 5 to 14 days. This persistence poses a challenge for the diagnosis of an early recurrent MI, for which the measurement of more rapidly cleared MB isoenzyme of creatine kinase (CK-MB) can be useful.

Other Laboratory Tests

On admission, routine assessment of complete blood count and platelet count, standard blood chemistry studies, a lipid panel, and coagulation tests (prothrombin time, partial thromboplastin time) are useful. Results assist in assessing comorbid conditions and prognosis and in guiding therapy. Hematologic tests provide a useful baseline before initiation of antiplatelet, anticoagulant, and fibrinolytic therapy or coronary angiography or angioplasty. Myocardial injury precipitates polymorphonuclear leukocytosis, thereby commonly resulting in an elevation of the white blood cell count to up to 12,000 to 15,000/µL, which appears within a few hours and peaks at 2 to 4 days. The metabolic panel provides a useful check on electrolytes, glucose, and renal function.

Serum lipid levels may fall in the first 24 to 48 hours after an MI, but a fasting lipid panel is recommended as a baseline for lipid-lowering (statin) therapy (Chapter 190). Unless carbon dioxide retention is suspected, finger oximetry is adequate to diagnose hypoxemia and titrate oxygen therapy. B-type natriuretic peptide, which increases with ventricular wall stress and relative circulatory fluid overload, may provide useful incremental prognostic information in the setting of acute MI.

Imaging

The rapid triage of ST-elevation MI patients to reperfusion therapy, most often for coronary angiography with intent to perform percutaneous intervention (PCI), should not be delayed by routine imaging studies. A chest radiograph is the only imaging test routinely considered in the emergency department for ST-elevation MI, and its usefulness is limited to selected patients with a concern for findings that might affect initial management. Although the chest radiograph is often normal, findings of pulmonary venous congestion, cardiomegaly, or a widened mediastinum can contribute importantly to diagnosis and management decisions. For example, a history of severe, "tearing" chest and back pain in association with a widened mediastinum should raise the question of a dissecting aortic aneurysm (Chapter 63). In such cases, fibrinolytic therapy must be withheld pending more definitive diagnostic imaging of the aorta, and the approach to angiography may be modified. Other noninvasive imaging (e.g., echocardiography [Chapter 43], cardiac nuclear scanning [Chapter 44], and other testing) may be performed later during the course of hospitalization to evaluate specific clinical issues, including suspected complications of acute MI, or for predischarge risk stratification. Coronary angiography (Chapter 59) is performed urgently as part of an interventional strategy for ST-elevation MI or later for risk stratification in higher-risk patients who are initially managed medically.

Echocardiography

Two-dimensional transthoracic echocardiography with color flow Doppler imaging is the most generally useful noninvasive test obtained during the hospital course (Chapter 43). Echocardiography efficiently assesses global and regional cardiac function and enables the clinician to evaluate suspected complications of acute MI. The sensitivity and specificity of echocardiography for regional wall motion assessment are high (>90%), although the age of the abnormality (new vs. old) must be distinguished clinically or by electrocardiography. Echocardiography is helpful in determining the cause of circulatory failure with hypotension (relative hypovolemia, left ventricular failure, right ventricular failure, or mechanical complication of acute MI). Echocardiography also can assist in differentiating pericarditis and perimyocarditis from acute MI. Doppler echocardiography is indicated to evaluate a new murmur and other suspected mechanical complications of acute MI (e.g., papillary muscle dysfunction or rupture, acute ventricular septal defect, and left ventricular free wall rupture with tamponade or pseudoaneurysm). Later in the course of acute MI, echocardiography may be used to assess the degree of recovery of stunned myocardium after reperfusion therapy, the degree of residual cardiac dysfunction and indications for angiotensin-converting enzyme (ACE) inhibitors and other therapies for heart failure, and the presence of left ventricular aneurysm and mural thrombus (requiring oral anticoagulants).

Radionuclide, Magnetic Resonance, and Other Imaging Studies

Radionuclide techniques generally are too time-consuming and cumbersome for routine use in the acute setting of definite or probable acute MI. More commonly, they are used in risk stratification before or after hospital discharge to augment exercise or pharmacologic stress testing (Chapter 44). Thallium Tl 201 or technetium Tc 99 m sestamibi nuclear scans or rubidium Rb 82 positron emission tomography scans can assess myocardial perfusion and viability as well as infarct size. Cardiac magnetic resonance imaging (Chapter 44) with late gadolinium enhancement also can assess infarct size as well as myocardial function during the convalescent phase. Computed tomography and magnetic resonance imaging also can be useful to evaluate patients with a suspected dissecting aortic aneurysm (Chapter 63). When a nonatherosclerotic cause of myocardial necrosis is suspected (e.g., perimyocarditis simulating acute MI), contemporary multislice (e.g., 64-256 slice) coronary computed tomography can assess coronary artery disease qualitatively and semiquantitatively as well as distinguish other causes of chest pain syndromes (Chapters 39 and 44).

TREATMENT

Prehospital Phase

Prehospital cardiac arrest (Chapter 50) and extensive necrosis are major causes of acute MI-associated morbidity and mortality. The first hour after the onset of symptoms represents the best opportunity for myocardial salvage with reperfusion therapy. Thus the primary goals of prehospital care are to recognize symptoms promptly and seek medical attention, deploy an emergency medical system trained in emergency cardiac care, and transport the patient expeditiously to a medical facility capable of advanced coronary care, including reperfusion therapy (primary PCI or fibrinolysis).[10] Guidelines set an average system time goal for first medical contact-to-device of 90 minutes or less. For patients who initially arrive at or are transported to a non–PCI-capable hospital, the system time goal to device is 120 minutes or less. The greatest time lag to reperfusion therapy is the patient's delay in calling for help. Public education efforts aimed at reducing this delay have yielded mixed results, and innovative approaches are needed.

Expert emergency medical system teams perform prehospital ECGs, communicate preliminary diagnoses, and transport patients preferentially to a PCI-capable hospital where an ST-elevation MI team is on alert. This approach results in more rapid primary PCI (average savings of about 15 minutes) and superior clinical outcomes. Direct triage to the catheterization laboratory rather than to the emergency department also may decrease time to reperfusion. However, as many as one third of initial activations of the ST-elevation MI-team may be false positives.

Aspirin (162 to 325 mg, chewed) and sublingual nitroglycerin (0.4 mg every 5 minutes for up to three doses) are administered at first medical contact where appropriate. Administering fibrinolytic therapy in the field by physician-directed systems is feasible when the expected transit time is long (i.e., >120 min), but this practice is rare in the United States. Prehospital antiplatelet therapy of ST-elevation MI patients with ticagrelor does not improve pre-PCI coronary reperfusion.

Emergency Department Phase

The goals of emergency department care are to identify patients with acute myocardial ischemia rapidly, to stratify them into acute ST-elevation MI versus other acute coronary syndromes (Fig. 58-3), to initiate a reperfusion strategy and other appropriate medical care, to assess risk (E-Fig. 58-1), and to triage them rapidly to inpatient care (patients with suspected acute coronary syndrome) or outpatient care (patients without suspected ischemia; see Fig. 57-2).

The evaluation of patients with chest pain and other suspected acute coronary syndromes begins with a 12-lead ECG (with a goal of within 10 minutes of hospital arrival) and continues with a focused history and a targeted physical examination. Continuous ECG monitoring is started, an intravenous line is established, and admission blood tests are drawn (including a troponin level). As rapidly as possible, the patient is stratified into acute ST-elevation MI, likely or definite non–ST-elevation acute coronary syndrome, possible non–ST-elevation acute coronary syndrome (Chapter 57), or noncardiac chest pain categories.

Emergent Therapeutic Measures and Early Inpatient Care

Although troponin assays are the "gold standard" for detecting myocardial necrosis, the decision to proceed with urgent reperfusion (primary angioplasty or fibrinolysis) in ST-elevation MI should be based on the patient's clinical history, and the initial ECG and not be delayed by troponin testing. Coronary reperfusion is accomplished by primary PCI (angioplasty and stenting) or by intravenous fibrinolytic therapy.[11]

Primary PCI

Prompt PCI (with a goal of <90 minutes from first medical contact) is the preferred approach at PCI-capable hospitals for ST-elevation MI patients within 12 hours of the onset of symptoms and is reasonable for ECG and clinical evidence of ongoing ischemia within 12 to 24 hours after the onset of symptoms (Table 58-4). The preferred access site for emergent PCI is the radial artery,[A1] because it results in lower mortality as well as less bleeding compared with a femoral artery approach. Primary PCI also is indicated in patients with cardiogenic shock (Chapter 93) or severe acute heart failure regardless of time delay. Advantages of primary PCI over fibrinolysis include lower rates of early mortality, reinfarction, and intracranial hemorrhage.[A2]

Current guidelines for ST-elevation MI support implantation of advanced-generation drug-eluting stents to provide the best outcomes.[A3] Aspiration thrombectomy does not provide incremental benefit[A4] and is not indicated as a routine strategy.

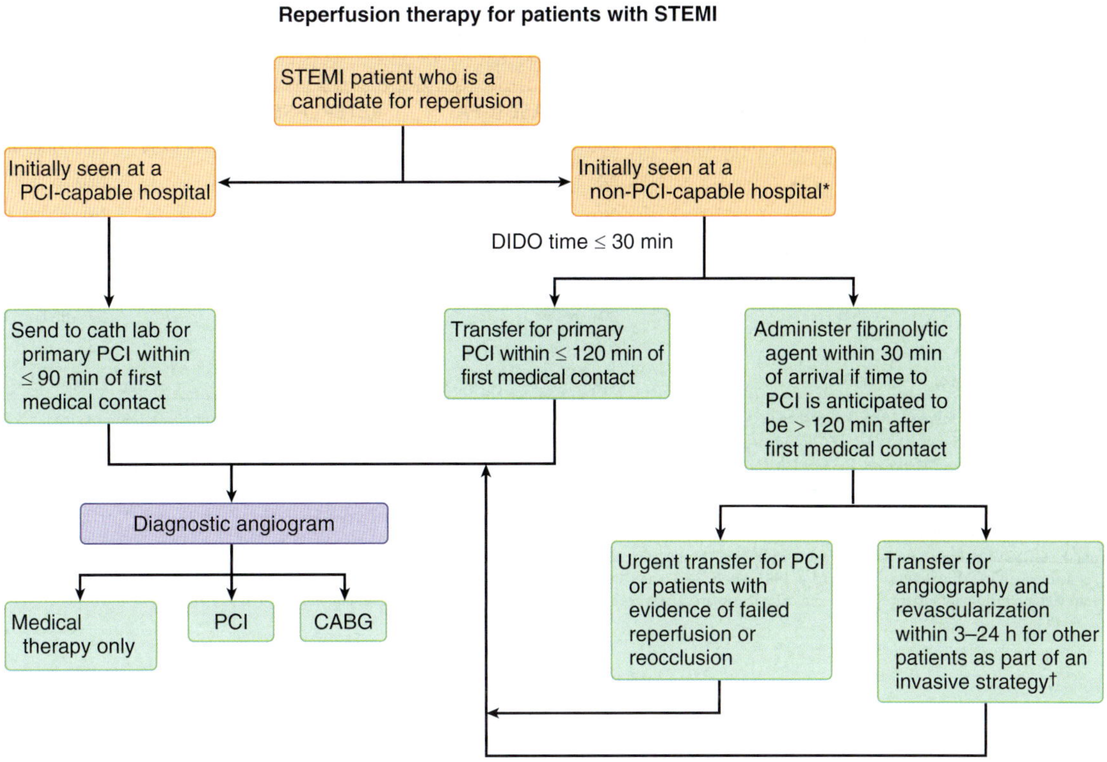

FIGURE 58-3. **Reperfusion therapy for patients with ST-segment elevation myocardial infarction (STEMI).** All eligible STEMI patients also are treated with dual antiplatelet therapy and an anticoagulant on admission (see text). *Patients with cardiogenic shock or severe heart failure initially seen at a non–PCI-capable hospital should be transferred for cardiac catheterization and revascularization as soon as possible, irrespective of time delay from the onset of the myocardial infarction. †Angiography and revascularization should not be performed within the first 2 to 3 hours after administration of fibrinolytic therapy. CABG = coronary artery bypass grafting; DIDO = door in–door out; PCI = percutaneous coronary intervention. (Modified from O'Gara PT, Kushner FG, Ascheim DD, et al. 2013 ACCF/AHA guideline for the management of ST-elevation myocardial infarction: a report of the American College of Cardiology/American Heart Association Task Force on Practice Guidelines. *Circulation*. 2013;127:e362-e425.)

TABLE 58-4 INDICATIONS FOR PRIMARY ANGIOPLASTY AND COMPARISON WITH FIBRINOLYTIC THERAPY

INDICATIONS
A preferred reperfusion strategy for ST segment elevation or LBBB acute MI within 12 hours of symptom onset (or >12 hours if symptoms persist)
Cardiogenic shock developing within 36 hours of ST-segment elevation/Q wave acute MI or LBBB acute MI in patients <75 years old who can be revascularized within 18 hours of the onset of shock
Recommended at centers performing >400 PCIs/year with backup cardiac surgery and for operators performing >75 PCIs/year
Primary PCI can be performed at centers without on-site cardiac surgery if performed on carefully selected patients by experienced operators and if arrangements are in place for rapid transfer to a surgery-capable center when needed
ADVANTAGES OF PRIMARY PCI
Higher initial reperfusion rates
Reduced risk of intracerebral hemorrhage
Less residual stenosis; less recurrent ischemia or infarction
Usefulness when fibrinolysis is contraindicated
Improvement in outcomes with cardiogenic shock
Evaluation of total burden of coronary artery disease
DISADVANTAGES OF PRIMARY PCI (COMPARED WITH FIBRINOLYTIC THERAPY)
Access, advantages restricted to high-volume centers and operators
Longer average time to treatment
Greater dependence on operators for results
Higher system complexity and costs

LBBB = left bundle branch block; MI = myocardial infarction; PCI = percutaneous coronary intervention (includes balloon angioplasty, stenting).

Randomized trials support that the emergent PCI address not only the infarct-related artery but also significant stenoses in "nonculprit" arteries,[A5] either at the time of the initial procedure or within the next month or so,[A6,A7] except in patients who are in cardiogenic shock.[A8] Such an approach reduces the need for repeat revascularization and also lowers the subsequent risk of recurrent MI and of cardiovascular death.[A9]

Thrombolysis

With the increasing availability of PCI-capable facilities, the use of fibrinolytic therapy (Table 58-5) has decreased. When PCI will be delayed by more than 120 minutes, however, fibrinolytic therapy, in the absence of contraindications, is indicated within 12 hours of the onset of symptoms. It should begin immediately in the emergency department (or ambulance, if available) with a goal of a door-to-needle time of less than 30 minutes. When PCI is not available, fibrinolysis also is reasonable for ECG and clinical evidence of ischemic injury within 12 to 24 hours of the onset of symptoms in patients who are hemodynamically unstable or have a large area of myocardium at risk (Fig. 58-3).

When fibrinolysis is used, an accelerated regimen of a tissue plasminogen activator (plus intravenous heparin) is preferred to streptokinase because the patency rate of the infarct-related artery at 90 minutes is higher and mortality is lower. Longer-acting variants of alteplase, given as single-bolus (tenecteplase) or double-bolus (reteplase) injections, now are more commonly used than alteplase in clinical practice because they are more convenient to administer, but they do not further improve survival.[A10]

The risk-to-benefit ratio should be assessed in each patient when fibrinolysis is considered and specific regimens are selected (Table 58-6). The major risk of fibrinolytic therapy is bleeding. Intracranial hemorrhage is the most serious and frequently fatal complication; its incidence rate is 0.5 to 1% with currently approved regimens. Older age (older than 70 to 75 years), female sex, hypertension, and higher relative doses of plasminogen activators and heparin increase the risk of intracranial hemorrhage. In patients over age 75 years, half-dose tenecteplase is as efficacious as full-dose tenecteplase and associated with less intracranial hemorrhage, thereby making it an attractive alternative.

If fibrinolysis fails to open the infarct-related artery, urgent transfer to a PCI-capable hospital for rescue PCI is more effective than repeated fibrinolysis.

TABLE 58-5 CHARACTERISTICS OF INTRAVENOUS FIBRINOLYTIC AGENTS APPROVED BY THE U.S. FOOD AND DRUG ADMINISTRATION

	STREPTOKINASE (SK)	ALTEPLASE (t-PA)	RETEPLASE (r-PA)	TENECTEPLASE (TNK–t-PA)
Dose	1.5 MU in 30-60 minutes	100 mg in 90 minutes*	10 U + 10 U, 30 minutes apart	30-50 mg† during 5 seconds
Circulating half-life (minutes)	≅20	≅4	≅18	≅20
Antigenic/Allergic reactions	Yes	No	No	No
Systemic fibrinogen depletion	Severe	Mild to moderate	Moderate	Minimal
Intracerebral hemorrhage	≅0.4%	≅0.7%	≅0.8%	≅0.7%
Patency (TIMI 2/3) rate, 90 minutes‡	≅51%	≅73-84%	≅83%	≅77-88%
Lives saved per 100 treated	≅3§	≅4‖	≅4	≅4
Cost per dose (approximate U.S. dollars)	300	1800	2200	2200

*An accelerated alteplase regimen is given as follows: 15-mg bolus, then 0.75 mg/kg during 30 minutes (maximum, 50 mg), then 0.50 mg/kg during 60 minutes (maximum, 35 mg).
†TNK–t-PA is dosed by weight (supplied in 5-mg/mL vials): <60 kg = 6 mL; 61-70 kg = 7 mL; 71-80 kg = 8 mL; 81-90 kg = 9 mL; >90 kg = 10 mL.
‡TIMI = Thrombolysis in Myocardial Infarction. Data from Granger CB, Califf RM, Topol EJ. Thrombolytic therapy for acute myocardial infarction: a review. *Drugs.* 1992;44:293-325; and Bode C, Smalling RW, Berg G, et al. Randomized comparison of coronary thrombolysis achieved with double-bolus reteplase (recombinant plasminogen activator) and front-loaded, accelerated alteplase (recombinant tissue plasminogen activator) in patients with acute myocardial infarction: the RAPID II Investigators. *Circulation.* 1996;94:891-898.
§Patients with ST-segment elevation or bundle branch block, treated <6 hours.
‖Based on the finding from the GUSTO trial that t-PA saves one more additional life per 100 treated than does SK. Data from The GUSTO Investigators. An international randomized trial comparing four thrombolytic strategies for acute myocardial infarction. *N Engl J Med.* 1993;329:673-682; and Simes RJ, Topol EJ, Holmes DR Jr, et al. Link between the angiographic substudy and mortality outcomes in a large randomized trial of myocardial reperfusion: importance of early and complete infarct artery reperfusion. GUSTO-I Investigators. *Circulation.* 1995;91:1923-1928.

Even for patients successfully reperfused, rapid transfer to a PCI-capable facility, where angiography and PCI are performed as early as feasible within the window of 3 to 24 hours after fibrinolysis, can reduce the risk for recurrent ischemia, reinfarction, heart failure, cardiogenic shock, or death by about 35%.

Acute Hospital Phase

Ancillary and Other Therapies

General Medical Management

Beyond prompt initiation of reperfusion and other antithrombotic therapy, initial management includes bedrest (i.e., for 12 hours or until ischemia has been relieved and hemodynamic parameters have stabilized) with ECG monitoring. Routine oxygen supplementation does not benefit normoxemic patients.[A11,A12] Oxygen should be used in doses just sufficient to avoid hypoxemia (e.g., initially at 2 to 4 L/minute by nasal cannula; fingertip oximetry may be used to monitor effect) in patients with hypoxemia (oxygen saturation <90%), respiratory distress, or other high-risk features for hypoxemia. Initiation or continuation of high-intensity statin therapy (i.e., atorvastatin 80 mg/day or rosuvastatin 20 or 40 mg/day), beginning on admission, is supported by clinical trials.

Patients with ischemic chest discomfort or pain should be given sublingual nitroglycerin (0.4 mg every 5 minutes for up to three doses). Subsequently, intravenous (IV) nitroglycerin, titrated to symptom relief and blood pressure effects, may be considered to treat ongoing discomfort, uncontrolled hypertension, or heart failure. Bradycardia is a relative contraindication for nitrates, particularly in the setting of acute inferior ST-elevation MI, in which it may slow the heart rate even more. Persistent ischemic pain may be treated with titrated intravenous doses of morphine (i.e., 1 to 4 mg intravenously, repeated in 5 to 30 minutes as needed to relieve pain).

Routine IV β-blocker therapy does not benefit ST-elevation MI patients treated with primary PCI.[A13] However, selected patients (e.g. with hypertension, persistent chest pain, left ventricular dysfunction) may benefit. In such cases, titrated oral β-blockers (e.g., metoprolol tartrate, 12.5 mg orally every 6 hours, increased to 25 to 50 mg every 6 hours as tolerated) can be started, beginning within the first 24 hours if there are no contraindications. For hypertension, intravenous therapy (e.g., metoprolol tartrate, 5 mg every 2 to 5 minutes, up to three doses, transitioning to oral therapy, e.g., 25 to 50 mg every 8 hours) may be used. β-Blockers should be avoided in patients with active heart failure or cardiogenic shock. However, β-blockade, preferably with carvedilol, should be considered in patients with a left ventricular ejection fraction <40% once the heart failure has resolved.

In the absence of contraindications (e.g., hypotension), ACE inhibitors (e.g., initially captopril 6.25 mg every 8 hours or lisinopril 2.5 mg twice daily, titrated upward as tolerated) or angiotensin receptor blockers (e.g., losartan 12.5 to 25 mg once or twice daily, titrated upward as tolerated) should be started within 24 hours in patients with an anterior MI, left ventricular dysfunction, or heart failure. Subsequently (e.g., at 3 to 14 days), patients with an ejection fraction ≤40% and either symptomatic heart failure or diabetes become candidates for the addition of an aldosterone antagonist (i.e., eplerenone; initially, 25 mg once daily) or spironolactone (12.5 to 25 mg twice daily.)

The optimal systolic blood pressure range during acute MI is generally 100 to 140 mm Hg. Excessive hypertension usually responds to titrated nitroglycerin, β-blocker therapy, and morphine. Relative hypotension could require discontinuation of these medications, fluid administration, and/or other measures as appropriate to the hemodynamic subset (Table 58-7). Atropine (0.5 to 1.5 mg intravenously) should be available to treat symptomatic bradycardia and hypotension related to hypervagotonia.

Antiplatelet Therapy

Given the critical role of coronary thrombosis in the precipitation of acute MI, antithrombotic therapy, supplemental to primary PCI or fibrinolysis, plays a key role in management of ST-elevation MI (Fig. 58-4; Table 58-7).

Aspirin (162 to 325 mg, non–enteric-coated) should be given on presentation to all patients unless it is contraindicated (see Fig. 58-4). A daily maintenance aspirin dose of 81 to 325 mg is then given and continued indefinitely. An 81 mg maintenance dose of aspirin is required with ticagrelor and preferred with prasugrel. However, a higher initial dose (325 mg daily for 30 days) of aspirin may be preferred with clopidogrel.

In addition to aspirin, a loading dose of an adenosine diphosphate receptor (*$P2Y_{12}$*) inhibitor (i.e., clopidogrel 600 mg, prasugrel 60 mg, or ticagrelor 180 mg)

TABLE 58-6 INDICATIONS FOR AND CONTRAINDICATIONS TO FIBRINOLYTIC THERAPY

INDICATIONS

Ischemic-type chest discomfort or equivalent for 30 minutes–12 hours with new or presumed new ST-segment elevation in two contiguous leads of ≥2 mm (≥0.2 mV) in leads V_1, V_2, or V_3 or ≥1 mm in other leads
New or presumed new left bundle branch block with symptoms consistent with myocardial infarction
Absence of contraindications

CONTRAINDICATIONS, ABSOLUTE

Active bleeding or bleeding diathesis (menses excluded)
Prior hemorrhagic stroke, ischemic stroke within 3 months, except acute ischemic stroke within 3-4.5 hours
Intracranial or spinal cord neoplasm or arteriovenous malformation
Suspected or known aortic dissection
Closed head or facial trauma within 3 months

CONTRAINDICATIONS, RELATIVE

Severe, uncontrolled hypertension by history or on presentation (>180/110 mm Hg)
Anticoagulation with therapeutic or elevated international normalized ratio (>2-3)
Old ischemic stroke (>3 months ago); intracerebral disease other than above
Recent (<3 weeks) major trauma/surgery or prolonged (>10 minutes) cardiopulmonary resuscitation or internal bleeding
Active peptic ulcer
Recent noncompressible vascular punctures
Pregnancy
For streptokinase/anistreplase: prior exposure (especially if >5 days ago) or allergic reaction

Modified from Kushner FG, Hand M, Smith SC Jr, et al. 2009 Focused updates: ACC/AHA guidelines for the management of patients with ST-elevation myocardial infarction and the ACC/AHA/SCAI guidelines on percutaneous coronary intervention. *Circulation.* 2009;120:2271-2306.

TABLE 58-7 IN-HOSPITAL DOSING OF SELECTED ANTITHROMBOTIC DRUGS

DRUG	INITIAL DOSE	MAINTENANCE DOSE
Abciximab	0.25 mg/kg IV bolus	0.125 μg/kg/min (maximum, 10 μg/min) for up to 12 hr
Aspirin	162-325 mg	81 mg[*]-325 mg/day
Clopidogrel	PCI: 300-600 mg[*] Fibrinolysis and age >75: 75-150 mg	75 mg/day (optional: 150 mg/day × 1 wk)
Eptifibatide	180 μg/kg IV bolus × 2[†]	2.0 μg/kg/min for up to 18 hr reduce rate by 50% for CrCl < 50 mL/min
Prasugrel	60 mg	10 mg/day
Ticagrelor	180 mg	90 mg bid (given with aspirin 81 mg/day)
Tirofiban	25 μg/kg IV bolus	0.15 μg/kg/min for up to 12 to 18 hr; reduce rate by 50% for CrCl < 30 mL/min
UFH	PCI[‡]: 70-100 U/kg IV bolus Fibrinolytic[§]: 60 U/kg IV bolus (max, 4000 U)	Repeat to achieve, maintain target ACT 12 U/kg/hr (max, 1000 U/hr) initial adjust aPTT to 1.5-2.0 × control (~50-70 sec)
Bivalirudin	PCI[‡]: 0.75 mg/kg IV bolus Additional 0.3 mg/kg PRN	1.75 mg/kg/hr infusion 1 mg/kg/hr for CrCl < 30 mL/min
Enoxaparin	Fibrinolytic[§]: 30 mg IV bolus Age >75: no bolus	1 mg/kg SQ at 15 min and q12h (max, 100 mg) 0.75 mg/kg SQ q12h (max, 75 mg) All ages, CrCl <30 mL/min: 1 mg/kg q24h
Fondaparinux	Fibrinolytic[§]: 2.5 mg IV	2.5 mg SQ daily, starting the next day Contraindicated if CrCl < 30 mL/min

[*]Generally preferred dose.
[†]Boluses are separated by 10 minutes.
[‡]Anticoagulants are generally stopped following uncomplicated PCI.
[§]Given for the index hospitalization (up to 48 hr [UFH] or up to 8 days [enoxaparin or fondaparinux]) or until revascularization.
ACT = activated clotting time; bid = twice daily; CrCl = creatinine clearance; IV = intravenous; max = maximum; PCI = percutaneous coronary intervention (e.g., stenting); SQ = subcutaneous; UFH = unfractionated heparin.

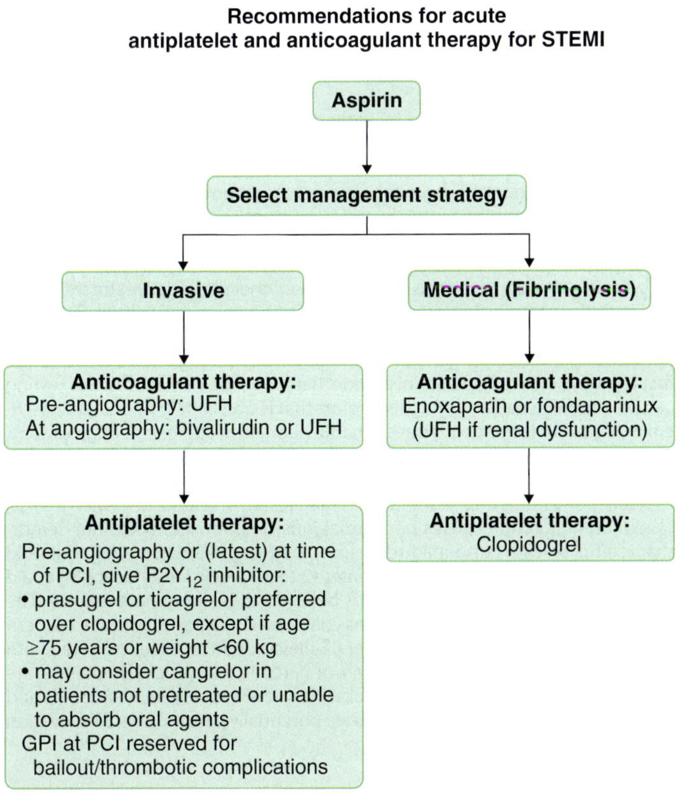

FIGURE 58-4. **Recommendations for antiplatelet and anticoagulant therapy for ST-segment elevation myocardial infarction (STEMI). See text for doses. GPI = glycoprotein IIb/IIIa inhibitor; UFH = unfractionated heparin.**

should be given as early as possible or at the time of primary PCI to ST-elevation MI patients for whom an invasive approach is planned, followed by a daily maintenance dose for at least 1 year. The more potent prasugrel and ticagrelor are preferred over clopidogrel for ST-elevation MI patients undergoing primary PCI when their bleeding risk is acceptable, with data suggesting that prasugrel is more effective and equally safe.[A14] By comparison, clopidogrel is preferred in patients with a history of a stroke or transient ischemic attack, and it also is recommended for at least 14 days and up to 1 year after fibrinolytic therapy. *Cangrelor*, a short-acting IV $P2Y_{12}$ inhibitor (given as a 30 μg/kg IV bolus followed immediately by a 4 μg/kg/min infusion for at least 2 hours or until the end of the procedure), has a rapid onset/offset of action (3- to 6-minute half-life) and is better than clopidogrel for preventing ischemic events, but at the cost of increased bleeding.

Glycoprotein (GP) IIb/IIIa inhibitors (Table 58-7) can provide a rapid onset of antiplatelet activity in the precatheterization laboratory setting or for the prevention and treatment of periprocedural thrombotic complications. Otherwise, their use is now limited.

Anticoagulant Therapy

Inhibition of thrombin generation is crucial to the management of occluding coronary thrombi in ST-elevation MI. Initiation of a parenteral anticoagulant thrombin inhibitor is recommended at the time of presentation for all ST-elevation MI patients (Fig. 58-4). Intravenous unfractionated heparin and bivalirudin are comparably effective alternatives for the composite end point of death, recurrent MI, and major bleeding in supporting PCI and intensive antiplatelet therapy.[A15] Anticoagulants are generally stopped after an uncomplicated PCI. Recommended options to support fibrinolytic therapy include unfractionated heparin, enoxaparin, and fondaparinux (see Table 58-7).

Combined Oral Anticoagulant and Antiplatelet Therapy

Based on limited evidence, current guidelines recommend dual antiplatelet therapy combined with an oral anticoagulant in post-MI patients with high-risk atrial fibrillation (AF; Chapter 52), a mechanical heart valve (Chapter 60), venous thromboembolism (Chapter 68), or hypercoagulable disorders (Chapter 67) but that the duration of such triple therapy be as short as possible (usually 1 week to 1 month). Warfarin (INR goal 2.0 to 2.5) is indicated as the anticoagulant for patients with a mechanical heart valve or left ventricular thrombus, typically combined with clopidogrel. For patients with AF or a history of venous thromboembolism, a direct-acting oral anticoagulant is preferred: options include low-dose rivaroxaban (15 mg daily) plus a $P2Y_{12}$ inhibitor (primarily clopidogrel), apixaban 2.5 or 5 mg twice daily (depending on renal function) plus a $P2Y_{12}$ inhibitor (primarily clopidogrel),[A16] or very-low-dose rivaroxaban (2.5 mg twice daily) plus dual antiplatelet therapy with aspirin plus a $P2Y_{12}$ inhibitor.[A17]

Coronary Intensive Care

Prompt reperfusion therapy has dramatically lowered the prevalence of MI-related ventricular arrhythmias. After early successful primary PCI, patients who have small infarcts and who are hemodynamically and electrically stable may be transferred to a telemetry step-down unit within 24 hours.

In the contemporary care of patients with an ST-elevation MI, the primary role of coronary intensive care unit admission (Table 58-8) is to manage patients with or at risk for complications of acute MI. The goals of the coronary intensive care unit include continuous electrocardiographic monitoring and therapy for serious arrhythmias (e.g., rapid defibrillation of ventricular fibrillation [VF]; Chapter 53), monitoring the success of the primary PCI, monitoring or continuing fibrinolytic therapy, initiating or continuing other acute medical therapies (as discussed earlier), appropriate hemodynamic assessment and monitoring, and diagnosis and treatment of mechanical and physiologic complications of acute MI.

General care measures in the coronary intensive care unit include attention to activity, diet and bowels, education, reassurance, and sedation. Bedrest is encouraged for the first 12 hours. In the absence of complications, dangling, bed-to-chair, and self-care activities can begin within 24 hours or earlier after successful reperfusion therapy. When stabilization has occurred, usually within 1 to 3 days, patients may be transferred to a step-down unit for progressive ambulation. The risk for emesis and aspiration or the anticipation of angiography or other procedures usually dictates nothing by mouth or clear liquids for the first 4 to 12 hours. Thereafter, a heart-healthy diet in small portions is recommended. In patients at high risk for bleeding gastric stress ulcers, a proton pump inhibitor or an H2-receptor antagonist is recommended. Many patients benefit from an analgesic (see Tables 26-4 and 26-6) to relieve ongoing pain and an anxiolytic or sedative during the acute phase. A benzodiazepine (Table 362-9) is frequently selected, but routine use of anxiolytics is neither necessary nor recommended. Sedatives should not substitute for education and reassurance from concerned caregivers to relieve emotional distress and improve behavior. Constipation often occurs with bedrest and narcotics; stool softeners and a bedside commode are advised.

The ECG should be monitored continuously during the entire hospital course to detect serious arrhythmias and to guide therapy. Measures to limit infarct size (i.e., coronary reperfusion) and to optimize hemodynamics also stabilize the heart electrically. Routine antiarrhythmic prophylaxis (e.g., with lidocaine

TABLE 58-8 SAMPLE ADMISSION ORDERS FOR ST-SEGMENT ELEVATION ACUTE MYOCARDIAL INFARCTION

Diagnosis	Acute ST-segment elevation myocardial infarction
Admit	Coronary care unit with telemetry
Condition	Serious
Vital signs	q½h until stable, then q1-4h and PRN; pulse oximetry × 24 hr; notify if heart rate <50 or >100; respiratory rate <8 or >20; SBP <90 or >150 mm Hg; O_2 saturation <90%
Activity	Bedrest × 12 hr with bedside commode; thereafter, light activity if stable
Diet	NPO except for sips of water until pain free and stable; then 2 g sodium, heart-healthy diet as tolerated, unless on call for catheterization (or other test requiring NPO)
Laboratory tests*	Troponin I or T at 2 hours, then q8h × 3; comprehensive blood chemistry, magnesium, CBC with platelets; PT/INR, aPTT; BNP; lipid profile (fasting in morning); portable CXR
IV therapy	D_5W or NS to keep vein open (increase fluids for relative hypovolemia); second IV if IV medication given
Reperfusion therapy*	Emergency primary coronary angioplasty or fibrinolysis (if appropriate and if not already performed) 1. Primary angioplasty (preferred if available within 90 minutes) 2. Tenecteplase, reteplase or alteplase (preferred); or streptokinase (see Table 58-6 for doses), if primary PCI is unavailable within 90-120 minutes
Medications	1. Nasal O_2 at 2 L/min if with or at risk of hypoxemia, titrated to keep O_2 saturation >90% 2. Aspirin 162-325 mg chewed on admission, then 81-365 mg PO daily 3. IV heparin, 60-U/kg bolus (maximum, 4000 U) and 12 U/kg/hr (maximum, 1000 U/hr), titrate to target aPTT 1.5-2.0 × control (about 50-70 seconds); *or* enoxaparin (preferred with fibrinolytic), 30 mg IV, then 1 mg/kg SQ q12h (maximum SQ doses, 100 mg on day 1; reduce to 0.75 mg/kg for age ≥75 years, increase interval to q24h for CrCl <30 mL/min); *or* bivalirudin (with primary PCI), 0.75-mg/kg IV bolus, then 1.75 mg/kg/hr (delay 30 minutes if heparin given) 4. Metoprolol, 12.5 PO q6h, incremented to 25-50 mg q6h as tolerated (hold for SBP < 100 mm Hg, pulse <50 beats/min, asthma, heart failure); may consider IV metoprolol if immediate effect required (tachyarrhythmia, severe hypertension, unrelieved pain) in the absence of heart failure 5. Consider IV nitroglycerin drip × 24-48 hr (titrated to SBP 100-140 mm Hg) 6. Morphine sulfate, 1-4 mg IV and increment at 5-30 minutes PRN for unrelieved pain 7. Stool softener 8. Anxiolytic or hypnotic if needed 9. ACE inhibitor for hypertension, anterior acute MI, or LV dysfunction, in low oral dose (e.g., captopril, 6.25 mg q8h), begun within 24 hours or when stable (SBP > 100 mm Hg) and adjusted upward 10. Lipid-lowering therapy (i.e., high-intensity statin) regardless of LDL: target LDL reduction of ≥50%; give atorvastatin 80 mg PO or rosuvastatin 20-40 mg PO on admission (pre-cath) and continue daily. 11. Antiplatelet therapy: Ticagrelor, 180 mg PO on admission, then 90 mg bid *or* prasugrel, 60 mg PO on admission, then 10 mg PO daily with a primary PCI strategy (preferred to clopidogrel if acceptable bleeding risk); *or* clopidogrel, 600 mg PO on admission for a primary PCI strategy, or 300 mg PO with fibrinolytic, then 75 mg PO daily. For specific treatments for hemodynamic subgroups, see Table 58-9.

*If not ordered in the emergency department.

ACE = angiotensin-converting enzyme; aPTT = activated partial thromboplastin time; BNP = brain natriuretic peptide; CABG = coronary artery bypass graft surgery; CBC = complete blood count; CrCl = creatinine clearance; CXR = chest radiograph; D_5W = 5% dextrose in water; daily = once daily; INR = international normalized ratio; IV = intravenous; LDL = low-density lipoprotein; LV = left ventricle; MI = myocardial infarction; NPO = nothing by mouth; NS = normal saline; PCI = percutaneous coronary intervention; PO = orally; PRN = as needed; PT = prothrombin time; SBP = systolic blood pressure; SQ = subcutaneous.

or amiodarone) is not indicated, but specific arrhythmias require treatment (see later text).

Hemodynamic evaluation is helpful in assessing prognosis and in guiding therapy (see Table 58-9). Clinical and noninvasive evaluation of vital signs is adequate for normotensive patients without pulmonary congestion. Patients with pulmonary venous congestion are at high risk and must be carefully monitored in terms of fluid status, oxygenation, and urine output (Chapter 46). Invasive hemodynamic monitoring is appropriate only when the cause of circulatory failure is uncertain or when titration of intravenous therapies depends on hemodynamic measurements (e.g., pulmonary capillary wedge pressure and cardiac output). Arterial catheters are appropriate and useful in clinically unstable, hypotensive patients who do not respond to intravenous fluids to replete or to expand intravascular volume (see the later discussion of complications).

Management of Complications

Complications of acute MI have declined with early reperfusion and modern medical therapy, but they remain an important cause of morbidity and mortality.

Recurrent Chest Pain

Recurrent chest pain can be caused by post-infarction ischemia of the border zones of the infarcted territory, acute closure of the treated infarct-related artery, non–infarct-related coronary lesions, mechanical complications (see later), and pericarditis. Characterization of the pain, physical examination, electrocardiography, echocardiography, and cardiac marker determinations assist in the differential diagnosis. Treatment should be specific to the cause.

Postinfarction angina developing spontaneously during hospitalization for acute MI despite medical therapy may indicate infarct extension or reinfarction and usually merits coronary angiography. Infarct expansion implies circumferential slippage with thinning of the infarcted myocardium. Infarct expansion can be associated with chest pain but without recurrent elevation of cardiac markers. Expansive remodeling can lead to a left ventricular aneurysm. The risk for remodeling is reduced by early reperfusion therapy and administration of ACE inhibitors. β-Blockers and nitroglycerin are recommended medical therapies.

Pain with recurrent ST-segment elevation or recurrent elevation of cardiac markers may be due to acute closure (e.g., stent thrombosis) of the treated infarct-related artery. An invasive approach is recommended and preferred to relieve discomfort that occurs hours to days after an acute MI and that is associated with objective signs of reinfarction. Other potential treatment strategies include readministration of thrombolytic therapy or a GP IIb/IIIa inhibitor, along with nitroglycerin, β-blockade, and heparin. Streptokinase, which induces neutralizing antibodies, generally should not be readministered beyond the first few days of an initial administration. Radionuclide perfusion stress testing can be helpful in patients with discomfort that is transient or of uncertain ischemic origin. For lesions with questionable degrees of stenosis at angiography, coronary pressure gradient (fractional flow reserve) or Doppler velocimetry or intracoronary ultrasound can determine whether PCI is warranted.

Acute pericarditis most commonly is manifested on days 2 to 4 when a large, transmural infarction causes pericardial inflammation. On occasion, hemorrhagic effusion with tamponade develops, so excessive anticoagulation should be avoided. Pericarditis developing later (2 to 10 weeks) after acute MI could represent Dressler syndrome, which is believed to be immune mediated. The incidence of this post-MI syndrome has decreased dramatically in the modern reperfusion era. Pericardial pain after ST-elevation MI is usually treated with aspirin, but colchicine, acetaminophen, or narcotic analgesics (Chapter 62) are reasonable if aspirin (even in high doses) is not effective. Glucocorticoids and nonsteroidal anti-inflammatory drugs are potentially harmful after ST-elevation MI and should be avoided.

Rhythm Disturbances

Ventricular Arrhythmias

Acute MI and subsequent reperfusion are associated with a proarrhythmic environment that includes heterogeneous myocardial ischemia, heightened

TABLE 58-9 HEMODYNAMIC SUBSETS OF ACUTE MYOCARDIAL INFARCTION

	BLOOD PRESSURE (RELATIVE)	TYPICAL PHYSICAL FINDINGS	CARDIAC INDEX (L/min/m²)	PA WEDGE PRESSURE (mm Hg)	SUGGESTED INTERVENTIONS
Normal	Normal	$\pm S_4$	>2.5	≤12	None required
Hyperdynamic	Normal or high	Anxious	>3	<12	Control pain, anxiety; β-blocker; treat SBP to <140 mm Hg
Hypovolemia	Low	Dry	≤2.7	≤9	Add fluids to maintain normal pressure; can develop pulmonary edema if hypotension is caused by unrecognized LV failure
Mild LV failure	Low to high	Rales, $\pm S_3$	2-2.5	>15	Diuresis; nitrates, ACE inhibitor; consider low-dose β-blocker
Severe LV failure	Low to normal	Above $+S_3$, ± ↑ JVP, ± edema	<2	>20	Diuresis; nitrates; low-dose ACE inhibitor; avoid β-blockers; consider inotropes, urgent revascularization
Cardiogenic shock	Very low	Above + cool, clammy; ↓ mental or renal function	≤1.5	>25	Avoid hypotensive agents; place intra-aortic balloon pump or LV assist device; urgent revascularization if possible
RV infarct	Very low	↑ JVP with clear lungs	<2.5	≤12	Give IV fluids; avoid nitrates and hypotensive agents; dobutamine if refractory to fluids

↑ = increased; ↓ = decreased; ACE = angiotensin-converting enzyme; IV = intravenous; JVP = jugular venous pressure; LV = left ventricle; PA = pulmonary artery; RV = right ventricle; SBP = systolic blood pressure.
Modified from Forrester JS, Diamond G, Chatterjee K, et al. Medical therapy of acute myocardial infarction by application of hemodynamic subsets (second of two parts). *N Engl J Med.* 1976;295:1404-1413.

adrenergic tone, intracellular electrolyte disturbance, lipolysis and the production of free fatty acids, and the generation of oxygen free radicals. Micro-reentry likely is the most common electrophysiologic mechanism of early-phase arrhythmias, although enhanced automaticity and triggered activity also are observed in experimental models.

Accelerated idioventricular rhythm (60 to 100 beats per minute) frequently occurs within the first 12 hours and is generally benign (i.e., is not a risk factor for more serious ventricular arrhythmias). Indeed, accelerated idioventricular rhythm frequently heralds successful reperfusion. Antiarrhythmic therapy is not indicated except for sustained, hemodynamically compromising accelerated idioventricular rhythm.

Primary ventricular fibrillation (Chapter 50) is associated with a higher rate of 24-hour in-hospital and short-term mortality, but the longer-term risk of recurrent ventricular tachycardia or ventricular fibrillation and mortality is largely unaffected in survivors. Polymorphic ventricular tachycardia (Chapter 53) and, less commonly, monomorphic ventricular tachycardia are associated life-threatening arrhythmias that can occur in almost 6% of patients in the early phase of acute MI. Clinical features (including warning arrhythmias) are not adequately specific or sensitive to identify patients at risk for sustained ventricular tachyarrhythmias, so all patients should be continuously monitored. Prophylactic lidocaine, which reduces primary ventricular fibrillation but does not decrease (and may increase) mortality, is not recommended.

In comatose ST-elevation MI patients resuscitated from out-of-hospital cardiac arrest due to ventricular fibrillation or pulseless ventricular tachycardia, body temperature management to avoid hyperthermia is beneficial and should be considered as soon as possible after hospital arrival (Chapter 50).

Electrical cardioversion is required for ventricular fibrillation and sustained polymorphic ventricular tachycardia (unsynchronized shock) and for sustained monomorphic ventricular tachycardia (synchronized shock) that causes hemodynamic compromise (Chapters 53 and 54). Brief intravenous sedation is given to conscious, "stable" patients. For slower, stable ventricular tachycardia and nonsustained ventricular tachycardia requiring therapy, intravenous amiodarone or intravenous lidocaine is commonly used. After episodes of ventricular tachycardia or ventricular fibrillation, infusions of antiarrhythmic drugs may be given for 6 to 24 hours; the ongoing risk for arrhythmia then is reassessed. Electrolyte and acid-base imbalance and hypoxia should be corrected. β-Blockade is useful in patients with frequent polymorphic ventricular tachycardia associated with adrenergic activation ("electrical storm"). Additional, aggressive measures should be considered to reduce cardiac ischemia (e.g., emergency PCI or CABG) and to address left ventricular dysfunction (e.g., intra-aortic balloon pump or left ventricular assist device) in patients with recurrent polymorphic ventricular tachycardia despite the use of β-blockers or amiodarone or both.

Late ventricular fibrillation, which develops more than 48 hours after the onset of acute MI, portends a worse prognosis and deserves aggressive therapy (see below). Monomorphic ventricular tachycardia resulting from re-entry in the context of a recent or old MI also can appear late after MI, and patients may require long-term therapy (see below). An implantable cardioverter-defibrillator (ICD; Chapter 54) is indicated in patients with ventricular fibrillation or hemodynamically significant sustained ventricular tachycardia occurring more than

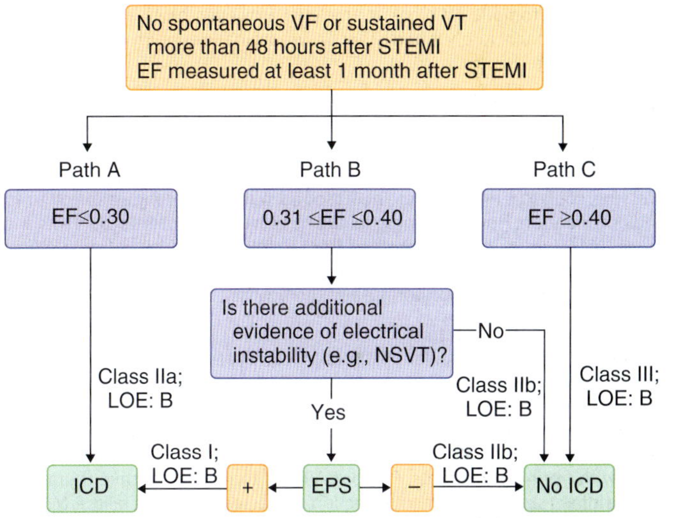

FIGURE 58-5. **Algorithm to aid in selection of implantable cardioverter-defibrillator (ICD) in patients with ST-segment elevation myocardial infarction (STEMI) and diminished ejection fraction (EF). The appropriate management path is selected on the basis of left ventricular EF measured at least 1 month after STEMI. All patients, whether an ICD is implanted or not, should receive medical therapy. EPS = electrophysiologic studies; LOE = level of evidence; NSVT = nonsustained ventricular tachycardia; VF = ventricular fibrillation; VT = ventricular tachycardia. (Modified from Antman EM, Anbe DT, Armstrong PW, et al. 2004 Update: ACC/AHA guidelines for the management of patients with ST-elevation myocardial infarction—executive summary. A Report of the American College of Cardiology/American Heart Association Task Force on Practice Guidelines [Writing Committee to Revise the 1999 Guidelines for the Management of Patients with Acute Myocardial Infarction].** ***Circulation.*** **2004;110:588-636.)**

2 days after ST-elevation MI and not due to a transient or reversible cause (e.g., ischemia, reinfarction, metabolic abnormalities; Figure 58-5).

Atrial Fibrillation and Other Supraventricular Tachyarrhythmias

Atrial fibrillation (AF), which is an important and relatively common acute MI-related arrhythmia, occurs in 5 to 10% of patients with an acute MI, often within the first day (Chapter 52). The incidence of atrial flutter and other supraventricular tachyarrhythmias is much lower. The risk for AF increases with age, larger MIs, heart failure, pericarditis, atrial infarction, hypokalemia, hypomagnesemia, hypoxia, pulmonary disease, and hyperadrenergic states. The incidence of AF is reduced by effective early reperfusion. Hemodynamic compromise with rapid rates and systemic embolism (in about 2% of cases) are adverse consequences of AF. Systemic embolism can occur on the first day, so prompt anticoagulation with heparin is indicated.

Recommendations for management of AF include electrical cardioversion for patients with hemodynamic compromise or ischemia; rate control with an intravenous β-blocker (e.g., metoprolol, 5 mg over 2 minutes to a total of 15 mg over 10 to 15 minutes) in patients without clinical ventricular dysfunction, with intravenous digoxin for patients with ventricular dysfunction (i.e., give 1.0 mg, half initially and half in 4 hours), or with intravenous diltiazem or verapamil in hemodynamically compensated patients with a contraindication to β-blockers; and anticoagulation with heparin (or low-molecular-weight heparin). Amiodarone, which is generally reserved for patients with or at high risk for AF recurrence, may be started and continued for 6 weeks if sinus rhythm is restored and maintained. Long-term chronic anticoagulation may not be necessary thereafter unless other indications exist.

Bradycardias, Conduction Delays, and Heart Block

Bradycardias caused by sinus or atrioventricular (AV) nodal delay, typically owing to increased parasympathetic tone associated with an inferior wall MI, are common and usually benign. Atropine (0.5 to 1.5 mg IV) is useful for symptomatic cases (e.g., heart rates generally <50 beats per minute associated with hypotension, ischemia, or escape ventricular arrhythmias). Temporary pacing is needed rarely. By comparison, atropine can worsen infranodal AV block (usually observed in association with anterior MI and a wide-complex escape rhythm), so it is important to differentiate the two (Chapter 52).

New-onset infranodal AV, intraventricular, and bundle branch blocks predict a four-fold to six-fold increase in in-hospital mortality, but this increase is related more to extensive myocardial damage than to the heart block itself. Temporary pacing usually is indicated, but it only modestly improves survival. Fortunately, the incidence of these arrhythmias has declined markedly in the reperfusion era (from 10 to 20% to ~4%).

Indications for permanent pacing after acute MI depend on the prognosis of the AV block and not solely on symptoms. Indications include even transient second- or third-degree AV block in association with bundle branch block and ongoing symptomatic AV block at any level. However, block at the AV nodal level (Wenckebach) rarely is persistent or symptomatic enough to warrant permanent pacing.

Heart Failure and Other Low-Output States

Of all serious acute MI-related complications, heart failure (Chapters 45 and 46) is the most common and is the leading cause of in-hospital acute MI-related death.[12] Manifestations of circulatory failure can include a weak pulse, low blood pressure, cool extremities, a third heart sound, pulmonary congestion, oliguria, and obtundation. However, pump failure has several distinct mechanisms and causes, which must be distinguished from each other as well as from volume depletion as the cause of a low cardiac output state. Each requires a specific approach to diagnosis, monitoring, and therapy (see Table 58-7).

Left Ventricular Dysfunction

The degree of left ventricular dysfunction correlates well with the extent of acute ischemia and infarction. Hemodynamic compromise becomes evident when impairment involves 20 to 25% of the left ventricle, and cardiogenic shock occurs with impairment of 40% or more (Chapter 93). Pulmonary congestion and S_3 and S_4 gallops are the most common physical findings. Early reperfusion (with fibrinolytic agents, PCI, or CABG) is the most effective therapy to reduce infarct size, ventricular dysfunction, and associated heart failure. Medical treatment of heart failure related to the ventricular dysfunction of acute MI is otherwise generally similar to that of heart failure in other settings (Chapter 46) and includes adequate oxygenation and diuresis (begun early, blood pressure permitting, and continued on a long-term basis if needed). Morphine sulfate (i.e., 1 to 4 mg intravenously, with increments as needed after 5 to 30 minutes or more) is useful for patients with pulmonary congestion. Titrated oral ACE inhibitor therapy (e.g., captopril, incremented from 3.125 to 6.25 mg three times daily to 50 mg twice daily as tolerated, or lisinopril, 1.25 to 2.5 mg once or twice daily, titrated as tolerated up to 10 to 20 mg twice daily) also is indicated for heart failure and pulmonary edema unless excessive hypotension (systolic blood pressure <100 mm Hg) is present. Nitroglycerin reduces preload as well as afterload and effectively relieves congestive symptoms; treatment can be begun sublingually (0.4 mg every 5 minutes times three), and then transition can be made to intravenous therapy (initially 5 to 10 μg/minute, incrementing by 5 to 20 μg/minute until symptoms are relieved or until mean arterial pressure falls by 10% in normotensive patients or 30% in hypertensive patients but not <90 mm Hg or >30 mm Hg lower than baseline).

Volume Depletion

Relative or absolute hypovolemia is a frequent cause of hypotension and circulatory failure and is easily corrected if it is recognized and treated promptly. Poor hydration, vomiting, diuresis, and disease- or drug-induced peripheral vasodilation can contribute to this condition. Occult gastrointestinal and/or access site bleeding should also be considered. Hypovolemia should be identified and corrected with intravenous fluids before more aggressive therapies are considered. An empirical fluid challenge may be tried in the appropriate clinical setting (e.g., for hypotension in the absence of congestion, for inferior or right ventricular infarction, and for hypervagotonia). If filling pressures are measured, cautious fluid administration to a pulmonary capillary wedge pressure 15 to 20 mm Hg may optimize cardiac output and blood pressure without impairing oxygenation.

Right Ventricular Infarction

Right ventricular ischemia and infarction occur with proximal occlusion of the right coronary artery (before the take-off of the right ventricular branches). Ten percent to 15% of inferior acute ST-elevation MIs show classic hemodynamic features, and these patients form the highest-risk inferior MI subgroup for morbidity and mortality (25 to 30% vs. <6% hospital mortality). Improvement in right ventricular function commonly occurs over time if short-term management is successful.

Hypotension in patients with clear lung fields and elevated jugular venous pressure in the setting of inferior or inferoposterior acute MI should raise the suspicion of right ventricular infarction. The Kussmaul sign (distention of the jugular veins on inspiration) is relatively specific and sensitive in this setting. ST-segment elevation in lead V_1 and in right precordial lead V_4R (Chapter 42), particularly in the first 24 hours, is the most sensitive electrocardiographic marker of right ventricular infarction. Echocardiography is helpful in confirming the diagnosis. (Right ventricular dilation and dysfunction are observed.) When right-sided heart pressures are measured, a right atrial pressure of 10 mm Hg or greater and 80% or more of the pulmonary capillary wedge pressure are relatively sensitive and specific for right ventricular ischemic dysfunction.

Management of right ventricular infarction consists of early maintenance of preload with intravenous fluids, reduction of right ventricular afterload (i.e., treatment of pulmonary congestion), early reperfusion, short-term inotropic support if needed, and avoidance of venodilators (e.g., nitrates) and diuretics used for left ventricular failure (they may cause marked hypotension). Volume loading with normal saline solution alone is often effective. If the cardiac output fails to improve after 0.5 to 1 L of fluid, inotropic support with intravenous dobutamine (starting at 2 μg/kg/minute and titrating to hemodynamic effect or tolerance, up to 20 μg/kg/minute) is recommended. High-grade AV block is common, and restoration of AV synchrony with temporary AV sequential pacing can lead to substantial improvement in cardiac output. Because the onset of AF (in up to one third of right ventricular infarcts) can cause severe hemodynamic compromise, it requires prompt cardioversion. In rare circumstances, a right ventricular assist device may be required if shock from right ventricular failure persists despite optimized hemodynamic parameters and rhythm control. Early coronary reperfusion with PCI or fibrinolysis markedly improves outcomes.

Cardiogenic Shock

Cardiogenic shock (Chapter 93) is a form of severe left ventricular failure characterized by marked hypotension (systolic pressures <90 mm Hg) and reductions in cardiac index (to <1.8 L/minute/m^2) despite high left ventricular filling pressure (pulmonary capillary wedge pressure >18 mm Hg). The cause is loss of a critical functional mass (>40%) of the left ventricle. Risk factors include age, large (usually anterior) acute MI, previous MI, and diabetes. The treatment and prognosis of cardiogenic shock are discussed in Chapter 46.

Mechanical Complications

Mechanical complications of acute MI may occur throughout the hospital course and include acute mitral valve regurgitation (often caused by papillary muscle dysfunction or rupture), ventricular septal defect, and left ventricular free wall rupture.[13,14] These mechanical complications are much less common after early reperfusion therapy: in ST-elevation MI patients treated with primary PCI, current risks are about 0.5% for free wall rupture, 0.2% for ventricular septal defect, and 0.3% for papillary muscle rupture, for a total mechanical complication rate of 1% or less. Prompt diagnosis and early surgery, although still associated with a high mortality rate, lead to better outcomes than delayed diagnosis and medical therapy alone

A left ventricular aneurysm can develop after a large, most commonly anterior, acute MI and create mechanical and electrical complications. If refractory heart failure, ventricular tachycardia, or systemic embolization occurs despite medical therapy and PCI, aneurysmectomy with CABG is indicated.

Thromboembolic Complications

Arterial thromboembolism, typically arising from the left ventricle or left atrium, is very unusual in ST-elevation MI patients who are treated with early reperfusion and aggressive antithrombotic therapies. Arterial embolism can cause dramatic clinical events, such as hemiparesis (Chapter 376), loss of a pulse, ischemic bowel (Chapter 129), or sudden changes in blood pressure, depending on the regional circulation involved.

Left ventricular mural thrombosis occurs typically in the setting of a large (especially anterior) acute ST-elevation MI and heart failure. The risk for embolism is particularly high when a mural thrombus is detected by echocardiography. Thus, in patients with anterior acute ST-elevation MI and in other high-risk patients, echocardiography should be performed during hospitalization; if results are positive, oral anticoagulation (e.g., apixiban 5 mg twice daily) should be started and continued for 3 to 6 months.[15,16]

Pulmonary emboli, which commonly arise from thrombi in leg veins, are highly unusual unless patients are immobilized for several days. Deep venous thrombosis can be prevented by lower extremity compression therapy, by limiting the duration of bedrest, and by the use of subcutaneous heparin (in patients at risk and not receiving intravenous heparin) until patients are fully ambulatory (Chapter 68).

As noted in more detail previously (see Combined Oral Anticoagulant and Antiplatelet Therapy), adding a direct-acting oral anticoagulant to aspirin and a $P2Y_{12}$ inhibitor for the prevention of venous thromboembolic disease (Chapters 67 and 68) or the prevention of systemic embolization in patients with AF (Chapter 52) is indicated for up to about 1 month in an ST-elevation MI patient with AF and a high risk of systemic emboli, recent venous thromboembolism, or a hypercoagulable disorder. For patients with a mechanical heart valve or left ventricular mural thrombus (Chapter 70), warfarin, usually to an international normalized ratio of 2.0 to 2.5, should be added to dual antiplatelet therapy for 3 months. To minimize bleeding, careful attention must be paid to the appropriate selection and doses of antithrombotic regimens based on age, weight, renal function, and other comorbid conditions.

Late Hospital Phase

Transfer from coronary intensive care to a step-down unit usually occurs within 1 to 3 days, when the cardiac rhythm and hemodynamics are stable. The duration of this late phase of hospital care is usually an additional 1 to 3 days in uncomplicated cases. Activity levels should be increased progressively under continuous electrocardiographic monitoring. Medical therapy should progress from parenteral and short-acting agents to oral medications appropriate and convenient for long-term outpatient use. Risk stratification and functional evaluations are critical to assess prognosis and to guide therapy as the time for discharge, which may be as early as 2 to 3 days in uncomplicated, successfully reperfused patients. Functional evaluation also can be extended to the early period after hospital discharge. Education must be provided about diet, activity, smoking, and other risk factors (e.g., lipids, hypertension, and diabetes—see later).

Risk Stratification after Myocardial Infarction

Risk stratification is a continuous process that begins on admission and continues through hospital discharge. The goals of risk stratification before and early after discharge for acute MI are to assess ventricular and clinical function, latent ischemia, and arrhythmic risk; to use this information for patient education and prognostic assessment; and to guide therapeutic strategies (E-Fig. 58-1).

Cardiac Functional Assessment

An echocardiogram should be obtained to assess resting left ventricular function before discharge in all patients. Patients who initially have a reduced left ventricular ejection fraction and who are possible candidates for ICD therapy should have the ejection fraction re-evaluated 40 days or more after discharge.

Risk stratification during hospitalization or around the time of discharge should include an assessment of exertional capacity. This assessment can be formally addressed with submaximal exercise stress testing at 4 to 6 days after the infarction or limited stress testing at 2 to 6 weeks after discharge (to peak heart rate of 120 to 130 beats per minute or 70% of the predicted maximum) unless patients have unstable post-MI angina, uncompensated heart failure, or serious cardiac arrhythmias. Alternatively, patients may undergo symptom-limited stress testing at 2 to 6 weeks before they return to work or resume other increased physical activities. Abnormal test results include not only ECG ST-segment depression but also low functional capacity, exertional hypotension, and serious arrhythmias. Patients with positive test results should be considered for coronary angiography if coronary anatomy had not been previously defined. Imaging-enhanced stress testing with radionuclide perfusion tests (Chapter 44), echocardiography (Chapter 43), or cardiac magnetic resonance (Chapter 44) can increase the sensitivity for detecting latent ischemia compared with stress ECG tests, can provide information about ejection fraction and infarct size, and should be used for patients with ECG changes that preclude accurate ECG interpretation during stress. For patients unable to exercise, pharmacologic stress testing can be performed with adenosine, a long-acting bolus analogue of adenosine (e.g., regadenoson), or by dipyridamole scintigraphy.

Discharge and Post-Hospital Phase

Secondary Prevention

Advances in secondary prevention have resulted in increasingly effective measures to reduce recurrent MI and cardiovascular death. Secondary prevention should be conscientiously applied after acute MI (Table 58-10).

Lipid Reduction

A fasting lipid profile is recommended within 24 hours of admission, and high-intensity lipid-lowering therapy with a statin should start in the hospital, preferably on admission, and be continued as outpatient therapy in all patients with ST-elevation MI and no contraindication to its use (e.g., atorvastatin, 80 mg daily or rosuvastatin 20 to 40 mg daily; Chapter 190). Ezetimibe (10 mg daily) or a PCSK9 inhibitor can be considered in patients who have not achieved an LDL-cholesterol goal of 70 mg/dL or lower.

Continued smoking doubles the subsequent mortality risk after acute MI, and smoking cessation reduces the risk for reinfarction and death within 1 year (Chapter 363). An individualized smoking cessation plan should be formulated, including pharmacologic aids (nicotine gum and patches, bupropion, or varenicline).

Antiplatelet and Anticoagulation Therapies

Antiplatelet therapy (Chapter 70) is indicated in all patients, and some patients require concomitant anticoagulant therapy. After PCI for ST-elevation MI, at

TABLE 58-10 DISCHARGE MEDICATION CHECKLIST AFTER MYOCARDIAL INFARCTION*

MEDICATION	DOSES	REASONS NOT TO USE	COMMENTS
Aspirin	81 (preferred) to 325 mg daily	High bleeding risk	Reduces mortality, reinfarction, and stroke
Clopidogrel *Or*	75 mg daily	High bleeding risk; suboptimal antiplatelet response	Indicated after PCI for at least 1 year (shorter time for BMS if high bleeding risk); also reduces vascular events when added to aspirin in non–ST-segment elevation acute MI (also useful on the basis of clinical trials after ST-segment elevation acute MI) Genetic variants (CYP2C19) may reduce response Controversial interaction with proton pump inhibitors (e.g., omeprazole)
Prasugrel *Or*	10 mg daily	High bleeding risk	Avoid with history of prior stroke or TIA
Ticagrelor	90 mg bid		Consider 5 mg prasugrel daily in patients >75 years or <60 kg Avoid if history of intracranial bleed Limit daily aspirin dose to 81 mg
β-Blocker (e.g., metoprolol, carvedilol)	Metoprolol: 25-200 mg daily Carvedilol: 6.25-25 mg bid	Asthma, bradycardia, heart failure	Reduces mortality, reinfarction, sudden death, arrhythmia, hypertension, angina, atherosclerosis progression
ACE inhibitor (e.g., ramipril, lisinopril) or ARB (e.g., valsartan, losartan)	Ramipril: 2.5-10 mg daily Lisinopril: 5-10 mg daily Valsartan: 80-160 mg daily-bid Losartan: 50-100 mg daily	Hypotension, allergy, hyperkalemia	Reduces mortality, reinfarction, stroke, heart failure, diabetes, atherosclerosis progression
Lipid-lowering agent (i.e., a high-intensity statin; e.g., atorvastatin, rosuvastatin)	Atorvastatin: 80 mg daily Rosuvastatin: 20-40 mg daily	Myopathy, rhabdomyolysis, hepatitis	Goal = LDL ≥50% reduction (statins also can benefit patients with lower LDL[†])
Nitroglycerin sublingual	0.4 mg SL PRN for angina	Aortic stenosis; sildenafil (Viagra) use	Instruct on PRN use and appropriate need for medical attention

*Medications given at hospital discharge improve long-term compliance. All are oral except for nitroglycerin.

[†]Heart Protection Study (*Lancet.* 2002;360:7); and PROVE-IT study (*N Engl J Med.* 2004;350:1495).

ACE = angiotensin-converting enzyme; ARB = angiotensin receptor blocker; bid = twice daily; BMS = bare metal stent; daily = once daily; LDL = low-density lipoprotein; MI = myocardial infarction; PCI = percutaneous coronary intervention; PRN = as needed; SL = sublingual; TIA = transient ischemic attack.

least 1 year of dual antiplatelet therapy generally has been indicated (usually aspirin [81 mg/day] plus a $P2Y_{12}$ inhibitor) to reduce ischemic events and stent thrombosis, with treatment beyond 1 year providing additional anti-ischemic benefit but at the expense of more bleeding.[A18] However, accumulating evidence with second-generation polymer-free, drug-eluting stents (Chapter 59) suggests safety with just 1 month of dual antiplatelet therapy, because stent thrombosis now is less common,[A19,A20] and that the duration and strength of antiplatelet therapy should be individualized (Chapter 59) based on bleeding and thrombotic risks. For patients who are not at a high risk of bleeding, prasugrel (10 mg/day) or ticagrelor (90 mg twice daily) is the preferred $P2Y_{12}$ inhibitor rather than clopidogrel (75 mg daily) because of greater efficacy, and prasugrel appears to be superior to ticagrelor. A genotype-guided approach to the selection of prasugrel versus clopidogrel at discharge is of uncertain benefit.[A21]

For patients with AF (Chapter 52), recent trials support a shortened period of triple antithrombotic therapy (i.e., ≤1 month) followed by dual antithrombotic therapy consisting of a direct-acting oral anticoagulant and a $P2Y_{12}$ inhibitor (e.g., dabigatran [110 or 150 mg twice daily] plus clopidogrel or ticagrelor or apixaban plus clopidogrel),[A22,A23] with clopidogrel usually preferred over ticagrelor because of its lower bleeding risk. Patients with venous thromboembolic disease (Chapter 68) can be treated similarly. For other hypercoagulable states (Chapter 67), data are sparse, but generally the antiplatelet therapy would be added to the background anticoagulant therapy. By comparison, patients with a left ventricular thrombus require a direct-acting oral anticoagulant (e.g., apixaban 5 mg twice daily), and patients with a mechanical heart valve require careful chronic warfarin anticoagulation in addition to antiplatelet therapy.

Prevention and Treatment of Heart Failure

ACE inhibitor therapy can prevent adverse myocardial remodeling after acute MI and can reduce heart failure and death; it is strongly indicated for long-term use in patients with anterior acute MI or an left ventricular ejection fraction less than 40%. ACE inhibitors also reduce recurrent MI in patients with an ejection fraction greater than 40%, except in patients who have stable coronary disease and are at low risk for a recurrent coronary event (i.e., without heart failure, hypertension, or glucose intolerance). Recommended ACE inhibitors include ramipril (2.5 mg titrated to 10 mg/day) or lisinopril (2.5 to 5 mg titrated to 10 mg/day). An angiotensin-receptor blocker (e.g., valsartan, 80 to 160 mg twice daily, or losartan, 50 to 100 mg/day) should be substituted in patients who cannot tolerate an ACE inhibitor (Chapter 46). Overt heart failure requires careful treatment (Chapter 46) titrated to symptoms and tolerance. Sacubitril plus valsartan is no better than ramipril alone in this setting.[A24]

Anti-Ischemic Therapies

Long-term β-blocker therapy does not benefit patients who have a preserved ejection fraction when added to standard modern therapy during the first year after acute MI, but it is recommended for MI survivors who have a reduced ejection fraction without other contraindications. Options include metoprolol (20 to 200 mg/day) or carvedilol (6.25 to 25 mg twice daily). However, chronic β-blocker therapy in patients at low subsequent cardiovascular risk (normal ventricular function, successful reperfusion, absence of arrhythmias) currently is viewed as reasonable but not mandatory.

Nitroglycerin (0.4 mg) is commonly prescribed for sublingual or buccal administration for acute anginal attacks (Chapter 56), although this long-standing practice has never been fully evaluated. Longer-acting oral therapy (isosorbide mononitrate, 30 to 60 mg orally every morning, or dinitrate, 10 to 40 mg orally two or three times daily) or topical nitroglycerin (e.g., start with 0.5 inch; can be titrated up to 2 inches every 6 hours for 2 days) may be added to treatment regimens for angina or heart failure (in combination with hydralazine) in selected patients.

Calcium-channel blockers are negatively inotropic and are not routinely given on a long-term basis. However, they may be used in selected patients who do not have left ventricular dysfunction (ejection fraction >0.40), who are intolerant of β-blockers, and who require these drugs for antianginal therapy (e.g., amlodipine, 5 to 10 mg/day orally, or diltiazem, 120 to 480 mg/day orally as sustained-release preparations or in divided doses; see Chapter 56) or for control of heart rate in AF (e.g., diltiazem, 120 to 480 mg/day orally, or verapamil, 180 to 480 mg/day orally, as sustained-release preparations or in divided doses). Short-acting nifedipine should be avoided.

If these medical approaches do not control post-infarction angina and complete revascularization was not performed during an acute PCI, coronary angiography should be considered in patients whose symptoms would warrant it (Chapter 56).[17]

Anti-Inflammatory Therapy

In patients who have survived an MI and have a high-sensitivity C-reactive protein level of 2 mg/L or greater, the use of canakinumab, a monoclonal antibody against interleukin-1β (150 mg subcutaneously every 3 months) reduced the risk of subsequent nonfatal MI, nonfatal stroke, or cardiovascular death.[A25] Colchicine (0.5 mg daily) also can reduce the risk of subsequent cardiovascular events in patients who have survived a myocardial infarction,[A26] especially if begun within 3 days of the MI.[A27] Whether these therapies will become a part of routine post-MI medical care is yet to be determined.

Antiarrhythmic Therapy

In patients who do not require an acute ICD (see Ventricular Rhythms, earlier), an ICD is recommended for those with severe left ventricular dysfunction (ejection fraction ≤0.30) at least 40 days after ST-elevation MI and 3 months after CABG, even without spontaneous or induced ventricular tachycardia or ventricular fibrillation.[A28] Antiarrhythmic drugs are not generally recommended after acute MI, and class I antiarrhythmic agents can increase the risk for sudden death. Class III drugs (amiodarone, sotalol, dofetilide) may be used as part of the management strategy for specific arrhythmias (e.g., AF, ventricular tachycardia) (Chapters 52 and 53).

Other Medical Therapies

Hypertension (Chapter 64) and diabetes mellitus (Chapter 210) must be assessed and tightly controlled in patients after an acute MI. ACE inhibitors or β-blockers as described earlier are usually the first-choice therapies for hypertension, with ARBs indicated when ACE inhibitors are not tolerated. ACE inhibitors and ARBs also can reduce the long-term complications of diabetes. Such drugs should be titrated to a goal blood pressure of less than 130/80 mm Hg, which is equivalent to an office goal of 120/80 mm Hg (Chapter 64).

Hormone replacement therapy (Chapter 222) with estrogen with or without progestin is not begun after an acute MI because it increases thromboembolic risk and does not prevent reinfarction. For women already receiving hormone replacement, therapy should be discontinued unless it is being given for a compelling indication.

Antioxidant supplementation (e.g., vitamin E, vitamin C) does not benefit patients after acute MI and is not recommended. The role of fish oil and related supplements is unclear, but purified agents such as eicosapentoic ethyl appear to decrease cardiovascular events in chronic coronary heart disease.

Patient Education and Rehabilitation

The hospital stay provides an important opportunity to educate patients about their MI and its treatment, coronary risk factors, and behavioral modification. Education should begin on admission and continue to and beyond discharge. At hospital discharge, a detailed, evidence-based plan of care should emphasize the importance of a healthy lifestyle, including diet (Chapter 13), exercise (Chapter 14), smoking cessation (Chapter 363), and compliance with medications. Timely outpatient health care follow-up also should be scheduled and a rehabilitation program referral provided. Exercise-based cardiac rehabilitation may reduce reinfarction by about 50% and overall mortality by about 25%, with home-based programs being as safe and effective as center-based programs.[A29] Many hospitals use case managers and prevention specialists to augment physicians and nurses, to provide educational materials, to review important concepts, to assist in formulating and actualizing individual risk reduction plans, and to ensure proper and timely outpatient follow-up. This follow-up should include early return appointments with the patient's physician (within 2 to a few weeks), which may be facilitated with virtual platforms. Instructions on activities also should be given before discharge.

PROGNOSIS

With the broad application of reperfusion and other contemporary therapies, the prognosis often myocardial infarction continues to improve.[18] The 30-day mortality after ST-elevation MI is now less than 6%, and the 1-year mortality rate is 7 to 8%. Since reductions in mortality can be directly related to the number of evidence-based therapies given, patients treated at high-performing hospitals live about 1 year longer than do patients treated at low-performing hospitals. Of note is that the long-term survival is similar in patients who do and do not have evidence of obstructive coronary disease on acute coronary arteriography.[19]

GENERAL REFERENCES

For the General References and other additional features, please visit Elsevier eBooks+ at https://ebooks.health.elsevier.com.

Grade A References

A1. Valgimigli M, Frigoli E, Leonardi S, et al. Radial versus femoral access and bivalirudin versus unfractionated heparin in invasively managed patients with acute coronary syndrome (MATRIX): final 1-year results of a multicentre, randomized controlled trial. *Lancet*. 2018;392:835-848.

A2. Thrane PG, Kristensen SD, Olesen KKW, et al. 16-year follow-up of the Danish Acute Myocardial Infarction 2 (DANAMI-2) trial: primary percutaneous coronary intervention vs. fibrinolysis in ST-segment elevation myocardial infarction. *Eur Heart J*. 2020;41:847-854.

A3. Sabaté M, Brugaletta S, Cequier A, et al. Clinical outcomes in patients with ST-segment elevation myocardial infarction treated with everolimus-eluting stents versus bare-metal stents (EXAMINATION): 5-year results of a randomised trial. *Lancet*. 2016;387:357-366.

A4. Jolly SS, Cairns JA, Yusuf S, et al. Randomized trial of primary PCI with or without routine manual thrombectomy. *N Engl J Med*. 2015;372:1389-1398.

A5. Engstrom T, Kelbaek H, Helqvist S, et al. Complete revascularization versus treatment of the culprit lesion only in patients with ST-segment elevation myocardial infarction and multivessel disease (DANAMI-3-PRIMULTI): an open-label randomized controlled trial. *Lancet.* 2015;386:665-671.

A6. Wood DA, Cairns JA, Wang J, et al. Timing of staged nonculprit artery revascularization in patients with ST-segment elevation myocardial infarction: COMPLETE trial. *J Am Coll Cardiol.* 2019;74:2713-2723.

A7. Bainey KR, Engstrøm T, Smits PC, et al. Complete vs culprit-lesion-only revascularization for ST-segment elevation myocardial infarction: a systematic review and meta-analysis. *JAMA Cardiol.* 2020;5:881-888.

A8. Thiele H, Akin I, Sandri M, et al. One-year outcomes after PCI strategies in cardiogenic shock. *N Engl J Med.* 2018;379:1699-1710.

A9. Pavasini R, Biscaglia S, Barbato E, et al. Complete revascularization reduces cardiovascular death in patients with ST-segment elevation myocardial infarction and multivessel disease: systematic review and meta-analysis of randomized clinical trials. *Eur Heart J.* 2020;41:4103-4110.

A10. Jinatongthai P, Kongwatcharapong J, Foo CY, et al. Comparative efficacy and safety of reperfusion therapy with fibrinolytic agents in patients with ST-segment elevation myocardial infarction: a systematic review and network meta-analysis. *Lancet.* 2017;390:747-759.

A11. Hofmann R, Witt N, Lagerqvist B, et al. Oxygen therapy in ST-elevation myocardial infarction. *Eur Heart J.* 2018;39:2730-2739.

A12. Hofmann R, James SK, Jernberg T, et al. Oxygen therapy in suspected acute myocardial infarction. *N Engl J Med.* 2017;377:1240-1249.

A13. Roolvink V, Ibáñek B, Ottervanger JP, et al. Early intravenous beta-blockers in patients with ST-segment elevation myocardial infarction before primary percutaneous coronary intervention. *J Am Coll Cardiol.* 2016;67:2705-2715.

A14. Schüpke S, Neumann F-J, Menichelli M, et al. Ticagrelor or prasugrel in patients with acute coronary syndromes. *N Engl J Med.* 2019;381:1524-1534.

A15. Erlinge D, Omerovic E, Frobert O, et al. Bivalirudin versus heparin monotherapy in myocardial infarction. *N Engl J Med.* 2017;377:1132-1142.

A16. Lopes RD, Heizer G, Aronson R, et al. Antithrombotic therapy after acute coronary syndrome or PCI in atrial fibrillation. *N Engl J Med.* 2019;380:1509-1524.

A17. Gibson CM, Mehran R, Bode C, et al. Prevention of bleeding in patients with atrial fibrillation undergoing PCI. *N Engl J Med.* 2016;375:2423-2434.

A18. Bonaca MP, Bhatt DL, Cohen M, et al. Long-term use of ticagrelor in patients with prior myocardial infarction. *N Engl J Med.* 2015;372:1791-1800.

A19. Mehran R, Baber U, Sharma SK, et al. Ticagrelor with or without aspirin in high-risk patients after PCI. *N Engl J Med.* 2019;381:2032-2042.

A20. Windecker S, Latib A, Kedhi E, et al. Polymer-based or polymer-free stents in patients at high bleeding risk. *N Engl J Med.* 2020;382:1208-1218.

A21. Pereira NL, Farkouh ME, So D, et al. Effect of genotype-guided oral P2Y12 inhibitor selection vs conventional clopidogrel therapy on ischemic outcomes after percutaneous coronary intervention: the TAILOR-PCI randomized clinical trial. *JAMA.* 2020;324:761-771.

A22. Cannon CP, Bhatt DL, Oldgren J, et al. Dual antithrombotic therapy with dabigatran after PCI in atrial fibrillation. *N Engl J Med.* 2017;377:1513-1524.

A23. Khan SU, Osman M, Khan MU, et al. Dual versus triple therapy for atrial fibrillation after percutaneous coronary intervention. *Ann Intern Med.* 2020;172:474-483.

A24. Pfeffer MA, Claggett B, Lewis EF, et al. Angiotensin receptor-neprilysin inhibition in acute myocardial infarction. *N Engl J Med.* 2021;385:1845-1855.

A25. Ridker PM, Everett BM, Thuren T, et al. Antiinflammatory therapy with canakinumab for atherosclerotic disease. *N Engl J Med.* 2017;377:1119-1131.

A26. Tardif JC, Kouz S, Waters DD, et al. Efficacy and safety of low-dose colchicine after myocardial infarction. *N Engl J Med.* 2019;381:2497-2505.

A27. Bouabdallaoui N, Tardif J-C, Waters DD, et al. Time-to-treatment initiation of colchicine and cardiovascular outcomes after myocardial infarction in the colchicine cardiovascular outcomes trial (COLCOT). *Eur Heart J.* 2020;41:4092-4099.

A28. Kolodziejczak M, Andreotti F, Kowalewski M, et al. Implantable cardioverter-defibrilators for primary prevention in patients with ischemic or nonischemic cardiomyopathy: a systematic review and meta-analysis. *Ann Intern Med.* 2017;167:103-111.

A29. Anderson L, Sharp GA, Norton RJ, et al. Home-based versus centre-based cardiac rehabilitation. *Cochrane Database Syst Rev.* 2017;6:CD007130.

59

INTERVENTIONAL DIAGNOSIS AND TREATMENT OF CORONARY ARTERY DISEASE

PAUL S. TEIRSTEIN AND AJAY J. KIRTANE

Percutaneous coronary intervention (PCI) and coronary artery bypass graft (CABG) surgery represent alternative and sometimes complementary approaches to coronary revascularization. Each has its relative indications, advantages, disadvantages, and contraindications.

CORONARY ARTERIOGRAPHY TO ASSESS CORONARY STENOSIS

For coronary angiography, catheters are inserted into the epicardial arteries of the heart to obtain radiographic images of the coronary vasculature and to define the site and severity of any lesions or anomalies, as well as any visible collateral blood vessels beyond arterial stenoses or occlusions. Coronary arteriography often is part of a more comprehensive catheterization to assess valvular (Chapter 60), congenital (Chapter 55), or myocardial diseases (Chapter 47) or to perform a variety of catheter-based interventions (E-Table 59-1).

THE PROCEDURE

Vascular access under local anesthetic is preferably via the radial artery,[1] which is associated with less bleeding and equivalent or better outcomes compared with femoral access.[A1] A specially shaped catheter is inserted over a guidewire to facilitate atraumatic passage to a coronary artery ostium (origin at the aorta) to inject radiographic contrast media for coronary arteriography. This process is performed twice, once for the left coronary ostium and once for the right, although each may be accompanied by more than one injection as needed. Hemodynamic data may be acquired to assist in the evaluation of cardiac function at rest or sometimes after stationary exercise.

After a radial procedure, the patient can ambulate immediately and may be discharged 2 to 4 hours later. After a femoral procedure, however, the patient must remain stationary in bed for 1 to 2 hours using a vascular closure device (or otherwise for 4 hours) and can be discharged after 4 to 6 hours of recovery.

ASSESSMENT OF CORONARY STENOSES

The patient's coronary arteriographic images are compared with normal anatomy (Fig. 59-1). The degree of stenosis in any vessel is based on a visual estimate of the percentage reduction in luminal diameter at the most severely narrowed coronary segment compared with the closest angiographically unobstructed vessel segment (Fig. 59-2). The degree of coronary collateralization, which is assessed qualitatively, correlates with longer chronicity of stenoses or complete occlusion and is associated with a more favorable prognosis.

Because these estimates of the severity of stenoses may vary, even among experienced angiographers, the importance of an intermediately severe lesion (i.e., a 40 to 90% stenosis) can be determined by passing a pressure sensor guidewire to measure the pressure gradient across the stenosis after injecting adenosine to maximize flow. The ratio of post-lesion pressure to aortic pressure during maximal flow (the fractional flow reserve) indicates the percentage of normal flow across the stenosis.[2] Stenoses with fractional flow reserve (a ratio of distal hyperemic pressure to aortic pressure) above 0.80 are considered nonischemic and typically do not require revascularization, whereas a lower fractional flow reserve typically warrants percutaneous coronary intervention (PCI).

COMPLICATIONS OF CARDIAC CATHETERIZATION

Diagnostic cardiac catheterization has few contraindications and a low but not trivial risk of serious complications (Table 59-1). In the United States, for example, the overall risk is less than 0.2% for death, less than 0.5% for myocardial infarction, less than 0.07% for stroke, less than 0.5% for serious arrhythmia, and less than 1% for major vascular complications (including thrombosis or cholesterol embolization [Chapter 110]), bleeding requiring transfusion, or pseudoaneurysm.[3,4] Vascular complications are less common with the radial artery approach.

For a diagnostic catheterization, patients are not routinely anticoagulated except for the radial approach, in which preexisting anticoagulation is typically maintained or heparin is given to reduce the occurrence of radial artery occlusion. For the femoral approach, anticoagulation may be uninterrupted or held for 2 to 3 days before the procedure. For a patient who is taking warfarin after a mechanical valve replacement, warfarin is withheld for 3 days before the procedure, with consideration of bridging heparin in high-risk cases.

Most medications should be continued up to and including the morning of the procedure. For diabetic patients, 50% of the usual morning dose of insulin is usually given; metformin should be withheld.

Contrast-induced acute kidney injury, which usually is not clinically evident until 2 to 3 days after the procedure,[5] is clinically significant in about 1.2% of patients,[6] but the risk is 3 to 5 times higher in patients who have diabetes or renal insufficiency or who are dehydrated. In such patients, preprocedural hydration with sodium chloride is usually indicated to increase urine output.[A2] An oral statin (e.g., rosuvastatin, either 40 mg on admission followed by 20 mg per day for patients with an acute coronary syndrome or 10 mg for two days before and three days afterward for patients with diabetes and

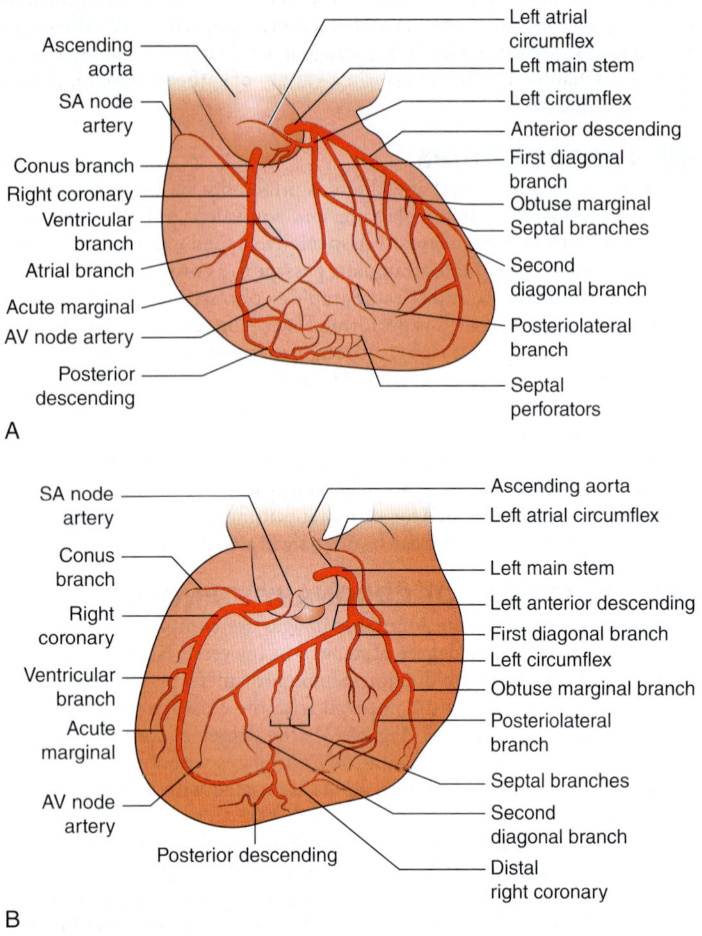

FIGURE 59-1. **Coronary vessels. The right anterior oblique (A) and left anterior oblique (B) views are shown. The major arteries are the left main, left anterior descending, circumflex, and right coronary arteries. AV = atrioventricular; SA = sinoatrial. (Modified from Yang SS, Bentivoglio LG, Maranhao V, et al, eds. From *Cardiac Catheterization Data to Hemodynamic Parameters*. Philadelphia: Oxford University Press; 1988.)**

TABLE 59-1 CARDIAC CATHETERIZATION: CONTRAINDICATIONS AND COMPLICATIONS

ABSOLUTE CONTRAINDICATIONS
Inadequate facilities
Patient refusal
RELATIVE CONTRAINDICATIONS
Severe uncontrolled hypertension
Ventricular arrhythmias
Recent acute stroke
Severe anemia
Active gastrointestinal bleeding
Allergy to radiographic contrast agents
Acute renal failure
Uncompensated heart failure (patient cannot lie flat)
Unexplained febrile illness or untreated active infection
Electrolyte abnormalities (e.g., hypokalemia)
Severe coagulopathy
Pregnancy
Uncontrolled arrhythmias, hypertension
Uncooperative patient or patient refusal
MAJOR COMPLICATIONS
Death
Cerebrovascular accident
Myocardial infarction, shock
Ventricular tachycardia or fibrillation
RARE BUT SERIOUS COMPLICATIONS
Aortic dissection
Cardiac perforation
Tamponade
Heart failure
Reaction to contrast agents, anaphylaxis
Nephrotoxicity
Arrhythmias, including heart block, asystole, supraventricular tachyarrhythmias
Hemorrhage, including local or retroperitoneal
Infection
Protamine reaction
Vascular complications, including thrombosis, embolus, vascular injury, pseudoaneurysm

Adapted from Kern MJ, Kirtane AJ. Catheterization and angiography. In: Goldman L, Schafer AI, eds. *Goldman-Cecil Medicine*. 26th ed. Philadelphia, PA: Elsevier; 2020.

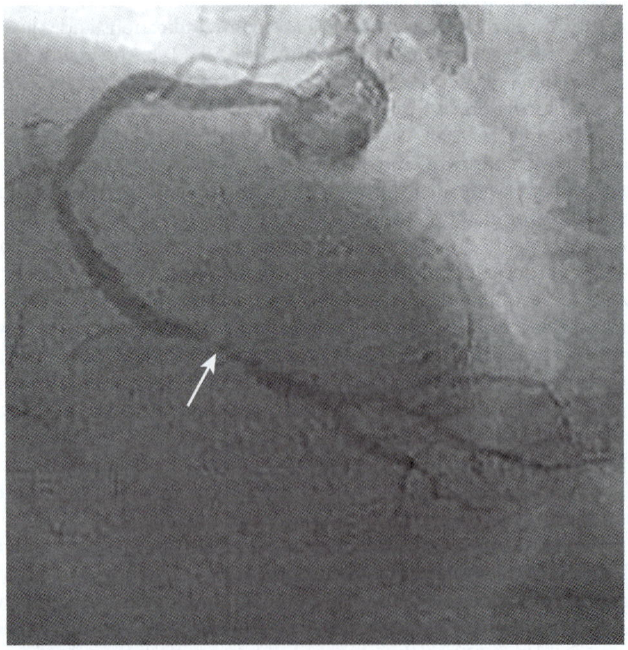

FIGURE 59-2. **Example of a significant stenosis (*arrow*) in the right coronary artery.** (Courtesy of Morton J. Kern, MD.)

chronic kidney disease) can reduce the risk of acute kidney injury by about 50%.[A3] Treatment with sodium bicarbonate or *N*-acetylcysteine (Mucomyst) is not of incremental value and is not routinely recommended.[A4,A5] In patients who have advanced chronic kidney disease and in whom radiocontrast is contraindicated, angiography can be avoided, with PCI guided by intravascular ultrasound and physiologic measurements.

Adverse reactions to contrast media are potentially serious but rare, with an overall incidence of 5% or less. However, adverse reactions occur in about 15% of patients with a previously reported allergic contrast reaction. Patients who have had a previous allergic reaction to contrast media should be premedicated with prednisone (60 mg orally the evening before and morning of the procedure) and diphenhydramine (25 to 50 mg orally the morning of the procedure).

Vasovagal hypotension, which is relatively common, is treated with intravenous fluids and atropine (0.5 to 1.0 mg intravenously). Hypotension that is accompanied by back pain is rare but suggests retroperitoneal bleeding and hematoma and requires emergency intervention. Hypotension also can be caused when perforation of a coronary artery leads to cardiac tamponade (Chapter 62); this emergency requires urgent pericardiocentesis and treatment of any coronary perforation. Pulmonary congestion, which may develop in patients with compromised left ventricular function or valvular heart disease, is treated with oxygen and diuretics (Chapter 46) or more intensive interventions if it progresses to cardiogenic shock (Chapter 93).

Chest pain is unusual during coronary angiography, but may be associated with myocardial ischemia and ST segment changes during PCI. Treatment (e.g., nitroglycerin, heparin, and antiplatelet medications) usually controls myocardial ischemia before revascularization (Chapter 57). Atrial or ventricular premature contractions or even brief episodes of supraventricular tachycardia are common and usually resolve spontaneously. Ventricular tachycardia and ventricular fibrillation are rare but require prompt defibrillation (Chapter 50).

PERCUTANEOUS CORONARY INTERVENTION

Percutaneous coronary intervention is applicable to most forms of coronary artery disease, including single- and double-vessel disease, but also can be performed for multivessel disease, total occlusions, saphenous vein graft disease, unstable angina (Chapter 57), and acute myocardial infarction (MI) (Chapter 58). An estimated 2 million PCIs are performed worldwide each year, making it one of the most widely used medical procedures. Its popularity is based largely on its simplicity, the need for only local anesthesia, a short (≈1 day or even outpatient) hospitalization, and negligible postprocedure recovery time. In the United States, PCI is a cornerstone of the treatment of acute coronary syndromes (Chapters 57 and 58), but the number of nonacute PCIs has declined by over one third since 2010.

MECHANISMS AND TECHNICAL CONSIDERATIONS

Under local anesthesia, a hollow-bore needle is inserted percutaneously into a peripheral artery (usually the radial or femoral artery). A guidewire is placed through this needle and advanced into the aorta. The needle is removed, leaving the guidewire, over which a small-caliber (≈3 mm), specially shaped catheter (called a guiding catheter) is advanced under fluoroscopic guidance into the ostium of the obstructed coronary artery. By use of radiographic contrast injections that provide fluoroscopic visualization of the coronary artery lumen, a thin (≈0.014 inch), highly steerable guidewire is directed down the coronary artery and across the stenotic lesion. This guidewire becomes a "rail" over which therapeutic tools such as inflatable balloons, stents, and atherectomy catheters are passed to the diseased segment (Fig. 59-3).

Balloon catheters (Fig. 59-4) typically have two lumens, one to allow passage over the guidewire and another to carry a mixture of saline and radiographic contrast material to inflate a balloon at the distal catheter tip. Under fluoroscopy, the balloon is centered across the lesion and inflated to typically 4 to 30 atmospheres of pressure. Balloon inflation widens the narrowed lumen by stretching the vessel and, in most cases, causing a tear (a therapeutic dissection) at the edges of the plaque, where the atheroma meets the nondiseased media. Atherectomy catheters, which also are passed over a guidewire to the diseased segment, remove plaque by a shaving, grinding, slicing, or suction mechanism. Coronary stents are metallic or polymeric scaffolding devices that are crimped onto a deflated balloon catheter before insertion into the diseased vessel (Videos 59-1, 59-2, and 59-3). During balloon inflation, the collapsed stent expands to support the vessel lumen (see E-Fig. 59-1 and Video 59-4). Although balloons and atherectomy devices create an adequate, albeit rough channel through diseased arteries, the supporting structure of the stent can widen the lumen to near its predisease dimensions. With a stent, tissue flaps are "pinned" against the wall, and recoil is limited (Video 59-5). Most stents are designed so that the metallic struts comprise only about 20% of the surface area, thereby allowing for endothelialization, which reduces the risk of thrombosis.[7] In some cases (e.g., PCI of saphenous vein grafts), filters deployed within a coronary vessel beyond the target lesion can limit distal embolization of plaque, platelet aggregates, and other "debris" can further reduce ischemic complications in vessels with a friable endothelium.

During the PCI procedure, the interventional cardiologist is able to assess the target vessel fluoroscopically by injections of contrast material through the guiding catheter (Fig. 59-5). A more detailed assessment of the target vessel is often obtained using intravascular imaging technologies, with catheters that use sound waves or light to produce an image of the lumen (channel for blood flow) and vessel walls (E-Fig. 59-2). When the coronary artery has been opened successfully, all catheters are withdrawn and the arterial access site is sealed by mechanical pressure, an absorbable plug, or an external suturing device. Patients without comorbidity ambulate in 2 to 6 hours. Discharge from the hospital usually occurs 2 to 6 hours later or the morning after the procedure, when stability of the arterial access site, cardiac biomarkers, and the electrocardiogram are confirmed.

SELECTION OF PATIENTS FOR PERCUTANEOUS CORONARY INTERVENTION

Any decision to perform PCI must include a comprehensive and detailed review of the coronary angiogram by an experienced interventional cardiologist to assess the lesion's technical suitability for the procedure. Coronary flow is not significantly obstructed until a stenosis narrows the coronary artery lumen by at least 60%. A pressure drop of more than 20% (which corresponds to a fractional flow reserve <0.80) predicts a clinical benefit from PCI[A6-A7] in stable chronic ischemic heart disease but not clearly for stenting a nonculprit lesion in a patient with a non–ST elevation acute myocardial infarction.[A8]

For each patient, the benefits of PCI must be weighed against the procedural risk. Patients whose lesions are characterized by longer length, tortuous vessels, calcification, or the presence of thrombus can be treated with PCI but are at increased risk. Other patient characteristics conveying increased risk include advanced age (i.e., >75 years), diabetes, smaller vessels that are often found in women, prior MI, significant impairment of left ventricular function, and renal insufficiency.

PROCEDURAL SUCCESS AND COMPLICATIONS

With use of modern techniques in appropriately selected patients, most PCI procedures have a greater than 95% success rate. The single exception is a chronic total coronary occlusion (100% obstruction of the lumen), in which the interventional cardiologist's ability to negotiate a guidewire through the blockage is only about 60% to 90% and varies substantially with the operator's expertise. With the increased use of coronary stents and adjunctive antiplatelet agents, acute coronary artery closure is rarely encountered. When PCI is performed by an experienced interventional cardiologist in appropriately selected patients, the risk of in-hospital death is less than 0.5%, but the risk of a type 4 MI (usually a small, non–ST segment elevation MI; Chapter 57) is not negligible, especially when assessed by sensitive biomarker assays.[8] The

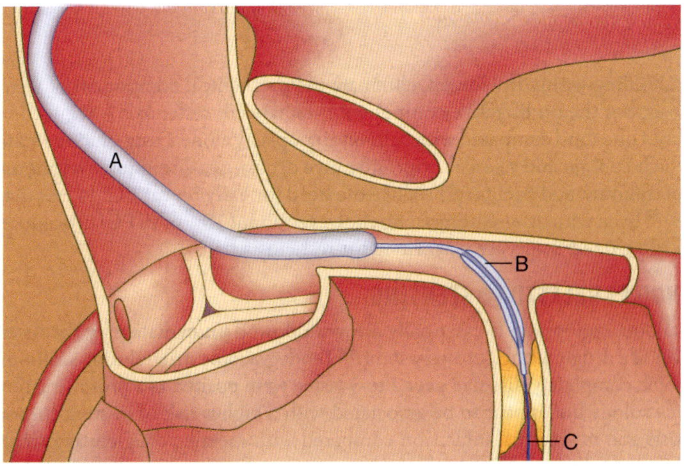

FIGURE 59-3. Schematic view of coronary angioplasty technique. A guide catheter (**A**) is inserted into the orifice of the coronary artery (in this figure, the left main artery), and a balloon catheter (**B**) is advanced over a thin guidewire (**C**) into the lesion. Balloon inflation dilates the stenotic region. (Modified from Baim DS. Percutaneous balloon angioplasty and general coronary intervention. In: Baim DS, ed. *Grossman's Cardiac Catheterization, Angiography, and Intervention*. 7th ed. Philadelphia: Lippincott Williams & Wilkins; 2005.)

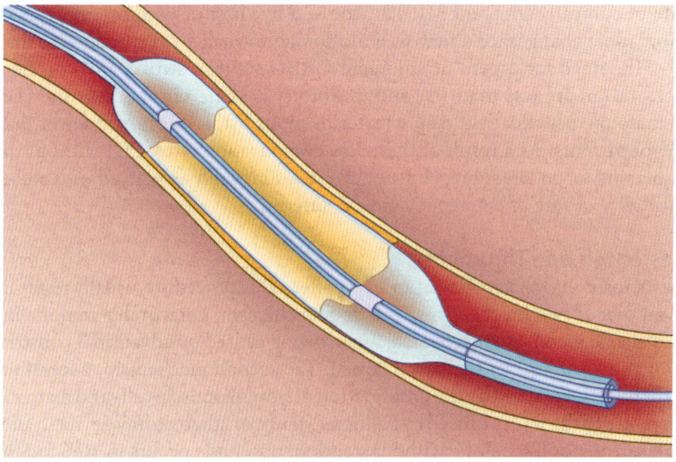

FIGURE 59-4. Balloon angioplasty catheter. The catheter consists of two lumens, an inflation lumen and a guidewire lumen. Two radiopaque markers, indicating the lateral balloon margins, aid in positioning of the balloon before inflation.

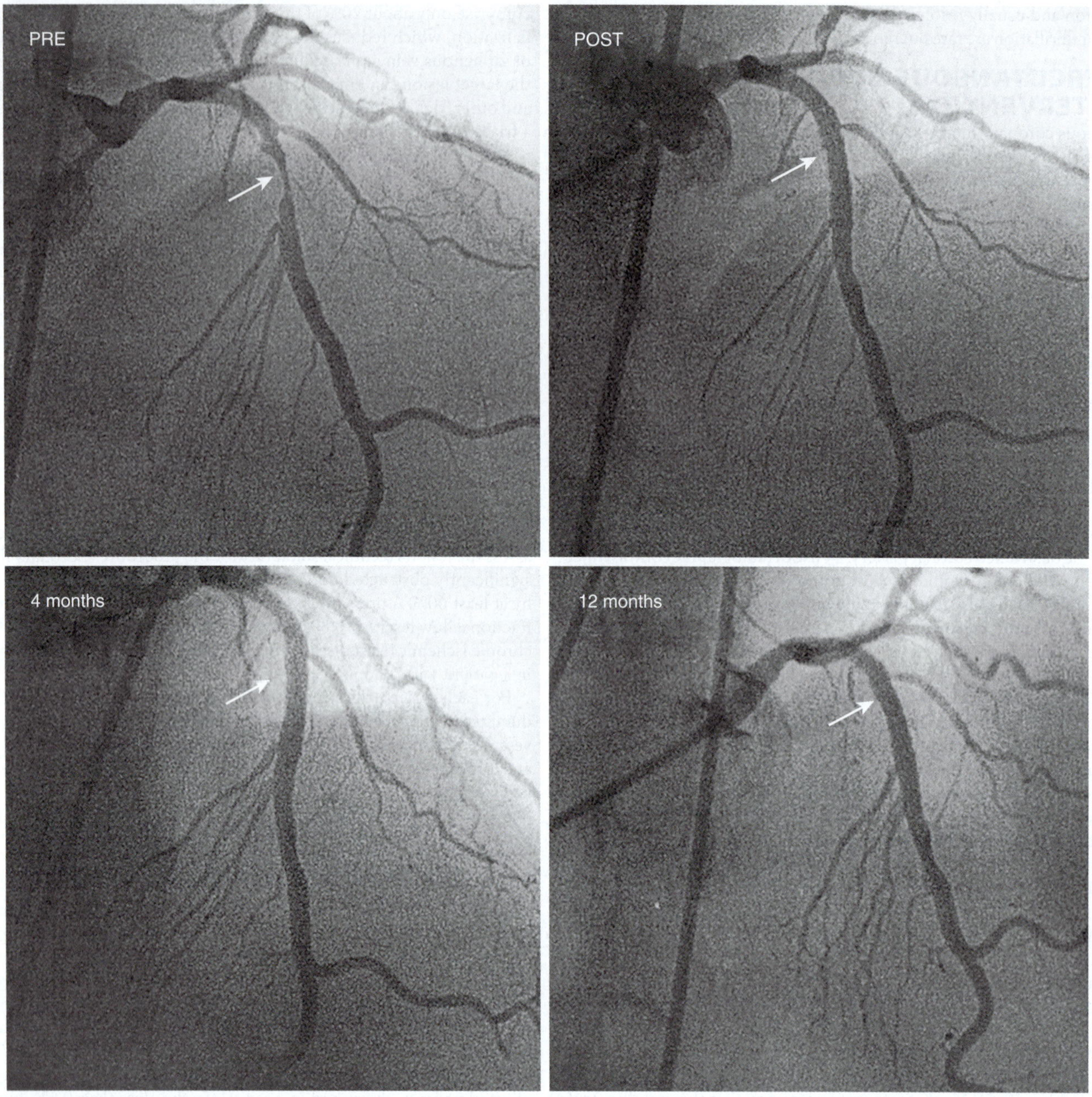

FIGURE 59-5. **Angiographic images before, after, and at late follow-up after placement of a drug-eluting stent.** The left anterior descending artery contains a tight stenosis *(arrow, upper left panel)*. After stent implantation *(upper right panel)*, the stenosis is abolished *(arrow)*. Follow-up at 4 and 12 months *(bottom panels)* reveals a completely open lumen with no evidence of restenosis *(arrows)*.

rate of clinically apparent MI characterized by chest discomfort, electrocardiographic changes, or a new wall motion abnormality is typically less than 2%. The need for urgent or emergent CABG surgery, stroke, and coronary perforation are less than 1%, and morbidity at the arterial access site (i.e., hematoma, pseudoaneurysm, or arteriovenous fistula) occurs in fewer than 5% of patients. As a result of these low complication rates, PCI without the availability of on-site surgery has not been demonstrably associated with higher mortality or rate of emergency CABG surgery.

Restenosis and Thrombosis

Restenosis[9] is a renarrowing of an artery after a PCI procedure, usually resulting from one of two mechanisms. The first mechanism, unfavorable remodeling and elastic recoil, is a mechanical renarrowing caused by adventitial constriction and shrinkage of the vessel lumen. The second mechanism, neointimal hyperplasia, is caused by the proliferation of smooth muscle cells and matrix in response to the injury caused by balloons, stents, or atherectomy devices. After balloon angioplasty alone without stenting, restenosis occurs in 10% to 50% of patients, usually within the first 6 months after the procedure, because of remodeling and recoil. Bare metal coronary stents, which provide a semi-rigid scaffolding within the lumen, eliminate the mechanical component of restenosis, but the proliferative component is enhanced; restenosis is reduced by about one third compared with balloon angioplasty alone. Drug-eluting stents, which contain and release antiproliferative drugs (e.g., sirolimus, everolimus, zotarolimus, and paclitaxel) reduce the need for early repeat PCI to less than 5%.[A9] Even with drug-eluting stents, however, about 10% of all PCI procedures in the United States are performed for restenosis.[10]

CHOICES RELATED TO STENTING

Balloon angioplasty is essentially always followed immediately by the insertion of a drug-eluting coronary stent.[A10] Biodegradable drug-eluting scaffolds, which completely dissolve over 2 to 3 years, were posited as a promising new technology but appear to be associated with a higher risk of in-stent thrombosis and myocardial infarction compared with metallic drug-eluting stents at 3-year follow-up.[A11]

The treatment of highly calcified vessels often requires rotational atherectomy or lithotripsy. Atherectomy (using a spinning catheter containing abrasive particles or laser energy) pulverizes plaque into microparticles that pass through the coronary microcirculation and is particularly helpful for the treatment of heavily calcified lesions. Intravascular lithotripsy catheters deliver localized pulsatile sonic pressure waves that disrupt calcified plaque by creating microfractures. After the calcium has been cracked by lithotripsy or pulverized by atherectomy, the artery can be more easily expanded, and a drug-eluting stent is usually implanted.

DISCHARGE ISSUES

Discharge planning after PCI represents an important opportunity to emphasize evidence-based medical treatment of atherothrombotic disease and coronary risk factor modification (Chapter 40). Prolonged use of lipid-lowering agents, angiotensin-converting enzyme inhibitors, and in some cases β-blockers should be considered on the basis of randomized trials showing improved long-term outcome, particularly in patients who present with unstable coronary syndromes (Chapters 57 and 58). Smoking cessation (Chapter 363), blood pressure control (Chapter 64), stress management, exercise, weight loss, changes in dietary habits, and strict blood glucose control for patients with diabetes (Chapter 210) also are important elements of the discharge plan.

All patients should receive aspirin (81 mg/day) indefinitely. For patients receiving bare metal stents, a minimum 2-week course of a $P2Y_{12}$ receptor inhibitor (e.g., clopidogrel 75 mg/day, prasugrel 10 mg/day, or ticagrelor 90 mg/day) is mandatory. If a drug-eluting stent is deployed, aspirin plus a $P2Y_{12}$ inhibitor historically was required for a minimum of 3 to 6 months if the stent was implanted in a stable patient and 6 to 12 months if stenting was performed due to an acute coronary syndrome (unstable angina or myocardial infarction),[A12] However, switching to $P2Y_{12}$ monotherapy can be safe and effective in selected high-risk patients after 1 to 3 months of dual antiplatelet therapy.[A13] In fact, with second-generation polymer-free drug-eluting stents,[11] 1 month of dual anti-platelet therapy followed by 11 months of clopidogrel alone is a potential option to limit bleeding in patients with higher risks of bleeding. [A14,A15] Extending dual antiplatelet therapy to 30 or 36 months reduces ischemic cardiovascular events but increases bleeding. In patients with atrial fibrillation (Chapter 52), dual therapy with a direct-acting oral anticoagulant (e.g., dabigatran 110 mg or 150 mg twice daily) plus a $P2Y_{12}$ receptor inhibitor carries similar ischemic protection with a lower risk of bleeding compared with triple therapy with aspirin, warfarin, and either clopidogrel or ticagrelor.[A16]

Activity restrictions after PCI are modest. If the femoral artery was instrumented, heavy lifting is discouraged for several days. Intense aerobic exercise is usually discouraged for 2 to 4 weeks (especially after stent implantation) because exercise can activate platelets and lead to formation of thrombus at the angioplasty site. Patients may return to work 1 or 2 days after the procedure if their occupation does not include heavy lifting or excessive physical exercise. There is usually no restriction on driving an automobile. Routine postoperative functional testing has not been shown to be beneficial.[A17]

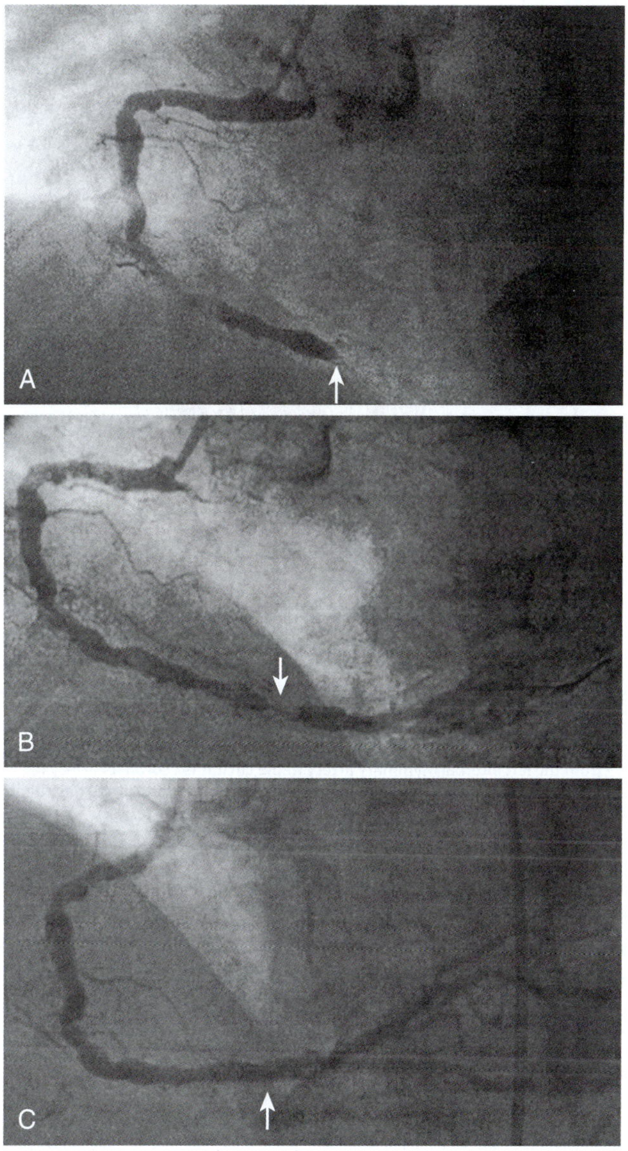

FIGURE 59-6. Primary coronary angioplasty for acute myocardial infarction. This 50-year-old man presented at midnight with 70 minutes of crushing substernal chest pressure accompanied by inferior ST segment elevation. Emergency angiography performed 45 minutes after arrival found 100% occlusion of the right coronary artery (**A**, *arrow*). Within 10 minutes, a guidewire was negotiated through the obstruction (presumably caused by fresh thrombus), allowing perfusion into the distal vessel and uncovering a high-grade stenotic lesion (**B**, *arrow*). After deployment of a coronary stent (**C**, *arrow*), the stenosis was abolished and significant myocardial damage aborted.

CORONARY ANGIOPLASTY VERSUS MEDICAL THERAPY

Percutaneous coronary intervention reduces angina and commonly leads to better treadmill exercise performance and improved quality-of-life measurements. However, in patients with stable angina, PCI has not been shown to reduce the risks of death, MI, or other major cardiovascular events compared with modern optimal medical therapy (Chapter 56).[A18-A22] In truly asymptomatic patients, significant ischemia first should be documented by functional testing, or a large quantity of myocardium should be supplied by the stenotic coronary artery. Patients experiencing acute MI such as ST segment elevation MI (Chapter 58) represent an important subgroup in whom PCI has proved beneficial compared with medical therapy (Fig. 59-6). In ST segment elevation MI, randomized trials have consistently shown a reduction in mortality, stroke, subsequent MI, and recurrent ischemia with immediate PCI compared with thrombolytic therapy or with initial thrombolytic therapy followed by rescue PCI as needed even if immediate PCI requires transfer to another hospital. For non–ST segment elevation MI and many patients with unstable angina, an early aggressive approach that includes either PCI or CABG in angiographically suitable patients is generally preferable to a conservative strategy except in lower risk patients (Chapter 57).[12]

CORONARY ARTERY SURGERY

Coronary artery bypass graft surgery is based on the premise that the morbidity and mortality associated with coronary atherosclerosis are largely related to atherosclerotic coronary stenoses that can be demonstrated by coronary angiography and that if grafts are constructed to route blood flow around these stenoses, myocardial blood supply can be improved or preserved, cardiac symptoms relieved, cardiac events diminished, and survival prolonged.

The most common types of grafts for coronary artery bypass have been reversed segments of saphenous vein and the internal thoracic arteries. Saphenous vein grafts are anastomosed to the aorta (proximal anastomosis) and to the coronary artery distal to the major obstruction (Fig. 59-7). Saphenous vein grafts have the advantages of availability, larger size than most coronary arteries, and favorable handling characteristics. With time, however, saphenous vein grafts may develop intrinsic pathologic changes, intimal fibroplasia, and vein graft atherosclerosis, each of which may lead to narrowing or occlusions. Modern treatment with platelet inhibitors and statins (Chapter 190) decreases the risk of vein graft failure but cannot eliminate it. Internal thoracic artery grafts, on the other hand, are resistant to the development of late atherosclerosis. When used as an in situ (subclavian origin intact) graft to the left anterior descending (LAD) coronary artery, the left internal thoracic artery graft has a more than 90% patency rate up to 20 years after operation. As a result, patients who receive a left internal thoracic artery to LAD graft, with or without saphenous vein grafts, have a better long-term survival rate, fewer reoperations, and fewer cardiac events compared with

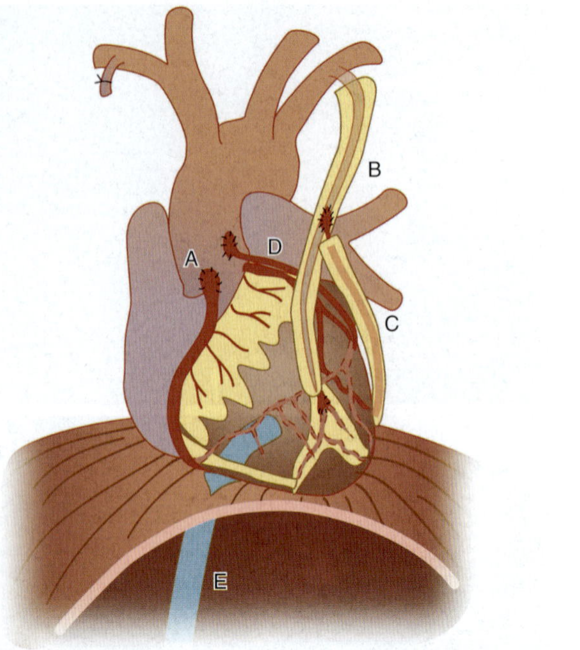

FIGURE 59-7. **Types of bypass grafts.** Bypass grafts include reversed saphenous vein graft from the aorta to the right coronary artery (**A**), in situ left internal mammary artery graft to the anterior descending coronary artery (**B**), Y graft of the right internal mammary artery from the left internal mammary artery to the circumflex coronary artery (**C**), radial artery graft from the aorta to the circumflex coronary artery (**D**), and in situ gastroepiploic graft to the posterior descending branch of the right coronary artery (**E**).

patients receiving only saphenous vein grafts. The right internal thoracic artery also may be used for revascularization as an in situ graft, as an aorta to coronary artery graft, or as a composite arterial graft from the left internal thoracic artery to a coronary artery. Despite its theoretical appeal, use of both internal thoracic arteries as grafts has not been proven to provide benefit over a single internal thoracic artery graft strategy and is associated with a higher rate of sternal infections and complications.[A23,A24] For the second graft, using the radial artery as another arterial conduit is preferred over a saphenous vein graft.[A25]

Most CABG operations are performed with a full median sternotomy incision, historically with the aid of cardiopulmonary bypass, aortic cross-clamping, and cardioplegic solution—techniques that allow exposure and arrest of the heart such that detailed microsurgical anastomoses can be constructed while myocardial function is effectively protected. By comparison, operations performed through smaller incisions (minimally invasive surgery) can be more challenging to perform without specialized training and have had limited application for coronary revascularizations. In randomized trials, beating heart ("off-pump") surgery without cardiopulmonary bypass has not consistently reduced morbidity, often has been associated with a lower rate of long-term graft patency, and does not provide better outcomes;[A26] as a result, it is usually reserved for carefully selected patients.

PERIOPERATIVE RISKS

The risk of mortality associated with CABG correlates with the extent of ischemia at the time of operation, left ventricular function, extent of coronary stenoses, noncardiac atherosclerosis, and comorbid conditions, as well as with the experience, skill, and judgment of the surgeon. Effective myocardial protection has diminished much of the incremental risk based on the severity of cardiac disease. For patients younger than 70 years without serious comorbid conditions, the mortality risk of primary CABG surgery is less than 1% in experienced hands. Nevertheless, CABG surgery in the presence of ongoing myocardial ischemia caused by acute MI, unstable angina, or acute vessel closure after PCI is still associated with increased risk. Noncardiac comorbid conditions (aortic atherosclerosis, renal function, chronic obstructive pulmonary disease, and coagulation system disorders) increase perioperative risk when these conditions are severe.

Aside from mortality, the most serious postoperative morbidity after CABG is stroke, often related to aortic or cerebrovascular atherosclerosis and atherosclerotic embolization. Heightened awareness of the importance of aortic and carotid atherosclerosis and improved management strategies appear to have decreased the risk of focal stroke in patients previously at high risk. Serious wound complications of median sternotomy are uncommon (1 to 2%).

INDICATIONS FOR BYPASS SURGERY

The goals of CABG are to relieve symptoms and to prolong life expectancy. On the basis of randomized trials and the emergence of alternative medical treatments and PCI, the surgical population has evolved toward patients who benefit most from CABG relative to other treatments: patients with complex conditions, often involving left main or triple-vessel disease, diffuse coronary stenoses, totally obstructed vessels, abnormal left ventricular function, and diabetes. Surgically treated patients with single-vessel disease usually have LAD stenoses or have failed alternative treatments, such as developing recurrent restenosis after PCI.

Relief of Symptoms

If patients who experience angina have severe stenoses in graftable coronary arteries that supply areas of myocardium ischemia at rest or with stress, CABG will reliably relieve angina. Randomized trials have shown that the relief of angina after CABG is more consistent than that achieved with alternative treatments. When intermittent heart failure symptoms represent an "anginal equivalent" that is also caused by ischemia, such symptoms also respond well to relief of that ischemia by CABG. For patients with symptoms of heart failure at rest, dobutamine echocardiography (Chapter 43), positron emission tomography (Chapter 44), and cardiac magnetic resonance imaging (Chapter 44) can identify segments of viable but hibernating myocardium (ischemic at rest) that may improve with bypass grafting, thus reducing symptoms of heart failure.

Survival

Chronic Stable Angina

In randomized trials of patients with mild to moderate chronic stable angina, an improved survival rate has been documented for patients treated with initial CABG compared with those treated with initial medical treatment in the presence of a left main stenosis of more than 50% of the diameter, triple-vessel disease, double-vessel disease with a proximal LAD lesion, abnormal left ventricular function, or a strongly abnormal exercise test result (Chapter 56). Meta-analysis of these randomized trials also suggests a survival benefit of CABG for any patient with a proximal LAD lesion and myocardial ischemia. These are subgroups of patients for whom bypass surgery should be strongly considered even in the absence of severe symptoms. During these trials, patients with severe angina were not randomized but were included in observational studies that noted improved survival rates with CABG for patients with double- and triple-vessel disease and normal or abnormal left ventricular function. Medical, interventional, and surgical treatments have all advanced substantially since these trials were completed.

Acute Coronary Syndrome and Ischemic Cardiomyopathy

Current data suggest an aggressive strategy, including CABG when indicated, in patients who have an acute coronary syndrome (unstable angina or non–ST segment elevation acute MI; Chapter 57). Patients who have coronary artery disease, heart failure, and severe left ventricular systolic dysfunction often can be controlled symptomatically with medications (Chapter 46). However, CABG added to guideline-directed medical therapy significantly reduces all-cause death, death from cardiovascular causes, and death from any cause or hospitalization for cardiovascular causes at 10 years,[A27] irrespective of whether it improves left ventricular function.[A28]

Other Ischemic Syndromes

ST Segment Elevation Acute Myocardial Infarction

For patients with ST segment elevation acute MI, CABG may be indicated in the acute setting when thrombolytic therapy or PCI has not been effective, ischemia is ongoing, and large areas of myocardium remain jeopardized. CABG after a completed MI may be indicated in patients in whom persistent ischemia in noninfarcted areas of myocardium produces post-infarction angina or hemodynamic instability. Mechanical complications of myocardial necrosis, including papillary muscle rupture, ventricular septal rupture, and myocardial free wall rupture, are acute life-threatening situations that usually require urgent operation for repair of the defect, often combined with CABG (Chapter 58).

Failed Percutaneous Coronary Intervention

Drug-eluting stents have decreased the need for emergency CABG to treat acute failure of PCIs. Current indications for emergency CABG include closure or threatened closure of a vessel supplying a significant amount of myocardium or recurrent restenosis despite several PCIs.

Coronary Bypass Reoperations

Patients in whom new stenoses develop in native arteries or in bypass grafts may have recurrent ischemic syndromes. Severe vein graft atherosclerosis is an unstable lesion that often leads to serious cardiac events, particularly if the LAD or multiple vessels are jeopardized; reoperation appears to improve the survival rate of these patients. Conversely, if the LAD coronary artery is supplied by a patent internal thoracic artery graft, reoperation does not appear to improve survival, although it may improve symptoms. Reoperations are more difficult and dangerous than primary procedures, but the risk now approaches that for primary procedures in institutions performing a large number of reoperations. PCI is often less-invasive and potentially a lower-risk alternative for the treatment of vein graft disease.

Late Outcomes

The late outcomes after CABG are related to age, severity of cardiac disease before operation, noncardiac comorbid conditions, progression of atherosclerosis, and the operation itself. For patients with severe coronary artery disease, CABG prolongs life expectancy. The achievement of complete revascularization (bypass grafts to all stenotic coronary vessels) and the use of internal thoracic artery grafts improve long-term survival rates and symptomatic status.

More than 80% of patients are alive more than 10 years after operation. Over the long term, control of the progression of atherosclerosis by lifestyle modifications, pharmacologic treatment of hypertension (Chapter 64) and lipids (Chapter 190), and platelet inhibitors (Chapter 70) appear to extend the benefits of CABG.[13]

COEXISTING CARDIAC DISEASE

During cardiac operations performed for valvular (Chapter 60) or aortic (Chapter 63) disease, the standard treatment is to perform bypass grafts to major coronary arteries with angiographic stenoses of more than 50% of the luminal diameter. No randomized trials have addressed this issue, and these indications, although logical given the natural history of atherosclerosis, remain practice patterns based on consensus but not on definitive data.

PERCUTANEOUS CORONARY INTERVENTION VERSUS CORONARY ARTERY BYPASS GRAFTING

The decision between PCI and CABG surgery is largely determined by clinical status and anatomic features, but some areas remain controversial. For patients with acute coronary syndromes, PCI is the preferred initial approach and has been shown to improve the survival rate of patients with ST segment elevation MI.[14] CABG is reserved for patients with failed acute PCI or residual myocardial ischemia. For patients who have chronic coronary syndromes, no data confirm that PCI prolongs life regardless of anatomy.

By comparison, randomized trials, albeit older trials, demonstrate that CABG prolongs the life expectancy of patients with severe coronary artery disease, particularly patients with left ventricular dysfunction or severe ischemia. Patients with more complex, multivessel coronary artery disease benefit most from CABG, including a clear improvement in survival rate, but patients with more limited coronary disease have equivalent survival outcomes with drug-eluting PCI.[A29] For patients with left main coronary artery disease[15] without extensive additional disease, PCI appears to be similar to CABG in terms of subsequent death, superior with respect to stroke, but inferior with respect to the need for repeat revascularization and out-of hospital myocardial infarction, and perhaps all-cause mortality.[A30-A33] Randomized trials also show that diabetic patients with multivessel coronary artery disease have better survival rates with CABG compared with PCI.[A34]

GENERAL REFERENCES

For the General References and other additional features, please visit Elsevier eBooks+ at https://ebooks.health.elsevier.com.

Grade A References

A1. Gargiulo G, Giacoppo D, Jolly SS, et al. Effects on mortality and major bleeding of radial versus femoral artery access for coronary angiography or percutaneous coronary intervention: meta-analysis of individual patient data from 7 multicenter randomized clinical trials. *Circulation.* 2022;146:1329-1343.
A2. Nijssen EC, Rennenberg RJ, Nelemans PJ, et al. Prophylactic hydration to protect renal function from intravascular iodinated contrast material in patients at high risk of contrast-induced nephropathy (AMACING): a prospective, randomised, phase 3, controlled, open-label, non-inferiority trial. *Lancet.* 2017;389:1312-1322.
A3. Wang N, Qian P, Yan TD, et al. Periprocedural effects of statins on the incidence of contrast-induced acute kidney injury: a systematic review and trial sequential analysis. *Int J Cardiol.* 2016;206:143-152.
A4. Weisbord SD, Gallagher M, Jneid H, et al. Outcomes after angiography with sodium bicarbonate and acetylcysteine. *N Engl J Med.* 2018;378:603-614.
A5. Subramaniam RM, Suarez-Cuervo C, Wilson RF, et al. Effectiveness of prevention strategies for contrast-induced nephropathy: a systematic review and meta-analysis. *Ann Intern Med.* 2016;164:406-416.
A6. Xaplanteris P, Fournier S, Pijls NHJ, et al. Five-year outcomes with PCI guided by fractional flow reserve. *N Engl J Med.* 2018;379:250-259.
A7. Xu B, Tu S, Song L, et al. Angiographic quantitative flow ratio-guided coronary intervention (FAVOR III China): a multicentre, randomised, sham-controlled trial. *Lancet.* 2021;398:2149-2159.
A8. Puymirat E, Cayla G, Simon T, et al. Multivessel PCI guided by FFR or angiography for myocardial infarction. *N Engl J Med.* 2021;385:297-308.
A9. Sabaté M, Brugaletta S, Cequier A, et al. Clinical outcomes in patients with ST-segment elevation myocardial infarction treated with everolimus-eluting stents versus bare-metal stents (EXAMINATION): 5-year results of a randomised trial. *Lancet.* 2016;387:357-366.
A10. Piccolo R, Bonaa KH, Efthimiou O, et al. Drug-eluting or bare-metal stents for percutaneous coronary intervention: a systematic review and individual patient data meta-analysis of randomised clinical trials. *Lancet.* 2019;393:2503-2510.
A11. Kim HS, Kang J, Hwang D, et al. Durable polymer versus biodegradable polymer drug-eluting stents after percutaneous coronary intervention in patients with acute coronary syndrome: the HOST-REDUCE-POLYTECH-ACS trial. *Circulation.* 2021;143:1081-1091.
A12. Hahn JY, Song YB, Oh JH, et al. 6-month versus 12-month or longer dual antiplatelet therapy after percutaneous coronary intervention in patients with acute coronary syndrome (SMART-DATE): a randomised, open-label, non-inferiority trial. *Lancet.* 2018;391:1274-1284.
A13. Mehran R, Baber U, Sharma SK, et al. Ticagrelor with or without aspirin in high-risk patients after PCI. *N Engl J Med.* 2019;381:2032-2042.
A14. Valgimigli M, Frigoli E, Heg D, et al. Dual antiplatelet therapy after PCI in patients at high bleeding risk. *N Engl J Med.* 2021;385:1643-1655.
A15. Smits PC, Frigoli E, Vranckx P, et al. Abbreviated antiplatelet therapy after coronary stenting in patients with myocardial infarction at high bleeding risk. *J Am Coll Cardiol.* 2022;80:1220-1237.
A16. Cannon CP, Bhatt DL, Oldgren J, et al. Dual antithrombotic therapy with dabigatran after PCI in atrial fibrillation. *N Engl J Med.* 2017;377:1513-1524.
A17. Park D-W, Kang D-Y, Ahn J-M, et al. Routine functional testing or standard care in high-risk patients after PCI. *N Engl J Med.* 2022;387:905-915.
A18. Al-Lamee R, Thompson D, Dehbi HM, et al. Percutaneous coronary intervention in stable angina (ORBITA): a double-blind, randomised controlled trial. *Lancet.* 2018;391:31-40.
A19. Maron DJ, Hochman JS, Reynolds HR, et al. Initial invasive or conservative strategy for stable coronary disease. *N Engl J Med.* 2020;382:1395-1407.
A20. Bangalore S, Maron DJ, Stone GW, et al. Routine revascularization versus initial medical therapy for stable ischemic heart disease: a systematic review and meta-analysis of randomized trials. *Circulation.* 2020;142:841-857.
A21. Spertus JA, Jones PG, Maron DJ, et al. Health-status outcomes with invasive or conservative care in coronary disease. *N Engl J Med.* 2020;382:1408-1419.
A22. Fearon WF, Zimmermann FM, De Bruyne B, et al. Fractional flow reserve-guided PCI as compared with coronary bypass surgery. *N Engl J Med.* 2022;386:128-137.
A23. Taggart DP, Altman DG, Gray AM, et al. Randomized trial of bilateral versus single internal-thoracic-artery grafts. *N Engl J Med.* 2016;375:2540-2549.
A24. Taggart DP, Benedetto U, Gerry S, et al. Bilateral versus single internal-thoracic-artery grafts at 10 years. *N Engl J Med.* 2019;380:437-446.
A25. Gaudino M, Benedetto U, Fremes S, et al. Association of radial artery graft vs saphenous vein graft with long-term cardiovascular outcomes among patients undergoing coronary artery bypass grafting: a systematic review and meta-analysis. *JAMA.* 2020;324:179-187.
A26. Quin JA, Wagner TH, Hattler B, et al. Ten-year outcomes of off-pump vs on-pump coronary artery bypass grafting in the Department of Veterans Affairs: a randomized clinical trial. *JAMA Surg.* 2022;157:303-310.
A27. Velazquez EJ, Lee KL, Jones RH, et al. Coronary-artery bypass surgery in patients with ischemic cardiomyopathy. *N Engl J Med.* 2016;374:1511-1520.
A28. Panza JA, Ellis AM, Al-Khalidi HR, et al. Myocardial viability and long-term outcomes in ischemic cardiomyopathy. *N Engl J Med.* 2019;381:739-748.
A29. Head SJ, Milojevic M, Daemen J, et al. Mortality after coronary artery bypass grafting versus percutaneous coronary intervention with stenting for coronary artery disease: a pooled analysis of individual patient data. *Lancet.* 2018;391:939-948.
A30. Giacoppo D, Colleran R, Cassese S, et al. Percutaneous coronary intervention vs coronary artery bypass grafting in patients with left main coronary artery stenosis: a systematic review and meta-analysis. *JAMA Cardiol.* 2017;2:1079-1088.
A31. Holm NR, Mäkikallio T, Lindsay MM, et al. Percutaneous coronary angioplasty versus coronary artery bypass grafting in the treatment of unprotected left main stenosis: updated 5-year outcomes from the randomised, non-inferiority NOBLE trial. *Lancet.* 2020;395:191-199.
A32. Sabatine MS, Bergmark BA, Murphy SA, et al. Percutaneous coronary intervention with drug-eluting stents versus coronary artery bypass grafting in left main coronary artery disease: an individual patient data meta-analysis. *Lancet.* 2021;398:2247-2257.
A33. Gaudino M, Hameed I, Farkouh ME, et al. Overall and cause-specific mortality in randomized clinical trials comparing percutaneous interventions with coronary bypass surgery: a meta-analysis. *JAMA Intern Med.* 2020;180:1638-1646.
A34. Wang R, Serruys PW, Gao C, et al. Ten-year all-cause death after percutaneous or surgical revascularization in diabetic patients with complex coronary artery disease. *Eur Heart J.* 2022;43:56-67.

60

VALVULAR HEART DISEASE

BLASE A. CARABELLO AND SUSHEEL KODALI

APPROACH TO THE PATIENT WITH VALVULAR HEART DISEASE

The cardiac valves permit unobstructed forward blood flow through the heart when they are open while preventing backward flow when they are closed. Most valvular heart diseases cause either valvular stenosis with obstruction to forward flow or valvular regurgitation with backward flow. Valvular stenosis imparts a pressure overload on the left or right ventricle because these chambers must generate higher than normal pressure to overcome the obstruction to pump blood forward. Valvular regurgitation imparts a volume overload on the heart, which now must pump additional volume to compensate for what is regurgitated. When valve disease is severe, these hemodynamic burdens can lead to ventricular dysfunction, heart failure, and sudden death (Table 60-1). In almost every instance, definitive therapy for severe valvular heart disease is mechanical restoration of valve function.

A careful history and physical examination are key to the evaluation of a patient with suspected or known valvular heart disease. Because the presence or absence of symptoms dramatically affects prognosis and hence the proper therapy in most valvular diseases, an intense effort must focus on the patient's symptomatic status. The physical examination should include not only careful auscultation but also a detailed assessment for evidence of heart failure (Chapter 45). Transthoracic echocardiography (Chapter 43), which is the mainstay of diagnosis, provides both anatomic and physiologic information regarding the lesion's type, cause, and severity. In cases in which transthoracic echocardiography fails to provide adequate information, transesophageal echocardiography, cardiac magnetic resonance imaging (MRI; Chapter 44), and cardiac computed tomography (CT) usually provide the additional needed information, but invasive hemodynamic measurements are still occasionally required.[1,2]

AORTIC STENOSIS

EPIDEMIOLOGY

Bicuspid and Other Congenitally Abnormal Aortic Valves

Approximately 0.8% of the population is born with a bicuspid aortic valve,[3] with a male preponderance (Chapter 55). Although this abnormality does not usually cause a hemodynamic disturbance at birth, bicuspid aortic valves tend to deteriorate with age. Approximately one third of these valves become stenotic, another third become regurgitant, and the remainder cause only minor hemodynamic abnormalities. A murmur is typically noted in childhood or adolescence, and congenital aortic stenosis from a bicuspid tricuspid valve can cause symptoms during childhood and require correction by adolescence (Chapter 55). However, bicuspid valves more commonly become symptomatic when patients are in their 40s, 50s, and 60s. Aortic aneurysms develop in nearly one-third of patients with bicuspid aortic valves, so careful screening is warranted, even in asymptomatic patients.

Tricuspid Aortic Valve Stenosis

The most common form of aortic stenosis is a calcific process that results from the deposition of calcium and the thickening of valve leaflets in patients with apparently normal tricuspid aortic valves. This disease process typically develops in the seventh to eighth decade of life. This type of aortic stenosis is not a degenerative process but rather arises from an active inflammatory process similar to that of coronary heart disease (Chapter 41), with hypertension and hyperlipidemia as risk factors.

Rheumatic Valvular Heart Disease

Rheumatic valve disease is now a rare cause of aortic stenosis in developed countries, but rheumatic fever and its sequelae remain an important issue in many developing countries (Chapter 269). In virtually every case, the mitral valve is also involved in the disease process.

PATHOBIOLOGY

The normal aortic valve area is 3 to 4 cm^2, and little hemodynamic disturbance occurs until the orifice is reduced to about half of normal, at which point a systolic gradient develops between the left ventricle and aorta. Typically left ventricular and aortic pressures are nearly equal during systole (E-Fig. 60-1A). In aortic stenosis, however, intracavitary left ventricular pressure must increase above aortic pressure to produce forward flow across the stenotic valve and to achieve acceptable downstream pressure (E-Fig. 60-1B). Each of the processes that cause aortic stenosis has a typical pathoanatomic configuration (Fig. 60-1). There is a geometric progression in the magnitude of the gradient as the valve area narrows. Given a normal cardiac output, the gradient rises rapidly from 10 to 15 mm Hg at valve areas of 1.5 to 1.3 cm^2 to about 25 mm Hg at 1.0 cm^2, 50 mm Hg at 0.8 cm^2, 70 mm Hg at 0.6 cm^2, and 100 mm Hg at 0.5 cm^2. The rate of progression of aortic stenosis varies widely from patient to patient; it may remain stable for many years or increase by more than 15 mm Hg per year.

A major compensatory response to the increased left ventricular pressure associated with aortic stenosis is the development of concentric left ventricular hypertrophy. The Laplace equation—Stress (s) = Pressure (p) × Radius (r)/2 Thickness (th)—indicates that the stress on the left ventricle (afterload) varies directly with intracavitary pressure and radius but inversely with wall thickness. As left ventricular pressure increases with increasing severity of aortic stenosis, it can be offset by increased left ventricular wall thickness (concentric hypertrophy). The determinants of the left ventricular ejection fraction are contractility, preload, and afterload. By normalizing afterload, the development of concentric hypertrophy helps preserve ejection fraction and cardiac output despite the pressure overload. Although hypertrophy may serve as a compensatory function, it also has a pathologic role and is in part responsible for the classic symptoms and the poor outcome of untreated symptomatic aortic stenosis.

Angina

In general, angina (Chapter 56) results from ischemia when myocardial oxygen (and other nutrient) demand exceeds supply, which is predicated on coronary blood flow. In normal subjects, coronary blood flow can increase five- to eight-fold under maximum metabolic demand, but in patients with aortic stenosis, this reserve is limited. Reduced coronary blood flow reserve may be caused by a relative diminution in capillary ingrowth to serve the needs of the hypertrophied left ventricle or by a reduced transcoronary gradient for coronary blood flow because of the elevated left ventricular end-diastolic pressure. Restricted coronary blood flow reserve is in part responsible for angina in many patients who have aortic stenosis despite normal epicardial coronary arteries, but angina also may be caused by increased oxygen demand when inadequate hypertrophy allows wall stress, a key determinant of myocardial oxygen consumption, to increase.

Syncope

Syncope (Chapters 39 and 49) generally occurs because of inadequate cerebral perfusion. In aortic stenosis, syncope is often related to exertion. It may result when exertion causes a fall in total peripheral resistance that cannot be offset by increased cardiac output because output is limited by the obstruction to outflow across the stenotic valve. Furthermore, patients with small left ventricular cavity size are more prone to syncope because of lower stroke volume. In addition, high left ventricular pressure during exercise may trigger a systemic vasodepressor response that lowers blood pressure and produces syncope. Any sudden drop in preload may precipitate syncope because the left ventricle is unable to maintain cardiac output. Finally, cardiac arrhythmias, often related to a dilated left atrium, can also result in hypotension and syncope.

Heart Failure

In aortic stenosis, contractile dysfunction (systolic failure) and failure of normal relaxation (diastolic failure) result in symptoms of heart failure (Chapter 45). The extent of ventricular contraction is governed by contractility and afterload. In aortic stenosis, contractility (the ability to generate force) is often reduced. The mechanisms of contractile dysfunction may include abnormal calcium handling, microtubular hyperpolymerization causing an internal viscous load on the myocyte, and myocardial ischemia (Chapter 41). In some cases, contractile function is normal, but the hypertrophy is inadequate to normalize wall stress and excessive afterload results. Excessive afterload inhibits ejection, reduces forward output, and leads to heart failure.

The increased wall thickness that helps normalize stress increases diastolic stiffness. Even if muscle properties remain normal, higher filling pressure is required to distend a thicker ventricle. As aortic stenosis advances, collagen deposition also stiffens the myocardium and adds to the diastolic dysfunction. These processes eventually result in elevated left atrial and pulmonary artery pressures.

TABLE 60-1 SUMMARY OF SEVERE VALVULAR HEART DISEASE

	AORTIC STENOSIS	MITRAL STENOSIS	MITRAL REGURGITATION	AORTIC REGURGITATION
Etiology	Idiopathic calcification of a bicuspid or tricuspid valve Congenital Rheumatic	Rheumatic fever Annular and leaflet calcification	Mitral valve prolapse Ruptured chordae Endocarditis Ischemic papillary muscle dysfunction or rupture Collagen vascular diseases and syndromes Secondary to LV myocardial diseases	Annuloaortic ectasia Hypertension Endocarditis Marfan syndrome Ankylosing spondylitis Aortic dissection Syphilis Collagen vascular disease
Pathophysiology	Pressure overload on the LV with compensation by LVH. As disease advances, reduced coronary flow reserve predisposes to angina. Hypertrophy and afterload excess lead to systolic and diastolic LV dysfunction.	Obstruction to LV inflow increases LA pressure and limits cardiac output, thus mimicking LV failure. Mitral valve obstruction increases the pressure work of the RV. Right ventricular pressure overload is augmented further when pulmonary hypertension develops.	Places volume overload on the LV. Ventricle responds with eccentric hypertrophy and dilation, which allow increased ventricular stroke volume. Eventually, however, LV dysfunction develops if volume overload is uncorrected.	*Chronic:* Total stroke volume causes hyperdynamic circulation, induces systolic hypertension, and causes pressure and volume overload. Compensation is by concentric and eccentric hypertrophy. *Acute:* Because cardiac dilation has not developed, hyperdynamic findings are absent. High diastolic LV pressure causes mitral valve preclosure and potentiates LV ischemia and failure.
Symptoms	Angina Syncope Dyspnea Heart failure	Dyspnea Orthopnea PND Hemoptysis Hoarseness Edema Ascites	Dyspnea Orthopnea PND	Dyspnea Orthopnea PND Angina
Signs	Systolic ejection murmur radiating to the neck Delayed carotid upstroke S_4, soft or paradoxical S_2	Diastolic rumble after an opening snap Loud S_1 RV lift Loud P_2	Holosystolic apical murmur radiating to the axilla, S_3 Displaced PMI	*Chronic:* Diastolic blowing murmur Hyperdynamic circulation Displaced PMI Quincke pulse de Musset sign Austin Flint murmur *Acute:* Short diastolic blowing murmur Soft S_1
Electrocardiogram	LAA LVH	LAA RVH	LAA LVH	LAA LVH
Chest radiograph	Boot-shaped heart Aortic valve calcification on lateral view	Straightening of left heart border Double density at right heart border Kerley B lines Enlarged pulmonary arteries	Cardiac enlargement	*Chronic:* Cardiac enlargement Uncoiling of the aorta *Acute:* Pulmonary congestion with normal heart size
Echocardiographic findings	Concentric LVH Reduced aortic valve cusp separation Doppler shows mean gradient ≥40 mm Hg in most severe cases	Restricted mitral leaflet motion Valve area ≤1.5 cm^2 LA enlargement Tricuspid Doppler may reveal pulmonary hypertension	LA enlargement LV enlargement and LV dysfunction in severe cases Doppler: large regurgitant jet	*Chronic:* LV enlargement Large Doppler jet with PHT <400 msec *Acute:* Small LV Mitral valve preclosure
Catheterization findings	Increased LVEDP Transaortic gradient 40 mm Hg AVA ≤0.8 in most severe cases	Elevated pulmonary capillary wedge pressure Transmitral gradient usually >5 mm Hg in severe cases MVA <1.5 cm^2	Elevated pulmonary capillary wedge pressure with prominent V waves Ventriculography shows regurgitation of dye into LA	Wide pulse pressure Aortography shows regurgitation of dye into LV
Medical therapy	Avoid vasodilators Avoid a decline in venous return (preload) Diuretics for symptom control in inoperable cases	Diuretics for mild symptoms Anticoagulation in atrial fibrillation Digitalis, β-blockers, verapamil, or diltiazem for rate control	Afterload reduction in acute MR—primarily with ACE inhibitors Blood pressure control	*Chronic:* Vasodilators in chronic asymptomatic disease with hypertension even if LV function is normal *Acute:* Vasodilators
Indications for surgery	Appearance of symptoms in patients with severe disease (see text) or asymptomatic LV dysfunction	Appearance of more than mild symptoms Development of pulmonary hypertension Appearance of persistent atrial fibrillation	Appearance of symptoms EF <0.60 ESD ≥40 mm	*Chronic:* Appearance of symptoms EF <0.50 ESD ≥50 mm *Acute:* Even mild heart failure Mitral valve preclosure

ACE = angiotensin-converting enzyme; AVA = aortic valve area; EF = ejection fraction; ESD = end-systolic diameter; LA = left atrial; LAA = left atrial abnormality; LV = left ventricle or left ventricular; LVEDP = left ventricular end-diastolic pressure; LVH = left ventricular hypertrophy; MR = mitral regurgitation; MVA = mitral valve area; PHT = pressure half-time; PMI = point of maximal impulse; PND = paroxysmal nocturnal dyspnea; RV = right ventricle or right ventricular; RVH = right ventricular hypertrophy.

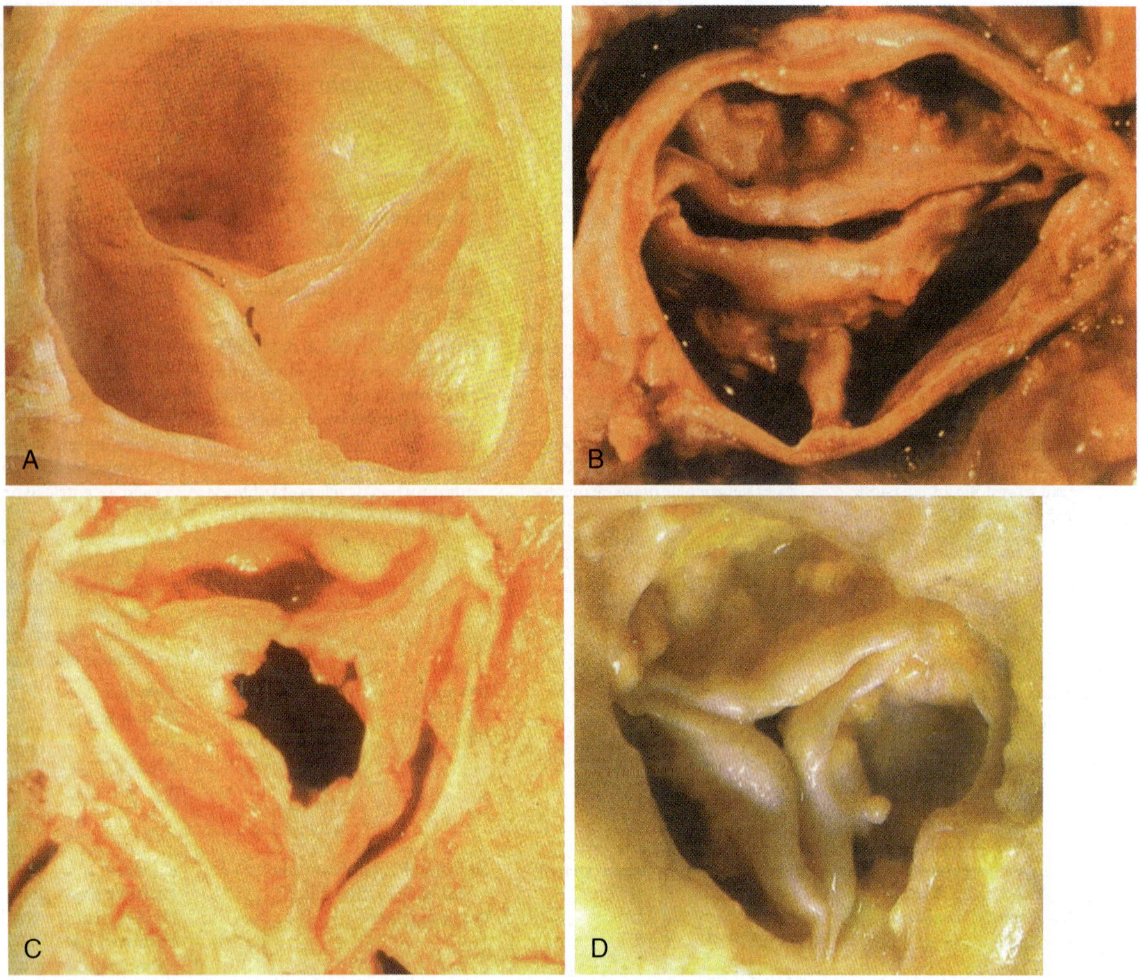

FIGURE 60-1. **Pathology of aortic stenosis. A, A normal aortic valve. B, A stenotic congenital bicuspid valve. C, Rheumatic aortic stenosis. D, A stenotic calcified tricuspid aortic valve.** (From Bonow RO, Braunwald E. Valvular heart disease. In: Zipes DP, Libby P, Bonow RO, Braunwald E, eds. *Heart Disease: A Textbook of Cardiovascular Medicine*. 7th ed. Philadelphia: WB Saunders; 2005:1583.)

CLINICAL MANIFESTATIONS

The diagnosis of aortic stenosis is usually first suspected when the classic systolic ejection murmur is heard during physical examination (Chapter 39) in an often asymptomatic individual. The murmur is loudest in the aortic area and radiates to the neck. In some cases, the murmur may disappear over the sternum and reappear over the left ventricular apex, thereby giving the false impression that a murmur of mitral regurgitation is also present (Gallavardin phenomenon). The intensity of the murmur increases with cycle length because longer cycles are associated with greater aortic flow. In mild disease, the murmur peaks in intensity in early systole or mid systole. As the severity of stenosis worsens, the murmur peaks progressively later in systole. Perhaps the most helpful clue to the severity of aortic stenosis by physical examination is the characteristic delay in the carotid pulse with a diminution in its volume (see Fig. 39-4 in Chapter 39); in elderly patients, however, increasing carotid stiffness may pseudonormalize the carotid upstrokes. The left ventricular apical impulse in aortic stenosis is not displaced but is enlarged and forceful. The simultaneous palpation of a forceful left ventricular apex beat and a delayed and weakened carotid pulse is a persuasive clue that severe aortic stenosis is present. S_1 in aortic stenosis is generally normal. In congenital aortic stenosis when the valve is not calcified, S_1 may be followed by a systolic ejection click. In calcific disease, S_2 may be single and soft when the aortic component is lost because the valve neither opens nor closes well. In some cases, delayed left ventricular emptying may create paradoxical splitting of S_2. An S_4 gallop is common. In advanced disease, pulmonary hypertension and signs of right-sided failure are common.

Because of the dire consequences of missing the diagnosis of aortic stenosis, the physician must have a low threshold for obtaining an echocardiogram whenever aortic stenosis cannot be excluded by physical examination, especially in patients with a history of angina, syncope, or heart failure. In asymptomatic patients with suspicious murmurs, early diagnosis allows the patient and physician to be more vigilant regarding possible early signs and symptoms.

Although exercise testing is contraindicated in symptomatic patients with aortic stenosis because of the high risk for complications, cautious exercise testing is reasonable in asymptomatic patients to detect latent symptoms or hemodynamic instability that is otherwise unrecognized. Exercise-induced hypotension (>10 mm Hg drop in systolic blood pressure from baseline) or symptoms are indications for aortic valve replacement in patients who have severe aortic stenosis; in patients who have only mild to moderate aortic stenosis, another source of exercise limitation should be sought.

DIAGNOSIS

Echocardiography (Chapter 43) performed in multiple views by an experienced sonographer is the primary modality for confirming the diagnosis of aortic stenosis (Fig. 60-2). Although the visual appearance of the valve leaflets is useful, the assessment of the severity of aortic stenosis relies on Doppler interrogation of the aortic valve. As blood flows from the body of the left ventricle across the stenotic valve, the flow rate must accelerate for the volume to remain constant. Doppler interrogation of the valve can be performed to detect this increase in velocity. If the peak aortic flow velocity is 3.0 m/second or less, symptoms are unlikely to develop in the next 5 years; by comparison, in patients with a flow velocity of 4.0 m/second or greater, symptoms usually develop within 2 years, and when the velocity exceeds 5 m/second, symptoms are likely to develop within 1 year. The modified Bernoulli equation (gradient = $4 \times \text{velocity}^2$) can calculate the peak gradient across the valve and estimate the aortic valve area (Chapter 43). In patients in whom there is discrepancy between the visual appearance of the aortic valve and the calculated valve area, transesophageal echocardiography can measure the valve area directly by tracing its opening, although the measured orifice area should not replace other ways to assess the severity of aortic stenosis.

When echocardiography shows severe aortic stenosis and the patient has one or more of the classic symptoms of the disease, cardiac catheterization to document the severity of the stenosis is not recommended. However, when the

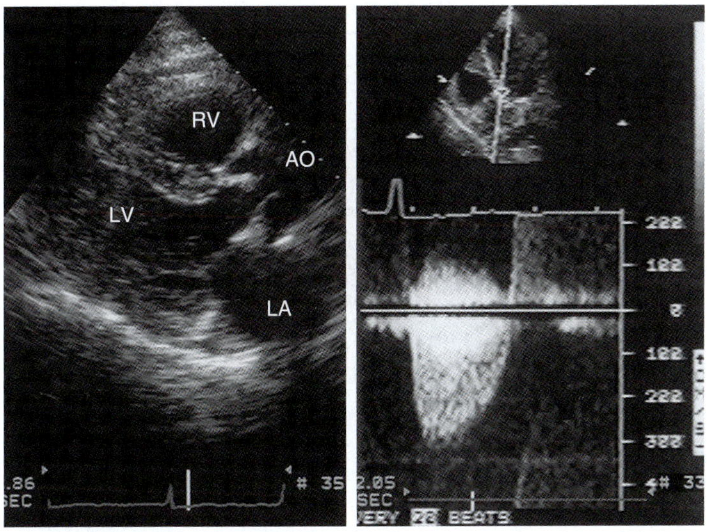

FIGURE 60-2. **Doppler echocardiogram from a patient with aortic stenosis. The *left panel* shows thickened aortic valve leaflets that dome into the aorta with restricted opening in systole. The *top right panel* shows a miniaturized apical four-chamber view at the top with a Doppler cursor through the aorta, and the *bottom right panel* shows a continuous-wave spectral Doppler signal with a peak velocity of 3 m/second. The peak valve gradient can be calculated as 4×3^2, or 36 mm Hg. AO = aorta; LA = left atrium; LV = left ventricle; RV = right ventricle. (Courtesy of Dr. Anthony DeMaria.)**

hemodynamic diagnosis is unclear, right- and left-sided heart catheterization should be performed to determine the transaortic valvular pressure gradient and cardiac output, which are used to calculate the aortic valve area by the Gorlin formula:

$$A = \frac{CO/SEP \times HR}{44.3\sqrt{h}}$$

where *CO* is the cardiac output (mL/minute), *SEP* is the systolic ejection period (seconds), *HR* is the heart rate, and *h* is the mean gradient. Coronary arteriography is commonly recommended before aortic valve surgery because most patients with aortic stenosis are of the age at which coronary disease is common.

The extent of valve calcification correlates with the severity of aortic stenosis, so quantification of valve calcification by CT scanning can occasionally be helpful. A calcium score greater than 1300 in women or greater than 2000 in men is consistent with severe aortic stenosis.

Brain natriuretic peptide levels may be higher in patients who will become symptomatic in a short time span and also have prognostic importance. Levels exceeding three to four times the normal value portend a poor prognosis and may be a criterion for referral for valve replacement.

The electrocardiogram (ECG) in patients with aortic stenosis usually shows left ventricular hypertrophy (Chapter 48). In some cases of even severe aortic stenosis, however, left ventricular hypertrophy is absent on the ECG, possibly because of the lack of left ventricular dilation. Left atrial abnormality is common because the stiff left ventricle increases left atrial afterload and causes the left atrium to dilate.

The chest radiograph in aortic stenosis is generally nondiagnostic. The cardiac silhouette is not usually enlarged but may assume a boot-shaped configuration. In advanced cases, there may be signs of cardiomegaly and pulmonary congestion; severe aortic valve calcification may be seen in the lateral view.

Low Flow, Low Gradient Aortic Stenosis

Two types of pathophysiology can reduce cardiac output and reduce the aortic gradient, thereby misleading the clinician into underestimating the severity and clinical gravity of aortic stenosis. The first type occurs in patients who have developed systolic dysfunction, typically from valvular heart disease or coronary artery disease. In such patients, the ejection fraction and stroke volume are reduced, as is the transvalvular gradient. Although these patients have a poorer prognosis than do patients with preserved left ventricular function, many still benefit from aortic valve replacement. The second type is patients who have severe left ventricular hypertrophy, which reduces left ventricular volume. Although the ejection fraction is normal, stroke volume and the valve gradient are reduced. Such patients also usually benefit from valve replacement.

In general, the diagnosis of severe aortic stenosis should not rely on a single diagnostic value or test, and current guidelines deemphasize valve area as the single gold standard of severity. Rather, the findings of the physical examination, jet velocity, transvalvular gradient, valve area, biomarkers, and valve calcium should be viewed in their totality.

Mixed Moderate Aortic Stenosis and Regurgitation

Some patients have combined moderate aortic stenosis and regurgitation, with neither condition by itself mandating therapy. However, symptomatic patients with combined moderate stenosis and moderate regurgitation have a prognosis similar to that of patients with pure severe aortic stenosis if their peak aortic jet velocity is 4.0 m/sec or greater. As a result, they should undergo aortic valve replacement.[4]

TREATMENT

Asymptomatic Patients

In asymptomatic patients, no medical treatment has been shown to delay the progression of stenosis, but careful blood pressure control (Chapter 64) is recommended to minimize pressure overload on the left ventricle. Close follow-up is very important to detect early symptoms, especially in elderly patients who may have other reasons to limit their exercise. In patients with severe asymptomatic aortic stenosis, the prognosis is poor, and data suggest that early aortic valve replacement improves outcomes.[A1,A2] For example, valve replacement may be considered in asymptomatic patients who have left ventricular dysfunction with very high jet velocities (>5 m/second), brain natriuretic peptide values three to four times normal, or positive exercise tolerance test results.

Symptomatic Patients

No accepted effective medical therapy is available for symptomatic aortic stenosis, and valve replacement should be performed as expeditiously as possible.[5] In patients who are awaiting surgery, diuretics can be used cautiously to relieve pulmonary congestion and nitrates may be used very cautiously to treat angina pectoris. However, vasodilation reduces pressure distal to the obstruction, often without increasing cardiac output, and may cause syncope. In rare situations in which surgery is impossible, diuretics can improve symptoms but will not improve life expectancy.

Aortic Valve Procedures

Balloon Aortic Valvuloplasty

Percutaneous balloon aortic valvuloplasty, by which a balloon is inserted via the femoral artery and inflated across the aortic valve to increase its mobility, can provide a temporary reduction in the aortic valve gradient for perhaps 6 to 12 months. This palliation may be useful in inoperable patients and is sometimes used in very advanced patients who have low flow and a low left ventricular ejection fraction to determine whether aortic valve replacement may be of benefit.

Valve Replacement Surgery

Surgical aortic valve replacement, which nearly always requires either a mechanical or bioprosthetic valve, is a proven effective therapy for symptomatic aortic stenosis and for selected asymptomatic patients (see earlier). The one exception is young patients with bicuspid valves, in whom the Ross procedure (an autograft by which the patient's own pulmonic valve is transplanted to the aortic portion and a prosthetic pulmonic valve is implanted) is the preferred operation.[6] Even octogenarians benefit from valve replacement unless other comorbid factors preclude surgery, so aortic valve replacement should not be denied simply on the basis of age. Class I indications for aortic valve replacement include the presence of symptoms or severe disease in patients who are undergoing another cardiac operation. Valve replacement also should not be denied because the ejection fraction is reduced, because the excess afterload imposed by the stenotic valve is relieved with valve replacement, and a depressed ejection fraction usually improves dramatically after surgery. The exception to this rule is a patient who has a severely reduced ejection fraction (<20%) and a low aortic valve gradient (<20 mm Hg); in this case, the severity of the aortic stenosis may be overestimated because the failing left ventricle has difficulty opening a mildly to moderately stenotic valve. In such patients, left ventricular dysfunction either has another cause or is often so severe that it does not recover after valve replacement. Even in this situation, however, patients who demonstrate increased cardiac output during dobutamine infusion may benefit from aortic valve replacement.

Transcatheter Aortic Valve Replacement

Percutaneous transcatheter aortic valve implantation[7] reduces the 1-year mortality rate by 45% (from 51 to 31%) in patients who have severe aortic stenosis and are too ill to undergo open surgery. In addition, outcomes, including mortality at up to 5 years, are as good as or better than standard surgical valve replacement in high-risk, intermediate-risk, and low-risk adults,[A3-A7] using either a balloon-expandable or self-expanding prosthesis. In intermediate-risk patients with noncomplex coronary artery disease, a percutaneous valve replacement with coronary stenting is as good as open valve replacement and coronary artery bypass surgery.[A8]

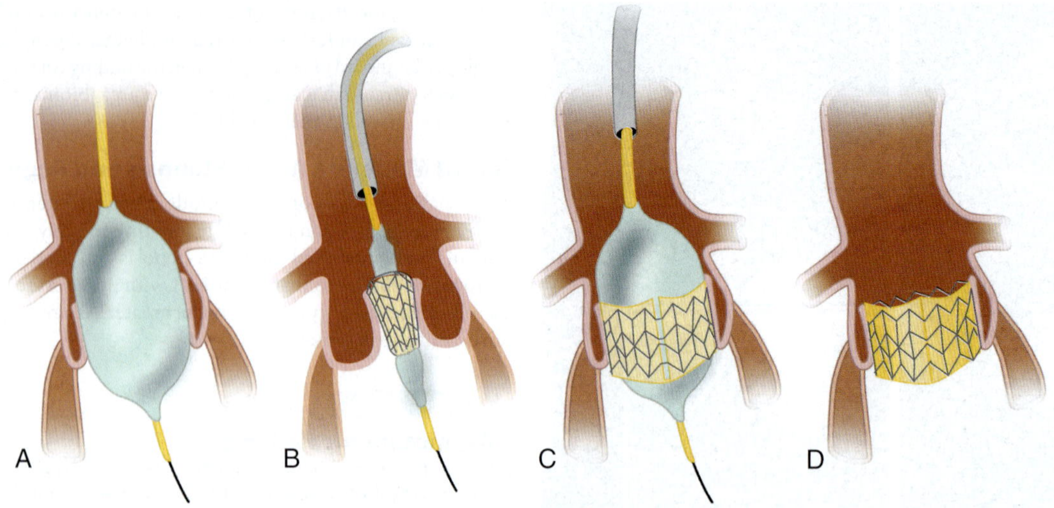

FIGURE 60-3. Steps for transcatheter aortic valve replacement. A, Dilation of the native stenotic valve. B, A crimped stented valve has been inserted over a guidewire into the aortic annulus. C, Inflation of the balloon deploys the valve. D, The balloon is deflated and removed with the aortic valve replaced. (Modified from Cleveland Clinic. Heart valve disease—percutaneous interventions. http://my.clevelandclinic.org/heart/percutaneous/percutaneousValve.aspx.)

It is important to note that major randomized trials of transcatheter aortic valve replacement have been limited to patients who have degenerated tricuspid aortic valves. Emerging data on current devices suggest equivalent outcomes in patients with bicuspid valves or rheumatic aortic disease,[8] but data are limited.

Two types of valves are available throughout much of the world, including the United States. One is a balloon-expandable, a bioprosthetic, stented valve that is crimped onto a balloon catheter, which is advanced across the aortic annulus (Fig. 60-3). The balloon is then inflated to expand the prosthesis and secure it in the native annulus while excluding the diseased valve. In the second type, the tissue valve is sewn into a self-expanding frame and crimped within a delivery catheter, which is advanced across the aortic valve and slowly withdrawn, thereby allowing the prothesis to expand and exclude the diseased valve.

The success of transcatheter aortic valve replacement has resulted in an estimated 100,000 such procedures being performed annually in the United States and exceeding the volume of surgical aortic valve replacement. Rates of stroke are lower with transcatheter aortic valve replacement than with surgical valve replacement; paravalvular regurgitation now occurs rarely. Finally, the rate of structural deterioration of newer transcatheter valves appears to be similar to that of surgical tissue valves, at least in the mid-term. After implantation, 3 months of aspirin alone is preferred over 3 months of dual-antiplatelet therapy in patients who do not have an indication for ongoing anticoagulation.[A9]

PROGNOSIS

In asymptomatic patients with normally functioning or minimally dysfunctional aortic valves, the survival rate is reasonably similar to age-matched control participants, and sudden death is rare, occurring in fewer than 1% of asymptomatic patients. However, mortality is increased with a valve gradient above 20 mm Hg, and about 25% of patients require surgery by 20 years after diagnosis. In adults with asymptomatic but hemodynamically significant aortic stenosis, symptoms typically develop within 5 years. A higher peak aortic jet velocity, heavy valve calcification, a positive exercise test result, severe left ventricular dysfunction, and high brain natriuretic peptide levels predict a worse prognosis and may warrant consideration of valve replacement in asymptomatic patients with severe disease.

The progression of mild to moderate aortic stenosis to severe disease is the key to the natural history of the disease and is quite variable. Aortic stenosis may remain mild for a decade or more in some patients, but it may progress to severe disease in as little as 5 years in other patients.

When symptoms develop, survival declines precipitously. Approximately 35% of patients with aortic stenosis are initially evaluated for angina. Of these, 50% are dead in 5 years unless aortic valve replacement is performed. Approximately 15% have syncope; of these, 50% are dead in only 3 years unless the aortic valve is replaced. Of the 50% with symptoms of heart failure, 50% are dead in 2 years without aortic valve replacement. In all, only 25% of patients with symptomatic aortic stenosis survive 3 years in the absence of valve replacement, and the annual risk for sudden death ranges from 10% in patients with angina to 15% with syncope to 25% with heart failure. After valve replacement surgery, prognosis improves to near normal, especially for patients older than 65 years at the time of valve implantation, presumably because older patients have fewer years at risk for valve-related complications.

MITRAL STENOSIS

EPIDEMIOLOGY

Traditionally the cause of acquired mitral stenosis has been rheumatic heart disease. Although it has become rare in developed countries because of the waning incidence of rheumatic fever, rheumatic mitral stenosis is still prevalent in developing nations, where rheumatic fever is common (Chapter 269). Rheumatic disease is three times more common in women and usually develops in their 40s and 50s. Although the vast majority of mitral stenosis worldwide still results from rheumatic disease, severe age-associated calcification of the mitral annulus and leaflet bases is an increasingly common cause of mitral stenosis in the absence of rheumatic involvement.[9]

PATHOBIOLOGY

At the beginning of diastole, a transient gradient between the left atrium and left ventricle normally initiates left ventricular filling. After early filling, left atrial and left ventricular pressures equilibrate. In mitral stenosis, obstruction to left ventricular filling increases left atrial pressure and produces a persistent gradient between the two chambers (E-Fig. 60-2). The combination of elevated left atrial pressure (and pulmonary venous pressure) and restriction of inflow into the left ventricle limits cardiac output. Although myocardial involvement from the rheumatic process occasionally affects left ventricular muscle function, the muscle itself is normal in most patients with mitral stenosis. However, in approximately one third of patients with mitral stenosis, left ventricular ejection performance is reduced despite normal muscle function because of reduced preload (from inflow obstruction) and increased afterload as a result of reflex vasoconstriction caused by reduced cardiac output.

Because the right ventricle generates most of the force that propels flow across the mitral valve, the right ventricle incurs the pressure overload of the transmitral gradient. In addition, secondary but reversible pulmonary vasoconstriction develops, thus further increasing pulmonary artery pressure and the burden on the right ventricle. As mitral stenosis worsens, right ventricular failure develops.

CLINICAL MANIFESTATIONS

Patients with mitral stenosis usually remain asymptomatic until the valve area is reduced to about one third its normal size of 4 to 5 cm^2. Then the symptoms typical of left-sided failure—dyspnea on exertion, orthopnea, and paroxysmal nocturnal dyspnea—develop. As the disease progresses and right ventricular failure occurs, ascites and edema are common. Hemoptysis, which is common in mitral stenosis but uncommon in other causes of left atrial hypertension, develops when high left atrial pressure ruptures the anastomoses of small bronchial veins. In some cases, a large left atrium may impinge on the left recurrent laryngeal nerve and cause hoarseness (Ortner syndrome) or may impinge on the esophagus and cause dysphagia.

Physical Examination

Although mitral stenosis produces typical and diagnostic findings on physical examination, the diagnosis is missed frequently because the auscultatory findings may be subtle. Palpation of the precordium finds a quiet apical impulse. If pulmonary hypertension and right ventricular hypertrophy have developed, the examiner notes a parasternal lift. S_1 is typically loud and may be the most prominent physical finding of the disease. A loud S_1 is present because the transmitral gradient holds the mitral valve open throughout diastole until ventricular systole closes the fully opened valve with a loud closing sound. In far-advanced disease, the mitral valve may be so damaged, however, that it neither opens nor closes well, so S_1 may become soft. S_2 is normally split; the pulmonic component is increased in intensity if pulmonary hypertension has developed. Left-sided S_3 and S_4 gallop sounds, which represent the ventricular and atrial components of rapid left ventricular filling, are exceedingly rare in mitral stenosis because obstruction at the mitral valve prevents rapid filling. S_2 is usually followed by an opening snap. The distance between S_2 and the opening snap provides a reasonable estimation of left atrial pressure and the severity of the mitral stenosis. The higher the left atrial pressure, the sooner the left atrial pressure and the falling left ventricular pressure of early ventricular relaxation equilibrate. At this equilibration point, the mitral valve opens, and the opening snap occurs. When left atrial pressure is high, the opening snap closely (0.06 second) follows S_2. Conversely, when left atrial pressure is relatively normal, the snap occurs later (0.12 second) and may mimic the cadence of an S_3 gallop. The opening snap is followed by the classic low-pitched early diastolic mitral stenosis rumble, which increases in length as the mitral stenosis worsens. This murmur may be inaudible if the patient has a relatively low resting cardiac output. Modest exercise, such as isometric handgrip, may accentuate the murmur's intensity. If the patient is in sinus rhythm, atrial systole may produce a presystolic accentuation of the murmur. If pulmonary hypertension has developed, the pulmonic component of S_2 increases in intensity to become as loud as or louder than the aortic component. With pulmonary hypertension, a diastolic blowing murmur of pulmonary insufficiency (Graham Steell murmur) is often heard, although in many cases, a coexistent murmur of mild aortic insufficiency is mistaken for this murmur. Neck vein elevation, ascites, and edema are present if right ventricular failure has developed.

DIAGNOSIS

Similar to other valvular lesions, an echocardiogram is the most important diagnostic tool in confirming the diagnosis (Fig. 60-4). Transthoracic echocardiography or, if necessary, transesophageal echocardiography makes the diagnosis in nearly 100% of cases and accurately assesses severity. Mitral stenosis, similar to aortic stenosis, can be quantified by assessing the transvalvular gradient with the modified Bernoulli principle. The stenosis is considered severe when the area is smaller than 1.5 cm^2 and very severe when the valve area is smaller than 1.0 cm^2. It is important to keep in mind that gradients are rate dependent. In patients with poorly controlled atrial fibrillation, gradients will be increased owing to decreased diastolic filling time. Therefore, it is important to assess multiple heart beats or obtain better rate control to assess mitral stenosis properly.

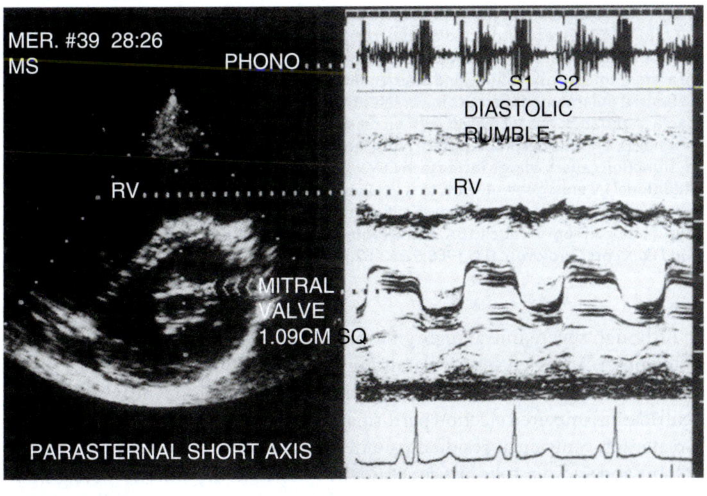

FIGURE 60-4. **Mitral stenosis. An *en face* view of a stenotic mitral valve in the short-axis view of the left ventricle is shown on the *left*. Planimetry for the mitral valve orifice yielded an area of 1.09 cm^2. The M-mode echocardiogram on the *right* has been aligned with the appropriate structures on the *left*. It shows the restricted opening of the mitral valve in diastole associated with the classic diastolic rumbling murmur. RV = right ventricle. (From Assey ME, Usher BW, Carabello BA. The patient with valvular heart disease. In: Pepine CJ, Hill JA, Lambert CR, eds. *Diagnostic and Therapeutic Cardiac Catheterization*. 3rd ed. Baltimore: Williams & Wilkins; 1998:709.)**

During echocardiography, the suitability of the valve for percutaneous balloon mitral valvotomy also can be assessed. Patients with pliable valves, minimal valvular calcification, limited involvement of the subvalvular apparatus, and less than moderate mitral regurgitation are ideal candidates.

In addition to evaluating the mitral valve, echocardiography can be used to evaluate pulmonary artery pressures by measuring the systolic gradient across the tricuspid valve. The elevation of pulmonary pressures is a poor prognostic sign in mitral stenosis and may drive treatment decisions.

Atrial fibrillation is common, especially in patients older than 50 years of age, but left atrial abnormality is generally present on the ECG if the patient is in sinus rhythm. If pulmonary hypertension has developed, there is often evidence of right ventricular hypertrophy.

On the chest radiograph, left atrial enlargement produces straightening of the left heart border and a double density at the right heart border as a result of the combined silhouettes of the right and left atria. Pulmonary venous hypertension produces increased vascularity. Kerley B lines, which represent thickening of the pulmonary septa secondary to chronic venous engorgement, also may be seen.

Invasive Evaluation

Cardiac Catheterization

Cardiac catheterization is usually unnecessary to assess the severity of mitral stenosis. Because many patients with mitral stenosis are of an age when coronary disease might be present, however, coronary arteriography is generally performed if cardiac surgery is anticipated or if the patient has coexistent angina. In these cases, it is common to perform left- and right-sided heart catheterization to confirm the transmitral gradient and to calculate the valve area from the Gorlin formula (see earlier).

PREVENTION, TREATMENT, AND PROGNOSIS

Mitral stenosis can be prevented by appropriate antibiotic treatment of β-hemolytic streptococcal infections (Chapter 269).

Medical Therapy

Asymptomatic patients with mitral stenosis and sinus rhythm require no therapy. Symptoms of mild dyspnea and orthopnea can be treated with diuretics alone. When symptoms worsen to more than mild or if pulmonary hypertension develops (resting pulmonary artery systolic pressure > 50 mm Hg), mechanical correction of the stenosis is preferable to medical therapy because it improves longevity in severely symptomatic patients. In patients in whom symptoms are not consistent with resting hemodynamics, exercise testing with either echocardiography or invasive hemodynamic monitoring is reasonable to assess exercise tolerance as well as the expected increases in gradients and pulmonary pressures with exercise.

Patients with mitral stenosis in whom atrial fibrillation develops usually decompensate because the rapid heart rate reduces diastolic filling time, increases left atrial pressure, and decreases cardiac output. The heart rate must be controlled promptly, preferably with an infusion of diltiazem, amiodarone, or esmolol for acute atrial fibrillation or with a β-blocker, a calcium-channel blocker, or oral digoxin in chronic atrial fibrillation (Chapter 52).

Conversion to sinus rhythm is routinely recommended either pharmacologically or with direct-current countershock (Chapter 52) after anticoagulation is therapeutic. It should be noted that patients with rheumatic atrial fibrillation have been excluded from trials of echocardiogram-guided cardioversion without anticoagulation and from trials of rate control versus rhythm control for the chronic management of atrial fibrillation. If sinus rhythm cannot be maintained, mechanical therapy for the mitral stenosis is generally recommended in the hope that sinus rhythm can be restored after the obstruction to atrial outflow is corrected. However, the cause of atrial fibrillation in patients with mitral stenosis probably includes atrial rheumatic inflammation, so restoration of sinus rhythm is unpredictable even after mechanical intervention.

Because patients with concomitant mitral stenosis and atrial fibrillation have an extraordinarily high risk for systemic embolism, they should undergo chronic anticoagulation with warfarin at an international normalized ratio (INR) target of 2.5 to 3.5 unless there is a serious contraindication to its use. It should be noted that atrial fibrillation with rheumatic mitral stenosis or a mechanical heart valve requires vitamin K antagonist anticoagulation instead of direct-acting oral anticoagulants (Chapter 70).

Mechanical Therapy

When symptoms occur with ordinary activity or if pulmonary hypertension develops, prognosis is worse unless the mitral stenosis is relieved. In contrast to aortic stenosis, the valve leaflets are fused at the commissures in mitral stenosis.

As a result, percutaneous balloon dilation produces a commissurotomy, thereby substantially increasing the valve area, and provides improvement comparable to that of open surgical commissurotomy for at least a decade in suitable patients. Even at 20 years, 30% of patients have durable functional benefit. In patients whose anatomy is not suitable for balloon dilation, usually because of significant mitral regurgitation, open surgery with placement of a bioprosthetic or mechanical valve is preferred.

Nonrheumatic mitral stenosis caused by mitral annular calcification does not respond to balloon valvotomy. The only effective mechanical therapy for this condition is surgical debridement of the mitral annulus followed by mitral valve replacement. Because this procedure carries up to a 30% risk, it should be reserved for highly symptomatic patients with an otherwise good life expectancy and performed only by surgeons with experience performing this operation. Clinical trials are ongoing to evaluate the role of transcatheter valve replacement as an option to open surgical therapy in this population.[10]

PRIMARY (ORGANIC) MITRAL REGURGITATION

EPIDEMIOLOGY

The mitral valve is composed of the mitral annulus, the leaflets, the chordae tendineae, and the papillary muscles. Abnormalities in any of these structures may lead to mitral regurgitation. In primary mitral regurgitation, valvular abnormalities cause the valve to leak; the resulting hemodynamic overload, if prolonged and severe, causes left ventricular damage, heart failure, and eventual death if untreated. This condition must be distinguished from secondary or functional mitral regurgitation, wherein disease of the left ventricle causes the valve to leak; this secondary mitral regurgitation is discussed later in this chapter.

The most common cause of primary mitral regurgitation in the United States is mitral valve prolapse, which is responsible for approximately 90% of all cases and comprises many diseases, including myxomatous degeneration of the valve (E-Fig. 60-3). Annular calcification, endocarditis, papillary muscle dysfunction or infarction, collagen vascular disease, and rheumatic heart disease are less common causes. Dopamine receptor agonists such as pergolide, cabergoline and ergot derivatives and serotonin receptor agonists such as fenfluramine when used in high doses and for prolonged periods of time may lead to mitral regurgitation.

Primary mitral regurgitation can be subdivided on the basis of chronicity. Common causes of severe acute mitral regurgitation include ruptured chordae tendineae and infective endocarditis. Chronic severe mitral regurgitation is more likely to be caused by myxomatous degeneration of the valve, rheumatic heart disease, or annular calcification.[11]

PATHOBIOLOGY

The pathophysiology of mitral regurgitation can be divided into three phases (Fig. 60-5). In acute mitral regurgitation of any cause, the sudden option for ejection of blood into the left atrium "wastes" a portion of the left ventricular stroke volume as backward rather than forward flow. The combined regurgitant and forward flow causes volume overload of the left ventricle and stretches the existing sarcomeres toward their maximum length. Use of the Frank-Starling mechanism is maximized, and end-diastolic volume increases concomitantly. The regurgitant pathway unloads the left ventricle in systole because it allows ejection into the relatively low-impedance left atrium and thereby reduces end-systolic volume. Although increased end-diastolic volume and decreased end-systolic volume act in concert to increase total stroke volume, forward stroke volume is subnormal because a large portion of the total stroke volume is regurgitated into the left atrium. This regurgitant volume increases left atrial pressure, so the patient experiences heart failure with low cardiac output and pulmonary congestion despite normal left ventricular contractile function.

In many cases, severe acute mitral regurgitation necessitates emergency surgical correction. By comparison, patients who can be managed through the acute phase or in whom the valve abnormalities develop more slowly may enter the phase of hemodynamic compensation. In this phase, eccentric left ventricular hypertrophy and increased end-diastolic volume, combined with normal contractile function, allow ejection of a sufficient total stroke volume to permit forward flow to return toward normal. At the same time, left atrial enlargement allows accommodation of the regurgitant volume while maintaining a lower left atrial pressure. In this phase, the patient may be relatively asymptomatic even during strenuous exercise. Although mitral regurgitation is often thought to reduce left ventricular afterload, reduced afterload occurs only in acute, severe, primary mitral regurgitation. In the chronic phase, the increased left ventricular radius returns afterload (wall stress) to normal, and impedance is decreased only in the most severe cases.

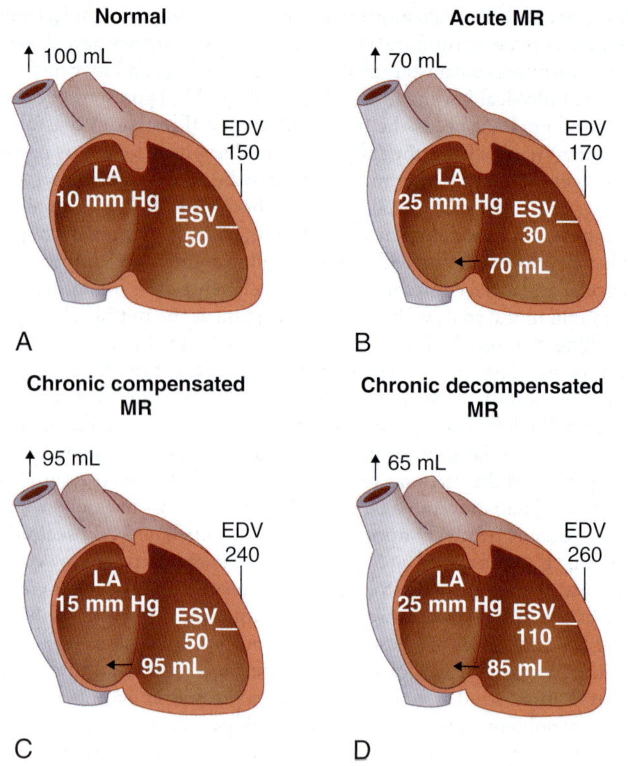

	Preload SL (μ)	Afterload ESS (kdyne/cm²)	CF	EF	RF	FSV (mL)
N	2.07	90	N	.67	.0	100
AMR	2.25	60	N	.82	.50	70
CCMR	2.19	90	N	.79	.5	95
CDMR	2.19	120	↓	.58	.57	65

FIGURE 60-5. **Mitral regurgitation (MR).** Normal physiology (N) **(A)** is compared with the physiology of acute mitral regurgitation (AMR) **(B)**. Acutely, the volume overload increases preload (sarcomere length [SL]), and end-diastolic volume (EDV) increases from 150 to 170 mL. Unloading of the left ventricle (LV) by the presence of the regurgitant pathway decreases afterload (end-systolic stress [ESS]), and end-systolic volume (ESV) falls from 50 to 30 mL. These changes result in an increase in the ejection fraction (EF). Because 50% of the total LV stroke volume (regurgitant fraction [RF]) is ejected into the left atrium (LA), however, forward stroke volume (FSV) falls from 100 to 70 mL. At this stage, contractile function (CF) is normal. **C,** Chronic compensated mitral regurgitation (CCMR). In CCMR, eccentric cardiac hypertrophy has developed, and EDV has increased substantially. Increased EDV, combined with normal contractile function, permits ejection of a larger total stroke volume and a larger forward stroke volume than in the acute phase. Left atrial enlargement permits lower left atrial pressure. Because the radius term in the Laplace equation has increased with increasing LV volume, afterload and ESV return to normal. **D,** Chronic decompensated mitral regurgitation (CDMR). In this stage, contractile dysfunction causes a large increase in ESV with a fall in total and forward stroke volume. Additional LV enlargement leads to worsening mitral regurgitation. The relatively favorable loading conditions in this phase still permit a normal EF, however, despite contractile dysfunction. (From Carabello BA. Mitral regurgitation: basic pathophysiologic principles. *Mod Concepts Cardiovasc Dis*. 1988;57:53-57.)

Although severe mitral regurgitation may be tolerated for many years, the lesion often causes left ventricular dysfunction, atrial fibrillation, or heart failure within 5 years of the detection of severe mitral regurgitation. The now damaged ventricle has impaired ejection performance, and end-systolic volume increases. Greater left ventricular residual volume at end systole increases end-diastolic volume and end-diastolic pressure, and the symptoms of pulmonary congestion may reappear. Additionally, left ventricular dilation may worsen the amount of regurgitation by causing further enlargement of the mitral annulus and displacement of the papillary muscles, thereby leading to malcoaptation of the mitral leaflets. Although there is substantial contractile dysfunction, the increased preload and the presence of the regurgitant pathway, which mitigates the increased afterload expected from ventricular enlargement, augment the ejection fraction and may maintain it in a relatively normal range.

The causes of left ventricular contractile dysfunction in patients with mitral regurgitation may relate to loss of contractile proteins and abnormalities in calcium handling. In at least some cases, contractile dysfunction is reversible by timely mitral valve surgery.

CLINICAL MANIFESTATIONS

In the medical history, the standard symptoms of left-sided heart failure should be sought (Chapter 45). An attempt to discover potential causes should be made by questioning for a history of a heart murmur or abnormal findings on cardiac examination (Chapter 39), rheumatic heart disease, endocarditis (Chapter 61), or the use of anorexigenic drugs.

Volume overload of the left ventricle displaces the apical impulse downward and to the left. S_1 may be reduced in intensity, whereas S_2 is usually physiologically split. In severe mitral regurgitation, S_2 is followed by S_3, which may not indicate heart failure but reflects rapid filling of the left ventricle by the large volume of blood stored in the left atrium during systole. The typical murmur of mitral regurgitation is a holosystolic apical murmur that often radiates toward the axilla (Chapter 39). There is a rough correlation between the intensity of the murmur and the severity of the disease, but this correlation is too weak to use in clinical decision making because the murmur may be soft when cardiac output is low. In contrast to aortic stenosis, murmur intensity does not usually vary with the RR interval. In acute mitral regurgitation, the presence of a large v wave may produce rapid equilibration of left atrial and left ventricular pressure, thereby reducing the driving gradient and shortening the murmur. Pulmonary hypertension may develop and produce right-sided signs, including an right ventricular lift, an increased P_2, and, if right ventricular dysfunction has developed, signs of right-sided heart failure.

DIAGNOSIS

The ECG usually shows left ventricular hypertrophy and left atrial abnormality. The chest radiograph typically shows cardiomegaly; the absence of cardiomegaly indicates either that the mitral regurgitation is mild or that it has not been chronic enough to allow cardiac dilation to occur.

Echocardiography shows the extent of left atrial and left ventricular enlargement (Chapter 43). Ultrasonic imaging of the mitral valve is excellent and offers clues to the mitral valve abnormalities responsible for the regurgitation. In some patients, three-dimensional echocardiography can add pathoanatomic information of potential use in aiding surgical repair of the valve. Color-flow Doppler interrogation of the valve (Fig. 60-6) helps assess the severity of regurgitation, but because this technique images flow velocity rather than actual flow, it is subject to errors in interpretation. The Doppler technique is excellent for excluding the presence of mitral regurgitation and for distinguishing between mild and severe degrees. Newer techniques may quantify regurgitation more precisely but are not applicable in every patient, and standard color-flow Doppler examination may not be sufficient for exact quantification of mitral regurgitation or to determine whether the severity of the lesion is sufficient to cause eventual left ventricular dysfunction. Cardiac MRI (Chapter 44), when available, can more precisely quantify the severity of the regurgitation. When the severity of mitral regurgitation is in doubt or if mitral valve surgery is being contemplated, cardiac catheterization (Chapter 59) can be helpful in resolving the severity of the lesion; coronary arteriography should be included in patients older than 40 years or with symptoms suggesting coronary disease (Chapter 56).

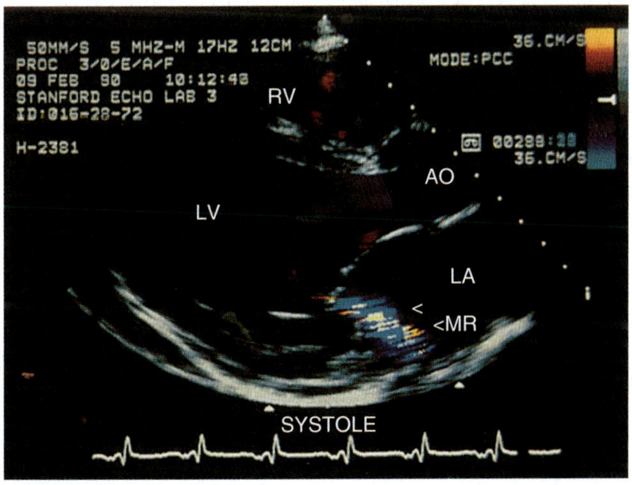

FIGURE 60-6. **Two-dimensional echocardiogram of mitral regurgitation with Doppler flow mapping superimposed on a portion of the image. The color information is represented in the sector of the imaging plane extending from the apex of the triangular plane to the two small *arrowheads* at the *bottom* of the image plane. Mitral regurgitation (MR) is indicated *(open arrows)* and extends from the mitral valve leaflets toward the posterior aspect of the left atrium (LA) during systole. The mosaic of colors representing the mitral regurgitant signal is typical of high-velocity turbulent flow. The low-intensity *orange-brown* signal represents flow directed away from the transducer on the chest wall, and the *blue* shades represent blood in the left ventricular outflow tract moving toward the transducer. AO = aorta; LV = left ventricle; RV = right ventricle.**

TREATMENT AND PROGNOSIS

Medical Therapy

Severe Acute Mitral Regurgitation

In severe acute mitral regurgitation, the patient is usually symptomatic with heart failure or even shock. The goal of medical therapy is to increase forward cardiac output while concomitantly reducing regurgitant volume (Chapter 46). Arterial vasodilators reduce systemic resistance to flow and preferentially increase aortic outflow and simultaneously decrease the amount of mitral regurgitation and left atrial hypertension. If hypotension already exists, vasodilators such as nitroprusside lower blood pressure further and cannot be used. In these cases, intra-aortic balloon counterpulsation (Chapter 93) is preferred if the aortic valve is competent. Counterpulsation increases forward cardiac output by lowering ventricular afterload while augmenting systemic diastolic pressure.

Chronic Symptomatic Mitral Regurgitation

In patients with *symptomatic* mitral regurgitation, angiotensin-converting enzyme (ACE) inhibitors (e.g., lisinopril, 20 mg/day) reduce left ventricular volume and improve symptoms but do not alter outcome and are reserved for inoperable patients. Observational evidence suggests that such patients may benefit from administration of β-blockers. Mitral valve surgery rather than medical therapy is indicated in most symptomatic patients with mitral regurgitation. When atrial fibrillation is present, anticoagulation is indicated.

Chronic Asymptomatic Mitral Regurgitation

Vasodilators have had little effect in reducing left ventricular volume or improving normal exercise tolerance in patients with mitral regurgitation, perhaps because afterload is not usually increased in chronic asymptomatic mitral regurgitation, so there is no definitive indication to begin afterload reduction before symptoms appear. However, hypertension, if present, should be treated with standard guideline-directed therapy (Chapter 64).

Surgical Therapy

The timing of mitral valve surgery must weigh the risks of the operation and placement of a prosthesis, if one is inserted, against the risk for irreversible LV dysfunction if surgery is delayed unwisely. In patients with mitral regurgitation, the native valve often can be repaired, and this option may influence the patient and physician towards earlier surgery.

Types of Mitral Valve Surgery

Mitral Valve Repair

When feasible, mitral valve repair (Fig. 60-7) is the preferred operation.[12] Repair restores valve competence, maintains the functional aspects of the apparatus, and avoids the insertion of a prosthesis. Repair is most applicable in cases of posterior chordal rupture; anterior involvement and rheumatic involvement make repair more difficult. Currently, the percentage of mitral valve surgeries that are valve repair average about 70% across the United States overall, with outcomes that are highly dependent on the skill and experience of the operating physician.

Percutaneous mitral valve repair, with implantation of a clip device via the femoral vein and a transseptal puncture, is less invasive than conventional mitral valve repair but is also less effective than open surgery for eliminating mitral regurgitation.[A10] Percutaneous repair, which is approved in the United States for primary mitral regurgitation in symptomatic patients who are at high risk for surgery, usually leaves the patient with mild to moderate residual regurgitation that does not usually worsen over time.[13]

Mitral Valve Replacement with Preservation of the Mitral Apparatus

In this procedure, a prosthetic valve is inserted, but continuity between the native leaflets and the papillary muscles is maintained. This procedure has the advantage of ensuring mitral valve competence while preserving the functional aspects of the mitral apparatus in the left ventricle. Even if only the posterior leaflets and chordae are preserved, the patient benefits from improved postoperative ventricular function and possibly better survival. Although the patient benefits from restored mitral valve competence and maintenance of left ventricular function, insertion of a prosthesis still carries all prosthesis-associated risks. Operative mortality with all mitral valve replacement operations is at least twice as high as with mitral valve repair.

Mitral Valve Replacement without Preservation of the Mitral Apparatus

When the native valve cannot be repaired or the chordae preserved, such as in severe rheumatic deformity, the mitral valve leaflets and its apparatus are

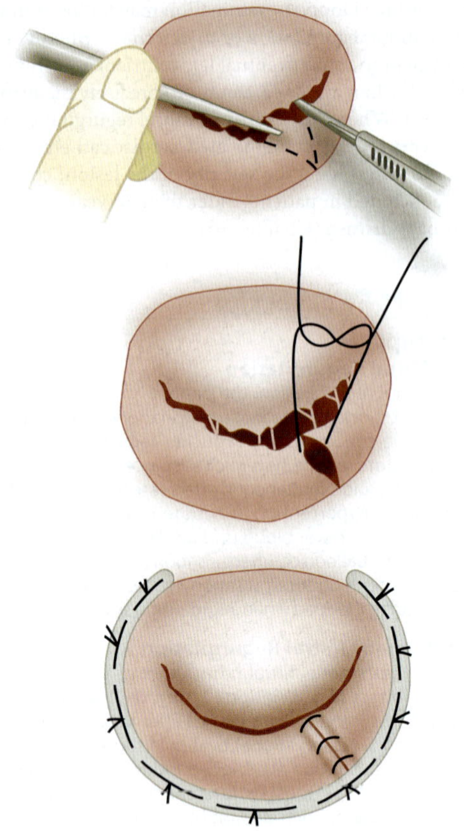

FIGURE 60-7. The stages of mitral valve repair. (Modified from Cleveland Clinic. Mitral valve repair. http://my.clevelandclinic.org/heart/disorders/valve/mvrepair.aspx.)

removed and a prosthetic valve is inserted. Although this operation almost guarantees mitral valve competence, the mitral valve apparatus is responsible for coordinating left ventricular contraction and for helping maintain the efficient prolate ellipsoid shape of the left ventricle. Destruction of the apparatus leads to a sudden fall in left ventricular function and a decline in postoperative ejection fraction that is often permanent.

Transcatheter Mitral Valve Replacement

Transcatheter mitral valve replacement has been used especially in patients who are unsuitable for repair, such as patients who have severe mitral annular calcification and have an extremely high operative risk.[14] Although the technical success rate has been promising, the procedure is still experimental.

Timing of Surgery

Symptomatic Patients

Most patients with symptoms of dyspnea, orthopnea, or fatigue should undergo surgery regardless of which operation is performed because they already have lifestyle limitations from their disease. The mere presence of symptoms worsens the prognosis despite relatively well-preserved left ventricular function. The onset or worsening of symptoms is a summary of the patient's pathophysiology and may give a broader view of cardiovascular integrity than possible with any single measurement of pressure or function. For patients with acute mitral regurgitation owing to flail mitral valve leaflets, earlier surgery appears to be better than prolonged medical management, but randomized trials have not been performed.

Asymptomatic Patients with Normal Left Ventricular Function

Surgery has increasingly been considered in asymptomatic patients who have normal left ventricular function but echocardiographic findings indicating that valve repair is likely to be successful. Although these patients are at low risk with continued medical therapy, early surgery reduces the risks of subsequent left ventricular dysfunction or atrial fibrillation and should be considered if the risk associated with valve repair is less than 1% because lifespan can be normal if successful repair is performed before left ventricular dysfunction has developed. This approach is sensible, however, only if it is certain that valve repair can be performed, because insertion of a prosthesis carries unacceptable risk in this low-risk group.

Asymptomatic Patients with Left Ventricular Dysfunction

The onset of left ventricular dysfunction in patients with mitral regurgitation may occur without causing symptoms. Early surgery is warranted to prevent the muscle dysfunction from becoming severe or irreversible. Regardless of whether valve repair or replacement is eventually performed, survival is prolonged if surgery is performed before the ejection fraction declines to less than 60% or the left ventricular end-systolic dimension increases beyond 40 mm. Elevated brain natriuretic peptide levels and deterioration of global longitudinal strain also may be considered as adjuncts to the decision for surgery. Patients with severe mitral regurgitation should be monitored yearly with a history, physical examination, and echocardiographic evaluation of left ventricular function. When the patient reports symptoms or echocardiography shows the onset of left ventricular dysfunction, surgery should be undertaken. However, it is not necessary to wait until these thresholds are reached to recommend surgery. If it is clear that valve repair is highly likely and the patient is approaching these indications for intervention, surgery should be considered at that time.

Asymptomatic Elderly Patients

Among Medicare recipients, the operative mortality rate is 4% for patients undergoing mitral valve repair and 9% for patients undergoing replacement. Even in patients who have no comorbid conditions, the mortality rates are 2% for repair and 4% for replacement. Patients older than 75 years of age may have poorer surgical results than younger patients, especially if coronary disease is present or if mitral valve replacement rather than repair must be performed. As a result, there is little compelling reason to commit elderly asymptomatic patients to a mitral valve operation.

MITRAL VALVE PROLAPSE

DEFINITION

Mitral valve prolapse occurs when one or both of the mitral valve leaflets prolapse during systole beyond the mitral valve annular plane and into the left atrium. The importance of mitral valve prolapse varies from patient to patient. In some cases, prolapse is simply a consequence of normal left ventricular physiology without significant medical impact, such as in situations that produce a small left ventricle (e.g., the Valsalva maneuver or an atrial septal defect), in which reduction of ventricular volume causes relative lengthening of the chordae tendineae and subsequent mitral valve prolapse. At the other end of the spectrum, severe redundancy and deformity of the valve, which occur in myxomatous valve degeneration, increase the risk for stroke, arrhythmia, endocarditis, and progression to severe mitral regurgitation.[15]

DIAGNOSIS

History

Most patients with mitral valve prolapse are asymptomatic. In some cases, however, mitral valve prolapse is associated with symptoms, including palpitations, syncope, and chest pain. In some cases, chest pain indicates true myocardial ischemia despite normal epicardial coronary arteries, perhaps because excessive tension on the papillary muscles increases oxygen consumption. Palpitations, syncope, and presyncope, when present, are linked to autonomic dysfunction (Chapters 39, 49, and 386), which appears to be more prevalent in patients with mitral valve prolapse.

Physical Examination

On physical examination, the mitral valve prolapse syndrome produces the characteristic findings of a midsystolic click and a late systolic murmur. The click occurs when the chordae tendineae are stretched taut by the prolapsing mitral valve in mid-systole. As prolapse occurs, the mitral leaflets move past their coaptation point, permit mitral regurgitation, and cause the late systolic murmur (see Table 39-7 in Chapter 39). Maneuvers that make the left ventricle smaller, such as the Valsalva maneuver, cause the click to appear earlier and the murmur to be more holosystolic and often louder (see Table 39-8 in Chapter 39). In some cases of echocardiographically proven mitral valve prolapse, neither the click nor the murmur is present; in other cases, only one of these findings is present.

Noninvasive Evaluation

Echocardiography is useful to prove that prolapse is present, to image the amount of regurgitation and its physiologic effects, and to discern the pathoanatomy of the mitral valve. Although an echocardiogram is not necessary to diagnose prolapse in patients with the classic physical findings, the echocardiogram adds significant prognostic information because it can detect patients who have specifically abnormal valve morphology and in whom most of the complications of the disease occur.

TREATMENT

Because most cases of mitral valve prolapse are asymptomatic, therapy is usually unnecessary and prophylaxis against infective endocarditis is not recommended (Chapter 61). In patients with palpitations and autonomic dysfunction, β-blockers are often effective in relieving symptoms. If severe mitral regurgitation or a flail mitral leaflet develops, the therapy is the same as for other causes of mitral regurgitation. If surgical valve repair is chosen, leaflet preservation and leaflet resection provide equivalent results.[A11]

PROGNOSIS

Most patients with mitral valve prolapse, even patients with redundant and misshapen mitral leaflets, have a benign clinical course. Approximately 10% of patients with thickened leaflets experience infective endocarditis, stroke, progression to severe mitral regurgitation, or sudden death. The progression to severe mitral regurgitation varies with gender and age, and men are approximately twice as likely to progress as women. By 50 years of age, only approximately 1 in 200 men requires surgery to correct mitral regurgitation. By the age of 70 years, the risk increases to approximately 3%.

SECONDARY (FUNCTIONAL) MITRAL REGURGITATION

DEFINITION

Secondary or functional mitral regurgitation is a very different disease than primary mitral regurgitation. In primary mitral regurgitation, treating the mitral regurgitation cures the patient. Conversely, secondary mitral regurgitation is typically a consequence of left ventricular myocardial dysfunction, usually caused by myocardial infarction or dilated cardiomyopathy,[16] but sometimes occurs when atrial fibrillation results in annular dilatation and leaflet malcoaptation.[17] Because treating secondary mitral regurgitation cannot reverse those entities, the role of valve therapy is often unclear.

EPIDEMIOLOGY

An estimated 6 million Americans have heart failure (Chapters 45 and 46), and about half of them have heart failure with a reduced ejection fraction. About 75% of these latter patients also have some degree of secondary mitral regurgitation, which is severe in about 20% of them.

PATHOBIOLOGY

In secondary mitral regurgitation, the valve itself is normal. Regurgitation occurs because of leaflet malcoaptation that results from either displacement of the papillary muscles in patients with left ventricular dysfunction or annular dilatation in patients with atrial fibrillation. Mitral closing is further impaired by mitral annular dilation and reduced closing force from the weakened myocardium.

CLINICAL MANIFESTATIONS

Because virtually all patients with secondary mitral regurgitation have heart failure, almost all complain of the symptoms of heart failure. Some may note a worsening of symptoms when more than mild secondary mitral regurgitation develops. Probably because the mitral valve itself is normal, as well as because of the weakened force of contraction, the murmur of functional mitral regurgitation may be unimpressive or even inaudible.

DIAGNOSIS

Echocardiography is the mainstay of the diagnosis. In addition to evaluating the severity of the mitral regurgitation itself, the echocardiogram is helpful in establishing the extent of the dilated cardiomyopathy or of the prior myocardial infarction that is responsible for causing the secondary mitral regurgitation.

TREATMENT AND PROGNOSIS

The presence of mitral regurgitation in patients with systolic dysfunction is associated with worsened prognosis, which in turn probably reflects both poorer left ventricular function and the imposition of an extra volume overload on an already weakened left ventricle.

Because almost all patients with secondary mitral regurgitation have heart failure, the primary treatment is standard treatment for heart failure (Chapter 46). For secondary functional mitral regurgitation owing to heart failure with left ventricular dilation, the combination of sacubitril/valsartan (49/51 mg twice daily, titrated as tolerated at 4-week intervals to a maximum dose of 97/103 mg twice daily) is better than valsartan alone for reducing regurgitation.[A12] Many patients with secondary mitral regurgitation also have conducting system abnormalities, and patients with left bundle branch block may benefit from cardiac resynchronization therapy (Chapters 46 and 54), which improves systolic function while often reducing secondary mitral regurgitation, sometimes even eliminating it. When these therapies fail to relieve symptoms, surgical treatment can be considered.[18]

For severe *ischemic mitral regurgitation,* mitral valve repair and chordal-sparing mitral valve replacement provide equivalent clinical outcomes at 1 and 2 years, although replacement results in less residual mitral regurgitation and is associated with less severe heart failure, fewer heart failure–related adverse events, and fewer cardiovascular admissions.[A13] For moderate ischemic mitral regurgitation, mitral valve repair does not clearly add benefit above and beyond the benefits of coronary artery bypass surgery.[A14]

For *mitral regurgitation secondary to heart failure,* several studies have shown percutaneous mitral repair to be no better than optimal medical therapy[A15] or open surgery,[A16] but one trial demonstrated better survival than medical therapy.[A17] However, the average survival rate at 5 years is about 50%, and this figure has not changed much over the past several decades.

AORTIC REGURGITATION

DEFINITION

Aortic regurgitation is caused either by abnormalities of the aortic leaflets or by abnormalities of the proximal aortic root. Leaflet abnormalities causing aortic regurgitation include a bicuspid aortic valve, infective endocarditis, and rheumatic heart disease. Dopamine receptor agonists and serotonin receptor agonists have also been implicated. Common aortic root abnormalities that cause aortic regurgitation include Marfan syndrome (Chapter 239), hypertension-induced annuloaortic ectasia, aortic dissection (Chapter 63), syphilis (Chapter 295), ankylosing spondylitis (Chapter 244), and psoriatic arthritis (Chapter 244). Acute aortic regurgitation is usually caused by infective endocarditis (Chapter 61) or aortic dissection.

PATHOBIOLOGY

As with mitral regurgitation, aortic regurgitation imparts a volume overload on the left ventricle because it must pump the forward flow entering from the left atrium and the regurgitant volume returning through the incompetent aortic valve. Also as with mitral regurgitation, the volume overload is compensated for by the development of eccentric cardiac hypertrophy, which increases chamber size and allows the ventricle to pump a greater total stroke volume and a greater forward stroke volume. Ventricular enlargement also accommodates the volume overload at a lower filling pressure. Because pulse pressure is proportional to stroke volume and elastance of the aorta, the increased stroke volume increases systolic pressure. Systolic hypertension leads to afterload excess, which does not generally occur in mitral regurgitation. Accordingly, ventricular geometry also differs between mitral and aortic regurgitation because the afterload excess in aortic regurgitation causes a modest element of concentric hypertrophy, as well as severe eccentric hypertrophy.

In acute aortic insufficiency, such as might occur in infective endocarditis, severe volume overload of the previously unprepared left ventricle results in a sudden fall in forward output while precipitously increasing left ventricular filling pressure. It is probably this combination of pathophysiologic factors that leads to rapid decompensation, presumably because the severely diminished gradient for coronary blood flow causes ischemia and progressive deterioration in left ventricular function. In acute aortic insufficiency, reflex vasoconstriction increases peripheral vascular resistance. In compensated chronic aortic insufficiency, vasoconstriction is absent, and vascular resistance may be reduced and contribute to the hyperdynamic circulation observed in these patients.

CLINICAL MANIFESTATIONS

The most common symptoms from chronic aortic regurgitation are those of left-sided heart failure (Chapter 45); that is, dyspnea on exertion, orthopnea, and fatigue. In acute aortic regurgitation, cardiac output and shock may develop rapidly. The onset of symptoms in patients with chronic aortic regurgitation usually heralds the onset of left ventricular systolic dysfunction. Some patients with symptoms have apparently normal systolic function, however, and the symptoms may be attributed to diastolic dysfunction. Other patients may have ventricular dysfunction yet remain asymptomatic.

Angina may also occur in patients with aortic insufficiency but less commonly than in patients with aortic stenosis. Coronary blood flow reserve is reduced in some patients because diastolic runoff into the left ventricle lowers aortic diastolic pressure while increasing left ventricular diastolic pressure; these two influences lower the driving pressure gradient for flow across the coronary bed. When angina occurs in aortic regurgitation, it may be accompanied by flushing. Other symptoms include carotid artery pain and an unpleasant awareness of the heartbeat.

DIAGNOSIS

Physical Examination

Chronic aortic regurgitation produces a myriad of signs because a hyperdynamic, enlarged left ventricle ejects a large stroke volume at high pressure into the systemic circulation. Palpation of the precordium finds a hyperactive apical impulse displaced downward and to the left. S_1 and S_2 are usually normal. S_2 is followed by a diastolic blowing murmur heard best along the left sternal border with the patient sitting upright. In mild disease, the murmur may be short and heard only in the beginning of diastole when the gradient between the aorta and the left ventricle is highest. As the disease worsens, the murmur may persist throughout diastole. A second murmur, a mitral valve rumble, is heard at the left ventricular apex in patients with severe aortic insufficiency. Although the cause is still debated, this Austin Flint murmur is probably produced as the regurgitant jet impinges on the mitral valve and causes it to vibrate.

In chronic aortic regurgitation, the high stroke volume and reduced systemic arterial resistance result in a wide pulse pressure, which may generate a number of signs, including Corrigan pulse (sharp upstroke and rapid decline of the carotid pulse), de Musset sign (head bobbing), Duroziez sign (combined systolic and diastolic bruits created by compression of the femoral artery with the stethoscope), and Quincke pulse (systolic plethora and diastolic blanching in the nail bed when gentle traction is placed on the nail). Perhaps the most reliable of physical signs indicating severe aortic regurgitation is Hill sign, an increase in femoral systolic pressure of 40 mm Hg or more compared with systolic pressure in the brachial artery.

In contrast to chronic aortic insufficiency with its myriad clinical signs, acute aortic insufficiency may have a subtle manifestation. The eccentric hypertrophy, which compensates for chronic aortic insufficiency, has not yet had time to develop, and the large total stroke volume responsible for most of the signs of chronic aortic insufficiency is absent. The only clues to the presence of acute aortic insufficiency may be a short diastolic blowing murmur and reduced intensity of S_1. This latter sign occurs because high diastolic left ventricular pressure closes the mitral valve early in diastole (mitral valve preclosure) so that when ventricular systole occurs, only the tricuspid component of S_1 is heard.

Noninvasive Evaluation

The ECG in patients with aortic insufficiency is nonspecific but almost always demonstrates left ventricular hypertrophy. The chest radiograph shows an enlarged heart, often with uncoiling and enlargement of the aortic root.

Echocardiography (Chapter 43) is the most important noninvasive tool for assessing the severity of aortic insufficiency and its impact on left ventricular geometry and function (Fig. 60-8). During echocardiography, the left ventricular end-diastolic dimension, end-systolic dimension, and fractional shortening are determined. Aortic valve anatomy and aortic root anatomy can be assessed, and the cause of the aortic regurgitation often can be determined. Color-flow Doppler examination of the aortic valve helps quantify the severity of aortic regurgitation by assessing the depth and width to which the diastolic jet penetrates the left ventricle. Another way to assess the severity of aortic regurgitation is the pressure half-time method: continuous-wave Doppler interrogation of the aortic valve displays the decay of the velocity of retrograde flow across the valve. In mild aortic insufficiency, the gradient across the valve is high throughout diastole, and its rate of decay is slow, with production of a long Doppler half-time (the time that it takes the velocity to decay from its peak to that value divided by the square root of 2). In severe aortic regurgitation, pressure in the aorta and pressure in the left ventricle equilibrate rapidly, and the Doppler half-time is short. In cases in which the severity of aortic insufficiency is in doubt, MRI can quantify regurgitant flow or catheterization with aortography can visualize regurgitant flow to resolve the issue.

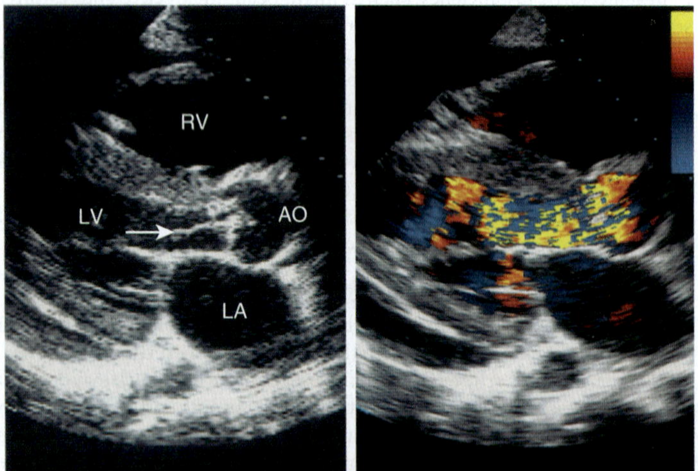

FIGURE 60-8. Echocardiogram of a patient with aortic regurgitation caused by infective endocarditis. The *left panel* shows a linear vegetation *(arrow)* prolapsing into the left ventricular (LV) outflow tract from the aortic valve leaflet in diastole. The *right panel* is a color-flow Doppler image exhibiting turbulent blood flow filling the LV tract during diastole. AO = aorta; LA = left atrium; RV = right ventricle. (Courtesy of Dr. Anthony DeMaria.)

TREATMENT AND PROGNOSIS

Acute Aortic Regurgitation

When any of the symptoms or signs of heart failure develop, even if mild, the medical mortality rate is high and approaches 75%. Echocardiographic evidence of preclosure of the mitral valve from high diastolic intracavitary left ventricular pressure is an especially ominous sign and an indication for urgent surgery. Therapy with vasodilators, such as nitroprusside, may temporarily improve the patient's condition before surgery but is never a substitute for surgery. In patients with acute aortic regurgitation caused by bacterial endocarditis (Chapter 61), surgery may be delayed to permit a full or partial course of antibiotics, but persistent, severe aortic regurgitation requires emergency valve replacement. Even when blood cultures have been positive recently and antibiotic therapy has been of brief duration, the valve reinfection rate is low, 0 to 10%, with valve replacement or valve repair. Emergency surgery should not be withheld simply because the duration of antibiotic therapy has been brief.

Chronic Aortic Regurgitation

Asymptomatic Patients

Because aortic regurgitation increases left ventricular afterload, which decreases cardiac efficiency, afterload reduction with nifedipine and other vasodilators, including ACE inhibitors, improves hemodynamics in the short term but does not reliably delay or reduce the need for aortic valve surgery. When hypertension accompanies aortic regurgitation, it should be treated according to standard guidelines (Chapter 64).

Asymptomatic patients who manifest evidence of left ventricular dysfunction benefit from surgery. When the left ventricular ejection fraction is less than 50% or the end-systolic dimension is greater than 50 mm, postoperative outcome is impaired, presumably because these markers indicate that left ventricular dysfunction has developed. Data suggest that surgery should be timed even before an end-systolic dimension of 45 mm has been reached.[19] A calculated regurgitant orifice above 30 mm^2 portends a poorer prognosis and may warrant surgery.

Symptomatic Patients or Patients with Left Ventricular Dysfunction

Patients who have symptoms or manifest left ventricular dysfunction should not be treated medically, except for short-term stabilization, but should undergo aortic valve surgery as soon as feasible before symptoms compromise their lifestyle. Although some patients may be able to undergo successful aortic valve repair to restore aortic valve competence, most patients require insertion of an aortic valve prosthesis.

TRICUSPID REGURGITATION

DEFINITION

As the population ages, the prevalence of tricuspid regurgitation has increased. Tricuspid regurgitation is usually caused by the hemodynamic load on the right ventricle, owing to pulmonary hypertension, an intracardiac shunt, left ventricular dysfunction, or mitral or aortic valve disease, rather than by a structural valve deformity. Because most of the force that is needed to fill the left ventricle is provided by the right ventricle, left ventricular dysfunction leading to elevated left ventricular filling pressure also places the right ventricle under a hemodynamic load and can eventually lead to right ventricular failure and tricuspid regurgitation. Another frequent cause of tricuspid regurgitation is atrial fibrillation, which can lead to annular dilatation and regurgitation on the right side similar to what happens on the left side with the mitral valve.[20] Less commonly, tricuspid regurgitation may be caused by pathology of the valve itself, usually from infective endocarditis, typically stemming from intravenous drug abuse and unsterile injections (Chapter 61). Other causes include trauma (especially from hitting the steering wheel or dashboard in motor vehicle accidents), carcinoid syndrome (Chapter 213), rheumatic involvement of the tricuspid valve, myxomatous degeneration, and right ventricular infarction. Pacemaker leads placed across the tricuspid valve can also lead to significant tricuspid regurgitation by tethering the leaflets and preventing leaflet coaptation.[21]

DIAGNOSIS

The traditional symptoms of tricuspid regurgitation are those of right-sided heart failure (Chapter 45), including ascites, edema, and occasionally right upper quadrant pain. However, some patients may present with atypical symptoms of low cardiac output such as fatigue and dyspnea. In elderly patients, these symptoms often can be difficult to attribute solely to the tricuspid valve because they often have other comorbid conditions that could be responsible.

On physical examination, tricuspid regurgitation produces jugular venous distention accentuated by a large v wave as blood is regurgitated into the right atrium during systole. Regurgitation into the hepatic veins causes hepatic enlargement and liver pulsation. Right ventricular enlargement is detected as a parasternal lift. Ascites and edema are common. The murmur of tricuspid regurgitation is a holosystolic murmur heard along the left sternal border, often increasing with inspiration. The murmur may be faint, and it usually can be heard only under the best auscultatory conditions.

The definitive diagnosis of tricuspid regurgitation is made by echocardiography. Doppler interrogation of the tricuspid valve shows systolic disturbance of the right atrial blood pool. Echocardiography (Chapter 43) also can be used to determine the severity of pulmonary hypertension, measure right ventricular dilation and function, and assess whether the valve itself is intrinsically normal or abnormal.

TREATMENT AND PROGNOSIS

Therapy for secondary tricuspid regurgitation is generally aimed at the cause of the lesion. If left ventricular failure has been responsible for right ventricular failure and tricuspid regurgitation, the standard therapy for improving left ventricular failure (Chapter 46) lowers left ventricular filling pressure, reduces secondary pulmonary hypertension, relieves some of the hemodynamic burden of the right ventricle, and partially restores tricuspid valve competence. If pulmonary disease is the primary cause, therapy is directed toward improving lung function. Medical therapy directed at tricuspid regurgitation is usually limited to diuretics because the vasodilators that are so useful in the treatment of left-sided heart failure are often ineffective in treating pulmonary hypertension. However, a number of options can improve late-stage symptoms that are primarily caused by the pulmonary hypertension itself (Chapter 69).

Transcatheter repair[22] of severe tricuspid regurgitation can improve quality of life.[A18] Open surgical intervention for the tricuspid valve is rarely entertained in isolation. However, if other cardiac surgery is planned in a patient with severe tricuspid regurgitation, concomitant ring annuloplasty or tricuspid valve repair is frequently attempted to ensure postoperative tricuspid competence. Because a second operation to address residual tricuspid regurgitation after successful left-sided valve surgery carries an unacceptably high mortality rate, concomitant tricuspid annuloplasty is now entertained for even mild to moderate tricuspid regurgitation during left-sided valve surgery if annular dilatation is present. For example, concurrent tricuspid valve repair at the time of mitral valve surgery for mitral regurgitation reduces the likelihood of progressive tricuspid regurgitation but has not been shown to reduce subsequent all-cause mortality.[A19,A20] Tricuspid valve replacement is often not well tolerated and is rarely performed except when severe deformity, as is often seen in endocarditis or carcinoid disease, precludes valve repair.

PULMONIC STENOSIS

DEFINITION

Pulmonic stenosis is a congenital disease resulting from fusion of the pulmonic valve cusps (Chapter 55). It is usually detected and corrected during childhood, but occasionally cases are diagnosed for the first time in adulthood. Symptoms of pulmonic stenosis include angina and syncope. Occasionally, symptoms of right-sided heart failure develop. During physical examination, the uncalcified valve in pulmonic stenosis produces an early systolic ejection click on opening. During inspiration, the click diminishes or disappears because increased flow into the right side of the heart during inspiration partially opens the pulmonic valve in diastole so that systole causes less of an opening sound. The click is followed by a systolic ejection murmur that radiates to the base of the heart. If the transvalvular gradient is severe, right ventricular hypertrophy develops and produces a parasternal lift.

The diagnosis of pulmonic stenosis is confirmed by echocardiography, which quantifies the transvalvular gradient and the degree of right ventricular hypertrophy and dysfunction.

TREATMENT AND PROGNOSIS

In asymptomatic patients with a gradient less than 25 mm Hg, no therapy is required. If symptoms develop or the gradient exceeds 50 mm Hg, balloon commissurotomy is effective in reducing the gradient, improving right ventricular function, and relieving symptoms.[23] Although long-term prognosis is not yet established, 90% of patients do not require reintervention 10 years after balloon therapy. If pulmonary valve replacement is required, the transcatheter approach generally provides excellent outcomes.[24]

CHOICES AMONG PROSTHETIC VALVES

Different types of prosthetic valves (Fig. 60-9) have different advantages and disadvantages (Table 60-2). At long-term follow-up, primary valve failure with resulting need for reoperation is much more common with bioprosthetic valves, and bleeding is generally more common with mechanical valves. For mitral valves, long-term survival is similar with bioprosthetic and mechanical valves. Survival after aortic valve replacement is probably better with mechanical valves, except for young patients with congenital bicuspid aortic stenosis, in whom the Ross procedure is preferred.[25]

In general, a tissue valve is recommended in patients who have a life expectancy of less than 15 years or who are unable or unwilling to maintain warfarin anticoagulation. The choice of tissue valve is left to the implanting surgeon because no randomized trials have compared tissue valves to each other. A mechanical valve is preferred in patients who already have another indication for anticoagulation or who have a longer life expectancy and want to minimize the risk of reoperation. Because many patients prefer the risk of reoperation to that of anticoagulation, the age at which bioprostheses are implanted has steadily declined, and many 60-year-old patients now request and receive a bioprosthetic valve.

Reoperations to replace prosthetic valves are required when the valve becomes stenotic or regurgitant. Prosthetic valve failure is much more common in bioprosthetic valves compared with mechanical valves. For unclear reasons, bioprosthetic failure occurs more rapidly in younger patients, especially patients younger than age 50 years. Transcatheter aortic valve replacement is an alternative to open surgery in patients with an uninfected, nonthrombosed prior aortic bioprosthesis that now needs replacement.[26] Emerging data also support the use of transcatheter mitral valve insertion in patients who have a dysfunctional but noninfected or thrombosed mitral bioprosthesis and are at high risk for repeat open surgery.[27]

POSTOPERATIVE CARE OF PATIENTS WITH SUBSTITUTE HEART VALVES

After a prosthetic valve has been inserted, a baseline echocardiogram should be obtained to provide a reference point in the event that valve dysfunction is suspected at a later date. Echocardiography does not need to be repeated unless the patient's clinical status or physical findings change. The major causes of mechanical valve dysfunction are infective endocarditis and thrombus formation. For bioprostheses, endocarditis is also a risk, but valve degeneration, which can cause either stenosis or regurgitation, is a major concern.

Whenever a patient with a prosthetic heart valve has a temperature higher than 100° F, endocarditis must be excluded by blood culture; for fever with signs of sepsis, broad-spectrum antibiotics must be begun while awaiting culture results. For patients with bioprosthetic valves, mechanical prostheses, and homografts, endocarditis prophylaxis should be instituted at the time of procedures that are associated with a high risk for bacteremia (Chapter 61). Whether prophylaxis is necessary for a pulmonary autograft after the Ross procedure is currently unclear, but physicians usually prescribe prophylaxis for these patients.

All patients with a mechanical heart valve require warfarin anticoagulation. Recommended INR values range from 2.0 (1.5 for the On-X aortic valve) for a young normotensive patient in sinus rhythm with an aortic valve prosthesis to 3.5 for a patient with atrial fibrillation and a mitral valve prosthesis. Aspirin 75 to 100 mg/day added to warfarin may be beneficial in patients who have a separate indication for antiplatelet therapy. Direct-acting anticoagulants such as dabigatran are associated with more thrombosis and bleeding in patients with mechanical prosthetic valves[A21] and should not be used. Direct-acting oral anticoagulants are, however, appropriate for patients who have atrial fibrillation in the setting of a bioprosthetic valve.[A22] When thrombosis occurs on a prosthetic

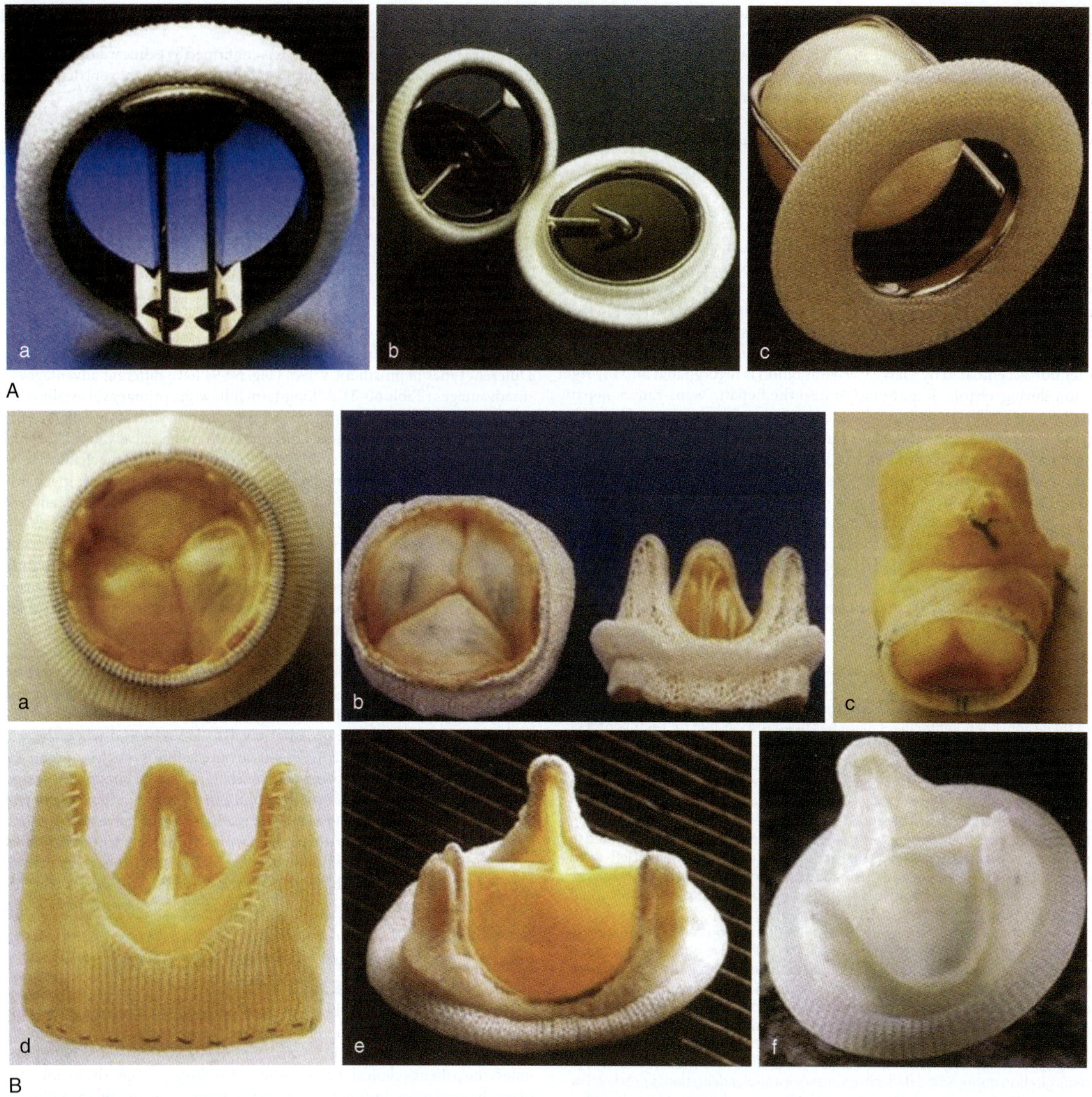

FIGURE 60-9. **Prosthetic aortic valves. A,** Common mechanical valves: *a,* a bileaflet St. Jude Medical valve; *b,* a Medtronic-Hall tilting disc valve; *c,* a Starr-Edwards ball cage valve (no longer manufactured but still in use). (From Antunes MJ, Burke AP, Carabello B. Valvular heart disease. In: Braunwald E, Rahimtoola SH, eds. *Essential Atlas of Heart Diseases*. 3rd ed. Philadelphia: Current Medicine Group; 2005:296-297.) **B,** Common bioprostheses: *a,* Hancock modified orifice stented valve; Carpentier-Edwards stented porcine valve; Medtronic Freestyle Stentless Valve; *d,* St. Jude Medical Toronto SPV stentless valve; *e,* Carpentier-Edwards pericardial valve; *f,* Autologous pericardial valve. (From Grunkemeier GL, Rahimtoola SH, Starr A. Prosthetic heart valves. In: Rahimtoola SH, ed. *Valvular Heart Disease*. Philadelphia: Current Medicine Group; 1997:13.9-13.11.)

TABLE 60-2 ADVANTAGES AND DISADVANTAGES OF SUBSTITUTE CARDIAC VALVES

TYPE OF VALVE	ADVANTAGES	DISADVANTAGES
Bioprosthesis (Carpentier-Edwards, Hancock)	Avoids anticoagulation in patients with sinus rhythm	Durability limited to 10-15 yr Relatively stenotic
Mechanical valves (St. Jude)	Good flow characteristics in small sizes	Require anticoagulation
Homografts and autografts	Anticoagulation not required Durability increased over that of bioprostheses	Surgical implantation technically demanding

valve, about 60% of patients can have restored valve function after intravenous infusion of a thrombolytic agent. In patients with periprosthetic paravalvular leaks, a percutaneous procedure can successfully close about 85% of the leaks.

GENERAL REFERENCES

For the General References and other additional features, please visit Elsevier eBooks+ at https://ebooks.health.elsevier.com.

Grade A References

A1. Kang D-H, Park S-J, Lee S-A, et al. Early surgery or conservative care for asymptomatic aortic stenosis. *N Engl J Med.* 2020;382:111-119.

A2. Banovic M, Putnik S, Penicka M, et al. Aortic valve replacement versus conservative treatment in asymptomatic severe aortic stenosis: the AVATAR trial. *Circulation*. 2022;145:648-658.
A3. Lazkani M, Singh N, Howe C, et al. An updated meta-analysis of TAVR in patients at intermediate risk for SAVR. *Cardiovasc Revasc Med*. 2019;20:57-69.
A4. UK TAVI Trial Investigators; Toff WD, Hildick-Smith D, Kovac J, et al. Effect of transcatheter aortic valve implantation vs surgical aortic valve replacement on all-cause mortality in patients with aortic stenosis: a randomized clinical trial. *JAMA*. 2022;327:1875-1887.
A5. Leon MB, Mack MJ, Hahn RT, et al. Outcomes 2 years after transcatheter aortic valve replacement in patients at low surgical risk. *J Am Coll Cardiol*. 2021;77:1149-1161.
A6. Makkar RR, Thourani VH, Mack MJ, et al. Five-year outcomes of transcatheter or surgical aortic-valve replacement. *N Engl J Med*. 2020;382:799-809.
A7. Forrest JK, Deeb GM, Yakubov SJ, et al. 2-Year outcomes after transcatheter versus surgical aortic valve replacement in low-risk patients. *J Am Coll Cardiol*. 2022;79:882-896.
A8. Søndergaard L, Popma JJ, Reardon MJ, et al. Comparison of a complete percutaneous versus surgical approach to aortic valve replacement and revascularization in patients at intermediate surgical risk: results from the randomized SURTAVI trial. *Circulation*. 2019;140:1296-1305.
A9. Brouwer J, Nijenhuis VJ, Delewi R, et al. Aspirin with or without clopidogrel after transcatheter aortic-valve implantation. *N Engl J Med*. 2020;383:1447-1457.
A10. Feldman T, Kar S, Elmariah S, et al. Randomized comparison of percutaneous repair and surgery for mitral regurgitation: 5-year results of EVEREST II. *J Am Coll Cardiol*. 2015;66:2844-2854.
A11. Chan V, Mazer CD, Ali FM, et al. Randomized, controlled trial comparing mitral valve repair with leaflet resection versus leaflet preservation on functional mitral stenosis: the CAMRA CardioLink-2 study. *Circulation*. 2020;142:1342-1350.
A12. Kang D-H, Park S-J, Shin S-H, et al. Angiotensin receptor neprilysin inhibitor for functional mitral regurgitation. *Circulation*. 2019;139:1354-1365.
A13. Goldstein D, Moskowitz AJ, Gelijns AC, et al. Two-year outcomes of surgical treatment of severe ischemic mitral regurgitation. *N Engl J Med*. 2016;374:344-353.
A14. Virk SA, Tian DH, Sriravindrarajah A, et al. Mitral valve surgery and coronary artery bypass grafting for moderate-to-severe ischemic mitral regurgitation: meta-analysis of clinical and echocardiographic outcomes. *J Thorac Cardiovasc Surg*. 2017;154:127-136.
A15. Obadia JF, Messika-Zeitoun D, Leurent G, et al. Percutaneous repair or medical treatment for secondary mitral regurgitation. *N Engl J Med*. 2018;379:2297-2306.
A16. Michler RE, Smith PK, Parides MK, et al. Two-year outcomes of surgical treatment of moderate ischemic mitral regurgitation. *N Engl J Med*. 2016;374:1932-1941.
A17. Stone GW, Abraham WT, Lindenfeld J, et al. Five-year follow-up after transcatheter repair of secondary mitral regurgitation. *N Engl J Med*. 2023. [Epub ahead of print.]
A18. Gammie JS, Chu MWA, Falk V, et al. Concomitant tricuspid repair in patients with degenerative mitral regurgitation. *N Engl J Med*. 2022;386:327-339.
A19. Sorajja P, Whisenant B, Hamid N, et al. Transcatheter repair for patients with tricuspid regurgitation. *N Engl J Med*. 2023. [Epub ahead of print.]
A20. Cardoso JL, Ferraz Costa GN, Neves F, et al. Tricuspid repair in mitral regurgitation surgery: a systematic review and meta-analysis. *J Cardiothorac Surg*. 2023;18:76.
A21. Dangas GD, Tijssen JGP, Wöhrle J, et al. A controlled trial of rivaroxaban after transcatheter aortic-valve replacement. *N Engl J Med*. 2020;382:120-129.
A22. Guimarães HP, Lopes RD, de Barros e Silva PGM, et al. Rivaroxaban in patients with atrial fibrillation and a bioprosthetic mitral valve. *N Engl J Med*. 2020;383:2117-2126.

61 INFECTIVE ENDOCARDITIS

VANCE G. FOWLER, JR., ARNOLD S. BAYER, AND LARRY M. BADDOUR

DEFINITION

Infective endocarditis is defined as an infection, usually bacterial, of the endocardial surface of the heart. Infective endocarditis affects primarily the cardiac valves, although in some cases the septa between the chambers, the mural endocardium, or cardiovascular implantable electronic devices (e.g., pacemakers) may be involved. In the past, infective endocarditis was categorized as "acute" or "subacute," based on the duration of symptoms before presentation. However, these strict categories have proven to be unreliable, so clinical classification considers the causative organism, the involved valve, and the "pace" of clinical disease.

EPIDEMIOLOGY

The true incidence of infective endocarditis is difficult to determine because of the different criteria for diagnosis and methods of reporting. An analysis based on strict case definitions reveals that only a relatively small proportion (≈20%) of clinically diagnosed cases are categorized as "definite." In 10 large surveys, infective endocarditis accounted for approximately one case per 1000 U.S. hospital admissions, with a range of 0.16 to 5.4 cases per 1000 admissions. Estimates from the American Heart Association (AHA) place the incidence of infective endocarditis in the United States at 10,000 to 20,000 new cases per year. Recent data also suggest that rates of *Staphylococcus aureus* infective endocarditis have increased significantly, in part due to an increase in injection drug use (Chapter 365) as part of the current opioid epidemic, as well as the increasing use of implantable cardiac devices.[1]

Men are more commonly affected than women (mean male : female ratio, 1.7 : 1 in 18 large series). However, in patients younger than 35 years, more cases occur in women. More than 50% of patients with infective endocarditis in the United States are now older than 50 years of age, due in part to the low incidence of acute rheumatic heart disease (Chapter 269) and a simultaneous rise in the prevalence of degenerative valvular heart disease in the aging population.

Although some patients have no clearly definable risk factors for endocarditis, cardiac conditions that cause turbulent flow at the endocardial surface or across a valve (Chapter 60) predispose patients to infective endocarditis (Table 61-1). The most commonly affected valves in descending order of prevalence are the mitral valve only, the aortic valve only, the mitral and aortic valves together, the tricuspid valve, mixed right- and left-sided infection, and the pulmonic valve.

Historically, rheumatic heart disease with valvular dysfunction was the most common underlying condition, although its contribution has diminished in the antibiotic era, especially in developed countries. Degenerative valvular disease is also associated with infective endocarditis, particularly in elderly patients; the increasing relevance of senile calcification as a risk factor is reflected in the increasing proportion of aortic valve involvement in infective endocarditis (e.g., calcific aortic stenosis). Most significant congenital heart defects (Chapter 55) confer an increased risk of infective endocarditis, particularly complex cyanotic disease such as single-ventricle states, transposition of the great vessels, and tetralogy of Fallot. Similarly, surgically constructed pulmonary–systemic shunts and ventricular septal defects are risk factors associated with infective endocarditis.

Mitral valve prolapse is currently the most common underlying cardiac condition in patients with infective endocarditis, a statistic that reflects its prevalence in the general population (4%). Notably, mitral valve prolapse is a risk only in patients with thickened mitral leaflets or significant regurgitation, in which case the risk of endocarditis increases by about 10-fold over that of the general population. In addition, patients with hypertrophic cardiomyopathy are at increased risk of infective endocarditis, particularly in the presence of outflow obstruction. Finally, previous endocarditis is among the highest risk factors for subsequent infective endocarditis cases.

Prosthetic cardiac valves represent an important risk factor for infective endocarditis. More than 150,000 heart valves are implanted annually worldwide, and prosthetic valve infective endocarditis develops in 1 to 4% of prosthetic valve recipients in the first year after valve replacement and in approximately 0.8% of recipients annually thereafter. Mechanical prosthetic valves may initially be more susceptible to infective endocarditis, but bioprosthetic valves are more likely to develop infective endocarditis after 1 year; overall, the rate is similar with either type of valve. Bioprosthetic valve endocarditis can also involve transcatheter-placed aortic, mitral, or pulmonic valve prostheses.

The incidence of infective endocarditis in injection drug users (Chapter 365) may be 30 times higher than in the general population and four times higher than in adults with rheumatic heart disease.[2] In some areas of the United States, injection drug use is the most common predisposing cause of infective endocarditis in patients younger than 40 years. *S. aureus* is the predominant organism, and tricuspid valve involvement is noted in 78% of cases, mitral involvement in 24%, and aortic involvement in 8%. More than

TABLE 61-1 PREDISPOSING CONDITIONS ASSOCIATED WITH INCREASED RISK OF ENDOCARDITIS

MORE COMMON	LESS COMMON
Mitral valve prolapse (especially with regurgitation)	Rheumatic heart disease†
Degenerative valvular disease	Idiopathic hypertrophic subaortic stenosis
Injection drug use*	Pulmonary–systemic shunts*
Prosthetic valves*	Coarctation of the aorta
Congenital (valvular heart disease or ventricular [especially uncorrected] septal defect)	Complex cyanotic congenital heart disease*
Previous endocarditis*	

*Indicates conditions with highest risk for endocarditis.
†Still common in developing countries.

one valve is infected in approximately 20% of cases, and some of these infections are polymicrobial.

Health care–associated infective endocarditis arises primarily as a consequence of invasive therapies, including intravenous (IV) catheters, hyperalimentation lines, pacemakers, other cardiovascular implantable electronic devices,[3] and hemodialysis devices.[4] In a recent prospective, multinational cohort study of more than 1600 non–drug-using patients with native valve endocarditis, more than one third of patients had health care–associated endocarditis, many cases of which originated in the community (e.g., in patients on outpatient hemodialysis). The emerging importance of health care–associated infective endocarditis in industrialized nations has also influenced the microbiology of the disease, with an increasing prevalence of *S. aureus* and a decreasing prevalence of viridans group streptococci in much of the industrialized world.

Implantable cardiovascular electronic devices can become infected at the time they are implanted, particularly if patients develop local pocket site complications, such as a hematoma, at the incision site or need the device to be revised or replaced. Other factors that increase the risk of device infection include older age, comorbid conditions (particularly dialysis-dependent renal failure), and a larger number of device leads.

Systemic medical conditions can predispose patients to the development of infective endocarditis. For example, HIV infection is an independent risk factor for the development of infective endocarditis in injection drug users, with the risk increasing as the CD4 count decreases. Vascular catheter–related bacteremia is an important risk factor for nosocomial infective endocarditis. Patients with end-stage renal disease, particularly those receiving long-term hemodialysis, and patients with diabetes mellitus are also at increased risk, presumably because of the recurrent vascular access–site infections associated with the former and the low-level immunosuppression associated with both conditions.

PATHOBIOLOGY

Experimental models of infective endocarditis have demonstrated that the disease follows a predictable sequence: endocardial damage; aggregation of platelets, fibrin, and other coagulation molecules to create a "sterile vegetation" *(nonbacterial thrombotic endocarditis)*; transient bacteremia resulting in seeding of the vegetation; microbial proliferation on and invasion of the endocardial surface; and metastatic infection to organs receiving high blood flow (e.g., kidneys, spleen, and brain). Such sterile vegetations can occur either on previously damaged native valves or at the sewing ring following prosthetic valve placement. Nonbacterial thrombotic endocarditis may also occur spontaneously in patients with systemic illnesses (e.g., the marantic endocarditis of malignancy [Chapter 47] or other wasting diseases or the Libman-Sacks marantic endocarditis of systemic lupus erythematosus [Chapter 245]).

When transient bacteremia occurs—for example, as a result of distant infection or gingival manipulations—the previously sterile vegetation may be seeded. Some bacterial species, such as staphylococci and streptococci, are more avidly adherent to vegetations, better able to evade innate endovascular host defenses, and, as a result, more frequently cause endocarditis. The bacteria then proliferate within the vegetation and may ultimately achieve an organism load of 10^9 to 10^{11} colony-forming units per gram of tissue. Lastly, the surfaces of cardiac valves and vegetations are avascular, thereby making antibiotic therapy and healing difficult. Implantable cardiac devices disrupt the endothelial surface and predispose to infection and the formation of biofilms, particularly early after their placement and before endothelialization and fibrosis occur.

CLINICAL MANIFESTATIONS

History

The initial presentation of infective endocarditis varies enormously from patient to patient. Some cases develop acutely, with symptoms progressing rapidly over days. Other cases develop insidiously and present with progressive but nonspecific symptoms for weeks to months. In patients suspected of having infective endocarditis, the initial history should include a complete review of systems, a travel history, exposures to pets or other animals, illicit drug use, and sexual activity. Most patients complain of fever and nonspecific constitutional symptoms such as fatigue, malaise, or weight loss. Nearly 50% of patients complain of musculoskeletal symptoms ranging from frank arthritis to diffuse myalgias. In about 5 to 10% of patients, low back pain is the chief complaint, even in the absence of osteomyelitis or epidural abscess. In IV drug users with tricuspid valve infective endocarditis and patients with venous or right heart implantable devices, endocarditis can present as pleuritic chest pain and multilobar pneumonia. Health care–associated infective endocarditis is more likely to be clinically occult and requires a high index of suspicion.

Physical Examination

A thorough physical examination should include a search for the prototypic stigmata of endocarditis (Table 61-2), which are very helpful when present but are less frequent than in the past, now that patients are diagnosed and treated more expeditiously. Although fever is present in up to 90% of patients, it is less common in elderly patients and in patients with renal or heart failure. A widened pulse pressure should alert the clinician to the possibility of acute aortic insufficiency (Chapter 60). The skin and nails should be carefully examined for evidence suggestive of embolic phenomena, such as petechiae (Fig. 61-1), Osler nodes, Janeway lesions, and splinter hemorrhages. Petechiae are most often found on the conjunctiva, palate, and extremities. Osler nodes are small, painful nodules found most often on the palmar surfaces of the fingers and toes; they frequently wax and wane (Fig. 61-2). Classically considered to be an immunologic phenomenon, Osler nodes may have an immune complex–mediated component but are most likely initiated by microemboli. Janeway

TABLE 61-2 PHYSICAL EXAMINATION AND LABORATORY FINDINGS IN INFECTIVE ENDOCARDITIS

FINDING	% OF CASES
Fever	96
Worsening of previous murmur	20
New murmur	48
Vascular embolic event	17
Splenomegaly	11
Splinter hemorrhages	8
Osler nodes	3
Janeway lesions	5
Roth spots	2
Elevated ESR	61
Hematuria	26
Positive rheumatoid factor	5
Abnormal chest radiography findings (effusion, infiltrate, septic emboli)	67-85 (right-sided infective endocarditis)

ESR = erythrocyte sedimentation rate.
Adapted from Murdoch DR, Corey GR, Hoen B, et al. Clinical presentation, etiology, and outcome of infective endocarditis in the 21st century: International Collaboration on Endocarditis—Prospective Cohort Study. *Arch Intern Med.* 2009;169:463-473.

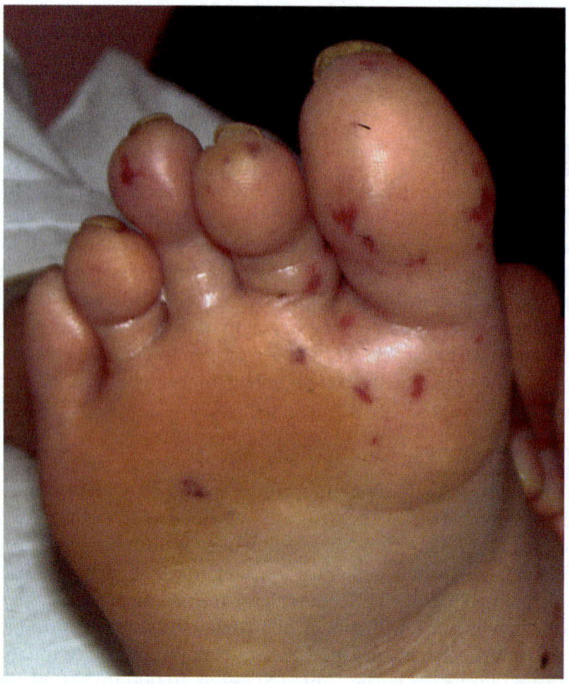

FIGURE 61-1. Petechiae in infective endocarditis.

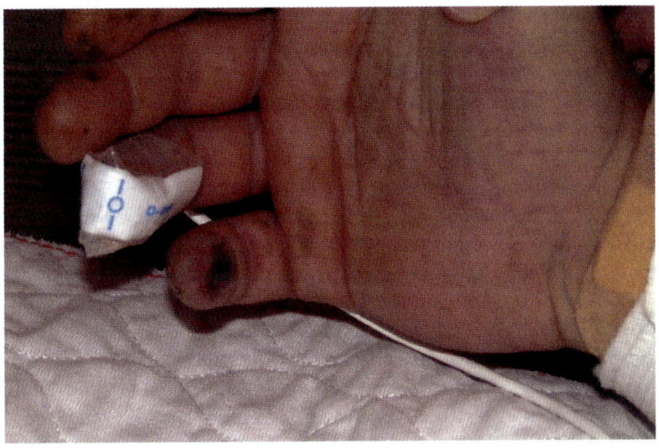

FIGURE 61-2. Osler node in infective endocarditis.

TABLE 61-3 MODIFIED DUKE CRITERIA FOR THE DIAGNOSIS OF INFECTIVE ENDOCARDITIS

MAJOR CRITERIA
1. Blood culture positive (a *OR* b)
a. Typical organism (α-hemolytic streptococcus, *Streptococcus gallolyticus*, HACEK organisms, or *Staphylococcus aureus*, or community-acquired *Enterococcus* species, without a primary focus) from two separate blood cultures *OR*
b. Persistent bacteremia with any organism (two positive cultures >12 hr apart or three positive cultures or a majority of ≥4 cultures positive >1 hr apart)
2. Evidence of endocardial involvement (a *OR* b)
a. Echocardiographic findings: mobile mass attached to valve or valve apparatus, abscess, or new partial dehiscence of prosthetic valve *OR*
b. New valvular regurgitation
3. Serology: single positive blood culture for *Coxiella burnetii* or anti–phase 1 *C. burnetii* IgG antibody titer ≥1 : 800
MINOR CRITERIA
1. Predisposing condition: IV drug use or predisposing cardiac condition
2. Fever ≥38° C
3. Vascular phenomena: arterial embolism, septic pulmonary emboli, mycotic aneurysm, intracranial hemorrhage, conjunctival hemorrhages, Janeway lesions
4. Immunologic phenomena: glomerulonephritis, Osler nodes, Roth spots, rheumatoid factor
5. Echocardiogram findings consistent with endocarditis but not meeting major criteria
6. Microbiologic evidence: positive blood cultures not meeting major criteria or serologic evidence of active infection consistent with endocarditis
DEFINITE INFECTIVE ENDOCARDITIS (1 *OR* 2)
1. Pathologically proven infective endocarditis *OR*
2. Clinical diagnosis defined by
a. Two major criteria *OR*
b. One major and three minor criteria *OR*
c. Five minor criteria
POSSIBLE INFECTIVE ENDOCARDITIS (1 *OR* 2)
1. One major criterion and one minor criterion *OR*
2. Three minor criteria
REJECTED INFECTIVE ENDOCARDITIS
1. Firm alternative diagnosis *OR*
2. Resolution of infective endocarditis syndrome with antibiotic therapy for ≤4 days *OR*
3. No pathologic evidence of infective endocarditis at surgery or autopsy with antibiotic therapy for ≤4 days *OR*
4. Does not meet criteria for possible infective endocarditis, as above

HACEK = *Haemophilus* spp, *Aggregatibacter* spp (formerly *Actinobacillus actinomycetemcomitans*), *Cardiobacterium hominis*, *Eikenella corrodens*, and *Kingella* spp; IgG = immunoglobulin G; IV = intravenous.

Adapted from Li JS, Sexton DJ, Mick N, et al. Proposed modifications to the Duke criteria for the diagnosis of infective endocarditis. *Clin Infect Dis*. 2000;30:633-638.

lesions (Fig. 39-10 in Chapter 39) are hemorrhagic, nonpainful macules also found primarily on the palms and soles; they are embolic in origin and are less frequently noted than the other cutaneous stigmata. Splinter hemorrhages (see Fig. 39-10 in Chapter 39) are nonblanching, linear, brownish red lesions in the nail beds parallel to the direction of nail growth; they are nonspecific and may also be found in a significant percentage of hospitalized patients without infective endocarditis.

Funduscopic examination should be performed to look for Roth spots (see Fig. 391-26 in Chapter 391), chorioretinitis, or endophthalmitis; the latter two are present in a substantial proportion of cases of fungal endocarditis (e.g., *Candida*). A careful cardiac examination (Chapter 39) should be performed to detect any murmurs, especially new-onset or worsening murmurs, as well as any evidence of heart failure, which is an ominous sign. Of note, patients with health care–associated infective endocarditis are less likely than others to have a pathologic murmur on initial presentation. The abdomen should be examined for evidence of splenomegaly (Chapter 154), which is more common in patients with subacute endocarditis. Finally, a thorough neurologic examination should be performed, both to assess for any focal neurologic deficits and to serve as a baseline during the patient's hospital stay. The neurologic examination may demonstrate evidence of major vessel embolism, cranial nerve palsies, visual field defects, or generalized toxic-metabolic encephalopathy with altered mental status. Up to 15 to 20% of patients with endocarditis initially have or develop a stroke or stroke-like symptoms (Chapter 375). Patients with device-related infective endocarditis often have local signs and symptoms of infection at the site of implantation.

DIAGNOSIS

The "gold standard" for the diagnosis of infective endocarditis is culture of a pathologic organism from a valve or other endocardial surface. However, unless the patient undergoes valve surgery or postmortem examination, the diagnosis is usually made clinically.[5] The most widely accepted clinical criteria are the modified Duke criteria (Table 61-3), which rely heavily on blood culture results and echocardiographic data and have an estimated 76 to 100% sensitivity and 88 to 100% specificity, with a negative predictive value of at least 92%.

Microbiology

When bacteremia is suspected,[6] at least three sets of blood cultures, each set consisting of one aerobic and one anaerobic bottle, should be obtained from separate sites, with careful attention to aseptic technique. Because some bacteria may not be eliminated by skin surface disinfection, the likelihood of a contaminant can be reduced by 50% if the blood culture is obtained after another tube of blood is collected with the same venipuncture.[A1] Starting antibiotics before blood cultures are drawn will reduce their sensitivity by about one third.[7] Ideally, blood cultures should be collected at least 1 hour apart to document continuous bacteremia, which is a characteristic of infective endocarditis and is not seen in many other infectious syndromes; however, when patients are critically ill, this approach, which requires that antimicrobial therapy be delayed, may not be feasible. In this latter circumstance, the three sets of blood cultures should be drawn without interim time delays.

Causative Organisms

About 90% of community-acquired, native valve infective endocarditis is caused by staphylococci, streptococci, or enterococci, which are normal inhabitants of the skin, oropharynx, urogenital, and gastrointestinal tracts, respectively. These organisms express specific receptors for attachment and adherence to damaged endothelial surfaces. Streptococcal species (Chapter 269) are the most common cause of community-acquired infective endocarditis in patients with no history of injection drug use or health care contact. In patients with either of these latter epidemiologic risk factors, *S. aureus* (Chapter 267) is the predominant cause of infective endocarditis. Because of the emergence of health care contact as the predominant risk factor for blood stream infections, *S. aureus* is now the most common cause of infective endocarditis in most industrialized regions of the world.

Viridans group streptococci (Chapter 269) are the most common streptococci implicated in native valve endocarditis. This group of organisms, which normally inhabit the oropharynx, includes species such as *Streptococcus sanguinis*, *Streptococcus mutans*, and *Streptococcus mitis/oralis*. Group B streptococci (β-hemolytic organisms that are normal oropharyngeal and urogenital flora, as well as skin flora in patients with diabetes) most frequently cause infective endocarditis in patients with cirrhosis or diabetes mellitus, as well as in injection drug users. In contrast, group A streptococci, although also β-hemolytic, rarely cause infective endocarditis. Among streptococcal species, the risk of developing endocarditis after blood stream infection is highest with *Streptococcus mutans*, *Streptococcus gordonii*, *Streptococcus sanguinis*, *Streptococcus gallolyticus* (previously known as *Streptococcus bovis*), and *Streptococcus mitis/oralis*, and it is lowest with *Streptococcus pneumoniae*.[8] *Streptococcus gallolyticus* is now a leading cause of infective endocarditis in some parts of the world; for example, its incidence in France has increased significantly in recent years. Its presence in blood cultures should prompt endoscopic evaluation for adenocarcinoma of the colon or other malignant lesions of the gastrointestinal tract.

S. aureus (Chapter 267) is the predominate pathogen among injection drug users and patients with health care contact. The clinical course of *S. aureus* endocarditis is typically acute, with a rapid progression over the course of days. Because about 10 to 15% of patients with *S. aureus* bacteremia have echocardiographic evidence of endocarditis even in the absence of classic stigmata, possible cardiac involvement should always be considered in any patient with *S. aureus* bacteremia but especially in patients with relapsing or persistent bacteremia or fever, community-acquired infection, or an implantable cardiac device. Coagulase-negative staphylococci are an uncommon cause of native valve endocarditis but are important pathogens in the setting of prosthetic valves or other intracardiac devices.

Enterococci are responsible for a significant number of cases of both community-acquired and nosocomial endocarditis, and the bulk (>90%) are due to *Enterococcus faecalis*. In most cases, the source of bacteremia is thought to be the genitourinary tract, and the presentation is usually subacute. Endocarditis, which develops in about 25% of patients with *E. faecalis* bacteremia, is suggested by community acquisition of infection, the absence of a clear source of infection, preexistent valvular heart disease, and the absence of polymicrobial bacteremia. As with *S. gallolyticus* endocarditis, gastrointestinal screening for colonic neoplasms is recommended.[9]

The HACEK group of gram-negative organisms (*Haemophilus* spp, *Aggregatibacter* spp [formerly *Actinobacillus actinomycetemcomitans*], *Cardiobacterium hominis, Eikenella corrodens,* and *Kingella* spp) accounts for about 5% of endocarditis cases. Because these fastidious organisms usually grow in blood cultures within 7 days using current methods, prolonged incubation is no longer required to isolate HACEK strains. Many other gram-negative bacilli can cause infective endocarditis but are even more unusual. Traditionally, injection drug use has been the primary risk factor for enteric aerobic gram-negative bacillary bacterial endocarditis. However, recent experience from large multinational studies shows that nosocomial health care contact, not injection drug use, is currently the most common risk factor for enteric gram-negative endocarditis.

Fungal endocarditis is often difficult to diagnose and treat; it is most commonly found in patients with a history of injection drug use, recent cardiac valve surgery, or prolonged use of indwelling vascular catheters, especially those used for total parenteral nutrition. The most common fungi found in infective endocarditis are *Aspergillus* and *Candida* spp. *Aspergillus* (Chapter 311) rarely grows in blood cultures and usually must be cultured from a pathologic specimen (either an embolic site or vegetation). Serodiagnostic strategies for antigen detection are often useful to diagnose *Aspergillus* endocarditis. By contrast, *Candida* spp (Chapter 310) frequently grow in blood cultures. Mortality is very high, and valve replacement surgery is usually necessary for fungal endocarditis.

Prosthetic valve endocarditis can be classified into one of two groups based on the time between valve surgery and disease onset: *early* (<2 months after surgery) and *late* (>2 months) (Table 61-4). Staphylococci, particularly *S. aureus,* predominate during the early postsurgery period, when most episodes of infective endocarditis are thought to be related to perioperative infection. In the late postsurgery period, the spectrum of organisms becomes more akin to that of community-acquired native valve endocarditis, in which *S. aureus* and viridans group streptococci predominate. Of note, among the coagulase-negative staphylococci, oxacillin resistance is frequently seen in these late cases. A transcatheter prosthetic valve placement (aortic, mitral, or pulmonic) procedure also can be complicated by endocarditis, with enterococci, *S. aureus,* and coagulase-negative staphylococci as the most common pathogens in the aortic valve position and *S. aureus* predominating in the pulmonic valve position.

Staphylococcal species account for the large majority (≥70%) of implantable cardiac device infections. The prevalence of oxacillin resistance among *S. aureus* strains varies but is generally in the 30 to 50% range; such resistance is even higher among coagulase-negative staphylococci.

TABLE 61-4 CAUSES OF PROSTHETIC VALVE ENDOCARDITIS*

EARLY (<2 mo POSTOPERATIVELY)	LATE (>2 mo POSTOPERATIVELY)
Staphylococcus aureus	Coagulase-negative staphylococci
Coagulase-negative staphylococci	*Staphylococcus aureus*
Gram-negative bacilli	Viridans group streptococci
Enterococci	Enterococci
Fungi	*Mycobacterium chimaera*†
Diphtheroids	

*Listed in order of relative frequency.

†May occur up to 4-5 years after valve replacement.

Adapted from Wang A, Athan E, Pappas PA, et al. Contemporary clinical profile and outcome of prosthetic valve endocarditis. *JAMA.* 2007; 297:1354-1361.

Endocarditis with Negative Blood Cultures

In most patients who have infective endocarditis and who have not received previous antibiotic therapy, every blood culture is positive. Blood cultures are truly negative in less than 5% of cases of endocarditis; however, prior antibiotic administration may decrease the yield of blood cultures by up to 35%. Accordingly, the large majority of "culture-negative" cases of endocarditis occur in patients who have recently received antimicrobial agents. These cases are probably caused by the same organisms responsible for most native valve endocarditis; viridans group streptococci and the HACEK organisms are the most "likely suspects" because they are much more fastidious than staphylococci and enterococci and are therefore more likely to be affected by previous antibiotic administration. Ultimately, however, when blood cultures are negative and endocarditis is suspected, especially when a history of recent antimicrobial treatment is lacking, consideration should be given to fastidious bacterial organisms, fungi, and noncultivatable organisms (Table 61-5), particularly when the patient's history suggests exposure to farm animals or unpasteurized milk (*Coxiella burnetii, Brucella* spp), cats (*Bartonella henselae*), body lice (*Bartonella quintana*), or pet birds (*Chlamydophila psittaci*). It is important to notify the microbiology laboratory that endocarditis is suspected because special culture techniques, including prolonged (>5 days) incubation of blood cultures, can occasionally increase the yield for nutritionally variant streptococci (*Abiotrophia* and *Granulicatella* spp), *Brucella* spp, *Legionella* spp, *Cutibacterium acnes,* and some fungi. Specific serologic tests can diagnose endocarditis related to *C. burnetii* (the agent of Q fever; Chapter 302), *Brucella* spp (Chapter 286), *Bartonella* spp (Chapter 291), and *C. psittaci* (Chapter 294). *Tropheryma whippelii,* the etiologic agent in Whipple disease (Chapter 305), and multiple other organisms may be diagnosed by broad-range polymerase chain reaction testing in plasma or especially on resected cardiac tissue.[10] Histopathologic features of resected tissue also can provide clues in the etiologic diagnosis of culture-negative endocarditis. If the search for a causative organism is fruitless, noninfectious causes such as marantic or Libman-Sacks endocarditis and atrial myxoma (Chapter 47) should be considered.

Laboratory Findings

Initial laboratory tests should include a complete blood count with differential, serum electrolytes, measurement of renal function, and urinalysis. Most patients with subacute infective endocarditis have the serum iron profile of "anemia of chronic disease" (Chapter 145). The peripheral white blood cell count is frequently elevated in acute infective endocarditis, particularly if *S. aureus* is the causative organism, but may not be elevated in more subacute forms. Microscopic hematuria is common, as is proteinuria.

Rheumatoid factor, which is an ancillary test that has been included in the modified Duke criteria as a "minor criterion" in the category of "immunologic phenomenon," may be positive in subacute or chronic endocarditis. Other ancillary tests, such as the erythrocyte sedimentation rate, the C-reactive protein level, and the procalcitonin level, are generally not helpful in establishing the diagnosis of endocarditis.

Imaging, Including Echocardiography

The chest radiograph is abnormal—demonstrating consolidation, atelectasis, pleural effusion, or clear septic emboli—in the overwhelming majority of patients with right-sided endocarditis. In others, it may show evidence of heart failure. The electrocardiogram (ECG) should be carefully examined for evidence of atrioventricular conduction blocks, especially a prolonged PR interval (see Figs. 51-4 through 51-9 in Chapter 51), suggestive of an aortic ring abscess or frank myocardial infarction (see Figs. 58-1 and 58-2 in Chapter 58).

Both transthoracic echocardiography and transesophageal echocardiography (Chapter 43) are highly specific tests for defining valvular vegetations (≈98%) when used as part of the diagnostic evaluation of suspected endocarditis. By contrast, transesophageal echocardiography has a much

TABLE 61-5 ORGANISMS CAUSING "CULTURE-NEGATIVE" ENDOCARDITIS*

ORGANISM	EPIDEMIOLOGY	DIAGNOSTIC TESTS
HACEK spp	Mostly oral flora, so often history of periodontal disease	May require up to 7 days to grow
Nutritionally variant streptococci	Slow and indolent course	Supplemented culture media or growth as satellite colonies around *Staphylococcus aureus* streak
Coxiella burnetii (Q fever)	Worldwide; exposure to raw milk, farm environment, or rural areas	Serologic tests (high titers of antibody to both phase 1 and phase 2 antigens); also PCR on blood or valve tissue
Brucella spp	Ingestion of contaminated milk or milk products; close contact with infected livestock	Bulky vegetations usually seen on echocardiography; blood cultures positive in 80% of cases with incubation time of 4-6 wk; lysis-centrifugation technique may expedite growth; serologic tests are available
Bartonella spp	*Bartonella henselae:* transmitted by cat scratch or bite or by cat fleas; *Bartonella quintana:* transmitted by human body louse; predisposing factors include homelessness and alcohol abuse	Serologic testing (may cross-react with *Chlamydophila psittaci*); PCR of valve or emboli is best test; lysis-centrifugation technique may be useful
Chlamydophila psittaci	Exposure to birds	Serologic tests available, but must exclude *Bartonella* spp because of cross-reactivity; monoclonal antibody direct stains on tissue may be useful; PCR now available
Tropheryma whippelii (Whipple disease)	Systemic symptoms include arthralgias, diarrhea, abdominal pain, lymphadenopathy, weight loss, CNS involvement; however, endocarditis may be present without systemic symptoms	Histologic examination of valve with PAS stain; valve cultures may be done using fibroblast cell lines; PCR on vegetation material
Legionella spp	Contaminated water distribution systems; often nosocomial outbreaks; usually prosthetic valves	Lysis-centrifugation technique; also periodic subcultures onto buffered charcoal yeast extract medium; serologic tests and PCR available
Aspergillus and other noncandidal fungi	Prosthetic valve	Lysis-centrifugation technique; also culture and direct examination of any emboli; serodiagnostic test for *Aspergillus* antigen
Mycobacterium chimaera	Following cardiac surgery with contaminated heater/cooler units used for cardiopulmonary bypass; often delayed months-years	PCR and mycobacterial cultures of blood and other sterile body sites

*Listed in approximate order of relative frequency.

CNS = central nervous system; HACEK = *Haemophilus* spp, *Aggregatibacter* spp, *Cardiobacterium hominis, Eikenella corrodens,* and *Kingella* spp; PAS = periodic acid–Schiff; PCR = polymerase chain reaction.

higher sensitivity (90 to 95%) in this setting than transthoracic echocardiography (48 to 63%). In most cases in which endocarditis is a serious diagnostic consideration, the evaluation should begin with initial transthoracic echocardiography followed by transesophageal echocardiography as soon as possible because both studies provide complementary information (Fig. 61-3). Because transesophageal echocardiography is a relatively noninvasive means of detecting perivalvular extension of infection, any patient with a new conduction system abnormality or persistent fever—clinical predictors of perivalvular extension—should be evaluated with it. Likewise, transesophageal echocardiography is strongly preferred in the evaluation of suspected prosthetic valve– or device–related endocarditis. Of note is that bland clots can occur on the leads of 5 to 10% of patients with intracardiac devices, and the finding of a "vegetation" on a lead is not specific for infection. The high sensitivity of transesophageal echocardiography in detecting valvular vegetations on native valves also may be used in combination with clinical parameters (e.g., prompt resolution of bacteremia and defervescence) to support the clinical decision to abbreviate therapy in patients with vascular catheter–associated *S. aureus* bacteremia. A vegetation greater than 10 mm is a significant predictor of an increased risk of peripheral embolization and mortality.[11]

A negative transesophageal echocardiography result has a negative predictive value of about 95%. Nevertheless, when clinical suspicion of endocarditis is high (e.g., persistent fever or embolic events) and the initial transesophageal echocardiography is negative, repeat transesophageal echocardiography in 3 to 5 days may reveal the diagnosis.

When echocardiographic results are negative or indeterminant, multislice computed tomography with or without angiography can be helpful in patients with possible prosthetic valve endocarditis or with a perivalvular extension of infection.[12] Positron emission tomography with computed tomography (PET/CT) scanning may be useful for identifying prosthetic valve endocarditis [13] and may sometimes identify a noncardiac primary source of infection, a metastatic site that requires a change in the therapeutic approach, or evidence of undiagnosed tumors. However, these tests should not be obtained routinely but rather should be reserved for difficult diagnostic situations.

The diagnosis of infective endocarditis complicating transcatheter aortic or pulmonic valve replacements can be difficult. Vegetations may not be detected with echocardiography, but leaflet thickening and an increased transvalvular gradient are often seen.

TREATMENT

Definitive antibiotic treatment of infective endocarditis (Table 61-6) is guided by antimicrobial susceptibility testing of the responsible pathogen isolated from clinical cultures.[14–16] Although it is often advisable to begin empiric treatment before definitive culture results are available, not all patients who are admitted because of possible endocarditis necessarily need to be treated empirically.[17] Patients who are clinically stable, with a subacute presentation syndrome and without evidence of heart failure or other end-organ complications, can be closely observed without antibiotics so that serial blood cultures can be obtained. Likewise, such stable patients who were started on empiric antibiotics before hospitalization and before blood was drawn for cultures can discontinue antibiotics so that blood cultures can be obtained, preferably as long as possible after stopping the antibiotics. A normal procalcitonin level does not exclude endocarditis, but procalcitonin-guided treatment may help reduce the duration of antibiotic treatment in patients with positive blood cultures.[A2] By contrast, acutely ill patients, patients with evidence of complications of endocarditis, and patients who are at high risk for endocarditis (e.g., prosthetic valve recipients)[18] should be treated empirically with antibiotics pending culture results. An infectious diseases specialist, as part of an multidisciplinary endocarditis team, is critical in guiding the diagnostic evaluation and designing an appropriate initial empiric (and subsequent definitive) antibiotic regimen. This consultation may guide molecular diagnostic testing by the hospital's microbiology laboratory or a reference laboratory to secure a specific etiologic diagnosis.

Empiric Therapy

Either of two regimens provides appropriate empirical coverage for patients with suspected native valve endocarditis when cultures have not revealed a specific organism: nafcillin (or oxacillin)–penicillin–gentamicin or vancomycin–gentamicin (Table 61-7). Some experts recommend a regimen of nafcillin–ceftriaxone–penicillin–gentamicin to cover for HACEK isolates that produce β-lactamase. If methicillin-resistant *S. aureus* (MRSA) is an important consideration, as in injection drug users and patients with health care contact, empirical therapy should consist of vancomycin–ceftriaxone–gentamicin. Patients with prosthetic valves should be empirically treated with vancomycin–gentamicin–rifampin for adequate coverage of the most important pathogens in this setting (MRSA, methicillin-sensitive staphylococci, and coagulase-negative staphylococci).

Treatment of Specific Organisms

When the organism is definitively identified, the antibiotic treatment must be narrowed accordingly, and validated regimens should be followed (see Table 61-6). Infectious disease consultation should be obtained in all cases of infective endocarditis as part of an "Endocarditis Team" approach, which has been shown to improve outcomes.

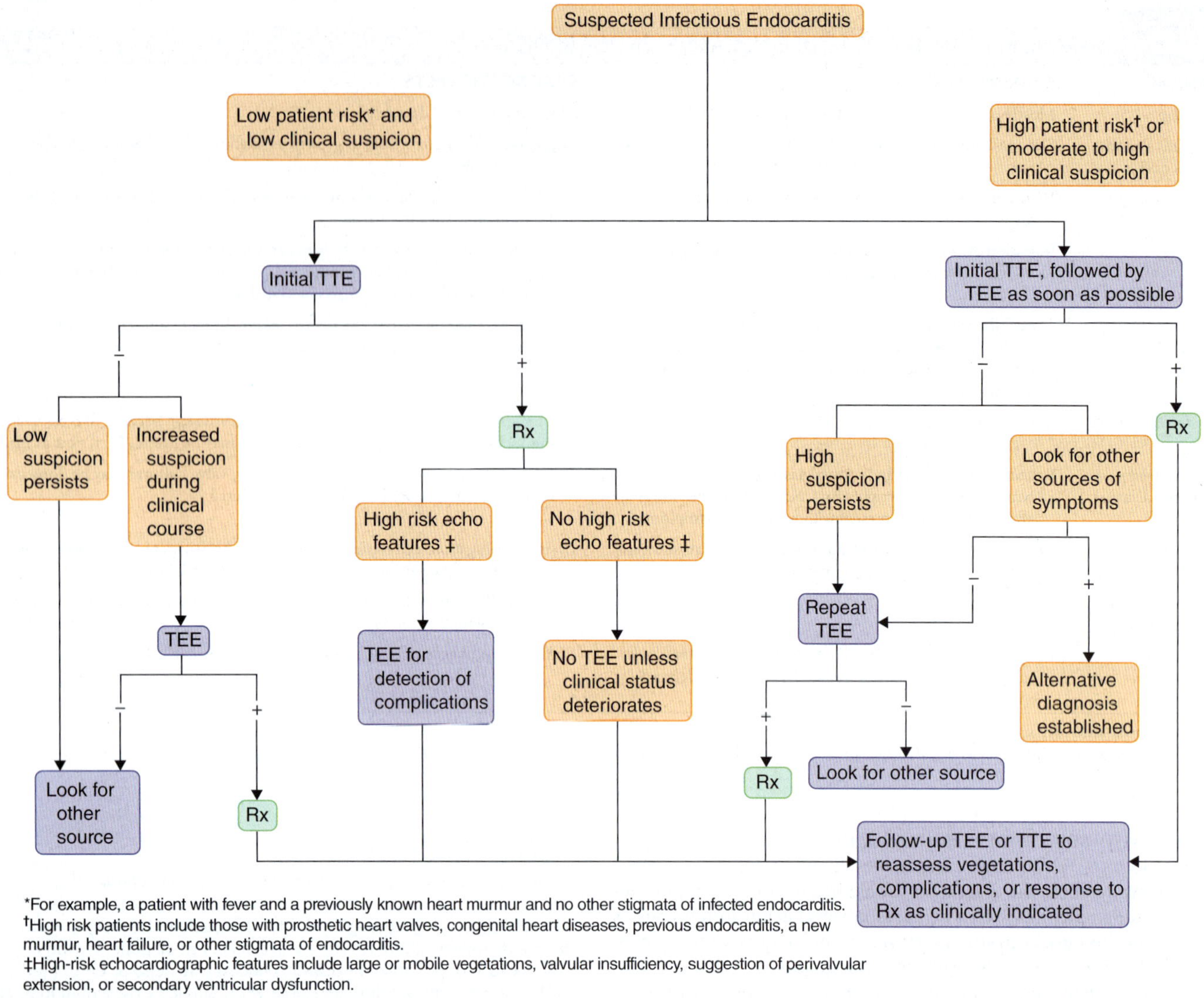

FIGURE 61-3. Approach to the diagnostic use of echocardiography (Echo). Rx = treatment, TEE = transesophageal echocardiography, TTE = transthoracic echocardiography. (Adapted from Baddour LM, Wilson WR, Bayer AS, et al. Infective endocarditis in adults: diagnosis, antimicrobial therapy, and management of complications: a scientific statement for healthcare professionals from the American Heart Association. *Circulation*. 2015;132:1435-1486.)

Many regimens recommend consideration of low-dose gentamicin to provide antibacterial synergy with a low risk of toxicity. However, aminoglycoside toxicity is a significant risk in elderly patients and in patients with preexisting renal disease or hearing impairment; even low-dose gentamicin increases the likelihood of a decrease in creatinine clearance by about three-fold. Among the organisms listed in Table 61-6, added gentamicin is critical for cure only in enterococcal endocarditis (when combined with penicillin). As a result of these risks and the minimal data supporting its benefit, initial low-dose gentamicin should not be routinely used.

In uncomplicated viridans group streptococcal endocarditis, outpatient therapy with once-daily ceftriaxone is as effective as more complex regimens, provided the patient has been observed in the hospital for the development of complications. The decision to administer antimicrobial therapy in the outpatient setting must, of course, take into account the patient's social situation, likelihood of compliance, and other risks involved with either an indwelling IV line or recurrent peripheral IV line placements.

Traditional therapy for infective endocarditis caused by fully susceptible enterococci includes penicillin or ampicillin plus gentamicin. Although gentamicin is preferred over streptomycin, the choice of a specific aminoglycoside should be based on in vitro susceptibility testing. Nonrandomized data suggest that the duration of aminoglycoside therapy can be limited to 2 to 3 weeks in combination with either penicillin, ampicillin, or vancomycin; an aminoglycoside can be avoided in favor of combination therapy with ampicillin plus high-dose (2 g IV every 12 hours) ceftriaxone in endocarditis that is due to *Enterococcus faecalis*. Optimal therapy for enterococci that are resistant to aminoglycosides or vancomycin is not well defined. Endocarditis caused by vancomycin-resistant enterococci may be treated with daptomycin, quinupristin–dalfopristin (7.5 mg/kg IV every 8 hours), or linezolid (600 mg orally or IV twice daily); however, clinical experience with these agents is limited. In this situation, relapse or failure rates are likely to be high, and many cases require surgical intervention (discussed later).

Semisynthetic penicillins, such as nafcillin, are advocated for endocarditis caused by methicillin-susceptible *S. aureus*. Cefazolin represents an alternative to semisynthetic penicillins in patients in whom the latter are not tolerated or feasible to administer. Although vancomycin is recommended in patients who are allergic to β-lactams, the microbiologic and clinical cure rates are less than those of β-lactam therapy. Because of this lower cure rate and the fact that over 90% of patients who report a history of penicillin allergy do not have it when skin tested, an allergy expert should be consulted. Daptomycin (6 mg/kg/day for 10 to 42 days, depending on the severity of infection) is as effective as either a semisynthetic antistaphylococcal penicillin or vancomycin for the treatment of *S. aureus* bacteremia and right-sided infective endocarditis caused by methicillin-susceptible *S. aureus* and MRSA; the combination of daptomycin plus fosfomycin may be slightly better than daptomycin alone.[A3] Non-randomized data suggest that higher-dose daptomycin regimens (8-10 mg/kg/d) are safe and may be superior for clearing bacteremia in *S. aureus* endocarditis. Ceftaroline, a fifth-generation cephalosporin, can be successful in patients with MRSA bacteremia and endocarditis, especially when combined with daptomycin.

Data suggest that after about 2 weeks of successful IV therapy, patients with stable left-sided endocarditis due to streptococcus, *Enterococcus faecalis*, *Staphylococcus aureus*, or coagulase-negative staphylococci have been safely switched from IV to oral antibiotics for the duration of their treatment,[A4] although experience with *S. aureus* endocarditis, especially MRSA, is relatively limited.

Rifampin or gentamicin can be added to either nafcillin or vancomycin for the treatment of prosthetic valve infection caused by methicillin-susceptible *S. aureus* or to MRSA, respectively. Gentamicin is administered for 2 weeks, and rifampin is given for the duration of either nafcillin or vancomycin therapy.

TABLE 61-6 DEFINITIVE THERAPY OF BACTERIAL ENDOCARDITIS

ORGANISM AND REGIMEN*	COMMENTS
PCN-SUSCEPTIBLE VIRIDANS STREPTOCOCCI (MIC ≤0.1 µg/mL) AND *STREPTOCOCCUS GALLOLYTICUS (formerly S. bovis)*	
1. Aqueous crystalline PCN G 2-3 million units IV q4h × 4 wk; 6 wk for prosthetic valve endocarditis	1. Also effective for other PCN-susceptible nonviridans streptococci
2. Ceftriaxone 2 g IV qd × 4 wk; 6 wk for prosthetic valve endocarditis	2. Useful in outpatient therapy and in patients with non-IgE-mediated PCN allergy
3. Aqueous crystalline PCN G 2-3 million units IV q4h × 2 wk plus gentamicin 3 mg/kg IV per 24 h in 1 dose × 2 wk	3. Uncomplicated infection with none of the following features: renal insufficiency, eighth cranial nerve deficit, prosthetic valve infection, CNS complications, severe heart failure, age >65 yr; also not acceptable for nutritionally variant streptococci; this option is not commonly used
4. Vancomycin 15-20 mg/kg IV q8-12h × 4 wk	4. For IgE-mediated PCN allergy; goal trough level of 15-20 mg/L
RELATIVELY PCN-RESISTANT VIRIDANS STREPTOCOCCI (MIC 0.12-<0.5 µg/mL)	
1. Aqueous crystalline PCN G 4 million units IV q4h × 4 wk plus gentamicin 3 mg/kg IV q24h × 2 wk	—
2. Vancomycin 15-20 mg/kg IV q8-12h × 4 wk	For IgE-mediated PCN allergy or to avoid gentamicin; goal trough level of 15-20 mg/L
ENTEROCOCCI[†] *ABIOTROPHIA*, AND *GRANULICATELLA* SPECIES, AND PCN-RESISTANT VIRIDANS STREPTOCOCCI (PCN MIC ≥0.5 µg/mL)	
1. Penicillin[‡] 18-30 million units IV per day in divided doses × 4-6 wk or ampicillin 12 g/24 hr IV in 6 equally divided plus gentamicin 3 mg/kg IV q24h × 4-6 wk	1. Increase duration of both drugs to 6 wk for prosthetic valve endocarditis or symptoms >3 mo in enterococcal infection
2. Vancomycin 15-20 mg/kg IV q8-12h × 6 wk plus gentamicin 1 mg/kg q8h × 6 wk[§]	2. For IgE-mediated PCN allergy; high risk of nephrotoxicity with this regimen
3. Ampicillin 12 g/24 h IV in 6 equally divided doses plus ceftriaxone 2 g IV q12h × 6 wk	3. An alternative to aminoglycoside-containing regimens in infective endocarditis due to *Enterococcus faecalis*, especially in patients with pre existing renal disease
STAPHYLOCOCCUS AUREUS	
1. Nafcillin 2 g IV q4h × 6 wk	1. Methicillin-susceptible strain; gentamicin discouraged for native valve endocarditis
2. Vancomycin 15-20 mg/kg IV q8-12h × 6 wk	2. PCN allergy (immediate hypersensitivity or anaphylaxis) or MRSA
3. Nafcillin 2 g IV q4h × 2 wk	3. Methicillin-susceptible strain; 2-wk regimen for use only in people who inject drugs and have uncomplicated tricuspid valve endocarditis
4. Nafcillin 2 g IV q4h × ≥6 wk plus gentamicin 1 mg/kg IV q8h × 2 wk plus rifampin 300 mg PO/IV q8h × ≥6 wk	4. Prosthetic valve endocarditis with methicillin-susceptible strain; use vancomycin instead of nafcillin for MRSA
5. Cefazolin 2 g IV q8h × 4-6 wk	5. Non-IgE-mediated PCN allergy
6. Daptomycin 6 mg/kg IV qd × 14-42 days	6. Daptomycin is FDA-approved for treatment of right-sided *S. aureus* infective endocarditis; for adults; some experts recommend up to 10 mg/kg IV qd
COAGULASE-NEGATIVE STAPHYLOCOCCI, PROSTHETIC VALVE INFECTION	
Vancomycin 15-20 mg/kg IV q8-12h × ≥6 wk plus gentamicin 1 mg/kg IV q8h × 2 wk plus rifampin 300 mg PO/IV q8h × ≥6 wk	Can substitute nafcillin in above listed doses for vancomycin if isolate is sensitive to methicillin
HACEK STRAINS	
1. Ceftriaxone 2 g IV qd × 4 wk; 6 wk for prosthetic valve endocarditis	This regimen is used in most patients
2. Ampicillin–sulbactam 3 g IV q6h × 4 wk; 6 wk for prosthetic valves	HACEK strains increasingly may produce β-lactamase
NON-HACEK GRAM-NEGATIVE BACILLI	
Enterobacteriaceae	
Extended-spectrum PCN or cephalosporin plus aminoglycosides for susceptible strains	Treat for a minimum of 6-8 wk; some species exhibit inducible resistance to third-generation cephalosporins; valve surgery is required for most patients with left-sided endocarditis caused by gram-negative bacilli
Pseudomonas aeruginosa	
High-dose tobramycin (8 mg/kg/day IV or IM in once-daily doses) with maintenance of peak and trough concentrations of 15 to 20 µg/mL and ≤2 µg/mL, respectively, in combination with an extended-spectrum PCN (e.g., ticarcillin, piperacillin, azlocillin); ceftazidime, cefepime, or imipenem in full doses; or imipenem	Treat for a minimum of 6-8 wk; early valve surgery usually required for left-sided *Pseudomonas* endocarditis
Fungi	
Treatment with a parenteral antifungal agent (usually a lipid-containing amphotericin B product, 3-5 mg/kg/day IV for at least 6 weeks) with or without flucytosine (25 mg/kg PO four times daily in patients with normal renal function) in patients with *Candida* infections; fluconazole, 400 mg daily PO is an alternative for susceptible yeasts; other azoles, such as voriconazole, may be required for resistant yeasts or molds	Combined with valve replacement and subsequent lifelong suppressive therapy with oral antifungal agents; for patients who are not candidates for surgery, lifelong oral suppressive therapy should follow completion of initial IV therapy.

[‡]Ampicillin 12 g/day can be used instead of PCN.

[§]The need to add an aminoglycoside has not been demonstrated for PCN-resistant streptococci.

*Dosages are for patients with normal renal function; for those with renal insufficiency, adjustments must be made for all drugs except nafcillin, rifampin, and ceftriaxone. Gentamicin doses should be adjusted to achieve a peak serum concentration of approximately 3 µg/mL 30 min after dosing and a trough gentamicin level of <1 µg/mL.

[†]Enterococci must be tested for antimicrobial susceptibility. These recommendations are for enterococci sensitive to PCN, gentamicin, and vancomycin.

HACEK = *Haemophilus* spp, *Aggregatibacter* spp (formerly *Actinobacillus actinomycetemcomitans*), *Cardiobacterium hominis, Eikenella corrodens*, and *Kingella* spp; ID = infectious diseases; IM = intramuscular; IV = intravenous; MIC = minimum inhibitory concentration; MRSA = methicillin-resistant *Staphylococcus aureus;* PCN = penicillin; PO = oral; q = every; qd = every day.

Consultation with an infectious diseases specialist is recommended in all cases of infective endocarditis.

Adapted from Baddour LM, Wilson WR, Bayer AS, et al. Infective endocarditis in adults. *Circulation.* 2015;132:1435-1486.

TABLE 61-7 EMPIRICAL TREATMENT OF ENDOCARDITIS

CHARACTERISTICS OF PATIENTS	TREATMENT REGIMEN*
Native valve, community-acquired infection, MRSA unlikely	Nafcillin 2 g IV q4h plus penicillin 4 million units IV q4h plus gentamicin 1 mg/kg IV q8h
Any of the following: health care–associated infection or other reason to suspect MRSA; severe penicillin allergy	Vancomycin 15-20 mg/kg IV q8-12h† plus gentamicin 1 mg/kg IV q8h
Prosthetic valve	Vancomycin 15-20 mg/kg IV q8-12h† plus gentamicin 1 mg/kg IV q8h plus rifampin 300 mg PO/IV q8h

*Dosages are for patients with normal renal function; for those with renal insufficiency, adjustments must be made for all drugs except nafcillin.
†Goal is trough level of 15-20 mg/L.
IV = intravenous; MRSA = methicillin-resistant *Staphylococcus aureus;* PO = oral; q = every.

Rifampin is never used as monotherapy because of the rapid development of resistance.

Fungal endocarditis is usually a consequence of extensive health care contact. Traditionally, fungal endocarditis was regarded as a primary indication for valvular surgery, and intravenous amphotericin B was considered the adjunctive treatment of choice (Chapter 307). However, selected patients with *Candida* endocarditis have been successfully treated medically (with azole-containing antimicrobial agents, with or without amphotericin B), particularly patients who have been deemed not to be surgical candidates. Importantly, the management of fungal endocarditis should always involve the collaboration of an experienced infectious diseases specialist.

Zoonotic endocarditis is usually culture-negative and most commonly caused by *Bartonella* spp (Chapter 291), *C. burnetii* (Chapter 302), or *Brucella* spp (Chapter 286). The treatments of choice for these fastidious pathogens are based on limited data, but documented *Bartonella* endocarditis is treated with doxycycline for 6 weeks plus gentamicin for the first 2 weeks.

In cases of presumed culture-negative endocarditis in which unusual organisms (see Table 61-5) and other infections have been reasonably excluded, an empirical course of treatment may be undertaken. The choice of antimicrobial therapy should be influenced by the specifics of the patient's presentation, and an infectious diseases consultation is recommended.

Continuing Care of the Patient with Endocarditis

In addition to antibiotics, appropriate inpatient care includes attention to other chronic medical issues. For endocarditis in people who inject drugs, early inpatient consultation with an addiction medicine specialist is strongly advised to optimize adherence to completion of antimicrobial therapy as well as to implement strategies to mitigate subsequent drug use and reduce harm in this high-risk population that is at risk of a variety of serious infectious diseases, including recurrent endocarditis (Chapter 365).[19,20]

Regular surveillance should assess the potential development of complications. A careful cardiac examination should be performed on a daily basis to assess for new regurgitant murmurs. Widening of the pulse pressure should alert the clinician to the possible development of acute aortic insufficiency (Chapter 60). New conduction delays on the ECG suggest a possible myocardial abscess.

Repeat echocardiography is recommended during therapy for patients with persistent fever, recurrent embolic events, a new murmur, widening of the pulse pressure, or signs or symptoms of heart failure. Repeat echocardiography is also recommended to look for periannular complications in prosthetic valve endocarditis. Although end-of-therapy echocardiography is not routinely recommended if patients respond adequately to antimicrobial therapy, serial echocardiography is usually suggested over the ensuing years to screen for long-term valvular dysfunction.

Routine serial ECGs are not recommended. ECG-documented conduction abnormalities are a late sign of perivalvular infections in patients with endocarditis; transesophageal echocardiography (TEE) is the screening method of choice if this complication is suspected.

Any new neurologic findings should prompt a search for evidence of central nervous system (CNS) complications such as embolic events, cerebral hemorrhage, mycotic aneurysm, or brain abscess. Renal function should be closely monitored so that antibiotic doses can be adjusted if necessary. If gentamicin is used for more than a few days, the patient should be alerted to watch for the signs and symptoms of vestibular or ototoxicity. Audiometric testing at baseline and periodically thereafter should be considered in patients at high risk for aminoglycoside-induced ototoxicity, including elderly patients, patients with preexisting renal dysfunction or hearing damage, patients receiving prolonged courses of gentamicin, and patients who also receive other potentially nephrotoxic agents. Serum gentamicin trough concentrations should also be assayed at regular intervals (e.g., twice weekly and more often if renal function is changing) and should be targeted for 1 to 3 μg/mL or less; higher concentrations should prompt either lower or less frequent dosing or both.

Serial blood cultures, especially early in the treatment course, are indicated in patients whose infective endocarditis is caused by virulent organisms that commonly fail first-line treatment, such as *S. aureus* or aerobic gram-negative bacilli. Positive follow-up blood cultures in this setting might suggest the need to change therapy, search for metastatic abscesses, or repeat echocardiography. Infectious disease consultation is highly recommended in this scenario.

Patients with infective endocarditis may continue to be febrile for some time after the institution of appropriate antibiotic treatment. About 50% of patients defervesce within 3 days of starting antibiotics, 75% by 1 week, and 90% by 2 weeks. Patients whose endocarditis is caused by *S. aureus*, aerobic gram-negative organisms, or fungi tend to defervesce more slowly than patients infected with other organisms. Prolonged fever (>1 week after the institution of appropriate antibiotics) should prompt repeat blood cultures. If such cultures are negative, several possibilities should be considered: myocardial abscess, extracardiac infection (e.g., mycotic aneurysm, psoas or splenic abscess, vertebral osteomyelitis, septic arthritis), immune complex–mediated tissue damage, or a complication of hospitalization and therapy (e.g., drug fever, nosocomial superinfection, pulmonary embolism). Appropriate studies might include TEE, CT scan of the abdomen, bone scan, and urinalysis with microscopy (to elicit evidence of interstitial nephritis). IV line sites should be carefully examined for evidence of infection, and indwelling central lines should be changed according to published guidelines.

Anticoagulation in individuals with infective endocarditis is controversial. Although new anticoagulation in the setting of native valve endocarditis does not appear to provide a benefit, continuing ongoing anticoagulation may be advisable. Some authorities recommend continuing anticoagulation in patients with mechanical prosthetic valve endocarditis. However, discontinuation of all anticoagulation for at least the first 2 weeks of antibiotic therapy is generally advised in patients who have *S. aureus* prosthetic valve endocarditis and who have experienced a recent CNS embolic event. This approach allows any CNS thrombus to organize and potentially prevents the acute hemorrhagic transformation of such embolic lesions. Reintroduction of anticoagulation in these patients must be cautious, and the international normalized ratio must be monitored carefully. The best option for patients with other indications for anticoagulation, such as deep vein thrombosis, major vessel embolization, or atrial fibrillation, is less clear and should be decided in a multidisciplinary fashion that balances the risks and benefits for each individual patient.

Initiation of high-dose (325 mg/day) aspirin in patients with infective endocarditis does not prevent subsequent embolic events and tends to increase the incidence of bleeding. Whether patients should remain on chronic, low-dose (81 mg) prophylactic aspirin if they develop subsequent infective endocarditis is uncertain, although nonrandomized data suggest such an approach is safe and may even reduce the risk of embolization from the infected valve.

Complications

The complications of infective endocarditis can be divided into four groups for ease of classification: direct valvular damage and consequences of local microbial invasion, embolic complications, metastatic infections from bacteremia, and immunologic phenomena. Local damage to the endocardium or myocardium may directly erode through the involved cardiac valve or adjacent myocardial wall, resulting in hemodynamically significant valvular perforations or intracardiac or extracardiac fistulae. Such local complications typically present clinically with the acute onset of heart failure and carry a poor prognosis, even with prompt cardiac surgery. Valve ring abscesses also require surgical intervention and are more frequent in patients with prosthetic valves. Although a conduction defect on ECG may suggest the diagnosis, TEE is the diagnostic technique of choice for detecting paravalvular abscess, valve perforation, or intracardiac fistulae. Frank myocardial abscesses are found in up to 20% of cases on autopsy, and *Aspergillus* endocarditis invades the myocardium in more than 50% of cases. Purulent pericarditis is rare and is usually associated with a concomitant myocardial abscess. Myocardial infarction (MI), thought to be caused by embolism of vegetative material into the coronary arteries, is seen in 40 to 60% of cases on autopsy, although most cases are clinically silent and lack characteristic ECG changes. However, up to 15% of elderly patients may present with clinical evidence of acute MI, with potentially disastrous complications if the MI is thought to be the primary event and the patient is given thrombolytic therapy. Heart failure is the leading cause of death in infective endocarditis, usually related to direct valvular damage.

About 35% of patients have at least one clinically evident embolic event. In fungal endocarditis, the majority of patients have at least one embolic event, frequently with a large embolus. The presence of large (>10 mm), mobile vegetations on the echocardiogram, particularly when the anterior mitral valve leaflet is involved, predicts a high risk of embolic complications. Systemic emboli most commonly lodge in the kidneys, spleen, large peripheral blood vessels, or especially in the CNS. Vegetations in right-sided endocarditis usually embolize to the lungs and cause abnormalities on the chest radiograph, although occasionally such emboli reach the left-sided circulation via a patent foramen ovale.

Renal abscesses are rare in infective endocarditis; however, bland renal infarction is a frequent, asymptomatic finding on abdominal CT scanning (about 50%

of cases at autopsy). Similarly, splenic infarction occurs in up to 44% of autopsy-confirmed cases. Such emboli may be asymptomatic but also can cause left upper quadrant pain radiating to the left shoulder, sometimes as the presenting symptom of infective endocarditis. A splenic infarction that progresses to form an abscess can cause persistent fever or bacteremia, so such patients should undergo abdominal CT to search for this complication.

Mycotic vascular aneurysms, which frequently occur at bifurcation points, are found in about 10 to 15% of cases at autopsy but may be clinically silent until they rupture (which may be months to years after apparently successful antibiotic treatment of infective endocarditis). Whereas peripheral mycotic aneurysms require surgical resection, intracerebral aneurysms can be resected or managed with intravascular techniques (e.g., coils) if they bleed, increase in size, and/or cause a mass effect (Chapter 377). For mycotic aneurysms of the abdominal aorta, endovascular repair may be preferable, but long-term antibiotics are generally recommended.

Many patients may have evidence of cerebrovascular emboli, which have a predilection for the middle cerebral artery distribution. Most emboli to the CNS occur early in the course of the disease, and are evident at the time of presentation or shortly thereafter. Embolic strokes may undergo hemorrhagic transformation, with a sudden worsening of the patient's neurologic status. Many patients with fungal endocarditis present with an embolic stroke or large emboli that occlude major vessels.

Some complications of infective endocarditis result when bacteremic seeding causes metastatic infection at a distant site. Patients may present with or develop osteomyelitis, septic arthritis, or epidural abscess. Purulent meningitis (Chapter 381) is a rare complication except in pneumococcal endocarditis, although many patients with *S. aureus* infective endocarditis who undergo lumbar puncture have a pleocytosis, without frank meningitis. Importantly, the finding of one metastatic complication of infective endocarditis does not exclude the possibility of additional sites of hematogenous infection, particularly in *S. aureus* endocarditis. Thus, the need for additional diagnostic evaluations should be guided by the patient's clinical course.

Immunologic phenomena complicating infective endocarditis are often directly related to high levels of circulating immune complexes. Renal biopsy results are usually abnormal in the setting of active infective endocarditis, especially in patients with renal impairment and abnormal urinalyses. Endocarditis classically causes a hypocomplementemia-related glomerulonephritis (Chapter 107). Histopathologically, the glomerular changes may be focal, diffuse, or membranoproliferative, or they may be akin to the immune complex disease found in systemic lupus erythematosus. In addition, many of the musculoskeletal conditions associated with infective endocarditis, including monoarticular and oligoarticular arthritides, are probably mediated by immune complexes. These immunologic phenomena usually abate with successful antimicrobial therapy.

Surgery

Some patients with infective endocarditis require surgical treatment, either to cure the infection or to address its complications (Table 61-8).[21] Most patients with evidence of direct extension of infection to myocardial structures, prosthetic valve dysfunction, or heart failure from endocarditis-induced valvular damage should undergo surgery. In addition, many cases of endocarditis caused by fungi, aerobic gram-negative bacilli, or multidrug-resistant organisms (e.g., vancomycin- or gentamicin-resistant enterococci) require surgical management. Progression of disease or persistence of fever and bacteremia for more than 7 to 10 days in the presence of appropriate antibiotic therapy also may indicate the need for valve surgery, although a thorough search must first be conducted to exclude other primary or metastatic foci of infection. In a randomized trial of patients with left-sided infective endocarditis, severe valve disease, and large vegetations (>10 mm), early valve surgery did not significantly reduce all-cause mortality at 6 months, but it markedly decreased the risk of systemic embolism, including stroke and MI. Surgical management also should be considered for patients who have recurrent (two or more) embolic events on appropriate antibiotic therapy and sometimes in patients who have large vegetations (>10 mm) on echocardiography plus one embolic event. The presence of *S. aureus* endocarditis involving the anterior mitral valve leaflet and large vegetations (>10 mm) may be a special circumstance calling for early surgical intervention to reduce the high risk of CNS emboli, especially when mitral valve repair, rather than valve replacement, can be accomplished. Unfortunately, only about 15 to 20% of these latter patients are judged to be candidates for valve repair at the time of valve surgery.

After 7 days of preoperative antibiotics, the risk of infection on a newly implanted valve is low.[22] Delaying surgery in patients with deteriorating cardiac function in an attempt to sterilize the affected valve is ill advised because the risk of progressive heart failure or further complications usually outweighs the relatively small risk of recurrent infective endocarditis after prosthetic valve implantation. Relative contraindications to valve replacement include recent large CNS emboli (>2 cm) or bleed (because of the risk of CNS bleeding in the perioperative period, when systemic anticoagulation is required), multiple prior valve replacements (because of the difficulty of sewing a new valve into tissue already weakened from previous surgeries), and ongoing injection drug use. On occasion, patients have both a compelling indication for valve replacement (e.g., acute heart failure) and a recent CNS embolic event. The risk of hemorrhagic transformation of such lesions during cardiac bypass–associated anticoagulation is controversial, but the greatest risk of such transformation is with larger (>2 cm) emboli, especially those that have exhibited a hemorrhagic component. In these latter scenarios, it is prudent to try to delay surgery for at least 2 to 4 weeks to allow organization and resolution of such emboli. However, there appears to be no survival benefit in delaying indicated valve replacement surgery (>7 days) after an ischemic stroke, especially in patients who have smaller CNS lesions.

After definitive surgical treatment, most patients should receive further antibiotic therapy unless a full course of antibiotics was administered before surgery and there is no evidence of ongoing infection. If the patient received antibiotics for less than 1 week before surgery or the culture from the operative site is positive, the patient should receive the equivalent of a full initial course of antibiotics appropriate for the organism. If the patient received antibiotics for 2 weeks or more and the culture result from the operative site is negative (regardless of whether valve histopathology shows inflammation or a positive Gram stain result), the patient should receive whatever remains of the originally planned course of appropriate antibiotic therapy.

In patients with infective endocarditis related to implanted cardiovascular devices, complete device removal is usually mandatory, regardless of the pathogen, if the goal is to cure the infection.[23] In patients who truly cannot tolerate device removal, chronic antibiotic therapy, sometimes delivered regionally in situ,[24] is the best alternative. If a replacement device needs to be implanted, the optimal timing for such a procedure is unclear. However, blood culture results should be negative, and any concomitant local or pocket site infection should be completely resolved.

The duration of antimicrobial therapy after device extraction depends on the device and the infection. For lead-related infective endocarditis, which is usually

TABLE 61-8 INDICATIONS FOR VALVE SURGERY IN ENDOCARDITIS

INDICATION	CLASS*
NATIVE VALVE ENDOCARDITIS	
Acute aortic insufficiency or mitral regurgitation with heart failure	I
Acute aortic insufficiency with tachycardia and pre-closure of the mitral valve on echocardiogram	I
Fungal endocarditis	I
Evidence of annular or aortic abscess, sinus or aortic true or false aneurysm, valvular dehiscence, rupture, perforation, or fistula	I
Evidence of valve dysfunction and persistent infection after a prolonged period (7-10 days) of appropriate therapy, provided there are no noncardiac causes of infection	I
Recurrent emboli after appropriate antibiotic therapy	I
Infection with enteric gram-negative organisms or organisms with a poor response to antibiotics in patients with evidence of valve dysfunction	I
Anterior mitral leaflet vegetation (especially with size >10 mm) or persistent vegetation after systemic embolization	IIa
Increase in vegetation size despite appropriate antimicrobial therapy	IIb
Early infections of the mitral valve that probably can be repaired, especially in the presence of large vegetations and/or recurrent emboli	III
Persistent fever and leukocytosis with negative blood cultures	III
PROSTHETIC VALVE ENDOCARDITIS	
Early prosthetic valve endocarditis (<2 mo after surgery)	I
Heart failure with prosthetic valve dysfunction	I
Nonstreptococcal/non-HACEK endocarditis	I
Evidence of perivalvular leak, annular or aortic abscess, sinus or aortic true or false aneurysm, fistula formation, or new-onset conduction disturbances	I
Persistent bacteremia after 7-10 days of appropriate antibiotic therapy, with noncardiac causes for bacteremia excluded	IIa
Recurrent peripheral embolus despite therapy	IIa

*Class I = conditions for which there is evidence or general agreement that a given procedure or treatment is useful and effective; class II = conditions for which there is conflicting evidence or a divergence of opinion about the usefulness or efficacy of a procedure or treatment; class IIa = weight of evidence or opinion is in favor of usefulness or efficacy; class IIb = usefulness or efficacy is less well established by evidence or opinion; class III = conditions for which there is evidence or general agreement that the procedure or treatment is not useful and in some cases may be harmful.

HACEK = *Haemophilus, Aggregatibacter, Cardiobacterium, Eikenella,* and *Kingella* spp.

Adapted from Otto CM, Nishimura RA, Bonow RO, et al. 2020 ACC/AHA guideline for the management of patients with valvular heart disease: a report of the American College of Cardiology/American Heart Association Joint Committee on Clinical Practice Guidelines. *Circulation.* 2021;143:e72-e227.

associated with blood stream infection, 2 weeks of therapy is recommended if there are no infection complications. For infection caused by *S. aureus*, therapy should be extended for up to 4 weeks.

Nearly 40% of patients with infective endocarditis related to implantable cardiovascular electronic devices have concomitant valve involvement, predominantly tricuspid valve infection, with in-hospital and 1-year mortality rates of 15% and 23%, respectively. Removal of the device appears to reduce the mortality rate by about 50% (from about 40% to about 20%). In such patients, 4 to 6 weeks of concomitant antibiotic therapy is recommended after complete removal of the device.

PREVENTION

No randomized clinical trials have addressed whether dental procedures predispose to infective endocarditis and whether antibiotic prophylaxis prevents it. However, data support a temporal association between invasive dental procedures and the subsequent development of infective endocarditis in high-risk patients,[25] and antibiotic prophylaxis is associated with reduced incidence of endocarditis following these procedures.[26] Based on these observational data, antibiotic prophylaxis is recommended by the American Heart Association (Table 61-9) when patients with the highest risk of endocarditis-related adverse outcomes undergo dental procedures that involve manipulation of the gingival tissue, the periapical region of teeth, or perforation of the oral mucosa.[27] Antibiotic prophylaxis is also recommended when high-risk patients undergo an invasive procedure of the respiratory tract, with incision or biopsy of the respiratory mucosa, such as tonsillectomy and adenoidectomy; or invasive procedures involving infected skin, skin structures, or musculoskeletal tissue (Table 61-10). Other consensus guidelines have also narrowed the indications for antibiotic prophylaxis with dental procedures. For example, guidelines from the European Society of Cardiology are largely consistent with American Heart Association guidelines. In contrast, guidelines in the United Kingdom state that no prophylaxis is routinely advised for any dental patient, regardless of underlying cardiac valvular conditions, while still giving dentists the latitude to prescribe antibiotic prophylaxis for selected patients. Since the recent publications of these more limited recommendations, follow-up surveys in these countries have generated mixed results without definitive evidence of cause-and-effect between reduction in the use of dental prophylaxis and any increased incidence of endocarditis due to viridans group streptococci.[28]

Amoxicillin is the usual first choice for prophylaxis of infective endocarditis in patients undergoing invasive dental procedures, but other options are likely equally given (Table 61-11). More than 90% of patients labeled as being "penicillin allergic" are not truly allergic by skin testing. If such patients require ongoing antibiotic prophylaxis, allergy evaluation (Chapter 234) is warranted so that appropriate patients can be "de-labeled" and receive amoxicillin in the future.

Patients with implanted electronic cardiovascular devices do not require antibiotic prophylaxis for dental or other invasive procedures, but such patients do require surgical site prophylaxis at the time of device placement. The recommended regimens for this latter scenario generally include a β-lactam (commonly cefazolin, 2 g IV 1 hour before device placement), regardless of whether a new device is being placed or a device is being revised. More aggressive prophylaxis with vancomycin, intraprocedural bacitracin pocket wash, and 2 days of postprocedural oral cephalexin does not significantly reduce infection rates.[A5] However, one randomized trial showed that use of an absorbable antibiotic-eluting envelope at the time

TABLE 61-9 UNDERLYING CONDITIONS FOR WHICH ANTIBIOTIC PROPHYLAXIS IS AND IS NOT SUGGESTED FOR DENTAL PROCEDURES

ANTIBIOTIC PROPHYLAXIS GENERALLY RECOMMENDED
Prosthetic cardiac valve or material
Presence of cardiac prosthetic valve
Transcatheter prosthetic valves
Cardiac valve repair with devices, including annuloplasty, rings, or clips
Left ventricular assist devices or implantable heart
Previous, relapsed, or recurrent infectious endocarditis
Congenital heart disease
Unrepaired cyanotic congenital congenital heart disease, including palliative shunts and conduits
Completely repaired congenital heart defect with prosthetic material or device, whether placed by surgery or by transcatheter during the first 6 mo after the procedure
Repaired congenital heart disease with residual defects at the site of or adjacent to the site of a prosthetic patch or prosthetic device
Surgical or transcatheter pulmonary artery valve or conduit placement
Cardiac transplant recipients who develop cardiac valvulopathy
ANTIBIOTIC PROPHYLAXIS NOT RECOMMENDED
Implantable electronic devices such as a pacemaker or similar devices
Septal defect closure devices when complete closure is achieved
Peripheral vascular grafts and patches, including those used for hemodialysis
Coronary artery stents or other vascular stents
Central nervous system ventriculoatrial shunts
Vena cava filters

Reprinted with permission *Circulation*. 2021;143:e963-e978 ©2021 American Heart Association, Inc.

TABLE 61-10 PROCEDURES FOR WHICH ENDOCARDITIS PROPHYLAXIS IS AND IS NOT RECOMMENDED

PROPHYLAXIS IS RECOMMENDED*
Dental: all dental procedures involving manipulation of gingival tissue, the periapical region of teeth, or perforation of the oral mucosa
Respiratory: procedures involving incision or biopsy of the respiratory mucosa, such as tonsillectomy and adenoidectomy
Other: procedures involving infected skin, skin structures, or musculoskeletal tissue prior to incision and drainage
PROPHYLAXIS IS NOT RECOMMENDED
Dental: routine anesthetic injections through noninfected tissue, dental radiographs, placement of removable prosthodontic or orthodontic appliances, adjustment of orthodontic appliances, placement of orthodontic brackets, shedding of deciduous teeth, bleeding from trauma to the lips or oral mucosa
Respiratory: procedures not involving incision or biopsy of the respiratory mucosa, including bronchoscopy (unless the procedure involves incision of the respiratory tract mucosa)
Genitourinary: antibiotic prophylaxis solely to prevent infective endocarditis is not recommended
Gastrointestinal: antibiotic prophylaxis solely to prevent infective endocarditis is not recommended

*Only in patients with underlying cardiac conditions associated with the highest risk for adverse outcome from endocarditis (listed in Table 61-9).

Reprinted with permission *Circulation*. 2021;143:e963-e978 ©2021 American Heart Association, Inc.

TABLE 61-11 ANTIBIOTIC REGIMENS FOR AN ADULT UNDERGOING A DENTAL PROCEDURE: SINGLE DOSE 30 TO 60 MINUTES BEFORE PROCEDURE*†

PATIENT CHARACTERISTICS	REGIMEN‡
Able to take oral medications	Amoxicillin 2 g PO
Unable to take oral medications	Ampicillin 2 g IV or IM; or cefazolin or ceftriaxone 1 g IM or IV
Allergic to penicillin or ampicillin and able to take oral medications	Cephalexin 2 g PO (or other first- or second-generation oral cephalosporin in equivalent adult doses); azithromycin 500 mg PO; or clarithromycin 500 mg PO; or doxycycline 100 mg PO
Allergic to penicillin or ampicillin and unable to take oral medications	Cefazolin or ceftriaxone 1 g IM or IV

*For the applicable procedures, see Table 61-10.

†For the applicable conditions, see Table 61-9.

‡Cephalosporins should not be used in an individual with a history of anaphylaxis, angioedema, or urticaria with penicillin or ampicillin.

Clindamycin is no longer recommended for antibiotic prophylaxis for a dental procedure.

IM = intramuscular; IV = intravenous; PO = oral.

Reprinted with permission *Circulation*. 2021;143:e963-e978 ©2021 American Heart Association, Inc.

of device placement, replacement, or pocket revision could significantly reduce infections without adverse effects.[A6]

PROGNOSIS

Untreated infective endocarditis is uniformly fatal. Aggressive medical and surgical management dramatically improves the outcome. The overall mortality rate from both native and prosthetic valve endocarditis remains fairly high, ranging from 17 to 36%. Whereas certain subgroups, such as patients with viridans group streptococcal endocarditis, have a lower risk of death, patients with *S. aureus,* fungal, aerobic gram-negative bacillary, and zoonotic endocarditis have higher mortality rates. Heart failure and CNS events are the most frequent causes of death.

Endocarditis recurs in about 12 to 16% of patients and is more common in injection drug users, elderly people, and patients with prosthetic valves. The rate of relapse also varies depending on the causative organism. Easily treated infections, such as those with viridans group streptococci, have a low rate of relapse (5%), but more difficult-to-eradicate organisms may have significantly higher rates.

GENERAL REFERENCES

For the General References and other additional features, please visit Elsevier eBooks+ at https://ebooks.health.elsevier.com.

Grade A References

A1. Zimmerman FS, Karameh H, Ben-Chetrit E, et al. Modification of blood test draw order to reduce blood culture contamination: a randomized clinical trial. *Clin Infect Dis.* 2020;71:1215-1220.

A2. Meier MA, Branche A, Neeser OL, et al. Procalcitonin-guided antibiotic treatment in patients with positive blood cultures: a patient-level meta-analysis of randomized trials. *Clin Infect Dis.* 2019;69:388-396.

A3. Pujol M, Miró JM, Shaw E, et al. MRSA Bacteremia (BACSARM) Trial Investigators. Daptomycin plus fosfomycin versus daptomycin alone for methicillin-resistant *Staphylococcus aureus* bacteremia and endocarditis: a randomized clinical trial. *Clin Infect Dis.* 2021;72:1517-1525.

A4. Iversen K, Ihlemann N, Gill SU, et al. Partial oral versus intravenous antibiotic treatment of endocarditis. *N Engl J Med.* 2019;380:415-424.

A5. Krahn AD, Longtin Y, Philippon F, et al. Prevention of arrhythmia device infection trial: the PADIT trial. *J Am Coll Cardiol.* 2018;72:3098-3109.

A6. Tarakji KG, Mittal S, Kennergren C, et al. Antibacterial envelope to prevent cardiac implantable device infection. *N Engl J Med.* 2019;380:1895-1905.

62

PERICARDIAL DISEASES

BRIAN D. HOIT AND JAE K. OH

The pericardium is a two-layered sac composed of visceral and parietal components. The visceral pericardium is a serosal cell monolayer that adheres firmly to the epicardium, reflects over the origin of the great vessels, and, together with a tough, fibrous parietal layer encases the heart. The pericardial space enclosed between the two serosal layers normally contains up to 50 mL of plasma ultrafiltrate. The pericardium is well innervated, so pericardial inflammation may produce severe pain and trigger vagally mediated reflexes.

As a result of its relatively inelastic physical properties, the pericardium limits acute cardiac dilation and enhances mechanical interactions of the cardiac chambers.[1] In response to chronic stretch, the pericardium dilates to allow a slowly accumulating pericardial effusion to become quite large without compressing the cardiac chambers and to allow left ventricular remodeling to occur without excessive pericardial restraint. Conversely, a scarred or thickened pericardium can limit the filling of the heart, resulting in pericardial constriction. Despite the important functions of the normal pericardium, congenital absence or surgical resection of the pericardium does not appear to have any major untoward effects.

ACUTE PERICARDITIS

EPIDEMIOLOGY AND PATHOBIOLOGY

Acute inflammation of the pericardium, with or without an associated pericardial effusion, can occur as an isolated clinical problem or as a manifestation of systemic disease. Although about 85% of isolated cases of acute pericarditis are idiopathic or viral, the list of other potential causes is quite extensive (Table 62-1). Viral causes include echoviruses, group B coxsackieviruses, and, recently, severe acute respiratory syndrome coronavirus 2 (Chapter 336),[2] but obtaining specific viral titers does not alter patient management. About 6% of cases are neoplastic in origin, about 4% are caused by tuberculosis, about 3% are caused by other bacterial or fungal infections, and about 2% are caused by collagen vascular disease. Patients with fever greater than 38° C or a subacute course or who fail to respond promptly to therapy are most likely to have pericarditis caused by a systemic autoimmune disease, malignancy, drugs (including checkpoint inhibitors [Chapter 164]),[3] or bacterial infection.

CLINICAL MANIFESTATIONS

Most patients with acute pericarditis experience sharp retrosternal chest pain (see Table 39-2 in Chapter 39), which can be quite severe and debilitating. In some cases, however, pericarditis is asymptomatic, such as when it accompanies rheumatoid arthritis. Pericardial pain is usually worse with inspiration and when supine, and it is generally relieved by sitting and leaning forward. Typically, pericardial pain is referred to the scapular ridge, presumably owing to irritation of the phrenic nerves, which provide sensory innervation to the pericardium. The chest pain of acute pericarditis must be differentiated from pulmonary embolism and myocardial ischemia or infarction (Table 62-2).

The pericardial friction rub is the classic finding in patients with acute pericarditis. A friction rub is a high-pitched, scratchy sound that can have one, two, or three components corresponding to ventricular ejection, rapid ventricular filling in early diastole, and atrial systole. A pericardial rub, which is differentiated from a murmur by its scratchy quality, is sometimes localized to a small area on the chest wall and may come and go spontaneously or with changes in position. To hear a rub, it may be necessary to auscultate the heart with the patient in multiple positions, especially using the diaphragm with the patient learning forward and not breathing after full expiration. The pericardial friction rub must be differentiated from a pleural rub, which is absent during suspended respiration, but the pericardial rub is unaffected.

DIAGNOSIS

A targeted evaluation (Table 62-3) can help distinguish pericarditis from other conditions as well as help establish the cause of true pericarditis (Table 62-4).[4] The diagnosis of acute pericarditis can be made with two of the following criteria: typical chest pain, pericardial friction rub, characteristic electrocardiogram (ECG) changes, and pericardial effusion. Early in the course of acute pericarditis, the ECG typically displays diffuse ST elevation in association with PR depression (Fig. 62-1). The ST elevation is usually present in all leads except for aVR, but the changes may be atypical in post–myocardial infarction (MI) pericarditis. Classically, the ECG changes of acute pericarditis evolve over several days; resolution of the ST elevation is followed by widespread T wave inversion that subsequently normalizes, although the temporal evolution of ECG changes is highly variable. Uremic pericarditis usually occurs without the typical ECG abnormalities.

Patients with acute pericarditis usually have evidence of systemic inflammation, including leukocytosis, an elevated erythrocyte sedimentation rate (ESR), and increased C-reactive protein (CRP) level. A low-grade fever is common, but a temperature greater than 38° C is unusual and suggests the possibility of bacterial pericarditis.

Troponin levels typically are minimally elevated in acute pericarditis owing to some involvement of the epicardium by the inflammatory process. An elevated troponin level in acute pericarditis usually returns to normal within 1 to 2 weeks and is not associated with a worse prognosis. Although the elevated troponin level may lead to the misdiagnosis of an ST elevation MI (Chapter 58), most patients with elevated troponin levels and acute pericarditis have normal coronary angiograms. An echocardiogram (Chapter 43) can help avoid a misdiagnosis of MI.

Echocardiography may demonstrate a small pericardial effusion in the presence of acute pericarditis, but a normal echocardiogram does not exclude the diagnosis of acute pericarditis. An echocardiogram is critical, however, in excluding the diagnosis of cardiac tamponade (see later). When the diagnosis of acute pericarditis is unclear, cardiac magnetic resonance imaging (MRI) can demonstrate pericardial inflammation as delayed enhancement of the pericardium (Fig. 62-2). Diagnostic pericardiocentesis is indicated in suspected purulent tuberculosis or malignant pericarditis or if the patient has cardiac tamponade.

TABLE 62-1 CAUSES OF PERICARDITIS: INFECTIOUS AND NONINFECTIOUS

INFECTIOUS PERICARDITIS (⅔ OF CASES)

Viral (most common): echovirus and coxsackievirus (usual), influenza, EBV, CMV, adenovirus, varicella, rubella, mumps, SARS-CoV-2, HBV, HCV, HIV, parvovirus B19, human herpesvirus 6
Bacterial: tuberculosis (4-5%)* and *Coxiella burnetii* (most common); other bacterial causes (rare) include pneumococcosis, meningococcosis, gonococcosis, *Haemophilus*, staphylococci, *Chlamydia, Mycoplasma, Legionella, Leptospira, Listeria*
Fungal (rare): histoplasmosis more likely in immunocompetent patients; aspergillosis, blastomycosis, candidiasis more likely in immunosuppressed patients
Parasitic (very rare): *Echinococcus, Toxoplasma*

NONINFECTIOUS PERICARDITIS (⅓ OF CASES)

Autoimmune Pericarditis (<10%)*
Pericardial injury syndromes: post–myocardial infarction syndrome; postpericardiotomy syndrome; posttraumatic pericarditis, including iatrogenic pericarditis (e.g., after percutaneous coronary interventions, pacemaker insertion, ablation)
Pericarditis in systemic autoimmune and autoinflammatory diseases: more common in systemic lupus erythematosus, Sjögren syndrome, rheumatoid arthritis, systemic sclerosis, systemic vasculitides, Behçet syndrome, sarcoidosis, familial Mediterranean fever
Autoreactive pericarditis†
Neoplastic Pericarditis (5-7%)*
Primary tumors (rare): pericardial mesothelioma
Secondary metastatic tumors (common): lung and breast cancer, lymphoma
Metabolic Pericarditis: Uremia, Myxedema (common); others rare
Traumatic Pericarditis (rare)
Direct injury: penetrating thoracic injury, esophageal perforation, iatrogenic
Indirect injury: nonpenetrating thoracic injury, radiation injury
Drug-related pericarditis (rare): procainamide, hydralazine, isoniazid, and phenytoin (lupus-like syndrome), penicillins (hypersensitivity pericarditis with eosinophilia), doxorubicin, and daunorubicin (often associated with cardiomyopathy; may cause pericardiopathy), immune checkpoint inhibitors (e.g., ipilimumab, pembrolizumab)

*Percentages refer to unselected cases.
†The diagnosis of autoreactive pericarditis is established using the following criteria: (1) increased number of lymphocytes and mononuclear cells >5000/μL (autoreactive lymphocytic) or the presence of antibodies against heart muscle tissue (antisarcolemmal) in the pericardial fluid (autoreactive antibody mediated), (2) signs of myocarditis on epicardial or endomyocardial biopsies by ≥14 cells/mm², and (3) exclusion of infections, neoplasia, and systemic and metabolic disorders.
CMV = cytomegalovirus; EBV = Epstein-Barr virus; HBV = hepatitis B virus; HCV = hepatitis C virus; HIV = human immunodeficiency virus; SARS-CoV 2 = severe acute respiratory syndrome coronavirus 2.
From Imazio M, Spodick DH, Brucato A, et al. Controversial issues in the management of pericardial diseases. *Circulation*. 2010;121:916-928.

TABLE 62-2 DIFFERENTIATION OF PERICARDITIS FROM MYOCARDIAL ISCHEMIA OR INFARCTION AND PULMONARY EMBOLISM

FINDINGS	MYOCARDIAL ISCHEMIA OR INFARCTION	PERICARDITIS	PULMONARY EMBOLISM
CHEST PAIN			
Character	Pressure-like heavy, squeezing	Sharp, stabbing, occasionally dull	Sharp, stabbing
Change with respiration	No	Worsened with inspiration	In phase with respiration (absent when the patient is apneic)
Change with position	No	Worse when supine; improved when sitting up or leaning forward	No
Duration	Minutes (ischemia); hours (infarction)	Hours to days	Hours to days
Response to nitroglycerin	Improved	No change	No change
PHYSICAL EXAMINATION			
Friction rub	Absent (unless pericarditis is present)	Present in most patients	Pleural friction rub may occur
ELECTROCARDIOGRAM			
ST segment elevation	Localized convex	Widespread concave	Limited to leads III, aVF, and V_1
PR segment depression	Rare	Frequent	None

Modified from Little WC, Freeman GL. Pericardial disease. *Circulation*. 2006;113:1622-1632.

TREATMENT

Patients who have manifestations of an underlying systemic process, such as an inflammatory disease, have high-risk features (i.e., fever >38° C, subacute course, failure to respond to treatment, an elevated troponin level with evidence of concomitant left ventricular dysfunction, a large pericardial effusion, incipient or established pericardial tamponade), or have suspected acute MI (Chapter 58) warrant hospitalization and further evaluation. Patients without these features can usually be followed as outpatients (Fig. 62-3).

If acute pericarditis is a manifestation of an underlying disease, such as a systemic rheumatologic condition, it often responds to treatment of the primary condition. Most cases of acute idiopathic or viral pericarditis are self-limited and respond to treatment with aspirin (650 mg every 6 hours) or another nonsteroidal anti-inflammatory drug (NSAID) such as ibuprofen (300 to 800 mg every 6 to 8 hours).[5] The dose of NSAID should be tapered after symptoms and any pericardial effusion have resolved, but the medication should be taken for at least 3 to 4 weeks to minimize the risk of recurrent pericarditis.

In addition, colchicine (0.6 to 1.2 mg/day for 3 months) should be started in all patients with acute pericarditis[6] to reduce the rate of persistent symptoms at 72 hours, reduce the likelihood of recurrent pericarditis from 55 to 24% at 18 months, and reduce the rate of subsequent hospitalization.[A1] The major side effect of colchicine is diarrhea. The lower dose of colchicine should be used in patients who weigh less than 70 kg or who have side effects with the higher dose. Colchicine should be avoided in patients with abnormal renal or hepatic function and in patients being treated with macrolide antibiotics, which alter its metabolism.

A proton pump inhibitor, such as omeprazole (20 mg/day), should be considered to improve the gastric tolerability of NSAIDs. Warfarin and heparin should be avoided to minimize the risk of hemopericardium, but anticoagulation may be required if the patient is in atrial fibrillation or has a prosthetic heart valve. It is prudent to avoid exercise until after the chest pain completely resolves. If pericarditis recurs, the patient can be reloaded with colchicine and intramuscular ketorolac (15 to 30 mg, once) and then continued on an oral NSAID and colchicine for at least 3 months.

TABLE 62-3 SELECTED DIAGNOSTIC TESTS IN ACUTE PERICARDITIS

IN ALL PATIENTS
Tuberculin skin test (plus control skin test to exclude anergy)
BUN and creatinine to exclude uremia
Erythrocyte sedimentation rate
Electrocardiogram
Chest radiograph
Echocardiogram
IN SELECTED PATIENTS
Cardiac magnetic resonance imaging
ANA and rheumatoid factor to exclude SLE or rheumatoid arthritis in patients with acute arthritis or pleural effusion
TSH and T_4 to exclude hypothyroidism in patients with clinical findings suggestive of hypothyroidism and in asymptomatic patients with unexplained pericardial effusion
HIV test to exclude AIDS in patients with risk factors for HIV disease or a compatible clinical syndrome
Blood cultures in febrile patients to exclude infective endocarditis and bacteremia
Fungal serologic tests in patients from endemic areas or in immunocompromised patients
ASO titer in children or teenagers with suspected rheumatic fever
Heterophil antibody test to exclude mononucleosis in young or middle-aged patients with a compatible clinical syndrome or acute fever, weakness, and lymphadenopathy

AIDS = acquired immunodeficiency virus; ANA = antinuclear antibody; ASO = antistreptolysin O; BUN = blood urea nitrogen; HIV = human immunodeficiency virus; SLE = systemic lupus erythematosus; T_4 = thyroxine; TSH = thyroid-stimulating hormone.

Modified from Nishimura RA, Kidd KR. Recognition and management of patients with pericardial disease. In: Braunwald E, Goldman L, eds. *Primary Cardiology*. 2nd ed. Philadelphia: WB Saunders; 2003:625.

Although acute pericarditis usually responds dramatically to systemic corticosteroids, observational studies strongly suggest that the use of steroids increases the probability of relapse in patients treated with colchicine. Except when needed to treat an underlying inflammatory disease, every effort should be made to avoid the use of steroids, reserving low-dose steroids for patients who cannot tolerate aspirin and other NSAIDs or whose recurrence is not responsive to colchicine and intravenous NSAIDs. If steroids are used, low-dose prednisone (0.2 to 0.5 mg/kg) appears to be as effective as higher doses and is less likely to be associated with recurrence. Steroids should be continued for at least 1 month before slow tapering, which can be guided by return of the CRP level to the normal range. Pericardiocentesis is not recommended unless purulent or tuberculous pericarditis is clinically suspected or the patient fails to respond to 2 to 3 weeks of NSAID therapy.

PROGNOSIS

The course of viral and idiopathic pericarditis is usually self-limited. Although most patients recover completely, the 5-year mortality after hospitalization for pericarditis is about 30% higher than in age-matched controls.

About 25% of patients, however, have recurrent pericarditis weeks to months later, probably caused by an immune response, and some patients may have multiple debilitating episodes.[7] Interestingly, in patients whose acute pericarditis is accompanied by myocarditis, as evidenced by elevation of serum troponin levels, the recurrence rate is closer to 10%. Recurrent pericarditis is more common in patients treated with steroids for the acute episode, especially during a rapid steroid taper. Prolonged high-dose NSAID treatment (e.g., ibuprofen 300 to 600 mg three times a day) plus colchicine (0.5 to 0.6 mg twice daily, reducing to once daily after 3 to 6 months) is effective for recurrent pericarditis.[A2] In patients who cannot tolerate colchicine or who have recurrent episodes despite colchicine and high-dose NSAID treatment (e.g., indomethacin 50 mg three times a day or ibuprofen 800 mg four times a day), oral steroids (e.g., prednisone 0.2 to 0.5 mg/kg/day for 2 to 4 weeks and then slowly tapered over several months) are generally recommended. The addition of an anti–interleukin 1 drug, such as rilonacept[A3] (after a 320-mg load, 160 mg subcutaneously once weekly) or anakinra[A4] (100 mg subcutaneously once daily), lowers the risk of recurrent pericarditis by over 90%.[A5] In patients with refractory, recurrent pericarditis, surgical pericardiectomy can be considered. Patients who have tuberculous or purulent pericarditis have the highest risk for progression to constrictive pericarditis (see later).

PERICARDIAL EFFUSION AND TAMPONADE

EPIDEMIOLOGY

A pericardial effusion can be caused by any disease that causes acute pericarditis (see Table 62-1), but a majority of cases are caused by conditions other than viral or idiopathic pericarditis (Table 62-5). For example, tamponade occurs in about 10 to 15% of patients with idiopathic pericarditis, but it develops in more than 50% of patients with malignant, tuberculous, or purulent pericarditis. Tuberculosis and neoplastic disease are typically associated with serosanguineous effusions, but such effusions also can be seen with typical viral or idiopathic pericarditis, with uremia, and after mediastinal irradiation. Hemopericardium is seen most commonly with trauma, myocardial rupture after MI, catheter-induced myocardial or epicardial coronary artery rupture, aortic dissection with rupture into the pericardial space, or primary hemorrhage in patients receiving anticoagulant therapy, often after cardiac valve surgery. Chylopericardium is rare and usually results from traumatic or surgical injury to, or neoplastic obstruction of, the thoracic duct.

PATHOBIOLOGY

Under normal conditions, the space between the parietal and visceral pericardium can accommodate only a small amount of fluid before the development of tamponade physiology. The clinical consequences of a pericardial effusion depend on the rate of increase. A rapidly accumulating effusion, as in hemopericardium caused by trauma or aortic dissection, may result in tamponade physiology with just 100 to 200 mL of fluid. It is not surprising, therefore, that cardiac perforation quickly results in tamponade. By comparison, a more slowly developing effusion gradually stretches the pericardium and shifts the normally steep pericardial pressure-volume relation to the right; this explains why large but slowly developing effusions may not produce tamponade.

Tamponade physiology occurs when fluid accumulation in the intrapericardial space is sufficient to compress the heart, resulting in impaired cardiac filling. The increased pericardial pressure in cardiac tamponade accentuates the interdependence among the cardiac chambers as the total cardiac volume is limited by the pericardial effusion. With normal inspiration, right ventricular filling is enhanced, the intraventricular septum is displaced toward the left ventricle, and left ventricular filling and the resulting stroke volume are reduced; these changes are reversed during expiration. In tamponade, these physiologic variations are enhanced and are responsible for the clinical finding of "paradoxical pulse." A small (<10 mm Hg) pulsus paradoxus, which is a decline in systemic blood pressure during inspiration, is normal and is related to the ventricles being confined within the pericardium and sharing a common septum. In cardiac tamponade, this phenomenon is exaggerated, and systemic blood pressure falls by more than 10 mm Hg during inspiration. A pulsus paradoxus also may be present with hypovolemic shock, chronic obstructive pulmonary disease, and bronchospasm.

CLINICAL MANIFESTATIONS

A slowly accumulating, isolated pericardial effusion is often completely asymptomatic. The physical examination results may be normal, but the heart sounds may be muffled. The diagnosis is usually suggested by a chest radiograph that shows cardiomegaly with a globular heart (Fig. 62-4; see also Fig. 44-5) or by an echocardiogram, computed tomography (CT) scan, or MRI performed for another indication. Patients with hypothyroidism, uremia, or collagen vascular disease may have asymptomatic effusions discovered during comprehensive evaluations.

Patients with tamponade are usually anxious and tachycardic, and they may complain of dyspnea, orthopnea, and chest pain. The increased venous pressure is usually apparent as jugular venous distention.[8] The x descent (during ventricular systole) is typically the dominant jugular venous wave, with little or no y descent (during early diastole) (Chapter 39). The heart sounds are classically soft or muffled, especially if there is a large pericardial effusion. In rapidly developing cardiac tamponade, especially hemorrhagic cardiac tamponade, the jugular veins may not be distended because the time course has been insufficient for a compensatory increase in venous pressure. Such "low-pressure" tamponade may also occur in volume-depleted patients. The patient may have signs of right heart failure, with peripheral edema, right upper quadrant pain caused by hepatic congestion, or abnormal liver enzymes and serum bilirubin level.

TABLE 62-4 PRESENTATION AND TREATMENT OF THE MOST COMMON CAUSES OF PERICARDITIS

TYPE	PATHOGENESIS OR ETIOLOGY	DIAGNOSIS	TREATMENT	COMPLICATIONS	COMMENTS
Viral	Coxsackievirus B Echovirus type 8 Epstein-Barr virus	Leukocytosis Elevated ESR Mild cardiac biomarker elevation	Symptomatic relief, NSAIDs, colchicine	Tamponade Relapsing pericarditis	Peaks in spring and fall
Tuberculous	*Mycobacterium tuberculosis*	Isolation of organism from biopsy fluid Granulomas not specific	Triple-drug antituberculosis regimen Pericardial drainage followed by early (4-6 wk) pericardiectomy if signs of tamponade or constriction develop	Tamponade Constrictive pericarditis	1-8% of patients with tuberculosis pneumonia; rule out HIV infection
Bacterial	Group A streptococcus *Staphylococcus aureus* *Streptococcus pneumoniae*	Leukocytosis with marked left shift Purulent pericardial fluid	Pericardial drainage by catheter or surgery Systemic antibiotics Pericardiectomy if constrictive physiology develops	Tamponade in one third of patients	Very high mortality rate if not recognized early
Post–myocardial infarction	12 hr–10 days after infarction	Fever Pericardial friction rub Echo: effusion	Aspirin Prednisone	Tamponade rare	More frequent in large Q wave infarctions Anterior > inferior
Uremic	Untreated renal failure: 50% Chronic dialysis: 20%	Pericardial rub: 90%	Intensive dialysis Indomethacin: probably ineffective Catheter drainage Surgical drainage	Tamponade Hemodynamic instability on dialysis	Avoid NSAIDs ≈50% respond to intensive dialysis
Neoplastic	In order of frequency: lung cancer, breast cancer, leukemia and lymphoma, others	Chest pain, dyspnea Echo: effusion CT, MRI: tumor metastases to pericardium Cytologic examination of fluid positive in 85%	Catheter drainage Subxiphoid pericardiectomy Chemotherapy directed at underlying malignant neoplasm	Tamponade Constriction	

CT = computed tomography; Echo = echocardiogram; ESR = erythrocyte sedimentation rate; HIV = human immunodeficiency virus; MRI = magnetic resonance imaging; NSAIDs = nonsteroidal anti-inflammatory drugs.

Modified from Malik F, Foster E. Pericardial disease. In: Wachter RM, Goldman L, Hollander H, eds. *Hospital Medicine*. 2nd ed. Philadelphia: Lippincott Williams & Wilkins; 2005:449.

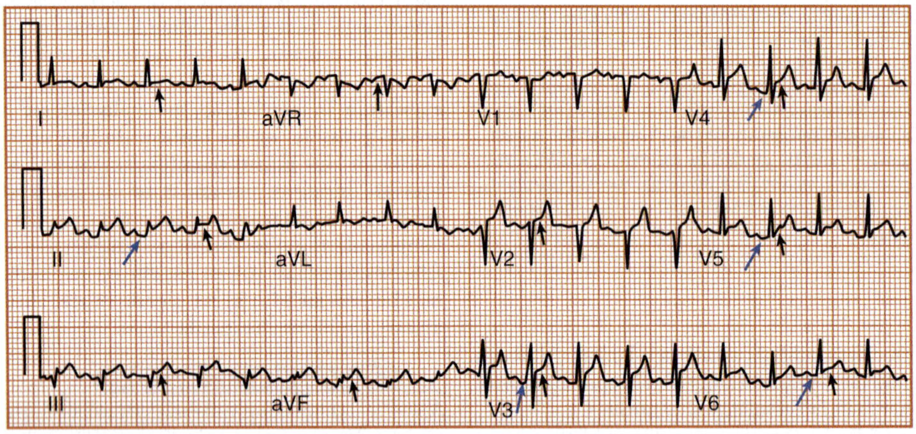

FIGURE 62-1. **Electrocardiogram demonstrating typical features of acute pericarditis on presentation.** There is diffuse ST elevation and PR depression, except in aVR, in which there is ST depression and PR elevation.

The hallmark of cardiac tamponade is a paradoxical pulse, which is defined as a drop of more than 10 mm Hg in inspiratory systolic arterial pressure (usually measured with a sphygmomanometer during slow inspiration). When severe, the paradoxical pulse may be apparent as the absence of a palpable brachial or radial pulse during inspiration. A paradoxical pulse can also occur when there are wide swings in intrathoracic pressure, pulmonary embolism (Chapter 68), or hypovolemic shock (Chapter 92). A paradoxical pulse may be difficult to recognize in the presence of severe shock.

DIAGNOSIS

Cardiac tamponade, which is a treatable cause of shock (Chapter 93), can be rapidly fatal if unrecognized. As such, cardiac tamponade should be considered in the differential diagnosis of any patient with shock or pulseless electrical activity.

Cardiac tamponade is usually suspected based on jugular venous distention, sinus tachycardia with hypotension, narrow pulse pressure, elevated (>10 mm Hg) pulsus paradoxus, and distant heart sounds.

The ECG often shows low voltage and sometimes electrical alternans (Fig. 62-5) when the heart swings within a large pericardial effusion. The chest radiograph shows a globular, enlarged cardiac shadow (see Fig. 44-5 and Fig. 62-6) without pulmonary venous congestion.

Echocardiography, which is the key diagnostic test for cardiac tamponade, must be performed without delay in any patient suspected of having this condition. Echocardiography detects pericardial effusions as an echo-free space around the heart (Fig. 62-4), demonstrates the size and distribution of the pericardial effusion, and reflects its hemodynamic consequences. The inferior vena cava is almost always enlarged, right atrial and right ventricular collapse indicates cardiac compression, and enhanced respiratory variation of ventricular filling is a manifestation of increased ventricular interdependence.

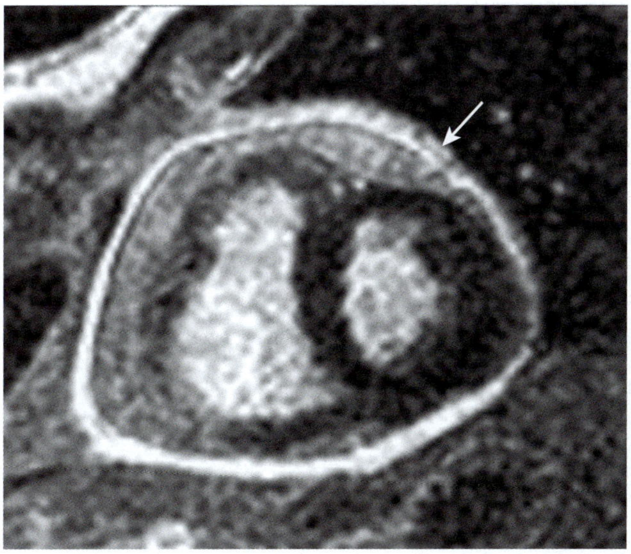

FIGURE 62-2. Cardiac magnetic resonance image of a patient with acute pericarditis shows late gadolinium hyperenhancement of the pericardium and epicardium.

TABLE 62-5 CAUSES OF MODERATE TO LARGE ASYMPTOMATIC PERICARDIAL EFFUSIONS

CAUSE	CASES (%)
Idiopathic or viral	37
Neoplastic	19
Iatrogenic or trauma	13
Tuberculous or purulent	6
Acute myocardial infarction	6
Collagen vascular disease	4
Heart failure	4
Uremia	4
Radiation induced	2
Aortic dissection	2
Hypothyroidism	1
Other	2

Modified from Nishimura RA, Kidd KR. Recognition and management of patients with pericardial disease. In: Braunwald E, Goldman L, eds. *Primary Cardiology*. 2nd ed. Philadelphia: WB Saunders; 2003:625.

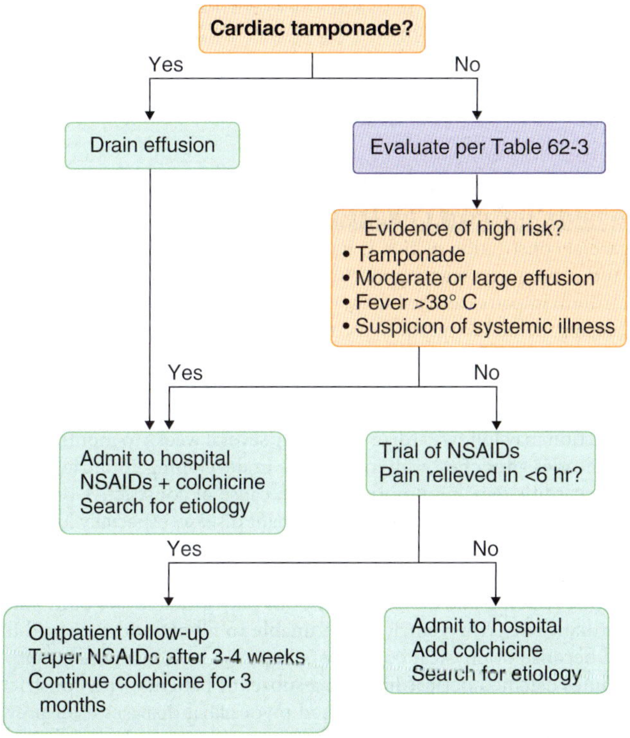

FIGURE 62-3. Initial management of patients with pericarditis. NSAID = nonsteroidal anti-inflammatory drug.

Right ventricular collapse is more specific for tamponade than is right atrial collapse, but the right-sided chambers may not collapse when tamponade occurs in patients with pulmonary hypertension. Cardiac tamponade can result from a loculated pericardial effusion after cardiac surgery or trauma and may present atypically. A loculated effusion may not be apparent on transthoracic echocardiography, but transesophageal echocardiography and thoracic CT or MRI can delineate loculated pericardial effusions.

On Doppler study, mitral inflow velocity (especially early diastolic velocity, designated as E velocity) normally increases with expiration and decreases with inspiration; the opposite respiratory variation is seen in tricuspid inflow velocity. Doppler findings for tamponade, which are more sensitive than two-dimensional echocardiography, include augmented respiratory variation of mitral and tricuspid inflow E velocities as a function of ventricular interdependence. These changes may be seen even before frank hemodynamic compromise caused by pericardial effusion. Although Doppler echocardiography provides important information, it must be emphasized that cardiac tamponade is ultimately a clinical diagnosis.

The routine evaluation should include an assessment of renal function, a thyroid-stimulating hormone level, a complete blood count with differential, a platelet count, coagulation parameters, and a tuberculin skin test. Common medications that can cause a pericardial effusion include cromolyn, isoniazid, phenytoin, hydralazine, and procainamide. Blood cultures are indicated if an infectious cause is suspected. Complement levels, antinuclear antibodies, and the ESR can suggest systemic lupus erythematosus (Chapter 245), which may initially present as an isolated pericardial effusion.

TREATMENT

Pericardial Effusion without Tamponade

Acute pericarditis is often accompanied by a small pericardial effusion that does not produce tamponade. If there is no hemodynamic compromise and the diagnosis can be established by other means, pericardiocentesis is not necessary (Fig. 62-7). Even small pericardial effusions may be related to underlying systemic illnesses such as systemic lupus erythematosus (Chapter 245), cardiac amyloid (Chapter 174), scleroderma (Chapter 246), hypothyroidism (Chapter 207), or AIDS, so it is important to consider and treat associated illnesses. Chylous pericardial effusion, which is usually related to obstruction of the thoracic duct, may require a surgical procedure for relief.

For suspected pericardial effusion, transthoracic echocardiography is the initial test of choice, although loculated effusions may be identified better by CT or MRI. If a small (0.5 to 1 cm) echolucent or "organized" pericardial effusion is observed, a follow-up echocardiogram in 1 to 2 weeks, or sooner if the patient deteriorates, is recommended. If the effusion is getting smaller, subsequent echocardiograms are not necessary unless the patient's clinical condition changes.

For moderate (1 to 2 cm) or large (>2 cm) effusions in patients who are hemodynamically stable and in whom tamponade is not suspected, a follow-up echocardiogram should be performed in 7 days and then every month until the effusion is minimal. If bacterial or malignant pericarditis is suspected, diagnostic pericardiocentesis should be performed immediately even in the absence of clinical instability or suggestion of tamponade; tuberculous pericarditis is diagnosed best by pericardial biopsy. Anticoagulation with heparin or warfarin should be discontinued unless the patient has a mechanical heart valve or atrial fibrillation.

In hypothyroidism (Chapter 207), the effusion and the coexistent cardiomyopathy respond to hormone replacement, sometimes over several months. Uremic pericardial effusions often respond to initiation of dialysis or more intensive dialysis (Chapter 117).

Cardiac Tamponade

The treatment of cardiac tamponade is urgent drainage of the pericardial effusion, especially when there is hemodynamic compromise. Fluid resuscitation may be of transient benefit if the patient is volume depleted (hypovolemic cardiac tamponade), but inotropic agents are usually ineffective because there is already intense endogenous adrenergic stimulation. The initiation of mechanical ventilation in a patient with tamponade may produce a sudden drop in blood pressure because the positive intrathoracic pressure further impairs cardiac filling.

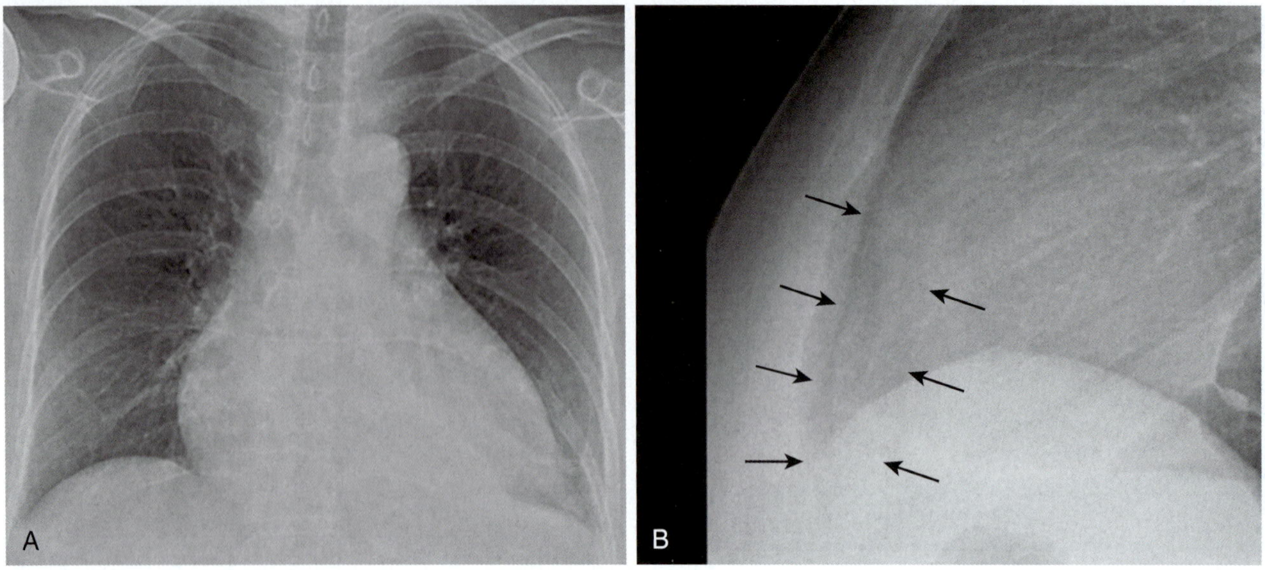

FIGURE 62-4. Chest radiographs in a patient with a large pericardial effusion. The cardiac silhouette on the posteroanterior view (**A**) is enlarged with a "water bag" configuration. The lateral view (**B**) shows a separation between the pericardial and epicardial fat stripes *(arrows)*.

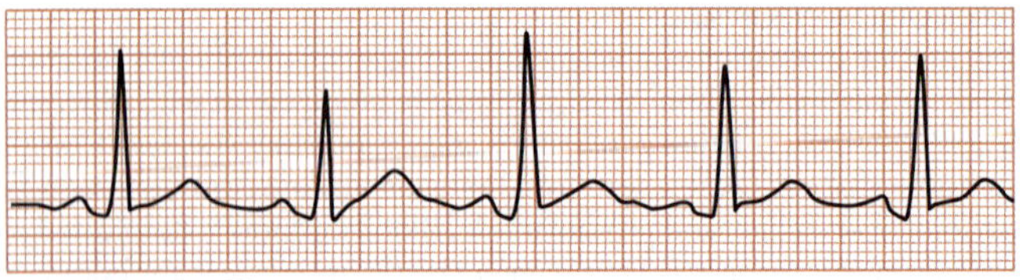

FIGURE 62-5. Electrical alternans. Lead V_5 rhythm strip from a patient with a large pericardial effusion and tamponade physiology. Note the relatively low voltage and electrical alternans.

Echocardiographic-guided percutaneous pericardiocentesis, which can be performed at the bedside by experienced operators (Fig. 62-8), is indicated if a patient is in dire circumstances and at least 1 cm of fluid is seen anterior to the mid-right ventricular free wall throughout diastole. The ideal entry site (usually near the apex) is defined using echocardiography as the minimal distance from the skin to pericardial fluid without intervening structures. The pericardial space is entered with a needle and then drained through a catheter. Although clinical and epidemiologic clues should tailor the extent of the diagnostic evaluation, pericardial fluid should be analyzed for lactate dehydrogenase, protein, cell count, cytology, polymerase chain reaction for tuberculosis, and culture for bacteria and tuberculosis. Continued drainage of the pericardial fluid through an indwelling catheter minimizes the risk of recurrent effusion. For hemodynamically significant effusions of less than 1 cm, organized or multiloculated effusions, and focal effusions, a limited thoracotomy-mediastinoscopy and creation of a pericardial window are advised.

Surgical drainage may be the preferred treatment if pericardial tissue is required for diagnosis or in the case of recurrent effusions or bacterial pericarditis. Malignant pericardial effusions frequently recur and, similar to other recurrent pericardial effusions, may necessitate the surgical creation of a pericardial window that allows the effusion to drain into the pleural space, preventing recurrence of cardiac tamponade. An attractive alternative in these patients, especially if their overall prognosis is poor from the malignancy, is the percutaneous creation of a pericardial window by balloon dilation. Hemorrhagic effusions related to cardiac trauma or aortic dissection are best managed by emergency surgery.

PROGNOSIS

A pericardial effusion may recur or persist. Symptoms are usually weight loss, fatigue, dyspnea on exertion, and whatever symptoms are associated with the specific cause. Treatment of chronic or recurrent idiopathic effusions is similar to the treatment of recurrent pericarditis. If medical therapy is unsuccessful, creation of a pericardial window is indicated.

A large idiopathic, asymptomatic effusion that persists for 6 months or longer can unpredictably result in tamponade in as many as 30% of patients over long-term follow-up; diagnostic pericardiocentesis occasionally detects a neoplastic or tuberculous cause. Pericardiocentesis with prolonged drainage resolves many chronic large pericardial effusions, but pericardiectomy is often required. The long-term prognosis depends on the cause of the effusion. With pericardial tamponade, the in-hospital mortality rate is less than 10%, but the subsequent mortality rate is about 75% with a malignant effusion compared with only a 3 to 5% subsequent annual mortality rate for other causes.

PERICARDIAL CONSTRICTION

EPIDEMIOLOGY AND PATHOBIOLOGY

Pericardial constriction, which is usually the result of pericardial inflammation and subsequent scarring, occurs when a scarred and usually thickened pericardium impairs cardiac filling, thereby limiting the total cardiac volume and causing venous congestion. As the pericardium thickens from its normal 2 mm or less, it may also calcify and adhere to the adjacent epicardium.

The most frequent causes in the developed world are previous cardiac surgery, chronic idiopathic or viral pericarditis, and mediastinal radiation. Constriction may follow cardiac surgery by several weeks to months and may occur decades after chest wall irradiation. In developing countries, tuberculous pericarditis remains a more common cause of constrictive pericarditis. Other less common causes include malignant disease, especially lung cancer, breast cancer, or lymphoma; histoplasmosis; rheumatoid arthritis; and uremia. However, a specific cause may not be identified in many patients.

Fibrous scarring and adhesions of both pericardial layers obliterate the pericardial cavity. The ventricles are unable to fill beyond the rapid filling period because of physical constraints imposed by a thickened, rigid, and sometimes calcified pericardium. In a subset of patients with constriction, especially patients with superimposed myocardial diseases after previous cardiac surgery or radiation therapy, the pericardium may be only minimally thickened and less calcified. The pathophysiologic hallmarks of pericardial constriction are exaggerated interventricular dependence and the dissociation of intracardiac and intrathoracic pressures.

CLINICAL MANIFESTATIONS

Patients with pericardial constriction typically present with manifestations of elevated systemic venous pressures and low cardiac output. Because there is equalization of all cardiac pressures (including right and left atrial pressures), systemic congestion is much more marked than pulmonary congestion. Typically, patients develop marked jugular venous distention, hepatic congestion, ascites, and peripheral edema, but their lungs usually remain clear, and patients with pericardial constriction are much more likely to have left-sided or bilateral pleural effusions than the right-sided effusions that are typically seen in heart failure (Chapter 45). The limited cardiac output typically presents as exercise intolerance and may progress to cardiac cachexia with muscle wasting. In long-standing pericardial constriction, lower extremity edema, ascites, and hepatic dysfunction may be prominent clinical features. Because of the prominent clinical symptoms of ascites and liver enzyme abnormalities, patients may be evaluated for hepatic disease before constrictive pericarditis

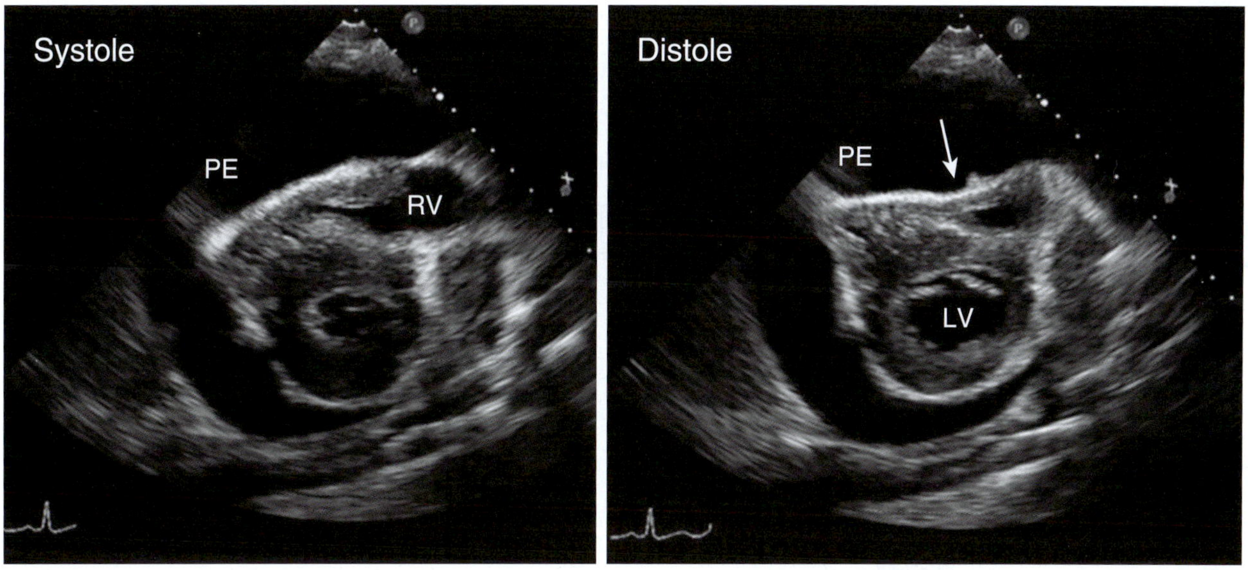

FIGURE 62-6. **Two-dimensional echocardiogram from a patient with cardiac tamponade.** A large pericardial effusion (PE) is apparent as an echo-free space surrounding the left ventricle (LV) and right ventricle (RV). In diastole, there is collapse of the right ventricle *(arrow)*.

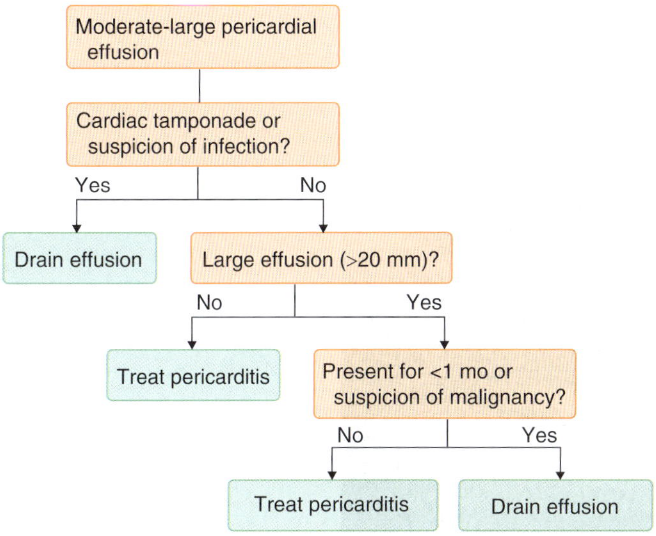

FIGURE 62-7. **Algorithm for managing patients with moderate to large pericardial effusions.** (Modified from Little WC, Freeman GL. Pericardial disease. *Circulation.* 2006;113:1622-1632.)

is recognized. If a patient has patent foramen ovale, hypoxemia from right to left shunting with increased right atrial pressure may be a presenting symptom of constrictive pericarditis.

The jugular veins are distended with prominent y descent. The normal inspiratory drop in jugular venous distention may be replaced by a rise in venous pressure (Kussmaul sign). The y descent, which is when rapid diastolic ventricular filling suddenly ceases, coincides with the timing of the classic auscultatory finding of pericardial constriction, which is an audible pericardial knock (Fig. 39-5)—a high-pitched sound early in diastole.

DIAGNOSIS

Pericardial constriction should be considered in any patient with unexplained systemic venous congestion or a low cardiac output syndrome. Pericardial calcification, seen best on the lateral plain chest radiograph, is a classic finding but is present in only 25% of patients with constrictive pericarditis, mostly in those with long-standing constriction.

Transthoracic echocardiography, which is usually the initial diagnostic tool, classically shows paradoxical interventricular dependence, with ventricular septal motion during inspiration; restrictive mitral inflow velocity, often with respiratory variation; normal or increased (≥8 cm/sec) medial mitral annulus e′ velocity; and reversal of diastolic flow in the hepatic vein during expiration (E-Fig. 62-1). In addition, the hepatic veins are plethoric, and cardiac morphology may be pear shaped, with the narrowest dimension at the atrioventricular grooves. Echocardiography also differentiates pericardial constriction from right heart failure caused by tricuspid valve disease or associated pulmonary hypertension (see later).

Most patients with pericardial constriction have a thickened pericardium (>2 mm) that can be imaged by echocardiography (better by transesophageal than transthoracic echocardiography), CT, and MRI (Fig. 62-9). It is important to recognize, however, that most patients with pericardial constriction present without pericardial calcification and, in about 20% of patients, without any obvious pericardial thickening.[9]

At cardiac catheterization, both cardiac tamponade and pericardial constriction impair diastolic ventricular filling and elevate venous pressure. However, the impairment in ventricular filling with constriction is minimal in early diastole until cardiac volume reaches the anatomic limit set by the noncompliant pericardium, at which time diastolic pressure rises abruptly and remains elevated until the onset of systole. The result is a prominent "y" descent with an elevated plateau of ventricular pressure, which has been termed the "square root" sign (E-Fig. 62-2) and which differentiates constriction from tamponade, in which the y descent is absent.

The pulmonary artery systolic pressure is typically less than 50 mm Hg, and the end-diastolic pressures of both ventricles are equalized. However, the best way to distinguish constrictive pericarditis from a restrictive cardiomyopathy (Chapter 47) is a discordant change in the systolic pressure of the left and right ventricles with respiration compared with a concordant change seen in restrictive cardiomyopathy. In restrictive pericarditis, the left ventricular systolic pressure decreases with inspiration, whereas the right ventricular systolic pressure increases; the opposite change occurs with expiration (E-Fig. 62-3). Stroke volume and cardiac output are reduced because of impaired filling, but the intrinsic systolic function of the ventricles is usually normal.

Differential Diagnosis

The most difficult differentiation is between pericardial constriction and restrictive cardiomyopathy (Chapter 47) (Fig. 62-10), the clinical manifestations of which may be very similar to those of pericardial constriction (Table 62-6).[10] Doppler echocardiography is the most useful method to distinguish constriction from restriction. Whereas patients with pericardial constriction usually have pronounced respiratory variation (>25%) of mitral inflow E velocity, patients with restrictive cardiomyopathies do not. In some patients with pericardial constriction and markedly elevated venous pressures, the respiratory variation may not be present unless preload can be decreased; for example, with head-up tilt. The tissue Doppler measurement of early diastolic septal mitral annular velocity (e′) is almost always reduced in patients with myocardial restriction due to abnormal myocardial relaxation, but it remains normal or increased in patients with

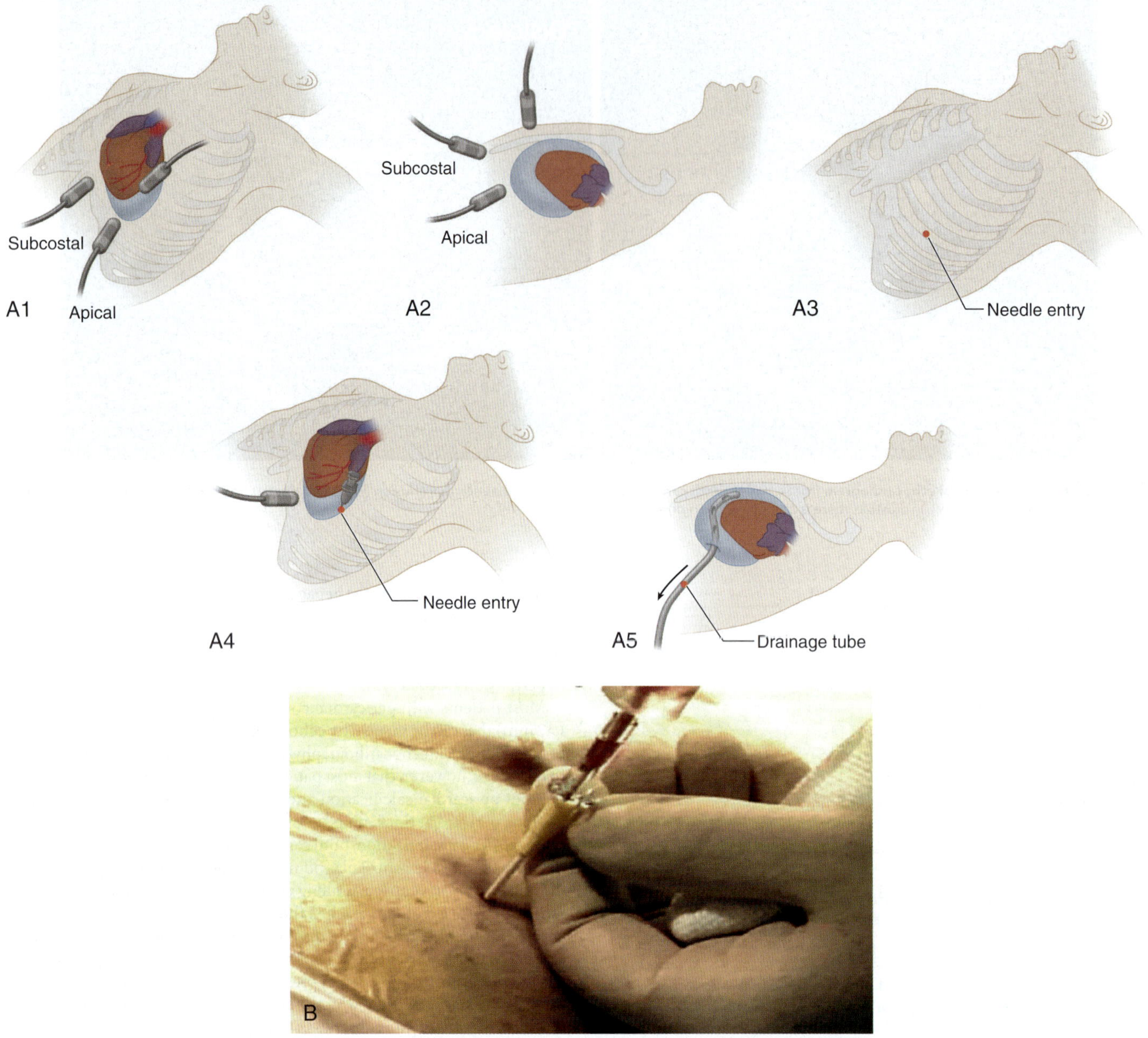

FIGURE 62-8. **Pericardiocentesis. A,** Schematic diagrams demonstrate steps of echocardiography-guided pericardiocentesis.
Step 1. Locate an area on the chest or subcostal region from which the largest amount of pericardial effusion can be visualized and mark it (**A1-A3**).
Step 2. Determine the depth of effusion and the optimal angulation from the marked position.
Step 3. After sterile preparation and local anesthesia, perform pericardiocentesis (**A4**).
Step 4. When in doubt about the location of the needle, inject saline solution through the needle and image it from a remote site to locate the bubbles.
Step 5. Monitor the completeness of the pericardiocentesis with repeat echocardiography.
Step 6. Place a 6 F or 7 F pigtail catheter in the pericardial space to minimize the reaccumulation of fluid (**A5**).
Step 7. Drain any residual fluid or fluid that has reaccumulated via the pigtail catheter every 4 to 6 hours. If after 2 to 3 days pericardial fluid has not reaccumulated by echocardiography, the pigtail catheter may be removed. Always have the pericardial fluid analyzed for cell counts, glucose and protein measurements, culture, and cytology. (Modified from Callahan JA, Seward JB, Tajik AJ, et al. Pericardiocentesis assisted by two-dimensional echocardiography. *J Thorac Cardiovasc Surg*. 1983:85:877-879. Used with permission.)
B, A photo of actual pericardiocentesis. Echocardiography determined the site and the angulation of needle insertion as well as anticipated depth of needle insertion. In this case, bloody fluid is being drained.

pericardial constriction. In addition, lateral e′, which is higher than septal or medial e′ velocity in normal and restrictive cardiomyopathy, is lower than septal e′ in most patients with constrictive pericarditis ("Annulus Reversus"). Whereas a prominent diastolic reversal of hepatic vein flow velocity during expiration is characteristic of constriction, the reversal flow velocity occurs during inspiration in patients with right heart failure from other causes. Patients with pericardial constriction usually have only minimally elevated (<200 pg/mL) brain natriuretic peptide (BNP), but BNP levels are typically markedly increased (<600 pg/mL) in patients with restrictive cardiomyopathy.

Confirmation of the diagnosis of constriction may require cardiac catheterization in patients whose noninvasive evaluation is not clear-cut. Traditional invasive hemodynamic findings of equalized end-diastolic pressures in the right and left ventricles and the "dip and plateau" pattern of left ventricular diastolic pressure do not reliably differentiate constriction from restrictive cardiomyopathy. More specific invasive hemodynamic features of constriction and restriction are based on the respiratory variation in ventricular filling; the simultaneous measurement of left and right ventricular pressures demonstrates discordant changes in their systolic pressures with respiration in constrictive pericarditis. By comparison, the direction of these pressures is concordant (both left and right sides increase with expiration and decrease with inspiration) in restrictive cardiomyopathy.

All patients with documented but otherwise unexplained pericardial constriction should be evaluated for potential tuberculosis.

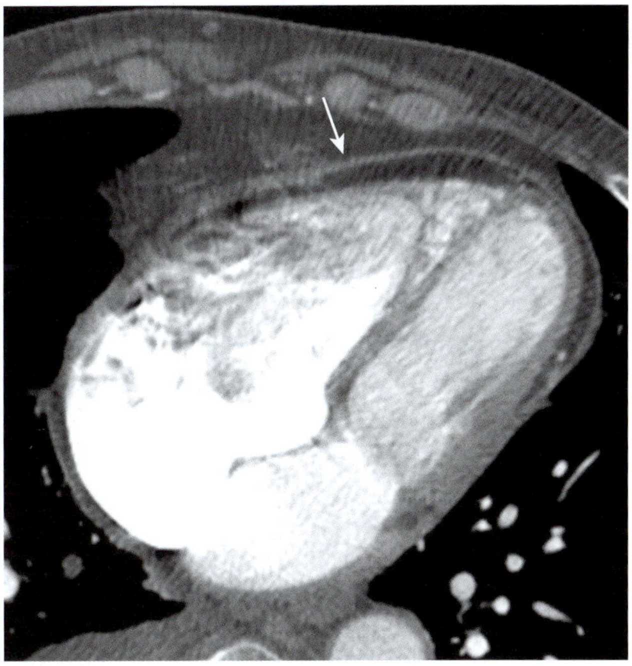

FIGURE 62-9. Computed tomography in a patient with constrictive pericarditis shows a thickened pericardium *(arrow)*.

TREATMENT AND PROGNOSIS

In some patients with pericardial constriction of less than 3 months' duration, the symptoms and constriction may resolve over several weeks with medical therapy consisting of NSAIDs (e.g., ibuprofen 300-800 mg every 6-8 hours), colchicine (0.6 mg once or twice daily), and the cautious use of diuretics. If the patient is severely compromised hemodynamically, steroid therapy (e.g., 0.5 to 1.0 mg/kg up to a maximum dose of 60 mg tapered slowly over 3 months as guided by the clinical response and normalization of the CRP) can be very effective. Patients with constriction who respond to medical therapy usually have high inflammatory biomarkers (ESR and CRP) and intense inflammation of the pericardium on cardiac MRI. For more chronic pericardial constriction or cases that do not respond to medical therapy, the definitive treatment is surgical pericardial decortication, with a wide resection of both the visceral and parietal pericardium. This operation is a major undertaking, but it can be undertaken with acceptable risk (about a 5% mortality rate in the most experienced centers).[11] In many patients, surgery does not immediately restore normal cardiac function; it may take weeks after removal of the constricting pericardium to return to normal. Empirical treatment of tuberculosis (Chapter 299) may be required in patients with constriction and a high suspicion of tuberculosis, even without a definitive diagnosis.

EFFUSIVE-CONSTRICTIVE PERICARDITIS

In about 10 to 20% of patients who present with cardiac tamponade, the elevated right atrial pressure and jugular venous distention do not resolve after removal of the pericardial fluid. In these patients, pericardiocentesis converts the hemodynamics from those typical of tamponade to those of constriction.[12] Thus, the restriction of cardiac filling is not only attributable to pericardial effusion but also to pericardial constriction, predominantly involving the visceral pericardium. Effusive-constrictive pericarditis[13] most likely represents an intermediate transition from acute pericarditis with pericardial effusion to pericardial constriction. Restrictive mitral inflow and plethora of the hepatic veins on echocardiography may be early predictors of which patients will progress to constriction.[14] Frequently, the symptoms resolve after several weeks of treatment with an NSAID (e.g., ibuprofen 300 to 800 mg every 6 to 8 hours). Pericardiectomy may be necessary if constrictive pericarditis persists.

SPECIFIC FORMS OF PERICARDIAL DISEASE

POSTPERICARDIOTOMY SYNDROME

The postcardiac injury syndromes comprise the postpericardiotomy syndrome, post–myocardial infarction pericarditis (Dressler syndrome), and post-traumatic pericarditis. The postpericardiotomy syndrome, like all of the post–cardiac injury syndromes, is initiated by the combination of damage to mesothelial pericardial cells and blood in the pericardial space, which releases cardiac antigens and stimulates an immune response. An inflammatory response is later generated by immune complexes that deposit in the pericardium, pleura, and lungs. This syndrome occurs several days to weeks after cardiothoracic surgery. It most commonly occurs after surgery involving the pericardium, but it can also occur after pacemaker lead implantation, coronary stenting, and other therapeutic misadventures. Patients have typical symptoms of acute pericarditis, which is associated with antimyocardial antibodies. Leukocytosis and elevated inflammatory markers are common laboratory findings. Pericardial effusions are commonly seen, but tamponade physiology is rare. Pleural effusions or pulmonary infiltrates may also be seen.

Treatment of postcardiotomy syndrome is similar to the treatment of acute pericarditis. One month of colchicine therapy (0.5 mg twice daily for patients weighing 70 kg or more; half that dose for smaller patients or patients with side effects) started 48 to 72 hours prior to cardiac surgery appears to reduce the rate of the postcardiotomy syndrome from about 30% to less than 20% but does not reduce the occurrence of atrial fibrillation.

Some patients who have undergone cardiac surgery develop late pericardial constriction without preceding acute pericarditis owing to bleeding in and around the open pericardium followed by inflammation, scarring, and fibrosis. If active inflammation is present, a trial of anti-inflammatory agents may be instituted; however, surgical removal of the blood clot, usually accompanied by more extensive pericardiectomy, is typically required.

UREMIC PERICARDITIS

Pericardial effusions develop in patients with severe renal failure, especially those on dialysis (Chapter 117). Aggressive dialysis may decrease the pericardial effusion, but sometimes the effusion persists and requires drainage or even pericardiectomy.

INFECTIOUS PERICARDITIS

BACTERIAL PERICARDITIS

Purulent bacterial pericarditis may result from direct extension of bacterial pneumonia, direct extension of pleural empyema, or, rarely, peritonitis or a subphrenic abscess. Most patients are acutely ill with systemic sepsis and develop acute tamponade. The most common organisms are streptococci, pneumococci, and staphylococci. Urgent pericardiocentesis, which is required for both diagnosis and therapy, shows leukocytosis and frank pus, and the fluid glucose level is markedly depressed. Persistent or recurrent drainage with an indwelling catheter or repeated taps combined with antimicrobial therapy leads to a high survival rate, but late constrictive pericarditis requiring pericardiectomy develops in 30 to 40% of patients.

TUBERCULOUS PERICARDITIS

Tuberculous pericarditis is common in developing countries but accounts for less than 5% of cases of acute pericarditis in developed countries, usually in patients who are immunosuppressed, including patients infected with the human immunodeficiency virus. Symptoms are often nonspecific, and acute painful pericarditis is rare. Most patients have an effusive-constrictive physiology or pericardial constriction. The chest radiograph suggests active pulmonary tuberculosis in about 30% of cases, and a pleural effusion is present in 40 to 60% of cases. The echocardiogram typically shows fibrinous strands in the pericardial effusion, with multiple echo densities adherent to the pericardial surface. Pericardiocentesis is mandatory if tuberculous pericarditis is suspected. About 75% of patients have a positive culture, and a pericardial fluid adenosine deaminase level of 40 U/L or greater is seen in 75% of patients. Polymerase chain reaction testing and pericardial biopsy are recommended when tuberculous pericarditis is strongly suspected but not otherwise confirmed.

Aggressive antituberculosis therapy (Chapter 299) yields a cure rate of about 85 to 90%. Neither corticosteroids nor adjunctive immunotherapy improves outcome.[A6] Empirical treatment may be required in patients with a consistent clinical picture but without a confirmed diagnosis.

Even with prompt treatment, 30 to 60% of patients develop constrictive pericarditis, for which surgical pericardiectomy is the treatment of choice. In cases of suspected tuberculous constriction, antituberculosis therapy (Chapter 299) should be administered before and after pericardial surgery.

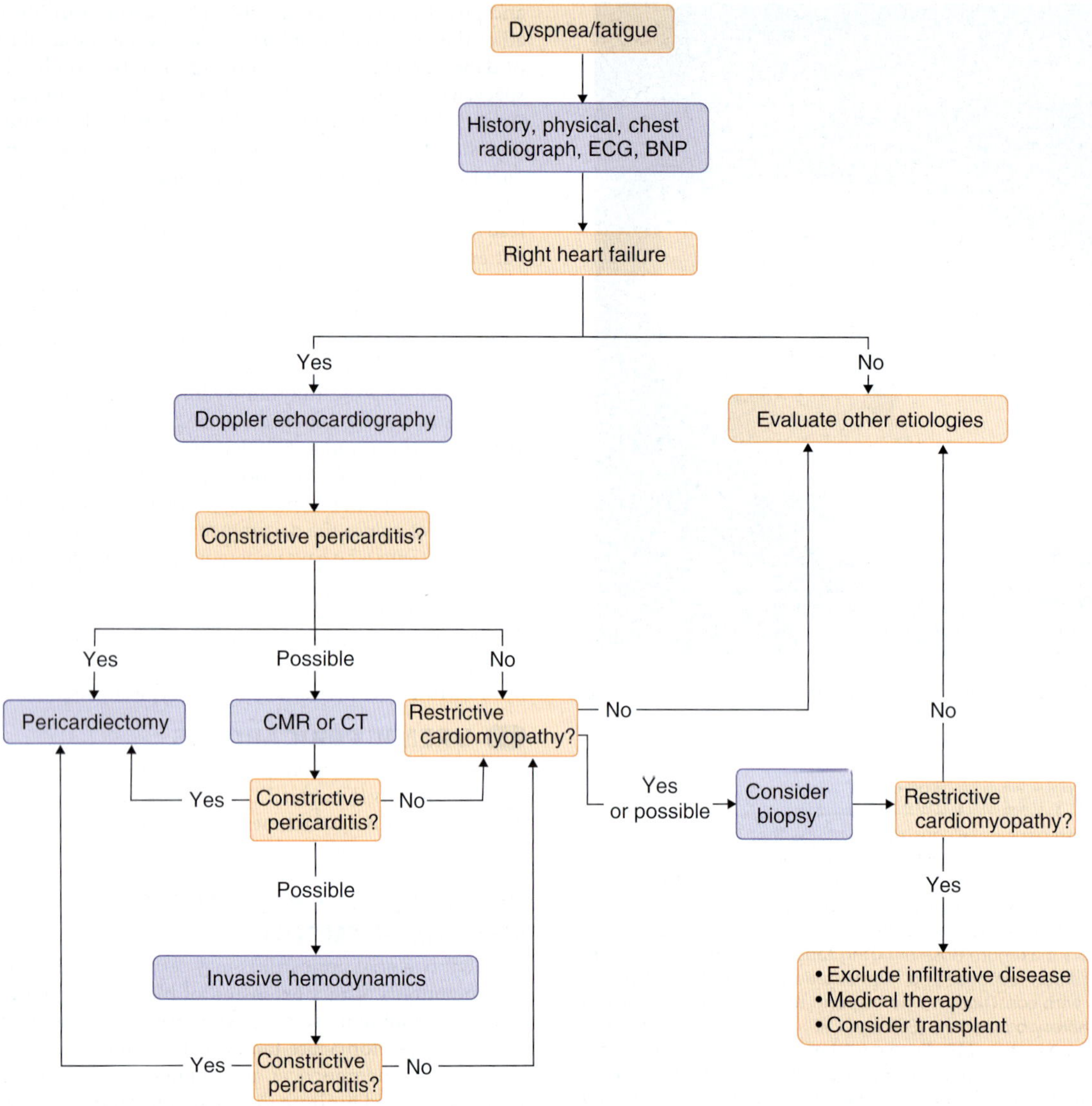

FIGURE 62-10. **Approach to the differentiation of constrictive pericarditis vs. restrictive cardiomyopathy.** BNP = brain natriuretic peptide; CMR = cardiovascular magnetic resonance; CT = computed tomography; ECG = electrocardiogram.

FUNGAL PERICARDITIS

The most common fungal pericarditis is histoplasmosis, which usually resolves in several weeks and can be treated successfully with NSAIDs. Specific antifungal therapy (Chapter 307) is recommended only in patients with disseminated histoplasmosis (Chapter 308).

MALIGNANT PERICARDITIS

About 6% of cases of acute pericarditis that initially have no obvious cause, and about 20% of cases of moderate to large pericardial effusions are related to malignant diseases; in patients with cardiac tamponade, the percentage is even higher. About 80% of malignant pericarditis is linked to breast cancer (Chapter 183), lymphoma (Chapters 171 and 172), and leukemia (Chapters 168, 169, and 170). Melanoma (Chapter 188) is an uncommon cause of malignant pericarditis, but a large proportion of patients with melanoma have pericardial involvement.

Most patients have direct tumor extension from an adjacent malignant lesion or a tumor from hematogenous or lymphatic spread.[15] Pericardial effusions also may be caused by pericardial irritation or compromised lymphatic drainage in patients with mediastinal lymphoma.

Pericardiocentesis is key to diagnosis and management. Fluid cytology results are positive in about 85% of patients. Complete drainage with an indwelling catheter for 2 or 3 days is the treatment of choice. Colchicine (0.6 mg twice daily for 6 months) may be useful,[16] and cancer chemotherapy may sometimes be helpful.[17] If the effusion does not resolve, pericardiectomy is generally recommended, but extended catheter drainage is also an option.[18]

The prognosis depends on the treatment of the underlying malignancy. The 1-year mortality rate is 80% or higher, but patients with breast cancer may have 1-year survival rates as high as 40%.

POSTRADIATION PERICARDITIS

Postradiation pericarditis develops in about 2% of patients after mantle radiation for Hodgkin disease (Chapter 172) and in 0.4 to 5% of patients after irradiation for breast cancer. Pericardial injury occasionally manifests during treatment, but it more commonly appears months or even a decade later. The initial pericarditis and effusion may resolve spontaneously, but constrictive pericarditis, adjacent myocarditis, and even coronary artery damage can develop. Pericardiocentesis is critical to distinguish postradiation pericarditis from malignant pericardial disease. Pericardiectomy is recommended for recurrent pericarditis and for large recurrent pericardial effusions.

AUTOIMMUNE PERICARDITIS

Pericarditis, often with an effusion, can complicate systemic rheumatologic conditions.[19] Up to 50% of patients with systemic lupus erythematosus (Chapter 245) have pericarditis, usually during an acute flare.[20] Patients usually present with acute pericarditis or an asymptomatic effusion; cardiac tamponade is uncommon, and constrictive pericarditis is rare. If purulent pericarditis is not suspected, pericardiocentesis is not usually required. The underlying disease should be treated aggressively.

Acute pericarditis or asymptomatic pericardial effusions also can develop in patients with advanced rheumatoid arthritis (Chapter 243), scleroderma

TABLE 62-6 DIFFERENTIATION OF PERICARDIAL CONSTRICTION FROM RESTRICTIVE CARDIOMYOPATHY

FINDINGS	PERICARDIAL CONSTRICTION	RESTRICTIVE CARDIOMYOPATHY
PHYSICAL EXAMINATION		
Pulmonary congestion	Usually absent	Usually present
Early diastolic sound	Pericardial knock	S_3 (low pitched)
ECHO/DOPPLER		
Respiratory variation in E wave (%)	>25	<20
Mitral septal annular early diastolic velocity (cm/sec)	>7	<7
CT/MRI		
Pericardial thickness	>2 mm (but <2 mm in 20%)	<2 mm
BIOMARKER		
B-type natriuretic peptide (pg/mL)	<200	>600
HEMODYNAMICS		
PA systolic pressure (mm Hg)	<60	>60
PCW-LV diastolic pressure	Respiratory variation with reduction in inspiration	No variation
Respiratory variation in RV/LV peak systolic pressure	Discordant	Concordant

CT = computed tomography; LV = left ventricular; MRI = magnetic resonance imaging; PA = pulmonary artery; PCW = pulmonary capillary wedge; RV = right ventricular.
Modified from Little WC, Freeman GL. Pericardial disease. *Circulation*. 2006;113:1622-1632.

(Chapter 246), or mixed connective tissue disease (Chapter 246). The process is usually self-limited or responds to aggressive treatment of the underlying disease, although cardiac tamponade can develop.

A wide variety of drugs and toxins may cause pericardial heart disease (see Table 62-1) by producing either drug-induced lupus, a hypersensitivity or idiosyncratic reaction, pericardial irritation, or hemorrhage. Immune checkpoint inhibitors are monoclonal antibodies that target a critical mechanism of immune evasion and thereby activate immune responses against tumor cells; cases of pericarditis, pericardial effusion, and cardiac tamponade can complicate cancer treatment with these drugs.

MYOPERICARDITIS

Concomitant myopericarditis (Chapter 47) may develop in patients with pericarditis, probably owing to direct extension of the inflammatory process. It is often manifested by ECG conduction delays, ventricular arrhythmias, and elevated troponin levels. No specific treatment is available.

Acute ventricular dilation and sudden or progressive heart failure develop in some patients after pericardiectomy for constrictive pericarditis or even after drainage of a large pericardial effusion. The syndrome may be due to an underlying myocarditis.

CONGENITAL ABNORMALITIES

Congenital total absence of the pericardium is asymptomatic and clinically unimportant. However, partial or localized absence of the pericardium around the left atrium can cause focal herniation and lead to strangulation. CT or MRI can establish the diagnosis. Patients may present with atypical chest pain or sudden death. Surgical repair is often recommended for a partial pericardial defect.

BENIGN CYSTS

Benign pericardial cysts are rare and are usually asymptomatic, but they can be associated with chest pain. They are typically seen as rounded or lobulated structures adjacent to the heart on the chest radiograph or adjacent to the right atrium on transthoracic echocardiography (Chapter 43). Thoracic CT and MRI are useful for the diagnosis. Cysts rarely rupture and do not require treatment unless they become symptomatic with chest pain. In this situation, the cyst can be removed surgically or drained percutaneously or with a thoracoscope.[21]

GENERAL REFERENCES

For the General References and other additional features, please visit Elsevier eBooks+ at https://ebooks.health.elsevier.com.

Grade A References

A1. Lutschinger LL, Rigopoulos AG, Schlattmann P, et al. Meta-analysis for the value of colchicine for the therapy of pericarditis and of postpericardiotomy syndrome. *BMC Cardiovasc Disord.* 2019;19:207.

A2. Li YL, Qiao SB, Wang JY, et al. Colchicine in addition to conventional therapy for pericarditis recurrence: an update meta-analysis. *Herz.* 2016;41:630-638.

A3. Klein AL, Imazio M, Cremer P, et al. Phase 3 trial of interleukin-1 trap rilonacept in recurrent pericarditis. *N Engl J Med.* 2021;384:31-41.

A4. Bracato A, Imazio M, Gattorno M, et al. Effect of anakinra on recurrent pericarditis among patients with colchicine resistance and corticosteroid dependence: the AIRTRIP randomized clinical trial. *JAMA.* 2016;216:1906-1912.

A5. Imazio M, Andreis A, Piroli F, et al. Anti-interleukin 1 agents for the treatment of recurrent pericarditis: a systematic review and meta-analysis. *Heart.* 2021;107:1240-1245.

A6. Wiysonge CS, Ntsekhe M, Thabane L, et al. Interventions for treating tuberculous pericarditis. *Cochrane Database Syst Rev.* 2017;9:CD000526.

IX

VASCULAR MEDICINE

63 DISEASES OF THE AORTA

JOSHUA A. BECKMAN

The aorta, which is the singular vascular recipient of cardiac output, facilitates the distribution of blood throughout the body. Anatomic landmarks that define its segments (Fig. 63-1A) include the aortic root, which arises from the aortic valve annulus; the ascending aorta, which extends to the branching of the innominate artery; the transverse aorta or arch segment, which begins at the innominate artery and ends at the left subclavian artery; the descending thoracic aorta, which extends from beyond the left subclavian artery to the diaphragm; and the abdominal aorta, which begins at the diaphragm and terminates at the iliac bifurcation.

The aorta comprises three layers: the intima, media, and adventitia. The intima is a single layer of endothelial cells delimited by the internal elastic lamina. The media, which represents approximately 80% of the aortic wall, is composed of vascular smooth muscle cells, collagen fibers, elastin fibers, and fibroblasts. The presence of elastin defines the aorta as an elastic artery and permits the compliance needed to absorb and distribute cardiac output and modulate vascular tone. The adventitia, which contains collagen fibers and fibroblasts, contains the aortic vascular supply (the vaso vasorum). Three pathologic processes comprise the majority of aortic disease encountered by the medical clinician: aneurysm, acute aortic syndromes, and vasculitis.

AORTIC ANEURYSM

DEFINITION

The normal aorta is at its largest at takeoff from the aortic annulus and decreases in size to reach its nadir in the distal abdominal aorta prior to its bifurcation. The normal diameter of the aorta varies by sex (Table 63-1). The normal diameter also increases directly in association with older age, heavier weight, taller height, and greater body surface area, especially for the thoracic aorta.

All segments of the aorta are at risk for the formation of aneurysms, which are defined as enlargement of a segment by more than 50% when compared with a more proximal segment. Below this amount, an increase in size is described as ectasia. Aneurysms may occur in two different morphologies: fusiform, which is a generalized expansion of the entire aortic segment, and saccular, which is a focal area of expansion or outpouching.

EPIDEMIOLOGY

Based on screening with computed tomographic (CT) scanning, the estimated prevalences of aortic aneurysms of the ascending aorta, aortic arch, descending aorta, and abdominal aorta at an average age of 68 years are 0.1%, <0.1%, 0.1%, and 3.7% in men and 0.1%, 0.0%, 0.1%, and 0.4% in women, respectively.[1] Other studies have shown similar results using abdominal ultrasound screening, with data showing abdominal aortic aneurysms above 3 cm in 3.6% of men and above 4 cm in 1.2% of men ages 50 to 79 years but above 3 cm in only 1.3% of women in this age range.

Risk Factors

Abdominal Aortic Aneurysm

The risk of an abdominal aortic aneurysm is largely determined by four risk factors: age, sex, cigarette smoking, and a family history. Abdominal aortic aneurysms are very uncommon in individuals under age 60 years, but the prevalence increases to 6% for persons ages 55 to 64 years and 18.5% for persons ages 75 to 84 years.

The prevalence of abdominal aortic aneurysms is significantly higher among men. Furthermore, about 75% of the abdominal aortic aneurysms found in women are small, between 3 and 3.9 cm.

The presence of an abdominal aortic aneurysm in a first-degree relative is a particularly powerful risk factor, with the increased risk ranging from three- to five-fold. Genome-wide association studies have identified multiple loci for the development of abdominal aortic aneurysm,[2] including a polygenic risk score that appears to be able to explain this familial tendency.

Among acquired risk factors, cigarette smoking (Chapter 363) increases the risk of all aneurysms by 2.7-fold and large abdominal aortic aneurysms by 5.6-fold; the risk is about 2.5-fold higher in current smokers compared with former smokers. Other cardiovascular risk factors, including hypertension (Chapter 64) and dyslipidemia (Chapter 190), also increase the risk of abdominal aortic aneurysm, albeit more modestly than smoking.

Thoracic Aortic Aneurysm

The factors that enhance the risk of abdominal aortic aneurysm are similar in thoracic aortic aneurysm, including hypertension (Chapter 64) and smoking (Chapter 363). The prevalence of thoracic aortic aneurysms in the general population is about 2.7%, and the presence of an aneurysm in one aortic segment is also strongly associated with aortic dilation in another segment. Predisposing conditions include heritable thoracic aortic diseases (Marfan syndrome [Chapter 239], vascular Ehlers-Danlos syndrome [Chapter 239], and familial bicuspid aortic valve syndrome) and inflammatory diseases (e.g., giant cell arteritis, Takayasu arteritis). Thoracic aortic dilatation, especially of the ascending segment, is also seen in Turner syndrome (Chapter 214), tertiary syphilis (Chapter 295), and rheumatoid vasculitis (Chapter 243). About 10% of thoracic aneurysms extend below the diaphragm and are designated as thoracoabdominal aortic aneurysms.

PATHOBIOLOGY

The mesoderm is the source of smooth muscle cells in the distal abdominal aorta, whereas neural crest cells give rise to smooth muscle cells in the thoracic aorta. Both thoracic and abdominal aortic aneurysms are associated with a reduction in the density of this medial smooth muscle cell layer, with evidence of apoptosis or reductions in structural proteins such as elastin, collagen, and glycosaminoglycans.

Four major interconnected processes have been identified in abdominal aortic aneurysm: dysregulation of matrix metalloproteinase, inflammation, activation of the renin-angiotensin pathway, and the increased elaboration of reactive oxygen species. Matrix metalloproteinases are enzymes that degrade extracellular matrix proteins and participate in cell proliferation, differentiation, and apoptosis. Multiple matrix metalloproteinases, including 1, 3 (stromelysin-1), 9, and 13 (collagenase-3), are elevated in the aorta and blood of patients with abdominal aortic aneurysms.[3] The normal source of these enzymes includes endothelial cells, smooth muscle cells, and adventitial fibroblasts, but inflammation may play an important role in the adverse expression of matrix metalloproteinases. Inflammatory cells serve as important additional sources of matrix metalloproteinases. Most major components of cellular immunity, including neutrophils, T cells, B cells, and macrophages, are thought to participate in the inflammatory process. The inflammation underlying the formation of an aneurysm may be coordinated by the production of adverse cytokines that infiltrate the aortic wall.

Oxidative stress increases many components of aneurysmal formation, including induction of proinflammatory genes, activation of matrix metalloproteinases, and apoptosis. Superoxide anion, which is a potent oxygen-derived free radical, is found in excess in the smooth muscle and inflammatory cells of abdominal aortic aneurysm specimens. Important enzymatic sources of oxidants include nicotinamide adenine dinucleotide phosphate (NADPH) oxidase and uncoupled endothelial nitric oxide synthase.

In contrast to the formation of aneurysms in the abdomen, thoracic aortic aneurysms may have a more varied explanation. Among patients with Marfan syndrome, for example, 92% of males and 84% of females have aortic root dilatation. In addition to systemic genetic syndromes (e.g., Marfan, Turner syndrome), familial nonsyndromic conditions (e.g., bicuspid aortic valve), infections (e.g., syphilis, mycotic aneurysm), or inflammatory conditions (e.g., rheumatoid vasculitis), about 20 genetic abnormalities that predispose to heritable causes of thoracic aortic aneurysms have been identified.[4]

CLINICAL MANIFESTATIONS

The hallmark of aneurysms, both in the thorax and abdomen, is asymptomatic clinical silence until dissection or rupture.

Abdominal Aortic Aneurysms

Abdominal aortic aneurysms are almost always asymptomatic and are discovered incidentally on routine abdominal palpation, on an imaging study obtained for another purpose, or as part of a screening program. Slowly progressive enlargement can very rarely cause nerve compression or vertebral erosion. When an abdominal aortic aneurysm begins to leak or rupture, however, patients may complain of hypogastric, flank, lower back, or hip pain associated with tenderness on physical examination. An expanding hematoma can compress or impair the blood supply to the bowel or the urinary tract, thereby causing constipation, bloating, or urinary retention for hours to a few days. Acute rupture and cardiovascular collapse may occur unless the aneurysm is repaired.

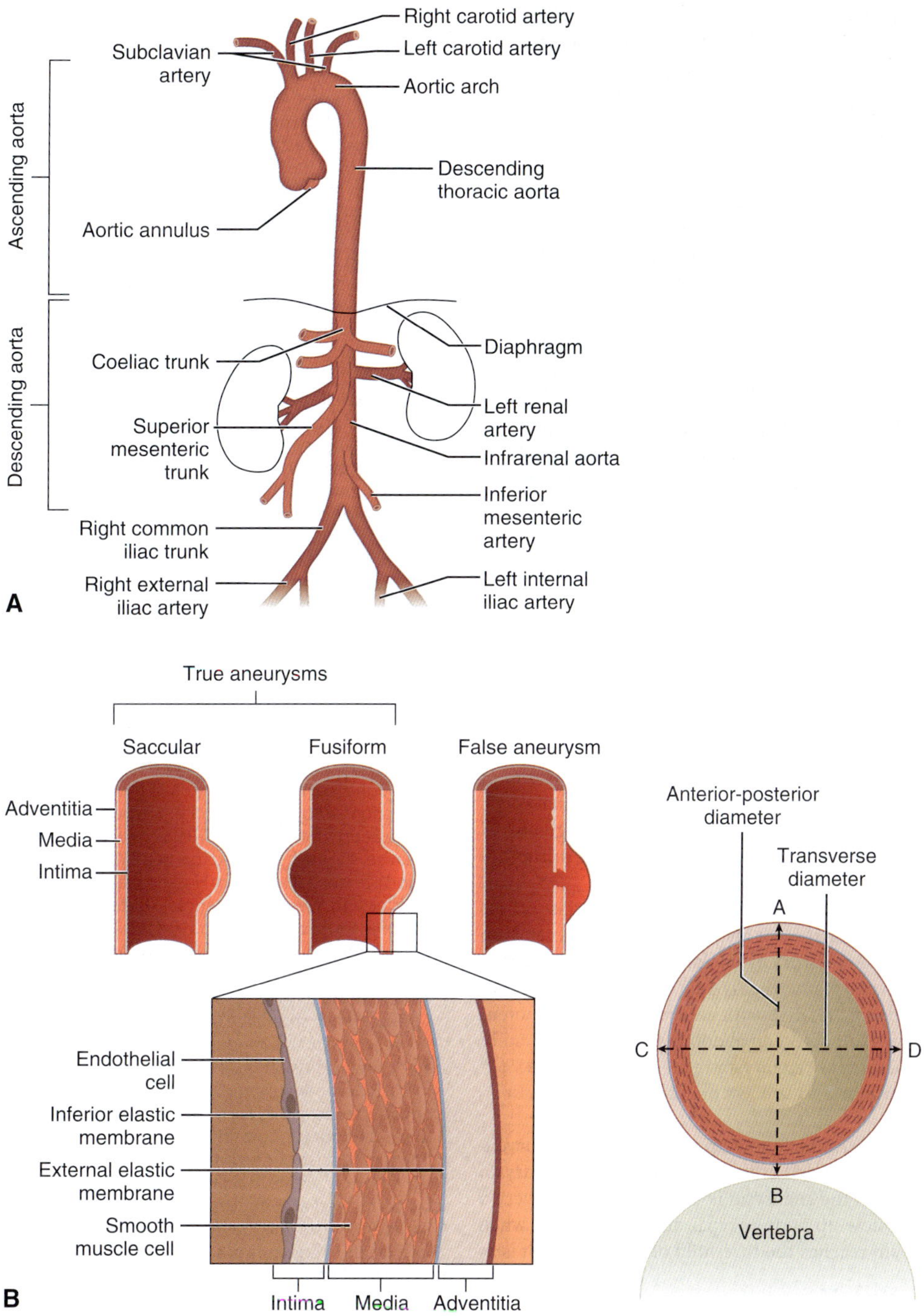

FIGURE 63-1. Schematic of the anatomy of the aorta. **A,** The aorta, which is divided into segments in the thorax and abdomen. **B,** The aorta has three layers: the intima, media, and adventitia. The formation of an aneurysm may occur in any segment. Fusiform aneurysms are a generalized expansion of the vessel, whereas saccular aneurysms represent a focal outpouching. (Reproduced from Sakalihasan N, Michel JB, Katsargyris A, et al. Abdominal aortic aneurysms. *Nat Rev Dis Primers*. 2018;4:34.)

TABLE 63-1 MEAN AORTIC DIMENSIONS FROM 15,000 NONCONTRAST CT SCANS

	MEN (N = 14,235)	WOMEN (N = 754)
Ascending aorta, mm	37.5 ± 4.1	34.1 ± 3.6
Aortic arch, mm	30.7 ± 2.9	28.1 ± 2.6
Descending aorta, mm	28.5 ± 2.7	25.2 ± 2.4
Abdominal aorta, mm	20.5 ± 4.8	16.6 ± 2.2

Adapted from Obel LM, Diederichsen AC, Steffensen FH, et al. Population-based risk factors for ascending, arch, descending, and abdominal aortic dilations for 60-74-year-old individuals. *J Am Coll Cardiol*. 2021;78:201-211.

Thoracic Aortic Aneurysms

As with abdominal aortic aneurysms, thoracic or thoracoabdominal aneurysms usually expand asymptomatically and are either discovered incidentally by echocardiography or thoracic imaging obtained for other reasons or are found on routine screening of patients with congenital causes. However, expanding thoracic aortic aneurysms, especially from systemic conditions such as syphilis, can sometimes compress adjacent mediastinal structures to cause chest pain, back pain, hoarseness, wheezing, coughing, and dysphagia. Rupture may present with chest or back pain, aortic valve insufficiency, and cardiovascular collapse.

DIAGNOSIS

Abdominal Aortic Aneurysms

An abdominal aortic aneurysm can often be palpated as a pulsatile mass a few centimeters cephalad from the umbilicus, which is at the level of the aortic bifurcation. By placing both hands with the palms down on the abdomen and an index finger at each side of the pulsation, the examiner can palpate the aneurysm and estimate its width. Any pulsatile abdominal mass that exceeds 2.5 to 3.0 cm by this method requires prompt abdominal ultrasonography for a more accurate measurement. An aortic diameter of 3 cm or more establishes the diagnosis of an aneurysm that requires ongoing surveillance.

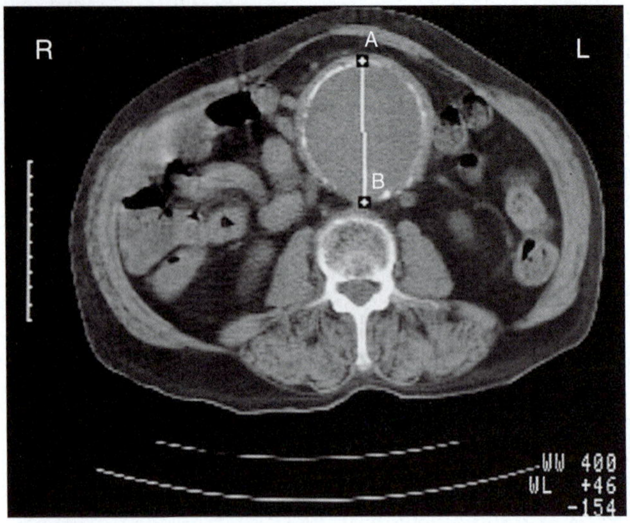

FIGURE 63-2. **Abdominal aortic aneurysm on computed tomography.** This sensitive imaging method allows precise measurement of size (*point A* to *point B*) and demonstrates the thickened wall of the aneurysm. (From Forbes CD, Jackson WF. *Color Atlas and Text of Clinical Medicine*. 3rd ed. London: Mosby; 2003.)

The diagnosis of a leaking or rupturing abdominal aortic aneurysm is a medical emergency. The classic findings of abdominal pain, hypotension, and a palpable pulsatile abdominal mass is insensitive, and any one of the three should be considered a warning sign, especially in older men with a history of smoking or in a patient with known aortic enlargement. An abdominal aortic aneurysm can be detected and measured by abdominal ultrasonography or by a CT scan (Fig. 63-2), but urgent CT is required when leaking or rupture is being considered.[5]

Because of the usual lack of symptoms, screening abdominal ultrasonography is uniformly recommended to assess for an abdominal aortic aneurysm in men ages 65 to 75 years with any history of smoking, and some guidelines recommend screening for men and women ages 65 to 75 years who have ever smoked or who have a first-degree relative with an abdominal aortic aneurysm. Such screening strategies can detect an abdominal aortic aneurysm in about 5.5% of examinations and reduce aneurysm-related mortality by 45%,[A1] although overall reductions in mortality are less dramatic because of associated comorbid conditions.[6]

Once the diagnosis is made, periodic follow-up ultrasonographic surveillance imaging is generally recommended every 2 to 3 years if the aneurysm is 3 to 3.9 cm, every 12 months if the aneurysm is 4.0 to 4.9 cm, and every 6 months if it is ≥5 cm. Such follow-up permits repair to be performed when an abdominal aortic aneurysm reaches the threshold of 5.5 cm, which is as safe as earlier repair.

Thoracic Aortic Aneurysms

Thoracic aortic aneurysms rarely can be palpated or detected on physical examination even when very large, so they are either found incidentally by a widened mediastinal silhouette or enlarged aortic knob on a chest radiograph or incidentally on an echocardiogram or a CT scan (Fig. 63-3) obtained for other indications.[7] Because of its low prevalence in the general population, routine screening is not recommended.

However, about 20% of thoracic aortic aneurysms are a result of genetic disorders, and screening transthoracic echocardiography is generally recommended in patients who have syndromes such as Marfan (Chapter 239), Loeys-Dietz, or vascular Ehlers-Danlos (Chapter 239), as well as in individuals who have a family history of aneurysmal disease or a first- or second-degree relative with a history of sudden or unexplained death at a young age. Screening should be repeated every 2 to 3 years if the size is normal.

Subsequent surveillance once an aneurysm is detected commonly requires CT imaging if the aorta is involved beyond the routine scanning range of echocardiography. A follow-up scan may be performed in 6 months and then every 6 to 24 months thereafter, based on the size of the aorta and the underlying condition. Surveillance imaging seeks to identify one of two criteria that would lead to referral for surgery: rapid growth or attainment of a specific size (see Treatment).

TREATMENT

Abdominal Aortic Aneurysm

The presence of an abdominal aortic aneurysm mandates aggressive risk modification (Chapter 40), including smoking cessation (Chapter 363), aggressive lowering of blood pressure (Chapter 64), and treatment of dyslipidemia (Chapter 190). Smoking cessation and treatment with high-intensity statins (Table 190-2), which may have some anti-inflammatory as well as hypolipidemic effects, have been associated with a reduced rate of aneurysmal growth and rupture in observational studies. No medical therapy has been proven to reduce the expansion of aneurysms.

Once an abdominal aortic aneurysm reaches the threshold for repair, intervention, whether by open surgical repair or endovascular repair,[8,9] reduces aneurysm-related mortality.[A2] The endovascular approach is preferable for reducing early morbidity and mortality, but both treatments are associated with similar survival after about 2 years and probably extending for at least a decade.[A3-A5] Unfortunately, endovascular repair is not worthwhile in patients whose overall surgical risk would exclude them from open repair because their all-cause mortality rate offsets any potential benefit from repair of the abdominal aortic aneurysm itself.[A6]

After open surgical repair, follow-up surveillance imaging is not needed. In contrast, the risk of late aortic rupture after endovascular repair is >5% over 8 years of follow-up, and current recommendations are for surveillance at 1 month, 12 months, and annually thereafter to delineate any potential endoleaks, stent migration, fracture, and noncontiguous aneurysms. Duplex ultrasound is recommended for surveillance if the first CT angiogram at 1 month does not demonstrate any endoleaks. Endoleaks may result in an abdominal aortic aneurysmal sac that is not depressurized by the placement of a graft. The two most worrisome are type 1 leaks, which occur as a result of an inadequate seal at the graft end, and type 2 leaks, in which the aneurysmal sac fills by a branch vessel (E-Fig. 63-1). Enlargement is a sign that the aneurysmal sac remains under increased or systemic pressure and may require repair.

Thoracic Aortic Aneurysm

Although data regarding medical therapies to reduce the rate of expansion, dissection, or rupture are limited, hypertension increases the risk of aortic dissection and rupture 2.7-fold. Patients with thoracic aortic aneurysm, regardless of cause, should be treated to a heart rate of 60 to 70 beats per minute, systolic blood pressure of ≤120 mm Hg, and diastolic pressure of ≤80 mm Hg by titrating a β-blocking agent (e.g., atenolol starting at 25 to 50 mg twice daily) and using angiotensin receptor blockers (e.g., irbesartan 150 mg daily increased to 300 mg daily as tolerated), or a combination of the two, based on data for the treatment of aortic enlargement in patients with Marfan syndrome.[A7] Isometric exercises, which can acutely increase peripheral arterial resistance and intrathoracic pressure, generally should be avoided.

In contrast to the standard size at which repair is recommended for abdominal aortic aneurysms, surgical recommendations vary depending on the cause of a thoracic aortic aneurysm. Upon diagnosis, a transthoracic echocardiogram is recommended to assess aortic diameters and aortic valvular function. In addition, the entire thoracic aorta should be imaged by CT scan because an aneurysm in one segment is a strong predictor of aneurysmal dilatation in another. Standard surveillance, with echocardiography if it can visualize the aneurysm, should be performed at 6 months after diagnosis and then annually. If the thoracic aortic aneurysm enlarges to within 0.5 cm of the size recommended for surgical referral, the frequency of surveillance imaging should increase to twice yearly.

Surgical repair of the aortic root or ascending aorta with resection of the aneurysm and an interposition graft replacement is recommended when an ascending or aortic root aneurysm reaches a diameter of 5.5 cm or greater or grows ≥5 mm in a single year in a nonsyndromic patient. In patients with a heritable cause of thoracic abdominal aneurysm (e.g., Marfan syndrome), the recommended size for repair is usually 5 cm, but it is 4.5 cm in patients who have high-risk features, including a family history of sudden death, rapid growth, or significant aortic valve regurgitation. In addition to size, the presence of symptoms arising from an aneurysm is an indication for repair. Urgent repair is required for severe pain or hemodynamic collapse.

For rare mycotic aortic aneurysms in patients who have survived bacterial endocarditis (Chapter 61), either open surgery or endovascular repair can be recommended. If endovascular repair is selected, long-term antibiotic treatment is recommended to prevent late recrudescence of infection.

PROGNOSIS

Aneurysms typically expand slowly over time, with an average growth in diameter of about 0.17 cm per year for abdominal aortic aneurysms,[10] and the risk of rupture increases accordingly. An abdominal aortic aneurysm below 5.5 cm in diameter has a 1% or lower annual rupture risk. For nonsyndromic thoracic aortic aneurysms, the 5-year rupture risk is essentially 0% if the aneurysm is below 4.0 cm in diameter but rises to about 15% for aneurysms 4.0 to 6.0 cm in diameter and about 30% if the aneurysm is larger than 6.0 cm in diameter in patients without inherited connective tissue disorders.[11]

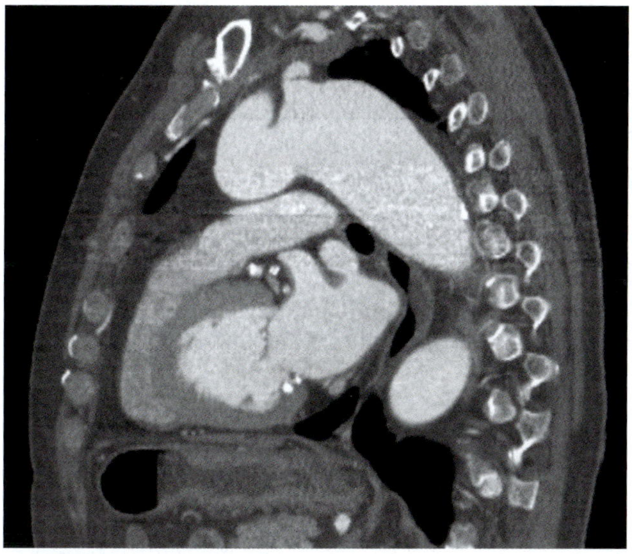

FIGURE 63-3. Sagittal plane computed tomographic image of a tortuous proximal descending aortic aneurysm.

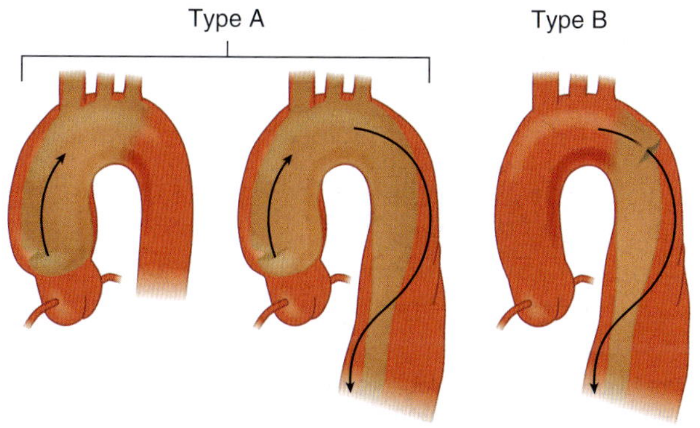

FIGURE 63-4. Schematic representation of types of aortic dissections by location.

The impact of an unruptured aneurysm, per se, on survival is modest, and there is no variation in survival whether an aneurysm is repaired at or below the recommended threshold size of 5.5 cm. However, life expectancy is reduced in patients who have an abdominal aortic aneurysm because of their higher rates of cardiovascular disease and cancer. In one study, for example, overall mortality was about 30% at 5 years and about 65% at 12 years.

When an aortic aneurysm leaks or ruptures, the mortality rate is about 75%, with about a 35% mortality rate even after emergent intervention. After endovascular repair, lifelong surveillance imaging is recommended, probably annually. The patient's prognosis is determined largely by risk factors and comorbid conditions rather than the aneurysm itself. Careful attention to blood pressure (Chapter 64) and lipid levels (Chapter 190) is indicated.

Survival in all-comers after repair of an ascending aortic aneurysm is 93% at 3 years and 80% at 8 years.[12] In patients with Marfan syndrome, results are similar after elective aortic root replacement.

ACUTE AORTIC SYNDROMES

DEFINITION

Acute aortic syndromes are an uncommon but life-threatening emergency. The three types of acute aortic syndrome are penetrating aortic ulceration, intramural hematoma, and aortic dissection.[13] Aortic dissection represents about 75% of all acute aortic syndromes.

EPIDEMIOLOGY

The incidence of acute aortic syndromes is likely underappreciated because as many as 1 in 15 out-of-hospital arrests may be due to aortic dissection, and an estimated 20 to 50% of patients die before the diagnosis can be made. In emergency departments, the incidence is about 5 to 8 cases per 100,000 patients per year.[14]

The peak age of incidence is between 50 and 70 years, and about two thirds of cases occur in men.[15] Key predisposing features include genetic abnormalities of the aorta (e.g., Marfan syndrome [Chapter 239]), arterial hypertension, a bicuspid aortic valve, advanced atherosclerosis, use of cocaine or methamphetamines, pregnancy,[16] prior known aortic aneurysm, aortitis, blunt trauma to the chest, heart surgery, and intraaortic catheter-based procedures.

PATHOBIOLOGY

Each of the acute aortic syndromes is characterized by a different mechanism of rupture in the aortic wall. The location of an acute aortic syndrome typically is defined by whether or not the site of dissection, origin of intramural hematoma, or penetrating aortic ulceration involves the ascending aorta (Fig. 63-4), because the initial lesion may propagate proximally as well as distally.

Aortic dissection is defined by the presence of an intimal tear that facilitates entry of the fully pressurized circulation into the media, thereby dividing it into two layers. The most common site of intimal tear is just beyond the level of the aortic valve for dissections that involve the ascending and/or transverse aorta (called type A dissections regardless of whether or not they extend into the descending aorta; see Fig. 63-5) and just beyond the insertion of the ligamentum arteriosum (where the mobile arch meets the fixed descending aorta) for dissections that are limited to the descending aorta (called type B dissections). The pulsatile blood flow propagates this separation, both distally and proximally, to create a false lumen or channel for blood flow. The false lumen may continue to extend, rupture back into the aortic true lumen, or rupture outward.

The complications of aortic dissection include rupture and end-organ malperfusion. Common sites of rupture include the pericardial space, thereby leading to cardiac tamponade in type A dissection and the left pleural space in type B dissection. Compromised blood flow to viscera or limbs may be the result of compression of the branch vessels by the hematoma within the false lumen, extension of the dissection within a branch vessel, or swinging movement of the dissection flap over the branch vessel.

Intramural hematoma, which is the second most common form of acute aortic syndrome, is usually found in 20 to 25% of cases in Western populations and as high as 40% of cases in Asian populations. In contrast to a dissection, the intramural hematoma is collection of blood in the wall of the aorta as a result of rupture of the vaso vasorum or an unappreciated intimal microtear. Unlike the linear tear seen on imaging with a dissection, an intramural hematoma appears as a round or crescent-shaped thickening without connection to the active circulation in the lumen. In Western populations, almost 50% of intramural hematomas progress to frank intimal tear and dissection, but intramural hematoma appears to carry a lower risk of morbidity and mortality than aortic dissection in East Asian populations.

A penetrating aortic ulcer, which probably represents about 5% of acute aortic syndromes, is initiated by ulceration of an atherosclerotic plaque. Disruption of the internal elastic lamina permits penetration of blood through the intima into the medial layers but, at least initially, no further. Because aortic atherosclerosis is most common in the descending aorta, this portion of the aorta is the most common segment for a penetrating aortic ulcer.

CLINICAL MANIFESTATIONS

For type A aortic dissections, which involve the ascending aorta, the vast majority of patients present as an acute aortic syndrome, with the sudden onset of severe anterior chest pain that is described as the most severe or worst pain ever experienced. Pain often radiates to the neck or jaw with an ascending aortic dissection and to the back and sometimes to the abdomen if the dissection extends to the descending aorta (Table 63-2). Tearing or ripping pain, once thought to be common, is reported in fewer than half of patients. In up to 20% of patients, however, syncope is the presenting symptom.

For type B dissection, severe pain is reported by more than 90% of patients. Back pain is reported in 55 to 80% of patients, but chest or abdominal pain is also common. Syncope is present in less than 5% of patients.

Other symptoms and signs can indicate compromise of aortic branch blood vessels and malperfusion or impingement on adjacent structures. For example, the presence of abdominal pain may indicate mesenteric ischemia (Chapter 129). Severe dyspnea or collapse may arise when retrograde extension causes aortic valve regurgitation or when rupture into the pericardial space causes cardiac tamponade. Paraplegia may be a result of spinal vascular malperfusion. Oliguria or hematuria can be the direct result of involvement of the renal arteries. Cerebral malperfusion, sometimes with a stroke, occurs in 6

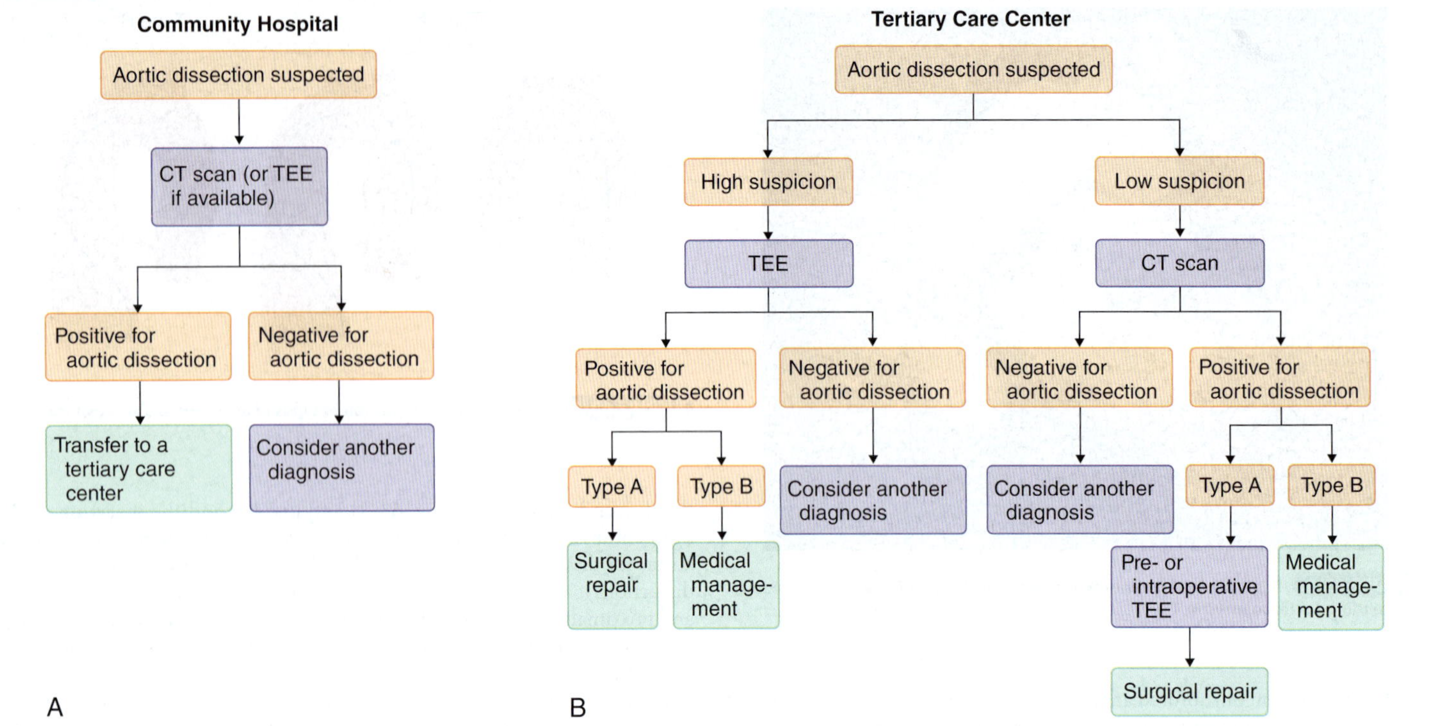

FIGURE 63-5. **Algorithms for the evaluation of suspected acute aortic dissection. A,** This approach is used in many community hospitals where cardiac surgery is not performed. **B,** This approach is used in many tertiary care centers where transesophageal echocardiography (TEE) and cardiac surgery are available. CT = computed tomography. (Courtesy of Eric M. Isselbacher, MD.)

TABLE 63-2 HIGH-RISK CHARACTERISTICS FOR ACUTE AORTIC DISSECTION

High-Risk Predisposing Conditions • Marfan syndrome • Family history of aortic disease • Known aortic valve disease • Recent aortic manipulation • Known thoracic aortic aneurysm
High-Risk Pain Chest, back, or abdominal pain described as the following: • Abrupt in onset • Severe in intensity • Ripping or tearing

High-Risk Physical Examination
• Evidence of perfusion deficit
  • Pulse deficit
  • Systolic blood pressure differential
  • Focal neurologic deficit (in conjunction with pain)
• Murmur of aortic insufficiency (new or not known to be old and in conjunction with pain)
• Hypotension or shock state

Adapted from Rogers AM, Hermann LK, Booher AM, et al. Sensitivity of the aortic dissection detection risk score, a novel guideline-based tool for identification of acute aortic dissection at initial presentation: results from the international registry of acute aortic dissection. *Circulation.* 2011;123:2213-2218.

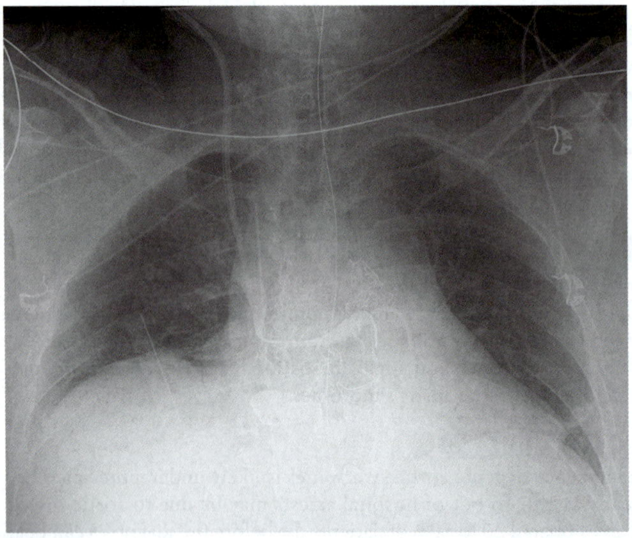

FIGURE 63-6. **Chest radiograph in ascending aortic dissection. Note the widened mediastinum.**

to 14% of proximal aortic dissection patients because of a partial or complete occlusion of the great vessels.

DIAGNOSIS

The significant early mortality associated with acute aortic syndromes can be reduced with rapid clinical evaluation and imaging (Fig. 63-5). The physical examination should include a complete cardiac and vascular inspection. Key high-risk findings include pulse deficits, a murmur of aortic valvular insufficiency, hypotension, and a focal neurologic deficit (particularly with pain). If patients have two of three high-risk characteristics (predisposing conditions, typical pain, suspicious findings on physical examination; see Table 63-2), emergent aortic imaging is required. If patients have one of the features, any chest pain syndrome (see Table 39-2) without clear evidence of an alternative diagnosis should prompt consideration of urgent imaging, especially if the chest radiograph shows any evidence of aortic widening.

Chest radiographs show a widened mediastinum (Fig. 63-6) in about 50% of type A dissections but are rarely diagnostic. Electrocardiography is also commonly abnormal and can show an inferior or anterior wall myocardial infarction if retrograde dissection compromises the ostium of the right or left coronary artery, respectively; in large series each of the two coronary ostia is equally likely to be compromised.[17] Transthoracic echocardiography has an 85 to 90% sensitivity for diagnosing aneurysms of the ascending aorta and can provide additional information about ventricular and valvular function, but it is not accurate for type B dissection. Transesophageal echocardiography (Fig. 63-7) raises the sensitivity for detecting a type A dissection to about 98% and may show the luminal tear but again is not very accurate for type B dissection. As a result, CT angiography, which is available in many emergency departments, is usually the test of choice for detecting proximal (Fig. 63-8) or distal (Fig. 63-9) aortic dissection, intramural hematoma (Fig. 63-10), or penetrating

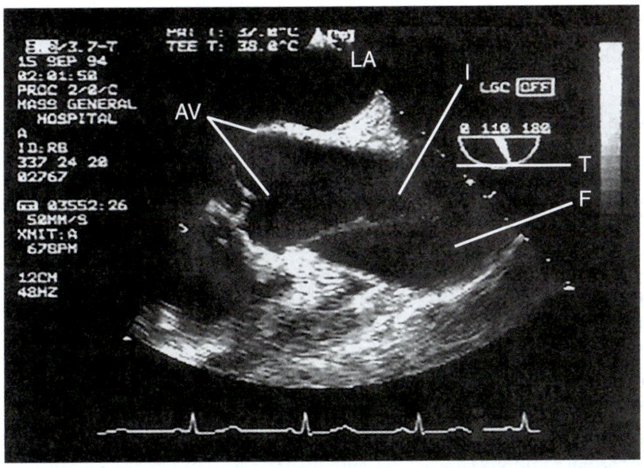

FIGURE 63-7. **Transesophageal echocardiogram of the ascending aorta in the long axis in a patient with type A aortic dissection.** The aortic valve (AV) is on the *left*, and the ascending aorta extends to the *right*. Within the aorta is an intimal flap (I) that originates at the level of the sinotubular junction. The true (T) and the false (F) lumens are separated by the intimal flap. LA = left atrium. (From Isselbacher EM. Diseases of the aorta. In: Braunwald E, Zipes DP, Libby P, Bonow RO, eds. *Braunwald's Heart Disease: A Textbook of Cardiovascular Medicine*. 7th ed. Philadelphia: Saunders; 2004:1423.)

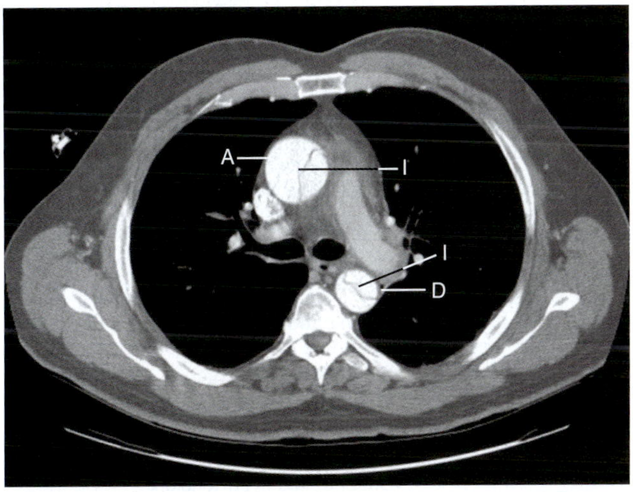

FIGURE 63-8. **Aortic dissection.** Contrast-enhanced computed tomography scan of the chest at the level of the pulmonary artery shows an intimal flap (I) separating the two lumens of the ascending (A) and descending (D) thoracic aorta in a type A aortic dissection. (Courtesy of Eric M. Isselbacher, MD.)

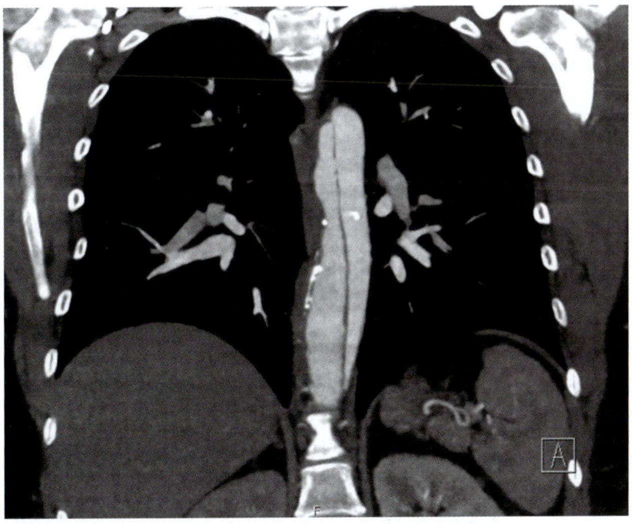

FIGURE 63-9. **Coronal plane computed tomography angiogram of a type B aortic dissection.**

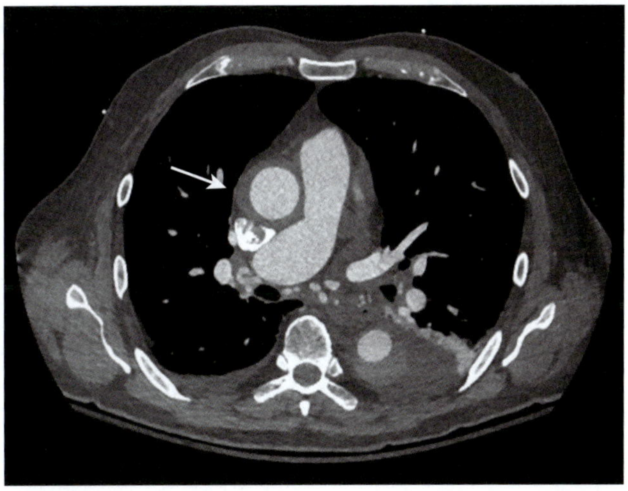

FIGURE 63-10. **Axial plane computed tomography angiographic of an ascending aorta intramural hematoma.** The *arrow* identifies the crescenteric wall thickening.

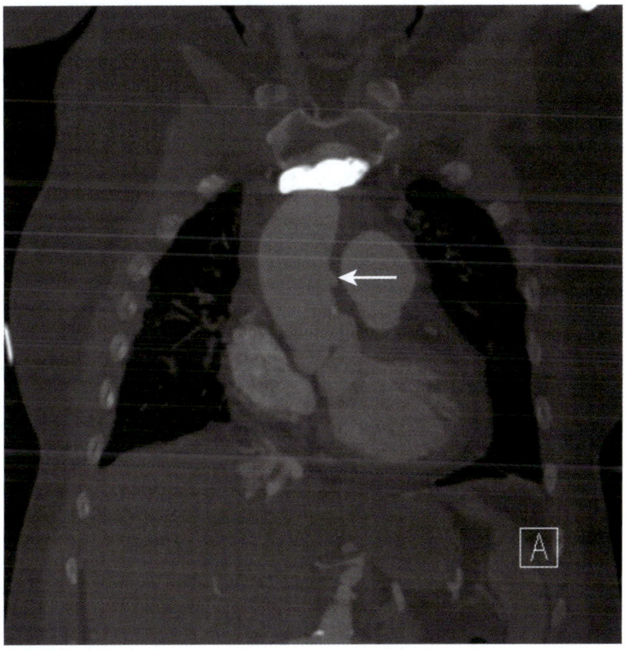

FIGURE 63-11. **Computed tomographic angiogram showing a penetrating aortic ulcer.** Coronal plane computed tomography angiographic image of an ascending aorta penetrating ulcer. The *arrow* identifies the outpouching of the ulceration.

aortic ulcer (Fig. 63-11). Magnetic resonance (MR) angiography is equally accurate but typically requires significantly more time in a poorly supervised setting for a critically ill patient. As a result, it is more commonly used as a second-line examination when clinical suspicion requires additional testing.

TREATMENT

Acute Type A Aortic Dissection and Intramural Hematoma

As soon as the diagnosis of a type A aortic dissection or intramural hematoma is made, surgical consultation should be obtained and arrangements should be made to transfer the patient to a high-volume facility if possible. In the meantime, acute medical management requires aggressive blood pressure control with agents that also decrease cardiac inotropy (Fig. 63-12). The goal of medical therapy is a systolic blood pressure of 100 to 120 mm Hg with a heart rate of 60 to 70 beats per minute. The first line of therapy is an intravenous β-adrenergic blocker, such as esmolol, labetalol, or metoprolol (Table 63-3). Should blood pressure control not be achieved despite realizing heart rates ≤60 beats per minute, intravenous vasodilators should be administered as second-line therapy. In addition to hemodynamic therapy, narcotic analgesia (Table 26-6) should be provided for treatment of pain. In the setting of spontaneous hypotension, pseudohypotension resulting from limb vascular compromise must be excluded, the cause must be ascertained, and hemodynamic support should be provided en route to emergency surgery (Chapter 93).

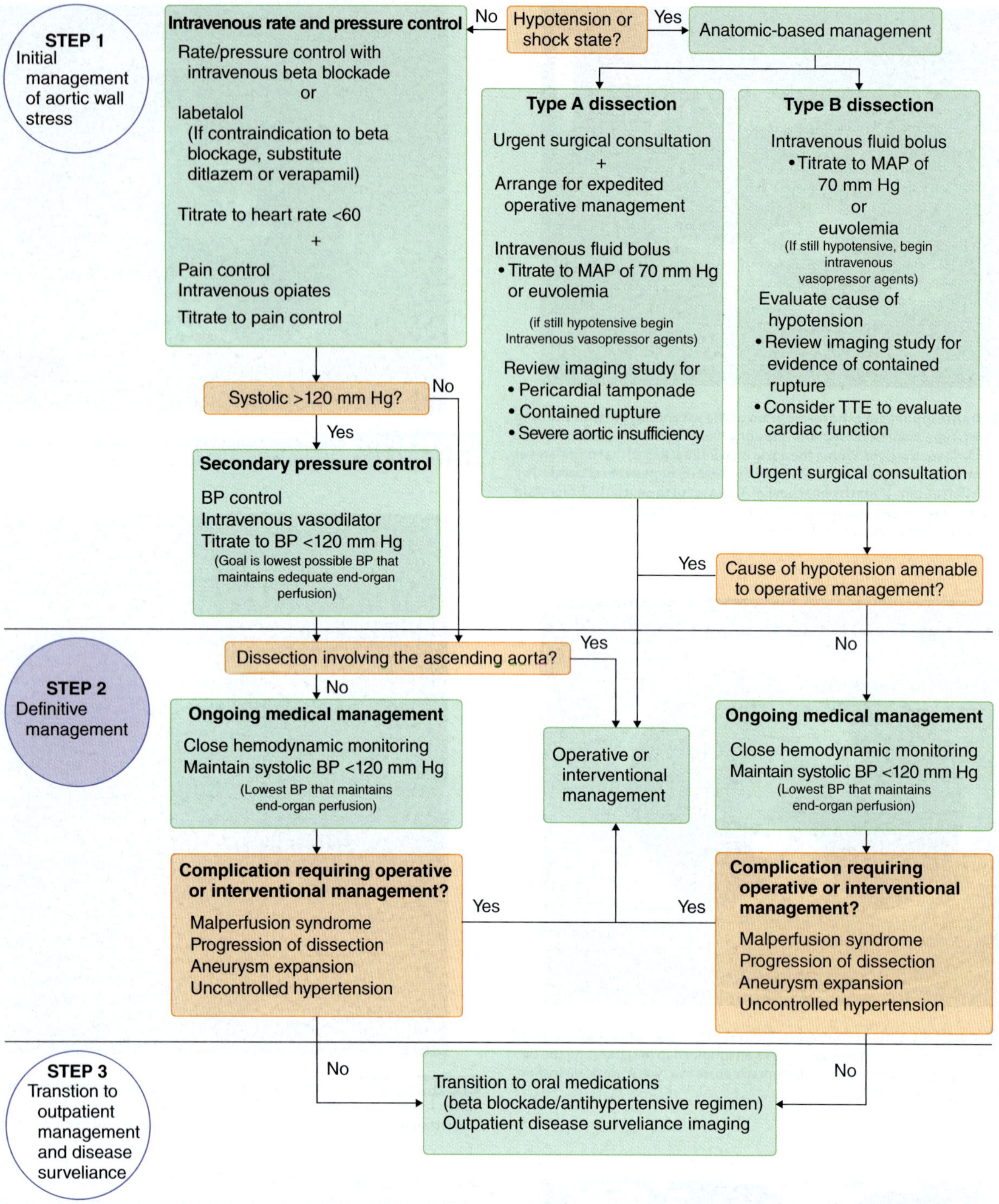

FIGURE 63-12. **Management pathway for acute aortic dissection.** AoD = aortic dissection; BP = blood pressure; MAP = mean arterial pressure. (Adapted from Hiratzka LF, Bakris GL, Beckman JA, et al. 2010 ACCF/AHA/AATS/ACR/ASA/SCA/SCAI/SIR/STS/SVM guidelines for the diagnosis and management of patients with thoracic aortic disease: executive summary. A report of the American College of Cardiology Foundation/American Heart Association Task Force on Practice Guidelines, American Association for Thoracic Surgery, American College of Radiology, American Stroke Association, Society of Cardiovascular Anesthesiologists, Society for Cardiovascular Angiography and Interventions, Society of Interventional Radiology, Society of Thoracic Surgeons, and Society for Vascular Medicine. *J Am Coll Cardiol*. 2010;55:e27-e129.)

For type A aortic dissection or intramural hematoma, prompt surgical repair of the ascending aorta is indicated, if possible, even in the setting of complications such as cardiac tamponade, aortic rupture, or stroke. For type A aneurysms, urgent surgical repair reduces death by more than 50% compared with medical therapy alone.[18,19] In patients who have malperfusion syndromes of the abdomen or lower extremity, repair of the ascending aorta should be performed first.

Acute Type B Aortic Dissection or Intramural Hematoma

The acute treatment of aortic dissections that do not involve the ascending aorta and of intramural hematomas is more nuanced. In the absence of ongoing pain, malperfusion syndromes, or rupture, type B aortic dissections usually should be treated medically, initially with an approach similar to the approach for type A lesions (Table 63-3). Interventional treatment is recommended, however, for type B aortic dissections with complications such as rupture, ongoing extension of the dissection, unremitting pain, or a visceral or peripheral malperfusion. For type B aortic dissection, endovascular stent grafting, including the placement of stent grafts or the creation of a channel through the dissection flap to decompress a hypertensive false lumen, is preferred over surgical repair.

Once blood pressure and pulse have been acutely controlled, the patient should be weaned from intravenous medications and switched to an oral regimen. The oral regimen should emphasize β-blockers[20] with adjunctive angiotensin-converting enzyme inhibitors or angiotensin receptor blockers (see Table 64-7).

Penetrating Aortic Ulcers

The acute medical management of a symptomatic penetrating aortic ulcer mirrors that of type A aortic dissection (Table 63-3). Ascending aortic penetrating atherosclerotic aortic ulcers should be repaired when they are associated with symptoms. Symptomatic penetrating aortic ulcers of the descending aorta are usually managed medically as for type B dissections. However, stable penetrating ulcers of the descending aorta and isolated asymptomatic penetrating aortic ulcers identified on CT angiographic scanning have a low (<4%) risk of progressing and should be managed medically as for a stable type B dissection.[21]

TABLE 63-3 ACUTE MEDICAL THERAPY FOR AORTIC DISSECTION*

Intravenous β-Blocker (Preferred Negative Inotrope)
- Esmolol: 250-500 μg/kg IV bolus followed by a 50-200 μg/kg/min infusion, titrated to effect
- Labetalol: 20 mg IV bolus over 2 min, followed by 20-80 mg IV every 10 min, then 0.5-2 mg/min IV fusion
- Metoprolol: 2.5-15 mg IV bolus followed by 2.5-15 mg IV every 3-6 hr

Intravenous Vasodilator (After Initiation of Negative Inotrope)
- Clevidipine: Start at 1-2 mg/hr, up to maximum of 16-32 mg/hr
- Sodium nitroprusside: Start at 0.25-0.5 μg/kg/min, up to a maximum of 8-10 μg/min (only in presence of β-blockers to avoid tachycardia and with careful observation to avoid thiocyanate toxicity with prolonged perfusion, especially in patients with renal impairment)
- Nicardipine: 2.5-5 mg/hr (to a maximum of 15 mg/hr)
- Nitroglycerin: 5 μg/min infusion (to a maximum 200 μg/min)
- Enalaprilat: 1.25 mg, then 1.25-5 mg IV every 6 hr
- Fenoldopam: Start at 0.1 μg/kg/min and titrate up to a maximum of 1.6 μg/kg/min

*Goal of therapy is heart rate less than 70 beats/min and blood pressure 100-120 mm Hg or as low as possible without compromising organ perfusion.

Adapted from Braverman AC, Schermerhorn M. Diseases of the aorta. In: Libby P, Bonow RO, Mann DL, Tomaselli GF, Bhatt D, Solomon SD, Braunwald E, eds. *Braunwald's Heart Disease: A Textbook of Cardiovascular Medicine*, 12th ed. Philadelphia: Elsevier; 2022.

PROGNOSIS

Mortality for type A dissections and intramural hematoma is 1 to 2% per hour in untreated patients, peaks within the first 24 hours, remains quite high from days 2 to 7 but is lower from days 8 to 30 and chronically thereafter (E-Fig. 63-2). Despite the delay, however, interfacility transfer from a low-volume hospital to a high-volume hospital is associated with a better short- and long-term outcome. For type B dissections, the acute mortality is lower, but the time pattern of mortality is similar.

The unadjusted 1-year survival for type A aortic dissection is 96% after repair compared with 89% with medical therapy, and the mortality curves continue to separate over time, with deaths about 2.5-fold more likely in patients who are treated medically. Predictors of death included older age, a history of atherosclerosis, prior cardiac surgery, and poorer control of blood pressure.

The survival for patients with type B aortic dissection is about 80% at 3 years. Predictors of mortality include older age, female sex, a history of prior aortic aneurysm, a history of atherosclerosis, in-hospital renal failure, and hypotension or shock. Surveillance imaging after hospitalization is recommended at 1, 6, and 12 months and annually thereafter. Adherence to careful follow-up and good control of blood pressure is associated with better outcomes.[22]

AORTIC VASCULITIS

Two large-vessel inflammatory diseases involve the aorta—giant cell arteritis and Takayasu arteritis (E-Fig. 63-3).[23]

GIANT CELL ARTERITIS

Giant cell arteritis, which is the most common vasculitis in the United States (Chapter 250), has an age-adjusted prevalence of 204 per 100,000 among persons older than age 50 years, with similar frequencies in White and Black patients. Giant cell arteritis commonly involves aortic branch vessels but may involve the aorta itself in up to 30% of cases. Markers of inflammation, such as the erythrocyte sedimentation rate (ESR) and C-reactive protein level, are increased in the vast majority of patients. The primary risk for adverse outcomes is the development of aortic aneurysm or dissection, with these risks about double that of unaffected individuals.

CLINICAL MANIFESTATIONS AND DIAGNOSIS

The hallmark clinical manifestations of aortic involvement are related to vascular insufficiency, commonly including fatigue and claudication of the upper extremities and sometimes of the lower extremities. Patients may complain of headache, fatigue, muscle aches, jaw claudication, and amaurosis fugax. On physical examination, diminished or absent pulses and diminished blood pressure are noted in the upper extremities. The temporal artery may also be tender and tortuous. Bruits may be audible over the involved arteries, and vigorous exercise of the involved extremity may reveal pallor from diminished circulation.

The diagnosis of giant cell arteritis is based on the presence of three of five criteria including age over 50 years, ESR ≥50 mm/hour, a temporal artery abnormality (tenderness), new-onset headache, and/or temporal artery biopsy showing mononuclear or granulomatous inflammation, commonly with giant cell infiltrates (see Chapter 250).[24] Ultrasonographic imaging of the temporal artery or one of its branches[25] with a hypoechoic halo sign around the lumen is also a useful diagnostic sign.[26] The extent of aortic involvement can be determined by CT angiography or MR angiography.

TREATMENT

In patients with visual symptoms, treatment should be started even while awaiting biopsy results. Otherwise, medical therapy with 40 to 60 mg per day of prednisone (or its equivalent) should be started as soon as the diagnosis is established. The dose can be tapered based on clinical response and normalization of the ESR.[27] After the patient is stabilized, tocilizumab (an anti-interleukin 6 receptor antibody at 162 mg subcutaneously weekly) should be started, and corticosteroids usually can be tapered or discontinued within about 6 months.[A8] Methotrexate (15 to 25 mg per week) also has modest benefit.[A9] Adding abatacept (10 mg/kg on days 1, 15, and 29 and week 8) to prednisone also can reduce the risk of relapse.[A10]

Endovascular intervention may be required for severe stenoses. Should a large aneurysm be diagnosed and surgical repair deemed necessary, surgery should be delayed, if possible, until remission of the active inflammatory state has been achieved to avoid surgical complications.

TAKAYASU ARTERITIS

Takayasu arteritis, which is the most common cause of aortitis in persons under age 40 years, is more common in women than in men. It occurs in 2 to 3 persons per million in the United States, is most prevalent in East Asia, but is seen worldwide. Takayasu arteritis typically affects the major aorta branch vessels, including the innominate, carotid, and subclavian arteries, but it also can affect the thoracic and abdominal aorta.[28]

Takayasu arteritis is a panarteritis in which all layers of the artery are involved. In its early stages, the aorta and its branches show active inflammation. As the disease progresses, a sclerotic stage with intimal hyperplasia, medial degeneration, and obliterative changes is common. Takayasu arteritis also can occasionally involve the pulmonary artery. Most arterial lesions are stenotic, but aneurysms may also be seen.

CLINICAL MANIFESTATIONS AND DIAGNOSIS

The presentation of Takayasu arteritis may include constitutional symptoms (e.g., fevers, night sweats, weight loss, myalgias, arthralgias), but arterial occlusive disease is the predominant manifestation, with aortic symptoms and signs similar to giant cell arteritis. Aneurysms form in less than 5% of patients.

Pulses may be diminished or absent in the upper extremities, and blood pressure may be different in the two arms. Bruits may be audible over affected arteries. More than 50% of patients are hypertensive because of renal artery involvement, but hypertension may be obscured on routine examination because of the diminished pulses. Involvement of the proximal aorta can cause aortic valve insufficiency. Involvement of the coronary ostia can cause angina or myocardial infarction. Cerebral ischemia or stroke may result from involvement of the carotid artery, and compromise of the mesenteric circulation may cause abdominal angina.

Laboratory abnormalities include an elevated C-reactive protein level, an elevated ESR, anemia, mild leukocytosis, and elevated immunoglobulin levels. Diagnostic criteria include age <40 years at onset, claudication of extremities, a decreased brachial artery pulse, a systolic blood pressure difference >10 mm Hg between arms, a bruit over subclavian arteries or aorta, and an arteriographic abnormality on CT or MR angiography or contrast aortography. On imaging, Takayasu arteritis can be diffuse or patchy, and it is usually most prominent at aorta branch points and in the abdominal aorta.

TREATMENT

Corticosteroid therapy (e.g., prednisone 40 to 60 mg daily or the equivalent) is the foundation of therapy to reduce the inflammation and arrest the inflammatory process. Methotrexate (15 to 25 mg/week) is commonly given as an adjunct to corticosteroid therapy. Tofacitinib 5 mg twice daily may be as good as or better than methotrexate.[29] Tocilizumab is also used, but the supporting data are not as strong as in giant cell arteritis.[A11] Routine follow-up with monitoring of disease activity, both by blood-based markers and imaging, is recommended. Percutaneous stent-based treatments are effective and can be repeated if needed.[30] As with giant cell arteritis, endovascular and surgical procedures have better outcomes when performed in periods of disease remission.

PROGNOSIS

About 50% of patients relapse within 10 years. The 15-year survival rate is about 95% in patients without major complications but only about 65% in patients with major complications. The predominant causes of morbidity and mortality are cardiovascular, including myocardial infarction, heart failure, pulmonary hypertension, and aortic aneurysm rupture.

GENERAL REFERENCES

For the General References and other additional features, please visit Elsevier eBooks+ at https://ebooks.health.elsevier.com.

Grade A References

A1. Guirguis-Blake JM, Beil TL, Senger CA, et al. Primary care screening for abdominal aortic aneurysm: updated evidence report and systematic review for the US Preventive Services Task Force. *JAMA*. 2019;322:2219-2238.
A2. Takagi H, Ando T, Umemoto T. Abdominal aortic aneurysm screening reduces all-cause mortality. *Angiology*. 2018;69:205-211.
A3. van Schaik TG, Yeung KK, Verhagen HJ, et al. Long-term survival and secondary procedures after open or endovascular repair of abdominal aortic aneurysms. *J Vasc Surg*. 2017;66:1379-1389.
A4. Lederle FA, Kyriakides TC, Stroupe KT, et al. Open versus endovascular repair of abdominal aortic aneurysm. *N Engl J Med*. 2019;380:2126-2135.
A5. Patel R, Sweeting MJ, Powell JT, et al. Endovascular versus open repair of abdominal aortic aneurysm in 15-years' follow-up of the UK endovascular aneurysm repair trial 1 (EVAR trial 1): a randomised controlled trial. *The Lancet*. 2016;388:2366-2374.
A6. Sweeting MJ, Patel R, Powell JT, et al. Endovascular repair of abdominal aortic aneurysm in patients physically ineligible for open repair: very long-term follow-up in the EVAR-2 randomized controlled trial. *Ann Surg*. 2017;266:713-719.
A7. Wang Z, Deng X, Kang X, et al. Angiotensin receptor blockers vs. beta-blocker therapy for Marfan syndrome: a systematic review and meta-analysis. *Ann Vasc Surg*. 2022;82:347-361.
A8. Spiera R, Unizony SH, Bao M, et al. Tocilizumab vs placebo for the treatment of giant cell arteritis with polymyalgia rheumatica symptoms, cranial symptoms or both in a randomized trial. *Semin Arthritis Rheum*. 2021;51:469-476.
A9. Song GG, Lee YH. Methotrexate for treating polymyalgia rheumatica: a meta-analysis of randomized controlled trials. *Int J Clin Pharmacol Ther*. 2021;59:366-371.
A10. Langford CA, Cuthbertson D, Ytterberg SR, et al. A randomized, double-blind trial of abatacept (CTLA-4Ig) for the treatment of giant cell arteritis. *Arthritis Rheumatol*. 2017;69:837-845.
A11. Singh A, Danda D, Hussain S, et al. Efficacy and safety of tocilizumab in treatment of Takayasu arteritis: a systematic review of randomized controlled trials. *Mod Rheumatol*. 2021;31:197-204.

64

ARTERIAL HYPERTENSION

JOHN M. FLACK

DEFINITION

Obtaining accurate blood pressure readings in any setting requires observer training, use of validated and calibrated devices, and adherence to a rigorous measurement protocol. The current threshold for diagnosing arterial hypertension is 130/80 mm Hg or greater.[1] The diagnosis should be confirmed by averaging multiple blood pressure readings over several temporally spaced visits, with confirmation by home measurements or by ambulatory blood pressure readings.

However, the cardiovascular risk associated with blood pressure begins at a systolic blood pressure of 100 mm Hg, and every increase of 10 mm Hg above that level is associated with about a 50% higher risk for atherosclerotic vascular disease.[2] Since risk rises at blood pressure levels that are well below the threshold for initiating pharmacologic therapies or the goals of therapy, primordial prevention of hypertension is key for mitigating the risk for pressure-related complications in the nonhypertensive population. In clinical trials, a treatment target of less than 120 mm Hg systolic is the most beneficial, but an office blood pressure target of 130/80 mm Hg or less is reasonable because blood pressures that are measured without standard protocols in most clinical settings are systematically higher than blood pressure readings obtained in clinical trials or on home monitoring.

EPIDEMIOLOGY

Aging and Pulse Pressure

In industrialized societies, systolic blood pressure rises with advancing age, whereas diastolic blood pressure plateaus in the sixth decade of life and declines thereafter (Fig. 64-1). Both systolic and diastolic blood pressure are important cardiovascular risk factors, but systolic blood pressure accounts for most of the pressure-related cardiovascular risk after middle age.

Arterial hypertension, defined at a threshold of 140/90 mm Hg, affects nearly 1.4 billion adults worldwide, with approximately three-quarters of all hypertensive individuals living in low- and middle-income countries, where the incidence of hypertension is rising much faster than in high-income countries.[3] Worldwide, hypertension is the leading cause of preventable death and is the number one reason for ambulatory office visits. In the United States, the prevalence of hypertension at the 140/90 mm Hg threshold has been declining since 2000, but its prevalence at the 130/80 mm Hg threshold is 45%, thereby affecting more than 115 million U.S. adults aged 20 years and older. In the United States, the prevalence of hypertension is higher in men (49%) than women (43%), but women have a higher prevalence than men after age 65 years.

The worldwide prevalence of hypertension varies considerably by geography. It is highest in Eastern Europe and Central Asia and lowest in South Asia. In high-income countries, hypertension is more prevalent in rural than in urban areas, but its prevalence is greater in urban than in rural areas in low- and middle-income countries. In the United States, the prevalence of hypertension is inversely related to educational attainment.

The relationship between blood pressure and cardiovascular risk begins at systolic blood pressure levels greater than 100 mm Hg, and most incident cardiovascular disease events occur in adults whose blood pressures are less than 140/90 mm Hg, whether naturally or while taking antihypertensive medications. Systolic blood pressure is a more important determinant of cardiovascular risk than diastolic blood pressure, at least for persons who are middle-aged and older.

In recent years, U.S. rates of control of hypertension to less than 140/90 mm Hg has begun to worsen after many decades of incrementally better control.[4] Since most blood pressure–related cardiovascular events occur in adults whose blood pressure levels are lower than levels that qualify for initial pharmacologic treatment (140/90 mm Hg), pharmacologic therapy of preexisting hypertension will never suffice to ameliorate the population burden of pressure-related complications.

Sex, Race, and Ethnicity

The prevalence of hypertension varies by race and ethnicity. In the United States, the prevalence is higher in non-Hispanic Blacks (59% of men, 56% of women) than in non-Hispanic Whites (48% of men, 41% of women), Asians (46% of men, 36% of women), and Hispanics (47% of men, 41% of women).[5] Not only is hypertension more prevalent in non-Hispanic Black adults relative to any other race-ethnicity group, it is also more severe and is preceded by higher blood pressure levels beginning in childhood. The prevalence of hypertension is higher in Black Americans who reside in the southeastern United States than in those living outside of that geographic region. A southern U.S.

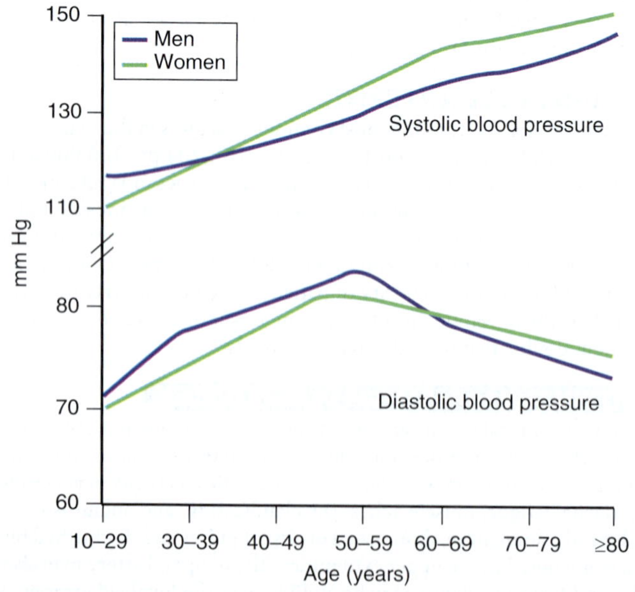

FIGURE 64-1. Aging and blood pressure. Age-dependent changes in systolic and diastolic blood pressure in the United States. (From Burt V, Whelton P, Rocella EJ, et al. Prevalence of hypertension in the U.S. adult population: results from the Third National Health and Nutrition Examination Survey, 1988-1991. *Hypertension*. 1995;25:305-313.)

dietary pattern appears to account for nearly one third (women) to half (men) of the excess risk of developing hypertension in Black compared with White Americans.[6] Pressure-related complications, such as stroke and heart failure, also occur disproportionately in non-Hispanic Black Americans, and their age-adjusted death rates are approximately two-fold higher compared with those of non-Hispanic White Americans. Black Americans who move from high to low segregation census tracts have significantly lower blood pressures than do those who remain in highly segregated areas.

Black populations do not invariably have higher blood pressure than White populations. The prevalence of hypertension is higher in several predominantly White European countries than in non-Hispanic Black Americans or Black Africans (E-Fig. 64-1). The prevalence of hypertension is similar in Black and non-Black Hispanic Cuban adults.

PATHOBIOLOGY

Normal Circulatory Physiology

Systole accounts for about one third of the cardiac cycle, and the cardiac stroke volume (the amount of blood propelled forward from the left ventricle with each heartbeat) is primarily ejected during the first half of systole (Chapter 41). However, blood flow is continuous throughout the cardiac cycle. A compliant aorta readily expands during systole and partially stores stroke volume. After the conclusion of active cardiac systole, the elastic recoil of the aorta provides a mechanical advantage to the pumping heart by propelling the stored blood volume forward, thereby damping the fall in blood pressure during diastole. Reflected pressure waveforms from the peripheral resistance arterioles normally arrive back at the aorta during diastole, thereby augmenting coronary artery perfusion, which occurs exclusively during diastole. Pulse pressure (systolic blood pressure minus diastolic blood pressure) is determined by the rise in pressure inside the arterial vasculature in response to the stroke volume that was ejected during systole.

Age-Related Changes

The development of hypertension is not an invariable consequence of normal aging. Age-related pathologic changes (e.g., vascular remodeling, endothelial dysfunction, atherosclerosis) reduce compliance and stiffen the aorta and large capacitance vessels, thereby resulting in less storage of the stroke volume in the aorta (E-Fig. 64-2). This change causes the forward pressure wave to travel faster and reflect back more quickly from the peripheral resistance arterioles, where it merges with the forward pressure wave, thereby augmenting systolic blood pressure. Accordingly, systolic blood pressure rises, diastolic blood pressure falls, and pulse pressure widens. The net result of wide pulse pressure hypertension is for cardiac systole to prolong, thereby increasing the work of the myocardium and its requirements for oxygen and blood supply. Because myocardial perfusion occurs during diastole, cardiovascular risk is greater in isolated systolic (e.g., 160/70 mm Hg) hypertension than in combined systolic/diastolic hypertension (e.g., 160/95 mm Hg) or isolated diastolic hypertension (e.g., 125/95 mm Hg).

Essential Hypertension

Approximately 85 to 90% of adults with hypertension have primary or essential hypertension for which no single reversible cause can be readily identified. At least 10% of hypertensive patients will, however, have an identifiable or secondary cause of their elevated blood pressure. Furthermore, essential and secondary hypertension are not mutually exclusive, and some patients who initially have essential hypertension may subsequently develop superimposed secondary hypertension. Risk factors for essential hypertension include multiple behaviors, such as lower levels of physical activity, high consumption of dietary sodium, low consumption of dietary potassium, and high caloric intake. The prevalence of hypertension parallels obesity as measured by body mass index. The primary vascular abnormality in essential hypertension is elevated systemic vascular resistance.

Behavioral Determinants of Human Blood Pressure Variation

Obesity, especially visceral fat, is linked to multiple physiologic derangements—augmented sympathetic nervous system activity, activation of the renin–angiotensin–aldosterone system, secretion of cytokines, insulin resistance, hyperinsulinemia, and the compression of the renal medulla—all of which impair renal-pressure natriuresis, thereby resulting in enhanced renal tubular absorption of sodium. Furthermore, obesity causes intrarenal vasodilation and hyperfiltration, which can injure the glomerulus. Obesity is also a risk factor for obstructive sleep apnea (Chapter 374), which contributes to nocturnal hypertension via repetitive arousals that further contribute to sympathetic nervous system activation.

Human hypertension is rare when the dietary sodium intake is less than 50 mmol per day, and virtually no age-related rise in blood pressure is seen in societies with very low dietary sodium intake. In patients with resistant hypertension, dietary sodium restriction promptly lowers blood pressure to a degree similar to the best single-drug add-on therapies.

People who smoke cigarettes (Chapter 363) tend to have lower blood pressures than nonsmokers, but cigarette smoking transiently raises blood pressure by 10 to 15 mm Hg for each cigarette smoked, and people who smoke a pack or more per day may have higher out-of-office than in-office blood pressures. Moderate alcohol consumption (Chapter 364) does not raise blood pressure, but heavy alcohol consumption (≥3 drinks per day; Chapter 364) results in the activation of the sympathetic nervous system in response to the withdrawal of alcohol. A polymorphism linked to increased enzymatic activity in the alcohol dehydrogenase gene is common in East Asians and raises systolic and diastolic blood pressure by 3/1 mm Hg per one drink per day in men but not women.

Genetic Determinants of Human Blood Pressure Variation

The concordance of blood pressure within a family is greater than that observed among unrelated individuals, and identical twins show greater blood pressure concordance than nonidentical twins. Adopted siblings have some, though less, blood pressure concordance than biologically related siblings, thereby suggesting that genetics is more important than shared environment.

The genetics of essential hypertension are complex, with multiple genetic alleles producing very small effects on blood pressure in the general population. However, several uncommon forms of hypertension caused by metabolic perturbations in salt metabolism are inherited as mendelian traits. For example, autosomal dominant Liddle syndrome, caused by a gain-of-function mutation in the *SCNN1A, SCNN1B*, or *SCNN1G* genes, causes hypertension by upregulation of the epithelial sodium channels (ENaCs) in the kidney. In autosomal dominant Gordon syndrome, disordered sodium metabolism is caused by increased activity of the sodium chloride transporter in the renal distal tubule. The autosomal recessive syndrome of apparent mineralocorticoid excess is caused by an inactivating mutation of the 11β-hydroxysteroid dehydrogenase type 2 enzyme that permits cortisol to bind to and activate the mineralocorticoid receptor. These uncommon forms of inherited hypertension highlight the important role of sodium metabolism in the genesis of hypertension.

CLINICAL MANIFESTATIONS

The vast majority of hypertensive individuals do not have symptoms that are attributable to hypertension per se. However, some patients may experience symptoms such as sleep disturbances and poor exercise tolerance.

The earliest sign of hypertension on physical examination is usually hypertensive retinopathy (Fig. 391-24). Cardiac (atrial and ventricular) enlargement on an electrocardiogram (ECG) or chest radiograph or an elevated serum creatinine level will often precede more serious end-organ damage such as stroke (Chapters 376 and 377), ischemic heart disease (Chapters 56, 57, and 58), heart failure (Chapters 45 and 46), or kidney damage (Chapters 116 and 117). Since the advent of effective antihypertensive drug therapies, hypertensive emergencies, defined as severe blood pressure elevations typically at least 180/110 mm Hg in conjunction with new or worsening pressure-related end-organ injury (see later), has become an uncommon initial clinical presentation in industrialized societies.

DIAGNOSIS

The three major goals for the initial evaluation of individuals with known or suspected hypertension are: an accurate determination of blood pressure levels; identification of non-blood-pressure cardiovascular risk factors so as to estimate global cardiovascular risk; and in selected patients, a screen for secondary forms of hypertension (Fig. 64-2). If blood pressure is elevated, the clinician must screen for orthostatic hypotension and identify any behavioral, lifestyle, or social determinants that will influence the choice of drug therapies.

GOAL 1: ACCURATE MEASUREMENT OF BLOOD PRESSURE

Blood pressure can be measured in the office by auscultation or by an oscillometric device, or outside of the office, either intermittently (typically by an oscillometric device) or continuously (by an ambulatory monitor). Potential hypertension is almost always first suspected by an office measurement but then should be confirmed by measurement outside of the office. The blood pressure thresholds for diagnosing hypertension in each of these settings (Table 64-1)

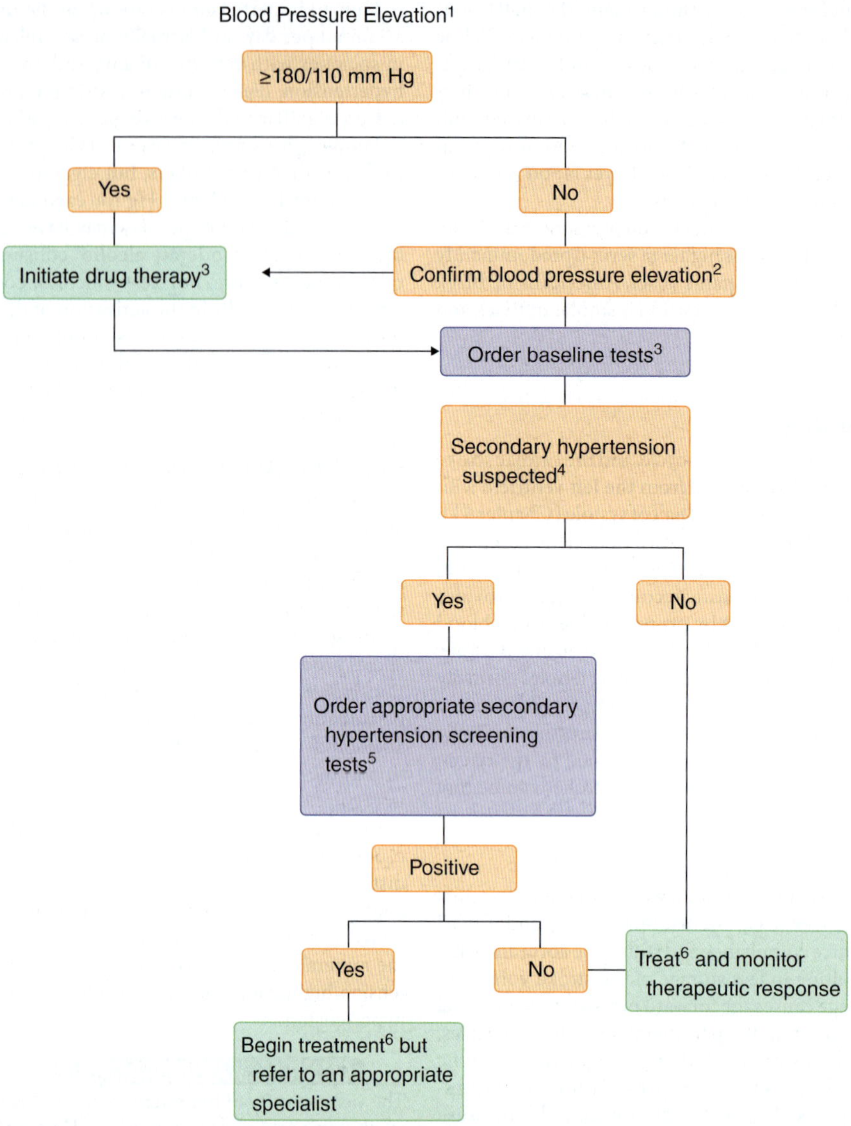

FIGURE 64-2. Evaluation of new-onset elevated blood pressure. [1]Obtain multiple (≥2) blood pressure readings using a standard protocol with validated/calibrated devices. [2]Blood pressure elevation should be confirmed by repeat office blood pressure measurement as well as by home blood pressure or ambulatory monitor readings. [3]Fasting glucose, hemoglobin A_{1C}, serum creatinine ratio, urinalysis, urine albumin: creatinine ratio, electrolyte panel, electrocardiogram test. [4]Abrupt hypertension onset of worsening of previously controlled blood pressure, resistant or refractory hypertension, hypertension in <25-yr-old, diastolic hypertension in ≥60-yr-old individuals, spontaneous hypokalemia or excessive hypokalemia in diuretic treated patients. [5]See text. Primary aldosteronism (AM plasma renin activity and aldosterone), renovascular (renal artery duplex scan), Cushing syndrome (overnight dexamethasone suppression test), pheochromocytoma (serum metanephrine levels). [6]Diet and lifestyle modifications should be used in all patients, to the degree possible, who initiate antihypertensive drug therapy (see Tables 64-6, 64-7, and 64-8).

TABLE 64-1 DEFINITIONS OF HYPERTENSION

CATEGORY	SYSTOLIC (mm Hg)		DIASTOLIC (mm Hg)
Auscultatory office blood pressure	≥130	and/or	≥80
Automated oscillometric blood pressure*	≥130	and/or	≥80
Home blood pressure	≥130	and/or	≥80
Ambulatory blood pressure			
• Daytime (awake)	≥130	and/or	≥80
• Nighttime (asleep)	≥110	and/or	≥65
• 24-hour	≥125	and/or	≥75

*Can be attended or unattended.

Adapted from Whelton PK, Carey RM, Aronow WS, et al. 2017 ACC/AHA/AAPA/ABC/ACPM/AGS/APhA/ASH/ASPC/NMA/PCNA guideline for the prevention, detection, evaluation, and management of high blood pressure in adults. *J Am Coll Cardiol.* 2018;71:e127-e248.

requires a careful approach that yields accurate readings.[7,8] For each modality, a standardized protocol should be followed by trained individuals.

AUSCULTATORY OFFICE BLOOD PRESSURE

Auscultatory office blood pressure measurement is still a method commonly used by medical personnel, unfortunately with varying degrees of training and standardization. As a result, this method is the least accurate relative to average daytime ambulatory blood pressure measurements. The patient should be instructed to empty their bladder and should rest in a quiet room with no distractions for at least 5 minutes before the initial blood pressure measurement. Caffeine and tobacco should not be consumed within 30 minutes of measurement. An appropriately sized cuff should be placed on a bare arm. While in the seated position, the back and measurement arm (at heart level) should be supported, and the legs should be uncrossed and supported on the floor. Two to three blood pressure readings should be taken, with 30 seconds to 1 minute of rest between readings, then averaged; a set of averaged blood pressure readings will typically be lower than a solitary reading. At the initial visit, blood pressure should be measured in both arms as well as in both the seated and upright positions (after 1 minute standing). Most patients with orthostatic hypotension do not have symptoms, and most patients with orthostatic dizziness do not have orthostatic hypotension. Differences in blood pressure levels between arms can be caused by coarctation of the aorta (Chapter 55), upper extremity arterial occlusion (Chapters 63 and 65), or possibly by external compression of the aorta. Subsequent blood pressure determinations should always be obtained from the arm with the higher reading at the initial visit. To make the diagnosis of hypertension, the readings taken on at least two temporally spaced visits should be averaged.

OSCILLOMETRIC OFFICE BLOOD PRESSURE

Oscillometric office blood pressure readings, obtained with a standard measurement protocol on validated and calibrated devices by trained observers, are the most accurate way to measure blood pressure in the office setting. These devices typically can be programmed to allow a 5-minute rest period before the initial measurement, as well for 1-minute intervals between the subsequent measurements. Unattended automated office blood pressure measurement (without medical personnel in the room) minimizes but does not completely eliminate the white coat reaction and is considered ideal; however, attended office blood pressure measurement is a reasonable alternative. Hypertension is diagnosed when oscillometric blood pressure is 130/80 mm Hg or higher.

HOME BLOOD PRESSURE

Home blood pressure measurement, typically with semi-automated oscillometric devices, is a reasonable alternative to the less widely available and less well-tolerated 24-hour ambulatory blood pressure monitoring. Home blood pressure readings, which may be either self-measured by the patient or obtained by another observer, are typically lower than office blood pressure readings. However, when office and home blood pressure readings are obtained using standard protocols with validated and calibrated devices, their difference will be minimized. The patient or observer should be instructed on a standard protocol for blood pressure measurement. Multiple readings should be obtained before any diagnostic or therapeutic decisions are made. A suggested approach is to obtain blood pressure readings over at least 3 days, both in the morning and the evening, with two readings at each time of measurement made 1 minute apart that are averaged.[9] Carefully obtained home blood pressure readings are at least as good, if not better, than ambulatory monitoring blood pressures. For example, 1 week of averaged home blood pressure readings better correlates with left ventricular mass than either three averaged office blood pressure measurements or two averaged 24-hour ambulatory blood pressure recordings. Newer devices have the capability of storing blood pressure measurements as well as for measuring blood pressure at night. Home blood pressure readings should be used to confirm office readings when diagnosing hypertension as well as for monitoring its therapeutics. Hypertension is diagnosed when home blood pressure is 130/80 mm Hg or higher.

AMBULATORY BLOOD PRESSURE MONITORING

Ambulatory blood pressure monitoring, which is the gold standard for noninvasive blood pressure measurement, provides multiple blood pressure readings through the day and night, typically over a 24- to 48-hour recording period (E-Fig. 64-3). However, this approach is less widely available and less well tolerated than is home blood pressure measurement. Ambulatory blood pressure monitoring predicts pressure-related cardiovascular events as accurately as home measurements predict such events and better than usual office blood pressure readings predict them.[10] Normally, the ambulatory blood pressure and pulse rate are 10 to 20% lower at night than during the daytime. When the nocturnal decline in blood pressure is less than 10% of the daytime level, this "non-dipping" phenomenon is often associated with obstructive sleep apnea (Chapter 374), disturbed sleep patterns, diabetes mellitus (Chapter 210), or autonomic dysfunction (Chapter 386). Non-dipping occurs in 10 to 30% of White Americans and in at least twice as many Black Americans. This aberrant ambulatory blood pressure phenotype is also associated with a greater risk for pressure-related end-organ damage and cardiovascular events. Hyper-dipping, which is defined as a nocturnal decline in blood pressure to a level that is more than 20% lower than daytime levels, is also seen in patients with autonomic dysfunction (Chapter 386). Hypertension is diagnosed when the average ambulatory blood pressure level is 125/75 mm Hg or greater.

WHITE COAT AND MASKED HYPERTENSION

Patients who have an elevated office blood pressure (≥130/80 mm Hg) with normal home (<130/80 mm Hg) or ambulatory blood pressure (<125/75 mm Hg) have white coat hypertension if they are not taking antihypertensive medication or white coat effect if they are taking drug therapy. White coat hypertension or effect is the result of a short-lived adrenergic response to blood pressure measurement in the office. The prevalence of white coat hypertension among patients with an elevated office blood pressure is 15 to 30% when 24-hour ambulatory blood pressure is used to confirm out of office blood pressure levels; an even higher percentage of drug-treated hypertensive patients will manifest white coat effect. Also, the prevalence of white coat hypertension/effect rises dramatically with age. The use of a standard blood pressure measurement protocol in conjunction with unattended automated oscillometric office blood pressure measurements minimizes the likelihood of white coat hypertension/effect. Patients who have white coat hypertension have minimal, if any, excess cardiovascular risk. However, 1 to 5% of individuals with white coat hypertension progress annually to sustained hypertension.

Patients who have normal office blood pressure measurements (<130/80 mm Hg) but elevated home (≥130/80 mm Hg) or ambulatory blood pressure (≥125/75 mm Hg) have masked hypertension if they are not taking antihypertensive medication or masked uncontrolled hypertension if they are taking antihypertensive drug therapy. This phenomenon occurs when frequently encountered daily stressors evoke hyperactivity of the sympathetic nervous system, but these stressors actually decrease when the individual is in the clinical setting. However, a potential cause of erroneously diagnosed masked hypertension is when measurements are obtained under nonstandard conditions and/or with inaccurate devices, thereby resulting in inflated home blood pressure readings. The prevalence of masked hypertension among persons with an office blood pressure more than 140/90 mm Hg ranges between 15 and 30%. Masked hypertension, which occurs more often in older persons and in patients who have diabetes mellitus, chronic kidney disease, and/or obstructive sleep apnea (E-Fig. 64-4), portends a similar risk for cardiovascular events as does sustained hypertension. However, no randomized control trial data have, as of yet, demonstrated benefit from drug therapy in patients who have masked hypertension or masked uncontrolled hypertension.

STAGING HYPERTENSION

The degree of confirmed blood pressure elevation by validated methods permits blood pressure to be categorized into one of four stages (Table 64-2). For nearly 70% of hypertensive individuals, the drug treatment threshold is 140/90 mm Hg, whereas higher risk and older hypertensive individuals qualify for treatment at 130/80 mm Hg.

GOAL 2: CARDIOVASCULAR RISK STRATIFICATION

Cardiovascular disease risk increases incrementally at higher levels of blood pressure, beginning well within the normal range, but the absolute level of cardiovascular risk also depends on the presence of other modifiable and nonmodifiable risk factors (Table 64-3). Initial diagnostic testing (Table 64-4) allows the clinician to estimate global cardiovascular risk in hypertensive patients (see http://tools.acc.org/ASCVD-Risk-Estimator).

GOAL 3: IDENTIFICATION AND TREATMENT OF SECONDARY (IDENTIFIABLE) CAUSES OF HYPERTENSION

Although a detailed search for secondary causes is neither prudent or cost-effective in all hypertensive patients, screening (Table 64-5) is important in younger patients and in patients who have suggestive findings on the history, physical examination, laboratory parameters, or imaging, regardless of the severity of their hypertension.

PRIMARY ALDOSTERONISM

Primary aldosteronism, which is the most common form of surgically curable secondary hypertension, has a prevalence that ranges from approximately 11%

TABLE 64-2 STAGES OF BLOOD PRESSURE

	SYSTOLIC (mm Hg)	DIASTOLIC (mm Hg)
Normal	<120	<80
Slightly elevated systolic	120-129	<80
Stage 1	130-139	80-89
Stage 2	≥140	≥90
Hypertensive urgency	≥180	>120

Adapted from Whelton PK, Carey RM, Aronow WS, et al. 2017 ACC/AHA/AAPA/ABC/ACPM/AGS/APhA/ASH/ASPC/NMA/PCNA guideline for the prevention, detection, evaluation, and management of high blood pressure in adults. *J Am Coll Cardiol.* 2018;71:e127-e248.

in normotensive individuals to 22% of patients who have either stage 2 or resistant/refractory hypertension.[11] Fewer than 40% of patients with primary aldosteronism are hypokalemic, so a serum potassium level alone is not adequate for screening. Approximately 60% of cases of primary aldosteronism result from bilateral adrenal gland hypersecretion. The aldosterone and epithelial sodium channel (ENaC) receptors in the distal nephron/collecting duct are stimulated by aldosterone, thereby resulting in sodium retention, kaliuresis, and expansion of the plasma volume. In many cases, hypertension can be severe and accompanied by extensive hypertension-related target-organ injury.

This diagnosis should be considered in patients who have refractory or resistant hypertension and especially patients in whom the plasma renin activity is suppressed (<1 μg/L), because the prevalence of primary aldosteronism in such patients is approximately 50%. Primary aldosteronism should also be suspected in the setting of a hypertensive emergency, sleep apnea, severe hypertension-related target-organ injury, a family history of primary aldosteronism, an incidentally detected adrenal adenoma, unprovoked (i.e., not associated with a diuretic) hypokalemia, or excessive hypokalemia (i.e., <3.0 mmol/L) when treated with a diuretic.

TABLE 64-3 COMMON CARDIOVASCULAR DISEASE RISK FACTORS IN PATIENTS WITH HYPERTENSION

MODIFIABLE RISK FACTORS	RELATIVELY FIXED RISK FACTORS
• Cigarette smoking, secondhand smoke	• Low socioeconomic status/educational attainment
• Pre-diabetes/diabetes mellitus	• Male sex
• Dyslipidemia/hypercholesterolemia	• Obstructive sleep apnea
• Overweight/obesity	• Known cardiovascular disease
• Physical inactivity/low fitness	• Psychosocial stress
• Unhealthy diet	• Chronic kidney disease
	• Family history
	• Increased age

Adapted from Whelton PK, Carey RM, Aronow WS, et al. 2017 ACC/AHA/AAPA/ABC/ACPM/AGS/APhA/ASH/ASPC/NMA/PCNA guideline for the prevention, detection, evaluation, and management of high blood pressure in adults. *J Am Coll Cardiol.* 2018;71:e127-e248.

TABLE 64-4 DIAGNOSTIC TESTING FOR ESSENTIAL HYPERTENSION

Fasting blood glucose level
Hemoglobin A_{1C}
Serum creatinine level with estimated glomerular filtration rate
Serum levels of sodium, potassium, and calcium
Complete blood count
Lipid profile
Thyroid-stimulating hormone
Urine albumin to creatinine ratio (spot morning urine)
Urinalysis
Electrocardiogram

OPTIONAL

Serum uric acid
Echocardiogram

Adapted from Arnett DK, Blumenthal RS, Albert MA, et al. 2019 ACA/AHA guideline on the primary prevention of cardiovascular disease: executive summary. *Circulation.* 2019;140:e563-595.

DIAGNOSIS

Serum aldosterone levels and a plasma renin activity level should be measured in a potassium replete state (a concentration of at least 3.5 Eq/L and preferably 4.0 mEq/L) in the early morning hours when aldosterone levels are at their highest. Although a usually defined upper limit of normal for a single serum aldosterone level is 15 ng/dL, about 25% of patients with primary aldosteronism have a serum aldosterone level less than 10 ng/dL. However, most patients with primary aldosteronism have suppressed renin activity, so patients should be further evaluated if their serum aldosterone level is greater than 10 ng/dL, if their renin level is low, or if they have other suggestive characteristics. The diagnostic hallmark of primary aldosteronism is excessive autonomous aldosterone secretion that does not suppress adequately (<12 μg/24 hour) during high levels (>150 mmol/day) of dietary sodium intake.[12] If the patient is at least willing to consider laparoscopic adrenalectomy, they should undergo adrenal computed tomographic scanning, with subsequent referral to an experienced interventional radiologist for bilateral adrenal vein sampling.

Most incidentally discovered adrenal adenomas, often termed incidentalomas (Chapter 208), do not secrete any detectable hormones, so they cannot be assumed to contribute to a patient's hypertension. Nevertheless, when an adenoma is discovered in hypertensive patients, the absence of hormone secretion (e.g., cortisol, catecholamines, and aldosterone) should be confirmed. However, an extensive diagnostic evaluation need not be performed prior to adrenalectomy in young (age <35 years) patients who have unprovoked hypokalemia and a typical appearing unilateral adenoma (<10 Hounsfield units of attenuation) on a computed tomographic (CT) scan.

TREATMENT

If adrenal vein sampling shows unilateral hypersecretion of aldosterone, laparoscopic adrenalectomy is the treatment of choice even if thin-slice CT scans of the affected adrenal gland show no detectable adenoma. Adrenalectomy cures the hypertension in just over 50% of cases. Catheter-based adrenal ablation is another alternative but is less likely to result in complete biochemical remission.[13] However, an appreciable percentage of patients with diagnosed primary aldosteronism likely also have underlying essential hypertension.

In patients who have bilateral adrenal gland hypersecretion or who choose to forego adrenalectomy for unilateral hypersecretion, dietary restriction, especially reductions in dietary sodium intake to less than 1500 mg per day, and intensive medical therapy are essential (see later). Aldosterone antagonists (e.g., spironolactone and eplerenone), an ENaC inhibitor (e.g., amiloride), and a thiazide-like diuretic (e.g., chlorthalidone and indapamide) should be combined with an angiotensin-converting enzyme (ACE) inhibitor or an angiotensin receptor blocker, a calcium-channel antagonist, and occasionally β-blockers. Nonrandomized data suggest better clinical outcomes in medically managed patients with primary aldosteronism when medical therapies and restriction of dietary sodium result in a rise in plasma renin activity to greater than 1 μg/L.

TABLE 64-5 GUIDE TO EVALUATION OF SECONDARY CAUSES OF HYPERTENSION

SUSPECTED DIAGNOSIS	CLINICAL CLUES	DIAGNOSTIC TESTING
Primary aldosteronism (Chapter 208)	Resistant or refractory hypertension, hypertensive emergency, severe hypertensive target-organ injury, hypokalemia, adrenal adenoma	Plasma renin and serum aldosterone, 24-hour urinary aldosterone excretion, adrenal vein sampling
Chronic kidney disease (Chapter 116)	Estimate GFR <60 mL/min/1.73 m^2 and/or urine albumin:creatinine ratio ≥300 mg/g	Serum creatinine, urine albumin : creatinine ratio
Renovascular disease (Chapter 110)	Azotemia, transient rise in creatinine when BP is lowered and/or with ACE or ARB therapy, flash pulmonary edema, abdominal/flank bruit	Renal artery duplex scan, CT or MR or invasive angiography, CO_2 angiography
Coarctation of the aorta (Chapter 55)	Arm pulses > leg pulses, arm BP > leg BP, chest bruits, rib notching on chest radiography	MR angiography, TEE, invasive angiography
Cushing syndrome (Chapter 208)	Adrenal adenoma, central obesity, pigmented abdominal striae, easy bruising, muscle weakness, cervical buffalo hump	Overnight dexamethasone suppression test, adrenal CT
Pheochromocytoma (Chapter 209)	Adrenal mass, paroxysms of hypertension, palpitations, sweating, pallor, orthostatic hypotension	Serum metanephrines, 24-hour fractionated urinary metanephrines, abdominal CT or MR imaging

ACE = angiotensin-converting enzyme; ARB = angiotensin receptor blocker; BP = blood pressure; CT = computed tomography; CO_2 = carbon dioxide; GFR = glomerular filtration rate; MR = magnetic resonance imaging; TEE = transesophageal echocardiography.

From Victor RG. Arterial hypertension. In: Goldman L, Schafer AI, eds., *Goldman-Cecil Medicine*. Philadelphia: Elsevier; 2020:443-456.

RENAL PARENCHYMAL HYPERTENSION

Hypertension affects at least 85% of patients who have chronic kidney disease (Chapter 116). Cardiovascular events, not kidney failure, are the predominant cause of morbidity and mortality, thereby highlighting the need for good blood pressure control. Mechanisms responsible for blood pressure elevations in these patients include impaired natriuresis, expansion of plasma volume, endothelial dysfunction, impaired arterial vasodilation, and arterial vasoconstriction as a consequence of activation of the sympathetic nervous system and renin–angiotensin system.

The serum creatinine level alone is not an adequate marker of kidney function but should be measured for inclusion in equations used to generate the estimated glomerular filtration rate (see Table 100-1 and Fig. 100-2). An estimated glomerular filtration rate below 60 mL/min/1.73 m^2 is considered reduced kidney function or chronic kidney disease. A spot urinary protein or, preferably, urinary albumin excretion should be measured, because chronic kidney disease is diagnosed when the urine albumin : creatinine ratio is greater than 300 mg/g irrespective of the estimated glomerular filtration rate. Quantification of protein or albumin excretion over 24 hours is not recommended.

TREATMENT

Patients who have chronic kidney disease typically have relatively resistant hypertension and require intensive multidrug therapy to slow the progressive decline in kidney function and also to lower the risk of nonrenal cardiovascular complications. An ACE inhibitor or angiotensin receptor blocker should be preferentially included in the treatment regimen, especially if the urine albumin : creatinine ratio is greater than 300 mg/g, because these agents most prominently slow the progressive decline in kidney function in patients who have significant proteinuria. If a thiazide-like diuretic is being used, indapamide maintains effectiveness down to an estimated glomerular filtrate rate of 30 mL/min/1.73 m^2 whereas chlorthalidone effectively lowers blood pressure in patients with an average estimated glomerular filtration rate in the low 20s. Nevertheless, loop diuretics (e.g., furosemide) are generally preferred if the estimated glomerular filtration rate is less than 40 mL/min/1.73 m^2. When patients develop end-stage renal disease and require dialysis (Chapter 117), tight blood pressure control is not warranted and may be dangerous, especially if blood pressure is too low pre-dialysis. An inter-dialytic systolic blood pressure less than 90 mm Hg or low enough to evoke symptoms should be avoided.[14]

RENOVASCULAR HYPERTENSION

Among patients with renovascular hypertension (Chapter 110), the cause is atherosclerotic renal artery obstruction in approximately 85% of cases, with fibromuscular dysplasia accounting for nearly all of the remainder. Atherosclerotic renal artery obstruction typically affects middle-aged to older patients, more commonly men who usually have evidence of advanced atherosclerosis, whereas fibromuscular dysplasia typically presents at a younger age and is more common in women. Atherosclerotic renal artery obstruction, which can be unilateral or bilateral, can raise blood pressure and cause ischemic nephropathy. Bilateral critical renal artery stenosis is a volume-dependent form of hypertension that, unlike unilateral renal artery stenosis, can cause azotemia.

CLINICAL MANIFESTATIONS

Critical atherosclerotic renal artery stenosis can present clinically with accelerating, resistant, or refractory hypertension and, especially if bilateral, with flash pulmonary edema, recurrent heart failure, and/or ischemic nephropathy.

DIAGNOSIS

When renal artery stenosis is suspected, its diagnosis should be pursued in patients who have characteristics that predict the failure of medical therapy and responsiveness to renal artery revascularization. Such patients have refractory hypertension, ischemic nephropathy, flash pulmonary edema, or recurrent heart failure. Young to middle-aged women with signs or symptoms suggestive of fibromuscular dysplasia should be screened. The most commonly used screening test is renal artery duplex scanning, but this test is highly operator-dependent and is technically difficult in obese patients. A positive duplex scan can be confirmed by direct renal angiography or by CT, MRI, or carbon dioxide angiography. Gadolinium-enhanced MRI should be avoided in patients who have acute kidney injury, an estimated glomerular filtration rate less than 30 mL/min/1.73 m^2, or are on dialysis because of the risk of a systemic fibrotic reaction (Chapter 246).

Fibromuscular dysplasia classically causes a "string of beads" sign in the midportion of the renal artery (see Fig. 64-3A), although it may occasionally present as a focal lesion. Atherosclerotic renal artery obstruction is more discrete, with a predilection for the proximal renal artery near the ostia (see Fig. 64-3B). However, simply documenting critical renal artery stenosis does not invariably prove that it is substantively affecting the blood pressure level.

TREATMENT

Angioplasty without stenting is the treatment of choice for fibromuscular dysplasia, and it resolves hypertension in about 45% of cases (Chapter 110). For atherosclerotic renal artery stenosis, however, renal artery revascularization may reduce the intensity of required medical therapy but does not lead to better control.[A1] Accordingly, medical therapy is preferred for most hypertensive patients with atherosclerotic renal artery obstruction, except it is reasonable to consider renal artery revascularization in patients who have refractory hypertension, ischemic nephropathy, heart failure, or recurrent episodes of pulmonary edema.

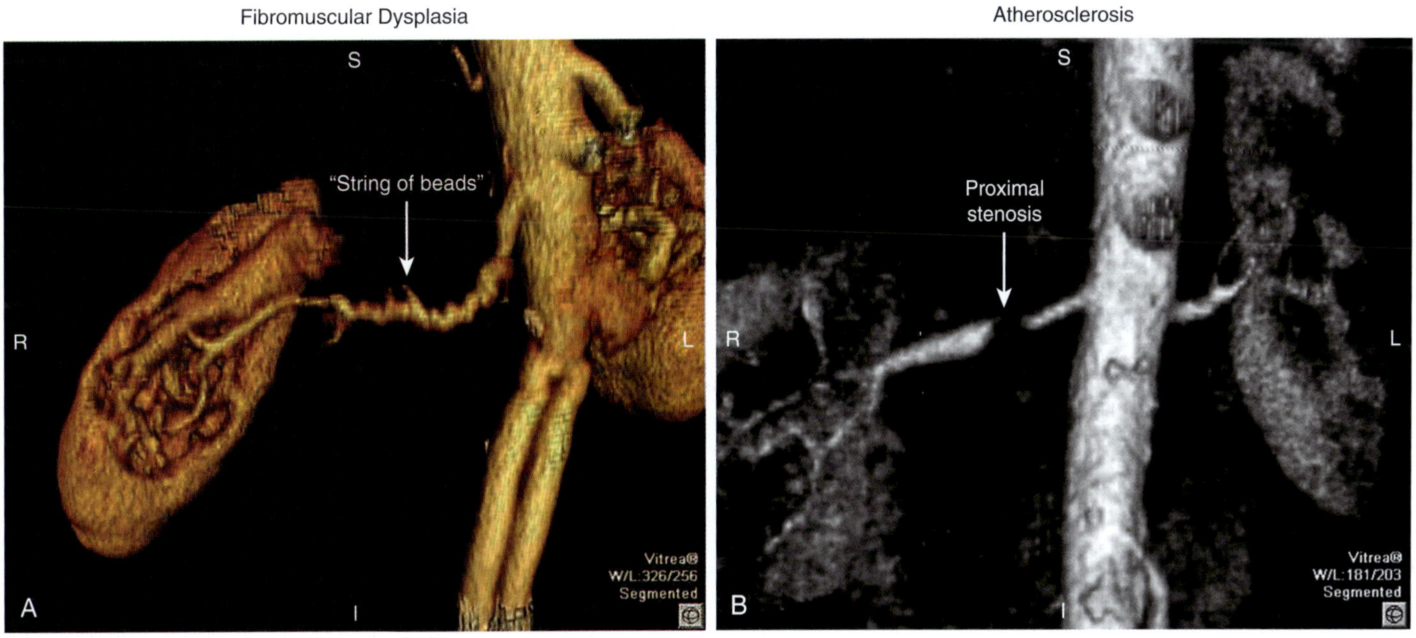

FIGURE 64-3. **Computed tomographic angiogram with three-dimensional reconstruction. A, The classic "string of beads" lesion of fibromuscular dysplasia (bilateral in this patient). B, A severe proximal atherosclerotic stenosis of the right renal artery and mild stenosis of the left renal artery. (Images courtesy of Bart Domatch, MD, Radiology Department, University of Texas Southwestern Medical Center, Dallas, Texas.)**

PHEOCHROMOCYTOMA AND PARAGANGLIOMA

Pheochromocytoma and paraganglioma are rare, histologically indistinguishable catecholamine-producing neuroendocrine tumors that are differentiated solely on the basis of their anatomic location (Chapter 209). This diagnosis should be suspected in patients who have suggestive symptoms, such as often paroxysmal headache, palpitations, profuse sweating, and anxiety, as well as weight loss. Patients who have proven pheochromocytoma can sometimes be misdiagnosed as having neuroses, anxiety, or panic disorders. Most (98%) of pheochromocytomas are intra-abdominal, with the majority occurring in the adrenal gland; the remaining 2% are paragangliomas that are found in the neck and thorax. Some pheochromocytomas are part of multiple endocrine neoplasia syndromes (Chapter 212). The best screening test is plasma fractionated metanephrines. Because these catecholamine-secreting tumors are exceedingly rare, most positive metanephrine tests are false-positive results, but elevations greater than 3 times the upper limit of normal rarely represent false-positive elevations. The diagnosis can be confirmed by measurement of fractionated metanephrines and catecholamines in a 24-hour urine specimen, followed by localization studies (Chapter 209).

TREATMENT

See Chapter 209.

OTHER SECONDARY CAUSES OF HYPERTENSION

Causes of neurogenic hypertension that can mimic pheochromocytoma include the use of sympathomimetic substances (cocaine, methamphetamine; Chapter 365), untreated obstructive sleep apnea (Chapter 374) and baroreflex failure. A history of surgery and/or radiation for head and neck tumors (Chapter 176) can damage baroreceptor reflexes and cause widely fluctuating blood pressure levels. Snoring and daytime sleepiness are suggestive of sleep apnea. Continuous positive airway pressure can modestly lower blood pressure in patients with sleep apnea.

In coarctation of the aorta (Chapter 63), which occurs in 0.4% of live births, an anatomic narrowing of the left subclavian artery distal to its origin results in paradoxically weaker pulses and lower blood pressure in the lower than the upper extremities. Intercostal collateral arteries can result in audible bruits on physical examination as well as notching of the ribs on a chest radiograph.

Hyperthyroidism (Chapter 207) can cause systolic hypertension with a wide pulse pressure, whereas hypothyroidism is associated with isolated diastolic hypertension. Hyperparathyroidism (Chapter 227) also has been linked to hypertension. Calcineurin inhibitors (cyclosporine more than tacrolimus), which are used predominantly to reduce rejection after solid organ transplantation, raise blood pressure, presumably by increasing sympathetic nervous system activity. Multiple oncologic drugs raise blood pressure, including vascular endothelial growth factor (VEGF) inhibitors (salt-sensitive hypertension), poly-ADP ribose polymerase inhibitors (niraparib), Bruton tyrosine kinase inhibitors, mammalian target of rapamycin (mTOR) inhibitors, inhibitors of androgen synthesis (mineralocorticoid effect), proteosome inhibitors, and rearranged during transfection (REF) inhibitors. Mendelian forms of salt-sensitive hypertension (Chapter 113) are typically uncovered when screening for primary aldosteronism shows suppressed levels of urinary renin (<1 μg/L/hour) and plasma level aldosterone (<5 ng/dL).

TREATMENT OF ESSENTIAL HYPERTENSION

Optimal management of hypertension is ideally undertaken by an experienced team of health care professionals, often though not always led by a knowledgeable physician, who accurately measure blood pressure, diligently diagnose hypertension, prescribe adequate evidence-based medical therapies, avoid therapeutic inertia, and build effective rapport with patients and their families.

LIFESTYLE MODIFICATION

Diet and lifestyle modifications (Table 64-6) are core strategies for primordial prevention of hypertension as well as for treating adults with elevated blood pressure or established hypertension. Lifestyle modifications can lower systolic blood pressure by 7 to up to 15 mm Hg and can be tried before embarking on drug therapy. However, lifestyle changes are more effective for delaying the need for drug therapy or reducing the intensity of drug therapy than for avoiding it altogether.

TABLE 64-6 DIET AND LIFESTYLE RECOMMENDATIONS TO LOWER BLOOD PRESSURE IN ADULTS WITH ELEVATED BLOOD PRESSURE OR HYPERTENSION

DIET
1. Recommended dietary patterns (see Fig. 13-1 and Table 13-4): High in fresh fruits, vegetables, legumes, fish, low-fat dairy products, nuts, and whole grains Low in energy-dense foods such as refined carbohydrates and sugar-sweetened beverages, total and saturated fats Reduce dietary sodium intake to <1500 mg per day or at least a reduction of 1000 mg per day
PHYSICAL ACTIVITY
2. Increased physical activity as part of a structured exercise program Aerobic or dynamic resistance 90 to 150 min/wk
ALCOHOL INTAKE
3. ≤2 drinks per day (men) or ≤1 drink per day (women)

Adapted from Whelton PK, Carey RM, Aronow WS, et al. 2017 ACC/AHA/AAPA/ABC/ACPM/AGS/APhA/ASH/ASPC/NMA/PCNA guideline for the prevention, detection, evaluation, and management of high blood pressure in adults. *J Am Coll Cardiol.* 2018;71:e127-e248.

The Mediterranean diet (Fig. 13-1; fresh fruit, vegetables, fatty fish, canola/olive oil) and the Dietary Approaches to Stop Hypertension diet (Table 13-4; fresh fruits, vegetables, low-fat dairy products) can effectively lower blood pressure by about 6 mm Hg systolic without limiting the intake of calories or sodium. The average U.S. adult consumes about 3400 mg of sodium per day (148 mmol). Reduction of dietary sodium intake minimally to less than 2000 mg/day (87 mmol) and preferably to less than 1500 mg/day (65 mmol) is advisable because reductions in dietary sodium lower blood pressure[A2] and cardiovascular risk.[A3] Approximately 70% of dietary sodium intake is from processed food, so most adults cannot achieve sodium targets just by eliminating the discretionary addition of salt to their food.

Moderate intensity regular physical activity (Chapter 14), consisting of aerobic and/or dynamic resistance, will lower blood pressure approximately 4 to 8 mm Hg in hypertensive patients. Stress management techniques, such as meditation, biofeedback, and breathing exercises, can also lower blood pressure, but the durability and magnitude of their effect has not been firmly established (Chapter 30). People who smoke cigarettes should be counseled to quit (Chapter 363). Alcohol should be limited to no more than the equivalent of two drinks per day in men and one drink per day in women.

MEDICAL THERAPY

Pharmacologic treatment of hypertension can lower risk for cardiovascular disease (e.g., stroke [Chapters 375, 376, and 377], heart failure [Chapters 45 and 46], myocardial infarction [Chapters 57 and 58], chronic kidney disease [Chapters 116 and 117], atrial fibrillation [Chapter 52], peripheral vascular disease [Chapter 65]), with each 5–mm Hg reduction in systolic blood pressure corresponding to about a 10% reduction in events,[A4] as well as the risks of dementia (Chapter 371)[A5] and premature mortality, even in elderly persons.[A6] Nevertheless, successfully treated hypertensive patients have residual cardiovascular risk, with an absolute risk that remains higher than the risk of untreated patients with the same blood pressure level. As a result, reduction of global cardiovascular disease risk requires identification and treatment of non–blood-pressure risk factors, such as dyslipidemia (Chapter 190) and diabetes (Chapter 210).

In most patients, effective antihypertensive drug therapy requires two or more drugs, ideally with complementary mechanisms of action.[15] The overwhelming majority of patients with established hypertension require lifelong drug therapy.[16] Desirable antihypertensive drug combinations not only effectively lower blood pressure but they also mitigate the potential side effects of high-dose monotherapy.[17]

Clinicians should tailor and simplify drug regimens, often by using single-pill, preferably once-daily, combinations that patients can afford and tolerate. Adherence to prescribed drug therapies is problematic, however, as reflected by the reality that approximately 20% of new prescriptions for antihypertensive medications in the United States are never filled and, even when filled initially, up to 50% of prescriptions are no longer filled by 1 year.

CLASSES OF ORAL ANTIHYPERTENSIVE MEDICATIONS

More than 100 drugs from multiple classes are approved for the treatment of hypertension (Table 64-7). Each has contraindications and potential side effects, and many have preferred indications for certain subsets of patients (Tables 64-8 and 64-9).

First-Line Drugs for Hypertension

Guidelines recommend initiating antihypertensive drug therapy with two or more of three groups of antihypertensive medication: calcium-channel blockers, ACE inhibitors or angiotensin receptor blockers or thiazide or thiazide-like diuretics.

TABLE 64-7 SELECTED ORAL ANTIHYPERTENSIVE MEDICATIONS

DRUG	TYPICAL DOSE RANGE (mg/day)	DOSING FREQUENCY
PRIMARY AGENTS		
Thiazide or Thiazide-like Diuretics		
Chlorthalidone	12.5-25	1
Hydrochlorothiazide	25-50	1
Indapamide	1.25-2.5	1
Metolazone	2.5-5	1
ACE Inhibitors		
Benazepril	10-40	1 or 2
Captopril	12.5-150	2 or 3
Enalapril	5-40	1 or 2
Fosinopril	10-40	1
Lisinopril	10-40	1
Moexipril	7.5-30	1 or 2
Perindopril	4-16	1
Quinapril	10-80	1 or 2
Ramipril	2.5-20	1 or 2
Trandolapril	1-4	1
Angiotensin Receptor Blockers		
Azilsartan	40-80	1
Candesartan	8-32	1
Eprosartan	600-800	1 or 2
Irbesartan	150-300	1
Losartan	50-100	1 or 2
Olmesartan	20-40	1
Telmisartan	20-80	1
Valsartan	80-320	1
CCB—Dihydropyridines		
Amlodipine	2.5-10	1
Felodipine	2.5-10	1
Isradipine	5-10	2
Nicardipine SR	60-120	2
Nifedipine LA	30-90	1
Nisoldipine	17-34	1
CCB—Nondihydropyridines		
Diltiazem ER	120-360	1
Verapamil IR	120-360	3
Verapamil SR	120-480	1 or 2
Verapamil—delayed-onset ER	100-300	1 (in the evening)
SECONDARY AGENTS		
Diuretics—Loop		
Bumetanide	0.5-2	2
Ethacrynic acid	25-80	2
Furosemide	20-80	2
Torsemide	5-10	1
Diuretics—Potassium Sparing (ENaC Channel Inhibitors)		
Amiloride	5-10	1 or 2
Triamterene	50-100	1 or 2
Diuretic—Aldosterone Antagonists		
Eplerenone	50-100	1 or 2
Spironolactone	12.5-100	1

DRUG	TYPICAL DOSE RANGE (mg/day)	DOSING FREQUENCY
β-Blockers—Cardioselective		
Atenolol	25-100	2
Betaxolol	5-20	1
Bisoprolol	2.5-10	1
Metoprolol tartrate	100-200	2
Metoprolol succinate	50-200	1
β-Blockers—Cardioselective and Vasodilatory		
Nebivolol	5-40	1
β-Blockers—Noncardioselective		
Nadolol	40-120	1
Propranolol IR	80-160	2
Propranolol LA	80-160	1
Timolol	10-20	2
β-Blockers—Intrinsic Sympathomimetic Activity		
Acebutolol	200-800	2
Carteolol[*]	2.5-10	2.5
Penbutolol	10-40	1
Pindolol	10-60	2
β-Blockers—Combined α- and β-Receptor		
Carvedilol	12.5-50	2
Carvedilol phosphate	20-80	1
Labetalol	200-800	2
Direct Renin Inhibitor		
Aliskiren	150-300	1
α-1 Blockers		
Doxazosin	1-16	1
Prazosin	2-20	2 or 3
Terazosin	1-20	1 or 2
α-1 and 2 Blockers		
Phenoxybenzamine	20-120	2 or 3
Central α_2-Agonist and Other Centrally Acting Drugs		
Clonidine oral	0.1-0.8	2
Clonidine patch	0.1-0.3	1 weekly
Guanabenz	8-32	2
Guanfacine	0.5-2	1
Methyldopa	250-1000	2
Reserpine	0.1-0.25 0.05-0.125[†]	1 1
Hydralazine	100-200	2 or 3
Minoxidil	5-100	1-3
Angiotensin–Neprilysin Inhibitor		
Sacubitril/valsartan	Initial dose[†] 24/26 Initial dose[§] 49/51 Maintenance dose[‖] 97/103	2 2 2
Fixed-Dose Combinations		
Aliskiren/HCTZ	75-300/12.5-25	1
Amiloride/HCTZ	5/50	1
Amlodipine/benazepril	2.5-5/10-20	1
Amlodipine/olmesartan	5-10/20-40	1
Amlodipine/perindopril	3.5/2.5	1
Amlodipine/telmisartan	5/20-10/80	1

TABLE 64-7 SELECTED ORAL ANTIHYPERTENSIVE MEDICATIONS—cont'd

DRUG	TYPICAL DOSE RANGE (mg/day)	DOSING FREQUENCY
Amlodipine/valsartan	5-10/160-320	1
Atenolol/chlorthalidone	20-100/25	1
Azilsartan/chlorthalidone	40-80/12.5-25	1
Benazepril/HCTZ	5-20/6.25-25	1
Bisoprolol/HCTZ	2.5-10/6.25	1
Candesartan/HCTZ	16-32/12.5-25	1
Captopril/HCTZ	25/15	1
Enalapril/HCTZ	5-10/25	1
Eprosartan/HCTZ	600/12.5-25	1
Fosinopril/HCTZ	10-20/12.5	1
Irbesartan/HCTZ	150-300/12.5-25	1
Lisinopril/HCTZ	10-20/12.5	1
Losartan/HCTZ	50-100/12.5-25	1
Metoprolol succinate/HCTZ	25-200/12.5-25	1
Metoprolol tartrate/HCTZ	100-200/25-50	1 or 2
Moexipril/HCTZ	7.5-15/12.5-25	1
Olmesartan/HCTZ	20-40/12.5	1
Olmesartan/amlodipine/HCTZ	20-40/5-10/12.5-25	1
Quinapril/HCTZ	10-20/12.5	1
Spironolactone/HCTZ	25/25	½
Telmisartan/HCTZ	40-80/12.5-25	1
Trandolapril/verapamil	2-4/180-240	1
Triamterene/HCTZ	37.5/25	½
Valsartan/HCTZ	80-160/12.5-25	1
Valsartan/amlodipine/HCTZ	80-160/5-10/12.5-25	1

*No longer commercially available in the United States.
†This dose range is indicated when given with a diuretic.
‡In patients taking a high-dose of an ACE-I or ARB.
§In patients previously not taking or taking a low dose of an ACE-I or ARB.
¶Double initial dose every 2 to 4 weeks as tolerated to reach the maintenance dose.
ACE = angiotensin-converting enzyme; CCB = calcium-channel blocker; ER = extended release; HCTZ = hydrochlorothiazide; IR = immediate release; LA = long-acting; SR = sustained release.
Adapted from the Whelton PK, Carey RM, Aronow WS, et al. 2017 ACC/AHA/AAPA/ABC/ACPM/AGS/APhA/ASH/ASPC/NMA/PCNA guideline for the prevention, detection, evaluation, and management of high blood pressure in adults: a report of the American College of Cardiology/American Heart Association Task Force on clinical practice guidelines. *J Am Coll Cardiol.* 2018;71:e127-e248.

Calcium-Channel Blockers

Mechanism of Action

Dihydropyridine and non-dihydropyridine calcium-channel blockers inhibit opening of voltage-gated calcium channels in vascular smooth muscle and the myocardium, thereby resulting in arterial dilatation. The dihydropyridine calcium-channel blockers (e.g., amlodipine) more potently lower blood pressure than do the non-dihydropyridine calcium-channel blockers (e.g., diltiazem, verapamil).

Clinical Use

Calcium-channel blockers effectively lower blood pressure when used alone or in combination with other antihypertensive drugs, especially ACE inhibitors, angiotensin receptor blockers, and thiazide diuretics. These agents are useful for the treatment of angina pectoris, are the most effective drug class for the primary prevention of stroke, and are equally useful in Black patients and other ethnic groups. Amlodipine, which is the prototype dihydropyridine calcium-channel blocker to treat hypertension, is comparable to chlorthalidone for reducing cardiovascular events other than heart failure. Unlike the other first-line antihypertensive drug classes, the antihypertensive effects of calcium-channel blockers are independent of dietary sodium intake and of concurrent use of nonsteroidal anti-inflammatory drugs. In patients with chronic kidney disease, dihydropyridine calcium-channel blockers should be prescribed only after the initiation of either an ACE inhibitor or an angiotensin receptor blocker. Non-dihydropyridine calcium-channel blockers typically should be avoided when β-blockers are concurrently prescribed because both drug classes share negative inotropic and chronotropic effects. Short-acting calcium-channel blockers (e.g., nifedipine) are effective to reduce blood pressure rapidly in a hypertensive urgency but should not be used chronically because it causes prominent, precipitous, and short-lived arterial vasodilation (and blood pressure lowering) that reflexively activates the sympathetic nervous system.

Side Effects

A common dose-dependent side effect of dihydropyridine calcium-channel blockers, especially in women, is lower extremity edema, which typically is worse later in the day after hours of upright posture. ACE inhibitors are the best antidote for this dose-dependent edema, whereas diuretics should not be used for this purpose. Gingival hyperplasia, which is an uncommon but serious side effect with both dihydropyridine and non-dihydropyridine calcium-channel blockers, occurs more often with dihydropyridines and diltiazem than with verapamil. The signature side effect for verapamil is constipation. All calcium channel antagonists can depress the sinoatrial node, so they should be avoided in patients who have the sick sinus syndrome (Chapter 51) unless they have a functioning ventricular pacemaker.

Renin–Angiotensin System Inhibitors: ACE Inhibitors, Angiotensin Receptor Blockers, and Direct Renin Inhibitors

Mechanisms of Action

ACE inhibitors inhibit the conversion of angiotensin 1 by angiotensin-converting enzyme (ACE) to its vasoactive form, angiotensin 2, while also inhibiting the degradation of bradykinin. Angiotensin receptor blockers antagonize the action of angiotensin 2 by blocking the angiotensin 1 receptor, thereby allowing angiotensin 2 to bind preferentially to the angiotensin 2 receptor instead. Direct renin inhibitors block conversion of pro-renin to renin, thereby inhibiting the renin–angiotensin system at its first metabolic step.

Clinical Use

All inhibitors of the renin–angiotensin system have relatively flat dose–response curves. ACE inhibitors and angiotensin receptor blockers lower blood pressure to a similar degree. Although both agents are less effective as monotherapy in Black compared with White patients, the efficacy of combination therapy, which is now routinely recommended with these drugs, appears to be equivalent in Black and White patients. ACE inhibitors provide equal protection against coronary events, lesser protection against stroke, and better protection against heart failure compared with calcium-channel blockers.

Angiotensin receptor blockers do not cause dose-related side effects and generally are the best tolerated of all hypertensive drug classes. Unlike ACE inhibitors, angiotensin receptor blockers do not cause cough or angioedema. Azilsartan is the most potent angiotensin receptor blocker for blood pressure reduction, and several long-acting agents (e.g., olmesartan, telmisartan, and irbesartan) lower blood pressure more effectively than does losartan.[A7]

Either an ACE inhibitor or an angiotensin receptor blocker is indicated in patients with chronic kidney disease, especially when the urine albumin : creatinine ratio is greater than 300 mg/g, because they slow the progressive loss of kidney function, particularly in patients who have significant proteinuria. ACE inhibitors and angiotensin receptor blockers should not be used concurrently, nor should either drug class be used concurrently with aliskirin because of the heightened risk of renal injury and hyperkalemia.

Side Effects

Because of the risk of fetal injury, all renin–angiotensin system inhibitors are contraindicated in women who are of childbearing age and who are not using an effective form of contraception, in women who are planning to become pregnant, or in women who are pregnant (Chapter 221). ACE inhibitors inhibit kininase II, thereby resulting in the accumulation of bradykinin, which stimulates bradykinin 2 receptors that lead to vasodilation, extravasation of plasma into the interstitial space, and release of substance P. These physiologic derangements appear to underly both the dry cough (seen in 10 to 15% of patients) and angioedema (<1% of patients) that are associated with their use. However, angioedema is more common in women, Black patients, patients who smoke, and patients who are older than age 65 years, have seasonal allergies, have a history of drug rashes or drug allergies, or are taking immunosuppressive drugs. In patients who experience angioedema during treatment with an ACE inhibitor, the ACE inhibitor should be discontinued and an angiotensin receptor blocker can be substituted if patients have a clear indication for blockade of the renin–angiotensin system.

Hyperkalemia is a potential complication of all of these agents, especially in patients who have chronic kidney disease (Chapter 116), diabetes (Chapter 210), or hyporeninemic hypoaldosteronism (type IV renal tubular acidosis; Chapter 104). Although these agents are reno-protective, some patients have an increase in the serum creatinine level that may require their discontinuation, most likely related to sluggish renal autoregulation but also associated with bilateral renal artery stenosis. The serum creatinine level and serum electrolytes should be measured within 1 to 2 weeks after initiating therapy with these agents.

TABLE 64-8 MAJOR CONTRAINDIATIONS AND SIDE EFFECTS OF ANTIHYPERTENSIVE DRUGS

DRUG CLASS	MAJOR CONTRAINDICATIONS	SIDE EFFECTS
DIURETICS		
Thiazides	Gout	Insulin resistance, new-onset type 2 diabetes Hypokalemia, hyponatremia, hypomagnesemia Triglyceride increase Hyperuricemia, precipitation of gout Erectile dysfunction Potentiates nondepolarizing muscle relaxants Photosensitivity dermatitis Skin cancer (mostly squamous cell)
Loop diuretics	Hepatic coma	Interstitial nephritis Hypokalemia Potentiate succinylcholine Potentiate aminoglycoside ototoxicity
Potassium-sparing diuretics	Serum potassium concentration >5.5 mEq/L GFR <45 mL/min, but may be used in patients with heart failure down to eGFR ~30 mL/min/1.73 m^2	Hyperkalemia
ACE inhibitors	Pregnancy Bilateral renal artery stenosis Hyperkalemia History of angioedema	Cough Hyperkalemia Angioedema Leukopenia Fetal toxicity Cholestatic jaundice (rare fulminant hepatic necrosis if the drug is not discontinued)
Dihydropyridine CCBs	As monotherapy in CKD with proteinuria Sick sinus syndrome	Headaches (vascular) Flushing Ankle edema Heart failure Gingival hyperplasia Esophageal reflux
Nondihydropyridine CCBs	Heart block Systolic heart failure Sick sinus syndrome Bradycardia	Bradycardia, AV block (especially with verapamil) Constipation (with verapamil) Worsening of systolic function, heart failure Gingival edema or hypertrophy Increase cyclosporine and tacrolimus blood levels Esophageal reflux
Angiotensin receptor blockers, direct renin inhibitors	Pregnancy Bilateral renal artery stenosis Hyperkalemia	Hyperkalemia Angioedema Fetal toxicity
β-Adrenergic blockers	Heart block Asthma Depression Cocaine and methamphetamine abuse	New-onset type 2 diabetes (especially in combination with a thiazide) Erectile dysfunction Heart block, acute decompensated heart failure Bronchospasm Depression, nightmares, fatigue Cold extremities, claudication (β_2 effect) Stevens-Johnson syndrome Rebound hypertension with abrupt cessation Weight gain
α-Adrenergic blockers	Orthostatic hypotension Systolic heart failure Left ventricular dysfunction	Orthostatic hypotension Drug tolerance (in the absence of diuretic therapy) Fluid retention Heart failure First-dose effect (hypotension) Potentiate hypotension with PDE-5 inhibitors (e.g., sildenafil)
Central sympatholytics	Orthostatic hypotension Bradycardia	Depression, dry mouth, lethargy Rebound hypertension with abrupt cessation Coombs test–positive hemolytic anemia and elevated liver enzymes with α-methyldopa
Direct vasodilators	Use prior to late add-on therapy	Reflex tachycardia Fluid retention Hirsutism, pericardial effusion with minoxidil Lupus with hydralazine

ACE = angiotensin-converting enzyme; AV = atrioventricular; CCBs = calcium-channel blocker; CKD = chronic kidney disease; GFR = glomerular filtration rate; NSAIDs = nonsteroidal anti-inflammatory drugs; PDE-5 = phosphodiesterase-5.

From Victor RG. Arterial hypertension. In: Goldman L, Schafer AI, eds. *Goldman-Cecil Medicine*. Philadelphia: Elsevier; 2020:443-456.

TABLE 64-9 PREFERRED ANTIHYPERTENSIVE DRUG CLASSES FOR SPECIFIC CONDITIONS

CONDITION	DRUG CLASSES
Hypertension (general)	ACE inhibitor or angiotensin receptor blocker and/or calcium-channel blocker or diuretic
Diabetes mellitus	ACE inhibitor or angiotensin receptor blocker and/or calcium-channel blocker or diuretic
Diabetes mellitus with nephropathy*	ACE inhibitor or angiotensin receptor blocker and calcium-channel blocker or diuretic
Chronic kidney disease	ACE inhibitor or angiotensin receptor blocker and calcium-channel blocker or diuretic
Kidney transplantation	Calcium-channel blocker
Heart failure (reduced ejection fraction)	β-Blocker, aldosterone antagonist, angiotensin receptor–neprilysin inhibitor, and diuretic† (congestive symptoms)
Heart failure (preserved ejection fraction)	Angiotensin receptor–neprilysin inhibitor and diuretic† (congestive symptoms)
Stable ischemic heart disease	GDMT β-blocker and ACE inhibitor or angiotensin receptor blocker plus dihydropyridine calcium-channel blocker for persistent angina or thiazide diuretic and/or mineralocorticoid receptor for blood pressure control
Aortic disease	β-Blocker
Atrial fibrillation	ACE inhibitor or angiotensin receptor blocker plus β-blocker or nondihydropyridine calcium-channel blocker (rate control)
Pregnancy	Methyldopa, β-blocker (labetalol), calcium-channel blocker (nifedipine)

*Urine albumin : creatinine >300 mg/g.
†Diuretics should be added to control volume overload and/or for additional blood pressure lowering.
ACE = angiotensin-converting enzyme; β-blockers = carvedilol, metoprolol tartrate, metoprolol succinate, nadolol, bisoprolol, propranolol, timolol; GDMT = guideline directed medical therapy.
Adapted from Whelton PK, Carey RM, Aronow WS, et al. 2017 ACC/AHA/AAPA/ABC/ACPM/AGS/APhA/ASH/ASPC/NMA/PCNA guideline for the prevention, detection, evaluation, and management of high blood pressure in adults: a report of the American College of Cardiology/American Heart Association Task Force on clinical practice guidelines. *J Am Coll Cardiol.* 2018;71:e127-e248; Tomson CRV, Cheung AK, Mann JFE, et al. Management of blood pressure in patients with chronic kidney disease not receiving dialysis: synopsis of the 2021 KDIGO clinical practice guideline. *Ann Intern Med.* 2021;174:1270-1281.

Diuretics

Mechanism of Action

During diuretic therapy, the circulating blood volume falls initially, but gradually returns toward baseline over the ensuing weeks. Over time, the predominant effect of thiazide or thiazide-like diuretics is to reduce systematic vascular resistance. Loop diuretics are more potent diuretics than thiazide or thiazide-like diuretics, but the latter are preferred to treat hypertension until the estimated glomerular filtration rate is significantly reduced (<40 mL/min/1.73 m^2).

Clinical Use

Hydrochlorothiazide (HCTZ) is by far the most common thiazide diuretic used to treat hypertension and may be equivalent to chlorthalidone, which is a thiazide-like diuretic, for reducing cardiovascular risk with less hypokalemia.[A8] Kidney function is an important determinant of which diuretics are likely to be effective options. Thiazide diuretics must cause an effective natriuresis to lower blood pressure. HCTZ does not predictably cause a natriuresis when the estimated glomerular filtrate rate is less than 45 mL/min/1.73 m^2, whereas indapamide, which is also a thiazide-like diuretic, effectively evokes a diuresis at an estimated glomerular filtration rate as low as 30 mL/min/1.73 m^2 and chlorthalidone is effective down to an average estimated glomerular filtration rate in the low 20s.[A9] HCTZ has a clear dose-response curve between 6.25 to 50 mg per day, whereas thiazide-like diuretics tend to have a flat dose-response curve. Chlorthalidone has a 1.5- to 2.5-day duration of action, which is a beneficial characteristic for the chronic treatment of hypertension.

Side Effects

Thiazide diuretics can cause dose-related hypokalemia (Chapter 103), worsened glucose tolerance (Chapter 210), hypomagnesemia (Chapter 105), hyperuricemia (Chapter 252), raised serum lipid levels, photosensitivity skin reactions, skin cancer (mostly squamous cell carcinoma), and erectile dysfunction. These agents can also cause serious hyponatremia (Chapter 102), particularly in older patients, by impairing free water clearance both with and without volume depletion. Over-diuresis is more likely with the more potent diuretic chlorthalidone than with HCTZ.

Add-On Drugs for Difficult-to-Treat Hypertension

Potassium-Sparing Diuretics

Mechanism of Action

Spironolactone and eplerenone, both of which are aldosterone receptor antagonists, prevent aldosterone and glucocorticoids from binding and subsequently activating the mineralocorticoid receptor in the distal nephron and collecting duct (as well as in the heart and vascular endothelium) and thereby inhibit the activation of ENaC channels. Increased reabsorption of sodium proximal to the collecting duct reduces the urinary secretion of potassium and, as a result, raises the serum potassium level because less sodium is presented to the collecting duct for exchange with potassium. Baxdrostat, which inhibits aldosterone synthase, is an experimental drug that has shown promise for resistant hypertension.[A10]

Clinical Use and Side Effects

These agents are very effective adjuncts in patients on complex drug regimens for resistant hypertension. Potassium-sparing diuretics should generally be avoided when the estimated glomerular filtration rate is less than 45 mL/min/1.73 m^2 to prevent potentially dangerous hyperkalemia. Eplerenone is a more specific inhibitor of the mineralocorticoid receptor than is spironolactone, so it less frequently activates sex hormone receptors and causes less gynecomastia, menstrual irregularities, and erectile dysfunction. However, spironolactone lowers blood pressure more effectively than eplerenone. Amiloride, which is a direct inhibitor of the ENaC channel, is at least as, if not more, potent than spironolactone. The risk of hyperkalemia is higher in patients who are treated concurrently with ACE inhibitors or angiotensin receptor blockers.

β-Adrenergic Blockers

Mechanism of Action

A heterogenous variety of β-blockers lower blood pressure to a relatively similar degree. When β-blocker therapy is initiated, the reduction in cardiac output is countered by an increase in systemic vascular resistance, but this reaction wanes over time, thereby allowing blood pressure to fall. The reduction of blood pressure is due to a reduction in cardiac output, decreased release of renin, and a decreased release of norepinephrine. Cardioselective β_1-blockers (which include metoprolol, atenolol, acebutolol, and bisoprolol) tend to lose some of their cardioselectivity at higher doses. Propranolol is a nonselective β-blocker that occupies both β_1 and β_2 receptor sites. Labetalol and carvedilol, which are combined α- and β-blockers, and nebivolol, which is a β-blocker that stimulates the endogenous production of nitric oxide, are collectively known as vasodilating β-blockers.

Clinical Use and Side Effects

β-Blockers are no longer recommended as part of the initial drug regimen for hypertension because they are generally less effective for lowering blood pressure and are less protective against stroke compared with first-line antihypertensive agents. β-Blockers can, however, be useful adjunctive antihypertensive agents and are part of evidence-based treatment in patients with heart failure or ischemic heart disease. Vasodilating β-blockers may cause fewer side effects, such as cold extremities and claudication.

Fatigue and reduced exercise tolerance are common side effects that contribute to the poor overall tolerability of β-blockers. Weight gain and acute bronchospasm can occur in patients with underlying lung disease, and these agents are the antihypertensive drug class most likely to cause erectile dysfunction. β-Blockers should be gradually tapered over several weeks when being discontinued, and they should be avoided in patients with suspected or known nonadherence because their abrupt cessation can result in rebound hypertension.

α-Adrenergic Blockers

Mechanism of Action

α-Adrenergic blockers block the effect of norepinephrine on vascular adrenergic receptors, thereby resulting in vasodilation and lowering of blood pressure. α-Adrenergic blockers improve both insulin sensitivity (by augmenting skeletal muscle blood flow; Chapter 210) and symptoms of bladder outlet obstruction (dilatation of urethral smooth muscle; Chapter 114). Prazosin, doxazosin, terazosin, and phentolamine block α-1 adrenergic receptors, whereas phenoxybenzamine blocks α-1 and α-2 adrenergic receptors.

Clinical Use and Side Effects

Phenoxybenzamine is very useful for the preoperative management of pheochromocytoma (Chapter 209), for which blockade of α-adrenergic receptors should be undertaken before administering β-blockers so as to prevent unopposed stimulation of the α-adrenergic receptor. α-1 Adrenergic receptor inhibitors are not recommended for first-line therapy because they do not lower blood pressure nor do they reduce the risk for cardiovascular events as well as first-line drugs, and they also can precipitate heart failure. α-Adrenergic agents are usually limited to late add-on therapy in men who have hypertension and symptoms of bladder outlet obstruction (Chapter 114), preferably combined with a diuretic to block their salt- and water-retaining properties. Orthostatic hypotension is a frequent adverse effect, and these agents must be used cautiously with phosphodiesterase-5 (PDE) inhibitors because of the risk of precipitous and profound drops in blood pressure.

Central Sympatholytics

Mechanism of Action

Central sympatholytic drugs stimulate the postsynaptic α-2 adrenergic or imidazoline receptors in the brain, thereby reducing the release of norepinephrine from peripheral sympathetic nerves, lowering sympathetic nervous system activity, and, as a result, lowering blood pressure.

Clinical Use and Side Effects

These drugs are limited to late add-on therapy for the treatment of resistant hypertension, in part because of their sedating side effects. These agents also cause orthostatic hypotension, which may go undetected if blood pressure is not measured in both the seated and standing positions. Clonidine is a rapidly acting oral agent, but it does not appear to have any discernable clinical benefit for acutely lowering blood pressure in patients who have a hypertensive urgency. Central sympatholytic drugs should be avoided in patients who have suspected or known nonadherence to prescribed drug therapy because of the possibility of rebound hypertension after their abrupt cessation. When these drugs are discontinued, they should be gradually tapered over several weeks.

Other Vasodilators

Mechanism of Action

Minoxidil and hydralazine work primarily by opening ATP-sensitive potassium channels in the resistance arterioles.

Clinical Use and Side Effects

These drugs are reserved for very late add-on therapy in the treatment of resistant hypertension. They cause profound arterial vasodilation that reflexively activates the sympathetic nervous system, thereby causing tachycardia. The use of either minoxidil or hydralazine necessitates the concurrent use of a potent diuretic to prevent the retention of salt and water, as well as a β-blocker to prevent reflex tachycardia. Hydralazine has also been linked to a lupus-like syndrome. Hirsutism, which is a common side effect of minoxidil therapy, can be particularly troubling in women. Endothelin antagonists, which are widely used for pulmonary hypertension (Chapter 69), are an experimental option for drug resistant hypertension.[A11]

ANTIHYPERTENSIVE DRUG INTERACTIONS

Nonsteroidal anti-inflammatory drugs (NSAIDs; Table 26-4) raise blood pressure and negatively affect kidney function. Of currently available NSAIDs, sulindac and celecoxib appear to have minimal, if any, effect on blood pressure levels in patients with hypertension. Acetaminophen can also raise blood pressure[A12] via unknown mechanisms. Grapefruit can cause excessive vasodilation for up to 24 hours in patients who are taking dihydropyridine calcium-channel blockers other than amlodipine by inactivating intestinal cytochrome P-450 3A4 (CYP34A) and possibly by inhibiting intestinal/hepatic p-glycoprotein (P-gp), thereby resulting in increased drug bioavailability. Verapamil and diltiazem are potent CYP3A4 inhibitors and can significantly raise the exposure to drugs such as simvastatin, atorvastatin, and fluvastatin that are all metabolized via CYP3A4; as a result, these drugs should be used at lower than the usually recommended reduced doses (Table 190-2), for both the initiation and maintenance of therapy, when patients are treated with verapamil or diltiazem. By comparison, amlodipine has more modest effects, but the dose of simvastatin still should not exceed 20 mg daily in amlodipine-treated patients. Rosuvastatin is a potent statin that does not inhibit CYP3A4 and can be used in its usual doses (Table 190-2). Cyclosporine and tacrolimus are also potent inhibitors of the CYP3A4 enzyme system and can significantly raise the blood levels of several statins that are metabolized via this pathway. Patients who are prescribed rivaroxaban, which is significantly metabolized via CYP3A4, should be monitored closely for bleeding. A lower than usual dose (see Table 70-6) is often preferred in patients who are treated with verapamil or diltiazem, particularly in the setting of renal impairment. In pregnant women requiring drug treatment for hypertension, iron supplementation reduces the absorption of methyldopa by 50%.

EVIDENCE-BASED MANAGEMENT OF HYPERTENSION

HOW FAR TO LOWER BLOOD PRESSURE?

U.S. guidelines recommended a blood pressure target of less than 130/80 mm Hg for most hypertensive patients, including less than 130 mm Hg systolic for patients ages 65 years and older (E-Table 64-1). However, published data demonstrate a mortality and cardiovascular benefit when middle-aged and older high-risk hypertensive patients are treated to a blood pressure target of less than 120 mm Hg systolic, including persons ages 75 years and older, even if they are frail, provided that they are not institutionalized.[A13,A14] The apparent contradiction is because clinical trials utilize rigorous standard protocols to measure blood pressure, and these protocols yield systolic blood pressure readings that, on average, are at least 10 mm Hg lower than are measurements that are obtained in routine clinical practice. In settings that use standard protocols to measure blood pressure, the recommended target blood pressure should be less than 120 mm Hg systolic.[18] In patients with diabetes, the currently recommended blood pressure target is less than 130/80 mm Hg, although guidelines suggest considering a goal of less than 120/80 mm Hg for patients who are at higher risk for complications of hypertension but at low risk for adverse effects from medications to lower blood pressure.[19]

WHICH DRUGS FOR WHICH PATIENTS?

Preferred antihypertensive drugs should be prescribed to patients who have specific indications (Table 64-9) because of their proven clinical benefit and safety. However, preferred antihypertensive agents often will be insufficient to control blood pressure without additional drugs.

Hypertensive Patients in General

The modern hypertension treatment paradigm emphasizes carefully selected combinations of antihypertensive drugs to control blood pressure. The selection of drugs should be guided by patient's clinical characteristics using combinations that have complementary efficacy and do not share adverse effects. Effective combinations include an ACE inhibitor or angiotensin receptor blocker combined with either a calcium-channel blocker (e.g., amlodipine) or a thiazide-like diuretic (e.g., chlorthalidone or indapamide). A single pill with quarter-doses of four medications (irbesartan 37.5 mg, amlodipine 1.25 mg, indapamide 0.625 mg, and bisoprolol 2.5 mg) is a potential simple alternative.[A15] However, β-blockers are not recommended for initial therapy in uncomplicated hypertension because they do not lower blood pressure nor protect against stroke as well as other first-line drugs. The combined use of any two renin–angiotensin system inhibitors (e.g., an ACE inhibitor, an angiotensin receptor blocker, or a dopamine reuptake inhibitor) should be avoided because of minimal incremental blood pressure lowering as well as a high risk of renal impairment and hyperkalemia.

Systolic Hypertension in Elderly Patients

Isolated systolic hypertension is the predominant phenotype in hypertensive patients ages 65 years and older. Randomized controlled trials have unequivocally proven that pharmacologic blood pressure lowering reduces premature mortality, morbid and fatal cardiovascular events, and dementia in such patients, even after age 80 years and even in the frail elderly. One caveat in such patients is a higher risk of orthostatic hypotension. Fortunately, intensive treatment to low blood pressure targets does not specifically cause orthostatic hypotension.[20] Older patients may not tolerate reductions in blood pressure as well as younger patients, so drug therapy should start with low doses of medications. Older patients are also more likely to have white coat hypertension or effect as well as masked or masked uncontrolled hypertension, thereby highlighting the need for home and/or ambulatory blood pressure measurements to assist therapeutic decision-making to prevent overtreatment as well as undertreatment. Older patients, particularly patients who have orthostatic hypotension, are also prone to developing postprandial hypotension (E-Fig. 64-5) because their splanchnic circulation dilates, thereby resulting in the pooling of blood. Postprandial home blood pressure measurements and/or ambulatory blood pressure monitoring is the best way to confirm this condition, which can be managed by consuming smaller and more frequent meals with a low glycemic index, drinking coffee with meals, and avoiding alcohol as well as hot showers.

Other potential problems in older persons include their higher risk for thiazide-induced hyponatremia, poorer adherence to medications, and polypharmacy with a greater probability of deleterious drug-drug interactions. The antihypertensive drug regimen should be simplified as much as possible, and medication refills should be synchronized with their pharmacy to the greatest degree possible.

Patients with Hypertensive Heart Disease

Left ventricular hypertrophy, which is an undesirable maladaptive myocardial response to uncontrolled blood pressure (Chapter 41), is a risk factor for atrial fibrillation, heart failure, ventricular arrhythmias, sudden death, and stroke. Most antihypertensive drug classes that successfully lower blood pressure will also lead to some degree of regression of left ventricular hypertrophy, but angiotensin receptor blockers and ACE inhibitors may be the best for this purpose. For patients who have a reduced left ventricular ejection fraction, guideline-directed medical therapy emphasizes β-blockers, aldosterone antagonists, and combination angiotensin receptor neprilysin inhibitors.

In patients with stable ischemic heart disease, a β-blocker combined with an ACE inhibitor or an angiotensin receptor blocker is first-line therapy. If such patients require further medication to control angina (Chapter 56), a dihydropyridine calcium-channel blocker should be added. If, however, the medical issue is resistant blood pressure, then an aldosterone antagonist or a thiazide-like diuretic is first-line add-on therapy.

Diabetes and Normal Renal Function

Approximately 80% of patients with type 2 diabetes (Chapter 210) have hypertension. Although no compelling evidence suggests that any particular first-line medications are preferred, treatment usually begins with an ACE inhibitor or angiotensin receptor blocker plus a calcium-channel blocker, or perhaps a thiazide-like diuretic.

Chronic Diabetic Kidney Disease

Diabetic nephropathy (Chapter 109) is characterized by albuminuria (≥300 mg/g), dysfunctional renal autoregulation, depressed glomerular filtration capacity, elevated blood pressure, and a high risk for cardiovascular–renal events. ACE inhibitors and angiotensin receptor blockers are indicated for patients who have chronic diabetic kidney disease to slow the progressive loss of kidney function. In addition to sodium–glucose cotransporter-2 inhibitors, combination drug therapy should be initiated with an ACE inhibitor or angiotensin receptor blocker plus a calcium-channel blocker, often with a thiazide-like diuretic, preferably chlorthalidone. However, a loop diuretic may be substituted for a thiazide-like diuretic when the estimated glomerular filtration rate is less than 25 mL/mm/1.73 m^2.

Secondary Stroke Prevention

Prior stroke (Chapters 376 and 377) is a major risk factor for recurrent stroke, disability, mortality, and cardiovascular events. In patients who have survived a stroke or a transient ischemic attack, oral medications should be started or restarted a few days post-stroke if possible. The blood pressure threshold for starting antihypertensive drug therapy is uncertain, but drug therapy is usually initiated when the blood pressure exceeds 140/90 mm Hg. Preferred drugs in this high-risk group include thiazide-like diuretics (especially indapamide), ACE inhibitors, and angiotensin receptor blockers. The magnitude of cardiovascular protection likely relates to the degree of blood pressure reduction. For example, lowering blood pressure to less than 130/80 mm Hg after a lacunar infarction reduces the risk for subsequent hemorrhagic stroke (Chapter 377).

Hypertension In Black Americans

Hypertension in Black Americans, relative to White Americans, has an earlier onset, is more prevalent and severe, and is accompanied by a greater risk for pressure-related target-organ injury, including left ventricular hypertrophy, heart failure, stroke, and death. Reductions in dietary sodium intake not only lower blood pressure but also reduce the intensity of antihypertensive drug therapy required to control blood pressure. However, hypertensive Black Americans have higher prevalences of several characteristics that confer resistance to antihypertensive drug therapy, including obesity, chronic kidney disease, and diabetes mellitus. As a result, more intense pharmacotherapy is typical required. Nevertheless, excellent responses can be provided by carefully selected combination drug therapy (anchored by either an ACE inhibitor or angiotensin receptor blocker plus a thiazide or thiazide-like diuretic or a calcium-channel blocker). Pharmacist-led treatment programs in barbershops are a useful strategy for controlling blood pressure in Black men with previously uncontrolled hypertension.[A16]

Hypertension Associated with Oral Contraceptives and Estrogen Replacement

Hypertension occurs in up to 8.5% of women who use oral contraception, especially with higher-dose ethinyl estradiol preparations (>50 mcg; see Table 220-2), and is directly related to the duration of therapy. By comparison, progestin-only contraceptives do not appear to raise blood pressure. Risk factors for oral contraceptive–associated hypertension include prior hypertensive disorders of pregnancy, smoking, older age, obesity, diabetes mellitus, chronic kidney disease, and Black race. Hormonal contraception (e.g., estrogen and estrogen/progestin combinations) is best avoided in women who have poorly controlled blood pressure, whereas progestin-only preparations are acceptable. If hypertension develops during use of estrogen-containing hormonal contraception, it should be discontinued and replaced with a nonhormonal or progestin-only form of contraception. Data are inconclusive as to whether postmenopausal estrogen therapy (Chapter 222) modestly raises or reduces blood pressure.

Hypertension in Pregnancy

Hypertension during pregnancy is an important cause of maternal and fetal morbidity. It is discussed in detail in Chapter 221.

Drug-Resistant Hypertension

Many patients with hypertension are treated with two or fewer antihypertensive drugs, so most patients who have persistent hypertension despite treatment have not been treated intensively enough to be categorized as having resistant or refractory hypertension. Many of these patients have pseudo-resistance (Table 64-10), and most will be effectively treated with appropriate multidrug regimens (Fig. 64-4). Among patients who are treated with multiple antihypertensive drugs, poor control may be a result of suboptimal or ineffective treatment regimens rather than true resistance.

Resistant hypertension is defined as persistent hypertension (≥130/80 mm Hg) despite prescribing three or four antihypertensive medications, one of which is a diuretic, or controlled blood pressure (<130/80 mm Hg) that requires four or more antihypertensive drugs, one of which is a diuretic. The prevalence of resistant hypertension in U.S. adults is about 15%. Refractory hypertension is defined as uncontrolled blood pressure despite five or more antihypertensive medications, one of which is a diuretic. The prevalence of refractory hypertension in U.S. drug-treated adults is 0.8%. Resistant and refractory hypertension are more common in Black Americans, older persons, and persons with chronic kidney disease, primary aldosteronism (Chapter 208), renal artery stenosis, pheochromocytoma, diabetes, known cardiovascular disease, obesity, high sodium intake, low levels of physical activity,[21] and low household income.

Among patients who have apparent treatment-resistant hypertension, nonadherence to medication is highly prevalent.[22] Long-acting antihypertensive agents (e.g., chlorthalidone, amlodipine) should be favored because they will provide better efficacy if some doses are missed.[23] Other strategies to maximize the effectiveness of antihypertensive drug regimens include using thiazide-like diuretics (e.g., indapamide or chlorthalidone) rather than HCTZ and adding an aldosterone antagonist (spironolactone, eplerenone) or an ENaC channel inhibitor (amiloride) in patients who have adequate kidney function (eGFR ≥45 mL/min/1.73 m^2). Counseling that successfully reduces dietary sodium intake rapidly lowers blood pressure in resistant or refractory hypertension

TABLE 64-10 CAUSES OF PSEUDORESISTANT AND TRULY RESISTANT HYPERTENSION

PSEUDORESISTANT HYPERTENSION	TRULY RESISTANT HYPERTENSION

• Ineffective medical regimen
• Heavy arterial calcification
• Medication nonadherence
• Pressor substances
  • Most nonsteroidal anti-inflammatory drugs
  • Calcineurin inhibitors (e.g., cyclosporine, tacrolimus)
  • Glucocorticoids
  • Herbs (e.g., yohimbine, St. John's wort)
  • Sympathomimetics (e.g., phenylephrine, sibutramine, methylphenidate)
  • Antipsychotic agents (e.g., clozapine, thioridazine)
  • Antidepressant agents (e.g., venlafaxine, fluoxetine)
  • Anxiolytic agents (e.g., buspirone)
	• Primary aldosteronism
	• Chronic kidney disease
	• Obesity
	• Obstructive sleep apnea
	• Other causes of secondary hypertension
	  • Pheochromocytoma
	  • Cushing syndrome
	  • Atherosclerotic renal artery stenosis
	  • Fibromuscular dysplasia
	  • Coarctation of the aorta
	  • Hyperthyroidism
	  • Hypothyroidism
	  • Hyperparathyroidism
	  • Severe essential hypertension

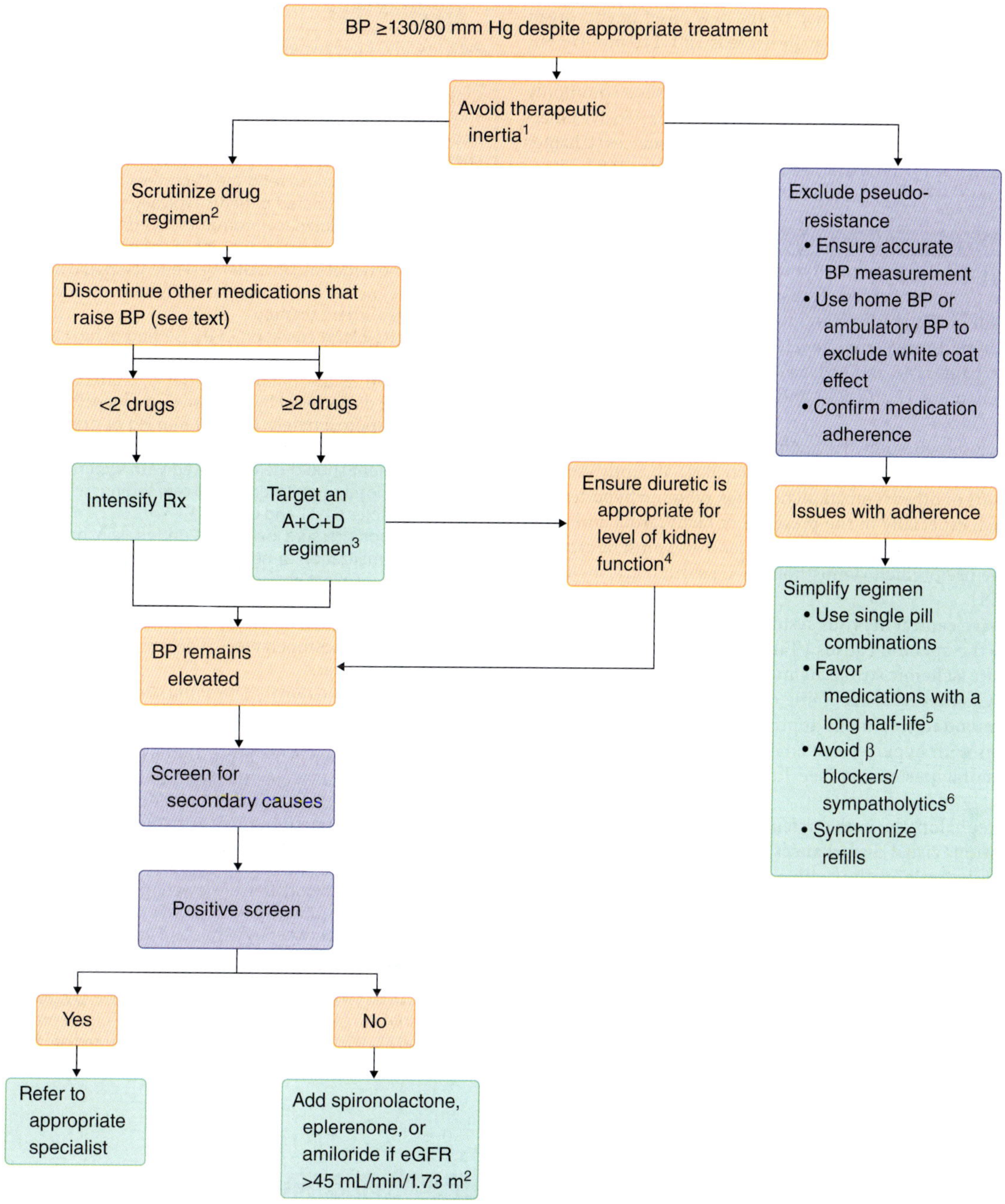

FIGURE 64-4. Algorithm for evaluating and treating residual hypertension. A = angiotensin-converting enzyme inhibitor or angiotensin receptor blocker; BP = blood pressure; C = calcium-channel blocker; D = diuretic; eGFR = estimated glomerular filtration rate; Rx = treatment. [1]Regimen should include comorbidity-indicated drugs (see Table 64-8). [2]Documenting office blood pressure elevations but taking no action(s) to intensify drug treatment or initiate treatment if unmediated. [3]3-Drug treatment with A: an angiotensin-converting enzyme inhibitor or an angiotensin receptor blocker, C: a calcium-channel blocker, and D: a diuretic (see Table 64-7). [4]eGFR ≥45 mL/min/1.73 m^2 (chlorthalidone, indapamide, hydrochlorothiazide); eGFR 30-45 (chlorthalidone, indapamide, loop diuretics); and eGFR <30 (loop diuretics or metolazone). [5]Drugs such as chlorthalidone, amlodipine, azilsartan, olmesartan. [6]Because their abrupt discontinuation can lead to rebound hypertension.

to a degree that exceeds the blood pressure reductions with most add-on single drug therapies.

Second-generation catheter-based electrode renal denervation modestly lowers blood pressure, whereas first-generation attempted treatments did not.[A17] Ultrasound renal denervation is another experimental option.[A18] To date, however, renal artery denervation has not received FDA approval for widespread use in the United States, and its future role remains unclear.

PREVENTION

Effective primordial prevention of hypertension is not principally dependent on medical care but rather on the widespread adoption of a prudent diet (Chapter 13) and lifestyle changes to reduce the intake of excess calories, sodium, and alcohol (Chapter 364), as well as to increase physical activity (Chapter 14) and prevent obesity (Chapter 201). Although these issues represent individual choices, societal barriers to the adoption of these guidelines include the limited availability and higher cost of healthy foods and safety concerns that limit outdoor physical activity in some geographic areas. Primary prevention depends on screening,[A19] which should be performed at least every 2 years or so in adults.[24]

Acute Severe Hypertension

Hypertensive urgencies and emergencies occur in approximately 1% and 0.3%, respectively, of all emergency department visits.[25] Most patients have an exacerbation of previously diagnosed but typically poorly controlled hypertension, but new-onset hypertension also can present as an urgency or emergency, especially in vulnerable populations and in middle- and low-income countries.[26]

A hypertensive urgency is defined as a blood pressure level of 180/110 mm Hg or greater without new or worsening pressure-related target-organ injury, such as myocardial or cerebral ischemia, aortic dissection,[27] or acute heart failure. A hypertensive emergency is defined by the new onset of end-organ damage with a blood pressure level that usually exceeds 180/110 mm Hg but may be substantially higher.

Nonadherence to prescribed antihypertensive medications is a commonly encountered cause of precipitous rises in blood pressure. Hypertensive emergencies also can occur after ingestion of sympathomimetic substances (Chapter 365), eclampsia (Chapter 221), traumatic head injuries (Chapter 368), extensive body burns (Chapter 97), and postoperatively.

CLINICAL MANIFESTATIONS AND DIAGNOSIS

Patients with a hypertensive urgency are typically asymptomatic. However, some patients with hypertensive urgency present with minimal vague symptoms but striking high blood pressure elevations (e.g., 220/120 mm Hg). The most common hypertensive emergencies include heart failure/acute pulmonary edema (Chapters 45 and 46), acute coronary syndromes/myocardial infarction (Chapters 57 and 58), and severe blood pressure elevations after surgery.

Patients should be closely questioned regarding their adherence to prescribed antihypertensive medications. In patients who may have abruptly stopped taking either β-blockers or other sympatholytic drugs, rebound hypertension should be considered, especially in the presence of tachycardia and other signs of sympathetic nervous system activation. Patients also must be carefully questioned about the use of illicit sympathomimetic substances, including cocaine (Chapter 365).

In patients who have central nervous system manifestations of a hypertensive emergency, the specific causes (Table 64-11; e.g., hypertensive encephalopathy, acute ischemic stroke, hemorrhagic stroke, and subarachnoid hemorrhage [Chapter 377; see Table 64-10]) must be determined because the recommended treatment approaches vary significantly. All patients who present with hypertensive emergencies should be screened for secondary forms of hypertension (see Table 64-4) while hospitalized, if possible.

Hypertensive encephalopathy is characterized by severe blood pressure elevations, obtundation, visual disturbances, altered sensorium, seizures, and marked hypertensive retinopathy (with or without papilledema; see Fig. 391-25), but an absence of focal neurologic findings. Brain imaging with CT or MRI is useful to exclude intracranial hemorrhage and acute ischemic stroke. An important subset of patients with hypertensive encephalopathy have the posterior leukoencephalopathy syndrome, which is characterized by symmetrical vasogenic edema in the posterior occipital regions of the brain, most readily visualized on MRI. Such patients can have focal neurologic signs that can be difficult to distinguish from an evolving stroke (Chapter 376).

TREATMENT

Patients who have hypertensive urgencies are often initially seen in ambulatory settings and are then subsequently referred to an emergency department, despite little evidence that such transfer is beneficial or that hospital admission should be required. Patients who present with severe blood pressure elevations above the threshold for diagnosing hypertensive urgency should have any discontinued blood pressure medications restarted or be switched to longer-acting drugs that do not cause rebound hypertension if they are abruptly discontinued. Previously untreated patients typically should be started on routine oral therapy and scheduled for prompt follow-up. However, rapid blood pressure reductions via either the oral or intravenous route run the short-term risk of precipitating target-organ ischemia. Patients should be observed long enough to be confident that they do not have any new or worsening target-organ injury that requires urgent therapy.

No precise blood elevation in the setting of new and worsening pressure-related target-organ injury (e.g., obtundation, confusion, focal neurologic signs, seizures, heart failure, pulmonary edema, blurred vision, severe retinopathy) confirms the diagnosis of hypertensive emergency. Nevertheless, when blood pressure is approximately 180/110 mm Hg or greater, the blood pressure is high enough to be the likely cause of the new/worsening target-organ injury and the patient should be diagnosed with hypertensive emergency and be treated in a closely monitored critical care settings with intravenous medications (Fig. 64-5; Tables 64-11 and 64-12).

When blood pressure lowering is undertaken, however, rapid reductions to achieve normalization or near normalization of blood pressure is not recommended except in patients who have aortic dissection (Chapter 63), cardiogenic pulmonary edema (Chapter 46), an acute coronary syndrome (Chapter 57), or hemorrhagic stroke (Chapter 377). Immediate blood pressure lowering is also indicated in postoperative patients to prevent bleeding, particularly from vascular suture lines.

Immediate blood pressure lowering can be accomplished with rapid-onset intravenous drugs such as clevidipine and nicardipine outside of the intensive care setting. In other hypertensive emergencies that do not necessitate a more immediate reduction in blood pressure, a prudent approach is to reduce blood pressure by 10 to 15% over the first 1 to 2 hours, then by another 10 to 15% over the ensuing 12 to 24 hours. The rationale for allowing blood pressure to remain in the hypertensive range is to prevent iatrogenic hypoperfusion and ischemia of pressure-sensitive target organs. For example, in severely hypertensive patients with acute ischemic stroke (Chapter 376), care must be taken to avoid overzealous blood pressure lowering because the cerebral autoregulation of blood flow is disrupted in the ischemic penumbra and is entirely dependent on the difference between systemic and intracranial pressures to sustain blood flow to vulnerable brain tissue in watershed areas.

Oral Medications for Hypertensive Urgencies

The overwhelming majority of patients with blood pressure levels above the threshold of 180/110 mm Hg will not require immediate blood pressure lowering with oral medications in the office nor in the hospital setting and do not require

TABLE 64-11 HYPERTENSIVE EMERGENCIES REQUIRING IMMEDIATE LOWERING OF BLOOD PRESSURE

CLINICAL PRESENTATION	TIMELINE AND TARGET BLOOD PRESSURE	PREFERRED TREATMENT	ALTERNATIVE
Malignant hypertension with or without thrombotic microangiopathy or acute renal failure	Several hours, MAP −20 to −25%	Labetalol OR nicardipine	Nitroprusside Urapidil
Hypertensive encephalopathy	Immediate, MAP −20 to −25%	Labetalol OR nicardipine	Nitroprusside
Acute ischemic stroke and BP >220 mm Hg systolic or >120 mm Hg diastolic (Chapter 376)	1 hour, MAP −15%	Labetalol OR nicardipine	Nitroprusside
Acute ischemic stroke with indication for thrombolytic therapy and BP >185 mm Hg systolic or >110 mm Hg diastolic (Chapter 376)	1 hour, MAP −15%	Labetalol OR nicardipine	Nitroprusside
Acute hemorrhagic stroke and systolic BP >180 mm Hg (Chapter 377)	Immediate, systolic BP 130 to 180 mm Hg	Labetalol OR nicardipine	Urapidil
Acute coronary event (Chapters 57 and 58)	Immediate, systolic BP <140 mm Hg	Nitroglycerin OR labetalol	Urapidil
Acute cardiogenic pulmonary edema (Chapter 46)	Immediate, systolic BP <140 mm Hg	Nitroprusside OR nitroglycerin (with a loop diuretic)	Urapidil (with loop diuretic)
Acute aortic disease (Chapter 63)	Immediate, systolic BP <120 mm Hg and heart rate <60 beats per minute	Esmolol PLUS nitroprusside OR nitroglycerin plus nicardipine	Labetalol OR metoprolol
Eclampsia and severe preeclampsia/HELLP (Chapter 221)	Immediate, systolic BP <160 mm Hg and diastolic BP <105 mm Hg	Magnesium sulfate PLUS labetalol OR nicardipine	

BP = blood pressure; HELLP = hemolysis, elevated liver enzymes and low platelets; MAP = mean arterial pressure.

Adapted from van den Born BH, Lip GYH, Brguljan-Hitij J, et al. ESC Council on hypertension position document on the management of hypertensive emergencies. *Eur Heart J Cardiovasc Pharmacother.* 2019;5:37-46; Victor RG. Arterial hypertension. In: Goldman L, Schafer AI eds. *Goldman-Cecil Medicine.* Philadelphia: Elsevier; 2020:443-456.

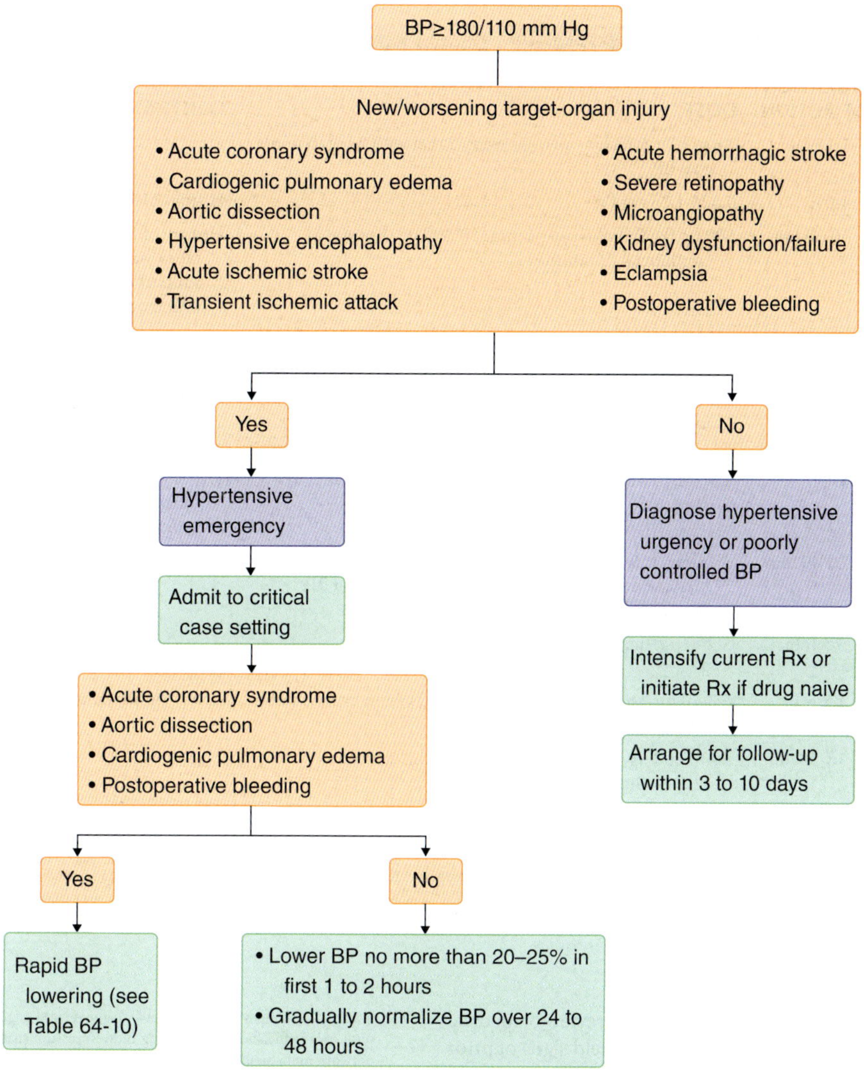

FIGURE 64-5. **Algorithm for diagnosing and treating hypertensive emergency.** BP = blood pressure; Rx = treatment.

referral to an emergency department. The one important exception, however, is patients who have abruptly discontinued β-blockers or sympatholytic drugs and who present with rebound hypertension with overt signs of sympathetic nervous system activation (e.g., tachycardia). Initiating intravenous labetalol (e.g., 20 mg initially then 20 mg to 80 mg every 10 minutes until the clinical manifestations of sympathetic nervous system hyperactivity have lessened) or oral clonidine (0.1 to 0.2 mg initially, then up to 0.1 mg hourly up to 0.7 mg total dose) to diminish sympathetic nervous system activity is reasonable in this situation. Other patients should have their discontinued medications restarted or their prescribed regimen intensified. If patients have not previously been treated, treatment should be initiated with two-drug therapy consisting of either a thiazide-like diuretic or calcium antagonist plus either an ACE inhibitor or an angiotensin receptor blocker.

Intravenous Medications for Hypertensive Emergencies

For a hypertensive emergency, labetalol (Table 64-12) is usually the favored drug, especially when treating severe blood pressure elevations in patients who have an acute ischemic stroke, because it has a reasonably quick onset of action and minimally reduces cerebral blood flow. However, labetalol has a delayed offset of action, thereby making it harder to titrate the blood pressure response, particularly if blood pressure falls too rapidly during the infusion. Conversely, nitroprusside has a near-immediate onset and offset of action, so near-instantaneous blood pressure titration can be obtained. A disadvantage of nitroprusside is that it does not preserve cerebral blood flow as well as labetalol as blood pressure is lowered. Nicardipine has a nearly identical onset of action as labetalol, but, importantly, has a much faster offset of action.

After gradual reduction of blood pressure into the target ranges for the various types of hypertensive emergencies, patients must be weaned from intravenous medications and transitioned to oral antihypertensive drugs so they can be transferred out of the intensive care unit. Patients should be transitioned to carefully selected combination drug therapies (e.g., calcium-channel blocker or thiazide-like diuretic plus an ACE inhibitor or angiotensin receptor blocker, depending on their comorbid conditions; see Tables 64-5 and 64-7). However, immediate blood pressure normalization is not the goal. A 20- to 40-mg dose of intravenous furosemide (repeated, if needed no sooner than 2 hours later) can enhance the blood pressure response to oral medications, especially because saline-containing intravenous fluid infusions and the profound vasodilation from intravenous antihypertensive drugs can expand the plasma volume and extracellular fluid volume, and thereby attenuate the response to antihypertensive drugs.

INCIDENTAL BLOOD PRESSURE ELEVATIONS IN THE EMERGENCY DEPARTMENT

Blood pressure elevations are commonly encountered in patients who present to emergency departments for a variety of complaints and conditions. The vast majority of these patients truly do have hypertension, but its severity is often overestimated because of pain, stress, and poor blood pressure measurement

TABLE 64-12 INTRAVENOUS DRUGS FOR HYPERTENSIVE EMERGENCIES

DRUG	ONSET OF ACTION	DURATION OF ACTION	DOSE	CONTRAINDICATIONS	ADVERSE EFFECTS
Clevidipine	2-3 min	5-15 min	2 mg/h IV infusion, increase every 2 min with 2 mg/h until goal BP		Headache and reflex-tachycardia
Enalaprilat	5-15 min	4-6 h	0.625-1.25 mg IV	History of angioedema	
Esmolol	1-2 min	10-30 min	500 µg/kg IV bolus over 1 min; 50-300 µg/kg/min as continuous IV infusion	History of 2nd- or 3rd-degree AV block (in the absence of rhythm support), systolic heart failure, asthma, and bradycardia	Bradycardia
Fenoldopam	5-15 min	30-60 min	0.1 µg/kg/min IV infusion, increase every 15 min until goal BP is reached with 0.05-0.1 µg/kg/min increments		
Labetalol	5-10 min	3-6 h	0.25-0.5 mg/kg IV bolus; 2-4 mg/min continuous infusion until goal BP is reached, thereafter 5-20 mg/h	History of 2nd- or 3rd-degree AV block, systolic heart failure, asthma, and bradycardia	Bronchoconstriction and fetal bradycardia
Metoprolol	1-2 min	5-8 h	2.5-5 mg IV bolus over 1 min; may repeat every 5 min to a maximum dose of 15 mg	History of 2nd- or 3rd-degree AV block, systolic heart failure, asthma and bradycardia	Bradycardia
Nicardipine	5-15 min	30-40 min	5-15 mg/h as continuous IV infusion, starting dose 5 mg/h, increase every 15-30 min with 2.5 mg until goal BP, thereafter decrease to 3 mg/h	Liver failure	Headache and reflex-tachycardia
Nitroglycerin	1-5 min	3-5 min	5-200 µg/min, 5 µg/min increase every 5 min		Headache and reflex-tachycardia
Nitroprusside	Immediate	1-2 min	0.3-10 µg/kg/min, increase by 0.5 µg/kg/min every 5 min until goal BP	Liver/kidney failure (relative)	Cyanide intoxication
Phentolamine	1-2 min	10-30 min	500-1000 µg/kg IV bolus OR 50-300 µg/kg/min as continuous IV infusion		Tachyarrhythmias and chest pain
Urapidil	3-5 min	4-6 h	12.5-25 mg IV bolus, 5-40 mg/h as continuous infusion		

1000 µg = 1 mg; AV = atrioventricular; BP = blood pressure; IV = intravenous.
Adapted from van den Born BH, Lip GYH, Brguljan-Hitij J, et al. ESC Council on hypertension position document on the management of hypertensive emergencies. *Eur Heart J Cardiovasc Pharmacother.* 2019;5:37-46.

techniques. Even in a busy emergency department, a careful review of medical records, clinical examination, and review of the ECG can yield signs of prior chronic blood pressure elevations. To the degree possible, patients should receive referral to a medical physician for follow-up and further evaluation. In patients who have severe blood pressure elevations and evidence of target-organ injury, consideration should be given to referral to a hypertension specialist.

GENERAL REFERENCES

For the General References and other additional features, please visit Elsevier eBooks+ at https://ebooks.health.elsevier.com.

Grade A References

A1. Piaggio D, Bracale U, Pecchia L, et al. Endovascular treatment versus medical therapy for hypertensive patients with renal artery stenosis: an updated systematic review. *Ann Vasc Surg.* 2019;61:445-454.

A2. Filippini T, Malavolti M, Whelton PK, et al. Blood pressure effects of sodium reduction: dose–response meta-analysis of experimental studies. *Circulation.* 2021;143:1542-1567.

A3. Neal B, Wu Y, Feng X, et al. Effect of salt substitution on cardiovascular events and death. *N Engl J Med.* 2021;385:1067-1077.

A4. The Blood Pressure Lowering Treatment Trialists' Collaboration. Pharmacological blood pressure lowering for primary and secondary prevention of cardiovascular disease across different levels of blood pressure: an individual participant-level data meta-analysis. *Lancet.* 2021;397:1625-1636.

A5. Hughes D, Judge C, Murphy R, et al. Association of blood pressure lowering with incident dementia or cognitive impairment: a systematic review and meta-analysis. *JAMA.* 2020;323:1934-1944.

A6. The Blood Pressure Lowering Treatment Trialists' Collaboration. Age-stratified and blood-pressure-stratified effects of blood-pressure-lowering pharmacotherapy for the prevention of cardiovascular disease and death: an individual participant-level data meta-analysis. *Lancet.* 2021;398:1053-1064.

A7. Wang J-G, Zhang M, Feng Y-Q, et al. Is the newest angiotensin-receptor blocker azilsartan medoxomil more efficacious in lowering blood pressure than the older ones? A systematic review and network meta-analysis. *J Clin Hypertens.* 2021;23:901-914.

A8. Ishani A, Cushman WC, Leatherman SM, et al. Chlorthalidone vs. hydrochlorothiazide for hypertension—cardiovascular events. *N Engl J Med.* 2022;387:2401-2410.

A9. Agarwal R, Sinha AD, Cramer AE, et al. Chlorthalidone for hypertension in advanced kidney disease. *N Engl J Med.* 2021;385:2507-2519.

A10. Freeman MW, Halvorsen Y-D, Marshall W, et al. Phase 2 trial of baxdrostat for treatment-resistant hypertension. *N Engl J Med.* 2023;388:395-405.

A11. Schlaich MP, Bellet M, Weber MA, et al. Dual endothelin antagonist aprocitentan for resistant hypertension (PRECISION): a multicentre, blinded, randomised, parallel-group, phase 3 trial. *Lancet.* 2022;400:1927-1937.

A12. MacIntyre IM, Turtle EKJ, Farrah TE, et al. Regular acetaminophen use and blood pressure in people with hypertension: the PATH-BP trial. *Circulation.* 2022;145:416-423.

A13. SPRINT Research Group, Lewis CE, Fine LJ, et al. Final report of a trial of intensive versus standard blood-pressure control. *N Engl J Med.* 2021;384:1921-1930.

A14. Zhang W, Zhang S, Deng Y, et al. Trial of intensive blood-pressure control in older patients with hypertension. *N Engl J Med.* 2021;385:1268-1279.

A15. Chow CK, Atkins ER, Hillis GS, et al. Initial treatment with a single pill containing quadruple combination of quarter doses of blood pressure medicines versus standard dose monotherapy in patients with hypertension (QUARTET): a phase 3, randomized, double-blind, active-controlled trial. *Lancet.* 2021;398:1043-1052.

A16. Victor RG, Lynch K, Li N, et al. A cluster-randomized trial of blood-pressure reduction in black barbershops. *N Engl J Med.* 2018;378:1291-1301.

A17. Bhatt DL, Vaduganathan M, Kandzari DE, et al. Long-term outcomes after catheter-based renal artery denervation for resistant hypertension: final follow-up of the randomised SYMPLICITY HTN-3 Trial. *Lancet.* 2022;400:1405-1416.

A18. Kirtane AJ, Sharp ASP, Mahfoud F, et al. Patient-level pooled analysis of ultrasound renal denervation in the sham-controlled RADIANCE II, RADIANCE-HTN SOLO, and RADIANCE-HTN TRIO trials. *JAMA Cardiol.* 2023. [Epub ahead of print.]

A19. Guirguis-Blake JM, Evans CV, Webber EM, et al. Screening for hypertension in adults: updated evidence report and systematic review for the US Preventive Services Task Force. *JAMA.* 2021;325:1657-1669.

65

ATHEROSCLEROTIC PERIPHERAL ARTERIAL DISEASE

CHRISTOPHER J. WHITE

DEFINITION

Lower extremity atherosclerotic peripheral arterial disease is one subset of a larger group of peripheral vascular diseases that includes all noncoronary vascular disorders that may affect the arterial, venous (Chapters 66 and 68), or lymphatic circulation. Atherosclerotic arterial diseases are characterized by arterial narrowing or occlusion caused by the accumulation of atherosclerotic plaque elements in the vessel wall. Atherosclerotic vascular disease can also lead to aneurysm formation, which is the pathologic enlargement of arterial segments, and may result in rupture, dissection, or thromboembolism (Chapter 63).

EPIDEMIOLOGY

The prevalence of lower extremity peripheral arterial disease in the United States, Europe, and Asia continues to increase as the population ages and is exposed to atherosclerotic risk factors (Chapter 40). The presence of peripheral arterial disease is defined as an ankle-brachial index (ABI)—the ratio of the highest systolic blood pressure in the ankle divided by the highest systolic blood pressure in the arm (Fig. 65-1)—less than 0.90. Among individuals age 40 years and older, the prevalence is 4.3% (95% confidence interval [CI], 3.1 to 5.5%), but the prevalence in individuals with diabetes ranges from 20 to 30%.[1]

Risk factors for atherosclerosis (Chapter 40) increase the likelihood of developing lower extremity peripheral arterial disease (Table 65-1). More than 95% of individuals with peripheral arterial disease have at least one traditional cardiovascular risk factor, and most have multiple risk factors. More than one third of patients with peripheral arterial disease have significant coronary disease, and up to one quarter have carotid artery disease. As a result, the risk of heart attack, stroke, and death are increased several-fold in patients with peripheral arterial disease.

Among conventional atherosclerotic risk factors, cigarette smoking is two to three times more likely to cause lower extremity peripheral arterial disease than to cause coronary artery disease. Hypertension is also associated with lower extremity peripheral arterial disease. The development of peripheral arterial disease is more likely in patients with lipid abnormalities (elevated total and low-density lipoprotein [LDL] cholesterol, decreased high-density lipoprotein [HDL] cholesterol, and hypertriglyceridemia), and the risk increases by 5 to 10% for each 10 mg/dL increase in total cholesterol. Increased homocysteine levels are associated with a two- to three-fold increased risk for developing atherosclerotic peripheral arterial disease. Diabetes mellitus increases the risk of lower extremity peripheral arterial disease by two- to four-fold, and the risk of developing lower extremity peripheral arterial disease is proportional to the severity and duration of diabetes. Tight control of diabetes is important because the risk of developing peripheral arterial disease increases by 28% for every 1% increase in glycosylated hemoglobin (Chapter 210). Patients with diabetes who have lower extremity peripheral arterial disease are seven- to 15-fold more likely to undergo a major amputation than nondiabetics with lower extremity peripheral arterial disease.

Peripheral arterial disease disproportionately affects older individuals, non-Hispanic Blacks, current smokers, individuals with diabetes, and those with abnormal renal function. The overall prevalence of peripheral arterial disease in the United States among persons age 70 years and older is 14.5% (95% CI, 10.8 to 18.2%), which corresponds to approximately 4 million individuals.

TABLE 65-1 PATIENTS AT RISK FOR PERIPHERAL ARTERIAL DISEASE

- Age ≥65 yr
- Age 50-64 yr with risk factors for atherosclerosis (e.g., diabetes mellitus, history of smoking, hyperlipidemia, hypertension; see Chapter 40) or family history of peripheral arterial disease
- Age <50 yr with diabetes mellitus and 1 additional risk factor for atherosclerosis
- Known atherosclerotic disease in another vascular bed (e.g., coronary, carotid, subclavian, renal, mesenteric artery stenosis, or abdominal aortic aneurysm)

Adapted from Gerhard-Herman MD, Gornik HL, Barrett C, et al. 2016 AHA/ACC guideline on the management of patients with lower extremity peripheral artery disease: executive summary: a report of the American College of Cardiology/American Heart Association Task Force on Clinical Practice Guidelines. *J Am Coll Cardiol.* 2017;69:1465-1508.

PATHOBIOLOGY

Acute Limb Ischemia

Acute limb ischemia occurs when blood flow to an extremity is abruptly halted or markedly diminished, resulting in hypoperfusion that threatens the viability of the limb. Acute limb ischemia is most commonly caused by either thrombosis

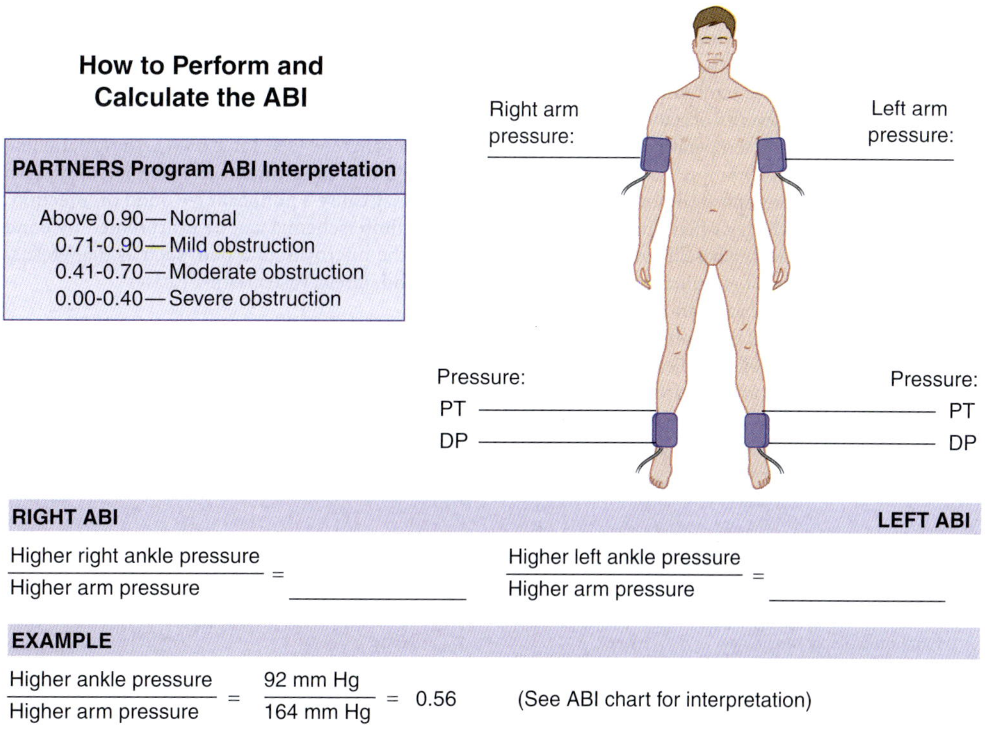

FIGURE 65-1. **Performing pressure measurements and calculating the ankle-brachial index (ABI). To calculate the ABI, systolic pressures are determined in both arms and both ankles with the use of a handheld Doppler instrument. The higher reading in either the dorsalis pedis (DP) or the posterior tibial (PT) arteries of the right foot and the left foot is divided by the higher systolic blood pressure reading in either the right or left arm to calculate the index. PARTNERS = PAD (peripheral arterial disease) Awareness, Risk, and Treatment: New Resources for Survival.**

or embolism. Most emboli originate from the heart as a mural thrombus from a recent myocardial infarction (MI; Chapter 58) or from the atrial appendage in a patient with atrial fibrillation (Chapter 52). A less common cause of lower extremity emboli is an abdominal aortic aneurysm (Chapter 63) that serves as the source of cholesterol emboli (Chapter 66).

Arterial in situ thrombosis as a result of plaque rupture usually represents the final stage of a chronically diseased artery, most commonly the femoral or popliteal artery. If native artery thrombosis occurs in the absence of a preexisting stenosis, a thorough search for a hypercoagulable state or undetected atrial fibrillation should be undertaken. A vascular ultrasound may reveal thrombosis of a popliteal aneurysm presenting as acute limb ischemia.

Chronic Limb Ischemia

Lower extremity peripheral artery disease may be manifest as either chronic stable disease[2] or as critical limb ischemia.[3] Peripheral arterial disease is most commonly caused by atherosclerosis, but it also may be caused by thromboembolism, inflammatory disease, trauma, aneurysmal disease, adventitial cysts, entrapment syndromes, or congenital abnormalities. Aneurysms may be associated with atherosclerosis, or they may be caused by underlying hereditary (familial) or acquired (e.g., smoking or trauma) causes.

Patients with critical limb ischemia have inadequate blood flow to sustain viability in the distal tissue bed. Critical limb ischemia is most often caused by atherosclerosis, but it also can be caused by atheroembolic or thromboembolic disease, vasculitis, in situ thrombosis related to hypercoagulable states, thromboangiitis obliterans, cystic adventitial disease, popliteal entrapment, or trauma. Patients presenting with critical limb ischemia typically have multisegment disease along the length of the limb.

Inflammation plays a fundamental role in the development and progression of atherosclerosis. Elevated levels of C-reactive protein (CRP) are strongly associated with the development of peripheral arterial disease. Markers of inflammation such as interleukin-6, tumor necrosis factor-α, CRP, and platelet activation are increased compared with normal subjects.

No specific genetic markers have been confirmed for peripheral arterial disease, although one study identified a linkage on chromosome 1p. The proportion of low ABIs attributable to heritability is estimated at 20%. Concordance rates among twins are about 33% for monozygotic pairs and about 31% for dizygotic pairs, suggesting a limited role for heritability. Taken together, these data suggest a modest but significant heritability factor for peripheral arterial disease.

CLINICAL MANIFESTATIONS

Acute Limb Ischemia

A patient with acute limb ischemia presents with a cool, painful extremity (Table 65-2). Typically, the major muscle groups below the level of obstruction are symptomatic. The absence of a pulse may help localize the site of occlusion, but pulses may be normal in cases of microemboli or cholesterol emboli (Chapter 66). Venous and capillary filling is an indicator of the severity of acute limb ischemia. The leg should be carefully examined for color and temperature abnormalities. Pallor is seen early on, but with time, cyanosis is common. Poikilothermia, or coolness, is an important finding, particularly if the opposite limb is warm. A transition level for color and temperature changes, which is often clinically obvious, should be correlated with the pulses and denoted as a baseline reference at the initial examination for comparison with subsequent examinations.

Sensory changes include numbness and paresthesias. Paralysis indicates that ischemia had advanced to jeopardize the survival of the limb unless the patient undergoes urgent revascularization. Any motor deficit indicates tissue anoxia and implies a very poor prognosis. Motor deficits progress from distal to more proximal muscle groups, so early motor weakness is seen in the intrinsic foot muscles. Complete motor paralysis is a late symptom that suggests irreversible injury. With irreversible ischemia, paralysis progresses to rigor.

TABLE 65-3 FONTAINE'S AND RUTHERFORD'S CLINICAL CLASSIFICATIONS OF CHRONIC LOWER LIMB ISCHEMIA

FONTAINE		*RUTHERFORD*		
STAGE	**CLINICAL**	**GRADE**	**CATEGORY**	**CLINICAL**
I	Asymptomatic	0	0	Asymptomatic
IIa	Mild claudication	I	1	Mild claudication
IIb	Moderate to severe claudication	I	2	Moderate claudication
		I	3	Severe claudication
III	Rest pain	II	4	Rest pain
IV	Ulceration or gangrene	III	5	Minor tissue loss
		IV	6	Ulceration or gangrene

Adapted from Norgren L, Hiatt WR, Dormandy JA, et al. Inter-society consensus for the management of peripheral arterial disease (TASC II). *Eur J Vasc Endovasc Surg.* 2007;33(Suppl):S1-S75.

Chronic Stable Lower Limb Ischemia

Among patients with chronic stable lower extremity peripheral arterial disease, 50% of patients are asymptomatic despite abnormal pulse examinations, the presence of a vascular bruit, or an abnormal ABI (see Fig. 65-1). About 40% of patients have atypical symptoms (e.g., leg tiredness or fatigue), and only about 10% of patients have classic symptoms of intermittent claudication.

Claudication is defined as exertional discomfort, relieved with rest, in specific muscle groups at risk for ischemia during exercise (Table 65-3). Symptoms usually begin one segment below the level of the arterial narrowing. For example, whereas vascular obstructions (occlusions or stenoses) of the iliac vessels typically cause hip, thigh, and calf pain, femoral and popliteal artery obstructions typically cause symptoms in the calf and foot muscles. Claudication, which is a specific vascular syndrome, must be distinguished from other conditions that cause exertional leg pain, which have been termed *pseudoclaudication* (Table 65-4).

Symptoms in individual patients are remarkably variable despite similar degrees of vascular stenosis, in part owing to collateral vessel formation. A patient with superficial femoral artery occlusion but robust collateral formation via the deep femoral artery and geniculate collaterals, which supply blood to the infrapopliteal vessels, may have minimal or no symptoms. Another patient with similar anatomy but poor collaterals may have severe functional limitation.

Chronic Critical Lower Limb Ischemia

Critical limb ischemia, which develops in about 10% of all patients with peripheral arterial disease, presents as resting limb pain, nonhealing lower extremity ulcers, or gangrene (see Table 65-3). These patients' limbs are in jeopardy, and even the most minor trauma from a poorly fitting shoe or a carelessly clipped toenail may cause a nonhealing wound or infection that leads to amputation. Critical limb ischemia can be exacerbated by conditions that reduce blood flow to the microvascular bed, such as diabetes; severe low cardiac output states; and, rarely, vasospastic diseases.

DIAGNOSIS

Acute Limb Ischemia

In patients with acute limb ischemia, the history and physical examination are the most important steps, not only for assessing the cause and severity of ischemia but also for determining the diagnostic and therapeutic path. Upon

TABLE 65-2 CLINICAL CATEGORIES OF ACUTE LIMB ISCHEMIA

CATEGORY	DESCRIPTION	SENSORY LOSS	MUSCLE WEAKNESS	ARTERIAL DOPPLER	VENOUS DOPPLER
I. Viable	Not immediately threatened	None	None	Audible	Audible
IIa. Threatened marginally	Salvageable if promptly treated	Minimal or none	None	Inaudible	Audible
IIb. Threatened immediately	Salvageable if immediately treated	More than toes, associated with rest pain	Mild to moderate	Inaudible	Audible
III. Irreversible	Major tissue loss inevitable	Profound, anesthetic	Profound, paralysis, rigor	Inaudible	Inaudible

Adapted from Rutherford RB, Baker JD, Ernst C, et al. Recommended standards for reports dealing with lower extremity ischemia: revised version. *J Vasc Surg.* 1997;26:517-538.

TABLE 65-4 DIFFERENTIATION OF TRUE CLAUDICATION FROM PSEUDOCLAUDICATION

	INTERMITTENT CLAUDICATION	SPINAL STENOSIS	ARTHRITIS	VENOUS CONGESTION	COMPARTMENT SYNDROME
Character of discomfort	Cramping, tightness, or tiredness	Same as claudication or tingling, weakness, clumsiness	Aching	Tightness, bursting pain	Tightness, bursting pain
Location of discomfort	Buttock, hip, thigh, calf, foot	Buttock, hip, thigh	Hip, knee	Groin, thigh	Calf
Exercise-induced discomfort	Yes	Variable	Variable	After walking	Excessive exercise
Walking distance to discomfort	Reproducible	Variable	Variable	Variable	Excessive exercise
Occurs with standing	No	Yes	Yes, but positional	Yes, but positional	Yes, but positional
Relief of discomfort	Rapid relief with rest	Relief with sitting or changing position	Slow relief with avoidance of weight bearing	Slow relief with leg elevation	Slow relief with leg elevation
Other	Associated with atherosclerosis and decreased pulses	History of lower back problems	Discomfort at joint	History of deep vein thrombosis, signs of venous congestion	Typical in athletes

From White C. Intermittent claudication. *N Engl J Med.* 2007;356:1241-1250.

completion of the history and physical examination, the physician should be able to answer the following questions about the severity of acute limb ischemia: Is the limb viable? Is the limb's viability immediately threatened? Are there already irreversible changes that may preclude salvage of the limb? Three findings that help differentiate "threatened" from "viable" extremities are the presence of persistent pain, sensory loss, and muscle weakness.

Chronic Limb Ischemia

The clinical severity of chronic stable and chronic critical limb ischemia can be semiquantitatively assessed using either the Fontaine or the Rutherford classification (see Table 65-3). The clinician must distinguish intermittent claudication from nonvascular causes that may mimic claudication (i.e., pseudoclaudication), such as neurogenic pain from spinal stenosis or nerve root compression (Chapter 369), musculoskeletal or arthritic pain, or discomfort from venous congestion or a compartment syndrome (see Table 65-4). A typical history of claudication has a low sensitivity but a high specificity for peripheral arterial disease.

Patients presenting with peripheral arterial disease should be assessed for atherosclerotic risk factors (blood pressure, serum lipid and glucose levels, renal function) and undergo a complete vascular physical examination with their shoes and socks removed. A diminished palpable peripheral pulse is insufficiently sensitive to exclude the diagnosis, so measurement of the ABI (see Fig. 65-1) is required.[4] ABI results should be uniformly reported, with noncompressible values defined as greater than 1.40, normal values defined as 1.00 to 1.40, borderline values as 0.91 to 0.99, and abnormal values as 0.90 or less.[5]

Imaging

Duplex imaging combines ultrasound imaging and Doppler blood velocity measurements to localize vascular obstructions and estimate lesion severity. The sensitivity and specificity of duplex ultrasonography for the diagnosis of a 50% stenosis or greater in the lower extremity is 90% or higher.

Computed tomography angiography (CTA) and magnetic resonance angiography (MRA) offer cross-sectional images that can be reconstructed into a three-dimensional angiogram (Fig. 65-2). Whereas CTA requires iodinated intravenous contrast material and ionizing radiation, MRA uses gadolinium contrast and does not expose the patient to ionizing radiation but cannot be used in patients with ferromagnetic metallic implants such as pacemakers or defibrillators. The major toxicity of gadolinium is a rare but potentially debilitating systemic disorder called nephrogenic systemic fibrosis or nephrogenic sclerosing dermopathy (Chapter 246); a glomerular filtration rate of 60 mL/minute or less is a risk factor.

An advantage of CTA over MRA is its ability to visualize metallic stents and stent grafts (Fig. 65-3). CTA requires only about one-fourth the radiation required for invasive digital angiography, and it can be performed more quickly and with less pretreatment planning than MRA. Vascular calcification may be a source of artifact with CTA but is inconsequential with MRA. MRA tends to overestimate lesions at the ostia of arteries owing to turbulent flow.

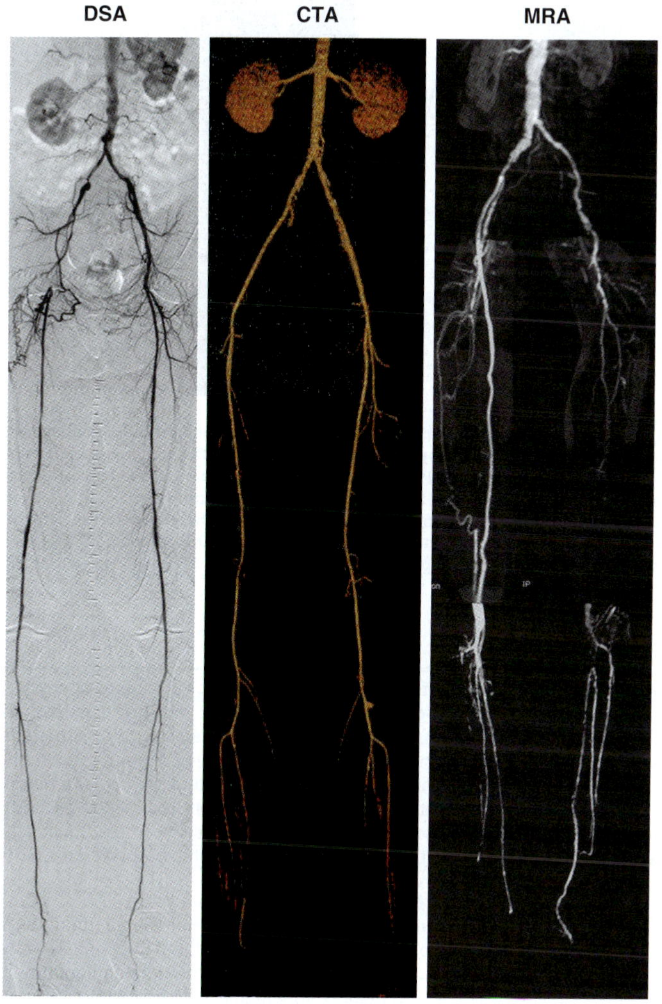

FIGURE 65-2. **Aortography with distal run-off in three different patients by three different methods: digital subtraction angiography (DSA), computed tomography angiography (CTA), and magnetic resonance angiography (MRA).** (From White C. Intermittent claudication. *N Engl J Med.* 2007;356:1241-1250.)

Invasive digital subtraction angiography remains the "gold standard" for the diagnosis and evaluation of peripheral arterial disease despite the need for iodinated contrast material and the exposure to ionizing radiation. Invasive angiographic procedures (Chapter 59) are associated with a relatively small but nontrivial rate of complications, including severe contrast allergy in 0.1%, access-related bleeding complications, and contrast-induced nephropathy.

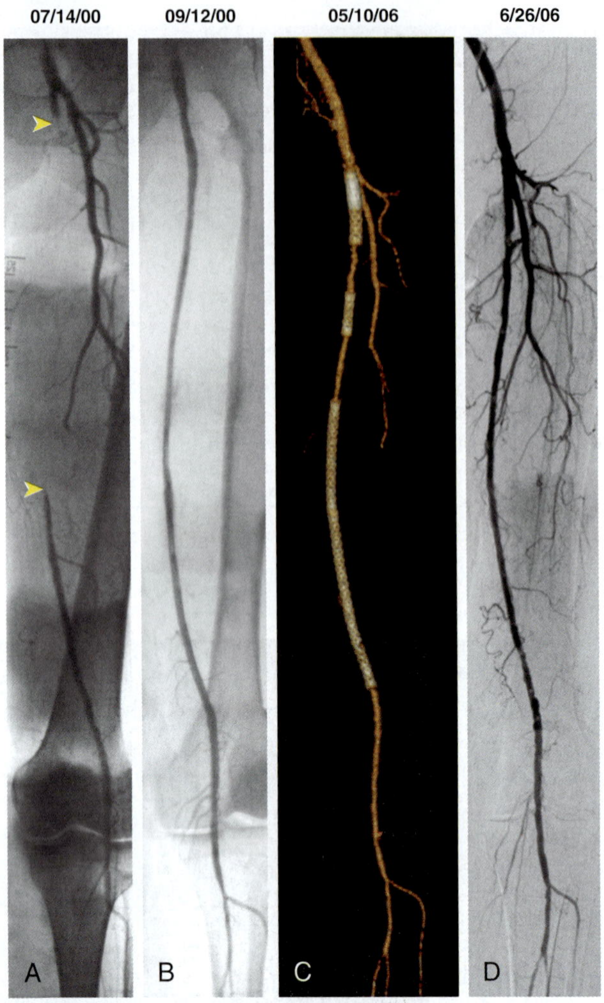

FIGURE 65-3. Pre- and postprocedural angiograms in a patient with peripheral arterial disease. A, Baseline angiogram of left leg showing occlusion (arrowheads) of the femoral-popliteal segment. B, Post-treatment angiogram after balloon angioplasty and stent placement. C, More than 5 years later, the patient returns with claudication and a reduced ankle-brachial index. Follow-up computed tomography angiogram shows narrowing of the superficial femoral artery between the two stents. D, Final angiogram following balloon angioplasty and stent placement.

TREATMENT

The primary treatment of patients with atherosclerotic lower extremity peripheral arterial disease is guideline-directed medical therapy to reduce the patient's risk for life-threatening cardiovascular complications of atherosclerosis.[6,7] Structured exercise therapy with or without revascularization strategies improves functional status such as walking distance.[A1] Revascularization strategies to improve walking distance and avoid amputation have shifted from open surgical approaches to percutaneous, catheter-based endovascular treatments because of the relative safety, success, and durability of stenting and drug-coated balloons.

Acute Limb Ischemia

Patients with irreversible limb ischemia (nonviable limb) should not undergo angiography and should be scheduled for amputation (Fig. 65-4). All other patients with acute limb ischemia should undergo emergent angiography to define the culprit lesion and to treat it endovascularly if possible.

The options for prompt revascularization include (1) endovascular therapies, with intra-arterial thrombolysis (e.g., recombinant tissue plasminogen activator 0.05 to 0.1 mg/kg/hr intra-arterially) and/or catheter-based thrombectomy and stenting, or (2) open surgical thrombectomy with or without arterial bypass. In general, endovascular therapy is recommended for patients with an onset of acute symptoms less than 14 days earlier, and surgical revascularization is recommended for patients with a duration of symptoms longer than 14 days.

Chronic Lower Limb Ischemia

The approach to patients with claudication is directed at both the limb disease itself (preserving the limb and improving walking distance), as well as to reducing the patient's risk for life-threatening cardiovascular complications of atherosclerosis (Fig. 65-5). Risk factor modification (e.g., aggressive treatment of elevated LDL cholesterol levels [Chapter 190] and blood pressure [Chapter 64], as well as smoking cessation [Chapter 363]), an exercise prescription, antiplatelet agents (Chapter 70), and medical therapy to reduce claudication are the basic elements of treating chronic stable peripheral arterial disease[8] (Fig. 65-5).

Risk Factor Modification

Patients with known peripheral arterial disease should be encouraged to modify or eliminate atherosclerotic risk factors such as diabetes (Chapter 210), tobacco use (Chapter 363), hyperlipidemia (Chapter 190), and hypertension (Chapter 64) and to exercise regularly (Chapter 14).[9]

Patients who are smokers or former smokers should be asked about their status of tobacco use at every visit. Smokers should receive counseling, usually be offered pharmacotherapy (e.g., nicotine replacement therapy, sometimes with varenicline or bupropion), and be considered for referral to a smoking cessation program (Chapter 363). For patients with severe peripheral arterial disease and elevated CRP levels, statin therapy, and especially high-intensity therapy to reduce LDL cholesterol levels to 70 mg/dl or lower, reduces the risk of both amputation and death. In patients who have peripheral arterial disease and are already on statin therapy, the proprotein convertase subtilisin/kexin type 9 (PCSK9) inhibitors further reduce LDL cholesterol levels, cardiovascular events, and the risk of major adverse limb events.[A2] Blood pressure control is very important, especially in patients with coexisting diabetes. β-Blockers are effective antihypertensive therapy and are not contraindicated in peripheral arterial disease.

Exercise Therapy

Patients should be reassured that exercising, even though it may precipitate their claudication symptoms, is not harmful and is the preferred initial treatment.[10] A meta-analysis comparing supervised with unsupervised exercise therapy demonstrated superior improvement in claudication with supervised exercise,[A3] but home-based exercise does not appear to be as useful even if combined with a wearable activity monitor and telephone coaching.[A4,A5] Improvement in walking distance often can be achieved with pharmacologic management; discontinuation of tobacco use; and a regular, supervised exercise program. For example, a randomized trial of patients with aortoiliac peripheral arterial disease who underwent a supervised exercise program showed greater improvement in walking performance compared with those who underwent primary stent therapy or home walking with cilostazol.

Antiplatelet and Antithrombotic Therapy

Antiplatelet therapy with aspirin (usually 75 to 325 mg/day) has an established role in the secondary prevention of cardiovascular events in all patients with peripheral arterial disease because they are at high risk of MI, stroke, and vascular death, whether they are being managed medically, have had prior endovascular or surgical revascularization, or have had prior amputation. The addition of low-dose rivaroxaban (2.5 mg twice daily) to aspirin (100 mg daily) can further reduce major cardiovascular events, limb events,[A6] and all-cause mortality,[A7,A8] despite an increase in bleeding events.[A9]

The thienopyridines, such as clopidogrel (usually 75 mg/day), are indicated only if aspirin is not tolerated, based on clopidogrel's efficacy compared with aspirin among patients with peripheral arterial disease. Recent evidence suggests that another thienopyridine, ticagrelor (usually 90 or 60 mg twice daily), is not more effective than clopidogrel as monotherapy for reducing cardiovascular events,[A10] but ticagrelor on a background of low-dose aspirin therapy does reduce major cardiac events compared with aspirin alone in patients who have also had an MI.[A11] A promising novel protease-activated receptor-1 antagonist, vorapaxar, may significantly reduce the incidence acute limb ischemia and the need for revascularization in patients with peripheral arterial disease.[A12]

Pharmacology

Cilostazol, a phosphodiesterase inhibitor, at 50 to 100 mg twice daily, improves maximal walking distance by 40 to 50% compared with placebo[A13] and has been shown to reduce restenosis after femoral artery revascularization.[A14] Cilostazol is contraindicated in patients with heart failure. Oral vasodilating prostaglandins, vitamin E, and chelation therapy with ethylenediaminetetraacetic acid (EDTA) have not been effective in improving either symptoms or walking distance.

Revascularization

The decision to perform an endovascular or surgical revascularization procedure for the relief of claudication in a patient with chronic stable lower limb ischemia is based upon a risk-to-benefit assessment that weighs the patient's disability and discomfort against the estimated short- and long-term benefits and risks of the procedure. Because very few patients with claudication are in danger of losing their limbs, the primary goal of revascularization is durable functional improvement, not limb salvage. Patients selected for revascularization to relieve symptoms of intermittent claudication should have significant lifestyle limitation or be unable to work and should have failed to respond to medications and to a structured exercise program.[11,12]

Superficial femoral and popliteal artery stenoses or occlusions (E-Fig. 65-1) are commonly associated with calf claudication. Revascularization with endovascular techniques or surgery is indicated for the relief of vocational or lifestyle-limiting claudication in patients who have failed to respond to exercise and pharmacologic therapy.

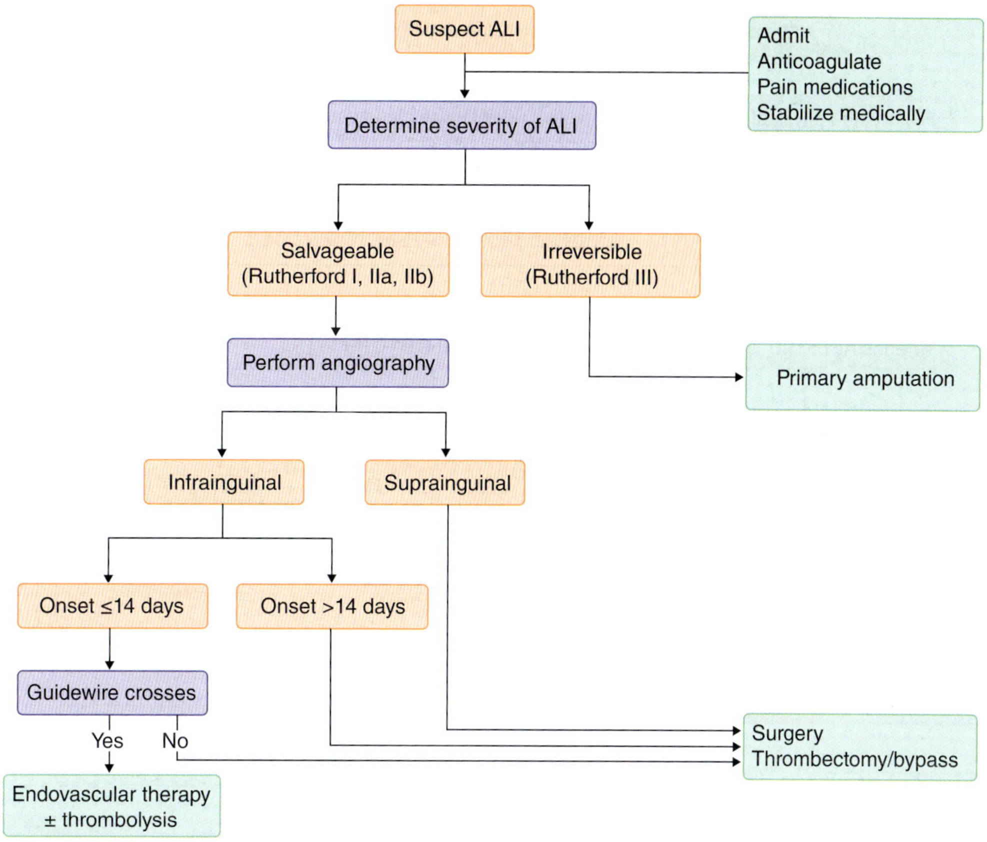

FIGURE 65-4. **Treatment algorithm for acute limb ischemia (ALI). (Modified from Gray BH, Conte MS, Dake MD, et al. Atherosclerotic Peripheral Vascular Disease Symposium II: lower-extremity revascularization: state of the art. *Circulation*. 2008;118:2864-2872.)**

In patients with claudication, the combination of a structured exercise program plus balloon angioplasty is superior to supervised exercise therapy alone for improving the ABI, walking distance and quality of life.[A15] Randomized trials comparing surgery with angioplasty show similar rates of mortality, amputation, and patency at 4 years in patients with lower extremity ischemia.[A16] Percutaneous therapy is preferred in amenable lesions because of its lower periprocedural mortality and morbidity. Angioplasty is more cost effective than surgery if the expected 5-year patency rate of the treated vessel is 30% or greater.

Drug-eluting stents and drug-coated balloons,[13] which appear to be equivalent to each other,[A17] safely provide a superior and more durable benefit for claudication caused by femoral-popliteal disease than do angioplasty and stenting alone.[A18,A19] Adjunctive angioplasty devices such as atherectomy, cryotherapy, and the cutting balloon have not been meaningfully tested in any population, and there are few data to support their use.

For chronic critical lower limb ischemia, the therapeutic goal is urgent revascularization to reestablish pulsatile, straight-line flow to the distal extremity and to reduce the rate of amputation. Surgical bypass using the great saphenous vein provides the best outcomes, but endovascular therapy is as good as open surgery if an adequate saphenous vein is not available. It also is reasonable to attempt a percutaneous therapy first if a patient is a candidate for either surgery or angioplasty, particularly if the patient's life expectancy is less than 2 years. In tibial arteries, coronary drug-eluting stents and drug-coated balloons are superior to conventional therapies,[A20,A21] but the two approaches may produce similar results for the treatment of critical limb ischemia in below-the-knee arteries.[A22]

Nevertheless, primary amputation is indicated in patients who have extensive necrosis or infectious gangrene with rest pain, are not ambulatory, and are not candidates for revascularization. Cellular therapies and growth factor therapy are being investigated for limb salvage, but none have yet proven clinically effective.

PROGNOSIS

Peripheral arterial disease is a major cause of acute and chronic illness associated with impaired functional capacity, reduced quality of life, limb loss, and increased risk of death (E-Fig. 65-2). About 18% of patients who undergo peripheral arterial revascularization have an unplanned readmission within 30 days.[14]

Approximately two thirds of patients with peripheral arterial disease have at least one severely diseased coronary artery, and up to one quarter of patients have significant carotid artery stenosis. Consequently, patients with peripheral arterial disease face an increased risk of cardiovascular ischemic events such as MI, ischemic stroke, and death. It is estimated that coronary and cerebrovascular adverse events occur two- to four-fold more commonly than do limb adverse events in patients with peripheral arterial disease. Outcomes are improved when guideline-recommended therapy is followed.

The annual mortality rate for patients with peripheral arterial disease is about 5%, but it is higher for patients with severe disease. For example, the estimated 1-year mortality rate for patients with critical limb ischemia is 25%, but this can climb to 45% for patients requiring amputation; in contrast, the annual mortality rate for patients with intermittent claudication is only 1 to 2%. For patients presenting with acute limb ischemia, the 30-day amputation rate is as high as 40%, and mortality rates up to 30% have been reported.

Patients with lower extremity claudication should be reassured that the risk of limb loss is low. Moreover, a history of claudication by itself only slightly increases the risk of amputation after 10 years. However, a reduced ABI and diabetes mellitus are associated with the development of ischemic rest pain and ischemic ulceration, which may lead to limb loss. Among patients with peripheral arterial disease, those who have diabetes are 15 times more likely to have an amputation than are patients without diabetes, whose annual amputation rate is less than 1%.

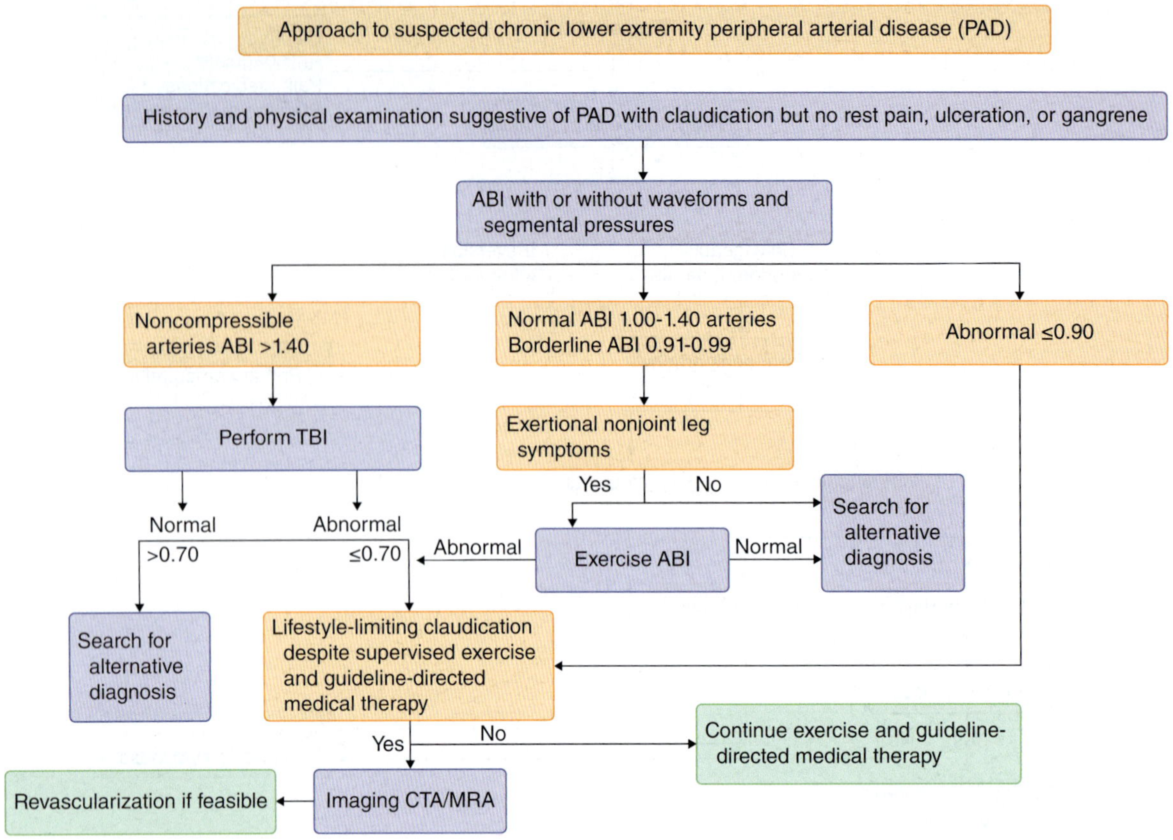

FIGURE 65-5. Approach to suspected chronic lower extremity peripheral arterial disease. ABI = ankle brachial index; CTA = computed tomographic angiography; MRA = magnetic resonance angiography; TBI = toe brachial index.

GENERAL REFERENCES

For the General References and other additional features, please visit Elsevier eBooks+ at https://ebooks.health.elsevier.com.

Grade A References

A1. Fakhry F, Spronk S, van der Laan L, et al. Endovascular revascularization and supervised exercise for peripheral artery disease and intermittent claudication: a randomized clinical trial. *JAMA*. 2015;314:1936-1944.

A2. Bonaca MP, Nault P, Giugliano RP, et al. Low-density lipoprotein cholesterol lowering with evolocumab and outcomes in patients with peripheral artery disease: insights from the FOURIER trial (further cardiovascular outcomes research with PCSK9 inhibition in subjects with elevated risk). *Circulation*. 2018;137:338-350.

A3. Pandey A, Banerjee S, Ngo C, et al. Comparative efficacy of endovascular revascularization versus supervised exercise training in patients with intermittent claudication: meta-analysis of randomized controlled trials. *JACC Cardiovasc Interv*. 2017;10:712-724.

A4. McDermott MM, Spring B, Berger JS, et al. Effect of a home-based exercise intervention of wearable technology and telephone 6 coaching on walking performance in peripheral artery disease: the HONOR randomized clinical trial. *JAMA*. 2018;319:1665-1676.

A5. McDermott MM, Spring B, Tian L, et al. Effect of low-intensity vs high-intensity home-based walking exercise on walk distance in patients with peripheral artery disease: the LITE randomized clinical trial. *JAMA*. 2021;325:1266-1276.

A6. Anand SS, Caron F, Eikelboom JW, et al. Major adverse limb events and mortality in patients with peripheral artery disease: the COMPASS trial. *J Am Coll Cardiol*. 2018;71:2306-2315.

A7. Hess CN, Debus ES, Nehler MR, et al. Reduction in acute limb ischemia with rivaroxaban versus placebo in peripheral artery disease after lower extremity revascularization: insights from VOYAGER PAD. *Circulation*. 2021;144:1831-1841.

A8. Eikelboom JW, Bhatt DL, Fox KAA, et al. Mortality benefit of rivaroxaban plus aspirin in patients with chronic coronary or peripheral artery disease. *J Am Coll Cardiol*. 2021;78:14-23.

A9. Bonaca MP, Bauersachs RM, Anand SS, et al. Rivaroxaban in peripheral artery disease after revascularization. *N Engl J Med*. 2020;382:1994-2004.

A10. Hiatt WR, Fowkes FG, Heizer G, et al. Ticagrelor versus clopidogrel in symptomatic peripheral artery disease. *N Engl J Med*. 2017;376:32-40.

A11. Bonaca MP, Bhatt DL, Storey RF, et al. Ticagrelor for prevention of ischemic events after myocardial infarction in patients with peripheral artery disease. *J Am Coll Cardiol*. 2016;67:2719-2728.

A12. Bonaca MP, Creager MA, Olin J, et al. Peripheral revascularization in patients with peripheral artery disease with vorapaxar: insights from the TRA 2°P-TIMI 50 trial. *JACC Cardiovasc Interv*. 2016;9:2157-2164.

A13. Brown T, Forster RB, Cleanthis M, et al. Cilostazol for intermittent claudication. *Cochrane Database Syst Rev*. 2021;6:CD003748.

A14. Desai K, Han B, Kuziez L, et al. Literature review and meta-analysis of the efficacy of cilostazol on limb salvage rates after infrainguinal endovascular and open revascularization. *J Vasc Surg*. 2021;73:711-721.e3.

A15. Fakhry F, Fokkenrood HJP, Spronk S, et al. Endovascular revascularization versus conservative management for intermittent claudication. *Cochrane Database Syst Rev*. 2018;3:CD010512.

A16. Goueffic Y, Della Schiava N, Thaveau F, et al. Stenting or surgery for de novo common femoral artery stenosis. *JACC Cardiovasc Interv*. 2017;10:1344-1354.

A17. Liistro F, Angioli P, Porto I, et al. Drug-eluting balloon versus drug-eluting stent for complex femoropopliteal arterial lesions: the DRASTICO study. *J Am Coll Cardiol*. 2019;74:205-215.

A18. Schneider PA, Laird JR, Tepe G, et al. Treatment effect of drug-coated balloons is durable to 3 years in the femoropopliteal arteries: long-term results of the IN.PACT SFA randomized trial. *Circ Cardiovasc Interv*. 2018;11:1-8.

A19. Nordanstig J, James S, Andersson M, et al. Mortality with paclitaxel-coated devices in peripheral artery disease. *N Engl J Med*. 2020;383:2538-2546.

A20. Farber A, Menard MT, Conte MS, et al. Surgery or endovascular therapy for chronic limb-threatening ischemia. *N Engl J Med*. 2022;387:2305-2316.

A21. Zeller T, Micari A, Scheinert D, et al. The IN.PACT DEEP clinical drug-coated balloon trial: 5-year outcomes. *JACC Cardiovasc Interv*. 2020;13:431-443.

A22. Patel A, Irani FG, Pua U, et al. Randomized controlled trial comparing drug-coated balloon angioplasty versus conventional balloon angioplasty for treating below-the-knee arteries in critical limb ischemia: the SINGA-PACLI trial. *Radiology*. 2021;300:715-724.

66

OTHER PERIPHERAL ARTERIAL DISEASES

JOHN R. BARTHOLOMEW

POPLITEAL ARTERY ENTRAPMENT SYNDROME

Popliteal artery entrapment syndrome, which is a cause of intermittent claudication in young and often athletic patients, can be anatomic or functional. Anatomic popliteal artery entrapment syndrome results from extrinsic compression on the popliteal artery by muscles or ligaments within or surrounding the popliteal fossa. In a functional version of popliteal artery entrapment, the medial head of the gastrocnemius, plantaris, or soleus muscle becomes hypertrophied and occludes the popliteal artery without a true fixed anatomic abnormality.[1] The popliteal vein and nerve can also can be involved.

Anatomic evidence of entrapment can be found on physical examination or imaging performed for unrelated reasons in up to 4% of apparently normal individuals and imaging evidence for popliteal artery compression with provocative maneuvers in as many of 80% of asymptomatic individuals. Clinically evident popliteal artery entrapment syndrome is rare, with one study showing a prevalence of approximately 0.16% among military recruits.

CLINICAL MANIFESTATIONS AND DIAGNOSIS

Symptoms of popliteal artery entrapment syndrome include exertional limb pain, cold feet after exercise, ischemic rest pain, and even tissue necrosis if undiagnosed cases progress to arterial degeneration with thromboembolization. Entrapment of the popliteal vein results in swelling and discoloration of the calf, heaviness, varicosities, nocturnal or exertional calf cramping, and even deep vein thrombosis (Chapter 68). Nerve involvement can cause paresthesias.

The diagnosis of popliteal artery entrapment syndrome is suggested by demonstration of popliteal artery compression on active pedal plantar flexion against resistance. This compression is manifested by a decrease in the intensity of the pedal arterial pulse on physical examination and loss of the continuous-wave Doppler signal over the pedal arteries. Pulse volume recordings and segmental limb pressures should be measured at rest with the knee extended and the ankle in the neutral, dorsiflexed, and plantar-flexed positions. Exercise treadmill studies also may demonstrate diminished limb arterial pressure after exercise in the symptomatic limb. Arterial duplex ultrasonography, dynamic computed tomographic (CT) arteriography, or magnetic resonance (MR) arteriography may confirm the diagnosis, whereas CT or MR arteriography also define the structure that causes the entrapment. The differential diagnosis includes compartment syndrome, stress fracture, cystic adventitial disease, and arterial embolism.

TREATMENT AND PROGNOSIS

Treatment of structural popliteal artery entrapment is largely surgical, with relief of the entrapment by resection or translocation of the compressing elements. If popliteal artery entrapment syndrome is not identified until after the artery has been injured, arterial reconstruction or surgical bypass, ideally with a venous autologous graft, may be required. In functional popliteal artery entrapment, exertional symptoms may respond to injection of botulinum toxin A into the popliteal space. In patients whose functional entrapment symptoms persist, resection or translocation of the medial head of the gastrocnemius muscle is recommended. If therapy is offered early in the course of the syndrome, patients may expect full recovery with complete resolution of symptoms.

CYSTIC ADVENTITIAL DISEASE OF THE LOWER EXTREMITY ARTERIES

In cystic adventitial disease, a mucinous cyst develops within the adventitial layers of the arterial wall and encroaches on the arterial lumen.[2] Cystic adventitial disease most commonly affects the popliteal artery, thereby resulting in intermittent claudication, classically in middle-aged men. However, the external iliac, femoral, axillary, brachial radial, and ulnar arteries can be involved. The exact cause of cystic adventitial disease is unknown.

CLINICAL MANIFESTATIONS AND DIAGNOSIS

Intermittent claudication is the most common symptom of cystic adventitial disease. However, limb discomfort may persist for up to 20 minutes after the cessation of activity, unlike the classic relief of limb pain on cessation of activity in atherosclerotic peripheral artery disease (Chapter 65). The limb symptoms of cystic adventitial disease also tend to be inconsistent, often reappearing without obvious precipitants and resolving without an obvious explanation. Acute limb ischemia (Chapter 65) secondary to arterial compression and thrombosis also can occur.

The diagnosis is suspected when pedal pulses disappear with passive knee flexion and occasionally with exercise. However, cystic adventitial disease is most often confirmed with MR angiography. By comparison, arteriography may demonstrate only compression of the arterial lumen without identifying the cyst. The finding of eccentric compression of the popliteal arterial lumen, known as the scimitar sign, is considered pathognomonic for cystic adventitial disease (Fig. 66-1).

TREATMENT AND PROGNOSIS

Image-guided aspiration of the cyst may be attempted, but recurrence is likely. Balloon angioplasty is unlikely to be an effective and durable therapy and is not advised. Surgical resection of the cyst, potentially with placement of a venous interposition graft, is the primary therapy. When this condition is identified early, patients may anticipate complete resolution of claudication after resection of the cyst.

ENDOFIBROSIS OF THE ILIAC ARTERY

Endofibrosis of the iliac artery represents stenosis of the external iliac artery, thought to be due to repetitive trauma in highly functioning and competitive athletes.[3] This condition, which is increasingly being diagnosed, commonly occurs in cyclists, football players, or long-distance runners 30 to 50 years of age.

Endofibrosis results from intimal hyperplasia and fibrosis of the arterial wall. Smooth muscle cell proliferation and medial and intimal proliferation also may occur.

CLINICAL MANIFESTATIONS AND DIAGNOSIS

Symptoms include exercise-interfering, intermittent thigh claudication and leg weakness accompanied by a sensation of swelling or paresthesia in the proximal lower limb at the time of maximal exercise. Physical examination may be normal at rest, although a bruit may be heard over the ipsilateral pelvic fossa or inguinal region.

Diagnostic imaging includes preexercise and postexercise Doppler ankle pressure measurements at the time of maximal, symptom-limiting treadmill exercise. Ultrasound imaging and contrast angiography, preferably when the leg is flexed at the hip in the cycling position, will reveal concentric stenosis, often with lengthening of the affected iliac artery. Intravascular ultrasound and intra-arterial translesional pressure gradients may be helpful.

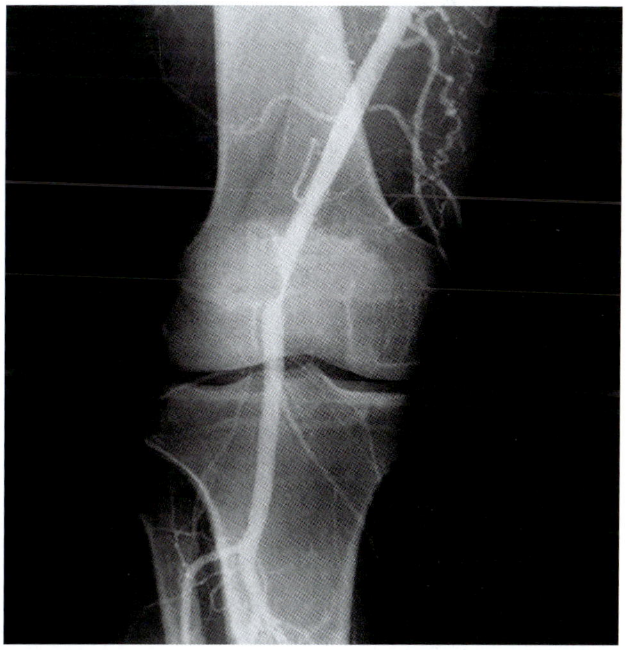

FIGURE 66-1. The finding of eccentric compression of the popliteal artery lumen known as the scimitar sign is considered pathognomonic for cystic adventitial disease.

TREATMENT AND PROGNOSIS

The first line of treatment is to avoid activities that aggravate the symptoms. If intervention is required, angioplasty results in high restenosis rates, and endovascular stenting is complicated by the risk of stent fracture. As a result, surgical revascularization with vein patch angioplasty or interposition grafts is the recommended treatment and usually ameliorates the symptoms. With continued trauma to the arterial segment, however, careful surveillance for recurrence is warranted.

FIBROMUSCULAR DYSPLASIA

Fibromuscular dysplasia (Chapter 110) is a noninflammatory, nonatherosclerotic arterial disease that most commonly involves the medial layer of the artery wall and can affect any artery in the body.[4] It is most commonly seen in women 20 to 60 years of age, with a mean age at onset of 52 years but a range of 5 to 83 years. Its true prevalence is unknown, but a series of potential renal donors showed a prevalence as high as almost 4%.

Fibromuscular dysplasia is multifocal in 90% of cases and focal in 10% of cases. Multifocal fibromuscular dysplasia results in the classic "string of beads" appearance on contrast arteriography (Fig. 66-2). Pathology shows alternating segments of thinning and thickening of the arterial media, but the adventitia or intima may be predominantly affected, thereby resulting in an angiographic appearance different from that for medial fibroplasia. Other types of fibromuscular dysplasia include an intimal variant that causes a single focal, weblike stenosis within the affected artery.

CLINICAL MANIFESTATIONS AND DIAGNOSIS

The clinical presentation of patients with fibromuscular dysplasia depends on the arteries involved, and sometimes it may be incidentally discovered without any symptoms when imaging is performed for other reasons. Although most symptoms are related to stenoses, about 20% of patients develop aneurysms, about 25% develop dissections, and rare patients develop occlusions.

The renal arteries are affected in almost 60% of cases (Chapter 110), and the extracranial carotid and vertebral arteries are involved in almost 40% of cases. Not surprisingly, hypertension (Chapter 64) and recurrent headaches (especially migraine type; Chapter 367) represent the two most common signs and symptoms. Less common symptoms and signs include dizziness, pulsatile tinnitus, and cervical bruits. Additional clinical clues include a transient ischemic attack or stroke in a patient under 60 years of age, an aneurysm in an intracranial vessel, subarachnoid hemorrhage, or renal infarction.[5] Fibromuscular dysplasia may occasionally affect the brachial, iliac, femoral, or popliteal arteries, and it also can be associated with spontaneous coronary artery dissection (Chapter 58).[6]

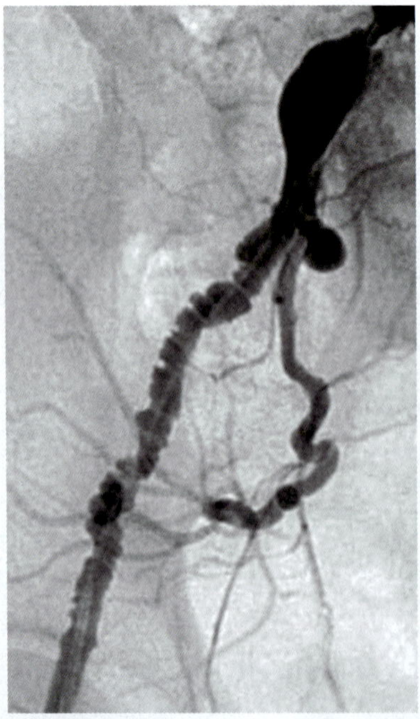

FIGURE 66-2. Angiogram showing a typical "string of beads" pattern, typical of the medial type in fibromuscular dysplasia, in the external iliac artery. Also note the aneurysm proximal to the area of dysplasia. (Courtesy Dr. Jeffrey W. Olin.)

The diagnosis of fibromuscular dysplasia relies on a combination of clinical and imaging findings. Duplex ultrasound, MR angiography, and CT angiography can identify fibromuscular dysplasia and assess possible aneurysms, but contrast angiography and intravascular ultrasound are the best diagnostic tests. Because fibromuscular dysplasia may involve several vascular beds, patients should initially undergo comprehensive MR or CT imaging of their intracranial arteries, the extracranial carotid arteries, the thoracic and abdominal aorta and its branches, and the renal arteries. Nearly 13% of patients have intracranial aneurysms detectable by imaging. If arterial aneurysms or dissections are identified without clear evidence of fibromuscular dysplasia, a genetic collagen disorder should be considered.

TREATMENT AND PROGNOSIS

Treatment of fibromuscular dysplasia depends on the clinical presentation and extent of arterial involvement.[7] Asymptomatic patients are empirically prescribed aspirin. In young patients with sudden onset of hypertension and renal artery fibromuscular dysplasia, percutaneous transluminal angioplasty can cure the hypertension that is often found (Chapter 110). Renal and intracranial artery aneurysms should be followed closely for expansion and may require surgery. The decision about repair is often based on the size of the aneurysm, its rate of expansion, and the presence of associated symptoms. Carotid artery fibromuscular dysplasia is generally treated with antiplatelet therapy (e.g., aspirin 81 to 325 mg/day) or 3 to 6 months of warfarin anticoagulation in the case of carotid artery dissection. Percutaneous transluminal angioplasty is reserved for patients with hemispheric cerebral ischemic symptoms and progressive dissection. Peripheral artery percutaneous transluminal angioplasty is recommended only for patients with symptoms of intermittent claudication.

In general, patients with fibromuscular dysplasia have an excellent outcome. After percutaneous transluminal angioplasty of the renal arteries, approximately one third of patients with hypertension will have normal blood pressures and most others will have substantial improvement. Optimal antiplatelet therapy (e.g., aspirin 81 to 325 mg/day) is recommended for the majority of patients with fibromuscular dysplasia. The most feared complications, which occur in less than 5% of patients, are stroke owing to progressive carotid dissection, rupture of an intracranial arterial aneurysm, or rupture of a visceral artery aneurysm.

THROMBOANGIITIS OBLITERANS (BUERGER DISEASE)

Thromboangiitis obliterans is a nonatherosclerotic, segmental inflammatory disorder that affects small and medium-sized arteries, veins, and nerves, most often but not exclusively of the lower extremities.[8] Thromboangiitis obliterans is typically found in men who are under the age of 50 years and who smoke, chew tobacco, or use cannabis.

Although rarely performed, biopsy of affected digits demonstrates highly cellular inflammatory thrombi with sparing of the artery wall. Thromboangiitis obliterans is one of the few vascular disorders that affects both arteries and veins, so superficial thrombophlebitis can also develop.

CLINICAL MANIFESTATIONS AND DIAGNOSIS

Patients classically present with digital or extremity pain with digital ischemia, distal limb claudication (such as in the arch of the foot or arm), and digital ulcerations (Fig. 66-3). More than 40% of patients have Raynaud phenomenon.

Clinicians must maintain a high degree of clinical suspicion in young smokers with distal extremity ischemia and pain without evidence of atherosclerosis. Many patients will demonstrate an abnormal Allen test, in which one of two of the major arteries to the hand (radial or ulnar) does not fill after the examiner compresses the other artery, as well as absent peripheral arterial pulses. The ankle-brachial index (Chapter 65) is classically abnormal, even though plethysmographic studies demonstrate essentially normal proximal artery circulation. Serologic results show no evidence for inflammatory vasculitis (Chapter 249), and proximal sources of arterial emboli are not found. Contrast arteriography is often needed to demonstrate distal arterial involvement with the absence of atherosclerosis. Segmental arterial occlusions with corkscrew collaterals are commonly found but are not pathognomonic.

TREATMENT AND PROGNOSIS

The cornerstone of treatment is complete abstinence from tobacco (preferably confirmed by urinary testing for cotinine) and cannabis.[9] Patients who cannot abstain commonly have unremitting pain, recurrent tissue necrosis, and the need for progressive limb amputation.

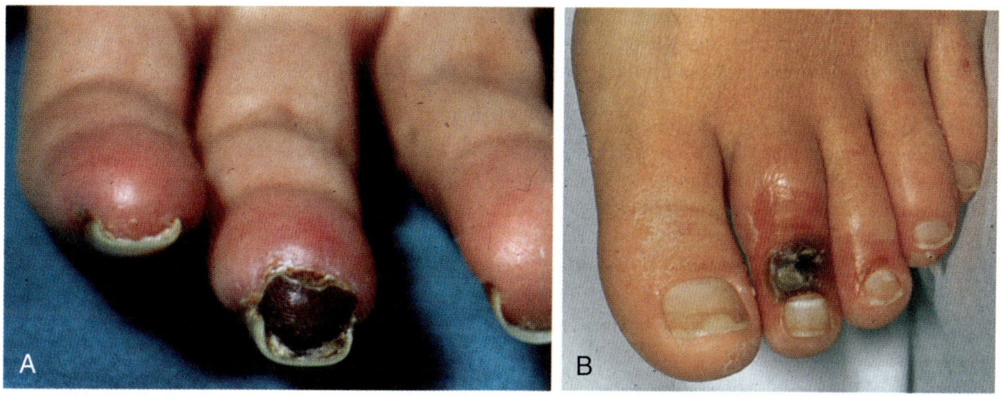

FIGURE 66-3. **Buerger disease.** Ischemic finger of a young male patient (**A**) and ischemic toe of a 28-year-old woman (**B**) with Buerger disease. (Courtesy Dr. Jeffrey W. Olin.)

Antiplatelet therapy (e.g., aspirin 81 to 325/day) is commonly prescribed, though usually with no more than modest benefit. A 28-day course of the prostacyclin analogue iloprost (1 ng/kg/minute intravenously for 6 hours daily) may be tried off-label by experts to improve pain and accelerate wound healing compared with aspirin or lumbar sympathectomy.[A1] There are no data demonstrating benefit with vasodilators such as calcium-channel antagonists, peripheral α-blockers, or sildenafil. Digital sympathectomy, bosentan, spinal cord stimulators, and intermittent pneumatic compression have all been tried with variable success. Angioplasty may be effective in preserving the limb and preventing amputation,[10,11] with stenting generally reserved for bail-out procedures or for more proximal disease.

LIVEDO RETICULARIS AND LIVEDO RACEMOSA

Livedo reticularis, which typically involves the lower extremities, is an ischemic dermopathy caused by an increased prominence of venous beds owing to obstruction of arterial inflow, venous dilation, or blockage of venous outflow. It is a vasospastic disorder that appears as a violaceous or reddish-blue netlike or mottled discoloration surrounding a pale central area of skin (Fig 66-4).

Primary livedo reticularis is a benign condition exacerbated by cold temperatures, tobacco, or emotional upset, whereas the secondary form, referred to as livedo racemosa (Fig. 66-5), is a pathologic variant seen in association with a number of disorders (Table 66-1). Primary livedo reticularis is commonly found in healthy women during their second to fifth decade of life. The secondary form may be associated with antiphospholipid antibodies (Chapter 67). Livedo reticularis is rare in males, in whom its presence warrants investigation for possible secondary causes such as antiphospholipid syndrome (Chapter 160), other hypercoagulable syndromes (Chapter 67), vasculitis (Chapter 249), and infections.

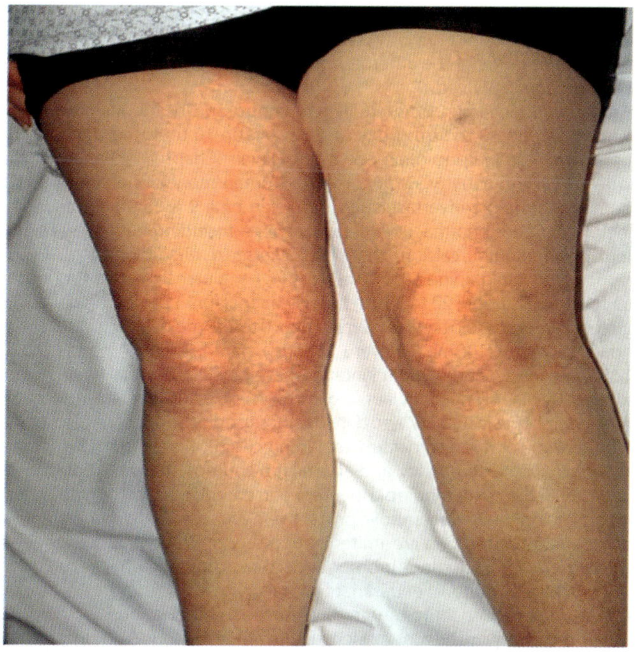

FIGURE 66-4. **Livedo reticularis.** Livedo reticularis appearing as a violaceous or reddish-blue netlike or mottled discoloration surrounding a pale central area of skin.

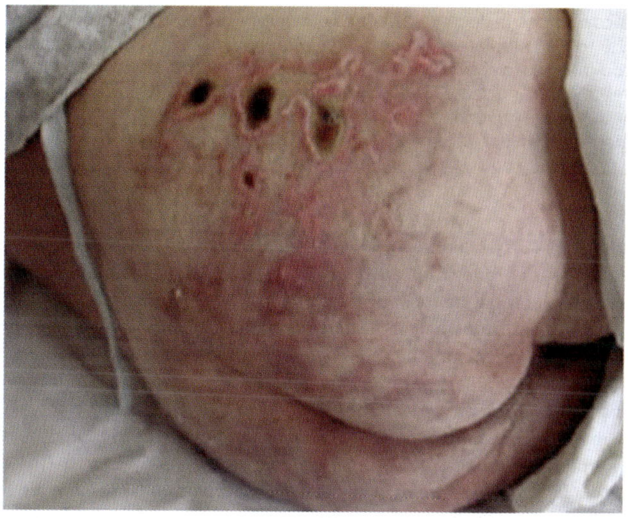

FIGURE 66-5. **Livedo racemosa.** Livedo racemosa with ischemic ulcerations and violaceous, netlike, and broken patterns in a patient who developed atheromatous embolization after cardiac catheterization on the buttocks.

TABLE 66-1 DISORDERS ASSOCIATED WITH LIVEDO RACEMOSA

Polyarteritis nodosa, systemic lupus erythematosus, rheumatoid arthritis, Sjögren syndrome, scleroderma
Atheromatous embolization, atrial myxoma
Antiphospholipid syndrome, Sneddon syndrome
Infections
Polycythemia vera, essential thrombocythemia, cryoglobulinemia, cryofibrinogenemia, cold agglutinin disease
Calciphylaxis, hyperoxaluria
Medications: Amantadine, amphetamines, ergotamines, vasopressors (epinephrine, norepinephrine, dopamine), heparin, minocycline, gemcitabine

Livedo reticularis and livedo racemosa have been reported in patients with coronavirus disease 2019 (Chapter 336). In such patients, livedo reticularis lesions are frequently mild and transient, whereas the racemosa form can be associated with an acute coagulopathy.[12]

CLINICAL MANIFESTATIONS AND DIAGNOSIS

The legs and, to a lesser extent, arms are most commonly involved in primary livedo reticularis, whereas the face, trunk, buttocks, and extremities may be involved with livedo racemosa. The discoloration of livedo reticularis is worsened by dependency and improves with elevation, but livedo racemosa does not show such postural changes. It is important to differentiate the usually painless, symmetrical, unbroken vessel network of primary livedo reticularis from the frequently painful, irregular, asymmetrical, and broken pattern observed in livedo racemosa.

A thorough history should focus on exacerbating conditions. Laboratory investigation is usually not necessary for the primary form, but specific testing for antiphospholipid antibodies should be performed to diagnose the secondary forms (i.e., circulating lupus anticoagulant, anticardiolipin antibodies) and P and C antineutrophil cytoplasmic antibodies. A skin biopsy may be necessary when serologies are indeterminate and the diagnosis remains unclear. The differential diagnosis includes erythema ab igne, retiform purpura, livedoid vasculopathy (a rare subtype of livedo racemosa), and acrocyanosis.

TREATMENT AND PROGNOSIS

Cold temperatures, tobacco, and stressful conditions should be avoided. Primary livedo reticularis does not require treatment, although calcium-channel blockers (e.g., nifedipine 10 to 20 mg PO every 6 hours or amlodipine 2.5 to 10 mg/day PO) may be beneficial for patients who are uncomfortable with their appearance. Treatment for livedo racemosa should focus on the underlying disorder. Anticoagulants, including warfarin to provide an international normalized ratio of 2.0 to 3.0, antiplatelet therapy (e.g., aspirin 81 to 325 mg/day), or both are recommended for livedo racemosa associated with antiphospholipid syndrome, cerebrovascular disease (Sneddon syndrome), or both. The prognosis is excellent for primary livedo reticularis but depends on the underlying disorder for patients with livedo racemosa.

ATHEROMATOUS EMBOLIZATION

Atheromatous embolization, also known as cholesterol crystal embolization, atheroembolic renal disease, or blue or purple toe syndrome, refers to the showering of multiple small cholesterol crystals or fibrin-platelet aggregates to the extremities or any organ. The exact incidence of atheromatous embolization is unknown, in part because it is often poorly recognized. In unselected autopsy series, the prevalence ranges from 0.18 to 2%, although it is reported to be much higher in individuals who have undergone aortic manipulation, arteriography, or cardiac or vascular procedures. As many as 5 to 10% of all cases of acute renal failure may result from atheroembolism (Chapter 110). Atheromatous embolization is more common in elderly individuals with advanced atherosclerosis but is less commonly diagnosed in Blacks, largely owing to a failure to recognize the classic dermatologic feature because of their skin pigmentation.

Atheromatous embolization usually originates from ulcerated or stenotic atherosclerotic plaques or aneurysms of both large and small arteries. Precipitating factors include arteriography, endovascular procedures (cerebral, coronary, or peripheral), surgery, trauma, or anticoagulation.[13] The risk after a cardiovascular interventional procedure is about 4 per 10,000 patients.[14] Atheroembolism also may occur spontaneously. Light microscopy demonstrates multiple biconvex, needle-shaped cholesterol crystals that lodge in arterioles and result in a foreign body inflammatory response in which polymorphonuclear leukocytes, macrophages, and multinucleated giant cells are observed days to weeks after the initiating event. This process eventually leads to end-organ damage owing to intraluminal obliteration, ischemia, and even often infarction.

CLINICAL MANIFESTATIONS AND DIAGNOSIS

Dermatologic findings involving the lower extremities are the most common clinical presentation (see Fig. 66-5), but atheromatous embolization may be seen in any organ (Table 66-2). Atheromatous embolization is frequently overlooked or misdiagnosed because the signs and symptoms are nonspecific and diverse. Once suspected, the diagnosis usually can be made on clinical grounds alone. The clinical triad of a history of a precipitating event, acute renal failure, and cutaneous or retinal findings should raise suspicion for the diagnosis. In some cases, the definitive diagnosis may require biopsy of the skin, kidney, or gastrointestinal tract. Patients may have elevated markers of inflammation (erythrocyte sedimentation rate, C-reactive protein) or transient eosinophilia. Elevations in amylase, hepatic aminotransferase, blood urea nitrogen, serum creatinine, or serum creatinine kinase levels may be seen with involvement of the pancreas, liver, kidney, or muscle, respectively. The urine is generally nonspecific, but eosinophiluria can be seen.

Invasive diagnostic angiographic procedures should be avoided. Noninvasive procedures, including multidetector CT angiography, MR angiography, or transesophageal echocardiography, may be helpful if they reveal a markedly irregular and shaggy aorta.

TABLE 66-2 CLINICAL MANIFESTATIONS OF ATHEROMATOUS EMBOLIZATION

Skin	Purple or blue toes Gangrenous digits Livedo reticularis or livedo racemosa Petechiae Ulcers, nodules Splinter hemorrhages
Kidney	Uncontrolled hypertension Advanced renal disease End-stage renal disease
Neurologic	Amaurosis fugax Hollenhorst plaque Transient ischemic attack or stroke Confusion, organic brain syndrome Spinal cord infarction
Gastrointestinal	Abdominal pain Diarrhea Gastrointestinal bleeding Ischemic bowel Acute pancreatitis Acute gangrenous cholecystitis
Cardiac	Angina pectoris Myocardial infarction
Constitutional symptoms	Fever Weight loss Malaise, myalgias Anorexia, nausea, vomiting

The differential diagnosis, which depends on the end organ involved, includes contrast-induced nephropathy (Chapters 59 and 106), polyarteritis nodosa (Chapter 249), leukocytoclastic vasculitis (Chapters 249 and 406), cryoglobulinemia (Chapter 173), antiphospholipid syndrome (Chapter 67), and thrombotic thrombocytopenia purpura (Chapter 158). An underlying malignancy must be considered in patients who present with constitutional symptoms such as anorexia and weight loss. Cardiac sources such as nonbacterial thrombotic endocarditis (Chapter 61), infective endocarditis (Chapter 61), or atrial myxoma (Chapter 47) should be excluded.

TREATMENT AND PROGNOSIS

The most important aspect of treatment is prevention and avoidance of recurrent atheroembolism. Smoking cessation (Chapter 363) and aggressive control of hypertension (Chapter 64), diabetes (Chapter 210), and hyperlipidemia (Chapter 190) should be instituted to prevent progression of the disease. In the absence of data from randomized trials, therapy is directed toward prescribing aggressive lipid-lowering treatment, avoiding recurrent embolization, removing the source of the atheroemboli, and providing symptomatic care of the end organ(s) involved.

Patients with ischemic ulcers require pain control and local wound care. Statins (e.g., atorvastatin 10 to 80 mg/day or rosuvastatin 10 to 40 mg/day to obtain optimal low-density lipoprotein cholesterol levels [Chapter 190]) may provide plaque-stabilizing activity. Evolocumab, a human monoclonal antibody that targets anti-protein convertase subtilisin/kexin type 9 (PCSK9) antibody, may be helpful.[15] Other pharmacologic approaches—including antiplatelet agents (aspirin or clopidogrel), calcium-channel blockers (e.g., nifedipine 10 to 20 mg PO every 6 hours or amlodipine 2.5 to 10 mg/day PO), angiotensin-converting enzyme inhibitors (e.g., lisinopril 20 to 30 mg per day or enalapril 10 to 40 mg per day), or angiotensin receptor blockers (e.g., valsartan 80 to 160 mg daily or losartan 50 mg per day), cilostazol (100 mg PO every 12 hours), pentoxifylline (400 mg PO every 8 hours), and intravenous prostaglandins—have been tried with varying degrees of success. The use of anticoagulants is controversial because of concerns that they may lead to plaque instability, and data do not support the use of corticosteroids.

Nonpharmacologic approaches, including chemical or surgical sympathectomy, a spinal cord stimulator, and arterial flow pumps, may help control pain. Endovascular therapies (angioplasty, stent placement, atherectomy, or covered stent grafts and the use of embolic protective devices) may help prevent future embolic events, but studies are limited and further clinical evaluation is needed. Surgical therapies, including thromboendarterectomy, aortobiiliac or aortobifemoral bypass grafting, or extra-anatomic reconstruction, may be necessary to eliminate the embolic source and reduce further embolization.

Patients with advanced atherosclerosis and atheromatous embolization have a poor prognosis. The estimated 1-year mortality rate is approximately 15% even with optimal medical care.

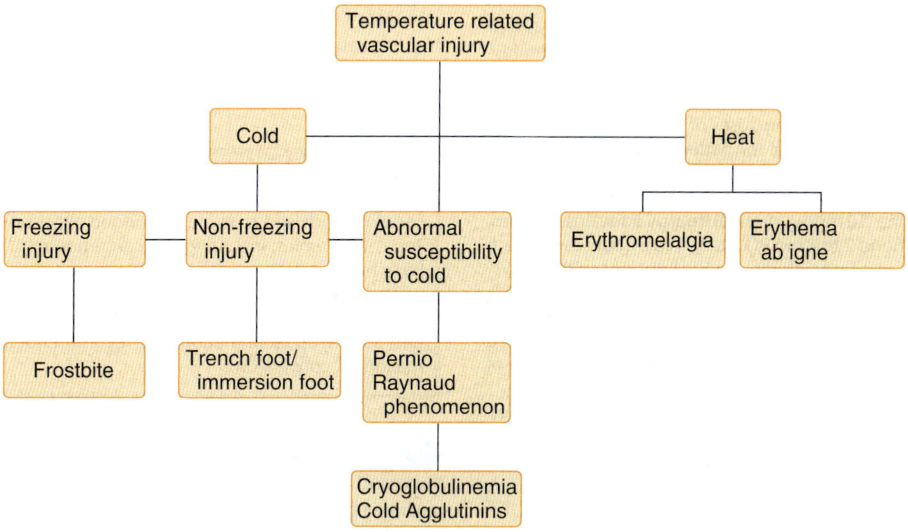

FIGURE 66-6. Clinical syndromes caused by heat or cold.

THERMAL DISORDERS

A variety of clinical syndromes can be caused by heat or cold (Fig. 66-6).

ERYTHROMELALGIA

The term *erythromelalgia* is derived from the Greek words *erythros* ("red"), *melos* ("extremities"), and *algos* ("pain"). It is characterized by episodic periods of erythema, increased warmth, and intense burning pain of the extremities.

Erythromelalgia is an uncommon disorder that affects younger to middle-aged women, adolescents, and children. The exact incidence is not known but has been reported at 1.3 per 100,000 living in Olmsted County, Minnesota. Erythromelalgia has been reported to occur in nearly 30% of patients with polycythemia vera (Chapter 152).

Both primary (familial and sporadic/idiopathic) and secondary forms occur. The primary trigger is heat exposure or increased ambient temperature. The familial form is autosomal dominant, with symptoms most often beginning in childhood. The pathophysiology is believed to be due to a small and large fiber neuropathy and vasculopathy. Although the exact cause of primary erythromelalgia is unknown, it is a neuropathic disorder with neuronal hyperexcitability owing to sodium-channel abnormalities because of a mutation of the gene *(SCN9A)* that encodes the Nav1.7v sodium channel (located on 2q). The causes of secondary erythromelalgia (Table 66-3) are not as well understood but are thought to be due to neuropathologic and microvascular functional changes caused by the underlying condition.

CLINICAL MANIFESTATIONS AND DIAGNOSIS

A triad of clinical findings including erythema, increased warmth, and intense burning pain of the extremities is usually observed (Fig. 66-7). The lower limbs (soles or entire foot) are more often affected than the hands. Involvement of the knees, elbows, ears, and face has been reported. Symptoms are generally bilateral and paroxysmal. An attack, which may last for several minutes or hours to days, is generally aggravated by dependency, alcohol, warm rooms, summer heat, exercise, or simply wearing shoes and socks or gloves. Attacks may also be more frequent at night. Erythromelalgia is often a disabling condition, and ulceration or even gangrene can occur in secondary forms.

TABLE 66-3 CAUSES OF SECONDARY ERYTHROMELALGIA

Myeloproliferative neoplasms: Essential thrombocythemia, polycythemia vera, chronic myelogenous leukemia, myelodysplastic syndrome
Drugs: Calcium-channel blockers, cyclosporine, bromocriptine, pergolide
Infectious diseases: Human immunodeficiency virus, hepatitis B vaccine, influenza vaccine, infectious mononucleosis, varicella virus
Connective tissue diseases: Systemic lupus erythematosus, rheumatoid arthritis
Neuropathic: Diabetic neuropathy, peripheral neuropathies, neurofibromatosis, Riley-Day syndrome, multiple sclerosis, spinal cord disease
Neoplastic: Paraneoplastic syndrome, astrocytoma, malignant thymoma, colorectal cancer, lung cancer, and thyroid cancer
Others: Mushroom ingestion, mercury poisoning

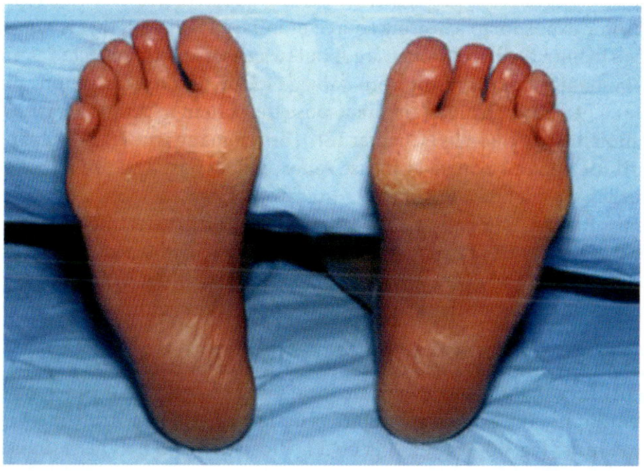

FIGURE 66-7. **Erythromelalgia.** Note the erythema of the feet. The patient also had pain and increased warmth on physical examination.

The history and physical examination are keys to the diagnosis. The physical examination is usually normal unless the patient is examined during an attack. A thorough vascular and neurologic examination should include demonstration of color changes and measurement of elevated skin temperatures during an attack. In between attacks, the affected area may be purple or cyanotic when dependent, consistent with acrocyanosis. A complete blood count is essential to exclude an underlying myeloproliferative disorder, and periodic blood counts are recommended because a myeloproliferative disorder (Chapter 152) may develop several years after the onset of symptoms. Electromyography and nerve conduction studies, autonomic and small fiber nerve testing, and vascular studies may help exclude other disorders. The quantitative sudomotor axon reflex test is useful to assess for small fiber neuropathy. Genetic testing is helpful for diagnosing primary erythromelalgia.

The differential diagnosis includes complex regional pain syndrome (Chapter 26), cellulitis (Chapter 408), peripheral neuropathy (Chapter 388), osteomyelitis (Chapter 251), Raynaud syndrome, acrocyanosis, peripheral arterial disease (Chapter 65), and gout (Chapter 252).

TREATMENT AND PROGNOSIS

Patients must avoid aggravating conditions, such as warm environments, exercise, tight shoes, and alcohol intake, as well as learn to cool their involved areas without causing tissue damage.[16] Patients seek relief by cooling the affected area with a fan, cold towels, cooling blankets, or immersion in ice water for short periods of time. These approaches may be helpful, but care must be taken not to overuse these methods. Elevation of the feet may help. Medications aimed at treatment of both the neuropathy and vasculopathy are often tried. Intravenous iloprost (at varying doses for up to 6 hours per day on 3 consecutive days) can significantly reduce symptoms and sympathetic dysfunction in about 60% of patients. In the genetic form, a small trial showed benefit from orally administered XEN402 (an inhibitor of Nav1.7 that is designated as an orphan drug by the U.S. Food and Drug Administration). Patients with an infectious, traumatic, or surgical precipitant may respond to varying doses of glucocorticoids if given early in their course. Aspirin may be helpful for patients with an underlying myeloproliferative disorder (Chapter 152). Tricyclic antidepressants (e.g., nortriptyline 25 to 100 mg/day PO), anticonvulsants (e.g., pregabalin 50 to 100 mg PO three times daily), mexiletine (10 mg/kg/day PO), topical lidocaine patches, and opioids (e.g., hydromorphone 2 to 8 mg PO every 4 to 6 hours as needed) have been used with benefit in some patients. Topical options without systemic side effects include lidocaine patches, a gel of 1% amitriptyline and 0.5% ketamine, capsaicin, and 1% diclofenac. Small case series have reported some success with the peripheral acting alpha-1 agonist midodrine (0.2% applied topically in a moisturizing cream three times daily) and with local injection of botulinum toxin.

Other methods, including a pain rehabilitation program, biofeedback, sympathectomy, spinal cord stimulator, and epidural blocks, have been tried with varying degrees of success. Patients have a reduced quality of life, and life expectancy is also reduced, primarily owing to suicide.

ERYTHEMA AB IGNE

Erythema ab igne is a hyperpigmented skin condition that results from repeated or chronic exposure to a heating source or infrared radiation that is not warm enough to burn the skin. Women are about twice as frequently affected as men.[17]

Skin manifestations result from damage to the dermis and venous plexus system. Dysplastic changes can predispose the patient to actinic keratosis and squamous cell carcinomas (Chapter 188). Erythema ab igne is an occupational hazard for persons whose arms are repeatedly exposed to fire in bakeries, foundries, or kitchens. It can also result from repeated application of a hot water bottle, heating pads, or electric blankets for the treatment of chronic pain. It also may be seen in persons who sit on heated seats or too close to space heaters, wood burning stoves, or car heaters, and it has been reported to involve the anterior thighs of persons using laptop computers.

CLINICAL MANIFESTATIONS AND DIAGNOSIS

Patients may report a slight burning or itching sensation but generally have no symptoms. The skin discoloration is described as reticular, erythematous, or brownish (Fig. 66-8 and E-Fig. 66-1). Ulceration and bullous lesions have been reported in chronic cases.

The diagnosis is made clinically based solely on dermatologic findings and on the history of exposure to a heating source or infrared radiation, so laboratory tests should be avoided. A biopsy must be obtained if signs such as hyperkeratotic, hyperpigmented papular or nodular lesions suggest a malignant transformation. The differential diagnosis includes livedo reticularis and livedo racemosa.

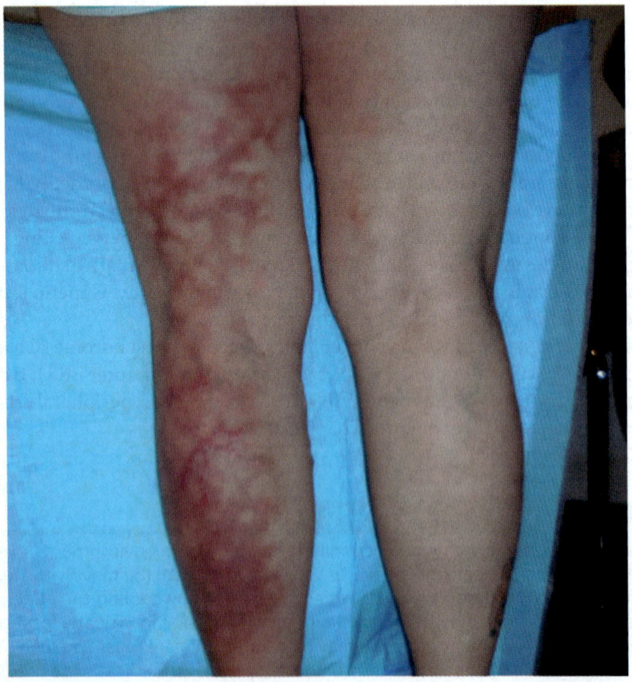

FIGURE 66-8. **Erythema ab igne. Note the hyperpigmentation and livedo reticularis pattern.**

TREATMENT AND PROGNOSIS

Removing the offending heat source is essential for treatment, and patients should be advised to avoid prolonged exposure to any form of infrared heat. Topical therapies, including topical tretinoin (0.05% cream) or hydroquinone, have been used to reduce the hyperpigmentation.

The prognosis is favorable once the source is removed, but the condition can be chronic and progressive if prolonged and repeated exposure continues. Follow-up examinations are recommended because of the potential for malignant conversion.

RAYNAUD PHENOMENON

Raynaud phenomenon is defined as episodic attacks of discoloration (white or blue) of the digits brought on by cold or emotional stimuli and resulting in a characteristic triphasic color change from white to blue to red. Raynaud phenomenon affects 3 to 5% of the U.S. population and is seen more often in young women, in whom it is reported to have a prevalence as high as 5 to 15%. The prevalence is higher in cooler northern climates and in smokers. Family history (as many as 30 to 50% of patients with primary Raynaud have a first-degree relative with this condition), estrogen exposure, and emotional stress are commonly associated with Raynaud phenomenon in women.

The pathophysiology of the vasoconstriction in Raynaud phenomenon is not well understood. It includes abnormalities of the blood vessel wall, neural control mechanisms, and intravascular factors, including platelet activation and oxidative stress. As the arterial vasoconstriction subsides, postcapillary venular constriction leads to deoxygenation of the blood and the cyanotic appearance. On rewarming, blood flow increases as a result of vasodilation, which leads to the red or hyperemic appearance of the digits.

Primary Raynaud phenomenon is a benign vasospastic disorder, whereas a number of conditions are associated with the secondary form (Table 66-4). Several clinical features can help distinguish between these two forms (Table 66-5).

TABLE 66-4 UNDERLYING CONDITIONS ASSOCIATED WITH SECONDARY RAYNAUD PHENOMENON

Rheumatologic: Scleroderma, systemic lupus erythematosus, rheumatoid arthritis, Sjögren syndrome, mixed connective tissue disorders
Obstructive arterial disease: Atherosclerosis, thromboangiitis obliterans, arterial embolism
Occupational/environmental disorders: Hypothenar hammer syndrome, hand-arm vibration syndrome, frostbite
Endocrine: Hypothyroidism
Hematologic: Polycythemia vera, multiple myeloma, cryoglobulinemia, cryofibrinogenemia, cold agglutinins
Drugs: Amphetamines, cocaine, β-blockers, clonidine, ergot preparations, oral contraceptives, cyclosporine, certain antineoplastic agents
Infections: Hepatitis B and C antigenemia
Thoracic outlet syndrome, subclavian artery aneurysm
Complex regional pain syndrome
Arteriovenous fistula
Lead and arsenic poisoning

TABLE 66-5 FEATURES SUGGESTIVE OF PRIMARY OR SECONDARY RAYNAUD PHENOMENON

CLINICAL FEATURE	PRIMARY	SECONDARY
Sex	Female	Female or male
Age	<40 yr	≥40 yr
Involvement	Bilateral	Unilateral or bilateral
Ischemic digits or ulcerations	Absent	±
Underlying cause	Absent	Present
Systemic complaints	Absent	±

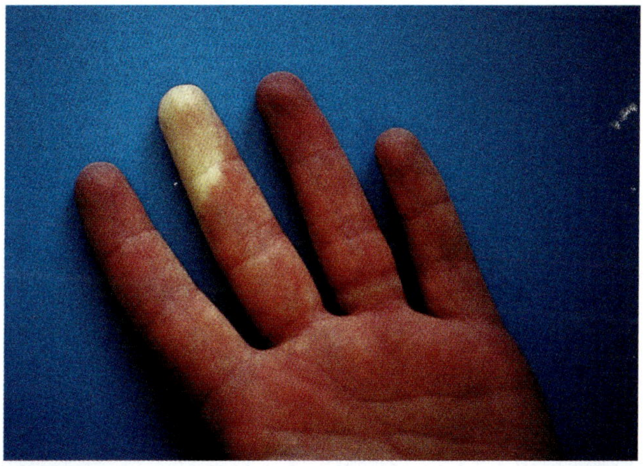

FIGURE 66-9. **Unilateral Raynaud phenomenon.** (From Forbes CD, Jackson WF. *Color Atlas and Text of Clinical Medicine*, 3rd ed. London: Mosby; 2003.)

CLINICAL MANIFESTATIONS AND DIAGNOSIS

Raynaud phenomenon is characterized by triphasic color change of the digits, pallor, cyanosis, and rubor after exposure to cold or stressful stimuli (Fig. 66-9 and E-Fig. 66-2). All three color changes are not seen in most individuals, and pallor may be the only finding. The middle and ring fingers are most commonly involved, whereas the thumb may be entirely spared. Raynaud phenomenon also can affect the toes, nose, ears, tongue, knees, or nipples. Patients may experience paresthesias and clumsiness of the hand during an attack.

A thorough history and physical examination is essential, but it may be normal in primary Raynaud phenomenon unless there is an ongoing attack. Secondary Raynaud findings may include ulceration or necrosis of the fingertips. Raynaud phenomenon is often the presenting symptom of an underlying connective tissue disorder, especially systemic sclerosis (Chapter 246).[18]

Routine laboratory testing should include a complete blood count, erythrocyte sedimentation rate, C-reactive protein level, thyroid function tests, antinuclear antibody, serum protein electrophoresis, urinalysis, and chest radiograph to evaluate for secondary causes. If the antinuclear antibody is positive or if the patient's history and physical examination indicate an underlying rheumatologic disorder, specific autoantibodies should be ordered (Chapter 237). Other tests including cryoglobulin levels, cryofibrinogen, and cold agglutinins may be helpful, depending on the clinical presentation (Chapter 236).

A number of noninvasive tests may help differentiate primary and secondary Raynaud phenomenon and evaluate the extent of vasospasm, including photoplethysmography, pulse volume recordings, laser Doppler flux, duplex ultrasonography, and nail-fold capillary microscopy. The presence of abnormal nail-fold capillaries on capillaroscopy (or video capillaroscopy) is useful for distinguishing patients with primary Raynaud phenomenon from those with secondary causes, and it can be an early predictor of systemic sclerosis. MR angiography or contrast angiography may be necessary, and the latter can help determine the cause of ischemia.

TREATMENT AND PROGNOSIS

Lifestyle modifications, including avoidance of cold exposure (such as when moving from a warm to an air-conditioned environment) and known stressful stimuli (with an emphasis on keeping the body core temperature and extremities warm), are essential for preventing attacks.[19] Raynaud phenomenon can be treated with both pharmacologic and nonpharmacologic approaches (Table 66-6). Topical nitroglycerin is effective for both primary and secondary Raynaud phenomenon.[A2]

For primary Raynaud phenomenon, calcium-channel blockers (e.g., nifedipine 10 to 20 mg orally every 6 hours or amlodipine 2.5 to 10 mg/day) can reduce attacks and the severity of symptoms.[A3] For patients with secondary Raynaud phenomenon, aggressive treatment of the underlying condition is essential, and the addition of calcium-channel blockers also may be beneficial. If the symptoms of ischemia persist or side effects are not tolerable, the addition of phosphodiesterase type 5 inhibitors (e.g., sildenafil 20 mg orally up to three times daily or tadalafil 5 mg orally daily) may help.[A4] Additional options include an endothelin-1 inhibitor (e.g., bosentan 62.5 to 125 mg orally twice daily) or a prostanoid infusion (e.g., iloprost 1 ng/kg/minute for 6 hours intravenously daily). Pain control with narcotics, chemical or surgical sympathectomy, and spinal cord stimulation may be necessary in the most severe cases, particularly in situations of nonhealing digital ulceration and tissue loss.

The prognosis for primary Raynaud phenomenon is excellent, whereas the prognosis for secondary Raynaud phenomenon depends on the underlying condition.

TABLE 66-6 PHARMACOLOGIC AND NONPHARMACOLOGIC THERAPIES FOR RAYNAUD PHENOMENON

NONPHARMACOLOGIC THERAPIES
Educate and reassure patients about their condition
Avoid cold exposure or other triggering factors
Use warm clothing to maintain core body temperature (cover the entire body and wear a hat and scarf)
Teach how to terminate attacks: Exit from cold, warming techniques
Avoid nicotine
Biofeedback
PHARMACOLOGIC THERAPIES
Nitroglycerin topical 1 inch q6h
Calcium channel blockers (nifedipine 10-20 mg q6h or amlodipine 2.5-10 mg q24h
Phosphodiesterase-5 inhibitors (sildenafil 25-50 mg three times daily, tadalafil 5-20 mg three times daily) and phosphodiesterase-3 inhibitors (cilostazol 100 mg twice daily)
Angiotensin-converting enzyme inhibitors/angiotensin-receptor blockers (especially for scleroderma-associated Raynaud phenomenon)
Others: Hydralazine 10-50 mg four times daily; reserpine 0.1-0.25 mg/day PO; bosentan 125 mg PO twice daily
Prostaglandins: Iloprost, epoprostenol, alprostadil, beraprost
Antithrombotics/anticoagulants: (aspirin 81-325 mg/day, dipyridamole 75 mg three times daily, heparin [via weight-based nomogram; see Table 68-6 in Chapter 68], low-molecular-weight heparin [e.g., enoxaparin 1 mg/kg q12h; see Table 70-3 in Chapter 70])
Botulinum toxin A

PERNIO

Pernio, also known as chilblains, is a cold-induced vasospastic inflammatory process that affects the skin after exposure to nonfreezing temperatures or damp climates. Pernio is seen more commonly in the northern United States and northwestern Europe. It is most common in individuals with a low body mass and in young women between the ages of 15 and 30 years, although it also can occur in children and in the elderly.

The cause is unknown but is likely a result of cold-induced vasoconstriction that induces inflammation and ischemia of vessels and surrounding tissue. It has been seen as a complication of coronavirus disease 2019 (COVID-19; Chapter 336), often with elevated D-dimer levels and significantly increased levels of interferon-alpha after in vitro stimulation.[20] The histopathologic findings include dermal edema, keratinocyte necrosis, a deep dermal lymphocytic infiltrate, thickening of venule walls, and pericyte hyperplasia.

Pernio can be classified as acute or chronic. Acute pernio develops a few hours after exposure, whereas chronic pernio develops after repeated exposures to nonfreezing cold or damp conditions.

CLINICAL MANIFESTATIONS AND DIAGNOSIS

Pernio occurs most frequently in late fall to early spring in wet or nonfreezing cold environments. Acute pernio is characterized by intense itching, numbness, or a burning sensation that develops shortly after exposure to cold or damp conditions and disappears within a few weeks.

Pernio is generally symmetrical. It usually involves the toes and fingers and less commonly involves the nose, ears, or cheeks. Pernio may also affect the thighs of horse riders, young women wearing tight slacks, motorcycle riders, or people who frequently apply ice packs. Pernio is associated with single or multiple erythematous, brownish or red, purple-blue skin lesions (macules, papules, or plaques) that may progress to blisters or ulcers (Fig. 66-10 and E-Fig. 66-3).

Chronic pernio develops after repeated cold exposure and results in cyanotic papules, macules, or nodules. Patients often report a history of similar episodes that develop each year during the cold months and typically resolve with warmer temperatures.

The diagnosis is based on the history and physical examination (Table 66-7). Patients generally have a normal arterial examination. Pulse volume recordings may reveal vasoconstriction, but capillaroscopy is usually normal. A skin biopsy may be necessary to differentiate pernio from other disorders, such as Raynaud phenomenon, frostbite, acrocyanosis, atheromatous embolization, erythema nodosum (Chapter 407), erythema induratum (Chapter 407), lupus erythematosus (Chapter 245), sarcoidosis (Chapter 83), or atherosclerosis (Chapter 65). Laboratory testing is important to exclude an underlying collagen vascular disease. Up to 35 to 40% of patients may have cold agglutinins as a precipitating cause (Chapter 236).

PREVENTION

Patients susceptible to pernio should be advised to avoid cold exposure. If they must go outside in cold or damp weather, they should dress appropriately with layered outdoor clothing, insulated footgear, gloves, scarf, and hat.

Pernio is usually self-limiting in the acute state. Chronic pernio can lead to scarring, atrophy, and chronic occlusive vascular disease.

TREATMENT AND PROGNOSIS

Treatment begins by warming and drying the affected areas. Topical corticosteroids (e.g., 0.025% fluocinolone acetonide) may be tried, and oral calcium-channel blockers (nifedipine 20 to 60 mg/day or amlodipine 2.5 to 10 mg/day) may reduce symptoms. Nifedipine may also be given in a topical gel form. Pentoxifylline (400 mg three times daily)[A5] and capsaicin have also been reported to be helpful. Tissue loss is uncommon.

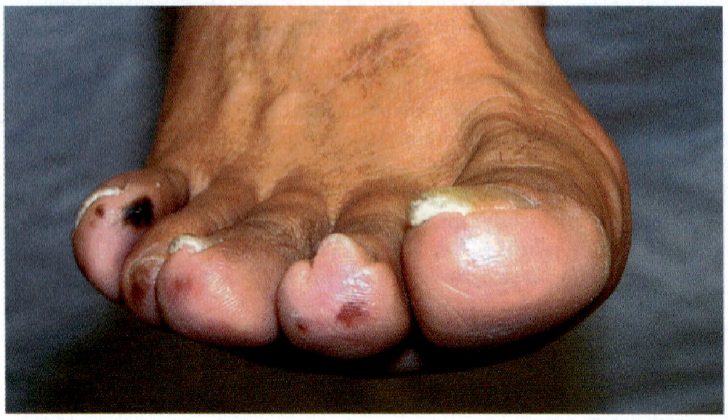

FIGURE 66-10. **Pernio on the toes of the right foot.** The lesions on the second, third, and fourth toes are the typical red, brown, and yellow scaling lesions. The lesion on the fifth toe can be confused with atheromatous embolization.

TABLE 66-7 PROPOSED DIAGNOSTIC CRITERIA OF PERNIO

MAJOR CRITERIA
Localized erythema and swelling involving acral sites and persisting for >24 hours
MINOR CRITERIA
Onset and/or worsening in cooler months (between November and March)
Skin biopsy consistent with pernio (dermal edema with superficial and deep perivascular lymphocytic infiltrate) without findings of lupus erythematosus.
Response to conservative treatments (warming and drying of affected areas)

FROSTBITE

Frostbite is a local cold-induced injury (Chapter 95) that occurs when persons are exposed to temperatures below the freezing point of intact skin or in above-freezing temperatures in association with wet environments, high altitudes, and strong winds.

Frostbite is more common in individuals 30 to 49 years who participate in winter outdoor sports and in individuals who are homeless, have psychiatric illnesses (Chapter 362), survive outdoor trauma (Chapter 97), consume excess alcohol (Chapter 364), or use illegal drugs (Chapter 365). Patients with peripheral arterial disease (Chapter 65), a smoking history (Chapter 363), younger or older age, or diabetes (Chapter 210) are also at increased risk. Frostbite injury involves three pathophysiologic components: tissue injury from extracellular and intracellular ice crystal formation, intracellular dehydration, and ischemia.

CLINICAL MANIFESTATIONS AND DIAGNOSIS

The severity of frostbite relates to the absolute temperature and to the duration of exposure. The digits of the hands and feet account for most injuries, although the ears, nose, and cheeks may be affected. Patients complain of numbness or paresthesias and report clumsiness and lack of fine coordination if the hands are involved. The numbness may persist even after rewarming. The skin may be pale, waxy, and cool to touch, and the patient may have mild to extensive swelling depending on the severity of the frostbite. Large, clear or hemorrhagic blisters often appear (Fig. 66-11), followed by black scabs. Damage to the muscles, tendons, cartilage, joints, and bones occur in severe frostbite. Pain is often severe during the rewarming process.

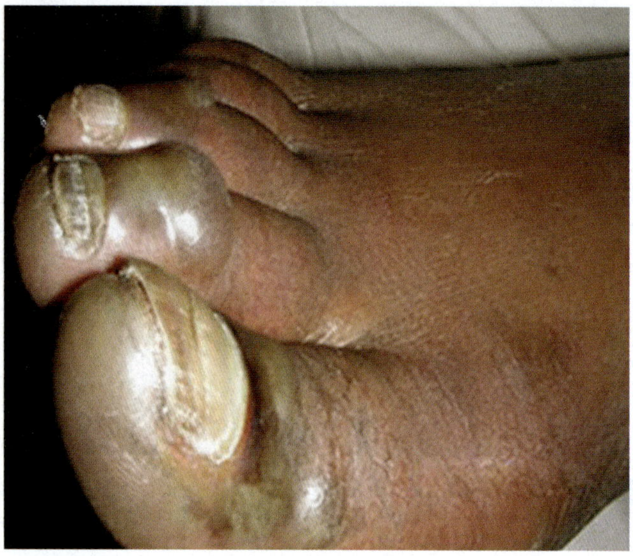

FIGURE 66-11. **Blisters in a patient with frostbite.**

The diagnosis of frostbite is made by the exposure history and physical examination. The differential diagnosis includes peripheral arterial disease, pernio, trench foot, or thermal burns.

TREATMENT AND PROGNOSIS

Proper recognition of frostbite and removal from cold exposure is essential. Local rewarming should begin only if refreezing will not occur while the patient is being transferred to a hospital. Uninterrupted rapid rewarming in a water bath of between 40 and 42° C for 15 to 30 minutes is critical to help minimize tissue loss. Removal of wet or damp clothing and jewelry is important, but rubbing or massage should be avoided. Splinting and elevation of the affected limb can help minimize swelling and improve perfusion. Patients should receive tetanus toxoid and analgesics (e.g., hydromorphone 2 to 8 mg either orally or parenterally every 3 to 4 hours as needed) for pain. Ibuprofen (12 mg/kg) divided in twice-daily doses to inhibit the release of harmful prostaglandins should also be administered unless contraindicated.[21,22] Broad-spectrum antibiotics should be given only to patients with significant trauma, other potential infectious sources, or signs and symptoms of cellulitis or sepsis. Daily cleansing in a warm whirlpool bath and physical therapy are important. Clear blisters should be left alone, but ruptured blisters should be covered with a topical antibiotic, such as neomycin/bacitracin/polymyxin B ointment.

For severe frostbite, the combination of intravenous iloprost (not available in the United States) plus aspirin is superior to the combination of aspirin plus buflomedil (an α-blocker) or the combination of aspirin plus iloprost plus tissue plasminogen activator (tPA) for reducing the amputation rate. The Wilderness Medical Society Clinical Practice guidelines for the prevention and treatment of frostbite recommend tPA (intravenous or intra-arterial) be initiated within 24 hours of injury if appropriate monitoring capabilities are available and iloprost cannot be obtained promptly. If possible, surgical débridement and amputation should be avoided until complete demarcation occurs.

Patients subjected to frostbite are more susceptible to future cold injuries, including frostbite arthritis of the small joints of the hands or feet. They also are susceptible to chronic pain, complex regional pain syndrome (Chapter 26), cold hypersensitivity, and a reduced sensitivity to touch.

ACROCYANOSIS

DEFINITION

Acrocyanosis is a poorly defined and often misunderstood clinical condition that manifests as painless, symmetrical, bluish or cyanotic discoloration affecting the hands, the feet, or both.[23] Acrocyanosis occurs in primary and secondary forms. Primary acrocyanosis is generally a benign condition seen most often in young women during their second to fourth decades of life. It may be more common in cooler temperatures, and a familial predisposition has been reported. The overall incidence is not known, but its prevalence has been reported to be approximately 20 to 40% in persons with anorexia nervosa (Chapter 200) and up to 25% of all patients with cancer.

Acrocyanosis was originally thought to be a vasospastic disorder that develops when small cutaneous arteries and arterioles constrict and reduce blood flow, dilation, and oxygen desaturation in the venules. More recent data suggest that low pressures and sluggish flow result in capillary constriction.

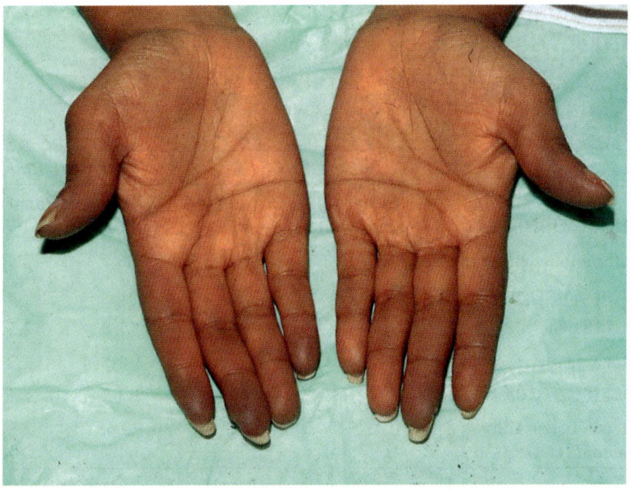

FIGURE 66-12. Acrocyanosis. Persistent, painless, symmetrical bluish discoloration (of different shades) in a patient with acrocyanosis.

The underlying cause of primary acrocyanosis is unknown, but a role for estrogen is suggested. Some of the secondary causes of acrocyanosis can be associated with a number of conditions, including Ehlers-Danlos syndrome (Chapter 239), hypoxemia (Chapter 90), cryoglobulins (Chapter 173), cryofibrinogens, cold agglutinins, antiphospholipid antibodies (Chapter 160), malignancy, spinal cord injury (Chapter 368), arsenic poisoning (Chapter 20), eating disorders (including anorexia nervosa [Chapter 200] and chronic starvation), and some medications (vasopressors and tricyclic antidepressants). It is also seen with "puffy hand syndrome," a finding unique to injection drug users (Chapter 365) who inject into their hands or fingers.

CLINICAL MANIFESTATIONS AND DIAGNOSIS

Persistent, painless, symmetrical bluish discoloration (of different shades) (Fig 66-12) involves the hands and feet but also can affect the forearms, nose, ears, and even nipples. Acrocyanosis may be exacerbated by cold exposure, emotional stress, or dependency of the limbs. It improves with elevation. Patients also report clamminess and hyperhidrosis of their hands and feet. Secondary acrocyanosis may be asymmetrical and associated with pain, ulceration, or tissue loss or gangrene.

The diagnosis of acrocyanosis is based on the history and physical examination. Laboratory evaluation should include a complete blood count, metabolic profile, and levels of antiphospholipid antibodies, cold agglutinins, cryofibrinogens, and cryoglobulins, as well as testing for connective tissue disorders (Chapter 236).

The differential diagnosis includes Raynaud phenomenon, pernio, erythromelalgia, and peripheral cyanosis. Acrocyanosis can be differentiated from peripheral cyanosis by the presence of cyanosis on the mucous membranes and hypoxia on an arterial blood sample.

TREATMENT AND PROGNOSIS

No treatment is necessary for primary acrocyanosis other than reassurance and avoidance of cold and damp exposures. Wearing gloves and avoiding tobacco may be helpful. A trial of α-adrenergic blocking agents such as prazosin (3 mg/daily) may be considered. Calcium-channel blockers, including amlodipine or nifedipine, are generally not helpful. Bioflavonoids and nicotinic acid derivatives have been reported beneficial in some cases, and sympathetic nerve block and sympathectomy may be tried for more severe cases. Treatment for secondary acrocyanosis depends on the underlying cause.

The prognosis of primary acrocyanosis is excellent. The prognosis of secondary acrocyanosis depends on the underlying cause.

GENERAL REFERENCES

For the General References and other additional features, please visit Elsevier eBooks+ at https://ebooks.health.elsevier.com.

Grade A References

A1. Cacione DG, Macedo CR, do Carmo Novaes F, et al. Pharmacological treatment for Buerger's disease. *Cochrane Database Syst Rev.* 2020;5:CD011033.
A2. Curtiss P, Schwager Z, Cobos G, et al. A systematic review and meta-analysis of the effects of topical nitrates in the treatment of primary and secondary Raynaud's phenomenon. *J Am Acad Dermatol.* 2018;78:1110-1118.
A3. Rirash F, Tingey PC, Harding SE, et al. Calcium channel blockers for primary and secondary Raynaud's phenomenon. *Cochrane Database Syst Rev.* 2017;12:CD000467.
A4. Roustit M, Giai J, Gaget O, et al. On-demand sildenafil as a treatment for Raynaud phenomenon: a series of n-of-1 trials. *Ann Intern Med.* 2018;169:694-703.
A5. Al-Sudany NK. Treatment of primary perniosis with oral pentoxifylline (a double-blind placebo-controlled randomized therapeutic trial). *Dermatol Ther.* 2016;29:263-268.

67 THROMBOTIC DISORDERS: HYPERCOAGULABLE STATES

ANDREW I. SCHAFER

The hypercoagulable states, also referred to as thrombophilias, encompass a group of inherited or acquired conditions that are associated with an increased risk for thrombosis. The primary hypercoagulable states are quantitative or qualitative prothrombotic abnormalities in specific coagulation proteins. Most of these disorders involve inherited mutations and polymorphisms that lead to either a deficiency of a physiologic antithrombotic factor (typically associated with a loss-of-function mutation) or an increased level of a prothrombotic factor (typically associated with a gain-of-function mutation) (Table 67-1).[1] Particularly when they are combined with other inherited prothrombotic mutations (multigene interactions), these primary hypercoagulable states are associated with a lifelong predisposition to thrombosis.

The secondary hypercoagulable states, which are a diverse group of mostly acquired conditions, cause a thrombotic tendency by more complex, often multifactorial mechanisms. The trigger for a discrete, clinical thrombotic event is often of one of the acquired secondary hypercoagulable states superimposed on an inherited state of hypercoagulability (E-Fig. 67-1).[2]

PRIMARY HYPERCOAGULABLE STATES

Antithrombin III Deficiency

EPIDEMIOLOGY AND PATHOBIOLOGY

Inherited quantitative or qualitative deficiency of antithrombin III leads to increased accumulation of fibrin and a lifelong propensity to thrombosis (Chapter 157). Antithrombin is the major physiologic inhibitor of thrombin and other activated coagulation factors, so its deficiency leads to the increased formation of fibrin.[3]

The frequency of asymptomatic heterozygous antithrombin deficiency in the general population is 1 in 350 (Table 67-2). Most of these individuals have clinically silent mutations and never have thrombotic manifestations. The frequency of symptomatic antithrombin deficiency in the general population has been estimated to be between 1 in 2000 and 1 in 3000. Among all patients seen with venous thromboembolism (VTE), antithrombin deficiency is detected in only about 1 to 2%, but it is found in approximately 2.5% of selected patients with recurrent thrombosis or the onset of thrombosis at a younger age (<45 years).

Patients with type I antithrombin deficiency have proportionately reduced plasma levels of antigenic and functional antithrombin because of a quantitative deficiency of the normal protein. Impaired synthesis, defective secretion, or instability of antithrombin in type I antithrombin-deficient individuals is caused by major gene deletions, single nucleotide changes, or short insertions or deletions in the antithrombin gene. Patients with type II antithrombin deficiency have normal or nearly normal plasma antigen levels but low activity

TABLE 67-1 PRIMARY HYPERCOAGULABLE STATES

DEFICIENCY OF ANTITHROMBOTIC FACTORS
Antithrombin (III) deficiency
Protein C deficiency
Protein S deficiency
INCREASED PROTHROMBOTIC FACTORS
Factor Va (activated protein C resistance; factor V Leiden)
Prothrombin (prothrombin G20210A mutation)
Factor IX Padua (factor IX R338L mutation)
Factors VII, XI, IX, VIII; von Willebrand factor; fibrinogen (epidemiologic data; molecular mechanisms unknown)

levels, thereby indicating a functionally defective molecule. Type II deficiency is usually caused when specific point mutations lead to single amino acid substitutions that produce a dysfunctional protein.

The pattern of inheritance of antithrombin deficiency is autosomal dominant. Most affected individuals are heterozygotes whose antithrombin activity levels are typically about 40 to 60% of normal. These individuals may have the full clinical manifestations of lifelong hypercoagulability. Rare homozygous antithrombin-deficient patients generally have type II deficiency with reduced heparin affinity (and consequently heparin resistance), a variant that is associated with a low risk for thrombosis in its heterozygous form. Other forms of homozygous antithrombin deficiency, however, are probably incompatible with life due to thrombosis-related intrauterine demise.

PROTEIN C DEFICIENCY

Protein C deficiency leads to the unregulated generation of fibrin because of impaired inactivation of factors VIIIa and Va, two essential cofactors in the coagulation cascade.[4]

EPIDEMIOLOGY AND PATHOBIOLOGY

The prevalence of heterozygous protein C deficiency in the general population is about 1 per 200 to 500. Protein C deficiency is found in 2 to 5% of all patients with VTE (Table 67-2).

As with antithrombin deficiency, two general forms of protein C deficiency are recognized: type I, in which quantitative deficiency of the protein is associated with a proportionate decrease in protein C antigen and activity, and type II, in which qualitative defects in protein C are associated with disproportionately reduced protein C activity relative to antigen. In the more common type I deficiency, frameshift, nonsense, or missense mutations cause premature termination of synthesis or loss of protein C stability. In type II deficiency, different mutations can cause abnormalities in the activation or function of protein C. The mode of inheritance of protein C deficiency is autosomal dominant. As in antithrombin deficiency, most affected individuals are heterozygotes. Neonatal purpura fulminans, a very rare complication involving widespread and sometimes fatal thrombosis, occurs in homozygous protein C– or protein S–deficient individuals.

PROTEIN S DEFICIENCY

Protein S is the principal cofactor of activated protein C, and its deficiency mimics that of protein C deficiency in causing loss of regulation of fibrin generation because of impaired inactivation of factors VIIIa and Va.[5] Reduced levels of free protein S and total protein S only marginally increase the risk for venous thrombosis; only levels far below the normal range cause increase thrombosis risk two-fold to five-fold.

EPIDEMIOLOGY AND PATHOBIOLOGY

Protein S deficiency is estimated to occur in about 1 in 500 in the general population. Its frequency in all patients evaluated for VTE (1 to 3%) is comparable to that of protein C deficiency.

Protein S circulates in plasma partly in complex with C4b-binding protein; only free protein S, which normally constitutes about 35 to 40% of total protein S, can function as a cofactor of activated protein C. As in deficiencies of antithrombin and protein C, quantitative (type I) and qualitative (type II) forms of inherited protein S deficiency are known. In addition, type III protein S deficiency is characterized by normal plasma levels of total protein S but low levels of free protein S. Most mutations involve frameshift, nonsense, or missense point variants.

ACTIVATED PROTEIN C RESISTANCE (FACTOR V LEIDEN)

EPIDEMIOLOGY AND PATHOBIOLOGY

The factor V Leiden mutation is remarkably frequent (3 to 8%) in healthy White populations of European ancestry but is far less prevalent in certain Black and Asian populations. The factor V Leiden mutation causes activated protein C resistance and an increased risk of VTE.[6] In various studies, activated protein C resistance has been found in a wide range of frequencies (10 to 64%) in patients with VTE.

Almost all subjects with functional activated protein C resistance have a single specific point mutation in the gene for factor V, which is a critical target of the physiologic anticoagulant action of activated protein C. In this mutation, termed factor V Leiden, guanine is replaced with adenine at nucleotide 1691 (G1691A), and this mutation leads to the amino acid substitution of Arg504 by Gln and renders factor Va incapable of being inactivated by activated protein C. Heterozygosity factor V Leiden mutation increases the risk for thrombosis by a factor of 5 to 10, whereas homozygosity increases the risk by a factor of 50 to 100.

TABLE 67-2 MOST COMMON INHERITED HYPERCOAGULABLE STATES (THROMBOPHILIAS): EPIDEMIOLOGY AND RISK OF VENOUS THROMBOEMBOLISM (VTE)

	PREVALENCE (%)		RELATIVE RISK	
THROMBOPHILIA	General Population*	Unselected VTE	First VTE	Recurrent VTE
Antithrombin deficiency	0.02-0.3	1-2	5-8	2.5
Protein C deficiency	0.2-0.5	2-5	5-8	2.5
Protein S deficiency	0.5	1-3	1.7-8	2.5
Factor V Leiden	3-8	10-65	5-10†	1.3
Factor II G20210A	1-6	3-8	1.5-3.8	1.4
Factor V Leiden and factor II G20210A	0.01	—	20-60	2.5

*Data refer to White populations. The prevalence of factor V Leiden and factor II G20210A is much lower in African, African American, and Asian populations.
†Relative risk of first VTE with homozygous factor V Leiden is up to 10-fold higher (50-100).
Modified from Coppola A, Tufano A, Cerbone AM, et al. Inherited thrombophilia: implications for prevention and treatment of venous thromboembolism. *Semin Thromb Hemost*. 2009;35:683-694.

PROTHROMBIN GENE MUTATION (PROTHROMBIN G20210A)

The substitution of G for A at nucleotide 20210 of the prothrombin gene is associated with elevated plasma levels of prothrombin and an increased risk for venous thrombosis. The allele frequency for this gain-of-function mutation is 1 to 6% in White populations, but it is much less prevalent in other racial groups. The prothrombin G20210A mutation is found in 3 to 8% of all patients with VTE.

OTHER PRIMARY HYPERCOAGULABLE STATES

X-linked thrombophilia is caused by a gain-of-function mutation in the gene for coagulation factor IX (factor IX Padua). Hereditary thrombosis can be caused by a missense mutation in the prothrombin gene (prothrombin Yukuhashi) that results in impaired inhibition of its mutant thrombin product by antithrombin. Elevated levels of factor VIII coagulant activity are a significant risk factor for venous thrombosis and its recurrence, and family studies suggest that high factor VIII levels are often genetically determined. Increased levels of factor VII, factor IX, factor XI, fibrinogen, von Willebrand factor, and thrombin-activatable fibrinolysis inhibitor, as well as very low levels of tissue factor pathway inhibitor, may also confer increased risk. Mutations in *STAB2*, which codes for stabilin-2, may raise levels of procoagulant von Willebrand factor.[7]

Many other inherited abnormalities of specific physiologic antithrombotic systems may be associated with a thrombotic tendency. Most of these conditions are limited to case reports or family studies, their molecular genetic bases are less well defined, and their prevalence rates are unknown but are probably much lower than those of the disorders described earlier. These uncommon hereditary disorders include heparin cofactor II deficiency, dysfunctional thrombomodulin, and many fibrinolytic disorders that lead to impaired fibrin degradation, including hypoplasminogenemia, dysplasminogenemia, plasminogen activator deficiency, and certain dysfibrinogenemias that cause a thrombotic rather than a bleeding diathesis.

CLINICAL MANIFESTATIONS

The primary hypercoagulable states are associated with predominantly venous thromboembolic complications (see Table 157-3). Deep venous thrombosis (DVT) of the lower extremities and pulmonary embolism (Chapter 68) are the most frequent clinical manifestations. Venous thromboses occurring in more unusual sites include superficial thrombophlebitis and splanchnic and cerebral venous thrombosis (see Table 157-3). Arterial thrombosis involving the coronary, cerebrovascular, and peripheral circulations is not generally linked to any of the primary hypercoagulable states.[8] However, venous thrombosis can result in arterial occlusion by paradoxical embolism across a patent foramen ovale. Also, epidemiologic studies have revealed increased overall risk of arterial thrombotic and atherosclerotic vascular disease in patients with a history of VTE and vice versa. Recurrent pregnancy loss is probably increased in primary hypercoagulable states, but this association is not as strongly established as it is in antiphospholipid syndrome (see later under Secondary Hypercoagulable States).

The initial episode of VTE can occur at any age in patients with primary hypercoagulable states, but it typically is seen in early adulthood. Positive family histories of thrombosis can frequently be elicited. Recurrent VTE, especially at a young age, and VTE in unusual sites (e.g., splanchnic or cerebral veins) are also suggestive of an underlying primary hypercoagulable state. The risk for thrombosis varies among the individual primary hypercoagulable states and is highest in patients with deficiencies of antithrombotic factors (Table 67-2); it is also markedly increased with the coexistence of multiple prothrombotic mutations. Patients with homozygous deficiency states tend to have more severe thrombotic complications.

In most patients with primary hypercoagulable states, discrete clinical thrombotic complications appear to be provoked by acquired prothrombotic events (e.g., pregnancy, use of oral contraceptives, surgery, trauma, immobilization), many of which are the secondary hypercoagulable states (see E-Fig. 67-1). For example, thrombosis complicates pregnancy, especially during the puerperium, in about 30 to 60% of women with antithrombin deficiency, 10 to 20% with protein C or protein S deficiency, and almost 30% with activated protein C resistance (factor V Leiden) unless prophylactic anticoagulation is administered during this period.

Whether or not an episode of VTE has been "provoked" by a precipitating event is presently considered pivotal in determining the recommended duration of anticoagulation and possibly even the extent of the required evaluation for an underlying thrombophilia. Whereas active cancer, immobilization, oral contraceptives or hormone replacement therapy, pregnancy, and the postoperative state at the time of VTE are clearly "provoking" factors, many weak transient risk factors for thrombosis (e.g., minor soft tissue injury to a leg) or risk factors that preceded VTE by some length of time are less certainly related events. Furthermore, many acquired triggers for VTE are subclinical or undisclosed by the patient. Therefore, the notion of a straightforward binary distinction between "provoked" versus "unprovoked" VTE can be challenged as a primary determinant of diagnostic testing or the duration of anticoagulant therapy.

DIAGNOSIS

Who to Test

The diagnostic approach to a patient with a documented episode of VTE includes a thorough history (including inquiry about changes in activity or medications, trauma, immobility, surgical procedures, use of oral contraceptive agents or hormone replacement therapy in the months leading up to the VTE and family history of thrombosis), physical examination (especially signs that suggest an occult malignancy), and basic laboratory tests to search for possible precipitating conditions or triggers for the acute event and to exclude underlying acquired causes of hypercoagulability. No randomized trial data are available to determine whether testing for a primary hypercoagulable state is worthwhile after a first episode of thrombosis. Guidelines commonly recommend against detailed testing for inherited thrombophilia after a first VTE in adults if the VTE occurred in the presence of major transient risk factors (Fig. 67-1).[9]

A reasonable diagnostic approach is to screen patients after an initial episode of VTE with a documented event before 40 years of age, a positive family history, or unprovoked or recurrent VTE. However, thrombophilia testing is not routinely recommended indiscriminately in all patients after a first VTE episode or in patients with overt provoking factors. Although indefinite anticoagulation is recommended for patients who have had two or more VTE events, regardless of whether a primary hypercoagulable state is found, testing of these individuals for thrombophilia can still be useful to guide family screening strategies (see Fig. 67-1).

Individuals with arterial thrombosis generally should not be tested for any of these disorders because primary hypercoagulable states are not clearly associated with an increased risk for arterial thrombosis. In contrast, some of the secondary hypercoagulable states, including hyperhomocysteinemia and antiphospholipid syndrome (see later), are associated with an increased risk for arterial as well as venous thrombosis (Table 67-3).

When to Test

In general, testing for primary hypercoagulable states is not recommended immediately after a major thrombotic event, particularly because these test results are very unlikely to alter initial management. Testing ideally should be performed in clinically stable patients after completion of oral anticoagulation at least 3 to 6 months after a thrombotic episode because active thrombosis may transiently consume and deplete some of the antithrombotic proteins in plasma and lead to the erroneous diagnosis of inherited antithrombin, protein C, or protein S deficiency. In addition to acute thrombosis, pregnancy, estrogen use, liver disease, and disseminated intravascular coagulation may cause acquired deficiencies of antithrombin, protein C, or protein S.

Anticoagulation may also interfere with some of the functional tests for primary hypercoagulable states. Heparin treatment can cause a decline in antithrombin levels to the deficiency range even in normal individuals. In contrast, warfarin can elevate antithrombin levels into the normal range in patients who do have an inherited deficiency state. Warfarin therapy, by its very mode of action, also predictably reduces the functional levels and, less prominently, the immunologic levels of protein C and protein S. Active warfarin treatment thereby potentially leads to a misdiagnosis of inherited deficiency. The direct oral anticoagulants can interfere with testing for lupus anticoagulant (see later). To avoid interference of oral anticoagulants with functional tests of hypercoagulable states or interpretation of their results, blood should be

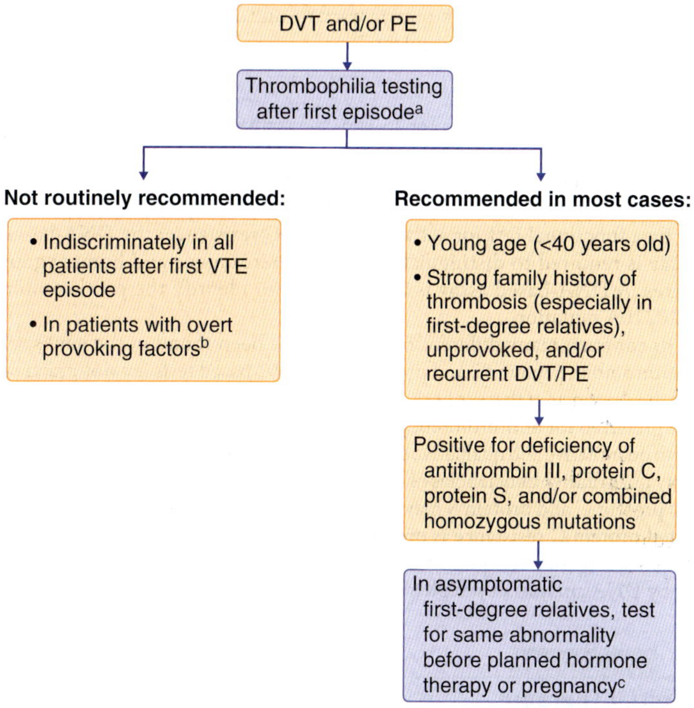

FIGURE 67-1. Algorithm for thrombophilia testing after a first episode of deep venous thrombosis (DVT) or pulmonary embolism (PE) and in asymptomatic, first-degree relatives. In the absence of strong evidence-based guidelines (see text), decisions about thrombophilia testing should be individualized, ranging from "not routinely recommended" to "recommended in most cases." VTE = venous thromboembolism. [a]Thrombophilia testing to include antithrombin III, protein C, protein S, factor V Leiden, prothrombin 20210A gene mutation, and lupus anticoagulant/antiphospholipid antibodies. [b]Provoking factors include active malignant disease, postoperative state, immobilization, trauma, active chronic inflammatory disease (e.g., extensive psoriasis), myeloproliferative neoplasm, pregnancy, oral contraceptives, and hormone replacement therapy. [c]In asymptomatic first-degree relatives of such individuals, avoidance is an alternative to testing.

TABLE 67-3 LONG-TERM MANAGEMENT OF PATIENTS WITH PRIMARY HYPERCOAGULABLE STATES*

RISK CLASSIFICATION	MANAGEMENT
High risk ≥2 spontaneous thromboses 1 spontaneous life-threatening thrombosis 1 spontaneous thrombosis at an unusual site (e.g., mesenteric, cerebral venous) 1 spontaneous thrombosis in the presence of antiphospholipid syndrome, antithrombin deficiency, or more than a single hypercoagulable state	Indefinite or lifelong anticoagulation
Moderate risk 1 thrombosis with an acquired prothrombotic stimulus	Vigorous prophylaxis during high-risk situations
Asymptomatic	

*Beyond initial period of thromboprophylaxis.

Modified from Bauer K. Approach to thrombosis. In: Loscalzo J, Schafer AI, eds. *Thrombosis and Hemorrhage*. 3rd ed. Philadelphia: Lippincott Williams & Wilkins; 2003:330-342.

drawn at least 2 weeks after stopping warfarin and at least 48 to 72 hours after stopping a direct oral anticoagulant.

How to Test

Laboratory diagnosis (Chapter 157) of the primary hypercoagulable states requires testing for each of the disorders individually because no general screening test is currently available to determine whether a patient may have such a condition.[10] Factor V Leiden can be diagnosed by a DNA-based assay or by a functional test for activated protein C resistance; the DNA-based assay is required to distinguish between heterozygous and homozygous states. A DNA-based assay is also required to identify the prothrombin G20210A mutation.

In contrast, many different mutations have been found in the genes for antithrombin, protein C, and protein S, so DNA-based tests are not practical for the diagnosis of these inherited deficiency states. Functional activity assays are preferred for antithrombin, protein C, and protein S because they detect both quantitative and qualitative defects; antigenic (immunologic) assays detect only quantitative deficiencies of these proteins. Functional coagulation assays for protein C and protein S may yield spuriously low values, however, if activated protein C resistance is present. Activated protein C resistance can be diagnosed by newer high-sensitivity and high-specificity coagulation assays or by DNA analysis of peripheral blood for the factor V Leiden mutation.

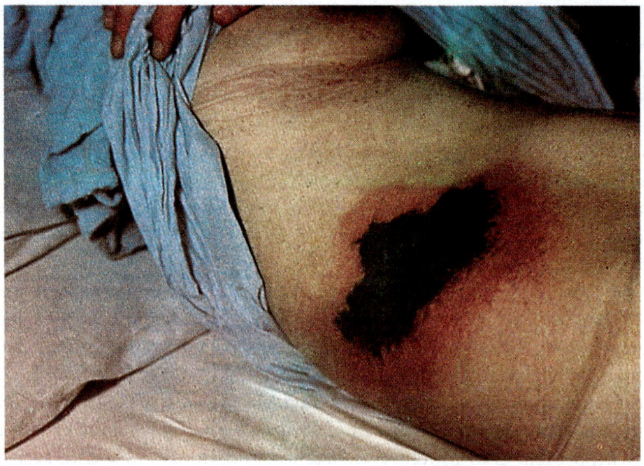

FIGURE 67-2. Acute skin necrosis in a patient with previously not known protein C deficiency who was given prophylactic warfarin for prevention of deep venous thrombosis after elective hip surgery. Warfarin treatment was withdrawn and anticoagulation continued with heparin. Skin grafting of the affected area was required. (From Forbes CD, Jackson WF. *Color Atlas and Text of Clinical Medicine*. 3rd ed. London: Mosby; 2003.)

TREATMENT

Initial Therapy

The initial treatment of acute deep venous thrombosis or pulmonary embolism in patients with primary hypercoagulable states is not different from that in patients without genetic defects (Chapter 68). As in patients without known thrombophilia, thrombolytic therapy should be considered after massive venous thrombosis or pulmonary embolism.

In most patients, direct oral anticoagulants (e.g., rivaroxaban, edoxaban, apixaban, and dabigatran) can be used for both acute treatment (at higher doses) and long-term prophylaxis against recurrence of venous thromboembolism (see Table 70-6). In addition to the convenience of fixed dosing, these medications are at least as effective and safer in terms of bleeding complications compared with warfarin. Even in patients who have cerebral venous thrombosis, anticoagulation with a direct-acting anticoagulant leads to similar clinical and imaging outcomes and has a more favorable safety profile when compared with warfarin.[A1]

However, warfarin is still preferred in some special circumstances. In patients who have prosthetic heart valves or high-risk antiphospholipid syndrome, however, treatment with heparin followed by warfarin is superior to direct oral anticoagulants[11] (Chapters 68 and 70). Acute management is initiated with at least 5 days of unfractionated or low-molecular-weight heparin or fondaparinux (see Tables 70-1 and 70-3). Oral anticoagulation with warfarin can be started on the first day of parenteral anticoagulation use (see Table 70-4) and continued for at least 6 months in patients with a first episode of VTE in the absence of triggering factors (e.g., postoperative state), with regulation of the dose to maintain an international normalized ratio of the prothrombin time between 2.0 and 3.0. This approach is especially preferred for secondary prevention of VTE in the antiphospholipid syndrome, particularly for patients who are "triple positive" (two positive IgG antiphospholipid antibodies plus lupus anticoagulant).[A2]

Warfarin-induced skin necrosis (Fig. 67-2) infrequently complicates the initiation of the anticoagulant in patients with heterozygous protein C or protein S deficiency. Because both these proteins depend on vitamin K for normal function, their plasma levels in patients with inherited deficiency states may drop to nearly zero within a few days of starting therapy with warfarin (which is a vitamin K antagonist) and lead to a transient prothrombotic imbalance and skin necrosis caused by dermal vascular thrombosis, especially in patients who are started on higher doses of warfarin without concurrent heparin. Acutely, the patient can be switched to heparin, but case reports suggest that switching to a direct-acting anticoagulant such as rivaroxaban is safe and effective for long-term antithrombotic prophylaxis in these individuals.

Duration of Therapy

Continuing oral anticoagulant prophylaxis beyond the initial 6 to 12 months after an acute episode of VTE must weigh the risk of bleeding with continued treatment against the significant risk of recurrent VTE after stopping anticoagulant prophylaxis. The risk of recurrence after an unprovoked episode of VTE following discontinuation of anticoagulation is greatest during the first 6 months and then decreases linearly by 4 to 5% per year, whereas the risk of major bleeding with continued anticoagulation is low and decreases linearly by less than 2% per year. Among patients with a first episode of unprovoked pulmonary embolism who received 6 months of anticoagulation, an additional 18 months of treatment with warfarin reduced the rate of recurrent VTE compared with placebo, although that benefit was not maintained after discontinuation of anticoagulation prophylaxis. These findings, which are consistent with earlier studies, highlight the fact that unprovoked VTE is a chronic, often recurrent, disease in the absence of prophylaxis. Patients with primary hypercoagulable states who have had two or more thrombotic events should receive indefinite or lifelong prophylactic oral anticoagulation (Chapter 70). Indefinite or lifelong anticoagulation is probably also indicated for individuals with recurrent thrombosis even in the absence of an identifiable primary hypercoagulable state (Table 67-3).

Asymptomatic Individuals

Asymptomatic individuals who have known thrombophilia but who have not had previous thrombotic complications do not require prophylactic anticoagulation except during periods of high risk for thrombosis. Because about half of the first-degree relatives of a patient with a primary hypercoagulable state should be affected, these individuals should be counseled about the implications of testing and potentially making a diagnosis.

Pregnancy

Management of pregnancy in women with primary hypercoagulable states requires special consideration because of the high risk for thrombosis, particularly during the puerperium. Women who have thrombophilia and who have previously had thrombosis—and probably also asymptomatic women with thrombophilia—should receive prophylactic anticoagulation throughout pregnancy and for at least the high-risk 6 weeks postpartum. Coumarin derivatives cross the placenta and have the potential to cause both bleeding and teratogenic effects in the fetus. The safety to the fetus of the direct oral anticoagulants has not yet been established. Therefore, oral anticoagulants should not be used during pregnancy. Heparin does not cross the placenta and does not cause these fetal complications. Fixed-dose, low-molecular-weight heparin (Table 70-3) is the anticoagulant of choice during pregnancy. Neither warfarin nor heparin induces an anticoagulant effect in a breast-fed infant when the drug is given to a nursing mother, so either can be given safely when indicated in the postpartum period. The same is not yet established for the direct oral anticoagulants.

Heparin Resistance

Antithrombin concentrate purified from normal human plasma or human recombinant antithrombin may be a useful adjunct to anticoagulation in "heparin-resistant" patients, who represent unusual cases of type II antithrombin deficiency, and in antithrombin-deficient patients with recurrent thrombosis despite adequate anticoagulation. Infusion of antithrombin concentrate can also be considered in some perioperative or obstetric settings in which anticoagulation poses an unacceptable bleeding risk.

SECONDARY HYPERCOAGULABLE STATES

DEFINITION

The secondary hypercoagulable states are diverse, mostly acquired disorders that predispose patients to thrombosis by complex, multifactorial pathophysiologic mechanisms. Many of these conditions also represent the acquired provocative stimuli for clinical thrombotic events in individuals with a genetic predisposition (primary hypercoagulable states; Table 67-4). Although each disorder causes thrombosis primarily through abnormalities in blood flow (rheology), the composition of blood (coagulation factors and platelet function), or the vessel wall, multiple overlapping mechanisms are operative in many of them.

TABLE 67-4 CAUSES OF SECONDARY HYPERCOAGULABLE STATES (PROVOKING FACTORS FOR VENOUS THROMBOEMBOLISM)

Immobilization
Surgery (postoperative state)*
Trauma*
Estrogen-mediated medications
Oral contraceptives*
Hormone replacement therapy*
Tamoxifen
Pregnancy (including early postpartum period)
Assisted reproductive technologies*
Ovarian hyperstimulation syndrome
Malignancy*
Myeloproliferative neoplasms*
Polycythemia vera
Essential thrombocythemia
Paroxysmal nocturnal hemoglobinuria*
Hyperviscosity states
Sickle cell disease and trait
Other hemolytic anemias
Corticosteroid excess
Therapeutic corticosteroids
Cushing syndrome
Nephrotic syndrome
Drugs
Lenalidomide, thalidomide*
L-asparaginase*
Cisplatin*
Bevacizumab*
Anabolic steroids (testosterone derivatives)*
Heparin (heparin-induced thrombocytopenia and thrombosis)*
Erythropoiesis-stimulating agents*
Intravenous immunoglobulin
Antifibrinolytics
Cocaine*
Systemic inflammatory states* (see Table 67-5)

*In these disorders there is also increased risk of arterial thrombosis.

HYPERHOMOCYSTEINEMIA

Hyperhomocysteinemia (Chapter 193) is an elevated blood level of homocysteine, a sulfhydryl amino acid derived from methionine by a transmethylation pathway (E-Fig. 67-2). Homocysteine is remethylated to methionine or catabolized to cystathionine. The major remethylation pathway requires folate and cobalamin (vitamin B_{12}) and involves the action of methylenetetrahydrofolate reductase (MTHFR); a minor remethylation pathway is mediated by betaine–homocysteine methyltransferase. Alternatively, homocysteine is converted to cystathionine in a trans-sulfuration pathway catalyzed by cystathionine β-synthase, with pyridoxine used as a cofactor.

Homozygous cystathionine β-synthase deficiency states that lead to severe hyperhomocysteinemia (homocystinuria) (Chapter 193) cause premature arterial atherosclerotic disease and VTE as well as mental retardation, neurologic defects, lens ectopy, and skeletal abnormalities. By comparison, adults with heterozygous cystathionine β-synthase deficiency have only mild to moderate hyperhomocysteinemia but still are at risk for venous or arterial thrombotic manifestations. Hyperhomocysteinemia resulting from inherited remethylation pathway defects usually involves reduced activity of MTHFR. In some homozygous individuals with the autosomal recessive C677T mutation of the *MTHFR* gene, which occurs in 15% of certain populations, moderate hyperhomocysteinemia may occur, but the mutation by itself does not appear to be related to the risk of venous thrombosis in the absence of coexisting hyperhomocysteinemia. Acquired causes of hyperhomocysteinemia in adults most commonly involve nutritional deficiencies of the cofactors required for homocysteine metabolism, including pyridoxine, cobalamin, and folate. Hyperhomocysteinemia is correctable with folic acid, pyridoxine, and cobalamin (Chapter 193), but treatment of nonhomozygous adults has not proven beneficial in reducing serious adverse events or death.[A3]

MALIGNANT DISEASE

Multiple abnormalities of hemostasis are involved in the hypercoagulable state in cancer patients, many of which initiate a systemic process of chronic disseminated intravascular coagulation (Chapter 161). The thrombotic tendency of patients with cancer may also be related to mechanical factors, such as immobility, indwelling central venous catheters, or a bulky tumor mass compressing vessels, and to comorbid conditions, such as sepsis, surgery, liver dysfunction secondary to metastases, and the prothrombotic effects of certain antineoplastic agents

The incidence of thrombotic complications in cancer patients depends in part on the type of malignant disease. Hypercoagulability is most prominent in patients with pancreatic cancer (Chapter 180), adenocarcinoma of the gastrointestinal tract (Chapters 178 and 179), lung cancer (Chapter 177), ovarian cancer (Chapter 184), prostate cancer (Chapter 186), and hematologic malignant neoplasms. The presence of underlying malignant disease compounds the independent risk for thrombosis in the postoperative state. There is a two-fold increase in the risk of postoperative thrombosis (see later section, Postoperative State, Immobilization, and Trauma) in cancer patients compared with noncancer patients. Thrombosis most commonly occurs in patients with established or concurrently diagnosed malignant disease. In these patients, the risk of venous thrombosis has been found to be highest in the first few months after the diagnosis of malignant disease, then decreases progressively during the subsequent 15 years.

The increased risk of harboring an occult malignant neoplasm in patients who present with VTE is now well established. The overall prevalence of undiagnosed cancer in patients with unprovoked VTE is approximately 3.5 to 6% at the time of thrombosis and 5 to 10% within the first year after thrombosis.[12] Because of the relatively low prevalence of occult cancer among adults with a first unprovoked VTE, routine screening with computed tomography (CT) of the abdomen and pelvis[A4] or with F-fluorodeoxyglucose positron emission tomography/CT[A5] is generally not recommended. However, focused screening with a complete blood count, serum electrolytes, tests of renal and liver function, and a chest radiograph are indicated (Fig. 67-3). A mammogram should be obtained in women, and a prostate-specific antigen level should be checked in men. Suspicious results on these basic tests should be pursued with CT scans or other appropriate diagnostic tests. In the absence of suggestive findings on these basic tests, decisions about screening must be individualized based on factors such as age or family history.

The most frequent thrombotic manifestations in patients with neoplasms are DVT and pulmonary embolism, but more unusual and distinctive thrombotic complications are also found. Trousseau syndrome (Chapter 68), characterized by migratory superficial thrombophlebitis of the upper or lower extremities, is strongly linked to cancer. Of patients with nonbacterial thrombotic endocarditis (Chapter 61), 75% have underlying malignant neoplasms at autopsy. Trousseau syndrome and nonbacterial thrombotic endocarditis are highly associated with adenocarcinomas. The occurrence of either syndrome in patients without known cancer demands a more vigorous search for occult malignant disease than in other patients with DVT or pulmonary embolism. Thrombotic microangiopathy (Chapter 158) occurs in about 5% of patients with metastatic carcinomas, most commonly patients with gastric (Chapter 178), lung (Chapter 177), and breast (Chapter 183) primary sites.

Some antineoplastic agents themselves increase the risk of thrombosis in cancer patients. For example, the antiangiogenic agents thalidomide and lenalidomide increase the risk of VTE, whereas bevacizumab, sunitinib, and sorafenib increase the risk of arterial thrombosis. Newly diagnosed, treatment-naïve patients with multiple myeloma are at significant risk of thrombosis, and therapy with immunomodulatory agents such as lenalidomide and thalidomide markedly increases that risk (Chapter 173).[13] Other thrombogenic chemotherapeutic agents include all-*trans*-retinoic acid and arsenic trioxide, particularly when used as induction chemotherapy for acute promyelocytic leukemia (Chapter 168); cis-platin (causing both venous and arterial thrombosis); L-asparaginase (which can also cause bleeding); and methotrexate (Table 67-3).

TREATMENT

Treatment of acute VTE in cancer patients should be initiated as in other patients, but subsequent prophylactic anticoagulation generally should be continued while active malignant disease is present.[14,15] In some patients, however, complete resolution of the VTE may allow treatment to be stopped safely.

Anticoagulation can be challenging in many cancer patients because of nausea, vomiting, low platelet counts, and bleeding into tumors. Long-term treatment of cancer patients with edoxaban (60 mg daily) or other direct-acting oral anticoagulants is as good as low-molecular-weight heparin (LMWH) overall, with insignificantly lower rates of recurrent VTE balanced against insignificantly higher rates of bleeding, without differences in overall mortality.[A6,A7] If direct-acting oral anticoagulants cannot be tolerated, LMWH is preferred over warfarin.

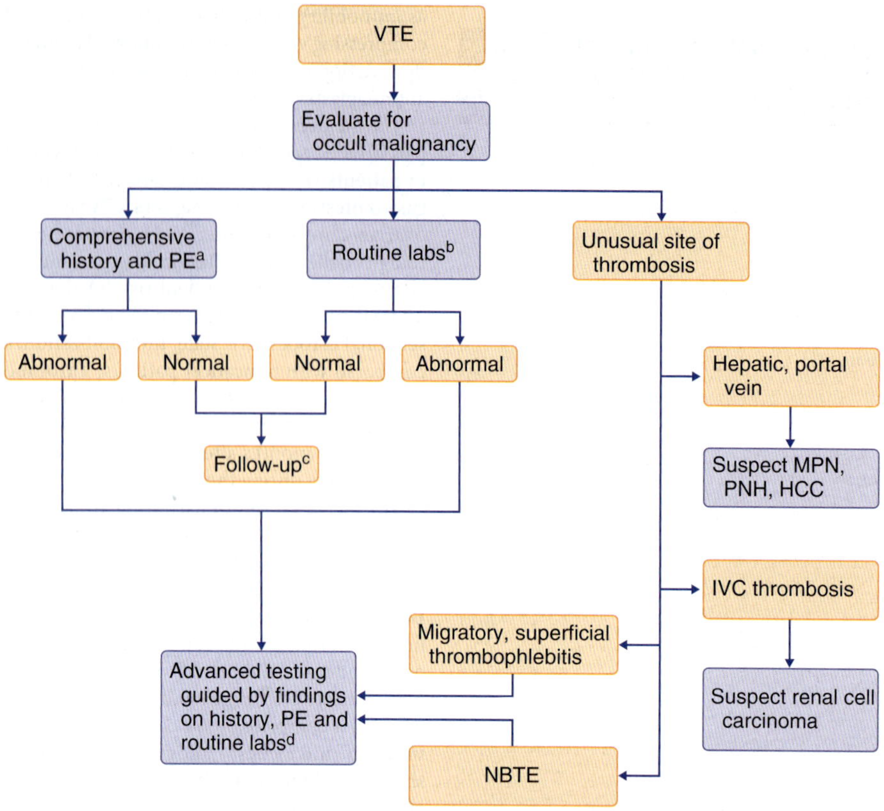

FIGURE 67-3. **Algorithm for evaluating a patient for occult malignant neoplasm after an unprovoked episode of deep venous thrombosis or pulmonary embolism or thrombosis at an unusual site.** HCC = hepatocellular carcinoma; IVC = inferior vena cava; MPN = myeloproliferative neoplasm; NBTE = nonbacterial thrombotic endocarditis; PE = physical examination; PNH = paroxysmal nocturnal hemoglobinuria; VTE = venous thromboembolism. [a]Physical examination to include rectal (with stool sample for occult blood) and breast and pelvic examinations for women. [b]Routine laboratory evaluations to include chest radiography, complete blood count, basic chemistries, calcium concentration, tests of liver and renal function, and a mammogram in women and a prostate-specific antigen level in men. [c]Follow-up suggested at 6 to 12 months. [d]Advanced testing could include advanced imaging, endoscopies, cytologies, and the like.

PREVENTION

For primary prevention of venous thrombosis in patients with cancer, rivaroxaban (10 mg daily) and apixaban (2.5 mg twice daily) are safe and effective as prophylaxis against a first VTE in patients who are at very high risk (pancreas, gastric, brain malignancies) or high risk (gynecologic and genitourinary cancers and lymphoma), especially in patients who have advanced disease.[A8–A10] LMWH is also an option if a direct-acting oral anticoagulant cannot be tolerated or is unsuccessful.[A11] However, prophylaxis is not recommended in low-risk patients.[16]

PROGNOSIS

Although treatment of cancer-associated thrombosis is usually successful, thrombosis generally portends poor prognosis. Venous thromboembolism is associated with increased mortality in cancer patients, especially within the first year after the thrombotic event.

MYELOPROLIFERATIVE NEOPLASMS AND PAROXYSMAL NOCTURNAL HEMOGLOBINURIA

Thrombosis and, apparently paradoxically, bleeding are major causes of morbidity and mortality in patients with chronic myeloproliferative neoplasms (Chapter 152)[17,18] and the related bone marrow stem cell disorder paroxysmal nocturnal hemoglobinuria (Chapter 146). In uncontrolled polycythemia vera, increased whole blood viscosity contributes to the thrombotic tendency. Thrombocytosis, abnormal platelet function, and other less well-understood factors are also probably involved in the hemostatic defect of myeloproliferative neoplasms and paroxysmal nocturnal hemoglobinuria.

In addition to DVT and pulmonary embolism, some distinctive thrombotic manifestations are seen. Hepatic vein thrombosis (Budd-Chiari syndrome) and portal and other intra-abdominal venous thromboses (Chapter 129) are associated with myeloproliferative neoplasms and paroxysmal nocturnal hemoglobinuria (Chapter 146) and may be the initial manifestations of the disease. Myeloproliferative neoplasms, particularly polycythemia vera (Chapter 152) and essential thrombocythemia (Chapter 152), may cause erythromelalgia (Chapter 66). Erythromelalgia is a syndrome of microvascular thrombosis manifested by intense pain accompanied by warmth, duskiness, and mottled erythema, sometimes resembling livedo reticularis. It is seen in a patchy distribution on the extremities, most prominently in the feet, and digital microvascular ischemia can progress to vascular insufficiency and gangrene (Chapter 66). A wide spectrum of neurologic manifestations may be caused by cerebrovascular ischemia, especially in patients with essential thrombocythemia.

TREATMENT

Treatment of VTE in patients with myeloproliferative neoplasms and paroxysmal nocturnal hemoglobinuria should be initiated as in patients without these hematologic disorders. In patients with thrombosis associated with polycythemia vera (Chapter 152), the hematocrit should be maintained in the normal range with phlebotomies or chemotherapy, or with both. Patients maintained at a hematocrit target of less than 45% have a significantly lower rate of cardiovascular death and major thrombosis than do those with hematocrit targets of 45 to 50%. Low-dose aspirin (100 mg daily) can prevent thrombotic complications without increasing the incidence of major bleeding in patients who have polycythemia vera and no contraindications to such treatment. In patients with essential thrombocythemia and high risk or previous history of thrombosis, cytoreduction of the elevated platelet count should be achieved with chemotherapy.

Patients with paroxysmal nocturnal hemoglobinuria (Chapter 146) benefit from treatment with a complement inhibitor that targets terminal complement. Options include eculizumab (600 mg IV weekly as the initial dose, followed by maintenance dosing with expert consultation) and ravulizumab (single loading dose of 2400 to 3000 mg depending on weight, followed by maintenance dosing with expert consultation).[A12] These drugs also reduce the risk of thrombosis.[A13,A14]

ANTIPHOSPHOLIPID SYNDROME

Antiphospholipid syndrome (Chapter 160) is characterized by venous and arterial thrombosis, recurrent spontaneous pregnancy loss (which may also be due to thrombosis), thrombocytopenia, and a variety of neuropsychiatric manifestations.[19] The syndrome is associated with a heterogeneous group of autoantibodies that bind to anionic phospholipid-protein complexes, a protein cofactor of which is β_2-glycoprotein I. Patients with this syndrome have any combination of positive tests for different plasma antiphospholipid-protein antibodies (e.g., anticardiolipin, beta-2-glycoprotein I antibodies) and phospholipid-based clotting tests (lupus anticoagulants; Chapter 245).[20] The predominant prothrombotic effects of these antibodies are probably directed to the vessel wall.

DVT and pulmonary embolism are the most frequent venous thrombotic events in these patients. Cerebrovascular events, which are the most common arterial thrombotic complications, are manifested as stroke, transient ischemic attacks (Chapter 376), multi-infarct dementia (Chapter 371), or retinal artery occlusion (see Fig. 391-27). Peripheral and intra-abdominal vascular occlusion is encountered more rarely. About one third of these patients have nonbacterial heart valve vegetations (Libman-Sacks endocarditis; Chapter 61). The most prominent obstetric complications are recurrent spontaneous pregnancy loss and fetal growth retardation, which are probably due to thrombosis of placental vessels. Patients are occasionally seen with "catastrophic" antiphospholipid syndrome involving a series of acute and sometimes fatal vascular occlusive events, or "thrombotic storm." Thrombotic complications are limited largely to patients with primary antiphospholipid syndrome and patients in whom the antibodies are associated with collagen vascular disease, not with drugs or infections.

TREATMENT AND PREVENTION

Acute management of thrombosis in patients with antiphospholipid syndrome is essentially the same as in other individuals with thrombosis. Monitoring of heparin anticoagulation is difficult in patients with a lupus anticoagulant because they already have a prolonged activated partial thromboplastin time at baseline; the use of low-molecular-weight heparin, which does not require monitoring, can circumvent this problem. Warfarin is effective in preventing recurrent thrombosis but usually requires prolonged or indefinite therapy with doses to achieve an international normalized ratio of 2.0 to 3.0. Unlike most other situations, direct oral anticoagulants are not as effective as warfarin in patients with the antiphospholipid syndrome.[A15,21] Whereas laboratory evidence of antiphospholipid antibodies in patients with a first episode of VTE is still usually considered an indication for indefinite anticoagulant therapy, the data supporting this strategy are limited. No established treatment of women with the antiphospholipid syndrome has been shown to prevent recurrent fetal loss.

PROGNOSIS

Patients with the lupus anticoagulant have a six-fold higher risk of future thrombosis, a two- to four-fold increased risk of recurrent thrombosis, and 12% increased 10-year mortality.[22]

PREGNANCY, ASSISTED REPRODUCTIVE TECHNOLOGIES, ORAL CONTRACEPTIVES, AND HORMONE REPLACEMENT THERAPY

Activation of the coagulation system is initiated locally in the maternal uteroplacental circulation, where the placenta is the source of increased generation of thrombin. Platelet activation and increased platelet turnover also occur during normal pregnancy, and about 8% of healthy women have mild thrombocytopenia at term. Simultaneously, the fibrinolytic system is progressively blunted throughout pregnancy because of the action of placental plasminogen activator inhibitor type 2. The net effect of these coagulation changes is creation of a state of hypercoagulability. These systemic alterations are compounded by prothrombotic mechanical and rheologic factors in pregnancy, including venous stasis in the legs (especially the left lower extremity) caused by the gravid uterus, pelvic vein injury during labor, and the trauma of cesarean section. Increasing age, increasing parity, cesarean delivery, prolonged bedrest or immobilization, obesity, and previous thromboembolism are additional prothrombotic risk factors in pregnant women. Most thrombotic events associated with pregnancy occur in the peripartum period, especially after delivery. Special considerations for anticoagulation in the setting of pregnancy are noted in the section on treatment of primary hypercoagulable states.

Assisted reproductive technologies, mainly in vitro fertilization (IVF), confer an increased risk of venous thromboembolism, although the absolute magnitude is quite low. With IVF, the incidence of VTE is approximately 0.1 to 0.5% per treatment cycle. Ovarian hyperstimulation syndrome (Chapter 218), which is an iatrogenic and potentially fatal complication of IVF, represents an important risk factor for thrombosis.

Oral contraceptives induce a prothrombotic state by increasing procoagulant effects and decreasing physiologic anticoagulant effects. The use of oral contraceptives is associated with an increased risk for venous thrombosis, myocardial infarction, stroke, and peripheral arterial disease, particularly during the first year of use (Chapter 220). Unexpectedly, third-generation oral contraceptives, which contain less estrogen and a different progestin, double the risk for VTE

TABLE 67-5 SOME PROTOTYPICAL SYSTEMIC INFLAMMATORY STATES THAT ARE ASSOCIATED WITH INCREASED THROMBOSIS RISK

Immune-mediated rheumatic and cutaneous inflammatory states
Rheumatoid arthritis
Systemic lupus erythematosus
Ankylosing spondylitis
ANCA-associated vasculitis
Psoriasis
Infections
Human immunodeficiency virus (HIV)
Cytomegalovirus
COVID-19
Acute pneumonia or urinary tract infection
Autoinflammatory disorders
Familial Mediterranean fever
Behçet disease
Systemic-onset juvenile idiopathic arthritis
Obesity
Sarcoidosis
Autoimmune gastrointestinal diseases
Ulcerative colitis
Crohn disease
Celiac disease
Pancreatitis

ANCA = anti-neutrophil cytoplasmic antibody; COVID-19 = coronavirus disease-2019.

in comparison to second-generation preparations. Postmenopausal hormone replacement increases the risk for deep VTE by a factor of 2 to 3.5, at least during the first year. Combined hormone replacement therapy with an estrogen and a progestin has no beneficial effect and possibly even a detrimental effect on the risk for arterial disease (Chapter 222),[A16] but low-dose estrogen monotherapy may reduce the risk of arterial thrombosis.[A17]

DVT and pulmonary embolism are the most common thrombotic complications of pregnancy and of the use of oral contraceptives or hormone replacement therapy. Coexisting primary hypercoagulable states are an at least additive risk factor in all these settings. In the absence of a clear family history of clinical VTE or a strongly thrombophilic mutation in a first-degree relative, there is little justification, however, to screen for prothrombotic mutations with pregnancy or before starting hormone replacement therapy or oral contraceptives.

SYSTEMIC INFLAMMATION

Diseases that cause systemic inflammation (Table 67-5) may be involved in the pathogenesis of VTE because of inflammation and damage to vessel walls as well as systemic hypercoagulability. Patients with autoimmune connective tissue diseases, particularly rheumatoid arthritis (Chapter 243), juvenile rheumatoid arthritis, and systemic lupus erythematosus (Chapter 245), are at increased risk of VTE. Psoriasis (Chapter 405), an immunoinflammatory disease that is associated with cardiovascular risk and atherothrombotic events, carries an increased risk of VTE, especially in younger patients with severe psoriasis. Other autoimmune skin diseases have not been associated with VTE.

In hospitalized patients with severe acute respiratory syndrome coronavirus 2 (SARS-CoV-2) and coronavirus disease 2019 (COVID-19) infection (Chapter 336), the overall thrombosis rate has been reported to be 9.5%.[23] About 20% of patients with SARS-CoV-2 and COVID-19 have a prolonged aPTT, of which about 90% are caused by a lupus anticoagulant. This finding should not, however, be considered a barrier to anticoagulation when it is otherwise appropriate (see Chapter 337). Intermediate-dose (enoxaparin 1 mg/kg daily) anticoagulation does not reduce venous or arterial thrombosis compared with standard-dose (enoxaparin 40 mg daily) prophylactic anticoagulation.[A18]

POSTOPERATIVE STATE, IMMOBILIZATION, AND TRAUMA

Postoperative thrombosis (Chapter 401) is caused by a combination of local mechanical factors, including decreased venous blood flow in the lower extremities, as well as systemic changes in coagulation. The level of risk for postoperative thrombosis depends largely on the type of surgery performed. However, the risk is increased in the presence of coexisting risk factors, such as an underlying inherited primary hypercoagulable state or malignant disease (see earlier sections), advanced age, and prolonged procedures. Postoperative

DVT and pulmonary embolism, which are the most common thrombotic complications, are often asymptomatic and detectable only by imaging. The incidence of DVT after general surgical procedures is about 20 to 25%, with almost 2% of these patients having clinically significant pulmonary embolism. Without prophylaxis, the risk for DVT after hip surgery and knee reconstruction ranges from 45 to 70%, and clinically significant pulmonary embolism occurs in 20% of patients undergoing hip surgery. Although the process of thrombosis generally begins intraoperatively or within a few days of surgery, the risk for this complication can extend to at least 6 weeks beyond the time of discharge from the hospital, particularly in hip replacement patients.

Patients who are bedridden or experiencing prolonged air travel (Chapter 265) are at increased risk for VTE. VTE is also one of the most common causes of morbidity and mortality in survivors of major trauma (Chapter 97), and asymptomatic DVT of the lower extremities has been detected by venography in more than 50% of hospitalized trauma patients. The risk for venous thrombosis after trauma is increased by advanced age, need for surgery or transfusions, and the presence of lower extremity fractures or spinal cord injury.

PREVENTION

Mechanical methods of prophylaxis against VTE are recommended in high-risk postoperative patients and bedridden patients with medical conditions (see Chapter 68).[24] Such methods include graduated compression stockings, intermittent pneumatic compression devices, and venous foot pumps. In-hospital anticoagulant prophylaxis is recommended for 10 to 14 days after major hip or limb surgery and in medical inpatients whose mobility is likely to be reduced for 72 hours or longer (see Chapter 68).[25] When anticoagulation is contraindicated in a severely injured patient, prophylactic placement of an inferior vena cava (IVC) filter does not reduce the incidence of symptomatic pulmonary embolism or 90-day mortality.[A19]

For long-distance travelers at increased risk of VTE (Chapter 265), including individuals with previous VTE or hypercoagulable states, current recommendations include frequent ambulation, nonalcoholic hydration, calf muscle exercises, and the use of properly fitted, below-knee graduated compression stockings providing 15 to 30 mm Hg of pressure at the ankle during travel; compression stockings are not recommended for other long-distance travelers. Aspirin or anticoagulants to prevent VTE are often used but not recommended for long-distance travelers at increased risk of VTE.

GENERAL REFERENCES

For the General References and other additional features, please visit Elsevier eBooks+ at https://ebooks.health.elsevier.com.

Grade A References

A1. Yaghi S, Shu L, Bakradze E, et al. Direct oral anticoagulants versus warfarin in the treatment of cerebral venous thrombosis (ACTION-CVT): a multicenter international study. *Stroke.* 2022;29:728-738.
A2. Pengo V, Hoxha A, Andreoli L, et al. Trial of rivaroxaban in antiphospholipid syndrome (TRAPS): two-year outcomes after the study closure. *J Thromb Haemost.* 2021;19:531-535.
A3. Martí-Carvajal AJ, Solà I, Lathyris D, et al. Homocysteine-lowering interventions for preventing cardiovascular events. *Cochrane Database Syst Rev.* 2017;8:CD006612.
A4. Robertson L, Yeoh SE, Broderick C, et al. Effect of testing for cancer on cancer- or venous thromboembolism (VTE)-related mortality and morbidity in people with unprovoked VTE. *Cochrane Database Syst Rev.* 2018;11:CD010837.
A5. Robin P, Le Roux PY, Planquette B, et al. Limited screening with versus without (18) F-fluorodeoxyglucose PET/CT for occult malignancy in unprovoked venous thromboembolism: an open-label randomised controlled trial. *Lancet Oncol.* 2016;17:193-199.
A6. Raskob GE, van Es N, Verhamme P, et al. Edoxaban for the treatment of cancer-associated venous thromboembolism. *N Engl J Med.* 2018;378:615-624.
A7. Mulder FI, Bosch FTM, Young AM, et al. Direct oral anticoagulants for cancer-associated venous thromboembolism: a systematic review and meta-analysis. *Blood.* 2020;136:1433-1441.
A8. Khorana AA, Soff GA, Kakkar AK, et al. Rivaroxaban for thromboprophylaxis in high-risk ambulatory patients with cancer. *N Engl J Med.* 2019;380:720-728.
A9. Carrier M, Abou-Nassar K, Mallick R, et al. Apixaban to prevent venous thromboembolism in patients with cancer. *N Engl J Med.* 2019;380:711-719.
A10. Agnelli G, Becattini C, Meyer G, et al. Apixaban for the treatment of venous thromboembolism associated with cancer. *N Engl J Med.* 2020;382:1599-1607.
A11. Rutjes AW, Porreca E, Candeloro M, et al. Primary prophylaxis for venous thromboembolism in ambulatory cancer patients receiving chemotherapy. *Cochrane Database Syst Rev.* 2020;12:CD008500.
A12. Hillmen P, Szer J, Weitz I, et al. Pegcetacoplan versus eculizumab in paroxismal nocturnal hemoglobinuria. *N Engl J Med.* 2021;382:1028-1037.
A13. Kulasekararaj AG, Hill A, Rottinghaus ST, et al. Ravulizumab (ALXN1210) vs eculizumab in C5-inhibitor-experienced adult patients with PNH: the 302 study. *Blood.* 2019;133:540-549.
A14. Lee JW, Sicre de Fontbrune F, Wong Lee Lee L, et al. Ravulizumab (ALXN1210) vs eculizumab in adult patients with PNH I to complement inhibitors: the 301 study. *Blood.* 2019;133:530-539.
A15. Khairani CD, Bejjani A, Piazza G, et al. Direct oral anticoagulants vs vitamin K antagonists in patients with antiphospholipid syndromes: meta-analysis of randomized trials. *J Am Coll Cardiol.* 2023;81:16-30.
A16. Gartlehner G, Patel SV, Feltner C, et al. Hormone therapy for the primary prevention of chronic conditions in postmenopausal women: evidence report and systematic review for the US Preventive Services Task Force. *JAMA.* 2017;318:2234-2249.
A17. Prentice RL, Aragaki AK, Chlebowski RT, et al. Randomized trial evaluation of the benefits and risks of menopausal hormone therapy among women 50-59 years of age. *Am J Epidemiol.* 2021;190:365-375.
A18. Bikdeli B, Talasaz AH, Rashidi F, et al. Intermediate-dose versus standard-dose prophylactic anticoagulation in patients with COVID-19 admitted to the intensive care unit: 90-day results from the INSPIRATION randomized trial. *Thromb Haemost.* 2022;122:131-141.
A19. Ho KM, Rao S, Honeybul S, et al. A multicenter trial of vena cava filters in severely injured patients. *N Engl J Med.* 2019;381:328-337.

68 VENOUS THROMBOSIS AND EMBOLISM

JEFFREY I. WEITZ AND JOHN W. EIKELBOOM

DEFINITIONS

Venous thromboembolism (VTE) includes deep vein thrombosis (DVT) and pulmonary embolism. DVT usually involves the deep veins of the legs or arms, but it can occur in other sites. Occlusion of the deep veins in a limb by thrombus impairs drainage of blood, thereby leading to pain and swelling distal to the obstruction. Pulmonary embolism refers to an obstruction of a pulmonary artery by thrombus that has traveled from elsewhere in the body, through the blood stream, and to the lungs. DVT in the legs or, less commonly, the arms is by far the leading source of pulmonary embolism.

Chronic complications of DVT and pulmonary embolism include post-thrombotic syndrome and chronic thromboembolic pulmonary hypertension, respectively. Post-thrombotic syndrome, which occurs in up to 40% of patients with extensive DVT, is characterized by dependent swelling and discomfort in the affected limb and in severe cases can lead to venous ulcers. The syndrome is caused by venous hypertension because of venous obstruction by residual thrombus and reflux of blood because of incompetent venous valves. Chronic thromboembolic pulmonary hypertension, which complicates up to 4% of cases of pulmonary embolism, occurs when emboli in the major pulmonary arteries fail to resolve and are replaced by fibrous tissue that becomes incorporated into the vessel walls, thereby narrowing or obstructing them. Obstruction of the pulmonary vascular bed increases pulmonary arterial resistance and can lead to right heart failure.

Thrombosis also can occur in superficial veins. Although benign and self-limiting when veins in the hand or antecubital fossa are involved as a complication of blood collection, intravenous catheters, or drug delivery, superficial vein thrombosis in the lower extremities can extend into the deep veins, thereby leading to DVT and pulmonary embolism.

EPIDEMIOLOGY

A first episode of VTE occurs in about 1 to 2 persons per 1000 each year in the United States. The incidence rises with age, with 5 to 10 cases per 1000 persons per year by the age of 80 years. Although men and women are affected equally, the incidence is four times higher in high-income than low-income countries.

Approximately one third of patients with symptomatic VTE present with pulmonary embolism, whereas the remainder present with DVT. Pulmonary embolism accounts for an estimated 15% of deaths in hospitalized patients and is responsible for about 150,000 deaths each year in the United States. As a result, VTE is the third most common cause of vascular death after myocardial infarction and stroke.

PATHOBIOLOGY

Heritable and acquired risk factors determine the intrinsic risk of VTE (E-Fig. 68-1).[1] Heritable risk factors include abnormalities associated with hypercoagulability of the blood (Chapter 67), the most common of which are factor V Leiden and the prothrombin G20210A gene mutation. Acquired risk factors include advanced age, history of previous VTE, obesity, and active cancer, which limit mobility and may be associated with hypercoagulability. Superimposed on this background risk, VTE often occurs in the presence of triggering factors, which increase the risk above a critical threshold. Triggering factors such as surgery, trauma, and pregnancy or estrogen therapy lead to endothelial cell activation, stasis, and hypercoagulability, which are the components of the Virchow triad.

Up to half of patients with a first episode of VTE have no identifiable risk factors and are described as having unprovoked or idiopathic VTE. The

TABLE 68-1 ALTERNATIVE DIAGNOSES IN 87 CONSECUTIVE PATIENTS WITH CLINICALLY SUSPECTED DEEP VEIN THROMBOSIS AND NORMAL VENOGRAMS

DIAGNOSIS	PATIENTS (%)
Muscle strain	24
Direct twisting injury to the leg	10
Leg swelling in paralyzed limb	9
Lymphangitis, lymphatic obstruction	7
Venous reflux	7
Muscle tear	6
Baker cyst	5
Cellulitis	3
Internal abnormality of the knee	2
Unknown	26

remainder develop VTE secondary to risk factors; these episodes are considered provoked. Risk factors for VTE can be classified according to their magnitude and duration as major or minor and transient or persistent, respectively. Major transient risk factors include surgery or trauma, whereas active cancer is an example of a major persistent risk factor. Minor transient risk factors include estrogen therapy or prolonged travel, whereas obesity, a past or family history of VTE, and thrombophilic defects such as the factor V Leiden or prothrombin gene mutation are examples of minor persistent risk factors (Chapter 67).

Coronavirus disease 2019 (COVID-19) caused by the severe acute respiratory syndrome coronavirus 2 (SARS-CoV-2) is a major transient risk factor for VTE and other thrombotic events (Chapter 336). The risk of VTE is greatest in patients who are hospitalized with moderate or severe COVID-19 disease and who develop a hypercoagulable state characterized by marked elevation of D-dimer levels. Symptomatic VTE occurs in about 10% of patients hospitalized with COVID-19, and its incidence is four-fold higher in patients who are in intensive care units compared with non–intensive care settings.[2]

DVT can occur in either leg. However, DVT in pregnancy involves the ileofemoral veins of the left leg in 90% of cases and typically spares the calf and popliteal veins. Localization to this site reflects compression of the left iliac vein by the enlarging uterus, an exaggeration of the so-called May-Thurner syndrome, in which venous webs and compression of the left iliac vein by the overlying right iliac artery reduce blood flow and can lead to DVT.

Most pulmonary emboli originate from DVT in the lower limbs, and pulmonary embolism can be detected in about 40% of patients with proximal DVT. Likewise, at least 50% of patients with proven pulmonary embolism have demonstrable DVT. Upper extremity DVT involving the axillary or subclavian veins also can give rise to pulmonary embolism but only in 10 to 15% of such patients. Upper extremity DVT most often occurs in patients with cancer (Chapter 164), particularly patients with indwelling central venous catheters. Spontaneous upper extremity DVT, usually involving the dominant arm, can occur with strenuous effort—the so-called Paget-Schroetter syndrome.

CLINICAL MANIFESTATIONS

Patients with DVT typically present with swelling, pain, warmth, and redness in the involved extremity (Fig. 68-1).[3] However, some patients may have minimal symptoms. The differential diagnosis includes trauma, infection, a ruptured Baker cyst (Chapter 243; Table 68-1), peripheral artery disease (Chapter 65), and other venous diseases such as chronic venous insufficiency; DVT may coexist with these disorders.

DVT usually starts in the calf veins, where it remains isolated in about 15% of such patients. Most cases of isolated calf DVT resolve spontaneously, but in about 20% of such patients the thrombus extends into the proximal veins, usually within a week after the onset of symptoms. Once thrombi extend into the proximal veins of the leg, they can dislodge and cause pulmonary embolism.

The most common symptoms and signs of pulmonary embolism include dyspnea on exertion,[4] often pleuritic chest pain, tachypnea, and cough. Many patients with pulmonary emboli have concomitant symptoms and signs of DVT. Less common symptoms and signs include fever, hemoptysis, cyanosis, hypotension, and shock. Other nonspecific symptoms include palpitations, anxiety, and light-headedness.

Patients with extensive pulmonary emboli often have dyspnea at rest and hypotension, and they may present with syncope (Chapters 39 and 49) because

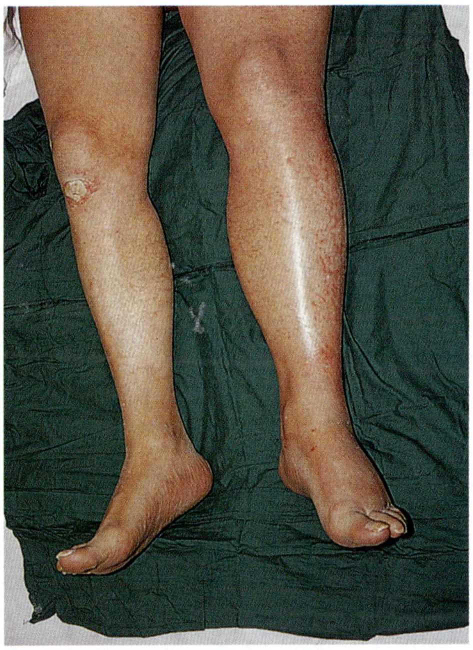

FIGURE 68-1. **Deep vein thrombosis (DVT) manifesting as an acutely swollen left leg.** Note the dilation of the superficial veins. The leg was hot to the touch, and there was tenderness along the course of the left popliteal and femoral veins. Fewer than 50% of patients with DVT present with these findings, and other conditions may mimic DVT, so further investigation is always indicated. Note the coincidental psoriatic lesion below the right knee. (From Forbes CD, Jackson WF. *Color Atlas and Text of Clinical Medicine*, 3rd ed. London: Mosby; 2003.)

of hypoxemia and low cardiac output. Central and peripheral cyanosis can occur, and a gallop rhythm may develop as a consequence of heart failure. The jugular veins may be distended if right heart failure develops. The second heart sound can be widely split, and the pulmonic component may be loud because of delayed emptying of the right ventricle. A right ventricular heave may be present with massive pulmonary embolism and acute pulmonary hypertension. The combination of hypotension, hypoxemia, and increased cardiac workload may trigger angina (Chapter 56) or overt myocardial infarction (Chapters 57 and 58).

When patients present with chest symptoms suggestive of pulmonary embolism, the differential diagnosis includes pulmonary disorders, such as pneumonia (Chapter 85), an exacerbation of chronic obstructive lung disease (Chapter 76), or asthma (Chapter 75); pleurisy secondary to connective tissue disease (Chapter 86); cardiac disorders, such as heart failure (Chapter 45), acute coronary syndrome (Chapter 57), or pericarditis (Chapter 62); and musculoskeletal disorders, such as rib fracture.

DIAGNOSIS

By itself, the clinical diagnosis of DVT or pulmonary embolism is inaccurate because no individual symptom or sign is sufficiently predictive for confirming or excluding the diagnosis. In patients with symptoms suggestive of DVT, the diagnosis is confirmed in up to 25%.

Therefore, diagnosis starts with determination of the pretest probability using validated risk assessment models for DVT (Table 68-2) or pulmonary embolism (Table 68-3).[5] Although these clinical assessment tools categorize patients according to their pretest probability of VTE with reasonable accuracy, they should not be used in isolation. Instead, risk assessment models should be combined with laboratory testing such as the D-dimer, which, if normal, can be used to exclude the diagnosis of VTE in patients with low to moderate pretest probability. If the D-dimer test is positive or if the pretest probability is high, the diagnosis of DVT or pulmonary embolism should be confirmed using venous compression ultrasonography or computed tomography pulmonary angiography (CTPA), respectively (Fig. 68-2).

Laboratory Tests

D-Dimer

A plasmin-derived degradation product of cross-linked fibrin, D-dimer can be measured in whole blood or plasma and is a biomarker that reflects ongoing activation of the coagulation system. D-dimer assays vary in their sensitivity and specificity for the diagnosis of VTE. Enzyme-linked immunosorbent and advanced turbidimetric D-dimer assays have sensitivities over 95%, but they are not specific for the diagnosis of VTE. D-dimer levels can be elevated with

TABLE 68-2 PREDICTION RULE FOR LIKELIHOOD OF DEEP VEIN THROMBOSIS

CLINICAL CHARACTERISTIC	SCORE*
Active cancer (treatment ongoing within previous 6 months or receiving palliative care)*	1
Paralysis, paresis, or recent plaster immobilization of the lower extremities	1
Recent bedrest of >3 days or major surgery within 3 months requiring anesthesia	1
Localized tenderness of the deep veins of the leg	1
Entire leg swollen	1
Calf swelling of >3 cm larger than asymptomatic side measured 10 cm below tibial tuberosity	1
Pitting edema confined to the symptomatic leg	1
Collateral superficial veins (not varicose)	1
Previously documented deep vein thrombosis	1
Alternative diagnosis as likely as or more likely than deep vein thrombosis	−2

*A score of 0 or less indicates low probability, 1 or 2 indicates moderate probability, and 3 or more indicates high probability. Non-melanoma skin cancer is not a risk factor.

Modified from Wells PS, Anderson DR, Bormanis J, et al. Value of assessment of pretest probability of deep-vein thrombosis in clinical management. *Lancet.* 1997;350:1795-1798.

TABLE 68-3 PREDICTION RULE FOR LIKELIHOOD OF PULMONARY EMBOLISM

VARIABLE	POINTS
PREDISPOSING FACTORS	
Previous VTE	1.5
Recent surgery or immobilization	1.5
Cancer	1
SYMPTOMS	
Hemoptysis	1
SIGNS	
Heart rate >100 beats/min	1.5
Clinical signs of DVT	3
CLINICAL JUDGMENT	
Alternative diagnosis less likely than PE	3
CLINICAL PROBABILITY	**TOTAL POINTS***
Low	<2
Moderate	2-6
High	>6

*This rule also can be used to classify patients into two groups in which a score of 4 or less indicates low probability and a score of more than 4 indicates high probability. When this approach is used, D-dimer testing should be considered in those with low probability.

DVT = deep vein thrombosis; PE = pulmonary embolism; VTE = venous thromboembolism.

Adapted from Wells PS, Ginsberg JS, Anderson DR, et al. Use of a clinical model for safe management of patients with suspected pulmonary embolism. *Ann Intern Med.* 1998;129:997-1005.

advanced age, chronic inflammatory conditions, and malignancy. In addition, hospitalized patients are more likely to have elevated D-dimer levels than outpatients. Because of this lack of specificity, the value of the D-dimer assay resides with its high negative predictive value. A normal D-dimer level in a patient with a low or moderate pretest probability of DVT or pulmonary embolism essentially excludes the diagnosis, thereby obviating the need for further diagnostic testing[6] without increasing the risk of a missed VTE.[A1]

Compression Ultrasonography

Compression ultrasonography with or without Doppler imaging is the most widely used noninvasive test for diagnosis of DVT because of its accuracy for detecting thrombus involving the popliteal or more proximal veins. Noncompressibility (Fig. 68-3) of the proximal leg veins on ultrasonography is diagnostic of DVT in symptomatic patients and is an indication for treatment. The sensitivity of ultrasonography for detecting calf DVT is lower than for detecting proximal DVT; consequently, some centers examine only the veins above the trifurcation in the calf, whereas others examine both the proximal and calf veins. A normal whole-leg ultrasound excludes the diagnosis of DVT. If only the proximal veins are examined, the ultrasound should be repeated in 1 week to identify the 20% of patients who initially have isolated calf vein thrombosis but whose thrombus subsequently extends into the proximal veins.

Contrast Venography

Although ascending contrast venography remains the gold standard for diagnosis of DVT, the test is rarely performed because of its expense, discomfort to the patient, and potential for complications. A constant intraluminal filling defect is diagnostic of acute thrombosis (Fig. 68-4), and DVT can be excluded in patients who have a normal, adequately performed venogram. Minor side effects, including local pain, nausea, and vomiting, are not uncommon, whereas more serious adverse reactions, such as anaphylaxis or other allergic manifestations, are rare.

Computed Tomographic Pulmonary Angiography

Multidetector CT pulmonary angiography has largely replaced ventilation-perfusion lung scanning for diagnosing pulmonary embolism because of its wide availability, the rapidity of its results, and a sensitivity and specificity sufficient for its use as a stand-alone test. In contrast to lung scanning, CT pulmonary angiography not only permits direct visualization of thrombi in the pulmonary arteries of patients with pulmonary embolism (Fig. 68-5) but also provides an alternative diagnosis in many of those who prove not to have pulmonary embolism. A CT pulmonary angiogram showing thrombus in pulmonary arteries up to the segmental level provides evidence of pulmonary embolism, whereas a negative CT pulmonary angiogram excludes pulmonary embolism and is associated with subsequent clinical outcomes that are at least as good as those in patients with negative lung scans. Compared with lung scanning, CT pulmonary angiography detects more isolated subsegmental thrombi in about 1 to 5% of patients, but it is unclear whether isolated subsegmental defects are benign or associated with outcomes like those of more proximal thrombi. A normal bilateral venous compression ultrasound examination of the lower extremities to exclude DVT in this setting may help to identify patients with a low thrombus burden who do not require anticoagulation.

CT pulmonary angiography can be combined with CT venography so that the diagnosis of pulmonary embolism and DVT can be established with a single test and only one injection of contrast dye. Compared with CT pulmonary angiography alone, combining it with CT venography increases the sensitivity for diagnosing pulmonary embolism from 83 to 90%, but the specificity remains unchanged, thereby resulting in only a modest increase in negative predictive value. CT venography adds significant radiation exposure and only marginally increases the overall detection rate. Therefore, venous compression ultrasonography is preferred over CT venography for the diagnosis of DVT because it provides the same information without exposing patients to ionizing radiation.

Ventilation-Perfusion Lung Scanning

This two-part test consists of a ventilation phase and a perfusion phase. The ventilation phase involves inhalation of an aerosol form of radioactive isotopes of xenon or technetium to assess air delivery to the various parts of the lung. In contrast, the perfusion phase involves the intravenous injection of technetium-labeled macroaggregates of albumin, which enables assessment of blood flow within the lungs once the aggregates lodge in the pulmonary microcirculation. Images for both parts of the test are acquired using a gamma counter. Areas of lung affected by pulmonary embolism do not light up on the perfusion scan because the macroaggregates of albumin fail to reach sites where the pulmonary arteries are occluded (Fig. 68-6). By comparison, areas with abnormal perfusion because of pulmonary embolism will ventilate normally, yielding a ventilation-perfusion mismatch.

A normal ventilation-perfusion lung scan effectively excludes the diagnosis of pulmonary embolism, but only 25% of patients with suspected pulmonary embolism have a normal scan. One or more segmental or larger perfusion defects that ventilate normally characterize a high-probability lung scan, which establishes the diagnosis of pulmonary embolism. However, even with single-photon emission CT technology, only about 10% of patients with suspected pulmonary emboli have a high-probability lung scan. The remaining 65% of lung scans exhibit smaller areas of mismatch or matched defects and fall within the non–high-probability category. Because up to 40% of patients with non–high-probability scans have pulmonary emboli, such patients require additional investigations to exclude the diagnosis.

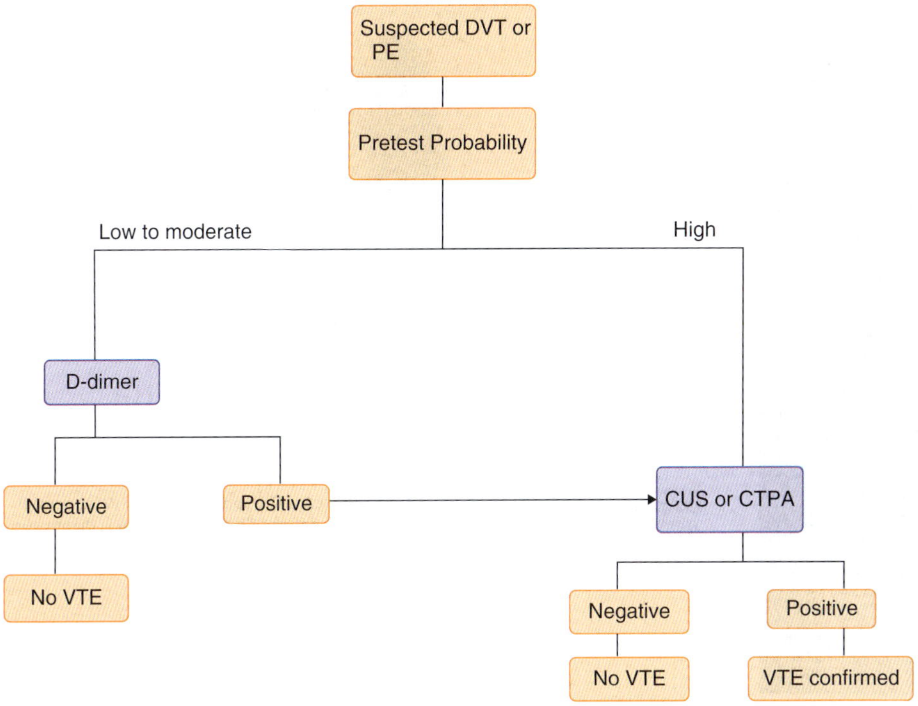

FIGURE 68-2. **Clinical approach in patients with suspected deep vein thrombosis (DVT) or pulmonary embolism (PE).** CTPA = computed tomographic pulmonary angiogram; CUS = compression ultrasound; VTE = venous thromboembolism.

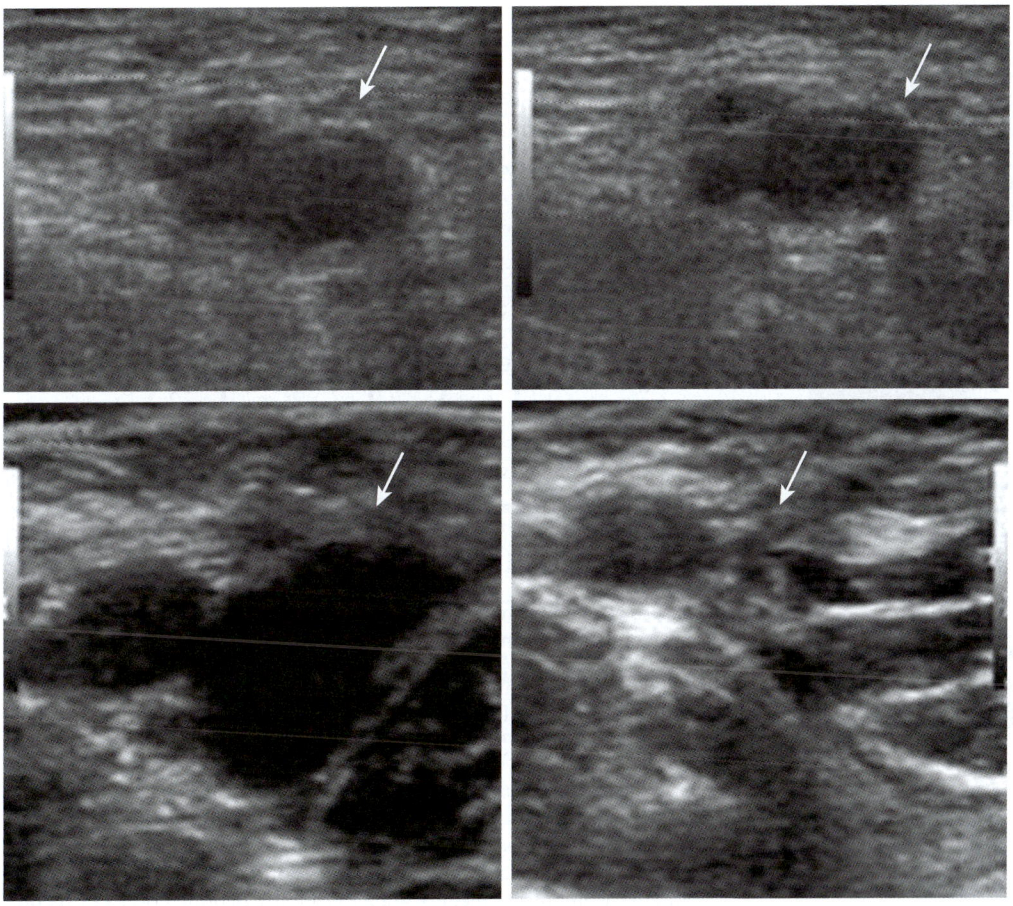

FIGURE 68-3. **Compression ultrasonography demonstrates thrombosis in the popliteal vein.** The sonograms in the *top row* demonstrate examination without *(left side)* and with *(right side)* probe compression of the skin overlying the popliteal vein. The lack of compressibility is diagnostic of deep vein thrombosis. The *bottom row* shows analogous views of the femoral vein, which shows partial compressibility.

Although CT pulmonary angiography has largely replaced lung scanning for the diagnosis of pulmonary embolism, the lung scan is the diagnostic test of choice for patients with renal impairment or a history of allergy to angiographic contrast media and for women younger than 40 years to reduce radiation exposure to the breasts. For the diagnosis of pulmonary embolism in pregnancy, lung scanning produces less maternal and fetal radiation exposure and is sometimes preferred over CT pulmonary angiography. However, the incremental value of a ventilation-perfusion scan is low in patients with a nondiagnostic CT pulmonary angiogram.

Magnetic Resonance Imaging

In contrast to CT pulmonary angiography, gadolinium-enhanced magnetic resonance imaging (MRI) does not subject patients to ionizing radiation, and gadolinium can safely be given to patients with a history of allergy to contrast dye but not to patients with renal impairment. The combination of MR pulmonary angiography with MR venography has a higher sensitivity than MR pulmonary angiography alone for the diagnosis of pulmonary embolism, and MRI can be especially useful for diagnosing recurrent ipsilateral DVT.[7] However, MR angiography and venography protocols are technically

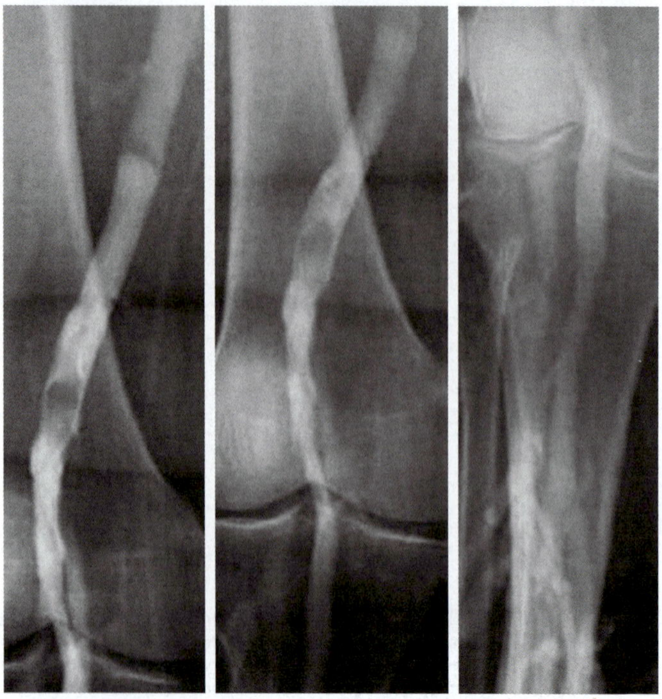

FIGURE 68-4. **Ascending venography.** The venogram demonstrates a persistent (two or more different views) intraluminal filling defect in the popliteal vein.

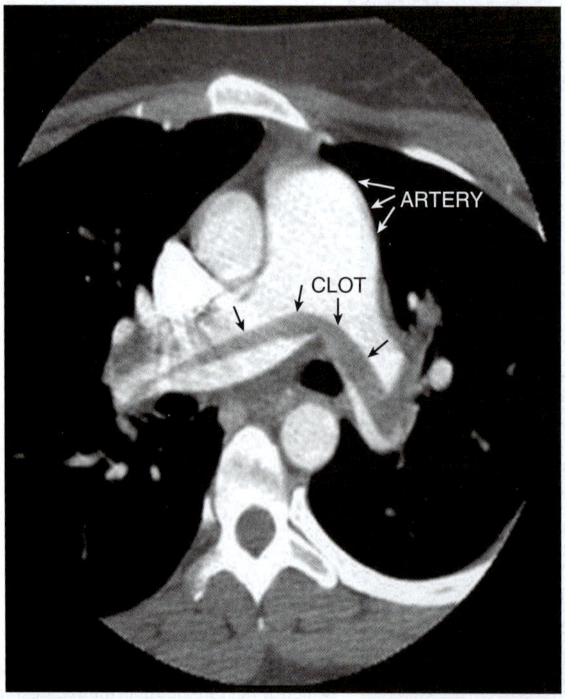

FIGURE 68-5. **Computed tomographic pulmonary angiography.** The scan demonstrates a saddle pulmonary embolus in the main pulmonary artery.

demanding, so MRI should be used to diagnose pulmonary embolism only in experienced centers and in patients for whom standard tests are contraindicated.

Interventional Contrast Pulmonary Angiography

Pulmonary angiography requires direct contrast injection into the pulmonary arteries, followed by imaging using digital subtraction technology. Presence of a thrombus, which appears as a filling defect or as a sudden cutoff of blood flow in a pulmonary arterial branch, establishes the diagnosis of pulmonary embolism. Although direct angiography allows visualization of small thrombi in subsegmental pulmonary arteries, high interobserver variability in the interpretation of isolated filling defects at this level limits the specificity of this finding. As an invasive test, the mortality rate associated with pulmonary angiography is 0.2%, with deaths usually occurring in patients with hemodynamic compromise or respiratory failure.

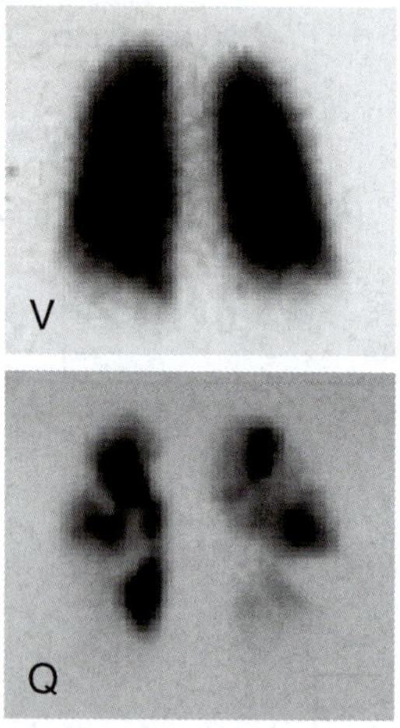

FIGURE 68-6. **Ventilation-perfusion lung scan.** The ventilation scan (V) is normal, whereas the perfusion scan (Q) shows multiple defects. This combination is diagnostic of pulmonary embolism.

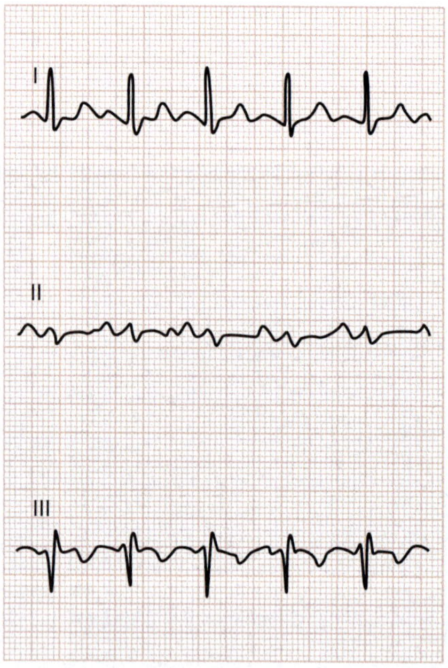

FIGURE 68-7. **Classic electrocardiogram findings with pulmonary embolism.** Note the S waves in lead I and the Q waves and inverted T waves in lead III, findings that comprise the S_1, Q_3, and T_3 pattern.

Because of its associated risks and because CT pulmonary angiography offers similar or better information, direct pulmonary angiography is rarely performed.

Other Tests

Routine blood tests in patients with suspected or diagnosed VTE should include a complete blood count, including a platelet count, and a baseline international normalized ratio (INR) and activated partial thromboplastin time (aPTT). Serum creatinine and blood urea nitrogen levels are needed to help guide the choice of anticoagulant therapy and the suitability for diagnostic testing using angiographic dyes; serum electrolytes and liver enzymes also may provide useful information.

Blood markers of right ventricular dysfunction, which occurs with extensive pulmonary embolism, include brain natriuretic peptide (BNP) or its precursor, N-terminal pro-BNP, which are released in response to myocardial stretching (Chapter 45). Elevated levels of troponin I or T provide evidence of myocardial injury (Chapter 57). Although these markers are associated with a worse prognosis in patients with pulmonary embolism, their positive predictive value for making the diagnosis is low.

The ECG may show new changes suggestive of right ventricular strain, such as T wave inversion in leads V_1 to V_4; the classic S_1, Q_3, and T_3 pattern (Fig. 68-7); and complete or incomplete right bundle branch block. However, these ECG changes have limited sensitivity and are mainly found in patients with more extensive pulmonary emboli.

Echocardiographic findings suggestive of right ventricular dysfunction include right ventricular dilation or hypokinesis, increased right ventricular diameter relative to that of the left ventricle, and increased velocity of the jet of tricuspid regurgitation. Echocardiography may also detect a right-to-left shunt through a patent foramen ovale (Chapter 55) and may provide evidence of right ventricular thrombus, both of which are associated with increased mortality in patients with pulmonary embolism. With no universal criteria for the diagnosis of right ventricular dysfunction, however, the utility of routine echocardiography remains uncertain. In general, routine echocardiography is recommended only in patients with severe hypoxemia or other evidence to suggest hemodynamic compromise.

TREATMENT

Outpatient treatment is as safe as routine inpatient treatment for most patients with DVT and for low-risk patients with acute pulmonary embolism.[8,9] In pulmonary embolism patients at intermediate risk, such as patients with right ventricular enlargement, outpatient management can be considered, but brief admission to hospital may be a safer approach. Therefore, rapid risk stratification is crucial to help guide treatment. Patients who have contraindications to anticoagulant therapy may require insertion of a retrievable inferior vena cava filter.

Anticoagulation is the cornerstone of treatment for VTE and should be initiated immediately in patients with suspected pulmonary embolism or DVT even while awaiting the results of confirmatory tests. Although anticoagulant therapy remains the main treatment for pulmonary embolism, patients with severe hemodynamic compromise may benefit from reperfusion therapy or surgical thrombectomy to restore blood flow rapidly to the pulmonary arteries and to reduce pulmonary artery pressure.

The risk of recurrent VTE is highest in the first few weeks after diagnosis and progressively decreases thereafter. Consequently, VTE treatment has been divided into three stages: initial therapy for the first 1 to 3 weeks, the goals of which are to prevent thrombus extension and fatal pulmonary embolism; therapy for the subsequent 3 months, which is often termed long-term therapy and is given to treat the VTE and to reduce the risk of complications, such as post-thrombotic syndrome and chronic thromboembolic pulmonary hypertension; and extended therapy beyond 3 months, which is administered when the risk of recurrent VTE without anticoagulant therapy is high and exceeds the risk of major bleeding with continued anticoagulant therapy.[10]

High-Risk Pulmonary Embolism

High-risk patients can be identified at the bedside based on the presence of hemodynamic compromise. Such patients also may have right ventricular dysfunction and elevated levels of biomarkers (i.e., troponin and BNP). The most common cause of death in patients with severe pulmonary embolism is acute right ventricular failure, which causes low systemic output. To prevent this complication, patients who present with hemodynamic compromise require circulatory and respiratory support. Patients with right ventricular failure often require modest fluid expansion and may need inotropic agents, such as dobutamine, dopamine, or norepinephrine, for severe hypotension or shock (Chapter 93). Emerging data raise the possibility that endothelin antagonists and phosphodiesterase-5 inhibitors may attenuate the pulmonary hypertension in patients with severe pulmonary embolism (Chapter 69).

Patients with pulmonary embolism frequently have hypoxemia and hypocapnia. Hypoxemia can usually be reversed with nasal oxygen. Measures to reduce fever and agitation with acetaminophen and mild sedation may help minimize oxygen consumption. In patients who have severe pulmonary embolism and who require mechanical ventilation, low tidal volumes should be used, and positive end-expiratory pressure should be applied with caution because it can reduce venous return and worsen right ventricular failure (Chapter 91).

Patients with pulmonary embolism associated with hypotension or shock also may benefit from pharmacologic, mechanical, or surgical reperfusion therapy. Pharmacologic reperfusion therapy involves the systemic administration of a fibrinolytic agent (Table 68-4), preferably within 48 hours of the onset of symptoms, but later treatment still may be of benefit. Up to 13% of patients who receive fibrinolytic therapy experience a major bleed, and the rate of intracranial or fatal bleeding can reach 1.8%. Consequently, fibrinolytic therapy currently is justified only in patients who have severe pulmonary embolism and no contraindications (Table 68-5). In patients at intermediate risk, fibrinolytic therapy prevents hemodynamic deterioration but increases bleeding and stroke. If patients with severe pulmonary embolism are not treated with reperfusion therapy, they should generally be treated with heparin (Table 68-6) or low-molecular-weight heparin (LMWH) (Table 68-7). LMWH is preferred in the majority of patients, including patients with a creatinine clearance of 15 to 30 mL/min, whereas heparin remains the treatment of choice in patients who have end-stage renal disease (creatine clearance <15 mL/min) and patients who are on dialysis.

TABLE 68-4 APPROVED REGIMENS FOR INTRAVENOUS FIBRINOLYTIC THERAPY FOR TREATMENT OF SEVERE PULMONARY EMBOLISM

AGENTS	RECOMMENDED REGIMENS
Streptokinase	250,000 IU as a loading dose over 30 min, followed by 100,000 IU/hr over 12 to 24 hr
Tissue plasminogen activator	100 mg over 2 hr or 0.6 mg/kg over 10 to 15 min (maximal dose of 50 mg)

TABLE 68-5 CONTRAINDICATIONS TO FIBRINOLYTIC THERAPY

ABSOLUTE CONTRAINDICATIONS

Any hemorrhagic stroke or stroke of unknown origin
Central nervous system damage or neoplasm
Major trauma, surgery, or head injury in past 3 weeks
Gastrointestinal bleeding in past month
Significant ongoing bleeding

RELATIVE CONTRAINDICATIONS

Ischemic stroke or transient ischemic attack in past 6 months
Treatment with a direct oral anticoagulant or a vitamin K antagonist
Pregnancy or within 1 week of delivery
Noncompressible puncture site
Traumatic resuscitation
Advanced liver disease
Infective endocarditis
Active peptic ulcer disease

TABLE 68-6 WEIGHT-BASED NOMOGRAM FOR INITIAL INTRAVENOUS HEPARIN THERAPY

aPTT	DOSE (IU/kg)
Initial dose	80 bolus, then 18/hr
<35 sec (<1.2×)*	80 bolus, then 4/hr
35-45 sec (1.2-1.5×)	40 bolus, then 2/hr
46-70 sec (1.5-2.3×)	No change
71-90 sec (2.3-3×)	Decrease infusion rate by 2/hr
>90 sec (>3×)	Hold infusion 1 hr, then decrease infusion rate by 3/hr

*Figures in parentheses show comparison with control.
aPTT = activated partial thromboplastin time. In general, with contemporary aPTT reagents, the target therapeutic range is two to three times control.
Modified from Raschke RA, Reilly BM, Guidry JR, et al. The weight-based heparin dosing nomogram compared with a "standard care" nomogram: a randomized controlled trial. *Ann Intern Med.* 1993;119:874-881.

TABLE 68-7 SUBCUTANEOUS DOSING REGIMENS FOR VARIOUS LOW-MOLECULAR-WEIGHT HEPARIN PREPARATIONS

AGENT	DOSE	INTERVAL
Enoxaparin	1 mg/kg 1.5 mg/kg	Twice daily Once daily
Dalteparin	100 IU/kg 200 IU/kg	Twice daily Once daily
Tinzaparin	175 IU/kg	Once daily

IU = international unit (note that 1 mg of enoxaparin = 100 IU).

Mechanical reperfusion includes percutaneous catheter thrombectomy, an approach that avoids the need for fibrinolytic drugs altogether, or catheter-directed fibrinolytic therapy (without or with ultrasound assistance), which requires lower doses of fibrinolytic agents than are used for systemic administration. In some centers, surgical pulmonary embolectomy may be an option for patients who have severe pulmonary embolism, such as a saddle embolus occluding the main pulmonary artery (see Fig. 68-5), and who are at high risk for bleeding with systemic fibrinolytic therapy or who have failed such treatment. Mechanical and surgical techniques require skilled operators and should only be performed in high-volume centers.

DVT and Low-Risk Pulmonary Embolism

Most patients with DVT and low-risk patients with pulmonary embolism are treated as outpatients.[11] The principal indications for admission include clinical instability, the inability to adhere to outpatient therapy, or the need for interventions to treat massive pulmonary embolism or extensive iliofemoral DVT.

Guidelines favor direct oral anticoagulants (Table 70-6) for the treatment of VTE based on their efficacy and safety, as well as the ease of fixed dosing without the need for monitoring. Treatment typically starts with an oral factor Xa inhibitor (e.g., rivaroxaban 15 mg twice daily or apixaban 10 mg twice daily).[12] Four direct oral anticoagulants are licensed for VTE treatment: dabigatran, which inhibits thrombin, and rivaroxaban, apixaban, and edoxaban, which inhibit factor Xa (Chapter 70). These agents are as effective as LMWH followed by warfarin but are associated with less bleeding.[A2]

In patients suitable for treatment with direct oral anticoagulants, apixaban (begin at 10 mg twice daily for 7 days followed by 5 mg twice daily thereafter) and rivaroxaban (begin at 15 mg twice daily for 21 days followed by 20 mg once daily thereafter) can be started as soon as the diagnosis is established.[13] If dabigatran or edoxaban is chosen, a minimum 5-day course of treatment with a parenteral anticoagulant (see below) is needed before their initiation because these agents have not yet been evaluated for the initial treatment of VTE. Dabigatran is given at a dose of 150 mg twice daily, whereas edoxaban is given at a dose of 60 mg once daily. The dose of edoxaban is reduced to 30 mg once daily in patients who have a creatinine clearance of 15 to 50 mL/min, weigh 60 kg or less, or are taking potent P-glycoprotein inhibitors.

Patients who require thrombolytic therapy for massive pulmonary embolism or pharmacomechanical treatment for extensive DVT are usually started on heparin or LMWH but can be switched to a direct oral anticoagulant (see later) when their condition stabilizes. Direct oral anticoagulants should be avoided in patients with renal impairment (creatinine clearance <15 mL/min for rivaroxaban, apixaban, and edoxaban and <30 mL/min for dabigatran), in patients with severe hepatic impairment associated with coagulopathy, and in women who are pregnant or breast-feeding.

Parenteral Anticoagulation Followed by Warfarin

Direct oral anticoagulants should be used with caution in patients who weigh more than 150 kg because data on their efficacy in such patients are limited. The recommended role for warfarin is now limited to situations in which direct oral anticoagulants are contraindicated. Direct oral anticoagulants should be avoided if the patient is taking multiple medications that may interact with the direct oral anticoagulants (including strong inhibitors of P-glycoprotein, such as verapamil or dronedarone, or potent inducers or inhibitors of both P-glycoprotein and cytochrome P450 A34 isoenzymes, such as carbamazepine, phenytoin, rifampin, itraconazole, or ketoconazole). Warfarin also is the treatment of choice for VTE patients with a creatinine clearance less than 15 mL/min and for patients with antiphospholipid syndrome (Chapter 67).[A3] When warfarin is chosen, it must be combined with parenteral anticoagulant therapy such as unfractionated heparin, LMWH, or fondaparinux, given for at least 5 days and overlapped with warfarin.

Unfractionated heparin is the parenteral agent of choice for patients with a creatinine clearance less than 30 mL/min because LMWH and fondaparinux are cleared by the kidneys. Heparin should be administered by continuous intravenous infusion and dosed using a weight-based nomogram (see Table 68-6). Typically, a heparin bolus is followed by an infusion, and subsequent doses are adjusted based on the results of the activated partial thromboplastin time (aPTT). The aPTT is determined 6 hours after starting heparin or after changing the infusion rate. Once-daily aPTT determination is sufficient after a therapeutic value is achieved. Rapid achievement and maintenance of therapeutic aPTT values are important to reduce the risk for recurrent VTE.

Up to 25% of patients with acute VTE have resistance to unfractionated heparin, which is defined as a requirement for higher-than-expected doses (e.g., >40,000 units in 24 hours) to achieve a therapeutic aPTT.[14] If available, anti–factor Xa monitoring is recommended in place of aPTT monitoring in such patients. In addition to coagulation monitoring, the platelet count should be measured at least two or three times per week because of the risk for heparin-induced thrombocytopenia (Chapter 158).

LMWH is administered using weight-based dosing, and the use of prefilled syringes simplifies its delivery. Dosage regimens differ for the various LMWH formulations (see Table 68-7), but once-daily LMWH administration appears to be as safe and effective as twice-daily administration. Anti–factor Xa monitoring should be considered for three types of patients: patients with severe renal impairment (creatinine clearance 15 to 30 mL/min), patients with morbid obesity (e.g., BMI >40 or weight >150 kg) because the volume of distribution of LMWH in such patients might render weight-adjusted dosing inappropriate, and pregnant women because the dose may require adjustment as their weight changes. Anti–factor Xa levels are usually determined on blood samples drawn 4 hours after subcutaneous injection; therapeutic ranges of 0.5 to 1.0 IU/mL for twice-daily dosing and 1.0 to 1.8 IU/mL for once-daily dosing have been proposed.

Fondaparinux is a synthetic analogue of the pentasaccharide sequence required for the binding of heparin to antithrombin. The drug is given subcutaneously once daily in a weight-adjusted manner: 5 mg for a body weight below 50 kg, 7.5 mg for body weights of 50 to 100 kg, and 10 mg for body weights greater than 100 kg.

Warfarin can be started on the same day that parenteral anticoagulant therapy is initiated. Parenteral anticoagulant therapy should be continued for at least 5 days and should be stopped only when the INR has been within the therapeutic range of 2 to 3 for at least 48 hours. Initiation of warfarin therapy should be delayed in patients with massive pulmonary embolism or extensive DVT; such patients should receive only a parenteral anticoagulant until they have stabilized. Pharmacogenetic factors influence the relatively wide range of warfarin dose requirements among different populations, but their ability to guide warfarin dosing and increase the percentage of time that patients have INR values within the therapeutic range is limited. Warfarin requirements also vary over time in individual patients (Chapter 70), and it is unclear whether dosing algorithms enhance the efficacy or safety of warfarin therapy.

Although LMWH and fondaparinux are effective and safe, they require daily subcutaneous injection, which is difficult for some patients. Warfarin also is problematic because it requires frequent monitoring and dose adjustments, which are cumbersome for patients and physicians and costly for health care systems. The use of direct oral anticoagulants circumvents these problems.

Thrombolytic Therapy for DVT

Although catheter-directed thrombolytic therapy with or without mechanical intervention can increase early patency rates in patients with proximal DVT, such therapy has not been shown to reduce the subsequent rate of post-thrombotic syndrome. Therefore, thrombolysis is recommended only for patients whose proximal DVT is associated with extensive leg swelling or incipient venous gangrene.

Evaluation for Underlying Malignancy

Once treatment is underway, the possibility of an underlying malignancy must be considered, especially in patients with apparently unprovoked VTE. Age- and sex-specific cancer screening tests (e.g., colonoscopy and mammography) can be considered to exclude a previously undiagnosed malignancy as the precipitant. If these tests are negative and a comprehensive history, physical examination, and routine testing (blood counts, serum chemistries, chest radiography, urine analysis, stool for blood) are unrevealing or if their abnormalities are evaluated further without pathologic findings, the likelihood of finding occult cancer within a year of diagnosis is about 5%.[15] Therefore, routine abdominal and pelvic CT scanning or positron emission tomography is not recommended because such testing is expensive and does not increase the rate of cancer diagnosis or improve outcome.[A4,A5]

Long-Term Anticoagulant Therapy

All VTE patients require anticoagulant therapy for at least 3 months, when a decision should be made as to whether to stop or to extend it based on the balance between the risk of recurrence if treatment is discontinued and the risk of bleeding if it is not.[16] Patient preference also is an important factor to consider.

A 3-month course of treatment is sufficient for patients whose VTE was provoked by major transient and reversible risk factors, such as surgery or trauma, provided that these risk factors have resolved. The risk of recurrence after stopping anticoagulation treatment in such patients is about 1% at 1 year and 5% at 5 years. Women who develop VTE with estrogen therapy also can be treated for 3 months if hormonal treatment is withdrawn.

Patients who have an unprovoked VTE or persistent major risk factors, such as active cancer, are at higher risk for recurrence if anticoagulant therapy is stopped and therefore are expected to benefit from extended treatment unless they are at high risk for bleeding. Patients with pulmonary embolism are more likely to have recurrent pulmonary emboli, which are associated with a two-fold higher case-fatality rate than is DVT. Patients with a history of prior VTE have a 1.5-fold higher risk of recurrence than after a first VTE. Patients with recurrent DVT also are at higher risk for the post-thrombotic syndrome and may benefit from extended anticoagulation.

An elevated D-dimer level 1 month after stopping anticoagulant therapy identifies patients at higher risk for recurrence. Even with a normal D-dimer level, however, men have a 1-year risk of recurrence of about 9%, which typically is too high to justify stopping anticoagulation. The risk of recurrence in women with a normal D-dimer level 1 month after stopping anticoagulant therapy is about 5%, but the only women who probably should stop treatment are those who are younger than age 65 years, are not obese, have no evidence of post-thrombotic syndrome, and have either a normal D-dimer level 1 month after stopping anticoagulant therapy or a D-dimer level <250 μg/L while still on anticoagulant therapy.

For anticoagulation therapy extended beyond 6 months, the dose of apixaban can be reduced from 5 mg twice daily to 2.5 mg twice daily and the dose of rivaroxaban can be reduced from 20 mg once daily to 10 mg once daily without compromising efficacy and with the potential of reducing the risk of bleeding. Anticoagulation therapy is superior to aspirin for secondary VTE prevention and is not associated with an increased risk of major bleeding.[A6] It remains unclear whether the lower-dose regimens of apixaban or rivaroxaban are as effective as the higher-dose regimens for prevention of recurrent VTE in patients with active cancer. The higher-dose regimens should be resumed if patients develop recurrent VTE when the dose is lowered.

If warfarin is used for extended anticoagulation therapy, the target INR remains between 2.0 and 3.0. For patients with erratic INR values, consideration should be given to switching to a direct oral anticoagulant. Switching also can be considered for patients who find INR testing and warfarin dose adjustment burdensome, such as patients who have limited mobility or travel frequently.

Side Effects of Anticoagulants

Bleeding is the most common side effect of anticoagulant therapy.[17] Factors such as recent surgery, trauma, and concurrent aspirin or thrombolytic therapy increase the risk for bleeding.

Major bleeding—such as intracranial (Chapter 377), gastrointestinal (Chapter 121), or retroperitoneal bleeding—leads to transfusion or death in approximately 2% of patients treated with intravenous unfractionated heparin for acute VTE. The risk for major bleeding with direct oral anticoagulants is about 40% lower than the 1 to 3% per year risk of adjusted-dose warfarin targeted to an INR of 2.0 to 3.0. The risk for major bleeding increases with older age, the presence of comorbid conditions (e.g., diabetes, hypertension, renal insufficiency, previous gastrointestinal bleeding, or cancer), and the use of concomitant drugs, particularly antiplatelet agents.

Dabigatran can be rapidly reversed with idarucizumab (Chapter 70), a monoclonal antibody fragment that binds it with high affinity. Andexanet alfa, a recombinant variant of factor Xa that competes with native factor Xa for binding these drugs, can reverse apixaban and rivaroxaban (Chapter 70). If these drugs are unavailable, four-factor prothrombin complex concentrate is suggested for life-threatening bleeding[18] (Chapter 70). If serious bleeding occurs with heparin or LMWH, protamine sulfate (Chapter 70) completely reverses the anticoagulant effect of heparin but only partially reverses that of LMWH because protamine fails to bind to shorter LMWH chains. For serious bleeding with warfarin, vitamin K should be given by slow intravenous infusion along with four-factor prothrombin complex concentrate to replenish the missing vitamin K–dependent clotting factors (Chapter 70).

Heparin-induced thrombocytopenia (Chapter 158), which is a relatively common nonhemorrhagic complication of unfractionated heparin but a very uncommon complication with LMWH or fondaparinux, typically presents with thrombocytopenia and new thrombosis (Chapter 158). Monitoring of the platelet count is recommended at least two to three times per week in patients who receive therapeutic unfractionated heparin but is not routinely recommended with LMWH or fondaparinux.

When Medications Fail or Are Contraindicated

Therapeutic strategies to manage patients in whom symptomatic VTE recurs while they are receiving direct oral anticoagulants or conventional-intensity warfarin include LMWH, higher direct oral anticoagulant doses, higher-intensity warfarin (INR range of 3.0 to 4.0), or insertion of a vena cava filter. However, the optimal management of such patients is unknown because few randomized studies have been performed.

Inferior vena cava filters, which are inserted percutaneously, are usually placed below the level of the renal veins but can be placed higher if thrombus extends higher into the inferior vena cava. Both permanent and retrievable filters reduce the risk of recurrent pulmonary embolism[19] but do not reduce mortality, in part because permanent filters can be associated with long-term complications, including inferior vena cava occlusion because of thrombus, recurrent DVT, and post-thrombotic syndrome.[A7] Retrievable filters, designed to be removed within 2 to 4 weeks of implantation, can circumvent these long-term complications, but device migration or thrombosis occurs in up to 10% of patients with such filters because many are not removed. Because of these potential problems, vena cava filters should be used only in patients who are at high risk for pulmonary embolism and who have an absolute contraindication for anticoagulation therapy, such as patients who develop extensive DVT after major surgery, patients who experience major bleeding with anticoagulant therapy, and pregnant women who suffer a DVT shortly before delivery. Retrievable filters should be used in these cases, and the devices should be removed as soon as anticoagulant therapy safely can be administered. Laser-assisted removal may be useful in difficult cases. Permanent filters are suitable for patients who have ongoing contraindications to anticoagulation.

Specific Patient Subgroups

Patients with VTE in the setting of active cancer and women who suffer a VTE during pregnancy require special treatment.

Cancer-Associated VTE

Active cancer (Chapter 67) and its treatment with chemotherapy, radiation therapy, growth factors or other biologic agents, or immunotherapy increase the risk for VTE (Chapter 164). Patients with advanced cancer often have limited mobility, and venous compression by tumor adds to their risk for VTE. In addition, central venous access catheters or ports can trigger upper extremity DVT, which can lead to pulmonary embolism. Therefore, the index of suspicion should be high in cancer patients who present with symptoms and signs suggestive of VTE. With advances in diagnostic imaging, incidental pulmonary emboli may be discovered on CT scans performed for staging purposes or for monitoring response to treatment. Incidental pulmonary emboli or calf DVTs involving segmental or more proximal veins should be treated because of the risk of recurrence or extension.

In patients with active cancer, apixaban, edoxaban, and rivaroxaban are associated with similar or lower risks of recurrent VTE compared with subcutaneous LMWH, but edoxaban and rivaroxaban have been associated with more bleeding.[A8–A10] Most of the excess bleeding with edoxaban and rivaroxaban is from the gastrointestinal tract and occurs in patients with gastrointestinal cancers, particularly unresectable tumors of the upper gastrointestinal tract such as esophageal or gastric cancers. Warfarin is less effective in these patients and is not recommended.[20] As a result, apixaban, edoxaban, and rivaroxaban are suitable alternatives to LMWH for treatment of cancer-associated VTE, but they should be used with caution in patients with intact cancers involving the gastrointestinal or genitourinary tract and should be avoided in patients with a platelet count below 50,000/μL.

Apixaban (2.5 mg twice daily) and rivaroxaban (10 mg daily) are also effective for preventing a first VTE in intermediate and high-risk cancer patients, but they are associated with about a two-fold increase in major bleeding.[A11–A13] Therefore, when used for primary thromboprophylaxis, careful patient selection is important.[21]

VTE in Pregnancy

The management of pregnant women with VTE (Chapter 221) is problematic because direct oral anticoagulants and warfarin cross the placenta. Consequently, LMWH or unfractionated heparin, which do not cross the placenta and are safe for the fetus, are the agents of choice for treatment of VTE in pregnancy. The easiest approach is to initiate therapy with weight-adjusted treatment doses of LMWH (see Table 68-7), which is continued for the duration of the pregnancy. As pregnancy progresses, women gain weight and generally require higher doses of LMWH to achieve an anti–factor Xa level like that achieved at the time of diagnosis. The adequacy of the dose can be assessed by measuring the anti–factor Xa level 4 hours after injection and adjusting the dose to achieve a level of 0.5 to 1.0 IU/mL for twice-daily LMWH and 0.8 to 1.5 IU/mL for once-daily LMWH. Alternatively, the dose of LMWH can simply be adjusted based on weight.

Subcutaneous unfractionated heparin is less attractive than LMWH because it must be given twice daily and is associated with a greater reduction in bone density and a higher risk of heparin-induced thrombocytopenia than LMWH. Unfractionated heparin can be initiated by continuous intravenous infusion in doses adjusted to maintain an aPTT in the therapeutic range (see Table 68-6) or simply with 12-hourly subcutaneous injections throughout the course of pregnancy. The subcutaneous dose should be adjusted to achieve a therapeutic aPTT 6 hours after its injection.

Pregnant women with VTE should be treated for the duration of pregnancy and for at least 6 weeks postpartum. If the VTE occurs early in pregnancy, elective induction of delivery at approximately 37 weeks with discontinuation of the heparin 24 hours earlier is recommended. If the VTE occurs in the latter part of the third trimester, intravenous heparin should be administered by continuous infusion until approximately 6 hours before the expected time of delivery.

Subcutaneous LMWH should be started postpartum as soon as hemostasis has been achieved. Warfarin is safe for nursing mothers because neither the parent drug nor its metabolites are secreted into breast milk. Consequently, warfarin can be started after delivery, with bridging using LMWH or unfractionated heparin for a minimum of 5 days and until the INR is 2.0 or higher. Direct oral anticoagulants should not be used in nursing mothers because small amounts may pass into the breast milk and it is uncertain whether this may cause harm.

PROGNOSIS

At 30 days, the mortality rates in patients with DVT and pulmonary embolism are about 6% and 12%, respectively. Many of these deaths are due to concomitant diseases rather than to the VTE. Death rates are about 75% higher if the pulmonary embolism was associated with syncope.[22] If anticoagulation therapy is stopped after 3 months, patients whose VTE was provoked by a major transient risk factor such as surgery or trauma have the lowest risk of recurrence (about 1% at 1 year and 5% at 5 years), whereas those with unprovoked VTE are at higher risk (about 10% at 1 year and 25% at 5 years).[23] Patients whose VTE was provoked by minor nonsurgical risk factors such as prolonged travel or short-term immobility are at intermediate risk for recurrent VTE (about 5% at 1 year and 15% at 5 years), whereas those with major persistent risk factors such as active cancer (particularly brain, pancreatic, or colorectal cancer) are at highest risk of recurrence (at least 15 to 20% at 1 year). Therefore, when evaluating patients with VTE, it is important to determine whether the episode was unprovoked and, if provoked, whether the provoking factor was major or minor and transient or persistent.

LONG-TERM COMPLICATIONS OF VTE

The post-thrombotic syndrome, recurrent VTE, and chronic thromboembolic pulmonary hypertension are potential long-term complications of VTE.

POST-THROMBOTIC SYNDROME

The initial pain and swelling in patients with DVT are caused by venous obstruction and the inflammation that accompany venous thrombosis. After anticoagulant therapy is initiated, the acute obstruction usually resolves as recanalization occurs and collateral venous channels develop, thereby leading to a reduction in the pain and swelling. However, venous hypertension can occur if there is residual venous obstruction and incompetence of the venous valves. Venous hypertension is the hallmark of post-thrombotic syndrome, which develops in up to 50% of patients with proximal DVT, usually 6 months to 2 years after the event. The syndrome is characterized by dependent pain and swelling that is worse at the end of the day and is relieved with elevation of the legs.

Evidence regarding compression stockings to prevent post-thrombotic syndrome is conflicting,[24] and they are not routinely recommended. Lifestyle alterations such as frequent leg elevation, avoidance of prolonged standing or sitting, and occasional use of analgesics relieve symptoms of the post-thrombotic syndrome in many patients. If symptoms are severe, a lightweight stocking (e.g., support hose) can be helpful until the edema improves. A stocking that applies 30 to 40 mm Hg of pressure at the ankle can be prescribed if symptoms persist or worsen despite these measures. However, if symptoms subside or have little or no impact on quality of life, most patients opt to avoid the use of stockings.

Venous ulcers, which are the most severe complication of post-thrombotic syndrome, typically occur in the perimalleolar area of the leg. The best management is prevention by application of graduated compression stockings if skin changes develop in association with leg swelling. Treatment of ulcers consists of an emollient cream such as a moisturizer, with or without a low-dose topical corticosteroid (Table 404-2), and regular leg wrapping. After the ulcer heals, graduated compression stockings should be prescribed. Surgical closure or removal of the incompetent saphenous veins does not accelerate healing time in patients with chronic venous ulcers compared with dressing management alone, but surgery can significantly reduce the rate of recurrent ulceration.[A14]

SUSPECTED RECURRENT VTE

Approximately 10% of patients with unprovoked VTE will experience a recurrent thromboembolic event in the first year after stopping anticoagulant therapy. The diagnosis of recurrent DVT is complicated by the fact that many patients with prior DVT have positional leg swelling and pain because of the post-thrombotic syndrome. This syndrome and other venous disorders such as chronic venous insufficiency can produce symptoms that are similar to those of acute DVT, so accurate diagnostic testing to confirm recurrence is mandatory. Residual venous abnormalities on ultrasound are common in patients with a history of proximal DVT and are found in approximately 80% of patients at 3 months and in 50% of patients at 1 year after the event. Therefore, comparison with previous ultrasound images is required in patients with suspected recurrence. Although an increase in vein diameter of 4 mm or more in the compressed vein segment suggests recurrent DVT, a new noncompressible proximal venous segment is the most reliable criterion for the diagnosis of recurrence. A normal D-dimer test result helps to exclude recurrent DVT.

For patients with suspected recurrent pulmonary embolism, the diagnosis is confirmed by finding new thrombi on CT pulmonary angiography. Comparison with previous tests is important, particularly if ventilation-perfusion lung scanning is performed because residual perfusion defects are common in patients with a history of pulmonary embolism. As with suspected recurrent DVT, a normal D-dimer test helps to exclude the diagnosis. The treatment of recurrent VTE is the same as for a first event, except that most patients with recurrent VTE that is either unprovoked or provoked by minor risk factors require extended anticoagulation therapy.

CHRONIC THROMBOEMBOLIC PULMONARY HYPERTENSION

A rare complication of pulmonary embolism, chronic thromboembolic pulmonary hypertension develops in 0.5 to 5% of patients over the course of months or years when emboli in major pulmonary arteries are replaced by fibrous tissue that becomes incorporated into the vessel walls, thereby narrowing or obstructing them.[25] Chronic obstruction of the pulmonary vascular bed increases pulmonary arterial resistance and can lead to right heart failure. Although patients initially may be asymptomatic, they experience increasing dyspnea on exertion and hypoxemia as the disease progresses. Chronic thromboembolic pulmonary hypertension[26] should be suspected in patients who have pulmonary hypertension (Chapter 69), and the diagnosis can be established with a combination of echocardiography and lung scanning or CT pulmonary angiography.

Medical therapy focuses on treatment of right heart failure and the use of vasodilating agents (Chapter 69). Riociguat, a soluble guanylate cyclase stimulator (starting at 0.5 to 1 mg three times daily and titrated up to 2.5 mg three times per day as tolerated) is the only licensed medication for medical treatment of chronic thromboembolic pulmonary hypertension.[A15] A lower starting riociguat dose of 0.5 mg three times daily is suggested for patients at risk for hypotension. Riociguat may be of limited utility, however, because of the fibrotic nature of the obstructing material. Therefore, definitive treatment involves surgical thromboendarterectomy to remove the occluding material from the pulmonary arteries. For patients who are too sick for surgery, balloon pulmonary angioplasty can be effective and, in selected patients, provides excellent outcomes. This procedure is associated with a perioperative mortality rate that can be as high as 4%, depending on the severity of the disease, and a 3-year survival rate of about 80%. In patients with residual pulmonary hypertension after endarterectomy, pulmonary artery denervation is a potential option to reduce the pressure and improve functional capacity.[27]

VENOUS THROMBOSIS OF THE UPPER EXTREMITIES

DVT of the upper extremities (including the axillary, subclavian, and internal jugular veins, as well as the superior vena cava) is much less common than DVT of the legs, but it is not rare, especially among critically ill adults in intensive care units.[28] Factors associated with upper extremity DVT include central venous catheters, pacemakers, acquired or hereditary thrombophilias (Chapter 67), and anatomic (cervical rib) and physiologic (muscular individuals) impingement of the vein. The incidence of clinically important post-thrombotic syndrome is not high if patients receive anticoagulant therapy.

Contrast venography is the gold standard for the diagnosis of upper extremity DVT, but venous ultrasonography is accurate and less invasive. Because it is not feasible to test for compression of the subclavian vein, a diagnosis of subclavian DVT by ultrasonography is based on flow abnormalities or direct visualization of thrombus by B-mode ultrasonography. Upper extremity DVT can cause pulmonary emboli, although the exact frequency is unknown. Controversy exists about the management of patients in whom DVT develops in association with a central venous catheter. If the line is no longer required or is nonfunctional, some experts recommend removing the line without subsequent anticoagulant therapy, whereas most recommend full-dose anticoagulant therapy. If the line is functional and is needed for drug delivery or venous access, full-dose anticoagulant therapy should be given. Such therapy should be given to all patients whose upper extremity DVT was not triggered by a central venous catheter or port. The medications, doses, regimens, and treatment durations generally are identical to those for treatment of DVT of the leg.[29]

SUPERFICIAL VEIN THROMBOSIS

Superficial vein thrombosis usually manifests with pain, swelling, redness, and tenderness of superficial veins. Thrombosed varicose veins (Fig. 68-8) can be red, warm, and clustered in a circumscribed area. When superficial vein thrombosis involves the greater or lesser saphenous veins, a tender cord often follows the course of the involved vein in the thigh or medial aspect of calf, respectively. Superficial vein thrombosis also can occur at the insertion site of intravenous catheters. Approximately 25% of patients with superficial vein thrombosis in the lower extremity have concurrent DVT at the time of presentation, and approximately 3% of the others will subsequently develop DVT or pulmonary embolism in the next 3 months, with a subsequent risk of about 1% per year thereafter.[30] Therefore, compression ultrasonography should be performed to exclude DVT in patients with superficial vein thrombosis in the lower extremity.

Treatment with nonsteroidal anti-inflammatory drugs (NSAIDs), moderate or full doses of LMWH, fondaparinux, or rivaroxaban is approximately 70% more effective than placebo for treating superficial vein thrombosis. LMWH relieves symptoms more quickly and prevents thrombotic extension more effectively than do NSAIDs. Fondaparinux, 2.5 mg/day for 45 days, reduces the risk of DVT or pulmonary embolism from approximately 1.3 to 0.2% without notable adverse effects. A 45-day course of rivaroxaban (10 mg once daily) is as effective and safe as fondaparinux.[A16] Thus, it is reasonable to use these moderate doses of rivaroxaban, fondaparinux, or LMWH to treat symptomatic superficial vein thrombosis, particularly

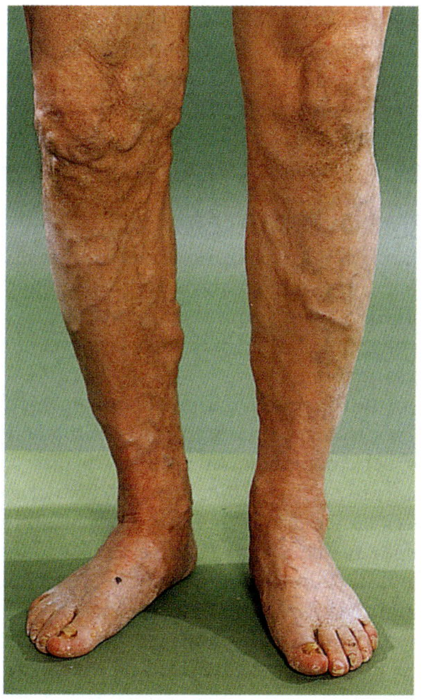

FIGURE 68-8. **Varicose veins.** Varicose veins are a risk factor for superficial and deep vein thrombosis. (From Forbes CD, Jackson WF. *Color Atlas and Text of Clinical Medicine*, 3rd ed. London: Mosby; 2003.)

in patients with severe symptoms, proximal saphenous vein thrombosis, recurrent disease, or underlying cancer or thrombophilia. For less severe cases, topical or systemic NSAIDs can be prescribed. For treatment of varicose veins, laser and surgical treatments appear to be superior to liquid or foam sclerotherapy.[A17]

PREVENTION OF VTE

At least half of all outpatients with newly diagnosed VTE have a history of recent hospitalization, and many failed to receive thromboprophylaxis during their hospital stay. Consequently, pulmonary embolism is thought to be a common preventable cause of death in hospitalized patients in the United States. Therefore, every patient admitted to hospital should be assessed for their risk of VTE and, if indicated, appropriate thromboprophylaxis should be administered.

Despite the plethora of large, randomized trials demonstrating the efficacy and safety of mechanical and pharmacologic measures in reducing the risk for VTE in a wide range of hospitalized populations of patients, prophylaxis remains underused. Factors that increase the risk for DVT include surgery (particularly major orthopedic surgery and neurosurgery [Chapters 255 and 399]), major trauma (Chapter 97), prolonged bedrest or immobilization, history of VTE, presence of malignant disease, paralysis or paresis, morbid obesity, chronic heart failure, and advanced age. Interestingly, statins and inhibition of proprotein convertase subtilisin/kexin type 9 (PCSK9) to lower low-density lipoprotein levels also reduce the risk of venous thromboembolism, perhaps owing to their effects on lowering Lp(a).[A18,A19]

In general, mechanical prophylaxis (graded compression stockings and intermittent pneumatic compression) should be used as a stand-alone prophylaxis in patients at high risk for bleeding. Pneumatic compression or stockings are often added to pharmacologic thromboprophylaxis, but a randomized trial showed no increased value of adding pneumatic compression to such medications in critically ill patients.[A20] Early prophylactic placement of a vena cava filter is of no benefit in severely injured patients who have a contraindication to pharmacologic thromboprophylaxis.[A21]

For general medical patients admitted to the hospital with a major illness and in whom mobility is likely to be reduced for 72 hours or longer, a 45-day course of rivaroxaban (10 mg once daily) can reduce the risk of symptomatic VTE after hospital discharge without a significant increase in major bleeding.[A22]

For patients hospitalized with COVID-19 (Chapter 337), standard-dose prophylaxis (e.g., enoxaparin 40 mg daily or rivaroxaban 15 to 20 mg daily) is preferred over intermediate therapeutic doses,[A23,A24] but therapeutic-dose heparin may be better than prophylaxis in non–critically ill hospitalized patients.[A25]

In patients who undergo major hip or knee surgery, oral rivaroxaban (10 mg once daily), apixaban (2.5 mg twice daily), warfarin (dose-adjusted to achieve an INR of 2.0 to 3.0), subcutaneous LMWH, or subcutaneous fondaparinux (2.5 mg/day) should generally be administered for 10 to 14 days postoperatively. In lower risk patients undergoing knee or hip arthroplasty, a 5-day course of rivaroxaban (10 mg once daily) followed by a 9- or 30-day course of aspirin (81 mg daily) appears to be as effective and safe as an extended course of rivaroxaban.[A26] In patients with continued immobility, prophylaxis should be extended until full mobility is regained.

Compared with inhibition of factor Xa, less is known about the clinical utility of inhibiting factor XIa. However, a single postoperative dose of intravenous monoclonal antibody against factor XIa appears to be as effective as enoxaparin or apixaban for preventing venous thromboembolism after knee arthroplasty.[A27,A28] The oral factor XIa inhibitor milvexian (50 mg twice daily) appears to be as safe and more effective compared with enoxaparin (40 mg once daily) to prevent VTE in patients undergoing knee arthroplasty.[A29] Whether this approach will be widely applicable, however, must await further studies.

NONTHROMBOTIC PULMONARY EMBOLISM

DEFINITION

Nonthrombotic material that can embolize to the lungs includes fat, air, amniotic fluid, tumor cells, talc in intravenous drug abusers, and medical devices.

FAT EMBOLISM SYNDROME

EPIDEMIOLOGY

Fat embolism syndrome usually occurs in the setting of trauma, particularly after fracture of long bones or the pelvis. The risk increases with the number of fractured bones, and the syndrome occurs more often with closed fractures than with open ones. Fat embolism also can complicate orthopedic surgery or trauma to tissues rich in fat, such as may occur with liposuction.

PATHOBIOLOGY

Characterized by a combination of respiratory, neurologic, hematologic, and cutaneous manifestations, fat embolism syndrome reflects a combination of vascular obstruction by fat globules (E-Fig. 68-2) as well as the deleterious effects of free fatty acids released from these fat globules by the action of lipoprotein lipases. These free fatty acids increase vascular permeability, induce a capillary leak syndrome, and can trigger platelet aggregation.

CLINICAL MANIFESTATIONS

Symptoms typically develop 24 to 72 hours after trauma or surgery. Patients often complain of vague chest pain and shortness of breath. Tachypnea and fever associated with disproportionate tachycardia are common. The syndrome can rapidly progress to severe hypoxemia that requires mechanical ventilation. Neurologic manifestations, which often start after the respiratory distress, include drowsiness, confusion, decreased level of consciousness, and seizures. Patients may have petechiae, particularly involving the conjunctiva, oral mucosa, and upper half of the body.

DIAGNOSIS

Fat embolism syndrome should be suspected when respiratory distress occurs a day or more after major trauma or orthopedic surgery, particularly when there are associated neurologic defects and petechiae.[31] The chest radiograph may reveal diffuse alveolar infiltrates. Although fat droplets may be found in bronchoalveolar lavage fluid (Chapter 73), this finding lacks specificity for the fat embolism syndrome.

PREVENTION, TREATMENT, AND PROGNOSIS

Early stabilization of long bone fractures reduces the risk for fat embolization. Supportive treatment should be provided, including oxygen and mechanical ventilation. The utility of corticosteroids remains controversial.

Although mortality rates as high as 10% have been reported, most patients fully recover without residual deficits.

VENOUS AIR EMBOLISM

EPIDEMIOLOGY

Venous air embolism, which involves entrapment of environmental air or exogenous gas in the venous system, requires direct communication between the air and a vein, as well as a pressure gradient that favors entry of the air into the vein. Air can be introduced through indwelling central venous catheters as a consequence of invasive surgical or medical procedures or after barotrauma.

PATHOBIOLOGY

Large venous air emboli obstruct the right ventricular pulmonary outflow tract, whereas mixtures of air bubbles and fibrin thrombi can obstruct pulmonary arterioles. In either case, right ventricular failure can result. With a patent foramen ovale (Chapter 55), venous air emboli can enter the coronary, cerebral, or systemic circulation.

CLINICAL MANIFESTATIONS

Symptoms and signs depend on the volume of air and the rapidity of its entry into the circulation. Large, rapid boluses of air are tolerated less well than slow entry of smaller amounts. Small air emboli may be asymptomatic. With larger emboli, patients often complain of dyspnea and retrosternal chest discomfort, and they may feel lightheaded. Physical findings include tachypnea, tachycardia, and evidence of respiratory distress. Patients may have signs of right heart failure. A continuous, drum-like, mill-wheel murmur, which reflects air in the right ventricle, may be heard.

PREVENTION AND TREATMENT

All catheters should be removed using techniques that minimize air embolism, air should be removed from syringes before injection, and care should be taken during surgery to ensure that air bubbles do not form in blood vessels. To avoid air embolism associated with barotrauma, divers require training in how to dive and surface safely (Chapter 82).

The source of any air embolism should be identified so that further embolism can be prevented. Left lateral decubitus positioning may benefit patients who have a large air bubble trapped in the right ventricular outflow tract; such positioning places the outflow tract below the right ventricular cavity, thereby allowing the air bubble to migrate into a nonobstructing position. Aspiration of the right ventricle through a central venous catheter also may be of benefit. Patients should receive high-flow supplemental oxygen, and hyperbaric oxygenation should be considered for patients with cardiac or neurologic dysfunction.

DIAGNOSIS

Patients may present with ECG evidence of right ventricular dysfunction associated with elevated levels of troponin, indicative of myocardial injury. Echocardiography or chest CT may reveal air in the right ventricle. Patients may have hypoxemia and hypercapnia, and the platelet count may be low.

PROGNOSIS

The outcome depends on the extent of air embolism. With good supportive care, the mortality rate can be less than 10%, even in patients with major air emboli. However, residual neurologic defects often persist.

AMNIOTIC FLUID EMBOLISM

EPIDEMIOLOGY AND PATHOBIOLOGY

Amniotic fluid embolism is a rare but catastrophic complication of pregnancy, occurring in about 1 in 8000 to 1 in 80,000 pregnancies.[32] The syndrome develops when amniotic fluid and fetal cells enter the maternal blood stream through small tears in the uterine veins during labor. Emboli to the heart and lungs (E-Fig. 68-3) cause cardiac dysfunction and respiratory distress. In addition, amniotic fluid and other debris activate the coagulation system, and the resultant thrombin then triggers fibrin formation and platelet activation to induce disseminated intravascular coagulation (Chapter 161).

CLINICAL MANIFESTATIONS AND DIAGNOSIS

The syndrome often starts with the abrupt onset of dyspnea, cyanosis, and hypotension that can rapidly progress to cardiovascular collapse and death. Patients who survive this stage often develop manifestations of disseminated intravascular coagulation (Chapter 161) characterized by diffuse bleeding, petechiae, and ecchymoses.

The diagnosis should be suspected in women late in pregnancy, often in labor, who present with sudden onset of respiratory distress followed by cyanosis, hypotension, and shock. These findings are often associated with confusion or reduced level of consciousness, seizures, and evidence of a consumptive coagulopathy.

TREATMENT

Supportive measures include oxygen, mechanical ventilation, and hemodynamic support. Fresh-frozen plasma, cryoprecipitate, and platelets transfusion can be given to replace consumed clotting factors and platelets. Heparin, often in low therapeutic doses, may be useful in some cases. If amniotic fluid embolism occurs before or during delivery, the fetus often has a poor outcome. As soon as the mother stabilizes, therefore, every attempt should be made to deliver the fetus.

PROGNOSIS

Although rare, amniotic fluid embolism remains the leading cause of maternal death during labor and the first few hours after delivery. Despite advances in critical care management, maternal and fetal mortality rates continue to be about 60% and 20%, respectively, with up to half of the survivors, both mother and baby, suffering from permanent hypoxia-induced neurologic dysfunction.

OTHER EMBOLIC MATERIAL

Many substances, such as talc, starch, and cellulose, are used as fillers in the manufacture of illicit drugs. Some of these drugs are ground up by drug users (Chapter 365), mixed in liquids, and then injected intravenously. The filler particles can then be trapped in the pulmonary vasculature, where they can induce granuloma formation.

Tumor emboli[33] in the lung can mimic pneumonia, tuberculosis, or interstitial lung disease on the chest radiograph. Cancers of the prostate and breast are the most common sources of such emboli, followed by hepatocellular cancer and cancers of the stomach and pancreas. Although found in up to 26% of autopsies in patients with advanced cancer, tumor emboli are infrequently identified before death.

Various types of intravascular devices can embolize to the lungs, including vena cava filters, broken catheter tips, guidewires, stent fragments, and coils used for embolization. Many of these devices lodge in the right atrium, right ventricle, or pulmonary arteries. Intravascular retrieval can recover most of these devices; open surgery may be required for the remainder.

GENERAL REFERENCES

For the General References and other additional features, please visit Elsevier eBooks+ at https://ebooks.health.elsevier.com.

Grade A References

A1. Freund Y, Chauvin A, Jimenez S, et al. Effect of a diagnostic strategy using an elevated and age-adjusted D-dimer threshold on thromboembolic events in emergency department patients with suspected pulmonary embolism: a randomized clinical trial. *JAMA.* 2021;326:2141-2149.

A2. Sterne JA, Bodalia PN, Bryden PA, et al. Oral anticoagulants for primary prevention, treatment and secondary prevention of venous thromboembolic disease, and for prevention of stroke in atrial fibrillation: systematic review, network meta-analysis and cost-effectiveness analysis. *Health Technol Assess.* 2017;21:1-386.

A3. Khairani CD, Bejjani A, Piazza G, et al. Direct oral anticoagulants vs vitamin K antagonists in patients with antiphospholipid syndromes: meta-analysis of randomized trials. *J Am Coll Cardiol.* 2023;81:16-30.

A4. van Es N, Le Gal G, Otten HM, et al. Screening for occult cancer in patients with unprovoked venous thromboembolism: a systematic review and meta-analysis of individual patient data. *Ann Intern Med.* 2017;167:410-417.

A5. Robin P, Le Roux PY, Planquette B, et al. Limited screening with versus without 18f-fluorodeoxyglucose PET/CT for occult malignancy in unprovoked venous thromboembolism: an open-label randomised controlled trial. *Lancet Oncol.* 2016;17:193-199.

A6. Weitz JI, Lensing AWA, Prins MH, et al. Rivaroxaban or aspirin for extended treatment of venous thromboembolism. *N Engl J Med.* 2017;376:1211-1222.

A7. Mismetti P, Laporte S, Pellerin O, et al. Effect of a retrievable inferior vena cava filter plus anticoagulation vs anticoagulation alone on risk of recurrent pulmonary embolism: a randomized clinical trial. *JAMA.* 2015;313:1627-1635.

A8. Raskob GE, van Es N, Verhamme P, et al. Edoxaban for the treatment of cancer-associated venous thromboembolism. *N Engl J Med.* 2018;378:615-624.

A9. Frere C, Farge D, Schrag D, et al. Direct oral anticoagulant versus low molecular weight heparin for the treatment of cancer-associated venous thromboembolism: 2022 updated systematic review and meta-analysis of randomized controlled trials. *J Hematol Oncol.* 2022;15:69.

A10. Mulder FI, Bosch FTM, Young AM, et al. Direct oral anticoagulants for cancer-associated venous thromboembolism: a systematic review and meta-analysis. *Blood.* 2020;136:1433-1441.

A11. Khorana AA, Soff GA, Kakkar AK, et al. Rivaroxaban for thromboprophylaxis in high-risk ambulatory patients with cancer. *N Engl J Med.* 2019;380:720-728.

A12. Carrier M, Abou-Nassar K, Mallick R, et al. Apixaban to prevent venous thromboembolism in patients with cancer. *N Engl J Med.* 2019;380:711-719.

A13. Agnelli G, Becattini C, Meyer G, et al. Apixaban for the treatment of venous thromboembolism associated with cancer. *N Engl J Med.* 2020;382:1599-1607.

A14. Gohel MS, Heatley F, Liu X, et al. A randomized trial of early endovenous ablation in venous ulceration. *N Engl J Med.* 2018;378:2105-2114.

A15. Ying M, Song J, Gu S, et al. Efficacy and safety of riociguat in the treatment of chronic thromboembolic pulmonary arterial hypertension: a meta-analysis. *Medicine (Baltimore).* 2021;100:e26211.

A16. Beyer-Westendorf J, Schellong SM, Gerlach H, et al. Prevention of thromboembolic complications in patients with superficial-vein thrombosis given rivaroxaban or fondaparinux: the open-label, randomised, non-inferiority SURPRISE phase 3b trial. *Lancet Haematol.* 2017;4:e105-e113.

A17. Brittenden J, Cooper D, Dimitrova M, et al. Five-year outcomes of a randomized trial of treatments for varicose veins. *N Engl J Med.* 2019;381:912-922.

A18. Marston NA, Gurmu Y, Melloni GEM, et al. The effect of PCSK9 (proprotein convertase subtilisin/kexin type 9) inhibition on the risk of venous thromboembolism. *Circulation.* 2020;141:1600-1607.

A19. Joseph P, Glynn R, Lonn E, et al. Rosuvastatin for the prevention of venous thromboembolism: a pooled analysis of the HOPE-3 and JUPITER randomized controlled trials. *Cardiovasc Res.* 2022;118:897-903.

A20. Arabi YM, Al-Hameed F, Burns KEA, et al. Adjunctive intermittent pneumatic compression for venous thromboprophylaxis. *N Engl J Med.* 2019;380:1305-1315.

A21. Ho KM, Rao S, Honeybul S, et al. A multicenter trial of vena cava filters in severely injured patients. *N Engl J Med.* 2019;381:328-337.

A22. Spyropoulos AC, Ageno W, Albers GW, et al. Rivaroxaban for thromboprophylaxis after hospitalization for medical illness. *N Engl J Med.* 2018;379:1118-1127.
A23. Investigators REMAP-CAP, ACTIV-4a Investigators, Investigators ATTACC, et al. Therapeutic anticoagulation with heparin in critically ill patients with Covid-19. *N Engl J Med.* 2021;385:777-789.
A24. Lopes RD, de Barros E, Silva PGM, et al. Therapeutic versus prophylactic anticoagulation for patients admitted to hospital with COVID-19 and elevated D-dimer concentration (ACTION): an open-label, multicentre, randomised, controlled trial. *Lancet.* 2021;397:2253-2263.
A25. Investigators ATTACC, Investigators ACTIV-4a, Investigators REMAP-CAP, et al. Therapeutic anticoagulation with heparin in noncritically ill patients with Covid-19. *N Engl J Med.* 2021;385:790-802.
A26. Anderson DR, Dunbar M, Murnaghan J, et al. Aspirin or rivaroxaban for VTE prophylaxis after hip or knee arthroplasty. *N Engl J Med.* 2018;378:699-707.
A27. Weitz JI, Bauersachs R, Becker B, et al. Effect of osocimab in preventing venous thromboembolism among patients undergoing knee arthroplasty: the FOXTROT randomized clinical trial. *JAMA.* 2020;323:130-139.
A28. Verhamme P, Yi BA, Segers A, et al. Abelacimab for prevention of venous thromboembolism. *N Engl J Med.* 2021;385:609-617.
A29. Weitz JI, Strony J, Ageno W, et al. Milvexian for the prevention of venous thromboembolism. *N Engl J Med.* 2021;385:2161-2172.

69 PULMONARY HYPERTENSION

MARIUS M. HOEPER AND VALLERIE MCLAUGHLIN

DEFINITION

The normal pulmonary vasculature is a low-pressure system, with less than one tenth the resistance to flow observed in the systemic vasculature. Pulmonary hypertension refers to the hemodynamic state in which the pressure in the pulmonary artery is elevated above a mean of 20 mm Hg.[1] A specific type of pulmonary hypertension, pulmonary arterial hypertension, also requires that the left-sided heart filling pressure (pulmonary capillary wedge pressure, left ventricular end-diastolic pressure, or left atrial pressure) be 15 mm Hg or less and that the calculated pulmonary vascular resistance be greater than 2 Wood units (Wood unit = [pulmonary artery pressure minus mean pulmonary capillary wedge pressure] divided by cardiac output). The syndrome of pulmonary arterial hypertension (Table 69-1) results when blood flow through the pulmonary circulation is restricted, thereby leading to pathologic increases in pulmonary vascular resistance and, ultimately, to right ventricular failure. Pulmonary hypertension may also be a consequence of many other chronic diseases, including left-sided heart failure (Chapter 45), a variety of parenchymal lung diseases, and thromboembolic disease (Chapter 68).

EPIDEMIOLOGY

Normal pulmonary blood pressure is 20/10 (mean, 15) mm Hg at rest at sea level, rising to 30/13 (mean, 20) mm Hg with mild exercise. Pressures rise with altitude, and at an altitude of about 15,000 feet, normal resting pulmonary artery pressures are about 38/14 (mean, 20) mm Hg. Pulmonary arterial systolic pressure rises gradually with age, and each increase of 10 mm Hg is associated with a 2.7-fold greater risk for mortality.

Idiopathic pulmonary arterial hypertension, formerly called primary pulmonary hypertension, is the prototype of group 1 pulmonary arterial hypertension. This disease affects women more than men in a 1.5 : 1 ratio. It may be manifested at any age, with a mean age at onset in the fourth to sixth decade of life. The prevalence of pulmonary arterial hypertension is between 15 and 50 per million persons. Heritable pulmonary arterial hypertension occurs in a familial context, most often (70%) due to a mutation in the bone morphogenetic protein receptor type 2. (See Pathobiology.)

Drug- and toxin-induced pulmonary arterial hypertension has been most clearly linked to anorexigens, including aminorex, fenfluramine, and dexfenfluramine. Although these agents are no longer used, observational studies link amphetamines, methamphetamines, interferons, and L-tryptophan to pulmonary arterial hypertension. Tyrosine kinase inhibitors (dasatinib and bosutinib) also have been associated with the development of pulmonary arterial hypertension.

One of the most common types of group 1 pulmonary arterial hypertension occurs in the setting of connective tissue diseases.[2] In patients with systemic sclerosis (Chapter 246),[3] for example, the prevalence of pulmonary arterial hypertension is in the range of 7 to 12%. It is less common in systemic lupus erythematosus (Chapter 245), rheumatoid arthritis (Chapter 243), and other systemic vasculitides (Chapter 249). Pulmonary arterial hypertension is a rare but well-established complication of human immunodeficiency virus (HIV) infection (Chapter 359), and its prevalence of 0.5% in such patients has not changed with the widespread use of highly active antiretroviral therapy. Prospective hemodynamic studies show that 2 to 6% of patients with portal hypertension (Chapter 139) develop pulmonary arterial hypertension, although the reason for the association is not clear.

A significant proportion of patients with untreated systemic-to-pulmonary shunts, commonly due to congenital heart disease (Chapter 55), develop pulmonary arterial hypertension. Persistent exposure of the pulmonary vasculature to increased blood flow and pressure leads to an elevated pulmonary vascular resistance. In some cases, Eisenmenger syndrome (Chapter 55), with a reversal of flow across the defect, results in right-to-left shunting. Pulmonary veno-occlusive disease (Chapter 68) and pulmonary capillary hemangiomatosis[4] are rare disorders that directly affect the pulmonary vasculature. The presentation of each is often similar to pulmonary arterial hypertension, but the prognosis is particularly poor.

Pulmonary hypertension due to left-sided heart disease (group 2) probably represents the most frequent cause of pulmonary hypertension seen in practice (group 2 patients).[5] Left-sided ventricular (Chapter 45) or valvular (Chapter 60) disease may increase left atrial pressure, which then is transmitted back to the pulmonary vasculature. The pulmonary vascular resistance is often normal (isolated postcapillary pulmonary hypertension). In such cases, optimal treatment of the left-sided heart disease may result in reduction of the left-sided heart filling pressures and, consequently, a reduction in the pulmonary artery pressures. However, some patients have a pulmonary vascular resistance greater than 3 Wood units in the setting of left-sided heart disease (combined post- and

TABLE 69-1 CLINICAL CLASSIFICATION OF PULMONARY HYPERTENSION

GROUP 1
Pulmonary arterial hypertension
Idiopathic pulmonary arterial hypertension
Heritable pulmonary arterial hypertension
Mutations in *BMPR2*, *BMPR1B*, *ALK1*, endoglin, *SMAD9*, *CAV1*, *KCNK3*
Unknown
Drug- and toxin-induced pulmonary hypertension
Associated with
Connective tissue diseases
HIV infection
Portal hypertension
Congenital heart diseases
Schistosomiasis
Pulmonary veno-occlusive disease
Pulmonary capillary hemangiomatosis
GROUP 2
Pulmonary hypertension due to left heart disease
Heart failure with preserved LVEF
Heart failure with reduced LVEF
Valvular heart disease
Congenital/acquired cardiovascular conditions leading to postcapillary pulmonary hypertension
GROUP 3
Pulmonary hypertension due to lung diseases and/or hypoxia
Obstructive lung disease
Restrictive lung disease
Other lung diseases with mixed restrictive/obstructive pattern
Hypoxia without lung disease
Developmental lung disorders
GROUP 4
Chronic thromboembolic pulmonary hypertension
Other pulmonary artery obstructions
GROUP 5
Pulmonary hypertension with unclear and/or multifactorial mechanisms
Hematologic disorders
Systemic and metabolic disorders
Complex congenital heart disease

ALK1 = activin receptor-like kinase type 1; *BMPR1B* = bone morphogenetic protein receptor type 1B; *BMPR2* = bone morphogenetic protein receptor type 2; *CAV1* = caveolin-1; HIV = human immunodeficiency virus; *KCNK3* = potassium two pore domain channel subfamily K member 3; LVEF = left ventricular ejection fraction.

Adapted from Simonneau G, Montani D, Celermajer DS, et al. Haemodynamic definitions and updated clinical classification of pulmonary hypertension. *Eur Resp J.* 2019;53:1801913.

precapillary pulmonary hypertension); such patients may have pulmonary vascular remodeling owing to persistently elevated left-sided filling pressures.

Group 3 patients have pulmonary hypertension due to lung diseases or hypoxia.[6] The most common underlying conditions are chronic obstructive lung disease (Chapter 76), interstitial lung disease (Chapter 80), and chronic hypoventilation syndromes (Chapters 74 and 374). Echocardiography-based observations have suggested that up to 80% of patients with advanced chronic obstructive lung disease and idiopathic pulmonary fibrosis have elevated pulmonary artery pressures. Most often, the elevations in pulmonary artery pressures are modest, but a small proportion of patients develop severe pulmonary hypertension, defined by a pulmonary vascular resistance greater than 3 Wood units.

Group 4 patients have chronic thromboembolic pulmonary hypertension (Chapter 68),[7] which must be differentiated from the other groups because the treatment is different. Approximately 2 to 3% of patients who have suffered an acute pulmonary embolism progress to development of chronic thromboembolic pulmonary hypertension. About one third of patients who are ultimately diagnosed with chronic thromboembolic pulmonary hypertension do not have a known history of an acute pulmonary embolism.

PATHOBIOLOGY

The pathobiology of pulmonary arterial hypertension is complex and incompletely elucidated (E-Fig. 69-1). The pulmonary arterial hypertension phenotype is characterized by endothelial dysfunction, a decreased ratio of apoptosis to proliferation in pulmonary artery endothelial and smooth muscle cells, and a thickened, disordered adventitia in which adventitial metalloproteases are excessively activated. The evolution of pulmonary vascular disease frequently originates with the interaction of a predisposing state and one or more inciting stimuli, a concept referred to as the multiple-hit hypothesis.

In group 1 pulmonary arterial hypertension, patients have a vasculopathy that predominantly affects the small pulmonary arterioles. It is characterized by a variety of arterial abnormalities, including intimal hyperplasia, medial hypertrophy, adventitial proliferation, thrombosis in situ, varying degrees of inflammation, and plexiform lesions. An individual patient may manifest all or some of these lesions, and the distribution of the lesions may be diffuse or focal.

The genetic defect best characterized in heritable pulmonary arterial hypertension is that of the bone morphogenetic protein receptor type 2, a member of the transforming growth factor-β (TGF-β) signaling family.[8] Less commonly, mutations in activin receptor–like kinase type 1, or endoglin, have been identified in patients with pulmonary arterial hypertension, predominantly with coexistent hereditary hemorrhagic telangiectasia (Chapter 159). Mutations in other genes (i.e., *BMPR1B*, *CAV1*, and *SMAD9*), all of which are involved in the TGF-β signaling pathway, are considerably less common. A novel channelopathy of KCNK3, which has been identified in familial and idiopathic cases of pulmonary arterial hypertension, is the first indication that the disease may involve factors apparently independent of the TGF-β signaling pathway.

The imbalance in the production or metabolism of vasoactive mediators in the pulmonary vasculature includes a reduction in prostacyclin and nitric oxide, which have vasodilator and antiproliferative properties, and an increase in thromboxane and endothelin, which are vasoconstrictors as well as mitogens. The reduction in nitric oxide synthase in pulmonary arterial hypertension diminishes nitric oxide and, subsequently, cyclic guanosine monophosphate production. Upregulation of phosphodiesterase-5 further diminishes the intracellular concentration of cyclic guanosine monophosphate. Endothelin-1 is a potent vasoconstrictor and smooth muscle mitogen that may contribute to the development of pulmonary arterial hypertension. Prostacyclin synthase is reduced in pulmonary arterial hypertension, resulting in an inadequate production of prostacyclin, which is a vasodilator with potent antiproliferative effects. Other aberrations include those of the voltage-dependent potassium channels and serotonin pathways. Disorders of inflammatory and coagulation pathways have also been described.

Chronic changes in the pulmonary vasculature also occur as a result of other types of pulmonary hypertension. Chronic elevation of left-sided heart filling pressures causes a backward transmission of pressure to the pulmonary venous system and triggers vasoconstriction in the pulmonary arterial bed. On histologic evaluation, the veins are thickened abnormally, and a neointima is formed. As secondary features, medial hypertrophy and thickening of the neointima on the arterial side of the pulmonary circulation occur. These changes can be partly reversed with therapies that result in chronic reduction of left-sided heart filling pressures.

In parenchymal lung disease, changes in the distal pulmonary arterial vessels consist of muscularization of the distal vessels and medial hypertrophy of the more proximal vessels. Neither neointima formation nor the development of plexiform lesions is observed.

The pathologic process of chronic thromboembolic pulmonary hypertension is distinct from idiopathic pulmonary arterial hypertension. The lesions are more variable, with some arterial pathways that appear relatively unaffected and others that show recanalized vascular thromboses. However, the involvement of distal microvessels, particularly when thromboses have occurred in subsegmental arteries, can resemble idiopathic pulmonary arterial hypertension, even with the formation of plexiform lesions.

Pathophysiology

The normal pulmonary vasculature bed has a remarkable capacity to dilate and recruit unused vasculature to accommodate increases in pulmonary blood flow. In pulmonary hypertension, the pulmonary artery pressure and pulmonary vascular resistance are increased at rest and further increase with exertion. In response to this increased afterload, the normally very thin right ventricle hypertrophies and eventually dilates. Early in the process, the right ventricle may be capable of maintaining normal cardiac output at rest, although it may fail to augment cardiac output with exercise, thereby leading to exertional dyspnea. As the disease progresses, the right ventricular dysfunction may progress to the point that resting cardiac output is impaired. Right ventricular function is a major determinant of functional capacity and prognosis in pulmonary arterial hypertension. Although the left ventricle is not directly affected by pulmonary vascular disease itself, progressive right ventricular dilation can impair left ventricular filling and lead to left-sided diastolic dysfunction. The pathophysiologic mechanism of pulmonary hypertension related to left-sided heart and lung disease is further complicated by those underlying disorders.

Right ventricular failure, as evidenced by elevated jugular venous pressure, lower extremity edema, and occasionally ascites, may also be accompanied by evidence of poor forward flow due to inadequate filling of the left ventricle. Hypotension, hypoperfusion, and renal insufficiency may result.

CLINICAL MANIFESTATIONS

History

Dyspnea, which is the most common symptom of pulmonary hypertension, typically is insidious in onset and gradually progressive. Dyspnea is classified by the World Health Organization (WHO) system, which is similar to the New York Heart Association classification system for angina and heart failure (see Table 39-5), and may progress to dyspnea with minimal physical activity.

Other common symptoms of pulmonary hypertension include fatigue, lightheadedness, chest pain (Chapter 39), and palpitations (Chapters 39 and 49). Syncope (Chapter 49), which may be an ominous finding, is often exertional in nature; it signifies the inability of the right ventricle to augment cardiac output as needed for physical activity. Symptoms of right-sided heart failure, including extended jugular veins, edema, and ascites, signify advanced disease.

The nonspecific symptoms of pulmonary hypertension often explain its delayed recognition. In various reviews, the delay from onset of symptoms to diagnosis can be as long as 2 years.

Patients with group 2 pulmonary hypertension may also exhibit paroxysmal nocturnal dyspnea and orthopnea. Patients with group 3 disease may have cough, sputum production, or wheezing. Patients with group 4 chronic thromboembolic pulmonary hypertension may have a history of venous thromboembolism, edema, and hemoptysis.

Physical Examination

Distention of jugular veins (see Fig. 39-2) may signify right ventricular failure, and prominent *v* waves (see Fig. 39-3) may be a result of tricuspid regurgitation.[9] The amplitude of the carotid upstroke may give some insight into the cardiac output. The classic physical examination finding in pulmonary hypertension is a loud pulmonic component to the second heart sound, which reflects high pulmonary pressures that increase the force of the pulmonic valve closure. A palpable left parasternal heave may be caused by the hypertrophied, pressure-overloaded right ventricle. A right ventricular fourth heart sound reflects diastolic filling of the hypertrophied, noncompliant right ventricle, akin to the left-sided fourth heart sound in a patient with systemic hypertension and left ventricular hypertrophy. The murmur of tricuspid regurgitation, which is holosystolic, located at the left lower sternal border, and augments with inspiration, is common in patients with moderate to severe pulmonary hypertension. Other findings on auscultation may include an early systolic click and the murmur of pulmonic regurgitation. A right ventricular third heart sound often signifies advanced disease and right-sided heart failure. Other signs consistent with right ventricular failure include hepatomegaly, peripheral edema (see Fig. 39-6), ascites, hypotension, diminished pulse pressure, and cool extremities.

Other physical examination findings may give some insight into the etiology of the pulmonary hypertension. For example, central cyanosis and clubbing may suggest an intracardiac shunt and Eisenmenger physiology. Sclerodactyly, digital ischemia (see Fig. 246-2), telangiectasias (see Fig. 159-3), arthritis, Raynaud phenomenon (see Fig. 66-9), and rashes may increase the suspicion of an underlying connective tissue disease. Splenomegaly, spider angioma, palmar erythema (see Fig. 132-2), icterus (see Fig. 132-1), and caput medusae may suggest portal hypertension as an etiology. Signs of left-sided heart disease, such as pulmonary congestion, left-sided third heart sound, or findings of mitral or aortic valve disease on auscultation, may signify pulmonary hypertension as a result of left-sided heart disease. Fine rales, crackles, accessory muscle use, wheezing, protracted expiration, and productive cough may denote group 3 pulmonary hypertension as a result of lung disease.

DIAGNOSIS

Initial assessments should include measurement of serum N-terminal fragment of pro–brain natriuretic peptide (NT-proBNP), an electrocardiogram, and chest radiograph.[10] NT-proBNP is frequently elevated in patients who have pulmonary hypertension, but normal values do not exclude its presence. The electrocardiogram may show right axis deviation, right ventricular enlargement, right atrial enlargement, and ST- and T-wave changes across the anterior precordium that reflect right ventricular strain (Fig. 69-1). The chest radiograph may demonstrate enlarged proximal pulmonary arteries (see Fig. 44-4) with peripheral tapering or pruning of the pulmonary vasculature (Fig. 69-2A). The lateral radiograph may reveal the reduction in retrosternal air space as a result of right ventricular enlargement (Fig. 69-2B). Notably, normal electrocardiographic and radiographic findings do not exclude the presence of pulmonary hypertension.

If pulmonary hypertension is suspected, a series of diagnostic evaluations should follow (Fig. 69-3), usually beginning with an echocardiogram and with further testing guided by the patient's subtype.[11,12] The echocardiogram gives insight not only into the presence of pulmonary hypertension but also into the presence of common disorders of the left side of the heart that may result in pulmonary hypertension. Two-dimensional echocardiographic findings reflective of elevated pulmonary artery pressures include right atrial enlargement, right ventricular enlargement, flattening of the intraventricular septum, and underfilled left ventricle (Fig. 69-4). The right ventricular systolic pressure may be estimated on the basis of the velocity of the tricuspid regurgitant jet by the modified Bernoulli equation (Chapter 43) (Fig. 69-5), although a reliable estimate of right ventricular systolic pressure is not always obtainable, and this measurement is prone to error, particularly in patients with parenchymal lung disease.

The echocardiogram is also useful to assess for left-sided heart causes of pulmonary hypertension, such as systolic dysfunction, diastolic dysfunction, and valvular heart disease. On occasion, a previously unknown congenital heart defect is discovered during this evaluation. In approximately 25% of patients, a previously trivial patent foramen ovale may shunt blood from the right atrium to the left atrium because of the high pulmonary vascular resistance and thereby worsen systemic oxygenation.

In a patient with unexplained dyspnea and evidence of pulmonary hypertension on echocardiography, chronic thromboembolic pulmonary hypertension must be excluded. The study of choice for this assessment is the ventilation-perfusion (V/Q) scan (see Fig. 68-6), which often shows multiple perfusion defects that are not matched on ventilation. Although computed tomography is excellent for the assessment of acute pulmonary embolus, it sometimes fails to detect chronic thromboembolic disease. If either of these studies detects an abnormality, further evaluation with pulmonary angiography may be required to determine whether chronic thromboembolic disease is the diagnosis and, if so, whether it is surgically accessible.

Pulmonary function tests in patients with pulmonary arterial hypertension may show a mild restrictive or obstructive pattern and (usually) a mildly reduced diffusing capacity for carbon monoxide. Pulmonary function tests may disclose evidence of obstructive or restrictive lung disease; further evaluation with chest computed tomography may be necessary. Polysomnography may be required to evaluate for obstructive sleep apnea (Chapter 374).

Recommended serologic testing includes an antinuclear antibody test and HIV serology in addition to liver function tests. A study of functional capacity, most commonly the 6-minute walk test, is useful to assess the severity of disease and to establish a baseline against which to assess subsequent changes in exercise capacity as a result of medical interventions. The high prevalence of pulmonary arterial hypertension in patients with scleroderma (Chapter 246) serves as an opportunity for screening of this high-risk population using pulmonary function testing, biomarkers, and echocardiography to make an early diagnosis.

If pulmonary arterial hypertension is suspected on the basis of the noninvasive evaluation, the diagnosis must be confirmed with a right-sided heart catheterization that measures right atrial pressure, right ventricular pressure, pulmonary artery (systolic, diastolic, and mean) pressures, pulmonary arterial wedge pressure (reflective of left ventricular end-diastolic pressure or left atrial pressure), cardiac output and index, heart rate, systemic blood pressure, and oxygen saturations in the superior vena cava, inferior vena cava, pulmonary artery, and a systemic artery. From this information, pulmonary vascular resistance and systemic vascular resistance may be calculated, right ventricular

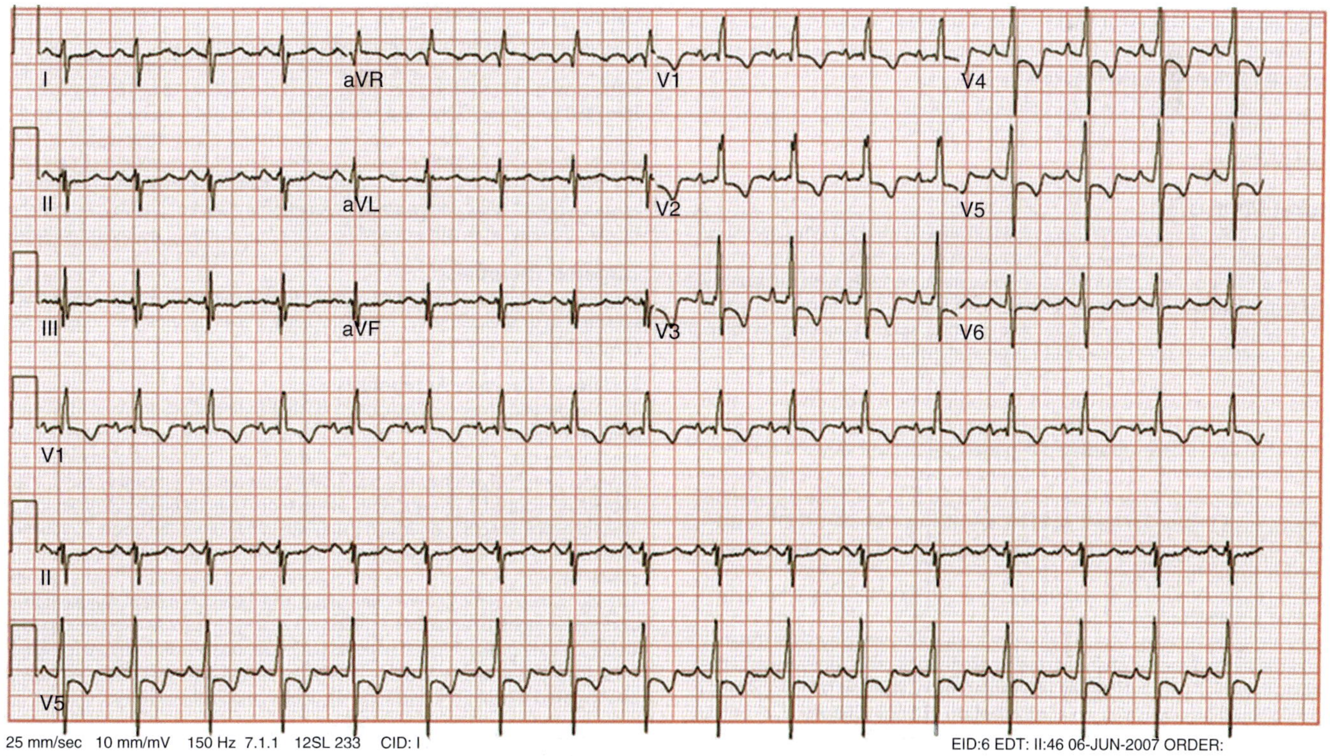

FIGURE 69-1. Electrocardiogram demonstrating sinus rhythm, right axis deviation, and right ventricular hypertrophy with a strain pattern.

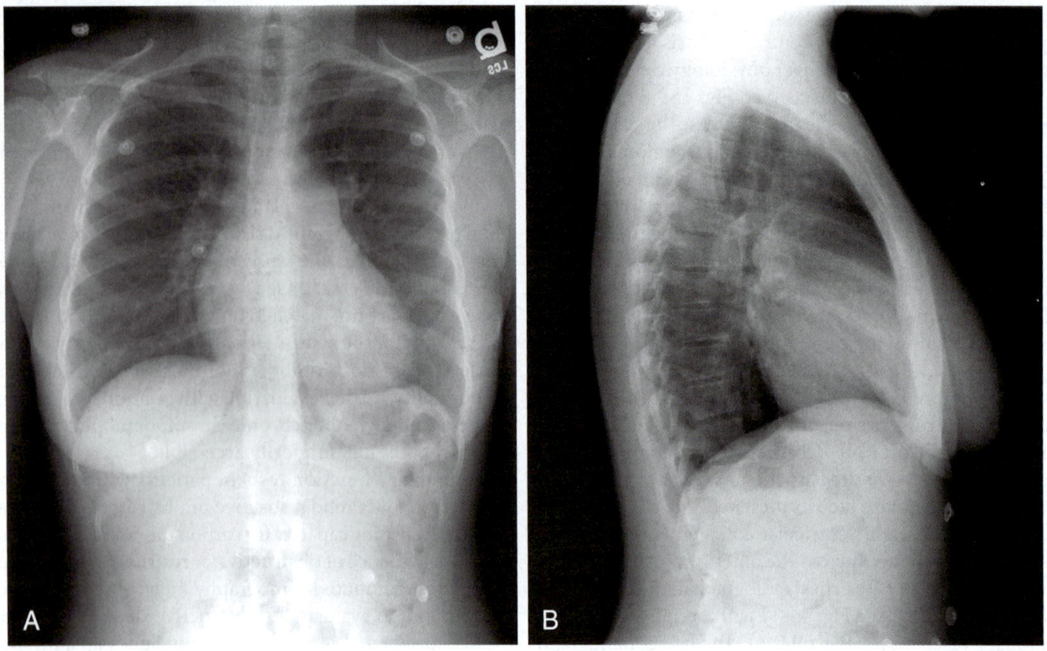

FIGURE 69-2. Posterior-anterior (A) and lateral (B) chest radiographs demonstrating enlarged proximal pulmonary arteries and right ventricular enlargement.

performance can be ensured, and an intracardiac or intrapulmonary shunt can be confirmed or excluded.

Measurement of the wedge pressure, a surrogate for left atrial pressure in the absence of pulmonary vein obstruction, is useful to exclude pulmonary hypertension caused by left-sided heart disease. If an optimal wedge pressure tracing cannot be obtained, or if there is any question about the accuracy of the wedge pressure tracing, a left ventricular end-diastolic pressure should be obtained. At the time of the initial right-sided heart catheterization, acute vasodilator testing is recommended in patients with idiopathic pulmonary arterial hypertension to identify patients who might be candidates for therapy with calcium-channel blockers.

The three agents most commonly used for acute vasodilator testing in the cardiac catheterization laboratory are inhaled nitric oxide, intravenous epoprostenol, and inhaled iloprost. A positive response to an acute vasodilator is a decrease in mean pulmonary artery pressure by at least 10 mm Hg to a mean pulmonary artery pressure of less than 40 mm Hg, without a decrease in cardiac output. If a patient meets these criteria, it is reasonable to administer a trial of oral calcium-channel blockers.

TREATMENT

General Measures

Patients with pulmonary arterial hypertension should always be treated at or in collaboration with a pulmonary hypertension center. Basic counseling and education are important components in the care of patients with pulmonary arterial hypertension. Patients are encouraged to avoid strenuous activities but to engage in low-level graded aerobic exercise, such as walking, as tolerated, and to enroll in specialized pulmonary rehabilitation programs, which can improve hemodynamic metrics and exercise tolerance.[A1] Exposure to high altitudes should be avoided because it may aggravate hypoxemia and cause hypoxic pulmonary vasoconstriction. A sodium-restricted diet (<2400 mg/day) and restricted fluid intake are advised in patients with right ventricular failure. Routine immunizations, such as for influenza (Chapter 332), pneumococcal pneumonia (Chapter 268), and severe acute respiratory syndrome coronavirus 2 (SARS-CoV-2; Chapter 337), are advised. In patients with persistent oxygen saturations below 90%, supplemental oxygen is recommended. In patients with intracardiac shunting and Eisenmenger physiology (Chapter 55), supplementary oxygen is recommended only if it produces a consistent increase in oxygen saturations and relief of symptoms.

Women with pulmonary arterial hypertension are advised to avoid pregnancy because the hemodynamic changes during pregnancy, labor, delivery, and the postpartum period are potentially life-threatening. Women of childbearing potential should be counseled on contraception options (Chapter 220) at the time of diagnosis. If women with pulmonary arterial hypertension consider pregnancy or become pregnant, prompt counseling by an experienced center is recommended.

Background Therapy

Diuretics (e.g., furosemide, initiated at 20 mg and titrated as needed, optionally in combination with other diuretics, such as spironolactone 25 mg; Table 102-4) are indicated to manage right ventricular volume overload; serum electrolytes and renal function must be closely monitored. Anticoagulation is not recommended in patients with pulmonary arterial hypertension unless other indications for anticoagulation are present.

Medical Therapy

Medical therapy for pulmonary arterial hypertension (Fig. 69-6) is based on the patient's characteristics and a comprehensive risk assessment (Table 69-2).[13,14] Reaching and maintaining a low-risk profile (determined by a 6-minute walking distance >440 meters, functional class I or II, and normal or near-normal NT-proBNP) is a key objective when treating a patient with pulmonary arterial hypertension. Unfortunately, this goal is not always achievable, especially in older patients with comorbid conditions.

Calcium-Channel Blockers

Approximately 7% of adult patients with idiopathic pulmonary arterial hypertension have a favorable response to acute vasodilator testing and an excellent prognosis with calcium-channel blockers. Long-acting nifedipine (90 to 180 mg daily), diltiazem (360 to 720 mg daily), and amlodipine (10 to 20 mg daily) are the most commonly used calcium-channel blockers. Because of its potential negative inotropic effects, verapamil should be avoided. Patients must be observed closely for both the safety and efficacy of this therapy. If a patient who meets the definition of an acute response does not improve to functional class I or II with calcium-channel blocker therapy, alternative or additional therapies should be instituted (see later).

Targeted Therapies

Targeted therapies for pulmonary arterial hypertension can be directed against endothelin or the pathways for nitric oxide, cyclic guanosine monophosphate (GMP), and prostacyclin.

Endothelin Receptor Antagonists

The endothelin receptor antagonist bosentan (initiated orally at 62.5 mg twice daily and titrated up to 125 mg twice daily after 1 month) improves hemodynamic measurements, exercise capacity, and the clinical course of pulmonary arterial hypertension.[A2] Liver enzymes must be monitored on a monthly basis; the dose should be reduced if liver enzymes rise to more than three to five times the upper limits of normal and discontinued if they rise to five times the upper limit of normal. Ambrisentan (administered orally at doses of either 5 mg or 10 mg once daily) has similar benefits, but liver function monitoring is not mandated.[A3] Other side effects include lower extremity edema, headache, and nasal congestion. Macitentan, a dual endothelin receptor antagonist (10 mg once daily), improves exercise capacity and delays disease progression in patients with pulmonary arterial hypertension.[A4] The most frequent adverse events are headache, nasopharyngitis, and anemia, without an increased rate of peripheral edema or elevated liver enzymes.

Phosphodiesterase Type 5 Antagonists

The phosphodiesterase type 5 antagonists sildenafil (20 mg three times daily) and tadalafil (40 mg once daily) improve hemodynamic measurements and

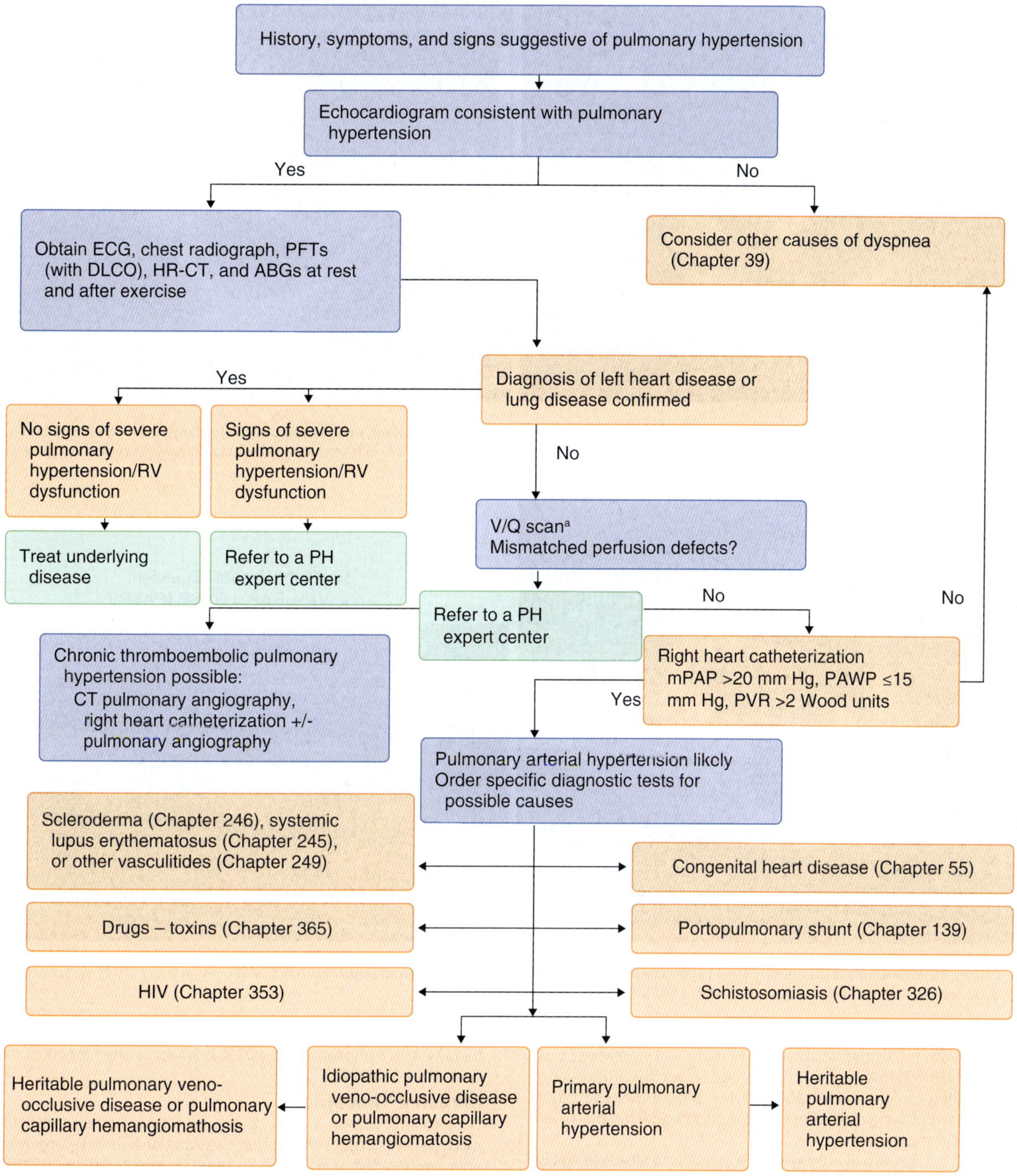

FIGURE 69-3. Diagnostic algorithm for pulmonary hypertension. [a]CT pulmonary angiography alone may miss diagnosis of chronic thromboembolic pulmonary hypertension. ABG = arterial blood gas; CT = computed tomography; DLCO = carbon monoxide diffusing capacity; ECG = electrocardiogram; HIV = human immunodeficiency virus; HR-CT = high resolution CT; mPAP = mean pulmonary arterial pressure; PAWP = pulmonary artery wedge pressure; PFT = pulmonary function test; PH = pulmonary hypertension; PVR = pulmonary vascular resistance; RV = right ventricular; V/Q = ventilation/perfusion. (Adapted from Galie N, Humbert M, Vachiery JL, et al. 2015 ESC/ERS guidelines for the diagnosis and treatment of pulmonary hypertension: the Joint Task Force for the Diagnosis and Treatment of Pulmonary Hypertension of the European Society of Cardiology [ESC] and the European Respiratory Society [ERS]: endorsed by: Association for European Paediatric and Congenital Cardiology [AEPC], International Society for Heart and Lung Transplantation [ISHLT]. *Eur Heart J*. 2016;37:67-119.)

exercise capacity in patients with pulmonary arterial hypertension.[A5] The most common side effects of these medications are headache, back pain, flushing, dyspepsia, and epistaxis.

Guanylate Cyclase Stimulation

Riociguat, which is a soluble guanylate cyclase stimulator, directly stimulates soluble guanylate cyclase independent of nitric oxide and thereby increases the sensitivity of soluble guanylate cyclase to nitric oxide. Riociguat (1.0 mg up to 2.5 mg three times daily) significantly improves 6-minute walking distance as well as pulmonary vascular resistance, brain natriuretic peptide levels, functional class, and time to clinical worsening, including in patients who were previously treated with endothelin receptor antagonists or nonparenteral prostanoids.[A6] The most common adverse events include headache, dyspepsia, peripheral edema, and hypotension. Riociguat should not be used concurrently with a phosphodiesterase type 5 inhibitor.

Prostanoids

Intravenous epoprostenol improves functional class, exercise endurance, hemodynamics, and survival in patients with idiopathic pulmonary arterial hypertension,[A7] and it also improves exercise tolerance and hemodynamics in patients with pulmonary arterial hypertension related to the scleroderma spectrum of diseases. Epoprostenol must be delivered by continuous intravenous infusion, commonly initiated in the hospital at a dose of 2 ng/kg/minute, with the dose titrated up on the basis of symptoms of pulmonary arterial hypertension and side effects of the therapy. Each patient must learn the techniques of sterile preparation of the medication, operation of the ambulatory infusion pump, and care of the central venous catheter. Although dosing must be highly individualized, maintenance doses in the range of 25 to 40 ng/kg/minute are typically needed. Common side effects include headache, jaw pain, flushing, nausea, diarrhea, rash, and musculoskeletal pain. Infections and infusion interruption can be life-threatening.

Subcutaneous treprostinil provides a modest but statistically significant improvement in exercise tolerance. Subcutaneous treprostinil is often started in the home, with the dose titrated on the basis of symptoms and side effects. Treprostinil is less potent than epoprostenol, and higher doses are required to achieve the desired efficacy. The main limitation of this therapy is pain and erythema at the site of the subcutaneous infusion, a complication that occurs in 85% of patients. Treprostinil may also be delivered as a continuous intravenous infusion via a fully implantable pump.[15] Oral treprostinil

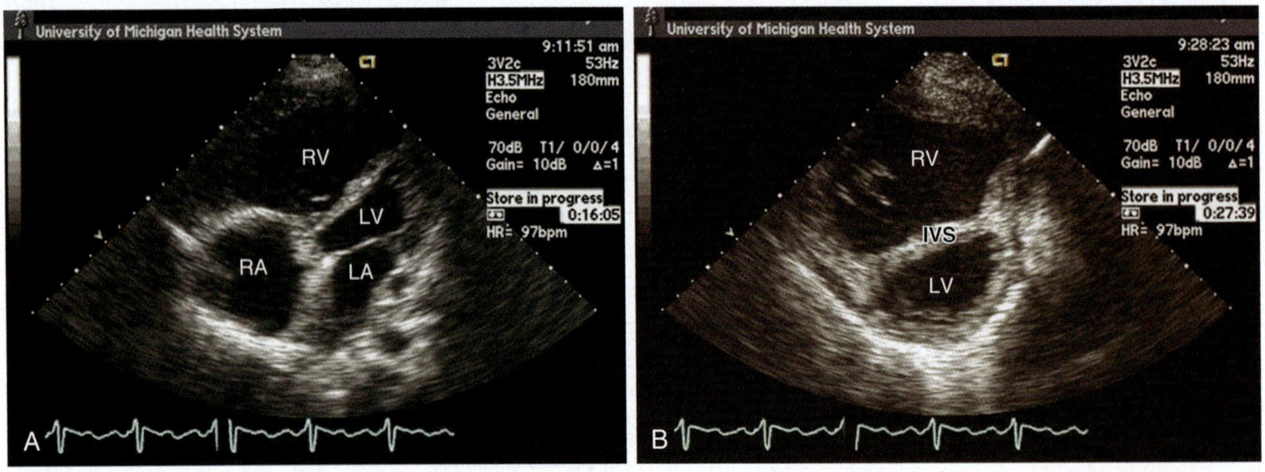

FIGURE 69-4. Echocardiographic images of the heart. A, Four-chamber view. Right atrial (RA) enlargement, right ventricular (RV) enlargement. The left atrium (LA) and left ventricle (LV) are small and underfilled. B, Short-axis view. RV enlargement is present. Flattening of the intraventricular septum (IVS) results from pressure and volume overload of the RV.

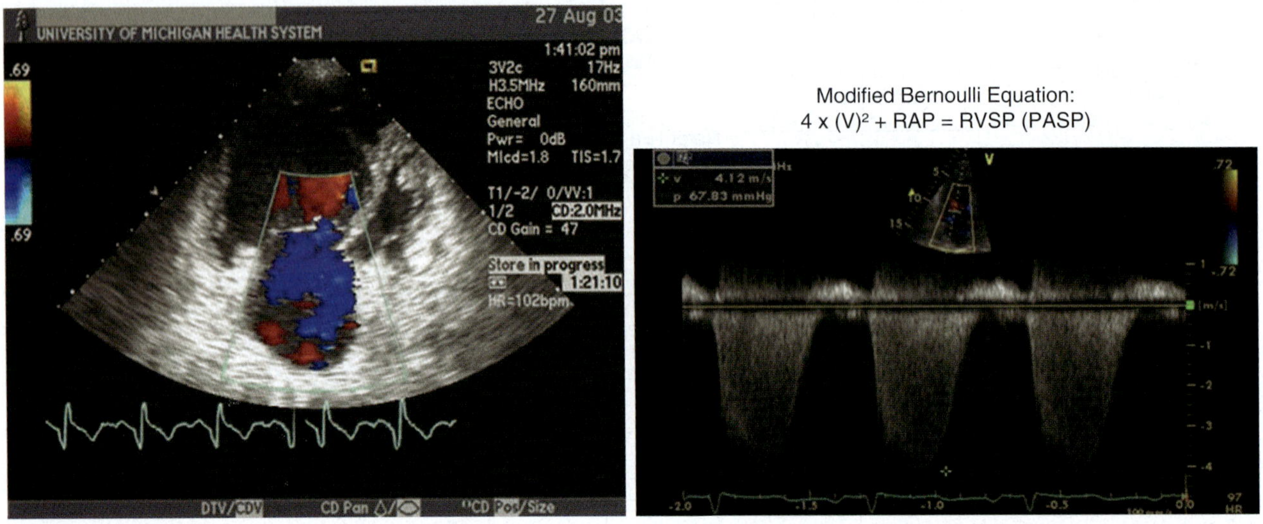

FIGURE 69-5. Calculation of estimated pulmonary artery pressure based on the velocity of the tricuspid regurgitant jet. PASP = pulmonary artery systolic pressure; RAP = right atrial pressure; RVSP = right ventricular systolic pressure; V = tricuspid jet velocity (m/sec).

(starting at 0.25 mg with meals two to three times daily and increased to as high as 12 mg two to three times daily as tolerated) delays the progression of disease when added to other medications.[A8] For subcutaneous or oral therapy, other prostanoid-type side effects, including headache, diarrhea, rash, and nausea, also occur.

Inhaled treprostinil four times daily and inhaled iloprost six to nine times daily also provide modest improvements in exercise capacity, including in patients with pulmonary hypertension owing to interstitial lung disease.[A9] Cough is an additional side effect with this method of administration.

Another option is selexipag, which is a selective prostacyclin receptor agonist, at a maximum dose of 1600 µg orally twice daily. Selexipag can significantly reduce the risk of the composite end point of death from any cause or a complication related to pulmonary arterial hypertension, but it has not been shown to reduce mortality per se significantly.[A10]

Targeting BMP

Sotatercept (a fusion protein designed to help regulate bone morphogenetic protein pathway signaling, given as 0.3 to 0.7 mg/kg subcutaneously every 3 weeks) also can reduce pulmonary vascular resistance in patients already on other therapies for pulmonary arterial hypertension.[A11,A12] It also reduces brain natriuretic peptide levels and increases walking distance.

Combination Therapy

Combination therapy[16] targeting different pathways is increasingly used in patients with pulmonary arterial hypertension. For example, initial combination therapy[A13] with ambrisentan plus tadalafil is more effective in improving exercise and preventing disease progression than monotherapy with either drug alone.[A14] In newly diagnosed patients whose pulmonary arterial hypertension is not associated with comorbid conditions, initial combination therapy with a phosphodiesterase-5 inhibitor plus an endothelin receptor antagonist has become the preferred treatment. Initial oral triple therapy has not been shown to be superior to double therapy.[A15] In contrast, in newly diagnosed patients who have other cardiopulmonary comorbid conditions, oral monotherapy is preferred, and initial therapy with a phosphodiesterase-5 inhibitor is often the most commonly used class of medications (Fig 69-6).

Invasive Therapies

Despite advances in medical therapies for pulmonary arterial hypertension, many patients experience progressive functional decline, largely related to worsening right-sided heart failure. In carefully selected patients, atrial septostomy may improve symptoms. Atrial septostomy creates a right-to-left interatrial shunt, thereby decreasing right-sided heart filling pressures and improving right-sided heart function and left-sided heart filling. Although the right-to-left shunting decreases systemic arterial oxygen saturation, the anticipated improvement in cardiac output will result in overall augmentation in systemic oxygen delivery. Because of its high morbidity and mortality as well as its limited benefit, atrial septostomy is rarely performed in the United States and should be considered only by experienced operators in specialized centers.

Bilateral lung (Chapter 87) or heart-lung (Chapter 46) transplantation remains an option for selected patients with pulmonary arterial hypertension when medical therapy fails. Transplantation should be discussed with selected patients at the time of diagnosis, although timing of referral is challenging. The International Society for Heart and Lung Transplantation recommends that patients with pulmonary arterial hypertension be referred for transplantation evaluation if they have persistent functional class III or IV symptoms despite optimized medical therapy, including prostanoids. Patients who are otherwise good transplant candidates should be referred when they have an unsatisfactory response to medical therapies. In some instances, advanced circulatory support may be required as a bridge to transplantation.

Special Populations

Group 2: Pulmonary Venous Hypertension

No specific therapy is currently approved for the treatment of pulmonary hypertension caused by left heart disease. Treatment should focus on the treatment of the heart failure itself (Chapter 46), with the goal of lowering pulmonary venous pressure and, as a result, pulmonary arterial pressure as well.

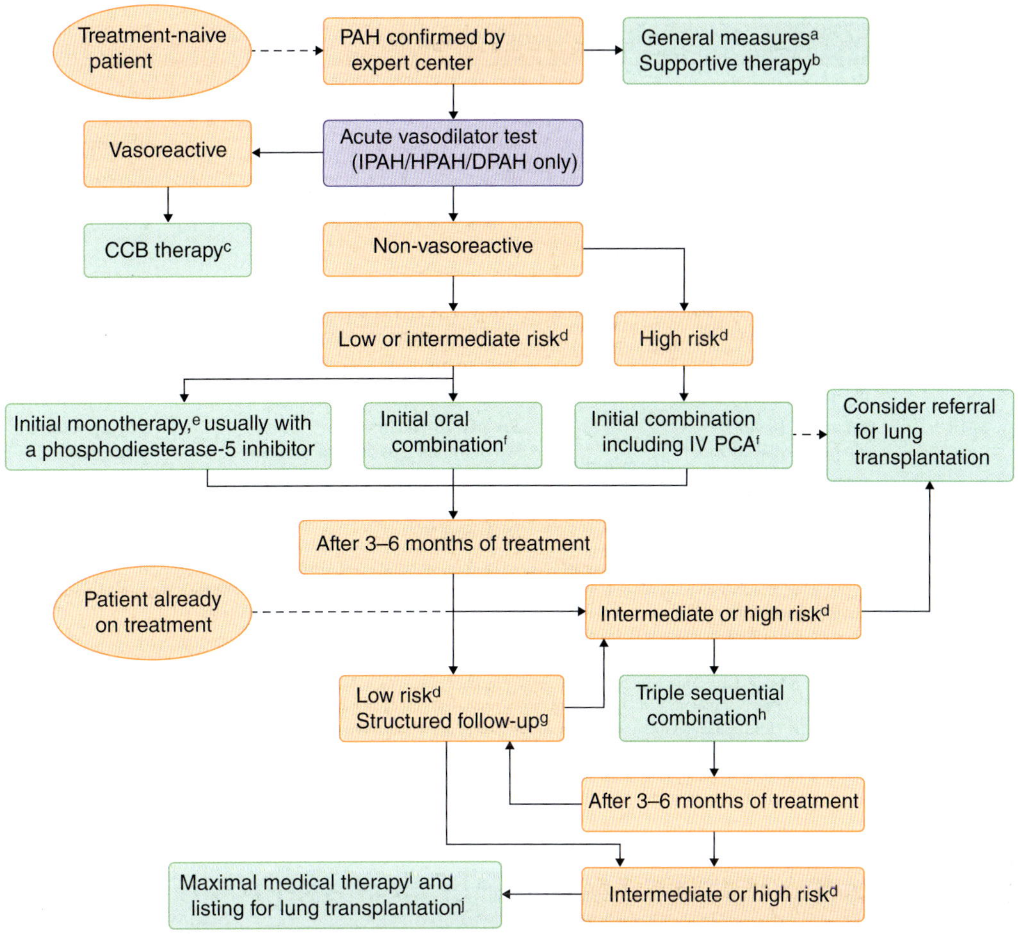

FIGURE 69-6. Pulmonary hypertension treatment algorithm. CCB = calcium channel blocker; DPAH = drug-induced pulmonary arterial hypertension; HIV = human immunodeficiency virus; HPAH = hereditary pulmonary arterial hypertension; IPAH = idiopathic pulmonary arterial hypertension; IV = intravenous; PAH = pulmonary arterial hypertension; PCA = prostacyclin analogues.

a. General measures include psychosocial support, supervised rehabilitation, and avoidance of excessive physical activity.
b. Supportive therapy includes the use of diuretics and oxygen as needed.
c. Calcium-channel blocker treatment is recommended for patients with idiopathic, hereditary, or drug-induced pulmonary arterial hypertension who have a positive vasoreactivity test.
d. Risk assessment should be done using established and validated risk stratification tools.
e. Initial monotherapy is recommended for patients with pulmonary arterial hypertension and cardiopulmonary comorbid conditions and for patients with distinct forms of pulmonary arterial hypertension (portopulmonary hypertension, pulmonary arterial hypertension associated with congenital heart disease, and human immunodeficiency virus–associated pulmonary arterial hypertension).
f. In patients with idiopathic, hereditary, or drug-induced pulmonary arterial hypertension and pulmonary arterial hypertension associated with connective tissue disease without cardiopulmonary comorbid conditions who present at a low or intermediate risk of death, initial oral combination therapy with an endothelin receptor antagonist and a phosphodiesterase type 5 inhibitor is recommended; if such patients present at a high risk of death, initial combination therapy with an endothelin receptor antagonist, a phosphodiesterase type 5 inhibitor, and an intravenous or subcutaneous prostacyclin analogue is recommended.
g. Regular follow-up at a pulmonary hypertension center, including risk assessment, is advised.
h. Addition of oral or parenteral prostacyclin pathway agents as determined by risk assessment and other clinical variables, such as comorbid conditions and patients' preferences, is recommended.
i. Optimized medical therapy, usually including an endothelin receptor antagonist, a phosphodiesterase type 5 inhibitor, and/or a soluble guanylate cyclase stimulator, plus an intravenous or subcutaneous prostacyclin analogue, is recommended.
j. Potentially eligible patients who do not reach a low-risk profile with optimized medical therapy should be referred for transplant evaluation; active listing should be considered if these patients present with a high risk profile. (Adapted from Galiè N, Channick RN, Frantz RP, et al. Risk stratification and medical therapy of pulmonary arterial hypertension. *Eur Resp J.* 2019;53:1801889.)

Group 3: Primary Lung Disease

For primary lung disease, treatment of the underlying disorder is indicated. Inhaled treprostinil can be effective in patients with interstitial lung disease (Chapter 80) and pulmonary hypertension, but other medications that are helpful for pulmonary arterial hypertension are usually not recommended for the treatment of pulmonary hypertension due to lung disease. However, in patients who have severe pulmonary hypertension but only mild lung disease, individualized decisions should be made in consultation with a specialized pulmonary hypertension center.

Group 4: Chronic Thromboembolic Hypertension

For patients with chronic thromboembolic pulmonary hypertension, pulmonary endarterectomy (E-Fig. 69-2) is the treatment of choice and is a potentially curative procedure.[17] Balloon pulmonary angioplasty is an option for patients who are not surgical candidates owing to distal disease.[18] Riociguat (1.0 up to 2.5 mg three times daily) improves 6-minute walking distance, pulmonary vascular resistance, NT-proBNP level, and functional class[A16] in patients with either inoperable chronic thromboembolic pulmonary hypertension or persistent pulmonary hypertension after pulmonary endarterectomy. If these options fail, pulmonary artery denervation may be helpful.[19] Indefinite anticoagulation is also recommended.

Group 5: Other Causes

Group 5 pulmonary hypertension consists of several forms for which the cause is unclear or multifactorial. Among these conditions are a number of hematologic, systemic, and metabolic disorders (see Table 69-1). No treatments are of proven value, but patients who have evidence of severe pulmonary hypertension should be referred to a pulmonary hypertension center for individualized treatment.

Assessing Response to Therapy

Given the complexity of the disease, the variable response to therapy, and the goal of optimizing and individualizing care, patients with pulmonary arterial hypertension must be observed closely (Table 69-3). Consensus recommendations rely on the routine assessment of important prognostic indicators, such as WHO functional class, 6-minute walking distance, NT-proBNP, and echocardiographic and hemodynamic parameters (Table 69-2).

Collaborative Care

Due to the rare and complex nature of pulmonary arterial hypertension, optimal care requires collaboration among multiple disciplines. At pulmonary hypertension centers, this collaboration helps patients receive high-quality specialty care for a rare disease while also coordinating with the patient's local primary care doctor and specialists.

TABLE 69-2 RISK ASSESSMENT IN PULMONARY ARTERIAL HYPERTENSION

DETERMINANTS OF PROGNOSIS* (ESTIMATED 1-YEAR MORTALITY)	LOW RISK <5%	INTERMEDIATE RISK 5-10%	HIGH RISK >10%
Clinical signs of right heart failure	Absent	Absent	Present
Progression of symptoms	No	Slow	Rapid
Syncope	No	Occasional syncope†	Repeated syncope‡
WHO functional class	I, II	III	IV
6MWD	>440 m	165-440 m	<165 m
Cardiopulmonary exercise testing	Peak VO_2 > 15 mL/min/kg (>65% pred.) VE/VCO_2 slope < 36	Peak VO_2 > 11-15 mL/min/kg (35-65% pred.) VE/VCO_2 slope 36-44.9	Peak VO_2 > 11 mL/min/kg (<35% pred.) VE/VCO_2 slope > 45
BNP or NT-proBNP plasma levels	BNP < 50 ng/L NT-proBNP < 300 ng/L	BNP 50-300 ng/L NT-proBNP 300-1400 ng/L	BNP > 300 ng/L NT-proBNP < 300 ng/L
Imaging (echocardiography, CMR imaging)	RA area < 18 cm² No pericardial effusion	RA area 18-26 cm² No or minimal pericardial effusion	RA area > 26 cm² Pericardial effusion
Hemodynamics	RAP < 8 mm Hg CI ≥ 2.5 L/min/m² SvO_2 > 65%	RAP 8-14 mm Hg CI 2.0-2.4 L/min/m² SvO_2 60-65%	RAP > 14 mm Hg CI < 2.0 L/min/m² SvO_2 < 60%

*Most of the proposed variables and cutoff values are based on expert opinion. They may provide prognostic information and may be used to guide therapeutic decisions, but application to individual patients must be done carefully. Most of these factors have been validated primarily for idiopathic pulmonary arterial hypertension, and the cutoff levels used above may not necessarily apply to other forms of pulmonary arterial hypertension. Furthermore, the use of approved therapies and their influence on the variables should be considered in the evaluation of the risk.

†Occasional syncope during brisk or heavy exercise, or occasional orthostatic syncope in an otherwise stable patient.

‡Repeated episodes of syncope, even with little or regular physical activity.

6MWD = 6-minute walking distance; BNP = brain natriuretic peptide; CI = cardiac index; CMR = cardiac magnetic resonance; NT-proBNP = N-terminal pro-brain natriuretic peptide; pred. = predicted; RA = right atrium; RAP = right atrial pressure; SvO_2 = mixed venous oxygen saturation; VE/VCO_2 = ventilatory equivalents for carbon dioxide; VO_2 = oxygen consumption; WHO = World Health Organization.

Adapted from Galie N, Humbert M, Vachiery JL, et al. 2015 ESC/ERS guidelines for the diagnosis and treatment of pulmonary hypertension: the Joint Task Force for the Diagnosis and Treatment of Pulmonary Hypertension of the European Society of Cardiology (ESC) and the European Respiratory Society (ERS): endorsed by: Association for European Paediatric and Congenital Cardiology (AEPC), International Society for Heart and Lung Transplantation (ISHLT). *Eur Heart J*. 2016;37:67-119.

TABLE 69-3 SUGGESTED ASSESSMENT AND TIMING FOR THE FOLLOW-UP OF PATIENTS WITH PULMONARY ARTERIAL HYPERTENSION

	AT BASELINE	EVERY 3-6 MONTHS*	EVERY 6-12 MONTHS*	3-6 MONTHS AFTER CHANGES IN THERAPY*	IN CASE OF CLINICAL WORSENING
Medical assessment and determination of functional class	+	+	+	+	+
Electrocardiogram	+	+	+	+	+
6MWT/Borg dyspnea score	+	+	+	+	+
Cardiopulmonary exercise testing	+		+		+‖
Echocardiography	+		+	+	+
Basic laboratory tests†	+	+	+	+	+
Extended laboratory tests‡	+		+		+
Blood gas analysis§	+		+	+	+
Right heart catheterization	+		+¶	+‖	+‖

*Intervals to be adjusted according to patient needs.

†Basic lab includes blood count, INR (in patients receiving vitamin K antagonists), serum creatinine, sodium, potassium, ASAT/ALAT (in patients receiving ERAs), bilirubin, and BNP/NT-proBNP.

‡Extended lab includes TSH, troponin, uric acid, iron status (iron, ferritin, soluble transferrin receptor), and other variables according to individual patient needs.

§From arterial or arterialized capillary blood; may be replaced by peripheral oxygen saturation in stable patients or if BGA is not available.

‖Should be considered.

¶Some centers perform RHCs at regular intervals during follow-up.

6MWT = 6-minute walking test; ALAT = alanine aminotransferase; ASAT = aspartate aminotransferase; BGA = blood gas analysis; BNP = brain natriuretic peptide; ERAs = endothelin receptor antagonists; FC = functional class; INR = international normalized ratio; lab = laboratory assessment; NT-proBNP = N-terminal pro–brain natriuretic peptide; RHC = right heart catheterization; TSH = thyroid-stimulating hormone.

Adapted from Galie N, Humbert M, Vachiery JL, et al. 2015 ESC/ERS guidelines for the diagnosis and treatment of pulmonary hypertension: the Joint Task Force for the Diagnosis and Treatment of Pulmonary Hypertension of the European Society of Cardiology (ESC) and the European Respiratory Society (ERS): endorsed by: Association for European Paediatric and Congenital Cardiology (AEPC), International Society for Heart and Lung Transplantation (ISHLT). *Eur Heart J*. 2016;37:67-119.

PROGNOSIS

Even mild pulmonary hypertension on echocardiography, as evidenced by an estimated pulmonary artery systolic pressure of 27 to 39 mm Hg, is associated with a significant increase in mortality.[20] The natural history of symptomatic idiopathic pulmonary arterial hypertension is a median survival of 2.8 years with 1-, 3-, and 5-year survival rates of 68%, 48%, and 34%, respectively. In the era of targeted therapies, survival has improved but remains suboptimal, with 1-, 2-, and 3-year survival of approximately 90%, 70%, and 55%, respectively, for incident cases. The most frequent cause of death in patients with advanced pulmonary hypertension is progressive right ventricular failure.

Several clinical factors are correlated with prognosis (see Table 69-2). Patients who have better functional, echocardiographic, and hemodynamic parameters or who improve on these parameters with treatment have a better prognosis than patients who do not achieve these goals or who experience pulmonary hypertension–related morbidities.[21,22] For example, achieving a 6-minute walk of more than 440 meters, functional class I or II symptoms, and a normal brain natriuretic peptide level is associated with excellent survival.[23]

Patients with pulmonary arterial hypertension related to the scleroderma spectrum of diseases tend to have a poorer prognosis than that of patients with idiopathic pulmonary arterial hypertension, whereas patients with pulmonary arterial hypertension related to congenital heart disease tend to have a better prognosis, perhaps because they have better right ventricular function. The natural history of patients with groups 2, 3, and 4 pulmonary hypertension is influenced by their left-sided heart and lung disease. In most cases, the presence of pulmonary hypertension in addition to the underlying disease portends a poor prognosis.

GENERAL REFERENCES

For the General References and other additional features, please visit Elsevier eBooks+ at https://ebooks.health.elsevier.com.

Grade A References

A1. Grünig E, MacKenzie A, Peacock AJ, et al. Standardized exercise training is feasible, safe, and effective in pulmonary arterial and chronic thromboembolic pulmonary hypertension: results from a large European multicentre randomized controlled trial. *Eur Heart J*. 2021;42:2284-2295.

A2. Kuang H-Y, Li Q, Du H-A, et al. Efficacy and safety of long-term oral bosentan in different types of pulmonary arterial hypertension: a systematic review and meta-analysis. *Am J Cardiovasc Drugs*. 2021;21:181-191.

A3. Zhao Q, Guo N, Chen J, et al. Comparative assessment of efficacy and safety of ambrisentan and bosentan in patients with pulmonary arterial hypertension: a meta-analysis. *J Clin Pharm Ther*. 2022;47:146-156.

A4. Mehta S, Sastry BKS, Souza R, et al. Macitentan improves health-related quality of life for patients with pulmonary arterial hypertension: results from the randomized controlled seraphin trial. *Chest*. 2017;151:106-118.

A5. Barnes H, Brown Z, Burns A, et al. Phosphodiesterase 5 inhibitors for pulmonary hypertension. *Cochrane Database Syst Rev*. 2019;1:CD012621.

A6. Zhao R, Jiang Y. Influence of riociguat treatment on pulmonary arterial hypertension: a meta-analysis of randomized controlled trials. *Herz*. 2019;44:637-643.

A7. Barnes H, Yeoh HL, Fothergill T, et al. Prostacyclin for pulmonary arterial hypertension. *Cochrane Database Syst Rev*. 2019;5:CD012785.

A8. White RJ, Jerjes-Sanchez C, Bohns Meyer GM, et al. Combination therapy with oral treprostinil for pulmonary arterial hypertension. A double-blind placebo-controlled clinical trial. *Am J Respir Crit Care Med*. 2020;201:707-717.

A9. Waxman A, Restrepo-Jaramillo R, Thenappan T, et al. Inhaled treprostinil in pulmonary hypertension due to interstitial lung disease. *N Engl J Med*. 2021;384:325-334.

A10. Sitbon O, Channick R, Chin KM, et al. Selexipag for the treatment of pulmonary arterial hypertension. *N Engl J Med*. 2015;373:2522-2533.

A11. Humbert M, McLaughlin V, Gibbs JSR, et al. Sotatercept for the treatment of pulmonary arterial hypertension. *N Engl J Med*. 2021;384:1204-1215.

A12. Humbert M, McLaughlin V, Gibbs JSR, et al. Sotatercept for the treatment of pulmonary arterial hypertension: PULSAR open-label extension. *Eur Respir J*. 2023;61:2201347.

A13. Lajoie AC, Lauzière G, Lega JC, et al. Combination therapy versus monotherapy for pulmonary arterial hypertension: a meta-analysis. *Lancet Respir Med*. 2016;4:291-305.

A14. Galie N, Barbera JA, Frost AE, et al. Initial use of ambrisentan plus tadalafil in pulmonary arterial hypertension. *N Engl J Med*. 2015;373:834-844.

A15. Chin KM, Sitbon O, Doelberg M, et al. Three- versus two-drug therapy for patients with newly diagnosed pulmonary arterial hypertension. *J Am Coll Cardiol*. 2021;78:1393-1403.

A16. Ying M, Song J, Gu S, et al. Efficacy and safety of riociguat in the treatment of chronic thromboembolic pulmonary arterial hypertension: a meta-analysis. *Medicine (Baltimore)*. 2021;100:e26211.

70

ANTITHROMBOTIC AND ANTIPLATELET THERAPY

RICHARD C. BECKER AND THOMAS L. ORTEL

Antithrombotic therapy is a key component of the prevention and treatment of cardiovascular, cerebrovascular, and peripheral vascular diseases. These therapies include anticoagulation, which targets secondary hemostasis; antiplatelet agents, which target primary hemostasis; and fibrinolysis, which enhances natural fibrinolytic mechanisms. The therapies may be used individually or in combination, depending on the clinical setting.

ANTICOAGULANT THERAPY

Anticoagulant therapies are used for the prevention and treatment of venous and arterial thromboembolic events. Parenteral agents include heparin and related compounds, as well as two direct thrombin inhibitors (Table 70-1). Oral therapies include the vitamin K antagonists and direct oral anticoagulants (DOACs; Table 70-2).

PARENTERAL ANTICOAGULANTS

Parenteral anticoagulants include heparin, low-molecular-weight heparins, and fondaparinux.

Heparin

Unfractionated heparin, which is prepared from porcine intestine or bovine lung, is a heterogeneous mixture of negatively charged polysulfated glycosaminoglycans that range in size from 3000 to 30,000 daltons. Anticoagulant activity depends on a specific sequence of five sugar residues within the polysaccharide chain. Up to two thirds of the chains lack this sequence, however, and have minimal to no anticoagulant effect.

Heparin binds to the natural anticoagulant antithrombin through the pentasaccharide sequence, thereby inducing a conformational change that markedly enhances antithrombin's ability to inhibit thrombin, factor Xa, and other hemostatic proteinases. Factor Xa inhibition requires the pentasaccharide sequence only. In contrast, thrombin inactivation requires the pentasaccharide sequence and a minimal chain length of 18 sugar units to provide an essential docking surface for both inhibitor and enzyme. Unfractionated heparin binds

TABLE 70-1 PARENTERAL ANTICOAGULANT THERAPIES

	UNFRACTIONATED HEPARIN	LOW-MOLECULAR-WEIGHT HEPARIN*	FONDAPARINUX	BIVALIRUDIN	ARGATROBAN
Mechanism of action	Enhances AT-mediated inactivation of thrombin, factor Xa, and other serine proteinases	Primarily enhances AT-mediated inactivation of factor Xa with less effect on thrombin	Enhances AT-mediated inactivation of factor Xa with no effect on thrombin	Direct inhibition of thrombin	Direct inhibition of thrombin
Typical dosing	Treatment: 80 U/kg IV bolus then 15-18 u/kg/hr (see Table 68-6) Prophylaxis: 5000 U SQ 2 to 3 times daily	See Table 70-3	Treatment: 7.5 mg SQ daily (5 mg if <50 kg, 10 mg if >100 kg) Prophylaxis: 2.5 mg SQ daily (avoid if <50 kg)	Treatment: 0.75 mg/kg IV bolus, then 1.75 mg/kg/hr (for PCI)	Treatment: For heparin-induced thrombocytopenia, start at 2 μg/kg/min IV
Laboratory monitoring	aPTT, anti-factor Xa activity; ACT for selected indications	Usually not necessary, but can use anti-factor Xa activity	Usually not necessary, but can use anti-factor Xa activity	aPTT; dilute thrombin time	aPTT; dilute thrombin time
Plasma half-life	1-2 hr	See Table 70-3	17 hr	25 min	45 min
Reversal therapy	Protamine	Protamine partially effective	Protamine ineffective; factor VIIa can be used to treat the hemorrhagic event	Discontinue anticoagulant; no specific reversal agent available	Discontinue anticoagulant; no specific reversal agent available

*Includes enoxaparin and dalteparin.
ACT = activated clotting time; aPTT = activated partial thromboplastin time; AT = antithrombin; IV = intravenous; PCI = percutaneous coronary intervention; SQ = subcutaneous.

TABLE 70-2 ORAL ANTICOAGULANT THERAPIES

	WARFARIN	DABIGATRAN	RIVAROXABAN	APIXABAN	EDOXABAN
Mechanism of action	Vitamin K antagonist	Direct thrombin inhibition	Direct factor Xa inhibition	Direct factor Xa inhibition	Direct factor Xa inhibition
Bioavailability	Essentially 100%	6%	80%	50%	55%
Plasma half-life	~40 hr	14-17 hr	7-11 hr	8-14 hr	8-10 hr
Plasma protein binding (%)	99%	35%	92-95%	87%	40-59%
Clearance	Hepatic, primarily through CYP2C9	80% renal	~2/3 renal (half as unchanged drug and half metabolized by CYP 3A4); ~1/3 fecal	25% renal; remainder metabolized by CYP 3A4	50% renal (primarily unchanged)
Laboratory monitoring	Regular monitoring of the PT/INR required	Not necessary, but can check for drug with a modified thrombin time	Not necessary, but can check for drug with an anti-factor Xa assay	Not necessary, but can check for drug with an anti-factor Xa assay	Not necessary, but can check for drug with an anti-factor Xa assay
Drug interactions	Multiple*	Inducers/inhibitors of P-gp	Inducers/inhibitors of P-gp or CYP3A4	Inducers/inhibitors of P-gp or CYP3A4	Inducers/inhibitors of P-gp
Reversal therapy	Vitamin K, PCC, FFP	Idarucizumab	Andexanet-alfa	Andexanet-alfa	Andexanet-alfa

*Drugs associated with an increase in the INR, listed by class: antibiotics (azithromycin, clarithromycin, erythromycin, ciprofloxacin, levofloxacin, moxifloxacin, metronidazole, sulfamethoxazole, isoniazid); antifungal agents (fluconazole, itraconazole, voriconazole, miconazole); cardiovascular drugs (amiodarone, propafenone, propranolol, diltiazem, simvastatin, fluvastatin, fenofibrate, gemfibrozil, fish oil); central nervous system agents (sertraline, paroxetine, fluoxetine, fluvoxamine, citalopram, escitalopram, venlafaxine, desvenlafaxine, duloxetine, ropinirole, phenytoin); gastrointestinal medications (cimetidine, omeprazole); pain medications (aspirin, diclofenac, etodolac, ibuprofen, indomethacin, ketoprofen, naproxen, piroxicam, sulindac, nabumetone, celecoxib, acetaminophen); other agents (e.g., tamoxifen, testosterone, methotrexate); and herbal supplements (e.g., gingko biloba, garlic). Drugs associated with a decrease in the INR, listed by class: antibiotics (nafcillin, rifampin); central nervous system agents (carbamazepine, trazodone, phenobarbital, phenytoin); and herbal supplements (e.g., ginseng, St. John wort).
FFP = fresh frozen plasma; INR = international normalized ratio; PCC = prothrombin complex concentrate; P-gp = P-glycoprotein; PT = prothrombin time.

to multiple other circulating proteins and cell surfaces, thereby contributing to its variable anticoagulant effect.

DOSAGE AND MONITORING. Heparin is an effective anticoagulant for the prevention and initial treatment of venous thromboembolism (Chapter 68) and for the treatment of the acute coronary syndrome (Chapter 57) and myocardial infarction (Chapter 58). Prophylactic unfractionated heparin uses a fixed dose, typically 5000 units, administered subcutaneously two or three times a day, without laboratory monitoring. In contrast, therapeutic anticoagulation is administered intravenously using a weight-based algorithm, with an initial bolus of 80 units/kg followed by an infusion of 15 to 18 units/kg/hour. Therapeutic unfractionated heparin requires monitoring, typically with an activated partial thromboplastin time (aPTT) range of approximately 50 to 70 seconds for patients with the acute coronary syndrome or acute myocardial infarction but determined in each clinical laboratory to correlate with 0.3 to 0.7 anti-factor Xa units/mL in an assay specific for heparin for venous thromboembolism.

Heparin is also an effective anticoagulant for patients undergoing surgical procedures that require cardiopulmonary bypass, during vascular surgery, during extracorporeal membrane oxygenation (ECMO), with intra-aortic balloon pumps, and with coronary angioplasty and placement of a coronary stent. In these settings, the activated clot time is the best way to monitor heparin therapy.

ADVERSE EFFECTS. The most common complication associated with unfractionated heparin is bleeding, which is influenced by the dose and duration of therapy as well as by any additional risk factors specific to the patient (e.g., concomitant thrombocytopenia or coagulopathy, recent surgery, presence of ex vivo circuits such as ECMO). Major bleeding is rarely encountered in patients who receive prophylactic unfractionated heparin, but it occurs in up to 3% of patients who receive therapeutic unfractionated heparin.

Less common complications associated with unfractionated heparin are heparin-induced thrombocytopenia and osteopenia. Heparin-induced thrombocytopenia (Chapter 158), which is an immune complication that develops in response to circulating complexes of heparin and platelet factor 4, is associated with the development of thrombotic complications despite the thrombocytopenia. Osteoporosis can develop in patients who receive unfractionated heparin over a prolonged period of time, such as women during the course of a pregnancy.

REVERSING THE ANTICOAGULANT EFFECT. Protamine sulfate is a positively charged protein that forms a complex with heparin, thereby neutralizing its anticoagulant effect. Protamine sulfate (1 mg per 100 units of unfractionated heparin, with a maximum dose of 50 mg) has a short half-life (about 7 minutes), and repeated doses may be necessary for complete reversal. Protamine sulfate can be associated with a hypersensitivity reaction, including anaphylaxis, in patients with recurrent exposures, fish allergies, or prior exposure to protamine-containing drugs (e.g., NPH insulin).

Low-Molecular-Weight Heparins

The low-molecular-weight heparins (LMWHs) are smaller fragments produced by chemical or enzymatic depolymerization of unfractionated heparin. Chain lengths range from 4 to 22 monosaccharide units, so these agents primarily inhibit factor Xa and have less effect on thrombin. The LMWHs also exhibit reduced binding to plasma proteins and endothelial surfaces, thereby resulting in increased bioavailability compared with unfractionated heparin. The LMWHs are administered subcutaneously, have a half-life of 3 to 5 hours, and are primarily excreted by the kidney (Table 70-3).

The LMWHs are safe and effective for the prevention and treatment of venous thromboembolism (Chapter 68). For cancer-associated venous thromboembolism (Chapters 67 and 68), they are safer and more effective compared with warfarin and are somewhat less effective but safer than direct oral anticoagulants.[A1,A2] They also have been used in patients with acute coronary syndrome and acute myocardial infarction (Chapter 57). LMWHs do not cross the placenta and are therefore safe and effective during pregnancy. Patients who receive LMWHs are significantly less likely to develop heparin-induced thrombocytopenia than are patients who receive unfractionated heparin, but LMWH should not be used in patients who have acutely developed heparin-induced thrombocytopenia while receiving unfractionated heparin because of the risk of cross-reactive antiplatelet factor 4/heparin antibodies.

Laboratory monitoring is typically not necessary for patients treated with LMWHs, although anti-factor Xa testing may be useful in select situations (e.g., patients with renal insufficiency or to confirm adherence). Protamine sulfate partially reverses the anticoagulant effect of LMWH, but protamine sulfate is less effective in reversing the anticoagulant effect of LMWH compared with unfractionated heparin.

Fondaparinux

Fondaparinux is a synthetic pentasaccharide designed for the binding sequence of antithrombin. Fondaparinux binds antithrombin with high affinity and inactivates factor Xa; because of its short chain length, it has no inhibitory activity against thrombin. Fondaparinux is administered once daily subcutaneously (7.5 mg for a 50- to 100-kg patient; 5 mg if lighter, 10 mg if heavier), has a

TABLE 70-3 ANTICOAGULANT PROFILES, MOLECULAR WEIGHTS, PLASMA HALF-LIVES, AND RECOMMENDED DOSES OF COMMERCIAL LOW-MOLECULAR-WEIGHT HEPARINS AND HEPARINOID

		RECOMMENDED DOSE (INTERNATIONAL ANTI-XA UNITS)§		
AGENT	PLASMA HALF-LIFE (MIN)	GENERAL SURGERY PROPHYLAXIS	ORTHOPEDIC SURGERY PROPHYLAXIS	ACUTE TREATMENT
Enoxaparin	130-180	4000 U SQ daily	4000 U SQ daily or 3000 U SQ bid	7000 U SQ bid*† or 10,500 U SQ daily*
Dalteparin	120-139	5000 U SQ daily	2500 U SQ bid or 5000 U SQ daily	8400 U SQ bid for acute coronary syndromes or 7000 U SQ bid or 14,000 U SQ daily for venous thromboembolism*
Nadroparin	130-162	2850 U SQ daily	2700 U SQ daily,* 4000 U SQ daily* from day 4	13,300 U SQ daily*
Tinzaparin	110	3500 U SQ daily	3500 U SQ daily* or 4500 U SQ daily*	12,250 U daily*
Ardeparin	200	50 U/kg SQ bid		
Danaparoid‡	1100	750 U SQ bid	750 U SQ bid	2500 U IV, then 4 hr each of 400 U/hr and 300 U/hr, then 200 U/hr; or 2000 U SQ bid

*Weight-adjusted dose; stated dose for 70-kg patient.
†The twice-daily dose is for acute coronary syndromes; either twice-daily (preferred) or once-daily dosing is for venous thromboembolism.
‡Danaparoid sodium is a heparinoid.
§Dosing of low-molecular-weight heparins and heparinoid is based on international units (IU or U), representing anti-Xa activity. In the case of enoxaparin only, the conversion of U to mg is simple: 1 mg inhibits 100 anti-Xa units, so dosing of enoxaparin can be prescribed as either 1 mg or 100 U, for example.
bid = twice daily; IV = intravenously; SQ = subcutaneously.
From Schulman S, Levin GN. Antithrombotic and antiplatelet therapy. In: Goldman L, Schafer AI, eds. *Goldman-Cecil Medicine*. 26th ed. Philadelphia: Elsevier; 2020:496.

bioavailability of 100%, has a long terminal half-life (17-21 hours), and is primarily excreted by the kidney (see Table 70-1).

Fondaparinux is approved for the prevention of venous thromboembolism in surgical patients and treatment of acute deep venous thrombosis and pulmonary embolus (Chapter 68).[A3] Off-label, it can be used in patients with heparin-induced thrombocytopenia,[1] although rare cases of fondaparinux-induced thrombocytopenia have been described. Laboratory monitoring is typically not necessary, but an anti-factor Xa assay can be used to detect circulating drug. Protamine sulfate is not effective in reversing the anti-factor Xa effect of fondaparinux. Recombinant factor VIIa has been used in patients with fondaparinux-related bleeding, but there is an increased risk for thromboembolic complications with this approach.

PARENTERAL DIRECT THROMBIN INHIBITORS

The direct thrombin inhibitors inhibit thrombin without the need for antithrombin (see Table 70-1). Argatroban, which is a synthetic molecule derived from the amino acid L-arginine, reversibly inhibits thrombin by binding to the enzyme's active site. Argatroban is useful for prophylaxis or treatment of thrombosis in patients who have developed heparin-induced thrombocytopenia.[2] It is administered intravenously (starting at 2 µg/kg/min for heparin-induced thrombocytopenia) and monitored by the aPTT. The drug is primarily cleared by the liver and should be used with caution, or avoided, in patients with hepatic insufficiency. Argatroban can be used in patients with renal failure.

Bivalirudin is an analog of hirudin, which is a thrombin inhibitor isolated from leeches. Bivalirudin binds to both the active and fibrin-binding sites of thrombin in patients undergoing percutaneous coronary intervention who have, or are at risk for, heparin-induced thrombocytopenia. Bivalirudin has also been used as an alternative to heparin in patients who require mechanical circulatory support. It is administered intravenously (typically starting with an intravenous bolus of 0.75 mg/kg followed by 1.75 mg/kg/hour for percutaneous coronary intervention) and monitored by an aPTT targeted to a ratio of 1.5 to 2.5 times the patient's baseline or the upper boundary of the reference range. Bivalirudin is primarily cleared by the kidneys and by enzymatic degradation; it can be used in patients with hepatic insufficiency.

Argatroban and bivalirudin have short half-lives, and their anticoagulant effects resolve quickly once the infusion is discontinued. No specific reversal agents are available.

ORAL ANTICOAGULANTS

Vitamin K Antagonists

Vitamin K is an essential cofactor for post-translational γ-carboxylation of glutamate residues that are located within the vitamin K–dependent proteins. This post-translational modification is necessary for normal function of coagulation factors II, VII, IX, and X, as well as proteins C, S, and Z. The vitamin K antagonists interfere with the cyclic conversion of vitamin K and its 2,3-epoxide by vitamin K epoxide reductase, thereby inhibiting the regeneration of the reduced form of vitamin K and blocking post-translational γ-carboxylation. The resulting coagulation factors are dysfunctional, thereby resulting in the observed anticoagulant effect.

Warfarin, which is the most commonly used vitamin K antagonist, is rapidly absorbed in the proximal gastrointestinal tract and has a circulating half-life of about 40 hours. The duration of its anticoagulant effect depends on the synthesis of new coagulation proteins. Factor VII has the shortest half-life (about 4 to 6 hours), so its level drops first after the initiation of warfarin. In contrast, factor II (also called prothrombin), has a half-life of 2 to 3 days, and its level does not begin to decrease until after several days of therapy. Since decreased factor II levels are most important for clinical efficacy, warfarin's benefits are delayed for several days after it is initiated.

Warfarin is an effective anticoagulant for the prevention and treatment of thromboembolism for multiple clinical indications, including venous thromboembolism and thromboembolic events originating from atrial fibrillation or cardiac valve replacement. However, the direct oral anticoagulants (DOACs) have largely replaced warfarin, except for patients who have prosthetic cardiac valves or conditions such as high-risk antiphospholipid syndrome, for which vitamin K antagonists are still the anticoagulant of choice.

DOSAGE AND MONITORING. Warfarin has a narrow therapeutic index, and its effects must be monitored to prevent recurrent thromboembolism if subtherapeutic or bleeding if supratherapeutic. Monitoring is performed with the prothrombin time (PT), reported as an international normalized ratio (INR). The target INR for most clinical indications is 2.5 (range, 2 to 3), but the target INR is 3.0 (range, 2.5 to 3.5) for patients with a mechanical prosthetic heart valve in the mitral position. The PT can be checked on a blood sample drawn by phlebotomy or on a capillary specimen obtained by fingerstick. A typical starting dose would be 5 mg daily with an initial INR level checked at 3 days after initiation of therapy, then daily depending on the result until the INR is in range (with dose modifications as needed; Table 70-4), then in 1 to 2 weeks, and then every 4 weeks when a stable dose is reached. Polymorphisms in the genes encoding for vitamin K epoxide reductase complex 1 (*vitamin K epoxide reductase C1*) and the CYP2C9 enzyme are associated with lower dosage requirements, but dosing based on such data has been no better than standard therapy.[A4]

The INR, which is most sensitive to the level of factor VII, usually can reach its therapeutic range before the level of factor II, which is most important for efficacy, has declined sufficiently for true therapeutic efficacy. As a result, 4 to 5 days of therapy are typically required to achieve a full therapeutic effect. Patients who are started on warfarin for the treatment of acute thromboembolism must be started concomitantly on heparin, which should be continued until the INR is in the target therapeutic range for 2 days.

Factors that can adversely impact the INR include adherence, changes in the intake of vitamin K, other medications (see Table 70-2, footnote), and comorbid conditions. Accurate point-of-care testing using capillary blood obtained by fingerstick has enabled more frequent self-testing, more time in therapeutic range, and likely better clinical outcomes.

ADVERSE EFFECTS. The median rate of major bleeding for patients who are taking a vitamin K antagonist for atrial fibrillation therapy is about 2.51 bleeds per 100 patient years, and the most common bleeding site is the gastrointestinal tract. The risk of bleeding associated with the use of a vitamin K antagonist increases as the INR becomes increasingly supratherapeutic. The risk of bleeding also increases in patients whose INR results are difficult to manage, patients who concomitantly take aspirin or other antiplatelet therapies, older patients, and patients with comorbid conditions such as liver disease or thrombocytopenia.

REVERSING THE ANTICOAGULANT EFFECT. For asymptomatic patients with an isolated elevated INR, simply decreasing the dose or withholding the vitamin K antagonist for 1 to 2 days is appropriate (Table 70-5). Since this approach depends on the synthesis of new factors, it takes a few days to have an impact on the INR. For INR results that are markedly elevated, reversal can be augmented by supplementation with vitamin K (2.5 to 5.0 mg orally). For patients with hemorrhagic complications, urgent normalization can be achieved by augmenting vitamin K therapy with 4-factor prothrombin complex concentrates (pretreatment INR 2 to <4, 25 units/kg, not to exceed 2500 units; pretreatment INR 4 to 6, 35 units/kg, not to exceed 3500 units; pretreatment INR >6, 50 units/kg, not to exceed 5000 units), which contain factors VII, IX, X, and II, and which are more effective than fresh frozen plasma for this purpose.

TABLE 70-4 WARFARIN DOSE PROTOCOL

1. ACHIEVING A THERAPEUTIC RANGE

DAY	INR	RECOMMENDED DOSE (MG)
1		5
2		5
3	<1.5	10
	1.5-1.9	5
	2.0-3.0	2.5
	>3.0	0
4	<1.5	10
	1.5-1.9	7.5
	2.0-3.0	5
	3.0-4.0	2.5
	>4.0	0
5	<1.5	10
	1.5-1.9	7.5
	2.0-3.0	5
	3.0-4.0	2.5
	>4.0	0
6	<1.5	12.5
	1.5-1.9	10
	2.0-3.0	5
	3.0-4.0	2.5
	>4.0	0

2. INR-INTERNATIONAL NORMALIZED RATIO GOAL

2 to 3	target 2.5	Venous thromboembolism (treatment and prevention), atrial fibrillation, bioprosthetic heart valve
2.5 to 3.5	target 3.0	Mechanical prosthetic heart valve (except low-risk patients with bileaflet aortic valves) Anti-phospholipid syndrome with recurrent thromboembolism

INR = international normalized ratio.

Direct Oral Anticoagulants

The direct oral anticoagulants (DOACs) are small molecules that specifically inhibit either thrombin or factor Xa (Table 70-2). Because of their efficacy, safety, and ease of use, direct oral anticoagulants, often with dose adjustments, have largely replaced warfarin for most clinical indications.[3,4]

Direct Thrombin Inhibitors

Dabigatran etexilate is an oral prodrug that is rapidly converted by serum esterases to dabigatran, which is a potent, reversible, direct thrombin inhibitor (Table 70-6). It has a rapid onset of action, a 14- to 17-hour half-life, and is predominantly cleared by the kidney. Dabigatran's serum concentration may be affected by drugs that induce or inhibit the P-glycoprotein transporter (e.g., dronedarone, systemic ketoconazole), but the interactions are generally minor.

Dabigatran is non-inferior to warfarin for the prevention of stroke and systemic thromboembolism in patients with non-valvular atrial fibrillation,[5] with less bleeding at the 110-mg daily dose. Dabigatran is as effective as warfarin for the treatment of acute venous thromboembolism. In this setting, treatment should start with a parenteral anticoagulant (e.g., unfractionated heparin or LMWH) for 5 days prior to starting therapy with dabigatran (see Table 70-6). Dabigatran is also effective for extended prevention of recurrent venous thromboembolism, and it is as effective as enoxaparin for the prevention of venous thromboembolism in patients undergoing total hip arthroplasty or total knee arthroplasty, with a similar safety profile. As with other direct oral anticoagulants, however, dabigatran cannot substitute for warfarin in patients with prosthetic cardiac valves. Dabigatran should generally be avoided in patients who have atrial fibrillation and renal insufficiency (creatinine clearance <30 mL/minute), although a lower dose (75 mg twice daily) is available for patients with a creatinine clearance of 15-30 mL/minute.

DOSAGE AND MONITORING. Dabigatran is taken twice daily without regard to food, but the dose varies by indication. Dabigatran is primarily absorbed in the lower stomach and duodenum, and bariatric gastric bypass procedures may decrease absorption.[6] Laboratory monitoring is not necessary. The INR and aPTT may be prolonged, but the degree of prolongation correlates poorly with the drug concentration. The thrombin time is the most useful screening assay for detection of an anticoagulant effect (e.g., suspected drug overdose, acute trauma, need for emergent surgery).

ADVERSE EFFECTS. Dyspepsia, which is a frequent side effect, can be decreased by taking the drug with food. The risk for major bleeding, particularly for intracranial bleeding, is less than with warfarin and is comparable to the bleeding risk associated with the other direct oral anticoagulants. Gastrointestinal bleeding occurs more frequently with dabigatran, possibly related to the pill's tartaric acid content, which is designed to increase absorption.

REVERSAL OF THE ANTICOAGULANT EFFECT. Idarucizumab, which is a humanized monoclonal antibody fragment developed to specifically reverse

TABLE 70-5 REVERSAL STRATEGIES FOR ANTICOAGULANT THERAPY WITH VITAMIN K ANTAGONISTS

INR	CLINICAL MANIFESTATIONS	INTERVENTION
<5.0	None	Decrease or withhold 1 dose, recheck INR within 1-2 weeks
5.0-9.9	None	Decrease or withhold 1-2 doses, recheck INR within 1-2 weeks
≥10	None	Withhold VKA, consider oral vitamin K (2.5 to 5.0 mg), and recheck INR within 2-3 days; resume VKA when INR in therapeutic range with an appropriate dose adjustment
Any	Serious bleeding	Withhold VKA, give vitamin K (10 mg IV or orally), and consider supplementation with 4-factor PCCs (pretreatment INR 2 to <4, 25 units/kg, not to exceed 2500 units; pretreatment INR 4 to 6, 35 units/kg, not to exceed 3500 units; pretreatment INR >6, 50 units/kg, not to exceed 5000 units), FFP, or recombinant factor VIIa*; recheck INR within 24 hours
Any	Life-threatening bleeding	Withhold VKA, administer 4-factor PCCs (same as above), FFP (1-2 units), or recombinant factor VIIa (approximately 16 μg/kg),* supplemented with vitamin K (10 mg IV or orally)

*Recombinant factor VIIa can be associated with thromboembolic events when used in this setting and should be used only when PCCs or FFP are not available.

FFP = fresh frozen plasma; INR = international normalized ratio; IV = intravenously; PCCs = prothrombin complex concentrates; VKA = vitamin K antagonist.

Adapted from Ansell J, Hirsh J, Hylek E, et al. Pharmacology and management of the vitamin K antagonists: American College of Chest Physicians Evidence-Based Clinical Practice Guidelines (8th edition). *Chest.* 2008;133:160S-198S.

TABLE 70-6 DIRECT-ACTING ORAL ANTICOAGULANTS

	DABIGATRAN	RIVAROXABAN	APIXABAN	EDOXABAN
Mechanism of action	Direct factor IIa (thrombin) inhibitor	Direct factor Xa inhibitor	Direct Xa inhibitor	Direct factor Xa inhibitor
DOSING				
Acute phase (within the first 1-3 weeks of diagnosis)	Initial therapy with a parenteral anticoagulant for at least 5 days	Initial therapy is 15 mg twice daily for 21 days	Initial therapy is 10 mg twice daily for 7 days	Initial therapy with a parenteral anticoagulant for 5-10 days
Treatment phase (following acute phase, and continuing for 3-6 months from diagnosis	150 mg twice daily	20 mg daily	5 mg twice daily	60 mg once daily (30 mg once daily if weight ≤60 kg)
Extended thromboprophylaxis (following treatment phase and typically lasting indefinitely)	Same as for treatment phase	10 or 20 mg daily	2.5 or 5 mg twice daily	Same as for treatment phase
Atrial fibrillation (indefinite duration)	150 mg or 110 mg twice daily	20 mg daily	5 mg twice daily	60 mg or 30 mg daily
VTE prevention after knee or hip replacement surgery (14-30 days)	110 mg (initial dose) then 220 mg daily	10 mg daily	2.5 mg twice daily	Not applicable
RENAL ADJUSTMENT				
Creatinine clearance in mL/min				
>95	No dose adjustment	No dose adjustment	No dose adjustment	Avoid
50-95	"	"	"	No dose adjustment
30-49	"	"	2.5 mg twice daily for AF	"
15-29	Avoid	Avoid	"	30 mg
<15	"	"	"	Avoid
KEY DRUG INTERACTIONS				
Increase levels	Amiodarone, quinidine, azole antifungals (e.g., ketoconazole), ritonavir	Azole antifungals (e.g., ketoconazole), ritonavir, clarithromycin		
Decrease levels	Rifampin	Anticonvulsants (e.g., phenytoin, carbamazepine), rifampin		
Antidote	Idarucizumab (5 gm intravenously)	Andexanet alfa (see Table 70-7)		
Laboratory monitoring	Not necessary, but can check for drug with a modified thrombin time	Not necessary, but can check for drug with an anti-factor Xa assay		

the effect of dabigatran,[7] irreversibly binds dabigatran, with an affinity about 350-fold higher than the affinity of dabigatran for thrombin. Administration of idarucizumab (5 g intravenously, provided as two separate vials of 2.5 g/50 mL infused consecutively) normalizes dabigatran-induced prolongation of the thrombin time within minutes in a dose-dependent fashion.

Direct Factor Xa Inhibitors

Several direct oral anticoagulants that specifically target factor Xa include rivaroxaban, apixaban, and edoxaban (see Table 70-6). Although these agents share some characteristics, each also has unique characteristics that may make one more attractive than the others in certain situations.

Each of the factor Xa inhibitors is as effective as warfarin for the treatment of acute venous thromboembolism, with a risk for bleeding that ranges from similar to slightly lower than with warfarin.[8] These agents are also effective for the treatment and secondary prophylaxis of venous thromboembolism in patients with cancer, in which they are more effective than LMWH but associated with somewhat more bleeding.[A5,9] The factor Xa inhibitors also are noninferior or superior to warfarin for the prevention of ischemic stroke and systemic thromboembolism in patients with non-valvular atrial fibrillation,[10] except edoxaban is not as good as warfarin for patients with a creatinine clearance greater than 95 mL/min.

Rivaroxaban (10 or 20 mg daily) and apixaban (2.5 or 5.0 mg twice daily) are effective for extended thromboprophylaxis in patients with venous thromboembolism. Rivaroxaban (10 mg daily) and apixaban (2.5 mg twice daily) are effective for thromboprophylaxis following total hip or total knee arthroplasty (duration for a minimum of 10 to 14 days, extending up to 35 days). In patients with stable coronary artery disease, rivaroxaban (2.5 mg twice daily) combined with aspirin can decrease the frequency of major vascular events compared to aspirin alone, although it is associated with an increased risk for major bleeding,[A6] and this combination also is better than aspirin alone in preventing adverse limb events in patients with lower extremity peripheral arterial disease (Chapter 65).[A7] For hospitalized medically ill patients, an extended post-discharge course of rivaroxaban (10mg daily for 45 days) decreases the risk for fatal and major thromboembolic events without significantly increasing major bleeding.[A8] Rivaroxaban, apixaban, and dabigatran have all been used off-label as an alternative anticoagulant for patients with heparin-induced thrombocytopenia. Rivaroxaban is less effective than warfarin in high-risk patients with antiphospholipid syndrome, however.[A9]

DOSAGE AND MONITORING. Rivaroxaban is administered once daily for all indications, except during the first 21 days of treatment of acute venous thromboembolism and for patients with coronary artery disease or peripheral arterial disease, in whom it is administered twice daily. The drug is rapidly absorbed, primarily in the stomach and small intestine, with a time to peak effect of 2 to 4 hours. It is best absorbed when taken with food. It is metabolized by CYP3A4 and should be avoided in patients being treated with strong inducers or inhibitors of P-glycoprotein or CYP3A4, such as carbamazepine, phenytoin, rifampin, systemic ketoconazole, or ritonavir. Approximately two thirds of the drug is excreted in the urine (half unchanged and half as inactive metabolites), so it should be avoided in patients with severe renal insufficiency (creatinine clearance <15-30 mL/min). Rivaroxaban is highly protein-bound in the circulation and is not removed by hemodialysis.

Apixaban is administered twice daily for all clinical indications and can be taken with or without food. It is rapidly absorbed, primarily in the upper gastrointestinal tract, with a time to peak effect of 3 to 4 hours. It is primarily eliminated by metabolism by CYP3A4 and other cytochromes to inactive metabolites, and it should be avoided in patients being treated with strong inhibitors or inducers of the P450 system. Approximately 25% of the drug is excreted in the urine, the remainder in the feces. For the prevention and treatment of venous thromboembolism, no dose adjustment is necessary for renal insufficiency. For the treatment of atrial fibrillation,

TABLE 70-7 DOSING AND ADMINISTRATION OF ANDEXANET ALFA*

		TIME FROM LAST DOSE OF FACTOR XA INHIBITOR	
FACTOR XA INHIBITOR	LAST DOSE OF FACTOR XA INHIBITOR	<8 HOURS OR UNKNOWN	≥8 HOURS
Apixaban	≤5 mg >5 mg or unknown	Low-dose andexanet alfa High-dose andexanet alfa	Low-dose andexanet alfa
Rivaroxaban	≤10 mg >10 mg or unknown	Low-dose andexanet alfa High-dose andexanet alfa	

*Low-dose andexanet alfa: initial 400 mg IV bolus administered at a target rate of about 30 mg/min, followed within 2 minutes by continuous IV infusion of 4 mg/min for up to 120 minutes.
High-dose andexanet alfa: initial 800 mg IV bolus administered at a target rate of about 30 mg/min, followed within 2 minutes by continuous IV infusion of 8 mg/min for up to 120 minutes.
For patients receiving edoxaban, enoxaparin, or other low-molecular-weight heparins, the high-dose andexanet alfa dosing has been used.

TABLE 70-8 ANTIPLATELET AGENTS

DRUG	CLOPIDOGREL	PRASUGREL	TICAGRELOR	CANGRELOR	TIROFIBAN	EPTIFIBATIDE	VORAPAXAR
Prodrug	Yes	Yes	No	No	No	No	No
Route	Oral	Oral	Oral	Intravenous	Intravenous	Intravenous	Oral
Mechanism of action	$P2Y_{12}$ inhibition	$P2Y_{12}$ inhibition	$P2Y_{12}$ inhibition	$P2Y_{12}$ inhibition	GPIIb/IIIa inhibition	GPIIb/IIIa inhibition	PAR-1 inhibition
Onset of action	2–6 hr	30 min	30 min	2 min	<15 min	<15 min	1–2 hr
Duration of action	3-10 days	7-10 days	3-5 days	1-2 hr	4-8 hr	4-8 hr	2-3 wk
Withdrawal before surgery	5 days	7 days	5 days	1 hr	8 hr	8 hr	12 hr
Loading dose	300-600 mg	60 mg	180 mg	30 μg/kg	25 μg/kg	180 μg/kg	NA
Regular dose	75 mg daily	10 mg daily	90 mg twice daily	4 μg/kg/min infusion	0.15 μg/kg/min infusion	2 μg/kg/min infusion	2.5 mg twice daily

GP = glycoprotein.

the dose should be reduced to 2.5 mg twice daily for patients with a serum creatinine ≥1.5 mg/dL and either age ≥80 years or body weight ≤60 kg. As with rivaroxaban, apixaban is highly protein-bound and not removed by hemodialysis.

Edoxaban is administered once daily and can be taken with or without food. It is rapidly absorbed, primarily in the proximal small intestine, with a time to peak effect of 1 to 2 hours. Absorption is dependent on acidic solubility. Edoxaban has negligible CYP450 metabolism, but inducers or inhibitors of P-glycoprotein (e.g., rifampin, systemic ketoconazole, and clarithromycin) can affect serum concentrations. Approximately 50% of the drug is excreted by the kidney, primarily unchanged. The dose should be reduced in patients with moderate renal insufficiency (creatinine clearance 15 to 50 mL/minute), and edoxaban should be avoided in patients with severe renal insufficiency (creatinine clearance <15 mL/minute).

Several notable differences must be noted among these three direct oral anticoagulants when initiating therapy. As for dabigatran, edoxaban requires an initial lead-in phase with heparin or a LMWH before starting it for an acute indication. In contrast, rivaroxaban and apixaban do not require co-therapy with LMWH or heparin if started at a higher dose for 7 days (apixaban) or 21 days (rivaroxaban).

ADVERSE EFFECTS. Other than bleeding, the direct factor Xa inhibitors are associated with relatively few adverse events. Compared with warfarin, the risk for major bleeding is less, particularly for intracranial bleeding, but the risk of gastrointestinal hemorrhage is increased with rivaroxaban[11] and the risk of menstrual bleeding is increased, particularly with rivaroxaban.[12]

REVERSAL OF THE ANTICOAGULANT EFFECT. For most patients who have bleeding complications with the factor Xa inhibitors, simply withholding the drug and providing supportive measures is sufficient. For severe hemorrhagic complications, however, andexanet alfa (a modified recombinant form of factor Xa that is enzymatically inactive but binds to and rapidly neutralizes the factor Xa inhibitors) is effective within 12 hours against the oral factor Xa inhibitors as well as against enoxaparin and fondaparinux (Table 70-7).[13] If andexanet alfa is not available, 4-factor prothrombin complex concentrates (2000 units once, or 25 to 50 units/kg once) can be used as a nonspecific pro-hemostatic alternative.[14]

Anticoagulant Strategies in Development

Several promising strategies that target factor XI are in development based on the concept that factor XI is important for thrombosis but not hemostasis.[15] Decreasing factor XI levels with an antisense oligonucleotide provides effective prophylaxis against postoperative venous thromboembolism in patients undergoing elective primary unilateral total knee arthroplasty.[A10] Direct inhibition of factor Xia with a fully human monoclonal antibody[A11] or with a small molecule inhibitor[A12] also can prevent postoperative venous thromboembolism in patients undergoing total knee arthroplasty.

ANTIPLATELET THERAPY

The development of antiplatelet drugs for clinical use has closely followed an understanding of platelet surface receptors that, under specific conditions, are activated, thereby resulting in platelet adhesion and aggregation, assembly of coagulation proteins, and the formation of thrombus encased in a fibrin meshwork (Table 70-8). No direct antagonist can reverse their effects, so treatment of bleeding relies on platelet transfusions (usually 1 U platelets, except 2 U for P2Y12 inhibitors and glycoprotein [GP] IIb/IIIa inhibitors) and desmopressin (0.3 μg/kg every 12 hours). Cryoprecipitate (1 unit per 10 kg body weight) also can be administered in GP IIb/IIIa-related bleeding.

Aspirin

Aspirin represents a mainstay for the prevention and treatment of atherosclerotic vascular events, including ischemic stroke (Chapter 376), acute coronary syndrome (Chapter 57), chronic coronary disease (Chapter 56), and peripheral arterial disease (Chapter 65).

PHARMACOLOGY. Aspirin irreversibly acetylates cyclooxygenase (COX), thereby impairing the metabolism of prostaglandin and the synthesis of thromboxane A_2. Aspirin is rapidly absorbed in the stomach and duodenum, and it achieves peak levels within 15 to 20 minutes and platelet inhibition within 40 to 60 minutes after administration. Despite the drug's rapid clearance (20 minutes), platelet inhibition persists for the platelet's life span (7 ± 2 days) owing to aspirin's irreversible inactivation of COX-1. For cardiovascular protection, 81 mg per day[A13] is as effective as higher doses and is associated with less bleeding.

USES. Although all patients may achieve reasonably similar relative benefits from aspirin for preventing vascular events, the risks of bleeding increase with age. Aspirin's net beneficial effect is determined by the patient's absolute risk of vascular events and of bleeding based on patient-specific underlying conditions. Patients who have a low absolute risk derive minimal absolute benefit, whereas patients at high risk (e.g., with acute coronary syndrome, chronic coronary syndrome, percutaneous coronary intervention, or ischemic stroke) derive greater benefit. Aspirin (81 mg) is also useful to reduce the likelihood of developing colorectal cancer (Chapter 179).A14

PRIMARY PREVENTION OF VASCULAR EVENTS. The benefit-to-risk ratio for aspirin at a dose of 75 to 100 mg daily becomes favorable when the 10-year atherosclerotic cardiovascular disease risk ≥10%, despite the increased risk of bleeding.[16] As a result, aspirin may be beneficial for the primary prevention of MI and stroke in persons who have not achieved optimal control of risk factors for atherosclerotic cardiovascular disease. However, prophylactic aspirin is not recommended for primary prevention in adults over age 70 years because of the risks of bleeding.A15

SECONDARY PREVENTION OF VASCULAR EVENTS. Aspirin is a first-line antiplatelet agent for secondary presentation and a routine component of dual antiplatelet regimens that are useful after an acute coronary syndrome (Chapter 57), with or without percutaneous coronary intervention (Chapter 59).A16

Acute Coronary Syndrome. The duration of dual antiplatelet therapy after an acute coronary syndrome (Chapter 57) is based on the risk of ischemic compared with the risk of bleeding.[17] In general, patients who are at low and intermediate risk for bleeding are often treated up to 12 months, whereas patients at high or very high risk for bleeding may be treated for 1 to 3 months. Extended dual antiplatelet therapy beyond 1 year should be considered for patients at high risk for ischemic and thrombotic events, including patients with diabetes mellitus, recurrent myocardial infarction, concomitant inflammatory or autoimmune disease, chronic kidney disease, left main coronary artery disease, bifurcating stents, or a history of stent thrombosis.

Chronic Coronary Artery Syndrome. Aspirin can reduce vascular events in a wide variety of high-risk patients. Antiplatelet therapy (predominantly aspirin) reduces nonfatal myocardial infarction and non-fatal stroke by approximately one-third and vascular death by about 25%.

Coronary Artery Bypass Grafting and Percutaneous Coronary Intervention. Aspirin is recommended after internal thoracic and other coronary arterial bypass grafting. Dual antiplatelet therapy is recommended after off-pump CABG.[18] Recommendations for percutaneous coronary intervention include aspirin prior to and after the procedure. For patients unable to tolerate aspirin, pretreatment with clopidogrel (600 mg oral loading dose followed by 75 mg daily) is suggested. Dual antiplatelet therapy with aspirin and a P2Y12 receptor agonist is now usually recommended for only 1 to 3 months after insertion of a polymer-free drug-eluting stent.

Peripheral Artery Disease. Although proven to reduce cardiovascular mortality in atherosclerotic cardiovascular disease, the data for aspirin in peripheral arterial disease (Chapter 65) are less robust. Current recommendations are antiplatelet therapy with aspirin alone (75 to 325 mg per day) or clopidogrel alone (75 mg per day) to reduce MI, stroke, and vascular death in patients with symptomatic peripheral arterial disease.

ADVERSE EFFECTS. The principal adverse effect of aspirin is bleeding, especially upper gastrointestinal bleeding. These risks are lower with lower doses of aspirin (75 to 100 mg daily) and with aspirin monotherapy compared with dual antiplatelet therapy. Bleeding risks are higher in patients who have a prior history of acid-peptic disease or gastrointestinal bleeding or who have a coagulopathy, thrombocytopenia, chronic kidney or liver disease, or poorly controlled hypertension. Salicylate toxicity (Chapter 96), whether an intentional overdose or unintentional, is a life-threatening emergency.

Platelet $P2Y_{12}$ Receptor Antagonists

The density of $P2Y_{12}$ receptors on the platelet surface, coupled with their active role in platelet activation and aggregation makes this receptor an attractive target for pharmacologic inhibition. Clopidogrel (75 mg once daily), prasugrel (10 mg once daily), and ticagrelor (90 mg twice daily) are oral inhibitors of the platelet-stimulatory ADP receptor ($P2Y_{12}$), whereas cangrelor is administered intravenously. Clopidogrel and prasugrel bind irreversibly to platelet $P2Y_{12}$ receptor, whereas ticagrelor and cangrelor bind to it reversibly.

PHARMACOLOGY. Clopidogrel is rapidly absorbed following oral administration with peak levels of the predominant circulating metabolite occurring 60 minutes later. As a pro-drug, it is extensively metabolized in the liver to an active compound with a plasma elimination half-life of 7.7 ± 2.3 hours. Dose-dependent inhibition of ADP-mediated platelet aggregation is observed several hours after a single oral dose of clopidogrel.

Prasugrel is a prodrug that undergoes rapid de-esterification to an intermediate thiolactone, which is then converted to the active metabolite via a single CYP-dependent step. Maximal concentrations of prasugrel's active metabolite are reached within 0.5 hours after oral administration. After discontinuation, platelet aggregation returns to pretreatment levels within 7 to 10 days.

Ticagrelor, unlike clopidogrel and prasugrel, does not require metabolic activation or conversion for platelet inhibition. It is rapidly absorbed, and 60 to 80% inhibition of ADP-induced platelet aggregation is achieved 2 to 4 hours after a 180 mg loading dose. Its plasma half-life is 6 to 13 hours, so twice-daily administration is required.

Cangrelor intravenously acts within 20 minutes to achieve high-level inhibition of ADP-induced platelet aggregation. Cangrelor occupies the platelet $P2Y_{12}$ binding site, thereby precluding the binding and pharmacodynamic effect of clopidogrel and prasugrel but not of ticagrelor. Following rapid dephosphorylation, it is excreted in urine (58%) and feces (35%), with an average half-life of 3 to 6 minutes.

CLINICAL USES. Monotherapy with $P2Y_{12}$ inhibition provides essentially the same benefit and risks as aspirin monotherapy. As a result, $P2Y_{12}$ monotherapy is generally limited to patients who have an aspirin allergy or situations in which dual antiplatelet therapy is indicated for secondary prevention in patients with established cardiovascular disease. Ticagrelor and prasugrel are more potent antiplatelet inhibitors than clopidogrel, so they tend to provide more antithrombotic protection but at a higher risk of bleeding. Clopidogrel is therefore generally preferred in patients who have a high underlying bleeding risk.

SECONDARY PREVENTION

Acute Myocardial Infarction and Stent. Clopidogrel or ticagrelor added to aspirin for up to 12 months improves outcomes in patients who have survived an ST-elevation myocardial infarction compared with aspirin alone. Ticagrelor plus aspirin for 30 days is also more effective than aspirin alone in patients who have had an ischemic stroke or transient ischemic attack.A17,A18

Acute Coronary Syndrome and Post–Percutaneous Coronary Intervention. Aspirin plus clopidogrel is superior compared with aspirin alone in patients who have an acute coronary syndrome, despite carrying a higher risk of bleeding.[19] Prasugrel is even (about 20%) more effective than clopidogrel but with yet a higher risk of bleeding.

Cangrelor is used as an adjunct to percutaneous coronary intervention to reduce the risk of periprocedural MI, repeat coronary revascularization, and stent thrombosis in patients who have not been treated with a GPIIb/IIIa antagonist.[20] When transitioning from cangrelor to an oral $P2Y_{12}$ receptor antagonist, ticagrelor can be administered during cangrelor administration, but clopidogrel should be administered after cessation of cangrelor and prasugrel.

After percutaneous coronary intervention, 12 months of dual treatment with aspirin plus either clopidogrel or prasugrel reduces the risk of in-stent thrombosis and major adverse cardiovascular events, but at the expense of an increased risk of bleeding. By comparison, in patients with an acute coronary syndrome, ticagrelor monotherapy (180 mg loading dose, 90mg twice daily thereafter) is preferred over clopidogrel monotherapy to reduce subsequent coronary events. Aspirin plus ticagrelor may reduce the incidence of ischemic events in patients with diabetes and known coronary artery disease but without a history of MI or stroke, especially after prior percutaneous coronary intervention,A19 but the modest benefit (absolute reduction <1%) comes with an increased risk of major bleeding (absolute increase 2.2%). Clopidogrel and ticagrelor are equivalent in patients with peripheral arterial disease.A20

Dual antiplatelet therapy after percutaneous coronary intervention reduces the risk of ischemic events compared with monotherapy but increases the risk of bleeding.A21 With modern polymer-free drug-eluting stents, one to at most 3 months of dual antiplatelet therapy followed by continual treatment with aspirin or clopidogrel appears to be the preferred option. Clopidogrel may be favored over aspirin for monotherapy.

Intracardiac Procedures. Current guidelines recommend the use of dual antiplatelet therapy with aspirin and clopidogrel for 3 to 6 months in patients who have undergone transcatheter aortic valve replacement (Chapter 60),[21] although the incremental benefit of dual antiplatelet therapy over single antiplatelet therapy is unproven. After transcutaneous mitral valve replacement or insertion of a mitral valve clip, monotherapy with aspirin 81 to 325 mg daily for 6 months is reasonable (Chapter 60).A22 For edge-to-edge mitral repair, either a short course (30 days) of dual antiplatelet therapy followed by aspirin or monotherapy (aspirin or clopidogrel) for about 6 months is recommended. In patients undergoing percutaneous closure of an atrial

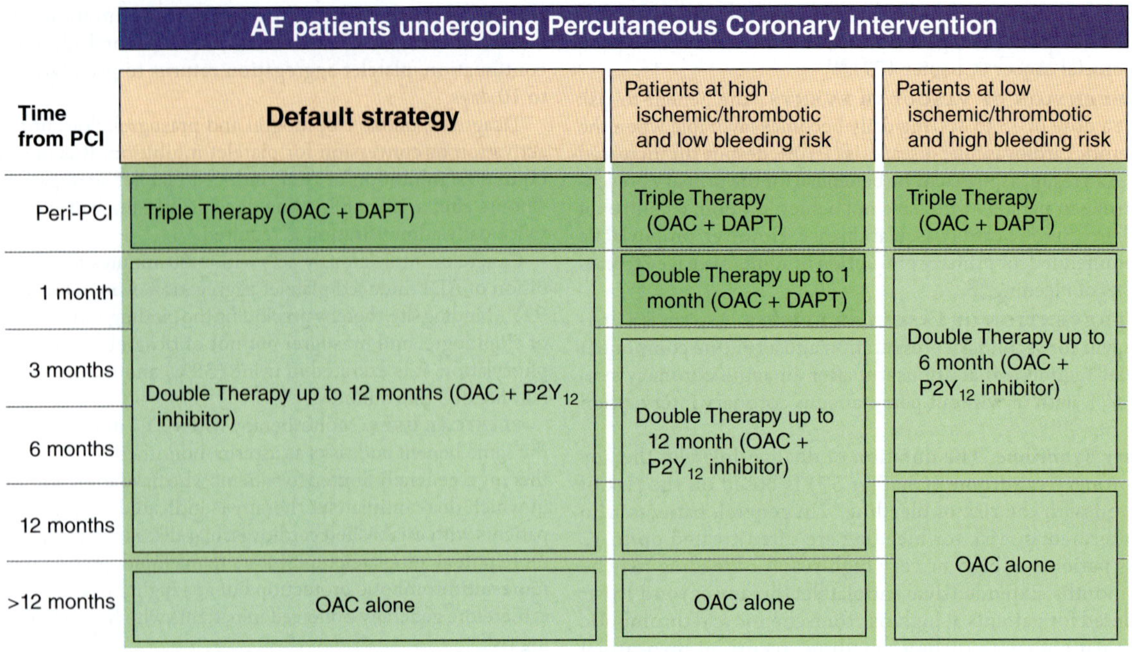

FIGURE 70-1. **Management of antiplatelet therapy in patients with atrial fibrillation (AF) undergoing percutaneous coronary intervention (PCI) treated with an oral anticoagulant: 2018 North American Consensus Update.** A double-therapy regimen, consisting of oral anticoagulant therapy plus a $P2Y_{12}$ inhibitor, should be considered for most patients immediately after the peri-PCI period (default strategy). Aspirin should be used during the peri-PCI period, defined as inpatient stay until time of discharge, generally 1 to 2 days after PCI, and in some patients continued for 1 week after PCI. A non–vitamin K antagonist direct-acting oral anticoagulant (DOAC) should be preferred over a vitamin K antagonist unless contraindicated. Clopidogrel is the $P2Y_{12}$ inhibitor of choice; ticagrelor may be an alternative in patients with high thrombotic and acceptable bleeding risk; prasugrel should be avoided. It is reasonable to continue aspirin for up to 1 month after PCI (i.e., triple therapy) in patients at high thrombotic risk and who have an acceptable risk of bleeding. Extending aspirin therapy beyond 1 month after PCI is not recommended. $P2Y_{12}$-inhibiting therapy should be discontinued at 1 year in most patients; earlier discontinuation (e.g., 6 months) can be considered in patients at low ischemic or high bleeding risk; continuation of antiplatelet therapy beyond 1 year should be considered only in select patients with high risk for ischemic recurrences and low bleeding risk. DAPT = dual antiplatelet therapy; OAC = oral anticoagulant. (From Angiolillo DJ, Bhatt DL, Cannon CP, et al. Antithrombotic therapy in patients with atrial fibrillation treated with oral anticoagulation undergoing percutaneous coronary intervention: a North American perspective: 2021 update. *Circulation*. 2021;143:583-596. With permission.)

septal defect or patent foramen ovale (Chapter 55), the post-procedural antithrombotic therapy regimen typically includes a combination of aspirin 75 to 325 mg daily plus clopidogrel 75 mg daily for 1 to 3 months followed by aspirin monotherapy for an additional 3 to 5 months. After closure (or exclusion) of a left atrial appendage, up to 6 months of dual antiplatelet therapy is generally administered after the procedure, followed by long-term aspirin monotherapy.

ADVERSE EFFECTS. Idiopathic thrombocytopenic purpura and thrombotic thrombocytopenic purpura (Chapter 158) have rarely been reported with clopidogrel. Prasugrel causes more major bleeding, life-threatening bleeding, and fatal bleeding compared with clopidogrel. Prasugrel is contraindicated in patients who have a history of transient ischemic attacks or stroke and generally is not recommended in patients age 75 years or older. Ticagrelor can be reversed with the monoclonal antibody bentracimab under expert oversight.

COMBINATION ANTICOAGULANT AND ANTIPLATELET THERAPY. In patients with stable cardiovascular disease (Chapter 56), the combination of rivaroxaban plus aspirin can reduce the composite end point of cardiovascular death, stroke, or myocardial infarction, but at a cost of a higher rate of major bleeding. In patients who have atrial fibrillation and who have an acute coronary syndrome, evidence supports the safety and benefit of dual therapy,[A23] although monotherapy with an oral anticoagulant may be sufficient 1 year after percutaneous coronary intervention in some patients[A24] (Fig. 70-1).

Patients with stable ischemic coronary artery disease and a clinical indication for time-limited anticoagulation, such as a venous thromboembolism, should receive triple therapy for up to 3 months, at which time the anticoagulant therapy can be discontinued. Aspirin should be continued in combination with clopidogrel for another 3 to 6 months, followed by aspirin monotherapy. In patients with acute coronary syndrome, the same strategy for anticoagulant therapy and aspirin is recommended, but clopidogrel is recommended for 12 months unless there is a high-to-very-high risk for bleeding. For patients who have an indefinite indication for anticoagulant therapy, anticoagulation with a reduced prophylactic dose (see Table 70-6) is recommended in combination with a $P2Y_{12}$ receptor inhibitor (clopidogrel is preferred) for 3 to 6 months followed by either a $P2Y_{12}$ receptor inhibitor or aspirin for 6 to 12 months; antiplatelet therapy can be stopped at 12 months.[22]

Intravenous Platelet GPIIb/IIIa Receptor Antagonists

The two intravenous GPIIb/IIIa receptor antagonists are tirofiban and eptifibatide. These agents are generally used only by interventional cardiologists in situations of no-reflow (patency without perfusion) or a thrombotic complication after a percutaneous coronary intervention. The duration of platelet inhibition with these agents is about 4 hours following cessation of tirofiban and eptifibatide.

Phosphodiesterase Inhibition: Cilostazol

PHARMACOLOGY. Cilostazol, a quinolinone derivative, and several of its metabolites inhibit phosphodiesterase III activity and suppress the degradation of cyclic adenosine monophosphate. The resultant increase in cyclic adenosine monophosphate in platelets and blood vessels leads to inhibition of platelet aggregation and vasodilation, respectively.

Metabolism occurs via the hepatic cytochrome P-450 enzymes, and most of the metabolites are excreted in the urine (75% of overall clearance). Cilostazol and its active metabolites have elimination half-lives of about 11 to 13 hours. Short-term coadministration of aspirin with cilostazol inhibits ADP- and arachidonic acid-induced platelet aggregation by about 30% and 25%, respectively, compared with cilostazol alone.

CLINICAL USES

Peripheral Artery Disease. Cilostazol is approved for the treatment of intermittent claudication (Chapter 65). Cilostazol should not be considered a substitute for aspirin or clopidogrel in patients with acute coronary syndrome and concomitant peripheral arterial disease.

ADVERSE EFFECTS. The most common adverse effect associated with cilostazol is headache. Other relatively frequent causes of drug discontinuation include palpitations, ventricular tachycardia, and diarrhea. Cilostazol is contraindicated in patients with heart failure of any severity.

Direct Thrombin Inhibition: Vorapaxar

PHARMACOLOGY. Vorapaxar, which is a tricyclic himbacine-derived selective inhibitor of the thrombin receptor, inhibits platelet aggregation through reversible antagonism. Vorapaxar is rapidly absorbed after oral administration, with peak concentrations at about 1 hour. Vorapaxar is primarily eliminated as its metabolite M19 through the feces (91.5%), and partially eliminated in the urine (8.5%). It has an effective half-life of 3 to 4 days and an apparent terminal half-life of 8 days.

CLINICAL USES. Vorapaxar is indicated for reducing the incidence of thrombotic cardiovascular events in patients with a history of MI or with peripheral arterial disease.

ADVERSE EFFECTS. Vorapaxar is associated with an increased risk of major bleeding, including intracranial hemorrhage. It should not be used in patients with prior intercranial hemorrhage.

FIBRINOLYTIC AND ANTITHROMBIN AGENTS

Fibrinolytic Therapy

Fibrinolytic agents directly or indirectly activate plasminogen to plasmin, which then degrades fibrin to soluble fragments, thereby lysing a thrombus. Both streptokinase, which indirectly activates plasminogen by binding to the zymogen and triggering a conformational change that leads to its activation, and urokinase, which directly activates plasminogen, degrade fibrinogen as well as fibrin.

These first-generation plasminogen activators have been largely replaced by newer agents, particularly alteplase, which is a second-generation plasminogen activator that possesses greater fibrin specificity, is not allergenic or antigenic, and has a short half-life of about 3.5 minutes. Third generation plasminogen activators, such as reteplase and tenecteplase, have been engineered to improve various structural and functional properties, thereby resulting in a longer half-life, resistance to inhibitors, improved safety profiles, and/or enhanced fibrin specificity.

CLINICAL USES. For acute ischemic stroke (Chapter 376), alteplase has been the mainstay of treatment,[23] but tenecteplase[A25] provides better recanalization rates and early neurologic improvement than alteplase. Fibrinolytic therapy is recommended for patients within 12 hours of an ST-elevation myocardial infarction (Chapter 58) when primary percutaneous coronary intervention is not available. Intra-arterial, catheter-directed fibrinolytic therapy is an effective treatment for acute limb ischemia within 14 days of the acute onset of symptoms (Chapter 65). Fibrinolytic therapy followed by anticoagulant therapy is recommended over anticoagulant therapy alone when a pulmonary embolism causes acute hemodynamic compromise (Chapter 68).[24] Dosing of the fibrinolytic agents varies for the different clinical indications. Laboratory monitoring is not necessary for most patients.

Reversal of fibrinolytic therapy is most directly achieved by discontinuing the fibrinolytic agent, and if the fibrinogen level is low, replacing fibrinogen, either with cryoprecipitate or fibrinogen concentrate. For patients with significant bleeding complications, antifibrinolytic agents, such as aminocaproic acid (4 to 5 g loading dose, oral or intravenous, followed by 1 g/hour for 8 hours or until bleeding is controlled) or tranexamic acid (1 g [or 10 to 15 mg/kg] once intravenously, not to exceed 100 mg/minute), can inhibit the fibrinolytic effect.

GENERAL REFERENCES

For the General References and other additional features, please visit Elsevier eBooks+ at https://ebooks.health.elsevier.com.

Grade A References

A1. Li A, Garcia DA, Lyman GH, et al. Direct oral anticoagulant (DOAC) versus low-molecular-weight heparin (LMWH) for treatment of cancer associated thrombosis (CAT): a systematic review and meta-analysis. *Thromb Res.* 2019;173:158-163.

A2. Rutjes AW, Porreca E, Candeloro M, et al. Primary prophylaxis for venous thromboembolism in ambulatory cancer patients receiving chemotherapy. *Cochrane Database Syst Rev.* 2020;12:CD008500.

A3. Brandao GM, Junqueira DR, Rollo HA, et al. Pentasaccharides for the treatment of deep vein thrombosis. *Cochrane Database Syst Rev.* 2017;12:CD011782.

A4. Belley-Cote EP, Hanif H, D'Aragon F, et al. Genotype-guided versus standard vitamin K antagonist dosing algorithms in patients initiating anticoagulation. *Thromb Haemost.* 2015;114:768-777.

A5. Giustozzi M, Agnelli G, Del Toro-Cervera J, et al. Direct oral anticoagulants for the treatment of acute venous thromboembolism associated with cancer: a systematic review and meta-analysis. *Thromb Haemost.* 2020;120:1128-1136.

A6. Connolly SJ, Eikelboom JW, Bosch J, et al. Rivaroxaban with or without aspirin in patients with stable coronary artery disease: an international, randomised, double-blind, placebo-controlled trial. *Lancet.* 2018;391:205-218.

A7. Anand SS, Caron F, Eikelboom JW, et al. Major adverse limb events and mortality in patients with peripheral artery disease: the COMPASS trial. *J Am Coll Cardiol.* 2018;71:2306-2315.

A8. Spyropoulos AC, Ageno W, Albers GW, et al. Post-discharge prophylaxis with rivaroxaban reduces fatal and major thromboembolic events in medically ill patients. *J Am Coll Cardiol.* 2020;75:3140-3147.

A9. Pengo V, Denas G, Zoppellaro G, et al. Rivaroxaban vs warfarin in high-risk patients with antiphospholipid syndrome. *Blood.* 2018;132:1365-1371.

A10. Buller HR, Bethune C, Bhanot S, et al. Factor XI antisense oligonucleotide for prevention of venous thrombosis. *N Engl J Med.* 2015;372:232-240.

A11. Verhamme P, Yi BA, Segers A, et al. Abelacimab for prevention of venous thromboembolism. *N Engl J Med.* 2021;385:609-617.

A12. Weitz JI, Strony J, Ageno W, et al. Milvexian for the prevention of venous thromboembolism. *N Engl J Med.* 2021;385:2161-2172.

A13. Jones WS, Mulder H, Wruck LM, et al. Comparative effectiveness of aspirin dosing in cardiovascular disease. *N Engl J Med.* 2021;384:1981-1990.

A14. Burn J, Sheth H, Elliott F, et al. Cancer prevention with aspirin in hereditary colorectal cancer (Lynch syndrome), 10-year follow-up and registry-based 20-year data in the CAPP2 study: a double-blind, randomised, placebo-controlled trial. *Lancet.* 2020;395:1855-1863.

A15. Zheng SL, Roddick AJ. Association of aspirin use for primary prevention with cardiovascular events and bleeding events: a systematic review and meta-analysis. *JAMA.* 2019;321:277-287.

A16. Chiarito M, Sanz-Sánchez J, Cannata F, et al. Monotherapy with a P2Y12 inhibitor or aspirin for secondary prevention in patients with established atherosclerosis: a systematic review and meta-analysis. *Lancet.* 2020;395:1487-1495.

A17. Johnston SC, Amarenco P, Denison H, et al. Ticagrelor and aspirin or aspirin alone in acute ischemic stroke or TIA. *N Engl J Med.* 2020;383:207-217.

A18. Amarenco P, Denison H, Evans SR, et al. Ticagrelor added to aspirin in acute ischemic stroke or transient ischemic attack in prevention of disabling stroke: a randomized clinical trial. *JAMA Neurol.* 2020;78:1-9.

A19. Bhatt DL, Steg PG, Mehta SR, et al. Ticagrelor in patients with diabetes and stable coronary artery disease with a history of previous percutaneous coronary intervention (THEMIS-PCI): a phase 3, placebo-controlled, randomised trial. *Lancet.* 2019;394:1169-1180.

A20. Kinlay S, Young MM, Sherrod R, et al. Long-term outcomes and duration of dual antiplatelet therapy after coronary intervention with second-generation drug-eluting stents: the Veterans Affairs Extended DAPT Study. *J Am Heart Assoc.* 2023;12:e027055.

A21. Gragnano F, Mehran R, Branca M, et al. P2Y12 inhibitor monotherapy or dual antiplatelet therapy after complex percutaneous coronary interventions. *J Am Coll Cardiol.* 2023;81:537-552.

A22. Kang J, Park KW, Lee H, et al. Aspirin versus clopidogrel for long-term maintenance monotherapy after percutaneous coronary intervention: the HOST-EXAM Extended Study. *Circulation.* 2023;147:108-117.

A23. Gargiulo G, Cannon CP, Gibson CM, et al. Safety and efficacy of double vs. triple antithrombotic therapy in patients with atrial fibrillation with or without acute coronary syndrome undergoing percutaneous coronary intervention: a collaborative meta-analysis of non-vitamin K antagonist oral anticoagulant-based randomized clinical trials. *Eur Heart J Cardiovasc Pharmacother.* 2021;7:f50-f60.

A24. Yasuda S, Kaikita K, Akao M, et al. Antithrombotic therapy for atrial fibrillation with stable coronary disease. *N Engl J Med.* 2019;381:1103-1113.

A25. Oliveira M, Fidalgo M, Fontao L, et al. Tenecteplase for thrombolysis in stroke patients: Systematic review with meta-analysis. *Am J Emerg Med.* 2021;42:31-37.

X

RESPIRATORY DISEASES

71

APPROACH TO THE PATIENT WITH RESPIRATORY DISEASE

MONICA KRAFT

Respiratory symptoms, which are among the most common reasons why patients seek medical care, are responsible for approximately 20% of office visits to a primary care physician. In addition to a careful history, a systematic physical examination is critical for accurate diagnosis. Even in young adults, persistent respiratory symptoms are associated with a greater likelihood of developing chronic lung disease.[1]

A careful pulmonary examination complements the cardiac physical examination (Chapter 39). Inspection may reveal an elevated jugular pressure, indicative of right heart failure owing to cor pulmonale (Chapter 69). Cervical or supraclavicular adenopathy (Chapter 154) may be the first clue to suggest a thoracic malignancy (Chapter 177) or mycobacterial infection (Chapter 299). Unilateral arm swelling can be caused by venous thrombosis (Chapter 68), whereas venous engorgement of the head and neck can be caused by a tumor that results in superior vena cava syndrome (see Fig. 86-8 in Chapter 86). On the cardiac examination, a loud pulmonic second heart sound is suggestive of pulmonary hypertension, which also can result in a murmur of tricuspid (see Table 39-7 in Chapter 39) or pulmonic valve insufficiency.

Inspection of the chest may show hyperinflation and reduced diaphragmatic excursion, typical of chronic obstructive pulmonary disease (COPD; Chapter 76), chest wall abnormalities such as kyphoscoliosis (Chapter 86), or diaphragmatic muscle wall weakness as in many hypoventilation syndromes (Chapter 74). Percussion may reveal dullness in patients with pleural effusions or with lung that has been consolidated by pneumonia.

Auscultation of the lungs includes listening at both apices and over both upper and lower lobes, anteriorly and posteriorly, and during inspiration and expiration. Normal lung sounds are heard during inspiration and early expiration as soft and non-musical sounds (Table 71-1).[2,3] *Bronchial breath sounds,* which sound similar to but often somewhat harsher than normal lung sounds, are heard throughout expiration as well as inspiration, similar to what would be heard by placing a stethoscope over the trachea.

The term *rales* is no longer used and has been replaced by the term *crackles.* Fine crackles are non-musical and heard typically in late inspiration; they are most commonly a sign of heart failure (Chapter 45) or interstitial lung disease (Chapter 80). By comparison, coarse crackles, which, unlike fine crackles, tend to be transmitted through the mouth and cleared by coughing, are typical of bronchitis (Chapter 84) and COPD (Chapter 76). *Wheezes* are high-pitched, musical sounds heard during expiration and sometimes inspiration, most commonly in asthma (Chapter 75) and sometimes in COPD (Chapter 76). When these diseases are severe, however, the degree of airflow may be insufficient to produce wheezes. A *rhonchus* is a musical, low-pitched sound typically heard in expiration and sometimes during inspiration; it often resolves with coughing. Like coarse crackles, rhonchi are common in bronchitis (Chapter 84) and COPD (Chapter 76). A *pleural friction rub,* which classically occurs during inspiration but sometimes also during expiration, is heard in a fraction of patients with inflammatory diseases or malignancies involving the pleura (Chapters 86 and 177). *Stridor* is a musical, high-pitched sound that may be audible without a stethoscope and that indicates upper airway obstruction, such as found with acute inflammatory or chronic degenerative diseases of the larynx (Chapter 397) or obstruction of the trachea, as may be caused by intrathoracic malignant diseases (Chapter 177). An absence of breath sounds would be noted if the lung is not ventilated because of a complete bronchial obstruction or if it is displaced by a pleural effusion.

Tactile fremitus, which is a vibratory sensation noted during breathing, is increased in patients who have consolidated lung from pneumonia, because the vibratory sensation conducts better through such lung tissue and is diminished in patients with pleural effusion. *Egophony,* by which a patient's recitation of the long E sound is heard on auscultation as a long A sound, is another indication of consolidation typical of pneumonia.

Evaluation of the abdomen may show a readily palpable liver, sometimes mistaken for hepatomegaly, in patients with COPD whose pulmonary hyperinflation results in a low diaphragm. Examination of the extremities may reveal cyanosis in patients who are hypoxemic, usually with a partial pressure of oxygen less than 55 mm Hg, although it also may be observed in patients with methemoglobinemia (Chapter 144). Clubbing (Chapter 39) is indicative of chronic hypoxemia, as seen in patients with chronic right-to-left-shunting from congenital heart disease (Chapter 55) or other causes of long-standing hypoxemia (Chapters 76 and 80), but it also may be indicative of pleural-based diseases (Chapter 86) as part of the syndrome of hypertrophic pulmonary osteoarthropathy (Chapters 164 and 254).

In patients with suspected hypoxemia, careful analyses of arterial blood gases can help determine its severity and guide therapy (Chapter 89). In patients in whom it is difficult to distinguish heart failure from a pulmonary cause of hypoxemia, an elevated brain natriuretic peptide level may point to a cardiac cause (Chapter 45). Chest imaging (Chapter 72) is a crucial part of the evaluation of many potential pulmonary complaints, and pulmonary function testing (Chapter 73) can be extremely helpful in distinguishing among causes of acute and chronic lung disease.

Among the most common respiratory complaints are cough, wheezing, dyspnea, and hemoptysis. Each can and should be approached in a systematic way.

TABLE 71-1 DIAGNOSTIC UTILITY OF LUNG AUSCULTATION

AUSCULTATORY FINDING	CLINICAL CORRELATION
Bronchial breathing	Pneumonia or interstitial lung disease
Fine crackle	Heart failure, interstitial lung disease, alveolar filling disorders
Coarse crackle	Bronchitis
Wheeze	Asthma, COPD, bronchomalacia
Rhonchus	Bronchitis, COPD
Stridor	Upper-airway obstruction from laryngeal or tracheal inflammation, mass lesions, or external compression
Pleural friction rub	Pleural inflammation or tumors

COPD = chronic obstructive pulmonary disease.

APPROACH TO THE PATIENT WITH COUGH

Cough is the single most common respiratory complaint for which patients seek care. Referrals of patients with persistently troublesome chronic cough of unknown cause account for 10 to 38% of outpatient visits to respiratory specialists.

For acute cough, defined as coughing that has been present for less than 8 weeks, a careful medical history and physical examination will usually reveal the diagnosis[4] (Table 71-2). Although most acute coughs are of minor consequence,[5] cough occasionally can be a sign of a potentially life-threatening illness, such as pulmonary embolism (Chapter 68), pneumonia (Chapter 85), or heart failure (Chapter 46).

Up to 98% of all cases of chronic cough, defined as a cough that persists for more than 8 weeks, in immunocompetent adults are caused by eight common conditions: postnasal drip syndrome from a variety of rhinosinus conditions often termed the "upper airway cough syndrome" (asthma; Chapter 75), gastroesophageal reflux disease (GERD; Chapter 124), chronic bronchitis (Chapter 76), eosinophilic bronchitis, bronchiectasis (Chapter 78), use of angiotensin-converting enzyme (ACE) inhibitors, and postinfectious cough. Postinfectious cough is usually nonproductive and generally persists for 3 to 8 weeks after an upper respiratory tract infection; patients have a normal chest radiograph. Environmental and occupational factors can also contribute to chronic cough and should be assessed. Cough in athletes is usually due to reactive airway disease, exercise-induced asthma, rhinitis, respiratory tract infections, and environmental exposures. Uncommon causes of chronic cough include bronchogenic carcinoma (Chapter 177), chronic interstitial pneumonia (Chapter 80), sarcoidosis (Chapter 83), left ventricular failure (Chapter 45), and aspiration (Chapter 82).[6] Cough itself also can cause complications, sometimes life-threatening, involving many organ systems, thereby providing further rationale for its diagnosis and treatment.[7]

DIAGNOSIS

In chronic cough (Fig. 71-1), the character and timing are not of diagnostic help. A chest radiograph should be obtained in all patients, but other tests should not be ordered in current smokers or patients taking ACE inhibitors

TABLE 71-2 SPECTRUM OF CAUSES AND FREQUENCIES OF COUGH IN IMMUNOCOMPETENT ADULTS

COMMON	LESS COMMON
ACUTE COUGH	
Common cold	Asthma exacerbation
Acute bacterial sinusitis	Pneumonia
Pertussis	Heart failure
Exacerbations of COPD	Aspiration syndromes
Allergic rhinitis	Pulmonary embolism
Environmental irritant rhinitis	Exacerbation of bronchiectasis
SUBACUTE COUGH	
Postinfectious cough	
Pertussis	
CHRONIC COUGH	
Rhinosinus conditions/UACS	Bronchiolitis
Asthma	Occupational and environmental
Non-asthma eosinophilic bronchitis	Aspiration Bronchogenic carcinoma
Bronchiectasis	Drug-induced cough
Gastroesophageal reflux	Tuberculosis
Chronic bronchitis/COPD	Interstitial lung disease

COPD = chronic obstructive pulmonary disease; UACS = upper airway cough syndrome.

until the response to smoking cessation or discontinuation of the drug for at least 4 weeks can be assessed.[8] Sinus radiographs, barium esophagography, methacholine challenge, esophageal pH, and bronchoscopy can be ordered as part of the initial evaluation, depending on the history and physical examination (Table 71-3; see Fig. 71-1). If a test points toward a possible diagnosis, a trial of treatment for that condition is needed to confirm the diagnosis. The diagnosis of psychogenic cough is often a diagnosis of exclusion.

TREATMENT

The specific cause of cough can be diagnosed and treated successfully 84 to 98% of the time, so nonspecific therapy aimed to suppress the cough per se is rarely indicated.[9,10] There is no strong evidence that nonspecific therapies such as antitussives, mucolytics, decongestants, or antihistamine-decongestant combinations are efficacious for acute cough in the setting of an upper respiratory tract infection. For nonspecific persistent cough, effective treatment of chronic gastroesophageal reflux disease with a proton pump inhibitor (Chapter 124) provides no more than modest benefit, with approximately one in five patients improving. Inhaled corticosteroids can reduce cough but should be used only after evaluation by chest radiography and often spirometry.[A1] Dextromethorphan and codeine-containing cough suppressants can reduce chronic cough by approximately 40%. In adults with refractory chronic cough without active respiratory disease or infection, gabapentin (up to a maximum daily dose of 1800 mg) or pregabalin (300 mg daily) significantly improves cough-specific quality of life compared with placebo.[A2] For chronic refractory cough despite comprehensive evaluation and opioid therapy, a combination of education, speech and language intervention, which includes cough suppression techniques, and counseling can significantly reduce cough and its negative impact on quality of life.[A3] Gefapixant, a P2X3 inhibitor that has shown promise in improving unexplained or chronic cough in randomized trials,[A4,A5] is currently undergoing FDA review.

APPROACH TO THE PATIENT WITH WHEEZING

Wheeze is a continuous musical sound that lasts longer than 80 to 100 msec, likely generated by flow through critically narrowed collapsible bronchi. Although expiratory wheezing is a common physical finding in asthma (Chapter 75), the many causes of wheezing (Table 71-4) (e.g., COPD [Chapter 76], pulmonary edema [Chapter 45], bronchiolitis [Chapter 80], bronchiectasis [Chapter 78], and less common entities such as carcinoid [Chapter 213] and parasitic infections) often can be distinguished based on the history, physical examination, and pulmonary function testing (Chapter 73).[11]

TABLE 71-3 TESTING CHARACTERISTICS OF DIAGNOSTIC PROTOCOL FOR EVALUATION OF CHRONIC COUGH

TESTS	DIAGNOSIS	POSITIVE PREDICTIVE VALUE, %	NEGATIVE PREDICTIVE VALUE, %
Sinus radiograph	Sinusitis	57-81	95-100
Methacholine inhalation challenge	Asthma	60-82	100
Modified barium esophagography	GERD, esophageal stricture	38-63	63-93
Esophageal pH*	GERD	89-100	
Bronchoscopy	Endobronchial mass/lesion	50-89	100

*24-Hour esophageal pH monitoring.
GERD = gastroesophageal reflux disease.

DIAGNOSIS

On pulmonary function testing, the shape of inspiratory and expiratory flow-volume loops provides key information about the presence of airway obstruction and whether the obstruction is extrathoracic or intrathoracic (E-Fig. 71-1). An important cause of extrathoracic obstruction is vocal cord lesions (Chapter 176). Variable intrathoracic obstruction can be caused by tracheomalacia, whereas fixed upper airway obstruction can be caused by a proximal tracheal tumor.

TREATMENT

Treatment of the specific cause will usually lead to complete or at least partial resolution of wheezing. However, treatment of associated asymptomatic or minimally symptomatic gastroesophageal reflux disease is not beneficial.

APPROACH TO THE PATIENT WITH DYSPNEA

Dyspnea is the sensation of difficult, labored, or unpleasant breathing. The word *unpleasant* is very important to this definition because the labored or difficult breathing encountered by healthy individuals while exercising does not qualify as dyspnea because it is at the level expected for the degree of exertion. The sensation of dyspnea is often poorly or vaguely described by the patient. The physiology of dyspnea remains unclear, but multiple neural pathways can be involved in processes that lead to dyspnea.

In acute dyspnea, or shortness of breath of sudden onset, the history, physical examination, and laboratory testing must first focus on potential life-threatening conditions, including pulmonary embolism (Chapter 68), pulmonary edema (Chapters 45 and 46), acute airway obstruction from anaphylaxis or foreign bodies, pneumothorax (Chapter 86), or pneumonia (Chapter 85). For chronic dyspnea, specific conditions to consider include COPD (Chapter 76), asthma (Chapter 75), interstitial lung disease (Chapter 80), heart failure (Chapter 45), cardiomyopathy (Chapter 47), GERD (Chapter 124), other respiratory diseases, or hyperventilation syndrome (Table 71-5).[12]

DIAGNOSIS

Dyspnea is often underdiagnosed unless patients are specifically questioned, especially in critical care settings. In addition to an appropriate history and physical examination, a chest radiograph, electrocardiogram (ECG), pulmonary function testing, and an exercise test with electrocardiographic monitoring and pulse oximetry at rest and during exercise[13] are key tests to assess patients with unexplained dyspnea (Fig. 71-2). For acute dyspnea, B-type natriuretic peptide testing can be extremely helpful in distinguishing heart failure from other causes.[14] Point-of-care ultrasound[15] by appropriately trained clinicians can improve the sensitivities of standard diagnostic pathways to detect heart failure, pneumonia, pulmonary embolism, pleural effusion, or pneumothorax.[A6] The utility of more detailed pulmonary testing with maximal inspiratory and

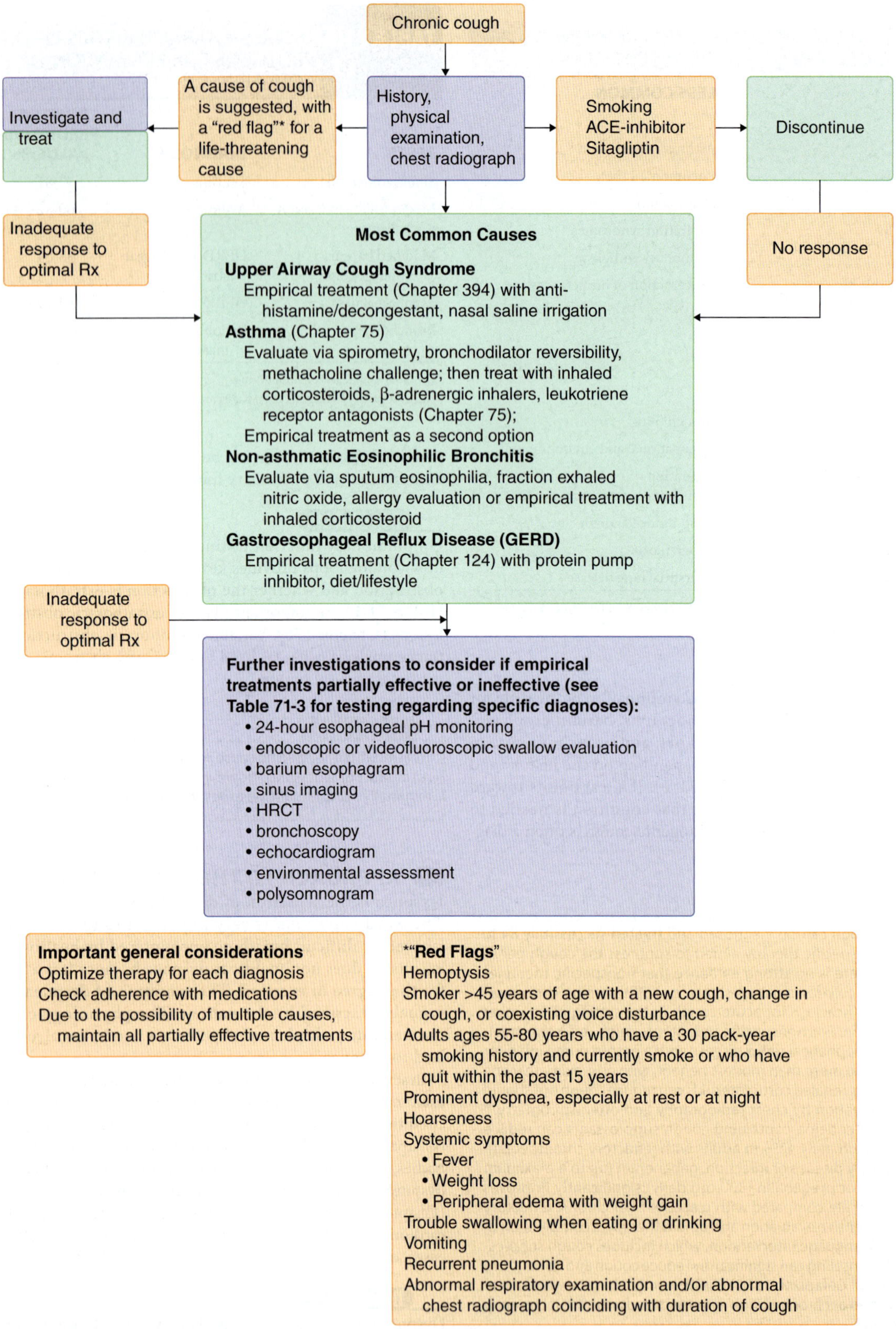

FIGURE 71-1. **Algorithm for the management of selected causes of chronic cough that persists for longer than 8 weeks.** ACE = angiotensin-converting enzyme; HRCT = high-resolution computed tomography; Rx = prescription. (Based on recommendations in Irwin RS, French CL, Chang AB, et al. Classification of cough as a symptom in adults and management algorithms: CHEST guideline and expert panel report. *Chest.* 2018;153:196-209.)

expiratory pressures; flow-volume loops, with or without methacholine challenge (Chapter 73); computed tomographic screening of the chest; and echocardiography depends on history and physical examination and the results of these tests. When GERD is a suspected cause of dyspnea, a modified barium esophagogram or 24-hour esophageal pH monitoring, or both, should be considered (Chapter 124). Other more invasive tests such as cardiac catheterization or lung biopsy may be indicated when the results of less invasive tests have not been conclusive.

TREATMENT AND PROGNOSIS

Whenever possible, the final determination of the cause of dyspnea is made by observing which specific therapy eliminates it. Dyspnea may be simultaneously the result of more than one condition, each of which may need to be treated. In patients with chronic exertional dyspnea, exercise-induced pulmonary hypertension is a predictor of a worse outcome.[16] In cases of refractory dyspnea despite maximally treated chronic heart and lung disease, judicious use of opioids can curb air hunger.[17]

APPROACH TO THE PATIENT WITH HEMOPTYSIS

Hemoptysis is the expectoration of blood from the lung parenchyma or airways. Hemoptysis may be scant, with just the appearance of streaks of bright red blood in the sputum, or massive, with the expectoration of a large volume of blood. Massive hemoptysis, which is defined as the expectoration of at least 600 mL of blood in 24 to 48 hours, may occur in 3 to 10% of patients with hemoptysis. Dark red clots also may be expectorated when the blood has been present in the lungs for days.

Pseudohemoptysis, which is the expectoration of blood from a source other than the lower respiratory tract, may cause diagnostic confusion when patients cannot clearly describe the source of the bleeding. Pseudohemoptysis can occur when blood from the oral cavity, nares, pharynx, or tongue clings to the back of the throat and initiates the cough reflex or when patients who have hematemesis aspirate into the lower respiratory tract. When the oropharynx is colonized with *Serratia marcescens,* a red pigment–producing aerobic gram-negative rod, the sputum also can be red and can be confused with hemoptysis.

TABLE 71-4 DIAGNOSIS OF SELECTED WHEEZING ILLNESSES OTHER THAN ASTHMA

DISEASES	DISTINGUISHING FEATURES
UPPER AIRWAY DISEASES	
Postnasal drip syndrome	History of postnasal drip, throat clearing, nasal discharge; physical examination shows oropharyngeal secretions or cobblestone appearance to mucosa.
Epiglottitis	History of sore throat out of proportion to pharyngitis. Evidence of supraglottitis on endoscopy or lateral neck radiographs.
Vocal cord dysfunction syndrome/ paradoxical vocal fold movement	Lack of symptomatic response to bronchodilators, presence of stridor plus wheeze in absence of increased $P(A\text{-}a)O_2$; extrathoracic variable obstruction on flow-volume loops; paradoxical inspiratory and/or early expiratory adduction of vocal cords on laryngoscopy during wheezing. This syndrome can masquerade as asthma, be provoked by exercise, and often coexists with asthma.
Retropharyngeal abscess	History of stiff neck, sore throat, fever, trauma to posterior pharynx; swelling noted by lateral neck or CT radiographs.
Laryngotracheal injury due to tracheal cannulation	History of cannulation of the trachea by endotracheal or tracheostomy tube; evidence of intrathoracic or extrathoracic variable obstruction on flow-volume loops, neck and chest radiographs, laryngoscopy, or bronchoscopy.
Neoplasms	Bronchogenic carcinoma, adenoma, or carcinoid tumor is suspected when there is hemoptysis, unilateral wheeze, or evidence of lobar collapse on chest radiograph or combinations of these; diagnosis is confirmed by bronchoscopy.
Anaphylaxis	Abrupt onset of wheezing with urticaria, angioedema, nausea, diarrhea, and hypotension, especially after insect bite, in association with other signs of anaphylaxis such as hypotension or hives, or administration of drug or IV contrast, or family history.
LOWER AIRWAY DISEASES	
COPD	History of dyspnea on exertion and productive cough in cigarette smoker. Because productive cough is nonspecific, it should only be ascribed to COPD when other cough-phlegm syndromes have been excluded, forced expiratory time to empty more than 80% of vital capacity is >4 sec, and there is decreased breath sound intensity, unforced wheezing during auscultation, and irreversible, expiratory airflow obstruction on spirometry.
Pulmonary edema	History and physical examination consistent with passive congestion of the lungs, ARDS, impaired lung lymphatics; abnormal chest radiograph, echocardiogram, radionuclide ventriculography, cardiac catheterization, or combinations of these.
Aspiration	History of risk for pharyngeal dysfunction or gastroesophageal reflux disease; abnormal modified barium swallow, 24-hr esophageal pH monitoring, or both.
Pulmonary embolism	History of risk for thromboembolic disease, positive confirmatory tests.
Bronchiolitis	History of respiratory infection, connective tissue disease, transplantation, ulcerative colitis, development of chronic airway obstruction over months to a few years rather than over many years in a nonsmoker; mixed obstructive and restrictive pattern on PFTs and hyperinflation; may be accompanied by fine nodular infiltrates on chest radiograph.
Cystic fibrosis	Combination of productive cough, digital clubbing, bronchiectasis, progressive COPD with *Pseudomonas* sp colonization and infection, obstructive azoospermia, family history, pancreatic insufficiency, and two sweat chloride determinations of >60 mEq/L; some patients are not diagnosed until adulthood, in one instance as late as age 69 yr; when sweat test is occasionally normal, definitive diagnosis may require nasal transepithelial voltage measurements and genotyping.
Carcinoid syndrome	History of episodes of flushing and watery diarrhea; elevated 5-hydroxyindoleactic acid level in 24-hr urine specimen.
Bronchiectasis	History of episodes of productive cough, fever, or recurrent pneumonias; suggestive chest radiographs or typical chest CT findings; ABPA should be considered when bronchiectasis is central.
Endobronchial sarcoidosis	Consider in patient with history of sarcoidosis with bilateral lymphadenopathy on chest radiography with wheezing and dyspnea out of proportion to findings on imaging. Confirmation required by bronchoscopy with biopsies.
Lymphangitic carcinomatosis	History of dyspnea or prior malignancy; reticulonodular infiltrates with or without pleural effusions; suggestive high-resolution chest CT scan; confirmed by bronchoscopy with biopsies.
Parasitic infections	Consider in a nonasthmatic patient who has traveled to an endemic area and complains of fatigue, weight loss, fever; peripheral blood eosinophilia; infiltrates on chest radiograph; stools for ova and parasites for nonfilarial causes; blood serologic studies for filarial causes.

ABPA = allergic bronchopulmonary aspergillosis; ARDS = acute respiratory distress syndrome; COPD = chronic obstructive pulmonary disease; CT = computed tomography; IV = intravenous; $P(A\text{-}a)O_2$ = alveolar-arterial oxygen tension gradient; PFTs = pulmonary function tests.

TABLE 71-5 DISEASES THAT CAUSE DYSPNEA GROUPED BY PHYSIOLOGIC MECHANISMS OF ACTION*

INCREASED RESPIRATORY DRIVE
Stimulation of Chemoreceptors

Conditions leading to acute hypoxemia
  Impaired gas exchanger (e.g., asthma, pulmonary embolism, pneumonia, congestive heart failure[†])
  Environmental hypoxia (e.g., altitude, contained space with fire)
Conditions leading to increased dead space, acute hypercapnia
  Impaired gas exchanger (e.g., acute, severe asthma; exacerbation of COPD; severe pulmonary edema)
  Impaired ventilator pump (e.g., muscle weakness, airflow obstruction)
Metabolic acidosis
  Renal disease (e.g., renal failure, renal tubular acidosis)
Decreased oxygen carrying capacity (e.g., anemia)
  Decreased release of oxygen to tissues (e.g., hemoglobinopathy)
Decreased cardiac output

Stimulation of Pulmonary Receptors (Irritant, Mechanical, Vascular)[‡]
Interstitial lung disease Pleural effusion (compression atelectasis) Pulmonary vascular disease (e.g., thromboembolism, idiopathic pulmonary hypertension) Heart failure Mild asthma
Behavioral Factors
Hyperventilation syndrome, anxiety disorders, panic attacks
VENTILATORY PUMP: INCREASED EFFORT OR WORK OF BREATHING
Muscle Weakness
Myasthenia gravis, Guillain-Barré syndrome, spinal cord injury, myopathy, postpoliomyelitis syndrome
Decreased Compliance of the Chest Wall
Severe kyphoscoliosis, obesity, pleural effusion
Airflow Obstruction (including increased resistive load from narrowing of the airways and increased elastic load from hyperinflation)
Asthma, COPD, laryngospasm, aspiration of foreign body, bronchitis

*Some diseases appear in more than one category, because they act via several physiologic mechanisms.
[†]Heart failure includes both systolic and diastolic dysfunction. Systolic dysfunction may produce dyspnea at rest and with activity. Diastolic dysfunction typically leads to symptoms primarily with exercise. In addition to the mechanisms noted above, systolic heart failure may produce dyspnea via metaboreceptors, which are postulated to exist in muscles and be stimulated by changes in the metabolic milieu when oxygen delivery does not meet oxygen demand.
[‡]These conditions probably produce dyspnea by a combination of increased ventilator drive and primary sensory input from the receptors.
COPD = chronic obstructive pulmonary disease.

Hemoptysis can be caused by a wide variety of disorders. Virtually all causes of hemoptysis (Table 71-6) may result in massive hemoptysis, but massive hemoptysis is most frequently caused by infection (e.g., tuberculosis [Chapter 299], bronchiectasis [Chapter 78], lung abscess [Chapter 78], and cancer [Chapter 177]).[18] Infections with aspergilloma (Chapter 311) and in patients with cystic fibrosis (Chapter 77) also are associated with massive hemoptysis. Iatrogenic causes of massive hemoptysis include rupture of a pulmonary artery after less than 0.2% of cases of balloon-guided flotation catheterization and tracheal artery fistula as a complication of tracheostomy.

In nonmassive hemoptysis, the cause is bronchitis in more than one third of cases (Chapter 84), bronchogenic carcinoma (Chapter 177) in one fifth of cases, tuberculosis (Chapter 299) in 7%, pneumonia (Chapter 85) in 5%, and bronchiectasis in 1% (Chapter 78). Using a systematic diagnostic approach (see later), the cause of hemoptysis can be found in 68 to 98% of cases. The remaining 2 to 32% have idiopathic or central hemoptysis, which occurs most commonly in men between 30 and 50 years of age. Prolonged follow-up of idiopathic hemoptysis almost always fails to reveal the source of bleeding, even though 10% continue to have occasional episodes of hemoptysis.

DIAGNOSIS

The diagnostic evaluation for hemoptysis begins with a detailed medical history and a complete physical examination.[19] Information on the amount of bleeding should be obtained, as well as details about the frequency, timing, and duration of hemoptysis. For example, repeated episodes of hemoptysis occurring over a period of months to years suggest a bronchial adenoma or bronchiectasis as the cause, whereas small amounts of hemoptysis occurring every day for weeks are more likely to be caused by bronchogenic carcinoma. A travel history can suggest coccidioidomycosis (Chapter 308) and histoplasmosis (Chapter 308) in the United States, paragonimiasis and ascariasis (Chapter 327) in the Far East, and schistosomiasis (Chapter 326) in South America. Orthopnea and paroxysmal nocturnal dyspnea suggest heart failure (Chapter 45), especially from mitral stenosis (Chapter 60). In patients who have occupational exposure to trimellitic anhydride, which occurs when heated metal surfaces are sprayed with a corrosion-resistant epoxy resin, hemoptysis can be part of the postexposure syndrome, sometimes referred to as reactive airways dysfunction syndrome (Chapter 81). In a patient with the triad of upper airway disease, lower airway disease, and renal disease, granulomatosis with polyangiitis (Chapter 249) should be suspected. Pulmonary hemorrhage also may be a presenting manifestation of systemic lupus erythematosus (Chapter 245). Goodpasture syndrome, which typically occurs in young men, is also associated with renal disease (Chapter 107). Diffuse alveolar hemorrhage occurs in 20% of cases during autologous bone marrow transplantation (Chapter 163) and should be suspected in patients who have undergone recent bone marrow transplantation when they present with cough, dyspnea, hypoxemia, and diffuse pulmonary infiltrates.

On physical examination, inspection of the skin and mucous membranes may show telangiectasias suggesting hereditary hemorrhagic telangiectasia (Chapter 159) or ecchymoses and petechiae, suggesting a hematologic abnormality (Chapter 158). Pulsations transmitted to a tracheostomy cannula should heighten suspicion of a tracheal artery fistula. Inspection of the thorax should show evidence of recent or old chest trauma, and unilateral wheeze or crackles may herald localized disease such as a bronchial adenoma or carcinoma. Although pulmonary embolism (Chapter 68) cannot be definitively diagnosed on physical examination, tachypnea, phlebitis, and pleural friction rub suggest this disorder. If crackles are heard on the chest examination, heart failure as well as other diseases causing diffuse pulmonary hemorrhage (see earlier) or idiopathic pulmonary hemosiderosis (Chapter 80) should be considered. Careful cardiovascular examination may help diagnose mitral stenosis (Chapter 60), pulmonary artery fistulas, or pulmonary hypertension (Chapter 69).

Routine laboratory studies should include a complete blood count, urinalysis, and coagulation studies. The complete blood count may suggest an infection, hematologic disorder, or chronic blood loss. Urinalysis may reveal hematuria and suggest the presence of a systemic disease (e.g., Wegener granulomatosis, Goodpasture syndrome, systemic lupus erythematosus) associated

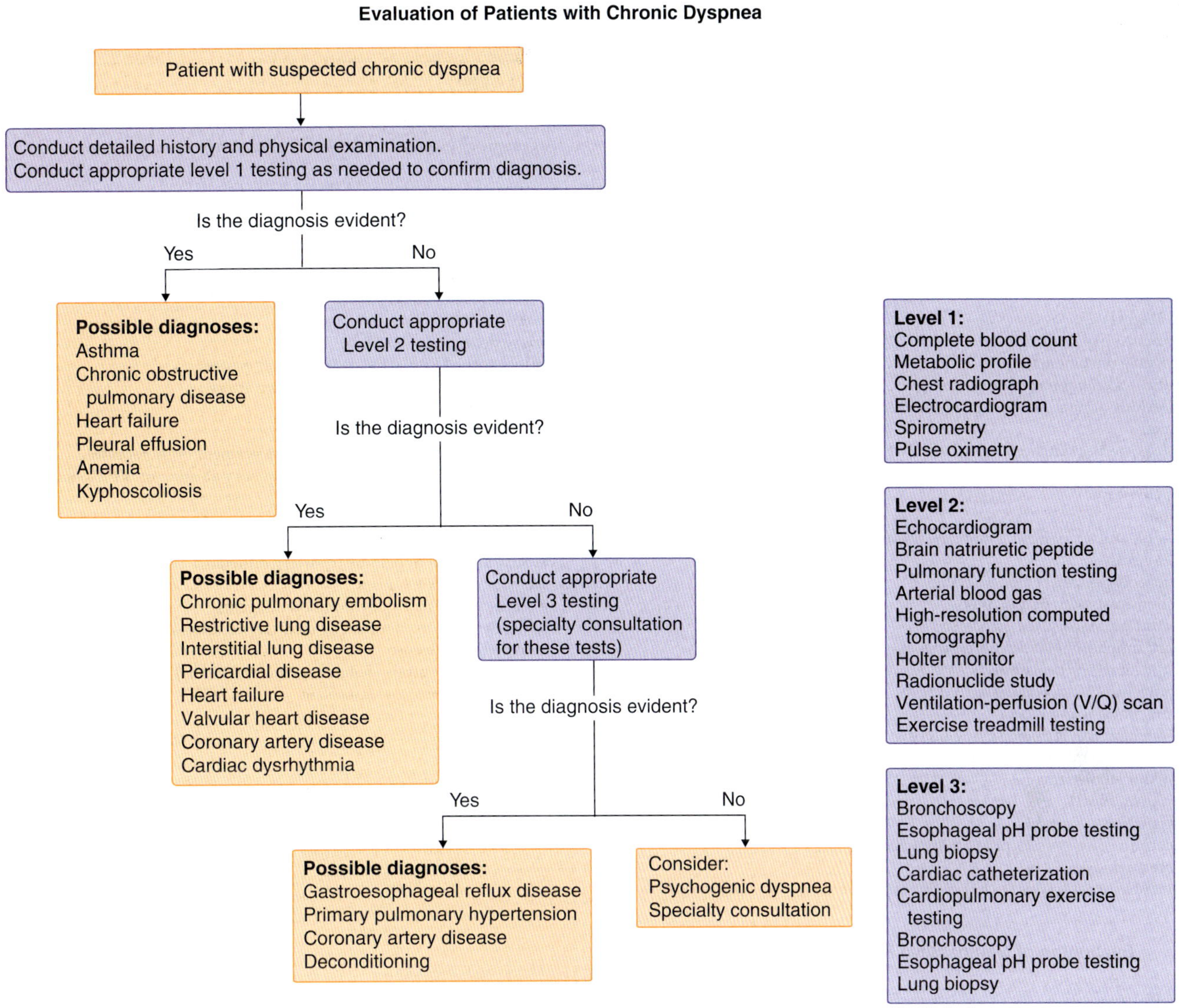

FIGURE 71-2. **Algorithm outlining the approach to selected causes of chronic dyspnea.** (Modified from Karnani NG, Reisfield GM, Wilson GR. Evaluation of chronic dyspnea. *Am Fam Phys*. 2005;71:1529-1537.)

with renal disease. Coagulation studies may uncover a hematologic disorder that is primarily responsible for hemoptysis or that contributes to excessive bleeding from another disease. The ECG may help suggest the presence of a cardiovascular disorder. Although as many as 30% of patients with hemoptysis have a normal chest radiograph, a routine chest radiograph is the beginning of the diagnostic process (Fig. 71-3).

Bronchoscopy can localize the bleeding site in up to 93% of patients by fiberoptic bronchoscopy and in up to 86% with rigid bronchoscopy. It may establish sites of bleeding different from those suggested by the chest radiograph. The best results are obtained when bronchoscopy is performed during or within 24 hours of active bleeding, and rates of diagnosis fall to approximately 50% by 48 hours after bleeding. When there is no active bleeding, bronchoscopy with bronchoalveolar lavage can be helpful in patients thought to have diffuse intrapulmonary hemorrhage. Typical findings include bright red or blood-tinged lavage fluid from multiple lobes in both lungs or a substantial number of hemosiderin-laden macrophages (i.e., at least 20% of the total number of alveolar macrophages).

Depending on the results of the initial evaluation and the likely categories of hemoptysis, additional diagnostic tests can be helpful (Table 71-7). Bronchoscopy may not be needed in patients who have stable chronic bronchitis (Chapter 76) with one episode of blood streaking or who have acute tracheobronchitis (Chapter 76). Bronchoscopy also may not be needed with obvious cardiovascular causes of hemoptysis, such as heart failure and pulmonary embolism.

TABLE 71-6 COMMON CAUSES OF HEMOPTYSIS

Cardiovascular	Drugs and Toxins
Arteriovenous malformation	Anticoagulants
Congenital heart disease	Anti-platelet medications
Pulmonary embolism (fat, septic, thrombotic)	Argemone alkaloid (e.g., contaminated cooking oil)
Heart failure, especially from mitral stenosis	Bevacizumab
Pulmonary Vascular Disease	Cocaine use
Pulmonary veno-occlusive disease	Nitrogen dioxide toxicity
Pulmonary artery rupture following catheterization	Trimellitic anhydride
Tricuspid endocarditis	Trauma
Pulmonary Infection	Blunt chest trauma (bronchial rupture, lung contusion)
Anthrax	Penetrating lung injury
Lung abscess	Iatrogenic
Mycetoma/fungal infection	Airway stent
Necrotizing pneumonia	Aortobronchial fistula due to aortic graft or stent
Parasitic (e.g., *Paragonimus westermani*)	Erosion of tracheal tube into innominate artery
Tuberculosis or nontuberculous mycobacterial disease	Erosion of airway stent
Tularemia	Lung transplantation
Viral (e.g., herpes simplex)	Pulmonary laceration from chest tube placement or thoracentesis
Yersinia pestis (plague)	Pulmonary vein stenosis after radiofrequency ablation of the AV node
Rheumatic Disease	Thrombolytic therapy
Amyloid	Transbronchial biopsy or cryobiopsy
Anti–glomerular basement membrane disease (Goodpasture)	Transthoracic needle aspiration
Behçet disease	Vascular injury from pulmonary artery catheter
Genetic collagen defect (Ehlers-Danlos)	Miscellaneous and Rare Causes
Granulomatosis with polyangiitis	Systemic coagulopathy or thrombolytic agents
Idiopathic pulmonary hemosiderosis	Platelet dysfunction/antiplatelet medications/thrombocytopenia
Primary antiphospholipid syndrome	von Willebrand disease
Systemic lupus erythematosus	Catamenial hemoptysis (pulmonary endometriosis)
Tracheobronchial/Airway Diseases	Leukemia/bone marrow transplant
Bronchogenic carcinoma	
Bronchiectasis, including cystic fibrosis	
Bronchitis, acute and chronic	
Bullous emphysema	
Broncholithiasis	
Bronchovascular fistula	
Dieulafoy disease (subepithelial bronchial artery)	
Foreign body	
Metastatic cancer to bronchus or trachea	

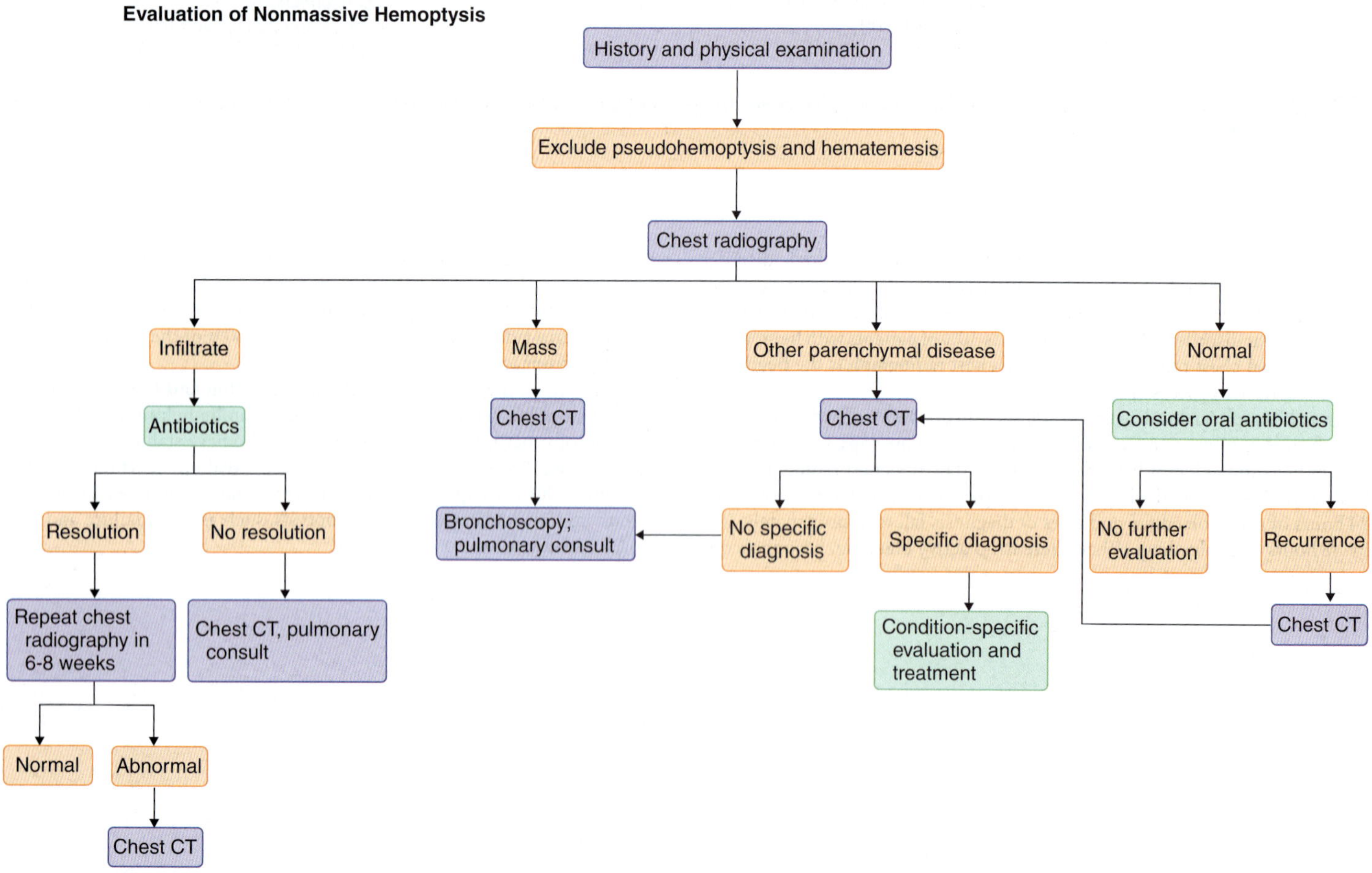

FIGURE 71-3. **Algorithm for evaluation of nonmassive hemoptysis.** CT = computed tomographic scan. (Adapted from Earwood JS, Thompson TD. Hemoptysis: evaluation and management. *Am Acad Fam Physicians*. 2015;91:243-249.)

TABLE 71-7 EXAMPLES OF SPECIAL EVALUATIONS FOR HEMOPTYSIS ACCORDING TO CATEGORY OF DISEASE*

TRACHEOBRONCHIAL DISORDERS
Expectorated sputum for TB, parasites, fungi, and cytology
Bronchoscopy (if not done previously)
High-resolution chest CT scan
LOCALIZED PARENCHYMAL DISEASES
Expectorated sputum for TB, parasites, fungi, and cytology
Chest CT scan
Lung biopsy with special stains
DIFFUSE PARENCHYMAL DISEASES
Expectorated sputum for cytology
Blood for BUN, creatinine, ANA, RF, complement, cryoglobulins, ANCA, anti-GBM antibody
High-resolution chest CT scan
Lung or kidney biopsy with special stains
CARDIOVASCULAR DISORDERS
Echocardiogram
Arterial blood gas on 21% and 100% oxygen
Ventilation-perfusion scans
Chest CT with contrast
Aortogram
HEMATOLOGIC DISORDERS
Coagulation studies
Bone marrow

*This table is not meant to be all-inclusive.

ANA = antinuclear antibody; ANCA = antineutrophil cytoplasmic antibody; BUN = blood urea nitrogen; CT = computed tomography; GBM = glomerular basement membrane; RF = rheumatoid factor; TB = tuberculosis.

TREATMENT

Treatment is targeted toward the cause of hemoptysis. Bronchoscopic approaches (Chapter 87) are increasingly used for endobronchial lesions, as is bronchial artery embolization[20] for the emergency treatment of hemoptysis and the treatment of hemoptysis associated with bronchiectasis.[21] In nonmassive hemoptysis, inhaled tranexamic acid (500 mg by nebulizer, three times daily) can safely and effectively control bleeding.[A7]

GENERAL REFERENCES

For the General References and other additional features, please visit Elsevier eBooks+ at https://ebooks.health.elsevier.com.

Grade A References

A1. Lee SE, Lee JH, Kim HJ, et al. Inhaled corticosteroids and placebo treatment effects in adult patients with cough: a systematic review and meta-analysis. *Allergy Asthma Immunol Res.* 2019;11:856-870.

A2. Vertigan AE, Kapela SL, Ryan NM, et al. Pregabalin and speech pathology combination therapy for refractory chronic cough: a randomized controlled trial. *Chest.* 2016;149:639-648.

A3. Chamberlain Mitchell SA, Garrod R, Clark L, et al. Physiotherapy, and speech and language therapy intervention for patients with refractory chronic cough: a multicentre randomised control trial. *Thorax.* 2017;72:129-136.

A4. Smith JA, Kitt MM, Morice AH, et al. Gefapixant, a P2X3 receptor antagonist, for the treatment of refractory or unexplained chronic cough: a randomised, double-blind, controlled, parallel-group, phase 2b trial. *Lancet Resp Med.* 2020;8:775-785.

A5. McGarvey LP, Birring SS, Morice AH, et al. Efficacy and safety of gefapixant, a $P2X_3$ receptor antagonist, in refractory chronic cough and unexplained chronic cough (COUGH-1 and COUGH-2): results from two double-blind, randomised, parallel-group, placebo-controlled, phase 3 trials. *Lancet.* 2022;399:909-923.

A6. Gartlehner G, Wagner G, Affengruber L, et al. Point-of-care ultrasonography in patients with acute dyspnea: an evidence report for a clinical practice guideline by the American College of Physicians. *Ann Intern Med.* 2021;174:967-976.

A7. Wand O, Guber E, Guber A, et al. Inhaled tranexamic acid for hemoptysis treatment: a randomized controlled trial. *Chest.* 2018;154:1379-1384.

72

IMAGING IN PULMONARY DISEASE

PAUL STARK

IMAGING OF THE LUNGS, MEDIASTINUM, AND CHEST WALL

EPIDEMIOLOGY

Worldwide, chest radiography is the most commonly performed imaging procedure; more than 75 million chest radiographs are performed every year in the United States alone. Chest radiographs provide useful information about the patient's anatomy and disease at a minimal monetary cost and with radiation exposure that most experts agree is negligible (0.05 to 0.1 mSv; Chapter 18). Although many novel imaging techniques are available, the conventional chest radiograph remains invaluable in the initial assessment of disorders of the lung, pleura, mediastinum, and chest wall.

IMAGING TECHNIQUES

The standard chest radiograph is performed at 2 m from the x-ray tube focal spot to the image detector, in frontal and lateral projections. If possible, the radiographs should be obtained with the patient inhaling to total lung capacity. These images, which provide views of the lungs, mediastinum, and chest wall simultaneously, are typically acquired, stored, and distributed digitally.

Bedside Radiography

Although bedside radiography accounts for a large number of chest radiographs, especially in the intensive care unit (ICU), the images obtained are generally of lower technical quality, cost more, and are more difficult to interpret. Lung volumes are low, thereby leading to crowding of vascular structures, and the low kilovoltage technique required for the mobile equipment yields radiographs with overexposed lungs and an underpenetrated mediastinum. The anteroposterior projection and the slightly lordotic angulation of the x-ray beam combine to distort the basal lung structures and magnify the cardiac silhouette. Recumbent studies also make recognition of pleural effusions or pneumothoraces more difficult. In the ICU, chest radiography can be ordered selectively rather than as a daily routine, without compromising care.

Computed Tomography

Computed tomography (CT) has multiple advantages over conventional radiography. It displays cross-sectional anatomy free of superimposition, with a 10-fold higher contrast resolution. Multislice CT scanners acquire a continuous, volumetric, near-isotropic data set with possibilities for high-quality two-dimensional or three-dimensional reformatting (volume rendering) in any plane. High-resolution CT of the lung parenchyma is an important application; narrow collimation of the beam combined with an edge-enhancing high spatial frequency algorithm results in exquisite detail of normal and abnormal lungs, and correlation with pathologic anatomy is high. CT angiography is also a key component of the evaluation of suspected pulmonary embolism (Chapter 68) and coronavirus disease 2019 (COVID-19).[1]

Magnetic Resonance Imaging

Magnetic resonance imaging (MRI) depends on the magnetic properties of hydrogen atoms. Magnetic coils and radio frequency coils lead to induction, excitation, relaxation, and eventual readout of magnetized protons. The molecular environment of hydrogen atoms will affect the rate at which they release energy; this energy yields a spatial distribution of signals that is converted into an image by computer algorithms, similar to CT. Because of its soft tissue specificity, MRI has applications in the assessment of chest wall invasion, mediastinal infiltration, and diaphragmatic involvement by lung cancer or malignant mesothelioma.

Positron Emission Tomography

Fluorodeoxyglucose positron emission tomography (FDG-PET) uses labeled fluorodeoxyglucose to image the glycolytic pathway of tumor cells or other metabolically active tissues with affinity for glucose. This technique has proved helpful in studying intrathoracic tumors and has facilitated the work-up of solitary pulmonary nodules. Integrated PET-CT scans have improved the diagnosis and staging of intrathoracic tumors.

Ultrasonography

Outside the heart, ultrasonography traditionally has played only a limited role in thoracic imaging. Its primary use has been to localize pleural effusions and guide their drainage (Chapter 86). However, some data suggest that lung ultrasound can be used as a preliminary screen for pneumonia (Chapter 85), pulmonary edema (Chapter 45),[2] or pneumothorax (Chapter 86). In the intensive care setting, ultrasound also may help with the diagnosis of ventilator-associated pneumonia (Chapter 85), pneumothorax (Chapter 86), and diffuse alveolar damage (Chapter 79).

EVALUATION OF CHEST IMAGES

Images of the chest are best evaluated by examining regions of the lung for specific findings and relating these findings to known diagnostic groups.[3] A number of critical radiographic features should be considered, with an appreciation for the known causes of these changes. Artificial intelligence is a promising method to aid in the clinical interpretation of chest images.

Diffuse Lung Disease

Diffuse lung disease is an overall term for a number of related abnormal parenchymal radiographic patterns. Although radiologists have attempted to separate alveolar (Chapter 79) from interstitial lung disease (Chapter 80) radiographically, this distinction is no longer recommended because the correlation between the radiographic localization to a compartment and the actual histopathologic findings is relatively poor. For example, nodular patterns can be produced by either interstitial or alveolar disease. Conversely, so-called alveolar disease processes can induce an interstitial reaction. Ground-glass opacities can be induced by either alveolar or interstitial disease. Air bronchograms, the presumed paradigm of air space disease, can be identified in a small percentage of patients with predominantly interstitial lung disease (Chapter 80), such as sarcoidosis, pulmonary lymphoma, and pulmonary calcinosis.

Because of such limitations, a graphically descriptive approach that combines analysis of predominant opacities, assessment of lung expansion, and distribution and profusion of disease yields a differential diagnosis. The term *infiltrate* should be avoided; instead, the term *pulmonary opacities* should be used, with opacities further classified as large (i.e., >1 cm in the largest dimension) or small (i.e., <1 cm in diameter).

Large Opacities

Large opacities (Table 72-1) are characterized according to their distribution. Diffuse homogeneous opacities are typical for diffuse alveolar damage (Fig. 72-1); increased permeability (noncardiogenic) pulmonary edema; diffuse viral pneumonia (see Fig. 72-1B), including COVID-19 (E-Fig 72-1; see Chapter 336)[4,5]; or *Pneumocystis jirovecii* pneumonia. Multifocal patchy opacities (see Fig. 72-1C) are found in bacterial multifocal bronchopneumonia, recurrent aspiration with multifocal pneumonia or abscesses (Chapter 78), COVID-19 pneumonia in the organizing phase (E-Figs. 72-2 to 72-6), and vasculitis (E-Fig. 72-7). Lobar opacities without atelectasis are typically seen in lobar pneumonia (Fig. 72-2, E-Figs. 72-8 and 72-9). Lobar opacities with atelectasis often result from obstruction of a lobar bronchus by foreign bodies, tumors, or mucous plugs. Perihilar opacities are seen in hydrostatic pulmonary

TABLE 72-1 CLASSIFICATION OF LARGE PULMONARY OPACITIES

Diffuse homogeneous
Multifocal patchy
Lobar without atelectasis
Lobar with atelectasis
Perihilar
Peripheral

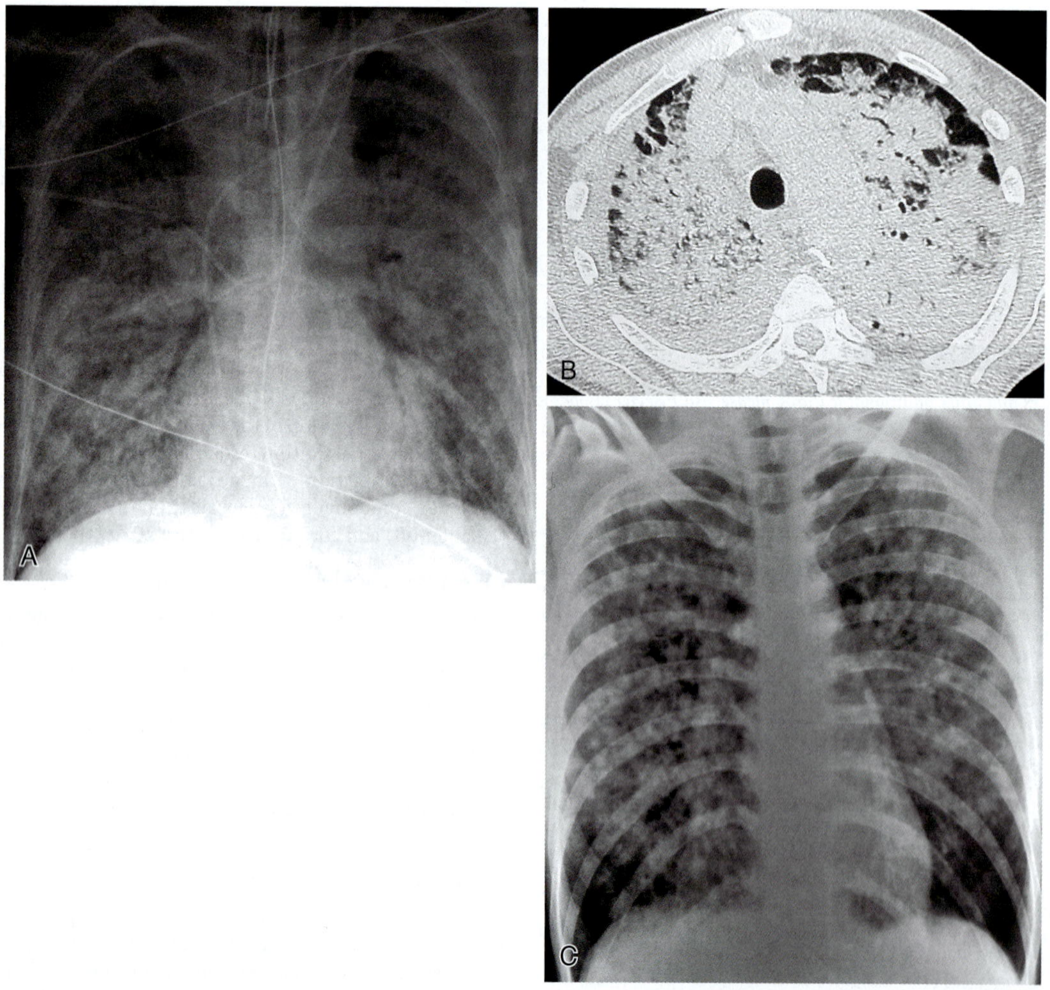

FIGURE 72-1. Diffuse alveolar damage. A, Chest radiograph shows diffuse homogeneous opacification of both lungs with clearly visible air bronchograms. **B,** Computed tomographic scan demonstrates diffuse consolidation with air bronchograms extending to the periphery of both lungs in a patient with community-acquired pneumonia. **C,** Patient with acute varicella pneumonia. Chest radiograph demonstrates multiple acinar nodules with tendency for confluence, yielding multifocal, patchy parenchymal opacification.

edema as a result of left-sided heart failure (Figs. 72-3A and B), renal failure, volume overload, or pulmonary hemorrhage. Subacute or chronic peripheral opacities are described in eosinophilic lung disease. Acute, rounded, large, ground-glass peripheral, subpleural opacities are characteristic of the acute, exudative, and early organizing phase of COVID-19 pneumonia (Fig. 72-4). Similar patterns may also be seen in e-cigarette or vaping use–associated lung disease (Chapter 82).

Small Opacities

In contrast to the large pulmonary opacities, a number of radiographic patterns characterize small pulmonary opacities in diffuse lung disease. It is helpful to differentiate small nodular, linear, reticular, or combined patterns (Table 72-2).

Nodular Patterns

Micronodular opacities, which include nodules 1 mm and smaller in diameter, can result from talc granulomatosis (excipient lung disease) in intravenous drug abusers (Chapter 365), alveolar microlithiasis, rare cases of silicosis, talcosis, coal workers' pneumoconiosis (Chapter 81), and beryllium-induced lung diseases (Chapter 81), as well as from occasional cases of sarcoidosis (Chapter 83) or hemosiderosis. The nodular pattern includes nodules up to 1 cm in diameter. Frequent causes include infections or inflammatory granulomata such as miliary tuberculosis (Chapter 299), sarcoidosis (Chapter 83), fungal diseases, hypersensitivity pneumonitis (Chapter 82), and Langerhans cell histiocytosis (Chapter 80).[6]

Linear Patterns

Linear patterns, also called Kerley lines, are mostly a reflection of thickened interlobular septa. Kerley A lines, which radiate 2 to 4 cm from the hilum toward the pulmonary periphery and particularly toward the upper lobes (Fig. 72-5), reflect thickening of the axial interstitial compartment and can be a feature of left ventricular failure or allergic reactions. Kerley B lines, which reflect thickening of the subpleural interstitial compartment, typically are approximately 1 cm in length and 1 mm in thickness and usually found in the periphery of the lower lobes, abutting the pleura. The B lines are characteristic of subacute and chronic left ventricular failure (Chapter 45), mitral valve disease (Chapter 60), lymphangitic carcinomatosis, viral pneumonia, and pulmonary fibrosis (Chapter 80). Kerley C lines, which are rarely diagnosed by radiologists, result from thickening of the lung parenchymal interstitium and form a reticular pattern on chest radiographs.

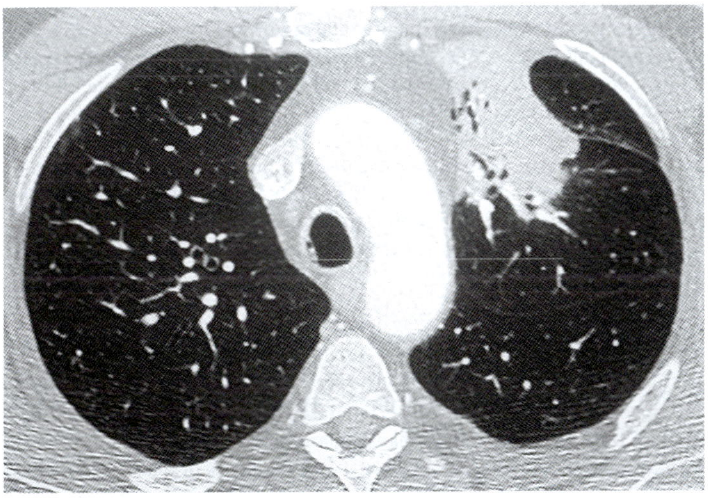

FIGURE 72-2. **Bacterial pneumonia in the left upper lobe.** Computed tomographic scan demonstrates segmental consolidation of the anterior segment of the left upper lobe with air bronchograms.

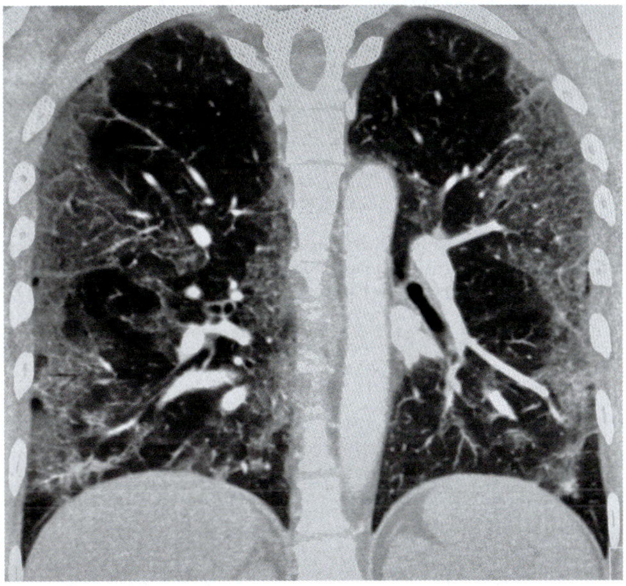

FIGURE 72-4. **Computed tomographic scan in a patient with COVID-19 pneumonia.** Image with coronal reformation shows extensive bilateral subpleural, peripheral ground-glass opacification with interlobular and intralobular septal thickening forming a "crazy pattern" indicative of organizing pneumonia.

TABLE 72-2 PATTERNS OF SMALL PULMONARY OPACITIES

Micronodular
Acinar
Linear
Reticular
Bronchial
Arterial
Destructive

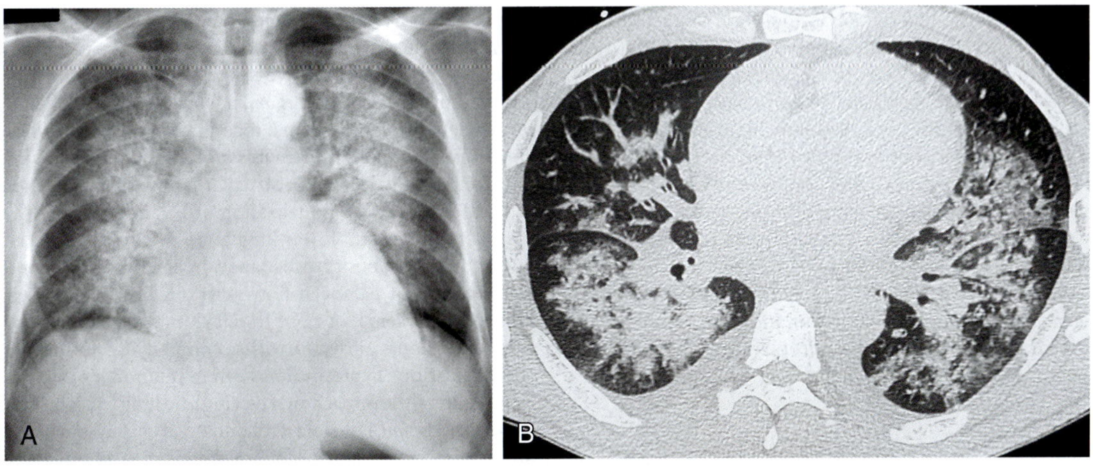

FIGURE 72-3. **A,** Pulmonary edema. Chest frontal radiograph demonstrates classic "batwing" distribution of hydrostatic pulmonary edema. **B,** Computed tomographic scan shows bilateral perihilar consolidations and a small right pleural effusion in a patient with pulmonary edema.

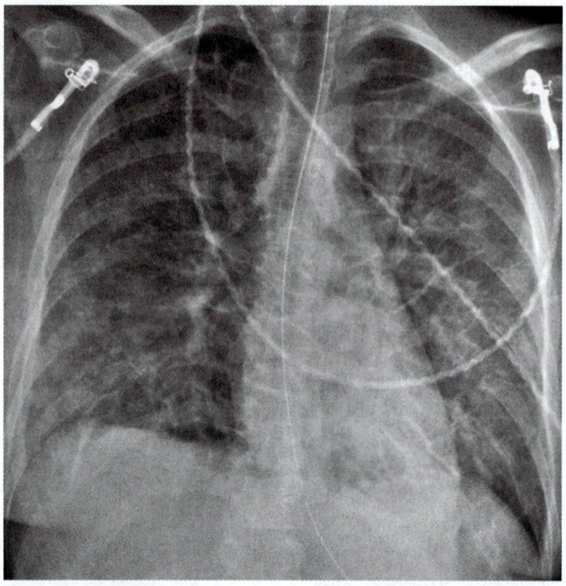

FIGURE 72-5. **Patient with known transfusion reaction.** Chest radiograph displays ground-glass opacification of both lungs and bilateral Kerley A lines, presenting as long linear structures extending from the hilar regions into the pulmonary periphery.

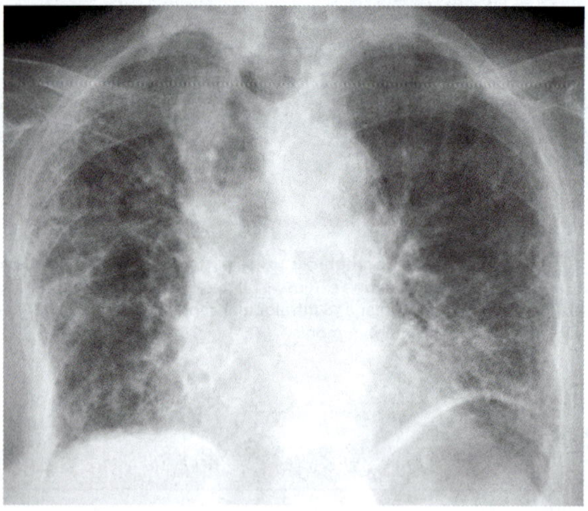

FIGURE 72-6. **Diffuse reticular lung disease.** Chest radiograph in a 94-year-old patient with diffuse reticular opacities (due to idiopathic pulmonary fibrosis with honeycombing) and multiple areas with traction bronchiectasis. The lung volumes are typically reduced by a decreased pulmonary compliance.

Reticular Patterns

Reticular patterns are small polygonal, irregular, or curvilinear opacities on chest radiographs (Fig. 72-6). The differential diagnosis varies according to the timeline of the pathologic change. Acute onset of a reticular pattern can occur in interstitial pulmonary edema (e.g., due to left-sided heart failure), atypical pneumonias (e.g., viral or mycoplasmal pneumonia), early exudative changes in a connective tissue disorder (e.g., systemic lupus erythematosus; Chapter 245), and acute allergic reactions (e.g., transfusion reactions [Chapter 162] or reactions to *Hymenoptera* stings). The common chronic processes resulting in a reticular pattern are idiopathic interstitial pneumonias (Chapter 80), connective tissue diseases (particularly scleroderma and rheumatoid lung), asbestosis (Chapter 81), radiation fibrosis (Chapter 80), end-stage hypersensitivity pneumonitis (Chapters 81 and 82), drug reactions, lymphangitic spread of cancer, end-stage granulomatous infection, lymphoma in its bronchovascular form, Kaposi sarcoma in its bronchovascular manifestation, and sarcoidosis.

Honeycombing

Honeycombing, which is an indication of end-stage interstitial lung disease (Chapter 80), reflects a restructuring of pulmonary anatomy with subpleural cysts, accompanied by bronchiolectasis. Honeycombs (Fig. 72-7) form a

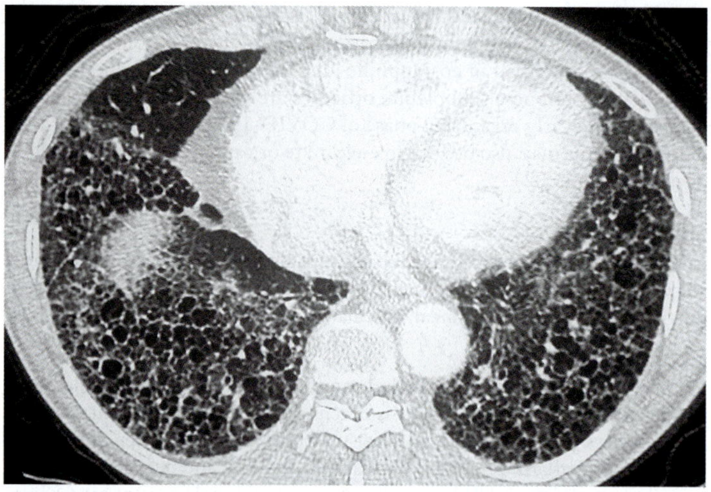

FIGURE 72-7. **Honeycombing in a patient with idiopathic pulmonary fibrosis and usual interstitial pneumonia.** Computed tomographic scan shows multiple bibasal reticular opacities with honeycombing and traction bronchiectases.

multilayer of small subpleural spaces between 3 and 10 mm in diameter. They can be distinguished from paraseptal emphysema by their thicker wall and multiple layers.

Alveolar Pattern

An alveolar (Chapter 79) or air space pattern is characterized by acinar nodules, 0.6 to 1 cm in diameter. These nodules encompass more than the acinus, in the strict anatomic sense, with surrounding peribronchiolar lung tissue. Other patterns include ground-glass opacities (a reflection of incomplete alveolar filling), coalescent large opacities, consolidation involving whole lobes or segments, opacification in a bronchocentric distribution, air bronchograms, and air alveolograms. These radiographic features are helpful in placing a disease into a particular radiologic category, but the radiographic pattern called *alveolar* does not simply correspond to exclusive histologic alveolar filling because the interstitial compartment is involved as well in most cases. A more accurate description is parenchymal rather than alveolar opacification or consolidation.

Bronchial Patterns

Bronchial patterns, as best depicted by diffuse bronchiectasis (Chapter 78), are seen on conventional radiographs as linear, tubular, or cystic lucencies and opacities that follow the expected path of bronchi, so-called tramlines because they resemble tram tracks. Mucoid impaction, as seen in patients with asthma, allergic bronchopulmonary aspergillosis, or plastic bronchitis,[7] leads to opacities described as toothpaste, cluster of grapes, or finger-in-glove. The "dirty lung" pattern seen in smokers with chronic bronchitis (Chapter 76) results from bronchial wall thickening, peribronchial fibrosis, respiratory bronchiolitis, and pulmonary arterial hypertension.

Vascular Patterns

Arterial patterns reflect changes in pulmonary perfusion. The term *caudalization* reflects the normal blood flow distribution pattern in an upright person in which the basal pulmonary vessels are two to three times wider than the upper lobe vasculature. *Cephalization*, in which the ratios of diameters of vessels are reversed, is frequently seen in recumbent persons, in whom it may be considered normal; however, when it is present in individuals imaged in the upright position, it indicates left ventricular failure (Fig. 72-8), mitral valve disease, or basal emphysema. Equalization or balanced flow with well-demonstrated vessels to upper and lower lung zones is found in hyperkinetic circulation due to anemia, obesity, pregnancy, hyperthyroidism, or left-to-right shunts. Equalization or balanced flow with oligemia can be seen in hypovolemia, diffuse emphysema, or right-to-left shunts. Centralization reflects dilation of central pulmonary arteries, with accompanying normal or diminished peripheral circulation. Typically, it is seen in pulmonary arterial hypertension (Fig. 72-9). Lateralization of flow, favoring one lung over the other, also called *asymmetrical perfusion*, is visible with unilateral emphysema, unilateral bronchiolitis obliterans (Swyer-James-McLeod syndrome), or unilateral obstruction of the pulmonary artery. Locally dilated pulmonary vessels occur adjacent to affected oligemic lung regions in patchy emphysema, multiple pulmonary emboli,

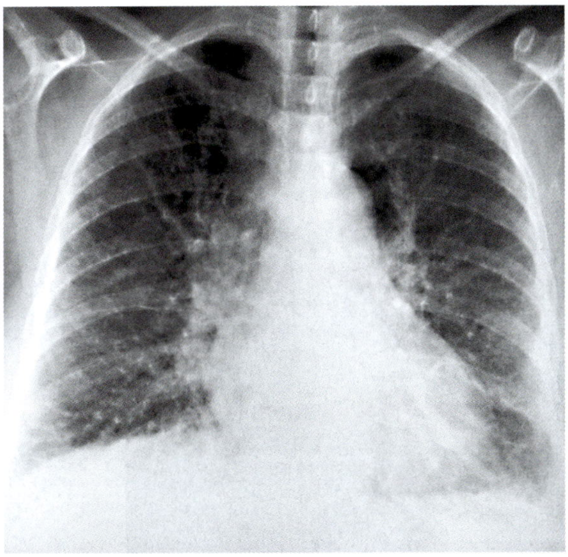

FIGURE 72-8. **Patient with left ventricular failure.** Chest frontal radiograph shows cephalization of pulmonary blood flow.

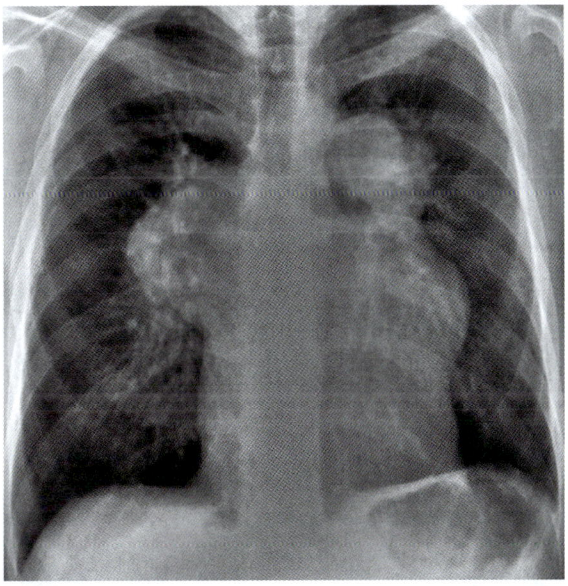

FIGURE 72-9. **Patient with primary pulmonary arterial hypertension.** Chest frontal radiograph shows centralization of flow with pulmonary artery aneurysms and peripheral pulmonary oligemia.

arteriovenous malformations, and nonuniform bronchiolitis obliterans. This pattern produces mosaic attenuation on high-resolution CT scanning. Focal oligemia with vascular deficiency is characteristically seen in emphysema but also can occur after pulmonary embolism (Westermark sign). Centrilobular emphysema (Chapter 76), paraseptal emphysema, and bullous lung disease have a predilection for the upper lung regions, whereas panlobular emphysema induces basal oligemia with vascular deficiency.

Lung Volume

Conventional radiographs and CT scans are performed during a breath hold at full inspiration and total lung capacity. Low lung volumes are inferred by the high position of the diaphragm and the crowding of basal vascular structures (Table 72-3). Lung volumes larger than expected are commonly found in patients with diffuse emphysema (Fig. 72-10; Chapter 76), chronic or severe acute asthma (Chapter 75), or diffuse bronchiolitis obliterans and in highly trained athletes. With a few rare exceptions, chronic diffuse infiltrative lung diseases (Chapter 80) lead to loss of volume.

Anatomic Distribution

The anatomic distribution of disease can often guide the approach to diagnosis (Table 72-4 and Fig. 72-11). Upper zone lung disease predominates in

TABLE 72-3 CONDITIONS ASSOCIATED WITH VARIOUS LUNG VOLUMES IN PATIENTS WITH AN UNDERLYING DIFFUSE LUNG DISEASE PATTERN

LARGE LUNG VOLUMES
Emphysema
Chronic or severe asthma
Diffuse bronchiolitis obliterans
Highly trained athletes
Lymphangioleiomyomatosis
SMALL LUNG VOLUMES
End-stage lung fibrosis
Bilateral diaphragmatic paralysis
Massive ascites
NORMAL LUNG VOLUMES
Sarcoidosis
Langerhans cell histiocytosis
Neurofibromatosis
Combined pulmonary fibrosis and emphysema

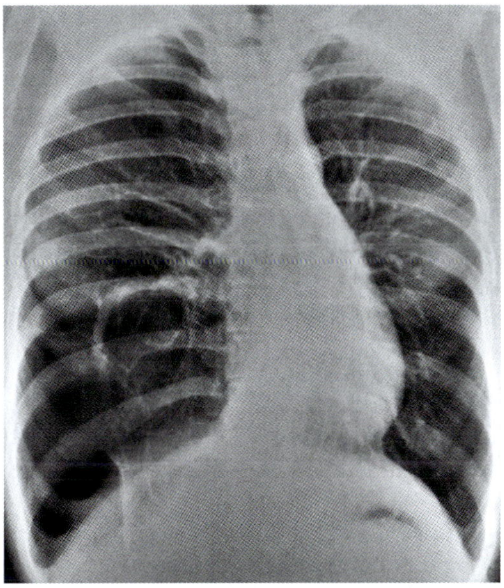

FIGURE 72-10. **Patient with severe emphysema.** Chest radiograph shows hyperexpansion of both lungs with bullous changes at the right lung base and leftward mediastinal shift.

TABLE 72-4 CONDITIONS ASSOCIATED WITH DISEASE DISTRIBUTION PATTERNS

UPPER ZONE LUNG DISEASE
Bullous lung disease
Centrilobular and paraseptal emphysema
Tuberculosis
Fungal disease
Sarcoidosis
Pneumoconiosis
Langerhans cell histiocytosis
Cystic fibrosis
End-stage hypersensitivity pneumonitis
Ankylosing spondylitis
Radiation pneumonitis
BASAL LUNG DISEASE
Panlobular emphysema
Bronchiectasis
Aspiration
Drug reactions
Interstitial pulmonary fibrosis, nonspecific interstitial pneumonia, desquamative interstitial pneumonia, cryptogenic organizing pneumonia (also called bronchiolitis obliterans with organizing pneumonia)
Asbestosis
Scleroderma

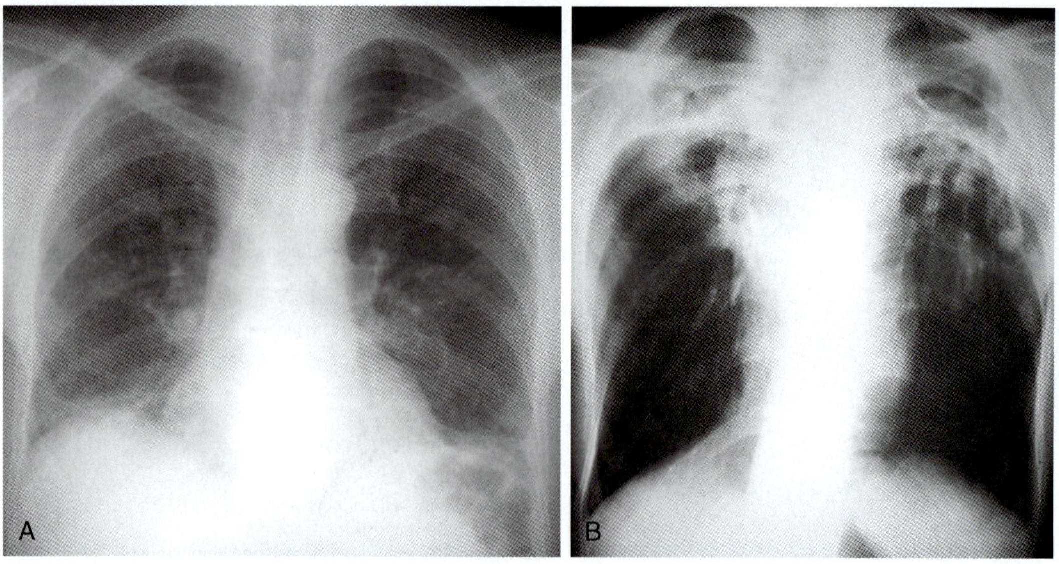

FIGURE 72-11. A, Basal pulmonary disease. Chest radiograph in a 48-year-old patient with known scleroderma. Bibasal fine reticular opacities and parenchymal bands are visible in both lower lobes. B, Apical lung disease. Chest radiograph in a 42-year-old patient with ankylosing spondylitis. Severe architectural distortion with cicatrizing atelectasis of both upper lobes, retraction of both pulmonary arteries cephalad, and bilateral bulla formation containing fungus balls are evident.

TABLE 72-5 DISEASES AFFECTING THE LUNG PERIPHERY

Chronic eosinophilic pneumonia
Cryptogenic organizing pneumonia
Idiopathic interstitial fibrosis (usual interstitial pneumonia)
Bronchioloalveolar cell carcinoma (rare)
Pseudo-alveolar sarcoidosis (rare)
COVID-19 pneumonia
E-cigarette or vaping product use-associated lung injury

TABLE 72-6 CONDITIONS ASSOCIATED WITH HILAR AND MEDIASTINAL LYMPH NODE ENLARGEMENT

Sarcoidosis
Lymphoma
Fungal disease
Tuberculosis
Metastatic cancer
Silicosis, coal worker's pneumoconiosis, beryllium lung

tuberculosis, fungal disease, sarcoidosis, pneumoconiosis (except asbestosis), Langerhans cell histiocytosis, ankylosing spondylitis, cystic fibrosis, cystic *P. jirovecii* pneumonia, radiation pneumonitis, and end-stage hypersensitivity pneumonitis. Basal lung disease is preferentially found in bronchiectasis (Chapter 78), aspiration pneumonia, desquamative interstitial pneumonia, nonspecific interstitial pneumonia, usual interstitial pneumonia (Chapter 80), drug reactions, asbestosis, scleroderma (Chapter 246), and rheumatoid arthritis (Chapter 243). Peripheral lung disease is seen in the initial exudative and early organizing phase of COVID-19 pneumonia (Chapter 336)[8]; in eosinophilic pneumonia, cryptogenic organizing pneumonia, usual interstitial pneumonia, bronchioloalveolar cell carcinoma, adenocarcinoma in situ or minimally invasive adenocarcinoma (Chapter 177); and in occasional patients with so-called alveolar sarcoidosis (Table 72-5). However, any diffuse lung process will eventually progress to involve both lungs irrespective of zonal boundaries.

Lymph Nodes

Enlarged lymph nodes that are visible on chest CT scans and, when larger, on chest radiographs can provide diagnostic information (Table 72-6). The following entities can be associated with diffuse lung disease and concurrent enlarged lymph nodes: sarcoidosis (Chapter 83); lymphoma; fungal disease; tuberculosis (Chapter 299); pneumoconiosis (Chapter 81), particularly silicosis and beryllium-associated lung disease; lung cancer; and metastatic malignant disease other than lung cancer.

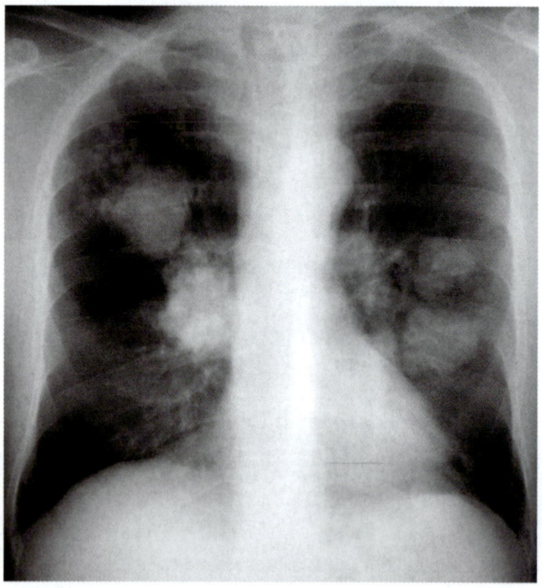

FIGURE 72-12. **Multifocal pulmonary opacities.** Chest radiograph in a 70-year-old patient with known carcinoma of the thyroid gland shows widening of the superior mediastinum, displacing the cervical trachea to the right. Bilateral large and small pulmonary nodules and masses due to metastatic tumor are present.

Pulmonary Nodules

Deep-learning models are increasingly being pilot-tested to help determine whether pulmonary nodules are likely to be benign or malignant.[9] The detailed approach to evaluating solitary pulmonary nodules is covered in Chapter 177.

Most patients with multiple pulmonary nodules larger than 1 cm in diameter have metastatic disease from primary cancers either within or outside the lung (Fig. 72-12). These lesions have a predilection for subpleural lung regions, including the lung subtending the interlobar fissures. In patients with human immunodeficiency virus infection, Kaposi sarcoma and lymphoma can induce the formation of such nodules. Infectious processes that present with multiple nodules include multiple abscesses from recurrent aspiration (Chapter 82) or septic emboli (Chapter 61); tuberculous and nontuberculous mycobacterial granulomata (Chapters 299 and 300); fungal processes, including histoplasmosis (Chapter 308), coccidioidomycosis (Chapter 308), and cryptococcosis (Chapter 309); and infestation with flukes, such as *Paragonimus westermani* (Chapter 326). Noninfectious inflammatory conditions that can present with multiple pulmonary nodules include granulomatosis with polyangiitis (Chapter 249), rheumatoid nodules (Chapter 243), sarcoidosis (Chapter 83), and amyloidosis (Chapter 174).

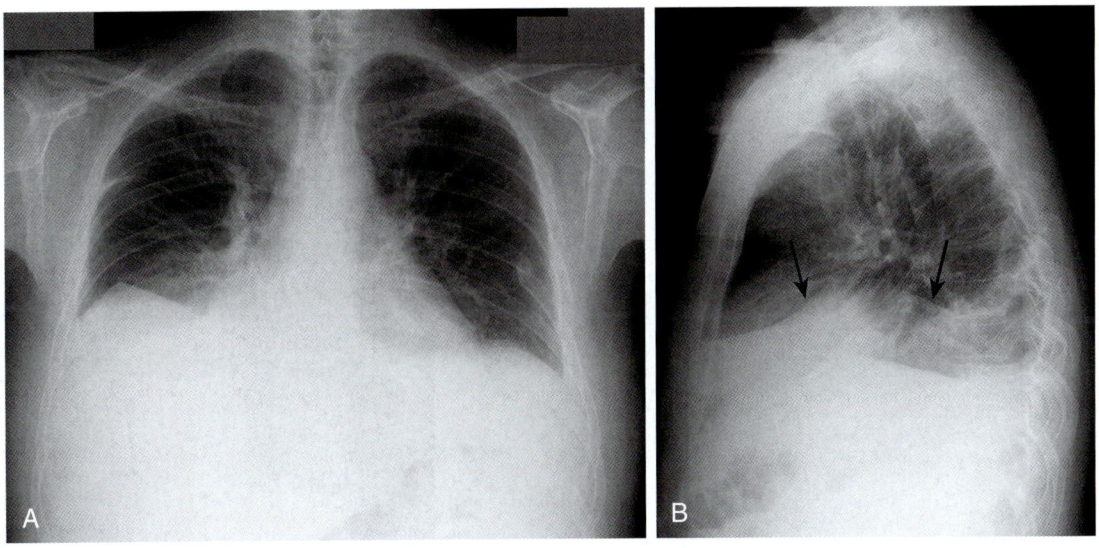

FIGURE 72-13. **Bilateral subpulmonic pleural effusions.** Chest frontal (**A**) and lateral (**B**) views. Both lung bases are elevated, with lateralization of the lung base curvature that mimics an elevated diaphragm. In the lateral projection, the configuration of the interface between the effusion and the aerated lung mimics the shape of the Rock of Gibraltar (*arrows*).

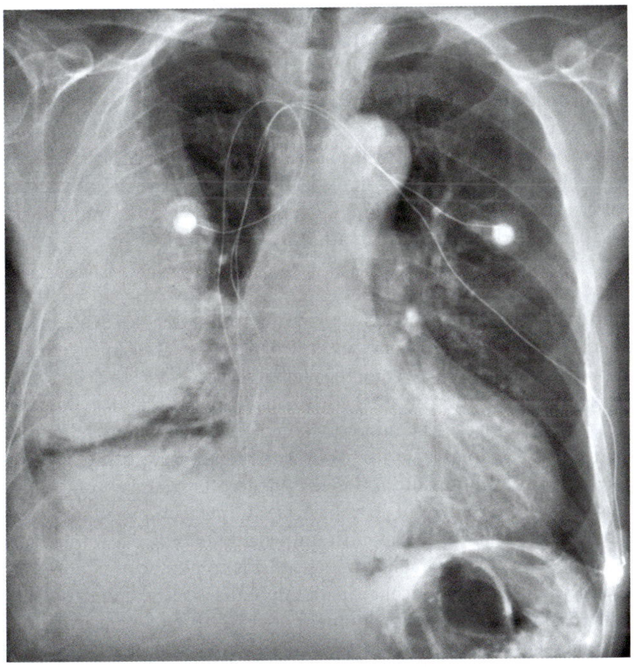

FIGURE 72-14. **Loculated right-sided pleural effusion.** Chest frontal view. A right-sided peripheral pleural mass is seen with characteristic obtuse angles of interface toward the chest wall, with tapered borders and sharp contour toward the lung. These findings localize the mass to the pleural or extrapleural compartment and not to the lung parenchyma. This loculated effusion proved to be an empyema.

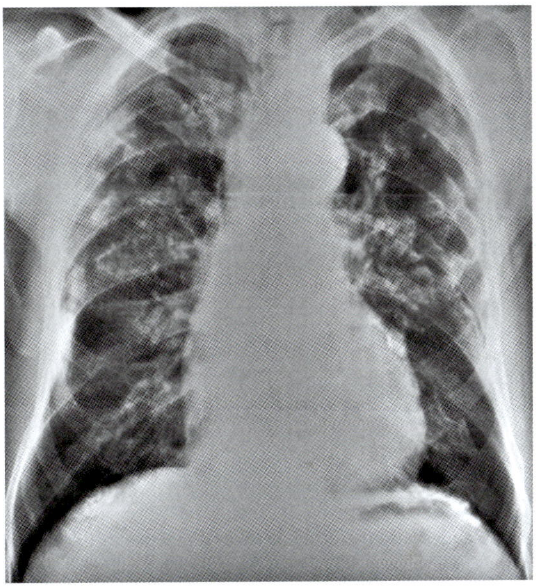

FIGURE 72-15. **Patient with known prior occupational asbestos exposure.** Chest radiograph shows extensive bilateral calcified pleural plaques seen en face, in profile, and along the diaphragmatic contour.

Pleural Disease

Abnormalities of the pleural space (Chapter 86) can be displayed effectively by conventional radiographic methods supplemented by CT scanning. The volume of a pleural effusion (see Figs. 86-3 and 86-4 in Chapter 86) can be reliably estimated on standard frontal upright chest radiograph: 75 mL obscures the posterior costophrenic sulcus, 150 mL obscures the lateral costophrenic sulcus, 200 mL produces a rind of 1 cm in thickness on decubitus radiographs, 500 mL obscures the diaphragm and is visible on supine radiographs, and 1000-mL effusions reach the level of the fourth anterior rib on upright chest radiographs. An effusion of 200 mL or more can be sampled by thoracentesis. The smallest amount visible on decubitus radiographs is 10 mL. With care, as little as 175 mL of effusion can be detected on supine images. Free-layering pleural effusions produce a veil of opacity or filter effect superimposed on the aerated lung; pulmonary vessels are clearly visible through the added opacity generated by the effusion, and air bronchograms are absent.

Subpulmonic and Loculated Pleural Effusions

Subpulmonic pleural effusions elevate the lung base, mimicking a high-riding hemidiaphragm. The highest curvature point of the pseudodiaphragm is shifted laterally with an abrupt lateral descent, the so-called Rock of Gibraltar sign; it also can be seen in the lateral projection (Fig. 72-13). Large pleural effusions can lead to diaphragmatic inversion. Separation of the lung base from the gas-containing stomach is indicative of a subpulmonic effusion, particularly when the stomach gas bubble is displaced inferomedially.

Loculated pleural effusions suggest the presence of pleural adhesions or indicate an underlying parenchymal lung abnormality with a focal decrease in adjacent pleural pressure. Such encapsulated collections have obtuse angles of interface with the chest wall, tapered borders that are incomplete toward the chest wall, and a sharply defined contour with the adjacent lung (Fig. 72-14).

Pleural Plaques

Pleural plaques result from parietal pleural accumulation of hyalinized collagen fibers (Fig. 72-15); their presence suggests asbestos exposure (Chapter 81). Plaques preferentially involve the parietal pleura adjacent to ribs six through nine and the diaphragm. They are less pronounced in the intercostal spaces and spare the costophrenic sulci as well as the apices. Calcifications are visible on chest radiographs in 20% and on CT scans in 50% of individuals with pleural plaques. Imaged in

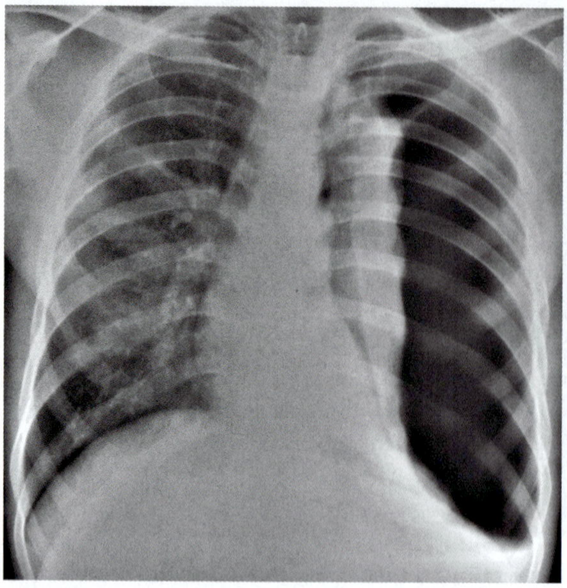

FIGURE 72-16. **Patient with spontaneous tension hydropneumothorax.** Chest radiograph shows complete atelectasis of the left lung with a large pneumothorax and a left basal gas-liquid level. The patient had primary tuberculosis.

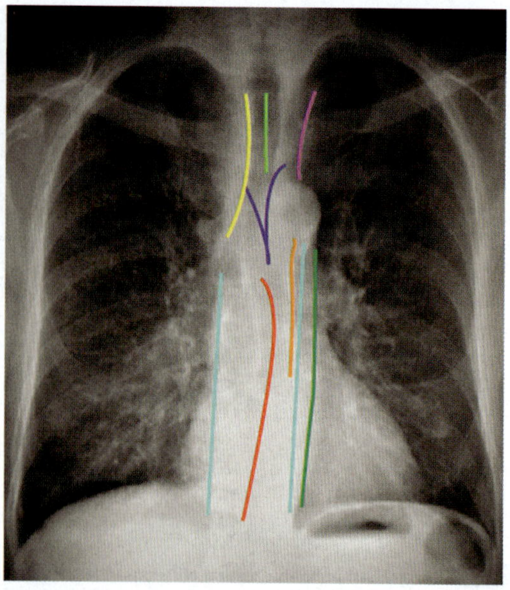

FIGURE 72-17. **Chest radiograph with superimposed mediastinal stripes.** *Yellow:* Right paratracheal stripe. *Light blue:* Right and left paraspinal stripes. *Red:* Azygoesophageal stripe. *Brown:* Pleuroesophageal stripe. *Purple:* Anterior junction line complex. *Pink:* Left subclavian artery border. *Light green:* Posterior-superior junction line. *Dark green:* Para-aortic line.

TABLE 72-7 CLASSIFICATION OF MEDIASTINAL COMPARTMENTS

ANTERIOR MEDIASTINUM
Retrosternal: Prevascular compartment
MIDDLE MEDIASTINUM: VISCERAL COMPARTMENT
Subcarinal space Paratracheal region Retrotracheal space Aortopulmonic window Retrocardiac space
POSTERIOR MEDIASTINUM: PARAVERTEBRAL COMPARTMENT
Paraspinal region

profile, pleural plaques produce focal areas of apparent pleural thickening. Over the diaphragm, they appear as curvilinear calcifications or scalloping. Pleural plaques viewed en face can simulate lung disease. Their appearance has been likened to holly leaves, sunburst patterns, or geographic patterns and, when calcified, to a dripping candle, rolled margins, or stippled or irregular structures. Rare visceral pleural plaques that occur in interlobar fissures can mimic pulmonary nodules.

Diffuse Pleural Thickening

Diffuse thickening of the parietal and visceral pleurae is a response observed after exposure to any of a number of stimuli, including infection, inflammation, trauma, tumor, thromboembolism, radiation, and asbestos. Severe involvement results in formation of a generalized pleural peel with smooth margins, usually less than 2 cm in thickness. Radiologically diffuse pleural thickening is characterized by a smooth, noninterrupted pleural opacity involving at least one fourth of the chest wall circumference, obliterating the costophrenic sulci and encompassing also the apices. The CT criteria for diffuse pleural thickening include a thickness of at least 3 mm.

Pleural Tumors

Malignant tumors of the pleura are more common than benign ones, and metastatic disease is more frequent than primary pleural mesothelioma. Primary tumors originate from pleural membranes. Pleural invasion by lung cancer, subpleural plaques in lymphoma, hematogenous dissemination to the pleura, and direct pleural seeding are other mechanisms of pleural involvement by tumor. Benign pleural tumors include lipomas, fibrous tumors, and neurogenic tumors. Lipomas are most common; their diagnosis is facilitated by CT scanning. Fibrous tumors of the pleura originate from pluripotent mesenchymal cells found in the visceral pleura or, less commonly, in the parietal pleura. Fibrous tumors can induce paraneoplastic syndromes, such as hypertrophic osteoarthropathy (Chapter 164) or hypoglycemia (Doege-Potter syndrome), but they rarely invade or metastasize. In nearly half of affected patients, the tumor can be on a pedicle and be mobile as a patient changes position. Torsion of this pedicle can, on rare occasions, lead to tumor necrosis with accumulation of gas in the mass. Post-traumatic splenosis can lead to multiple pleural masses, particularly in the left hemithorax.

Pneumothorax

Pneumothorax, which means gas in the pleural space (Chapter 86), can be open or closed. An open pneumothorax results when a penetrating injury of the chest wall allows atmospheric air to enter the pleural space, whereas a closed pneumothorax is the accumulation of air that originated in the respiratory system within the pleural space. A closed pneumothorax can be simple, where the air pressure within the pneumothorax is similar to that in the adjacent alveolar space, or under tension, where the air pressure within the pneumothorax is substantially above the air pressure in the adjacent alveolar space and can compress lung tissue and great vessels (Chapter 86). The most important radiologic feature of a pneumothorax is a visceral pleural line or edge that is convex or straight toward the chest wall and produces a lucent separation of the visceral and parietal pleura (Fig. 72-16). In most cases, no pulmonary vascular structures are visible beyond the visceral pleura. On upright chest radiographs, gas is primarily found in the apicolateral pleural space. Expiratory chest radiographs are not necessary for the detection of small pneumothoraces because all pneumothoraces are visible on inspiratory studies. On supine chest radiographs, pleural gas accumulates in a subpulmonic location; it outlines the costophrenic sulcus, forming the deep sulcus sign. A tension pneumothorax leads to a marked shift of the mediastinum to the contralateral side and to flattening or inversion of the ipsilateral hemidiaphragm. In supine patients with a hydropneumothorax, a veil of opacity can be seen with a gradient of decreasing attenuation toward the apex of the affected hemithorax. Post-traumatic, open pneumothorax can lead to mediastinal flutter with wide respiratory excursions. After evacuation of a pneumothorax, unilateral pulmonary edema can occur in the re-expanded lung (E-Fig. 72-10).

IMAGING OF THE MEDIASTINUM

The mediastinum encompasses midline thoracic structures that are delineated by mediastinal pleura, the diaphragm, the sternum, the spine, and the thoracic inlet. The mediastinum is commonly divided into an anterior prevascular compartment, a visceral middle compartment, and a paraspinal, posterior mediastinal compartment (Table 72-7). Each compartment contains specific pathologic entities.

IMAGING TECHNIQUES

On well-penetrated chest radiographs, the anterior junction line, the posterior-superior junction line, the azygoesophageal stripe, the pleuroesophageal stripe, the paratracheal stripe, and the para-aortic and the paraspinal stripes or lines should be assessed (Fig. 72-17). Mediastinal masses need to be detected and

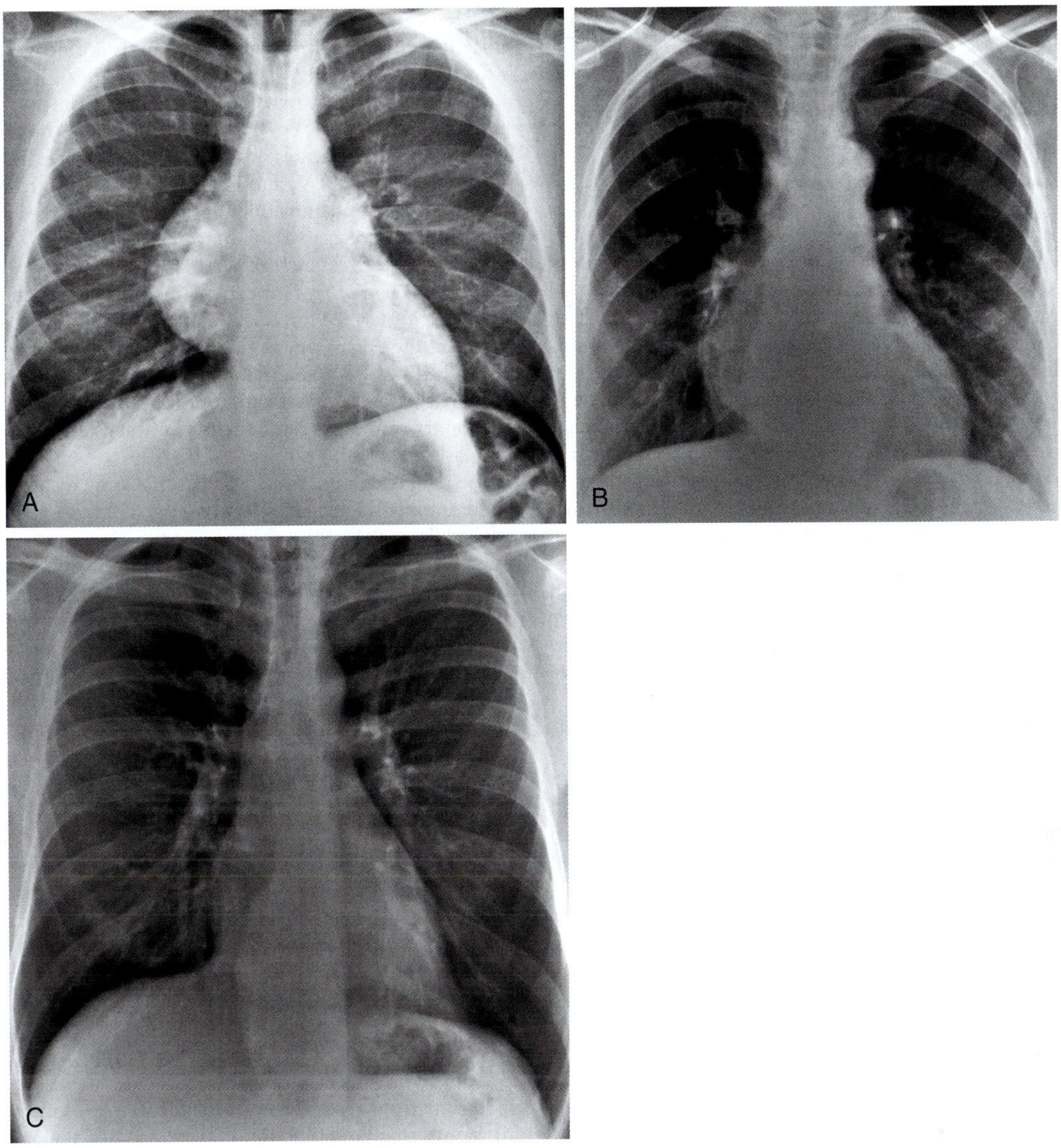

FIGURE 72-18. **Mediastinal findings on chest radiographs. A, Patient with anterior mediastinal teratoma. Chest radiograph shows a mediastinal contour abnormality due to projection of the mass into the right hemithorax. Note the obtuse angle of interface formed by the pleura covering the mass with the mediastinum. The right descending pulmonary artery is visible through the mass, thereby proving that the mass is mediastinal and not hilar. This finding is called the hilum overlay sign. B, Patient with Castleman giant lymph node hyperplasia. Chest frontal radiograph shows large subcarinal middle mediastinal mass that projects lateral to the right atrium. C, Patient with paraspinal ganglioneuroma. Chest radiograph shows right lower paraspinal contour abnormality widening the right paraspinal region and encompassing the height of three thoracic vertebrae.**

localized first. Their obtuse angles of interface with the mediastinal pleura, incomplete border toward the mediastinum, sharp contour toward the lung, and extension into both hemithoraces indicate the mediastinal origin of such lesions.

CT facilitates localization of a mass to a specific mediastinal compartment. When it is known whether the mass is predominantly fatty or cystic, contains soft tissue, or is calcified, the differential diagnosis can be limited. MRI of the mediastinum has a role in diagnosis of vertebral disease or neurogenic tumors with extension into the spinal canal. It is equivalent to CT in diagnosis of aortic aneurysms and dissections (Chapter 63).

MEDIASTINAL COMPARTMENTS

The anterior mediastinum or prevascular compartment is actually a potential space that may contain the fatty replaced thymus and small normal lymph nodes. Space-occupying lesions in this compartment typically include thymomas, lymphomas, teratomas, and other germ cell tumors; substernal thyroid goiters; lipomas; and other connective tissue tumors, as well as hemangiomas or lymphangiomas (Fig. 72-18).

The middle mediastinum or visceral compartment is subdivided into the subcarinal space, paratracheal region, retrotracheal region, aortopulmonic window region, cardiac space, and retrocardiac space. Characteristic lesions are enlarged lymph nodes and bronchopulmonary foregut malformations (see Fig. 72-18B).

In the retrotracheal region, aberrant right subclavian arteries, posterior descending goiters, esophageal tumors, diverticula, or thoracic duct cysts can be found. In the aortopulmonic window, enlarged lymph nodes, ductus diverticula, bronchopulmonary foregut malformations, and aortic or pulmonic artery aneurysms can form compartment-specific space-occupying lesions. Pericardial cysts, pericardial tumors, and cardiac masses are the common space-occupying lesions in the cardiac space. Hiatal hernias are common masses in the retrocardiac region.

The paraspinal region or paravertebral compartment is considered radiologically to belong to the posterior mediastinum. Important masses in that space include neurogenic tumors that originate from the sympathetic chain or from segmental nerve roots (see Fig. 72-18C). Extramedullary hematopoiesis in patients with severe anemia can result in paravertebral masses formed by hypertrophied bone marrow that extrudes from ribs or vertebral bodies. Enlarged lymph nodes due to lymphoma or metastatic disease are occasionally seen in a paraspinal location. Vertebral disease, including bacterial or tuberculous spondylitis, tumors, and post-traumatic hematomas, can widen the paraspinal region and produce contour abnormalities.

GENERAL REFERENCES

For the General References and other additional features, please visit Elsevier eBooks+ at https://ebooks.health.elsevier.com.

73

RESPIRATORY TESTING AND FUNCTION

PAUL D. SCANLON AND ALEXANDER S. NIVEN

Pulmonary function testing has been used in the medical evaluation of patients with respiratory issues since Hutchinson's 1846 demonstration that vital capacity, the largest volume of air that can be exhaled, is an important measure of health. Lung function is one of the most important predictors of all-cause mortality. Environmental exposures, especially exposure to tobacco smoke, and diseases affect pulmonary function, as do genetic and socioeconomic factors, especially during periods of lung growth. Pulmonary function is central to our understanding of pulmonary disorders; many are classified as "obstructive" or "restrictive" disorders in acknowledgement of their pulmonary function pattern. Change or stability of pulmonary function is a key outcome in many clinical trials of respiratory medications.

Pulmonary function can also be an important outcome after an acute respiratory infection. For example, about 70% of survivors of moderate to severe, but not critical, coronavirus-2019 (COVID-19; Chapter 336) pneumonia have pulmonary diffusion abnormalities on pulmonary function testing 6 weeks after discharge, about 25% have obstructive findings, and about 20% have restrictive findings.[1]

Measures of lung function include assessments of respiratory mechanics, for example, the volume of gas that is contained by the lung in various circumstances, the inspiratory and expiratory flow rates across the vital capacity, the pressures that can be generated by inspiratory and expiratory efforts, and the resistance to airflow, as well as calculations of gas exchange. Exertional symptoms often correlate poorly with resting physiologic measurements, and cardiopulmonary exercise testing can be a valuable tool to measure the degree of functional impairment.[2] The analysis of bronchoalveolar lavage fluid, obtained by bronchoscopy, can also provide important insights into pulmonary disease.

SPIROMETRY

The simplest, most commonly performed pulmonary function test is spirometry (Table 73-1).[3,4] This test measures the forced vital capacity (FVC), which is the amount of air that can be forcefully expelled from the lungs, beginning at maximal inhalation (termed total lung capacity [TLC]) and ending with the lungs emptied to their minimal volume (residual volume [RV]). Many secondary measures are derived from the FVC maneuver, including volume exhaled in a given time, termed the forced expiratory volume (FEV), with a subscript indicating the number of seconds during which this measurement is made (e.g., FEV_1, FEV_3). The ratio of the FEV_1/FVC is the proportion of the total vital capacity that can be expelled in the first second of a maximal expiratory effort; a low (<70%) FEV_1/FVC ratio (below the predicted lower limit of normal) indicates obstructive lung disease. In patients with asthma (Chapter 75), the FEV_1 and FEV_1/FVC ratio will often vary based on the degree of airway inflammation. By comparison, a fixed low ratio is consistent with chronic obstructive pulmonary disease (COPD; see Chapter 76) and is associated with an increased risk for future hospitalization or mortality.[5] In addition, expiratory flow can be measured at specific portions of exhaled vital capacity, termed forced expiratory flow (FEF), followed by a number to represent the percentage of the FVC at which the flow was measured (e.g., FEF_{75}, FEF_{50}, FEF_{25}). Expiratory flow can also be measured over a volume range (e.g., $FEF_{25\text{-}75}$). With appropriate coaching and modest patient effort, spirometry results are reproducible between test sessions, thereby allowing comparisons over time.

The data from a maximal exhalation can be displayed using a spirogram (volume-time tracing) or a flow-volume curve (Fig. 73-1A), which depicts exhaled flow at any given volume as a function of exhaled volume. The flow-volume curve has a unique shape for any individual at any given time. It can reflect airflow obstruction (Fig. 73-1B and C), such as is seen in asthma (Chapter 75) and chronic obstructive lung disease (COPD; Chapter 76), or lung restriction (Fig. 73-1D and E), such as is seen in many interstitial lung diseases (Chapter 80). A restrictive disorder may be indicated by a decreased FEV_1 and FVC but a preserved or even an increased FEV_1/FVC ratio. It also may demonstrate less common abnormalities, including variable extrathoracic (Fig. 73-1F) or intrathoracic (Fig. 73-1G) obstruction, fixed central airway obstruction (Fig. 73-1H), or severe muscle weakness (Chapter 74; Fig. 73-1I).

The FVC, FEV_1, FEV_1/FVC ratio, and shape of the flow-volume curves are highly reproducible measures of lung function if the tested individual makes an expiratory effort above a certain, easy-to-obtain level in a pulmonary function laboratory with modern spirometry equipment and trained staff. In the absence of quality assurance, however, measurements of lung function are often neither accurate nor reproducible; poor-quality pulmonary function testing results are biased to lower values, thereby giving an incorrect impression of disease where none may exist. In many but not all cases, poor performance can be identified from inspection of the flow-volume curve (Fig. 73-1L).[6] Poor performance should be noted by the interpreter to avoid erroneous diagnoses.

Spirometry is recommended for the diagnosis of respiratory symptoms, for monitoring lung function in response to a therapeutic intervention or potentially harmful drug exposure, for objective quantification of physiologic impairment, for disability evaluations, and for preemployment and lung health monitoring for at-risk occupations. Use of spirometry as a screening test for asymptomatic persons thought to be at risk for development of lung disease, such as current or former smokers, should be used with caution. Unfortunately, an abnormal spirometry result has not been shown to improve the likelihood that such at-risk individuals will quit smoking, and a normal screening spirometry test result might be misinterpreted to indicate that an individual may continue smoking without risk.

Spirometry is often performed before and after administration of an inhaled bronchodilator, either a selective β_2-agonist (e.g., albuterol/salbutamol), a muscarinic antagonist (e.g., ipratropium), or both, especially if it shows changes consistent with airflow obstruction. The degree of improvement after administration of a bronchodilator indicates the degree of airflow responsiveness, which is generally more in asthma (Chapter 75) and less in COPD (Chapter 76). Unfortunately, the measured response to a bronchodilator on spirometry varies with the dose of drug used in the test, is poorly repeatable from test to test, and is not a good predictor of the clinical response to bronchodilator therapy in an individual patient.

TABLE 73-1 PULMONARY FUNCTION TESTS

LUNG VOLUMES	
TLC	Total lung capacity (volume of gas in lungs at the end of maximal inspiration)
FRC	Functional residual capacity (volume of gas in the lungs at relaxation, when the inward pull of lungs is balanced by the outward pull of the relaxed chest wall)
RV	Residual volume (FRC – ERV, volume of gas left in lungs after maximal exhalation)
IC	Inspiratory capacity (volume of gas inspired from FRC to TLC)
EXPIRATORY FLOW	
FEV_1	Forced expiratory volume (in 1 second)
FVC	Forced vital capacity
FEV_1/FVC	FEV_1/FVC ratio (can be expressed as a ratio or as a percentage)
DIFFUSING CAPACITY	
DLCO	Diffusing capacity of lungs for carbon monoxide
ARTERIAL BLOOD GASES	
PaO_2	Partial pressure of oxygen in arterial blood
$PaCO_2$	Partial pressure of carbon dioxide in arterial blood
pH	Negative log of hydrogen ion concentration in a solution

OTHER TESTS OF VENTILATION

Maximal voluntary ventilation (MVV) is an indication of the maximal ventilation a patient can perform, expressed in liters per minute. MVV estimates a person's upper limit of ventilatory capacity. Reductions in MVV may be due to central airway obstruction, muscle weakness, or poor performance. Because MVV is effort dependent, it may be a better predictor of postoperative respiratory complications (Chapter 401) than is FEV_1. Concomitant measurement of inspiratory flows can be useful for patients in whom there is a suspicion of upper airway disease, such as a patient who has stridor or a patient whose MVV is reduced out of proportion to the FEV_1.

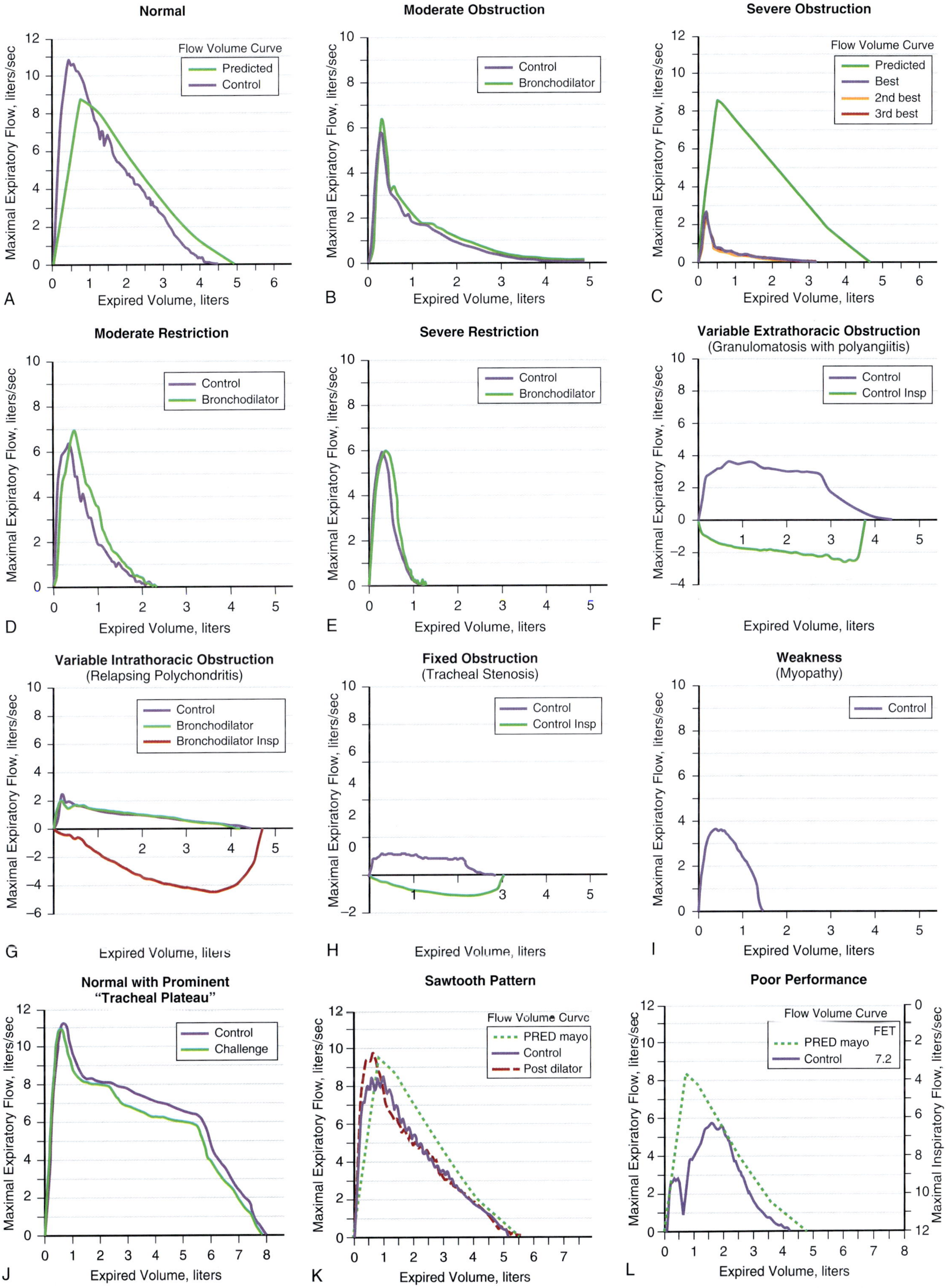

FIGURE 73-1. Common patterns of flow-volume curve. A, Normal. B, Moderate obstruction. C, Severe obstruction. D, Moderate restriction. E, Severe restriction. F, Variable extrathoracic obstruction (granulomatosis with polyangiitis). G, Variable intrathoracic obstruction (relapsing polychondritis). H, Fixed obstruction (tracheal stenosis). I, Weak effort (myopathy). J, Normal but with a prominent tracheal plateau. K, Sawtooth curve associated with obstructive sleep apnea. L, Poor-quality maneuver with both delay in peak flow and cough within the first second. Challenge = methacholine challenge; Control = patient's baseline performance; Insp = inspiration.

REFERENCE EQUATIONS

Normal lung size varies from person to person as a function of height, age, sex, and a wide variety of environmental and socioeconomic factors that impact lung development and function over time. Differences historically attributed to ethnic origin have been replaced by race-neutral equations.[7,8] Therefore, values obtained from pulmonary function testing are compared with those of normal individuals with similar characteristics. Results are expressed as a percentage of a reference value calculated with those factors.

LUNG VOLUMES

The volume of air in the lung at any given time can be partitioned (Fig. 73-2). The air that remains in the lung after a maximal expiratory effort is the residual volume. The difference between functional residual capacity (FRC) and residual volume is the expiratory reserve volume (ERV). The volume exhaled in a normal breath is the tidal volume (TV). The volume that can be inhaled above tidal volume is the inspiratory reserve volume (IRV).

A series of *capacities* consist of the sum of two or more different volumes. FRC, which is the sum of expiratory reserve volume plus residual volume, represents the resting level at which the opposing forces of lung and chest wall elastic recoil are equal in the absence of volitional inspiratory or expiratory efforts. Inspiratory capacity (IC) is the sum of tidal volume plus inspiratory reserve volume. A low IC is strongly associated with chronic dyspnea, reduced exercise capacity, and increased mortality in patients with COPD. Vital capacity (VC) is the sum of tidal volume plus inspiratory reserve volume plus expiratory reserve volume. Total lung capacity is the sum of residual volume plus expiratory reserve volume plus tidal volume plus inspiratory reserve volume.

Three volumes (tidal volume, inspiratory reserve volume, expiratory reserve volume) can be measured with a spirometer. Measurement of residual volume or any of the capacities that include it (so-called *absolute lung volumes*) requires more sophisticated methods, such as body plethysmography, the inert gas dilution technique, or the nitrogen washout technique.

BODY PLETHYSMOGRAPHY

Body plethysmography, the preferred method for measuring lung volumes, is based on Boyle's law: at a given temperature, the product of the pressure and volume of a quantity of gas at one time will be equal to the product of the pressure and volume of the gas at another time ($P1 \times V1 = P2 \times V2$). The body plethysmograph, which is a sealed box in which the patient sits, measures FRC while the patient pants against a closed shutter to compress and to rarify gas in the chest. During panting, the pressure measured at the mouth represents the pressure changes within the lung during these volume changes. A similar panting maneuver with the shutter open is used to calculate airway resistance, which is another method used to measure airway function Although body plethysmography is generally the most accurate method for measurement of lung volumes, particularly in patients with airway obstruction, it can overestimate lung volumes if panting is too rapid. A plethysmographic total lung capacity greater than 150% of the reference value should be viewed with suspicion.

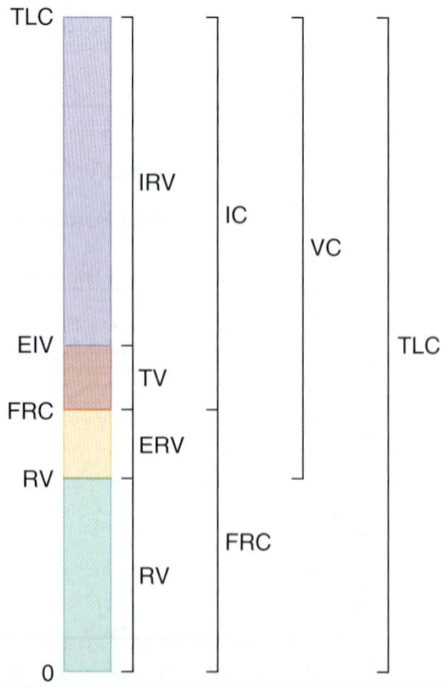

FIGURE 73-2. A schematic diagram showing lung volume partitions as measured in lung function tests. EIV = end-inspiratory volume; ERV = expiratory reserve volume; FRC = functional residual capacity; IC = inspiratory capacity; IRV = inspiratory reserve volume; RV = residual volume; TLC = total lung capacity; TV = tidal volume; VC = vital capacity.

INERT GAS DILUTION TECHNIQUE

Lung volumes also can be measured by having the patient breathe from a device containing a known volume and concentration of an inert gas (e.g., helium, neon, argon, or methane), which does not react with elements in the blood or tissues, until equilibrium is achieved. The final concentration of inert gas equals the initial inert gas concentration times the initial gas volume of the device divided by the final volume of the lungs plus the device, adjusting for oxygen consumption and carbon dioxide production during the test. This equation can be solved for lung volume. This method underestimates lung volumes when portions of the lung communicate poorly with the central airways, particularly in patients who have severe obstructive lung disease and emphysematous bullae.

NITROGEN WASHOUT TECHNIQUE

The air that we breathe consists of approximately 21% oxygen, 1% argon, 0.04% carbon dioxide, and a variable amount of water vapor. The remainder is nitrogen. Exhaled air contains a lower concentration of oxygen, usually 14 to 16%, plus 3 to 5% carbon dioxide and water. For the nitrogen washout technique, the individual being tested inhales 100% oxygen beginning at FRC. As the subject breathes, exhaled gas is collected until the concentration of nitrogen reaches a plateau. Knowing that the initial concentration of exhaled nitrogen is approximately 75% and measuring the final concentration and volume of gases collected, the initial volume of gas in the lungs at FRC can be calculated. As with the inert gas dilution technique, this method also underestimates lung volumes in patients with poorly communicating air spaces.

Absolute lung volumes, as determined by body plethysmography, inert gas dilution, or nitrogen washout, can refine the spirometric evaluation of both obstructive and restrictive disorders. In obstructive disorders, air trapping or hyperinflation can be inferred when a residual volume, total lung capacity, or residual volume/total lung capacity (RV/TLC) ratio is above the upper limit of normal.[9] However, in patients who have chest wall limitations or neuromuscular weakness, residual volume may be increased—not because of true airway trapping, but because of limitation to expiratory chest wall movement, so the term *air trapping* should be used with caution.

A restrictive disorder can be inferred from a spirometry pattern that shows a reduced FVC with a normal or increased FEV_1/FVC ratio. To confirm the presence of true restriction, lung volumes are required to demonstrate a TLC less than the lower limit of normal. If TLC is normal, these findings are called a nonspecific pattern (see online supplement).

DIFFUSING CAPACITY

The single-breath diffusing capacity for carbon monoxide (DLCO, also referred to as transfer factor or TLCO) measures the capacity of the lungs to exchange gas.[10] The maneuver for measurement of DLCO requires breathing out to residual volume and then quickly inhaling a mixture of known concentrations of an inert gas (e.g., helium or methane) and of carbon monoxide. After inhaling to total lung capacity, patients hold their breath for 10 seconds. During this time, the tracer gases mix with other gases occupying the lungs, and a portion of the carbon monoxide diffuses across the alveolar-capillary membrane and binds to hemoglobin with strong affinity. After the 10-second breath-hold, the remaining gas mixture is exhaled. The concentration of inert gas is used to calculate the volume of the lungs (alveolar volume); the concentration of carbon monoxide is used to calculate the absorption of carbon monoxide, expressed in volume per minute per unit of pressure (mL/min per mm Hg).

A normal value for DLCO indicates relatively normal gas exchange, which requires a normal pulmonary gas-exchange surface, normal capillary blood volume, and relatively homogeneous ventilation-perfusion relationships. A low DLCO is indicative of impaired gas exchange. Among patients with obstructive disorders (Chapters 75 and 76), impaired gas exchange occurs most commonly in patients with COPD as opposed to asthma. In restrictive disorders, impaired gas exchange is seen most commonly in patients with interstitial disease rather than patients with chest wall disorders. Patients with pulmonary vascular disorders typically have a low DLCO and may have restriction or normal lung mechanics (Chapter 80). An isolated reduction in DLCO (i.e., in association with normal total lung capacity, vital capacity, and FEV_1) can indicate a pulmonary vascular disorder, but is more commonly seen in association with emphysema (Chapter 76), interstitial disease (Chapter 80), or a combination of the two.

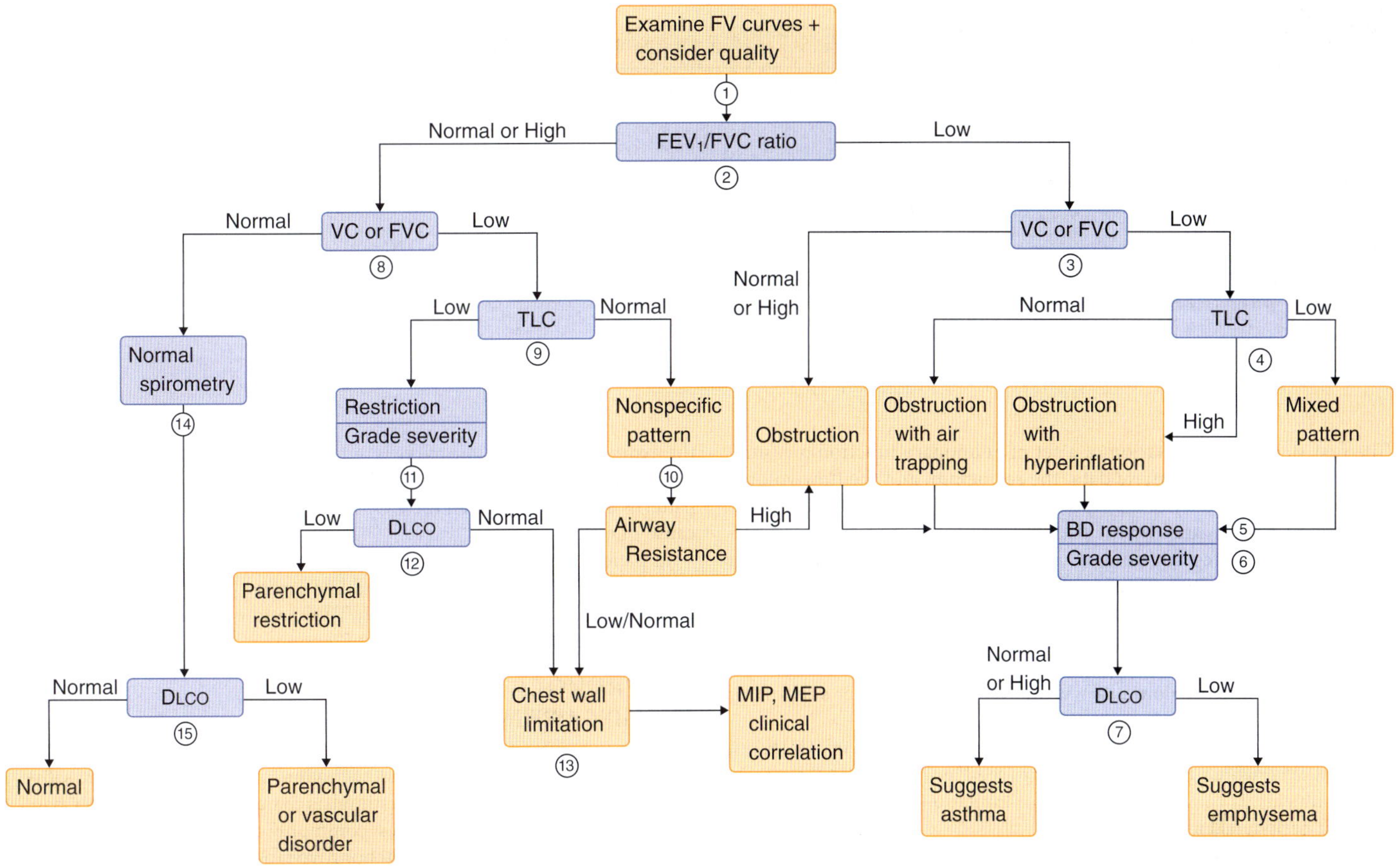

FIGURE 73-3. **An algorithm for interpreting pulmonary function tests in which spirometry, lung volumes, and DLCO are measured.** If only spirometry is available, interpretation is more limited. The legend keys refer to numbered branch points in the algorithm. BD = bronchodilator; DLCO = diffusing capacity of the lung for carbon monoxide; FEV$_1$ = forced expiratory volume in one second; FVC = forced vital capacity; MEP = maximal expiratory pressure; MIP = maximal inspiratory pressure; TLC = total lung capacity; VC = vital capacity.

1. Inspect the data and flow-volume (FV) curve to assess test quality and then consider the basic type of abnormality (e.g., obstruction vs. restriction).
2. A reduced FEV$_1$/FVC ratio suggests obstruction, and the obstruction algorithm on the right side should be followed. If the FEV$_1$/FVC ratio is normal or high, the restriction side (left side) of the algorithm should be followed.
3. If FEV$_1$/FVC is low and the VC or FVC is normal or high, simple obstruction is present. If VC or FVC is low, TLC should be measured.
4. If TLC is normal, simple obstruction is present. If TLC is high, obstruction with hyperinflation is present. If TLC is low, a mixed obstructive/restrictive pattern is present. (Note that the inert gas dilution and nitrogen washout methods commonly underestimate TLC in the presence of obstruction and can give a false impression of a mixed disorder.)
5. Bronchodilator responsiveness (BD) may be assessed to determine whether the change in FEV$_1$ or FVC is significant (i.e., a ≥12% improvement and at least a 200 mL absolute increase) and to determine the degree of positivity.
6. The severity of obstruction should be graded based on the FEV$_1$ percentage predicted. Some algorithms grade severity based on post-bronchodilator values.
7. In current or former smokers with obstruction, a low DLCO suggests emphysema or other pulmonary parenchymal or vascular disorders. A normal DLCO may suggest asthma or chronic bronchitis.
8. If FEV$_1$/FVC is normal or high, the restriction (left) side of the algorithm is followed. If VC or FVC is normal, spirometry is generally normal (occasional patients have an isolated abnormality of FEV$_1$ of uncertain significance). If VC or FVC is low, TLC should be checked.
9. If TLC is low, a restrictive disorder is present. If TLC is normal, the "nonspecific pattern" is present.
10. If the nonspecific pattern is identified, airway resistance (Raw) can be measured. An increased Raw suggests obstruction. A normal Raw suggests an alternative cause (see #13).
11. If true restriction is present, grade severity on the basis of the reduction in TLC percentage predicted.
12. If restriction is demonstrated, DLCO should be measured next. If abnormal, it indicates a pulmonary parenchymal restrictive process. If normal, it suggests an extraparenchymal or nonpulmonary cause of restriction.
13. Restriction with a normal DLCO or a nonspecific pattern with normal Raw suggests an alternative cause (chest wall limitation, weakness, heart failure, poor performance). Consider measurement of maximal respiratory pressures and review the study for test performance.
14. If spirometry is normal, lung volumes are rarely useful, but DLCO is sometimes helpful.
15. If DLCO is normal, gas exchange can be considered normal. An isolated reduction in DLCO is seen most often in patients with emphysema, pulmonary fibrosis, or both. It less commonly indicates a pulmonary vascular disorder, such as primary pulmonary hypertension, or an obliterative vasculopathy, as is sometimes seen in systemic sclerosis.

An increased DLCO is relatively uncommon and is most often seen in individuals with asthma (Chapter 75) or obesity (Chapter 201). It can also be seen in association with polycythemia (Chapter 152), left-to-right intracardiac shunt (Chapter 55), or acute pulmonary hemorrhage (Chapter 79). It can also be seen during or after exercise or when the patient is in the supine position.

MAXIMAL RESPIRATORY PRESSURES

Maximal respiratory pressures help identify muscle weakness, which can cause a restrictive disorder, a nonspecific pattern, or an isolated reduction in MVV relative to FEV$_1$. Maximal respiratory pressures do not distinguish muscle weakness from poor test performance (Fig. 73-3).

INTERPRETATION OF LUNG FUNCTION TESTS

Interpretation of pulmonary function tests uses the data obtained to infer a physiologic diagnosis and to categorize the nature and magnitude of the impairment of lung function (Table 73-2).[11] The four broad categories of physiologic abnormalities include obstructive disorders, such as asthma and COPD (Chapters 75 and 76); restrictive disorders of the lung, such as pulmonary fibrosis (Chapter 80) or restriction due to factors outside the lung, such as chest wall limitation due to obesity, pleural disease, or musculoskeletal disorders,[12] or weak chest wall (Chapter 86), such as Guillain-Barré syndrome (Chapter 388); and disorders resulting in impaired gas exchange, which are often associated with an obstructive or restrictive disorder, but in some cases can be found in patients who have normal mechanical function of the lungs, such as pulmonary embolism (Chapter 68). Some patients have mixed physiologic defects, such as a combined restrictive and obstructive defect (see Fig. 73-3), or more than one cause of restriction (e.g., pulmonary fibrosis plus obesity or heart failure).

Spirometry screening of the U.S. adult population shows evidence of airflow obstruction in about 13.5% of individuals and evidence of restriction in about 6.5%. Of individuals with spirometric evidence of restriction, about 50% have true restriction when lung volumes are measured, whereas the other 50% have a nonspecific pattern.

TABLE 73-2 COMMON CHANGES ASSOCIATED WITH PATTERNS OF LUNG FUNCTION ABNORMALITY

	FORCED EXPIRATORY VOLUME IN 1 SECOND (FEV_1)	FORCED VITAL CAPACITY (FVC)	FEV_1/FVC RATIO	RESIDUAL VOLUME	TOTAL LUNG CAPACITY	MAXIMAL RESPIRATORY PRESSURES
Normal	Normal*	Normal	Normal	Normal	Normal	Normal
Obstructive	↓	Normal to ↓	↓	↑ to ↑↑	Normal to ↑↑	Normal
Restrictive	↓	↓ to ↓↓	Normal or ↑	Normal or ↓	↓ to ↓↓	Normal
Weak chest wall	↓	↓ to ↓↓	Normal or ↑	↑	Normal or ↓	↓

*Normal or abnormal values are determined by comparing the measured values with those predicted from regression equations based on the patient's sex, age, height, and race. The normal range for FEV_1/FVC also varies, mainly with age, ranging from 0.70 to 0.80 among 25-year-olds to 0.63 to 0.68 among 65-year-olds.

The first step in interpretation of a set of pulmonary function measurements is to inspect the numeric data, the spirogram, and the flow-volume curve to assess the quality of the test. A poor-quality test result, whether it is due to poor performance by the patient or poor coaching by the technician, may have an irregular flow-volume curve (see Fig. 73-1L) or poor reproducibility of results from one effort to another. Once good quality is affirmed, the presence of an abnormal pattern (e.g., obstruction or restriction) can be determined. If so, attention then turns to assessing the severity, subtleties of the flow-volume curve, and other physiologic data (e.g., total lung capacity, residual volume, MVV, and DLCO) that either support or supplement the initial impression.

The normal flow-volume curve is roughly triangular (see Fig. 73-1A). A *tracheal plateau*, which is a normal variant (see Fig. 73-1J) usually seen in younger subjects, is caused by normal flow limitation in the trachea in the absence of peripheral airway obstruction.

In obstructive diseases, the degree of pulmonary functional impairment can be classified on the basis of the FEV_1. Patients with obstructive disorders typically have a reduced FEV_1/FVC ratio and a flow-volume curve with a "scooped" appearance (see Fig. 73-1B and C). Atypical patients may have unusually shaped flow-volume curves or unusual patterns of obstruction (e.g., abnormal airway resistance despite a normally shaped flow-volume curve and normal FEV_1/FVC ratio). If a patient has what appears to be obstruction, the next step is to determine the degree to which the obstruction can be reversed by administration of a bronchodilator. Hyperinflation or air trapping can be identified by an increase in total lung capacity, residual volume, or the RV/TLC ratio. The adequacy of gas exchange can be assessed by measuring DLCO and oximetry. For individuals with normal spirometry and alveolar volume (from the DLCO), measurement of total lung capacity can be avoided to save unnecessary expense.

Patients with restrictive disorders have reduced lung volumes and typically have a flow-volume curve with a "witch's hat" shape—a tall peaked curve (see Figs. 73-1D and E). Restriction may be due to either reduced lung compliance or mechanical changes to the chest wall and tissues surrounding the lungs (e.g., obesity, muscle weakness, chest wall deformity, pregnancy, pleural effusion, or heart failure). For many restrictive diseases, the severity can be graded with use of the total lung capacity as a percentage of the predicted value, and changes in VC and TLC measured over time are helpful in predicting prognosis.

In patients with restriction caused by interstitial lung disease, the total lung capacity and the vital capacity or FVC are usually reduced by a similar proportion. In some patients with restriction, however, the total lung capacity and the vital capacity percentages of predicted values are quite different (>10% difference). The usual cause is the presence of more than one restrictive process, such as a parenchymal restrictive disorder plus obesity, respiratory muscle weakness, atelectasis, or occult obstruction.

Some patients have a mixed disorder with evidence of both obstruction and restriction. Common causes include cystic fibrosis (Chapter 77), sarcoidosis (Chapter 83), and heart failure (Chapters 45 and 46) as well as cases in which the causes of the obstructive disorder and the restrictive disorder are unrelated.

Disorders of the central airways can cause characteristic patterns of abnormality. In a "fixed airway obstruction" such as tracheal stenosis (see Fig. 73-1H), flows are typically reduced on both inspiration and expiration. In contrast, in a variable extrathoracic (upper) airway obstruction (see Fig. 73-1F), inspiratory flow is disproportionately reduced; expiration is often abnormal, but merely less so. Likewise, in variable intrathoracic obstruction (e.g., relapsing polychondritis, tracheomalacia, or a dynamic intrathoracic tracheal tumor), the expiratory flow-volume curve is reduced but often in a pattern unlike that seen in asthma or COPD (see Fig. 73-1G). These central airway obstructive patterns are often mistaken for COPD but may signify a localized, treatable cause of obstruction.

In patients with heart disease, a decline in FEV_1/FVC ratio is associated with underfilling of the left heart and low cardiac output. By comparison, a decline in FVC with preserved FEV_1/FVC ratio is associated with left ventricular hypertrophy and diastolic dysfunction.

PROVOCATIVE TESTING

ASSESSING AIRWAY RESPONSIVENESS

Hyperresponsiveness of airways to the smooth muscle–contracting effect of pharmacologic agents (such as methacholine, mannitol, hypertonic saline), cold air, dry air, and other physical stimuli is characteristic of asthma (Chapter 75). Hyperresponsiveness is also less commonly observed in COPD and other obstructive airway diseases. Bronchoprovocation studies, in which graded doses of a stimulus are used to elicit airway constriction, are performed to measure airway responsiveness. A responsive airway (i.e., one in which a small stimulus leads to a fall in FEV_1 to 15 to 20% below starting values) may be used to confirm the diagnosis of asthma (Chapter 75). Fractional concentration of exhaled nitric oxide (FE_{NO}), which is a marker of eosinophilic airway inflammation, also can be used to predict the likelihood that airflow obstruction will improve with corticosteroid treatment.

CARDIOPULMONARY EXERCISE TESTS

Some patients have dyspnea (Chapter 71) or exercise limitation that is not adequately explained by the clinical examination, standard pulmonary function testing, and chest imaging. For such patients, laboratory testing of physiologic performance during exercise can be enlightening.

Cardiopulmonary exercise testing, which is usually performed on a cycle ergometer or treadmill, includes monitoring of the heart rate, electrocardiography, and pulse oximetry as well as breath-by-breath measurement of tidal volume, breathing rate, oxygen consumption, and carbon dioxide production. Optional measurements include but are not limited to arterial blood gases and noninvasive cardiac output. Outcomes include peak oxygen uptake, maximal workload, maximal heart rate, ventilation parameters during exercise, and measurements of gas exchange. Results are analyzed to determine if anaerobic metabolism occurs when the study subject reaches maximal effort and to determine what limits the ability of a patient to exercise—a gas exchange abnormality, ventilatory limitation, cardiac limitation, or deconditioning.

Simple tests of exercise performance, such as the 6-minute walk test, can quantify and serially assess exercise performance. This test measures the maximum distance that a patient can walk at their own pace in an indoor corridor 30 meters long during a 6-minute interval. The result, which provides a global assessment of functional capacity, is commonly used to monitor responses to therapeutic interventions and pulmonary rehabilitation in patients with significant functional impairment. The 6-minute walk test also has prognostic significance in cardiac and pulmonary diseases.[13]

BRONCHOALVEOLAR LAVAGE

Bronchoalveolar lavage is most commonly used to diagnose opportunistic infections in immunocompromised hosts (Chapter 260), ventilator-associated pneumonia (Chapters 85 and 261), diffuse alveolar hemorrhage (Chapter 79), atypical pulmonary infections in immunocompetent individuals, or peripheral malignancies. Bronchoalveolar lavage also can be useful in patients with acute respiratory failure,[14] but its utility in the evaluation of interstitial lung disease (Chapter 80) is less clear.[15]

The differential cell count on a normal bronchoalveolar lavage specimen includes 85% macrophages or more, 10 to 15% lymphocytes, 3% neutrophils or less, 1% eosinophils or less, 1% mast cells or less, and less than 5% squamous epithelial cells (which are an indicator of contamination from the upper airway). Individuals who smoke may have higher cell counts and a higher percentage of neutrophils. Increased lymphocyte counts are seen in sarcoidosis (Chapter 83), hypersensitivity pneumonitis (Chapter 82), nonspecific interstitial pneumonitis (Chapter 80), collagen vascular diseases (Chapter 80), radiation pneumonitis (Chapter 82), cryptogenic organizing pneumonia (Chapter 80), and lymphoproliferative disorders. Increased neutrophil counts are seen in idiopathic pulmonary fibrosis (Chapter 80), collagen vascular diseases (Chapter 80), infectious pneumonia (Chapter 85), aspiration pneumonia (Chapter 85), acute respiratory distress syndrome (Chapter 90), diffuse alveolar damage (Chapter 79), acute interstitial pneumonia (Chapter 80), and asbestosis (Chapter 81). Increased eosinophils can be seen in asthma (Chapter 75), bronchitis (Chapter 84), allergic bronchopulmonary aspergillosis (Chapter 311), eosinophilic granulomatosis with polyangiitis (Chapter 249), Hodgkin lymphoma (Chapter 172), and drug-induced lung disease (Chapter 82). If eosinophils are more than 25%, eosinophilic pneumonia is likely (Chapter 156). If lymphocytes are increased and the clinical differential diagnosis includes sarcoidosis (Chapter 83) or hypersensitivity pneumonitis (Chapter 82), analysis of T-cell populations may be helpful; the CD4:CD8 ratio is typically increased in sarcoidosis but reduced in hypersensitivity pneumonitis. If more than 20% of macrophages stain positive for hemosiderin, diffuse alveolar hemorrhage is considered likely (Chapter 79), particularly if lavage fluid is progressively bloody in successive aliquots.

Cellular constituents of bronchoalveolar lavage are usually stained for cytologic analysis for malignant cells and viral inclusions. If Langerhans cell histiocytosis (Chapter 80) is considered possible, 5% or more CD1a–positive cells support the diagnosis. If chronic beryllium disease or beryllium sensitization is possible, a lymphocyte proliferation test in response to exposure to beryllium salts can be helpful (Chapter 81). Staining of solid material from the bronchoalveolar lavage with periodic acid–Schiff (PAS) stain for the presence of PAS-positive material is essential to the diagnosis of pulmonary alveolar proteinosis (Chapter 79). A diagnosis of lipoid pneumonia (Chapter 82), caused by the aspiration of oil, can be confirmed by an excess of lipid-laden macrophages from bronchoalveolar lavage. The presence of asbestos bodies or silica is not diagnostic of lung disease related to these substances (Chapter 81) but does indicate significant exposure.

COMPLEX DISORDERS

Approximately 3 to 5% of pulmonary function tests have more than one physiologic defect, such as a combination of restriction plus obstruction, or more than one cause of restriction (e.g., pulmonary fibrosis plus obesity or heart failure). These cases do not fit neatly into standard interpretive patterns of typical obstruction or restriction, yet they can be described, and their patterns suggest a differential diagnosis.

A *mixed disorder* is a combination of both restriction, as indicated by a reduced TLC, plus obstruction, as indicated by a reduced FEV_1/FVC ratio. Although it is widely recognized, it only occurs in 1 to 2% of pulmonary function tests. A mixed disorder may be due to a combination of a restrictive disorder plus an unrelated obstructive disorder, such as an interstitial disease plus COPD, but several disorders typically produce a mixed pattern, including cystic fibrosis (Chapter 77), sarcoidosis (Chapter 83), Langerhans cell histiocytosis (Chapter 155), and heart failure (Chapters 45 and 46). In a mixed pattern, the degree of severity of restriction can be determined from the TLC percent predicted. The overall impairment can be determined from the FEV_1 percent predicted. The severity of the obstructive component can be inferred from the FEV_1 percent predicted divided by the TLC percent predicted.

Reduced lung volumes are the sine qua non of the diagnosis of restriction. However, about half of patients whose spirometry suggests restriction (reduced vital capacity with normal FEV_1/FVC ratio, also called preserved ratio impaired spirometry or PRISM) have a normal total lung capacity, so they do not have true restriction, but rather what is called the *nonspecific pattern*. The nonspecific pattern is very common, occurring in 9 to 10% of all complete pulmonary function tests. It is approximately as frequent as true restriction. Patients with the nonspecific pattern commonly have evidence of an obstructive disorder, not restriction, as indicated either by increased airway resistance, a response to a bronchodilator, or other clinical indicator of obstruction. It can be argued that the clinical utility of the measurement of airway resistance is limited to patients with the nonspecific pattern of whom about half have an increased airway resistance. Some patients with a nonspecific pattern do not have evidence of airway obstruction but are obese or have other chest wall limitations, neuromuscular weakness, poor performance, heart failure, pleural effusion, or a variety of other conditions.

In typical cases of restrictive lung disease, including most cases of interstitial lung disease, lung volumes are reduced in proportion to the severity of the interstitial disease. For example, TLC might be reduced to 60% of the predicted value and FVC would be similarly reduced to about 60% of the predicted value. In such a case, grading the severity of restriction is easy. One should be cautious not to overlook the fact that the gas exchange abnormality may be more or less severe, depending on the underlying pathology. In contrast, about one third of patients with restrictive diseases have reductions in FEV_1 and FVC that are disproportionate (lower by >10% of predicted value) to the reduction in TLC. The discrepancy may be large; for example, TLC may be 70% predicted while FVC is only 25% predicted. Interpreting physicians sometimes disagree whether to grade severity of restriction based on TLC percent predicted or FVC percent predicted. In such a case, the impairment might be called either mild or very severe. Cases of "typical restriction" are seen in association with interstitial lung disease, and hence weighted toward older men, whereas patients with "complex restriction" are more often women; younger; either underweight or obese; have slightly less severe reductions in D_{LCO}; and more often have atelectasis, a mosaic pattern on computed tomography, diaphragmatic dysfunction, or neuromuscular disease.

PULMONARY FUNCTION IN OBESITY

The epidemic of obesity is manifested in many organ systems, including the respiratory system. Dyspnea, exercise limitation, and respiratory failure are more common in obese persons than in the nonobese. Asthma is more common and more severe in obese patients. The effects of obesity on lung function are usually relatively modest among ambulatory patients with a body mass index (BMI) less than 40. The most commonly observed effect of obesity on lung function is a reduction in expiratory reserve volume (the amount of air exhaled between FRC and residual volume), which is substantially reduced even in persons who are overweight (BMI 25 to 30) or mildly obese (BMI 30 to 35). Vital capacity is reduced in obesity, but the effect is modest, usually within the normal range, and highly variable. In large studies, vital capacity or FVC is reduced on average by 0.5 to 0.8% for each unit increase in BMI above 25. Effects of obesity on total lung capacity and FEV_1 are somewhat smaller. The FEV_1/FVC ratio and D_{LCO} actually increase slightly with increasing BMI.

In exercise studies, the effects of obesity among ambulatory outpatients are likewise modest. Such patients have an increased work of breathing and decreased external work efficiency related to the work of moving their own body mass, but peak oxygen uptake is often normal.

GENERAL REFERENCES

For the General References and other additional features, please visit Elsevier eBooks+ at https://ebooks.health.elsevier.com.

74

DISORDERS OF VENTILATORY CONTROL

ATUL MALHOTRA AND FRANK POWELL

DEFINITIONS AND PATHOGENESIS

Ventilatory Control

Ventilation is controlled by complex interactions between central chemoreceptors, which respond mainly to arterial carbon dioxide tensions, and peripheral chemoreceptors, which respond to arterial carbon dioxide and oxygen tensions. These reflexes modulate the underlying respiratory rhythm, and disorders of ventilatory control are caused by derangements in these control systems.

HYPOVENTILATION SYNDROMES

Hypoventilation syndromes are defined by a lack of adequate alveolar ventilation to maintain a normal arterial carbon dioxide tension of 40 mm Hg. The two most common clinical settings that result in chronic hypoventilation are severe chronic obstructive pulmonary disease (COPD; Chapter 76) and morbid obesity (Chapters 374 and 201); less common causes are chronic opiate therapy, neuromuscular weakness (Chapters 389 and 390), and severe kyphoscoliosis (Chapter 86). The epidemiology of these hypoventilation syndromes is poorly studied, but about 15 to 30% of patients with severe COPD or morbid obesity have an elevated $Paco_2$. Regardless of the cause, patients with hypoventilation frequently have further worsening of their ventilation at the onset of sleep due to loss of the wakefulness stimulus, which is the normal drive to breathe while awake, and some degree of upper airway collapse after the onset of sleep (Chapter 374).

Patients with central sleep apnea (Chapter 374), which is a group of conditions in which cessation of airflow occurs because of a lack of respiratory effort, are classified into those with inadequate ventilatory drive and those with excessive drive (Table 74-1).[1] The apparent paradox of how excessive drive leads to central apnea is explained by the concept of loop gain. A negative feedback control system with a high loop gain is prone to instability that leads to periods of excessive breathing followed by periods of apnea. The prototype of a condition with high loop gain is periodic breathing or Cheyne-Stokes breathing (Fig. 74-1). Hypercapnic diseases include acquired diseases and the central congenital hyperventilation syndrome (Table 74-2).

CHEYNE-STOKES BREATHING

Cheyne-Stokes breathing is a waxing and waning pattern of breathing, which is classically described as crescendo-decrescendo and often includes periods of central apnea. Cheyne-Stokes is seen most commonly during sleep in patients with heart failure.

EPIDEMIOLOGY

Cheyne-Stokes breathing is a form of ventilatory instability that occurs in 20 to 40% of patients with left ventricular systolic dysfunction.[2] Male sex, advanced age, low baseline $Paco_2$, and atrial fibrillation are risk factors for Cheyne-Stokes breathing among patients with heart failure. Controversy remains regarding whether this breathing pattern itself is deleterious or whether it is simply a marker of the underlying severity of cardiac disease. Cheyne-Stokes breathing represents about 5 to 10% of all cases of sleep apnea (Chapter 374) and is uncommon among patients who do not have heart failure.

PATHOBIOLOGY

Individuals with Cheyne-Stokes breathing have robust chemosensitivity, as evidenced by marked increases in ventilation with small increases in $Paco_2$. The drive to breathe may be further increased by neural reflexes that are triggered by extravascular lung fluid and an elevated left atrial pressure. Intermittent hypoxemia and catecholamine surges, which are frequent in these patients, contribute to oxidative stress and neuroendocrine activation, both of which are thought to contribute to worsening of the underlying heart failure.

CLINICAL MANIFESTATIONS AND DIAGNOSIS

Patients with Cheyne-Stokes breathing can sometimes be diagnosed at the bedside by careful observation of their breathing pattern. During sleep or exercise, breathing becomes dependent primarily on metabolic stimuli. Patients may complain of fatigue or sleepiness because arousals from sleep tend to occur during the hyperpneic phase. Paroxysmal nocturnal dyspnea, a classic symptom of heart failure (Chapter 45), most commonly reflects underlying Cheyne-Stokes breathing. Patients often are diagnosed in the sleep laboratory while undergoing investigation for possible obstructive sleep apnea. However, in contrast to obstructive sleep apnea, Cheyne-Stokes breathing usually resolves during rapid eye movement (REM) sleep, and arousals on the electroencephalogram typically occur during the hyperpneic phase. Furthermore, Cheyne-Stokes breathing generally does not resolve immediately when nasal continuous positive airway pressure (CPAP) is applied.

TREATMENT

Medical management of Cheyne-Stokes breathing most often is treatment of the underlying heart failure (Chapter 46). After optimization of medical management, the Cheyne-Stokes breathing pattern frequently resolves. CPAP can improve breathing indices but is no better than standard medical therapy from the standpoint of mortality. Results have been similar with other ventilator techniques.[A1,3] An implantable phrenic nerve stimulator has been approved by the U.S. Food and Drug Administration, but definitive outcome data are still lacking.[4]

CENTRAL CONGENITAL HYPOVENTILATION SYNDROME

DEFINITION AND EPIDEMIOLOGY

Central congenital hypoventilation syndrome is a rare congenital condition, previously referred to as Ondine's curse, characterized by a diminished ventilatory response to carbon dioxide. The central congenital hypoventilation syndrome was traditionally diagnosed in neonates, but more subtle forms of disease are increasingly noted in older children and adults.

PATHOBIOLOGY

The syndrome is now defined by a mutation in the *PHOX2B* gene, located on chromosome 4p12. The *PHOX2B* gene is a highly conserved homeobox gene

TABLE 74-1 CLASSIFICATION OF CENTRAL SLEEP APNEA

CENTRAL SLEEP APNEA SYNDROME	MECHANISM	THERAPY
Sleep transition apneas	Carbon dioxide fluctuations during transitions from sleep to wake to sleep	Reassurance, occasionally hypnotics or oxygen
Chronic narcotic therapy	Lack of central drive	Reduce narcotic dose Consider positive-pressure device
Cheyne-Stokes breathing	High loop gain from robust chemosensitivity and ventilatory drive	Optimize medical therapy for heart failure; consider PAP device
Idiopathic central apnea	Unknown	Supportive, bilevel PAP; consider ventilatory stimulants
Treatment of emergent central apnea or "complex apnea"	Lowering upper airway resistance at CPAP initiation improves efficiency of carbon dioxide excretion	Reassurance, generally resolves spontaneously
Sleep hypoventilation syndromes	Fall in drive with loss of wakefulness stimulus, loss of accessory muscle activity during REM sleep	Noninvasive ventilation

CPAP = continuous positive airway pressure; PAP = positive airway pressure; REM = rapid eye movement.

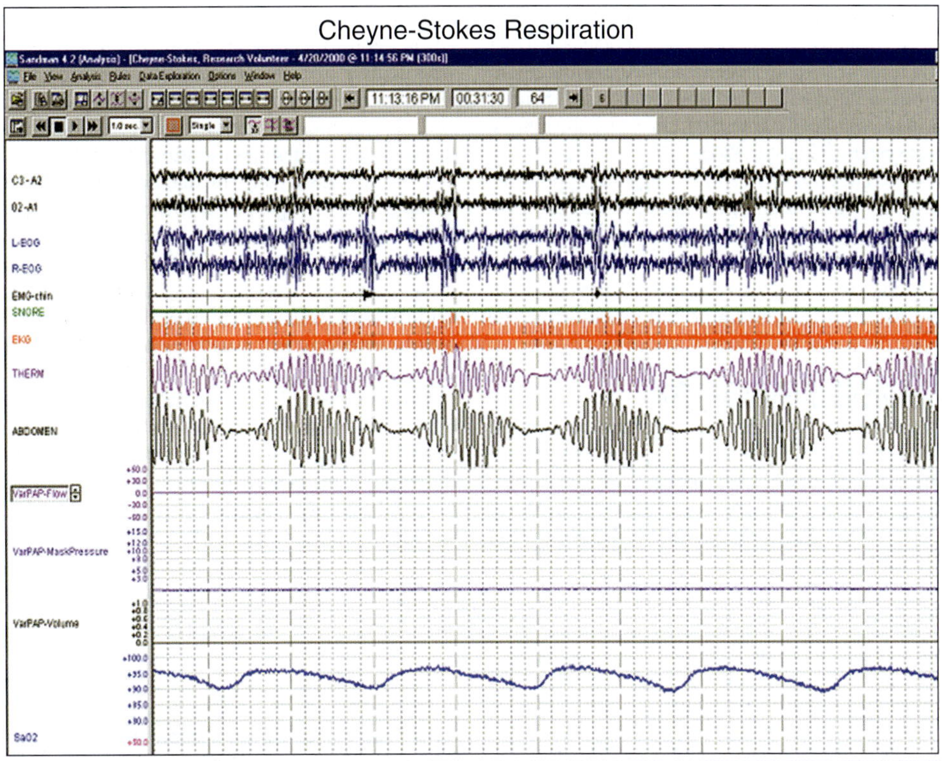

FIGURE 74-1. Cheyne-Stokes breathing with crescendo-decrescendo pattern of breathing. The thermistor detects air temperature changes at the mouth and nose. Note absences in airflow without respiratory effort seen in the abdominal belts. This breathing pattern leads to intermittent desaturations, arousals from sleep, and bursts of tachycardia. The loop gain concept can be understood by considering the thermostat analogy in which a control system is working to regulate a stable room temperature (e.g., 20° C). By analogy, the respiratory control system is working primarily to maintain a stable $Paco_2$ of 40 mm Hg and stable pH. Situations in which marked fluctuations in room temperature might occur would include one in which the thermostat is excessively sensitive (i.e., furnace turns on if room temperature falls to 19.999° C); if the furnace is too powerful, a marked overshoot in room temperature will be followed by a prolonged period when the furnace does not run. In the analogy to Cheyne-Stokes breathing, carbon dioxide is equated to room temperature and would be predicted to be unstable if chemosensitivity (i.e., the thermostat) were excessively robust (i.e., a marked increase in ventilation for a small change in carbon dioxide) or if the efficiency of carbon dioxide excretion were high (i.e., marked fall in $Paco_2$ with increased ventilation). Situations that increase the propensity for carbon dioxide fluctuations lead to elevated loop gain and thus increase the risk for Cheyne-Stokes breathing. C3-A2 and O2-A1 = leads for electroencephalogram; EKG = electrocardiogram; EMG = electromyogram; EtCO2 = end-tidal carbon dioxide; L and R-EOG = left and right electrooculogram; SaO2 = oxygen saturation; Therm = thermistor.

TABLE 74-2 CLASSIFICATION OF HYPERCAPNIC DISEASES

HYPERCAPNIC DISEASES	MECHANISM	DIAGNOSIS	TREATMENT
ACQUIRED DISEASE			
Narcotic overdose	Reduced central drive	History, narcotized pupils, toxicology	Supportive care, naloxone
Acute severe asthma (Chapter 75)	Severe airflow obstruction, high dead space	Typical history, wheezing on examination, low FEV_1/FVC	Bronchodilators, anti-inflammatories, mechanical ventilation (usually invasive)
Acute exacerbation of COPD (Chapter 76)	Airflow obstruction, high dead space	History, cigarette smoking, low FEV_1/FVC, infectious etiology	Bronchodilators, anti-inflammatories, noninvasive ventilation
Obesity-hypoventilation syndrome	Low respiratory system compliance, high upper airway resistance, low central drive	High BMI, lack of other diagnoses; blunted carbon dioxide response	Weight loss, nocturnal bilevel positive airway pressure
Neuromuscular disease (e.g., myasthenia gravis, polymyositis, GBS/AIDP, ALS; Chapters 248, 387, and 390)	Lack of respiratory muscle force	Immediate orthopnea, low VC, low MIPs/MEPs	Underlying cause, nocturnal noninvasive ventilation, supportive care
Severe parenchymal lung disease (e.g., COPD)	Lack of alveolar surface area; high pulmonary dead space and work of breathing	Typical history, smoking, low FEV_1 and FEV_1/FVC	Bronchodilator, anti-inflammatory therapy, possible nocturnal noninvasive ventilation, smoking cessation
Kyphoscoliosis (Chapter 86)	Low respiratory system compliance	Physical examination	Supportive care, noninvasive ventilation
CONGENITAL DISEASE			
Central congenital hypoventilation syndrome	*PHOX2B* mutation, lack of central drive	Genetic testing	Supportive care, mechanical ventilation (usually noninvasive)

AIDP = acute inflammatory demyelinating polyneuropathy; ALS = amyotrophic lateral sclerosis; BMI = body mass index; COPD = chronic obstructive pulmonary disease; FEV_1 = forced expiratory volume in 1 second; FVC = forced vital capacity; GBS = Guillain-Barré syndrome; MEPs = maximal expiratory pressures; MIPs = maximal inspiratory pressures; VC = vital capacity.

that is expressed in cardiopulmonary reflex pathways, including central CO_2-sensitive chemoreceptors that are located in the retrotrapezoid nucleus and that provide excitatory input to the respiratory pattern generator. Abnormalities in *PHOX2B* genes have also been associated with Hirschsprung disease (Chapter 122), neural crest tumors, cardiac asystole (Chapter 50), and other abnormalities of the autonomic nervous system (Chapter 386).

Because most parents of affected children with central congenital hypoventilation syndrome do not carry a *PHOX2B* mutation, the mutations are de novo. About 90% of patients are heterozygous for a polyalanine repeat expansion mutation, in which the affected allele has 24 to 33 alanines rather than the normal 20 alanines. The remaining 10% of central congenital hypoventilation syndrome patients have missense, nonsense, or frameshift mutations in the *PHOX2B* gene.[5]

CLINICAL MANIFESTATIONS AND DIAGNOSIS

Neonates can present with cyanosis at birth, recurrent central apneas, or both. Adults can present with idiopathic central sleep apnea, unexplained hypercapnia, or autonomic abnormalities (Chapter 386).[6] The degree of oxygen desaturation during ventilatory and orthostatic challenges correlates with measures of neurocognition.[7] Confirmation of the diagnosis requires the demonstration of an abnormality in the *PHOX2B* gene.

TREATMENT

There are currently no specific therapies for central congenital hypoventilation syndrome beyond supportive care. Genetic counseling is required for afflicted individuals and their families, given the autosomal dominant pattern of inheritance. Patients must be cautioned against the use of sedatives, which could precipitate respiratory failure. Mechanical ventilation during sleep either invasively (through tracheostomy) or noninvasively (through bilevel positive airway pressure support [Chapter 374]) is required in most patients. Some patients remain fully ventilator dependent. Diaphragmatic pacing can sometimes be effective, but ventilatory stimulants are generally ineffective.

ACQUIRED HYPOVENTILATION SYNDROMES

DEFINITION AND EPIDEMIOLOGY

Patients with hypoventilation syndromes cannot maintain adequate minute ventilation to keep their Pa_{CO_2} at 40 mm Hg. Patients can be classified into those who lack central ventilatory drive and those who have a pulmonary mechanical or neuromuscular abnormality that prevents adequate gas exchange (see Table 74-2). The case frequency is unknown, but hypercapnic respiratory failure is one of the more common admission diagnoses in intensive care units.

PATHOBIOLOGY

Patients with conditions characterized by the lack of central drive have reasonably normal lungs and respiratory muscle function but lack adequate response to carbon dioxide and hypoxia. In contrast, most patients with mechanical or neuromuscular abnormalities have a larger work of breathing compared with normal individuals; the most common underlying conditions are severe COPD (Chapter 76) and morbid obesity (Chapter 201) with obesity-hypoventilation syndrome. Such individuals have diminished but not absent chemoresponsiveness, which may be an acquired trait or may relate to an as yet unknown genetic predisposition. Another cause of inadequate gas exchange is neuromuscular disease; common causes include disorders of neuromuscular transmission (Chapter 390), severe muscle weakness (Chapter 389), the residua from poliovirus infection (Chapter 349), Guillain-Barré syndrome (Chapter 388), and acute poisoning (Chapter 96). Although coronavirus disease 2019 (COVID-19) was thought to involve impaired hypoxic sensing, data now suggest chemosensitivity is not systematically impaired in afflicted patients (Chapter 336).[8,9]

CLINICAL MANIFESTATIONS AND DIAGNOSIS

Patients with hypoventilation have myriad presentations ranging from asymptomatic abnormalities in laboratory testing (e.g., elevated Pa_{CO_2}, unexplained low Sa_{O_2}, or elevated serum bicarbonate level) to respiratory failure in the intensive care unit (e.g., respiratory infection with laboratory evidence of chronic abnormalities, such as acute-on-chronic respiratory acidosis). Patients who acutely overdose on sedative-hypnotic or narcotic agents may present with acute respiratory acidosis and loss of consciousness. Patients who take chronic narcotics may present with central sleep apnea-hypopnea or otherwise unexplained oxygen desaturation at night.

Once it is suspected, the diagnosis of hypoventilation is confirmed by the finding of Pa_{CO_2} higher than 42 mm Hg on analysis of an arterial blood sample. If the increase in Pa_{CO_2} is of short duration so that renal compensation has not yet occurred (Chapter 104), the serum bicarbonate level is increased by 1 mEq/L for every rise of 10 mm Hg in Pa_{CO_2}. By comparison, if the respiratory acidosis is of sufficient duration for renal compensation to occur, the serum bicarbonate level will usually be increased by 4 mEq for every rise of 10 mm Hg in Pa_{CO_2} (Fig. 74-2).

Once an elevated Pa_{CO_2} is established, it is appropriate to distinguish patients who "can't breathe" from those who "won't breathe." "Can't breathe" implies that a respiratory mechanical problem or neuromuscular weakness is causing the elevation in Pa_{CO_2}. Abnormalities in pulmonary function testing (e.g., a very low vital capacity) suggest a parenchymal or chest wall disorder. Ultrasound can identify phrenic neuropathy causing diaphragmatic dysfunction. Patients who "won't breathe" have central nervous system abnormalities that affect central drive, chemosensitivity, or both.

TREATMENT AND PROGNOSIS

The treatment of hypoventilation should focus on the underlying cause. Acute poisonings can be managed supportively or, in some cases, with specific antidotes (Chapter 96). Chronic conditions can be treated by addressing the underlying cause, such as weight loss in obesity-hypoventilation syndrome[10] or cholinesterase inhibitors in myasthenia gravis (Chapter 390). For parenchymal lung disease, treatment is directed at the underlying cause, if possible (Chapters 76 and 80).

Sedative medications should be used cautiously because they can occasionally precipitate acute respiratory failure.[11] Although profound hypoxemia can clearly be deleterious, oxygen occasionally can precipitate severe acute respiratory acidosis, particularly in patients with acute exacerbations of COPD (Chapter 76). As a result, hypoventilating patients with COPD require cautious management, including the careful administration of supplemental oxygen, which should be titrated to an arterial oxygen saturation of 90% or an arterial oxygen tension of 60 mm Hg.

Severe hypoventilation requires mechanical ventilation (Chapter 91), such as noninvasive ventilation for an acute exacerbation of COPD. For other presentations in which the Pa_{CO_2} is believed to be acutely elevated, endotracheal intubation and mechanical ventilation are frequently used, especially in patients with impaired consciousness.

For chronic hypoventilation in hypercapnic COPD, noninvasive bilevel positive airway pressure through a face mask during sleep can maintain alveolar ventilation, but there is no definitive evidence that noninvasive positive-pressure ventilation can prolong life or reduce hospitalizations in patients with COPD and chronic respiratory failure. In addition, the considerable difficulty of adhering to nocturnal bilevel therapy in COPD emphasizes the need for discussions with patients and families regarding its risks and benefits. For obesity hypoventilation syndrome without severe obstructive sleep apnea, noninvasive ventilation improves Pa_{CO_2} and reduces daytime sleepiness, as well as improving health-related quality of life.[A2] If such patients also have severe obstructive sleep apnea, noninvasive ventilation and continuous positive airway pressure (CPAP) are equally effective,[A3,A4] but CPAP is easier and less expensive to implement. If noninvasive ventilation is chosen, nasal and oronasal masks are equally effective and tolerated.[A5] In patients with central sleep apnea and heart failure, adaptive servo-ventilation, which provides inspiratory pressure support in addition to expiratory positive airway, was not helpful.[A6]

Other chronic hypoventilation syndromes are also commonly treated with bilevel positive airway pressure, although data are not compelling. In some chronic conditions, such as motor neuron disease (Chapter 387), tracheostomy should be discussed, although the impact of such interventions on quality of life should be carefully considered. Regardless of the underlying cause, an elevation in the Pa_{CO_2} level is considered a poor prognostic sign. End-of-life discussions are also important in such cases because the prognosis of patients with chronic respiratory failure is generally poor.

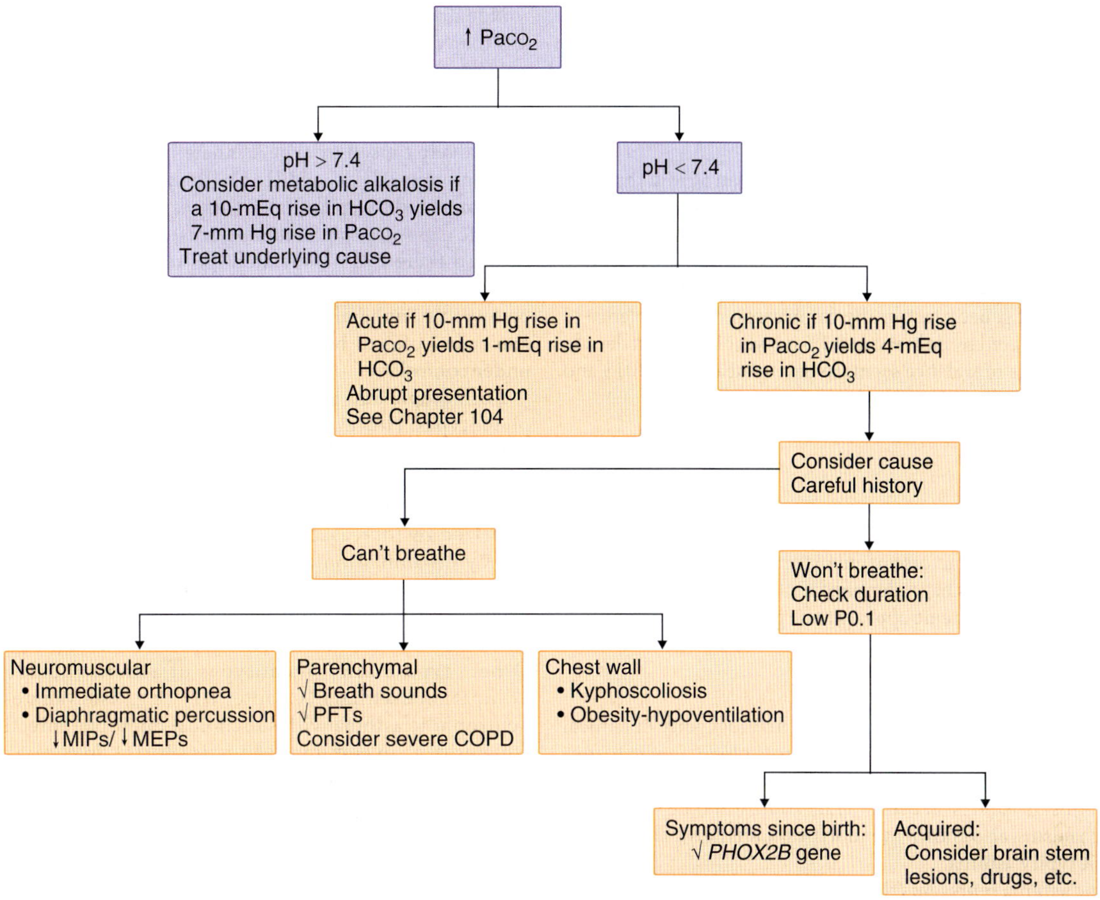

FIGURE 74-2. **A flowchart of a systematic approach to hypercapnia and various causes of hypoventilation.** The change in pH can help determine the cause and chronicity. A careful history and physical examination, coupled with pulmonary function testing, can help classify patients into those who "can't breathe" because of neuromuscular or mechanical abnormalities of the respiratory system compared with those who "won't breathe" because of central nervous system disease. COPD = chronic obstructive pulmonary disease; MEPs = maximal expiratory pressures; MIPs = maximal inspiratory pressures; P0.1 = the negative mouth pressure generated during the first 100 msec of an occluded inspiration; PFTs = pulmonary function tests.

GENERAL REFERENCES

For the General References and other additional features, please visit Elsevier eBooks+ at https://ebooks.health.elsevier.com.

Grade A References

A1. Tamisier R, Damy T, Bailly S, et al. Adaptive servo ventilation for sleep apnoea in heart failure: the FACE study 3-month data. *Thorax*. 2022;77:178-185.

A2. Zheng Y, Yee BJ, Wong K, et al. A pilot randomized trial comparing CPAP versus bilevel PAP spontaneous mode in the treatment of hypoventilation disorder in patients with obesity and obstructive airway disease. *J Clin Sleep Med*. 2022;18:99-107.

A3. Masa JF, Mokhlesi B, Benítez I, et al. Long-term clinical effectiveness of continuous positive airway pressure therapy versus non-invasive ventilation therapy in patients with obesity hypoventilation syndrome: a multicentre, open-label, randomised controlled trial. *Lancet*. 2019;393:1721-1732.

A4. Masa JF, Mokhlesi B, Benítez I, et al. Echocardiographic changes with positive airway pressure therapy in obesity hypoventilation syndrome. Long-term Pickwick randomized controlled clinical trial. *Am J Respir Crit Care Med*. 2020;201:586-597.

A5. Lebret M, Léotard A, Pépin JL, et al. Nasal versus oronasal masks for home non-invasive ventilation in patients with chronic hypercapnia: a systematic review and individual participant data meta-analysis. *Thorax*. 2021;76:1108-1116.

A6. O'Connor CM, Whellan DJ, Fiuzat M, et al. Cardiovascular outcomes with minute ventilation-targeted adaptive servo-ventilation therapy in heart failure: the CAT-HF trial. *J Am Coll Cardiol*. 2017;69:1577-1587.

75

ASTHMA

JEFFREY M. DRAZEN AND ELISABETH H. BEL

DEFINITION

Asthma is a clinical syndrome of unknown etiology characterized by recurrent episodes of airway obstruction that resolve spontaneously or as a result of treatment. These changes occur in the setting of various types of airway inflammation that are thought to reflect specific endotypes of this clinical syndrome. Although airway obstruction is largely reversible, some changes that lead to obstruction in the asthmatic airway may be irreversible.

EPIDEMIOLOGY

Asthma is an extremely common disorder affecting boys more commonly than girls and, after puberty, women more commonly than men (rate ratio women : men is 1.8); approximately 8% of the adult population of the United States has signs and symptoms consistent with a diagnosis of asthma. Although most cases begin before the age of 25 years, new-onset asthma may develop at any time throughout life. An estimated 340 million people worldwide suffer from asthma, with 420,000 annual deaths attributed to the disease.[1]

The worldwide prevalence of asthma increased more than 50% in the latter half of the 20th century. During that period, the greatest increases in the prevalence of asthma occurred in countries that adopted an "industrialized" lifestyle without contact with farm animals. In contrast, being raised in a farming environment in close contact with cows is associated with a much lower risk of asthma, independent of genetic factors. By comparison, the prevalence of wheezing in children increased by only about 0.1% per year in the first decade of the 21st century, and the prevalence seems to have plateaued by 2015 and stabilized since then.

PATHOBIOLOGY

Genetics

In twin studies, asthma has about 60% heritability, thereby indicating that both genetic and environmental factors are important in its etiology. Multiple genome-wide association studies have identified multiple genetic loci associated with asthma; the common theme appears to be genes related to immune mechanisms.[2]

Pathology

The asthma syndrome is characterized by marked heterogeneity in clinical expression, environmental triggers, and immunopathologic mechanisms. Traditionally, clinicians identified only two forms of asthma, atopic and nonatopic asthma, but this division is an oversimplification. Multiple underlying pathobiologic mechanisms, also known as endotypes, underlie the classic signs and symptoms that typify asthma.

Atopic or allergic asthma represents the most common and most studied subtype of asthma. It is characterized by the presence of immunoglobulin E (IgE)-mediated sensitization to environmental allergens and can be observed in almost all school-aged children with asthma and about half of adult asthmatics. Inflammation and remodeling of the airways are characteristic pathologic features of atopic asthma. Remodeling changes include epithelial fragility, edema, and hyperemia of the mucosa, as well as thickening of the subepithelial reticular basement due to deposition of collagen types III and IV. In more severe chronic asthma, the airway wall thickens as a result of hyperplasia of airway smooth muscle, hypertrophy of mucus secreting glands, and subepithelial angiogenesis. Infiltration of the airway wall with inflammatory cells including adaptive T helper-2 (T_H2) cells, mast cells, and eosinophils is a general finding, and occurs even in the mildest cases of atopic asthma.

T_H2 cells initiate and propagate the inflammatory cascade associated with allergy by producing a variety of cytokines, including interleukin (IL)-4, IL-5, and IL-13. IL-4 induces B-cell proliferation and is capable of stimulating these cells to produce IgE. IL-13 has similar effects of those to IL-4 with respect to B-cell stimulation and IgE production but, in addition, induces airway hyperresponsiveness, goblet cell metaplasia, and mucus hypersecretion. IL-5 plays a major role in the regulation of eosinophil formation, maturation, recruitment, and survival. Increased production of IL-5 may be related to the pathogenesis of severe eosinophilic asthma.

Mast cells are found in close association with airway smooth muscle cells and are classically activated by allergens when IgE is bound to the high-affinity IgE receptor. IgE-mediated mast cell degranulation and activation results in the release of histamine and in the generation of cysteinyl leukotrienes and prostaglandins, which contribute to bronchoconstriction and airway hyperresponsiveness.

Eosinophils accumulate in the airways after sensitized persons are exposed to allergens. Elevated numbers of circulating eosinophils are now considered a key biomarker indicating that a patient has a form of asthma that is likely to respond to inhaled glucocorticoids and, in more severe cases, to treatment with antibodies against aspects of the T_H2 inflammatory pathway. Upon activation, eosinophils release toxic granule products (e.g., major basic protein and eosinophil cationic protein) that damage airway epithelium and nerves. These cells also produce lipid mediators such as leukotrienes and platelet activating factor, as well as a range of cytokines, growth factors, and chemokines.

Nonatopic or intrinsic asthma develops in adulthood and accounts for less than 5% of cases of asthma. It is not associated with allergies, is often accompanied by chronic rhinosinusitis and nasal polyposis, and is poorly responsive to inhaled glucocorticoids. The eosinophilic airway inflammation observed in this type of asthma is not dependent on adaptive immunity but is likely caused by type 2 innate lymphoid cells (ILC2) that produce high amounts of IL-5 and IL-13. The growth and maturation of ILC2 cells are stimulated by epithelial cytokines ("alarmins"), which are induced by chronic exposure to pollutants, viruses, or fungi. ILC2 cells produce little IL-4, so there is no associated IgE response from B cells. Patients with intrinsic asthma often have a severe form of asthma with elevated eosinophil counts in peripheral blood, and generally require high doses of systemic glucocorticoids or biologics aimed at IL-5 or IL-13 to keep their asthma under control.

Both atopic and intrinsic asthma are so called "type-2-high" asthma phenotypes. However, cluster analyses of large cohorts of adult patients with asthma have identified at least three subtypes of asthma that are not characterized by the presence of type 2 cytokines or eosinophilic airway inflammation. These "type-2-low" subtypes of asthma are characterized by increased numbers of neutrophils in the airway or by no airway inflammation at all. One increasingly recognized "type-2-low" asthma phenotype is obesity-associated asthma. This type of asthma occurs later in life, usually in female patients without prior airway disease. The mechanism of obesity-associated asthma is not well understood. Other "type-2-low" phenotypes of asthma include certain forms of occupational asthma (Chapter 81) (e.g., isocyanate-induced asthma), neutrophilic asthma with subclinical microbial infection, and asthma in athletes (e.g., in endurance aquatic sports). In clinical practice in adults, different asthma phenotypes can coexist and interact within the same patient, thereby underscoring the need for a personalized and targeted approach to diagnosis and management.

Physiological Changes in Asthma

Increased resistance to airflow is the physiological hallmark of asthma; it is due to airway obstruction that results from smooth muscle constriction, thickening of the airway epithelium, and free secretions within the airway lumen. Obstruction to airflow is manifested by increased airway resistance and decreased flow rates throughout the vital capacity. At the onset of an exacerbation of asthma, obstruction occurs at all airway levels; as the exacerbation resolves, these changes are reversed—first in the large airways (i.e., mainstem, lobar, segmental, and subsegmental bronchi) and then in the more peripheral airways. This anatomic sequence of onset and reversal is reflected in the physiological changes observed during resolution of an asthmatic episode. Specifically, as an exacerbation of asthma resolves, flow rates first normalize at volumes high in the vital capacity and only later at volumes low in the vital capacity. Because asthma is largely an airway disease rather than an air space disease, no primary changes occur in the static pressure-volume curve of the lungs. However, during an acute exacerbation of asthma, airway narrowing may be so severe as to result in airway closure, with individual lung units closing at a volume that is near their maximal volume. This closure results in a change of the pressure-volume curve such that for a given contained gas volume within the thorax, elastic recoil is decreased, which in turn further depresses expiratory flow rates.

Exercise-induced bronchoconstriction, which is the transient narrowing of the airways after exercise, occurs frequently among athletes who may not have asthma or even have any respiratory symptoms. The mechanism is uncertain, but the key stimulus is probably airway dehydration because of increased ventilation.

Additional factors influence the mechanical behavior of the lungs during an exacerbation of asthma. During inspiration in this setting, the maximal inspiratory pleural pressure becomes more negative than the subatmospheric pressure of 4 to 6 cm H_2O usually required for tidal airflow. The expiratory phase of respiration also becomes active as the patient tries to force air from the lungs. As a consequence, expiratory peak pleural pressures, which normally are, at most, only a few centimeters of water above atmospheric pressure, may be as high as 20 to 30 cm H_2O above atmospheric pressure. The low pleural pressures during inspiration tend to dilate airways, whereas the high pleural pressures during expiration tend to narrow airways. During an exacerbation of asthma, the wide pressure swings, coupled with alterations in the mechanical properties of the airway wall, lead to a much higher resistance to expiratory airflow than to inspiratory airflow.

The respiratory rate is usually rapid during an acute exacerbation. This tachypnea is driven not by abnormalities in arterial blood gas composition but rather by stimulation of intrapulmonary receptors with subsequent effects on central respiratory centers. One consequence of the combination of airway narrowing and rapid airflow rates is a heightened mechanical load on the ventilatory pump. During a severe exacerbation, the load can increase the work of breathing by a factor of 10 or more and can predispose to fatigue of the ventilatory muscles. With respect to gas exchange, the patchy nature of asthmatic airway narrowing results in a maldistribution of ventilation ($\dot{V}$) relative to pulmonary perfusion (Q). A shift occurs from the normal preponderance of ($\dot{V}/Q$) units, with a ratio of near unity, to a distribution with a large number of alveolar-capillary units, with a ($\dot{V}/Q$) ratio of less than unity. The net effect is to induce modest arterial hypoxemia with Pa_{O_2} values commonly in the 60 mm Hg range while the patient is respiring ambient air at sea level. In addition, the hyperpnea of asthma is reflected as hyperventilation with a low arterial P_{CO_2}.

CLINICAL MANIFESTATIONS

History

During an acute exacerbation of asthma, often referred to as an asthma exacerbation, patients seek medical attention for shortness of breath accompanied by cough, wheezing, and anxiety. The degree of breathlessness experienced by the patient is not closely related to the degree of airflow obstruction but is often influenced by the acuteness of the exacerbation. Dyspnea may occur only with exercise (exercise-induced asthma), after treatment with agents inhibiting the actions of cyclooxygenase 1 (aspirin-exacerbated respiratory disease),[3] after exposure to a specific known allergen (extrinsic asthma), or for no identifiable reason (intrinsic asthma). Variants of asthma exist in which cough, hoarseness, or inability to sleep through the night is the presenting symptom. Identification of a provoking stimulus through careful questioning helps establish the diagnosis of asthma and may be therapeutically useful if the stimulus can be avoided. Most patients with asthma complain of shortness of breath when they are exposed to rapid changes in the temperature and humidity of inspired air. For example, during the winter months in less temperate climates, patients commonly become short of breath on leaving a heated house; in warm humid climates, patients may complain of shortness of breath on entering a cold dry room, such as an air-conditioned theater.

An important factor to consider in taking a history from a patient with asthma is the potential for occupational exposures (Chapter 81). Asthma that is triggered by occupational exposures is termed occupational asthma; preexisting asthma that is exacerbated by workplace exposures is termed workplace-exacerbated asthma. In reactive airway dysfunction syndrome, a single large exposure leads to a persistent asthma-like phenotype in a previously normal individual.

Physical Examination

Vital Signs

Common features noted during an exacerbation of asthma include a rapid respiratory rate (often 25 to 40 breaths per minute), tachycardia, and pulsus paradoxus (an exaggerated inspiratory decrease in the systolic pressure). The magnitude of the pulsus is related to the severity of the exacerbation; a value greater than 15 mm Hg indicates an exacerbation of moderate severity. Pulse oximetry, with the patient respiring ambient air at sea level, commonly reveals an oxygen saturation near 90%.

Thoracic Examination

Inspection may reveal that patients experiencing acute asthma exacerbations are using their accessory muscles of ventilation; if so, the skin over the thorax may be retracted into the intercostal spaces during inspiration. The chest is usually hyperinflated, and the expiratory phase is prolonged relative to the inspiratory phase. Percussion of the thorax demonstrates hyperresonance, with loss of the normal variation in dullness due to diaphragmatic movement; tactile fremitus is diminished. Auscultation reveals wheezing, which is the cardinal physical finding in asthma but does not establish the diagnosis (Chapter 71). Wheezing, commonly louder during expiration but heard during inspiration as well, is characterized as polyphonic in that more than one pitch may be heard simultaneously (Video 75-1). Accompanying adventitious sounds may include rhonchi, which are suggestive of free secretions in the airway lumen, or rales, which should raise the suspicion of an alternative diagnosis and are indicative of localized infection or heart failure. The loss of intensity or the absence of breath sounds in a patient with asthma, the so-called quiet chest, is an indication of severe airflow obstruction.

DIAGNOSIS

Laboratory Findings

Pulmonary Function Findings

A decrease in airflow rates throughout the vital capacity is the cardinal pulmonary function abnormality during an asthmatic episode.[4] The peak expiratory flow rate (PEFR), the forced expiratory volume in the first second (FEV_1), and the maximal mid-expiratory flow rate (MMEFR) are all decreased in asthma (Chapter 73). In severe asthma, dyspnea may be so severe as to prevent the patient from performing a complete spirogram. In this case, if 2 seconds of forced expiration can be recorded, reasonable estimates for PEFR and FEV_1 can be obtained. Gradation of the severity of the exacerbation (Table 75-1) must be assessed by objective measures of airflow; no other methods yield accurate and reproducible results. As the exacerbation resolves, the PEFR and the FEV_1 increase toward normal together while the MMEFR remains substantially depressed; as the episode resolves further, the FEV_1 and the PEFR may normalize while the MMEFR remains depressed (Fig. 75-1). Even when the exacerbation has fully resolved clinically, residual depression of the MMEFR is not uncommon; this depression may resolve during a prolonged course of treatment. If the patient is able to cooperate such that more complete measurements of lung function can be made, lung volume measurements made during an exacerbation demonstrate an increase in both total lung capacity and residual volume; the changes in total lung capacity and residual volume often, but not always, resolve with treatment. Because of the extra cooperation needed for this testing, it is not advised during an acute asthma exacerbation but is indicated before discharge in a patient hospitalized for such treatment or between exacerbations.

Pulmonary function testing obtained when the patient is relatively stable, for example, a month or more after a clinical exacerbation,[5] usually demonstrates airway obstruction, as indicated by low FEV_1 (as a percentage of the patient's predicted value), low forced vital capacity, and slightly elevated total lung capacity and residual volume values. These results may fully normalize after administration of a bronchodilator. In a patient with suspected asthma, a "bronchodilator response" is canonically defined as a 12% increase in the FEV_1, provided it is at least 200 mL (Fig. 75-2).

Exhaled NO•

The fraction of NO• in the exhaled air (Fe_{NO}) is elevated in patients with asthma. Although the exact concentration considered "elevated" will vary with the details of the technique used to obtain the gas sample, a concentration of 20 to 25 parts per billion is a convenient and reliable

TABLE 75-1 RELATIVE SEVERITY OF AN ASTHMATIC EXACERBATION AS INDICATED BY PEFR, FEV_1, AND MMEFR

TEST	PREDICTED VALUE (%)	SEVERITY OF ASTHMA
PEFR	>80	
FEV_1	>80	No spirometric abnormalities
MMEFR	>80	
PEFR	>80	
FEV_1	>70	Mild asthma
MMEFR	55-75	
PEFR	>60	
FEV_1	45-70	Moderate asthma
MMEFR	30-50	
PEFR	<50	
FEV_1	<50	Severe asthma
MMEFR	10-30	

FEV_1 = forced expiratory volume in the first second; MMEFR = maximal mid-expiratory flow rate; PEFR = peak expiratory flow rate.

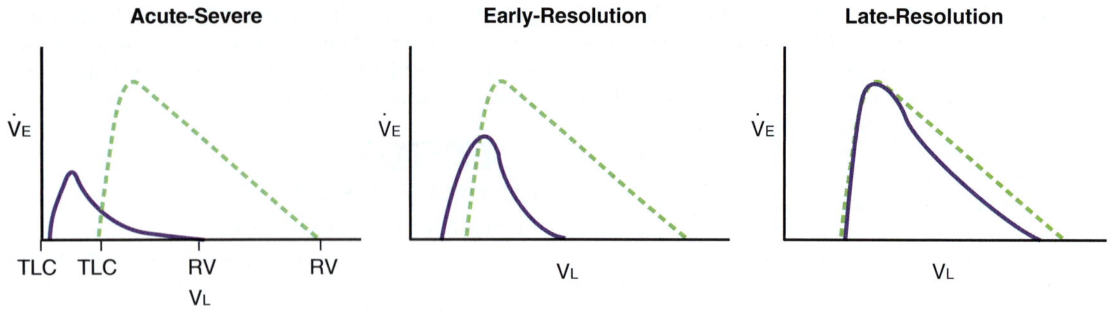

FIGURE 75-1. Schematic flow-volume curves in various stages of asthma. In each figure, the *dashed line* depicts the normal flow-volume curve. Predicted and observed total lung capacity (TLC) and residual volume (RV) are shown at the extremes of each curve. V̇E = expiratory flow rate; VL = lung volume.

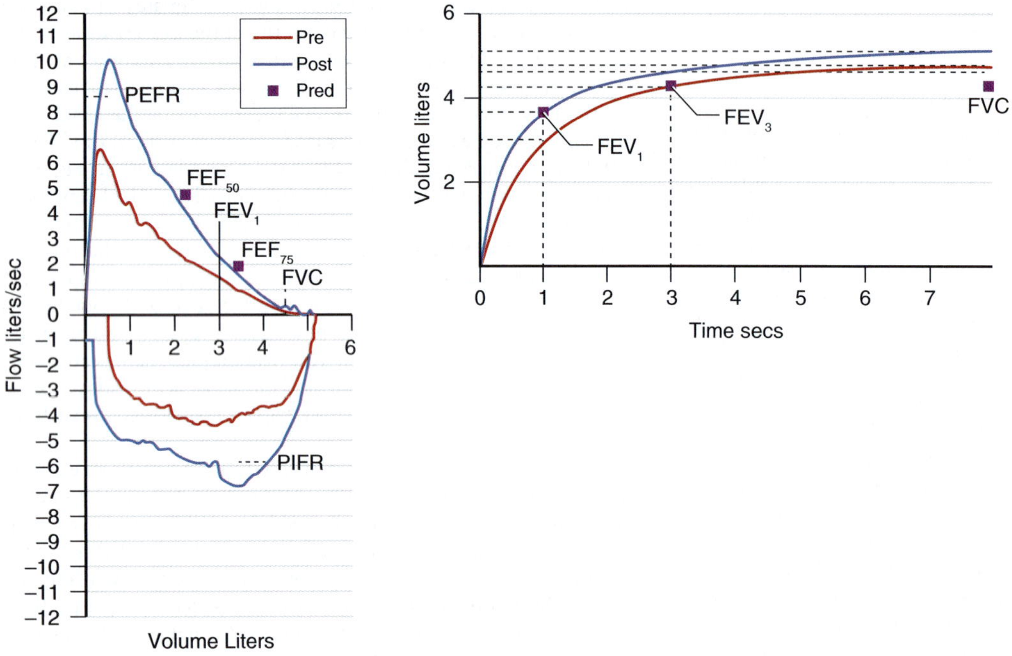

Spirometry (BTPS)

		Pre Bronchodilator			Predicted Range		Post Bronchodilator	Percent
		Actual	%Pred	Mean	95% CI	Actual	%Pred	Change
FVC	(L)	4.78	105	4.51	3.46	5.12	113	7
FEV_1	(L)	3.01	80	3.75	2.89	3.70	98	22
FEV_1/FVC	(%)	63.00	75	83.00	75.00	72.00	86	14
FEF_{25-75}	(L/s)	1.87	46	4.03		2.64	65	41
PEFR	(L/s)	6.64	75	8.74		10.17	116	53
FET	(sec)	7.89				7.89		

FIGURE 75-2. Lung function test results of a patient with asthma before (*red line*) and after (*blue line*) treatment with inhaled albuterol. BTPS = body temperature, pressure, water vapor saturated; FEF_{25-75} = forced expiratory flow rate of the middle 50% of expiration; FET = forced expiratory time; FEV_1 = forced expiratory volume in the first second; FVC = forced vital capacity; PEFR = peak expiratory flow rate; PIFR = optimal peak inspiratory flow rate; Pred = predicted.

level that can be used to distinguish people without asthma from patients with untreated asthma.

Arterial Blood Gases

Blood gas analysis need not be undertaken in individuals with mild asthma. If the asthma is of sufficient severity to merit prolonged observation, however, blood gas analysis is indicated[6]; in such cases, hypoxemia and hypocapnia are the rule. With the patient breathing ambient air near sea level, the PaO_2 is usually between 55 and 70 mm Hg and the $PaCO_2$ between 25 and 35 mm Hg. At the onset of the exacerbation, an appropriate pure respiratory alkalemia is usually evident; with exacerbations of prolonged duration, the pH returns toward normal as a result of a compensatory metabolic acidemia. A normal $PaCO_2$ in a patient with a history of several days of moderate to severe airflow obstruction is reason for concern because it may indicate that the mechanical load on the respiratory system is greater than can be sustained by the ventilatory muscles and that respiratory failure is imminent. When the $PaCO_2$ increases in such settings, the pH decreases quickly because the bicarbonate stores have become depleted as a result of renal compensation for the prolonged preceding respiratory alkalemia. Because this chain of events can take place rapidly, close observation is indicated for asthmatic patients with "normal" $PaCO_2$ levels and a history of several days of moderate to severe airflow obstruction.

Other Blood Findings

Patients with asthma are frequently of the "type-2-high" phenotype; thus, blood eosinophilia is common but not universal. The number of eosinophils in a microliter of blood has been used as a method to forecast a given patient's response to anti-cytokine treatment in asthma (see later). In addition, elevated serum levels of immunoglobulin E (IgE) are often documented and are part of the indication for treatment with anti-IgE monoclonal antibodies. If indicated by the patient's history, specific immunosorbent tests, which measure IgE directed against specific offending antigens, can be conducted. Epidemiologic studies indicate that asthma is unusual in subjects with low IgE levels, but some patients with severe asthma have high blood eosinophil levels with low IgE levels.

Radiographic Findings

The chest radiograph of a patient with asthma is often normal. Severe asthma is associated with hyperinflation, as indicated by depression of the diaphragm and abnormally lucent lung fields. Complications of severe asthma, including

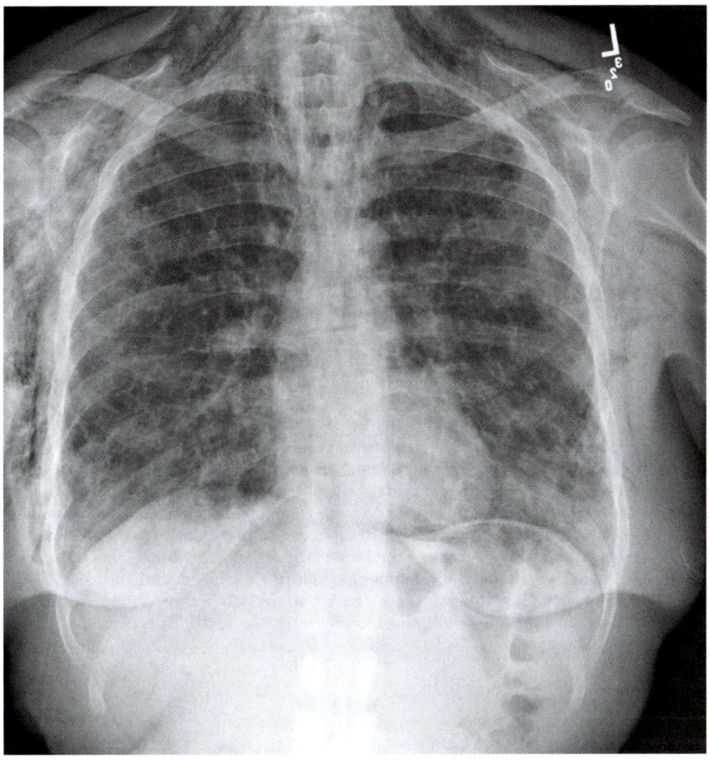

FIGURE 75-3. Chest radiograph showing substantial subcutaneous emphysema and pneumomediastinum in a patient with a severe asthma exacerbation. (Radiograph courtesy Christopher Fanta, MD.)

subcutaneous emphysema, pneumomediastinum (Fig. 75-3), and pneumothorax, may be detected radiographically. In mild to moderate asthma without adventitious sounds other than wheezing, a chest radiograph need not be obtained; if the asthma is of sufficient severity to merit hospital admission, a chest radiograph is advised.

Electrocardiographic Findings

The electrocardiogram, except for sinus tachycardia, is usually normal in acute asthma. However, right axis deviation, right bundle branch block, "P pulmonale," or even ST-T wave abnormalities may arise during severe asthma and resolve as the exacerbation resolves.

Sputum Findings

The sputum of the asthmatic patient may be either clear or opaque with a green or yellow tinge. The presence of color does not invariably indicate infection, and examination of a Gram-stained and Wright-stained sputum smear is indicated. The sputum often contains eosinophils, Charcot-Leyden crystals (crystallized eosinophil lysophospholipase), Curschmann spirals (bronchiolar casts composed of mucus and cells), or Creola bodies (clusters of airway epithelial cells with identifiable cilia that, in fresh samples, often can be seen to beat), which can affect color without the presence of infection. Asthma specialists may examine induced sputum samples to help identify specific asthma endotypes.

DIAGNOSIS

Differential Diagnosis

Asthma is easy to recognize in a young patient without comorbid medical conditions who has exacerbating and remitting airway obstruction accompanied by blood eosinophilia. A rapid symptomatic and laboratory response to bronchodilator treatment is usually all that is needed to establish the diagnosis. However, in the patient with cryptic episodic shortness of breath, an elevated FE_{NO} can help establish a diagnosis of asthma. However, in the absence of an elevated FE_{NO}, other causes of wheezing (see Table 71-4 in Chapter 71) should be investigated. It is important to note that cigarette smoking and the use of inhaled glucocorticoids can lower measured FE_{NO} values, and this information should be used when interpreting this laboratory test. Epidemiologic studies show that up to one-third of patients who have physician-diagnosed asthma may not actually have asthma when they are studied systematically.[7]

TREATMENT

The treatment of asthma is directed at two distinct facets of the disease: the control of symptoms and the prevention of exacerbations.

Symptomatic control is graded by the severity and frequency of asthmatic symptoms during the day, including limitations of activities of daily life, the need to use "rescue" inhaler treatments, and asthmatic symptoms that wake the patient from sleep. The prevention of exacerbations is less linked to symptoms than to levels of lung function, so management must include objective measures of lung function. The best measure is FEV_1, but measures of PEFR can be substituted, especially because inexpensive and easy-to-use peak flowmeters make this measurement feasible in virtually all cases.

Treatment of asthma has two components. The first is the use of acute treatments when the patient has symptoms consistent with airway obstruction; these are known as *rescue treatments*. The second is the use of *controller treatments,* which modify the asthmatic airway environment so that acute exacerbations occur less frequently.[8]

In a given individual, the intensity of asthma treatment is adjusted, for the most part, to achieve five goals:

1. to allow the patient to pursue the activities of her or his daily life without excessive interference from asthma,
2. to allow the patient to sleep without awakening because of asthmatic symptoms,
3. to minimize the use of rescue treatments,
4. to prevent the need for unscheduled medical care, and
5. to maintain lung function reasonably near normal.

The treatment of asthma is divided into five steps ranging from step 1 with minimal treatment to step 5 with very intensive treatment. Based on a patient's history and lung function values, the clinician must decide if the patient's asthma is "in control" or not and note the current treatment step. A patient who is "in control" should stay at their current step or can attempt to step down after about 3 months of stability at a given treatment step. By comparison, a patient whose disease is "out of control" should have their treatment stepped up (Fig. 75-4).

Asthma Medications

Although some chronic asthma treatments are oral, the core of treatment relies on inhaled medications to provide effects directly on the airways and thereby to avoid systemic toxicity.

Using an Inhaler

With all pressurized propellant-driven inhalers (Fig. 75-5), patients should be instructed to exhale to a comfortable volume and to actuate the inhaler as they breathe in very slowly (such as they would when sipping hot soup). Inspiration to near total lung capacity is followed by holding the breath for 10 seconds to allow the deposition of smaller aerosol particles in more peripheral airways (Video 75-2). Patients should be asked to demonstrate their ability to use inhalers correctly and instructed if they are not. Aerosol "spacers" can help patients who have difficulty in coordinating their inspiratory effort and inhaler actuation. For dry-powder inhalers, the manufacturer's directions must be followed because each inhaler differs. With nebulized treatments, patients fill the nebulizer reservoir with the appropriate medication and breathe the generated aerosol quietly until the reservoir is empty.

Inhaled Glucocorticoids

Inhaled glucocorticoids, which have less systemic impact than systemic steroids for a given level of therapeutic effect, are effective controller treatments for improving lung function and preventing asthmatic exacerbations in patients with persistent asthma; inhaled glucocorticoids do not change the long-term natural history of asthma.[9] Inhaled glucocorticoids are combined with inhaled β-agonists for the treatment of acute asthmatic symptoms controller and reliever treatment in which the immediate benefits of bronchodilation with inhaled β-agonists are accompanied by the disease-controlling effects of inhaled glucocorticoids.

All available inhaled glucocorticoids (Table 75-2) are effective treatments for asthma but differ in terms of cost, the magnitude of adrenal suppression, and the potential for systemic effects, including loss of bone mineralization, cataracts, and glaucoma. Overall, no convincing data are available to suggest that there is reason to prefer one glucocorticoid to the others. Adverse effects common to all inhaled glucocorticoids are oral thrush and hoarseness (attributed to myopathy of the laryngeal muscles); the risk and severity can be reduced by aerosol spacers and good oropharyngeal hygiene (i.e., rinsing out the mouth by gargling with drinking water after dosing).

Patients whose disease can be categorized as being in control most of the time without any regularly scheduled treatment are categorized as mild asthma and represent the largest number of asthmatic patients. They are on step 1 of the treatment staircase, and they should use controller and reliever therapy only when they have asthmatic symptoms.[A1-A3]

β_2-Adrenergic Agents

β_2-Adrenergic agonists (Table 75-3) can be classified as short-acting or long-acting. Therapy with β_2-adrenergic agonists always must be accompanied by an inhaled glucocorticoid. Short-acting agonists are used to treat an acute asthmatic exacerbation in patients who are on step 4 or 5 of the treatment staircase and who are already using inhaled glucocorticoids. By comparison, either short

Asthma Treatment Staircase. See legend to understand how to apply	STEP 1	STEP 2	STEP 3	STEP 4	STEP 5
CONTROLLER MEDICATIONS to prevent exacerbations: Primary options	No controller except as needed for symptoms using controller and reliever therapy*	Daily low-dose IGC	Daily low-dose IGC-LABA	Daily high-dose IGC-LABA	Daily high-dose IGC-LABA plus seek expert consultation for anti-cytokine Rx or anti-IgE Rx
Secondary options		LTRA	Daily medium-dose IGC	Daily high-dose IGC, add-on tiotropium	Add oral glucocorticoids at as low a dose as possible
RELIEVER MEDICATIONS to treat symptoms	Controller and reliever therapy*			SABA	

FIGURE 75-4. Asthma treatment algorithm. To use this staircase, determine what treatment your patient is receiving and then if their asthma is "in control" as noted in the text. If the patient's asthma is in control (e.g., with all five stability indicators noted in the text for 2 to 3 months), leave the patient at the current treatment level or decrease one step as indicated in the figure. If the patient's asthma is not in control, increase it from the current level of treatment by one or two steps depending on overall control. If it is not possible to get the patient's asthma in control while using step 4 treatment, it is prudent to refer the patient to a specialty asthma center for evaluation by an asthma expert. Treatments such as asthma biologics (monoclonal antibodies) or daily oral glucocorticoids should be monitored by such a specialist. At steps 1-3, the patient should be instructed to use controller and reliever therapy (termed CART) in which a patient uses an inhaled glucocorticoid and a β_2 selective bronchodilator (either in separate inhalers or as a combined product) to treat bothersome asthmatic symptoms at step 1 or "breakthrough" symptoms in steps 2 and 3. See text for more details of controller and reliever therapy. Ig = immunoglobulin; IGC = inhaled glucocorticoid; IL4r = interleukin-4 receptor; IL5/5r = interleukin-5 or its receptor; LABA = long-acting β_2-agonist; LTRA = leukotriene receptor antagonist; Rx = prescription; SABA = short-acting β_2-agonist. *See legend for an explanation of controller and reliever therapy. (Modified from National Asthma Education and Prevention Program, Update December 2020. https://www.nhlbi.nih.gov/health-topics/all-publications-and-resources/2020-focused-updates-asthma-management-guidelines.)

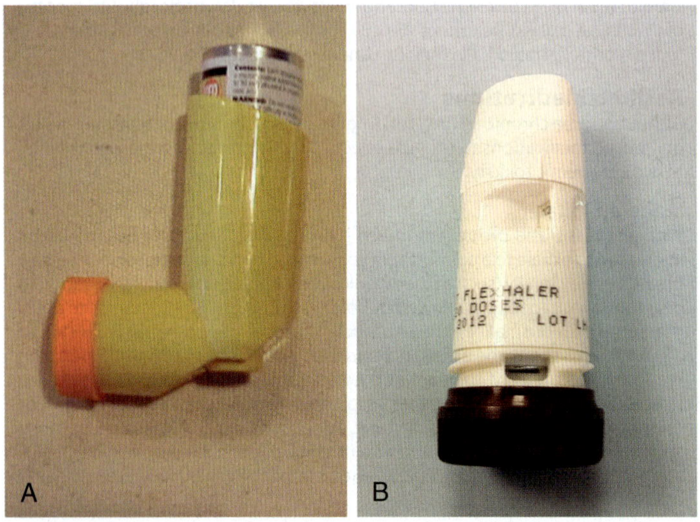

FIGURE 75-5. Commonly used inhalers. A, A pressurized metered-dose inhaler for a branded form of albuterol. Such inhalers propel the medication by means of a pressurized gas; many inhalers use propellants that do not harm the ozone layer, but recent concerns have arisen about greenhouse effects of such gases. **B,** One of many types of dry powder inhalers; the one shown is a Flexhaler and dispenses budesonide. When this type of inhaler is activated, the active agent is released as a dry powder into a chamber. The patient creates the energy for airflow by means of an inspiratory effort that is directed through the device and that entrains medication into the inhaled airway. As a result, effectiveness can be impaired in patients whose airflow is extremely limited.

or long-acting β_2-adrenergic agonists can be used with an inhaled glucocorticoid as part of controller and reliever therapy (see below) when patients are on step 1, 2, or 3 of the treatment staircase.

Short-Acting β-Adrenergic Agents (SABA)

These agents, given by inhalation, are an important part of treatment for asthma. Constricted airway smooth muscle relaxes in response to stimulation of β_2-adrenergic receptors. Short-acting β-adrenergic agonists with varying degrees of β_2-selectivity, onset of action, and duration of response are available for routine use in inhaled (or oral preparations, only in parts of the world where cost or availability limits the use of inhalers) and for emergent use as parenteral preparations.

Long-Acting β-Agonists (LABA)

Long-acting β-agonists should not be used in patients with asthma unless they are given as concomitant treatment with an inhaled glucocorticoid. To avoid inappropriate monotherapy, patients should be prescribed a dual inhaler that contains both an inhaled glucocorticoid and a long-acting β-agonist together so that the treatments with these two agents cannot be separated. Triple inhalers contain an inhaled glucocorticoid, a long-acting β_2-agonist, and a long-acting muscarinic antagonist (see later) in the same aerosol device. Although the combination inhalers are convenient and effective,[A4] they generally are not recommended because of their expense and the problem that "stepping down" treatment requires the patient to switch to entirely different inhalers. When choosing among the many dual combination (i.e., a β_2-agonist and an inhaled glucocorticoid) inhalers available, the selection should be driven by the lowest inhaled dose of glucocorticoid (fluticasone, budesonide, beclomethasone, mometasone, or others) that the patient requires and then identifying a combination product that will also deliver the long-acting β_2-agonist when given as 2 puffs twice per day or less. Prescribing physicians also must consider cost and availability.

Randomized trials demonstrate that, when used with inhaled glucocorticoids, long-acting β_2-agonists do not result in a higher frequency of severe asthmatic events compared with inhaled glucocorticoids alone.[A5]

Antimuscarinic Agents

Agents that inhibit the effects of acetylcholine, which is released from the intrapulmonary motor nerves that run in the vagus nerve and innervate airway smooth muscle, are useful as add-on asthma treatment in step 5. Ipratropium bromide is available in a metered-dose inhaler; the recommended dose is 2 puffs from a metered-dose inhaler every 4 to 6 hours. In adults, inhaled tiotropium (2.5 μg by metered dose inhaler every morning) can be added to an inhaled glucocorticoid as a controller treatment. In patients who have asthma and a low sputum eosinophil level, treatment with tiotropium bromide, 5 μg once-daily, can provide a salutary effect that is equivalent to an inhaled glucocorticoid.[A6] Although other antimuscarinic agents have also been used in the treatment of chronic obstructive pulmonary disease (see Chapter 76), their use in asthma is not evidence based and not recommended.

Antileukotrienes

Agents with the capacity to inhibit the synthesis of the leukotrienes (zileuton, 600 mg four times a day, or controlled-release [Zyflo CR], 1200 mg twice daily) or the action of leukotrienes at the $CysLT_1$ receptor (montelukast [Singulair], 10 mg once a day; pranlukast [Onon, Ultair], 225 mg twice a day, not available in the United States; and zafirlukast [Accolate], 20 mg twice a day) are effective oral controller medications for some patients with mild or moderate persistent asthma. In older patients with asthma, leukotriene inhibitors are equivalent to low-dose inhaled glucocorticoids.[A7] In patients treated with zileuton, alanine aminotransferase levels should be monitored for the first 3 to 6 months; if levels rise to more than three times the upper limit of normal, the drug should be stopped. Theophylline metabolism is slowed by zileuton, so monitoring of levels is indicated if both are prescribed. These treatments can be used on their own for mild persistent asthma or in combination with inhaled glucocorticoids for more severe asthma.

Systemic Glucocorticoids

Systemic glucocorticoids are effective for the treatment of moderate to severe persistent asthma as well as for occasional severe exacerbations of asthma in a patient with otherwise mild asthma. No consensus has been reached on the specific type, dose, or duration of glucocorticoid to be used in the treatment of asthma. In non-hospitalized patients with asthma refractory to standard therapy, a steroid "pulse" of prednisone (40 mg/day for 5 days without a taper)

TABLE 75-2 GLUCOCORTICOID INHALERS USED FOR THE TREATMENT OF ASTHMA

AGENT	COMMON BRAND NAMES*	INHALER TYPES	LOW DOSE	HIGH DOSE	COMMENTS
Beclomethasone dipropionate Standard particle size For extrafine particle size-use half the standard particle size dose	Beclovent, Clenil, Qvar, Asmabec	Comes in both MDI and DPI inhalers with amounts per puff varying from 40-400 µg	1-2 puffs twice a day of low strength	5-6 puffs twice a day of high strength	Inhaled glucocorticoid with the longest use record. Although medication is generic, the inhaler type and propellant may be proprietary. Dose adjustments for patients in renal or hepatic failure are not needed
Budesonide	Budelin, Pulmicort	Inhalers are all DPIs with amounts per dose 100-400 µg. Solution for nebulization is also available with amount of drug per treatment varying between 0.5 and 1.0 mg	1-2 puffs twice a day of the 100 µg strength	1-2 puffs twice a day of the 400-µg strength The maximum DPI dose is two puffs twice daily of the 400-µg strength. The maximum nebulized dose is 4 mg/day.	Dose adjustments for patients in renal or hepatic failure are not needed
Ciclesonide	Alvesco	MDIs delivering 80 or 160 µg	1 puff of the 80-µg strength twice daily	2 puffs of the 160-µg strength twice daily. The maximum dose is 2 puffs twice daily of the highest strength	Dose adjustments for patients in renal or hepatic failure are not needed
Fluticasone propionate	Flovent, Flixotide	MDIs with 50, 125, 250 µg dose strengths; DPIs 50, 100, 250 µg; packets for nebulization at 0.25 and 1.0 mg/mL	1-2 puffs twice/day of 50 µg/puff dose strength With nebulizer, 1 mL of 0.25 mg/mL twice a day	1-2 puffs twice/day of 250-µg/puff dose strength-the maximum dose is two puffs twice daily of the 250 µg/puff dose With nebulizer, 1 mL of 1.0 mg/mL twice a day, which is the maximum dose	Dose labels vary depending on whether it is the amount loaded in the metering chamber (outside of United States [U.S.]) vs. the dose leaving the inhaler (U.S.). The three strengths are generally equal to low, medium, and high doses Dose adjustments for patients in renal failure not needed. In patients with hepatic failure, patients should be carefully monitored for steroid side effects and dose adjusted appropriately
Fluticasone furoate (DPI)	Arnuity Ellipta	DPIs with strengths of 50, 100 and 200 µg/dose	1 puff daily of the 50-µg/dose	1 puff daily of the 200-µg/dose The above is the maximum recommended dose	Once-daily dosing
Mometasone furoate	Asmanex	MDI with strengths of 100 and 200-µg/dose DPIs with strengths of 100 and 200 µg/dose	1 puff low strength daily	2 puffs high strength twice a day	Dose adjustments for patients in renal failure not needed. In patients with hepatic failure, patients should be carefully monitored for steroid side effects and dose adjusted appropriately

*Not all products marketing each medication are listed.
DPI = dry powder inhaler; MDI = metered dose inhaler.

TABLE 75-3 SELECTED SHORT-ACTING INHALED β-ADRENERGIC AGONISTS FOR ASTHMA†

GENERIC NAME	TRADE NAME*	DOSE/PUFF	DOSE AS PUFFS	COMMENTS
Albuterol-MDI‡	AccuNeb, Proair HFA, Proventil HFA, Ventolin HFA, Airomir HFA, Salamol HFA	Varies from 90-200 μg	2 puffs as needed for asthma symptoms. Can be repeated every 4 hr. 10-12 puffs in 24 hr is the maximum dose. Use of more than 6 puffs/day should prompt medical consultation for asthma control.	All are metered-dose inhalers that deliver a fixed amount of medication per puff
Albuterol-DPI	Ventolin, Asmasal, Salbulin	100 or 200 μg	1 puff as needed, otherwise same as albuterol MDI	All are dry powder inhalers that deliver a fixed amount of medication per inhalation
Albuterol solution	—	Varies from 0.63 mg/mL to 5 mg/mL	Inhale while breathing till solution consumed. Need for more than 6 home treatments/day should prompt medical consultation.	This solution is for use with a liquid nebulizer driven by compressed gas. Mix the dose with a volume of sterile normal saline to achieve a nebulizer concentration of 0.63 mg/mL
Levalbuterol-MDI	Xopenex HFA		Same as albuterol-MDI	The isolated R-isomer of albuterol. Some studies show superiority to the racemic albuterol found in the MDIs listed above
Levalbuterol-solution	Xopenex inhalation solution	0.63 mg/mL	Same as albuterol solution	Nebulizer solution as noted for albuterol above
Terbutaline-DPI	Bricanyl	250 or 500 μg	Same as albuterol-MDI	Dry powder inhaler, uses patient-generated effort to achieve airflow to disperse and deposit medication
Terbutaline solution	Bricanyl inhalation solution	2.5 mg/mL	Same as albuterol	The per dose amount is 2 mL with sterile saline added to achieve the requisite volume for the nebulizer used

*Not all products marketing each medication are listed.
†All have onset of effect 5 to 10 minutes and duration of effect 4 to 8 hours. All patients with asthma should have a short-acting bronchodilator as a rescue inhaler to use for rescue from signs of airway obstruction.
‡The generic names albuterol and salbutamol are synonyms. Albuterol is used in the United States and salbutamol in many other countries.
DPI = dry powder inhale; HFA = hydrofluoroalkane; MDI = metered dose inhaler.

is recommended.[A8] When patients cannot stop taking steroids without having recurrent uncontrolled bronchospasm, referral to an asthma specialist for biologic treatment is indicated. For patients whose asthma requires in-hospital treatment but is not considered life-threatening, an initial intravenous bolus of 2 mg/kg of hydrocortisone, followed by continuous infusion of 0.5 mg/kg/hour, has been shown to be beneficial within 12 hours. In exacerbations of asthma that are considered life-threatening, the use of intravenous methylprednisolone (125 mg every 6 hours) has been advocated. As the patient improves, oral steroids are substituted for intravenous steroids, and the oral dose is tapered during 1 to 3 weeks; addition of inhaled steroids is strongly recommended when oral steroids are started. Patients whose asthma requires oral glucocorticoid treatment to maintain control are prime candidates for monoclonal antibody treatment.

Monoclonal Antibody Treatment

Monoclonal antibodies are effective in carefully selected patients under expert guidance,[10-12] but they are quite expensive. Most insurance companies require specific clearance before these drugs can be administered, and they should be prescribed only by an asthma specialist who is familiar with their use.

Omalizumab (Xolair), a humanized murine monoclonal antibody that binds circulating IgE, is associated with decreased serum free (not total) IgE levels. In patients who have moderate to severe allergic asthma with elevated levels of serum IgE and who are receiving inhaled glucocorticoids, omalizumab treatment improves asthma control even as doses of inhaled steroids are decreased.[13] Dosing is guided by weight and by pretreatment IgE levels: a monthly subcutaneous dose of 0.016 mg × body weight (kg) × IgE level (IU/mL). Dosing calculators can be found online (e.g., https://www.xolairhcp.com/starting-treatment/dosing.html). Treatment with anti-IgE antibodies can reduce asthma exacerbations and improve quality of life in patients with severe allergic asthma; it is also useful in patients with aspirin-exacerbated respiratory disease (see later), but omalizumab's place in treatment schema has not been fully established. Because of the potential for anaphylaxis, all patients need to be monitored for 30 to 60 minutes after injection.

Mepolizumab (Nucala) is a humanized monoclonal antibody directed against IL-5. In randomized trials, it reduces asthma exacerbations by about 50% among patients who have severe asthma and who still have blood eosinophils greater than 150 cells/μL despite treatment with oral or high-dose inhaled glucocorticoids. In patients requiring daily oral glucocorticoid therapy to maintain asthma control, mepolizumab has a significant glucocorticoid-sparing effect.[A9] The dose is 100 mg subcutaneously every 4 weeks.

Reslizumab (Cinqair), which is another humanized monoclonal antibody against circulating IL-5 for patients with severe eosinophilic asthma, has benefits similar to mepolizumab. At 3 mg/kg intravenously every 4 weeks, it can reduce the frequency of exacerbations by about 50% in patients who had asthma and elevated blood eosinophil counts and who were inadequately controlled on inhaled glucocorticoid-based therapy.[A10]

Benralizumab (Fasenra) is a humanized monoclonal antibody against the α subunit of the IL-5 receptor that induces near-complete depletion of eosinophils and basophils in the circulation and lung tissue. In randomized trials, benralizumab (30 mg subcutaneously every 4 to 8 weeks) reduced exacerbations by 50% and improved lung function in patients with severe eosinophilic asthma, often despite a reduced dose of oral glucocorticoids.[A11]

Dupilumab (Dupixent), a monoclonal antibody against the α subunit of the shared interleukin-4 and interleukin-13 receptor (at 300 mg subcutaneously every 2 weeks), can improve the control of moderate to severe asthma and allow the dose of inhaled and oral glucocorticoids to be reduced, oftentimes with an improvement in lung function as well.[A12]

Tezepelumab, a human monoclonal antibody specific for the epithelial-cell-derived cytokine thymic stromal lymphopoietin (at 210 mg given subcutaneously every 4 weeks), reduces asthma exacerbations among patients treated with medium-to-high doses of inhaled glucocorticoids and at least one additional controller medication with or without oral glucocorticoids,[A13] regardless of their blood eosinophil level, although efficacy is greater when patients have a higher percentage of eosinophils in their peripheral blood.

Theophylline

Theophylline, and its more water-soluble congener aminophylline, are moderately potent bronchodilators. Because of potential toxicity and the availability of other regimens, they are not recommended for routine outpatient treatment. An exception is that aminophylline, given intravenously, can be helpful for the treatment of status asthmaticus.

Other Medical and Procedural Options

Vaccination for Seasonal Influenza, Pneumococcal Disease, and COVID-19

Vaccination (Chapter 15) for seasonal influenza (Chapter 332), pneumococcal disease (Chapter 268), and COVID-19 (Chapter 337) is recommended because all are efficacious, safe, and not associated with enhanced risk of asthmatic exacerbations. No worsening of any component of asthma has been identified with any of the vaccines.

Antibiotics

Azithromycin (500 mg 3 times a week for 48 weeks) added to standard step 4 treatment (Fig. 75-4) in patients with persistent symptomatic asthma can reduce exacerbations and improve quality of life in patients with persistent symptoms but at the expense of more diarrhea and an unknown risk of selecting resistant organisms.[A14] The electrocardiographic QT-C interval should be monitored to detect a risk of potentially serious cardiac arrythmias.

Suppression of Gastric Acid

Proton-pump inhibitor treatment had been advocated based on the concern that asthma could be caused by silent gastroesophageal reflux disease, even in the absence of gastrointestinal symptoms. Adequately powered clinical studies suggest that this approach provides no benefit for asthma control.

Radio Frequency Ablation of Airway Smooth Muscle

A proprietary system to ablate airway smooth muscle by delivery of radio frequency energy through a bronchoscopically placed probe has reduced exacerbations of asthma in sham-controlled trials among patients whose asthma remained out of control despite the use of multiple controller medications. Although a device for such treatment has been approved by the FDA, specific recommendations with respect to its use are not available, and it should be considered only at specialized centers.

Treatment of Specific Clinical Scenarios

Consensus guidelines recommend a stepped approach to the treatment of asthma (Fig. 75-4).

Minimally Symptomatic Patients

At the mild end of the spectrum (i.e., step 1 of the staircase), a patient who has rare limitations in activities of daily life, has nearly normal lung function, and sleeps without interruption from asthma can be prescribed a combination inhaler with a rapid-onset, long-acting β-agonist (e.g., formoterol plus a glucocorticoid; see Table 75-4) to use as a rescue inhaler on an as-needed basis or be prescribed a combination inhaler with a short-acting β-agonist plus a glucocorticoid (e.g., 180 μg albuterol/160 μg budesonide, with 2 puffs given up to 6 times a day). If a combination inhaler is not available or is cost prohibitive, the patient should use their short-acting β-agonist inhaler and their glucocorticoid inhaler one after the other up to 6 times per day.[A15-A18] Alternatively, for the patient who uses nebulized treatment on an intermittent basis, treatment with a short-acting β-agonist should ALWAYS be accompanied a treatment with an inhaled glucocorticoid. If a patient has a requirement for such rescue treatment more than twice weekly (excluding events brought on by exercise), they should progress to step 2 of the staircase with maintenance controller treatment with an inhaled glucocorticoid (see Table 75-2) or an anti-leukotriene (should be added, starting at the lowest dose recommended for the particular drug). For inhaled glucocorticoids, treatment can be escalated either by increasing the number of puffs or the strength per puff until control is achieved—this approach cycles the patient through low-, medium-, and high-dose inhaled glucocorticoid therapy (see Fig. 75-4) and will move the patient "up the staircase" to steps 3 and 4.

Rescue for Acute Exacerbations

All patients who have asthma should be prescribed a rescue treatment to be used if they develop symptoms consistent with acute asthmatic airway obstruction.[14] Rescue treatment should always include a rapid-acting inhaled β-agonist (Table 75-4). If appropriate dual-medication inhalers containing both drugs are not available, patients should be instructed to use sequential separate inhalers or nebulizer treatments, one containing a short-acting β_2-selective agonist and another containing an inhaled glucocorticoid, taken one after the other. For the patient who is already using low to medium doses of inhaled glucocorticoids (i.e., those on step 2 or 3 of therapy; see Fig. 75-4) and who then develops an exacerbation, a self-directed quadrupling of the inhaled glucocorticoid can abort the exacerbation and reduce the number of severe exacerbations by about 30%.[A19]

Patients Not on Chronic Asthma Medication

Most patients with mild asthma do not require regularly scheduled treatment, but should be treated with controller and reliever therapy when they develop asthmatic symptoms. Controller and reliever therapy with formoterol plus budesonide or albuterol plus budesonide (see Table 75-4) can potentially be used as up to 12 inhalations (6 treatments of 2 puffs each) from a combination inhaler per day without toxicity, although most patients use this combination at much lower frequencies. (This use of combination formoterol-inhaled glucocorticoid for "as-needed" asthma treatment is approved in many other countries around the world but is *off-label* for budesonide-formoterol in the United States. An albuterol plus budesonide combination inhaler is approved in the United States.)

For all IGC-containing inhalers after inhalation, the patient should rinse his/her mouth with water without swallowing to help reduce the risk of oropharyngeal candidiasis.

Concurrent Pulmonary Infection

In some patients, acute exacerbations of asthma may be due to concurrent infection, which requires targeted therapy (Chapters 76, 78, and 85). In patients with suspected or known infection with severe acute respiratory syndrome coronavirus-2 (Chapter 336), all asthma treatments should be continued as prescribed, including inhaled or systemic glucocorticoids.

Aspirin-Exacerbated Respiratory Disease (Previously Termed Aspirin-Induced Asthma)

Approximately 5% of patients with moderate to severe persistent asthma develop asthma when they ingest agents that inhibit cyclooxygenase, such as aspirin and other nonsteroidal anti-inflammatory drugs.[15] Inhibitors of cyclooxygenase 2 are less likely to cause these reactions, but aspirin-type reactions have been reported in sensitive patients treated with selective cyclooxygenase 2 inhibitors. The physiological manifestations of a laboratory-based aspirin challenge can be blocked by inhibitors of the leukotriene pathway and by omalizumab, but only omalizumab has been shown to prevent clinical disease.[A20] For most patients with this disorder, avoidance of aspirin and other nonsteroidal anti-inflammatory drugs is the first-line therapy, but omalizumab (see Monoclonal Antibody Treatment above for dosing) is indicated if that approach is not successful.

Exercise-Induced Asthma

Patients who develop asthmatic symptoms most prominently with exercise are said to have exercise-induced asthma.[16] In such patients preexercise treatment is recommended. Although 2 puffs of an inhaler containing a short-acting β-agonist had been the standard of care, expert opinion now suggests using a combination formoterol-budesonide inhaler before exercise for this purpose.

Allergic Bronchopulmonary Aspergillosis

Some patients with asthma as well as some patients with cystic fibrosis (Chapter 77), develop a phenotype characterized by wheezing, sputum containing brown sputum plugs, intermittent hemoptysis, fleeting pulmonary infiltrates, high levels of serum IgE, (often >1000 IU/mL), positive skin test reactions to *Aspergillus fumigatus* (Chapter 311), and positive IgG titers to *A. fumigatus*. When this combination of findings is present, the diagnosis is allergic of bronchopulmonary is established.[17]

Treatment with oral prednisone at (0.5 mg/kg a day for 4 weeks, then reducing the dose by 50% for 4 weeks, and finally reducing the dose by 50% for another 4 weeks before discontinuing it). Monotherapy with voriconazole (200 mg twice daily for 4 months) is usually successful and is as effective as prednisolone (dosed as noted earlier) for preventing exacerbations.[A21]

Occupational Asthma

Occupational asthma is discussed in Chapter 81.

Asthma in the Emergency Department

When a patient with asthma presents for acute emergency care, objective measures of the severity of the exacerbation, including quantification of pulsus paradoxus and, if the patient's dyspnea allows it, measurement of airflow rates (PEFR or FEV_1), should be evaluated in addition to the usual vital signs. If the exacerbation has been prolonged and failed to respond to treatment with bronchodilators (e.g., albuterol by metered-dose inhaler, two puffs every 2 to 3 hours) and high-dose inhaled glucocorticoids (see Table 75-2) before arrival at the emergency department, high-dose inhaled glucocorticoids should be continued[A22] and intravenous glucocorticoids (40 to 60 mg of methylprednisolone or its equivalent) should be administered. If the patient has not been receiving treatment with a leukotriene receptor antagonist, such agents should be administered (10 mg of montelukast or 20 mg of zafirlukast) as soon as possible. Treatment with inhaled β-agonists (either nebulized albuterol, 0.5 mL of a 0.5% solution repeated at 20- to 30-minute intervals, or albuterol by metered-dose inhaler, 2 puffs every 30 minutes) should be used until the PEFR or FEV_1 increases to greater than 40% of the predicted values or the patient shows obvious signs of clinical improvement, such as a slowed respiratory rate, a decrease in the magnitude of pulsus paradoxus, or less use of accessory muscles of ventilation. If this point is not reached within 2 hours, admission to the hospital for further treatment is strongly advocated.

When patients have PEFR and FEV_1 values that are greater than 60% of their predicted value on arrival in the emergency department, treatment with inhaled β_2-agonists alone, albuterol (0.5 mL of an albuterol 0.083% solution) or equivalent, is likely to result in an objective improvement in airflow rates. If significant improvement takes place in the emergency department, such patients can usually be treated as outpatients with inhaled β_2-agonists and a controller agent (see Fig. 75-4). A good strategy is to add inhaled glucocorticoids if the patient has not been receiving this treatment or has been using a single controller therapy.

For patients whose PEFR and FEV_1 values are between 40 and 60% of the values predicted at the time of initial evaluation in the emergency care setting, a plan of treatment varying in intensity between these two plans is indicated. Failure to respond to treatment by objective criteria (e.g., respiratory rate, PEFR or FEV_1) within 2 hours of arrival at the emergency department is an indication for the use of systemic glucocorticoids.

Status Asthmaticus

Status asthmaticus is defined as a PEFR or FEV_1 that does not increase to greater than 40% of the predicted value with treatment, an increasing $Paco_2$ without improvement of indices of airflow obstruction, or the development of a major complication, such as pneumothorax, pneumomediastinum, acute myocardial ischemia (Chapter 57), or a cardiac tachyarrhythmia other than sinus tachycardia (Chapter 52). Patients who have status asthmaticus should be admitted to the hospital for close monitoring. Frequent treatments with inhaled β-agonists (0.5 mL of an albuterol 0.083% solution every 2 hours), intravenous aminophylline (at doses to yield maximal acceptable plasma levels, that is, 15 to 20 μg/mL; 500- to 1000-mg loading dose given during an hour followed by an infusion of 30 to 60 mg/hour), and high-dose intravenous steroids (methylprednisolone, 40 to 60 mg every 4 to 6 hours) are indicated. Oxygen should be administered by face mask or nasal cannula in amounts sufficient to achieve Spo_2 values between

TABLE 75-4 SELECTED COMBINED INHALED FDA-APPROVED INHALED MEDICATIONS FOR MAINTENANCE TREATMENT OF ASTHMA

GENERIC NAME	TRADE NAME*	DOSE/PUFF	DOSE AS PUFFS	COMMENTS
COMBINATION INHALERS THAT CAN BE USED AT ALL ASTHMA STEPS				
IGC = budesonide LABA = formoterol	Symbicort, Generic	Available only as MDIs. Each strength contains the same fixed dose of LABA with varying amounts of IGC. Exact amounts vary by inhaler type.	Start with one puff twice daily at the lowest dose of IGC that is effective for asthma control. Titrate up and down as symptom control requires. Max dose is 4 puffs of highest strength per day.	Dose adjustments for patients in renal or hepatic failure are not needed. When used as both regular maintenance and controller and reliever therapy, which is not FDA approved, the maximum dose is 12 puffs a day. This is the only LABA-IGC combination that can be used with this frequency.
IGC = budesonide SABA = albuterol	Airsupra	MDI containing 180 μg of albuterol and 160 μg of budesonide	FDA approved for use when asthma symptoms require treatment as 2 puffs per treatment; 6 treatments (12 puffs) is the maximum daily dose.	If available a formoterol/IGC combination is preferred. Dosing is not adjusted for renal or hepatic failure.
IGC = fluticasone propionate LABA = salmeterol	Advair Diskus, Advair HFA, AirDuo Digihaler, AirDuo RespiClick, Wixela Inhub, Generic	Available as MDIs or DPIs. Each type contains the same fixed dose of LABA with varying amounts of IGC. Exact amounts vary by inhaler type.	Start with one puff twice daily at the lowest dose of IGC that is effective for asthma control. Titrate up and down as symptom control requires. Max dose is 4 puffs of highest strength per day.	Dose adjustments for patients in renal failure not needed. In patients with hepatic failure, patients should be carefully monitored for steroid side effects and dose adjusted appropriately.
IGC = mometasone LABA = formoterol	Dulera	Available only as MDIs. Each strength contains a 5-μg dose of formoterol with 50, 100, or 200 μg doses of mometasone.	Start with one puff twice daily at the lowest dose of IGC that is effective for asthma control. Titrate up and down as symptom control requires. Max dose is 4 puffs of highest strength per day.	Dose adjustments for patients in renal or hepatic failure are not needed.
IGC = fluticasone furoate LABA = vilanterol	Breo Ellipta	All forms contain 25 μg of vilanterol with 100 (low strength) or 200 μg (high strength) of fluticasone furoate-once daily dosing.	Adjust IGC dose to achieve asthma control with a dose of 1 puff once/day.	Bronchodilator effect of vilanterol onsets in about 15 min. Maximum dose is 1 puff of high strength per day. Dose adjustments for patients in renal failure not needed. In patients with hepatic failure, patients should be carefully monitored for steroid side effects and dose adjusted appropriately.
TRIPLE COMBINATION INHALERS CONTAINING AN IGC, A LABA, AND A LONG-ACTING MUSCARINIC ANTAGONIST (LAMA)*				
IGC = fluticasone furoate LABA = vilanterol trifenatate LAMA = umeclidinium bromide	Trelegy Ellipta†	Products are DPIs. All inhalers contain per puff 62.5 μg of umeclidinium bromide and 25 μg of vilanterol trifenatate with either 100 or 200 μg of fluticasone furoate with once-daily dosing.	Adjust IGC dose to achieve asthma control with a dose of 1 puff once/day.	Bronchodilator effect of vilanterol onsets in about 15 min. Maximum dose is 1 puff of high strength per day. Dose adjustments for patients in renal failure not needed. In patients with hepatic failure, patients should be carefully monitored for steroid side effects and dose adjusted appropriately. Urinary retention may occur. Close monitoring for glaucoma and cataracts is warranted; use in patients with patients with narrow angle glaucoma may require ophthalmologic consultation.
IGC = budesonide LABA = formoterol fumarate LAMA = glycopyrrolate	Breztri Aerosphere‡	Product is an MDI containing a combination 160 μg of budesonide, 9 μg of glycopyrrolate and 4.8 μg of formoterol fumarate per inhalation.	Adjust dose to achieve asthma control using 1-2 puffs twice daily. Maximum dose is 2 puffs twice daily.	Dose adjustments for patients in renal or hepatic failure are not needed. Urinary retention may occur. Close monitoring for glaucoma and cataracts is warranted; use in patients with patients with narrow-angle glaucoma may require ophthalmologic consultation.

*Not all products marketing each medication are listed. Only products containing formoterol as the LABA should be used for rescue treatment.

†FDA approved for asthma.

‡Not FDA approved for asthma—thus use is off label. This is a scheduled maintenance treatment; acute symptoms should be treated with a SABA + IGC or LABA + formoterol at steps 1 and 2 and a SABA alone at steps 4 and 5.

DPI = dry powder inhaler; FDA = U.S. Food and Drug Administration; HFA = hydrofluoroalkane; IGC = inhaled glucocorticoid; LABA = long-acting β-agonist; LAMA = long-acting muscarinic antagonist; MDI = metered dose inhaler; SABA = short-acting β-agonist.

92% and 94%; a higher FIO_2 promotes absorption atelectasis and provides no therapeutic benefit. If objective evidence of an infection is present, appropriate treatment should be given for that infection. If no improvement is seen with treatment and if respiratory failure appears imminent, bronchodilator treatment should be intensified to the maximum tolerated by the patient as indicated by the maximum tolerated heart rate, usually 130 to 140 beats per minute. If indicated, intubation of the trachea and mechanical ventilation can be instituted; in this case, the goal should be to provide a level of ventilation just adequate to sustain life but *not sufficient to normalize arterial blood gases*. For example, a $PaCO_2$ of 60 to 70 mm Hg, or even higher, is acceptable for a patient in status asthmaticus.

Asthma in Pregnancy

Asthma may be exacerbated, remain unchanged, or remit during pregnancy (Chapter 221), and the ordinary management of asthma need not be changed during pregnancy.[18] The only potential difference is that one randomized trial suggests that, unlike in other settings, measurement of the fraction of exhaled nitric oxide can improve the management of asthma during pregnancy.

Good asthma control is beneficial to both the mother and the fetus, and key medications (inhaled glucocorticoids, β_2-agonists, montelukast, and theophylline) are not associated with an increased incidence of fetal abnormalities, but long-acting muscarinic antagonists should be avoided to prevent fetal tachycardia. Most importantly, no unnecessary medications should be administered; systemic steroids should be used sparingly to avert fetal complications, and certain drugs should be avoided: ipratropium bromide and tiotropium, which may cause fetal tachycardia; terbutaline, which is contraindicated during active labor because of its tocolytic effects; and tetracycline, which should not be used as a treatment of intercurrent infection. Biologic therapies for asthma have not been assigned a pregnancy risk category, so the risks and benefits of treatment should be weighed under expert care, and such agents should be used only if their benefit outweighs the risk to the fetus. Conversely, use of prostaglandin $F_{2\alpha}$ as an abortifacient should be avoided in asthmatic patients because of the potential for bronchoconstriction due to these agents.

PROGNOSIS

Asthma is a chronic relapsing disorder. Most patients have recurrent exacerbations without a major loss in lung function for many years. A minority of patients experience a significant irreversible loss in lung function over and above the normal pulmonary senescence. Risk factors for death from asthma include the need for emergent intensive care in the prior year, overuse of short-acting β-adrenergic agonists, poor adherence to medications, and comorbid conditions such as diabetes, cardiac arrhythmias, and psychiatric disease.

GENERAL REFERENCES

For the General References and other additional features, please visit Elsevier eBooks+ at https://ebooks.health.elsevier.com.

Grade A References

A1. Bateman ED, Reddel HK, O'Byrne PM, et al. As-needed budesonide-formoterol versus maintenance budesonide in mild asthma. *N Engl J Med*. 2018;378:1877-1887.

A2. Papi A, Chipps BE, Beasley R, et al. Albuterol-budesonide fixed-dose combination rescue inhaler for asthma. *N Engl J Med*. 2022;386:2071-2083.

A3. Israel E, Cardet JC, Carroll JK, et al. Reliever-triggered inhaled glucocorticoid in Black and Latinx adults with asthma. *N Engl J Med*. 2022;386:1505-1518.

A4. Kim LHY, Saleh C, Whalen-Browne A, et al. Triple vs dual inhaler therapy and asthma outcomes in moderate to severe asthma: a systematic review and meta-analysis. *JAMA*. 2021;325:2466-2479.

A5. Busse WW, Bateman ED, Caplan AL, et al. Combined analysis of asthma safety trials of long-acting β2-agonists. *N Engl J Med*. 2018;378:2497-2505.

A6. Lazarus SC, Krishnan JA, King TS, et al. Mometasone or tiotropium in mild asthma with a low sputum eosinophil level. *N Engl J Med*. 2019;380:2009-2019.

A7. Hong SH, Kang HR, Nam JH, et al. A comparison of leukotriene receptor antagonists to low-dose inhaled corticosteroids in the elderly with mild asthma. *J Allergy Clin Immunol Pract*. 2019;7:2642-2652.e3.

A8. Rowe BH, Kirkland SW, Vandermeer B, et al. Prioritizing systemic corticosteroid treatments to mitigate relapse in adults with acute asthma: a systematic review and network meta-analysis. *Acad Emerg Med*. 2017;24:371-381.

A9. Khatri S, Moore W, Gibson PG, et al. Assessment of the long-term safety of mepolizumab and durability of clinical response in patients with severe eosinophilic asthma. *J Allergy Clin Immunol*. 2019;143:1742-1751.

A10. Bernstein JA, Virchow JC, Murphy K, et al. Effect of fixed-dose subcutaneous reslizumab on asthma exacerbations in patients with severe uncontrolled asthma and corticosteroid sparing in patients with oral corticosteroid-dependent asthma: results from two phase 3, randomised, double-blind, placebo-controlled trials. *Lancet Respir Med*. 2020;8:461-474.

A11. Nair P, Wenzel S, Rabe KF, et al. Oral glucocorticoid-sparing effect of benralizumab in severe asthma. *N Engl J Med*. 2017;376:2448-2458.

A12. Rabe KF, Nair P, Brusselle G, et al. Efficacy and safety of dupilumab in glucocorticoid-dependent severe asthma. *N Engl J Med*. 2018;378:2475-2485.

A13. Menzies-Gow A, Corren J, Bourdin A, et al. Tezepelumab in adults and adolescents with severe, uncontrolled asthma. *N Engl J Med*. 2021;384:1800-1809.

A14. Undela K, Goldsmith L, Kew KM, et al. Macrolides versus placebo for chronic asthma. *Cochrane Database Syst Rev*. 2021;11:CD002997.

A15. Crossingham I, Turner S, Ramakrishnan S, et al. Combination fixed-dose β agonist and steroid inhaler as required for adults or children with mild asthma: a Cochrane systematic review. *BMJ Evid Based Med*. 2021;5:CD013518.

A16. Hardy J, Baggott C, Fingleton J, et al. Budesonide-formoterol reliever therapy versus maintenance budesonide plus terbutaline reliever therapy in adults with mild to moderate asthma (PRACTICAL): a 52-week, open-label, multicentre, superiority, randomised controlled trial. *Lancet*. 2019;394:919-928.

A17. O'Byrne PM, FitzGerald JM, Bateman ED, et al. Inhaled combined budesonide-formoterol as needed in mild asthma. *N Engl J Med*. 2018;378:1865-1876.

A18. Beasley RW, Holliday M, Reddel HK. Controlled trial of as-needed budesonide/formoterol in mild adult asthma. *N Engl J Med*. 2019;380:2020-2030.

A19. McKeever T, Mortimer K, Wilson A, et al. Quadrupling inhaled glucocorticoid dose to abort asthma exacerbations. *N Engl J Med*. 2018;378:902-910.

A20. Hayashi H, Fukutomi Y, Mitsui C, et al. Omalizumab for aspirin hypersensitivity and leukotriene overproduction in aspirin-exacerbated respiratory disease. A randomized controlled trial. *Am J Respir Crit Care Med*. 2020;201:1488-1498.

A21. Agarwal R, Dhooria S, Sehgal IS, et al. A randomised trial of voriconazole and prednisolone monotherapy in acute-stage allergic bronchopulmonary aspergillosis complicating asthma. *Eur Respir J*. 2018;52:1801159.

A22. Kearns N, Maijers I, Harper J, et al. Inhaled corticosteroids in acute asthma: a systemic review and meta-analysis. *J Allergy Clin Immunol Pract*. 2020;8:605-617.

76

CHRONIC OBSTRUCTIVE PULMONARY DISEASE

JOHN REILLY

DEFINITION

Chronic obstructive pulmonary disease (COPD) is an umbrella term for a number of conditions that result in fixed airway obstruction and dyspnea on exertion. COPD is characterized by persistent respiratory symptoms and airflow limitation that is due to airway or alveolar abnormalities usually caused by significant exposure to noxious particles or gases. Nearly all patients have both the air space destruction associated with emphysema as well as the pathologic airway changes that are consistent with chronic bronchitis. However, subsets of the COPD population can differ in terms of natural history and response to therapeutic intervention. Daily cough and sputum for 3 months for 2 or more years is the qualifying definition for chronic bronchitis.

Airflow limitation is defined as a ratio of forced expiratory volume in 1 second (FEV_1) and the forced vital capacity (FVC) of less than 0.7 ($FEV_1/FVC < 0.7$) (Chapter 73). Classification systems can also incorporate other characteristics that are independent predictors of symptoms and mortality (Fig. 76-1).

EPIDEMIOLOGY

COPD is a disease of adults, typically presenting in the sixth decade of life or later, with an estimated global prevalence of 175 million. The estimated annual 3.2 million deaths from COPD make it the third leading cause of death worldwide.[1] Given the lag time between the initiation of smoking and the development of clinical disease, the global prevalence of cigarette smoking and the aging of the population imply that the number of cases will continue to increase. In the United States, the costs associated with COPD are estimated to be about $50 billion annually: $30 billion in direct medical costs and $20 billion in indirect costs.

Epidemiologic data support the concept that habitual cigarette smoking is the major risk factor for the development of COPD.[2] At the population level, the smoking "dose," as measured in pack-years (the product of the number of packs of cigarettes smoked per day and the number of years with the habit at this intensity), is inversely related to FEV_1. Factors that impair full lung growth, including childhood respiratory infections, result in lower peak lung function in adulthood; subsequent decline, whether accelerated or not, can result in the development of COPD (E-Fig. 76-1). Cigarette smoking is by far the major contributor to the development of COPD, but other implicated exposures include combustion of biomass fuels, especially in poorly ventilated spaces where such materials are used for cooking food and heating.[3] The role of environmental air pollution is less clear. Cough, sputum, and permanent loss of lung function may also occur among individuals who are exposed to workplace dust in mines, grain-handling facilities, and cotton mills. Although data show that increased pollution levels are temporally associated with increased mortality in patients with established COPD, it is less clear whether air pollution alone

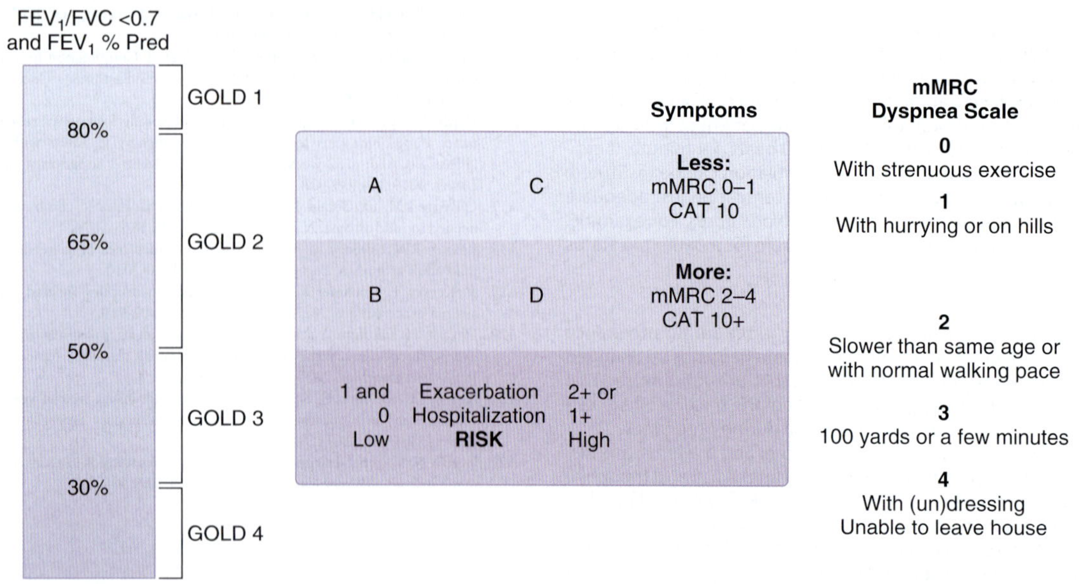

FIGURE 76-1. **GOLD Classification System for COPD. In addition to airflow obstruction, as defined by an FEV_1/FVC ratio of less than 0.7 and quantified by the FEV_1 as a percent of the predicted value *(box on the left)*, it incorporates symptoms and risk of exacerbation to create four categories: GOLD 1, GOLD 2, GOLD 3, and GOLD 4. These in turn are used to recommend therapy and estimate prognosis. CAT = COPD Assessment Test (scores range from 0-40, with higher numbers more severe dyspnea); FEV_1 = forced expiratory volume in 1 second; FVC, forced vital capacity; mMRC = modified Medical Research Council Dyspnea Score (scores range 0-4, with higher numbers more severe dyspnea); Pred = predicted.**

is a substantial risk factor for the disease. Whether prior respiratory infections produce residual effects on adult lung function is unclear.

PATHOBIOLOGY

Pathology

The pathology of COPD includes parenchymal destruction characteristic of emphysema as well as inflammation and fibrosis in the small airways. The relative contributions of these distinct components vary from individual to individual. The parenchymal destruction, which is characterized by a loss of alveolar walls and their associated capillary beds, can be demonstrated by a reduction in the diffusing capacity for carbon monoxide (DLCO) on pulmonary function testing (Chapter 73) and by areas of reduced tissue density on computed tomographic (CT) scanning of the lung.

Pathogenesis

Data suggest important roles for the airways, the lung parenchyma, and the pulmonary vasculature in patients with COPD. The relative importance of these mechanisms varies among patients and contributes to the heterogeneity of disease presentation and response to therapy.[4]

The most widely accepted paradigm for the development of emphysema is the protease-antiprotease theory. This theory postulates that emphysema develops when elastolytic protease activity is in excess compared with antiprotease levels. The prototype for this theory is that individuals deficient in α_1-antiprotease are at higher risk for developing emphysema. α_1-Antiprotease is a member of the serpin (serine protease inhibitor) superfamily and is the major inhibitor of neutrophil elastase. Proteases that degrade elastin can produce emphysema. In addition to neutrophil elastase, macrophage elastases can produce emphysema. Cigarette smoking induces an influx of inflammatory cells into the lung, including neutrophils and macrophages. Quantitatively, macrophages are the largest component of this response. Experimental data also support the hypotheses that vascular mechanisms and apoptosis may contribute to the development of emphysema.

Small airway inflammation with the presence of pigmented macrophages is a consistent finding in cigarette smokers. CD8+ lymphocytes and neutrophils also are important components of the inflammatory response. In COPD, in contrast to many patients with asthma, eosinophils are a relatively small component of the inflammatory response, but a subpopulation of patients with COPD manifest sputum and peripheral eosinophilia. The signaling that promotes this inflammatory response may involve oxidative stress and the production of reactive oxygen species. However, attempts to block various inflammatory pathways with monoclonal antibodies have generally been disappointing.

In patients with COPD, the inflammatory response in the lung persists after smoking cessation. This observation, coupled with documented changes in the microbiome and the demonstration of autoimmunity in subjects with COPD, provides a potential mechanism for the clinical observation of the continued progression of disease despite smoking cessation.

In patients with emphysema, cigarette smoking induces intimal thickening and smooth muscle proliferation in the endothelium of the pulmonary vasculature, with decreased expression of vascular endothelial growth factor (VEGF) and apoptosis of endothelial cells in septal vessels. Manipulating VEGF expression in animal models can produce emphysema, thereby suggesting that pulmonary vascular changes may be a primary driving event in some patients with COPD. Data also suggest that inhibiting the expression of transforming growth factor-beta by blocking the angiotensin pathway may slow the loss of lung tissue that is characteristic of emphysema.[5] In addition, chronic hypoxemia produces pulmonary vascular constriction that leads to the development of pulmonary hypertension (Chapter 69). Hypertrophied bronchial mucous glands, an expanded epithelial goblet cell population, and increased airway mucin concentration all correlate with symptoms of cough and excess sputum production in chronic bronchitis but do not correlate with airflow obstruction.

Pathophysiology

By definition, COPD is characterized by obstruction of expiratory airflow. The anatomic site of this flow limitation is in the small airways (<2 mm). Obstruction may result from a variety of mechanisms: airway smooth muscle constriction; small airway inflammation, wall thickening, and scarring; loss of small airways owing to parenchymal destruction; and dynamic airway collapse owing to the loss of parenchymal tethering secondary to the parenchymal destruction that is characteristic of emphysema. A concomitant alteration may be a decreased driving force owing to loss of elastic recoil in the setting of parenchymal destruction. This airflow obstruction results in a prolonged expiratory time, which can be measured as lower flow rates over time on a spirogram and which produces a characteristic "coving" of the expiratory portion of the flow volume loop. When the expiratory time is shortened owing to an increased respiratory rate, the previous tidal volume is incompletely exhaled prior to the initiation of the next inspiration. This phenomenon, termed dynamic hyperinflation, results in an increase in end-expiratory lung volume to a level at which expiratory flow rates increase enough to achieve complete exhalation of the prior tidal volume. The increase in end-expiratory lung volume can produce a sensation of dyspnea independent of hypoxemia.

In its pure form, emphysema results in dynamic expiratory airway collapse owing to a loss of tethering, a loss of small airways because of parenchymal destruction, and a loss of alveolar gas exchange surface. Chronic bronchitis, in contrast, is characterized by airway inflammation, increased airway reactivity with resultant dynamic airway smooth muscle constriction, mucous gland hypertrophy, and hypersecretion. The result of this is airflow obstruction and a chronic productive cough with sputum. Clinical observation, pathologic studies, physiologic measurements, and imaging studies have shown neither of these entities typically exist in isolation; almost all patients with COPD have elements of both emphysema and chronic bronchitis, although the relative contributions of each process vary from patient to patient.

Genetics

The most common monogenic trait associated with COPD is α_1-antitrypsin deficiency.[6] α_1-Antitrypsin is encoded by the *SERPINA1* gene; the gene product is a serine protease inhibitor synthesized and secreted by the liver. The most common mutations associated with deficiency result in polymerization of α_1-antitrypsin in the liver and the inability to secrete a functional protein product. Circulating levels of α_1-antitrypsin are decreased to about 15% of normal, a level that is associated with an increased incidence of emphysema and bronchiectasis (Chapter 78), as well as liver disease (Chapter 132) in some individuals. Very uncommon in non-White populations, the allele frequency of mutations in the White population is as high as 4 to 5%. Because fewer patients are diagnosed with COPD and α_1-antitrypsin deficiency than would be expected based on mathematical calculations, other factors, especially cigarette smoking,[7] presumably influence whether clinically significant organ damage results from these mutations. Whether patients who are heterozygous for a mutant allele are at increased risk for lung disease is controversial.

Several other genetic syndromes include emphysema or airflow obstruction. Among these genes are cutis laxa (*ATP7A*, *elastin*, *fibulin 4*, and *fibulin 5*), Ehlers-Danlos syndrome (Chapter 239; collagen type 3 α_1), and Marfan syndrome (Chapter 239; fibrillin 1).

The observations that COPD clusters in families and that many smokers do not develop COPD have led to the hypothesis that genetic factors explain the differential response to cigarette smoke. A number of genes have been implicated, including *MMP-12*, *Serpin E2*, and the interleukin-33 pathway, which is also implicated in asthma, but such findings have been inconsistent. Ongoing longitudinal studies may potentially provide more evidence concerning genetic contributions to COPD.[8]

CLINICAL MANIFESTATIONS

The hallmark symptom of COPD is breathlessness with exertion. Because maximal exertion typically is not limited by ventilatory capacity, individuals can develop significant COPD before becoming symptomatic. The gradual progression of disease, coupled with the fact that other factors such as cardiac disease, obesity, and deconditioning can also result in dyspnea on exertion, often results in patients being symptomatic for months to years before the diagnosis of COPD is made.[9]

In many instances, the diagnosis of COPD is made when a patient presents with an exacerbation manifested by increased dyspnea, increased cough, and an increase or change in character of sputum production; it may or may not be accompanied by fever and constitutional symptoms suggestive of infection. The development of these symptoms may prompt the patient to seek medical evaluation, at which time the history may reveal exposure(s) that increase the risk of COPD (typically chronic cigarette smoking) and antecedent dyspnea on exertion. In a subset of patients, an important component of the natural history of COPD is recurrent exacerbations.

By definition, COPD with chronic bronchitis includes chronic cough and sputum. Hemoptysis may occur in patients with chronic bronchitis, particularly in the context of an exacerbation. Clubbing (Fig. 39-9) is not a manifestation in COPD, and its presence should prompt an evaluation for other conditions, notably lung cancer (Chapter 177) or pulmonary fibrosis (Chapter 80).

Patients with more advanced disease may develop hypoxemia or hypercarbia. Hypoxemia, which is usually documented by pulse oximetry, can produce cyanosis. Hypercarbia, which may be suggested by an elevated serum bicarbonate level, requires an arterial blood gas measurement for confirmation.

COPD also can have systemic manifestations, including arrhythmias such as atrial fibrillation.[10] Patients with emphysema lose body mass and may develop sarcopenia. Pulmonary hypertension (Chapter 69) may develop and be associated with a significant limitation in exercise. Depression (Chapter 362) is a frequent comorbidity with COPD.

DIAGNOSIS

History and Physical Examination

Elements of the history relevant to establishing the diagnosis include a history of cigarette smoking, other inhalational or environmental exposures, a childhood history of recurrent lung infections or premature birth, cough (chronicity, frequency), and sputum production. Particular emphasis should be placed on the degree to which limitations are caused by dyspnea because patients may gradually restrict activity over time to avoid the uncomfortable sensation of being out of breath and may not report dyspnea during their daily activities. Patients should be asked about any family history of lung disease and about the presence of comorbid conditions.

The physical findings seen in COPD include whether or not the patients have evidence of cyanosis, use of pursed lip breathing, use of accessory muscles of respiration, or other signs of respiratory distress. The chronic hyperinflation associated with COPD may result in a large anteroposterior thoracic dimension (barrel chest), use of the arms to fix the shoulder girdle to allow the use of accessory muscles of respiration (tripod position, history of less dyspnea when pushing a cart than when walking), and, in advanced cases, retraction of the lower rib cage with inspiration owing to the altered biomechanics of flattened diaphragms (Hoover sign). The presence of paradoxical abdominal wall motion with inspiration suggests respiratory muscle fatigue. Percussion of the chest may reveal increased resonance. Auscultation may reveal decreased breath sounds in patients who primarily have emphysema; asymmetry raises the possibility of a pneumothorax. Patients with airway disease may exhibit rhonchi with inspiration and wheezing with forced exhalation.

Cardiac findings related to COPD mainly relate to chest wall geometry and right heart function. Heart sounds may be diminished owing to increased retrosternal airspace. Elevated jugular venous pressure (Fig. 39-2), an accentuated pulmonic valve closure sound (P2), a right ventricular heave, hepatic congestion, and peripheral edema all raise the possibility of pulmonary hypertension (cor pulmonale; Chapter 69). Given that cigarette smoking is also a risk factor for lung cancer and that patients with COPD have about a twofold increased risk of lung cancer compared with smokers without COPD, hemoptysis should prompt an evaluation to determine whether the patient has lung cancer. Patients whose COPD is manifested primarily as emphysema may develop weight loss and sarcopenia, evident on physical examination.

Diagnostic Testing

Spirometry demonstrating airflow obstruction (Fig. 76-2) establishes the diagnosis (Chapter 73). The hallmark of obstruction on spirometry is a reduction in the FEV_1/FVC ratio to less than 0.7, with lower ratios commonly expressed as a percent of predicted calculated from reference data gathered for a normal population (standardized by age, sex, height, and ethnic background), indicating greater severity (Table 76-1). Lung volumes may demonstrate an elevated residual volume (RV) and total lung capacity (TLC). In patients with emphysema or pulmonary hypertension, the DLCO may be reduced, consistent with the degree of loss of pulmonary capillary vessels participating in gas exchange.

All adults with COPD or bronchiectasis should be tested for alpha-1 antitrypsin deficiency, although the patients most at risk have a family history of COPD, lower lobe predominant emphysema, or presentation at a relatively young age. The evidence for screening family members of patients with α_1-antitrypsin is not as strong, although the case can be made that such screening

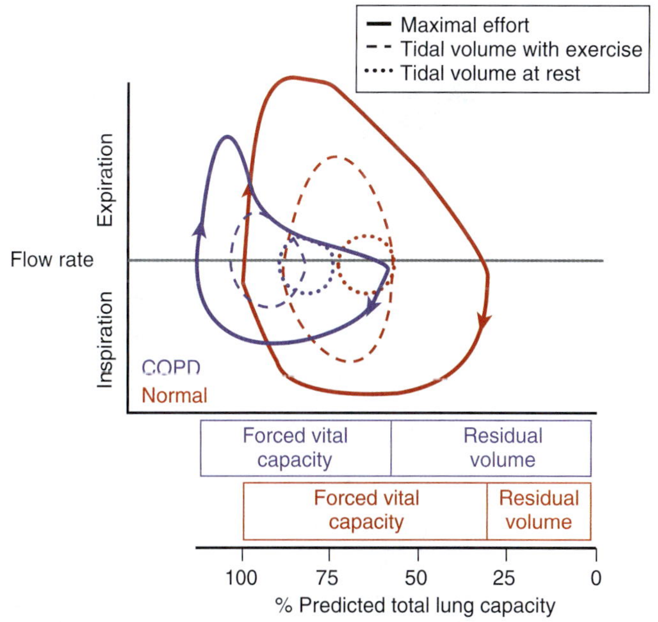

FIGURE 76-2. Representative flow-volume loops in normal subjects *(red)* and COPD *(blue)*. Flow-volume tracings are shown at rest, with exercise (*dashed lines*), and with maximal effort. The normal tracings demonstrate that the metabolic demands generated by exercise can be met with increased tidal volumes and frequency without reaching flow limitation and that lung volumes do not change. In contrast, the patient with COPD has flow limitation during tidal breathing. Increasing tidal volumes and frequency limit expiratory time, and the flow limitation results in a failure to reach resting end-expiratory lung volume. The resulting increases in lung volumes, termed dynamic hyperinflation, are associated with an increased work of breathing and, hence, dyspnea. COPD = chronic obstructive pulmonary disease.

allows for an intensified focus on avoiding inhalational exposures, including smoking, and careful observation for the development of early signs of disease so that replacement therapy can be considered.

In patients for whom pharmacotherapy is being considered, a peripheral blood eosinophil count may help guide decisions regarding inhaled glucocorticoids.

Imaging

Chest radiographs may demonstrate hyperinflation as evidenced by a flattened diaphragmatic silhouette, increased retrosternal air space on the lateral image, decreased parenchymal markings, and bullae in patients with emphysema (Fig. 76-3). In patients with a suspected COPD exacerbation, the chest radiograph may show an infiltrate suggestive of pneumonia (Chapter 85).

Chest CT (Fig. 76-4) provides a more detailed assessment of parenchymal characteristics and is more sensitive than plain chest radiographs for demonstrating parenchymal loss consistent with emphysema, bullae, and pulmonary vascular changes suggestive of pulmonary hypertension. It is now the tool of choice for screening for lung cancer (Chapter 177) in an at-risk population that includes most patients with COPD and a significant smoking history. Although CT scanning provides information about the presence and extent of emphysema and airway abnormalities, most available therapeutic options are prescribed regardless of the relative contributions of emphysema and chronic bronchitis. Hence, CT scanning has little role in guiding therapy in COPD, with the exception of instances in which surgical intervention (discussed later) or replacement therapy for alpha-1 antitrypsin deficiency is being considered.

TABLE 76-1 SEVERITY OF AIRFLOW OBSTRUCTION IN COPD ACCORDING TO POSTBRONCHODILATOR SPIROMETRY

STAGE AND SEVERITY	DEFINITION
I: Mild	$FEV_1/FVC < 0.70$, $FEV_1 \geq 80\%$ of predicted
II: Moderate	$FEV_1/FVC < 0.70$, $50\% \leq FEV_1 < 80\%$ of predicted
III: Severe	$FEV_1/FVC < 0.70$, $30\% \leq FEV_1 < 50\%$ of predicted
IV: Very severe	$FEV_1/FVC < 0.70$, $FEV_1 < 30\%$ of predicted or $FEV_1 < 50\%$ of predicted plus chronic respiratory failure

COPD = chronic obstructive pulmonary disease; FEV_1 = forced expiratory volume in the first second; FVC = forced vital capacity.

MRI has little clinical role in the assessment of COPD because the presence of air adversely impacts the ability to generate detailed images of lung parenchyma. Echocardiography can noninvasively quantify pulmonary artery pressures by assessing the velocity of any tricuspid regurgitant jet (Chapter 43), but imaging may be compromised by retrosternal hyperinflation between the ultrasound probe and the heart. Transthoracic ultrasound is primarily used to assess for the presence of pleural effusion (Chapter 86) and to guide thoracentesis.

Arterial Blood Gases and Oximetry

Hypoxemia can be assessed by oximetry or arterial blood gases, whereas the diagnosis of hypercarbia requires an arterial blood gas sample. Chronic hypercarbia is typically accompanied by a respiratory acidosis with a compensatory elevation in the serum pH and the serum bicarbonate level that incompletely corrects the acidemia (Chapter 89).

Differential Diagnosis

The differentiation of COPD from asthma (Chapter 75) has become less important as the treatments for the two conditions have become more similar. Clinical manifestations suggestive of asthma rather than COPD include the onset of symptoms at a young age, atopy, no history of smoking, varying symptoms over time, and airflow obstruction that is largely reversible. However, elderly people can develop new-onset asthma, some patients with asthma smoke, many asthmatics do not have a history of atopy, and long-standing, severe asthma may result in some degree of fixed airflow obstruction. Furthermore, many COPD patients have asthma-like features.[11]

In bronchiectasis (Chapter 78), which is characterized by chronic inflammation and results in abnormal airway dilation, clinical manifestations are dominated by cough and purulent sputum. Bronchiectasis can be distinguished from COPD by high-resolution chest CT imaging that demonstrates abnormally widened and thickened airways that have irregular walls and do not taper in the periphery of the lung.[12]

In bronchiolitis obliterans, cicatricial narrowing of distal airways is associated with severe and irreversible airflow obstruction. Bronchiolitis obliterans can develop in patients with collagen vascular diseases (Chapters 243 and 245), and it is common after lung transplantation (Chapter 87). A similar disorder can be caused by industrial inhalants, such as diacetyl, which is a butter-like flavoring used with microwavable popcorn (Chapter 81). In nonsmokers, bronchiolitis obliterans can be reliably diagnosed based on a careful history and the presence of irreversible airflow obstruction in the absence of emphysema or other explanations on a chest CT. In smokers, however, the diagnosis is more difficult to make because exposure to diacetyl produces abnormalities similar to those caused by cigarette smoke.

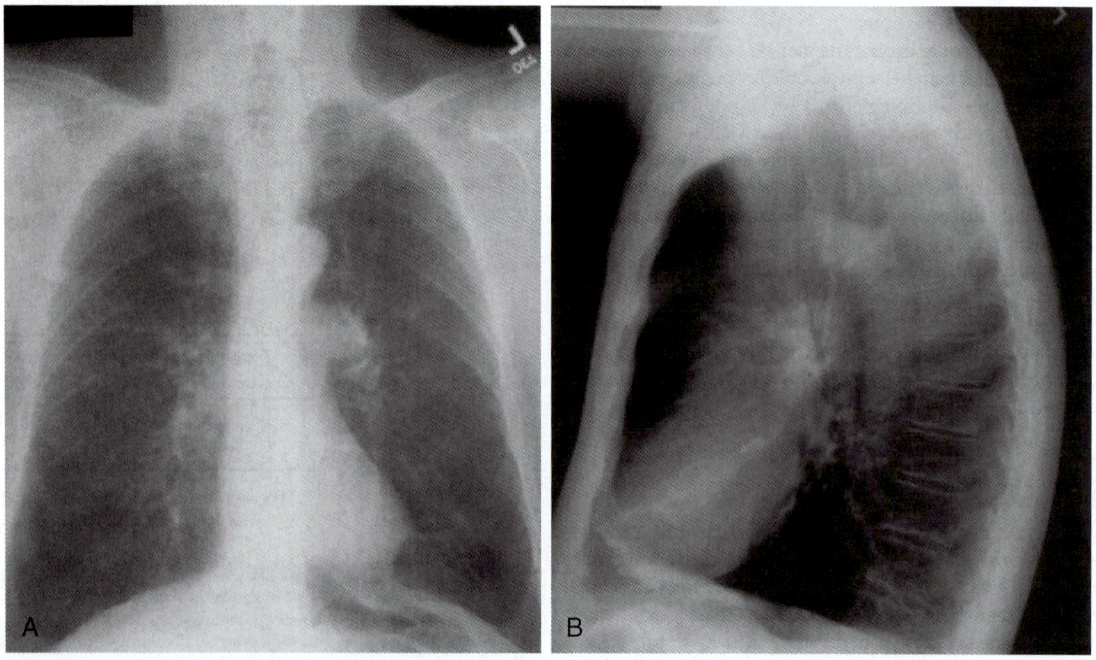

FIGURE 76-3. Posteroanterior (A) and lateral (B) radiographs of the thorax in a patient with emphysema. The most obvious abnormalities are those associated with increased lung volume. The lungs appear dark because of their increased air relative to tissue. The diaphragms are caudal to their normal position and appear flatter than normal. The heart is oriented more vertically than normal because of caudal displacement of the diaphragm, and the transverse diameter of the rib cage is increased; as a result, the width of the heart relative to the rib cage on the posteroanterior view is decreased. The space between the sternum and heart and great vessels is increased on the lateral view.

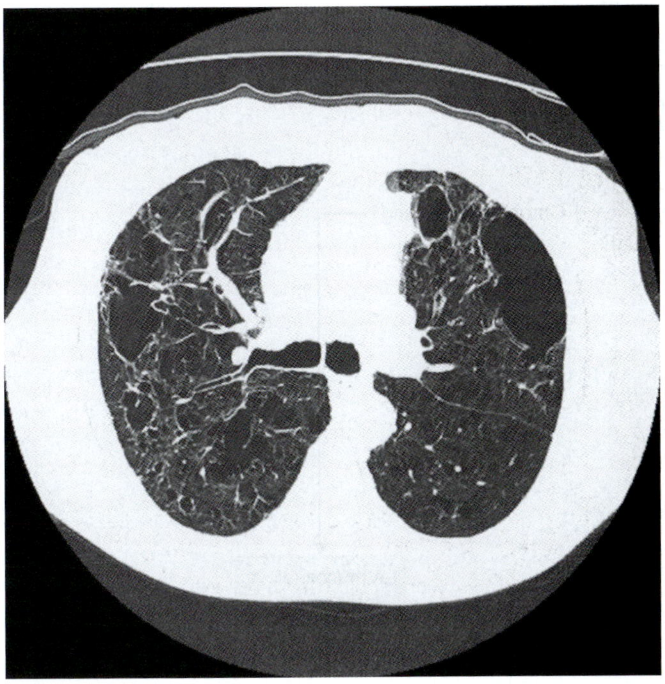

FIGURE 76-4. Computed tomographic (CT) scan demonstrating emphysema. High-resolution CT scan of the thorax at the level of the tracheal carina in a patient with emphysema. The left lung is seen on the right. There are multiple areas of confluent parenchymal loss (bullae) that appear as black areas with no parenchymal markings. There are additional small areas of parenchymal loss consistent with emphysema. The right upper lobe bronchus is seen entering the lung; its walls are thickened, thereby suggesting chronic inflammation. (Courtesy Bruce Maycher, MD.)

TREATMENT

No intervention other than lung transplantation can reverse or cure COPD, so treatment focuses on modifying its natural history, improving symptoms, minimizing complications, and reducing mortality.[13,14]

Modifying the Natural History of COPD

Smoking cessation reduces the rate of decline in FEV_1 and overall long-term mortality, including mortality attributable to lung cancer and cardiovascular disease. By comparison, pharmacotherapy has not been conclusively demonstrated to alter the rate of decline of FEV_1. An inhaled anticholinergic, ipratropium bromide, can provide a small initial increase in FEV_1, but it does not impact the subsequent rate of decline. Inhaled tiotropium, another anticholinergic agent, can modestly reduce the rate of decline in post-bronchodilator FEV_1 when used regularly in patients with early-stage COPD.[A1] Multiple other studies of inhaled β-agonists, anticholinergic agents, and glucocorticoids have not consistently demonstrated an impact on the rate of decline in FEV_1. Based on these disappointing results, the United States Preventative Services Task Force has reinforced their recommendation against screening of asymptomatic individuals for COPD because of the lack of data to support a substantial beneficial effect of intervention in such individuals.[15] Nevertheless, emerging data suggest that aggressive combination therapy can prolong survival in well-established disease (see Combined Treatment).

Oxygen Therapy

For patients with serious resting hypoxemia, defined as an arterial oxygen saturation less than 88% or a PaO_2 less than 56 mm, continuous supplemental oxygen for 24 hours/day can significantly reduce mortality. In patients with persistent stable hypercapnia, home high-flow nasal cannula oxygen[A2] or adding noninvasive ventilation to oxygen therapy can reduce future hospital admissions and delay death.[A3,16] The oxygen flow rate should be titrated in 1-L/minute increments every 15-minute interval to provide a resting oxygen saturation that is consistently above 90%. Long-term oxygen may decrease polycythemia and pulmonary hypertension, and it also can improve neuropsychiatric function.

For patients with COPD and moderate resting hypoxemia (SaO_2 88 to 93%) accompanied by exertional desaturation or nocturnal desaturation that does not fall below an SaO_2 of 80%, however, oxygen supplementation does not alter the time to first hospitalization or mortality.[A4] In patients who are normoxemic or minimally hypoxemic at rest while breathing ambient air but develop oxygen desaturation with exercise, ambulatory oxygen can modestly improve dyspnea, lactic acidosis with exercise, and dynamic hyperinflation, but activities of daily living are rarely improved,[A5] so these benefits do not routinely justify the expense and inconvenience of chronic supplemental oxygen therapy.[17]

Improving Symptoms

Interventions directed at improving COPD symptoms include pharmacotherapy, rehabilitation, and surgery.

Pharmacotherapy

For chronic symptoms, the mainstay of therapy is inhaled medications (Fig. 76-5), which fall into three classes: β-agonists, muscarinic antagonists, and glucocorticoids (Table 76-2). Within each of these three classes, medications differ primarily by their pharmacokinetics and dosing intervals.

Each class of long-acting bronchodilators is about 15 to 20% more effective than placebo for reducing exacerbations, and only about six patients need to be treated to prevent one exacerbation per year. The adverse events of long-acting bronchodilators are generally minor in patients with COPD.

Inhaled β-agonists

Although COPD is defined by airflow obstruction that is not completely reversible, many patients have a measurable increase in expiratory flow rates in response to inhaled β-agonists. *Short-acting β-agonists* have a rapid onset of action and a duration of action of 4 to 6 hours. The most commonly prescribed is albuterol (salbutamol), which produces modest increases in FEV_1 and reduces symptoms in patients with moderate to severe COPD. Side effects include tachycardia and tremor. These agents require frequent dosing, so they are typically used to relieve acute symptoms and to treat exacerbations.

Long-acting β-agonists, including salmeterol and formoterol, have a duration of action of about 12 hours, whereas indacaterol has a 24-hour duration of action. These agents modestly increase FEV_1 and improve quality of life, with indacaterol perhaps having the largest improvement on quality of life. These agents also reduce the frequency of exacerbations by about 20%, although this benefit may be muted in patients who are also taking inhaled glucocorticoids. These agents can cause tachycardia and tremor. Whether they may increase the risk of cardiovascular events in patients with COPD remains unresolved.[18]

Muscarinic Antagonists

Muscarinic antagonists, which are used in the same way as β-agonists in patients with COPD, produce modest improvements in FEV_1 and significant improvements in health-related quality of life and also reduce the risk of exacerbations. The primary short-acting muscarinic antagonist is ipratropium bromide, which can be used both acutely and chronically in symptomatic patients with COPD. However, its chronic use has largely been supplanted by the long-acting muscarinic antagonists, which have a more convenient dosing schedule. Muscarinic antagonists are useful in patients with chronic symptoms and/or a history of recurrent exacerbations. These agents are generally well tolerated, with the most common side effects being related to anticholinergic activity: dry mouth, urinary retention, and constipation, without any significant increase in cardiac risk.

Inhaled Glucocorticoids

Inhaled glucocorticoids reduce COPD exacerbations and the rate of decline in quality of life. However, they do not reliably improve measured lung function, reduce the rate of decline in FEV_1, or decrease mortality. They are best prescribed in addition to a long-acting adrenergic agonist or muscarinic antagonist rather than as the sole treatment for COPD (see Table 76-2). Inhaled corticosteroids produce marginal improvements in lung function and respiratory health status in COPD patients, and they reduce COPD exacerbation rates by about 15 to 20% in relative terms.[19] Retrospective analyses of interventional studies suggest that the benefit of inhaled corticosteroids for reducing exacerbations is higher when the peripheral blood eosinophil count is ≥300 cells/μL.

Side effects are oropharyngeal candidiasis and dysphonia, as well as an apparent increase in the risk of pneumonia. Therefore, the decision to use inhaled corticosteroids in COPD should weigh the anticipated benefit against the small but significant risk of side effects.

Combined Treatment

Inhaled corticosteroids combined with an inhaled long-acting β_2-agonist (e.g., vilanterol, formoterol, fumarate, or indacaterol) safely provide incremental benefit compared with either monotherapy.[A6] The combination of a long-acting β_2-adrenergic agonist inhaler plus a long-acting anticholinergic inhaler or the combination of a once-daily inhaled glycopyrronium (a long-acting antimuscarinic agent at 50 μg) plus long-acting indacaterol (110 μg) is also more effective than single-agent treatment.[A7] Furthermore, once- or twice-daily triple therapy, which combines a long-acting muscarinic antagonist with a long-acting β-agonist and a corticosteroid (e.g., adding umeclidinium [62.5 μg] to vilanterol [25 μg] plus fluticasone furoate [100 μg] or adding glycopyrrolate [18 μg] to formoterol [9.6 μg] plus budesonide [160 or 320 μg]) is even more effective for preventing COPD exacerbations and hospitalizations than double therapy[A8–A10] and can reduce all-cause mortality.[A11,A12]

Phosphodiesterase 4 (PDE4) Inhibitors

Roflumilast and cilomilast are oral phosphodiesterase-4 inhibitors that reduce COPD exacerbations and result in modest improvements in lung function and quality of life, with benefits similar to those seen with inhaled corticosteroids. Oral roflumilast (500 μg once daily) can increase FEV_1 by about 50 mL and can reduce both exacerbations and hospital admissions in patients who have severe COPD and who have had severe or frequent exacerbations despite using inhaled corticosteroids and long-acting β_2-agonists, even in combination with tiotropium.[A13] However, these agents generally have more side effects than inhaled corticosteroids, including nausea,

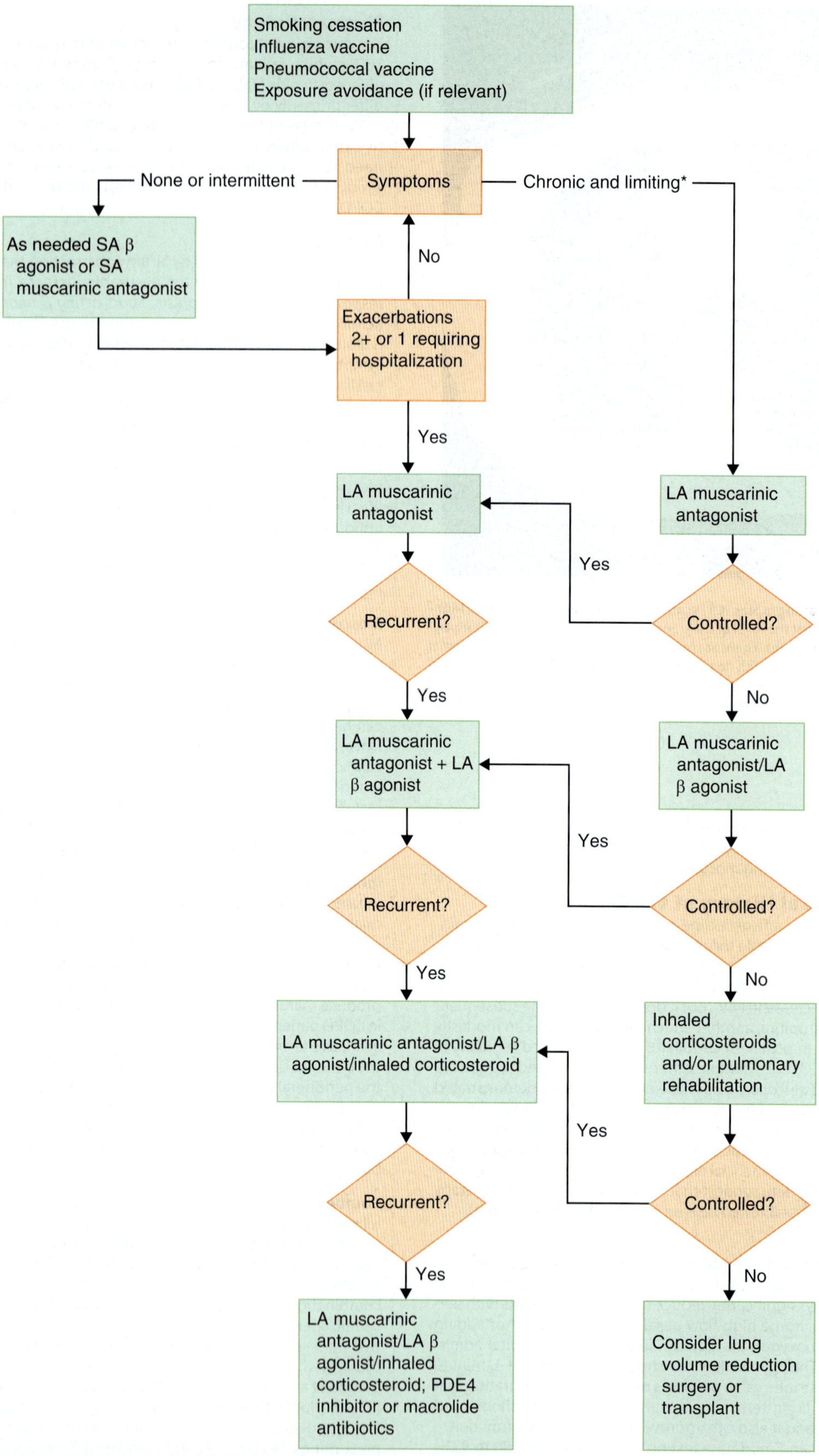

FIGURE 76-5. **Approach to the patient with chronic obstructive pulmonary disease.** *Dyspnea causes the patient to walk slower than patients of the same age or to stop to catch their breath when walking at their own pace; patient stops for breath after walking 100 yards or less or after a few minutes; or patient is breathless when dressing or housebound due to dyspnea. COPD = chronic obstructive pulmonary disease; LA = long acting; PDE = phosphodiesterase; SA = short acting.

TABLE 76-2 MEDICATIONS FOR CHRONIC OBSTRUCTIVE PULMONARY DISEASE

DRUG(S)	FREQUENCY/FORMULATION	DOSAGE	SIDE EFFECTS OF EACH CLASS OF DRUGS
β-AGONISTS			
Salmeterol	bid/DPI	50 μg	Palpitations, hypokalemia
Formoterol	bid/nebulizer	20 μg	
Indacaterol	qd/DPI	75 μg	
Olodaterol	qd/MDI	5 μg (2.5 μg/puff)	
MUSCARINIC ANTAGONISTS			
Aclidinium bromide	bid/DPI	400 μg	Dry mouth, constipation, aggravation of narrow angle glaucoma
Tiotropium bromide	qd/MDI or DPI	5 μg (MDI), 18 μg (DPI)	
Glycopyrronium	bid/DPI	15.6 μg	
Umeclidinium	qd/DPI	62.5 μg	
Ipratropium bromide	qid/MDI	34 μg (17 μg/puff)	
INHALED CORTICOSTEROIDS			
Fluticasone	bid/DPI	88-500 μg	Oropharyngeal candidiasis and hoarseness, and risk of pneumonia
Budesonide	bid or qd/nebulizer	360-1600 μg daily total	
Beclomethasone	bid/MDI	40-320 μg bid	
Mometasone	qd/DPI bid/MDI	220-440 μg 200-800 μg	
Flunisolide	bid/MDI	160-320 μg bid	
PHOSPHODIESTERASE-4 INHIBITORS			
Roflumilast	qd/pill	500 μg	Diarrhea, nausea, and weight loss
COMBINATION INHALERS			
*Combination Long-acting β-Agonist/Long-acting Muscarinic Antagonist**			
Formoterol/glycopyrrolate	bid/MDI	9.6 μg formoterol/18 μg glycopyrrolate	Side effects of each constituent
Indacaterol/glycopyrrolate	bid/DPI	27.5 μg indacaterol/15.6 μg glycopyrrolate	
Olodaterol/tiotropium	qd/MDI	5 μg of each (2 puffs)	
Vilanterol/umeclidinium	qd/DPI	25 μg vilanterol/62.5 μg umeclidinium	
Combination Short-acting β-Agonist/Short-acting Muscarinic Antagonist			
Albuterol/ipratropium	q4-6h/MDI or nebulizer	100 μg albuterol/20 μg ipratropium	Side effects of each constituent
Combination Long-acting β-Agonist/Inhaled Corticosteroids			
Salmeterol/fluticasone	bid/MDI	25 μg salmeterol/115 μg fluticasone; 2 inhalations bid	Side effects of each constituent
	bid/DPI	50 μg salmeterol/250 μg fluticasone; 1 inhalation bid	
Formoterol/budesonide	bid/MDI	9 μg formoterol/160-320 μg budesonide (two strengths available)	
Formoterol/mometasone	bid/MDI	5 μg formoterol/100 or 200 μg mometasone; 2 inhalations per administration	
Vilanterol/fluticasone	qd/DPI	25 μg vilanterol/100 μg fluticasone; 1 inhalation	
Combination Long-acting β-Agonist/Long-acting Muscarinic Antagonist/Inhaled Corticosteroids			
Vilanterol/umeclidinium/fluticasone	qd/DPI	25 μg vilanterol/62.5 μg umeclidinium/100 μg fluticasone	Side effects of each constituent
Formoterol/glycopyrrolate/budesonide	bid/MDI	9 μg formoterol/4.8 μg glycopyrrolate/160 μg budesonide; 2 inhalations bid	Side effects of each constituent

* = dose labeling (i.e., the amount of drug per puff varies across the world but the doses, either loaded in the dosing chamber or delivered from the inhaler, are generally within 10% of each other).
bid = twice daily; DPI = dry powder inhaler; MDI = metered dose inhaler; qd = once daily; qid = four times daily.

diarrhea, and weight loss. Although these side effects tend to abate over time, patients often discontinue these drugs shortly after starting therapy. As a result, phosphodiesterase-4 inhibitors are recommended only in COPD patients who experience persistent symptoms or recurrent exacerbations despite treatment with long-acting muscarinic antagonists, long-acting β-agonists, and inhaled corticosteroids.

Eosinophilic COPD

Some patients have substantial eosinophilia in their sputum or blood. In such patients, treatment with mepolizumab, a monoclonal antibody directed against interleukin-5, as 100 mg subcutaneously every 4 weeks for 1 year can reduce exacerbations.[A14]

Alpha-1 Antitrypsin Replacement Therapy

Patients with α_1-antitrypsin deficiency and signs of lung disease may benefit from replacement therapy, with weekly infusion of Prolastin (a proprietary mix of protease inhibitors) at 60 mg/kg.[20] Replacement therapy is not recommended for heterozygous patients.

Pulmonary Rehabilitation

Rehabilitation does not demonstrably change lung function, but education and exercise training can significantly improve quality of life, patients' sense of mastery of their disease, and exercise performance as assessed by ergometry and the 6-minute walk. In all patients with COPD, these effects are, on average, comparable to or greater than the benefit achievable with pharmacotherapy.[A15]

Surgical Therapy

Three principal surgical interventions have been used in selected patients with COPD: bullectomy, lung volume reduction, and lung transplantation (Chapter 87).

Bullectomy

A bulla is defined as a contiguous air space measuring more than 1 cm, and a giant bulla is defined as occupying more than 30% of a hemithorax. Bullectomy is a consideration in patients who have a giant bulla and who have persistent symptoms or exercise limitations despite medical therapy and rehabilitation. The likelihood of benefit and magnitude of risk for surgical intervention are largely dictated by an assessment of the characteristics of the parenchyma in the nonbullous lung. Patients with diffuse emphysema in addition to bullous disease are at higher risk for perioperative mortality and are less likely to experience substantial benefit than are those with relatively normal surrounding lung that is underexpanded due to the volume occupied by the giant bulla.

Lung Volume Reduction

Lung volume reduction is based on the premise that reducing the increase in lung volume that develops in patients with emphysema would help promote better diaphragmatic mechanics, reduce dyspnea associated with thoracic hyperinflation, and improve parenchymal tethering of airways during exhalation, thereby leading to improved expiratory flow rates. Two general interventions attempt to achieve these goals: lung volume reduction surgery and bronchoscopic interventions designed to produce regional volume loss (Chapter 87). Lung volume reduction surgery, most typically performed via a thoracoscopic approach, can reduce mortality in patients with predominantly upper lobe disease but not in patients with non–upper-lobe–predominant emphysema. Patients with FEV_1 less than 20% predicted and either low exercise capacity or a DLCO less than 20% are at high risk for perioperative mortality and should not be offered surgery.

The bronchoscopic approach eliminates the need for a chest wall incision. Emphysematous lung regions can be deflated by endoscopic placement of one-way bronchial valves, endobronchial coils, or transbronchial stents. Such procedures can provide modest benefit, primarily in patients with heterogeneous emphysema, intact interlobar fissures, and no collateral interlobar ventilation (Chapter 87).[A16] These procedures also may benefit patients with homogeneous emphysema but no collateral ventilation. Other devices, including airway bypass conduits, are under evaluation.

Lung Transplantation

Lung transplantation (Chapter 87) is an option for a broad variety of advanced lung diseases, including COPD. Initially, single-lung transplantation was recommended for patients with COPD, but emerging data suggest better long-term survival in those receiving bilateral lung transplants, so about 75% of transplants are currently bilateral procedures. COPD now accounts for about 25% of the lung transplants done in the United States. Median survival after lung transplant for COPD is 5.8 years.

PREVENTION

Given that the vast majority of those with COPD develop it as the result of inhalational exposures, avoiding such exposures will reduce the incidence of the disease.[21] The most commonly identified inhalational exposure associated with COPD is cigarette smoking, and smoking cessation, which slows the rate of decline in measured lung function, is critical (Chapter 363).

ACUTE EXACERBATIONS OF COPD

An acute exacerbation of COPD is defined as an increase in dyspnea over the patient's usual state, an increase in cough, or increase and change in character of mucus production. Acute exacerbations of COPD carry a short-term mortality of about 10%, have an independent detrimental effect on quality of life, and are responsible for about 60% of the direct medical costs of COPD.

EPIDEMIOLOGY

The risk of acute exacerbation of COPD increases with increasing chronic airflow obstruction, but there is substantial heterogeneity in the frequency of exacerbations at any degree of airflow obstruction. The best predictor of patients likely to have recurrent exacerbations is a history of recurrent exacerbations. Exacerbations exhibit a seasonality, with the highest frequency being during the winter months.

PATHOBIOLOGY

The final common pathway for an exacerbation, regardless of the initial stimulus, is an inflammatory response characterized by airway inflammation, mucus hypersecretion, and airway smooth muscle constriction that combine to produce the classic triad of dyspnea, cough, and sputum. Viral or bacterial pathogens can be implicated in 75 to 80% of acute exacerbations of COPD. The most frequently implicated viruses are rhinovirus (Chapter 329), influenza (Chapter 332), parainfluenza (Chapter 331), respiratory syncytial virus (Chapter 330), coronaviruses (Chapter 334), and adenovirus (Chapter 333). Many patients with chronic bronchitis are chronically colonized with bacterial species that have also been implicated in exacerbations, notably *Streptococcus pneumoniae* (Chapter 268), *Haemophilus influenza* (Chapter 277), *Moraxella catarrhalis* (Chapter 277), and, to a lesser extent, *Pseudomonas aeruginosa* (Chapter 282). In cohort studies of patients with chronic colonization, acquisition of a new genotype of these species is associated with an increased risk of exacerbation and the development of new strain-specific antibodies that contribute to the inflammatory response characteristic of an exacerbation. Additional support for the hypothesis that exposure to infectious agents is a likely source of exacerbations of COPD comes from the observation that such exacerbations decreased in frequency during social distancing and widespread use of face masks to help control the spread of illness during the severe acute respiratory syndrome coronavirus 2 pandemic.

Other environmental exposures also likely contribute, particularly in the 20 to 25% for which no pathogen or infectious exposure is identified. For example, emergency department visits for respiratory symptoms in patients with COPD increase during times of higher ambient air pollution.

CLINICAL MANIFESTATIONS AND DIAGNOSIS

Because acute exacerbations of COPD are often accompanied by fever or occur after contact with other sick individuals, the symptoms are generally similar to those of acute bronchitis (Chapter 84). The patient should be questioned about acute symptoms, prior history of exacerbations, presence of comorbidities such as heart disease, any infectious exposures, baseline functional status, past response to therapy (if any), and the presence of somnolence or confusion that may suggest hypercarbia. In addition to acute exacerbations of COPD, other possibilities that should be considered include decompensated heart failure (Chapter 45), pneumonia (Chapter 85), pulmonary embolism (Chapter 68), and pneumothorax (Chapter 86). Less likely is a tumor of the large airways.[22]

The physical examination should include assessment of vital signs and signs of respiratory distress (i.e., use of accessory muscles, intercostal retractions, tachypnea, and the inability to speak in complete sentences). The cardiac examination should assess the presence of tachycardia, irregular rhythm, and signs of left or right heart failure, including bibasilar rales, an elevated jugular venous pressure, hepatic congestion, peripheral edema, and an S3 gallop. Abnormal mental status should raise concerns for hypercarbia.

Laboratory evaluation should include oximetry and, in patients in respiratory distress or other reasons to suspect hypercarbia, an arterial blood gas. Given that tachycardia, elevated jugular venous pressure, and peripheral edema can be seen in both left and right heart failure, measurement of the circulating level of brain natriuretic peptide in patients may help identify patients with significant left heart failure (Chapter 45). Point-of-care testing of C-reactive protein to guide the prescribing of antibiotics can reduce antibiotic prescriptions with no evidence of harm.[A17]

A chest radiograph will demonstrate abnormalities in about 15% of patients but likely alter therapy in only about 5% of cases. A chest radiograph should always be obtained in any patient with chest pain, leukocytosis, a history of heart disease, or other complicating comorbidity. A chest CT scan is not routinely indicated, but a contrast-enhanced CT scan is the preferred mode of evaluation for patients in whom pulmonary embolism (Chapter 68) is a serious consideration. In most circumstances, a sputum culture is unlikely to influence therapy.

TREATMENT

Antibiotics and corticosteroids are beneficial for patients with an acute exacerbation of COPD.[A18] Indications for hospitalization include hypercarbia, acidemia, or significant respiratory distress despite bronchodilator therapy. In other cases, the decision is subjective and requires consideration of the patient's living situation, social support, transportation, reliability, and ability to perform activities of daily living. Similarly, in patients who are admitted for inpatient treatment, the timing of discharge depends on these same considerations.

Bacterial infection is involved in about 50% of cases of acute exacerbations of COPD. Antibiotics, which should be selected based on the need to cover the most common pathogens (i.e., *Streptococcus pneumoniae, Haemophilus influenza*, and *Moraxella catarrhalis*) reduce the duration of symptoms, particularly in patients with the triad of cough, increased dyspnea, and sputum (Table 76-3). In patients with severe COPD, a history of recent hospitalization or prior colonization with *Pseudomonas aeruginosa*, an antibiotic with anti-pseudomonal activity should be considered, such as levofloxacin 750 mg orally daily for 7 to 10 days. The specific choice of agent should take into account the local antibiotic resistance patterns of these species, but examples include azithromycin (500 mg orally daily) or amoxicillin-clavulanate (875 mg/125 mg orally twice daily) for 5 days. Continuing low-dose azithromycin (250 mg every 2 days) for 3 months after an infection can significantly reduce the likelihood of treatment failure.[A19]

Glucocorticoids (e.g., 40 mg daily by mouth for 5 days) should be administered to patients with symptoms severe enough to present for emergency

TABLE 76-3 HOSPITAL MANAGEMENT OF EXACERBATIONS OF COPD*

Diagnostic testing	Chest radiograph, oximetry, ABGs, and ECG Other testing as warranted by clinical indication
Bronchodilator therapy	Inhaled short-acting β_2-agonist Consider ipratropium if inadequate clinical response
Antibiotics	Recommended if (1) increases in dyspnea, sputum volume, and sputum purulence all are present; (2) increase in sputum purulence along with increase in either dyspnea or sputum volume; or (3) need for assisted ventilation Initial empirical therapy with amoxicillin plus clavulanic acid (875 mg/125 mg orally twice daily for 5 to 7 days), a macrolide antibiotic (e.g., azithromycin 500 mg orally daily for 5 days), or doxycycline (100 mg orally twice daily for 5 to 7 days) based on local bacterial resistance patterns Subsequent therapy based on sputum and blood cultures
Systemic corticosteroids	Daily oral prednisolone 30-40 mg (or its equivalent) for 5 days
Supplemental oxygen	Maintain oxygen saturation 88-92% Monitor ABGs for hypercapnia and acidosis
Assisted ventilation	Indications for NPPV include respiratory acidemia (arterial pH ≤7.35) or severe dyspnea with clinical signs of respiratory muscle fatigue or increased work of breathing

*Data from http://goldcopd.com.
ABGs = arterial blood gases; COPD = chronic obstructive pulmonary disease; ECG = electrocardiogram; ICU = intensive care unit; NPPV = noninvasive positive-pressure ventilation.

care, and parenteral corticosteroids are no more effective and are associated with potential complications and morbidity.[A20] Patients should be treated with a short-acting bronchodilator to help alleviate their dyspnea; β-agonists and antimuscarinics are equally efficacious in this setting. Methylxanthines are not recommended.

Patients with hypoxemia should be treated with supplemental oxygen at a dose sufficient to maintain an SaO_2 of above 90%. Some patients may experience a modest increase in P_{CO_2} owing to changes in their respiratory pattern and V/Q matching, but this phenomenon should not be a reason to withhold supplemental oxygen. In patients with persistent respiratory distress, acute hypercarbia, or acidemia, noninvasive positive-pressure ventilation (NIPPV) (Chapter 91) can improve these parameters and reduce the need for invasive mechanical ventilation, the number of ICU days, and mortality.[A21] For patients who have refractory hypoxemia, progressive hypercarbia, or acidemia despite NIPPV, endotracheal intubation and mechanical ventilator support (Chapter 91) are indicated if such an intervention is consistent with the patient's wishes. Care should be used to prescribe a relatively low respiratory rate to avoid dynamic hyperinflation ("auto-PEEP") in the setting of expiratory airflow obstruction. If evaluation demonstrates the presence of auto-PEEP, exogenous PEEP can be used to reduce the chest wall muscle work associated with initiating inspiration.

PREVENTION

Annual influenza vaccination (Chapter 332) reduces COPD-related hospitalization. Data are less clear for polyvalent pneumococcal vaccination (Chapter 15), but recommendations are to administer it in patients over 65 years of age, patients with heart disease or other comorbidities, and patients with severe COPD.

Patients who have an exacerbation requiring corticosteroid therapy are at increased risk for additional exacerbations in the year following the initial episode. Consideration should be given to the interventions demonstrated to decrease this risk.

The commonly prescribed inhaled agents (i.e., long-acting β-agonists, long-acting muscarinic antagonists, inhaled corticosteroids) reduce exacerbations by about 20% in patients with a history of exacerbations. There is modest additive benefit, and recommendations are to add inhaled corticosteroids to single or double inhaled bronchodilator therapy in patients who are still experiencing exacerbations. For patients who continue to have exacerbations on this regimen, a phosphodiesterase-4 inhibitor (roflumilast in patients with chronic bronchitis and recurrent exacerbations) or azithromycin (250 mg orally daily) can be added to reduce the risk of exacerbations by about 25% in patients with a history of COPD exacerbation.[A22] Patients who receive chronic azithromycin require assessment of their electrocardiographic QT interval and have a low (about 5%) but appreciable risk of reversible hearing loss on therapy. Unfortunately, other prophylactic antibiotics have generally failed to reduce exacerbations.[A23] Oral glucocorticoid therapy, with or without concomitant theophylline, is also ineffective.[A24]

PROGNOSIS

In patients with COPD, post-bronchodilator spirometry (see Table 76-1 and Fig. 76-1), typically assessed as FEV_1 (% predicted), predicts mortality and other important health outcomes. The body mass index, airflow obstruction, dyspnea, and exercise capacity index (BODE) index has more predictive value for mortality than the FEV_1 percent predicted alone. It incorporates patient-reported dyspnea, spirometry results, 6-minute walk distance, and body mass index to generate a score ranging between 0 and 10, with higher scores indicating a higher risk of death and scores ranging from 7 to 10 having a 48-month mortality of about 80%.

Exacerbations are independent determinants of health-related quality of life and are associated with an increase in short-term mortality (about 10% for patients hospitalized with an exacerbation) and longer-term mortality (43% at 1 year, 49% at 2 years). Resting hypoxemia, weight loss, a low body mass index, more severe dyspnea, and low exercise tolerance are independent predictors of mortality in patients with COPD.[23] A diagnosis of COPD is also a risk factor for lung cancer (Chapter 177). Given that most patients with COPD have a significant smoking history, the prevalence of cardiovascular disease (Chapter 40) is also increased. If β-blocking agents are indicated for cardiovascular disease, they can be used safely in patients with COPD while reducing cardiovascular risk.[24]

Pharmacotherapy can blunt the usual annual reduction in FEV_1 by about 5 mL per year.[A25] For patients with resting hypoxemia, supplemental oxygen therapy reduces mortality. For patients with significant exercise limitation in the setting of upper-lobe predominant emphysema, lung volume reduction surgery (Chapter 87) reduces mortality. End-of-life care for advanced COPD includes palliative care and the judicious use of opioids for dyspnea (Chapter 3).[25]

GENERAL REFERENCES

For the General References and other additional features, please visit Elsevier eBooks+ at https://ebooks.health.elsevier.com.

Grade A References

A1. Zhou Y, Zhong NS, Li X, et al. Tiotropium in early-stage chronic obstructive pulmonary disease. *N Engl J Med.* 2017;377:923-935.
A2. Nagata K, Horie T, Chohnabayashi N, et al. Home high-flow nasal cannula oxygen therapy for stable hypercapnic COPD: a randomized clinical trial. *Am J Respir Crit Care Med.* 2022;206:1326-1335.
A3. Murphy PB, Rehal S, Arbane G, et al. Effect of home noninvasive ventilation with oxygen therapy vs oxygen therapy alone on hospital readmission or death after an acute COPD exacerbation: a randomized clinical trial. *JAMA.* 2017;317:2177-2186.
A4. Lacasse Y, Sériès F, Corbeil F, et al. Randomized trial of nocturnal oxygen in chronic obstructive pulmonary disease. *N Engl J Med.* 2020;383:1129-1138.
A5. Prieur G, Delorme M, Lebret M, et al. Nasal high-flow during exercise in patients with COPD: a systematic review and meta-analysis. *Ann Am Thorac Soc.* 2022;19:291-302.
A6. Oba Y, Keeney E, Ghatehorde N, et al. Dual combination therapy versus long-acting bronchodilators alone for chronic obstructive pulmonary disease (COPD): a systematic review and network meta-analysis. *Cochrane Database Syst Rev.* 2018;12.
A7. Wedzicha JA, Banerji D, Chapman KR, et al. Indacaterol-glycopyrronium versus salmeterol-fluticasone for COPD. *N Engl J Med.* 2016;374:2222-2234.
A8. Lipson DA, Barnhart F, Brealey N, et al. Once-daily single-inhaler triple versus dual therapy in patients with COPD. *N Engl J Med.* 2018;378:1671-1680.
A9. Papi A, Vestbo J, Fabbri L, et al. Extrafine inhaled triple therapy versus dual bronchodilator therapy in chronic obstructive pulmonary disease (TRIBUTE): a double-blind, parallel group, randomised controlled trial. *Lancet.* 2018;391:1076-1084.
A10. Rabe KF, Martinez FJ, Ferguson GT, et al. Triple inhaled therapy at two glucocorticoid doses in moderate-to-very-severe COPD. *N Engl J Med.* 2020;383:35-48.
A11. Chen H, Deng Z-X, Sun J, et al. Association of inhaled corticosteroids with all-cause mortality risk in patients with COPD: a meta-analysis of 60 randomized controlled trials. *Chest.* 2023;163:100-114.
A12. Martinez FJ, Rabe KF, Ferguson GT, et al. Reduced all-cause mortality in the ETHOS trial of budesonide/glycopyrrolate/formoterol for chronic obstructive pulmonary disease. A randomized, double-blind, multicenter, parallel-group study. *Am J Respir Crit Care Med.* 2021;203:553-564.
A13. Janjua S, Fortescue R, Poole P. Phosphodiesterase-4 inhibitors for chronic obstructive pulmonary disease. *Cochrane Database Syst Rev.* 2020;5.
A14. Pavord ID, Chanez P, Criner GJ, et al. Mepolizumab for eosinophilic chronic obstructive pulmonary disease. *N Engl J Med.* 2017;377:1613-1629.
A15. Burge AT, Cox NS, Abramson MJ, et al. Interventions for promoting physical activity in people with chronic obstructive pulmonary disease (COPD). *Cochrane Database Syst Rev.* 2020;4.
A16. van Agteren JE, Hnin K, Grosser D, et al. Bronchoscopic lung volume reduction procedures for chronic obstructive pulmonary disease. *Cochrane Database Syst Rev.* 2017;2.
A17. Butler CC, Gillespie D, White P, et al. C-reactive protein testing to guide antibiotic prescribing for COPD exacerbations. *N Engl J Med.* 2019;381:111-120.
A18. Dobler CC, Morrow AS, Beuschel B, et al. Pharmacologic therapies in patients with exacerbation of chronic obstructive pulmonary disease: a systematic review with meta-analysis. *Ann Intern Med.* 2020;172:413-422.

A19. Vermeersch K, Gabrovska M, Aumann J, et al. Azithromycin during acute chronic obstructive pulmonary disease exacerbations requiring hospitalization (BACE). A multicenter, randomized, double-blind, placebo-controlled trial. *Am J Respir Crit Care Med.* 2019;200:857-868.
A20. Walters JA, Tan DJ, White CJ, et al. Different durations of corticosteroid therapy for exacerbations of chronic obstructive pulmonary disease. *Cochrane Database Syst Rev.* 2018;3.
A21. Osadnik CR, Tee VS, Carson-Chahhoud KV, et al. Non-invasive ventilation for the management of acute hypercapnic respiratory failure due to exacerbation of chronic obstructive pulmonary disease. *Cochrane Database Syst Rev.* 2017;7:CD004104.
A22. Vermeersch K, Gabrovska M, Aumann J, et al. Azithromycin during acute chronic obstructive pulmonary disease exacerbations requiring hospitalization (BACE). A multicenter, randomized, double-blind, placebo-controlled trial. *Am J Respir Crit Care Med.* 2019;200:857-868.
A23. Janjua S, Mathioudakis AG, Fortescue R, et al. Prophylactic antibiotics for adults with chronic obstructive pulmonary disease: a network meta-analysis. *Cochrane Database Syst Rev.* 2021;1:CD013198.
A24. Jenkins CR, Wen FQ, Martin A, et al. The effect of low-dose corticosteroids and theophylline on the risk of acute exacerbations of COPD: the TASCS randomised controlled trial. *Eur Respir J.* 2021;57:2003338.
A25. Celli BR, Anderson JA, Cowans NJ, et al. Pharmacotherapy and lung function decline in patients with chronic obstructive pulmonary disease. A systematic review. *Am J Respir Crit Care Med.* 2021;203:689-698.

77

CYSTIC FIBROSIS

HARTMUT GRASEMANN

DEFINITION

Cystic fibrosis, which is among the most common life-shortening autosomal recessive genetic diseases in White populations, is caused by absent or reduced function of the cystic fibrosis transmembrane conductance regulator (CFTR) protein. CFTR, which is expressed at the mucosal surfaces of the aerodigestive tract, sweat glands, and vas deferens, conducts the flow of chloride, bicarbonate, and thiocyanate ions across cell membranes. The loss of CFTR function in the airways of patients with cystic fibrosis leads to progressive lung disease.

EPIDEMIOLOGY

In Northern Europe and the Americas, the incidence of cystic fibrosis is approximately 1 : 2500 to 1 : 3000 live births. The worldwide prevalence of cystic fibrosis is about 1 in 60,000, with about 100,000 total cases, but the prevalence in the United States is about 1 : 10,000 (resulting in about 35,000 cases). Although most patients are of European ancestry, the disease is also seen in Hispanic Americans (about 1 : 7000), African Americans (about 1 : 12,000), and infrequently in Native Americans. The disease is rarely diagnosed in Africa or Asia. With improved treatment and prognosis, affected adults now outnumber children and adolescents.[1]

PATHOBIOLOGY

Absent or deficient CFTR function causes dehydration of mucosal surfaces and viscous secretions that obstruct the impacted luminal compartments and ducts.

Sweat Glands

Sweat gland sodium chloride (NaCl) concentrations are initially isotonic with plasma, but CFTR function normally reclaims NaCl to minimize salt loss as the sweat travels to the skin surface. In cystic fibrosis, sweat chloride concentrations are 60 mEq/L or more, a level that is used in the case definition, compared with sweat chloride concentrations that are almost always less than 20 mEq/L in nonaffected individuals. Because the sweat of individuals with cystic fibrosis is almost isotonic with plasma, patients become dehydrated in conditions that cause substantial sweating. However, because their plasma sodium levels do not rise, they perceive less of a sense of thirst compared with when normal individuals sweat heavily.

Sinuses and Lungs

CFTR dysfunction in the airways results in reduced chloride and bicarbonate secretion by the respiratory epithelium into the airway lumen. In addition, sodium absorption by the airway epithelial cells is increased. This imbalance in ion transport leads to airway surface dehydration. Reduction in height of the airway surface liquid layer causes impaired mucociliary clearance and, subsequently, mucus plugging of airways.

For reasons that are not entirely clear, cystic fibrosis airways represent an ecologic niche that favors infections with pathogens such as *Staphylococcus* and *Pseudomonas* species. The infection is often characterized by the formation of biofilms, in which cells are mostly nondividing; as a result, antibiotics are less effective than they would be for traditional infections. These microorganisms activate both innate and adaptive immune responses in the airway mucosa (E-Fig. 77-1). Unfortunately, chronic polymorphonuclear neutrophils cannot obliterate the biofilm, but their enzymes (especially neutrophil elastase) do cause collateral damage that leads to inflammation, destruction of the airway wall, and bronchiectasis (Chapter 78).

Exacerbations of cystic fibrosis lung disease are believed to occur when the increased metabolic activity in the biofilm results in the recruitment of more neutrophils into the airway. These neutrophils do not rapidly apoptose but instead disintegrate and form neutrophilic extracellular traps that activate local macrophages that then increase the inflammatory response. This process leads to more airway obstruction and a measurable decrease in the forced expiratory volume in one second (FEV_1) on pulmonary function testing.

Pancreas

In classic cystic fibrosis, the inability of the exocrine pancreatic ducts to secrete bicarbonate and chloride leads to pancreatic autodigestion. Whereas the normal pancreas secretes about 1 to 1.5 L of bicarbonate- and chloride-rich fluid daily, patients with cystic fibrosis secrete less than half of that volume because the exocrine pancreas is replaced by fatty infiltration and chronic inflammation. In many cases, this inflammation also leads to loss of pancreatic endocrine function, thereby resulting in cystic fibrosis–related diabetes mellitus.

Liver

In the biliary tract, the absence of CFTR-mediated hydration leads to obstruction of the biliary canaliculi, which can then cause cirrhosis (Chapter 139) and its complications. In many patients with cystic fibrosis, mildly elevated aminotransferase levels are the only hepatic abnormality, but about 5% of patients progress to hepatic failure that requires transplantation (Chapter 140). Liver disease often presents in childhood, and the SERPINA1 Z allele may lead to genetic predisposition.

Other Organs

The small intestine secretes about 1.8 L of fluid each day (per 70 kg body mass). Abnormal CFTR-mediated secretion leads to inadequate hydration of small bowel contents, which in turn can lead to obstipation and intussusception, principally in the ileum and appendix.

Other associated conditions include short stature, delayed sexual maturation, clubbing of the digits (see Fig. 39-9 in Chapter 39), wrinkling of the hands and feet, hypochloremic hypokalemic alkalosis (Chapter 104), gastric reflux (Chapter 124), and esophagitis (Chapter 124).

Genetics

Although over 2000 CFTR variants have been described, about 70% of all patients with cystic fibrosis have at least one copy of F508del—the gene that encodes CFTR is missing the codon for phenylalanine at position 508. The origin is thought to be a founder mutation about 52,000 years ago in the Middle East.

The various cystic fibrosis–causing CFTR variants can interfere with virtually every aspect of protein expression (Tables 77-1 and 77-2). A limitation of the current classification system is that some mutations—including W1282X,

TABLE 77-1 CLASSIFICATION OF CYSTIC FIBROSIS–CAUSING VARIANTS

	CFTR DYSFUNCTION	COMMON VARIANTS
Class I	Severe reduction or absence of synthesis	W1282X, G542X, R563X
Class II	Protein misfolding, premature degradation	F508del, N1303K
Class III	Disordered regulation, ATP binding, and hydrolysis	G551D, G551S, G1349D
Class IV	Defective chloride conductance or gating	R117H, R334W, R347P
Class V	Reduced transcripts, promoter or splicing	2789 +5 G>A, A445E
Class VI	Accelerated turnover from cell surface	120del23, rescued F508del, N287Y

CFTR = cystic fibrosis transmembrane conductance regulator.

TABLE 77-2 CYSTIC FIBROSIS–ASSOCIATED VARIANTS WITH A FREQUENCY OF >1%

VARIANT (>1%)	PERCENTAGE OF ALL VARIANTS	ORIGIN
F508del	66%	Middle East
G542X	2.4%	Spain
G551D	1.6%	England
N1303K	1.3%	Italy
W1282X	1.2%	Ashkenazi Jewish

Data from http://www.genet.sickkids.on.ca/resource/Table1.html.

F508del, and R117H—display combinatorial molecular defects, which may explain some of the variability seen in response to CFTR modulator therapies.

Patients with the most severe CFTR variants (Class I to III) usually develop pancreatic insufficiency, but other patients may retain some pancreatic function. Genome-wide association studies suggest that variants in genes encoding mucin and alternative ion channels could explain some of the variation in lung, sinus, pancreatic, and hepatobiliary diseases. For example, patients who are homozygotic for the F508del mutation but who nevertheless have stable lung function into the fifth or sixth decade of life often have variants in the epithelial sodium channel.

CLINICAL MANIFESTATIONS

Lung Disease

Pulmonary manifestations include chronic productive cough and crackles on auscultation. Mucus retention and airway inflammation may cause chronic wheezing. Even in children diagnosed by newborn screening, bronchiectasis (Chapter 78) can be detected on chest computed tomography imaging in up to 30% of infants at 3 months of age, increasing to about 60% at 3 years of age even in the absence of clinically apparent lung disease.

As in asthma (Chapter 75) and chronic obstructive pulmonary disease (Chapter 76), an exacerbation of cystic fibrosis lung disease is frequently preceded by a viral respiratory infection. Exacerbations are characterized by increased cough, dyspnea, and often changes in sputum color and viscosity. Fever is uncommon, but hypoxemia may develop. During the social isolation imposed by the severe acute respiratory syndrome coronavirus 2 pandemic, rates of pulmonary exacerbations of cystic fibrosis actually decreased, thereby suggesting that an underlying exogenous infectious cause is responsible for a substantial fraction of exacerbations.

In cystic fibrosis, secondary polymicrobial endobronchial colonization is dominated by *Staphylococcus aureus* (including multidrug-resistant *Staphylococcus aureus*) and *Pseudomonas aeruginosa*. *Burkholderia* species, *Stenotrophomonas*, and anaerobes are less common but can be associated with a greater inflammatory response. *Aspergillus* and *Candida* infections also can develop.

During an exacerbation, the FEV_1 usually decreases by at least 10% from the previous baseline. Pulmonary function testing also typically shows a decreased mid-expiratory flow rate (MEFR 25 to 75) or an increase in the lung clearance index (Chapter 73). Over time, repeated exacerbations lead to a progressive loss in pulmonary function and to bronchiectasis (Chapter 78), predominantly in the upper lobes (Fig. 77-1). Radiographic evidence of sinusitis is common, as are nasal polyps, but only a minority of patients with cystic fibrosis have chronic sinus disease (Chapter 394) manifested with pain, anosmia, congestion, and discharge.

Gastrointestinal Disease

Infants with cystic fibrosis are susceptible to meconium ileus and small bowel obstruction that may necessitate life-saving surgery at birth. In many patients, inadequate hydration leads to distal intestinal obstruction syndrome, which may result in ileo-ileal intussusception (Chapter 128) that can require emergent surgery. Bulky, inadequately hydrated stools may also cause chronic obstipation, abdominal pain, hemorrhoids, and rectal prolapse.

Up to 90% of patients with cystic fibrosis develop pancreatic insufficiency (Chapter 130) with resulting fat malabsorption that leads to deficiencies in fat-soluble vitamins D, A, K, and E. Osteopenia and coagulopathies are common sequelae of these deficiencies.[2] The minority of patients who initially retain pancreatic sufficiency usually have milder Class IV or V mutations but still are subject to chronic pancreatitis (Chapter 130) that may lead to eventual

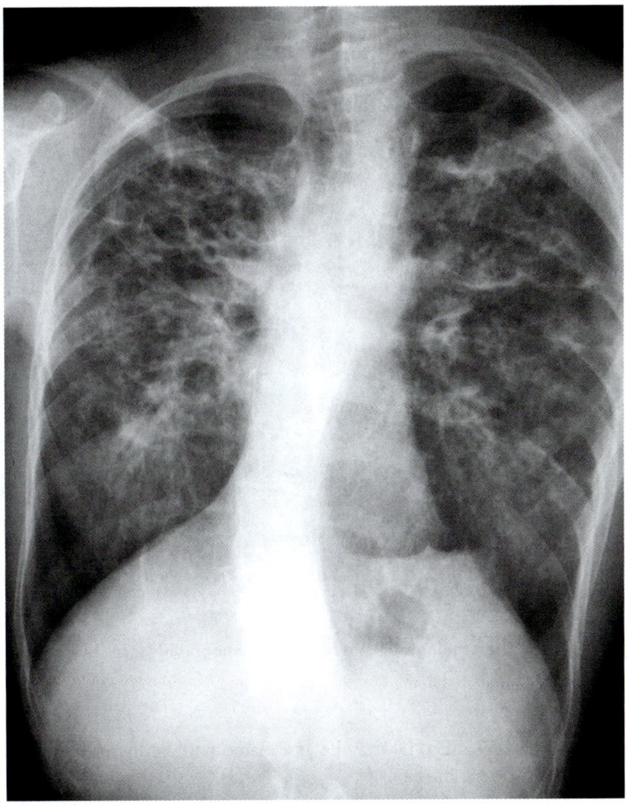

FIGURE 77-1. **Cystic fibrosis.** Chest radiograph shows cystic bronchiectasis preferentially involving both upper lobes with accompanying bilateral apical bullae. Bilateral upper lobe loss of volume with retraction of the hilar regions cephalad. (Courtesy of Paul Stark, MD.)

pancreatic insufficiency. Many patients with cystic fibrosis suffer from reflux esophagitis (Chapter 124). Portal hypertension owing to liver involvement[3] increases the risk for esophageal varices.

Reproductive Issues

Some men are diagnosed with cystic fibrosis after evaluation for infertility (Chapter 216). Sperm production is normal, but virtually all men with cystic fibrosis have congenital bilateral absence of the vas deferens. Many females with cystic fibrosis may have difficulty conceiving due to blockage of the cervix with viscid mucus.

Additional Manifestations

By 30 years of age, approximately one third of patients have cystic fibrosis–related diabetes (Chapter 210). Although ketoacidosis rarely develops, the microvascular and macrovascular complications of diabetes mellitus can occur. The risks of osteoporosis (Chapter 225), osteopenia, and fracture also increase in frequency with age.

Patients who have cystic fibrosis are also predisposed to short stature, developmental delay, atypical mycobacterial infections (Chapter 300), obstructive sleep apnea (Chapter 374), pulmonary hypertension (Chapter 69), gallstones (Chapter 141), amenorrhea (Chapter 218), cystic fibrosis–related rheumatoid arthritis (Chapter 243), erythema nodosum (Chapter 407), renal calculi (Chapter 111), and chronic renal insufficiency (Chapter 116).

DIAGNOSIS

In the United States, routine newborn screening for cystic fibrosis is performed by measuring immunoreactive trypsinogen from a heel stick at birth. This test is highly sensitive but relatively less specific. For babies who have initially positive results, most hospitals perform genetic mutation analysis as the next step. For patients whose genetic testing is negative using a panel of the 40 or so most common CFTR mutations, sequencing of the gene, which may not be available in all centers, is required. In patients who are suspected of having cystic fibrosis but who have only a single identified mutation, sweat testing is required to establish the diagnosis. Even if patients have two CFTR mutations, pilocarpine iontophoresis sweat testing is the gold-standard diagnostic test. Chloride values equal to or greater than 60 mEq/L are diagnostic of cystic fibrosis, and values lower than 30 mEq/L are normal. Borderline results

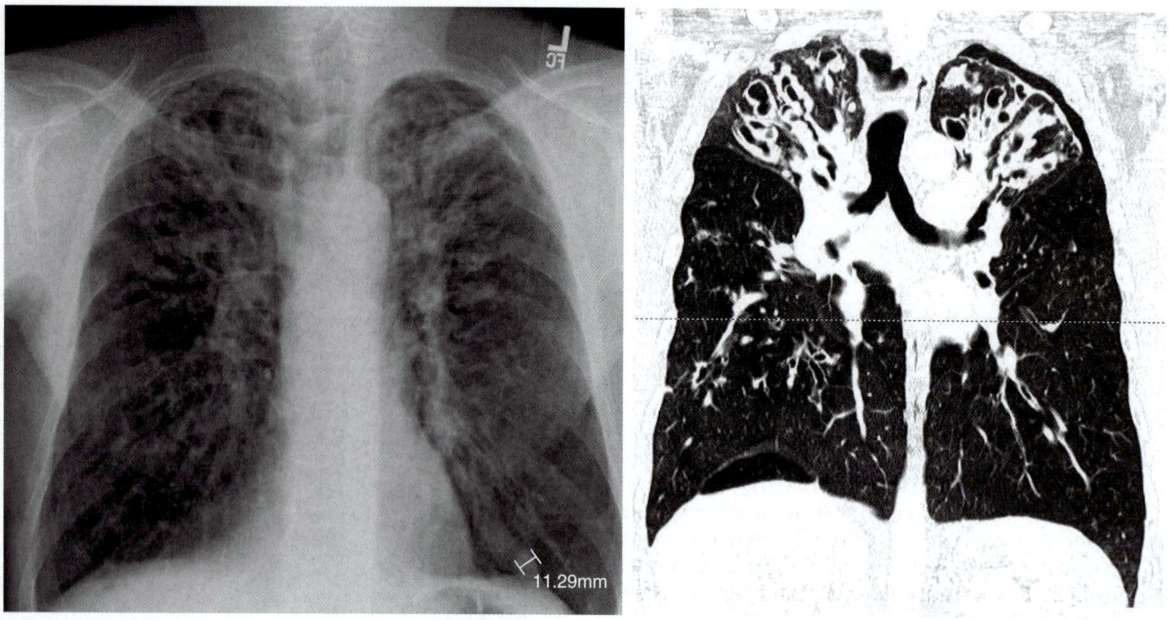

FIGURE 77-2. Chest radiograph and computed tomographic scan show bronchiectasis in a patient with cystic fibrosis.

(between 30 and 59 mEq/L) may be associated with milder CFTR variants and *forme fruste* cystic fibrosis.

In infants with steatorrhea or failure to thrive, CFTR variant genetic analyses should supplement standard testing. The sweat test can be falsely positive in patients who have nephrogenic diabetes insipidus (Chapter 206), malnutrition (Chapter 197), Addison disease (Chapter 208), or hypoparathyroidism (Chapter 227).

In an occasional patient, cystic fibrosis can present in adulthood. Nearly all such patients have chronic rhinosinusitis (Chapter 394), and many have recurrent respiratory infections (including bronchitis [Chapter 84] and bronchiectasis [Chapter 78]), abdominal pain, and pancreatitis (Chapter 130).[4] If the sputum culture reveals *Pseudomonas*, *S. aureus*, atypical mycobacteria, or fungi, the physician should suspect possible cystic fibrosis. The clinical evaluation should include spirometry, computed tomographic scanning of the sinuses and chest, and sweat testing. The chest radiograph typically shows evidence of cystic bronchiectasis, especially involving the upper lobes (see Fig. 77-1), most evident in a computed tomographic scan (Fig. 77-2). In advanced cases, pulmonary hypertension can also develop (E-Fig. 77-2).

DIFFERENTIAL DIAGNOSIS

Conditions that can mimic cystic fibrosis include bronchiectasis (Chapter 78), chronic aspiration, tuberculosis (Chapter 299), primary or secondary immunodeficiencies (Chapter 231), Crohn disease (Chapter 127), and connective tissue diseases (such as rheumatoid arthritis [Chapter 243] and Sjögren syndrome [Chapter 247]), primary ciliary dyskinesia (Chapter 78), and Shwachman-Diamond syndrome (Chapter 231).

In some patients who have a clinical phenotype that suggests cystic fibrosis, the diagnosis cannot be established, either because their sweat test is normal or because two genetic mutations cannot be identified. Such patients have what is now termed CFTR-related disorder. In some such patients, comprehensive analysis of the CFTR coding and flanking regions may help establish the diagnosis of cystic fibrosis.

TREATMENT

In the United States, nearly every patient with cystic fibrosis receives care by a highly specialized multidisciplinary care team at a Cystic Fibrosis Foundation–accredited center, where better outcomes are achieved compared with treatment in other settings.[5] Standard supportive therapy involves airway clearance, mucolytic drugs, bronchodilators, treatment of infections, anti-inflammatory therapy, pancreatic enzyme replacement, and bowel clearance. CFTR potentiators and correctors can substantially benefit patients with certain CFTR mutations.[6]

Airway Clearance

The clearance of viscid mucus from the airways is facilitated by exercise[A1] as well as chest physical therapy, including postural drainage, percussion, and external vests that utilize vibration. Chest physical therapy is optimally performed two to three times a day. A positive-pressure expiratory mask, autogenic drainage, and the forced expiratory technique are also useful. Airway clearance can be improved by using mucolytics, including human recombinant DNase (dornase alfa, 2.5 mg once daily by inhalation),[A2] N-acetyl cysteine (10% solution, 10 to 30 mL every 6 hours), and osmotic drugs (e.g., 7% hypertonic saline solution, 4 mL nebulized twice daily) immediately prior to these airway clearance techniques.

For nasal sinus symptoms, nasal saline irrigation with or without xylitol (12 mg dissolved into 240 mL water in a sinus irrigation bottle for 10 days) and topical corticosteroids (e.g., betamethasone 100 μg twice daily for 6 weeks) are efficacious. Nasal polyposis and sinus ostia blockage can also be treated surgically (Chapter 394).

Treatment of Infection

Antibiotic therapy should focus on the microorganisms identified in the sputum or on throat swab. Typical organisms include *Staphylococcus* sp. (Chapter 267), *Pseudomonas aeruginosa* (Chapter 282), and atypical mycobacteria (Chapter 300). Multidrug-resistant *Staphylococcus aureus* are increasingly observed, and multidrug-resistant *Burkholderia* species (Chapter 282) are associated with high morbidity and mortality.

Outpatient therapies for chronic *Pseudomonas* infection include nebulized tobramycin solution (300 mg twice daily for 28 days on-off cycles), inhaled tobramycin powder (112 mg twice daily for 28 days on-off cycles), aerosolized colistin (1 to 2 million units twice daily), or inhaled aztreonam (75 mg inhaled every 8 hours for 28 days).[A3] For *Staphylococcus aureus* infections, by comparison, there is insufficient evidence for chronic antimicrobial therapy.

For exacerbation of lung disease, oral antibiotics are usually prescribed for 2- to 3-week courses.[7] Depending on culture and sensitivity results, options include ciprofloxacin (500 to 750 mg twice daily), trimethoprim/sulfamethoxazole (1 double-strength tablet twice daily), amoxicillin (1 gram three times daily), linezolid (600 mg twice daily), erythromycin (500 mg four times a day), and clarithromycin (500 mg twice daily) (Chapters 78 and 266).[8] Other options include doxycycline, tetracycline, minocycline, and tigecycline (Chapter 266).

For severe exacerbations, patients may require intravenous antibiotics: options include penicillins, cephalosporins, aminoglycosides, macrolides, vancomycin, carbapenems, aztreonam, colistin, sulfa drugs, and quinolones (Chapter 266). For atypical mycobacterial infections, combination therapy is required (Chapter 300).

Unfortunately, many of these antimicrobial agents have significant side effects, including nephrotoxicity; dosing must be tailored to renal function. Antibiotic resistance is frequent and can complicate choices among antibiotic options.

Bronchodilators

Clinically important airway hyperresponsiveness, presumably caused by chronic airway inflammation, is nearly universal among patients with cystic fibrosis (Chapter 75). Treatment with inhaled β-adrenergic bronchodilators may include albuterol (aerosol or dry powder 90 to 180 μg every 4 to 6 hours, or 3 mL of a 0.083% solution [2.5 mg] nebulized three to four times daily) and salmeterol (50 μg inhalation twice daily). A β-adrenergic agent is typically combined with an anticholinergic agent, such as ipratropium bromide (17 μg two puffs twice daily) or tiotropium (1.25 μg inhaled daily). Combination inhalers (such as ipratropium bromide 20 μg/albuterol sulfate 120 μg [Combivent Respimat], 1 inhalation four times daily or ipratropium bromide 0.5 mg/albuterol sulfate 3.0 mg [DuoNeb], 3-mL vial nebulized four times daily) may be easier for patients to use.

Anti-Inflammatory Agents

Macrolide antibiotics have antimicrobial and immunomodulatory properties. Azithromycin in subinhibitory doses (250 to 500 mg three times weekly) can improve lung function and weight gain and is often recommended regardless of whether patients have chronic *Pseudomonas aeruginosa* infection.[9] Because chronic azithromycin may result in bacterial resistance, patients should be screened for nontuberculous mycobacterium (Chapter 300) before starting it and then at 6- or 12-month intervals; azithromycin should be withheld in the presence of active nontuberculous mycobacterial infection.

High-dose ibuprofen (800-mg tablets titrated to achieve serum concentrations between 50 and 100 μg/mL) can slow the rate of decline in FEV_1 and is recommended for patients who are under 18 years of age and who have an FEV_1 lower than 60% of predicted. The narrow therapeutic window and side effects limit the clinical utility of this treatment.

Corticosteroids, both inhaled (e.g., beclomethasone, fluticasone, budesonide; see Chapter 75) and oral (e.g., prednisone up to 1 mg/kg on alternate days with close attention to adverse effects), are recommended for patients who have asthma or allergic bronchopulmonary aspergillosis (Chapter 311). Allergic bronchopulmonary aspergillosis should be treated with prednisone (0.5 to 2.0 mg/kg/day for 1 to 2 weeks, then hopefully tapered over 1 to 3 months). Itraconazole (5 mg/kg/day, up to a maximum of 400 mg per day, for 3 to 6 months) can be added if patients with bronchopulmonary aspergillus have a slow or poor response to corticosteroids or if they relapse; it is also recommended if patients develop steroid toxicity.

CFTR Correctors and Potentiators

In patients who have gating mutations (including G551D, which affect about 4% of the cystic fibrosis population), ivacaftor (a CFTR potentiator at 150 mg twice daily) can increase FEV_1, as well as decrease the sweat chloride concentration, increase weight, and decrease the rate of hospitalization.[10,11] Ivacaftor is currently approved for patients with at least 1 of 38 CFTR gating or splice mutations.

For the nearly 50% of cystic fibrosis patients who are homozygous for F508del alleles, a combination of a CFTR corrector (lumacaftor 400 mg daily) plus ivacaftor (250 mg twice daily) can modestly improve FEV_1 and increase the interval between hospitalizations.[A4,A5] The combination of tezacaftor (100 mg once daily) plus ivacaftor (150 mg twice daily) also improves FEV_1 and reduces pulmonary exacerbation rates with an acceptable side effect profile in patients who are homozygous for F508del.[A6,A7] The three-drug combination of the CFTR corrector elexacaftor (200 mg once daily) plus tezacaftor (100 mg once daily) and ivacaftor (150 mg twice daily) can improve FEV_1 in patients homozygous for F508del by 10% compared to tezacaftor plus ivacaftor and by 14% in patients who are heterozygous for F508del and a minimal function mutation, thus extending such therapy to about 90% of patients.[A8-A11] However, CFTR modifier treatment can cause serious side effects, and dosing must be reduced in patients who have hepatic failure or who are taking CYP3A inhibitors such as itraconazole or clarithromycin.

Improving CFTR function can benefit even patients with advanced lung disease,[11] but it may not halt the ongoing inflammatory response in chronically infected and bronchiectatic airways. Ion channel modulator agents may therefore need to be started as early as perinatally to prevent lung disease and potentially other organ manifestations, including exocrine pancreatic insufficiency and cystic fibrosis–related diabetes.

Despite more than two decades of research since the discovery of CFTR, gene therapy is not currently an effective therapeutic option. Whether nucleic acid technologies, antisense oligonucleotides, CRISPR/Cas9, or induced pluripotent stem cell therapy will become clinically useful is currently unknown.

Pancreatic Enzyme Replacement Therapy

The replacement of pancreatic enzymes (Chapter 130) is an essential component of the treatment of patients with cystic fibrosis. Dosing (see Table 130-5 in Chapter 130) should aim for the near elimination of steatorrhea. Oral pancreatic enzymes are inactivated by stomach acid. Enteric-coated capsules or acid-resistant microspheres are preferred over acid suppression with H_2 blockers or proton pump inhibitors (see Table 124-1 in Chapter 124), in part because protein pump inhibitors may increase the risk of pneumonia. The absorption of fat-soluble vitamins (D, A, K, and E) may be inadequate despite pancreatic enzyme therapy, so the blood levels of these vitamins should be monitored, and vitamins should be supplemented as needed.[12]

Gastrointestinal Agents

Virtually all patients with cystic fibrosis should receive an empiric bowel regimen to avoid obstipation. Mineral oil (e.g., 15 to 45 mL/day depending on the product), senna (17.2 to 34.4 mg per day), and osmotic stool softeners (e.g., polyethylene glycol 3350 at 0.5 to 1 g/kg/day to a maximum of 40 g/day) are routinely used. Lactulose is another alternative, but it may cause flatulence or abdominal pain in high doses.

A more serious complication is distal intestinal obstructive syndrome, which may occur with dehydration or the use of opioid analgesics. This complication usually requires hospitalization, intravenous rehydration, and administration via a nasogastric tube of iso-osmotic polyethylene glycol 3350 plus an electrolyte solution (20 to 40 mL/kg/h up to a maximum of 1 L/h over 8 hours) or diatrizoate (Gastrografin). Surgical consultation is often required if small bowel obstruction persists.

Other Organ Systems

Sweating may cause excessive salt loss with resulting dehydration and hypotension. Adolescents and adults with cystic fibrosis require about 6000 mg (3 teaspoons) of salt per day. Foods naturally high in salt are recommended, but prophylactic sodium chloride tablets are often added.

Because pancreatic damage can lead to cystic fibrosis–related diabetes, annual glucose tolerance testing is recommended beginning at age 10 years for all patients who do not have diagnosed diabetes. Treatment is similar to type 1 diabetes (Chapter 210). The need for insulin therapy may be delayed by diet and exercise.

Women with cystic fibrosis can have children, but intrauterine insemination may be required if the cervix is blocked with viscid mucus. In men, epididymal sperm aspiration is needed because of the ubiquitous absence of the vas deferens. Patients with cystic fibrosis should be routinely screened for depression and anxiety (Chapter 362) and referred to mental health professionals as appropriate.

Lung Transplantation

Lung transplantation (Chapter 87), which is a life-saving therapy in patients with end-stage lung disease, results in improved quality of life because of better lung function, even though disease progresses in other organs.[13] Current survival rates for adult lung transplant recipients with cystic fibrosis are about 75% at 5 years and 50% at 10 years. In recipients with risk factors such as *Burkholderia cepacia* complex infection or retransplantation, however, outcomes are less favorable. Long-term (>5 years) survival is limited by chronic lung allograft dysfunction (bronchiolitis obliterans and restrictive allograft syndrome) and by reinfection of donor lungs with opportunistic pathogens.

PREVENTION

Genetic counseling should be offered to all at-risk couples prior to pregnancy. Antenatal screening, especially if a previous child was diagnosed with cystic fibrosis, can identify whether future offspring may be affected as well. Prenatal screening can make the diagnosis in utero. Parents also can choose to undergo in vitro fertilization with an embryo that has undergone preimplantation screening for cystic fibrosis.

PROGNOSIS

Factors that influence the outcome of patients with cystic fibrosis include the initiation of effective treatment early in life, the number of hours per day each patient spends in physical therapy, adherence to an often-complicated medical regimen, transition from parental care to self-care, insurance, and psychosocial coping. Although life expectancy for people born with cystic fibrosis has increased over recent years, respiratory failure and death still often occur before the fourth decade of life.

GENERAL REFERENCES

For the General References and other additional features, please visit Elsevier eBooks+ at https://ebooks.health.elsevier.com.

Grade A References

A1. Radtke T, Nevitt SJ, Hebestreit H, et al. Physical exercise training for cystic fibrosis. *Cochrane Database Syst Rev.* 2017;11:CD002768.

A2. Yang C, Montgomery M. Dornase alfa for cystic fibrosis. *Cochrane Database Syst Rev.* 2021;3:CD001127.

A3. Smith S, Rowbotham NJ, Regan KH. Inhaled anti-pseudomonal antibiotics for long-term therapy in cystic fibrosis. *Cochrane Database Syst Rev.* 2018;3:CD001021.

A4. Taylor-Cousar JL, Jain M, Barto TL, et al. Lumacaftor/ivacaftor in patients with cystic fibrosis and advanced lung disease homozygous for F508del-CFTR. *J Cyst Fibros.* 2018;17:228-235.

A5. Graeber SY, Dopfer C, Naehrlich L, et al. Effects of lumacaftor-ivacaftor therapy on cystic fibrosis transmembrane conductance regulator function in Phe508del homozygous patients with cystic fibrosis. *Am J Respir Crit Care Med.* 2018;197:1433-1442.

A6. Taylor-Cousar JL, Munck A, McKone EF, et al. Tezacaftor-ivacaftor in patients with cystic fibrosis homozygous for Phe508del. *N Engl J Med.* 2017;377:2013-2023.

A7. Donaldson SH, Pilewski JM, Griese M, et al. Tezacaftor/ivacaftor in subjects with cystic fibrosis and F508del/F508del-CFTR or F508del/G551d-CFTR. *Am J Respir Crit Care Med.* 2018;197:214-224.

A8. Sutharsan S, McKone EF, Downey DG, et al. Efficacy and safety of elexacaftor plus tezacaftor plus ivacaftor versus tezacaftor plus ivacaftor in people with cystic fibrosis homozygous for F508del-CFTR: a 24-week, multicentre, randomised, double-blind, active-controlled, phase 3b trial. *Lancet Respir Med.* 2022;10:267-277.

A9. Davies JC, Moskowitz SM, Brown C, et al. VX-659-tezacaftor-ivacaftor in patients with cystic fibrosis and one or two Phe508del alleles. *N Engl J Med.* 2018;379:1599-1611.

A10. Middleton PG, Mall MA, Dřevínek P, et al. Elexacaftor-tezacaftor-ivacaftor for cystic fibrosis with a single Phe508del allele. *N Engl J Med.* 2019;381:1809-1819.

A11. Barry PJ, Mall MA, Álvarez A, et al. Triple therapy for cystic fibrosis Phe508del-gating and -residual function genotypes. *N Engl J Med.* 2021;385:815-825.

78

BRONCHIECTASIS, ATELECTASIS, AND CAVITARY OR CYSTIC LUNG DISEASES

ANNE E. O'DONNELL

BRONCHIECTASIS

DEFINITION

Bronchiectasis is an abnormal permanent dilation of the bronchi and bronchioles caused by repeated cycles of airway infection and inflammation. The distal airways become thickened; the mucosal surfaces develop edema, inflammation, and suppuration; and ultimately there is neovascularization of the adjacent bronchial arterioles. Bronchiectasis, which can be focal or diffuse, is triggered by a variety of genetic, anatomic, and systemic processes. Abnormalities of cilia, mucus clearance, mucus rheology, airway drainage, and host defenses can result in bronchiectasis.[1] Regardless of the cause, patients with bronchiectasis develop chronic infections, which may lead to progressive lung destruction.

EPIDEMIOLOGY

Based on insurance claims reviews, an estimated 110,000 or more patients in the United States are receiving treatment for bronchiectasis that is not related to cystic fibrosis (Chapter 77), and these numbers appear to be increasing.[2] Similar findings have been reported in the United Kingdom and in other parts of the world. Recent U.S. data showed a prevalence of 4.2 per 100,000 persons aged 18 to 34 years and 272 per 100,000 among those older than 75 years. In the older age category, women are disproportionally represented. Other epidemiologic surveys suggest that there is increased risk for the development of bronchiectasis in individuals with reduced access to health care and higher rates of pulmonary infection in childhood.

PATHOBIOLOGY

In up to one third of cases, the cause of bronchiectasis is not identified. Other cases are related to pulmonary infections, genetic causes, anatomic abnormalities, and immune and autoimmune diseases.[3] Hyperconcentrated airway mucous is a characteristic pathogenic abnormality.

Pulmonary Infections

Approximately one third of patients with bronchiectasis have an infectious trigger, usually years before the onset of the disease. Childhood viral infections, such as pertussis (Chapter 289) and bacterial infection, can cause permanent damage to the airways, leading to bronchiectasis years after the initial infection. Mycobacterial tuberculosis with its resultant granulomatous inflammation of the airway, lung parenchyma, and lymph nodes can cause subsequent bronchiectasis (Chapter 299), and nontuberculous mycobacterial infections have been recognized as an increasing cause and complication of bronchiectasis, particularly in White women older than 55 years (Chapter 300). Nontuberculous mycobacterial–related bronchiectasis typically involves the right middle lobe and lingula and can be associated with the "tree-in-bud" pattern of bronchiolar involvement on computed tomography (CT) scans (see later section on imaging).

Genetics

Cystic fibrosis (Chapter 77) is characterized by bilateral diffuse bronchiectasis. Although many cystic fibrosis patients are diagnosed in childhood with multisystem disease, older patients may present with only pulmonary or pulmonary and sinus manifestations. Some patients with bronchiectasis may have subtle defects in the cystic fibrosis transmembrane conductance regulator channel without a clear-cut diagnosis of cystic fibrosis.

In primary ciliary dyskinesia, abnormalities in the dynein arms prevent normal ciliary beating. Patients with primary ciliary dyskinesia generally have significant sinopulmonary disease and infertility, and approximately half of these patients have Kartagener syndrome with situs inversus (Chapter 55). Patients with α_1-antitrypsin deficiency also may develop bronchiectasis.

Anatomic Causes

Patients with chronic abnormalities of their swallowing mechanism or with esophageal dysfunction may develop focal or diffuse bronchiectasis with lower lobe predominance (Chapter 124). Direct lung injury caused by acid or particulate matter aspiration or recurrent pneumonia may lead to bronchiectasis.

Severe asthma (Chapter 75) and chronic obstructive pulmonary disease (COPD; Chapter 76) are sometimes complicated by bronchiectasis.[3] Allergic bronchopulmonary aspergillosis (Chapter 311) can cause a distinct "finger-in-glove" central bronchiectasis observed on CT scans owing to chronic inflammation and mucous plugging. Airway abnormalities such as endobronchial tumors (Chapter 177), extrinsic compression by lymph nodes (right middle lobe syndrome), and foreign bodies are also rare causes of focal bronchiectasis. Tracheobronchomegaly (Mounier-Kuhn syndrome) is associated with distal bronchiectasis.

Immune and Autoimmune Diseases

Primary hypogammaglobulinemia (Chapter 231) leads to recurrent pulmonary infections that may result in bronchiectasis. Patients with immunoglobulin G subclass deficiencies may develop bronchiectasis if the deficiency leads to reduction in antibody production. Defects of neutrophil adhesion and chemotaxis (Chapter 153) have been found to cause bronchiectasis. Patients with human immunodeficiency virus infection (Chapter 359) have a higher prevalence of bronchiectasis than individuals with a normally functioning immune system.

Bronchiectasis is an increasingly recognized complication of collagen vascular diseases, particularly rheumatoid arthritis (Chapter 243) and Sjögren syndrome (Chapter 247). The airway injury is likely attributable to chronic inflammation or esophageal dysfunction. Inflammatory bowel disease (Chapter 127) also causes bronchiectasis by undetermined mechanisms.

CLINICAL MANIFESTATIONS

Patients present with chronic cough and usually have mucopurulent or purulent sputum production. Occasionally, a dry nonproductive cough is the primary manifestation. Other symptoms include dyspnea, intermittent hemoptysis, and pleuritic chest pain. Weight loss, malaise, and fatigue sometimes develop. When patients have infectious exacerbations, they may develop fever as well as an increase in their baseline symptoms. Physical findings in patients with bronchiectasis are nonspecific and include an abnormal chest examination with wheezing, crackles, or both. Clubbing of the digits is rare.

The clinical course of patients with bronchiectasis is variable. Some patients have few to no symptoms, others have daily cough with sputum production, and some patients have occasional to frequent exacerbations. A slow decline in pulmonary function is seen with bronchiectasis; the decline is more rapid in patients infected with *Pseudomonas aeruginosa* (Chapter 282) and in patients who have more frequent exacerbations.

DIAGNOSIS

Imaging Studies

Although the diagnosis may be suspected by plain chest radiography, high-resolution computed tomography (HRCT) is the current "gold standard" for confirming bronchiectasis. The characteristic CT findings are lack of bronchial tapering, bronchi visible in the peripheral 1 cm of the lungs, and an internal bronchial diameter greater than the diameter of the accompanying bronchial artery.[4] Other associated HRCT findings are cysts off the end of a bronchus, tree-in-bud irregular branching lines (E-Fig. 78-1) indicating mucus impaction (E-Figs. 78-2 and 78-3), volume loss (E-Fig. 78-4), and occasionally associated consolidation (Fig. 78-1). The location of the bronchiectatic airways may suggest the cause: upper lobe predominance is seen in cystic fibrosis and lower lobe predominance in aspiration syndromes (E-Fig. 78-5). Whereas right middle lobe and lingula involvement suggests the presence of nontuberculous mycobacterial infection (Fig. 78-2 and E-Figs. 78-6A and 78-6B), central bronchiectasis is seen with allergic bronchopulmonary aspergillosis (Fig. 78-3).

Pulmonary function testing, which should be performed on all patients with suspected bronchiectasis, usually shows airflow obstruction as measured by the ratio between the forced expiratory volume in 1 second (FEV_1) and forced vital capacity (FVC) (Chapter 73). The severity of the airflow obstruction and the rate of decline correlate with radiographic extent of disease and frequency of exacerbation. Bronchoscopy will detect airway abnormalities, including tumors, structural deformities, and foreign bodies, and hence should be considered in the evaluation of localized bronchiectasis.

Cultures of sputum and of bronchoalveolar lavage when expectorated sputum is not available have an important role in assessing the infectious complications of bronchiectasis. Molecular techniques have recently demonstrated diverse polymicrobial communities in the lungs of patients with bronchiectasis, both when they are clinically stable and also during an exacerbation.[5]

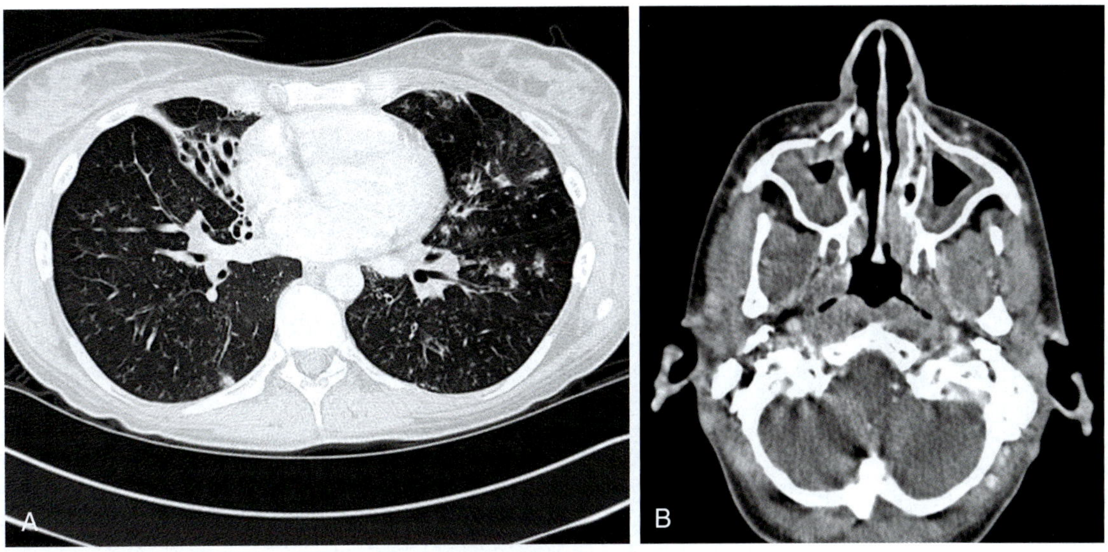

FIGURE 78-1. **Bilateral bronchiectasis. A and B, High-resolution computed tomography images of bilateral bronchiectasis in a patient with primary ciliary dyskinesia.**

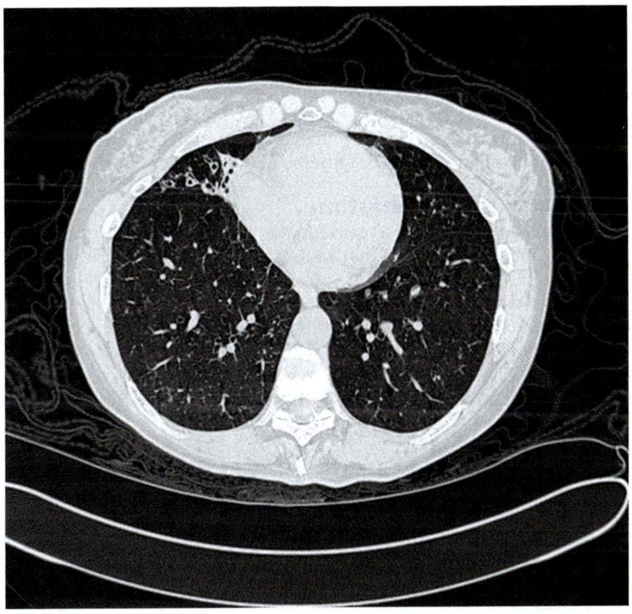

FIGURE 78-2. **High-resolution computed tomography image of nodular bronchiectasis caused by a nontuberculous mycobacterium infection.**

The dominant organisms are *P. aeruginosa* and *Haemophilus influenzae*, but anaerobic organisms also may be detected. The presence of *P. aeruginosa* portends a worse prognosis and more frequent exacerbations. Patients with no identifiable pathogens have the mildest disease. *Staphylococcus aureus* in the airway may suggest cystic fibrosis as the cause of the bronchiectasis. Nocardia and fungi, particularly aspergillus and candida, are sometimes cultured from bronchiectasis patients but do not always require treatment. Nontuberculous mycobacteria are found with increasing frequency in the airways of patients with bronchiectasis, usually as a complication of preexisting bronchiectasis but occasionally as its primary cause. The laboratory evaluation of patients with bronchiectasis should be individualized. All patients should have sputum cultures for bacterial, fungal, and mycobacterial testing. Other tests that should be considered include measurement of serum immunoglobulin levels and screening for genetic diseases, particularly in patients with diffuse bronchiectasis. Cystic fibrosis (Chapter 77) is diagnosed by elevated sweat chloride levels and by genetic testing. Primary ciliary dyskinesia can be evaluated by measurement of nasal nitric oxide levels, ciliary beat frequency and pattern testing, and electron microscopy studies. α_1-Antitrypsin deficiency is diagnosed by measuring levels and performing phenotyping (Chapter 76). Screening for rheumatoid arthritis (Chapter 243) or Sjögren syndrome (Chapter 247) also may be reasonable in patients with diffuse bronchiectasis.

TREATMENT

The goals of treatment are to reduce the frequency of exacerbations and potentially to improve quality of life, reduce symptoms, and alter the natural history of the disease (Table 78-1).[6–8] Multimodality maintenance treatment for patients with more advanced or symptomatic disease may include airway clearance and anti-inflammatory therapies. Long-term antibiotic therapy, which reduces markers of airways and systemic inflammation, should be considered in patients who have two to three or more exacerbations per year. Pulmonary rehabilitation also is efficacious. Exacerbations are treated based on clinical acuity. Because patients are heterogeneous and therapeutic trials are few, therapy is commonly individualized, especially because no therapies are currently approved by the U.S. Food and Drug Administration for non–cystic fibrosis bronchiectasis and because the proven treatments for cystic fibrosis are often not effective in this patient population.

Preventing Exacerbations

The 23-valent pneumococcal vaccination (Chapter 15) is recommended for patients with bronchiectasis. Routine seasonal influenza vaccination is also standard. At present, no vaccines are available for prevention of the other infectious complications of bronchiectasis. Of note, is that infectious exacerbations appear to have decreased during the coronavirus-19 (COVID-19) pandemic, presumably attributed to social distancing and masking.[9]

Treatment of the Underlying Etiology

For treatable conditions, such as immunoglobulin deficiency or α_1-antitrypsin deficiency (Chapter 76), replacement therapy (Chapter 231) should be considered even though there are few data on whether those therapies alter the natural history of the bronchiectasis and resultant infections. Patients with allergic bronchopulmonary aspergillosis (Chapter 311) should be treated with steroids to mitigate the inflammatory process that leads to the bronchiectasis.

Airway Clearance

Chest physiotherapy and the use of devices to aid mucociliary clearance appear to be beneficial in non–cystic fibrosis bronchiectasis. Patients should be taught airway clearance maneuvers that they can perform independently.[10] Twice-daily use of an oscillatory positive expiratory pressure device (Acapella) can improve sputum volume and quality of life. Other techniques that also may have a role for airway clearance include traditional chest physical therapy with postural drainage and high-frequency chest wall oscillator vests. Formal pulmonary rehabilitation and exercise likely benefit patients with bronchiectasis. Personalizing the treatment yields the best compliance and results.

Inhaled therapy with nebulized hypertonic saline (3 to 7%) may enhance airway clearance, decrease exacerbations, and improve lung function as well as quality of life.[A1] A novel neutrophil elastase inhibitor, brensocatib (10 to 25 mg orally daily), can improve clinical outcomes, including prolonging the time to first exacerbation, in patients who have non–cystic fibrosis bronchiectasis and who have had two or more exacerbations in the prior year.[A2] Although recombinant human DNase is efficacious in cystic fibrosis bronchiectasis, a large clinical trial showed it had deleterious effects when given as maintenance therapy in patients with non–cystic fibrosis bronchiectasis, so it should not be used. Other mucolytic agents are of unproven benefit.

No randomized trials support the use of routine short-acting β-agonist or anticholinergic bronchodilators in bronchiectasis. However, a subset of patients with airway reactivity likely benefits from use of these agents (Chapter 75).

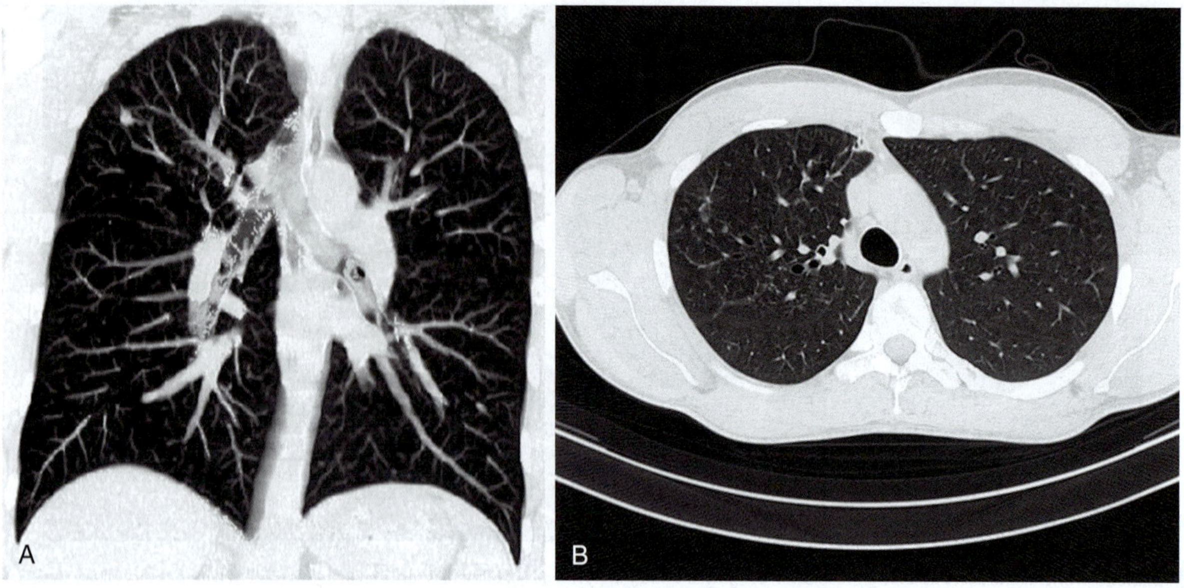

FIGURE 78-3. A and B, High-resolution computed tomography images of finger-in-glove central bronchiectasis caused by allergic bronchopulmonary aspergillosis; best shown in the coronal display of panel A.

TABLE 78-1 POTENTIAL THERAPIES FOR BRONCHIECTASIS

Treatment of underlying condition, if possible
Mobilization of secretions
Pharmacologic
Mechanical
Anti-inflammatory therapy
Inhaled steroids
Macrolides
Antimicrobial therapy
Pathogen specific
Surgery
Localized or refractory disease
Transplantation
End-stage disease

Adapted from O'Donnell A. Bronchiectasis. *Chest*. 2008;134:815-823.

Reduction of Airway Inflammation

Inhaled medium-dose budesonide, when combined with formoterol, is safe and more effective than high-dose budesonide in treating patients with non–cystic fibrosis bronchiectasis. Oral steroids, although occasionally used in patients with bronchiectasis, have never been evaluated in a clinical trial. A small case series suggested potential benefit from mepolizumab in patients who have severe uncontrolled asthma complicated by bronchiectasis.[11]

Antimicrobial Therapy

At present, there is no firm evidence to support the use of routine maintenance antibiotics, although such therapy may be considered in patients with frequent exacerbations and progressive lung destruction. When mycobacterial species are cultured from patients with bronchiectasis, decisions regarding whether to treat and which antimicrobial agents to use are based on published guidelines (Chapters 299 and 300).[12]

Chronic low-dose oral macrolide therapy (e.g., azithromycin 500 mg three times per week or 250 mg/day or erythromycin ethylsuccinate 400 mg twice daily) can reduce exacerbations in patients with non–cystic fibrosis bronchiectasis.[A3] Whether patients will develop resistant organisms is of concern, and the respiratory microbiota is clearly changed by the chronic use of macrolides. Macrolide monotherapy should not be used in patients coinfected with nontuberculous mycobacteria.

Targeted inhaled antimicrobial therapies are also an option, particularly in patients infected with *Pseudomonas* spp. For example, nebulized gentamicin (80 mg twice daily) for 12 months can provide sustained bacteriologic and clinical benefit. Inhaled tobramycin can reduce bacterial colony forming units, but adverse respiratory side effects limit its use.[A4] Inhaled colistin, 1 million IU twice daily delivered by nebulizer, also is safe and possibly effective in adherent patients with bronchiectasis and *P. aeruginosa* infection. Two large trials of inhaled aztreonam lysine showed no clinical improvement, but there may be a benefit in patients with the most severe baseline symptoms. Randomized controlled trials of dry powder ciprofloxacin and nebulized liposomal ciprofloxacin have shown mixed results.[A5] Other off-label antibiotic strategies include prolonged intravenous antibiotics targeted at the specific cultured pathogens.

Surgery and Transplantation

Resectional surgery may have a role for patients who have focal disease or for patients who have hemoptysis that cannot be controlled by embolization of the bleeding vessels (Chapter 87). Surgical resection can also benefit some patients who have diffuse bronchiectasis unresponsive to conventional therapy and some patients infected with nontuberculous mycobacteria. Double-lung transplantation (Chapter 87) has been successfully performed in patients with end-stage lung disease caused by non–cystic fibrosis bronchiectasis, and the clinical outcomes parallel those seen with transplantation for other end-stage lung diseases.

Treatment of Acute Exacerbations of Bronchiectasis

When a patient with bronchiectasis experiences an acute exacerbation, antimicrobial treatments should be aimed at the chronic infecting organisms.[13] Mild to moderate exacerbations can be treated with oral antibiotics, targeted to the results of the sputum culture, for 2 to 3 weeks. Viruses, including coronavirus, rhinovirus, and influenza A and B viruses also cause exacerbations. More severe exacerbations or exacerbations caused by resistant organisms generally require intravenous antibiotics administered in the hospital or at home. No benefit has yet been demonstrated by adding an inhaled antibiotic to systemic therapy for an acute exacerbation. Patients experiencing an acute exacerbation likely benefit from airway clearance modalities and the other nonantibiotic therapies discussed previously.

PROGNOSIS

Non–cystic fibrosis bronchiectasis is a heterogeneous disease with a widely variable prognosis. Patients with more severe obstructive and restrictive findings on pulmonary function tests, poor gas transfer, and chronic pseudomonal infection have the worst prognosis. Independent predictors of future hospitalization include prior hospital admissions, advanced dyspnea, FEV_1 less than 30% predicted, *P. aeruginosa* colonization, colonization with other pathogenic organisms, and three or more lobes involved on HRCT. Comorbidities, including COPD and rheumatoid arthritis, increase the risk for mortality. Radiographic extent of disease, hypoxemia, hypercapnia, and evidence of right heart failure are also predictors of outcome. Bronchiectasis patients who are admitted to an intensive care unit for respiratory failure have been reported to have a 60% 4-year survival rate.

ATELECTASIS

DEFINITION

Atelectasis, or collapse, is caused by hypoventilation of lung units. Atelectasis may involve an entire lung or a lobe, segment, or subsegment. Atelectasis can be caused by intrinsic obstruction of an airway or external compression from lymph nodes, parenchymal masses, or other entities. When lung units are atelectatic, ventilation-perfusion mismatch leads to hypoxemia. Infection may result from sustained atelectasis.

EPIDEMIOLOGY AND PATHOBIOLOGY

The lung bases and posterior segments are vulnerable to dependent atelectasis, which is caused by inadequate ventilation, particularly in an immobilized or postoperative patient. Patchy atelectasis is caused by alveolar filling processes, such as hemorrhage and edema (Chapter 79). Passive, relaxation, or compression atelectasis occurs when the lung recoils to a smaller volume because of fluid or air in the adjacent pleural space.

Obstructive or resorptive atelectasis is caused by bronchial block to the entry of air, with resultant retractile consolidation. Intrinsic airway obstruction may be caused by mucous plugs, foreign bodies, or tumors in the airway. Extrinsic airway obstruction results from compression of the airway owing to peribronchial lymph node enlargement or other masses impinging on the airway.

Rounded atelectasis is caused by pleural thickening that invaginates and traps adjacent lung. Any chronic pleural disease can cause rounded atelectasis, particularly asbestos-related pleural disease.

CLINICAL MANIFESTATIONS AND DIAGNOSIS

Atelectasis is typically asymptomatic and diagnosed on chest imaging or bedside ultrasound; it may cause dyspnea and tachypnea and result in hypoxemia.[14] In postoperative patients, atelectasis may be a cause of low-grade fever. An arterial oxygen saturation of 96% or less after breathing oxygen through a Venturi mask for 30 minutes is a moderately sensitive and specific test for diagnosing postoperative atelectasis.

Plain chest radiography shows loss of lung volume and the displacement of the lobar fissure, mediastinum, or diaphragm toward the involved lung unit (Fig. 78-4). Platelike or discoid atelectasis manifests as horizontal or curvilinear lines on plain chest radiography. Rounded atelectasis (Fig. 78-5) is an ovoid masslike density abutting the pleura. Secondary atelectasis can be seen in association with a mass lesion (E-Figs. 78-7A and 78-7B). The type and cause of atelectasis can sometimes be elucidated by CT or ultrasonography. Bronchoscopy is required to confirm intrinsic versus extrinsic compression in obstructive-resorptive atelectasis and to determine the exact pathology of the obstruction.

At the bedside, a measurement of arterial oxygen saturation can help assess the severity of the atelectasis and overall lung dysfunction.

PREVENTION AND TREATMENT

Incentive spirometry is commonly prescribed to prevent or treat atelectasis in patients with limited mobility because of recent surgery, neuromuscular weakness, or any prolonged immobilization, but no randomized controlled trials have proved its effectiveness. Preoperative inspiratory muscle training and recruitment maneuvers may reduce atelectasis in patients undergoing upper abdominal or cardiac surgery,[A6] and prophylactic use of noninvasive ventilation may reduce pulmonary dysfunction after lung resection surgery. Other modalities such as positive expiratory pressure devices, high-frequency chest wall oscillation airway clearance, and pharmacologic agents are of no proven benefit.

Patchy atelectasis is treated by addressing the underlying disease process in the lung parenchyma. Compression atelectasis is treated by alleviating the pleural space process.

Obstructive or resorptive atelectasis often requires bronchoscopy for diagnosis and treatment. In patients with obstruction owing to retained secretions, multiple bronchoscopies are sometimes required, but the mucus often rapidly reaccumulates and will resolve only when the patient's overall status improves.

Rounded atelectasis does not require treatment. CT is helpful in distinguishing rounded atelectasis from parenchymal tumor.

CAVITARY LUNG DISEASES

DEFINITION

A lung cavity is a gas-filled space with a well-defined wall (greater than 4 mm thick) within a nodule, mass, or area of parenchymal consolidation. Cavities can be acute or subacute, and they may be solitary or multiple. A cavity that is more than 2 cm in largest diameter, is caused by liquefactive necrosis of the lung tissue, and that contains necrotic debris or fluid as a result of microbial infection is a lung abscess.[15]

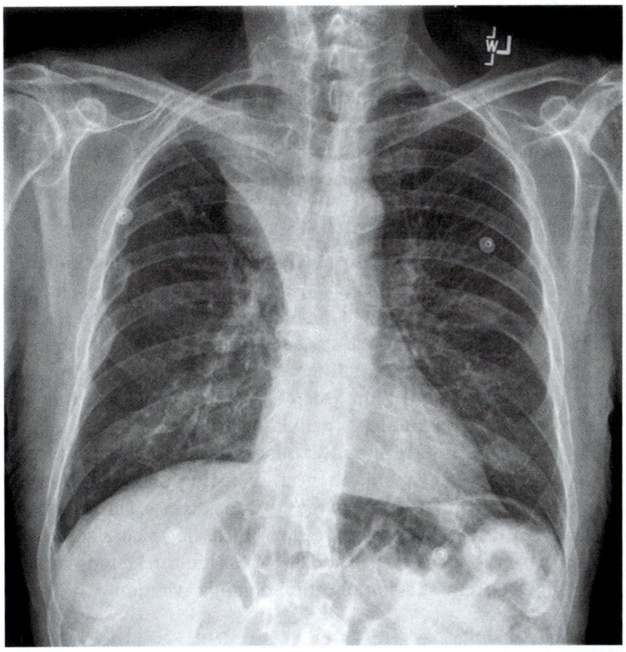

FIGURE 78-4. Plain chest radiograph demonstrating right upper lobe atelectasis (caused by an endobronchial tumor).

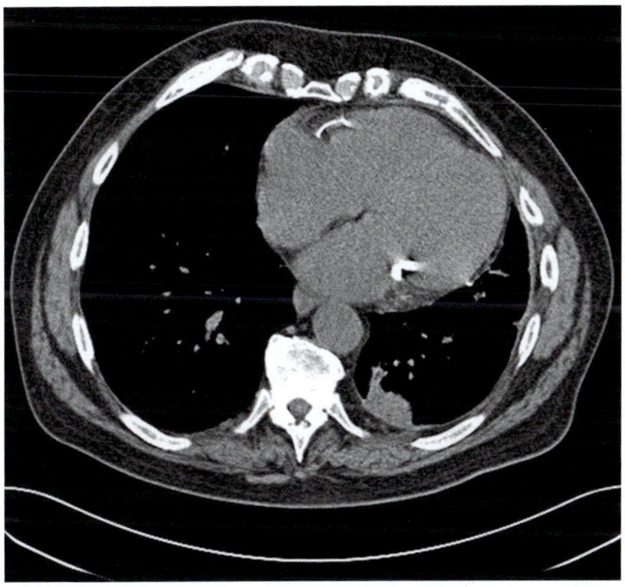

FIGURE 78-5. Computed tomography image of rounded atelectasis.

EPIDEMIOLOGY

The incidence and prevalence of cavitary lung disease is unknown. Lung cavitation can occur across a wide range of underlying diseases, including pulmonary infection, vascular pulmonary disease, malignancy, and autoimmune disorders (Table 78-2).

PATHOBIOLOGY

A lung cavity forms when necrosis and subsequent liquefaction of lung tissue is followed by removal of that debris via the bronchial tree. Bacterial, fungal, mycobacterial, and parasitic infections can cause cavitation. Bacterial infections also can result from aspiration of oral bacteria, especially in patients who have chronic aspiration but also in healthy immunocompetent individuals as a result of dental procedures. Infections that spread hematogenously (septic pulmonary emboli; Chapter 61) may result in multiple areas of cavitation. Organisms associated with lung necrosis include gram-negative and anaerobic bacteria, *Staphylococcus aureus* (Chapter 267), aspergillus (Chapter 311), tuberculous and nontuberculous mycobacteria (Chapters 299 and 300), paragonimus

(Chapter 326), and echinococcus (Chapter 325). Lung abscesses also have been reported as a complication of severe acute respiratory syndrome coronavirus-2 (SARS-CoV-2) pneumonia. Noninfectious causes of lung cavities include autoimmune diseases such as rheumatoid arthritis (Chapter 243) and granulomatosis with polyangiitis (Chapter 249), as well as malignancy (e.g., carcinoma or lymphoma). Sometimes lung cavitation is a consequence of cancer treatment, especially radiation therapy.

CLINICAL MANIFESTATIONS

Patients with cavitary lung disease generally have a productive cough, often with purulent or bloody sputum. Chest pain is occasionally present, particularly if the lung abscess has resulted in pleural effusion or empyema (Chapter 86). Other manifestations include systemic symptoms such as fever, rigors, and weight loss. Subacute presentations (3 months or less of symptoms) are more typical of bacterial infection, whereas more chronic symptoms suggest fungal, mycobacterial, vasculitic, or neoplastic causes.

Cavitary lung disease due to noninfectious causes may be less likely to present with these symptoms, but patients often have constitutional complaints as well as extrapulmonary manifestations of the systemic disease. Untreated cavitary lung disease may lead to local complications, including pleural infection, and may also cause sepsis or even sepsis shock. Rarely, life-threatening hemoptysis (Chapter 71) can occur as a complication of lung cavitation.

DIAGNOSIS

Cavitary lung disease is diagnosed by chest imaging (Fig. 78-6). Plain chest radiographs may demonstrate areas of cavitation; whereas CT imaging is often helpful in documenting the extent of disease and detecting features that may suggest the etiology of the cavities.[16] If prior imaging studies are available, they may also provide clues as to the cause of the cavitation. Further diagnostic evaluation includes cultures of sputum and blood. If septic emboli are suspected, echocardiography may be helpful to assess for valvular vegetations indicative of endocarditis. Inflammatory markers and testing for autoimmune diseases may also provide clues, especially when there are no clinical signs to suggest infection. When malignancy is suspected, positron emission tomography (PET) scanning may be helpful to look for evidence of extrathoracic disease. Image-guided aspiration for culture or needle biopsy[17] is often required to make a definitive diagnosis.

TABLE 78-2 CAUSES OF CAVITARY LUNG LESIONS

INFECTIOUS

Bacterial aspiration/pneumonia
  Anaerobic bacteria
  Aerobic bacteria
Bacterial embolic
  Especially *Staphylococcus aureus*
Mycobacteria
  Often multifocal
Fungi
Parasites
  Especially *Echinococcus* or *Paragonimus westermani*

VASCULITIS
Especially rheumatoid arthritis or granulomatosis with polyangiitis
MALIGNANT
Necrotizing carcinoma Lymphoma

TREATMENT

Treatment of cavitary lung disease must be aimed at the underlying cause. Necrotizing pneumonia due to bacterial, mycobacterial, fungal, and parasitic infections often responds to prolonged (6 weeks) systemic antibiotic therapy,[18] targeted against the pathogen diagnosed by cultures of blood, bronchoalveolar lavage fluid, or needle aspiration. Percutaneous tube drainage of a lung abscess can speed the resolution of infection and decrease hospital length-of-stay.[A7] Occasionally, salvage surgery is needed to remove areas of persistent necrosis. Patients who have lung cavitation owing to autoimmune disease or malignancy generally resolve the cavities with successful systemic treatment of the underlying process.

PREVENTION

Infectious cavitary lung disease can be prevented in some patients by improving oral hygiene and preventing aspiration of oral and gastric contents. Prompt treatment of endocarditis and removal of infected intravascular devices may also prevent cavitary infections owing to septic pulmonary emboli.

PROGNOSIS

The prognosis of cavitary lung disease depends upon the cause. Successful treatment of primary infections will often cure the areas of cavitation. Likewise, cavitary lung disease caused by autoimmune disease and malignancy may resolve if those underlying diseases are successfully treated.

CONGENITAL CYSTIC DISEASES OF THE THORAX

Thoracic cysts,[19] which are exceedingly rare, develop because of abnormal development or branching of the foregut. Cysts may develop in the mediastinum at an early stage of gestation or in the lung parenchyma at a later stage. Abnormalities include bronchogenic cysts (mediastinal and parenchymal), congenital pulmonary airway malformation, and pulmonary sequestrations. The cysts are lined with airway and alveolar epithelium but do not communicate in a normal fashion with the airways or lung tissue. Congenital lung malformations may be due to disruptions in Ras or phosphatidylinositol 3-kinase-AKT-mammalian target of rapamycin signaling pathways.

Most patients with thoracic cysts present in childhood, but the cysts can remain asymptomatic and unnoticed until adulthood. In the absence of symptoms, these cystic lesions sometimes present as an incidental finding on chest imaging performed for another indication. Congenital cystic diseases can cause recurrent pneumonia, hemoptysis, or compression of normal structures.

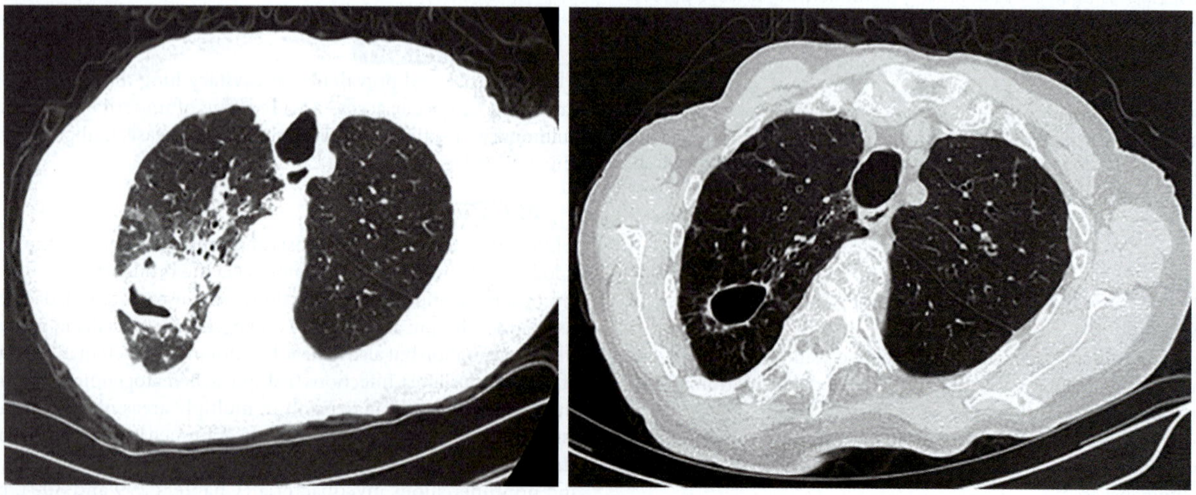

FIGURE 78-6. Cavitary pneumonia due to *Mycobacterium* abscess (left slice pre-treatment; right slice post-treatment).

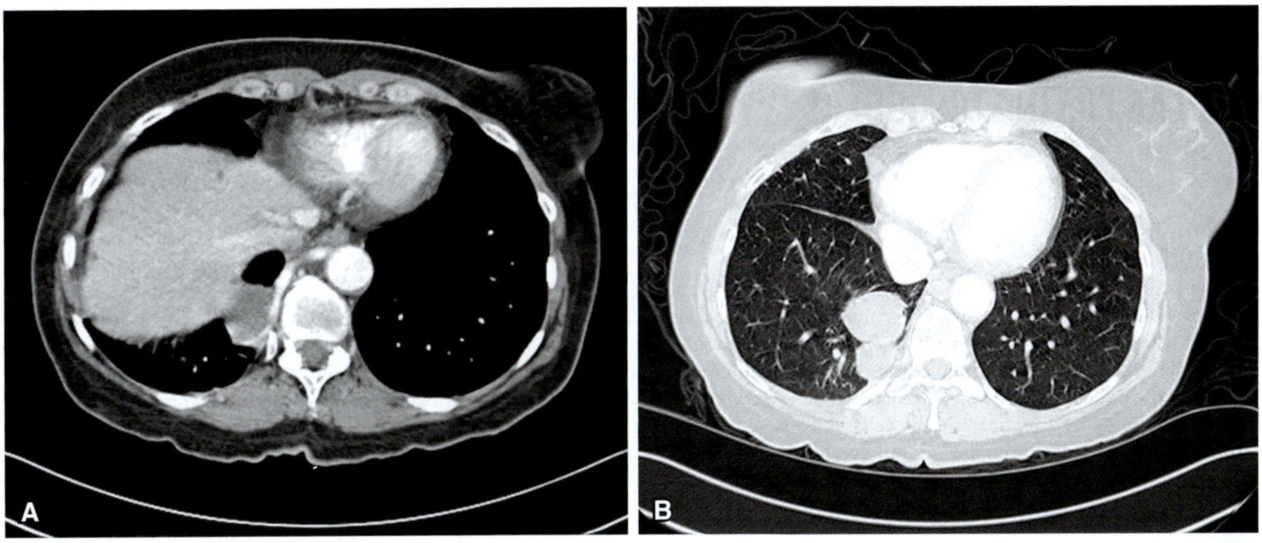

FIGURE 78-7. Pulmonary sequestration. A, Computed tomography image of pulmonary sequestration in right lower lobe. B, Feeding vessel visible arising from the aorta.

CT angiography can usually detect congenital cystic lesions of the thorax, but pulmonary or bronchial angiography is sometimes necessary to define the blood flow to the lesion.

Bronchogenic cysts are usually found in the right paratracheal or subcarinal areas of the mediastinum but are occasionally seen in the lung parenchyma. These cysts are often asymptomatic, but they can cause wheezing, dyspnea, and cough when they compress adjacent structures. Secondary infection may develop in the cysts, and there are a few case reports of malignant transformation. Complete surgical resection is generally recommended, but partial excision with de-epithelization of the cysts also has been performed. Observation is also an option when the cysts are asymptomatic.

Congenital pulmonary airway malformation, previously called *congenital cystic adenomatoid malformation of the lung*, is an exceedingly rare abnormality with reported incidence of 1 in every 25,000 to 35,000 pregnancies. The abnormality is caused by arrested development of the bronchial tree. Most patients are diagnosed prenatally by ultrasonography, but the condition may rarely first present in adulthood with complications, including pneumothorax and air embolism. Treatment is anatomic surgical resection.

Pulmonary sequestrations are areas of nonfunctioning pulmonary parenchyma with no communication to the tracheobronchial tree and abnormal arterial supply and venous drainage (Fig. 78-7). Intralobar sequestration, which accounts for about 75% of cases, does not have visceral pleura and is generally found in a lower lobe, the left more frequently than the right. Extralobar sequestrations have their own visceral pleura, are separate from the normal lobes, and even may be found below the diaphragms. Sequestrations usually have a feeding vessel that arises from the aorta. Sequestrations may be asymptomatic, but patients sometimes develop recurrent infections and/or hemoptysis. Surgical excision with special care for the management of the feeding vessel is curative. Embolization of the feeding vessel is sometimes a successful treatment option.

Hyperlucent lungs are diagnosed by a paucity of vascular and interstitial markings noted on chest imaging. Lung parenchymal air collections can be caused by congenital parenchymal cysts, congenital lobar emphysema (almost exclusively diagnosed in infancy), giant bullous emphysema (vanishing lung syndrome), or Swyer-James syndrome. Lung parenchymal cysts may be a bullous alveolar type or may contain bronchial wall elements such as cartilage, smooth muscle, and glands. They may become infected and may rupture to cause pneumothorax. Surgical resection is generally recommended unless the lesions are small. Congenital lobar emphysema, otherwise known as *congenital large hyperlucent lobe,* may cause severe respiratory distress in infants owing to compression of surrounding lung tissue. Giant bullous emphysema is a rare condition that usually affects the upper lobes of young male smokers. Compression of normal lung parenchyma from these overdistended lobes may require surgical resection.

Birt-Hogg-Dubé syndrome is caused by an autosomal dominant condition of germline mutations in the folliculin gene. It is characterized by pulmonary cysts, recurrent pneumothoraces, renal cell carcinomas, and skin fibrofolliculomas.

Swyer-James-Macleod syndrome, which is characterized by unilateral lucency of an entire lung, is caused by childhood bronchiolitis obliterans owing to viral or bacterial infection or toxic inhalation. CT shows air trapping and hyperlucency of the affected lung, with a normal contralateral lung. No therapy is required.

ACQUIRED CYSTIC LUNG DISEASES

High-resolution CT scans can detect a variety of acquired cystic lung diseases.[20] Cysts typically represent as subpleural emphysema or bullae in the lung parenchyma. Causes of multifocal cysts include lymphocytic interstitial pneumonia (Chapter 80), Birt-Hogg-Dubé syndrome, tracheobronchial papillomatosis, and primary and metastatic cancers. Multifocal cysts with associated nodules are seen in lymphocytic interstitial pneumonia (Chapter 80), light chain deposition disease (Chapter 173), amyloidosis (Chapter 174), and Langerhans cell histiocytosis (Chapter 155) and are associated with ground-glass opacities in *Pneumocystis jiroveci* pneumonia (Chapter 313) and desquamative interstitial pneumonia (Chapter 80). Emphysema (Chapter 76) and cystic bronchiectasis also can mimic cystic disease. A careful noninvasive evaluation can usually determine the cause, but bronchoalveolar lavage or even lung biopsy may be required.

GENERAL REFERENCES

For the General References and other additional features, please visit Elsevier eBooks+ at https://ebooks.health.elsevier.com.

Grade A References

A1. Anuradha KWDA, Gunathilaka PKG, Wickramasinghe VP. Effectiveness of hypertonic saline nebulization in airway clearance in children with non-cystic fibrosis bronchiectasis: a randomized control trial. *Pediatr Pulmonol.* 2021;56:509-515.

A2. Chalmers JD, Haworth CS, Metersky ML, et al. Phase 2 trial of DPP-1 inhibitor brensocatib in bronchiectasis. *N Engl J Med.* 2020;383:2127-2137.

A3. Chalmers JD, Boersma W. Long-term macrolide antibiotics for the treatment of bronchiectasis in adults: an individual participant data meta-analysis. *Lancet Respir Med.* 2019;10:845-854.

A4. Loebinger MR, Polverino E, Chalmers JD, et al. Efficacy and safety of TOBI Podhaler in *Pseudomonas aeruginosa* infected bronchiectasis patients: iBEST study. *Eur Respir J.* 2021;57:2001451.

A5. Wang S, Zhang A, Yao X. Meta-analysis of efficacy and safety of inhaled ciprofloxacin in non-cystic fibrosis bronchiectasis patients. *Intern Med J.* 2021;51:1505-1512.

A6. Hu MC, Yang YL, Chen TT, et al. Recruitment maneuvers to reduce pulmonary atelectasis after cardiac surgery: a meta-analysis of randomized trials. *J Thorac Cardiovasc Surg.* 2022;164:171-181.e4.

A7. Lin Q, Jin M, Luo J, et al. Efficacy and safety of percutaneous tube drainage in lung abscess: a systematic review and meta-analysis. *Expert Rev Respir Med.* 2020;14:949-956.

79

ALVEOLAR FILLING DISORDERS

STEPHANIE M. LEVINE

DEFINITION

Alveolar filling disorders (Table 79-1) are characterized by chest radiographic findings of alveolar involvement ranging from a ground-glass appearance to consolidation; the pathologic process shows primary involvement of the alveolar air spaces distal to the terminal bronchioles. For example, in pulmonary alveolar proteinosis, the alveoli are filled by proteinaceous fluid. By comparison, the alveolar walls are lined by adenocarcinoma cells in invasive mucinous adenocarcinoma and lepidic predominant nonmucinous adenocarcinoma, formerly called bronchioloalveolar cell cancer. In acute interstitial pneumonia, exudative organizing fibroproliferative infiltrates fill the alveolar space; in the alveolar hemorrhage disorders, blood fills the alveolar space. Alveolar spaces filled with acute inflammatory cells, as in bacterial pneumonia (Chapter 85); water, as in cardiogenic or hydrostatic pulmonary edema (Chapter 45); or high-protein fluid, as in noncardiogenic or increased permeability pulmonary edema (Chapter 90), are also part of the radiographic differential diagnosis of alveolar filling disorders and must be excluded.

TABLE 79-1 ALVEOLAR FILLING DISORDERS

DISEASES	PATHOPHYSIOLOGY	RADIOGRAPHIC FINDINGS
Pulmonary alveolar proteinosis	Impaired processing of surfactant by alveolar macrophages caused by defects in GM-CSF signaling	Bilateral alveolar opacities with "crazy paving" and diffuse areas of ground-glass attenuation on CT scan
Acute interstitial pneumonia	Diffuse alveolar damage with temporal uniformity	Diffuse alveolar filling process similar to acute respiratory distress syndrome
Diffuse alveolar hemorrhage	Bleeding from the pulmonary microcirculation, usually from the capillaries	Acute development of bilateral alveolar opacities
Invasive mucinous adenocarcinoma and lepidic predominant nonmucinous adenocarcinoma (formerly called bronchioloalveolar cell carcinoma)	Cancer cells growing along the alveolar septa	Pneumonic opacities, consolidation with air bronchograms, ground-glass opacities (either solitary or multiple)

CT = computed tomography; GM-CSF = granulocyte-macrophage colony-stimulating factor.

A general approach to these suspected alveolar filling diseases (Fig. 79-1) can be stratified by the time elapsed since the onset of symptoms. The typical patient may present with the onset of cough (usually dry) and dyspnea of variable duration, depending on the disease process. Hemoptysis is a frequent presenting symptom in the alveolar hemorrhagic disorders. With the exception of acute interstitial pneumonia, symptoms suggesting an acute infectious process such as fever, leukocytosis, and productive cough are usually absent. If the initial chest radiograph or chest computed tomography (CT) is consistent with a possible alveolar filling process (Chapter 72) and acute pneumonia and pulmonary edema are excluded, bronchoscopy with bronchoalveolar lavage (Chapter 73) and transbronchial biopsy should be performed, particularly if pulmonary alveolar proteinosis, invasive mucinous adenocarcinoma, lepidic predominant nonmucinous adenocarcinoma (Chapter 177), or alveolar hemorrhage is suspected. When these tests are nondiagnostic, and in many cases of suspected acute interstitial pneumonia, a surgical lung biopsy obtained by thoracoscopy or an open surgical procedure may be indicated to establish a firm diagnosis.

PULMONARY ALVEOLAR PROTEINOSIS

EPIDEMIOLOGY

Pulmonary alveolar proteinosis is a rare alveolar filling disease caused by the accumulation of phospholipoproteinaceous surfactant material in the alveoli. The incidence is estimated to be 3.7 cases per million people. Pulmonary alveolar proteinosis is a primary acquired, autoimmune disorder in more than 90% of cases,[1] but similar histopathologic features may be found with identifiable secondary causes, such as acute silicosis (silicoproteinosis; Chapter 81), aluminum dust exposure (Chapter 81), indium dust exposure, immunodeficiency disorders (e.g., immunoglobulin G monoclonal gammopathy and severe combined immunodeficiency syndrome), hematologic malignant neoplasms (particularly myeloid leukemias; Chapters 168 and 170), and certain infections (e.g., *Pneumocystis jiroveci* pneumonia and severe acute respiratory syndrome coronavirus 2 [Chapter 336]).[2] Pulmonary alveolar proteinosis has also been described after bone marrow transplantation (Chapter 163). A congenital form also usually presents in infancy.

PATHOBIOLOGY

The pathogenesis of pulmonary alveolar proteinosis is related to impaired processing of surfactant by alveolar macrophages caused by defects in granulocyte-macrophage colony-stimulating factor (GM-CSF) signaling. This impairment

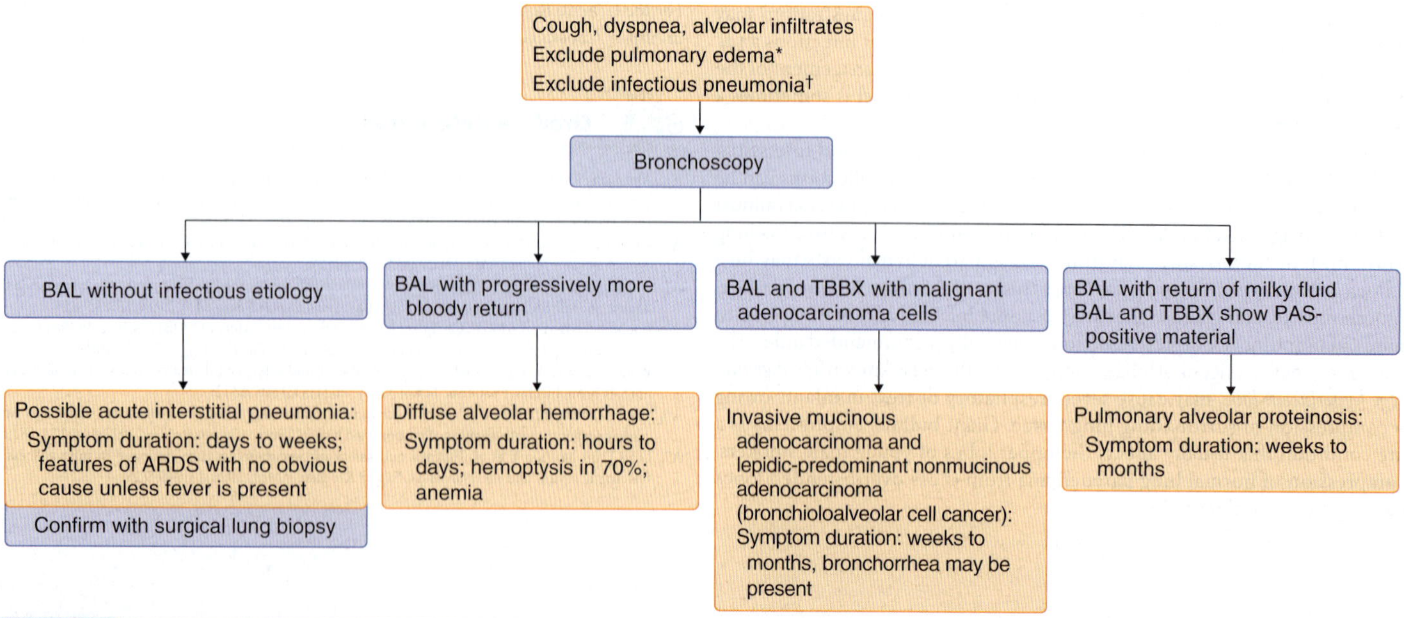

FIGURE 79-1. **A general approach to the alveolar filling disorders.** *See Chapter 45. †See Chapter 85. ARDS = acute respiratory distress syndrome; BAL = bronchoalveolar lavage; PAS = periodic acid–Schiff; TBBX = transbronchial biopsy.

may be caused by autoantibodies against GM-CSF or GM-CSF receptor gene mutations, which are found in 90% of cases. The secondary forms are caused by a relative GM-CSF deficiency, leading to macrophage dysfunction and reduced surfactant clearance. The autosomal recessive congenital form of pulmonary alveolar proteinosis, caused by a mutation in the genes encoding surfactant protein B or C, or the GM-CSF receptor results in abnormal surfactant function and severe respiratory distress in homozygous infants. The result of this impairment is accumulation of surfactant-rich material and progressive dysfunction in phagocytosis caused by excessive production or diminished clearance of surfactant by alveolar macrophages.

Histologic examination in pulmonary alveolar proteinosis reveals alveoli filled with lipoproteinaceous material that stains pink (positive reaction) with periodic acid–Schiff stain. Classically, there is no destruction of alveolar architecture. Electron microscopy reveals lamellar (phospholipid-containing) myelin bodies.

CLINICAL MANIFESTATIONS

Pulmonary alveolar proteinosis presents in patients in the third to fourth decade of life with a 2 : 1 male predominance. Most patients (72%) are smokers. Patients present with the insidious onset of dyspnea and cough, which may be dry or occasionally productive of grayish material.[3] The duration of symptoms before diagnosis is typically 6 weeks to 6 to 8 months. Low-grade fevers, malaise, and weight loss may also be present. Hemoptysis is unusual. On physical examination, rales are present in 50% of cases. Clubbing is an unusual finding until later stages of disease.

DIAGNOSIS

Mildly elevated leukocyte counts and mildly to moderately elevated lactate dehydrogenase (LDH) levels may be found in the blood in more than 80% of patients; LDH levels may correlate with the severity of disease. Polycythemia and hypergammaglobulinemia may also be present. The chest radiograph (Fig. 79-2) and chest CT scans demonstrate a diffuse symmetrical alveolar filling process with predominance in the lower two thirds of the lung fields; the radiographic appearance may mimic pulmonary edema. The characteristic CT pattern is often described as "crazy paving," which is attributable to scattered or diffuse areas of ground-glass attenuation with thickening of intralobular structures and interlobular septa in polygonal shapes (Fig. 79-3 and E-Fig. 79-1), sometimes with a subpleural sparing pattern.[4] This radiographic pattern is not specific for this disorder and can be seen in a variety of pulmonary disorders, including but not limited to acute respiratory distress syndrome (ARDS; Chapter 90), *P. jiroveci* pneumonia (Chapter 313), adenocarcinomas formerly described as bronchioloalveolar carcinoma (Chapter 177), lipoid pneumonia (Chapter 82), sarcoidosis (Chapter 83), organizing pneumonia, drug reactions, pulmonary hemorrhage, cardiogenic pulmonary edema (Chapter 46), and acute interstitial pneumonias. Pulmonary function tests often, but not always, show a restrictive pattern with a reduced diffusing capacity. Arterial blood gas analyses reveal hypoxemia.

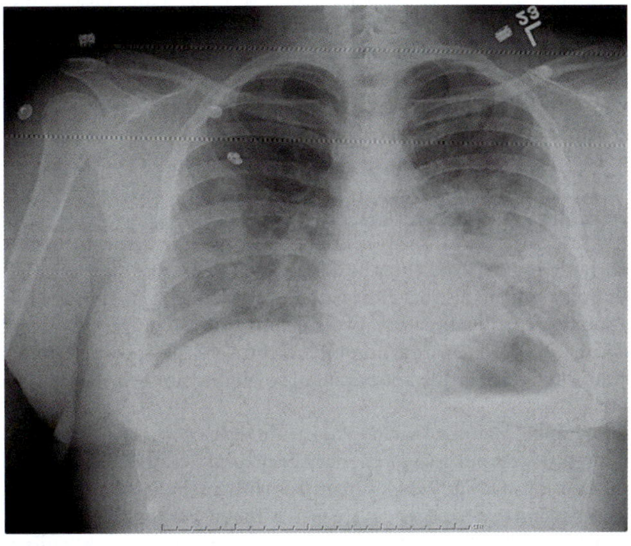

FIGURE 79-2. A chest radiograph showing bilateral alveolar opacities in a patient with pulmonary alveolar proteinosis.

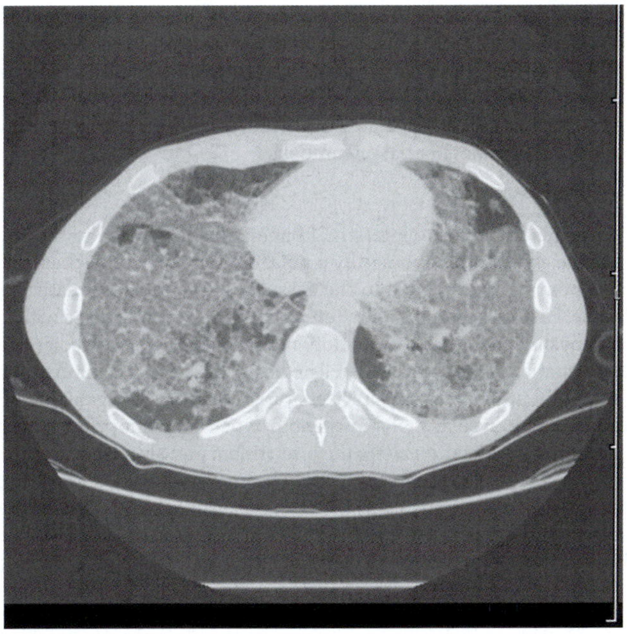

FIGURE 79-3. A chest computed tomography scan showing the "crazy paving" pattern characteristic of pulmonary alveolar proteinosis.

Bronchoscopy should be the initial procedure when pulmonary alveolar proteinosis is suspected. The diagnosis of pulmonary alveolar proteinosis can be established in most cases by the recovery of milky white to sandy-colored or light brown fluid on bronchoalveolar lavage. When it is subjected to cytologic analysis, the lavage fluid has a positive reaction on periodic acid–Schiff staining and reveals alveolar macrophages filled with positive staining material. Transbronchial biopsy or thoracoscopic biopsy can confirm the diagnosis by providing tissue that has similar staining characteristics. Serologic analysis for GM-CSF antibodies is now often performed to support the diagnosis. GM-CSF autoantibody levels may be obtained and are thought to be 100% sensitive and specific for the autoimmune form of pulmonary alveolar proteinosis. There does not appear to be a correlation between antibody levels and the severity of disease.

TREATMENT

About 8 to 30% of cases of pulmonary alveolar proteinosis resolve spontaneously, and smoking cessation may contribute to spontaneous resolution. A second group of patients will progress to respiratory failure. The remainder will have stable disease. Superinfection with *Nocardia* spp, atypical mycobacteria, fungi, and other opportunistic organisms can occur in more than 15% of patients as a result of macrocyte phagocytic dysfunction.

Therapy depends on the severity of symptoms. Corticosteroids are ineffective and may be deleterious. Treatment of severely symptomatic patients with dyspnea and hypoxemia[5] begins with multistage or sequential whole-lung lavage performed under general anesthesia with a double-lumen endotracheal tube. The recovered fluid initially has an opaque, sandy-colored appearance (E-Fig. 79-2). This procedure may have to be repeated at variable intervals. Asymptomatic patients should be observed and followed closely. Mildly symptomatic patients should receive supportive therapy with supplemental oxygen as needed. Case reports suggest that inhaled GM-CSF can improve quality of life, oxygenation, pulmonary function, and exercise capacity in about half of treated patients who cannot undergo whole-lung lavage or who have failed standard treatment with whole-lung lavage. One randomized trial of this experimental therapy in patients with mild to moderate disease showed no clinical benefits despite modest improvements in arterial saturation and chest radiography,[A1] but another showed improvement in clinical symptoms as well as in arterial saturation, especially with continuous daily therapy.[A2] Isolated case series have reported variable responses to CD-20 monoclonal antibody, rituximab, or plasmapheresis. Corticosteroids are not routinely used. Lung transplantation can be performed, but recurrent pulmonary alveolar proteinosis has been reported.

Survival rates at 5 years approach 75%.

ACUTE INTERSTITIAL PNEUMONIA

DEFINITION

Acute interstitial pneumonia, also referred to as *Hamman-Rich syndrome*, is a rare and often fatal disease that mimics ARDS (Chapter 90). The etiology is unknown, and acute interstitial pneumonia is sometimes defined as the development of ARDS in the absence of known triggers. A similar acute presentation may be seen in patients with an acute exacerbation of idiopathic pulmonary fibrosis (Chapter 80), but most investigators believe that acute interstitial pneumonia is a separate disease process with no histologic evidence of underlying usual interstitial pneumonia.

PATHOBIOLOGY

The pathogenesis of acute interstitial pneumonia is damage to the epithelium of the alveolar membranes by a neutrophil-mediated mechanism; the result is pouring of exudate into the air space in the initial exudative phase of disease. Histologic examination reveals diffuse alveolar damage with intra-alveolar hyaline membrane formation, interstitial and intra-alveolar edema, acute inflammation, and epithelial cell necrosis with a nonspecific distribution and temporal uniformity. This process progresses to the organizing phase, characterized by alveolar septal thickening, type II pneumocyte hyperplasia, and fibroblast proliferation along the interstitium and alveolar spaces. In situ thrombi of small pulmonary arteries may be present. Finally, a fibrotic phase occurs with alveolar septal thickening from organizing fibrosis. One of the key pathologic findings in acute interstitial pneumonia is the temporal uniformity of the diffuse alveolar damage and of organizing and proliferating connective tissue. This uniformity supports a single acute injury at a particular point in time. Long-standing fibrosis is not a typical pathologic finding in acute interstitial pneumonia.

CLINICAL MANIFESTATIONS

Acute interstitial pneumonia manifests with equal frequency in men and women, typically in previously healthy individuals in the 50- to 55-year age range. It develops acutely to subacutely during a few days to a few weeks. The mean duration of symptoms is 7 to 15 days. Dry cough, shortness of breath, malaise, and fever (in 75% of patients) are typical clinical findings. A virus-like prodrome period has been described. Pulmonary rales are heard on physical examination, and hypoxemia is characteristic. Clubbing is rare. Leukocytosis may be present. Acute interstitial pneumonia often progresses to hypoxemic respiratory failure, and intensive care unit admission with mechanical ventilation is usually required. Early mortality rates are high. Radiographic features of acute interstitial pneumonia are diffuse alveolar opacities and air space consolidation similar to the appearance of ARDS (Fig. 79-4 and E-Fig. 79-3); CT scans reveal bilateral air space consolidation with areas of ground-glass opacities with little honeycombing. Septal thickening and a subpleural distribution of the opacities may also be present.

DIAGNOSIS

The diagnosis of acute interstitial pneumonia is made in the appropriate clinical setting in a patient who has a clinical presentation compatible with ARDS but without a clear etiology. The differential diagnosis histologically and clinically includes other causes of ARDS (Chapter 90), such as severe infection, trauma, and sepsis, as well as other causes of acute lung injury (Chapter 82), such as drug toxicity, inhalation injury, and collagen vascular diseases. The presentation is clinically and radiographically similar to that of diffuse alveolar hemorrhage, acute hypersensitivity pneumonitis, acute exacerbation of pulmonary fibrosis, acute eosinophilic pneumonia, and cryptogenic organizing pneumonia. Bronchoscopy with bronchoalveolar lavage is often performed to exclude alveolar hemorrhage, eosinophilic pneumonias, and infectious causes of lung injury. In a small number of cases, transbronchial biopsy may yield the diagnosis, but definitive diagnosis in most cases of acute interstitial pneumonia requires a surgical lung biopsy revealing diffuse alveolar damage.

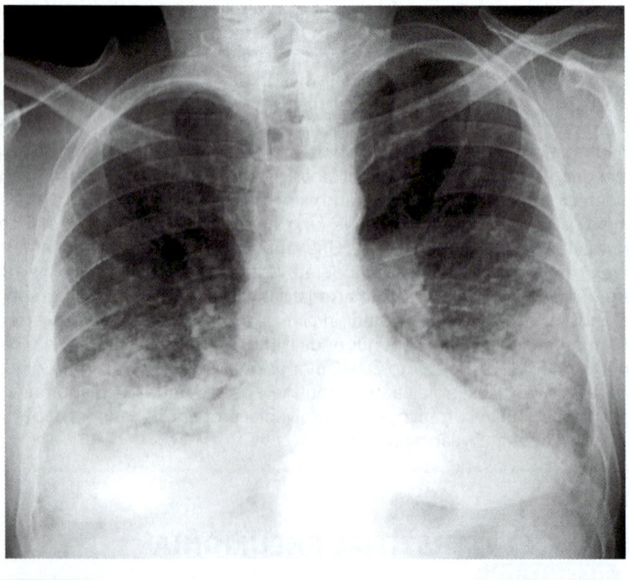

FIGURE 79-4. Acute interstitial pneumonia (AIP), also called idiopathic ARDS. Chest radiograph shows perihilar, right middle lobe, and bibasal consolidations with air bronchograms. (From Dr. Stark with courtesy of Paul Stark, MD.)

TREATMENT

Treatment includes supportive intensive care unit management. In small case series, corticosteroids (up to 1 g of methylprednisolone in divided doses intravenously per day for 3 consecutive days, followed by prednisone or the equivalent at 1 mg/kg/day with a taper over several weeks to months, with or without cyclophosphamide) may be of benefit, but the mortality rate remains higher than 70%. Patients also can have recurrences in months to years. Some cases of acute interstitial pneumonia may resolve without sequelae, but in some series, more than 50% of survivors may be left with residual fibrosis.

DIFFUSE ALVEOLAR HEMORRHAGE

DEFINITION

The alveolar hemorrhage syndromes cause alveolar filling disease, usually with an acute onset and often with life-threatening severity. They can be associated with antineutrophil cytoplasmic antibody (ANCA)–associated vasculitides such as microscopic polyangiitis (Chapter 249) and granulomatosis with polyangiitis (Chapter 249)[6]; immunologic diseases, such as Goodpasture syndrome (anti–glomerular basement membrane antibody disease; Chapter 107)[7]; collagen vascular diseases,[8] such as systemic lupus erythematosus (Chapter 245); cocaine inhalation (Chapter 365); drugs (including penicillamine, mitomycin C, trimellitic anhydride inhalation, all-*trans* retinoic acid, propylthiouracil, and isocyanates); hematopoietic cell transplantation[9] (Chapter 163); coagulopathy (Chapter 160); and mitral stenosis (Chapter 60). A small percentage of idiopathic and recurrent cases are termed idiopathic pulmonary hemosiderosis.[10] In Goodpasture syndrome, there is a strong association with tobacco use and a male predominance, with young men most frequently affected. A viral syndrome and exposure to hydrocarbons may simulate Goodpasture disease. Idiopathic pulmonary hemosiderosis most often occurs in children and young adults.

PATHOBIOLOGY

Alveolar hemorrhage is caused by bleeding from the pulmonary microcirculation, including the capillaries, arterioles, and venules. It may be associated with injury or neutrophilic inflammation of the alveolar walls and adjacent interstitial capillaries (i.e., a capillaritis), usually when it is associated with collagen vascular or vasculitic processes. In Goodpasture syndrome, for example, the circulating anti–glomerular basement membrane antibodies are directed against the α_3 chain of type IV collagen in the glomerular basement membrane, where they cause glomerulonephritis; these core antibodies can cross-react with the alveolar capillary basement membranes, resulting in alveolar hemorrhage. Alternatively, alveolar hemorrhage may be associated with relatively bland pathologic changes with red blood cells in the alveolar spaces. Idiopathic pulmonary hemosiderosis can be an example of bland hemorrhage.

CLINICAL MANIFESTATIONS

Patients present acutely (usually in hours to a week) with dyspnea, shortness of breath, hemoptysis (which may be absent in up to one third of patients), and cough. Some patients also have low-grade fever. Lung examination reveals rales.

Laboratory examination may reveal anemia, and arterial blood gases reveal hypoxemia. In Goodpasture syndrome and the ANCA-associated vasculitides, hematuria and renal insufficiency caused by glomerulonephritis are typically present.

Radiographic features[11] include the acute development of bilateral alveolar filling disease similar to pulmonary edema but without cardiomegaly or pleural effusions (E-Fig. 79-4), sometimes with a subpleural sparing pattern. Rapid remission and recurrences are seen with repeated episodes of bleeding, which also may result in chronic interstitial changes on the chest radiograph. Pulmonary function testing may reveal an increase in the diffusion capacity for carbon monoxide because of the presence of hemoglobin in the alveolar spaces.

DIAGNOSIS

The diagnosis of alveolar hemorrhage is usually made in the appropriate clinical setting by the triad of diffuse alveolar opacities (Fig. 79-5), hemoptysis (in two thirds of patients), and anemia. In immunosuppressed patients, the most frequent causes of diffuse alveolar hemorrhage are hematologic neoplasms, hematopoietic stem cell or solid organ transplantation, drug reaction or infection, and associated HIV infection. Bronchoalveolar lavage typically demonstrates the return of progressively more bloody aliquots of fluid (E-Fig. 79-5), and cytologic analysis reveals that more than 20% of the macrophages are hemosiderin laden. Although rarely recommended, lung biopsy is the gold standard for diagnosing diffuse alveolar hemorrhage and pulmonary capillaritis. Goodpasture syndrome is diagnosed by circulating anti–glomerular basement membrane antibodies, which are present in more than 90% of patients, or by the demonstration of linear deposition of immunoglobulin G antibodies along the alveolar or renal capillary basement membrane tissue when it is viewed by direct immunofluorescence. Cytoplasmic antineutrophil cytoplasmic antibody (c-ANCA)–associated vasculitis causes a focal, segmental, necrotizing glomerulonephritis and is associated with the presence of proteinase 3 antineutrophilic cytoplasmic antibodies in 90% of active cases of granulomatosis with polyangiitis (Chapter 249). Necrotizing granulomatous inflammation is often found in the upper airway in addition to the lungs and kidneys. A perinuclear myeloperoxidase antineutrophilic antibody is often present in association with microscopic polyarteritis (Chapter 249). Patients with systemic lupus erythematosus usually have antinuclear antibodies (Chapter 245). Patients using illicit drugs such as cocaine may have a positive drug screen. Idiopathic pulmonary hemosiderosis is a diagnosis of exclusion after other causes of diffuse alveolar hemorrhage have been eliminated.

TREATMENT

Treatment of alveolar hemorrhage varies according to its underlying cause. Massive hemoptysis (Chapter 71) from any cause of alveolar hemorrhage should be managed as needed. In the case of anticoagulation-, drug-, or toxin-related alveolar hemorrhage, the offending agent should be withdrawn, and supportive care is indicated. In Goodpasture syndrome, the ANCA-associated vasculitides, and other vasculitides (Chapter 249), treatment typically includes immunosuppressant agents such as corticosteroids (methylprednisolone, 500 to 1000 mg/day in divided doses for 3 to 5 days followed by a prednisone taper beginning at 1 mg/kg/day during the next 6 to 9 months) and cyclophosphamide (2 mg/kg/day orally or 0.5 g/m^2 to 0.75 g/m^2 intravenously for one dose) and then, if needed, every 2 weeks or change to oral therapy. Plasmapheresis (3 to 14 exchanges) to remove the offending circulating antibody is a mainstay of therapy for Goodpasture syndrome and may also be used in alveolar hemorrhage caused by systemic lupus erythematosus. However, plasmapheresis is not beneficial for ANCA-associated vasculitis.[A3] In patients with ANCA-associated vasculitis, rituximab (375 mg/m^2 once a week for 4 weeks) is at least as good as cyclophosphamide (2 mg/kg adjusted for renal function) followed by azathioprine (2 mg/kg) for 12 to 15 months for inducing and maintaining remission (≈50% at 12 months and about 40% at 18 months), and rituximab (at 500 mg on days 0 and 14 and at 6, 12, and 18 months) is better than azathioprine for maintaining remission and improving quality of life at 5 years.[A4]

PROGNOSIS

Alveolar hemorrhage can result in acute respiratory failure and death. Recurrent alveolar hemorrhage from any cause, such as idiopathic pulmonary hemosiderosis, can be associated with the development of pulmonary fibrosis. Alveolar hemorrhage related to collagen vascular disease, vasculitides, and idiopathic pulmonary hemosiderosis can have mortality rates ranging from 25 to 50%. With Goodpasture syndrome, renal failure is common, and the degree of renal impairment may correlate with outcome.

INVASIVE MUCINOUS ADENOCARCINOMA AND LEPIDIC PREDOMINANT NONMUCINOUS ADENOCARCINOMA (FORMERLY CALLED BRONCHIOLOALVEOLAR CELL CARCINOMA)

DEFINITION

In 2011, a multidisciplinary committee eliminated the term *bronchioloalveolar cell carcinoma* and divided pulmonary adenocarcinomas into five types: adenocarcinoma in situ, minimally invasive adenocarcinoma, lepidic predominant nonmucinous adenocarcinoma, invasive mucinous adenocarcinoma, and invasive adenocarcinoma and its subtypes. The types that would most likely be correlated with an alveolar filling appearance pathologically and on chest imaging are invasive mucinous adenocarcinoma, in which consolidation and air bronchograms may be present, and lepidic-predominant nonmucinous adenocarcinoma, in which a ground-glass appearance is characteristic. Both of these types of adenocarcinoma are among those formally characterized as bronchioloalveolar cell carcinoma. In general, these tumors are characterized by malignant cells lining the alveolar cell wall (Chapter 177). Among bronchogenic carcinomas, these subtypes are the least associated with tobacco use, and patients with these cancers are more likely to be nonsmokers. Unlike other non–small cell lung cancers, the sex ratio approaches 1:1 or may be slightly female predominant, and younger patients may be affected.

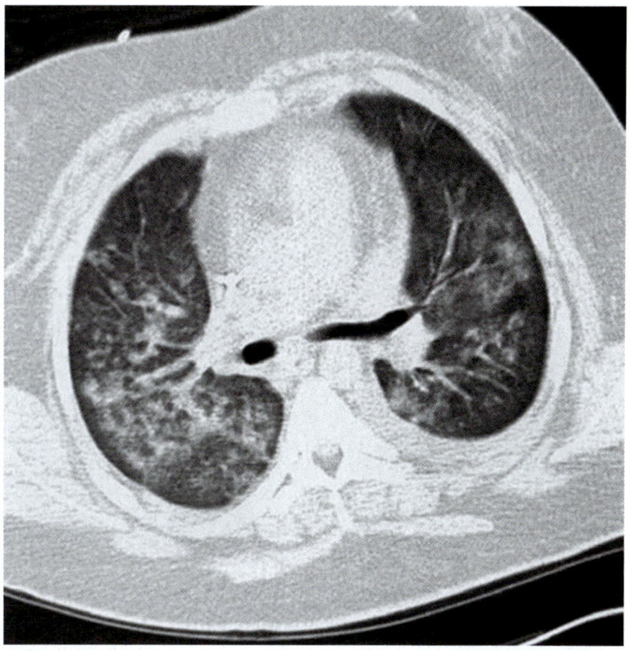

FIGURE 79-5. A chest computed tomography scan showing alveolar opacities in a patient with diffuse alveolar hemorrhage.

PATHOBIOLOGY

These types of adenocarcinoma usually arise in the periphery of the lung and may be characterized by lepidic growth, which means contiguous growth along the intact alveolar septa, with varying degrees of stromal, pleural, vascular, or lymphatic invasion and without a known primary adenocarcinoma elsewhere. The mucinous type is thought to derive from respiratory goblet cells and columnar cells, and the nonmucinous type from type II pneumocytes or Clara cells.

CLINICAL MANIFESTATIONS

Patients present with a gradual onset of shortness of breath and cough. The duration of symptoms is usually several months. Constitutional symptoms such as malaise and weight loss may be present. Hemoptysis may occur. An unusual but unique clinical finding is bronchorrhea, with patients reporting the production of copious amounts of clear sputum daily. This finding is more common in the invasive mucinous form of the disease.

DIAGNOSIS

Radiographic patterns vary and can include localized disease with peripheral solitary or multiple nodules or masses in 60% of cases or a persistent pneumonic pattern in 40% of cases. The radiographic findings of consolidation with air bronchograms are often initially thought to be consistent with acute pneumonia (Fig. 79-6), but the typical clinical presentation is that of a nonresolving peripheral density on chest radiograph (E-Fig. 79-6).[12] In addition, CT may show areas of ground-glass attenuation. Positron emission tomography may be normal because of the low glucose uptake of these tumors. The diagnosis of invasive mucinous adenocarcinoma and lepidic predominant

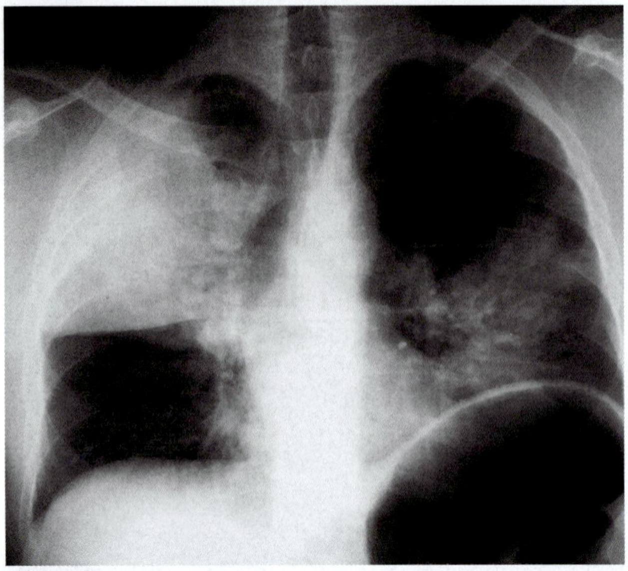

FIGURE 79-6. **Mucinous adenocarcinoma (bronchioloalveolar carcinoma). Chest radiograph shows right upper lobe complete consolidation with air bronchograms as well as left lower lobe consolidation. The findings mimic extensive lobar pneumonia. Eventration of the left hemidiaphragm and gastric distention are unrelated. (From Dr. Stark with courtesy of Paul Stark, MD.)**

nonmucinous adenocarcinoma is most often made by bronchoscopy with transbronchial biopsy.

TREATMENT

For staging and treatment, these types of adenocarcinoma are approached like other types of non–small cell lung cancers (Chapter 177).[13] Testing for epidermal growth factor receptor (EGFR) mutations should be performed, and chemotherapy planned accordingly. In general, the invasive mucinous adenocarcinomas are KRAS positive and EGFR negative. The lepidic predominant nonmucinous type tends to be EGFR positive. Bilateral lung transplantation has been performed, but recurrence in the transplanted lungs has been reported.

PROGNOSIS

Prognosis correlates with stage, histology, and genetics. Patients who undergo surgical resection for adenocarcinoma in situ or minimally invasive adenocarcinoma with a single focus of disease have a better prognosis than patients with other adenocarcinomas of like stage, with the 5-year survival rate approaching 100%. Lepidic pattern adenocarcinomas generally present at an early stage and have a better prognosis than do solid/micropapillary patterns that usually present at a higher stage with a worse prognosis. More advanced forms likely have a prognosis similar to that of other adenocarcinomas. Mutations in *EGFR*, the epidermal growth factor receptor gene, are a poor prognostic factor.[14]

GENERAL REFERENCES

For the General References and other additional features, please visit Elsevier eBooks+ at https://ebooks.health.elsevier.com.

Grade A References

A1. Tazawa R, Ueda T, Abe M, et al. Inhaled GM-CSF for pulmonary alveolar proteinosis. *N Engl J Med.* 2019;381:923-932.

A2. Trapnell BC, Inoue Y, Bonella F, et al. Inhaled molgramostim therapy in autoimmune pulmonary alveolar proteinosis. *N Engl J Med.* 2020;383:1635-1644.

A3. Walsh M, Merkel PA, Szpirt WM, et al. Plasma exchange and glucocorticoids in severe ANCA-associated vasculitis. *N Engl J Med.* 2020;382:622-631.

A4. Terrier B, Pagnoux C, Perrodeau É, et al. Long-term efficacy of remission-maintenance regimens for ANCA-associated vasculitides. *Ann Rheum Dis.* 2018;77:1150-1156.

80 INTERSTITIAL LUNG DISEASE

GANESH RAGHU AND FERNANDO J. MARTINEZ

DEFINITION

In an apparently immunocompetent host, *interstitial lung disease* is a clinical term for a heterogenous group of acute and chronic lower respiratory tract disorders with many potential causes.[1] Clinical and physiologic features commonly include cough, exertional dyspnea, absence of pulmonary infection or neoplasm, and abnormal pulmonary physiology, including a restrictive pattern on pulmonary function testing (Chapter 73), coexistent airflow obstruction, decreased diffusing capacity (DLCO), and increased alveolar-arterial oxygen difference (PAO_2-PaO_2) (Chapter 89) at rest or during exertion. Interstitial lung diseases include acute and chronic lung disorders with variable degrees of pulmonary inflammation and/or fibrosis (Table 80-1). The term *interstitial* is a misnomer because the pathologic processes are not restricted to the interstitium, which is the microscopic space bounded by the basement membranes of epithelial and endothelial cells. All of the cellular and soluble constituents that make up the gas exchange units (alveolar wall, capillaries, alveolar space, and acini) and the bronchiolar lumen, terminal bronchioles, and pulmonary parenchyma beyond the gas exchange units (as well as the pleura and lymphatics and sometimes the lymph nodes) may be involved in the pathogenesis and manifestations of interstitial lung disease.

EPIDEMIOLOGY

Among persons 18 years or older, the prevalence of all interstitial lung diseases in the United States is about 80 per 100,000 men and 70 per 100,000 women. The overall incidence is higher in men (31.5 per 100,000 per year) than in women (26.1 per 100,000 per year).[2] Moreover, the prevalence of undiagnosed or early interstitial lung disease is estimated to be 10 times that of clinically recognized disease; as physicians' awareness of these entities increases, it is expected that the frequency of the diagnosis will rise. Among the interstitial lung diseases, the two most common are idiopathic pulmonary fibrosis and connective tissue–associated disease. In the United States, the annual incidence of idiopathic pulmonary fibrosis is 94 per 100,000 in the Medicare population, with a mean age of onset of 79 years. Recent data suggest that more than 5000 new cases are diagnosed each year in the United Kingdom.

Although idiopathic pulmonary fibrosis is the prototypical progressive interstitial lung disease, up to one third of patients with interstitial lung diseases other than idiopathic pulmonary fibrosis (e.g., interstitial lung disease associated with systemic sclerosis or associated with hypersensitivity pneumonitis) also develop the progressive phenotype. This clinical phenotype, which is agnostic to etiology, is now termed progressive pulmonary fibrosis, and its prevalence is estimated to be 70.3 per 100,000 patients.

PATHOBIOLOGY

Interstitial lung diseases are thought to result from an unknown tissue injury and attempted repair in the lung of a genetically predisposed person. Numerous genetic variants have been associated with subsets of familial pulmonary fibrosis and with some sporadic cases. These variants include the *MUC5B* gene, genes related to immune function (*TOLLIP, TLR3, IL1RN, IL8, TGFβ1*), epithelial cell function (*DSP, DPP9*), the maintenance of telomeres (*TERT, TERC, OBFC1, TINF2, DKC1, RTEL1, PARN*), the production of surfactant (SFTPC, SFTPA1, ABCA3), and cell cycle regulation (*KIF15, MAD1L1, CDKN1A*).[3] About 3 to 4% of patients treated with programmed cell death-1 inhibitors can develop interstitial lung diseases.[4]

In *idiopathic pulmonary fibrosis*, varying degrees of acute, subacute, and chronic fibrinous proliferation are present in the lungs. Ultimately, progressive fibrosis results in honeycombing, an end-stage finding that is often associated with increased pulmonary vascular resistance and secondary pulmonary hypertension. As a reflection of these dynamic processes, histopathologic examination of lung tissue often reveals highly heterogeneous findings within the same biopsy specimen.

CLINICAL MANIFESTATIONS

Interstitial lung diseases are typically characterized by cough and progressive dyspnea. Pleuritic chest pain may occur with certain connective tissue or

TABLE 80-1 CLINICAL CLASSIFICATION OF INTERSTITIAL LUNG DISEASE

IDIOPATHIC INTERSTITIAL PNEUMONIAS
Chronic Fibrosing Interstitial Pneumonias
Idiopathic pulmonary fibrosis Nonspecific interstitial pneumonia
Smoking-Related Interstitial Pneumonias
Respiratory bronchiolitis–interstitial lung disease Desquamative interstitial pneumonia
Acute or Subacute Idiopathic Interstitial Pneumonias
Cryptogenic organizing pneumonia Acute interstitial pneumonia Lymphoid and lymphocytic interstitial pneumonia
Rare Interstitial Pneumonias
Histologic pattern of acute fibrinous and organizing pneumonia Histologic pattern of interstitial pneumonias with a bronchiolocentric distribution Pleuroparenchymal fibroelastosis
INTERSTITIAL LUNG DISEASE ASSOCIATED WITH CONNECTIVE TISSUE DISEASE
Progressive systemic sclerosis Rheumatoid arthritis Systemic lupus erythematosus Dermatomyositis and polymyositis Sjögren syndrome Mixed connective tissue disease Ankylosing spondylitis
HYPERSENSITIVITY PNEUMONITIS
Occupational and environmental factors (e.g., farmer's lung, bird fancier's lung) Iatrogenic
DRUG-INDUCED AND IATROGENIC INTERSTITIAL LUNG DISEASE
See Table 80-2
ALVEOLAR FILLING DISORDERS (Chapter 79)
Goodpasture syndrome Pulmonary alveolar proteinosis Pulmonary hemosiderosis Alveolar hemorrhage syndromes Chronic eosinophilic pneumonia
INTERSTITIAL LUNG DISEASE ASSOCIATED WITH PULMONARY VASCULITIS
Pulmonary capillaritis Granulomatosis with polyangiitis (formerly known as Wegener granulomatosis) Churg-Strauss syndrome
OTHER SPECIFIC FORMS OF INTERSTITIAL LUNG DISEASE
Sarcoidosis Langerhans cell histiocytosis (histiocytosis X) Lymphangioleiomyomatosis Coronavirus-19 disease associated
INHERITED FORMS OF INTERSTITIAL LUNG DISEASE
Familial idiopathic pulmonary fibrosis Familial pulmonary fibrosis or interstitial pneumonia Tuberous sclerosis Neurofibromatosis Gaucher disease Niemann-Pick disease Hermansky-Pudlak syndrome

drug-induced forms; acute pleuritic chest pain with dyspnea may represent a spontaneous pneumothorax (Chapter 86) in association with lymphangioleiomyomatosis, tuberous sclerosis (Chapter 385), neurofibromatosis, or Langerhans cell histiocytosis. Hemoptysis suggests a diffuse alveolar hemorrhagic syndrome, systemic lupus erythematosus (SLE) (Chapter 245), lymphangioleiomyomatosis, granulomatosis with polyangiitis (Chapter 249), or Goodpasture syndrome (Chapter 107); it is rare in other interstitial lung diseases. In patients with existing disease, new hemoptysis should prompt consideration of a superimposed malignancy, pulmonary embolus, or infection such as aspergillosis.

In some patients, the first and the only clue to the presence of an interstitial lung disease may be the incidental finding of parenchymal abnormalities in computed tomography (CT) images of the chest or rales (crackles) on lung auscultation. A history of wheezing suggests the coexistence of occult hyperactive airways and airflow obstruction, thereby raising the possibility of allergic bronchopulmonary aspergillosis (Chapter 311), eosinophilic granulomatosis with polyangiitis (Chapter 249), chronic eosinophilic pneumonia (see later), or parasitic infection (Chapter 315). In some patients, the initial presentation may be with peripheral cyanosis, clubbing, or the signs and symptoms of an underlying systemic disease (see later).

DIAGNOSIS

The first key in patients is to establish the syndromic diagnosis and then pursue the differential diagnosis of its specific cause (Fig. 80-1). However, a conclusive cause often may not be identified despite an exhaustive medical history and invasive diagnostic interventions, including bronchoalveolar lavage and bronchoscopic or surgical lung biopsy specimens. Thus, the cause of several of the interstitial lung diseases, even when diagnosed as specific entities, remains unknown.

History

The patient's age, sex, and cigarette smoking history may provide useful clues to the diagnosis. Idiopathic pulmonary fibrosis is an adult disorder that usually occurs in patients older than 50 years. Pulmonary sarcoidosis (Chapter 83), in contrast, is more common in young and middle-aged adults. Whereas pulmonary Langerhans cell histiocytosis (Chapter 155) characteristically occurs in young cigarette-smoking men, lymphangioleiomyomatosis occurs exclusively in women of childbearing age. Respiratory bronchiolitis–associated interstitial lung disease is seen almost exclusively in cigarette smokers but occurs in both men and women of all ages.

The medical history should include a careful assessment of environmental and occupational exposures, as well as medication and drug use (Chapters 81 and 82). A family medical history should address possible familial disease. Environmental risk factors that may suggest the diagnosis of hypersensitivity pneumonitis include farming or exposure to overt or occult avian antigens at or in the close vicinity of home; bird droppings or feather duvets; visible molds; unkempt recreational hot tubs; dusty homes; unchanged filters in furnaces; unkempt ventilatory systems at home, in the workplace, other frequently visited places or in automobiles; water leaks or humidifiers in the domestic and/or work environment; and changes in environmental exposures (hypersensitivity to thermophilic actinomycetes, *Aureobasidium pullulans*). At-risk occupations include mining (pneumoconioses), machine tool grinding, sandblasting and working with granite (silicosis), welding, as well as working in a shipyard (asbestosis) or the aerospace or electronic industries (berylliosis) (Chapters 81 and 82). Because of the long interval between the exposure and the onset of symptoms in many occupations, it is important to take a detailed, lifelong occupational history (Chapter 16) as well as to establish the interval between exposure and the onset of symptoms. Because the list of medications known to cause interstitial lung disease is long and continues to grow (Table 80-2), a careful history regarding recent use of prescription and over-the-counter products is essential. Risk factors for immunosuppression, including infection with human immunodeficiency virus, raise the possibility of opportunistic lung infections (Chapter 359), neoplasm (Chapter 177), and transplant-related pulmonary complications. Infection with severe acute respiratory syndrome coronavirus 2 (SARS-CoV-2; Chapter 336) can result in a clinical syndrome (COVID-19) that includes diffuse parenchymal damage with features of organizing pneumonia, interstitial pneumonitis, and fibrosing interstitial lung disease.

Particular attention should be paid to the onset and duration of symptoms, the rate of disease progression, and association with hemoptysis, fever, or extrathoracic symptoms. Symptoms that persist 4 weeks or less and the presence of fever suggest infection, cryptogenic organizing pneumonia, drug-induced pulmonary injury, or acute hypersensitivity pneumonitis. Idiopathic pulmonary fibrosis, interstitial lung disease associated with connective tissue diseases, and Langerhans cell histiocytosis tend to have a more subacute onset. Extrapulmonary symptoms suggest that the interstitial lung disease may be associated with systemic disorders (e.g., sarcoidosis; Chapter 83), and symptoms such as dysphagia, dry eyes or mouth, skin rash, or arthritis may suggest a connective tissue disorder (Chapters 245 to 249). Proximal muscle aches or weakness suggests the possibility of polymyositis or dermatomyositis (Chapter 248), and recurrent sinusitis suggests granulomatosis with polyangiitis (Chapter 249). Extrathoracic manifestations present in tuberous sclerosis (Chapter 385) include hematuria, epilepsy, and developmental delay.

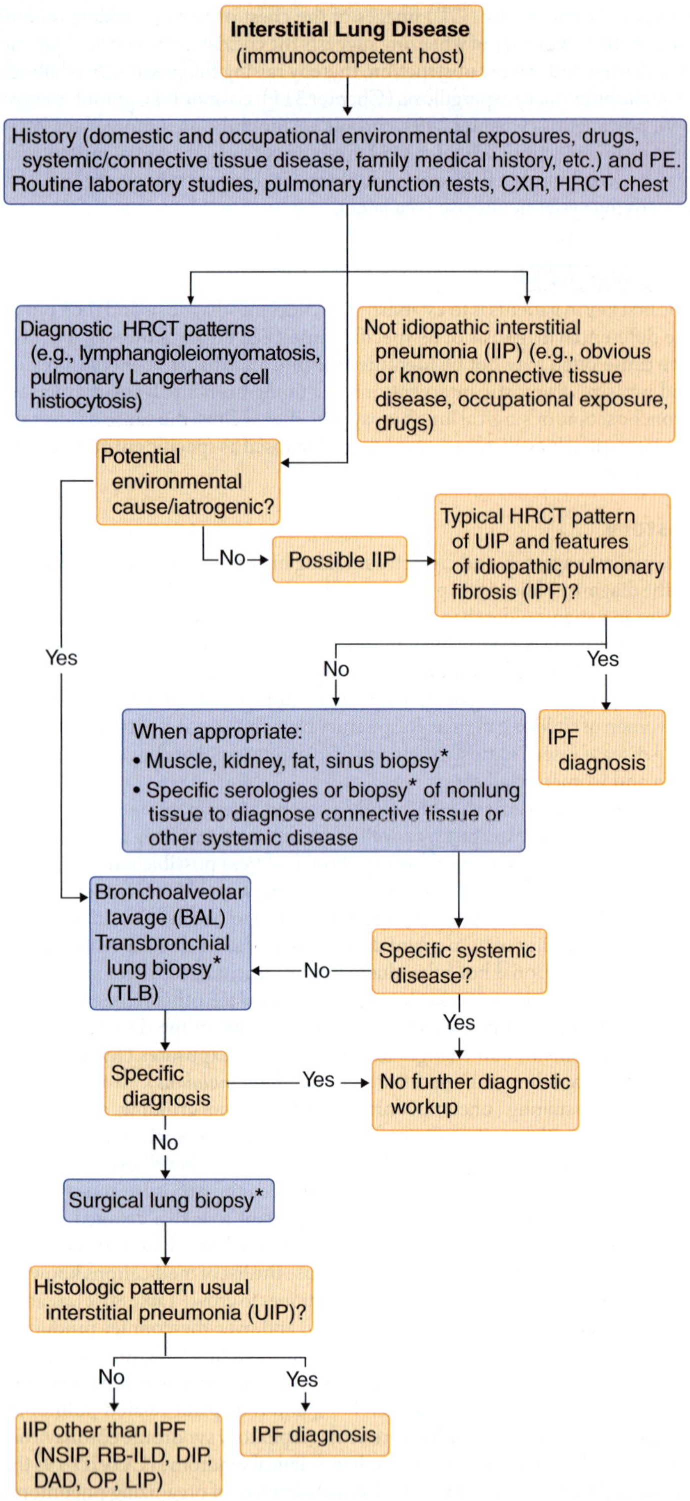

FIGURE 80-1. **A diagnostic approach to interstitial lung disease.** The evaluation commonly should include multidisciplinary discussions with experts in interstitial lung disease, including a pulmonologist, chest radiologist, thoracic surgeon, pathologist, and rheumatologist. *Surgical lung biopsy is not indicated in patients with a probable UIP pattern on HRCT if all other features of IPF are typical, and lung biopsy is considered a last resort in patients who have a significant risk of surgical complications; CXR = chest radiograph; DAD = diffuse alveolar damage; DIP = desquamative interstitial pneumonia; HRCT = high-resolution computed tomography; IIP = idiopathic interstitial pneumonia; IPF = idiopathic pulmonary fibrosis; LIP = lymphoid interstitial pneumonia; NSIP = nonspecific interstitial pneumonia; OP = organizing pneumonia; PE = physical examination; RB-ILD = respiratory bronchiolitis–associated interstitial lung disease; TLB = transbronchial lung biopsy; UIP = usual interstitial pneumonia. (Adapted from American Thoracic Society/European Respiratory Society: International multidisciplinary consensus classification of idiopathic interstitial pneumonias. *Am J Respir Crit Care Med*. 2002;165:277-304; Raghu G, Collard HR, Egan JJ, et al. Diagnosis of idiopathic pulmonary fibrosis. An official ATS/ERS/JRS/ALAT clinical practice guideline. *Am J Respir Crit Care Med*. 2018;198:e44-e68.)

TABLE 80-2 DRUG-INDUCED AND IATROGENIC INTERSTITIAL LUNG DISEASE*

ANTIMICROBIAL AGENTS
Cephalosporins
Isoniazid
Nitrofurantoin
Penicillins
Sulfonamides
ANTI-INFLAMMATORY AGENTS
Aspirin
Everolimus
Gold
Methotrexate
Nonsteroidal anti-inflammatory agents
D-Penicillamine
Phenylbutazone
Sirolimus
Tensirolimus
Zafirlukast
CARDIOVASCULAR DRUGS
Amiodarone
Angiotensin-converting enzyme inhibitors
β-Blockers
Hydralazine
Hydrochlorothiazide
Procainamide
Protamine sulfate
Tocainide
IMMUNE MODULATING, ANTINEOPLASTIC, AND CHEMOTHERAPEUTIC AGENTS
Atezolizumab
Bleomycin
Busulfan
Chlorambucil
Cyclophosphamide
Durvalumab
Erlotinib
Gefitinib
Gemcitabine
Imatinib
Ipilimumab
Melphalan
Mercaptopurine
Methotrexate
Mitomycin
Nitrosoureas
Nivolumab
Pembrolizumab
Procarbazine
Tumor necrosis factor-α–modulating agents
CENTRAL NERVOUS SYSTEM DRUGS
Carbamazepine
Chlorpromazine
Imipramine
Phenytoin
ORAL HYPOGLYCEMIC AGENTS
Chlorpropamide
Tolazamide
Tolbutamide
ILLICIT DRUGS
Cocaine
Heroin
Methadone
Propoxyphene
OTHER AGENTS
Antithymocyte globulin
All-*trans*-retinoic acid
Colony-stimulating factors
Interferon-α and -β
Irradiation
Mycophenolate mofetil
High fraction of inspired oxygen (FIO_2) with mechanical ventilation

*This list contains examples only and is not meant to be inclusive. An exhaustive list is available at www.pneumotox.com.

TABLE 80-3 CHARACTERISTIC CHEST RADIOGRAPHIC PATTERNS IN PATIENTS WITH INTERSTITIAL LUNG DISEASE

PATTERN	SUGGESTED DIAGNOSES*
Decreased lung volumes	Idiopathic pulmonary fibrosis, nonspecific interstitial pneumonia, desquamative interstitial pneumonia, connective tissue disease, chronic eosinophilic pneumonia, asbestosis, chronic hypersensitivity pneumonitis, or drug-induced interstitial lung disease (ILD)
Increased or preserved lung volumes	Idiopathic pulmonary fibrosis with emphysema, respiratory bronchiolitis–associated ILD, cryptogenic organizing pneumonia, hypersensitivity pneumonitis, lymphangioleiomyomatosis, Langerhans cell histiocytosis, sarcoidosis, neurofibromatosis, tuberous sclerosis
Micronodules	Infection, hypersensitivity pneumonitis, sarcoidosis, respiratory bronchiolitis–associated ILD
Septal thickening	Malignancy, infection, chronic congestive heart failure, pulmonary veno-occlusive disease
Honeycombing	Idiopathic pulmonary fibrosis, fibrotic nonspecific interstitial pneumonia, connective tissue disease, asbestosis, chronic hypersensitivity pneumonitis, sarcoidosis
Recurrent infiltrates	Cryptogenic organizing pneumonia, chronic eosinophilic pneumonia, drug- or radiation-induced ILD
Migratory or fleeting infiltrates	Cryptogenic organizing pneumonia, hypersensitivity pneumonitis, eosinophilic granulomatosis with polyangiitis, Löffler syndrome, allergic bronchopulmonary aspergillosis
Pleural disease	Connective tissue disease, asbestosis, malignancy, radiation-induced ILD, amyloidosis, sarcoidosis, lymphangioleiomyomatosis, nitrofurantoin-induced ILD
Pneumothorax	Langerhans cell histiocytosis, lymphangioleiomyomatosis, tuberous sclerosis, neurofibromatosis
Mediastinal or hilar adenopathy	Lymphocytic interstitial pneumonia, connective tissue disease, silicosis, chronic berylliosis, malignancy, infection, sarcoidosis, amyloidosis, Gaucher disease
Normal (rare)	Cellular nonspecific interstitial pneumonia, respiratory bronchiolitis–associated interstitial lung disease, connective tissue disease, hypersensitivity pneumonitis, sarcoidosis
LOCATION OF RADIOGRAPHIC ABNORMALITY	**SUGGESTED DIAGNOSES***
Mid to upper lung zone	Hypersensitivity pneumonitis, chronic berylliosis, ankylosing spondylitis, silicosis, Langerhans cell histiocytosis, sarcoidosis, pleuroparenchymal fibroelastosis, cystic fibrosis
Lower lung zone	Idiopathic pulmonary fibrosis, nonspecific interstitial pneumonia (fibrotic), connective tissue disease, asbestosis, chronic hypersensitivity pneumonitis
Peripheral	Idiopathic pulmonary fibrosis, nonspecific interstitial pneumonia (fibrotic), cryptogenic organizing pneumonia, chronic eosinophilic pneumonia

*This list is not intended to be comprehensive.
Adapted from Raghu G, Brown K. Clinical issues: patient evaluation. In: Baughman RP, du Bois RM, eds. *Diffuse Lung Disease: A Practical Approach*. New York: Oxford University Press; 2004.

Physical Examination

Physical examination of the respiratory system is rarely helpful in the diagnostic evaluation because findings such as rhonchi and rales on auscultation and digital clubbing are nonspecific. An accentuated P_2, a right ventricular heave, or tricuspid insufficiency on the cardiac examination suggest pulmonary hypertension (Chapter 69) and cor pulmonale in patients with advanced lung disease. However, extrathoracic findings such as skin abnormalities, peripheral lymphadenopathy, and hepatosplenomegaly may be more specifically associated with underlying sarcoidosis (Chapter 83); muscle tenderness and proximal muscle weakness may point to coexisting polymyositis (Chapter 248); and signs of arthritis may indicate connective tissue disease (Chapters 243, 245, and 249) or sarcoidosis (Chapter 83). Characteristic rashes occur in several connective tissue diseases, disseminated Langerhans cell histiocytosis, tuberous sclerosis, and neurofibromatosis. Ophthalmologic findings (Chapter 391) such as iridocyclitis, uveitis, or conjunctivitis may be a clue to the diagnosis of sarcoidosis or a connective tissue disease. Central nervous system abnormalities may be present in sarcoidosis, SLE, Langerhans cell histiocytosis, or tuberous sclerosis.

Laboratory Testing

Routine laboratory testing should include a complete blood count, leukocyte differential, erythrocyte sedimentation rate, C-reactive protein, chemistry panel (calcium, liver enzymes, electrolytes, creatinine), serologies for connective tissue disease, and urinalysis. Although these data rarely yield a specific diagnosis, they may provide helpful clues. Routine serology for occult connective tissue diseases (Chapter 237) may reveal typical findings of SLE (e.g., antinuclear antibodies), rheumatoid arthritis (rheumatoid factor, anti–citrullinated peptide antibody), scleroderma (ScL 70), dermatomyositis or polymyositis (creatine kinase, aldolase, myositis panel [Chapter 248], and anti–Jo-1 antibody), granulomatosis with polyangiitis (antineutrophil cytoplasmic antibodies), Sjögren syndrome, and Goodpasture syndrome (anti-basement membrane antibodies).

Mild hypoxemia is typically present on arterial blood gas analysis because of abnormal ventilation-perfusion ratios, especially in moderate to severe cases. However, carbon dioxide retention is rare and suggests possible coexisting emphysema (Chapter 76) or a hypoventilatory disorder (Chapter 74).

Noninvasive Evaluation

Chest Radiograph

The distribution and appearance of radiographic abnormalities (Chapter 72) may prove useful in differentiating among the clinicopathologic syndromes in patients with interstitial lung disease (Table 80-3). Comparison of previous chest radiographs with the current one is important in establishing the rate of progression of the patient's disease. A diffuse ground-glass pattern is often observed early in the course of disease followed by progression to reticular (linear) infiltrates with nodules (reticulonodular infiltrates) or, in the case of alveolar filling disorders, ill-defined nodules (acinar rosettes) with air bronchograms. Most interstitial lung diseases cause infiltrates in the lower lung zones, but upper lobe predominance is typically present in sarcoidosis, berylliosis, Langerhans cell histiocytosis, silicosis, chronic hypersensitivity pneumonitis, cystic fibrosis, and ankylosing spondylitis. The middle and lower lung zones show the most prominent abnormalities in lymphangitic carcinomatosis, idiopathic pulmonary fibrosis, subacute eosinophilic pneumonia, asbestosis, and pulmonary fibrosis caused by rheumatoid arthritis or progressive systemic sclerosis. Hilar adenopathy and mediastinal adenopathy are not common; their presence should suggest sarcoidosis, berylliosis, silicosis, lymphocytic interstitial pneumonia, amyloidosis, or Gaucher disease. A pattern of peripherally located pulmonary infiltrates in the upper and middle lung zones with relatively clear perihilar and central zones is a clue to chronic eosinophilic pneumonia. Recurrent infiltrates raise the possibility of cryptogenic organizing pneumonia, chronic eosinophilic pneumonia, or drug- or radiation-induced pneumonitis, and fleeting or migratory infiltrates may occur in eosinophilic granulomatosis with polyangiitis, cryptogenic organizing pneumonia, allergic bronchopulmonary aspergillosis, tropical eosinophilic pneumonia, or Löffler syndrome. Whereas localized pleural plaques may indicate asbestosis, diffuse pleural thickening can result from asbestosis, rheumatoid arthritis, progressive

TABLE 80-4 RADIOGRAPHIC FEATURES OF IDIOPATHIC INTERSTITIAL PNEUMONIAS

CLINICAL DIAGNOSIS	USUAL RADIOGRAPHIC FEATURES	TYPICAL FINDINGS ON HRCT
Idiopathic pulmonary fibrosis	Basal-predominant abnormality with volume loss	Pattern of usual interstitial pneumonia—peripheral, basal, subpleural reticulation; honeycombing, traction bronchiectasis
Nonspecific interstitial pneumonia	Ground-glass and reticular opacification	Peripheral, basal, subpleural, symmetrical ground-glass attenuation with irregular lines and consolidation; occasional subpleural sparing
Cryptogenic organizing pneumonia	Patchy bilateral consolidation	Subpleural or peribronchial patchy consolidation or nodules
Acute interstitial pneumonia	Diffuse ground-glass density or consolidation	Diffuse consolidation and ground-glass opacification, often with lobular sparing and late traction bronchiectasis
Desquamative interstitial pneumonia	Ground-glass opacity	Peripheral, lower lung zone ground-glass attenuation with reticulation and/or small cysts
Respiratory bronchiolitis–associated interstitial lung disease	Bronchial wall thickening, ground-glass opacification	Diffuse bronchial wall thickening with poorly defined centrilobular nodules and patchy ground-glass opacification
Lymphocytic interstitial pneumonia	Reticular opacities and nodules	Diffuse centrilobular nodules, ground-glass attenuation, septal and bronchovascular wall thickening, and thin-walled cysts

HRCT = high-resolution computed tomography.

Adapted from American Thoracic Society/European Respiratory Society. International multidisciplinary revised classification of the idiopathic interstitial pneumonias. *Am J Respir Crit Care Med.* 2002;165:277-304; Travis WD, Costabel U, Hansell DM, et al. An official American Thoracic Society/European Respiratory Society statement: update of the international multidisciplinary classification of the idiopathic interstitial pneumonias. *Am J Respir Crit Care Med.* 2013;188:733-748; Raghu G, Remy-Jardin M, Myers JL, et al. Diagnosis of idiopathic pulmonary fibrosis. An official ATS/ERS/JRS/ALAT clinical practice guideline. *Am J Respir Crit Care Med.* 2018;198:e44-e68.

systemic sclerosis, radiation pneumonitis, nitrofurantoin, or malignancy. In the absence of left ventricular failure, the presence of a pleural effusion (Chapter 86) raises the possibility of rheumatoid arthritis, SLE, acute hypersensitivity pneumonitis, sarcoidosis, asbestosis, amyloidosis, lymphangioleiomyomatosis, or lymphangitic carcinomatosis. A reduction of lung volumes is typical in most interstitial lung diseases; the presence of preserved lung volumes or hyperinflation should raise suspicion for chronic hypersensitivity pneumonitis, Langerhans cell histiocytosis, lymphangioleiomyomatosis, neurofibromatosis, sarcoidosis, the combination of idiopathic pulmonary fibrosis and emphysema, or tuberous sclerosis. However, plain chest radiographs may be normal in about 10% of patients with interstitial lung disease.

High-Resolution Computed Tomography

Because of its increased sensitivity and ability to distinguish ground-glass changes, which are generally considered to be reversible areas of lung disease, from irreversible fibrotic and honeycomb changes, high-resolution computed tomography (HRCT) is essential in both the diagnosis and staging of interstitial lung disease. Although microscopic interstitial lung disease cannot be excluded by a normal HRCT result, HRCT allows recognition of abnormalities not apparent in plain chest radiographs and may lead to an earlier diagnosis, help narrow the differential diagnosis patterns (Table 80-4), aid in selecting the site or sites for bronchoalveolar lavage and lung biopsy, assist in choosing among therapeutic options, and allow monitoring the response to treatment. Whereas a normal HRCT excludes the diagnosis of pulmonary fibrosis, the presence of patchy subpleural reticular and basilar septal fibrosis, traction bronchiectasis, and honeycombing increases the level of diagnostic confidence for the pattern of usual interstitial pattern, which is characteristic of idiopathic pulmonary fibrosis. The finding of lung cysts, including their size, configuration, distribution, and appearance, helps differentiate among lymphangioleiomyomatosis, tuberous sclerosis, pulmonary Langerhans cell histiocytosis, Birt-Hogg-Dube syndrome, Erdheim-Chester disease, and lymphocytic interstitial pneumonia. HRCT can detect interstitial lung disease despite normal chest radiographs in patients with asbestosis, silicosis, sarcoidosis, and scleroderma. Patients with respiratory bronchiolitis–associated interstitial lung disease typically have patchy ground-glass attenuation on HRCT in concert with bilateral interstitial prominence, fine nodular radiographic opacities, and normal lung volumes. Images obtained in the supine and prone positions help to differentiate fibrosis from atelectasis. Images obtained on deep inspiration and exhalation sometimes aid in identifying areas of air trapping, which reflect airway abnormalities.

Pulmonary Function Tests

The most characteristic physiologic abnormalities in patients with interstitial lung disease, regardless of etiology, are a restrictive lung defect and decreased DLCO (see Table 73-1 in Chapter 73). Forced expiratory volume in 1 second (FEV_1) and forced vital capacity (FVC) are decreased proportionally such that the ratio of the two remains normal or may even be increased. Both total lung capacity (TLC) and lung volumes measured by body plethysmography are reduced. Pulmonary function tests (PFTs) may be useful in monitoring the progression of disease, assessing the response to therapy, and estimating prognosis; significant changes in FVC or DLCO (corrected to hemoglobin) at 1 year after diagnosis portend a worse survival in patients with idiopathic pulmonary fibrosis.

Certain PFT findings may also aid in the differential diagnosis. A mixed obstructive–restrictive pattern occurs in patients with eosinophilic granulomatosis with polyangiitis syndrome, allergic bronchopulmonary aspergillosis, endobronchial sarcoidosis, hypersensitivity pneumonitis, cryptogenic organizing pneumonia, tropical pulmonary interstitial eosinophilia, coexisting chronic obstructive pulmonary disease or asthma, or secondary bronchiectasis. Diseases associated with respiratory muscle weakness, such as polymyositis, progressive systemic sclerosis, and SLE, may exhibit a decrease in maximal voluntary ventilation and increased residual volume out of proportion to the decrease in total lung capacity.

Exercise Testing

The magnitude of the increase in PAO_2-PaO_2 on exercise correlates well with the severity of disease and the degree of pulmonary fibrosis in patients with idiopathic pulmonary fibrosis. Other exercise-induced physiologic abnormalities in interstitial lung disease include a decrease in work rate and maximal oxygen consumption, abnormally high minute ventilation at submaximal work rates, decreased peak minute ventilation, and failure of tidal volumes to increase at submaximal levels of work while the respiratory rate increases disproportionately. The 6-minute walk test, performed on a flat surface, can provide quantitative data on exercise capacity and on oxygen desaturation with exercise and can justify use of supplemental oxygen based on clinical and physiologic needs. It also provides prognostic information in patients with idiopathic pulmonary fibrosis.

Invasive Evaluation

A collegial interaction and multidisciplinary discussions among the clinician, chest radiologist, thoracic surgeon, pathologist, and rheumatologist can help determine the best diagnostic approach for an individual patient (see Fig. 80-1). Findings on bronchoalveolar lavage can be diagnostic in some patients and can narrow the differential diagnosis in others (Chapter 73). For example, a lymphocyte-predominant cellular pattern raises the possibility of sarcoidosis or hypersensitivity pneumonitis in the appropriate clinical setting. Eosinophils may be seen in pulmonary Langerhans cell granulomatosis or eosinophilic pneumonia, an asbestos body count greater than 1 fiber per milliliter of bronchoalveolar lavage fluid may be seen in asbestosis, and specially staining surfactant material may be seen in pulmonary alveolar proteinosis. A transbronchial lung biopsy may reveal noncaseating granulomas in sarcoidosis, "loose" noncaseating granulomas in hypersensitivity pneumonitis, giant cell granulomas in hard metal pneumoconiosis, or smooth muscle proliferation in lymphangioleiomyomatosis. However, failure to establish a diagnosis despite bronchoalveolar lavage and transbronchial lung biopsy does not exclude these entities. Transbronchial cryobiopsy, a procedure which requires highly specific training, can yield diagnostic histopathology in about 80% of cases.[5] In cases in which the imaging pattern suggests usual interstitial pneumonia, a genomic classifier has proven valuable in identifying a pattern of usual interstitial pneumonia regardless of HRCT imaging features.[6]

Video-assisted thoracoscopic biopsy (Chapter 87) or open lung biopsy may be required to obtain an adequate sample for histologic evaluation of a patient with unexplained signs and symptoms when other studies have failed to establish a diagnosis. The mortality rate is generally less than 2% when the procedure is performed electively.

TREATMENT

When the cause of the interstitial lung disease is clearly known (e.g., acute or subacute hypersensitivity pneumonitis, occupational interstitial lung disease, iatrogenic), further avoidance of the inciting agent or agents is essential (Chapter 81). Although systemic corticosteroids are generally indicated and are associated with a favorable response in some interstitial lung diseases, the dosage and duration are unclear and essentially based on anecdotal experience (Table 80-5).

Supportive oxygen supplementation is dictated by clinical needs. For selected patients with end-stage interstitial lung diseases, such as those associated with significant pulmonary fibrosis and pulmonary hypertension, lung transplantation (Chapter 87) may be a viable option. Treatments for pulmonary hypertension associated with interstitial lung diseases (Chapter 69) are indicated in patients with connective tissue diseases, but their clinical benefit for patients with other interstitial lung diseases has been disappointing.

TABLE 80-5 INTERSTITIAL LUNG DISEASE: CLINICAL RESPONSE TO SYSTEMIC CORTICOSTEROIDS ALONE*

GENERALLY RESPONSIVE	UNRESPONSIVE†
Sarcoidosis	Idiopathic interstitial pneumonia
Acute hypersensitivity pneumonitis	Idiopathic pulmonary fibrosis (usual interstitial pneumonia)
Drug induced	Desquamative interstitial pneumonia (subset)
Environmental causes (some)	Chronic secondary and advanced pulmonary fibrosis
Idiopathic interstitial pneumonia	Fibrotic hypersensitivity pneumonitis (subset)
Cryptogenic organizing pneumonia	Chronic radiation fibrosis
Nonspecific interstitial pneumonia (cellular)	Cryptogenic organizing pneumonia (subset)
Respiratory bronchiolitis–associated ILD	Acute interstitial pneumonia (?)
Lymphocytic interstitial pneumonia	Chronic pulmonary hemorrhage syndromes
Desquamative interstitial pneumonia (subset)	Pulmonary veno-occlusive disease
Acute interstitial pneumonia (some)	Environmental (e.g., asbestosis, pneumoconiosis)
Acute pulmonary capillaritis	End-stage ILDs, pulmonary fibrosis coexisting or associated with pulmonary hypertension
Eosinophilic pneumonia (acute and chronic)	Pulmonary Langerhans cell granulomatosis
Acute radiation pneumonitis‡	Lymphangioleiomyomatosis
Organizing pneumonia associated with connective tissue diseases	ILD in inherited disorders (?)

*The dosage plus duration of corticosteroids used is variable and based on anecdotal experience, individual expert opinion, clinical judgment, and response as judged by objective measurements (clinical, radiologic, or physiologic). Oral prednisone or prednisolone is the most common corticosteroid used. Most patients who respond during the first few weeks of 20 to 60 mg of prednisone per day require maintenance low-dose oral prednisone at 5 to 10 mg/day beyond 6 months. Some patients who require maintenance of oral prednisone doses higher than 20 mg/day beyond 4 to 6 months may tolerate lower doses of prednisone if other immune-modulating agents (e.g., azathioprine, mycophenolate) are used in combination. There is no evidence to recommend a specific regimen. Patients should be monitored carefully and regularly for known side effects of corticosteroid use (e.g., osteoporosis, glucose intolerance), and preventive and therapeutic measures must be undertaken appropriately.

†Some patients unresponsive to oral corticosteroids alone may respond to combined treatment with corticosteroids and other immune-modulating drugs (e.g., azathioprine, mycophenolate).

‡Although most patients respond to modest doses of oral prednisone (initially, 40-60 mg/day), it is important to taper the prednisone very slowly to reach a maintenance dose of 5 to 10 mg/day beyond 6 months; rapid taper of oral prednisone has been associated with "rebound," which is an exaggerated lung injury beyond the irradiated segment of the lung and in the contralateral lung.

ILD = interstitial lung disease.

SPECIFIC TYPES OF INTERSTITIAL LUNG DISEASE

IDIOPATHIC INTERSTITIAL PNEUMONIAS

Idiopathic interstitial pneumonias, which are a subset of acute or chronic interstitial lung diseases of unknown etiology, are characterized by the presence of varying degrees of interstitial and alveolar inflammation and fibrosis. Distinct clinicopathologic forms of idiopathic interstitial pneumonia include chronic fibrosing interstitial pneumonias (idiopathic pulmonary fibrosis and nonspecific interstitial pneumonia), smoking-related interstitial pneumonias (respiratory bronchiolitis–interstitial lung disease and desquamative interstitial pneumonia), and acute or subacute idiopathic interstitial pneumonias (cryptogenic organizing pneumonia and acute interstitial pneumonia). Rare histologic patterns of acute fibrinous and organizing pneumonia and interstitial pneumonias with a bronchiolocentric distribution and pleuroparenchymal fibroelastosis have been recently recognized. In some patients, mixed histopathologic features are evident in different segments of the same lung. When the distinct pathologic forms are not evident, the diagnosis of unclassifiable interstitial pneumonia has been recently recognized. The accuracy of the diagnosis of idiopathic interstitial pneumonias is increased by multidisciplinary discussions among expert pulmonologists, radiologists, and pathologists familiar with interstitial lung diseases and idiopathic interstitial pneumonias.

Although the clinical severity may vary, the idiopathic interstitial pneumonias tend to manifest as an insidious onset of exertional dyspnea and a nonproductive cough. Chest pain and systemic symptoms such as weight loss and fatigue may be present. Bibasilar end-inspiratory crackles are often heard on auscultation. Clubbing, although not specific, is found in 25 to 50% of patients with idiopathic pulmonary fibrosis. Findings on the chest radiograph are most often nonspecific, and the presence of normal lung markings on the chest radiograph does not exclude interstitial lung disease. On HRCT, many pathologic entities have characteristic image patterns that have greatly aided diagnosis (see Table 80-4). The clinical course of idiopathic pulmonary fibrosis is heterogeneous.

CHRONIC FIBROSING INTERSTITIAL PNEUMONIA

Idiopathic Pulmonary Fibrosis

Idiopathic pulmonary fibrosis accounts for 50 to 60% of all idiopathic interstitial pneumonias. Idiopathic pulmonary fibrosis occurs in adult men and women with a mean age at onset of 62 years. Some patients have familial disease, likely autosomal dominant with variable penetrance. Numerous genes have been associated with familial disease as well as some sporadic disease. Examples include the *MUC5B* gene, genes related to immune function, epithelial cell function, maintenance of telomeres, surfactant production, and cell cycle regulation.

Idiopathic pulmonary fibrosis is limited to the lungs in adults, usually older than 60 years, and generally occurs in men with a history of cigarette smoking. Most often patients have otherwise been in good health and have no known connective tissue disease or exposure to drugs or environmental factors known to cause pulmonary fibrosis, although patients with significant cigarette smoking history may have coexisting emphysema. Typical clinical manifestations include a gradual onset and progression of exertional dyspnea, restrictive abnormalities on PFTs (Chapter 73), and a distinct pattern of bilateral pulmonary fibrosis on HRCT.[7]

DIAGNOSIS

Chest radiographs typically show basal-predominant reticular abnormalities with low lung volumes (Fig. 80-2). Compared with the other idiopathic interstitial pneumonias, the HRCT appearance of idiopathic pulmonary fibrosis is distinguished by the presence of fibrotic abnormalities, predominantly in the bases of the lower lobes (E-Fig. 80-1), by subpleural reticulations (E-Fig. 80-2), and by its hallmark honeycombing (E-Fig. 80-3) and traction bronchiectasis (E-Fig. 80-4). These features on HRCT are diagnostic in the appropriate clinical setting (Fig. 80-3A). Radiographs are notable for the absence of extensive ground-glass opacification, micronodules, cysts, consolidation, significant air trapping in multiple lobes, pleural plaques, pleural effusion, and extensive mediastinal adenopathy, all of which are inconsistent with the radiographic pattern of usual interstitial pneumonia.

PFTs usually show a progressive restrictive pattern. However, patients with milder disease may have normal lung volumes and a decreased DLCO; rarely, PFT results may be normal.

The cellular pattern in bronchoalveolar lavage fluid, which is nonspecific, is marked by an excess of neutrophils in proportion to the extent of reticular change on HRCT; the percentage of eosinophils may be mildly increased. The histopathologic pattern of usual interstitial pneumonia consists of patchy interstitial changes alternating with zones of honeycombing, fibrosis, minimal inflammatory cells, collagen deposition, and normal lung (Fig. 80-3B). Subepithelial fibroblastic foci, small aggregates of myofibroblasts, and fibroblasts within myxoid matrix are invariably present and represent areas of active fibrosis. The presence of temporal heterogeneity, or areas at different stages of fibrosis transitioning with normal areas and honeycomb cysts, along with fibrotic foci within the lung, is an essential feature of usual interstitial pneumonia that distinguishes it from other processes such as nonspecific interstitial pneumonia. Interstitial cellular inflammation is minimal in usual interstitial pneumonia. Although usual interstitial pneumonia characterizes the microscopic abnormality in idiopathic pulmonary fibrosis, the same histologic and radiologic pattern also can be seen in patients with rheumatologic lung diseases, chronic hypersensitivity pneumonitis, and asbestosis (Chapter 81). In the appropriate clinical setting (and after definitive exclusion of other known clinical conditions associated with interstitial lung disease) (see later), a definitive diagnosis of idiopathic pulmonary fibrosis is based on the presence of a pattern of usual interstitial pneumonia on HRCT or surgical lung biopsy (Table 80-6).

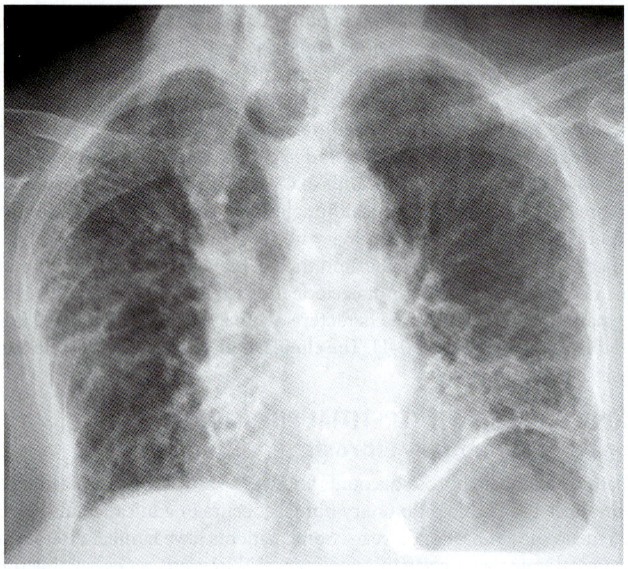

FIGURE 80-2. **Idiopathic pulmonary fibrosis.** Chest radiograph shows low lung volumes with coarse diffuse bilateral reticular opacities and honeycombing. Traction tracheomegaly is also present. (Courtesy of Paul Stark, MD.)

TREATMENT

Antifibrotic therapy[8,9] with pirfenidone (up to 2403 mg per day) slows the rate of decline in forced vital capacity[A1] and the number of respiratory-related hospitalizations[A2] in patients who have idiopathic pulmonary fibrosis and mild to moderate impairment in pulmonary function, with pooled data suggesting an improvement in survival.[A3] Treatment with nintedanib (a tyrosine kinase inhibitor) at 150 mg orally twice daily also reduces the decline in FVC in patients with idiopathic pulmonary fibrosis and mild to moderate impairment in pulmonary function by a similar amount.[A4] Data suggest that both pirfenidone and nintedanib reduce mortality to a similar extent.[10]

Abnormal acid gastroesophageal reflux (Chapter 124) is very common in patients with idiopathic pulmonary fibrosis. Treatment with standard doses of proton pump inhibitors, H_2 receptor antagonists, or both as used for gastroesophageal reflux disease (Chapter 124) may alleviate symptoms, but observational data do not suggest a benefit for survival[11] and their routine use is not recommended.[12]

Warfarin increases respiratory hospitalizations and death in patients with idiopathic pulmonary fibrosis. Prophylactic antibiotics,[A5] interferon-γ1b, cyclophosphamide, colchicine, D-penicillamine, simtuzumab, dual endothelin receptor antagonists (bosentan and macitentan), *N*-acetylcysteine, oral corticosteroids as monotherapy or in combination with azathioprine or cyclophosphamide, sildenafil alone or in combination with nintedanib or pirfenidone[A6] are not beneficial.

Despite the absence of data, patients who require hospitalization and intensive care for an acute exacerbation with loss of respiratory function in the absence of infection or other complications are often treated with empirical intravenous corticosteroids (e.g., methylprednisolone 1.0 g intravenously as a pulse dose once a day for 3 days and followed by hydrocortisone, 125 mg every 6 hours for another 3 to 5 days), with further dosing dependent on the clinical response. Ancillary treatment measures, including supplemental oxygen (based on clinical and physiologic needs), prompt detection and treatment of respiratory tract infections and pulmonary embolism (Chapter 68), pulmonary rehabilitation,[A7] and immunization for influenza, herpes zoster, and pneumococcus, are all appropriate. Treatment of acute exacerbations of idiopathic pulmonary fibrosis with pulse cyclophosphamide is not beneficial.[A8]

Pulmonary hypertension, if present, may be treated (Chapter 69) with inhaled treprostonil (72 mg four times daily), which can significantly improve exercise capacity.[A9] However, endothelin receptor antagonists (e.g., ambrisentan, bosentan, or macitentan) should not be used because of clear data that ambrisentan is harmful in all patients with idiopathic pulmonary fibrosis, even those who have pulmonary hypertension.

Lung transplantation (Chapter 87) is indicated in selected patients, but most patients with idiopathic pulmonary fibrosis are older than age 65 years, an age that is a relative contraindication to lung transplantation. Nevertheless, lung transplantation should be considered in selected patients who are younger than 70 years of age. Palliative care measures should be discussed and instituted before patients reach the terminal stages of the disease.

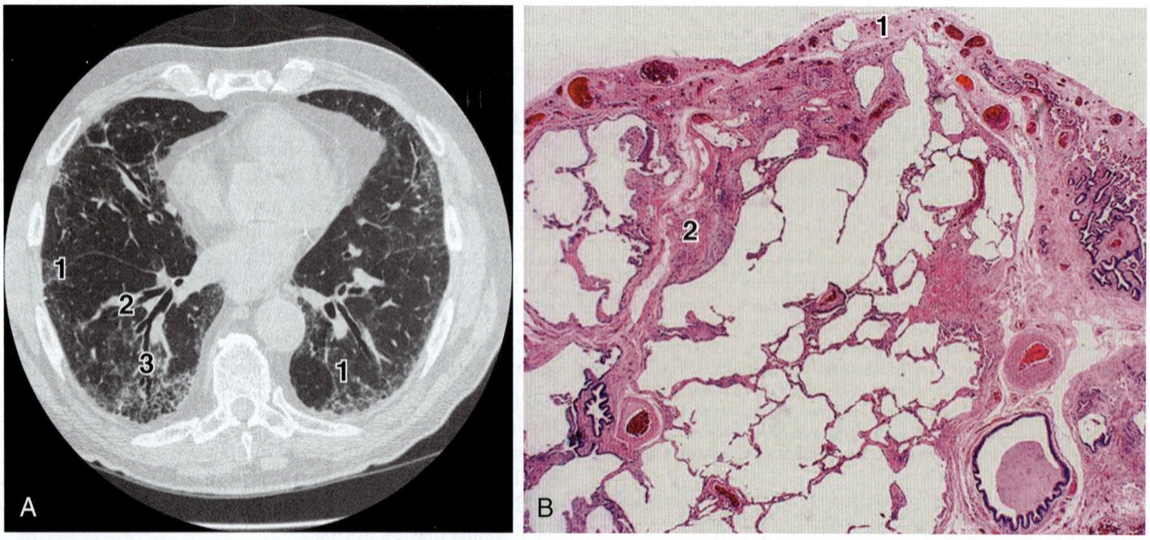

FIGURE 80-3. **Diagnosis of idiopathic pulmonary fibrosis. A,** The usual interstitial pneumonia pattern of idiopathic pulmonary fibrosis in the lower lobes on high-resolution computed tomography consists of (1) subpleural fibrotic changes with (2) traction bronchiectasis and (3) honeycomb cysts in the lower lobes. **B,** Usual interstitial pneumonia pattern of idiopathic pulmonary fibrosis. Note the presence of (1) subpleural fibrosis with (2) fibroblastic foci and temporal heterogeneity of microscopic abnormalities at low magnification. (Courtesy of Dr. Kevin Leslie.)

TABLE 80-6 DIAGNOSIS CRITERIA FOR IDIOPATHIC PULMONARY FIBROSIS

The diagnosis of idiopathic pulmonary fibrosis requires the exclusion of other known causes of interstitial lung disease (e.g., domestic, occupational, and environmental exposures; connective tissue disease; and drug toxicity) AND either #1 or #2:

1. the presence of HRCT pattern of usual interstitial pneumonia (UIP)
2. specific combinations of HRCT patterns and histopathology patterns of UIP in patients subjected to lung tissue sampling[†]

HRCT FEATURES OF UIP	HISTOPATHOLOGIC FEATURES OF UIP
• Subpleural, basal predominance • Reticular abnormality • Distribution is often heterogeneous • Honeycombing with or without peripheral traction bronchiectasis or bronchiolectasis • Absence of peribronchovascular predominance, extensive ground-glass abnormality, diffuse micronodules, discrete cysts, diffuse mosaic attenuation, or consolidation	• Marked fibrosis/architectural distortion, +/− honeycombing in a predominantly subpleural/paraseptal distribution • Patchy parenchymal lung fibrosis • Fibroblast foci • No features suggesting an alternative diagnosis*

*Based on data from Raghu G, Remy-Jardin M, Myers JL, et al. Diagnosis of idiopathic pulmonary fibrosis. An official ATS/ERS/JRS/ALAT clinical practice guideline. *Am J Respir Crit Care Med.* 2018;198:e44-e68.

[†]See above article by Raghu G et al. for specific criteria for patterns of probable UIP, indeterminate for UIP, and alternate diagnosis and combinations.

HRCT = high-resolution computed tomography.

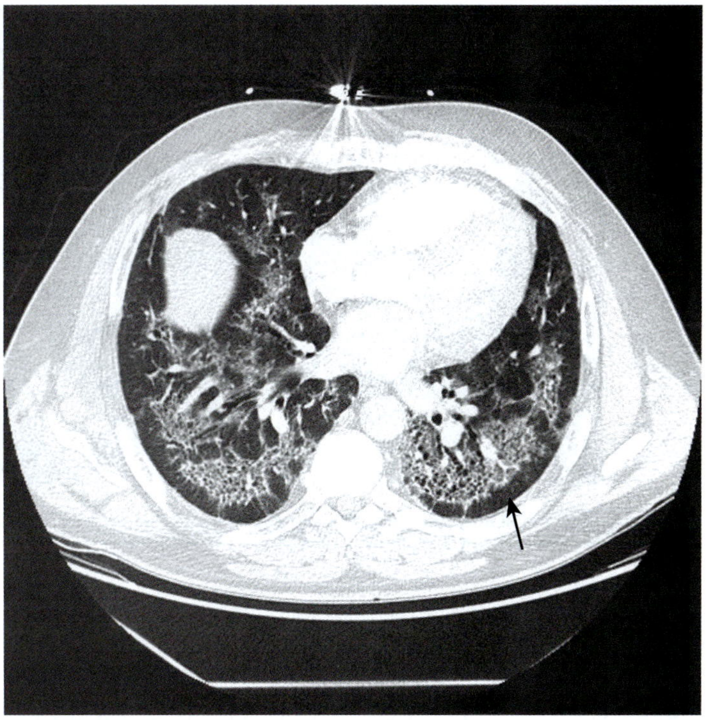

FIGURE 80-4. Nonspecific interstitial pneumonia. Computed tomography scan showing characteristic subpleural sparing (*arrow*).

PROGNOSIS

The natural course of idiopathic pulmonary fibrosis is heterogeneous. Most patients exhibit a slow and steady decline, as measured by FVC (at a rate 150 to 200 mL at the end of first year of follow-up), with a mortality rate of about 7% at 1 year and 14% at 2 years after diagnosis. Treatment with antifibrotic agents appears to reduce mortality by up to 50% at 1 year, but its long-term benefit remains to be determined.

A small subset of patients declines rapidly over several months, but another subset of patients remains stable over several years before declining. Progressive impairment of lung function and gas exchange ultimately is fatal unless the patient undergoes lung transplantation. Patients who survive longer generally have less fibrosis on HRCT, less functional impairment, no evidence of pulmonary hypertension, and no significant oxygen desaturation during a modified version of the 6-minute walk test. Patients with coexisting emphysema, pulmonary hypertension, or episodes of acute exacerbation have even shorter survival times.

Nonspecific Interstitial Pneumonia

Nonspecific interstitial pneumonia is often associated with connective tissue diseases, but idiopathic nonspecific interstitial pneumonia is also recognized as a distinct clinical entity. It typically occurs in middle-aged, nonsmoking women with an average age at diagnosis of about 50 years. The prevalence of nonspecific interstitial pneumonia has been estimated at 1 to 9 per 100,000.

Two subgroups have been described, cellular and fibrotic. Because the average age at onset is about 10 years earlier in nonspecific interstitial pneumonia than in idiopathic pulmonary fibrosis and because the clinical features of idiopathic fibrotic nonspecific interstitial pneumonia are very similar to early cases of idiopathic pulmonary fibrosis, questions persist as to whether idiopathic fibrotic nonspecific interstitial pneumonia is a separate clinical entity or represents an early form of idiopathic pulmonary fibrosis.

DIAGNOSIS

Chest radiographs show bilateral patchy pulmonary infiltrates with lower lung zone predominance. HRCT reveals a predominant ground-glass pattern of attenuation, usually bilateral and often associated with reticulation and subpleural sparing (Fig. 80-4), and loss of volume in the lower lobe. In cellular nonspecific interstitial pneumonia, HRCT shows ground-glass opacification, consolidation, or both, but the biopsy shows mild to moderate lymphoplasmacytic interstitial chronic inflammation. The major differential diagnosis to consider as an alternative to cellular nonspecific interstitial pneumonia is acute or subacute hypersensitivity pneumonitis, so a thorough history regarding environmental exposures is crucial. In contrast, fibrotic nonspecific interstitial pneumonia has a bilateral lower lobe distribution with architectural derangement on HRCT; histopathologically, it has uniformly dense interstitial fibrosis and may sometimes be difficult to distinguish from idiopathic pulmonary fibrosis and usual interstitial pneumonia in the early clinical stages. In these circumstances, the diagnosis of fibrotic nonspecific interstitial pneumonia can be ascertained only by the histologic features in a surgical lung biopsy specimen.

TREATMENT AND PROGNOSIS

Patients with cellular nonspecific interstitial pneumonia usually respond to treatment with corticosteroids (see Table 80-5), and their prognosis is generally better than that of patients with idiopathic pulmonary fibrosis. Nonetheless, some patients progress over several years, and some manifest acute exacerbations similar to patients with idiopathic pulmonary fibrosis. Nintedanib (150 mg orally twice daily) can attenuate the loss of lung function in patients with progressive nonspecific interstitial pneumonia.[A10,A11] Immune-modulating drugs, including prednisone, azathioprine, and mycophenolate, have been used empirically, with their doses based on clinical response as assessed by clinicians and not on evidence with randomized clinical trials.

SMOKING-RELATED INTERSTITIAL PNEUMONIAS

Respiratory Bronchiolitis–Associated Interstitial Lung Disease

This interstitial lung disease is almost invariably associated with cigarette smoking and usually manifests clinically during the fourth or fifth decade of life. However, it also may be detected incidentally on radiographs in relatively younger and asymptomatic persons with a previous history of cigarette smoking or in people passively exposed to chronic cigarette smoke.

DIAGNOSIS

Pulmonary function tests show varying degrees of airway obstruction, mildly decreased or preserved TLC, and decreased DLCO. The chest radiograph typically reveals bronchial wall thickening and areas of ground-glass attenuation. HRCT reveals centrilobular nodules with an upper lobe predominance, patchy ground-glass attenuation, and peribronchial alveolar septal thickening (Fig. 80-5A). Areas of hypoattenuation (mosaic attenuation) represent air trapping as a result of small airways disease. The characteristic finding on bronchoalveolar lavage is numerous brown-pigmented alveolar macrophages,

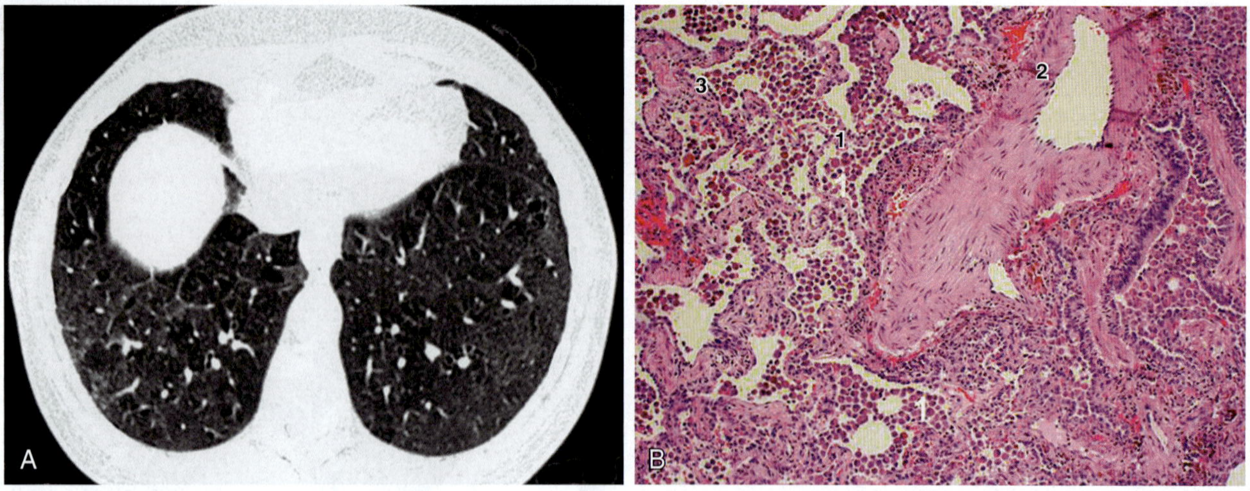

FIGURE 80-5. **Respiratory bronchiolitis–associated interstitial lung disease. A,** Ground-glass attenuation with a mosaic pattern on high-resolution computed tomography. **B,** Note the dense aggregates of (1) pigmented macrophages present in the air spaces around the terminal airways with (2) variable bronchiolar metaplasia and (3) interstitial fibrosis.

often with a modest increase in neutrophils. Lung biopsy is rarely needed, but its hallmark histopathologic feature is the accumulation of pigmented alveolar macrophages with glassy eosinophilic cytoplasm and granular pigmentation within respiratory bronchioles, typically with a chronic inflammatory cell infiltrate in the bronchioles and surrounding alveolar walls (Fig. 80-5B). Fibroblastic foci and honeycomb change are not present, but centrilobular emphysema is frequent.

TREATMENT AND PROGNOSIS

Progression to honeycomb lung and end-stage fibrosis seldom occurs if patients completely cease smoking. Total discontinuation of cigarette smoking is essential, and the prognosis is good. Patients who discontinue cigarette smoking may benefit from low-dose corticosteroids (e.g., prednisone, 10 to 20 mg/day) for a few months.

Desquamative Interstitial Pneumonia

Desquamative interstitial pneumonia is a rare entity (<3% of all interstitial lung diseases) that may represent a form of respiratory bronchiolitis–associated interstitial lung diseases extending into the alveolar spaces and alveolar walls. Although most affected individuals are cigarette smokers, the histologic pattern of desquamative interstitial pneumonia may also occur in pneumoconiosis, rheumatologic disease, and drug-associated interstitial lung disease. Patients are often initially seen with advanced disease and striking hypoxemia. The histopathology features of desquamative interstitial pneumonia are characterized by accumulation of pigmented alveolar macrophages within the alveoli. Histologic changes within the respiratory bronchioles and within the alveolar spaces can coexist and represent a histopathologic spectrum of alveolar macrophage accumulation, with a variable degree of interstitial fibrosis.[13]

DIAGNOSIS

PFTs reveal a restrictive lung defect and decreased DLCO with or without coexisting airway obstruction. The chest radiograph shows patchy basal consolidation with a lower lobe and peripheral predominance (Fig. 80-6). HRCT shows bilateral symmetrical ground-glass opacities with a predominantly basal and peripheral distribution as well as diffuse alveolar septal thickening (Fig. 80-7A). Irregular linear opacities, typically associated with traction bronchiectasis, may be noted. The finding of small discrete cysts, believed to represent trapped air in dilated bronchioles, within areas of ground-glass changes (E-Fig. 80-5) and intervening normal lung parenchyma is highly suggestive of desquamative interstitial pneumonia. Fluid recovered from bronchoalveolar lavage quite often shows increased numbers of pigmented alveolar macrophages, frequently with increased neutrophils. Histopathologic findings on biopsy include diffuse alveolar septal thickening, hyperplasia of type II pneumocytes, and intense accumulation of intra-alveolar granular pigmented macrophages in a uniform manner (Fig. 80-7B); fibrosis is minimal.

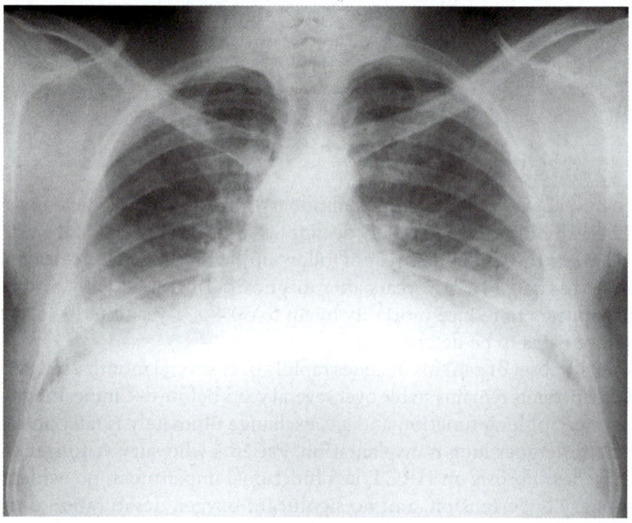

FIGURE 80-6. **Desquamative interstitial pneumonia (DIP).** Chest radiograph shows homogeneous bilateral perihilar ground-glass opacification and basal predominant consolidation. (Courtesy of Paul Stark, MD.)

TREATMENT AND PROGNOSIS

With total cessation of smoking and administration of oral corticosteroid therapy (see Table 80-5), outcomes are generally good, with an estimated overall survival rate of 70% at 10 years. However, a subset of patients may progress despite cessation of cigarette smoking, and a trial of corticosteroid therapy with or without immune-modulating agents and lung transplantation is an appropriate consideration for selected patients.

ACUTE OR SUBACUTE IDIOPATHIC INTERSTITIAL PNEUMONIA

Acute Interstitial Pneumonia

Acute interstitial pneumonia is seen in otherwise healthy persons usually after an apparent acute viral upper respiratory infection (Fig. 80-8). The syndrome, historically known as Hamman-Rich syndrome (Chapter 79), mimics acute respiratory distress syndrome (Chapter 90). Acute interstitial pneumonia is a rare and fulminant idiopathic interstitial pneumonia that presents with acute symptoms and leads to respiratory distress or failure.

Cryptogenic Organizing Pneumonia

Cryptogenic organizing pneumonia,[14] previously referred to as bronchiolitis obliterans organizing pneumonia (BOOP) of unknown cause, is an idiopathic form of organizing pneumonia. Organizing pneumonia affects the small airways, including the distal bronchioles, respiratory bronchioles, alveolar ducts, and

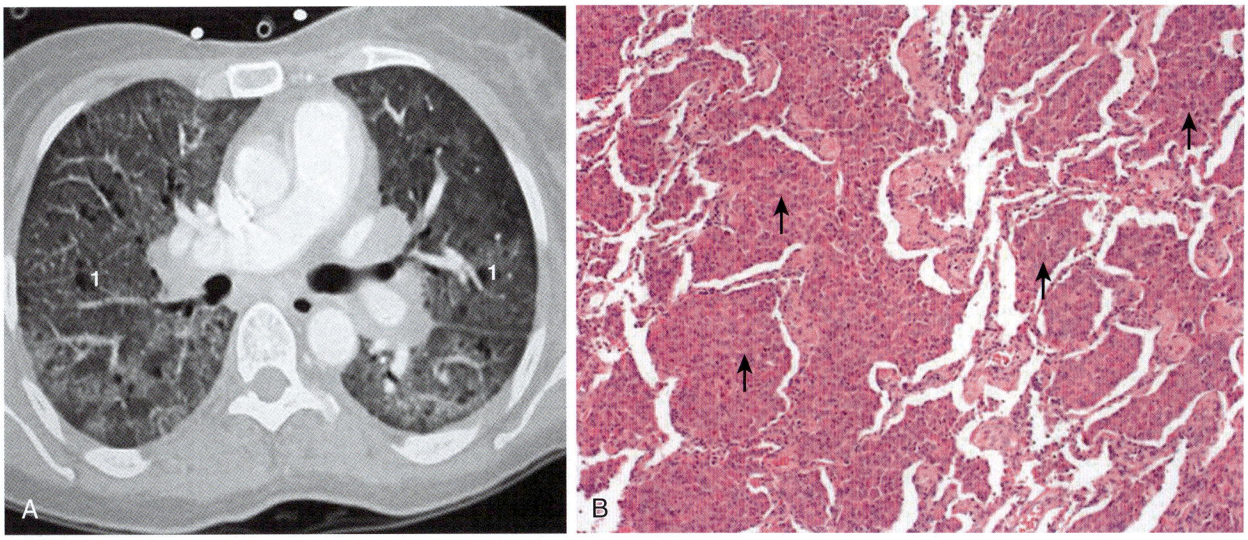

FIGURE 80-7. **Desquamative interstitial pneumonia. A, Ground-glass attenuation with cystic spaces on high-resolution computed tomography. B, Note that the alveolar spaces are densely filled with macrophages *(arrowheads)*.**

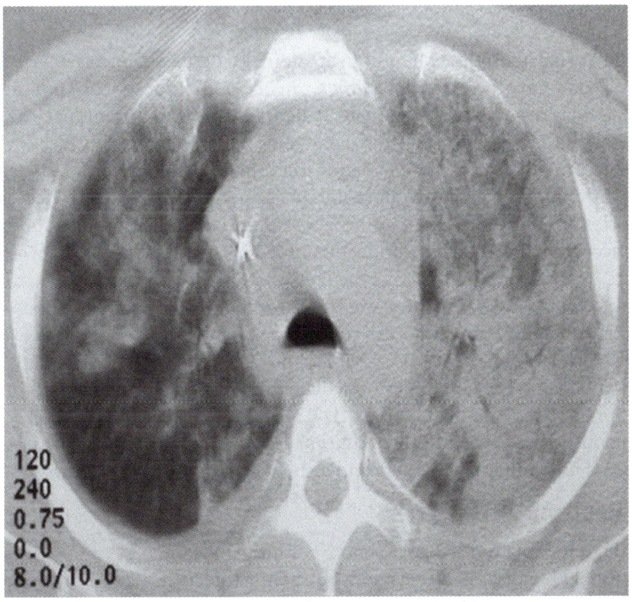

FIGURE 80-8. **Acute interstitial pneumonia with diffuse alveolar damage histologically. Note the dense air space consolidation.**

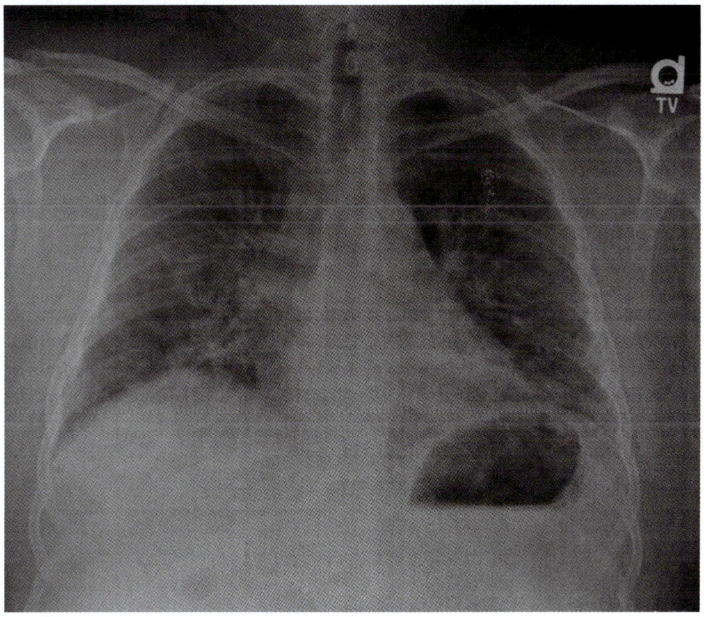

FIGURE 80-9. **Chest radiograph showing cryptogenic organizing pneumonia. Note the bilateral patchy air space opacities.**

alveolar walls. Although the incidence and prevalence of cryptogenic organizing pneumonia are unknown, the estimated annual incidence in the United States is 6 to 7 cases per 100,000. The mean age at presentation is about 60 years, and there is no sex predominance.

DIAGNOSIS

Cryptogenic organizing pneumonia most commonly manifests as a flulike illness with a nonproductive cough followed by exertional dyspnea. This scenario has been reported to occur following SARS-CoV-2 infection. PFTs show a restrictive defect, but 20% of patients, most of whom are current or past smokers, also have an obstructive defect. Chest radiography reveals patchy unilateral or bilateral alveolar opacities that may be peripheral or migratory; small nodular opacities are seen in 10 to 50% of cases (Fig. 80-9). In about 90% of patients, HRCT shows areas of air space consolidation with lower lung zone predominance, frequently in a subpleural or peribronchial distribution (Fig. 80-10); other features include small nodules along bronchovascular bundles and ground-glass attenuation. Bronchoalveolar lavage is nonspecific; increased lymphocytes, neutrophils, and eosinophils may be seen. On biopsy, key histologic features are excessive proliferation of granulation tissue within the small airways and alveolar ducts as well as chronic inflammation in the surrounding alveoli.

TREATMENT AND PROGNOSIS

Most patients recover rapidly and completely when treated with oral corticosteroids (see Table 80-5) for 6 months but may relapse after discontinuation and require oral corticosteroids for longer periods and sometimes indefinitely, often with adjunct immunomodulating agents such as azathioprine or mycophenolate. Some data suggest that clarithromycin (250 to 500 mg daily) is an alternative for patients whose PFTs are reasonably normal (forced vital capacity >80% of predicted). A small subset of patients in whom pulmonary fibrosis develops despite corticosteroids and immune-modulating agents progress to pulmonary fibrosis and behave similarly to patients with idiopathic pulmonary fibrosis. Spontaneous remissions are known to occur.

Lymphoid and Lymphocytic Interstitial Pneumonia

This condition is more common in women, especially in the fifth decade of life, but it may occur at any age. Patients should be evaluated for concurrent connective tissue disease, an autoimmune disorder (especially Sjögren syndrome; Chapter 247), or common variable immunoglobulin deficiency (Chapter 231) because idiopathic LIP is very rare. Symptoms are nonspecific and include a gradual onset of cough and exertional dyspnea. Lymphoid and LIP is within the spectrum of benign lymphoproliferative

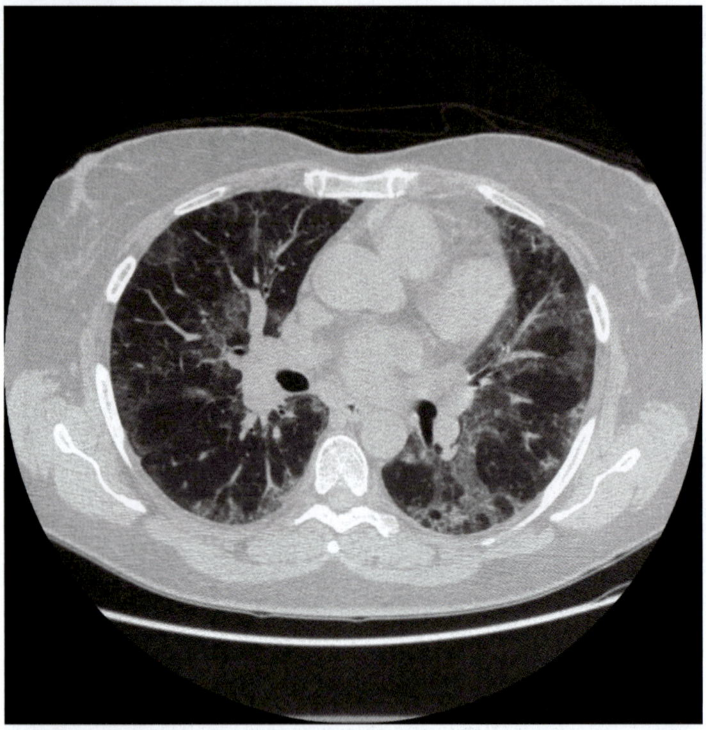

FIGURE 80-10. Peripheral ground-glass opacities in a patient with cryptogenic organizing pneumonia.

disorders, and some patients manifest pseudolymphoma or lymphoma as a complication.

DIAGNOSIS

Chest radiographs show a reticular or reticulonodular pattern predominantly involving the lower lung zones. HRCT reveals bilateral ground-glass attenuation, small or large nodules, and scattered cysts; perivascular honeycombing and reticular abnormalities also may be seen (E-Fig. 80-6). Increased numbers of lymphocytes are found on bronchoalveolar lavage, and biopsy reveals a dense interstitial lymphocytic infiltrate.

TREATMENT AND PROGNOSIS

Some patients respond to or stabilize with oral corticosteroids (see Table 80-5). The prognosis is variable, with more than one third of patients progressing to diffuse pulmonary fibrosis.

INTERSTITIAL LUNG DISEASE ASSOCIATED WITH CONNECTIVE TISSUE DISEASE

Many of the connective tissue diseases, including progressive systemic sclerosis (Chapter 246), rheumatoid arthritis (Chapter 243), SLE (Chapter 245), dermatomyositis and polymyositis (Chapter 248), Sjögren syndrome (Chapter 247), and mixed connective tissue disorder (Chapter 246), may have interstitial lung disease as one of their manifestations.[15] In fact, up to 20% of patients with connective tissue diseases may initially be thought to have an interstitial lung disease alone. Therefore these diagnoses must be considered in patients with interstitial lung disease, even in the absence of extrathoracic findings. Conversely, because pulmonary involvement is a major cause of death in patients with connective tissue diseases, the presence of interstitial lung disease should be carefully sought in affected patients.[16] All forms of interstitial pneumonia can occur in patients with connective tissue diseases. The natural history of interstitial lung disease complicating connective tissue diseases is variable, especially because coexisting pulmonary vascular disease or nonparenchymal pulmonary involvement may be present.

PROGRESSIVE SYSTEMIC SCLEROSIS

Of the connective tissue diseases, progressive systemic sclerosis is most frequently associated with interstitial lung disease.[17] Pulmonary symptoms may antedate cutaneous or digital manifestations of the disease by several years. Most patients affected have nonspecific interstitial pneumonia, with a minority

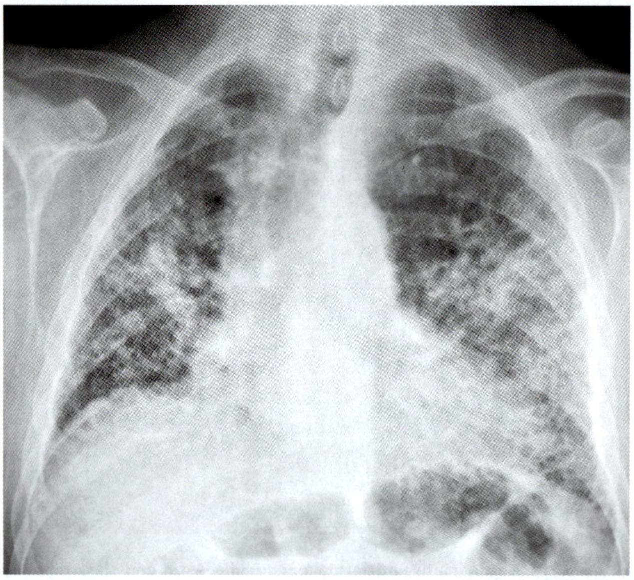

FIGURE 80-11. Rheumatoid interstitial lung disease with usual interstitial pneumonia pattern. Chest radiograph shows low lung volumes, diffuse reticular opacities, and honeycombing with basal predominance. (Courtesy of Paul Stark, MD.)

having a usual interstitial pneumonia pattern. DLCO levels correlate with mortality. Pulmonary hypertension, which can occur in the absence of pulmonary fibrosis, may result in cor pulmonale. Patients with chronic pulmonary fibrosis also have an increased risk for bronchogenic carcinoma, usually either bronchoalveolar cell carcinoma or adenocarcinoma. For scleroderma-associated interstitial lung disease, mycophenolate (target dose 1500 mg twice daily) provides similar physiologic improvement and stabilization of pulmonary function compared with cyclophosphamide (2.0 mg/kg/day) with fewer side effects,[A12] so mycophenolate is now considered first-line therapy. Rituximab (two cycles of a 1000 mg intravenous infusion, 2 weeks apart) has been used as an alternate immunosuppressive regimen of interstitial lung disease associated with systemic sclerosis.[18] Nintedanib (150 mg orally twice daily) can attenuate the loss of lung function when administered alone or in addition to mycophenolate.[A13] Tocilizumab, an IL-6 receptor blocker (162 mg weekly subcutaneously), also can mitigate decline in lung function in patients with elevated systemic inflammatory markers and a short duration of systemic disease.[A14]

RHEUMATOID ARTHRITIS

Although rheumatoid arthritis is more common in women (2 : 1 to 4 : 1 ratio), interstitial lung disease associated with rheumatoid arthritis is more common in men (3 : 1 ratio). Most cases occur at 50 to 60 years of age, and pulmonary symptoms follow the onset of arthritis in about 75% of cases.[19] Lung involvement in rheumatoid arthritis may take many forms, but bronchiectasis, bronchiolitis, idiopathic interstitial pneumonias (Fig. 80-11), and pleural effusions or pleural thickening are some of the most common. Early in the course, the histologic changes are similar to those of idiopathic interstitial pneumonias, including pulmonary fibrosis, but are distinguished by a prominent lymphocytic infiltrate that may contain germinal follicles adjacent to vessels and airways. As the disease progresses, the infiltration becomes less pronounced and is replaced by fibrous tissue, honeycomb changes, or both. Other pulmonary manifestations include pulmonary nodules, vasculitis, pulmonary hypertension, and Caplan syndrome (progressive upper lobe nodular pulmonary fibrosis in a coal miner with rheumatoid arthritis) but are relatively rare. Patients with usual interstitial pneumonia pattern on HRCT have worse prognosis than those with a nonspecific interstitial pneumonia pattern. Treatment is directed at the underlying rheumatoid arthritis (Chapter 243), but methotrexate therapy is generally avoided since one of its potential toxicities is the development of interstitial lung disease. Nintedanib (150 mg orally twice daily) can attenuate the decline in lung function in patients with progressive inherited lung disease.

SYSTEMIC LUPUS ERYTHEMATOSUS

Pulmonary abnormalities complicating SLE (Chapter 245) may vary greatly. Pleural disease or pleural effusions (or both) are commonly present in lung disease that complicates SLE. Acute lupus pneumonitis may mimic acute interstitial pneumonia, with widespread ground-glass attenuation admixed with consolidation, or it may manifest as diffuse alveolar hemorrhage.

Chronic interstitial lung disease may also occur. Infection must always be considered in acutely ill patients who have received steroids or other immunosuppressive therapy. Rarely, the restrictive lung defect, which may be predominantly a result of diaphragmatic weakness, leads to a chest radiographic pattern of small-appearing lungs that may look progressively smaller over time. This so-called "shrinking lung" is generally resistant to corticosteroids or other immunosuppressive agents used to treat SLE. Otherwise, treatment of the interstitial lung disease is similar to treatment of the underlying SLE.

DERMATOMYOSITIS AND POLYMYOSITIS

In contrast to progressive systemic sclerosis, the pattern of lung involvement in dermatomyositis and polymyositis is more heterogeneous. Usual interstitial pneumonia, nonspecific interstitial pneumonia, and organizing pneumonia have all been reported. Most patients have an anti–Jo-1 antibody or anti-PL-7 antibody, and the disease is typically progressive over time.[20] An acute interstitial pneumonia–like syndrome occurs in a subset of patients and is associated with high mortality rate despite aggressive immunosuppressive agents and high-dose corticosteroids. Interstitial lung disease may precede the muscular manifestations by months to years or be superimposed on established muscle disease. The severity of the muscular disease does not correlate with that of the interstitial lung disease. Treatment is directed at the underlying disease (Chapter 248).

SJÖGREN SYNDROME

Interstitial lung disease is seen in patients with Sjögren syndrome, particularly those with the primary form of the disease. LIP is the most frequent subtype, but cryptogenic organizing pneumonia also may be present. Respiratory infections and bronchiectasis are common in advanced stages, perhaps because of inspissated mucus. Response to corticosteroid or immunosuppressive therapy is usually good (Chapter 247).

MIXED CONNECTIVE TISSUE DISEASE

This overlap syndrome (Chapter 246) combines features of progressive systemic sclerosis, SLE, rheumatoid arthritis, and polymyositis or dermatomyositis. Pulmonary disease is common, but it is most often subclinical and identified only radiographically. Treatment includes corticosteroids and other immune-modulating agents for the underlying disease.

ANKYLOSING SPONDYLITIS

The most common pulmonary manifestation of ankylosing spondylitis (Chapter 244) is upper lobe bilateral reticulonodular infiltrates with cyst formation as a result of parenchymal destruction. There is no known effective therapy for this apical fibrobullous disease.

HYPERSENSITIVITY PNEUMONITIS

PATHOBIOLOGY

Hypersensitivity pneumonitis, which is an inflammatory and/or fibrotic disease affecting the lung parenchyma and small airways, is a syndrome caused when sensitized individuals repeatedly inhale specific antigens from occupational or environmental exposure (Chapters 81 and 82). Within a short period after inhalation of an inciting agent, patients develop a nonspecific diffuse pneumonitis with inflammatory cell infiltration of the bronchioles, alveoli, and interstitium, sometimes associated with a pleural effusion. Loosely formed, noncaseating, epithelioid cell granulomas and a mononuclear infiltrate may be dispersed in the interstitium. Hypersensitivity pneumonitis can occur with exposure to a wide range of inhaled antigens (Chapters 81 and 82). Some of the more common exposures are farmer's lung, bird fancier's lung, parakeet keeper's lung, and pigeon breeder's lung. The avian antigen may be related to overt exposure to birds, bird droppings, or bird nests or to occult exposures to bird feeders or bird feather components used in beddings, down comforters, duvets, or jackets. Despite a thorough evaluation, the source and/or the inciting agent/antigen may not be identified in a substantial number of patients who meet the diagnostic criteria for HP. Hobbies (woodworker's lung) and recreational activities (sauna taker's lung; hot tub) may be implicated as well as occupations.

CLINICAL MANIFESTATIONS

The clinical features and severity of symptoms vary according to the frequency and intensity of exposure. The index of clinical suspicion for hypersensitivity pneumonitis should be high in every patient with new-onset interstitial lung disease. This should prompt a detailed history of exposure to potential agents or changes in the domestic and other environments (or both) (Chapters 16 and 81). The interval between exposure to the antigen and the clinical manifestations of lung disease is unknown, although symptoms can occur as soon as 4 to 12 hours after exposure. In such cases, fever and chills are common symptoms, are often temporally related to the workplace or to hobbies, and may actually disappear on vacations or during absence from the site of exposure, only to recur when exposure is resumed. In more chronic and low-level exposures, however, the onset is insidious. Some patients with fibrotic hypersensitivity pneumonitis owing to many years of exposure may manifest clinical features similar to those of patients with idiopathic pulmonary fibrosis.

DIAGNOSIS

Findings on chest radiography are diverse, with focal patchy consolidation or a diffuse ground-glass appearance in nonfibrotic hypersensitivity pneumonitis (E-Fig. 80-7), micronodular and reticular shadowing, and diffuse, predominantly upper lung zone reticulation with honeycombing in the fibrotic form. Chest radiograph results may be normal in up to 30% of patients with significant physiologic abnormalities.

On HRCT, small centrilobular ill-defined nodules of ground-glass densities are seen, along with evidence of mosaic attenuation (trapped air) as a result of concomitant bronchiolitis and upper lobe predominance of the parenchymal abnormalities (E-Fig. 80-8). Chronically, findings of lung fibrosis may be indistinguishable from the patterns seen in usual interstitial pneumonia and idiopathic pulmonary fibrosis (E-Fig. 80-9).

Precipitating serum antibodies for potential causes of hypersensitivity pneumonitis confirm exposure but not cause and effect. The absence of antibodies does not exclude hypersensitivity pneumonitis. In some cases, a thorough investigation of the patient's home and workplace by an industrial hygienist may reveal occult molds, spores, *Thermoactinomycetes* spp, *Aureobasidium pullulans*, and other precipitating causes. When such exposures are evident and suspected to be the cause of the manifested interstitial lung disease, further diagnostic interventions such as bronchoalveolar lavage may be quite helpful by showing the most marked increase in T lymphocytes and an increased number of plasma cells. The characteristic histologic triad in hypersensitivity pneumonitis is cellular nonspecific interstitial pneumonia, cellular bronchiolitis, and granulomatous inflammation; however, this triad is seen in no more than 75% of affected patients. Differentiation from cellular nonspecific interstitial pneumonia may be challenging. Prompted by an elicited history of environmental exposure for an attributable antigen, bronchochallenge testing with the suspected antigen in experienced laboratories may provide further clues for the diagnosis of hypersensitivity pneumonitis in a patient otherwise suspected to have idiopathic pulmonary fibrosis. A subset of patients who meet the diagnostic criteria for idiopathic pulmonary fibrosis may be subsequently diagnosed as having fibrotic hypersensitivity pneumonitis after careful evaluation by experts who are familiar with hypersensitivity pneumonitis. Hypersensitivity pneumonitis can be diagnosed with high confidence in patients in whom an exposure has been identified by history or by serum IgG antibodies against associated antigens or a specific inhalation challenge, a typical pattern on HRCT imaging, and lymphocytosis on bronchoalveolar lavage.[21]

TREATMENT AND PROGNOSIS

A thorough investigation must be undertaken to identify the antigen in the patient's environment. Sometimes an industrial hygienist is needed to obtain samples for culture from potential sources in the patient's domestic or workplace environment. The identified antigen must be eradicated from the patient's environment. Avoidance of exposure to the identified antigen or antigens and treatment with corticosteroids (see Table 80-5) are important if improvement is to be obtained. However, despite thorough searches, the antigen may remain undetected in a substantial number of patients who have hypersensitivity pneumonitis confirmed by lung biopsy. Corticosteroids (0.5 to 1 mg/kg daily) and immune-modulating agents (e.g., mycophenolate usually at 1000 to 1500 mg bid and azathioprine usually at 100 to 150 mg daily) are useful for patients with nonfibrotic hypersensitivity pneumonitis. Continued exposure to the unidentifiable antigens, prolonged exposure to antigens, or both can lead to chronic pneumonitis and irreversible fibrosis that may not respond to any treatment regimen. In the fibrotic stages, the prognosis and clinical course may be similar to those of idiopathic pulmonary fibrosis, and antifibrotic agents used for idiopathic pulmonary fibrosis may slow the progression of the disease.

OCCUPATIONAL INTERSTITIAL LUNG DISEASES

Interstitial lung diseases associated with specific occupations generally involve the inhalation and deposition of dust in the lungs followed by a tissue reaction that ultimately results in fibrosis. Examples include silicosis (inhalation of silica in crystalline form or silicon dioxide as quartz, cristobalite, or tridymite; at-risk occupations include sandblasting and working with granite), coal workers' pneumoconiosis (inhalation of coal dust), asbestosis (deposition of fibers during mining, milling, or other handling of asbestos; welding and working in a shipyard are two at-risk occupations), berylliosis (seen in aerospace workers and in electronic industries), and hard metal disease (Chapter 81). Radiographic features vary depending on the inciting inhalant. Cessation of the exposure is important, but the fibrosis is generally irreversible.

DRUG-INDUCED INTERSTITIAL LUNG DISEASE

More than 300 drugs, biomolecules, or homeopathic remedies (see Table 80-2) can cause acute, subacute, or chronic interstitial lung disease, and the list continues to increase as new medications are introduced (https://www.pneumotox.com). The clinical and radiographic manifestations are quite varied. Examples of known syndromes include chronic nitrofurantoin-induced interstitial lung disease that mimics idiopathic pulmonary fibrosis (and is fatal in ≈8% of cases), granulomatous pneumonitis secondary to methotrexate (<5%), sarcoid-like granulomatous interstitial lung disease induced by interferon-α and tumor necrosis factor–modulating agents, nonspecific bilateral alveolar and interstitial inflammatory and fibrotic abnormalities caused by bleomycin, immune-modulating agents and other chemotherapeutic agents, and alveolar and interstitial abnormalities and nodular densities in acute and chronic amiodarone pulmonary toxicity. Most drug-induced interstitial lung disease is reversible if recognized early and if use of the responsible drug is discontinued. In addition to discontinuing the implicated drug, treatment with corticosteroids (see Table 80-5) is indicated in patients with moderate to severe functional impairment.

ALVEOLAR FILLING DISORDERS

In alveolar filling disorders (Chapter 79), air spaces distal to the terminal bronchioles are filled with blood, lipid, protein, water, or inflammatory cells. The radiographic appearance is that of an alveolar infiltrate with small nodular densities and ill-defined margins; hence, the radiographic picture is similar to an interstitial lung disease, and virtually all the alveolar filling disorders may result in interstitial lung disease, including Goodpasture syndrome, pulmonary alveolar proteinosis (primary and secondary), alveolar hemorrhage syndromes (Chapter 79), acute interstitial pneumonia, and bronchoalveolar cell carcinoma (Chapter 177).

IDIOPATHIC PULMONARY HEMOSIDEROSIS

This rare disorder of children and young adults (Chapter 79) is characterized by intermittent, diffuse alveolar hemorrhage without evidence of vasculitis, inflammation, granulomas, or necrosis. The etiology is poorly understood. Anemia and hepatosplenomegaly may be present. Hemosiderin-laden macrophages in bronchoalveolar lavage fluid and lung tissue are part of the diagnostic picture. The chest radiograph reveals diffuse, bilateral alveolar infiltrates. A chronic interstitial infiltrate may develop after repeated episodes, infrequently with hilar and mediastinal adenopathy. Systemic corticosteroids (see Table 80-5) may be beneficial in treating acute disease.

CHRONIC EOSINOPHILIC PNEUMONIA

The clinical manifestation of chronic eosinophilic pneumonia varies over a wide spectrum, from asymptomatic to respiratory failure. The disease often occurs in women in the second to fourth decades of life; such women often manifest constitutional symptoms of fevers, sweats, weight loss, fatigue, dyspnea, and cough. Peripheral blood eosinophilia (Chapter 156), usually at levels of 10 to 40%, is common but may be absent in up to one third of affected patients at initial evaluation. On chest radiography and HRCT, the cardinal feature is peripheral multifocal consolidation, predominantly in the upper and mid lung zones. These dense peripheral infiltrates, which have sometimes been called the "photographic negative of pulmonary edema," often resolve dramatically after treatment with corticosteroids. Ground-glass attenuation commonly accompanies the consolidation. Bronchoalveolar lavage fluid may show greater than 40% eosinophils during exacerbations. Treatment with corticosteroids (see Table 80-5) results in a rapid response, frequently within hours; in fact, such a dramatic resolution of symptoms with radiographic clearance of infiltrates shortly after initiation of corticosteroid therapy is considered "diagnostic." However, the rate of relapse is high, so most patients require prolonged treatment with low-dose corticosteroids (prednisone, 5 to 10 mg/day) to stay in remission.

INTERSTITIAL LUNG DISEASE ASSOCIATED WITH PULMONARY VASCULITIDES

GRANULOMATOSIS WITH POLYANGIITIS

Granulomatosis with polyangiitis (Chapter 249) is the most common form of vasculitis that involves the lung. The systemic necrotizing granulomatous inflammation and small-vessel vasculitis are often manifested first in the upper respiratory tract as chronic rhinitis or sinusitis (or both), epistaxis, oropharyngeal ulcerations, gingival hyperplasia with clefting, or serous otitis media. Destruction of the nasal cartilage may lead to septal perforation or a saddle nose deformity. Ulcerative lesions of the tracheobronchial tree, cavitating nodules within the lung parenchyma, and diffuse alveolar hemorrhage caused by pulmonary capillaritis are lower respiratory tract manifestations. Focal segmental necrotizing glomerulonephritis is the most common extrathoracic manifestation, although pulmonary involvement may occur without renal disease. Chest radiography usually reveals multiple nodular or cavitating infiltrates, but single nodules may be found as well. The diagnosis is most commonly made serologically, with demonstration of antineutrophil cytoplasmic antibodies, although a negative test result does not exclude the disease. Treatment is usually with cyclophosphamide (50 to 100 mg/day or 2 mg/kg of ideal body weight per day but not more than 150 mg/day) in conjunction with oral corticosteroids (prednisone, 10 to 40 mg/day). Initial remission occurs in more than 90% of patients, but most patients require treatment for several years. Relapses may occur in up to 30% of patients, especially when treatment is tapered; such patients may need treatment indefinitely. Rituximab has become a first-line therapy for anti-neutrophil cytoplasma antibody (ANCA) associated vasculitis (remission-induction dose of 375 mg/m^2 body-surface area typically infused once a week for 4 weeks) (Chapter 249). Prophylaxis for *Pneumocystis jiroveci* infection is indicated in patients receiving chronic treatment.

EOSINOPHILIC GRANULOMATOSIS WITH POLYANGIITIS

This systemic necrotizing vasculitis, previously known as Churg-Strauss syndrome (Chapter 249), affects both the upper and lower respiratory tracts and is almost invariably preceded by allergic disorders such as asthma, allergic rhinitis, sinusitis, or a drug reaction. Peripheral and lung eosinophilia, bronchospasm, increased immunoglobulin E levels, and rashes are common manifestations. The pulmonary radiographic findings are bilateral patchy, fleeting infiltrates; diffuse nodular infiltrates; or diffuse reticulonodular disease. Histopathologic examination of lung tissue is generally diagnostic with features of granulomatous angiitis or vasculitis. Although treatment with corticosteroids is indicated, the dosage and duration are unclear (see Table 80-5). Response rates are high when mepolizumab (an anti-IL-5 monoclonal antibody at a dose of 300 mg administered subcutaneously every 4 weeks) is added to standard care.[A15] Additional immunosuppression, usually with cyclophosphamide (2 mg/kg/day orally or an initial intravenous pulse dose of 15 mg/kg or 0.6 g/m^2 to maximum dose of 1.2 g), is often used to achieve disease control particularly in severe disease.

IDIOPATHIC PULMONARY CAPILLARITIS

Idiopathic pulmonary capillaritis may involve the pulmonary vasculature within the alveolar walls and be manifested as interstitial lung disease. Patients may also have subclinical alveolar hemorrhage, often associated with the presence of perinuclear antineutrophilic cytoplasmic antibodies. Corticosteroids are the mainstay of treatment, but the doses and duration of treatment are unclear. Frequently, patients need adjunctive treatment with cyclophosphamide or rituximab, similar to patients with vasculitis and granulomatosis with polyangiitis (Chapter 249).

OTHER FORMS OF INTERSTITIAL LUNG DISEASE

SARCOIDOSIS

See Chapter 83.

PULMONARY LANGERHANS CELL HISTIOCYTOSIS

Langerhans cell histiocytosis is an idiopathic, granulomatous interstitial lung disease that typically occurs in the second or third decade of life, with a male preponderance (Chapter 155). The currently accepted term is pulmonary Langerhans cell histiocytosis. It is rare, with an estimated incidence of two to five cases per million population. The large majority (about 90%) of affected individuals are male smokers, and current evidence suggests that the disorder results from an abnormal immune response to a component or derivative of cigarette smoke. The disease is thought to be a myeloid neoplasm, with a high proportion of cells carrying somatic mutations in the *BRAF* gene and/or in the *NRAS*, *KRAS*, and *MAP2K1* genes.

CLINICAL MANIFESTATIONS

The clinical findings are variable and range from an abnormal chest radiograph in an asymptomatic patient to progressive dyspnea with a nonproductive cough. Systemic symptoms of malaise, fever, and weight loss may be present. Hemoptysis is rare. Spontaneous pneumothorax, which occurs in approximately 25% of patients and is caused by rupture of subpleural cysts, may be an initial finding. Langerhans cell histiocytosis may be confined to the lung or may be a component of a multisystem disease that includes painful cystic bone lesions and diabetes insipidus (Chapter 206).

DIAGNOSIS

The chest radiograph shows diffuse symmetrical reticulonodular opacities superimposed on multiple small cysts in the upper and mid lung zones. HRCT reveals subpleural nodules, scattered ground-glass densities, and irregular cysts of varying number, size, and configuration in both lungs, with sparing of the lung bases (E-Fig. 80-10). In the appropriate clinical setting, this pattern may be pathognomonic.[22] As the disease progresses, the increase in fibrosis and cysts may lead to honeycombing of the lung. PFTs are characterized by a mixed restrictive and obstructive pattern, including a reduction in diffusing capacity. Vital capacity is disproportionately reduced compared with TLC because of air trapping within the cysts; the result is an increased residual volume. Bronchoalveolar lavage reveals Langerhans cells (atypical histiocytes) that have the characteristic "x body" (i.e., Birbeck granule) on electron microscopy; immunostaining shows CD1 antigen on the cell surface and S-100 protein in the cytoplasm. However, the absence of these findings does not exclude the diagnosis. The diagnosis is usually made by transbronchial biopsy or surgical lung biopsy, which reveals interstitial and peribronchiolar collections of histiocytes, eosinophils, and lymphocytes; peribronchiolar nodules; and cysts with areas of central stellate fibrosis.

TREATMENT AND PROGNOSIS

Although definitive regression after discontinuation of smoking has not been proved, small series report improvement, so patients should be encouraged to discontinue smoking.[23] The prognosis in pulmonary Langerhans cell histiocytosis is usually favorable, with approximately 75% of patients improving or stabilizing, especially with cessation of smoking; some patients, however, may progress to end-stage lung disease. In patients with progressive disease, corticosteroids (see Table 80-5) with or without vincristine, vemurafenib in patients with *BRAF* V600 mutations, arabinoside, cyclosporine, cyclophosphamide, and azathioprine have been used with some anecdotal reports of success. Lung transplantation has been performed, but recurrent disease has been reported in the allograft.

LYMPHANGIOLEIOMYOMATOSIS

This rare interstitial lung disease is limited to women, primarily of childbearing age. The two clinical forms are sporadic disease and tuberous sclerosis complex–associated disease (Chapter 385).[24] The disorder is thought to reflect tuberous sclerosis complex 1 or 2 mutations that regulate the mammalian target of rapamycin (mTOR) pathway. Proliferation of abnormal smooth muscle around bronchioles leads to bilateral small cysts (E-Fig. 80-11), which give an appearance of interstitial lung disease on chest radiographs, and progressive impairment of lung function. Hemoptysis, pneumothorax (from rupture of subpleural cysts), and chylothorax (from lymphatic obstruction) may be initial symptoms that distinguish this disorder from other diffuse lung diseases. Although lymphangioleiomyomatosis is usually limited to the lungs, angiomyolipomas of the mediastinal and retroperitoneal lymph nodes and kidney can mimic the manifestations of tuberous sclerosis (Chapter 385). Coarse reticulonodular infiltrates, often with cysts or bullae, are typically seen on chest radiographs. In contrast to most other interstitial lung diseases, increased lung volumes may be present and should prompt consideration of this diagnosis in a nonsmoking woman of reproductive age. HRCT shows characteristic diffuse thin-walled cysts, generally less than 2 cm in diameter. For women who have cystic changes on HRCT of the chest but have no additional clinical, radiologic, or serologic features of lymphangioleiomyomatosis, a clinical diagnosis is based on a combination of characteristic HRCT features plus one or more of the following: presence of tuberous sclerosis complex, angiomyolipomas, chylous effusions, lymphangioleiomyomas, or an elevated serum vascular endothelial growth factor-D (VEGF-D) level of 800 pg/mL or higher. When a definitive diagnosis is required in patients who have characteristic parenchymal cysts on HRCT but no additional confirmatory features, transbronchial lung biopsy should be considered before a surgical lung biopsy.

Bronchoalveolar lavage may show occult alveolar hemorrhage. Lung biopsy reveals abnormal smooth muscle cells lining the airways, lymphatics, and blood vessels, with concurrent airflow obstruction and replacement of the lung parenchyma with cysts.

TREATMENT AND PROGNOSIS

Sirolimus, an inhibitor of rapamycin signaling, initially at 2 mg/day and titrated to maintain trough levels between 5 and 15 ng/mL, can safely stabilize lung function. Treatment with progesterone or tamoxifen has been tried, but no randomized trials support the use of interventions to alter the estrogen–progesterone balance. Although lung transplantation is indicated as the patient reaches severe functional impairment, the disease may recur in the transplanted lung. Most patients currently die of respiratory failure about 10 years after the onset of symptoms.

INHERITED DISORDERS

Several rare genetic disorders are associated with interstitial lung disease and pulmonary fibrosis. Inheritance is autosomal dominant with variable penetrance for most cases of familial idiopathic pulmonary fibrosis and familial idiopathic interstitial pneumonia and for tuberous sclerosis (Chapter 385), neurofibromatosis (Chapter 385), and familial hypocalciuric hypercalcemia (Chapter 227). Inheritance is autosomal recessive for Gaucher disease (Chapter 192), Niemann-Pick disease (Chapter 192), and Hermansky-Pudlak syndrome (Chapter 192). The congenital form of the alveolar filling disorder pulmonary alveolar proteinosis also is inherited in an autosomal recessive manner.

Tuberous sclerosis (Chapter 385), an autosomal dominant disease of variable penetrance, is characterized pathologically by the presence of hamartomas in multiple organs. The most well-known clinical manifestations include epilepsy, developmental delay, adenoma sebaceum, and renal angiomyolipomas. Interstitial lung disease occurs in only 1% of patients with tuberous sclerosis, usually in women older than 30 years with little or no mental retardation. The pulmonary involvement, which is indistinguishable from lymphangioleiomyomatosis both radiographically and histopathologically, may be manifested as exertional dyspnea, recurrent pneumothorax, and hemoptysis. HRCT reveals thin-walled cysts and a diffuse reticulonodular infiltrate. Recurrent parenchymal hemorrhage may lead to hemosiderin deposition and interstitial pulmonary fibrosis. There is no cure, and treatment is supportive.

Neurofibromatosis (Chapter 385) may affect all age groups and both sexes. Type 1 (von Recklinghausen disease) is characterized by café au lait spots, neurofibromas, optic glioma, and bony lesions; the rarer type 2 is associated with bilateral acoustic neuromas. Diffuse interstitial lung disease is manifested as bilateral lower lobe fibrosis as well as bullae or cystic changes. Interstitial fibrosis and alveolitis with thickening of the alveolar septa, accompanied by a cellular infiltrate, are seen on lung biopsy. Management is as for idiopathic pulmonary fibrosis.

Gaucher disease (Chapter 192), a lysosomal glycolipid storage disorder, has a predilection for the Ashkenazi Jewish population. Pulmonary manifestations, which occur most frequently in type 2 disease, may be a result of interstitial infiltration by Gaucher cells with fibrosis, alveolar consolidation, and filling of alveolar spaces; capillary plugging by Gaucher cells may cause secondary pulmonary hypertension. Treatment is as for the systemic disease, and the general approaches for idiopathic interstitial pneumonias and pulmonary arterial hypertension may be followed for these patients.

Niemann-Pick disease (Chapter 192) is a rare lipid storage disease that may cause infiltration of the characteristic "foam cell" throughout the pulmonary lymphatics, the pulmonary arteries, and the pulmonary alveoli. Patients with type B may survive into adulthood. Treatment is as for the systemic disease.

Hermansky-Pudlak syndrome (Chapter 192) is characterized by oculocutaneous albinism, a bleeding diathesis, and ceroid inclusions in macrophages. Most patients are of Puerto Rican ancestry, and women are affected more frequently than men. Pulmonary fibrosis, with onset in the third or fourth decade, is slowly progressive. Treatment principles and interventions are largely supportive and extrapolated from other related conditions, especially idiopathic pulmonary fibrosis.

Short telomere syndromes are a group of rare genetic disorders that are caused by mutations of the telomere complex, including the telomerase reverse transcriptase *(TERT)*, the telomerase RNA component *(TERC)*, poly(A)-specific ribonuclease *(PARN)*, regulator of telomere elongation helicase 1 *(RTEL1)*, and TERF1 interacting nuclear factor 2 *(TINF2)*.[25] The prevalence of telomerase mutations in lung disease makes the short telomere syndromes the most-common premature aging disorders, with an estimated 10,000 affected adult individuals in the United States alone. The most common short telomere syndromes are interstitial lung diseases, including idiopathic pulmonary fibrosis. Approximate 10 to 25% of patients with familial pulmonary fibrosis have mutations in a telomerase enzyme gene, as do a smaller percentage of sporadic cases. Although specific criteria are evolving, genetic testing for telomere variants has been suggested in patients with a family history of interstitial lung disease, patients with early-onset idiopathic pulmonary fibrosis (<50 years), and patients who have extrapulmonary features suggesting a telemeropathy.[26]

GENERAL REFERENCES

For the General References and other additional features, please visit Elsevier eBooks+ at https://ebooks.health.elsevier.com.

Grade A References

A1. Ghazipura M, Mammen MJ, Bissell BD, et al. Pirfenidone in progressive pulmonary fibrosis: a systematic review and meta-analysis. *Ann Am Thorac Soc.* 2022;19:1030-1039.
A2. Ley B, Swigris J, Day BM, et al. Pirfenidone reduces respiratory-related hospitalizations in idiopathic pulmonary fibrosis. *Am J Respir Crit Care Med.* 2017;196:756-761.
A3. Nathan SD, Albera C, Bradford WZ, et al. Effect of pirfenidone on mortality: pooled analyses and meta-analyses of clinical trials in idiopathic pulmonary fibrosis. *Lancet Respir Med.* 2017;5:33-41.
A4. Ghazipura M, Mammen MJ, Herman DD, et al. Nintedanib in progressive pulmonary fibrosis: a systematic review and meta-analysis. *Ann Am Thorac Soc.* 2022;19:1040-1049.
A5. Martinez FJ, Yow E, Flaherty KR, et al. Effect of antimicrobial therapy on respiratory hospitalization or death in adults with idiopathic pulmonary fibrosis: the CleanUP-IPF randomized clinical trial. *JAMA.* 2021;325:1841-1851.
A6. Behr J, Nathan SD, Wuyts WA, et al. Efficacy and safety of sildenafil added to pirfenidone in patients with advanced idiopathic pulmonary fibrosis and risk of pulmonary hypertension: a double-blind, randomised, placebo-controlled, phase 2b trial. *Lancet Respir Med.* 2021;9:85-95.
A7. Reina-Gutiérrez S, Torres-Costoso A, Martínez-Vizcaíno V, et al. Effectiveness of pulmonary rehabilitation in interstitial lung disease, including coronavirus diseases: a systematic review and meta-analysis. *Arch Phys Med Rehabil.* 2021;102:1989-1997.e3.
A8. Naccache JM, Jouneau S, Didier M, et al. Cyclophosphamide added to glucocorticoids in acute exacerbation of idiopathic pulmonary fibrosis (EXAFIP): a randomised, double-blind, placebo-controlled, phase 3 trial. *Lancet Respir Med.* 2022;10:26-34.
A9. Waxman A, Restrepo-Jaramillo R, Thenappan T, et al. Inhaled treprostinil in pulmonary hypertension due to interstitial lung disease. *N Engl J Med.* 2021;384:325-334.
A10. Flaherty KR, Wells AU, Cottin V, et al. Nintedanib in progressive fibrosing interstitial lung disease. *N Engl J Med.* 2019;381:1718-1727.
A11. Wells AU, Flaherty KR, Brown KK, et al. Nintedanib in patients with progressive fibrosing interstitial lung diseases-subgroup analyses by interstitial lung disease diagnosis in the INBUILD trial: a randomized, double-blind, placebo-controlled, parallel-group trial. *Lancet Respir Med.* 2020;8:453-460.
A12. Tashkin DP, Roth MD, Clements PJ, et al. Mycophenolate mofetil versus oral cyclophosphamide in scleroderma-related interstitial lung disease (SLS II): a randomised controlled, double-blind, parallel group trial. *Lancet Respir Med.* 2016;4:708-719.
A13. Distler O, Highland KB, Gahlemann M, et al. Nintedanib for systemic sclerosis-associated interstitial lung disease. *N Engl J Med.* 2019;380:2518-2528.
A14. Khanna D, Lin CJF, Furst DE, et al. Tocilizumab in systemic sclerosis: a randomized, double-blind, placebo-controlled, phase 3 trial. *Lancet Respir Med.* 2020;8:963-974.
A15. Wechsler ME, Akuthota P, Jayne D, et al. Mepolizumab or placebo for eosinophilic granulomatosis with polyangiitis. *N Engl J Med.* 2017;376:1921-1932.

81 OCCUPATIONAL LUNG DISEASE

SUSAN M. TARLO AND CARRIE A. REDLICH

Occupational lung diseases include a wide spectrum of respiratory disorders with symptoms, signs, and diagnostic test results that often present with features similar to nonoccupational diseases (Table 81-1). For example, adult-onset asthma (Chapter 75) may be occupational asthma. An acute infection may result from occupational exposures (e.g., to severe acute respiratory syndrome coronavirus 2 [SARS-CoV-2] infection).[1] Undiagnosed underlying silicosis predisposes patients to tuberculosis. Presumed sarcoidosis (Chapter 83) may actually be chronic beryllium disease, apparent idiopathic pulmonary fibrosis may be asbestosis, or a suspected viral pneumonia (Chapter 85) may be hypersensitivity pneumonitis from an occupational cause such as contaminated metal-working fluid.

When evaluating any respiratory disease, the clinician should consider the possibility of an occupational cause or contribution (see E-Fig. 16-1; see Table 81-1).[2] The onset of disease after an occupational exposure may occur with a short latency period, as for an acute toxic inhalation injury, or over a period of months to years, as for occupational asthma or hypersensitivity pneumonitis. Latency can be 20 years or more for pneumoconioses such as asbestosis or silicosis, for chronic beryllium disease, or for lung cancer from asbestos or other carcinogens. The most relevant job and occupational exposure history will therefore depend in part on the type of lung disease: for acute syndromes, the recent job exposure is most relevant; for asthma or hypersensitivity pneumonitis, the exposures at the onset of symptoms and ongoing exposures are most relevant; but for chronic diseases or diseases that may result from a long latency exposure, a full working history is essential. Consideration also should be given to potentially relevant exposures that may be related to a patient's hobbies or avocations (e.g., woodworking, model building, or insect collecting).

The clinical relevance of a correct occupational attribution is most apparent for diseases with a close temporal relationship between exposure and the onset of symptoms because intervention to reduce or remove exposure may reverse the disease or prevent progression. In addition, interventions in the workplace may reduce or prevent disease in other workers. However, even for diseases with a potential long latency, such as chronic beryllium disease, identification of disease in one worker should be regarded as a sentinel event that can lead to investigation of the workplace exposures and introduction of preventive measures. The implementation of occupational health interventions can reduce adverse pulmonary events.[3] With the assistance of their physicians, workers with occupational lung diseases also often can qualify for workers' compensation.

EPIDEMIOLOGY

Work-related lung diseases frequently go unrecognized and unreported, so no reliable figures exist for the total incidence or prevalence of occupational lung diseases. Furthermore, regional variations in occupations and exposures are substantial. Nevertheless, work-related asthma has become the most common chronic occupational lung disease in developed countries, where occupational asthma (asthma caused by work) accounts for about 15% of all adult-onset asthma, and work-exacerbated asthma occurs in 25 to 52% of asthmatic workers. The occupational contribution of workplace dusts, fumes, and gases to chronic obstructive pulmonary disease (COPD) is estimated at 15%.[4]

Pneumoconiosis from silica or coal dust, although more important in developing countries,[5] still persists in developed countries. For example, although the total number of cases of coal miners with pneumoconiosis has fallen in the United States substantially since the 1970s, since about 2000 the prevalence of coal workers pneumoconiosis has risen from approximately 5% to over 10% nationally and to over 20% in some regions, especially among long-tenured (>25 years) underground coal miners. In some regions, mortality rates have also started to rise again, especially in smaller mines, and silicosis continues to occur in industries such as construction and sandblasting where exposures can be more challenging to monitor and control. Newer work settings that can cause silicosis include the textile industry's use of jet silica blasting of denim jeans, the use of artificial stone for kitchen counters, and hydraulic fracturing (fracking) to extract oil and gas from subterranean deposits. Because of the persistence of silicosis in the United States, standards were implemented in 2018[6] to lower the permissible exposure limit and to mandate medical surveillance of workers who have exposures above this limit.

Newly recognized asbestos-related cases continue to occur, owing to the long latency period between exposure and clinical disease, despite the declining exposure to asbestos in developed countries. Although annual deaths from asbestosis have now reached a plateau in North America and will likely decline, asbestosis continues to increase worldwide,[7] and new cases of mesothelioma, which has a latency of up to 35 years or more, are expected to plateau in the next few years.

SPECIFIC OCCUPATIONAL LUNG DISORDERS

Occupational lung diseases are often misdiagnosed as other common nonoccupational diseases, but a careful history and appropriate investigations can lead to a correct diagnosis. For many occupational lung diseases, the diagnosis

TABLE 81-1 EXAMPLES OF OCCUPATIONAL RESPIRATORY DISEASES THAT COULD BE MISDIAGNOSED AS COMMON NONOCCUPATIONAL RESPIRATORY DISEASE

DISEASE THAT IS MIMICKED	POSSIBLE OCCUPATIONAL DISEASE	EXAMPLES OF FEATURES THAT SUPPORT AN OCCUPATIONAL DIAGNOSIS
Asthma	Occupational asthma from a work sensitizer	Asthma symptoms begin and are worse during a working period, with some improvement on days or weeks off work. Exposure to a workplace sensitizer
	Occupational asthma—irritant induced, including reactive airways dysfunction syndrome	Asthma begins within days after a high-level (accidental) workplace exposure or begins months to years after repeated more moderate levels of exposures (less definitive)
	Work-exacerbated asthma	History of prior asthma. Severity is worse at work and/or improves away from work and work exposures
COPD	Occupational COPD	Prolonged exposure at work to dusts, fumes, or gases regardless of smoking status
Pneumonia	Acute hypersensitivity pneumonitis	Symptoms typically resolve within days and recur on re-exposure to the same work trigger (e.g., metal-working fluid, moldy hay, humidifiers)
Acute viral respiratory illness or pneumonia	Humidifier fever, organic dust toxic syndrome, metal fume fever, polymer fume fever, cotton dust fever	Work exposures trigger the episodes
Sarcoidosis	Chronic beryllium disease	History of exposure to beryllium dust or fumes up to 30 years or more before onset of disease
	Silicosis	History of exposure; typical radiographic findings of rounded opacities with upper lobe predominance and/or progressive massive fibrosis
Idiopathic pulmonary fibrosis	Asbestosis	History of moderate or high asbestos exposure and appropriate latency period, often with pleural plaques
	Chronic hypersensitivity pneumonitis	± Work exposure to a known trigger, ± improvement during periods away from exposure
	Hard metal disease	History of exposure to hard metal (e.g., tungsten, cobalt), with giant cell pneumonitis noted on lung biopsy
	Flock-worker's lung	Lymphocytic bronchiolitis and interstitial lung disease from nylon/synthetic textile microfibers
Pulmonary fibrosis or alveolar proteinosis	Silicoproteinosis, indium lung	Exposure to silica, exposure to indium–tin oxide in making of flat screens
Pulmonary chest infections	Occupational causes of chest infections (e.g., SARS-CoV-2 or TB in health care workers, TB in miners, histoplasmosis in construction workers, anthrax in wool workers or farmers)	History of relevant occupation and/or work exposures
Pleural effusion	Asbestos-related benign pleural effusion	History of previous asbestos exposure with appropriate latency; pleural plaques may be present
Incidental pulmonary nodule	Rounded atelectasis from asbestos	History of previous asbestos exposure with appropriate latency; pleural plaques commonly present
Multiple nodules	Silicosis or pneumoconiosis	History of silica or other causative dust exposure, distribution of nodules, presence of progressive massive fibrosis
Lung cancer	Occupational lung cancer	History of work exposure to lung carcinogens (e.g., asbestos, radon, chromium, diesel exhaust fumes) with an appropriate latency period
Bronchiolitis obliterans	Popcorn lung; bronchiolitis in military personnel	History of working with microwave popcorn or flavorings; history of deployment in Southeast Asia with exposure to burn pits and other irritants

COPD = chronic obstructive pulmonary disease; SARS-CoV-2 = severe acute respiratory syndrome coronavirus 2; TB = tuberculosis.

can significantly improve prognosis and lead to measures to prevent illness in other workers.

WORK-RELATED ASTHMA

Work-related asthma includes both occupational asthma that is caused by work and asthma that is not caused by work but is exacerbated by work exposures.

SENSITIZER-INDUCED OCCUPATIONAL ASTHMA

EPIDEMIOLOGY

Occupational asthma is most commonly associated with a specific immune response to a high- or low-molecular-weight sensitizer[8] (Table 81-2). Sensitizer-induced occupational asthma usually affects no more than 5 to 20% of workers exposed to the sensitizing agent, but exposure to complex platinum salts or detergent enzymes may result in symptoms in about 50% of highly exposed workers. In most studies, higher levels of exposure are associated with higher rates of sensitization in the exposed populations, but there is no clear threshold exposure below which all workers are protected from the risk for sensitization. Overall, work exposures may cause or worsen about 10 to 15% of cases of adult asthma.[9]

PATHOBIOLOGY

Genetic factors increase the risk for sensitization, but the risks appear to be polygenic and may differ for different allergens and sensitizers. Underlying atopy, as exemplified by a history of allergy or positive skin tests to common environmental allergens (Chapter 230), carries an increased risk for sensitization to the high-molecular-weight allergens, and smoking (Chapter 363) has been reported as a risk factor for sensitization to complex platinum salts. Currently, no host factors are sufficiently specific to justify exclusion of workers from settings with exposure to potential sensitizers. Occupational asthma from a high-molecular-weight allergen is associated with specific immunoglobulin E (IgE) antibody production. Low-molecular-weight sensitizers may act as haptens or may induce neoantigens by reacting with proteins in vivo, but specific IgE antibodies have been demonstrated with only a few low-molecular-weight sensitizers, such as complex platinum salts, acid anhydrides used in epoxy compounds, and sometimes with isocyanates used to make polyurethane coatings, foam, and adhesives.[10]

CLINICAL MANIFESTATIONS

Sensitizer-induced occupational asthma has a latency period ranging from weeks to several years before it develops, but most patients develop symptoms within the first few years of exposure. After a patient has become sensitized

TABLE 81-2 COMMON OCCUPATIONS AT RISK FOR WORK-RELATED ASTHMA AND CAUSATIVE EXPOSURES

SELECTED OCCUPATIONS AT RISK	
SENSITIZER-INDUCED OCCUPATIONAL ASTHMA	**ALLERGEN, SENSITIZER**
Bakers	Wheat, rye, fungal amylase in flour
Laboratory workers	Animal allergens (e.g., proteins in rat urine, mouse or rabbit dander), chemical sensitizers (e.g., glutaraldehyde, anhydrides, diamines)
Detergent making, medical instrument cleaning, pharmaceuticals	Enzymes (e.g., *Bacillus subtilis*, pancreatic enzymes)
Farmers	Grains, plant, and animal allergens; mites, fungi
Greenhouse workers, florists, woodworkers	Pollen, fungi, mites, wood dusts
Food workers	Airborne food allergens (e.g., powdered milk or eggs and vegetables)
Health care workers	Cleaning products (e.g., quaternary ammonium compounds, glutaraldehyde), latex, aerosolized medications
Factory or other industrial workers	Chemical sensitizers (e.g., isocyanates, epoxies) in spray paints, glues, polyurethane, coatings, spray foam insulation, and adhesives
Electronic workers, machinists	Soldering flux with colophony, metal-working fluids
WORK-EXACERBATED ASTHMA	**TRIGGERS**
Any occupation with exposure to asthma triggers at work (e.g., office workers, teachers, factory workers, construction workers, transportation workers)	Typical asthma triggers (irritants and allergens), including dusts, fumes, smoke, mold, dampness, common environmental allergens, cleaning products, perfumed products, extreme temperatures

and has developed asthma, even very small subsequent exposures can trigger asthma, sometimes including exposures that may be below the limit of measurable detection. Pulmonary function and histologic changes are similar to those in nonoccupational asthma (Chapter 75). Sensitizer-induced occupational asthma from a high-molecular-weight agent sensitizer typically causes a prompt asthmatic response within minutes after exposure with or without a late asthmatic response starting 4 to 6 hours after exposure. By comparison, responses to low-molecular-weight sensitizers typically start 4 to 6 hours after exposure.

DIAGNOSIS

The diagnosis of sensitizer-induced occupational asthma is clinically suspected by history and should be considered in all cases of new-onset asthma in patients who work.[11] Supportive features include symptomatic improvement when away from work, such as weekends off work or holidays but not necessarily in the evenings after a work shift, when symptoms from a late asthmatic response may occur. In patients who are exposed to high-molecular-weight sensitizers, allergic rhinitis or conjunctivitis associated with work frequently appears before the development of asthma. A detailed occupational history (Chapter 16) or review of Material Safety Data Sheets or occupational hygiene reports may reveal a known occupational sensitizer. However, more than 300 occupational respiratory sensitizers are currently known, and new agents or exposures are reported each year; as a result, the absence of a recognized sensitizer does not exclude occupational asthma.

Although the history can be very helpful, the evaluation should also include objective pulmonary function testing (Chapter 73) to confirm asthma, either when the patient has symptoms or within 24 hours of the typical suspected work exposure (Fig. 81-1). Allergy skin-prick tests, blood samples, or both should be obtained to test for specific IgE antibodies to any relevant sensitizer if feasible. Serial monitoring of peak expiratory flow rates, symptom diaries, or use of rescue inhalers can provide supportive information. The results of a methacholine challenge test (Chapter 75) toward the end of a typical work week can help when compared with results after 10 days or more without exposure. A comparison of eosinophil counts in induced sputum at work and after a period away from exposure, showing higher levels when exposed, provides supportive diagnostic information. If the diagnosis is still in doubt, a carefully controlled specific inhalation challenge with the suspected workplace sensitizer can be performed in a specialized referral center. Each investigation can be falsely positive or negative, so a combination of investigations is advised while the patient continues to work until the diagnosis is confirmed. Given the specialized nature of many of these studies, consultation with a specialist is recommended. The main differential diagnosis for patients with confirmed asthma is the coincidental onset of asthma with subsequent work-exacerbated asthma. Other conditions, such as vocal cord dysfunction, may explain symptoms or may coexist with asthma and confound the diagnosis.

TREATMENT AND PREVENTION

The optimal management of patients with sensitizer-induced occupational asthma includes complete removal from further exposure to the sensitizer and cross-reacting agents combined with the usual pharmacologic approach to the treatment of asthma (Chapter 75) and advocacy for appropriate workers' compensation. Consideration of the other exposed workers typically includes communication with the workplace or public health officials, in the hope that measures may be instituted to protect other workers from similar exposures and symptoms. Recommendations for primary prevention have been to reduce exposures to occupational sensitizers as far as possible, removing unnecessary sensitizing agents (e.g., removing high-powdered and high-protein latex gloves), and limiting exposures to sensitizers with occupational hygiene measures.[12,13] Ongoing medical surveillance measures in the workplace also may be of value.

PROGNOSIS

Outcome is best if an early diagnosis results in removal from further exposure while asthma is relatively mild. Improvement may continue to occur up to 10 years after removal from exposure, but asthma does not completely resolve in most patients. For patients with occupational asthma from natural rubber latex, use of powder-free, low-protein latex gloves by coworkers and direct avoidance of natural rubber products by the sensitized worker usually result in improvement that is similar to the improvement in patients who are completely removed from work.

WORK-EXACERBATED ASTHMA

EPIDEMIOLOGY AND CLINICAL MANIFESTATIONS

Work-exacerbated asthma is defined as asthma that is not caused by work but is aggravated or exacerbated by work conditions. Asthma may have been present before starting employment or may begin coincidentally during employment, but it is not caused by work. Work exposures that commonly exacerbate asthma include extreme temperature or humidity, exertion, dusts, fumes, and gases. Patients may be exposed at work to common environmental allergens (e.g., fungal allergens in an office setting or dust mites or animals in domestic settings) that exacerbate asthma in patients who are sensitized to these allergens. Symptoms of work-exacerbated asthma may occur transiently with an unusual work exposure (e.g., during renovation in a work building) or may occur on a daily basis (e.g., daily exposure to fumes while performing physical exertion in an industrial setting).

DIAGNOSIS AND TREATMENT

Work-exacerbated asthma is commonly diagnosed on the basis of the history of work exposures and the associated increase in asthmatic symptoms, medication requirements, or unscheduled physician visits. The recommended evaluation of patients with daily or frequent work exacerbations of asthma is similar to that for patients with suspected occupational asthma. Work-related changes in serial peak flow recordings can mimic those seen in occupational asthma, but sputum eosinophil counts typically show less of a work-related increase than is observed with occupational asthma. If the workplace exposure includes a potential work sensitizer, immunologic testing or a controlled challenge exposure may confirm whether respiratory sensitization has occurred.

Management includes the same pharmacologic measures as for non–work-related exacerbations, including the optimization of pharmacologic asthma management (Chapter 75) and, when needed, adjusting the work exposures to avoid ongoing exacerbations. Occupational hygiene measures can reduce exposures, but some patients require a change in job description or work area. Workers' compensation may be available for some patients who have work-related exacerbations of their asthma.

TREATMENT AND PROGNOSIS

Treatment principles are the same as for nonoccupational hypersensitivity pneumonitis (Chapter 82).[18] Removal from exposure to the causative agent is the primary treatment measure. As with occupational asthma from a sensitizer, the removal must be complete and often requires a change in work if the causative agent cannot be removed. Reduction of exposure by use of respiratory protective devices is generally not practical and not effective, with the exception of air-supplied respirators for occasional short-term exposures. Patients with acute (nonfibrotic) hypersensitivity pneumonitis may not require any medications in addition to removal from antigen exposure, but if acute episodes are severe, they may need supportive measures, including corticosteroids (e.g., 20 to 60 mg of prednisone orally per day), supplemental oxygen, and, rarely, intensive care (Chapter 82). Chronic hypersensitivity pneumonitis, also termed fibrotic or nonfibrotic hypersensitivity pneumonitis (Chapter 80), may require additional oral corticosteroid treatment (e.g., 60 mg of prednisone orally per day, tapering down to <20 mg per day) similar to what is recommended for nonoccupational chronic hypersensitivity pneumonitis. Immunosuppressive agents of potential use to reduce the required dose of corticosteroids include azathioprine (e.g., 125 mg per day orally) or mycophenolate mofetil (e.g., 1000 mg orally twice daily), with doses dependent on the patient's weight, response to and duration of prior treatment and response to the new agent. However, more evidence is needed to guide the use of these medications and for antifibrotic agents (e.g., pirfenidone or nintedanib) that are used for idiopathic pulmonary fibrosis (Chapter 80).

Prognosis is better with early diagnosis and complete removal from exposure to the causative agent. Despite treatment, severe end-stage fibrosis may require lung transplantation. Preventive measures include occupational hygiene to reduce inhalational allergen exposures and use of appropriate protective respiratory devices.

CHRONIC BERYLLIUM DISEASE

EPIDEMIOLOGY AND PATHOBIOLOGY

Acute toxic pneumonitis, first described in workers who had high exposure to beryllium in the manufacture of fluorescent light bulbs, is now rare, but chronic beryllium disease remains a problem in many countries (Table 81-4). Chronic hypersensitivity beryllium disease has a strong genetic association with *HLA-DPB1* gene variants that code for Glu69. *HLA-DPB1* genotyping for the number of E69-containing alleles and the calculated surface electronegativity of the *HLA-DPB1* allele has predictive value, but the utility of using this information in future job selection is not known.[19]

CLINICAL MANIFESTATIONS

The pulmonary clinical features of chronic beryllium disease are similar to those of sarcoidosis (Chapter 83), ranging from asymptomatic histologic or imaging findings, to potential progression, to severe granulomatous restrictive lung disease. Onset can occur up to 20 years or more after exposure to beryllium, even if the patient no longer is exposed. The clinical history in all patients with apparent sarcoidosis must include inquiry about possible beryllium exposure, even many years ago.

DIAGNOSIS AND TREATMENT

The chest radiograph shows changes that appear identical to sarcoidosis with enlarged hilar or mediastinal lymph nodes or multiple lung nodules or both (Fig. 81-2). Sensitization to beryllium can be detected by a beryllium lymphocyte proliferation test that demonstrates the presence of sensitized lymphocytes in blood or bronchoalveolar lavage fluid. This test also can detect sensitization to beryllium among asymptomatic exposed workers, who can then be evaluated to assess possible chronic beryllium disease and provided with advice for reducing or eliminating further work exposures.

After disease develops, removal from exposure is advised, but the disease may still worsen. Progressive deterioration in lung function is treated similarly to sarcoidosis (Chapter 83), with oral corticosteroids and supportive measures.

ASBESTOS-RELATED DISEASES

Although the use of asbestos has declined and better protective equipment has been mandated, asbestos-related disease has continued to occur owing to the long latency between exposure and disease. Chrysotile asbestos has less effect on the lungs than other forms of asbestos; that is, amphiboles. Effects of exposure include benign and malignant disease.[20]

Benign asbestos disease is often asymptomatic and identified on chest imaging. Pleural thickening and pleural plaques, commonly with calcification, can occur 20 to 30 years after first exposure and may initially appear on the chest radiograph as calcified linear opacities over the hemidiaphragms and cardiac border (see Fig. 72-15 in Chapter 72). If extensive, it may be difficult to exclude intrapulmonary opacities except by CT scan. Pleural plaques are a marker of asbestos exposure but do not occur in all workers with significant asbestos exposure. Plaques generally do not cause significant changes in

TABLE 81-4 POTENTIAL OCCUPATIONAL EXPOSURES TO BERYLLIUM

Metal and alloy production (alloys of aluminum, copper, and nickel; recently includes golf clubs and metal pen clips)
Ceramic manufacturing
Metal casting, including dental technicians (crowns, bridges)
Electronics, including computer components, transistors, microwave and x-ray windows, heat sinks, telecommunications
Aerospace and atomic engineering (rocket fuels, heat shields, nose cones, and metal parts)
Aircraft manufacture and repair
Nuclear reactors, nuclear weapons, and defense industry
Coating of cathode ray tubes for radar and similar installations
Laboratories
Extraction of beryllium from ore
Metal reclamation and recycling

From Tarlo SM, Rhee K, Powell E, et al. Marked tachypnoea in siblings with chronic beryllium disease due to copper-beryllium alloy. *Chest.* 2001;119:647-650.

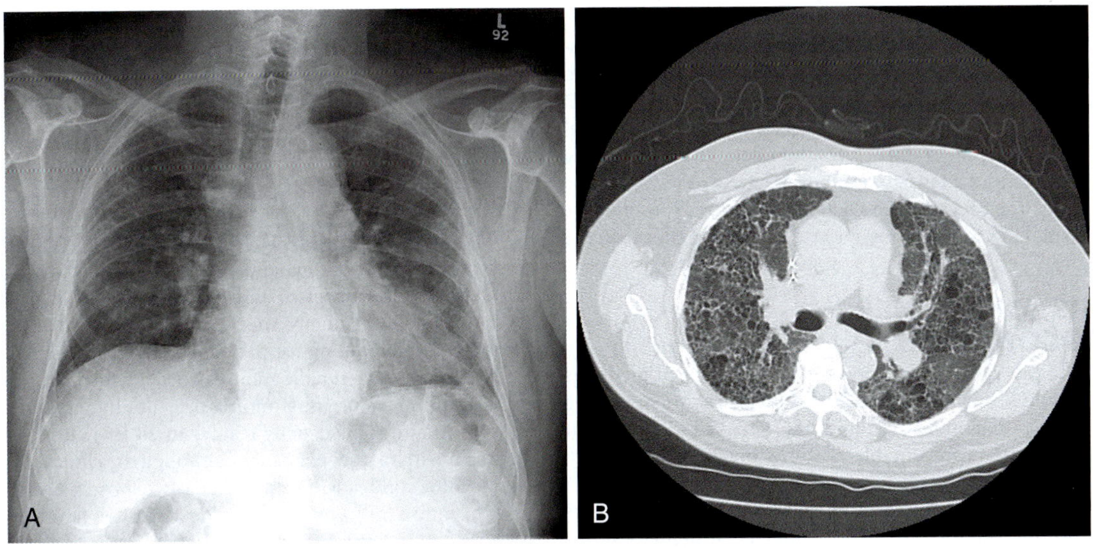

FIGURE 81-2. **Posteroanterior chest radiograph (A) and high-resolution computed tomography scan (B) from patients with chronic beryllium disease.** The chest radiograph demonstrates hilar adenopathy and infiltrates, and the scan shows air space destruction and infiltrates.

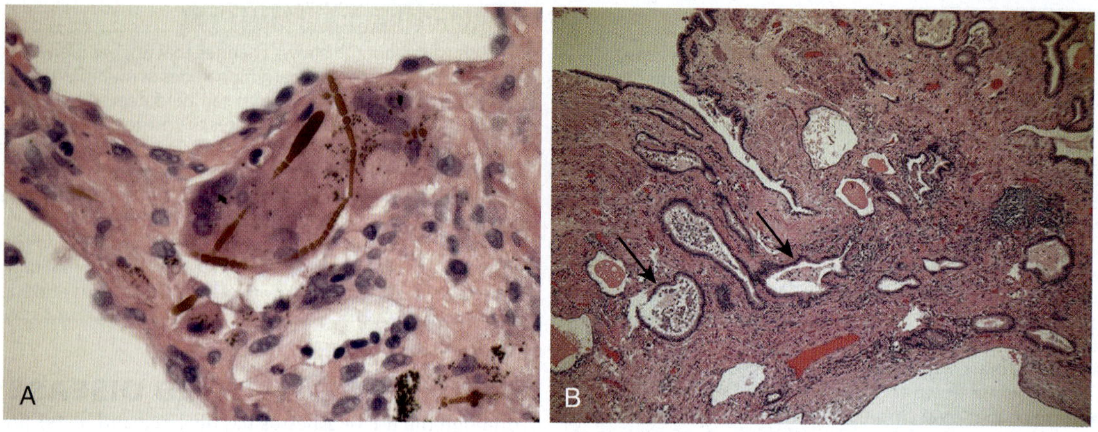

FIGURE 81-3. **Histology from a lung biopsy showing asbestos bodies. (A, higher power, B, low power) Ferruginous bodies consisting of asbestos fibers coated by iron-protein-mucopolysaccharide material with typical golden-brown, beaded appearance. The two longest asbestos bodies, at the center of figure A, are present within a multinucleated giant cell. (Hematoxylin and eosin stain, ×400.) (Courtesy of Dr. David Hwang, Toronto General Hospital.)**

lung function, except that diffuse pleural thickening may result in exertional dyspnea and extrapulmonary restrictive lung disease. Pleural thickening may cause rounded atelectasis (Chapter 78) when encasement of a portion of the peripheral lung tissue by thickened pleura causes an apparent lung nodule, typically with a "comet sign" showing the thickened pleura. Benign pleural effusion can develop, usually about 10 to 15 years after asbestos exposure. It requires further investigation because the differential diagnosis includes malignant pleural effusion (Chapter 86).

Asbestosis is the term for interstitial lung disease caused by asbestos. The clinical presentation is usually with dry cough and dyspnea on exertion. Physical examination usually reveals digital clubbing and basal crackles on lung auscultation. Chest imaging shows basal interstitial lung disease, with or without additional pleural changes as described earlier. Pulmonary function testing shows restrictive lung disease (Chapter 73), and histologic findings are the same as in usual interstitial pneumonia (Chapter 80). Findings supporting the diagnosis of asbestosis rather than usual interstitial pneumonia include a significant duration and level of exposure to asbestos, an appropriate latency of usually 20 to 40 years after first exposure, and/or the finding of ferruginous asbestos bodies in sputum, bronchoalveolar fluid, or lung tissue (Fig. 81-3).[21] Unfortunately, pharmacologic treatment is not effective, and the lung disease may progress to end-stage fibrosis. Management is supportive, including supplemental oxygen and consideration for lung transplantation (Chapter 87). As with the other diseases of long latency, preventing exposure is paramount.

Mesothelioma (Chapter 177), a malignant tumor of the pleura, peritoneum, or both, is the one complication of asbestos exposure that can occur after even relatively minor exposure, such as second-hand exposure from dust on clothing in the families of those working with exposure. It typically occurs 30 to 40 years after exposure to asbestos and may present incidentally on chest imaging or with chest pain or weight loss. Radiographs show pleural thickening, and a pleural effusion may be present. Mesothelioma often is difficult to distinguish from benign pleural thickening without a biopsy. No treatment has proved effective (Chapter 177), so routine screening to detect mesothelioma in exposed persons is not currently recommended. The risk for lung cancer (Chapter 177) increases after significant exposure to asbestos, with a usual latency period of 20 to 30 years. Smoking and asbestos exposure have additive effects, and smoking and asbestosis have even greater effects on the risk for lung cancer.

SILICOSIS AND OTHER PNEUMOCONIOSES

The incidences of silicosis[22] and other inorganic dust diseases of the lungs (Table 81-5) have declined substantially in recent decades, in part owing to better worksite protection in mines, sandblasting, and other settings, but silicosis remains an important preventable pneumoconiosis worldwide.[23] Silicosis is associated with the development of mycobacterial infection[24] and of collagen vascular disease, especially rheumatoid arthritis. Patients with pneumoconiosis and rheumatoid arthritis may be at higher risk for developing rheumatoid nodules in the lung, so-called Caplan syndrome, and mycobacterial infections.

TABLE 81-5 JOBS THAT CAN LEAD TO SILICOSIS

Mining: surface or underground mining (tunneling)
Milling: ground silica for abrasives and filler
Quarrying
Sandblasting: e.g., of buildings, preparing steel for painting
Pottery: ceramic or clay work
Grinding and polishing using silica wheels
Stone work
Foundry work: grinding, molding, chipping
Refractory brick work
Glass making: to polish and as an abrasive
Boiler work: cleaning boilers
Manufacture of abrasives

Patients may initially be identified incidentally during a medical surveillance program or by a chest radiograph that shows multiple small lung nodules, often with enlarged mediastinal lymph nodes that can mimic sarcoidosis (Fig. 81-4).[24] Nodules can coalesce and lead to progressive massive fibrosis, especially in the upper lungs, sometimes mimicking malignancy, and can be positive on positron emission tomography scanning owing to their metabolic activity. There can be compensatory emphysema in the lower lung fields. On chest imaging, mediastinal lymph nodes may have a characteristic "eggshell" calcification in silicosis. Treatment is supportive. Patients with exposure to silica or coal dust may develop COPD from the dust exposure or dust-related diffuse fibrosis. Patients who develop end-stage lung disease may be considered for lung transplantation.

ACUTE FEBRILE SYNDROMES

A variety of occupational exposures can cause acute febrile respiratory syndromes that may mimic acute viral respiratory illnesses (Table 81-6). The mechanism of these syndromes is incompletely understood, but they are associated with systemic neutrophilia and cytokine activation, often with increased interleukin-6 (IL-6) and IL-8.

CLINICAL MANIFESTATIONS AND DIAGNOSIS

Typically, chills, fever, malaise, dry cough, and chest tightness start about 6 to 8 hours after onset of an exposure at work and generally resolve by the next day. Occasionally, shortness of breath and other respiratory symptoms are severe enough for patients to seek emergency medical attention. Infiltrates on the chest radiograph can occur with neutrophilia and hypoxemia that can mimic acute pneumonia or acute hypersensitivity pneumonitis. Symptoms and signs usually resolve in 24 to 48 hours without antibiotics and recur with further exposures, although the clinical manifestations generally become milder with repeated daily exposures (e.g., Monday morning fever in cotton mill workers). Workers are often familiar with the syndrome because it commonly affects up to 30% of exposed workers. If the diagnosis is not provided by the patient, however, careful elicitation of potential work exposures is needed.

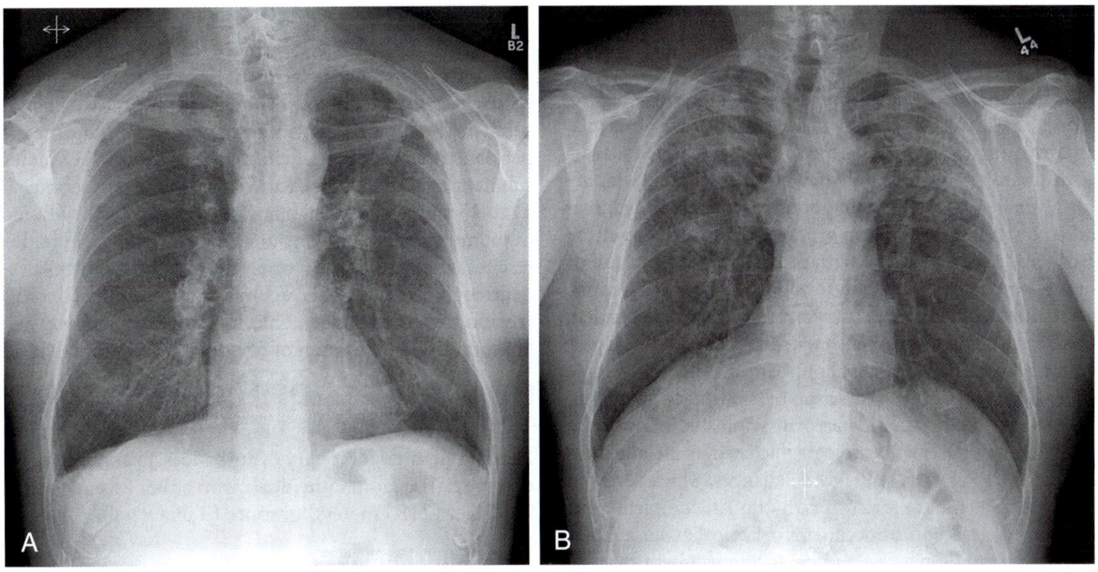

FIGURE 81-4. Posteroanterior chest radiographs from two patients with silicosis. **A**, Small nodules and eggshell calcification of hilar lymph nodes. **B**, Progressive massive fibrosis of the upper lung zones with compensatory emphysema.

TABLE 81-6 OCCUPATIONAL CAUSES OF AN ACUTE FEBRILE SYNDROME

SYNDROME	CAUSE
Polymer fume fever or Teflon fever	Polytetrafluoroethylene and other fluorocarbon polymer fumes
Metal fume fever	Zinc fumes from welding of galvanized steel, less commonly other metal fumes
Cotton mill fever	Dust and endotoxins from bacterial contamination of unprocessed cotton, flax, and hemp
Humidifier fever	Microorganisms found in reservoirs (e.g., humidifiers, air conditioners, aquariums); the differential diagnosis includes acute hypersensitivity pneumonitis
Organic dust toxic syndrome	Grain dust, moldy wood chips; the differential diagnosis includes acute hypersensitivity pneumonitis

TREATMENT

Treatment is supportive. If the causative exposure can be removed (e.g., cleaning a contaminated humidifier), symptoms can be prevented. If the cause cannot be removed and symptoms are severe, the patient may need reduction or change of the work exposure.

OCCUPATIONAL LUNG CANCER

A significant duration and level of exposure to a recognized carcinogen such as asbestos, hexavalent chromium (as in chromate production and the pigment industry), soluble radon compounds or radon gas, polycyclic aromatic hydrocarbons, chloromethyl ethers, arsenic, diesel exhaust, or silica[25,26] can increase the risk for lung cancer (Chapter 177). Such a history should be elicited in all patients, and exposure to these agents represents a risk factor when considering whether to recommend patients for CT screening for lung cancer (Chapter 177).[27]

GENERAL REFERENCES

For the General References and other additional features, please visit Elsevier eBooks+ at https://ebooks.health.elsevier.com.

82

PHYSICAL AND CHEMICAL INJURIES OF THE LUNG

DAVID C. CHRISTIANI AND LISA A. MAIER

SUBMERSION INCIDENTS: DROWNING

DEFINITION

Drowning is defined as the process of experiencing respiratory impairment from submersion/immersion in liquid. The term *near-drowning* was previously used to describe individuals who survived a submersion incident, at least temporarily, but it has been abandoned on the basis of recommendations of the First World Congress of Drowning in Amsterdam in 2002.

EPIDEMIOLOGY

The estimated annual number of deaths worldwide due to drowning is about 400,000, mostly in low- and middle-income countries. About 4200 persons are treated per year for nonfatal drowning in U.S. emergency departments, and about another 3400 suffer fatal drowning. Alcohol use, age younger than 4 years, and male gender are associated with increased rates of both nonfatal and fatal drowning.

PATHOBIOLOGY

The physiology of drowning is complex and relates to two different events: immersion (upper airway above water) and submersion (upper airway under water). Immersion involves integrated cardiorespiratory responses to skin and deep body temperature, including cold shock, physical incapacitation, and hypovolemia, as precursors of collapse and submersion. The initial response to submersion/immersion is apnea, followed almost invariably by aspiration. Laryngospasm may result in aspiration of a variable quantity of liquid medium into the lungs. Hypoxemia, hypercapnia, and acidemia develop acutely. Aspiration of either fresh or salt water results in occlusion of the airway, reduced surfactant activity, direct alveolar injury, and bronchospasm. Acute lung injury or acute respiratory distress syndrome (ARDS)—associated with noncardiogenic pulmonary edema, respiratory failure, and severe hypoxemia—may develop hours or days after the incident. Acute renal failure may also occur. Alcohol consumption also increases the risk for hypothermia. Changes to serum electrolytes with drowning in either fresh water or salt water are not clinically significant.

The most serious secondary consequence of hypoxemia is anoxic brain injury. Fortunately, a reduction of brain temperature by 10°C during drowning decreases adenosine triphosphate (ATP) consumption by approximately 50%, thereby doubling the duration of time that the brain can survive. Mortality is primarily due to the cardiovascular sequelae of severe early or late hypoxemia.

CLINICAL MANIFESTATIONS

The initial presentation of a drowning victim varies widely. Hypothermia, which is common in drowning victims, may be associated with bradycardia or cardiac arrest due to asystole or ventricular fibrillation. Tachypnea, tachycardia, and low-grade fever are typical in nonhypothermic patients. Cyanosis may be present, and a coughing patient may produce pink frothy sputum. Neurologic evaluation may reveal agitation with or without intoxication or coma. The patient should be examined carefully for signs of associated trauma.

Expected laboratory findings include mild electrolyte abnormalities independent of whether submersion occurs in salt water or fresh water, moderate leukocytosis, and slight decrease in hematocrit in the first 24 hours or slight increase in free hemoglobin with a stable hematocrit in fresh water submersion due to hemolysis, severe hypoxemia, and metabolic acidosis. Evidence of disseminated intravascular coagulation (DIC) may occur. Initial electrocardiographic changes include sinus tachycardia and nonspecific ST segment and T wave changes, which revert to normal within hours. Life-threatening ventricular arrhythmias, complete heart block, or evidence of myocardial infarction can occur early or late in the course. Chest radiographs may initially be normal, despite severe respiratory impairment. Bilateral patchy alveolar infiltrates, which indicate progression to ARDS, may develop.

DIAGNOSIS

The diagnosis of drowning is made on clinical history of submersion in liquid medium with resulting respiratory impairment. Patients with unusual presenting circumstances should be carefully examined for evidence of trauma or assault.

PREVENTION

Drowning incidents are largely preventable, particularly in children. Pool fencing is a proven, effective strategy to prevent drowning. The primary cause of drowning of infants and toddlers is lack of adult supervision, and supervision of all young children near any form of water is strongly recommended. The role of alcohol in teenage and adult drowning incidents is substantial, and all individuals participating in water-based activities should restrict alcohol intake. The use of personal flotation devices is recommended for children and adults.

TREATMENT

When the victim has been recovered from submersion, treatment should focus on basic life support, including notification of emergency response personnel, establishment of an adequate airway, and cardiopulmonary resuscitation,[1] if necessary (Chapter 50). If the victim is apneic, rescue breathing should occur immediately, even before removal from the water. Cervical spine stabilization is needed if there is a history of diving, use of a water slide, signs of injury, or signs of alcohol intoxication. Spinal cord injury (Chapter 368) is otherwise unlikely, and cervical spine stabilization techniques and equipment may impede timely and effective treatment. Attempts to remove water from the airway are unnecessary. Cardiac arrhythmias should be treated with Advanced Cardiac Life Support protocols, including the use of automated external defibrillators when appropriate (Chapter 50). A majority of drowning victims who receive cardiopulmonary resuscitation or rescue breathing will vomit; if vomiting occurs, the head should be turned to the side, and any visible vomitus remaining in the oral cavity should be removed with a finger. When vomiting occurs in patients who may have spinal cord injury, log-rolling techniques are recommended for turning the patient to the side.

All victims of a submersion incident should be transported to a hospital for further evaluation, treatment of potential respiratory failure (Chapter 90), and monitoring for up to 24 hours. Bronchoscopy may be required to evaluate localized wheezing or persistent atelectasis. Prophylactic antibiotics are not useful, but evidence of pneumonia (Chapter 85) should be treated with appropriate antibiotics. Because unusual microorganisms may be isolated from the lower airways, efforts should be made to identify specific microbial flora pertinent to the locus of the drowning incident. Randomized controlled trials of specific ventilator strategies have not been conducted, but lung-protective ventilation (i.e., a tidal volume of 4 to 6 mL/kg ideal body weight) with sufficient positive end expiratory pressure of 5 to 10 cm H_2O to avoid atelectasis is commonly recommended.

Treatment of neurologic injury is focused on supportive care while the extent of cerebral edema is minimized. To decrease cerebral edema and intracranial pressure, intravenous hypertonic saline (7.5 to 23% to target serum sodium values of 145 to 155 mmol/L) or mannitol (1-g/kg bolus of 20% mannitol, with repeat dosing every 6 to 8 hours as necessary to target serum osmolality of less than 300 to 320 mOsm/kg) may be used, although their benefit in this setting is unproved. Hyperventilation to a $Paco_2$ of 34 to 36 mm Hg may be helpful. Intracranial pressure may increase in response to shivering or purposeless movements, which should be reduced. Maintaining targeted normothermia (temperature < 37.8°C)[A1] improves neurologic outcome after cardiac arrest (Chapter 50). Hyperthermia should be avoided at all times.

PROGNOSIS

Most drownings are fatal. The mortality rate for drowning victims who present alive to an emergency department is about 25%. Long-term neurologic deficits persist in approximately 6% of nonfatal drowning victims. Prolonged duration of submersion is associated with a worse prognosis, and the risk for death or severe permanent neurologic deficits increases from 10% after less than 5 minutes of submersion, to about 55% with 6 to 10 minutes of submersion, nearly 90% with 11 to 25 minutes of submersion, and nearly 150% with more than 25 minutes of submersion. However, young children who are hypothermic when they are rescued after submersion times of up to 60 minutes have recovered without neurologic damage. Other factors associated with poor prognosis include hypotension, persistent apnea, coma, more than a 10-minute delay in receiving basic life support, and duration of resuscitation of more than 25 minutes.

DISEASES OF HIGH ALTITUDE

DEFINITION

Neurologic and pulmonary disturbances, primarily due to direct tissue effects of hypoxia, occur in individuals who either ascend to or reside at altitudes of 7000 feet (2133 meters) or more (Table 82-1).

EPIDEMIOLOGY

Acute mountain sickness is the most common high-altitude syndrome. It occurs in approximately 20% of individuals who ascend to altitudes of 7000 to 9000 feet, 40% at 10,000 to 14,000 feet, and more than 50% above 14,000 feet.[2] The incidence of chronic mountain sickness, also known as Monge disease, is thought to be between 5 and 18%. More severe neurologic disturbances due to high-altitude cerebral edema are rare, occurring in approximately 1 to 2% of individuals who ascend to altitudes above 15,000 feet. High-altitude pulmonary edema occurs in approximately 2 to 6% of otherwise healthy individuals who ascend to altitudes of 8000 to 15,000 feet. However, the incidence in individuals with a prior history of high-altitude pulmonary edema may be as high as 60%, or higher during rapid ascents. The occurrence of high-altitude retinal hemorrhage is approximately 33% among individuals who ascend to very high altitudes (up to 19,000 feet) and is thought to be common at lower altitudes as well. High-altitude retinal hemorrhage is not associated with high-altitude cerebral edema or long-term visual consequences.

PATHOBIOLOGY

Clinically significant hypoxemia is the underlying factor in all high-altitude diseases. The decrease in barometric pressure during an ascent to altitude causes a decrease in the alveolar pressure of oxygen (Pao_2). For example, Pao_2 drops from 105 mm Hg at sea level to 60 mm Hg at 10,000 feet and to 40 mm Hg at 18,000 feet. Below 60 mm Hg, oxygen dissociates from hemoglobin more readily (see Fig. 144-1 in Chapter 144), thereby decreasing oxygen saturation and oxygen delivery to tissues. The effect is even more noticeable in patients with impaired diffusion capacity, such as occurs in emphysema, interstitial lung diseases, or heart failure. Furthermore, increased ventilatory drive induces an acute respiratory alkalosis. In the brain, tissue hypoxia causes cerebral vasodilation, whereas hypobaria causes cerebral vasoconstriction. In severe hypoxemia, vasodilation is the likely cause of cerebral edema in susceptible individuals. The response to hypoxemia in the lungs is primarily increased pulmonary

TABLE 82-1 HIGH-ALTITUDE SYNDROMES

SYNDROME	CLINICAL DESCRIPTION
Acute mountain sickness	Common after recent ascent to altitudes above 7000 feet; symptoms include headache, anorexia, and malaise
Chronic mountain sickness	Occurs in 5-18% of people dwelling above 10,000 feet; symptoms include headache, fatigue, dyspnea, and digestive disturbances
High-altitude pulmonary edema	Occurs in 2-6% of people above 9500 feet; symptoms include dyspnea, cough, and tachycardia
High-altitude retinal hemorrhage	Common above 15,000 feet; asymptomatic or reversible vision changes
High-altitude cerebral edema	Occurs in 1-2% of people above 15,000 feet; symptoms include confusion, ataxia, hallucinations, coma, or death

arterial pressures due to hypoxic pulmonary vasoconstriction, which results in reversible injury to pulmonary capillaries, increased capillary permeability, and eventually pulmonary edema. Reduced oxygen consumption also occurs, perhaps because of impaired mitochondrial function. Sleep disordered breathing has also been noted but has minimal, if any, clinical significance.

CLINICAL MANIFESTATIONS

Symptoms of acute mountain sickness begin 2 to 3 hours after ascent and include breathlessness, lightheadedness, fatigue, nausea, anorexia, headache, and insomnia. Most symptoms resolve within 2 to 3 days, although insomnia may persist. Chronic symptoms of headache, fatigue, sleep disturbances, dyspnea, and digestive complaints are seen with chronic mountain sickness in individuals residing at higher elevations. Chronic mountain sickness may be associated with polycythemia (hemoglobin concentrations above 21 g/dL). Severe neurologic symptoms with high-altitude cerebral edema include ataxia and confusion that may progress to coma or death. Symptoms of high-altitude pulmonary edema that usually begin 2 to 4 days after ascent to higher altitudes include dyspnea, cough, and tachycardia. Funduscopic changes of flame-shaped hemorrhages are seen with high-altitude retinal hemorrhage.

DIAGNOSIS

Diagnosis of most high-altitude disease is made on the basis of clinical manifestations at high altitude. Diagnosis of chronic mountain sickness, and a milder form often termed subacute mountain sickness, is more challenging because it may mimic other cardiopulmonary, neurologic, or psychiatric disease. Individuals with chronic mountain sickness typically have higher hemoglobin concentrations, higher serum erythropoietin levels, higher nocturnal heart rates, lower nocturnal oxygen saturation, and higher systolic and diastolic arterial pressure than do normal individuals living at similar altitude.

PREVENTION

Prevention of high-altitude disease can be achieved by avoidance in high-risk individuals, such as young children and persons with a history of high-altitude disease. Gradual ascent and acclimatization are crucial to prevention of high-altitude illness, particularly at extreme altitudes. At altitudes up to 10,000 feet, 2 to 3 days or more may be needed for adjustment to the effects of hypoxemia. For mountaineers, current recommendations are to ascend no more than approximately 984 feet (300 meters) per day at altitudes higher than 9843 feet (3000 meters).

When rapid ascent is unavoidable, such as flights to high-altitude locales, the carbonic anhydrase inhibitor acetazolamide (125 mg orally twice daily)[2] provides effective prophylaxis of acute mountain sickness,[A2,A3] and 125 mg at night may improve sleep[A4] (Table 82-2). Other medications shown to be effective in the prevention of acute mountain sickness in randomized, controlled trials include dexamethasone (2 mg every 6 hours or 4 mg every 12 hours), prednisolone (20 mg daily), ibuprofen (600 mg three times daily), and sumatriptan (50 mg orally once after ascent), although a head-to-head comparison showed that ibuprofen was not as effective as acetazolamide.[A5] Inhaled budesonide (200 μg inhaled twice daily) may be useful for prevention of mild but not severe acute mountain sickness if acetazolamide or oral corticosteroids cannot be used.[A6] For prevention of high-altitude pulmonary edema in susceptible individuals, options include the long-acting β-adrenergic agonist salmeterol (125 μg inhaled twice daily), the phosphodiesterase inhibitor tadalafil (10 mg twice daily), the calcium-channel blocker nifedipine (20 mg of slow-release formulation every 8 hours, or 30 mg of slow-release formulation every 12 hours), and dexamethasone (8 mg twice daily).

TREATMENT

For acute, life-threatening symptoms such as high-altitude pulmonary edema and high-altitude cerebral edema, the best treatment is immediate descent, if possible, combined with supplemental oxygen therapy and, if needed, use of a portable hyperbaric chamber. For individuals who develop less severe symptoms, acetazolamide (250 mg twice daily) or dexamethasone (4 mg every 6 hours) is useful.[A7,A8] Sildenafil (50 mg, one-time dose) can increase exercise capacity at altitude by 10 to 35%. Increasing inspired oxygen concentrations in high-altitude working facilities also improves productivity and quality of sleep. Sustained-release theophylline (300 mg daily) significantly reduces the symptoms of acute mountain sickness compared with placebo. Milder forms of acute mountain sickness, such as headache, can be treated with typical doses of nonsteroidal anti-inflammatory medications, including aspirin or acetaminophen.

TABLE 82-2 RECOMMENDED MEDICATION FOR THE PREVENTION AND TREATMENT OF ALTITUDE SICKNESS

MEDICATION	INDICATION	ROUTE	DOSE
Acetazolamide	Prevention of AMS, HACE	Oral	62.5 mg or 125 mg twice per day Pediatrics: 2.5 mg/kg every 12 hr
	Treatment of AMS*	Oral	250 mg twice per day Pediatrics: 2.5 mg/kg every 12 hr
Dexamethasone	Prevention of AMS, HACE	Oral	2 mg every 6 hr or 4 mg every 12 hr Pediatrics: should not be used for prophylaxis
	Treatment of AMS, HACE	Oral, IV, IM	AMS: 4 mg every 6 hr HACE: 8 mg once then 4 mg every 6 hr Pediatrics: 0.15 mg/kg/dose every 6 hr
Nifedipine	Prevention of HAPE	Oral	30 mg SR version every 12 hr, *or* 20 mg of SR version every 8 hr
	Treatment of HAPE	Oral	30 mg SR version every 12 hr, *or* 20 mg of SR version every 8 hr
Tadalafil	Prevention of HAPE	Oral	10 mg twice per day
Salmeterol	Prevention of HAPE	Inhaled	125 μg twice per day†

*Acetazolamide can also be used at this dose as an adjunct to dexamethasone in HACE treatment, but dexamethasone remains the primary treatment for that disorder.
†Should not be used as monotherapy and should only be used in conjunction with oral medications.
AMS = acute mountain sickness; HACE = high-altitude cerebral edema; HAPE = high-altitude pulmonary edema; IM = intramuscular; IV = intravenous; SR = sustained release.

PROGNOSIS

Symptoms of high-altitude disease respond rapidly to immediate descent. However, high-altitude cerebral edema and high-altitude pulmonary edema can be fatal, particularly at extreme altitudes and weather when descent may be impossible.

DECOMPRESSION ILLNESS: DECOMPRESSION SICKNESS, BAROTRAUMA, AND ARTERIAL GAS EMBOLISM

DEFINITION

Exposures to changes in ambient pressure cause a spectrum of illness, either by increasing or decreasing the volume of gas in air-filled body cavities or by causing the release of inert gas bubbles from solution in tissues or blood vessels. Symptoms associated with decreasing ambient pressure, which occur most commonly with ascent from depth during recreational or occupational diving, are known as decompression illness. The most common form of decompression illness is decompression sickness, which is classified as either type I (mild symptoms, such as general fatigue or joint pain) or type II (more severe neurologic or cardiopulmonary disturbances). Life-threatening forms of decompression illness include pulmonary barotrauma and arterial gas embolism syndromes. During the descent of a dive, increasing ambient pressure may cause mild symptoms of facial or sinus pain, often called "the squeezes."

EPIDEMIOLOGY

In addition to the approximately 9 million recreational divers in the United States, aviators, astronauts, and compressed air workers are also exposed to changes in ambient pressure that may cause decompression illness. Among recreational divers, the annual incidence rate for either type I or type II decompression sickness is estimated at 1 case per 5000 to 10,000 dives. Approximately 1000 episodes of decompression illness severe enough to warrant recompression therapy occur each year, up to 10% of which are fatal. Well-recognized risk factors for decompression illness include long duration of dives, deep dives, repetitive dives, heavy exertion at depth, cold water, and rapid ascent. Additional risk occurs in individuals who experience further decreases in ambient pressure after the dive, such as on commercial or private aircraft or driving over mountainous areas.

PATHOBIOLOGY

The principles of Boyle's law and Henry's law describe the properties of gases during changes in ambient pressure. Boyle's law states that the volume of a gas varies inversely to changes in pressure, $P_1V_1 = P_2V_2$. During the descent of a dive, pain due to the "squeezes" is caused by increasing ambient pressures that are not equalized by a compensatory increase in gas volume. The resulting negative pressure causes a vacuum effect in the mask associated with engorgement of the blood vessels in adjacent tissues, such as periorbital and ocular vessels, and may result in swelling, pain, and subconjunctival hemorrhages. Facial sinuses, the middle ear, and the external auditory canals may also be affected.

Barotrauma in sinus, otic, or pulmonary tissues may be due to changes in ambient pressures and the resulting increase or decrease in the volume of gas. During descent, the decreasing volume of gas causes vascular engorgement in the sinuses and otic compartments and may result in rupture of the tympanic or inner ear membranes. During ascent, breath holding, particularly with compressed air devices (SCUBA diving), and the presence of obstructive lung disease with delayed exhalation times and air trapping impair equilibration and increase the risk for pulmonary barotrauma (E-Fig. 82-1). If the expanding volume of gas causes a pressure gradient between the alveoli and pulmonary interstitium that exceeds the compliance of the lung, alveolar rupture will lead to pulmonary interstitial emphysema. Further extension of gas along pulmonary tissues may cause additional barotrauma, leading to pneumothorax, mediastinal emphysema, pneumopericardium, and soft tissue emphysema.

Arterial gas embolism, which is a serious consequence of pulmonary barotrauma, results in the development of free gas in the pulmonary arterial circulation. The resulting bubbles may then enter the systemic circulation by overwhelming the filtering mechanism of the pulmonary capillaries or through a right-to-left intracardiac shunt (Chapter 55), such as a patent foramen ovale. Bubbles may then migrate to the brain, spinal cord, heart, lung, or kidney and lead to tissue ischemia or infarct.

Henry's law states that the solubility of a gas in liquid is proportional to the partial pressure of that gas above the liquid. An increase in partial pressure of gases during descent will therefore cause the amount of gas dissolved in the pulmonary capillaries to increase. Dissolved oxygen is used during normal body metabolism; however, inert nitrogen, which is abundant in inspired air, becomes dissolved in the blood and tissues, particularly in fat, where it is five-fold more soluble than in water. During ascent, decreasing ambient pressure causes tissues to become supersaturated with nitrogen, and nitrogen is subsequently released into blood vessels and tissues as gas bubbles. Decompression-induced gas bubbles cause decompression illness by either mechanical compression of tissues or embolization through blood vessels to end organs. Bubbles that obstruct capillaries or venules damage the endothelium and cause tissue ischemia, which leads to activation of inflammatory mediators or tissue reperfusion injury. Although not well understood, toxic effects due to increased partial pressure of gases also are likely to contribute to symptoms of decompression illness, possibly by denaturing proteins and releasing fatty acids from cell membranes.

CLINICAL MANIFESTATIONS AND DIAGNOSIS

Symptoms of decompression illness can occur within minutes and up to 24 hours or more after exposure to changes in ambient pressure associated with dives of 20 feet in depth or more. The severity of symptoms depends on the rate and the magnitude of the change of ambient pressure and can vary among individuals. Diagnosis is based on clinical manifestations, which can be classified according to whether they are caused by formation of inert nitrogen gas bubbles or the localized toxic effects of gas (associated with decompression sickness), barotrauma associated with descent (sinus or otic barotrauma), barotrauma associated with ascent (pulmonary barotrauma), or more severe arterial gas embolism syndromes.

Symptoms vary according to location of bubble formation. For example, type I decompression sickness, also known as the bends or caisson disease, is typically associated with pain in the joints, from mild to severe, and numbness of the extremities. Rashes and lymphedema may also occur. Symptoms of type II decompression sickness may be systemic (fatigue, hypovolemic shock), cardiopulmonary (cough, substernal chest pain, tachypnea, asphyxia), otic (vertigo, hearing loss), or neurologic (ataxia, aphasia, speech disturbances, incontinence, confusion, personality changes, depression, paralysis, and loss of consciousness).

Otic barotrauma, which typically occurs during descent, can affect the external, middle, or inner ear (Chapter 394). External ear symptoms, such as a sensation of ear fullness or otalgia, are caused by a blockage of the canal, for example, with the use of ear plugs or presence of cerumen. Middle ear symptoms of otalgia, vertigo, tinnitus, transient conductive hearing loss, and facial nerve palsy occur when inadequate equalization of pressures results from blocked eustachian tubes, typically in association with allergic rhinitis or upper respiratory infections. Inner ear barotrauma, which is a more serious form of otic barotrauma, is associated with elevated intracranial pressure and rupture of the inner ear membrane. Inner ear barotrauma causes symptoms of sensorineural deafness, tinnitus, vertigo, nausea, and vomiting. Sinus barotrauma typically occurs during descent, is associated with facial pain and epistaxis, and occurs more frequently in individuals with mucosal inflammation from allergies or infection.

Pulmonary barotrauma, which is the second leading cause of death among divers, should be suspected in postdive individuals, particularly at-risk individuals, with symptoms of sudden pleuritic pain, dyspnea, or coughing. Physical examination findings include tachypnea, subcutaneous emphysema, and dullness to percussion or decreased breath sounds over a pneumothorax. Development of tension pneumothorax (Chapter 86) or severe pneumomediastinum may lead to decreased venous return of systemic blood and reduced cardiac preload, a situation that is characterized by hypotension and may lead to refractory shock or cardiac arrest. Chest and neck radiographs are recommended for diagnosis, particularly because pneumothoraces must be treated with chest tube thoracostomy before recompression therapy.

Because arterial gas embolism syndromes are caused by pulmonary barotrauma, careful neurologic assessment is critical. The neurologic findings are similar to those of an acute stroke (Chapter 376), with manifestations of focal or unilateral motor deficits, visual disturbances, sensory deficits, speech difficulties, and cognitive disturbances, including loss of consciousness. Symptoms typically occur within 10 minutes after ascent. Delayed neurologic symptoms are more likely to be due to type II decompression sickness.

PREVENTION

Education is the most effective method of preventing decompression illness.[3] Before participation in diving-related activities, all individuals should undergo a thorough and intensive training program. Instruction of proper pressure equalization techniques is critical in the prevention of decompression illness. Persons with asthma who wish to dive should be assessed by a physician (preferably knowledgeable in the field of diving medicine), have no wheezing on physical examination, and have normal spirometry before and after exercise. The presence of structural lung disease (e.g., lung cysts or bullae) is associated with a significant increase in the risk for pneumothorax and is a contraindication to diving. Presence of a known right-to-left intracardiac shunt, such as a patent foramen ovale, is not an absolute contraindication to diving, although conservative diving is recommended, and patients should be cautioned that they are at increased risk for decompression illness.

TREATMENT

Symptoms of decompression illness at altitude should be treated with supplemental oxygen and return to the lowest attainable altitude. Serious decompression illness associated with diving requires immediate medical evaluation by emergency personnel, including basic and advanced life support (Chapter 50) when hemodynamic instability is present. Pneumothorax (Chapter 86) should be treated immediately with needle decompression or chest tube thoracostomy. Symptoms that persist for more than 2 hours or increase in intensity require recompression therapy, preferably with 100% oxygen or transfer to a facility with a hyperbaric chamber,[4] where standard protocols should be followed. The only two randomized controlled trials to evaluate recompression therapy found that the addition of tenoxicam (20 mg daily, not available in the United States) or a helium-oxygen mixture (rather than pure oxygen) decreases the number of recompression treatments needed in divers with decompression illness, but neither improved the overall effectiveness of recompression treatment.

PROGNOSIS

Survival of patients with decompression illness depends on prompt medical evaluation and treatment. Immediate hyperbaric oxygen therapy per standard protocols is associated with resolution of symptoms in 95% of cases. However, symptoms of decompression illness, even neurologic deficits, may respond to recompression therapy after delays of 24 hours or more.

INHALATION INJURIES

Smoke Inhalation and Thermal Injury

DEFINITION

Pulmonary complications, largely caused by smoke inhalation, occur in a large proportion of burn victims (Chapter 97) and account for a substantial number of deaths in these patients. Even patients who do not sustain surface burns in a fire can inhale sufficient smoke to result in injury to the lungs or airways.

EPIDEMIOLOGY

Modern building codes and the widespread presence of firefighting personnel in communities have decreased the importance of fire as a cause of death in the United States. However, fire continues to cause several thousand deaths annually. Also, larger-scale fires with mass casualties and wildfires that affect large geographic areas still occur occasionally.

PATHOGENESIS

Smoke loses heat rapidly as it traverses the upper airway, so direct thermal injury is often limited to the mucosa of the supraglottic airway. A notable exception is steam inhalation, which can produce thermal injury throughout the airways. Smoke inhalation injury affects the entire respiratory tract. The pathogenesis of smoke inhalation is complicated by the wide variety of pulmonary irritants in smoke, many of which are directly toxic to respiratory epithelial or alveolar cells: aldehydes such as acrolein, acetaldehyde, and formaldehyde; acids such as hydrochloric, hydrofluoric, and hydrocyanic acid; and ammonia, nitrogen oxides, and phosgene.

Irritants can rapidly induce intense neutrophilic inflammation, which evolves during 12 to 24 hours after injury and is characterized by mucosal edema and ulceration; abnormally increased permeability of pulmonary capillaries with resultant capillary leak; and epithelial, alveolar, and immune cellular dysfunction. Bronchospasm or bronchorrhea may occur, and the processes may result in ARDS. In addition, because oxygen is consumed in fires, breathing of hypoxic air for prolonged periods may potentiate other injuries or cause clinically significant hypoxemia in its own right.

CLINICAL MANIFESTATIONS

Thermal injury to upper airway mucosa can cause airway compromise, particularly due to laryngeal edema, sometimes rapidly and sometimes over the first 12 to 24 hours. Burns to the face, mouth, and neck can externally damage and distort structures of the upper airway and cause airway compromise, both subacutely and late in the course. Inhalation injury manifests primarily with bronchospasm and bronchorrhea, which cause cough, dyspnea, or wheezing and may progress rapidly to respiratory failure. Accumulation of secretions, failure of mucociliary clearance and immune mechanisms, and epithelial necrosis predispose to pulmonary infection, particularly 3 to 5 days after injury. Late pulmonary complications can also be caused indirectly by eschar formation and restriction of thoracic motion.

DIAGNOSIS

Patients with apparent or suspected burn injuries (Chapter 97) should be assessed emergently for airway patency. Head or neck burns, respiratory distress, stridor, or visibly erythematous or edematous oral mucosa should prompt immediate laryngoscopic evaluation of the oropharynx and supraglottic airway. Hypoxemia may develop and may be severe enough to meet criteria for ARDS. Chest radiography should be performed serially to detect the evolution of lung injury or superinfection.

TREATMENT

All patients should receive supplemental oxygen, with the goal of providing a high fractional concentration of inspired oxygen (FiO_2) to reverse the effects of hypoxemia and carbon monoxide inhalation (see later). If airway patency is threatened, endotracheal intubation should be performed immediately.[5] Delay can result in increased edema and greater technical difficulty of intubation. Patients who cannot be intubated should have emergent tracheostomy performed surgically. Because of the risk for ARDS, mechanical ventilation with a goal tidal volume of 4 to 6 mL/kg of ideal body weight should be considered. Extracorporeal membrane oxygenation may occasionally be life saving.[6] Whether inhaled anticoagulants mitigate the development of acute lung injury is unproven. Pulmonary toilet is essential to clear secretions in the face of bronchorrhea and epithelial sloughing. Because of the risk for superinfection, surveillance for infection should be vigilant, including diagnostic bronchoscopy if ventilator-associated pneumonia is suspected.

PROGNOSIS

Patients who survive burns and recover generally do not have long-term pulmonary sequelae. Tracheostomies placed at the time of injury can usually be removed later, unless airway structures are damaged or distorted. Impaired pulmonary function is uncommon but may be manifested as airway hyperresponsiveness that has been termed reactive airway dysfunction syndrome.

E-CIGARETTES/VAPING

Electronic nicotine delivery systems (ENDSs; see Chapter 363) include an e-liquid cartridge, a heating element, and a battery. The e-liquid solution can have variable amounts of nicotine (0 to 26 mg/mL) mixed with flavoring agents. The inhaled e-liquid can irritate the mouth and throat and cause dry coughing. Most concerning, however, is vaping-associated acute lung disease (E-VALI), in which cough, fever, and sometimes severe acute lung injury are typically associated with constitutional and gastrointestinal symptoms.[7-9] Vitamin E acetate, which was commonly added to vaping products that contained tetrahydrocannabinol or cannabidiol, or its breakdown products appears to be a primary cause. E-VALI is now very uncommon since the removal of vitamin E acetate from vaping products, although illicit formulations may still contain it, and cases have been reported since the original outbreak.

Chest radiographs usually show bilateral infiltrates, consistent with ARDS.[9] Bronchoalveolar lavage shows lipid-laden macrophages.

After excluding infection, cessation of exposure and systemic corticosteroids usually lead to clinical improvement, but the steroid dose is uncertain in the absence of clinical trials. However, a substantial proportion of patients have residual abnormalities on their chest radiographs or pulmonary function tests, and the mortality rate is about 2%.[10]

CARBON MONOXIDE POISONING

DEFINITION AND EPIDEMIOLOGY

Carbon monoxide is a colorless, odorless gas produced by the combustion of carbon-based fuels. Because of the ubiquity of these substances, carbon monoxide inhalation is often coincident with smoke inhalation in fires or may occur accidentally in association with malfunctioning equipment or improper venting of emissions from heaters, stoves, combustion motors, or other similar devices. In addition, intentional inhalation of carbon monoxide is a method commonly used in suicide attempts. Carbon monoxide inhalation is the leading cause of death from poisoning (Chapter 96) worldwide.

PATHOBIOLOGY

Carbon monoxide readily diffuses across the alveolar-capillary interface and binds to hemoglobin with extremely high affinity. When the resulting carboxyhemoglobin molecule undergoes an allosteric change at oxygen-binding sites, the ability of bound oxygen to dissociate and to be delivered to peripheral tissues is greatly reduced. This tissue hypoxia can cause severe functional impairment and ischemic injury of oxygen-sensitive tissues, particularly in the brain and heart.

CLINICAL MANIFESTATIONS

Mild carbon monoxide intoxication may go unrecognized because the symptoms are nonspecific and may include headache, nausea, malaise, fatigue, and dizziness. With more severe intoxications, neuropsychiatric symptoms may range from minor disturbances in attention and cognition to agitation, confusion, hallucination, or, in the worst intoxications, seizures or frank coma. Physical findings, which are generally nonspecific, can include tachycardia or hyperthermia. The classic "cherry-red" skin thought to be associated with carbon monoxide intoxication is rarely seen. Other manifestations of severe intoxications may include lactic acidosis, cardiac dysfunction with arrhythmia or ischemia, pulmonary edema, and rhabdomyolysis.

DIAGNOSIS

A high index of suspicion is required for diagnosis because clinical findings are nonspecific. All patients known to have been involved in fires, suicide attempts, or other scenarios compatible with exposures should have arterial carboxyhemoglobin levels checked by co-oximetry. Although levels do not correlate well with clinical findings or risk for complications, symptoms generally occur at carboxyhemoglobin concentrations of 10% or higher.

TREATMENT

All patients should be treated with 100% supplemental oxygen, which competes with carbon monoxide for hemoglobin-binding sites and gradually eliminates it from the blood. If patients require mechanical ventilation because of a depressed neurologic status or respiratory problems, 100% oxygen should be administered by endotracheal tube. Rigorously conducted randomized controlled trials are lacking, but most expert guidelines endorse treatment with hyperbaric oxygen at a pressure of 2.5 to 3.0 atm, which can increase the dissolved oxygen content of blood by more than 10-fold.[11] At least one treatment of approximately 2 hours should be considered in severe cases to reverse the effects of acute intoxication; three hyperbaric oxygen treatments within 24 hours of diagnosis reduce neurocognitive sequelae.

PROGNOSIS

The mortality rate is highly variable according to the severity of intoxication but can approach 30% in severe cases. Approximately two thirds of patients who survive acute intoxication will recover without sequelae. However, the presence of acute brain abnormalities in magnetic resonance imaging portends long-term neuropsychiatric symptoms,[12] including cognitive dysfunction, abnormal mood or affect, memory disturbances, and other motor or sensory abnormalities, which can often occur within the first month but may be delayed for up to 6 to 9 months.

CYANIDE AND OTHER GASES

PATHOBIOLOGY

In addition to carbon monoxide and pulmonary irritants, cyanide gas may be formed when a number of commonly found substances, particularly plastics and textiles, are combusted. This gas is highly toxic and can rapidly cause morbidity and death by binding to cytochrome enzymes and inhibiting cellular respiration.

Other inhaled gases that can injure the lungs in occupational settings include ammonia, chlorine, nitrogen dioxide, organic dust, paraquat, phosgene (which has also been used as a chemical weapon), sulfur dioxide, and toxic metal fumes such as cadmium and mercury.

CLINICAL MANIFESTATIONS AND DIAGNOSIS

Cyanide intoxication typically includes shock, lactic acidosis, and coma; it can rapidly lead to death before results of laboratory studies are available. In the setting of possible exposure, an elevated venous oxygen saturation indicates that cyanide is preventing cells from extracting oxygen from arterial blood.

Other inhaled gases that can produce potent irritant responses include ammonia, chlorine, and nitrogen dioxide ("silo-filler's lung"). Phosgene is notable for its propensity to cause delayed symptoms up to 24 hours after exposure. Other inhalants may produce an acute chemical pneumonitis with respiratory distress (Chapter 81). A diverse group of inhaled toxins can cause syndromes of inhalational fever, including heavy metal fumes, polymer fumes, and organic dust aerosols that contain thermophilic bacteria, gram-negative bacteria and their associated endotoxins, and fungal elements. These inhalations are characterized by fever and malaise with mild respiratory symptoms and are also notable for tachyphylaxis with repeated exposure (and thus are referred to as Monday morning fever in some occupational settings).

TREATMENT

Cyanide intoxication preferably is treated using hydroxocobalamin intravenously (usually 5 mg once, can be repeated for a total of 10 mg) to bind cyanide directly. If no clinical improvement is noted, sodium thiosulfate (12.5 g one-time dose) can be added via a separate intravenous line to detoxify cyanide to less harmful thiocyanate ions.

If hydroxocobalamin is not available, induction of methemoglobinemia, usually with intravenous sodium nitrate (300 mg to induce 15 to 20% methemoglobinemia) is another strategy. Nithiodote, which contains both sodium nitrite and sodium thiosulfate, is a cyanide antidote kit available in the United States. If carboxyhemoglobinemia is present (e.g., due to carbon monoxide poisoning) or the patient has heart disease or lung disease, sodium nitrate is contraindicated because of the additive toxicity of methemoglobinemia.

The mainstay for treatment of other irritating inhalations is to remove the patient immediately from the toxic environment and to provide supportive care for respiratory injury. Depending on the intensity and duration of exposure, most patients will recover completely without sequelae.

OXYGEN TOXICITY

DEFINITION

Hypoxemic respiratory failure often requires treatment with supplemental oxygen to maintain tissue oxygenation. In some settings, such as ARDS, patients may require high FIO_2 for prolonged periods to combat severe hypoxia. However, it has long been recognized that oxygen may be toxic to the lungs when it is present in concentrations higher than those found in ambient air.

PATHOBIOLOGY

When the concentration of oxygen in the airways is high, formation of reactive oxygen species and free radicals is increased. Under normal circumstances, innate antioxidant mechanisms in airway epithelia and alveoli are sufficient to abrogate the effect of these molecules. However, under conditions of critical illness, prolonged exposure to increased concentrations of these toxins may overwhelm these defenses. Superoxide, hydrogen peroxide, and hydroxyl radicals may directly oxidize cellular components. Cellular damage potentiates inflammation and may be synergistic with inflammatory processes already underway in the diseased lung; the result can be alveolar edema, formation of hyaline membranes, hypoxemia, and progression to fibrosis and obliteration of alveolar and capillary structures. In addition, washout of nitrogen from air spaces can result in absorptive atelectasis if oxygen is removed by the circulation faster than it can be replenished by ventilation (especially in the setting of ventilation-perfusion mismatch). Hyperoxia can also worsen hypercapnia through multiple mechanisms, as occurs in patients with chronic obstructive pulmonary disease who suffer from carbon dioxide retention.

CLINICAL MANIFESTATIONS AND DIAGNOSIS

Although the exact levels of hyperoxia that cause lung injury are unclear, injury appears to occur with exposure to FIO_2 of 50 to 60% after exposures as short as 6 hours in duration.[13] Because of the high flow of supplemental oxygen required to deliver this FIO_2, oxygen toxicity is observed primarily in mechanically ventilated patients who are being treated for hypoxemic respiratory failure. This level of exposure can cause a clinically detectable tracheobronchitis, demonstrable by symptoms of cough and dyspnea, as well as airway erythema that is visible macroscopically on bronchoscopy. This syndrome may impair mucociliary clearance and result in impaction of secretions, especially in conjunction with absorptive atelectasis.

Patients who may be susceptible to oxygen toxicity generally already have a significant degree of parenchymal injury from other processes. Thus, although some patients may appear to display a syndrome of worsening air space disease, atelectasis, consolidation, hypoxemia, and diffuse alveolar damage, it is not clear when these changes are related to oxygen therapy or merely occur as part of the acute lung injury from other causes.

TREATMENT

Because the threshold level for oxygen toxicity is unknown, a general guideline for treatment of hypoxemic respiratory failure (Chapter 90) is that patients be ventilated with the lowest possible FIO_2 that is required to restore an acceptable oxygen saturation. An SaO_2 of 90%, which corresponds to PaO_2 of 55 to 60 mm Hg, is generally considered the minimum acceptable level, and targeting a PaO_2 of 60 mm Hg is as safe and efficacious as targeting a PaO_2 of 90 mm Hg in intensive care unit patients who require an inspired oxygen concentration of at least 50%.[A9] Unfortunately, under conditions of severe hypoxemia, such as ARDS, patients often require an FIO_2 approaching 100% to achieve this oxygen level. Maneuvers to improve oxygenation without increasing FIO_2 include paralysis with continuous infusions of neuromuscular blocking agents; inhaled pulmonary vasodilators; red blood cell transfusions to improve the delivery of oxygen; alternative ventilatory strategies, such as high-frequency oscillatory ventilation, airway pressure-release ventilation, inverse-ratio ventilation, and prone positioning; and alveolar recruitment maneuvers using positive end-expiratory pressure or transiently increased inflation pressures (Chapter 91).

PROGNOSIS

Patients who sustain oxygen toxicity in the setting of prior bleomycin exposure may be left with residual pulmonary fibrosis. In other patients, the incremental impact of oxygen toxicity on prognosis is unknown.

LUNG INJURY

Radiation Lung Injury

DEFINITION

Accidental or occupational radiation exposures (Chapter 18) are generally characterized by systemic toxicity that outweighs any injury to the lungs. As such, radiation lung injury refers to a pneumonitis that can progress to pulmonary fibrosis and that results from therapeutic use of ionizing radiation, usually in the treatment of malignant neoplasms.

EPIDEMIOLOGY

As many as 50% of patients receiving thoracic radiation will display radiographic abnormalities after treatment; duration and dose of therapy affect the odds for development of lung injury. However, most of these patients will never have clinically significant radiation lung injury. For unclear reasons, the incidence of lung injury appears to vary by the type of underlying malignant disease and modality of treatment, with lung cancer carrying the greatest risk. The highest frequency is in lung cancer (10 to 20%).

PATHOBIOLOGY AND CLINICAL MANIFESTATIONS

The pathogenesis of radiation lung injury is often divided into three or four phases on the basis of time course. Typically, the early phase occurs immediately after exposure and is characterized by injury to alveolar cells, resulting in mild alveolitis, recruitment of inflammatory cells, capillary leak, and pulmonary edema. These changes are usually asymptomatic; patients do not usually come to clinical attention, although the chest radiograph will be abnormal if it is performed. In most patients, these changes resolve without progression within 1 to 3 months.

A minority of patients will progress to the next phase, in which alveolar cells desquamate and the air spaces fill with protein-rich fluid. In this phase, referred to as radiation pneumonitis, patients will complain of cough, dyspnea, and occasionally fever or pleuritic chest pain. Severe cases may present with hypoxemic respiratory failure. This phase generally resolves within 3 to 6 months after exposure and is followed by an organizing phase, in which alveolar edema resolves and the damaged alveoli heal. Clinically, patients generally show improvement in symptoms during this period. However, this phase is also characterized by fibroblast proliferation and deposition of collagen in the lung. In a minority of patients, this process will proceed unchecked and result in clinically significant fibrosis, with progressive loss of alveolar-capillary surface and development of restrictive lung disease.

DIAGNOSIS

Clinical history and radiographic evaluation are often sufficient for diagnosis of radiation lung injury, because patients typically present with respiratory symptoms and opacities on chest radiography after undergoing radiation therapy. Radiography may show air space disease with alveolar filling or consolidation during the pneumonitis phase, which may progress to an interstitial pattern and eventual honeycombing with parenchymal distortion in the chronic phase.[14] Because radiation characteristically causes injury only within directly affected lung tissue, radiography may show opacities that are well delineated and form straight lines that cross anatomically distinct regions of lung. This finding is rarely, if ever, seen in other conditions.

The differential diagnosis may include pneumonia, recurrence, and metastatic malignant disease. On occasion, invasive evaluation with bronchoalveolar lavage or even biopsy is required to exclude these possibilities if the clinical history and imaging do not provide a diagnosis.

TREATMENT AND PREVENTION

Corticosteroids, such as prednisone 1 mg/kg body weight per day for 2 to 4 weeks followed by a slow taper over several weeks or months, are the mainstay of therapy for radiation pneumonitis.[15] Patients often show a dramatic response to treatment, and symptoms may recur after treatment is discontinued. Other immunosuppressive agents have been used successfully in case reports of patients who failed to respond to corticosteroids. No treatments are currently available for radiation fibrosis.

Reduction in radiation dose and volumes are the best approach to reduce incidence and severity of radiation-induced lung injury. Prophylactic amifostine, a cytoprotective agent, at 340 mg/m^2 IV daily prior to irradiation significantly reduces the risk for radiation pneumonitis but does not improve survival in patients who receive radiation treatment for lung cancer. Side effects, including hypotension, nausea, and vomiting, limit its use.

PROGNOSIS

Within 2 years after initial exposure, progression will usually slow, and symptoms and lung function will stabilize or improve. After this time, further improvement or worsening is uncommon. In severe cases that become chronic, patients may develop features of advanced interstitial lung disease, including pulmonary hypertension and hypoxic respiratory failure.

ASPIRATION INJURY

DEFINITION AND EPIDEMIOLOGY

Aspiration, which is defined as the inhalation of any nongaseous foreign substance into the lungs, generally refers specifically to the inhalation of gastric contents or secretions from the oropharynx. Aspiration is a common occurrence, and in most cases it resolves spontaneously without clinical manifestations. Clinically significant aspiration can range from acute pneumonitis and respiratory failure caused by a single massive aspiration to chronic symptoms of respiratory disease caused by recurrent small-scale aspiration. These syndromes may overlap with pneumonia that occurs when the lungs are exposed to bacteria from the gastrointestinal tract (Chapter 85).

PATHOBIOLOGY

The common element of clinically significant aspiration is impairment of normal airway protective mechanisms. Under normal circumstances, the airway is protected by the normal swallowing mechanism, the cough reflex, and the anatomy of the supraglottic airway. However, even healthy individuals experience microaspiration despite having functional protective mechanisms. These secretions are handled by normal pulmonary clearance mechanisms.

Any disturbance of these protective mechanisms can result in aspiration injury to the lungs. An altered level of consciousness can impair normal swallowing and suppress the cough reflex. Even in patients who are alert, neurologic injury can result in dysphagia and concomitant aspiration, as in patients who have bulbar neurologic deficits in association with ischemic stroke. Patients with altered airway or oropharyngeal anatomy, such as patients who have received surgical or radiation therapy for head and neck malignant neoplasms, may also be highly susceptible to aspiration of oral secretions.

The nature of the aspirated material is also important in determining whether an injury occurs. Materials with a pH lower than 2.5, such as acidic gastric contents, are much more likely to cause a significant chemical pneumonitis. Particulate matter also increases the likelihood for development of clinically significant inflammation. A large-volume aspiration with distribution throughout the lungs is more likely to produce an acute, severe pneumonitis.

When material has been aspirated into the lungs, the injury that occurs is similar to a chemical burn. Acid rapidly injures airway epithelial and alveolar cells; within hours, cells become dysfunctional and capillary leak occurs, resulting in profound noncardiogenic pulmonary edema. In severe cases, diffuse alveolar damage may result.

CLINICAL MANIFESTATIONS

The classic eponym applied to aspiration pneumonia is Mendelsohn syndrome, which refers to a single, large-volume aspiration of gastric contents followed by rapidly progressive hypoxemic respiratory failure that develops within hours. Patients may suffer from cough, dyspnea, fever, and respiratory distress. Physical examination may reveal diffuse crackles, wheezing, cyanosis, and hypotension. Chest radiography may show a pattern of alveolar filling with diffuse bilateral involvement or involvement of dependent regions, particularly the right lower lobe if the patient is upright at the time of aspiration. In many patients, this period of acute deterioration is followed by stabilization and resolution within 2 or 3 days. In other patients, deterioration may continue, and patients may meet clinical criteria for ARDS. If the volume of aspirated material is large enough, the initial aspiration may be sufficient to cause tracheal obstruction and asphyxiation.

In patients who initially improve, a small percentage will show further deterioration after 2 or 3 days. This deterioration should prompt an investigation for bacterial superinfection.

DIAGNOSIS

The clinical history and presentation are generally sufficient for diagnosis of aspiration pneumonitis. Bacterial pneumonia and other causes of ARDS also should be considered, as should cardiogenic pulmonary edema. Airway erythema and edema on bronchoscopy can be suggestive of aspiration. Bronchoalveolar lavage may help evaluate for the presence of bacterial infection.

PREVENTION

Prevention should focus on identification of patients who are at risk for aspiration[16] and then use of strategies to minimize the risk. Patients with swallowing dysfunction or airway abnormalities can work with speech pathologists to learn effective strategies for swallowing. Patients who are unsuccessful or not suitable for this approach may benefit from tracheostomy or enteral tube feedings, which do not prevent microaspiration but can prevent large-volume aspiration. However, the risk for aspiration pneumonia is no different among patients with nasogastric tubes compared with patients who have percutaneous endoscopy gastrostomy tubes. In hospitalized patients, particularly patients with an altered mental status due to illness or sedation, simple strategies such as avoidance of oral feeding and semirecumbent positioning can effectively reduce the risk for aspiration. Use of histamine-2 blockers or proton pump inhibitors (Chapter 125) can alter gastric pH to reduce the risk for injury from acidic secretions.

TREATMENT

Because of the acuity and severity of aspiration pneumonitis, immediate attention should be paid to maintaining a patent airway. The oropharynx and trachea should be suctioned to clear any potentially obstructing material, and endotracheal intubation should be performed if necessary (Chapter 91). Bronchoscopy is often performed to clear residual particulate or solid matter, but it cannot remove acidic secretions, which damage airways and parenchyma quickly and then are rendered neutral. Oxygen supplementation should be provided as needed for hypoxia. Corticosteroids have not been shown to be beneficial. Antibiotics should be reserved for patients who appear to have developed bacterial superinfection (Chapter 85).

PROGNOSIS

For patients with severe respiratory failure or ARDS, mortality can be high. In others, improvement should be expected within days. If the underlying factor that led to aspiration is irreversible, patients have an increased likelihood of recurrent episodes.

LIPOID PNEUMONIA

DEFINITION

Lipoid pneumonia is a chronic inflammatory reaction of the lungs to the presence of lipid substances. Exogenous lipoid pneumonia results from the aspiration of vegetable, animal, or (most commonly) mineral oils.

PATHOBIOLOGY

The most frequently implicated agent is mineral oil used as a laxative and to reduce dysphagia, either in clear liquid form or as petroleum jelly. Mineral oil is bland and, when introduced into the pharynx, can enter the bronchial tree without eliciting the cough reflex. It also mechanically impedes the ciliary action of the airway epithelium. The risk for mineral oil aspiration is increased in debilitated or senile patients, in those with neurologic disease that interferes with deglutition, and in patients with esophageal disease. Mineral oil taken as nose drops to relieve nasal dryness can also cause lipoid pneumonia. Inhalation of mineral oil mist by airplane and automobile mechanics has also been implicated as a cause.

Mineral oils, which cannot be hydrolyzed in the body, provoke a chronic inflammatory reaction that may not become clinically overt until years later. In the alveolar spaces, macrophages accumulate and phagocytose the emulsified oil. Some macrophages disintegrate, releasing their lysosomal enzymes and oil. The alveolar septa become thickened and edematous, containing lymphocytes and lipid-laden macrophages. Oil droplets are seen in the pulmonary lymphatics and hilar nodes. Later, fibrosis develops, and the normal lung architecture is effaced. A single pathologic specimen may include both the early inflammatory and the later fibrotic picture, in keeping with repetitive aspirations during many months or years. Nodular lesions may grossly resemble tumor and be called paraffinomas.

CLINICAL MANIFESTATIONS

Most patients are asymptomatic and come to the physician's attention because of an abnormal chest radiograph. When patients are symptomatic, cough and exertional dyspnea are the most frequent complaints. Chest pain (sometimes pleuritic), hemoptysis, fever (usually low grade), chills, night sweats, and weight loss may occur. Findings on physical examination may be completely normal, but fever, tachypnea, dullness on percussion of the chest, bronchial or bronchovesicular breath sounds, rales, and rhonchi may be found. Clubbing and cor pulmonale are rare.

DIAGNOSIS

In mild lipoid pneumonia, arterial blood gas values may be normal with the patient at rest but may show hypoxemia after exercise. In more severe disease, resting hypoxemia, hypocapnia, and mild respiratory alkalosis develop. Pulmonary function testing reveals a restrictive ventilatory defect; lung compliance is decreased. The only specific laboratory finding is the presence in sputum of macrophages with clusters of vacuoles that are 5 to 50 µm in diameter and that stain deep orange with Sudan IV; extracellular droplets may stain similarly.

On radiographic examination, the earliest abnormalities are air space infiltrates, most often in the dependent portions of the lung.[17] The infiltrates may be unilateral or bilateral, localized or diffuse. Air bronchograms may be seen. Hilar adenopathy and pleural reaction are rare. As fibrosis develops, volume loss occurs, and linear and nodular infiltrates appear. A solid lesion that closely resembles bronchogenic carcinoma may develop. High-resolution computed tomography usually shows consolidated areas of low attenuation and "crazy paving" (Fig. 82-1).

The differential diagnosis is extensive, particularly in the late phase, when multiple other causes of pulmonary fibrosis must be considered. The key to the correct diagnosis before biopsy is the history of chronic oral or intranasal use of an oil- or a lipid-based product or an occupational exposure to oil mists. The presence of lipid-laden macrophages in sputum or bronchoalveolar lavage fluid also can be used to confirm the diagnosis, particularly in conjunction with typical findings on high-resolution computed tomography.

TRANSFUSION-RELATED ACUTE LUNG INJURY

DEFINITION

The syndrome of transfusion-related acute lung injury (TRALI; Chapter 162) involves the rapid onset of respiratory distress within minutes to hours after the transfusion of blood products (fresh-frozen plasma, platelets, and red blood cells). The initial clinical picture is indistinguishable from acute lung injury or ARDS due to other causes, such as sepsis, multiple trauma, and lung injury. TRALI may similarly be confused with pulmonary edema due to volume overload (Chapter 45).

TREATMENT AND PREVENTION

When the diagnosis has been made and the aspiration stopped, the subsequent course is variable. Because the only way the lung can dispose of mineral oil is by expectoration, the patient should be instructed in coughing exercises to be performed many times each day for months. Expectorants have not been shown to help. In some uncontrolled case reports, systemic corticosteroids have been used successfully at varying doses and length, but the literature suggests that they cannot be routinely recommended for treatment.

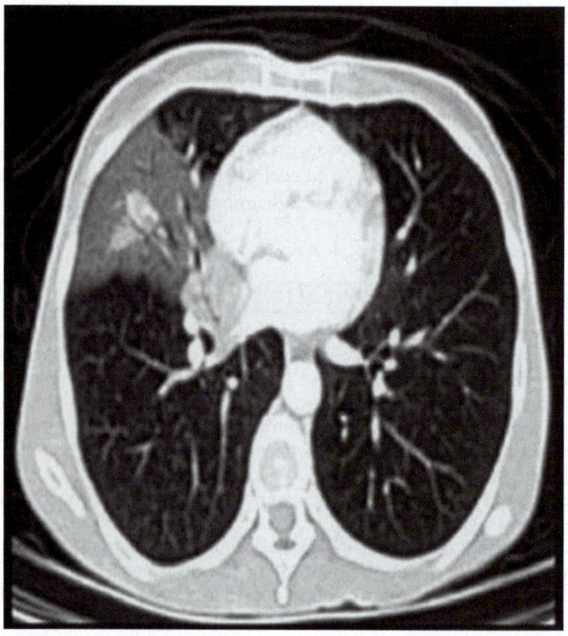

FIGURE 82-1. Lipoid pneumonia on a computed tomographic scan.

EPIDEMIOLOGY

The true incidence of TRALI is unknown; incidence rates are underestimated because of the difficulty in distinguishing TRALI from other causes of acute respiratory failure and the labor-intensive and costly diagnostic evaluation required. Reported incidences range from 1 in 1000 to 1 in 100,000 units of blood products transfused. The risk for TRALI varies according to the volume and type of blood product transfused, with pooled products associated with a higher incidence. In fact, risk factors for TRALI (pre-existing positive fluid balance, shock, severe multisystem disease) are the same as for noncardiogenic pulmonary edema (Chapter 90).[18] Only 8 to 21 TRALI-related deaths are reported to the U.S. Food and Drug Administration annually, and even liberal estimates accounting for underreporting suggest the number may be only as high as 300 per year of an estimated 25 million transfusions in the United States.

PATHOBIOLOGY

The physiologic manifestations of TRALI are caused by alveolar filling with fluid and protein.[19] This alveolar process is the result of increased microvascular permeability due to pulmonary endothelial damage mediated by either leukocyte antibodies or the priming and activation of neutrophils in the pulmonary circulation by bioactive substances.

TRALI most commonly occurs when human leukocyte antigen (HLA) type I or II or neutrophil-specific antigen antibodies from the donor attach to the recipient's leukocytes, leading to the release of injurious oxidative and nonoxidative products. Development of HLA antibodies occurs commonly in women during pregnancy, and increasing parity in female blood donors is associated with an increased risk for TRALI.

Episodes of TRALI occurring in patients without HLA or neutrophil-specific antigen antibodies in either the donor or recipient are thought to be caused by a two-hit process of neutrophil priming and activation. Neutrophils are primed and sequestered in the lung by conditions that often occur in patients requiring blood products, such as multiple trauma, surgery, or sepsis. Primed neutrophils are then activated by bioactive lipids and cytokines stored in the blood products, thereby leading to lung injury and alveolar damage. Levels of these bioactive lipids or cytokines may increase after prolonged storage of blood products.

CLINICAL MANIFESTATIONS

Although most cases of TRALI present within 1 to 2 hours after the transfusion of blood products, tachypnea, hypoxemia, cyanosis, dyspnea, and fever can develop during the transfusion or up to 6 hours later. Hypertension or hypotension commonly occurs, depending on the severity of the reaction. Copious amounts of pink, frothy edema fluid may be present. Lung auscultation generally reveals bilateral crackles and decreased breath sounds in dependent lung zones.

DIAGNOSIS

Bilateral patchy infiltrates consistent with alveolar edema are found on plain chest radiographs, typically without effusions. Arterial blood gas analysis demonstrates reduced PO_2, and further laboratory testing may reveal thrombocytopenia or a transient leukopenia. Diagnosis of TRALI type I requires the presence of the following: acute onset of hypoxemia with PaO_2/FIO_2 of less than 300 mm Hg or room air oxygen saturation of less than 90% during or within 6 hours after a transfusion, bilateral infiltrates on the chest radiograph, no evidence of left atrial hypertension, no preexisting acute lung injury before transfusion, and no temporal relationship to an alternative risk factor for acute lung injury.

The diagnosis of TRALI type II (formerly known as possible TRALI) is made in patients who had an acute lung injury within 6 hours of transfusion, had a stable respiratory status for 12 hours before transfusion, but also had either another concurrent risk factor for acute lung injury or a pre-existing mild acute lung injury.[20] In these situations, a prior inflammatory lung condition may predispose the patient to develop TRALI.

TREATMENT

Most cases are self-limited and resolve within hours to days with supplemental oxygen and supportive care. Volume resuscitation, with or without vasopressors, is required for hypotension. Mechanical ventilation should be managed as for any other case of acute lung injury, with the implementation of a low tidal volume ventilation strategy to prevent further ventilator-induced lung injury. Diuresis should be attempted cautiously and may even be detrimental because intravascular filling pressures are often low.

PROGNOSIS

The mortality of TRALI is approximately 5%. If an implicated donor can be identified, the recipient should not receive any further transfusions from that donor, but patients are not at increased risk for further episodes of TRALI from nonimplicated donor transfusions.

GENERAL REFERENCES

For the General References and other additional features, please visit Elsevier eBooks+ at https://ebooks.health.elsevier.com.

Grade A References

A1. Dankiewicz J, Cronberg T, Lilja G, et al. Hypothermia versus normothermia after out-of-hospital cardiac arrest. *N Engl J Med.* 2021;384:2283-2294.

A2. McIntosh SE, Hemphill M, McDevitt MC, et al. Reduced acetazolamide dosing in countering altitude illness: a comparison of 62.5 vs 125 mg (the RADICAL trial). *Wilderness Environ Med.* 2019;30:12-21.

A3. Lipman GS, Jurkiewicz C, Burnier A, et al. A randomized controlled trial of the lowest effective dose of acetazolamide for acute mountain sickness prevention. *Am J Med.* 2020;133:e706-e715.

A4. Nieto Estrada VH, Molano Franco D, Medina RD, et al. Interventions for preventing high altitude illness: part 1. Commonly-used classes of drugs. *Cochrane Database Syst Rev.* 2017;6:CD009761.

A5. Burns P, Lipman GS, Warner K, et al. Altitude sickness prevention with ibuprofen relative to acetazolamide. *Am J Med.* 2019;132:247-251.

A6. Nepal G, Yadav JK, Rehrig JH, et al. Efficacy and safety of inhaled budesonide on prevention of acute mountain sickness during emergent ascent: a meta-analysis of randomized controlled trials. *BMC Emerg Med.* 2020;20:38.

A7. Sharma S, Gralla J, Ordonez JG, et al. Acetazolamide and N-acetylcysteine in the treatment of chronic mountain sickness (Monge's disease). *Respir Physiol Neurobiol.* 2017;246:1-8.

A8. Simancas-Racines D, Arevalo-Rodriguez I, Osorio D, et al. Interventions for treating acute high altitude sickness. *Cochrane Database Syst Rev.* 2018;6:CD009567.

A9. Schjørring OL, Klitgaard TL, Perner A, et al. Lower or higher oxygenation targets for acute hypoxemic respiratory failure. *N Engl J Med.* 2021;384:1301-1311.

83 SARCOIDOSIS

MICHAEL C. IANNUZZI

DEFINITION

Sarcoidosis, a systemic granulomatous disease of unknown cause, is characterized by a variable clinical presentation and course. More than 90% of patients exhibit thoracic involvement with mediastinal and hilar lymph node enlargement or parenchymal lung disease, but any organ may be involved. The presentation and course vary from asymptomatic disease with spontaneous resolution to organ system failure and even death.

EPIDEMIOLOGY

Sarcoidosis occurs worldwide, affects people of all racial and ethnic groups, and may present at any age. Sarcoidosis usually develops before the age of 50 years, with the incidence peaking at 20 to 39 years. The incidence of sarcoidosis fluctuates throughout the world, most likely because of differences in the disease presentation and the surveillance methods used. The annual incidence of sarcoidosis is highest in Northern European countries, where it is 5 to 40 cases per 100,000 people. The incidence in Japan is about 1 to 2 cases per 100,000 people. In the United States, the adjusted annual incidence among Black Americans is about 3.5 times higher than among White Americans (35.5 cases per 100,000 compared with 10.9 per 100,000). Regardless of ethnic or racial group, sarcoidosis affects women more often. The reportedly low incidence in certain regions such as Africa, China, India, and Russia may be due to decreased access to health care, minimal surveillance, and misdiagnosis of sarcoidosis as tuberculosis or leprosy.

Black women in the United States have the highest lifetime risk for developing sarcoidosis (2.7%). In both Black men and women, sarcoidosis occurs later in life, peaks in the fourth decade, and is more likely to be chronic and fatal. Socioeconomic status does not affect the incidence of sarcoidosis, but low income and other financial barriers to care are associated with more severe sarcoidosis, even after adjustment for age, sex, and race or ethnic group.

Sarcoidosis clusters in families.[1] A Scandinavian registry study of 210 twin pairs identified an 80-fold increased risk for sarcoidosis in monozygotic compared with a 7-fold increase in dizygotic twins. Familial sarcoidosis occurs in 10% of cases from the Netherlands, 7.5% from Germany, 6% from the United Kingdom, 4.7% from Finland, and 0.8% from Spain. In the United States, sarcoidosis patients are five times as likely to have siblings or parents with sarcoidosis as control subjects. However, less than 1% of the first-degree relatives of patients with sarcoidosis are affected, so screening for disease in asymptomatic relatives is ineffective.

PATHOBIOLOGY

The development and accumulation of granulomas represent the basic pathologic abnormality in sarcoidosis (E-Fig. 83-1). Sarcoidal granulomas are tightly organized collections of macrophages and macrophage-derived epithelioid cells encircled by lymphocytes. Fused epithelioid cells, which become multinucleated giant cells, are often found scattered throughout the granuloma. This structural appearance suggests that the granuloma is assembled to contain an inciting agent.

Granuloma formation begins with HLA-mediated processing of antigens by macrophages. T-cell activation follows, with oligoclonal expansion of $CD4^+$ (helper-inducer) lymphocytes. These $CD4^+$ cells, primarily of the T_H1 phenotype, produce interleukin-2 (IL-2) and interferon-γ (IFN-γ). A complex interplay of cytokines, along with macrophage-derived tumor necrosis factor-α, organizes the inflammatory cells into granulomas. Additional T-cell phenotypes, T_H17 and T-regulatory cells (Treg), help to orchestrate the formation, perpetuation, and resolution of sarcoidal granulomas.[2] Treg cell activity, which can abolish IL-2 production and inhibit T-cell proliferation, is likely responsible for the immune paradox that exists in sarcoidosis. Patients often develop anergy, as indicated by a suppressed response to tuberculin, despite active granulomatous inflammation. Although sarcoidosis is predominantly a T-cell–driven disease, the presence of polyclonal hyperglobulinemia, increased numbers of circulating B cells, and a clinical response to anti–B-cell therapies indicates that B lymphocytes also play a role.

In some cases, likely due to unbridled inflammation, fibroblasts and collagen encase the granulomas and lead to fibrosis, which in part may be due to a noninflammatory healing response to epithelial injury. The fibrotic process irreversibly alters organ architecture and function.

Multiple inciting agents rather than a single pathogen are likely to cause sarcoidosis. Airborne antigens are suspected because the lungs, followed by the eyes and skin, are the most commonly involved organs. A microbial origin of the antigens is favored because sarcoidosis occurs sporadically in clusters and is worldwide. Sarcoidosis may recur in transplanted organs and can develop in recipients of tissues from donors with sarcoidosis. Several environmental exposures are modestly associated with the risk for sarcoidosis, each with odds ratios of about 1.5: mold or mildew, musty odors at work, agricultural employment, and pesticide-using industries. Epidemiologic studies suggest a potential causal association between sarcoidosis and occupational exposure to specific agents.[3] Mycobacteria and propionibacteria have long been candidates as causative sarcoidal antigens,[4] but an infectious cause for sarcoidosis remains to be firmly demonstrated.

Major histocompatibility complex (MHC) genes and non-MHC genes located on the short arm of chromosome 6p have been implicated as genetic risk factors for sarcoidosis HLA-DQB1*0201, and HLA-DRB1*0301 alleles are strongly associated with acute disease and good prognosis. The HLA-DRB1*1501/DQB1*0602 haplotype predicts a chronic course and severe pulmonary sarcoidosis.[5] Genome-wide scans and whole-genome sequencing have identified several gene candidates including *ANXA11* (annexin A11), *BTNL2* (butyrophillin-like 2 gene), *Notch 4* (neurogenic locus notch homolog protein 4), *Rab-23* (Ras-related protein), *XIAP*-associated factor (*XAF1*), Janus kinase 2 (*Jak2*), BTB domain and CNC homology 2 (*BACH2*), and neutrophil cytosolic factor 1 (*NCF1*).[6]

CLINICAL MANIFESTATIONS

Patients may present with any organ involved, with or without concomitant intrathoracic involvement. The severity of symptoms and organ dysfunction also varies, and as many as 30 to 50% of patients have no symptoms at the time of diagnosis. Clinical manifestations also vary by ethnicity, race, and sex, as well as by the particular organ system predominantly affected.

Sarcoidosis often first comes to attention during routine screening when enlarged mediastinal and hilar lymph nodes are detected on a chest radiograph (Figs. 83-1 and 83-2). Symptomatic individuals commonly experience night sweats and weight loss. Fatigue, which may be related to inflammation, depression, small fiber neuropathy, and corticosteroid use, often remains a prominent problem and can lead to impaired quality of life.

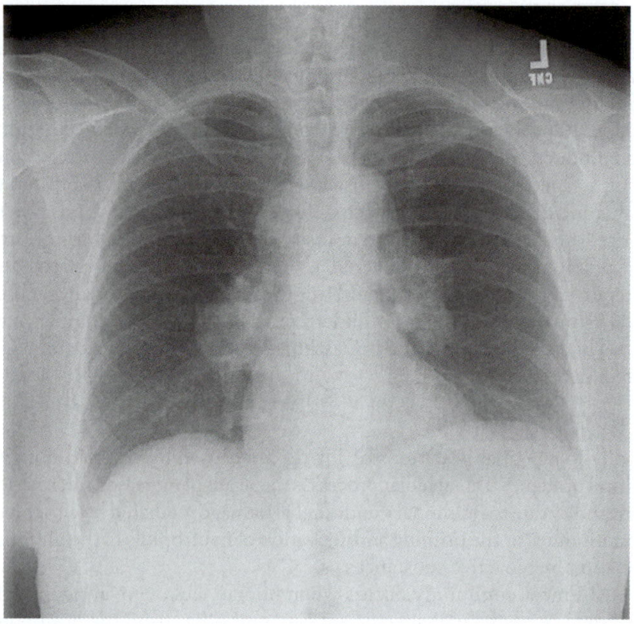

FIGURE 83-1. Chest radiograph demonstrating a stage 1 disease with enlarged mediastinal and hilar lymph nodes.

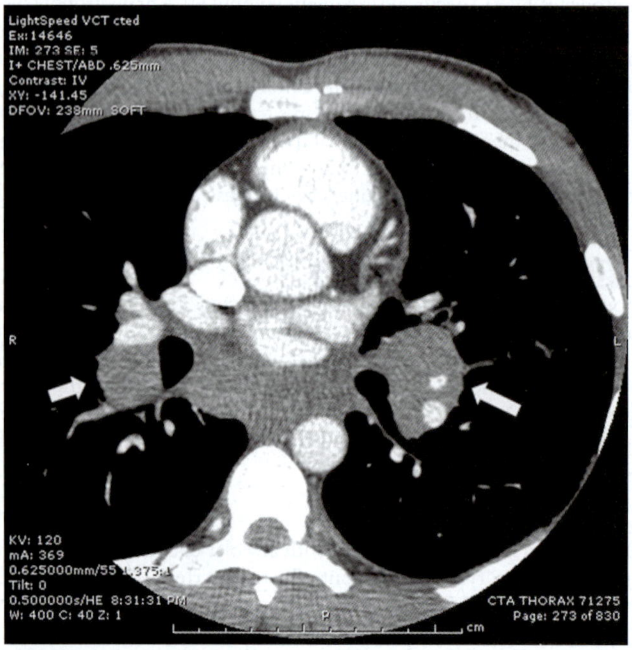

FIGURE 83-2. Chest computed tomographic scan showing typical hilar adenopathy *(arrows)*, which correlates with stage 1.

Symptomatic sarcoidosis may present insidiously or as an acute illness. Löfgren syndrome, an acute form of the disease, consists of erythema nodosum (see Fig. 407-24), arthritis, and bilateral hilar adenopathy. Fever and uveitis may also accompany Löfgren syndrome. Erythema nodosum occurs predominantly in women, whereas arthritis predominates in men.

Respiratory System Disease

More than 90% of patients have respiratory tract involvement, sometimes with symptoms and sometimes with asymptomatic radiographic abnormalities. The most common respiratory symptoms are dry cough and dyspnea. Chest pain, when present, is vague and nonspecific.

Upper respiratory tract involvement occurs in 2 to 6% of patients, with most having nasal mucosal involvement. Severe upper respiratory tract disease may lead to anosmia, erosion of septal cartilage, and nasal deformity. Supraglottic and glottic involvement can lead to stridor, dysphonia, cough, and dysphagia.

TABLE 83-1 CHEST RADIOGRAPHIC STAGING

Stage 0: Normal
Stage 1: Bilateral hilar adenopathy, often with right paratracheal adenopathy
Stage 2: Bilateral hilar adenopathy and parenchymal infiltration
Stage 3: Parenchymal infiltration without lymphadenopathy
Stage 4: Advanced parenchymal disease demonstrating fibrosis and possibly including honeycombing, cysts, bullae, and traction bronchiectasis

Examination of the chest often reveals few or no findings. Localized wheezing suggests endobronchial granulomatous disease, whereas diffuse wheezing suggests hyperreactive airways disease. Crackles may be heard when bronchiectasis and fibrosis are present. Hemoptysis may occur with bronchiectasis or cavitary disease.

The most common radiographic finding is intrathoracic lymph node enlargement with or without parenchymal lung involvement. Mediastinal lymphadenopathy without hilar adenopathy is extremely rare. Hilar lymph node enlargement is usually symmetrical, and less than 3% of patients have unilateral enlargement. Concurrent enlargement of right paratracheal and aortic-pulmonary window lymph nodes is common.

The chest radiograph is traditionally categorized into five stages (Table 83-1), but these stages do not necessarily denote the severity or chronologic progression of disease, particularly when extrathoracic involvement is present. Furthermore, 50 to 94% of patients will have hilar or mediastinal lymphadenopathy on computed tomography (CT) scans irrespective of their stage on a plain chest radiograph.

Chest CT may demonstrate nodules, ground-glass opacities, bronchiectasis, cysts, and thickening of the pleural surface (Fig. 83-3). In more advanced cases, patients develop fibrotic changes (Fig. 83-4) and evidence of pulmonary hypertension (Fig. 83-5). CT, however, generally adds little to diagnosis and management, particularly for those with a stage 1 chest radiograph. No evidence exists that CT changes help to guide therapy. CT can be justified when atypical clinical and chest radiographic findings are present, a normal chest radiograph is found during the evaluation of suspected extrathoracic disease, or complications are suspected.

Endobronchial sarcoidosis may lead to bronchial stenosis and recurrent obstructive pneumonias. Pleural effusions on plain radiography are uncommon (1 to 3% of patients). Pulmonary hypertension (Chapter 69) may complicate sarcoidosis, particularly when pulmonary fibrosis is present.

Skin Disease

Skin involvement occurs in 25 to 35% of patients, but lesions are commonly misdiagnosed because they can present as macules, papules, plaques, subcutaneous lesions, areas of increased or decreased pigmentation, and ulcerations.[7] Lesions are commonly found on the upper back, the nape of the neck, and extremities (Fig. 83-6) and have a predilection for scars and tattoos. The most common skin manifestation is a maculopapular eruption, consisting of firm, flesh-colored to violaceous lesions that have a predilection for the eyelids and perioral area. Scalp involvement with alopecia may occur. Skin lesions in Black American patients frequently leave hyperpigmented scars and pale or depigmented areas.

Erythema nodosum occurs in about 10% of patients and commonly occurs as part of Löfgren syndrome. It presents as raised, red, hot, tender subcutaneous nodular lesions, most commonly on the shins but sometimes also on the arms and buttocks (see Fig. 407-24). Lesions persist for 1 to 3 weeks and may recur. The lesions of erythema nodosum typically show nonspecific septal panniculitis without sarcoidal granulomas, so biopsy is not usually helpful. Erythema nodosum portends a good prognosis, with up to 85% of patients resolving their sarcoidosis within 2 years.

Lupus pernio (Fig. 83-7) consists of chronic, lumpy, violaceous, indurated plaques and nodules distributed around the nose, cheeks, lips, and ears; it is specific to sarcoidosis. Patients with lupus pernio more commonly have a chronic course, fibrotic lung disease, and upper respiratory tract involvement.

Eye Disease

More than 25% of patients have ocular involvement (Chapter 391), and any part of the eye and adnexa may be involved. Women are more likely to develop ocular involvement. Dry eyes, the most common ocular manifestation, usually do not affect vision. Lacrimal gland enlargement and conjunctival involvement are common. Conjunctival involvement consists of pale yellow nodules, which demonstrate granulomas on biopsy. Corneal involvement is rare. Acute anterior uveitis presents with pain, photophobia, lacrimation, and redness.

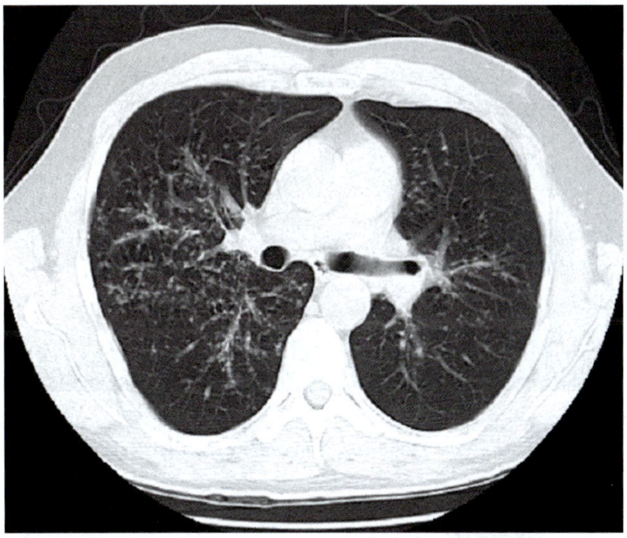

FIGURE 83-3. High-resolution chest computed tomographic scan demonstrating numerous small nodules in a predominantly bronchovascular distribution.

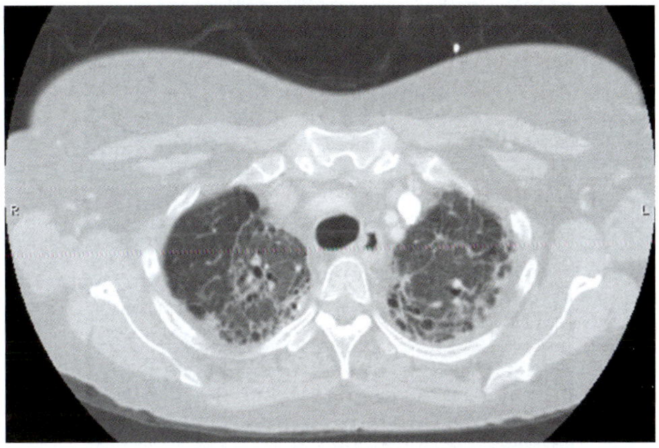

FIGURE 83-4. Chest computed tomographic scan showing fibrotic changes in the upper lobes with bronchiectasis.

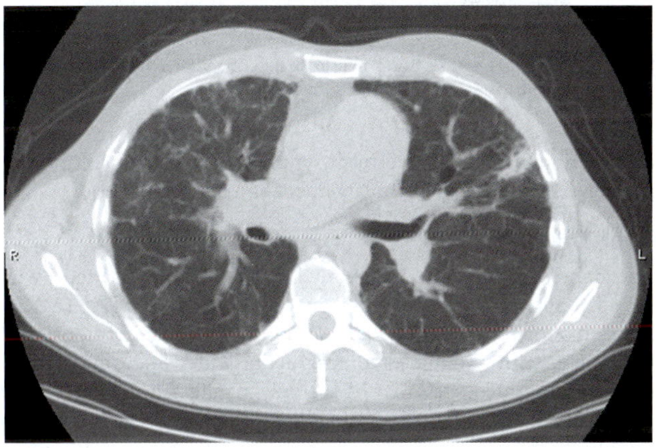

FIGURE 83-5. Chest computed tomographic scan showing diffuse bilateral fibrosis along with severe pulmonary artery enlargement consistent with pulmonary hypertension.

Chronic anterior uveitis, which is more common than acute uveitis, may have minimal symptoms. Posterior uveitis, which occurs in about 30% of patients with ocular sarcoidosis, is frequently accompanied by central nervous system involvement. Choroidal lesions may occur anywhere in the fundus and may be multifocal. In 10 to 15% of patients with uveitis, both the anterior and posterior segments are affected.

Uveitis can herald the nonocular signs of sarcoidosis and may precede the diagnosis of sarcoidosis by decades. Chronic anterior uveitis may lead

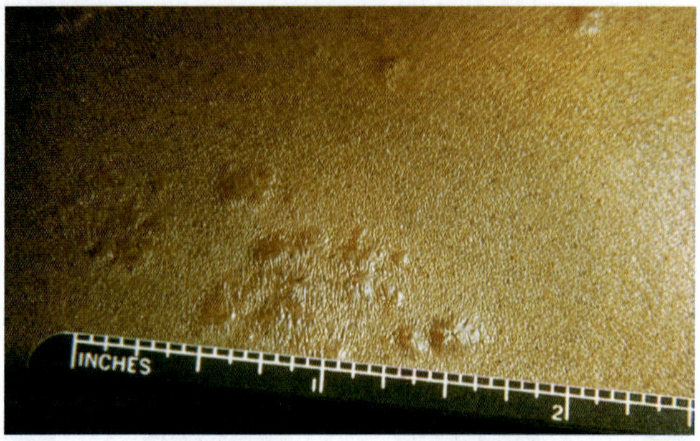

FIGURE 83-6. **Skin lesions of sarcoidosis.** Sarcoidal lesions may occur at any site. This patient's papules have a waxy appearance and are located on the upper part of the back.

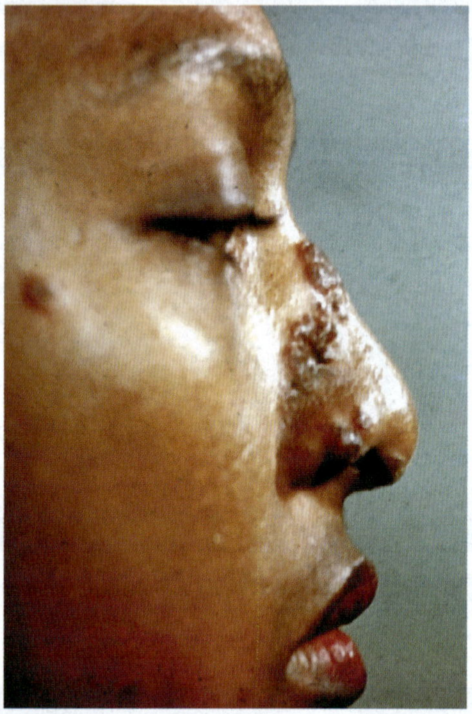

FIGURE 83-7. ***Lupus pernio*** **is the term used to describe infiltrative skin lesions affecting the nose, cheeks, and ears in chronic sarcoidosis.**

to cataracts and glaucoma. Heerfordt syndrome consists of anterior uveitis accompanied by parotid gland enlargement and fever.

Cardiac Disease

Cardiac granulomas are found in about 25% of sarcoidosis patients who are examined at autopsy, and cardiac magnetic resonance imaging (MRI) and positron emission tomography (PET) scans reveal cardiac sarcoidosis in 25 to 30% of patients with systemic sarcoidosis in the United States and nearly 60% in Japan. Cardiac sarcoidosis may be the only manifestation of sarcoidosis in about 25% of patients. In cardiac sarcoidosis (Chapter 47), granulomas most often infiltrate the left ventricular free wall. Next most frequently, sarcoidal granulomas infiltrate the intraventricular septum, where they often involve the conduction system. Cardiac manifestations include atrioventricular block, ventricular arrhythmias, left ventricular dysfunction, and sudden death.[8]

Neurologic Disease

Nervous system granulomas are found in up to 25% of sarcoidosis patients who undergo autopsy, but only 10% of patients present with neurologic symptoms (Table 83-2). In patients with neurologic involvement, the neurologic signs or symptoms precede the diagnosis of sarcoidosis in up to 75% of patients and may be the only manifestation of sarcoidosis.[9]

Neurosarcoidosis has a predilection for the base of the brain, hypothalamus, and pituitary gland. When the pituitary gland is involved, the most common abnormalities are deficiencies in gonadotropins (Chapter 205) and thyroid-stimulating hormone, as well as hyperprolactinemia. Myelopathy may occur anywhere in the spinal cord and carries a poor prognosis. Peripheral neuropathy (Chapter 388) may manifest as mononeuropathy or polyneuropathy.

TABLE 83-2 NEUROSARCOIDOSIS

Cranial neuropathies
VII—Facial nerve palsy (unilateral, bilateral)
II—Optic nerve (unilateral and bilateral)
VIII—Hearing loss
Other cranial neuropathies
Myelopathy (sensory and motor)
Seizure
Basilar meningitis
Central diabetes insipidus
Panhypopituitarism
Intraparenchymal mass
Hydrocephalus
Peripheral neuropathy

Liver and Spleen

Liver involvement is twice as common in Black Americans as in White Americans.[10] Symptoms due to liver disease are infrequent, but abdominal pain and pruritus are the most common symptoms. Fever, weight loss, and jaundice are present in less than 5% of those with liver involvement. About 20% of patients will have hepatomegaly on physical examination, and 35% will have an elevated serum aminotransferase or alkaline phosphatase level. Sarcoidosis can rarely (<1%) cause progressive liver disease that leads to portal hypertension with variceal bleeding; hepatopulmonary syndrome, with refractory hypoxemia, cirrhosis, and liver failure, may also occur.

Splenomegaly is found on physical examination in 5 to 15% of patients with sarcoidosis. Massive splenomegaly is rare.

Bone and Joint

Most patients complain of arthralgias, but only about 35% develop arthritis. Acute sarcoid arthritis (Chapter 254) consists of large joint periarthritis, particularly involving the ankles and knees, and commonly occurs with Löfgren syndrome.[11] These patients often report difficulty walking related to joint pain. Acute sarcoid arthritis usually persists for up to 3 months but is self-limited. Chronic sarcoid arthritis with direct granulomatous synovial infiltration is rare. Osseous sarcoidosis occurs in 3 to 13% of patients and usually does not produce symptoms.

Calcium Metabolism

Increased 1-α hydroxylase activity in macrophages within granulomas and the alveoli converts 25-hydroxyvitamin D to the biologically active form, 1,25-dihydroxyvitamin D (calcitriol), resulting in increased intestinal absorption of calcium in up to 50% of patients and may result in renal stones (Chapter 111), nephrocalcinosis with renal insufficiency, and hypercalciuria (urine calcium > 300 mg/24 hours) with or without hypercalcemia (Chapter 227). In chronic sarcoidosis, 10 to 14% of patients have at least one symptomatic renal stone.

Renal Involvement

Renal involvement, other than as a result of dysregulated calcium metabolism, occurs in less than 1% of patients. Renal disease may include granulomatous interstitial nephritis, glomerular disease, renal tubular dysfunction, renal vascular disease, and obstructive uropathy. Granulomatous interstitial nephritis is more common in White men.

DIAGNOSIS

The diagnosis of sarcoidosis is often delayed because it can be confused with infections, tumors, or autoimmune conditions.[12] The diagnosis should be based on compatible clinical and radiographic findings supported by histologic evidence of noncaseating granulomas in one or more organs in the absence of any foreign particles or organisms.[13] An occupational history consistent with beryllium exposure (Chapter 81), such as employment in the aerospace, automotive, ceramic, or computer industries, requires further investigation because chronic beryllium disease cannot be clinically or histologically distinguished from sarcoidosis.

A diagnosis of sarcoidosis is reasonably certain even without histologic confirmation in patients who present with Löfgren syndrome.[14] In all other cases, a biopsy specimen from an involved organ should be obtained. The organ for which biopsy is safest, such as the skin, peripheral lymph nodes, lacrimal glands, or conjunctiva, should be sampled.

Up to 65% of patients will have granulomas on liver biopsy, but hepatic granulomas (Chapter 137) occur commonly with other disorders such as infection and drug-induced hepatitis. As a result, the diagnosis of sarcoidosis should not be based solely on detection of hepatic granulomas.

If diagnosis requires intrathoracic sampling, fine-needle aspiration of enlarged intrathoracic lymph nodes guided by endobronchial ultrasound has become the preferred procedure, with a diagnostic yield of 80% or higher. Endobronchial ultrasound visualizes mediastinal structures, including the subcarinal region, the paraesophageal space, and the aortopulmonary window. Wherever available, rapid-onsite cytologic evaluation should be performed to assess the adequacy of the sample and guide the need for additional needle aspirates or endobronchial or transbronchial biopsies. Bronchoscopy and endobronchial ultrasound-guided fine-needle aspiration have generally replaced more invasive approaches, such as mediastinoscopy or video-assisted thoracoscopic surgical biopsies.

Bronchoalveolar lavage sampling demonstrates lymphocytosis with normal or low granulocyte counts in more than 85% of patients (Chapter 73). The CD4/CD8 ratio is increased in bronchoalveolar lavage in about 50% of patients with sarcoidosis, but bronchoalveolar lavage findings are nonspecific and should not be used to diagnose sarcoidosis. Bronchoalveolar lavage findings cannot predict prognosis or responsiveness to corticosteroid therapy.

Sarcoidal granulomas produce angiotensin-converting enzyme (ACE). Although serum ACE levels are elevated in 60% of patients with sarcoidosis, the value of a serum ACE level in diagnosing sarcoidosis remains limited because positive and negative predictive values are only about 84% and 74%, respectively.

Patients should routinely undergo pulmonary function testing, which often does not correlate with the chest radiographic stage. For example, pulmonary function tests may be abnormal even in patients with a normal chest radiograph. Diffusion capacity for carbon monoxide (DLCO) is usually the first abnormality detected and the last to normalize on remission. A DLCO of less than 50% of predicted is associated with exercise-induced oxygen desaturation and should prompt formal oxygen saturation testing with exercise.

About two thirds of patients have airflow limitation at presentation. Spirometry usually indicates restrictive ventilatory dysfunction with a reduced forced vital capacity (FVC) and reduced forced expiratory volume in 1 second (FEV_1). At least 50% of patients have concurrent obstructive airway disease. Airway hyperreactivity, as measured by increased responsiveness to methacholine, occurs in up to 83% of patients. In patients with abnormal spirometric findings at diagnosis, spirometry returns to normal in 80%. Alterations in cardiopulmonary exercise testing have been reported in nearly 50% of patients with sarcoidosis. Abnormalities, including a ventilatory limitation with exercise and a widened alveolar-arterial O_2 gradient, may be present. FVC is the single best test for following respiratory involvement and correlates well with FEV_1, total lung capacity, and DLCO.

Because ocular involvement is common and vision loss may occur, complete ocular evaluation with slit lamp and funduscopic examinations should be routinely performed during the initial evaluation and then annually in patients with active systemic disease.

An electrocardiogram (ECG) should be performed at the initial encounter. Screening for cardiac symptoms (palpitations, dizziness, and syncope) should be performed during the initial evaluation and routinely during follow-up visits if the disease is active. Any cardiac symptoms or abnormalities on the ECG should prompt further cardiac event monitoring (Chapter 49) and testing by echocardiography (Chapter 43).

PET with use of the marker ^{18}F-FDG combined with CT (PET/CT) may demonstrate uptake in metabolically active macrophages within granulomas. This approach has proven to be highly sensitive for diagnosing sarcoidosis, and it can demonstrate active granulomas in patients who have stage 0 chest radiographs, as well as in patients with marked fibrosis.[15]

If cardiac involvement is suspected, PET scanning (see E-Fig. 44-3) or cardiac MRI with contrast should be performed, separately or simultaneously.[16] Endomyocardial biopsy, which can be considered in highly suspected cases with nondiagnostic imaging results, has less than 20% diagnostic yield because cardiac involvement is patchy and is usually most dense in the left ventricle and basal ventricular septum where endomyocardial biopsies are avoided. Targeted endomyocardial biopsy guided by real-time cardiovascular MRI may reduce sampling error.

A definite diagnosis of neurosarcoidosis requires histologic confirmation of noncaseating granulomas in affected tissue. A probable diagnosis of neurosarcoidosis requires compatible MRI findings and clinical presentation, exclusion of other neurologic disease, and histologic confirmation of sarcoidosis elsewhere. Histologic confirmation of disease elsewhere, which may be detected by PET scan, supports the diagnosis of neurosarcoidosis. Cerebrospinal fluid (CSF) analysis typically demonstrates nonspecific lymphocytic inflammation (Chapter 381). The CSF glucose can be as low as 14 mg/dL, with a white blood cell count as high as 350 cells/μL and a protein concentration as high as 670 mg/dL. CSF ACE levels are neither sensitive nor specific. CSF oligoclonal immunoglobulin bands are elevated in one third of patients, thereby making it difficult to differentiate sarcoidosis from multiple sclerosis (Chapter 380).

On plain radiographic images, most skeletal lesions of sarcoidosis are seen in the small bones of the hands and feet. MRI and PET scanning show much greater involvement of the axial skeleton and long bones, and osseous sarcoidosis may appear similar to metastatic disease on a PET scan.

Drug-Induced Sarcoidosis and Sarcoidosis-like Reaction

Type 1 interferons, IFN-α and IFN-β, used to treat viral hepatitis (Chapter 135), multiple sclerosis (Chapter 380), and autoimmune and malignant disease, may increase the T_H1 cytokines, IFN-γ, and IL-2 and rarely (<1 to 5%) result in sarcoidosis.[17] Most reported cases of interferon-induced sarcoidosis occur within 6 months of therapy and manifest primarily with lung and skin involvement. Paradoxically, patients receiving anti-TNF-α biologics for various autoimmune diseases also have developed sarcoidosis. Sarcoidosis-like syndrome has also been reported with monoclonal immunomodulators such as tocilizumab and adalimumab, as well as with the use of checkpoint inhibitors (antiprogrammed cell death [PD-1]) to treat metastatic melanoma.[18]

TREATMENT

Because the inciting agent has not yet been identified nor genetic risk factors firmly established, no means exist to prevent sarcoidosis. Most patients with sarcoidosis are not disabled by their illness, so the decision to recommend treatment should weigh the risks of using corticosteroids (Chapter 28), which are the most common treatment, against potential benefits (Table 83-3).[19,20] Hypercalcemia, cardiac disease, and neurologic disease are indications for treatment, and immediate treatment is appropriate whenever organ function is threatened or when symptoms are severe. Detection of granulomatous inflammation on physical examination, biopsy, or imaging or the presence of an elevated serum ACE level is not a mandate to provide treatment.

Pulmonary Sarcoidosis

Treatment is recommended for patients who have a progressive decline in their pulmonary function, which sometimes is accompanied by progressive changes on chest imaging. Oral prednisone at a dose of 20 to 40 mg per day for 3 months is usually the initial recommended therapy. Response to treatment is indicated by improvement in symptoms or objective measures, such as decreased size and number of skin lesions, increased FVC, or a reduction of detectable cardiac or brain lesions. For pulmonary involvement, steroids improve symptoms, pulmonary function test results, and chest radiographic findings. If a response is noted at 3 months, the prednisone dose should be tapered to 10 to 15 mg per day for an additional 6 to 9 months and then tapered off.

Fatigue and poor quality of life often accompany active sarcoidosis. A small randomized trial found that low-dose dexamethasone (1 mg once daily) may improve fatigue and quality of life.[A1] Inhaled corticosteroids should be used only in patients with bronchial hyperreactivity or persistent cough. As with other chronic respiratory diseases, pulmonary rehabilitation should be considered, particularly for patients with pulmonary fibrosis (stage 4 chest imaging).[A2]

Because recurrence after discontinuing therapy may occur in from 30 to 80% of patients, patients should be followed closely for 1 to 2 years after discontinuing treatment. The indications for restarting treatment are the same as those used to begin treatment. When treatment or retreatment is indicated, short courses of high-dose steroids (burst and taper over a few weeks) are unlikely to result in sustained benefit. Lack of response after a 3-month trial suggests nonadherence to therapy, an inadequate dose of prednisone, or irreversible fibrotic disease. Repository drugs may help mitigate poor adherence. One potential option is repository corticotropin, 40 units injected subcutaneously twice weekly; in a small study, this approach was prednisone-sparing and associated with improvement in lung function, PET scan parameters, and patient-reported outcomes. However, cost and limited availability may restrict the use of parenteral corticotropin. In a small randomized trial of patients with fibrotic sarcoidosis, roflumilast (a phosphodiesterase-4 inhibitor at 500 μg orally daily) reduced the risk of exacerbations, but further studies are needed to determine its role in sarcoidosis.[A3] Treatment of advanced pulmonary sarcoidosis is mostly based on expert consensus, because of limited evidence-based data.[21]

Hypercalcemia

Moderate doses of corticosteroids (15 to 20 mg prednisone) reduce elevated serum and urinary calcium levels within a few days of starting treatment. Failure of serum calcium to normalize within 2 weeks should alert the clinician to an alternative diagnosis such as hyperparathyroidism or malignancy (Chapter 227). With treatment, most patients with granulomatous interstitial nephritis regain renal function but are often left with chronic kidney disease of varying severity.

Neurosarcoidosis

Neurologic disease generally requires much higher doses (80 to 100 mg prednisone a day). If neurosarcoidosis is not sufficiently responsive to corticosteroids alone, early immunosuppressive treatment with azathioprine, methotrexate, or infliximab (see Table 83-3) may improve clinical outcomes.[22]

Despite the absence of definitive randomized trials, cytotoxic and immunosuppressive drugs have been used to treat patients who do not respond to corticosteroid therapy or who cannot tolerate it (see Table 83-3), and both methotrexate and azathioprine appear to have significant steroid-sparing effects. Corticosteroids should be continued for at least 1 month after the addition of immunosuppressive agents. Generally, 3 to 6 months of cytotoxic and immunosuppressive treatment are required to determine whether a response has occurred. For patients who respond, the duration of treatment should be 9 to 12 months.

Cardiac Sarcoidosis

For cardiac sarcoidosis, corticosteroid doses of 30 to 40 mg per day are as good as higher doses. In patients who have arrhythmias, decreased ventricular function, or septal involvement detected on MRI or PET, electrophysiologic studies should be considered, and the need for an automatic implantable cardioverter-defibrillator (ICD) should be evaluated (Chapters 53 and 54).[23] For patients with pulmonary hypertension, bosentan (up to 125 mg daily) can reduce pulmonary arterial pressure[24] but has not been shown to improve exercise tolerance in patients with sarcoidosis.

Steroid-Dependent Sarcoidosis

In patients who are steroid dependent but have ongoing disease, TNF-α antagonists may be useful despite their potential side effects. The addition of infliximab (3 to 5 mg/kg for 24 weeks) can be efficacious for extrapulmonary disease.[25] Other options include adalimumab 40 mg subcutaneously once a week for 6 to 12 months, especially for uveitis and for skin lesions.

Transplantation

Less than 1% of heart and liver and about 3% of lung transplantations are performed in patients with sarcoidosis. The 1- and 5-year graft survival rates for lung, liver, and heart transplantations in patients with sarcoidosis compare favorably with the results obtained for patients with other disorders.

TABLE 83-3 TREATMENT

ORGAN	CLINICAL FINDINGS	TREATMENT
Respiratory	Dyspnea, persistent cough, FVC < 70%	Prednisone, 20-40 mg/day
	Mild cough, wheezing	Inhaled corticosteroid
Skin	Lupus pernio	Prednisone, 20-40 mg/day Hydroxychloroquine, 400 mg/day Methotrexate, 10-15 mg/wk Infliximab, 3-5 mg/kg every 2-4 wk
	Maculopapular eruptions	Topical corticosteroid Hydroxychloroquine, 400 mg/day Prednisone, 20-40 mg/day
	Erythema nodosum	NSAID*
Eyes	Anterior uveitis	Topical corticosteroid
	Posterior uveitis	Prednisone, 20-40 mg/day
Cardiac	Complete heart block, ventricular arrhythmias	AICD, prednisone, 20-40 mg/day
	Decreased LVEF (<35%)	AICD, prednisone, 20-40 mg/day
Central nervous system	Cranial nerve palsies	Prednisone, 20-40 mg/day
	Myelopathy	Prednisone, 40-60 mg/day, and azathioprine, 150 mg/day (or methotrexate 10-15 mg/wk or mycophenolate mofetil, 1000-2000 mg/day, or cyclophosphamide, 1-5 mg/kg/day)
	Intracerebral involvement	Prednisone, 40-60 mg/day, and azathioprine, 150 mg/day (or methotrexate 10-15 mg/wk or mycophenolate mofetil, 1000-2000 mg/day, or cyclophosphamide, 1-5 mg/kg/day)
Liver	Cholestatic hepatitis	Prednisone, 20-40 mg/day
Bone and joint	Arthralgias	NSAID
	Granulomatous arthritis	Prednisone, 20-40 mg/day Methotrexate, 10-15 mg/wk
	Bone destruction/pain	Prednisone, 20-40 mg/day Methotrexate, 10-15 mg/wk
Hypercalciuria and hypercalcemia	Kidney stones	Prednisone, 20-40 mg/day Hydroxychloroquine, 400 mg/day

*For example, ibuprofen, 200-800 mg three times a day.

AICD = automatic implantable cardioverter-defibrillator; FVC = forced vital capacity; LVEF = left ventricular ejection fraction; NSAID = nonsteroidal anti-inflammatory drug.

PROGNOSIS

Patients with Löfgren syndrome have a good prognosis characterized by spontaneous resolution with few consequences. Overall, spontaneous remission with few or no consequences occurs in more than 50% of patients within 3 years of diagnosis and in two thirds of patients within a decade. After 1 or more years of remission without treatment, recurrence occurs in less than 5% of patients. Up to one third of patients have unrelenting disease that leads to significant organ impairment, but less than 5% of patients die from sarcoidosis. Black Americans tend to have a worse prognosis with more chronic disease and more extrathoracic involvement of the eyes, liver, bone marrow, extrathoracic lymph nodes, and skin. In the absence of extrathoracic disease, patients with stage 1 radiographs generally have the best prognosis. Pulmonary function testing is more reliable in determining prognosis than is radiograph staging. Patients with neurologic and cardiac involvement have a poorer prognosis. Sarcoidosis-associated pulmonary hypertension is a harbinger for poor prognosis. For cardiac sarcoidosis, for example, estimates for 1-, 5-, and 10-year transplantation-free cardiac survival are 97%, 90%, and 83%, respectively, but heart failure at presentation predicts a poorer outcome, with a 10-year transplantation-free cardiac survival of only 53%.

GENERAL REFERENCES

For the General References and other additional features, please visit Elsevier eBooks+ at https://ebooks.health.elsevier.com.

Grade A References

A1. Vis R, vad de Gard EMW, Meek B, et al. Randomised, placebo-controlled trial of dexamethasone for quality of life in pulmonary sarcoidosis. *Respir Med.* 2020;165:105936.

A2. Wallaert B, Kyheng M, Labreuche J, et al. Long-term effects of pulmonary rehabilitation on daily life physical activity of patients with stage IV sarcoidosis: a randomized controlled trial. *Respir Med Res.* 2020;77:1-7.

A3. Baughman RP, Judson MA, Culver DA, et al. Roflumilast (Daliresp) to reduce acute pulmonary events in fibrotic sarcoidosis: a multi-center, double blind, placebo controlled, randomized clinical trial. *Sarcoidosis Vasc Diffuse Lung Dis.* 2021;38:e2021035.

84 ACUTE BRONCHITIS AND TRACHEITIS

GONZALO M. BEARMAN AND RICHARD P. WENZEL

DEFINITION

The term *acute bronchitis and tracheitis* defines a self-limited (1 to 3 weeks) inflammation of the large airways of the lung that extends to the tertiary bronchi (E-Fig. 84-1). In patients with a primary symptom of cough (Chapter 71), the diagnosis is made if there is no clinical or imaging evidence of pneumonia. At the bedside, the absence of criteria for systemic inflammatory response syndrome (Chapter 94) suggests bronchitis and tracheitis and makes a diagnosis of pneumonia (Chapter 85) unlikely. The criteria for the systemic inflammatory response syndrome are met if the patient has more than two of the following: temperature lower than 36° C or higher than 38° C, pulse greater than 90 beats per minute, respiratory rate higher than 20 breaths per minute, or white blood cell count less than 4000 cells/μL or higher than 12,000 cells/μL or with greater than 10% bands.

The definition of acute bronchitis and tracheitis also seeks to differentiate the illness from acute inflammation of the small airways (bronchiolitis), even though the accompanying symptoms with the former may include sputum production, wheezing, and shortness of breath. Among patients with primarily small airways disease, some might be expected to have prominently decreased breath sounds in the areas involved. Acute bronchitis and tracheitis is also different from bronchiectasis (Chapter 78), which is associated with permanent dilation of bronchi and a chronic cough. Furthermore, a diagnosis of chronic bronchitis (Chapter 76) is reserved for patients who have prolonged cough and sputum production: at least 3 months of the year for 2 consecutive years.

EPIDEMIOLOGY

Occurring at a rate of 44 per 1000 adults per year, acute bronchitis and tracheitis affects approximately 5% of adults annually. A higher incidence is observed in the winter and fall than in the summer and spring. In the United States, acute bronchitis and tracheitis is the ninth most common illness in outpatients as reported by physicians.

The disorder is thought to be viral in origin almost all the time. However, viruses have been isolated in only 8 to 37% of patients. Thus, the true causes of the illness are unknown in most cases. Nevertheless, at least 70% of patients with acute bronchitis and tracheitis in the United States receive antibacterial antibiotics after visiting a physician. Importantly, although the same bacteria that are commonly implicated in community-acquired pneumonia are also isolated from the sputum in half the patients, their role in the pathobiology of acute bronchitis and tracheitis or its attendant symptoms is unclear, and bronchial biopsies have not shown bacterial invasion.

PATHOBIOLOGY

Infections of the epithelium of the bronchi and trachea are thought to incite an inflammatory response. Pathologically, there is an accompanying microscopic thickening of bronchial and tracheal mucosa corresponding to the inflamed areas. Such pathologic findings are also consistent with the occasional case report of upper airway inflammation confined to the bronchi and trachea detected by ^{18}F-labeled fluorodeoxyglucose positron emission tomography (FDG-PET).

In various studies, specific pathogens have been found in more than half of patients with acute bronchitis. These pathogens include common respiratory viruses, typical respiratory bacteria, and atypical bacteria. At least three variables can influence the yield of specific pathogens: the presence of epidemics, the season of the year, and the population's influenza vaccination status. Furthermore, there are probably wide variations in the anatomic distribution of all pathogens causing acute bronchitis and tracheitis, extending from the nasal mucosa to the bronchiolar epithelium.

The viruses implicated in acute bronchitis and tracheitis include influenza A and B (Chapter 332), parainfluenza (Chapter 331), respiratory syncytial virus (Chapter 330), coronavirus (Chapters 334 and 335), adenovirus (Chapter 333), and rhinoviruses (Chapter 329), usually in this order from the most to the least common, with the pandemic spread of severe acute respiratory syndrome coronavirus 2 (SARS-CoV-2; Chapter 336) as a striking anomaly. Human metapneumovirus (Chapter 329) also has been identified as an etiologic agent. In children, bronchiolitis has been associated with respiratory syncytial virus, influenza virus, parainfluenza virus, and metapneumovirus.

Typical bacteria implicated in acute bronchitis include *Haemophilus influenzae* (Chapter 277) and *Moraxella catarrhalis* (Chapter 277). Severe bronchiolitis has also been reported with *Mycoplasma pneumoniae* (Chapter 293), even though this pathogen is usually associated with either pneumonia or acute bronchitis and tracheitis in adults. Up to 25% of cases of acute bronchitis and tracheitis may be due to "atypical" bacteria: *Bordetella pertussis* (Chapter 289), *Chlamydophila (Chlamydia) pneumoniae* (Chapter 294), and *Mycoplasma pneumoniae* (Chapter 293).

CLINICAL MANIFESTATIONS

The cardinal clinical symptom is cough (Chapter 71) of recent onset. Because most upper respiratory infections resolve within 1 week, a more extended period of cough is useful for considering the diagnosis of acute bronchitis. Patients usually seek care from their physician after 4 to 7 days of coughing that is not resolving. With acute bronchitis, there is often a continued cough and sometimes a worsened cough that lasts an initial 1 to 3 weeks. Associated symptoms vary and include sputum production, fever, malaise, wheezing, and dyspnea. Adults with pertussis may exhibit paroxysms of coughing, whooping, or vomiting, although less commonly than seen in children with this infection. Pertussis can infrequently lead to a cough lasting months, but data are lacking on the prevalence of pertussis among adults with chronic cough.

DIAGNOSIS

Acutely ill patients may not be able to distinguish their early symptoms from those accompanying very mild upper respiratory infections. However, with acute bronchitis and tracheitis, a protracted phase of coughing persists beyond 1 to 5 days, during which time a substantial proportion of patients will have significant declines in forced expiratory volume in 1 second (FEV_1) (Chapter 73).

When "atypical" bacteria are identified by culture or serology, patients tend to be seen later in the course of their illness than patients with viral causes and more often have wheezing. In some studies, 12 to 32% of patients with coughing that persists for longer than 1 week have pertussis. In other studies, however, pertussis has been confirmed in only 1% of such patients.

Because a major issue is whether symptoms are caused by an organism that could be responsive to antibiotics, the differentiation between bacterial infection compared with viral infection is often more important than determining the precise organism primarily responsible for the infection.

Rapid molecular diagnostic tests can identify specific bacteria or viruses linked to acute bronchitis and tracheitis. However, their major value lies in identifying a virus for which there is therapy or avoiding antibacterial antibiotics if a pathogenic virus is identified.[1]

Measurement of serum levels of procalcitonin, which is the prohormone of calcitonin and an inflammatory marker suggesting bacterial infection, also can help guide the initiation or discontinuation of antibacterial antibiotics.[2] A level lower than 0.1 ng/L makes bacterial infection highly unlikely, and limiting treatment to patients with levels higher than 0.25ng/L can markedly reduce the use of antibiotics without adverse clinical outcomes[A1] in some settings but not in emergency departments of U.S. hospitals with high adherence rates to pneumonia guidelines.[A2,A3] If the test is available, the finding of very low levels may help the clinician decide against prescribing antibiotics.

For diagnosing specific bacterial causes, polymerase chain reaction (PCR) testing of nasopharyngeal swabs or aspirates is the easiest and most sensitive way to diagnose infections by *B. pertussis, M. pneumoniae*, and *C. pneumoniae;* most experts recommend calcium alginate swabs for pertussis because cotton inhibits growth. Dacron swabs with aluminum handles are preferred for specimens used to diagnose *Chlamydophila* because cotton, calcium alginate, and the wooden shaft can all inhibit growth of the organism. Cultures for *M. pneumoniae* are slow and insensitive. In general, testing for atypical organisms should not be done because of the cost of PCR and both the insensitivity and slowness of cultures. However, if the clinician suspects an outbreak in the community or the likelihood of pertussis, rapid testing with PCR may be quite beneficial.

TREATMENT

For acute cough thought to be caused by acute bronchitis in an immunocompetent adult, no further tests or treatments are routinely recommended.[3] Nevertheless, although fewer than 50% of cases of acute bronchitis are probably caused by bacterial pathogens, antibiotics are used in 50 to 85% of cases worldwide and in about 45% of elderly patients with nonbacterial upper respiratory infections in the United States.[4] In a meta-analysis of randomized trials of antibacterial antibiotics for acute bronchitis, patients receiving antibiotics were significantly less likely to have a cough, but their 0.58 fewer days with cough, 0.46 fewer days of productive cough, and 0.64 fewer days of feeling ill were not statistically significant and were generally offset by the adverse effects of the antibiotics themselves.[A4] Electronic feedback, integrated into clinical practice workflow, can reduce antibiotic prescribing without adverse consequences.[A5]

When antibiotics are prescribed, azithromycin (500 mg daily for 3 days) is probably better than other alternatives. Another option is to delay the initiation of antibiotics and to use them only in patients with persistent symptoms. This strategy substantially reduces antibiotic use, slightly reduces patient satisfaction, but has had no detectable adverse clinical implications.[A6] Of note is that discolored sputum per se does not appear to predict responsiveness to antibiotics. Based on such data, guidelines suggest that antibiotics generally should be reserved for patients with suspected pneumonia.

Antibiotics may be used in patients with known atypical pathogens, but even then their effect on outcomes is not clear except to limit the spread of pertussis, especially during a defined outbreak. In adults suspected of having pertussis, erythromycin, 500 mg four times a day for 14 days, is thought to be most effective. However, many patients cannot tolerate erythromycin, and either doxycycline, 100 mg every 12 hours, or a newer macrolide such as azithromycin, 500 mg on day 1 and 250 mg/day thereafter, is effective. The latter two drugs are also active against *C. pneumoniae* and *M. pneumoniae*, although the optimal duration of therapy for acute bronchitis is unknown. A useful range is 5 to 14 days.

During influenza season, anti-influenza agents may be useful in decreasing symptoms by approximately 1 day and may lead to a 0.5-day earlier return to normal activity in patients with influenza. The first-generation drugs amantadine and rimantadine are ineffective against H3N2 influenza A viruses and are not recommended. Second-generation drugs such as zanamivir (two inhalations of 5 mg each, twice a day) or oseltamivir (75 mg twice a day) can be given for 5 days. Up to 20% of patients given oseltamivir will have nausea or vomiting.

Antihistamines and over-the-counter antitussives and expectorants have no apparent value. Although some subsets of patients with bronchial hyperresponsiveness may benefit from inhaled selective β_2-agonists at doses commonly used to treat asthma (see Chapter 75), overall they appear to confer no benefit. No data support the routine use of inhaled steroids. Mucolytic agents may be of small benefit.

In experimental rhinovirus colds, nonsteroidal drugs, alone or in combination with antihistamines, reduce the severity of symptoms, including cough. However, the widespread use of either type of drug alone or as a combination in naturally occurring, community-acquired bronchitis and tracheitis has not been evaluated.

In patients who do not have an established diagnosis of asthma (Chapter 75), oral corticosteroids are not helpful[A7] and should not be used. In patients with acute bronchitis, various alternative medicines include *Pelargonium sidoides* (a herbaceous perennial widely used in Europe), extracts of thyme herb and primrose root, Spicae atheroleum phytomedicine from the flowering tops of *Lavandula latifolia*,[A8] and a combination of medicinal plants[A9] have shown some benefit compared with placebo in acute bronchitis, but their true effectiveness is uncertain and they cannot be recommended until large, well-controlled, randomized trials are completed.[5]

Because antibiotics are overused and probably lead to community-wide alterations in antibiotic resistance,[6] interventions to reduce overuse can potentially have substantial long-term benefits while also reducing health care costs.[7] The increasing availability of multiplex PCR testing, which commonly includes detection of SARS-CoV-2, should help decrease the use of empiric antibiotics in the emergency department setting. Antibiotic use also can be safely reduced by physician education, peer review, and feedback,[A10] and the combination of education plus feedback is better than education alone.[A11]

PROGNOSIS

Coughing usually lasts 10 to 14 days, during which time the illness causes significant transient decrements in vitality and social functioning. Limited data on short- and long-term outcomes show that up to 20% of patients have persistent or recurrent symptoms for a month. Antibiotics may reduce symptoms by a fraction of a day, but they do not reduce return visits to the emergency department.[8] Furthermore, side effects, the emergence of antibiotic resistance, and cost must be weighed against their modest benefits.

GENERAL REFERENCES

For the General References and other additional features, please visit Elsevier eBooks+ at https://ebooks.health.elsevier.com.

Grade A References

A1. Schuetz P, Wirz Y, Sager R, et al. Effect of procalcitonin-guided antibiotic treatment on mortality in acute respiratory infections: a patient level meta-analysis. *Lancet Infect Dis.* 2018;18:95-107.
A2. Huang DT, Yealy DM, Filbin MR, et al. Procalcitonin-guided use of antibiotics for lower respiratory tract infection. *N Engl J Med.* 2018;379:236-249.
A3. Huang DT, Yealy DM, Angus DC. Longer-term outcomes of the ProACT trial. *N Engl J Med.* 2020;382:485-486.
A4. Smith SM, Fahey T, Smucny J, et al. Antibiotics for acute bronchitis. *Cochrane Database Syst Rev.* 2017;6:CD000245.
A5. Gulliford MC, Prevost AT, Charlton J, et al. Effectiveness and safety of electronically delivered prescribing feedback and decision support on antibiotic use for respiratory illness in primary care: REDUCE cluster randomised trial. *BMJ.* 2019;364:l236.
A6. de la Poza Abad M, Mas Dalmau G, Moreno Bakedano M, et al. Prescription strategies in acute uncomplicated respiratory infections: a randomized clinical trial. *JAMA Intern Med.* 2016;176:21-29.
A7. Hay AD, Little P, Harnden A, et al. Effect of oral prednisolone on symptom duration and severity in nonasthmatic adults with acute lower respiratory tract infection: a randomized clinical trial. *JAMA.* 2017;318:721-730.
A8. Kahler C, Derezinski T, Bocian-Sobkowska J, et al. Spicae aetheroleum in uncomplicated acute bronchitis: a double-blind, randomised controlled trial. *Win Med Wochenschr.* 2019;169:137-148.
A9. Yoon SW, Park JM, Rhee CK, et al. HL301 in the treatment of acute bronchitis: a phase 2b, randomized, double-blind, placebo controlled, multi-center study. *Korean J Intern Med.* 2020;35:133-141.
A10. Meeker D, Linder JA, Fox CR, et al. Effect of behavioral interventions on inappropriate antibiotic prescribing among primary care practices: a randomized clinical trial. *JAMA.* 2016;315:562-570.
A11. Du Yan L, Dean K, Park D, et al. Education vs clinician feedback on antibiotic prescriptions for acute respiratory infections in telemedicine: a randomized controlled trial. *J Gen Intern Med.* 2021;36:305-312.

85 OVERVIEW OF PNEUMONIA

LINDSEY R. BADEN, MARIE R. GRIFFIN, AND MICHAEL KLOMPAS

Hospital-acquired pneumonia and ventilator-acquired pneumonia are more frequently caused by *Staphylococcus aureus* or gram-negative bacilli. Pneumonia in immunocompromised hosts can be caused by a wide range of pathogens depending on the nature of the immune impairment, so early diagnosis and treatment are critical.

DEFINITION

Pneumonia is an acute infection of the lung parenchyma associated with at least one respiratory symptom (e.g., cough, dyspnea, chest pain) and abnormal opacities on lung imaging, with or without fever, in the absence of an alternative diagnosis. Pneumonia may be community-acquired pneumonia (CAP) or hospital-acquired pneumonia (HAP). In patients with immunocompromising conditions (e.g., inherited or acquired immunodeficiencies, neutropenia, human immunodeficiency virus (HIV) infection with a suppressed CD4 count, a solid organ or hematopoietic stem cell transplant, or conditions that require immunosuppressive agents), the causes of pneumonia include common organisms but also a number of organisms that are uncommon in hosts who have normal immunity.

COMMUNITY-ACQUIRED PNEUMONIA

EPIDEMIOLOGY

Community-acquired pneumonia is one of the most common serious health conditions and the most common infectious cause of hospitalization and death in the United States. It accounts for about 7 annual health care visits per 1000 young adults but 96 health care visits per 1000 adults ages 85 years and older. Hospitalization rates increase exponentially with age, from about 1 to 2 per 1000 in young adults to about 15 to 20 per 1000 individuals ages 65 to 84 years and almost 40 per 1000 among persons ages 85 years and older. About 35% of hospitalizations for community-acquired pneumonia among U.S. adults[1] occur in patients with recent exposures to health care settings, and about 25% occur in patients with immunocompromising conditions.

In the United States, pneumonia hospitalizations and deaths increase in November through March, coincident with the seasonal increases in influenza (Chapter 332) and other respiratory viruses, with the degree of excess morbidity and mortality depending on the circulating viral strains. Respiratory illness associated with influenza, human metapneumovirus (Chapter 330), respiratory syncytial virus (Chapter 330), *Staphylococcus aureus* (Chapter 267), and *Streptococcus pneumoniae* (Chapter 268) also peak during winter months. The seasonality of the novel pandemic severe acute respiratory syndrome coronavirus-2 (SARS-CoV-2; Chapter 336) has yet to be determined, but during the pandemic it became the leading cause of death owing in large part to pneumonia and respiratory failure.

Risk factors for developing pneumonia include male sex, smoking (Chapter 363), poor dental hygiene, crowded living conditions (including institutional settings), and more underlying comorbid conditions, especially malnutrition (Chapter 198), alcohol use disorder (Chapter 364), chronic immunosuppression, chronic lung disease, and neurologic disease, particularly dementia or conditions that compromise the normal gag reflex.[2] Medications associated with an increased risk of pneumonia include opioids, proton pump inhibitors,[3] corticosteroids, and other immunosuppressive drugs. Both inherited and acquired genetic disorders also can result in an increased frequency and/or severity of pneumonia. Examples include disorders of white cell production or function (Chapter 153), common variable immunodeficiency (Chapter 231), multiple myeloma (Chapter 173), and cystic fibrosis (Chapter 77).

PATHOBIOLOGY

Even in healthy adults, the lungs receive a continuous barrage of diverse microbes from inhaled air and from subclinical microaspiration of microbes that colonize the oropharynx. In healthy lungs, dominant bacteria, which most closely resemble those in the mouth, include *Prevotella, Veillonella,* and *Streptococcus* species. The lung microbiome includes both microbial elements (bacteria, viruses, phages, and fungi) and the normal host response. The mucosa of the upper respiratory tract is in direct communication with that of the lungs, so no region of the respiratory tract can be considered sterile.

Because bacterial pathogens can be found in low quantities in the healthy lung, pneumonia can be viewed as an alteration of homeostasis such that one (or more) pathogens can become dominant in the microbiome and stimulate a host response that results in inflammation (inflammatory markers and migration of cells into the lung), thereby resulting in the clinical picture of pneumonia. Infectious agents also can reach the lungs by hematogenous spread.

The total microbial burden and the frequency of specific types of bacteria in the lung depend on three factors: immigration, elimination, and relative reproduction rates. Lipid-rich and bacteriostatic surfactant, which lines the alveoli, other local conditions (e.g., pH, oxygen tension, temperature, microbial competition), and host defenses limit reproduction of pathogenic bacteria in the healthy lung. Inhaled and aspirated bacteria are eliminated by ciliated epithelial cells, which propel microbes entrapped in the mucous layer toward the upper airway, coughing, and both innate and adaptive immune defenses. Factors that increase microbial immigration (e.g., increased oropharyngeal colonization, supine position, more frequent mini-aspiration events, or gastrointestinal reflux), decrease the elimination of microbes (e.g., decreased cough, impaired ciliary function, obstructing lesions in the airways), or change the micro-environment (e.g., immunosuppression, destruction of lung surface area) contribute to infection.

Aging is the strongest risk factor for both the incidence and severity of pneumonia. Even among healthy adults, aging is associated with loss of adult stem cell reservoirs, mitochondrial dysfunction, oxidative stress, and shortening of telomeres, all of which interfere with the regeneration and repair needed to maintain homeostatic balance in the lung.[4] Chronic cumulative damage from exposure to atmospheric pollution, cigarette smoke, and other airborne substances are amplified by these changes. Chronic inflammation upregulates epithelial cell surface receptors that may increase bacterial adhesion in the aging lung and increase susceptibility to pneumonia. Decreased clearance mechanisms, including cough and mucociliary dysfunction, and structural lung changes may also increase susceptibility. Patients who have chronic lung conditions (e.g., chronic obstructive pulmonary disease [Chapter 76], cystic fibrosis [Chapter 77], or bronchiectasis [Chapter 78]) commonly have exacerbations that are triggered by bacterial or viral infections that cause inflammation and reduce lung function.

Whereas microaspiration is the presumed primary mechanism for most bacterial pneumonias, bacterial infections such as *Mycobacterium tuberculosis* (Chapter 299) and *Bacillus anthracis* (Chapter 272) are typically acquired by the direct inhalation of aerosols. Some bacteria, such as *Staphylococcus aureus* and *Escherichia coli,* can infect the lung via hematogenous spread. Any organism that causes vascular infection, especially right-sided endocarditis, also can seed the lungs and cause pneumonia.

Viruses are not typically part of the normal oropharyngeal flora but rather tend to be transmitted from infected persons by aerosols or by fomites. Viruses then replicate and spread through respiratory epithelial cells. Although viruses can cause pneumonia in the absence of bacterial infection,[5] some viruses (e.g., influenza, parainfluenza, respiratory syncytial virus) also may facilitate bacterial coinfection.

CLINICAL MANIFESTATIONS

Most patients with bacterial, COVID-19, or influenza pneumonia are acutely ill, but patients with *Mycoplasma, Chlamydia* pneumonia, or other viral pneumonias may not appear very ill. Pulmonary symptoms associated with pneumonia include cough (with or without purulent sputum), tachypnea, shortness of breath (dyspnea), and chest pain, which may be pleuritic. The classic triad of fever, dyspnea, and productive cough is absent in more than 40% of older adults with community-acquired pneumonia.[6] Instead, older adults and frail individuals often have atypical presentations, including malaise, changes in mental status, general fatigue, a decrease in functional status, urinary incontinence, and falls. Hypoxemia can cause confusion, but any neurologic symptoms should raise suspicion for meningitis.

DIAGNOSIS

The diagnosis of pneumonia requires compatible clinical manifestations combined with new opacities detected on chest imaging. Clinical judgement is paramount to avoid overtreatment that may result from the lack of an alternative diagnoses as well as the fear of potential negative consequences of withholding antibiotics from a patient with a bacterial pneumonia.

Physical Examination

Systemic signs include fever or hypothermia and tachycardia; hypotension suggests sepsis (Chapter 94). The respiratory rate may be increased, and a rate above 25 breaths per minute or an oxygen saturation below 92% suggests respiratory compromise. On the pulmonary examination, crackles are generally heard over the affected area (in bacterial pneumonia). Bronchial breath sounds and egophony (the patient says "a" but the clinician hears "e" on auscultation over the affected area) strongly suggest pneumonia with lobar consolidations but often are not heard. Dullness to percussion is consistent with consolidation or a pleural effusion. Increased tactile fremitus (a feeling of vibration over the affected area when the patient speaks) may be noted in an area with a pulmonary infiltrate but not over a pleural effusion. If the diaphragm does not move by percussion, an effusion is likely. Unfortunately, none of these findings on physical examination is sufficiently sensitive or specific to avoid the need for imaging for radiographic validation.

Radiology

The diagnosis of pneumonia requires a chest radiograph; thus, the first decision in the outpatient setting is often whether someone with cough or other respiratory symptoms needs an imaging study to confirm the diagnosis. Normal vital signs, especially if accompanied by lack of abnormal findings on physical examination of the chest, identify patients who have a sufficiently low risk of pneumonia such that imaging will likely not be useful. Rhinorrhea and sore throat suggest an upper respiratory process rather than pneumonia.

Chest radiographic abnormalities (Chapter 72) associated with community-acquired pneumonia include lobar consolidation, cavitation, and/or interstitial infiltrates (Fig. 85-1). Although consolidation or cavitation make a bacterial (or mycobacterial if cavitation is seen in the upper lobes) cause more likely, the radiographic presentation cannot reliably differentiate among pathogens. Parapneumonic effusions (Chapter 86) occur in up to 60% of patients with community-acquired pneumonia. Lung ultrasound is an attractive point-of-care option in experienced hands,[7] but standardized ultrasonographic criteria do not exist, and ultrasound does not avoid the need for a chest radiograph.

Chest computed tomography (CT) scanning (see Figs. 72-2 and 72-4) has higher sensitivity and specificity than a chest radiograph but is not ideal as an initial test because of its limited availability, cost, and radiation exposure. CT also can help distinguish whether an abnormal chest radiograph is being caused by an exacerbation of COPD or heart failure (see Fig. 72-3). Other conditions that should be included in the differential diagnosis in patients who have abnormalities on chest imaging include interstitial lung diseases (Chapter 80), lung cancer (Chapter 177), vasculitis (Chapter 249), pulmonary embolus (Chapter 69), or pulmonary hemorrhage (Chapter 69). In a patient who has symptoms and signs consistent with pneumonia, the absence of an infiltrate suggests an acute exacerbation of chronic obstructive pulmonary disease (Chapter 76), asthma (Chapter 75), or bronchitis (Chapter 84), or a viral infection such as pertussis (Chapter 289).

Radiographic abnormalities unfortunately are not particularly helpful in determining the cause of the pneumonia. Dense consolidation of a segment or lobe (see Fig. 85-1A1-1A3) suggests a bacterial cause, especially *S. pneumoniae, Klebsiella,* and often *Legionella.* Viral pneumonias other than COVID-19 usually cause diffuse

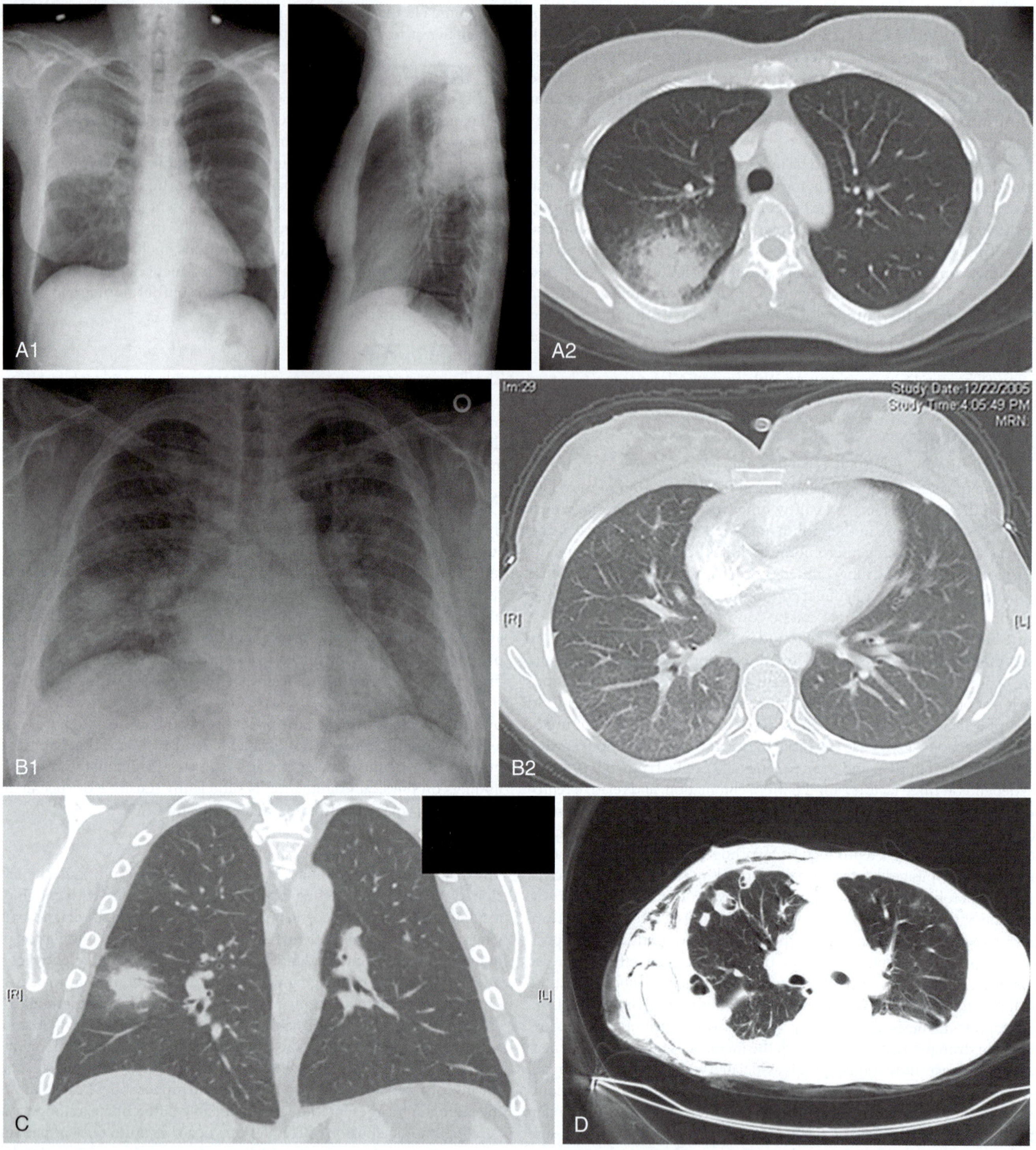

FIGURE 85-1. **Chest radiographic findings in pneumonia. A,** Lobar Infiltrate: Right upper lobe infiltrate in patient with pneumococcal pneumonia. 1. Anteroposterior chest radiograph. 2. Lateral chest radiograph. **B,** Diffuse or "patchy" interstitial infiltrates. 1. Anteroposterior chest radiograph. Bilateral patchy infiltrates in a patient with coronavirus pneumonia. 2. Computed tomographic scan. Diffuse interstitial infiltrates in a patient with *Pneumocystis jiroveci* pneumonia. **C,** Nodular Infiltrates. Computed tomographic scan. **D,** Cavitation. Computed tomographic scan. Cavitation in a patient with staphylococcal pneumonia. (From Musher DM. Overview of pneumonia. In: Goldman L, Schafer AI, eds. *Goldman-Cecil Medicine.* 26th ed. Philadelphia: Elsevier; 2020.)

infiltration (see Fig. 85-1B1) but may present with segmental or lobar consolidation, particularly when complicated by bacterial superinfection.[8] Subsegmental infiltration (see Fig. 85-1B2) can be seen with *Mycoplasma, Chlamydia,* and viruses. Hematogenous spread of *S. aureus* typically causes 1- to 3-cm round lesions that frequently cavitate (see Fig. 85-1D). A cavitary upper lobe lesion without a fluid level is typical of tuberculosis (Chapter 299), nontuberculous *Mycobacterium* (Chapter 300), or nocardiosis (Chapter 306). *Aspergillus* (Chapter 311) can cause a cavity with a distinctive intracavitary mycetoma (fungus ball; Fig. 311-2).

Diagnosing the Causative Agent

Polymerase chain reaction (PCR) testing of a nasopharyngeal swab is the best and most sensitive method for detecting viral pneumonias, which tend to have a presentation similar to that of atypical bacterial pneumonia. The SARS-CoV-2 (Chapter 336) and the disease it causes (COVID-19) have been the dominant causes of pneumonia worldwide during the recent pandemic, but other viruses such as rhinovirus (Chapter 329), influenza virus (Chapter 332), parainfluenza virus (Chapter 331), respiratory syncytial virus (Chapter 330), human metapneumovirus (Chapter 330), pre-2019 coronavirus (Chapter 334), and adenovirus (Chapter 333) also must be considered. Although a positive result may reflect colonization rather than infection, PCR is sensitive and specific for organisms that do not normally colonize the upper airways (e.g., *Chlamydia, Mycoplasma,* SARS-CoV-2, other coronaviruses, influenza, parainfluenza, respiratory syncytial virus, human metapneumovirus, and adenovirus). PCR testing should be done routinely for both SARS-CoV-2 and influenza when these viruses are circulating in the community, at least for patients who are eligible for antiviral treatment and for patients who will be hospitalized.

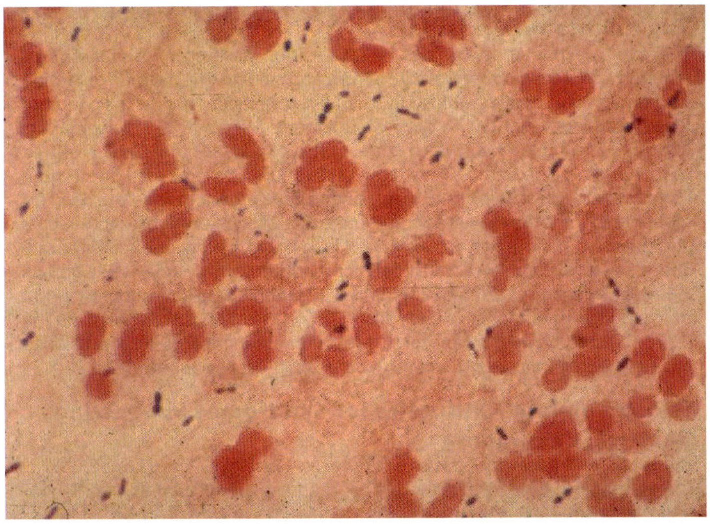

FIGURE 85-2. Gram stain of sputum from a patient with pneumococcal pneumonia shows large numbers of polymorphonuclear leukocytes and many lancet-shaped gram-positive cocci with no epithelial cells, indicating that this specimen originated in the lower airways. Such a specimen is diagnostic of pneumococcal pneumonia, although it cannot exclude coinfection by an organism such as a virus that is not seen by Gram stain. (From Musher DM. Overview of pneumonia. In: Goldman L, Schafer AI, eds. *Goldman-Cecil Medicine*. 26th ed. Philadelphia: Elsevier; 2020.)

Guidelines recommend against obtaining a sputum Gram stain (Fig. 85-2) and culture in most adults with community-acquired pneumonia because of their low sensitivity, the difficulty in obtaining adequate specimens, and the low likelihood that the results will change the choice of antibiotic treatment.[9] However, pretreatment Gram stain and culture of respiratory samples should be obtained in patients who are hospitalized with disease that meets the definition of severe pneumonia (Table 85-5, later) or who have risk factors for methicillin-resistant *Staphylococcus aureus* (MRSA) or *Pseudomonas aeruginosa*.[10] Blood cultures have a low yield and are not recommended, except in patients who meet criteria for severe pneumonia (Table 85-5, later) or who have risk factors for methicillin-resistant *Staphylococcus aureus* (MRSA) or *Pseudomonas aeruginosa*.[11]

In the recent pre-coronavirus-2019 (COVID-19) era, more than 50% of adults diagnosed and hospitalized with community-acquired pneumonia had no identifiable pathogen despite PCR testing of respiratory samples for viruses and atypical bacteria; culture of blood, sputum, and pleural fluid; and urinary assays for antigens (*Legionella* and *Streptococcus pneumoniae*). Bacteria were identified in 15 to 30% of cases, with *Streptococcus pneumoniae* (5 to 16%; Chapter 268), *Haemophilus influenzae* (<1 to 7%; Chapter 277), *Staphylococcus aureus* (2 to 5%; Chapter 267) and *Pseudomonas* (<1 to 3%; Chapter 282) being the most frequent (Table 85-1). Atypical bacteria each were responsible for less than 3%, even when routinely included in the testing protocol. In the pre-coronavirus-19 (COVID-19) era, routine multiplex PCR detected respiratory viruses in 20 to 27% of patients, with rhinoviruses (5 to 13%; Chapter 329) and influenza viruses (1 to 9%; Chapter 332) being the most common and all other viruses accounting for only 1 to 4% of cases. Other rare pathogens included mycobacteria (Chapter 300), nocardia (Chapter 306), and fungi.

Laboratory Testing

Many patients with community-acquired pneumonia do not require additional diagnostic testing other than a chest radiograph to confirm the diagnosis of pneumonia, a pulse oximetry measurement (with a saturation of 95% or higher indicating normal oxygenation), plus PCR testing for SARS-CoV-2 and, during flu season, for influenza. Additional routine testing for hospitalized patients to assess clinical stability should include a complete blood count, glucose level, and a measure of renal function. If the patient is tachypneic, an arterial blood gas should be obtained.

Laboratory findings include an elevated white blood cell count with neutrophilia in bacterial pneumonia, but viral infections and overwhelming bacterial infections can present with leukopenia. Inflammatory markers (e.g., the erythrocyte sedimentation rate, the C-reactive protein level, and, in bacterial infections, the procalcitonin level) may be elevated, especially with more severe bacterial pneumonias. Specific additional diagnostic testing is recommended for patients in whom admission is being contemplated (see Fig. 85-4) or in whom MRSA or *Pseudomonas aeruginosa* is suspected. Guidelines recommend against routine testing of urine for pneumococcal or *Legionella* antigens except in patients who have severe community-acquired pneumonia, or during *Legionella* outbreaks. If a *Legionella* outbreak is suspected, culture of respiratory secretions on selective media is also recommended.

TABLE 85-1 BACTERIAL AND VIRAL PATHOGENS IN COMMUNITY-ACQUIRED PNEUMONIA IN THE PRE-SARS-COV-2 ERA

PATHOGEN	PERCENT*
TYPICAL BACTERIA	**15-30**
Streptococcus pneumoniae	5-16
Staphylococcus aureus	3-5
Haemophilus influenzae	<1-7
Pseudomonas aeruginosa	<1-3
Escherichia coli	<1
Klebsiella pneumoniae	<1
Moraxella catarrhalis	<1
Other streptococci	<1
Acinetobacter baumannii	<1
ATYPICAL BACTERIA	**4**
Mycoplasma pneumoniae	1-2
Legionella spp	1
Chlamydia pneumoniae	1-2
VIRUSES	**20-27**
Human rhinoviruses	9-13
Influenza A and B viruses	1-6
Human metapneumovirus	2-4
Respiratory syncytial virus	2-3
Parainfluenza viruses 1-3	2-3
Other coronaviruses (229E, HKU1, NL63, and OC43)	2-3
NO PATHOGEN IDENTIFIED	**55-66**

*Percents based on various studies since 2010.
SARS-CoV-2 = severe acute respiratory syndrome coronavirus-2.

Unusual Causes of Pneumonia

Epidemiologic clues may be useful, especially for prompt consideration of unusual causes of pneumonia (Table 85-2), including *Coccidioides immitis* (southwest United States; Chapter 308), *Histoplasma capsulatum* (Midwest and South-Central United States; Chapter 308), *Francisella tularensis* (exposure to rabbits; Chapter 287), *Chlamydia psittaci* (exposure to parrots and parakeets; Chapter 294), *Cryptococcus neoformans* (exposure to pigeons; Chapter 302), and *Coxiella burnetii* (exposure to farm animals; Q fever; Chapter 302). Tuberculosis (Chapter 299) and nontuberculous mycobacterial infection (Chapter 300) must be considered in patients who have lived in endemic areas, have been incarcerated or homeless, have bronchitis (Chapter 78), or have extensive lung scarring owing to emphysema (Chapter 76).

Differential Diagnosis

Fever, cough, sputum production in the absence of infiltrate or a chest radiograph is consistent with acute bronchitis (Chapter 84). Persistent cough for several weeks in the absence of a fever or sputum should raise suspicion for pertussis (Chapter 289) but is also seen after a viral infection such as adenovirus (Chapter 333) or respiratory syncytial virus (Chapter 330).

About 15 to 20% of patients who are admitted to the hospital for suspected pneumonia have noninfectious causes for their symptoms. Acute heart failure (Chapter 45), which is the most likely noninfectious cause in older patients, may be suspected based on the history, physical examination, and radiographic findings, and it often can be confirmed by an elevated B-natriuretic peptide level. Pulmonary emboli with infarction (Chapter 68) can cause pleuritic chest pain and pulmonary infiltrates. Lung cancer (Chapter 177) can present with fever and a pulmonary infiltrate from a postobstructive pneumonia. The acute respiratory distress syndrome (Chapter 90), which can be the result of

TABLE 85-2 CONDITIONS SUGGESTING VARIOUS CAUSES OF PNEUMONIA

UNDERLYING CONDITION	ASSOCIATED MICROORGANISM
Pandemic condition	SARS-CoV-2
Aspiration/poor dentition	Microaerophilic and anaerobic mouth flora; *Candida* spp
Gross aspiration, bedridden person	*Staphylococcus aureus*, gram-negative rods
Travel to southwestern United States	*Coccidioides immitis*
Residence in Mississippi River basins, exposure to bats	*Histoplasma capsulatum*
Exposure to birds	Cryptococcus neoformans, *H. capsulatum*
Exposure to sick psittacine birds	*Chlamydia psittaci*
Exposure to rabbits	*Francisella tularensis*
Exposure to farm animals	*Coxiella burnetii* (Q fever)
Influenza active in community	Influenza virus, *S. aureus, S. pneumoniae, H. influenzae, Streptococcus pyogenes*
Bronchiectasis, cystic fibrosis	*Pseudomonas aeruginosa, Burkholderia cepacia, S. aureus, Aspergillus* spp, nontuberculous mycobacteria
Cavitary lung lesion	Microaerophilic and anaerobic mouth flora, *S. aureus*, tuberculous and nontuberculous mycobacteria, endemic fungi
Intravenous drug use	*S. aureus, Mycobacteria tuberculosis, S. pneumoniae*
Endobronchial obstruction	Microaerophilic and anaerobic mouth flora, gram-negative bacilli, *S. aureus*
Recent antibiotic therapy	Antibiotic-resistant *S. pneumoniae*
HIV (early)	*S. pneumoniae, H. influenzae, M. tuberculosis*
HIV/AIDS	Pathogens listed for early HIV infection, plus *Pneumocystis jiroveci, Cryptococcus, Histoplasma, Aspergillus, Mycobacterium kansasii, Mycobacterium avium* complex, *P. aeruginosa*
Travel to Middle East	Middle East respiratory syndrome (MERS) coronavirus
Bioterrorism	*Bacillus anthracis* (anthrax), *Yersinia pestis* (plague), *Francisella tularensis* (tularemia)

AIDS = acquired immunodeficiency syndrome; HIV = human immunodeficiency virus; SARS-CoV-2 = severe acute respiratory syndrome coronavirus 2; spp = species.

Data from Infectious Diseases Society of America/American Thoracic Society. Consensus guidelines on the management of community-acquired pneumonia in adults. *Clin Infect Dis*. 2007;44:S27-S72. From Musher DM. Overview of pneumonia. In: Goldman L, Schafer AI, eds. *Goldman-Cecil Medicine*. 26th ed. Philadelphia: Elsevier; 2020;592-603.

a serious nonpulmonary infection, may have clinical manifestations that are difficult to distinguish from pneumonia. Noninfectious interstitial pneumonia (Chapter 80), especially cryptogenic organizing pneumonia, eosinophilic pneumonia, and sarcoidosis (Chapter 83), are frequently initially misdiagnosed as community-acquired pneumonia.

TREATMENT

Initial Treatment

If SARS-CoV-2 is identified by point-of-care PCR testing, antibacterial agents should not be given unless bacterial coinfection is suspected, but antiviral agents and/or antibody treatments should be used in higher risk patients (see Chapter 337). When PCR testing documents influenza infection, antiviral treatment (see Chapter 332 and Table 85-6, later) is recommended in addition to empirical treatment for community-acquired pneumonia, due to possible coinfection with a bacterial pathogen.

Otherwise, empirical treatment (Table 85-6, later) for community-acquired pneumonia often begins before a specific etiologic diagnosis is established because the early administration of antibiotics improves outcomes for patients who have bacterial pneumonia. Antibiotic treatment can then be tailored if and when a pathogen is identified.[12] Despite some promising data, professional societies recommend against the use of procalcitonin levels to determine whether to administer antibiotics.

The Admission Decision

The severity of pneumonia guides the key decision of whether hospitalization is required and, if so, what level of care is most appropriate. The decision regarding hospital admission can be guided by validated approaches such as the pneumonia severity index along with clinical judgement. A score of 90 or fewer points (Fig. 85-3 and Table 85-3), which corresponds to classes I to III, indicates that outpatient management is likely to be safe in nonhypoxemic patients. Higher scores should alert clinicians to increasingly grave prognoses and the need for higher levels of care, as well as communication of such prognoses to patients and their designees when appropriate. If laboratory testing is not readily available to make the decision about admission, another severity index, the CURB-65 (Table 85-4), is a less preferred alternative. In patients who have more than 130 points on the pneumonia severity score (Fig. 85-3), more than 3 points on the CURB-65 score, or meet criteria for severe pneumonia (Table 85-5), admission to an intermediate care unit or intensive care unit is usually appropriate.

Choices among Antibiotics for Syndromes Suggesting Bacterial Pneumonia

Antibiotic treatments depend on the site of care (see Fig. 85-4 and Table 85-3),[13,14] the presence or absence of comorbid conditions (see Fig. 85-4), and epidemiologic clues (see Table 85-2).

Treatment should be altered as appropriate when a specific organism and its antimicrobial sensitivities are identified. Patients must be reevaluated if clinical stability is not achieved, and treatment must be discontinued in a timely and appropriate way.

Outpatient Antimicrobial Therapy

For otherwise healthy adults with community-acquired pneumonia in the outpatient setting, monotherapy is recommended for 5 days[15] with amoxicillin, doxycycline, or azithromycin (see Table 85-6). For outpatient adults who have chronic conditions that may both increase the risk of acquiring a drug-resistant organism, as well as the consequences of insufficient antibiotic coverage, the recommended antibiotic regimens include monotherapy with a respiratory fluoroquinolone or the combination of one of amoxicillin/clavulanate, cefpodoxime, or cefuroxime plus azithromycin, clarithromycin, or doxycycline (see Table 85-6). For patients who will not be hospitalized, there is no evidence for or against an initial dose of a parenteral antibiotic before sending the patient home.[16]

Inpatient Antimicrobial Therapy

For inpatients who have nonsevere community-acquired pneumonia without risk factors for MRSA or *P. aeruginosa*, antibiotic choices include monotherapy with a respiratory fluoroquinolone or the combination of a β-lactam plus either a macrolide or doxycycline (see Table 85-6).[A1,A2] In clinically stable patients (temperature 37.8° C or less, heart rate less than 100 beats per minute, respiratory rate less than 24 breaths per minute, oxygen saturation 90% or higher, systolic blood pressure 90 mm Hg or higher, and normal mental status), 3 days of intravenous treatment need not be followed by oral treatment.[A3] Newer options found noninferior to fluoroquinolone monotherapy are omadacycline monotherapy[A4] and lefamulin monotherapy[A5,A6] (see Table 85-6). Alternatives to fluoroquinolones should be strongly considered because of the association of fluoroquinolones with the development of *Clostridioides difficile* infection, tendinopathy/tendon rupture, mental status changes, and peripheral neuropathy. Fluoroquinolones are contraindicated in patients who have a prolonged QT interval, and lefamulin is contraindicated in patients who have a prolonged QT interval as well as in patients who have moderate to severe liver disease.

Patients who are hospitalized with severe community-acquired pneumonia should receive dual therapy with a β-lactam and either a macrolide or a respiratory fluoroquinolone[17] (see Table 85-6). The risk of infection with MRSA or *Pseudomonas* is increased in patients who have received parenteral antibiotics in the prior 90 days and who have had infection with these organisms previously. If treatment is being considered to cover MRSA, a rapid negative nasal PCR test has high predictive value and suggests a different etiology; a positive test has a low predictive value but warrants empirical treatment in patients who have severe community-acquired pneumonia or who are at high risk for MRSA in the absence of other etiology. Anaerobic coverage such as with clindamycin is not routinely recommended unless a lung abscess or empyema is suspected.

Antibiotics generally should be continued for a minimum of 5 days for most patients, for 7 days for patients with suspected MRSA or *Pseudomonas*, but longer if needed to achieve clinical stability (i.e., resolution of vital sign abnormalities, toleration of oral intake, and normal mentation). In patients whose community-acquired pneumonia does not require an intensive care unit (ICU); however, 3 days of intravenous treatment that includes a β-lactam can be adequate if they are clinically stable.

All hospitalized patients who test positive for influenza should receive anti-influenza treatment regardless of the duration of illness before diagnosis. Such patients also should receive adjunctive antibiotic treatment given the high prevalence of bacterial coinfection.

Adjunctive Therapy and Supportive Care

Guidelines recommend against the use of corticosteroids in most adults with community-acquired pneumonia, except in patients who have refractory septic shock (Chapter 94). However, corticosteroids (e.g., hydrocortisone 200 mg for 4 or 8 days

Sex

- ○ M (0 points)
- ○ F (–10 points)

Demographic factors

- ▭ Age
- ☐ Nursing home resident (10 points)

Comorbid illnesses

- ☐ Cancer, not of skin (30 points)
- ☐ Active chronic liver disease (20 points)
- ☐ Heart failure (10 points)
- ☐ Cerebrovascular disease (10 points)
- ☐ Renal disease (10)

Physical examination findings

- ☐ Altered mental status (20 points)
- ☐ Respiratory rate ≥30/minute (20 points)
- ☐ Temperature <35° C or ≥40° C (15 points)
- ☐ Pulse ≥125/minute (10 points)

Laboratory and radiographic findings

- ☐ Arterial pH <7.35 (30 points)
- ☐ Blood urea nitrogen ≥30 mg/dL (11 mmol/L) (20 points)
- ☐ Serum sodium <130 mEq/L (20 points)
- ☐ Serum glucose ≥250 mg/dL (14 mmol/L) (10 points)
- ☐ Hematocrit <30 percent (10 points)
- ☐ Partial pressure of arterial oxygen <60 mmHg or oxygen saturation <90% (10 points)
- ☐ Pleural effusion on chest radiograph (10 points)

FIGURE 85-3. **Community-Acquired Pneumonia Severity Index for Adults. Compute total point score (see Table 85-3).**

TABLE 85-3 MORTALITY AT 30 DAYS BASED ON THE SCORE ON THE COMMUNITY-ACQUIRED PNEUMONIA SEVERITY INDEX (SEE FIG. 85-3)

POINT SCORE	CLASS	APPROXIMATE 30-DAY MORTALITY
≤70	II	<1-3%
71-90	III	3-4%
91-130	IV	8%
>130	V	25%

From Fine MJ, Auble TE, Yealy DM, et al. A prediction rule to identify low-risk patients with community-acquired pneumonia. *N Engl J Med.* 1997;336:243-250; and Musher DM, Roig IL, Cazares G, et al. Can an etiologic agent be identified in adults who are hospitalized for community-acquired pneumonia: results of a one-year study. *J Infect.* 2013;67:11-18.

TABLE 85-4 CURB-65 SCORING SYSTEM FOR PNEUMONIA

CLINICAL FACTOR	POINTS
Confusion	1
Blood urea nitrogen ≥ 20 mg/dL	1
Respiratory rate ≥ 30 breaths per minute	1
Systolic blood pressure < 90 mm Hg or Diastolic blood pressure ≤ 60 mmHg	1
Age ≥ 65 years	1
Total points:	

One point given for the presence of each of the factors. Higher scores indicate a greater risk of death. A score of >2 points generally suggests that hospital admission is required, and a score of >3 points suggests that admission to an intensive care unit is advisable.

Data from Eccles S, Pincus C, Higgins B, et al. Diagnosis and management of community and hospital acquired pneumonia in adults: summary of NICE guidance. *BMJ.* 2014;349:g6722.

depending on clinical improvement, then tapered for a total of 8 or 14 days) improve outcomes in severe community-acquired pneumonia,[A7] and corticosteroids (e.g., dexamethasone) also benefit severely ill patients who have COVID-19 and who are receiving supplemental oxygen or are on ventilatory support (Chapter 337).

Supportive Care

Supportive care will depend on severity of pneumonia and site of care. Patients should remain active as tolerated, but hospitalized patients may require assistance to ambulate safely. Frequent monitoring of vital signs and oxygenation should alert clinicians to important clinical deterioration in a timely way. At discharge, some patients may require supplemental oxygen, but often only temporarily. Patients should be warned of the cardiovascular complications that frequently accompany or follow pneumonia (including arrhythmias, heart failure, and acute coronary syndrome) and seek care if they do not continue to improve or develop new symptoms.

Failure to Improve

A follow-up chest radiograph is not routinely recommended to ensure resolution because radiograph clearance may require weeks. However, failure to achieve clinical stability within 5 to 7 days should prompt consideration of empyema (Chapter 86), lung abscess (Chapter 78), or an alternative diagnosis that requires repeat imaging and merits alternative specific management (Table 85-7).

Most parapneumonic effusions (Chapter 86) resolve with resolution of the pneumonia and do not require drainage. If appropriate antibiotic treatment is not timely; however, an uncomplicated parapneumonic effusion may progress to a fibrinopurulent stage (complicated pleural effusion or empyema), which carries significant morbidity. In patients with a complicated parapneumonic effusion, bacteria are identified in fewer than 20% of cases by culture, but by PCR testing in 93% of cases. When bacteria are identified, viridans streptococci are the most frequent pathogens, followed by *Fusobacterium* and *Streptococcus pneumoniae*.

TABLE 85-5 INFECTIOUS DISEASES SOCIETY OF AMERICA/AMERICAN THORACIC SOCIETY CRITERIA FOR DEFINING SEVERE COMMUNITY-ACQUIRED PNEUMONIA*

Major criteria
Septic shock with need for vasopressors
Respiratory failure requiring mechanical ventilation
Minor criteria
Hypotension requiring aggressive fluid resuscitation
Hypothermia (core temperature <36° C)
Respiratory rate ≥30 breaths/min
Pa_{O_2}/Fi_{O_2} ratio ≤250
Confusion/disorientation
Multilobar infiltrates
White blood cell count <4000 cells/μL†
Thrombocytopenia (platelet count <100,000/μL)
Renal impairment (blood urea nitrogen level ≥20 mg/dL)

*Validated definition includes either one major criterion or three or more minor criteria.
†Due to infection alone (i.e., not chemotherapy-induced).
Reprinted with permission of the American Thoracic Society. Copyright © 2023 American Thoracic Society. All rights reserved. Metlay JP, Waterer GW, Long AC, et al. 2019, Diagnosis and treatment of adults with community-acquired pneumonia. An official clinical practice guideline of the American Thoracic Society and Infectious Diseases Society of America. *Am J Respir Crit Care Med.* 2019;200:e45-e67.

PREVENTION

Smoking cessation, avoidance of drugs known to increase the risk of pneumonia (e.g., opioids, proton pump inhibitors, corticosteroids, and other immunosuppressive agents) and control of the blood sugar in patients with diabetes can help prevent pneumonia and its morbidity. Masks, social distancing, and good ventilation have a substantial benefit for preventing SARS-CoV-2 (Chapter 336) and may also decrease rates of infection with influenza and respiratory syncytial virus. Individuals who have acute respiratory symptoms should avoid close contact with others, practice good hand hygiene, and may consider using appropriate face masks while symptomatic.

Influenza vaccine is recommended annually for all persons age 6 months and older (Chapter 15) and is especially important for individuals who have chronic health conditions, pregnant women, and older adults. SARS-CoV-2 vaccines (Chapter 15) are currently recommended for all adults and children ages 6 months and older. Pneumococcal conjugate vaccines protect against pneumonia, bacteremia, and meningitis caused by pneumococcal serotypes 15 (PCV15) and 20 (PCV20). Either of these vaccines is recommended for all adults ages 65 years and older and for adults age 19 through 64 years with certain medical conditions or risk factors (e.g., chronic heart; liver, lung, or kidney disease; diabetes mellitus; alcohol use disorder; cigarette smoking; cerebrospinal fluid leak; cochlear implant; or an immunocompromising

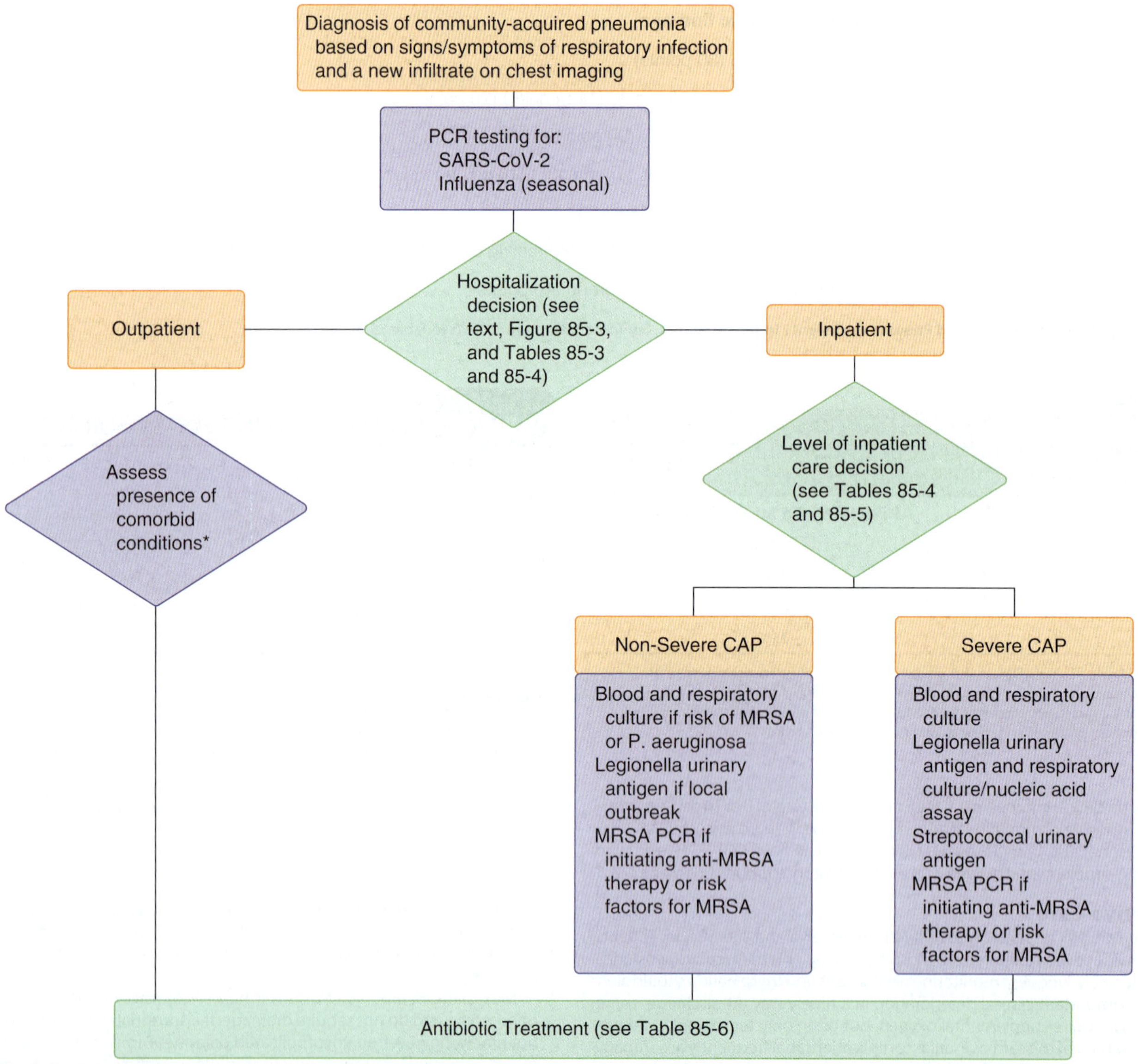

FIGURE 85-4. Diagnostic approach to community-acquired pneumonia management pathway for community-acquired pneumonia (CAP). *Comorbid conditions: chronic heart, lung, liver or renal disease; diabetes mellitus, alcoholism, malignancy; or asplenia. MRSA = methicillin-resistant *Staphylococcus aureus; P. aeruginosa = Pseudomonas aeruginosa;* PCR = polymerase chain reaction; SARS-CoV-2 = severe acute respiratory syndrome coronavirus-2. (Data from Jones BE, Herman DD, Dela Cruz CS, et al. Summary for clinicians: clinical practice guideline for the diagnosis and treatment of community-acquired pneumonia. *Ann Am Thorac Soc.* 2020;17:133-138.)

TABLE 85-6 RECOMMENDED ANTIMICROBIAL REGIMENS AND DOSING (ORAL FOR OUTPATIENTS, INTRAVENOUS FOR INPATIENTS)

I. FOR OUTPATIENT SYNDROMES SUGGESTING BACTERIAL PNEUMONIA
- A. Healthy outpatient adults with no comorbid conditions or risk factors for MRSA or *P. aeruginosa:*
  1. Amoxicillin 1 g three times daily
  2. Or doxycycline 100 mg twice daily),
  3. Or a macrolide (azithromycin 500 mg on first day then 250 mg daily or clarithromycin 500 mg twice daily or clarithromycin extended-release 1000 mg daily)
- B. Outpatient adults with comorbid conditions (e.g., chronic heart, lung, liver, or renal disease; diabetes mellitus; alcohol use disorder; malignancy; or asplenia)
  1. Combination therapy: amoxicillin/clavulanate (500 mg/125 mg three times daily or 875 mg/125 mg twice daily, or 2000 mg/125 mg twice daily) or a cephalosporin (cefpodoxime 200 mg twice daily or cefuroxime 500 mg twice daily); PLUS a macrolide (azithromycin 500 mg daily, or clarithromycin 500 mg daily or extended-release 1000 mg once daily), or doxycycline (100 mg twice daily)
  2. OR: Monotherapy: respiratory fluoroquinolone (levofloxacin 750 mg daily, or moxifloxacin 400 mg daily, or gemifloxacin 320 mg daily)

II. FOR OUTPATIENT SYNDROMES SUGGESTING VIRAL PNEUMONIA
- A. For SARS-CoV-2 (see Chapter 337)
- B. For syndromes suggesting influenza pneumonia:
  1. Oseltamivir (75 mg twice daily for 5 days)
  2. Treat as above for possibility of bacterial coinfection

III. FOR SYNDROMES SUGGESTING VIRAL PNEUMONIA OTHER THAN INFLUENZA, treat for possibility of bacterial coinfection

IV. FOR INPATIENT SYNDROMES SUGGESTING BACTERIAL PNEUMONIA
- A. Inpatient adults with nonsevere community-acquired pneumonia without risk factors for MRSA or *P. aeruginosa*:
  1. Combination therapy: a β-lactam (ampicillin 1 sulbactam 1.5-3 g every 6 hr, cefotaxime 1-2 g every 8 hr, ceftriaxone 1-2 g daily, or ceftaroline 600 mg every 12 hr) plus a macrolide (azithromycin 500 mg daily or clarithromycin 500 mg twice daily)
  2. Monotherapy: a respiratory quinolone (levofloxacin 750 mg daily, moxifloxacin 400 mg daily, or gemifloxacin 320 mg daily)
  3. For adults hospitalized with community-acquired pneumonia and contraindications to both macrolides and fluoroquinolones: combination therapy with a β-lactam (ampicillin sulbactam, cefotaxime, ceftaroline, or ceftriaxone; doses as earlier) plus doxycycline (100 mg twice daily)
  4. New monotherapies: omadacycline (100 mg every 12 hours × 2 then every 24 hours, substituting 300 mg by oral route on or after 3 days); lefamulin (150 mg every 12 hours, substituting 600 mg by oral route on or after 3 days)
- B. Adults hospitalized with severe community-acquired pneumonia (specific agents and doses are the same as earlier):
  1. A β-lactam plus a macrolide or a β-lactam plus a respiratory fluoroquinolone
  2. If MRSA is a consideration (see text): vancomycin (15 mg/kg every 12 hr, adjust based on levels) or linezolid (600 mg every 12 hr).
  3. If *P. aeruginosa* is a consideration: piperacillin-tazobactam (4.5 g every 6 hr), cefepime (2 g every 8 hr), ceftazidime (2 g every 8 hr), aztreonam (2 g every 8 hr), meropenem (1 g every 8 hr), or imipenem (500 mg every 6 hr)

V. FOR INPATIENT SYNDROMES SUGGESTING VIRAL PNEUMONIA
- A. If SARS-CoV-2:
  1. (See Chapter 337)
- B. If influenza is likely, bacterial coinfection may coexist:
  1. Oseltamivir (75 mg twice daily for 5 days) PLUS
  2. As per IV A and B
- C. For other viral pneumonias, bacterial coinfection may coexist, so patients should be treated as per IV A and B

MRSA = methicillin-resistant *Staphylococcus aureus; P. aeruginosa* = *Pseudomonas aeruginosa.*
Data from Jones BE, Herman DD, Dela Cruz CS, et al. Summary for clinicians: clinical practice guideline for the diagnosis and treatment of community-acquired pneumonia. *Ann Am Thorac Soc.* 2020;17:133-138.

TABLE 85-7 REASONS FOR FAILURE OF ANTIMICROBIAL THERAPY IN TREATING PNEUMONIA

Correct organism, but inappropriate antibiotic choice or dose
- Organism not susceptible
- Wrong dosage (e.g., morbidly obese or fluid-overloaded patient)

Correct organism and antibiotic, but infection is loculated
- Empyema (the most common)
- Obstruction (e.g., lung cancer, foreign body)

Causative organism not susceptible to chosen antibiotics

Noninfectious condition
- Pulmonary embolism
- Malignancy
- Inflammatory noninfectious lung disease (see text)
- Heart failure

Adapted from Musher DM. Overview of pneumonia. In: Goldman L, Schafer AI, eds. *Goldman-Cecil Medicine.* 26th ed. Philadelphia: Elsevier; 2020;592-603.

condition). Pneumococcal polysaccharide vaccine (PPSV23), which protects against serious pneumococcal disease from 23 serotypes of the pneumococcus, is recommended for all adults ages 19 years and older who receive PCV15 but is unnecessary for people who receive PCV20 (Chapter 15). When both vaccines are given, the conjugate vaccine should be given first, followed by the polysaccharide vaccine 1 year later. Vaccines for RSV may be available soon.[18]

PROGNOSIS

For patients who are treated as outpatients, the prognosis for full recovery is excellent. However, close follow-up is required to ensure that clinical stability is achieved and maintained.

About 85% of hospitalized patients respond within 7 days in terms of improved cough and shortness of breath, becoming afebrile, and tolerating of oral intake; such patients have only a 1% in-hospital mortality and 5% 30-day mortality. Characteristics associated with a failure to improve include the need for initial intensive care, obesity, diabetes, and an active malignancy. Overall, all-cause mortality is about 6% for hospitalized patients during their acute hospital stay and is about 13% at 30 days, 23% at 6 months, and 30% at 1 year, partly owing to the pneumonia itself and partly as a reflection of comorbid conditions and underlying frailty. For example, nearly 25% of patients experience at least one new cardiovascular event, including decompensated heart failure, atrial fibrillation or flutter, an acute coronary syndrome or stroke,[19] within the first 3 days of hospitalization. Mortality depends to a large degree on achievement of clinical stability.

Among hospitalized patients, about 70% are ultimately discharged home (including one-third of whom require home health follow-up), whereas about 30% are discharged to a nursing home or rehabilitation care facility. The overall readmission rate is about 15% at 30 days but is higher among patients who are discharged with a need for home health care.

HOSPITAL-ACQUIRED PNEUMONIA IN THE IMMUNOCOMPETENT HOST

Hospital-acquired pneumonia, which is defined as pneumonia that develops 48 hours or more after hospital admission, is typically divided into ventilator-associated pneumonia (VAP) and nonventilator hospital-acquired pneumonia (NV-HAP) depending on whether or not the patient was treated with mechanical ventilation in the 48 hours preceding the onset of pneumonia.

EPIDEMIOLOGY

Hospital-acquired pneumonia, which is the most common and morbid health care–associated infection (Chapter 261), affects approximately 1 in every 100 hospitalized patients. Incidence rates differ markedly, however, in different populations: about 3.5% of ventilated patients (Chapter 91) develop pneumonia compared with about 0.5% of nonventilated patients.[20] Nonetheless, many more hospitalized are nonventilated, so most hospital-acquired pneumonia is not ventilator-associated. The incidence of hospital-acquired pneumonia rises with age and most commonly affects patients on medical, surgical, oncology, and neurology services. Key risk factors include impaired consciousness, dysphagia, and feeding by an oral or nasogastric tube.

PATHOBIOLOGY

Hospital-acquired pneumonia, like community-acquired pneumonia, is thought to be due largely to microaspiration or macroaspiration events when perturbations of the oral microbiome permit pathogenic organisms to proliferate. Microscopic and microbial evaluations of material obtained at autopsy note scattered, heterogenous areas of inflammation at various stages of injury and recovery, some with microorganisms and some without. Chemical analyses of tracheal aspirates and bronchoalveolar lavage specimens identify gastrin and/or pepsin in up to two thirds of intubated patients. These findings collectively suggest that patients routinely aspirate oral and gastric secretions, thereby leading to scattered local areas of inflammation of various degrees of severity throughout the lungs. Some affected areas remain subclinical and resolve spontaneously, whereas others progress to frank infection and clinically overt pneumonia.

CLINICAL MANIFESTATIONS

After a median interval from hospital admission until the onset of pneumonia of 4 to 7 days,[21] the cardinal symptoms and signs of hospital-acquired pneumonia are fever, tachypnea, increased respiratory secretions, leukocytosis, a decline in oxygen saturation, measured by pulse oximetry, new radiographic infiltrates, and positive lower respiratory tract cultures. However, none of these findings is particularly sensitive or specific for hospital-acquired pneumonia[22] (Table 85-8). For example, the combination of a radiographic infiltrate and any two of fever, purulent secretions, and leukocytosis has a sensitivity and specificity of 69 and 75%, respectively, for histologically confirmed ventilator-associated pneumonia. The combination of a radiographic infiltrate plus fever, purulent secretions, and leukocytosis, increases the specificity to 92% but decreases sensitivity to 23%.

DIAGNOSIS

The diagnosis of hospital-acquired pneumonia is subjective because of the limited accuracy of clinical manifestations, and experienced clinicians often disagree. Furthermore, bacteria and viruses can colonize the respiratory tract without causing an invasive infection, so a positive PCR assay, Gram stain, or culture does not necessarily mean that the identified organism is the cause of the patient's respiratory syndrome. Procalcitonin, which is the most frequently used biomarker, has a sensitivity that ranges from 60 to 70% and a specificity that ranges from 24 to 80%, but current guidelines recommend against its routine use to diagnose hospital-acquired pneumonia and ventilator-associated pneumonia. Bronchoalveolar lavage cultures are positive in only about one third of patients with clinically suspected ventilator-associated pneumonia. Blood cultures can be positive in up to 10% of hospital or ventilator associated pneumonia, depending on its severity, and should be obtained.

The organisms that are typically associated with ventilator-associated pneumonia (Table 85-9) and nonventilator hospital-acquired pneumonia are similar.[23] *Staphylococcus aureus* (Chapter 267) predominates and accounts for approximately 30 to 40% of pneumonias in which an organism is recovered. Fortunately, the incidence of staphylococcal infections that are resistant to methicillin has declined by 50% in recent years. *Pseudomonas* (Chapter 282), which is the second

TABLE 85-8 ACCURACY OF CLINICAL SIGNS TO DIAGNOSE VENTILATOR-ASSOCIATED PNEUMONIA, DERIVED FROM A META-ANALYSIS OF 25 STUDIES, INCLUDING 1639 PATIENTS*

SIGN	SENSITIVITY	SPECIFICITY	POSITIVE LIKELIHOOD RATIO	NEGATIVE LIKELIHOOD RATIO	DIAGNOSTIC ODDS RATIO
Fever	66%	54%	1.4	0.6	2.3
Purulent secretions	77%	39%	1.3	0.6	2.1
Leukocytosis	64%	59%	1.6	0.6	2.6
Infiltrate on chest radiograph	89%	26%	1.2	0.4	2.8
Endotracheal aspirate culture ($\geq 10^5$ CFU/mL)	76%	68%	2.4	0.4	6.6
Bronchoalveolar lavage culture ($\geq 10^4$ CFU/mL)	71%	80%	3.5	0.4	9.6

*Histopathology is used as reference standard.
CFU = colony-forming units.
From Fernando SM, Tran A, Cheng W, et al. Diagnosis of ventilator-associated pneumonia in critically ill adult patients—a systematic review and meta-analysis. *Intensive Care Med.* 2020;46:1170-1179.

TABLE 85-9 ORGANISMS AND ANTIBIOTIC SUSCEPTIBILITY RATES ASSOCIATED WITH 6131 CULTURE-POSITIVE EPISODES OF VENTILATOR-ASSOCIATED PNEUMONIA IN THE UNITED STATES, 2015-2017

	APPROXIMATE FREQUENCY	SUSCEPTIBILITY RATES TO COMMON ANTIBIOTICS
Staphylococcus aureus (Chapter 267)	30-40%	Methicillin or oxacillin 63%
Pseudomonas aeruginosa (Chapter 282)	15-20%	Aminoglycosides 86% Antipseudomonal cephalosporins 74% Fluoroquinolones 73% Carbapenems 73% Piperacillin-tazobactam 78%
Klebsiella pneumoniae (Chapter 281)	10%	Antipseudomonal cephalosporins 85% Carbapenems 94%
Escherichia coli (Chapter 280)	5-10%	Antipseudomonal cephalosporins 77% Carbapenems 99% Fluoroquinolones 67%
Enterobacter spp (Chapter 281)	5-10%	Cefepime 93% Carbapenems 96%
Acinetobacter baumannii (Chapter 283)	3%	Carbapenems 58%

spp = species.
From Weiner-Lastinger LM, Abner S, Edwards JR, et al. Antimicrobial-resistant pathogens associated with adult healthcare-associated infections: summary of data reported to the National Healthcare Safety Network, 2015-2017. *Infect Control Hosp Epidemiol.* 2020;41:1-18.

most common organism, accounts for 15 to 20% of culture-positive hospital acquired pneumonias. Other organisms include *Klebsiella* species (10%; Chapter 281), *Enterobacter* species (5 to 10%; Chapter 281), *Escherichia coli* (5 to 10%; Chapter 280), *Haemophilus influenzae* (5%; Chapter 277), *Streptococcus* species (5%; Chapter 268), and *Acinetobacter* species (3%; Chapter 283).

A substantial proportion, perhaps 20 to 25%, of hospital-acquired pneumonia may be attributable solely to respiratory viruses, including rhinovirus (Chapter 329), influenza (Chapter 332), parainfluenza (Chapter 331), metapneumovirus (Chapter 330), and non–SARS-CoV-2 coronaviruses (Chapter 334). Another 15% or so may be caused by coinfection with both a virus and a bacterium. Large nosocomial clusters of hospital-onset respiratory viral infections, including SARS-CoV-2 and influenza, also have been reported.

The clinical signs associated with pneumonia are also common in hospitalized patients who have pulmonary edema (Chapter 45), exacerbations of chronic obstructive lung disease (Chapter 76), thromboembolic disease (Chapter 68), mucous plugging, and atelectasis (Chapter 78). As a result, clinicians should aggressively search for these alternative explanations for patients' clinical manifestations. CT scanning, especially with contrast, can help differentiate among atelectasis, pulmonary edema, pneumonitis, and pneumonic consolidation. An elevated BNP level is suggestive of heart failure.

TREATMENT

Antibiotics can generally be withheld in clinically stable patients unless and until the diagnosis is confirmed.[24] Conversely, immediate treatment is mandatory in clinically unstable patients whose oxygenation is rapidly deteriorating (Chapter 90) or who are hypotensive.

Despite the popular perception that antibiotic-resistant organisms are common in hospital-associated pneumonia, the majority of culture-positive hospital-onset bacterial pneumonias are caused by organisms susceptible to common first-line agents (see Table 85-9),[25] and antimicrobial susceptibility rates have generally been increasing in the United States.

Guidelines recommend tailoring treatment regimens to each individual patient's risk factors for potentially drug-resistant pathogens, including both individual risk factors (e.g., recent exposure to intravenous antibiotics, prior history of resistant organisms) and the local distribution and antibiotic resistance profiles of organisms associated with hospital or ventilator associated pneumonia. Initial empirical treatment (Table 85-10) typically includes an agent active against methicillin-resistant *Staphylococcus aureus* (MRSA) (e.g., linezolid or vancomycin) plus one or two agents active against *Pseudomonas aeruginosa* and other gram-negative organisms (e.g., cefepime, ceftazidime, piperacillin-tazobactam, imipenem, meropenem, imipenem-relebactam, ceftolozane-tazobactam, ceftazidime-avibactam, ciprofloxacin, levofloxacin, aztreonam, colistin, cefidorocol). Key risk factors for drug-resistant pathogens include a prior history of infection or colonization with drug-resistant organisms and a history of receiving intravenous antibiotics within the preceding 90 days. If PCR on a nasal swab or bronchoalveolar lavage is negative for MRSA, specific coverage for MRSA can be withheld in patients who do not have a history of drug-resistant organisms and in patients who are admitted to hospitals with a low prevalence of MRSA (typically <20% of *Staphylococcus aureus* isolates). In such cases, the regimen should still include coverage active against MSSA (e.g., cefazolin, ceftriaxone, cefepime, piperacillin-tazobactam, imipenem, meropenem, or levofloxacin. Similarly, one gram-negative agent may be adequate for patients who do not have risk factors for multidrug-resistant pathogens and who are receiving care in hospitals with a low prevalence of such organisms. For gram-negative nosocomial pneumonia, adding cefiderocol (2 g every 8 hours for 7 to 10 days) to linezolid (600 mg every 12 hours for at least 5 days) is as good as adding meropenem (also 2 g every 8 hours for 7 to 10 days) to linezolid.[A8]

Once the causative pathogen and its antibiotic susceptibilities have been established, the antibiotic regimen should immediately be narrowed to a single active agent so as to reduce the risk of adverse effects. Treatment is usually for 7 to 8 days. If patients fail to improve clinically after several days of therapy, additional diagnostic studies (e.g., computed tomography or bronchoalveolar lavage) are advised to identify possible causes, such as the development of pyogenic complications that require drainage or prolonged treatment (e.g., empyema [Chapter 86] or abscess [Chapter 78]), superinfection with a drug-resistant pathogen, and/or a noninfectious diagnosis (e.g., pulmonary edema, pulmonary embolism, atelectasis, pneumothorax, etc.). Serial measurement of procalcitonin values every day or every other day can help decrease treatment courses to less than 7 days in patients who are clinically improving. Antibiotics can generally be safely discontinued when the procalcitonin value drops to normal or 20% or less of its peak value.[A9]

PREVENTION

The most important step to prevent ventilator-associated pneumonia is to try to avoid tracheal intubation, whenever safe and possible, and to minimize time spent on mechanical ventilation when tracheal intubation is required. Potential strategies to avoid tracheal intubation include the use of high-flow oxygen by nasal cannula or noninvasive positive pressure ventilation (Chapters 90 and 261). Strategies to reduce exposure to mechanical ventilation include minimizing sedation by using propofol or dexmedetomidine rather than benzodiazepine, trials of spontaneous breathing (Chapter 91), and mobilization.

For nonventilated patients, bundling interventions such as oral care, having patients sit up in a chair to eat, compulsive care of feeding tubes, and patient education may decrease the use of antibiotics and the rate of hospital-acquired pneumonia (Chapter 261).[26] Prevention of hospital acquired pneumonia should also focus on preventing aspiration by elevating the head of the bed, exercising dysphagia precautions when feeding patients with impaired swallowing or impaired attention, and mobilizing patients to prevent deconditioning and delirium. Enhancing the frequency and rigor of oral care may also decrease hospital-acquired pneumonia and ventilator-associated pneumonia by decreasing the microbial burden in the mouth and in aspirated secretions. Toothbrushing twice a day is recommended. Oral care with antiseptics, by contrast, is discouraged because aspiration may lead to pneumonitis.[A10] The combination of oral and digestive decontamination with a slurry of oral antibiotics (typically a combination of an aminoglycoside, polymyxin, and amphotericin) plus a 4-day course of intravenous cefotaxime has been associated with lower mortality rates in the Netherlands but has not been widely adopted because it has not been proven to be beneficial in settings with higher baseline rates of antibiotic utilization and drug-resistant pathogens (Chapter 261).[A11] Probiotics are not helpful for prevention.[A12]

Modifications to endotracheal tubes and cuffs can reduce microbial colonization, prevent the formation of biofilm, and decrease aspiration around the cuff. Unfortunately, none of these innovations has consistently led to earlier extubation or lower mortality rates.

PROGNOSIS

Crude mortality rates for patients with ventilation-associated pneumonia and nonventilation hospital-acquired pneumonia range from 15 to 30%. Mortality rates appear to be similar regardless of whether the infection was viral, bacterial, or both. The median length-of-stay for patients who develop hospital-acquired pneumonia is 15 to 30 days compared with approximately 5 days for hospitalized patients who do not develop hospital-acquired pneumonia.

The extent to which these adverse events reflect patients' underlying conditions and baseline severity of illness as compared with incremental morbidity from pneumonia itself is uncertain, especially for ventilator-associated pneumonia. For example, some estimates suggest that eliminating ventilator-associated pneumonia would reduce overall ICU mortality by only about 2%.[27] Non–ventilator-associated hospital-acquired pneumonia, however, may increase mortality rates by two-fold or more compared with similar patients who do not develop it.

ASPIRATION PNEUMONIA

EPIDEMIOLOGY AND PATHOBIOLOGY

Although microaspiration is the most common cause of all pneumonias, gross aspiration of oropharyngeal contents is a different clinical syndrome. Predisposing factors include alcohol use disorder, poor dental hygiene, dental procedures, homelessness, drug overdose, seizures, an inadequate gag reflex, acute or chronic changes in mental status, poststroke paralysis, neuromuscular diseases, esophageal obstruction, and severe esophageal reflux. Oftentimes the pneumonia is not infectious but rather a chemical response to gastric acid or gastric contents.

CLINICAL MANIFESTATIONS

Gross aspiration pneumonia usually presents acutely[28] and then leads to progressive fever, dyspnea, purulent sputum, and leukocytosis. Hypoxemia may evolve over several days. A common complication is a lung abscess (Chapter 78), which often causes sputum with a foul taste and odor. Lung abscesses (Chapter 78), which most often results from a large volume aspiration, are typically associated with impaired consciousness.

Physical examination generally reveals evidence of the underlying precipitating condition as well as coarse rhonchi in the lower lobes or dependent lung regions.

DIAGNOSIS

Aspiration pneumonia commonly causes a parenchymal bronchopneumonia process, typically in areas of the lung that are dependent when the patient is supine: the superior segment of the right lower lobe and the posterior segment of the upper lobes.[29] However, aspiration can involve any part of the lung except the apices depending on the patient's position during aspiration. A thick-walled abscess with a fluid level (Chapter 78) can confirm the diagnosis.

TABLE 85-10 EMPIRICAL ANTIBIOTIC TREATMENT OF HOSPITAL-ACQUIRED PNEUMONIA, VENTILATOR-ASSOCIATED PNEUMONIA, AND HEALTH CARE–ASSOCIATED PNEUMONIA

GROUP A: PATIENTS WITH EITHER HOSPITAL-ACQUIRED PNEUMONIA OR VENTILATOR-ASSOCIATED PNEUMONIA, WITHOUT RISK FACTORS FOR MULTIDRUG-RESISTANT PATHOGENS, AND WITH EARLY-ONSET PNEUMONIA	
POTENTIAL PATHOGENS	**RECOMMENDED THERAPY**
Streptococcus pneumoniae *Haemophilus influenzae* Methicillin-sensitive *Staphylococcus aureus* Antibiotic-sensitive enteric gram-negative bacilli *Escherichia coli* *Klebsiella pneumoniae* *Enterobacter* spp *Proteus* spp *Serratia marcescens*	Ceftriaxone, 1-2 g IV/IM every 12-24 hr, maximum of 2 g/day* *Or* Levofloxacin, 750 mg IV every day, or ciprofloxacin, 400 mg IV every 8 hr, or moxifloxacin, 400 mg IV or orally every 24 hr* *Or* Ampicillin-sulbactam, 1.5-3 g (1-2 g ampicillin and 0.5-1 g sulbactam) IV/IM every 6 hr, maximum of 4 g/day sulbactam, depending on type and severity of infection* Ertapenem, 1 g IV/IM once a day*
GROUP B: HOSPITALIZED PATIENTS WITH LATE-ONSET PNEUMONIA OR WITH RISK FACTORS FOR MULTIDRUG-RESISTANT PATHOGENS	
ORGANISMS	**THERAPY (SELECT TWO AGENTS IF >20% OF LOCAL PSEUDOMONAS ISOLATES ARE RESISTANT TO PROPOSED MONOTHERAPY)**
S. pneumoniae *H. influenzae* Methicillin-sensitive *S. aureus* Antibiotic-sensitive enteric gram-negative bacilli *E. coli* *K. pneumoniae* *Enterobacter* spp *Proteus* spp *S. marcescens* Multidrug-resistant pathogens *Pseudomonas aeruginosa* *K. pneumoniae* (extended spectrum β-lactamase producing) *Acinetobacter* spp Methicillin-resistant *S. aureus* *Legionella pneumophila*	Antipseudomonal cephalosporin (ceftazidime, 2 g IV every 8 hr; cefepime, 1-2 g every 8-12 hr; ceftazidime/avibactam [2.5 g IV every 8 hr], ceftolozane/tazobactam [3 g IV every 8 hr]; or cefiderocol [3 g IV every 8 hr] depending on renal function)* *Or* Antipseudomonal carbapenems (meropenem, 1 g every 8 hr; imipenem, 500 mg every 6 hr or 1 g every 8 hr; or imipenem-relebactam 1.25 g every 6 hr)* *Or* β-Lactam/β-lactamase inhibitor (piperacillin-tazobactam, 4.5 g IV every 6 hr)* *Or* Antipseudomonal fluoroquinolone (levofloxacin, 750 mg IV every day, or ciprofloxacin, 400 mg IV every 8 hr).* This choice is increasingly limited by antibiotic resistance. *Plus* Vancomycin (15 mg/kg IV every 12 hr, with monitoring to maintain trough at 10-15 μg/mL and duration dependent on clinical response and individualized) or linezolid (600 mg IV every 12 hr)*

*Dosing requires modification if renal function impaired. Duration of treatment typically 7 days but should be individualized depending on the clinical response.

IM = intramuscular; IV = intravenous; spp = species.

Data from American Thoracic Society. Guidelines modified from Kalil AC, Metersky ML, Klompas M, et al. Executive summary: management of adults with hospital-acquired and ventilator-associated pneumonia: 2016 clinical practice guidelines by the Infectious Diseases Society of America and the American Thoracic Society. *Clin Infect Dis.* 2016;63:575-582. From Musher DM. Overview of pneumonia. In: Goldman L, Schafer AI, eds. *Goldman-Cecil Medicine.* 26th ed. Philadelphia: Elsevier; 2020.

Lung abscesses are polymicrobial infections that reflect oral flora and often include anaerobic bacteria.

Aspiration can cause a purely chemical pneumonia without infection that is often self-resolving but occasionally leads to ARDS. Some aspiration episodes, however, lead to a polymicrobial infection with purulent sputum and mixed bacteria. Cultures usually show normal respiratory flora, and lung abscesses typically show mouth organisms (e.g., microaerophilic streptococci and staphylococci, *Bacteroides* species, *Fusobacterium* species, and *Prevotella* species). However, aspiration in hospitalized patients and residents of long-term care facilities often involves gram-negative bacteria, *P. aeruginosa*, and *S. aureus*.

TREATMENT

Community-acquired aspiration pneumonia should be treated empirically with parenteral ampicillin-sulbactam (1.5 to 3 g intravenously every 6 hours) or clindamycin (600 mg intravenously every 8 hours) for at least 5 days. If cultures reveal organisms not sensitive to this regimen, other antibiotics should be added based on sensitivity results while continuing to provide anaerobic coverage. When the patient is stable, oral therapy (e.g., clindamycin 600 mg three times daily or ampicillin-sulbactam 750 mg three times daily) can be used to complete a 7 to 10 day course. In patients with a lung abscess (Chapter 78), however, therapy typically must be continued until the cavity is no longer detectable.

For health care–acquired aspiration pneumonia, the initial therapy should be ceftriaxone (1 to 2 g IV every 12 hours),[30] intravenous piperacillin-tazobactam (3.375 g intravenously every 6 hours), meropenem (1 g intravenously every 8 hours), or imipenem (1 g intravenously every 6 to 8 hours). If the clinical syndrome resolves within 24 hours, then antibiotics typically can be stopped. Otherwise, antibiotics should be continued for at least 5 to 7 days.

For a lung abscess, clindamycin (600 mg every 8 hours if hospitalized followed by 150 to 300 mg orally 4 times daily) typically results in improvement within 7 to 10 days. Treatment is usually continued for 3 weeks or until substantial resolution. Drainage may be necessary in 20% of cases.

Cultures are critical in patients who fail to improve rapidly so as to identify potentially resistant organisms that may require expanded or alternative treatment regimens (e.g., coverage for MRSA or *Pseudomonas*). Therapy can be modified based on microbiologic results.

The most common serious complication of anaerobic pneumonia or a lung abscess is the development of an empyema (Chapter 86). In patients with otherwise untreatable recurrent aspiration, a gastrostomy or jejunostomy feeding tube (Chapter 198) can provide palliative nutrition, fluids, and medications.

PROGNOSIS

The mortality rate for hospitalized aspiration pneumonia is 15 to 30%, including about 20% for a lung abscess. Prognosis is largely determined by precipitating underlying conditions rather than by the aspiration itself.

PNEUMONIA IN IMMUNOCOMPROMISED HOSTS

EPIDEMIOLOGY

Patients with weakened immune systems are at risk for pneumonic routine community acquired organisms, geographically restricted (e.g., coccidiomycosis and histoplasmosis [Chapter 308] organisms), and nosocomial (Chapter 261) infections. In such patients, a lower inoculum of any given organism may be sufficient to establish infection. In addition, however, immunocompromised patients are at risk for a variety of opportunistic pathogens (e.g., *Pneumocystis jiroveci* [Chapter 313], cryptococcus [Chapter 309], legionella [Chapter 290], and nocardia [Chapter 306]) and geographically restricted organisms (e.g., coccidiomycosis, talaromycosis [Chapter 308]) (Table 85-11).[31] The risk for various lower virulence organisms is a function of the overall net-state of immunosuppression, which changes based on time from immunosuppressive events, and the interval since the receipt of cancer chemotherapy, or a hematopoietic stem cell or solid organ transplant. Latent

TABLE 85-11 RESPIRATORY PATHOGENS THAT MAY CAUSE COMMUNITY-ACQUIRED PNEUMONIA IN IMMUNOCOMPROMISED HOSTS

GRAM-POSITIVE BACTERIA	GRAM-NEGATIVE BACTERIA	"ATYPICAL" BACTERIA	RESPIRATORY VIRUSES	MYCOBACTERIA	FUNGI	PARASITES
Streptococcus pneumoniae (Chapter 268) *Staphylococcus aureus* (MRSA and MSSA) (Chapter 267) *Streptococcus pyogenes* (Chapter 269) Other streptococci (Chapter 269) *Rhodococcus equi* (Chapter 272)	*Haemophilus influenzae* (Chapter 277) Nonfermenting gram-negative bacilli (e.g., *Pseudomonas* or *Acinetobacter*) (Chapter 282) *Moraxella catarrhalis* (Chapter 277) Enterobacteriaceae (e.g., *Klebsiella* spp [Chapter 281], *Escherichia coli* [Chapter 280])	*Legionella pneumophila* (Chapter 290) *Chlamydophila pneumoniae* (Chapter 294) *Mycoplasma pneumoniae* (Chapter 293) *Coxiella burnetii* (Chapter 302)	Influenza virus (Chapter 332) Parainfluenza virus (Chapter 331) Coronavirus (Chapter 334) Respiratory syncytial virus (Chapter 330) Rhinovirus (Chapter 329) Adenovirus (Chapter 333) Human metapneumovirus (Chapter 330) Cytomegalovirus (Chapter 347) Herpes simplex virus (Chapter 345) Varicella-zoster virus (Chapter 346)	*Mycobacterium tuberculosis* (Chapter 299) Nontuberculous mycobacteria (Chapter 300)	*Pneumocystis jiroveci* (Chapter 313) *Aspergillus* spp (Chapter 311) *Mucorales* spp (Chapter 312) *Histoplasma* spp (Chapter 308) *Cryptococcus* spp (Chapter 309) *Blastomyces* spp (Chapter 308) *Coccidioides* spp (Chapter 308) *Talaromycosis* spp [Chapter 308])	*Toxoplasma gondii* (Chapter 320) *Strongyloides stercoralis* (Chapter 327)

MRSA = methicillin-susceptible *Staphylococcus aureus;* MSSA = methicillin-resistant *Staphylococcus aureus;* spp = species.
Adapted from Ramirez JA, Musher DM, Evans SE, et al. Treatment of community-acquired pneumonia in immunocompromised adults: a consensus statement regarding initial strategies. *Chest.* 2020; 158:1896-1911.

organisms, which may have been previously controlled, may reactivate (e.g., *Mycobacteria tuberculosis* [Chapter 299], coccidiomycosis, and herpes group viruses [Chapters 345 to 348]), or patients may develop hyperinfection from a previous low-level infection (e.g., *Strongyloides stercoralis;* Chapter 327). In patients undergoing an organ transplant, donor-derived infection also should be considered.

PATHOBIOLOGY

The nature of the immunocompromising process or processes substantially affects the risk for pneumonia. Risk factors include impairments of T cells (e.g., advanced HIV infection; use of medications such as calcineurin inhibitors, glucocorticoids, and T cell–depleting agents), of B cells (e.g., lymphomas and medications such as anti-CD19 and 20 agents), neutrophils (e.g., chronic granulomatous disease and severe neutropenia), and of mucosal integrity (e.g., cytotoxic chemotherapy). In patients who are receiving B cell–depleting agents, such as anti-CD19 or 20 agents, the ability to form antibodies to neopathogens is significantly impaired for months after treatment, so encapsulated organisms such as pneumococcus become greater concerns.

CLINICAL MANIFESTATIONS

In immunocompromised hosts, many of the typical symptoms and signs of inflammation may be attenuated or absent (Chapter 260) and may not readily localize to the chest. For example, classic physical examination findings of pneumonia may be absent. However, cough, fever, and dyspnea are often noted and associated with hypoxemia and pulmonary infiltrates.

DIAGNOSIS

Although a chest radiograph can show abnormal pulmonary opacities, a chest CT scan is often required to detect lobar, interstitial, and nodular or cavitary abnormalities (see Fig. 85-1).[32] Lobar infiltrates often indicate bacterial infections, sometimes postobstructive in etiology. Interstitial patterns are suggestive of pneumocystis, viral, and atypical bacterial pathogens. Nodular or cavitary images are consistent with bacterial, fungal, or hematogenous processes. However, the many noninfectious conditions that can mimic pneumonia include hypersensitivity reactions, cardiogenic or non-cardiogenic pulmonary edema, medication reactions, or lung injury due to the primary underlying diagnosis.

Given the broad differential diagnosis of potential pathogens that cause pneumonia in immunocompromised patients, a specific etiologic diagnosis is critical to minimize unnecessary toxicity from empirical therapy (Fig. 85-5). Blood cultures and samples collected via fine needle aspirate, biopsy, or bronchoscopy are more likely to represent the infecting pathogens than is examination of expectorated sputum.

Multiple molecular technologies (e.g., PCR and nucleic acid testing) of nasopharyngeal swabs can aid in the identification of suspected pathogens. Serum markers (e.g., antigen testing for cryptococcus, aspergillus, and other fungi) may be helpful to avoid more invasive diagnostic testing. Serology is of very limited value because many immunocompromised patients may have a limited ability to generate antibody responses.

TREATMENT

Treatment requires not only the correct antimicrobial agent for the infecting organism but also, if possible, efforts to improve the host's immunity by lowering the dose of any immunosuppressive agents. In patients who are seriously ill or at risk of rapid deterioration, prompt antibiotic therapy targeting the likely infecting pathogen(s), if known, are warranted. However, antibiotic therapy typically must be initiated as an urgent diagnostic evaluation is begun.[33] When no obvious pathogen is evident, the radiographic pattern and the nature of the host's immunodeficiency will further inform the diagnostic evaluation and empirical therapy. For an interstitial pattern, broad-spectrum antibacterial agents (e.g., a carbapenem or respiratory fluoroquinolone) are recommended, along with consideration of treatment for *Pneumocystis jiroveci* (Chapter 313). For a nodular or cavitary process, broad-spectrum antibacterial agents are recommended, with consideration for nocardia (Chapter 306), and antifungal treatment (Chapter 307).

In appropriate circumstances, other bacteria (e.g., mycobacteria), parasites (e.g., *Toxoplasma, Strongyloides*), and fungal pathogens (e.g., *Cryptococcus, Aspergillus,* and *Mucorales* sp.) must be considered. For certain infections, such as severe *Pneumocystis jiroveci* pneumonia with hypoxemia, adjunctive glucocorticoids may be warranted. As soon as the infecting organism is identified, antibiotics should be narrowed to reduce the risk of adverse effects, or the acquisition of antimicrobial-resistant organisms.

PREVENTION

Principles of prevention include minimizing exposure to pathogens of concern, augmenting immunity, and pharmacologic prophylaxis. Immunosuppressive treatments should be limited to the lowest dose for the shortest duration possible. Vaccinations (Chapter 15) to measles, *Streptococcus pneumoniae*, SARS-CoV-2, and influenza should be updated before the initiation of immunosuppression or at a time when immunosuppression is the lowest to allow the strongest possible immune response.

Antimicrobials should be used to prevent infections associated with immunosuppression. Effective prophylaxis against *Pneumocystis jiroveci* includes trimethoprim-sulfamethoxazole (either a single-strength tablet once a day or a double-strength tablet 3 times a week), atovaquone (1500 mg orally once daily), pentamidine (aerosolized or intravenous), and dapsone (100 mg orally once daily). Of these regimens trimethoprim-sulfamethoxazole, is the most efficacious and preferred. Prophylaxis should be continued until immunosuppression is decreased, such as lowering the prednisone dose to less than 20 mg per day. When possible, treatment for latent tuberculosis (e.g., isoniazid) is warranted in patients with prior exposure to tuberculosis before initiating immunosuppression when possible (Chapter 299). In patients who have potential exposure to geographically

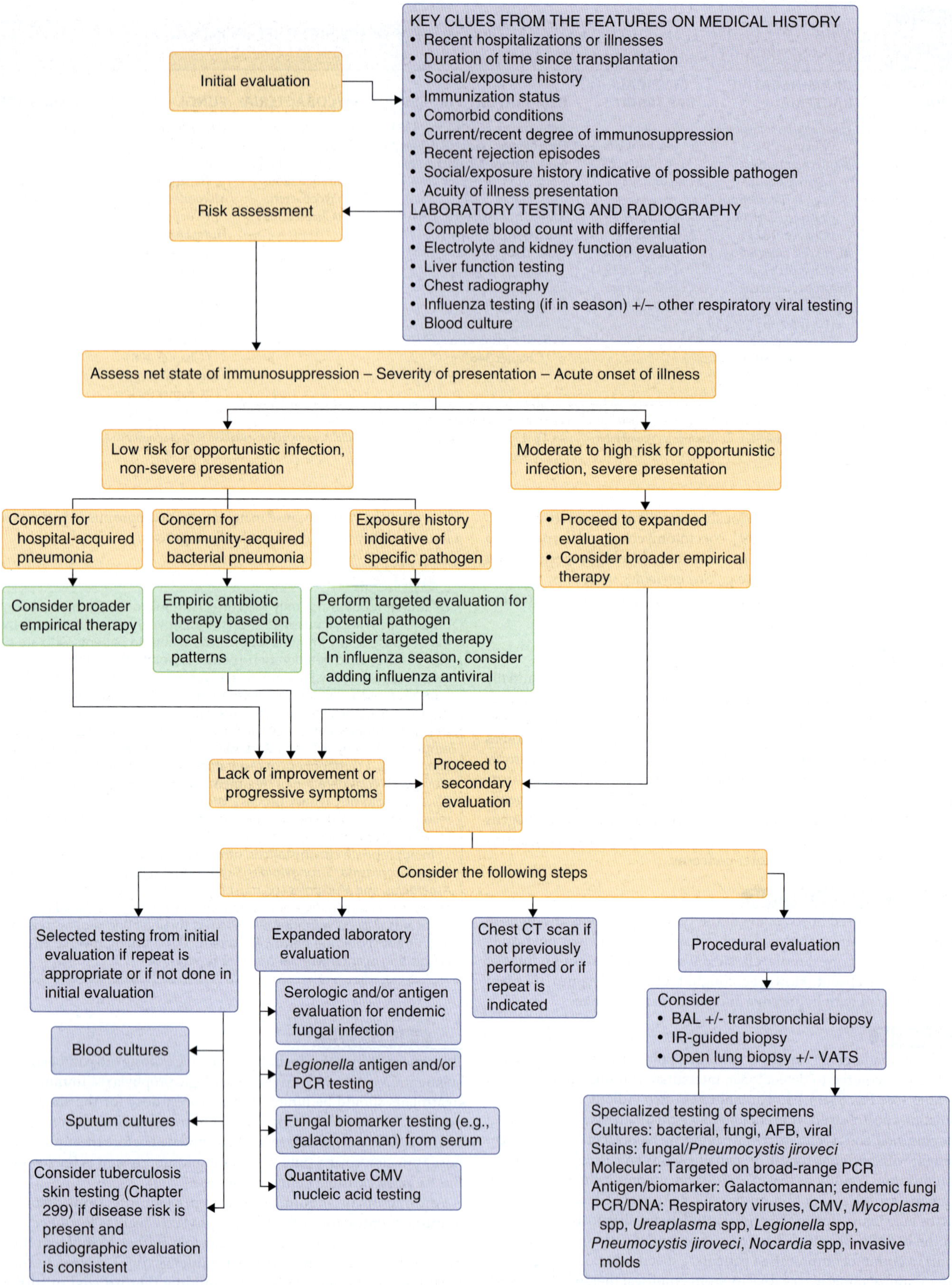

FIGURE 85-5. Evaluation of pneumonia in the immunocompromised host. AFB = acid fast bacillus; BAL = bronchoalveolar lavage; CMV = cytomegalovirus; CT = computed tomography; IR = interventional radiology; PCR = polymerase chain reaction; spp = species; VATS = video-assisted thoracic surgery. (Adapted from Dulek DE, Mueller NJ; AST Infectious Diseases Community of Practice. Pneumonia in solid organ transplantation: guidelines from the American Society of Transplantation Infectious Diseases Community of Practice. *Clin Transplant*. 2019;33:e13545.)

restricted organisms, consideration for the assessment of their presence and secondary prophylaxis is warranted (e.g., ivermectin for strongyloides [Chapter 327], fluconazole for *Coccidioides immitis* or *Coccidioides posadasii* [Chapter 308]).

PROGNOSIS

The response to treatment depends on diagnosing the etiologic pathogen as early as possible, before more serious complications develop. With targeted antimicrobial therapy, drug-drug interactions and significant perturbations in healthy microbial flora can be minimized.

GENERAL REFERENCES

For the General References and other additional features, please visit Elsevier eBooks+ at https://ebooks.health.elsevier.com.

Grade A References

A1. Choi S-H, Cesar A, Snow TAC, et al. Efficacy of doxycycline for mild-to-moderate community-acquired pneumonia in adults: a systematic review and meta-analysis of randomized controlled trials. *Clin Infect Dis.* 2022;76:683-691.

A2. Montes-Andujar L, Tinoco E, Baez-Pravia O, et al. Empiric antibiotics for community-acquired pneumonia in adult patients: a systematic review and a network meta-analysis. *Thorax.* 2021;76:1020-1031.

A3. Dinh A, Ropers J, Duran C, et al. Discontinuing β-lactam treatment after 3 days for patients with community-acquired pneumonia in non-critical care wards (PTC): a double-blind, randomised, placebo-controlled, non-inferiority trial. *Lancet.* 2021;397:1195-1203.

A4. Torres A, Garrity-Ryan L, Kirsch C, et al. Omadacycline vs moxifloxacin in adults with community-acquired bacterial pneumonia. *Int J Infect Dis.* 2021;104:501-509.

A5. File TM, Goldberg L, Das A, et al. Efficacy and safety of intravenous-to-oral lefamulin, a pleuromutilin antibiotic, for the treatment of community-acquired bacterial pneumonia: the phase III lefamulin evaluation against pneumonia (LEAP 1) trial. *Clin Infect Dis.* 2019;69:1856-1867.

A6. Alexander E, Goldberg L, Das AF, et al. Oral lefamulin vs moxifloxacin for early clinical response among adults with community-acquired bacterial pneumonia: the LEAP 2 randomized clinical trial. *JAMA.* 2019;322:1661-1671.

A7. Dequin PF, Meziani F, Quenot JP, et al. Hydrocortisone in severe community-acquired pneumonia. *N Engl J Med.* 2023. [Epub ahead of print.]

A8. Wunderink RG, Matsunaga Y, Ariyasu M, et al. Cefiderocol versus high-dose, extended-infusion meropenem for the treatment of gram-negative nosocomial pneumonia (APEKS-NP): a randomised, double-blind, phase 3, non-inferiority trial. *Lancet Infect Dis.* 2021;21:213-225.

A9. de Jong E, van Oers JA, Beishuizen A, et al. Efficacy and safety of procalcitonin guidance in reducing the duration of antibiotic treatment in critically ill patients: a randomised, controlled, open-label trial. *Lancet Infect Dis.* 2016;16:819-827.

A10. Dale CM, Rose L, Carbone S, et al. Effect of oral chlorhexidine de-adoption and implementation of an oral care bundle on mortality for mechanically ventilated patients in the intensive care unit (CHORAL): a multi-center stepped wedge cluster-randomized controlled trial. *Intensive Care Med.* 2021;47:1295-1302.

A11. Wittekamp BH, Plantinga NL, Cooper BS, et al. Decontamination strategies and bloodstream infections with antibiotic-resistant microorganisms in ventilated patients: a randomized clinical trial. *JAMA.* 2018;320:2087-2098.

A12. Johnstone J, Meade M, Lauzier F, et al. Effect of probiotics on incident ventilator-associated pneumonia in critically ill patients: a randomized clinical trial. *JAMA.* 2021;326:1024-1033.

86

DISEASES OF THE DIAPHRAGM, CHEST WALL, PLEURA, AND MEDIASTINUM

F. DENNIS MCCOOL

DIAPHRAGM

The diaphragm is the major muscle of ventilation. It is a dome-shaped structure that separates the thorax from the abdomen. It consists of a central tendon and a muscular component that inserts into the rib cage laterally along the inner surface of the lower six ribs, anteromedially along the costal cartilages, and posteriorly along the upper three lumbar vertebral bodies. The diaphragm is innervated by the phrenic nerve, which originates from cervical nerve roots 3 through 5.

DIAPHRAGMATIC WEAKNESS AND PARALYSIS

EPIDEMIOLOGY AND PATHOBIOLOGY

When activated, the diaphragm contracts and descends caudally. The downward descent of the diaphragm expands the anterior abdominal wall and lower rib cage, lowers pleural pressure, and thereby promotes lung inflation. It is the major muscle of inspiration, and its action accounts for approximately 70% of the inspired tidal volume in the normal individual. Diaphragm function can be impaired by disorders that affect the brain (Chapter 368), spinal cord, and peripheral nerves (Chapter 388), neuromuscular junction (Chapter 390), and muscle itself (Chapter 389). The incidence and prevalence of diaphragmatic paralysis and weakness are unknown.

CLINICAL MANIFESTATIONS

Diaphragmatic weakness or paralysis can involve either one or both hemidiaphragms.[1] With unilateral diaphragmatic paralysis, patients are generally asymptomatic at rest but may have dyspnea with exertion or when supine, especially with comorbid conditions such as obesity. If they are asymptomatic, the abnormality may be discovered as an incidental finding of an elevated hemidiaphragm on chest radiography.

Bilateral diaphragmatic paralysis is less common than unilateral paralysis. The disability with bilateral paralysis is more dramatic than with unilateral paralysis, and orthopnea is an especially prominent symptom.[2] Other symptoms include dyspnea with exertion or when bending and lifting objects. These individuals also are at an increased risk of hypoventilation during sleep, especially during rapid eye movement (REM) sleep. Occasionally patients may present with symptoms related to nocturnal hypoventilation, including frequent nocturnal awakenings, nocturia, vivid nightmares, night sweats, daytime hypersomnolence, depression, and morning headaches.

The physical examination is remarkable for use of accessory muscles of inspiration and paradoxical inward motion of the abdominal wall during inspiration, particularly in patients with bilateral diaphragmatic paralysis. This finding is especially noticeable when these individuals are supine. Chest wall percussion during inspiration and expiration can detect the absence of diaphragmatic movement.

DIAGNOSIS

Disorders that can cause unilateral diaphragmatic weakness or paralysis (Table 86-1) include traumatic phrenic nerve injury, neuropathies such as neuralgic amyotrophy (Chapter 388), herpes zoster (Chapter 346), cervical spinal

TABLE 86-1 CAUSES OF DIAPHRAGMATIC WEAKNESS AND PARALYSIS

TRAUMA
Cardiac surgery with cold cardioplegia
Blunt trauma
Spinal cord injury
Cervical manipulation
Scalene and brachial nerve block
TUMOR COMPRESSION
Lung cancer
Metastatic mediastinal tumor
METABOLIC
Diabetes
Vitamin deficiency (B_6, B_{12}, folate)
Hypothyroidism
Acid maltase deficiency
INFLAMMATORY NEURITIS
Neuralgic amyotrophy (Parsonage-Turner syndrome)
Mononeuritis multiplex
Vasculitis
Paraneoplastic
MUSCULAR DYSTROPHIES
Limb-girdle
Duchenne and Becker
MISCELLANEOUS
Amyloidosis
Malnutrition
Radiation injury
Cervical spondylosis
Poliomyelitis
Amyotrophic lateral sclerosis
IDIOPATHIC

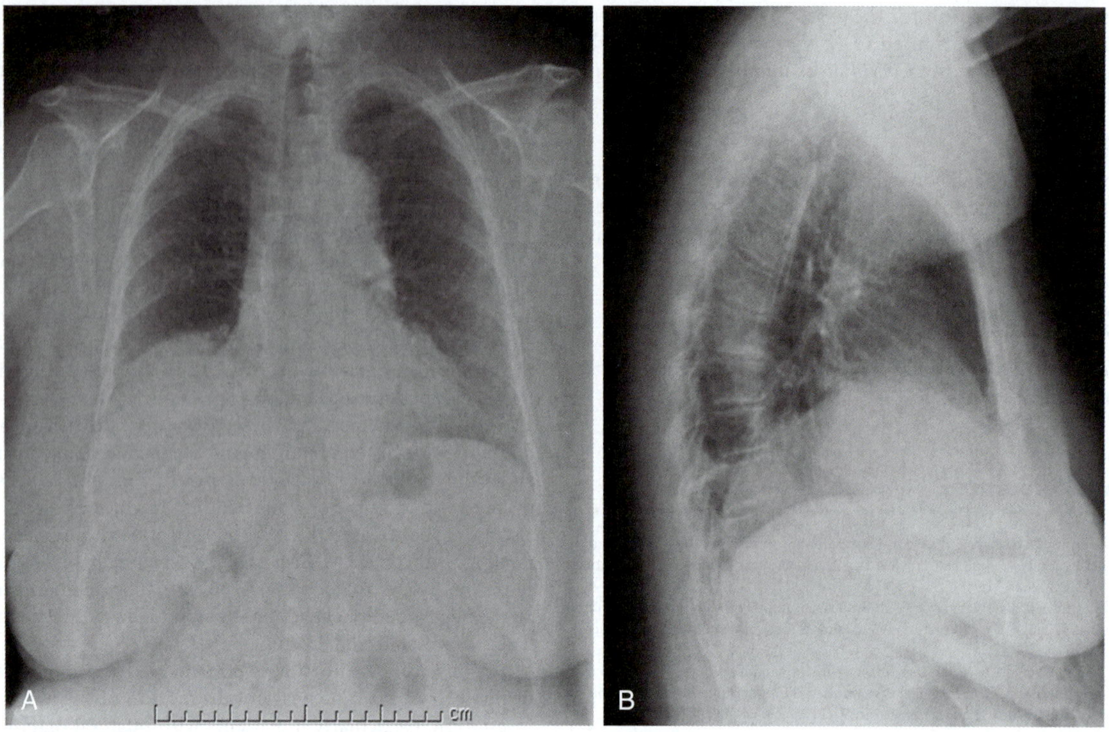

FIGURE 86-1. **Paralysis of the right hemidiaphragm.** Patient with paralysis of the right hemidiaphragm as seen on the posteroanterior radiograph of the chest (**A**) and lateral radiograph of the chest (**B**).

disease (Chapter 369), compressive tumors, and phrenic nerve injury related to cardiac or thoracic surgery or prolonged mechanical ventilation. Neuralgic amyotrophy has been linked to the *SEPT9* gene and may occasionally be an extrahepatic manifestation of hepatitis E (Chapter 135). Diagnosis of diaphragmatic dysfunction is often suggested by elevation of a hemidiaphragm on a chest radiograph (Fig. 86-1). The diagnosis of unilateral paralysis can be confirmed by performing a "sniff test" using fluoroscopy or ultrasound, in which paradoxical (cephalad) movement of the hemidiaphragmatic dome occurs during a sniff maneuver.

Bilateral diaphragmatic paralysis is more difficult to diagnose than unilateral paralysis. Chest radiography typically shows elevation of both hemidiaphragms. This finding may be interpreted as a "poor inspiratory effort" or "low lung volumes." Routine pulmonary function testing (Chapter 73) is nonspecific; it typically demonstrates moderate to severe restriction, with both the vital capacity and total lung capacity reduced to 30 to 60% of predicted. A more specific test for diaphragmatic paralysis is the measurement of supine vital capacity. A decline of 20% or greater when supine is consistent with diaphragmatic paralysis. Maximal static inspiratory pressure measured at the airway opening (PI_{max}) is reduced to 20 to 30% of predicted in individuals with bilateral diaphragmatic paralysis, but maximal static expiratory pressure may be preserved in individuals with isolated diaphragm paralysis.[3]

The diagnosis of unilateral or bilateral diaphragmatic paralysis can be confirmed using ultrasound. Absence of diaphragmatic thickening during inspiration indicates paralysis. A more invasive test is the measurement of transdiaphragmatic pressure (the pressure difference between the thoracic and abdominal cavity), which requires the patient to swallow a balloon for manometry. With diaphragmatic paralysis, there is no increase in transdiaphragmatic pressure during inspiration. Diaphragm electromyography and phrenic nerve conduction studies may be useful to distinguish neuropathy or myopathy. If the diagnosis of bilateral diaphragmatic paralysis is confirmed, the patient should be evaluated for nocturnal hypoventilation (Chapter 374). Computed tomography (CT) of the chest may be needed to exclude a mediastinal mass, and magnetic resonance imaging (MRI) of the neck may be necessary to evaluate the spinal cord and nerve roots (E-Fig. 86-1).

TREATMENT AND PROGNOSIS

Bilateral diaphragmatic paralysis may not be reversible unless the underlying cause is treatable. For example, myopathies (Chapter 389) related to metabolic disturbances may be improved by correcting electrolyte imbalances or replacing thyroid hormone. Toxic or metabolic disturbances related to diabetes, alcohol, or viral infections may resolve with treatment of the underlying disease. Idiopathic diaphragmatic paralysis or paralysis due to neuralgic amyotrophy may spontaneously improve or resolve completely in approximately 60% of individuals, but recovery can take 18 months to 3 years. Phrenic nerve damage related to cardiac surgery usually resolves spontaneously but may persist if the phrenic nerve is transected. For a high spinal cord injury, in which the phrenic nerve roots remain intact (injury above C3), phrenic nerve pacing can provide ventilation.

Noninvasive positive-pressure ventilation (NPPV) is the preferred method of treatment for patients with diaphragmatic paralysis because it can improve both symptoms and physiologic derangements related to nocturnal hypoventilation (E-Table 86-1 and Chapter 374). NPPV also may reverse the brain's adaptation to high levels of CO_2 by "resetting" chemoreceptors in the medulla toward normal. When patients with unilateral paralysis have severe symptoms, surgical plication of the paralyzed hemidiaphragm may improve vital capacity, but this intervention has no role in bilateral diaphragmatic paralysis. Phrenic nerve reconstruction is a promising treatment that has been associated with symptomatic relief and improved respiratory function at 1- to 2-year follow-up.[4]

MISCELLANEOUS DIAPHRAGMATIC DISORDERS

Diaphragmatic eventration results from localized atrophy of the diaphragm muscle or from part of the diaphragm being replaced with fibroelastic tissue. Eventration most often results in an elevation of the right anteromedial portion of the diaphragm. Metastatic tumors to the diaphragm usually are related to direct extension of lung cancer. Primary tumors of the diaphragm are very rare. Lipomas are the most common benign tumor, and fibrosarcomas are the most common malignant neoplasm.

CHEST WALL

The chest wall is a key component of the "inspiratory pump" and allows for maintenance of normal alveolar ventilation. It consists of the bony structures of the rib cage, the articulations between the ribs and the vertebrae, the diaphragm, intercostal muscles, and abdomen. Disorders that affect any of the components of the chest wall can impair breathing.

KYPHOSCOLIOSIS

EPIDEMIOLOGY AND PATHOBIOLOGY

Kyphoscoliosis is a common spinal disorder that affects approximately 1 in 1000 individuals, about 1 in 10,000 of whom has a severe spinal deformity. Deformities include excessive spinal curvature in the coronal (scoliosis) and sagittal (kyphosis) planes as well as rotation of the spinal axis. The most common form is idiopathic, but kyphoscoliosis also can be caused by congenital vertebral malformations or be secondary to neuromuscular disorders

(Chapter 390). Adult degenerative scoliosis is an increasing affliction as the population ages.[5]

A familial predilection may be related to the chromatin-remodeling gene family *(CHD7)*. Kyphoscoliosis typically becomes more prominent in late childhood or early adolescence, with a female-to-male ratio of 4 : 1.

CLINICAL MANIFESTATIONS

Kyphoscoliosis may be classified as mild, moderate, or severe based on the angle of spinal deformity. In younger individuals with milder spinal deformities, the physical findings may be subtle. Individuals with mild to moderate kyphoscoliosis may have complaints of back pain and have psychosocial problems related to the spinal deformity. Adolescents with mild idiopathic kyphoscoliosis usually have normal exercise capacity, whereas those with moderate idiopathic kyphoscoliosis have reduced exercise capacity with additional exercise limitations owing to deconditioning. With severe deformities, patients may experience dyspnea with minimal exertion or at rest.

Typical findings of severe kyphoscoliosis are the dorsal hump, which is due to the angulated ribs and shoulder asymmetry and the presence of tilted hips. With severe kyphoscoliosis, signs of right heart failure (Chapter 45) may be present.

DIAGNOSIS

Severe kyphoscoliosis can be readily diagnosed on physical examination, whereas mild or moderate degrees of kyphoscoliosis may be noted only on chest radiographs. The Adams forward bend test, in which the examiner observes for thoracic or lumbar region asymmetry while the patient bends forward at the waist until the spine becomes parallel to the floor, can help detect minor deformities. The degree of spinal deformity should be calculated based on the angle of spinal curvature (the Cobb angle) from radiographs (E-Fig. 86-2). Angles more than 100 degrees are severe and are usually associated with respiratory symptoms such as dyspnea.

Kyphoscoliosis reduces the internal volume and mobility of the rib cage, thereby producing a restrictive respiratory impairment, with total lung capacity and vital capacity reduced to as low as 30% of predicted values. As the degree of spinal angulation increases, the degree of restriction worsens. The patient's age, sex, degree of spinal rotation, presence of respiratory muscle weakness, and involvement of the thoracic vertebrae are all factors that promote the restrictive process.

TREATMENT

Patients should be encouraged to remain physically active to improve quality of life.[A1] In addition, general supportive measures, including immunizations against influenza and pneumococci (Chapter 15), smoking cessation (Chapter 363), maintenance of a normal body weight (Chapter 201), and treatment of respiratory infections in a timely fashion should be instituted. Patients with severe kyphoscoliosis and Cobb angles of more than 100 degrees should be monitored closely for respiratory complications and nocturnal hypoventilation.

Because sleep-related abnormalities and their effects on cardiorespiratory function are potentially treatable, individuals with kyphoscoliosis should be evaluated for nocturnal hypoventilation (Chapter 374), which typically precedes findings of daytime hypercapnia and hypoxemia. Indications for instituting NPPV include symptoms of nocturnal hypoventilation or signs of cor pulmonale (Chapter 45), with either an elevated daytime $Paco_2$ (≥45 mm Hg) or nocturnal oxygen saturation of 88% or less for 5 consecutive minutes while breathing ambient air. Supplemental oxygen is needed if hypoxemia persists despite correction of hypoventilation. NPPV can reduce the number and duration of hospitalizations and improve gas exchange, daytime blood gases, quality of life, and survival (see E-Table 86-1).

Surgical and nonsurgical (back-brace) treatments are useful in growing children and adolescents with Cobb angles between 25 and 40 degrees,[6] whereas surgery has been used for adolescents with a Cobb angle of more than 45 degrees. Although screening radiographs can detect otherwise asymptomatic scoliosis, there is no evidence to support screening for scoliosis in adults.[7]

PROGNOSIS

Individuals with mild kyphoscoliosis have an overall benign course. Patients with moderate or severe deformities are at higher risk for developing respiratory complications. Cobb angles more than 120 degrees can be associated with respiratory failure. Factors associated with progression of the spinal deformity include inspiratory muscle weakness, a large spinal curvature at the time of presentation, skeletal immaturity, and a thoracic location of the curve apex. For a given degree of spinal deformity, individuals with inspiratory muscle weakness and kyphoscoliosis are more prone to develop respiratory failure than those with kyphoscoliosis and normal inspiratory muscle strength. Treatment with NPPV improves prognosis compared to treatment with oxygen alone.

In secondary kyphoscoliosis, early age of onset, rapid curve progression during growth, progression of scoliosis after skeletal maturity, large curves at the time of presentation, and a thoracic rather than a thoracolumbar or lumbar location of the curve apex are risk factors for respiratory complications. When cor pulmonale develops (Chapter 45), the prognosis is poor, and death may occur within 1 year without therapy.

PECTUS EXCAVATUM

EPIDEMIOLOGY AND PATHOBIOLOGY

Pectus excavatum (funnel chest) is a common congenital chest wall deformity that occurs in approximately 0.5 to 2% of the population. It is characterized by excessive depression of the sternum and its adjacent costal cartilages. It affects males more than females (4 : 1), and a family history is common.

CLINICAL MANIFESTATIONS AND DIAGNOSIS

Cosmetic concerns are the usual reason for seeking medical attention. Pectus excavatum typically produces minimal respiratory impairment, and it is occasionally associated with mild reductions in vital capacity and total lung capacity. Individuals with the most severe pectus deformities may exhibit a mild reduction in maximal exercise capacity. On physical examination, sternal depression is readily apparent. Rib cage excursion is normal during inspiration. A mild degree of scoliosis may be present in 40 to 60% of individuals.

Pectus excavatum is readily diagnosed by inspecting the rib cage. On the chest radiograph, the anteroposterior diameter is reduced (Fig. 86-2). The severity of the deformity is best assessed with a chest CT. A transverse-to-anteroposterior diameter ratio greater than 3.5 signifies a significant pectus deformity.

TREATMENT AND PROGNOSIS

Surgical correction of the deformity is considered for patients with a transverse to anteroposterior rib cage ratio of more than 3.0 to 3.5 in conjunction with symptoms of dyspnea or laboratory evidence of cardiac or pulmonary restriction. However, there is no convincing evidence that correction of the deformity improves either cardiopulmonary function or exercise capacity. Minimally invasive approaches use rods to force the sternum outward gradually. The overall prognosis is excellent in individuals who have mild deformities and in patients whose more severe deformities have been corrected. A multidisciplinary team composed of thoracic surgeons, radiologists, and cardiologists can provide recommendations for surgery by not only assessing the severity of chest wall deformity by CT scan but also by assessing echocardiographic findings such as interventricular dependence, compression of the tricuspid annulus, and exercise-related systolic and diastolic function.[8] The risk of complications is similar following either open or minimally invasive repair of the pectus excavatum.[9]

FLAIL CHEST

EPIDEMIOLOGY AND PATHOBIOLOGY

Flail chest occurs following chest trauma (Chapter 97) in which there have been either double fractures of three or more contiguous ribs or combined sternal and rib fractures. The result is an unstable segment of the chest wall, which moves paradoxically inward with inspiration and outward with expiration. In adults, flail chest is most commonly a consequence of blunt chest wall trauma owing to automobile accidents or falls. Pulmonary contusion may be present and contribute to hypoxemia.

CLINICAL MANIFESTATIONS

The vital capacity may be acutely reduced by 50% or more. Flail-related changes in respiratory muscle function can lead to acute respiratory failure (E-Fig. 86-3). The causes are an increase in the work of breathing (owing to excessive diaphragmatic shortening) in concert with reduced oxygen supply to the diaphragm (owing to pulmonary contusion or hypoventilation) and impaired cough (owing to pain associated with the rib fractures as well as paradoxical motion of the flail segment). Appropriate diagnostic studies should be undertaken to determine if the patient has a concomitant pneumothorax or hemothorax.

DIAGNOSIS

Bedside inspection looking for paradoxical motion of the flail segment is key to the diagnosis. Gentle palpation of the rib cage and abdomen may reveal the characteristic paradoxical movement of the flail segment. Chest radiographs will confirm the presence of multiple rib fractures, but a three-dimensional reconstruction of a thoracic CT can provide better visualization of thoracic injuries, including lung contusion. The diagnosis may be less apparent in a sedated mechanically ventilated patient, in whom paradoxical motion of a segment of the rib cage may not occur because the positive alveolar and pleural pressures act as a "pneumatic splint" and allow for uniform inflation of the chest wall.

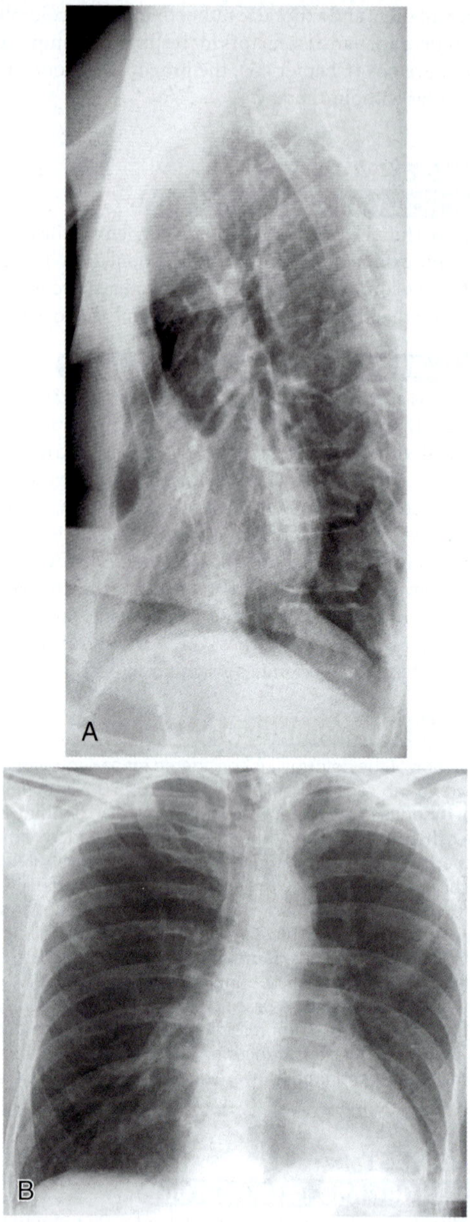

FIGURE 86-2. Pectus excavatum deformity. A, Chest lateral radiograph. The pectus excavatum deformity is marked by dorsal displacement of the cardiac structures and a narrow anterior-posterior diameter of the chest measuring less than 8 cm from the posterior cortex of the sternal body to the anterior cortex of the lower thoracic vertebrae. B, Chest frontal radiograph. The right heart border is obscured, mimicking right middle lobe disease. The cardiac silhouette is slightly rotated and shifted into the left hemithorax. (Courtesy of Paul Stark, MD.)

TREATMENT

Nonsurgical management of flail chest consists of adequate analgesia, clearance of bronchial secretions, and mechanical ventilatory assistance if needed. Pain relief (Chapter 26), which is crucial for averting atelectasis and achieving an effective cough, can be accomplished by oral medications (Table 26-4), patient-controlled analgesic pumps, intercostal nerve blocks, or epidural anesthesia. NPPV delivered by a nasal or face mask to patients who are spontaneously breathing improves gas exchange, can stabilize the flail segment, and may allow for early mobilization and access to physical therapy. If respiratory failure ensues despite NPPV, intubation and positive-pressure ventilation will stabilize the flail segment and enhance gas exchange. Surgical fixation of the flail segment may be needed for patients who are unable to wean from mechanical ventilation, patients with significant chest wall deformities, and patients who are undergoing thoracotomy for concomitant injuries. Surgical stabilization of flail chest may reduce the incidence of pneumonia as well as length-of-stay in the intensive care unit and hospital. Surgical stabilization of non-flail rib fractures reduces the need for narcotic medications to control pain but does not have other proven benefits.[A2]

PROGNOSIS

A flail chest is a marker of increased mortality, both in patients with isolated chest wall trauma and in patients with multiple sites of trauma, with an overall mortality ranging from 7 to 16%. Mortality from rib fractures increases after age 45 years, and 60% of patients over age 60 years who die from chest trauma have at least one rib fracture. Patients who have flail chest without a concomitant lung contusion may have restrictive impairment that typically resolves, with the vital capacity returning to baseline values within 6 months. By contrast, patients who have both flail chest and a concomitant lung contusion often have impairment of pulmonary function that may persist for up to 4 years after injury. If concomitant lung contusion and flail chest are present, the mortality rate increases further and may be as high as 70%, in part due to the coexistence of other injuries.

ANKYLOSING SPONDYLITIS

EPIDEMIOLOGY AND PATHOBIOLOGY

Ankylosing spondylitis (Chapter 244) is a chronic progressive inflammatory disease that involves the ligamentous structures of the spine, sacroiliac, and large peripheral joints. It affects men more than women, with the most common age of onset between 15 and 25 years. There is a genetic predisposition, with the HLA-B27 antigen present in 95% of Whites with ankylosing spondylitis. Chronic inflammation of the spine and peripheral joints may cause fibrosis and ossification of structures adjacent to the spine. Fusion of the costovertebral and sternoclavicular joints produces relative fixation of the rib cage in an inspiratory position. This limited motion may produce mild restrictive respiratory impairment with the degree of restriction proportional to disease duration and activity, as well as to the degree of spinal and rib cage immobility. Concomitant kyphosis, which may occur in advanced disease or be secondary to osteoporosis, will further impair respiratory function. Because the rib cage is less distensible, the diaphragm shortens to a greater degree for a given tidal volume, thereby increasing the work performed by the diaphragm. Intercostal muscle atrophy secondary to decreased rib cage mobility may cause inspiratory muscle weakness.

Fibrobullous upper lobe disease, which is one of the extra-articular manifestations of ankylosing spondylitis (Chapter 244), occurs in roughly 1 to 4% of patients. The cause of this apical disease is unknown, but its presence may impair gas exchange. Occasionally, individuals with ankylosing spondylitis develop nonapical interstitial lung disease (Chapter 80). When these complications occur, lung compliance, which otherwise is usually normal despite a pronounced reduction in rib cage mobility, may be reduced.

CLINICAL MANIFESTATIONS AND DIAGNOSIS

Ankylosing spondylitis is diagnosed when there is a history of low back pain and stiffness for more than 3 months, limited chest wall expansion (<2.5 cm at the fourth intercostal space), limited lumbar spine motion in the sagittal and frontal planes, and radiographic evidence of sacroiliitis. Radiographic findings include calcifications and ossifications of the vertebrae and paravertebral tissues. Low back pain and spinal stiffness are the most common presenting symptoms. Dyspnea may be present as the disease progresses and chest wall expansion becomes more restricted. Physical examination may reveal loss of lateral flexion of the lumbar spine, tenderness over the sacroiliac joints, and kyphosis. Respiratory function may be further impaired and kyphosis worsened by fractures involving the rigid spine. Endotracheal intubation should be performed with caution because hyperextension of a rigid cervical spine may lead to fracture because of frequent involvement of the cricoarytenoid joint.

TREATMENT AND PROGNOSIS

Exercise and physiotherapy programs can enhance cardiorespiratory fitness and spinal mobility.[A3] When ankylosing spondylitis is treated with nonsteroidal anti-inflammatory agents and biologic agents, such as tumor necrosis factor antagonists (Chapter 29), rib cage expansion can also improve. A high index of suspicion for possible reactivation of latent tuberculosis is required for patients treated with anti–tumor necrosis factor-α (anti-TNF-α) agents. Corticosteroids do not prevent the progression of fibrobullous disease, which can be complicated by major hemoptysis. Thoracic surgery may be indicated for hemoptysis, but surgical intervention carries major risk, with 50 to 60% of patients developing bronchopleural fistulas. Ankylosing spondylitis rarely leads to pulmonary disability unless individuals develop fibrobullous disease.

OBESITY

Obesity (Chapter 201) can be accompanied by changes in pulmonary function or alterations in respiratory control. Obesity characteristically reduces functional reserve capacity and expiratory reserve volume. Total lung capacity and vital capacity may be normal or only mildly reduced, except in the most severe cases. Obesity-hypoventilation is characterized by alterations in respiratory control, thereby resulting in elevated levels of $Paco_2$ (Chapter 74).

Dyspnea and exercise intolerance, which are the most frequent respiratory complaints of obese individuals, may be related to disordered chest wall mechanics, altered respiratory control, or the presence of inflammatory mediators, such as those linking obesity to airway hyper-responsiveness. The increase in intra-abdominal pressure when supine will further reduce functional residual capacity, impair lung emptying, increase auto–positive end-expiratory pressure, and contribute to orthopnea. The worsening of respiratory mechanics in the supine position must be considered when evaluating the risk for general anesthesia in obese patients. Weight loss (Chapter 201) is the optimal therapy, and it improves lung volumes, respiratory muscle performance, gas exchange, dyspnea, and sleep apnea.[10] In individuals with obesity-hypoventilation syndrome (Chapter 74), NPPV can reverse abnormalities in gas exchange.

PLEURA

The pleura is a thin membrane that covers the inner surfaces of the thoracic cavity. It consists of a layer of mesothelial cells supported by a network of connective and fibroelastic tissue. The visceral pleura lines the lung, whereas the parietal pleura lines the rib cage, diaphragm, and mediastinal structures. The closed space between the visceral and parietal pleura is referred to as the pleural space. The vascular supply of the parietal pleural surface is from the systemic circulation, and it contains sensory nerves and lymphatics. By contrast, the visceral pleura is supplied with blood vessels from the pulmonary circulation and has no sensory nerves.

PLEURAL EFFUSION

EPIDEMIOLOGY AND PATHOBIOLOGY

The overall frequency of pleural effusion on a chest radiograph ranges from 0.3 to 1% but varies widely depending on the underlying disease. Pleural effusions can be caused by a vast number of disease processes and are most frequently seen in patients with pneumonia (Chapter 85) and heart failure (Chapter 45).[11]

Normally, a small amount of fluid in the pleural space forms a thin layer between the visceral and parietal pleural surfaces and acts as a lubricant to minimize friction between the chest wall and lung as they move against each other during inspiration and expiration. There is continual movement of fluid into and out of the pleural space. This flux of fluid depends on the oncotic and hydrostatic pressures within the parietal and visceral pleura as well as the pressure within the pleural space itself. Hydrostatic pressure in the parietal pleura is similar to systemic circulation (30 cm H_2O), whereas that of the visceral pleura is similar to the pulmonary circulation (10 cm H_2O). Accordingly, most fluid in the pleural space is filtered from the higher pressure vascular structures in the parietal pleura. Because the pressure within the pleural space itself is more subatmospheric at the apex than at the base, most of the fluid filters in from the upper lung zones. Fluid is drained out primarily through lymphatic stomas on the surface of the parietal pleura. The normal turnover of fluid within the pleural space is 10 to 20 mL/day, with only 0.2 to 1 mL remaining in the pleural space. Excess fluid can accumulate in the pleural space because of decreased removal (owing to obstruction of pleural lymphatics) or increased production (owing to an increase in hydrostatic pressure, a decrease in oncotic pressure, decreased pressure in the pleural space, or increased pleural membrane permeability; Table 86-2).

An increase in hydrostatic pressure or decrease in oncotic pressure will result in a low-protein collection of pleural fluid characterized as *transudates* (Table 86-3). Heart failure (Chapter 45) can produce transudates by increasing hydrostatic pressure in the pulmonary venous system, atelectasis (Chapter 78) can promote transudates by making pleural pressure more subatmospheric, and occasionally, oncotic pressure may be sufficiently reduced to cause transudates (e.g., with hypoalbuminemia). Changes in pleural membrane permeability can produce high-protein effusions, which are characterized as *exudates* and can be seen in malignancy or inflammatory states such as pneumonia, tuberculosis, or rheumatoid arthritis. Tumors can disrupt the integrity of the mesothelial layer or the integrity of the capillary epithelium, thereby resulting in exudative effusions, or they may block

TABLE 86-2 MECHANISMS PROMOTING PLEURAL FLUID ACCUMULATION

MICROVASCULAR CIRCULATION
Increased hydrostatic pressure (heart failure)
Decreased oncotic pressure (severe hypoalbuminemia)
Increased permeability (pneumonia)
PLEURAL SPACE
Decreased pressure (lung collapse)
LYMPHATICS
Impaired lymphatic drainage (malignant effusion)
DIAPHRAGM
Movement of fluid from the peritoneal space (hepatic hydrothorax)

TABLE 86-3 CONDITIONS THAT CAUSE PLEURAL EFFUSION

TRANSUDATES
Heart failure
Nephrotic syndrome
Hepatic hydrothorax
Superior vena cava syndrome
Peritoneal dialysis
Atelectasis
Urinothorax
EXUDATES
Parapneumonic effusions
Simple
Complicated
Empyema
Infections
Tuberculosis
Fungal
Parasites
Nocardia
Esophageal rupture
Malignancy
Carcinoma
Lymphoma
Mesothelioma
Metastatic disease
INFLAMMATORY DISORDERS
Connective tissue disease
Rheumatoid arthritis
Systemic lupus erythematosus
Churg-Strauss syndrome (now termed eosinophilic granulomatosis with polyangiitis)
Wegener granulomatosis (now termed granulomatosis with polyangiitis)
Familial Mediterranean fever
Abdominal disease
Subdiaphragmatic abscess (hepatic, splenic)
Pancreatitis, pancreatic pseudocyst
Postoperative
Iatrogenic
Drug induced
Misplacement of enteral feeding tube
Esophageal endoscopic interventions
Miscellaneous
Asbestos exposure
Atelectasis
Cholesterol effusion
Chylothorax
Dressler syndrome
Meigs syndrome
Pulmonary embolus
Radiation
Sarcoidosis
Trapped lung
Uremia
Yellow nail syndrome

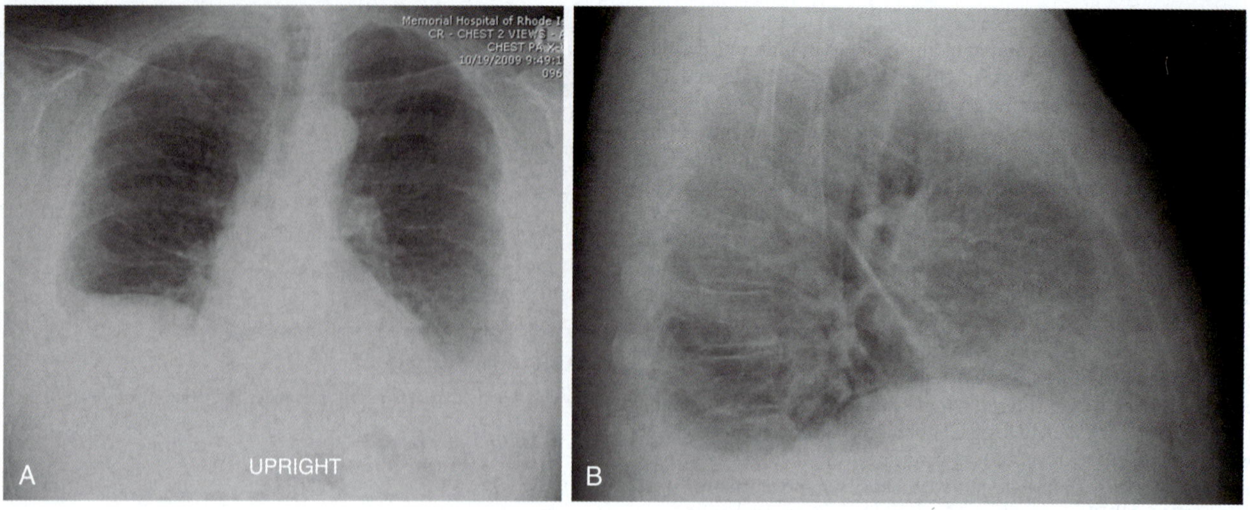

FIGURE 86-3. Patient with bilateral pleural effusions as seen on the posteroanterior radiograph of the chest (A) and lateral radiograph of the chest (B).

lymphatic drainage either through interference with stomal openings into the pleural space or obstruction of lymphatic channels. Pleural effusions also may be caused from transdiaphragmatic movement of intra-abdominal fluid related to hepatic or pancreatic disease.

CLINICAL MANIFESTATIONS

Patients with pleural effusions may be asymptomatic, experience dyspnea, or have pleuritic chest pain that is generally unilateral and sharp. At times, effusions may be sufficiently large to contribute to respiratory failure. Physical findings include dullness to percussion in the area of the effusion, along with diminished breath sounds and absent tactile fremitus.

DIAGNOSIS

Chest radiography (Chapter 72) is often the first imaging method used to detect an effusion (Fig. 86-3). The volume of fluid in the pleural space needs to exceed 250 mL to be visualized on a standing posteroanterior chest radiograph. When an effusion is present, there is blunting of the costophrenic angle on the posteroanterior chest radiograph (see Fig. 86-3), and a meniscus can be seen posteriorly on the lateral chest radiograph (see Fig. 86-3B). Fluid may also collect in either the minor or major fissures. Occasionally, pleural fluid collections in the major or minor fissures may appear as a pulmonary mass and are referred to as *pseudotumors*. Apparent elevation or changes in the contour of the diaphragm on a posteroanterior chest radiograph may signify a subpulmonic effusion, which does not distort the general shape of the diaphragm but will be evident on the lateral film. A lateral decubitus chest radiograph can determine whether fluid is free flowing or loculated. Chest CT can detect much smaller amounts of pleural fluid and determine if an effusion is loculated. It also can identify pleural and parenchymal abnormalities that may be causing the effusion, differentiate between atelectatic lung and fluid, and distinguish a loculated effusion from lung abscess (Fig. 86-4). Ultrasound can detect as little as 5 to 10 mL of fluid and is usually used to guide needle placement when performing a thoracentesis (Fig. 86-5). Positron emission tomography (PET) CT demonstrating pleura uptake of fluorodeoxyglucose is suggestive of pleural malignancy.

Pleurocentesis is required to determine whether an effusion is a transudate or exudate, as well as to determine its specific cause. The tests needed to diagnose the cause of the effusion require a relatively small amount of fluid (30 to 50 mL). Larger volumes of fluid (1 to 1.5 L) can be removed in an attempt to alleviate symptoms. Removing volumes greater than 1.5 L may result in re-expansion pulmonary edema. Relative contraindications to a diagnostic thoracentesis include a bleeding diathesis, a very small volume of pleural fluid, and a low benefit-to-risk ratio.

The fluid can be classified as either a transudate or exudate (Table 86-4).[12,13] Pleural fluid is an exudate if one of the following criteria is met: the pleural fluid–to–serum protein ratio is greater than 0.5, the pleural fluid–to–serum lactate dehydrogenase (LDH) ratio is greater than 0.6, or the pleural fluid LDH level is greater than two-thirds the normal serum LDH level. When all three criteria are met, the sensitivity, specificity, and positive predictive value exceed 98% for defining an exudative effusion. An exudate also can be defined if the pleural fluid cholesterol level is greater than 45 mg/dL in conjunction with a pleural fluid protein level greater than 2.9 g/dL and LDH level greater than 0.45 the upper limit of normal.

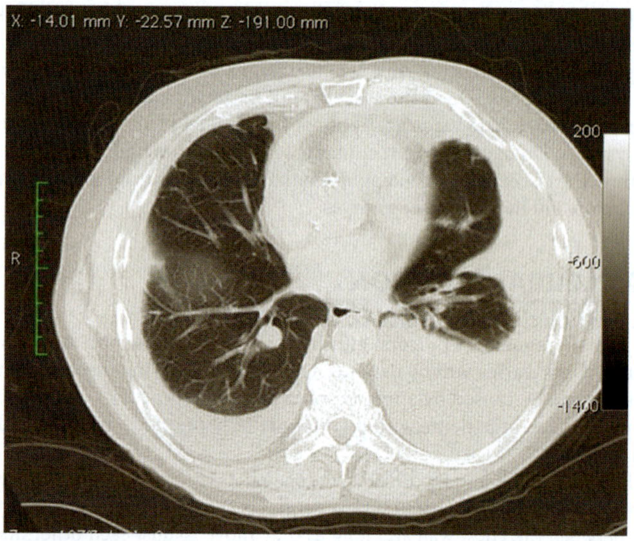

FIGURE 86-4. Chest computed tomography showing pleural effusion in the same patient as in Fig. 86-3.

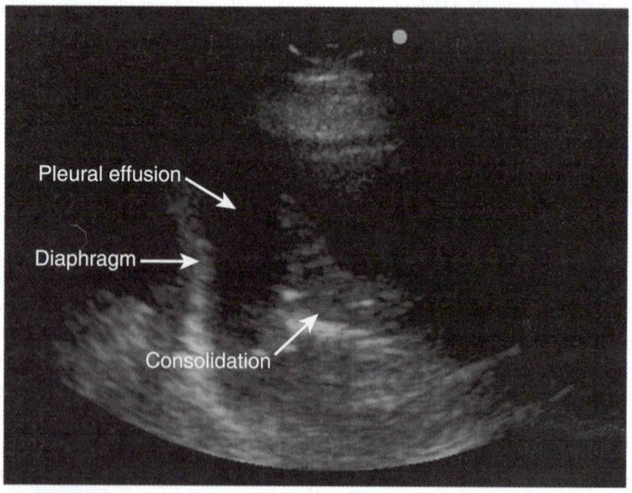

FIGURE 86-5. A right-sided pleural effusion as seen on ultrasound. The ultrasound can be performed at the bedside to aid in needle placement for thoracentesis.

Transudates

Effusions that accumulate owing to changes in osmotic and hydrostatic forces usually form transudates. Transudative effusions are most commonly due to heart failure, in which the effusions are often bilateral or, if unilateral, preferentially involve the right hemithorax. Effusions caused by heart failure are usually related to elevated

TABLE 86-4 PLEURAL FLUID CHARACTERISTICS OF EXUDATES

LIGHT CRITERIA	
Protein	>0.5 pleural fluid/serum value
LDH	>0.6 pleural fluid/serum value
LDH	>⅔ upper limit of normal serum value

LDH = lactate dehydrogenase.

TABLE 86-5 CORRELATION OF THE CHARACTERISTICS OF PLEURAL EXUDATES WITH SPECIFIC DISEASE

TEST	DISEASE
pH < 7.2	Empyema, malignancy, esophageal rupture; rheumatoid, lupus, and tuberculous pleuritis
Glucose (<60 mg/dL)	Infection, rheumatoid pleurisy, tuberculous and lupus effusions, esophageal rupture
Amylase (>200 μg/dL)	Pancreatic disease, esophageal rupture, malignancy, ruptured ectopic pregnancy
RF, ANA, LE cells	Collagen vascular disease
↓ Complement	SLE, RA
RBCs (>5000/μL)	Trauma, malignancy, pulmonary embolus
Chylous effusion (triglycerides > 110 mg/dL)	Tuberculosis, disruption of thoracic duct (trauma, malignancy)
Cytology or biopsy (+)	Malignancy
ADA (>50 μg/L)	Tuberculosis

ADA = adenosine deaminase; ANA = antinuclear antibody; RA = rheumatoid arthritis; RBC = red blood cell; RF, rheumatoid factor; SLE = systemic lupus erythematosus.

left and right heart pressures (Chapter 45), although right heart failure alone (such as seen in advanced pulmonary arterial hypertension) may rarely cause an effusion. Transudates also may be seen in cirrhosis (Chapter 139), nephrotic syndrome (Chapter 107), myxedema (Chapter 207), pulmonary embolism (Chapter 68), superior vena caval obstruction, and peritoneal dialysis (Chapter 117). With cirrhosis, ascites may cross from the peritoneum into the pleural space through small defects in the diaphragm (hepatic hydrothorax; see Table 86-3). Unusual causes of transudates include peritoneal dialysis and atelectasis. Although malignancy typically causes an exudate, it can occasionally produce a transudate.

Urinothorax, which is a rare cause of transudate, results from obstruction of the urinary system. Urinothorax typically has a pleural fluid/serum creatinine ratio greater than 1.0 and may be associated with a pleural fluid pH less than 7.40. Occasionally, aggressive diuresis for heart failure may elevate the pleural fluid protein level sufficiently for the effusion to be classified as an exudate; in such cases, an N-terminal pro–brain natriuretic peptide (BNP) level should be greater than 1500 pg/mL.

Exudates

Exudative effusions, which occur because of an alteration in vascular permeability and/or pleural fluid resorption, can be seen in inflammatory states, infection, or neoplasm. Pleural fluid analysis helps distinguish among the causes of pleural exudates (Table 86-5). In some cases, however, definitive diagnosis may require the procurement of pleural tissue via a CT-guided needle biopsy or a video-assisted thoracoscopic pleural biopsy.

TREATMENT

Treatment should be directed at the underlying cause of the effusion. Unless the effusion is clearly related to heart failure, the first step is thoracentesis to identify whether the effusion is a transudate or exudate and whether it is infected or malignant. Nonmalignant effusions may be treated with thoracentesis if the patient is symptomatic. If the fluid reaccumulates, repeat thoracentesis may be needed. However, thoracentesis must be performed carefully if the lung is nonexpandable (trapped lung); in this circumstance, pleural pressure may become excessively negative as the fluid is withdrawn, thereby resulting in complications such as chest discomfort and re-expansion pulmonary edema. Pleural manometry does not appear to safeguard against these complications.[A4] For a refractory effusion, an indwelling pleural catheter may provide relief of dyspnea but may be associated with complications in patients with hepatic hydrothorax.[14] Other options for refractory effusion include talc or chemical pleurodesis.

SPECIFIC CAUSES OF PLEURAL EFFUSIONS

Parapneumonic Effusions and Empyemas

Parapneumonic effusions, which are the most common type of exudative pleural effusion, occur in up to 40% of patients with pneumonia, typically in patients with bacterial pneumonia (Chapter 85). In an uncomplicated parapneumonic effusion, the pH is generally greater than 7.3, the glucose content greater than 60 mg/dL, and the pleural fluid LDH less than 1000 IU/L. Complicated effusions are characterized by a pH less than 7.2 and often have a glucose content less than 60 mg/dL.

An empyema is present when frank pus is aspirated from the pleural space, when the Gram stain of the fluid is positive for bacteria, or when bacteria are cultured from the fluid. Patients with empyema often report pleuritic chest pain and have refractory fevers several days or more into the course of their pneumonia. Immunocompromised patients may develop empyema sooner and more rapidly. Pneumonia caused by *Streptococcus pneumoniae* (Chapter 268) or *Staphylococcus aureus* (Chapter 267) infection can cause empyema. Patients who aspirate are at high risk for empyema caused by anaerobic organisms, and patients with tuberculosis (Chapter 299) can develop a tuberculous empyema. Methicillin-resistant staphylococci, *Klebsiella* species pneumonia, and *Pseudomonas* species infections may cause an empyema that is difficult to treat. Uncommon infectious causes of effusions include *Actinomyces* species (Chapter 304), *Nocardia* species (Chapter 306), amebiasis (Chapter 323), *Echinococcus* species (Chapter 325), and paragonimiasis (Chapter 326).

TREATMENT

Uncomplicated parapneumonic effusions are usually free flowing, do not require drainage, and will respond to the same antibiotic therapy as the pneumonia itself (Chapter 85). However, in comparison, uncomplicated effusions can transition rapidly to complicated effusions, sometimes within 24 hours. Complicated parapneumonic effusions and empyemas require not only appropriate antibiotics for the particular infection (see Chapter 85) but also prompt drainage by tube thoracostomy to cure the infection as well as prevent cutaneous fistulas, bronchopleural fistulas, or a thick pleural peel (fibrothorax).[A5]

The combination of intrapleural t-PA (10 mg) and DNase (5 mg) therapy can improve chest tube drainage in patients with parapneumonic pleural infections and emyema.[A6] These agents may reduce treatment failure but do not significantly change mortality.[A7] If chest tube drainage is unsuccessful, video-assisted thoracic surgery (Chapter 87) is preferred.[A8] Occasionally, empyema requires thoracotomy and decortication.

MALIGNANT EFFUSION

Malignant effusions, which may account for up to 35% of exudative pleural effusions,[15] may be due to seeding of the parietal or visceral pleura with malignant cells that change vascular permeability and/or impede resorption. Tumor cells also may amplify the production of mediators that promote leakage of fluid into the pleural space. Rarely, a malignant effusion may be transudative. Lung cancer (Chapter 177) is the most frequent cause of malignant pleural effusion, and other malignancies that can involve the pleural space include breast cancer (Chapter 183), ovarian cancer (Chapter 184), gastric cancer (Chapter 178), and lymphoma (Chapters 171 and 172). When malignancy involves the pleural space, the prognosis is poor. However, the finding of a pleural effusion in an individual with underlying malignancy does not necessarily imply that there is a metastatic malignant process involving the pleural space, because effusions in patients with underlying malignancy also may be due to atelectasis, postobstructive pneumonia, hypoalbuminemia, pulmonary emboli (Chapter 68), lymphatic obstruction, and complications from radiation (Chapter 18) or chemotherapy. For this reason, it is critical to obtain a sample of pleural fluid in these individuals. The diagnosis of malignant pleural effusion is established by demonstrating malignant cells in the pleural fluid. Approximately 60% of malignant pleural effusions can be diagnosed with one thoracentesis, and the yield increases to 80% with repeat thoracenteses. A chest CT may show a pleural mass, and pleural biopsy, obtained either by medical or surgical thoracoscopy (Chapter 87), may be helpful in difficult cases.

TREATMENT

Treatment options for malignant pleural effusion include observation and treatment of the underlying malignancy.[16–18] Malignant effusions with a tendency to respond to generalized chemotherapy include those related to breast cancer (Chapter 183), small cell carcinoma of the lung (Chapter 177), and lymphomas (Chapters 171 and 172) with obstruction of lymphatic drainage of the pleural space. The other options are chemical pleurodesis (with tetracycline derivatives, talc poudrage, or talc slurry[A9]) and placement of an indwelling pleural catheter. These two options are equivalent initial options for relieving patient-reported dyspnea, with catheter-based treatment shortening hospital length of stay[A10] but also producing more adverse effects. A complete response occurs in perhaps 50% of patients, but a low pleural fluid pH (<7.2) portends a poorer response to chemical pleurodesis. For patients with recurrent malignant effusions, symptom-guided drainage is generally as good as more aggressive approaches.[A11] The tunneled placement of an indwelling pleural catheter can permit outpatient talc administration, which increases the likelihood of successful resolution of the effusion,[A12] as well as a way to perform intermittent drainage to relieve symptoms. Daily drainage via an indwelling catheter is more effective than every-other-day drainage.[A13] Indwelling pleural catheters can be left in place for several weeks and can induce spontaneous pleurodesis in about 40% of patients.[19] The value of injecting intrapleural urokinase to facilitate treatment of a nondraining malignant pleural effusion is uncertain.

Tuberculous Effusions

Tuberculosis (Chapter 299) can cause pleural effusion in up to 30% of patients who reside in locations endemic for tuberculosis. The pleural effusion typically is not due to direct mycobacterial infection but rather to increased vascular permeability of the pleural membrane because of a hypersensitivity reaction to mycobacterial proteins. The pleural fluid is generally lymphocyte predominant and culture negative for acid-fast bacilli. Adenosine deaminase levels greater than 50 U/L may be helpful in identifying tuberculous pleural effusions, especially when the effusion is lymphocytic. A tuberculous empyema, which is distinct from a tuberculous effusion, is characterized by direct extension of the infection from thoracic lymph nodes or hematogenous spread of tuberculosis into the pleural space.

TREATMENT

Tuberculous effusions typically respond to initial drainage followed by appropriate antitubercular therapies (Chapter 299), whereas tuberculous empyemas require treatment as noted earlier for other bacterial empyemas.

Systemic Inflammatory Disorders

Effusions may be seen in as many as 15% of patients with rheumatoid arthritis (Chapter 243), with a male preponderance. Effusions typically appear after the onset of disease but may precede joint disease. Rheumatoid factor in the pleural fluid is often greater than 1 : 320, and pleural fluid glucose is low (<60 mg/dL, or the pleural fluid–to–serum glucose ratio is <0.5). Other causes of low pleural fluid glucose levels include complicated parapneumonic effusions or empyema, malignant effusions, tuberculous pleurisy, lupus pleuritis, and esophageal rupture, with the lowest concentrations typically seen in rheumatoid arthritis and empyema. Pleural effusions can be seen in 15 to 50% of patients with systemic lupus erythematosus (Chapter 245) and may be characterized by the presence of lupus erythematosus cells, low levels of complement (C3 and C4), and a pleural fluid antinuclear antibody titer greater than 1 : 160. Pleural fluid ANA titers ≥1 : 160 in patients with systemic lupus erythematosus generally indicates that the fluid is a result of lupus pleuritis rather than from other causes. Granulomatosis with polyangiitis (Chapter 249), Sjögren syndrome (Chapter 247), and sarcoidosis (Chapter 83) are less common causes of pleural effusions.

TREATMENT

For inflammatory effusion, treatment of the underlying disease is key, with anti-inflammatory agents and corticosteroids as needed (Chapters 243 and 245).[20] Thoracentesis is useful for symptomatic control, but local measures cannot be expected to resolve the effusion.

PANCREATITIS

Patients with pancreatitis or pancreatic pseudocysts (Chapter 130) may develop exudative pleural effusions that often involve the left hemithorax. A pleural fluid amylase concentration that is greater than the upper limit of normal for serum amylase is consistent with the diagnosis. Extremely high amylase levels have been reported in effusions due to pancreaticopleural fistulas. Amylase also may be seen in the pleural fluid with an esophageal rupture or malignancy. Pancreatic disease is associated with pancreatic isoenzyme amylase, whereas malignancy and esophageal rupture are characterized by a predominance of salivary amylase isoenzymes.

TREATMENT

Large pleural effusions secondary to pancreatitis (Chapter 130) may be evacuated by thoracentesis. General measures to reduce pancreatic stimulation, including the use of octreotide (100 μg subcutaneously three times daily for 7 days) may prevent further fluid accumulation. For chronic effusions, endoscopic or surgical procedures to correct a pancreaticopleural fistula may be required.

Chylous Effusions

A chylothorax has a milky-white appearance and is characterized by high levels of triglycerides (>110 mg/dL) and chylomicrons. A chylothorax is caused by leakage of lymph from the thoracic duct into the pleural space, most commonly related to mediastinal malignancy but also occurring after trauma to the thoracic duct. Major complications from a chylothorax are malnutrition and immunologic compromise when fat, protein, and lymphocytes are depleted by repeated thoracentesis or chest tube drainage. Chylous effusions must be distinguished from pseudochylous effusions, which have a white appearance but are devoid of chylomicrons, and are indicative of a chronic long-standing effusion.

TREATMENT

For chylous effusions, transpedal interstitial magnetic resonance lymphangiography can visualize the central lymphatic system and help guide interventional radiologic or surgical approaches to correct chylous leaks.[21] Treatment of chylothorax includes tube thoracostomy or repeated thoracentesis, combined with dietary restriction of fat intake, although fat malnutrition may ensue. Attempts to decrease chyle formation can be accomplished by intravenous hyperalimentation, and the intake of medium- and light-chain fatty acids, which are absorbed directly into the portal circulation. Ligation of the thoracic duct should be considered for traumatic chylous effusions.[22] Thoracic duct embolization has been performed successfully for nontraumatic chylous effusion.

Hemothorax

A hemothorax has a pleural fluid hematocrit that is at least half that of the circulating hematocrit. By contrast, a bloody pleural effusion will appear red but have a lower hematocrit. A bloody effusion often suggests a malignant process. Other causes include trauma, pulmonary infarction (Chapter 68), tuberculosis (Chapter 299), collagen vascular disease (Chapters 243 and 245), and hematologic disorders. Generally, blood removed from the pleural space does not clot, whereas blood resulting from the trauma of the thoracentesis itself will clot when collected. Because blood in the pleural space does not clot, it can be removed by lymphatics if the volume is small. Larger hemothoraces that impair ventilatory function may require chest tube drainage.

Asbestos Exposure

Pleural effusion may occur after exposure to asbestos. The effusion is often small, unilateral, and serosanguineous, and it generally contains less than 6000 cells/mL. The effusion tends to resolve within a year, resulting in pleural plaques that may calcify over time. Malignant mesothelioma (see later) should be excluded in these individuals.

Other Causes of Pleural Exudates

Meigs syndrome is the triad of ovarian tumor (Chapter 184), ascites, and pleural effusion. The effusion, which is usually large and on the right side, is formed when fluid moves from the abdomen to the pleural space through diaphragmatic defects. Meigs syndrome usually occurs in postmenopausal women and resolves following removal of the tumor.[23] Dressler syndrome may occur from 3 to 30 days after open heart surgery or myocardial infarction. The patient usually experiences pleuritic pain and has a small to moderate left-sided effusion. Pleural effusions that accompany acute idiopathic pericarditis are exudates, typically left-sided, usually occupy less than one third of the hemithorax, and have a predominance of lymphocytes. Treatment is as for the accompanying pericardial effusion (Chapter 62).

Uremia (Chapter 116), which can cause a polyserositis with effusion, must be distinguished from the transudate that commonly is seen in the nephrotic syndrome. Treatment is intensified dialysis, but repeated drainage may sometimes be required (Chapter 117).

Subdiaphragmatic processes, such as hepatic or splenic abscesses (Chapter 137), may cause effusions that typically resolve with resolution of the underlying cause. Trapped lung occurs when a lobe or segment is unable to re-expand owing to a restrictive visceral pleural peel or an endobronchial mass. Increased negative intrapleural pressures associated with trapped lung promote the formation of an effusion.

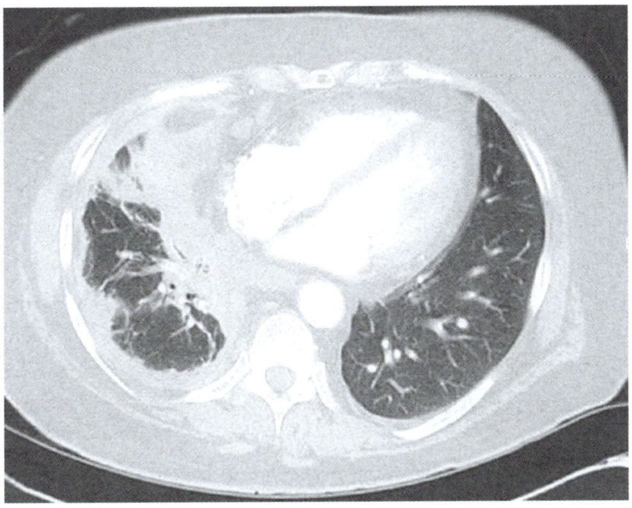

FIGURE 86-6. **Computed tomographic angiogram of the chest in a patient with mesothelioma.** There is diffuse thickening of the pleura and pericardium on the right with a rind-like appearance.

A number of drugs, including amiodarone, bleomycin, dantrolene, hydralazine, isoniazid, methotrexate, methysergide, mitomycin, procainamide, and procarbazine, can cause pleural effusions. Treatment consists of discontinuing the offending agent, although treatment with oral corticosteroids may be needed (Chapter 234).

MESOTHELIOMA

EPIDEMIOLOGY AND PATHOBIOLOGY

Malignant mesotheliomas arise from the serosal membrane of body cavities and usually originate in the pleural space. Patients are typically male, older than age 60 years, and have a distant history (30 to 40 years) of air- or waterborne exposure to asbestos. Smoking is not a risk factor for developing mesothelioma, but smoking in concert with asbestos exposure increases the risk for lung cancer. Mesothelioma is rare, with approximately 3000 cases annually in the United States. The annual incidence in the United States peaked in the early 1990s at 1.5 cases per 100,000 and has been decreasing as a result of better control of occupational exposure. However, the incidence may still be increasing in other countries that have fewer occupational regulations.

CLINICAL MANIFESTATIONS AND DIAGNOSIS

Patients with mesothelioma may complain of dyspnea, loss of appetite, night sweats, weight loss, and chest pain. CT findings of malignant mesothelioma may include localized or circumferential pleural thickening, various amounts of calcified pleural plaque, a pleural based mass, and varying degrees of pleural effusion (Fig. 86-6). The diaphragm or the lung parenchyma also may be involved. The pleural fluid level of hyaluronic acid may be elevated, but pleural fluid cytology frequently is insufficient for diagnosis; as a result, a CT-guided video-assisted thoracoscopic biopsy is commonly needed. A PET-CT can assess mediastinal nodes for staging purposes. Pleural fluid biomarkers such as fibulin-3 and soluble mesothelin-related peptides may help detect mesothelioma at an earlier stage and distinguish it from other malignancies involving the pleura.

A fraction of mesotheliomas are benign. Benign mesotheliomas are usually large and often pedunculated at the time of diagnosis.

TREATMENT AND PROGNOSIS

Benign mesotheliomas should be surgically resected. In highly selected patients with localized malignant disease and no comorbid illnesses, surgical resection or radical extrapleural pneumonectomy may be attempted, although the benefits are uncertain. With more extensive disease, pleural decortication may be preferred over radical extrapleural pneumonectomy.[24,25] Radiation therapy can provide symptom palliation and has been used following attempts at curative surgery. Combination checkpoint inhibitor immunotherapy,[26] such as nivolumab plus ipilimumab, can provide an additional 4 months of median survival compared with standard platinum-based chemotherapy.[A14] Gemcitabine plus ramucirumab is a potentially useful second-line option.[A15] Palliative therapy includes pleurodesis with talc or pleurectomy. Even with the addition of chemotherapy, the prognosis is poor, with a median survival of only 8 to 12 months. However, the presence of tissue biomarkers ERCC1 and RRM1 predict better patient outcomes.[27]

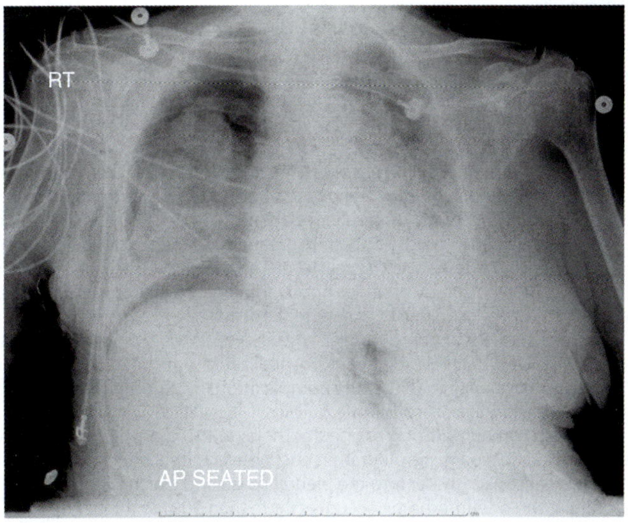

FIGURE 86-7. **A portable anteroposterior chest radiograph demonstrating a right-sided pneumothorax.** Note that the right lung has collapsed to less than half the size of the right hemithorax. In addition, there is a pneumoperitoneum best seen as a collection of air under the right hemidiaphragm.

PNEUMOTHORAX

Pneumothorax refers to the accumulation of air in the pleural space between the parietal pleura lining the rib cage and visceral pleura lining the lung (see Fig. 72-16). Normally, the pressure within the pleural space is slightly subatmospheric, but more than a very small amount of air within the pleural space causes positive pressure that compresses the underlying lung. A primary spontaneous pneumothorax occurs with no precipitating event in a person without underlying lung disease, whereas a secondary pneumothorax is a complication of underlying lung disease or trauma.[28]

EPIDEMIOLOGY AND PATHOBIOLOGY

Spontaneous primary pneumothorax is more common in tall, young, thin men, presumably as a result of rupture of preexisting apical blebs. It is associated with Marfan syndrome (Chapter 239) and Birt-Hogg-Dube syndrome. Secondary pneumothorax may be associated with a number of lung diseases, including but not limited to emphysema (Chapter 76), cystic fibrosis (Chapter 77), granulomatous inflammation, necrotizing pneumonia, pulmonary fibrosis (Chapter 80), eosinophilic granulomatous disease (Chapter 156), sarcoidosis (Chapter 83), necrotizing pneumonia, and lung cancer (Chapter 177). Patients with underlying lung disease undergoing mechanical ventilation (Chapter 91) may acutely develop a pneumothorax when high local pressures disrupt lung tissue, thereby leading to a leak. Blunt or penetrating trauma (Chapter 97) can cause pneumothorax. Catamenial pneumothorax occurs in patients who have subpleural and diaphragmatic endometriosis (Chapter 218); rupture of the endometrial nodules at the time of menstruation causes pneumothorax.

CLINICAL MANIFESTATIONS AND DIAGNOSIS

Symptoms typically include acute shortness of breath and sharp chest pain. Physical examination is characterized by tachycardia, tachypnea, decreased breath sounds, decreased tactile fremitus, a pleural friction rub, subcutaneous emphysema, hyper-resonance to percussion, and a tracheal shift toward the uninvolved hemithorax.

Diagnosis can be made by obtaining an upright chest radiograph, and rapid assessment with point-of-care ultrasound can be used as well. Air within the pleural space appears as an area of lucency on the chest radiograph (Fig. 86-7). With a small pneumothorax, the lucency is best appreciated at the lung apex when the patient is upright. An end-expiratory radiograph is particularly helpful in diagnosing a small pneumothorax. When a portable chest radiograph is obtained with the patient in the supine position, such as a patient in an intensive care unit, the lucent area may be most noticeable over the lower rib cage (superior sulcus sign). Ultrasound may be more sensitive than the chest radiograph for detecting a small pneumothorax, especially in the intensive care unit setting.

A *tension pneumothorax* is associated with a contralateral mediastinal shift and hemodynamic compromise, usually because high intrathoracic pressures compress the vena cava and atrium. This physiology implies an ongoing leak of air into the pleural space.

TREATMENT AND PROGNOSIS

Small unilateral pneumothoraces (<3 cm of air between the lung and chest wall on the chest radiograph) and pneumothoraces that are not associated with physiologic impairments typically resolve on their own. Analgesics, preferably nonopioid (see Table 26-4) but opioids if required (see Table 26-6), may be given for pain control. Moderate to large unilateral pneumothoraces without physiologic impairment also can be managed initially with careful observation (with pain medication and supplemental oxygen if the oxygen saturation is <92%), with interventional therapy reserved for patients who develop a systolic blood pressure less than 90 mm Hg, a pulse rate greater than their systolic blood pressure, a respiratory rate above 30 breaths per minute, or an oxygen saturation below 90%. Such a strategy provides good radiologic and symptomatic resolution at 8 weeks with less risk of later recurrence or adverse events, including just a 1% risk of subsequent pneumothorax.[A16] Another option is to place a device with a one-way valve, which can decrease hospitalizations at the expense of more short-term but usually manageable complications.[A17] Supplemental oxygen may help the pleural air resorb more quickly.

For a tension pneumothorax or pneumothorax with initial physiologic impairment or intractable pain, the pleural air must be evacuated, preferably by inserting a thoracentesis catheter into the pleural space and evacuating the air with a syringe. If the pneumothorax occupies more than 50% of the hemithorax or a tension pneumothorax develops, management requires insertion of a thoracostomy tube, suction, and water-seal drainage.[A18,A19]

If a leak continues despite tube thoracostomy, a bronchopleural fistula may be suspected. In this instance, chemical pleurodesis or surgical correction, usually by video-assisted thoracoscopic surgery, may be necessary (Chapter 87). For recurrent pneumothorax, which may occur in up to 50% of patients with primary spontaneous pneumothorax, pleurodesis is safe and effective.

MEDIASTINUM

The mediastinum, which is the central part of the thoracic cavity, lies between the right and left lungs. It contains the heart and aorta, esophagus, trachea, lymph nodes, thymus, and great vessels. It is bordered by the two pleural cavities laterally, the diaphragm inferiorly, and the thoracic inlet superiorly.

MEDIASTINAL MASSES

PATHOBIOLOGY

The mediastinum can be divided into three compartments: anterior, middle, and posterior (E-Fig. 86-4). The anterior compartment contains the thymus, substernal extensions of the thyroid, blood vessels, pericardium, and lymph nodes. The middle compartment contains the heart, great vessels, trachea, main bronchi, lymph nodes, and the phrenic and vagal nerves. The posterior compartment contains the vertebrae, descending aorta, esophagus, thoracic duct, azygous and hemizygous veins, lower portion of the vagus, sympathetic chain, and lymph nodes.

CLINICAL MANIFESTATIONS

Mediastinal masses usually are not accompanied by symptoms, and most masses are incidentally found on either a chest radiograph or a chest CT scan. If present, however, symptoms may be related to compression of normal mediastinal structures or to systemic effects. Symptoms include chest pain, cough, hoarseness, stridor, dysphasia, dyspnea, fever, and night sweats. One third of patients with a mediastinal thymoma have symptoms or weakness owing to myasthenia gravis (Chapter 390), and individuals with mediastinal lymphoma (Chapters 171 and 172) may have systemic symptoms such as fever, night sweats, and weight loss. Occasionally, a mass may compress the superior vena cava, causing partial obstruction and resulting in facial edema and dilated neck and chest veins (Fig. 86-8).

DIAGNOSIS

When a mass is identified by chest radiography or chest CT, further evaluation is mandatory. Chest CT can usually provide resolution sufficient to determine the tissue composition of the mass and the presence of fluid, fat, or calcifications.[29] If a benign process is suspected, follow-up CT may be indicated. If a malignant process is suspected, radiologic evaluation may include angiography, PET scan, or MRI. A technetium scan may be useful if a goiter is suspected. Biopsies can be obtained by mediastinotomy, ultrasound-guided transbronchial needle aspiration biopsy, or transthoracic CT-guided needle aspiration. Biopsy should be avoided if thymoma is suspected because of potential seeding of tumor cells.

The evaluation and differential diagnosis of mediastinal masses are guided by the compartment in which they arise (Table 86-6). The *anterior mediastinal compartment* includes lesions such as thymomas, germ cell tumors (teratomas), lymphomas, and intrathoracic thyroid tissue. Thymomas make up about 30% of mediastinal neoplasms in adults, in whom they are the most common anterior mediastinal primary neoplasm. Patients with systemic lymphoma often have involvement of the mediastinum, but only 5 to 10% of patients with lymphoma present with primary mediastinal lesions. Teratomas, which account for most mediastinal germ cell tumors, are benign but may undergo malignant transformation. They may contain squamous cells, hair follicles, sweat glands, cartilage, and linear calcifications; about one third are malignant. Intrathoracic goiters (Chapter 207) (Fig. 86-9) may compress the trachea and cause stridor, cough, dyspnea, and, occasionally, superior vena

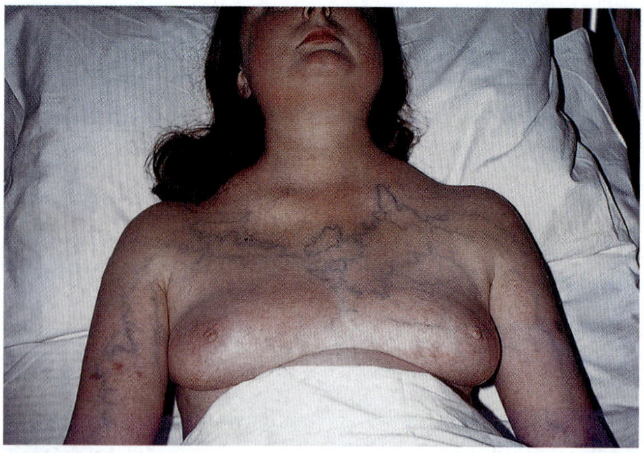

FIGURE 86-8. **Superior vena cava obstruction in bronchial carcinoma.** Note the swelling of the face and neck and the development of collateral circulation in the veins of the chest wall.

TABLE 86-6 CAUSES OF MEDIASTINAL MASSES

ANTERIOR	MIDDLE	POSTERIOR
Teratoma	Pericardial cyst	Neurogenic tumor
Thymoma	Lymph node hyperplasia	Esophageal tumor
Thyroid tumor	Bronchogenic tumor	Bronchogenic tumor
Goiter	Bronchogenic cyst	Bronchogenic cyst
Aneurysm	Aneurysm	Aneurysm
Lymphoma	Lymphoma	Lymphoma
Parathyroid tumor		Meningocele
Lipoma		Enteric cyst
Morgagni diaphragm hernia		Esophageal diverticula
		Bochdalek diaphragm hernia

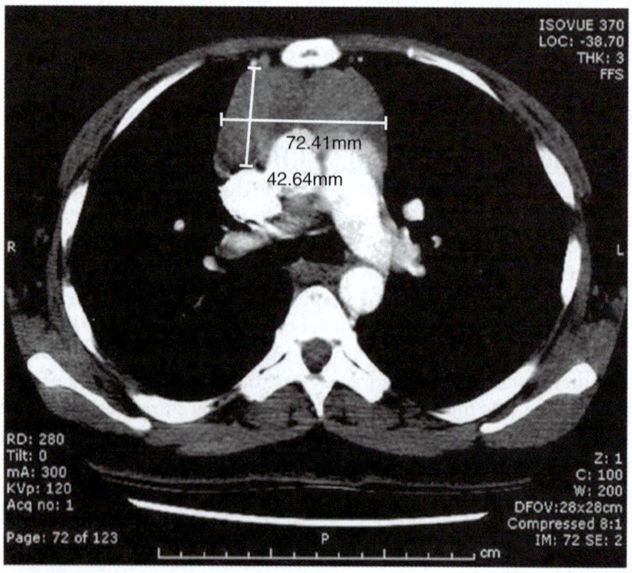

FIGURE 86-9. **Chest computed tomography of a patient with an anterior mediastinal mass that proved to be a substernal goiter.**

cava obstruction. Anterior masses in the right cardiophrenic angle, which are rare and may be associated with pericardial defects or obesity, may be due to herniation of liver or intestinal contents through the foramina of Morgagni. Lymphadenopathy related to sarcoid, lung cancer, or lymphoma accounts for most middle mediastinal masses.

Neurogenic tumors are the most common lesions that cause posterior mediastinal masses. CT or MRI can help distinguish schwannomas greater than 10 cm, which often show cystic degeneration, from other neoplasms.[30] Many of these tumors are benign and originate in the nerve sheath or sympathetic ganglion cells (schwannoma or ganglioneuroma). Posterior mediastinal masses also include cysts, meningoceles, and lymphomas (Chapters 171 and 172). Aortic aneurysm (Chapter 63) and esophageal disorders (Chapter 124) such as diverticula and neoplasm may be seen in the middle or posterior mediastinum. Herniation of abdominal contents into the thorax can result in posterior mediastinal masses. Herniation of abdominal contents through the foramina of Bochdalek results in a mass in the posterolateral area of the diaphragm, usually on the left side; it is the most common congenital hernia and may contain spleen or kidney. Herniation of the stomach through the esophageal hiatus (Chapter 124), which is the most common type of diaphragmatic herniation, produces a mass posterior to the heart, often with an air-liquid level.

Benign cysts can occur in the anterior, middle, or posterior compartments. They can arise in the pericardium, bronchi, thymus, thoracic duct, esophagus, and stomach and can produce compressive symptoms. Pericardial cysts, which are often located in the cardiophrenic angle, contain clear liquid. Bronchogenic cysts occur in the middle or posterior compartments and are filled with liquid and lined with respiratory epithelium; they often develop around the paratracheal area or carina and do not communicate with the tracheal bronchial tree.

TREATMENT

The treatment of a mediastinal mass depends on the underlying pathology. Some lesions, such as thymomas, teratomas, cysts, neurogenic tumors, and hernias, require surgical resection. Others, such as lymphoma, are treated with radiation or chemotherapy.

MEDIASTINITIS

Acute mediastinal infections, which are uncommon, are usually complications after oropharyngeal and odontogenic infections, cardiothoracic or other thoracic surgical procedures (e.g., sternotomy), or procedures involving the esophagus or tracheobronchial tree. Rupture of the esophagus or trachea from trauma or tissue necrosis can cause mediastinitis.[31] Treatment of acute mediastinitis requires antibiotics, pleural drainage, and evacuation of necrotic tissue.[32] Fibrosing mediastinitis is a rare, progressive illness that may be idiopathic or can be caused by chronic granulomatous infection (histoplasmosis), radiotherapy, autoimmune disease, immunoglobulin (Ig)G4–related diseases, or drugs (e.g., methysergide). Patients with fibrosing mediastinitis remain asymptomatic until vascular or neurologic structures are affected. When respiratory structures are involved, tracheobronchial narrowing is the most common presentation. The diagnosis and treatment often require surgical exploration. In patients with fibrosing mediastinitis, catheter-based treatment of pulmonary vein stenosis may sometimes provide relief. The prognosis is poor and treatment ineffective unless it is related to tuberculosis (Chapter 299) or autoimmune disease.

PNEUMOMEDIASTINUM

Pneumomediastinum occurs when air infiltrates the mediastinal structures. Air leaks owing to alveolar rupture or less commonly esophageal tears will dissect into the hilum and mediastinal space because the pressure in the mediastinum is more negative than the pulmonary parenchymal pressure. Loss of esophageal or tracheal integrity often results from trauma, whereas leaks from alveoli may result from trauma, occur spontaneously, or can be a complication of mechanical ventilation (Chapter 91). Pneumomediastinum rarely is seen as a complication of an exacerbation of asthma (Chapter 75), violent coughing, or emesis. Pneumomediastinum may present as a sore throat, neck pain, or shortness of breath. A chest radiograph or CT scan will reveal thin columns of hyperlucency between mediastinal structures. Mediastinal air can dissect into the subcutaneous tissues of the neck and chest wall, where it results in subcutaneous emphysema with characteristic palpable crepitus. Spontaneous pneumomediastinum generally resolves without treatment. When more severe collections of subcutaneous air occur, surgical decompression may be warranted.

GENERAL REFERENCES

For the General References and other additional features, please visit Elsevier eBooks+ at https://ebooks.health.elsevier.com.

Grade A References

A1. Zhou Z, Liu F, Li R, et al. The effects of exercise therapy on adolescent idiopathic scoliosis: an overview of systematic reviews and meta-analyses. *Complement Ther Med.* 2021;58:102697.

A2. Pieracci FM, Leasia K, Bauman Z, et al. A multicenter, prospective, controlled clinical trial of surgical stabilization of rib fractures in patients with severe, nonflail fracture patterns (Chest Wall Injury Society NONFLAIL). *J Trauma Acute Care Surg.* 2020;88:249-257.

A3. Pecourneau V, Degboe Y, Barnetche T, et al. Effectiveness of exercise programs in ankylosing spondylitis: a meta-analysis of randomized controlled trials. *Arch Phys Med Rehabil.* 2018;99:383-389.

A4. Lentz RJ, Lerner AD, Pannu JK, et al. Routine monitoring with pleural manometry during therapeutic large-volume thoracentesis to prevent pleural-pressure-related complications: a multicentre, single-blind randomised controlled trial. *Lancet Respir Med.* 2019;7:447.

A5. Redden MD, Chin TY, van Driel ML. Surgical versus non-surgical management for pleural empyema. *Cochrane Database Syst Rev.* 2017;3:CD010651.

A6. Chong WH, Hu K, Saha BK, et al. Comparing the outcomes of intrapleural fibrinolytic and DNase therapy versus intrapleural fibrinolytic or DNase therapy: a systematic review and meta-analysis. *Pulm Pharmacol Ther.* 2021;24:102081.

A7. Altmann ES, Crossingham I, Wilson S, et al. Intra-pleural fibrinolytic therapy versus placebo, or a different fibrinolytic agent, in the treatment of adult parapneumonic effusions and empyema. *Cochrane Database Syst Rev.* 2019;2019:CD002312.

A8. Kheir F, Thakore S, Mehta H, et al. Intrapleural fibrinolytic therapy versus early medical thoracoscopy for treatment of pleural infection. Randomized controlled clinical trial. *Ann Am Thorac Soc.* 2020;17:958-964.

A9. Dipper A, Jones HE, Bhatnagar R, et al. Interventions for the management of malignant pleural effusions: a network meta-analysis. *Cochrane Database Syst Rev.* 2020;4:CD010529.

A10. Iyer NP, Reddy CB, Wahidi MM, et al. Indwelling pleural catheter versus pleurodesis for malignant pleural effusions: a systematic review and meta-analysis. *Ann Am Thorac Soc.* 2019;16:124-131.

A11. Muruganandan S, Azzopardi M, Fitzgerald DB, et al. Aggressive versus symptom-guided drainage of malignant pleural effusion via indwelling pleural catheters (AMPLE-2): an open-label randomised trial. *Lancet Respir Med.* 2018;6:671-680.

A12. Bhatnagar R, Keenan EK, Morley AJ, et al. Outpatient talc administration by indwelling pleural catheter for malignant effusion. *N Engl J Med.* 2018;378:1313-1322.

A13. Wahidi MM, Reddy C, Yarmus L, et al. Randomized trial of pleural fluid drainage frequency in patients with malignant pleural effusions. The ASAP trial. *Am J Respir Crit Care Med.* 2017;195:1050-1057.

A14. Baas P, Scherpereel A, Nowak AK, et al. First-line nivolumab plus ipilimumab in unresectable malignant pleural mesothelioma (CheckMate 743): a multicentre, randomised, open-label, phase 3 trial. *Lancet.* 2021;397:375-386.

A15. Pinto C, Zucali PA, Pagano M, et al. Gemcitabine with or without ramucirumab as second-line treatment for malignant pleural mesothelioma (RAMES): a randomised, double-blind, placebo-controlled, phase 2 trial. *Lancet Oncol.* 2021;22:1438-1447.

A16. Brown SGA, Ball EL, Perrin K, et al. Conservative versus interventional treatment for spontaneous pneumothorax. *N Engl J Med.* 2020;382:405-415.

A17. Hallifax RJ, McKeown E, Sivakumar P, et al. Ambulatory management of primary spontaneous pneumothorax: an open-label, randomised controlled trial. *Lancet.* 2020;396:39-49.

A18. Carson-Chahhoud KV, Wakai A, van Agteren JE, et al. Simple aspiration versus intercostal tube drainage for primary spontaneous pneumothorax in adults. *Cochrane Database Syst Rev.* 2017;9:CD004479.

A19. Lee JH, Kim R, Park CM. Chest tube drainage versus conservative management as the initial treatment of primary spontaneous pneumothorax: a systematic review and meta-analysis. *J Clin Med.* 2020;9:3456.

87

INTERVENTIONAL AND SURGICAL APPROACHES TO LUNG DISEASE

DAVID J. FELLER-KOPMAN AND MALCOLM M. DECAMP

Interventional pulmonology and minimally invasive thoracic surgery have drastically changed the approach to the diagnosis and staging of lung cancer, the management of central airway obstruction, and the treatment of patients with pleural disease.

BRONCHOSCOPIC PROCEDURES

Flexible bronchoscopy and endobronchial ultrasound have revolutionized the evaluation of airway and parenchymal diseases, the approach to hilar and mediastinal adenopathy, and the staging of lung cancer. New technologies offer bronchoscopic treatment for patients with severe asthma and emphysema.

ENDOBRONCHIAL ULTRASOUND

Bronchoscopy is a standard component of the evaluation and staging of patients with thoracic tumors. Convex-probe endobronchial ultrasound uses a curvilinear ultrasound probe (E-Fig. 87-1), which is incorporated into the tip of the bronchoscope, to visualize structures outside of the airway and sample hilar and mediastinal lymph nodes under direct, real-time imaging. This approach has largely replaced mediastinoscopy in the staging of patients with lung cancer and in the diagnosis of sarcoidosis (Chapter 83) and mediastinal lymphomas. Adding endobronchial ultrasound to surgical staging improves the sensitivity for finding nodal metastases and can reduce the unnecessary thoracotomy rate from 18 to 7%. Additionally, endobronchial ultrasound–guided biopsies can provide adequate tissue for identification of "tumor markers," which are now required to guide lung cancer treatment. It also reduces complications as well as the need for additional procedures for molecular marker analysis compared with computed tomography (CT)-guided transthoracic needle aspiration. It is important to note, however, that the sensitivity of endobronchial ultrasound is not 100%, so nondiagnostic samples must be confirmed as true negatives with either surgical staging or clinical and radiologic follow-up.

In radial-probe endobronchial ultrasound, an ultrasound probe is passed through the working channel of the bronchoscope to visualize parenchymal lesions as well as to discriminate tumor invasion compared with compression of the central airways. When used with smaller bronchoscopes and advanced navigational technologies, such as electromagnetic navigation or virtual bronchoscopic navigation, this technique can improve the diagnostic yield when sampling pulmonary nodules.

BRONCHIAL THERMOPLASTY

Bronchial thermoplasty uses radio frequency energy to ablate airway smooth muscle in patients whose severe asthma (Chapter 75) remains symptomatic despite medical therapy. The patient must undergo three bronchoscopic procedures to treat all of the visible airways. The right lower lobe is treated during the first procedure, the left lower lobe in the second, and both upper lobes in the third (the right middle lobe is not treated). Although asthma may be exacerbated in the immediate peritreatment period, this approach can significantly improve asthma-related quality of life, days lost from work or school, and emergency department visits in carefully selected patients.[A1]

BRONCHOSCOPY FOR CENTRAL AIRWAY OBSTRUCTION

A variety of malignant and nonmalignant diseases can obstruct the central airways (Table 87-1). Malignant causes include bronchogenic carcinoma (Chapter 177) or metastatic malignancy to the airways, as well as extrinsic compression from adenopathy. Nonmalignant causes include granulation tissue arising after an intubation or tracheostomy, adenopathy from sarcoidosis (Chapter 83), inflammatory conditions such as relapsing polychondritis (Chapter 254), amyloidosis (Chapter 174), and infectious causes such as tuberculosis (Chapter 299) and respiratory papillomatosis.

TABLE 87-1 CAUSES OF CENTRAL AIRWAY OBSTRUCTION

NONMALIGNANT	MALIGNANT
Congenital vascular sling	Primary airway tumors (e.g., bronchogenic, mucoepidermoid, adenoid cystic carcinoid)
Cartilage	Tumors metastatic to the airway (e.g., bronchogenic, renal cell, breast, melanoma, thyroid, colon, esophageal)
Relapsing polychondritis	External compression
Tracheobronchomalacia	Lymphadenopathy from any malignancy
Lymphadenopathy	Mediastinal tumors (e.g., thyroid, thymus, germ cell, lymphoma)
Infectious (e.g., histoplasmosis, tuberculosis)	
Sarcoidosis	
Granulation tissue associated with artificial airways, airway stenosis, aspirated foreign bodies, surgical anastomosis	
Inflammatory lesions (e.g., granulomatosis with polyangiitis, amyloidosis, papillomatosis)	
External compression (e.g., goiter)	
Internal	
Secretions	
Blood clot	

Adapted from Feller-Kopman D, Shojaee S. Therapeutic bronchoscopy: interventional techniques. In: Mason RJ, Broaddus VC, Martin T, et al, eds. *Murray and Nadel's Textbook of Respiratory Medicine*. 7th ed. Philadelphia, PA: Elsevier; 2022.

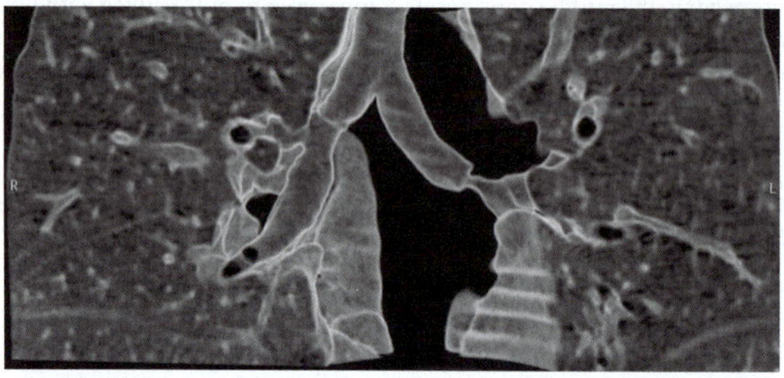

FIGURE 87-1. Three-dimensional reconstruction of a computed tomographic scan in a 20-year-old woman after bilateral lung transplantation. The image clearly shows the high-grade stenosis at the level of the left mainstem anastomosis. The right-sided airways are normal.

CLINICAL MANIFESTATIONS AND DIAGNOSIS

A high index of suspicion is essential because significant airway obstruction can be present before the development of symptoms or the characteristic abnormalities on the inspiratory and expiratory flow-volume curves (Chapter 73). Patients with central airway obstruction often develop exertional dyspnea when the tracheal lumen is less than 8 mm in diameter (normal is about 18 to 20 mm) but do not develop stridor, which usually is a sign of impending respiratory failure and the need for urgent intervention, until the tracheal diameter is less than 5 mm.

Hemoptysis (Chapter 71) may be present in patients with malignancies but is also seen in infectious and inflammatory conditions. Some patients may present with a postobstructive pneumonia that responds poorly to antibiotic treatment. Most patients, however, present with nonspecific symptoms including dyspnea and cough.

Patients who have risk factors for chronic airway obstruction and present with symptoms consistent with obstruction unresponsive to conventional therapy should undergo airway imaging by CT (Fig. 87-1) and flexible bronchoscopy (Fig. 87-2). Because loss of airway patency can be lethal, evaluation of these patients should be performed by individuals experienced in the management of critical airway disorders.

TREATMENT

Relief of airway obstruction requires a multidisciplinary approach by expert physicians. Techniques for achieving a patent airway include coring out the tissue with the barrel of the rigid bronchoscope; laser treatment to vaporize the tissue; electrocautery or argon plasma coagulation to carbonize the tissue, so it will later slough; cryotherapy; and mechanical débridement with forceps or a microdebrider. In the absence of definitive randomized trials, the choice of modality is often left to the expertise and resources of the bronchoscopist.

In contrast to endobronchial disease, airway stenting, preferably with silicone stents,[1] is the primary treatment for airway obstruction caused by extrinsic compression. Because airway stents can be associated with long-term complications, including stent fractures, the formation of granulation tissue, infection, and migration, they are primarily a palliative approach for malignant diseases and should be used sparingly in patients with nonmalignant airway obstruction.

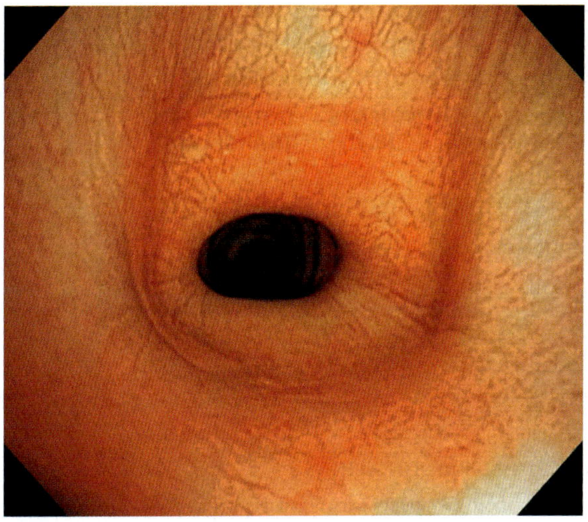

FIGURE 87-2. Bronchoscopic view of the proximal trachea in a 54-year-old man with shortness of breath and stridor. Significant circumferential narrowing is noted in the subglottic space, consistent with gastric reflux–induced subglottic stenosis.

PROGNOSIS

Successful endoscopic treatment can significantly improve the quality of life of patients with malignant airway obstruction and improve their survival rates to be the equivalent of similar stage patients without airway obstruction. Patients with nonmalignant disease similarly experience significant improvements in physiology (pulmonary function), exercise capacity, and quality of life.

SURGICAL PROCEDURES

Open Approaches

Thoracotomy has been the standard approach to evaluate the contents of the pleural space, lung parenchyma, pulmonary hilum, and ipsilateral mediastinum and diaphragm. Selective lung ventilation, achieved by use of a double-lumen endotracheal tube or mainstem bronchial blocker, allows one lung to be collapsed and visualized. The precision and accuracy of preprocedure CT and magnetic resonance imaging (MRI) now allow many procedures to be performed using smaller targeted incisions, with a muscle-sparing technique that allows specific access to regional pathology.

Minimally Invasive Approaches

Point-of-care ultrasound can guide catheter drainage of an effusion, hemothorax, empyema, or pneumothorax with persistent air leak. Thoracoscopy or video-assisted thoracoscopic surgery (VATS) and robotic-assisted thoracic surgery require between two and four port incisions to place a camera, light source, and instruments in almost any intercostal space. With a VATS or robotic approach, recovery is shorter than after an open thoracotomy because little if any muscle is divided and no mechanical rib spreading retractors are used.

A variety of benign lung diseases present as focal parenchymal lesions or diffuse processes that require a tissue biopsy for diagnosis. Thoracoscopy has essentially replaced a limited thoracotomy and wedge resection for this purpose. VATS provides a more complete view of the ipsilateral hemithorax, including the visceral, parietal, and mediastinal pleura, as well as access to all lung lobes. In addition, nodules within 1 to 2 cm of the pleura can be identified so that representative excisional biopsies can be performed.

SPONTANEOUS PNEUMOTHORAX

Although most spontaneous pneumothoraces (Chapter 86) are uncomplicated, up to 20% of patients with pneumothoraces experience complications such as tension pneumothorax, persistent air leak despite tube drainage, or recurrent pneumothoraces either ipsilaterally or contralaterally. If the patient is clinically stable and has an oxygen saturation of 92% or higher on room air or supplemental oxygen, a spontaneous pneumothorax can be managed with observation, a single aspiration, or an ambulatory device with a one-way valve alone.[A2,A3] Such conservative therapy can safely reduce invasive procedures and the duration of hospitalization. More complicated patients typically require continuous in-hospital drainage. Patients in whom a second pneumothorax develops have a 70 to 80% chance of a third recurrence within 2 years. The current surgical approach to the treatment of recurrent pneumothoraces is VATS resection of the subpleural blebs responsible for the pneumothorax, usually combined with mechanical abrasion of the parietal pleura, a parietal pleurectomy, or chemical pleurodesis (e.g., with 300 mg of minocycline or with insufflated talc) to induce an inflammatory reaction that will cause the visceral and parietal pleural surfaces to fuse, thereby preventing subsequent recurrence.

MALIGNANT LUNG DISEASE

Solitary Pulmonary Nodules

Most small pulmonary nodules (see Fig. 177-2 in Chapter 177) present in the periphery of the lung beyond the reach of diagnostic bronchoscopy. Nevertheless, advanced techniques such as electromagnetic navigation[2] and robotic bronchoscopy[3] can significantly increase the diagnostic yield to about 75% even for nodules smaller than 2 cm. If peripheral nodules are not amenable to a bronchoscopic approach, VATS excisional biopsy (Video 87-1) of a small pulmonary nodule leads to a definitive diagnosis in almost all cases and is generally preferred over transthoracic needle biopsy. Furthermore, thoracoscopy can allow concurrent nodal staging should a primary malignancy (Chapter 177) be confirmed. In the absence of regional adenopathy, patients with primary malignant lesions can undergo definitive resection at the same time.

Primary Lung Cancer

In patients with node-negative primary lung cancer and adequate pulmonary reserve, lobectomy or pneumonectomy is indicated to obtain optimal survival and to decrease the risk for local recurrence. Similar oncologic outcomes can be achieved by performing an open thoracotomy via VATS or robotic assistance, and either of these minimally invasive approaches generally is associated with fewer complications, less pain, a shorter hospitalization, and a speedier recovery.[4] Lobectomy is preferred because sublobar resection (segmentectomy or wedge) for stage I lung cancers is historically associated with a two- to three-fold higher incidence of locoregional recurrence.

Metastatic Cancer

The lung is a frequent site of metastatic recurrence. Common histologies include colorectal cancer (Chapter 179), renal cell carcinoma (Chapter 182), sarcoma (Chapter 187), melanoma (Chapter 188), breast cancer (Chapter 183), and head and neck cancer (Chapter 176). VATS is often the diagnostic procedure of choice to locate and excise nodules that are too small for reliable percutaneous biopsy.

The role of pulmonary metastectomy as therapy for advanced disease remains controversial. Five-year survival rates of 20 to 30% have been reported for selected patients, especially if the disease-free interval from original diagnosis to lung metastasis is greater than 2 to 3 years.

PROCEDURES FOR EMPHYSEMA

LUNG VOLUME REDUCTION SURGERY

Emphysema (Chapter 76) is the most common chronic progressive disabling lung disease treated by pulmonologists and thoracic surgeons. In eligible patients (Table 87-2), lung volume reduction surgery confers durable symptomatic, physiologic, and survival benefits compared with medical therapy (E-Fig. 87-2) for patients who have severe emphysema but who do not have a forced expiratory volume in 1 second (FEV_1) measure of less than 20% of predicted with either a homogeneous distribution of emphysema on CT or a diffusing capacity of less than 20% of predicted.[A4] However, subgroup analyses suggest that the benefit is mainly in patients with upper lobe predominant disease.

For eligible patients, most programs require a 6- to 10-week period of preoperative pulmonary rehabilitation followed by a cardiopulmonary exercise test to assess the risks and benefits of surgery. Patients with upper lobe predominant emphysema and a low preoperative exercise capacity have a nearly 50% lower risk for death after lung volume reduction surgery compared with continued medical therapy. Lung volume reduction surgery also can reduce systemic blood pressure, allow for weight gain, and reduce exacerbations of chronic obstructive pulmonary disease (COPD). In experienced centers, bilateral stapled resection approaches yield nearly twice the physiologic benefit of unilateral lung volume reduction surgery without adversely affecting operative morbidity or mortality. High-risk patients with severe airflow obstruction ($FEV_1 < 20\%$) should be assessed for lung transplantation unless their disease is localized to the upper lobes and their gas exchange as defined by diffusing capacity is preserved (Table 87-3).

Most patients with COPD have diffuse parenchymal disease, but a small number of patients with COPD have dominant or giant bullae that may occupy 50% or more of the volume of the hemithorax and that compress relatively preserved lung parenchyma. The indications for bullectomy include progressive symptoms with demonstrated disability, obstructive spirometry (Chapter 73),

TABLE 87-2 INCLUSION AND EXCLUSION CRITERIA FOR LUNG VOLUME REDUCTION SURGERY

INCLUSION CRITERIA
Radiographic evidence of emphysema, especially involving upper lobes
Hyperinflation evidenced by TLC > 100% predicted and RV > 150% predicted
FEV_1 > 20 and <45% predicted (after bronchodilator)
DLCO > 20% predicted
Severe dyspnea
Restricted activities of daily living
Decreased quality of life
Abstinence from tobacco
EXCLUSION CRITERIA
Active smoking
Bronchiectasis
Pulmonary nodule requiring evaluation
Excessive daily sputum production
Previous thoracotomy
Obvious pleural disease
Active or inducible coronary ischemia
Pulmonary hypertension
Depressed LVEF (<45%)
Obesity (BMI > 32)
Unable or unwilling to participate in pulmonary rehabilitation
Systemic steroids, ≥20 mg prednisone/day

BMI = body mass index; DLCO = diffusion capacity for carbon monoxide; FEV_1 = first second forced expiratory volume; LVEF = left ventricular ejection fraction; RV = residual capacity; TLC = total lung capacity.

Adapted from DeCamp MM Jr, McKenna RJ Jr, Deschamps CC, et al. Lung volume reduction surgery: technique, operative mortality and morbidity. *Proc Am Thorac Soc.* 2008;5:442-446; and DeCamp MM Jr, Lipson D, Krasna M, et al. The evaluation and preparation of the patient for lung volume reduction surgery. *Proc Am Thorac Soc.* 2008;5:427-431.

TABLE 87-3 DECISION GUIDE FOR SELECTION OF LUNG VOLUME REDUCTION SURGERY VERSUS TRANSPLANTATION FOR SEVERE CHRONIC OBSTRUCTIVE PULMONARY DISEASE

FACTORS FAVORING LVRS	FACTORS FAVORING TRANSPLANTATION
Age > 65 yr	FEV_1 ≤ 20% predicted
Upper lobe predominant disease	DLCO ≤ 20% predicted
Chronic medical conditions	Homogeneous or lower lobe distribution of disease
Hepatitis B and/or C	TLC < 100% predicted
HIV infection	RV < 150% predicted
Renal insufficiency	$Paco_2$ > 60 mm Hg
Cirrhosis	Pao_2 < 45 mm Hg
Neuropathy	6 MWD < 140 m or <3 min unloaded pedaling cycle ergometer
Poorly controlled diabetes	Pulmonary hypertension
Osteoporosis	Bronchiectasis
Severe GERD	Recurrent pulmonary infections
Poor esophageal motility	
Malignancy	
Unable to maintain long-term follow-up	
Psychiatric issues limiting compliance	
Insufficient social support	

6 MWD = 6-minute walk distance; DLCO = diffusion capacity of carbon monoxide; FEV_1 = first second forced expired volume; GERD = gastroesophageal reflux disease; HIV = human immunodeficiency virus; LVRS = lung volume reduction surgery; RV = residual volume; TLC = total lung capacity.

Adapted from Patel N, DeCamp M, Criner GJ. Lung transplantation and lung volume reduction surgery versus transplantation in chronic obstructive pulmonary disease. *Proc Am Thorac Soc.* 2008;5:447-453.

and a single or dominant bullous lesion with radiographic demonstration of compression of surrounding preserved lung parenchyma. Either excision or plication can remove the bullous lesion.

ENDOSCOPIC MANAGEMENT OF EMPHYSEMA

Endoscopic approaches to lung volume reduction may offer a less invasive way to achieve some of the benefits of surgical lung volume reduction for patients with severe emphysema.[5,6] As with surgical lung volume reduction, the goals of these technologies are to reduce the magnitude of overdistended and poorly perfused lung tissue, thereby increasing elastic recoil, diminishing dynamic hyperinflation, and redistributing airflow to better perfused areas of the lung. Unilateral lobar occlusion with endobronchial valves can significantly improve lung function, exercise capacity, and quality of life in patients who have heterogeneous emphysema with intact interlobar fissures and no interlobar collateral ventilation,[A5-A6] as well as in patients who have homogeneous emphysema without collateral ventilation.[A7-A8] Overall, the preponderance of evidence from randomized trials supports meaningful 1-year symptomatic benefit[A9-A11] but uncertain mortality benefit.[A12]

TABLE 87-4 INDICATIONS AND CONTRAINDICATIONS FOR LUNG TRANSPLANTATION

SINGLE-LUNG TRANSPLANT	PATIENTS (%)	DOUBLE-LUNG TRANSPLANT	PATIENTS (%)
INDICATIONS			
COPD	39	CF, bronchiectasis	26
Pulmonary fibrosis, sarcoid	46	Emphysema	26
α_1-Antitrypsin deficiency	4	α_1-Antitrypsin deficiency	5
PPH, Eisenmenger	1.2	PPH, Eisenmenger	6
CF, bronchiectasis	1.5	Pulmonary fibrosis, sarcoid	30
Retransplantation	5	Retransplantation	3.6
ABSOLUTE CONTRAINDICATIONS			
Untreatable advanced extrapulmonary organ dysfunction (e.g., heart, liver, kidney)			
CAD not amenable to PCI or bypass			
Poor LV function (could consider heart-lung transplantation)			
Malignancy within 2 years (excludes cutaneous squamous or basal cell carcinoma)			
5-year disease-free interval preferred			
Noncurable extrapulmonary infection			
Infection with human immunodeficiency virus			
Hepatitis B antigen positivity			
Hepatitis C with histologic evidence of active liver disease			
Active substance abuse (including cigarettes)			
Severe musculoskeletal disease affecting the thorax			
Documented noncompliance			
Untreatable psychiatric condition that impairs compliance			
Absence of consistent and reliable social support			
RELATIVE CONTRAINDICATIONS			
Physiologic age > 65 yr			
Poor nutritional status (BMI < 18 kg/m²)			
Severe obesity (BMI > 30 kg/m²)			
Symptomatic osteoporosis			
Colonization with highly virulent and/or highly resistant fungi, mycobacteria, or bacteria			
Requirement for invasive ventilation and/or circulatory support			
Uncontrolled chronic medical conditions (e.g., diabetes, hypertension, GERD)			
Severely limited functional status with poor rehabilitation potential			
Psychosocial problems likely to affect the outcome adversely			
High-dose (>20 mg of prednisone daily) corticosteroid use			

BMI = body mass index; CAD = coronary artery disease; CF = cystic fibrosis; COPD = chronic obstructive pulmonary disease; GERD = gastroesophageal reflux disease; LV = left ventricle; PCI = percutaneous coronary intervention; PPH = primary pulmonary hypertension.

Adapted from Weill D, Benden C, Corris PA, et al. A consensus document for the selection of lung transplant candidates: 2014—an update from the Pulmonary Transplantation Council of the International Society for Heart and Lung Transplantation. *J Heart Lung Transplant.* 2015;34:1-15.

LUNG TRANSPLANTATION

More than 160 worldwide lung transplant centers perform nearly 4500 transplantations per year.[7] Lung transplantation is now an accepted therapy for all forms of advanced lung disease.[8] The use of ex vivo perfusion to resuscitate lungs considered unsuitable for transplant by traditional procurement criteria appears to be expanding the availability of donor organs.

The most common indications for transplantation (Table 87-4) are diseases or conditions that share the following features: they produce extreme disability in affected patients, they are unresponsive to medical therapy, and they are responsible for limited life expectancy in affected patients. With the exception of a small number of cases of sarcoidosis and lymphangioleiomyomatosis, the original lung disease does not usually recur after lung transplantation.

TYPES OF PROCEDURES

Currently, four types of lung transplantation procedures are performed. *Bilateral lung transplantation* is performed in a sequential fashion that is functionally equivalent to two single-lung transplantations completed during a single operation, most commonly through a transverse bilateral sternothoracotomy ("clamshell") incision. It is the procedure of choice for patients with bilaterally infected lungs and is also performed in certain patients with emphysema, primary pulmonary hypertension, and other diseases (see Table 87-4). Bilateral transplantation is preferred for nearly all indications because a double-lung recipient can expect a 7.4-year 50% survival compared with 4.6 years for a single-lung recipient. As a result, about 80% of the world's reported lung transplants are now bilateral.

Single-lung transplantation is typically performed through a posterolateral thoracotomy incision. The contralateral lung is not removed, so single-lung transplantation is not appropriate for patients with bilaterally infected lungs (e.g., patients with cystic fibrosis or bronchiectasis) (see Table 87-4).

Heart-lung transplantation is now performed in only about 60 cases per year. It is performed in patients with advanced lung disease and coexistent irreparable cardiac disease, usually associated with fixed pulmonary hypertension, and in those with Eisenmenger syndrome (Chapter 55).

Living donor lobar transplantation involves the removal of a lower lobe from each of two living donors. One is implanted into each hemithorax of the recipient in a manner similar to bilateral lung transplantation.

EVALUATION OF POTENTIAL TRANSPLANT RECIPIENTS

The ideal candidate for lung transplantation has lung disease unresponsive to medical therapy but is in otherwise good health. Patients who experience critical illness as a result of lung disease often have poor nutritional status, coexistent major organ dysfunction, refractory infection, or other contraindications to transplantation. The specific evidence-based recommendations for referral for transplant evaluation vary with the underlying disease.

In the United States, the lung allocation score system is based on expected disease-specific and patient-specific survival during the waiting period and after engraftment, thereby reflecting net transplant benefit. Evaluations of the lung allocation score system, which was introduced in 2005, indicate shorter waiting times, an increase in the total number of transplants performed, a decreased waitlist mortality, and unchanged overall survival after transplantation.

POST-TRANSPLANTATION ISSUES

Most of the medical issues that patients and physicians face after lung transplantation are the consequence of the transplanted lung(s) and post-transplantation medication rather than the underlying disease for which the transplantation was performed. Examples include toxicities of immunosuppression, infections and their prophylaxis, acute allograft rejection, chronic allograft rejection, and nonpulmonary complications of transplantation.

Immunosuppression

The standard chemotherapeutic regimen for immunosuppression after lung transplantation consists of a calcineurin inhibitor such as cyclosporine or tacrolimus, an antimetabolite such as azathioprine or mycophenolate mofetil, and corticosteroids (Chapter 28). More than 50% of centers add a monoclonal or polyclonal antilymphocyte antibody preparation in the first days after transplantation, and this practice has led to a small but statistically significant improvement in long-term survival.

Infections and Prophylaxis after Lung Transplantation

Lung transplant recipients are at high risk for bacterial, viral, fungal, and protozoal infections; infections are the leading causes of death during the early post-transplantation period. In the first 3 months after transplantation, bacterial infections are responsible for most deaths. In approximately one third of patients, pneumonia is diagnosed in the first weeks after transplantation, with gram-negative organisms as the cause in 75% of cases. Colonization and recurrent infections, usually with *Pseudomonas* species, often develop in patients with chronic rejection.

Among potential viral pathogens, *cytomegalovirus* (CMV; Chapter 347) is the most important in lung transplant recipients. Seronegative patients who receive an allograft from a seropositive donor are at particularly high risk for the development of a clinically significant CMV infection. Seronegative patients who have a seronegative donor are at low risk for infection if they are treated with seronegative blood products. Epstein-Barr virus (EBV) has been associated with the development of post-transplantation lymphoproliferative disorder.

Aspergillus species are the most common cause of invasive fungal infection (Chapter 311). Colonized patients and those deemed at risk may receive prophylactic inhaled amphotericin B.

Because of the nature of the immunosuppressive chemotherapeutic regimen used, patients are at high risk for infection by the protozoan *Pneumocystis jirovecii* (Chapter 313). The use of trimethoprim-sulfamethoxazole prophylaxis (typically 1 double-strength tablet three times weekly indefinitely) has virtually eliminated *Pneumocystis* pneumonia.

Acute Rejection

Histologically, the initial manifestation of acute rejection is a lymphocyte-predominant inflammatory response, usually centered on blood vessels, airways, or both. By convention, acute rejection is graded histologically from 0 (normal) to 4 (severe), with subclasses defined by the presence or absence of airway inflammation.

The risk for acute allograft rejection is highest in the early months after transplantation and declines with time. Multiple episodes of acute rejection are the major risk factor for the subsequent development of chronic rejection.

Clinically, patients may have fever, cough, and exertional dyspnea. Evaluation may demonstrate crackles or rhonchi on chest examination, a decline in pulmonary function by spirometry, leukocytosis, opacities on chest radiography, and exertional desaturation. The clinical manifestation is often indistinguishable from infectious pneumonia, and the clinical impression is accurate in only 50% of cases. Histologic confirmation by a transbronchial biopsy is mandatory.

Treatment of acute rejection most often consists of high-dose corticosteroids (typically 500 to 1000 mg/day of methylprednisolone administered intravenously for 3 days).

CHRONIC REJECTION

PATHOBIOLOGY

The bronchiolitis obliterans syndrome, also termed chronic lung allograft dysfunction, is thought to be a manifestation of chronic rejection. Risk factors include the number of acute rejection episodes and, in some series, previous symptomatic CMV infection. Pathologically, "early" lesions demonstrate inflammation and disruption of the epithelium of small airways, followed by growth of granulation tissue into the airway lumen and subsequent complete or partial obstruction. The granulation tissue then organizes in a stereotypical pattern with resultant fibrosis that obliterates the lumen of the airway.

CLINICAL MANIFESTATIONS

Clinically, bronchiolitis obliterans is accompanied by nonspecific symptoms. Progressive exertional breathlessness typically develops, and pulmonary function testing usually demonstrates evidence of progressive airflow obstruction (Chapter 73). Bronchiolitis obliterans is classified according to the FEV_1: 0 (no significant abnormality) if FEV_1 is greater than 80% of baseline, 1 (mild) if FEV_1 is 65 to 80% of baseline, 2 (moderate) if FEV_1 is 50 to 65% of baseline, and 3 (severe) if FEV_1 is 50% or less of baseline. Later stages of bronchiolitis obliterans may include a syndrome of bronchiectasis with chronic productive cough and airway colonization with *Pseudomonas* species.

DIAGNOSIS

The diagnosis of bronchiolitis obliterans or chronic lung allograft dysfunction is made on both clinical and pathologic grounds. Transbronchial biopsy has a low yield for demonstrating histologic evidence of bronchiolitis obliterans, but when such evidence is seen, it is diagnostic. In patients with a compatible clinical syndrome, exclusion of anastomotic stenosis and occult pulmonary infection is sufficient to establish the diagnosis.

TREATMENT

A variety of therapies have been tried for chronic rejection, including pulse corticosteroids, antilymphocyte antibodies, total lymphoid irradiation, photopheresis, and nebulized cyclosporine, but none has been clearly established as effective. Most patients with bronchiolitis obliterans experience a progressive decline in pulmonary function despite immunosuppression.

PROGNOSIS

Bronchiolitis obliterans is the leading cause of late mortality after lung transplantation. Half of lung transplant recipients surviving to 5 years will have either clinically diagnosed or biopsy-proven bronchiolitis obliterans.

Nonpulmonary Medical Complications of Lung Transplantation

Most of the nonpulmonary medical complications that arise in patients after lung transplantation are the result of immunosuppressive therapy.[9] One or more of these complications develop in virtually all lung transplant recipients.

Osteoporosis (Chapter 225) is common because of the long-term use of corticosteroids and cyclosporine. Bone density should be monitored periodically, and pharmacologic therapy should be instituted if excessive bone loss is identified.

Chronic renal insufficiency (Chapter 116) is common and is the result of therapy with the calcineurin inhibitors cyclosporine or tacrolimus, both of which affect afferent vascular tone in the kidneys and result in an average 50% drop in the glomerular filtration rate in the first 12 months after lung transplantation. Systemic arterial hypertension is also common and is caused by corticosteroids and cyclosporine. Calcium-channel blockers, which are often used to treat hypertension, raise serum cyclosporine levels; appropriate monitoring and dose adjustment are needed when starting such therapy. Both corticosteroids and tacrolimus contribute to the development of diabetes mellitus and hyperlipidemia.

Solid organ transplantation is associated with an increased incidence of malignancy, thought to be due to pharmacologic immunosuppression and alteration in immune surveillance. Patients are at increased risk for lymphoproliferative malignancies and other types of cancers. Post-transplantation lymphoproliferative disorders occur in about 4% of patients after organ transplantation; most are associated with EBV. These syndromes can be polyclonal or monoclonal. Reduction in immunosuppression is sometimes therapeutic in those with polyclonal disease. The prognosis in patients with monoclonal disease is poor, with little response to modification of immunosuppression or antineoplastic chemotherapy. Patients are also at increased risk for skin, bladder, lung, cervical, and hepatobiliary malignancy after solid organ transplantation.

Currently, the annual mortality rate following lung transplantation is 7 to 10% per year, largely owing to the bronchiolitis obliterans syndrome. The median survival after lung transplantation averages 6.2 years but varies between 4.8 to 7.8 years[10] depending on both the type of operation performed and the indication for transplant (E-Fig. 87-3).

GENERAL REFERENCES

For the General References and other additional features, please visit Elsevier eBooks+ at https://ebooks.health.elsevier.com.

Grade A References

A1. Goorsenberg AWM, d'Hooghe JNS, Srikanthan K, et al. Bronchial thermoplasty induced airway smooth muscle reduction and clinical response in severe asthma. The TASMA randomized trial. *Am J Respir Crit Care Med.* 2021;203:175-184.

A2. Hallifax RJ, McKeown E, Sivakumar P, et al. Ambulatory management of primary spontaneous pneumothorax: an open-label, randomised controlled trial. *Lancet.* 2020;396:39-49.

A3. Brown SGA, Ball EL, Perrin K. Conservative versus interventional treatment for spontaneous pneumothorax. *N Engl J Med.* 2020;382:405-415.

A4. Van Agteren JE, Carson KV, Tiong LU, et al. Lung volume reduction surgery for diffuse emphysema. *Cochrane Database Syst Rev.* 2016;10:CD001001.

A5. Davey C, Zoumot Z, Jordan S, et al. Bronchoscopic lung volume reduction with endobronchial valves for patients with heterogeneous emphysema and intact interlobar fissures (the BeLieVeR-HIFi study): a randomised controlled trial. *Lancet.* 2015;386:1066-1073.

A6. Klooster K, ten Hacken NH, Hartman JE, et al. Endobronchial valves for emphysema without interlobar collateral ventilation. *N Engl J Med.* 2015;373:2325-2335.

A7. Valipour A, Slebos DJ, Herth F, et al. Endobronchial valve therapy in patients with homogeneous emphysema. Results from the IMPACT study. *Am J Respir Crit Care Med.* 2016;194:1073-1082.

A8. Kemp SV, Slebos DJ, Kirk A, et al. A multicenter randomized controlled trial of zephyr endobronchial valve treatment in heterogeneous emphysema (TRANSFORM). *Am J Respir Crit Care Med.* 2017;196:1535-1543.

A9. Patel M, Chowdhury J, Zhao H, et al. Meta-analysis and systematic review of bronchoscopic lung volume reduction through endobronchial valves in severe emphysema. *J Bronchology Interv Pulmonol.* 2022;29:224-237.

A10. Dransfield MT, Garner JL, Bhatt SP, et al. Effect of Zephyr endobronchial valves on dyspnea, activity levels, and quality of life at one year. Results from a randomized clinical trial. *Ann Am Thorac Soc.* 2020;17:829-838.

A11. Eberhardt R, Slebos DJ, Herth FJ, et al. Endobronchial valve (zephyr) treatment in homogeneous emphysema: one-year results from the IMPACT randomized clinical trial. *Respiration.* 2021;100:1174-1185.

A12. Xu W, Wang J, Xiang H, et al. Bronchoscopic lung volume reduction procedures for emphysema: a network meta-analysis. *Medicine (Baltimore).* 2020;99:e18936.

XI

CRITICAL CARE MEDICINE

88

APPROACH TO THE PATIENT IN A CRITICAL CARE SETTING

DEBORAH J. COOK

THE INTENSIVIST-LED INTERPROFESSIONAL TEAM

Unlike many other specialties, critical care medicine is not limited to a particular population, disease, diagnosis, or organ system. Patients with critical illness in the intensive care unit (ICU) usually require advanced life support, such as invasive or noninvasive mechanical ventilation, vasopressors, inotropic agents, or renal replacement therapy. Morbidity associated with critical illness includes complications of both acute and chronic diseases, nosocomial and iatrogenic consequences, slow recovery, and impaired quality of life among survivors. Patients who are critically ill are at a higher risk of death than any other hospital population. Accordingly, the goals of critical care are to reduce morbidity and mortality, to maintain organ function, and to restore health. The care of surviving critically ill patients often follows a trajectory of resuscitation, stabilization, improvement, and rehabilitation.

One model for staffing of ICUs uses critical care physicians, who are often referred to as *intensivists*, who provide mandatory consultations or principal ongoing care. Specialist care by intensivists is associated with a significantly reduced ICU and hospital mortality and reduced ICU and hospital lengths of stay compared with other staffing models. The addition of nighttime intensivist staffing appears to reduce mortality by about 40% in ICUs with low-intensity daytime staffing but not in centers with high-intensity daytime staffing, such as academic ICUs. These findings emphasize the value of the on-site availability of trained physicians who are dedicated to appropriate triaging, diagnosis, monitoring, treatment, and palliation of critically ill patients.

Daily rounds by an ICU physician who leads the coordinated work of nurses, pharmacists, respiratory therapists, physiotherapists, dietitians, chaplains, and other physicians appear to improve outcomes. Observational studies suggest that a standardized, goal-oriented approach to care delivered by multidisciplinary clinicians, with explicitly defined roles, an interprofessional perspective, and best practices checklists, can help improve the quality of ICU rounds. Critical care can be optimized by interprofessional leadership, communication, and a positive organizational culture.[1] However, although processes of care may be improved by multifaceted quality improvement interventions with explicit-goal setting and daily checklists, such approaches have not been shown to reduce hospital mortality.[A1] Furthermore, ICU admission is not beneficial for all seriously ill patients, and attempts to increase the use of ICUs for frail elderly patients do not necessarily improve outcomes.[A2]

FLUID RESUSCITATION AND ACUTE KIDNEY INJURY

Intravenous fluids to maintain or to restore intravascular volume are an important component of ICU therapy. Both crystalloid and colloid solutions are in widespread use. Crystalloids are readily available and inexpensive, whereas colloids generally require less volume to achieve a specific physiologic goal.[2]

Fluid replacement with either normal saline or 4% albumin results in similar rates of death, organ failure, and other clinical outcomes, but crystalloids may lower mortality for patients with traumatic brain injury (Chapter 368). Fluid management with hydroxyethyl starch increases the need for renal replacement therapy and increases mortality compared with crystalloid infusions. On the basis of these data, either crystalloid- or albumin-based colloid fluid resuscitation is recommended for most critically ill patients, crystalloids are recommended for head-injured patients, and starches are not recommended.

However, crystalloids differ regarding their pH, tonicity, and osmolality. Hypertonic saline is not recommended for general ICU patients. The most commonly used isotonic crystalloid is 0.9% (normal) saline, which contains a supraphysiologic concentration of chloride. Other isotonic crystalloids, referred to as balanced crystalloids, contain an organic anion (e.g., lactate as in Ringer lactate) and, because their lower chloride content resembles that in human plasma, result in lower chloride concentrations and higher base excess. Data from various randomized trials have not shown a significantly lower all-cause mortality, reduction in ventilator-free days, or decrease in the need for renal replacement therapy with the use of balanced crystalloids.[A3-A5]

The early initiation of renal replacement therapy in critically ill patients with acute kidney injury does not reduce mortality compared with standard therapy.[A6,A7] Furthermore, intensive dialytic renal support therapy is no better than standard dialytic therapy, and intermittent hemodialysis and continuous renal replacement therapy lead to similar clinical outcomes in acute renal failure. It also is important to verify that the prescribed dialysis is received and that standardized measures of the intensity of dialysis are achieved. Some patients—especially patients in an increased catabolic state, trauma patients, and patients receiving glucocorticoids—may require dialysis more than three times per week to achieve adequate therapy (Chapter 117). Neither furosemide nor low-dose dopamine infusions improve outcome, even though low-dose dopamine may temporarily improve metrics of renal physiology.

OXYGEN INTUBATION, SEDATION, ANALGESIA

Critically ill patients commonly require high-flow oxygen, noninvasive mechanical ventilation, or invasive mechanical ventilation. In patients with hypoxemic respiratory failure (Chapter 90), high-flow nasal oxygen by cannula is associated with a lower risk of requiring escalation of oxygen therapy or endotracheal intubation compared with conventional oxygen therapy. However, using high-flow nasal oxygen does not reduce length of stay in the ICU or mortality.[A8]

Among critically ill general medical inpatients, oxygen to maintain a median oxyhemoglobin saturation of 96% is preferred to a median saturation below 94% and is associated with lower rates of mortality, shock, liver failure, and bacteremia than values between 97% and 100%.[A9] In patients with acute respiratory failure requiring at least 10 L of oxygen per minute, a target PaO_2 of 60 mm Hg is as good as a target of 90 mm Hg.[A10] In patients with septic shock (Chapter 94), hyperoxia achieved by administration of FIO_2 of 1.0 also may increase the risk of death.[A11]

Endotracheal intubation, central venous catheterization, postoperative pain management, and other ICU procedures typically require that most patients receive sedation, analgesia, or both. Sedatives (e.g., propofol 5 to 50 μg titrated to effect) and analgesics (e.g., hydromorphone, 0.5 to 2 mg loading dose followed by 0.5 to 3 mg/hour titrated to effect) are used to ensure ongoing tolerance to invasive mechanical ventilation, particularly in patients with shock or severe acute respiratory distress syndrome (ARDS). If pain[3] and anxiety can be well treated, bolus injections are preferred to continuous infusions because of emerging concerns about drug accumulation drug-induced delirium and delayed weaning from the ventilator. Co-analgesics (e.g., acetaminophen up to 3 g/day assuming normal hepatic function) can provide cost-effective pain control and decrease exposure to opiates in critically ill patients.[A12] If patients are receiving drug infusions, daily interruption of sedatives and analgesics, by protocols that provide an opportunity for the patient to be observed safely in a less sedated state, are associated with a shorter duration of mechanical ventilation and ICU length of stay than continuous infusions. A second key component of managing sedation and analgesia is to use a drug titration protocol and nurse-led sedation scale; in these situations, daily interruption of sedation infusions may confer no additional benefit.

Discontinuation of ventilation is affected by sedation and analgesic infusions and vice versa. A daily sedation vacation followed by a spontaneous breathing test increases the days of breathing without assistance and shortens ICU stay and hospital stay compared with usual sedation management plus a daily spontaneous breathing test. In the year after enrollment, patients who were treated with a "wake up and breathe" protocol, which linked daily sedation vacation periods with daily spontaneous breathing trials, had a 32% better survival rate. On the basis of these data, a nurse-implemented sedation and analgesic management scale with daily drug interruption and daily spontaneous breathing trials is recommended for mechanically ventilated critically ill patients.

Following endotracheal extubation, high-flow oxygen via a nasal cannula decreases the risk of reintubation and postextubation respiratory failure compared with conventional oxygen therapy, but it does not decrease ICU length of stay or mortality.[A13]

LONG-TERM OUTCOMES FOR SURVIVORS

Biomarkers of inflammation, residual organ dysfunction, and functional disabilities persist in most ICU survivors even after transfer out of the ICU. Treatments administered in the ICU also have serious sequelae. For example, neuromuscular blockers and corticosteroids may contribute to critical illness polyneuropathy. These problems have particularly serious adverse consequences for frail patients who are deconditioned before hospitalization.

Although highly selected patients may be discharged home directly from intensive care,[4] the large majority of patients require further hospital care. Although ICU discharge and hospital discharge are milestones in a patient's trajectory, sequelae of critical illness have rarely resolved completely when patients are on the regular hospital unit. For example, over 50% of survivors have new physical, mental, or cognitive problems 1 year after admission,[5] and their caregivers are at risk for anxiety and mood disorders. Residual muscle weakness is common, even 5 years after ICU discharge.

APPLYING EVIDENCE TO PREVENT COMPLICATIONS OF CRITICAL ILLNESS

About 50% of ICU patients have suspected or proven infection. An ICU-acquired infection increases mortality rates by about 30% compared with community-acquired infection.[6] The Surviving Sepsis Campaign has developed evidence-based guidelines that are periodically updated to incorporate recent literature.[7] The proactive implementation of these performance-based improvement strategies at the systems level is associated with better outcomes and lower costs. Evidence-based initial management of a patient with sepsis (Chapter 94) and ARDS (Chapter 90) includes rapid administration of antimicrobial agents when infection is suspected, a target mean arterial pressure of greater than 65 mm Hg,[A14] initial resuscitation with crystalloids, avoidance of starches for resuscitation, initial inotrope infusion of norepinephrine, and corticosteroids for refractory shock.[A15] For patients who are endotracheally intubated, other proven management strategies include low tidal volume ventilation, targeting low plateau pressures below 30 mm H_2O (Chapter 91), head of bed elevation, early enteral small bowel nutrition (Chapter 198), oral antisepsis with chlorhexidine (Chapter 261), thromboprophylaxis with low-molecular-weight heparin (Table 70-3), and insulin therapy aimed at avoiding marked hyperglycemia but not achieving normoglycemia (Chapters 90 and 91). Treatment should avoid early high-frequency oscillation, high positive end-expiratory pressure (unless patients have ARDS), routine use of paralytic agents (Chapter 90),[A16] and antioxidants. Stress ulcer prophylaxis (e.g., pantoprazole 40 mg intravenously daily) can reduce the risk of gastrointestinal bleeding but not overall complications or mortality.[A17] Antimicrobial stewardship is important to reduce the risk of nosocomial infection (Chapter 261) and renal injury.[8]

In mechanically ventilated adults, a strategy of obtaining chest radiographs based on clinical need provides clinical outcomes equivalent to a strategy of routine radiographs, despite about one-third fewer radiographs. Later during the stabilization and recovery phase of critical illness, evidence-based management includes targeted protocol-driven sedation, daily interruption of sedation infusions, and daily spontaneous breathing trials. Low-dose (starting at 0.2 μg/kg/hour and titrated to sedation and agitation) nocturnal intravenous dexmedetomidine can help prevent ICU delirium.[A18]

Neuromuscular weakness is a common complication of ICU care.[9] Physical rehabilitation interventions delivered in the ICU can hasten and improve overall recovery in some patients but have not been shown to reduce mortality. Active mobilization and rehabilitation improves muscle strength at ICU discharge, the probability of walking without assistance at hospital discharge, and the number of days alive and out of the hospital; however, it does not improve quality of life, reduce the duration of mechanical ventilation or length of stay in the ICU or hospital, or change the discharge destination.[A19]

Potential barriers to applying evidence in fast-paced ICUs include a perceived lack of responsibility, unclear decisional authority, and errors of omission. Passive dissemination of information, whether written or verbal, is generally ineffective in modifying physicians' behaviors. More effective strategies to encourage the implementation of evidence-based recommendations are interactive education, audit and feedback, reminders (written or computerized), involvement of local opinion leaders, and multifaceted approaches. In the high-acuity ICU setting, preprinted physician orders may help guide (but not dictate) management (Table 88-1). For example, a statewide intervention coached local safety teams to lead multidisciplinary education about central venous catheter management strategies known to decrease infection risk, including a procedural checklist that incorporated handwashing, full barrier precautions for catheter insertion, chlorhexidine skin cleansing, avoidance of the femoral site, and removal of unnecessary catheters. A multimethod approach including video conferencing, education, provision of algorithms, audit, and feedback can increase adoption of beneficial management strategies in community ICUs.

TABLE 88-1 ICU ADMISSION ORDERS: EXAMPLE FOR A PATIENT WITH UROSEPSIS AND ARDS

MANAGEMENT STRATEGY	ORDERS	REEVALUATE
ACUTE PHASE		
Mechanical ventilation	Target TV 5-7 mL/kg of ideal body weight, PC 16 cm, rate 12, FIO_2 0.7, PEEP 16 cm, plateau pressure <35 cm	PRN
Maintenance fluid	Lactated Ringer 75 mL/hr IV	PRN
Norepinephrine	Titrate to mean arterial pressure >65 mm Hg	PRN
Corticosteroids	Hydrocortisone 50 mg IV q6h while vasopressor dependent	Daily
Sedation	Midazolam 2-8 mg/hr IV, bolus 2-4 mg PRN	PRN
Analgesia	Morphine 1-4 mg IV PRN	PRN
Red blood cell transfusion	Transfuse 1 unit of packed red blood cells if hemoglobin <70 g/L	PRN
Antibiotics	Ampicillin 2 g IV q6h	Daily
Head of bed	45-Degree elevation from horizontal	PRN
Oral antisepsis	Chlorhexidine 15 mL q6h	Daily
Enteral nutrition	10 mL/hr of a commercial balanced feed containing about 1 kcal/mL; increase by 20 mL q4h to 70 mL/hr as tolerated	Daily
Bowel protocol	Individualized for constipation management	PRN
Stress ulcer prophylaxis	Pantoprazole 40 mg IV daily	Daily
Thromboprophylaxis	Dalteparin 5000 U SQ daily	Daily
Intensive insulin therapy if blood glucose >180 mg/dL	50 U insulin in 50 mL NS; start at 0.5 U/hour, repeat glucose q1h for 4 hours, and reassess; target 110-150 mg/dL	Daily
Glucometer calibration	Calibrate glucose from glucometer and central laboratory every morning	Daily
Tests	Glucose q4h when stable, ABG with each ventilator change, other tests as per ICU team	PRN
Monitoring	Arterial catheter for systolic blood pressure, central venous catheter for central venous pressure and mixed venous oxygen saturation, ECG, oximetry, ABGs, sedation scale, Foley catheter, others as per ICU monitoring protocols	PRN
STABILIZATION AND RECOVERY PHASES		
Sedation vacation	Daily interruption of sedation from 7 AM until 9 AM; restart at half prior infusion rate at 9 AM if necessary; aim to discontinue infusion as soon as possible	Daily
Spontaneous breathing trials	Spontaneous breathing trial when weaning readiness criteria met	Daily
Early mobility	Individualized, graduated physiotherapy and occupational therapy	Daily

ABG = arterial blood gas; ARDS = acute respiratory distress syndrome; ECG = electrocardiogram; FIO_2 = fraction of inspired oxygen; ICU = intensive care unit; IV = intravenous; NS = normal saline; PC = pressure control; PEEP = positive end-expiratory pressure; PRN = as needed; SQ = subcutaneous; TV = tidal volume.

PREDICTIONS, PREFERENCES, AND PALLIATIVE CARE

The prognosis of many critically ill patients improves once they are in the ICU. For others, treatment responsiveness is delayed or not realized, organ dysfunction evolves but does not resolve, and complications arise. Despite best efforts of the multidisciplinary ICU team, critical illness proves fatal to between 5% and 40% of adults. Approximately 2% of ICU patients discharged to a general inpatient service are readmitted to an ICU within 48 hours and about 4% within 120 hours. When a therapeutic trial of critical care is started, and particularly when it is failing, it is crucial to discuss prognosis openly with families (Chapter 3). Among medical ICU patients older than 80 years at one tertiary care university hospital, ICU mortality was 46%, hospital mortality was 55%, and mortality among hospital survivors was 53% at 2 years. About 15% of patients who are admitted to an ICU have clinical courses that probably should generate discussion about palliative care. Families bring key information about the patient's prior function and preferences.

In the shared decision-making model dominant in many settings today, these exchanges often result in plans to withhold or to withdraw basic or advanced life support. Physicians and the entire health care team must be well trained to discuss prognosis with surrogate decision-makers, to address requests for potentially inappropriate therapies, and to manage any resulting discordance. Mechanical ventilation is the most frequent life support administered to and withdrawn from critically ill patients. Ventilator withdrawal very often precedes death in the ICU. Patients undergoing ventilator withdrawal or who die while mechanically ventilated have a shorter ICU stay than patients successfully weaned from the ventilator. When life support modalities are withdrawn because their further use would be futile, each can be discontinued or weaned, with attendant considerations and cautions (Table 88-2 and E-Table 88-1).

TABLE 88-2 CONSIDERATIONS AND CAUTIONS IN THE WITHDRAWAL OF LIFE SUPPORT

ISSUE	RISKS	OTHER CONSIDERATIONS
Weaning from inotropes or vasopressors	No risk of physical distress	May prolong the dying process, particularly if patient requires low doses and this is the only life support withdrawn
Discontinuation of inotropes or vasopressors	No risk of physical distress	Death may not occur quickly if the patient requires low doses, particularly if mechanical ventilation is ongoing Death may occur quickly if the patient requires high doses, with or without withdrawal of mechanical ventilation
Weaning from mechanical ventilation	Low risk of dyspnea	May prolong the dying process, particularly if the patient requires low pressure settings or low oxygen levels and this is the only life support withdrawn
Discontinuation of mechanical ventilation	Risk of dyspnea	Death may not occur quickly if the patient requires low pressure settings or low oxygen levels Death may occur quickly if the patient requires high pressure settings or high oxygen levels Preemptive sedation is typically needed to blunt air hunger due to rapid changes in mechanical ventilation
Extubation	Risk of dyspnea Risk of stridor (steroids) Risk of airway obstruction (jaw thrust) Risk of noisy breathing (glycopyrrolate)	Avoids discomfort and suctioning of endotracheal tube Can facilitate oral communication Informing families about possible physical signs after extubation can prepare and reassure them Allows for the most natural appearance Not advised if the patient has hemoptysis
Discontinuation of renal replacement therapy	Low risk of physical distress	Death may take several days if this is the only advanced life support withdrawn

Reprinted with permission from Cook D, Rocker G. Dying with dignity in the intensive care unit. *N Engl J Med.* 2014;370:2506-2514. Copyright © 2014 Massachusetts Medical Society.

Withdrawal may be guided by the severity of the illness and other physiological characteristics, but it is more heavily influenced by the contemporary life support model that is attentive to a patient's values and the physician's predictions about future quality of life. A patient's status at ICU discharge, particularly orders to limit subsequent medical therapy, is the major predictor of hospital survival. This complexity underscores the need for ICU teams to be expert communicators, sensitive in eliciting patients' preferences (often through family members), timely in relieving suffering, and compassionate in providing dignity to the dying. In today's pluralistic society, administering culturally competent, patient-centered, and family-centered end-of-life care, including respect and expressions of spirituality, is paramount. During the coronavirus disease 2019 (COVID-19) pandemic, this holistic approach to family-centered end-of-life care was particularly challenged by severe restrictions on visitors. Family-support interventions also can reduce ICU length of stay.[A20] A death with dignity in the ICU infers that whereas some treatments may be foregone, care can be enhanced as death ensues. Fundamental to maintaining dignity is the need to understand a patient's unique perspectives on what gives life meaning in a setting replete with depersonalizing devices. The goal is caring for patients in a manner consistent with their age,[10] comorbid conditions, and values at a time of incomparable vulnerability, when they cannot speak for themselves.[11] For patients who are unrepresented (i.e., they lack capacity, do not have an advance directive, do not have an available surrogate decision-maker), a multidisciplinary committee rather than the treating physicians should guide end-of-life care.[12]

GENERAL REFERENCES

For the General References and other additional features, please visit Elsevier eBooks+ at https://ebooks.health.elsevier.com.

Grade A References

A1. Cavalcanti AB, Bozza FA, Machado FR, et al. Effect of a quality improvement intervention with daily round checklists, goal setting, and clinician prompting on mortality of critically ill patients: a randomized clinical trial. *JAMA.* 2016;315:1480-1490.

A2. Guidet B, Leblanc G, Simon T, et al. Effect of systematic intensive care unit triage on long-term mortality among critically ill elderly patients in France: a randomized clinical trial. *JAMA.* 2017;318:1450-1459.

A3. Finfer S, Micallef S, Hammond N, et al. Balanced multielectrolyte solution versus saline in critically ill adults. *N Engl J Med.* 2022;386:815-826.

A4. Semler MW, Self WH, Wanderer JP, et al. Balanced crystalloids versus saline in critically ill adults. *N Engl J Med.* 2018;378:829-839.

A5. Zampieri FG, Machado FR, Biondi RS, et al. Effect of slower vs faster intravenous fluid bolus rates on mortality in critically ill patients: the BaSICS randomized clinical trial. *JAMA.* 2021;326:830-838.

A6. Yang XM, Tu GW, Zheng JL, et al. A comparison of early versus late initiation of renal replacement therapy for acute kidney injury in critically ill patients: an updated systematic review and meta-analysis of randomized controlled trials. *BMC Nephrol.* 2017;18:1-14.

A7. STARRT-AKI Investigators, Canadian Critical Care Trials Group, Australian and New Zealand Intensive Care Society Clinical Trials Group, et al. Timing of initiation of renal-replacement therapy in acute kidney injury. *N Engl J Med.* 2020;383:240-251.

A8. Rochwerg B, Granton D, Wang X, et al. High flow nasal cannula compared with conventional oxygen therapy for acute hypoxemic respiratory failure: a systematic review and meta-analysis. *Intensive Care Med.* 2019;45:563-572.

A9. Chu DK, Kim LH, Young PJ, et al. Mortality and morbidity in acutely ill adults treated with liberal versus conservative oxygen therapy (IOTA): a systematic review and meta-analysis. *Lancet.* 2018;391:1693-1705.

A10. Schjørring OL, Klitgaard TL, Perner A, et al. Lower or higher oxygenation targets for acute hypoxemic respiratory failure. *N Engl J Med.* 2021;384:1301-1311.

A11. Asfar P, Schortgen F, Boisrame-Helms J, et al. Hyperoxia and hypertonic saline in patients with septic shock (HYPERS2S): a two-by-two factorial, multicentre, randomized, clinical trial. *Lancet Respir Med.* 2017;5:180-190.

A12. Wheeler KE, Grilli R, Centofanti JE, et al. Adjuvant analgesic use in the critically ill: a systematic review and meta-analysis. *Crit Care Explor.* 2020;2:e0157.

A13. Granton D, Chaudhuri D, Wang D, et al. High-flow nasal cannula compared with conventional oxygen therapy or noninvasive ventilation immediately postextubation: a systematic review and meta-analysis. *Crit Care Med.* 2020;48:e1129-e1136.

A14. Lamontagne F, Richards-Belle A, Thomas K, et al. Effect of reduced exposure to vasopressors on 90-day mortality in older critically ill patients with vasodilatory hypotension: a randomized clinical trial. *JAMA.* 2020;323:938-949.

A15. Rochwerg B, Oczkowski SJ, Siemieniuk RAC, et al. Corticosteroids in sepsis: an updated systematic review and meta-analysis. *Crit Care Med.* 2018;46:1411-1420.

A16. National Heart, Lung, Blood Institute PETAL Clinical Trials Network, Moss M, Huang DT, et al. Early neuromuscular blockade in the acute respiratory distress syndrome. *N Engl J Med.* 2019;380:1997-2008.

A17. Krag M, Marker S, Perner A, et al. Pantoprazole in patients at risk for gastrointestinal bleeding in the ICU. *N Engl J Med.* 2018;379:2199-2208.

A18. Skrobik Y, Duprey MS, Hill NS, et al. Low-dose nocturnal dexmedetomidine prevents ICU delirium. A randomized, placebo-controlled trial. *Am J Respir Crit Care Med.* 2018;197:1147-1156.

A19. Tipping CJ, Harrold M, Holland A, et al. The effects of active rehabilitation in ICU on mortality and function: a systematic review. *Intensive Care Med.* 2017;43:171-183.

A20. White DB, Angus DC, Shields AM, et al. A randomized trial of a family-support intervention in intensive care units. *N Engl J Med.* 2018;378:2365-2375.

89

RESPIRATORY MONITORING IN CRITICAL CARE

JAMES K. STOLLER AND NICHOLAS S. HILL

PHYSICAL EXAMINATION

The physical examination can provide important information about the patient's ventilation and oxygenation. Ventilation can be assessed by recording the respiratory rate (normally 12 to 20 breaths/minute in adults) as well as by closely inspecting the pattern of chest wall movement during inspiration and by noting the use of accessory inspiratory muscles (e.g., the scalene, trapezius, and sternocleidomastoid muscles). Hypopnea (shallow or slow breathing) or a slowed respiratory rate (bradypnea) can indicate decreased ventilation. Shallow breathing may relate to muscle weakness (Chapter 389) or increased lung stiffness, which is commonly accompanied by a compensatory increase in the respiratory rate to maintain ventilation. Bradypnea may relate to a suppressed respiratory drive (e.g., excessive use of narcotics, slowing the respiratory rate). Conversely, sustained tachypnea (e.g., >35 breaths/minute in an adult) can indicate ongoing increased work of breathing, impending respiratory failure, and the need for mechanical assistance, such as noninvasive ventilation or intubation and mechanical ventilation, depending on the etiology of the respiratory failure.

Contraction of the sternocleidomastoid muscles or scalene muscles, often with a seated, bent posture, is called the tripod sign (E-Fig. 89-1). This response indicates inadequate diaphragmatic function, most commonly in the setting of emphysema with associated diaphragmatic flattening, which causes a mechanical disadvantage of diaphragmatic contraction. In this circumstance, patients may demonstrate Hoover sign, which is inspiratory retraction of the rib cage at the level of the zone of apposition, where the diaphragm inserts on the chest wall.

The physical examination of the nail beds and lips may also reveal cyanosis, which suggests hypoxemia. Cyanosis occurs when saturation falls, but it requires the presence of 5 g of desaturated hemoglobin. As such, polycythemic patients may show cyanosis with relatively high oxyhemoglobin saturation values, whereas patients with profound anemia may not demonstrate cyanosis even in the face of low values of oxyhemoglobin saturation.

SYSTEMIC ARTERIAL BLOOD GAS ANALYSIS

Sampling of arterial blood, either through a percutaneous arterial puncture or by withdrawal of blood from an indwelling arterial catheter, provides important information about the patient's oxygenation and ventilation status as well as the acuity of and compensation for derangements. The partial pressure of carbon dioxide ($Paco_2$) reflects ventilation, the elimination of carbon dioxide. In many but not all cases, $Paco_2$ is close to the mixed alveolar $Paco_2$. The $Paco_2$ in the arterial blood is closely related to the ratio of metabolic carbon dioxide production to alveolar ventilation:

$$Paco_2 = (K)(CO_2 \text{ production rate})/(\text{alveolar ventilation } [V_A]) \quad (1)$$

The partial pressure of oxygen (Pao_2) reflects the level of oxygenation. Normal levels of oxygenation are defined by the alveolar-arterial oxygen gradient, $P(A\text{-}a)o_2$, which is calculated as

$$P(A\text{-}a)o_2 = Fio_2(P_B - P_{H_2O} \text{ at standard pressure and body temperature}) - (Pao_2 + Paco_2/\text{respiratory quotient}) \quad (2)$$

where the respiratory quotient equals the number of moles of carbon dioxide produced for each mole of oxygen consumed (generally ~0.8 under normal metabolic conditions at rest but variable with dietary intake and metabolic rate). The normal value of the alveolar-arterial oxygen gradient varies with age and position and can be approximated by the simple equation

$$P(A\text{-}a)o_2 = (\text{age}/4) + 4 \quad (3)$$

Normal age-related values of Pao_2 in the sitting position can be determined by the equation

$$Pao_2 \text{ sitting} = 104.2 - (0.27 \times \text{age in years}) \quad (4)$$

Normal values of Pao_2 are generally in the range of 70 to 95 mm Hg, depending on the patient's age. Nevertheless, a goal of a Pao_2 of 60 mm Hg is as good as a goal of 90 mm Hg in intensive care unit (ICU) patients who have acute hypoxemic respiratory failure that requires at least 10 liters of oxygen per minute.[A1]

The $Paco_2$ helps assess the adequacy of the patient's ventilation. At sea level, normal values of $Paco_2$ range from 35 to 45 mm Hg. Values of $Paco_2$ below 35 mm Hg indicate hyperventilation, either as a primary respiratory event (e.g., with anxiety) or in response to another insult (e.g., hypoxemia, sepsis, liver disease). Similarly, values of $Paco_2$ exceeding 45 mm Hg indicate hypoventilation, hypercapnia, and respiratory acidosis, which may result either from suppression of the ventilatory drive (Chapter 74) (e.g., excess narcotics; Chapter 365) or from respiratory insufficiency (e.g., respiratory muscle weakness; Chapter 389).

Assessment of the patient's bicarbonate level (HCO_3^-) helps define the chronicity of changes in the patient's $Paco_2$, where the value of bicarbonate is defined by the Henderson-Hasselbalch equation:

$$pH = 6.1 + \log_{10}[HCO_3^-]/0.003\,Paco_2 \quad (5)$$

Acute increases in $Paco_2$ drive the normal kidney to retain bicarbonate (Chapter 104), whereas acute decreases in $Paco_2$, as in hyperventilation from anxiety or liver disease, would be expected to cause the normal kidney to waste bicarbonate to preserve the body's pH (normally 7.35 to 7.45).

The clinician can also assess whether the patient's ventilatory response to metabolic acidosis is appropriate or inadequate by the Winter equation, which predicts the expected $Paco_2$ in the face of a decreased bicarbonate from a metabolic acidosis (Eq. 6). Specifically, a measured $Paco_2$ above the expected value indicates an inadequate ventilatory response, whereas a value of $Paco_2$ that falls within the expected range indicates an expected, appropriate ventilatory response to the metabolic derangement (i.e., the acidosis).

$$Paco_2 = (1.5[HCO_3^-] + 8) \pm 2 \quad (6)$$

When the patient is hypercapnic and hypoxemic, a useful step is to calculate the ambient air $P(A\text{-}a)o_2$ and to determine whether it is normal or increased for the patient's age. Of the six mechanisms of hypoxemia, only two (hypoventilation and breathing decreased ambient oxygen, as at altitude or from a hypoxic gas mixture) are associated with a preserved $P(A\text{-}a)o_2$ (Table 89-1). Under clinical circumstances at sea level, hypoxemia in the face of a normal $P(A\text{-}a)o_2$ indicates that the patient's hypoxemia is caused by hypoventilation and should prompt the clinician to consider the various causes of suppressed respiratory drive (Chapter 74) or respiratory insufficiency that interferes with a normal ventilatory response (e.g., respiratory muscle weakness; Chapter 389).[1]

Increasingly, venous blood gases (VBGs) are being used instead of arterial blood gases (ABGs) because they are easier and safer to obtain.[2] Peripheral venous blood may be used, but central VBGs are considered more accurate. The correlation with arterial pH has been good, with venous pH averaging about 0.03 lower; $Pvco_2$ and $Paco_2$ correlate less well, with $Pvco_2$ averaging 3 to 8 mm Hg higher and not being reliably comparable to $Paco_2$. VBGs are considered unacceptably inaccurate in hypotensive patients and patients with severe hypercapnia, but a normal $Pvco_2$ may be used to exclude hypercapnia.

TABLE 89-1 PHYSIOLOGIC MECHANISMS OF HYPOXEMIA AND ACCOMPANYING VALUES OF THE ALVEOLAR-ARTERIAL OXYGEN GRADIENT ON BREATHING OF ROOM AIR

MECHANISM/ PHYSIOLOGIC PROCESS	EXAMPLE	ALVEOLAR-ARTERIAL OXYGEN GRADIENT ON ROOM AIR
Ventilation-perfusion mismatch	Pneumonia	Increased
Diffusion impairment	Interstitial lung disease	Increased
Anatomic right-to-left shunt	Pulmonary arteriovenous malformation	Increased
Hypoventilation	Neuromuscular weakness	Normal
Breathing decreased ambient oxygen (from either hypobaric conditions [e.g., altitude] or breathing a gas mixture with decreased inspired oxygen fraction)	Altitude exposure	Normal
Diffusion-perfusion impairment	Hepatopulmonary syndrome	Increased

PULSE OXIMETRY

Pulse oximetry is a noninvasive method to assess arterial blood oxygenation.[3] The percentage of hemoglobin that is oxygenated is measured by passing light of two different wavelengths (660 nm [for deoxyhemoglobin] and 940 nm [for oxyhemoglobin]) through a blood-carrying tissue (e.g., finger, earlobe, forehead), identifying the pulsatile component (which contains arterial blood and background tissue elements), and subtracting the nonpulsatile component to isolate the arterial component. The device can estimate the percentage of oxygenated hemoglobin over the range of 100% to about 75%. By comparison smart phone pulse oximeters have, to date, been unreliable.[4]

Clinicians must be aware of the diagnostic accuracy of pulse oximetry in assessing hypoxemia and, in particular, the risk that pulse oximetry measurements may overestimate true arterial oxygenation. In one large series of over 48,000 paired measurements of pulse oximetry and arterial blood gases, the prevalence of "occult hypoxemia" (i.e., a pulse oximetry measurement of 92% to 96% with a paired arterial oxygen saturation of <88%) was more frequent among Black individuals (12% to 17%) than among White individuals (3.6% to 6.2%), apparently because darker skin affects the accuracy of the devices. Blue or green nail polish may have the same effect.[5,6] Thus, clinicians must remain vigilant for hypoxemia even when pulse oximetry measurements appear acceptable, especially in Black patients. Concern about occult hypoxemia should prompt obtaining an arterial blood gas.

Most clinicians also regard the output of pulse oximeters to be inaccurate for percentage saturation values of less than 70%, although the probability of a low saturation should not be discounted (Fig. 89-1). Pulse oximetry measurements may help identify significant drops in PaO_2 below 60 to 65 mm Hg but are relatively insensitive to changes in PaO_2 from 90 to 65 mm Hg.

Prolonged hypoxemic episodes are common in postoperative patients after noncardiac surgery, but it is not clear whether routine continuous monitoring will improve clinical outcomes. Similarly, the true value of pulse oximetry for decision making in the emergency department setting remains uncertain, although even asymptomatic hypoxemia by pulse oximetry appears to be a poor prognostic sign in patients with coronavirus disease 2019 (COVID-19).[7] When patients are markedly tachypneic, a reasonably normal pulse oximetry should not be reassuring because of the patient's difficulty in maintaining oxygenation.

CARBON DIOXIDE MONITORING: CAPNOMETRY AND TRANSCUTANEOUS CARBON DIOXIDE MEASUREMENT

The fraction of carbon dioxide in exhaled air can be measured in real time by infrared capnometry.[8] Partial pressures can then be calculated on the basis of knowledge of atmospheric pressure. The expiratory capnogram (E-Fig. 89-2) represents a continuous plot of exhaled PCO_2 versus time or exhaled volume and reflects the sequential appearance of gas from various compartments (e.g., the endotracheal tube, central airways, and finally the alveoli, where the PCO_2 is in equilibrium with end-capillary blood). The shape of the capnogram provides clues to the presence of chronic obstructive pulmonary disease, in that emptying of areas of lung with increased dead space (see later) can cause the capnogram to have a rising contour (E-Fig. 89-2A), whereas the attainment of a so-called alveolar plateau on the normal capnogram (E-Fig. 89-2B) indicates that alveolar gas is composed of a mix with a relatively small contribution from areas of increased dead space. The value of $PECO_2$ measured at the end of expiration on the capnometer (i.e., the highest value recorded) represents the end-tidal $PETCO_2$. Notably, the value of $PETCO_2$ is always below the $PaCO_2$ because there is a normal component of dead space ventilation (VD/VT) related to the anatomic dead space of the conducting airways (i.e., the trachea and airways to the level of gas-exchanging alveolar ducts and alveoli). The numeric difference between the $PaCO_2$ and the mixed exhaled carbon dioxide tension ($PECO_2$, defined as the partial pressure of carbon dioxide that would be measured in a balloon in which the entire exhaled volume is gathered) is related to the magnitude of dead space ventilation (i.e., areas of the lung that are ventilated without accompanying blood flow, normally ~0.3 to 0.4) as defined by the Bohr equation:

$$VD/VT = (PaCO_2 - PECO_2)/PaCO_2 \qquad (7)$$

The difference between $PaCO_2$ and $PECO_2$ may be as low as several millimeters of mercury, but changing conditions of ventilation-perfusion matching (e.g., with pulmonary embolism [Chapter 68], atelectasis [Chapter 78]) may change the gradient over time. Measurement of the $PETCO_2$ can be clinically useful to assess trends, to help detect esophageal intubation, to detect disconnection from the ventilator, and to detect perfusion during cardiopulmonary resuscitation, but it is not a reliable surrogate for $PaCO_2$. Furthermore, measurement of the dead space fraction has prognostic value in patients with early acute respiratory distress syndrome (Chapter 90), in whom rising dead space is linearly related to increased mortality risk. Measurement of transcutaneous PCO_2 by heated probes applied to the skin is an alternative noninvasive method for estimating PCO_2, especially during anesthesia or sleep studies. However, these measures are not reliable for determining absolute values or trends in ICU settings, where patients are unstable hemodynamically or have respiratory failure owing to parenchymal lung disease.

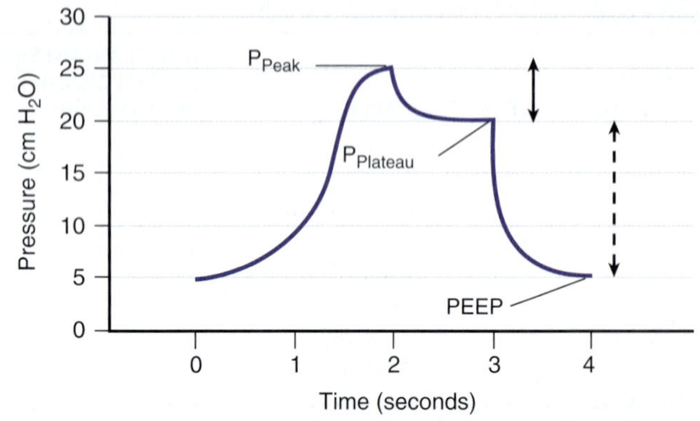

FIGURE 89-1. Illustration of inspiratory hold maneuver to determine plateau pressure ($P_{plateau}$). Airway pressure during volume-targeted mechanical ventilation rises as the tidal volume is delivered and reaches a peak. An inspiratory hold is initiated at peak pressure that prevents exhalation, so pressure falls to a "plateau" of about 20 cm H_2O. The drop in pressure reflects the pressure needed to overcome airway resistance. After slightly more than 1 second, the inspiratory hold is released, and airway pressure falls to positive end-expiratory pressure (PEEP). The difference between $P_{plateau}$ and PEEP is used to calculate static compliance by dividing the difference into the tidal volume.

ARTERIAL OXYGEN CONTENT AND SYSTEMIC OXYGEN DELIVERY

Arterial (CaO_2) and venous oxygen content (CvO_2) are used to calculate cardiac output by the Fick equation (Eq. 8), which is an alternative to determining cardiac output by the thermodilution method with a flow-directed pulmonary artery (Swan-Ganz) catheter (Chapter 59). The Fick equation is

$$\text{Oxygen consumption (mL } O_2/\text{min)} = \text{cardiac output} \times (CaO_2 - CvO_2) \qquad (8)$$

where oxygen content (C) has the units of milliliters of oxygen per 100 mL of blood and hemoglobin units are grams per 100 mL of blood, and is calculated as:

$$\text{Oxygen content} = 1.34\,(\text{hemoglobin})(\%\ \text{saturation}) + 0.0031(PaO_2) \qquad (9)$$

Under normal conditions (with, for example, an arterial percentage saturation of 95% and a hemoglobin level of 15 g/100 mL and an oxygen consumption of 250 mL/minute), arterial oxygen content is about 20 mL/100 mL, and because mixed venous oxygen saturation is about 75%, central venous oxygen content is about 15 mL/100 mL, making the normal arteriovenous oxygen content difference with a normal cardiac output about 5 mL/100 mL.

Systemic oxygen transport defines the amount of oxygen delivered to the tissues and multiplies the arterial oxygen content by the cardiac output:

$$\text{Systemic oxygen transport (mL/min)} = \text{cardiac output} \times CaO_2 \qquad (10)$$

where the normal value is about 1000 mL/minute.

MEASURING VENTILATION: MINUTE VENTILATION AND ALVEOLAR VENTILATION

Minute ventilation ($\dot{V}E$), which is the amount of gas exhaled from the airway per minute, is the product of the respiratory rate times the exhaled tidal volume, measured at body temperature and standardized to barometric pressure at sea level, saturated with water vapor (BTPS). The BTPS is a standard condition under which many measurements for most pulmonary function equipment and mechanical ventilators are made. These devices use an airflow meter to measure exhaled airflow and integrate the signal to derive tidal volume. An alternative way to measure tidal volume in an intensive care setting is respiratory impedance plethysmography, which uses calibrated magnetic coils in belts strapped around the chest and abdomen to monitor respiratory frequency and changes in thoracic volume.

Alveolar ventilation is the rate of gas delivery in liters per minute to gas-exchanging areas of the lung (i.e., the alveoli and alveolar ducts). The portion of minute ventilation that fails to undergo gas exchange is dead space ventilation ($\dot{V}D$) and is determined by Eq. 7. Minute, alveolar ($\dot{V}A$), and dead space ventilation are related as follows:

$$\dot{V}E = \dot{V}A + \dot{V}D \qquad (11)$$

It follows that conditions such as acute lung injury and acute respiratory distress syndrome (ARDS; Chapter 90) that are associated with very high dead space ratios require high VE to achieve a sufficient VA. Conversely, conditions that cause neuromuscular weakness (Chapter 389) are associated with small tidal volumes and have a high VD/VT ratio because the anatomic dead space is fixed and constitutes a higher fraction of the diminished tidal volume.

MEASURING CARBON DIOXIDE PRODUCTION

Measurement of carbon dioxide production is sometimes referred to as indirect calorimetry because it provides an index of metabolic rate and permits estimation of calorie requirements. Metabolic "carts" that simultaneously measure not only carbon dioxide production but also oxygen consumption and respiratory quotient are commonly used clinically to estimate metabolic needs to prescribe nutritional repletion (Chapter 198). The normal baseline carbon dioxide production is in the range of 200 mL/minute but is subject to wide variation because of hypermetabolic states commonly encountered in critically ill patients, such as sepsis and systemic inflammatory response syndrome.

The respiratory quotient also gives insight into the composition of feedings because carbohydrates yield a respiratory quotient of 1, whereas fatty acids yield a ratio of 0.8 and amino acids a ratio of 0.7. Thus, balanced nutrition should yield a respiratory quotient of approximately 0.85. A respiratory quotient of 1 in combination with a high carbon dioxide production suggests that the dietary proportion of carbohydrates is excessive.

MEASURING RESPIRATORY COMPLIANCE

Respiratory compliance is the change in respiratory system volume induced by a change in applied pressure (i.e., inspiratory pressure) and is the mathematical inverse of elastance. Compliance diminishes in conditions like lung injury and ARDS (Chapter 90) or pulmonary fibrosis (Chapter 80), in which diffuse inflammation and scarring alter lung structure and contribute to increased lung "stiffness." Static respiratory compliance is measured in patients receiving volume-limited mechanical ventilation by imposing a brief inspiratory hold at end inspiration. Assuming the patient has no spontaneous breathing effort, the airway pressure measured when airflow ceases is referred to as the plateau pressure ($P_{plateau}$). The difference between this pressure and the positive end-expiratory pressure (PEEP) is taken as the driving pressure required to deliver the tidal volume (see Fig. 89-1). Static respiratory system compliance (CRS) is then calculated as

$$C_{RS} = \Delta V(\text{exhaled tidal volume})/\Delta P\,(P_{plateau} - \text{PEEP}) \qquad (12)$$

This compliance not only reflects the status of the lung but also includes contributions of the chest wall and abdomen. Thus, patients with chest wall deformities or morbid obesity have lower values of respiratory compliance even in the absence of lung abnormalities (Chapter 86). The normal respiratory compliance is in the range of 50 to 70 mL/cm H_2O, and patients with ARDS usually have values of CRS of less than 30 cm H_2O. If respiratory compliance is below 20 to 25 cm H_2O, weaning from mechanical ventilation (Chapter 91) is difficult or impossible because of the high work of breathing requirements (see later).

MEASURING RESPIRATORY DRIVE

The respiratory center, located in the pons and medulla, regulates respiratory drive.[9] Hypercapnia is a strong stimulus to ventilation (Chapter 74). This response may be blunted by chronic carbon dioxide retention or by drugs like narcotics. Hypoxemia is a weaker ventilatory stimulus that is potentiated by hypercapnia and blunted by hypocapnia.

Thus, respiratory drive can be assessed as the response to carbon dioxide in the blood in the hypercapnic ventilatory response. In one technique to measure respiratory drive, the patient rebreathes his or her exhaled air while minute ventilation and P_{ETCO_2} are monitored; a graph relating P_{ETCO_2} with minute ventilation is used to measure respiratory drive. However, this technique is impractical in an ICU setting. Another technique is to measure the negative swing in airway pressure during the first 100 msec of inspiration (P_{100}). This technique avoids the problem of diminished ventilatory response due to airway obstruction, but it is still subject to blunting by some drugs and still underestimates drive in patients with respiratory muscle weakness, a common problem in the ICU. In patients who are failing to be weaned from mechanical ventilation, a practical way to assess the integrity of respiratory drive is to determine whether the respiratory rate increases, usually into the range of 30 to 40 breaths/minute, as Pa_{CO_2} rises after the patient is removed from ventilatory support.

MEASURING RESPIRATORY MUSCLE STRENGTH

Respiratory muscle weakness has long been recognized as a contributor to respiratory failure and failure to be weaned from mechanical ventilation in the ICU (Chapter 91). This recognition has intensified in recent years with the increased awareness of ICU-acquired weakness after critical illness. However, measurement of respiratory muscle strength remains challenging because of the need to differentiate between actual weakness and reduced muscle performance due to inability to cooperate or to exert a full inspiratory effort.

The most commonly used measures of respiratory muscle strength are the maximal inspiratory and expiratory pressures (PImax or MIP and PEmax or MEP). These values are obtained by measuring the pressure change with a manometer when the patient inhales with maximal force from residual volume and exhales with maximal force from total lung capacity. Normal MIP is usually more negative than −75 cm H_2O, and normal MEP is usually more positive than 125 cm H_2O. When the value for MIP is less negative than −20 or −30 cm H_2O, weaning from mechanical ventilation may be difficult, and values less positive than 60 cm H_2O suggest cough insufficiency. However, these values have poor predictive value for weaning of mechanically ventilated patients because many of these patients are unable to cooperate. This problem may be addressed by attaching a one-way valve to the end of an endotracheal tube that permits exhalation but not inhalation and then measuring the inspiratory pressure efforts for 20 to 25 seconds.

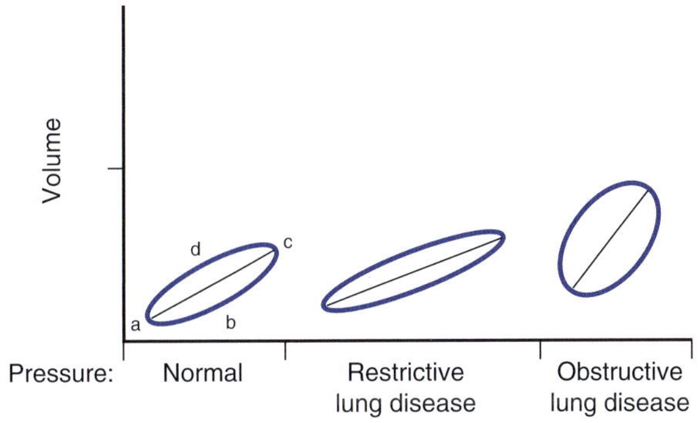

FIGURE 89-2. Pressure-volume curves illustrating components of work in a normal subject and in patients with restrictive or obstructive disease. The line between *a* and *c* represents elastic work as the lung expands, but this work is a net zero because static forces return the lung to its neutral position. The restrictive curve is flatter than normal because the lung is stiffer and volume changes less for a given unit change in pressure. The obstructive curve has a greater slope because (e.g., in emphysema) the lung is more compliant and starts inhalation from a higher volume. The *abc* curve represents resistive work during inspiration, and *cda* represents resistive work during exhalation. Resistive work during exhalation is greater in patients with obstructive lung disease.

MEASURING WORK OF BREATHING

Work of breathing is the product of pressure and volume for each breath (Fig. 89-2). The components include work needed to overcome elastic recoil of the lung and to displace the chest wall and abdomen as well as work needed to overcome airway resistance and lung viscosity and work needed to overcome inertia. With restrictive lung diseases, the inspiratory work of breathing is increased because of the decreased lung elasticity. With obstructive diseases, the work of breathing is increased because of increased airway resistance.

In clinical settings, a more practical way to assess the inspiratory work of breathing is to calculate the pressure-time product (in cm H_2O-seconds). The pressure-time product can be calculated by the decrease in airway pressure during inspiration, esophageal pressure (measured with an esophageal balloon manometer), or transdiaphragmatic pressure (measured with esophageal and gastric balloon manometers) as an index of diaphragmatic work. The work can be calculated as work of breathing per breath or as work of breathing per minute by multiplying the work per breath by the respiratory frequency. Commercially available devices using esophageal manometry automatically calculate the inspiratory work of breathing, which may be of some value in assessing the likelihood of weaning from mechanical ventilation. If the drop in inspiratory pressure necessary to achieve an adequate tidal volume is too large, the calculated work of breathing will be high, and the likelihood of successful weaning will be reduced.

GENERAL REFERENCES

For the General References and other additional features, please visit Elsevier eBooks+ at https://ebooks.health.elsevier.com.

Grade A Reference

A1. Schjørring OL, Klitgaard TL, Perner A, et al. Lower or higher oxygenation targets for acute hypoxemic respiratory failure. *N Engl J Med.* 2021;384:1301-1311.

90 ACUTE RESPIRATORY FAILURE

MICHAEL A. MATTHAY AND LORRAINE B. WARE

DEFINITION

Acute respiratory failure occurs when dysfunction of the respiratory system results in abnormal gas exchange that is potentially life-threatening. Each element of this definition is important to understand. The term *acute* implies a relatively sudden onset (from hours to days) and a substantial change from the patient's baseline condition. *Dysfunction* indicates that the abnormal gas exchange may be caused by abnormalities in any element of the respiratory system (e.g., a central nervous system abnormality affecting the regulation of breathing or a musculoskeletal thoracic abnormality affecting ventilation [Chapter 71]) in addition to abnormalities of the lung itself. The term *respiration* refers, in a broad sense, to the delivery of oxygen (O_2) to metabolically active tissues for energy use and the removal of carbon dioxide (CO_2) from these tissues (Table 90-1). Respiratory failure is a failure of the process of delivery of O_2 to the tissues or removal of CO_2 from the tissues.[1] Abnormalities in the periphery (e.g., cyanide poisoning, circulatory shock, pathologic distribution of organ blood flow in sepsis) can lead to tissue hypoxia; although these conditions represent forms of respiratory failure in the broadest terms, this chapter focuses on respiratory failure resulting from dysfunction of the lungs, chest wall, and control of respiration.

PATHOBIOLOGY

Abnormal gas exchange is the physiologic hallmark of acute respiratory failure, which can be classified in several ways (Table 90-2). Although gas exchange can be abnormal for either oxygenation or CO_2 removal, significant hypoxemia is nearly always present when patients with acute respiratory failure breathe ambient air. If CO_2 is retained at a potentially life-threatening level under these conditions, it will be accompanied by significant hypoxemia (see later). The *life-threatening* aspect of the condition places the degree of abnormal gas exchange in a clinical context and calls for urgent treatment.

The diagnosis of acute respiratory failure requires a significant change in arterial blood gases or arterial oxygen saturation from baseline. Many patients with chronic respiratory problems can function with blood gas tensions that would be alarming in a physiologically normal individual. Over time, patients with so-called chronic respiratory failure or chronic respiratory insufficiency develop mechanisms to compensate for inadequate gas exchange. Conversely, chronic respiratory failure makes patients vulnerable to respiratory insults (e.g., pneumonia, heart failure) that could be easily tolerated by a previously healthy individual.

In acute respiratory failure, the O_2 content in the blood (available for tissue use) is reduced to a level at which the possibility of end-organ dysfunction, as a result of inadequate oxygen delivery, increases. The value of the partial pressure of O_2 in the arterial blood (Pao_2) that demarcates this vulnerable zone is often considered to be the point of the oxyhemoglobin dissociation relationship at which any further decrease in the Pao_2 results in sharp decreases in the amount of hemoglobin saturated with O_2 (Sao_2) and in the arterial blood O_2 content (Cao_2). Thus, acute respiratory failure is often defined in practice as occurring when the Pao_2 is less than about 55 to 60 mm Hg (Fig. 90-1). However, it is important to note that the oxyhemoglobin dissociation curve of whole blood, which governs the partial pressure at which O_2 is unloaded to the tissues, is a critical determinant of how much O_2 is available for the cells and their mitochondria at a given Pao_2. Conditions such as fever or acidosis can shift the curve rightward. Other than under conditions of an extremely hypoxic environment (e.g., in utero or on the summit of Mt. Everest), however, the enhanced ability to unload O_2 at the tissue level more than compensates for small decreases in the amount of O_2 picked up in the lungs when the oxyhemoglobin dissociation curve is shifted rightward. With a leftward shift in the curve, O_2 is bound more tightly to hemoglobin, so less O_2 is available for tissue delivery.

These physiologic and clinical considerations imply that any definition of acute respiratory failure based on an absolute level of Pao_2 is arbitrary. A healthy, young, conditioned individual climbing at high altitude may have a Pao_2 of less than 50 mm Hg because of the reduction in inspired O_2 pressure. This individual is not in acute respiratory failure, even though the Pao_2 may be in the low 40s. A patient who has chronic obstructive pulmonary disease (COPD) and whose usual range of Pao_2 is 50 to 55 mm Hg would not be considered to be in acute respiratory failure if the Pao_2 was 50 mm Hg. However, if a patient's usual Pao_2 is 80 mm Hg, a sudden drop to a Pao_2 of 50 to 55 mm Hg could be associated with a substantial risk for a further life-threatening reduction in oxygenation; this patient should be considered to have acute respiratory failure.

Traditionally, the level of arterial CO_2 partial pressure ($Paco_2$) that defines acute respiratory failure has been 45 mm Hg or greater, if it is accompanied by arterial acidosis with a pH of less than about 7.35. The $Paco_2$ is linked to

TABLE 90-1 ABBREVIATIONS COMMONLY USED IN ACUTE RESPIRATORY FUNCTION

ABG	Arterial blood gas or arterial blood gas analysis
ARDS	Acute respiratory distress syndrome
ARF	Acute respiratory failure
cm H_2O	Centimeters of water
Cao_2	Content of oxygen in arterial blood
Cco_2	Content of oxygen in end-capillary blood
CO_2	Carbon dioxide
COPD	Chronic obstructive pulmonary disease
CPAP	Continuous positive airway pressure (used when positive pressure during exhalation is applied with spontaneous ventilation)
Cvo_2	Content of oxygen in mixed venous blood
Fio_2	Fraction of inspired oxygen
g/dL	Grams per deciliter
HbO_2	Saturation of hemoglobin by oxygen
L/min	Liters per minute
mL/kg	Milliliters per kilogram
mL/min	Milliliters per minute
mm Hg	Millimeters of mercury
NIPPV	Noninvasive positive-pressure ventilation
O_2	Oxygen
$P(A\text{-}a)o_2$	Difference of partial pressure of oxygen between mean alveolar gas and arterial blood (alveolar-to-arterial oxygen difference)
P_{ACO_2}	Partial pressure of carbon dioxide in alveolar gas
$Paco_2$	Partial pressure of carbon dioxide in arterial blood
P_{AO_2}	Partial pressure of oxygen in alveolar gas
Pao_2	Partial pressure of oxygen in arterial blood
Pao_2/Fio_2	Ratio of partial pressure of oxygen in arterial blood to fraction of inspired oxygen
PBW	Predicted body weight
Pc_{co2}	Partial pressure of carbon dioxide in end-capillary blood
Pco_2	Partial pressure of carbon dioxide
Pc_{o2}	Partial pressure of oxygen in end-capillary blood
PEEP	Positive end-expiratory pressure (used when positive pressure during exhalation is applied with mechanical ventilation)
P/F	Pao_2/Fio_2 ratio
Pio_2	Partial pressure of oxygen in inspired gas
Po_2	Partial pressure of oxygen
$Pvco_2$	Partial pressure of carbon dioxide in mixed venous blood
Pvo_2	Partial pressure of oxygen in mixed venous blood
$\dot{Q}$	Blood flow or perfusion
RR	Respiratory rate
Sao_2	Percentage of saturation of hemoglobin by oxygen in arterial blood
$\dot{V}$	Ventilation
$\dot{V}/\dot{Q}$	Ventilation-perfusion ratio
Vt	Tidal volume

TABLE 90-2 SYSTEMS TO CLASSIFY HYPOXEMIC VERSUS HYPERCAPNIC ACUTE RESPIRATORY FAILURE

Common Causes of Primary Hypoxemic Acute Respiratory Failure	Mechanisms of Hypoxemia
ARDS Pneumonia Acute lobar atelectasis Cardiogenic pulmonary edema Pulmonary embolism Lung contusion	**Normal P(A-a)O_2*** ↓PIO_2 High altitude; inadvertent administration of low FIO_2 gas mixture Hypoventilation See causes of hypercapnic-hypoxemic acute respiratory failure earlier
Common Causes of Primary Hypercapnic Acute Respiratory Failure	**Increased P(A-a)O_2***
Pulmonary disease COPD Asthma: advanced, acute, severe asthma Drugs causing respiratory depression Neuromuscular Guillain-Barré syndrome Acute myasthenia gravis Metabolic derangements causing weakness (including hypophosphatemia, hypomagnesemia) Obesity hypoventilation syndrome (with additional acute, superimposed abnormality as cause of acute respiratory failure)	Ventilation-perfusion ($\dot{V}/\dot{Q}$) mismatch (in severe disease $\dot{V}/\dot{Q}$ mismatch can act like a shunt) Airway disease Vascular disease, including pulmonary thromboembolism ARDS Cardiogenic pulmonary edema Pneumonia Parenchymal lung disease Pulmonary infarction Shunt Intracardiac right to left shunt Intrapulmonary shunt (e.g., A-V malformation/trauma) Decreased mixed venous oxygen concentration (PvO_2) (e.g., heart failure or hypovolemia)

*Calculated by the alveolar-air equation; see text for description.

ARDS = acute respiratory distress syndrome; A-V = arteriovenous; COPD = chronic obstructive pulmonary disease; FIO_2 = fraction of inspired oxygen; P(A-a)O_2 = alveolar-to-arterial oxygen difference; PIO_2 = partial pressure of inspired oxygen: $\dot{V}/\dot{Q}$ = ventilation-perfusion ratio.

pH in this definition because of the general belief that acidosis is what leads to tissue dysfunction and symptoms. Patients with severe COPD may have chronic CO_2 retention, but renal compensation for the respiratory acidosis protects them against acidosis related to the elevation in CO_2. A further acute rise in $PaCO_2$ can precipitate symptoms and other organ dysfunction; however, even severe respiratory acidosis (pH 7.1) seems to be better tolerated than metabolic acidosis of the same pH in most previously healthy individuals if arterial and tissue oxygenation is adequate.

Pathophysiology

Six mechanisms can lead to a reduction in PaO_2: (1) decreased inspired partial pressure of O_2 (PIO_2) (e.g., at high altitude or when breathing a reduced percentage O_2 mixture); (2) hypoventilation; (3) ventilation-perfusion mismatch; (4) shunting of blood from the pulmonary to systemic circulation, thereby bypassing the alveoli anatomically or functionally; in essence, a shunt is an extreme $\dot{V}/\dot{Q}$ mismatch in which blood perfuses alveoli with *no* ventilation, and it is differentiated clinically from other $\dot{V}/\dot{Q}$ mismatching by the response to breathing supplemental O_2 (see later); (5) any barrier for diffusion of O_2 from the alveoli into the capillary blood; and (6) a decrease in the concentration of oxygen in the mixed venous blood in the pulmonary artery.

If only hypoventilation is present, the resulting hypoxemia is associated with a normal difference between the calculated alveolar and the measured arterial oxygenation levels [P(A-a)O_2]. In this setting, an elevated $PaCO_2$ suggests disease processes that affect nonpulmonary respiratory function (e.g., central respiratory depression resulting from drug overdose, neuromuscular diseases such as Guillain-Barré syndrome, or chest wall disease such as flail chest; Chapter 74). In contrast, $\dot{V}/\dot{Q}$ mismatch and shunting are associated with an elevated P(A-a)O_2, which may or may not coexist with hypoventilation. The normal value for P(A-a)O_2 varies as a function of the fraction of inspired O_2 (FIO_2), increasing as FIO_2 increases.

When $\dot{V}/\dot{Q}$ mismatch or shunting is the cause of hypoxemia, some alveolar regions have increased levels of PCO_2 and associated reduced levels of PO_2; the blood in the vessels perfusing these alveoli reflects these abnormal gas tensions. The resulting increased arterial PCO_2 ($PaCO_2$) usually can be reversed by increasing overall ventilation, but this increased ventilation usually does not correct the decreased arterial PO_2 (PaO_2).

$\dot{V}/\dot{Q}$ mismatch is distinguished from shunting by assessing the PaO_2 response to enhanced O_2 administration. Hypoxemia caused by $\dot{V}/\dot{Q}$ mismatch can be corrected to a nearly complete O_2 saturation of the hemoglobin in most patients by a relatively small increase in FIO_2, such as from 0.24 to 0.28 by face mask or 1 to 2 L/minute O_2 by nasal prongs, in patients with acute exacerbations of COPD. If the airways to poorly ventilated alveoli remain open and the enriched O_2 mixture is administered for an adequate length of time (ranging from a few minutes to about 20 minutes, depending on the degree of $\dot{V}/\dot{Q}$ inequality), the increased PIO_2 is reflected by an increased PAO_2 and an increased PaO_2. When a shunt is present (no ventilation but continued perfusion), a relatively small increase in the FIO_2 has little or no effect on the PaO_2, and even large increases in FIO_2 up to 1.0 result in only modest increases in PaO_2 (Fig. 90-2).

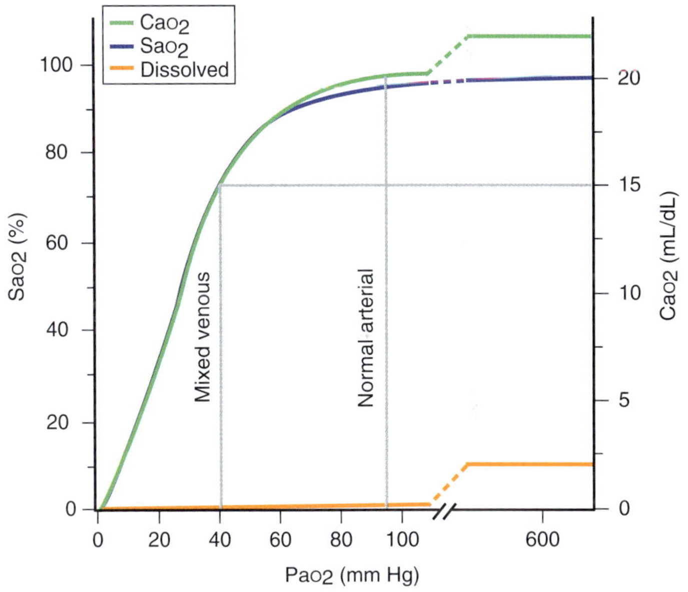

FIGURE 90-1. **Oxyhemoglobin association-dissociation curve. The axis for oxygen saturation in the arterial blood (SaO_2) is on the left, and the axis for arterial content of oxygen (CaO_2) is on the right. CaO_2 is the sum of the oxygen dissolved in plasma (denoted as "Dissolved" in the figure) plus the oxygen bound to hemoglobin. With a normal hemoglobin, most of the oxygen is carried bound to hemoglobin, with only a relatively small amount of oxygen dissolved in plasma. When the value of the arterial partial pressure of oxygen (PaO_2) is on the "flat" portion of the curve ($PaO_2 \geq 60$ to 65 mm Hg, normal partial pressure of arterial carbon dioxide [$PaCO_2$], and normal pH), raising the PaO_2 further has relatively little effect on total oxygen content. Increases in temperature, PCO_2, hydrogen ion concentration, or 2,3-diphosphoglycerate cause a rightward shift in the oxyhemoglobin association-dissociation curve.**

For clinical purposes, diffusion abnormalities are not usually important causes of hypoxemia at sea level because there is sufficient time for adequate diffusion of O_2 during the transit of a red blood cell through the pulmonary capillary bed, even in the presence of severe lung disease. When diffusion

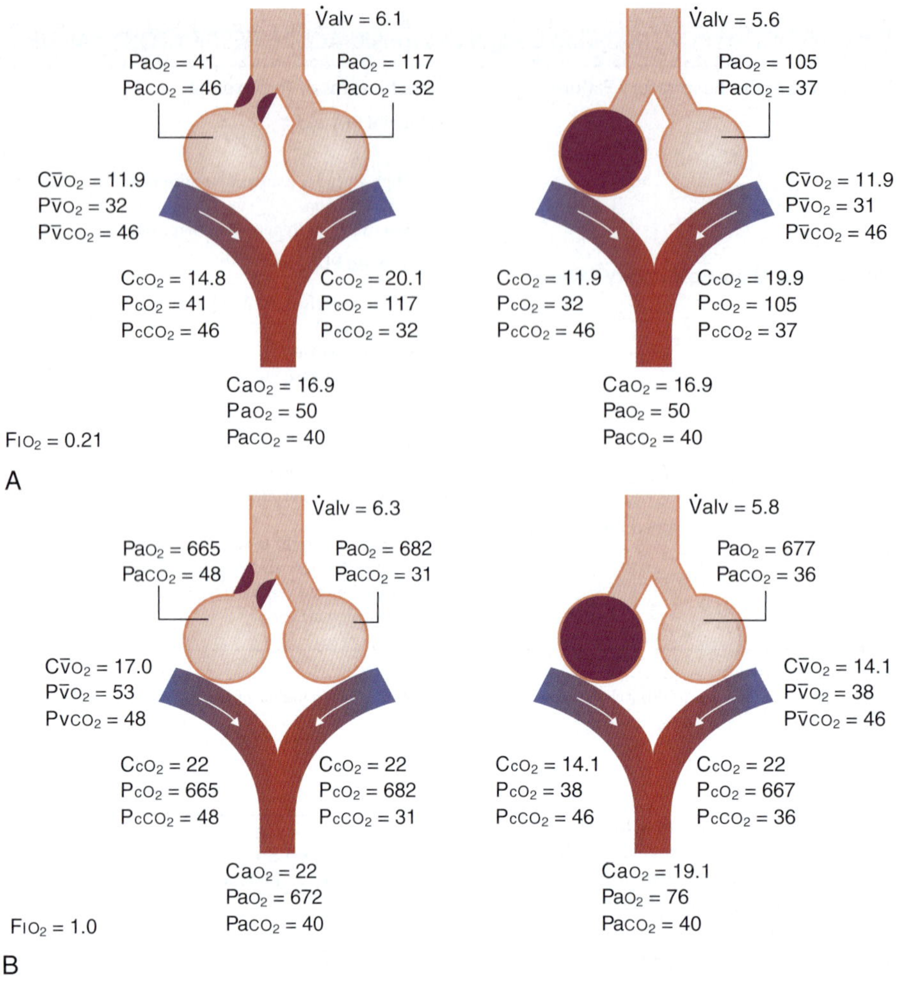

FIGURE 90-2. Arterial oxygenation. Comparison of the effect on arterial oxygenation of increasing the fraction of inspired oxygen (FIO_2) from breathing of ambient air ($FIO_2 = 0.21$) (**A**) to breathing of 100% oxygen ($FIO_2 = 1.0$) (**B**) with a low ventilation-perfusion ratio ($\dot{V}/\dot{Q}$) (*left*) and a shunt (*right*), using a two-compartment lung model. Shunting and decreased $\dot{V}/\dot{Q}$ can lead to identical arterial blood gases (partial pressure of oxygen in arterial blood [PaO_2] = 50 mm Hg; partial pressure of carbon dioxide in arterial blood [$PaCO_2$] = 40 mm Hg). The response to supplemental oxygen administration is markedly different. Hypoxemia is only partially corrected by breathing of 100% oxygen when a shunt is present because arterial oxygenation represents an average of the end-capillary oxygen content (CcO_2) from various parts of the lung, not an average of the partial pressures of oxygen (partial pressure of carbon dioxide in the end-capillary blood [$PcCO_2$]). When the CcO_2 values are mixed, the PaO_2 is determined from the resultant content of oxygen in the arterial blood (CaO_2) by the oxyhemoglobin association-dissociation relationship (see Fig. 90-1). With low $\dot{V}/\dot{Q}$ (as is often the case in patients with chronic obstructive pulmonary disease), an increase in FIO_2 increases the alveolar partial pressure of oxygen (PO_2) of the low $\dot{V}/\dot{Q}$ unit and leads to a marked increase in arterial PO_2. The values in this figure were generated from modeling to result in the same $PaCO_2$ (40 mm Hg) for all four situations shown; this is the reason for slight changes in alveolar ventilation (V) for some of the conditions. Several assumptions are made: no diffusion limitation is present; oxygen consumption = 300 mL/minute, and CO_2 production = 240 mL/minute; cardiac output = 6.0 L/minute; the low $\dot{V}/\dot{Q}$ regions in the left panels represent 60% of the cardiac output perfusing alveoli with a $\dot{V}/\dot{Q}$ 25% of normal; and the shunts in the right panels represent a 37% shunt (i.e., 37% of the cardiac output is perfusing alveoli with no ventilation).

abnormalities are present and contribute to hypoxemia, $\dot{V}/\dot{Q}$ mismatch nearly always coexists with the shunting, and this mismatch is an important cause of hypoxemia. Except at high altitude or when a person is breathing a gas mixture low in O_2, hypoventilation, $\dot{V}/\dot{Q}$ mismatch, and shunting are the dominant causes of hypoxemia.

The sixth cause of arterial hypoxemia, a reduced mixed venous oxygen concentration, usually reflects a reduction in cardiac output, with increased oxygen extraction from the blood in the periphery leading to a decrease in oxygen content of blood returning to the heart. The most common causes are heart failure (Chapter 45) or hypovolemia, but it is also a common cause of arterial hypoxemia immediately after resuscitation from cardiac arrest (Chapter 50).

CLINICAL MANIFESTATIONS

The hallmark of acute respiratory failure is the inability to maintain adequate oxygenation or the inability to maintain an appropriate $PaCO_2$. Patients are typically dyspneic and tachypneic, unless progressive respiratory failure causes fatigue—sometimes leading to respiratory arrest—or a drug overdose or neuromuscular condition prevents an appropriate respiratory response to hypoxemia or hypercapnic acidosis. Neurologic function may deteriorate, and myocardial ischemia (Chapter 57) or even infarction (Chapter 58) may be precipitated by hypoxemia; other organ dysfunction such as acute kidney injury (Chapter 106) may also occur. In addition, each cause has its own specific manifestations (see later).

DIAGNOSIS

As part of the diagnosis of acute respiratory failure, the physician has three objectives: (1) to confirm the clinical suspicion that acute respiratory failure is present; (2) to classify the type of acute respiratory failure as primary hypoxemia or primary hypercapnia (Table 90-2) (e.g., hypoxemia caused by $\dot{V}/\dot{Q}$ mismatch or shunting, as compared with hypoxemia caused by hypoventilation); and (3) to determine the specific cause. Defining the type of acute respiratory failure and determining the specific cause are prerequisites to optimal management.

The initial approach to diagnosis consists of considering information from four sources: (1) clinical history and physical examination; (2) physiologic abnormalities, particularly arterial blood gas derangements, which help establish the mechanisms of hypoxemia; (3) chest radiographic findings; and (4) other tests aimed at elucidating specific causes. In many cases, the clinical picture from the history is so clear that the presumptive type of acute respiratory failure (and sometimes the cause) is obvious, so treatment can be started while confirmatory laboratory studies are ordered. In other cases, a clinician may be asked to see a patient because of an abnormal chest radiograph, abnormal oxygen saturation, or abnormal arterial blood gases ordered by someone else and may elicit the pertinent history based on these clues. When the degree of hypoxemia is life-threatening, therapeutic decisions must be made quickly, even if data are limited. The clinician must obtain updated information continually and should view most therapeutic decisions as therapeutic trials, with careful monitoring to assess for benefits and possible detrimental effects.

TABLE 90-3 CLINICAL MANIFESTATIONS OF HYPOXEMIA AND HYPERCAPNIA

HYPOXEMIA	HYPERCAPNIA
Tachycardia	Somnolence
Tachypnea	Lethargy
Anxiety	Restlessness
Diaphoresis	Tremor
Altered mental status	Slurred speech
Confusion	Headache
Cyanosis	Asterixis
Hypertension	Papilledema
Hypotension	Coma
Bradycardia	Diaphoresis
Seizures	
Coma	
Lactic acidosis*	

*Usually indicates additional reduction in oxygen delivery because of inadequate cardiac output, severe anemia, or redistribution of blood flow.

Clinical Evaluation

The presentation often reflects one of three clinical scenarios: (1) the systemic effects of hypoxemia or respiratory acidosis, (2) the local effects of primary (e.g., pneumonia) or secondary (e.g., heart failure) diseases on the lungs, and (3) the nonpulmonary effects of the underlying disease process (e.g., shock from sepsis). The clinical effects of hypoxemia and respiratory acidosis are manifested mainly in the central nervous system (e.g., irritability, agitation, anxiety, changes in personality, depressed level of consciousness, coma) and the cardiovascular system (e.g., arrhythmias, hypotension, hypertension) (Table 90-3). In patients with underlying COPD (Chapter 76) with a gradual onset of acute respiratory failure, central nervous system abnormalities may be the major presenting findings. Cyanosis, which requires at least 5 g/dL of unsaturated hemoglobin to be detectable, may not be present before serious tissue hypoxia develops, especially in patients with underlying anemia.

Pulmonary symptoms and signs often reflect the respiratory disease causing the acute respiratory failure. Examples include cough and sputum with pneumonia (Chapter 85) or pleuritic chest pain from pulmonary thromboembolism with infarction (Chapter 68). Dyspnea and respiratory distress are nonspecific reflections of the respiratory system's difficulty in meeting the increased demands from both pulmonary and nonpulmonary diseases.

Physical findings may be associated with a particular pathologic lung process, such as pneumonia (Chapter 85), which often results in bronchial breath sounds, egophony, and crackles on auscultation, or cardiogenic pulmonary edema (Chapter 45), which commonly is associated with crackles (rales) or an S_3 heart sound. Abnormal findings may be minimal or absent in patients with ARDS or pulmonary thromboembolism (Chapter 68).

In some patients, the clinical picture is dominated by the underlying disease process, particularly with diseases that cause ARDS, such as sepsis (Chapter 94), severe pneumonia (Chapter 85), aspiration of gastric contents (Chapter 82), and trauma. In these conditions, the physical examination findings are often nonspecific, with no obvious clues except, for example, fever with sepsis or pneumonia and hypotension with septic shock.

Assessment of Physiologic Abnormalities

The clinical suspicion of acute respiratory failure must be addressed by arterial blood gas analysis to answer several questions.

Is hypoxemia present? The answer is based largely on the FIO_2 and the PaO_2 or SaO_2. The degree of the hypoxemia not only confirms the diagnosis of acute respiratory failure but also helps define its severity.

Is hypoventilation present? If the $PaCO_2$ is elevated, alveolar hypoventilation is present.

Does the degree of hypoventilation fully explain the hypoxemia? If the $P(A-a)O_2$ is normal, hypoventilation fully explains the presence and degree of hypoxemia. When this is the case, the most likely causes of acute respiratory failure are central nervous system abnormalities or a chest wall abnormality. If the $P(A-a)O_2$ is increased such that hypoventilation does not fully explain the hypoxemia, another condition must be present; common diagnoses include COPD (Chapter 76), severe asthma (Chapter 75), pneumonia (Chapter 85), and early stages of ARDS.

If hypoxemia exists without hypoventilation, an elevated $P(A-a)O_2$ should be confirmed, and the response to breathing of an enhanced O_2 mixture would answer this question: *Is the increase in $P(A-a)O_2$ primarily the result of a $\dot{V}/\dot{Q}$ abnormality or of shunting?* If hypoxemia is primarily the result of a $\dot{V}/\dot{Q}$ abnormality, the likely cause is an airway disease, either COPD or acute severe asthma, or a vascular disease, such as pulmonary thromboembolism. If effective shunting (lung units with very low but not zero $\dot{V}/\dot{Q}$ values) is the major explanation for the hypoxemia, processes that fill the air spaces (e.g., cardiogenic pulmonary edema, noncardiogenic pulmonary edema or severe ARDS, or purulent pulmonary secretions in acute pneumonia) or, less commonly, an intracardiac or anatomic intrapulmonary shunt is the likely cause. In the setting of pulmonary edema of any cause, $\dot{V}/\dot{Q}$ mismatch and intrapulmonary shunting usually coexist. Conditions that fill air spaces should be confirmed by abnormal findings on a chest radiograph; if the radiograph is normal, the possibility of intracardiac shunt (Chapter 55) or thromboembolism (Chapter 68) should be evaluated. If there is a reduction in the mixed venous oxygen saturation, causes of a reduced cardiac output should be considered, including acute or chronic heart failure or hypovolemia.

Chest Radiography

The chest radiograph in acute respiratory failure is likely to show one of three patterns (Fig. 90-3): (1) normal (or relatively normal), (2) localized alveolar filling opacities, or (3) diffuse alveolar filling opacities. Diffuse interstitial opacities are also possible, but diseases that cause this pattern usually have a more gradual onset and are associated with chronic respiratory failure. If the chest radiograph is normal (i.e., it is clear or relatively clear), airway diseases, such as COPD and asthma, or pulmonary vascular diseases, such as thromboembolism, are more likely. If a localized alveolar filling abnormality is present, pneumonia is the major consideration, but pulmonary embolism with infarction should also be considered. When diffuse (bilateral) alveolar filling abnormalities (E-Fig. 90-1) are present, cardiogenic pulmonary edema and ARDS (e.g., as seen after sepsis, trauma, and pneumonia, including coronavirus disease 2019 [COVID-19] pneumonia [Chapter 336], or aspiration of gastric contents) are the major considerations. The combination of the chest radiograph and the arterial blood gas interpretation can be helpful. The finding of a significant shunt may suggest ARDS in a patient in whom this diagnosis was not clinically obvious; the chest radiograph should help confirm that possibility.

Other Evaluations

All patients with acute respiratory failure should have a complete blood count including a platelet count, routine blood chemistry tests, prothrombin time, and urinalysis to screen for possible underlying causes and comorbid conditions. Other blood tests should be guided by the clinical picture. Examples include a serum lipase level if pancreatitis is a possible cause of ARDS and thyroid indices if severe hypothyroidism is a possible cause of hypoventilation. Blood cultures are recommended when an infectious cause such as sepsis is suspected. Sputum Gram stain and cultures can be useful if bacterial pneumonia is suspected, but nucleic acid testing for viruses is recommended when severe acute respiratory syndrome coronavirus 2 (SARS-CoV-2; Chapter 337), influenza, and other respiratory viruses are suspected. A urine toxicology screen is recommended if drug overdose is a possibility. Any abnormal fluid collections, especially pleural effusion (Chapter 86), should usually be aspirated for diagnostic purposes.

Other specific tests should be directed by the history, physical examinations, arterial blood gas levels, and chest radiograph. An abdominal computed tomography (CT) scan may be indicated to search for the source of infection in a patient with sepsis and ARDS. A chest CT scan may help define pulmonary disease if the chest radiograph is not definitive. CT arteriography of the pulmonary circulation may diagnose pulmonary thromboembolism (Chapter 68). An electrocardiogram should be obtained routinely and be supplemented by cardiac troponin levels and echocardiography if a primary cardiac cause of pulmonary edema (Chapter 45) is suspected. A head CT scan may be indicated if a stroke involving the respiratory center is suspected. Routine blood chemistry studies can detect diabetic ketoacidosis (Chapter 210) or renal failure (Chapter 106) as contributing causes.

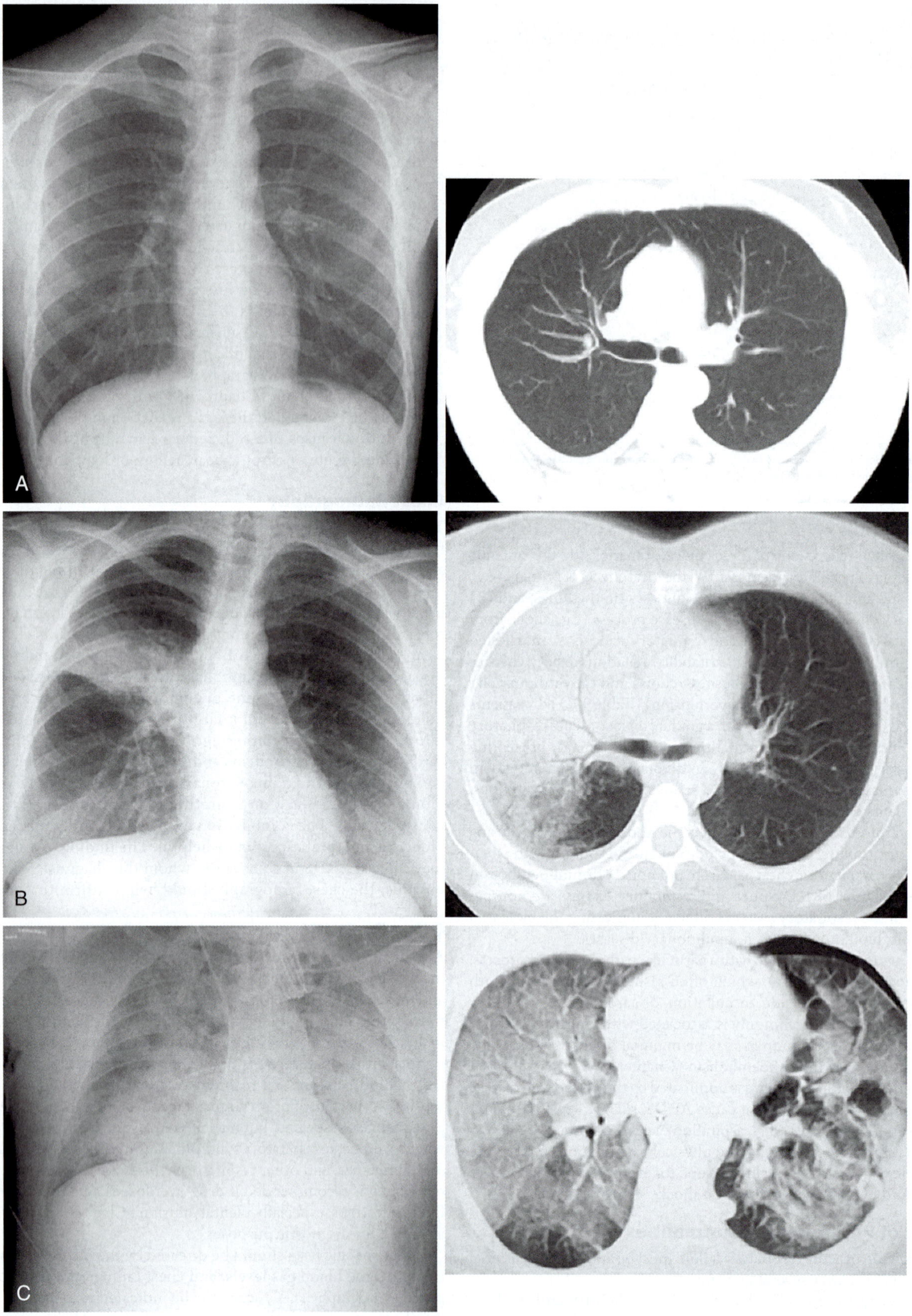

FIGURE 90-3. **Chest radiographs (*left*) and computed tomography scans (*right*) of the three most common findings in diseases causing acute respiratory failure. A,** Relatively clear chest, consistent with an acute exacerbation of airway disease (e.g., asthma, chronic obstructive pulmonary disease) or a central nervous system or neuromuscular disease as the cause of acute respiratory failure. **B,** Localized alveolar filling opacity, most commonly seen with acute pneumonia. **C,** Diffuse bilateral alveolar filling opacities consistent with acute respiratory distress syndrome or cardiogenic pulmonary edema. The computed tomography scan in C shows a small left pneumothorax and cavities or cysts that are not apparent on the anteroposterior chest radiograph.

TREATMENT

General Measures

The management of acute respiratory failure depends on its cause, its clinical manifestations, and the patient's underlying status.[2] Certain goals apply to all patients: improvement of the hypoxemia to eliminate or markedly reduce the acute threat to life; improvement of the acidosis if it is considered life-threatening; maintenance of cardiac output or improvement if cardiac output is compromised; treatment of the underlying disease process; and avoidance of predictable complications.

The precise methods for improving hypoxemia depend on the cause of the acute respiratory failure. However, an increase in the inspired O_2 concentration is a cornerstone of treatment for nearly all patients, even though it may not produce a marked increase in $Pa{O_2}$ in patients whose underlying pathophysiologic process involves a significant amount of lung with low ventilation-perfusion ratios or true shunting. Earlier treatment is preferred. For example, continuous positive airway pressure (CPAP) begun in the prehospital setting can reduce subsequent intubation rates and mortality. Often, however, initial oxygen therapy alone is as good as early noninvasive ventilation. Conservative oxygen therapy is as good as more liberal therapy, and the peripheral $Sa{O_2}$ goal should not be above 94 to 96%.[A1,A2]

The level of acidosis that requires treatment other than for the underlying disease process is a matter of debate. Although normalization of the arterial pH was suggested in the past, respiratory acidosis seems to be well tolerated in many patients with severe ARDS, so a patient with a pH of 7.15 or higher may not require bicarbonate therapy. If the acidemia coexists with clinical complications, such as cardiac arrhythmias or a decreased level of consciousness, that have no other obvious cause, treatments to increase pH should be considered. The therapeutic goal is alleviation or reduction of the accompanying complications by improving the level of acidosis; normalization of the pH usually is not indicated (Chapter 104).

The maintenance of cardiac output is crucial for O_2 delivery in acute respiratory failure, especially because mechanical ventilation and positive end-expiratory pressure (PEEP) may compromise cardiac output. Placement of a pulmonary artery catheter allows measurement of cardiac output and filling pressures, but most patients who have these catheters do no better than similar patients managed without them. Nevertheless, selective use of diagnostic pulmonary artery catheterization can help determine the cause of the pulmonary edema (cardiogenic vs. noncardiogenic) and the physiologic basis for shock (sepsis, hypovolemia, or decreased cardiac output from impaired cardiac function) in selected patients in whom the diagnosis is not clear.

Many therapeutic interventions that improve short-term physiologic measures may worsen long-term, clinically important outcomes. For example, transfusing all patients to maintain a hemoglobin greater than 10 g/dL *increases* mortality in critically ill patients who have not had an acute myocardial infarction and do not have unstable angina, even though the O_2-carrying capacity of the blood is acutely increased. Use of a relatively large tidal volume (e.g., 12 mL/kg predicted body weight, which is equivalent to approximately 10 to 10.5 mL/kg measured body weight in patients who are somewhat overweight) *increases* mortality in patients with ARDS compared with a lower tidal volume (6 mg/kg predicted body weight), even though it raises $Pa{O_2}$ more in the short term than does a lower tidal volume. When vasopressors are no longer required to support the systemic blood pressure in ARDS, liberal use of fluids to optimize organ perfusion is usually detrimental to lung function and increases the duration of mechanical ventilation and intensive care.

Improvements in oxygenation, acid-base status, and cardiac output are of no more than temporary benefit unless the underlying disease processes are diagnosed and treated properly. In patients with ARDS, untreated or suboptimally treated sepsis may worsen injury to the lung and other organs despite optimal supportive care, so careful attention should be given to control the source of any infectious process. Similarly, if the precipitating cause of acute respiratory failure in a patient with COPD is not identified and treated, supportive care is likely to be futile. Complications may arise from the physiologic effects of the gas exchange abnormality, from the disease processes causing the acute respiratory failure, from being critically ill and its associated incursions on homeostasis (e.g., sleep deprivation), from limited mobility (critical illness myopathy and/or neuropathy), or from iatrogenic complications of therapy.

Therapy to Improve Oxygenation

The preferred approach to providing adequate oxygenation depends on the severity of disease and the patient's response to progressive intensification of therapy (Fig. 90-4). An initial step-wise approach begins with low-flow nasal oxygen (starting with 2 L/min and advancing to 6 L/min). If hypoxemia persists, therapy should be advanced to high-flow nasal oxygen (initially at 15 to 20 L/min but can be increased to higher flow rates of 40 to 60 L/min). The fraction of oxygen can be adjusted between 50% and 100% as well to achieve an arterial oxygen saturation of approximately 90 to 97%. If adequate oxygenation cannot be achieved with nasal oxygen, then therapy can be advanced to CPAP or NIPPV, if possible, before proceeding to endotracheal intubation and mechanical ventilation.

A $Pa{O_2}$ greater than 60 mm Hg is usually adequate to produce an $Sa{O_2}$ in the low to middle 90s and to provide an adequate oxygen content of the blood for tissue oxygenation. The $Pa{O_2}$ can be increased by the administration of supplemental O_2, by pharmacologic manipulations (e.g., diuretics to reduce pulmonary edema [see Fig. 46-2]), by CPAP, by mechanical ventilation with or without maneuvers such as PEEP, and by the prone position. PEEP, pharmacologic manipulations, and prone positioning are used primarily in patients with ARDS (see later).

The initial choice of the concentration and amount of supplemental O_2 is based on the severity of the hypoxemia, the clinical diagnosis, the likely mechanism causing the hypoxemia, and the O_2 delivery systems available. For the tracheal $F{IO_2}$ to be the same as the delivered $F{IO_2}$, the O_2 delivery system must deliver a flow that matches the patient's peak inspiratory flow rate with gas of a known $F{IO_2}$.

Simple face masks, non-rebreather masks, and partial rebreather masks use a simple regulator that mixes room air with O_2 from a wall unit or tank, with resulting flows that are frequently unable to match the patient's peak inspiratory flow rate. The patient entrains more air from the environment, and the resulting tracheal $F{IO_2}$ or partial pressure of oxygen in inspired gas ($Pa{O_2}$) is unknown. The amount of air entrained depends on the patient's inspiratory pattern and minute ventilation. Although the resulting $F{IO_2}$ is unknown, these systems are satisfactory if the delivery is constant and if they result in adequate arterial O_2 saturation, as monitored by arterial blood gases or oximetry.

Nasal and Face Mask Oxygen

Standard nasal prongs can deliver a tracheal $F{IO_2}$ of approximately 0.50, and non-rebreather masks can deliver 50 to 100% O_2; in both cases, this concentration depends on the inspiratory pattern and flow rate. If only hypoventilation or $\dot{V}/\dot{Q}$ mismatch is present, a small increment in $F{IO_2}$ (e.g., an $F{IO_2}$ of 0.24 or 0.28 delivered by a Venturi principle face mask or by mechanical ventilation; or 1 to 2 L/minute O_2 delivered by nasal prongs) is likely to be sufficient to restore normoxia. By comparison, if marked shunting or many lung units with low but not zero $\dot{V}/\dot{Q}$ are the cause of hypoxemia, a considerably higher $F{IO_2}$ (e.g., >0.7) may be required, and even this high $F{IO_2}$ may not reverse the hypoxemia. A common practice when a significant shunt is suspected is to give an $F{IO_2}$ of 1.0, then adjust the $F{IO_2}$ downward as guided by the resulting $Pa{O_2}$ or $Sa{O_2}$.

A low concentration of supplemental O_2 can be administered by nasal prongs or nasal cannula, which most patients find comfortable and allows them to cough, speak, eat, and drink while receiving O_2. When the nasal passages are open, the $P{IO_2}$ does not depend too much on whether the patient breathes through the nose or the mouth because O_2 is entrained from the posterior nasal pharynx during a breath taken through the mouth. The level of O_2 can be adjusted by the flow rate to the nasal prongs. In patients with COPD, flows as low as 0.5 to 2 L/minute are usually adequate unless an intrapulmonary shunt is contributing to the hypoxemia, as usually occurs in acute pneumonia. At flows greater than approximately 6 L/minute, only a small further augmentation in the $P{IO_2}$ can be achieved.

Because gas flow through the nose has a drying and irritating effect, a face mask should be considered at high flow rates. O_2 face masks using the Venturi principle allow the regulation of $F{IO_2}$ and can be particularly useful when COPD is suspected, and it is important to avoid the CO_2 retention that can be associated with the unregulated administration of O_2. A higher $F{IO_2}$ of 0.5 to nearly 1.0 can be administered through a non-rebreathing face mask with an O_2 reservoir.

High-Flow Nasal Oxygen

High-flow O_2 blenders deliver humidified nasal oxygen at rates as high as 60 L/minute or more to a nonintubated spontaneously breathing patient. These systems require a large flow of O_2 (from a wall unit or tank), however, and are not universally available.

This method of oxygen delivery provides a low level of positive end-expiratory airway pressure (about 2 to 3 cm H_2O) and a modest increase in the elimination of carbon dioxide.[3] High-flow nasal oxygen may reduce subsequent rates of intubation compared with conventional oxygen delivery with a face mask[A3] but not in comparison with noninvasive ventilation,[A4] except in immunocompromised patients with acute hypoxemic respiratory failure.[A5]

The O_2 concentration that is toxic to the lungs in critically ill patients is not known, but prior injury may provide tolerance to O_2 toxicity, whereas prior exposure to conditioning agents, such as bleomycin, may enhance oxidative

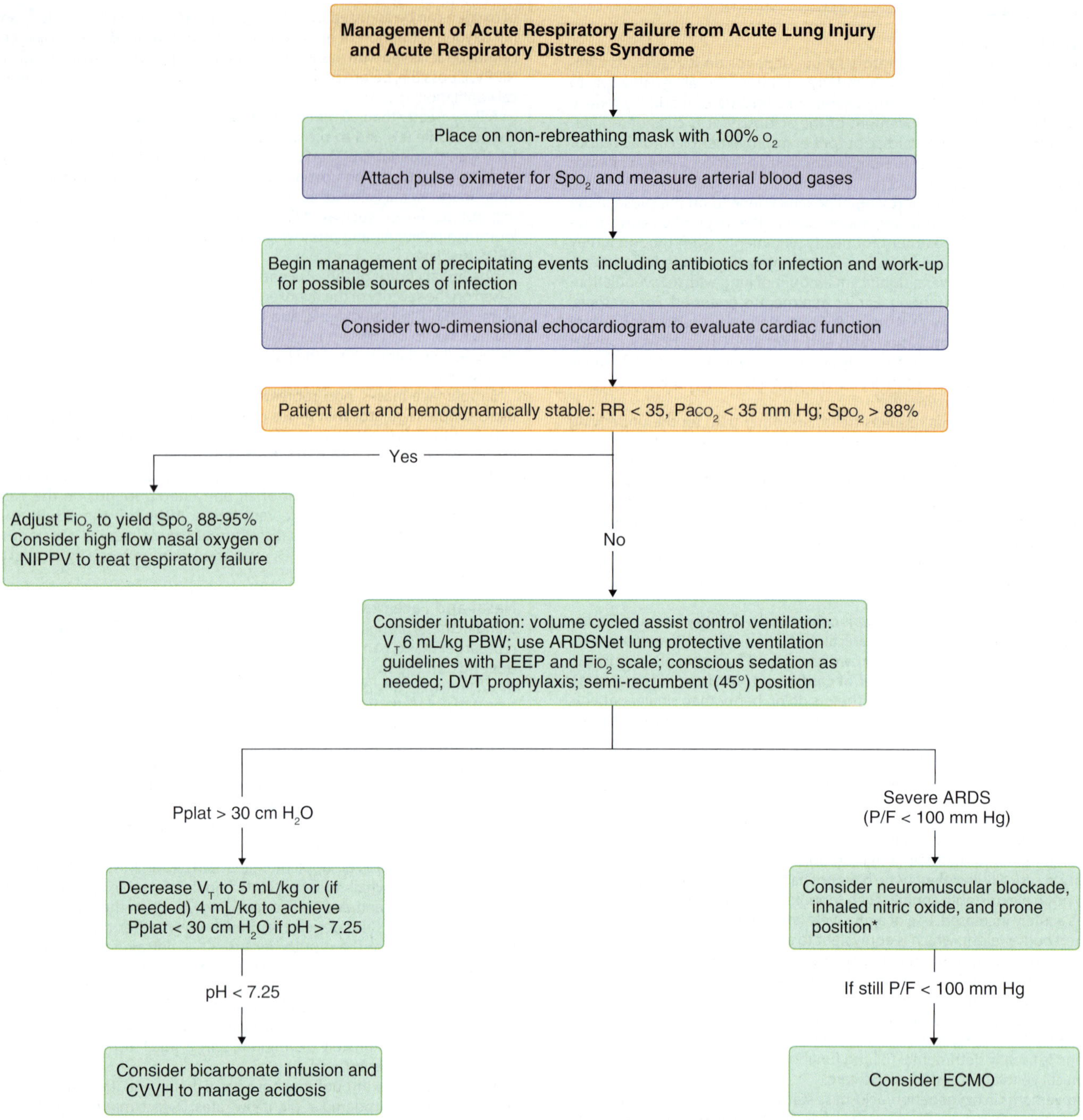

FIGURE 90-4. Management of acute respiratory failure from acute lung injury and acute respiratory distress syndrome. *Prone positioning can be considered when P/F < 150 mm Hg if clinically indicated. ARDS = acute respiratory distress syndrome; CVVH = continuous veno-venous hemofiltration; DVT = deep venous thrombosis; ECMO = extracorporeal membrane oxygenation; Fio_2 = fraction of inspired oxygen; NIPPV = noninvasive positive pressure ventilation; PBW = predicted body weight; PEEP = positive end-expiration pressure; P/F = Pao_2/Fio_2; Pplat = plateau airway pressure; RR = respiratory rate; Spo_2 = arterial oxygen saturation; V_T = tidal volume.

injury. An Fio_2 of 0.7 or higher is generally considered potentially injurious to the normal human lung. Because it is unknown what lower concentration is safe, however, patients should be given the lowest Fio_2 that provides an adequate Sao_2 (≥90%). If an Fio_2 equal to or greater than 0.5 to 0.7 is required for adequate oxygenation, other measures, especially PEEP or CPAP, should be considered. Even a lower Fio_2 of about 0.5 may be associated with impaired ciliary action in the airways and impaired bacterial killing by alveolar macrophages, but the clinical importance of these effects is not known.

Pressure-Assisted Ventilation

CPAP refers to the maintenance of positive pressure during the respiratory cycle while breathing spontaneously.[4] PEEP refers to the maintenance of positive pressure throughout the expiratory cycle when it is applied together with mechanical ventilation (Chapter 91). CPAP and PEEP can result in recruitment of microatelectatic regions of the lung that are perfused but were not previously ventilated, thus contributing substantially to hypoxemia. CPAP and PEEP have the theoretical advantage of keeping some of these regions open during exhalation, thus preventing cyclic closure and reopening of lung units, which may result in alveolar wall stress and injury.

Ventilatory maneuvers that may increase arterial oxygenation include mechanical ventilation itself and the administration of PEEP or CPAP, all of which allow ventilation of areas of the lung that were previously poorly ventilated or unventilated. Although large tidal volumes with mechanical ventilation may open areas of atelectasis and may improve oxygenation initially, these higher tidal volumes can cause ventilator-induced lung injury, particularly if the lung has already been injured (Chapter 91).

If the patient has refractory hypoxemia, acidosis, or a high work of breathing, then endotracheal intubation should be considered to provide positive-pressure ventilation. Indications for placement of an artificial airway in a patient with acute respiratory failure are to protect the airway against aspiration of gastric contents, to deliver an increased FIO_2, to facilitate ventilation, and possibly to aid in the control of respiratory secretions (Chapter 91).

Supportive Measures

Every patient with acute respiratory failure is at risk for deep venous thrombosis, pulmonary thromboembolism, gastric stress ulceration, acute delirium, and deconditioning/weakness. Prophylactic anticoagulation to prevent venous thrombosis (Chapter 68) is recommended in patients who are not at high risk for bleeding complications; sequential leg compression therapy may be preferred for high-risk patients. Nutrition is important to maintain strength needed for weaning. In patients with ARDS, limited enteral feeding for up to 6 days is as good as full enteral feeding in terms of ventilator-free days, 60-day mortality, and infectious complications, and limited feedings induce less gastrointestinal intolerance.

The best means of preventing gastric stress ulceration is not known, but current evidence indicates that the use of an H_2-receptor blocker is superior to the gastric administration of sucralfate on the basis of a large randomized, controlled trial that found a higher incidence of significant bleeding in patients receiving sucralfate than in those receiving ranitidine. Evidence also indicates that proton pump inhibitors may be useful in the acute care setting, although there is concern that more complete acid suppression with these agents may lead to a higher incidence of ventilator-associated pneumonia (Chapter 85) and *Clostridium difficile* infection (Chapter 271).

Current evidence supports maintaining the head of the bed at a 45-degree angle to reduce aspiration and the risk of ventilator-associated pneumonia in critically ill patients. Attempts should be made to ensure a normal day-night sleep pattern, including minimizing activity and reducing direct lighting at night. The patient should change position frequently, including sitting in a chair and walking short distances if possible, even while receiving mechanical ventilatory support. Mobilization can enhance the removal of secretions, help maintain musculoskeletal function, reduce the risk of deep venous thrombosis, and provide psychological benefits.

To facilitate early mobilization and weaning from the ventilator, sedating agents should be minimized and benzodiazepines should be avoided because of their potential to induce or exacerbate delirium in critical illness. Daily awakening and spontaneous breathing trials in mechanically ventilated patients facilitate weaning, reduce time on the ventilator, and improve survival (Chapter 91).

SPECIFIC ACUTE RESPIRATORY FAILURE SYNDROMES

Chronic Obstructive Pulmonary Disease

EPIDEMIOLOGY AND PATHOBIOLOGY

The epidemiology and pathobiology of COPD are discussed in Chapter 76.

CLINICAL MANIFESTATIONS

When patients with COPD develop acute respiratory failure, they commonly have a history of increasing dyspnea and sputum production. Acute respiratory failure may also present with a change in mental status, arrhythmias, or other cardiovascular abnormalities. Acute respiratory failure must be considered whenever patients with COPD have significant nonspecific clinical changes.

DIAGNOSIS

The diagnosis can be confirmed by an arterial blood gas that reveals alveolar hypoventilation with an elevated $PacO_2$ and an acidemic pH. The pH is helpful in assessing whether the hypoventilation is partly or exclusively acute. The pH declines by approximately 0.08 for each rise of 10 mm Hg in the $PacO_2$ in acute respiratory acidosis without renal compensation. By comparison, in chronic respiratory acidosis with normal renal compensation, the pH declines by only about 0.03 for each 10 mm Hg rise in the $PacO_2$.

TREATMENT

General Care

As soon as acute respiratory failure is confirmed in a patient with COPD, attention must focus on identifying the precipitating events (Table 90-4), including increased airway resistance, caused by bronchospasm or increased secretions, often associated with an upper respiratory viral infection; atelectasis, pneumonia, or pulmonary edema; decreased ventilatory drive, secondary to oversedation; decreased muscle strength or function, often related to electrolyte abnormalities, including hypophosphatemia and hypomagnesemia; decreased chest wall elasticity, possibly related to rib fracture, pleural effusion, ileus, or ascites; or increased metabolic O_2 requirements that may be associated with a systemic infection. Some of these abnormalities can impair the cough mechanism and diminish the clearance of airway secretions.

TABLE 90-4 PRINCIPLES IN THE MANAGEMENT OF CHRONIC OBSTRUCTIVE PULMONARY DISEASE PATIENTS WITH ACUTE RESPIRATORY FAILURE

1. Monitor and treat life-threatening hypoxemia (these measures should be performed simultaneously)
   a. Assess the patient clinically, and measure oxygenation by arterial blood gases and/or oximetry
      (1) If the patient is hypoxemic, initiate supplemental oxygen therapy with nasal prongs (low flows [1to 2 L/min] are usually sufficient) or by Venturi face mask (24 or 28% oxygen delivered)
      (2) If the patient needs ventilatory support, consider noninvasive ventilation
      (3) Determine whether the patient needs to be intubated; this is almost always a clinical decision. Immediate action is required if the patient is comatose or severely obtunded
   b. A reasonable goal in most patients is a PaO_2 of 55 to 60 mm Hg or SaO_2 of 88 to 90%
   c. After changes in FIO_2, check blood gases and check regularly for signs of carbon dioxide retention and worsening respiratory acidosis
2. Start to correct life-threatening acidosis
   a. The most effective approach is to correct the underlying cause of acute respiratory failure (e.g., bronchospasm, infection, heart failure)
   b. Consider ventilatory support, based largely on clinical considerations
   c. With severe acidosis, the use of bicarbonate is often ineffective, and there is little evidence of a clinical benefit
3. If ventilatory support is required, consider noninvasive mechanical ventilation.
   a. The patient must have intact upper airway reflexes and be alert, cooperative, and hemodynamically stable
   b. Careful monitoring is required; if the patient does not tolerate the mask, becomes hemodynamically unstable, or has a deteriorating mental status or worsening acidosis, consider intubation
4. Treat airway obstruction and the underlying disease process that triggered the episode of acute respiratory failure
   a. Treat airway obstruction with pharmacologic agents: systemic corticosteroids and bronchodilators (ipratropium and β-adrenergic agents)
   b. Improve secretion clearance: encourage the patient to cough; administer chest physical therapy if cough is impaired and a trial appears effective
   c. Treat the underlying disease process (e.g., antibiotics, diuretics)
5. Prevent complications of the disease process and minimize iatrogenic complications
   a. Pulmonary thromboembolism prophylaxis: use intermittent pneumatic compression or use subcutaneous low-dose unfractionated heparin or low-molecular-weight heparin if no contraindications exist
   b. Gastrointestinal complications: administer prophylaxis for gastrointestinal bleeding in patients requiring mechanical ventilation
   c. Hemodynamics: if the patient is ventilated, monitor and minimize auto-PEEP, which can cause hypotension and barotrauma
      (1) Treat the underlying airway obstruction
      (2) Decrease the respiratory rate to allow adequate expiratory time; may require sedation and controlled hypoventilation
      (3) Use small tidal volumes (6 to 8 mL/kg/PBW); increase the inspiratory flow rate to decrease the inspiratory time and lengthen the expiratory time
   d. Cardiac arrhythmias: maintain oxygenation and normalize electrolytes

FIO_2 = fraction of inspired oxygen; PaO_2 = partial pressure of oxygen in arterial blood; PBW = predicted body weight; PEEP = positive end-expiratory pressure; SaO_2 = oxygen saturation

Infection

The most common specific precipitating event is airway infection, especially acute bronchitis. The role played by viral agents, *Mycoplasma pneumoniae*, chronic colonizers of the lower airway such as *Haemophilus influenzae* and *Streptococcus pneumoniae*, and other acute pathogens is difficult to determine. Acute exacerbations of COPD commonly result from new infections rather than from reemergence of an infection by preexisting colonization. Antibiotics modestly shorten the duration of the exacerbation, with no significant increase in toxicity, compared with placebo; the impact of antibiotics on the subsequent emergence of resistant organisms is not known. It is standard practice to use antibiotics to treat a patient with COPD who has an exacerbation severe enough to cause acute respiratory failure and who has evidence consistent with acute tracheobronchitis (Chapters 76 and 84). Pneumonia may account for 10 to 20% of cases of acute respiratory failure in patients with COPD. Compared with the physiologically normal population, patients with COPD who have community-acquired pneumonia are more likely to have gram-negative enteric bacteria or *Legionella* infections and are more likely to have antibiotic-resistant organisms.

Other Precipitating Causes

Other common precipitating causes of acute respiratory failure include heart failure and worsening of the underlying COPD, often related to noncompliance with medications. Pulmonary thromboembolism must also be considered, particularly if no other cause of acute respiratory failure is identified.

Mechanical Ventilation

The decision to institute mechanical ventilation in patients with COPD and acute respiratory failure must be made on clinical grounds and is not dictated by any particular arterial blood gas values. In general, if the patient is alert and is able to cooperate with treatment, mechanical ventilation often is not necessary. If ventilatory support is required (Chapter 91), the decision is whether to use NIPPV therapy (i.e., ventilatory support through a mask without endotracheal intubation) or endotracheal intubation with positive-pressure ventilation. A number of clinical trials have demonstrated that NIPPV is preferred for patients with COPD and can decrease mortality if it is applied in appropriate patients with no characteristics that are likely to lead to complications, such as a markedly decreased mental status, hypotension, or an inability to tolerate the tight-fitting face mask that is required for NIPPV. A trial of therapy with NIPPV requires close monitoring. If the patient develops worsening acidosis (pH < 7.25), a decline in mental status, or worsening oxygenation, then endotracheal intubation is indicated. In most patients, improvement in the pH and the $Paco_2$ within 30 minutes to 2 hours predicts success. Most patients with acute respiratory failure caused by an exacerbation of COPD require treatment in an intensive care unit where appropriate physician, nursing, and respiratory care are available (Chapter 76).

PROGNOSIS

Acute respiratory failure in patients with severe COPD is associated with an in-hospital mortality rate of 6 to 20%. The severity of the underlying disease and the severity of the acute precipitating illness are important determinants of hospital survival. Hospital mortality is higher if the respiratory failure is associated with a pH lower than 7.25 and if the patient requires invasive mechanical ventilation. However, the pH, the $Paco_2$, and other clinical characteristics are not reliable in predicting a particular patient's chances of survival to hospital discharge.

ACUTE RESPIRATORY DISTRESS SYNDROME

DEFINITION

ARDS is the abrupt onset of diffuse lung injury characterized by severe hypoxemia (shunting) and bilateral pulmonary infiltrates not explained by left-sided cardiac failure (Table 90-5).[4] The severity of ARDS is determined on the basis of the Pao_2 divided by the Fio_2 (Pao_2/Fio_2, also called the P/F ratio). These oxygenation categories require positive-pressure ventilation with at least 5 cm H_2O positive end-expiratory pressure.

One limitation of this definition is that it does not include patients who have ARDS-like acute respiratory failure but who are not receiving positive-pressure ventilation, including patients who initially are profoundly hypoxemic but can be sufficiently oxygenated with high-flow nasal oxygen.[5] Such early acute lung injury can be diagnosed in spontaneously breathing patients who have bilateral pulmonary infiltrates and in whom the inspired Fio_2 can be estimated and the Pao_2 measured.[6,7] In addition, pulse oximetric oxygen saturation (Spo_2) can be substituted for the directly measured Pao_2 in most patients to estimate the P/F ratio. If patients with early acute lung injury can be identified prior to the need for positive-pressure ventilation, they can be treated with strategies, such as high-flow nasal oxygen, that might reduce the progression of their acute respiratory failure.

EPIDEMIOLOGY

ARDS is a clinical syndrome triggered most commonly by pulmonary or nonpulmonary infections, aspiration of gastric contents, or severe trauma (Table 90-6). The annual incidence of ARDS is about 80 cases per 100,000 in the U.S. adult population, with a high frequency in intensive care units worldwide. These numbers have increased dramatically with the SARS-CoV-2 (Chapter 336) COVID-19 pandemic.[8,9] The underlying precipitating factor may affect and injure the lungs directly, such as in diffuse pneumonia or aspiration of gastric contents, or it may affect the lungs indirectly, as in severe sepsis from a nonpulmonary source (Chapter 94) or severe nonthoracic trauma associated with shock (Chapter 97). Sepsis is the most common precipitating cause of ARDS worldwide. The organisms vary widely, ranging from gram-negative and gram-positive bacteria and viruses (e.g., H1N1 influenza [Chapter 332] in 2009; SARS-CoV-2 infection [Chapter 337] in 2020-2021) to leptospiral infections (Chapter 298) or malaria (Chapter 316).

TABLE 90-5 BERLIN DEFINITION OF THE ACUTE RESPIRATORY DISTRESS SYNDROME

CRITERIA			
Timing	Within 1 week of a known clinical insult or new/worsening respiratory symptoms		
Chest imaging	Bilateral opacities—not fully explained by effusions, lobar/lung collapse, or nodules		
Origin of edema	Respiratory failure not fully explained by cardiac failure or fluid overload Need objective assessment (e.g., echocardiography) to exclude hydrostatic edema		
	MILD	**MODERATE**	**SEVERE**
Oxygenation	$200 < Pao_2/Fio_2 \le 300$ with PEEP or CPAP ≥ 5 cm H_2O	$100 < Pao_2/Fio_2 \le 200$ with PEEP ≥ 5 cm H_2O	$Pao_2/Fio_2 \le 100$ with PEEP ≥ 5 cm H_2O

CPAP = continuous positive airway pressure; Fio_2 = fraction of inspired oxygen; Pao_2 = partial pressure of oxygen in arterial blood; PEEP = positive end-expiratory pressure.
Ranieri VM, Rubenfeld GD, Thompson BT, et al. Acute respiratory distress syndrome: the Berlin Definition. *JAMA*. 2012;307:2526-2533.

TABLE 90-6 DISORDERS ASSOCIATED WITH ACUTE RESPIRATORY DISTRESS SYNDROME

COMMON

Sepsis (gram-positive or gram-negative bacterial, viral, fungal, or parasitic infection; Chapter 94)
Diffuse pneumonia (bacterial, viral, or fungal; Chapters 85, 336)
Aspiration of gastric contents
Trauma (usually severe; Chapter 97)

LESS COMMON

Drowning (fresh or salt water; Chapter 82)
Drug overdose
- Acetylsalicylic acid (Chapter 96)
- Heroin and other narcotic drugs (Chapter 365)

Transfusion-associated lung injury (Chapter 162)
Massive blood transfusion (likely a marker of severe trauma, but also seen with severe gastrointestinal bleeding, especially in patients with severe liver disease; Chapter 162)
Inhalation of smoke or corrosive gases (usually requires high concentrations; Chapter 82)
Acute pancreatitis (Chapter 130)
Fat embolism (Chapter 68)
Cardiopulmonary bypass (Chapter 59)

PATHOBIOLOGY

Pathology

Despite the variety of underlying disease processes leading to ARDS, the lung's response to these insults results in similar clinical findings, physiologic changes, and morphologic abnormalities. The pathologic abnormalities in ARDS are nonspecific and are described as *diffuse alveolar damage* by pathologists. Ultrastructural studies with electron microscopy usually show endothelial and alveolar epithelial injury. Routine histology shows acute inflammation, usually with neutrophils predominating in the alveolar edema fluid. Hyaline membranes are present in some, but not all, patients, similar to those seen in premature infants with infant respiratory distress syndrome, presumably related to a procoagulant environment in the injured alveoli. Large-molecular-weight plasma proteins, including fibrinogen, accumulate, and inflammatory factors lead to fibrin deposition. Alveolar flooding impairs surfactant, which is abnormal in quantity and quality. The result is microatelectasis, which may be associated with impaired immune function. The resolution of ARDS depends in part on restoration of a functional alveolar epithelial barrier that is capable of removing alveolar edema fluid by sodium-dependent vectorial fluid transport. Pulmonary fibrosis may occur, particularly in the setting of injurious mechanical ventilation (Chapter 91). However, lung function tends to improve over time in survivors of ARDS, and the fibrosis is often reversible.

Pathophysiology

The physiologic abnormalities are dominated by severe hypoxemia with shunting, decreased lung compliance, decreased functional residual capacity, increased pulmonary dead space, and increased work of breathing. Initially, the $PaCO_2$ is low or normal, usually associated with increased minute ventilation. The initial abnormalities in oxygenation are thought to be related to alveolar flooding and collapse, which create a physiologic shunt. As the lung injury progresses, especially in patients who require ventilatory support, fibroproliferation may develop; the lungs (including alveoli, blood vessels, and small airways) remodel and scar, with a loss of microvasculature. Pulmonary microvascular thrombosis may also occur. In some patients, these changes may lead to pulmonary hypertension and increased pulmonary dead space; marked elevations in minute ventilation are sometimes required to achieve a normal $PaCO_2$, even as oxygenation abnormalities are improving.

CLINICAL MANIFESTATIONS

In most cases of ARDS, the onset either coincides with or occurs within 72 hours of the onset of the underlying disease process; the mean time from onset of the underlying cause to onset of ARDS is 12 to 24 hours. The onset may be more protracted in patients with viral pneumonia, such as COVID-19 pneumonia due to SARS-CoV-2 infection (Chapter 337). The presenting clinical picture is dominated by respiratory distress and the accompanying findings of severe hypoxemia, tachypnea, an increase in minute ventilation, and generalized alveolar infiltrates or opacities on the chest radiograph. The clinical presentation may also reflect manifestations of the underlying disease process, such as severe sepsis with hypotension and other manifestations of systemic infection.

DIAGNOSIS

The key to diagnosis is to distinguish ARDS from pure cardiogenic pulmonary edema (Table 90-7). No specific blood test or bronchoalveolar lavage finding (Chapter 73) is sufficiently specific to be useful for diagnosing ARDS. Furthermore, ARDS may coexist with left ventricular failure or intravascular volume overload, and as many as 30% of ARDS patients can have an elevated pulmonary arterial wedge pressure at some point during their clinical course (Table 90-7).

TABLE 90-7 FEATURES ASSOCIATED WITH NONCARDIOGENIC AND CARDIOGENIC PULMONARY EDEMA*

NONCARDIOGENIC PULMONARY EDEMA (ARDS)	CARDIOGENIC PULMONARY EDEMA/VOLUME OVERLOAD
PRIOR HISTORY	
No history of heart disease	Prior history of heart disease
Appropriate fluid balance (difficult to assess after resuscitation from shock or trauma)	Hypertension, chest pain, new-onset palpitations; positive fluid balance
PHYSICAL EXAMINATION	
Flat neck veins	Elevated neck veins
Hyperdynamic pulses	Left ventricular enlargement, lift, heave, dyskinesis
Early diastolic gallop	S_3 and S_4; gallops
Absence of edema	Edema: flank, presacral, legs
ELECTROCARDIOGRAM	
Sinus tachycardia, nonspecific ST-T wave changes	Evidence of prior or ongoing ischemia, supraventricular tachycardia, left ventricular hypertrophy
CHEST RADIOGRAPH	
Normal heart size	Cardiomegaly
Peripheral distribution of abnormal opacities	Central or basilar abnormal opacities peribronchial and vascular congestion Cephalization of great vessels
Air bronchograms common (80%)	Septal lines (Kerley lines), air bronchograms (25%), pleural effusion
HEMODYNAMIC MEASUREMENTS	
Pulmonary artery wedge pressure < 15 mm Hg, cardiac index > 3.5 L/min/m^2	Pulmonary capillary wedge pressure > 18 mm Hg, cardiac index < 3.5 L/min/m^2 with ischemia, may be >3.5 L/min/m^2 with volume overload
ECHOCARDIOGRAM	
Transthoracic echocardiogram showing a left ventricular ejection fraction >50%	Transthoracic echocardiogram showing a decreased left ventricular ejection fraction
LABORATORY VALUES	
B-type natriuretic peptide < 100 pg/mL	B-type natriuretic peptide > 500 pg/mL

*These features are neither highly sensitive nor specific. Although the findings are more commonly associated with the type of pulmonary edema as listed, they do not have high positive or negative predictive value.
ARDS = acute respiratory distress syndrome.

TREATMENT

Treatment of ARDS consists predominantly of respiratory support and treatment of the underlying disorder (see Fig. 90-4).[10–12] Sepsis, which is a common predisposing condition for the development of ARDS, must be treated promptly (Chapter 94).

Because infection is the most common cause of ARDS, it is very important to identify the pulmonary or extrapulmonary source of infection. The differential diagnosis of pneumonia (Chapter 85) should be carefully considered, including determining whether the patient is immunosuppressed and, as a result, susceptible to a wider variety of infectious agents. Viral pneumonia from influenza (Chapter 332), respiratory syncytial virus (Chapter 330), or other viruses should be considered. A recent travel history should inform the patient's exposure to malaria (Chapter 316), leptospirosis (Chapter 298), ehrlichiosis (Chapter 302), or fungal infections such as coccidiomycosis (Chapter 308) or blastomycosis (Chapter 308). If the patient has an abdominal source of infection, then appropriate diagnostic imaging and surgical approaches are needed to establish a diagnosis and drain the infection. Any coexisting left heart failure or intravascular volume overload should be treated promptly (Chapter 46).

Current recommendations for lung-protective mechanical ventilation by endotracheal intubation in ARDS (Table 90-8) emphasize lower tidal volumes based on the patient's predicted body weight (Chapter 91).[A6] This approach also includes achieving a plateau airway pressure less than 30 cm H_2O. PEEP is a mainstay in the ventilatory strategy for ARDS. Although the method for determining the optimal level of PEEP has not been established, moderately high PEEP levels in the range of 12 to 20 cm H_2O may be beneficial compared with lower levels, but routine use of very high PEEP levels (greater than 20 cm H_2O) and large recruitment maneuvers is potentially detrimental.[A7] PEEP may allow a lower FIO_2 to provide adequate oxygenation, thereby reducing the risk of O_2 toxicity. It also may prevent the cyclic collapse and reopening of lung units, a process that is thought to be a major cause of ventilator-induced lung injury, even when adequate oxygenation can be obtained at relatively low levels of FIO_2. Routine early neuromuscular blockade does not appear to be beneficial,[A8] but it can be used to obtain patient-ventilator synchrony if deep sedation is not sufficient. In patients with severe ARDS who do not respond to standard therapy but otherwise have a reasonable life expectancy and do not have multiorgan failure, extracorporeal membrane oxygenation is an acceptable rescue therapy[13,14] that can be reserved for patients who require it for severe refractory hypoxemia.[A9] Data also indicate that prone positioning[15] reduces mortality in patients with moderate to severe ARDS (initial P/F < 150 mm Hg).[A10]

In patients with ARDS, a conservative fluid strategy decreases the duration of positive pressure ventilation[A11] and can be instituted if a patient is not in shock, as defined by the need for vasopressors to support systemic blood pressure. The primary principle of a conservative fluid strategy is to achieve a daily net negative fluid balance of 0.5 to 2 liters, usually by limiting intravenous fluids and administering diuretics at least twice daily, though more frequent dosing may be required. Measurement of pulmonary artery or central venous pressure is not of major value for guiding fluid balance in most cases.

PROGNOSIS

Case-fatality rates are 30 to 50% and are highly dependent on disease severity, the underlying predisposing condition, and the presence of comorbid diseases. Based on the degree of hypoxemia (mild, 200 mm Hg < PaO_2/FIO_2 < 300 mm Hg; moderate, 100 mm Hg < PaO_2/FIO_2 < 200 mm Hg; and severe, PaO_2/FIO_2 < 100 mm Hg), inpatient mortality rates are about 27%, 32%, and 45%, respectively, not including patients with severe underlying conditions, such as end-stage cancer. Patients who require higher driving pressures while intubated

TABLE 90-8 ARDS NETWORK VENTILATORY MANAGEMENT PROTOCOL FOR TIDAL VOLUME AND PLATEAU AIRWAY PRESSURE

Calculate PBW (in kg):
 Male PBW: 50 + 2.3 (height in inches − 60) or 50 + 0.91 (height in centimeters − 152.4)
 Female PBW: 45.5 + 2.3 (height in inches − 60) or 45.5 + 0.91 (height in centimeters − 152.4)
Select assist control mode
Set initial Vt at 8 mL/kg PBW
Reduce Vt by 1 mL/kg at intervals <2 hr until Vt = 6 mL/kg PBW
Set initial RR to approximate baseline minute ventilation (maximum RR = 35/min)
Set inspiratory flow rate higher than patient's demand (usually >80 L/min)
Adjust Vt and RR further to achieve P_{plat} and pH goals
 If P_{plat} >30 cm H_2O: decrease Vt by 1 mL/kg PBW (minimum = 4 mL/kg PBW)
 If pH ≤7.30, increase RR (maximum = 35)
 If pH <7.15, increase RR to 35; consider sodium bicarbonate administration or increase Vt

ARDS = acute respiratory distress syndrome; PBW = predicted body weight; P_{plat} = plateau pressure (airway pressure at the end of delivery of a tidal volume breath during a condition of no airflow); RR = respiratory rate; Vt = tidal volume.
See the ARDSNet website (http://www.ardsnet.org) for further details about the protocol, including the approach for setting positive end-expiratory pressure and fraction of inspired oxygen.

also have a worse prognosis. Memory, verbal fluency, and executive function are impaired in about 13%, 16%, and 49% of long-term survivors after ARDS.

ACUTE RESPIRATORY FAILURE WITHOUT LUNG DISEASE

Acute respiratory failure without pulmonary abnormalities (see Table 90-2) develops in patients with depressed ventilatory drive secondary to central nervous system dysfunction and in patients with severe neuromuscular disease. The prototypical patient with suppressed ventilatory drive has taken an overdose of a sedative or tranquilizing medication (Chapter 96). The prototypical patient with neuromuscular disease has Guillain-Barré syndrome (Chapter 388). The treatment for both types of patients is supportive. In the case of a patient with a sedative overdose, the threshold for intubation with mechanical ventilatory support should be low because this temporary condition is quickly reversible when the responsible drug is eliminated. In addition, such a patient may require intubation for airway protection against aspiration of gastric contents regardless of whether acute respiratory failure has developed.

Patients with Guillain-Barré syndrome (Chapter 388) or other forms of progressive neuromuscular disease should be monitored with serial measurements of vital capacity and of their ability to cough and swallow. In general, when the vital capacity decreases to less than 10 to 15 mL/kg body weight and the patient's normal upper airway reflexes are impaired for protection against aspiration of oropharyngeal or gastric contents, then intubation and mechanical ventilatory support should be considered without regard to the patient's $Paco_2$.

GENERAL REFERENCES

For the General References and other additional features, please visit Elsevier eBooks+ at https://ebooks.health.elsevier.com.

Grade A References

A1. Schjørring OL, Klitgaard TL, Perner A, et al. Lower or higher oxygenation targets for acute hypoxemic respiratory failure. *N Engl J Med*. 2021;384:1301-1311.
A2. Chu DK, Kim LH, Young PJ, et al. Mortality and morbidity in acutely ill adults treated with liberal versus conservative oxygen therapy (IOTA): a systematic review and meta-analysis. *Lancet*. 2018;391:1693-1705.
A3. Baldomero AK, Melzer AC, Greer N, et al. Effectiveness and harms of high-flow nasal oxygen for acute respiratory failure: an evidence report for a clinical guideline from the American College of Physicians. *Ann Intern Med*. 2021;174:952-966.
A4. Ferreyro BL, Angriman F, Munshi L, et al. Association of noninvasive oxygenation strategies with all-cause mortality in adults with acute hypoxemic respiratory failure: a systematic review and meta-analysis. *JAMA*. 2020;324:57-67.
A5. Azoulay E, Lemiale V, Mokart D, et al. Effect of high-flow nasal oxygen vs standard oxygen on 28-day mortality in immunocompromised patients with acute respiratory failure: the HIGH randomized clinical trial. *JAMA*. 2018;320:2099-2107.
A6. Sud S, Friedrich JO, Adhikari NKJ, et al. Comparative effectiveness of protective ventilation strategies for moderate and severe acute respiratory distress syndrome: a network meta-analysis. *Am J Respir Crit Care Med*. 2021;203:1366-1377.
A7. Cavalcanti AB, Suzumura EA, Laranjeira LN, et al. Effect of lung recruitment and titrated positive END-expiratory pressure (PEEP) vs low PEEP on mortality in patients with acute respiratory distress syndrome: a randomized clinical trial. *JAMA*. 2017;318:1335-1345.
A8. Moss M, Huang DT, Brower RG, et al. Early neuromuscular blockade in the acute respiratory distress syndrome. *N Engl J Med*. 2019;380:1997-2008.
A9. Combes A, Hajage G, Capellier A, et al. Extracorporeal membrane oxygenation for severe acute respiratory distress syndrome. *N Engl J Med*. 2018;378:1965-1975.
A10. Park SY, Kim HJ, Yoo KH, et al. The efficacy and safety of prone positioning in adults patients with acute respiratory distress syndrome: a meta-analysis of randomized controlled trials. *J Thorac Dis*. 2015;7:356-367.
A11. Silversides JA, Major E, Ferguson AJ, et al. Conservative fluid management or deresuscitation for patients with sepsis or acute respiratory distress syndrome following the resuscitation phase of critical illness: a systematic review and meta-analysis. *Intensive Care Med*. 2017;43:155-170.

91 MECHANICAL VENTILATION

LAURENT BROCHARD AND ARTHUR S. SLUTSKY

Mechanical ventilation is a life-sustaining therapy in which a mechanical device (the ventilator) provides partial or full support for patients with respiratory failure (Chapter 90). The main goals of ventilatory support are to maintain adequate gas exchange, to rest the respiratory muscles, and to decrease the oxygen cost of breathing, while minimizing iatrogenic consequences of ventilation. To achieve these goals, the clinician can use a variety of modes of ventilation and can alter the inspired oxygen fraction, the pressure at the end of a breath, and other facets of the volume or pressure time pattern generated by the ventilator.

Modern ventilation strategies focus on minimizing its iatrogenic consequences, such as hyperinflation (from endogenously derived positive pressure at the end of a breath; i.e., auto-PEEP), infection, oxygen toxicity, injury to the respiratory muscles (e.g., disuse atrophy or injury due to excessive loading), and ventilator-induced lung injury. A major goal of current ventilatory strategies is to protect the ventilated aerated lung and, to some extent, to protect the respiratory muscles. In some patients, the physician should be willing to accept arterial blood gases that are not in the normal range to avoid these complications, by using lower levels of minute ventilation or smaller tidal volumes than those required to normalize gas exchange.[1] As a result, targeting normal values of blood gases is not always preferred for critically ill patients in the intensive care unit (ICU). For example, a conservative protocol for oxygen therapy (e.g., a goal Pao_2 between 70 and 100 mm Hg or arterial oxyhemoglobin saturation between 94% and 98%) is at least as good as more aggressive or liberal oxygen therapy (e.g., Pao_2 up to 150 mm Hg or arterial oxyhemoglobin saturation between 97% and 100%).[A1,A2] However, further reducing the target Pao_2 to 55 to 75 mm Hg or an oxyhemoglobin saturation goal of 90% is not beneficial.[A3,A4] Other trade-offs include the acceptable level of $Paco_2$ and pH versus the minute ventilation and the risks related to excessive energy delivered to the lungs, and the degree of spontaneous breathing versus the risks of injury to the respiratory muscles from disuse atrophy or excessive loading.[2]

POSITIVE-PRESSURE VENTILATION

Modern mechanical ventilation delivers gas to the lung with positive-pressure ventilation applied through an endotracheal tube, a tracheostomy, or a tight-fitting mask. The approach using a mask is termed noninvasive ventilation (NIV).[3]

The most basic positive pressure mode is controlled ventilation, in which a pre-set tidal volume (volume-controlled) or a pre-set inspiratory pressure (pressure-controlled) is delivered at a predetermined rate and insufflation time, regardless of the patient's effort. This form of ventilation is used in patients who cannot initiate spontaneous breaths (e.g., heavily sedated or paralyzed patients) and/or in patients who need full ventilatory support because of extremely severe pulmonary (e.g., severe acute respiratory distress syndrome [ARDS]) or cardiovascular disease (e.g., severe shock).

A disadvantage of this approach is that respiratory muscle atrophy can occur relatively rapidly, since there is no respiratory muscle contraction. Another disadvantage is that gas exchange may not be optimal because the distribution of ventilation is altered compared with spontaneous breathing. This altered ventilation is an indirect effect of deep sedation, with or without paralysis, and the patient's supine position, both of which promote atelectasis in the dorsal regions of the lungs. For these reasons, it is best to limit the time that a patient is paralyzed and receiving controlled ventilation.

Assisted ventilation is a general term that describes mechanical ventilation in which the patient's spontaneous ventilatory effort triggers the ventilator to deliver a breath, rather than having the breaths delivered by the ventilator at a fixed rate. Assist-control ventilation (in pressure or volume control mode) uses settings similar to controlled ventilation for the delivery of each breath, but breaths can be triggered by the patient's spontaneous ventilatory effort; it will provide a baseline ventilatory rate if the patient fails to trigger the ventilator. The back-up rate is set to allow the patient to breathe at a faster rate than set on the ventilator. Assist-control is the most frequently used mode of ventilation at the early phase of mechanical ventilation.

Positive End-Expiratory Pressure

A key characteristic that can be combined with most ventilatory modes is the pressure level at end expiration. Positive end-expiratory pressure (PEEP) is used in patients with diffuse pulmonary diseases (e.g., pulmonary edema or ARDS) to prevent atelectasis, to reopen collapsed lung units or closed airways, or, more precisely, to help ensure that collapsed alveolar regions opened during inspiration remain open during expiration, so as to redistribute ventilation to dependent, atelectatic lung regions. All these changes can increase end-expiratory lung volume above the natural functional residual capacity and improve the matching of ventilation to perfusion, thereby frequently improving oxygenation and allowing the fractional inspiratory concentration of oxygen (FIO_2) to be reduced. In addition, when PEEP is able to keep part of the lung reopened, the tidal volume can be delivered into a larger lung volume, thereby potentially reducing the risk of injury. PEEP does not usually improve alveolar ventilation and, in fact, it may increase dead space by overdistending alveoli, with a concomitant decrease in alveolar capillary blood flow in certain regions of the lung. The major risks of PEEP are overdistention of the lung (or regions of the lung) and hemodynamic consequences, such as decreasing cardiac output by decreasing venous return or increasing right ventricular afterload. The main limitation of titrating PEEP as a single pressure delivered to the whole lung is that the distribution of lung injury and collapse in patients with hypoxemia is influenced by gravity. Therefore, a certain level of positive pressure may effectively reopen the dorsal (dependent) lung region but excessively distend the ventral (nondependent lung).

Volume- and Pressure-Controlled Ventilation

Volume-controlled ventilation (or volume-limited ventilation) refers to mechanical ventilation in which the tidal volume (and usually the peak flow) is pre-set. The major advantage is that the delivered tidal volume is maintained even if lung mechanics change, thereby ensuring a more constant partial pressure of arterial carbon dioxide ($PaCO_2$). If respiratory mechanics deteriorate, higher pressures may be required to achieve the tidal volume goal. In volume-controlled ventilation, an upper limit to applied airway pressure is commonly used for safety reasons.

With pressure-controlled ventilation, the ventilator delivers pressure-limited breaths to the patient. The delivered volume is variable and depends on the pre-set pressure, the ventilatory rate, the inspiratory time, and the patient's respiratory mechanics (resistance, compliance, and auto-PEEP). The ventilation resulting from volume and pressure-controlled ventilation is very similar in passive conditions.

Assist-control ventilation can accompany either volume-limited ventilation or pressure-limited ventilation. Pressure-controlled breaths are often considered more comfortable for the patient because they do not limit the flow or delivered volume in response to patient's demand. The disadvantage is that tidal volume is more difficult to control because it is greatly influenced by patient effort. With volume assist-control, the volume is strictly controlled, but local overdistention can still occur when the patient is breathing with high intensity and a high respiratory drive. In this latter case, high inspiratory peak flows are required to allow the ventilator to meet the patient's volume demands to minimize the work of breathing required by the patient.

Intermittent Mandatory Ventilation

Intermittent mandatory ventilation (IMV) is a mode in which the patient receives some pre-set (and thus mandatory) volume or pressure-limited breaths from the ventilator but in which the patient also breathes spontaneously with different or no support above a certain rate. The so-called mandatory breaths are triggered by the patient and are synchronized (synchronized IMV), and spontaneous breaths are often aided by pressure-support ventilation. This mode has fallen into disfavor, based on clinical studies showing that it leads to longer durations of ventilation.

Pressure-Support Ventilation

Pressure-support ventilation is a pressure-limited, patient-triggered form of assisted ventilation. The patient triggers each ventilator breath by creating either a small negative pressure or a low inspiratory flow at the airway opening, and the ventilator switches to inspiratory mode and provides the airflow needed to maintain a pre-set level of pressure. In contrast to pressure-controlled ventilation, the inspiratory time is not fixed and terminates when the inspiratory airflow decreases to a threshold level (a level that is often adjustable by the person responsible for the ventilator). This mode provides flexibility for the patient with respect to tidal volume, inspiratory flow, respiratory rate, and ratio of time allowed for inspiration compared with expiration. Tidal volume depends on the patient's effort, respiratory system mechanics, and the level of pressure set for support. It is considered to be comfortable for the patient.

The disadvantage of pressure-support ventilation is that it is easy to over-assist the patient because a minimal ventilation (determined by pressure and compliance) is always delivered regardless of the patient's effort.[4] It can thereby deliver breaths that exceed a patient's needs, both in terms of volume and inspiratory duration, and often result in patient-ventilator asynchrony. Pressure-support ventilation has been used to help wean patients because it provides a simple way of reducing the magnitude of mechanical support as the patient assumes a larger fraction of the ventilatory work. It also has become the most frequently used mode of ventilation when the patient begins to stabilize.

High-Frequency Ventilation

High-frequency ventilation refers to modes of ventilation delivered at frequencies that are substantially greater than those used during normal breathing. During high-frequency ventilation, tidal volumes may be less than the dead space, so adequate gas transport takes place by various convective and diffusive mechanisms. Interest in these modes of ventilation has waned for adult patients because it appears to be no better or even worse than conventional ventilation for adults with ARDS.

Proportional Assist Ventilation and Neurally Adjusted Ventilatory Assist

Two major difficulties in providing assisted ventilation are ensuring adequate synchrony between the patient's respiratory pattern and the delivery of the ventilator's breaths and adapting to the patient's variable demand over time. The first point is particularly of concern for patients with markedly abnormal respiratory mechanics, including significant auto-PEEP. Two modes of ventilation, proportional assist ventilation and neurally adjusted ventilatory assist, can partly address these concerns. Both modes deliver ventilation (and pressure) in direct proportion to the instantaneous effort of the patient. However, neither approach is in widespread use because they are not available on all ventilators and because of limited clinical data. Nevertheless, some evidence suggests that these modes may reduce the time spent on the ventilator.[A5]

Noninvasive Positive-Pressure Ventilatory Support

Positive-pressure ventilation can be provided through a mask rather than through an endotracheal tube. This method, which has been termed noninvasive because the patient is not intubated, is conceptually simple but requires appropriate implementation and monitoring for successful application. Of particular importance are patient selection and training of hospital personnel. Patients must be alert, cooperative, and hemodynamically stable. Patients must also have intact upper airway reflexes to prevent aspiration, and they must not have facial trauma that precludes the use of a mask. Once patients are started on noninvasive ventilation, they should be carefully monitored, and noninvasive ventilation should be discontinued if the patient's clinical condition deteriorates, if the patient develops cardiovascular instability, or if it appears that the patient is likely to aspirate. Noninvasive ventilation also can be delivered through a "helmet," thereby avoiding some of the problems associated with use of face masks.[A6]

Noninvasive ventilation offers advantages compared with invasive ventilation because it can avoid many complications associated with intubation and sedation; patients are able to speak and to eat if they are sufficiently stable to remove the mask for short periods, and they are probably able to sleep better. Noninvasive ventilation is also relatively simple to apply, and it can be used for short intervals because it can be started and stopped easily.

However, noninvasive ventilation has limitations and risks. Adequate implementation can be labor intensive, and the time course of correction of blood gases is slower than usually occurs if patients are intubated and ventilated. Data strongly support the use of noninvasive ventilation for patients with chronic obstructive pulmonary disease (COPD; see Chapter 76) or cardiogenic pulmonary edema with elevated CO_2. It is uncertain whether noninvasive ventilation improves outcomes or unduly delays intubation in patients who have hypoxemic respiratory failure and who do not also have concomitant ventilatory failure (i.e., hypoxemic, nonhypercapnic, respiratory failure).

PEEP also can be administered to spontaneously breathing patients by a technique termed continuous positive airway pressure (CPAP). In patients with exacerbations of COPD, PEEP and CPAP can overcome some of the negative mechanical consequences of auto-PEEP (see later) and minimize the work of breathing, provided that the magnitude of the PEEP is sufficiently low that it does not cause additional hyperinflation. CPAP is very effective for relieving the respiratory distress associated with cardiogenic pulmonary edema, in which it has clinical benefits similar to those of noninvasive ventilation. Both noninvasive ventilation and CPAP also can be useful in the postoperative period after thoracic or abdominal surgery to prevent reintubation.

High-flow nasal oxygen (HFNO) therapy offers an attractive alternative for supporting patients who have hypoxemic respiratory failure.[A7] Heated and fully humidified gas at adjustable levels of oxygen concentration is delivered through the nose to the upper airways. This technique generates low levels of positive pressure, washes out the upper airway dead space, and is associated with reduced mortality in patients with acute hypoxemic respiratory failure.[A8]

COMPLICATIONS OF MECHANICAL VENTILATION

INTUBATION, SEDATION, AND BED IMMOBILIZATION

Endotracheal intubation can act as a conduit to deliver gas from the ventilator to the patient, secure a patient's airway, prevent aspiration, and help with pulmonary toilet. However, intubation can be associated with complications, including a risk of aspiration or hypoxemia during insertion of the endotracheal tube, difficulty in swallowing and communicating, disruption of normal host defense mechanisms, and upper airway trauma. Pressure from the cuff of the endotracheal tube that provides a pneumatic seal between the tube and trachea can lead to tracheal ischemia and may eventually cause tracheal stenosis. Bag-mask ventilation during tracheal intubation can maintain better oxygen saturation concentrations and reduce the risk of severe hypoxemia.[A9]

The upper airway is normally an effective means of heating and humidifying inspiratory gases. This natural system is bypassed by an endotracheal tube; inadequately humidified inspiratory gases reduce mucociliary clearance and can lead to inspissation of tracheal secretions and occlusion of the endotracheal tube.

Intubation increases the likelihood of nosocomial pneumonia (Chapters 85 and 261) by a number of mechanisms. Cough involves an increase in airway pressure as respiratory muscles contract against a closed glottis; this mechanism is impaired in the presence of the tube. A cuffed endotracheal tube helps prevent gross aspiration, but pharyngeal secretions that pool at the top of the cuff often seep into the lungs. Endotracheal tubes often become colonized with the microorganisms that cause ventilator-associated pneumonia (Chapter 85). Silver-coated tubes may reduce this risk in selected patients but are considerably more expensive than conventional endotracheal tubes and are unlikely to be used routinely for initial intubation. Endotracheal tubes with a port that allows suctioning of secretions above the cuff may also reduce the incidence of ventilator-associated pneumonia, although results of studies have been mixed.

Endotracheal intubation is often not well tolerated in awake patients, in whom the tube is more likely to be inadvertently dislodged—a complication that can have tragic consequences. Sedation reduces these problems and also prevents or treats dyssynchronies between the patient's respiratory drive and the delivery of gas from the ventilator. Modern strategies focus on reducing sedation as much as possible, thereby facilitating early mobilization of the patient even while ventilated but still allowing for patient-ventilator synchrony. Daily interruption of sedation, light sedation, or no sedation have all been tested with various results in terms of ICU length of stay and mortality.[A10] Studies suggest that adjunctive dexmedetomidine can reduce the time on the ventilator and decrease the incidence of delirium[A11] compared with benzodiazepines, but it has not been shown to impact mortality, and patients may require more supplemental sedation.[A12] Endotracheal intubation, sedation, and paralysis can lead to atelectasis and can reduce functional residual capacity by at least 20%, even in patients with normal lungs.

To decrease sedation, enhance patient mobilization, and improve oral care and feeding, a tracheostomy can be performed. However, tracheostomy is associated with its own complications, and performing a tracheostomy in the first week is frequently no better than waiting until the patient has been ventilated for about 10 to 15 days, in part because clinicians cannot accurately predict which patients will require prolonged ventilatory support. As a result, a common practice is to consider tracheostomy when a patient has been intubated for at least 2 weeks.

HEMODYNAMIC COMPROMISE

Cardiovascular instability, which is the most common peri-intubation complication, may occur in up to 40% of emergency intubations.[5] The subsequent major mechanical determinants of cardiovascular hemodynamics during mechanical ventilation are intrathoracic pressure, changes in lung volume, and the patient's circulatory volume status. An increase in lung volume can be beneficial if it opens lung units that had been closed (thereby leading to a decrease in pulmonary vascular resistance), or it can be detrimental if the resulting pulmonary overdistention leads to compression of alveolar vessels and increased pulmonary vascular resistance. One complication of mechanical ventilation with high pressures is therefore excessive right ventricular loading and acute cor pulmonale.

Positive pressure can affect cardiovascular hemodynamics through its effect on pleural pressure, an effect that is related to changes in lung volume and chest wall stiffness but not necessarily directly reflected in measurements of airway pressure. For example, in a patient with low lung compliance (e.g., ARDS), a given increase in airway pressure will lead to a much lower increase in lung volume than in a patient with COPD, so the increase in pleural pressure will be much lower. As a result, patients with ARDS tolerate relatively higher PEEP levels compared with patients with COPD. At high lung volumes, a direct effect of the pressure of the lung on the heart can increase pericardial pressure and can thereby decrease cardiac filling. Obese patients can tolerate PEEP levels on average 8 cm H_2O above those used in non-obese patients because obese patients have higher intrathoracic pressures generated by the load of the chest wall and abdomen.[6]

AUTO-PEEP, DYNAMIC HYPERINFLATION, AND AIRWAY CLOSURE

A key factor that affects cardiovascular hemodynamics and other physiologic variables is the development of auto-PEEP, defined as the difference between alveolar pressure and airway opening pressure at end expiration. The auto-PEEP is associated with dynamic hyperinflation, which is an increase in the end-expiratory lung volume above the value that would be obtained if there was complete exhalation to the static functional residual capacity. This phenomenon occurs whenever time is insufficient for complete exhalation to occur. The major determinants of auto-PEEP and hence dynamic hyperinflation are high minute ventilation, increased expiratory airway resistance, increased respiratory system compliance, and decreased expiratory time. In addition, expiratory flow limitation may further aggravate hyperinflation in patients with small airway pathology. The auto-PEEP phenomenon is a reason to reduce the tidal volume delivered to patients' lungs.

Auto-PEEP is not detected at the airway opening during the ventilator cycle, because the pressure drop occurs across the airways upstream of where the airway pressure is measured in the ventilatory circuit. When patients are not making spontaneous breathing efforts, auto-PEEP can be easily assessed as the difference in pressure between the set PEEP and the pressure obtained when the airway opening is occluded at the end of expiration (E-Fig. 91-1). If it is considered safe for the patient, a rapid estimate of the effect of auto-PEEP on cardiovascular hemodynamics can be obtained by a prolonged expiration to atmosphere. Matching the alveolar pressure, referred to as total PEEP, is especially important when the patient triggers the ventilator. Reliable measurements of auto-PEEP, however, are more difficult to obtain in spontaneously breathing patients.

If auto-PEEP is not considered in the interpretation of respiratory mechanics, measurements of respiratory system compliance can be falsely low. Dynamic hyperinflation can be measured as the volume of gas that is released during a prolonged expiration (20 to 30 seconds).

Auto-PEEP should be suspected whenever flow at end expiration remains detectable or when a patient fails to trigger the ventilator consistently with inspiratory efforts. This failure to trigger the ventilator occurs because the patient must generate sufficient pressure to overcome the level of auto-PEEP before a negative deflection of pressure or generation of inspiratory flow (either of which may be used by the ventilator to detect the onset of inspiration) is sensed at the airway opening. These failed attempts are referred to as ineffective efforts, and they occur in more than 10% of breathing efforts in about 25% of patients who receive pressure support ventilation, usually because the patients receive ventilatory volume in excess of the expiratory capacity of the patient's respiratory system. As a result, the respiratory rate of the ventilator may be considerably lower than the patient's real respiratory rate.

Auto-PEEP and the attendant dynamic hyperinflation have detrimental consequences. In a patient who is not breathing spontaneously, dynamic hyperinflation increases pleural pressure and right atrial pressure, thereby leading to a decrease in the driving pressure for venous return. This effect can be magnified immediately after intubation and initiation of mechanical ventilation because compensatory mechanisms to enhance venous return are impaired by pharmacologic agents used for intubation, which itself also reduces venous and arterial tone.

Auto-PEEP is more likely to occur in patients with airway obstruction, especially when expiratory flow limitation is present. Minimizing auto-PEEP, which is a fundamental principle in ventilating patients who have severe airway obstruction, can best be achieved by decreasing minute ventilation, increasing expiratory time, and decreasing airway resistance (e.g., using bronchodilators, when appropriate).

Another phenomenon that can affect ventilation, especially in patients with ARDS or obesity, is referred to as airway closure, in which some airways are either continuously closed or cyclically open and close during ventilation. Although an airway is closed, the lung distal to the closure still may be inflated. The pressure needed to reopen the airways during each insufflation may reach more than 20 cm H_2O. Airway closure, which occurs in 30 to 60% of patients with ARDS,[7] can be visualized by performing a low-flow inflation pressure-time (or pressure-volume) maneuver.[8]

VENTILATOR-INDUCED LUNG INJURY

The forces generated during mechanical ventilation can cause lung injury (E-Fig. 91-2). High levels of inspired oxygen concentrations can cause oxygen toxicity.

Barotrauma refers to pulmonary air leaks, such as pneumothorax and pneumomediastinum. Other forms of pressure injury include diffuse alveolar damage presenting as pulmonary edema and biotrauma. For these types of injury, the critical factor is the degree of overdistention of the lung, which is related to the transpulmonary pressure, defined as airway pressure minus pleural pressure, when airway flow is zero. Esophageal pressure (Pes), measured with an esophageal balloon, is used clinically to estimate pleural pressure.

A high peak pressure does not necessarily indicate an increased propensity to overdistention. For example, use of a smaller endotracheal tube will increase peak pressure, but the danger of pulmonary overdistention is no greater than would be present if the patient was ventilated with a larger-bore tube and a lower peak pressure, provided there is no auto-PEEP. The plateau pressure, which is the airway pressure at the end of an end-inspiratory pause (usually after 0.2 to 0.5 seconds), is an easy-to-measure direct estimate of peak alveolar pressure. As a first approach in patients with ARDS, the plateau pressure should be kept below 30 cm H_2O to minimize the risks of distention. If the patient is breathing spontaneously, however, pleural pressure will be negative, and overdistention may occur even with a plateau pressure much lower than 30 cm H_2O because the transpulmonary pressure distending the lung could be high during the patient's inspiratory effort. Conversely, in a patient who is not making ventilatory efforts and who has a stiff chest wall (e.g., owing to obesity, ascites, abdominal compartment syndrome, pregnancy), much of the pressure increase will be dissipated across the chest wall, and a high plateau pressure may not be indicative of lung distention.

An even better prediction of risk of ventilator-induced lung injury may be the driving pressure, termed δP, which is equal to plateau pressure minus PEEP (or total PEEP). Values above 15 cm H_2O are associated with increased mortality.

During mechanical ventilation, some areas of the lung may undergo cyclic recruitment and de-recruitment, a process termed atelectrauma. Prevention of this type of injury provides part of the rationale for the use of PEEP to maintain recruitment of lung units during tidal ventilation (Video 91-1).

Ventilatory strategies that promote overdistention and atelectrauma can lead to an inflammatory response in the lung, a mechanism of injury termed biotrauma. The release of proinflammatory cytokines and chemokines and can potentially lead to dysfunction of other organs (E-Fig. 91-3), thereby suggesting that optimal ventilatory strategies are important not only to maintain lung function but also to prevent the development of multiple-organ dysfunction (Chapter 90). This hypothesis may explain the lower mortality when patients with ARDS are treated with a strategy designed to minimize ventilator-induced lung injury.

Lung injury also can occur in patients who have high respiratory drive. This drive can translate into large negative intrathoracic pressures that lead to injury that has been termed "patient self-inflicted lung injury," which can occur whether the patient is being ventilated or not. An increased respiratory rate can also contribute to ventilator-induced lung injury, albeit to a lesser degree.[9]

TABLE 91-1 STEPS AND GUIDELINES FOR INITIATION OF MECHANICAL VENTILATION*

1. Ventilatory mode
   Unintubated patients
   - NIV for patients with COPD and acute hypercapnic respiratory failure, if patient is cooperative and hemodynamically stable
   - NIV not routinely recommended for acute hypoxemic respiratory failure; high-flow oxygen therapy may be initiated in these patients, or the patients may be intubated

   Intubated patients
   - Assist/control volume-limited ventilation or PCV as initial mode
   - PSV: consider as soon as patient's effort are reasonable, respiratory mechanics are such that pressure support levels of 10-15 can be used, ventilatory needs are moderate to low, and the patient is more comfortable during PSV trial than while receiving full ventilatory support
   - Oxygenation:
     - If there are infiltrates on chest radiograph, begin with F_{IO_2} 0.8 (avoid 1.0 if possible), reduce rapidly according to Sp_{O_2}; PEEP: begin with 5 cm H_2O, but use rapidly higher levels if oxygenation is poor and Pplat high (i.e., up to 15 cm H_2O in severe ARDS). Adapt according to Pa_{O_2} or Sp_{O_2}, F_{IO_2} requirements, and hemodynamic effects; consider PEEP/F_{IO_2} "ladder" or estimate of recruitability (recruitment to inflation ratio; see Fig. 91-1); goal of Sp_{O_2} >90% and ≤96% (except in the case of acute myocardial infarction), F_{IO_2} adapted to Sp_{O_2}
     - If no infiltrates on chest radiograph (COPD, asthma, PTE), start at F_{IO_2} 0.4 and adjust according to Sp_{O_2} (consider starting higher if pulmonary embolism is strongly suspected)
     - Tidal volume: begin with 8 mL/kg PBW (see Fig. 91-1 for formulas); decrease to 6 mL/kg PBW over a few hours if ARDS present (see Fig. 91-1); inspiratory flow rate of 50-60 L/min
     - Rate: begin with 10-20 breaths/min (10-15 if not acidotic; 20-30 if acidotic or ARDS and small volumes); adjust for pH; goal pH > 7.3 with maximal rate of 35; may accept higher Pa_{CO_2} and lower pH goal if minute ventilation high
2. Secondary modifications
   - Triggering: in assisted modes, minimize diaphragm inactivity
   - Assessment of auto-PEEP, especially in patients with increased airways obstruction (e.g., asthma, COPD)
3. Monitoring
   - Clinical: blood pressure, ECG, observation of ventilatory pattern including assessment of dyssynchrony, minimal effort or work by the patient (as measured by the pressure at the airway opening of 2-4 cm H_2O or less when flow is occluded for 100 msec), assessment of airflow throughout the expiratory cycle
   - Ventilator: tidal volume, minute ventilation, airway pressures (including auto-PEEP), total compliance
   - Arterial blood gases, pulse oximetry

*Decisions within this algorithm will be influenced by the specific conditions of the individual patient.

ARDS = acute respiratory distress syndrome; COPD = chronic obstructive pulmonary disease; ECG = electrocardiogram; F_{IO_2} = fraction of inspired oxygen; HFOV = high-frequency oscillatory ventilation; I/E ratio = inspiratory-to-expiratory ratio; NIV = noninvasive ventilation; Pa_{CO_2} = arterial partial pressure of carbon dioxide; Pa_{O_2} = partial pressure of oxygen in arterial blood; PBW = predicted body weight; PCV = pressure-controlled ventilation; PEEP = positive end-expiratory pressure; Pplat = plateau pressure; PSV = pressure-support ventilation; PTE = pulmonary thromboembolism; Sp_{O_2} = arterial oxygen saturation by pulse oximetry.

Finally, mechanical ventilation can also lead to diaphragmatic weakness and dysfunction after a few days of mechanical ventilation. Respiratory muscle weakness is strongly associated with difficulties in weaning the patient from ventilator support.[10]

SPECIFIC COMMON TREATMENT SCENARIOS

INITIATION OF MECHANICAL VENTILATION

The initiation of mechanical ventilation involves several steps in clinical decision making (Table 91-1). Each patient must be evaluated for specific factors that could modify the recommendation or mandate an alternative.

ACUTE RESPIRATORY DISTRESS SYNDROME

Patients with ARDS (Chapter 90) have noncardiogenic pulmonary edema, with a reduced functional residual capacity and a mortality rate that commonly exceeds 30%. Although therapy may be available for the underlying disease process that led to the development of ARDS (e.g., antibiotics for a predisposing pneumonia), and corticosteroids may reduce subsequent damage, no therapy directly reverses diffuse alveolar damage. These patients require mechanical ventilation as a life-supportive therapy to improve oxygenation decrease the work of breathing and reduce the associated oxygen cost of breathing until their lungs recover from the primary insult that led to the alveolar damage. The

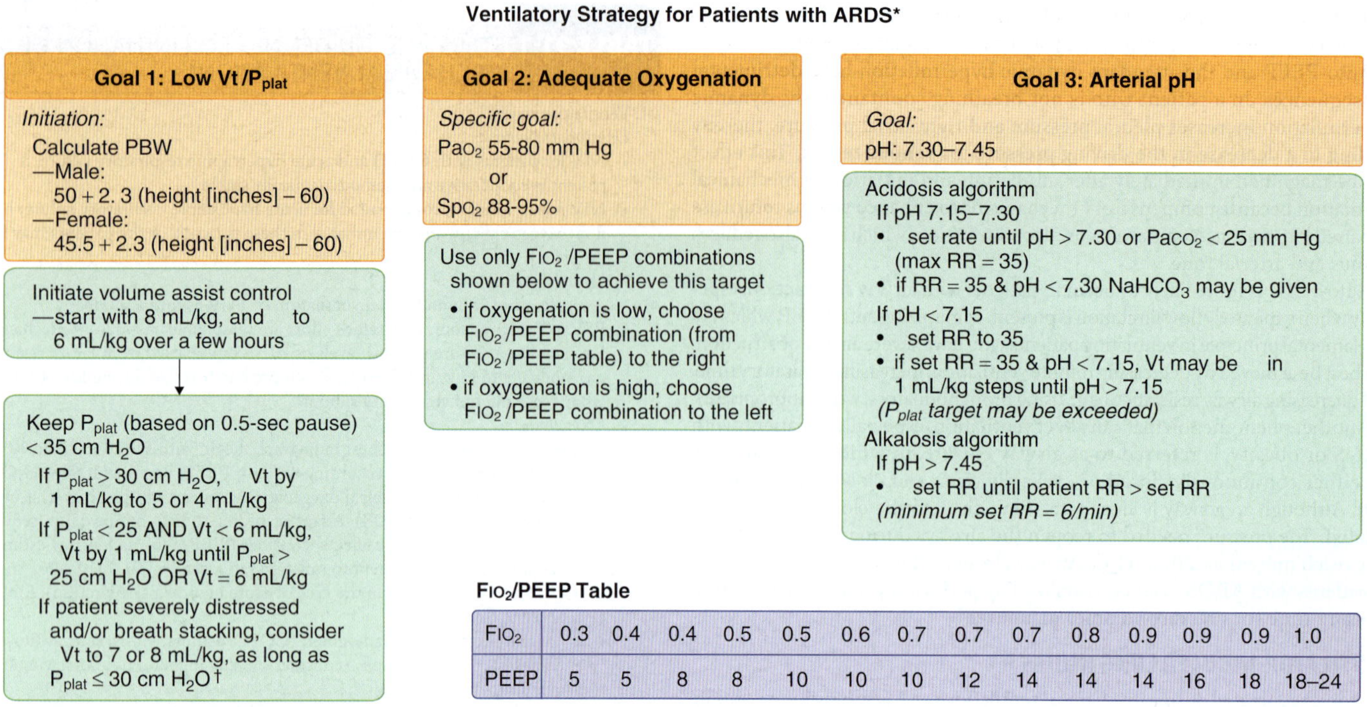

FIO₂	0.3	0.4	0.4	0.5	0.5	0.6	0.7	0.7	0.7	0.8	0.9	0.9	0.9	1.0
PEEP	5	5	8	8	10	10	10	12	14	14	14	16	18	18–24

*Based on ARDS Network Algorithm
†If compliance of the chest wall is markedly decreased (e.g., massive ascites), it may be reasonable or necessary (if the patient is very hypoxemic) to allow a P_{plat} >30 cm H_2O.

FIGURE 91-1. Ventilatory strategy for patients with the acute respiratory distress syndrome (ARDS) as proposed by the ARDSNetwork. FIO_2 = fraction of inspired oxygen; $PaCO_2$ = arterial partial pressure of carbon dioxide; PaO_2 = arterial partial pressure of oxygen; PBW = predicted body weight; Pplat = plateau pressure; RR = respiratory rate; SpO_2 = oxygen saturation based on pulse oximeter; Vt = tidal volume.

major therapeutic goal is to provide adequate gas exchange while ensuring that damaged lungs are not further injured by the ventilatory strategy and/or by spontaneous breathing. The ventilatory approaches used to achieve this goal are termed lung-protective ventilation or lung-protective strategies.

Lung-Protective Ventilation Strategies

Because the heavy, edematous lung in ARDS behaves like a sponge, the distribution of lesions is influenced by gravity: most patients have a dependent zone that is either consolidated and fluid filled or atelectatic and recruitable; a nondependent, often small zone that looks normal; and a middle zone with poorly aerated regions that can be recruited to resemble the nondependent regions. Alveolar recruitment, which can occur during ventilation, is facilitated by PEEP or by transient high levels of airway pressure. Gas exchange can often be improved by high tidal volumes but at the expense of regional overdistention of lung units that were not affected by the disease process itself—a treatment strategy that can lead to worse lung injury and poorer clinical outcomes.

Ventilator-induced lung injury can be minimized by strategies that avoid or diminish regional lung overdistention. For example, the use of lower tidal volumes (6 mL/kg predicted body weight) along with plateau pressure less than 30 cm H_2O can decrease mortality by about 20% (from an absolute value of about 40% to about 30%) compared with 12 mL/kg predicted body weight, even though larger tidal volumes provide higher values of PaO_2 (see Fig. 91-1). Lung-protective strategies also may be useful in ventilated patients who are intubated for reasons other than ARDS (e.g., intubated ICU patients, patients undergoing major abdominal surgery, and patients with brain death whose lungs may subsequently be donated for transplantation).

Several caveats should be considered in using the low tidal volume strategy. First, the protocols mandate a tidal volume of 6 mL/kg or less of predicted body weight if the plateau pressure is greater than 30 cm H_2O and allow small increases in tidal volume if the patient is severely distressed and develops breath stacking (i.e., unintended high tidal volumes that occur as a consequence of incomplete exhalation between consecutive inspiratory cycles delivered by the ventilator). Driving pressure may better reflect the risk of injury, and larger tidal volumes may be used safely in patients with higher compliance,[11] so as to avoid the detrimental consequences of low tidal volumes (e.g., respiratory acidosis, further atelectasis, lower PaO_2, poor patient-ventilator synchrony, and increased need for sedation). Second, respiratory acidosis can be treated with increasingly aggressive strategies depending on the arterial pH. Third, in specific patients with a stiff chest wall or with elevated intrathoracic pressures owing to obesity, it is reasonable for the plateau pressure to increase to greater than 30 cm H_2O.

Positive End-Expiratory Pressure

Some level of PEEP is necessary to reduce lung injury by recruiting lung units and keeping them open. PEEP also may be used to keep airways open in cases of airway closure.[12] The critical issue, however, is how to set the optimum PEEP level in an individual patient and to determine whether procedures to recruit lung units and keep them open are more harmful than allowing the lung units to remain de-recruited. A bedside index of lung recruitability, termed the recruitment-to-inflation ratio, measures the change in expired volume when PEEP is abruptly reduced from 15 to 5 cm H_2O and calculates the compliance of the recruited lung by dividing the change in volume by the effective pressure change.[13]

Data suggest that higher PEEP levels (about 12 to 13 cm H_2O) may be better than lower levels (about 8 cm H_2O),[A13,A14] and PEEP levels are often individualized on the basis of the relationship of PEEP to FIO_2 (see Fig. 91-1). Higher PEEP levels are probably associated with decreased mortality in severe and moderate ARDS (PaO_2/FIO_2 <200 mm Hg) but not in patients with mild ARDS with higher PaO_2/FIO_2 ratios; very high PEEP associated with recruitment maneuvers and an open-lung strategy can be harmful.[A15] PEEP guided by esophageal pressures has not been shown to improve outcomes when used in all patients, but possible benefits have been suggested in less severe disease and in obese patients.[A16]

Adjunctive Approaches for Ventilating ARDS Patients

The routine use of neuromuscular blockers is not recommended in patients with moderate-severe ARDS,[A17] but the judicious use of these agents may be beneficial in selected patients (e.g., patients with patient-ventilator asynchrony that leads to breath stacking or patients with very large inspiratory efforts). Use of prone rather than the supine position in patients with ARDS improves oxygenation, permits a more even distribution of pleural pressure and distribution of ventilation, reduces ventilator-induced lung injury because of a more optimal distribution of ventilation, and decreases mortality by about 15% in ARDS patients with PaO_2/FIO_2 less than 150 mm Hg.[A18] This life-saving procedure should be used irrespective of its effect on oxygenation in any given patient.

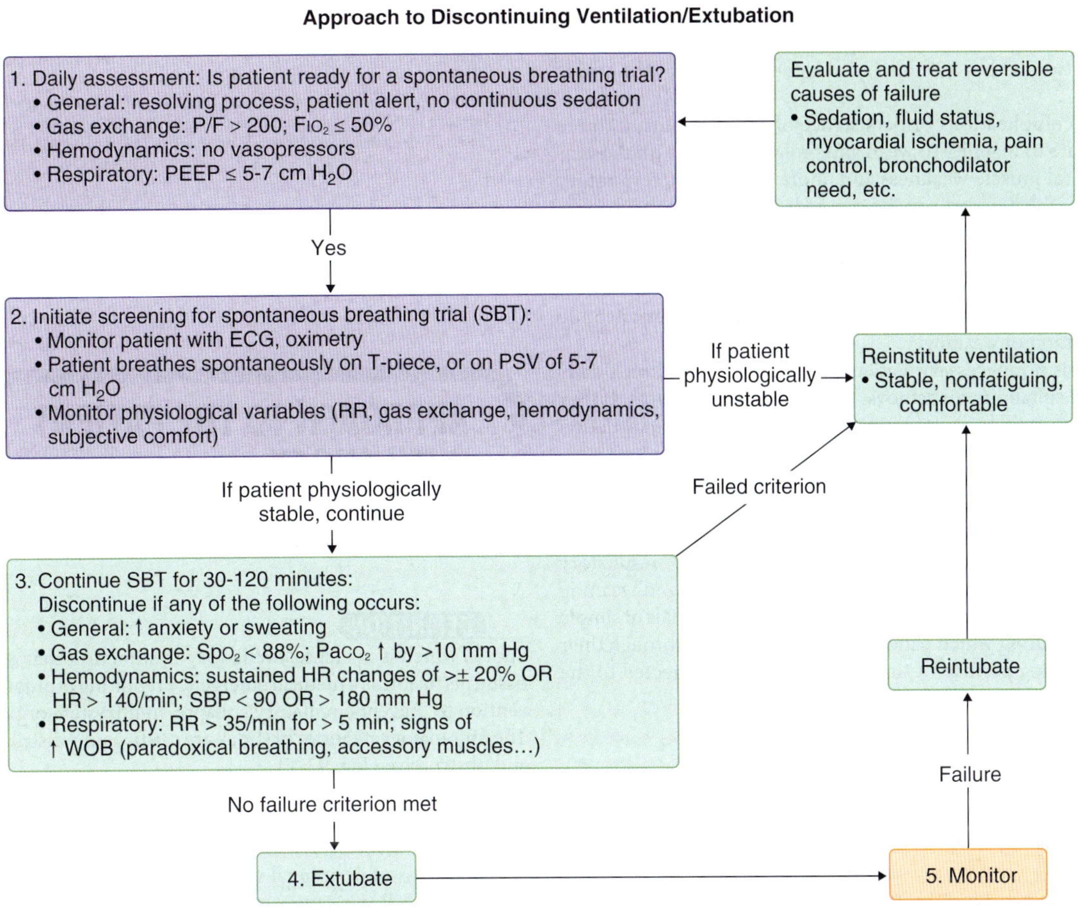

FIGURE 91-2. **Algorithm for assessing whether a patient is ready to be liberated from mechanical ventilation and extubated.** ECG = electrocardiogram; HR = heart rate; $Paco_2$ = arterial partial pressure of carbon dioxide; PEEP = positive end-expiratory pressure; P/F = Pao_2/Fio_2 ratio; PSV = pressure support ventilation; RR = respiratory rate; SBP = systolic blood pressure; Spo_2 = oxygen saturation based on pulse oximeter; WOB = work of breathing.

OBSTRUCTIVE AIRWAYS DISEASES

The major physiologic abnormality in patients with obstructive airways diseases (e.g., COPD, asthma) is an increase in airway resistance with limitation in tidal expiratory airflow. The result is dynamic hyperinflation, which is associated with numerous complications. The first goal in the ventilatory support of these patients is to avoid intubation by using noninvasive ventilation. If the patient is hemodynamically stable and does not need to be intubated to protect the airway, this strategy is usually applied using pressure support and positive end-expiratory airway pressure.

OTHER CONDITIONS

If patients require intubation, it is important to minimize auto-PEEP, maintain reasonable ventilation (normalizing pH more than $Paco_2$), and rest the respiratory muscles to decrease the oxygen cost of breathing, while simultaneously minimizing the iatrogenic complications of mechanical ventilation. These strategies allow time for the diagnosis and treatment of the primary cause of the exacerbation (Chapters 75 and 76). When the patient is being assisted by the ventilator and the patient has an intrinsic PEEP higher than the external PEEP, adding external PEEP to match the patient's intrinsic PEEP is essential to reduce the work of breathing.

Intubation and Ventilation

The key goal after intubation of patients with airway obstruction is to minimize the detrimental effects of dynamic hyperinflation. The most effective approach is to minimize the delivered minute ventilation, even if this strategy does not normalize $Paco_2$. Judicious use of sedation may decrease the production of carbon dioxide and improve patient-ventilator synchrony, but the avoidance of sedation can reduce the duration of ventilation and hospitalization.

In patients who have COPD and who are spontaneously breathing, the addition of external (set) PEEP at a level that is just less than what is necessary to overcome the auto-PEEP will not increase hyperinflation and may decrease the inspiratory effort that the patient needs to generate to initiate inspiratory airflow. This strategy does not appear to be as effective in patients with status asthmaticus, however.

Noninvasive ventilation or even simple CPAP is extremely useful for patients with respiratory distress related to cardiogenic pulmonary edema. Patients who are obese or have sleep disorders may require higher PEEP levels.

DISCONTINUATION OF MECHANICAL VENTILATION

From the moment that mechanical ventilation is instituted, it is important to start planning for its eventual discontinuation. A key aspect of this approach is serial evaluation, with aggressive treatment of the factors that contribute to the patient's ventilator dependence.

Readiness for extubation requires clinical stability (e.g., hemodynamic stability with no or minimal need for vasopressors and oxygen requirements that can be met by face mask after extubation)[14] (Fig. 91-2). One way to assess whether the patient is ready to be extubated is the use of the rapid shallow breathing index, which is the ratio of tidal volume in liters to the respiratory rate in breaths per minute, measured after 2 minutes of spontaneous breathing. If this ratio is not elevated (<105 breaths/min/L), a spontaneous breathing trial is recommended (see Fig. 91-2).

Spontaneous breathing trials assess the ability of the patient to be separated from the ventilator, but they do not accurately predict the outcomes of extubation,[A19] which are often related to a weak cough, abundant secretions, microaspirations, and limited wakefulness. For example, a strategy that pairs spontaneous awakening, based on the daily interruption of sedatives, with spontaneous breathing trials can improve extubation rates, reduce ICU length of stay, and decrease mortality at 1 year. However, early active physiotherapy is not beneficial in intubated patients.[A20] The advantages of early discontinuation must be balanced against the detrimental consequences if patients require urgent reintubation. Within 3 to 5 days, approximately 15% of patients require reintubation, which is associated with a higher mortality rate that may be partly precipitated by the failed extubation itself. A majority of patients (between 60 and 75%) will be successfully extubated after the first spontaneous breathing trial, whereas others will need repeated attempts. Patients with a high pre-test probability of success (e.g., postoperative patients) may not need a formal spontaneous breathing trial and may be extubated as soon as they are awake. Noninvasive ventilation,[15] especially in obese patients,[16] or high-flow nasal oxygen after extubation can reduce the risk of reintubation within 72 hours, and a combination of the two is even better.[A21]

Apart from new complications or persistence of the initial insult, three factors that contribute to inability to wean and prolong the time on the ventilator include general muscle weakness and, more specifically, respiratory muscle dysfunction, which in part may be caused by the ventilatory process; cardiovascular factors and volume status that may lead to weaning-induced pulmonary edema via diastolic dysfunction or ischemia; and neurologic factors including residual sedation or inability of patients to protect their airways. A fluid management strategy based on measurement of brain natriuretic peptide may reduce the duration of weaning.

Gradual weaning is not necessary. Patients should be assessed on a daily basis regarding their suitability for removal from ventilatory support. If they are not ready, a comfortable, nonfatiguing form of mechanical ventilation should be used between assessments.

Despite repeated trials of spontaneous breathing, about 10 to 15% of patients will continue to be ventilator-dependent even after one week of weaning attempts. In these patients, a global approach including mobilization, nutrition, and therapies focused on psychological factors can be crucial,[17] respiratory muscle rehabilitation may be of potential benefit, and specialized weaning centers may be useful.[18] For patients who have a tracheostomy, trials of simple tracheostomy masks, during which patients breathe unassisted through their tracheostomy for varying periods of time before being reconnected to the ventilator, may be the preferred approach for weaning.

GENERAL REFERENCES

For the General References and other additional features, please visit Elsevier eBooks+ at https://ebooks.health.elsevier.com.

Grade A References

A1. Girardis M, Busani S, Damiani E, et al. Effect of conservative vs conventional oxygen therapy on mortality among patients in an intensive care unit: the oxygen-ICU randomized clinical trial. *JAMA*. 2016;316:1583-1589.
A2. Chu DK, Kim LH, Young PJ, et al. Mortality and morbidity in acutely ill adults treated with liberal versus conservative oxygen therapy (IOTA): a systematic review and meta-analysis. *Lancet*. 2018;391:1693-1705.
A3. ICU-ROX Investigators and the Australian and New Zealand Intensive Care Society Clinical Trials Group, Mackle D, Bellomo R, et al. Conservative oxygen therapy during mechanical ventilation in the ICU. *N Engl J Med*. 2020;382:989-998.
A4. Semler MW, Casey JD, Lloyd BD, et al. Oxygen-saturation targets for critically ill adults receiving mechanical ventilation. *N Engl J Med*. 2022;387:1759-1769.
A5. Kacmarek RM, Villar J, Parrilla D, et al. Neurally adjusted ventilatory assist in acute respiratory failure: a randomized controlled trial. *Intensive Care Med*. 2020;46:2327-2337.
A6. Grieco DL, Menga LS, Cesarano M, et al. Effect of helmet noninvasive ventilation vs high-flow nasal oxygen on days free of respiratory support in patients with COVID-19 and moderate to severe hypoxemic respiratory failure: the HENIVOT randomized clinical trial. *JAMA*. 2021;325:1731-1743.
A7. Rochwerg B, Einav S, Chaudhuri D, et al. The role for high flow nasal cannula as a respiratory support strategy in adults: a clinical practice guideline. *Intensive Care Med*. 2020;46:2226-2237.
A8. Frat JP, Thille AW, Mercat A, et al. High-flow oxygen through nasal cannula in acute hypoxemic respiratory failure. *N Engl J Med*. 2015;372:2185-2196.
A9. Casey JD, Janz DR, Russell DW, et al. Bag-mask ventilation during tracheal intubation of critically ill adults. *N Engl J Med*. 2019;380:811-821.
A10. Olsen HT, Nedergaard HK, Strom T, et al. Nonsedation or light sedation in critically ill, mechanically ventilated patients. *N Engl J Med*. 2020;382:1103-1111.
A11. Skrobik Y, Duprey MS, Hill NS, et al. Low-dose nocturnal dexmedetomidine prevents ICU delirium. A randomized, placebo-controlled trial. *Am J Respir Crit Care Med*. 2018;197:1147-1156.
A12. Shehabi Y, Howe BD, Bellomo R, et al. Early Sedation with dexmedetomidine in critically ill patients. *N Engl J Med*. 2019;380:2506-2517.
A13. Algera AG, Pisani L, Serpa Neto A, et al. Effect of a lower vs higher positive end-expiratory pressure strategy on ventilator-free days in ICU patients without ARDS: a randomized clinical trial. *JAMA*. 2020;324:2509-2520.
A14. Santa Cruz R, Villarejo F, Irrazabal C, et al. High versus low positive end-expiratory pressure (PEEP) levels for mechanically ventilated adult patients with acute lung injury and acute respiratory distress syndrome. *Cochrane Database Syst Rev*. 2021;3:CD009098.
A15. Writing Group for the Alveolar Recruitment for Acute Respiratory Distress Syndrome Trial I, Cavalcanti AB, Suzumura EA, et al. Effect of lung recruitment and titrated positive end-expiratory pressure (PEEP) vs low PEEP on mortality in patients with acute respiratory distress syndrome: a randomized clinical trial. *JAMA*. 2017;318:1335-1345.
A16. Beitler JR, Sarge T, Banner-Goodspeed VM, et al. Effect of titrating positive end-expiratory pressure (PEEP) with an esophageal pressure-guided strategy vs an empirical high PEEP-Fio2 strategy on death and days free from mechanical ventilation among patients with acute respiratory distress syndrome: a randomized clinical trial. *JAMA*. 2019;321:846-857.
A17. National Heart, Lung, and Blood Institute PETAL Clinical Trials Network, Moss M, Huang DT, et al. Early neuromuscular blockade in the acute respiratory distress syndrome. *N Engl J Med*. 2019;380:1997-2008.
A18. Mushni L, Del Sorbo L, Adhikari NJ, et al. Prone position for acute respiratory distress syndrome. A systematic review and meta-analysis. *Ann Am Thorac Soc*. 2017;14:S280-S288.
A19. Thille AW, Gacouin A, Coudroy R, et al. Spontaneous-breathing trials with pressure-support ventilation or a T-piece. *N Engl J Med*. 2022;387:1843-1854.
A20. Hodgson CL, Bailey M, Bellomo R, et al. Early active mobilization during mechanical ventilation in the ICU. *N Engl J Med*. 2022;387:1747-1758.
A21. Thille AW, Muller G, Gacouin A, et al. Effect of postextubation high-flow nasal oxygen with noninvasive ventilation vs high-flow nasal oxygen alone on reintubation among patients at high risk of extubation failure: a randomized clinical trial. *JAMA*. 2019;322:1465-1475.

92 APPROACH TO THE PATIENT WITH SHOCK

DEREK C. ANGUS

DEFINITION

Shock, which is an acute circulatory dysfunction that results in inadequate tissue perfusion, is a medical emergency requiring prompt diagnosis and intervention to prevent circulatory collapse, multisystem organ failure, and death. The four major categories of shock are cardiogenic, distributive, hypovolemic, and obstructive (Fig. 92-1).

Cardiogenic shock (Chapter 93) is due to pump failure caused most commonly by acute myocardial ischemia but also by acute valvular dysfunction, arrhythmias, myocarditis, or ventricular wall rupture. Distributive shock is caused by loss of peripheral vasomotor tone, most commonly due to sepsis (Chapter 94). Rarer causes of distributive shock include neurogenic shock, typically following major spinal cord injury (Chapter 368), and anaphylaxis (Chapter 233). Hypovolemic shock is caused by loss of circulating volume from dehydration, profound vascular leakage (e.g., secondary to the toxin-mediated endothelial leak of dengue fever), or hemorrhage (e.g., secondary to trauma, perioperative, or gastrointestinal bleeding, or rupture of an aortic aneurysm). Obstructive shock, which is less common, is caused by intrinsic blockage of a major vessel, such as saddle pulmonary embolus (Chapter 68), or extrinsic compression, such as cardiac tamponade (Chapter 62), status asthmaticus (Chapter 75), or tension pneumothorax.

Patients also can present with combined forms of shock. For example, septic shock can include loss of autonomic tone (distributive), myocardial depression (cardiogenic), and loss of vascular volume (hypovolemic) owing to dehydration and vascular leak.

EPIDEMIOLOGY

In the United States, an estimated 500,000 incident cases of shock occur each year. Septic shock, which is the most common cause, accounts for more than 250,000 cases per year. Hemorrhagic shock accounts for 60,000 deaths each year in the United States, predominantly owing to trauma.[1] Of the 650,000 cases per year of acute myocardial infarction, about 25,000 (4%) develop cardiogenic shock (Chapter 93).[2] Of the 200,000 or so patients who suffer a clinically significant pulmonary embolus each year, about 25,000 (13%) present in shock (or cardiac arrest). Thus, over half of all shock is due to sepsis (primarily distributive), one fifth is due to trauma (primarily hypovolemic),[3] one tenth is due to coronary artery disease (cardiogenic), and the remaining (approximately 20%) is due to other causes. Shock occurs in both sexes, all age groups, and all racial and ethnic groups, with its incidence depending on the frequency of precipitating conditions within these populations.

PATHOBIOLOGY

Shock is classically described in terms of cardiovascular pathophysiology when oxygen delivery to tissues is inadequate because of reduced cardiac output (hypovolemic, cardiogenic, or obstructive) or impaired vasomotor tone (distributive). However, these macrocirculatory changes are often accompanied by important pathobiologic changes in the cells and tissue beds of vital organs.

Cardiovascular Pathophysiology

In *hypovolemic shock* a decrease in circulating blood volume decreases venous return and thus cardiac preload. As preload decreases, the heart shifts left on the

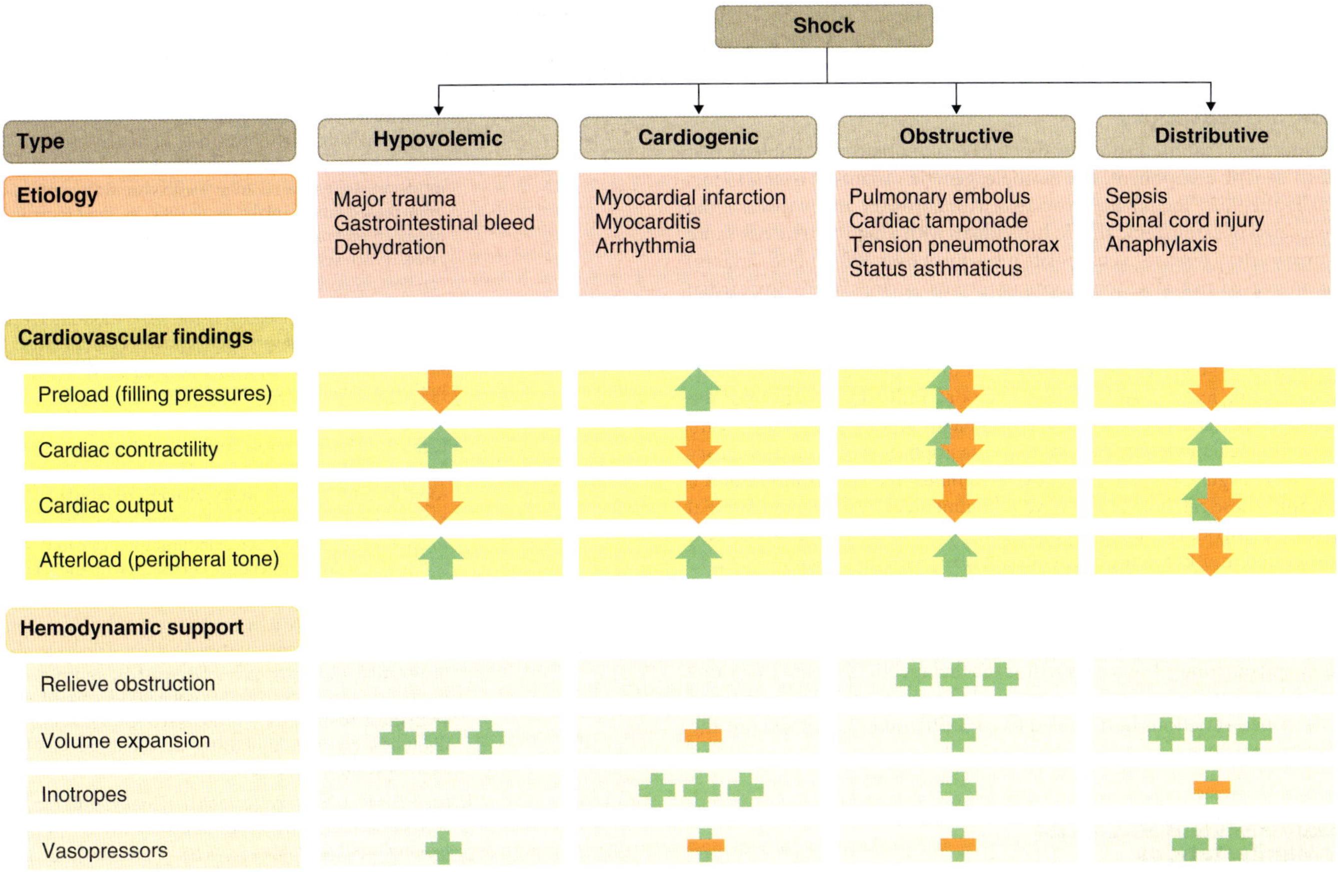

FIGURE 92-1. **The causes, cardiovascular findings, and hemodynamic support for different types of shock. Under cardiovascular findings, bidirectional *arrows* indicate variation in findings among patients with the particular type. Under hemodynamic support, the number of + signs indicate the importance of therapy. A combined + and – indicates that the intervention could help some patients but must be used with caution.**

Starling curve to the point that stroke volume and, hence, both cardiac output and oxygen delivery fall. Decreases in cardiac output and oxygen delivery are detected by a complex system of baroreceptors and chemoreceptors that stimulate autonomic and endocrine-mediated compensatory changes in the heart and vasculature. Peripheral vasomotor tone is increased in arterial and venous capacitance vessels, thereby reducing total capacitance and effectively increasing the circulating volume, venous return, and preload. Selective autoregulatory changes also redistribute blood flow preferentially to vital organs (e.g., heart and brain) at the expense of the splanchnic, muscle, and skin vascular beds. In addition, sympathetic stimulation of the heart generates tachycardia and increases inotropy to increase cardiac output. The tradeoff initially sustains effective oxygen delivery. However, as blood volume decreases, compensation fails, and tissue hypoperfusion of vital organs ensues.

In *cardiogenic shock* (Chapter 93), cardiac output falls because of primary pump failure rather than reduced preload. When left ventricular failure predominates, accompanying pulmonary edema (Chapter 46) can lead to arterial hypoxemia, which further compromises oxygen delivery. Peripheral and central compensatory mechanisms are similar to those in hypovolemic shock, with the caveat that increasing sympathetic drive to increase myocardial contractility has limited effect.

In *obstructive shock*, the mechanism that reduces cardiac output depends on the cause: massive pulmonary embolus (Chapter 68) increases right ventricular afterload but reduces left ventricular preload, whereas tension pneumothorax (Chapter 86) and cardiac tamponade (Chapter 62) principally reduce cardiac output via reduced preload, akin to hypovolemic shock. As with cardiogenic shock, obstructive shock can be accompanied by impaired oxygenation, thereby further compromising oxygen delivery.

In *distributive shock*, the autoregulation of peripheral vasomotor tone is impaired. For example, neurogenic shock following acute spinal cord injury (Chapter 368) arises owing to loss of sympathetic tone, thereby leading to dilatation of capacitance vessels, increased arterial-venous shunting, and loss of selective autoregulation. Preload is reduced, but afterload is also reduced. Compensatory mechanisms, such as reflex tachycardia, will depend on the level of the cord injury. Thus, the effects on cardiac output are variable (and cardiac output can even be increased), but effective oxygen delivery to vital organs can still be compromised. Septic shock (Chapter 94) is primarily a form of distributive shock triggered initially by the release of circulating mediators that have local effects on peripheral vessels, thereby causing both vasodilation and vascular leak. These effects impair autoregulation, increase capacitance, and reduce the absolute and effective circulating blood volume, thereby reducing preload and afterload, with variable effects on cardiac output. Inflammatory mediators released in sepsis also have direct myocardial depressant effects. Importantly, because of both impaired redistribution of flow and impaired tissue oxygen extraction (discussed later), distributive shock can persist despite a seemingly adequate oxygen delivery, and blood returning from the peripheral beds can have a normal or elevated oxygen content.

Cellular and Organ Pathobiology

As oxygen delivery falls, hypoperfused tissue beds increase oxygen extraction, which decreases venous oxygen content but preserves aerobic metabolism. With further reduction in oxygen delivery, cells switch to glycolysis, thereby generating lactic acid and a base deficit. An acid environment helps oxygen dissociate from hemoglobin, partially offsetting the consequences of reduced oxygen delivery. Cells also decrease mitochondrial activity, a form of protective hypometabolism to decrease oxygen demand. However, these compensatory mechanisms can be overwhelmed, thereby resulting in deepening ischemia and acidosis.

When cells are stressed or injured by ischemia, they release molecules that signal via damage-associated molecular pattern (DAMP) receptors, which stimulate innate immune cells (Chapters 35 and 36) to release a cascade of inflammatory mediators that alter endothelial function and permeability, coagulation and fibrinolysis, and leukocyte recruitment and activity. These changes disrupt microvascular flow and increase tissue edema and hypoxia. Tissue hypoxia also directly stimulates release of vasoactive mediators, such as nitric oxide and adenosine, thereby further contributing to vasomotor dysregulation. Reduced mitochondrial activity can also be maladaptive, with impaired oxygen utilization exacerbating cellular injury. After prolonged ischemia, reperfusion can aggravate these effects via reactive oxygen species, which induces local tissue ischemia-reperfusion injury. Thus, regardless of the initial cause of shock, prolonged tissue ischemia generates local changes characteristic of distributive shock, and these changes can persist for hours or days after resuscitation.

Untreated, prolonged ischemia eventually exhausts stores of adenosine triphosphate (ATP); as a result, tissue cells undergo bioenergetic failure, which triggers widespread apoptotic and necrotic cell death.

Genetic Susceptibility

Many conditions that predispose to shock have a multifactorial etiology that includes a genetic component. For example, genetic variants at over 243 loci (especially the 9p21 locus) are associated with coronary artery disease, the principal cause of cardiogenic shock. Individuals with a high genetic risk score for coronary artery disease (a composite measure of over 300 genetic variants) have an increased risk of serious coronary events, such as acute myocardial infarction, heart failure, or premature death. Susceptibility and outcome of septic shock have also been linked to genetic variations, such as variable number tandem repeats in genes involved in the detection of microbial products (e.g., mannose binding lectin-2 and toll-like receptor [TLR]-4), activation of the inflammatory cascade (e.g., tumor necrosis factor-alpha), and downstream events, such as leukocyte recruitment (e.g., macrophage migration inhibitory factor-1) and coagulation activation (e.g., plasminogen activator inhibitor-1). For example, these relationships are well-documented in sibling and familial studies of meningococcal disease (Chapter 274). Genetic variation has also been described in other components of the host response to shock, such as the sympathetic receptors in the peripheral vasculature that are responsible for regulating vasomotor tone (e.g., alpha 1B adrenergic receptor gene) and a broad set of innate immune cell functions.[4] These variations may affect the trajectory and outcome of shock, as well as the therapeutic response to various agents, such as adrenergic vasopressors, used to treat shock. However, none of the described variations have yet led to a specific clinical approach for the management of shock.

CLINICAL MANIFESTATIONS

Early Manifestations

Before the overt expression of shock, the dominant clinical features are those of the inciting event, such as the chest pain of an acute myocardial infarction (Chapter 58) or the fever, cough, and purulent sputum production of a worsening pneumonia (Chapter 85). During these early phases, the body's compensatory mechanisms to ensure adequate oxygen delivery will produce only subtle nonspecific signs and symptoms (Chapter 7). For example, the respiratory rate will typically rise to generate a compensatory respiratory alkalosis to the incipient metabolic acidosis. Sympathetic autonomic responses to absolute or relative hypovolemia include tachycardia, sometimes a temporary increase in blood pressure, and peripheral vasoconstriction, which can result in cool skin, peripheral cyanosis, and sluggish capillary refill. However, in patients with impending distributive shock, impaired vasomotor control may paradoxically present as warm, flushed peripheries.

Overt Shock

The cardinal features of overt shock are hypotension together with evidence of inadequate perfusion (Table 92-1). Typically, a systolic blood pressure lower than 90 mm Hg or mean blood pressure lower than 60 mm Hg overwhelms autoregulatory mechanisms so that selective vasoconstriction no longer can preserve adequate blood flow to vital organs. With decreased cerebral perfusion, confusion, disorientation, altered consciousness, or coma develop; focal or localizing signs are atypical and suggest an alternative diagnosis or preexisting cerebrovascular disease (Chapter 375) sensitive to low-flow states. Oliguria develops but may not be noted immediately. Skin changes will be more apparent, and the patient will typically appear cold, clammy, and cyanotic, with loss or diminution of peripheral pulses (Chapter 7). Hypothermia is common, even in septic shock.

Reliance of hypoperfused tissue beds on anaerobic metabolism leads to hyperlactatemic metabolic acidosis (Chapter 104), which stimulates increased respiratory effort; as the patient fatigues or mental status worsens, however, air hunger may give way to agonal breathing. Similarly, although tachycardia is typical, worsening hypotension and myocardial ischemia in advanced shock can result in paroxysmal bradycardia. Although peripheral cyanosis is a common early feature, central cyanosis is also common in cardiogenic and obstructive shock. Even in hypotensive or septic shock, profound oxygen extraction coupled with compromised respiration may promote central cyanosis. All organs are compromised, even if not clinically evident. For example, splanchnic and hepatic flow is severely diminished, often resulting in ileus and hepatic ischemia (Chapter 129).

TABLE 92-1 PHYSICAL EXAMINATION AND SELECTED LABORATORY SIGNS IN SHOCK

Central nervous system	Acute delirium, restlessness, disorientation, confusion, and coma, which may be secondary to decreased cerebral perfusion pressure (mean arterial pressure minus intracranial pressure). Patients with chronic hypertension or increased intracranial pressure may be symptomatic at normal blood pressures. Cheyne-Stokes respirations may be seen with severe decompensated heart failure. Blindness can be a presenting complaint or complication.
Temperature	Hyperthermia results in excess tissue respiration and greater systemic oxygen delivery requirements. Hypothermia can occur when decreased systemic oxygen delivery or impaired cellular respiration decreases heat generation.
Skin	Cool distal extremities (combined low serum bicarbonate and high arterial lactate levels) aid in identifying patients with hypoperfusion. Pallor, cyanosis, sweating, and decreased capillary refill and pale, dusky, clammy, or mottled extremities indicate systemic hypoperfusion. Dry mucous membranes and decreased skin turgor indicate low vascular volume. Low toe temperature correlates with the severity of shock.
General cardiovascular	Neck vein distention (e.g., heart failure, pulmonary embolus, pericardial tamponade) or flattening (e.g., hypovolemia), tachycardia, and arrhythmias. Decreased coronary perfusion pressures can lead to ischemia, decreased ventricular compliance, and increased left ventricular diastolic pressure. A "mill wheel" heart murmur may be heard with an air embolus.
Heart rate	Usually elevated. However, paradoxical bradycardia can be seen in patients with preexisting cardiac disease and severe hemorrhage. Heart rate variability is associated with poor outcomes.
Systolic blood pressure	May actually increase slightly when cardiac contractility increases in early shock and then fall as shock advances. A single episode of undifferentiated hypotension with a systolic blood pressure <80 mm Hg carries an in-hospital mortality of 18%.
Diastolic blood pressure	Correlates with arteriolar vasoconstriction and may rise early in shock and then fall when cardiovascular compensation fails.
Pulse pressure	Defined as systolic minus diastolic pressure and related to stroke volume and the rigidity of the aorta. Increases early in shock and decreases before systolic pressure decreases.
Pulsus paradoxus	An exaggerated change in systolic blood pressure with respiration (systolic blood pressure declines >10 mm Hg with inspiration) seen in asthma, cardiac tamponade, and air embolus.
Mean arterial blood pressure	Diastolic blood pressure + [pulse pressure/3]
Shock index	Heart rate/systolic blood pressure. Normal = 0.5 to 0.7. A persistent elevation of the shock index (>1.0) indicates impaired left ventricular function (as a result of blood loss or cardiac depression) and is associated with increased mortality.
Respiratory	Tachypnea, increased minute ventilation, increased dead space, bronchospasm, hypocapnia with progression to respiratory failure, acute lung injury, and adult respiratory distress syndrome.
Abdomen	Low-flow states may result in abdominal pain, ileus, gastrointestinal bleeding, pancreatitis, acalculous cholecystitis, mesenteric ischemia, and shock liver.
Renal	Because the kidney receives 20% of cardiac output, low cardiac output reduces the glomerular filtration rate and redistributes renal blood flow from the renal cortex toward the renal medulla, thereby leading to oliguria. Paradoxical polyuria in early sepsis may be confused with adequate hydration.
Metabolic	Respiratory alkalosis is the first acid-base abnormality, but metabolic acidosis occurs as shock progresses. Hyperglycemia, hypoglycemia, and hyperkalemia may develop.

Courtesy of Emanuel P. Rivers, MD.

Cryptic Shock

In some patients, signs of hypoperfusion and hyperlactatemia develop despite blood pressure that is temporarily normal, either because of pronounced vasoconstriction at the expense of compromised flow and hypoperfusion or because the patient's preexisting hypertension is masking an important decline relative to baseline blood pressure.

Untreated Shock

The length of time that a patient can survive in shock before diagnosis and intervention depends on the patient's underlying fitness and the magnitude of the inciting event. For example, a patient with shock from major arterial hemorrhage may only survive minutes. A patient who suffers a massive acute myocardial infarction with ensuing cardiogenic shock may survive only a few hours. Similarly, gram-negative septic shock in patients with chemotherapy-induced neutropenia may also be fatal within hours. However, other patients may survive for several days with altered mental status, borderline hypotension, and oliguria. Regardless of the rate of decline, untreated shock progresses to catastrophic ischemia, acidemia, vital organ failure, and death. The patient will lapse into coma, potentially with seizures typical of anoxic brain injury; worsening myocardial ischemia will accelerate pump failure and potentially cause fatal arrhythmias; and ventilation will degenerate to agonal breaths or apnea.

Typical Progression of Treated or Partially Treated Shock

A period of prolonged tissue hypoperfusion can compromise the function of any vital organ or tissue bed. Thus, even if the patient is resuscitated, sequelae that may blossom over the following hours and days include acute kidney injury (Chapter 106), shock liver (Chapters 133 and 140), intestinal ileus and ischemia (Chapter 129), anoxic brain injury (Chapter 373), and acute respiratory distress syndrome (Chapter 90).

DIAGNOSIS

Discerning That the Patient Is in Shock

Shock, which is a syndrome with multiple causes, lacks unambiguous diagnostic criteria. Instead, the diagnosis is based on a constellation of features not otherwise explained by other causes (see Table 92-1). Three principles dominate the diagnosis of shock. First, the clinical context is critical to inform the index of suspicion, especially regarding the inciting event. Second, because shock requires immediate treatment, the emphasis must focus on establishing a presumptive diagnosis; if in doubt, the patient should be presumed to be in shock until proven otherwise. Third, other conditions (e.g., an acute cerebrovascular accident [Chapter 376], drug overdose or poisoning [Chapter 96], or diabetic ketoacidosis [Chapters 104 and 210]) can mimic shock yet be present concomitantly; their presence should not be inferred as evidence that shock is absent.

Shock is diagnosed when the patient is hypotensive (systolic blood pressure <90 mm Hg or mean arterial pressure <60 mm Hg) with signs of hypoperfusion not otherwise explained by another diagnosis. Even if other conditions could explain the clinical features, shock must be presumed to be present until definitively excluded, given its gravity and need for immediate intervention. These blood pressure cut-points reflect population norms and are somewhat arbitrary. Thus, borderline values should be interpreted in light of other findings. If blood pressure is normal despite signs suggestive of hypoperfusion, a serum lactate level should be checked immediately[5]; values above 2 mmol/L are clearly consistent with hypoperfusion and shock. In the appropriate clinical setting, however, any patient who has elevated serum lactate levels not explained by another cause (e.g., metformin-induced hyperlactatemia or recent seizure) should be presumed to have shock. Although the magnitude of hypoperfusion broadly correlates with the serum lactate level and although even a minor elevation within the normal range (typically <2 mmol/L) can portend an increased risk of death, a mild elevation in the lactate level is not specific for shock. A sensitive but nonspecific cut-point for suspected shock is any value greater than 1 or greater than 1.5 mmol/L, though a less sensitive but more specific cut-point of 4 mmol/L also can be used to establish the diagnosis.

Differential Diagnosis

Acute emergencies that resemble shock include altered mental status owing to a variety of intoxications and drug overdoses (Chapter 96), acute metabolic derangements (e.g., hypoglycemia or diabetic ketoacidosis; Chapter 210), seizures (Chapter 372), or nonlocalizing stroke or intracranial hemorrhage (Chapters 376 and 377). Similarly, acute hypoxemic respiratory failure (Chapter 90) due to any cause may present as respiratory distress, tachycardia, and cyanosis and thus mimic shock.

Shock is caused by inadequate oxygen delivery owing to cardiovascular compromise, so conditions that impair the oxygen delivery/oxygen demand relationship via other mechanisms are not shock. For example, acute hypoxemic respiratory failure (Chapter 90) or severe anemia (Chapter 144) can cause tissue hypoxia, but they are not shock states. Rare conditions, such as cyanide poisoning (Chapters 82 and 96), in which oxygen is unavailable to the tissues because it cannot be released from hemoglobin, or carbon monoxide poisoning (Chapter 82), in which carbon monoxide competitively blocks the binding of oxygen to hemoglobin, are not examples of true shock.

Discerning the Type of Shock

The history and physical examination provide strong clues to the type of shock. If the patient arrives following trauma (Chapter 97), gastrointestinal bleeding (Chapter 121), or several days of severe diarrhea (Chapter 126), hypovolemic shock will be most likely. If the presentation suggests an acute myocardial infarction (Chapter 58), then cardiogenic shock (Chapter 93) is most likely, and so on. In addition to a physical examination focused on features of potential inciting events, attention should be paid to the skin color and turgor, peripheral pulses, and signs suggestive of obstruction or pump failure, such as jugular venous distension, tachypnea, cyanosis, and late inspiratory basilar crackles (Chapters 39 and 71). A chest radiograph may help by demonstrating evidence of cardiomegaly and pulmonary edema (see Fig. 44-2 in Chapter 44) in cardiogenic shock or oligemic lung fields in massive pulmonary embolus or status asthmaticus. However, the most useful rapid imaging study is bedside ultrasound (Chapter 44) to assess the size, filling, and contractility of cardiac chambers to suggest cardiogenic shock (Chapter 93); the presence of a pericardial effusion (Chapter 62) to suggest obstructive shock; and the collapsibility of the inferior vena cava to suggest hypovolemic shock (Table 92-2).

TABLE 92-2 RAPID ULTRASOUND IN SHOCK (RUSH) PROTOCOL*

RUSH EVALUATION	HYPOVOLEMIC SHOCK	CARDIOGENIC SHOCK	OBSTRUCTIVE SHOCK	DISTRIBUTIVE SHOCK
Heart	Hypercontractile LV Small LV chamber size	Hypocontractile or dilated LV	Hypercontractile LV Pericardial effusion Cardiac tamponade RV strain Cardiac thrombus	Hypercontractile LV in early sepsis, hypocontractile LV in late sepsis
Fluid status	Flat IVC Flat jugular veins Peritoneal fluid (fluid loss) Pleural fluid (fluid loss)	Distended IVC Distended jugular veins Pulmonary edema Pleural or peritoneal fluid (fluid loss)	Distended IVC Distended jugular veins Pneumothorax	Normal or small IVC in early sepsis Peritoneal or pleural fluid (fluid loss)
Extracardiac circulatory system	Abdominal aneurysm Aortic dissection	Normal	DVT	Normal

*Data from Perera P, Mailhot T, Riley D, et al. The RUSH exam: Rapid Ultrasound in SHock in the evaluation of the critically ill. *Emerg Med Clin North Am.* 2010;28:29-56.

DVT = deep venous thrombosis; IVC = inferior vena cava; LV = left ventricle; RV = right ventricle.

TREATMENT

The First Hour

When resuscitating a patient with shock, the goal is to restore adequate tissue perfusion as quickly as possible—a task that usually requires initiation of treatment before a definitive diagnosis and cause are established (Fig. 92-2). The first steps focus on establishing adequate oxygen delivery by ensuring adequate preload, cardiac output, and arterial oxygenation. Therefore, resuscitation begins with intravenous access to administer fluids (including blood products when indicated) and vasoactive agents (typically vasopressors), as well as the institution of ventilatory support (supplemental oxygen or mechanical ventilation [Chapter 91]). Optimal body positioning (e.g., the Trendelenburg position—elevation of the legs and feet to increase venous pressure) and other emergency procedures (e.g., needle thoracostomy to relieve a tension pneumothorax) are also recommended, depending on the clinical situation.

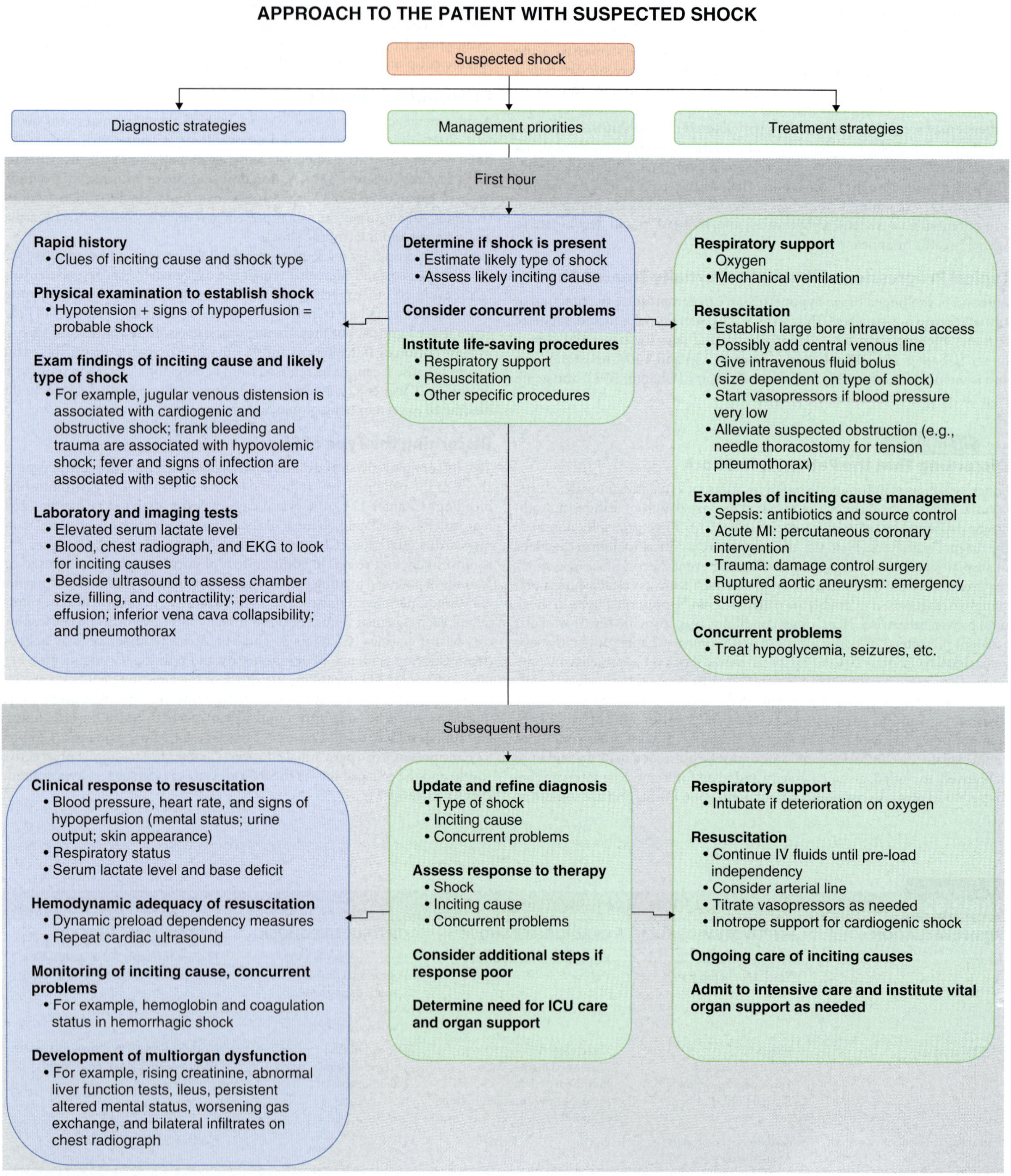

FIGURE 92-2. Management principles for the diagnosis and treatment of shock. Examples are intended to be representative. Further detail is provided in the corresponding text. BP = blood pressure; EKG = electrocardiogram; ICU = intensive care unit; IV = intravenous; MI = myocardial infarction.

Intravenous Access

Because all key treatment interventions are administered intravenously, intravenous access is a priority. If large-volume resuscitation is anticipated (hypovolemic or distributive shock), large-bore intravenous access (e.g., two #16 gauge peripheral catheters in case one malfunctions) will facilitate rapid resuscitation. Central venous catheterization, typically into a subclavian or internal jugular vein and ideally using ultrasound guidance,[A1,A2] is preferred for the administration of vasopressors. Of note, central access does not necessarily facilitate more rapid fluid infusion, because central lines are longer and infusion rates are a function of both diameter and length. If a central line is inserted for rapid infusion, a short #8.5 French catheter is ideal. Central venous access should be obtained with appropriate attention to sterile technique; a femoral vein can be used, albeit with a higher risk of infection.

Intravenous Fluids

Intravenous fluids are the primary method to ensure adequate preload—the point on the Starling curve (see Fig. 41-3 in Chapter 41) where further increases in preload do not increase output (preload independence). Intravenous fluids should ideally be given until the heart is preload independent but not to the point that the heart is overfilled and pushed too far to the right on the Starling curve, with subsequent cardiac decompensation, pulmonary edema, and worsening oxygen delivery.[6] The volume chosen for the initial bolus of fluids must be made somewhat empirically, but a challenge dose of 500 mL of crystalloids (e.g., normal saline, lactated Ringer solution) over 20 to 30 minutes is typically used, and infusion rates of 333 mL/hour and 1 L/hour produce equivalent outcomes.[A3] Of note, even in cardiogenic shock, where a patient typically has high preload pressures, a small bolus of intravenous fluid (e.g., 125 to 250 mL) can sometimes improve cardiac output and oxygen delivery.

When the clinician can be confident that the ventricles are underfilled (e.g., major hemorrhage, severe dehydration, or septic shock), resuscitation begins with a large volume of fluid—20 to 30 mL/kg administered as a bolus.[7] However, when pulmonary edema or cardiogenic shock is evident, a smaller amount (e.g., a 250-mL bolus) is more prudent.

Broadly speaking, there is no clear advantage of colloid over crystalloid solutions,[A4] so crystalloids, which are less expensive, are preferred. Crystalloids have a greater volume of distribution than colloids, so the effective intravascular volume expansion is less once fluid redistributes. However, there is no evidence that use of colloids during the initial resuscitation improves patient outcomes. "Balanced" crystalloids, such as PlasmaLyte or lactated Ringer solution, have a lower chloride content than normal saline, but their potential advantage over saline for improving outcomes is uncertain.[A5–A7] Hetastarches are never recommended because they are associated with worse outcomes.

Blood and Blood Products

Hemorrhagic shock can be classified by the degree of blood loss (Table 92-3). In trauma-induced hemorrhagic shock (Chapter 97), guidelines suggest commencing with 1 to 2 L of intravenous crystalloid but augmenting resuscitation of patients with massive hemorrhage by also administering plasma, platelets, and packed red blood cells in a ratio of 1 : 1 : 1 until bleeding is controlled.[8] Some advocate a similar approach for massive nontraumatic hemorrhage, such as from upper gastrointestinal bleeding (Chapter 121), though data to support this approach are scant.

TABLE 92-3 CLASSIFICATION OF HEMORRHAGIC SHOCK*

	CLASS I	CLASS II	CLASS III	CLASS IV
Blood loss (mL)	Up to 750	750-1500	1500-2000	>2000
% Volume	Up to 15	15-30	30-40	>40
Pulse rate (per minute)	<100	>100	>120	>140
Blood pressure	Normal	Normal	Decreased	Decreased
Pulse pressure	Normal or increased	Decreased	Decreased	Decreased
Respiratory rate (per minute)	14-20	20-30	30-40	>35
Urine output (mL/hr)	>30	20-30	5-15	Negligible
Mental status	Slightly anxious	Mildly anxious	Anxious, confused	Confused, lethargic
Fluid replacement	Crystalloid	Crystalloid	Crystalloid and blood	Crystalloid and blood

*Estimates based on a 70-kg patient.

From Committee on Trauma of the American College of Surgeons. *Advanced Trauma Life Support for Doctors*. Chicago: American College of Surgeons; 1997:108.

In septic shock, patients frequently become anemic—primarily because the considerable volume expansion with intravenous fluids leads to dilutional anemia, although hemolysis, coagulopathy-induced bleeding, and marrow suppression can all contribute over time. Anemia can compromise oxygen delivery, but transfusion of packed red blood cells beginning at a hemoglobin level of 7 g/dL is as good as beginning at a level of 9 g/dL.[A8] Unlike hemorrhagic shock, there is no role for the routine use of platelets or other blood products in the resuscitation of septic shock.

Transfusion of blood products in cardiogenic shock (Chapter 93) runs the risk of exacerbating pulmonary edema and worsening heart failure. For patients with acute myocardial infarction, a transfusion threshold of 8 g/dL is as safe as 10 g/dL,[A9] but maintaining myocardial oxygen supply is critical. When transfusing a patient with cardiac ischemia and cardiogenic shock, the patient must be monitored carefully for signs of worsening failure. Blood and blood products are not typically required in obstructive shock.

Vasopressors

Because fluid alone may be inadequate to restore blood pressure, especially in distributive shock, vasopressors (Table 92-4) are often required.[9–11] Vasopressors increase afterload, so adequate hydration is important to optimize their effects. Vasopressors may have to be started concomitantly with fluid resuscitation, and they often can be reduced after adequate fluid resuscitation. In patients with vasodilatory shock, such as with sepsis, postresuscitation strategies that restrict fluids, so as to rely more on vasopressors, yield similar outcomes to those that restrict vasopressors, so as to rely more on fluid administration.[A10,A11] In vasodilatory shock, permissive hypotension to a target mean arterial pressure of 60 to 65 mmHg by reducing vasopressor doses does not appear to be preferable to standard care.[A12]

The preferred vasopressor for distributive shock is norepinephrine,[8] because it is a strong vasoconstrictor with enough beta-adrenergic effects to increase myocardial contractility and to protect the heart against the increased afterload posed by vasoconstriction. Dopamine offers the theoretical advantage of selective vasodilation of the renal and splanchnic beds, but it has not provided renal protection in clinical practice; dopamine also had more side effects than norepinephrine in a large study of septic shock.

Vasopressin is not superior to norepinephrine as a single agent for septic shock[A13] but is useful as a second-line vasopressor when blood pressure remains inadequate despite high doses of norepinephrine. Vasopressin may also be a useful alternative to norepinephrine in nonseptic distributive shock.[A14] A synthetic angiotensin II pharmacologic agent has adrenergic vasopressor-sparing effects in distributive shock and may prove to be a useful alternative, but it cannot be recommended now based on available data.

Vasopressors play less of a role in cardiogenic shock (Chapter 93) but may be required temporarily in hypovolemic or obstructive shock until adequate cardiac output and blood pressure are restored. All vasopressors increase afterload, thereby potentially worsening cardiac failure, and can cause severe vasoconstriction, thereby leading to worsening acidosis and ischemia of the gut or limb.

Other Vasoactive Agents

Adrenergic (e.g., dobutamine) and nonadrenergic (e.g., milrinone) inotropic agents are used in cardiogenic shock (Chapter 93) but are not useful as routine agents in other forms of shock. Vasodilator therapy may be useful in cardiogenic shock, where it can increase cardiac output by reducing afterload without increasing myocardial oxygen demand (Chapter 93). However, the risk is worsened by hypotension, so it is not a routine treatment for other forms of shock. Some data suggest that beta-blockade might be useful in some patients in whom overstimulation by synthetic agents causes myocardial dysfunction akin to what is seen in patients with pheochromocytoma, but the clinical utility of such an approach is speculative at this time.

Respiratory Support

Although the primary cause of inadequate oxygen delivery is cardiovascular failure, supplemental oxygen can raise arterial oxygen content, thereby ameliorating tissue hypoxia. Supplemental oxygen by face mask is encouraged for all patients in suspected shock, with a greater emphasis placed on invasive mechanical ventilation (Chapter 91) via endotracheal intubation for patients with significant respiratory distress or severe hypotension or acidosis. A patient who is in shock and who is struggling to breathe despite supplemental oxygen should be intubated without a trial of noninvasive ventilation because it can be difficult to implement effectively, does not provide airway protection, and is less effective than invasive ventilation at reducing the work of breathing, facilitating gas exchange, and recruiting alveoli (Chapter 90). Invasive mechanical ventilation (Chapter 91) protects the airway, reduces the risk of aspiration, decreases the work of breathing (and therefore decreases oxygen demand), and improves gas exchange (to increase oxygen delivery and facilitate compensatory respiratory alkalosis). In cardiogenic shock (Chapter 93), mechanical ventilation provides the added benefit of improving alveolar recruitment and increasing transmural pressure on the heart, thereby reducing cardiac afterload and facilitating ventricular function.

The major complication of initiating mechanical ventilation in patients with shock is inadvertent worsening of cardiac output and hypotension because the positive intrathoracic pressure associated with mechanical ventilation retards

TABLE 92-4 VASOPRESSOR AGENTS

		PERIPHERAL VASCULATURE		CARDIAC EFFECTS			
AGENT	**IV DOSE RANGE**	**VASOCONSTRICTION**	**VASODILATION**	**HEART RATE**	**CONTRACTILITY**	**DYSRHYTHMIAS**	**TYPICAL USE**
Dopamine	1-4 μg/kg/min	0	1+	1+	1+	1+	"Renal dose" does not improve renal function; may be used with bradycardia and hypotension
	5-10 μg/kg/min	1-2+	1+	2+	2+	2+	
	11-20 μg/kg/min	2-3+	1+	2+	2+	3+	Vasopressor range
Vasopressin	0.04-0.1 units/min	3-4+	0	0	0	1+	Septic shock, post–cardiopulmonary bypass shock state, no outcome benefit in sepsis
Phenylephrine	20-200 μg/min	4+	0	0	0	1+	Vasodilatory shock; best for supraventricular tachycardia
Norepinephrine	1-20 μg/min	4+	0	2+	2+	2+	First-line vasopressor for septic shock, vasodilatory shock
Epinephrine	1-20 μg/min	4+	0	4+	4+	4+	Refractory shock, shock with bradycardia, anaphylactic shock
Dobutamine	1-20 μg/kg/min	1+	2+	1-2+	3+	3+	Cardiogenic shock, septic shock
Milrinone	37.5-75 μg/kg bolus followed by 0.375-0.75 μg/min	0	2+	1+	3+	2+	Cardiogenic shock, right-sided heart failure, dilates pulmonary artery; caution in renal failure

IV = intravenous.
Courtesy of Emanuel P. Rivers, MD.

right ventricular filling. This complication is most likely in patients with hypovolemic shock (who are most dependent on preload), but distributive shock, obstructive shock due to extrinsic compression, and some instances of cardiogenic shock can all be preload-dependent. Many sedation agents typically used during intubation, such as etomidate or short-acting benzodiazepines, cause vasodilation and hypotension, thereby potentially exacerbating this problem. A bolus of intravenous fluids (e.g., 500 mL normal saline) before or during intubation will frequently be necessary, together with judicious use of sedation agents, avoidance of excessive positive-pressure ventilation, and a potential increase in the dose of vasopressors.

Body Positioning

If the patient is very hypotensive, cardiac filling and cerebral perfusion can be augmented by having the patient lie flat or with the legs elevated (Trendelenburg position), especially patients in hypovolemic or distributive shock. Intubation and central line access are also facilitated by these positions. However, patients in severe respiratory distress, especially owing to pulmonary edema, usually cannot tolerate lying flat, and their hypoxemia may worsen. Similarly, until the airway is secured, a patient at risk of vomiting blood or gastric contents will be at higher risk of aspiration when managed flat. Furthermore, if a patient is suspected of having increased intracranial pressure (e.g., following major intracranial hemorrhage [Chapter 377], fulminant hepatic failure [Chapter 140], or traumatic brain injury [Chapter 368]), lying flat or in the Trendelenburg position could paradoxically worsen cerebral perfusion.

Other Emergency Procedures

A variety of other procedures must be initiated immediately in specific situations. For example, obstructive shock owing to cardiac tamponade (Chapter 62) will require emergency pericardial drainage, and a tension pneumothorax will require emergent drainage of the air. A trauma patient (Chapter 97) may require a pelvic binder or other tourniquet, a bedside ultrasound to evaluate possible intra-abdominal bleeding, and an emergency computed tomographic scan or exploratory laparotomy, depending on the findings. Similarly, a patient with an obvious major upper gastrointestinal bleed (Chapter 121) requires emergent endoscopy. Patients with septic shock and right upper quadrant pain require intravenous antibiotics and an urgent ultrasound followed by endoscopic retrograde cholangiopancreatography if dilated biliary ducts or stones are seen (Chapter 141). Patients with cardiogenic shock (Chapter 93) may require emergent percutaneous coronary intervention (Chapter 59). In addition, problems that can frequently co-occur with shock, such as generalized seizures (Chapter 372), acute alcohol intoxication (Chapter 364), drug overdose (Chapter 96), and hyperglycemia (Chapter 210), require emergency evaluation and treatment.

Monitoring the Adequacy of Resuscitation

After the initial appraisal and management, the subsequent hours are crucial to confirm the diagnosis and cause of shock, as well as to monitor the effectiveness of resuscitation. Simple measures of the adequacy of resuscitation include restoration of normal blood pressure, improvement in the clinical signs of hypoperfusion (e.g., sustained production of urine output and improved mental status), and improvement in base deficit and hyperlactatemia.

Although blood pressure can be measured by cuff manometry, the unreliability of this method in patients who are in profound shock commonly requires placement of an arterial line if the patient does not improve rapidly. However, restoration of blood pressure does not mean that oxygen delivery has improved or that tissue perfusion has been restored. Clinical and biochemical improvement may lag improvement in oxygen delivery by hours, or it may be obfuscated either by medical treatment, such as the need for sedating agents, or the blossoming of acute organ dysfunction despite successful resuscitation.

A pulmonary artery catheter can monitor right and pulmonary capillary wedge pressures, stroke volume, cardiac output, and mixed venous oxygen saturation. In shock states, inadequate oxygen delivery leads to increased peripheral oxygen extraction and low venous oxygen saturation for venous blood returning to the right heart. However, multiple clinical trials failed to demonstrate better outcomes based on therapy guided by a pulmonary artery catheter, and it is no longer recommended in the routine management of shock.[12]

One way to assess the adequacy of fluid resuscitation is to determine the responses to maneuvers that increase preload. Examples include passive leg raising or administering a fluid challenge (e.g., 500 mL of 0.9% saline or Ringer lactate solution) over 30 minutes.

Several multicenter trials of early goal-directed therapy, which specifically tries to improve measures of hemoglobin and oxygenation, have failed to demonstrate benefit beyond standard care. For example, a low central venous pressure suggests hypovolemia, but treatment of septic shock based on central venous pressure readings and blood pressure targets does not improve outcomes.[A15] Current recommendations therefore emphasize an early suspicion for shock, a low threshold to check a serum lactate level, prompt antibiotics if sepsis is a possible cause (Chapter 94), and an initial bolus of 20 to 30 mL/kg of intravenous fluids, followed by close monitoring of the adequacy of resuscitation using the clinical examination, serial blood lactate assessments, or measures of preload dependency, such as a passive leg raise test.

Ongoing Supportive Care

Unless a patient has advanced directives to limit care, shock should be treated with the goal of saving the patient's life. Patients who do not rapidly improve are typically admitted to an intensive care unit, where vital organ function can be monitored and appropriate support can be instituted.

As soon as the patient is able or family members are available, conversations to understand preferences for cardiopulmonary resuscitation (Chapter 7), mechanical ventilation (Chapter 91), and other aspects of intensive care are extremely important (Chapter 3). The physician should provide the best possible information about the diagnosis, potential course, and prognosis.

PREVENTION

Shock can be prevented by preventing the events that cause it (e.g., trauma, sepsis, myocardial infarction) or intervening promptly in sick patients to prevent their progression to shock. Many hospitals have instituted early warning systems to deploy rapid response teams for patients with abnormal vital signs (Chapter 7). Such programs can facilitate early assessment and treatment, and they may also improve outcomes.

PROGNOSIS

Mortality from shock is now about 25%. The degree to which blood pressure, cardiac output, and measures of hypoperfusion, such as serum lactate, are responding to resuscitation is prognostic, and early evidence of multiorgan dysfunction is predictive of the need for prolonged intensive care and higher mortality. For patients who survive, the long-term prognosis is variable but is a function of age, chronic health, the natural history of the inciting event, and the duration and intensity of the hospital course. Interestingly, acute features of the shock itself (e.g., degree of hypotension) predict short-term mortality but are less predictive of long-term outcomes.

GENERAL REFERENCES

For the General References and other additional features, please visit Elsevier eBooks+ at https://ebooks.health.elsevier.com.

Grade A References

A1. Brass P, Hellmich M, Kolodziej L, et al. Ultrasound guidance versus anatomical landmarks for subclavian or femoral vein catheterization. *Cochrane Database Syst Rev*. 2015;1:CD011447.

A2. Brass P, Hellmich M, Kolodziej L, et al. Ultrasound guidance versus anatomical landmarks for internal jugular vein catheterization. *Cochrane Database Syst Rev*. 2015;1:CD006962.

A3. Zampieri FG, Machado FR, Biondi RS, et al. Effect of slower vs faster intravenous fluid bolus rates on mortality in critically ill patients: the BaSICS randomized clinical trial. *JAMA*. 2021;326:830-838.

A4. Lewis SR, Pritchard MW, Evans DJ, et al. Colloids versus crystalloids for fluid resuscitation in critically ill people. *Cochrane Database Syst Rev*. 2018;8:CD000567.

A5. Finfer S, Micallef S, Hammond N, et al. Balanced multielectrolyte solution versus saline in critically ill adults. *N Engl J Med*. 2022;386:815-826.

A6. Zampieri FG, Machado FR, Biondi RS, et al. Effect of intravenous fluid treatment with a balanced solution vs 0.9% saline on mortality in critically ill patients: the BaSICS randomized clinical trial. *JAMA*. 2021;326:818-829.

A7. Hammond NE, Zampieri FG, Di Tanna GL, et al. Balanced crystalloids versus saline in critically ill adults—a systematic review with meta-analysis. *NEJM Evidence*. 2022;1.

A8. Hirano Y, Miyoshi Y, Kondo Y, et al. Liberal versus restrictive red blood cell transfusion strategy in sepsis or septic shock: a systematic review and meta-analysis of randomized trials. *Crit Care*. 2019;23:262.

A9. Ducrocq G, Gonzalez-Juanatey JR, Puymirat E, et al. Effect of a restrictive vs liberal blood transfusion strategy on major cardiovascular events among patients with acute myocardial infarction and anemia: the REALITY randomized clinical trial. *JAMA*. 2021;325:552-560.

A10. Meyhoff TS, Hjortrup PB, Wetterslev J, et al; CLASSIC Trial Group. Restriction of intravenous fluid in ICU patients with septic shock. *N Engl J Med*. 2022;386:2459-2470.

A11. Shapiro NI, Douglas IS, Brower RG, et al. Early restrictive or liberal fluid management for sepsis-induced hypotension. *N Engl J Med*. 2023;388:499-510.

A12. Lamontagne F, Richards-Belle A, Thomas K, et al. Effect of reduced exposure to vasopressors on 90-day mortality in older critically ill patients with vasodilatory hypotension: a randomized clinical trial. *JAMA*. 2020;323:938-949.

A13. Gordon AC, Mason AJ, Thirunavukkarasu N, et al. Effect of early vasopressin vs norepinephrine on kidney failure in patients with septic shock: the VANISH randomized clinical trial. *JAMA*. 2016;316:509-518.

A14. Hajjar LA, Vincent JL, Barbosa Gomes Galas FR, et al. Vasopressin versus norepinephrine in patients with vasoplegic shock after cardiac surgery: the VANCS randomized controlled trial. *Anesthesiology*. 2017;126:85-93.

A15. Rowan KM, Angus DC, Bailey M, et al. Early, goal-directed therapy for septic shock—a patient-level meta-analysis. *N Engl J Med*. 2017;376:2223-2234.

93

CARDIOGENIC SHOCK

STEVEN M. HOLLENBERG AND CLYDE W. YANCY

DEFINITION

Cardiogenic shock occurs when the heart is unable to deliver enough blood to maintain adequate tissue perfusion. Cardiogenic shock is a hemodynamic syndrome defined by sustained systemic hypotension (systolic BP less than 90 mm Hg), high pulmonary capillary wedge pressure (PCWP greater than 18 mm Hg), and low cardiac index (less than 2.2 L/minute/m^2) (Table 93-1). The diagnosis of cardiogenic shock is often made on clinical grounds—hypotension combined with signs of poor tissue perfusion, including oliguria, clouded sensorium, and cool extremities, all in the setting of myocardial dysfunction. To make the diagnosis, it is important to document myocardial dysfunction and to exclude or correct factors such as hypovolemia, hypoxemia, and acidosis.

EPIDEMIOLOGY

The classic cause of cardiogenic shock (Fig. 93-1) is left ventricular failure secondary to an extensive acute myocardial infarction (MI), often with a mechanical complication of MI (Chapter 58).[1] However, recent data suggest the epidemiology is shifting, with an increased proportion of cases related to acute decompensated chronic heart failure (Chapter 46).[2] Other causes include arrhythmia, valvular heart disease, and prolonged cardiopulmonary bypass (Table 93-2).[3] Fulminant myocarditis and stress-induced (takotsubo) cardiomyopathy may also present with cardiogenic shock (Chapter 47). Cardiac tamponade (Chapter 62) and massive pulmonary embolism (Chapter 68) with acute right ventricular failure can cause shock without pulmonary edema. An important consideration is that some cardiogenic shock may have an iatrogenic component. Early diagnosis of impending shock and identification of patients at high risk for development of shock is essential, both to speed intervention and to avoid therapies that may worsen hemodynamics.

After a decline over the past two decades, the incidence of cardiogenic shock complicating various acute clinical syndromes appears to be increasing, albeit for unclear reasons. The mortality associated with cardiogenic shock continues to decline, because effective early treatment and more widespread adoption of early revascularization have improved outcomes.

Only about 25% of patients who develop cardiogenic shock in the setting of an MI are in shock at initial presentation; in the others, shock usually evolves over several hours, thereby suggesting that early treatment may prevent shock. Patients with early and late shock show similar demographic, historical, clinical, and hemodynamic characteristics.

Risk factors for the development of cardiogenic shock in MI parallel those for LV dysfunction and the severity of coronary artery disease (CAD). Patient characteristics include older age, anterior MI, diabetes, hypertension, multivessel CAD, previous MI, and peripheral vascular or cerebrovascular disease. Clinical risk factors include decreased ejection fraction, larger infarctions, and lack of compensatory hyperkinesis in myocardial territories remote from the infarction. Clinical harbingers of impending shock include the degree of hypotension and tachycardia at hospital presentation. The factors that predict

TABLE 93-1 DIAGNOSIS OF CARDIOGENIC SHOCK

CLINICAL SIGNS
Hypotension
Oliguria
Clouded sensorium
Cool and mottled extremities
HEMODYNAMIC CRITERIA
Systolic blood pressure < 90 mm Hg or >30 mm Hg decrease from baseline for >30 minutes
Cardiac index < 2.2 L/min/m^2
Pulmonary capillary wedge pressure > 18 mm Hg
OTHER
Documented myocardial dysfunction
Exclusion of hypovolemia, hypoxemia, and acidosis

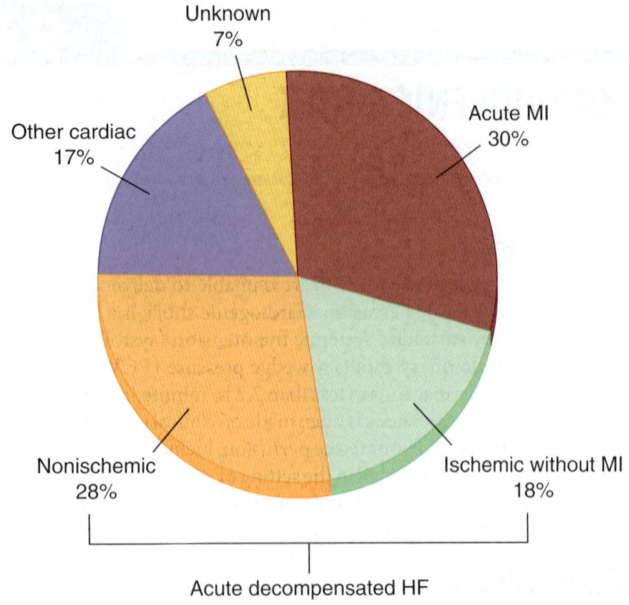

FIGURE 93-1. Causes of cardiogenic shock from the Critical Care Trial Network registry. HF = heart failure; MI = myocardial infarction. (Berg DD, Bohula EA, van Diepen S, et al. Epidemiology of shock in contemporary cardiac intensive care units. *Circ Cardiovasc Qual Outcomes*. 2019;12:e005618.)

TABLE 93-2 CAUSES OF CARDIOGENIC SHOCK

ACUTE MYOCARDIAL INFARCTION
Pump failure
Large infarction
Smaller infarction with preexisting left ventricular dysfunction
Infarct extension
Reinfarction
Infarct expansion
Mechanical complications
Acute mitral regurgitation due to papillary muscle rupture
Ventricular septal defect
Free wall rupture
Pericardial tamponade
Right ventricular infarction
CARDIOMYOPATHY
Myocarditis
Peripartum cardiomyopathy
End-stage low-output heart failure
Hypertrophic cardiomyopathy with outflow tract obstruction
Stress cardiomyopathy
VALVULAR HEART DISEASE
Acute mitral regurgitation (chordal rupture)
Acute aortic regurgitation
Aortic or mitral stenosis with tachyarrhythmia or other comorbid condition causing decompensation
Prosthetic valve dysfunction
TACHYARRHYTHMIA
OTHER CONDITIONS
Prolonged cardiopulmonary bypass
Septic shock with severe myocardial depression
Penetrating or blunt cardiac trauma
Orthotopic transplant rejection
Massive pulmonary embolism
Pericardial tamponade

mortality after cardiogenic shock reflect the severity of the acute insult as well as comorbid conditions.

Coronary angiography most often demonstrates multivessel CAD, with left main stenosis in 30% of patients and three-vessel coronary disease in 60%. Multivessel CAD may help explain failure to develop compensatory hyperkinesis in remote myocardial segments.

PATHOBIOLOGY

Cardiogenic shock is characterized by a downward cascade in which myocardial dysfunction reduces stroke volume, cardiac output, and blood pressure; these changes compromise myocardial perfusion, exacerbate ischemia, and further depress myocardial function, cardiac output, and systemic perfusion. Concomitant diastolic dysfunction increases left atrial pressure, which leads to pulmonary congestion and hypoxemia that can exacerbate myocardial ischemia and impair ventricular performance.

Compensatory mechanisms include sympathetic stimulation, which increases heart rate and contractility, thereby raising cardiac output but also increasing myocardial oxygen demand. Compensatory vasoconstriction can increase blood pressure, but it also increases myocardial afterload, further impairing cardiac performance and increasing myocardial oxygen demand. In the face of inadequate perfusion, this increased demand can worsen ischemia and perpetuate a vicious circle that, if unbroken, may culminate in death. Interruption of this circle of myocardial dysfunction and ischemia is the basis for therapeutic regimens for cardiogenic shock.

Patients with cardiogenic shock do not always have severe left ventricular dysfunction, so mechanisms other than primary pump failure are often operative. Furthermore, systemic vascular resistance is not always elevated, suggesting that compensatory vasoconstriction is not universal. Inflammatory responses may contribute to vasodilation and myocardial dysfunction in cardiogenic shock.

Patients in cardiogenic shock may have areas of nonfunctional but viable myocardium because of myocardial stunning, or postischemic dysfunction that persists despite restoration of normal blood flow. Some patients have hibernating myocardial segments with persistently impaired function at rest owing to severely reduced coronary blood flow. Although conceptually distinct, the two conditions may overlap; repetitive episodes of myocardial stunning can occur in areas of viable myocardium subtended by a critical coronary stenosis. Contractile function of hibernating myocardium improves with revascularization, and the severity of the antecedent ischemic insult determines the intensity of stunning, thereby providing a rationale for the early reestablishment of coronary patency in cardiogenic shock. The notion that some myocardial tissue may recover function emphasizes the importance of measures to provide hemodynamic support and minimize myocardial necrosis in patients with shock.

CLINICAL MANIFESTATIONS

The physical examination should be geared toward characterizing the patient's hemodynamic profile by evaluating congestion ("wet" or "dry") and systemic perfusion ("cold" or "warm") (Table 93-3). Signs of left-sided congestion (Chapter 45) include pulmonary rales, whereas jugular venous distention (see Fig. 39-1), peripheral edema, and ascites may indicate right-sided congestion.

Most patients with cardiogenic shock present "wet" and "cold," but a mixed shock profile, with congestion and vasodilation ("wet" and "warm") also occasionally can be seen. Patients with shock are usually ashen or cyanotic, and they have faint pulses, cool skin, and mottled extremities. Cerebral hypoperfusion may cloud the sensorium. Jugular venous distention and pulmonary rales are usually present, although their absence does not exclude the diagnosis. A precordial heave resulting from left ventricular dyskinesis may be palpable. The heart sounds may be distant, and third and/or fourth heart sounds are usually present. A systolic murmur of mitral regurgitation or a ventricular septal defect may be heard, but either complication can occur without an audible murmur (Chapter 58). Signs or symptoms of kidney, liver, intestinal, and cognitive dysfunction may be observed.

DIAGNOSIS

After recognizing the clinical manifestations of apparent cardiogenic shock, the clinician must confirm its presence and assess its cause while simultaneously initiating supportive therapy before irreversible organ damage ensues. The clinician must balance overzealous pursuit of an etiologic diagnosis before achieving stabilization with overzealous empirical treatment without adequate characterization of the underlying pathophysiologic process.

An electrocardiogram (ECG) should be performed immediately. In cardiogenic shock caused by acute MI, the ECG most commonly shows ST elevation, but ST depression or nonspecific changes are found in 25% of cases. If RV infarction is suspected, ST elevation in modified right-sided leads may be diagnostic (Chapter 58). An ECG showing Q waves or bundle branch block may suggest extensive disease.

Other initial diagnostic tests include a chest radiograph, complete blood count, and measurement of arterial blood gases, electrolytes, and cardiac biomarkers. Metabolic acidosis with elevated serum lactate levels may indicate

TABLE 93-3 SIGNS AND SYMPTOMS OF VOLUME STATUS AND PERFUSION

SIGNS AND SYMPTOMS OF CONGESTION
Orthopnea, paroxysmal nocturnal dyspnea
Jugular venous distention
Abdominojugular reflux
Rales
Hepatomegaly
Edema
Right upper quadrant tenderness
POSSIBLE EVIDENCE OF LOW PERFUSION
Hypotension
Narrow pulse pressure
Obtundation
Cool extremities
Cachexia, muscle loss
Decreased exercise tolerance
Renal/hepatic dysfunction

global hypoperfusion. A point-of-care ultrasound examination[4] or chest radiograph may demonstrate pulmonary edema and or suggest an alternative diagnosis, as when a widened mediastinum indicates aortic dissection (Chapter 63).

Echocardiography

Echocardiography is an indispensable tool for confirming the diagnosis of cardiogenic shock[5] and should be performed as early as possible, preferably with Doppler (Chapter 43). Echocardiography provides information about overall and regional systolic function, diastolic function, and valvular disease, and it can rapidly diagnose mechanical causes of shock, such as papillary muscle rupture, acute ventricular septal defect, and free wall rupture, and tamponade (Chapter 58).

Right Heart Catheterization

If the history, physical examination, chest radiograph, and echocardiogram demonstrate systemic hypoperfusion, low cardiac output, and elevation of venous pressures, right heart catheterization may not be necessary for diagnosis. If there is any uncertainty, however, invasive hemodynamic monitoring can be quite useful to characterize hemodynamics and to exclude volume depletion, right ventricular infarction, and mechanical complications.

Right heart catheterization is most useful, however, to optimize therapy in unstable patients. In such patients, clinical estimates of filling pressures can be unreliable, and optimal filling pressures may be higher than expected in individual patients with left ventricular diastolic dysfunction. Changes in myocardial performance or therapeutic interventions, including revascularization, can change cardiac output and filling pressures precipitously. Concomitant right ventricular dysfunction is often underrecognized in patients with cardiogenic shock, and its importance underappreciated; right heart catheterization is the best and most expeditious way to assess right-sided hemodynamics in these patients. Measurement of cardiac output and mixed venous oxygen saturation can assess cardiac performance and help select patients for inotropic and/or mechanical circulatory support. Some data suggest that, in contrast to patients with other forms of shock or with straightforward heart failure, the use of hemodynamic monitoring is associated with improved outcomes in patients with cardiogenic shock.[6]

TREATMENT

Initial Management

Initial stabilization of the patient with suspected cardiogenic shock includes venous access, supplemental oxygen, and continuous ECG monitoring (Fig. 93-2).[7,8] Management by a dedicated shock team is associated with better outcomes.[9] Many patients require endotracheal intubation and mechanical ventilation (Chapter 91), not only to improve gas exchange but also to reduce the work of breathing and facilitate sedation. Electrolyte abnormalities should be corrected. Relief of pain and anxiety with opiates (Chapter 58) can reduce excessive sympathetic activity, as well as decrease oxygen demand, preload, and afterload. Arrhythmias (Chapter 52) can reduce cardiac output and should be corrected promptly with antiarrhythmic drugs (see Table 52-2 in Chapter 52), cardioversion, or pacing (Chapter 54).

If the cause is likely an acute MI, aspirin and heparin should be given immediately (Chapter 58). Some therapies routinely used in acute MI (e.g., nitrates, β-blockers, renin-angiotensin system blockers) have the potential to exacerbate hypotension in cardiogenic shock and have been associated with poorer outcomes in hypotensive patients. Consequently, these agents should be avoided in patients with tenuous hemodynamic status until they stabilize.[10]

An initial assessment of fluid status and systemic perfusion should be performed.[11] Ischemia produces diastolic dysfunction, so high filling pressures may be necessary to maintain stroke volume in some patients. Some patients may benefit from rapid bolus infusions of 100 to 200 mL of crystalloid titrated to clinical end points. Patients who do not respond rapidly to initial treatment should be considered for invasive hemodynamic monitoring to identify the filling pressure at which cardiac output is maximized. Maintenance of adequate preload is particularly important in patients with right ventricular infarction.

Following initial stabilization and restoration of adequate blood pressure, tissue perfusion should be assessed. If tissue perfusion is adequate but significant pulmonary congestion remains, diuretics (e.g., intravenous furosemide as a 20 to 40 mg bolus) may be employed. If tissue perfusion remains inadequate, inotropic support and/or mechanical support should be initiated.

Vasopressors and Inotropes

Maintenance of adequate blood pressure is essential to break the vicious circle of progressive hypotension and further myocardial ischemia. When arterial pressure remains inadequate, therapy with vasopressor agents, titrated not only to blood pressure but also to clinical indices of perfusion and mixed venous oxygen saturation, may be required.[12] Norepinephrine (0.02 to 1.0 μg/kg/minute) acts primarily as a vasoconstrictor, has only a relatively mild inotropic effect, and increases coronary flow. It is preferable to dopamine,[A1,A2] which acts as both an inotrope (at 3 to 10 μg/kg/minute) and vasopressor (at 10 to 20 μg/kg/minute). Epinephrine (at 0.05 to 2 μg/kg/minute) increases both vascular tone and cardiac output, but it is associated with more refractory shock and more metabolic derangement when compared to norepinephrine.[A3] Vasopressin (at 0.02 to 0.04 U/min) may raise blood pressure in patients who are refractory to catecholamines. Vasopressor infusions must be titrated carefully in patients with cardiogenic shock to maximize coronary perfusion pressure with the least possible increase in myocardial oxygen demand. Invasive hemodynamic monitoring with an arterial line and temporary right heart catheterization are advisable during the initial titration of vasoactive agents.

If tissue perfusion remains inadequate despite norepinephrine, inotropic therapy should be initiated. Dobutamine (2.5 to 20 μg/kg/minute), a selective β1-adrenergic receptor agonist, can improve myocardial contractility and increase cardiac output. Dobutamine is the initial agent of choice in patients with systolic blood pressures greater than 90 mm Hg, but it may exacerbate hypotension in some patients, and can precipitate tachyarrhythmias. Milrinone (a phosphodiesterase inhibitor at 0.125 to 0.75 μg/kg/minute without a loading dose) has fewer chronotropic and arrhythmogenic effects than catecholamine but also has a long half-life and can cause hypotension. Milrinone is equivalent to dobutamine in patients who are in cardiogenic shock.[A4]

Intra-Aortic Balloon Pumps

Intra-aortic balloon pumps reduce systolic afterload and augment diastolic perfusion pressure without increasing oxygen demand, but do not significantly improve blood flow distal to a critical coronary stenosis. Despite a hemodynamic rationale for their use, randomized trials have shown no improvement in 30-day, 1-year, or 6-year mortality with intra-aortic balloon pump insertion in patients who have cardiogenic shock and who undergo early revascularization for acute MI.[A5] Whether intra-aortic balloon insertion may still be reasonable to support occasional patients through a critical period of shock until definitive therapy undertaken is not known. Failure of an intra-aortic balloon to reverse hypoperfusion, however, is a poor prognostic sign, and such patients should be considered for more aggressive mechanical support, e.g., a left ventricular assist device.

Cardiogenic Shock Complicating Acute MI

Reperfusion

Supportive therapy may improve blood pressure and cardiac output in cardiogenic shock, but rapid restoration of myocardial blood flow is the cornerstone of therapy for patients with cardiogenic shock due to MI (Chapter 58). Prompt revascularization is the only intervention that consistently reduces mortality rates in patients with cardiogenic shock that complicates an acute MI,[13] and randomized trials suggest that about 13 patients will be saved at 1 year for each 100 patients treated. Furthermore, most survivors will have good functional status.

Outcomes are best when PCI is performed within 6 hours after the onset of symptoms, but survival benefits are still demonstrable up to 18 hours after the onset of shock. In patients with multivessel disease, data suggest that stenting of the culprit lesion only is as good as immediate multivessel PCI, with a lower risk that the patient will require renal replacement therapy.[A6] Patients over 75 years of age who are suitable for aggressive therapy also appear to benefit.[14]

CABG surgery is more likely to provide complete revascularization and achieves long-term survival rates comparable to PCI, often despite worse coronary anatomy and a higher prevalence of diabetes. In practice, however, emergency CABG is performed less than 10% of the time.

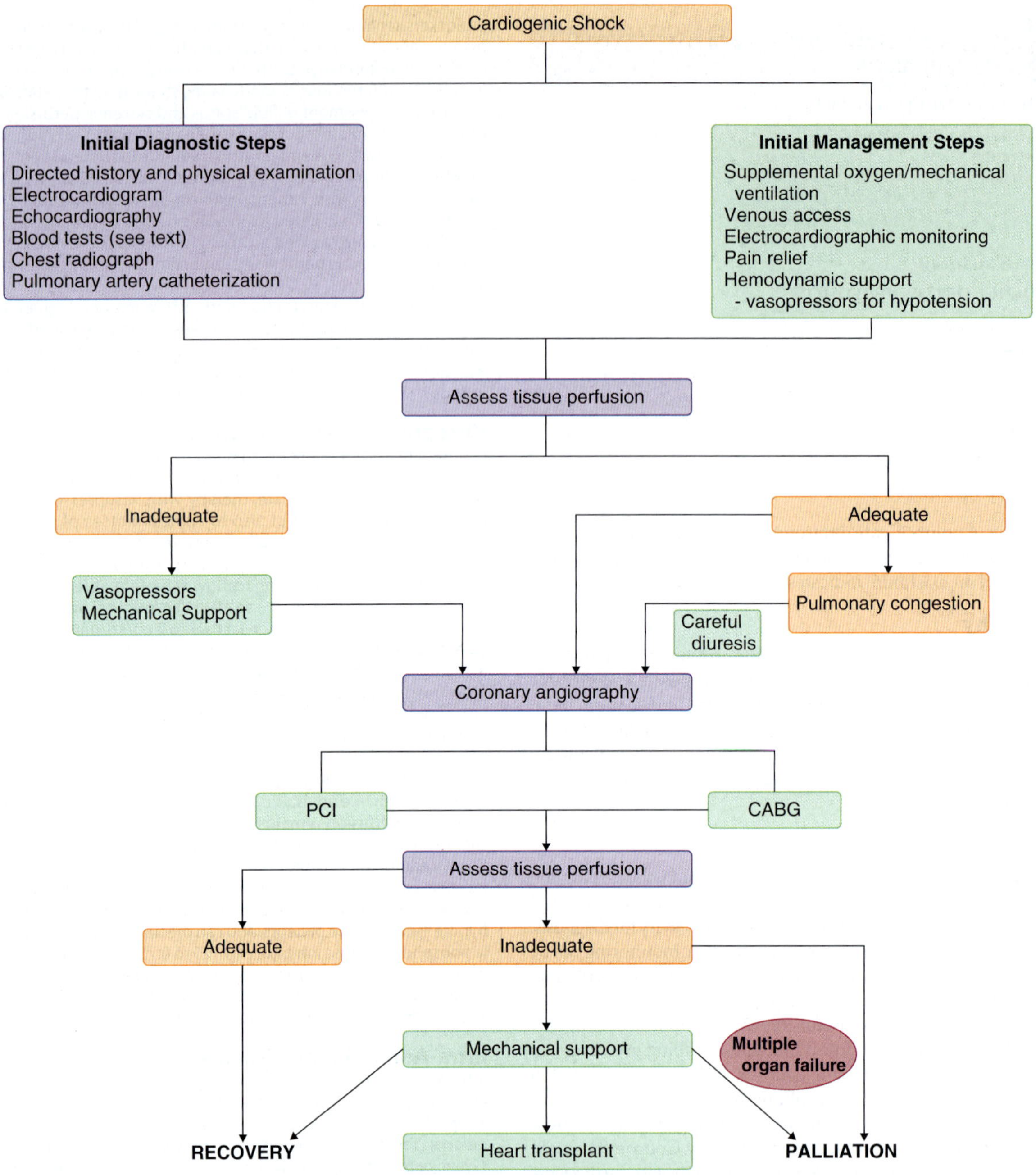

FIGURE 93-2. **Approach to the diagnosis and treatment of cardiogenic shock caused by myocardial infarction. Right ventricular infarction and mechanical complications are discussed in the text. CABG = coronary artery bypass graft; LVAD = left ventricular assist device; PCI = percutaneous coronary intervention.**

When cardiogenic shock results from mechanical complications of MI (Chapter 58), surgery is recommended when feasible. For acute mitral regurgitation owing to papillary muscle rupture, vasoactive and mechanical support are temporizing measures; definitive therapy requires expeditious surgical valve repair or replacement (Chapter 60). Although mortality is 20 to 40%, surgical results are improving, and both survival and ventricular function are improved compared with medical therapy.

Timely surgery is also critical in patients whose cardiogenic shock results from ventricular septal or free wall rupture. Because perforations are exposed to shear forces, the rupture site can expand abruptly. Repair can be technically difficult owing to the need to suture in areas of necrosis. Surgical mortality is 20 to 50% and is especially high for serpiginous inferoposterior ruptures, which are typically less well circumscribed than anteroapical ruptures. Right ventricular function is an important determinant of outcome in this setting. Timing of surgery has been controversial, but guidelines now recommend that operative repair be undertaken early, within 48 hours of the rupture. Placement of a septal occluding device may be helpful in selected patients.

Mechanical Circulatory Support

Percutaneous mechanical circulatory support devices can potentially interrupt the downward spiral of myocardial dysfunction, hypoperfusion, and ischemia in cardiogenic shock, thereby allowing time for myocardial recovery.[15] These devices, to different extents, increase arterial pressure and cardiac output, reduce left ventricular filling pressures and afterload, and support coronary perfusion. They can provide short-term support as a bridge to recovery or to transplantation,[16] and they are sometimes used as destination therapy when transplantation cannot be performed.[17] For cardiogenic shock in acute MI, however, these devices improve hemodynamic function but have not been shown to reduce morbidity.[A7]

Extracorporeal membrane oxygenation (ECMO) provides cardiopulmonary support for both heart and lungs using a membrane oxygenator and an arterial return catheter. ECMO reduces right ventricular and left ventricular preload but increases left ventricular afterload, and it can be useful for refractory cardiogenic shock,[18,19] including otherwise-refractory sepsis-induced cardiogenic shock, although its optimal timing and use remain uncertain.[A8,20]

A key issue in choosing among mechanical support options is right ventricular function. Some patients with both right and left heart failure might benefit from initial biventricular support with addition of right ventricular support. The left ventricle rarely fails alone for long, and assessment of right ventricular hemodynamics with invasive hemodynamic monitoring can be important to optimize mechanical support strategies.

Cardiogenic Shock Not Related to Acute MI

At the end stage of a dilated or restrictive cardiomyopathy (Chapter 47), low cardiac output can result in cardiogenic shock.[21] A search for reversible precipitating causes should be undertaken. Some patients will respond to inotropic therapy and will have a brief period of relative improvement. Appropriate candidates should be referred for evaluation for possible cardiac transplantation (Chapter 46) or mechanical support. A fully magnetically levitated circulatory pump can provide an 85% survival rate free of device surgery or disabling stroke in appropriately selected patients at 6 months.[A9] Left ventricular assist devices can be used either as a bridge to transplantation or as destination therapy. A discussion about end-of-life care is also warranted.

Acute myocarditis (Chapter 47) can take a fulminant course leading to shock in 10 to 15% of cases. Patients with acute myocarditis are typically younger than those with cardiogenic shock due to MI, and more commonly present with dyspnea rather than chest pain. Echocardiography usually shows global left ventricular dysfunction. Supportive therapy is indicated; some patients may require circulatory support and even consideration of cardiac transplantation. Immunosuppressive therapy has not been shown to improve outcome in fulminant myocarditis.

Patients with hypertrophic cardiomyopathy (Chapter 47) may sometimes present with severe outflow tract obstruction and shock. In such patients, diuretic and inotropic therapy typically worsen the obstruction. Careful volume resuscitation and use of a pure α-agonist, such as phenylephrine (0.1 to 0.3 mg/kg/minute), can reduce obstruction by increasing afterload and cavity size.

Stress (takotsubo) cardiomyopathy (Chapter 47) presents with chest pain and ECG changes similar to acute MI; exclusion of significant coronary obstruction and characteristic apical hypokinesis with basal sparing establish the diagnosis. Some patients may have left ventricular dysfunction severe enough to produce shock. Treatment is supportive. Most patients recover left ventricular function within days to weeks, and long-term prognosis is excellent.

Acute mitral regurgitation (Chapter 60) presents with pulmonary edema and decreased forward cardiac output. Causes include posterior papillary muscle rupture in acute MI, spontaneous chordal rupture, infective endocarditis (Chapter 61), and trauma (Chapter 97). The diagnosis is best made by echocardiography. Immediate stabilization may include inotropic or vasopressor therapy or mechanical support to support cardiac output and blood pressure. Definitive therapy, however, entails surgical valve repair or replacement (Chapter 60).

Acute aortic regurgitation most commonly results from infective endocarditis (Chapter 61) with leaflet destruction, but it may also be due to traumatic injury (Chapter 97) or acute aortic dissection (Chapter 63). The pulse pressure is usually narrow, indicating decreased forward stroke volume, and the bounding pulsations seen with chronic aortic regurgitation are typically absent. Temporizing measures include afterload reduction, with vasopressor and inotropic support as needed. Intra-aortic balloon pump is contraindicated, and excessive slowing of the heart rate may worsen hemodynamics by prolonging diastole. Definitive therapy is surgical.

PROGNOSIS

Cardiogenic shock is still the most common cause of death in acute MI. Survival rates are improving as advances in supportive therapy and reperfusion are used in appropriately selected patients. Lower systolic blood pressure, acidosis, and higher serum lactate and alanine aminotransferase levels are associated with a poorer prognosis.[22] Age and time to revascularization independently predict survival, but the benefits of revascularization are seen at every level of risk. Better myocardial perfusion at the capillary level, as determined by postrevascularization angiography, predicts better prognosis.[23] Average 1 year survival after early revascularization is 50 to 55%, and the survival benefit is maintained at follow-up, with 5-year survival approaching 45%. The quality of life in survivors is usually excellent; 83% of patients are either asymptomatic or have only mildly symptomatic heart failure. For patients with end-stage nonischemic myocardial disease, the prognosis is very poor in the absence of heart transplantation or long-term mechanical support.[24]

GENERAL REFERENCES

For the General References and other additional features, please visit Elsevier eBooks+ at https://ebooks.health.elsevier.com.

Grade A References

A1. Schumann J, Henrich EV, Strobl H, et al. Inotropic agents and vasodilator strategies for the treatment of cardiogenic shock or low cardiac output syndrome. *Cochrane Database Syst Rev.* 2018;1:CD009669.

A2. Rui Q, Jiang Y, Chen M, et al. Dopamine versus norepinephrine in the treatment of cardiogenic shock: a PRISMA-compliant meta-analysis. *Medicine (Baltimore).* 2017;96:e8402.

A3. Levy B, Clere-Jehl R, Legras A, et al. Epinephrine versus norepinephrine for cardiogenic shock after acute myocardial infarction. *J Am Coll Cardiol.* 2018;72:173-182.

A4. Mathew R, Di Santi P, Jung RG, et al. Milrinone as compared with dobutamine in the treatment of cardiogenic shock. *N Engl J Med.* 2021;385:516-525.

A5. Thiele H, Zeymer U, Thelemann N, et al. Intraaortic balloon pump in cardiogenic shock complicating acute myocardial infarction: long-term 6-year outcome of the randomized IABP-SHOCK II trial. *Circulation.* 2019;139:395-403.

A6. Thiele H, Akin I, Sandri M, et al. One-year outcomes after PCI strategies in cardiogenic shock. *N Engl J Med.* 2018;379:1699-1710.

A7. Ouweneel DM, Eriksen E, Sjauw KD, et al. Percutaneous mechanical circulatory support versus intra-aortic balloon pump in cardiogenic shock after acute myocardial infarction. *J Am Coll Cardiol.* 2017;69:278-287.

A8. Ostadal P, Rokyta R, Karasek J, et al. Extracorporeal membrane oxygenation in the therapy of cardiogenic shock: results of the ECMO-CS randomized clinical trial. *Circulation.* 2023;147:454-464.

A9. Mehra MR, Naka Y, Uriel N, et al. A fully magnetically levitated circulatory pump for advanced heart failure. *N Engl J Med.* 2017;376:440-450.

94 SHOCK SYNDROMES RELATED TO SEPSIS

ANTHONY C. GORDON AND JAMES A. RUSSELL

DEFINITION

Sepsis is life-threatening organ dysfunction caused by a dysregulated host response to infection. Organ dysfunction is defined as an acute change of two or more points in the total Sequential Organ Failure Assessment (SOFA) score[1] (Table 94-1). In addition to the full SOFA, a briefer quick SOFA—defined by respiratory rate of 22/min or more, altered mentation, and systolic blood pressure lower than 100 mm Hg—provides simple bedside criteria to screen quickly for sepsis. *Bacteremia* is defined as the growth of bacteria in blood cultures, but infection does not have to be proved to diagnose sepsis at the onset. *Septic shock* was also redefined in 2016 as a subset of sepsis with persisting hypotension requiring vasopressors to maintain a mean arterial pressure of 65 mm Hg or higher accompanied by a serum lactate level greater than 18 mg/dL (2 mmol/L), despite adequate volume resuscitation.[2]

EPIDEMIOLOGY

More than 750,000 cases of severe sepsis or septic shock occur every year in the United States, and more than 48 million cases are estimated to occur globally each year. Sepsis, which is diagnosed in 6% of adult U.S. hospitalizations, causes as many deaths as acute myocardial infarction, and septic shock and its complications are the most common causes of death in noncoronary intensive care units (ICUs). Worldwide, the age-standardized incidence and mortality rates of sepsis have been declining substantially over the past three decades, although less so in sub-Saharan Africa.[3] The medical care costs associated with sepsis are approximately $20 billion a year in the United States alone. The incidence of septic shock is increasing as physicians perform more aggressive surgery, as more resistant microorganisms are present in the environment, and as the prevalence of immune compromise resulting from disease and immunosuppressive drugs increases. Risk factors for septic shock include age, underlying chronic conditions (e.g., chronic obstructive pulmonary disease, cancer), and immunosuppressive drugs. Studies suggest that African Americans have a higher incidence of sepsis than Whites (6.0 vs. 3.6 per 1000 population) and a higher mortality in ICUs (32% vs. 29%) even after adjusting for poverty levels. The mechanisms of this apparent difference in risk for and mortality from sepsis are not known.

Gram-positive or gram-negative bacteria, fungi, and, very rarely, protozoa or rickettsia can cause septic shock. Increasingly common causes of septic shock are antibiotic-resistant gram-positive bacteria, especially methicillin-resistant *Staphylococcus aureus*, vancomycin-resistant enterococci, and penicillin-resistant *Streptococcus pneumoniae*, as well as sometimes multidrug-resistant gram-negative bacilli.

The most common infections causing septic shock are pneumonia (about half of cases), peritonitis, pyelonephritis, abscess (especially intra-abdominal), primary bacteremia, cholangitis, cellulitis, necrotizing fasciitis, and meningitis. Nosocomial pneumonia is the most common cause of death from nosocomial infection. Blood cultures are positive in only about one third of patients with septic shock, and 20 to 30% of cases are culture negative from all sites.

TABLE 94-1 SCREENING FOR SEPSIS AND SEPTIC SHOCK

Step 1. Screen for sepsis using Quick SOFA (Sepsis-related Organ Failure Assessment): One point is given for each adverse finding as follows:
1. Respiratory rate ≥22/minute
2. Altered mentation—Glasgow Coma Score less than 15
3. Systolic blood pressure ≤100 mm Hg

Step 2. Diagnose sepsis as a 2-point increase in SOFA as follows:
Sequential SOFA

Step 3. Diagnose septic shock by the following:
Use of vasopressors (e.g., norepinephrine, epinephrine, phenylephrine) to maintain a mean arterial pressure ≥65 mm Hg
PLUS
Serum lactate >18 mg/dL (2 mmol/L) despite adequate volume resuscitation

SEQUENTIAL (SEPSIS-RELATED) ORGAN FAILURE ASSESSMENT (SOFA) SCORE

	SCORE				
SYSTEM	**0**	**1**	**2**	**3**	**4**
Respiratory (PaO_2/FIO_2)	≥400	<400	<300	<200	<100
Coagulation (platelet count × $10^3/\mu L$)	≥150	<150	<100	<50	<20
Liver (bilirubin mg/dL [μmol/L])	<1.2 (20)	1.2-1.9 (20-32)	2.0-5.9 (33-101)	6.0-11.9 (102-204)	>12 (204)
Cardiovascular	MAP ≥70 mm Hg	MAP <70 mm Hg	Dopa <5 (or any dose dob*)	Dopa 5.1-15 or epi ≤0.1 or norepi ≤0.1	Dopa >15 or epi >0.1 or norepi >0.1
CNS (Glasgow Coma Scale)†	15	13-14	10-12	6-9	<6
Renal (creat mg/dL [μmol/L])	<1.2 (100)	1.2-1.9 (110-170)	2.0-3.4 (171-299)	3.5-4.9 (300-400)	>5 (440)
Urine output, mL/d				<500	<200

*Catecholamine doses are given as μg/kg/minute for at least 1 hour.
†Glasgow Coma Scale scores range from 3 to 15; higher score indicates better neurological function.
CNS = central nervous system; Dob = dobutamine; Dopa = dopamine; epi = epinephrine; FIO_2 = fraction of inspired oxygen; MAP = mean arterial pressure; norepi = norepinephrine; PaO_2 = partial pressure oxygen.
Adapted from Singer M, Deutschman CS, Seymour CW, et al. The third international consensus definitions for sepsis and septic shock (Sepsis-3). *JAMA*. 2016;315:801-810.

Septic shock occurs in about 20 to 30% of patients hospitalized with coronavirus disease 2019 (COVID-19; Chapter 336), likely with a similar pathophysiology as other causes of septic shock. In addition, however, severe acute respiratory syndrome coronavirus 2 (SARS-CoV-2), which is the causative agent of COVID-19, binds and downregulates angiotensin-converting enzyme 2, which normally degrades angiotensin II (a very potent vasoconstrictor and permeability-inducing agent) to angiotensin 1-7 (a vasodilator). This effect appears to enhance lung damage (Chapter 335) and increase the risk of septic shock.

PATHOBIOLOGY

At its onset, septic shock activates inflammation, as evidenced by neutrophilia and a shift to immature neutrophils and a procoagulant phenotype (detected by an increased international normalized ratio and thrombocytopenia) owing to enhanced coagulation, activated platelets, and diminished fibrinolysis. An immunosuppressed state may emerge and may contribute to death. Several pathways amplify one another: inflammation triggers coagulation, coagulation triggers inflammation, and tissue hypoxia amplifies both inflammation and coagulation, thereby resulting in positive pro-inflammatory and procoagulant feedback loops. Many mediators critical to homeostatic control of infection are also injurious to the host (e.g., tumor necrosis factor-α [TNF-α], interleukin-1 [IL-1]), perhaps in part explaining why therapies that neutralize such mediators have generally been ineffective to date.

Widespread endothelial injury is an important feature of septic shock; an injured endothelium is more permeable. Consequently, protein-rich edema fluid fluxes into tissues such as the lung, where it leads to acute respiratory distress syndrome (ARDS). In septic shock, injured endothelial cells release nitric oxide, a potent vasodilator. Septic shock also injures epithelial cells of the lung and intestine. Intestinal epithelial injury increases intestinal permeability and the epithelial translocation of intestinal bacteria and endotoxin, thereby further augmenting the inflammatory phenotype of septic shock.

Early Infection, the Innate Immune Response, Inflammation, and the Endothelium

Bacteria have cell surface endotoxins (lipopolysaccharide [LPS] and lipoteichoic acid [LTA] of gram-negative and gram-positive bacteria, respectively) that are major ligands for innate immune receptors, mainly on various immune cells that launch the septic inflammatory response. Endotoxins are shuttled from high-density lipoprotein (HDL) to low-density lipoprotein (LDL) (E-Fig. 94-1) and are cleared mainly by the liver via the LDL receptor—the same receptor that clears LDL cholesterol—and then are excreted harmlessly in bile (E-Fig. 94-2). Endotoxin clearance is modulated by proprotein convertase subtilisin/kexin type 9 (PCSK9); lower PCSK9 activity increases recycling of the LDL receptor to the hepatocyte cell surface, thereby increasing hepatic endotoxin clearance.

Host defense is organized into innate and adaptive immune responses. The innate immune system uses pattern recognition receptors (e.g., toll-like receptors [TLRs], C-type lectin receptors, retinoic acid inducible gene 1–like receptors, and nucleotide-binding oligomerization domain–like receptors) to bind pathogen-associated molecular patterns, which are extremely well-conserved molecules of microorganisms. LPS and LTA of gram-negative and gram-positive bacteria, respectively, bind to TLR-4 and TLR-2, respectively (see E-Fig. 94-2; E-Fig. 94-3). TLR-4 and TLR-2 binding initiates an intracellular signaling cascade that causes nuclear transport of the transcription factor nuclear factor κB (NF-κB), which in turn initiates transcription of cytokines such as TNF-α and IL-6. Nucleotide-binding oligomerization domain–like receptors are important in the inflammasome response to sepsis. IL-3 also amplifies acute inflammation and is a potential therapeutic target in sepsis.

Cytokines upregulate adhesion molecules of neutrophils and endothelial cells, and neutrophil activation leads to bacterial killing. However, cytokines also directly injure host endothelial cells, as do activated neutrophils, monocytes, and platelets. Inhibition of early cytokine mediators of sepsis, such as TNF-α and IL-1β, has not proved successful, probably because TNF-α and IL-1β peak and then decline quickly, before these antagonist therapies can be applied clinically.

After the early cytokine inflammatory response, immune cells, including macrophages and neutrophils, release later mediators, such as high-mobility group box 1 (HMGB-1). HMGB-1 activates neutrophils, monocytes, and endothelium. Unlike TNF-α antagonists, inhibitors of HMGB-1 decrease mortality even when they are given 24 hours after the induction of experimental peritonitis.

Autophagy is a self-degradative housekeeping cellular process in many tissues and is increased in sepsis in immune cells, heart, lung, kidney, and liver. Autophagy removes damaged mitochondria in hepatocytes, regulates inflammasome activation of immune cells (see E-Fig. 94-3), and is a pro-survival mechanism of cardiomyocytes. Dysregulated autophagy is associated with decreased survival in septic models. Autophagy research suggests that modulation of autophagy in sepsis may prove beneficial. The inflammatory response to septic shock varies according to the organism load, host genotype, underlying conditions, and prior immunosuppressing drugs.

Endothelial Injury

In septic shock, widespread endothelial injury is common and leads to increased endothelial permeability with loss of protein and fluid to the interstitial space. Endothelial permeability is a final common pathway for widespread tissue injury. Cytokines and other inflammatory mediators induce intercellular endothelial cell gaps by disrupting intercellular junctions, by changing cytoskeletal structure, or by direct damage to endothelial cells. Several pathways of altered endothelial permeability have been implicated in sepsis, including protease-activated receptor 1 (PAR-1) and disruption of the intercellular VE-cadherin, β-catenin, and p120-catenin complex. PAR-1 binding by activated protein C and low-dose thrombin is cytoprotective, whereas PAR-1 stimulation by high-dose thrombin increases endothelial permeability. Binding of Slit to Robo4 maintains the integrity of the intercellular VE-cadherin, β-catenin, and p120-catenin complexes and thus maintains healthy endothelial permeability. Mediators of increased permeability in sepsis include heparin-binding protein, soluble thrombomodulin, angiopoietin-2, sphingosine-1 phosphate, and natriuretic peptides.

Adaptive Immunity Adds Specificity and Amplifies the Immune Response

Microorganisms stimulate specific humoral and cell-mediated adaptive immune responses that amplify innate immunity. B cells release immunoglobulins that bind to microorganisms and thereby facilitate delivery of microorganisms to natural killer cells and neutrophils. In sepsis, type 1 helper T (T_H1) cells generally secrete pro-inflammatory cytokines (TNF-α, IL-1β), and type 2 helper T (T_H2) cells secrete anti-inflammatory cytokines (IL-4, IL-10).

Coagulation Response to Infection

Septic shock activates the coagulation system, thereby causing sepsis-associated coagulopathy (E-Fig. 94-4), and ultimately converts fibrinogen to fibrin, which binds to platelets to form microvascular thrombi. A marked or sustained procoagulant response to septic shock can lead to disseminated intravascular coagulation (DIC; Chapter 161) and widespread tissue injury, including loss of digits and limbs. The three main features of sepsis-associated coagulopathy are increased procoagulant activity and decreased anticoagulant and fibrinolytic activity. Microvascular thrombi amplify endothelial injury by the release of inflammatory mediators and by tissue hypoxia because of obstruction to blood flow.

Normally, natural anticoagulants (protein C, protein S, antithrombin, and tissue factor pathway inhibitor) dampen coagulation, enhance fibrinolysis, and remove microthrombi. Thrombin-α binds to thrombomodulin, which activates protein C when protein C is bound to the endothelial protein C receptor (EPCR). Activated protein C dampens the procoagulant phenotype because it inactivates factors Va and VIIIa and inhibits the synthesis of plasminogen activator inhibitor 1 (PAI-1). Activated protein C also decreases apoptosis, leukocyte activation and adhesion, and production of cytokines. Endothelial thrombomodulin expression is decreased in meningococcemia (Chapter 274), thereby explaining in part the profound DIC characteristic of meningococcemic shock.

Septic shock decreases the levels of the natural anticoagulants protein C, protein S, antithrombin, and tissue factor pathway inhibitor. Furthermore, lipopolysaccharide and TNF-α decrease the expression of thrombomodulin and EPCR, thereby further limiting the activation of protein C. Lipopolysaccharide and TNF-α also increase levels of PAI-1, inhibiting fibrinolysis. The coagulation system is linked to the inflammatory response by protease activated receptors (PARs), especially PAR-1.

Tissue Hypoxia in Septic Shock

Tissue hypoxia independently activates inflammation (by activation of NF-κB and cytokines, synthesis of nitric oxide, and activation of HMGB-1); induces coagulation (through tissue factor and PAI-1); and activates neutrophils, monocytes, and platelets. Hypoxia disinhibits hypoxia-inducible factor-1α (HIF-1α), which upregulates erythropoietin, and vascular endothelial growth factor (VEGF). Erythropoietin is protective to brain and other tissues. VEGF inhibits fibrinolysis and increases inducible nitric oxide synthase, thereby increasing nitric oxide–induced vasodilation. Nitric oxide's other injurious effects include inhibiting the beneficial actions of HIF-1α (e.g., upregulating synthesis of erythropoietin) during hypoxia. Tissue hypoxia also causes release of damage-associated molecular patterns (alarmins), which are ligands for the pattern recognition receptors described earlier, thereby increasing the inflammation in septic shock.

Endocrine Responses Relevant to Cardiovascular Support

Complex interactions of several endocrine systems modulate vascular tone, heart rate, and other noncardiovascular functions such as immune function. The main axes stimulated to increase hormone production are the adrenal medullary release of norepinephrine and epinephrine (Chapter 209), hypothalamic-posterior pituitary release of vasopressin (Chapter 204), the hypothalamic-anterior pituitary-adrenal cortex release of corticosteroids (such as cortisone) (Chapter 208), and the renin-angiotensin-aldosterone (RAAS) release of angiotensin II (E-Fig. 94-5). Norepinephrine binds to α1 receptors, vasopressin binds to V1a receptors, and angiotensin II similarly binds to angiotensin II receptors on smooth muscle to stimulate calcium-mediated vasoconstriction. Cortisone modulates α1 receptor density. Deficiencies in each of these hormone levels and the downregulation of relevant receptors (such as V1a) in part explain the need for vasopressor(s)—such as first-line norepinephrine, and second-line epinephrine, vasopressin, and possibly angiotensin II—to increase vascular tone by producing vasoconstriction in patients who do not respond to volume resuscitation.

Immunosuppression and Apoptosis of Immune and Epithelial Cells

Septic shock can initiate an immunosuppressed state that can exceed the pro-inflammatory response starting soon after the onset of septic shock and can be fatal. Patients move through the balance of pro- versus anti-inflammatory/immunosuppressed states at different rates, likely accounting for the wide variability in the clinical progression and recovery from septic shock. Immunodepression occurs in the humoral, cellular, and neural regulation of immunity. Immunosuppression is suggested by anergy, lymphopenia, a decreased CD-4 level, hypothermia, and nosocomial infection (E-Fig. 94-6). Multiple organ dysfunction may be an immunodepressed phenotype because of the apoptosis of immune (B and T cells as well as dendritic cells), epithelial, and endothelial cells. Activated $CD4^+$ T cells evolve into either a T_H1 pro-inflammatory (TNF-α, IL-1β) or a T_H2 anti-inflammatory (IL-4, IL-10) phenotype. Sepsis leads to migration from a T_H1 to a T_H2 phenotype; for example, persistent elevation of IL-10 is associated with an increased risk of death. Immunosuppression also develops because of apoptosis of lymphocytes. Pro-inflammatory cytokines, activated B and T cells, and glucocorticoids induce lymphocyte apoptosis, whereas TNF-α and endotoxin induce apoptosis of lung and intestinal epithelial cells. Other late features of septic shock include expansion of regulatory T cells and myeloid suppressor cells, decreasing inflammation, but impaired phagocytosis. The vagus nerve activates the splenic nerve, thereby causing CD4+ T cells to release acetylcholine, which further attenuates inflammation.

Septic patients can be divided into subgroups based on transcriptomic signatures in blood and the key differences in gene expression related to immunosuppression.[4] These subgroups may respond differently to treatment such as corticosteroids, thereby paving the way for personalized medicine approaches in septic shock.

Death from infectious disease appears to be highly heritable. Sepsis is a prime example of a polygenic disease related to the interaction of multiple genes and an environmental insult (infection). Single-nucleotide polymorphisms of cytokines (TNF-α, IL-6, IL-10), coagulation factors (protein C, fibrinogen-β), the catecholamine pathway (β-adrenergic receptor), and innate immunity genes (CD14, TLR-1, TLR-2) have been variably associated with an increased risk of death from sepsis. To date, none of these findings have evolved into actionable diagnostic or prognostic biomarkers for clinical use.

Cardiovascular Dysfunction

The main features of cardiovascular dysfunction in septic shock are vasodilation, hypovolemia, decreased ventricular contractility, and increased vascular permeability. Inadequate tissue perfusion and tissue hypoxia are the cardinal features of all types of shock. Peripheral levels of catecholamines are dramatically increased in septic shock, but peripheral vasodilation indicates decreased responsiveness to these endogenous vasoconstrictors. Vasodilation in sepsis is mediated mainly by increased synthesis of nitric oxide and prostacyclin. Nitric oxide is increased by a calcium-independent nitric oxide synthase induced by endotoxin interaction with vascular endothelial cells. Prostacyclin is released by endothelial cells in response to both endotoxin and inflammatory cytokines. Adrenomedullin, which is a pleiotropic vasodilating hormone and cardiac depressant, is increased in septic shock. Early in septic shock, most patients have sinus tachycardia and, by definition, a need for vasopressor(s) because of decreased blood pressure (<90 mm Hg systolic, a decrease of ≥40 mm Hg from baseline systolic pressure, or mean arterial pressure <65 mm Hg; see Table 94-1). Septic shock is the classic form of distributive shock (Chapter 92), characterized by increased pulse pressure (bounding pulses), decreased systemic vascular resistance (warm, flushed skin), and functional hypovolemia (low jugular venous pressure). Distributive shock means that the distribution of systemic blood flow is abnormal, with areas of low flow (and low venous oxygen saturation) and high flow (and high venous oxygen saturation) present. Nevertheless, about one third of patients with septic shock initially present with findings more typical of hypovolemic shock (low central venous pressure, low central venous oxygen saturation, and cold, poorly perfused limbs) because the clinical features depend on the stage and severity of septic shock as well as on the degree of fluid resuscitation that has occurred. After fluid resuscitation, patients typically develop the characteristic clinical and hemodynamic features of classic distributive shock.

Vascular volume and ventricular preload are commonly decreased in early septic shock for several reasons. First, patients may be volume depleted because of decreased fluid intake and because of increased fluid losses due to fever, vomiting, and diarrhea if gastrointestinal disease is present. Second, fluid loss from the intravascular to the interstitial space (capillary leak) is caused by mediators that induce widespread endothelial injury, which increases capillary permeability. Increased capillary permeability leads to loss of protein-rich edema fluid into the interstitial space. The increased vascular permeability exacerbates transmural vascular leak at any given transmural hydrostatic pressure, thereby creating a vicious cycle. Sicker patients have greater increases in endothelial permeability, yet sicker patients have greater third-space fluid losses, so they need more fluid input. If, however, fluid input increases transmural hydrostatic pressure even modestly, then sicker patients will have greater fluid leakage into tissues, with increasing organ edema, organ dysfunction, and mortality.

In the lung, increased capillary permeability is a key component of ARDS (Chapter 90). Ventricular preload is also decreased in septic shock because of venodilation induced by mediators such as nitric oxide. Venodilation increases venous capacitance and relative volume depletion, thereby compounding absolute volume depletion. Ventricular afterload is decreased because of excessive release of potent vasodilators such as nitric oxide, prostaglandin I_2, adenosine diphosphate, and other vasodilators.

In addition to abnormal vasodilation, patients have concurrent microvascular vasoconstriction. Microvascular vasoconstriction may not be apparent clinically but can cause tissue hypoxia, detected by increased arterial lactate concentrations. Microvascular vasoconstriction is caused by increased norepinephrine, thromboxanes, and other local vasoconstrictors. Microvascular vasoconstriction-induced focal hypoxia is exacerbated by microvascular obstruction by platelets and leukocytes.

The abnormal mismatch of oxygen delivery to oxygen demand disturbs the global relationship of oxygen delivery to oxygen consumption. Normally, oxygen consumption is independent of oxygen delivery over a wide range. When oxygen delivery decreases to less than the critical oxygen delivery level, oxygen consumption decreases and leads to a state in which oxygen consumption depends on oxygen delivery. At levels lower than the critical oxygen delivery level, blood lactate increases as a result of tissue hypoxia, explaining in part why an elevated serum lactate level is a component of the diagnosis of septic shock. The clinical implication is that oxygen delivery should be increased (e.g., by increasing cardiac output by volume resuscitation, infusion of dobutamine, or transfusion of erythrocytes) to more than the critical level.

Cardiovascular function is further compromised in septic shock because of decreased ventricular contractility.[5] Within minutes of recognizing bacteria, cardiomyocytes secrete pro-inflammatory cytokines and chemokines that recruit inflammatory cells. Cardiomyocytes concurrently express cell-surface-adhesion molecule ICAM-1, which interacts with actin filaments within the cell to reduce contractile efficiency. Decreased ventricular contractility may be difficult to detect clinically and may be diagnosed only by hemodynamic or echocardiographic assessment. Numerous circulating mediators of sepsis, including endotoxin, cytokines (e.g., IL-6, TNF-α), and nitric oxide (locally released into the coronary circulation), decrease contractility. Endotoxin signals through TLRs to upregulate the expression of proteins such as two small calcium-regulated molecules (S110A8 and S100A9) to cause a receptor for advanced glycation end products (RAGE)–dependent decrease in calcium flux, thereby decreasing the ejection fraction. Coronary ischemia resulting from microvascular obstruction is another mechanism of decreased contractility.

Early in septic shock, patients who ultimately survive have increased left ventricular end-diastolic volume to help maintain cardiac output despite decreased contractility. In contrast, nonsurvivors do not increase their left ventricular end-diastolic volume, so cardiac output is compromised. In some patients with septic shock, concurrent ARDS causes secondary pulmonary hypertension, which increases right ventricular afterload and shifts the interventricular septum from right to left. This septal shift decreases left ventricular end-diastolic volume, thereby further limiting cardiac output.

CLINICAL MANIFESTATIONS

Patients in septic shock have a systolic pressure of 100 mm Hg or less, often accompanied by an elevated respiratory rate (>22/minute) or altered mental status. About 80% of patients are febrile, but patients can be normothermic or even hypothermic (in about 20% of cases). On initial presentation, the source of infection may be obvious, especially if patients have previous evidence of a specific site of infection such as pneumonia or a surgical site infection, or can be occult.

The cardiovascular dysfunction in septic shock is characterized by decreased preload (because of decreased intake, fluid losses, third spacing resulting from increased permeability, and venodilation), decreased afterload, and often decreased ventricular contractility. Decreased ventricular volume is detected clinically by low jugular venous pressure and hemodynamically by decreased central venous pressure. Left ventricular resistance, or afterload, is also commonly decreased and is detected clinically by warm, flushed skin and hemodynamically by decreased systemic vascular resistance.

DIAGNOSIS

The initial assessment of a critically ill patient must focus on the airway (need for intubation), breathing (respiratory rate, respiratory distress, pulse oximetry), circulation (heart rate, blood pressure, jugular venous pressure, skin perfusion), and the rapid initiation of warranted resuscitation (Fig. 94-1).[6] Arterial blood gases and lactate levels are useful especially since an elevated lactate level is a component of the clinical diagnosis of septic shock.

A secondary survey is designed to determine the source of infection and the status of organ function. Pneumonia (Chapter 85) is suggested by cough, sputum, and respiratory distress; empyema (Chapter 86) is suggested by pleuritic chest pain. Signs of peritonitis (Chapter 128), an abdominal mass (Chapter 118), and tenderness (Chapter 141) suggest abdominal sepsis (Chapter 118). Pyelonephritis (Chapter 263) is likely in patients with dysuria and costovertebral angle tenderness. Integumentary assessment for erythema (cellulitis), erythema at the vascular access site (line sepsis), tenderness (necrotizing fasciitis; Chapter 271), crepitus (anaerobic myonecrosis), and petechiae and purpura (meningococcemia; Chapter 274) can be illuminating. Headache, stiff neck, and signs of meningismus raise the suspicion of meningitis (Chapter 381). Focal neurologic signs suggest brain abscess (Chapter 382).

Laboratory investigations that are helpful to identify the source of infection include appropriate cultures and Gram stains (blood, sputum, urine, fluids, and cerebrospinal fluid). Blood cultures are positive in about 30 to 40% of patients with septic shock, but they are positive one-third less often if antibiotics were administered before the cultures were drawn.[7] In patients with negative cultures, RNA gene-targeted metagenomic sequencing can find a likely pathogenic organism in about 40% of cases.[8] The chest radiograph aids in the diagnosis of pneumonia, empyema, and the acute respiratory distress syndrome.

Direct visualization of the heart by transthoracic bedside echocardiography can immediately estimate the left ventricular ejection fraction. It can also be used to assess intravascular volume status (diagnosed by collapse of the inferior vena cava) and valvular dysfunction. Echocardiographic features of decreased ventricular contractility include decreased right and left ventricular ejection fractions and increased end-diastolic and end-systolic volumes. Early in septic shock, the left ventricular ejection fraction is decreased, and it remains low in nonsurvivors. In survivors, the left ventricular ejection fraction usually returns to normal during 5 to 10 days.

In early septic shock, central venous pressure is usually low and increases in response to volume resuscitation. Central venous oxygen saturation, cardiac output, and ventricular filling pressures may be determined. Central venous pressure measurement is recommended in patients who require vasopressors because their hypotension is not responsive to fluids alone. Pulmonary artery pressure is usually normal but may be increased because septic shock can cause pulmonary hypertension. Pulmonary artery occlusion (or wedge) pressure is

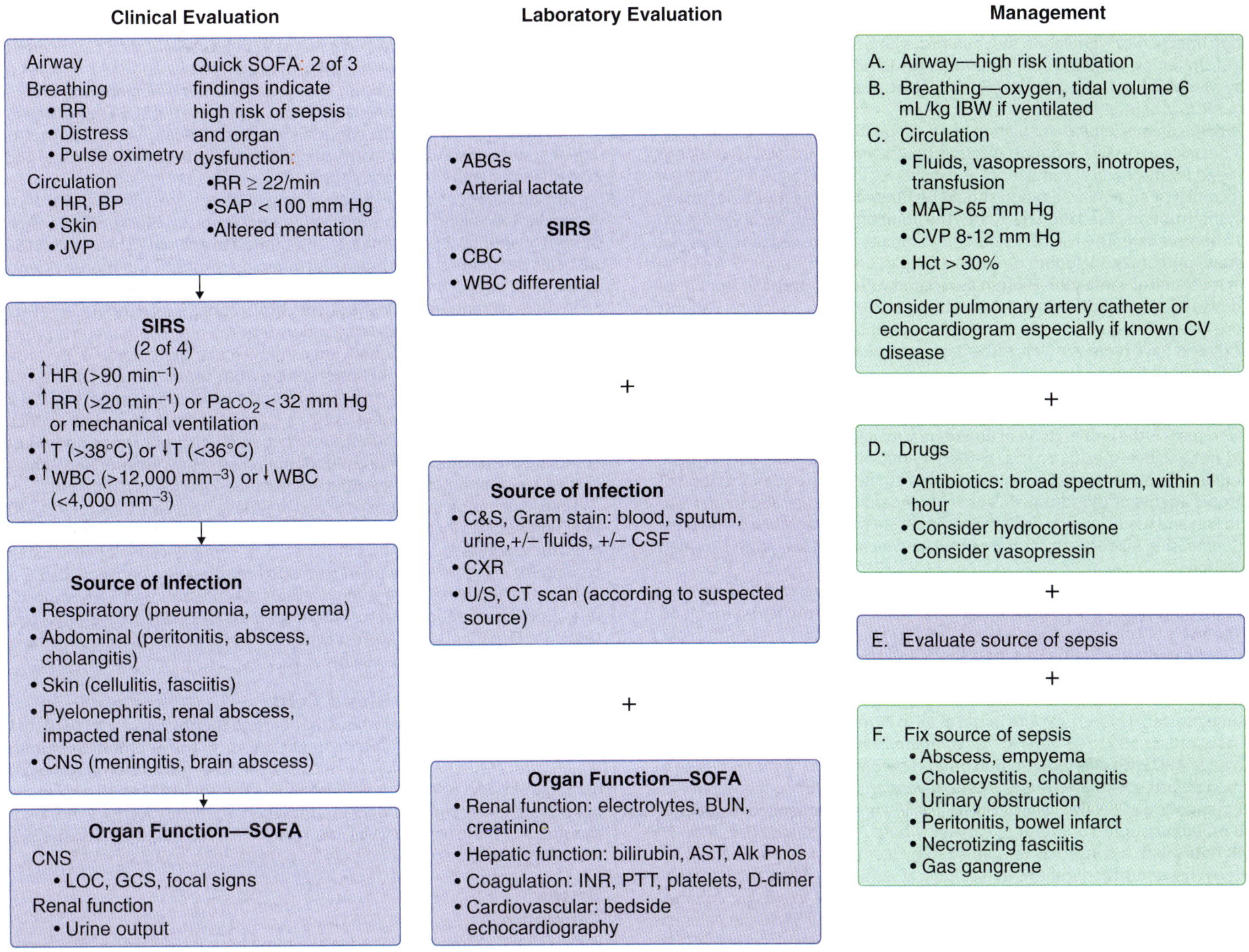

FIGURE 94-1. **Algorithm for the clinical and laboratory evaluation and management of septic shock.** ABGs = arterial blood gases; Alk Phos = alkaline phosphatase; AST = aspartate aminotransferase; BP = blood pressure; BUN = blood urea nitrogen; C&S = culture and sensitivity; CBC = complete blood count; CNS = central nervous system; CSF = cerebrospinal fluid; CT = computed tomography; CV = cardiovascular; CVP = central venous pressure; CXR = chest radiograph; GCS = Glasgow Coma Scale; Hct = hematocrit; HR = heart rate; IBW = ideal body weight; INR = international normalized ratio; JVP = jugular venous pressure; LOC = level of consciousness; MAP = mean arterial pressure; $Paco_2$ = partial pressure of carbon dioxide; PTT = partial thromboplastin time; RR = respiratory rate; SAS = systolic arterial pressure; $Scvo_2$ = central venous oxygen saturation; SIRS = systemic inflammatory response syndrome; SOFA = Sequential Organ Failure Assessment; T = temperature; U/S = ultrasound; WBC = white blood cell count.

usually low before resuscitation, but it may be normal or increased if the patient has underlying preexisting heart disease (e.g., heart failure, prior myocardial infarction) or if left ventricular contractility is decreased by sepsis. Cardiac output may be low or normal before fluid resuscitation and typically increases to higher than normal after fluid resuscitation. If fluid resuscitation increases central venous pressure and pulmonary artery occlusion pressure but cardiac output does not increase, left ventricular dysfunction is presumably present.

Vital signs and the leukocyte count quickly establish whether the patient has the systemic inflammatory response syndrome (SIRS). Abdominal ultrasound and computed tomography are indicated if abdominal sepsis is suspected. Renal, hepatic, and coagulation function tests are helpful to evaluate acute kidney injury, hepatic dysfunction, and sepsis-associated coagulopathy, respectively. After determining the source of sepsis, the clinician must address source control by draining abscesses and empyemas; using image-directed procedures or open surgery to correct urinary tract obstruction; and surgically managing peritonitis, bowel infarction, cholecystitis, cholangitis, necrotizing fasciitis, and gas gangrene.

Differential Diagnosis

The major differential diagnoses of septic shock are acute pancreatitis (Chapter 130), the acute respiratory distress syndrome (Chapter 90), aspiration pneumonitis (Chapter 82), multiple trauma (Chapter 97), cytokine storm,[9] and recent major surgery without infection (Chapter 401). Other causes of distributive shock to consider are anaphylactic shock (suggested by angioedema and hives; Chapter 407), spinal shock (recent trauma and paraplegia; Chapter 368), acute adrenal insufficiency ("tanned skin," hyperkalemia, metabolic alkalosis; Chapter 208), and acute or acute-on-chronic hepatic failure (jaundice, ascites, encephalopathy; Chapter 139).

The differential diagnosis of septic shock must include the other causes of shock: hypovolemic, cardiogenic, and obstructive shock (Chapters 92 and 93). Patients with hypovolemic shock (e.g., from internal or external fluid losses or hemorrhage) present with a suggestive history and signs of hypovolemia (low jugular venous pressure) and skin hypoperfusion (cool and clammy skin, peripheral cyanosis, slow capillary refill). Cardiogenic shock (e.g., owing to myocardial infarction, heart failure, or post–cardiovascular surgery) is suggested by the history, signs of increased filling pressure (increased jugular venous pressure, crackles, S_3, pulmonary edema, cardiomegaly), and skin hypoperfusion (Chapter 93). Some patients who have acute myocardial infarction and cardiogenic shock have features of SIRS, with excessive vasodilation in the absence of infection. Obstructive shock (e.g., pulmonary thromboembolism [Chapter 68], cardiac tamponade [Chapter 62], pneumothorax [Chapter 86]) manifests similarly to cardiogenic shock.

TREATMENT

Respiratory Therapy

All patients in septic shock require oxygen initially, and many require mechanical ventilation because acute respiratory distress syndrome (ARDS) is the most common complication of septic shock.[10] Endotracheal intubation of the patient in septic shock can be complicated by worsening hypotension, but a 500 mL intravenous bolus of normal saline prior to intubation does not improve outcomes in critically ill patients undergoing intubation.[A1] Lung-protective ventilation (mechanical ventilation that minimizes lung injury by using a combination of strategies, including a set tidal volume, such as 6 to 8 mL/kg of predicted body weight [when using volume-cycled ventilatory assist]) decreases mortality from ARDS (Chapter 91).

Patients on mechanical ventilation need adequate, but not excessive, sedation because excessive sedation worsens hemodynamic instability, prolongs the need for mechanical ventilation, and increases the risk for development of nosocomial pneumonia. Sedation should be titrated by objective assessment. Daily interruption of sedation decreases the duration of mechanical ventilation and intensive care. The use of dexmedetomidine to induce sedation does not improve outcomes, including delirium, compared with propofol.[A2] Weaning from mechanical ventilation is often associated with fluid overload from prior fluid resuscitation and from the reduction in intrathoracic pressure. Patients whose weaning is guided by brain natriuretic peptide levels are weaned more quickly and have more ventilator-free days because they receive more aggressive diuretic therapy.

Circulatory Therapy

Early therapy is the cornerstone of emergency management, but such therapy need not achieve specific central hemodynamic or oxygen-delivery targets, or require the placement of a central venous catheter or the administration of inotropic agents or blood transfusions.[A3] Standard therapies aim to increase perfusion and tissue oxygen delivery by increasing profoundly low blood pressure, increasing inadequate cardiac output, and increasing low arterial oxygen saturation.

The overall goal is to achieve adequate mean arterial pressure (>65 mm Hg) and other indices of perfusion such as urine output (>0.5 mL/kg/hour), blood lactate levels (<2 mmol/L), mental status, and skin perfusion. To assess the adequacy of early resuscitation of septic shock and to guide ongoing therapy, a central venous oxygen saturation goal greater than 70% or a lactate clearance of at least 10% is equivalent.[11]

A mean arterial blood pressure target of 65 to 70 mm Hg generally is as effective as a target of 80 to 85 mm Hg[A4] or compared with usual care.[A5] In patients who have ARDS, no difference in outcomes is seen with management using a pulmonary artery catheter versus a central venous catheter, so measurement and monitoring of central venous pressure (CVP) is recommended in patients who require vasopressor infusion. Patients whose ARDS is managed after 24 to 48 hours with a conservative fluid strategy (compared with a liberal fluid strategy) have shorter durations of mechanical ventilatory assist and ICU stay.

Fluids must be administered in an adequate but not excessive volume. Restrictive and liberal fluid strategies result in similar mortality rates for patients in septic shock,[A6,A7] but the restrictive fluid approach requires strict protocols for identifying and treating hypovolemia to avoid more prevalent and longer duration vasopressor support. Fluids (30 mL/kg of intravenous crystalloid, either 0.9% saline or a balanced solution such as lactated Ringer solution) should be given over the first 3 hours followed by additional fluids to achieve and maintain central venous pressure at 8 to 12 mm Hg and adequate tissue perfusion (e.g., mentation, urine output). In critically ill adults, balanced crystalloids are often used instead of sodium chloride because of lower rates of acute kidney injury, less need for renal replacement therapy, and fewer deaths,[A8] but a recent double-blind trial comparing a balanced solution with saline found no difference in outcomes in a diverse group of ICU patients, including the subgroup who had sepsis.[A9] There are no convincing data indicating that albumin is better than crystalloid solutions.[A10] Hetastarch should not be used in septic shock. Excess fluid resuscitation is associated with increased mortality from septic shock, and an increased CVP may indicate fluid overload and a higher risk of developing pulmonary edema. Heart failure with a decreased ejection fraction is common in patients with sepsis,[12] and lesser amounts of fluid administration (i.e., below guideline recommended volumes) are safer and associated with no difference in risk-adjusted mortality compared with patients with normal ejection fractions.[13]

Vasopressors (e.g., first-line: norepinephrine, 1 to 50 μg/minute; alternative: epinephrine, 1 to 30 μg/minute) should be added if the mean arterial pressure is less than 65 mm Hg despite adequate fluid resuscitation,[14] and earlier administration concomitant with fluid resuscitation appears to improve the early control of septic shock but not clearly reduce septic shock mortality.[A11] Norepinephrine is slightly, but not significantly, better than dopamine for reducing mortality when used as the first-line vasopressor for patients with septic shock; however, norepinephrine is associated with a lower rate of arrhythmias, especially atrial fibrillation. Norepinephrine and vasopressin are similar for preventing acute kidney failure in patients with septic shock.[A12] These accumulated data suggest that norepinephrine is the preferred first-line vasopressor in septic shock.

Although vasopressin deficiency and downregulation of vasopressin receptors are common findings in septic shock, a low-dose vasopressin infusion added to norepinephrine is not significantly better than a norepinephrine infusion alone in septic shock. Vasopressin (up to 0.03 U/min) may be added in patients not responding adequately to norepinephrine to increase mean arterial pressure and to decrease norepinephrine dose, but selepressin (a vasopressin agonist) has no incremental value when added to norepinephrine.[A13] Whether vasopressin infusion may be beneficial in patients with less severe shock is uncertain.

Angiotensin II infusion (20 ng/kg/minute initially, adjusted upward to a maximum of 200 ng/kg/minute) can decrease early norepinephrine requirements and improve the cardiovascular component of the SOFA score. However, it does not significantly reduce mortality. Levosimendan, which is an inotropic agent and mild vasodilator with anti-inflammatory properties, is not of added benefit in patients with septic shock.

Some patients, especially younger patients, have excessive tachycardia that limits diastolic filling time. Short-acting intravenous β-blockers (e.g., esmolol started at about 0.2 μg/kg/minute and titrated to a targeted heart rate of 80 to 90 beats per minute) have shown encouraging results,[A14] but more evidence is required before recommending this approach for routine clinical use.

In some patients in septic shock, the cardiac index is inadequate, as reflected by a low mixed venous oxygen saturation despite a high central venous pressure (>12 mm Hg) because of underlying cardiovascular dysfunction or because of acute left ventricular dysfunction resulting from sepsis. In such patients, clinicians can consider use of an inotropic agent (e.g., dobutamine, initially 2 to 5 μg/kg/minute and increasing to 20 μg/kg/minute) to increase left ventricular contractility and raise cardiac output. In patients with septic shock, however, the combination of norepinephrine plus dobutamine results in a mortality similar to that with epinephrine alone, with no differences in organ dysfunction.

Fever is common in septic shock and may have beneficial effects for resisting infection but also increases oxygen demand. Reducing fever can decrease the need for vasopressors and possibly the risk of septic encephalopathy. External cooling for 48 hours to maintain core body temperature between 36.5°C and 37°C is safe and can decrease the need for vasopressors and 14-day mortality rates. Cooling to reduce fever to normothermia is especially promising for febrile septic shock patients who are receiving high doses of vasopressors or inotropic agents, or who have marked tachycardia.

Transfusion of Red Blood Cells

Anemia is common in septic shock, but red cell transfusion can increase risk of nosocomial infection and other complications, so the appropriate hemoglobin level for resuscitation has been controversial. A transfusion threshold of a hemoglobin level of 7 g/dL is equivalent to a threshold of 9 to 10 g/dL in terms of the need for life support, or death, and such a goal can decrease the need for transfusion.[A15] The freshest available, compatible red blood cells are no better than standard-issue red blood cells for patients with septic shock.[A16]

Drugs

Antibiotics

Early antibiotic administration, ideally within 1 hour, is highly recommended and allows the duration of antibiotic administration to be shortened without increasing resistance or the subsequent need for additional antibiotics.[15] Meropenem alone is equivalent to the combination of meropenem and moxifloxacin in terms of mortality rates and organ dysfunction. Adding empirical fluconazole treatment does not result in better outcomes in critically ill, non-neutropenic patients. Continuous infusion of beta-lactam antibiotics results in higher clinical cure rates 14 days after cessation of antibiotics, better pharmacokinetic/pharmacodynamic target attainment, and more ventilator-free days compared with an intermittent bolus of antibiotics but does not improve 30-day survival.[A17]

The infected site and infecting organisms of septic shock are often not known initially, and clinicians often must select an empirical antibiotic regimen before knowing culture results. After appropriate culture specimens are obtained, intravenous broad-spectrum antibiotics as guided by an infectious disease consultation should be administered within 1 hour (while considering host factors such as immune and allergic status) complemented by control of the infectious source based on an anatomic diagnosis, which may require radiologic investigations (Chapters 259 and 260; see Fig. 94-1). Emergency, empirical antibiotic therapy (Table 94-2) should be guided by the greater frequency of gram-positive bacteria, the possibility of resistant organisms, and the local bacteriologic features. In a meta-analysis, the efficacies of empirical antibiotic monotherapies and combination antibiotic therapy appear to be equivalent for the treatment of sepsis.[A18]

Broad-spectrum antibiotics should be used for as short a time as possible. If a causative organism is identified, the antibiotic regimen should be quickly narrowed within 3 to 5 days to decrease the emergence of resistant organisms. The duration of antibiotics should be guided by the cause of septic shock, reviewed regularly, but patients generally require 7 to 10 days of therapy. Compared with usual care, procalcitonin-guided use of antibiotics (e.g., a ≥80% reduction in the procalcitonin level or a level ≤0.5 μg/L on day 5 or later) in critically ill patients can decrease the duration of antibiotic therapy and hospitalization, but its effect on more important outcomes is less clear.[A19,A20]

Corticosteroids

Corticosteroids administered before antibiotics can decrease the neurologic sequelae of bacterial (especially pneumococcal) meningitis (Chapter 381). Although corticosteroids are not effective for preventing septic shock in patients who have sepsis but are not in shock, the combination of 50 mg intravenous hydrocortisone every 6 hours (200 mg daily) plus 50 μg fludrocortisone (orally via a nasogastric tube) once daily for 7 days can improve 90-day all-cause mortality in patients with septic shock.[A21] By comparison, hydrocortisone (200 mg intravenously daily) treatment alone is associated with a shorter duration of shock but no reduction in 90-day mortality,[A22] and no benefit from the combination of hydrocortisone, vitamin C, and thiamine has been seen in randomized clinical trials.[A23,A24] Current sepsis guidelines suggest that corticosteroids not be used if fluid resuscitation and vasopressors can restore hemodynamic stability, but low-dose corticosteroids (200 mg hydrocortisone per day) or the combination of hydrocortisone plus fludrocortisone may be added if hemodynamic stability cannot be achieved. The one exception is COVID-19 (Chapter 337), for which corticosteroids (e.g., dexamethasone 6 mg intravenously once daily) decrease the need for ventilation and mortality by about 30% in patients who require oxygen.[A25] Enthusiasm for steroid therapy must be tempered by the risk of complications such as superinfection, neuromyopathy, hyperglycemia, immune suppression, and impaired wound healing.

Hyperglycemia and Intensive Insulin Therapy

Hyperglycemia and insulin resistance are common in septic shock, but intensive insulin therapy to control blood glucose levels tightly is not beneficial in patients in medical ICUs because of significantly higher rates of hypoglycemia and perhaps increased mortality. Aggressive insulin therapy to address the hyperglycemia that often accompanies corticosteroid treatment is no better than usual glucose control.

Renal Dysfunction and Dialysis

Acute kidney injury is an important complication of septic shock because of its associated morbidity, mortality, and resource use (Fig. 94-2). In critically ill patients who have acute kidney injury, hemodialysis six times per week is no better than conventional hemodialysis, and intensive renal replacement therapy is no better than standard therapy overall or in patients who have sepsis.

Continuous renal replacement therapy may be preferable to intermittent hemodialysis in patients with septic shock who remain hemodynamically unstable. The use of regional citrate for anticoagulation increases the filter's life span during renal replacement therapy and reduces the risk of bleeding.[A26]

The timing for initiation of renal replacement therapy in the critically ill remains uncertain. The largest trials have not shown any benefit in mortality when renal replacement therapy is started earlier than with standard criteria.[A27] Venoarterial extracorporeal membrane oxygenation may be beneficial for patients with sepsis-induced cardiogenic shock (Chapter 93).

Low-dose dopamine (2 to 4 μg/kg/minute) does not decrease the need for renal support, does not improve outcomes, and is not recommended. Lactic acidosis is a common complication of septic shock, but administration of sodium bicarbonate for lactic acidosis does not improve hemodynamics or the response to vasopressors.

Other Therapies

Deep venous thrombosis prophylaxis with low-molecular-weight heparin (LMWH) may be superior to low-dose unfractionated heparin because it may decrease the risk of pulmonary emboli in the critically ill. LMWH is recommended for patients who do not have active bleeding, coagulopathy, or a contraindication to heparin (see Fig. 94-2). Stress ulcer prophylaxis with proton pump inhibitors or H_2-receptor antagonists decreases the risk of gastrointestinal hemorrhage.

Adding vitamin C and thiamine does not add benefit to corticosteroids alone,[A28] and, as noted earlier, the three-drug combination may be no better than placebo. Enteral nutrition is generally safer and more effective than total parenteral nutrition (Chapter 198), but total parenteral nutrition is sometimes required in patients with abdominal sepsis, surgery, or trauma. Initial trophic feeding, which provides about 25% of normal calorie requirements, is comparable to full enteral feeding after stabilization of patients in septic shock. The use of sedation, neuromuscular blocking agents, and corticosteroids should be minimized because they can exacerbate septic encephalopathy and the polyneuropathy or myopathy of sepsis. Neutropenic patients may benefit from granulocyte colony-stimulating factor (Chapter 153). The risk of nosocomial infection is decreased by narrow-spectrum antibiotics, early weaning from ventilation, and periodic removal and replacement of catheters (Chapter 261).

TABLE 94-2 POTENTIAL ANTIBIOTIC REGIMENS FOR PATIENTS WITH SEPTIC SHOCK*

SOURCE OF SEPSIS	INITIAL ANTIBIOTIC REGIMEN	ALTERNATIVE ANTIBIOTIC REGIMEN
Community-acquired pneumonia	Third-generation cephalosporin (e.g., cefotaxime 2 g IV q6h; ceftriaxone 2 g IV q12h; ceftizoxime 2 g IV q8h) *plus* fluoroquinolone (e.g., ciprofloxacin 400 mg IV q12h, levofloxacin 750 mg IV q24h, moxifloxacin 400 mg IV q24h) *or* macrolide (azithromycin 500 mg IV q24h)	Piperacillin-tazobactam (3.375 g IV q6h) *plus* fluoroquinolone (e.g., ciprofloxacin 400 mg IV q12h, levofloxacin 750 mg IV q24h, moxifloxacin 400 mg IV q24h) *or* macrolide (azithromycin 500 mg IV q24h)
Hospital-acquired pneumonia	Vancomycin (15 mg/kg IV q 8-12h, if increased risk of MRSA) *or* linezolid (600 mg IV q12h, if increased risk of MRSA) *plus* carbapenem (e.g., imipenem 0.5 g IV q6h *or* meropenem 1 g IV q8h) *plus* fluoroquinolone (e.g., ciprofloxacin 400 mg IV q12h, levofloxacin 750 mg IV q24h)	Fluoroquinolone (e.g., ciprofloxacin 400 mg IV q12h, levofloxacin 750 mg IV q24h) *plus* vancomycin (1.5 g IV q12h) *plus* piperacillin-tazobactam (3.375 g IV q6h) *or* ceftazidime (2 g IV q8h) *or* aztreonam (2 g IV q8h)
Spontaneous bacterial peritonitis	Ceftriaxone (1 g IV q12h)	Moxifloxacin (400 mg IV q24h)
Gastrointestinal perforation	Piperacillin-tazobactam (3.375 g IV q6h) *or* carbapenem (e.g., imipenem 0.5 g IV q6h, meropenem 1 g IV q8h)	Cefepime (1 g IV q8h) *plus* metronidazole (500 mg IV q8h) *or* Metronidazole (500 mg IV q8h) *plus* fluoroquinolone (e.g., ciprofloxacin 400 mg IV q12h)
Urinary tract	Third-generation cephalosporin (e.g., cefotaxime 2 g IV q6h, ceftriaxone 2 g IV q12h, or ceftizoxime 2 g IV q8h)	Ampicillin (2 g IV q4h) *plus* gentamicin (1.5 mg/kg IV q8h) *or* ertapenem (1 g IV q24h, if ESBL)
Necrotizing fasciitis	Vancomycin (15 mg/kg IV q8-12h) *plus* piperacillin-tazobactam (3.375 g IV q6h) *plus* clindamycin (600 mg IV q8h)	Vancomycin (15 mg/kg IV q8-12h) *plus* ciprofloxacin (400 mg IV q12h) *plus* clindamycin (600 mg IV q8h)
Primary bacteremia (normal host)	Piperacillin-tazobactam (3.375 g IV q6h) *plus* vancomycin (1.5 g IV q12h)	Carbapenem (e.g., imipenem 0.5 g IV q6h, meropenem 1 g IV q8h) *plus* vancomycin (1.5 g IV q12h)
Primary bacteremia (intravenous drug user)	Vancomycin (1.5 g IV q12h) *plus* fluoroquinolone (e.g., ciprofloxacin 400 mg IV q12h)	Piperacillin-tazobactam (3.375 g IV q6h) *plus* vancomycin (1.5 g IV q12h)

TABLE 94-2 POTENTIAL ANTIBIOTIC REGIMENS FOR PATIENTS WITH SEPTIC SHOCK*—cont'd

SOURCE OF SEPSIS	INITIAL ANTIBIOTIC REGIMEN	ALTERNATIVE ANTIBIOTIC REGIMEN
Catheter-related bloodstream infection (CR-BSI)	Vancomycin (1.5 g IV q12h) +/− cefepime (2 g IV q8h)	Vancomycin (1.5 g IV q12h) +/− carbapenem (e.g., imipenem 0.5 g IV q6h, meropenem 1 g IV q8h)
If gram-positive cocci in clusters ≥2 blood cultures	Vancomycin (1.5 g IV q12h)	Piperacillin-tazobactam (3.375 g IV q6h) *or* ceftazidime (2 g IV q8h) *or* aztreonam (2 g IV q8h)
Febrile neutropenia	Cefepime (2 g IV q8h) *plus* vancomycin (1.5 g IV q12h)	Aztreonam (2 g IV q8h) *plus* gentamicin (1.5 mg/kg q8h) *or* Cefepime (2 g IV q8h) *plus* gentamicin (1.5 mg/kg q8h) *or* Piperacillin-tazobactam (3.375 g IV q6h) *plus* gentamicin (1.5 mg/kg q8h) *or* Carbapenem (e.g., imipenem 0.5 g IV q6h, meropenem 1 g IV q8h) *plus* gentamicin (1.5 mg/kg q8h) If beta-lactam allergy: Vancomycin (1.5 g IV q12h) *plus* gentamicin (1.5 mg/kg q8h) *plus* ciprofloxacin (400 mg IV q12h)
Bacterial meningitis	Ceftriaxone (2 g IV q12h) *plus* ampicillin (3 g IV q6h) *plus* vancomycin (1.5 g IV q12h) *plus* dexamethasone (0.15 mg/kg IV q6h for 2-4 days)	Gram-positive cocci: vancomycin (1.5 g IV q12h) *plus* ceftriaxone (2 g IV q12h) Gram-negative diplococci: cefotaxime (2 g IV q4-6h) *or* ceftriaxone (2 g IV q12h) Gram-positive bacilli: ampicillin (3 g IV q6h) *plus* gentamicin (1.5 mg/kg IV q8h) Gram-negative bacilli: ceftazidime (2 g IV q8h) *plus* gentamicin (1.5 mg/kg IV q8h) *or* cefepime (1 g IV q8h) All above *plus* dexamethasone (0.15 mg/kg IV q6h for 2-4 days)
Cellulitis†	Severe: Vancomycin (1.5 g IV q12h) *plus* piperacillin-tazobactam (3.375 g IV q6h)	Moderate: Cefazolin (1-2 g IV q8h) *or* ceftriaxone (2 g IV q12h) *or* clindamycin (600 mg IV q8h)

*Most antibiotic doses must be adjusted if there is hepatic or renal dysfunction. Some antibiotics require adjustment based on levels (e.g., gentamicin). In selecting a drug, carefully consider the patient's history of antibiotic (especially penicillin) allergy.

†Assess for necrotizing fasciitis and consider surgical consultation; raise extremity.

ESBL = gram-negative organisms including those that produce extended spectrum β-lactamases (ESBL); IV = intravenous; MRSA = methicillin-resistant *S. aureus*.

PREVENTION

Measures to prevent sepsis include caregiver handwashing before and after patient contact, elevation of the head of the bed to help prevent aspiration, sterile techniques for the insertion of catheters, and possibly the use of antibiotic-impregnated catheters. New catheter insertion sites for catheter changes, isolation of patients who have resistant organisms, and isolation of significantly immunocompromised patients may also prevent infection.

Preventing the progression from sepsis to septic shock requires early diagnosis and aggressive resuscitation.[16] Early intravenous antibiotics (within 1 hour),[17] fluid resuscitation, and lung-protective ventilation are critical therapies in early septic shock (Table 94-3). In patients with severe community-acquired pneumonia (Chapter 85), hydrocortisone (200 mg intravenously daily for 4 to 8 days) can reduce the need for vasopressors.[A29]

PROGNOSIS

The survival and quality of life after hospital discharge after septic shock remain poorer than expected for at least the next 10 years. For example, the 28-day mortality of septic shock is about 20% in academic centers, where early initiation of appropriate therapies, especially antibiotics, is routine.[18] Deaths in the first 72 hours are usually due to refractory septic shock despite increasing life support. Later deaths (after day 3) are usually due to multiple organ dysfunction, nosocomial infection, or both. The number of dysfunctional organs is a marker of poor prognosis, especially in patients who do not improve or have progressive organ dysfunction. Other markers of poor prognosis include delays in achieving adequate resuscitation and antibiotics, increased age, underlying chronic comorbidities, more severe critical illness, increased arterial lactate, and the need for high doses of vasopressors. Patients who have an episode of acute kidney injury during septic shock also have a significantly decreased long-term survival than patients without it.

The increasing numbers of septic shock survivors highlight the importance of long-term sequelae, such as depression, cognitive dysfunction, and post-traumatic stress disorder. Septic shock survivors have about a 35% risk of hospital readmission within 6 months, higher than that of patients who are discharged after an acute myocardial infarction, heart failure, or chronic obstructive pulmonary disease.

Quality of life is frequently impaired in survivors of septic shock. For example, survivors of septic shock accompanied by ARDS (Chapter 90) can have neuromuscular dysfunction (weakness) and dyspnea on exertion or other persistent organ dysfunction. Unfortunately, a trial of more intensive postdischarge therapy compared with usual care found no difference in mental health–related quality of life.[A30]

B. Breathing—Oxygen, with a tidal volume 6 mL/kg IBW if ventilated. Wean according to ARDSNet protocol (Chapters 90 and 91)

C. Circulation

- Fluids, vasopressors, inotropes, transfusion; goals include:
  - MAP >65 mm Hg
  - CVP 8-12 mm Hg
  - Hgb 7.0-9.0 g/L

Consider pulmonary artery catheter or echocardiogram especially if known cardiovascular disease; goals include:

- Wedge pressure 8-15 mm Hg
- Cardiac index: normal or increased

D. Drugs:

- Antibiotics: Narrow spectrum to cause of infection

Consider:

- Hydrocortisone (see text): hydrocortisone 50 mg intravenously every 6 hours daily for 7 days
- Vasopressin 0.01–0.03 units/minute intravenously

Other Organ Support

- Renal function: Continuous renal replacement
- DVT prophylaxis: (e.g., low molecular weight heparin [e.g., dalteparin 5000 IU subcutaneously daily])
- Stress ulcer prophylaxis: PPI (e.g., pantoprazole 40 to 80 mg intravenously once or twice daily) or H_2-receptor antagonist (e.g., ranitidine 50 mg intravenously every 8 hours)
- Nutrition: Enteral preferred
- Sedation: Intermittent with daily awakening

FIGURE 94-2. **Ongoing critical care support and management in septic shock.** ARDSNet = The US National Institute of Health Acute Respiratory Distress Syndrome; CVP = central venous pressure; DVT = deep venous thrombosis; Hgb = hemoglobin; IBW = ideal body weight; MAP = mean arterial pressure; NG = nasogastric; PPI = proton pump inhibitor; $Scvo_2$ = central venous oxygen saturation.

TABLE 94-3 HEMODYNAMIC VARIABLES, ABBREVIATIONS, AND NORMAL VALUES

Arterial pressure: systolic pressure (SAP) (>100 mm Hg), diastolic pressure, pulse pressure, mean arterial pressure (MAP) (>65 mm Hg)
Central venous pressure (CVP): normal, 6-12 mm Hg
Pulmonary artery pressure (PAP): normal, 25/15 mm Hg
Pulmonary vascular resistance (PVR): normal, 150-250 dynes*sec/cm^5

$$\left(=\frac{\text{PAP}-\text{PAOP}}{\text{CO}}\times 80\right)$$

Pulmonary artery occlusion pressure (PAOP) or pulmonary artery wedge pressure (PAWP): normal, 8-15 mm Hg
Systemic vascular resistance (SVR): normal, 900-1400 dynes*sec/cm^5

$$\left(=\frac{\text{PAP}-\text{CVP}}{\text{CO}}\times 80\right)$$

Cardiac output (CO): normal, 5 L/min
Left ventricular stroke work index (LVSWI): normal, (60-100 grams × meters/beats) = (SV × [MAP − PAWP] × 0.0136)
Oxygen delivery (Do_2): normal, 1 L/min (= CO × [Hb × 1.38 × Sao_2] + [0.003 × Po_2])
Oxygen consumption ($\dot{V}o_2$): normal, 250 mL/min (= CO × Hb × 1.38 × [Sao_2 − Svo_2] + [0.003 × (Pao_2 − Pvo_2)])
Oxygen extraction ratio: normal, 0.23-0.32 (= $\dot{V}o_2/Do_2$)
Hemodynamic variables are often normalized to account for different body mass by dividing by body surface area (BSA)
Pulmonary vascular resistance index (PVRI): normal (= PVR/BSA)
Systemic vascular resistance index (SVRI): normal (= SVR/BSA)
Cardiac index (CI): normal, 2.5-4.2 L/min/m^2 (= CO/BSA)
Left ventricular stroke work index (LVSWI): normal (= LVSW/BSA)
Oxygen delivery index (Do_2I): normal, 460-650 mL/min/m^2 (= Do_2/BSA)
Oxygen consumption index ($\dot{V}o_2I$): normal, 95-170 mL/min/m^2 (= $\dot{V}o_2$/BSA)
Hb = hemoglobin concentration in grams/liter: Normal value is 12 to 15 mg/dL in females and about 10% higher in males.

GENERAL REFERENCES

For the General References and other additional features, please visit Elsevier eBooks+ at https://ebooks.health.elsevier.com.

Grade A References

A1. Russell DW, Casey JD, Gibbs KW, et al. Effect of fluid bolus administration on cardiovascular collapse among critically ill patients undergoing tracheal intubation: a randomized clinical trial. *JAMA*. 2022;328:270-279.
A2. Hughes CG, Mailloux PT, Devlin JW, et al. Dexmedetomidine or propofol for sedation in mechanically ventilated patients with sepsis. *N Engl J Med*. 2021;384:1424-1436.
A3. Rowan KM, Angus DC, Bailey M, et al. Early, goal-directed therapy for septic shock—a patient-level meta-analysis. *N Engl J Med*. 2017;376:2223-2234.
A4. Lamontagne F, Day AG, Meade MO, et al. Pooled analysis of higher versus lower blood pressure targets for vasopressor therapy septic and vasodilatory shock. *Intensive Care Med*. 2018;44:12-21.
A5. Lamontagne F, Richards-Belle A, Thomas K, et al. Effect of reduced exposure to vasopressors on 90-day mortality in older critically ill patients with vasodilatory hypotension: a randomized clinical trial. *JAMA*. 2020;323:938-949.
A6. Shapiro NI, Douglas IS, Brower RG, et al. Early restrictive or liberal fluid management for sepsis-induced hypotension. *N Engl J Med*. 2023;388:499-510.
A7. Meyhoff TS, Hjortrup PB, Wetterslev J, et al. Restriction of intravenous fluid in ICU patients with septic shock. *N Engl J Med*. 2022;386:2459-2470.
A8. Semler MW, Self WH, Wanderer JP, et al. Balanced crystalloids versus saline in critically ill adults. *N Engl J Med*. 2018;378:829-839.
A9. Zampieri FG, Machado FR, Biondi RS, et al. Effect of intravenous fluid treatment with a balanced solution vs. 0.9% saline solution on mortality in critically ill patients. The BaSICS randomized clinical trial. *JAMA*. 2021;326:818-829.
A10. Lewis SR, Pritchard MW, Evans DJ, et al. Colloids versus crystalloids for fluid resuscitation in critically ill people. *Cochrane Database Syst Rev*. 2018;8:CD000567.
A11. Permpikul C, Tongyoo S, Viarasilpa T, et al. Early use of norepinephrine in septic shock resuscitation (CENSER). A randomized trial. *Am J Respir Crit Care Med*. 2019;199:1097-1105.
A12. Nagendran M, Russel JA, Walley KR, et al. Vasopressin in septic shock: an individual patient data meta-analysis of randomised controlled trials. *Intensive Care Med*. 2019;45:844-855.
A13. Laterre PF, Berry SM, Blemings A, et al. Effect of selepressin vs placebo on ventilator- and vasopressor-free days in patients with septic shock: the SEPSIS-ACT randomized clinical trial. *JAMA*. 2019;322:1476-1485.
A14. Lee YR, Seth MS, Soney D, et al. Benefits of beta-blockade in sepsis and septic shock: a systematic review. *Clin Drug Investig*. 2019;39:429-440.
A15. Hirano Y, Miyoshi Y, Kondo Y, et al. Liberal versus restrictive red blood cell transfusion strategy in sepsis or septic shock: a systematic review and meta-analysis of randomized trials. *Crit Care*. 2019;23:262.
A16. Cooper DJ, McQuilten ZK, Nichol A, et al. Age of red cells for transfusion and outcomes in critically ill adults. *N Engl J Med*. 2017;377:1858-1867.
A17. Vardakas KZ, Voulgaris GL, Maliaros A, et al. Prolonged versus short-term intravenous infusion of antipseudomonal beta-lactams for patients with sepsis: a systematic review and meta-analysis of randomised trials. *Lancet Infect Dis*. 2018;18:108-120.
A18. Sjövall F, Perner A, Møller MH. Empirical mono- versus combination antibiotic therapy in adult intensive care patients with severe sepsis—a systematic review with meta-analysis and trial sequential analysis. *J Infect*. 2017;74:331-344.
A19. Kynazopoulou E, Liaskou-Antoniou L, Adamis G, et al. Procalcitonin to reduce long-term infection-associated adverse events in sepsis. A randomized trial. *Am J Respir Crit Care Med*. 2021;203:202-210.
A20. Meier MA, Branche A, Neeser OL, et al. Procalcitonin-guided antibiotic treatment in patients with positive blood cultures: a patient-level meta-analysis of randomized trials. *Clin Infect Dis*. 2019;69:388-396.
A21. Annane D, Renault A, Brun-Buisson C, et al. Hydrocortisone plus fludrocortisone for adults with septic shock. *N Engl J Med*. 2018;378:809-818.
A22. Venkatesh B, Finfer S, Cohen J, et al. Adjunctive glucocorticoid therapy in patients with septic shock. *N Engl J Med*. 2018;378:797-808.
A23. Moskowitz A, Huang DT, Hou PC, et al. Effect of ascorbic acid, corticosteroids, and thiamine on organ injury in septic shock: the ACTS randomized clinical trial. *JAMA*. 2020;324:642-650.
A24. Sevransky JE, Rothman RE, Hager DN, et al. Effect of vitamin C, thiamine, and hydrocortisone on ventilator- and vasopressor-free days in patients with sepsis: the VICTAS randomized clincial trial. *JAMA*. 2021;325:742-750.
A25. WHO Rapid Evidence Appraisal for COVID-19 Therapies (REACT) Working Group. Association between administration of systemic corticosteroids and mortality among critically ill patients with COVID-19: a meta-analysis. *JAMA*. 2020;324:1330-1341.
A26. Zarbock A, Kullmar M, Kindgen-Milles D, et al. Effect of regional citrate anticoagulation vs. systemic heparin anticoagulation during continuous kidney replacement therapy on dialysis filter life span and mortality among critically ill patients with acute kidney injury. A randomized clinical trial. *JAMA*. 2020;324:1629-1639.
A27. The STARRT-AKI Investigators. Timing of initiation of renal-replacement therapy in acute kidney injury. *N Engl J Med*. 2020;383:240-251.
A28. Fujii T, Luethi N, Young PJ, et al. Effect of vitamin C, hydrocortisone, and thiamine vs hydrocortisone alone on time alive and free of vasopressor support among patients with septic shock: the VITAMINS randomized clinical trial. *JAMA*. 2020;323:423-431.
A29. Dequin PF, Meziani F, Quenot JP, et al. Hydrocortisone in severe community-acquired pneumonia. *N Engl J Med*. 2023. [Epub ahead of print.]
A30. Schmidt K, Schwarzkopf D, Baldwin LM, et al. Long-term courses of sepsis survivors: effects of a primary care management intervention. *Am J Med*. 2020;133:381-385. e5.

95

DISORDERS DUE TO HEAT AND COLD

MICHAEL N. SAWKA AND FRANCIS G. O'CONNOR

TEMPERATURE REGULATION

Body temperature is regulated through two parallel processes that modify body heat balance: behavioral (clothing, shelter, physical activity) and physiologic (skin blood flow, sweating, shivering). Both peripheral (skin) and central (core) thermal receptors provide afferent input to a central nervous system integrator (hypothalamic thermoregulatory center), and any deviation between the controlled variable (body temperature) and a theoretical reference variable ("set point" temperature) results in a heat loss or conservation response.

Humans normally regulate body (core) temperature at about 37° C (98.6° F), and fluctuations within the narrow range of 35° to 41° C (95° to 105.8° F) can be tolerated by healthy acclimatized persons; core temperatures outside this range can induce morbidity and mortality. By one estimate, about 8% of worldwide mortality can be attributed to high or low ambient environmental temperatures, with cold-attributable mortality exceeding heat-attributable mortality by a wide margin worldwide.[1]

There is no single core temperature because it varies at different deep body sites, during rest and physical exercise, and with different measurement techniques.[2] Arterial blood temperature, which provides the best invasive measurement of core temperature, is slightly lower than brain temperature. The most accurate noninvasive index of core temperature is esophageal temperature, followed in order of preference by rectal, gastrointestinal tract (telemetry pill), and oral temperature. Ear (tympanic and auditory meatus) or scanned temporal artery temperature should not be relied on for clinical judgment. Rectal temperatures are most commonly recommended because they are easy to measure and are not biased by environmental conditions.

HEAT ILLNESS

DEFINITION

Minor heat-related illnesses include miliaria rubra, heat syncope, and heat cramps. Serious heat illness represents a spectrum from heat exhaustion to heat injury and heatstroke.

EPIDEMIOLOGY

Heat illness, which is increasing because of global warming, accounts for considerable morbidity and mortality in the world today.[3] Serious heat illness is associated with a variety of individual factors, health conditions, drugs, and environmental factors (Table 95-1). Exertional heat illness is among the leading causes of death in young athletes, and its incidence appears to be increasing in the United States, particularly in vulnerable (e.g., homeless) populations.[4] Classic heat illness caused by high environmental temperatures remains a problem, especially in homebound elderly persons without air conditioning.[5] Anticholinergic and sympathomimetic poisoning (Chapter 96) can induce hyperthermia. Malignant hyperthermia (Chapter 400) is a rare disorder occurring in genetically predisposed individuals. Rapid and massive skeletal muscle contraction from exposure to certain volatile anesthetic agents (most commonly halothane, sevoflurane, desflurane, isoflurane, or enflurane) or depolarizing muscle agent relaxants (e.g., succinylcholine) can trigger core temperature elevations well above 43° C (110° F). However, some speculate that heat disorders with extreme exercise may represent a similar syndrome. Neuroleptic malignant syndrome (Chapter 402) is an idiosyncratic hyperthermic reaction caused by skeletal muscle rigidity from treatment with neuroleptic medications (e.g., antipsychotics, antidepressants, antiemetics, and L-dopa. Both malignant hyperthermia and neuroleptic malignant syndrome are potentially fatal without prompt recognition and early intervention.

Heat illness can also occur in low-risk individuals who have taken appropriate precautions relative to situations to which they have been exposed in the past. Historically, such unexpected cases were attributed to dehydration (which impairs thermoregulation and increases hyperthermia and cardiovascular strain), but it is now suspected that a previous heat exposure or a concurrent event (e.g., sickness or injury) might make these individuals more susceptible to serious heat illness. One theory is that previous heat injury or illness primes the acute phase response and augments the hyperthermia of exercise, inducing unexpected serious heat illness. Another theory is that previous infection produces proinflammatory cytokines that deactivate the cells' ability to protect against heat shock.

TABLE 95-1 FACTORS PREDISPOSING TO SERIOUS HEAT ILLNESS

INDIVIDUAL FACTORS
Lack of acclimatization
Low physical fitness
Excessive body weight
Dehydration
Advanced age
Young age
Toll-like receptor-4 polymorphisms
HEALTH CONDITIONS
Inflammation and fever
Viral or bacterial infection
Cardiovascular disease
Diabetes mellitus
Gastroenteritis
Rash, sunburn, and previous burns to large areas of skin
Seizures
Thyroid storm
Neuroleptic malignant syndrome
Malignant hyperthermia
Sickle cell trait
Cystic fibrosis
DRUGS
Anticholinergic properties (atropine)
Antiepileptic (topiramate)
Antihistamines
Anti-Parkinsonian medications
Glutethimide
Phenothiazines
Tricyclic antidepressants
Amphetamines, cocaine, ecstasy [3,4-methylenedioxy-methamphetamine (MDMA)]
Ergogenic stimulants (e.g., ephedrine, ephedra)
Lithium
Diuretics
β-Blockers
Ethanol
Nonsteroidal anti-inflammatory drugs
ENVIRONMENTAL FACTORS
High temperature
High humidity
Little air motion
Lack of shade
Heat wave
Physical exercise
Heavy clothing
Prior compromised heat exposures

PATHOBIOLOGY

Body temperature can increase from a number of mechanisms: exposure to environmental heat (impeded heat dissipation), physical exercise (increased heat production), fever from systemic illness (elevated set point with subsequent activation of shivering), and medications (neuroleptic malignant syndrome and malignant hyperthermia). In addition, febrile persons have accentuated elevations in core temperature when they are exposed to high ambient temperature, physical exercise, or both. Environmental temperature and humidity, medications, and exercise heat stress in turn challenge the cardiovascular system to provide high blood flow to the skin, where blood pools in warm, compliant vessels such as those found in the extremities. When blood flow is diverted to the skin, reduced perfusion of the intestines and other viscera can result in ischemia, endotoxemia, and oxidative stress. Several common mutations in toll-like receptor 4 are associated with endotoxin hypo-responsiveness. In addition, excessively high tissue temperatures (heat shock: >41° C [105.8° F]) can produce direct tissue injury; the magnitude and duration of the heat shock influence whether cells respond by adaptation (acquired thermal tolerance), injury, or death (apoptotic or necrotic). Heat shock, ischemia, and systemic inflammatory responses can result in cellular dysfunction, disseminated intravascular coagulation, and multiorgan dysfunction syndrome (E-Fig. 95-1). Furthermore, reduced cerebral blood flow, combined with abnormal local metabolism and coagulopathy, can lead to dysfunction of the central nervous system.

CLINICAL MANIFESTATIONS AND DIAGNOSIS

Minor heat illness is common and can be recognized by its clinical features. Miliaria rubra (heat rash) results from the occlusion of eccrine sweat gland ducts and can be complicated by secondary staphylococcal infection. Heat syncope (fainting) is caused by temporary circulatory insufficiency as a result of blood pooling in the peripheral veins, especially the cutaneous and lower extremity veins. Skeletal muscle cramps most commonly occur during and after intense exercise and are probably related to dehydration, loss of sodium or potassium, and neurogenic fatigue rather than to overheating itself.

Serious heat illness includes heat exhaustion, heat injury, and heatstroke, with some individuals progressing along this spectrum. Patients who exhibit symptoms (e.g., dizziness, unsteady gait, ataxia, headache, confusion, weakness, fatigue, nausea, vomiting, diarrhea) should have an immediate assessment of their mental status, core (rectal) temperature, and other vital signs. The most common heat-related causes of hospital admission are fluid and electrolyte disorders (Chapters 102 and 103), acute kidney injury (Chapter 106), urinary tract infection (Chapter 263), and heatstroke. Until proven otherwise, heatstroke should be the initial working diagnosis in anyone who is a heat casualty and has an altered mental status.

Heat exhaustion is defined as a syndrome of hyperthermia (temperature at time of event usually ≤40° C or 104° F) and debilitation that occurs during or immediately after exertion in the heat, accompanied by no more than minor central nervous system dysfunction (headache, dizziness, mild confusion), which resolves rapidly with intervention. It is primarily a cardiovascular event (insufficient cardiac output) frequently accompanied by sweaty hot skin, dehydration, and collapse.

Heat injury is a moderate to severe illness characterized by evidence of damage to end organs (e.g., liver, renal, gut) and tissues (e.g., rhabdomyolysis) without sufficient neurologic symptoms to be diagnosed as heatstroke. It is usually associated with body temperatures above 40° C (104° F).

Heatstroke is a severe illness characterized by profound mental status changes with high body temperatures usually, but not always, higher than 40.5° C (104.9° F).[6] However, patients with a core temperature higher than 40.5° C do not universally have a heat injury or heatstroke, and core temperatures this high can be seen transiently after stressful exercise in the heat. To establish the diagnosis of heatstroke, the entire clinical picture, including mental status and laboratory results, must be considered. Heatstroke is often categorized as classic or exertional; classic heatstroke is observed primarily in otherwise sick and compromised individuals, and exertional heatstroke is observed during or after vigorous exercise (Table 95-2).

Severe heatstroke evolves clinically through three distinct phases, more commonly seen in exertional heatstroke than in classic heatstroke: a hyperthermic-neurologic acute phase, a hematologic-enzymatic phase, and a late renal-hepatic phase. In the hyperthermic-neurologic acute phase, the marked elevation in tissue and organ temperatures is associated with gastrointestinal and central nervous system dysfunction. In the hematologic-enzymatic phase, manifestations range from mild activation of coagulation and fibrinolysis to severe disseminated intravascular coagulation with elevated aminotransferase and creatine kinase levels. The late renal-hepatic phase is characterized by diffuse end-organ failure. In fulminant heatstroke, patients have the full spectrum of abnormalities associated with the systemic inflammatory response syndrome (Chapter 94).

TREATMENT AND PREVENTION

Heat illness can be prevented by heat acclimatization and acquired thermal tolerance, maintenance of adequate hydration, and avoidance of overwhelming heat exposure.[7] Adequate fluid intake is critical, and oral rehydration solutions should contain sodium and other electrolytes to restore both intracellular and extracellular fluid.

Management of serious heat illness, which should begin in the field setting, includes cooling, rehydration, and monitoring (Table 95-3).[8] The first priority should be immediately to initiate whole-body cooling and to continue cooling until the core temperature falls below 38.8° C (102° F). Body cooling lowers skin temperatures, thereby facilitating conduction and convection from the core to the shell, and reduces cardiovascular stress by causing arterial and venous constriction that redirects blood back to the heart. Immersion or soaking of the skin in cool or ice water with skin massage is the most effective method,[9] but other effective methods include soaking of the skin followed by accelerated evaporation with fans or the use of ice sheets and ice packs. These noninvasive treatments can be supplemented with the infusion of chilled (≈4° C) normal saline. Cooling can induce shivering, which is usually not sufficient to increase body temperature, so shivering need not be treated.

Hospital care of exertional heat stroke, while largely supportive, can rapidly escalate to the complex management of fulminant multiorgan failure.[10] The highest priority for patient care remains urgent cooling, including cold intravascular fluid. Cooling is usually discontinued at a core temperature of 38° to 39° C to avoid overcooling, but this practice is not based on data from controlled trials.[11]

Patients who are unconscious are at risk of poor airway control and may require endotracheal intubation to prevent aspiration. Fluid and electrolyte deficits should be corrected; restoration of plasma volume with isotonic fluids (e.g., normal saline) sufficient to sustain adequate perfusion, as judged by carefully monitored urine output, is also a priority. Rapid overcorrection of serum electrolytes (e.g., sodium) should be avoided. If rhabdomyolysis (Chapter 99) and myoglobinuria are present, maintaining urine flow helps minimize renal injury.

TABLE 95-2 COMPARISON OF CLASSIC AND EXERTIONAL HEATSTROKE

PATIENT CHARACTERISTICS	CLASSIC	EXERTIONAL
Age	Young children or elderly	15-55 years
Health	Chronic illness	Usually healthy
Fever	Unusual	Common
Prevailing weather	Frequent in heat waves	Variable
Activity	Sedentary	Strenuous exercise
Drug use	Diuretics, antidepressants, anticholinergics, phenothiazines	Ergogenic stimulants or cocaine
Sweating	Often absent	Common
Acid-base disturbances	Respiratory alkalosis	Lactic acidosis
Acute renal failure	Uncommon	Common (≈15%)
Rhabdomyolysis	Uncommon	Common (≈25%)
CK	Mildly elevated	Markedly elevated (500-1000 U/L)
ALT, AST	Mildly elevated	Markedly elevated
Hyperkalemia	Uncommon	Common
Hypocalcemia	Uncommon	Common
DIC	Mild	Marked
Hypoglycemia	Uncommon	Common

ALT = alanine aminotransferase; AST = aspartate aminotransferase; CK = creatine kinase; DIC = disseminated intravascular coagulation.

TABLE 95-3 MANAGEMENT OF HEAT ILLNESS

HEAT EXHAUSTION

- Rest and shade
- Loosen and remove clothing
- Supine position and elevate legs
- Actively cool skin
- Fluids by mouth
- Monitor core temperature
- Monitor mental status

HYPERTHERMIA

- Protect the airway
- Insert at least two large-bore intravenous lines
- Monitor core temperature; options include rectal, pulmonary artery, esophageal probe
- Actively cool the skin until core temperature reaches <39° C (<102.2° F)
- Ice baths or cool water (≈22° C [71.6° F]) immersion
- Wetting with water (avoid alcohol rubs)
- Continuous fanning
- Exposure to cool environment
- Axillary or perineal ice packs and ice sheets
- Infusion of room-temperature saline
- Gastric or colonic iced saline lavage
- Peritoneal lavage with iced normal saline
- Monitor electrocardiogram for arrhythmia
- Obtain serial diagnostic studies*

*Electrocardiogram, chest radiograph, complete blood count with differential, platelet count, urinalysis, aminotransferases, alkaline phosphatase, bilirubin, creatine kinase, blood urea nitrogen, creatinine, phosphate, calcium, glucose, electrolytes, uric acid, prothrombin time and partial thromboplastin time, D-dimer, fibrinogen, arterial blood gases, toxicology screen.

The hematologic-enzymatic and renal-hepatic phases should be anticipated, because they may require appropriate subspecialty care. Patients should be carefully monitored to detect possible metabolic abnormalities (e.g., hyperkalemia; Chapter 103), renal or hepatic failure (Chapters 116 and 140), disseminated intravascular coagulation (Chapter 161), cardiac arrhythmias (Chapters 51 to 53), and acute respiratory failure (Chapter 90). Management of these complications is largely supportive, with specific therapies as indicated for any critically ill patient. Medications to be avoided include antipyretics and sedatives with hepatic toxicities. Lorazepam (1 to 2 mg administered intravenously during a 2- to 5-minute period, repeated if necessary), which is a safe sedative because of its low hepatotoxicity and rapid metabolism, may be indicated in patients who are combative or exhibit seizure activity.

For exercise-induced and environmental heat illness, no pharmacologic interventions have been proved to augment cooling. For patients with malignant hyperthermia, however, dantrolene should be administered as a loading bolus of 2.5 mg/kg intravenously, with subsequent bolus doses of 1 to 2.5 mg/kg every 5 minutes intravenously as needed (up to a maximum total loading dose of 10 mg/kg) until the signs have abated.

PROGNOSIS

A single episode of heat exhaustion does not imply a predisposition to heat illness, and most patients recover within several hours after cooling and rehydration. For patients who present to a hospital with heatstroke, however, mortality rates can range from 26 to 63%. Mortality in both classic and exertional heatstroke correlates directly with the magnitude and duration of temperature elevation, the delay in time to initiation of cooling, and the number of organ systems affected. The likelihood of survival to discharge can be estimated based on prehospital severity as determined by a respiratory rate 22/minute or higher, a Glasgow coma score (Table 368-1) below 15, a systolic blood pressure below 100 mm Hg, a heart rate above 100/minute, a body temperature of 38° C or higher, and age 65 years or above.[12] Although most patients who survive a heatstroke event will have a full recovery, some can sustain permanent organ damage.[13] Neurologic injury with cerebellar dysfunction is the most common clinical picture. Patients who have recovered from heatstroke with organ damage have a higher long-term mortality from cardiovascular, liver, and digestive diseases.

Patients who have suffered heat injury or heatstroke should not be re-exposed to heat until recovery is complete, which can be many weeks or months, and about 10% of heatstroke patients remain intolerant of heat. Return to physical activity should be a gradual process of increased physical activity without heat exposure and then combined with heat exposure.[14]

COLD INJURY

DEFINITION

Cold injuries are classified as hypothermia and peripheral cold injuries. Hypothermia is whole-body cooling, whereas peripheral cold injuries are localized to the extremities and exposed skin. Hypothermia is further divided into three categories: mild (≈33° C to ≈35° C), moderate (≈27° C to ≈32° C), and profound (<27° C). Peripheral cold injuries can be divided into nonfreezing (chilblain, trench foot) and freezing (frostbite). Both hypothermia and peripheral cold injuries often occur simultaneously, and treatment priority should be given to rewarming in moderate and profound hypothermia.

EPIDEMIOLOGY

Accidental hypothermia can occur in most climates, but exposure to cold, wet conditions pose the greatest risk.[15] A variety of individual factors, health conditions, medications, and environmental factors are associated with a predisposition to cold injury (Table 95-4). Homeless persons are at increased risk owing to climatic exposure, which is often exacerbated by the concomitant use of alcohol and other intoxicating substances. In trauma patients (Chapter 97), hypothermia is associated with increased morbidity and mortality. Unwarmed anesthetized patients (Chapter 400) typically become 1° to 2° C hypothermic because of an internal redistribution of body heat from the core to the periphery, so warming should be considered to maintain normothermia

TABLE 95-4 FACTORS PREDISPOSING TO COLD INJURY

INDIVIDUAL FACTORS
Inadequate clothing and shelter
Lean and low body fat
Low physical fitness
Prior exhaustive physical exercise
Advanced age
Young age
Black race (men and women)
HEALTH CONDITIONS
Burns
Diabetes mellitus
Hypoglycemia
Neurologic lesions
Dementia
Hypoadrenalism, hypopituitarism, hypothyroidism
Prior frostbite or trench foot
Raynaud phenomenon
Sickle cell trait
Trauma
Spinal cord injury
DRUGS
Alcohol
Anesthetics
Antidepressants
Antipsychotics
Antithyroid agents
Sedatives and narcotics
ENVIRONMENTAL FACTORS
Cold temperatures
High air motion
Rain and immersion
Skin contact with metal and fuels
Repeated cold exposure
Physical fatigue
Immobility
High-altitude and low-oxygen-tension environments

PATHOBIOLOGY

Cold exposure elicits peripheral vasoconstriction to reduce heat transfer between the body's core and shell (skin, subcutaneous fat). If sufficiently cold, the underlying tissues (e.g., muscle) constrict to thicken the isolative shell while reducing the body's core area. This vasoconstrictor response defends core temperature but at the expense of declining peripheral tissue temperatures, which contribute to peripheral cold injuries. Hypothermia depresses enzymatic activity, interferes with physiologic functions (e.g., clotting, respiration, cardiac conduction and rhythm), impairs the expression of cytokines, and can induce cellular injury and death.

The pathophysiologic mechanism of frostbite includes four overlapping pathologic phases: prefreeze, freeze-thaw, vascular stasis, and late ischemic. The prefreeze phase consists of tissue cooling with accompanying vasoconstriction and ischemia but does not involve actual ice crystal formation. In the freeze-thaw phase, intracellular ice crystals form, thereby causing protein and lipid derangement, cellular electrolyte shifts, cellular dehydration, cell membrane lysis, and subsequent cell death. In the vascular stasis phase, vessels may fluctuate between constriction and dilation; blood may leak from vessels or coagulate within them. The late ischemic phase results from progressive tissue ischemia and infarction due to a cascade of inflammatory cytokines and prostaglandins, intermittent vasoconstriction with continued thrombus formation, and secondary reperfusion injury.

CLINICAL MANIFESTATIONS AND DIAGNOSIS

Hypothermia is a core temperature below 35° C (95° F), and clinical manifestations are related to the core temperature achieved (Table 95-5). The classic J wave on the electrocardiogram (Fig. 95-1) appears at a core temperature below about 33.8° C (93° F).

Chilblain (Chapter 66) appears as localized inflammatory lesions of the skin, most often involving the dorsal surface of fingers but also involving the ears, face, and exposed shins. Trench foot is caused by prolonged cold, wet exposure (e.g., wet socks or gloves), which can cause skin breakdown and nerve damage. Trench foot is often accompanied by infection and increased sensitivity to pain.

Frostbite (Chapter 66),[16] which is actual freezing of tissues, has traditionally been categorized as first degree (superficial, "frostnip"), second degree (full skin) with superficial skin vesiculation, third degree (subcutaneous tissue) with hemorrhagic blisters, and fourth degree (extensive tissue and bone). For patients with frostbite, early surgical consultation is advised.

TABLE 95-5 HYPOTHERMIA: STAGES AND ASSOCIATED CLINICAL MANIFESTATIONS

STAGE	CORE TEMPERATURE °F	CORE TEMPERATURE °C	CLINICAL MANIFESTATIONS
Normothermia	98.6	37.0	
Mild hypothermia	95.0	35.0	Cold diuresis, maximal shivering
	93.0	33.8	Ataxia, poor judgment, ECG J wave
	91.0	32.7	Amnesia, blood pressure difficult to measure
Moderate hypothermia	89.0	31.6	Stupor, pupils dilated
	87.0	30.5	Shivering ceases
	85.0	30.0	Cardiac arrhythmias, insulin inactive
	82.0	27.8	Unconsciousness, ventricular fibrillation likely
	80.0	26.6	No muscle reflexes
Profound hypothermia	78.0	25.5	Acid-base disturbances, no response to pain
	75.0	23.8	Pulmonary edema, hypotension
	73.0	22.7	No corneal reflexes
	66.0	18.8	Heart standstill
	62.0	16.6	Isoelectric electrocardiogram
	57.6	14.2	Lowest infant survival from accidental hypothermia
	48.2	9.0	Lowest adult survival from accidental hypothermia

ECG = electrocardiogram.

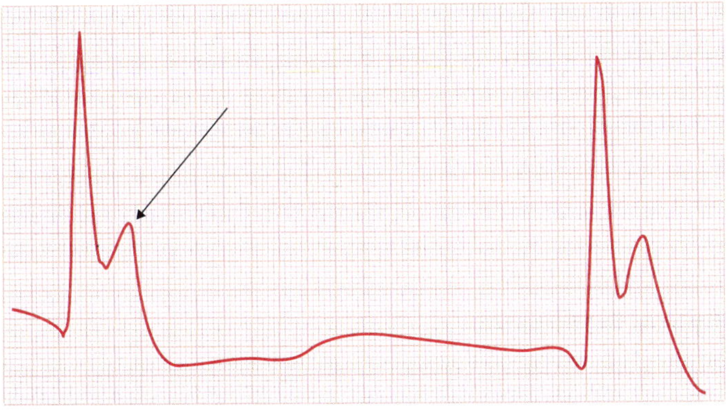

FIGURE 95-1. J (Osborne) wave.

PREVENTION AND TREATMENT

Humans demonstrate minimal cold acclimatization, so prevention depends primarily on avoiding cold exposure and having adequate protection and caloric intake to support metabolism.[17,18] Management of hypothermia depends on the core temperature (Table 95-6). Patients' wet clothing should be removed, and they should be provided with dry insulation. Shivering is an effective physiologic rewarming mechanism and should not be pharmacologically suppressed.

Moderately and profoundly hypothermic patients require active rewarming. Rewarming of the hypothermic patient includes both passive (insulation of the patient to prevent further heat loss) and active core (e.g., warmed saline and warmed humidified oxygen) and external (e.g., warmed water bottles, electric blankets) techniques. Rewarming at a rate of 0.5° to 1.0° C (0.9° to 1.8° F) per hour is acceptable in most cases, except that aggressive rewarming is warranted in patients with significant trauma (because coagulation is hindered by hypothermia) or cardiac arrest.

Complications commonly associated with rewarming of the hypothermic individual include both afterdrop (reduction of core temperature by cold blood returning to the circulation from the periphery) and aftershock (hypotension caused by peripheral vasodilation). Another potential complication of rewarming is ventricular fibrillation, which is more difficult to treat in the presence of moderate or profound hypothermia. If ventricular tachycardia or ventricular fibrillation develops, defibrillation should be attempted (Chapter 50). If ventricular tachycardia or ventricular fibrillation persists after a single shock, additional defibrillation attempts should be made, concurrent with rewarming but without waiting for the patient to warm to a particular target body temperature. Standard resuscitation approaches generally should be followed (Chapter 50). Extracorporeal life support is an option for refractory hypothermia-induced cardiac arrest.[19]

Body cooling induces cold diuresis, so plasma volume must be reestablished to support adequate perfusion. Patients should receive an intravenous infusion of 250 to 1000 mL of heated (40° to 42° C [104° to 108° F]) 5% dextrose in normal saline. Lactated Ringer solution should be avoided because the liver cannot metabolize lactate efficiently during hypothermia. Patients should be monitored for disturbances in potassium and glucose. If hypoglycemia, alcohol, or opiate intoxication is contributing to hypothermia, intravenous glucose (50 to 100 mL of 50% dextrose), thiamine (100 mg), or naloxone (0.4 to 2 mg intramuscularly or intravenously), respectively, may be indicated.

The treatment of frostbite is detailed in Chapter 66.

TABLE 95-6 TREATMENT OF HYPOTHERMIA

STAGE	MANAGEMENT	BODY REWARMING
Mild hypothermia	Monitor vital signs Warm intravenous saline Oxygen Monitor electrocardiogram for arrhythmia	Insulate Shivering Warm bath Active warming blanket
Moderate hypothermia	Diagnostic studies* Intensive care Anticipate infection and multiorgan dysfunction	Prevent extra heat loss by supplementing with airway rewarming Colonic irrigation Peritoneal dialysis
Profound hypothermia	Diagnostic studies*	Central rewarming

*See Table 95-3. Also lactate dehydrogenase, serum lactate, cortisol, thyroid-stimulating hormone, T3, and T4.

PROGNOSIS

Although noninvasive imaging with technetium pyrophosphate or magnetic resonance imaging can often predict the likelihood of tissue viability, it may take weeks to determine the precise demarcation of tissue that will require amputation. As morbidity may result from premature or unnecessary surgical intervention, consultation with a surgeon with experience evaluating and treating frostbite should be obtained to assess the need for and the timing of any amputations.

HYPOTHERMIC SYNDROMES

Exercise-induced bronchospasm (Chapter 75) can be triggered by exercise in cold air, particularly in patients with asthma. Livedo reticularis is patchy mottling of the limbs with cold exposure. Cryoglobulinemia (Chapter 173) occurs when immunoglobulins (IgM, IgG) reversibly precipitate after being cooled and contribute to impaired capillary blood flow in hypothermic tissues. Cold urticaria (Chapters 232 and 407) is the development of localized and general erythema and wheals in skin exposed to cold. Paroxysmal hypothermia is periodic lowering of the thermoregulatory set point and is often associated with hypothalamic abnormalities. Raynaud phenomenon (see Fig. 66-9 in Chapter 66) is intense vasoconstriction with sensitivity to pain in limbs exposed to cold.

TRAUMA HYPOTHERMIA

In trauma patients (Chapter 97), unintended hypothermia (<34° C [93° F]) is associated with increased morbidity and mortality due to impaired coagulation, peripheral vasoconstriction, respiratory depression, and increased risk for cardiac arrhythmias. Shivering aggravates perfusion problems by requiring blood flow to support increased metabolism in contracting muscles. Trauma patients become hypothermic because of heat loss from exposed cavities, environmental exposure, infusion of cool fluids, and ischemia, which depletes cell energy stores. Body temperature should be measured, and appropriate actions, as noted earlier, should be taken to restore normothermia during the early treatment of trauma patients.

THERAPEUTIC HYPOTHERMIA AND HYPERTHERMIA

THERAPEUTIC HYPOTHERMIA

For adults after an out-of-hospital cardiac arrest (Chapter 50), therapeutic cooling (a goal of 36° C for 24 to 48 hours) to prevent the usual hyperthermia can improve survival and neurologic outcomes[A1,A2] but is no better than therapeutic normothermia (<37.8° C).[A3] However, in-hospital hypothermia does not improve outcomes for patients after brain trauma, patients with intracranial hypertension,[A4] patients after an in-hospital arrest, patients who have undergone decompressive hemicraniectomy for malignant middle cerebral artery stroke,[A5] or patients with convulsive status epilepticus (Chapter 372).[A6]

THERAPEUTIC HYPERTHERMIA

Hyperthermia treatment (whole body or regional) is an experimental technique used as an adjunct to chemotherapy or radiation therapy in patients with advanced cancer. Hyperthermia (40° to 43° C [104° to 109° F]) alone can damage or kill cancer cells but, more important, hyperthermia might potentiate the effectiveness of chemotherapy and radiation by softening the tumor tissue, thus reducing its interstitial pressure.

Externally applied radiant heat, microwaves, or extracorporeal circulation usually induces local, regional, or whole-body hyperthermia. Target tissue temperatures are achieved and maintained based upon the specific cancer protocol, then followed by a passive cooling phase. Patients are usually sedated while core and skin temperatures are monitored. In regional hyperthermia, the part of the body where the tumor is located is heated while being perfused or bathed by a warmed solution containing anticancer drugs. The potential benefit of regional hyperthermia as an adjunct treatment of advanced prostate cancers is currently under investigation.

GENERAL REFERENCES

For the General References and other additional features, please visit Elsevier eBooks+ at https://ebooks.health.elsevier.com.

Grade A References

A1. Holgersson J, Meyer MAS, Dankiewicz J, et al. Hypothermic versus normothermic temperature control after cardiac arrest. *NEJM Evidence*. 2022;1.

A2. Lascarrou JB, Merdji H, Le Gouge A, et al. Targeted temperature management for cardiac arrest with nonshockable rhythm. *N Engl J Med*. 2019;381:2327-2337.

A3. Dankiewicz J, Cronberg T, Lilja G, et al. Hypothermia versus normothermia after out-of-hospital cardiac arrest. *N Engl J Med*. 2021;384:2283-2294.

A4. Cooper DJ, Nichol AD, Bailey M, et al. Effect of early sustained prophylactic hypothermia on neurologic outcomes among patients with severe traumatic brain injury: the POLAR randomized clinical trial. *JAMA*. 2018;320:2211-2220.

A5. Neugebauer H, Schneider H, Bösel J, et al. Outcomes of hypothermia in addition to decompressive hemicraniectomy in treatment of malignant middle cerebral artery stroke: a randomized clinical trial. *JAMA Neurol*. 2019;76:571-579.

A6. Legriel S, Lemiale V, Schenck M, et al. Hypothermia for neuroprotection in convulsive status epilepticus. *N Engl J Med*. 2016;375:2457-2467.

96 ACUTE POISONING

LEWIS S. NELSON AND DIANE P. CALELLO

EPIDEMIOLOGY

Each year, more than 4 million poisoning cases, suspected or verified, and 300,000 related hospital admissions occur in the United States. Poison centers provide support and collect data on more than 2 million of these exposures annually.[1] Poisoning-related deaths now total about 10,000 annually, and the number of opioid-related deaths has tripled since 2000. Poisonings are the leading cause of injury-related death in the United States, where approximately 90% of these deaths involve drugs, predominantly opioids (75%), such as heroin, fentanyl, and prescription analgesics.[2] Worldwide, however, pesticides, insecticides, caustics, and snakebites (Chapter 98) are also common causes. The incidence of recurrent, purposeful self-poisoning is 12 to 18%, with most events occurring within 3 months of the original attempt. To reduce fatalities and repeated attempts, an emphasis must be placed on measures to improve the safety of prescription drugs, including appropriate prescribing and aggressive treatment of poisoned patients with early psychiatric intervention for suicidal behavior (Chapter 362).

DIAGNOSIS

Despite the vast array of toxins to which a patient may be exposed, the clinical manifestations of poisoning are fairly limited. In most cases, it is less important to predict exactly which toxin is responsible for the acute poisoning than it is to create a differential diagnosis based on a careful history and physical examination as well as basic laboratory assays. The recognition of the specific toxic syndrome, or *toxidrome*, guides the clinician toward the likely diagnosis based on reasonably solid evidence. On this basis, treatment, including initial stabilization, critical care, decontamination, and even the empirical administration of antidotes, can be guided by an understanding of the pharmacology and physiology of the patient's toxidrome. More advanced care, such as methods to enhance the elimination of specific toxicants, commonly requires serial examinations, additional history, and subsequent laboratory testing. Even then, however, the clinical picture is often clouded by exposures to multiple toxicants and an ill-defined time course since the initial exposure.

History

Details elicited about toxic exposures should include the involved drugs and other toxicants, their estimated or known amounts, the time and routes of exposure, the patient's symptoms and signs, and any treatment already administered. Poisoning may result from acute, chronic, or acute-on-chronic exposure. A *toxicant* is defined as a chemical capable of harming a biologic organism; this definition encompasses toxins, which are derived from living organisms (such as plants, bacteria, and venoms), as well as synthetic substances, such as medications, drugs of abuse, and industrial and other chemicals.[3] Determination of chronicity is important because signs and symptoms of chronic exposure (Chapter 20) can differ from those of acute and acute-on-chronic exposure. For example, a history of acute multisystem organ failure narrows the toxicant possibilities to a few gases, chemicals, and drugs. A listing of available medications (e.g., those of the patient, spouse, relatives, or friends), nonprescription medications and herbals, dietary supplements, or ethnic remedies and occupational and avocational activities should be obtained. Occupational and avocational histories should include present and all past jobs and hobbies, with a focus on chemicals, metals, and gases. Known medical conditions may suggest classes of medications available to the patient. The patient's history, which may be incomplete or inaccurate if the patient is confused or suicidal, should be correlated with the clinical manifestations and course. Corroborative history from relatives and friends and findings from the scene as reported by the transporting emergency medical services personnel may be relevant.

Physical Examination

The physical examination should focus on vital signs; the eye, ear, nose, and throat examination; and the neurologic, cardiopulmonary, gastrointestinal, and dermatologic systems. Findings can suggest certain toxidromes, which are clusters of signs and symptoms typical of a specific class of poison. Among the dozens of toxidromes that assist in patient assessment and guide management, those due to adrenergic, anticholinergic, cholinomimetic, opioid, and sedative-hypnotic agents are most relevant to the emergency management of poisoned patients (Table 96-1). Patients may have some or all of these signs and symptoms; an incomplete clinical picture does not exclude a particular toxidrome, and it can still assist the clinician in identifying the correct category of toxicant involved.

Vital Signs

Tachycardia, which can occur with numerous toxicants, is most prominent in patients with anticholinergic and sympathomimetic toxidromes. However, because tachycardia also may occur with anxiety and other nontoxicologic conditions, it is not generally a helpful finding. The differential diagnosis for toxicant-induced *bradycardia* is more limited and includes β-adrenergic receptor antagonists, L-type calcium-channel antagonists (diltiazem or verapamil), cardioactive steroids, peripheral α-adrenergic receptor agonists (e.g., phenylephrine, whose effects are mediated by baroreceptor reflexes), central α_2-agonists such as clonidine, γ-hydroxybutyric acid, opioids, sedative-hypnotics, baclofen, organophosphorus and carbamate pesticides, muscarine-containing mushrooms (*Clitocybe*, *Inocybe* sp), plant- and animal-derived toxins (e.g., aconitine, andromedotoxin, ciguatoxin, and veratridine, all of which open sodium channels in the myocardium), therapeutic cholinesterase inhibitors (e.g., physostigmine), and some antiarrhythmic drugs (e.g., procainamide, flecainide, and other class IA, IC, and III drugs, such as amiodarone and sotalol). Bradycardia also is a preterminal sign for many highly lethal toxicants, such as cyclic antidepressants and cyanide.

TABLE 96-1 TOXIDROMES AND ASSOCIATED DRUGS AND TOXICANTS

	SYNDROME FEATURES		
TOXIDROME	**VITAL SIGNS**	**END ORGAN**	**REPRESENTATIVE DRUGS AND TOXICANTS**
Adrenergic	Hypertension, hyperthermia, tachycardia, tachypnea	Agitation, dysrhythmias, diaphoresis, mydriasis, seizures	Amphetamines, caffeine, cathinone derivatives, cocaine, ephedrine, pseudoephedrine, *Ephedra* sp, phenylephrine,* synthetic cannabinoids, theophylline
Anticholinergic	Hyperthermia, tachycardia, blood pressure generally normal	Agitation, delirium, decreased or absent bowel sounds, dry flushed skin and mucous membranes, mydriasis or blurred vision, seizures, urinary retention	First-generation H_1-receptor antagonists (e.g., diphenhydramine), belladonna alkaloids (e.g., scopolamine, atropine) from plants (e.g., *Datura* sp—deadly nightshade, henbane), benztropine, cyclic antidepressants, dicyclomine, muscle relaxants (e.g., orphenadrine, cyclobenzaprine), trihexyphenidyl
Cholinomimetic	Tachycardia or bradycardia†	Agitation, delirium, coma; bronchorrhea, bronchospasm; diaphoresis; fasciculations; lacrimation; miosis; urination; diarrhea, vomiting; seizures	Carbamate cholinesterase inhibitors (e.g., physostigmine, neostigmine), organophosphorus compounds including pesticides (e.g., diazinon, malathion) and nerve agents (e.g., soman, sarin, VX, novichok), *Inocybe* or *Clitocybe* mushroom spp
Opioid	Bradypnea or apnea, bradycardia, hypotension (late), hypothermia	CNS depression; hypotonia; miosis	Fentanyl, fentanyl analogs, heroin, hydrocodone, oxycodone, morphine, buprenorphine, central α_2-agonists (e.g., clonidine, guanfacine)
Sedative-hypnotic	Generally near normal with benzodiazepines, but bradypnea or apnea, mild hypotension, and mild hypothermia can occur	Ataxia, CNS depression, hyporeflexia, slurred speech, stupor, or coma	Barbiturates, benzodiazepines, bromides, ethanol, gamma-hydroxybutyrate and its precursors, meprobamate, propofol, zolpidem

*Reflex bradycardia can occur as a result of a pure α-adrenergic agonist effect.
†Depending on the specific toxicant, tachycardia can occur early as a result of a preganglionic nicotinic effect; as toxicity progresses, postganglionic muscarinic effects may predominate, and bradycardia develops.
CNS = central nervous system.

Many toxicants cause *hypotension* (Chapter 7). The primary mechanisms are decreased peripheral vascular resistance, decreased myocardial contractility, hypovolemia secondary to gastrointestinal or dermal loss of intravascular volume, and, occasionally, dysrhythmias. Common causes of *hypertension* (Chapter 64), which is generally due to vasoconstriction with or without enhanced inotropy, include amphetamines, cocaine, ephedrine and similar agents, ergots, phencyclidine, nicotine, phenylephrine, thyroid hormones, yohimbine, and chronic lead toxicity. Blood pressure can rise early in poisoning with central α_2-adrenergic agonists and monoamine oxidase inhibitors, but subsequent hypotension should be expected and is more concerning.

Hyperthermia (Chapter 95) occurs with toxicants that cause agitation or excessive psychomotor activity (e.g., cocaine, phencyclidine, monoamine oxidase inhibitors, strychnine), uncouple oxidative phosphorylation (e.g., salicylates, 2,4-dinitrophenol), increase the metabolic rate (e.g., thyroid hormones), impair sweating (e.g., first-generation antihistamines, anticholinergics, phenothiazines), cause vasoconstriction (e.g., amphetamines, cocaine, ephedrine), or alter perception of heat (e.g., cocaine). Other toxicant-induced states associated with hyperthermia include malignant hyperthermia, neuroleptic malignant syndrome, serotonin syndrome, metal fume fever, and aspiration pneumonitis. Toxicant-induced *hypothermia* is typically due to sedative-hypnotics, opioids, barbiturates, ethanol, phenothiazines, or hypoglycemic agents (such as insulin, sulfonylureas, and meglitinides) or rarely to unripe ackee fruit. Oxygen saturation (see Fig. 90-1 in Chapter 90), as measured by *pulse oximetry,* decreases with true hypoxemia (see Table 90-3 in Chapter 90) or methemoglobinemia (not proportionally to concentration) (Chapter 144) but remains normal or may be increased in patients with carbon monoxide or cyanide poisoning (Chapter 82).

Eyes, Ears, Nose, and Throat

Toxicant-induced bilateral miosis (Fig. 96-1) has a limited differential diagnosis that includes central α_2-agonists such as clonidine, guanfacine, and the imidazolines; olanzapine; opioids; organophosphorus compounds or carbamates; therapeutic cholinesterase inhibitors (e.g., pyridostigmine); topical miotic ophthalmic drugs (e.g., pilocarpine, carbachol); and, variably, phencyclidine, phenothiazines, ethanol, and some sedative-hypnotics (Chapter 392). Pontine hemorrhage is a major nontoxicologic diagnosis to consider in a comatose patient with miotic pupils (Chapter 377). Mydriasis is a nonspecific finding. A unilateral dilated pupil may be due to topical ocular application of sympathomimetics (e.g., phenylephrine), antihistamines, or anticholinergic agents (e.g., inhaled anticholinergics such as ipratropium or tiotropium, dust or sap from *Datura* sp) and can be caused by a postauricular scopolamine patch. Failure of topical 4% pilocarpine ophthalmic drops to constrict the pupil supports the diagnosis of pupillary dilation from a topical mydriatic agent. Visual disturbances, including partial or total blindness as a result of systemic toxicity, have been reported with anticholinergic agents, carbon monoxide, digitalis, ethambutol, methanol, methyl bromide, quinine, and agents that are associated with pseudotumor cerebri, including antimicrobials (e.g., ampicillin, metronidazole, nalidixic acid, nitrofurantoin, sulfa drugs, tetracycline), glucocorticosteroids, lead, lithium, oral contraceptives, phenothiazines, phenytoin, and vitamin A. Nonarteritic anterior ischemic optic neuropathy has developed after the use of sildenafil and other related drugs (Chapter 216); the causal relationship is unknown.

Neurologic Signs

Many toxicants affect the central nervous system (CNS) and can produce agitated delirium,[4] decreased level of consciousness,[5] or seizures (Table 96-2). Distinguishing features of various toxicants may assist in making the correct diagnosis. Patients who are withdrawing from opioids because of abstinence (as opposed to after being administered naloxone) are alert and oriented, whereas patients withdrawing from alcohol, barbiturates, benzodiazepines, and other sedative-hypnotics are often disoriented. Initial CNS depression can also develop with large ingestions of acetaminophen or ibuprofen. Isoniazid and theophylline are noted for producing seizures refractory to the usual doses of benzodiazepines and barbiturates. Pyridoxine treats isoniazid-induced seizures by increasing CNS γ-aminobutyric acid, synthesis of which is inhibited by isoniazid. Bupropion can cause seizures at both therapeutic doses and overdoses. Phenytoin is relatively ineffective for the majority of toxicant-induced seizures, perhaps because of the absence of a discrete seizure focus in most poisoned patients. Plant or mushroom ingestion can also produce CNS depression (e.g., *Rhododendron* sp, *Solanum* [bittersweet], *Taxus* [yew], *Sophora* [mescal bean]), CNS stimulation (e.g., *Catha edulis* [khat], *Strychnos nux-vomica* [contains strychnine], *Cicuta* sp [water hemlock], *Ephedra* [Mormon tea]), atropine-like effects (e.g., *Atropa belladonna* [deadly nightshade], *Datura* sp [jimsonweed]), and cholinomimetic effects (e.g., *Nicotiana* genus [tobacco], *Conium maculatum* [poison hemlock], *Inocybe* and *Clitocybe* mushrooms). Seizures can also occur with many of these plants and with mushrooms that contain gyromitrins (e.g., false morel, *Gyromitra* sp) and muscimol (e.g., *Amanita muscaria, Amanita pantherina*).

Distal axonopathy, a primary degeneration of peripheral nervous system axons with secondary degeneration of the myelin sheath, is the predominant type of toxicant-induced peripheral neuropathy. It usually is insidious in onset

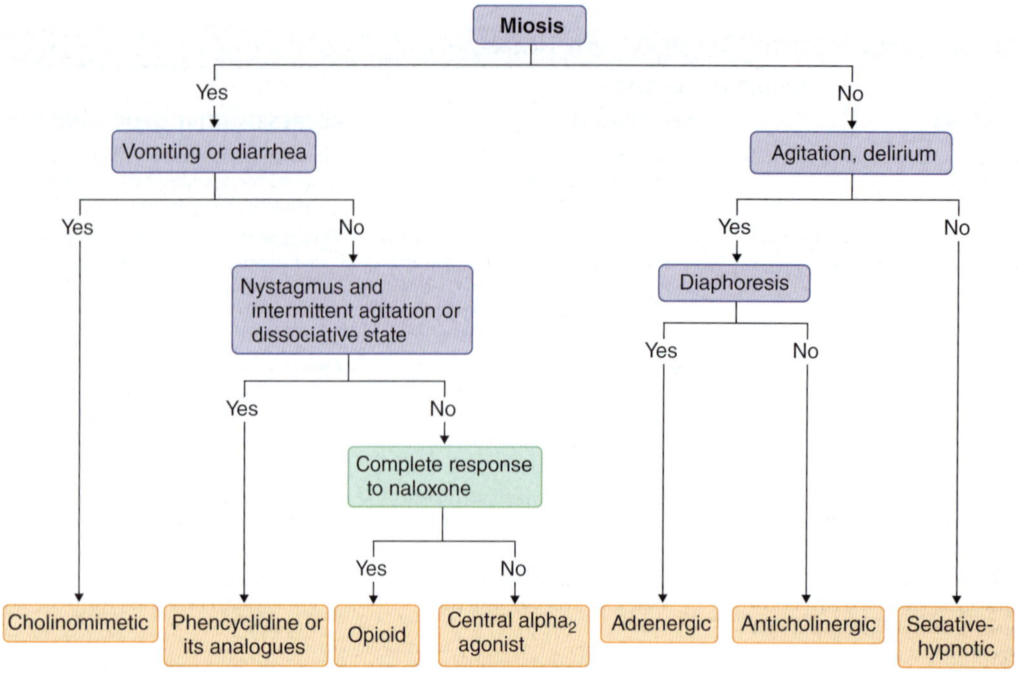

FIGURE 96-1. **Diagnostic algorithm for assessing toxicant-induced bilateral miosis.** Note that atypical toxidromes are common because of mixed toxicant exposures, so the examiner can be misled if relying only on this sign.

and follows chronic exposure; there is often slow recovery following termination of exposure, but, depending on the exposure and extent of neuronal damage, the clinical effects may be permanent. Neuropathy may be sensory, motor, or mixed. Common causative agents include acrylamide monomer, allyl chloride, arsenic (inorganic), capsaicin, carbon disulfide, chloramphenicol, cisplatin, colchicine, cyanate, dapsone, dideoxycytidine, dideoxyinosine, disulfiram, ethambutol, ethanol, ethylene oxide, gold salts, hexachlorophene, *n*-hexane, hydralazine, interferon, isoniazid, lead, linezolid, mercury, methyl bromide, methyl *n*-butyl ketone, metronidazole, nitrofurantoin, nitrous oxide, some organophosphorus compounds, phenol, platinum, podophyllotoxin, polychlorinated biphenyls, pyridoxine, tacrolimus, taxoids, thalidomide, thallium, vidarabine, vinca alkaloids, and vinyl chloride. Amiodarone, arsenic, and trichloroethylene can produce a demyelinating neuropathy, whereas pyridoxine can produce a sensory, sometimes painful, neuropathy. In addition, the neuropathy may be multifactorial in nature, such as vitamin deficiency associated with chronic ethanol consumption (Chapter 384). Neuronal transmission can be altered by aminoglycosides; the venom of *Latrodectus* species (widow spiders; see also Chapter 98 on envenomation and related injuries), scorpions (only the bark scorpion, *Centruroides sculpturatus*, in the United States), and crotaline (e.g., rattlesnakes) and elapid snakes; brevetoxin (shellfish) and ciguatoxin (various fish); neuromuscular blocking drugs; nicotine and related alkaloids; paralytic shellfish toxins; saxitoxin (shellfish); organophosphorus compounds and carbamates; tetrodotoxin (puffer fish [fugu], blue-ringed octopus, salamanders, newts, and others); and veratridine (e.g., false hellebore). Cranial nerves can be affected by carbon disulfide, ciguatoxin, domoic acid (shellfish), elapid venom, ethylene glycol metabolites, paralytic shellfish toxins, bark scorpion, saxitoxin, tetrodotoxin, thallium, and trichloroethylene. Mononeuropathies and vasculitic neuropathies are unlikely to be induced by toxicants (Chapter 98).

Cardiopulmonary Effects

The examination should focus on blood pressure, heart rate, electrocardiographic abnormalities (e.g., rhythm, conduction, depolarization, repolarization), and pulmonary findings, including pulse oximetry. Drugs and other toxicants that can cause dysrhythmias or conduction abnormalities include β-adrenergic receptor antagonists, butyrophenones (e.g., haloperidol), L-type calcium-channel antagonists, cardioactive steroids (e.g., bufadienolides, found in toxic toad venom and incorporated into some illicit aphrodisiacs; cardenolides, such as digoxin,[6] found in plants such as foxglove, oleander, and lily of the valley), halogenated hydrocarbons, chloroquine, cocaine, cyclic antidepressants, ethanol, halogenated hydrocarbons (e.g., halothane, trichloroethylene), magnesium salts, potassium salts, propoxyphene, thioridazine or mesoridazine, bupropion, and antiarrhythmics and other agents that affect the myocardial voltage-gated sodium channels (e.g., bupivacaine, chloroquine, cocaine, cyclic antidepressants, flecainide, mexiletine, quinidine, procainamide, propafenone) and potassium channels (e.g., typical and atypical antipsychotics, citalopram/escitalopram, erythromycin [especially when taken concomitantly with cytochrome P-450 A inhibitors; Chapter 25], quinidine, sotalol, terfenadine). Bedside echocardiography may reveal depressed myocardial contractility as a result of agents that block the myocardial voltage-gated sodium channel, β-adrenergic receptor antagonists, calcium-channel antagonists, cyclic antidepressants, magnesium salts, arsenic salts, ciguatoxin, cyanide, ethanol, iron salts, and scorpion venom.

Toxicants can produce myriad pulmonary effects, including airway irritation, parenchymal and pleural diseases, vascular diseases, and barotrauma. Typical syndromes and etiologic agents include pulmonary edema (β-adrenergic receptor antagonists, calcium-channel antagonists, antiarrhythmics, daunorubicin, doxorubicin), acute respiratory distress syndrome (Chapter 90) (amphetamines, cadmium, chlorine, cocaine, ethchlorvynol, methotrexate, opioids, heroin, paraquat, salicylates; inhalation of smoke, zinc chloride, methyl bromide, methyl chloride, and hydrocarbons), and rapidly developing pulmonary fibrosis or bronchiolitis obliterans (oxides of nitrogen, paraquat). For organophosphorous nerve agent and insecticide poisoning, acute respiratory failure is the most common primary cause of death, but some patients develop delayed neuromuscular junction dysfunction (i.e., intermediate syndrome), aspiration pneumonia, and acute respiratory distress syndrome.[7]

Gastrointestinal Effects

Symptoms of nausea, vomiting, diarrhea, and abdominal pain are nonspecific and must be interpreted in the context of other findings. Agents that produce severe or life-threatening toxicity with early gastrointestinal findings include acid or large alkali ingestions; cardioactive steroids; colchicine and other microtubular toxicants (e.g., podophyllin, vincristine); metal salts such as arsenic, iron, mercury salts, and thallium; mushrooms containing amanitin (*Amanita phalloides, Amanita virosa, Amanita verna, Lepiota chlorophyllum*), gyromitrins (*Gyromitra esculenta*), orellanines (*Cortinarius orellanus*), or allenic norleucine (*Amanita smithiana*); nicotine; organophosphorus compounds; and theophylline. Caustic damage is found with ingestion of alkalis (e.g., ammonium hydroxide, sodium hydroxide, potassium hydroxide, or sodium hypochlorite), acids (e.g., acetic acid, hydrochloric acid, oxalic acid, phosphoric acid, selenous acid, sulfuric acid, or hydrofluoric acid), and other agents (e.g., benzalkonium chloride, hydrogen peroxide, phenol, and zinc chloride).[8] Severe abdominal pain and rigidity can occur with lower extremity envenomation by *Latrodectus* species (widow spiders), unrelated to any direct organ injury. Hepatotoxicity can occur as an adverse effect of the therapeutic use of many drugs; in the United States, acetaminophen and ethanol are the most common causes of toxicant-induced hepatotoxicity (Chapter 136). For acetaminophen overdose,

TABLE 96-2 CENTRAL NERVOUS SYSTEM EFFECTS OF TOXICANTS

	CNS EFFECTS		
TOXICANT CATEGORIES AND AGENTS	**AGITATED DELIRIUM**	**DECREASED LEVEL OF CONSCIOUSNESS**	**SEIZURES**
CLASSES			
Anticholinergic agents	+	+	+
Anticonvulsants	+	+	+ (paradoxical with some agents)
Antipsychotic drugs		+	+
β-Adrenergic receptor antagonists	+	+	+ (theophylline/caffeine)
Hallucinogenic agents	+	+	+ (MDMA, substituted amphetamines)
Monoamine oxidase inhibitors	+	+	+
Opioids	+ (withdrawal, tramadol)	+	+ (meperidine, tramadol, dextromethorphan)
Sedative-hypnotics	+ (rare, paradoxical)	+	
Antidepressants	+ (serotonin syndrome)	+	+ (bupropion, venlafaxine)
AGENTS			
Amphetamines, cocaine	+	+ (following binge use)	+
Antidepressants (non SSRI)	+ (MAOI)	+	+
Antihistamines (first generation, e.g., diphenhydramine)	+	+	+
Barbiturates		+	
Benzodiazepines	+ (rare, paradoxical)	+	
Cytochrome oxidase inhibitors (e.g., carbon monoxide, cyanide, hydrogen sulfide, azides)		+	+
Ephedra alkaloids and similar agents	+	+	+
Ethylene glycol, methanol		+	+
γ-Hydroxybutyrate and precursors	+ (paradoxical, withdrawal)	+	+ (vs. myoclonus, withdrawal)
Lithium	+	+	+ (rare)
Organophosphorus compounds (e.g., diazinon, malathion, nerve agents) and carbamates (e.g., carbaryl, physostigmine)	+	+	+
Salicylates	+ (delirium)	+	+ (often pre-terminal)
SSRIs/SRIs/SNRI antidepressants	+ (serotonin syndrome)	+	+
Withdrawal from alcohol, barbiturates, benzodiazepines, other sedative-hypnotics	+		+
Withdrawal from opioids	+		+ (only in neonates)

CNS = central nervous system; MAOI = monamine oxidase inhibitor; MDMA = 3,4,-Methylenedioxymethamphetamine, also known as ecstasy or Molly; SNRIs = serotonin and norepinephrine re-uptake inhibitors; SRIs = serotonin re-uptake inhibitors; SSRIs = selective serotonin re-uptake inhibitors.

early measurement of the concentration of acetaminophen-protein adducts can predict the likelihood of hepatotoxicity.[9] Other notable hepatotoxicants include aflatoxins (in food contaminated with *Aspergillus flavus*), anabolic steroids, arsenicals, carbon tetrachloride, copper sulfate, cyclopeptide mushrooms (e.g., *Amanita phalloides*),[10] *Ephedra* species (e.g., ma huang), iron salts, methamphetamine, pennyroyal oil, pyrrolizidine alkaloids (various plant species used in herbal teas), and vitamin A in chronic excessive doses.

Dermatologic Signs

The skin, hair, nails, and mucous membranes should be examined for evidence of intravenous drug use; the presence or absence of skin and mucous membrane moisture; abnormal skin coloration, including erythema and cyanosis; alopecia; and nail abnormalities. Bullous skin lesions have been reported with chronic barbiturate use, glutethimide, carbon monoxide, meprobamate, methadone, and valproic acid. Sulfur mustard gas produces large yellow bullae on affected skin. Bluish discoloration may be dermal in origin (as with argyria from excessive exposure to colloidal silver) or due to cyanosis. Cyanosis may reflect hypoxemia or methemoglobinemia. Commonly used agents that can cause methemoglobinemia include aniline dyes, benzocaine and other amide anesthetics, dapsone, naphthalene, nitrates, nitrites, phenazopyridine, rifampin, and sulfonamides. Skin erythema or flushing occurs with anticholinergic agents, boric acid ingestion, monosodium glutamate, niacin, scombroid toxicity as a result of the ingestion of inadequately refrigerated fish with a high histidine content (e.g., tuna, mahi-mahi, amberjack), vancomycin, and interactions between ethanol and numerous agents that produce disulfiram or disulfiram-like reactions (e.g., carbon disulfide, some cephalosporins, *Coprinus atramentarius* mushroom, disulfiram, griseofulvin, metronidazole, thiuram herbicides, trichloroethylene).

Specific Toxicants

Some common toxicants can be suspected from their characteristic manifestations (Table 96-3). These suspicions should guide specific diagnostic and therapeutic strategies that complement general decontamination and supportive treatments.

Diagnostic Tests

Drug testing should be guided by the history and physical examination, with emphasis on tests that can influence management. Rapid qualitative urine drug screening tests are readily available in most hospitals, but their clinical value is limited by the number of drugs that can be tested and the reliability of the tests themselves. Although such testing may be valuable for subsequent psychiatric evaluation, it is less reliable for urgent diagnosis and therapy. For example, a positive test result may be unrelated to the patient's condition because drug analytes may be detectable for days after drug use, depending on the drug, dose, and frequency of use. In addition, both false-positive and false-negative results occur (Table 96-4), so the screening result must be verified with a

TABLE 96-3 PATHOPHYSIOLOGY, CLINICAL EFFECTS, AND MANAGEMENT OF SPECIFIC DRUGS AND TOXICANTS

DRUG OR TOXICANT	PATHOPHYSIOLOGY	TOXIC EFFECTS	LABORATORY	SPECIFIC THERAPY
Acetaminophen	NAPQI (toxic metabolite) binds hepatic and renal tubular cells, where it causes oxidant tissue damage; acetaminophen itself induces transient decrease in functional coagulation factor VII and can increase INR	Initial: nausea, vomiting, coma, lactic acidosis in severe cases Days 1-3: elevated INR, aminotransferase levels; RUQ tenderness; increased creatinine level in severe cases Days 4-14: gradual recovery or continued increase in INR and creatinine, lactic acidosis, coma, cerebral edema, death	Potentially toxic level ≥150 μg/mL 4 hours after single acute ingestion* INR may be transiently elevated in first 24 hours because of decrease in functional factor VII, and further increases indicate hepatic necrosis; elevated serum lactate levels and acidosis correlate with severity, but elevated aminotransferase and bilirubin levels are not predictive of hepatic failure Creatinine elevated in severe cases	N-acetylcysteine (see dosing guidelines in Table 96-6); NAC can increase INR but not aPTT†
Amphetamines (also cathinones, which are a class of keto substituted amphetamines)	Increased release of presynaptic norepinephrine and dopamine Increased serotonin release (especially MDMA, cathinones, other novel psychoactive drugs)	Mild: euphoria, decreased appetite, repetitive behavior, hallucinations Moderate: vomiting, agitation, hypertension, tachycardia, mydriasis, bruxism, diaphoresis Severe: hypertension or hypotension, dysrhythmias, hyperthermia, seizures, coma, multisystem organ failure, hyponatremia (SIADH), cerebral infarction or hemorrhage	Not helpful; many false-positives and false-negatives on screening tests (see Table 96-4)	IV crystalloids External cooling Benzodiazepines to control agitation or seizures Benzodiazepines for hypertension See SSRIs/SRIs for features and treatment of serotonin syndrome
β-Adrenergic receptor antagonists[11]	Blocks catecholamines from β-adrenergic receptors Additional actions: • α- and β-adrenergic receptor antagonism: carvedilol, labetalol • Delayed rectifier potassium-channel blockade: sotalol	Bradydysrhythmias (with high doses), decreased myocardial contractility, hypotension, respiratory depression, decreased consciousness with seizures or coma (lipophilic agents, e.g., propranolol), prolonged QT interval (sotalol)	ECG No specific tests	Regular insulin, 1 U/kg by IV bolus followed by 1 U/kg/hr (plus dextrose, usually needed within 20-30 min to maintain euglycemia), with upward titration every 10 min to max of 10 U/kg/hr. Other options include (1) IV glucagon (3-5 mg over 2-minute period; if no increase in BP or HR, can repeat up to 10 mg); if effective, immediately start continuous infusion at 2-10 mg/hr; or (2) norepinephrine infusion titrated to desirable BP and HR (less predictable) Electrical pacing, IABP, or intravenous lipid emulsion therapy in refractory cases
Calcium-channel antagonists	Blocks L-type voltage-sensitive calcium channels, thereby decreasing calcium entry into myocardial (verapamil, diltiazem) and vascular smooth muscle cells (all, but predominant effect of dihydropyridines) Decreases pancreatic insulin release and increases insulin resistance	Bradydysrhythmias (verapamil, diltiazem), hypotension, hyperglycemia Tachycardia and hypotension (dihydropyridines such as amlodipine, nifedipine)	ECG No specific tests	3 g (30 mL of 10% calcium gluconate solution) over 10 minutes (60 seconds if in extremis). Repeat in 10-20 minutes up to three times as needed. Alternative preferably via a central line: calcium chloride 10%, 10 mL (1 g) over 10 minutes (60 seconds if in extremis). Ionized Ca^{2+} levels should not exceed 2× normal (severe cases will be refractory to calcium therapy). Glucagon, high-dose insulin and dextrose, catecholamines, and milrinone (as for β-adrenergic antagonists). Intravenous lipid emulsion therapy for verapamil and diltiazem, unclear for dihydropyridines; indicated only for moribund patients.

TABLE 96-3 PATHOPHYSIOLOGY, CLINICAL EFFECTS, AND MANAGEMENT OF SPECIFIC DRUGS AND TOXICANTS—cont'd

DRUG OR TOXICANT	PATHOPHYSIOLOGY	TOXIC EFFECTS	LABORATORY	SPECIFIC THERAPY
Cardioactive steroids, including digoxin, bufadienolides (toxic toad venom), and cardenolides (e.g., oleander, lily of the valley, dogbane)	Inhibits Na^+,K^+-ATPase Decreased CNS sympathetic output Decreased baroreceptor sensitivity Increased vagal acetylcholine discharge	Bradydysrhythmias, including second- and third-degree AV block and asystole Ventricular ectopy, tachycardia, fibrillation Junctional tachycardia, paroxysmal atrial tachycardia with block Weakness, visual disturbances, nausea, vomiting	ECG Serum digoxin level Serum potassium (hyperkalemia occurs in acute poisoning and is prognostic for poor outcome without Fab; hypokalemia may be present in chronic poisoning due to concomitant medications such as furosemide), magnesium, and creatinine levels	Digoxin-specific antibody fragments (Fab) indicated if patient has rhythm disturbances such as sinus bradycardia, Mobitz II, or third-degree AV block, ventricular ectopy, serum potassium ≥5 mEq/L if acute overdose, ingestion of bufadienolide- or cardenolide-containing agents, or renal insufficiency Empiric dose: Acute: 10-20 vials Chronic: 3-6 vials Calculated dose: Acute: number of vials = 2 × oral digoxin dose (mg) × 0.8. Correcting the hyperkalemia with standard interventions is not helpful. Do not give calcium salts. If hypokalemic (generally chronic overdose), replete serum potassium. Chronic: number of vials = serum digoxin level (ng/mL) × wt (kg)/100
Cyclic antidepressants	Myocardial sodium- and potassium-channel blockade Blockade of α-adrenergic and cholinergic muscarinic receptors Inhibition of norepinephrine re-uptake	Decreased level of consciousness (can develop rapidly), myoclonus, seizures, coma Anticholinergic toxidrome (see Table 96-1) Sinus tachycardia, ventricular conduction delays, ventricular dysrhythmias, asystole Hypotension	Serum levels not helpful in management	Intermittent IV boluses of $NaHCO_3$ (1 mEq/kg) to narrow QRS to <100 msec; infusion of $NaHCO_3$ is less effective; maintain arterial pH at 7.5 because alkalemia and sodium ions can improve cardiovascular performance Contraindicated drugs: types IA and IC antiarrhythmic agents, physostigmine, flumazenil
Ethylene glycol, methanol (e.g., antifreeze, window cleaners, camping stove fuels)[12]	Ethylene glycol: toxic metabolites (glycolate and oxalate) produce cytotoxicity in CNS, kidneys, lungs, heart, liver, muscles; metabolic acidosis is due to glycolate accumulation; oxalate complexes with calcium, so hypocalcemia can develop Methanol: metabolized to formic acid, which is responsible for metabolic acidosis and inhibition of cytochrome *aa*$_3$; target organs include retina, optic nerve, CNS	Ethylene glycol: CNS depression, cerebral edema, seizures, anion gap metabolic acidosis, renal failure with acute tubular necrosis, pulmonary edema, myositis Methanol: nausea, vomiting; cerebral edema, hemorrhage, infarcts; necrosis of thalamus and putamen; anion gap metabolic acidosis; visual disturbances, papilledema, hyperemic optic disc, nonreactive pupils	Serum ethylene glycol and methanol levels; levels may be low or undetectable if significant metabolism has occurred Osmolar gap must be interpreted with caution, but a very high value (>50) more likely indicates the presence of a toxic alcohol Ethylene glycol: serum calcium, creatinine, BUN levels; examine urine for calcium oxalate crystals; false hyperlactatemia occurs with certain analyzers using L-lactate oxidase, which cross-reacts with glycolic and glyoxylic acid metabolites	For both: fomepizole[13] (inhibits alcohol dehydrogenase and blocks formation of toxic metabolites), 15 mg/kg IV loading dose, then 10 mg/kg IV every 12 hours for four doses during the next 48 hours, then 15 mg/kg for subsequent doses; interval dosing is q12h (q4h during hemodialysis, with dosing interval adjustments at start and finish); continue until ethylene glycol or methanol is no longer detectable Treatment with ethanol is no longer recommended Hemodialysis: initiate if level is ≥25 mg/dL or metabolic acidosis with end-organ toxicity; continue until acidosis resolves and serum level of ethylene glycol or methanol is undetectable (if available) Monitor for cerebral edema with possible herniation Ethylene glycol: IV calcium for symptomatic hypocalcemia Methanol: folic acid 1-2 mg/kg (50-75 mg) IV q4h × 24 h; extra dose at completion of hemodialysis; continue until methanol not detectable and acidosis cleared
γ-Hydroxybutyrate (GHB) and its precursors (γ-butyrolactone and 1,4-butanediol)	Agonist effect on CNS GHB receptors; indirect action with opioid receptors (may increase proenkephalins); metabolized to GABA, interacts with $GABA_B$ receptors; decreases dopamine release	CNS: rapid loss of consciousness, myoclonus/seizure, with recovery typical within 2-4 hours Respiratory depression; bradycardia; nausea, vomiting	No specific tests for acute management. Forensic testing available	Supportive care, including respiratory support as needed Withdrawal resembles sedative-hypnotic withdrawal and can be treated with benzodiazepines or phenobarbital

TABLE 96-3 PATHOPHYSIOLOGY, CLINICAL EFFECTS, AND MANAGEMENT OF SPECIFIC DRUGS AND TOXICANTS—cont'd

DRUG OR TOXICANT	PATHOPHYSIOLOGY	TOXIC EFFECTS	LABORATORY	SPECIFIC THERAPY
Lithium	Decreases brain inositol; alters CNS serotonin, dopamine, and norepinephrine; inhibits adenylate cyclases, including those that mediate vasopressin-induced renal concentration and thyroid function	Chronic toxicity usually more severe than acute toxicity: tremor, hyperreflexia, drowsiness, incoordination, clonus, confusion, ataxia; in severe cases, seizures (rare), coma, death (very rare); recovery may take weeks, and CNS deficits may persist (common) Sinus node dysfunction, QT prolongation, T wave abnormalities, U waves Nephrogenic diabetes insipidus, hypothyroidism, hyperthyroidism, hypercalcemia, pseudotumor cerebri Acute toxicity: nausea, vomiting, diarrhea, and milder neurologic findings	Peak serum levels: Normal dose, 2-3 hours; up to 5 hours for sustained-release lithium Acute overdose: peak may be delayed ≥4-12 hours	Replenish intravascular volume, maintain urinary output at 1-2 mL/kg/hr Consider gastrointestinal decontamination with oral or NG polyethylene glycol electrolyte solution within 1-2 hours after acute overdose of sustained-release drug Hemodialysis‡ in patients with altered mental status, ataxia, seizures, or coma or in patients with mild symptoms in the setting of acute overdose or renal insufficiency Ineffective or contraindicated therapies include oral activated charcoal, diuretics
Opioids (e.g., opiate [natural]: morphine, codeine; semisynthetic: heroin, oxycodone, hydrocodone; synthetic: methadone, fentanyl and fentanyl analogs such as carfentanil and acetylfentanyl)	Agonist effect at CNS μ, κ, and δ opioid receptors; result is cell hyperpolarization and decreased neurotransmitter release	CNS depression, respiratory depression, miosis (see Table 96-1) Nearly all fatalities due to respiratory depression, highlighting the importance of assessing and managing based on oxygenation and ventilation Seizure risk with tramadol, meperidine QTc prolongation and torsades de pointes with methadone	Rapid urine drug screens detect morphine, poorly detect semisynthetic opioids, and do not detect synthetic opioids at all; some interferents/irrelevants (see Table 96-4)	Ventilate and oxygenate IV naloxone, 0.04 mg initial dose and titrate every 2-3 minutes in patients with likely opioid dependence; in patients known to be naïve, start 0.4 mg; repeat in frequent, escalating doses up to 10 mg if no response Continuous infusion for recurrent symptoms or sustained-release opioid ingestion; give 50% of dose that produces desired effect 15 minutes after initial effect is obtained, then infuse two thirds of this dose every hour; infusion rate can be increased or decreased to maintain normal ventilation and to avoid withdrawal symptoms Contraindicated therapies: naltrexone should not be used for acute opioid reversal Intranasal naloxone (2-4 mg) can be given if IM/IV not possible
Organophosphorus compounds and carbamates (e.g., diazinon, mevinphos, fenthion, aldicarb); nerve agents (e.g., sarin); medicinals (pyridostigmine for myasthenia gravis and donepezil for Alzheimer disease)	Inhibits acetylcholinesterase, resulting in excessive acetylcholine stimulation of nicotinic and muscarinic receptors in autonomic and somatic motor nervous systems and CNS	Nicotinic-mediated effects: tachycardia, mydriasis, hypertension, delirium, coma, seizures, muscle weakness, fasciculations Muscarinic-mediated effects: salivation, lacrimation, urination, vomiting, defecation, miosis, bronchorrhea, bronchospasm, bradycardia Muscarinic or nicotinic effects may be mixed and unpreditable in an individual patient	Plasma (butyrylcholinesterase) or RBC (acetylcholinesterase) activity <50% of normal (see Table 96-6) Clinical recovery occurs before plasma cholinesterase levels normalize	Atropine, 1-2 mg by initial IV bolus; double the dose every 5 minutes (2 mg, 4 mg, 8 mg, 16 mg, and so on) until drying of bronchial secretions and adequate oxygenation is achieved or progress ceases; continuous infusion at 10-20% of total stabilizing dose per hour; stop infusion when patient develops concerning signs or symptoms of anticholinergic toxidrome (see Table 96-1); restart infusion at lower rate when signs or symptoms abate Pralidoxime chloride 30 mg/kg (maximum 2 g) IV over 30 minutes, then 8-10 mg/kg/hr (maximum 650 mg/hr) continuous infusion; administer as soon as possible after poisoning; continue 12-24 hours after atropine no longer required and symptoms resolve§ Benzodiazepines for agitation or seizures Magnesium sulfate (4 g IV over 30minutes upon ICU admission) can decrease the need for atropine, the need for intubation, and the length of ICU stay[A1] Treatment not generally needed for overdose of Alzheimer medications

TABLE 96-3 PATHOPHYSIOLOGY, CLINICAL EFFECTS, AND MANAGEMENT OF SPECIFIC DRUGS AND TOXICANTS—cont'd

DRUG OR TOXICANT	PATHOPHYSIOLOGY	TOXIC EFFECTS	LABORATORY	SPECIFIC THERAPY
Salicylates[14]	Inhibit cyclooxygenase; decrease formation of prostaglandins and thromboxane A_2; stimulate CNS medullary respiratory center and chemoreceptor trigger zone; impair platelet function; disrupt carbohydrate metabolism; uncouple oxidative phosphorylation; increase vascular permeability	Acute toxicity Mild: nausea, vomiting, diaphoresis, tinnitus, decreased hearing, hyperpnea, tachypnea Moderate-severe: confusion, delirium, coma, seizures, hyperthermia, ARDS; death can occur within hours of overdose Chronic toxicity: same as acute, but may not have diaphoresis or vomiting Consider diagnosis in patients with new-onset confusion, anion gap metabolic acidosis, or acute lung injury	Serum salicylate level: acute: toxic ≥30 mg/dL; level ≥100 mg/dL indicates life-threatening toxicity with possible sudden, rapid clinical deterioration; in chronic toxicity, levels may be minimally elevated (>30 mg/dL), and clinical evaluation is more reliable for gauging degree of toxicity Arterial blood gases: respiratory alkalosis with metabolic acidosis Anion gap metabolic acidosis Prolonged PT and PTT, ketonuria, ketonemia	Multidose activated charcoal q2-3h in acute overdose Frequent monitoring of salicylate level and acid-base status Alkalinization of serum and urine with IV $NaHCO_3$ Hemodialysis with progressive clinical findings, particularly neurologic, hyperthermia, renal failure, ARDS, with any moderately elevated salicylate level or salicylate level >100 even with minor clinical findings
SSRIs/SRIs	Inhibit re-uptake of serotonin SRIs have additional effects (e.g., duloxetine inhibits norepinephrine re-uptake, nefazodone inhibits serotonergic 5-HT_2 receptors, trazodone inhibits peripheral α-adrenergic receptors, venlafaxine inhibits norepinephrine and dopamine re-uptake)	Vomiting, blurred vision, CNS depression, tachycardia Seizures and coma rare except with bupropion Torsades de pointes reported with citalopram Serotonin syndrome: clonus, agitation, tremor, diaphoresis, hyperreflexia; hyperthermia and hypertonicity in severe cases	No specific tests If serotonin syndrome suspected: electrolytes, BUN, glucose, liver enzymes, coagulation panel, blood gases, chest radiograph	Respiratory support as needed Benzodiazepines for agitation or seizures Serotonin syndrome: consider cyproheptadine, 4-12 mg PO initial dose, then 2 mg PO q2h (to a maximum of 32 mg/day) until symptoms resolve Critical therapies for hyperthermia, rhabdomyolysis, DIC, ARDS, renal and hepatic dysfunction, torsades de pointes; dantrolene not indicated

*A nomogram to evaluate the potential toxicity of levels drawn more than 4 hours after ingestion is available at: https://en.wikipedia.org/wiki/Rumack–Matthew_nomogram.

†Intravenous *N*-acetylcysteine (NAC) has generally replaced oral NAC for the majority of cases, largely because of convenience, not efficacy. The full 21-hour course of intravenous NAC should be administered in most situations in which it is used. Oral NAC, which remains an acceptable alternative, can be discontinued in patients with uncomplicated disease after a loading dose plus six maintenance doses if hepatic aminotransferase levels are normal and acetaminophen is not detected; otherwise, the full regimen should be administered.

‡Continue hemodialysis until the serum lithium level is less than 1 mEq/L. Recheck the level 4 to 8 hours after dialysis, and restart hemodialysis if the level rebounds significantly or if clinical findings of lithium toxicity are present. Repeat this cycle until the serum lithium level remains low or the patient remains clinically well.

§Randomized, placebo-controlled trials of pralidoxime in acute organophosphorus poisoning have not found a significant difference in mortality rates or need for intubation.

aPTT = activated partial thromboplastin time; ARDS = acute respiratory distress syndrome; AV = atrioventricular; BP = blood pressure; BUN = blood urea nitrogen; CNS = central nervous system; DIC = disseminated intravascular coagulation; DOB = 4-bromo-2,5-dimethoxyamphetamine; ECG = electrocardiogram; GABA = γ-aminobutyric acid; HR = heart rate; IABP = intra-aortic balloon counterpulsation; ICU = intensive care unit; INR = international normalized ratio; IV = intravenous, MDMA = 3,4-methylenedioxymethamphetamine, also known as ecstasy or Molly; Na^+,K^+-ATPase = sodium, potassium adenosine triphosphatase; NAC = *N*-acetylcysteine; NAPQI = *N*-acetyl-*p*-benzoquinone imine; NG = nasogastric; NMDA = *N*-methyl-D-aspartate; PMA = paramethoxyamphetamine; PO = orally; PT = prothrombin time; PTT = partial thromboplastin time; QT = QT interval from an electrocardiogram, QTc = rate-corrected QT interval from an electrocardiogram; RBC = red blood cell; RUQ = right upper quadrant (abdomen); SIADH = syndrome of inappropriate antidiuretic secretion; SRIs = serotonin re-uptake inhibitors; SSRIs = selective serotonin re-uptake inhibitors.

TABLE 96-4 QUALITATIVE URINE DRUG SCREENS: CAUSES OF ERRONEOUS RESULTS*

DRUG/TOXICANT	INTERFERENTS/CROSS-REACTIONS†	COMMENTS
Amphetamines	Amantadine, bupropion, chlorpromazine, ephedrine, pseudoephedrine, desoxyephedrine, ephedra alkaloids (from *Ephedra* sp), mexiletine, phenylephrine, phenylpropanolamine, selegiline, trazodone	Many false-positives from medicinal sympathomimetics or true positives from prescribed stimulants; nasal inhaler (desoxyephedrine) and selegiline cause positive GC-MS findings; chiral confirmation is required; newer immunoassays have reduced false rates but also lower sensitivity for the class of amphetamines
Benzodiazepines	Oxaprozin, sertraline	Most assays directed against oxazepam; poor detection of benzodiazepines without the oxazepam metabolite (e.g., alprazolam, lorazepam, triazolam)
Cocaine	Coca leaf teas (clinical false-positive; still considered illicit use)	Few analytical false-positives; urine is reliable for detecting true positives
Opioids	Poppy seeds (contain morphine)	Assay directed against morphine; poorly detects semisynthetic opioids and does not detect synthetic opioids (e.g., fentanyl, meperidine, methadone, propoxyphene, oxycodone, buprenorphine)
Phencyclidine	Dextromethorphan, diphenhydramine, doxylamine, ibuprofen, ketamine, tramadol, venlafaxine	Can be used, although not reliably, to identify dextromethorphan or ketamine
Tetrahydrocannabinol	Dronabinol, efavirenz, proton pump inhibitors	Positive result is seldom clinically relevant and does not indicate recent use; synthetic cannabinomimetics (e.g., spice, K2) are not reliably detected
Tricyclic antidepressants	Carbamazepine, cyclobenzaprine, cyproheptadine, diphenhydramine, phenothiazines, quetiapine	

*Advances in drug screening and variability in immunoassay results should be considered by the clinician when interpreting qualitative drug screening results. There are many marketed assays, so consultation with the testing laboratory is advised. Positive screening results are considered presumptive and should be verified by GC-MS or another advanced analytical methodology.

†Cross-reactants are agents causing true-positive but clinically irrelevant results on laboratory screening tests; they vary, depending on the screening method.

GC-MS = gas chromatography–mass spectrometry.

TABLE 96-5 CLINICALLY IMPORTANT QUANTITATIVE DRUG LEVELS

	LEVELS	
DRUG OR TOXICANT	**THERAPEUTIC**	**TOXIC***
SOURCE: BLOOD OR SERUM		
Acetaminophen[†]	10-30 μg/mL	≥150 μg/mL 4 hours after ingestion[‡]
Carbamazepine	4-12 μg/mL	>15 μg/mL
Carboxyhemoglobin	Nonsmoker: 0.5-1.5% Smoker: 4-9%	>20%[§]
Cholinesterase[‖] Serum (butyrylcholinesterase) Red blood cell (acetylcholinesterase)	 3100-6500 U/L 26.7-49.2 U/g of hemoglobin	 <50% of normal value <50% of normal value
Digoxin (≥6 hours after oral dose for long-term therapy)	0.8-2.0 ng/mL[¶]	>2.0 ng/mL
Ethanol	None measured	>80 mg/dL[**]
Ethylene glycol	None measured	>25 mg/dL
Iron	50-175 μg/dL	>350 g/dL
Lead	<5 μg/dL	>25 μg /dL
Lithium	0.6-1.2 mEq/L	>1.2 mEq/L[††]
Methanol	None measured	>25 mg/dL
Methemoglobin	1-2%	>15%
Phenobarbital	15-40 μg/mL	>40 g/mL
Phenytoin	10-20 μg/mL	>20 g/mL
Salicylate	≤30 mg/dL	>30 mg/dL
Theophylline	8-20 μg/mL	>20 g/mL
Valproic acid	50-100 μg/mL	>100 g/mL
	NORMAL	**TOXIC***
SOURCE: URINE		
Arsenic	<50 μg/day	>100 g/24-hr urine[††]
Mercury	<20 μg/L	>20 g/L[††]
Thallium	<5.0 μg/L	>200 g/L[††]

*The "toxic" level is provided for perspective. For many toxicants, simply being above this value does not imply a specific need for therapy or a necessarily poor prognosis. It does, however, generally suggest a need for additional evaluation, observation, or monitoring. Similarly, depending on the clinical context, levels below the "toxic" range may still be consequential.

†False-positive levels of 16 to 28 μg/mL have been reported in patients with bilirubin levels greater than 17 mg/dL.

‡Levels drawn more than 4 hours after ingestion should be plotted on the nomogram provided by Rumack and Matthew (Rumack BH, Matthew H. Acetaminophen poisoning and toxicity. *Pediatrics.* 1975;55:871-876) to assess the potential for toxicity.

§Lower levels may be toxic in pregnant patients and in those with prolonged exposure to carbon monoxide.

‖Consult a reference laboratory for normal values; results are assay dependent.

¶Some patients may require levels above the therapeutic range to control symptoms.

**The value of 80 mg/dL (0.08 g/dL) for ethanol is the statutory limit for operating a motor vehicle, but not for other activities. Consequential clinical effects other than inebriation are uncommon with concentrations below 200 mg/dL, even in ethanol-naïve patients.

††Lower values may indicate toxicity if appropriate clinical findings are present. For mercury and arsenic, both inorganic and organic levels should be measured when total levels are elevated.

second method, such as gas chromatography–mass spectrometry. The type of drug use in a population should be considered in determining the drugs to be screened to decrease the incidence of false-positive results. A test with 99% specificity for a drug with a prevalence of 0.1% in a population would produce 10 false-positive results for every true-positive result. Clinically irrelevant true-positive findings also occur, such as when poppy seeds produce a positive opiate assay result. Failure to consider these limitations of drug screens can result in misdiagnosis.

For a limited number of drugs and toxicants, levels in blood or urine are useful for diagnosis, therapy, or monitoring (Table 96-5). Threshold levels of certain toxicants indicate the need for specific therapies: acetaminophen (*N*-acetylcysteine), ethylene glycol (fomepizole and hemodialysis), iron (deferoxamine), methanol (fomepizole and hemodialysis), methemoglobin (methylene blue), and salicylates (urine alkalinization and hemodialysis). In chronic poisoning with some drugs, such as salicylates or theophylline, these therapies may be indicated at lower drug levels. In general, any end-organ toxicity that is evident or anticipated (on the basis of the toxicant, amount ingested, and time required to produce toxic effects) is more important than a specific level in determining the need for treatment.

Occult acetaminophen ingestion with toxic serum levels occurs in 0.3 to 1.9% of intentional ingestions. Given that these patients may be asymptomatic until hepatotoxicity develops and that administration of an antidote can prevent this hepatotoxicity, the current recommendation is to test the serum for acetaminophen in all patients with intentional self-harm ingestions.

Other Blood Tests

Anion gap metabolic acidosis resulting from primary lactic acidosis can be caused by cyanide, hydrogen sulfide, iron, isoniazid, metformin, nucleoside reverse transcriptase inhibitors, phenformin, sodium azide, and, rarely, acetaminophen with high serum levels. Anion gap metabolic acidosis not related to lactic acidosis occurs with diethylene glycol, ethylene glycol, nonsteroidal anti-inflammatory drugs, methanol, salicylates, and toluene. In poisonings resulting from ibuprofen, methanol, propylene glycol, and salicylates, lactic acid can also be produced, but the level is insufficient to account for the anion gap. Anion gap metabolic acidosis can also develop in patients with ongoing agitation, hyperthermia, and muscle rigidity, such as in neuroleptic malignant syndrome (Chapter 402), or in some cases of rhabdomyolysis (Chapter 99) secondary to toxicants such as doxylamine, phencyclidine, strychnine, cocaine, and amphetamines. Elevated serum creatinine and blood urea nitrogen levels indicative of declining renal function may be seen with numerous toxicants. Direct renal toxicity occurs with acetaminophen, aminoglycosides, cadmium, Chinese weight-loss botanicals containing *Stephania tetrandra* or *Magnolia officinalis*, chromium, *Crotalus durissus* venom, diethylene glycol, diquat, ethylene glycol, fluorinated anesthetics, gold, heroin, lithium (diabetes insipidus), mercury salts, mushrooms (*Amanita smithiana* and *Cortinarius* sp), paraquat, radiocontrast agents, solvents (e.g., carbon tetrachloride, trichloroethylene, tetrachloroethylene, toluene), and sulfonamides. Agents that decrease glomerular perfusion by reducing renal blood flow include amphotericin, angiotensin-converting enzyme inhibitors, angiotensin receptor blockers, cocaine, cyclosporine, mannitol (excessive chronic doses), methotrexate, and nonsteroidal anti-inflammatory drugs.

Imaging

A computed tomographic scan of the head can detect life-threatening cerebral edema secondary to toxicant-induced hepatic failure, ethylene glycol, and methanol. It also detects intracranial bleeding caused by anticoagulants, scorpion venom, and sympathomimetics (e.g., amphetamines, cocaine, phenylpropanolamine). An abdominal radiograph can reveal radiopaque ferrous sulfate tablets, drug-filled packets in illicit drug smugglers (body packers), or metals such as arsenic, lead, mercury, and thallium.

Diagnostic Syndromes

Given the myriad combinations of signs, symptoms, and laboratory findings, making the correct diagnosis in a noncommunicative patient can be daunting. A thorough history from bystanders, friends, and prehospital medical personnel may yield crucial information. In addition, the diagnostic possibilities can be narrowed by findings that can narrow the differential diagnosis with modest certainty. For example, consider a patient with sudden loss of consciousness, anion gap metabolic acidosis, and bradycardia without hypoxemia. Among the relevant possible causes from the list of toxicants that cause an anion gap metabolic acidosis (see earlier) along with sudden loss of consciousness are hydrogen sulfide, cyanide, and sodium azide.

TREATMENT

Initial Stabilization

Intubation and Respiratory Support

Appropriate airway management should be instituted to correct hypoxemia and respiratory acidosis and to protect against pulmonary aspiration (Fig. 96-2); intubation should be considered if the patient has depressed consciousness and a decreased gag reflex.[15] Rapid-sequence intubation facilitates airway management. Anatomic difficulties should be anticipated in patients with caustic ingestions (e.g., hypopharyngeal burns that may perforate); angioedema caused by angiotensin-converting enzyme inhibitor therapy or envenomation by some rattlesnakes, such as the canebrake (*Crotalus horridus atricaudatus*) and eastern diamondback (*Crotalus adamanteus;* Chapter 98); and swelling secondary to direct tissue injury (e.g., huffing compressed hydrocarbons, smoking crack) or secondary to anaphylactoid and anaphylactic reactions. Endotracheal intubation by flexible fiberoptic nasopharyngoscopy may be indicated in these cases. Hypoxemia can occur with toxicants that produce CNS depression, such as opioids, antidepressants, barbiturates, sedative-hypnotics, and central α_2-adrenergic receptor agonists (clonidine), or agents causing peripheral neuromuscular impairment, such as nicotine, organophosphorus compounds, tetrodotoxin (puffer fish, blue-ringed octopus), botulinum, or envenomation from elapids (coral snake), Mojave rattlesnakes, or certain coelenterates (box jellyfish; Chapter 98).

Respiratory acidosis can rapidly worsen the toxicities of cyclic antidepressants and salicylates; sedation of these patients should be accompanied by immediate airway placement and ventilatory support to match the patient's intrinsic minute ventilation. Intoxicated patients may have an increased risk for pulmonary aspiration because of concomitant CNS depression, attenuated airway reflexes, full stomachs, and delayed gastric emptying.

Succinylcholine can cause prolonged paralysis in patients with organophosphorus poisoning and can exacerbate hyperkalemia from cardioactive steroids (e.g., digoxin), hydrofluoric acid, or rhabdomyolysis (Chapter 99). Rhabdomyolysis has been reported with adrenergic agents, doxylamine, phencyclidine, heroin, carbon monoxide, *Tricholoma equestre* mushrooms, and envenomation by crotaline snakes, scorpions, or widow spiders (*Latrodectus* sp); short-acting nondepolarizing agents, such as vecuronium and rocuronium, are preferable in these cases.

Advanced Life Support

Standard emergency cardiovascular care algorithms (Chapter 50) must be modified for effects caused by specific poisons. Atropine often does not reverse bradycardia secondary to β-adrenergic receptor antagonists, L-type calcium-channel antagonists, or cardioactive steroids, and it may actually impair the ability to perform adequate gastrointestinal decontamination. In these cases, more specific therapy with intravenous calcium (calcium-channel antagonists), high doses of glucagon (β-adrenergic receptor antagonists, calcium-channel antagonists), or digoxin-specific Fab antibody (cardiac glycosides) is indicated. High-dose insulin-glucose therapy can successfully reverse myocardial depression and conduction abnormalities in humans poisoned with β-adrenergic receptor antagonists and calcium-channel antagonists (Table 96-6). Intravenous sodium bicarbonate may reverse cardiac conduction delays caused by antiarrhythmic drugs with sodium-channel blockade recovery rates of greater than 1 second (Vaughn-Williams classification IA and IC), cocaine, cyclic antidepressants, diphenhydramine, and quinine. β-Adrenergic receptor antagonists are relatively contraindicated in patients with acute cocaine-induced myocardial ischemia because they can result in unopposed α-adrenergic–mediated vasoconstriction, but phentolamine can reverse the agonistic effects of cocaine on α-adrenergic receptors (see Table 96-6). Benzodiazepines can reverse the significant sinus tachycardia seen with sympathomimetic agents by reducing autonomic outflow from the CNS. Calcium may also be life-saving in systemic hydrofluoric acid poisoning and severe hypermagnesemia, and it is indicated for symptomatic hypocalcemia caused by ethylene glycol toxicity (see Table 96-6). Drug-induced hypertension may be transitory; nitroprusside, phentolamine, or labetalol should be used if treatment is clinically indicated. (See Table 96-6.) Conversely, vasopressor infusions may be indicated in drug-induced hypotension (Chapter 92). In patients with toxicant-induced circulatory collapse refractory to maximal therapy, intravenous lipid emulsion therapy should be administered to those poisoned by lipophilic toxicants (e.g., calcium-channel blockers), and circulatory assist devices may support the patient until sufficient toxicant is eliminated (see Table 96-6 for dosing details) (Chapter 93).

Decontamination

Activated Charcoal

Activated charcoal consists of pyrolysis products that have been specially cleaned to produce an internal pore structure to which substances can adsorb, thereby limiting their systemic absorption. Single-dose activated charcoal without prior gastric emptying has been the preferred method of treatment for the ingestion of substances that have the potential to cause moderate to life-threatening toxicity and are known to adsorb to activated charcoal. The decision to administer activated charcoal should be based on a risk/benefit assessment that includes nature of the exposure, clinical effects displayed during evaluation, and abilities of the medical facility and staff. For patients likely to have a good outcome without decontamination, charcoal administration introduces unnecessary inconvenience and risk. Its use is justified in patients who present early (1 to 2 hours) after exposures to a large amount of a concerning toxin that is likely to be adsorbed to charcoal or to an unknown toxin that has presented with a concerning clinical picture. However, the documented efficacy of activated charcoal for reducing toxicant blood levels has not translated into a reduction in mortality.[A2]

The oral dose is approximately 1 g/kg body weight, with a maximum single dose of 100 g. Activated charcoal can be administered with antiemetic drugs or given through a nasogastric tube, when necessary. Efficacy in preventing toxicant absorption declines with time, so activated charcoal should be given as soon as possible after ingestion.

Activated charcoal should not be used in patients at risk for aspiration until the airway is secure to minimize aspiration; the patient's head should also be elevated unless it is contraindicated. Activated charcoal is contraindicated in patients with a perforated bowel, functional or mechanical bowel obstruction, ingestion of a pure aliphatic hydrocarbon such as gasoline or kerosene (no benefit and increased risk for aspiration), and ingestion of caustic acid and alkali (no benefit and obscures endoscopy). Certain agents, such as lithium, iron, and metal salts and ethanol, do not adsorb significantly to activated charcoal, but its use is not precluded if the patient has ingested other toxicants that do adsorb to activated charcoal. Pulmonary aspiration and bowel obstruction from inspissated activated charcoal are the most common complications; both occur more frequently when multidose activated charcoal is administered, but they can be avoided by withholding treatment in patients who have suboptimal bowel function or decreased fecal elimination.

Gastric Emptying

Two methods of gastric emptying, syrup of ipecac and orogastric lavage through a large-bore tube, are no longer routinely used; both are relatively ineffective therapies that potentially increase the risk for aspiration. Syrup of ipecac is no longer recommended, and no well-designed study has documented any benefit of gastric lavage compared with the use of activated charcoal alone. Nevertheless, gastric emptying may be of benefit in patients who have ingested toxicants that do not adsorb to activated charcoal and are known to produce significant morbidity or for which aggressive decontamination may offer the best chance for survival (e.g., colchicine, sodium azide, sodium fluoroacetate). Removal of a liquid toxicant, such as ethylene glycol, may be accomplished by simple aspiration of gastric contents (without lavage) through a nasogastric tube. Contraindications to gastric emptying include those for activated charcoal, a bleeding diathesis, and the ingestion of sharp objects. Placement of a cuffed endotracheal tube before gastric lavage may be necessary to protect the airway in patients who have a decreased level of consciousness and impaired gag reflex, but it is not required in all cases. Major complications of gastric emptying include pulmonary aspiration, esophageal tears and perforations, and laryngospasm (with lavage).

Whole Bowel Irrigation

Whole bowel irrigation with a nonabsorbable polyethylene glycol solution has been recommended for iron and sustained-release medications, for agents not

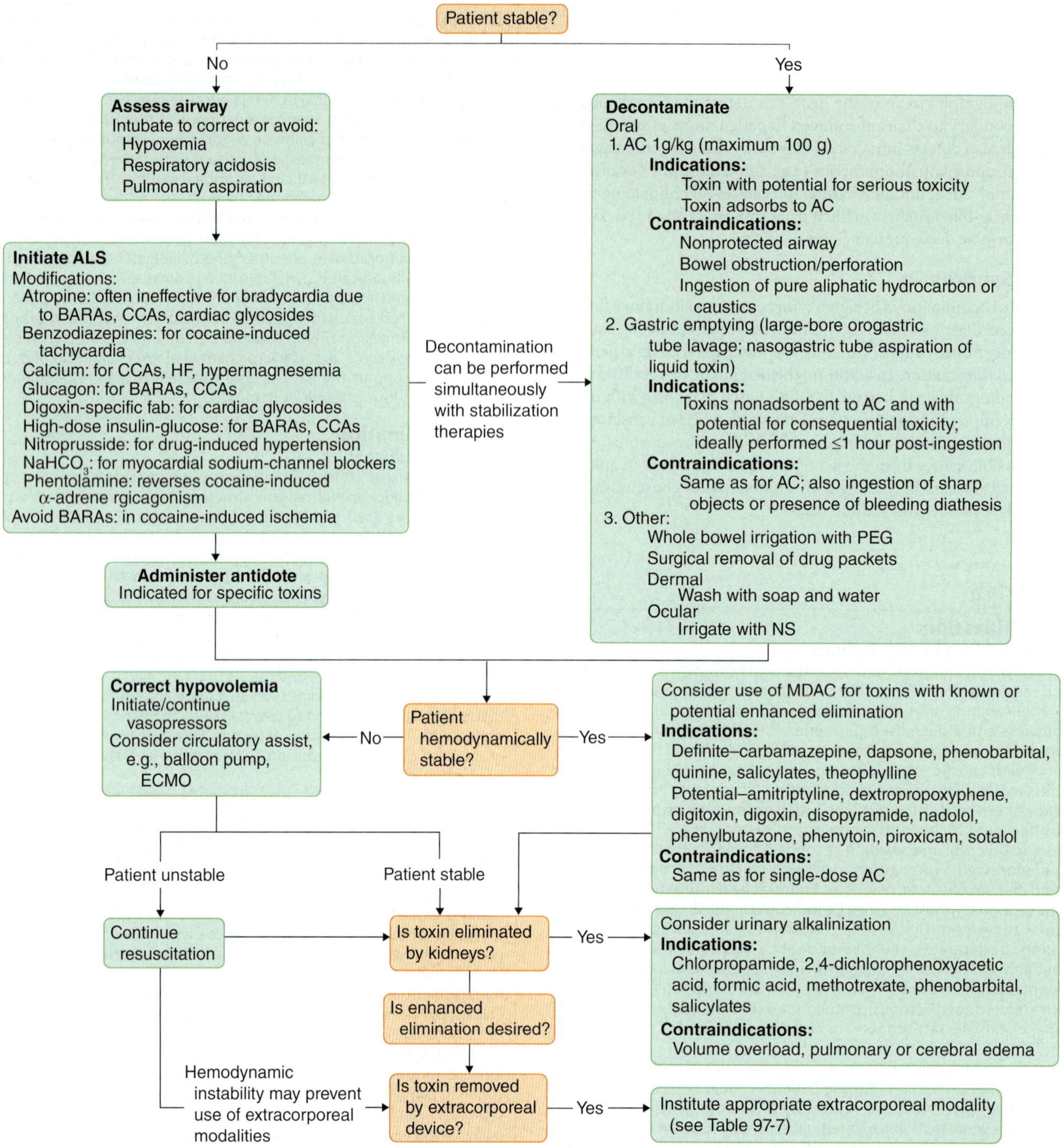

FIGURE 96-2. Algorithm for the management of acute poisoning. AC = activated charcoal; ALS = advanced life support; BARAs = β-adrenergic receptor antagonists; CCAs = L-type calcium-channel antagonists; ECMO = extracorporeal membrane oxygenation; HF = hydrofluoric acid; MDAC = multidose activated charcoal; NS = 0.9% saline solution; PEG = nonabsorbable polyethylene glycol solution.

adsorbed to activated charcoal, and for body packers (smugglers who swallow packets of illicit drugs, usually heroin or cocaine). The most common complication is vomiting, and whole bowel irrigation is contraindicated in patients with bowel perforation, obstruction, hemorrhage, or hemodynamic or respiratory instability. The initial recommended dose is 500 mL/hour given orally or by nasogastric tube, with titration to 2000 mL/hour as tolerated; treatment continues until the rectal effluent clears. Rarely, surgery may be necessary to remove packets in smugglers who have symptoms of cocaine toxicity or are obstructed; heroin toxicity is usually adequately managed with naloxone. Endoscopic removal of cocaine packets should never be attempted because of the risk of packet rupture.

Antidotes

Few toxicants have specific therapies (see Table 96-6). Although antidotes may be essential in treating patients exposed to certain toxicants, their use does not preclude the need for ongoing supportive care and, in some cases, extracorporeal elimination.

Enhanced Elimination

Methods to accelerate the elimination of toxicants or drugs from the body include multiple doses of activated charcoal, urinary alkalinization, and extracorporeal removal. Another method, using the oral ion exchange resins sodium polystyrene sulfonate and cholestyramine, has experimentally enhanced the elimination of lithium, digoxin, digitoxin, and organochlorines but has limited clinical usefulness.

Multiple Doses of Oral Activated Charcoal

The rationale for administering multiple doses of oral activated charcoal includes the adsorption of any toxic agent remaining in the gastrointestinal tract (e.g., sustained-release drugs or drugs that retard their absorption, such as anticholinergics), interference with the enterohepatic and enteroenteric recirculation of toxicants, and enhancement of the elimination of drugs with a long half-life, a volume of distribution less than 1 L/kg body weight, and low protein binding (termed gastrointestinal dialysis). The existing evidence shows enhanced elimination of carbamazepine, dapsone, phenobarbital, quinine, salicylates, and theophylline, but multiple doses of activated charcoal may also be effective for amitriptyline, dextropropoxyphene, digitoxin, digoxin, disopyramide, nadolol, phenytoin, piroxicam, and sotalol. Whether enhanced elimination provided by repeated doses of activated charcoal translates into decreased morbidity and mortality has not been adequately examined in large controlled clinical trials, except for yellow oleander and organophosphate ingestion, for which it has shown no benefit. The usual recommendations are an average dose of 12.5 g of activated charcoal (after the initial dose of 1 g/kg body weight, with a maximum single dose of 100 g) administered every 4 to 6 hours after the previous dose. The contraindications to single-dose activated charcoal also apply to multidose activated charcoal. Reported complications include pulmonary aspiration, bowel obstruction from inspissated charcoal, and fluid and electrolyte imbalance from multiple doses of a simultaneously administered cathartic.

Urinary Alkalinization

Alkalinization of the urine, which increases the renal elimination of weak acids, is used primarily to enhance the elimination of salicylates, but the elimination of chlorpropamide, 2,4-dichlorophenoxyacetic acid, formic acid, methotrexate, and phenobarbital may be increased with this method. Urinary alkalinization is accomplished by an intravenous bolus of 1 to 2 mEq of sodium bicarbonate per kilogram body weight, followed by three ampules (150 mL) of sodium bicarbonate (44 mEq/50 mL) in 850 mL of 5% dextrose in water infused at two to three times the normal maintenance fluid rate. Urinary pH should be checked hourly, and the infusion should be adjusted to maintain a urine pH of 7.5 to 8.0. Potassium should be administered simultaneously to avoid hypokalemia, which prevents urinary alkalinization because the distal tubule excretes hydrogen ion in exchange for potassium (Chapters 103 and 104). Serum pH should be monitored and kept below 7.55 to avoid excessive alkalemia. Contraindications to this therapy include volume overload and cerebral or pulmonary edema. Urinary acidification is not recommended to enhance the elimination of weak bases, such as amphetamines, because of the danger of precipitating tubular myoglobin in patients with rhabdomyolysis.

Extracorporeal Removal

Extracorporeal techniques enhance the elimination of a few drugs and toxicants, especially those that exist in the blood and are otherwise poorly eliminated.[17,18] Such drugs generally have single-compartment kinetics, a volume of distribution less than 1 L/kg, and endogenous clearance of less than 4 mL/minute/kg (Table 96-7). For hemodialysis, the toxicant must be water soluble, have a small molecular weight, and exhibit low protein binding. For continuous renal replacement therapy, the toxicant must have a molecular weight less than the permeability limit of the filter membrane. As a group, these latter forms of elimination are slow and likely to be of limited benefit to most patients with acute poisoning. Rarely, extracorporeal removal has been used for aminoglycosides, atenolol, bromide, carbamazepine, diethylene glycol, isopropanol, magnesium, metformin, methotrexate, *N*-acetylprocainamide, phenobarbital, procainamide, sotalol, and trichloroethanol (chloral hydrate).

TABLE 96-6 ANTIDOTES AND INDICATIONS FOR USE[§]

ANTIDOTE	INDICATION FOR USE	DOSE*	TREATMENT END POINT	COMMENTS
Antivenom, *Crotalidae* (Fab)[†,§] A3	Crotaline snake (e.g., rattlesnakes, copperhead; see Chapter 98)	Variable (several products available); initial dose followed by repeated doses as needed	Halt in progression of circumferential and proximal swelling Resolving systemic effects	Better safety profile than historical equine-derived antivenom Repetitive dosing indicated for recurrent soft tissue swelling Less effective at correcting hematologic (i.e., coagulation and platelet) disorders
Antivenom, *Latrodectus* (equine)[†,§]	Black widow spider (*Latrodectus* sp)	1 vial diluted in 50-100 mL NS, infused over 1 hour; can repeat	Resolution of symptoms, vital signs normal	Dilution and slow infusion rate are **critical** to avoid anaphylactoid reaction Indications include severe pain unresponsive to opioids and severe hypertension Serum sickness can occur IV calcium is ineffective
Atropine	Carbamates Nerve agents Organophosphorus compounds	2 mg IV; double the dose every 5 minutes to achieve atropinization and hemodynamic stability; then start continuous infusion of 10-20% of total stabilizing dose per hour	Cessation of excessive oral and pulmonary secretions, >80 beats/min, systolic blood pressure >80 mm Hg	Doubling of the dose every 5 minutes (e.g., 2 mg, 4 mg, 8 mg, 16 mg) estimated to achieve atropinization within 30 minutes Stop infusion when patient develops concerning signs or symptoms of anticholinergic toxidrome (see Table 96-1); restart infusion at lower rate when signs or symptoms abate
Calcium salt[‡]	Calcium-channel antagonists	Calcium gluconate 10%, 30 mL (3 g) over 10 minutes; can be given in 1 minute if critically ill Calcium chloride 10%, 10 mL (1 g) over 10 minutes; can be given in 1 minute if critically ill	Reversal of hypotension; may not reverse bradycardia	*All indications:* Monitor ionized calcium levels IV extravasation causes tissue necrosis, especially with calcium chloride Can administer at faster than stated rates for immediate life-threatening conditions (i.e., in 1 minute) Calcium chloride contains three times more elemental calcium than calcium gluconate does
	Hydrofluoric acid	Systemic toxicity: calcium gluconate 10%, 1-3 g (10-30 mL) per dose IV over 10-minute period; repeat as needed every 5-10 minutes Topical toxicity: calcium chloride 10%, 1 g (10 mL) mixed into water-soluble lubricant	Reversal of life-threatening manifestations of hypocalcemia and hyperkalemia Topical: reversal of severe neuropathic pain from dermal exposure	Can dilute and give intra-arterially or IV with a Bier block for extremity exposures and burns Topical: apply to skin under occlusive dressing
	Hyperkalemia (except due to cardiac glycosides)	Calcium gluconate 10%, 1 g (10 mL) per dose IV over 10-minute period; repeat as needed every 5-10 minutes	Reversal of myocardial depression and conduction delays	May precipitate ventricular dysrhythmias
	Hypermagnesemia	Calcium gluconate 10%, 1-2 g (10-20 mL) per dose IV over 10-minute period; repeat as needed every 5-10 minutes	Reversal of respiratory depression, hypotension, and cardiac conduction blocks	Simultaneous therapies to increase magnesium elimination should be instituted
	Hypocalcemia (e.g., ethylene glycol)	Calcium gluconate 10%, 0.5-1.0 g (5-10 mL) per dose over 10-minute period; repeat as needed every 10 minutes	Reversal of tetany	Correct symptomatic hypocalcemia; avoid excessive administration that may increase production of calcium oxalate crystals in ethylene glycol poisoning

TABLE 96-6 ANTIDOTES AND INDICATIONS FOR USE[§]—cont'd

ANTIDOTE	INDICATION FOR USE	DOSE*	TREATMENT END POINT	COMMENTS
L-Carnitine	Valproate-induced hyperammonemia or hepatotoxicity	100 mg/kg (maximum 6 g) IV over 30 minutes, then 15 mg/kg IV over 30-minute period q4h (maximum 6 g/day)	Treat until clinical improvement occurs	Levocarnitine is active form Adjust dose for end-stage renal disease
Cyanide antidote kit Hydroxocobalamin (preferred) Sodium thiosulfate	Cyanide	Hydroxocobalamin 5 g IV over 5 minutes (15 mL/min); second dose of 5 g if needed; the entire cyanide antidote kit is rarely indicated if hydroxocobalamin is available. Sodium thiosulfate 25%: 50 mL (12.5 g) IV over 10-minute period	Resolution of lactic acidosis and moderate to severe clinical signs and symptoms: seizures, coma, dyspnea, apnea, hypotension, bradycardia	Hydroxocobalamin causes red discoloration of urine and blood, may interfere with laboratory testing for carbon monoxide and lactate Sodium thiosulfate dosing can be repeated (the other components of the "cyanide antidote kit" cause methemoglobinemia and should not be administered to patients with possible carbon monoxide poisoning; e.g., fire exposure)
Deferoxamine	Iron salts	Initiate at 5 mg/kg/hr, titrate to 15 mg/kg/hr IV (maximum 8 g/day) Mild to moderate: administer for 6-12 hours Severe toxicity: administer for 24 hours	Resolution of clinical signs and symptoms Urine may appear rose-colored but is not a reliable marker for iron clearance Laboratory testing is unreliable while antidote is being received	Indications: symptomatic patients with lethargy, severe abdominal pain, hypovolemia, acidosis, shock; any symptomatic patient with peak serum iron level >350 g/dL Rate-related hypotension may occur Prolonged therapy can cause pulmonary toxicity
Digoxin-specific antibody fragments (Fab)	Digoxin Digitalis and related plants (e.g., oleander, lily of the valley) Other cardiac glycosides (e.g., bufadienolides [Bufo toads])	Unknown digoxin dose or serum level acute toxicity—10 vials; chronic toxicity—3-6 vials Digoxin dose known: number of vials = 2 × oral digoxin dose (mg) × 0.8 Digoxin serum level known: number of vials = [serum level (ng/mL) × weight (kg)] ÷ 100 Infuse dose over 30 minutes Plant or toad source of cardioactive steroid; 10-20 vials	Resolution of hyperkalemia, symptomatic bradydysrhythmias, ventricular dysrhythmias, Mobitz II or third-degree heart block	Each vial binds 0.5 mg of digoxin or digitoxin Monitor ECG and potassium levels Digoxin serum levels unreliable after antidote administered unless test is specific for free serum digoxin
Dimercaprol (BAL)	Arsenic salts Lead salts Mercury, elemental and inorganic salts	Inorganic arsenic: 3-5 mg/kg IM q4h for 48 hours and then q12h for 7 to 10 days Lead: 75 mg/m^2 (4 mg/kg) IM q4h for 5 days Inorganic mercury: 5 mg/kg IM, then 2.5 mg/kg IM q12h for 10 days or until patient is clinically improved	Arsenic: 24-hour urinary arsenic <50 μg/L Lead: encephalopathy resolved, blood lead level <100 μg/dL, and succimer therapy can be started Mercury, elemental and inorganic: 24-hour urinary mercury <20 μg/L	Formulated in peanut oil; painful IM injection is painful and is contraindicated in patients with peanut allergy Maximum adult dose is 3 g/day BAL started 4 hours before initiation of concomitant $CaNa_2EDTA$ for lead encephalopathy Dosing not well established for arsenic and elemental or inorganic mercury toxicity; not used for organic mercury poisoning Adverse effects: painful injections, fever, diaphoresis, agitation, headache, salivation, nausea and vomiting, hemolysis in G6PD-deficient patients, chelation of essential metals Check essential metal levels if chelation is prolonged Succimer is replacing BAL for many indications except lead encephalopathy Treatment end points for arsenic and mercury include improving clinical condition
Edetate calcium disodium ($CaNa_2EDTA$)	Lead	1500 mg/m^2/24 hr (maximum 3 g) by continuous infusion	Treat for 5 days, followed by 2-day hiatus; repeat until encephalopathy resolved, lead level <100 μg/dL, and succimer therapy can be started	Use in patients with lead encephalopathy or lead level >100 g/dL Administer BAL 4 hours before initiating $CaNa_2EDTA$ Hydrate patient and establish good urinary output before starting therapy Avoid thrombophlebitis by diluting in NS or D_5W to a concentration ≤0.5% Substitution of Na_2EDTA can cause fatal hypocalcemia

TABLE 96-6 ANTIDOTES AND INDICATIONS FOR USE§—cont'd

ANTIDOTE	INDICATION FOR USE	DOSE*	TREATMENT END POINT	COMMENTS
Flumazenil[A4]	Benzodiazepines	0.1 mg/min IV to a total dose of 1 mg Alternative: 0.2 mg IV over 2 min; repeat with 0.3 mg, then 0.5 mg. Total dose remains at 1.0 mg	Reversal of coma	Limit use to reversal of inadequate ventilation in benzodiazepine-toxic patients Acute benzodiazepine withdrawal may occur in patients dependent on benzodiazepines Increases intracranial pressure and risk for seizures in presence of underlying seizure disorder or ingestion of seizure-producing toxicants Monitor for resedation up to 2 hours after last dose
Folinic acid (tetrahydrofolic acid [leucovorin])	Methanol Methotrexate	Methanol intoxication: 50 mg IV q4h Methotrexate overdose: 100 mg/m^2 IV over 15-30 minutes q3-6h; dosing lower when used as "rescue" in chemotherapy	Methanol: methanol undetectable, metabolic acidosis cleared Methotrexate: serum level <1 × 10^{-8} mol/L	Essential therapy for both toxicants Little concern with excessive dosing when used for methotrexate overdose Methotrexate: large overdoses may require increased dose If indicated, glucarpidase administered 2-4 hours before or after folinic acid
Fomepizole	Ethylene glycol Methanol	Initial dose: 15 mg/kg IV bolus 10 mg/kg IV q12h for four doses (48 hr) All subsequent doses: 15 mg/kg IV q12h When hemodialysis (HD) performed: HD initiation: additional dose if >6 hours since last dose HD ongoing: q4h End of HD (based on time of last dose): <1 hour, no dose until next scheduled dose immediately after HD completion; 1-3 hours, 50% dose; >3 hours, 100% dose	For both: serum level <25 mg/dL and metabolic acidosis resolved	Start immediately if toxic alcohol suspected, without waiting for confirmatory levels Dose amount is not affected by interval timing of doses
Glucagon	β-Adrenergic receptor antagonists Calcium-channel antagonists	Bolus of 3-5 mg IV; can repeat to achieve clinical effect, then infusion of 2-10 mg/hr	Reversal of hypotension and bradycardia; taper infusion	Can precipitate vomiting; be prepared to protect airway Mild hyperglycemia occurs Maximum dosing amounts unknown; bolus doses up to 30 mg reported Duration of effect is 15 minutes; thus, infusion must be started immediately
Hydroxocobalamin	Cyanide	Initial: 5 g IV over 15-minute period Second dose: 5 g IV over 15 minutes to 2 hours; maximum total dose is 10 g Follow each hydroxocobalamin dose with sodium thiosulfate 25%: 50 mL (12.5 g) IV over 10-minute period	Resolution of lactic acidosis and moderate to severe clinical signs and symptoms: seizures, coma, dyspnea, apnea, hypotension, bradycardia	Can be administered IV push if patient is in cardiac arrest Do not give hydroxocobalamin and sodium thiosulfate through the same IV line Adverse effects: red discoloration of plasma, urine, mucous membranes, skin; transient hypertension Interference with laboratory colorimetric assays: Levels increased: bilirubin; creatinine; glucose; hemoglobin; magnesium; co-oximetry total Hb, COHb%, MetHb% Levels decreased: AST, ALT, creatinine, co-oximetry O_2Hb%
Hyperbaric oxygen (HBO)	Carbon monoxide COHb >25% independent of symptoms, 15% if pregnant Serious symptoms or findings with any elevated COHb concentration	3.0 atm pressure for 60 minutes (25 minutes O_2, 5 minutes air, 25 minutes O_2, 5 minutes air), then 2.0 atm for 65 minutes (30 minutes O_2, 5 minutes air, 30 minutes O_2), then "surface" to 1.0 atm	One treatment Repeated treatment controversial	Carbon monoxide: treatment protocols may vary HBO indicated for loss of consciousness; seizures; cerebellar dysfunction; impaired cognition; headache, nausea/vomiting persisting after 4 hours of O_2 therapy regardless of repeat carboxyhemoglobin level
Insulin-glucose (hyperinsulinemic euglycemic therapy)	Calcium-channel antagonists β-Adrenergic receptor antagonists	Regular insulin, 1 U/kg IV bolus, followed by 0.5-1 U/kg/hr; titrate up to 10 U/kg/hr as needed Titrate 50% dextrose IV to avoid hypoglycemia and replete serum potassium as needed	Reversal of myocardial depression	Initiate early to reverse myocardial depression Monitor glucose and potassium; hypoglycemia can occur during and after therapy Hyperglycemia results from calcium-channel antagonist–induced insulin resistance, and initial dextrose requirements may be less than anticipated Recovery may be heralded by normalization of glucose levels, with increased dextrose required to avoid hypoglycemia

TABLE 96-6 ANTIDOTES AND INDICATIONS FOR USE§—cont'd

ANTIDOTE	INDICATION FOR USE	DOSE*	TREATMENT END POINT	COMMENTS
Lipid emulsion	Cardiac toxicity from local anesthetics (e.g., bupivacaine, ropivacaine) and other lipophilic toxicants Provisional: verapamil, diltiazem, tricyclic antidepressants, bupropion, propranolol and other lipophilic toxicants	Use 20% formulation Initial bolus: 1.5 mL/kg IV during 1 minute, followed immediately by infusion of 0.25 mL/kg/min for 30-60 minutes Can repeat bolus for asystole	Return of hemodynamic stability	Use for other than bupivacaine based on animal experiments and human case reports Use if advanced life support measures fail and generally only if the patient is moribund; continue CPR as needed during drug administration
Methylene blue	Methemoglobin-producing agents	1-2 mg/kg body weight (0.1-0.2 mL/kg of 1%) methylene blue IV over 5-minute period; repeat dose for persistent or recurrent symptoms or signs	Resolution of dyspnea and altered mental status	Use if patient is symptomatic (i.e., dyspneic, altered mental status) Maximum dose should not exceed 7 mg/kg (0.7 mL/kg) Contraindicated in G6PD-deficient patients; may cause hemolysis Some toxicants (e.g., dapsone) may require prolonged therapy
N-Acetylcysteine (NAC)	Acetaminophen[A5] Other hepatotoxins: carbon tetrachloride, chloroform, pennyroyal oil, amatoxin[16]	Intravenous (preferred) Load: 150 mg/kg over 1-hour period Maintenance infusion: 12.5 mg/kg/hr over 4-hour period, then 6.25 mg/kg/hr over 16 hours as continuous infusion Oral (total 72 hours) Load: 140 mg/kg Maintenance (starting 4 hours after load): 70 mg/kg q4h × 17 doses IV (total 21 hours)	At the end of therapy, repeat AST and APAP levels: if AST normal and APAP not detected, treatment complete; if AST normal and APAP detected, continue NAC; if AST elevated, continue NAC After patient has received full course of NAC therapy, if INR ≥2.0 or severe hepatotoxicity present (AST > 1000 U/L), continue NAC until INR <2.0 and aminotransferases normalize	Most effective if initiated within 8 hours after acetaminophen ingestion; may be started any time after ingestion and is beneficial in patients with severe hepatotoxicity Longer duration of treatment may be required in patients with persistently elevated acetaminophen levels or ongoing hepatotoxicity Treatment end points simplified for ease of use INR result not valid indicator if fresh frozen plasma recently administered
Naloxone	Opioids	Possible opioid dependence: 40-50 μg (0.04-0.05 mg) IV titrated upward to reverse symptoms while providing respiratory support if needed and cautiously avoiding withdrawal Opioid dependence not likely: 0.4 mg by any route and titrate up to 10 mg Intranasal naloxone (2-4 mg) may be given if IM/IV not possible Continuous infusion: establish bolus dose required to reverse respiratory depression; begin infusing two thirds of reversal dose every hour and titrate to maintain adequate respirations; repeated bolus with half of reversal dose 15 minutes after reversal of respiratory depression	Initial: reversal of respiratory depression with resolution of hypoxemia and hypercapnia Final: resolution of CNS and respiratory depression Avoid rapid and full awakening in opioid-dependent patients to avoid precipitating opioid withdrawal Since the duration of naloxone is shorter than most opioids, re-sedation may occur—so several hours of observation is optimal	Pre-ventilate patients with respiratory depression by bag-valve-mask or intubation before administration Use smaller doses in opioid-dependent patients Some opioids (e.g., buprenorphine) may require larger doses of naloxone (fentanyl does not) Use continuous infusion for recurrent symptoms and prolonged action of some formulations (e.g., sustained-release morphine, methadone) Re-sedation can occur Do not use naltrexone to reverse acute toxicity
Octreotide	Sulfonylurea-induced hypoglycemia	50 μg SQ q6h	Resolution of hypoglycemia and dextrose no longer required to maintain euglycemia	Maintain dextrose infusion as needed Not for insulin-induced hypoglycemia
Physostigmine	Anticholinergic agents (e.g., diphenhydramine, jimsonweed [*Datura* sp], scopolamine)	1-2 mg IV during 5-minute period; can repeat in 5 minutes if no effect and cholinergic effects do not occur	Reversal of anticholinergic effects	Duration of effect is 60-90 minutes Benzodiazepine used for subsequent treatment of agitation and seizures; additional physostigmine used rarely (e.g., refractory seizures or agitation) Adverse effects include seizures, excessive oral secretions, bradydysrhythmias; contraindicated in cyclic antidepressant toxicity

TABLE 96-6 ANTIDOTES AND INDICATIONS FOR USE[§]—cont'd

ANTIDOTE	INDICATION FOR USE	DOSE*	TREATMENT END POINT	COMMENTS
Pralidoxime chloride	Organophosphorus compounds Nerve agents: sarin, VX	30 mg/kg IV bolus (maximum 2 g) over 30 minutes, followed by continuous infusion of 8-10 mg/kg/hr (maximum 650 mg/hr)	Resolution of signs and symptoms, atropine no longer required	Can give initial dose over 2-minute period for life-threatening clinical events Administer early when diagnosis known or strongly suspected Efficacy variable, depending on the organophosphate Fat-soluble organophosphates may require prolonged treatment
Pyridoxine	Ethylene glycol Isoniazid Monomethylhydrazine (*Gyromitra esculenta* mushrooms)	100 mg IV (ethylene glycol) 5 g IV, repeat for refractory seizures	One dose Resolution of seizures	Efficacy theoretical for ethylene glycol to enhance elimination of toxic metabolites Pyridoxine may be required even with benzodiazepines to stop seizures, but patient can remain comatose (isoniazid, *Gyromitra* mushrooms) Excessive dosing can cause neuropathy
Sodium bicarbonate ($NaHCO_3$)	Reversal of myocardial sodium-channel blockers (e.g., cyclic antidepressants, cocaine, sodium-channel–blocking antiarrhythmics with $\tau_{recovery}$ >1 second, piperidine phenothiazines (thioridazine, mesoridazine)	1-2 mEq $NaHCO_3$/kg by intermittent IV bolus; repeat as needed	Narrowing of prolonged QRS, resolution of ventricular dysrhythmias, reversal of hypotension	Monitor blood pH (optimal pH approximately 7.50); avoid pH > 7.55
	Altered tissue distribution or enhanced elimination of salicylates; may be used for chlorophenoxy herbicides, formic acid, methotrexate, phenobarbital	1-2 mEq $NaHCO_3$/kg, followed by 3 ampules (150 mL) $NaHCO_3$ (44 mEq per 50 mL) in 850 mL of D_5W, infused at two to three times normal maintenance fluid rate	Serum salicylate <30 mg/dL and patient clinically stable	Target blood pH: 7.50-7.55 Monitor urinary pH hourly; adjust infusion to maintain urine pH of 7.5-8.0 (avoid blood pH >7.55) Monitor ABGs Maintain normokalemia to allow urinary alkalinization
Succimer (DMSA)	Arsenic Lead Mercury, all forms	10 mg/kg/dose q8h for 5 days, followed by q12h for 14 days Drug holiday for 2 weeks; repeat if treatment end point not reached	Arsenic: 24-hour urinary arsenic <50 µg/L Lead: resolution of encephalopathy, gastrointestinal symptoms, neuropathy, nephropathy, arthralgias, myalgias, and blood lead level <70 µg/dL Mercury, elemental and inorganic: 24-hour urinary mercury <20 µg/L Mercury, organic: end point not well established	Oral chelator; adverse effects include rash, transient AST and alkaline phosphatase elevations, and gastrointestinal distress; minimal chelation of essential metals occurs Dosing for arsenic and mercury not well established Therapeutic end point for organic mercury not established; neurotoxicity not responsive to chelation therapy; suggest chelation until blood mercury level within normal value range for reference laboratory
Vitamin K	Vitamin K antagonist anticoagulants (e.g., warfarin, long-acting anticoagulant rodenticides [LAARs]) (note this is not for normalizing a supratherapeutic INR in patients prescribed warfarin)	Subcutaneous: phytonadione (K_1), 10-25 mg, repeat every 6-12 hours until oral vitamin K_1 started Oral: 25-50 mg q6h; larger doses may be required	INR is normal 48-72 hours after stopping vitamin K_1 therapy Can also monitor factor VII activity	Anaphylactoid reaction can occur with rapid IV administration Severe bleeding may also require FFP, prothrombin protein concentrate (off-label), or factor concentrates Base decision to treat on finding of elevated INR; do not administer prophylactic vitamin K_1 Oral therapy may be required for months with LAAR poisoning because of lipophilicity of toxicant, with slow body clearance

*Dose concentrations and infusion times are not given. Drug dosages may require adjustment in patients with renal or hepatic failure.
[†]Administer antivenom in a monitored setting; antivenom must be reconstituted and then diluted; initially infuse at a rate of 2 to 5 mL/hr, and double the infusion rate every 5 minutes as tolerated to administer antivenom during a 1-hour period.
[‡]Ten percent calcium chloride solution = 100 mg/mL (27.2 mg/mL elemental calcium); 10% calcium gluconate solution = 100 mg/mL (9 mg/mL elemental calcium).
[§]See also Chapter 98.
[¶]Given the relative infrequency of use of these antidotes, it is prudent that, when possible, the indications, alternatives, and doses for these antidotes should be confirmed if possible with a poison control center or medical toxicologist.
ABGs = arterial blood gases; ALT = alanine aminotransferase; APAP = acetyl-*p*-aminophenol (acetaminophen); AST = aspartate aminotransferase; BAL = British antilewisite; CNS = central nervous system; COHb% = percentage carboxyhemoglobin; CPR, cardiopulmonary resuscitation; D_5W = 5% dextrose in water; DMSA = 2,3-dimercaptosuccinic acid; ECG = electrocardiogram; FFP = fresh-frozen plasma; G6PD = glucose-6-phosphate dehydrogenase; Hb = hemoglobin; HD = hemodialysis; INR = international normalized ratio; IV = intravenous; MetHb% = percentage methemoglobinemia; NS = normal saline; $O_2Hb\%$ = percentage oxyhemoglobin; SQ = subcutaneous; $\tau_{recovery}$ = drug blockade recovery rate.

TABLE 96-7 COMMON TOXICANTS REMOVED BY HEMODIALYSIS

TOXICANT	INDICATIONS	COMMENTS
Ethylene glycol	Serum level ≥50 mg/dL, or lower levels with concomitant metabolic acidosis and evidence of end-organ toxicity, or if fomepizole not available	Not routinely required in a patient with normal creatinine clearance and acid-base status who is receiving fomepizole
Lithium*	Clinical indications, primarily CNS toxicity (e.g., decreased level of consciousness, ataxia, coma, seizures) in patients with an elevated blood lithium concentration	Use dialysate containing bicarbonate to decrease Na^+/K^+ antiporter intracellular sequestration of lithium
Methanol	Serum level ≥50 mg/dL, or lower levels with concomitant metabolic acidosis and evidence of end-organ toxicity, or if fomepizole not available	Usually required because of slow elimination half-life in presence of fomepizole (mean, 52 hours; range, 22-87 hours), even in patients with no metabolic acidosis or evidence of end-organ toxicity
Phenobarbital	Clinical indications (e.g., deep coma)	Rarely necessary except when a patient is hemodynamically unstable despite aggressive support
Salicylates	Acute toxicity: serum level ≥100 mg/dL without clinical abnormality or <100 mg/dL in the presence of a clinical indication. Chronic toxicity: any clinical indication, typically altered mental status	Serum protein binding decreases with increasing toxic levels, increasing the amount of free salicylate available for HD removal; clinical indications are one or more of the following: impaired kidney function, altered mental status, seizures, pulmonary edema, intractable acidosis
Valproic acid	Severe intoxication with serum concentration >900 mg/L	Clinical indications include hepatic dysfunction; coma, especially with hyperammonemia; deteriorating clinical status despite aggressive support

*Hemodiafiltration removes lithium; the clinical benefit of this technique is unknown.
CNS = central nervous system; HD = hemodialysis.

PROGNOSIS

Almost all patients who reach the hospital alive survive with appropriate care. Inpatient mortality rates are 0.2 to 0.5%.

GENERAL REFERENCES

For the General References and other additional features, please visit Elsevier eBooks+ at https://ebooks.health.elsevier.com.

Grade A References

A1. Vijayakumar HN, Kannan S, Tejasvi C, et al. Study of effect of magnesium sulphate in management of acute organophosphorous pesticide poisoning. *Anesth Essays Res*. 2017;11:192-196.

A2. Juurlink DN. Activated charcoal for acute overdose: a reappraisal. *Br J Clin Pharmacol*. 2016;81:482-487.

A3. Gerardo CJ, Quackenbush E, Lewis B, et al. The efficacy of crotalidae polyvalent immune fab (ovine) antivenom versus placebo plus optional rescue therapy on recovery from copperhead snake envenomation: a randomized, double-blind, placebo-controlled, clinical trial. *Ann Emerg Med*. 2017;70:233-244.e3.

A4. Razavizadeh AS, Zamani N, Ziaeefar P, et al. Protective effect of flumazenil infusion in severe acute benzodiazepine toxicity: a pilot randomized trial. *Eur J Clin Pharmacol*. 2021;77:547-554.

A5. Chiew AL, Gluud C, Brok J, et al. Interventions for paracetamol (acetaminophen) overdose. *Cochrane Database Syst Rev*. 2018;2:CD003328.

97 MEDICAL ASPECTS OF TRAUMA AND BURNS

ROBERT L. SHERIDAN

Injured or burned patients are complex to manage not only because of the vast number of potential anatomic derangements but also because of the complex physiologic cascades triggered by injury. Although most intense after extensive burns, stereotypical physiologic derangements are a characteristic of all injuries. As a result, needed interventions are often predictable regardless of the mechanism of injury.

EPIDEMIOLOGY

In the United States alone each year, about 2.5 million people are injured and about 35,000 to 40,000 are killed in automobile crashes, whereas about 120,000 are injured and about 40,000 are killed by gunshots. Burns and falls follow in frequency. Worldwide, injury by trauma and burns is the leading cause of death in children and young adults.[1] In the United States, injury follows only cancer and heart disease as a cause of death. Many long-term survivors of trauma and burns have high degrees of disability, which creates a particularly difficult and expensive problem given the young age of many victims.

The time of death after injury has a trimodal distribution. At least 50% of fatalities occur within minutes of the injury as a result of massive hemorrhage or nonsurvivable brain injury. Approximately one third of deaths occur within a few hours of injury, usually by hemorrhage, anoxia, or progressive brain trauma. This interval provides an opportunity for emergent intervention. Later fatalities are usually the result of multisystem organ dysfunction or overwhelming infection in the days and weeks after the injury. The likelihood of surviving a severe injury is better in communities that are closer to major trauma centers.[2]

PATHOBIOLOGY

Early Local Response to Injury

The local response to blunt, penetrating, electrical, crush, thermal, blast, or other injury varies with the energy transferred. All are associated with some degree of secondary injury by progressive microvascular thrombosis, progressive edema, and secondary compromise of perfusion. The most common preventable mechanisms are related to progressive edema beneath an inelastic eschar or fascial compartments or direct injury to vascular inflow or outflow.

Early Systemic Response to Injury

The early systemic response to burns and local trauma is driven by fluid loss and release of vasoactive mediators from injured tissue. In more severe injuries, including surface burns greater than about 20% of the body surface, interstitial edema develops in unburned skin as well as in distant organs and soft tissues. These distant microvascular effects, which can compromise the function of organs that were not directly injured, explain the frequent occurrence of pulmonary and other organ dysfunctions in patients with large burns.

The capillary leak syndrome, in which the leak is typically proportional to the scope of the injury, is caused by the release of vasoactive substances from the injured and reperfused tissue. As a result, during the first 18 to 24 hours after a serious burn, both electrolytes and large colloid molecules freely diffuse into the interstitial space.

Late Local Response to Injury

At about 72 hours after the initial trauma, local wound issues are particularly important in patients who have extensive soft tissue damage, especially after burns or crush injury with extensive volumes of devitalized tissue. Tissue that has been crushed or suffered reduced blood flow is subject to progressive necrosis. As bacteria multiply in the avascular tissue during the succeeding days, proteases liquefy the eschar and necrotic tissue, which then separates and leaves a bed of granulation tissue. In healthy patients with

TABLE 97-1 INJURY CLASSES

INJURY CLASS	CLINICAL IMPLICATIONS	COMMON ERRORS
Blunt	Graded soft tissue and bone injury, edema Occult vascular or visceral injury	Delayed consequences of edema Missed visceral injury and secondary consequences
Penetrating	Soft tissue and bone injuries vary with energy of injuring object (e.g., knife vs. fragment vs. bullet) Occult vascular or visceral injury	Missed vascular or visceral injury Secondary consequences of missed vascular injury
Thermal	Graded soft tissue injury (first- to fourth-degree burns) Capillary leak phenomenon	Inadequate appreciation of capillary leak phenomenon and consequent under-resuscitation Inaccurate wound evaluation and over-resuscitation Unanticipated local injury progression
Electrical	Range of soft tissue injury with increasing voltage and contact duration and quality	Occult cardiac and muscle injury Secondary compartment syndrome complications
Crush	Graded soft tissue, bone, and visceral injury with secondary consequences of edema and of reperfusion	Underappreciation of injury severity Missed muscle ischemia due to primary ischemia and to reperfusion edema
Blast	Graded injury severity (primary to quaternary injury patterns) Occult visceral injury	Underappreciation of secondary, tertiary, and quaternary components of injury Missed associated visceral injury
Fragmentation injury	Multiple unpredictable penetrations with associated visceral and vascular injury	Missed visceral and vascular injury Associated blast trauma

smaller wounds and burns (<20% of the body surface), this septic process is usually tolerated. When injuries are larger, however, systemic infection results and explains the rare survival of patients who have burns in excess of 40% of body surface area or who have massive soft tissue injuries with incomplete early wound excision.

Late Hypermetabolic Systemic Response to Injury

Successfully resuscitated patients with large burns or major non-burn trauma demonstrate an initial decrease in cardiac output and metabolic rate. After successful resuscitation, a hypermetabolic response occurs, with a near doubling of cardiac output and resting energy expenditure during the next 24 to 72 hours. The magnitude of the response, which becomes greater with larger burns and more severe injuries, peaks at up to twice the normal metabolic rate in otherwise healthy patients with burn involving 60% or more of the body surface area. This hypermetabolic response is characterized by enhanced gluconeogenesis, insulin resistance, and increased protein catabolism. Although the causes of these physiologic changes are not well understood, they seem to involve the systemic release of bacterial products, the breakdown of gastrointestinal barrier dysfunction with translocation of bacteria and their byproducts into the circulation, and increases in the secretion of glucagon, cortisol, and catecholamines.

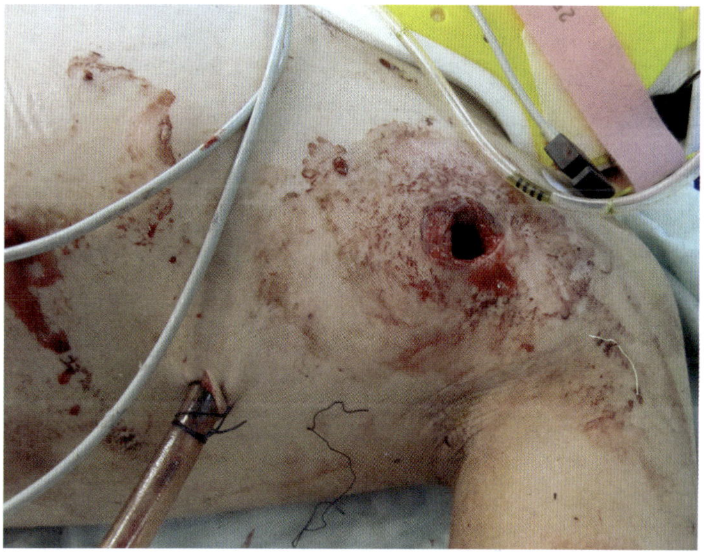

FIGURE 97-1. Penetrating injury often is associated with visceral and bone trauma.

CLINICAL MANIFESTATIONS

Common mechanisms of injury include blunt, penetrating, electrical, thermal, blast, and crush (Table 97-1), often in combination. For example, patients crushed in building collapses frequently suffer a concomitant penetrating component, and patients who suffer high-voltage injury frequently fall from a height, such as a utility pole. In all mechanisms, edema or vascular injury can compromise perfusion and lead to secondary injury.

Blunt injury is commonly seen in motor vehicle accidents and falls. Injuries are often multisystem. Penetrating soft tissue injuries vary widely (Fig. 97-1), but the overarching concern is the possibility of occult injury to vascular, bone, or visceral structures. The degree of trauma is directly related to the energy of the injury. For example, high-velocity gunshots cause greater injury than lower velocity rounds because they create a local blast effect, called cavitation, along their trajectory.

Thermal injury (Fig. 97-2) by whatever mechanism (flame, scald, contact) is associated with a graded soft tissue injury described in degrees. As thermal injuries increase beyond about 15% of the body surface, a diffuse capillary leak phenomenon occurs that continues for 18 to 24 hours after injury and involves both burned and unburned tissue. This phenomenon can result in cardiovascular collapse and is the key physiologic derangement underlying the shock state accompanying burns.[3]

The severity of electrical injuries (Fig. 97-3) varies with voltage, current flow, and contact quality. Low-voltage injuries are rarely associated with distant sequelae, whereas high-voltage injuries are commonly associated with compartment syndromes, cardiac complications, pigmenturia, and other trauma.

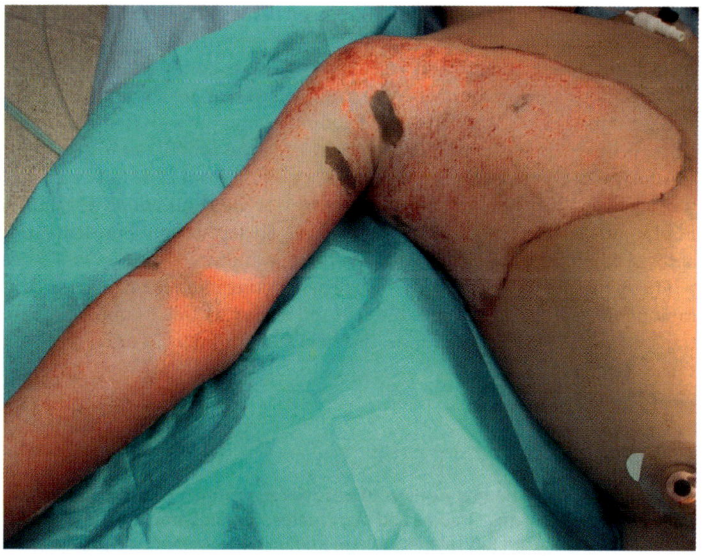

FIGURE 97-2. **Thermal injury is of variable depth.** Initial evaluation usually underestimates this depth.

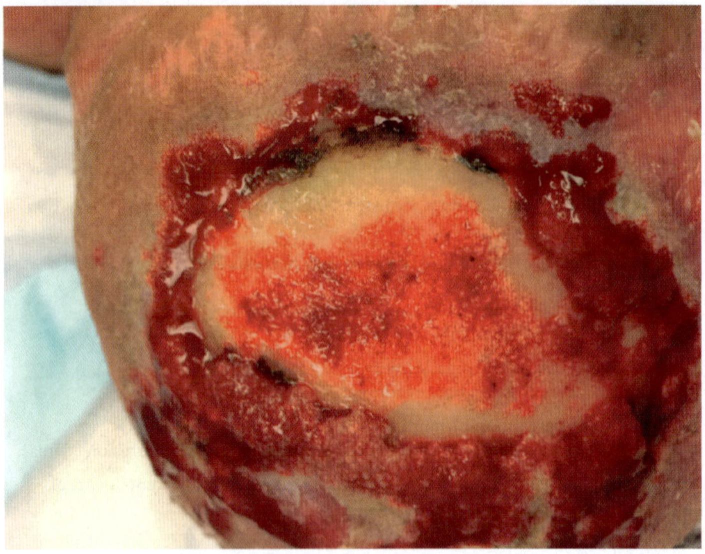

FIGURE 97-3. Electrical injury can be associated with a number of systemic sequelae, depending on current strength and pattern of flow.

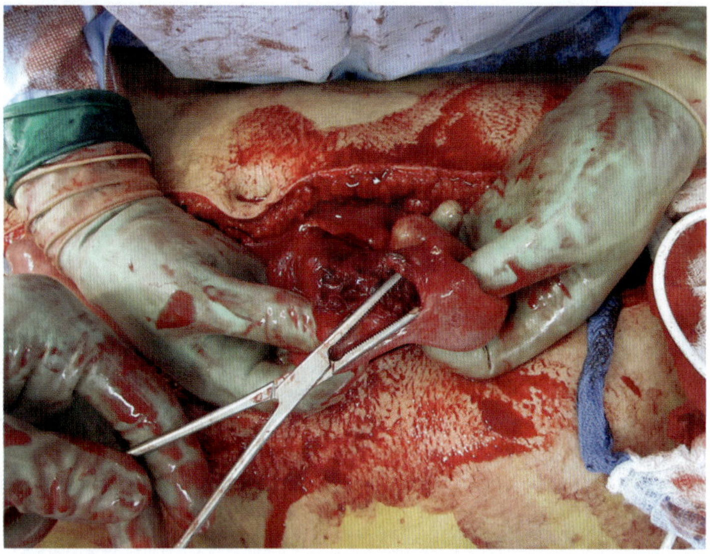

FIGURE 97-5. Blast injury is a complex of four injury subtypes. Missed injuries are common.

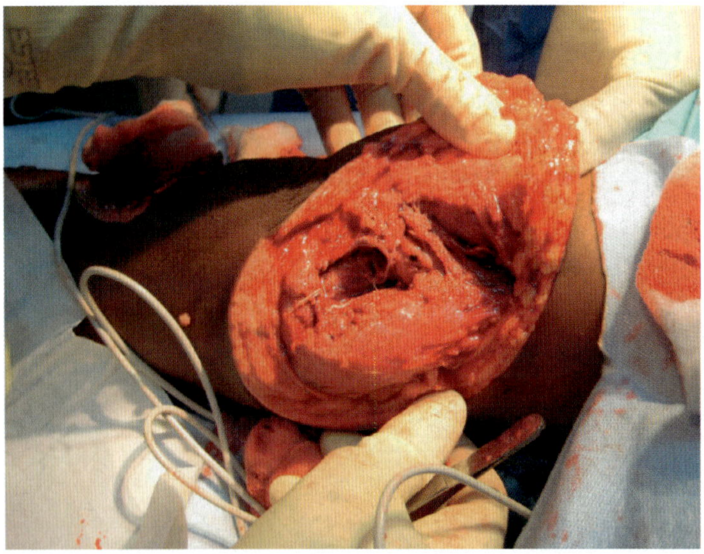

FIGURE 97-4. Crush injury is often associated with underappreciated deep muscle injury.

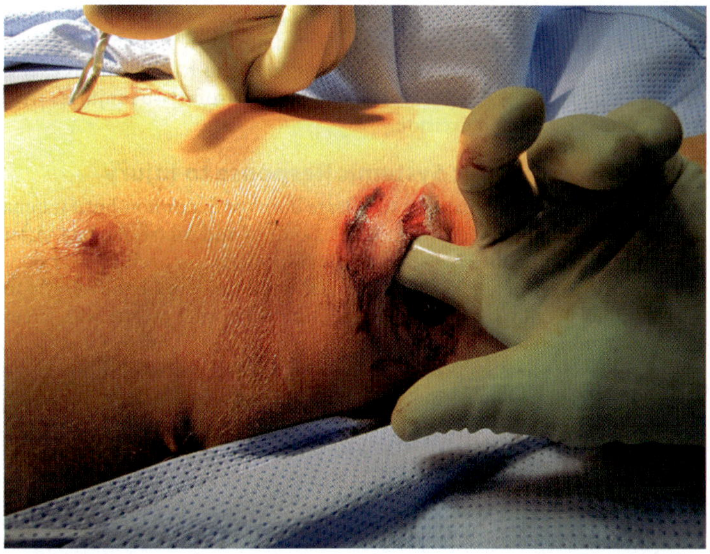

FIGURE 97-6. Fragmentation injury is a particular form of penetrating injury frequently associated with missed injuries.

Crush injuries (Fig. 97-4) include direct soft tissue injuries as well as secondary ischemic damage due to a compartment syndrome or ischemia-reperfusion. Associated bone, visceral, and vascular injuries are common. Major septic complications are common when necrotic soft tissues are left unexcised.

Blast injuries (Fig. 97-5) are graded complex injuries with four characteristics: primary injury to air-filled structures and the central nervous system, secondary injury from flying debris, tertiary injury from collisions with stationary objects, and quaternary injury from associated crush or other trauma. Blast injuries of all types can be subtle or have a delayed clinical presentation, and visceral injuries often are not diagnosed promptly.

Fragmentation injuries (Fig. 97-6) are penetrating injuries characterized by multiple foreign bodies of variable size and energy as well as unpredictable trajectories. As with blast injuries, the full extent of injury is often underestimated initially.

DIAGNOSIS AND TREATMENT

Complex burns and trauma are most successfully and cost-effectively managed in high-volume programs.[4] Trauma and burn center programs emphasize the comprehensive nature of injury care, including community involvement with injury prevention programs, thorough prehospital care, early resuscitation and surgery, and long-term rehabilitation and reconstruction. Most programs include embedded specialty intensive care units and operating rooms. Multidisciplinary staff include physicians, physician assistants, nurse practitioners, nurses, physical and occupational therapists, respiratory therapists, psychiatrists, social workers, and nurse administrators. Coordination and scheduled communication are essential.

Care of individual patients with serious multisystem injury is complex and requires a longitudinal four-phase approach.[5] Phase One, which describes the initial evaluation and resuscitation, generally is completed in the first 24 hours. Phase Two includes initial wound excision for burn patients and initial resuscitative surgery and fracture stabilization for non-burn trauma patients. This phase frequently overlaps with Phase One but is usually completed within 72 hours. Phase Three involves definitive wound closure for burns and the completion of surgery for trauma patients. The duration of this phase varies greatly with injury but is usually complete at the time of discharge. Phase Four describes the sometimes long process of reconstruction, rehabilitation, and reintegration. This phase of care commonly spans the later part of the acute hospitalization, inpatient rehabilitation, and variable amounts of time in the home-based setting.

Prehospital Care and Interhospital Transport

When prehospital and interhospital transfers are being arranged, key issues include control of the airway, secure venous access, placement of bladder and nasogastric catheters, maintenance of body temperature, fluid administration if transport time will be more than 1 hour, documentation of the events of the injury from personnel who will not be available to the receiving facility, efforts to notify family members, and clear documentation of all interventions.

Hypothermia (Chapter 95) is a particular problem in burn patients because of their evaporative heat losses. Transporting vehicles and emergency department receiving areas should be heated before the patient's arrival. Initial burn dressings should be dry, clean sheets rather than wetted dressings. Cooling of a wound involving less than 15% of the body surface within minutes of injury may help limit burn depth without causing systemic hypothermia, whereas cooling after a few minutes is generally unhelpful.

Phase One: Initial Evaluation and Resuscitation

Primary Survey

The organized approach to the initial evaluation of injured patients requires primary and subsequent patient surveys. The primary survey is an initial look for major aberrations in airway, circulatory, or neurologic status that justify emergent intervention. The airway is controlled with intubation if needed. Clinically obvious pneumothoraces (Chapter 86) should be decompressed, and hemothoraces must be diagnosed and drained. In suspicious cases, pericardial tamponade (Chapter 62) can usually be documented or excluded by handheld bedside ultrasonography. Vascular access is obtained and fluid resuscitation started. A very brief neurologic assessment (Chapter 366), including use of the Glasgow Coma Scale, is critical.

Secondary Survey

The secondary survey includes a much more detailed head-to-toe physical examination after the patient has a reliable airway and has been hemodynamically stabilized. The physical examination should assess for evidence of closed head injury, skull and facial fractures, and eye and ear injuries, with a low threshold for a head computed tomography (CT) scan. The neck must be stabilized and assessed for possible injury. Burns should be categorized as first-degree burns, involving only the epidermis; second-degree burns, involving variable amounts of dermis; third-degree burns, involving the entire dermis; and fourth-degree burns, involving fat, muscle, and bone.

A constant concern is the potentially missed injury. In the chaos of initial care, major issues can be missed if they do not have a dramatic initial presentation. Unfortunately, many injuries, such as epidural hematoma and small bowel perforations, are initially subtle and become catastrophic hours or days later. The best way to deal with this difficult reality is to have a highly organized approach that includes both a detailed initial evaluation and subsequent reevaluation so that all potential injuries are considered and reasonably excluded.

Projectiles often follow an unpredictable course through tissue and bone, thereby increasing the likelihood of missed injury. Missed visceral injury is also common with fragmentation injuries, especially because surgical exploration of all potential sites of injury is often impractical. Selected exploration is guided by initial and serial examination and by imaging when available.

Appropriate laboratory and imaging studies should be obtained. The fundamental goal is to consider carefully the injury mechanism and to exclude all potential occult injuries to a reasonable level of confidence. High-energy injuries, such as electrical burns, motor vehicle crashes, and blasts, are notorious for generating significant injuries that are missed during the initial evaluation. Bedside ultrasonography has emerged as a routine, rapid, and repeatable method to assess for abdominal fluid, usually blood. CT scanning of the head, chest, abdomen, and pelvis is justified if the mechanism of injury is consistent with head or abdominal trauma, and conventional imaging with selective CT scanning is as good as immediate total-body CT scanning.[A1] Rapid imaging has largely supplanted operative exploration for diagnostic purposes, except in unstable patients, in whom immediate operative exploration is performed for ongoing hemorrhage.

Chest Injuries

Tension pneumothorax (Chapter 86), hemothorax, cardiac tamponade (Chapter 62), flail chest, open pneumothorax, and disruption of the thoracic aorta (Chapter 63) are among the life-threatening injuries that should be considered during the primary and secondary surveys. All trauma patients should have a supine chest radiograph to examine the lung fields, mediastinal contour, and chest wall. Thoracic aortic injury is usually an immediately fatal complication of severe acceleration-deceleration injury, but some patients may have a contained mediastinal hematoma that requires urgent diagnosis and medical or surgical management.

Myocardial contusion should be suspected in patients with blunt trauma, especially if they have a sternal fracture or anterior rib fractures. Such blunt cardiac injuries can result in electrocardiographic abnormalities, ventricular arrhythmias, and cardiogenic shock. Coronary artery injuries are uncommon, although lacerations and dissections can occur and require emergent percutaneous coronary intervention similar to a typical ST elevation myocardial infarction (Chapter 58).

Commotio cordis is sudden cardiac arrest (Chapter 50) after acute blunt chest trauma from softballs, baseballs, hockey pucks, or collisions. The trauma presumably occurs during an electrically vulnerable period between 30 and 15 msec before the T-wave peak and produces ventricular fibrillation. Death is essentially universal unless the victim receives immediate cardiopulmonary resuscitation.

Abdominal Injuries

The liver and spleen are the most frequently injured intra-abdominal organs. Suggested findings on physical examination include lower rib fractures, upper

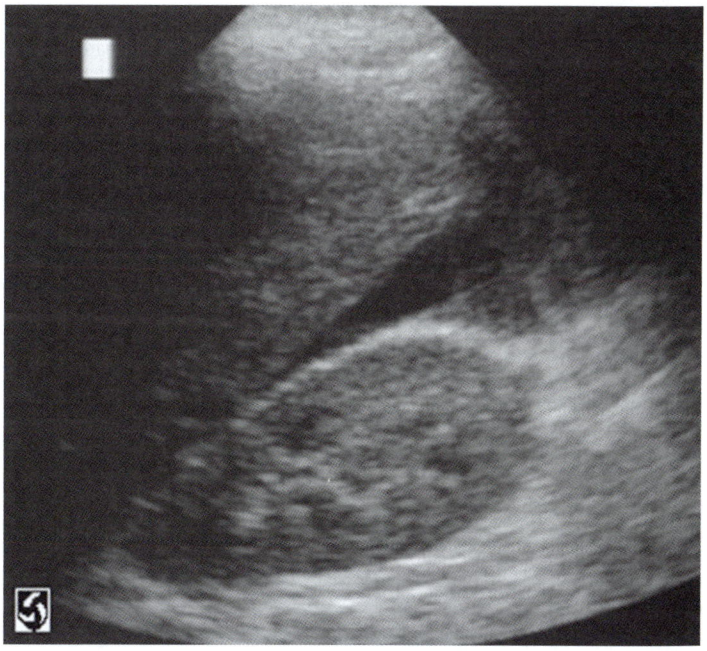

FIGURE 97-7. Positive focal abdominal sonography in trauma (FAST) study. There is a collection of fluid that shows up as a black strip between the liver and kidney. The white appearance is fat around the kidney. These findings are consistent with a fluid collection in the Morison pouch. (Courtesy Robert H. Demling, MD.)

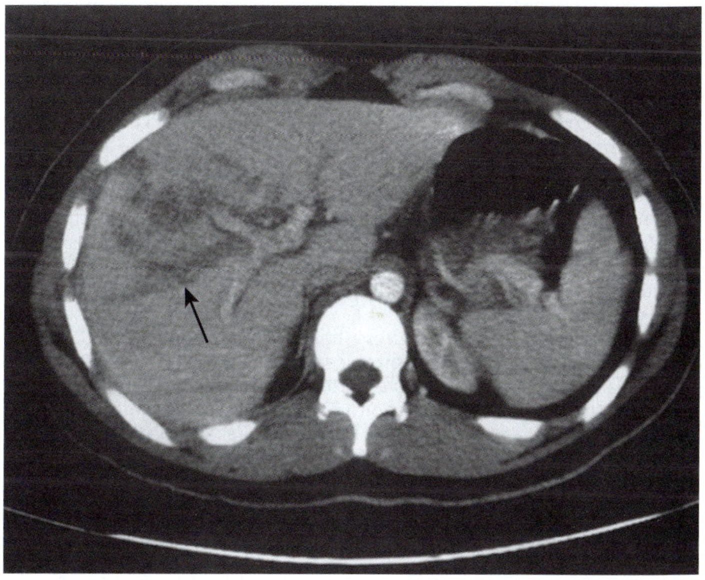

FIGURE 97-8. Abdominal injury. An abdominal computed tomography scan shows an injury to the right lobe of the liver (*arrow*). (Courtesy Robert H. Demling, MD.)

quadrant pain or tenderness, and pain referred to the shoulder secondary to diaphragmatic irritation. CT scanning is the test of choice. High-grade injuries require surgery, but most lesser injuries can be managed nonoperatively. Focused abdominal sonography has a sensitivity of 95% for detection of free blood in the abdomen (Fig. 97-7) but is not usually able to identify the source. An alternative in unstable patients or in austere environments is diagnostic peritoneal aspiration or lavage. Abdominal CT is a reliable determinant of both intraperitoneal and retroperitoneal injury (Fig. 97-8) and is preferable to diagnostic aspiration or lavage in stable patients. For selected stable patients whose blunt liver or spleen injury is originally treated nonoperatively, discharge on day 3 may be as safe as discharge on day 5, provided that the patient is stable and does not have other indications for continued hospitalization.[A2]

Head and Spine Injuries

Neurologic issues often dominate the quality of long-term outcome. The initial evaluation of the neurotrauma patient focuses on detection of reversible causes of elevated intracranial pressure or reduced perfusion (Chapter 368), but routine measurement of intracranial pressures does not improve outcome.[6] Although many outcomes are fixed from the time of injury, opportunities for early intervention should not be missed. It is particularly important to avoid secondary neurologic injury, most commonly due to reduced perfusion from hypotension and cerebral edema.

Prevention of spinal cord injury (Chapter 368) and evaluation of the spine for bone and ligamentous disruption are also important components of the early evaluation. Multidetector CT images can be obtained quickly to detect occult spinal injuries, and routine magnetic resonance imaging is rarely clinically indicated.[7]

A multidisciplinary approach to the evaluation and management of pain and anxiety in injured patients has important short- and long-term benefits. An organized approach facilitates dealing with the inevitable pain and anxiety in an organized and consistent manner and allows the unit to determine the effectiveness of new interventions.

Tertiary Survey

The tertiary survey is a planned repeat physical examination, usually 1 or 2 days after admission, often accompanied by focused imaging tests.[8] The goal is to exclude missed subtle injuries that might otherwise cause significant long-term morbidity. Examples include minor fractures of the wrist or foot, small deep lacerations of the scalp, subtle eye injuries, and some abdominal injuries, particularly retroperitoneal duodenal or colonic perforations. Such injuries can become the patient's dominant source of long-term morbidity if they are missed during initial evaluation and treatment.

Key Management Issues

Fluid Resuscitation and Transfusion

The clinical goal is to administer adequate, but not excessive, fluid[9] while ensuring that soft tissues are not rendered ischemic by increasing pressure beneath inelastic eschar or tense muscle compartments. The severity of hemorrhagic shock should be assessed and treated appropriately (Table 97-2).

For burn patients, several formulas based on weight, surface area, and burn size have been developed over the years. These are general guides, and physiologic monitoring is needed with individual titration of infusions to meet set resuscitation end points, such as urine output, base deficit, and vital signs (E-Table 97-1).[10]

In well-resuscitated trauma and burn patients, capillary integrity generally returns at 18 to 24 hours, and fluid requirements decrease to approximately 1.5-fold maintenance in most patients. With the reduction in the infusion rate of isotonic crystalloid, topical care of large wounds will have a major impact on serum electrolytes. Wounds treated with nonaqueous topical antimicrobials, such as silver sulfadiazine cream or mafenide acetate cream, promote transeschar water loss and generate a free water requirement. By comparison, wounds treated with aqueous topical agents are associated with electrolyte leaching and secondary hyponatremia (Chapter 102). Serum levels of potassium, calcium, and magnesium (Chapters 103-105 and 227) should be monitored frequently and replaced as needed. In most patients, enteral feedings (Chapter 198) can be started.

Current fluid resuscitation practices in trauma patients emphasize initial "permissive hypotension" to reduce early bleeding (Chapters 90 and 92). Patients with mean systemic arterial pressures in the range of 60 to 80 mm Hg are resuscitated initially to modest hypotension (i.e., the range of 80 to 90 mm Hg) if they are otherwise alert and well perfused. They are then taken expeditiously to the operating room for surgical control before targeting a normotensive state. Early use of blood products such as fresh-frozen plasma and red cells rather than crystalloid can minimize the coagulopathy and improve outcomes in rapidly hemorrhaging patients. Among patients with severe trauma and major bleeding, early administration of plasma, platelets, and red blood cells in a 1 : 1:1 ratio of infusion units is better than a 1 : 1:2 ratio for achieving hemostasis and reduces early death due to exsanguination.[A3] Liberal use of tourniquets and compressive dressings before surgery further improves outcome by reducing blood loss. Among the various crystalloids, none seem to have any obvious advantages or disadvantages for treatment of hemorrhage. Tranexamic acid (e.g., loading dose of 1g during 10 minutes, then infusion of 1 g during 8 hours), which inhibits thrombolysis, beginning within 8 hours of injury may reduce bleeding and improve survival in selected patients who require massive transfusion.[A4]

Pigmented urine is commonly seen in the setting of high-voltage, crush, blast, or very deep thermal injury. Myoglobin and hemoglobin that are liberated from lysed muscle (Chapter 99) and red cells cause the pigmentation. To avoid renal tubular injury (Chapter 106), crystalloids should be administered to achieve a urine output of 2 mL/kg/hour (Chapter 99).

Decompression Procedures

An important component of the initial evaluation of the trauma and burn patient is to find and to rectify compartment syndromes before irreversible tissue ischemia occurs.[11] Perfusion of the extremities can be compromised by inelastic near-circumferential burns, and the normal fascial envelopes of major muscle groups can cause high soft tissue pressure if muscles are injured by crush, thermal, or electrical injury or in association with major fractures. Extremities at risk should be dressed simply to facilitate frequent assessment for temperature, pliability, voluntary motion, pain with passive motion, detectable pulsations, and low-pressure flow by capillary refill and Doppler signals in the digital vessels and digital pulp. In assessing capillary refill, it is important to elevate the extremity, as even a mottled nonperfused extremity will demonstrate venous refill when it is dependent. Measurement of compartment pressures may be valuable in selected patients, with decompression recommended when measured pressures are above 30 cm H_2O. In most situations, serial clinical examination is sufficient to determine the need for escharotomy or fasciotomy, thereby avoiding the risk of bacterial seeding posed by passing pressure-monitoring catheters through contaminated wounds. Compromised extremities should be promptly decompressed by escharotomy or fasciotomy before the development of irreversible tissue necrosis (E-Fig. 97-1).

Abdominal Compartment Syndrome

If abdominal viscera become extremely edematous, abdominal compartment syndrome may result.[12] This syndrome, which is usually caused by edema of the bowel wall, occurs after abdominal trauma or after the gut is reperfused by resuscitative therapies. When intra-abdominal pressures exceed 25 mm Hg (34 cm H_2O), renal blood flow, inferior vena cava blood return, and diaphragmatic excursion are impaired. This syndrome typically is manifested with oliguria, hypotension, and difficult ventilation. Diagnosis is by physical examination and measurement of bladder pressure. Treatment is by laparotomy with temporary abdominal closure.

Phase Two: Initial Surgical Care

Phase Two includes initial wound excision for burn patients and initial resuscitative surgery and fracture stabilization for non-burn trauma patients. This phase frequently overlaps with Phase One but is usually completed within 72 hours. Multiple subspecialty surgical teams may need to be coordinated by a trauma surgeon who directs overall care and reconciles conflicting priorities.

Early Wound Excision

Excisional débridement of nonviable soft tissues or deep burns during the first days following injury, before heavy microbial colonization occurs, will reduce the incidence and severity of sepsis from burns, crush, or other soft tissue trauma.

TABLE 97-2 CATEGORIZATION AND INITIAL TREATMENT OF HEMORRHAGIC SHOCK*

	CLASS I	CLASS II	CLASS III	CLASS IV
Blood loss (mL)	≤750	750-1500	1500-2000	≥2000
Blood loss (% of blood volume)	≤15	15-30	30-40	≥40
Pulse rate	<100	>100	>120	≥140
Blood pressure	Normal	Normal	Decreased	Decreased
Capillary refill test	Normal	Positive	Positive	Positive
Respiratory rate	14-20	20-30	30-40	>35
Urine output (mL/hr)	≥30	20-30	5-15	Negligible
Mental status	Slightly anxious	Mildly anxious	Anxious and confused	Confused and lethargic
IV fluid replacement (3 : 1 rule)	Crystalloid	Crystalloid	Crystalloid + blood	Crystalloid + blood

*Based on a 70-kg adult.
IV = intravenous.
From Demling RH, Gates JD. Medical aspects of trauma and burn care. In: Goldman L, Schafer AI, eds. *Goldman's Cecil Medicine*. 24th ed. Philadelphia: Saunders-Elsevier; 2012.

Damage Control Surgery

Damage control surgery identifies the most important surgical tasks that must be done to save the patient's life, and only these tasks are performed initially, thereby allowing a more stable patient to return to the operating room later for a subsequent definitive and often time-consuming operation. The prototypical example is for abdominal trauma, when bleeding and gastrointestinal contamination are addressed initially but the abdomen is left open so a warmed and more stable patient can return to the operating room in 12 to 36 hours for a definitive bowel anastomosis and abdominal closure. This concept can also be applied to the trauma care system. If multiple patients need to share limited operating room resources, truncating individual operations allows more patients to be treated urgently.

Early Fracture Fixation

Early surgical fixation of long bone fractures benefits injured patients by reducing the complications of immobilization, enhancing rehabilitation, and likely reducing the systemic inflammatory state and proclivity to thromboembolic complications.

Prophylaxis for Thromboembolic Complications, Gastrointestinal Hemorrhage, and Infection

Trauma incites a hypercoagulable state, and seriously injured patients are prone to deep venous thrombosis and pulmonary embolism. Prophylaxis using low-molecular-weight heparin and/or automatic compression stockings has become routine in most trauma programs.

During the early hypodynamic phase with reduced splanchnic blood flow, gastrointestinal hemorrhage may occur in the seriously injured or burned patient. This complication can be sharply reduced with routine pharmacologic prophylaxis, including proton pump inhibitors or histamine-2 receptor blockers.

Prophylactic antibiotics are not recommended[A5] except perhaps in patients who have severe burns and require mechanical ventilation or who have undergone split-thickness skin grafting, because they can promote the growth of resistant organisms.[13] However, careful observation and prompt cultures in febrile patients are critical for optimal management.

Critical Care of the Injured or Burned

Many injured patients require transient intubation and mechanical ventilation (Chapter 91) to facilitate resuscitation, evaluation, and initial care. Some will go on to develop respiratory failure (Chapter 90) requiring protracted ventilator support.

Multiple mechanical and injury factors contribute to respiratory insufficiency in trauma patients, including chest wall trauma and pulmonary contusion. In patients with more severe injuries, including flail chest, rib fixation is a useful intervention.

In burn patients, inhalation injury (Chapter 82) is an important cause of respiratory failure. The diagnosis of inhalation injury is best made by history and clinical examination revealing singed nasal vibrissae and carbonaceous debris in the mouth and pharynx (E-Fig. 97-2). Chest radiographs are usually normal initially. Airway management is challenging but generally is similar to non-burn patients.[14] Carbon monoxide poisoning (Chapter 82) can be seen in conjunction with inhalation injury; the standard of care is 100% oxygen at the prevailing atmospheric pressure for 6 hours, with hyperbaric oxygen reserved for patients with a carboxyhemoglobin level above 30% or neurologic changes.

Pneumonia (Chapter 85) or tracheobronchitis (Chapter 84) occurs in about 30% of burn patients with inhalation injury. Acute respiratory distress syndrome (Chapter 90) also is common in burn and trauma patients, particularly those who go on to develop sepsis, pneumonia, and multiple organ failure. Antibiotic therapy is directed by sputum Gram stain and cultures and should not be prolonged beyond a 7- to 10-day therapeutic course. Vigorous pulmonary toilet, with directed bronchoscopy to clear secretions in selected patients, is an important component of therapy.

Post-Resuscitation Metabolic Issues

In the days that follow successful resuscitation, a hyperdynamic state predictably occurs, characterized by a high cardiac output and low peripheral resistance. Excision of necrotic tissue, prevention of tissue ischemia by repair of vascular injuries, and prompt management of compartment syndromes will minimize the burden of necrotic tissue and reduce post-injury infection and hypermetabolism (E-Fig. 97-3).

Several formulas have been devised to predict non-protein calorie needs (E-Table 97-2). A very rough estimate of calorie needs is a range of 25 to 35 kcal/kg/day, with the lower number applying to more stable and older patients and the upper number applying to more seriously injured and younger patients. Protein administration of 2 to 3 g per kilogram per day will adequately support the needs of most injured patients.

The route of nutritional support is ideally enteral (Chapter 198), with tube feeding beginning during resuscitation. However, some patients, particularly those with very severe and abdominal injuries or those with intervening sepsis, will not tolerate enteral feedings at goal rates and will require supplemental parenteral nutrition to ensure delivery of all needed nutrients (Chapter 198).

Safe and reliable modification of adverse components of the hypermetabolic response, particularly protein catabolism, has proved an elusive goal. Anabolic agents such as recombinant human growth hormone and anabolic steroids may help restore positive nitrogen balance but are not universally used because of their complications, expense, and conflicting data regarding the efficacy. Other attempted interventions, such as enteral glutamine,[A6] antipyretics, β-adrenergic blockade, β-adrenergic supplementation, nonsteroidal anti-inflammatory agents, recombinant growth hormone, insulin-like growth factor-I, and anabolic steroids, have been tried, but available data are inadequate to support any of these therapies as standard care.

Septic Complications and Multiple Organ Failure

Injured patients are at elevated risk for a multitude of infectious complications (Chapter 261). Multiple organ dysfunction and septic shock (Chapter 94) are manifestations of uncontrolled systemic inflammation for severe infection.

Phase Three: Definitive Surgical Care

Phase Three involves definitive wound closure for burns and completion surgery for trauma patients. In non-burn trauma patients, this phase may involve removal of vacuum wound dressings and definitive closure, closure of fasciotomy sites, and fixation of facial fractures. The duration of this phase varies greatly with injury, but it is usually complete at the time of acute hospital discharge. For example, in burn patients, this phase of care is defined by replacement of temporary membranes with permanent grafts and the important but time-consuming grafting of hands and face.

Phase Four: Rehabilitation and Reintegration

Phase Four describes the sometimes long process of reconstruction, rehabilitation, and reintegration.[15] This phase of care may begin in an inpatient rehabilitation setting and progress into the home environment. Depending on the specifics of the injury, the process may be a few weeks to months or years. Daily passive range-of-motion movements, splinting, anti-deformity positioning, and strengthening can reduce the frequency of these complications.

The environment of recovery is an important therapeutic consideration. Data suggest that specific qualities of the family have a major impact on multiple aspects of recovery, some that can potentially be modified. Community resources can be used to enhance recovery and are an important part of discharge planning. Attempts to reduce opiod use during the acute phase may reduce overall opiod use during the hospital course and afterwards.[A7]

REHABILITATION OF THE INJURED PATIENT

REHABILITATION IN THE CRITICALLY ILL PATIENT

Passive range-of-motion movement, splinting, and anti-deformity positioning will minimize the capsular contraction and shortening of tendon and muscle groups that otherwise occur with protracted immobilization.

Emotional recovery after severe trauma can be limited by neurologic injury and post-traumatic stress. These issues can be anticipated and their adverse effects blunted by early and continuous involvement of emotional supports for the family and patient. Ideally, psychiatric, social service, and psychological resources are available.

SPECIAL CONSIDERATIONS

Electrical Injury

Cardiopulmonary arrest can be caused by low-voltage electrical injury but is more common with high-voltage electrical injury. Extensive tissue necrosis may also liberate enough potassium to cause cardiac dysfunction. Because cardiac arrhythmias may recur after resuscitation or develop 24 to 48 hours after injury, all patients who have sustained high-voltage electrical injury should undergo continuous electrocardiographic monitoring for at least 24 to 48 hours after the last documented arrhythmia.

Deep muscle necrosis can be initially inapparent, so many patients benefit from serial operative evaluation and débridement. Recovery of function after direct electrical nerve damage is rare. Conversely, the nerves that are not injured directly commonly recover. Rarely, a polyneuritic syndrome of relatively late onset can cause deficits in the function of peripheral nerves far removed from the points of contact. Among patients hospitalized with serious high-voltage electrical injuries, about 8% die and another 22% have permanent neurologic deficits despite optimal care. Most patients with low-voltage injuries, such as can be caused by electrical flash burns, also develop long-term sequelae, including neurologic (memory loss, numbness, headache, chronic pain, weakness) and musculoskeletal (pain, reduced range of motion, contracture) symptoms.

FIGURE 97-9. The "flowers of Lichtenberg" is an evanescent cutaneous phenomenon commonly seen in lightning-struck patients.

Lightning Injury

Cardiopulmonary arrest is common in patients struck by lightning.[16] The "flowers of Lichtenberg" is an evanescent cutaneous phenomenon commonly seen in lightning-struck patients (Fig. 97-9). Coma is also common acutely but typically resolves in a few hours. Keraunoparalysis, which is lightning-induced paralysis, is characterized by usually transient paresthesias and paralysis that develop during several days and typically involve the lower limbs. Ruptured tympanic membranes and hearing loss may also occur. With immediate cardiopulmonary resuscitation, about two thirds of lightning victims survive, and persistent neurologic deficits are relatively uncommon.

Considerations at the Extremes of Age

Injured patients at the extremes of age bring with them a number of important physiologic and psychosocial issues that directly affect their care (E-Table 97-3). Older adults do not have the depth of physiologic reserve of the young (Chapter 24). Cardiopulmonary function may be compromised, and peripheral vascular disease is common. Muscle mass and respiratory muscle strength are often reduced. Reduced renal reserve increases sensitivity to nephrotoxic drugs. The skin is relatively atrophic and consequently tolerates burning and donor harvest poorly. Nutritional needs are not well predicted by standard equations.

As a result, a major injury is often the event that changes the subsequent living condition of an elderly person. Injuries are often the result of cognitive or functional changes (Chapter 361) and may be associated with syncopal episodes (Chapter 49) that need to be concurrently evaluated. Resuscitation should be carefully considered if burns are very large or trauma is severe. Data suggest that mortality is nearly 90% in patients who are older than 60 years, have burns of more than 40% of their body surface, and have concomitant inhalation injury. Patients may have advanced directives, interested families, or health care proxies who should be consulted as early as possible in the care of such patients (Chapter 3).

Older adults bring unique psychosocial issues to the trauma and burn center. They may live alone or have a spouse who cannot meet their discharge care needs for wound care, transportation, or general support. Children may live far away and be unable to support them. Discharge planning can be very involved, requiring orchestration of many community resources, and must be started early.

Emotional Consequences of Injury

Most patients who suffer significant injury will develop some degree of acute stress disorder characterized by anxiety, hypervigilance, fear, and re-experiencing the event.[17] This normal reaction can become pathologic and debilitating as post-traumatic stress disorder (Chapter 362). Early recognition and emotional support can blunt this progression and enhance both short-term rehabilitation and long-term recovery.

GENERAL REFERENCES

For the General References and other additional features, please visit Elsevier eBooks+ at https://ebooks.health.elsevier.com.

Grade A References

A1. Sierink JC, Treskes K, Edwards MJ, et al. Immediate total-body CT scanning versus conventional imaging and selective CT scanning in patients with severe trauma (REACT-2): a randomised controlled trial. *Lancet*. 2016;388:673-683.
A2. Kumar V, Mishra B, Joshi MK, et al. Early hospital discharge following non-operative management of blunt liver and splenic trauma: a pilot randomized controlled trial. *Injury*. 2021;52:260-265.
A3. Holcomb JB, Tilley BC, Baraniuk S, et al. Transfusion of plasma, platelets, and red blood cells in a 1:1:1 vs a 1:1:2 ratio and mortality in patients with severe trauma: the PROPPR randomized clinical trial. *JAMA*. 2015;313:471-482.
A4. Karl V, Thorn S, Mathes T, et al. Association of tranexamic acid administration with mortality and thromboembolic events in patients with traumatic injury: a systematic review and meta-analysis. *JAMA Netw Open*. 2022;5:e220625.
A5. Ramos G, Cirnistein W, Cerino GT, et al. Systemic antimicrobial prophylaxis in burn patients: systematic review. *J Hosp Infect*. 2017;97:105-114.
A6. Heyland DK, Wibbenmeyer L, Pollack JA, et al. A randomized trial of enteral glutamine for treatment of burn injuries. *N Engl J Med*. 2022;387:1001-1010.
A7. Harvin JA, Albarado R, Truong VTT, et al. Multi-modal analgesic strategy for trauma: a pragmatic randomized clinical trial. *J Am Coll Surg*. 2021;232:241-251.e3.

98 ENVENOMATION, BITES, AND STINGS

STEVEN A. SEIFERT†, RICHARD C. DART, AND JULIAN WHITE

EPIDEMIOLOGY

Envenomation (e.g., snakebite, spider bite, scorpion stings, jellyfish stings) may seem to be a rare medical problem, but envenomation affects millions of humans annually and results in hundreds of thousands of deaths (Table 98-1). For example, the annual number of venomous snakebites is estimated to be in excess of 2.5 million per year, with more than 100,000 fatalities and hence a case fatality rate of about 1 : 25. Another common envenomation, jellyfish stings, affects more than 1 million people per year, with a case fatality rate of about 1 : 10,000. The epidemiology of envenomations will differ by region. In Australia, for example, spider bites cause nearly twice as many hospital visits as compared with snakebites. In the United States, spider bites reported to poison centers are roughly equal to the number of venomous snakebites (about 5000 to 10,000 per year),[1] whereas reports of scorpion envenomations are nearly double that number.

PATHOBIOLOGY

Envenomation occurs when a venomous animal, usually via a bite or sting, injects a physiologically impactful quantity of venom into a target animal. A venomous animal may bite or sting without injecting enough venom to cause effects (a "dry bite"),[2] so signs of envenomation will not always develop. The rate of dry bites will vary by species and other circumstances. In the United States, for example, viperid bites have about a 20% dry bite rate, whereas elapid bites have about a 50% rate. Some snake species lack the capacity to envenomate because they have no venom apparatus.

Venom is an often complex mixture of a number of substances, including toxins. Venoms can be produced in specialized glands (e.g., venomous snakes, scorpions, spiders, cone snails, venomous stinging fish, stingrays) or cell structures (e.g., jellyfish nematocysts), or they can be acquired from the environment and concentrated in specific glands/organs (e.g., venomous octopuses). The function of venom is to assist the animal as a predator and/or in defense against predation.

CLINICAL MANIFESTATIONS AND DIAGNOSIS

Most envenomations are accompanied by dermatologic findings, commonly at the site of the bite or sting (Fig. 98-1), starting with the puncture mark(s) of

†Deceased.

TABLE 98-1 ESTIMATED ANNUAL GLOBAL IMPACT OF SOME SELECTED MAJOR GROUPS OF VENOMOUS ANIMALS AFFECTING HUMANS

VENOMOUS ANIMAL GROUP	ESTIMATED NUMBER OF NEW CASES PER YEAR	ESTIMATED NUMBER OF FATAL CASES PER YEAR
Venomous snakes	>2.5 million	>100,000
Scorpions	>1 million	<5000
Stinging insects	>1 million	>1000 (mostly due to anaphylactic reaction to venom in sting)
Jellyfish	>1 million	<100
Spiders	>100,000	<100
Venomous spiny fish and stingrays	>100,000	<10
Paralysis ticks	>1000	<10
Venomous mollusks (blue-ringed octopus, cone snails)	<1000	<10

the biting or stinging apparatus. Local tissue injury might result from mechanical effects and/or cytotoxic venom components that produce tissue edema, which may remain local, spread, or progress to necrosis. Snakes, scorpions, spiders, and jellyfish commonly have venoms that can injure tissue.

Systemic effects may include nausea and vomiting, bleeding, thrombosis, renal impairment, neurotoxicity, and even pituitary abnormalities or more specific end-organ effects, such as hematologic derangements, vascular toxicity, nephrotoxicity,[3] or neurotoxicity. For example, some snake, scorpion, and caterpillar venoms can produce thrombosis or uncontrolled bleeding. Snake, tick, blue-ringed octopus, and cone snail venoms are all capable of impairing transmission at the neuromuscular junction and causing paralysis (Table 98-2). Some scorpions, spiders, and jellyfish have venoms that can cause excitatory neurotoxicity, with pain, sweating, autonomic effects, cardiotoxicity, and pulmonary edema.

Key points of the history include time, place, and circumstances of the bite or sting; whether the patient was bitten/stung once or multiple times; a description of the offending animal if witnessed; the type and timing of first aid application; the type and time of onset of any symptoms; relevant past medical history; and any medications used. Some envenomation scenarios (e.g., attempting to capture or kill an offending animal, collections of venomous animals, multiple stings by a colony of marine animals) may include multiple bites or stings and may include multiple envenomating animals. Any symptoms of specific toxic effects (e.g., symptoms of progressive paralysis, neuroexcitation, myolysis, coagulopathy, cardiotoxicity, acute kidney injury, allergy) and systemic effects (e.g., headache, nausea/vomiting, abdominal pain, collapse, convulsions) should be sought. Examination should similarly target specific venom effects, including careful examination of the bite or sting site and a careful neurologic examination (Chapter 366).

Laboratory tests will vary depending on the likely animal and the consequent likely risks (e.g., a coagulation profile for venomous snakes). Clinical venom identity testing is available only for Australian snakebites. Hematologic tests typically should include a complete blood and platelet count, a fibrinogen level, and an international normalized ratio (INR). In some locations, the 20-minute whole-blood clotting test may be useful.

TREATMENT

Envenomation may be an obvious diagnosis or a cryptic presentation in which a bite/sting may not be suspected. Many cases of venomous bites/stings result in only mild effects, but clinical events can progress rapidly and require similarly time-sensitive treatment. The best approach is to assume every case may develop into severe envenomation and to ensure urgent and context-sensitive initial assessment, followed by ongoing reassessment over the major at-risk period. It is often very important to reassess all patients at 10- to 15-minute intervals for 8 to 12 hours to detect any developing symptoms, signs, and laboratory abnormalities.

The first aid provided to an envenomated patient before reaching definitive medical care may significantly impact final outcome. Bites and stings are traumatic wounds and should undergo thorough cleansing, evaluation for retained foreign bodies (e.g., teeth, fangs), and tetanus prophylaxis as for any contaminated wound (Chapter 15). In general, prophylactic antibiotics are not effective at preventing infection, and there is no role for glucocorticoids, antihistamines, or other allergy treatments unless the patient is having an acute allergic reaction. In addition, many commonly used first-aid methods, such as tourniquets, incisions, suction devices, electric shock, and snake stones, are ineffective or dangerous and should not be used. Key worthwhile first aid includes immobilizing the bitten limb and the patient if possible; anticipation of swelling with removal of jewelry and loosening or removal of tight-fitting clothing; support of airway, breathing, and circulation (Chapters 7, 50, 90, 92) as needed; and rapid transport to medical care. Local cryotherapy reduces the local inflammatory response and may reduce the needed dose of antivenom therapy and length of hospitalization.[A1] For snakebites by species that do not cause significant local tissue damage (e.g., Australian snakes, sea snakes, coral snakes, kraits, non-necrotic cobras, and South American rattlesnakes) and for Australian funnel web spider bites, the Australian pressure bandage and immobilization technique (E-Fig. 98-1)—which involves wrapping the entire extremity with a bandage, achieving lymphatic obstructive pressures of 40 to 70 mm Hg in the upper extremity and 55 to 70 mm Hg in the lower extremity, followed by immobilization to retard venom absorption—obstructs lymphatic flow but requires substantial training to apply effectively. Box jellyfish stings should be copiously irrigated with distilled ("white") vinegar (5 to 8% acetic acid), whereas all other jellyfish stings and fish/stingray stings respond to immersion in hot water (up to 45° C).

Some types of envenomation are associated with acute coagulopathy, so potentially problematic cannulations and injections should be avoided until any coagulopathy has been corrected. Hemolysis may result in insufficient oxygen-carrying capacity. The risk of spontaneous hemorrhage increases with platelet counts below 50,000/μL, and uncontrolled hemorrhage or thrombosis may occur with complete or near-complete consumption of fibrinogen. Consumption of clotting factors in the coagulation cascade may also increase the risk of spontaneous hemorrhage with an INR greater than 3.

In many cases of suspected envenomation, an intravenous fluid bolus (e.g., normal saline or a balanced salt solution, 10 to 20 mL/kg in the first hour of treatment) may be helpful, particularly in patients with fluid losses from subcutaneous edema, diarrhea, or decreased intake.

A swollen limb should be elevated with frequent monitoring to exclude severe rhabdomyolysis or an acute compartment syndrome (Chapter 97). Other than for bites by snakes with particularly long fangs, such as Gaboon vipers, tissue compartments bounded by rigid fascia are generally deeper than most venomous animals' fangs can reach. An exception is the anterior tibial compartment, which is relatively close to the surface. Nevertheless, elevated tissue pressures may result from subcutaneous deposition of venom and local fluid accumulation that extends to the elastic limits of the skin. Surgical intervention may be considered for patients with directly measured increases in tissue pressures despite adequate antivenom, elevation, and 20% mannitol (1 to 2 g/kg, IV over 1 to 2 hours), but animal studies have shown superior outcomes with antivenom alone. Similarly, dèbridement of necrotic tissue should generally be delayed until after acute envenomation problems have resolved, and it should be delayed for weeks for recluse spider bites.

In patients with evidence for neurotoxic paralysis, intubation and mechanical ventilation may be required (Chapter 91). Antivenom may reverse postsynaptic paralytic neurotoxicity, but an anticholinesterase (neostigmine, 35 μg/kg IV) may also be useful as adjunctive treatment. Patients who respond convincingly to the initial dose of neostigmine may receive repeated doses (up to 35 μg/kg every 1 to 3 hours, and up to 140 μg/kg per 24 hours), together with atropine as needed to block its muscarinic side effects. However, antivenom may not reverse established respiratory paralysis caused by presynaptic neurotoxins. Acute kidney injury may require dialysis (Chapter 117) for days to weeks, but renal function usually recovers. For important venomous animals without a corresponding effective antivenom, non-antivenom treatments must be used.

Antivenom

Antivenom is made by hyperimmunizing an animal (most commonly a horse, but also sheep, goats, dogs, and rabbits) against the venom, harvesting the antibody, and refining it into the final product.[4] The product may be whole IgG, or its $F(ab')_2$ or Fab fractions, and these products may further undergo purification by various methods to reduce adverse effects.

If the identity of the venomous animal is known, a monovalent genus- and/or species-specific antivenom should be administered. If the identity of the animal is uncertain, a polyvalent antivenom or mixture of antivenoms is preferred. Geographically appropriate, species-specific antivenom should be sought, but a paraspecific antivenom, which was produced for a different genus or species, occasionally may be effective. Antivenoms are typically dosed by the vial, as specified in the products' package inserts, because their neutralizing power varies from product to product. Since the amount of venom to be neutralized is not based on the victim's size, children may require the same or even higher doses of antivenom and may also require that the antivenom be reconstituted in a smaller volume to help manage the fluid load.

Adverse effects of antivenom include type 1 hypersensitivity reactions, with immediate or early onset of pruritus, urticarial rash, wheezing, laryngeal edema, hypotension, and other signs of an anaphylactoid reaction

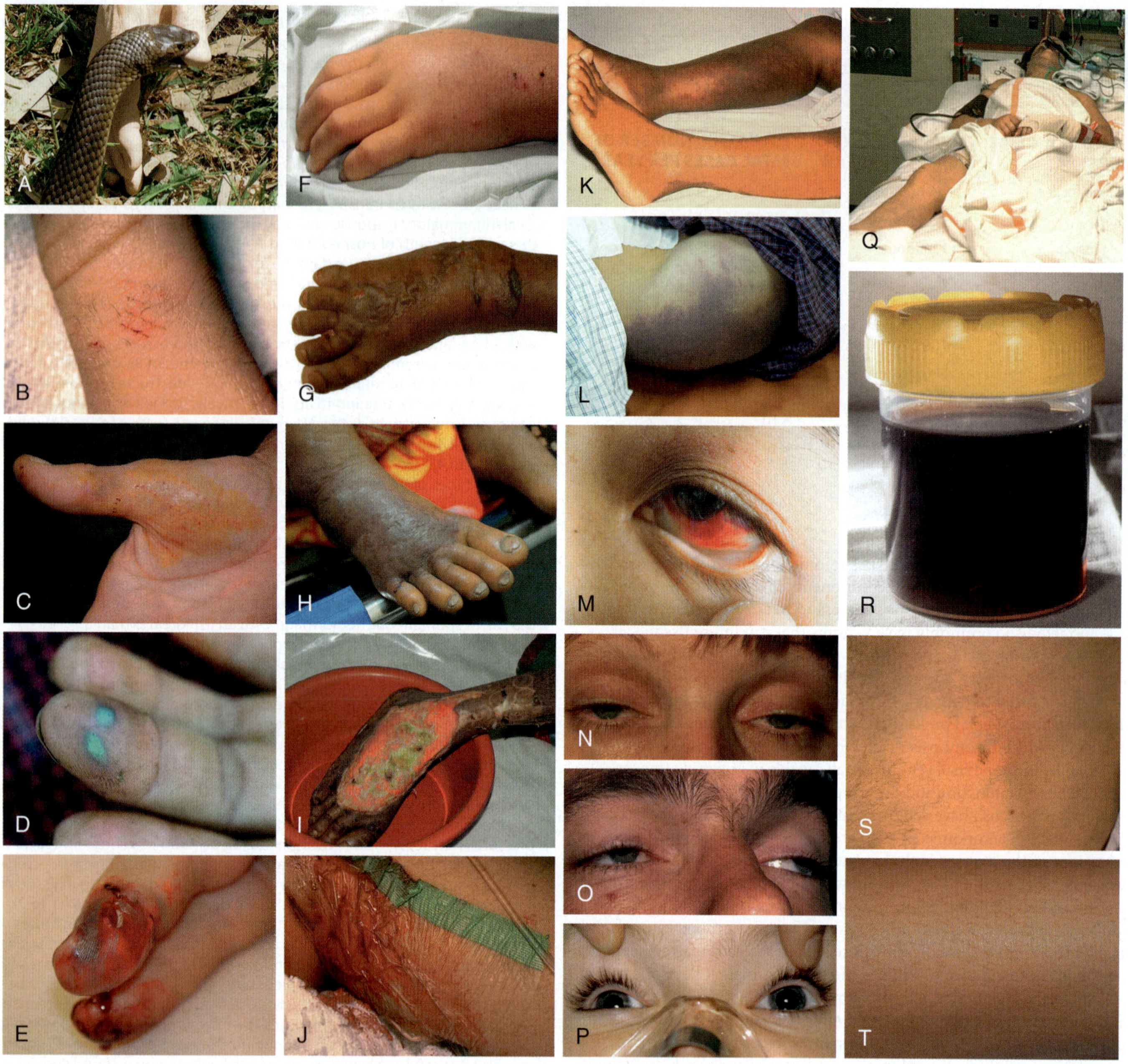

FIGURE 98-1. Clinical signs of envenomation. A, Snake biting thumb (brown snake, *Pseudonaja affinis*). **B,** Bite and scratch marks on thumb, with minimal local reaction (brown snake, *Pseudonaja textilis*). **C,** Python bite with large number of teeth marks (nonvenomous). **D,** Reaction in the first few hours to a bite from a Russell viper (*Daboia siamensis*). Blue discoloration from early hemorrhagic blister formation. **E,** Local oozing and ecchymosis (puff adder, *Bitis arietans*). **F,** Local swelling of bitten hand (mulga snake, *Pseudechis australis*). **G,** Developing skin damage around bite site (jararaca, *Bothrops jararaca*). **H,** Developing skin necrosis around bite site (Russell viper, *Daboia siamensis*), with blue discoloration from bruising/bleeding into the soft tissues. **I,** Extensive full-thickness necrosis days post-bite (Russell viper, *Daboia siamensis*). **J,** Blood ooze from around IV site indicative of active coagulopathy (inland taipan, *Oxyuranus microlepidotus*). **K,** Extensive bruising in bitten limb indicative of coagulopathy (green pit viper, *Trimeresurus albolabris*). **L,** Massive bruising distant from bite site indicative of severe coagulopathy (Russell viper, *Daboia siamensis*). **M,** Chemosis indicative of developing capillary leak syndrome (Russell viper, *Daboia siamensis*). **N,** Incomplete bilateral ptosis indicative of early developing neurotoxic flaccid paralysis (tiger snake, *Notechis scutatus*). **O,** Incomplete bilateral ptosis plus lateral ophthalmoplegia indicative of progressing neurotoxic flaccid paralysis (death adder, *Acanthophis antarcticus*). **P,** Fixed dilated pupils indicative of progressive neurotoxic flaccid paralysis in snakebite, not intracranial pathology (tiger snake, *Notechis scutatus*). **Q,** Complete snakebite neurotoxic flaccid paralysis requiring intubation and ventilation (taipan, *Oxyuranus scutullatus*). **R,** Myoglobinuria indicative of severe systemic rhabdomyolysis (mulga snake, *Pseudechis australis*). **S,** Widow spider bite with central blanching and surrounding erythema (red back spider, *Latrodectus hasseltii*). **T,** Widespread diaphoresis secondary to widow spider bite (red back spider, *Latrodectus hasseltii*). (All images copyright © Prof. Julian White; reproduced with permission.)

or anaphylaxis (Chapter 233). Skin testing for sensitivity to antivenom, a dangerous and unreliable practice, is no longer recommended in the United States. Non–IgE-mediated reactions, which are nonspecific and related to the rate of infusion, are usually easily managed by slowing or stopping the infusion, treating with H_1 and H_2 receptor antagonists (e.g., diphenhydramine, 25 to 50 mg IV, and ranitidine 25 to 50 mg IV) as needed, and restarting the infusion at a slower rate. IgE-mediated reactions are usually seen in patients who previously have been exposed to antivenom or components from the source animal. IgE-mediated reactions, which are usually more severe, require cessation of the infusion, treatment with H_1 and H_2 receptor antagonists (as noted earlier), and possibly the addition of epinephrine (see Chapter 233).

Type 3 hypersensitivity reactions ("serum sickness"), with rash, fever, myalgia, and arthralgias, may be seen 5 to 21 days following antivenom treatment (Chapter 230). These effects are usually easily managed with H_1 and H_2 receptor antagonists (see earlier for dosing recommendations), analgesia, and temperature control (acetaminophen, 1 g every 6 hours as needed); oral glucocorticoids (e.g., prednisone, 5 to 60 mg per day) are helpful if other treatments do not relieve signs or symptoms.

When the identity of the animal is unknown, particularly for venomous snakes, a characteristic clinical picture may indicate the most likely culprit. This process can be enhanced using diagnostic algorithms, which are available for Australia and parts of Asia (e.g., see http://www.toxinology.com or https://apps.who.int/bloodproducts/snakeantivenoms/database/).

TABLE 98-2 A FUNCTIONAL CLASSIFICATION OF SELECTED MAJOR VENOM EFFECTS IMPACTING HUMANS AND SELECTED ANIMAL GROUPS IN WHICH ACTIVITY MAY BE PRESENT

TOXIN ACTIVITY AND TARGET SITE	CLINICAL EFFECTS	PRINCIPAL CLINICAL MANIFESTATIONS	ANIMAL GROUPS
Paralytic neurotoxicity	Progressive descending or ascending flaccid paralysis (may be presynaptic, postsynaptic, or intrasynaptic [e.g., fasciculins])	Descending type: initial cranial nerve paresis commencing with bilateral ptosis, progressing to limb weakness, loss of upper airway protection, finally respiratory paralysis Ascending type: initial ataxia, progressive paralysis, finally respiratory paralysis	• Some snakes (descending) • Paralysis ticks (ascending) • Blue-ringed octopus (descending) • Some cone snails (descending)
Excitatory neurotoxicity	Rapid development of neuroexcitation	Local pain, sweating, autonomic/catecholamine storm effects, cardiotoxicity, pulmonary edema	• Some scorpions • Some spiders • Some jellyfish
Myotoxicity	Progressive systemic damage of skeletal muscles throughout body OR locally adjacent to bite site	Systemic: muscle pain, weakness, tenderness, grossly elevated blood creatine kinase, myoglobinuria; potential secondary acute kidney injury and hyperkalemic cardiac toxicity Local: local pain, swelling, potential compartment syndrome	• Some snakes
Hemostasis: procoagulant or anticoagulant/antiplatelet	Activation and/or consumption of clotting components, or inhibition of clotting	Varies depending on toxin target: consumption of fibrinogen and/or platelets causing bleeding tendency, *OR* inhibition of hemostasis causing bleeding tendency, *OR* formation of thrombi with embolic infarction	• Some snakes • Iranian scorpion (*Hemiscorpius*) • *Lonomia* caterpillars
Hemorrhagins: blood vessel wall	Direct damage to vessel wall allowing increased vascular permeability	Local swelling, bruising, bleeding Systemic vascular damage, capillary leak syndrome	• Some snakes
Cardiotoxins	Direct or indirect cardiac damage	Acute cardiac collapse or insufficiency	• Some snakes • Some scorpions • Some spiders • Box jellyfish
Nephrotoxins	Direct or indirect renal damage	Acute kidney injury; varies from mild rise in blood creatinine to full anuric renal failure	• Some snakes • Massed bee/wasp stings
Local necrotoxins	Progressive local skin/tissue injury	Skin discoloration, may progress to blister formation *AND/OR* skin necrosis and/or necrosis of underlying tissues	• Some snakes • Iranian scorpion (*Hemiscorpius*) • Recluse spiders • Some jellyfish • Stingrays
Allergy-stimulating toxins	Can induce acute allergic response, usually on subsequent bites/stings	Varies from local immune reaction (swelling, erythema, pruritus) through to full anaphylaxis	• Potentially all venomous animals • Particular problem for bees, wasps, and stinging ants

SPECIFIC ENVENOMATION SYNDROMES

SNAKES

Snakes are the most important global cause of human envenomation.[5] Venom composition varies not only between genera and species but also can vary between individuals of the same species and even within a given individual over time.

CLINICAL MANIFESTATIONS

The rate of dry bites varies among snake species, as do the average fang length, venom volume, venom toxicity, and range of clinical effects seen with envenomation (see www.toxinology.com or https://apps.who.int/bloodproducts/snakeantivenoms/database/ and E-Table 98-1). Some African and Asian cobra species have specially evolved fangs that allow them to spit a tightly direct stream of venom forward up to 2 to 3 m away. They specifically aim for the eyes, where the venom causes instant severe pain, blepharospasm, and temporary blindness, thereby incapacitating the victim and allowing the snake to escape. Venom spit ophthalmia requires prompt, copious irrigation, followed by inspection for corneal injury. Venom spit ophthalmia can result in permanent blindness, but it does not cause systemic envenomation and does not require antivenom.

Neurotoxic Paralysis

Pre- and postsynaptic snake venom neurotoxins target the neuromuscular junction and cause a progressive descending flaccid paralysis. In the United States, neurotoxic snakebite is often associated with coral snake bites (elapids), but some rattlesnake species also cause neurotoxicity. Once damaged by presynaptic neurotoxins, the axon must regrow, a process that can take days to weeks. It is critical that the earliest signs of developing paralysis be detected and antivenom given prior to more extensive damage, which antivenom cannot reverse. In contrast, postsynaptic neurotoxins bind to the acetylcholine receptor on the muscle end plate at the neuromuscular junction, external to the cell, so antivenom may reverse this type of paralysis.

Myotoxicity

Some snake venoms contain myotoxins that target muscle, either systemically (mainly skeletal muscle) or locally in the adjacent bitten limb. The former can cause severe progressive myotoxicity, often peaking more than 24 hours postbite, with muscle pain and rhabdomyolysis, as well as with occasionally massive elevations of serum creatine kinase levels (>100,000 IU/L), and myoglobinuria; acute kidney injury and hyperkalemic cardiotoxicity (see Chapter 99) may ensue. Local myotoxicity contributes to tissue injury in the bitten limb.

Coagulopathy

A consumptive coagulopathy reduces fibrinogen levels and may result in bleeding, but venoms also may inhibit coagulation or interfere with platelet function. Some species also have hemorrhagins that damage blood vessels, thereby allowing extravasation of blood, swelling, and the potential for local necrosis or shock. The Martinique viper and related species of *Bothrops* have procoagulant toxins that cause thrombosis, thereby resulting in embolic infarction (e.g., brain, heart, lungs).

Local Tissue Injury

Many snake venoms cause significant tissue injury at and adjacent to the bite site. The resulting necrosis, fluid shift, and secondary shock can be the most medically important effect of the bite. Secondary infection is mainly from streptococcus and staphylococcus species, but gram-negative organisms, mainly Enterobacteriaceae and enterococci, are common in South Africa. Prophylactic treatment with amoxicillin clavulanate is not effective in preventing secondary infection.

Other Envenomation Effects

Russell viper venom can cause direct nephrotoxicity and acute kidney injury (Chapter 106). The same species may cause hypopituitarism owing to anterior pituitary infarction (Chapter 205) and may also cause severe capillary leak syndrome. A number of other snake species may cause secondary acute kidney injury (Chapter 106), which is usually reversible, but rarely produces irreversible renal cortical necrosis.

SNAKEBITE TREATMENT IN PARTICULAR REGIONS

NORTH AMERICA

In the United States, an estimated 6000 to 8000 venomous snakebites occur per year. Pit vipers (i.e., Viperidae, subfamily Crotalinae, which includes rattlesnakes of the *Crotalus* and *Sistrurus* genera, and *Agkistrodon* species, which include the copperhead and cottonmouth) comprise the vast majority of bites (E-Fig. 98-2). Coral snakes, the only native elapid (mainly *Micrurus* species), are responsible for fewer than 100 bites per year. Approximately 50 non-native snake envenomations occur per year, primarily in private collections and zoos.

Viperid Bites

Ready availability of species-specific antivenom to viperids native to this region and a highly developed health care system has resulted in fewer than 10 deaths per year. Because the viperid antivenoms (a Fab antivenom, CroFab™ and a $F(ab')_2$ antivenom, Anavip™) are effective against all North American viperid snake species and because differentiation from coral, nonvenomous, and non-native snakebites is usually clear from description and context, the snake does not need to be identified. In the United States, expert assistance can be obtained through regional poison centers (1-800-222-1222).

CLINICAL MANIFESTATIONS AND DIAGNOSIS

Envenomation occurs in approximately 80% of viperid bites, invariably with tissue injury that manifests as proximal progression of edema, ecchymosis, and occasionally tissue loss.[6] Pain is variable but is often severe. Swelling may be difficult to appreciate in certain areas of the body (e.g., the thigh), and patients should be observed for 8 to 12 hours to be certain that no local signs of envenomation are developing. Subcutaneous, circumferential extremity swelling may reach the elastic limits of the skin, thereby resulting in increased tissue pressures. Extravascular fluid loss from extensive edema may compromise circulating blood volume and cause hypotension or shock.

Hematologic effects, including thrombocytopenia, hypofibrinogenemia, or prolongation of INR and partial thromboplastin time (PTT), may occur, singly or in combination, usually beginning within 1 to 2 hours after the bite and peaking several hours later. Bleeding is more likely to occur and be more severe with rattlesnake bites but can also occur with copperhead and cottonmouth envenomations. Other systemic effects, including nausea, vomiting, diaphoresis, hypotension, and muscle fasciculation, may also occur. Muscle fasciculation and weakness may be seen with Mojave (*C. sculpturatus*), Southern Pacific (*C. helleri*), and other species; they rarely progress to respiratory compromise but may cause increased serum levels of creatine kinase. Rattlesnake envenomations are typically more severe than copperhead or cottonmouth envenomations. Elevation, antivenom, and mannitol (20% mannitol, 1 to 2 g/kg intravenously over 1 to 2 hours) reduce local tissue pressures. Fasciotomy is generally neither indicated nor beneficial.

TREATMENT

Jewelry and tight-fitting clothing should be removed, the bitten body part should be loosely splinted, and standard wound care should be applied. Immobilization of the bitten body part at the level of the heart is recommended. Aggressive but appropriately monitored resuscitation with normal saline infusion may be needed, guided by signs of shock (Chapter 92).

Antivenom treatment is usually initiated for any evidence of local envenomation, especially in patients with worsening significant thrombocytopenia (<100,000/μL) or hypofibrinogenemia (<100 mg/dL). When antivenom is indicated, it should be initiated as soon as possible after the bite. Isolated prolongation of the INR usually does not require antivenom, but significant prolongation (>6) may be a marker for profound hypofibrinogenemia.

Two antivenoms are available in the United States. One is ovine Fab, the other an equine Fab2. Both have been approved for use in all types of crotalid snakebites (rattlesnake, copperhead snake, water moccasin), and both begin with an initial infusion to achieve control followed by additional doses as indicated by signs and symptoms.

For the Fab antivenom, a typical initial dose is 4 to 6 vials, over 1 hour, with additional doses of 4 to 6 vials as needed for progressive or worsening symptoms or signs. Following initial control, maintenance doses of 2 vials over 1 hour (infused slowly over the first 10 minutes) are given every 6 hours for three additional doses. Local effects and coagulation factors should be measured after treatment, predischarge, and about 4 to 8 days later (Table 98-3).[A2]

F(ab')2 antivenom starts with an initial infusion of 10 vials over 1 hour, followed by 10 additional vials to achieve initial control. If further doses are needed based on signs and symptoms, 4 vial boluses are administered. Maintenance doses are not needed for persistent local control. Late hematologic abnormalities are substantially less with F(ab')2 than with Fab.[A3] Patients should be monitored for local effects and coagulation factors after treatment, predischarge, and about 4 to 8 days later (Table 98-3).[7]

Complete resolution and return of function may require several weeks or months. Copperhead and water moccasin bites usually do not require additional antivenom after initial control is achieved. Rarely, additional antivenom is required for persistent, recurrent, or late-onset coagulopathy.

Type 1 hypersensitivity reactions to antivenom are uncommon, usually mild, and rate related. When they occur, antivenom should be stopped. H_1 (e.g., starting with diphenhydramine, 25 to 50 mg IV every 4 to 6 hours, maximum daily dose 400 mg) and H_2 receptor antagonists (e.g., starting with cimetidine, 300 mg IV every 6 to 8 hours, maximum daily dose 2400 mg), and beta-adrenergic agents (e.g., albuterol by inhalation) should be titrated for reactive airway symptoms. Epinephrine may be given as needed for symptoms and signs of anaphylaxis. If antivenom is still thought to be needed, it can be tried at an infusion rate between one half and one tenth the initial rate, depending on the speed and severity of the initial reaction. A type 3 hypersensitivity reaction ("serum sickness"), usually mild and managed symptomatically with diphenhydramine (25 to 50 mg orally every 6 hours with or without prednisone, 5 to 60 mg orally daily for 5 days), may develop in 5 to 15% of patients treated with antivenom between 5 and 21 days post-treatment. The $F(ab')_2$ antivenom has similar rates of hypersensitivity reactions.

Infection is uncommon, and prophylactic antibiotics are not indicated to prevent infection. The inflammatory effects of venom (erythema, warmth, lymphangitic erythema) may mimic infection after the first 24 hours, and antibiotics may reasonably be given at that time or if frank necrosis develops. The spectrum of organisms in snakebite, when infection does occur, appears to be similar to that in other contaminated wounds, mainly streptococcus and staphylococcus, but organisms may vary by geographic location.

Coral Snake Bites

Because of their smaller size and short fangs, coral snakes (Elapid snakes) cause an envenomation in only about 50% of bites. Local effects in coral snake envenomation are variable—pain and swelling occur in less than 50% of cases, so their absence cannot exclude envenomation.

Approximately 40% of patients will have local tissue edema, but necrosis is unusual. Systemic effects may include euphoria, perioral paresthesia, hypersalivation, nausea, and vomiting. Neurologic effects include progressive, descending paralysis, beginning with bulbar muscles (ptosis, diplopia, dysphagia). Respiratory muscles may be involved and cause ventilatory insufficiency and death. Symptoms may be delayed in onset but progress rapidly once bulbar muscle symptoms have begun. No routine laboratory monitoring is needed. An effective antivenom is available for North American coral snake envenomation at https://www.pfizer.com/products/product-detail/north_american_coral_snake_antivenin. Hematologic effects do not occur.

TREATMENT

A pressure-immobilization bandage or blood pressure cuff inflated to impede lymphatic flow (upper extremity: 50 mm Hg; lower extremity: 70 mm Hg) may be considered if the transport time will be long or there will be a considerable delay in administering antivenom. The pressure-immobilization technique is not recommended for North American crotaline snakebites, but it may be useful for North American coral snake bites. Antivenom can be administered in cases with likely envenomation (e.g., evidence of fang penetration and prolonged contact time) before neurologic effects are seen. Alternatively, treatment can be withheld unless and until neurologic signs appear if patients are observed very closely for 24 hours.

MEXICO, CENTRAL AND SOUTH AMERICA

Snake envenomation causes more morbidity and mortality in Mexico, Central America, and South America than in North America. The viperids of major importance include species of the *Bothrops, Crotalus*, and *Lachesis* genera (see E-Table 98-1). *Bothrops* spp, which are the predominant cause of medically significant snakebite throughout most of South and Central America, can cause local tissue swelling, blistering, necrosis, fluid shifts, and systemic effects such as coagulopathy. A number of larger *Micrurus* (coral snake) species can produce neurotoxicity, which manifests as a descending paralysis that can result in respiratory compromise and arrest. Coral snake envenomations are

TABLE 98-3 LABORATORY INVESTIGATIONS FOR NORTH AMERICAN CROTALINAE BITES

Baseline tests:
- Platelet count, fibrinogen level, INR, PTT
- CK, if signs of muscle injury, fasciculation, or elevated tissue pressures

Follow-up tests:
- Platelet count, fibrinogen level, INR after the initial dose of antivenom
- Add D-dimer × 1
- Platelet count, fibrinogen level, and INR after each antivenom dose given for hematologic indications
- Predischarge fibrinogen level, INR
- Platelet count, fibrinogen level, INR at 4 and 8 days after envenomation
- Repeat as needed if values severely abnormal or worsening trend

CK = creatine kinase; INR = international normalized ratio; PTT = partial thromboplastin time.

assessed and managed similarly to North American coral snake envenomations. Appropriate antivenoms are available for most species at http://apps.who.int/bloodproducts/snakeantivenoms/database/snakeframeset.html.

Other viperid pit-viper genera (including *Agkistrodon, Atropoides, Bothriechis, Cerrophidion, Ophryacus,* and *Porthidium*), particularly in Central America, can cause significant envenomation similar to *Bothrops* spp. Compared with North American rattlesnakes, South American rattlesnakes (*Crotalus* spp) typically cause less swelling, blistering, and necrosis but more systemic envenomation, particularly neurotoxicity (descending paralysis), systemic rhabdomyolysis with secondary renal damage, and procoagulant coagulopathy.

EUROPE

The medically important European snakes are the native vipers, mostly in Southern Europe and the Balkans, but also in parts of Scandinavia and in the United Kingdom. Several major species can cause severe, even lethal, envenomation, especially in children.

Local swelling can be extensive with fluid shifts and secondary shock, particularly in children. Coagulopathy may develop with bleeding and extensive bruising. Cardiac problems and even acute kidney injury have been reported. The venom of some populations of vipers, particularly *Vipera ammodytes* and *V. aspis*, contains neurotoxins that can cause paralytic effects, primarily to the cranial nerves such as ptosis.

Significant adder/viper bites in Europe warrant antivenom.[8] The dose depends on the type of antivenom, the type of snake, and the degree of severity of envenomation. Acute and ongoing fluid management is important. Poison centers are available in several countries and should be utilized where available.

ASIA

Asia is home to many venomous vipers (including pit vipers) and elapids, with sea snakes in coastal marine waters (see E-Table 98-1). Snakebite and its consequences are more common in Asia than anywhere else in the world, with snakebites predominantly an occupational disease of rural workers. Contributing explanations include the diversity of snake fauna, the size of the human population, and the extent of rural exposure without access to good health care. In India alone, at least 45,000 people die annually following snakebites. In adjacent river delta regions of Bangladesh, snakebites are the second most common cause of death during flooding events—less than drowning but more than all infectious and other diseases. In Myanmar, snakebite accounts for more than 70% of all cases of acute kidney injury. In Sri Lanka, up to 40,000 snakebites are recorded per year.

A variety of different snake envenomation syndromes can help guide diagnosis, which relies on a targeted history and physical examination, as well as simple tests for coagulopathy (20-minute whole-blood clotting test), and kidney damage (dipstick urine test, hourly urine output measurement; E-Table 98-2).

Antivenom is the mainstay of treatment (www.toxinology.com, or https://apps.who.int/bloodproducts/snakeantivenoms/database/), but the availability and quality of the antivenom are often an issue. Because some regional antivenoms have high rates of adverse reactions, including anaphylaxis, premedication with subcutaneous epinephrine (for adults, 0.25 mL of a 1 : 1000 solution, subcutaneously) is recommended to reduce overall risk. Corticosteroids, even intravenously, are not helpful, nor is the administration of fresh frozen plasma for coagulopathy in Russell viper envenomation.[A4] The mortality after snakebites is related to delayed access to treatment and suboptimal care.[9]

AFRICA

Africa is an important global region for snakebite,[10] but epidemiologic statistics are not widely available. Examples of known risks include saw scaled viper bites in West Africa as well as puff adder bites and cobra bites throughout much of sub-Saharan Africa. In the more arid areas of North Africa, scorpion stings may surpass snakebites as the leading cause of envenomation.

Key African snake species include viperids (e.g., puff adders and relatives, saw scaled vipers, night adders, bush vipers, desert horned adders, Persian horned vipers, vipers; there are no pit vipers endemic to Africa) and elapids (e.g., cobras, some of which are spitters; coral snakes; mambas; rhinkals; desert cobras). Unique to Africa and the Middle East are the side fanged burrowing asps. A few non–front-fanged-colubrid African snakes can cause fatal envenomation (e.g., boomslang, vine snakes). Rarely the pelagic sea snake (*Pelamis platurus*) reaches East African coastal waters.

The clinical effects vary with the genus and species (see E-Table 98-1). Puff adders and their close relatives may cause local bleeding but rarely a detectable coagulopathy.

TREATMENT

Treatment principles are similar to other regions, but antivenom is unavailable or unaffordable in most of sub-Saharan Africa. When available, antivenom is useful for saw scaled viper bites, but antivenoms may not be effective for coagulopathy caused by some other *Echis* and *Cerastes* spp. In that setting, clotting replacement factor may be helpful. For the rare cases of severe coagulopathy caused by boomslang and vine snake bites, particularly for vine snake bites for which there is no antivenom, blood products and clotting factor concentrates may be useful.

Spitting cobra venom spat into the eye can cause permanent blindness if inadequately treated. Urgent copious irrigation of the affected eye(s) with water, saline, Ringer solution, buffered commercial eye wash, or other bland fluid is required, with analgesia/anesthesia as needed, followed by assessment for corneal injury and appropriate treatment. Antivenom should not be instilled into the eye. Systemic envenomation is not expected after venom spit into the eye.

AUSTRALIA AND NEW GUINEA

EPIDEMIOLOGY

All venomous snakes of medical significance in Australia and New Guinea are elapids, which account for more than about 1000 annual venomous snakebites in Australia and 3300 in Papua New Guinea.[11] In Australia, up to several hundred patients will require antivenom, and two to four patients typically die each year, primarily from prehospital cardiac collapse. In Papua New Guinea, as many as 900 fatalities occur each year, most outside of the hospital system.

CLINICAL MANIFESTATIONS AND DIAGNOSIS

Each individual snake may have a distinct venom. Significant local effects are uncommon for most species, except for genus *Pseudechis*, whose bites may cause local swelling and pain, without necrosis.

The combination of systemic and local effects can be interpreted using diagnostic algorithms to help determine the type of snake and, therefore, which type of antivenom to use. (See http://www.toxinology.com or https://apps.who.int/bloodproducts/snakeantivenoms/database/.)

The venom detection kit can help determine which type of antivenom to use in a systemically envenomed patient. Laboratory tests should include coagulation studies (INR, PTT, fibrinogen, D-dimer, platelet count, whole-blood clotting time), electrolytes, serum creatinine and blood urea nitrogen levels, and creatinine kinase levels repeated serially in asymptomatic cases for at least 12 hours after the snakebite or after any symptoms or laboratory abnormalities have appeared.

TREATMENT

Antivenom for developing or established systemic envenomation is the mainstay of treatment for Australian and New Guinea snakebites. Monovalent antivenoms are preferred if the type of snake can be determined. Otherwise, a polyvalent antivenom covering all land snake species is available. Sea snakes require sea snake–specific antivenom, but if this is unavailable, tiger snake antivenom may provide some benefit. Antivenom is typically given as one vial diluted and infused intravenously over 20 to 30 minutes.

Although antivenom may neutralize circulating toxins, it cannot replenish consumed clotting factors, which should be replaced only in patients who have potentially life-threatening bleeding despite antivenom. For patients who develop microangiopathic hemolytic anemia (Chapter 146) with intravascular hemolysis, thrombocytopenia, and acute kidney injury, platelet infusions and dialysis may be required. Plasmapheresis is not of proven benefit.

SNAKE HANDLERS AND EXOTIC SNAKEBITE

Any person regularly exposed to venomous snakes, even without being bitten, is at risk of developing allergies to snakes or their venom, a situation accelerated by a history of past bites. Thus, snake keepers and handlers may present with major, even life-threatening anaphylactic reactions that may eclipse the effects of the envenomation itself. Similarly, some may develop allergies to antivenom. Exotic snakebites or snakebites from non-native species[12] should always result in early consultation with experts in this area (e.g., www.toxinology.com), preferably a clinical toxinologist at a regional poison center.

ARTHROPODS

SPIDERS

Data from Australia indicate that spider bites result in nearly twice as many hospital visits as do snakebites, but very few spider species harm humans (E-Fig. 98-3), and fatalities are extremely rare.

Widow spiders, principally of genus *Latrodectus*, are globally distributed and likely cause more significant bites than any other spider group. The venom contains α-latrotoxin, a potent neuroexcitatory toxin. Envenomation results in a classic syndrome, termed latrodectism, characterized by localized pain and sweating, followed in more severe cases by regional and sometimes systemic involvement, with generalized pain, sweating, hypertension, and malaise that can persist for days or longer. Fatalities occur rarely. Treatment of latrodectism is controversial. Specific antivenom was efficacious in one U.S. study but not in an Australian study. Only a minority of patients develop major latrodectism, but pain control may be difficult. An appropriate approach is to use analgesia first and to reserve antivenom for severe symptoms that do not respond adequately to conservative treatment within 2 hours.

Recluse spiders, genus *Loxosceles*, have venomous toxins that cause both local tissue damage and necrosis (necrotic arachnidism), as well as potentially lethal systemic envenoming, with intravascular hemolysis, coagulopathy, and multiorgan failure. The bite is often painless, but local necrosis slowly develops and may become extensive. However, necrotic arachnidism is often overdiagnosed in regions where the spider is not indigenous.[13] Treatment is supportive, with surgical intervention avoided if possible because early dèbridement can spread venomous effects and necrosis. A specific antivenom is available in Brazil, but evidence for its effectiveness is equivocal.

Funnel web and *mouse spiders*, which are limited to Australia, have venom that contains potent neuroexcitatory toxins and can kill humans, but most of their bites are minor. Bites are generally painful and the spider often hangs on. The patient may develop systemic envenomation rapidly (minutes), similar to a catecholamine storm, with death occurring within 60 minutes in some cases. A specific antivenom is very effective, and no known fatalities have been reported since its availability.

Armed or banana spiders, genus *Phoneutria*, are native to South America, especially Brazil, but are occasionally transported accidentally to other regions. They are large (body length of 17 to 48 mm and a leg span of 13 to 18 cm), wandering spiders whose venom contains neuroexcitatory toxins, with effects somewhat similar to latrodectism, though less severe. Pain and autonomic stimulation dominate the clinical picture, with priapism a common finding in boys. A specific antivenom is available in Brazil, where bites by this genus are one of the most common forms of spider bite. Antivenom should be reserved for the most severe cases, with other cases treated with analgesia and, where appropriate, local anesthetic agents.

The goliath tarantula, with a body length of up to 13 cm and a weight of up to 175 g, is found in upland rain forests of northern South America. It can bite humans but, if envenomation occurs, produces only mild effects similar to a wasp sting. Its urticating hairs also may produce intense mucosal irritation.

Other spider species, mostly larger spiders, can occasionally bite humans and cause variable effects such as local pain of limited duration. Treatment is supportive and symptomatic, with no antivenoms available.

SCORPIONS

Scorpions cause more worldwide cases of significant envenomation of humans than any other venomous animal group, except snakes.[14] In Mexico alone, for example, more than 300,000 scorpion stings are treated annually. *Buthid scorpion* venom is rich in peptide neuroexcitatory toxins, particularly ion channel toxins, some of which produce substantial pain. Immediate severe local pain can be followed quickly by autonomic stimulation, including sweating, tachycardia or bradycardia, hypertension, and, for some species, cardiac toxicity and pulmonary edema. A sting can be lethal in children but rarely in adults. North American bark scorpions can cause unusual features such as dystonic eye movements, athetoid limb movements, and reduced consciousness.

A few species can cause lethal effects, particularly in children, but the advent of effective antivenoms, preferably administered intravenously,[A5] has greatly reduced fatality rates. Oral prazosin (30 μg/kg/dose at 3-hour intervals until resolution of the clinical syndrome) is useful as an adjunct therapy in *Hottentotta tamulus* envenomations.[A6] Dobutamine may be helpful when scorpion envenomation leads to pulmonary edema and shock.[15]

Hemiscorpius lepturus is a scorpion found particularly in Iran, where it is responsible for severe and fatal cases. Unlike Buthid scorpions, this species has a cytotoxic venom, similar in clinical effects to *Loxosceles* spider venom. Stings cause minimal local pain, but an initially painless local necrosis develops over subsequent hours to several days, can be extensive, and may be associated with a systemic illness with potentially lethal intravascular hemolysis, coagulopathy, and multiorgan failure. An antivenom is available in Iran.

TICKS

Ticks are parasitic arachnid arthropods that feed on other animals, often with a complex life history involving multiple potential host species. A few tick species produce venom that contains paralytic neurotoxins, but the major medical significance of ticks and mites is as a vector for disease transmission (Chapter 297, 298, 303, and 324) or as a direct cause of disease.

Paralysis ticks, both hard-bodied Ixodid species and soft-bodied Argasid ticks, produce venomous saliva that can cause progressive ascending and potentially fatal flaccid paralysis. The most toxic ticks, genus *Ixodes* from Australia, have caused more fatalities than either funnel web spiders or widow spiders in that country. However, most paralysis ticks cause local irritation, sometimes a local allergic reaction, without detectable neurotoxicity. When neurotoxicity occurs, it usually starts as an ataxic gait and may progress to more generalized paralysis, including ventilatory muscle paralysis. Sometimes the paralysis can be localized, such as a Bell palsy (Chapter 388), after a tick attaches behind the ear near the seventh cranial nerve.

Treatment consists of removing all attached ticks, searching carefully in the scalp, behind and in ears, and in body folds. No antivenom is available. Patients with signs of neurotoxicity should be observed closely for 24 hours (in Australia for at least 48 hours) and provided supportive care, including mechanical ventilation if indicated.

MITES

SCABIES

Human scabies is caused by *Sarcoptes scabiei* variant *hominis*. This mite is an obligate human pathogen. Scabies, which has a worldwide prevalence that ranges from about 0.2% to 71.4%, is most common in Latin America and the Pacific regions, but all regions of the world, except Europe and the Middle East, have populations with prevalences over 10%.[16] In all parts of the world, the infection is seen much more often in children and adolescents than in adults.

PATHOBIOLOGY

After mating on the skin surface, the female mite burrows and lays eggs that hatch over 3 to 4 days. The larvae molt into adults 30 to 60 days later. Mites of all stages can penetrate the skin, and they may reach staggering proportions in immunosuppressed individuals.

CLINICAL MANIFESTATIONS

In immunocompetent adults, the infection causes severe pruritus on both affected and unaffected skin, with a symmetrical erythematous, papulovesicular eruption, especially in the interdigital web spaces, wrists, anterior axillary folds, periumbilical area, the areolae in females, and the penis and scrotum in males. In nodular scabies, patients have intensely pruritic red-brown nodules that range from 2 to 20 mm in the axillary region, groin, buttocks, and genitalia; these nodules represent hypersensitivity to mite products and do not contain mites. The mite burrow—a short serpiginous gray to white keratotic line that is 1 to 4 mm in length—is most common on the hands and feet. Crusted scabies manifests in immunosuppressed individuals as silver to white crusts on any part of the body but especially the hands and ears. Elderly patients may have subtle manifestations with mild pruritus and papules on the trunk and extremities.

DIAGNOSIS

The diagnosis is established by directly identifying mites, mite pellets, or eggs on microscopy (Fig. 98-2). The diagnosis also can be established by videodermoscopy or by using polymerase chain reaction (PCR) and enzyme-linked immunosorbent assay (ELISA) for mite products or specific immunoglobulin E (IgE).

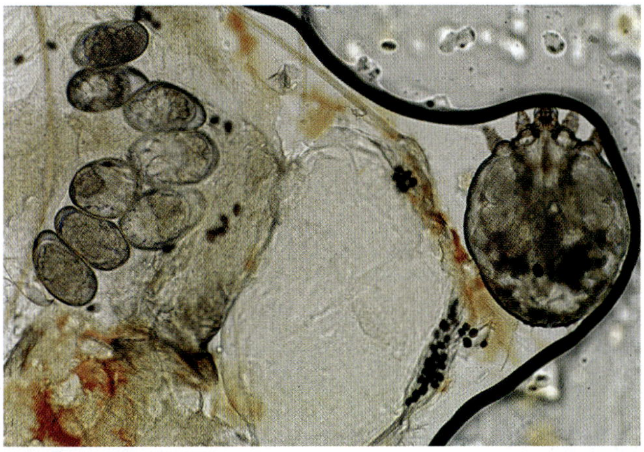

FIGURE 98-2. **Scabies preparation demonstrating an adult mite, ova, and feces.** (Courtesy of Dirk M. Elston, MD.)

TREATMENT AND PREVENTION

Topical options include permethrin 5% and precipitated sulfur 2 to 10% in petrolatum, benzyl benzoate 10 to 25%, monosulfiram 5 to 25%, malathion 0.5%, and esdepallethrin 0.63%. Topical crotamiton 10% is a weak antiscabic agent but an effective antipruritic; it also has antibacterial activity. Oral ivermectin (200 to 400 μg/kg given as a single dose, then repeated in 10 days) is an effective alternative to topical therapy, and mass administration of ivermectin can control scabies in endemic areas,[A7] with benefits persisting for at least 3 years.[17] Clothes and bed linens should be machine-washed at 60° C or higher followed by heated drying.

OTHER MITES

Mites are ubiquitous and frequently cause a dermatitis that can be a papular, vesicular, urticarial, or morbilliform eruption. Chigger mites, which commonly involve the lower legs, the edges of underwear, and the genitalia, can cause summer penile syndrome with tender to itchy papules of the glans and scrotum resembling a scabies infection. In Asia and South America, chigger mites are vectors for scrub typhus (Chapter 302). In urban areas, house mouse mites can transmit rickettsial pox (Chapter 302). In endemic areas, an eschar in an acutely febrile patient strongly suggests a mite-borne rickettsial infection. Most mite-induced rashes can be treated symptomatically either with topical corticosteroids or with camphor and menthol lotion.

CENTIPEDES

Centipedes are multilegged arthropods that possess pincers with fangs and associated venom glands at their head end. Human bites by some species, especially larger centipedes, can result in a locally painful reaction and sometimes broken skin, which can uncommonly lead to secondary infection. The pain is short-lived, systemic envenomation is unusual, and symptomatic treatment is rarely required, unless a secondary infection develops.

MILLIPEDES

Millipedes are multilegged arthropods that possess venom glands in their body segments. Human skin contact may result in exudation of toxins, thereby resulting in either a local irritant ache, a residual odor, or skin staining. The latter can mimic skin necrosis or bruising. No treatment is available or generally required.

LICE

Lice, which are obligate ectoparasites, cause three syndromes: *Pediculus humanus capitis* (the head louse), *Pediculus humanus* (the body louse), and *Pthirus pubis* (the crab louse).

HEAD LICE

Head lice affect 6 to 12 million people annually in the United States. Worldwide, the prevalence is much higher, especially in children ages 3 to 12 years. Transmission is via direct contact or close contact with scarves and hats.

Head lice should be suspected in a child who has pruritus of the scalp accompanied by cervical adenopathy. Nits can be seen on visual inspection, especially behind the ears. On the scalp, small bites and crusting blood are commonly seen. Definitive diagnosis requires that at least one live louse be found on the scalp.

TREATMENT

Ulesfia lotion contains benzyl alcohol to kill the louse by stunning and occluding its respiratory spiracle. Ivermectin (0.5% lotion in one 10-minute application at home) is 95% effective at 1 day, 85% effective at 7 days, and 74% effective at 14 days after treatment. For refractory infestations in children, oral ivermectin (400 μg/kg, twice at a 7-day interval) is superior to topical malathion 0.5% lotion. In epidemic settings, dimethicone is efficacious,[A8] but two applications of a shampoo-based neem extract is more ovicidal than typical dimethicone.[A9]

BODY LICE

Infestation with body lice is common among homeless people as well as in refugee situations and wars. The louse can serve as a vector for *Bartonella quintana* (which causes trench fever and endocarditis; Chapter 291), *Rickettsia prowazekii* (which causes epidemic typhus; Chapter 302), and *Borrelia recurrentis* (which causes louse-borne relapsing fever; Chapter 297).

Body lice produce a widespread rash that can be confused with allergic contact dermatitis, atopic dermatitis, a viral exanthema, or scabies. The diagnosis is made on physical examination by identifying bluish-hued maculae ceruleae (Fig. 98-3). This finding should then prompt a detailed search for body lice or nits, especially in the seams of clothing.

Lice are killed by washing and hot drying or ironing of the patient's clothing. Permethrin also can be applied to clothing but may not be necessary.

CRAB LICE

Crab louse infestation is a sexually transmitted disease, often concurrently with chlamydial (Chapter 294) or gonorrheal (Chapter 275) infection. Patients present with intense itching. Lice and nits may be found on pubic hairs and chest, abdominal, leg, and head hair. Infestation of the eyelashes can cause phthiriasis palpebrarum infection.

Treatment includes topical agents as used to treat head lice. Oral ivermectin (200 to 400 μg/kg, repeated in 10 days) is an alternative.

HEMIPTERA: BEDBUGS

Bedbugs are increasingly recognized in homes, hotels, and college campuses, and bedbugs can be introduced into buildings by birds, bats, and luggage. They hide in cracks and crevices of beds, particularly along the seams of mattresses. A bedbug is red-brown and about the size of a small tick (Fig. 98-4). Their bites, which characteristically are on the face, neck, and arms, typically present as a string of bites (Fig. 98-5). Symptomatic treatment is with topical corticosteroids (see Table 407-10), but disinfestation requires that all bedding be washed and dried in a hot setting and that the mattress and box spring be placed in a zippered plastic case.[18]

INSECTS

Insects have the largest diversity of species of any animal group, but few are venomous or medically significant. Myiasis, an ectoparasitic infestation by the dipterous larvae of flies, is commonly acquired during travel to areas of animal farming. The larvae must be surgically removed.

VENOMOUS INSECTS

Only two orders of venomous species are of major medical importance: Hymenoptera (ants, including fire ants, bees, wasps) and Lepidoptera (moths and butterflies).

Hymenoptera have a modified ovipositor apparatus that functions as a sting to inject venom produced in an intra-abdominal venom gland. Hymenopteran venom contains highly allergenic peptides, and acute allergy, particularly anaphylaxis (Chapter 233), is the major risk. Fatal anaphylaxis to bee, wasp, or ant stings causes as many or more deaths as true envenomation in most developed countries. Hymenoptera typically cause local effects such as pain, erythema, swelling, blistering, and even minor ulceration. However, massed attacks involving 500 or more stings can cause major envenomation, often characterized by hemolysis, acute renal failure, cardiac complications, and other organ failure. Treatment of systemic hymenopteran envenomation is supportive and symptomatic, commencing with urgent and rapid removal of any remaining embedded stings (honeybee mass attacks only). If an individual has a history of a significant prior type 1 hypersensitivity reaction (e.g., hypotension, airway edema), epinephrine should be carried to environments where exposure may occur. No antivenom is currently available. Any symptoms of anaphylaxis require urgent treatment (Chapter 233).

Lepidoptera larvae (caterpillars) pose a risk to humans because their hairs or spines can cause intense local skin irritation. Hairs may be removed by

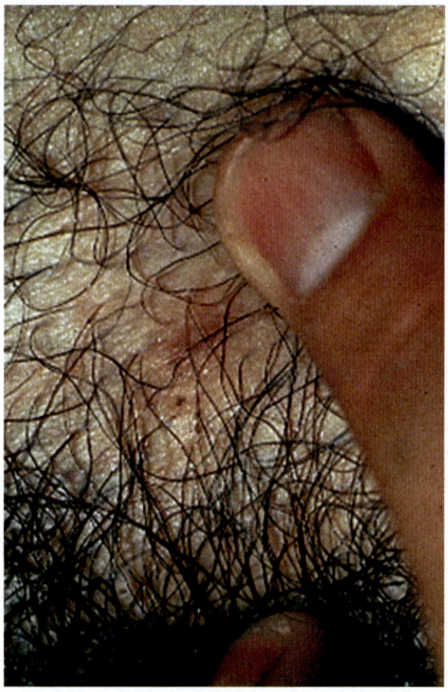

FIGURE 98-3. Maculae ceruleae are bluish-red spots that represent sites where body lice have fed. (Courtesy of Dirk M. Elston, MD.)

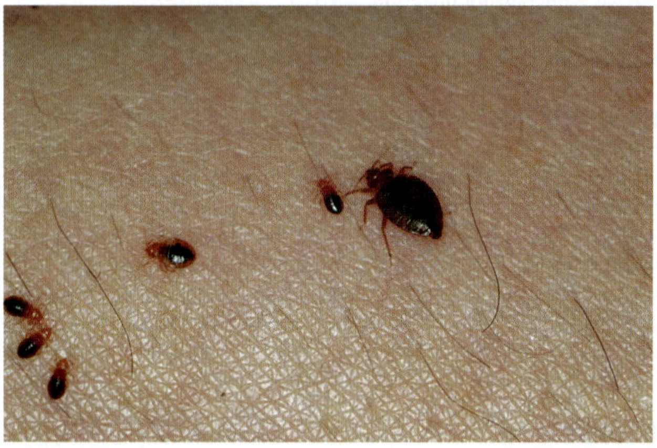

FIGURE 98-4. Bedbugs are red-brown and about the size of small ticks (~3 mm). (Courtesy of Dirk M. Elston, MD.)

application of duct or masking tape to the exposed area. For pain after envenomation by megalopygidae (moth larvae), local anesthesia alone or combined with oral analgesics is better than analgesics alone.[19] The venom of *Lonomia* caterpillar, found in the greater Amazon basin, includes a potent procoagulant that induces a consumptive coagulopathy and can result in severe and fatal bleeding. A specific anti-*Lonomia* antivenom is available in Brazil.

MARINE ANIMALS

Minor venomous interactions with marine animals probably occur frequently, but major envenomation is far less common, and fatalities are rare.[20] Some marine envenomation-related infections may involve organisms not otherwise commonly encountered, including *Vibrio* spp, *Aeromonas* spp, *Mycobacterium marinum*, *Streptococcus iniae*, and other organisms.

Jellyfish cause envenomation using a stinging organelle (nematocyst) located on its tentacles or main body. When the trigger hair makes contact with a biologic membrane, it fires the stinging tubule, which everts and injects venom into the victim within a fraction of a second.

Fortunately, most jellyfish venom causes local pain, erythema, and mild blistering without systemic effects. However, jellyfish venom can be allergenic in some people, thereby resulting in allergic reactions when stung on a subsequent occasion.

The box jellyfish (*Chironex fleckeri* and *Malo kingi*), so named for their cube-shaped medusae, produce potent venom. Stings are generally very painful and may be fatal by causing cardiac arrest within 5 minutes of envenomation. Other jellyfish can also produce severe envenomation. A large jellyfish like an Australian or Pacific species may have millions of nematocysts, each able to inject venom in microseconds, with some entering capillaries and causing rapid systemic envenomation. However, most stings have smaller areas of skin contact with insufficient venom injected to cause life-threatening effects. Even small jellyfish such as the Australian irukandji can deliver a potentially lethal dose of venom.

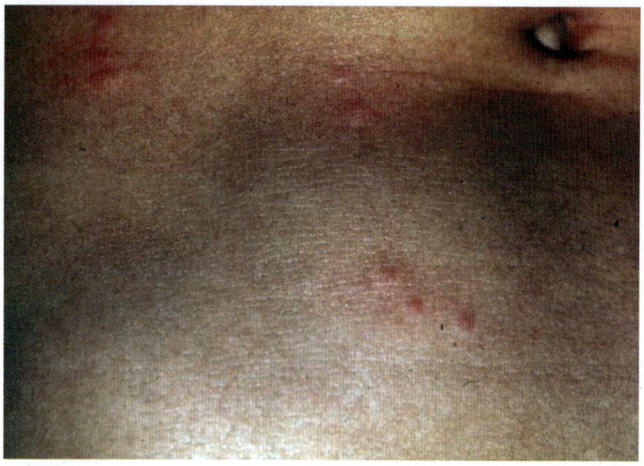

FIGURE 98-5. Bedbug bites are often arranged in a characteristic "breakfast, lunch, and dinner" pattern. (Courtesy of Dirk M. Elston, MD.)

TREATMENT

Treatment of most jellyfish stings is supportive and symptomatic, but application of hot water (no more than 45° C), preferably as a hot shower, will often provide rapid and lasting relief. The bluebottle or Portuguese-man-o-war jellyfish occurs globally. It causes local pain and welt formation and is occasionally associated with allergic reactions. Treatment is supportive and symptomatic (e.g., a hot water shower). No antivenom is available.

For box jellyfish stings, prolonged cardiopulmonary resuscitation (Chapter 50) should be provided for cardiac collapse because cardiotoxicity is likely to resolve within 60 minutes. An antivenom is available, but its effectiveness in severe cases is unclear. For less severe cases, supportive and symptomatic care is indicated. Any local tentacle track necrosis should be treated like a burn injury.

Irukandji syndrome, which is caused by a near-painless sting, is characterized by the onset of severe cramping muscle pains, notably in the back, about 15 to 60 minutes after the sting. Sweating, hypertension, and even cardiac compromise with elevated troponin levels and pulmonary edema may develop. Death is rare. No antivenom is available.

VENOMOUS STINGING FISH AND STINGRAYS

SPINY VENOMOUS FISH

Many fish species have evolved venomous spines that, upon skin puncture, release venom, which causes immediate intense local pain. Systemic effects are unusual. Treatment involves removing any residual spines from the wound. Hot water immersion (not more than 45° C) may provide adequate analgesia, but oral pain medications, including opioids (e.g., oxycodone, 5 to 15 mg orally every 4 to 6 hours) or even nerve block, may be necessary. An effective specific antivenom is available for the Australian stonefish.

VENOMOUS STINGRAYS

The sting of a venomous stingray causes intense local pain but not systemic envenomation. Treatment includes hot water immersion (no more than 45° C),[21] but parenteral analgesia (e.g., morphine, 4 to 10 mg IV every 4 hours) or a regional nerve block may be needed. For extensive wounds, exploration and removal of any residual sting debris, followed by copious irrigation, are appropriate. Stings to the abdomen or chest potentially can result in immediately lethal internal injury or fatal necrosis developing internally over a number of days. Such penetrating injuries warrant careful examination and, where appropriate, exploration and cleaning of the wound track to remove all necrotic tissue.

VENOMOUS MOLLUSKS

A few venomous *octopus species* have a potent paralytic neurotoxin, tetrodotoxin, which causes rapid (5 to 20 minutes) onset of flaccid paralysis, including respiratory paralysis, that generally persists for a few hours. The actual bite is often painless and thus may go unrecognized. Treatment is supportive and focused on providing respiratory support until the paralysis resolves several hours later. No antivenom is available.

Cone snails can fire tiny venom-inoculated darts into prey. Humans may note instant pain or no significant pain, usually followed by the rapid onset of flaccid paralysis and, in severe cases, ventilatory paralysis. Treatment is supportive. No antivenom is available.

Sea urchins possess numerous sharp spines that can result in both a mechanical injury and a local envenomation. The result is usually intense pain without systemic effects. Retained spines can act as a nidus for secondary infection. Treatment is symptomatic (analgesia; hot water immersion at no more than 45° C), antibiotics if a secondary infection develops, and careful search for and surgical removal of embedded spines.

Many *corals* may cause cuts or abrasions and potentially a local envenomation from coral nematocysts. Fire coral cuts may cause intense immediate pain and later local skin necrosis. Coral wounds may also be contaminated by microorganisms, and coral debris can act as a nidus for infection. Although the initial injury may appear trivial, it can progress to a more significant problem if left untended. Treatment includes standard wound care, analgesia as required, and antibiotics for secondary infection.

Sea anemone stings may cause envenomation with the rapid onset of severe local pain, which may progress to vesiculation and even ulceration or necrosis. The pain may persist for hours to days or even weeks. Treatment is symptomatic and supportive.

POISONING BY MARINE ANIMALS

TETRODOTOXIN POISONING

Tetrodotoxin is a small, highly potent, nonpeptide, paralytic neurotoxin. It is produced by microorganisms and then acquired and accumulated as a venom by certain marine animals for defensive purposes (e.g., fugu fish) or offensive purposes (e.g., blue-ringed octopus). Tetrodotoxin is not destroyed by cooking, so it may remain in contaminated animals prepared as human food. Competent preparation of these fish (i.e., removal of tissues and organs with high concentrations of the toxin) may reduce, but not completely eliminate, the risk of lethal poisoning.

Mild (grade 1) poisoning causes only perioral numbness, paresthesia, and nausea. Grade 2 poisoning includes facial and tongue numbness, mild generalized paresis, incoordination, and slurred speech. More severe poisoning is defined by generalized flaccid paralysis with inability to speak, fixed dilated pupils, and respiratory compromise, often with respiratory paralysis.[22] Progression and death can occur within 60 minutes. Treatment is supportive and focused on cardiopulmonary support until the toxin degrades within a few hours.

CIGUATERA POISONING

Ciguatera is a nonpeptide, small toxin produced by dinoflagellates and concentrated up the food chain. As a result, it accumulates in larger predatory fish, without any apparent effect on them. When the larger fish are eaten by humans, however, ciguatera poisoning may occur. Cooking does not destroy the toxin. Fish such as shark, barracuda, bass, and other predatory species are predominantly involved. Ciguatera poisoning is detected only when an outbreak occurs because the fish appear healthy and taste normal.

Clinical symptoms first appear about 6 to 12 hours after eating. Gastrointestinal effects include nausea, vomiting, diarrhea, and abdominal pain. Systemic symptoms, which can be variable in onset and delayed for hours, may include myalgia, arthralgia, circumoral parasthesiae, fatigue, generalized pruritus, headaches, and abnormal sensitivity to temperature. These effects can persist for days to months and are exacerbated in some patients by consumption of alcohol or any subsequent fish meal.[23] Fatalities are rare and associated with acute-phase dehydration, cardiac failure, or cerebral edema.

Ciguatera is notoriously resistant to treatment, and no specific antidote is available. Mannitol (one dose of 1 g/kg, IV) has been recommended, but trial results are conflicting. Amitriptyline (e.g., 25 mg, orally twice daily) has been used with anecdotal success. Indomethacin (25 mg orally three times daily) may assist with arthralgias.

PALYTOXIN POISONING

Palytoxin poisoning is similar to ciguatera poisoning, except the toxin is produced by zoanthid corals in the Pacific and Mediterranean. A recent problem in the Mediterranean is that massive dinoflagellate blooms can release sea spume (aerosolized palytoxin), which exposes humans onshore, thereby resulting in skin irritation, dyspnea, and airway obstruction. Some beaches and even seaside communities have been closed during intense spume events. Cleaning of tropical aquaria can also result in the aerosolysed release of palytoxin and subsequent poisoning. Treatment is symptomatic and supportive.

SHELLFISH POISONING

Shellfish poisoning can result from the contamination of shellfish fisheries by toxin-producing blooms of dinoflagellates.

Paralytic shellfish toxins are saxitoxin and gonyautoxins. Numbness (of fingertips, lips, tongue), abdominal pain, and nausea develop 30 to 120 minutes after ingestion, followed by progressive flaccid paralysis that may extend to full respiratory paralysis. Patients also may have vertigo, ataxia, transient blindness, headache, and back pain. No specific treatment is available. Management is symptomatic and supportive. Fatalities have occurred.

Neurotoxic shellfish poisoning is caused by brevetoxin, which particularly affects clams and oysters. Clinical manifestations seen several hours after ingestion include gastrointestinal effects (nausea, vomiting, diarrhea, abdominal pain) followed by paresthesias and incoordination but not paralysis. The poisoning is generally a self-limiting nonfatal disease treated with symptomatic and supportive care.

Amnesic shellfish poisoning is caused by domoic acid, which accumulates predominantly in mussels. Gastrointestinal effects begin 6 or more hours after ingestion, but days to weeks later some patients develop encephalopathy, delirium, permanent memory loss, and, less commonly, hypotension, increased pulmonary secretions, cardiac dysrhythmias, hemiplegia, seizures, and coma. Fatalities occur. Treatment is symptomatic and supportive.

Diarrheic shellfish poisoning is caused by polycyclic ethers such as okadaic acid derivatives, which stimulate excessive intraintestinal fluid accumulation. Patients present hours after ingestion with severe gastrointestinal effects, which can persist for days, and dehydration. Symptoms may mimic those of bacterial contaminants (e.g., vibrio parahaemolyticus [Chapter 278] and norovirus [Chapter 350]). Fatalities rarely occur. Treatment is symptomatic and supportive.

Scombroid poisoning is caused by histamine, which is produced by the degradation of histidine in dead fish that are poorly stored. Scombroid is a food processing/storage problem rather than a true toxin-based disease. Clinically it presents within 1 hour of ingestion with a rash, flushing, tachycardia, and, in more severe cases, headache, gastrointestinal symptoms, bronchospasm, hypotension, angioedema, and airway compromise. It usually resolves spontaneously in 6 to 12 hours or, at most, 36 hours. Fatalities have been reported. Treatment includes use of antihistamines (see Table 404-3), beta-2 androgenic inhalers (e.g., albuterol as needed), corticosteroids (see Chapter 28), and intramuscular epinephrine (0.25 mL of a 1 : 1000 solution).

GENERAL REFERENCES

For the General References and other additional features, please visit Elsevier eBooks+ at https://ebooks.health.elsevier.com.

Grade A References

A1. Canul-Caamal MA, Madrigal-Anaya JDC, Pastelin-Palacios RP, et al. Cryotherapy as a coadjuvant in crotaline snakebite management with F(ab')$_2$ antivenom: a randomized pilot study. *Complement Ther Med.* 2020;54:102569.

A2. Gerardo CJ, Quackenbush E, Lewis B, et al. The efficacy of Crotalidae polyvalent immune Fab (ovine) antivenom versus placebo plus optional rescue therapy on recovery from copperhead snake envenomation: a randomized, double-blind, placebo-controlled, clinical trial. *Ann Emerg Med.* 2017;70:233-244.

A3. Bush SP, Ruha AM, Seifert SA, et al. Comparison of F(ab')$_2$ versus fab antivenom for pit viper envenomation: a prospective, blinded, multicenter, randomized clinical trial. *Clin Toxicol (Phila).* 2015;53:37-45.

A4. Isbister GK, Jayamanne S, Mohamed F, et al. A randomized controlled trial of fresh frozen plasma for coagulopathy in Russell viper (Daboia russelii) envenoming. *J Thromb Haemost.* 2017;15:645-654.

A5. El-Asheer OM, Hammad EEM, Mohamad IL, et al. A randomized comparative study between intravenous and intramuscular scorpion antivenom regimens in children. *Toxicon.* 2019;159:45-49.

A6. Rodrigo C, Gnanathasan A. Management of scorpion envenoming: a systematic review and meta-analysis of controlled clinical trials. *Syst Rev.* 2017;6:1-12.

A7. Lake SJ, Kaldor JM, Hardy M, et al. Mass drug administration for the control of scabies: a systematic review and meta-analysis. *Clin Infect Dis.* 2022;75:959-967.

A8. Kassiri H, Fahdani AE, Cheraghian B. Comparative efficacy of permethrin 1%, lindane 1%, and dimeticone 4% for the treatment of head louse infestation in Iran. *Environ Sci Pollut Res Int.* 2021;28:3506-3514.

A9. Semmler M, Abdel-Ghaffar F, Gestmann F, et al. Randomized, investigator-blinded, controlled clinical study with lice shampoo (Licener®) versus dimethicone (Jacutin® Pedicul Fluid) for the treatment of infestations with head lice. *Parasitol Res.* 2017;116:1863-1870.

99

RHABDOMYOLYSIS

FRANCIS G. O'CONNOR AND PATRICIA A. DEUSTER

DEFINITION

Rhabdomyolysis, an acute, potentially fatal clinical syndrome, reflects the dissolution and disintegration of striated muscle, with the release of muscle cell contents into the systemic circulation.[1] Myoglobinemia and myoglobinuria are common sequelae. Other substances released from affected muscle cells (e.g., calcium, potassium) can cause systemic effects. Prerenal azotemia, complicated by the toxicity of free myoglobin on the renal tubules, may lead to acute kidney injury (Chapter 106), which exacerbates other metabolic abnormalities. At the extreme, arrhythmias, caused by the release of intracellular potassium and organic acids, coupled with hypocalcemia may be fatal.

EPIDEMIOLOGY

In the absence of a widely accepted laboratory definition or clinical diagnostic criteria, the true incidence of rhabdomyolysis is unclear, but about 26,000 hospitalized cases are seen each year in the United States. The U.S. military also reports over 500 annual cases of exertional rhabdomyolysis.[2] Among patients with rhabdomyolysis, anywhere from 13 to 67% may develop acute kidney injury, which accounts for 5 to 10% of all cases of acute kidney failure in the United States. Moreover, acute kidney injury secondary to rhabdomyolysis is independently associated with both longer hospitalizations and higher mortality.[3]

Rhabdomyolysis is a complex and multifactorial clinical disorder, with multiple potential inherited and acquired causes (Table 99-1).[4] In urban adults, abuse of alcohol and other drugs, muscle compression, and status epilepticus are common causes of rhabdomyolysis. Various viral infections, including influenza A and B, herpes simplex, adenovirus, echovirus, human immunodeficiency virus, cytomegalovirus, and most recently severe acute respiratory syndrome coronavirus 2 (SARS-CoV-2), which causes coronavirus disease 2019 (COVID-19), can cause rhabdomyolysis. In pediatric patients, the most common cause is trauma, followed by nonketotic hyperosmolar coma, viral myositis, dystonia, and malignant hyperthermia. However, exertional rhabdomyolysis from repetitive exercise is also a concern in young athletes. Importantly, children and adolescents with recurrent rhabdomyolysis are increasingly being recognized as possibly having inherited metabolic disorders.

Drugs and Intoxications

Among intoxications, the most frequent illegal drug-associated causes are cocaine and heroin (Chapter 365), with nearly 20% of cocaine overdoses complicated by rhabdomyolysis. Other recreational drugs, such as "bath salts" (of which methylenedioxypyrovalerone is the primary ingredient) and synthetic cannabinoids (or "spice"), have been associated with rhabdomyolysis. Other substances that can induce rhabdomyolysis include ethanol (Chapter 364), amphetamines, phenylalkylamine derivatives, antipsychotics, caffeine, and statins.[5] Up to 10% of patients taking statins (Chapter 190) may experience myalgias, but reported rates of statin-induced rhabdomyolysis range from 0 to 2.2 cases per 1000 person-years,[6] with cerivastatin being associated with the highest rates. Statins can also induce an autoimmune anti-HMG-CoA antibody myopathy with proximal muscle weakness and profound creatine kinase elevations. Dietary supplements, in particular those with combinations of stimulants, have also been associated with exertional rhabdomyolysis. Rhabdomyolysis can also be seen when severe hyponatremia is rapidly corrected.

Exertional Rhabdomyolysis

Rhabdomyolysis can be a consequence of exertion in sports (e.g., baseball, football, track, wrestling, endurance sports[7]), military, and recreational exercise settings, and especially with high-intensity, resistance-exercise training. For example, in one series of patients with rhabdomyolysis (defined as a creatine kinase [CK] level of greater than 25,000 units/L), 35% of patients had exertional rhabdomyolysis, with most of them related to high-intensity resistance training. In another series, 35 of 225,000 emergency department visits to an urban tertiary care center were for exertional rhabdomyolysis; the average CK level was 40,000 U/L, but no patient developed acute kidney injury.

According to data from the military, the incidence rate for exertional rhabdomyolysis is higher among Black, non-Hispanic men (60.0 cases per 100,000 person-years) than for all other ethnic groups. Additionally, individuals with sickle cell trait have a slightly higher risk of exertional rhabdomyolysis than those without sickle cell trait, although their subsequent clinical courses are not different.[8] Consistent risk factors for exertional rhabdomyolysis are low levels of physical fitness and early introduction of high-intensity repetitive exercises (e.g., squats, push-ups, sit-ups). Multiple case reports in athletes and the military identify both over-motivation and leadership (e.g., drill sergeant, coach, trainer) as important risk factors. Although most cases are self-limited, with no long-term evidence of kidney or muscle injury, patients who demonstrate systemic signs, generalized clinical findings, or acute kidney injury may have an underlying metabolic myopathy. Importantly, 25% of all heatstroke cases in the military between 1980 and 2000 were associated with exertional rhabdomyolysis; acute kidney injury developed in 33%.

The extreme exertion characteristics of military service carry over to the population of correctional inmates and civil servant first responders. Unsupervised repetitive exercise in prison populations can lead to exertional rhabdomyolysis. Among New York City firefighters, 32 of 16,506 candidates (0.2%) were hospitalized for exertional rhabdomyolysis after a physical fitness test, with 4 requiring hemodialysis. In a group of 50 prospective police officers from Massachusetts, 13 trainees were hospitalized with exertional rhabdomyolysis and had CK levels higher than 32,000 U/L; 6 required dialysis, and 1 died 44 days later as a result of complications of exertional rhabdomyolysis, heatstroke, and kidney and hepatic failure.

PATHOBIOLOGY

Pathophysiology

The final common pathway for all cases of rhabdomyolysis is from direct or indirect injury or destruction of muscle cells, with displacement of their intracellular contents into extracellular fluid, the circulation, or both (E-Fig. 99-1).

TABLE 99-1 INHERITED AND ACQUIRED CAUSES OF RHABDOMYOLYSIS

INHERITED	ACQUIRED
Glycolytic/glycogenolytic (e.g., McArdle disease [myophosphorylase deficiency])	Exertion (e.g., exercise, status epilepticus, delirium, electrical shock, status asthmaticus, cardiopulmonary resuscitation; see also Table 99-2)
Fatty acid oxidation (e.g., carnitine palmitoyltransferase II deficiency)	Crush (e.g., external weight, prolonged immobility, bariatric surgery)
Krebs cycle (e.g., aconitase deficiency)	Ischemia (e.g., arterial occlusion, compartment syndrome, sickle cell disease, disseminated intravascular coagulation)
Pentose phosphate pathway (e.g., glucose-6-phosphate dehydrogenase deficiency)	Extremes of body temperature (e.g., fever, exertional heatstroke, burns, malignant hyperthermia, hypothermia, lightning)
Purine nucleotide cycle (e.g., myoadenylate deaminase deficiency)	Metabolic (e.g., hypokalemia, hypernatremia or hyponatremia, hypophosphatemia, pancreatitis, diabetic ketoacidosis, renal tubular acidosis, hyperthyroidism or hypothyroidism, nonketotic hyperosmolar states)
Mitochondrial respiratory chain (e.g., succinate dehydrogenase deficiency)	Drugs or toxins (e.g., anticholinergics, amphetamines, antihistamines, arsenic, ethanol, opiates, statins, cocaine, succinylcholine, halothane, corticosteroids, cyclosporine, itraconazole, phenothiazines, bath salts, synthetic cannabinoids)
Malignant hyperthermia susceptibility (e.g., familial malignant hyperthermia [*RYR1*]) mutations, myotonic dystrophy, Duchenne and Becker dystrophies)	Infections (e.g., Epstein-Barr virus, human immunodeficiency virus, herpes simplex, influenza A and B, *Borrelia burgdorferi*, tetanus)
Other (e.g., familial recurrent myoglobinuria)	Inflammatory and autoimmune disorders (e.g., polymyositis, dermatomyositis)

Modified and reproduced with permission from Warren JD, Blumbergs PC, Thompson PD. Rhabdomyolysis: a review. *Muscle Nerve.* 2002;25:332-347.

Cell function is critically dependent on the relationship between intracellular calcium (Ca^{2+}) and sodium (Na^{+}) concentrations. Sarcolemmal Na^{+},K^{+}-ATPase regulates extracellular Ca^{2+} concentrations by exchanging Na^{+} for Ca^{2+} across the sarcolemma. A low intracellular Na^{+} concentration creates a gradient that actively results in efflux of Ca^{2+} as it is exchanged for Na^{+} ions. This process maintains intracellular Ca^{2+} levels at several orders of magnitude lower than extracellular Ca^{2+}.

When the cell is subjected to mechanical stress, stretch-activated channels in the sarcolemma can open and cause an influx of Na^{+} and Ca^{2+}. With excessive intracellular Ca^{2+}, several pathologic processes begin: persistent contraction of myofibers, depletion of adenosine triphosphate (ATP), production of free radicals, activation of vasoactive molecules, release of proteases, and, ultimately, cell death. Cell death is followed by an invasion of neutrophils, which amplify the damage by further release of proteases and increased production of free radicals. Rather than simple necrosis, a self-sustaining, inflammatory myolytic reaction develops. The activation of complement is a key contributor to the acute kidney injury.[9]

Rhabdomyolysis can be further complicated by reperfusion injury and compartment syndrome. In reperfusion injury, restoration of vascular flow after a prolonged period of ischemia results in the delivery of activated neutrophils in combination with an abundance of oxygen, which contributes to the development of highly reactive free radicals. Because most muscle groups are contained within rigid fascial compartments, rhabdomyolysis can quickly precipitate a secondary acute compartment syndrome. The swelling associated with traumatized tissue can also increase intracompartmental pressure and provoke additional damage by compromising both venous and arterial blood flow. Thus, compartment syndrome can also result in rhabdomyolysis.

Inherited and Acquired Rhabdomyolysis

Rhabdomyolysis can be classified as inherited or acquired (see Table 99-1).

Inherited Rhabdomyolysis

Patients who have recurrent episodes of high levels of CK in the blood triggered by low levels of stress or exertion should be evaluated for a metabolic myopathy. A number of pathways leading to the formation of ATP can be disrupted by genetic defects (e.g., inherited disorders of glycogenolysis, glycolysis, and lipid and purine metabolism).[10] In one series of 77 patients who underwent biopsy for idiopathic myoglobinuria, 47% were found to have enzymatic defects; the most common disorders were deficiencies of carnitine palmitoyltransferase II[11] and myophosphorylase. Mutations in the ryanodine receptor 1 gene also can cause rhabdomyolysis.[12] Carnitine palmitoyltransferase, acid maltase, and lipin deficiencies are other common causes of rhabdomyolysis. Malignant hyperthermia (Chapters 400 and 402) is a potentially fatal, heterogeneous, pharmacogenetic disorder that can be triggered by volatile anesthetics in predisposed individuals. When a susceptible patient is exposed to a triggering anesthetic agent, excessive release of Ca^{2+} into the myoplasm leads to a hypermetabolic state manifested by hypercapnia, tachycardia, and metabolic acidosis. A genetic predisposition to malignant hyperthermia may be linked to a predisposition to exertional rhabdomyolysis and exercise-induced heat injury via mutations in the ryanodine receptor 1 gene, but this association has not been proved.

Acquired Rhabdomyolysis

Drugs and Toxins

Drugs and toxins, also common causes of rhabdomyolysis, operate through a number of mechanisms, including direct membrane toxicity (e.g., herbicides), indirect metabolic derangements (e.g., anticholinergics), ischemia (e.g., cocaine), and agitation (e.g., hemlock). The most commonly cited drugs precipitating rhabdomyolysis are alcohol, statins, cocaine, amphetamines, and antipsychotics (phenothiazines), although new designer street drugs (known as spice and bath salts) are also implicated. Alcohol can induce rhabdomyolysis through a combination of mechanisms, including immobilization, direct myotoxicity, and electrolyte abnormalities. Statins, which inhibit 3-hydroxy-3-methylglutaryl-coenzyme A (HMG-CoA) reductase, can be directly myotoxic and appear to trigger sustained increases in intracellular Ca^{2+}. Although the precise mechanisms underlying statin-induced myopathy are currently incompletely understood, it can be aggravated by the concomitant administration of cytochrome P-450 3A4 inhibitors (e.g., itraconazole, erythromycin, cyclosporine, danazol) and fibrates, as well as by physical exercise, excessive alcohol intake, and preexisting comorbid medical conditions. Amphetamines and phenothiazines may lead to a clinical picture of rhabdomyolysis through the serotonin syndrome (Chapter 402) and the neuroleptic malignant syndrome (Chapter 386), respectively. The mechanism whereby bath salts lead to rhabdomyolysis may be direct muscle toxicity, severe hyperthermia, or electrolyte disorders.

Infections

Both viral and bacterial infections can trigger rhabdomyolysis. Either cellular invasion or generation of various toxins may precipitate infection-induced rhabdomyolysis. Influenza A and B (Chapter 332) are the most common viral causes, followed by human immunodeficiency virus (Chapter 355), coxsackievirus (Chapter 349), and Epstein-Barr virus (Chapter 348). SARS-CoV-2 infection (Chapter 336) also can be associated with myositis and rhabdomyolysis.[14] The most common bacterial organisms that induce rhabdomyolysis are *Legionella* species (Chapter 290), followed by *Francisella tularensis* (Chapter 287) and *Streptococcus pneumoniae* (Chapter 268). Acute kidney injury develops in approximately 57% (33 to 100%) and 34% (0 to 100%) of bacterial and viral cases of rhabdomyolysis, respectively.

Trauma

Trauma is the most common cause of rhabdomyolysis. Wars, natural disasters, and traffic and occupational accidents are frequent causes of trauma-induced "crush injury syndrome" (Chapter 97). Other less frequent causes of trauma- or compression-induced rhabdomyolysis include struggling against restraints, direct blows, child abuse, torture, prolonged immobilization (e.g., anesthesia, coma, drug- or alcohol-induced stupor), and bariatric and other forms of surgery. The primary mechanism of crush syndrome and compression-induced rhabdomyolysis is reperfusion of damaged tissue after a period of ischemia.

Muscle breakdown occurs in response to strenuous exercise in fit and unfit individuals, particularly eccentrically based activities (lengthening contractions, such as lowering a weight). However, it is important to note that muscle breakdown in response to exercise is expected and physiologic, whereas exertional rhabdomyolysis is pathophysiologic. Persons may present with delayed-onset muscle soreness 1 to 3 days after a bout of moderate to strenuous exercise. Key findings distinguishing exertional rhabdomyolysis from physiologic muscle breakdown and/or delayed-onset muscle soreness include (1) pain out of proportion to what one would normally expect; (2) muscle swelling; (3) significant limitation in active and passive range of motion; and (4) the presence of cola-colored urine.

External rhabdomyolysis can be triggered by exertion in combination with prolonged heat exposure (Chapter 95) and altitude, as well as by the use of medications (e.g., anticholinergics) or dietary supplements (e.g., ephedra, caffeine). It can range from a minor clinical event to a catastrophic collapse and death; underlying mechanisms may be mechanical or metabolic in nature, but all are associated with elevated myoplasmic Ca^{2+} concentrations.

A number of underlying genetic polymorphisms and inherited disorders are associated with exertional rhabdomyolysis (Table 99-2). Multiple mutations in the carnitine palmitoyl-transferase II and myophosphorylase genes have been found, and although each mutation has been associated with exercise-induced myoglobinuria, the mutations alone may not explain

TABLE 99-2 GENETIC MUTATIONS/VARIANTS ASSOCIATED WITH EXERTIONAL RHABDOMYOLYSIS

GENE	
Ryanodine receptor 1	*RyR1*
Myoadenylate deaminase	*AMPDA1*
Carnitine palmitoyltransferase II	*CPT2*
Myophosphorylase	*PYGM*
Phosphofructokinase	*PFKM*
Phosphorylase *b* kinase	*PHKA1*
Very long chain acyl–coenzyme A dehydrogenase	*ACAD9*
Phosphoglycerate mutase	*PGAMM*
Phosphoglycerate kinase	*PGK1*
Lactate dehydrogenase	*LDHA*
Cytochrome *c* oxidase	*COX I, II,* and *III*
Cytochrome *b* (complex III)	*CYTB*
Mitochondrial tRNA	*Mt-tRNA*
β-Sarcoglycan	*SGCB*
Mitochondrial DNA	*MT-CO2*

the clinical episodes. Mutations and variants in the ryanodine receptor 1 (*RYR1*) gene, which are common in malignant hyperthermia (Chapter 400), have also been found in persons with external rhabdomyolysis. Other single-nucleotide polymorphisms associated with severe exertional rhabdomyolysis are found in the genes encoding CK muscle isoform (*CKMM* NcoI), α-actinin-3 (*ACTN3* R577X), or myosin light chain kinase (*MYLK* C37885A). However, data are insufficient to use these or other variants to predict an individual's clinical susceptibility to infection-, toxin-, exertion-, or drug-induced rhabdomyolysis.

CLINICAL MANIFESTATIONS

The classic manifestations of rhabdomyolysis include acute myalgia and pigmenturia as a result of myoglobinuria in association with elevated serum muscle enzymes (CK in particular). Many clinical features are nonspecific, and the course and initial signs, symptoms, and laboratory abnormalities are clearly dependent on the underlying cause and severity of the event.[13]

Rhabdomyolysis can be accompanied by both local and systemic features. Local features, generally noted in the area of the traumatized muscle groups, can occur within hours of the trauma and include muscle pain, tenderness, and swelling. Systemic features include tea-colored urine, chills, fever, and malaise. In extreme cases, patients complain of nausea and vomiting and demonstrate confusion, agitation, or delirium. Whenever systemic features such as chills, fever, malaise, or generalized muscle involvement are observed, an underlying metabolic myopathy should be considered.

Clinical findings may also include compartment syndrome, which can occur in muscle groups encased by fascia, especially the lower leg, forearm, and thigh muscle groups. Pain with muscle group passive stretching and sensory abnormalities caused by nerve compression are early manifestations of compartment syndrome; the loss of a pulse as a result of vascular compromise is a later finding. If compartment syndrome is not addressed by surgical decompression within 6 to 8 hours, irreversible ischemic muscle and nerve damage may occur.

Laboratory findings are related to the degree of muscle involvement. Early findings include elevated blood levels of CK, myoglobin, potassium, urea, and phosphorus. CK levels typically peak 2 to 5 days after the initial insult; levels of 15,000 to 20,000 U/L are more likely to be associated with acute kidney injury than lower levels, particularly when it is "crush injury syndrome." Hypocalcemia, caused by the influx and deposition of Ca^{2+} in damaged muscle tissue, may accompany rhabdomyolysis. Also, an anion-gap metabolic acidosis may develop because of the release of organic acids from damaged muscle. With resolution of rhabdomyolysis, sequestered Ca^{2+} may be released back into the circulation and cause hypercalcemia.

DIAGNOSIS

Creatine Kinase Levels

A diagnosis of rhabdomyolysis is made when there is clinical evidence of myonecrosis and release into the systemic circulation of muscle cell contents, including myoglobin, creatinine, CK, organic acids, potassium, aldolase, lactate dehydrogenase, and hydroxybutyrate dehydrogenase. The skeletal muscle subtype CK-MM is abundantly present in skeletal muscle and released as a result of muscle destruction. Serum levels exceeding 100,000 U/L are not uncommon with rhabdomyolysis. Because CK remains in the circulation longer than myoglobin and can be detected easily and efficiently, it is the most frequently used marker to diagnose rhabdomyolysis. No universally accepted clinical or laboratory definition of rhabdomyolysis currently exists, but CK elevations ranging from more than 5 times to more than 50 times the upper limits of normal, as well as varying requirements for serum creatinine elevation, have been proposed. Importantly, sex, ethnicity, and baseline physical activity levels all affect individual baseline CK levels. For example, African American males and young athletic men have the highest baseline CK levels, whereas non–African American women have the lowest. Thus, modifying factors such as sex, ethnicity, and physical fitness must be considered when CK is used for the diagnosis of rhabdomyolysis. In general, CK levels in excess of at least five times normal, in combination with the appropriate clinical presentation, are accepted as evidence of muscle breakdown, which may be consistent with a diagnosis of rhabdomyolysis.

Myoglobin Testing

Because myoglobinuria does not occur in the absence of rhabdomyolysis, myoglobin should be the most specific marker of rhabdomyolysis. However, testing for serum or urine myoglobin is problematic and not always consistent. Because myoglobin is normally bound to plasma globulins, only a small fraction of the myoglobin that is released into the circulation reaches the glomeruli. In the presence of severe muscle damage, blood levels of myoglobin overwhelm the binding capacity of the circulating proteins, so free myoglobin reaches the glomeruli and eventually the renal tubules. Elevations in serum myoglobin occur before the rise in serum CK, but the elimination kinetics of serum myoglobin are more rapid than that of CK, which makes the often evanescent rise in serum myoglobin a less reliable marker of muscle injury. Furthermore, the liver can quickly metabolize myoglobin.

Because most laboratories will perform urine myoglobin testing no more often than once per day, urine myoglobin is neither a timely nor accurate predictor of acute kidney injury. Nevertheless, urine screening for rhabdomyolysis may be performed by dipstick. The orthotoluidine portion of urine dipsticks turns blue in the presence of hemoglobin or myoglobin, so if the urine sediment does not contain erythrocytes, one can assume, in the appropriate clinical setting, that a positive dipstick reading reflects the presence of myoglobin.

Other Laboratory Tests

Other associated laboratory findings in acute rhabdomyolysis can include hypocalcemia, hyperkalemia, hyperphosphatemia, metabolic (lactic) acidosis, thrombocytopenia, and disseminated intravascular coagulation. Muscle biopsy is not required to make a diagnosis of rhabdomyolysis, but it can be confirmatory, especially in cases of recurrent rhabdomyolysis or when the diagnosis is not clear. Histopathologic evaluation usually demonstrates muscle necrosis, loss of the cell nucleus, and muscle stria with the absence of inflammatory cells.

Differential Diagnosis

The clinical findings of acutely swollen muscles or muscle weakness (or both) with reddish-brown urine are not always the result of rhabdomyolysis, and the examining clinician must be careful to scrutinize all information. The differential diagnosis includes disorders that may indirectly affect myocytes, such as Guillain-Barré syndrome and periodic paralysis. Guillain-Barré syndrome (Chapter 388) differs from rhabdomyolysis in that it is characterized as a fulminant polyneuropathy, usually after an antecedent viral infection. Periodic paralysis (Chapter 389) is frequently associated with transient electrolyte disturbances and distinguished from rhabdomyolysis in that most cases follow periods of rest or sleep.

Myoglobinuria causes the urine to be reddish brown, but tea-colored (or cola-colored) urine does not necessarily indicate the presence of myoglobin. Other conditions associated with discoloration of urine include hemoglobinuria from hemolysis, intrinsic renal disease, porphyria, acute glomerulonephritis, "athletic pseudonephritis," and external factors such as ingestion of beets and various drugs (e.g., phenytoin, rifampin) or dietary supplements (riboflavin, or vitamin B_2).

The diagnosis of rhabdomyolysis is complete when the clinician determines the cause. This step, although it is frequently established during the history and physical examination, may require further diagnostic assessment after initiating clinical treatment during the acute phase. Individuals with recurrent rhabdomyolysis, a positive family history of rhabdomyolysis or malignant hyperthermia, low exercise tolerance, no apparent cause, or a fulminant form of rhabdomyolysis appear to warrant further testing.

Testing may include a nonischemic forearm test, which involves isometric exercise at 70% of maximal voluntary contraction for 30 seconds under nonischemic conditions; electromyography; more in-depth blood tests for muscle enzymes (e.g., mitochondrial myopathies [Chapter 389], fatty acid transport defects [Chapter 389], glycogen storage diseases [Chapter 191], diseases associated with myoglobinuria); muscle biopsy to investigate specific metabolic myopathies and other enzyme or genetic defects; or any combination of such testing. The forearm exercise test may help identify metabolic and genetic causes of rhabdomyolysis. Patients who have had an episode of malignant hyperthermia or exertional heat illness may be candidates for a caffeine halothane contracture test, which evaluates the force produced by biopsied muscle samples after separate exposures to caffeine, halothane, and caffeine/halothane in the laboratory (Chapter 400).

PREVENTION

Approaches for preventing rhabdomyolysis induced by infections, medications, and toxins may emerge in the future, but no definitive guidelines currently can be presented. Rhabdomyolysis secondary to heat stress or exercise is best prevented by adhering to recommended guidelines for acclimatization and exercise progression. To prevent further muscle injury, blood flow to ischemic areas must be promptly restored to minimize ischemia-reperfusion damage.

TREATMENT

Treatment of rhabdomyolysis begins with a careful history and physical examination to identify and manage any underlying illness. Vital signs, urine output, and serial electrolyte and CK levels should be obtained as soon as possible. Patients require aggressive early management to preserve renal function (Table 99-3).[15,16] Careful observation and treatment of potential early and late complications are critical, and intensive care monitoring may be required.[17]

Hydration

Hydration is the cornerstone of preserving kidney function in patients with rhabdomyolysis, and delaying fluid administration for more than 6 hours increases the risk for acute kidney injury. Inpatient hydration is indicated for victims of collapse, trauma, or exertional heat injury, as well as for patients who have moderate early symptoms; more than mild elevations in CK; or abnormal serum levels of creatinine, potassium, calcium, phosphate, or bicarbonate. In adults, the target urine output is 300 mL/hr for at least 24 hours to prevent acute kidney injury. Hydration is accomplished by the aggressive administration of isotonic intravenous fluids at a rate that results in a urine output of 200 to 300 mL/hour until CK levels begin to decline. If fluid resuscitation fails to correct intractable hyperkalemia and acidosis, renal replacement therapy should be considered (Chapter 106). By comparison, adults with mild symptoms and serum CK levels less than 3000 U/L are considered to be at low risk and may be treated as outpatients with vigorous oral hydration, limited physical activity, and careful follow-up.

Specific Therapeutic Measures

Alkalinization of the urine decreases cast formation, minimizes the toxic effects of myoglobin on the renal tubules, inhibits lipid peroxidation, and decreases the risk for hyperkalemia. However, bicarbonate therapy can cause calcium to precipitate in the soft tissues and contribute to a hyperosmolar state. Mannitol is an osmotic diuretic, volume expander, and free radical scavenger, but it should be used only after adequate kidney function is established and must be used with great caution in patients with marginal cardiac function. To date, no convincing evidence demonstrates that adding sodium bicarbonate or mannitol is superior to fluid therapy alone.[18] Mannitol should be used only when it is needed to maintain a target urine output.

Sodium bicarbonate should be used only in patients with evidence of systemic acidosis, and mannitol should be used only when it is needed to maintain a urine output of 300 mL/hour (see Table 99-3). Deposition of calcium, which occurs early in rhabdomyolysis, is directly related to the degree of muscle destruction and to the often unnecessary therapeutic administration of calcium given to correct asymptomatic hypocalcemia. Early therapeutic reversal of hypocalcemia can worsen ectopic calcification and exacerbate the exponent hypercalcemia during the resolution phase. Accordingly, hypocalcemia should be treated only when patients develop clinical symptoms, signs of tetany, or severe hyperkalemia.

Management of Compartment Syndrome

Compartment syndrome (Chapter 97) is a well-described late complication as well as a potential cause of rhabdomyolysis. Compartment syndrome can occur as a direct consequence of muscle injury associated with increased vascular permeability, aggressive fluid resuscitation, or restoration of reperfusion. Compartment syndrome should be suspected when the muscles are tense and swollen, previously declining CK levels start to rise, or neurovascular compromise occurs. In these cases, compartment pressures should be measured; if pressures exceed 30 mm Hg, prompt fasciotomy should be considered. However, because late fasciotomy (>12 hours after the onset of symptoms) can convert a closed injury into an open wound and thereby increase the risk of uncontrollable infection, late fasciotomy is relatively contraindicated.

Management of Crush Injury

For victims of crush injury (Chapter 97), aggressive on-site hydration with intravenous normal saline is recommended. For massive damage, amputation of the extremity may be required to protect the patient's overall health. The Mangled Extremity Severity Score can identify nonsalvageable extremities on the basis of the degree of skeletal and soft tissue injury, the patient's blood pressure, the presence of a detectable pulse, and age (see http://www.mdcalc.com/mangled-extremity-severity-score-mess-score/).

Malignant Hyperthermia

Rhabdomyolysis caused by malignant hyperthermia (Chapter 400) requires rapid diagnosis and aggressive management. Anesthetics should be discontinued, and the patient should be treated with dantrolene sodium, 2.5 to 4 mg/kg intravenously, followed by about 1 mg/kg every 4 hours for up to 48 hours to avoid recrudescence.

TABLE 99-3 STEPS IN THE PREVENTION AND TREATMENT OF RHABDOMYOLYSIS-INDUCED ACUTE KIDNEY INJURY

Check for extracellular volume status, central venous pressure, and urine output.*

Measure serum creatine kinase levels. Measurement of other muscle enzymes (myoglobin, aldolase, lactate dehydrogenase, alanine aminotransferase, aspartate aminotransferase) adds little information relevant to diagnosis or management.

Measure levels of plasma and urine creatinine, potassium, and sodium; blood urea nitrogen; total and ionized calcium, magnesium, and phosphorus; and uric acid and albumin. Evaluate acid-base status, blood cell count, and coagulation.

Perform a urine dipstick test and examine the urine sediment.

Identify and discontinue nephrotoxic and myotoxic medications.

Initiate volume repletion with IV normal saline promptly at a rate of approximately 400 mL/hr (200-1000 mL/hr, depending on the patient size, setting, and severity) and monitor the clinical course or central venous pressure.

Target urine output of approximately 3 mL/kg body weight/hr (200-300 mL/hr).

Maintain volume repletion until myoglobinuria is cleared (as evidenced by clear urine or urine dipstick test that is negative for blood).

Consider IV bicarbonate therapy for severe rhabdomyolysis. Check urine pH: if it is <6.5, alternate each liter of normal saline with 1 L 5% dextrose or 0.45% saline plus 100 mmol bicarbonate (2 ampules). Avoid potassium- and lactate-containing solutions.

Consider treatment with IV mannitol only if needed to maintain target urine output. If mannitol is utilized, 50 mL of 20 percent mannitol (1 to 2 g/kg per day [total, 120 g], given at a rate of 5 g per hour) should be added to each liter of fluid. Check for plasma osmolality and calculate the plasma osmolal gap (Chapter 106). Discontinue if diuresis (>20 mL/hr) is not established within a few hours.

Check serum potassium and calcium levels frequently; identify and manage metabolic abnormalities.

Correct hypocalcemia (Chapter 227) only if symptomatic (e.g., tetany, seizures) or severe hyperkalemia occurs.

Hyperkalemia should be treated with standard medical management (Chapter 103). Consider renal replacement therapy for resistant hyperkalemia (>6.5 mmol/L) that is symptomatic (as assessed by electrocardiography), rapidly rising serum potassium levels, oliguria (<0.5 mL of urine/kg/hr for 12 hours), anuria, volume overload, or resistant metabolic acidosis (pH < 7.1).

Investigate and treat the cause of rhabdomyolysis.

*In the case of crush syndrome (e.g., earthquake, building collapse, bariatric surgery), institute aggressive volume repletion promptly before evacuating the patient if creatine kinase level is >15,000 U/L.

IV = intravenous.

Modified from Bosch X, Poch E, Grau JM. Rhabdomyolysis and acute kidney injury. *N Engl J Med.* 2009;361:62-72.

PROGNOSIS

The most serious consequence of rhabdomyolysis is acute kidney injury, which occurs in up to 67% of all cases, regardless of cause. Predictors of the risk of needing renal replacement therapy or death in patients with rhabdomyolysis include age older than 50 years; a higher initial serum potassium level; initial serum creatinine level of 1.4 mg/dL or higher; initial serum calcium level below 7.5 mg/dL; initial serum phosphate level above 4.0 mg/dL[19]; initial serum bicarbonate level below 1 mEq/L; and a cause other than syncope, seizures, exercise, statins, or myositis (E-Table 99-1).

Long-term decline in renal function is best correlated with the serum myoglobin level.[20] A higher initial creatinine level but not a higher initial creatine kinase level also predicts acute kidney injury and mortality. Event rates range from 0% in patients with none of these criteria to 20% or more in patients with four or more criteria. For compartment syndrome, a poor prognosis is associated with an ischemic period lasting longer than 6 hours.

The prognosis of patients with rhabdomyolysis improves markedly when treatment is started soon after the diagnosis is made. With mild episodes, the prognosis is customarily excellent, and the patient can typically resume usual activities within several weeks after CK levels have normalized. However, some patients do not return to normal and continue to experience extreme fatigue and muscle pain on exertion. These patients require additional testing (nonischemic forearm test, electromyography, muscle disease enzyme panel, muscle biopsy; Chapter 389) to determine whether an underlying metabolic myopathy exists. The results of these tests will help determine future recommendations, but the patient's tolerance and response to light and more strenuous exercise are important factors. Most authorities agree that statin-induced rhabdomyolysis is an indication for discontinuation of their use.

GENERAL REFERENCES

For the General References and other additional features, please visit Elsevier eBooks+ at https://ebooks.health.elsevier.com.

XII

RENAL AND GENITOURINARY DISEASES

100 APPROACH TO THE PATIENT WITH RENAL DISEASE

ALI G. GHARAVI AND DONALD W. LANDRY

The prominent functions of the kidney include the excretion of nitrogenous waste; the regulated excretion of water, sodium, potassium, calcium, magnesium, phosphate, and acid; and the synthesis of a variety of hormones, including 1,25-dihydroxyvitamin D, erythropoietin, and renin. The kidney's elaboration of a protein-free and cell-free ultrafiltrate is uniquely responsible for the excretion of nitrogenous wastes. The approach to the patient with renal disease is largely focused on disordered ultrafiltration and not on defects in the isolated renal tubular processing of individual ions, molecules, water, or acids. A patient may, for example, present with an isolated defect in renal acid excretion (Chapter 104), but in this case the "approach to the patient" is framed for the evaluation of metabolic acidosis, an abnormality for which the kidney is only one among the many causes in a broad differential diagnosis. In contrast, acute kidney injury (Chapter 106) and chronic kidney disease (Chapter 116) refer specifically and exclusively to defects in the filtration function of the kidney. In the context of a diminished magnitude of filtration, many of the other individual functions of the kidney (e.g., hormone synthesis, electrolyte homeostasis) may fail as well.

Primary diseases of the tubules, such as acute tubular necrosis (Chapter 106) and tubulointerstitial disease (Chapter 108), also impair the rate of glomerular filtration and cause acute kidney injury and chronic kidney disease. In contrast, an impairment in ultrafiltration may, in early chronic kidney disease, be reflected solely in a decreased *quality* of glomerular filtration (e.g., the presence of albuminuria) rather than in a decreased *quantity* of filtrate with increased concentrations of nitrogenous waste. Similarly, the glomerular filtration rate (GFR) may be normal in nephrotic syndrome despite ultrafiltration defects that result in massive proteinuria. Defects in the filter can also allow passage of cells, such as red blood cells (RBCs), as is seen in the acute nephritic syndrome (Chapter 107), with or without heavy proteinuria. The paradox of glomerular hematuria without albuminuria is also possible. For example, in mild forms of immunoglobulin A (IgA) nephropathy (Chapter 107), relatively few defects in the glomerular filter will permit a detectable number of RBCs per high-power field in the urine despite a urine albumin level that still remains within normal limits (Fig. 100-1).

In this context, this chapter considers the approach to the patient with acute kidney injury, glomerular syndromes (nephrotic vs. nephritic), tubulointerstitial disease, vasculitis and vascular diseases of the kidney, papillary necrosis, and chronic kidney disease.

PATHOBIOLOGY

The approximately 2 million renal glomeruli normally filter about 180 L/day. The renal glomerulus is not simply a filter but rather a size- and charge-dependent ultrafilter that impedes not only cells but also proteins larger than 60 kD from entering the ultrafiltrate. Smaller proteins are variably filtered at the glomerulus and endocytosed in the proximal tubule so that the protein concentration of the urine is normally low. Kidney disease reflects a failure in the quantity or quality of the glomerular ultrafiltrate.

The normal GFR may decline in hours to days in acute kidney injury or during months to years in chronic kidney disease. An acute decline in glomerular filtration is the necessary and sufficient condition for the diagnosis of acute kidney injury, but abnormal urinary findings can assist with elucidating the etiology of the injury. Proteinuria, ranging from microscopic to nephrotic range (Chapter 107), and urinary findings, from a few cells per microscopic high-power field to gross hematuria or pyuria, may be the only evidence of the earliest stages of chronic kidney disease. As chronic kidney disease advances, the decline in the GFR progresses until dialysis or transplantation (Chapter 117) is required to forestall or to treat the syndrome of uremia.

DIAGNOSIS

Measuring Kidney Function

Although the most accurate method of evaluating kidney function is a formal measurement of GFR with iothalamate, iohexol, or similar markers, these

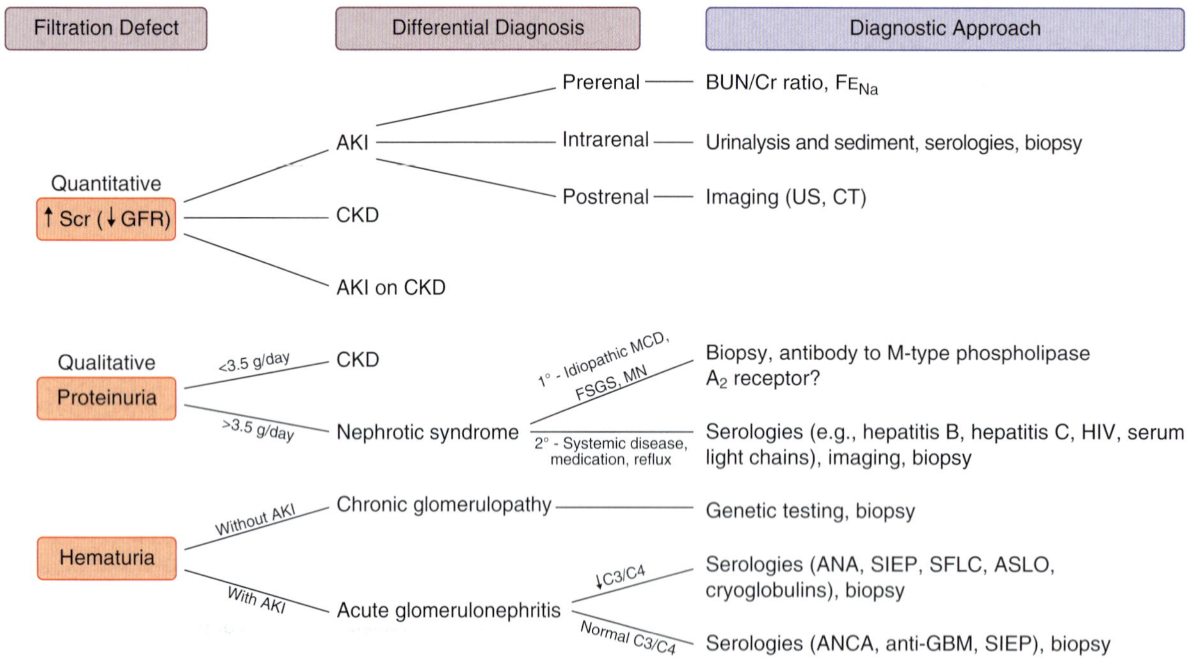

FIGURE 100-1. Overview of approach to kidney disease. Quantitative defects in filtration, manifested by elevated serum creatinine (Scr) and reduced glomerular filtration rate (GFR), should lead to a query into acute kidney injury (AKI) versus chronic kidney disease (CKD). AKI, in turn, is generally divided into prerenal, postrenal, and intrinsic causes. Qualitative defects in filtration, manifested by proteinuria or hematuria, can occur in the absence of changes in GFR and often require biopsy for diagnosis. Proteinuria of more than 3.5 g/day signals nephrotic syndrome, which may be idiopathic or secondary to systemic diseases, such as hepatitis B or C, human immunodeficiency virus (HIV) infection, or diabetes. Glomerular hematuria without AKI is consistent with a chronic glomerulopathy, such as IgA nephropathy, or familial diseases, such as thin basement membranes disease. When hematuria accompanies AKI, acute glomerulonephritis should be suspected and can diagnostically be divided into low-complement glomerulonephritides (immune complex–mediated lesions such as lupus nephritis, postinfectious glomerulonephritis, and cryoglobulinemic glomerulonephritis) and normocomplementemic glomerulonephritides (classically seen in the rapidly progressive glomerulonephropathies due to antineutrophil cytoplasmic antibody [ANCA] and anti–glomerular basement membrane [anti-GBM] antibody). ANA = antinuclear antibody; ASLO = antistreptolysin O; BUN = blood urea nitrogen; Cr = creatinine; CT = computed tomography; MCD = minimal change disease; Fe_{Na} = fractional excretion of sodium; FSGS = focal segmental glomerulosclerosis; MN = membranous nephropathy; SFLC = serum free light chain; SIEP = serum immunoelectrophoresis; US, ultrasonography.

tests are too expensive and time-consuming to be recommended for routine clinical practice. Currently, the most common methods used to estimate GFR are the serum creatinine concentration, the calculated creatinine clearance, and estimation equations based on serum creatinine.

Serum creatinine is, to a first approximation, neither secreted nor reabsorbed, so the amount appearing in the urine per unit time is a measure of the amount that was filtered at the glomerulus during that period. As a result, the rate of creatinine clearance is a reasonably close estimate of the GFR. A decrement in the GFR diminishes creatinine clearance but has no immediate effect on creatinine production by muscle; as a result, the serum creatinine concentration rises. The change in serum creatinine over time indicates the tempo of the renal disease and can distinguish acute injury from chronic kidney disease. The routine use of serum creatinine alone to infer GFR is ill-advised because of the differing rates of creatinine production among individuals, mainly related to variations in muscle mass. Women and the elderly can have deceptively low serum creatinine levels despite significant declines in GFR. In addition, the inverse relationship between GFR and serum creatinine (Fig. 100-2) has important and potentially easily overlooked clinical implications. An initial small absolute rise in creatinine usually reflects a marked fall in GFR, whereas seemingly large changes in the serum creatinine level in patients with more advanced chronic kidney disease (CKD) may reflect minor changes in GFR.

Approach to Diagnosis

The routine screening of asymptomatic adults without risk factors for kidney disease is not recommended. Most patients are diagnosed because other conditions lead to tests of kidney function.

Some kidney diseases may have clinical manifestations in their early stages (e.g., edema in the nephrotic syndrome [Chapter 107] or rash in IgA vasculitis [Chapter 249]). However, because of the kidney's large functional reserve, only significant impairments of kidney function result in clinical manifestations. Advanced renal failure (Chapter 116) is associated with anorexia, abnormal taste, nausea, vomiting, fatigue, sleep difficulties, and shortness of breath from volume overload. Physical examination and laboratory tests reveal malnutrition, hypertension, hypervolemia, anemia, hyperlipidemia, and bone disease. More advanced kidney disease results in the syndrome of uremia, which can manifest as impaired cognition, pericarditis, life threatening hyperkalemia, and acidosis, thereby necessitating renal replacement therapy (Chapter 117).

The serum creatinine level or cystatin C level to estimate and GFR plus additional tests (e.g., a formal 24-hour urine collection to measure creatinine clearance and proteinuria) can confirm the diagnosis of kidney disease. Calculation of creatinine clearance from a 24-hour urine collection can be cumbersome for patients and is prone to error because of inaccurate urine collection. To measure the creatine clearance accurately, the patient must be instructed to discard the first morning urine before initiating the collection and to conclude the collection by including the next morning void. The formula for calculating creatinine clearance is as follows:

$$CCr = (\text{urine Cr} \times V)/(\text{plasma Cr})$$

where *CCr* is creatinine clearance, *urine Cr* is urine creatinine concentration, *V* is urine flow rate, and *plasma Cr* is plasma creatinine. The normal value for GFR ranges from 120 to 140 mL/min/1.73 m^2.

Because of the logistical and practical limitations of a 24-hour urine collection for direct measurement of the GFR, several equations have been developed to estimate GFR based on the serum creatinine or cystatin C level[1–3] and levels of albuminuria (Table 116-2). Although useful for staging CKD, these estimating equations have limitations, particularly in the elderly and at the extremes in the distribution (Chapter 116).[4] For example, physiologic, age-related decline in the GFR in older individuals must be distinguished from a true reduction in the GFR due to kidney disease. All calculations of GFR assume that the patient is in a steady state (Table 100-1), and so values will be inaccurate in situations in which kidney function is changing rapidly (e.g., in acute kidney injury; Chapter 106). The creatinine clearance also overestimates GFR by about 10% owing to tubular secretion of creatinine. The calculations can be further influenced by drugs or conditions (i.e., the nephrotic syndrome or sickle cell disease) that can alter the secretion of creatinine. Cystatin C may provide a more accurate and prognostic measurement of GFR in patients whose creatinine levels are in the upper end of the normal range,[5] but it has not replaced estimated GFR measurements for most clinical purposes.

Urinalysis

Urinalysis can be a very useful test, although it can also be over-ordered in low-risk, asymptomatic individuals. The normal color of the urine is derived from urochromes, which are pigments excreted in the urine. Abnormal color or appearance of the urine may be explained by many conditions (Table 100-2). The basic analysis of the urine sample involves measurements with commercially available dipsticks or microscopic analyses.

Urine Dipstick

The *specific gravity* of the urine generally is related linearly with osmolality. However, it can be raised by the presence of molecules with relatively high molecular weight, such as glucose or contrast dye. A fixed specific gravity of 1.010, so-called isosthenuria, is characteristic of chronic kidney disease (Chapter 117).

Urine pH typically is 5 as a result of daily net acid excretion. An alkaline pH often is noted after meals, when an "alkaline tide" to balance gastric acid excretion increases urine pH. A high urine pH also is seen in patients who are on a vegetarian diet. An exceptionally high urine pH is indicative of an infection with a urea-splitting organism, such as *Proteus* species (Chapter 263). An inappropriately high urine pH in the setting of systemic non–anion gap metabolic acidosis may be seen in certain forms of renal tubular acidosis (Chapter 104). In a proximal renal tubular acidosis, the urine pH is high until the tubular reabsorption threshold for bicarbonate, which is abnormally low, is reached. At this point, the urine pH decreases to 5. In distal renal tubular acidosis, the inability to create a sufficient gradient for hydrogen ions results in a urine pH that is always higher than 5.5. In type 4 renal tubular acidosis, the urine pH is often 5, and the urine net charge is often positive, thereby confirming the

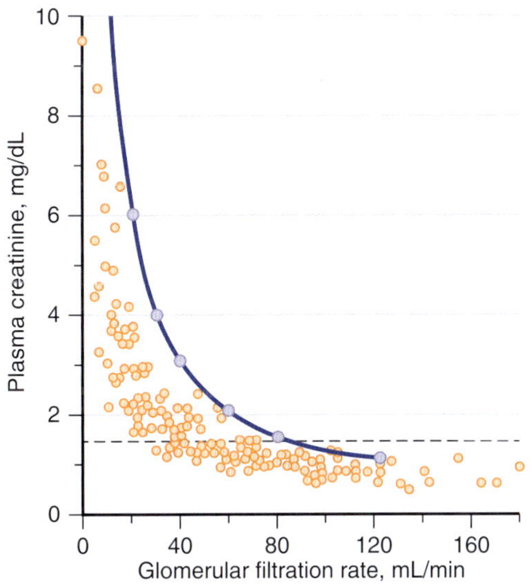

FIGURE 100-2. Relationship between plasma creatinine and glomerular filtration rate measured by inulin clearance in 171 patients (*circles*). The *continuous line* reflects the idealized relationship between these parameters if creatinine were excreted solely by glomerular filtration; the *dashed line* represents an upper limit of "normal" for the creatinine concentration of 1.4 mg/dL. (Redrawn from Shemesh O, Golbetz H, Kriss JP, et al. Limitations of creatinine as a filtration marker in glomerulopathic patients. *Kidney Int.* 1985;28:830-838.)

TABLE 100-1 CONSIDERATIONS FOR INTERPRETATION OF GFR VALUES

ASSUMPTIONS
Assumption of steady state
Assumption of complete 24-hour urine collection
FACTORS THAT ALTER CREATININE PRODUCTION OR SECRETION
Drugs that reduce creatinine secretion (cimetidine, trimethoprim, poly adenosine diphosphate-ribose polymerase inhibitors, tyrosine kinase inhibitors)
Diet (high protein meals can temporarily increase serum creatinine)
Muscle mass (higher muscle mass associated with increased production)
Rhabdomyolysis (increased release due to muscle injury)
Nephrotic syndrome and sickle cell disease (increased secretion)

GFR = glomerular filtration rate.

TABLE 100-2 MACROSCOPIC APPEARANCE OF URINE

APPEARANCE	CAUSE
Milky	Acid urine: urate crystals Alkaline urine: insoluble phosphates Infection: pus Spermatozoa Chyluria
Smoky pink	Hematuria (>0.54 mL blood/L urine)
Foamy	Proteinuria
Blue or green	*Pseudomonas* urinary tract infection Bilirubin Methylene blue
Pink or red	Aniline dyes in sweets Porphyrins (on standing) Blood, hemoglobin, myoglobin Drugs: phenindione, phenolphthalein Anthocyaninuria (beetroot, "beeturia")
Orange	Drugs: anthraquinones (laxatives), rifampicin Urobilinogenuria
Yellow	Mepacrine Conjugated bilirubin Phenacetin Riboflavin
Brown or black	Melanin (on standing) Myoglobin (on standing) Alkaptonuria
Green or black	Phenol Lysol
Brown	Drugs: phenazopyridine, furazolidone, L-dopa, niridazole Hemoglobin and myoglobin (on standing) Bilirubin

From Forbes CD, Jackson WF. *Color Atlas and Text of Clinical Medicine*. 3rd ed. London: Mosby; 2003.

absence of significant amounts of ammonium in the urine; this defect, which is most often present in patients with diabetic kidney disease, is exacerbated by the accompanying hyperkalemia.

Glucose in the urine is detected by an assay using dipsticks impregnated with the enzyme glucose oxidase. Glycosuria, which is seen in diabetes mellitus (Chapter 210), when pregnancy causes the tubular threshold for glucose reabsorption to change, and in tubular diseases that affect the proximal convoluted tubule and cause tubular glycosuria, is an independent risk factor for mortality. Evidence for pan–proximal tubular dysfunction (e.g., glycosuria, aminoaciduria, phosphaturia) indicates that Fanconi syndrome is present.

The dipstick for *protein* is a sensitive assay based on color change induced by the presence of proteins at a given pH. It is most sensitive to the presence of albumin[6] and is much less sensitive to other proteins, such as the light chains of Bence Jones protein (Chapter 173). The presence of 1+ protein correlates with about 30 mg/dL of albuminuria, and 3+ protein correlates with more than 500 mg/dL of proteinuria. Because the dipstick is not a quantitative measurement, small amounts of proteinuria in an oliguric patient may give the false appearance of high-grade proteinuria. The excretion of abnormal quantities of albumin below the level detectable by the urine dipstick is called *microalbuminuria*. Normal albumin excretion, which is less than 30 mg/day, is best detected by radioimmunoassay or enzyme immunoassay. Microalbuminuria is the earliest clinically detectable stage of diabetic nephropathy (Chapter 109). Proteinuria of increasing severity is associated with a more rapid decline in the GFR, regardless of the GFR and even after acute kidney injury,[7] except in minimal change disease (Chapter 107).

The dipstick for *heme* uses the peroxidase-like activity of hemoglobin and myoglobin molecules to detect the presence of heme pigment. The reaction occurs on exposure to hemoglobin, myoglobin, or intact RBCs. Urine dipstick testing is very sensitive (97%) and reasonably specific (75%) for the detection of hematuria. The presence of myoglobin, which is found in patients with rhabdomyolysis (Chapter 99), or free hemoglobin, which is seen in patients with intravascular hemolytic anemias (Chapter 147), is suspected if the heme reaction is intensely positive and there is a paucity of cellular elements in the sediment. Since RBCs lyse rapidly on storage, especially in a hypotonic urine, their absence on routine analysis of the urinary sediment is likely to provide false reassurance in the presence of a positive dipstick. Persistent, isolated, asymptomatic, microscopic hematuria is an independently significant risk factor for the subsequent development of end-stage renal disease (Chapter 116). Although gross asymptomatic hematuria is associated with cancer in 8 to 25% of cases, only about 2.5% of patients with dipstick-positive hematuria have cancer, including less than 0.5% of people under age 50 years.

The dipstick detection of *leukocytes* depends on the presence of leukocyte esterase. Leukocyte esterase is usually present in infections (Chapter 263) and in inflammatory conditions. When positive, it is reasonable to proceed directly to a urine culture without requiring confirmation of leukocytes on a microscopic examination of the urine.[8,9]

Urine Sediment

RBCs, white blood cells (WBCs), tubular cells, transitional cells, and squamous epithelial cells may be seen in the urine.[10] Casts are formed in tubules, may contain cells or cellular debris, or may be acellular.

Hematuria

RBCs may originate from intrarenal vessels, glomeruli, tubules, or anywhere in the urogenital tract (Fig. 100-3). Dysmorphic RBCs are cells that have been deformed by transit through the glomerulus and through the medullary interstitium, as opposed to RBCs from the remainder of the genitourinary tract (Figs. 100-4 and 100-5); these cells are often lysed and less refractile than nonglomerular RBCs. Dysmorphic RBCs often fragment with poikilocytosis and with blebs, forming so-called "Mickey Mouse" RBCs. Phase contrast microscopy aids in the identification of dysmorphic RBCs. The presence of a majority of dysmorphic RBCs in a urine sediment points to a glomerular origin of the hematuria. The presence of RBC casts is often conclusive evidence for the presence of glomerulonephritis.

In asymptomatic individuals with three or more RBCs per high-powered field in a properly collected urine specimen, formal evaluation of the lower and upper urinary tract is commonly indicated, regardless of whether or not patients are taking anticoagulants,[11] if infection, menstruation, and vigorous exercise can be excluded as causes. Lower urinary tract evaluation by cystoscopy should be performed in patients over age 35 years or with risk factors for urinary tract malignancies. Upper tract evaluation usually is performed by computed tomography (CT) or magnetic resonance (MR) imaging urography.[12] Findings suggestive of intrinsic parenchymal renal disease (dysmorphic RBCs, RBC casts, proteinuria, cellular casts) require nephrologic evaluation but do not preclude the need for a urologic evaluation.

Pyuria

WBCs are seen most commonly in bacterial urinary tract infections, but some patients with evident pyuria will have negative urine cultures. Infectious causes of sterile pyuria include tuberculosis (Chapter 299), gonorrhea (Chapter 275), chlamydia (Chapter 294), mycoplasma (Chapter 293) and ureaplasma (Chapter 293, 263, and 264), genital herpes (Chapter 345), trichomoniasis (Chapter 324), fungal infections (Chapter 307), and schistosomiasis (Chapter 326). Even when bacteriuria is confirmed, asymptomatic patients rarely require treatment (Chapter 263).[13,14]

WBCs also can be seen in acute interstitial nephritis, infections with *Legionella* (Chapter 290) and *Leptospira* (Chapter 298) species, allergic interstitial nephritis (Chapter 108), atheroembolic diseases (Chapter 110), granulomatous diseases such as sarcoidosis (Chapter 83), IgG4-related interstitial nephritis, and tubulointerstitial nephritis and uveitis syndrome (Table 100-3). Mononuclear cells often appear with transplant rejection. Tubular cells, which are seen in many conditions involving tubulointerstitial diseases, also are seen in ischemic and nephrotoxic injury, such as with myeloma kidney (Chapter 173) or cast nephropathy. Eosinophils require special stains, with the Giemsa stain being much less sensitive than the Hansel stain (Chapter 108). Urine eosinophils classically are seen in allergic interstitial nephritis (Chapter 108), but they also are seen in atheroembolic disease (Chapter 110), prostatitis (Chapter 114), and vasculitis.

Casts and Crystals

Casts, which are formed in tubules, are characterized by the arrangement of the cells in a clearly formed matrix composed of Tamm-Horsfall protein. Because casts are formed in the renal parenchyma, they may give a clue to the origin of accompanying cellular elements.

Hyaline casts are composed of Tamm-Horsfall proteins that are formed normally and are seen in increased numbers after exercise (Fig. 100-6). *Granular casts* are degenerated tubular cell casts that are seen in the setting of tubular

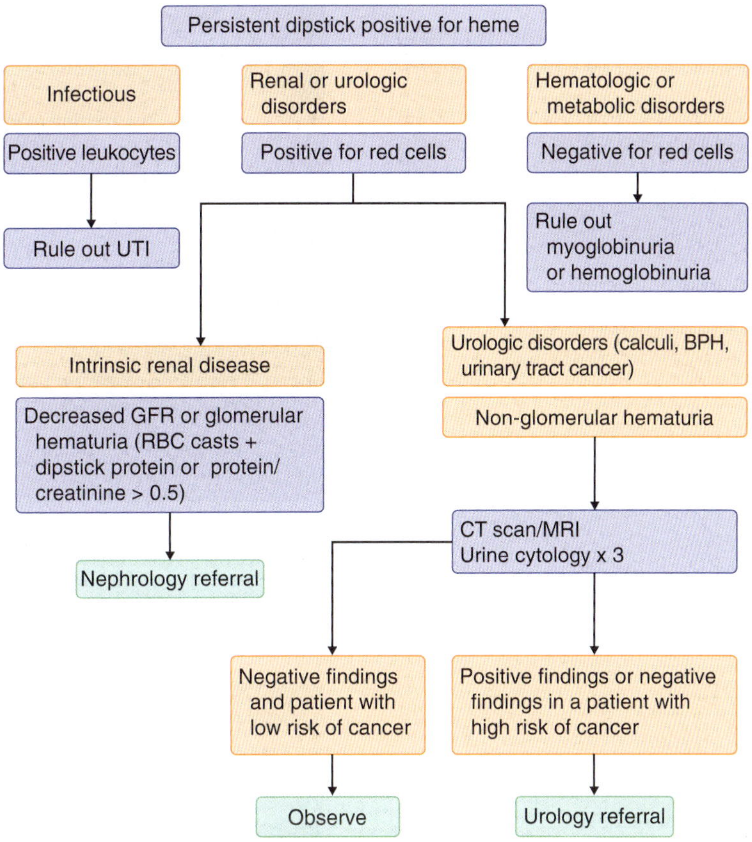

FIGURE 100-3. **Algorithm for the evaluation of asymptomatic hematuria.** BPH = benign prostatic hyperplasia; CT = computed tomography; GFR = glomerular filtration rate; MRI = magnetic resonance imaging; RBC = red blood cell; UTI = urinary tract infection. (Modified from Cohen RA, Brown RS. Microscopic hematuria. *N Engl J Med*. 2003;348:2330-2338.)

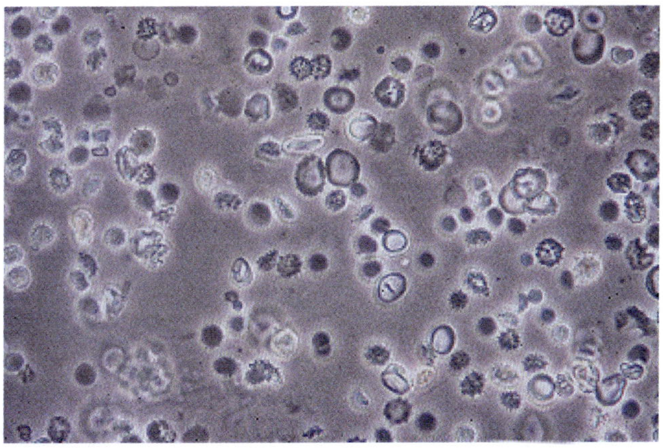

FIGURE 100-4. **Dysmorphic erythrocytes.** These dysmorphic erythrocytes vary in size, shape, and hemoglobin content and reflect glomerular bleeding. (From Johnson RJ, Feehally J. *Comprehensive Clinical Nephrology*. London: Mosby; 2000.)

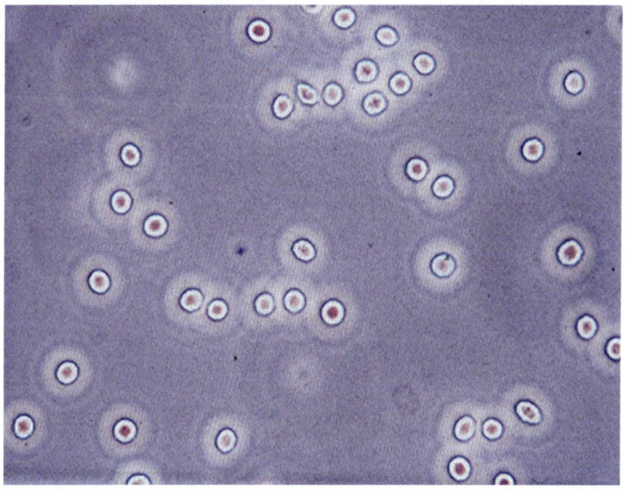

FIGURE 100-5. **Isomorphic erythrocytes.** These erythrocytes are similar in size, shape, and hemoglobin content. Isomorphic cells reflect nonglomerular bleeding from lesions such as calculi and papillomas or hemorrhage from cysts in polycystic renal disease. (From Johnson RJ, Feehally J. *Comprehensive Clinical Nephrology*. London: Mosby; 2000.)

injury (Fig. 100-7). *Pigmented granular casts* are seen in rhabdomyolysis (Chapter 99) with myoglobinuria or, rarely, hemoglobinuria. *RBC casts* (Fig. 100-8) are rarely seen in allergic interstitial nephritis and diabetic nephropathy, but they are frequently seen in acute glomerulonephritis (Chapter 107). The presence of RBC casts in a patient with microscopic hematuria can narrow the focus of the evaluation to a glomerular lesion. *WBC casts* are seen commonly in pyelonephritis (Chapter 263) and in acute and chronic nonbacterial infections. They also are seen in other conditions in which WBCs are associated with parenchymal renal processes, such as allergic interstitial nephritis (Chapter 108), atheroembolic diseases (Chapter 110), and granulomatous diseases such as sarcoidosis (Chapter 83). Rarely, WBC casts can be a dominant feature of many diseases that traditionally are thought of as glomerular diseases, such as lupus nephritis (Chapter 245) and antineutrophil cytoplasmic antibody (ANCA)–associated glomerulonephritis (Chapter 249). *Tubular cell casts* are seen with any acute tubular injury and are the dominant cellular casts in ischemic acute tubular necrosis (Chapter 106). They also can be seen with nephrotoxic injury, such as with aminoglycosides and cisplatin. Some casts may contain both leukocytes and tubule cells.

Crystals can be a normal finding in the urine or serve as clues to pathophysiologic processes. Certain crystals, such as the hexagonal crystals seen with cystinuria (Chapter 111), are always abnormal (Fig. 100-9). Others, such as the octahedral calcium oxalate crystals (Fig. 100-10), may be a normal finding or may be evidence for ethylene glycol intoxication (Chapter 96). Coffin lid–shaped triple phosphate crystals, which are composed of ammonium magnesium phosphate (Fig. 100-11), are seen in urinary tract infections with urea-splitting organisms (Chapter 263). Uric acid crystals, sodium urate

TABLE 100-3 CAUSES OF STERILE PYURIA

INFECTIOUS
Current use of antibiotics
Past treated urinary tract infection (within past 2 weeks)
Tuberculosis (Chapter 299)
Gonorrhea (Chapter 275) and chlamydia (Chapter 294)
Mycoplasma and ureaplasma (Chapter 293)
Genital herpes (Chapter 345)
Trichomoniasis (Chapter 324)
Fungal infections (Chapter 307)
Schistosomiasis (Chapter 326)
Prostatitis (Chapter 114)
Balanitis
Appendicitis (Chapter 128)
NONINFECTIOUS
Interstitial nephritis (e.g., analgesic nephropathy; Chapter 108)
Urinary tract stones (Chapter 111)
Polycystic kidney (Chapter 112)
Current or recent urinary tract manipulation
Catheter cystoscopy
Endoscopy
Foreign body such as surgical mesh in the urethra or a retained stent
Urinary tract neoplasm (Chapter 182)
Pelvic irradiation
Urinary fistula
Renal transplant rejection (Chapters 38 and 117)
Renal vein thrombosis (Chapter 110)
Papillary necrosis
Interstitial cystitis (Chapter 263)
Inflammatory diseases (e.g., systemic lupus erythematosus [Chapter 245] or Kawasaki disease [Chapter 249])

Adapted from Wise GJ, Schlegel PN. Sterile pyuria. *N Engl J Med*. 2015;372:1048-1054.

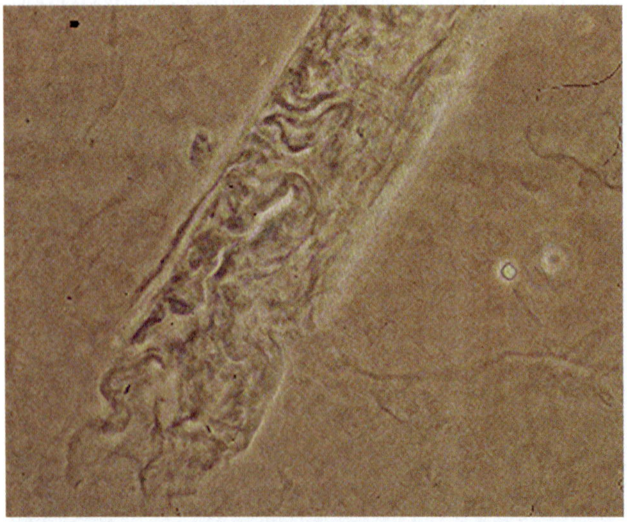

FIGURE 100-6. Hyaline cast of the type seen in small numbers in normal urine. (From Johnson RJ, Feehally J. *Comprehensive Clinical Nephrology*. London: Mosby; 2000.)

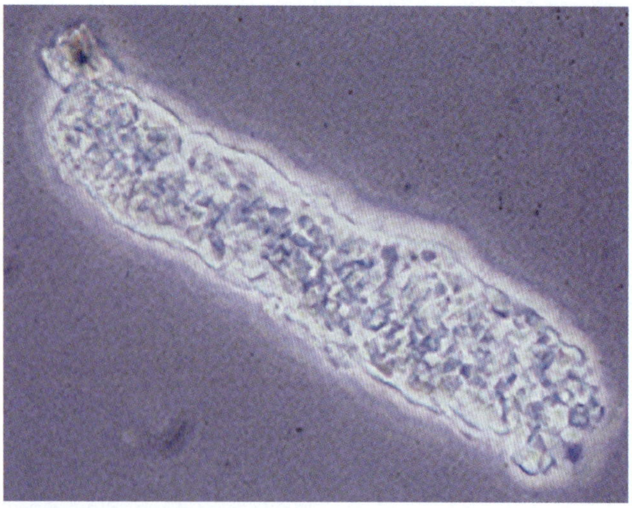

FIGURE 100-7. Number and type of granules and their density in the cast vary in different casts. The presence of erythrocytes in this cast may mean that the granules are derived partly from disrupted erythrocytes. (From Johnson RJ, Feehally J. *Comprehensive Clinical Nephrology*. London: Mosby; 2000.)

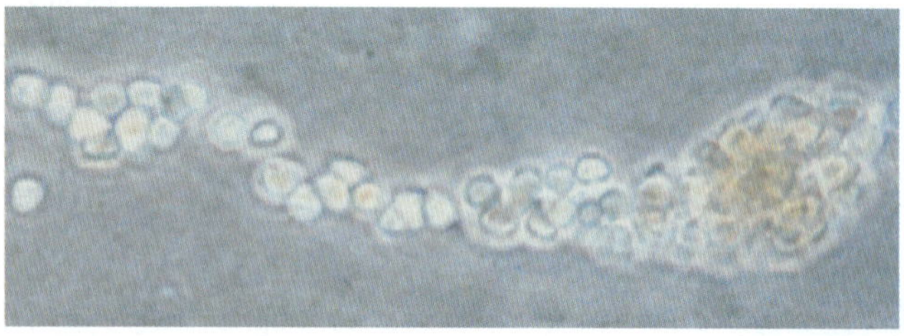

FIGURE 100-8. A cast composed entirely of erythrocytes reflects heavy hematuria and active glomerular disease. Crescentic nephritis is likely to be present if erythrocyte cast density is greater than 100/mL. (From Johnson RJ, Feehally J. *Comprehensive Clinical Nephrology*. London: Mosby; 2000.)

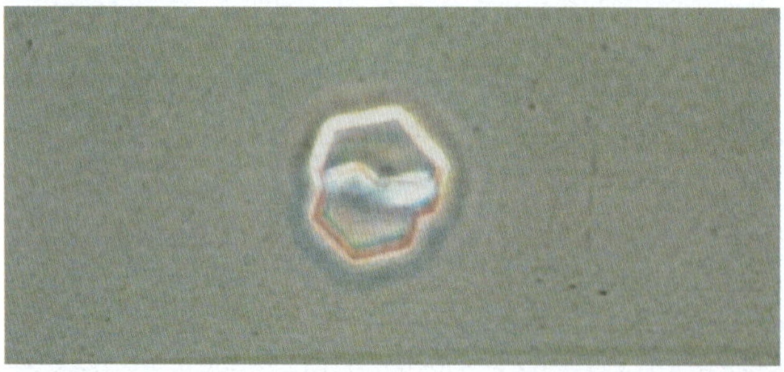

FIGURE 100-9. Typical hexagonal cystine crystal. A single crystal provides a definitive diagnosis of cystinuria. (From Johnson RJ, Feehally J. *Comprehensive Clinical Nephrology*. London: Mosby; 2000.)

crystals (Fig. 100-12), and calcium phosphate amorphous crystals are common and do not usually have pathologic significance.

Other Elements

Bacteria may be seen in the urine sediment. A spun urine sediment may show rods or cocci in chains, but bacteria are identified best by Gram staining of the urine sediment. Budding yeast forms (which are highly refractile), trichomonads, and spermatozoa also may be seen in the urinary sediment.

Disorders of Electrolytes

The kidneys mediate the homeostatic balance of a variety of electrolytes. Electrolyte disorders may accompany renal failure or may reflect isolated defects in tubular function or specific defects in ion transporters. The functional integrity of the renal tubules can be assessed by calculating the fractional excretion of an electrolyte X.

$$FE = \frac{(\text{urine}_X)/(\text{plasma}_X)}{(\text{urine}_{Cr})/(\text{plasma}_{Cr})} \times 100 = \frac{(\text{urine}_X) \times (\text{plasma}_{Cr})}{(\text{urine}_{Cr}) \times (\text{plasma}_X)} \times 100$$

Imbalances in renal sodium and water handling can lead to extracellular volume depletion or to the formation of edema (Chapter 102). Potassium homeostasis is regulated primarily at the distal nephron, but dietary intake, transcellular shifts, and gastrointestinal losses also contribute to balance (Fig. 100-13; Chapter 103). Calcium homeostasis is regulated by the actions of parathyroid hormone, calcitonin, and vitamin D on bone, intestine, kidney, and parathyroid tissue. Although Ca^{++} is also filtered and excreted by the kidney, the important role of these hormones generally places disorders of hypocalcemia and hypercalcemia within endocrinology (Chapter 227). Magnesium deficiency (Chapter 105) may be caused by decreased intake (either orally or by impaired intestinal absorption) or by increased losses via the gastrointestinal tract, kidneys, or skin. Conversely, hypermagnesemia

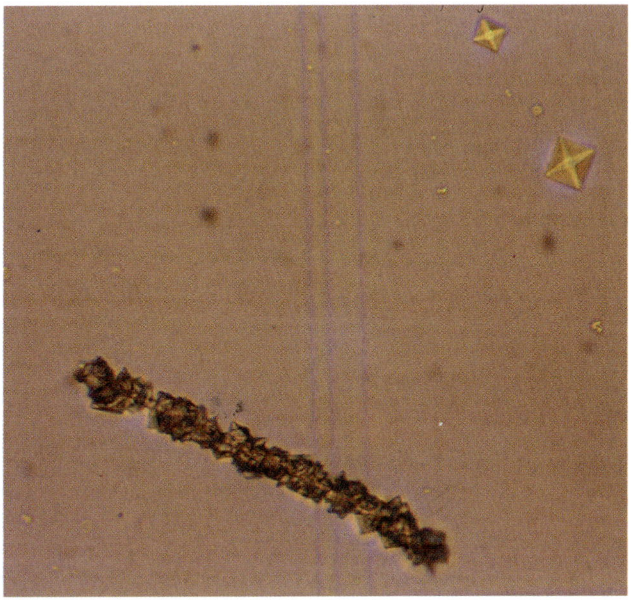

FIGURE 100-10. **Oxalate crystals.** A pseudocast of calcium oxalate crystals accompanied by crystals of calcium oxalate dehydrate. (From Johnson RJ, Feehally J. *Comprehensive Clinical Nephrology*. London: Mosby; 2000.)

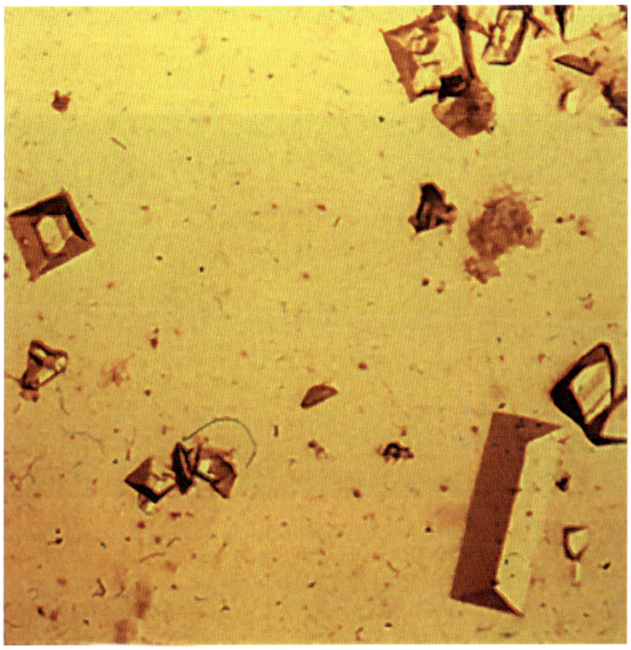

FIGURE 100-11. **Coffin lid crystals of magnesium ammonium phosphate (struvite).** (From Johnson RJ, Feehally J. *Comprehensive Clinical Nephrology*. London: Mosby; 2000.)

(Chapter 105) can rarely occur in individuals with a normal GFR when the rate of intake exceeds capacity of renal clearance (e.g., excessive use of Mg^{++}-based antacids or large parenteral doses given for preeclampsia). Similar to potassium, hyperphosphatemia (Chapter 105) can arise from reduced excretion (primarily chronic kidney disease), excessive intake, or redistribution of cellular phosphorus. Hypophosphatemia also can be caused by shifts into the intracellular compartment, or may occur from malnutrition or from renal losses. High urine phosphorus in the setting of hypophosphatemia suggests a renal tubule defect, hyperparathyroidism (Chapter 227), or a form of rickets (Chapter 226) and can be assessed by determining the fractional excretion.

SPECIFIC RENAL SYNDROMES

This chapter considers the approach to the patient with acute kidney injury (Chapter 106), glomerular syndromes (nephrotic vs. nephritic; Chapter 107), tubulointerstitial disease (Chapter 108), vasculitis and vascular diseases of

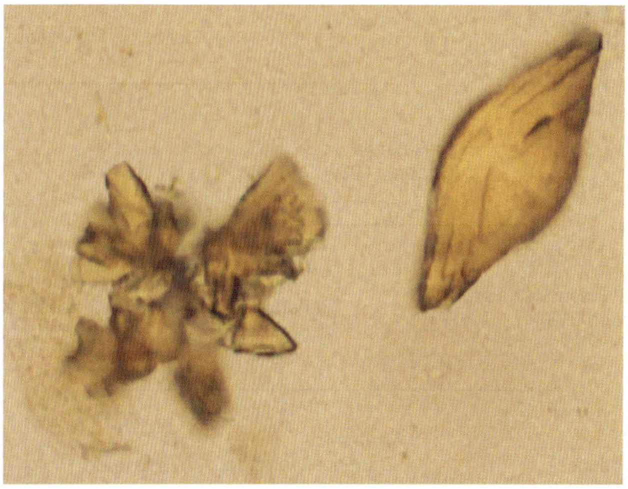

FIGURE 100-12. **Urate crystals.** Complex crystals suggestive of acute urate nephropathy or urate nephrolithiasis. (From Johnson RJ, Feehally J. *Comprehensive Clinical Nephrology*. London: Mosby; 2000.)

the kidney (Chapter 110), papillary necrosis, and chronic kidney disease (Chapter 116).

ACUTE KIDNEY INJURY

Acute kidney injury (Chapter 106) is a syndrome in which glomerular filtration declines during a period of hours to days. The serum creatinine level is elevated in both acute and chronic kidney disease, but an actively rising serum creatinine level confirms an acute or acute-on-chronic insult to kidney function. As a blood filtration organ, the kidney is susceptible to an acute compromise of renal arterial perfusion (Chapter 110), such as prerenal kidney injury, or blockage in urine outflow, such as urinary obstruction due to benign prostatic hypertrophy (Chapter 114). Thus, the patient with acute renal failure is best approached by evaluation for prerenal, renal, and postrenal causes. The intrarenal causes of acute kidney injury include acute tubular necrosis (Chapter 106), acute interstitial nephritis (Chapter 108), acute glomerulonephritis (Chapter 107), and acute vasculitis and vascular disease (Chapters 107, 110 and 249). The careful and systematic evaluation of the patient should start with a thorough history and physical examination, which should be followed by selected laboratory tests and often an imaging test, such as renal ultrasonography. Most cases of acute renal failure in the hospital have hemodynamic or toxic causes, so prerenal azotemia and acute tubular necrosis must be considered carefully and distinguished from one another.

DIAGNOSIS

Laboratory Testing

The normal concentration of blood urea nitrogen (BUN), which is a product of protein catabolism, is about 10-fold higher than the creatinine concentration. Because the BUN-to-creatinine ratio commonly rises with arterial underfilling, BUN typically is used as a marker of effective volume status. Classically, the BUN-to-creatinine ratio will be higher than 15 to 20 in prerenal azotemia but 10 or close to it in acute tubular necrosis. However, the BUN concentration (and hence its ratio to creatinine concentration) may be inappropriately high in other circumstances, such as with high protein intake, gastrointestinal bleeding, or the use of steroids or tetracyclines. The BUN concentration and its ratio to creatinine concentration may be low in patients who have a poor dietary intake of protein, malnutrition, or liver disease.

The excretion of sodium in the setting of oliguria and acute kidney injury (Chapter 106) often gives insight into the appropriateness of tubular function. The fractional excretion of sodium (FE_{Na}) is calculated as follows:

$$FE_{Na} = (\text{urine}_{Na}/\text{plasma}_{Na})/(\text{urine}_{Cr}/\text{plasma}_{Cr}) \times 100$$

where *Na* is the sodium concentration (in mmol/L) and *Cr* is the creatinine concentration (in mmol/L or mg/dL). In the setting of oliguria, FE_{Na} below 1% often denotes prerenal azotemia, whereas FE_{Na} above 1% suggests intrinsic renal damage. Although this measurement is generally useful, FE_{Na} below 1% may be seen without evidence of a prerenal component, including contrast nephropathy (Chapter 106), hepatorenal syndrome (Chapter 139), obstructive

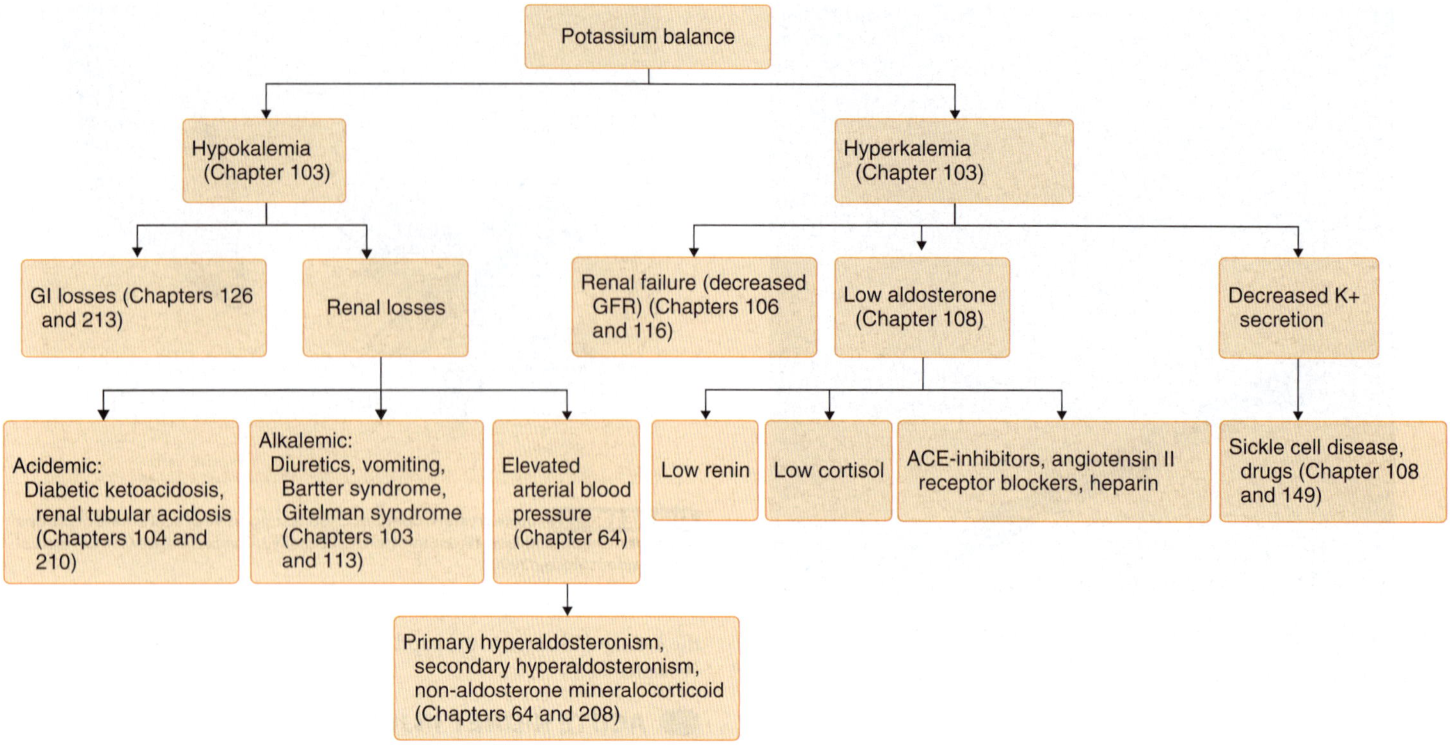

FIGURE 100-13. **Regulation of potassium balance.** ACE = angiotensin-converting enzyme; AKI = acute kidney injury; GI = gastrointestinal.

uropathy (Chapter 114), interstitial nephritis (Chapter 108), glomerulonephritis (Chapter 107), and rhabdomyolysis (Chapter 99). Conversely, a high FE_{Na} can be seen in cases in which there is a prerenal component, including diuretic use, adrenal insufficiency (Chapter 208), cerebral salt wasting, and salt-wasting nephropathy (Chapter 102). The FE_{Na} must be evaluated in the context of the clinical situation because it can be low or high in a normal patient or in a patient with chronic kidney disease. Ultimately, a patient's volume status is best evaluated at the bedside and should not be deduced solely from a measurement of electrolytes.

Imaging

Ultrasonography, which is the most commonly used renal imaging study (Fig. 100-14),[15] provides reliable information about obstruction, kidney size, presence of masses, and renal echotexture. Ultrasonography has only a 90% sensitivity for the detection of hydronephrosis and hence is not sufficient to exclude obstruction (Chapter 114) with certainty. In addition, its inability to detect stones in the ureters and bladder limits its utility in the evaluation for kidney stones (Chapter 111). Ultrasonography can detect vascular disease, and Doppler imaging permits evaluation of the renal vessels with resistive indices. Resistive indices are crucial in ascribing renal dysfunction to the detected vascular disease (Chapter 110). A high resistive index reflects parenchymal disease with scarring and indicates that intervention on the vascular disease itself is unlikely to improve renal function.

A CT scan stone protocol to assess the kidneys, ureters, and bladder is the study of choice for detecting kidney stones (Chapter 111) because of its ability to detect all types of stones, nonobstructing stones, and stones in the ureters (Fig. 100-15). Masses in the kidney can be evaluated with either contrast CT or a renal ultrasound examination. CT angiography with iodinated contrast material can assess possible renal artery stenosis (Chapter 110) with an accuracy comparable to that of MR angiography.

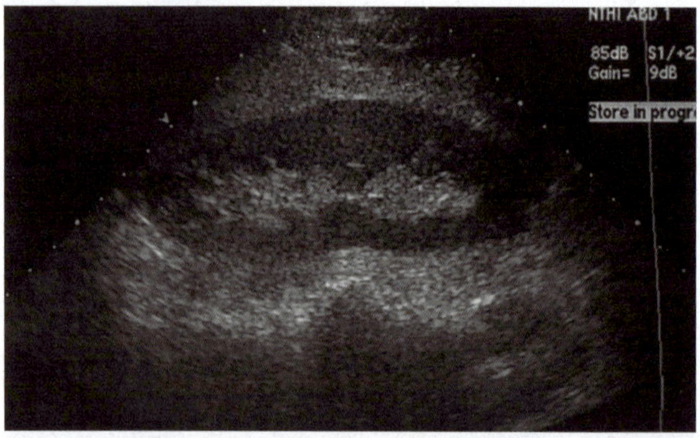

FIGURE 100-14. **Normal findings on sagittal renal ultrasound. The cortex is hypoechoic compared with the echogenic fat containing the renal sinus.** (From Johnson RJ, Feehally J. *Comprehensive Clinical Nephrology*. London: Mosby; 2000.)

GLOMERULAR SYNDROMES: NEPHROTIC VERSUS NEPHRITIC

The nephrotic syndrome (Chapter 107) is characterized by the presence of proteinuria of more than 3.5 g/day/1.73 m^2, with accompanying edema, hypertension, and hyperlipidemia. Other consequences include a predisposition to infection and hypercoagulability. In general, the diseases associated with nephrotic syndrome do not cause acute kidney injury, although acute kidney injury may be seen with minimal change disease, human immunodeficiency virus (HIV)–associated nephropathy, and bilateral renal vein thrombosis (Chapter 110). The causes of primary idiopathic nephrotic syndrome, in decreasing order of prevalence, are focal and segmental glomerulosclerosis, membranous nephropathy, minimal change disease, and membranoproliferative glomerulonephritis. Membranous nephropathy has been associated with antibodies to the M-type phospholipase A_2 receptor. Secondary causes of the nephrotic syndrome include diabetic nephropathy (Chapter 109), amyloidosis (Chapter 174), and membranous lupus nephritis (Chapters 107 and 245).

The acute nephritic syndrome is an uncommon but dramatic presentation of an acute glomerulonephritis (Chapter 107). The hallmark of the acute nephritic syndrome is the presence of dysmorphic RBCs and RBC casts, but their absence does not exclude the syndrome. The acute nephritic syndrome can be caused by any of the rapidly progressive glomerulonephropathies with ANCA-associated vasculitis (granulomatosis with polyangiitis, microscopic polyangiitis, and eosinophilic granulomatosis with polyangiitis), anti–glomerular basement membrane (anti-GBM) glomerulonephritis, and immune complex–mediated glomerulonephritis (including systemic lupus erythematosus, cryoglobulinemia, postinfectious glomerulonephritis, endocarditis, IgA nephropathy, and IgA vasculitis). The rapid decline in renal function often warrants urgent and usually inpatient evaluation.

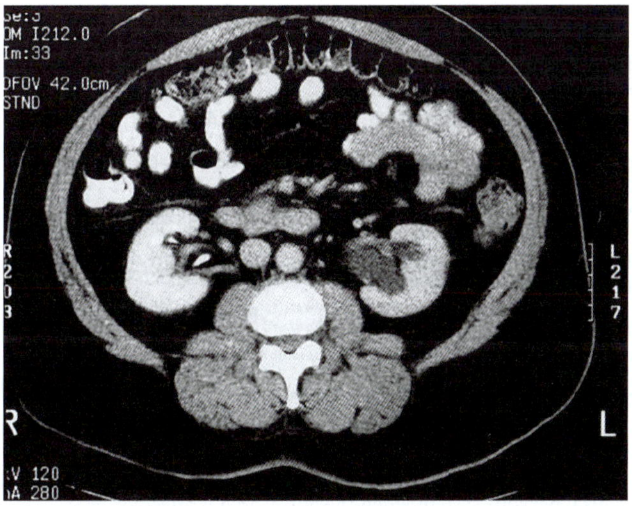

FIGURE 100-15. Delayed excretion in the left kidney secondary to a distal calculus. Contrast-enhanced computed tomography scan shows dilated left renal pelvis. (From Johnson RJ, Feehally J. *Comprehensive Clinical Nephrology*. London: Mosby; 2000.)

DIAGNOSIS

Laboratory Testing

Proteinuria (as albuminuria) of more than 3.5 g in 24 hours generally indicates glomerular disease (Chapter 107). Lesser quantities do not preclude glomerular disease, and electrophoresis gives valuable insight into the composition of the proteinuria (Chapter 173). On occasion, overflow proteinuria of a low-molecular-weight protein, such as light chains in Bence Jones proteinuria, can be higher than 3.5 g/day without any of the manifestations or implications of the nephrotic syndrome; a urine protein electrophoresis study is important in making the distinction. A comparison of the microalbumin-to-creatinine ratio with the protein-to-creatinine ratio will give an insight into the presence of Bence Jones protein because of the absence of albuminuria despite significant proteinuria. Collection must be done by discarding the first morning void and collecting all urine output for the next 24 hours, including the first morning void the next day.

The 24-hour urine collection for protein excretion is cumbersome and subject to inaccuracies. Instead, a spot urine sample for protein and creatinine can be used to estimate the amount of protein excreted. A protein-to-creatinine ratio of 3 translates to a 24-hour protein excretion of about 3 g. The ratio is most accurate when the first morning urine collection is used and may be inaccurate in patients with orthostatic proteinuria.

The evaluation of proteinuric renal dysfunction, particularly when glomerular diseases are suspected, should follow a stepwise progression from noninvasive serologic evaluation to a definitive or confirmatory diagnostic evaluation, such as a renal biopsy. Sometimes an expeditious diagnosis is needed, and a biopsy may be done relatively early in the evaluation.

Serologies

An *antinuclear antibody* (ANA) titer can be useful to evaluate glomerular disease in either nephrotic or nephritic presentations. A high ANA titer (e.g., 1 : 320), especially if it is accompanied by a more specific finding such as anti–double-stranded DNA antibody or anti-Smith antibody, can be highly specific for the diagnosis of lupus nephritis (Chapter 245), which usually requires a renal biopsy. Lower titers (e.g., 1 : 80 or 1 : 40) are nonspecific.

A *rheumatoid factor* titer will usually be elevated in patients with rheumatoid arthritis (Chapter 243), but vasculitis is a relatively late and rare event. Rheumatoid factor can be detected in some forms of cryoglobulinemia (Chapter 173); for example, IgM and occasionally IgG, which is present in type II and type III cryoglobulinemia, has rheumatoid factor activity. Rheumatoid factor also can be seen as a nonspecific finding in bacterial endocarditis (Chapter 61) and systemic vasculitis (Chapter 249).

The levels of *complement* components C3 and C4 and the 50% hemolyzing dose of complement (CH_{50}) usually are measured to evaluate suspected rapidly progressive glomerulonephritis (Chapter 107). Complement levels are usually low in active systemic lupus erythematosus (Chapter 245), post-streptococcal glomerulonephritis (Chapter 107), endocarditis (Chapter 61), membranoproliferative glomerulonephritis, cryoglobulinemia (Chapter 173), shunt nephritis with infection of a ventriculoatrial shunt, and glomerulonephritis associated with visceral abscesses. A particularly depressed C4 compared with C3 should raise the suspicion of cryoglobulinemia.

Serum immunoelectrophoresis will detect elevated polyclonal IgA levels in about 50% of cases of IgA nephropathy (Chapter 107) and IgA vasculitis (Chapter 107). Polyclonal elevation of IgG may occur in a variety of systemic diseases and is a nonspecific finding. The presence of a monoclonal protein in the serum should raise the suspicion for a monoclonal gammopathy–associated disease (Chapter 173). The differential diagnosis includes monoclonal gammopathy of uncertain significance, myeloma kidney, lymphomas (Chapter 171), amyloidosis (Chapter 174), light chain deposition disease, heavy chain deposition disease, immunotactoid glomerulonephritis, and cryoglobulinemia. These conditions, with the exception of monoclonal gammopathy of undetermined significance, have been collectively called monoclonal gammopathy of renal significance when they affect the kidney. The concentration of the monoclonal protein is higher when the diagnosis of multiple myeloma is made, but even small quantities of Bence Jones proteins in the serum can have clinical significance.

A *urine immunoelectrophoresis* always should be obtained if myeloma is suspected. Because a substantial fraction of multiple myelomas can have no heavy chain excretion and small quantities of light chains may be difficult to detect by serum immunoelectrophoresis, a urine immune electrophoresis test for Bence Jones protein should be obtained. In light chain myeloma, patients may have Bence Jones proteinuria even in the absence of an M component in the serum immunoelectrophoresis. Bence Jones proteinuria may be present in myeloma kidney, amyloidosis, light chain deposition disease, lymphoma, or, occasionally, monoclonal gammopathy of uncertain significance. However, some patients with systemic AL (light chain) amyloidosis have a normal serum immunoelectrophoresis and no Bence Jones proteinuria (Chapter 173). More sensitive assays for serum free light chains and an assessment of the ratio of κ to λ lights chains increase the sensitivity for detection of monoclonal gammopathies.

The *antineutrophil cytoplasmic antibody* (ANCA) assay has allowed earlier and more definitive recognition of vasculitic causes of rapidly progressive glomerulonephritis (Chapter 249), especially granulomatosis with polyangiitis, microscopic polyangiitis, and eosinophilic granulomatosis with polyangiitis, when it is confirmed by enzyme-linked immunosorbent assay. The antibodies cause two different patterns of staining: perinuclear staining (p-ANCA) and cytoplasmic staining (c-ANCA). Both antigens actually have a cytoplasmic distribution, and the perinuclear staining pattern is an artifact of the fixation method. In most cases, the antigen for p-ANCA is myeloperoxidase (MPO), whereas the antigen for c-ANCA is proteinase 3 (PR3). Anti-MPO antibodies are associated with microscopic polyangiitis, idiopathic crescentic glomerulonephritis, or Churg-Strauss syndrome (eosinophilic granulomatosis with polyangiitis; Chapter 249). Anti-PR3 antibodies often correlate with the classic disease of granulomatosis with polyangiitis (formerly known as Wegener granulomatosis) (Chapter 249).

Anti–glomerular basement membrane (anti-GBM) antibodies are autoantibodies to the Goodpasture antigen (Chapter 107), which resides in a domain of the α chain of type 4 collagen. An early and accurate diagnosis of Goodpasture syndrome can be made by immunofluorescence and confirmed by Western blot analysis. Anti-GBM antibody staining also may occur in the presence of a positive ANCA. In these cases, the theory is that exposure of the Goodpasture antigen, as a result of the glomerular injury, leads to anti-GBM antibody formation as a secondary process.

Cryoglobulins (Chapter 173) are thermolabile immunoglobulins. They are a single monoclonal type in type I cryoglobulinemia. In type II and type III cryoglobulinemia, however, the mixture of immunoglobulins includes one with rheumatoid factor activity against IgG. Type I and type II cryoglobulins are more likely to be associated with clinical disease, especially at higher titers. Type III cryoglobulinemia is often of less clinical significance. Type I cryoglobulinemia is seen with Waldenström macroglobulinemia and multiple myeloma (Chapter 173); type II with hepatitis C infection (Chapters 134 and 135), Sjögren syndrome (Chapter 247), lymphomas (Chapters 171 and 172), and systemic lupus erythematosus (Chapter 245); and type III with hepatitis C (Chapters 134 and 135), chronic infections, and inflammatory conditions. When cryoglobulinemia is associated with hepatitis C, the hepatitis C virus (HCV) RNA is concentrated in the cryoprecipitate as the antigen; the diagnosis can be made by an RNA assay of the cryoprecipitate at 37° C.

Membranous nephropathy is associated with chronic hepatitis B infection with hepatitis B surface antigenemia (Chapter 135). Classic polyarteritis nodosa (Chapter 249) occasionally is seen with chronic hepatitis B infection, often with surface antigenemia and hepatitis B e antigenemia. M-type phospholipase

A_2 receptor antibodies also have been detected as autoantibodies in about 70% of cases idiopathic membranous nephropathy and have diagnostic value. Antibodies to the thrombospondin type-1 domain-containing 7 A protein are detected in another 5 to 10% of cases.

Hepatitis C serology is associated with a variety of renal diseases, including cryoglobulinemia, membranoproliferative glomerulonephritis, and membranous nephropathy. The evaluation may include the antibody test and an assay for HCV RNA. On occasion, the HCV RNA analysis may have to be conducted on the cryoprecipitate at 37° C.

HIV-associated nephropathy (Chapter 107) is associated with nephrotic syndrome and acute kidney injury. In the appropriate clinical setting, HIV serology and viral titers are warranted tests for both clinical syndromes.

Streptococcal infection can be confirmed as the cause of postinfectious glomerulonephritis (Chapter 107) with an anti-DNase or antistreptolysin O assay. Acute and convalescent serology assays are used to confirm recent infection.

The erythrocyte sedimentation rate (ESR) is a relatively nonspecific test in the evaluation of renal disease. However, a high ESR often points to systemic vasculitis (Chapter 249), multiple myeloma (Chapter 173), or malignant disease as the underlying cause. However, the ESR often is elevated in the nephrotic syndrome (Chapter 107), including diabetic nephropathy (Chapter 109).

Renal Biopsy

No formal guidelines exist for the indications to perform a renal biopsy. Most nephrologists will perform a biopsy for adults with idiopathic nephrotic syndrome and for children with steroid-dependent or steroid-resistant nephrotic syndrome. In addition, acute kidney injury without an identifiable inciting cause is a clear indication for biopsy. Notably, patients with hospital-acquired kidney failure rarely meet this indication. Other abnormal clinical findings, such as gross or microscopic hematuria or subnephrotic proteinuria, often but not always lead to a kidney biopsy. Renal biopsy usually is performed percutaneously with real-time ultrasound or CT guidance. About 1 to 2% of patients without an underlying coagulopathy will develop bleeding that requires a transfusion. The transjugular approach can be used in patients in whom the risks for bleeding are high.

Genetic Testing

Inherited factors play an important role in kidney disease, and 25 to 30% of patients with CKD have a family history of nephropathy. Genetic testing can establish a genetic diagnosis in nearly 10% of patients with CKD and is useful even in patients who have had a renal biopsy.[16,17] The diagnostic yield is higher in patients who have a younger onset of disease, a family history of kidney disease, or multi-organ, syndromic features. The diagnostic yield is highest in patients with cystic kidney disorders (20 to 50%) and patients with nephrotic syndrome (5 to 25%), but full exome sequencing also has a diagnostic yield of about 20% in patients with CKD of unknown cause, thereby leading to the detection of many rare conditions spanning all major clinical categories of kidney disease (E-Fig. 100-1).[18]

TUBULOINTERSTITIAL DISEASES

Tubulointerstitial diseases (Chapter 108) vary in presentation from acute kidney injury to chronic kidney dysfunction that initially is manifested as asymptomatic mild renal insufficiency (Table 100-4). The urine sediment often contains small to moderate amounts of proteinuria, usually less than 1 g/day, as well as WBCs, RBCs, tubule cells, and WBC casts. RBC casts are rare in acute interstitial nephritis and more characteristic of glomerular disease.

TABLE 100-4 MAJOR CAUSES OF TUBULOINTERSTITIAL DISEASE

Ischemic and toxic acute tubular necrosis
Allergic interstitial nephritis
Interstitial nephritis secondary to immune complex–related collagen vascular disease, such as Sjögren disease or systemic lupus erythematosus
Granulomatous diseases: sarcoidosis, tubulointerstitial nephritis with uveitis
IgG4-related interstitial nephritis
Pigment-related tubule injury: myoglobinuria, hemoglobinuria
Hypercalcemia with nephrocalcinosis
Tubular obstruction: drugs such as indinavir, uric acid in tumor lysis syndrome
Myeloma kidney or cast nephropathy
Infection-related interstitial nephritis: *Legionella, Leptospira* species
Infiltrative diseases, such as lymphoma

Ig = immunoglobulin.

VASCULITIS AND VASCULAR DISEASES OF THE KIDNEY

Vascular diseases of the kidney can be divided into large-vessel obstruction and medium- to small-vessel diseases (Chapter 110). Renovascular disease is a common cause of hypertension, heart failure, and renal insufficiency. About 90% of renal artery stenosis is atherosclerotic in origin, with most of the remaining caused by fibromuscular dysplasia, which is more common in women 20 to 50 years of age. Medium-sized arterial vessel diseases include polyarteritis nodosa, which is seen in patients with hepatitis B (Chapters 134 and 135), HIV infection (Chapter 107), or, rarely, hepatitis C (Chapters 134 and 135). Symptoms include abdominal pain, hypertension, and mild renal insufficiency, often with a benign sediment; diagnostic findings include microaneurysms at the bifurcation of medium-sized arteries. Other diseases involving small vessels include atheroembolic disease (Chapter 110), which is seen after arteriography or surgery or, rarely, spontaneously. This syndrome typically affects the kidneys, gastrointestinal tract, and lower extremities, but it can also involve the central nervous system when the aortic arch is affected.

The thrombotic microangiopathies include hemolytic-uremic syndrome and thrombotic thrombocytopenic purpura (Chapter 158). Thrombotic thrombocytopenic purpura is associated with an acquired inhibitor to or the congenital inherited absence of a protease that cleaves large-molecular-weight von Willebrand multimers. The hemolytic-uremic syndrome is caused by endothelial injury. In diarrhea-positive (or typical) hemolytic-uremic syndrome, the endothelial injury is induced by Shiga toxin from *Escherichia coli* O157:H7 infection. In diarrhea-negative (atypical) hemolytic-uremic syndrome, dysregulation of the alternative complement pathway is the underlying cause of endothelial injury. The antiphospholipid antibody syndrome (Chapter 67) can cause large-vessel thrombosis and stenosis as well as a thrombotic microangiopathy with proteinuria, hypertension, and renal insufficiency. Scleroderma renal crisis, which is a manifestation of systemic sclerosis (Chapter 246), often leads to an inexorable progression to end-stage renal insufficiency if untreated.

A systemic vasculitis may be manifested in a variety of ways, including skin manifestations such as petechial rash, purpura, digital gangrene, and splinter hemorrhages. Otitis, sinusitis, epistaxis, hemoptysis, and nasal septal ulcers are common manifestations of granulomatosis with polyangiitis (Chapter 249). Pulmonary hemorrhage can be a catastrophic manifestation of Goodpasture syndrome (Chapter 107), anti-GBM disease, or ANCA-associated vasculitis (Chapter 249). Abdominal pain and tenderness and gastrointestinal hemorrhage may be observed in IgA vasculitis and classic polyarteritis nodosa (Chapter 249). Neurologic symptoms may be a manifestation of vasculitis, such as microscopic polyangiitis (Chapter 249) and cryoglobulinemia (Chapter 173).

DIAGNOSIS

Radiologic Evaluation

Magnetic resonance imaging (MRI) with MR angiography (Fig. 100-16) is highly sensitive for detecting atherosclerotic renovascular disease (Chapter 110), but it tends to overestimate the degree of stenosis. Its accuracy in detecting fibromuscular dysplasia, however, is less well validated. MRI also can be used to evaluate renal masses. MRI does not require iodinated contrast material, but gadolinium-based contrast agents for vascular studies are associated with the syndrome of nephrogenic systemic fibrosis in patients with advanced renal failure (Chapter 246).

Renal arteriography, which is the "gold standard" in the evaluation of renal artery stenosis (Chapter 110), also is used for the evaluation of arteriovenous malformations, polyarteritis nodosa, and other vascular lesions of the kidneys. This invasive study uses iodinated contrast material and incurs a small risk for atheroembolic disease (Chapter 110). Therapeutic angioplasty and stenting can be done at the time of angiography.

PAPILLARY NECROSIS

Acute necrosis of the renal papilla is associated with sickle cell anemia (Chapter 149), analgesic nephropathy (Chapter 108), diabetic nephropathy (Chapter 109), and obstructive pyelonephritis (Chapter 263). In sickle cell disease (Chapter 149), the hypoxic and hypertonic milieu of the inner medulla promotes sickling, and chronic sickling at the vasa recta results in medullary ischemia. Massive and prolonged consumption of analgesics, particularly the combination of aspirin, caffeine, and acetaminophen, is associated with chronic interstitial nephritis and a predisposition to papillary necrosis (Chapter 108); medullary ischemia is thought to be caused by inhibition of synthesis

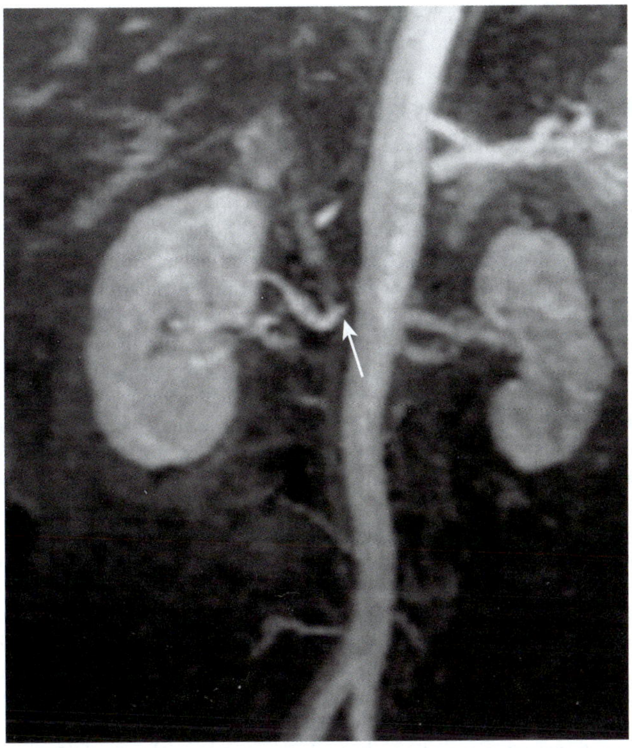

FIGURE 100-16. **Magnetic resonance angiography.** Coronal three-dimensional image shows right renal artery stenosis (*arrow*). (From Johnson RJ, Feehally J. *Comprehensive Clinical Nephrology*. London: Mosby; 2000.)

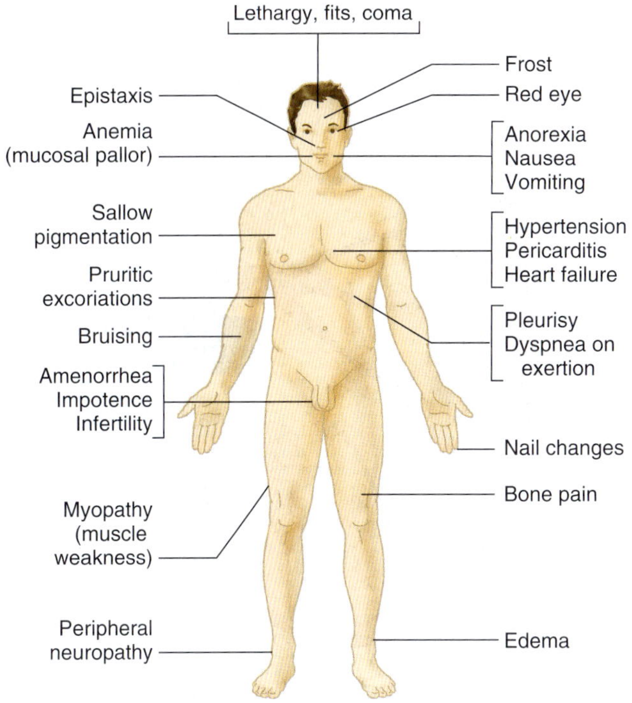

FIGURE 100-17. **Common symptoms and signs of chronic renal failure.** (Redrawn from Forbes CD, Jackson WF. *Color Atlas and Text of Clinical Medicine*. 3rd ed. London: Mosby; 2003.)

of vasodilatory prostaglandins by aspirin, and direct toxicity is attributed to metabolites of phenacetin. Similarly, medullary perfusion is thought to be compromised in diabetic nephropathy (Chapter 109) and obstructive pyelonephritis (Chapter 114).

The clinical manifestations of papillary necrosis can include flank pain and hematuria. If the papilla is sloughed, obstruction may occur at the renal pelvis or ureter of the affected kidney, with referred pain migrating from the flank to the groin. A sloughed papilla may precipitate frank renal failure if the function of the contralateral kidney is impaired or if obstruction occurs at the level of the bladder or urethra.

Classically, papillary necrosis is diagnosed on an excretory pyelogram as a calyceal defect after sloughing of a papilla, but CT with contrast enhancement is as good for advanced lesions. If the necrotic papilla is retained, however, the defect will be more subtle. Transitional cell carcinoma (Chapter 182) can occur in the setting of papillary necrosis or can mimic its appearance. Obstruction, if present, must be relieved, but treatment otherwise is limited to pain control and hydration.

CHRONIC KIDNEY DISEASE

Chronic kidney disease, which is defined as either kidney damage or a GFR of less than 60 mL/min/1.73 m^2 for longer than 3 months. Kidney damage is defined as pathologic abnormalities or markers of kidney damage, including abnormalities in the composition of blood or urine or abnormalities on imaging tests. The excretion of 30 to 300 mg of albumin in a 24-hour period defines microalbuminuria. CKD is classified according to underlying cause, level of GFR, and level of albuminuria (Fig. 116-2). An estimated 12% of the adult U.S. population has abnormal albumin excretion in the urine, and the frequency increases with age. Kidney failure is defined as either a GFR of less than 15 mL/min/1.73 m^2 that is accompanied by signs and symptoms of uremia or a need for initiation of kidney replacement therapy for treatment of complications of decreased GFR (Fig. 100-17). End-stage renal disease includes all cases requiring treatment by dialysis or transplantation regardless of the level of GFR.

Patients with chronic kidney disease warrant referral to a nephrologist. Care of these patients should focus on efforts to slow disease progression, to optimize medical management, and to make a seamless transition to renal replacement therapy (Chapter 116). The care should include optimal blood pressure control, use of angiotensin-converting enzyme inhibitors and angiotensin receptor blockers if indicated, dietary counseling, careful management of calcium and phosphorus levels, control of the parathyroid hormone level, and management of anemia with the use of erythropoietin and iron supplements. Early referral for placement of access for dialysis and initiation of transplant evaluation (Chapter 117) are important components of the care of patients with chronic kidney disease.

GENERAL REFERENCES

For the General References and other additional features, please visit Elsevier eBooks+ at https://ebooks.health.elsevier.com.

101 STRUCTURE AND FUNCTION OF THE KIDNEYS

QAIS AL-AWQATI AND JONATHAN BARASCH

The kidney regulates the ionic composition and volume of body fluids, the excretion of nitrogenous waste, the elimination of exogenous molecules (e.g., many drugs), the synthesis of a variety of hormones (e.g., erythropoietin), and the metabolism of low-molecular-weight proteins (e.g., insulin). Befitting such an array of responsibilities, the kidney receives 25% of the cardiac output. The gross anatomy of the kidney is notable for a weight of approximately 150 g and a characteristic bean shape with approximate dimensions of 11 × 6 × 2.5 cm. On bisection, a gross structure is evident with an outer cortex and a more central medulla that narrows to multiple papillae at the apices of so-called pyramids (Fig. 101-1).

Understanding renal physiology, however, requires an appreciation of the intricate microstructure that underlies its complex functions. Although the kidney is an organ, the *nephron* is actually the organ's independent filtration unit. On average, each human kidney is composed of 1 million essentially identical nephrons. All functions of the kidney are performed by each individual nephron, and to a first approximation, all nephrons are independent of each other because they have their own innervation and blood supply.

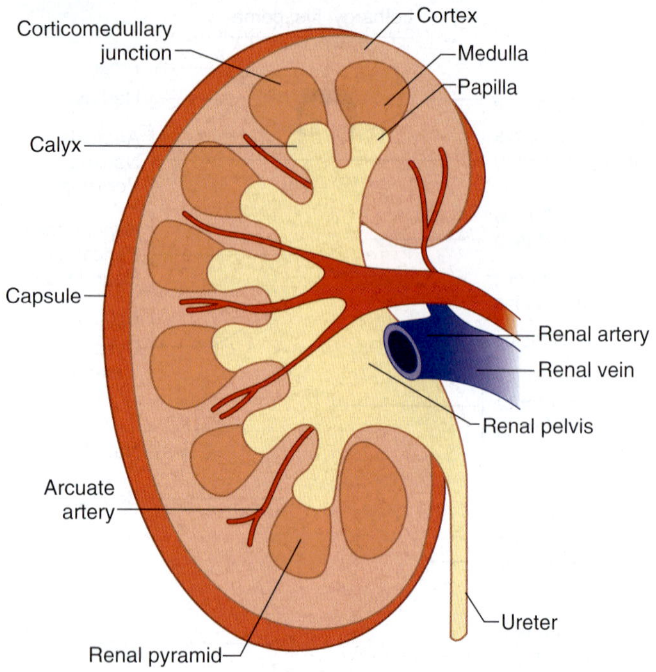

FIGURE 101-1. Sagittal section of the human kidney depicting gross anatomy and organization.

The nephron is made up of two functional subunits, the glomerulus and the tubules and ducts (Fig. 101-2). The glomerulus begins with the branching of the afferent arteriole, an end artery of the corresponding renal artery, into a tuft of capillaries. The glomerular capillaries invaginate an epithelium with the visceral epithelial cells adjacent to the capillary and the parietal epithelial cells outside this tuft. The space between the epithelial layers is the urinary space.[1] The fenestrated glomerular capillary endothelium, the intervening basement membrane, and the foot processes of the visceral epithelium, so-called podocytes, compose the glomerular filtration barrier. The balance of hydrostatic and oncotic pressures drives the extrusion of a protein-free filtrate through this barrier into the urinary space. The urinary space then leads to a series of tubules and ducts: the proximal tubule, the thin limb of the loop of Henle, the thick limb of the loop of Henle, the distal convoluted tubule, the cortical collecting duct, and the medullary collecting duct. The papillary collecting duct empties through the renal papilla into the renal pelvis and then to the ureter. The glomerular capillary bed coalesces to form the efferent arteriole, a vessel that is exquisitely sensitive to angiotensin II, and then the peritubular (proximal) capillaries. This system allows efferent arteriole constriction to regulate proximal tubule reabsorption, as described later.

The nephron regulates homeostasis by three actions. First, in the glomerulus, nephrons collectively produce as much as 120 mL/minute of an ultrafiltrate of blood. Second, different segments of the nephron change the composition of the filtrate by the transfer of nearly 99% of its components (e.g., glucose, NaCl, water) from the lumen to the blood. Third, additional electrolytes (e.g., NH_4^+, K^+, HCO_3^-) are secreted from the blood into the lumen.

To perform these functions, each nephron segment, with the exception of the connecting segment and the collecting ducts, is composed of a single epithelial cell type whose luminal or apical surface (facing the urine) and basolateral surface (facing the blood) differentially express various proteins and lipids. For example, the apical membrane often has microvilli or cilia, whereas the basolateral membrane does not. Polarized endocytosis and exocytosis are often important in the regulation of the number of transport proteins on the apical surface. In addition, epithelia are connected to one another by tight junctions, which confer a characteristic ionic permeability on the epithelial sheet. Transepithelial transport occurs largely through the cell, but transport also can occur through the tight junction (the *paracellular pathway*). For instance, sodium transport begins with entry at the luminal surface down an electrochemical gradient, whereas its exit at the basolateral surface is uphill and requires adenosine triphosphate (ATP) hydrolysis. The Na^+, K^+-ATPase is located at the basolateral surface of all epithelia, and all "active" energy-consuming transport is coupled directly or indirectly to it with the exception of H^+ transport by the H^+ATPase. Each segment has a distinct composition of channels, carriers, and ATPases, and each segment is regulated by different chemical and physical sensors, so the "final urine" contains the components that must be discarded to maintain constancy of body composition.

THE KIDNEY REGULATES EXTRACELLULAR FLUID VOLUME BY REGULATING SODIUM CONTENT

Filtration of 180 L/day of plasma containing 24,000 mEq of sodium is followed by the reabsorption of over 99% of the filtered sodium. Sodium reabsorption accounts for more than 90% of the oxygen consumed by the kidney. It is regulated by volume receptors that are located in the carotid artery and increase β-sympathetic output, which in turn releases renin, an aspartate protease from the granular cells of the juxtaglomerular apparatus, which is located near the afferent arteriole that supplies the glomerulus. Renin cleaves angiotensinogen to angiotensin I, which is then converted locally to angiotensin II. Angiotensin II binds to angiotensin receptors and constricts the efferent arteriole, thereby affecting glomerular hemodynamics. Increased hydrostatic pressure within the glomerular capillaries drives the formation of an ultrafiltrate of plasma. As filtration progresses, a protein-rich, oncotically active solution in the capillary opposes the glomerular capillary hydrostatic pressure until a pressure equilibrium is achieved before the efferent arteriole is reached. Consequently, angiotensin II may not change glomerular filtration rate (GFR) markedly, but it can increase proximal reabsorption by reducing the hydrostatic pressure and increasing the oncotic pressure in the peritubular capillaries that surround the proximal tubule in a plexus, thereby favoring reabsorption of water and solutes such as urea.

The glomerular filtrate next enters the tubules. Na^+ traverses the cell by entering the apical membrane either through a segment-specific cotransporter, counter-transporter, or sodium channel. The apical membrane of the proximal tubule contains an Na^+/H^+ (NHE3) exchanger, Na^+-coupled glucose carrier, and Na^+-coupled amino acid and phosphate cotransporter. Na^+ is then actively transported by the basolateral Na^+, K^+-ATPase into the paracellular space, thereby resulting in local hypertonicity, which causes osmosis through low-resistance tight junctions of the initial segments of the proximal tubule (E-Fig. 101-1).

In the thick ascending limb of Henle, Na^+ is absorbed by an Na-K-2Cl cotransporter. The driving force for this neutral carrier allows Na^+ and Cl^- to enter the cell, but then recycles K^+ across the apical membrane, thereby resulting in depolarization of the transepithelial membrane potential. In the distal convoluted tubule, Na^+ is absorbed by a thiazide-sensitive cotransporter, which conducts Na^+ and Cl^- in a strict 1 : 1 stoichiometry. Na^+ exits as usual by the Na^+, K^+-ATPase, but there is also a basolateral Na/Ca exchanger. In this short segment, the macula densa helps control the GFR by regulating renin release through secretion of adenosine and prostaglandins.

In the principal cells of the collecting duct, aldosterone, derived from the zona glomerulosa of the adrenal cortex, is the final critical regulator of Na^+ balance. Aldosterone increases reabsorption of the final 50 to 100 mEq/day of sodium remaining in the lumen by increasing the number of open sodium channels (ENaC) and by increasing the activity of the basolateral Na^+, K^+-ATPase.[2]

A number of the steps that regulate sodium reabsorption can be counteracted by atrial natriuretic peptide (ANP), which is released from the atria in response to volume overload. ANP increases filtration in the glomerulus by dilating the afferent arteriole, thereby increasing glomerular capillary pressure and lowering the oncotic pressure. In addition, ANP increases sodium excretion by inhibiting the release of renin, the production of aldosterone, and the tubular reabsorption of sodium in the terminal collecting duct.

THE KIDNEY CONTROLS BODY FLUID OSMOLARITY BY REGULATING WATER CONTENT

Water moves freely among all cells and compartments of the body via water-conducting channels called aquaporins. Osmolarity (the concentration of water) is strictly regulated to prevent cells from swelling or contracting via mechanisms that control the intake (thirst) and excretion of fluids, whereby the kidney can vary the osmolarity of urine. Channels in the thick ascending limb, distal tubule, and collecting duct absorb sodium without water to dilute the urine. The absorbed NaCl and urea provide a hyperosmotic region in the medulla, where the limited blood flow maintains an osmotic gradient. To concentrate the urine, water is removed from the filtrate by this osmotic gradient as it passes through the cortical and medullary collecting tubules.

Antidiuretic hormone (ADH), also called *vasopressin,* is a critical component of water reclamation. Changes of less than 1% in osmolarity induce cells in the neurohypophysis to shrink and, via activation of TRPV1 channels, to release ADH. In the kidney, ADH binds to the vasopressin type 2

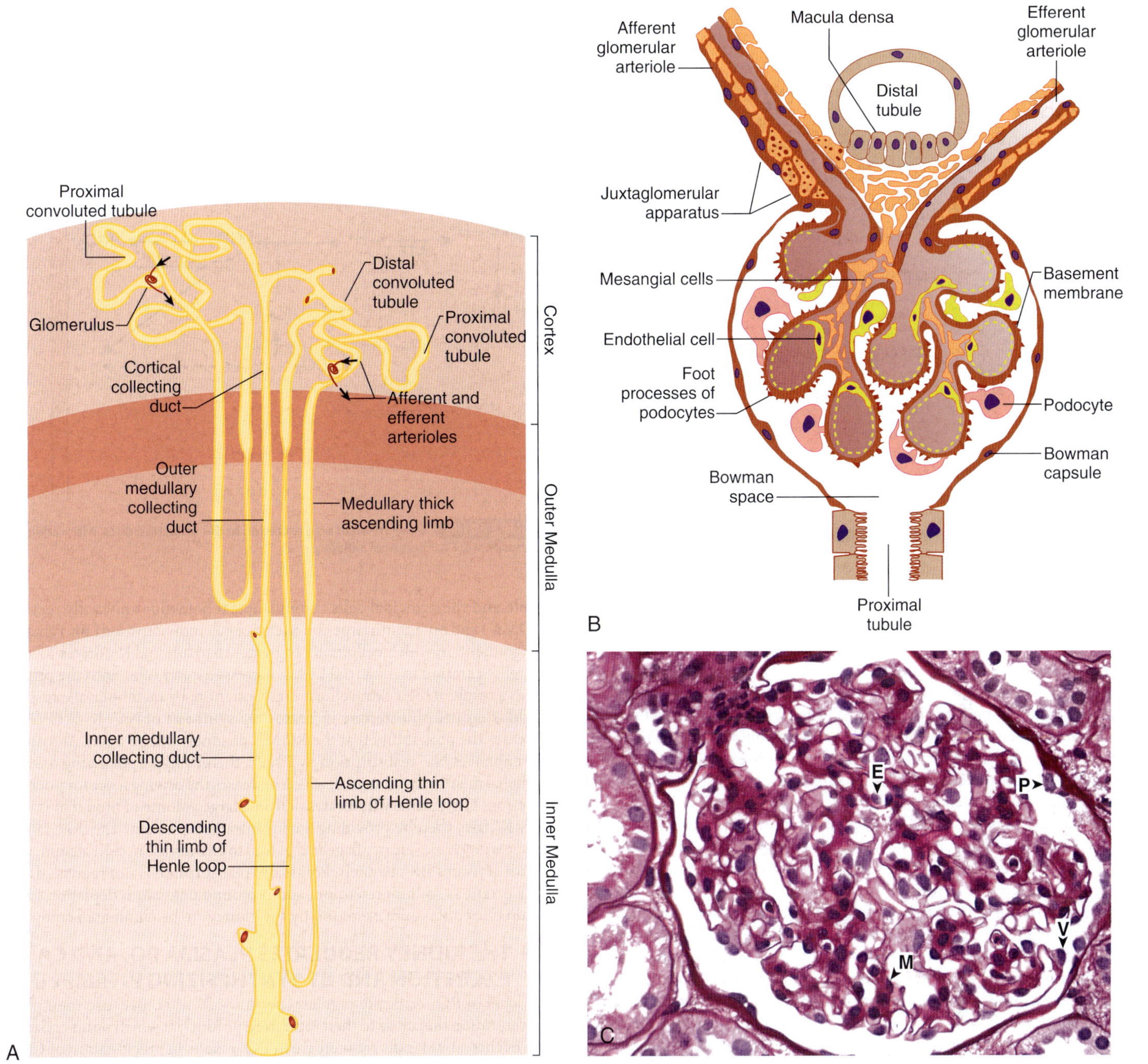

FIGURE 101-2. Structure of the nephron. A, Components of the cortical and juxtaglomerular nephrons. B, Anatomy of the glomerulus. C, Light micrograph of a human glomerulus. E = endothelial cell; M = mesangial cell; P = parietal epithelial cell; V = visceral epithelial cell. (C, Courtesy Dr. Glen Markowitz.)

receptor on collecting tubules and increases water permeability by reversibly inserting a water channel, called *aquaporin 2*, in the apical membrane.[3] During states of water deprivation, the dilute urine generated by the thick ascending limb enters vasopressin-sensitive segments in the cortical collecting tubule, where the bulk of the water is absorbed into the cortex to increase the osmolarity of the urinary filtrate to 300 mOsm, equivalent to plasma osmolarity. When it then travels through the medullary collecting duct, the urine becomes concentrated as it equilibrates with the osmolarity of the medulla (Fig. 101-3).[4]

THE KIDNEY REGULATES PLASMA pH BY REGULATING HCO_3^- CONTENT

The concentration of free H^+ in the intracellular and extracellular fluids is maintained at about 40 nM (pH 7.4) by the daily excretion of acid or base in amounts equal to what is generated by dietary intake and by cellular activity. The complete oxidation of carbohydrates and fats generates approximately 15 to 20 mol/day of the volatile acid CO_2, and nonvolatile acids generated by the metabolism of protein-rich diets account for 60 to 80 mEq/day. HCO_3^- is the most important buffer because it is consumed by metabolic acid, thereby producing CO_2 that can be exhaled, and because it can be regenerated by the kidney. The overall relationship of this buffer system is described by the Henderson-Hasselbalch equation:

$$pH = pK_a + \log[HCO_3^{\ -}]/\alpha P_{CO_2}$$

where pK_a is 6.1 and α represents the solubility coefficient of PCO_2 (which is 0.03). Because all the body buffers (e.g., bone, intracellular proteins) are in equilibrium, changes in the concentration of HCO_3^- regulate the pH of body fluids.

The kidney reabsorbs about 5000 mEq of HCO_3^- that is filtered daily. Beyond this task, it must replace the HCO_3^- that is lost as a consequence of the production of acid by oxidative metabolism. The proximal tubule reabsorbs luminal HCO_3^- by secreting H^+ through an apical Na^+/H^+ exchanger, which is directly stimulated by angiotensin II to secrete H^+ in strict 1 : 1 exchange for Na^+, thereby mediating both sodium absorption and H^+ secretion. An H^+-ATPase is also present in the apical membrane. H^+ secretion titrates filtered HCO_3 and, catalyzed by carbonic anhydrase, converts it to CO_2 and water, thereby allowing CO_2 reabsorption. H^+ secretion leads to an excess of OH^- in the cell, where it combines with this CO_2 to produce cellular HCO_3^-, which then exits across the basolateral membrane through an Na-HCO_3^- cotransporter (E-Fig. 101-2).

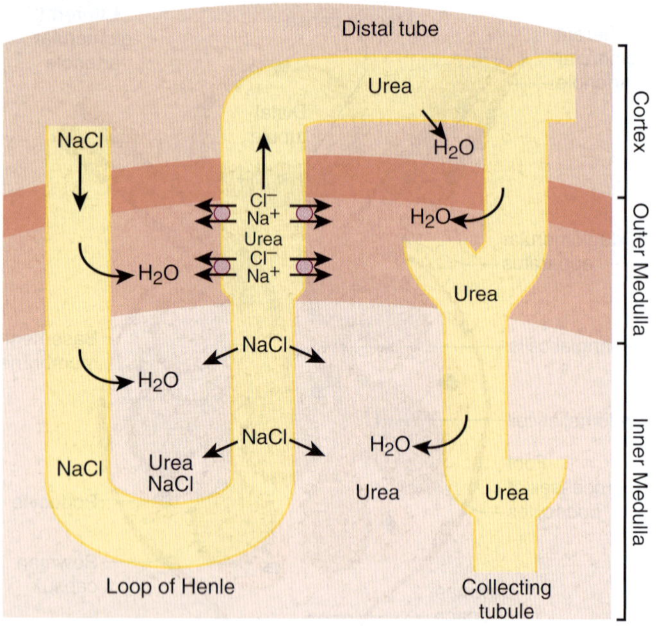

FIGURE 101-3. **Regulation of water content.**

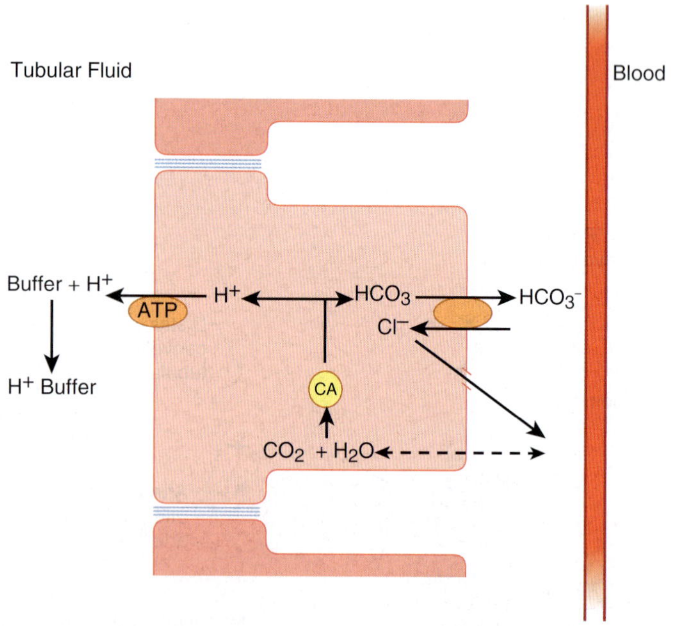

FIGURE 101-4. **Mechanism of acid secretion in the collecting duct.** ATP = adenosine triphosphate; CA = carbonic anhydrase.

Given that the proximal tubule regulates bicarbonate reabsorption, the collecting duct must produce "new" HCO_3 to replace what is lost during titration by nonvolatile acids. The cortical collecting tubules contain intercalated cells that mediate H^+ secretion (α-intercalated cell) and β-cell types that mediate the secretion of HCO_3, whereas only α cells are present in the medulla. In the α-intercalated cell, H^+ secretion is mediated by the H^+-ATPase that is delivered to the apical membrane by fusion of apical vesicles as stimulated by ambient Pco_2 (Fig. 101-4).

In a reaction catalyzed by carbonic anhydrase II, the excess OH^- is carboxylated by CO_2 to form HCO_3^-. HCO_3^- is subsequently transported across the basolateral surface in exchange for Cl^- by an alternately spliced form of the red cell anion exchanger (band 3). In contrast, β cells secrete HCO_3^- by an apical Cl/HCO_3 exchanger (pendrin) and a basolateral H^+-ATPase. An H^+, K^+-ATPase in the collecting tubule may also play a role in potassium absorption and perhaps in H^+ secretion.

The collecting tubule is a "tight epithelium" that can maintain electrical and concentration gradients. Secretion of H^+ reduces the pH of the filtrate; the maximal gradient is 3 pH units or 180 mV, but both the size of the pH gradient and its transepithelial membrane potential can be modified to fine-tune H^+ secretion. For example, Na^+ absorption by the principal cell hyperpolarizes the epithelium and can thus drive H^+ secretion. Aldosterone, in addition to regulating Na^+ absorption, independently can stimulate H^+ secretion; hence, it is the major hormone that stimulates acid secretion in the collecting tubule. Finally, chronic metabolic acidosis converts the β-intercalated cells into α-intercalated cells, preferentially increasing the number of acid-secreting cells and reducing the number of HCO_3^- secreting cells in this segment.

The secreted H^+ titrates urinary NH_3 and HPO_4^{2-}. NH_3, which is synthesized by the conversion of glutamine to α-ketoglutarate, is secreted into the proximal lumen. In the loop of Henle and distal segments, the protonated ammonium ion is transferred into the interstitium, from where it re-enters the nephron as ammonia gas. Once in the lumen, ammonia gas becomes reprotonated to ammonium, thus trapping a proton. The amount of NH_3 generated from glutamine increases up to four- to five-fold in the setting of metabolic acidosis. Net acid secretion is consequently urinary NH_4^+ plus titratable weak acids (such as HPO_4^{2-}) minus urinary HCO_3^-. Each of these components is regulated by the kidney.

THE KIDNEY REGULATES PLASMA POTASSIUM BY SECRETION AND THE CONTROL OF EXTRACELLULAR pH

Because the membrane potential of most cells is governed by the ratio of intracellular to extracellular potassium, the plasma potassium concentration must be tightly regulated. Most dietary potassium is pumped into the cell by the Na^+, K^+-ATPase, but about 90% of ingested potassium eventually must be excreted into the urine.[5] K^+ is filtered but is then reabsorbed by the proximal tubule and loop of Henle. K^+ is then secreted by the distal convoluted tubule and the principal cells through apical potassium inwardly rectifying (ROMK) and potassium large conductance calcium-activated (BK) channels. The gradient, in which cellular K^+ is greater than luminal K^+, drives K^+ out of the cell. Secretion is enhanced by the increased entry of K^+ into the principal cell as a result of high extracellular concentration, by metabolic alkalosis, and by aldosterone. Aldosterone increases the synthesis of Na^+, K^+-ATPase and increases the probability that the ROMK channels will be open. Aldosterone also enhances Na^+ reabsorption by ENaC, thereby hyperpolarizing the transepithelial membrane potential, which increases the driving force for potassium secretion. High urinary flow rates deliver a large volume of fluid that is essentially K^+ free, thereby providing a concentration gradient. The flow rate also activates mechanosensory flagella that lead to an increase in cell calcium, which in turn activates BK channels. Potassium reabsorption is not regulated to the same extent as sodium retention, and profound potassium depletion may be required for potassium excretion by the kidneys to be eliminated completely.

THE KIDNEY REGULATES PLASMA PO_4 AND CA^{2+} BY EXCRETION AND BY SYNTHESIZING VITAMIN D_3

The level of PO_4 critically regulates serum Ca^{2+} level. Because their plasma concentrations are close to their saturation product, at which point crystallization occurs, any significant increase in PO_4 results in precipitation of $CaPO_4$.

PO_4 concentration is regulated by glomerular filtration. Initially, about 85% is reabsorbed by the proximal tubule sodium-phosphate cotransporters NaPi-2a and NaPi-2c. Parathyroid hormone and the heteromeric receptor FGFR/Klotho, which binds fibroblast growth factor 23 (FGF23), inhibit the expression of NaPi and hence increase excretion of PO_4. Conversely, the proximal tubule generates vitamin D_3 (1,25-dihydroxycholecalciferol) by capturing 25-hydroxycholecalciferol, bound to its filterable transport protein with brush border megalin (E-Fig. 101-3), after which 1α-hydroxylation is stimulated by low Ca^{2+} and PO_4. 1,25-Vitamin D_3 inhibits parathyroid hormone and stimulates PO_4 reabsorption in gut and kidney, thereby counteracting parathyroid hormone and FGF23-Klotho. Nonetheless, Klotho signaling blocks 1,25-vitamin D_3 synthesis, thereby suggesting that it dominates the control of PO_4.[6]

The level of serum calcium is also regulated by the kidney. Approximately 60% of serum calcium is filtered, after which it is reabsorbed in the proximal tubule through the paracellular pathway. The tight junction protein claudin 2 is critical for calcium selectivity in this segment and mutations in it lead to hypercalciuria. Calcium is also absorbed paracellularly in the thick ascending limb driven by the positive membrane potential generated by the Na-K-2Cl/K recycling transporter. Mutations in the tight junction proteins claudin 14, 16 and 19, have been implicated in monogenic causes of hypercalciuria and nephrolithiasis.[7] In contrast, calcium and sodium are regulated independently in the distal convoluted tubule by parathyroid hormone and Klotho, which increase reabsorption. Phosphate and calcium metabolism is regulated by sodium reclamation, parathyroid hormone, 1,25-dihydroxycholecalciferol, and Klotho in different segments of the nephron.[8]

GENERAL REFERENCES

For the General References and other additional features, please visit Elsevier eBooks+ at https://ebooks.health.elsevier.com.

102 DISORDERS OF SODIUM AND WATER

QAIS AL-AWQATI AND JAI RADHAKRISHNAN

EPIDEMIOLOGY

Disturbances of water and sodium include hypovolemia, hypervolemia, hyponatremia, and hypernatremia.[1] Up to 15 to 20% of hospitalized patients may develop hyponatremia or hypernatremia. Among ambulatory individuals, these abnormalities are more common in the elderly and in patients who are treated with multiple medications. Patients may have combinations of abnormalities in extracellular osmolality and volume (Table 102-1). Hypovolemia, which can be caused by dehydration or bleeding, can cause postural symptoms (Chapter 7) or shock (Chapter 94). Common causes of fluid overload include heart failure (Chapters 45 and 46), renal dysfunction, and liver failure, commonly resulting in edema (Fig. 39-7).[2]

DISORDERS OF EXTRACELLULAR FLUID VOLUME

PATHOBIOLOGY

Control of Extracellular Fluid Volume

The regulation of circulating volume is one of the body's major homeostatic mechanisms, and perturbations in the regulation of volume can cause a number of clinical conditions that carry substantial morbidity and mortality. Water accounts for approximately 60% of body weight (Fig. 102-1). Two thirds of this water resides intracellularly, and the remainder constitutes the extracellular fluid space. The kidney regulates extracellular volume by adjusting the amount of sodium chloride it excretes. Additionally, the kidney's regulated excretion of water maintains serum osmolality within narrow limits. The kidney accomplishes this goal by balancing salt excretion with salt intake, even though the daily intake of salt is highly variable, owing to cultural, social, and personal factors.

In the steady state, the renal excretion of salt is essentially equal to the salt intake because other possible routes of salt loss from the body (e.g., sweat glands and the gastrointestinal tract) do not contribute significantly to the maintenance of salt balance. When the dietary intake of sodium is abruptly increased (Fig. 102-2), only about one half of the increment appears in the urine over the first day. The remainder of the dietary increment is retained as a positive sodium balance. On each successive day of the higher intake of sodium, a smaller fraction of the dietary increment is retained as the excretion of sodium progressively increases over 3 to 5 days to match the new intake. Weight

TABLE 102-1 PATHOGENIC PROCESSES LEADING TO DISORDERS OF BODY SODIUM AND FLUID HOMEOSTASIS

CLINICAL STATE	ECF VOLUME	BODY FLUID TONICITY	PATHOGENIC PROCESS
Normal	↔	↔	NA
Isonatremia			
• Hypovolemia	↓	↔	ECF depletion
• Hypervolemia	↑	↔	ECF overload
Hypernatremia			
• Hypovolemic	↓	↑	ECF depletion Na > H_2O
• Hypervolemic	↑		ECF overload Na > H_2O
Hyponatremia			Net loss of sodium in excess of water
• Normovolemic	↔	↓	
• Hypovolemic	↓		
• Hypervolemic	↑		

ECF = extracellular fluid; H_2O = water; Na = sodium.

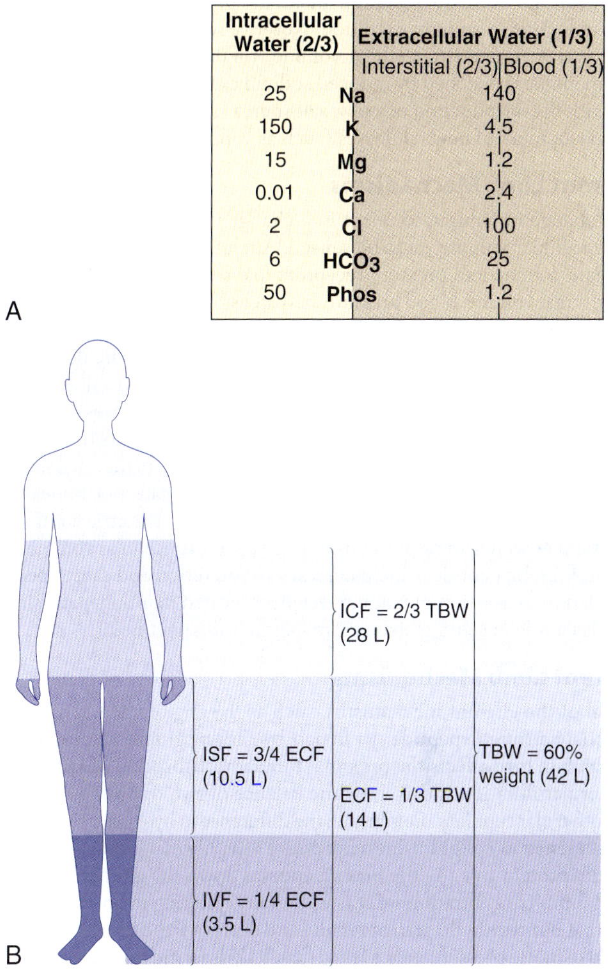

FIGURE 102-1. Composition of body fluid compartments. Schematic representation of (**A**) electrolyte composition of compartments in humans and (**B**) body fluid compartments. In **A**, electrolyte concentrations are in millimoles per liter; intracellular concentrations are typical values obtained from muscle. In **B**, shaded areas depict the approximate size of each compartment as a function of body weight. In a normally built individual, the total body water content is roughly 60% of body weight. Because adipose tissue has a low concentration of water, the relative water-to-total body weight ratio is lower in obese individuals. Relative volumes of each compartment are shown as fractions; in parentheses are shown approximate absolute volumes of the compartments (in liters) in a 70-kg adult. Ca = calcium; Cl = chloride; ECF = extracellular fluid; HCO_3 = bicarbonate; ICF = intracellular fluid; ISF = interstitial fluid; IVF = intravascular fluid; K = potassium; Mg = magnesium; Na = sodium; Phos = phosphate; TBW = total body water. (B from Verbalis JG. Body water osmolality. In: Wilkinson B, Jamison R, eds. *Textbook of Nephrology*. London: Chapman & Hall; 1997:89-94. Reproduced with permission of Hodder Arnold.)

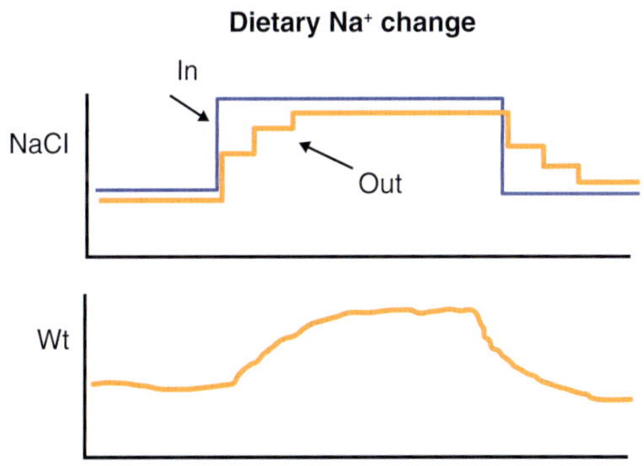

FIGURE 102-2. Time course of sodium excretion and weight change in humans following abrupt changes in daily sodium intake. Positive sodium balance continues for several days after salt intake is increased. As the volume of extracellular fluid increases, sodium excretion increases until the new lower intake of sodium is matched. It is this reduction of body sodium and extracellular fluid that provides the stimulus for diminishing the excretion of sodium. Na^+ = sodium; NaCl = sodium chloride; Wt = weight.

will increase because the retained Na will obligate the retention of an amount of water sufficient to maintain iso-osmolality. This positive balance of sodium and expansion of the extracellular water compartment stimulates a progressive increase in the excretion of sodium until the higher intake is matched by excretion. An abrupt decrease in sodium intake also does not result in an immediate equal reduction in sodium excretion. Negative sodium balance will continue for several days, and extracellular volume will diminish until the new, lower sodium intake is matched by reduced sodium excretion. Similar responses are seen with the introduction of a new salt source (such as intravenous fluids) or the development of new salt losses (such as vomiting or diarrhea).

Afferent Limb Mechanisms

For a change in volume to result in a change in salt excretion, the change in extracellular volume must be sensed. Alterations in extracellular volume stimulate volume and pressure receptors that sense concomitant changes in intravascular volume, blood pressure, or distension of a particular vascular bed. The juxtaglomerular apparatus is a renal volume sensor that releases renin when the perfusion pressure is reduced. In addition to increasing circulating levels of angiotensin II (see later), stimulation of these receptors leads to alterations in the local concentration of angiotensin, which profoundly decreases salt excretion. Volume receptors in the carotid sinus and aorta increase sympathetic output in response to hypotension. The increased sympathetic tone of the renal vasculature decreases salt excretion. Renal sympathetic nerves and catecholamines released from the adrenal medulla also stimulate renin release. The atria contain secretory granules which, in response to an increase in extracellular volume, release atrial natriuretic peptide, which increases salt excretion and causes peripheral vasodilation. Activation of volume receptors located in intrahepatic sinusoids may play a role in sensing changes in volume and salt content.

Efferent Limb Mechanisms

Several of the efferent mechanisms, such as the angiotensin/renin pathway and atrial natriuretic peptide, act in part by altering glomerular hemodynamics, which in turn affects the proximal tubular reabsorption of salt and water. Glomerular filtration is driven by the balance of two opposing forces across the glomerular capillary membrane: the difference in hydrostatic pressure and the difference in colloid osmotic pressure. The normal glomerular filtrate is virtually protein-free. As the plasma courses down the glomerular capillary, the albumin concentration increases, thereby resulting in an oncotic driving force that opposes hydrostatic pressure and decreases the filtration rate. When colloid osmotic pressure increases to match hydrostatic pressure (a condition called filtration pressure equilibrium), filtration ceases.

Because the efferent arteriole is a resistance vessel, the peritubular hydrostatic pressure is lower than the glomerular capillary pressure. Further, the peritubular capillary oncotic pressure is higher than the hydrostatic pressure because protein-free fluid has been removed by filtration. This balance of hydrostatic and oncotic forces in the peritubular capillary favors tubular reabsorption of fluid from the extracellular space of the tubules back into the capillaries. In this way, changes in glomerular hemodynamics can alter tubular reabsorption by changing the peritubular capillary oncotic and hydrostatic pressures.

Changes in glomerular and peritubular hemodynamics can influence the rate of net sodium reabsorption. Reabsorption of the filtered fluid occurs by active transport of sodium from the tubular lumen into the peritubular space. The proximal tubule is quite "leaky," so it cannot maintain large gradients of concentration or electrical potential. Sodium accumulates in the intercellular space, thereby resulting in local hypertonicity. Water is subsequently drawn in by osmosis through the cells and the leaky junctions. Removal of this fluid into the peritubular capillary occurs because the peritubular capillary has a higher protein concentration and a lower hydrostatic pressure than an ordinary capillary; these forces favor reabsorption of fluid from the intercellular space.

Filtered sodium is passively reabsorbed from the tubular lumen into the epithelial cell down a concentration gradient. It is then actively transported into the lateral intercellular channel, which communicates directly with the interstitial space. If the net force for uptake into the capillary is decreased, conductive and/or geometric changes in the tight junction complex may favor increased "back leak" of fluid into the tubular lumen, thereby diminishing net reabsorption. When those forces are in the opposite direction, the leak will decrease, thereby resulting in an increase in net reabsorption.

In principle, sodium excretion could be altered by either a change in the amount filtered or a change in the amount reabsorbed. In practice, both glomerular filtration rate and tubular reabsorption must be considered in analyzing the actions of atrial natriuretic peptide and angiotensin II.

Renin-Angiotensin II—Aldosterone

Renin is released from the juxtaglomerular apparatus in response to hypotension or to extracellular volume depletion in the absence of hypotension. Adrenergic innervation also stimulates renin release in response to the same stimuli. Additionally, prostaglandins, low plasma K^+, and increased Na^+ delivery to the macula densa also stimulate renin release. Circulating renin converts angiotensinogen, which is mainly produced by the liver and secreted into the blood, to angiotensin I. Angiotensin I in turn is converted by a converting enzyme located on the surface of endothelial cells to the active hormone, angiotensin II. Angiotensin II causes peripheral vasoconstriction and decreases salt excretion in the proximal and distal tubules.[3]

Angiotensin II increases the proximal tubule reabsorption of Na^+ by constricting the efferent arteriole, which increases the filtration fraction, which increases the peritubular capillary oncotic pressure, which increases the driving force for Na^+ reabsorption from the interstitial space into the capillary and decreases the backward leak. Increased reabsorption of sodium and water will result in a higher concentration of many solutes, including urea and uric acid, which are reabsorbed at a slower rate than are sodium and water. Based on their ability to be reabsorbed, these solutes will diffuse out of the tubule to a larger extent than normal. Since that diffusion is driven by a difference in concentration, the blood urea nitrogen (BUN) level will increase to a higher level than simply predicted by the reduction in filtration rates. Indeed, the serum ratio of BUN:creatinine is frequently elevated when angiotensin levels are increased. Angiotensin II also stimulates the Na:H exchanger, thereby causing a direct increase in Na reabsorption through the cells in the proximal tubule. Angiotensin II also directly stimulates Na^+ transporters in the thick ascending limb, the distal tubule, and the early collecting tubule.

A major effect of angiotensin II on Na+ reabsorption, however, is to stimulate the release of aldosterone from the zona glomerulosa of the adrenal cortex. In the collecting tubule and late distal tubule, aldosterone leads to an increase in the number of open Na^+ (and also K^+) channels, thereby leading to increased entry of Na^+ into the cell and, consequently, increased exit at the basolateral surface via the Na^+-K^+-ATPase, which is also stimulated by aldosterone. The Na^+ absorbed under the influence of aldosterone is estimated to be 50 to 100 mEq/day, amounting to less than 0.5% of that filtered. However, because it acts on the final 50 to 100 mEq that have escaped absorption, aldosterone has a critical effect on renal salt excretion and total body sodium balance. In the absence of aldosterone, such as in primary adrenal insufficiency (Chapter 209), patients will develop negative salt balance with severe salt depletion and shock unless their intake compensates for this loss of salt.

Interaction of Angiotensin II and Prostaglandins

In the setting of decreased renal perfusion, glomerular filtration is usually preserved. This effect is mediated by two vasoactive factors, angiotensin II and prostaglandins, which have opposing effects on the renal vasculature. Angiotensin II binds to receptor subtypes 1 A in the efferent arteriole and promotes vasoconstriction. Concomitantly, the release of vasodilating prostaglandins mitigates the constriction of the afferent arterioles. This combined effect of efferent arteriolar constriction and afferent arteriolar dilation maintains intraglomerular pressure. These factors also have opposite effects on salt handling: angiotensin II releases aldosterone to promote salt absorption in the distal nephron, whereas prostaglandins inhibit salt absorption in the loop of Henle. Inhibitors of the renin-angiotensin axis and nonsteroidal anti-inflammatory drugs (NSAIDs) may produce acute declines in glomerular filtration in the setting of low renal perfusion pressures (e.g., volume depletion, heart failure, and cirrhosis). Further, NSAIDs may induce salt retention in these circumstances (Chapter 106).

Atrial Natriuretic Peptide

Atrial natriuretic peptide is a 28–amino acid peptide that is released from granule stores of the right and left atria in response to volume overload with atrial distention or after an atrial tachyarrhythmia. Atrial natriuretic peptide inhibits renin release and thus indirectly inhibits the production of angiotensin II. Second, atrial natriuretic peptide inhibits aldosterone production regardless of the presence of angiotensin II, high plasma K^+, or elevated adrenocorticotropic hormone. Third, atrial natriuretic peptide increases the glomerular filtration rate and thus increases the amount of Na^+ available for excretion. Finally, atrial natriuretic peptide directly inhibits the tubular reabsorption of Na^+ in the terminal collecting duct.

Renal Nerves

Renal nerves directly increase afferent and efferent arterial tone, and the resulting decrease in renal plasma flow and glomerular filtration rate will favor Na^+

retention. Stimulation of these nerves also leads to release of renin and angiotensin, which results in salt retention. Sympathetic neurons also are present in apposition to the proximal tubule and thick ascending limb, where their stimulation results in an increase in proximal Na^+ absorption even when the filtration rate, renin, and angiotensin levels are not measurably changed.

HYPOVOLEMIA

Hypovolemia, which is a contraction of intravascular volume, can be caused by renal and nonrenal conditions (Table 102-2).

CLINICAL MANIFESTATIONS AND DIAGNOSIS

The clinical manifestations of hypovolemia depend on its magnitude, the rate at which it developed, and what fluid was lost.[4] A detailed history will usually reveal underlying bleeding, polyuria, gastrointestinal losses, medications, and diaphoresis. However, gradual volume loss with an intravascular volume contraction of less than 5% may be asymptomatic and associated with few physical findings. An intravascular volume contraction of 5 to 15% typically causes symptoms and signs, often including postural lightheadedness and weakness. Thirst is common as the volume loss worsens. Hemodynamic collapse (hypovolemic shock; Chapter 92) can occur with more rapid volume loss.

On physical examination, jugular venous pressure will generally be less than 5 cm H_2O in the absence of confounding factors. Findings such as reduced skin or eyeball turgor and dry mucous membranes are not reliable indicators of hypovolemia.

Relative intravascular hypovolemia also is seen with the vasodilation that typically accompanies sepsis (Chapter 94), even though no fluid has been lost outside of the body. Such patients can be critically ill, but typically they will have warm extremities unlike the cool extremities that are typical of patients in cardiogenic or true hypovolemic shock (Chapter 92). However, the diminished tissue perfusion in sepsis can reduce the level of consciousness and cause oliguria, acute kidney injury, and lactic acidosis.

In addition to oliguria with a high urine osmolality and a low urine sodium concentration (<20 mEq/L), hemoconcentration can raise the hemoglobin level unless the patient is bleeding. The BUN will rise, often out of proportion to the rise in the serum creatinine level. The serum albumin concentration often rises with gastrointestinal, urinary, or skin losses of albumin-free fluids but falls when accompanied by albumin loss (e.g., proteinuria, protein-losing enteropathy, and burns). Loss of hypotonic fluids with inadequate water ingestion or replacement results in hypernatremia. Hypokalemia with metabolic alkalosis frequently accompanies vomiting and hypovolemia induced by thiazide and loop diuretics. By comparison, diarrhea often is associated with a non–anion gap metabolic acidosis. Adrenal insufficiency is typically accompanied by hyperkalemia and mild metabolic acidosis.

An important goal is to assess volume responsiveness (i.e., the probability that the patient with suspected hypovolemia will respond to volume repletion), especially in critically ill patients in whom volume overload is equally, if not as, deleterious as volume depletion. A static assessment of intravascular volume by measuring central venous pressure or pulmonary arterial wedge pressure can be useful but does not provide a reliable measure of volume responsiveness. Dynamic techniques that more predictably indicate volume responsiveness include passive leg raising and respiratory variation in the diameter of the vena cava, pulse pressure, or left ventricular end-diastolic diameter.

TABLE 102-2 CAUSES OF ABSOLUTE AND RELATIVE HYPOVOLEMIA

RENAL
Absolute
Diuretics
Inherited sodium-wasting tubulopathies
Tubulointerstitial diseases
Partial urinary obstruction or postobstruction diuresis
Endocrine disorders (e.g., hypoaldosteronism, adrenal insufficiency)
Relative
Nephrotic syndrome
EXTRARENAL
Absolute
Bleeding
Gastrointestinal fluid loss (e.g., diarrhea, vomiting, ileostomy or colostomy secretions)
Fluid loss from skin (e.g., burns, sweat)
Respiratory fluid loss
Relative
Third space losses (e.g., sepsis, angioedema, pancreatitis, ileus, cirrhosis with ascites)

TREATMENT

Absolute Hypovolemia

The major goal in treating hypovolemia is to restore hemodynamic integrity and tissue perfusion (Chapter 92). The management approach includes treatment of the underlying disease state, assessment and replacement of the volume deficit, treating concomitant electrolyte and acid-base abnormalities, and maintaining volume in the face of continuing losses.[5]

The choice of fluid therapy includes isotonic crystalloids (0.9% and lactated Ringer solution), colloids (albumin), and packed red cells. Generally, crystalloids are used as first-line therapy. Buffered crystalloids (e.g., lactated Ringer solution or Plasmalyte-A) may have an advantage over 0.9% saline in avoiding the dilutional acidosis and the propensity to acute kidney injury that accompanies large-volume resuscitation in critically ill patients,[A1,A2] although data in critically ill patients are less clear.[A3,A4] Using albumin adds no benefit in essentially any situation other than cirrhosis (Chapter 139). Colloids such as hetastarch or dextran should not be used. In hemorrhagic shock, packed red cells are usually required to correct anemia after initial resuscitation with crystalloids.

The rate of fluid repletion depends on the severity of the volume deficit. In patients with hypovolemic shock (Chapter 92), rapid administration of a crystalloid is recommended until hemodynamic parameters are normalized. With lesser degrees of hemodynamic compromise, one or more boluses of crystalloids (e.g., 500 mL of saline followed by an assessment of the response)[A5] may be used. In uncertain situations in which avoidance of fluid overload is critical, dynamic assessment of fluid status (see Clinical Manifestations and Diagnosis) may be helpful.

For an accompanying metabolic acidosis (Chapter 104), hypertonic sodium bicarbonate can be added to half-isotonic saline or 5% dextrose to create an isotonic replacement fluid appropriate for the acid-base abnormality. Similarly, the addition of potassium chloride is indicated in patients with concomitant potassium depletion (Chapter 103).

Relative hypovolemia owing to peripheral vasodilation requires treatment of the underlying cause, such as sepsis (Chapter 94) or anaphylaxis (Chapter 233). While this treatment is being instituted, isotonic crystalloid is the mainstay of treatment until vascular resistance and capacitance are restored to normal. Such patients also may require vasopressors (Chapter 94).

HYPERVOLEMIA

Hypervolemia is an expansion primarily of extracellular volume owing to primary or secondary renal retention of sodium (Table 102-3).

PATHOBIOLOGY

Heart Failure

With heart failure (Chapters 45 and 46), a decrease in cardiac output activates baroreceptors (E-Fig. 102-1). The result is an increase in sympathetic activity, activation of the renin-angiotensin system, and increased levels of angiotensin II. Constriction of the efferent arteriole increases the glomerular capillary hydrostatic pressure but reduces renal plasma flow. In early heart failure, the filtration rate is maintained. In severe heart failure, the filtration rate may be reduced owing to a severe decline in renal plasma flow. However, the filtration fraction is always elevated because the decline in plasma flow is always greater than the decline in the filtration rate.

TABLE 102-3 PRIMARY AND SECONDARY RENAL SODIUM-RETAINING STATES

PRIMARY
Oliguric renal failure
Chronic kidney disease
Glomerular disease, including nephrotic syndrome
Severe bilateral renovascular obstruction
Mineralocorticoid excess
Inherited sodium-retaining tubulopathies
SECONDARY
Cardiac failure
Cirrhosis
Idiopathic edema

The lower peritubular capillary hydrostatic pressure (owing to reduced glomerular filtration) and elevated albumin concentration (owing to the elevated filtration fraction) favor increased absorption from the proximal tubule, which is the major cause of salt retention in heart failure. Angiotensin II also stimulates aldosterone release, which in turn stimulates Na^+ absorption in the more distal nephron.

Not all patients with heart failure continue to accumulate salt. After the initial salt retention, expansion of the extracellular volume may restore cardiac output to near-normal levels, albeit with a higher-than-normal extracellular volume. In this new state, the initial compensatory mechanisms will be largely deactivated: angiotensin and aldosterone levels will decrease, as will sympathetic tone. In this new steady state, salt excretion will equal salt intake. However, if heart failure worsens, owing, for example, to further myocardial damage, the cycle will be repeated. In severe heart failure, the patient will remain in the salt-retaining, high renin-angiotensin-aldosterone state despite massive extracellular volume expansion. The pathophysiology of heart failure therefore consists of two phases. The first is a salt-retaining, high-renin, high-angiotensin, and high-aldosterone state, in which the extracellular volume will continuously expand. The second phase is characterized by a normal renin-angiotensin-aldosterone axis, a higher-than-normal extracellular fluid volume, and external salt balance.

Cirrhosis

Cirrhosis of the liver (Chapter 139) is uniformly associated with disturbances in salt excretion and the consequent development of edema and ascites. Portal hypertension leads to transudation of fluid into the abdominal cavity, with consequent intravascular volume depletion. Peripheral vasodilation also causes a decrease in the "effective plasma volume," with consequent salt retention.

In general, salt retention appears to precede the development of ascites or portal hypertension. The main stimulus is the activation of volume receptors located in intrahepatic sinusoids. This increase in pressure appears to signal the kidney to retain salt and water, thereby causing volume expansion. At a time when the kidney is retaining Na^+, the glomerular filtration rate and renal plasma flow are normal, as are plasma levels of renin and angiotensin. Although total plasma volume is increased, the capacity of the splanchnic bed is much larger in cirrhotic patients than in normal individuals. If the extra-splanchnic plasma volume is depleted or effectively depleted owing to splanchnic vasodilation and increased capacity, then the mechanism for salt retention is the same as that induced by simple extracellular volume depletion.

Ascites (Chapter 132) is not only due to portal hypertension. As cirrhosis advances, progressive portal hypertension contributes to excessive transudation of fluid into the peritoneal cavity. Further, the albumin secreted by the hepatocytes enters the lymphatic system, which delivers it to the thoracic duct and then to the blood stream. In cirrhosis, however, the disturbed architecture of the hepatic lobules causes much of the albumin to be dumped directly into the ascitic fluid. Thus, although the albumin concentration in ascitic fluid is low enough to be classified as a transudate, it is actually much higher than the albumin concentration in the extravascular fluid elsewhere in the body. In addition, when the synthetic function of the liver deteriorates and the serum albumin concentration falls, the low oncotic pressure results in transudation of fluid into the interstitial space. Volume depletion from any of these causes promotes salt retention through an increase in angiotensin II and aldosterone.

Nephrotic Syndrome and Glomerulonephritis

Immunologic injury to the glomerulus results in proteinuria and, almost uniformly, in salt retention. When the proteinuria is especially severe, nephrotic syndrome (Chapter 107) develops.

In most adults with nephrotic syndrome, the plasma volume appears to be normal or even expanded, likely because of primary salt retention by the kidney. The increased glomerular permeability that causes proteinuria in these diseases also increases the filtration of circulating proteases, which activate the epithelial Na channel (ENaC) in the collecting tubule, thereby increasing Na reabsorption independent of aldosterone. In a minority of patients (usually children), low oncotic pressure leads to intravascular volume depletion and activation of the renin-angiotensin-aldosterone system, which may stimulate sodium retention by the kidney.

In patients with glomerulonephritis, the glomerular filtration rate is reduced; because salt excretion is dependent on the adequacy of the filtered load, the inability to excrete a salt load is common in advanced glomerulonephritis.

CLINICAL MANIFESTATIONS AND DIAGNOSIS

Clinical manifestations depend on the amount and relative distribution of accumulated fluid. Particularly harmful manifestations of hypervolemia include hypertension, pulmonary congestion, pleural effusions with compromised respiratory function, congestive hepatopathy, ascites, and peripheral edema that can be severe enough to compromise skin integrity and predispose the patient to cellulitis (Chapter 408).

On physical examination, left heart failure is associated with pulmonary venous congestion as manifested by pulmonary crackles (Chapter 45), and right heart failure is associated with jugular venous distention (Fig. 39-1), peripheral edema, hepatic congestion, and even ascites (see Fig. 132-4). Pitting peripheral edema (Fig. 39-6) usually does not develop until patients have at least 3 L of excess interstitial volume. Pleural effusions usually are a manifestation of combined right and left heart failure (Chapters 45 and 46). Relative hypotension suggests more severe heart failure or even cardiogenic shock (Chapter 94). When hypotension is caused by portal hypertension (as in cirrhosis) or hypoalbuminemia, the clinical manifestations may be similar to pure right heart failure, except the jugular venous pressure will be low, not high.

Laboratory tests can provide evidence of cardiac, pulmonary, or liver disease. An elevated brain natriuretic peptide (BNP) level is seen in heart failure and other states of central venous overload. Hypoalbuminemia is seen in both cirrhosis and nephrotic syndrome, but the latter is associated with marked proteinuria (Chapter 107). An elevated serum creatinine level suggests acute or chronic renal failure, which can be intrinsic or occur with advanced heart failure (cardiorenal syndrome) or hepatic cirrhosis (hepatorenal failure).

TREATMENT

Treatment must be targeted to the underlying cause to optimize hemodynamic parameters in heart failure (Chapter 46), improve liver function (Chapter 139), or treat nephrotic syndrome (Chapter 107). The reduction of excess volume requires a negative sodium balance, which can be achieved by diuretic therapy in combination with dietary sodium restriction. If these interventions are insufficient, extracorporeal fluid removal by ultrafiltration may be required.

Diuretics

Diuretics (Table 102-4) enhance urinary excretion of sodium by inhibiting its tubular reabsorption (E-Fig. 102-2).[6,7]

Loop Diuretics

Loop diuretics are the most potent diuretics, even in patients who have relatively compromised kidney function. Loop diuretics induce the loss of sodium by inhibiting the coupled entry of Na^+, Cl^-, and K^+ in the thick ascending limb of the loop of Henle, which is responsible for the reabsorption of about 25% of filtered sodium. Loop diuretics also cause hypercalciuria and are useful in some hypercalcemic states (Chapter 227). Side effects include hypokalemia and metabolic alkalosis.

Distal Tubule Diuretics

Distal tubule diuretics generally are used in the same conditions as loop diuretics, except for chronic kidney disease and disorders of calcium metabolism. Distal tubule diuretics block the sodium-chloride cotransport mechanism across apical plasma membranes in the distal tubule. Thiazide diuretics promote calcium retention and are useful in managing hypercalciuric states, including some forms of nephrolithiasis (Chapter 111). As with loop diuretics, thiazide diuretics may cause hypokalemia and metabolic alkalosis.

Collecting Duct Diuretics

Spironolactone and eplerenone compete with aldosterone and inhibit the absorption of sodium in the collecting duct, where they also suppress potassium secretion. Triamterene and amiloride, which directly block sodium uptake by collecting duct cells, also suppress potassium secretion. These collecting duct agents are used in combination with thiazide and loop diuretics to avoid hypokalemia, but hyperkalemia may complicate their injudicious use. Spironolactone and eplerenone are useful in managing disorders characterized by secondary hyperaldosteronism (e.g., cirrhosis with ascites), in promoting natriuresis in hypokalemic patients, and in competitively blocking nonepithelial mineralocorticoid receptors in patients with left ventricular dysfunction (Chapter 46).

Proximal Tubule Diuretics

Proximal tubule diuretics are rarely, if ever, used as primary therapy but are occasionally helpful as supplements to loop diuretics when loop diuretics alone are insufficiently effective. Acetazolamide, which is a carbonic anhydrase inhibitor, blocks the proximal reabsorption of sodium bicarbonate and can lead to hyperchloremic acidosis, in contrast to all other diuretics, which act at loci before the late distal nephron. Used alone, acetazolamide does not produce significant diureses since distal tubular absorption of sodium is maintained. It can, however, produce significant volume loss when used in combination with loop diuretics. Metolazone blocks sodium chloride absorption in the proximal tubule as well as in the early distal tubule, but it can cause phosphaturia.

TABLE 102-4 DIURETICS AND OTHER NATRIURETIC MEDICATIONS

CLASSES OF DIURETICS IN COMMON USE	DAILY DOSE RANGE	ADVERSE REACTIONS (CLASS)	COMMENTS (CLASS)
Thiazides (oral)		Rash, neutropenia, thrombocytopenia, hyperglycemia, hyperuricemia.	Usually not effective below GFR of 30-40 mL/mm (metolazone, 20-30 mL/mm)
Hydrochlorothiazide	25-100 mg		
Metolazone	2.5-5 mg		
Chlorthalidone	20-50 mg		
Loop diuretics (oral or iv)		Ototoxicity at high doses. Electrolyte disturbances.	Rapid onset, short duration Split doses in normal renal function; give intravenously in acute situations or if reduced gastrointestinal absorption Can use up to 500 mg furosemide (or equivalent) in severe renal insufficiency
Furosemide	20-320 mg		
Bumetanide	1-8 mg		
Torsemide	20-200 mg		
Potassium-sparing diuretics (oral)		Hyperkalemia	Not very potent
Spironolactone	25-400 mg		
Triamterene	25-100 mg		
Amiloride	5-20 mg		
Eplerenone	25-50 mg		
Vaptans		Constipation, increased thirst, hyperglycemia, hepatotoxicity	Used for hypervolemic hyponatremia
Tolvaptan (oral)	15-60 mg		
Conivaptan (IV)	20-40 mg IV		

GFR = glomerular filtration rate; IV = intravenous.

Combination Diuretic Therapy

Patients with severe degrees of renal sodium avidity can be resistant to conventionally recommended doses of loop diuretics and may require combinations that act at different sites along the nephron. Using various combinations of a loop diuretic with a thiazide diuretic, mineralocorticoid antagonist (e.g., spironolactone), or a proximal tubule diuretic (e.g., acetazolamide) can augment sodium loss as compared with a loop diuretic alone. Plasma concentrations of sodium, potassium, magnesium, calcium, and phosphate must be monitored carefully in such patients.

Sodium restriction does not clearly augment negative fluid balance over what can be achieved by furosemide alone. If dietary sodium is not restricted, however, patients will require higher doses of diuretics and can reaccumulate fluid. Sodium restriction to 50 to 100 mmol/day, which requires abstention from added salt as well as from foods rich in sodium, may be helpful. Sodium substitutes also can be useful, but they must be used with caution to avoid hyperkalemia if the salt substitute contains potassium. Caloric intake and nutrition must be monitored to ensure that a low-salt diet does not cause protein-energy malnutrition. Water restriction is not an appropriate therapy for hypervolemia unless hyponatremia develops. Similarly vasopressin V2-receptor antagonists, which may augment water loss, do not improve symptoms of heart failure but can raise the serum sodium concentration in patients who have hyponatremia (see Hyponatremia).

Extracorporeal Ultrafiltration

A small subset of patients have superimposed renal impairment or extreme resistance to the natriuretic actions of diuretics. Such patients may require the direct removal of excess volume by ultrafiltration, hemodialysis, or peritoneal dialysis (Chapter 117).

DISORDERS OF TONICITY OF BODY FLUIDS: HYPONATREMIA AND HYPERNATREMIA

PATHOBIOLOGY

Regulation of the Tonicity of Body Fluids

Osmotic pressure is a function of the sum of all solutes (in moles or equivalents) in a given volume of body fluids (osmolality). Tonicity is equal to the osmolality minus the concentration of ineffective solutes. Osmolality is a property of a particular solution and is independent of any membrane. Tonicity is a property of a solution in reference to a particular membrane. Tonicity (osmolality) is a highly regulated physiologic human parameter, and reasonable variations in daily water intake do not change osmolality by more than 0.5%. Water is freely permeable via water channels (aquaporins) through most cellular membranes, so no osmotic gradients exist among the body's fluid compartments. In contrast to water, sodium cannot travel freely across cell membranes. Thus, drinking a large volume of water is followed by a reduction in extracellular osmolality, thereby causing water to diffuse into the cell. This exchange causes an acute increase in cell volume, which is usually well tolerated except in cells that are encased in rigid compartments such as in the brain. Over time, compensatory mechanisms will decrease or increase intracellular osmoles in parallel with changes in extracellular osmolality, thereby restoring cell volume towards normal. The opposite phenomenon is seen when extracellular osmolality increases acutely (e.g., after consuming a high-salt diet).

A good approximation of osmolality can be obtained by measuring the serum or plasma sodium concentration, because sodium and its counter-ions (chloride and bicarbonate) comprise 90% of osmolality. With only a few exceptions, a normal Na concentration reflects normal osmolality. Thus, clinical states of low or high osmolality are frequently referred to as hyponatremia and hypernatremia, respectively.

Importantly, the regulation of osmotic pressure is entirely a function of the regulation of water content rather than sodium content. The total sodium *content* of the body fluids is most closely related to the total extracellular volume, whereas the sodium *concentration* is related to osmolality or water content. In hyponatremia, the total body sodium content may be high, low, or normal, but from the perspective of osmolar regulation, the water content is always too high relative to the sodium content.

The balance of water intake and excretion relative to sodium intake and excretion determines serum osmolality. Free water is the volume of electrolyte-free water. For example, 1.0 L of half-normal sodium chloride equals 0.5 L of normal saline and 0.5 L of free water, so infusion of 1.0 L of half-normal saline increases free water content by 0.5 L. When electrolytes other than sodium (e.g., potassium) are added to fluids, they reduce free water by corresponding amounts.

Body fluid tonicity (as measured in the serum) reflects the balance of free water input compared with free water output. Only the renal free water output is regulated; in the steady state, this renal free water output must equal free water input minus nonrenal water losses. Free water input equals oral intake plus intravenous intake. Nonrenal free water losses include cutaneous and respiratory insensible losses, as well as any water lost in the stool.

Oral intake varies with thirst and with habits. Thirst is stimulated by an increase in the osmotic pressure of the body fluids as well as by nonosmotic stimuli, such as hypotension or plasma volume depletion. These latter stimuli can dominate, and thirst, which is quenched only with hypotonic fluids, may be stimulated despite the presence of hypo-osmolarity. Insensible losses increase with increased ambient temperature, fever, or extensive damage to the skin, such as burns (Chapter 97). These variations can be very large; for example, the maximum rate of sweating is about 1 liter per hour.

The renal output of free water is a function of the urine volume and the concentration of the urinary solutes (E-Fig. 102-3). In the proximal tubule, where more than 60% of the glomerular filtrate is reabsorbed, water permeability is so high that the osmotic pressure at the end of the segment is similar to that of plasma. The volume of glomerular filtrate that reaches the loop of Henle varies with the glomerular filtration rate and the extent of proximal tubule reabsorption. As the fluid courses through the thick ascending limb, active salt reabsorption combined with low water permeability causes dilution of the tubular fluid. The salt that is reabsorbed (without much water) into the medulla establishes a hyperosmolar region. This gradient provides the driving force for water reabsorption from the collecting duct. As the thick ascending limb ends and the distal tubule, which is termed the cortical diluting segment, begins, salt reabsorption in the presence of low water permeability continues to reduce the tonicity of the urine to one third of that of plasma. The volume of hypotonic fluid reaching the collecting duct is about 25 L/day. If the collecting duct is relatively impermeable to water, then much of this volume can be excreted. At the other extreme, if the collecting duct is fully permeable to water and if the medullary concentration gradient is undisturbed, then water is maximally reabsorbed and only a small volume of concentrated urine is excreted (perhaps 0.5 L at 1200 mOsm/L). Arginine vasopressin, which is human antidiuretic hormone (ADH), regulates the collecting duct water permeability.

ADH is synthesized in the supraoptic and paraventricular nuclei and stored in the neurohypophysis. Thirst is mediated by adjacent cells intermingled with cells that synthesize ADH. Hypothalamic osmoreceptors modulate release of ADH in response to very small changes in the plasma osmolality. However, below a certain plasma osmolality, the ADH level does not decrease further. This set point, which is characteristic of each individual, represents the set point of the *osmostat*. ADH is released into the circulation, where it has a short half-life. ADH activates two types of G-protein coupled receptors, V1 that mediates vasoconstriction in vascular smooth muscle and V2 that is expressed in the principal cells of the collecting duct of the kidney. The luminal membrane of these cells is relatively impermeable to water. However, activation of the V2 receptors by ADH causes insertion of a specific water channel, aquaporin 2, into the luminal membrane of the cortical and medullary collecting duct, thereby leading to increased water absorption driven by the osmotic gradient.

Other factors can also stimulate ADH release. Low arterial filling in hypotension (Chapter 64), heart failure (Chapters 45 and 46), cirrhosis (Chapter 139), and intravascular volume depletion stimulate ADH release by activating the carotid sinus and left atrial receptors. Decreases in extracellular volume cause a decrease in the set point but an increase in the steepness of the relation between ADH secretion and osmolality. Compared with a normovolemic person, the same plasma osmolality in a volume-depleted person is associated with a higher ADH level.

HYPONATREMIA

DEFINITION

Hyponatremia is defined as a serum sodium below 135 mmol/L, which corresponds to a serum osmolality <280 mOsm/kg H_2O (Table 102-5). Hyponatremia generally indicates hypo-osmolarity, but with two exceptions. First, in marked hyperlipidemia (Chapter 190) or paraproteinemia (Chapter 173), the aqueous portion of a volume of plasma is reduced. Since Na^+ is present only in the aqueous phase, the Na^+ concentration appears to be low (pseudohyponatremia) even though the measured osmolality is normal. Second, the serum Na^+ concentration may be low in the presence of high concentrations of effective osmoles, such as seen with hyperglycemia (Chapter 210), alcohol ingestions, and mannitol. These molecules do not readily enter cells, but they withdraw water from cells, thereby leading to dilution of the serum Na^+ concentration and initially leading to a normal serum osmolality. However, severe dehydration in the presence of uncontrolled blood glucose elevations can lead to the hyperosmolar hyperglycemic syndrome (Chapter 210), in which the serum is hyperosmolar owing to the elevated concentration of these osmotically active substances.

TABLE 102-5 DEFINITIONS OF HYPONATREMIA

	SERUM SODIUM (mmol/L)	PLASMA OSMOLALITY (mOsm/kg H_2O)	ETIOLOGY
Hypo-osmolar	<135	Low (<280)	Volume depletion (true and effective)
Iso-osmolar	<135	Normal (280-295)	Hyperlipidemia, paraproteinemia, hyperglycemia, alcohols
Hyper-osmolar	<135	High (>295)	Hyperglycemia, alcohols (with severe dehydration)

EPIDEMIOLOGY

The incidence of hyponatremia (serum sodium concentration <135 mmol/L) is as high as 15 to 30% in hospitalized patients. Using a definition of serum sodium concentration <130 to 131 mmol/L, which may represent a more clinically significant threshold, the incidence is about 1 to 4%. In the nonhospitalized general population in the United States, the prevalence of hyponatremia (serum sodium concentration <133 to 136 mmol/L) is estimated to be 1.7%.

PATHOBIOLOGY

In every case of hypo-osmolar hyponatremia, either free water intake minus insensible losses is elevated, renal free water output is decreased, or both. Urine is diluted by the reabsorption of sodium in nephron segments with a low permeability to water. In the absence of antidiuretic hormone, such segments include the thick ascending limb of Henle, the distal tubule, and the collecting tubules. Urine is not diluted in the proximal tubule because reabsorption of sodium is isosmotic to plasma. For the kidney to generate a large volume of dilute urine, a sufficient volume must reach the distal nephron segments. Several mechanisms may impair the kidney's capacity to produce dilute urine, thereby leading to hyponatremia (Table 102-6).

Kidney Failure

In both acute (Chapter 106) and severe chronic renal failure (Chapter 116), a low glomerular filtration rate impairs the delivery of fluid to the distal cortical diluting segment of the nephron. Since the urine volume is relatively fixed, any increase in the intake of free water above the limited urine volume will lead to hyponatremia.

Primary Polydipsia

The capacity of the normal kidney to excrete free water under normal hemodynamic conditions is very large, about 20 L/day. Only rarely, such as in psychogenic polydipsia, can a patient become hyponatremic simply by increasing water intake. The hallmark of psychogenic polydipsia is hyponatremia with a maximally dilute urine (osmolality well below 100 mOsm/kg).[8]

Low Dietary Solute

A diet low in solutes will lead to decreased delivery of urine to the distal diluting segments. When this diet is combined with an increased intake of free water, hyponatremia ensues. For example, beer potomania syndrome occurs when patients consume large volumes of beer (rich in carbohydrates and water but poor in sodium and protein), thereby limiting urinary solutes and hence urinary water excretion. A similar phenomenon is noted with a diet of tea and toast.

Extracellular Volume Depletion

In true volume depletion, the genesis of hyponatremia involves two defects: antidiuretic hormone is secreted despite hypo-osmolarity and, to a lesser extent, inadequate delivery of tubular fluid to the diluting segment. The secretion of antidiuretic hormone is increased owing to the activation of volume receptors. If volume depletion is treated with hypotonic fluids, hyponatremia will ensue.

TABLE 102-6 MECHANISMS OF HYPONATREMIA

MECHANISM	EXAMPLES
Low GFR leading to decreased delivery to distal nephron	Acute or chronic kidney failure
Excessive free water intake exceeding kidney capacity to excrete free water	Primary polydipsia
Low dietary solute	"Beer potomania" and the "tea and toast diet"
True extracellular volume depletion	Diarrhea and vomiting, hypoadrenalism
Effective plasma volume depletion	Heart failure, cirrhosis
Syndrome of inappropriate ADH secretion (SIADH)	See Table 102-7
Multiple mechanisms	Thiazides, NSAIDs

ADH = antidiuretic hormone; GFR = glomerular filtration rate; NSAIDS = nonsteroidal anti-inflammatory drugs.

The urine sodium levels will be low and serum uric acid will be elevated in such conditions, with the exception of active use of diuretics, which will elevate urine sodium levels. Similar findings are seen in patients with a loss of effective intravascular volume (e.g., heart failure), but such patients will have edema.

Thiazide-induced hyponatremia, which is one of the most common causes of drug-induced hyponatremia, occurs in about 9% of treated patients,[9] especially in older female patients. The pathogenesis of hyponatremia is likely multifactorial, owing to an increased intake of water with an impaired capacity to excrete water. Thiazide diuretics reduce the generation of free water because they inhibit Na^+ reabsorption in the diluting segment. In addition, the mild volume depletion caused by thiazides induces a decrease in fluid delivery out of the proximal tubule, thereby further reducing the volume of dilute urine generated by the kidney. Finally, the collecting duct is more permeable to water, likely due in part to an increase in antidiuretic hormone induced by mild volume depletion. Hyponatremia is uncommon with the chronic use of loop diuretics because they abolish the medullary concentration gradient, which is maintained with thiazide diuretics.

Cerebral salt wasting occurs uncommonly after head injury, subarachnoid hemorrhage, and neurosurgical procedures. The pathogenesis is thought to result when proximal tubular salt wasting of unknown etiology leads to volume depletion and subsequent stimulation of antidiuretic hormone. Since uric acid is also lost from the proximal tubule defect, urinary concentrations of sodium and serum uric acid are unreliable markers of volume depletion.

Hypoadrenalism (Chapter 208) is typically associated with hyponatremia, in large part because of the extracellular volume depletion that is a feature of this disease. The volume depletion results from a decrease in salt reabsorption in the collecting duct owing to the absence of aldosterone. In contrast to other patients with extracellular volume depletion, urinary sodium excretion will be high in these patients. Glucocorticoid deficiency may also contribute to the development of hyponatremia (see later).

Effective Volume Depletion

In patients with heart failure (Chapters 45 and 46) and cirrhosis (Chapter 139), the intra-arterial volume is typically low despite total body hypervolemia. The urine sodium concentration is low and serum uric acid elevated, similar to what is seen in volume-depleted patients (in whom the urine sodium may not be low in the presence of diuretics).

Syndrome of Inappropriate Antidiuretic Hormone Secretion (SIADH)

In the presence of high concentrations of antidiuretic hormone, water is avidly reabsorbed in the collecting duct. If water intake is not curtailed, hyponatremia will result. A subclinical increase in the extracellular volume will lead to a decrease in the reabsorption of salt. Urine sodium levels will be high, and, as a result of decreased proximal tubular reabsorption of uric acid, the serum uric acid will be low.

The syndrome of inappropriate antidiuretic hormone (SIADH; Table 102-7)[10] is seen with a number of conditions, including tumors that secrete antidiuretic hormone, various pulmonary abnormalities and CNS disorders, and a number of medications (Table 102-8). Patients with tumor-induced SIADH have high antidiuretic hormone levels regardless of the plasma osmolality. Other patients seem to have a resetting of the osmostat (i.e., they are able to suppress antidiuretic hormone but at a lower plasma sodium concentration than normal). Still others seem to have a continuous low level of antidiuretic hormone secretion regardless of the plasma osmolality, as if there was a continuous leak of antidiuretic hormone from the posterior pituitary. A few others have perfectly normal responses, thereby implying that they might express another antidiuretic hormone.

The nephrogenic syndrome of inappropriate antidiuresis is a very rare condition that is clinically similar to SIADH. In this disorder, gene variants in *V2R* cause constitutive activation of the V2 receptor and result in antidiuresis. Unlike SIADH, plasma vasopressin levels are suppressed.

Isolated glucocorticoid deficiency occurs in association with anterior pituitary disorders (Chapter 205) that impair normal secretion of ACTH, thereby leading to secondary adrenal insufficiency. The deficiency of cortisol leads to failure to suppress vasopressin levels, and the hyponatremia resembles SIADH rather than classic primary adrenal insufficiency in which hypovolemia occurs consequent to a lack of aldosterone.

Other Causes

Hypothyroidism (Chapter 207) is rarely associated with hyponatremia. Patients typically have high antidiuretic hormone levels, perhaps owing to a decrease in cardiac output. However, hypo-osmolality is frequently out of proportion to the clinical signs of decreased cardiac output. Thyroid hormone also appears necessary to maintain the number of sodium pumps in the kidney; because salt reabsorption in the ascending limb of the loop of Henle is dependent on sodium pumping, more Na^+ will be lost in the urine.

Nonsteroidal anti-inflammatory drugs (NSAIDs) inhibit prostaglandin synthesis, and prostaglandins inhibit the effect of antidiuretic hormone on the collecting duct. Thus, NSAIDs increase the sensitivity of the tubule to ADH. This effect will not in and of itself impair free water absorption unless the vasopressin level is increased, as it often is in the setting of volume-depletion or heart failure. In addition, prostaglandins also enhance the effects of angiotensin II. When NSAIDs are administered to volume-depleted patients with elevated angiotensin II, the effect of angiotensin II is potentiated, the filtration fraction is increased, the proximal tubular reabsorption of water is

TABLE 102-7 CRITERIA FOR THE DIAGNOSIS OF THE SYNDROME OF INAPPROPRIATE ANTIDIURETIC HORMONE

Decreased effective osmolality of the extracellular fluid (plasma <275 mOsmol/kg H_2O). Inappropriate urinary concentration (Uosm >100 mOsmol/kg H_2O with normal renal function) at some level of plasma hypo-osmolality.
Clinical euvolemia, as defined by the absence of signs of hypovolemia (orthostasis, tachycardia, decreased skin turgor, dry mucous membranes) or hypervolemia (subcutaneous edema, ascites).
Elevated urinary sodium excretion (>20 to 30 mmol/L) while on normal salt and water intake.
Absence of other potential causes of euvolemic hypo-osmolality (e.g., severe hypothyroidism, hypocortisolism [glucocorticoid insufficiency]).
Normal renal function and absence of diuretic use, particularly thiazide diuretics.

TABLE 102-8 CAUSES OF THE SYNDROME OF INAPPROPRIATE ANTIDIURETIC HORMONE SECRETION

ECTOPIC ADH PRODUCTION FROM TUMORS
Bronchogenic carcinoma (Chapter 177) Adenocarcinoma of pancreas (Chapter 180) Adenocarcinoma of duodenum (Chapter 179) Carcinoma of the ureter (Chapter 182) Non-Hodgkin lymphoma (Chapter 171) Hodgkin disease (Chapter 172) Thymoma (Chapter 390)
PULMONARY DISEASE
Tuberculosis (Chapter 299) Pneumonia (Chapter 85) Aspergillosis with cavitation (Chapter 311) Lung abscess (Chapter 78) Chronic chest infections (e.g., bronchitis; Chapter 78) Positive pressure mechanical ventilation (Chapter 91)
CENTRAL NERVOUS SYSTEM DISEASE
Brain tumor (Chapter 175) Encephalitis (Chapter 383) Meningitis (Chapter 381) Brain abscess (Chapter 382) Head injury (Chapter 368) Subarachnoid hemorrhage (Chapter 377) Guillain-Barré syndrome (Chapter 380) Acute intermittent porphyria (Chapter 194) In response to stress (Chapter 97)
DRUG-INDUCED
AVP analogs: desmopressin (Chapter 206), oxytocin (Chapter 206) Alkylating agents/antimetabolites (Chapter 164) Anticonvulsants (Chapter 372) Antipsychotic agents (Chapter 362) Antidepressants (Chapter 362) Nicotine (Chapter 363) Opiates (Chapter 365) 3-4-Methylenedioxymethamphetamine (Ecstasy; Chapter 365)

AVP = arginine vasopressin.

increased, and the distal delivery of water is diminished. As a result, free water excretion is decreased.

CLINICAL MANIFESTATIONS AND DIAGNOSIS

Hyponatremia, which is a plasma sodium concentration of less than 136 mmol/L, is often an incidental finding on routine laboratory testing or is found as part of the investigation of other clinical syndromes. Hyponatremia may be hypertonic, isotonic, or hypotonic. Hypertonic hyponatremia is caused by an accumulation of non–sodium-containing effective solutes, such as very high concentrations of glucose in diabetic patients or exogenously administered mannitol or glycerol. Isotonic hyponatremia is not accompanied by any abnormalities in other electrolytes and nearly always reflects pseudohyponatremia from marked hyperlipidemia or hyperglobulinemia.

Hypotonic hyponatremia always reflects an important underlying disorder with abnormal retention of body water (see Table 102-6). Hypotonic hyponatremia can be further classified as hypervolemic (e.g., heart failure [Chapter 45], cirrhosis with ascites [Chapter 139], advanced renal failure [Chapter 116]) or hypovolemic hyponatremia (more sodium than water is lost through the gastrointestinal tract [diarrhea] or in the urine [e.g., thiazide diuretics], or ingested or administered replacement fluid is more hypotonic than the lost fluid).

The symptoms of hypotonic hyponatremia depend on its duration, severity, and rate of development.[11] When it develops over hours to days, acute brain swelling or cerebral edema may be manifested as headache, lethargy, seizures, and decreased levels of consciousness that can lead to coma and death, especially in women between menarche and menopause.[12] By comparison, if the rate of decline in the plasma sodium concentration is more gradual, osmotic adaptation may avoid serious clinical manifestations even with severe hyponatremia (plasma sodium concentration <120 mmol/L).

A careful evaluation, including a review of prior plasma sodium values, will help determine the rate of decline and provide important clues to the cause (Fig. 102-3). The physical examination should assess for hypervolemia (Chapters 7 and 39). Conversely, orthostatic hypotension and tachycardia suggest hypovolemia. The BUN, plasma electrolytes, glucose level, and osmolality should be checked to allow comparison of the measured with the calculated plasma osmolality according to the following equation:

$$\text{Plasma osmolality (mOsm/kg)} = 2\text{Na}^+\text{(mmol/L)} + (\text{blood urea nitrogen[mg/dL]}/2.8) + (\text{glucose[mg/dL]}/18)$$

Other laboratory tests in selected patients should include liver function tests and measurement of plasma creatinine, uric acid, thyroid-stimulating hormone, and cortisol concentrations; if indicated, an adrenocorticotropic hormone stimulation test should be performed (Chapter 209). Symmetrically elevated levels of both BUN and creatinine point to intrinsic renal disease, whereas a disproportionate elevation of BUN over creatinine suggests hypovolemia with a tendency to prerenal azotemia (Chapter 106). In contrast, very low levels of BUN and uric acid are typical of both SIADH and cerebral salt-wasting syndrome (see Normovolemic and Hypovolemic Hyponatremia).

About 85% of inpatients with hyponatremia have true hyponatremia, about 25% of whom are hypovolemic, about 25% of whom have an edematous state, about one third of whom are normovolemic, and the remainder of whom usually have renal failure. Since the plasma sodium concentration declines by approximately 1.6 mmol/L for each increase of 100 mg/dL (5.5 mmol/L) in plasma glucose concentration, marked elevation in the plasma glucose concentration can cause *hypertonic* hyponatremia. In contrast to hyperglycemia, an elevated BUN does not alter the plasma sodium concentration, even though urea contributes to the laboratory measurement of plasma osmolality; thus, a hyponatremic patient with a normal or elevated laboratory measurement of plasma osmolality that can be fully attributed to an increased BUN should be considered as having hypotonic hyponatremia.

A discrepancy in which measured plasma osmolality exceeds calculated plasma osmolality, even after accounting for glucose and urea, indicates the presence of an unidentified small solute (osmolar gap), including alcohols (e.g., ethanol, methanol, ethylene glycol, and isopropyl alcohol) and the organic anions of weak acids, which raise the plasma anion gap. Because these small

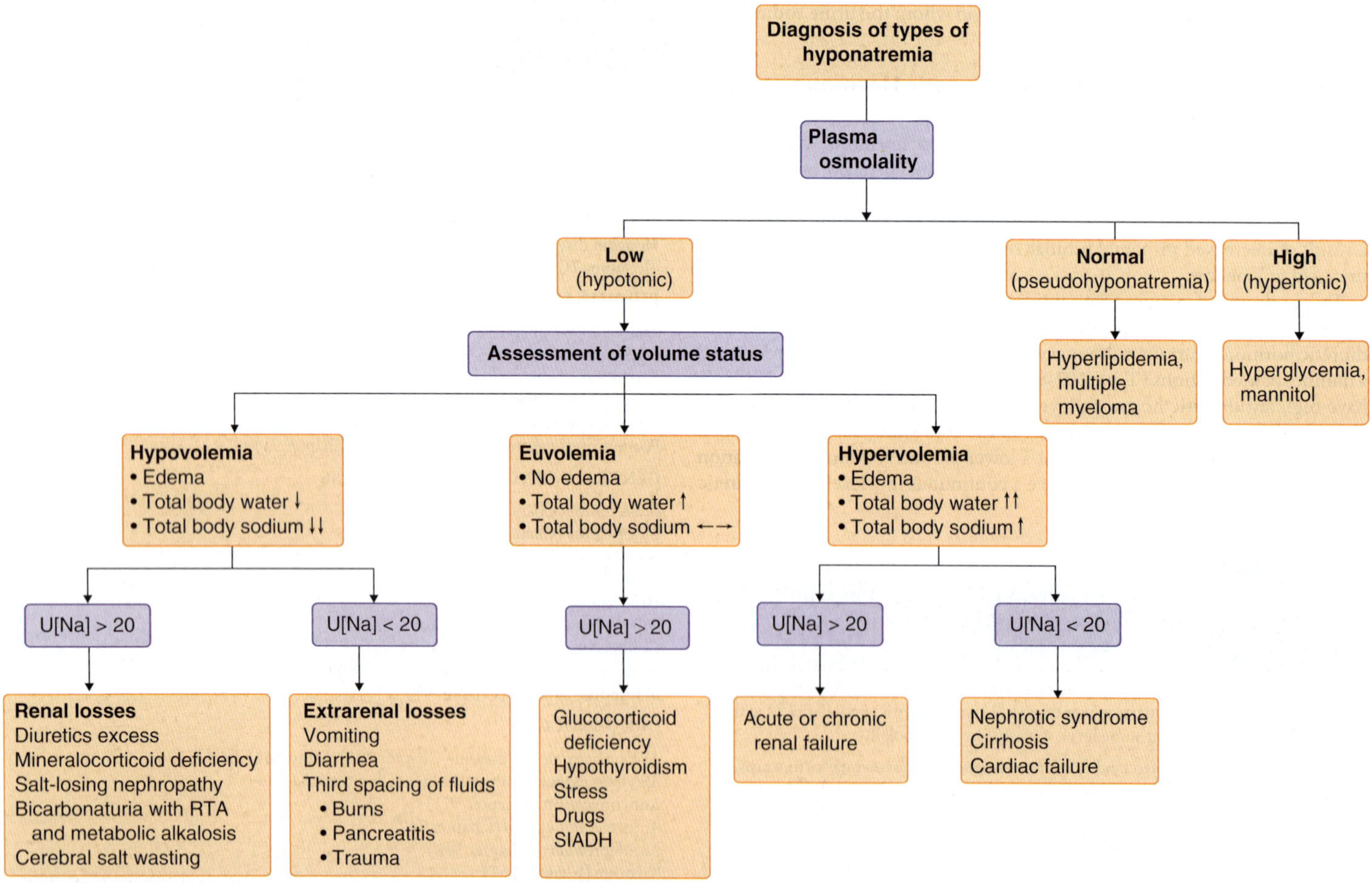

FIGURE 102-3. **Diagnostic approach to hyponatremia.** RTA = renal tubular acidosis; SIADH = syndrome of inappropriate antidiuretic hormone secretion; U[Na] = urinary sodium concentration. (Modified from Halterman R, Berl T. Therapy of dysnatremic disorders. In: Brady H, Wilcox C, eds. *Therapy in Nephrology and Hypertension*. Philadelphia: Saunders; 1999:256; and data from Cohen DM, Ellison DH. Evaluating hyponatremia. *JAMA*. 2015;313:1260-1261.)

molecules do not affect the movement of water, the patient's water balance is determined by the plasma sodium concentration. However, an osmolar gap should prompt a thorough investigation for poisoning, intoxication, or an organic acidosis (Chapter 104).

As soon as true hypotonic hyponatremia is established, the evaluation aims at classifying the cause into one of three categories based on the patient's volume status (see Fig. 102-3). Abnormal liver function test results can provide adjunctive support for hepatic disease and a hypervolemic hyponatremic state. The diagnosis of heart failure should be made clinically, but it can be assisted by a BNP level, chest radiograph, or echocardiography (Chapter 45).

In the absence of a clinically obvious edema, a low urine sodium concentration (<20 mmol/L) or a low fractional excretion of sodium (<1%) supports the diagnosis of hypovolemic hyponatremia secondary to extrarenal losses or past renal losses that have since abated. In hypovolemia caused by ongoing renal losses, the urine sodium concentration may remain high despite hypovolemia, but the fractional excretion of urea may also be low (<35%). A high urinary concentration of potassium is suggestive of potassium-depleting diuretic use, whereas the urinary potassium concentration of potassium is low (<20 mmol/L) if potassium is being lost because of diarrhea or vomiting.

The combination of hypotonic hyponatremia without hypovolemia, hypervolemia, hypothyroidism, or adrenal insufficiency combined with low plasma urea and uric acid concentrations strongly suggests SIADH. The urine sodium concentration typically is higher than 40 mmol/L, often higher than 100 mmol/L. Lack of sustained improvement after a salt-containing volume challenge further supports the diagnosis of SIADH and should prompt a search for its cause (see Table 102-8). A radiograph or chest computed tomography scan may help identify intrathoracic lesions that are associated with SIADH.

Hypervolemic Hyponatremia

In hypervolemic hyponatremia, both water and sodium are in excess, but the excess of water is greater than the excess of sodium. The most frequent causes are heart failure (Chapter 45), decompensated cirrhosis (Chapter 139) with ascites (Chapter 132), and advanced renal failure (Chapter 117), just as in hypervolemia without hyponatremia. The urine sodium concentration is less than 20 mmol/L and the fractional sodium excretion is less than 1% (despite obvious volume expansion, commonly with edema) unless it is altered by a diuretic-induced natriuresis.

Normovolemic and Hypovolemic Hyponatremia

Normovolemic and hypovolemic hyponatremia may be difficult to distinguish from each other because mild hypovolemia can be difficult to detect on the history and physical examination. A low urine sodium concentration and low fractional excretion of sodium are characteristic of extrarenal hypovolemia, but the urine sodium concentration is usually elevated when hypovolemia is due to urinary loss.

Hypovolemic hyponatremia always signifies past or ongoing sodium loss (often with potassium) accompanied by a lesser degree of water loss, with appropriately elevated ADH levels in response to the hypovolemia. In most cases, loss of sodium results in volume depletion, which activates thirst, thereby inducing the patient to drink water; because volume-mediated release of antidiuretic hormone is retained, hyponatremia develops. Hyponatremia is a common complication of diarrhea (Chapter 126) when the diarrheal fluid is secretory and rich in electrolytes. Sweating-induced hyponatremia occurs when individuals ingest high volumes of hypotonic fluid, often pure water, while losing sodium in sweat.

The renal causes of hypovolemic hyponatremia (see Fig. 102-3) include thiazide-induced hyponatremia and the cerebral salt-wasting syndrome. Thiazide-induced hyponatremia occurs when patients with impaired urinary diluting capacity excrete concentrated urine because thiazides do not affect the ability of the renal medulla to concentrate urine. Thiazide-treated patients are particularly susceptible to hyponatremia when they ingest or receive hypotonic solutions that exceed their maximal capacity to excrete electrolyte-free water in their urine. In cerebral salt wasting, patients who have suffered a head injury or intracranial hemorrhage have inappropriate renal sodium wasting; antidiuretic hormone levels rise and patients develop hyponatremia if hypotonic fluid is then ingested or administered. SIADH also is characterized by a high urine sodium concentration and hyponatremia, but a high fractional excretion of uric acid is found only in cerebral salt wasting.

In normovolemic hypotonic hyponatremia, urine containing sodium concentrations greater than 40 mmol/L usually indicate SIADH (Table 102-8),[13] but hypothyroidism (Chapter 207) and adrenal glucocorticoid insufficiency (Chapter 208) can be associated with hypotonic hyponatremia that mimics SIADH without clinically evident hypovolemia. Pregnancy, which also is associated with thirst as well as a reduction in the osmotic threshold for ADH release, results in mild hyponatremia (Chapter 221).

TREATMENT

Treatment of hyponatremia varies depending on the urgency of the clinical situation, its cause, and the underlying diagnosis (see Fig. 102-3). Some data suggest that a bolus of 3% saline (100 mL repeated up to two more times) may safely correct hyponatremia more rapidly than a continuous infusion. Hyponatremia should be approached from the perspective of free water intake compared with renal free water output.

The first principle is that the rate of correction should be guided by the patient's age, gender, and neurologic status and any information about recent and past plasma sodium concentrations or osmolality values. Delayed correction of hyponatremia can perpetuate cerebral edema and result in irreversible neurologic damage and death, especially in women of reproductive age and in patients whose hyponatremia developed at a pace that outstripped the rate of osmotic adaptation in the brain. In contrast, overly rapid correction or correction to a sodium concentration that is above the level needed to safeguard the patient from the neurologic sequelae of cerebral edema can result in the devastating and often irreversible *osmotic demyelination syndrome* (Chapter 384), which is characterized by fluctuating levels of consciousness, pseudobulbar palsy, ataxia, dysarthria, difficulty in swallowing, and characteristic abnormalities in the region of the brain stem on magnetic resonance imaging (MRI; see Fig. 384-3). Risk factors for the development of osmotic demyelination syndrome include severe hyponatremia (serum sodium concentration <105 mmol/L), hypokalemia, alcohol use disorder, malnutrition, and advanced liver disease.

The second principle is the importance of identifying and treating any underlying disorder, such as the hypervolemia of heart failure (Chapters 45 and 46). In hypovolemic patients, appropriate fluid administration can correct the hyponatremia.

Acute Symptomatic Hyponatremia

Acute symptomatic hyponatremia that requires urgent treatment includes self-induced acute water intoxication (e.g., psychiatric diseases such as acute psychosis or schizophrenia; endurance exercise), known hyponatremia with a duration <24 to 48 hours; hyponatremia from an intracranial cause (includes increased intracranial pressure); or hyponatremia accompanied by seizures or coma, regardless of chronicity. The goal is urgent correction by 4 to 6 mmol/L to prevent brain herniation and neurologic damage from cerebral ischemia.

For severe symptoms, 100 mL of 3% NaCl should be infused intravenously over 10 minutes, repeated twice as needed.[14] This rapid bolus approach is as good as a continuous infusion for correcting hyponatremia with a lower risk of overcorrection.[A6] For mild to moderate symptoms with a low risk of herniation, 3% NaCl should be infused at 0.5 to 2 mL/kg/hour. The rate of correction need not be restricted in patients who have true acute hyponatremia, nor should inadvertent overcorrection be reversed. If, however, the hyponatremia might be chronic rather than acute, the limits for correction of chronic hyponatremia should be followed.

Chronic Hyponatremia

Symptomatic hyponatremia or sodium concentrations below 125 to 130 mmol/L require specific treatment, but mild degrees of asymptomatic hyponatremia can be tolerated for long periods. When deciding treatment strategies in such patients who are known to have developed hyponatremia, the severity of symptoms, risk factors for osmotic demyelination syndrome, and the underlying cause of hyponatremia should be taken into consideration. Frequent monitoring of the plasma sodium concentration and osmolality is crucial. If the safe target rate of correction is exceeded, osmotic demyelination can be prevented by slowing the correction rate, by returning to a lower plasma sodium concentration with the judicious readministration of hypotonic solutions, or by administering vasopressin analogues (see later).

Patients who are at risk for osmotic demyelination syndrome have hyponatremia with serum [Na^+] <120 mmol/L of >48 hours' duration. Examples include outpatients who have been drinking conventional volumes of water, are treated with thiazide diuretics, or have hospital-acquired hyponatremia with a known duration of >48 hours.

To avoid osmotic demyelination syndrome in such patients, the goal of therapy is minimum correction of serum sodium concentration by 4 to 8 mmol/L per day, with a lower goal of 4 to 6 mmol/L per day if the risk of osmotic demyelination syndrome is high. The rate of correction should not exceed 8 mmol/L in any 24-hour period in patients who are at a high risk of osmotic demyelination syndrome, and it should not exceed 10 to 12 mmol/L in any 24-hour period (or 18 mmol/L in any 48-hour period) for patients at normal risk of osmotic demyelination syndrome.

If the correction of chronic hyponatremia has been inadvertently excessive, intervention is probably unnecessary if the starting serum sodium concentration was ≥120 mmol/L. However, if the starting serum sodium concentration was <120 mmol/L, the serum sodium should be lowered to the recommended level

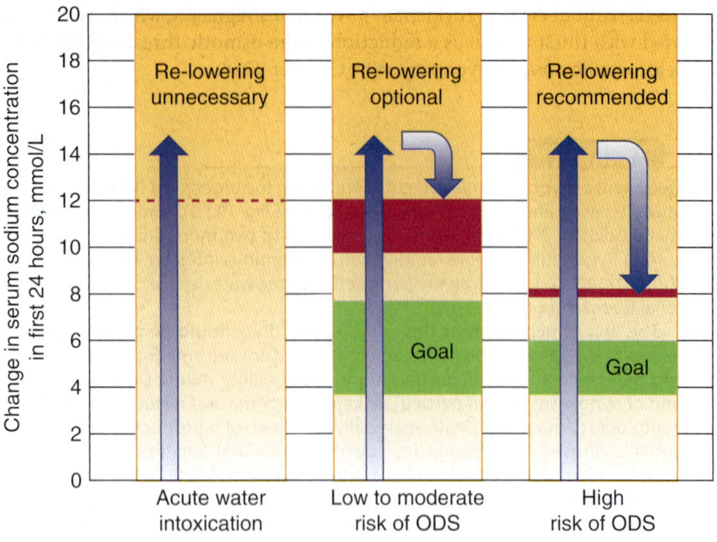

FIGURE 102-4. **Recommendations for relowering of serum sodium concentration ([Na]) to goals *(green)* for patients presenting with serum [Na] <120 mmol/L who exceed the recommended limits of correction *(red)* in the first 24 hours.** ODS = osmotic demyelination syndrome. (Reproduced with permission from Verbalis JG, Goldsmith SR, Greenberg A, et al. Diagnosis, evaluation, and treatment of hyponatremia: expert panel recommendations. *Am J Med.* 2013;126:S1-S42.)

if overcorrection occurs. To relower the serum sodium concentration (Fig. 102-4), desmopressin (2 to 4 mcg every 8 hours parenterally) should be administered to prevent further water losses, and water losses should be replaced with 5% dextrose in water intravenously at a rate of 3 mL/kg/hour. The next dose of a vasopressin antagonist should be withheld if the correction is >8 mmol/L. The serum sodium concentration should be checked hourly, and water replacement should be continued until the serum sodium concentration is reduced to goal. High-dose glucocorticoids (e.g., dexamethasone, 4 mg every 6 hours) for 24 to 48 hours is recommended if correction has occurred.

Hypervolemic Hyponatremia

In hypervolemic hyponatremia (e.g., heart failure), the goal is to remove salt and water, but relatively more of the latter. Water restriction is helpful but is often inadequate. Treatment with the AVP V_2-receptor antagonist tolvaptan (starting at 15 mg once daily, with a maximal dose of 60 mg once daily) increases the plasma sodium concentration significantly at 30 days in patients with euvolemic or hypervolemic hyponatremia,[A7] but it also increases the risk of overcorrection.[A8] Tolvaptan is not recommended in patients who have cirrhosis because of its potential liver toxicity.

Hypovolemic Hyponatremia

When hypovolemia is clearly evident (appropriate clinical history, orthostatic hypotension, low urine sodium concentration in the setting of extrarenal fluid losses, elevated plasma urea disproportionate to the rise in the serum creatinine level, and elevated uric acid concentrations), isotonic saline is the treatment of choice. However, caution should be exercised in the administration of isotonic saline to these patients because the administration of small volumes of isotonic saline can sometimes induce a brisk and rapid decrease in urine osmolality, an accompanying water diuresis, and an overly rapid correction of hyponatremia. Accordingly, hourly monitoring of urine output, urine osmolality, plasma sodium concentration, and plasma osmolality is required. A rapid drop in urine osmolality accompanied by water diuresis should prompt cessation of volume repletion and, in some cases, administration of hypotonic solutions or even analogues of vasopressin itself (see later) to bring the rise in sodium concentration to within the recommended guidelines. When hypovolemia is not clearly evident but cannot be excluded, a brisk drop in urine osmolality in response to a saline challenge confirms the suspicion of hypovolemia and simultaneously initiates therapy. In contrast, failure to induce such a response lends support to the diagnosis of normovolemic hyponatremia.

Normovolemic Hyponatremia

In patients with normovolemic hyponatremia, the appropriate therapeutic approach is to address the underlying hypothyroidism (Chapter 207), adrenal insufficiency (Chapter 208), or SIADH. If an underlying cause cannot be identified or reversed, treatment aims to generate a gradual net negative water balance. Fluid restriction is usually the first-line strategy.

Fluid restriction should address all intake that is consumed by drinking, not just water, aiming for an intake that is 500 mL/day below the 24-hour urine volume. Neither sodium nor protein intake should be restricted unless the patient has another indication for doing so. Unfortunately, fluid restriction may be insufficient in the setting of a high urine osmolality (e.g., >500 mOsm/kg H_2O), when the sum of the urine sodium and potassium concentrations exceeds the serum sodium concentration, when 24-hour urine volume is <1500 mL/day, or when the increase in serum sodium concentration is <2 mmol/L/day despite fluid restriction below 1 L/day for 24 to 48 hours. In such patients, titrated oral tolvaptan (beginning at 15 mg once daily and increasing to a maximum of 60 mg once daily) is indicated, especially in hospitalized patients, provided that the patient has an intact thirst mechanism to avoid polyuria or hypernatremia. When volume status is in doubt, however, these agents are better avoided.

Vaptans should not be used in patients who have hypovolemic hyponatremia, in conjunction with other treatments for hyponatremia, or immediately after the cessation of other treatments for hyponatremia, particularly 3% NaCl. For the first 24 to 48 hours after initiating treatment, the serum sodium concentration must be monitored every 6 to 8 hours, and ad libitum fluid intake should be maintained. Hyponatremia can correct too quickly if vaptans are given with coincidental fluid restriction in patients who have a defective or impaired thirst mechanism (e.g., intubated or unconscious patients), so sufficient fluid must be provided to prevent overly rapid correction owing to unopposed aquaresis. Vaptans should be discontinued if the patient develops complications that limit their ability to request, access, or ingest fluid. For severe, symptomatic hyponatremia or a serum sodium concentration below <120 mmol/L, treatment should be with 3% NaCl, which provides a quicker and more certain correction of the serum sodium concentration than do vasopressin antagonists. If overcorrection occurs, the serum sodium concentration can be relowered to safe limits as for acute hyponatremia.

Urea (typically starting at 15 g/day diluted in water and divided into two or three daily doses and with the dose increased to 90 g/day based on the patient's response) can increase the excretion of urinary solutes and thereby water excretion in patients with SIADH. Urea is well tolerated and can be used chronically in patients who have SIADH.

PROGNOSIS

Hyponatremia is a marker for worse outcomes among hospitalized patients. A serum sodium level <135 mmol/L is associated with about a 45% relative increased rate of intensive care unit admission.[15]

HYPERNATREMIA

Hypernatremia (a plasma sodium concentration higher than 144 mmol/L) always reflects a state of hypertonicity, with an increased concentration of osmotically active solutes throughout all body fluid compartments. Under normal conditions, the obligate daily loss of water is approximately 500 mL, consisting mostly of the water vapor in expired air and the loss due to insensible sweating. The minimal amount of water needed to keep the urinary solutes in solution is about 500 mL per day. However, sweating in hot, dry environments can lead to massive water losses as high as 1 L/hr. If the daily water intake is less than the obligate water loss, the osmotic pressure of the body fluids will increase.

CLINICAL MANIFESTATIONS AND DIAGNOSIS

Although hypernatremia can be diagnosed as an incidental laboratory abnormality, it most commonly occurs in the setting of a severe underlying disease with other accompanying disturbances to body fluid homeostasis (Table 102-9). Patients with hypovolemic hypernatremia have lost both sodium and water, but the net loss of water is disproportionately greater than the net loss of sodium.

The main clinical consequences of increased body fluid tonicity are confusion, seizures, focal neurologic deficits, and a progressively decreasing level of consciousness that can progress to coma. In the absence of an underlying neurologic problem or disturbance in the thirst mechanism, the patient would be expected to complain of thirst unless the neurologic injury has disturbed consciousness. Failure to replace hypotonic fluid losses generally reflects impairment in thirst, disability or infirmity that prevents the patient from responding to thirst, or failure of the clinician to recognize the need for hypotonic fluid replacement. Rarely, impaired thirst in patients who are awake and alert can be caused by damage to the hypothalamic osmoreceptors that control thirst perception and response, a condition known as *primary hypodipsia*. In patients with hypernatremia of sufficient duration to enable brain cells to undergo osmotic adaptation, few, if any, clinical manifestations are observed.

The causes of hypernatremia include loss of thirst or increased insensible loss of water, diabetes insipidus, or osmotic diuresis. Renal failure (Chapter 116)

TABLE 102-9 CAUSES OF HYPERNATREMIA CLASSIFIED BY EXTRACELLULAR FLUID VOLUME (TOTAL BODY SODIUM CONTENT)

Hypervolemia	Hypertonic saline excess Hypertonic sodium bicarbonate solutions
Hypertonicity with near normovolemia	Diabetes insipidus Febrile fluid loss
Hypovolemia	Gastrointestinal loss (diarrhea, vomiting) Skin fluid loss (burn, sweat) Loop diuretics Osmotic diuresis Impaired thirst perception

and tubulointerstitial disease (Chapter 108) cause relatively mild concentrating defects and tend not to be associated with significant hypernatremia, provided that a normal mechanism can readily compensate for it.

The laboratory diagnosis of hypernatremia should be repeated to confirm its accuracy and should be corroborated by an elevated plasma osmolality. The underlying cause is usually evident from the history and physical examination.

In hypovolemic hypernatremia with extrarenal fluid loss, urine output is usually less than 500 mL/day and urine osmolality is the maximum for age (>1000 mOsm/kg in young adulthood decreasing to >600 mOsm/kg by age 60 years). Polyuria with a submaximal urine osmolality suggests impaired urine-concentrating ability, owing to underlying intrinsic renal disease or diuretic agents. A spot urine osmolality less than 100 to 200 mOsm/kg or polyuria (>3 L/day) combined with 24-hour urine solute excretion less than 600 mOsm/day suggests diabetes insipidus (see later). In contrast, daily solute excretion greater than 800 to 1000 mOsm/day suggests an osmotic diuresis.

Hypervolemic hypernatremia is usually associated with prior administration of sodium-containing solutions, and the findings on physical examination are consistent with volume expansion. In the absence of underlying intrinsic renal disease or diuretic use, urine osmolality is high because the hypertonic stimulus to release vasopressin overrides the effects of hypervolemia.

TREATMENT

The management of serious symptomatic hypovolemic hypernatremia is challenging and includes rapid correction of the depleted volume followed by gradual replacement of the water deficit.[16] If volume contraction is severe, isotonic saline is generally the fluid of choice, and the volume and rate of administration should be guided by clinical parameters related to reversal of hypovolemia. After tissue perfusion has been restored, further fluid replacement aims to correct the estimated water deficit:

$$\text{Total body water deficit} = 0.4 \times \text{premorbid weight} \times ([\text{Na}]/140] - 1)$$

Unlike the initial isotonic fluid replacement, water replacement should be gradual over hours to days, so the rate of water replacement can match the rate at which brain intracellular solutes can be adaptively extruded or removed, unless the hypernatremia has itself clearly developed over minutes to hours. The estimated water deficit should be replaced at a rate that will lead to a reduction of approximately 0.5 to 1.0 mmol/L in measured plasma sodium concentration per hour and more than 6 mmol/L but no more than 10 to 12 mmol/L in 24 hours. In addition to the estimated water deficit, water replacement should consider estimated ongoing insensible water loss of at least 1 L per 24 hours, supplemented to account for ongoing water losses (renal or gastrointestinal) owing to the underlying disease process. Patients often require large volumes of water, sometimes reaching 5 to 10 L, for the duration of the correction period. This water requirement can be met by the dietary ingestion of tap water or administration of a hypotonic intravenous solution, such as D_5W or half-isotonic saline. The sodium concentration should be monitored at least every 4 hours, and the patient's volume status should be monitored to avoid hypervolemia.

The hypertonic state of uncontrolled diabetes with hyperglycemia (Chapter 210) requires insulin as well as fluid therapy.[17] Some hospitalized patients with hypervolemic hypernatremia require hypotonic solutions combined with a continuous infusion of loop diuretics or even extracorporeal removal of both the sodium and water excess. Once the sodium concentration has normalized, a patient with an intact thirst mechanism will generally correct the hypertonic state by spontaneous oral fluid intake.

TABLE 102-10 REASONS FOR POLYURIA

WATER DIURESIS
Diabetes insipidus
Central (neurogenic)
Inherited
Acquired (e.g., tumors, trauma, hypoxia)
Nephrogenic
Hypercalcemia
Amyloidosis
Drugs (e.g., lithium, foscarnet, cidofovir, vaptans)
Sjögren syndrome
Sickle cell disease
Inherited
Polydipsia
Primary (e.g., hypothalamic)
Psychogenic
SOLUTE DIURESIS
Sodium
Excess sodium intake (oral, enteral, parenteral)
Renal sodium wasting (e.g., inherited tubulopathies, interstitial nephritis, natriuretic drugs)
Anion based (sodium is usually the associated cation)
Chloride excretion (e.g., Bartter syndrome, loop diuretic)
Bicarbonate excretion (e.g., exogenous bicarbonate, carbonic anhydrase inhibition)
Glucose/keto acids
Diabetic ketoacidosis
Hyperglycemic-hyperosmolar syndrome
Renal glycosuria
Sugar alcohols
External loading (e.g., mannitol, glycerol)
Urea
Exogenous loading (e.g., urea, protein, amino acids)
Diuretic phase of acute kidney injury
Postobstructive diuresis
Hypercatabolic states
Hemoglobin/myoglobin driven (post-rhabdomyolysis or reabsorption of a hematoma)
Other
Radiocontrast agents

PROGNOSIS

Hypernatremia is associated with increased morbidity and mortality, both in the hospital and after discharge. Since hypernatremia in adults is typically associated with serious comorbid conditions, the mortality rates may reflect the severity of the underlying diseases rather than that of hypernatremia itself.

POLYURIA

Polyuria (Table 102-10),[18] which is defined as a urine output of more than 3 L/day, should be distinguished from urinary frequency, which can occur with frequent voiding of small volumes totaling less than this amount per day. Polyuria can be a water diuresis or a solute diuresis.

The evaluation for polyuria centers around the analysis of urine osmolality (Fig. 102-5). Urine osmolality <100 mOsm/kg suggests water diuresis, whereas a urine osmolality >300 mOsm/kg is typically related to solute diuresis.

DIABETES INSIPIDUS

The failure to release antidiuretic hormone is termed central diabetes insipidus (Chapter 206), whereas a lack of responsiveness to antidiuretic hormone is termed nephrogenic diabetes insipidus.[19] In diabetes insipidus, the urine becomes progressively dilute as it ascends in the loop of Henle, reaching osmolalities as low as 100 to 150 mOsm/kg in the distal tubule. In the absence of antidiuretic hormone, urine will be diluted further in the collecting tubules. The daily volume of this dilute urine can be as high as 20 liters.

Central diabetes insipidus (Chapter 206) results from destruction of the hypothalamus by tumor (Chapter 204), head injury (Chapter 368), hemorrhage (Chapter 375), surgical trauma, or congenital causes. If the involved area is extensive, the thirst mechanism will also be impaired. A few patients who manifest partial diabetes insipidus can concentrate their urine, though not to maximal levels.

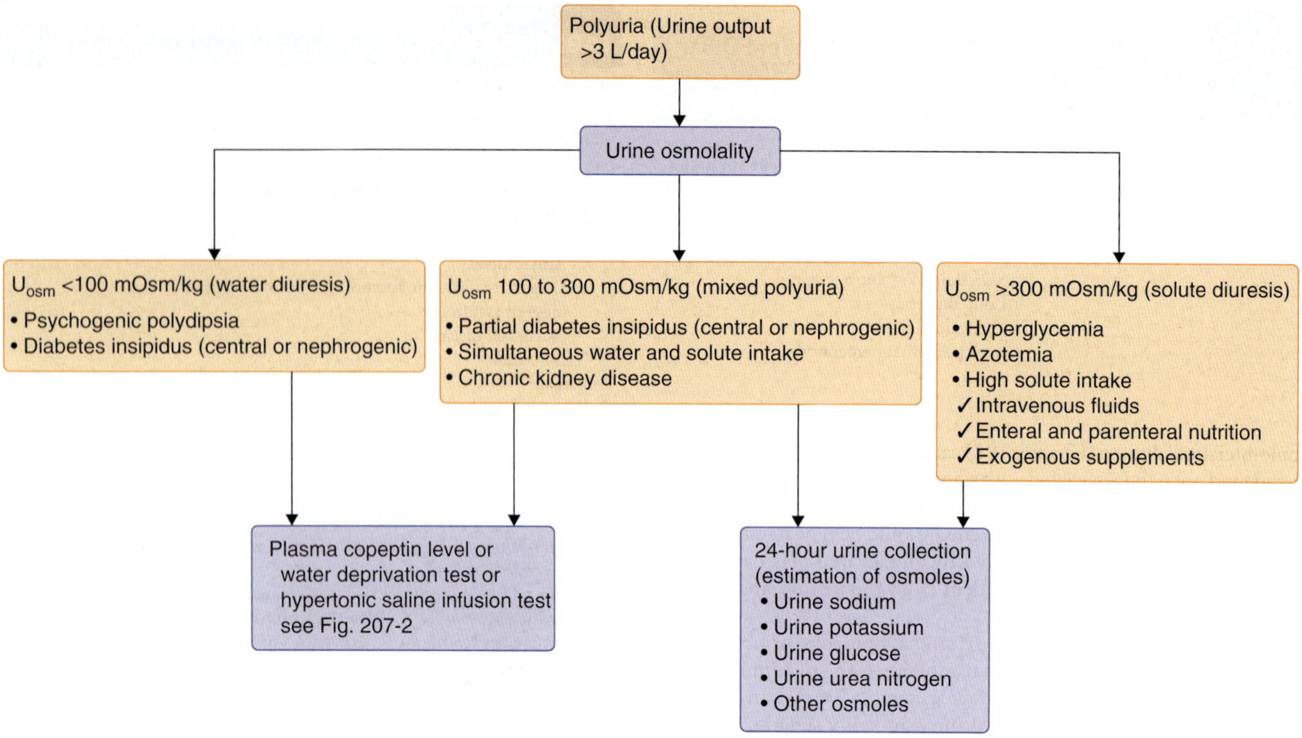

FIGURE 102-5. Diagnostic approach to polyuria. U_{osm} = urinary osmolality. (Adapted with permission from Bhasin B, Velez JCQ. Evaluation of polyuria: the roles of solute loading and water diuresis. *Am J Kidney Dis*. 2016;67:507-511.)

Nephrogenic diabetes insipidus can be caused by a mutation in the vasopressin V2 receptor or the aquaporin 2 water channel.[20] Drugs also can cause nephrogenic diabetes insipidus by interfering with the action of antidiuretic hormone, thereby preventing the insertion of aquaporin water channels into the luminal membrane of the principal cells of the collecting ducts. For example, lithium, used in the treatment of manic-depressive psychosis (Chapter 362), commonly causes polyuria, which can be quite severe. Demeclocycline, a tetracycline now rarely used in dermatologic conditions, also causes nephrogenic diabetes insipidus and is used to treat SIADH that cannot be controlled by water restriction.

Clinically, polyuria, which may be massive, is the hallmark of the disease. Although polyuria itself is not deleterious to health, it is a nuisance if the patient passes more than 6 or 7 liters of urine daily. It can be dangerous, however, if the thirst mechanism is depressed and hyperosmolarity supervenes. Repeated hyperosmolar episodes in such patients frequently lead to irreversible brain damage. If present from childhood, diabetes insipidus frequently leads to massive dilatation of the renal pelvis, ureters, and bladder.

OSMOTIC DIURESIS

Large volumes of urine can be excreted in the presence of large amounts of a poorly reabsorbed solute, most commonly glucose. For example, when the blood sugar concentration rises above the capacity of the kidney to reabsorb all of the filtered glucose, a large volume of glycosuria results. In fact, polyuria and polydipsia are the most common presenting features of diabetes mellitus (Chapter 210).

The more blood that flows through the medulla, the less concentrated it becomes. In some clinical situations, such as intravascular volume expansion and osmotic diuresis, medullary blood flow increases, thereby leading to a washout of the medullary gradient. Osmotic diuretics also impair water reabsorption at the collecting duct.

Osmotic diuresis also occurs after the relief of obstruction to the urinary tract. In this situation, the principal osmotic agent is urea, although other retained solutes also play a role in diuresis.

As the number of functioning nephrons is gradually reduced in renal failure, the amount of solutes added is also reduced; hence the inability to concentrate the urine, manifesting as nocturia and polyuria, is an early sign of renal failure. Direct damage to medullary tubules can also decrease the reabsorption of salt, particularly with tubulointerstitial kidney diseases (Chapter 108), such as analgesic nephropathy and sickle cell disease.

TREATMENT

The clinical manifestations and treatment of polyuria should address its underlying causes (Fig. 206-2). Depending on the nature of fluid intake and medication used at the onset of polyuria, a significant percentage of polyuric patients will have alterations in plasma sodium and volume, so treatment must also address these accompanying fluid and electrolyte abnormalities.

GENERAL REFERENCES

For the General References and other additional features, please visit Elsevier eBooks+ at https://ebooks.health.elsevier.com.

Grade A References

A1. Self WH, Semler MW, Wanderer JP, et al. Balanced crystalloids versus saline in noncritically ill adults. *N Engl J Med*. 2018;378:819-828.
A2. Semler MW, Self WH, Wanderer JP, et al. Balanced crystalloids versus saline in critically ill adults. *N Engl J Med*. 2018;378:829-839.
A3. Hammond DA, Lam SW, Rech MA, et al. Balanced crystalloids versus saline in critically ill adults: a systematic review and meta-analysis. *Ann Pharmacother*. 2020;54:5-13.
A4. Lewis SR, Pritchard MW, Evans DJ, et al. Colloids versus crystalloids for fluid resuscitation in critically ill people. *Cochrane Database Syst Rev*. 2018;8:CD000567.
A5. Zampieri FG, Machado FR, Biondi RS, et al. Effect of slower vs faster intravenous fluid bolus rates on mortality in critically ill patients: the BaSICS randomized clinical trial. *JAMA*. 2021;326:830-838.
A6. Baek SH, Jo YH, Ahn S, et al. Risk of overcorrection in rapid intermittent bolus vs slow continuous infusion therapies of hypertonic saline for patients with symptomatic hyponatremia: the SALSA randomized clinical trial. *JAMA Intern Med*. 2021;181:81-92.
A7. Bhandari S, Peri A, Cranston I, et al. A systematic review of known interventions for the treatment of chronic nonhypovolaemic hypotonic hyponatraemia and a meta-analysis of the vaptans. *Clin Endocrinol (Oxf)*. 2017;86:761-771.
A8. Zhou Y, Yang W, Liu G, et al. Risks of vaptans in hypernatremia and serum sodium overcorrection: a systematic review and meta-analysis of randomised controlled trials. *Int J Clin Pract*. 2021;75:e13939.

103 POTASSIUM DISORDERS

JULIAN LAWRENCE SEIFTER

DEFINITION

Maintenance of a normal and narrow range of blood plasma potassium concentration, [K^+], usually on the order of 3.5 to 5.0 mmol/L, is vital for health. *Hyperkalemia* refers to an increased plasma [K^+], and *hypokalemia* to a decreased plasma [K^+]. Within the human body, K^+ is not equally distributed in the total body water. Approximately two thirds of body water is intracellular, and K^+ is the major cation within that compartment, reaching concentrations as high as 140 mEq/L. Consequently, more than 98% of K^+ resides within cells. An *excess* of total body K^+ stores is less common than K^+ *depletion* unless renal function is compromised. K^+ *adaptation* defines changes in regulatory mechanisms resulting from K^+ excesses or deficits.

EPIDEMIOLOGY

Because K^+ is widely distributed in both plant and animal dietary sources, avoiding K^+ is difficult in the well-fed state. As a result, a healthy person on a regular diet is likely to require high rates of urinary K^+ losses, primarily by secretion in the cortical distal nephron, to prevent hyperkalemia. The ready availability of potassium in the diet also makes hypokalemia uncommon, unless excessive potassium is lost in gastrointestinal or renal body fluids. The kidney must be able both to eliminate and at other times conserve large amounts of potassium.

Disorders of K^+ balance are common in both inpatient and outpatient settings. Diets high in K^+ and low in Na^+ are associated with lower blood pressure and decrease the risk of cardiovascular disease, including stroke and chronic kidney disease. Mild decreases in plasma [K^+] are seen in healthy well-trained athletes and during normal pregnancy. Patients with chronic kidney disease (Chapter 116) and insulin-deficient diabetes (Chapters 109 and 210) have a tendency to develop hyperkalemia with high-K^+ diets or treatment with medications that interfere with the renin-angiotensin-aldosterone system.[1] Starvation, gastrointestinal disease, commonly used diuretics, and other medications may cause hypokalemia. Some renal disorders, such as tubular interstitial diseases and urinary tract obstruction, may be associated with hyperkalemia, whereas others, particularly if associated with Fanconi syndrome, result in hypokalemia. Some endocrine diseases, including adrenal insufficiency (Chapter 208), characteristically cause hyperkalemia, whereas hypokalemia is a common finding in patients who have hyperaldosteronism or tumors with ectopic secretion of adrenocorticotropic hormone (ACTH; Chapter 208).

Polyuric states may lead to K^+ depletion due to increased urinary flow rates over a period of time. However, chronic hypokalemia is itself a cause of polyuric nephrogenic diabetes insipidus (Chapter 102).

PATHOBIOLOGY

Potassium Balance

Most cells express sodium potassium adenosine triphosphatase (Na^+, K^+-ATPase) on the cell plasma membranes and thereby use metabolic energy in the form of ATP to develop gradients of Na^+ and K^+. As a result, cellular [K^+] may exceed extracellular concentrations 35-fold. These established electrochemical gradients enable normal muscle and neural function, as well as transcellular solute transport in intestinal and renal epithelia. K^+ entry into cells is balanced by extrusion by K^+ channels and transporters in a regulated and coordinated fashion.

The total body amount of K^+ is usually on the order of 50 mmol/kg of body weight, so a 70-kg individual has a store of about 3500 mmol of K^+, mostly in skeletal muscle. The potassium content of the total extracellular fluid is about 56 mmol, which may approximate the potassium content of a single meal. After a meal containing an 8-ounce steak, baked potato, 1 serving of spinach, and an 8-ounce glass of tomato juice, the plasma [K^+] might rise to 9.25 mmol/L, a likely fatal value, if it were not for the ability of potassium to distribute within minutes from the extracellular space to the intracellular space. The intracellular space, given its large volume and potassium content, can accommodate, or buffer, an extra load of potassium without significant changes in the plasma or cellular [K^+]. In contrast without the shift, K^+ would rise greatly in the extracellular fluid, and the large change in ratio would electrically cause serious arrhythmias. Fortunately, carbohydrate and amino acids in a meal increase the secretion of insulin, which increases the shifting of K^+ into cells. Within hours, renal elimination of potassium matches the dietary intake.

Discordance between total body stores and the plasma [K^+], owing to shifts between the intracellular and extracellular compartments, is the reason why total body potassium is poorly reflected by the plasma potassium concentration. Hyperkalemia may occur despite total body K^+ depletion (e.g., diabetic ketoacidosis with an osmotic diuresis causing urinary losses of Na^+ and K^+, a depletion in extracellular volume, and acute kidney injury), and hypokalemia may occur despite total body K^+ excess (e.g., acute diarrhea in a patient who has chronic kidney disease).

The Importance of Potassium

Potassium is essential for a number of critical body functions, including enzymatic reactions that regulate protein and glycogen synthesis, as well as cell growth and division. Within the normal dietary range, a higher intake of potassium and a lower intake of sodium are associated with a lower cardiovascular risk.[2]

The ability of cells to take up or to extrude potassium contributes to the regulation of cell volume during periods of osmotic stress. Because of the relative magnitudes of cellular and extracellular concentrations, larger percentage changes tend to occur in the extracellular potassium concentration, which consequently has the greatest impact on the electrical properties across cell membranes. In excitable cells, such as cardiac myocytes and skeletal muscle, the relationship of intracellular to extracellular potassium concentration contributes to the resting membrane potential. Hypokalemia hyperpolarizes these cells and decreases potassium conductance in some potassium channels required for repolarization (Chapter 48).

The increased potassium conductance in hyperkalemia antagonizes the normal slow depolarization and decrease in potassium conductance of pacemaker tissue, thereby making sinus bradycardia a common first sign of hyperkalemia. Certain muscle-depolarizing anesthetic agents, such as succinylcholine, may potentiate the effects of hyperkalemia.

Potassium is as important a body fluid osmole as sodium. Potassium losses, extracellular volume depletion, increased intake of water, and retained medullary urinary concentrating ability each contribute to thiazide diuretic–induced hyponatremia (Chapter 102). Summative iso-osmotic losses of potassium and sodium salts in watery diarrhea (Chapter 126) may result in isotonic extracellular volume depletion. Similarly, if potassium chloride is added to isotonic saline, the resultant hypertonic solution causes potassium to enter cells as sodium exits, thereby contributing to hypernatremia.

Potassium is also an important local mediator of vascular tone in muscle beds. During exercise, local interstitial fluid potassium concentrations may rise several-fold, thereby causing local vasodilation to allow more blood supply to the exercising muscle, but also resulting in sarcolemmal depolarization that creates muscle fatigue. Very little of that local tissue potassium enters the total extracellular fluid, so severe hyperkalemia does not usually occur with exercise. The trained athlete develops an adaptive increase in Na^+, K^+-ATPase to allow efficient reuptake of potassium into muscle cells but still may have chronically low plasma [K^+] or postexertional hypokalemia. Experienced marathoners know that their diet must provide adequate potassium stores needed for muscle endurance because overexertion during a state of potassium depletion can lead to rhabdomyolysis (Chapter 99).

Potassium excretion follows a circadian rhythm. This rhythm appears to include an intestinal feed-forward sensing mechanism that results in the highest level of urinary potassium excretion coinciding with the anticipated dietary intake of potassium. The relationship likely involves potassium sensing within the gastrointestinal tract or splanchnic or hepatic circulation. In healthy humans, potassium excretion is greatest during the daytime hours but can increase several-fold after a meal without requiring a noticeable change in the blood potassium level. Independent of aldosterone, a direct relationship between increased potassium and sodium excretion may account for the beneficial association of high-potassium diets with lower blood pressures. Additionally, increased dietary potassium may restore a nocturnal dip in blood pressure, thereby potentially reducing cardiac risk in hypertensive patients. The distribution of potassium between the extracellular and intracellular spaces shows a circadian variation that may contribute to the diurnal variance in cardiac arrhythmias and sudden death in patients at risk.

Renal Potassium Handling

In the kidney, potassium excretion begins with filtration. Because the extracellular concentration of potassium is approximately 4 mmol/L and that of sodium is 140 mmol/L, far less potassium is filtered than sodium. The renal proximal tubule reabsorbs potassium, primarily by the paracellular pathway, in the process of reabsorbing sodium and water. In the thick ascending limb of the loop of Henle, potassium is reabsorbed both by the apical sodium–potassium–2 chloride cotransporter (NKCC2) and, like calcium and magnesium, by paracellular reabsorption of the cation. The latter mechanism is a consequence of the development of an electropositive lumen that is created by the recycling of K^+ to the lumen through renal outer medullary potassium channels (ROMK) in the thick ascending limb of the loop of Henle. Barrter syndrome (Chapter 113) stems from loss-of-function mutations either in the NKCC2, ROMK, or in the chloride channel.

Potassium is neither appreciably reabsorbed nor secreted by the early distal convoluted tubular cells. Potassium that is reabsorbed downstream into the medullary collecting duct interstitium re-enters the tubular fluid by secretion into the thin descending limb in a process known as medullary potassium recycling. This decreased lumen-to-interstitial-fluid gradient facilitates high potassium excretion from the medullary collecting duct when required.

Luminal ammonium (NH_4^+) can substitute for potassium on the thick limb NKCC2; the resulting increase in medullary interstitial fluid NH_4^+ concentrations enhances medullary collecting duct net acid excretion. In hyperkalemic states, less NH_4^+ appears in the urine because the high concentration of luminal potassium competes with NH_4^+ for reabsorption in the thick limb. As a consequence, metabolic acidosis may develop in hyperkalemic states, and lowering of elevated plasma potassium levels helps treat acidosis.

In hypokalemia, whether through proximal tubule intracellular acidosis or other mechanisms, glutaminase enzymes are increased and more ammonia is produced. This ammonia leads to greater medullary interstitial fluid concentrations and therefore to enhanced net acid elimination. Ammonium production in hypokalemia allows potassium reabsorption to continue as cationic NH_4^+ accompanies excreted anions into the urine. The increase in ammonia production may have a deleterious effect in that it may contribute to the chronic tubulointerstitial nephritis of chronic hypokalemia.

By the time the tubular fluid reaches the distal tubule and collecting duct, more than 90% of filtered potassium and sodium has been reabsorbed. The absolute amount of sodium that needs to be reabsorbed far exceeds the amount of potassium that needs to be excreted. Therefore, the basolateral mechanism for potassium reabsorption is required to avoid potassium depletion. In potassium depletion, an increase in the apical membrane hydrogen-potassium ATPase (H^+, K^+-ATPase) of the collecting duct intercalated cell allows additional reabsorption of potassium from the urine. This process may sustain a metabolic alkalosis. It is unusual to see potassium concentrations in the urine lower than 5 to 10 mmol/L. In contrast, when dietary potassium is abundant, the reabsorption of 90% of filtered potassium by the proximal and distal nephron is followed by net potassium secretion in the collecting duct.

The secretion of potassium in the cortical collecting duct (E-Fig. 103-1), which may vary according to need by as much as 400%, is controlled by three major mechanisms: (1) apical membrane depolarization due to Na^+ current through epithelial Na^+ channels (ENaC) supporting K^+ secretion across the apical membrane; (2) regulated apical membrane secretory potassium channels; and (3) tubular fluid flow dependency. The urinary potassium most closely reflects potassium secreted by the distal nephron.

Early Sodium Reabsorption

The traditional view of regulating potassium secretion and therefore excretion has focused on the central role of aldosterone, the steroid hormone synthesized and secreted by the zona glomerulosa of the adrenal cortex. The renal effects of aldosterone show overlap of functions to conserve sodium and to eliminate potassium. Aldosterone is stimulated by angiotensin II in hyperreninemic states and independently by dietary potassium loading. In what has been called the *aldosterone paradox*, undesired losses of potassium are prevented when sodium retention (e.g., via the angiotensin II stimulus) is required to maintain extracellular volume. Conversely, undesired retention of sodium is prevented when potassium loading alone provides the stimulus to aldosterone secretion. The negative feedback that couples aldosterone with serum potassium is fundamental in potassium regulation. Hyperaldosteronism results in potassium loss, whereas hypokalemia reduces aldosterone production. Hyperkalemia stimulates aldosterone release, thereby facilitating urinary potassium.

The major site for potassium secretion resides in the aldosterone-sensitive distal nephron, which is composed primarily of the principal cells of the connecting tubule and the cortical collecting duct. Aldosterone regulates sodium reabsorption by the apical epithelial sodium channel. The reabsorption of sodium is dependent on the low intracellular sodium concentrations that result from the energy-requiring Na^+, K^+-ATPase on the basolateral membrane. Both increased intracellular Na^+ and extracellular K^+ stimulate the Na^+, K^+-ATPase.

To optimize potassium secretion, sodium must be delivered in ample amounts (depending on the flow rate and sodium concentration of the tubular fluid) to result in sodium reabsorption through the apical epithelial sodium channel in the cortical collecting duct cells. If sodium delivery is not limiting, reabsorption of the sodium cation creates a lumen-negative transepithelial potential difference. Aldosterone affects this transepithelial potential difference in several ways. The intracellular mineralocorticoid receptor functions to increase the activity and density of the epithelial sodium channel and of basolateral Na^+, K^+-ATPase enzymes. Cortisol, which is normally present in higher concentrations than aldosterone, has equal affinity for the aldosterone receptor and therefore could lead to increased epithelial sodium channel activity. However, the enzyme 11β-hydroxysteroid dehydrogenase type 2 is present in the principal cells and converts cortisol to inactive cortisone.

Role of Potassium Secretory Channels and Tubular Flow Rate

Potassium secretion requires adequate function of several types of potassium secretory channels on the luminal membranes of distal nephron cells. Two predominant potassium channels are present in the apical membranes of the collecting duct cells. The renal outer medullary potassium channel (ROMK), which is located on the apical membrane of the principal cell in the connecting tubule and cortical collecting duct, is aldosterone sensitive, is increased by dietary potassium loads, and likely subserves constitutive K^+ secretion under basal conditions. ROMK undergoes new synthesis and increased cycling to the apical membrane under the control of aldosterone. The principal cell also mediates vasopressin-responsive water reabsorption. Factors regulating ROMK channels include antidiuretic hormone (ADH) and intracellular pH. The increase in ROMK channel activity in response to ADH, combined with an ADH effect to increase epithelial sodium channel and osmotic water flow, allows the highest possible potassium concentration in the urine with the low tubular flow that accompanies antidiuresis. When ADH is suppressed, luminal potassium concentrations are lower, thereby favoring gradients for potassium secretion, but low ADH levels also suppress ROMK activity, thereby allowing independence of the regulation and the excretion of water and K^+. Cellular acidification inhibits potassium secretion through an effect on ROMK, thereby providing a renal mechanism for decreased electrogenic potassium secretion when proton secretion is necessary during metabolic and respiratory acidoses. In alkalosis, ROMK activity is increased, thereby favoring increased potassium secretion, but the result may be significant potassium loss.

Additional potassium channels, known as maxi-K or big-K channels, are prominent in the principal cells and intercalated cells of the cortical collecting duct, as the intercalated cell also has a role in potassium secretion. The big-K channels are highly regulated by tubular fluid flow rate. One mechanism by which flow rate influences this potassium secretory channel is by the deformation of the primary cilium of the principal cell, which leads to a secondary increase in cellular calcium that has both direct and indirect effects to enhance BK potassium secretion.

Excretion Mechanisms and Normal Function

Thiazide-sensitive NaCl cotransport is independent of aldosterone in the early distal convoluted tubule but is inhibited by sensors in those cells related to high potassium intake, gastrointestinal feed-forward sensing mechanisms, and clock genes associated with the circadian rhythm for potassium excretion. Decreased sodium reabsorption in the early distal convoluted tubule will increase delivery of sodium and water to the downstream aldosterone-sensitive distal nephron. Then, in response to increased plasma potassium-stimulated aldosterone release, the epithelial sodium channel is increased, thereby leading to greater potassium secretion. A network of protein kinases, including the "with no lysine" or WNK kinases, is central to regulated early distal convoluted tubule NaCl cotransporter function and the epithelial sodium channel. When the early aldosterone-insensitive distal convoluted tubule basolateral sensors detect a small drop in blood [K^+] during saline expansion, a regulatory "switch" provides crosstalk to the apical side in the form of phosphorylations, which activate NaCl cotransport and thereby increase the reabsorption of Na^+ in the distal convoluted tubule. The decreased delivery of Na^+ to the common collecting duct leads to less K^+ secretion. If the regulation of NaCl cotransport is incremental, the mechanism controlling NaCl reabsorption through the NaCl cotransporter and downstream K^+ secretion performs as a rheostat.

In states of avid sodium reabsorption, including hypovolemic states, hepatorenal syndrome (Chapter 139), and severe heart failure (Chapter 45), sodium delivery from more proximal sites may become the rate-limiting step for potassium secretion. In hypovolemia, sodium reabsorption is increased by angiotensin II in the proximal tubule, the early and late distal convoluted tubule, and the connecting tubule so that very little sodium is delivered to the principal cells of the cortical collecting duct. Potassium losses are diminished because of this decreased delivery of sodium, and an angiotensin II–induced switch involving WNK kinases decreases ROMK activity. Although aldosterone will still activate principal cell epithelial sodium channels, the decrease in sodium delivery and decreased potassium secretion (favoring chloride reabsorption instead) will allow greater NaCl reabsorption while limiting potassium loss. Sodium delivery may be increased by decreased angiotensin II during extracellular volume expansion, but the low aldosterone limits potassium losses.

Internal Potassium Balance and Associated Disorders

Because of the delay in hours before renal excretion matches dietary intake and because potassium first enters the extracellular fluid from the gastrointestinal tract, it is critical that the process of cellular buffering be effective (Table 103-1).[3] Essentially, increases in postprandial blood potassium are minimized before potassium is eliminated from the body. A major factor in this regulation after meals is the feedback loop involving insulin and potassium. An increase in serum potassium stimulates insulin release from the β-cells of the pancreatic islets. Insulin increases potassium uptake into cells, primarily muscle, independent of its effect on glucose uptake. Acutely, potassium uptake is chiefly the result of increased Na^+, K^+-ATPase activity, whereas chronically there is increased abundance in the plasma membranes in these cells.

Another important mechanism of regulating the distribution of potassium between extracellular and cellular spaces involves the sympathoadrenal system. β-Adrenergic activation, particularly through the $β_2$-receptor, increases potassium uptake into muscle and fat cells. As with insulin, potassium uptake is the consequence of increased Na^+, K^+-ATPase activity associated with increased intracellular cyclic adenosine monophosphate. The adrenergic effect is important in regulating the serum potassium concentration during exercise and is independent of the additional effect that catecholamines may have on blood glucose with the expected increases in insulin. In the trained athlete, a chronic increase in Na^+, K^+-ATPase on cell membranes may cause a transient lowering of the serum potassium concentration after exertion. By the same mechanism, a severe stress may contribute to hypokalemia, through both direct $β_2$ effects and insulin action secondary to the blood glucose rise.

Phenylephrine, an α-adrenergic agonist, increases serum potassium. Importantly, epinephrine, which also has α-adrenergic effects, is associated with a transient increase in potassium release from the liver before a more prolonged period of decreased serum potassium mediated by the $β_2$-receptor.

Metabolic acidosis raises the potassium level more than does respiratory acidosis; both metabolic alkalosis and respiratory alkalosis lower the potassium level. Anion gap acidosis does not raise the potassium level, probably because of the movement of the organic anion (e.g., lactate) from cells into the extracellular space with an accompanying proton. In contrast, the ingestion of chloride salts has the most profound effect on the potassium level because chloride concentration increases in the extracellular space. In hyperchloremic acidosis, chloride enters into cells through chloride-bicarbonate exchange and recycles back into the extracellular space in cotransport with potassium. The ingestion of excessive chloride salts of arginine and lysine is associated with hyperkalemic acidosis. ε-Aminocaproic acid has also been associated with hyperkalemia and is hypothesized to exchange for cellular potassium, much like the other cationic amino acids.

Just as a single blood pH measurement can reflect mixed acid-base disturbances, many processes that affect the net potassium concentration can coexist. Metabolic acidosis may be associated with diarrheal or urinary losses of potassium that are sufficient to result in hypokalemia. Metabolic acidosis in diabetes can also be associated with insulin deficiency and renal failure, and it can cause hyperkalemia despite osmotically driven urinary losses of potassium and total body potassium depletion.

Other hormonal effects on potassium include thyroid and growth hormone, but patients with disorders of these hormones do not usually have significant changes in their blood potassium levels. Some patients with hyperthyroidism may have mild hypokalemia, perhaps related to increased sympathetic activity. Growth states are associated with a greater need for potassium; for example, in normal pregnancy, the maternal potassium concentration may fall as the developing fetus grows.

Hypomagnesemia frequently accompanies hypokalemia. Both magnesium and potassium are found predominantly in cells, but the Na^+, K^+-ATPase requires magnesium to function. If magnesium is deficient, potassium distributes more to the extracellular fluid, thereby masking the degree of potassium deficiency. Moreover, magnesium deficiency leads to increased activity of renal potassium secretory channels, so potassium depletion is difficult to correct until magnesium is repleted.

TABLE 103-1 FACTORS REGULATING INTERNAL POTASSIUM BALANCE

Circadian rhythm
Insulin
β-Adrenergic activity
Acid-base balance
Magnesium
Aldosterone
Osmolality
Thyroid hormone
Extracellular potassium
Intracellular sodium

External Potassium Balance and Associated Disorders

Normally, no more than 10 to 20% of total potassium excretion is accomplished by the gastrointestinal tract, but colonic excretion is increased in renal failure, primarily through potassium-induced increases in epithelial Na^+, K^+-ATPase activity and aldosterone. In renal failure, the normal mechanisms to distribute potassium acquire increased importance.

Some conditions that cause the greatest losses of gastrointestinal potassium include secretory diarrheas of the colon, the result of infection or laxative abuse. Disorders of the small intestine, which may lead to large quantities of liquid stool with a low potassium concentration, engender favorable gradients for marked potassium secretion by the colon. A syndrome of watery diarrhea and hypokalemia is associated with neuroendocrine tumors (Chapter 213) that secrete vasoactive intestinal peptide. Rectosigmoid secretion of potassium may result in particularly high potassium losses, and potassium deficiency is seen in patients who have ureterosigmoidostomies. Potassium can be lost from a variety of other sources, including excess sweat or salivation.

Potassium can also be depleted by vomiting or diarrhea. In gastric alkalosis, the loss of potassium is in the urine. In renal tubular disorders, urinary losses may exceed intake when excessive quantities of osmotic or anionic products are excreted in the urine, or in patients who take diuretics.

Patients with pernicious anemia who receive vitamin B_{12} to stimulate erythropoiesis may deplete extracellular potassium and suffer from hypokalemia as a cost of producing new red blood cells. Leukemias with rapid growth rates (Chapter 168) also may cause a drop in the serum potassium level, and some forms of myelogenous leukemia are associated with a high level of lysozyme, which leads to urinary potassium loss.

It is unusual for hyperkalemia to be caused by excessive potassium intake unless the patient has renal dysfunction. However, in patients who have brisk hemolysis, internal hemorrhage, or rhabdomyolysis, particularly if the hemoglobinuria or myoglobinuria also results in acute kidney injury, life-threatening hyperkalemia can quickly develop by the rapid release of cellular potassium stores.

CLINICAL MANIFESTATIONS

Hypokalemia

Clinical manifestations of potassium depletion include hypertension, decreased growth, and muscle symptoms such as weakness, cramps, fasciculations, and even paralysis. In severe cases, the diaphragm may be paralyzed, leading to respiratory failure. Cardiac arrhythmias are a critical component of low potassium states and are usually seen when the serum potassium falls below 3 mmol/L or when ischemia, hypercalcemia, or drugs such as digoxin are simultaneously present. A patient who has a chronically low potassium level (e.g., from diuretic use) may be particularly vulnerable to supraventricular and ventricular tachyarrhythmias during periods of stress, such as head trauma, or during acute coronary syndrome,[4] to which cardiac ischemia also contributes. The prolonged cardiac repolarization phase of hypokalemia accounts for the characteristic electrocardiographic findings of broad, flattened T waves.

U waves are also indicative of this delay in repolarization (Fig. 103-1). In the intestine, hypokalemia may result in paralytic ileus, which may interfere with oral replacement.

In addition to these systemic effects of potassium imbalance, the kidney is particularly sensitive to depletion of potassium. Structural changes in the glomeruli and tubules lead to a decreased glomerular filtration rate, increased proximal tubule ammoniagenesis, increased sodium bicarbonate reabsorption, and net acid excretion, thereby causing and maintaining metabolic alkalosis. A condition of nephrogenic diabetes insipidus results when potassium depletion decreases expression of vasopressin-dependent water channels (aquaporin 2) in the collecting duct luminal plasma membranes. Hypokalemia diminishes insulin secretion and may be associated with glucose intolerance.

Hyperkalemia

Hyperkalemia can be a life-threatening emergency, especially if it develops rapidly. The depolarizing effect on the resting membrane potential and increased potassium channel conductance lead to the classic electrocardiographic changes of hyperacute peaked T waves associated with rapid repolarization (Fig. 103-2). Hyperkalemia commonly results in sinus bradycardia. Heart block, loss of P waves on the electrocardiogram, and prolonged QRS intervals are all seen in cases of severe hyperkalemia, usually in excess of 6 mmol/L. Although deep learning algorithms suggest that the electrocardiogram can be used to screen for hyperkalemia,[5] a standard reading of the electrocardiogram is not a sensitive indicator of severe hyperkalemia, and cardiac arrest may occur without clinical warning. Like hypokalemia, severe hyperkalemia can cause skeletal muscle paralysis; unlike hypokalemic paralysis, it is often ascending in nature.

DIAGNOSIS

The first clue to a disorder in potassium balance usually is an abnormal serum potassium concentration obtained as part of a laboratory evaluation, not because an abnormal potassium level itself is suspected. When the potassium concentration is elevated above normal, it is imperative to exclude common artifacts, known as pseudohyperkalemia. Hemolysis in the test tube is a common artifact; in cases of cold-induced hemolysis (Chapter 147), it is important to collect the blood and to allow it to clot in a warm environment. Some patients have pseudohyperkalemia resulting from high platelet counts, usually in excess of 1 million/μL, or myelogenous leukemia (Chapter 170); in such cases, potassium is released during clot formation in the test tube. Measurement of the plasma potassium level will avoid these artifacts. The serum potassium level may sometimes be elevated because of local ischemia related to application of the tourniquet and clenching of the fist.

A detailed medical history should focus on medications, family history, and sources of potassium excess or loss. The physical examination should pay particular attention to blood pressure, extracellular volume status, heart rate and rhythm, and muscle strength and reflexes.

Laboratory testing should include a complete blood count as well as serum levels of sodium, chloride, bicarbonate, creatinine, and blood urea nitrogen. In more serious cases, arterial blood gases and levels of creatine kinase and magnesium should be obtained. A 12-lead electrocardiogram also should be performed. A urinary potassium excretion rate in a timed urine test is the best measure of K+ excretion. In a hypokalemic patient, a urinary potassium concentration higher than 30 mEq/L suggests renal potassium wasting, whereas extrarenal losses are usually reflected by concentrations lower than 20 mEq/L. In a state of potassium excess, urinary potassium excretion should exceed about 35 mEq/L, unless urinary underexcretion was the cause of the hyperkalemia. A high aldosterone level causes a high urinary potassium-to-sodium ratio, whereas hypoaldosteronism may cause the opposite. Because water reabsorption complicates interpretation of the urinary K^+ concentration, distinguishing urinary loss or retention of K^+ in a hypokalemic or hyperkalemic state can

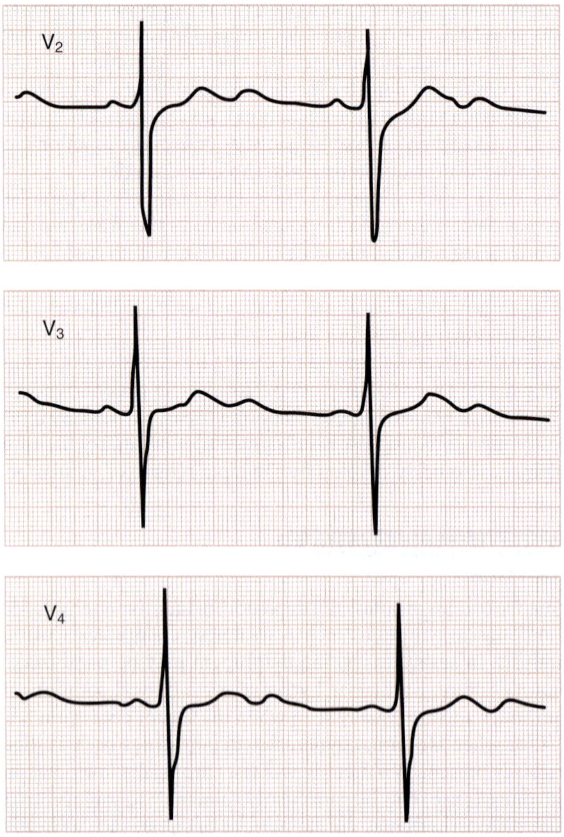

FIGURE 103-1. **The electrocardiographic manifestations of hypokalemia.** The serum potassium concentration was 2.2 mEq/L. The ST segment is prolonged, primarily because of a U wave following the T wave, and the T wave is flattened.

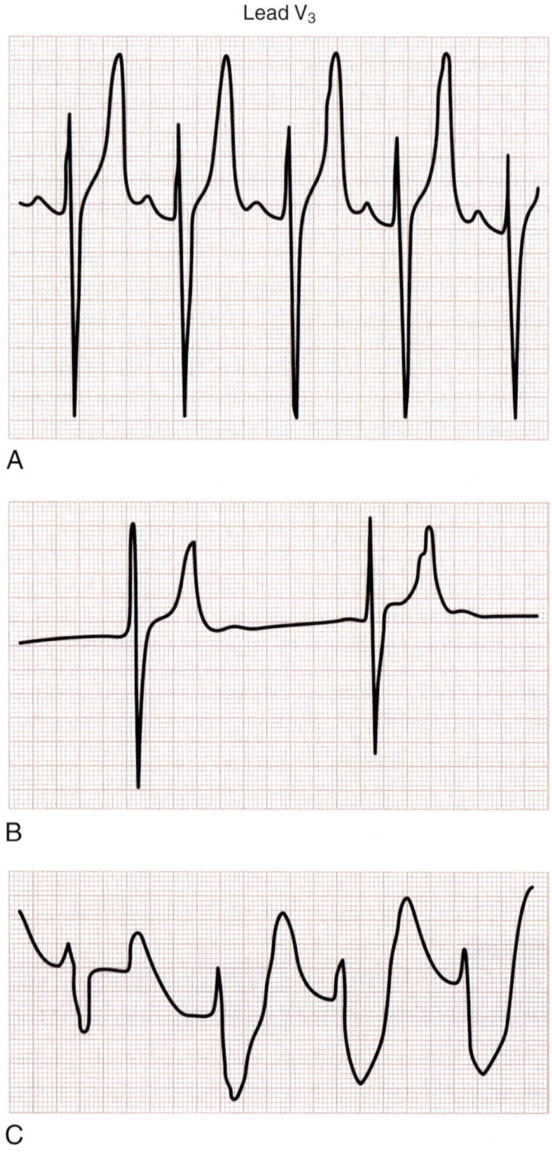

FIGURE 103-2. **The effects of progressive hyperkalemia on the electrocardiogram.** All of the illustrations are from lead V_3. **A,** Serum potassium concentration ($[K^+]$) = 6.8 mEq/L; note the peaked T waves together with normal sinus rhythm. **B,** Serum $[K^+]$ = 8.9 mEq/L; note the peaked T waves and absent P waves. **C,** Serum $[K^+]$ > 8.9 mEq/L; note the classic sine wave with absent P waves, marked prolongation of the QRS complex, and peaked T waves.

be made by measuring a urine $[K^+]:[Cr]$ ratio using 15 to 20 mEq per gram of creatinine as a cutoff.

Hypokalemic Disorders

The most common cause of hypokalemia (Table 103-2) in medical practice is the use of thiazide or loop diuretics.[6] Patients may have low, normal, or high blood pressures, depending on their volume status and whether the diuretics were prescribed for hypertension or heart failure. The most common acute causes of hypokalemia are diarrhea and vomiting (Fig. 103-3).

Hypokalemic Hypertensive Syndromes

Evaluation of plasma renin and aldosterone levels can help distinguish among specific diagnoses (see Table 103-2). Primary hyperaldosteronism is associated with low renin levels due to volume expansion.[7] If it is corrected for plasma potassium, an aldosterone-to-renin ratio of 30:1 suggests a primary adrenal cortical tumor (aldosteronoma) or hyperplasia (Chapter 208). However, such ratios must be used with caution, and the absolute value of aldosterone is important, especially when the renin and aldosterone levels are both low.

More sensitive measurements of renin have led to the increased recognition of primary hyperaldosteronism (Chapter 208), especially due to microadenomas or increased clusters of adrenal zona glomerulosa cells. At early stages, signs may be absent or manifest only by salt sensitivity and systemic hypertension, whereas more advanced stages typically are associated with a full blown syndrome of hypertension, metabolic alkalosis, hypomagnesemia, and hypokalemia.

The tubular delivery of large amounts of sodium chloride in a setting of volume expansion and nonsuppressible aldosterone results in hypokalemia, which improves after sodium restriction and worsens with the administration of intravenous saline. In congenital adrenal hyperplasia (Chapter 208), such as 11β-hydroxylase deficiency, hypokalemic alkalosis is associated with excessive androgen production. In patients with renin-secreting tumors or unilateral renal artery stenosis, high renin levels stimulate angiotensin II and then aldosterone secretion, with a resulting increase in sodium reabsorption, hypertension, and hypokalemic metabolic alkalosis.

In some patients with overproduction of ACTH, as in ectopic production from lung and other malignant neoplasms (Chapter 164), cortisol may overwhelm the aldosterone receptor and result in hypertensive, hypokalemic alkalosis. The patient may not show signs of Cushing syndrome in the short term. In glucocorticoid-remediable aldosteronism, which is a familial disorder in which episodes of hypokalemia and hypertension develop, a chimeric gene duplication couples the ACTH-responsive 11β-hydroxylase promoter to the coding region of aldosterone synthase.

Glycyrrhizic acid, which is found in licorice and anisette, inhibits the renal enzyme 11β-hydroxysteroid dehydrogenase and thereby causes hypokalemia, metabolic alkalosis, and hypertension. A rare genetic disorder known as apparent mineralocorticoid excess syndrome produces the same effect due to deficiency of 11β-hydroxysteroid dehydrogenase. The syndrome produces a high ratio of cortisol to cortisone; as a result, renin and aldosterone are suppressed by the volume expansion. Hypokalemia may be precipitated by ACTH stimulation of cortisol.

Activating mutations of ENaC cause increased sodium reabsorption (Liddle syndrome; Chapter 113). The syndrome can be distinguished from primary or secondary hyperaldosteronism by suppressed renin and aldosterone levels (see also Fig. 103-3 for an approach to the patient with hypokalemia and metabolic alkalosis).

Hypokalemic Hypotensive Syndromes

In contrast to the hypokalemic hypertensive syndromes, in which increased sodium reabsorption is a primary event, many hypokalemic alkaloses are associated with extracellular volume depletion. With a physiologic response to volume depletion, the potassium losses may be a result of appropriate sodium reabsorption; signs of hypotension or extracellular volume depletion will be observed. Secretory diarrheas, whether associated with hypochloremic alkalosis or hyperchloremic acidosis, lead to extracellular volume depletion and secondary increases in renin and aldosterone; the result is both gastrointestinal and urinary potassium losses. The urinary losses in alkalosis (e.g., vomiting or other chloride-wasting syndromes) result in greater degrees of potassium depletion because of the early bicarbonaturia and volume contraction.

Diuretic use, Bartter syndrome (Chapter 113), and Gitelman syndrome (Chapter 113) are renal tubular causes of extracellular volume depletion, hypotension, and hypokalemic, hypochloremic alkalosis; sodium and chloride are lost in the urine, and secondary rises in renin and aldosterone occur. Increased urinary flow rates are important contributors to the increased potassium losses in each of these examples. Bartter syndrome affects the function of the thick ascending limb through mutations in NKCC2 or in potassium or chloride channels, whereas Gitelman syndrome is characterized by inactivating mutations or dysregulation of the NaCl cotransporter in the distal tubule. The hypokalemia in Gitelman syndrome may be caused by secondary hyperaldosteronism, bicarbonaturia, and hypomagnesemia.

Classic type 1 distal renal tubular acidosis (Chapters 104 and 113) is often associated with hypokalemia, which may improve with correction of the acidemia. In contrast, proximal renal tubular acidosis, when it is corrected with bicarbonate, often results in worsening of the hypokalemia because of greater bicarbonate wasting associated with increases in the filtered bicarbonate load.

Acetazolamide, when it is given to an alkalotic patient, is a particularly potent kaliuretic agent. Volume depletion and hyperaldosteronism contribute to the potassium losses, as does the bicarbonate wasting, which appears to have a direct effect on potassium secretion.

Tubular toxins that may be associated with severe potassium losses include aminoglycosides, cisplatin, and ifosfamide. Amphotericin B results in significant potassium wasting accompanied by renal tubular acidosis. In many of these

TABLE 103-2 CAUSES OF HYPOKALEMIA AND INCREASED POTASSIUM EXCRETION

CAUSES OF INCREASED K^+ EXCRETION AND HYPOKALEMIA	RENIN	ALDOSTERONE	EXTRACELLULAR VOLUME OR BLOOD PRESSURE	ACID-BASE STATUS
Increased ENaC: Liddle syndrome	Low	Low	High	Alkalosis
Decreased β-hydroxysteroid dehydrogenase: apparent mineralocorticoid excess, licorice	Low	Low	High	Alkalosis
Adrenal tumor or hyperplasia	Low	High	High	Alkalosis
Ectopic ACTH: Cushing syndrome	Low	Low	High	Alkalosis
Congenital adrenal hyperplasia	Low	High	High	Alkalosis
Unilateral renal artery stenosis	High	High	High	Alkalosis
Renin-secreting tumor	High	High	High	Alkalosis
Diuretics				
Thiazides	High	High	Low	Alkalosis
Furosemide	High	High	Low	Alkalosis
Acetazolamide	High	High	Variable	Acidosis
Bartter syndrome	High	High	Low	Alkalosis
Gitelman syndrome	High	High	Low	Alkalosis
Fanconi syndrome	High	High	Low	Acidosis
Distal RTA	High	High	Low	Acidosis

ACTH = adrenocorticotropic hormone; ENaC = epithelial Na^+ channel; RTA = renal tubular acidosis.

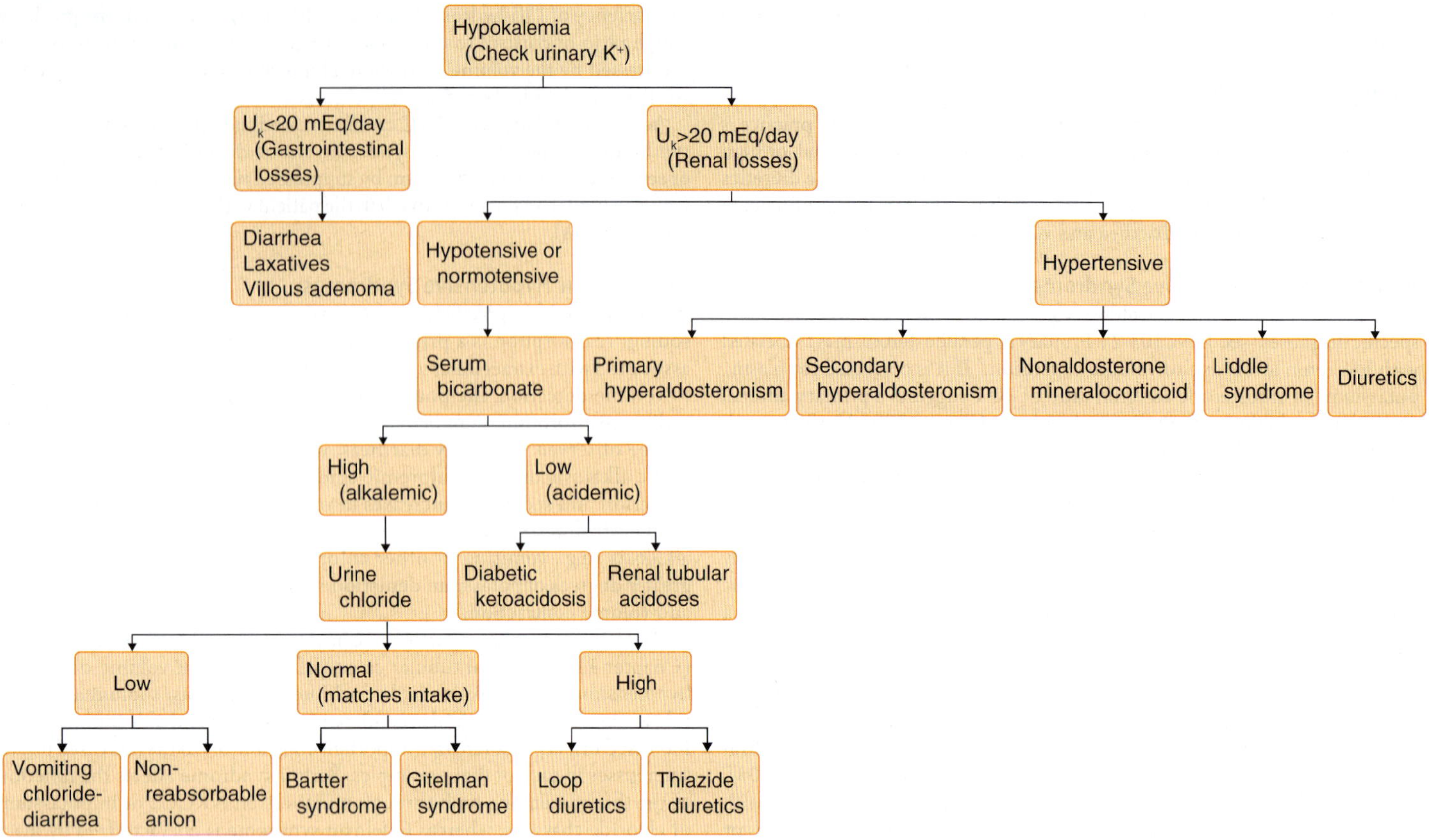

FIGURE 103-3. Causes of hypokalemia.

TABLE 103-3 CAUSES OF HYPERKALEMIA AND DECREASED POTASSIUM EXCRETION

CAUSE OF DECREASED K+ EXCRETION AND HYPERKALEMIA	RENIN	ALDOSTERONE	EXTRACELLULAR VOLUME OR BLOOD PRESSURE	ACID-BASE STATUS
Decreased ENaC Drugs: amiloride, triamterene, trimethoprim, lithium Pseudohypoaldosteronism type 1 autosomal recessive ENaC mutation	High	High	Low or normal	Normal or acidosis
Pseudohypoaldosteronism type 1 autosomal dominant MR mutation	High	High	Low	Acidosis
MR blockade: spironolactone, eplerenone, progesterone	High	High	Low	Acidosis
Hypoaldosteronism: adrenal insufficiency	High	Low	Low	Acidosis
Hyporenin-hypoaldosteronism: NSAIDs, β-blockers, autonomic neuropathy	Low	Low	Low	Acidosis
Pseudohypoaldosteronism type 2	Low	Low	High	Acidosis

ENaC = epithelial Na^+ channel; MR = mineralocorticoid receptor; NSAIDs = nonsteroidal anti-inflammatory drugs.

conditions, simultaneous use of amiloride may diminish potassium losses by as much as 50%.

Patients who present with unexplained hypokalemia and alkalosis with volume depletion should have urinary electrolytes measured to determine whether the urine chloride is low, as with vomiting or laxative abuse. If the urine contains chloride, a diuretic screen should be considered; Gitelman syndrome and Bartter syndrome are other possibilities.

Hyperkalemic Disorders

In clinical practice, acute hyperkalemia is seen most commonly with renal failure (Chapter 117), acidosis (Chapter 104), and acute muscle damage from rhabdomyolysis (Chapter 99) (Table 103-3). Chronic hyperkalemia is most commonly seen with medications that reduce potassium secretion and with renal tubular disorders.[8]

Hyperkalemic Hypotensive or Normotensive Syndromes

When classic type IV renal tubular acidoses (Chapter 104) are due to hypomineralocorticoidism or adrenal insufficiency, the urine will be able to acidify due to a defect in ammonium production. By comparison, type IV renal tubular acidoses that are associated with an inability to excrete sufficient acid in the urine are caused by diseases that disrupt distal nephron function, including systemic lupus erythematosus (Chapter 245), urinary tract obstruction, amyloidosis (Chapter 174), the nephropathy associated with kidney and bone marrow transplantation (Chapters 117 and 163), and sickle cell nephropathy (Chapter 149). Men who present with hyperkalemia and renal insufficiency of unknown cause should be evaluated for possible prostatic obstruction (Chapter 114). Each of these conditions also may be associated with failure to concentrate the urine (nephrogenic diabetes insipidus) or with a hyperchloremic metabolic acidosis caused by abnormalities in acid secretion.

Primary selective hypoaldosteronism or complete adrenal cortical deficiency (Chapter 209) is associated with elevated renin and low aldosterone. Secondary hypoaldosteronism may be seen in hyporenin states caused by β-blockers, renin antagonists, or nonsteroidal anti-inflammatory drugs (NSAIDs). Angiotensin-converting enzyme inhibitors and angiotensin receptor blockers increase renin and decrease aldosterone. Heparin, including low-molecular-weight and fractionated forms (Chapter 70), can lead to hyperkalemia even in small subcutaneous doses.

Disorders that affect the transepithelial potential difference and can result in hyperkalemia, acidosis, and extracellular volume depletion include inactivating mutations of ENaC (autosomal recessive pseudohypoaldosteronism type 1), which may be accompanied by high renin and aldosterone levels. The ENaC may also be inhibited by the potassium-sparing diuretics (i.e., amiloride and triamterene) and certain medications secreted by the proximal tubule organic cation transporters, such as trimethoprim and pentamidine, as well as by lithium. Inhibition of the aldosterone receptor may be the result of antagonists such as spironolactone and eplerenone.

Hyperkalemic Hypertensive Syndromes

NSAIDs can cause hyperkalemia, particularly in patients with renal disease, by decreasing sodium delivery, increasing water reabsorption, and decreasing renin and aldosterone. Hypertension with the NSAIDs is most likely caused by renal salt and water retention.

Cyclosporine or tacrolimus may produce a hyperkalemic acidosis. The mechanism may involve inhibition of cyclooxygenase-2 and therefore hyporeninhypoaldosteronism. There may also be a decrease in apical potassium secretion in the collecting duct. Familial hyperkalemic hypertension is a genetic disorder (pseudohypoaldosteronism type 2) associated with hyperkalemia, volume expansion, and metabolic acidosis. It is caused by activation of the thiazide-sensitive distal convoluted tubule NaCl cotransporter related to a dysfunction of the WNK kinase regulatory role.

TREATMENT

It may be difficult to determine the exact state of total body potassium stores from the serum potassium level because as much as 100 to 300 mmol of potassium may be lost from the body with a fall in serum potassium of only 1 mmol/L. As a result, therapy must be guided by careful assessment of the patient as well as the serum potassium level.[9,10]

Hypokalemia

The goal of acute therapy for hypokalemia is to prevent or to manage potentially life-threatening arrhythmias or paralysis. Patients at greatest risk are the elderly, patients with known liver disease or cardiac disturbances, and patients who have had an abrupt fall in serum potassium concentration to less than 2.5 mEq/L. Potassium must traverse the extracellular space before repleting intracellular stores, so it is dangerously easy to replete potassium too quickly. Oral potassium should be given, if possible. If the potassium level is greater than 3 mEq/L, an increase in dietary potassium can be considered, along with removal of the underlying cause of hypokalemia. Usual oral replacement is with potassium chloride at a dose of 40 to 100 mmol/day. The chloride salt has the advantage of treating concomitant metabolic alkalosis, but other available forms include potassium citrate (in the acidotic patient) and potassium phosphate (in patients with a phosphate deficit). Giving potassium with a non-reabsorbable anion, such as gluconate, may not replace the potassium deficit adequately. Intravenous potassium is reserved for patients who are unable to take enteral potassium and patients with symptomatic hypokalemia, paralysis, or cardiac arrhythmias. It is usually given as a solution of 20 to 40 mmol of potassium in 1 L of solution at a rate that does not exceed 10 to 20 mmol/hour. If the potassium level is less than 3 mmol/L or if more than 10 mmol/hour is to be delivered, the patient should be in a monitored setting to observe for cardiac complications. A central venous catheter may be required for these higher concentrations, and it is best to consult with a renal specialist and the pharmacy.

In patients who have prerenal azotemia associated with hyperglycemia or severe metabolic alkalosis, volume expansion with sodium chloride solutions alone can result in life-threatening potassium losses, despite improvement in the extracellular volume. Potassium must be given in anticipation of such events.

In a hypokalemic patient, care must be exercised when glucose-containing solutions are given because the resulting increase in insulin may further decrease the blood potassium level. Attention to the urine output and ongoing losses is crucial. If ongoing losses of potassium are severe, it may be necessary to provide a potassium-sparing diuretic (e.g., amiloride 5 to 10 mg orally) and to treat the cause of the ongoing losses (e.g., diarrhea). Magnesium causes further urinary excretion of potassium and should be repleted, if necessary (Chapter 105).

In the inpatient setting, hypokalemia is a common complication of intravenous fluid administration. In patients with normal renal function, a maintenance dose of intravenous potassium can avoid hypokalemia. In the outpatient setting, hypokalemia is a common side effect of diuretic therapy. Serum potassium should be maintained within the normal range (>3.5 mEq/L), especially in high-risk patients. Addition of 40 to 100 mmol of potassium per day as chloride salt is the usual treatment, depending on the patient's response.

Hyperkalemia

Emergent Treatment

If hyperkalemia is severe, concentration must be reduced rapidly by therapies that stabilize cardiac membranes (intravenous calcium) and shift potassium intracellularly (insulin, bicarbonate), while simultaneously instituting treatments that achieve net potassium loss (diuretics, potassium binders or hemodialysis).[11]

Cardiac Arrhythmias

If hyperkalemia is associated with cardiac arrhythmias, treatment in a monitored setting is warranted before the serum potassium level can be expected to decline, even with aggressive therapy. Calcium gluconate, 10 mL of a 10% solution (8.9 mg calcium) over 10 to 20 minutes, is often indicated to stabilize electrical effects on cardiac excitation. Calcium chloride (3 to 4 mL of a 10% solution) is an alternative, but it should be administered through a central access line because extravasation of the chloride salt may result in tissue necrosis. Gastrointestinal losses of potassium can also be achieved by use of potassium-binding drugs.

Lowering the Potassium Level

The administration of calcium does not lower the potassium concentration. Rapid-acting options to lower the potassium level acutely include an inhaled β_2-agonist or the intravenous combination of insulin plus glucose.

β_2-agonists are usually preferred because epinephrine can initially increase the release of K^+ from the liver. Albuterol by nebulizer (10 to 20 mg in 4 mL of saline during 10 minutes) can redistribute potassium acutely but should not be the sole treatment because some patients are not responsive. In some cases, intravenous β-adrenergic agonists (e.g., albuterol, 0.5 mg in 100 mL of 5% dextrose during 15 minutes) have been used to lower the serum potassium level by about 1 mmol/L within minutes to hours.

If insulin plus glucose is chosen, alternatives include 100 mL of 50% glucose alone or in combination with 10 units of regular insulin; the combination will, on average, provide a significantly greater reduction in the serum potassium level (0.8 mmol/L vs. 0.5 mmol/L) at 60 minutes, but about 20% of insulin-treated patients will develop hypoglycemia. Alternatively, 5 units of regular insulin can be given with 10% glucose solution during 1 hour for a total of 30 to 50 g in the normoglycemic patient. The blood glucose level should be monitored because an abrupt increase in plasma osmolality with glucose may worsen hyperkalemia if it causes potassium to leak from cells with osmotic water flow.

Sodium zirconium cyclosilicate (1.25 to 10 g three times a day), an oral crystalline agent with high binding affinity for potassium within the gastrointestinal tract, can reduce the serum potassium concentration within 1 hour, particularly in patients with heart failure.[A1] This potassium binder has been shown to be effective as an adjunct to glucose and insulin therapy.

Sodium bicarbonate, as an isotonic mixture calculated to correct acid-base status, should be reserved for acidemic patients who otherwise require alkalinization, while being careful to avoid hypocalcemia. Complications of sodium bicarbonate infusions include hypernatremia, volume expansion, and decreased ionized calcium, potentially resulting in tetany. Diabetic patients may be potassium depleted even though they present with hyperkalemia; as they are volume repleted, they typically require potassium replacement (Chapter 210).

If hyperkalemia occurs in the setting of volume contraction and oliguria, extracellular volume expansion with saline to achieve a rise in urine output may be adequate. If a patient is hyperkalemic and volume-expanded and not in renal failure, potassium-losing diuretics (e.g., furosemide 10 to 40 mg intravenously) may be effective.

The hyperkalemia of familial hyperkalemic hypertension is highly responsive to thiazide diuretics. In patients who have advanced or end-stage kidney failure, particularly in a volume-expanded hyperkalemic patient, hemodialysis (Chapter 117) will be required to remove potassium effectively from the body. However, patients who are dialyzed against zero K^+ dialysate may become rapidly hypokalemic.

Chronic Treatment

During the longer term, potassium loss may be sustained by use of cation exchange resins and a low-potassium diet.[12] Patiromer (4.2 to 8.4 g twice daily),[A2] a nonabsorbed calcium-potassium exchange resin that works in the colon, can decrease potassium levels for at least a year. It has been used successfully in patients with diabetic renal disease[A3] and in patients receiving potassium-retaining antihypertensive agents.[A4] Its major side effect is constipation, but hypomagnesemia, diarrhea, nausea, abdominal discomfort, and flatulence can also occur. To avoid potential interaction, no other orally administered medication should be taken at least 3 hours before or after patiromer. Zirconium cyclosilicate at 1.25 to 10 g three times daily[A5,A6] is also effective in managing hypokalemia. Sodium polystyrene sulfonate given orally or as an enema (Chapter 116) at a dose of 30 to 50 g can reduce potassium levels over several hours, but its use is limited by its many adverse effects, so it is now rarely used.

If the patient is volume expanded, furosemide (40 to 100 mg), chlorothiazide (500 mg), or, if the patient is also alkalotic, acetazolamide (250 to 500 mg) may enhance renal potassium clearance. If the patient is volume depleted, isotonic saline expansion may improve urine output and, with it, potassium excretion.

SPECIFIC CLINICAL SYNDROMES

Hypokalemic Periodic Paralysis

Familial hypokalemic periodic paralysis is an autosomal dominant disorder usually caused by mutations in certain voltage-gated skeletal muscle sodium channels or L-type calcium channels. Characteristically, periodic attacks of severe hypokalemia are precipitated by stimuli that usually induce mild hypokalemia by distributing potassium into cells. Precipitating factors include the increase in insulin levels after the ingestion of carbohydrates or postexercise, when the plasma potassium level falls because of ATPase reuptake of potassium. In affected individuals, these stimuli cause progressive and severe hypokalemia, enough to result in muscle paralysis due to hyperpolarization of the sarcolemma. The cause of the syndrome is an imbalance between outwardly directed K^+ current and inwardly directed cation leaks of Na^+ and Ca^{2+}. In the familial mutations, the cation depolarizing influx, normally very small under hyperpolarizing conditions, is instead increased and, when balanced with the outward K^+ current, results in a paradoxical depolarization. In turn, the depolarization inactivates the sodium channel needed for the rapid action potential, so the muscle cell is unexcitable. In nonfamilial hypokalemic periodic paralysis, a loss in function of outwardly directed potassium channels (Kir) accounts for paradoxical depolarization, inactivation of sodium channels, and decreased excitability.

The clinical presentation of hypokalemic periodic paralysis is usually in the teenage years or early adulthood.[13] In some familial cases, a progressive proximal myopathy (Chapter 389) may develop. Asian patients, usually males with hyperthyroidism (Chapter 207), have a decrease-in-function mutation of an outwardly directed potassium channel that causes them to develop episodic paralysis in response to high-carbohydrate meals or resting after exercise. In Anderson syndrome, which is another form of hypokalemic periodic paralysis, cardiac potassium channels are also affected, and serious cardiac arrhythmias may result.

TREATMENT

Hypokalemic periodic paralysis is treated by a high-potassium diet and cautious use of carbonic anhydrase inhibitors such as acetazolamide (125 to 500 mg/day) and dichlorphenamide (50 to 200 mg/day), which can significantly reduce the frequency of attacks. These medications work in part by creating a hyperchloremic acidosis that offsets the urinary potassium wasting they cause. β_2-Blockers (e.g., propranolol 20 to 40 mg twice daily) also may be used.

Insulin Deficiency

The abnormal distribution of potassium between cells and the extracellular space results in the hyperkalemia that is associated with acidosis, insulin-deficient states, and β_2-adrenergic blockade. Although it is not always possible, it is best to know the levels of serum glucose and potassium in an unconscious diabetic patient before infusing concentrated glucose solutions because of the risk of aggravating hyperkalemia.

Hyperkalemic Periodic Paralysis

Familial hyperkalemic periodic paralysis is a myopathy caused by a genetic defect in voltage-gated sodium channels in skeletal muscle. Exercise or dietary increases in plasma potassium result in mild depolarization of skeletal muscle that then unmasks the sodium channel defect, rendering the cells unexcitable. Treatment is frequent meals and acetazolamide (125 to 500 mg).

Digitalis Overdose

Potassium competes with digoxin-binding sites on the Na^+, K^+-ATPase, so that if hypokalemia coexists, digoxin will have an intensified effect and may lead to drug toxicity. In extreme cases of digitalis overdose (Chapter 96), severe hyperkalemia develops as a result of generalized blockade of Na^+, K^+-ATPase.

PROGNOSIS

The prognosis of patients with hypokalemia and hyperkalemia depends on the severity and underlying illness. Hypokalemia is associated with increased mortality, especially in patients with heart disease,[14] and hyperkalemic patients on renal dialysis have a higher cardiovascular mortality. Hypertensive patients with potassium levels either above or below the range of 4.1 to 4.7 mEq/L also appear to have an increased mortality,[15] but modest hyperkalemia (≤5.5 mEq/L) does not appear to have adverse effects on treated patients with heart failure.[16] Most hypokalemic cases are mild (potassium concentration 3 to 3.5 mEq/L). However, mortality of hospitalized patients with hypokalemia is increased 10-fold. Hyperkalemia is reported in 1 to 10% of hospitalized patients, of whom 10% have severe hyperkalemia (potassium concentration > 6.0 mEq/L). Hyperkalemia is associated with increased mortality (14 to 41%), and it accounts for 2 to 5% of deaths in patients with end-stage renal disease. Patients with electrocardiographic abnormalities are at highest risk, especially in the acute period before the serum potassium level is successfully reduced.

GENERAL REFERENCES

For the General References and other additional features, please visit Elsevier eBooks+ at https://ebooks.health.elsevier.com.

Grade A References

A1. Packham DK, Rasmussen HS, Lavin PT, et al. Sodium zirconium cyclosilicate in hyperkalemia. *N Engl J Med.* 2015;372:222-231.

A2. Meaney CJ, Beccari MV, Yang Y, et al. Systematic review and meta-analysis of patiromer and sodium zirconium cyclosilicate: a new armamentarium for the treatment of hyperkalemia. *Pharmacotherapy.* 2017;37:401-411.

A3. Bakris GL, Pitt B, Weir MR, et al. Effect of patiromer on serum potassium level in patients with hyperkalemia and diabetic kidney disease: the AMETHYST-DN randomized clinical trial. *JAMA.* 2015;314:151-161.

A4. Weir MR, Bakris GL, Bushinsky DA, et al. Patiromer in patients with kidney disease and hyperkalemia receiving RAAS inhibitors. *N Engl J Med.* 2015;372:211-221.

A5. Zhang Y, Xu R, Wang F, et al. Effects and safety of a novel oral potassium-lowering drug-sodium zirconium cyclosilicate for the treatment of hyperkalemia: a systematic review and meta-analysis. *Cardiovasc Drugs Ther.* 2021;35:1057-1066.

A6. Spinowitz BS, Fishbane S, Pergola PE, et al. Sodium zirconium cyclosilicate among individuals with hyperkalemia: a 12-month phase 3 study. *Clin J Am Soc Nephrol.* 2019;14:798-809.

104 ACID-BASE DISORDERS

JULIAN LAWRENCE SEIFTER

DEFINITION

The ability to regulate the H^+ ion concentration, or pH (defined as the negative logarithm of the hydrogen ion concentration), is essential to normal body function. Acid-base balance is assessed by measurements of arterial or venous blood. If arterial pH is below 7.35, *acidemia* is said to exist. If pH is above 7.45, *alkalemia* exists. However, several processes may simultaneously drive the pH upward or downward; these individual processes are known as alkaloses or acidoses, respectively. Because simultaneous alkalosis and acidosis of equal magnitude can coexist, an abnormal pH is not always noted in acid-base disturbances. Also, because pH is a function of the ratio of the blood bicarbonate concentration ($[HCO_3^-]$) to the partial pressure of carbon dioxide (Pco_2), the finding of an abnormal bicarbonate level alone cannot define acidemia or alkalemia.

EPIDEMIOLOGY

An acid-base disturbance should alert the clinician to the possible presence of an important underlying condition. Anion gap acidoses represent serious underlying metabolic disorders, ranging from sepsis (Chapter 94) to uremia (Chapter 116) to diabetic ketoacidosis (Chapter 210) to serious poisonings (Chapter 96). Specific renal abnormalities as well as diarrhea (Chapter 126) can cause hyperchloremic acidosis (Table 104-1). Metabolic alkaloses are commonly caused by diuretics or renal tubular abnormalities or the loss of acid from the stomach due to vomiting or nasogastric suction (Table 104-2). Respiratory acidosis and alkalosis are related to disturbances in ventilation, which is increased by conditions such as sepsis (Chapter 94) and anxiety, and is decreased in many pulmonary conditions and with depression of the central nervous system (CNS) (Chapters 71 and 89).

PATHOBIOLOGY

Growth, cell division, fertilization, and protein and glucose metabolism are examples of pH-sensitive intracellular processes. Acids are generated within cells during metabolism, and each cell must maintain a pH appropriate for its function. For example, cardiac contractility (Chapter 41) is reduced when cardiac myocytes are too acidic. Bone and muscle develop and grow poorly in an acidic environment. Intracellular pH may be lower than extracellular pH because cells are electronegative with respect to extracellular fluid, but they are not as acidic as they would be if H^+ reached electrochemical equilibrium with the extracellular fluid, which means that all cells utilize energy to extrude acid actively. Cells are capable of buffering an acid load, and intracellular vacuoles may use hydrogen adenosine triphosphatases (H^+-ATPases) to sequester excess acid before transport from the cell. The transport processes located on the plasma membranes can protect cells from both acid and alkaline loads. The specific mechanisms may differ from one cell type to another, but they are similar to those used by the excretory organs that finally eliminate the net acid produced by the body into the external world.[1,2]

In severe disease states, arterial pH may fall as low as 6.8 and rise as high as 7.7. Strenuous exercise with the metabolic production of lactic acid may transiently but severely lower pH, even in normal healthy individuals.

TABLE 104-1 EXAMPLES OF HYPERCHLOREMIC ACIDOSIS

TYPE	CAUSE
Renal with hypokalemia	Proximal RTA, type 2 Distal RTA, type 1 Some anion gap acidoses with high anion clearance
Renal with hyperkalemia	Type 4 RTA Hyporenin-hypoaldosteronism
Nonrenal with hypokalemia	Diarrhea Urinary diversions: ureteroileostomy, ureterosigmoidostomy
Nonrenal with hyperkalemia	NaCl, KCl, NH_4Cl, $CaCl_2$, Arg-HCl, Lys-HCl

RTA = renal tubular acidosis.

TABLE 104-2 EXAMPLES OF METABOLIC ALKALOSIS

TYPE	CAUSES
Renal, hypochloremic alkalosis with hypokalemia: chloride responsive with urine chloride concentration >20 mEq/L	Loop and distal tubule diuretics Bartter syndrome Gitelman syndrome Post-hypercapnic status
Nonrenal, hypochloremic alkalosis: chloride responsive with urine chloride concentration <20 mEq/L	Vomiting, nasogastric suction Congenital chloridorrhea Villous adenoma
Renal, alkalosis with extracellular expansion and hypokalemia: chloride unresponsive with urine chloride concentration >20 mEq/L	Hyperaldosteronism, primary and secondary to unilateral renal artery stenosis Liddle syndrome
Nonrenal alkalosis, chloride unresponsive	$NaHCO_3$, acetate, citrate, lactate. Minimal alkalosis will develop unless accompanied by a process such as hypokalemia or hypovolemia
Renal hypokalemic alkalosis	Excessive excretion of non-reabsorbable anions due to excretion of H^+ and K^+
Nonrenal alkalosis with decreased anion gap	Hypoalbuminemia

At a normal arterial blood pH, the hydrogen ion concentration is in the range of 40 nanoequivalents (nEq) per liter, a very small concentration in comparison to a normal plasma sodium concentration of 140 mEq/L. The hydrogen ion concentration of body fluids is in equilibrium with each of multiple weak acids or buffers, such as proteins and phosphate (the isohydric principle), but acid-base equilibria in the body are often described and analyzed by use of the CO_2/HCO_3^- system and the relationship of the proton concentration (thus pH) to the ratio of HCO_3^- to CO_2. The CO_2/HCO_3^- system is quantitatively the largest buffer system in the body, and it is the system whose parameters are most often measured clinically. The Henderson-Hasselbalch equation is a logarithmic expression of the relationship.

$$CO_2 + H_2O \leftrightarrow H_2CO_3 \leftrightarrow H^+ + HCO_3^-$$
$$pH = pK + \log[HCO_3]/0.03(P_{CO_2})$$

In this equation, p*K*, or the negative log of the dissociation constant for the reaction, is 6.1; 0.03 (mM/mm Hg) is the solubility factor for CO_2 in solution. The product of $0.03 \times P_{CO_2}$ represents dissolved CO_2; the "total CO_2" in plasma is the sum of HCO_3^-, normally about 25 mM, and $0.03 \times P_{CO_2}$, normally about 1.2 mM in arterial blood. It is important to emphasize that pH is a function of the *ratio* of HCO_3^- to P_{CO_2}. The HCO_3^- concentration in the numerator is regulated by the kidney, and P_{CO_2} is regulated by the lung.

Production of Carbonic Acid and the Elimination of Carbon Dioxide by the Lung

Volatile acid is the term used for the approximately 20,000 mmol/day of CO_2 produced, with an equimolar amount of water, by tissue respiration. This CO_2 is carried from tissues to the lung, where it is eliminated by alveolar ventilation. Steady-state arterial P_{CO_2} is normally 38 to 42 mm Hg.

Oxidation of carbohydrates, fat, and the carbon skeleton of amino acids results in the production of water and CO_2. To maintain a steady state, any acid (or base) produced per day must be equivalent to what is eliminated. If tissue CO_2 production exceeds CO_2 elimination by the lungs, respiratory acidosis characterized by a high P_{CO_2} will develop. If the rate of CO_2 eliminated exceeds production, respiratory alkalosis develops. The inverse relationship between alveolar ventilation (the clearance of CO_2) and P_{CO_2} is demonstrated as

$$\text{alveolar ventilation} \approx CO_2 \text{ elimination rate} \div P_{CO_2}$$

The circulation plays a critical role in transporting tissue CO_2 to the lungs. The process depends not only on cellular respiration but also on tissue capillary flow as well as diffusion of CO_2 into the blood and across red blood cell membranes, where it may react with hemoglobin and proteins to form carbamino compounds or combine with water for conversion to H^+ and HCO_3^- in a reaction catalyzed by carbonic anhydrase. The intracellular H^+ can combine with hemoglobin (the Bohr effect) and the HCO_3^- exchanged with plasma Cl^- through red cell anion exchangers. Most tissue CO_2 is brought to the lung as venous plasma HCO_3^-. Compared with arterial blood, venous blood has the characteristics of a respiratory acidosis. Venous pH is normally approximately 0.05 pH units more acid than arterial pH, its P_{CO_2} is 5 to 6 mm Hg higher than that of arterial blood, and its bicarbonate concentrations are normally greater than arterial concentrations.

In disease, changes in P_{CO_2} are most often caused by changes in alveolar ventilation rather than by production of CO_2. Thus, respiratory acidosis is a consequence of decreased pulmonary ventilation because of lung, skeletal muscle, or CNS disease. However, if alveolar ventilation is compromised, increased production of CO_2 will worsen CO_2 retention. Similarly, respiratory alkalosis develops because of hyperventilation rather than decreased CO_2 production. In either case, when the elimination rate of CO_2 (alveolar ventilation $\times P_{CO_2}$) again equals CO_2 production, a new steady-state P_{CO_2} will prevail, with no net retention or loss of carbonic acid.

Production of Acids and Excretion by the Kidney

Nonvolatile or fixed acid describes noncarbonic acids that are formed primarily from protein metabolism. The usual rate of formation is approximately 1 to 2 mEq of H^+ per kilogram of body weight per day. Most diets that contain animal protein metabolically produce a net positive quantity of nonvolatile acids, primarily sulfuric acid from the sulfur-containing amino acids cysteine and methionine. Other acids are produced in the form of phosphoric acid (from phosphoproteins, phospholipids, and phospho-nucleotides) and nonmetabolizable organic acids (e.g., uric acid), and hydrochlorides are produced from metabolism of the cationic amino acids lysine, arginine, and histidine. Conversely, HCO_3^- is generated from metabolism of organic anions absorbed from the diet (e.g., citrate, acetate).

From the Henderson-Hasselbalch equation, consider the addition of metabolic acid HA (where the anion A^- could be Cl^-, lactate$^-$, sulfite, or mono- or dihydrogen phosphate) to blood that contains Na^+ and HCO_3^-:

$$HA + NaHCO_3 \rightarrow Na^+ + A^- + H^+ + HCO_3^-$$

and

$$H^+ + HCO_3^- \leftrightarrow H_2CO_3 \leftrightarrow CO_2 + H_2O$$

The CO_2 produced by this process will not raise the blood P_{CO_2} if the system is well ventilated because the contribution of metabolic acid is a small part of the daily production of CO_2. Note that the addition of protons to body fluids by these acid end products consumes bicarbonate ("lost bicarbonate"), which then must be replenished by the kidney as it eliminates the proton and A^- in the urine. The process of excreting net H^+ and A^- is equivalent to producing a "new" HCO_3^- to restore the HCO_3^- that is lost by the addition of HA, the metabolic acid. The kidney must excrete any nonvolatile acid (or alkali) load to maintain a steady-state serum HCO_3^- concentration in the 22- to 28-mEq/L range.

When the diet requires the excretion of acids, the urine pH will fall to a value as low as 4.5 to 5.0, and the urine will become nominally free of bicarbonate. With an alkaline load, by comparison, the kidney will excrete excess filtered HCO_3^-, and the urine pH may approach a maximal value of 8.0 to 8.5. In most humans, particularly those who eat animal protein or an "acid-ash" diet, the requirement for net acid *excretion* predominates. However, some vegetarians may have an overall "alkaline-ash" diet, for which net alkali must be excreted to match intake.

Bicarbonate and the Kidney in Acid-Base Balance

The first role of the kidney in achieving acid excretion is to reabsorb all filtered HCO_3^- (E-Fig. 104-1). At a normal glomerular filtration rate (e.g., ≈180 L/day in an adult) and plasma HCO_3^- concentration of 25 mEq/L, about 4500 mEq of HCO_3^- is filtered in 1 day. Loss of even a small fraction of that amount would result in metabolic acidosis if not replaced by alkali (HCO_3^-) intake. Just as reabsorption of all filtered glucose does not add glucose to the body, reabsorption of all filtered HCO_3^- will maintain the status quo but will not fulfill the need to generate new HCO_3^-. Therefore, the kidney must perform two functions: reabsorb all filtered HCO_3^- and eliminate enough additional H^+ (producing HCO_3^- in the process) to replace HCO_3^- losses from acid that is generated by cellular metabolism. Urinary buffers are essential because urinary pH alone cannot be lowered enough to excrete the amount of acid needed for this purpose.

The Proximal Tubule

About 80 to 90% of HCO_3^- reabsorption is accomplished in the proximal tubule by a proton secretory process that renders the luminal fluid more acid (pH ≈ 6.5). The brush border membranes facing the lumen of the proximal tubule cell contain transporters known as Na/H exchangers (NHE3), which carry out the greatest proportion of acidification, and vacuolar H^+-ATPases, which provide a smaller contribution. Through the normal function of basolateral membrane Na^+, K^+-ATPase, cell Na^+ is kept at low concentration so that filtered Na^+ in the lumen will be favored to enter the cell in exchange for H^+ secreted into the lumen. This H^+ rapidly combines with filtered HCO_3^- to form H_2CO_3, which then rapidly dehydrates in the lumen to form CO_2 and H_2O. This process is greatly facilitated by the large surface area of microvillous membranes and by luminal carbonic anhydrase (CA_{IV}). The CO_2 enters the proximal cell by diffusion through apical water channels (aquaporin 1). CO_2 within the cell re-forms HCO_3^-, a reaction catalyzed by intracellular carbonic anhydrase (CA_{II}). The cell, more alkaline by apical H^+ secretion, favors the reaction $OH^- + CO_2$ to form HCO_3^- catalyzed by carbonic anhydrase. The HCO_3^- is then transported back toward the blood by an electrogenic sodium bicarbonate cotransporter (NBCel), which couples 1Na and $3HCO_3^-$, thereby completing net Na^+ and HCO_3^- reabsorption. The 1 : 3 net negative charge transport by NBC allows the inside negative membrane potential to drive outward movement of Na^+ and HCO_3^- against an adverse Na gradient in this reabsorptive process. NBC on the basolateral membrane protects the cell from an alkaline load, accomplishes HCO_3^- reabsorption, and mediates a component of Na^+ reabsorption without further direct requirement for adenosine triphosphate (ATP). The entire process requires a mitochondrial source of ATP for the Na^+/K^+ pump, intact NHE3 and NBC, and two isoforms of carbonic anhydrase. In addition, there must be favorable ion gradients for luminal Na^+ entry, H^+ secretion, and basolateral HCO_3^- transport. An inside negative potential depending on outwardly directed K^+ gradients explains how an increase in blood K^+ decreases the proximal reabsorption of HCO_3^- and the production of NH_4^+. Conversely, hypokalemia tends to stimulate the reabsorption of HCO_3^- and the production of ammonium. A disturbance in any of these factors may disrupt proximal HCO_3^- reabsorption and cause loss of HCO_3^- in urine. It is also clear that the acidifying process in the proximal tubule provides a significant mechanism for Na^+ reabsorption, consistent with the finding that HCO_3^- reabsorption is increased by angiotensin II and the sympathetic nervous system in the defense of extracellular volume.

Another 10 to 15% of filtered HCO_3^- is reabsorbed in the thick ascending limb of Henle, so that only small amounts of the filtered HCO_3^- are normally delivered to more distal nephron segments.

The Cortical Collecting Duct

The cortical connecting tubules and collecting ducts reabsorb less than 10% of the filtered HCO_3^-. In principal cells, Na^+ is reabsorbed from lumen to cell by the epithelial sodium channel (ENaC), driven by the inwardly directed Na^+ gradient and favorable electrical potential. With the reabsorption of Na^+, the lumen becomes electronegative, thereby favoring the secretion of both K^+, through potassium channels, and H^+, through vacuolar H^+-ATPases on the luminal surface of neighboring α-intercalated cells, which are acid-secreting cells. The secreted H^+ will combine with the remaining HCO_3^- in the lumen to generate CO_2, with subsequent reabsorption of CO_2, re-formation of cellular HCO_3^- with the help of cellular carbonic anhydrase (CA_{II}), and then exchange of HCO_3^- from cell to blood for entry of extracellular Cl^- through Cl^-/HCO_3^- exchangers, similar to the erythrocytic anion exchangers (AE1) that participate in blood CO_2 transport. The distal nephron, which has a smaller requirement for bicarbonate reabsorption than the proximal tubule, lacks both brush border and luminal carbonic anhydrase. It is at this distal site that tubular fluid pH starts to fall to levels below pH 6.0.

β-Intercalated cells comprise a population of collecting duct cells that have reverse polarity and secrete HCO_3^- into the lumen in exchange for Cl^- entry into the cell. In these, the H^+-ATPase faces the blood side of the cell. An elevated extracellular HCO_3^- concentration, as seen with an alkaline-ash diet or metabolic alkalosis, will increase HCO_3^- secretion by these cells through pendrin, which is the apical Cl^-/HCO_3^- anion exchanger.

The Medullary Collecting Duct

The medullary collecting duct continues to secrete protons into the luminal fluid, where the pH reaches its lowest values of 4.5 to 5.0. The mechanism is based on continued function of H^+-ATPases. In both the cortical and medullary collecting duct there is an additional role of an ATP-dependent K^+/H^+ exchanger, a member of the family of gastric and colonic ATPases.

Once the filtered HCO_3^- is fully reabsorbed, the kidney is still required to eliminate an additional net amount of acid equivalent to that produced in metabolism. Most of this net acid excretion is in the form of ammonium (NH_4^+), which is derived from the metabolism of glutamine in the proximal tubule and the titration of filtered phosphate to acid phosphate (titratable acidity).

$$NH_3 + H^+ \leftrightarrow NH_4^+ \quad pK\ 9.1$$

and

$$HPO_4^{2-} + H^+ \leftrightarrow H_2PO_4^- \quad pK\ 6.8$$

Urinary Buffers

As the collecting duct cells continue to secrete H^+ into urine with a diminishing luminal HCO_3^- concentration and decreasing pH, H^+ is captured by the urinary buffers. The resulting alkalinization of the cells after H^+ secretion results in the formation of cellular HCO_3^- ready for transport into blood. This process generates "new" HCO_3^- that is not a result of the reabsorption of filtered HCO_3^-. The amount of new HCO_3^- matches the amount of net acid eliminated and is also equal to each of the following: the amount of acid produced; the amount of body buffer consumed by that acid; and the amount of fixed acid anions, such as sulfate, phosphate, and Cl^-, that accompanied the H^+. The result is maintenance of normal acid-base equilibrium.

The ability of the kidney to lower urinary pH enables the buffers to capture a proton. Net acid excretion in urine is accomplished not simply by a decrease in urine pH but mostly by titration of these important urinary buffers. For example, a typical daily urine volume of 1 L at pH 5.0 contains only 10^{-5} molar hydrogen ion, or 0.01 mmol, a trivial amount compared with the amount of produced acid (≈1 mmol/kg/day). In chronic kidney disease, the failure to produce sufficient ammonium leads to a poorly buffered urine, thereby causing retention of acid while still consistent with reaching maximal urine acidity with respect to pH.

Regulation of Urinary Acid Secretion

Renal mechanisms of urinary acidification are adaptable. Transport processes such as H^+-ATPases, Na^+/H^+ exchange, and Cl^-/HCO_3^- exchange can increase or decrease their capacity to handle acid-base equivalents, depending on the challenge presented. Renal ammoniagenic mechanisms are also critically regulated to serve the acid-base needs of the individual. Metabolic acidosis and respiratory acidosis increase the capacity to reabsorb HCO_3^-, including increased expression of the transporters involved in acidifying the urine. At the same time, glutamine transport into proximal cells is stimulated, and increased production of ammonium facilitates acid excretion, as well as the generation of new HCO_3^- in the distal nephron. Metabolic alkalosis and respiratory alkalosis have the opposite effects.

Ammoniagenesis, which is a key element in urinary acid excretion, provides the major acceptor for protons. Ammonium is produced predominantly in the proximal tubule cell by mitochondrial glutaminase enzymes. Production is increased by increasing the metabolic acid load in the body, respiratory acidosis, and hypokalemia. NH_4^+ can preserve potassium in the hypokalemic state by serving as a cation needed for anion excretion. In response to metabolic acidosis, the kidney can excrete chloride with ammonium, thereby preserving the ability to retain Na^+.

Metabolic acidosis is a hypercatabolic state with increased cortisol, which increases proteolysis in muscle and increases the release of both glutamine and NH_3 into the circulation. In the liver, acidosis also decreases the activity of the urea cycle, which normally consumes NH_3 and HCO_3^- to form carbamoyl phosphate in the initial regulatory step in ureagenesis. In acidosis, NH_3 is favored to produce hepatic glutamine, which is also delivered to the proximal tubule cell, where mitochondrial enzymes remove NH_4 to assist in urinary net acid excretion. The associated increase in α-ketoglutarate provides a substrate for gluconeogenesis in the renal proximal tubule and results in the production of HCO_3^-.

Ammonium can be secreted by nonionic diffusion as NH_3 into the proximal fluid, where it will pick up a proton and re-form ammonium (NH_4^+), or it could form ammonium within the proximal tubule cell and be secreted by Na^+/NH_4^+ exchange, a mode of operation of the Na^+/H^+ exchanger. Ammonium is then reabsorbed by the thick ascending limb of Henle on the Na-K-2Cl transporter, where it can substitute for K^+. By countercurrent multiplication, NH_3/NH_4^+ concentrates in the medullary interstitial fluid rather than remaining in the ascending limb fluid as it reaches the highly perfused renal cortex, where it would otherwise dissipate into renal venous blood. The countercurrent mechanism also allows ammonia to diffuse into the medullary interstitium and ultimately the lumen of the medullary collecting duct, where it will be trapped as ammonium in the acid tubular fluid. Diffusion of NH_3 across membranes of collecting duct cells occurs by way of glycoproteins that are in the family of the Rh factor, red blood cell ammonia transporters. The efficient secretion of ammonium in the collecting duct and by acid trapping in the lumen is essential for excretion of acid from the body.

Regulation is accomplished at a number of levels. Hormones such as angiotensin II and catecholamines stimulate Na^+ reabsorption in the proximal tubule by increasing sodium-hydrogen exchange and $NaHCO_3$ cotransport. Aldosterone increases H^+-ATPase in the collecting duct cell and stimulates Na^+ reabsorption, thereby increasing proton secretion. Low extracellular fluid volume increases proximal HCO_3^- reabsorption, as does hypokalemia and high P_{CO_2}. Hyperkalemia (Chapter 103) may limit urinary acidification by decreasing the amount of NH_3 absorbed in the thick limb and, as a result, the amount entering the countercurrent multiplier in the loop of Henle. Hyperkalemia also decreases the secretion of H^+ in the collecting duct as the need to secrete K^+ predominates.

CLINICAL MANIFESTATIONS AND DIAGNOSIS

Assessment of clinical acid-base disturbances usually begins with measurement of arterial blood gases (Fig. 104-1 and Table 104-3). In some situations, venous blood can be used as an alternative.

It is useful to conceptualize acid-base disorders by a mass action shift of the variables to the right or left in the following relationship:

$$H^+ + HCO_3^- \leftrightarrow H_2CO_3 \leftrightarrow CO_2 + H_2O$$

The addition of CO_2, as in respiratory acidosis, will increase the hydrogen and bicarbonate concentrations (left shift). Removal of CO_2, as in respiratory alkalosis, will decrease CO_2, protons, and bicarbonate (shift right). The addition of protons with an anion other than HCO_3^-, as in metabolic acidosis, will lead to increased concentrations of protons and a decreased bicarbonate concentration. Removal of HCO_3^- with a cation such as Na^+, also a cause of metabolic acidosis, will increase the proton concentration and lower the HCO_3^- concentration. Metabolic alkalosis might be caused by the addition of $NaHCO_3$ with a resulting decrease in the proton concentration or by removal of H^+ with chloride, thereby leading to a decreased proton concentration and increased HCO_3^-. Because of the relationship of metabolic acidosis and alkalosis to the gain or loss of fluids and electrolytes, acid-base disorders can be considered a consequence of electrolyte imbalance.[3]

Compensatory Changes

Few patients have an isolated acid-base disturbance. In nearly all cases, a respiratory or renal compensation (or both) occurs in response to counteract a primary acid-base process.[4]

When functioning normally, the lungs may maintain a normal pH and P_{CO_2} during changes in volatile acid production. The kidneys will also maintain normal acid-base balance during changes in fixed acid production. Only excesses beyond the capacity to eliminate an acid or alkali load will lead to clinical disturbances. Patients with renal or lung disease may do less well in response to metabolic and respiratory disorders.

When an acid-base disturbance develops, the initial response to modulate its severity depends on the titration of various body buffer pairs. For example, phosphate, hemoglobin, and albumin change their protonated and unprotonated concentrations. The body will further attempt to correct the extracellular pH toward normal but usually not to normal. For metabolic disturbances caused by increased or decreased nonvolatile acid, the response is respiratory; for primary respiratory acidosis and alkalosis, the compensation is renal (Table 104-4). The direction of change in HCO_3^- and P_{CO_2} is the same when the primary disturbance is compensated; the ratio of HCO_3^- to

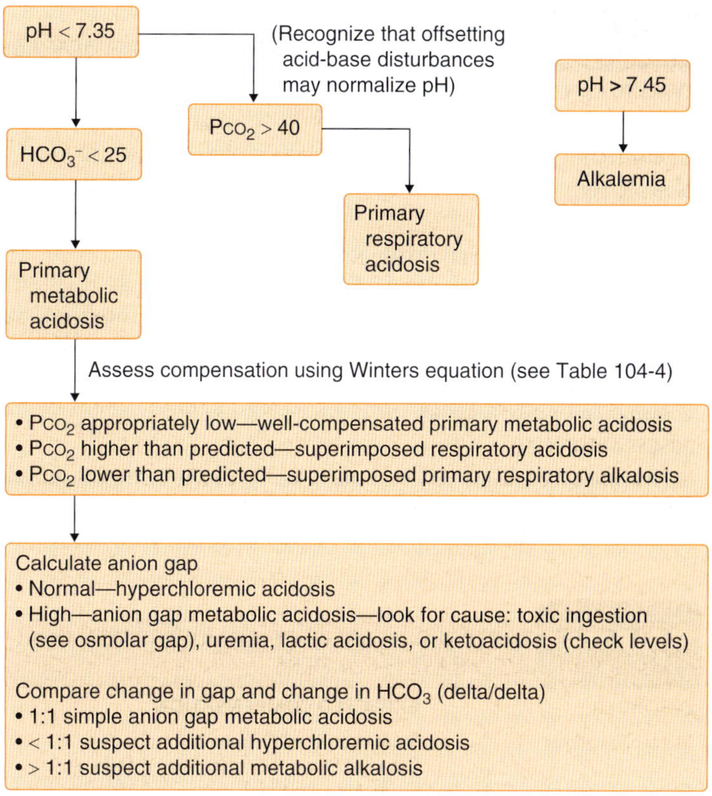

FIGURE 104-1. Evaluation of acidemia. In an anion gap acidosis, a simple 1 : 1 relationship is usually not present because organic anions are variably cleared by organs such as liver and kidney, and because the apparent volume of distribution of organic anions and bicarbonate may differ. In lactic acidosis, a 1 : 1 relationship is usually not present because of clearance of lactic acid from the circulation. In the Cori cycle, muscle lactic acid is taken up by liver cells via monocarboxylic acid transporters, and the lactate goes to re-form glucose via the gluconeogenic pathway. The glucose recycles to the muscle, where it is used for further energy. Another reason the ratio is not 1 : 1 is that lactate anion can be cleared with Na^+ by urinary excretion.

P_{CO_2} and thus pH become closer to normal. These compensations tend to take time, so acid-base disturbances, particularly the respiratory conditions requiring renal compensation, are classified as acute (lasting less than 24 to 48 hours) or chronic.

Peripheral blood does not demonstrate complete compensation for most acid-base disturbances, with the occasional exception of chronic respiratory alkalosis. Full compensation for metabolic acidosis would expend large amounts of respiratory muscle energy, which could limit a prolonged response. Full compensation for metabolic alkalosis would result in excessive hypoventilation and adverse effects on oxygenation. In both situations, the body requires an offset from "normal" to drive continued renal compensation. The degree of offset can be very close, or not that close, to normal. In contrast, the CNS closely regulates its pH, with nearly full correction within 1 to 2 days. Before this compensation occurs, acute alkalemia may be associated with cerebral vasoconstriction and ischemia, whereas acidemia may result in vasodilation and cerebral edema. Rapid changes in blood P_{CO_2} affect the CNS chemosensors more quickly than do changes in HCO_3^- because of more rapid movement of nonionic CO_2 across the blood-brain barrier. Increases in CNS CO_2 lead to acidification of the medullary center interstitial fluid and an increased ventilatory drive. Decreases in CNS CO_2 (alkalinization of the respiratory center) lead to hypoventilation. Acid-base changes are reflected in the composition of the cerebrospinal fluid (CSF).

In metabolic acidosis, peripheral chemosensors in the carotid body stimulate the CNS to increase ventilation to reduce P_{CO_2}. The fall in peripheral P_{CO_2} will lead to dissolved CO_2 leaving the CNS ahead of HCO_3^-; the alkalinization of the medullary center interstitial fluid will then slow the hyperventilatory response until a new steady state of hypocapnia is achieved. Patients may sense dyspnea or air hunger acutely with rapid and shallow respirations. In severe cases of metabolic acidemia, the respirations are deep and gasping, typical of Kussmaul breathing.

When the bicarbonate concentration increases as a result of metabolic alkalosis, a hypoventilatory response, signaled from the peripheral chemosensors, raises P_{CO_2}. As P_{CO_2} rises, the dissolved CO_2 will enter the CSF and acidify

TABLE 104-3 LABORATORY STEPS IN IDENTIFYING ACID-BASE DISORDERS

EVALUATE pH	ACIDEMIC	ALKALEMIC
Elevated Pco_2	Respiratory acidosis	Metabolic alkalosis
Elevated HCO_3	Respiratory acidosis	Metabolic alkalosis
Decreased Pco_2	Metabolic acidosis	Respiratory alkalosis
Decreased HCO_3	Metabolic acidosis	Respiratory alkalosis
EVALUATE FOR EXPECTED COMPENSATION		
Meets expectation: simple disorder with compensation or could be offsetting metabolic alkalosis and acidosis.		
Does not meet expectation: complex disorder, but pH indicates whether acidosis or alkalosis is dominant.		
If a metabolic disorder is dominant, a Pco_2 greater than predicted indicates an additional respiratory acidosis. A Pco_2 less than predicted indicates an additional respiratory alkalosis.		
If a respiratory disorder is dominant, an HCO_3 concentration greater than predicted indicates additional metabolic alkalosis. An HCO_3 concentration less than predicted indicates an additional metabolic acidosis.		
ASSESS ANION GAP		
Elevated: metabolic acidosis is present whether acidemic or alkalemic. If alkalemic, an additional metabolic or respiratory alkalosis is present.		
If the gap is greater than the fall in HCO_3, consider an additional metabolic alkalosis or respiratory acidosis.		
If the gap is less than the fall in HCO_3, consider an additional nongap acidosis or respiratory alkalosis.		

TABLE 104-4 EXPECTED DEGREES OF COMPENSATION IN ACID-BASE DISORDERS

DISORDER	EXPECTED COMPENSATION
Metabolic acidosis	Steady state in 12-36 hours Expected Pco_2 = 1.5 (measured HCO_3) + 8 ± 2 (Winters equation)
Metabolic alkalosis	Less predictable Expected Pco_2 increases 0.5 – 0.7 mm Hg per 1-mEq/L increase in HCO_3
Respiratory acidosis Acute Chronic, after 24-36 hours	 Expected 1-mEq/L increase in HCO_3 per 10-mm Hg rise in Pco_2 Expected 3- to 5-mEq/L increase in HCO_3 per 10-mm Hg rise in Pco_2
Respiratory alkalosis Acute Chronic, after 24-36 hours	 Expected 1- to 2-mEq/L fall in HCO_3 per 10-mm Hg fall in Pco_2 Expected 5-mEq/L fall in HCO_3 per 10-mm Hg fall in Pco_2

the medullary respiratory center. The stimulus to breathe will, in part, antagonize the peripheral signal until a steady state of hypoventilation is reached.

In respiratory acidosis, acute hypoventilation results in hypercapnia, because of the decreased clearance of carbon dioxide. The fall in blood pH and proximal tubular cell acidification results in compensatory ammoniagenesis and increased net renal acid excretion. When the Pco_2 reaches a new higher steady-state value, indicating that the production and elimination of carbonic acid have become equal at this low ventilatory rate, no further acid is retained, so further ammoniagenesis and net acid excretion are no longer required. However, the HCO_3^- produced during the period of high acid excretion persists at a high level because the high Pco_2 and hypochloremic volume depletion maintain proximal HCO_3^- reabsorption. The hypochloremia, brought about by the compensatory early excretion of NH_4Cl and elevated serum HCO_3^- and then maintained by the high Pco_2, persists until the extracellular volume is replaced with NaCl. An abrupt decrease in Pco_2, such as by mechanical ventilation, cannot correct the high HCO_3^- until chloride returns to its normal level. Reducing the Pco_2 before correcting the lost chloride results in post-hypercapnic metabolic alkalosis.

In respiratory alkalosis, the primary event is a fall in Pco_2 because of increased alveolar ventilation. On transition from acute to chronic respiratory alkalosis, the compensatory mechanisms that initially maintained a more normal systemic pH are no longer required as CO_2 production and elimination become equal. Thus, the initial compensatory decrease in renal acid excretion brought about by increased loss of filtered $NaHCO_3$ ceases, but low serum HCO_3^- and high serum Cl^- concentrations are maintained because the persistent hypocapnia induces proximal tubule bicarbonaturia. Once a lower steady-state level of HCO_3^- is achieved, net renal acid excretion returns to baseline.

In identifying whether an acid-base disturbance is simple (a single disturbance with its compensation) or complex (multiple primary processes simultaneously present), it is useful to compare the expected compensation for a simple process with the observed parameters of the blood gases (see Table 104-3). For example, if Pco_2 is lower than would be predicted by the Winters equation in a patient with a simple, compensated metabolic acidosis, an additional coexistent primary respiratory alkalosis must be driving the Pco_2 down. If Pco_2 is higher than would be predicted for a low bicarbonate level in a patient with metabolic acidosis, a coexistent respiratory acidosis is present.

METABOLIC ACIDOSIS

EPIDEMIOLOGY AND PATHOBIOLOGY

In metabolic acidosis, the primary change is a fall in serum bicarbonate.[5] The compensatory response is to increase ventilation to reduce Pco_2. Worsening acidosis elicits increasing alveolar ventilation.

Primary metabolic acidosis results from an imbalance between net acid production and net acid excretion in the form of urinary ammonium excretion and acid phosphate excretion. Increased excretion of acid phosphate and other weak acids is called total titratable acidity when measured in the urine. Consider the following relationship, where U_x represents the urinary concentration and the urinary flow rate $\dot{V}$:

$$NAE = (U_{NH4} \times \dot{V}) + (U_{TAphos} \times \dot{V}) - (U_{HCO_3^-} \times \dot{V})$$

In a normal steady-state condition, the rate of excretion of net acid must be equal to the rate of production. The normal production rate depends on diet. If net acid production is normal, metabolic acidosis could occur because of a failure to reabsorb bicarbonate or a failure to secrete adequate net acid, as is the case in renal failure and renal tubular acidosis. An inequality also could develop if net acid production were excessive or if large extrarenal bicarbonate losses were unable to be matched by maximal adaptive increases in net acid excretion. Endogenous sources of acid include ketoacidosis and lactic acidosis, whereas exogenous sources might be acid metabolic products of ingested ethylene glycol or methanol. On occasion, strong inorganic acids may be ingested. When net acid is retained, the serum bicarbonate concentration falls. However, maintenance of a constant low serum HCO_3^- concentration does not guarantee that there is a new steady state in which net acid production is equal to net acid excretion because body buffers such as carbonate salts of bone may become progressively depleted by relentless acid retention, as in chronic kidney disease and distal renal tubular acidosis.

The causes of metabolic acidosis are usually categorized according to the presence of either hyperchloremia or an elevated serum anion gap. The serum anion gap is the net charge difference when the sum of chloride and bicarbonate is subtracted from the serum sodium concentration.

$$\text{Anion gap} = [Na^+] - ([Cl^-] + [HCO_3^-])$$

The normal anion gap is due to the net unmeasured anionic charge associated predominantly with albumin. When acidemia is present, albumin is in a more protonated form, which lowers the normal gap. In alkalemia, the effect of pH is to increase the gap attributed to albumin. Each 1 g/dL of albumin contributes approximately 2.5 mEq/L to the normal anion gap. The anion gap may be low with hypoalbuminemia or with an increase in unmeasured cations, such as immunoglobulin G myeloma paraproteins, calcium, lithium, or magnesium. The anion gap may be high in the presence of unmeasured anions, including sulfates, bromides, iodides, and immunoglobulin A myeloma light chains. When the anion gap is increased above the normal value of 10 to 12 mEq/L by a non-chloride acid anion, an anion gap metabolic acidosis exists. The accompanying proton is responsible for lowering the serum bicarbonate concentration. The degree of increase in the anion gap, sometimes referred to as the *delta anion gap*, may be estimated by the difference between the observed anion gap and a normal value of 10 to 12 mEq/L. A similar calculation for a change in serum HCO_3^- can be made by subtracting the observed HCO_3^- from the normal value of about 25 mEq/L (the *delta* HCO_3^-). Comparison of the two values (the *delta-delta*) may help identify more complicated acid-base disorders. If the increase in the anion gap is larger than the decrease in serum HCO_3^-, an additional process is raising the HCO_3^- level. The patient may have a coexisting metabolic alkalosis or be compensating for chronic respiratory acidosis. If the decrease in serum HCO_3^- is larger than the increase in the anion gap, it is a sign of another process that raises the Cl^- while lowering the HCO_3^- level, such as an additional hyperchloremic acidosis or respiratory alkalosis. In most anion gap acidoses, the increase in anion gap and the decrease in HCO_3^- is not usually greater than 1 : 1 because the excretion of urinary anions with Na^+ results in a hyperchloremic component to the acidosis. (See Fig. 104-1 and its legend.) Conversely, any buffering of H^+ with non-HCO_3^- buffers will decrease the drop in HCO_3^- compared with the increase in anion gap. In severe cases of anion gap acidosis, Cl^- may be displaced into cells, thereby resulting in a higher anion gap compared with the decrease in HCO_3^-—a hypochloremic anion gap acidosis.

CLINICAL MANIFESTATIONS

The effects of metabolic acidosis depend on its rapidity of onset and severity. Patients often complain of fatigue, nausea, vomiting, shortness of breath, and dyspnea on exertion. Acutely, deep respirations, often labored with the use of accessory muscles, may be detected, but hyperventilation may be less notable with chronic metabolic acidemia. Metabolic acidemia also may be associated with vasodilation, tachycardia, and hypotension (Chapter 92). The negative inotropic effect of acidemia on the heart can exacerbate septic shock (Chapter 94). The stress of an underlying illness or an increase in adrenergic and corticosteroid activity associated with acidemia may elevate the peripheral white blood cell count and cause hyperglycemia. Other findings can include hyperkalemia (Chapter 103), hyperphosphatemia (Chapter 105), and hyperuricemia (Chapter 252) as well as hypocalcemia (Chapter 227) and markers of bone injury as a result of decreased renal synthesis of 1,25-dihydroxyvitamin D.

ANION GAP METABOLIC ACIDOSES

A variety of abnormalities can cause anion gap acidoses.[6] One mnemonic for the common ones is *gold mark*, for *g*lycols (ethylene and propylene), *o*xoproline, *L*-lactate, *D*-lactate, *m*ethanol, *a*spirin, *r*enal failure, and *k*etoacidosis. Because some causes are life-threatening, a rapid diagnosis is required. The osmolar gap should be calculated in all cases of anion gap acidosis (Table 104-5) because unmeasured toxic, nonionic alcohols will contribute to body osmolality but not to acidity. Although not acidic themselves, these alcohols oxidize to dangerous unmeasured organic acids with anions that contribute only to the anion gap. The osmolar gap is defined as the difference between the measured and the calculated serum osmolality. The serum osmolality should be measured by a freezing point depression technique and compared with the calculated osmolality.

$$\text{Calculated osmolality} = 2(\text{Na}^+) + (\text{Glucose [mg/dL]} \div 18) + (\text{Blood urea nitrogen [mg/dL]} \div 2.8)$$

UREMIC ACIDOSIS

The metabolic acidosis of advanced chronic kidney disease (Chapter 116) may be due to tubular leakage of HCO_3^-, but it is usually present when inadequate production of ammonium is unable to facilitate excretion of the normal metabolic acid load.[7] Because, of the low buffering capacity in the urine, many patients with renal failure maintain the ability to acidify their urine maximally. Many organic and inorganic anions, such as phosphate and sulfates, are retained at glomerular filtration rates of less than 25 mL/minute and constitute an increased anion gap in association with the metabolic acidosis. The magnitude of the gap is usually less than 20 mEq/L consisting of poorly filtered sulfates and phosphates and retention of anions that are suboptimally secreted. The renal patient who is maximally producing NH_3 to stay in balance with daily acid production may be unable to accommodate any further acid production, such as a metabolic or respiratory acidosis, that would require increased ammoniagenesis. The patient with poor glomerular filtration and an alkaline load will retain HCO_3^-, thereby worsening both

TABLE 104-5 CAUSES OF INCREASED ANION AND OSMOLAR GAPS

ANION GAP METABOLIC ACIDOSIS	OSMOLAR GAP
Uremia	No
Lactic acidosis	Variable/no
D-Lactic acidosis	No
Diabetic ketoacidosis	No
Starvation ketoacidosis	No
Alcoholic ketoacidosis	If ethanol is present
Ethylene glycol	Yes
Methanol	Yes
Salicylates	No
5-Oxoprolinuria (acetaminophen)	No

metabolic and respiratory alkalosis. For example, metabolic alkalosis commonly occurs instead of urinary alkalinization when HCO_3^- is used in the attempt to alkalinize the urine in a patient with kidney failure. The systemic acid-base disturbance in renal diseases with prominent tubular dysfunction is attributable to the kidney's inability to secrete hydrogen and to reabsorb and generate HCO_3^-. It is particularly pronounced in oliguric acute kidney injury and is exacerbated by hypercatabolic states such as infection. A significant metabolic acidosis disproportionate to the severity of chronic kidney disease of unknown cause should raise the possibility of tubular dysfunction due to urinary tract obstruction or chronic tubulointerstitial diseases (Chapter 108), including amyloidosis (Chapter 174), myeloma (Chapter 173), autoimmune disorders (Chapter 236), and analgesic nephropathy (Chapter 108).

It is important to treat the metabolic acidosis of chronic kidney disease.[8] Maintaining the serum HCO_3^- concentration above 20 to 22 mEq/L, by administering $NaHCO_3$ at a rate of 1 mEq HCO_3^-/kg/day, will slow the progression of chronic kidney disease, delay end-stage renal failure, and improve nutritional status.

PROGNOSIS

In population studies, a low serum bicarbonate level is associated with higher all-cause mortality. The relative risk of death is about 2.6-fold higher in patients with chronic kidney disease and about 1.7-fold higher even without it.

OVERPRODUCTION OF ENDOGENOUS ACIDS

Lactic Acidosis

EPIDEMIOLOGY AND PATHOBIOLOGY

Overproduction of lactic acid may occur with severe exertion, but true lactic acidosis (lactate level >4 mmol/L or >36 mg/dL) is frequently associated with critical illness, multiorgan failure, and increased mortality. Lactic acid, which is the final product in the anaerobic pathway of glucose metabolism, is produced from pyruvate in a reaction catalyzed by lactate dehydrogenase:

$$\text{NADH} + \text{pyruvate} + \text{H}^+ \rightarrow \text{lactate} + \text{NAD}^+$$

A high reduced nicotinamide adenine dinucleotide (NADH)/NAD ratio will favor the formation of lactate. Conversion of ethanol to acetaldehyde and conversion of β-hydroxybutyrate to acetoacetate use NAD and produce NADH. Alcohol metabolism may be associated with excessive β-hydroxybutyrate and lactic acidosis.

Lactic acidosis is caused by an imbalance in the rates of lactate production and its clearance, primarily in the liver. Lactic acidosis, which increases the anion gap, is most often due to circulatory failure, hypoxia, sepsis, and mitochondrial dysfunction that each increase anaerobic glycolysis and the rate of conversion of pyruvate to lactate (Table 104-6).[9] Sepsis (Chapter 94) is associated with an elevated lactate level because of poor clearance and impaired gluconeogenesis.[10] Lactic acidosis can also result from seizure activity (Chapter 372) when lactate is released from muscle cells that have sustained a period of anaerobic metabolism. Other causes include thiamine deficiency (Chapter 199), hypophosphatemia (Chapter 105), isoniazid toxicity (Chapter 96), and hypoglycemic states (Chapter 211). Metformin may cause lactic acidosis, particularly in elderly patients with cardiac, hepatic, or renal dysfunction.

TABLE 104-6 CAUSES OF LACTIC ACIDOSIS

Shock (Chapter 92): septic (Chapter 94), cardiogenic (Chapter 93), or hypovolemic
Advanced heart failure (Chapters 45 and 46)
Severe trauma (Chapter 97)
Severe hypoxemia (Chapter 90) with Pa_{O_2} <30 mm Hg
Carbon monoxide poisoning (Chapter 82)
Severe anemia (Chapter 144) with hemoglobin level <5 g/dL
Vigorous exercise, seizures (Chapter 372), or shivering (Chapter 95)
Diabetes mellitus (Chapter 210), usually in association with ketoacidosis
Cancer (especially lymphomas [Chapters 171 and 172], leukemias [Chapters 168,169 and 170], and solid tumors)
Liver disease with decreased lactate clearance (Chapter 140)
High plasma metformin levels
Nucleoside reverse-transcriptase inhibitors
Cocaine (Chapter 365)
Toxic alcohols, methanol, ethylene glycol, diethylene glycol (Chapter 96)
Propylene glycol (Chapter 96)
Salicylates (Chapter 70)
Cyanide (Chapter 96)
β_2-Agonists (Chapter 75)
Propofol (after prolonged high-dose infusion; Chapter 400)
Thiamine deficiency in children or adults receiving parenteral nutrition or those with fulminant beriberi (Chapters 198 and 199)

Adapted from Kraut JA, Madias NE. Lactic acidosis. *N Engl J Med*. 2014;371:2309-2319.

Nucleoside antivirals (Chapter 357), including zidovudine, may cause lactic acidosis and abnormal liver function as a result of toxic mitochondrial effects. Abnormal mitochondrial function is also a feature of aspirin overdose (Chapter 70) or toxicity with hypoglycin from ingestion of the unripe ackee fruit (Jamaican vomiting sickness). The antibiotic linezolid is another cause of lactic acidosis.

Lactic acidosis also can be caused by the overproduction of the acid, which may occur with severe exertion and malignant neoplasms, particularly with a large tumor burden from lymphoma or widely metastatic cancer. Malignant cells can upregulate glycolytic activity, which may increase their uptake of glucose and decrease their dependence on mitochondrion-derived energy. These tumors can use large amounts of available glucose and inorganic phosphate, thereby leading to a syndrome of hypoglycemia, hypophosphatemia, and lactic acidosis.

CLINICAL MANIFESTATIONS AND DIAGNOSIS

Lactic acidosis typically presents with a blood pH of 7.35 or lower and a serum HCO_3^- 20 mEq/L or lower. To make the diagnosis, however, the serum lactate level should be directly measured in any patient with an anion gap acidosis. Glucose, creatinine, and blood urea nitrogen levels also should be obtained. In cases in which a toxic ingestion is suspected (see Table 104-5), a screen for such toxins in the serum should be performed.

TREATMENT

Treatment of lactic acidosis is aimed at correction of the underlying cause. Central venous oxygen saturation should be increased, with a goal of at least 70%, by restoring tissue perfusion and ventilation. In general, the mean arterial pressure should be maintained at 65 to 70 mm Hg, the heart rate below 100 beats/minute, and the hemoglobin level over 7 g/dL.

Sodium bicarbonate can be considered when the arterial pH is below 7.0 or when acidemia has resulted in decreased cardiac inotropy or systemic vasodilation and shock. It is preferable to give $NaHCO_3$ as an isotonic mixture in 5% dextrose and water rather than as a hypertonic bolus, because the latter carries the risk of pulmonary edema and hypernatremia. The quantity of administered sodium bicarbonate to raise arterial pH to 7.2 should be estimated by multiplying the desired bicarbonate concentration minus the observed bicarbonate concentration by 50% of body weight. The calculated amount in patients with severe acidosis may require continuous dialytic methods to administer adequate amounts of bicarbonate without causing volume overload. Full correction should be avoided.

In patients with a metabolic acidosis after seizures (Chapter 372), the lactate is quickly metabolized to HCO_3^- by the liver and kidneys, and the acidosis often resolves within 60 minutes. The administration of HCO_3^- is usually unnecessary and may precipitate an overshoot metabolic alkalosis as the lactate is metabolized, which lowers the seizure threshold.

In patients with intestinal bacterial overgrowth (Chapter 126), a syndrome of disorientation, ataxia, and anion gap metabolic acidosis may develop after a carbohydrate meal because of bacterial production of D-lactate. This isomer of the mammalian L-lactate can be measured only by a specific D-lactate assay. The condition is treated with oral antibiotics and appropriate diet.

PROGNOSIS

Lactic acidosis, when severe, is associated with a high early mortality. When the pH is less than 7.2, only 17% of patients who are admitted to an intensive care unit are ultimately discharged from the hospital.

Diabetic Ketoacidosis

EPIDEMIOLOGY AND PATHOBIOLOGY

Diabetic ketoacidosis is defined as hyperglycemia with metabolic acidosis resulting from generation of the acids of the anions β-hydroxybutyrate (a hydroxy acid) and acetoacetate (a ketoacid) in response to insulin deficiency and elevated counter-regulatory hormones such as glucagon.[11] It is most commonly seen in cases of type 1 diabetes mellitus but can occasionally be seen in type 2 diabetes mellitus (Chapter 210). Diabetic ketoacidosis is more common in vulnerable populations with less access to quality medical care.

The lack of insulin increases lipolysis in adipose tissue; free fatty acids are transported to the liver, where hepatic mitochondria produce ketoacid anions, including acetoacetate, from acetyl coenzyme A. In the presence of high NADH/NAD ratio, the more reduced form of β-hydroxybutyrate is produced.

CLINICAL MANIFESTATIONS

Symptoms include nausea, vomiting, anorexia, polydipsia, and polyuria. Patients often exhibit Kussmaul respirations and volume depletion. Neurologic symptoms include fatigue and lethargy with depression of the sensorium. CSF exhibits a change in acid-base status with treatment of diabetic ketoacidosis. Even without bicarbonate administration, CSF pH falls as a result of the ventilatory response to the correction of acidosis and the sudden rise in P_{CO_2}. However, no correlation between decreased CSF pH and depression of sensorium has been established. Ketoacidosis is also seen in cases of starvation, in which it is generally mild and not associated with hyperglycemia.

Ketoacid anions in the urine may be accompanied by cations, including sodium and potassium, thereby contributing to an osmotic diuresis with depletion of volume and potassium. The overall electrolyte status in diabetic ketoacidosis may be relative chloride retention, a mixed anion gap, and hyperchloremic acidosis. The delta HCO_3^- may exceed the delta anion gap, especially if the glomerular filtration rate and the filtered load of ketoacid anions are high, thereby facilitating their excretion with sodium and potassium. The serum anion gap in general will be greatest when renal failure is present because the additional anions cannot be cleared from extracellular fluid.

DIAGNOSIS

The urinary dipstick nitroprusside test for ketones may underestimate the degree of ketosis because it does not detect β-hydroxybutyrate; in fact, the ketone test result may become more positive as treatment helps metabolize β-hydroxybutyrate to acetoacetate. This problem should be addressed by direct measurement of serum β-hydroxybutyrate. Diabetic patients also are more prone to lactic acidosis because an increase in NADH favors the formation of lactate from pyruvate, and pyruvate dehydrogenase is inhibited in the absence of insulin.

TREATMENT

Treatment of diabetic ketoacidosis (Chapter 210) consists of volume repletion, insulin administration with dextrose if necessary to avoid hypoglycemia, and potassium replacement (Chapter 103). Bicarbonate administration should be considered only if ketoacidosis is accompanied by shock or if arterial pH is less than 7.0 or 7.1, and bolus infusion should be avoided. The administration of bicarbonate occasionally results in cerebral edema significant enough to lead to loss of consciousness and even death.

PROGNOSIS

Most patients with diabetic ketoacidosis recover. In the less than 0.5% of patients who present with coma from cerebral edema, the mortality rate ranges from 20% to as high as 90%. The cerebral edema may be exacerbated by bicarbonate administration, which is discouraged in this situation.

Salicylate Intoxication

EPIDEMIOLOGY AND PATHOBIOLOGY

Salicylate intoxication can be caused by accidental overdose, therapeutic overdose, or a suicide attempt (Chapters 70 and 96).[12] Salicylate functions as an uncoupler of oxidative phosphorylation and consequently results in increased oxygen consumption and production of CO_2, as well as production of mixed organic acid, thereby causing an anion gap metabolic acidosis. However, the increase in alveolar ventilation resulting from stimulation of central chemoreceptors overcomes this increase in CO_2.

CLINICAL MANIFESTATIONS AND DIAGNOSIS

The most common clinical manifestation is a combined anion gap metabolic acidosis and respiratory alkalosis, although the condition also can be manifested as either one or the other only. Children are often seen with metabolic acidosis, whereas adults often have predominant respiratory alkalosis. Hypoglycemia, ketoacidosis, and lactic acidosis may result. Other manifestations of intoxication include hemorrhage, fever, nausea and vomiting, hyperventilation, diaphoresis, tinnitus, and occasionally polyuria followed by oliguria. Severe cases may lead to seizures, respiratory depression, and coma. Noncardiogenic pulmonary edema is sometimes seen in adults.

Respiratory alkalosis is the result of a direct stimulatory effect of salicylate on the medullary respiratory control center. Salicylate intoxication also increases the metabolic rate. Diagnosis is suspected by the clinical presentation and confirmed by the salicylate level (Chapters 70 and 96).

Treatment of salicylate intoxication (Chapter 96) is aimed at correction of the metabolic acidosis and removal of salicylate. Bicarbonate as a sodium salt should be administered according to an estimated calculation of the deficit if metabolic acidosis predominates. Salicylates are removed by alkaline diuresis because the less reabsorbable salicylate anion will predominate when the urine pH increases. Urinary alkalinization with acetazolamide should be used cautiously because carbonic anhydrase inhibition may impair CO_2 transport from tissue to blood and potentially worsen acidosis in the respiratory center. In severe intoxication (salicylate concentrations greater than 35 80 mg/dL) or when renal failure is present, dialysis may be required.

PROGNOSIS

The prognosis of salicylate toxicity is better with early diagnosis and prompt management, in which case most patients do well. Patients who ingest oil of wintergreen (methyl salicylate) may have more severe deterioration because of the high lipid solubility of the drug.

Alcoholic Ketoacidosis

EPIDEMIOLOGY AND PATHOBIOLOGY

Alcoholic ketoacidosis occurs in a patient who has been drinking very heavily without eating.[13] The pathophysiologic mechanism is based on the overproduction of the acids of β-hydroxybutyrate and, to a lesser extent, acetoacetate because of an increased production of free fatty acids from adipose tissue. Alcohol inhibits the conversion of lactate to glucose in the liver. The oxidation of ethanol increases the ratio of NADH to NAD^+ and favors the production of β-hydroxybutyrate from acetoacetate. Damage to mitochondria by alcohol can further elevate the ratio of β-hydroxybutyrate to acetoacetate by preventing reoxidation of NADH to NAD. The oxidative metabolism of ethanol favors the reaction of dehydrogenase enzymes to form β-hydroxybutyrate and lactate (opposing glucose production).

CLINICAL MANIFESTATIONS

Alcoholic ketoacidosis usually follows binge drinking and may be associated with withdrawal symptoms (Chapters 364 and 384) and the associated hyperadrenergic state. Alcoholic ketoacidosis is associated with abdominal pain, vomiting, starvation, and volume depletion. In contrast to diabetic ketoacidosis, coma is rare. Blood glucose levels are generally low or normal, and the insulin level is frequently low, with elevated glucagon (favoring ketogenesis) and cortisol levels. Some patients have hyperglycemia because of the increased catecholamine response.

DIAGNOSIS

Initially, patients typically have a high osmolar gap from ethanol or acetone. When serum alcohol or acetone levels become zero, the osmolar gap should disappear. A clue to the diagnosis of toxic alcohol ingestion is the simultaneous presence of an anion gap metabolic acidosis and an osmolar gap. The osmolar gap, if due to ethanol, should equal the ethanol concentration in milligrams per deciliter divided by 4.6. If this calculation does not yield the expected gap based on the ethanol level, ingestion of another alcohol, such as methanol, isopropanol, or ethylene glycol, should be suspected (see Table 104-2).

If possible, ethanol, ethylene glycol, propylene glycol, and methanol levels should be measured directly; each is associated with a metabolic acidosis. In contrast, isopropanol metabolizes to acetone and causes ketosis without acidosis. An osmolar gap may be present.

TREATMENT

Treatment of alcoholic metabolic acidosis consists of volume repletion with normal saline in dextrose; administration of thiamine (50 to 100 mg); treatment of hypoglycemia; and the correction of any hypophosphatemia (Chapter 105), hypokalemia (Chapter 103), and hypomagnesemia (Chapter 105) that may be present. The acid-base disturbance usually resolves after several hours. Both hypophosphatemia and thiamine deficiency, which may not be apparent until 12 to 24 hours after the initiation of treatment in an undernourished patient, are exacerbated by glucose administration and may contribute to an associated lactic acidosis.

PROGNOSIS

The prognosis of alcoholic ketoacidosis is usually favorable. The long-term outlook is more closely tied to other complications of continued alcohol abuse.

5-Oxoprolinuria

5-Oxoprolinuria, which is an acquired form of anion gap metabolic acidosis, is increasingly recognized in patients who have glutathione depletion associated with underlying chronic illness, malnutrition, diabetes, alcoholism, or cancer, especially in the context of a high therapeutic level or overdose of acetaminophen. It has been observed without concomitant hepatic failure. Glutathione, which is a tripeptide consisting of glutamate, cysteine, and glycine, has many functions, including protection from cellular toxins, combating of oxidative stress, and shuttling of amino acids into the cytosol by the γ-glutamyl transpeptidase pathway. Hereditary forms of 5-oxoprolinuria are associated with γ-glutamyl transpeptidase cycle enzyme deficiencies (5-oxoprolinase and glutathione synthase). The usual production of 5-oxoproline is by release of the transported amino acid from the γ-glutamyl–amino acid dipeptide. The enzyme 5-oxoprolinase re-forms glutamate to re-enter the cycle as glutamylcysteine. Acetaminophen causes further depletion of glutathione due to binding of an acetaminophen metabolite, *N*-acetyl-*p*-benzoquinone imine (NAPQI), to glutathione. Treatment with *N*-acetylcysteine, in doses similar to those used for acetaminophen toxicity (Chapter 96), should be considered to decrease further glutathione depletion.

Poisonings

A variety of acute poisonings (Chapter 96) can present as an anion gap acidosis.[14]

Ethylene Glycol

Ethylene glycol (Chapter 96) is commonly found in antifreeze and is used as an industrial solvent. It has a sweet taste, and patients occasionally ingest it as a substitute for ethanol. Although ethylene glycol itself is not particularly damaging, its highly toxic metabolites include the acids of glyoxylate and glycolate, oxalic acid, and ketoaldehydes. Glycolic acid appears to be primarily responsible for the metabolic acidosis observed in this condition. Further, glycolic acid may register as lactic acid in point-of-care measurements of whole blood by the lactic oxidase method, producing an artifactual high lactate level. However if an assay of lactate is performed in the laboratory by lactate dehydrogenase, the true lactate will be significantly less than the value from the lactic acid oxidase method. The difference between these two values, known as the lactate gap, represents glycolic acid.

Intoxication is characterized by profound CNS symptoms, including diplopia, seizures and coma, severe metabolic acidosis, cardiac failure, pulmonary failure, and renal failure. Patients are often dehydrated and hypernatremic because of osmotic diuresis from the renal excretion of the alcohol.

An increased anion gap is attributable to ethylene glycol metabolites. A high osmolar gap also will be present because of the uncharged alcohol. However, an osmolar gap may not be present if all of the alcohol has been converted to the toxic anionic forms. Calcium oxalate crystals in the urine may cause intratubular obstruction and inflammation with acute kidney injury. Treatment is aimed at rehydration with saline and correction of acidosis with $NaHCO_3$ based on an estimate of the bicarbonate deficit. When an osmolar gap exists, competitive inhibition of alcohol dehydrogenase should be initiated with fomepizole at a loading dose of 15 to 20 mg/kg intravenously in 100 mL normal saline during 30 minutes to 1 hour, followed by a maintenance dose of 10 mg/kg every 12 hours (Chapter 96). If ethanol is used, a solution of 10% ethanol in 5% dextrose can be given as a loading dose of 0.6 g/kg intravenously followed by a maintenance dose of 150 mg/kg per hour in alcoholic patients or 65 mg/kg per hour in nonalcoholic patients. The ethanol level should be maintained at 100 to 200 mg/dL. The goal of therapy is early recognition to prevent metabolism of the uncharged glycol to acidic products. Hemodialysis is required in severe cases. If the diagnosis is made promptly and appropriate therapy is instituted, outcomes are favorable. Renal failure may be reversible.

Methanol

Methanol, wood alcohol, is a component of shellac and windshield wiper fluid and is highly toxic to the CNS after metabolism to formaldehyde and formic acid. Some automotive fluids now contain the less toxic propylene glycol. Optic papillitis may cause blindness. Detection may be made easier if fluorescein has been added to the methanol-containing fluid.

Treatment consists of competitive inhibitors for alcohol dehydrogenase, including ethanol and fomepizole, in similar amounts as for ethylene glycol poisoning, to reduce the formation of acid anions and the anion gap while maintaining a higher level of methanol in the blood (Chapter 96). Hemodialysis may be necessary to increase elimination. Early diagnosis and treatment are associated with a favorable outcome, but visual loss may be permanent. Late presentation is associated with a poor prognosis, particularly if the amount consumed exceeds 30 mL. As with ethylene glycol, the simultaneous presence of ethanol on presentation may help slow the metabolism of methanol and improve outcome.

Isopropyl Alcohol

Toxic ingestion of isopropyl alcohol (Chapter 96), as in rubbing alcohol, does not cause an increased anion gap or ketoacidosis because the metabolite is acetone, but test results for ketones are positive, and a high osmolal gap will be present.

Propylene Glycol

On occasion, patients in the intensive care unit setting are given high doses of intravenous benzodiazepines, such as lorazepam or diazepam, that contain propylene glycol as a diluent. Other intravenous medications that also contain this diluent include phenobarbital, phenytoin, nitroglycerine, and esmolol. Propylene glycol also has been used as a less toxic substitute for methanol in windshield wiper fluid. A high osmolal gap may develop because of the propylene glycol and lead to a clinical picture of sedation, failure to be weaned from the respirator, and an increased lactate level. Propylene glycol can cause a severe lactic acidosis, and patients with this disorder can have a massive osmotic diuresis. Propylene glycol, a 3-carbon glycol, oxidizes to the acids of lactate and pyruvate. Treatment, which consists of early recognition and withdrawal of the offending agent, usually results in a favorable prognosis.

HYPERCHLOREMIC (NORMAL ANION GAP) ACIDOSIS

Hyperchloremic metabolic acidoses (see Table 104-1) can be caused by renal or nonrenal mechanisms and can be associated with an elevated, normal, or low serum potassium level (Fig. 104-2).

HYPERCHLOREMIC METABOLIC ACIDOSIS OF NONRENAL ORIGIN ASSOCIATED WITH NORMAL OR INCREASED POTASSIUM LEVEL

Hyperchloremic metabolic acidoses with a normal or elevated potassium concentration can develop with the administration of chloride salts such as NaCl, KCl, $CaCl_2$, NH_4Cl, arginine and lysine hydrochlorides, or HCl itself. If the quantity of Cl^- introduced exceeds the ability of the kidney to eliminate Cl^- salts in urine, hyperchloremia will develop. Electroneutrality is maintained by a decrease in the serum HCO_3^- concentration, and a hyperchloremic acidosis ensues. Renal production of NH_3 increases in an attempt to improve HCl (NH_4Cl) excretion. Hyperkalemia can occur because the acidemia favors the exit of K^+ from cells. Acidemia also inhibits K^+ secretion in the renal collecting duct.

HYPERCHLOREMIC METABOLIC ACIDOSIS OF NONRENAL ORIGIN ASSOCIATED WITH HYPOKALEMIA

Hypokalemic, hyperchloremic acidosis may result from loss of a body fluid that is low in Cl^- relative to Na^+ and K^+ compared with the ratio of Cl^- to Na^+ in extracellular fluid. For example, stool losses of Na^+, K^+, and HCO_3^- in small bowel diarrhea or organic acid anions of bacterial origin, such as butyrate, in colonic diarrhea lead to hyperchloremic acidosis (Chapter 126). Pancreatic secretions (Chapter 213) or heavy losses from ileostomy sites may lead to loss of bicarbonate-containing fluids. Secretagogues such as vasoactive intestinal peptide (VIP), which is associated with neoplasms of the pancreas or sympathetic chain (Chapter 213), cause large losses of HCO_3^- in stool, with a resulting hypokalemic, hyperchloremic metabolic acidosis. Concomitant gastric achlorhydria is part of the syndrome known as *watery diarrhea, hypokalemic, hypochlorhydric acidosis*. Urinary diversions, such as ureterosigmoidostomies and ileal loops, may increase chloride absorption in exchange for bicarbonate in the intestinal segment and lead to hyperchloremic acidosis. In the presence of urea-splitting bacteria, the net absorption of NH_4Cl can result in both hyperchloremic acidosis and hyperammonemia.

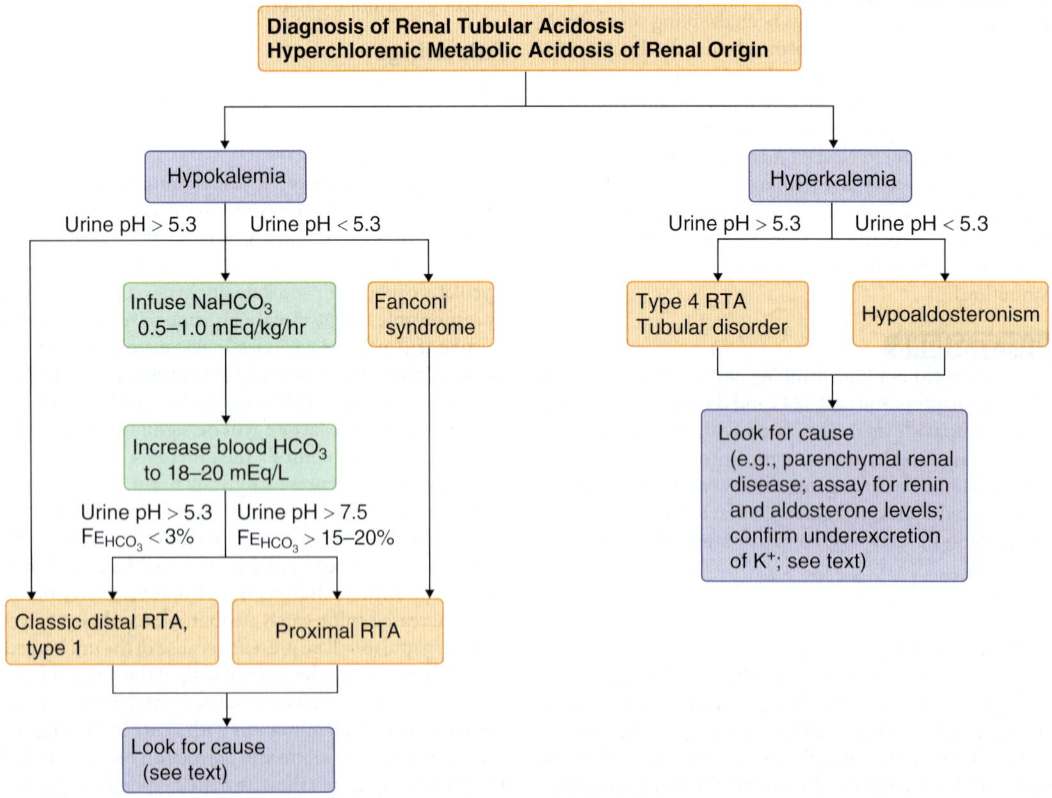

FIGURE 104-2. Evaluation of the patient with suspected renal tubular acidosis, hyperchloremic metabolic acidosis of renal origin. $FeHCO_3$ = fractional excretion of HCO_3^-; RTA = renal tubular acidosis.

RENAL TUBULAR ACIDOSIS TYPES 1 AND 2

Proximal Renal Tubular Acidosis

Renal tubular acidosis causes the cations Na^+ and K^+ to be lost in the urine with HCO_3^- rather than with Cl^-, thereby leading to hyperchloremia.[15] Proximal renal tubular acidosis (type 2) is characterized by a decreased threshold for bicarbonate reabsorption. HCO_3^- wasting and concomitant urinary losses of potassium occur until a lower level of serum bicarbonate reduces the filtered HCO_3^- to a level that the combined function of the dysfunctional proximal tubule and distal nephron can completely reabsorb. At that point, the urine becomes acid (pH < 5.3), and net acid production equals net acid excretion, with a steady-state low plasma HCO_3^-.

Isolated proximal renal tubular acidosis may result from mutations of specific transporters of the proximal tubule, such as the $NaHCO_3$ cotransporter, or from hereditary deficiency of carbonic anhydrase. More commonly, proximal renal tubular acidosis is associated with the Fanconi syndrome or generalized proximal tubule dysfunction. Causes (Table 104-7) include genetic diseases such as glucose-6-phosphatase deficiency (Chapter 147), cystinosis (Chapter 113), hereditary fructose intolerance (Chapter 189), and Wilson disease (Chapter 195). Multiple myeloma (Chapter 173) and Sjögren syndrome (Chapter 247) should be considered in an adult patient. Primary hyperparathyroidism (Chapter 227) results in proximal renal tubular acidosis and hypophosphatemia secondary to inhibition of Na^+/H^+ exchange and sodium phosphate cotransport in the proximal tubule by parathyroid hormone through cyclic adenosine monophosphate. Hyperparathyroidism is one of the few causes of metabolic acidosis with hypercalcemia. The Cl^-/phosphate ratio in plasma may be elevated. Drug toxicity with aminoglycosides, cisplatin, and ifosfamide may cause proximal tubule dysfunction. The antiretroviral drug tenofovir, a nucleotide analogue reverse transcriptase inhibitor, is a cause of the Fanconi syndrome. The syndrome also may be seen after kidney transplantation (Chapter 117).

Distal Renal Tubular Acidosis

In distal renal tubular acidosis (type 1), failure to excrete ammonium leads to an inability to excrete adequate net acid, thereby leading to continuous retention of acid in the body. The degree of acidemia is often severe, with pH reaching values as low as 7.2, whereas urine pH usually exceeds 5.3.[16]

Kindreds have been described in which mutations in genes for the distal vacuolar H^+-ATPase cause an autosomal recessive distal renal tubular acidosis with deafness. Mutations resulting in defective Cl^-/HCO_3^- exchange protein (AE1) have been linked to an autosomal dominant form of distal renal tubular acidosis.[17]

Distal renal tubular acidosis (see Table 104-7) is also associated with autoimmune disorders, including systemic lupus erythematosus (Chapter 245) and Sjögren syndrome (Chapter 247), and genetic diseases, including sickle cell anemia (Chapter 149), Wilson disease (Chapter 195), Fabry disease (Chapter 192), cystic kidney diseases (Chapter 112), and hereditary elliptocytosis (Chapter 147). Hypercalciuria and hyperoxaluria may cause distal renal tubular acidosis; nephrocalcinosis and nephrolithiasis may be present. Increased proximal tubular citrate reabsorption, as a consequence of the chronic acidosis, also leads to hypocitraturia, which is a risk factor for calcium nephrolithiasis (Chapter 111). A chronically alkaline urine is a risk for pure $CaHPO_4$ brushite stones and other calcium phosphate mixtures. Amyloidosis (Chapter 174) may be manifested as severe acidemia and other tubular dysfunction, including nephrogenic diabetes insipidus. Chronic tubulointerstitial diseases of the kidney (Chapter 108), including reflux nephropathy (Chapter 113) and urinary obstruction, may result in renal tubular acidosis with hypokalemia or hyperkalemia. Acute tubulointerstitial nephritis also may result in renal tubular acidosis. Drugs such as amphotericin B can cause hypokalemic distal renal tubular acidosis. Topiramate, used for migraines, is a carbonic anhydrase inhibitor that may cause mixed proximal and distal renal tubular acidosis.

HYPERCHLOREMIC METABOLIC ACIDOSIS OF RENAL ORIGIN ASSOCIATED WITH HYPERKALEMIA

Hyperkalemic, hyperchloremic acidosis (type 4) suggests dysfunction of the cortical collecting duct, where acidification of urine and disorders in potassium secretion may occur. Some patients with high blood potassium and hyperchloremic acidosis can lower urinary pH below 5.3, whereas others appear to have defects in both potassium balance and urinary acidification. Hyperkalemia itself may worsen metabolic acidosis by decreasing NH_3 accumulation by countercurrent multiplication in the medullary interstitium.

Causes include hyporenin-hypoaldosteronism, as seen in diabetic renal disease (Chapter 109); other tubulointerstitial diseases (Chapter 108), usually with some renal impairment; sickle cell anemia (Chapter 149); and the use of drugs such as β-blockers and nonsteroidal anti-inflammatory drugs. Low renin and aldosterone levels also can be found in cases of volume expansion with hypertension. Cyclosporine and tacrolimus may lead to decreased electrical driving forces for K^+ and H^+ secretion. Hyperkalemic acidosis with elevated renin and low aldosterone is found in adrenal insufficiency (Chapter 208), in isolated hypoaldosteronism (Chapter 208), and with the use of angiotensin-converting enzyme inhibitors, renin inhibitors, and angiotensin II receptor blockers. High renin and aldosterone levels are anticipated when the renal collecting duct cell is insensitive to aldosterone, as in urinary tract obstruction, sickle cell anemia, amyloidosis, and systemic lupus erythematosus. Inhibition of aldosterone action with spironolactone or eplerenone may cause hyperkalemic acidosis, as does ENaC inhibition by amiloride, triamterene, trimethoprim, and lithium.

Autosomal recessive pseudohypoaldosteronism type 1 is due to inactivating mutations of the sodium channel ENaC, whereas autosomal dominant pseudohypoaldosteronism type 1 is due to mutations of the mineralocorticoid receptor. Both cause hypovolemia, metabolic acidosis, and hyperkalemia with secondary increases in renin and aldosterone. In Gordon syndrome

TABLE 104-7 CAUSES OF RENAL TUBULAR ACIDOSIS*

HYPOKALEMIC DISTAL (TYPE 1) RTA
Hereditary tubule disorders
Vacuolar H^+-ATPase β-subunit gene mutations
Carbonic anhydrase type II deficiency
Cl^-/HCO_3^- exchanger (AE1) mutations
Genetic causes
Sickle cell anemia
Fabry disease
Wilson disease
Elliptocytosis
Paroxysmal nocturnal hemoglobinuria
Medullary cystic kidneys
Autoimmune disorders
Systemic lupus erythematosus
Sjögren syndrome
Multiple myeloma and amyloidosis
Drugs: amphotericin, cisplatinum, aminoglycosides
Nephrocalcinosis and hypercalcemic disorders
Tubulointerstitial diseases
Acute tubulointerstitial nephritis
Reflux nephropathy
Analgesic nephropathy
PROXIMAL (TYPE 2) RTA
Hereditary tubule disorders
$NaHCO_3$ cotransport (NBC) mutations
Carbonic anhydrase deficiency
Generalized proximal tubular dysfunction
Hereditary Fanconi syndrome
Genetic diseases: cystinosis, glycogen storage disease (glucose-6-phosphatase deficiency), Wilson disease
Hormonal: hyperparathyroidism, vitamin D deficiency
Multiple myeloma
Lysozymuria
Sjögren syndrome
Renal transplantation
Heavy metals: cobalt, mercury, lead
Drugs: ifosfamide, outdated tetracycline, tenofovir, tacrolimus, aminoglycosides
HYPERKALEMIC (TYPE 4) RTA
Renal diseases—aldosterone resistance
Diabetes mellitus
Amyloidosis
Systemic lupus erythematosus
Urinary tract obstruction
Hyporeninism
Autonomic neuropathy (diabetic)
Sickle cell anemia
Primary hypoaldosteronism
Adrenal insufficiency: Addison disease
Genetic disorders: pseudohypoaldosteronism
Drugs: potassium-sparing diuretics, amiloride, triamterene, spironolactone, nonsteroidal anti-inflammatory drugs, lithium, trimethoprim, cyclosporine, tacrolimus, renin inhibitors, angiotensin-converting enzyme inhibitors, angiotensin II receptor antagonists

*Type 3 renal tubular acidosis (RTA) is not listed separately because it is an overlap of proximal and distal dysfunction. Pure aldosterone deficiency will decrease the secretion of H^+ and K^+, thereby causing hyperkalemic acidosis. Also, renal diseases involving tubular cells may result in decreased urinary secretion of acid and potassium.

(pseudohypoaldosteronism type 2), increases in Na^+ and Cl^- reabsorption through increased activity of the distal thiazide-sensitive NaCl transporter lead to hypertension, hyperkalemic acidosis, volume expansion, and consequently low renin and aldosterone.

CLINICAL MANIFESTATIONS AND DIAGNOSIS

The urinary anion, or charge, gap helps distinguish renal tubular acidosis from extrarenal bicarbonate loss (e.g., from diarrhea).[18] Because the normal renal response to metabolic acidosis is an increase in ammoniagenesis, the urine should contain large amounts of NH_4Cl while the kidney retains sodium and potassium; the urinary charge gap, which is $(Na^+ + K^+) - Cl^-$, should be strongly negative because of the unmeasured NH_4^+.

In renal diseases such as distal renal tubular acidosis, however, the urinary anion gap will be zero or positive because of either inadequate excretion of ammonium or the excretion of sodium plus potassium with bicarbonate. With type 2 (proximal) renal tubular acidosis, patients often have Fanconi syndrome with glycosuria, phosphaturia, aminoaciduria, and uricosuria. In proximal renal tubular acidosis, the steady-state urine pH is usually less than 5.3, the acidosis is not severe (i.e., HCO_3^- usually not less than 16), and acid excretion may balance acid production at this new steady state.

In contrast to proximal renal tubular acidosis, distal renal tubular acidosis (type 1) is generally a more severe metabolic disorder that may be accompanied by hypercalciuria, nephrocalcinosis, calcium phosphate kidney stones (Chapter 111), and bone disease that includes rickets in children and osteomalacia in adults. Proximal and distal renal tubular acidoses usually can be distinguished by a careful clinical evaluation (see Fig. 104-2). Helpful findings include the presence of a urine pH greater than 5.3 in distal but not in proximal renal tubular acidosis during acidemia; a fractional excretion of bicarbonate as high as 10 to 15% in proximal renal tubular acidosis treated with alkali supplementation; and the lowering of serum potassium on correction of proximal but not of distal tubular acidosis.

In patients with an elevated serum anion gap, unmeasured anions such as keto acids and lactate, rather than NH_4^+, are present in urine, so a positive urinary anion gap does not indicate renal tubular acidosis. On occasion, the prompt renal excretion of organic anions with sodium and potassium may minimize the increase in the serum anion gap. In the metabolic acidosis of glue sniffers, hippurate, which is a product of toluene, is rapidly excreted, thus giving the appearance of a nongap metabolic acidosis with a positive urinary anion gap and mimicking a renal tubular acidosis. Similarly, if keto acids are completely cleared into the urine, ketoacidosis may be manifested as a hyperchloremic acidosis rather than as an anion gap acidosis.

TREATMENT

If possible, treatment of metabolic acidosis should focus on correction of the underlying cause, such as discontinuation of an offending drug, permitting the body's homeostatic mechanisms to correct the acid-base disturbance.[19]

Patients whose pH is less than 7.2 are typically treated with infusions of sodium bicarbonate,[20] guided by the estimated base deficit in milliequivalents, calculated by the serum HCO_3^- concentration in milliequivalents per liter:

$$\text{Amount of } HCO_3^- = (25 - [HCO_3^-]) \times \text{wt (kg)}/2$$

Such treatment appears to be especially beneficial in patients with acute kidney injury.[A1] In general, the correction of metabolic acidemia should be based on a calculated amount, with not more than 50% of the estimate given before recalculation. Moreover, this equation is used for deficit correction only; the ongoing losses of 1 to 2 mEq/kg per day, equivalent to the daily acid load, should be replaced in distal renal tubular acidosis with $NaHCO_3$ or $KHCO_3$, (depending on whether the patient has hypokalemia or hyperkalemia). Citrate salts (e.g., potassium citrate 60 to 90 mEq/day in divided doses) may be used to achieve a goal serum bicarbonate level of 22 to 24 mEq/L. Hypokalemia may accompany distal renal tubular acidosis and may improve with treatment. Citrate should be avoided as an alkalinizing salt in patients with low glomerular filtration rates because it may increase the gastrointestinal absorption of aluminum.

Proximal renal tubular acidosis in children may affect growth and require large quantities of bicarbonate in excess of 1 to 2 mEq/kg per day to correct the acidosis because ingested alkali is promptly excreted in alkaline urine. In adults, treatment is often deferred because the steady-state acidosis allows a normal acid excretion rate. Hypokalemia may worsen with bicarbonate treatment of proximal tubular acidosis.

In type 4 renal tubular acidosis, treatment of hyperkalemia with a low-potassium diet, thiazide or loop diuretics, or potassium-binding resins often improves urinary acidification without the use of bicarbonate salts. However, base supplements in the form of sodium bicarbonate or sodium citrate (0.5 to 0.8 mEq/kg, or 30 to 60 mEq per day) plus a diuretic aid in the excretion of potassium.

PROGNOSIS

The prognosis of renal tubular acidosis generally depends on the presence of an underlying systemic disease, such as myeloma (Chapter 173). In children, disorders such as medullary cystic kidney disease (Chapter 112) and cystinosis (Chapter 113) usually result in renal failure by the teenage years. These patients are candidates for renal replacement therapy, including transplantation. Chronic metabolic acidosis in children, if not well treated, is associated with rickets (Chapter 226) and short stature.

METABOLIC ALKALOSIS

EPIDEMIOLOGY AND PATHOBIOLOGY

In metabolic alkalosis, the primary event is elevation of the plasma bicarbonate concentration. In response to increased systemic pH, alveolar ventilation is decreased to increase P_{CO_2} and thereby decrease pH.[21] However, respiratory compensation is generally less effective in cases of metabolic alkalosis than in cases of metabolic acidosis. Contributing factors may include the fact that hypoventilation also decreases P_{O_2}, which is a potent stimulus for the peripheral chemoreceptors to increase alveolar ventilation when P_{O_2} falls below about 60 mm Hg. A second mechanism that may blunt respiratory compensation is intracellular acidosis in the brain in the setting of hypokalemia. In acute metabolic alkalosis, an initial paradoxical acidotic shift in CSF pH secondary to a sudden increase in P_{CO_2}, analogous to the alkaline shift in CSF pH in acute metabolic acidosis, may activate central chemoreceptors and increase ventilatory drive despite peripheral stimulation to decrease alveolar ventilation. In chronic metabolic alkalosis, CSF pH may return to normal, so respiratory drive is controlled entirely by the peripheral chemoreceptors. The result is that the ventilatory response to metabolic alkalosis is highly varied: many patients with metabolic alkalosis maintain nearly normal P_{CO_2} levels, and the level rarely rises above 60 mm Hg.

In the normal state, the renal response to metabolic alkalosis is greater filtration of bicarbonate, less proximal reabsorption of bicarbonate, and bicarbonate secretion in exchange for chloride. Metabolic alkalosis requires a generation phase, in which new HCO_3^- is added to the extracellular fluid, and a maintenance phase, in which the new elevated serum HCO_3^- concentration is sustained. Without the maintenance phase, a kidney with normal filtration and tubular function has a high capacity to excrete HCO_3^-, thereby preventing alkalosis. Maintenance of a high HCO_3^- concentration usually occurs because of volume depletion, reduced glomerular filtration rate, hypokalemia, or low chloride levels.

METABOLIC ALKALOSIS OF RENAL ORIGIN ASSOCIATED WITH VOLUME DEPLETION

Generation of metabolic alkalosis by the kidney can result from reduced renal tubular NaCl reabsorption due to diuretics or inherited disorders (e.g., Bartter or Gitelman syndromes). Metabolic alkalosis is usually associated with high urinary chloride levels, especially when diuretics inhibit reabsorption of Cl^- salts. The Cl^- loss results in hypochloremia, with a compensatory increase in plasma HCO_3^- to maintain electroneutrality. Extracellular volume depletion stimulates the renin–angiotensin–aldosterone pathway, and high aldosterone levels superimposed on increased distal Na delivery and urinary flow rates result in increased secretion of K^+, H^+, and $NH4^+$, with hypokalemia and hypokalemic metabolic alkalosis. The volume depletion and hypokalemia enhance proximal reabsorption of HCO_3^-, thereby maintaining the alkalosis, and the prerenal fall in the glomerular filtration rate limits the filtration of HCO_3^-.

Genetic syndromes characterized by urinary sodium chloride wasting include Bartter syndrome and Gitelman syndrome (Chapter 113). Bartter syndrome is an autosomal recessive salt-losing state associated with extracellular volume depletion and excessive urinary chloride loss that results in hypokalemia and hypochloremic metabolic alkalosis. Secondary increases of plasma renin and aldosterone occur, as does renal juxtaglomerular cell hyperplasia. The syndrome resembles the effects of furosemide on the thick ascending limb of Henle; gene mutations in the Na-K-2Cl cotransporter, the renal outer medullary potassium channel (ROMK), and voltage-gated CLC-Kb chloride channels mediating NaCl reabsorption have been described. Because calcium reabsorption occurs in the thick ascending limb of Henle, Bartter syndrome (Chapter 113), like furosemide, causes hypercalciuria and nephrocalcinosis as well as polyuria due to decreased urinary concentrating ability.

Gitelman syndrome is an autosomal recessive cause of extracellular volume depletion, urinary wasting of sodium chloride, and hypokalemic metabolic alkalosis. It is due to inactivating mutations in the *SLC12A3* gene encoding the thiazide-sensitive NaCl cotransporter of the renal distal tubule. Urinary concentrating ability is preserved, and patients are hypocalciuric because decreased

NaCl reabsorption in the distal tubule and volume depletion enhance the reabsorption of Ca^+ in the proximal tubule. Hypomagnesemia also may be severe owing to defective Mg^{2+} reabsorption in the distal convoluted tubule.

METABOLIC ALKALOSIS OF NONRENAL ORIGIN WITH EXTRACELLULAR VOLUME DEPLETION

Metabolic alkalosis may develop as a result of gastrointestinal loss of Cl^- or gain of HCO_3^- owing to vomiting, nasogastric suctioning, or some causes of secretory diarrhea. In such cases, extracellular volume is usually contracted, hypochloremia develops, and the urinary chloride level is usually less than 20 mEq/L.

In Zollinger-Ellison syndrome (Chapter 213), excessive gastrin-induced gastric acid secretion may result in an acidic stool with high chloride content. Diarrhea does not cause metabolic alkalosis unless the electrolyte relationship $[(Na^+ + K^+) - Cl^-]$ in the stool is less than plasma HCO_3^-.

Infectious gastroenteritis, congenital chloridorrhea, and villous adenomas also cause chloride losses in stool. Congenital chloridorrhea is an autosomal recessive disorder of defective intestinal apical Cl^-/HCO_3^- exchange associated with the downregulated adenoma *(DRA)* gene.

With vomiting, the initiating event is loss of HCl. This secretion of HCl into the stomach lumen by the parietal cell is coupled to the absorption of HCO_3^- in exchange for chloride at the basolateral membrane. When gastric acid is normally secreted, a mild increase in serum HCO_3^- spills into urine and causes an "alkaline tide." With vomiting, however, the net loss of HCl generates the alkalosis. With vomiting, the increased HCO_3^- is filtered by the glomeruli and excreted in urine, accompanied by Na^+ and K^+; volume and K^+ begin to be depleted. As vomiting continues, extracellular volume depletion worsens, glomerular filtration falls, HCO_3^- filtration is limited, the renin–angiotensin II–aldosterone system is stimulated, proximal reabsorption of fluid and HCO_3^- increases, distal reabsorption of Na^+ increases under the influence of aldosterone, and greater secretion of H^+ enhances the reabsorption of HCO_3^-. These effects reduce renal Na^+ loss but at the expense of maintaining the metabolic alkalosis. Significant urinary K^+ losses, which occur as a result of the bicarbonaturia and hyperaldosteronism, lead to hypokalemia, which is actually due to renal, not gastrointestinal, losses as a consequence of attempts to maintain extracellular volume. The hypokalemia further increases the proximal reabsorption of $NaHCO_3$, the distal secretion of H^+, and the reabsorption of K^+, all at the expense of further reabsorption of HCO_3^-. In the new steady state after vomiting or nasogastric suctioning ceases, the paradoxical aciduria of metabolic alkalosis develops as the reabsorption of HCO_3^- is complete, and the urine contains low levels of Na^+, K^+, and Cl^-. The patient may be hypovolemic, hypokalemic, and alkalemic, but because Na^+, K^+, and acid-base balance are intrinsically linked, life-threatening volume depletion, potassium depletion, and alkalemia are usually avoided.

Most nonrenal metabolic alkaloses with volume depletion are due to gastrointestinal losses. However, some patients with cystic fibrosis (Chapter 77) may develop hypochloremic alkalosis as a consequence of excessive sweat chloride related to the *CFTR* gene mutation.

The sweat gland, like the principal cell in the kidney, contains the aldosterone-sensitive epithelial sodium channel, so Na^+ absorption from the glandular duct renders the lumen electronegative. When the absorption of Cl^- is decreased in cystic fibrosis (Chapter 77), the lumen becomes more negative, thereby decreasing the absorption of Na^+, Cl^-, and fluid, as well as leading to salty sweat; the proportionally large Cl^- loss generates a hypochloremic metabolic alkalosis.

METABOLIC ALKALOSIS OF RENAL ORIGIN WITH VOLUME EXPANSION AND HYPERTENSION

The renal conditions that cause metabolic alkalosis and volume expansion are due to a proportionately greater increase in Na^+ reabsorption above what is required to maintain a steady state of Na^+ balance, rather than primary loss of the Cl^- anion. As Na^+ is reabsorbed, electroneutrality is maintained by an increase in plasma HCO_3^-. Cl^- appears in urine, but hypochloremia is not present except in cases of significant metabolic alkalosis. In the kidney, the loss of net acid as NH_4Cl in excess of the acid produced generates a metabolic alkalosis, in which the new bicarbonate generated is due to proton secretion by the distal nephron through H^+-ATPases. The H^+ then combines with NH_3 to form NH_4^+ in urine.

Na^+ is reabsorbed independently of Cl^- in the cortical collecting duct through the aldosterone-sensitive cells containing the ENaC. When Na^+ is reabsorbed by the principal cells of the cortical collecting duct, the tubular lumen becomes electronegative and stimulates the secretion of both K^+ and H^+ by the electrogenic H^+-ATPases. To the extent that HCO_3^- remains in the lumen, the secreted protons complete the reabsorption of HCO_3^-. Additional secreted protons combine with NH_3 and phosphates to lead to net acid excretion. Any increase in the distal H^+ secretory mechanism will produce more urinary net acid; more new HCO_3^- will be generated and returned to the now expanded extracellular fluid, and metabolic alkalosis will develop. The increased plasma HCO_3^- will be filtered, but in the absence of a stimulus to increase proximal HCO_3^- reabsorption, the HCO_3^- will flow distally to be reabsorbed by the increased secretion of H^+ in the collecting duct. At first, the alkalosis is mild, but increased Na^+ reabsorption in the cortical collecting duct will also lead to increased K^+ secretion and hypokalemia. Hypokalemia increases the capacity for the proximal reabsorption of HCO_3^-, thereby opposing the effect of volume expansion, so that the distal delivery of HCO_3^- decreases. The higher than normal distal H^+ secretion titrates urinary buffers, so further new HCO_3^- is formed in the presence of the high ENaC activity, thereby allowing the alkalosis to worsen. The alkalosis is maintained at a new steady state only when the distal secretion of H^+ results in the reabsorption of the remaining amount of filtered HCO_3^- in the collecting duct. Metabolic alkalosis in the hypermineralocorticoid syndromes is sustained by hypokalemia. The metabolic alkalosis in these syndromes is only mild if the patient is K^+ replete.

METABOLIC ALKALOSIS OF NONRENAL ORIGIN ASSOCIATED WITH NORMAL OR EXPANDED VOLUME

If an alkalotic patient is not hypochloremic, electroneutrality must be maintained either by depletion of an alternative anion or by an excessive concentration of a cation. An example of a metabolic alkalosis associated with depletion of a non-chloride anion is hypoproteinemic alkalosis, with hypoalbuminemia and a small anion gap. Chloride balance is normal and chloride appears in urine.

Alkalosis also may result from the administration of alkali salts of HCO_3 or metabolizable organic anions. The normal response to the ingestion of $NaHCO_3$ is rapid urinary alkalinization because of an unaltered threshold for the reabsorption of HCO_3^-. However, a marked excess of HCO_3^-, as may be administered in an attempt to alkalinize a patient's urine, expands volume and causes an alkalemia, especially in the presence of volume depletion or low glomerular filtration. Milk-alkali syndrome, usually seen when patients in renal failure ingest milk, excess vitamin D, or calcium antacids, is associated with hypercalcemia and alkalemia. Other situations in which intake of alkali salts results in metabolic alkalosis include infusion of large quantities of sodium salts of metabolizable organic anions, such as acetate, citrate, lactate, or bicarbonate; hyperalimentation with acetate salts; chronic peritoneal dialysis with acetate or lactate dialysate; and excessive transfusions or plasmapheresis, in which large quantities of citrate, used as an anticoagulant, are delivered.

CLINICAL MANIFESTATIONS

Mild metabolic alkalosis up to a pH of 7.50 is usually asymptomatic. When the pH exceeds 7.55, however, the alkalosis itself and the compensatory hypoventilation are frequently associated with metabolic encephalopathy. Symptoms include confusion, obtundation, delirium, and coma. The seizure threshold is lowered. Because more Ca^{2+} is protein-bound and less is ionized Ca^{2+}, tetany, paresthesias, muscle cramping, and other symptoms of low calcium are seen (Chapter 227). In patients with preexisting hypocalcemia, these signs may be seen at pH values above 7.45. Other findings include cardiac tachyarrhythmias and hypotension. The production of lactate increases as a result of the increased anaerobic glycolysis.

DIAGNOSIS

Measurement of urinary Cl can be very helpful in the diagnosis of the cause of metabolic alkalosis, and it is important to distinguish whether the condition is chloride responsive or chloride unresponsive. (See Table 104-2 and Fig. 104-3.) Chloride-responsive metabolic alkalosis with low urinary Cl^- is associated with depletion of extracellular fluid and chloride and is seen with loss of gastric fluid and prior use of diuretics. Chloride-responsive metabolic alkalosis with high urinary Cl^- is associated with Bartter or Gitelman syndrome or ongoing diuretic use. Chloride-unresponsive metabolic alkalosis with high urinary Cl^- is seen in volume-expanded states, such as primary hyperaldosteronism when metabolic alkalosis is primarily maintained by depletion of K^+. A diagnostic clue comes from the serum electrolytes. The HCO_3^- concentration is increased with a corresponding fall in serum chloride (hypochloremic alkalosis). Chloride-unresponsive metabolic alkalosis is seen in patients with extracellular fluid expansion in conditions such as primary aldosteronism and hypokalemia.

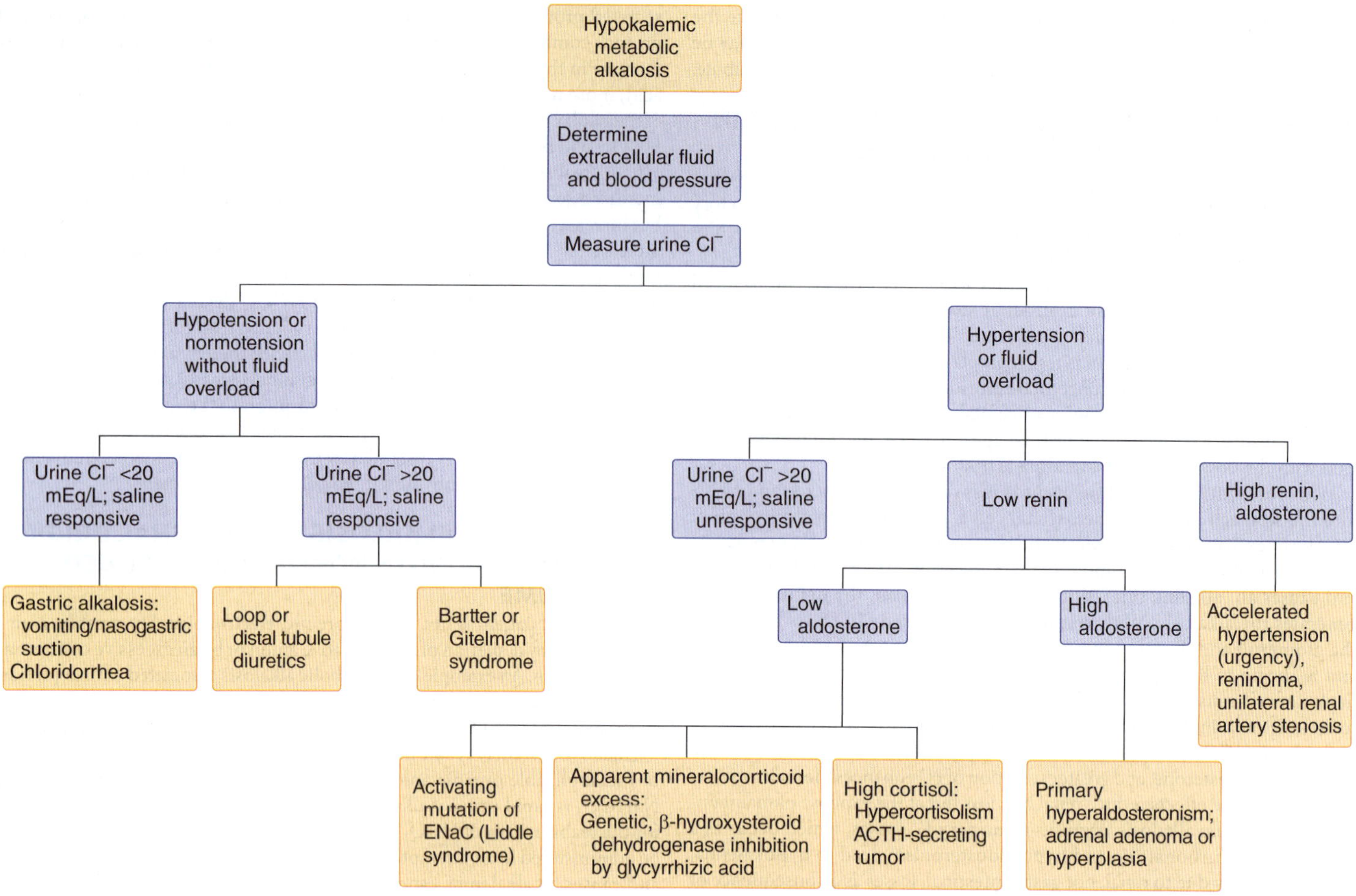

FIGURE 104-3. **Evaluation of the patient with hypokalemic metabolic alkalosis.** ACTH = adrenocorticotropic hormone; Cl = chloride; ENaC = epithelial sodium channel.

Vomiting, nasogastric suction, and diarrhea are usually obvious sources of metabolic alkalosis. However, the Zollinger-Ellison syndrome (Chapter 213), villous adenomas (Chapter 179), and VIPomas (Chapter 213) may be more difficult to diagnose unless the index of suspicion is high.

Patients who present with hypokalemic metabolic alkalosis (Fig. 104-3) with normal or low blood pressure and have urinary chloride concentrations above 25 mEq/L may be taking diuretics such as furosemide or thiazides surreptitiously; a diuretic screen can document the presence of the drug. If the screen is negative, Bartter or Gitelman syndrome (Chapter 113) should be considered. Bartter syndrome is less common, is usually more severe, and presents in young patients. The presence of hypercalciuria favors Bartter syndrome, whereas hypocalciuria and hypomagnesemia suggest Gitelman syndrome.

Specific causes of renal alkalosis with volume expansion and hypertension can be classified according to levels of renin and aldosterone. Primary increases in renin with secondary increases in aldosterone can be seen in patients with unilateral renal artery stenosis (Chapter 110), renin-secreting tumors of the kidney (Chapter 64), and malignant hypertension (Chapter 64). Low renin and elevated aldosterone levels are characteristic of primary hyperaldosteronism from an adrenal adenoma or hyperplasia (Chapter 208). A high cortisol level with volume expansion is seen in hypercortisolism and adrenocorticotropic hormone–secreting tumors (Chapter 208). Inhibition of the intracellular enzyme 11β-hydroxysteroid dehydrogenase type 2 will also result in low renin levels, low aldosterone levels, and hypokalemic alkalosis. Both genetic mutations (the apparent mineralocorticoid excess syndrome) and an excess consumption of glycyrrhizic acid found in licorice and anisette are causes of this enzymatic block. Another cause of hypertension with hypokalemic alkalosis but with low renin and aldosterone levels is Liddle syndrome (Chapter 113), in which an activating mutation in the cortical collecting duct sodium channel (ENaC) leads to increased Na^+ reabsorption.

Metabolic alkalosis may also develop without volume expansion when a non-reabsorbable anion is presented to the cortical collecting duct lumen. Nitrates, sulfates, and certain antibiotics such as nafcillin, carbenicillin, and ticarcillin may obligate the secretion of K^+ and H^+ as Na^+ is reabsorbed. Topical administration of silver nitrate to burn victims may result in alkalosis.

TREATMENT

In chloride-responsive patients who are volume-depleted, chloride-depleted, and most likely potassium-depleted (see Table 104-2), treatment is directed at ameliorating the factors that are maintaining the alkalosis. Providing saline and potassium chloride will increase bicarbonaturia and correct the metabolic alkalosis.[22] In patients with mild to moderate alkalosis, liberalizing NaCl intake and administering potassium chloride (20 to 80 mEq per day in divided doses) is effective in increasing the renal excretion of HCO_3^-. The K^+ deficit, though difficult to estimate from plasma [K^+], is likely to be at least 100 mEq for every 1 mEq/L decrease in plasma [K^+]. Unless potassium deficits are replenished simultaneously with extracellular volume expansion, the combination of increased bicarbonate filtration rate and an ongoing hypokalemia-induced increase in proximal tubular reabsorption of bicarbonate may severely worsen hypokalemia as bicarbonaturia develops and aldosterone's residual effects remain. Complete resolution of alkalosis will not occur until volume is restored and K^+ is normalized.

In a patient with renal failure and vomiting, the elevation in [HCO_3^-] may be more severe because of poor renal filtration of HCO_3^- and may require the administration of HCl or dialysis. If conditions such as volume expansion with decreased effective volume make the administration of NaCl unwise, potassium-sparing diuretics (Chapter 102) may help correct the alkalosis without increasing edema or potassium wasting. In the absence of renal failure, intravenous acetazolamide (250 to 500 mg every 8 hours) may be effective but may greatly increase renal losses of K^+. In patients who have edema and renal failure, acetazolamide treatment may be unsuccessful, so cautious administration of dilute solutions of HCl (0.1 N HCl) may be required. The amount of H^+, in milliequivalents, to be given may be calculated as the product of the desired change in serum HCO_3^- concentration (mEq/L) multiplied by 0.5 of body weight in kilograms. This calculation will likely overestimate the amount of acid needed for correction, so no more than one third of the amount should be given before recalculating to avoid metabolic acidosis. Full correction of HCO_3^- should not be the goal.

Chloride-unresponsive patients (see Table 104-2) include patients who have mineralocorticoid excess. In these patients, the metabolic alkalosis can be lessened by potassium replacement or by blocking Na^+ reabsorption with aldosterone antagonists such as spironolactone (starting with 25 mg orally) or amiloride (beginning with 5 mg orally). Indomethacin (75 mg per day) effectively treats Bartter syndrome (Chapter 113) by interfering with prostaglandin E_2 to allow greater reabsorption of NaCl in the thick ascending limb. Gitelman and Bartter syndromes are best treated with combinations of potassium chloride (40 to 160 mEq per day depending on the severity of the hypokalemia), a potassium-sparing diuretic (e.g., spironolactone 100 to 300 mg per day or eplerenone 150 mg per day), and magnesium if needed.

RESPIRATORY ACIDOSIS

Respiratory acidosis is characterized by a primary elevation in P_{CO_2} as reflected by reduced arterial pH with variable elevations in the HCO_3^- concentration. Respiratory acidosis is most frequently caused by a decrease in alveolar ventilation owing to pulmonary disease (Chapter 90), respiratory muscle fatigue, musculoskeletal abnormalities of the chest wall, or abnormalities in ventilatory control (Chapter 74).

CLINICAL MANIFESTATIONS

Clinical findings in respiratory acidosis are related to the degree and duration of the respiratory acidosis and whether hypoxemia is present. A precipitous rise in P_{CO_2} can lead to confusion, anxiety, psychosis, asterixis, seizures, and myoclonic jerks, with progressive depression of the sensorium and coma at an arterial P_{CO_2} greater than 60 mm Hg (CO_2 narcosis). Hypercapnia, which increases cerebral blood flow and volume, can lead to symptoms and signs of elevated intracranial pressure, including headaches and papilledema. Other findings in acute respiratory acidosis include signs of catecholamine release, such as skin flushing, diaphoresis, and increased cardiac contractility and output. Symptoms of chronic hypercapnia include fatigue, lethargy, and confusion, in addition to the findings seen in acute hypercapnia.

The slow time course of many of these diseases allows the kidney to compensate adequately by increasing its excretion of hydrogen ion as ammonium as well as by generating and reabsorbing bicarbonate to restore systemic pH toward normal values. This compensatory process is not maximal until 3 to 5 days after the onset of respiratory acidosis. Hypoxemia, hypercapnia with resulting chronic $NaHCO_3$ retention, and edema (cor pulmonale) often accompany chronic respiratory acidosis.

DIAGNOSIS

Disorders that cause a respiratory acidosis include central effects of drugs, strokes, and infections; airway obstruction; primary parenchymal processes, such as chronic obstructive pulmonary disease (Chapter 76) and acute respiratory distress syndrome (Chapter 90); disorders of ventilation (Chapter 74); and neuromuscular diseases, such as myasthenia gravis (Chapter 390) and muscular dystrophies (Chapter 389).

TREATMENT

Treatment of both chronic and acute respiratory acidosis aims primarily to correct the underlying cause and to ensure adequate ventilation. In acute respiratory acidosis, measures to relieve severe hypoxemia and acidemia should be instituted immediately, including intubation and assisted mechanical ventilation (Chapter 91) if necessary. Patients with myxedema coma require thyroid replacement (Chapter 207).

In patients with compensated chronic respiratory acidosis, rapid and complete correction of hypercapnia can result in post-hypercapnic metabolic alkalosis. Patients who are chronically hypercapnic and hypoxemic should receive necessary oxygen even though their P_{CO_2} will rise. The rise is not necessarily due to loss of a hypoxic drive to ventilation but may instead be because of release of CO_2 from hemoglobin in the presence of oxygen or because oxygen-induced pulmonary arteriolar vasodilation increases perfusion to poorly ventilated alveoli. Patients recovering from an acute-on-chronic respiratory acidosis should be monitored carefully to correct hypokalemia, hypochloremia, and hypovolemia so that adequate renal excretion of bicarbonate can occur.

Bicarbonate therapy is not indicated for respiratory acidosis unless the pH falls below 7.0 and the patient is about to be intubated.[23] Bicarbonate therapy has no role in patients with renal failure (Chapter 116), in whom adequate compensatory acid excretion cannot occur.

RESPIRATORY ALKALOSIS

EPIDEMIOLOGY AND PATHOBIOLOGY

In respiratory alkalosis, a primary decrease in P_{CO_2} is reflected by increases in the arterial pH and variable decreases in the plasma bicarbonate concentration. The most common cause is alveolar hyperventilation, not underproduction of CO_2.

Acute hypocapnia results in an initial increase in the pH of both the CSF and the brain's intracellular environment. The increased intracellular pH stimulates glycolysis, vasoconstriction, hypoxia, and an increased affinity of hemoglobin for oxygen, thereby offsetting the metabolic alkalosis by producing lactic acid. However, this increase in lactic acid is quickly offset because the renal compensation for decreased bicarbonate reabsorption will result in a lower blood bicarbonate level. The combination of increased oxygen demand and decreased oxygen delivery may contribute to adverse clinical outcomes in hypocapnic alkalosis.

Cerebral blood flow is significantly decreased by hypocapnia, which is a potent vasoconstrictor. As in respiratory acidosis, the CNS is immediately affected because of the blood-brain barrier's permeability to CO_2. In addition, as in respiratory acidosis, CSF and intracellular pH show an initial short-lived response that parallels the systemic increase in pH.

Renal compensation for sustained hypocapnia is complete in 36 to 72 hours. The mechanism rests primarily in the kidney's net reduction of hydrogen ion excretion, which is accomplished largely by decreasing the excretion of ammonium and titratable acid. The threshold for bicarbonate excretion is also lowered, and bicarbonaturia develops. As a result, systemic bicarbonate levels decrease, and arterial pH returns toward normal values.

Acute exposure to high altitude (Chapter 82) results in hypoxia-induced hyperventilation. Compensation requires several days and is characterized by a gradual further increase in hyperventilation, a steadily decreasing P_{CO_2}, and a recovering P_{O_2}. The effect of the hypoxic stimulus to ventilate is initially modulated by the effects of alkalosis, both peripherally and centrally. However, as HCO_3^- falls in the CSF, inhibition of the central stimulus to ventilate decreases. Once a steady state is achieved, the drive to ventilate is determined by the effects of hypoxemia and alkalemia on the peripheral chemoreceptors.

CLINICAL MANIFESTATIONS

The clinical manifestations of respiratory alkalosis depend on the degree and duration of the condition but are primarily those of the underlying disorder. Chronic hypocapnia does not appear to be associated with any significant clinical symptoms.

Symptoms of acute hypocapnia with P_{CO_2} below 30 mm Hg are largely attributable to the alkalemia and include dizziness, perioral or extremity paresthesias, confusion, asterixis, hypotension, seizures, and coma. Shortness of breath and chest wall pain, which frequently accompany hyperventilation because of pain or anxiety, do not appear to be related to hypocapnia itself.

DIAGNOSIS

Alveolar hyperventilation leading to respiratory alkalosis is seen with hypoxemia from pulmonary disease (Chapter 71), heart failure (Chapter 45), high altitudes (Chapter 82), or anemia. Mechanical ventilation (Chapter 91) is also a common cause of respiratory alkalosis. Rarely, patients have chronic hyperventilation syndrome without any detectable underlying disease.[24]

Another common cause of respiratory alkalosis is primary stimulation of the central chemoreceptor, as seen in sepsis (Chapter 94), hepatic cirrhosis (Chapter 139), salicylate intoxication (Chapters 70 and 96), correction of metabolic acidosis, hyperthermia (Chapter 95), and pregnancy, as well as cortical hyperventilation from anxiety and pain. In these situations, central signals override peripheral chemoreceptors until the primary stimulus is removed.

Primary neurologic diseases that can stimulate alveolar hyperventilation include acute stroke, infection, trauma, and tumors. Two patterns of respiration are seen: central hyperventilation and Cheyne-Stokes respiration (Chapter 74). Central hyperventilation, which is associated with lesions at the pontine-midbrain level, is regular but with an increased rate and tidal volume. Cheyne-Stokes breathing, which is characterized by periods of hyperventilation alternating with apnea, is seen in patients with bilateral cortical and upper pontine lesions and in patients with heart failure.

TREATMENT

Treatment of respiratory alkalosis must address the underlying cause of the disturbance. Hyperventilation syndrome is a diagnosis of exclusion, but patients who exhibit symptoms such as tetany and syncope and who do not have more serious causes of hyperventilation can be treated with a rebreathing mask. Hypophosphatemia can be seen, but usually improves with treatment of the alkalosis. Patients with respiratory alkalosis associated with mountain sickness can be pretreated with acetazolamide to induce metabolic acidosis (Chapter 82), thereby preventing extreme elevations in pH, but care must be taken to ensure adequate intake of K^+ to avoid hypokalemia.

GENERAL REFERENCES

For the General References and other additional features, please visit Elsevier eBooks+ at https://ebooks.health.elsevier.com.

Grade A Reference

A1. Jaber S, Paugam C, Futier E, et al. Sodium bicarbonate therapy for patients with severe metabolic acidaemia in the intensive care unit (BICAR-ICU): a multicentre, open-label, randomised controlled, phase 3 trial. *Lancet*. 2018;392:31-40.

105

DISORDERS OF MAGNESIUM AND PHOSPHORUS

ALAN S.L. YU

MAGNESIUM METABOLISM

Magnesium is an important mineral component of the bony skeleton, a cofactor for many metabolic enzymes, and a regulator of ion channels and transporters in excitable tissues.[1]

NORMAL MAGNESIUM METABOLISM

The majority of total body magnesium is intracellular or in bone, with only 1% in extracellular fluid. The normal serum magnesium concentration is 1.8 to 2.3 mg/dL (1.5 to 1.9 mEq/L). The average daily intake of magnesium is 300 mg, the main sources of which are green vegetables, nuts, whole grain cereals, milk, and seafood. Magnesium is absorbed mainly in the jejunum and ileum. In the kidney, 70 to 80% of serum magnesium is filtered at the glomerulus, with the majority being reabsorbed along the length of the tubule, particularly in the thick ascending limb of Henle. In states of magnesium deficiency or excess, renal tubule reabsorption is tightly regulated so that magnesium excretion is adjusted accordingly.[2]

MAGNESIUM DEFICIENCY

PATHOBIOLOGY

Magnesium deficiency is usually detected when hypomagnesemia becomes evident. However, because magnesium is stored primarily intracellularly, substantial depletion of total body magnesium can occur before serum magnesium levels drop appreciably.

Magnesium deficiency may be due to nutritional deficiency, intestinal malabsorption, redistribution into bone, or losses via cutaneous, lower gastrointestinal, or renal routes (Table 105-1). The recommended daily allowance of magnesium is 420 mg for males and 320 mg for females. Approximately 25% of alcoholics are chronically hypomagnesemic because of a combination of poor nutritional intake and increased renal loss. Magnesium deficiency can occur, rarely, in protein-calorie malnutrition and may be associated with acute hypomagnesemia during refeeding because of rapid cellular magnesium uptake. Fat malabsorption in conditions such as celiac disease, Crohn disease, and small intestinal resection causes magnesium deficiency because free fatty acids accumulate in the intestinal lumen, where they combine with magnesium to form insoluble soaps. Proton pump inhibitors also cause hypomagnesemia by inhibiting intestinal absorption, primarily in patients who are concurrently using diuretics.[3] Lower gastrointestinal tract secretions are rich in magnesium, so diarrhea of colonic origin is a common cause of hypomagnesemia. Sweat contains significant amounts of magnesium, and transient hypomagnesemia can occur after prolonged, intense exercise such as marathon runs. Magnesium is also lost from burned skin surfaces, and 40% of patients with severe burns (Chapter 97) are hypomagnesemic.

In patients with severe hyperparathyroidism (Chapter 227) and high bone turnover, continued sequestration of minerals within bone after parathyroidectomy causes transient hypocalcemia, hypomagnesemia, and hypophosphatemia. Renal magnesium losses can occur in the recovery phase of acute tubular necrosis or urinary tract obstruction. Hypomagnesemia is common in diabetes mellitus (Chapter 210), in which it is thought to be due to a combination of poor intestinal absorption, osmotic diuresis, and decreased renal tubule reabsorption. Inhibition of sodium reabsorption in the thick ascending limb of Henle by loop diuretics and in the distal convoluted tubule by thiazide diuretics inhibits tubular magnesium reabsorption and leads to urinary magnesium wasting. Tubular toxins that are common causes of renal magnesium wasting include cisplatin, carboplatin, amphotericin B, and aminoglycosides, which are often associated with hypokalemia and rarely with renal tubule acidosis, as well as calcineurin inhibitors such as cyclosporine and tacrolimus, which also cause hyperkalemia. Antibodies to the epidermal growth factor receptor, such as cetuximab and panitumumab, which are used to treat metastatic colorectal cancer, downregulate a distal tubule magnesium channel and cause isolated severe hypomagnesemia.

Inherited hypomagnesemia is usually caused by renal magnesium loss and can be subdivided into three main types, depending on the coexistence of other electrolyte disturbances: Bartter and Gitelman syndromes, which are associated with renal salt wasting and hypokalemic metabolic alkalosis; familial hypomagnesemia with hypercalciuria and nephrocalcinosis; and isolated hypomagnesemia, which is usually associated with hypocalcemia.

TABLE 105-1 CAUSES OF MAGNESIUM DEFICIENCY

Nutritional deficiency
Alcoholism*
Malnutrition
Refeeding syndrome
Intestinal malabsorption*
Proton pump inhibitors
Lower gastrointestinal losses
Colonic diarrhea*
Intestinal fistula
Laxative abuse
Cutaneous losses
Burns*
Exercise-induced sweating
Redistribution into bone
Hungry bone syndrome
Renal losses
Polyuria (including diabetes mellitus)*
Volume expansion
Hyperaldosteronism
Bartter and Gitelman syndromes
Hypercalcemia
Loop and thiazide diuretics*
Nephrotoxins (cisplatin, amphotericin, aminoglycosides, pentamidine, foscarnet, cyclosporine, tacrolimus)*
Epidermal growth factor monoclonal antibodies (cetuximab, panitumumab)*

*Common causes.

CLINICAL MANIFESTATIONS

Mild-to-moderate hypomagnesemia or magnesium deficiency is frequently asymptomatic. Manifestations of increased neuronal excitability are the most common symptoms, including paresthesias, tetany, and seizures. These may be associated with Chvostek sign (twitching of the cheek muscles in response to tapping the facial nerve in front of the ear) or Trousseau sign (carpal spasm induced by compressing the upper arm with a tourniquet or blood pressure cuff). Cardiac disturbances range from mild electrocardiographic abnormalities (nonspecific T wave changes, U waves, prolonged QT interval, and repolarization alternans) to ventricular tachycardia, torsades de pointes, and ventricular fibrillation (Chapter 53).

Coexistent hypokalemia is very common for two reasons: many of the causes of hypomagnesemia are also causes of potassium loss, and hypomagnesemia itself causes renal potassium wasting. Severe hypomagnesemia also impairs parathyroid hormone secretion and induces tissue resistance to its actions, thereby leading to hypocalcemia.

DIAGNOSIS

The cause of the magnesium deficiency is often obvious from the history. In difficult diagnostic cases, a random urine sample should be collected and the fractional excretion of magnesium (FE_{Mg}) determined.

$$FE_{Mg} = \frac{\text{Urine magnesium} \times \text{Serum creatinine}}{0.7 \times \text{Serum magnesium} \times \text{Urine creatinine}}$$

With extrarenal magnesium loss (usually diarrhea, malabsorption or laxative abuse), the FE_{Mg} is appropriately suppressed (<4%). Higher FE_{Mg} levels indicate renal magnesium wasting, often secondary to surreptitious diuretic use or one of the familial magnesium-wasting disorders.

TREATMENT

It is unclear whether mild, asymptomatic hypomagnesemia needs to be treated. Magnesium repletion is recommended in hypomagnesemic patients if they are symptomatic, have underlying cardiac or seizure disorders, exhibit concurrent severe hypocalcemia or hypokalemia, or have severe hypomagnesemia (<1.4 mg/dL). In mild cases or in the outpatient setting, oral magnesium salts such as magnesium oxide (250 to 500 mg four times daily) can be used for repletion, but these substances frequently cause diarrhea, particularly at high doses. In the inpatient setting, intravenous magnesium sulfate (1 to 2 g every 6 hours) can be used for repletion. Because the redistribution of magnesium from extracellular to intracellular compartments is relatively slow, the serum magnesium concentration may normalize before total body magnesium stores are replete. It is therefore prudent to continue intravenous magnesium for an additional 1 to 2 days after restoration of normomagnesemia. In patients with normal renal function, any excess magnesium is simply excreted renally. Adverse effects from intravenous magnesium administration are primarily due to transient hypermagnesemia and include flushing, hypotension, and flaccid paralysis. Amiloride (10 to 20 mg PO once daily) abrogates renal magnesium wasting in some patients.

PROGNOSIS

Hospitalized patients with hypomagnesemia have a higher 1-year mortality, presumably because it is a marker of more severe illness.[4] Low serum magnesium levels (<1.7 mg/dL) are also associated with about a 35% increase in all-cause mortality in the general population.[5] In patients with a self-limited cause of magnesium deficiency, repletion is easily accomplished. However, in patients with persistent magnesium wasting, such as in Gitelman syndrome (Chapter 113), it can be difficult to keep up with the ongoing losses with oral therapy. Fortunately, these individuals tend to adapt to their chronic hypomagnesemia and tolerate it fairly well.

HYPERMAGNESEMIA

Transient hypermagnesemia can occur in patients given large doses of intravenous magnesium, for example, in the setting of preeclampsia. It has also been reported in individuals taking large doses of magnesium-containing antacids or cathartics, particularly in settings in which intestinal absorption is enhanced, such as inflammatory bowel disease and intestinal obstruction. However, the kidney has a very large capacity to excrete excess magnesium. Thus, persistent hypermagnesemia is seen almost exclusively in patients who have a reduced glomerular filtration rate, as in chronic kidney disease (Chapter 116), and who are also taking excessive amounts of magnesium in the form of antacids, cathartics, or enemas.

CLINICAL MANIFESTATIONS

Magnesium toxicity is a serious and potentially fatal condition. Mild hypermagnesemia (serum magnesium level > 4 to 6 mg/dL) causes hypotension, nausea, vomiting, facial flushing, urinary retention, and ileus. Above serum levels of 8 to 12 mg/dL, flaccid skeletal muscle paralysis and hyporeflexia may ensue, along with bradyarrhythmias, respiratory depression, coma, and cardiac arrest. A low or even negative serum anion gap is sometimes seen.

TREATMENT

Mild hypermagnesemia in a patient with good renal function usually requires no treatment because renal clearance is rapid and the normal serum half-life of magnesium is approximately 1 day. In the event of serious toxicity, the effects of magnesium can be temporarily antagonized by the administration of intravenous calcium salts (5 to 10 mL of 10% calcium chloride). Renal magnesium excretion can be enhanced by administering furosemide (20 to 40 mg every 4 hours) together with a saline infusion (0.9% NaCl at 150 mL/hour, titrated to replace urinary losses). In patients with advanced renal insufficiency, the most effective method of magnesium removal is hemodialysis.

PROGNOSIS

Severe hypermagnesemia is potentially fatal. Lesser degrees of hypermagnesemia usually respond well to treatment, but hypermagnesemia at the time of hospital admission is associated with an increased 1-year mortality.[6]

PHOSPHORUS METABOLISM

Phosphorus has many critical roles. It is a major component of bone mineral, of phospholipids in cell membranes, and of nucleic acids. It forms high-energy phosphate bonds in compounds such as adenosine triphosphate (ATP), is post-translationally bound to proteins as an intracellular signal, and acts as a major pH buffer in serum and urine.

NORMAL PHOSPHORUS METABOLISM

Of the total body phosphorus content, 85% is in bone, 14% is in intracellular compartments, and only 1% is in extracellular fluid. The normal concentration of phosphorus in plasma is 3 to 4.5 mg/dL (1 to 1.5 mM). Daily intake of phosphorus is 800 to 1500 mg. Phosphorus is present in many foods, including dairy products, meats, and grains, and it is absorbed in the small intestine. The kidneys excrete excess phosphorus, which is the principal mechanism by which the body regulates extracellular phosphate balance. Ninety percent of serum phosphate is filtered at the glomerulus, of which 80 to 97% is reabsorbed along the nephron, primarily in the proximal tubule. Parathyroid hormone and fibroblast growth factor 23 increase renal phosphate excretion by inhibiting the sodium-phosphate cotransporter in the proximal tubule, whereas vitamin D enhances intestinal phosphate absorption.

HYPOPHOSPHATEMIA

PATHOBIOLOGY

Hypophosphatemia may be caused by decreased intake, impaired intestinal absorption, redistribution into cells or bone, and renal losses (Table 105-2, Fig. 105-1). Phosphate is frequently depleted in alcohol use disorder (Chapter 364) because of the intake of a carbohydrate-rich, phosphate-poor diet, as well as renal phosphate wasting. Divalent cation-containing antacids bind phosphate in the intestinal lumen to form insoluble salts, thereby preventing their absorption. Vitamin D deficiency also leads to decreased intestinal phosphate absorption and hence to hypophosphatemia. Acute respiratory (but not metabolic) alkalosis (Chapter 104), including that due to salicylate intoxication, may cause transient hypophosphatemia. In this disorder, intracellular pH is increased, thereby stimulating glycolysis, which depletes the intracellular inorganic phosphate pool and leads to a shift of phosphate into cells.

Insulin is also a strong stimulus for shifting phosphate into cells. Patients with diabetic ketoacidosis (Chapter 210) are often hyperphosphatemic because of a shift of phosphate out of cells under insulinopenic conditions, but their total body phosphate is actually depleted as a result of urinary losses. Subsequent treatment with insulin may uncover severe hypophosphatemia. Similarly, in malnourished patients (Chapter 197), whose total body phosphate stores may be depleted, overzealous intravenous refeeding with carbohydrate-rich fluids may stimulate insulin release and cause acute hypophosphatemia.[7] The tyrosine kinase inhibitors imatinib, sorafenib, and nilotinib, which are used in the treatment of various cancers (Chapters 164 and 170), can cause profound hypophosphatemia, which appears to be due either to inhibition of bone resorption or a partial Fanconi syndrome.

Renal phosphate wasting is usually due to impaired proximal tubule phosphate reabsorption. In primary hyperparathyroidism (Chapter 227), hypercalcemia is typically associated with hypophosphatemia. Fanconi syndrome is a generalized proximal tubule disorder characterized by hypophosphatemia in association with glycosuria, aminoaciduria, hypokalemia, and type II renal tubular acidosis; it can be caused by a variety of inherited metabolic disorders, multiple myeloma (Chapter 173), heavy metal intoxication (Chapter 20), intravenous iron therapy (Chapter 144),[8] and drugs such as ifosfamide, cidofovir, and tenofovir. Phosphaturia also can occur with diuretics, particularly carbonic anhydrase inhibitors, and with antimicrobial agents such as pentamidine and foscarnet.

TABLE 105-2 CAUSES OF HYPOPHOSPHATEMIA

Nutritional deficiency
Malnutrition/malabsorption
Alcoholism*
Impaired intestinal absorption
Antacids
Chronic diarrhea*
Vitamin D deficiency*
Redistribution into cells
Respiratory alkalosis*
Insulin*
Refeeding syndrome
Burns*
Redistribution into bone
Hungry bone syndrome
Tyrosine kinase inhibitors (imatinib, sorafenib, nilotinib)
Renal losses
Hyperparathyroidism*
Renal tubulopathy
Fanconi syndrome
Drugs (pentamidine, foscarnet, acetazolamide, toluene, acetaminophen overdose, intravenous iron)
Phosphatonin excess syndrome
Oncogenic osteomalacia
Familial hypophosphatemic rickets
Extracorporeal removal
Continuous venovenous hemodiafiltration

*Common causes.

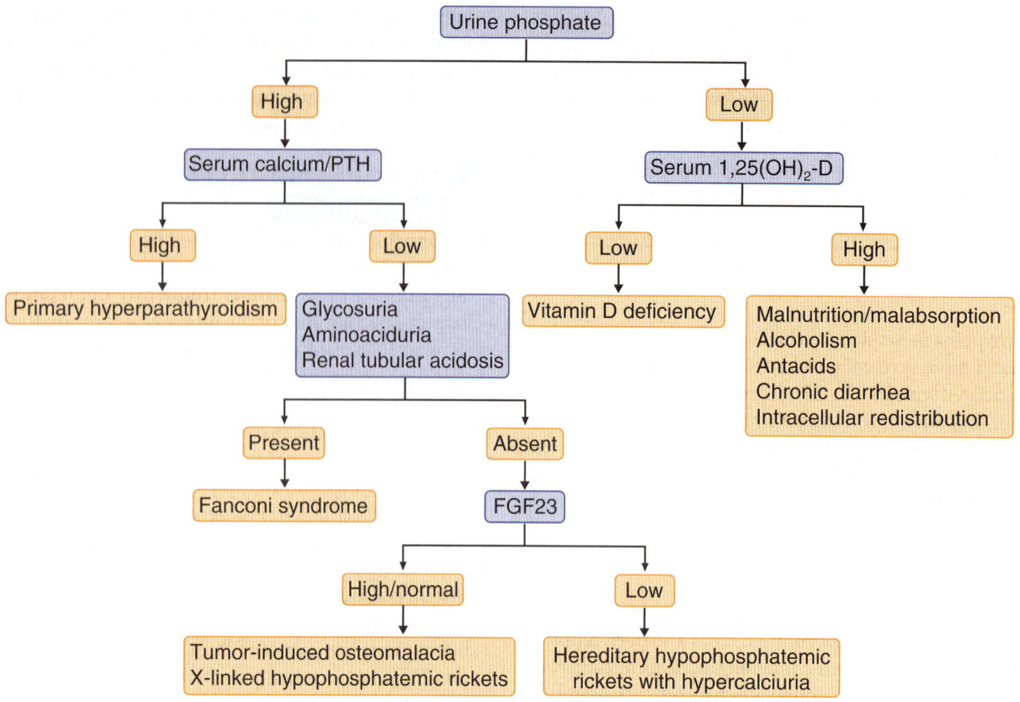

FIGURE 105-1. **Diagnostic approach to chronic hypophosphatemia.** 1,25(OH)$_2$-D = 1,25-Dihydroxyvitamin D; FGF23 = fibroblast growth factor 23; PTH = parathyroid hormone.

Oncogenic osteomalacia is a paraneoplastic syndrome (Chapters 164 and 226) associated primarily with mesenchymal tumors that secrete a variety of phosphaturic factors, including fibroblast growth factor 23, that are collectively known as phosphatonins.[9] A similar phenotype is found in X-linked, autosomal dominant and autosomal recessive hypophosphatemic rickets (Chapter 226), which are inherited disorders that are characterized by an increase in the levels or activity of fibroblast growth factor 23. Fibroblast growth factor 23 inhibits both renal tubular phosphate reabsorption and 1α-hydroxylation of 25-hydroxycholecalciferol, thereby leading to hypophosphatemia, rickets, or osteomalacia (Chapter 226) and inappropriately low serum levels of 1,25-dihydroxycholecalciferol. Finally, patients undergoing renal replacement therapy by continuous venovenous hemodiafiltration (Chapter 117) often become phosphate depleted and need ongoing replacement.

CLINICAL MANIFESTATIONS

Clinical complications, which are usually observed only with severe hypophosphatemia (<1 mg/dL), are thought to be due to the disruption of cell membrane composition, depletion of ATP (which particularly affects high energy–consuming tissues such as skeletal and cardiac muscle), and depletion of 2,3-diphosphoglycerate in erythrocytes, with impaired tissue oxygen delivery. Manifestations of severe hypophosphatemia include encephalopathy, dilated cardiomyopathy, generalized muscle weakness that can lead to respiratory failure, rhabdomyolysis, and hemolysis. Hypophosphatemia also impairs renal ammoniagenesis and reduces the availability of urinary buffer, thereby impairing renal acid excretion and causing metabolic acidosis. Chronic hypophosphatemia leads to resorption of bone and osteomalacia.

DIAGNOSIS

The cause of hypophosphatemia is often evident from the history and physical examination. If not, measurement of either 24-hour urinary phosphate excretion or fractional excretion of phosphate (FE_{PO4}) in a spot urine sample is often helpful.

$$FE_{PO4} = \frac{\text{Urine phosphate} \times \text{Serum creatinine}}{\text{Serum phosphate} \times \text{Urine creatinine}}$$

In the setting of hypophosphatemia, the normal response of the kidney is to reduce urinary phosphate excretion to less than 100 mg/day or to reduce FE_{PO4} to less than 5%. Higher values suggest one of the causes of renal phosphate wasting.

TREATMENT

Patients with asymptomatic mild-to-moderate hypophosphatemia, normal total body phosphorus stores, and minimal ongoing phosphorus losses (e.g., hypophosphatemia caused by acute respiratory alkalosis) do not require treatment. Phosphate should be repleted in patients who are symptomatic, are suspected of having severely depleted intracellular phosphorus stores (malnourished or alcoholic patients), have ongoing gastrointestinal or renal losses, or have severe hypophosphatemia (<1 mg/dL).[10] Oral repletion can be accomplished with sodium or potassium phosphate salts (1 to 2 g/day) or with skim milk. Intravenous phosphorus repletion at a dose of 0.16 to 0.64 mmol/kg over 4 to 8 hours is recommended for severe hypophosphatemia but is contraindicated in patients with renal insufficiency or hypercalcemia. Hypophosphatemia in patients on continuous venovenous hemodiafiltration can also be ameliorated by the use of phosphate-containing dialysate and replacement solutions. Complications of phosphate therapy include hypocalcemia, metastatic calcification, hypotension, acute renal failure, and arrhythmias, as well as concomitant hypernatremia or hyperkalemia, depending on which salt is administered.

PROGNOSIS

Most patients with hypophosphatemia respond well to treatment. However, hypophosphatemia is a marker of the severity of disease in patients who require intensive care.[11]

HYPERPHOSPHATEMIA

PATHOBIOLOGY

Pseudohyperphosphatemia may occur in blood specimens that are hemolyzed or hyperglobulinemic, such as in multiple myeloma (Chapter 173). True hyperphosphatemia is caused by excessive phosphate intake, increased intestinal absorption, redistribution from intracellular stores, or impaired renal excretion (Table 105-3 and Fig. 105-2). Overzealous phosphate repletion also can cause hyperphosphatemia. The phosphorus in some laxatives and enemas may be absorbed and cause hyperphosphatemia. Intoxication with vitamin D or its analogues increases intestinal absorption of both calcium and phosphorus. Conditions associated with massive cell lysis, such as rhabdomyolysis (Chapter 99) and tumor lysis syndrome (Chapter 164), release intracellular phosphate into the extracellular fluid, where it can bind calcium and result in hypocalcemia (Chapter 227). Patients with diabetic ketoacidosis (Chapter 210) are often hyperphosphatemic at initial evaluation because of the redistribution of phosphate out of cells in the insulin-deficient state. Decreased phosphate

TABLE 105-3 CAUSES OF HYPERPHOSPHATEMIA

Phosphate intake
Phosphate repletion
Phosphate-containing laxatives and enemas*
Increased intestinal absorption
Vitamin D toxicity
Redistribution from intracellular stores
Rhabdomyolysis*
Tumor lysis syndrome
Diabetic ketoacidosis
Decreased renal excretion
Renal failure*
Hypoparathyroidism
Pseudohypoparathyroidism
Familial tumoral calcinosis
Inhibitors of fibroblast growth factor receptor (e.g., erdafitinib, infigratinib, pemigatinib)

*Common causes.

TREATMENT

Acute hyperphosphatemia in an asymptomatic patient with normal renal function often resolves spontaneously as excess phosphate is excreted. In symptomatic patients and those with impaired renal function, phosphate can be removed by extracorporeal therapy. Because of the slow rate of phosphate mobilization from intracellular stores, continuous venovenous hemodiafiltration is considerably more effective than intermittent hemodialysis. Chronic hyperphosphatemia (Chapter 116) can be managed by minimizing the dietary intake of phosphorus and administering oral phosphate binders with meals. Current guidelines recommend minimizing the use of calcium salts in chronic kidney disease (Chapter 116), based on evidence that non–calcium-based phosphate binders and especially sevelamer (800 mg three times daily)[A1] may reduce all-cause mortality compared with calcium-based binders.[A2] Tenapanor (starting at 5 mg twice daily and titrating to as high as 30 mg twice daily if needed), which is an inhibitor of the paracellular absorption of phosphorus from the intestine, can lower serum phosphate levels.[A3] Cinacalcet (starting at 30 mg daily and titrated as high as 180 mg daily as needed), which is a calcimimetic used in patients with chronic kidney disease to treat secondary hyperparathyroidism, also reduces the serum phosphate concentration modestly and can be considered in refractory cases.

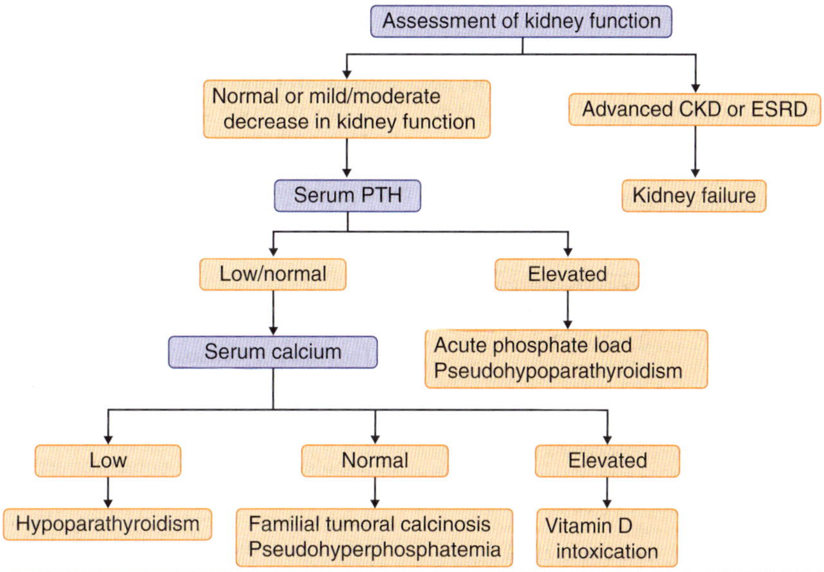

FIGURE 105-2. **Diagnostic approach to chronic hyperphosphatemia, a parathyroid hormone (PTH)–based diagnostic algorithm.** CKD = chronic kidney disease; ESRD = end-stage renal disease; PTH = parathyroid hormone. (Redrawn from Leaf DE, Wolf M. A physiologic-based approach to the evaluation of a patient with hyperphosphatemia. *Am J Kidney Dis.* 2013;61:330-336.)

excretion is most commonly due to acute or chronic kidney disease (Chapter 116). With a normal diet, serum phosphate levels can be maintained within the normal range until the glomerular filtration rate falls below 25 mL/minute. However, even mild degrees of renal insufficiency may predispose to hyperphosphatemia if there is a concurrent excessive intake of phosphate-containing compounds such as laxatives. Parathyroid hormone stimulates the excretion of phosphate in the proximal tubule, so primary hypoparathyroidism (Chapter 227) is often associated with mild hyperphosphatemia as well as hypocalcemia.[12] Oncologic drugs that inhibit fibroblast growth factor receptors (Chapters 164 and 166) also can cause hyperphosphatemia by antagonizing fibroblast growth factor 23.[13]

CLINICAL MANIFESTATIONS

Acute hyperphosphatemia increases the risk for the precipitation of calcium phosphate and subsequent metastatic calcification in soft tissues, including the kidney, in which it can cause acute kidney injury (Chapter 106).[14] For example, acute hyperphosphatemia is an independent risk factor for acute kidney injury in patients with rhabdomyolysis (Chapter 99).[15] The resultant hypocalcemia (Chapter 227) can cause tetany, hypotension, seizures, and cardiac arrhythmias. Hyperphosphatemia in chronic kidney disease (Chapter 116) is a risk factor for coronary and other vascular calcification and for increased mortality.

PROGNOSIS

Severe acute hyperphosphatemia can be life-threatening owing to metastatic calcification and multiorgan failure, but it generally responds well to prompt therapy. Chronic hyperphosphatemia in patients with chronic kidney disease (Chapter 116) is often fairly resistant to treatment, particularly in poorly compliant individuals, and is associated with increased long-term mortality.

GENERAL REFERENCES

For the General References and other additional features, please visit Elsevier eBooks+ at https://ebooks.health.elsevier.com.

Grade A References

A1. Lioufas NM, Pascoe EM, Hawley CM, et al. Systematic review and meta-analyses of the effects of phosphate-lowering agents in nondialysis CKD. *J Am Soc Nephrol.* 2022;33:59-76.
A2. Phannajit J, Wonghakaeo N, Takkavatakam K, et al. The impact of phosphate lowering agents on clinical and laboratory outcomes in chronic kidney disease patients: a systematic review and meta-analysis of randomized controlled trials. *J Nephrol.* 2022;35:473-491.
A3. Block GA, Rosenbaum DP, Yan A, et al. Efficacy and safety of tenapanor in patients with hyperphosphatemia receiving maintenance hemodialysis: a randomized phase 3 trial. *J Am Soc Nephrol.* 2019;30:641-652.

106

ACUTE KIDNEY INJURY

ANUPAM AGARWAL AND JONATHAN BARASCH

DEFINITION

Acute kidney injury (AKI), which is a clinical syndrome, is defined by a clinically evident defect in the kidney's clearance of waste materials within approximately 1 week after an injurious stimulus. Although formal definitions vary somewhat, the components include an increase in the serum level of the muscle metabolite creatinine by 0.3 mg/dL or greater (within 48 hours), an increase in the creatinine level to 1.5 times higher than a baseline value within 7 days or a fall in urine volume to less than 0.5 mL/kg/hour for 6 hours or longer (Table 106-1). The degree of the rise in serum creatinine or fall in urine output is typically reported in stages that describe progressive functional loss (Table 106-1).

EPIDEMIOLOGY

About 20 to 25% of hospitalized adults have an elevated serum creatinine level. Among patients admitted to the hospital from an emergency department, up to 45% present with an elevated serum creatinine level, and the rate is even higher (55 to 65%) among patients who are admitted to the intensive care unit (ICU). Because the serum creatinine level is insensitive for detecting tubular or vascular damage, the true incidence of acute kidney injury is probably even higher.[1] In contrast, community-acquired acute kidney injury is uncommon and estimated to have an annual incidence of less than 1%. The serum creatinine level can be elevated for a variety of reasons, including prerenal, intrarenal, and postrenal subtypes that are impossible to distinguish on the basis of a single measurement of the serum creatinine level (Fig. 106-1).

Prerenal azotemia, which is the most common cause of an elevated serum creatinine level, is found in 15% of patients admitted from the emergency department. Prerenal azotemia accounts for about 40% of hospital-acquired cases of acute kidney injury and as much as 60 to 70% of community-acquired cases, depending on its precise definition. Intrinsic acute kidney injury, defined as 7 days or longer of azotemia, is present in 5 to 6% of patients who are admitted from the emergency department in the United States and in as many as 60% of patients in the intensive care unit. Acute kidney injury is also common and underdiagnosed in low-resource settings worldwide.[2] Intrinsic acute kidney injury requiring dialysis has increased substantially over the past three decades. For postrenal acute kidney injury, the incidence depends on the patient's age and sex. Prostatic hypertrophy in older men (Chapter 114) is the leading cause.

TABLE 106-1 KIDNEY DISEASE IMPROVING GLOBAL OUTCOMES (KDIGO) ACUTE KIDNEY INJURY DEFINITIONS

STAGE	SERUM CREATININE	URINE OUTPUT
1	1.5-1.9 times baseline OR ≥0.3 mg/dL (≥26.5 µmol/L) increase	<0.5 mL/kg/hour for 6 to 12 hours
2	2.0-2.9 times baseline	<0.5 mL/kg/hour for ≥12 hours
3	3.0 times baseline OR Increase in serum creatinine to ≥4.0 mg/dL (≥353.6 µmol/L) OR Initiation of renal replacement therapy OR In patients <18 years of age, decrease in eGFR to <35 mL/min per 1.73 m^2	<0.3 mL/kg/hour for ≥24 hours OR Anuria for ≥12 hour

eGFR = estimated glomerular filtration rate.
Adapted from Molitoris BA. Acute kidney injury. In: Goldman L, Schafer AI, eds. *Goldman-Cecil Medicine*, 26th ed. Philadelphia: Saunders; 2020.

Prerenal Azotemia/Hypoperfusion

Prerenal azotemia is caused when hypoperfusion of the kidney reduces the clearance of serum creatinine and water, thereby limiting urine output. In prerenal azotemia, kidney function, including the serum creatinine level and urine output, can be corrected within hours of infusing volume, thereby stimulating cardiac output, or withdrawing vasoconstrictors (e.g., nonsteroidal anti-inflammatory drugs [NSAIDs], cyclosporine, radiocontrast agents). Although evidence of tubular injury may be limited, even 1 day of prerenal azotemia can result in hyponatremia, hyperkalemia, acidosis, and hence increased mortality (Fig. 106-2). Urinary biomarkers of acute kidney injury are not particularly elevated.

The causes of prerenal azotemia include true intravascular volume depletion because of limited oral intake, fever and sweating, burns, diarrhea, diuretic agents, and bleeding, as well as effective volume depletion from heart failure (Chapter 45) or liver failure (Chapter 140). In addition, a number of medications potentially reduce glomerular perfusion and raise the serum creatinine level, including NSAIDs, angiotensin-converting enzyme (ACE) inhibitors, and angiotensin receptor blockers. These medications can have a dramatic effect on the serum creatinine level when renal perfusion is compromised by volume depletion or other insults.

Intrinsic Acute Kidney Injury

Intrinsic acute kidney injury can involve any portion of the kidney or its vasculature. Central to the pathobiology is an abrupt decline in kidney function that cannot be restored for a number of days or even weeks owing to slow resolution of intensive vasoconstriction, tubular damage, and cell death, as well as interstitial inflammation with edema. Urinary biomarkers of tubular damage are particularly elevated. In contrast to prerenal azotemia, molecular

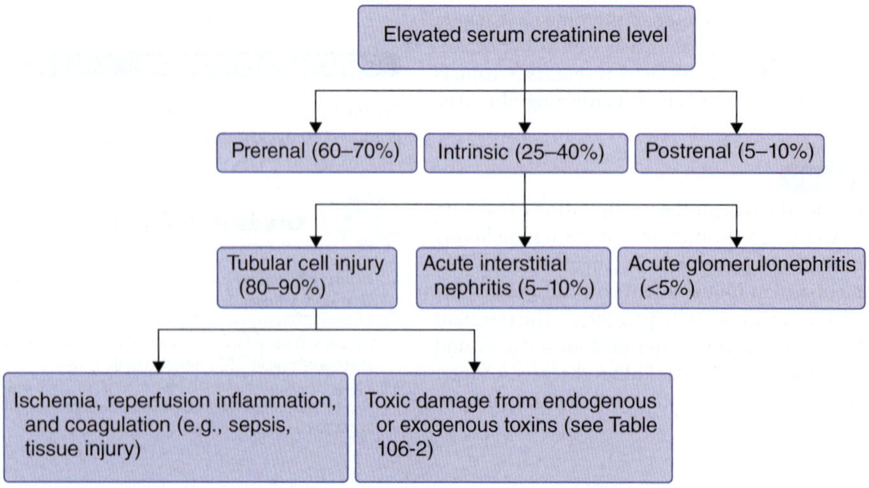

FIGURE 106-1. **Categories of acute kidney injury.** (Adapted from Molitoris BA. Acute kidney injury. In: Goldman L, Schafer AI, eds. *Goldman-Cecil Medicine*, 26th ed. Philadelphia: Saunders; 2020.)

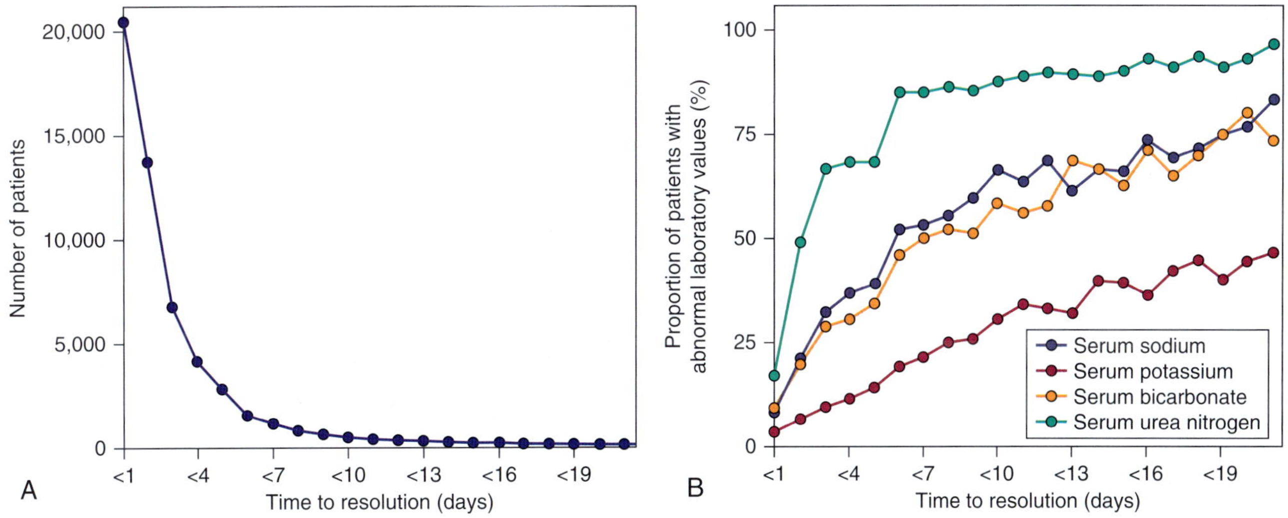

FIGURE 106-2. **Rapid resolution of an elevated serum creatinine in most patients with acute kidney injury. (A) In about one third of hospitalized patients, the condition resolves within 24 hours, about 60% by 48 hours, and about 70% by 72 hours after meeting criteria for acute kidney injury. (B) Electrolyte abnormalities correlate with a sustained elevation in the serum creatinine level. (Data from Xu K, Rosenstiel P, Paragas N, et al. Unique transcriptional programs identify subtypes of AKI. *J Am Soc Nephrol.* 2017;28:1729-1740.)**

TABLE 106-2 COMMON RENAL TUBULAR TOXINS

Antimicrobial agents
Acyclovir
Aminoglycosides
Amphotericin B
Foscarnet
Pentamidine
Sulfonamides
Tenofovir
Vancomycin
Calcium oxalate crystals
Cisplatin
Cocaine
Cyclosporine
Metals (e.g., iron, cadmium)
Methotrexate
Myoglobin/hemoglobin
Pancreatic enzymes (endogenous)
Radiocontrast agents
Tacrolimus
Toluene
Uric acid crystals
Ethylene glycol

Adapted from Molitoris BA. Acute kidney injury. In: Goldman L, Schafer AI, eds. *Goldman-Cecil Medicine*, 26th ed. Philadelphia: Saunders; 2020.

TABLE 106-3 MEDICATIONS ASSOCIATED WITH ACUTE INTERSTITIAL NEPHRITIS

ANTIMICROBIAL AGENTS
Acyclovir
Cephalosporins
Ciprofloxacin
Indinavir
Penicillin
Rifampin
Sulfonamides (e.g., trimethoprim-sulfamethoxazole)
Vancomycin
DIURETICS
Furosemide
Hydrochlorothiazide
Triamterene
OTHERS
Allopurinol
Checkpoint inhibitors
Cimetidine
Nonsteroidal anti-inflammatory drugs
Proton pump inhibitors
Salicylates (mesalamine)

Adapted from Molitoris BA. Acute kidney injury. In: Goldman L, Schafer AI, eds. *Goldman-Cecil Medicine*, 26th ed. Philadelphia: Saunders; 2020.

analysis demonstrates the activation of inflammatory, ischemic, and coagulation pathways.

The causes of intrinsic acute kidney injury[3] include ischemic hypoperfusion that results in cellular injury, septic injury,[4] inflammatory injury, and a myriad of renal toxins (Table 106-2), including intrinsic toxins (e.g., myoglobin, hemoglobin, calcium oxalate, uric acid, and endogenous pancreatic enzymes) and exogenous toxins (e.g., radiocontrast agents, antibiotics, and metals). Acute kidney injury does not develop in all patients who are exposed to potentially toxic agents, but patients with prior functional defects, such as elderly patients with chronic kidney disease or volume-depleted patients (e.g., due to diuretics, burns, heart failure, cirrhosis, or hypoalbuminemia), are more likely to suffer toxic tubular injury. For example, the risk of developing antibiotic nephrotoxicity is 10-fold higher in high-risk patients.

Injury to the renal interstitium or acute interstitial nephritis (Chapter 108) is found in about 15% of biopsy samples of patients who have an intrinsic acute kidney injury.[5] Implicated medications include sulfonamides, penicillins, cephalosporins, proton pump inhibitors, and NSAIDs (Table 106-3). In addition, checkpoint inhibitors trigger acute interstitial nephritis in about 5% of treated patients. Bacteria and viruses that can cause interstitial injury include *Legionella*, leptospirosis, *Yersinia*, streptococcus, *Mycobacterium tuberculosis*, Epstein-Barr virus, severe acute respiratory syndrome coronavirus 2 (SARS-CoV-2), and cytomegalovirus. Fungal infections, including histoplasmosis and coccidioidomycosis, as well as tuberculosis, are implicated in granulomatous acute interstitial nephritis. Interstitial nephritis also can be seen in patients who have systemic autoimmune diseases, including systemic lupus erythematosus (Chapter 245), Sjögren syndrome (Chapter 247), cryoglobulinemia (Chapter 173), and primary biliary cirrhosis (Chapter 141). Intratubular crystallization of compounds such as uric acid, calcium oxalate, acyclovir, sulfonamides, methotrexate, and myeloma light chains can result in tubular obstruction.

Postrenal Acute Kidney Injury

Postrenal acute kidney injury refers to obstruction of urinary outflow. Both kidneys (or a single solitary kidney) must be obstructed in order to cause postrenal acute kidney injury, because the serum creatinine level is too insensitive to detect kidney damage from partial or unilateral obstruction. Obstruction can occur in the lower tract owing to the constriction of the urethra or the base of the bladder by prostatic hypertrophy (Chapter 114) or cancer of the prostate (Chapter 186), cervix (Chapter 184), or bladder (Chapter 182). Patients with spinal cord disease or diabetes also can develop an elevated serum creatinine level because of functional obstruction from a neurogenic bladder. Obstruction of both ureters at the bladder trigone or along their course from the kidneys can be seen in retroperitoneal fibrosis (Chapter 246), endometriosis (Chapter 218), metastatic colon cancer (Chapter 179), and lymphomas (Chapters 171 and 172). Intraluminal blockade occurs when renal calculi (Chapter 111), papillary necrosis (Chapter 100), or blood clots obstruct both ureters.

PATHOBIOLOGY

Molecular processes that cause acute kidney injury can be categorized according to the principal site of disease activity. Such processes include decreased kidney perfusion, which can reduce the glomerular filtration rate (GFR) regardless of whether it causes acute cellular injury, a primary glomerular disease, an injury (toxic, septic, ischemic) to the nephron, or inflammation and edema of the tubules or interstitium (Fig. 106-3).

Prerenal Acute Kidney Injury

A reduction in extracellular or intravascular volume, commonly termed effective arterial volume, affects many segments of the kidney by activating the catecholamine–renin–angiotensin–aldosterone–antidiuretic hormone systems. These regulators determine afferent and efferent arteriolar tone in the glomerulus and hence the concentration of albumin and the reabsorption of Na^+ and water in the postglomerular capillary and in the nephron. The hormonal cascade is most active in the inner medulla, where the final capture of salt and water prevents further volume depletion. In addition, Na^+ recovery is a critical proinflammatory signal that defends the kidney from urinary infections during periods when urine flow rate is reduced.

In addition to regulating gene transcription via the hormonal axis, volume depletion also regulates oxygen tension in the medulla. Volume depletion reduces and volume expansion increases medullary partial pressure of oxygen (pO_2), without changing cortical pO_2. Severe and prolonged prerenal azotemia can damage the inner medullary tubules by hypoxia (Table 106-4). Conversely, volume resuscitation is needed to protect the kidney when a second insult, such as a nephrotoxic agent or radiologic contrast, may damage the kidney.

Prerenal acute kidney injury may also result from heart failure, called cardiorenal acute kidney injury. Both right-sided congestion, which can involve the renal vein, and left-sided failure with a decreased cardiac output, can reduce the effective arterial volume and, as a result, the filtration of creatinine.

Early in the course of heart failure (Chapter 45) and early in prerenal azotemia, the GFR remains relatively preserved, with only small increases in the serum creatinine level, because kidney hypoperfusion triggers a cascade of hormonal responses that dilate afferent arterioles and constrict efferent arterioles to maintain glomerular perfusion pressure and that stimulate the tubules to retain Na^+ and water. At later stages, however, intravascular volume expansion does not further improve kidney perfusion; rather, removal of volume

TABLE 106-4 CONDITIONS THAT LEAD TO ISCHEMIC ACUTE KIDNEY INJURY

MECHANISM	CONDITION
Severe volume depletion and hypotension	Severe hemorrhage; gastrointestinal, renal, and dermal losses
Severely decreased effective intravascular volume	Severe heart failure and cirrhosis, hepatorenal syndrome, peritonitis
Systemic vasodilation, renal vasoconstriction	Sepsis, hepatorenal syndrome
Large-vessel renal vascular disease	Renal artery thrombosis or embolism, intraoperative arterial cross-clamping, renal artery stenosis, cholesterol emboli
Small-vessel renal vascular disease	Sepsis, vasculitis, atheroembolism, hemolytic-uremic syndrome, malignant hypertension, scleroderma, preeclampsia, sickle cell anemia, hypercalcemia, transplant rejection
Impaired renal blood flow	Cyclosporine, tacrolimus, angiotensin-converting enzyme inhibitors, angiotensin receptor blockers, nonsteroidal anti-inflammatory drugs, radiocontrast agents

Adapted from Molitoris BA. Acute kidney injury. In: Goldman L, Schafer AI, eds. *Goldman-Cecil Medicine*, 26th ed. Philadelphia: Saunders; 2020.

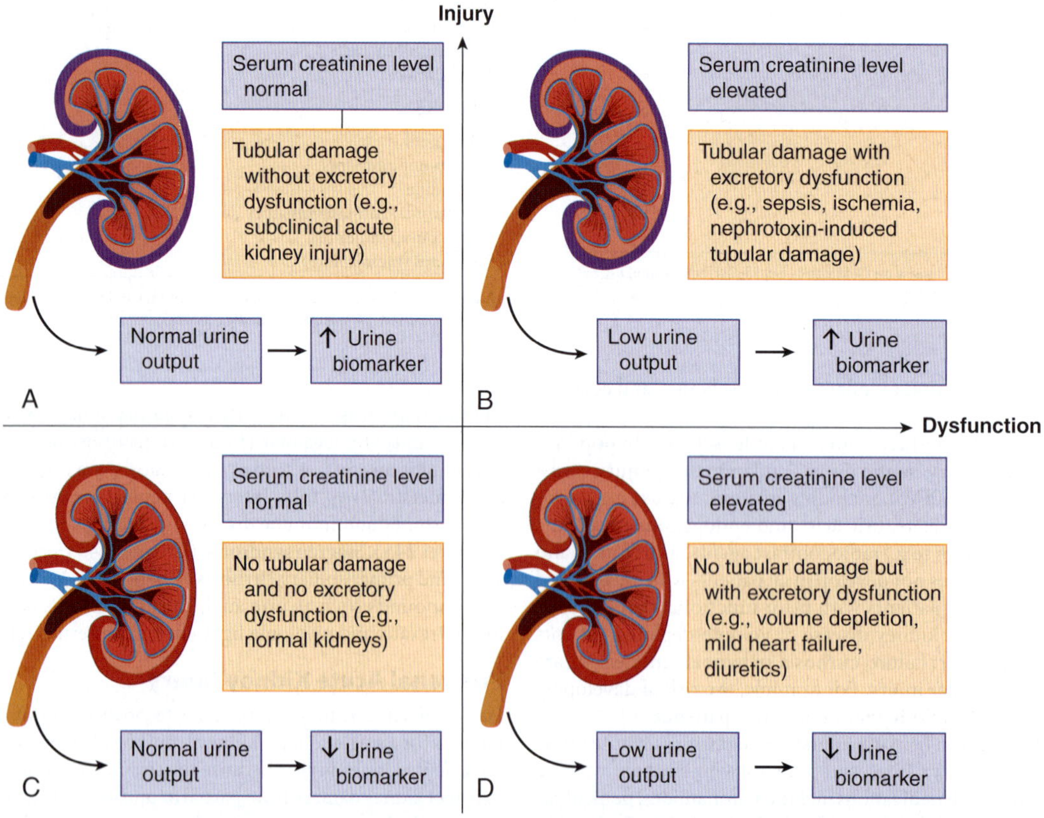

FIGURE 106-3. **Three forms of acute kidney injury based on the intersection of an elevated serum creatinine level and urinary biomarkers. (A) Partial damage is detected by biomarkers but not by the serum creatinine level. (B) Extensive damage detected by both biomarkers and the serum creatinine level. (C) Normal kidney. (D) Volume depletion detected by an elevated serum creatinine level without biomarker elevation. (Adapted from Desanti De Oliveira B, Xu K, Shen TH, et al. Molecular nephrology: types of acute tubular injury. *Nat Rev Nephrol*. 2019;15:599-612.)**

and reducing congestion in the pulmonary and renal veins is beneficial even as the serum creatinine level rises if tubular damage is not also present.

Progression of Prerenal to Intrinsic Acute Kidney Injury

Prerenal and intrarenal azotemia are distinct conditions, with different molecular pathways, including gluconeogenesis, lipid metabolism, and anti-inflammatory regulators in the prerenal state as compared with coagulation, inflammation, and epithelial remodeling in the intrarenal state. However, when a second insult, such as an inflammatory or toxic stimulus, is superimposed, volume depletion exacerbates the damage.[6] Without early volume repletion, prerenal azotemia may contribute to tubular epithelial injury.

Intrarenal Acute Kidney Injury

Intrinsic acute kidney injury can be classified by the primary site of injury: tubules, interstitium, vasculature, or glomerulus. Renal tubular injury, previously termed *acute tubular necrosis* (ATN) and now *acute tubular injury* (ATI), is typically found in the S3 segment of the proximal tubule and the medullary thick ascending limb of Henle, which are two segments that are located in the outer stripe of the medulla, where oxygen tension is limited. Different forms of ischemia preferentially target these segments: warm ischemia targets the proximal (S3) tubule, whereas cold ischemia, vasoconstrictors, contrast agents, gram-negative sepsis, myoglobinuria, and obstruction target the medullary thick ascending limb of Henle. The balance of injury may depend on the degree of injury-induced hypoxia (the proximal tubule is dependent on aerobic metabolism, whereas the medullary thick ascending limb of Henle can utilize anaerobic metabolisms) and on segmental variations in the activation of mitogen-activated protein kinases.

A very common cause of intrinsic acute kidney injury is sepsis. The initiation stage of sepsis-associated tubular injury is not fully elucidated, but lipopolysaccharide accumulates in proximal tubules and then in distal tubules. The uptake of lipopolysaccharide correlates with broadening of the distribution of toll-like receptors (TLRs), including TLR4, the lipopolysaccharide receptor, and its coreceptor (CD14) from distal tubules to proximal tubules in response to injury.

Tubular toxins initiate damage by binding endocytic receptors (megalin and cubilin) and trafficking to tubular lysosomes in the proximal tubule, similar to the pathway taken by lipopolysaccharide. The many endocytic toxins that may also undergo endocytosis by the megalin pathway include cadmium, aminoglycoside antibiotics, and other medicinal toxins such as intravenous radiocontrast agents and cisplatin (see Table 106-2).[7] The most important endocytic toxin is the endogenous molecule myoglobin (Chapter 99), which contains heme and iron and triggers ferroptosis and necroptosis. Tubular toxins also exacerbate kidney injury by inducing vasoconstriction. This phenomenon is linked to radiocontrast agents, NSAIDs, cyclosporine, and combinations of these agents with renin-angiotensin system inhibitors and diuretics.

In addition to direct cell toxicity and vasoconstriction, many toxins and metabolites can precipitate and thereby block tubular function. Endogenous compounds that can cause crystal nephropathy include calcium oxalate (both the common enteric form and the primary hyperoxaluric form), and uric acid. Exogenous compounds that create intratubular obstruction include acyclovir, sulfonamides (sulfadiazine and sulfamethoxazole), ciprofloxacin, vitamin C, ethylene glycol, methotrexate, protease inhibitors (e.g., indinavir, darunavir), and the light chains of multiple myeloma (Chapter 173).

Cellular Damage

Cellular dysfunction is typical in the proximal tubule, particularly in the S3 segment. In the initiation phase of renal ischemia, the apical membrane with the brush border sheds in blebs from the cells. Subsequently, the polarity of membrane proteins is lost, due to loss of function of cellular tight junctions. Retraction of tight junctions and loss of the epithelial cell barrier allow the back-leak of the glomerular filtrate into the interstitium, thereby reducing clearance of metabolic wastes. As the injury progresses, both live and necrotic proximal cells detach from the basement membrane and enter the tubular lumen, where they ultimately form casts in the distal tubule. Casts contribute to a reduction in GFR by obstructing the tubular flow of urine at the S3-thin limb of Henle junction,[8] thereby preventing further filtration into that nephron. The clearance of casts is necessary for recovery; it is mediated by proteases and by phagocytic proteins that bind intratubular casts. By day 3 after injury, casts are cleared from most of the nephron, but obstructing casts can linger at the S3 segment or descending limb of Henle.

During the phase of cellular death, endothelial dysfunction and an inflammatory endothelial response, particularly in the corticomedullary junction of the kidney, result from extensive signaling between the proximal tubular cells and adjacent endothelial cells. Leukocytes can block blood flow via cellular adhesion and rouleaux formation. Damage to the microvasculature in turn can generate coagulation abnormalities. When proximal tubular cells dedifferentiate, proliferate, and restore the nephron,[9] the kidney recovers and the GFR begins to improve.

In interstitial and vascular acute interstitial nephritis (Chapter 108), interstitial edema comprises an inflammatory infiltrate with T lymphocytes, eosinophils, monocytes, and macrophages invading the tubular basement membrane. In chronic interstitial nephritis, the characteristic findings are interstitial fibrosis and tubular atrophy, but inflammation can persist. Surprisingly, a greater degree of inflammation may portend a higher likelihood of resolution.[10]

Vascular Disease

Microvascular diseases (e.g., sepsis [Chapter 94], the hemolytic-uremic syndrome [Chapter 158], thrombotic thrombocytopenic purpura [Chapter 158], and the HELLP syndrome [*h*emolysis, *el*evated *l*iver enzymes, and *l*ow *p*latelet count; Chapters 132 and 221]) can also cause acute kidney injury by producing fibrin clots in the glomerulus and microvasculature. Acute kidney injury related to macrovascular disease is seen with embolism, including embolism of cholesterol plaques that occur especially after invasive vascular procedures (Chapter 110), and larger thromboembolism as in atrial fibrillation (Chapter 52). Vascular infarcts also can be seen with hypercoagulable states such as the nephrotic syndrome, antiphospholipid syndrome, and homocysteinemia, as well as with the use of oral contraceptive agents. Acute kidney injury also occasionally can be caused by glomerulonephritis (Chapter 107). Sometimes the glomerular injury is part of a systemic disease such as systemic lupus nephritis (Chapter 245), granulomatosis with polyangiitis (Chapter 249), polyarteritis nodosa (Chapter 249), Goodpasture syndrome (Chapter 107), Henoch-Schönlein purpura (Chapters 107 and 249), or the hemolytic-uremic syndrome (Chapter 158).

Postrenal Acute Kidney Injury

Postrenal acute kidney injury is caused by obstruction to luminal flow of the glomerular filtrate. In this condition, the GFR initially remains largely preserved because the glomerular afferent arteriole is dilated. If, however, the obstruction is not rapidly relieved, the release of angiotensin II and thromboxane causes vasoconstriction and reduces the GFR. If the obstruction persists for more than 12 to 24 hours, renal blood flow and intratubular pressure decline, and the GFR declines because of large underperfused areas of renal cortex. Subsequently, the kidney is invaded by macrophages, which stimulate fibrosis.

Acute Kidney Injury in the Setting of SARS-CoV-2

The SARS-CoV-2 virus that causes coronavirus disease 2019 (COVID-19) induces systemic responses, including a cytokine storm, immune and metabolic dysfunction, endothelial injury, coagulopathy, and microangiopathy (Chapter 336).[11] SARS-CoV-2 can directly infect kidney cells, where it causes dedifferentiation and activation of profibrotic pathways in the organoids.[12] Pathology reveals proximal tubular cell injury with loss of apical membrane and intracellular inclusions. In addition, nonviral mechanisms include hemodynamic factors, cardiac dysfunction, high levels of mechanical ventilation, hypovolemia, use of nephrotoxic drugs, and nosocomial sepsis.

CLINICAL MANIFESTATIONS

Acute kidney injury is usually clinically silent, and no specific symptoms are present in early stages of the injury. Some patients will rarely note a change in urine volume or color. Obstructive acute kidney injury due to a stone (Chapter 111) or papillary necrosis (Chapter 100) may result in hematuria and in flank pain radiating to the ipsilateral groin, but they also can be silent. Distal-type renal tubule acidosis (Chapter 104) is a common sequela of obstructive uropathy. In advanced states of acute kidney injury, uremic symptoms (Chapter 116) develop with anorexia, fatigue, nausea and vomiting, pruritus, and reversal of the sleep-wake cycle. Examination of the patient may reveal pulmonary edema and peripheral edema (Chapter 45), inflammatory complications such as a pericardial or pleural friction rub, and neurologic complications of uremia such as myoclonus and asterixis.

DIAGNOSIS

The diagnosis of acute kidney injury is based on a rise in the serum creatinine level and subsequently on elucidating the cause of the injury. Despite the utility of a single measurement of serum creatinine to demonstrate kidney dysfunction, a single elevated serum creatinine level measurement cannot accurately measure functional loss because it lacks the kinetic properties required to determine function in the absence of steady state. In addition, the serum creatinine level and urine output fail to detect kidney tubule injury in real time, to detect injury that involves less than one entire kidney, or to distinguish different clinical syndromes that elevate serum creatinine levels. Finally, serum creatinine levels are influenced by muscle mass, muscle damage, nutritional status, and medications that block the tubular transport of serum creatinine (e.g., cimetidine, trimethoprim, pyrimethamine, and salicylates), thereby raising serum creatinine in the absence of injury.[13]

All patients with an acutely elevated serum creatinine level should be evaluated with serum measurements of electrolytes, calcium, phosphorus, and a blood urea nitrogen level, as well as a complete blood count with differential. Urine dipstick and microscopy (Table 106-5) can detect blood, cells, and casts that are typical of different forms of intrarenal damage (Chapter 100). The urine and serum Na^+ and serum creatinine levels should be measured simultaneously to determine the fractional excretion of sodium (FE_{Na}), which measures the ability of the tubules to reabsorb Na^+, normalized for water reabsorption by measuring urine creatinine (Table 106-6).

$$FE_{Na} = \frac{\text{Urine Na} \times \text{Plasma Cr}}{\text{Plasma Na} \times \text{Urine Cr}} \times 100$$

In the setting of oliguria, an elevated FE_{Na} suggests tubular damage. Fractional excretion of chloride (FE_{Cl}) can substitute for FE_{Na} because urinary sodium can be elevated by systemic alkalosis when a high urinary bicarbonate level obligates the loss of sodium.

Prerenal azotemia can be diagnosed by evidence of dehydration and by its rapid resolution after a fluid challenge (e.g., 100 mL intravenously in 1 minute or up to 3 to 4 mL/kg over 5 minutes). In early true acute kidney injury, urine output of 100 mL within 1 hour after administering intravenous furosemide (1 or 1.5 mg/kg) can evaluate residual tubular function and can predict the subsequent rise in serum creatinine levels and mortality.[14] A renal ultrasound is key to exclude postrenal azotemia caused by stones, anatomic malformations, and bladder outlet obstruction.

TABLE 106-5 COMMON URINALYSIS FINDINGS IN ACUTE KIDNEY INJURY

CAUSE OF ACUTE KIDNEY INJURY	URINALYSIS
Prerenal	Normal or hyaline casts
Intrarenal	
Tubular cell injury	Muddy-brown, granular, epithelial casts
Interstitial nephritis	Pyuria, hematuria, mild proteinuria, granular and epithelial casts, eosinophils
Glomerulonephritis	Hematuria, marked proteinuria, red blood cell casts, granular casts
Vascular disorders	Normal or hematuria, mild proteinuria
Postrenal	Normal or hematuria, granular casts, pyuria

Adapted from Molitoris BA. Acute kidney injury. In: Goldman L, Schafer AI, eds. *Goldman-Cecil Medicine*, 26th ed. Philadelphia: Saunders; 2020.

TABLE 106-6 FE_{Na} VALUES FOR THE VARIOUS CAUSES OF ACUTE KIDNEY INJURY

CAUSE OF ACUTE KIDNEY INJURY	FE_{Na}	BUN-TO-SERUM CREATININE RATIO
Prerenal	<1%	>20
Intrarenal		<10-15
Tubular necrosis	≥1%	
Interstitial nephritis	≥1%	
Glomerulonephritis (early)	<1%	
Vascular disorders (early)	<1%	
Postrenal	≥1%	>20

FE_{Na} = fractional excretion of sodium.
Adapted from Molitoris BA. Acute kidney injury. In: Goldman L, Schafer AI, eds. *Goldman-Cecil Medicine*, 26th ed. Philadelphia: Saunders; 2020.

When the diagnosis appears to be true acute kidney injury, urine protein measurements for biomarkers (e.g., tissue inhibitor of matrix metalloproteinase 2–insulin-like growth factor–binding protein 7 [TIMP2-IGFBP7], kidney injury molecule 1 [KIM-1], neutrophil gelatinase–associated lipocalin [NGAL], and interleukin 18) can detect cell stress and damage that are typical of tubular injury rather than simple prerenal azotemia, even when the serum creatinine level has just started to rise because of a falling GFR.[15] Based on their sensitivity and specificity for tubular injury, some of these biomarkers may help guide the characterization of acute kidney injury (see Fig. 106-3), but their actual use in clinical practice has been limited.

Prerenal Azotemia

Prerenal azotemia is suggested by history of vomiting, diarrhea, hemorrhage, or poor oral intake. Heart failure indicates hypoperfusion either because of progressive disease or because of volume depletion due to diuretics. Medications such as NSAIDs, ACE inhibitors, and angiotensin-receptor blockers, can cause prerenal azotemia. Physical examination includes findings typical of underperfusion such as systemic or orthostatic hypotension, flat jugular veins, dry mucous membranes, and reflex tachycardia. Laboratory studies in patients with prerenal azotemia demonstrate elevated serum creatinine and blood urea nitrogen (BUN) levels. In prerenal azotemia, patients will typically have a ratio of BUN to serum creatinine of greater than 20 : 1. FE_{Na} is typically less than 1%. The FE_{Na} can provide reliable diagnostic information regarding acute kidney injury only if it is less than 1%, because elevated levels of FE_{Na} are seen in many diseases. In patients who are taking diuretics or in the presence of nonreabsorbable solutes such as glucose, a fractional excretion of urea (FE_{urea}) below 35% suggests prerenal acute kidney injury.

Intrarenal Acute Kidney Injury

In intrarenal acute kidney injury, significant hypotension, sepsis, and exposure to nephrotoxins (see Tables 106-2 and 106-3) are common. Physical examination is usually not revealing except for evidence of hypervolemia (Chapters 39 and 45). The skin examination may reveal embolic phenomenon or a rash consistent with allergic interstitial nephritis.

Laboratory testing will show elevated serum creatinine and BUN levels. Unlike prerenal azotemia, in which the elevation of the serum creatinine level tends to be modest and to plateau below 4 mg/dL, the serum creatinine level in intrarenal acute kidney injury may rise rapidly each day. The FE_{Na} is usually above 1 in acute injury, whereas it typically is below 1 in early sepsis, glomerulonephritis, radiocontrast-induced acute kidney injury, and vascular disorders. The urinalysis also can be helpful in making the diagnostic (see Table 106-6). In rare cases, acute interstitial nephritis may be associated with peripheral and urinary eosinophilia, but eosinophilia can also accompany cholesterol microemboli (Chapter 110). Urinary interleukin (IL)-9 and tumor necrosis factor (TNF)-α may be better markers for acute interstitial nephritis than are urinary findings.[16] Biomarkers can help detect intrarenal tubular injury within hours of the injury, and their levels in the urine can distinguish intrarenal (biomarkers are very elevated) from prerenal (biomarkers are not particularly elevated) forms of acute kidney injury.

Postrenal Acute Kidney Injury

Postrenal acute kidney injury should be suspected in patients who have a history of prostatic hypertrophy (Chapter 114), prostate cancer (Chapter 186), lymphoma (Chapter 171), cervical cancer (Chapter 184), or retroperitoneal disease. However, postrenal acute kidney injury also should be considered when patients have marked oliguria (urine output < 450 mL/day) or anuria (urine output < 100 mL/day). Renal ultrasound can diagnose bladder and upper tract disease, whereas a bladder catheterization showing a large residual is the best way to diagnose lower tract disease.

TREATMENT

Fluids and Supportive Care

The treatment of acute kidney injury initially focuses on optimizing intravascular volume and withdrawing any offending agents. Because the majority of cases of elevated serum creatinine levels result from reversible volume depletion, prompt volume resuscitation during the early phases of acute kidney injury provides the greatest opportunity for minimizing kidney injury (Fig. 106-4) and is critical to avoid progression to tubular damage (Chapter 92). However, aggressive volume resuscitation must be carefully monitored in elderly patients, patients who have a history of heart failure or cirrhosis, or septic patients because of the possibility of precipitating pulmonary and/or peripheral edema. Fluid status can be monitored by an estimation of central venous pressure on physical examination

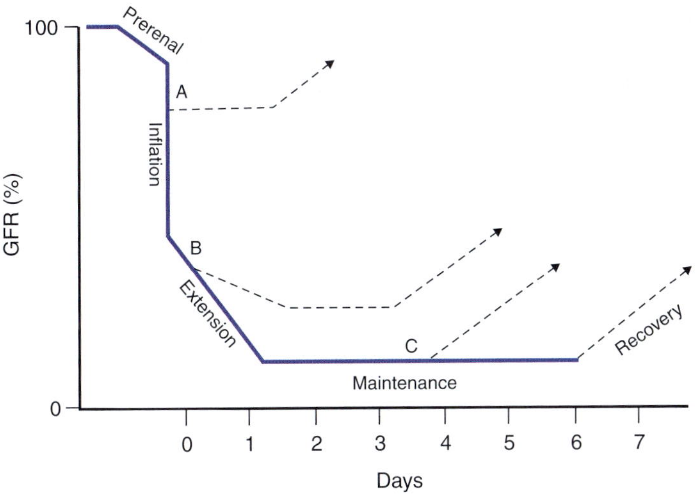

FIGURE 106-4. **Phases of acute kidney injury.** GFR = glomerular filtration rate. (From Sutton TA, Fisher CJ, Molitoris BA. Microvascular endothelial injury and dysfunction during ischemic acute renal failure. *Kidney Int*. 2002;62:1539-1549.)

(Chapters 39 and 45) as well as by monitoring the return of urine output and echocardiography (Chapter 43).

Postrenal obstructive uropathy from prostatic hypertrophy (Chapter 114) frequently can be corrected by insertion of a catheter into the bladder, often followed by definitive surgery. However, when outlet obstruction is caused by a tumor, a ureteral stent or a percutaneous nephrostomy tube usually is required.

For ischemic or septic tubular damage, no specific therapies are available, but general supportive measures include avoiding nephrotoxins, maintaining fluid balance, treating electrolyte abnormalities (with diets low in sodium, potassium, protein), and treating any comorbid or precipitating conditions aggressively. Volume overload is treated with daily diuretics (e.g., furosemide 40 to 80 mg intravenously) and a low-sodium diet. Hyperkalemia is generally treated with sodium zirconium cyclosilicate/lokelma or patiromer (see Chapter 103) and a low-potassium diet. Hyperphosphatemia is treated with oral binders (Chapter 105), hypocalcemia is treated with calcium tablets (Chapter 227), and acidosis is treated with $NaHCO_3$ tablets (Chapter 104). Intriguing experimental studies suggest that a deficiency of lipid β-oxidation and the production of β-hydroxybutyrate worsen the damage, and that treatment with niacinamide may prove to be beneficial.[17]

Immunosuppression

Intrarenal acute kidney injury resulting from glomerulonephritis (Chapter 107), vasculitis (Chapters 249), or systemic disease typically requires immunosuppressive therapy. For acute interstitial nephritis, an empiric trial of prednisone (often starting with 1 mg/kg for several days, followed by a gradual taper over 1 month) is usually tried (Chapter 108).

Dialysis

Acute hemodialysis is indicated in the setting of marked volume overload, hyperkalemia, acidosis, and uremic symptoms (e.g., changes in mentation, frank encephalopathy, myoclonus, asterixis, seizures, pleuritis, and pericarditis) that are unresponsive to dietary changes and other treatments.[18] Dialysis (Chapter 117) is generally begun when the serum creatinine level reaches about 10 mg/dL in symptomatic patients because starting it sooner is not of incremental benefit[A1,A2] and may result in unnecessary dialysis in some patients.[A3] In fact, delaying dialysis even longer (until the onset of important hyperkalemia, metabolic acidosis, or pulmonary edema) is as safe as initiating dialysis at a blood urea nitrogen level of 112 mg/dL or after 72 hours of oliguria.[A4,A5] The dose and modality of dialysis do not appear to affect the outcomes.

PREVENTION

Prevention begins with recognizing patients who are at the highest risk for developing acute kidney injury because they have known prior kidney disease or predisposing conditions, such as diabetes, atherosclerosis, hypertension, or heart failure. Consultation with a nephrologist before a potentially nephrotoxic exposure can reduce these risks. Key steps include maintaining adequate intravascular volume, avoiding nephrotoxic medications (e.g., NSAIDs and aminoglycosides), minimizing the use of radiocontrast material, and carefully monitoring urinary output and serum creatinine levels after interventions that might cause/induce acute kidney injury.

To prevent contrast-associated acute kidney injury, hydration with intravenous sodium chloride may be helpful, and the use of rosuvastatin (40 mg on admission then 20 mg/day or 10 mg/day for 2 days before and 3 days after the procedure) can reduce the risk of acute kidney injury in patients who have diabetes and chronic kidney disease.[A6] By comparison, neither intravenous sodium bicarbonate nor oral acetylcysteine reduces this risk.[A7-A9] In the intensive care unit, balanced crystalloid therapy (e.g., lactated Ringer solution) reduces the risk of acute kidney injury compared with normal saline[A10] but a similar benefit has not been demonstrated for noncritically ill adults.[A11]

PROGNOSIS

Prerenal acute kidney injury has the best prognosis. If it is diagnosed and treated early, the mortality rate is less than 10%, and most patients fully recover their kidney function. For postrenal acute kidney injury, prompt diagnosis and definitive treatment provide a high likelihood of full recovery of kidney function, but long-term prognosis depends on the cause of the obstruction.

By comparison, intrarenal acute kidney injury has a less favorable outcome, and even a 0.3 mg/dL rise in the serum creatinine level significantly increases risk, with mortality rates ranging from 30 to 80%. Mortality is higher in older patients who have hospital-acquired acute kidney injury and who are admitted to intensive care units. Acute kidney injury accelerates the progression of chronic kidney disease and is often the major reason why it progresses to end-stage kidney disease (Chapter 116). The outcomes of glomerulonephritis (Chapter 107) and vasculitis (Chapter 249) depend on the specific disease. More than 5% of patients who require hemodialysis recover enough renal function to discontinue it, but most patients (and especially patients who have prior underlying kidney disease) require chronic renal replacement therapy (Chapter 117).

GENERAL REFERENCES

For the General References and other additional features, please visit Elsevier eBooks+ at https://ebooks.health.elsevier.com.

Grade A References

A1. Barbar SD, Clere-Jehl R, Bourredjem A, et al. Timing of renal-replacement therapy in patients with acute kidney injury and sepsis. *N Engl J Med*. 2018;379:1431-1442.
A2. Bagshaw SM, Wald R, Adhikari NKJ, et al. Timing of initiation of renal-replacement therapy in acute kidney injury. *N Engl J Med*. 2020;383:240-251.
A3. Gaudry S, Hajage D, Benichou N, et al. Delayed versus early initiation of renal replacement therapy for severe acute kidney injury: a systematic review and individual patient data meta-analysis of randomised clinical trials. *Lancet*. 2020;395:1506-1515.
A4. Li X, Liu C, Mao Z, et al. Timing of renal replacement therapy initiation for acute kidney injury in critically ill patients: a systematic review of randomized clinical trials with meta-analysis and trial sequential analysis. *Crit Care*. 2021;25:15.
A5. Gaudry S, Hajage D, Martin-Lefevre L, et al. Comparison of two delayed strategies for renal replacement therapy initiation for severe acute kidney injury (AKIKI 2): a multicentre, open-label, randomised, controlled trial. *Lancet*. 2021;397:1293-1300.
A6. Wang N, Qian P, Yan TD, et al. Periprocedural effects of statins on the incidence of contrast-induced acute kidney injury: a systematic review and trial sequential analysis. *Int J Cardiol*. 2016;206:143-152.
A7. Weisbord SD, Gallagher M, Jneid H, et al. Outcomes after angiography with sodium bicarbonate and acetylcysteine. *N Engl J Med*. 2018;378:603-614.
A8. Valette X, Desmeulles I, Savary B, et al. Sodium bicarbonate versus sodium chloride for preventing contrast-associated acute kidney injury in critically ill patients: a randomized controlled trial. *Crit Care Med*. 2017;45:637-644.
A9. Timal RJ, Kooiman J, Sijpkens YWJ, et al. Effect of no prehydration vs sodium bicarbonate prehydration prior to contrast-enhanced computed tomography in the prevention of postcontrast acute kidney injury in adults with chronic kidney disease: the Kompas randomized clinical trial. *JAMA Intern Med*. 2020;180:533-541.
A10. Semler MW, Self WH, Wanderer JP, et al. Balanced crystalloids versus saline in critically ill adults. *N Engl J Med*. 2018;378:829-839.
A11. Self WH, Semler MW, Wanderer JP, et al. Balanced crystalloids versus saline in noncritically ill adults. *N Engl J Med*. 2018;378:819-828.

107 GLOMERULAR DISORDERS AND NEPHROTIC SYNDROMES

JAI RADHAKRISHNAN AND M. BARRY STOKES

GLOMERULAR DISORDERS

DEFINITION

Each *glomerulus,* the basic filtering unit of the kidney, consists of a tuft of anastomosing capillaries formed by the branching of the afferent arteriole. On average, 1 million glomeruli comprise approximately 5% of the weight of each kidney and provide almost 2 m^2 of glomerular capillary filtering surface. The glomerular basement membrane provides both a size- and charge-selective barrier to the passage of circulating macromolecules. Renal pathologic processes involving all glomeruli are called *diffuse* or *generalized;* if only some glomeruli are involved, the process is called *focal.* When dealing with the individual glomerulus, a process is *global* if the whole glomerular tuft is involved and *segmental* if only part of the glomerulus is involved. The descriptive terms *proliferative, sclerosing,* and *necrotizing* are often used (e.g., focal and segmental glomerulosclerosis; diffuse global proliferative lupus nephritis). Extracapillary proliferation or crescent formation is caused by the accumulation of macrophages, fibroblasts, proliferating epithelial cells, and fibrin within Bowman space. Such findings signify aggressive disease and consequently an adverse prognosis. Scarring of the tissue between the tubules and glomeruli, interstitial fibrosis, is also a poor prognostic sign.

EPIDEMIOLOGY

Glomerular disease is an important cause of end-stage kidney disease (Chapter 117), and diabetic kidney damage (Chapter 109) alone affects many millions of persons worldwide. Glomerular diseases associated with infectious agents such as malaria (Chapter 316), schistosomiasis (Chapter 326), human immunodeficiency virus (HIV; Chapter 355), and the hepatitis B and C viruses (Chapter 135) are major worldwide health problems. Manifestations of glomerular injury range from asymptomatic microhematuria and albuminuria to rapidly progressive oliguric kidney failure. Some patients develop massive fluid retention and edema at the onset of their glomerular disease, whereas others present with only the slow insidious signs and symptoms of chronic kidney failure (Chapter 117).

PATHOBIOLOGY

In a normal person, the urine contains no red blood cells (RBCs), the urinary excretion of albumin is less than 30 mg/day, and the total urinary excretion of protein is less than 140 mg/day. Glomerular diseases are characterized by breaks in the glomerular capillary wall, thereby leading to hematuria with proteinuria because of loss of the selective barrier to particles based on size and charge. Although increases in urinary protein excretion may come from the filtration of abnormal circulating proteins (e.g., light chains in multiple myeloma) or from the deficient proximal tubular reabsorption of normal, filtered low-molecular-weight proteins (e.g., β_2-microglobulin), the most common cause of proteinuria, and specifically albuminuria, is glomerular injury.

The nature of the initiating processes varies among different glomerular diseases. The nephrotic syndrome and glomerulonephritis (Table 107-1) are the key forms of glomerular disease. In the nephrotic syndrome (nephrosis), leakage of plasma proteins without inflammation is the primary pathogenic mechanism, whereas glomerulonephritis (nephritis) is characterized by glomerular inflammation that results in the passage of RBCs, white blood cells (WBCs), and plasma proteins into the urine. In some inflammatory diseases (e.g., lupus nephritis), nephrotic levels of proteinuria may be accompanied by cellular elements in a nephrotic-nephritic picture, whereas patients with milder involvement may have only isolated proteinuria or isolated hematuria.

In some conditions, such as diabetes and amyloidosis, structural and biochemical alterations are clearly present in the glomerular capillary wall. In others, immune-mediated kidney injury is caused by deposition of circulating immune complexes, in situ formation of immune complexes, or the localized effects of anti–glomerular basement membrane antibodies. Acquired defects in the glomerular podocytes in an increasingly recognized number of genetic glomerulopathies are also associated with proteinuria and progressive kidney dysfunction.

TABLE 107-1 TYPICAL FINDINGS IN NEPHROTIC SYNDROME VERSUS NEPHRITIS

NEPHROTIC SYNDROME	NEPHRITIS
KIDNEY INSUFFICIENCY ("AZOTEMIA")	
Uncommon at presentation	Common at presentation
PROTEINURIA	
Typically, high grade (>3 g/day)	Variable
Urine RBCs	
Few	Numerous (sometimes with RBC casts)
Urine RBC casts	
Unlikely	Likely

RBCs = red blood cells.

CLINICAL MANIFESTATIONS

Findings indicative of a glomerular origin of kidney disease include erythrocyte casts (Fig. 100-8) and dysmorphic RBCs in the urinary sediment, and abnormal amounts of albuminuria. Persistent urinary excretion of more than 500 to 1000 erythrocytes per milliliter (or more than 5 RBCs per high-power field on microscopy) is abnormal. Dysmorphic RBCs, which are deformed because of their passage through the glomerular capillary wall, as well as RBC casts, which are formed when these erythrocytes become enmeshed in a proteinaceous matrix in the lumen of the tubules, are also indicative of glomerular disease.

Proteinuria associated with glomerular disease may range from several hundred milligrams to more than 30 g daily. In some diseases, such as minimal change nephrotic syndrome, albumin is the predominant protein in the urine. In others, such as focal sclerosing glomerulonephritis and diabetes, the proteinuria, although still largely composed of albumin, is nonselective and contains many higher-molecular-weight proteins.

DIAGNOSIS

Some patients have asymptomatic microhematuria or proteinuria discovered by routine evaluations. Microscopic hematuria associated with deformed (dysmorphic) RBCs or RBC casts is likely to be glomerular in origin. Subnephrotic levels of proteinuria may arise from orthostatic proteinuria, exercise, hypertension, tubular disease, or glomerular damage.

In patients with asymptomatic urinary abnormalities of glomerular origin, the underlying kidney lesion may represent the early phase of a progressive glomerular disease or may be due to a benign, nonprogressive glomerular lesion. In general, if patients have less than 0.5 to 1.0 g of proteinuria daily or only glomerular microhematuria with a normal glomerular filtration rate (GFR) and no evidence of systemic disease, it is not necessary to proceed to a diagnostic kidney biopsy. Most of these patients need no immunosuppressive therapy. The patient can be followed closely, and biopsy need be performed only in patients with progressively increasing proteinuria or evidence of a decreasing GFR.[1]

THE NEPHROTIC SYNDROME

DEFINITION

The nephrotic syndrome (see Table 107-1) is defined by albuminuria of more than 3 to 3.5 g/day (or a ratio of 3.0 to 3.5 mg of protein per mg of creatinine in a random urine specimen) accompanied by hypoalbuminemia, edema, and hyperlipidemia. In practice, many clinicians refer to nephrotic range proteinuria regardless of whether patients have the other manifestations of the full syndrome.

EPIDEMIOLOGY

The annual incidence rate of the nephrotic syndrome in the U.S. is about 2 to 7 per 100,000 in children under age 16 years and about 3 per 100,000 among adults. The nephrotic syndrome may be primary and idiopathic (Table 107-2), or it may be caused by a known underlying condition, such as diabetes, amyloidosis, or systemic lupus erythematosus (Table 107-3). Although minimal change disease is the most common cause of nephrotic syndrome in children, idiopathic membranous nephropathy and focal segmental glomerular sclerosis

TABLE 107-2 SUBTYPES OF IDIOPATHIC NEPHROTIC SYNDROME IN ADULTS

SUBTYPE	INCIDENCE (%)
Minimal change disease	5-10
Focal segmental glomerulosclerosis	20-25
Membranous nephropathy	25-30
Membranoproliferative glomerulonephritis	5
Other proliferative and sclerosing glomerulonephritides	15-30

TABLE 107-3 NEPHROTIC SYNDROME ASSOCIATED WITH SPECIFIC CAUSES (SECONDARY NEPHROTIC SYNDROME)

SYSTEMIC DISEASES
Diabetes mellitus Systemic lupus erythematosus and other collagen vascular diseases* Amyloidosis (amyloid AL- or AA-associated)
INFECTIONS
Bacterial (congenital and secondary syphilis)* Viral (hepatitis B, hepatitis C, HIV infection, infectious mononucleosis, cytomegalovirus infection)* Parasitic (malaria, toxoplasmosis, schistosomiasis, filariasis)*
MEDICATION RELATED
Gold, mercury, and the heavy metals Penicillamine Nonsteroidal anti-inflammatory drugs, including COX2 inhibitors Lithium Captopril "Street" heroin Others: probenecid, chlorpropamide, rifampin, tolbutamide, phenindione, pamidronate
ALLERGENS, VENOMS, AND IMMUNIZATIONS
NEOPLASMS
Hodgkin lymphoma and leukemias/lymphomas (with minimal change lesion) Solid tumors (with membranous nephropathy)
HEREDITARY AND METABOLIC DISEASES
Alport syndrome* Fabry disease Sickle cell disease Diseases of the alternative complement pathway (C3 glomerulopathy and dense deposit disease)* Genetic subtypes resulting from mutations in genes encoding podocyte proteins or mitochondrial proteins (isolated or syndromic)
OTHER
Pregnancy related (includes preeclampsia) Chronic renal allograft nephropathy Serum sickness Accelerated hypertensive nephrosclerosis Renal artery stenosis Obesity Reflux nephropathy

*Indicates disorders that could also present as a nephritic-nephrotic syndrome (RBC, RBC casts with nephrotic-range proteinuria).
COX = cyclooxygenase; HIV = human immunodeficiency virus; RBC = red blood cells.

are the most common causes in adults, with the former being most common in Whites and the latter in Blacks.

PATHOBIOLOGY

Hypoalbuminemia, which is largely a consequence of urinary protein loss, also may be due to proximal tubular catabolism of filtered albumin, the redistribution of albumin within the body, and reduced hepatic synthesis of albumin. As a result, the relationship among urinary protein loss, the level of the serum albumin, and other secondary consequences of heavy albuminuria is inexact.

Salt and volume retention in the nephrotic syndrome may occur via at least two different major mechanisms. In a minority of patients, hypoalbuminemia reduces the oncotic pressure of plasma, the resulting intravascular volume depletion leads to activation of the renin–angiotensin–aldosterone axis, and this activation increases the retention of kidney sodium and fluid. However, primary salt retention in the distal nephron, which occurs independently of the renin–angiotensin–aldosterone axis, is likely the main reason for salt and water retention in nephrosis.

Thromboembolism (Chapters 67 and 68) often occurs in patients with the nephrotic syndrome. Explanations include urinary loss of antithrombin III, protein C, and protein S, which prevent thrombosis, as well as increased synthesis of acute phase reactants that promote thrombosis.

Hyperlipidemia (Chapter 190), sometimes extreme, is common in the nephrotic syndrome, likely because low oncotic pressures upregulate hepatic synthesis of apolipoproteins. Alterations in key regulatory enzymes of lipid synthesis also contribute to the lipid abnormalities. Hyperlipidemia may be absent with some causes of the nephrotic syndrome (e.g., systemic lupus erythematosus, HIV-associated nephropathy, and amyloidosis), either because of hepatic involvement or because of a systemic inflammatory state.

CLINICAL MANIFESTATIONS

Patients may present with weight gain, peripheral edema when sitting or standing, and with periorbital edema on awakening. Hypertension is common, and varying degrees of hematuria may be present. A 24-hour urine sample (or urine protein/creatinine ratio) usually shows more than 3 to 3.5 g of proteinuria. Nephrotic patients often have a hypercoagulable state (Chapter 67) and are predisposed to deep vein thrombosis (Chapter 68), pulmonary emboli (Chapter 68), and renal vein thrombosis (Chapter 110). Patients with nephrotic syndrome have increased risk for atherosclerotic complications because of the hypercoagulability and also because most nephrotic patients have elevated levels of total and low-density lipoprotein (LDL) cholesterol and lipoprotein(a), with low or normal high-density lipoprotein (HDL) cholesterol.

DIAGNOSIS

Initial evaluation of the nephrotic patient includes laboratory tests to define whether the patient has primary or idiopathic nephrotic syndrome (see Table 107-2), or a secondary cause related to a systemic disease, toxin, or medication (see Table 107-3). Common screening tests include fasting blood sugar and glycosylated hemoglobin tests for diabetes, and antinuclear antibody test for collagen vascular disease. In patients with the nephritic or nephrotic-nephritic syndrome, a low serum complement level, suggests an immune complex–mediated disease (Table 107-4). In selected patients, cryoglobulins, hepatitis B and C serologies, HIV testing, antineutrophil cytoplasmic antibodies (ANCAs), anti-GMB antibodies, serum protein and immunofixation, and other tests may be useful.

A kidney biopsy is often required in the adult nephrotic patient. Biopsy results in patients with heavy proteinuria and the nephrotic syndrome are likely to provide a specific diagnosis, determine prognosis, and guide therapy.

TREATMENT

Treatment varies by the specific cause.[2] Elevated lipid levels should be treated (Chapter 190). Chronic oral anticoagulation (Chapter 70) with warfarin is needed if thrombotic complications occur and is commonly recommended in patients with additional risk factors for thrombosis (e.g., a prior idiopathic thromboembolic event, immobilization, severe heart failure, or morbid obesity). Warfarin also may be considered in patients who have membranous nephropathy with hypoalbuminemia (<2.8 g/L) and who are at low risk for bleeding. Data are insufficient regarding the use of the direct-acting oral anticoagulants.

Edema is treated with a low-salt diet and loop diuretics (Table 102-4). Use of maximally tolerated doses of angiotensin-converting enzyme (ACE) inhibitors or angiotensin II receptor blockers (Table 64-7) often reduces proteinuria, increases the serum albumin level, and ameliorates the edema and hyperlipidemia. The combination of loop diuretics with intravenous albumin may be effective in patients with severe edema and signs of volume depletion.

IDIOPATHIC NEPHROTIC SYNDROME

MINIMAL CHANGE DISEASE

Minimal change disease, which is the most common pattern of nephrotic syndrome in children, accounts for only approximately 5 to 10% of cases of idiopathic nephrotic syndrome in adults. A similar histologic pattern may be seen as an adverse reaction to certain medications (e.g., nonsteroidal anti-inflammatory drugs [NSAIDs], lithium) or in association with certain malignancies (e.g., Hodgkin disease). The presence of autoantibodies to the podocyte protein nephrin indicates an autoimmune pathogenesis in at least some cases.[3]

TABLE 107-4 SERUM COMPLEMENT LEVELS IN NEPHRITIC SYNDROME

REDUCED COMPLEMENT LEVEL (TYPICALLY WITH NEPHRITIS)
Infection-related glomerulonephritis (e.g., streptococcal infections, endocarditis, shunt infections)
Systemic lupus erythematosus
Cryoglobulinemia
C3 glomerulopathies
NORMAL SERUM COMPLEMENT LEVEL
Immunoglobulin A nephropathy and Henoch-Schönlein purpura
Anti–glomerular basement membrane disease
Pauci-immune rapidly progressive glomerulonephritis (e.g., granulomatous polyangiitis and microscopic polyangiitis)

CLINICAL MANIFESTATIONS

Patients typically present with weight gain and periorbital and peripheral edema. Proteinuria in adult patients can average as much as 10 g/day, and subnephrotic levels are rare. Approximately 30% of adults are hypertensive and 30% have microscopic hematuria. However, an active urinary sediment with RBC casts is not seen. Many adult patients have mild-to-moderate azotemia, which may be related to hypoalbuminemia and intravascular volume depletion or to a reduction in glomerular permeability and filtration. Complement levels and serologic test results are normal.

DIAGNOSIS

In minimal change disease, histopathology typically reveals no glomerular abnormalities on light microscopy (Fig. 107-1). The tubules may show lipid droplet accumulation from absorbed lipoproteins (hence the older term *lipoid nephrosis*). Immunofluorescence staining and electron microscopy (Fig. 107-2) show no immune-type deposits. By electron microscopy, the glomerular basement membrane is normal and effacement of the visceral epithelial foot processes is noted along virtually the entire distribution of every capillary loop (Fig. 107-2).

TREATMENT

The course of minimal change disease is often one of remissions followed by relapses. About 75 to 85% of adults respond to a regimen of either daily prednisone (1 mg/kg, maximum 80 mg) or alternate-day therapy (2 mg/kg, maximum 120 mg), tapered after 2 months of treatment for a total of 5 to 6 months of therapy.[A1] Adults are not considered steroid-resistant until they have failed to respond to 16 weeks of treatment. Tapering of the steroid dose after remission should be gradual over 1 to 2 months.

Approximately 40% of adults relapse by 1 year. Infrequent relapses can be treated similarly to the initial episode.

However, in adults who have contraindications to corticosteroids, who relapse frequently, or who become corticosteroid-dependent (defined as being unable to decrease the prednisone dose without recurrent proteinuria), equivalently efficacious options include rituximab (1000 mg IV repeated in 2 weeks), cyclosporine (3 to 5 mg/kg/day for 4 months), tacrolimus (0.05 to 0.1 mg/kg/day),[A2] or mycophenolate mofetil (750 to 1000 mg twice daily). Because cyclosporine and tacrolimus are potentially nephrotoxic, trough blood levels must be monitored, and the lowest level that is associated with remission should be maintained. Cyclophosphamide (up to 2 mg/kg/day for 8 weeks) also may be used but is less desirable because of its potential for gonadal toxicity and bone marrow suppression.

PROGNOSIS

The prognosis of minimal change disease is excellent. More than 50% of patients with minimal change disease have relapses, and 10 to 20% may become steroid-dependent. Most patients who have a progressive decline in kidney function exhibit focal segmental glomerulosclerosis rather than minimal change disease on a subsequent kidney biopsy.

FOCAL SEGMENTAL GLOMERULOSCLEROSIS

Approximately 20% of adults with idiopathic nephrotic syndrome are found on biopsy to have focal segmental glomerulosclerosis. The incidence of focal segmental glomerulosclerosis is increasing in all races, but it is especially common in Black Americans.

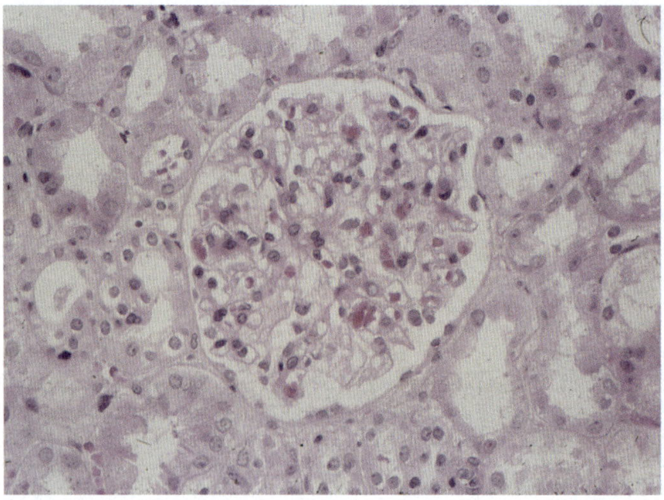

FIGURE 107-1. Unremarkable light microscopic appearance of minimal change disease glomerulopathy. Glomerular capillaries are patent and there is no glomerular hypercellularity.

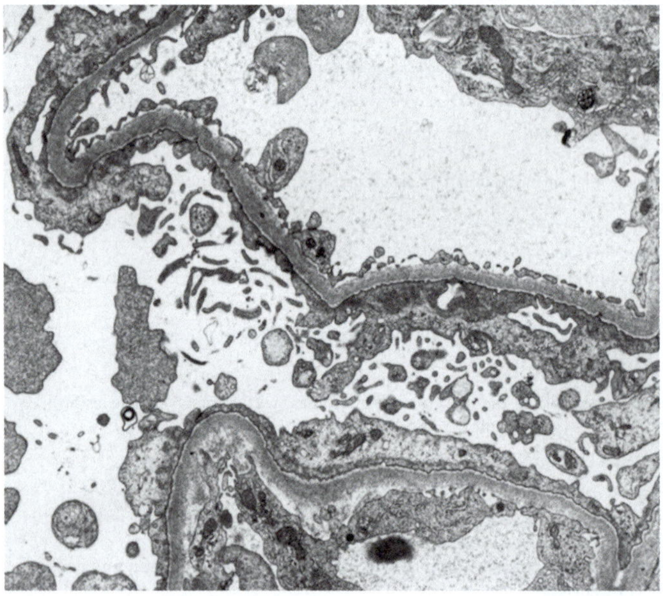

FIGURE 107-2. Minimal change disease. Electron micrograph shows widespread effacement of foot processes with microvillus transformation of the visceral epithelium. No electron-dense deposits are present (uranyl acetate, lead citrate stain; 6000×).

PATHOBIOLOGY

Several mechanisms are thought to underlie focal segmental glomerulosclerosis. In primary focal segmental glomerulosclerosis, glomerular permeability factors may cause direct injury to podocytes. In secondary focal segmental glomerulosclerosis, medications, viral infections,[4] or adaptive changes associated with glomerular hyperfiltration apparently cause the injury (Table 107-5).

Focal segmental glomerulosclerosis also can be associated with genetic variants in podocyte proteins. Pathogenic variants in collagen 4 appear to be emerging as the most common genetic form of focal segmental glomerulosclerosis. Other common defects include an autosomal recessive pattern caused by mutations in the structural protein podocin (*NPHS2*) and autosomal dominant forms caused by mutations in the structural protein α-actinin 4, the *TRPC6* glomerular slit diaphragm–associated channel, or *INF2*, which encodes a formin (actin-regulating protein). The predisposition of Black Americans to focal segmental glomerulosclerosis is partly related to two risk alleles of the apolipoprotein L1 (*APOL1*) gene, which apparently arose in high frequency because heterozygosity confers protection against African trypanosomiasis (Chapter 317), but for which biallelic inheritance increases the risk of focal segmental glomerulosclerosis by 10- to 20-fold. In the setting of severe acute respiratory syndrome coronavirus 2 (SARS-CoV-2) infection, the collapsing variant of focal segmental glomerulosclerosis has been associated with high-risk apolipoprotein L1 alleles in Black American patients.[5]

TABLE 107-5 CAUSES OF SECONDARY FOCAL SEGMENTAL GLOMERULOSCLEROSIS

SECONDARY TO ALTERATIONS OF GLOMERULAR EPITHELIAL CELLS	
Viral infections	Human immunodeficiency virus (established) Cytomegalovirus (probably) Parvovirus B19, Epstein-Barr virus, hepatitis C virus (possibly) Hemophagocytic syndrome (possibly) Severe acute respiratory syndrome coronavirus-2 (with *APOL1* risk genotype)
Drug-induced	Direct-acting antiviral therapy mTOR inhibitors Calcineurin inhibitors Anthracyclines Heroin (adulterants) Lithium Interferon Anabolic steroids Nonsteroidal anti-inflammatory drugs
SECONDARY TO ADAPTIVE CHANGES WITH GLOMERULAR HYPERTENSION	
Reduced number of nephrons	Reflux nephropathy Renal dysplasia Oligomeganephronia Sickle cell disease Age-related focal segmental glomerulosclerosis
Normal number of nephrons	Obesity-related glomerulopathy Primary glomerular diseases Systemic diseases (e.g., diabetic nephropathy, hypertensive nephrosclerosis)

APOL1 = apolipoprotein L1; mTOR = mammalian target of rapamycin.

CLINICAL MANIFESTATIONS

Patients with primary focal segmental glomerulosclerosis typically present with proteinuria, hypoalbuminemia, and edema. Absence of hypoalbuminemia is associated with focal segmental glomerulosclerosis secondary to adaptive changes to glomerular hyperfiltration as opposed to primary focal segmental glomerulosclerosis where patients show low serum albumin. Hypertension is found in 30 to 50% of patients, and microscopic hematuria occurs in approximately half of patients. The GFR is decreased at presentation in 20 to 30% of patients. Complement levels and other serologic test results are normal.

DIAGNOSIS

The diagnosis requires kidney biopsy. By light microscopy, only some glomeruli (focal) initially have areas of scarring involving only portions of a glomerulus (segmental) (Fig. 107-3).[6] As kidney function declines, repeat biopsy specimens show more widespread glomerular involvement with segmental sclerosing lesions and increased numbers of globally sclerotic glomeruli. By immunofluorescence staining, immunoglobulin M (IgM) and C3 commonly are trapped in the areas of glomerular sclerosis. Electron microscopy shows no immune-type deposits and only visceral epithelial cell foot process effacement. Typically, primary focal segmental glomerulosclerosis is associated with extensive, diffuse foot process effacement, whereas these findings are segmental in the adaptive type of focal segmental glomerulosclerosis.

TREATMENT

For primary focal segmental glomerulosclerosis, corticosteroids (e.g., prednisone, 1 mg/kg/day, maximum 80 mg, or 2 mg/kg every other day, maximum 120 mg, as tolerated) are used as initial therapy for a minimum of 3 to 4 months and slowly tapered for a total of 6 months of therapy if remission is noted. A complete or partial remission may be seen in up to 40 to 60% of patients, with preservation of long-term kidney function. Patients who do not show any improvement in 4 to 8 weeks are less likely to respond and may be switched to second-line therapy, rather than being continued on high doses of corticosteroids. Patients who do not achieve remission within 4 months are termed steroid-resistant.

In patients who are steroid-resistant, cyclosporine (5 to 6 mg/kg/day) or tacrolimus (0.05 to 0.1 mg/kg/day) is recommended.[A3] A minimum duration of 6 months is recommended before declaring resistance to calcineurin inhibitors. If remission occurs, a minimum of 12 months of therapy followed by a slow taper is suggested. Careful monitoring of kidney function and serum drug levels are necessary to avoid nephrotoxicity. Rituximab (e.g., two 1-g doses 1 week apart) has been used successfully in steroid-dependent or frequently relapsing patients,[7] but it is less effective in steroid-resistant patients.

Genetic forms of focal segmental glomerulosclerosis typically do not respond to immunosuppressive therapy. Treatment is conservative using ACE-inhibitors and angiotensin receptor blockers for blood pressure control (Table 64-7).

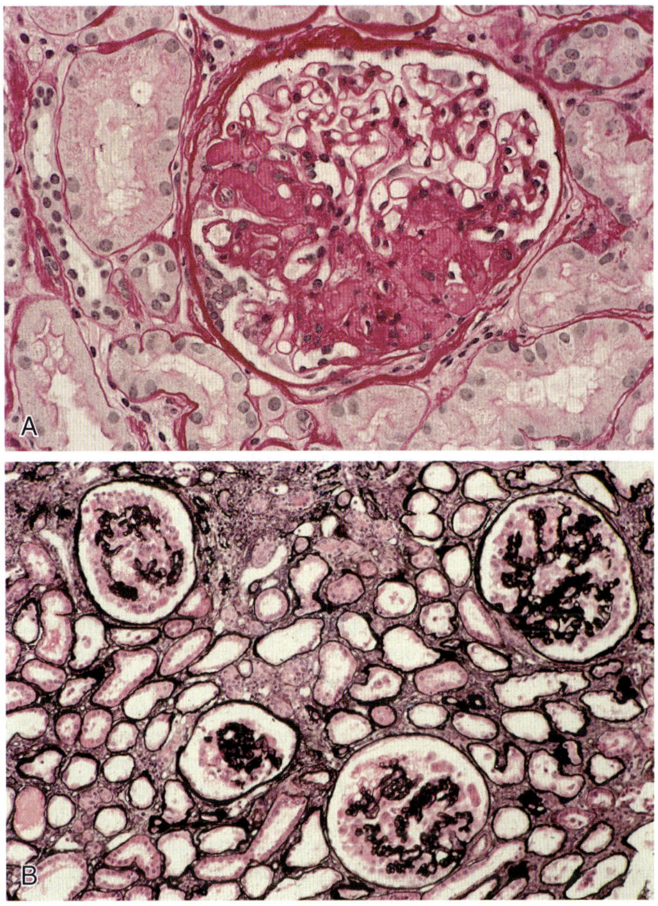

FIGURE 107-3. Focal segmental glomerulosclerosis. A, Segmental obliteration of glomerular capillaries by acellular matrix (sclerosis), which stains red with periodic acid–Schiff (PAS). **B,** Collapsing variant focal segmental glomerulosclerosis showing implosive collapse of the glomerular capillaries and hyperplasia of overlying epithelial cells (silver stain).

PROGNOSIS

The course of untreated focal segmental glomerulosclerosis is usually one of progressive proteinuria and declining GFR. The histopathologic variants of focal segmental glomerulosclerosis are associated with epidemiologic, clinical, and prognostic differences. For example, the "tip" variant has a relatively benign course, whereas the "collapsing" variant progresses more rapidly to kidney failure.

Only a minority of patients experience a spontaneous remission of proteinuria, and most untreated patients who do not remit eventually develop end-stage renal disease within 5 to 20 years. Patients with a sustained remission of their nephrotic syndrome are unlikely to progress to end-stage renal disease.

Most patients with genetic forms of focal segmental glomerulosclerosis are treatment-resistant, have a progressive course, and do not experience recurrences of the focal segmental glomerulosclerosis if they receive a kidney transplant. Primary focal segmental glomerulosclerosis recurs in the transplanted kidney in up to 30% of cases. Younger patients, those with a rapid course to kidney failure, and those with a prior recurrence are more likely to recur in the allograft.

MEMBRANOUS NEPHROPATHY

Membranous nephropathy is the most common pattern of idiopathic nephrotic syndrome in White patients. It also may be associated with infections (syphilis [Chapter 295], hepatitis B and C [Chapter 134]), systemic lupus erythematosus (Chapter 245), medications (gold salts, NSAIDs), and certain tumors (solid tumors and lymphomas). In most patients with primary membranous nephropathy, the antigen in the immune deposits is the M-type phospholipase receptor (PLA2R), which is present in podocytes.[8] Circulating PLA2R antibodies, which are highly specific for the diagnosis of primary membranous nephropathy, combine with this antigen to form in situ immune complexes on the epithelial side of the basement membrane, thereby leading to proteinuria. Other recently implicated antigens associated with primary membranous nephropathy include exostosin, NCAM-1 (neural cell adhesion molecule 1), NELL-1 (neural epidermal growth factor–like 1 protein), PCDH7 (protocadherin 7), and SEMA3B (semaphoring 3B).[9] About 10% of patients have circulating autoantibodies to the thrombospondin type-1 domain-containing 7 A (THSD7A), which has been associated with malignancy-related membranous nephropathy.

CLINICAL MANIFESTATIONS

Membranous nephropathy typically manifests with proteinuria and edema. Hypertension and microhematuria are not infrequent, but kidney function and GFR are usually preserved at presentation. Despite the finding of complement in the glomerular immune deposits, serum complement levels are normal. Membranous nephropathy is the most common pattern of the nephrotic syndrome to be associated with a hypercoagulable state and renal vein thrombosis (Chapter 110). The presence of sudden flank pain, deterioration of kidney function, or acute pulmonary symptoms in a patient with membranous nephropathy should prompt an investigation for renal vein thrombosis and pulmonary emboli. Conversely, the presence of otherwise unexplained thromboembolism should lead to a search for nephrotic syndrome.

DIAGNOSIS

A kidney biopsy is not required to confirm the diagnosis of membranous nephropathy in patients who have nephrotic syndrome, intact kidney function, absence of systemic disease, and a positive anti-PLA2R antibody test.[10] Otherwise, a kidney biopsy is required to make the diagnosis and to exclude other glomerulopathies.

On light microscopy, the glomerular capillary loops often appear rigid or thickened (Fig. 107-4), but cellular proliferation is not seen. Immunofluorescence staining and electron microscopy show immune deposits along the glomerular capillary loops beneath the visceral epithelial cell layer (Fig. 107-5). The presence of circulating antibodies to the M-type phospholipase A_2 receptor are highly sensitive and specific for idiopathic membranous nephropathy, as is the finding of PLA2R antigen in the immune deposits in the kidney.

In patients who do not have PLA2R or other recently described antibodies, membranous nephropathy may be the result of an underlying condition. In such patients, a search for systemic disease (e.g., systemic lupus erythematosus; Chapter 245), infection (e.g., syphilis [Chapter 295] and hepatitis B and C [Chapter 134]), and occult malignancy should be undertaken.

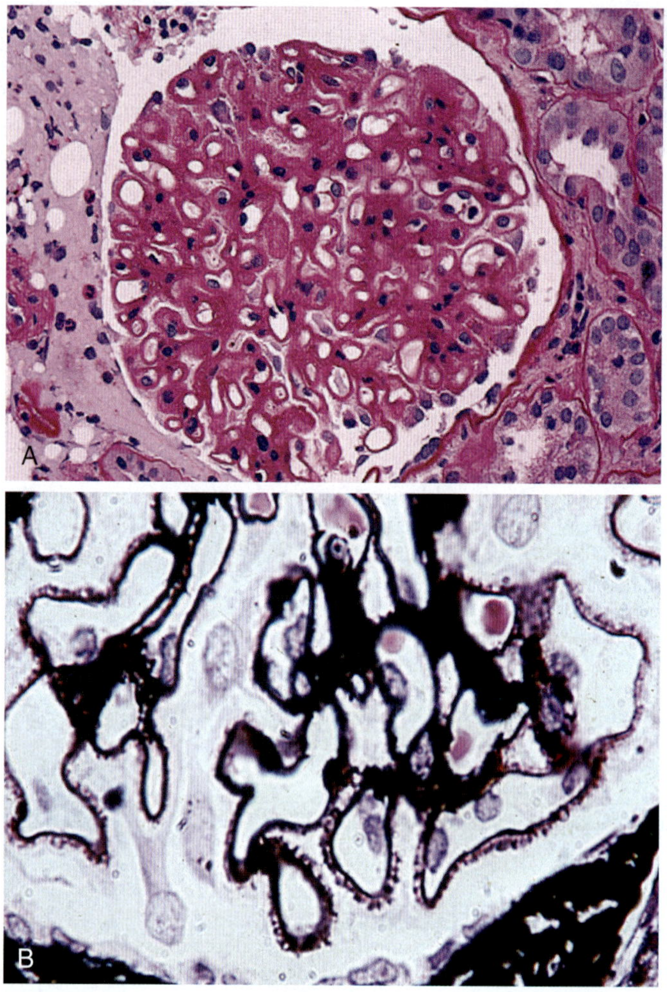

FIGURE 107-4. **Membranous nephropathy. A, Light micrograph of membranous nephropathy demonstrating thickening of the glomerular capillary wall but no hypercellularity. B, Silver stain of idiopathic membranous nephropathy showing spike formation along the outer aspect of the glomerular basement membrane corresponding to projections of the basement membrane between the epimembranous deposits.**

TREATMENT

All patients should receive optimal supportive care including blood pressure control and maximally tolerated doses of renin–angiotensin blockers (Table 64-7). Immunosuppressive therapy should be restricted to patients who are considered at risk for progressive kidney damage (Fig. 107-6).[A4,A5]

Cyclosporine (3.5 mg/kg/day adjusted to serum levels of 125 to 225 μg/L) plus prednisone (0.15 mg/kg/day up to a maximum of 15 mg/day) is the recommended initial therapy. Success with tacrolimus (0.05 to 0.10 mg/kg/day to target trough levels 3 to 8 ng/mL) has been similar to that with cyclosporine. Cyclosporine or tacrolimus should be used for a minimum of 4 months and withdrawn if there is no response. In the event of remission, treatment should be for a minimum of 12 months, usually with slow taper thereafter. Use of the anti-CD20 antibody rituximab (1000 mg IV × 2, 2 weeks apart then repeated at 6 months, if needed) has shown benefit in inducing remission.[A6] In patients at a high risk of progression, addition of rituximab after 6 months of treatment with cyclosporine is one alternative. However, the combination of corticosteroids (e.g., methylprednisolone, 1 g/day intravenously for 3 days, then prednisone, 0.5 mg/kg/day orally for 27 days, in months 1, 3, and 5) plus oral cytotoxic therapy (cyclophosphamide, 2 to 2.5 mg/kg/day, for 30 days in months 2, 4, and 6) is an alternative to rituximab[A7] for high-risk patients and is the suggested therapy for very high-risk patients.

Longitudinal monitoring of anti-PLA2R antibody levels at 6 months after the start of therapy may be useful for evaluating the response to treatment in patients, and can be used to guide adjustments to therapy.[11] Immunologic remission typical precedes proteinuric remission, and disappearance of the PLA2R antibody in patients who were positive allows discontinuation of immunosuppression despite persistent proteinuria.

In patients who do not respond to initial therapy, medications such as mycophenolate mofetil and adrenocorticotropic hormone may be attempted. However, nonresponsive patients should be referred to a specialized center with expertise in managing membranous nephropathy.

PROGNOSIS

In most large series, kidney survival in membranous nephropathy is more than 75% at 10 years, with a spontaneous remission rate of 20 to 30%. Patients with membranous nephropathy are at increased risk for developing renal vein thrombosis (Chapter 110), especially when their serum albumin levels decline.

In general, older patients, males, and those with heavy persistent proteinuria are most likely to progress to kidney failure and hence to benefit from therapy. Patients with primary membranous nephropathy and low levels of anti-*PLA2R* are more likely to have a spontaneous remission than are patients with high levels. Reductions of the circulating level of antibody to *PLA2R* precedes remission in most persons and may be a predictor of remission.

GLOMERULONEPHRITIS AND THE NEPHRITIC SYNDROME

EPIDEMIOLOGY AND PATHOBIOLOGY

The annual incidence of primary glomerulonephritis in U.S. adults is estimated to be between 0.2 to 2.5/100,000/year, with lower rates in children. The pathogenesis of glomerulonephritis includes infectious agents that activate the complement pathway. Glomerulonephritis also can be caused by the deposition of immune complexes in autoimmune diseases such as systemic lupus erythematosus (Chapter 245), IgA nephropathy, and from the effect of circulating antibodies directed against the glomerular basement membrane. Direct damage from activated white blood cells in the presence of antineutrophil cytoplasmic antibodies can also lead to the nephritic syndrome.

Invading neutrophils and monocytes, as well as resident glomerular cells, can damage the glomerulus through a number of mediators, including oxidants, chemoattractant agents, proteases, cytokines, and growth factors. Some

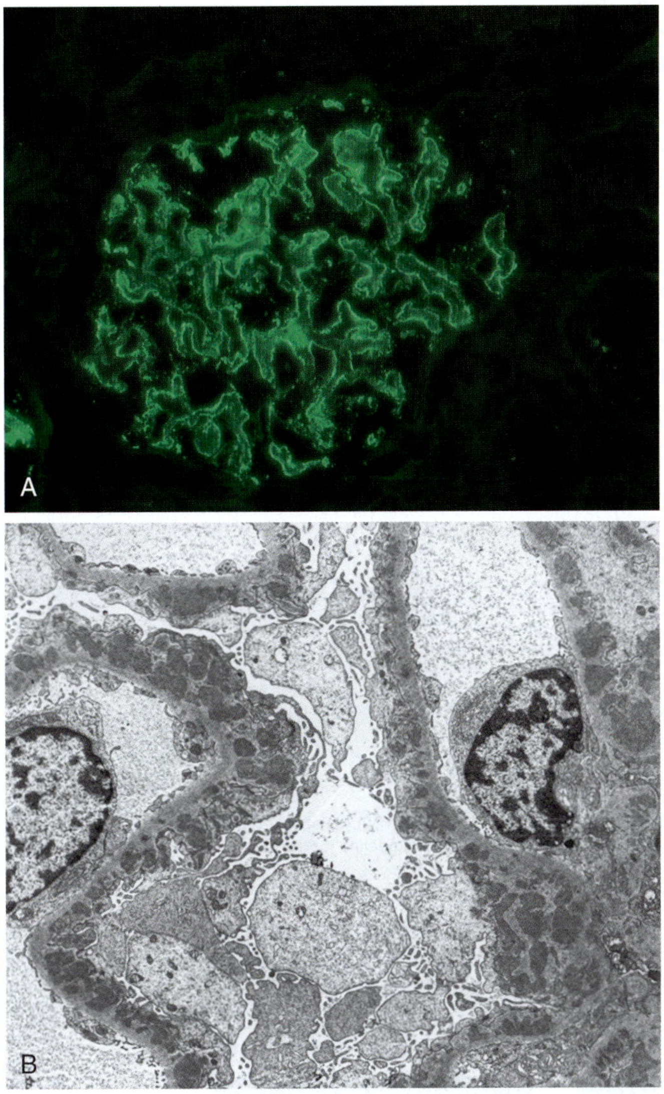

FIGURE 107-5. **Membranous glomerulopathy. A.** Granular capillary wall deposits of IgG on immunofluorescence microscopy. **B.** On ultrastructural examination, numerous, closely apposed epimembranous electron-dense deposits are separated by basement membrane spikes (uranyl acetate, lead citrate stain; 2500×).

factors, such as transforming growth factor-β, have been related to eventual glomerulosclerosis and chronic glomerular damage.

CLINICAL MANIFESTATIONS AND DIAGNOSIS

Patients with glomerulonephritis present with a nephritic picture characterized by a azotemia, oliguria, hypertension, and an active urinary sediment with hematuria and red blood cell casts (see Fig. 100-8 and Table 107-1).[12] Hypertension is common and is caused by intravascular volume expansion. Patients may note dark, smoky, or cola-colored urine or hematuria, and the urine sediment is typically composed of erythrocytes, leukocytes, and a variety of casts, including red blood cell casts. The degree of proteinuria is variable from subnephrotic to the nephrotic range. An impairment of the GFR is common. Serum complement levels may be low in the immune complex–related cause (Table 107-4). Regardless of the inciting cause, glomerulonephritis is characterized on light microscopy by hypercellularity of the glomerulus, which may be composed of infiltrating inflammatory cells, proliferation of resident glomerular cells, or both. The mechanisms associated with the various forms of glomerulonephritis are based on staining patterns on immunofluorescence microscopy (Fig. 107-7).

IMMUNOGLOBULIN A NEPHROPATHY

EPIDEMIOLOGY AND PATHOBIOLOGY

IgA nephropathy is the most frequent form of idiopathic glomerulonephritis worldwide; it represents 15 to 40% of primary glomerulonephritis in parts of Europe and Asia but is uncommon in people of African ancestry. In the United States, some centers report this diagnosis in up to 20% of all primary glomerulopathies. Males outnumber females, with peak occurrence in the second to third decades of life.

In IgA nephropathy, most patients and many of their direct blood relatives have elevated circulating levels of IgA molecules that are galactose deficient at the hinge region. The predominant form of IgA is composed of polymeric IgA1. Patients, but not relatives, have circulating IgG and IgA autoantibodies against this galactose-deficient IgA. It is thought that a second "hit" phenomenon (e.g., infection, oxidative stress, etc.) stimulates production of these antibodies, and then the resulting immune complexes deposit in the glomeruli, thereby leading to an inflammatory reaction and consequent glomerulosclerosis and interstitial fibrosis.

CLINICAL MANIFESTATIONS AND DIAGNOSIS

IgA nephropathy often presents either as asymptomatic microscopic hematuria with or without proteinuria (the most common presentation in adults) or as episodic gross hematuria after an upper respiratory tract infection or exercise (the most common presentation in children and young adults).[13,14] Approximately 20 to 50% of all patients have hypertension.

IgA nephropathy has no validated diagnostic serum or urine biomarkers. Serum complement levels are typically normal. The diagnosis of IgA nephropathy is established on kidney biopsy by finding dominant or codominant IgA deposits on immunofluorescence microscopy (Fig. 107-8). Deposits of C3 and IgG also are often found. Light microscopy varies from the most common pattern of mild mesangial proliferation to severe crescentic glomerulonephritis. By electron microscopy, immune-type dense deposits are typically found in the mesangial and paramesangial areas.

Secondary causes of IgA nephropathy include viral (HIV [Chapter 359], viral hepatitis [Chapter 135]), inflammatory bowel disease (Chapter 127), autoimmune diseases (Chapter 236), liver cirrhosis (Chapter 139), and IgA-dominant infection-related glomerulonephritis. Variant forms of IgA nephropathy that require specific intervention include IgA deposition with minimal change disease, IgA nephropathy with acute kidney injury, and IgA nephropathy with rapidly progressive glomerulonephritis.

TREATMENT

The main focus of treatment of primary IgA nephropathy is optimized supportive care,[A8] including optimizing blood pressure, with dietary sodium restriction and the use of renin angiotensin blockers at maximally tolerated doses (Table 64-7) for patients whose urine protein is greater than 0.5 g/day, regardless of whether hypertension exists. Patients who present with gross hematuria and acute kidney injury should be treated conservatively because the majority will recover without intervention. No specific dietary intervention has shown to affect progression.

In patients who are at high risk of progression (defined as proteinuria >0.75 to 1 g/day despite ≥90 days of optimized supportive care), immunosuppressive treatment should be considered, although its renal benefits are at least partly countered by its side effects.[A9] Corticosteroids are the preferred agents, typically with prednisone (1 mg/kg/day for 2 months followed by a tapering schedule over a total of 6 months).[A10] Targeted-release oral budesonide (16 mg/day) to the distal ileum, where mucosal immune dysfunction may be the precipitating cause of the IgA complexes, reduces proteinuria.[A11] Dapagliflozin (10 mg/day) is associated with a reduction in albuminuria and a slower rate of progression of kidney disease.[A12] Omega-3 fish oils are not of proven benefit and are not recommended. Mycophenolate analogs and hydroxychloroquine have shown efficacy in small trials in China.

Nephrotic syndrome with minimal IgA deposits resembles minimal change disease and should be treated as such (see earlier). Rapidly progressive glomerulonephritis with crescents (defined as ≥50% decline in eGFR over <3 months) may rarely occur with IgA nephropathy. Such patients should be treated with corticosteroids and cyclophosphamide, similar to the treatment of antineutrophil cytoplasmic antibody–associated vasculitis (see later).

PROGNOSIS

The course is variable, with some patients showing no decline in GFR over decades and others developing the nephrotic syndrome, hypertension, and kidney failure. The International IgAN Prediction Tool (https://qxmd.com/calculate/calculator_499/international-igan-prediction-tool-at-biopsy-adults?_branch_match_id=656546875419766679) is a valuable resource to quantify the risk of progression and to inform shared decision-making.[15]

Kidney survival rates are estimated at 80 to 85% at 10 years and 65% at 20 years. A significant percentage of transplant recipients have a morphologic recurrence in the allograft, but graft loss is uncommon.

Low risk	Moderate risk	High risk	Very high risk
• Normal eGFR, proteinuria <3.5 g/day, and serum albumin level >3.0 g/dL OR • Normal eGFR and proteinuria <3.5 g/day (or a decrease >50% after 6 months of conservative therapy with an angiotensin converting enzyme inhibitor or an angiotensin receptor blocker)	• Normal eGFR, proteinuria >3.5 g/day (and a failure decrease >50% after 6 months of conservative therapy with an angiotensin converting enzyme inhibitor or an angiotensin receptor blocker) AND • Not fulfilling high-risk criteria	• eGFR <60 mL/min/1.73 m^2 and/or proteinuria >8 g/day for >6 months OR • Normal eGFR, proteinuria >3.5 g/day, and no decrease >50% after 6 months of conservative therapy with an angiotensin converting enzyme inhibitor or an angiotensin receptor blocker AND at least one of the following: • Serum albumin level <2.5 g/dL • PLA2Rab >50 RU/mL • Urinary α_1-microglobulin >40 μg/min • Urinary IgG >1 μg/min • Urinary β_2-microglobulin >250 mg/day • Selectivity index >0.20	• Life-threatening nephrotic syndrome OR • Rapid deterioration of kidney function not otherwise explained
TREATMENT			
Wait and see	Wait and see OR rituximab OR calcineurin inhibitor ± corticosteroids	Rituximab OR cyclophosphamide + corticosteroids OR calcineurin inhibitor + rituximab	Cyclophosphamide + corticosteroids

FIGURE 107-6. **Risk-based treatment of membranous nephropathy.** eGFR = estimated glomerular filtration rate (see Table 106-1); PLA2Rab = M-type receptor antibodies. (Based on data from Kidney Disease: Improving Global Outcomes [KDIGO] Glomerular Diseases Work Group. KDIGO 2021 clinical practice guideline for the management of glomerular diseases. *Kidney Int.* 2021;100:S1-S276.)

Immune-complex glomerulonephritis	Anti-glomerular basement membrane disease	Anti-neutrophil cytoplasmic antibody/small vessel vasculitis
Granular deposits	**Linear deposits**	**No deposits**

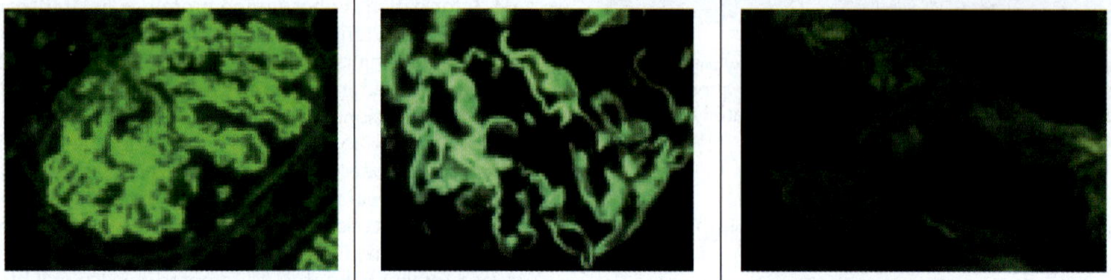

Immune-complex glomerulonephritis	Anti-glomerular basement membrane disease	Anti-neutrophil cytoplasmic antibody/small vessel vasculitis
• Infection-related glomerulonephritis • Lupus nephritis • C3 glomerulopathy • IgA nephropathy • Monoclonal gammopathy	• Renal limited • Lung limited • Renal plus lung involvement (Goodpasture syndrome)	• Polyangiitis with granulomatosis • Microscopic polyangiitis • Eosinophilic granulomatosis with polyangiitis

FIGURE 107-7. **Mechanisms of glomerulonephritis based on immunostaining patterns.**

IgA VASCULITIS (HENOCH-SCHÖNLEIN PURPURA)

IgA vasculitis, also called Henoch-Schönlein purpura (Chapter 249), is characterized by a small-vessel vasculitis with arthralgias, skin purpura, and abdominal symptoms, as well as a proliferative acute glomerulonephritis. IgA vasculitis is predominantly a disease of childhood, although cases occur at all ages.

CLINICAL MANIFESTATIONS AND DIAGNOSIS

The clinical manifestations of IgA vasculitis (Chapter 249) include dermatologic, gastrointestinal, rheumatologic, and renal findings.[16] Skin involvement typically starts with a macular rash that coalesces into purpuric lesions (see Fig. 249-2) on the ankles, legs, and occasionally arms and buttocks. Gastrointestinal symptoms include cramps, diarrhea, nausea, and vomiting, with melena and bloody diarrhea in the most severely involved cases. Although arthralgias of the knees, wrists, and ankles are common, true arthritis is uncommon. Symptoms of different organ system involvement may occur concurrently or separately, and recurrent episodes during the first year are not uncommon.

The clinical presentation resembles small vessel vasculitis and cryoglobulinemic vasculitis. As with IgA nephropathy, patients and their relatives have elevated levels of circulating IgA molecules that are galactose deficient. Kidney biopsies are identical to those seen in IgA nephropathy. Skin biopsies typically show a small-vessel leukocytoclastic angiitis with immune deposition of IgA. The presence of hypertension and degree of proteinuria influences the kidney prognosis especially if persistent over time. Treatment approaches are similar to IgA nephropathy.

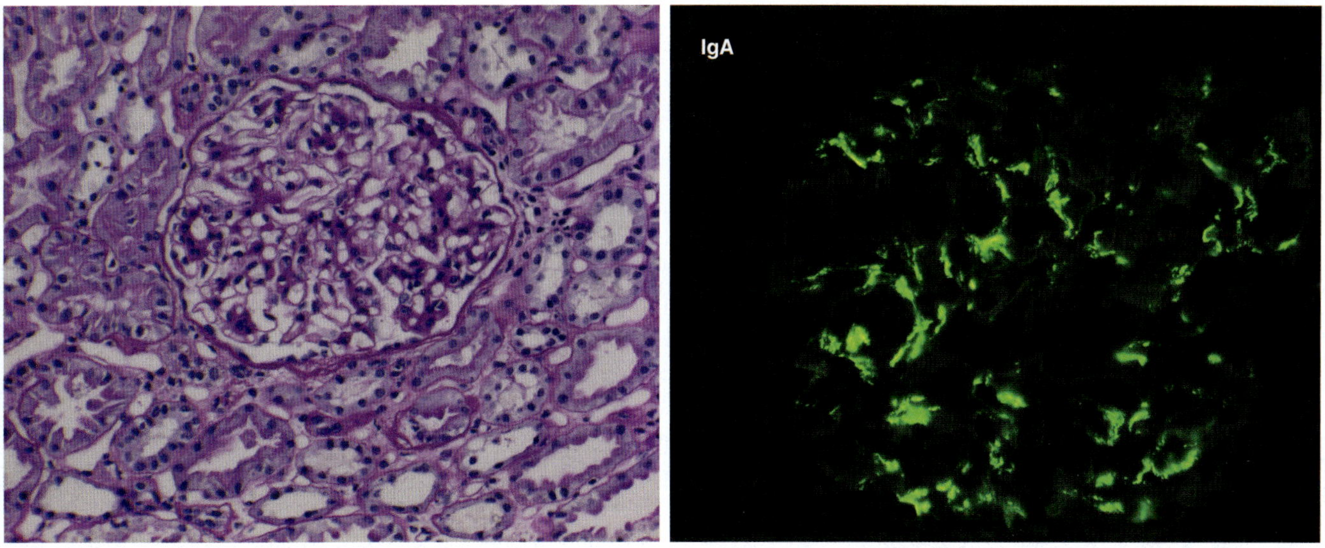

FIGURE 107-8. Immunoglobulin A (IgA) nephropathy with mesangial cell proliferation by light microscopy and IgA deposition on immunofluorescence.

POST-STREPTOCOCCAL GLOMERULONEPHRITIS

Acute post-streptococcal glomerulonephritis may occur in either an epidemic form or as sporadic cases after infection with nephritogenic strains of group A β-hemolytic streptococci (Chapter 269). Post-streptococcal glomerulonephritis is largely a disease of childhood, but severe disease in adults is well documented. The disease is most common after episodes of pharyngitis, but it can follow streptococcal infections at any site and subclinical cases greatly outnumber clinical cases. Post-streptococcal glomerulonephritis is an acute immune complex disease characterized by the formation of antibodies against streptococci with the localization of immune complexes and complement in the kidney. With improved socioeconomic conditions, the incidence of post-streptococcal glomerulonephritis has declined in developed nations. In adults, non-streptococcal bacterial infections are more common causes of infection-related glomerulonephritis.

CLINICAL MANIFESTATIONS AND DIAGNOSIS

Most cases manifest with hematuria, proteinuria, hypertension, and the nephritic syndrome (see Table 107-1) 10 days to several weeks after a streptococcal infection. Throat cultures and skin cultures of suspected sites of streptococcal involvement may no longer show group A β-hemolytic streptococci. A variety of antibodies (e.g., antistreptolysin O [ASLO], antihyaluronidase [AHT]) and a panel of antibodies against streptococcal antigens (which includes ASLO, AHT, antistreptokinase, and anti-DNase) often show high titers, but a change in titer over time is more indicative of a recent streptococcal infection. More than 95% of patients with post-streptococcal glomerulonephritis secondary to pharyngitis and 85% of patients with streptococcal skin infections have positive antibody titers. Complement C3 levels are decreased in more than 90% of patients during the episode of acute glomerulonephritis.

In a patient with a classic acute nephritic episode after a documented streptococcal infection, with a change in streptococcal antibody titer and a depressed serum complement level, a kidney biopsy adds little to the diagnosis. In other cases, a biopsy may be necessary to confirm the diagnosis. On light microscopy (Fig. 107-9), glomeruli are markedly enlarged and often fill the Bowman space. Glomeruli exhibit hypercellularity with infiltration of monocytes and polymorphonuclear cells and a proliferation of the glomerular cellular elements. The capillary lumens often are compressed. Some cases demonstrate extracapillary proliferation with crescents. On immunofluorescence microscopy, there is coarse granular deposition of IgG, IgM, and complement, especially C3, along the capillary wall. Electron microscopy shows large dome-shaped, electron-dense subepithelial deposits along the glomerular basement membrane.

TREATMENT AND PROGNOSIS

Therapy is symptomatic and directed at controlling the hypertension (see Table 64-7) and fluid retention with diuretic agents (Table 102-4) as needed. In most patients, this disease is self-limited, with recovery of kidney function and disappearance of hypertension in several weeks.[17] However, the presence of underlying kidney disease, especially diabetic nephropathy, is associated with a worse prognosis. Proteinuria and hematuria may resolve more slowly over months.

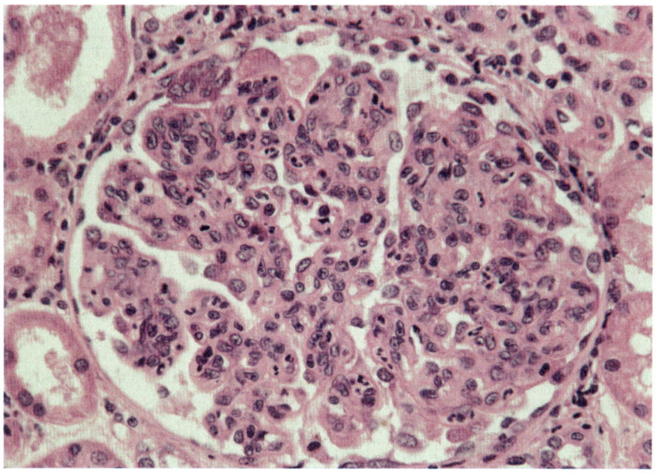

FIGURE 107-9. Post-streptococcal glomerulonephritis. A hypercellular glomerulus infiltrated by numerous polymorphonuclear leukocytes.

GLOMERULONEPHRITIS WITH ENDOCARDITIS, VISCERAL ABSCESSES, AND OTHER INFECTIONS

Various glomerular lesions are found in patients with acute and chronic bacterial endocarditis (Chapter 61). Although embolic phenomena can lead to glomerular ischemia and infarcts, a common finding is an immune complex glomerulonephritis. With *Streptococcus viridans* endocarditis, both focal or diffuse proliferative glomerulonephritis may be seen. With the increased incidence of *Staphylococcus aureus* endocarditis, 40 to 80% of patients have clinical evidence of an immune complex proliferative glomerulonephritis. Glomerulonephritis is now more common with acute than subacute bacterial endocarditis.[18]

Patients often have hematuria and urinary RBC casts, proteinuria ranging from less than 1 g/day to nephrotic levels, and progressive kidney failure. Serum complement C3 levels are usually reduced. Antineutrophil cytoplasmic antibodies (ANCA) occasionally may be positive, thereby leading to diagnostic confusion. Kidney insufficiency may be mild and reversible with appropriate antibiotic therapy, or it may be progressive and lead to dialysis and irreversible kidney failure.

A proliferative immune complex glomerulonephritis also can occur in patients with deep visceral bacterial abscesses and infections, such as empyema of the lung (Chapter 86) and osteomyelitis (Chapter 251). Immune complex forms of acute glomerulonephritis also have been noted in patients with bacterial pneumonias, including *Mycoplasma* (Chapter 293), and patients with chronically infected cerebral ventriculoatrial shunts for hydrocephalus. Many of these patients have nephrotic-range proteinuria and only mild kidney dysfunction. With appropriate antibiotic therapy, most glomerular lesions heal and kidney function recovers.

TABLE 107-6 CLASSIFICATION OF RAPIDLY PROGRESSIVE (CRESCENTIC) GLOMERULONEPHRITIS

PRIMARY
Anti–glomerular basement membrane antibody disease, Goodpasture syndrome (with pulmonary disease)
Immune complex–mediated
Pauci-immune (usually antineutrophil cytoplasmic antibody-positive)
SECONDARY
Membranoproliferative glomerulonephritis
IgA nephropathy, Henoch-Schönlein purpura
Post-streptococcal glomerulonephritis
Systemic lupus erythematosus

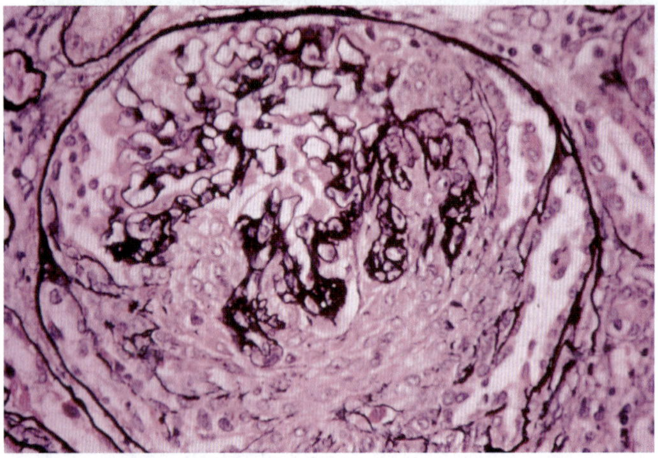

FIGURE 107-10. **Rapidly progressive glomerulonephritis.** A proliferation of cells in the Bowman space forming a crescent, with compression of the glomerular tuft.

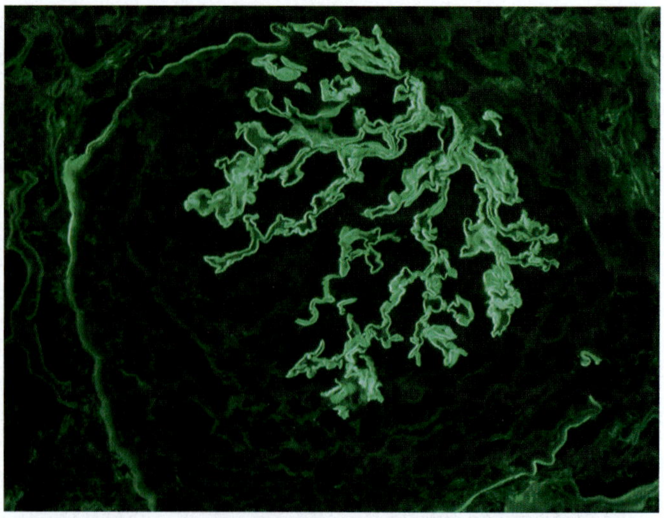

FIGURE 107-11. **Anti–glomerular basement membrane glomerulonephritis.** An immunofluorescence micrograph of a portion of a glomerulus with anti–glomerular basement membrane glomerulonephritis shows linear staining of glomerular basement membrane for immunoglobulin G (IgG) (fluorescein isothiocyanate anti-IgG stain, ×400).

TABLE 107-7 CLINICAL SYNDROMES OF KIDNEY DISEASES WITH CONCOMITANT PULMONARY DISEASES

DISEASE	MARKER
Goodpasture syndrome	+Anti–glomerular basement membrane antibodies
Small vessel vasculitis (granulomatous polyangiitis and microscopic polyangiitis)	+Antineutrophil cytoplasmic antibodies
Cryoglobulinemic vasculitis	Low C4 complement, +serum cryoglobulins
Systemic lupus erythematosus	+Anti-DNA antibodies, low complement
Nephrotic syndrome, renal vein thrombosis, pulmonary embolus	+Lung scan or +CT angiography
Pneumonia with immune complex glomerulonephritis	Low complement, circulating immune complexes
Uremic lung	Elevated creatinine level

CT = computed tomography.

An increased frequency of proliferative glomerulonephritis is also associated with staphylococcal infections in patients with diabetes. This glomerulonephritis is associated with IgA immune deposits (IgA-dominant infection related glomerulonephritis) in the glomeruli and has a poor prognosis.

RAPIDLY PROGRESSIVE GLOMERULONEPHRITIS

Rapidly progressive glomerulonephritis includes glomerular diseases that progress to kidney failure in a matter of weeks to months (Table 107-6).[19] The kidney biopsy shows extensive extracapillary proliferation manifested as crescent formation in the Bowman space (Fig. 107-10). The pathogenic mechanisms include linear anti–glomerular basement membrane antibodies, granular immune complex deposition (e.g., systemic lupus erythematosus, IgA vasculitis, infection-related glomerulonephritis), and pauci-immune, usually ANCA-positive, small vessel vasculitis.

ANTI–GLOMERULAR BASEMENT MEMBRANE DISEASE

Anti–glomerular basement membrane disease has two peaks of occurrence: in the third decade of life, predominantly in men, and after 60 years of age, predominantly in women. Anti–glomerular basement membrane disease (Fig. 107-11) is caused by circulating antibodies that are directed against the noncollagenous domain of the α_3 chain of type IV collagen. These antibodies damage the glomerular basement membrane, thereby resulting in an inflammatory response, breaks in the glomerular basement membrane, and the formation of a proliferative and often crescentic glomerulonephritis. If the anti–glomerular basement membrane antibodies cross-react with and damage the basement membrane of pulmonary capillaries, the patient develops pulmonary hemorrhage and hemoptysis, an association called Goodpasture syndrome and one of several diseases that can present with concomitant kidney and lung disease (Table 107-7).

CLINICAL MANIFESTATIONS AND DIAGNOSIS

Patients present with a nephritic picture (see Table 107-1). Kidney function may deteriorate from normal to dialysis-requiring levels in a matter of days to weeks.[20] Patients with pulmonary involvement may have life-threatening hemoptysis with dyspnea and with diffuse alveolar infiltrates on chest radiograph. The pathology of anti–glomerular basement membrane disease shows a proliferative glomerulonephritis, often with severe crescentic proliferation in the Bowman space (see Fig. 107-10). There is linear deposition of immunoglobulin (usually IgG) along the glomerular basement membrane by immunofluorescence (see Fig. 107-11), but electron microscopy does not show electron-dense deposits.

TREATMENT

Although the treatment of this anti–glomerular basement membrane disease has not been studied in large controlled trials, intensive immunosuppressive therapy is recommended with corticosteroids, cyclophosphamide, and plasmapheresis. Rapid treatment is necessary to prevent irreversible kidney damage and is also needed in patients with pulmonary hemorrhage. The possible exceptions to immunosuppression are patients who have 100% crescents or more than 50% global glomerulosclerosis in an adequate biopsy sample without pulmonary hemorrhage and who are treated with dialysis at presentation, because the prognosis for renal recovery is poor.

Corticosteroids are given as daily pulse methylprednisolone (15 to 30 mg/kg to a maximum dose of 1000 mg/day IV for three doses), followed by prednisone (1 mg/kg/day orally to a maximum of 60 to 80 mg/day), and slowly tapered over 6 months. Cyclophosphamide (2 to 3 mg/kg/day orally, dose adjusted to kidney function, age, and the granulocyte count) for 3 months is also given. Daily plasmapheresis (40 to 50 mL/kg) against albumin is also recommended until anti–glomerular basement membrane antibodies are negative, typically within 14 days. This combination therapy is effective in 90% of patients with lung hemorrhage. In patients who present with a serum creatinine less than 5.6 mg/dL, kidney survival is about 95% at 5 years. When the creatinine at presentation is greater than 5.6 mg/dL but the patient does not require immediate dialysis, renal survival is about 80% at 1 year and 50% at 5 years. In patients who present with an initial requirement for dialysis, however, renal recovery occurs only in about 8% of patients at 1 year. Relapses and recurrences are very rare after kidney transplantation.

IMMUNE COMPLEX RAPIDLY PROGRESSIVE GLOMERULONEPHRITIS

Rapidly progressive glomerulonephritis-associated immune complex–mediated glomerular damage can be seen with idiopathic glomerulopathies, such as IgA nephropathy, IgA vasculitis, and idiopathic membranoproliferative glomerulonephritis, or with systemic diseases, such as infection-related glomerulonephritis, cryoglobulinemic vasculitis, and systemic lupus erythematosus. Many cases of crescentic postinfectious glomerulonephritis resolve with successful treatment of the underlying infection. The treatments of others are as described elsewhere in this chapter.

PAUCI-IMMUNE AND VASCULITIS-ASSOCIATED RAPIDLY PROGRESSIVE GLOMERULONEPHRITIS

Pauci-immune rapidly progressive glomerulonephritis includes patients with and without evidence of systemic vasculitis. Most patients have circulating antineutrophil cytoplasmic antibodies (ANCAs) that are directed against components of neutrophil primary granules.[21] Clinical syndromes of ANCA-associated vasculitis include granulomatous polyangiitis (Chapter 249), microscopic polyangiitis, and eosinophilic granulomatosis with polyangiitis (Chapter 249).

CLINICAL MANIFESTATIONS AND DIAGNOSIS

Patients with ANCA-associated vasculitis often present with progressive kidney failure and a nephritic picture (see Table 107-1). Patients with microscopic polyangiitis often have circulating perinuclear ANCA (antibodies directed against granulocyte myeloperoxidase) and a systemic clinical picture (Chapter 249) with arthritis, dermal leukocytoclastic vasculitis, pulmonary disease, and constitutional and systemic signs. Patients with granulomatous polyangiitis often have circulating cytoplasmic ANCA (antibodies directed against a granulocyte serine proteinase, anti-PR3), upper and lower respiratory tract involvement by granulomatous angiitis, as well as pauci-immune glomerulonephritis (Chapter 249). However, there is considerable overlap among these groups, and some patients have both ANCA and anti–glomerular basement membrane antibodies. Patients with eosinophilic granulomatosis with polyangiitis usually have a history of asthma, pulmonary infiltrates, and circulating eosinophilia. If they are ANCA positive, they often have associated glomerular disease. Although there is no direct correlation between ANCA titers and disease activity, patients with high titers (especially high anti-PR3 titers) and patients with a major recent increase in titers are more likely to have flares of their disease.

TREATMENT

For induction therapy (Fig. 107-12), corticosteroids in combination with cyclophosphamide or rituximab should be used as initial treatment. Corticosteroids are typically administered as pulse methylprednisolone (10 to 15 mg/kg/day up to a maximum of 500 to 1000 mg/day IV for 3 days, followed by prednisone or equivalent, 1 mg/kg/day orally for the first week). By 6 months, prednisone should be tapered to 5 mg/day in cyclophosphamide-treated patients and withdrawn in rituximab-treated patients. Adjunctive therapy with avacopan (30 mg twice daily for 52 weeks in combination with standard therapy), which is an inhibitor of the C5a complement receptor and which may allow for lower cumulative corticosteroid exposure, is recommended for severe disease.[A13] Cyclophosphamide may be administered intravenously (15 mg/kg IV every 2 to 3 weeks for 6 to 10 doses) or orally (1.5 to 2 mg/kg/day for 3 to 6 months). Rituximab, a monoclonal antibody against CD20-positive B cells (375 mg/m^2 weekly for 4 weeks, or 1 g at 0 and 2 weeks), is effective and as safe as cyclophosphamide at 6 months or more. The role of plasmapheresis is controversial, but it may be considered for patients who have a serum creatinine level greater than 5.7 mg/dL (500 mmol/L), who require dialysis, or who have rapidly worsening renal function, as well as for patients who have diffuse alveolar hemorrhage with hypoxemia. Plasmapheresis is also commonly prescribed in the overlap syndrome of ANCA vasculitis and anti–glomerular basement membrane disease. In patients who have severe ANCA-associated vasculitis, cyclophosphamide may be added to rituximab.

The risk of relapse is significant when ANCA-associated vasculitis is treated with cyclophosphamide induction, so azathioprine (1.5 mg/kg/day) with or without low-dose corticosteroids (e.g., prednisone 5 mg/day) or rituximab (500 mg at months 6, 12, and 18) without corticosteroids should be used to prevent relapse (see Fig. 107-12). Mycophenolate mofetil or methotrexate also have been used in patients intolerant or unable to take rituximab or azathioprine. The optimal duration of maintenance therapy after achieving remission is not known but should be between 18 months and 4 years with azathioprine and 18 months after rituximab. Patients with relapsing disease should preferably be treated with rituximab in addition to corticosteroids.

PROGNOSIS

The prognosis of untreated ANCA-associated vasculitis is poor (Chapter 249), with a 90% mortality at 2 years. Despite treatment, the 5-year mortality is 25%, with infection and active vasculitis being the main causes of death. Fortunately, ANCA-associated vasculitis has a low chance of recurrence in a kidney allograft.

MEMBRANOPROLIFERATIVE GLOMERULONEPHRITIS

Membranoproliferative glomerulonephritis is classified based on immunofluorescence findings into immunoglobulin-mediated, complement-mediated and neither immunoglobulin or complement-mediated categories (Table 107-8).[22]

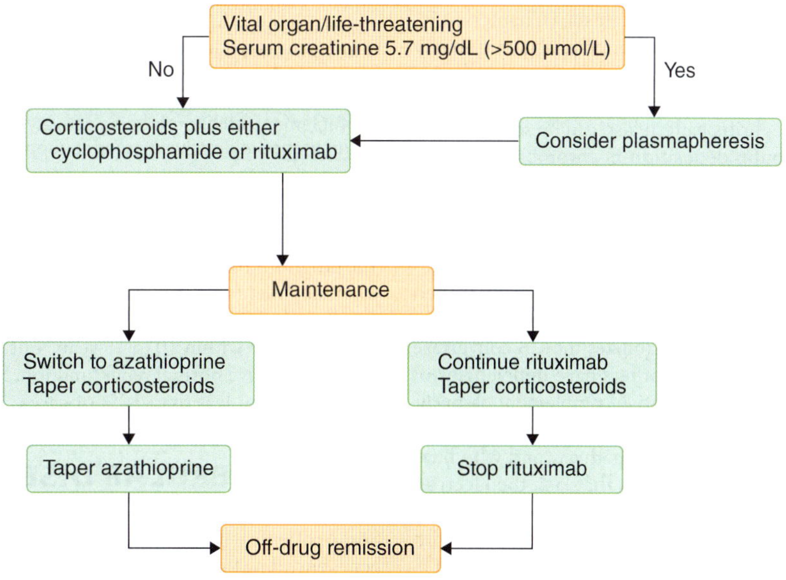

FIGURE 107-12. Treatment regimen for antineutrophil cytoplasmic antibodies–associated vasculitis. (Based on Kidney Disease: Improving Global Outcomes [KDIGO] Glomerular Diseases Work Group. KDIGO 2021 Clinical Practice Guideline for the Management of Glomerular Diseases. *Kidney Int.* 2021;100:S1-S276.)

TABLE 107-8 CAUSES OF A MEMBRANOPROLIFERATIVE PATTERN OF INJURY

Immunoglobulin-/immune complex–mediated	**Deposition of antigen–antibody immune complexes as a result of an infection:** • Viral: hepatitis C (including associated with mixed cryoglobulinemia), hepatitis B • Bacterial: endocarditis, infected ventriculo-atrial shunt, visceral abscesses, leprosy, meningococcal meningitis • Protozoa/other infections: malaria, schistosomiasis, mycoplasma, leishmaniasis, filariasis, histoplasmosis **Deposition of immune complexes as a result of an autoimmune disease:** • Systemic lupus erythematosus • Sjögren syndrome • Rheumatoid arthritis • Mixed connective tissue disease **Deposition of monoclonal Ig as a result of a monoclonal gammopathy due to a plasma cell or B cell disorder** **Fibrillary glomerulonephritis** **Idiopathic:** • None of the conditions above are present
Complement-mediated	**C3 glomerulonephritis and C3 dense deposit disease:** • Mutations in complement regulatory proteins: complement factor H, complement factor I, complement factor H–related protein 5 • Mutations in complement factors: C3 • Antibodies to complement factors: C3, C4, and C5 nephritic factors • Antibodies to complement regulatory proteins: complement factor H, complement factor I, complement factor B **C4 glomerulonephritis and C4 dense deposit disease**
Membranoproliferative pattern without immune complexes or complement	• Healing phase of hemolytic–uremic syndrome/thrombotic thrombocytopenic purpura • Antiphospholipid (anticardiolipin) antibody syndrome • POEMS syndrome • Radiation nephritis • Nephropathy associated with bone marrow transplantation • Drug-associated thrombotic microangiopathies • Sickle cell anemia and polycythemia • Dysfibrinogenemia and other prothrombotic states • Antitrypsin deficiency

POEMS = polyneuropathy, organomegaly, endocrinopathy, monoclonal protein, skin changes.

Common causes of immunoglobulin-mediated membranoproliferative glomerulonephritis include systemic lupus erythematosus (Chapter 245), infections such as hepatitis C (Chapter 134), and monoclonal gammopathy (Chapter 173). Complement-mediated membranoproliferative glomerulonephritis includes dense deposit disease and C3 glomerulonephritis. The membranoproliferative glomerulonephritis pattern also can be seen without either complement or immunoglobulin deposition in chronic thrombotic microangiopathies that are associated with endothelial cell injury. All these stimuli have been proposed to incite the glomerular mesangial cells to grow out along the capillary wall and split the glomerular basement membrane.

C3 glomerulopathies, which include dense deposit disease and C3 glomerulonephritis, are rare glomerular diseases characterized by uncontrolled systemic activation of the alternative complement pathway. Many patients have C3 nephritic factor, an autoantibody that stabilizes the C3 convertase of the alternate complement pathway, whereas others have deficiencies of factor H, factor I, or other inhibitors of the alternative complement pathway. Dense deposit disease may be associated with partial lipodystrophy. Patients who have activation of the alternative complement pathway and who have a proliferative glomerulonephritis with C3 deposits that lack the electron microscopic features of dense deposit disease have C3 glomerulonephritis.

Most patients with membranoproliferative glomerulonephritis present with proteinuria or the nephrotic syndrome.[23] Low serum complement levels (C3 and C4) are found intermittently in immunoglobulin-associated membranoproliferative glomerulonephritis, whereas only the C3 level is usually reduced in dense deposit disease. The diagnosis of dense deposit disease requires a kidney biopsy that shows complement C3 in a characteristic ribbon-like pattern around the capillary loops (Fig. 107-13). All patients with membranoproliferative glomerulonephritis on a biopsy should be evaluated for underlying disease (see Table 107-8). If no cause is found, an evaluation for a complement-related disorder (Chapter 37) should be undertaken if possible.

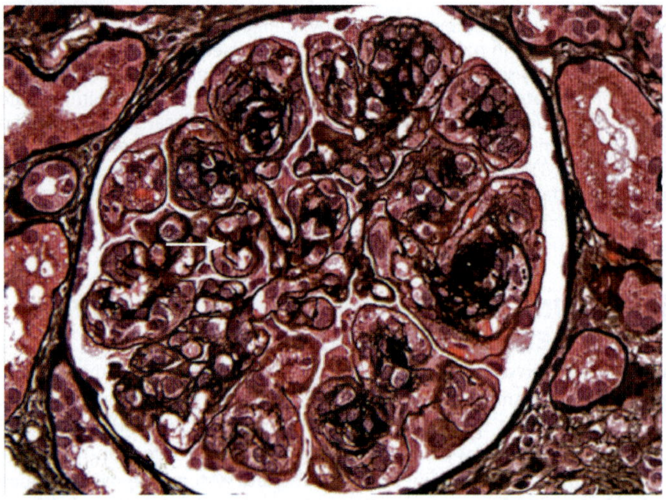

FIGURE 107-13. **Membranoproliferative glomerulonephritis. Note lobulation of the glomerular tuft and duplication of the basement membrane as seen by silver stain.**

TREATMENT

When the cause of immune complex membranoproliferative glomerulonephritis is determined, the initial approach to treatment should focus on the underlying pathologic process. For idiopathic immune complex membranoproliferative glomerulonephritis with proteinuria 3 g/day or less and normal kidney function, supportive care with blood pressure control, preferably with an ACE-inhibitor or angiotensin receptor blocker (Table 64-7), is adequate. For patients with abnormal kidney function but without crescentic involvements or an active urine sediment, with or without nephrotic-range proteinuria, corticosteroids and immunosuppressive therapy should be prescribed. Prednisone can be initiated at 1 mg/kg/day (maximum dose 60 to 80 mg/day) for 12 to 16 weeks. Mycophenolic acid analogs (e.g., mycophenolate mofetil 2 to 3 g/day) may be added for 6 to 12 months if a suboptimal response is seen after this time, with tapering of prednisone to 20 mg/day. In refractory patients, cyclophosphamide (2 mg/kg/day, maximum 200 mg/day) with prednisone (10 mg/day for 3 to 6 months) or rituximab (1 g × 2 doses 2 weeks apart, followed by a third dose in 6 months) may be given. For patients with rapidly progressive crescentic membranoproliferative glomerulonephritis, treatment with intravenous methylprednisolone (1 to 3 g) followed by oral corticosteroids and oral cyclophosphamide using a regimen similar to that used for patients with ANCA-associated vasculitis is suggested.

Patients who have C3 glomerulopathies (dense deposit disease and C3 glomerulonephritis) with moderate to severe disease (with proteinuria >1 g/day and hematuria or with declining kidney function) may be considered for immunosuppressive therapy with mycophenolic acid analogs plus corticosteroids, at doses similar to immune complex membranoproliferative glomerulonephritis. However, the evidence for efficacy for the latter is not established. The role of complement inhibitors is being actively investigated in both immune complex membranoproliferative glomerulonephritis and C3 glomerulopathies.

PROGNOSIS

The prognosis for membranoproliferative glomerulonephritis is dependent on whether patients achieve remission of proteinuria and stabilization of kidney function.[24] Up to 50 to 60% of untreated patients will progress to end-stage kidney disease within 10 to 15 years, but 25 to 40% of untreated patients will continue to have normal renal function. Spontaneous remission or improvement occurs in less than 10% of cases. With treatment, remission rates in observational studies have varied from 30 to 50%.

GLOMERULAR DISEASES ASSOCIATED WITH GENETIC DEFECTS

Some patients with focal segmental glomerulosclerosis have abnormalities in genes encoding for podocyte proteins, ion channels, or podocyte mitochondrial constituents. Other patients, often with a history of clinical kidney disease in siblings and other relatives, have other forms of hereditary nephritis.[25]

Alport Syndrome

Alport syndrome is a hereditary form of glomerulonephritis that often manifests with asymptomatic urinary findings. In approximately 85% of cases, it is an X-linked condition with hematuria and proteinuria, often in association with high-pitched hearing loss and abnormalities of the lens of the eye (lenticonus). X-linked form of disease are due to mutation in the α_5 chain of type IV collagen *(COL4A5)*. Mutations in the α_3 and α_4 chains of type IV collagen *(COL4A3, COL4A4)* cause dominant or recessive forms of disease.[26] Recessive forms of disease have severe, early-onset presentation, whereas dominant forms of disease have a very variable clinical course, ranging from normal, stable kidney function to progressive kidney failure. Patients with heterozygous pathogenic variants in *COL4A3/COL4A4* are often underdiagnosed and are frequently labeled as kidney disease of unknown cause. Although the light microscopy findings vary from mild mesangial proliferative to advanced sclerosing lesions depending on the stage of biopsy, electron microscopy typically shows areas of glomerular basement membrane thinning and other areas of glomerular basement membrane splitting with lamellations.

Use of ACE inhibitors (Table 64-7) at the onset of proteinuria delays progression of kidney failure, but males with X-linked Alport syndrome *(COL4A5)* often have progressive glomerulosclerosis and develop end-stage kidney disease. Owing to random X-inactivation, females with *COL4A5* mutations tend to have milder disease and may only progress to kidney failure late in life.

Fabry Disease

Fabry disease (Chapter 192), which is caused by an X-linked recessive genetic defect of α-galactosidase, leads to the deposition of ceramide trihexose in the kidneys and other organs. It may cause progressive proteinuria and kidney insufficiency in males and in some female carriers. It is associated with telangiectasias of the skin, typically in the bathing suit area, acroparesthesias, cardiac abnormalities, and eye changes. Replacement with intravenous recombinant enzyme agalsidase β is associated with clinical improvement.

Nail-Patella Syndrome

Nail-patella syndrome, associated with skeletal and nail deformities, is a rare cause of the nephrotic syndrome. It is due to an autosomal dominant mutation in the LMX1B transcription factor that regulates collagen, nephrin, and podocin gene expression. Progression to end-stage kidney disease is variable and estimated to be 1 to 15%. The use of maximally tolerated doses of ACE inhibitors or angiotensin receptor blockers (Table 64-7) may reduce proteinuria.

OTHER GLOMERULAR DISEASES

SYSTEMIC LUPUS ERYTHEMATOSUS

The pattern and degree of kidney involvement greatly influences the course and therapy of systemic lupus erythematosus (Chapter 245). Although the incidence of clinical kidney disease in systemic lupus erythematosus varies from 15 to 75%, histologic evidence of kidney involvement is found in most biopsy specimens.

The classification of lupus nephritis can provide a guide to therapy and prognosis (Table 107-9).[27] In general, patients with class I and II disease have mild lesions that require no therapy directed at the kidney, whereas all patients with class IV lesions (diffuse proliferative lupus nephritis) on biopsy (Fig. 107-14) require vigorous therapy. Many patients with class III (focal proliferative lupus nephritis) disease, especially patients who have active necrotizing lesions and large amounts of subendothelial deposits, also benefit from vigorous therapy. For patients with class V (membranous lupus nephritis) disease, the optimal therapy is less clear, and recommendations vary from uniform vigorous treatment to reserving such therapy for patients with serologic activity or more severe nephrotic syndrome.

TABLE 107-9 INTERNATIONAL SOCIETY OF NEPHROLOGY/RENAL PATHOLOGY SOCIETY CLASSIFICATION OF LUPUS NEPHRITIS

CLASS	CLINICAL FEATURES
I. Minimal mesangial lupus nephritis	Normal glomeruli by light microscopy but mesangial immune deposits by immunofluorescence
II. Mesangial proliferative lupus nephritis	Purely mesangial hypercellularity by light microscopy, with mesangial immune deposits
III. Focal lupus nephritis < 50% glomeruli involved A. Active A/C. Active and chronic C. Chronic	Active or inactive focal, segmental, or global endo- or extracapillary glomerulonephritis involving <50% of all glomeruli, typically with focal subendothelial immune deposits, with or without mesangial alterations
IV. Diffuse lupus nephritis (>50% glomeruli involved); all may be with segmental or global involvement (S or G) A. Active A/C. Active and chronic C. Chronic	Active or inactive diffuse, segmental or global endo- or extracapillary glomerulonephritis involving ≥50% of all glomeruli, typically with diffuse subendothelial immune deposits, with or without mesangial alterations
V. Membranous lupus nephritis glomerulonephritis	Global or segmental subepithelial immune deposits or their morphologic sequelae by light microscopy and by immunofluorescence or electron microscopy, with or without mesangial alterations
VI. Advanced sclerotic lupus nephritis	≥90% of glomeruli globally sclerosed without residual activity

Based on Weening JJ, D'Agati VD, Schwartz MM, et al. The classification of glomerulonephritis in systemic lupus erythematosus revisited. *J Am Soc Nephrol.* 2004;15:241-250; and Bajema IM, Wilhelmus S, Alpers CE, et al. Revision of the International Society of Nephrology/Renal Pathology Society classification for lupus nephritis: clarification of definitions, and modified National Institutes of Health activity and chronicity indices. *Kidney Int.* 2018;93:789-796.

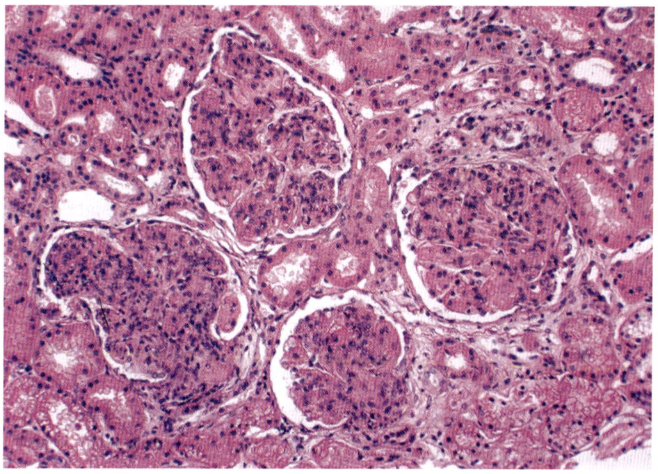

FIGURE 107-14. Diffuse proliferative lupus nephritis. Note involvement of all glomeruli.

TREATMENT

All patients with lupus nephritis should be treated with hydroxychloroquine (6.5 mg/kg ideal weight/day or 400 mg/day) or an equivalent antimalarial if there are no contraindications. For patients with class I or class II lupus nephritis with normal or low-grade proteinuria, no specific treatment is needed beyond what is given for extrarenal lupus. Patients who have class I/II lupus nephritis with nephrotic range proteinuria are considered to have lupus podocytopathy; treatment is as for minimal change disease (see earlier).

Initial therapy for patients with active class III or IV lupus nephritis, with or without a membranous component, is corticosteroids, with either low-dose intravenous cyclophosphamide or mycophenolic acid analogues (Fig. 107-15).[28] A novel calcineurin inhibitor, voclosporin (23.7 mg twice daily), has been used with a mycophenolic acid analog and corticosteroids in patients with eGFR ≥45 mL/min/1.73 m² with improved response rates.[A14] Similarly, the addition of belimumab, a monoclonal antibody that inhibits B-cell activating factor (at 10 mg/kg intravenously), to standard therapy increases the response rate when added to initial therapy.[A15]

After the induction period, the prednisone dose should be tapered to below 5 to 7.5 mg/day and other medications should be discontinued. For maintenance therapy, mycophenolate mofetil (1000 mg twice daily) is preferred over azathioprine (2 mg/kg/day). If neither is tolerated, alternatives include tacrolimus (trough approximately 4 to 6 ng/mL or 5 to 7.4 nmol/L) or cyclosporine A (trough approximately 60 to 100 ng/mL or 50 to 83 nmol/L) or mizoribine (3 mg/kg/day).

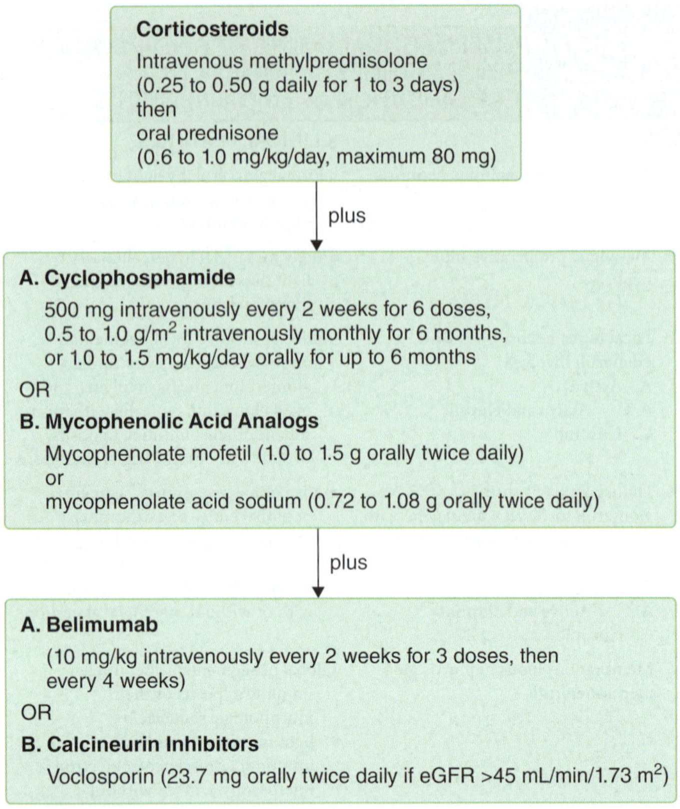

FIGURE 107-15. Initial therapy of active class III/IV with or without class V lupus nephritis. eGFR= estimated glomerular filtration rate. (Adapted from Kidney Disease: Improving Global Outcomes [KDIGO] Glomerular Diseases Work Group. KDIGO 2021 clinical practice guideline for the management of glomerular diseases. *Kidney Int.* 2021;100:S1-S276.)

Many patients with lupus nephritis (40 to 50%) produce autoantibodies against certain phospholipids, including anticardiolipin antibodies. Those patients who experience clotting in the glomeruli and arterioles require anticoagulation with either warfarin (Chapter 70) or antiplatelet agents (e.g., aspirin 81 to 325 mg/day) or with both, as well as immunosuppressive medications.

PROGNOSIS

Despite aggressive therapy, 10 to 30% of patients with lupus nephritis develop kidney failure. Moreover, patients with lupus nephritis have a higher risk for death compared with lupus patients without kidney involvement (Chapter 245). The risk of recurrence of lupus nephritis in kidney allografts is low.

DIABETES MELLITUS

Diabetic nephropathy, which is the most common form of glomerular disease in developed countries, is discussed in detail in Chapter 109.

MONOCLONAL GAMMOPATHY OF RENAL SIGNIFICANCE

Monoclonal gammopathy of renal significance refers to the association of B-cell or plasma-cell clonal disorders that per se do not fulfill criteria for cancer yet produce a nephrotoxic monoclonal immunoglobulin that leads to kidney disease. The toxicity of light chains results from multiple mechanisms, and kidney biopsy typically shows monotypic (single light and/or heavy chain) immunoglobulin deposition associated with a variety of morphologic patterns.[29]

AMYLOIDOSIS

Renal amyloid deposits, whether due to AL, AA, or hereditary-genetic forms of amyloid, are predominantly found within the glomeruli, where they often appear as amorphous eosinophilic extracellular nodules (Chapter 174). In all amyloidosis, proteins form β-pleated sheets, which are deposited in organs. All amyloid subtypes display apple-green birefringence under polarized light with the Congo red stain. By electron microscopy, amyloid appears as nonbranching rigid fibrils 8 to 10 nm in diameter. In AL amyloid,

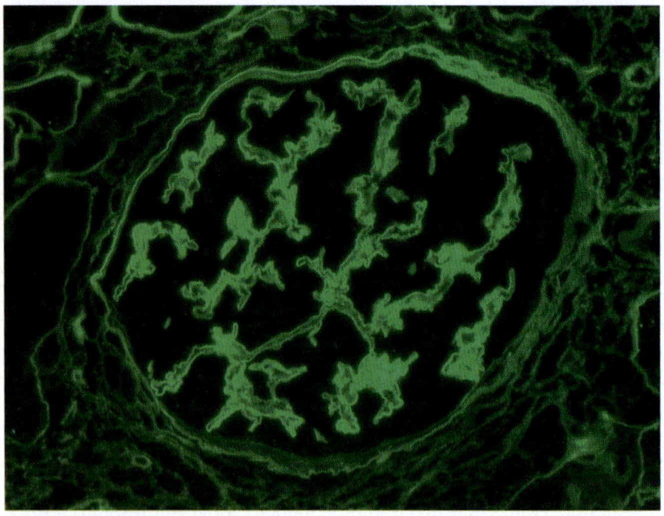

FIGURE 107-16. Light-chain deposition disease. Immunofluorescence shows linear staining of glomerular and tubular basement membranes for κ light chain.

overproduction of an abnormal light chain (λ 80%, κ 20%) can be detected by immunofluorescence staining that shows monotypic λ or κ light chains. Most patients have a clonal proliferation of plasma cells and do not meet criteria for multiple myeloma. In AA amyloid, antisera to the AA protein stain the glomeruli. Some patients with kidney amyloidosis have genetic variants that lead to the production of amyloidogenic proteins such as transthyretin, LECT2, and apolipoproteins.

Almost 80% of patients with AL amyloid have kidney disease. Kidney manifestations include albuminuria and renal insufficiency. Extrarenal amyloid involvement may cause cardiac disease (Chapter 47) or neuropathy (Chapter 388). Diagnosis may be made from organ biopsy other than the kidney (e.g., myocardial, rectal, or fat pad biopsy). Treatment strategies for kidney AL amyloidosis are similar to those for multiple myeloma and other plasma cell dyscrasias: stem cell transplantation and the use of anti-plasma cell agents such as proteasome inhibitors (bortezomib, carfilzomib, daratumumab), dexamethasone, and lenalidomide (Chapter 173).

AA amyloid is associated with chronic inflammatory conditions such as rheumatoid arthritis (Chapter 243), familial Mediterranean fever (Chapter 240), inflammatory bowel disease (Chapter 127), osteomyelitis (Chapter 251), and other chronic infections. Treatment is directed at the underlying inflammatory process. Specific therapy against the primary inflammatory disease (e.g., anti–tumor necrosis factor therapy in rheumatoid arthritis and colchicine in familial Mediterranean fever) can reduce the production of serum AA protein in patients with AA amyloid.

LIGHT-CHAIN DEPOSITION DISEASE

Light-chain deposition disease, like AL amyloidosis, is a systemic disease caused by the overproduction and extracellular deposition of a monoclonal immunoglobulin light chain (Chapter 173). However, the deposits do not form β-pleated sheets, do not stain with Congo red, and are granular rather than fibrillar. Most patients with light chain deposition disease have a lymphoplasmacytic B-cell disease similar to multiple myeloma (Chapter 173).

Albuminuria is common, and the nephrotic syndrome is found in half of patients at presentation, often accompanied by hypertension and kidney insufficiency. On light microscopy, most glomeruli contain eosinophilic mesangial glomerular nodules. Some biopsy samples show associated light-chain cast nephropathy with eosinophilic laminated and fracturing casts obstructing the tubules, as seen in myeloma. By immunofluorescence, a single class of immunoglobulin light-chain (κ in 80% of cases) stains in a diffuse linear pattern along the glomerular basement membrane, in the nodules and along the tubular basement membranes (Fig. 107-16). The treatment for most patients with light-chain deposition disease is chemotherapy similar to that for myeloma (Chapter 173).

FIBRILLARY GLOMERULOPATHY–IMMUNOTACTOID GLOMERULOPATHY

Some patients with kidney disease have glomerular lesions with deposits of nonamyloid fibrillar proteins ranging in size from 12 to more than 50 nm.

Patients with these lesions have been divided into two groups. Patients with fibrillary glomerulonephritis have fibrils of 20 nm in diameter that are deposited in a random fashion in the glomerular basement membrane and are associated with deposits of the DNAJB9 protein in deposits. Immunotactoid glomerulonephritis is a much rarer disease often associated with lymphoproliferative disorders, in which the fibrils are much larger (30 to 50 nm) and have a tubular substructure. Proteinuria is found in almost all patients, and hematuria, the nephrotic syndrome, and kidney insufficiency eventually develop in most patients. No therapy is of proven benefit for the fibrillary glomerulopathy per se, and a search for a treatable underlying B cell disorder is important.[30]

HUMAN IMMUNODEFICIENCY VIRUS–ASSOCIATED NEPHROPATHY

Infection with HIV (Chapter 355) is associated with a number of patterns of kidney disease, including acute kidney injury (Chapter 106) and a unique form of glomerulopathy now called HIV-associated nephropathy. HIV-associated nephropathy is characterized by heavy proteinuria and rapid progression to kidney failure. On light microscopy, biopsies show global collapse of the glomerular tufts, severe tubulointerstitial changes with interstitial inflammation, edema, microcystic dilation of tubules, and severe tubular degenerative changes. On electron microscopy, tubuloreticular inclusions can be seen in the glomerular endothelium.[31] The use of ACE inhibitors or angiotensin receptor blockers (see Table 64-7 in Chapter 64) and antiretroviral therapy may decrease proteinuria and slow the progression to kidney failure. In addition, corticosteroids (e.g., prednisone, 1 mg/kg for 1 month followed by a taper over several months) may be beneficial in selected patients with HIV-associated nephropathy.

COVID-19–ASSOCIATED NEPHROPATHY

Severe acute respiratory syndrome coronavirus 2 (SARS-CoV-2) and the coronavirus disease 2019 (COVID-19) that it causes can be associated with acute kidney injury. Postmortem examination in fatal cases shows diffuse acute tubular injury with a possible contribution of focal macrovascular and microvascular thrombi. Renal biopsies in patients with proteinuria and hematuria have demonstrated a glomerular-dominant pattern of injury, most notably a collapsing glomerulopathy similar to the findings seen in HIV-infected individuals with apolipoprotein L-1 (*APOL1*) risk allele variants. Other glomerular manifestations associated with COVID-19 include membranous nephropathy, ANCA-vasculitis, anti–glomerular basement membrane disease, and thrombotic microangiopathy.[32] Furthermore, acute flares of lupus nephritis, IgA nephropathy, and minimal change disease have been reported. SARS-CoV-2 vaccines have been rarely reported to be associated with relapsing or de novo glomerular disease, including IgA nephropathy, minimal change disease, ANCA-vasculitis, and others. The pathogenesis of glomerular disease associated with COVID-19 or vaccines is not understood, but is postulated to be related to immune activation.[33,34]

MIXED CRYOGLOBULINEMIA

Cryoglobulinemia (Chapter 173) is caused by the production of circulating immunoglobulins that precipitate on cooling and resolubilize on warming. Cryoglobulinemia may be found in association with infections, collagen vascular disease, and lymphoproliferative diseases such as multiple myeloma and Waldenström macroglobulinemia. Many patients with what was originally described as glomerulonephritis resulting from essential mixed cryoglobulinemia have been found to have hepatitis C–associated kidney disease. Some patients develop an acute nephritic picture with acute kidney insufficiency. Most patients have proteinuria, and approximately 20% present with the nephrotic syndrome. Hypocomplementemia, especially of the early components C1q to C4, is a characteristic finding in cryoglobulinemic glomerulonephritis, whether hepatitis C–related or idiopathic. Treatment of hepatitis C–associated cryoglobulinemia includes antiviral therapy (Chapter 135). When significant kidney disease is present, various combinations of corticosteroids with or without rituximab or cyclophosphamide or plasmapheresis have been used under expert guidance. Most patients with kidney disease have a slow, indolent course characterized by proteinuria, hypertension, hematuria, and renal insufficiency.

THROMBOTIC MICROANGIOPATHIES

A number of systemic diseases, including hemolytic-uremic syndrome (Chapters 110 and 158), thrombotic thrombocytopenic purpura (TTP; Chapter 158), and the antiphospholipid syndrome (Chapter 67), as well as microangiopathy associated with drugs such as mitomycin and cyclosporine, are characterized by microthromboses of the glomerular capillaries and small arterioles. The kidney findings may be dominant or only part of a more generalized picture of microangiopathy.

Kidney manifestations of the thrombotic microangiopathies may include gross or microscopic hematuria, proteinuria that is typically less than 2 g/day but may reach nephrotic levels, and renal insufficiency. Patients may have oliguric or nonoliguric acute kidney injury. In addition to glomerular chronic capillary thromboses, the histologic findings in all of the microangiopathies include a membranoproliferative glomerulonephritis pattern on light microscopy with no immune deposits or complement by immunofluorescence or electron microscopy, areas of ischemic damage, and intimal proliferation with luminal narrowing by thrombi of arterioles and small arteries.

In all thrombotic microangiopathies, treatment includes correcting hypovolemia, controlling hypertension, and the use of dialytic support for those with severe kidney failure. In TTP associated with an acquired or hereditary deficiency of the von Willebrand convertase ADAMTS-13 and in some other cases, plasmapheresis with fresh-frozen plasma is beneficial (Chapter 158).

In some patients whose hemolytic-uremic syndrome is not associated with Shiga toxin, defects in the alternate complement system are found. These patients with atypical hemolytic-uremic syndrome may benefit from eculizumab or ravulizumab, which inhibit complement C5 (Chapter 158). In the antiphospholipid syndrome, anticoagulation with heparin and then warfarin is useful (Chapter 67).

GENERAL REFERENCES

For the General References and other additional features, please visit Elsevier eBooks+ at https://ebooks.health.elsevier.com.

Grade A References

A1. Azukaitis K, Palmer SC, Strippoli GF, et al. Interventions for minimal change disease in adults with nephrotic syndrome. *Cochrane Database Syst Rev*. 2022;3:DC001537.

A2. Li X, Liu Z, Wang L, et al. Tacrolimus monotherapy after intravenous methylprednisolone in adults with minimal change nephrotic syndrome. *J Am Soc Nephrol*. 2017;28:1286-1295.

A3. Hodson EM, Sinha A, Cooper TE. Interventions for focal segmental glomerulosclerosis in adults. *Cochrane Database Syst Rev*. 2022;2:CD003233.

A4. von Groote TC, Williams G, Au EH, et al. Immunosuppressive treatment for primary membranous nephropathy in adults with nephrotic syndrome. *Cochrane Database Syst Rev*. 2021;11:CD004293.

A5. Bose B, Chung EYM, Hong R, et al. Immunosuppression therapy for idiopathic membranous nephropathy: systematic review with network meta-analysis. *J Nephrol*. 2022;35:1159-1170.

A6. Ou J-Y, Chen Y-W, Li T-L, et al. Evaluation of efficacy of rituximab for membranous nephropathy: a systematic review and meta-analysis of 11 studies. *Nephrol Ther*. 2022;18:104-112.

A7. Fernández-Juárez G, Rojas-Rivera J, Logt AV, et al. The STARMEN trial indicates that alternating treatment with corticosteroids and cyclophosphamide is superior to sequential treatment with tacrolimus and rituximab in primary membranous nephropathy. *Kidney Int*. 2021;99:986-998.

A8. Rauen T, Wied S, Fitzner C, et al. After ten years of follow-up, no difference between supportive care plus immunosuppression and supportive care alone in IgA nephropathy. *Kidney Int*. 2020;98:1044-1052.

A9. Lv J, Wong MG, Hladunewich MA, et al. Effect of oral methylprednisolone on decline in kidney function or kidney failure in patients with IgA nephropathy: the TESTING randomized clinical trial. *JAMA*. 2022;327:1888-1898.

A10. Rauen T, Eitner F, Fitzner C, et al. Intensive supportive care plus immunosuppression in IgA nephropathy. *N Engl J Med*. 2015;373:2225-2236.

A11. Fellström BC, Barratt J, Cook H, et al. Targeted-release budesonide versus placebo in patients with IgA nephropathy (NEFIGAN): a double-blind, randomized, placebo-controlled phase 2b trial. *Lancet*. 2017;389:2117-2127.

A12. Wheeler DC, Toto RD, Stefánsson BV, et al. A pre-specified analysis of the DAPA-CKD trial demonstrates the effects of dapagliflozin on major adverse kidney events in patients with IgA nephropathy. *Kidney Int*. 2021;100:215-224.

A13. Jayne DRW, Merkel PA, Schall TJ, et al. Avacopan for the treatment of ANCA-associated vasculitis. *N Engl J Med*. 2021;384:599-609.

A14. Rovin BH, Teng YKO, Ginzler EM, et al. Efficacy and safety of voclosporin versus placebo for lupus nephritis (AURORA 1): a double-blind, randomised, multicentre, placebo-controlled, phase 3 trial. *Lancet*. 2021;397:2070-2080.

A15. Furie R, Rovin BH, Houssiau F, et al. Two-year, randomized, controlled trial of belimumab in lupus nephritis. *N Engl J Med*. 2020;383:1117-1128.

108

INTERSTITIAL NEPHRITIS

CYBELE GHOSSEIN AND ERIC G. NEILSON

DEFINITION

Interstitial nephritis is characterized by an inflammatory infiltrate in the interstitium of the kidney. It can be primary and begin in the tubulointerstitium or appear as a secondary event and spread from blood vessels, including the glomerular capillaries. Injury to the tubulointerstitial compartment can be the result of autoimmunity, toxic insult, infection, or exposure to drugs. In all cases, however, the inflammatory process has an immunologic component that leads to the release of tissue cytokines, which attract T lymphocytes and other monocytes, which eventually convert tubular epithelia into fibroblasts to produce fibrosis.[1]

Interstitial nephritis can be arbitrarily divided into acute and chronic types. The acute form often begins abruptly. When inciting events subside, so does the nephritis. If this occurs in a matter of days/weeks, the glomerular filtration rate tends to normalize, with little residual damage except in patients with preexisting disease. Any cause of acute interstitial nephritis can transform into chronic interstitial nephritis.

Chronic interstitial nephritis is persistent and over time reduces the number of functioning nephrons by encasing and dismantling them with irreversible fibrosis. Sometimes acute and chronic injury is difficult to distinguish because global destruction of the tubulointerstitium can occur within a matter of weeks.

EPIDEMIOLOGY

Acute interstitial nephritis appears unexpectedly in otherwise healthy individuals from a variety of causes. Approximately 1% of patients with hematuria and proteinuria have acute interstitial nephritis, and it is seen in 1 to 15% of autopsy series. In recent decades its prevalence has increased in individuals over age 65 years, perhaps owing to their more frequent exposure to prescription drugs.

Although the most common cause of acute interstitial nephritis is the use of pharmaceuticals,[2,3] other important causes include infection and autoimmune diseases (Table 108-1). Almost any class of drugs can cause acute interstitial nephritis, but antibiotics, diuretics, proton pump inhibitors, immune checkpoint inhibitors, and nonsteroidal anti-inflammatory drugs (NSAIDs) top the list. NSAIDs cause both acute interstitial nephritis and chronic analgesic nephropathy. Diphtheria in children (Chapter 272), legionellosis (Chapter 290), leptospirosis (Chapter 298), histoplasmosis (Chapter 308), tuberculosis (Chapter 299), and DNA viruses, such as cytomegalovirus (Chapter 347), Epstein-Barr virus (Chapter 348), and severe acute respiratory syndrome coronavirus-2[4] (Chapter 336), are well-recognized causes of acute interstitial nephritis. Anti–tubular basement membrane disease is a rare cause of autoimmune interstitial nephritis.

Although sarcoidosis or the tubulointerstitial nephritis and uveitis syndrome can manifest as acute interstitial nephritis, they often quickly evolve into chronic disease. Initially described in the MesoAmerican region, a new entity named chronic interstitial nephritis in agricultural communities (CINAC) has become an epidemic in many parts of the world. Initially thought to be due to episodic heat-related volume depletion, evidence now suggests that pesticide exposure may be causative factor.[5]

All forms of injury to the kidney, regardless of origin, progress to end-stage renal disease through a terminal phase of chronic interstitial nephritis. A wide variety of kidney diseases, such as the glomerulonephritides (Chapter 107), cystic diseases (Chapter 112), and diabetes (Chapter 210), will start slowly in the tubulointerstitium and often go unrecognized until late in the course, when biopsy shows chronic interstitial nephritis.

Primary chronic interstitial nephritis can be caused by a variety of toxic, metabolic, hematologic, obstructive, and infectious processes (Table 108-2). Chronic ingestion of six or more tablets per day of acetaminophen, aspirin, and NSAIDs, in combination for at least 3 years, can also put patients at risk for analgesic nephropathy. Light chains can cause tubular injury in patients with multiple myeloma (Chapter 173). More recently, immune checkpoint inhibitors frequently have been associated with acute interstitial nephritis that may progress to severe acute kidney injury.[6,7]

TABLE 108-1 CAUSES OF ACUTE INTERSTITIAL NEPHRITIS

DRUGS
Antibiotics
Penicillins
Rifampin, ethambutol
Sulfa
Vancomycin
Cephalosporins
Erythromycin
Fluroquinolones
Trimethoprim-sulfamethoxazole
Acyclovir
Nonsteroidal Anti-Inflammatory Drugs
Selective and nonselective
Cyclooxygenase-2 inhibitors
Diuretics
Thiazides
Furosemide
Triamterene
Miscellaneous
Captopril
Ranitidine
Proton pump inhibitors
Phenobarbital
Phenytoin
Sodium valproate
Carbamazepine
Allopurinol
Interferon
Interleukin-2
All-*trans*-retinoic acid
Immune checkpoint inhibitors
Nucleotide polymerase inhibitors
Tyrosine kinase inhibitors
INFECTIONS
Bacteria
Legionella
Brucella
Diphtheria
Streptococcus
Staphylococcus
Yersinia
Salmonella
Escherichia coli
Campylobacter
Viruses
Epstein-Barr virus
Cytomegalovirus
Hantavirus
Herpes simplex virus
Hepatitis B virus
Severe acute respiratory syndrome coronavirus-2
Other
Mycoplasma
Rickettsia
Leptospira
Mycobacterium tuberculosis
Schistosoma mekongi
Toxoplasma
Chlamydia
AUTOIMMUNE DISEASES
Anti–tubular basement membrane disease
Tubulointerstitial nephritis and uveitis (TINU) syndrome
Kawasaki disease

PATHOBIOLOGY

Pathophysiology

Regardless of the origin of renal inflammation, the kidneys do not irreversibly fail until fibrosis and tubular atrophy develop. Chronic interstitial nephritis is the pathologic equivalent of clinical progression because it is the final common pathway to permanent tissue damage. The degree of reduction in the glomerular filtration rate correlates with the degree of interstitial injury. Urinary flow is impeded by

TABLE 108-2 CAUSES OF CHRONIC INTERSTITIAL NEPHRITIS

HEREDITARY DISEASES
Mitochondrial mutations Karyomegalic nephritis Autosomal dominant tubular interstitial kidney disease
METABOLIC DISTURBANCES
Hypercalcemia, nephrocalcinosis Hyperoxaluria Hypokalemia Hyperuricemia Cystinosis Methylmalonic acidemia
DRUGS AND TOXINS
Analgesics Cadmium Lead Health food botanicals, herbs Lithium Cyclosporine, tacrolimus Cisplatin, methotrexate Nitrosoureas Pesticides
AUTOIMMUNE DISEASES
Renal allograft rejection Granulomatosis with polyangiitis Immunoglobulin G4–related tubulointerstitial nephropathy Sjögren syndrome Systemic lupus erythematosus, vasculitis Tubulointerstitial nephritis and uveitis (TINU) syndrome Sarcoidosis
HEMATOLOGIC DISTURBANCES
Multiple myeloma, light chains Lymphoma Sickle cell disease
INFECTIONS
Complicated pyelonephritis Human immunodeficiency virus (HIV) Epstein-Barr virus Malakoplakia Xanthogranulomatous pyelonephritis
OBSTRUCTIVE NEPHROPATHY
Tumors Stones Outlet obstruction Vesicoureteral reflux
MISCELLANEOUS
Age-related vascular disease Hypertension Ischemia Balkan (endemic) nephropathy Radiation nephritis Oxalate nephropathy Cholesterol emboli

tubular obstruction. Increased vascular resistance causes progressive tubular injury and fibrosis. A net reduction in the cross-sectional area of peritubular vessels increases postglomerular resistance to the extent that the compensatory increase in glomerular hydrostatic pressure cannot fully restore filtration to normal levels. Tubuloglomerular feedback assumes increasing importance in the transition from acute to chronic glomerulonephritis when autoregulation of renal blood flow is disrupted by tubulointerstitial fibrosis. Loss of autoregulation by tubuloglomerular feedback results from the absence or insensitivity of the afferent arteriole. Perhaps more significant is the effect of interstitial pressure on the sensitivity of the feedback mechanism. Tubular atrophy may disrupt the normal renal osmotic gradient by decreasing sodium chloride transport along the proximal tubule or thick ascending loop of Henle. The result is poor abstraction of water from the filtrate, with hyposthenuria and polyuria. Such an increase in solute and water within the tubular fluid results in adaptive downregulation of the glomerular filtration process.

Patients with Fanconi syndrome exhibit proximal tubular epithelium alterations that variably impair transporter function in the area of injury. These tubular defects are classically and occasionally seen in light-chain myeloma, cystinosis, Lowe syndrome, and the tubulointerstitial nephritis and uveitis syndrome, as well as after exposure to selected drugs, such as tenofovir or ifosfamide.

The antigen targets engaging the inflammasome and the immune system in interstitial nephritis are slowly unfolding. Drugs act as haptens, mimic endogenous structures in the interstitium, alter regulation of the immune system, or function in some combination of the foregoing. Bacteria, fungi, and viruses can infect the kidney and cause mononuclear cell infiltration or activate toll-like receptors on tubular epithelia, which subsequently educate the adaptive immune response to events in the interstitium. Renal-specific autoimmune diseases such as anti–tubular basement membrane disease or spontaneous interstitial nephritis remain confined to the kidney, whereas systemic diseases spread to the kidney, where they cause persistent chronic interstitial nephritis.

Although the adaptive immune response is similar to that of other tissues, T-cell activation figures prominently in interstitial nephritis. Antibodies (e.g., anti–tubular basement membrane disease) and/or immune complex deposition along the tubular basement membrane (e.g., systemic lupus erythematosus) are rarely seen. Antigens presented by class II major histocompatibility complex molecules on macrophages, dendritic cells, and adjacent tubular epithelia, in conjunction with associative recognition molecules, engage the CD4/CD8 T-cell repertoires. The resultant cytokine and protease activity injures tubular nephrons and basement membranes and causes fibroblasts to form locally by epithelial-mesenchymal transition and to proliferate. Transforming growth factor-β (TGF-β), fibroblast growth factor 2, and platelet-derived growth factor are particularly active in this transition. If the nephritis persists, fibrogenesis dismantles nephrons and causes tubular atrophy; in late stages, the inflammatory reaction outgrows its survival factors and lymphocytes, and fibroblasts disappear by apoptosis and leave an acellular fibrotic scar.

Rarely, patients may have autosomal dominant tubulointerstitial kidney disease (Chapter 112)[8,9] caused by mutations in various genes, including uromodulin (*UMOD*), hepatocyte nuclear factor-1β (*HNF1B*), renin (*REN*), and mucin-1 (*MUC1*). Viruses, including Epstein-Barr virus, have been long suspected of contributing to idiopathic chronic interstitial nephritis. Malakoplakia and xanthogranulomatous pyelonephritis are probably not defects in nephrogenesis but rather are destructive responses to bacterial inflammation in the interstitium. Focal abnormalities in kidney structure can be a nidus for infections associated with perinephric, psoas, or peritoneal abscesses. Children with vesicoureteral reflux (Chapter 113) can have chronic or repeating episodes of pyelonephritis, but whether the reflux or the infection is more important to progression to renal failure is unclear. There is also no agreement on whether recurrent pyelonephritis by itself produces chronic interstitial nephritis in adults.

Pathology

Both kidneys are typically involved, except in cases of unilateral infection, obstruction, or trauma. The inflammatory reaction in acute interstitial nephritis consists mainly of T lymphocytes and monocytes, but neutrophils, plasma cells, and eosinophils can be present. The T cells are of a mixed phenotype with a distinct preference for $CD4^+$ lymphocytes. The infiltrative process is associated with interstitial edema, which displaces tubules away from one another and causes the kidneys to swell. The tubular basement membrane may be disrupted in more severe cases, but immune deposits are rarely found by immunofluorescence. In patients on anti-programmed cell death protein-1 (PD-1) and anti-programmed death ligand-1 (PD-L1) therapy, immunohistochemistry may show positive PD-1 or PD-L1 staining in patients with acute interstitial nephritis from these therapies.[10]

On gross inspection, the kidney in chronic interstitial nephritis has an irregular contour or contracted appearance. Pathologically, the tubular epithelia sit on thickened or disrupted tubular basement membranes and are often effaced against dilated lumens; the tubules eventually dismantle and atrophy. *Chronic* is a relative term, because fibrotic changes can be seen within 7 to 10 days of continuing inflammation. In primary interstitial nephritis, the glomerular compartment eventually succumbs to the ongoing fibrotic process; normal glomeruli are surrounded by periglomerular fibrosis and subsequently undergo segmental or global sclerosis. Chronic vascular thickening and glomerular changes are present in advanced stages of disease, so pathologic determination of the primary cause may be difficult in some biopsy samples. Progressive glomerular

TABLE 108-3 TYPICAL CLINICAL MANIFESTATIONS OF ACUTE INTERSTITIAL NEPHRITIS

History of drug hypersensitivity or recent infection and taking antibiotics
Sudden onset of fever lasting several days to weeks
Variable degrees of hypertension
Rise in creatinine with $FE_{Na} > 1.0$; no expected acute tubular necrosis or glomerulonephritis
Kidney size normal or increased
Hematuria with mild proteinuria (<1.0g)
Presence of WBC casts and WBCs on urinalysis; rarely eosinophils

FE_{Na} = fractional excretion of sodium; WBC = white blood cell.

sclerosis also occurs with aging and must be factored in when interpreting the biopsy findings.

A third pathologic category, granuloma formation, can be seen in either acute or chronic interstitial nephritis. In acute granulomatous interstitial nephritis, granulomas are sparse and non-necrotic and giant cells are rare. In chronic interstitial nephritis, granulomas contain an abundance of giant cells, and those caused by tuberculosis may become necrotic. Drugs are a common cause of this lesion in the acute setting, and most of the drugs associated with acute interstitial nephritis have been reported to cause granuloma formation. When numerous granulomas are present in the absence of drug exposure, sarcoidosis (Chapter 83), granulomatosis with polyangiitis (Chapter 249), histoplasmosis (Chapter 308), or tuberculosis (Chapter 299) should be considered, depending on the context. The kidney granulomas seen in granulomatosis with polyangiitis are almost always accompanied by glomerular and vascular pathology.

ACUTE INTERSTITIAL NEPHRITIS

CLINICAL MANIFESTATIONS

Most patients present with an asymptomatic rise in the serum creatinine level or an abnormal urinalysis, and it is important to consider acute interstitial nephritis in any patient with an unexplained precipitous diminution in kidney function.[11] Because kidney injury is often asymptomatic, patients already may have substantial kidney dysfunction on initial presentation. Patients also may present with nonspecific symptoms such as lethargy or weakness, and some patients may have fever. Oliguria may be present in patients who have severe acute kidney injury (Chapter 106).

Several features can distinguish acute interstitial nephritis from acute tubular necrosis (Chapter 106) or glomerulonephritis (Chapter 107; Table 108-3).[12] Fever and occasional flank pain, owing to acute distention of the kidney capsule, may occur in infection or with drug-induced acute interstitial nephritis. Allergic reactions can be associated with maculopapular rash, fever, and eosinophilia, but this triad is seen in less than 33% of all patients with acute interstitial nephritis; this triad is more common in antibiotic-related acute interstitial nephritis and is rarely seen when NSAIDs are the cause. These signs and symptoms of drug reaction have been codified and referred to as the DRESS syndrome (*d*rug *r*ash, *e*osinophilia, and *s*ystemic *s*ymptoms; Chapter 407), which is associated with interstitial nephritis in up to 40% of patients with persistent exposure to selected drugs.

The course of kidney failure in acute interstitial nephritis progresses over several days to weeks and follows the kinetics of the primary immune response. However, kidney failure can be precipitous, especially in patients re-exposed to a previous agent. Rarely, the course can be protracted, with the glomerular filtration rate declining over a period of months if the diagnosis is not recognized.

The onset of drug-induced nephritis ranges from days to weeks after the initiation of therapy, depending on previous drug exposure history. The classic setting for a drug reaction is a febrile patient with an infectious process and who defervesces while taking antibiotics but then develops recurrent fever several days later.

DIAGNOSIS

A careful history often points to the diagnosis (see Table 108-1). Urinalysis is particularly helpful. Mild-to-moderate proteinuria and hematuria are seen in most cases. The sediment typically shows red and white blood cells, as well as white blood cell casts. However, a bland urine sediment does not exclude the diagnosis of acute interstitial nephritis. A red blood cell cast (see Fig. 100-8) suggests a glomerular diagnosis. The finding of eosinophils in the urine supports the diagnosis of allergic interstitial nephritis, but the positive predictive value is low, even with more than 5% eosinophils in the urine, and the absence of eosinophiluria does not exclude the diagnosis of acute interstitial nephritis.

An elevated serum creatinine level is usually the first abnormal laboratory result in interstitial nephritis. The normal serum creatinine of 0.6 to 1.3mg/dL varies with muscle mass, age, and gender. Early recognition of acute interstitial nephritis requires a high degree of clinical suspicion because the serum creatinine level may be only mildly elevated even after the kidneys lose half their function.

Given the lack of glomerular involvement in acute interstitial nephritis, the degree of proteinuria is nearly always less than 3g per 24hours and is more typically less than 1g per 24hours. Nephrotic-range proteinuria is not seen except in the presence of a coexisting glomerular lesion, such as a concurrent minimal-change lesion, which can be seen in NSAID-induced interstitial nephritis. Many patients with acute interstitial nephritis also have a fractional excretion of sodium (FE_{Na}) greater than 1 and occasionally are oliguric.

Imaging is of little diagnostic value. The kidney in acute interstitial nephritis is usually normal or slightly increased in size on echographic or tomographic images. Increased cortical echogenicity may correlate with diffuse interstitial infiltrates on renal biopsy.

Differential Diagnosis

It is sometimes difficult to distinguish among nonoliguric acute tubular necrosis, acute interstitial nephritis, and glomerulonephritis without a biopsy.[13] Exposure to pharmaceuticals is responsible for most cases of acute interstitial nephritis, followed by infections and autoimmune disease. Selective tubular defects and tubular syndromes, such as proximal acquired Fanconi syndrome or distal renal tubular acidosis, can be seen in subacute or chronic interstitial nephritis but are unusual in acute interstitial nephritis.

Biopsy

Ultimately, the diagnosis can be established with certainty only by renal biopsy, which confirms and assesses the extent of acute interstitial inflammation. A biopsy should be performed in patients who have acute kidney failure, who have suggestive signs or symptoms of an interstitial process, and in whom prerenal azotemia and obvious acute tubular necrosis cannot be excluded on clinical grounds (Table 108-4). In primary acute interstitial nephritis, the biopsy demonstrates inflammatory cells that typically spare the glomeruli until late in the course (Fig. 108-1A). Lesions that reduce kidney function are usually diffuse, but drug-induced interstitial injury is often patchy and commonly begins deep in the cortex, closer to the corticomedullary junction, before spreading.

TABLE 108-4 WHEN TO CONSIDER A RENAL BIOPSY TO DIAGNOSE ACUTE INTERSTITIAL NEPHRITIS

The setting, history, or clinical findings do not support a diagnosis of acute tubular necrosis or volume depletion
The clinical setting warrants a tissue diagnosis to determine the type of lesion, the extent of involvement, or the degree of fibrosis
The patient is stable enough to undergo biopsy and receive immunosuppressive drugs
The physician believes that the choice of therapy or the length of treatment is partially determined by the type of tissue injury

TREATMENT

The principal intervention for acute interstitial nephritis is to remove the inciting drug or treat the underlying cause, whether it be infectious or autoimmune.[14] In observational series, patients treated with steroids seem to do somewhat better, so a trial of prednisone (starting at 0.75 to 1.0mg/kg/day orally) can be given daily for approximately 1 week, and the response can be assessed clinically. In patients whose autoimmune disease does not respond to steroids or who develop steroid toxicity, another immunosuppressive agent such as mycophenolate mofetil, azathioprine, or cyclophosphamide can be tried under expert guidance. These agents also can be used as steroid-sparing agents if long-term therapy is needed. High-dose immunosuppression should not be continued without some evidence of benefit because immunosuppressive drugs in patients with azotemia can lead to serious infection and even death. In such cases, these drugs can be reserved to use with kidney transplantation (Chapter 117) if the primary disease does not respond.

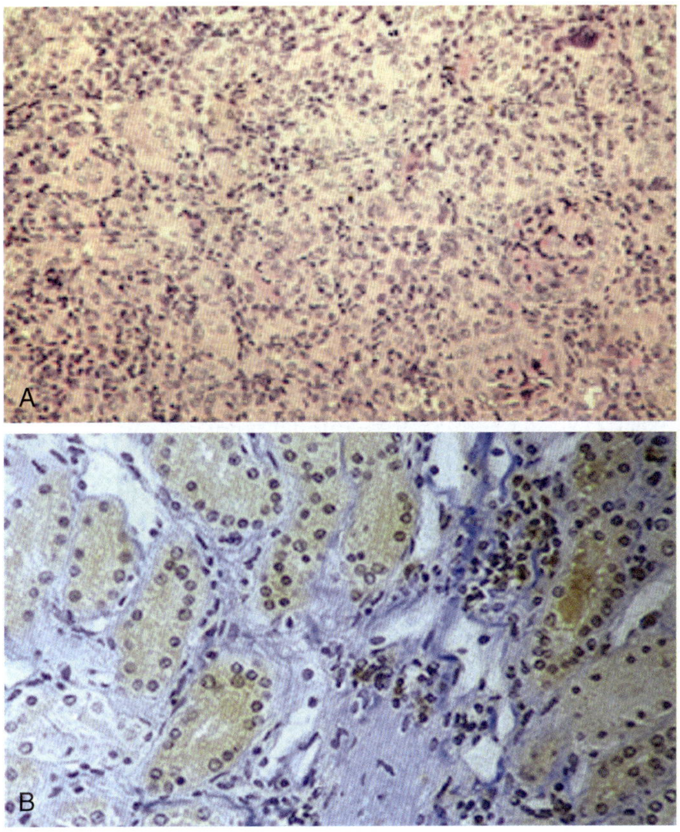

FIGURE 108-1. Interstitial nephritis on biopsy. **A,** Acute interstitial nephritis can be most aggressive when the interstitium is crowded with mononuclear cells and giant cells that destroy nearly all tubular nephrons (hematoxylin and eosin). **B,** Chronic interstitial nephritis is a slower process, with substantial collagen deposition (*blue color;* trichrome), tubular dropout, and fibroblasts in the interstitial spaces widened by fibrosis.

PROGNOSIS

The prognosis for acute interstitial nephritis is good if it is recognized early in the setting of minimal fibrosis.[15] Early removal of offending agents or prompt treatment of the underlying disorder when appropriate is essential. However, acute kidney tubular injury can be a catalyst for the development of chronic kidney disease.[16]

CHRONIC INTERSTITIAL NEPHRITIS

CLINICAL MANIFESTATIONS

Patients with primary chronic interstitial nephritis typically have elevated serum creatinine levels and signs and symptoms of kidney failure, including hematuria, isosthenuria or hyposthenuria, nocturia, fatigue, and nausea. Before the glomerular filtration rate falls below 25 to 30 mL/min, tubular acidosis is common. Anemia is often out of proportion to the degree of renal failure, and many patients have hypertension but only minimal edema until they develop advanced stages of kidney failure. Acquired Fanconi syndrome can be seen in patients with a serum creatinine level less than 2.5 mg/dL in the setting of drug exposure, myeloma, human immunodeficiency virus (HIV) infection, lead exposure, and herbal nephropathy.

DIAGNOSIS

A careful history including drug or toxin exposure, kidney imaging, and laboratory findings can often point to a probable diagnosis (see Table 108-2). As for any patient with evidence of kidney failure, the evaluation includes laboratory tests to determine possible causes and severity. These tests include measures of renal function (serum creatinine level and blood urea nitrogen level), as well as levels of serum electrolytes, calcium, phosphate, uric acid, and albumin. Urinalysis typically shows a fixed specific gravity of approximately 1.010, occasional glycosuria, and proteinuria (often <1 g/L); and red cells, white cells, and granular casts may be seen. Depending on the clinical situation, the search for specific causes may include serum and urine protein electrophoresis, blood and urine cultures, serologic tests for autoimmune diseases (e.g., cryoglobulin level, antinuclear antibodies, anti–neutrophil cytoplasmic antibody, and anti–glomerular basement membrane antibody levels [see Table 236-3]), or viral infection, particularly after renal transplantation (Chapter 117).

Selective tubular defects and tubular syndromes, such as proximal acquired Fanconi syndrome (bicarbonaturia with a plasma carbon dioxide [CO_2] content <20 mEq/L, aminoaciduria, phosphate wasting, uricosuria, and glycosuria) or distal renal tubular acidosis type 1 (urine pH >5.6, plasma CO_2 content <20 mEq/L, with low or high potassium) can be seen occasionally in subacute or chronic interstitial nephritis. Patients with Fanconi syndrome quickly develop an alkaline urine (pH >7.5) and increased fractional excretion of urine bicarbonate when the serum bicarbonate is elevated above 20 mEq/L by intravenous infusion.

Ultrasound images may show increased echogenicity and/or atrophic kidneys. Classic images of analgesic nephropathy on tomography are quite specific (Fig. 108-2) and show a decrease in overall kidney size, with atrophic scars and an irregular cortical contour, sometimes accompanied by papillary necrosis.

On biopsy (see Table 108-4), chronic interstitial nephritis is manifest by a cellular infiltrate that is eventually replaced by tubulointerstitial fibrosis (see Fig. 108-1B). Infiltrates of lymphocytes and rare neutrophils are scattered and less abundant than in acute interstitial nephritis. Genetic testing may detect a genetic tubulopathy (Chapters 108 and 113) in a substantial minority of patients.[17]

Specific Causes

Analgesics

Aspirin, acetaminophen, and NSAIDs in combination are a source of toxic metabolites and can induce medullary ischemia and papillary necrosis, sometimes with papillary calcification.[18] Uroepithelial malignancies also occur with increased frequency in this group of patients.

Aristolochic Acid Nephropathy

Aristolochic acid has been implicated as a cause of Balkan nephropathy and so-called Chinese herbal nephropathy. A growing number of people are taking vitamins and herbal preparations purchased from health food stores (Chapter 30), and some of these remedies contain botanicals that produce chronic interstitial nephritis. Patients who are dieting often use these remedies and are first seen when they already have late-stage disease, which increases the risk for uroepithelial malignancies (Chapter 182).

Human Immunodeficiency Virus Tubulointerstitial Nephropathy

Predominate tubulointerstitial nephropathy accounts for about 25% of the renal lesions seen on biopsy in HIV-infected patients (Chapter 359).[19] Biopsies show two general forms: a tubulopathy or an interstitial nephritis. In the tubulopathy, damage is to the proximal tubule. About 80% of cases are associated with drug exposure, particularly tenofovir (Chapter 357), but poorly controlled HIV is an even more important risk factor. Approximately 30% of patients improve with time. Patients in the tubulointerstitial nephritis group have a mononuclear infiltration and more persistent viral loads, but 50 to 60% recover.

Tubulointerstitial Nephritis with Uveitis Syndrome

Seen at any age but more commonly in young women and children, this syndrome may be idiopathic, genetic, or in response to pharmaceutical exposure.[20] Unilateral or bilateral anterior panuveitis (Chapter 391) may precede or follow evidence of interstitial nephritis that starts acutely but may persist as chronic kidney injury. If the renal function is not greatly impaired, concomitant Fanconi syndrome may suggest proximal tubular involvement.

Vascular Disease

Chronic renal ischemia from vascular injury can lead to interstitial nephritis, nephrosclerosis, and fibrosis, which are the classic renal lesions of untreated essential hypertension (Chapter 64). Similar injury is seen with aging, diabetes (Chapter 109), sickle cell disease (Chapter 149), and radiation nephritis (Chapter 18). This interstitial injury from vascular diseases is quite different from the aggressive necrosis seen with acute vasculitis. In patients who are taking calcineurin inhibitors such as cyclosporine or tacrolimus, renal ischemia from vasoconstriction can cause interstitial fibrosis that is sometimes difficult to distinguish from chronic allograft rejection (Chapter 117).

Immunoglobulin G4–Related Interstitial Nephritis

Immunoglobulin G4 (IgG4)-related interstitial nephritis is a systemic syndrome that presents in the kidney as inflammatory masses associated with

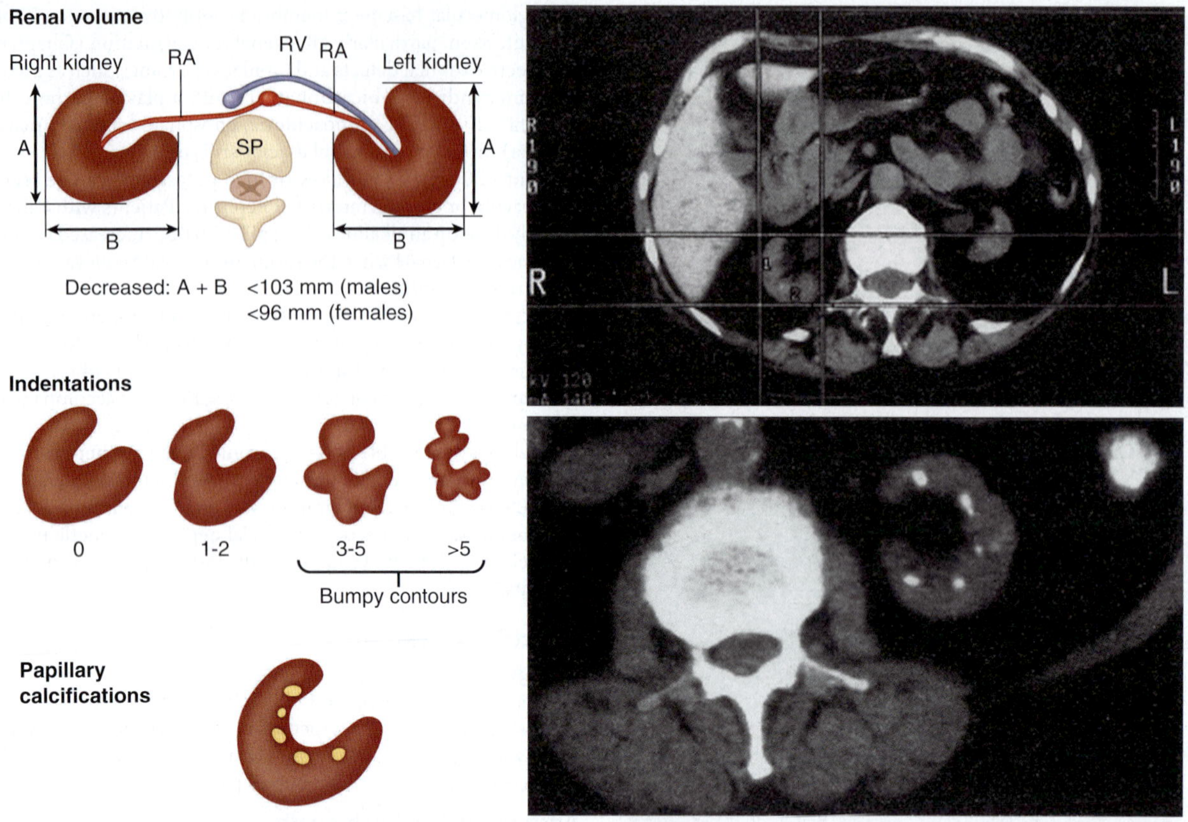

FIGURE 108-2. **Renal changes in analgesic nephropathy seen by tomographic imaging.** Structural changes, including reduced volume, nodularity, and calcifications, are seen on computed tomography. RA = right artery; RV = right vein; SP = spinal vertebra. (From Elseviers MM, De Schepper A, Corthouts R, et al. High diagnostic performance of CT scan for analgesic nephropathy in patients with incipient to severe renal failure. *Kidney Int*. 1995;48:1316.)

plasma cells, interstitial mononuclear cell infiltrates, and storiform fibrosis. Patients may have lesions in other organs, such as the liver, pancreas, parotids, thyroid, and myocardium.[21] Eosinophilia and low complement levels can be seen. Serum IgG4 levels and tissue plasma cells are increased, but it is not clear whether the IgG4 antibodies are a biomarker or causative. IgG4 is also separately associated with membranous nephropathy (Chapter 107) and nephrotic-range proteinuria.

Obstruction

Significant urinary obstruction, regardless of its etiology, is an important cause of chronic interstitial nephritis. Complete or partial urinary tract obstruction is accompanied by a decline in glomerular filtration and classic tubular abnormalities, including diminished reabsorption of solutes, impaired excretion of H^+ and K^+, and a vasopressin-resistant concentrating defect in the medulla. Obstruction is associated with a fall in the glomerular filtration rate because of reduced plasma flow and hydraulic pressure associated with the release of angiotensin II, leukotrienes, and nitric oxide, a process leading to mononuclear cell infiltration. Growth factors such as TGF-β, which is released by infiltrating cells, may contribute to the interstitial and glomerular fibrosis. Obstruction is more common in men than in women and is part of the routine assessment of kidney failure by kidney ultrasound (Chapters 106 and 114). Almost all obstructed kidneys eventually become infected if the obstruction is not relieved.

Hypercalcemia

Hypercalcemia can decrease glomerular filtration via renal vasoconstriction, a decrease in the glomerular ultrafiltration coefficient, and volume depletion as a result of a vasopressin-resistant concentrating defect associated with nephrocalcinosis and calcium deposition around the basement membranes of the distal tubules and collecting ducts. Such deposition secondarily leads to mononuclear cell infiltration and tubular death. Nephrocalcinosis also occurs in normocalcemic disorders of augmented calcium absorption through the gut (e.g., sarcoidosis [Chapter 83], vitamin D intoxication [Chapter 227]), skeletal breakdown (neoplasms or multiple myeloma [Chapter 173]), or classic distal renal tubular acidosis (Chapter 104).

Myeloma

The chronic kidney disease of multiple myeloma (Chapter 173) is caused by several mechanisms, including cast nephropathy ("myeloma kidney"), coexistent volume depletion, hypercalcemia (Chapter 227), nephrocalcinosis (Chapter 227), and uric acid nephropathy.[22] Proteinaceous casts form in dilated, atrophic distal nephron segments that are surrounded by multinucleated giant cells in interstitial infiltrates. The casts typically contain both Tamm-Horsfall protein and a pathologic light chain. Interstitial plasma cells and mononuclear infiltrates, calcifications in the interstitium, and amyloid deposits in the vessels and glomeruli are often present. Light chains are nephrotoxic by directly damaging tubular cells or by intrarenal obstruction because of the formation of casts. In the setting of excess production of light chains, the reabsorptive capacity of proximal tubule is overwhelmed, thereby leading to their urinary excretion as Bence Jones proteins. Proximal tubular damage may also lead to Fanconi syndrome.

Lead Toxicity

Epidemiologic analyses support the association between an excess burden of lead (Chapter 20) and chronic kidney disease. Blood lead levels reflect only recent, not chronic, exposure and can be normal in patients who have a significant burden of lead. Lead preferentially deposits in the proximal tubule, and nuclear inclusions within proximal tubular cells are characteristic of lead nephropathy. Ingestion of moonshine liquor, with its high lead content, as well as certain occupations, such as lead smeltering, can be an important historical clue to the diagnosis.

In adults, lead nephropathy produces chronic interstitial nephritis, fibrosis, and nephrosclerosis. Proximal tubular dysfunction may produce isolated tubule defects or a full Fanconi syndrome. Patients often have recurrent gout with gouty tophi, hyperuricemia, hypertension, and anemia. Some laboratories can measure δ-aminolevulinic acid dehydratase, which is inhibited by lead. Although chelation studies may document body lead burden, this test is difficult to perform in patients who have renal failure. X-ray fluorescent measurements of in vivo skeletal lead stores correlate well with ethylenediaminetetraacetic acid (EDTA) chelation tests and have the advantage of being rapid and noninvasive.

Cadmium Toxicity

Cadmium nephropathy (Chapter 20) is seen in regions where contamination from smelters results in prolonged low-level exposure. Cadmium is bound to metallothionein, and proximal tubular cells take up these complexes. The liver and kidney are the two major organs in which cadmium accumulates. Cadmium's half-life in the body is longer than 10 years. As with blood levels of lead, blood levels of cadmium fall after acute exposure because of extensive tissue deposition. Once a threshold of kidney deposition is exceeded, excess cadmium is excreted in urine. Cadmium intoxication produces irreversible proximal tubular dysfunction, hypercalciuria, nephrolithiasis, and metabolic bone disease with pain (called "ouch-ouch" disease in Japan).

Oxalate Nephropathy

Oxalate nephropathy results from the deposition of calcium oxalate in the tubular interstitium, thereby leading to mild secondary inflammation and tubular atrophy and fibrosis. Although oxalate nephropathy can occur in patients who have primary inborn errors of glycolate metabolism that lead to overproduction of oxalate (Chapter 189), more commonly it occurs in patients who have secondary causes of increased oxalate excretion (e.g., patients with roux-en-y gastric bypass, inflammatory bowel disease, or short bowel syndrome) because of increased intestinal availability and permeability of oxalate or decreased degradation of oxalate. Diagnosis requires a high index of suspicion. A 24-hour urine collection to measure oxalate excretion can help, but ultimately a kidney biopsy is needed to make the diagnosis.[23]

Autosomal Dominant Tubular Interstitial Diseases

Autosomal dominant tubular interstitial diseases are a rare group of inherited syndromes that lead to progressive chronic kidney disease and eventually lead to kidney failure (Chapter 112). The several subtypes of autosomal dominant tubular interstitial disease have an autosomal dominant inheritance pattern, present in late childhood or early adulthood, and are slowly progressive. Some patients may have early-onset gout. Kidney imaging may show small medullary cysts. Kidney biopsy will usually show nonspecific findings. A provisional diagnosis can made by obtaining a thorough family history in the appropriate clinical context. Genetic testing for mutations in uromodulin (*UMOD*) will confirm the clinical diagnosis in the majority of patients, whereas other patients will have mutations in renin (*REN*), hepatocyte nuclear factor-1β (*HNF1B*), or Mucin-1 (*MUC1*).

TREATMENT

Inciting factors such as obstruction, infection, drugs, or toxins should be removed whenever possible. Chronic interstitial fibrosis rarely responds to aggressive treatment. However, in immunoglobulin G4–related interstitial nephritis, the renal lesions in many patients respond briskly to corticosteroid treatment. In addition, treatment of tubulointerstitial nephritis with uveitis syndrome is with varying doses of methylprednisolone followed by oral prednisone under expert guidance may be beneficial in some patients. Varying durations of supplemental or steroid-sparing immunosuppression with mycophenolate mofetil or cyclophosphamide also have been used. Immunosuppression may also be helpful in sarcoidosis (Chapter 83).

Otherwise, the treatment is like that of other causes of chronic kidney disease. Angiotensin-converting enzyme inhibitors or angiotensin II receptor blockers (Table 64-7) are used early to slow disease progression, with a systolic blood pressure goal of 120/80 mm Hg (Chapters 64 and 117). Sodium glucose cotransporter-2 inhibitors (see Table 210-6) may be indicated in patients who have a glomerular filtration rate <75 mL/min (but not <45 mL/min for empagliflozin or <25 mL/min for dapagliflozin except in special circumstances under expert supervision) and an albumin to creatinine ratio >200 mg/g to slow the progression of kidney disease. Early treatment of acidosis with sodium bicarbonate (starting at 650 mg twice daily) is important to reach a goal bicarbonate level of 23 mEq/L. Other treatment goals include treatment of symptomatic anemia with erythropoiesis-stimulating agents to maintain a hemoglobin concentration between 10 and 11 g/L, treatment of hyperphosphatemia with oral phosphate binders, and hyperparathyroidism with activated vitamin D analogues (Chapters 116 and 117).

For certain specific causes of chronic interstitial nephritis, specific therapeutic approaches are warranted. For analgesic nephropathy, stopping analgesic use can help reduce progression. For hypercalcemia (Chapter 227), therapy is directed toward the primary disease—reduction of the serum calcium concentration, when appropriate, and correction of acid-base disturbances.

Appropriate therapy for presumed cast nephropathy in multiple myeloma includes chemotherapy to ameliorate excess production of light chains (Chapter 173), treatment of hypercalcemia (Chapter 227), alkalinization of the urine with the addition of bicarbonate to hypotonic fluids, and avoidance of radiocontrast agents, which may enhance the nephrotoxicity of light chains. Loop diuretics should be used with caution, particularly in the setting of volume depletion.

EDTA is advocated as chelation therapy for lead toxicity (Chapter 20). The goal of chelation is to normalize the EDTA mobilization test. In occasional patients, this treatment may arrest or reverse the progression of the kidney failure.

PROGNOSIS

Chronic interstitial nephritis tends to progress slowly. However, the prognosis is highly variable and depends on the underlying condition, the degree of fibrosis, the presence of glomerulosclerosis on kidney biopsy, and the patients' comorbid conditions, including cardiovascular disease and diabetes mellitus.

GENERAL REFERENCES

For the General References and other additional features, please visit Elsevier eBooks+ at https://ebooks.health.elsevier.com.

109 DIABETES AND THE KIDNEY

RAYMOND C. HARRIS

EPIDEMIOLOGY

In the industrialized world, diabetes mellitus is the single leading cause of end-stage renal disease (ESRD). Despite the improved care of patients with diabetes, both the incidence and prevalence of ESRD secondary to diabetes continue to rise. In the United States, almost 50% of patients undergoing either dialytic therapy or renal transplantation have ESRD as a result of diabetic nephropathy, and more than 40% of the new (incident) cases of ESRD are attributable to diabetes. Currently, more than 200,000 U.S. patients receive ESRD care as a result of diabetic nephropathy.

In the United States, Europe, and Japan, more than 90% of patients with diabetes have type 2 rather than insulinopenic type 1 diabetes (Chapter 210). In patients with type 1 and type 2 diabetes, the incidence rate of renal disease is equivalent when patients are monitored for an extended period of time, and more than 80% of the ESRD secondary to diabetes in the United States is seen in patients with type 2 diabetes. The demographics of ESRD secondary to type 2 diabetes mirror the prevalence of type 2 diabetes in the U.S. population, with a higher incidence in females and in Black Americans, Hispanic Americans, Native Americans, and Asian Americans, with a peak incidence in the fifth to seventh decades. Much of the increased mortality in both type 1 and type 2 diabetes is associated with the prevalence of nephropathy.

Given the global epidemic of obesity, the incidence of diabetic nephropathy is increasing worldwide.[1,2] Smoking, hypertension, and elevated blood cholesterol levels may be predisposing factors for the development of diabetic nephropathy in patients with type 2 diabetes.

PATHOBIOLOGY

Hyperglycemia

The metabolic sequelae of hyperglycemia appear to be the most important causative factor in the development of diabetic nephropathy.[3] Hyperglycemia leads to increased generation of reactive oxygen species; depletion of the reduced form of nicotinamide dinucleotide (phosphate); activation of the polyol pathway, which can lead to de novo synthesis of diacylglycerol and increased protein kinase C activity; alterations in the hexosamine pathway; and nonenzymatic protein glycation (advanced glycosylation end products). All of these pathways have been implicated in the development of diabetic nephropathy, and better glucose control generally reduces the risk of nephropathy and other microvascular diabetic complications.[4] For example, patients who have glucokinase mutations, which are associated with milder hyperglycemia (average hemoglobin A_{1c} [HbA_{1c}] levels 6.9%), have far less proteinuria, microalbuminuria, or nephropathy than patients who have long-standing type 2 diabetes with HbA_{1c} levels averaging 7.8%. Furthermore, randomized interventional studies clearly demonstrate that relatively better control of blood sugar decreases the development of nephropathy in type 1 diabetes, and observational studies with repeat renal biopsies show that the renal lesions of diabetic nephropathy may reverse after long-term functioning pancreas transplantation.

Hemodynamics

Patients with type 1 and, to a lesser extent, type 2 diabetes exhibit an increased glomerular filtration rate (GFR), so-called hyperfiltration, that is mediated by proportionately greater relaxation of the afferent arteriole than the efferent arteriole. This hyperfiltration leads to increased glomerular blood flow and elevated glomerular capillary pressure. With poorly controlled diabetes, patients also develop glomerular hypertrophy, with an increased glomerular capillary surface area. These intraglomerular hemodynamic and structural alterations may contribute to the development or progression (or both) of diabetic renal injury. Blockade of the renin-angiotensin system with angiotensin-converting enzyme (ACE) inhibitors or angiotensin receptor blockers and the use of sodium-glucose cotransporter-2 (SGLT2) inhibitors reduce this elevated intraglomerular capillary pressure in experimental animals, so this hyperfiltration hypothesis potentially explains how these medications slow the progression of diabetic nephropathy.

Hormones and Cytokines

A number of cytokines, hormones, and intracellular signaling pathways are implicated in the development and/or progression of diabetic nephropathy, notably transforming growth factor β, connective tissue growth factor, angiotensin II, vascular endothelial growth factor, endothelin, prostaglandins, and nitric oxide.[5] Because these factors have also been implicated in a variety of nondiabetic kidney diseases, they are not specific for diabetic nephropathy. However, agents that interrupt production and signaling of angiotensin II are very effective in slowing the progression of diabetic nephropathy.

Genetics

Although poor glycemic and blood pressure control undoubtedly contribute to the development of diabetic nephropathy, nephropathy may or may not occur in an individual patient even after many years of hypertension and hyperglycemia. Type 1 diabetic patients whose siblings have diabetic nephropathy have a greater than 70% lifetime risk of developing diabetic nephropathy themselves. Patients with type 2 diabetes also appear to have a hereditary predisposition for or against the development of diabetic nephropathy.

However, diabetic nephropathy is likely to be a polygenic disease, and its development and progression are likely related to the inheritance of multiple polymorphisms with variable effect sizes. For example, Black Americans with apolipoprotein-1 genetic risk genotypes do not have an increased predisposition to develop diabetic nephropathy, but nephropathy has an accelerated progression in such patients. In addition, the lack of nephropathy in patients with glucokinase mutations may be more pronounced than can be explained just by their relatively lower HbA_{1c} levels. Studies also suggest a long-term programming or memory effect in the development of diabetic kidney disease, such that patients whose type 1 diabetes was poorly controlled in the past will develop nephropathy at an increased rate despite subsequent excellent glycemic control. These findings suggest the possible role for epigenetic programming—such as for the glomerular expression of enzymes in glycolytic, sorbitol, methylglyoxal, and mitochondrial pathways—in type 1 diabetic patients who develop diabetic nephropathy.

CLINICAL MANIFESTATIONS

Diabetic kidney disease progresses through four stages at variable rates in different patients.[6,7]

Natural History

Diabetic nephropathy progresses through four relatively distinct stages (Fig. 109-1).

Stage I

In stage I, which commences soon after the overt manifestations of diabetes, renal blood flow and GFR increase by up to 50%, and the kidney's glomeruli and tubules hypertrophy compared with age- and weight-matched normal control subjects. Although patients with type 2 diabetes also tend to have an elevated GFR during the early course of their disease, the GFR increases are not usually as pronounced as seen with insulin-dependent diabetes mellitus. At this stage, macroalbuminuria (>300 mg per 24 hours) is not detectable, but transient microalbuminuria (30 to 300 mg per 24 hours) can occasionally be measured by radioimmunoassay, enzyme-linked immunosorbent assay, or special dipsticks, especially when induced by stress, physical exertion, concurrent illness, or poor glycemic control.[8] Hypertension is usually absent in the early stages in type 1 diabetic patients but is present in 10 to 25% of type 2 diabetic patients at initial evaluation.

Stage II

Approximately 30% of type 1 diabetic patients progress to stage 2, which is characterized by fixed microalbuminuria after a median of about 10 years of diabetes. Although the GFR either remains elevated or is within the normal range at this stage, renal histology becomes abnormal and is manifested as glomerular and tubular basement membrane thickening and the inception of mesangial matrix expansion. Microalbuminuria is more likely in patients who have evidence of other microvascular insults, especially proliferative retinopathy. Microalbuminuria is a more specific sign of diabetic nephropathy in type 1 diabetes than in type 2 diabetes because of the high incidence of hypertension, which itself may lead to microalbuminuria, in the latter.

Stage III

The majority of patients who are initially seen with fixed microalbuminuria progress to overt nephropathy (stage III) within 5 to 7 years. In this stage, patients have overt proteinuria (>500 mg of total protein per 24 hours) and macroalbuminuria, which are detectable with a routine urinary protein dipstick. With the onset of stage III, estimated glomerular filtration rate (eGFR) is usually below normal levels for age and continues to decrease as the disease progresses, but the serum creatinine level may remain in the normal range. Blood pressure begins to rise in type 1 diabetic patients with stage III nephropathy. In type 2 diabetic patients, who frequently have preexistent hypertension, blood pressure commonly becomes more difficult to control.

Stage IV

Stage IV, or advanced diabetic nephropathy, is characterized by a relentless decline in renal function and progression to ESRD. Patients typically have heavy or nephrotic-range proteinuria (>3.5 g/24 hr) and systemic hypertension but have no evidence of inflammatory glomerular (red blood cell casts) or tubulointerstitial (white blood cells, white blood cell casts) lesions. The kidneys may be inappropriately large for the observed degree of renal insufficiency. However, a subset of patients with type 2 diabetes develops chronic kidney disease without nephrotic-range proteinuria. Whether this difference represents a fundamental difference in the pathophysiology of the two conditions or represents the synergistic effects of other kidney injuries, such as hypertensive renal disease, is unclear.

Other Renal Complications

Patients with diabetes also have an increased rate of other kidney and genitourinary abnormalities. Type IV (hyporeninemic, hypoaldosteronemic) metabolic acidosis (Chapter 104) with hyperkalemia is commonly encountered in diabetic patients who have mild to moderate renal insufficiency. These patients should be carefully monitored for the development of severe hyperkalemia (Chapter 103) in response to volume depletion or after the initiation of drugs that interfere with the renin-angiotensin system, such as ACE inhibitors, angiotensin II receptor blockers, β-adrenergic blockers, nonsteroidal anti-inflammatory agents, and heparin, as well as potassium-sparing diuretics.

Patients with diabetes have an increased incidence of bacterial and fungal infections of the genitourinary tract (Chapter 263). In addition to lower urinary tract infections, they have an increased risk for pyelonephritis as well as for intrarenal and perinephric abscesses (Chapter 263).

Unilateral or bilateral renal artery stenosis (Chapter 110) occurs more frequently in the type 2 diabetic population than in age-matched nondiabetic individuals and should be considered if a diabetic patient has intractable hypertension or a rapidly rising serum creatinine level immediately after initiation of therapy with an ACE inhibitor or angiotensin receptor blocker. Other causes of acute deterioration in renal function include papillary necrosis with ureteral obstruction owing to sloughing of a papilla, obstructive uropathy caused by bladder dysfunction as a result of autonomic neuropathy, and contrast media–induced acute tubular necrosis (Chapter 106). In addition, prerenal azotemia or acute tubular necrosis may develop in diabetic patients as a result of heart failure or volume depletion owing to vomiting induced by gastroparesis (Chapter 210) or diarrhea from autonomic neuropathy.

DIAGNOSIS

The diagnosis of overt diabetic nephropathy[9] is made by three main criteria: the presence of proteinuria within an appropriate time frame, the presence of retinopathy (90 to 95% in type 1 and 60 to 65% in type 2), and the absence of other causes of nephrotic syndrome or renal insufficiency. For patients who have type 1 diabetes and who develop diabetic nephropathy, significant proteinuria is seen within 11 to 23 years of the onset of diabetes. Although microalbuminuria does not always progress to overt proteinuria in these patients, it always precedes overt proteinuria in the patients who do progress. All patients with type 1 diabetes should be screened for microalbuminuria 5 years after the diagnosis and yearly thereafter. Patients who have type 2 diabetes should be screened for microalbuminuria at the time of diagnosis and yearly thereafter.

	Stage I	Stage II	Stage III	Stage IV
Median year of onset	0	10	15-17	18-20
Patients with diabetes (%)	100	30-35	30	30

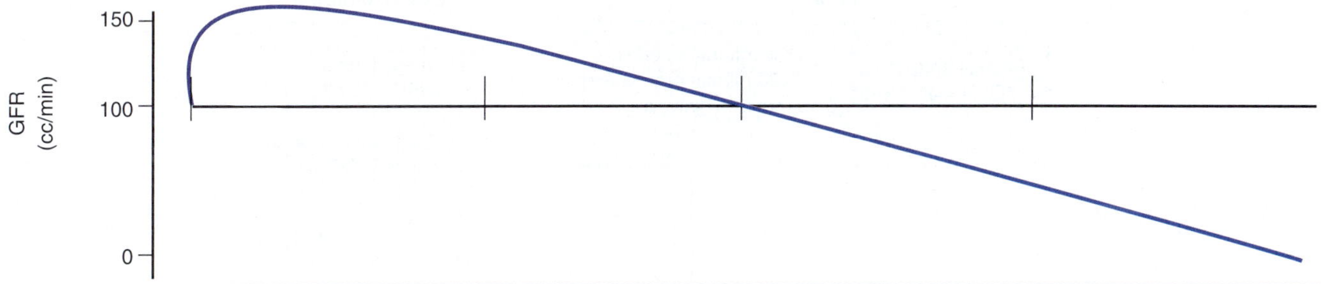

Urinary protein	Occasional and transient microalbuminuria	Fixed microalbuminuria	Proteinuria (>500 mg/24 hr) and microalbuminuria (200 mg/24 hr)	Nephrotic-range proteinuria (<3.5 g/24 hr)
Systemic manifestations	Hypertension: absent in type 1; often present in type 2	Hypertension: absent in type 1; typical in type 2	Hypertension: absent in type 1 and worsening in type 2	Manifestations of chronic renal insufficiency
Renal morphology and history	Kidney hypertrophy	Glomerular basement membrane thickening and mesangial matrix expansion	Focal glomerulosclerosis (± nodular or Kimmelstiel-Wilson lesions) Microvascular hyalinosis and tubulointerstitial fibrosis	Kidney may still be inappropriately large for level of renal insufficiency Global glomerulosclerosis and tubulointerstitial fibrosis

FIGURE 109-1. **Stages of diabetic nephropathy. GFR = glomerular filtration rate.**

Renal Biopsy

Renal biopsy is rarely required to make the diagnosis unless another cause of proteinuria and renal failure is suspected (Chapters 100, 107, and 108). If performed, the biopsy will reveal diffuse or nodular (Kimmelstiel-Wilson) glomerulosclerosis. Although the Kimmelstiel-Wilson lesion is considered pathognomonic of advanced diabetic nephropathy, only approximately 25% of patients manifest this lesion. A nodular pattern of glomerulopathy mimicking Kimmelstiel-Wilson lesions may also be seen in light chain nephropathy (Chapter 173). Nodular glomerular lesions can also be observed in amyloidosis (Chapter 174) and membranoproliferative glomerulonephritis type II (Chapter 107). An additional pathognomonic feature of diabetic nephropathy is the finding of both afferent and efferent arteriolar hyalinosis, which can be distinguished from the isolated afferent arteriolar lesion of essential hypertension. In overt diabetic nephropathy, tubular alterations owing to tubular hypoxia may mediate the progressive decline in renal function, and progressive tubulointerstitial fibrosis correlates most closely with the decline in renal function.

Stage I	Tight glucose control BP control—consider use of ACEI or ARB
Stage II	Tight glucose control BP control ACEI or ARB SGLT2 inhibitor* Finerenone Smoking cessation Weight reduction Exercise Annual eye examination
Stage III	BP control ACEI or ARB SGLT2 inhibitor or GLP-1 analogue* Finerenone Restriction of dietary protein (to 0.8 g/kg/day of ideal body weight) Antihyperlipidemic medications
Stage IV	BP control ACEI or ARB SGLT2 inhibitor or GLP-1 analogue† Finerenone Treat manifestations of nephrotic syndrome and chronic renal insufficiency Prepare for renal replacement therapy, including prevention of abnormalities in calcium and phosphorus metabolism and prevention of anemia by early use of erythropoietin

FIGURE 109-2. **Treatment of diabetic nephropathy.** ACEI = angiotensin-converting enzyme inhibitor; ARB = angiotensin-receptor blocker; BP = blood pressure; GLP-1 = glucagon-like peptide; SGLT2 = sodium glucose cotransporter 2. *SGLT2 inhibitor preferred, but GLP-1 analogue is the alternative if they cannot be used or are not tolerated †See text for adjustments/discontinuation in stage IV.

PREVENTION AND TREATMENT

Glycemic Control

Glycemic control significantly lessens the incidence of nephropathy in patients with type 1 diabetes for at least 20 or more years but does not completely eliminate the risk (Fig. 109-2).[10] In patients with type 2 diabetes, tight control reduces the progression of microvascular complications but appears to be less effective in reducing the risk of macrovascular complications. The goal of diabetic treatment is an HbA_{1c} of 7% or less unless patients have significant comorbid conditions or an increased risk for hypoglycemia.[A1,11]

In latent (stage II) and overt (stage III) diabetic nephropathy, renal function declines. With declining renal function, some oral hypoglycemic agents become contraindicated (Chapter 210). Because of the increased risk of prolonged hypoglycemia, use of sulfonylureas is contraindicated in patients with stage 3b chronic kidney disease or worse (e.g., a GFR <45). Because of the potentially increased risk of lactic acidosis with metformin therapy in patients who have renal insufficiency, treatment guidelines currently recommend not administering it to patients with serum creatinine of greater than 1.7. In addition, as GFR declines, insulin requirements may decrease owing to reduced insulin degradation and clearance by the failing kidney (Chapter 210).

The treatment of diabetic kidney disease has been revolutionized by the advent of SGLT2 inhibiting agents,[12,13] which reduce glucose levels without causing hypoglycemia.[A2] In multiple studies, treatment with canagliflozin (initial dose of 100 mg once daily, increasing to 300 mg starting from week 13),[A3] empagliflozin (10 or 25 mg once daily),[A4] or dapagliflozin (10 mg once daily)[A5] has reduced cardiovascular events, including the progression of renal disease, in patients with type 2 diabetes (Chapter 210).[A6] In addition to glycosuria, these inhibitors reduce intraglomerular pressure through tubuloglomerular feedback, promote an osmotic diuresis and natriuresis, and lower blood pressure. These agents increase the risk of urinary tract infections, and they are currently not approved for treatment of patients with type 1 diabetes because of the potential risk of developing ketoacidosis. Since the glucose-lowering effect of SGLT2

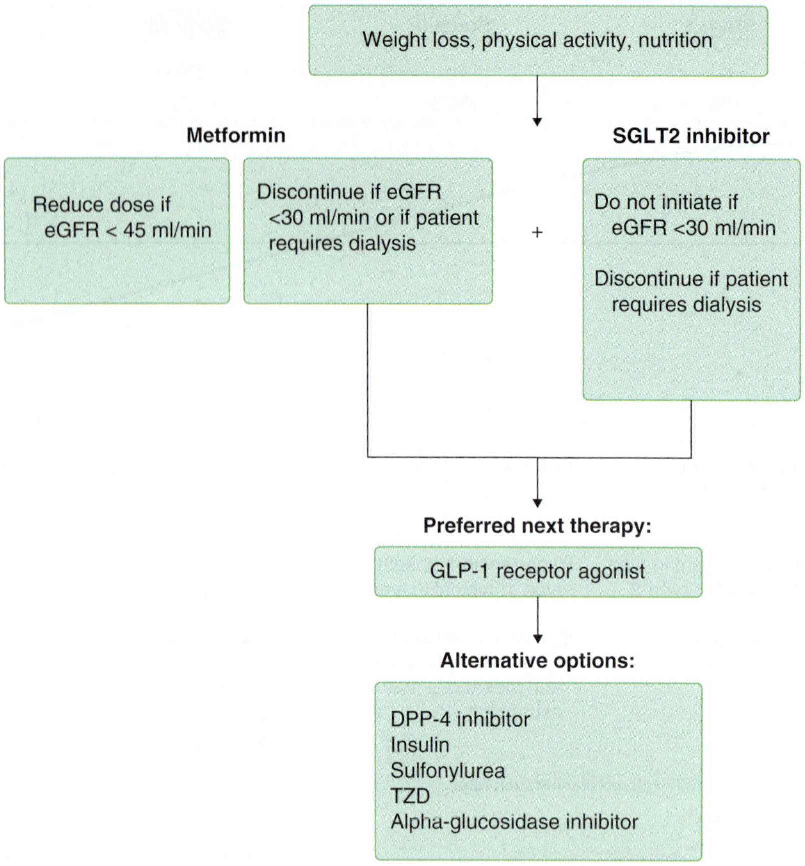

FIGURE 109-3. **Approach to oral hypoglycemic agents in type 2 diabetic kidney disease.** DPP-4 = dipeptidyl peptidase 4; eGFR = estimated glomerular filtration rate; GLP-1 = glucagon-like peptide 1; SGLT2 = sodium glucose cotransporter 2; TZD = thiazolidinedione.

inhibitors depends on glomerular filtration, the current recommendation is that they should be discontinued when the eGFR falls below 30 mL/min.

An alternative approach, especially when the GFR is too low to use SGLT2 inhibitors, is to use one of the subcutaneous glucagon-like receptor 1 (GLP-1) analogues (Fig. 109-3):[A7] liraglutide (1.2 or 1.8 mg once daily, added to basal insulin),[A8] semaglutide (starting dose of 0.25 mg for 4 weeks, then increasing to 0.5 mg for 4 weeks until a maintenance dose of 0.5 mg or 1.0 mg weekly is achieved),[A9] or dulaglutide (1.5 mg weekly).[A10] Efpeglenatide (4 to 6 mg subcutaneously weekly) is another experimental option.[A11] These agents also can slow the progression of diabetic nephropathy and reduce cardiovascular events in type 2 diabetes, and they can be continued until the GFR falls to 15 mL/min. These agents do not cause ketoacidosis but can induce hypoglycemia.

Blood Pressure Control

Elevated blood pressure is an important risk factor in the progression of diabetic nephropathy. To slow the progression of diabetic nephropathy, some guidelines recommend a blood pressure goal of <140/90 mm Hg whereas others recommend a target of <130/80 mm Hg.[14-16]

Medications that interfere with the renin-angiotensin system, either ACE inhibitors or angiotensin receptor blockers, are the preferred agents (see Tables 64-8 and 64-9), with calcium-channel antagonists as second-line therapy.[A12] SGLT2 inhibitors also lower blood pressure and can reduce the need for additional antihypertensive agents.[A13]

Because of the high prevalence of type IV renal tubular acidosis (Chapter 104) and renal artery stenosis (Chapter 110) associated with diabetic nephropathy, patients treated with ACE inhibitors or angiotensin receptor blockers should have their serum potassium and creatinine levels monitored closely in the first week after the initiation of therapy. If blood pressure control is not achieved with these agents, diuretics and other antihypertensive agents, including cardioselective β-blockers, α-blockers, and nondihydropyridine calcium-channel blockers, can be added (Chapter 64).[A14] Dihydropyridine calcium-channel blockers induce selective afferent arteriolar vasodilation and may increase intraglomerular capillary pressure, so they are usually reserved for patients who do not achieve blood pressure control with other agents.

Nonsteroidal Mineralocorticoid Antagonism

The addition of a nonsteroidal mineralocorticoid antagonist, finerenone (20 mg daily to standard of care with an ACE inhibitor or an angiotensin receptor blocker can significantly slow loss of kidney function[A15] and protect against cardiac complications in patients with type 2 diabetic nephropathy.[A16] Although hyperkalemia is a rare complication, careful monitoring and management of potassium levels are indicated when adding this agent.

General Measures

Because morbidity and mortality from cardiovascular disease are significantly increased in patients with diabetic nephropathy, physicians should encourage smoking cessation (Chapter 363) and should prescribe statins for patients with hyperlipidemia (Chapter 190). Judicial restriction of dietary protein to 0.8 g/kg of ideal body weight per day is also recommended. Although further dietary protein restriction may retard the progression of diabetic nephropathy, considerations of such restrictions must be balanced against the individual patient's nutritional requirements.

Renal Replacement Therapy

In general, the management of a diabetic patient nearing ESRD is similar to that of a nondiabetic patient (Chapter 116). Stage III patients should be under the care of a nephrologist, and planning should be initiated for the modality of dialysis. Although dialysis is generally initiated when the GFR declines to less than 10 mL/min, earlier initiation of dialysis is sometimes necessary in diabetic patients in whom issues such as volume-dependent hypertension or hyperkalemia may not otherwise be manageable without renal replacement therapy. Uremia and gastroparesis also can lead to malnutrition or uncontrollable recurrent emesis. More than 80% of patients with end-stage diabetic nephropathy receive dialysis as their modality of renal replacement therapy (Chapter 117), with about five times as many undergoing hemodialysis as compared with peritoneal dialysis (Chapter 117).

Approximately 25% of renal transplants performed in the United States are in diabetic patients. Pancreas and combined kidney-pancreas transplantation can significantly improve the quality of life of patients with diabetic nephropathy by improving autonomic neuropathy, by retarding or possibly correcting retinopathy, and by avoiding the potential complications of insulin administration. However, all transplantation options remain limited by organ availability.

PROGNOSIS

Diabetic nephropathy is relentlessly progressive, even though appropriate medical therapy may slow the progression. Epidemiologic data suggest that diabetic nephropathy is associated with about a 15-year reduction in life expectancy because of the microvascular and macrovascular complications of diabetes (Chapter 210) as well as the kidney disease itself.

Because of their associated cardiovascular, cerebrovascular, and peripheral vascular disease, as well as their increased risk for infection, the mortality of diabetic patients who receive dialysis (Chapter 117) is 1.5 to 2.0 times worse than in nondiabetic patients, corresponding to a 5-year survival rate of less than 20% in diabetic patients undergoing maintenance dialysis. Outcomes are worse in patients whose HbA_{1c} levels are above 8.5%. Long-term survival and quality of life are generally superior after kidney transplantation compared with chronic dialysis. However, the other microvascular complications (retinopathy, neuropathy) are not improved by renal transplantation alone.

GENERAL REFERENCES

For the General References and other additional features, please visit Elsevier eBooks+ at https://ebooks.health.elsevier.com.

Grade A References

A1. Ruospo M, Saglimbene VM, Palmer SC, et al. Glucose targets for preventing diabetic kidney disease and its progression. *Cochrane Database Syst Rev.* 2017;6:CD010137.

A2. Kaze AD, Zhuo M, Kim SC, et al. Association of SGLT2 inhibitors with cardiovascular, kidney, and safety outcomes among patients with diabetic kidney disease: a meta-analysis. *Cardiovasc Diabetol.* 2022;21:47.

A3. Perkovic V, Jardine MJ, Neal B, et al. Canagliflozin and renal outcomes in type 2 diabetes and nephropathy. *N Engl J Med.* 2019;380:2295-2306.

A4. Herrington WG, Staplin N, Wanner C, et al. Empagliflozin in patients with chronic kidney disease. *N Engl J Med.* 2023;388:117-127.

A5. Heerspink HJL, Stefánsson BV, Correa-Rotter R, et al. Dapagliflozin in patients with chronic kidney disease. *N Engl J Med.* 2020;383:1436-1446.

A6. Neuen BL, Young T, Heerspink HJL, et al. SGLT2 inhibitors for the prevention of kidney failure in patients with type 2 diabetes: a systematic review and meta-analysis. *Lancet Diabetes Endocrinol.* 2019;7:845-854.

A7. Kawai Y, Uneda K, Yamada T, et al. Comparison of effects of SGLT-2 inhibitors and GLP-1 receptor agonists on cardiovascular and renal outcomes in type 2 diabetes mellitus patients with/without albuminuria: a systematic review and network meta-analysis. *Diabetes Res Clin Pract.* 2022;183:109146.

A8. Mann JFE, Fonseca V, Mosenzon O, et al. Effects of liraglutide versus placebo on cardiovascular events in patients with type 2 diabetes mellitus and chronic kidney disease. *Circulation.* 2018;138:2908-2918.

A9. Marso SP, Bain SC, Consoli A, et al. Semaglutide and cardiovascular outcomes in patients with type 2 diabetes. *N Engl J Med.* 2016;375:1834-1844.

A10. Gerstein HC, Colhoun HM, Dagenais GR, et al. Dulaglutide and cardiovascular outcomes in type 2 diabetes (REWIND): a double-blind, randomised placebo-controlled trial. *Lancet.* 2019;394:121-130.

A11. Gerstein HC, Sattar N, Rosenstock J, et al. Cardiovascular and renal outcomes with efpeglenatide in type 2 diabetes. *N Engl J Med.* 2021;385:896-907.

A12. Nistor I, De Sutter J, Drechsler C, et al. Effect of renin-angiotensin-aldosterone system blockade in adults with diabetes mellitus and advanced chronic kidney disease not on dialysis: a systematic review and meta-analysis. *Nephrol Dial Transplant.* 2018;33:12-22.

A13. Ye N, Jardine MJ, Oshima M, et al. Blood pressure effects of canagliflozin and clinical outcomes in type 2 diabetes and chronic kidney disease: insights from the CREDENCE trial. *Circulation.* 2021;143:1735-1749.

A14. Huang R, Feng Y, Wang Y, et al. Comparative efficacy and safety of antihypertensive agents for adult diabetic patients with microalbuminuric kidney disease: a network meta-analysis. *PLoS ONE.* 2017;12:1-22.

A15. Bakdris GL, Agarwal R, Anker SD, et al. Effect of finerenone on chronic kidney disease outcomes in type 2 diabetes. *N Engl J Med.* 2020;383:2219-2229.

A16. Pitt B, Filippatos G, Agarwal R, et al. Cardiovascular events with finerenone in kidney disease and type 2 diabetes. *N Engl J Med.* 2021;385:2252-2263.

110 VASCULAR DISORDERS OF THE KIDNEY

THOMAS M. COFFMAN AND STEPHEN R. SMITH

Vascular disorders of the kidney include renal artery stenosis, atheromatous embolization, renal infarction, and renal vein thrombosis. Each of these abnormalities has characteristic clinical manifestations, but treatment options are limited, except for fibromuscular dysplasia. The kidneys also can be affected by systemic vasculitis, thrombotic thrombocytopenic purpura, malignant hypertension with fibrinoid necrosis, extrinsic compression of the renal vessels, trauma, dissection, and radiation-induced injury.

RENAL ARTERY STENOSIS

DEFINITION

Renal artery stenosis is defined as narrowing of one or both renal arteries, thereby resulting in reduction in blood flow to the kidney. The leading cause is atherosclerosis (about 90% of cases), followed by fibromuscular dysplasia. Although renal artery stenosis is often clinically silent, its major clinical sequelae are hypertension and reduced kidney function. A subset of patients with renal artery stenosis has renovascular hypertension, a diagnosis that can be confirmed when an intervention to correct renal artery stenosis results in a significant decline in blood pressure or a reduction in medications needed to control blood pressure.

EPIDEMIOLOGY

Some degree of renal artery stenosis is present in 10 to 20% of patients who have severe or therapy-resistant hypertension, recent-onset hypertension, hypertension developing at an early age, or hypertension with an abdominal bruit. A similar prevalence is observed in patients whose renal arteries are imaged during coronary arteriography for known or suspected coronary artery disease.

Atherosclerosis is the most common cause of renal artery stenosis, accounting for about 90% of clinically identified cases.[1,2] For atherosclerotic renal artery stenosis, epidemiologic risk factors mirror those of atherosclerotic vascular disease (Chapter 40), including risk factors such as hyperlipidemia (Chapter 190), diabetes (Chapter 210), hypertension (Chapter 64), smoking (Chapter 363), and increasing age. Most patients have evidence of widespread atherosclerosis involving the coronary, cerebral, and/or peripheral arteries.

Fibromuscular dysplasia (Chapter 66), which is a distinctly less frequent cause of renal artery stenosis compared with atherosclerosis, typically manifests between ages 20 to 60 years and is more common in women. Although its exact prevalence in the general population is not clear, mild, non-obstructive fibromuscular lesions are seen in about 4% of individuals undergoing renal arteriograms for evaluation as renal transplant donors. Although familial clusters of patients with fibromuscular dysplasia have been reported, most cases are sporadic, and no genetic associations have yet been identified.[3] Rare causes of renal artery stenosis include renal artery dissection, emboli, and extrinsic compression.[4]

PATHOBIOLOGY

The pathobiology of atherosclerotic renal artery stenosis is no different than for atherosclerosis in other arteries (Chapter 41). Fibromuscular dysplasia is an idiopathic, segmented, noninflammatory disease principally of medial layers of the artery (Chapter 63). Any artery can be involved, and about 90% of affected individuals have multifocal disease.

The pathobiologic sequelae of apparent renal artery stenosis depend on the extent and the acuity of the reduction of renal blood flow, as well as whether one or both renal arteries are affected. When the renal artery has a 70% or greater stenosis and a 20 to 25% peak systolic gradient across that stenosis, reduced perfusion pressure to the kidney triggers the release of renin by the juxtaglomerular apparatus, thereby activating the renin–angiotensin–aldosterone system and causing vasoconstriction, the retention of fluid and sodium, and hypertension, sometimes accompanied by flash pulmonary edema.

With bilateral renal artery stenosis or unilateral stenosis in a patient with a solitary functioning kidney, sustained reductions in the glomerular filtration rate can lead to chronic kidney disease, referred to as ischemic nephropathy. Although the kidneys are high-flow organs whose relatively low oxygen consumption provides some protection against the downstream consequences of reduced renal blood flow, critical stenosis sustained for prolonged periods can cause irreversible loss of kidney function. Non-hemodynamic mechanisms, such as activation of pro-inflammatory and pro-fibrotic pathways, also likely play a role. Impaired expression of angiogenic factors, such as vascular endothelial growth factor, results in pathologic remodeling of the renal microvasculature. These non-hemodynamic factors may explain, at least in part, why kidney function may not significantly improve after procedures that successfully restore a normal patency of the renal artery.

The nature of vascular disease in renal artery stenosis differs depending on the cause. With atherosclerosis, stenosis is caused by intrusion of atherosclerotic plaques, which may originate in the aorta, into the lumen of the main renal arteries. In atherosclerotic disease, the stenosis is commonly seen at the ostial segment at the origin of the renal artery, although stenoses can also occur along the entirety of one or both renal arteries. By contrast, fibromuscular dysplasia can be focal but more commonly is multifocal and characterized by areas of post-stenotic dilatation, thereby leading to the angiographic appearance of beads on a string. In fibromuscular dysplasia, lesions are typically located away from the origin of the renal artery, often in the midportion of the vessel or at the first arterial bifurcation.

CLINICAL MANIFESTATIONS

The clinical manifestations of renal artery stenosis may be minimal in many patients, and the diagnosis is often made incidentally during the course of unrelated vascular studies. The most common clinical manifestation of significant renal artery stenosis is arterial hypertension (Chapter 64). Flash pulmonary edema also can be observed and may be more common in patients who have had prior manifestations of heart failure.

Renovascular hypertension from fibromuscular dysplasia should be suspected in patients who have the onset of hypertension at an early age, especially in women, whereas atherosclerotic renal artery hypertension should be considered when an elderly patients or a patient with atherosclerosis in other organ systems develops new-onset hypertension or the sudden worsening of previously well-controlled existing hypertension. The presence of an abdominal bruit on physical examination should further increase the index of suspicion.

In renal artery stenosis caused by atherosclerosis, kidney damage (i.e., a reduction in the glomerular filtration rate) is generally slowly progressive without proteinuria or an active urinary sediment. By comparison, a progressive reduction in the glomerular filtration rate is uncommon with fibromuscular dysplasia. An acute precipitous decrease in the estimated glomerular filtration rate after initiating therapy with an inhibitor of the renin angiotensin system may indicate bilateral renal artery stenosis or unilateral stenosis in a patient with one functioning kidney.

TABLE 110-1 CLINICAL SITUATIONS IN WHICH STENTING OR SURGICAL REVASCULARIZATION IS LIKELY APPROPRIATE FOR ATHEROSCLEROTIC RENAL ARTERY STENOSIS

Flash pulmonary edema or recurrent acute coronary syndrome with hypertension and moderate or more renal artery stenosis with a resting translesional mean gradient ≥10 mm Hg
Stage IV chronic kidney disease with bilateral moderate renal artery stenosis and a resting translesional mean gradient ≥10 mm Hg and a kidney size >7 cm in pole-to-pole length
Stage IV chronic kidney disease and global renal ischemia with unilateral severe renal artery stenosis in a solitary kidney or bilateral severe renal artery stenosis without another explanation
Uncontrolled hypertension despite maximally tolerated doses of at least three antihypertensive agents, one of which is a diuretic agent, and bilateral or solitary severe renal artery stenosis

DIAGNOSIS

Since establishing the diagnosis of atherosclerotic renal artery principally influences the choice among medical therapies (Table 64-9) rather than guiding interventional therapies, specific diagnosis is helpful only in limited situations in which careful antihypertensive therapy is unsuccessful (Table 110-1).[5] By comparison, diagnosis and interventional treatment of fibromuscular muscle dysplasia can potentially cure hypertension and avoid its complications, so prompt diagnosis is important.

The diagnosis of renal artery stenosis requires an imaging study using Doppler ultrasound, computed tomographic angiography (CTA), magnetic resonance angiography (MRA), or conventional arteriography, with arteriography considered the gold standard for diagnosis. The choice among these options depends on the patient's characteristics, local imaging expertise, and whether the diagnosis would modify therapy. Doppler ultrasound requires a skilled operator and is typically less sensitive and specific than contrast-based approaches. CTA and MRA require exposure to iodinated or gadolinium-based contrast material, respectively, both of which can have toxicities, especially in individuals with reduced kidney function. Another option is MRA using ferumoxytol, which is an iron-containing contrast agent with no risk of nephrogenic sclerosis or nephrotoxicity but with somewhat lower resolution. However, noninvasive tests carry a significant likelihood of overestimating the degree of stenosis compared with conventional arteriography, so confirmatory catheter angiography is typically required for patients who are considered candidates for angioplasty or stenting.

Atherosclerotic stenoses are generally irregular and can be bilateral (Fig. 110-1), whereas stenoses of fibromuscular dysplasia typically show a "string of beads" appearance (Fig. 110-2). Isolated measurements of peripheral vein plasma renin activity are of limited utility in the diagnosis of renal artery stenosis, but measuring peripheral or renal vein plasma renin activity after a single dose of captopril may be of some value in determining whether an observed stenosis is hemodynamically significant.

TREATMENT

Atherosclerotic Renal Artery Stenosis

For atherosclerotic renal artery stenosis, neither percutaneous angioplasty nor stenting provide improved overall outcomes compared with best medical treatment.[A1,A2] Nevertheless, some individuals (i.e., patients whose severe hypertension requires three medications, who have had a recent acute decline in kidney function, or who have episodes of flash pulmonary edema) may have better subsequent blood pressure control or kidney function following stenting or surgical revascularization (see Table 110-1).[6–8]

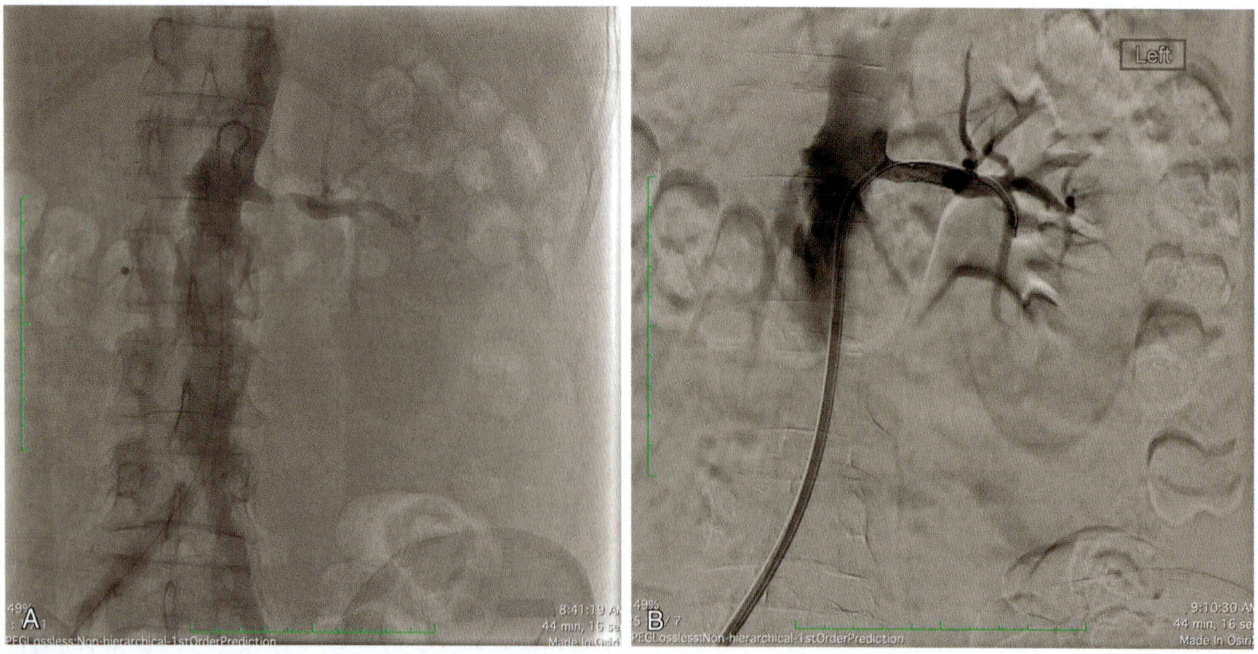

FIGURE 110-1. Renal artery atherosclerosis. **A,** Renal arteriogram showing moderate atherosclerotic stenosis of the left renal artery and total occlusion of the right renal artery in a patient with resistant hypertension and chronic kidney disease. **B,** Left renal artery with stent in place. The patient's blood pressure did not improve with stenting of the left renal artery but did improve dramatically with resection of the atrophic right kidney, not seen on the arteriogram.

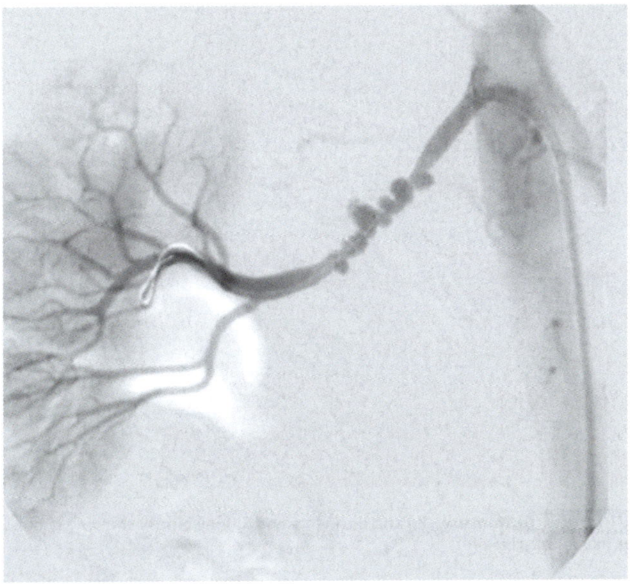

FIGURE 110-2. Right renal arteriogram showing "beads on a string" appearance of fibromuscular dysplasia.

As a result, medical management is the preferred therapeutic approach for the majority of individuals with atherosclerotic renal artery stenosis. The best medical therapy, based on expert opinion, includes smoking cessation (Chapter 363), management of hyperlipidemia (Chapter 190), aspirin (75 to 100 mg per day), and control of hypertension (Chapter 64) with inhibitors of the renin–angiotensin system (Tables 64-7 and 64-9) while carefully monitoring kidney function.

Fibromuscular Dysplasia

By comparison, nonrandomized data support a benefit from percutaneous angioplasty for patients who have fibromuscular dysplasia in terms of improved blood pressure control in 35 to 70% of patients.[9] Young women with severe hypertension may particularly benefit. Stenting is not generally required for lesions of fibromuscular dysplasia. Since fibromuscular dysplasia can be multifocal (Chapter 66), patients also may require angioplasty for lesions in other vascular beds or may need repeat renal angioplasty for recurrent disease in renal arteries years after successful angioplasty.

PROGNOSIS

Because atherosclerotic renal artery stenosis typically is a manifestation of severe systemic disease, it is a poor prognostic sign and patients are at markedly increased risk for ischemic events in other organs and the progression of renal insufficiency. For patients with fibromuscular dysplasia, prognosis depends on successful treatment of the hypertension as well as the severity and treatability of lesions in other vascular beds (Chapter 66).

ATHEROMATOUS EMBOLIZATION OF THE RENAL ARTERIAL SYSTEM

DEFINITION

Atheromatous cholesterol embolization (Chapter 66) is a multiorgan syndrome, which rarely can be caused by a spontaneous rupture of an atheromatous plaque but more commonly is a complication associated with interventional vascular procedures or the use of anticoagulants and thrombolytic agents. A shower of small particles, including cholesterol crystals from the larger central arteries to the distal circulation, can affect both native and transplanted kidneys. The clinical syndrome is distinct from arterial thromboembolism, in which larger thrombi lodge in downstream arteries and cause acute infarction.

EPIDEMIOLOGY

The precise incidence of renal atheromatous embolization is difficult to determine. Among patients known to have abdominal aortic aneurysms, the incidence is about 3% over 15 months, whereas the incidence is only 1% over 3 years in patients with thoracic aortic aneurysm.[10] Atheromatous embolization occurs in about 0.4% of patients undergoing left heart catheterization (Chapter 59),[11] and about two thirds of such cases affect the kidneys. Of patients who develop atheromatous embolization in the absence of a vascular procedure, about 7% have been taking anticoagulants or have received thrombolytic therapy. In patients over age 60 years who undergo a kidney biopsy for acute kidney injury (Chapter 106), about 5% have evidence of atheroembolic disease. Consistent with the epidemiology of atherosclerosis, atheroembolic disease is more commonly seen in older patients who have a high burden of systemic vascular disease.

PATHOBIOLOGY

Because of their small size, cholesterol emboli do not typically cause significant impairment of renal blood flow but instead tend to lodge and occlude smaller 100- to 200-μm arterioles such as arcuate and interlobular arteries and the glomerular capillaries. The presence of the crystals in vascular lumens leads to a complex inflammatory response with associated ischemia and necrosis. The glomerular lesion is presumably related to secondary effects of atheroembolization, including activation of immune and inflammatory mediators. The early phase of the inflammatory reaction includes neutrophils and eosinophils, but then a subsequent foreign body reaction is characterized by multinucleated giant cells and macrophages. The NLRP3 inflammasome has been implicated in the genesis of the inflammatory response. Complement is activated, as is the renin–angiotensin system, and some patients have reduced serum levels of complement. Emboli may be cleared over time by fibrinolysis and uptake by the endothelial cells, followed by their release into the perivascular space.

CLINICAL MANIFESTATIONS

Although a preceding invasive vascular procedure is an important precipitating event, the clinical manifestations can become apparent from days to months after the procedure. Involvement of other vascular beds is common and the presence of extrarenal atheroemboli such as livedo reticularis (Fig. 66-4), a petechial or purpuric rash (Chapter 66), ischemic toes, or amaurosis fugax with Hollenhorst plaques on fundoscopic examination strongly support the diagnosis.

The clinical presentation of atheromatous embolization to the kidneys is notoriously variable, but hypertension and slowly declining glomerular filtration rate are consistent features. Accordingly, the differential diagnosis is large and often includes acute tubular necrosis (Chapter 106), contrast nephrotoxicity (Chapter 59), allergic interstitial nephritis (Chapter 108), and vasculitis (Chapter 249).[12]

DIAGNOSIS

No pathognomonic laboratory tests are available, but peripheral blood eosinophilia may occur early in the course, and complement levels are low in a minority of cases. Inflammatory markers such as the erythrocyte sedimentation rate and the C-reactive protein level are typically elevated. Urinalysis is usually bland, but heavy proteinuria can occur. A urinary sediment with red cells is suggestive of acute glomerulonephritis and is rarely seen.

Tissue biopsy, typically of kidney, skin, or muscle, provides a definitive diagnosis but is not required in patients who have a history of a recent vascular procedure accompanied by physical findings suggestive of embolization. On kidney biopsy, the pathognomonic histologic feature on light microscopy is the presence of cholesterol crystal clefts (Fig. 110-3). The histopathologic process is patchy, and the sensitivity of kidney biopsy can be improved from about 75% with a single biopsy core to about 95% with the standard two cores. Focal segmental glomerulosclerosis is also seen in a substantial portion of biopsies.

TREATMENT

Although corticosteroids are often prescribed, no specific treatments are proven to be beneficial. Nevertheless, moderate- to high-dose statin therapy (Table 190-2) may be associated with better outcomes, whether at baseline or started after diagnosis. In the absence of effective medical therapy, prevention of further embolization emphasizes the avoidance, if possible, of anticoagulants and interventional vascular procedures. Blood pressure control, preferably with an angiotensin-converting enzyme inhibitor or angiotensin receptor blocker (Table 64-9), is recommended.

PROGNOSIS

Prognosis of patients with renal atheroembolism is poor.[13] Approximately 30% of patients progress to end-stage kidney disease that requires dialysis, although a minority of patients who initiate dialysis may eventually recover sufficient kidney function to discontinue dialysis. Median survival from the time of diagnosis is about 5.5 years, and most patients die from cardiovascular complications as a reflection of the severity of their underlying atherosclerotic vascular disease.

RENAL INFARCTION

Occlusion of a main or segmental renal artery is an uncommon occurrence, accounting for 0.004 to 0.007% of emergency department visits. The cause can usually be traced to one of three processes: thromboembolism, a renal vascular abnormality, or thrombosis in the setting of hypercoagulability (Chapter 67). Despite a rigorous evaluation,[14] up to 20 to 30% of cases have no identifiable cause.

The most common source of thromboembolism causing renal infarction is atrial fibrillation (Chapter 52), but thromboemboli to the kidney may also arise from endocarditis (Chapter 61), paradoxical embolus through a patent foramen ovale (Chapter 55), an atrial myxoma (Chapter 47), or aortic aneurysm (Chapter 63). Although renal infarction from thromboembolism usually affects only one kidney, bilateral disease also can be observed, and multiple segmental areas of infarction are typically seen.

The most common vascular abnormalities associated with renal infarction are spontaneous dissection of a renal artery aneurysm and fibromuscular dysplasia. However, infarction also can be seen after trauma and after endovascular procedures.

Hypercoagulable disorders associated with renal infarction, often bilateral, include thrombophilia (Chapter 67), the antiphospholipid syndrome (Chapter 160), the hypercoagulable state associated with nephrotic syndrome (Chapter 107), and in the setting of coronavirus-2019 (COVID-19)-associated hypercoagulability (Chapter 336).[15] Vasculitis (Chapter 249) is a very rare cause of renal infarction.

CLINICAL MANIFESTATIONS AND DIAGNOSIS

The clinical presentation of renal infarction can be fairly nonspecific and may resemble other more common disorders such as pyelonephritis (Chapter 263) or nephrolithiasis (Chapter 111).[16] Flank pain is the most common presenting symptom, sometimes accompanied by nausea and fever and often accompanied by increased blood pressure, which may be dramatically elevated. If the cause is embolic, symptoms ascribable to emboli in other vascular beds may be present. Leukocytosis and elevations in the erythrocyte sedimentation rate, C-reactive protein level, and lactate dehydrogenase level are common.

Diagnosis is confirmed by cross-sectional imaging, usually by a CT angiogram, which is rapid and accurate, showing typical findings of a segmental lack of enhancement indicative of infarction. In individuals with a reduced glomerular filtration rate, MRA imaging using a non–gadolinium-based contrast such as ferumoxytol is a safe alternative. If a lesion in the main renal artery is suspected, catheter-based contrast arteriography may be warranted.

TREATMENT

Treatment is based on the suspected cause of the infarction. If a renal artery is totally occluded by thrombus, intra-arterial infusion of a thrombolytic agent may be of benefit. If embolism from the heart is suspected, immediate systemic anticoagulation is indicated with unfractionated or low-molecular-weight heparin (Table 70-3) followed by long-term anticoagulation therapy. Whether direct-acting anticoagulants (see Table 70-6) are superior to warfarin over the long term in this condition is unknown. The long-term benefit of systemic anticoagulation in patients with idiopathic renal infarction is uncertain. Surgical or percutaneous intervention is usually limited to patients who have bilateral occlusions, occlusions to a solitary kidney, traumatic renal artery thrombosis, or procedure-related thrombosis.

PROGNOSIS

The prognosis in renal infarction correlates with the extent of the kidney parenchyma that is affected and whether treatment can re-establish perfusion within 60 to 90 minutes. Because the lesions are typically segmental, are self-limited, and do not involve the entire kidney, prospects for maintaining adequate kidney function are better than for patients with atheroembolic disease, in which the injury tends to be diffuse. By 60 months, about 45% of patients have hypertension and two-thirds have stage 3 or higher chronic kidney disease (Chapter 116).[17] Follow-up imaging often shows that the affected kidney is smaller in size and has reduced function compared with the unaffected contralateral kidneys, but most patients do not require dialysis.

RENAL VEIN THROMBOSIS

Complete or partial thrombotic occlusion of one or both renal veins is a rare condition that occurs almost exclusively when at least two of three of the Virchow triad are present: low blood flow or stasis, trauma to the endothelium, and hypercoagulability. Males are affected more often than females, and the left renal vein is involved more often than the right, rarely because of extrinsic compression of the left renal vein by the superior mesenteric artery and aorta.[18] The most common setting for renal vein thrombosis is the nephrotic syndrome (Chapter 107), in which severe hypoalbuminemia is associated with the urinary loss of inhibitors of

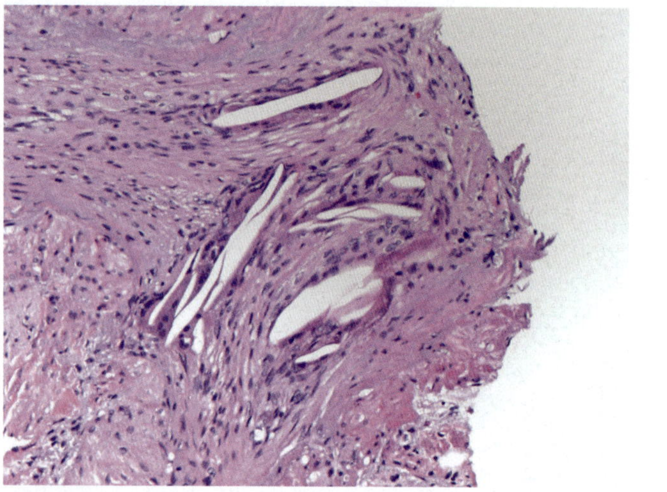

FIGURE 110-3. Hematoxylin and eosin–stained kidney biopsy showing cholesterol clefts in a renal arteriole.

coagulation (e.g., protein S and antithrombin III), an increase in procoagulant factors (e.g., fibrinogen and β-thromboglobulin), and low oncotic pressure. Of the causes of nephrotic syndrome, membranous glomerulopathy is most commonly associated with renal vein thrombosis, although the incidence of 1% is not high enough to warrant routine screening. Primary causes of hyper-coagulability (Chapter 67), such as factor V Leiden and antiphospholipid antibody syndrome, are also associated with renal vein thrombosis.[19,20] Trauma can cause renal vein thrombosis, most often after kidney transplantation when mechanical stress or kinking of the renal vein in combination with low post-transplant blood flow may cause thrombosis. Renal cell carcinoma (Chapter 182) invading the renal vein and inferior vena cava can induce thrombosis. Profound volume depletion can lead to low blood flow in the renal veins and rarely cause thrombosis.

CLINICAL MANIFESTATIONS AND DIAGNOSIS

Renal vein thrombosis may be asymptomatic, particularly if chronic. In the acute setting, however, flank pain, fever, nausea, and vomiting may occur along with gross hematuria. The differential diagnosis often includes pyelonephritis (Chapter 263) and nephrolithiasis (Chapter 111). If the left renal vein is involved, the gonadal vein may become distended, thereby causing the pelvic congestion syndrome in females and painful swelling of the left testicle in males.

Although Doppler ultrasound is a reasonable screening test and is often the study of choice for detecting renal vein thrombosis after kidney transplantation, the diagnosis is most readily made in native kidneys by CT angiography or MRI venography. Characteristic findings include enlargement of the kidney and renal vein, delayed excretion of contrast with a persistent nephrogram, and distortion of the renal pelvis and calyces. In more chronic cases, ureters may be notched by compressing venous varicosities.

TREATMENT

Patients who have asymptomatic unilateral renal vein thrombosis and good kidney function may not require anticoagulation. For patients with acute symptomatic renal vein thrombosis, anticoagulation with unfractionated or low-molecular-weight heparin (Table 70-3) should be followed by oral anticoagulation with warfarin to a target international normalized ratio of 2.0 to 3.0[21] to avoid further thromboembolic events and preserve kidney function, unless patients have contraindications to such treatment. Instillation of thrombolytic agents in the renal vein or, rarely, surgical thrombectomy is reserved for acute bilateral renal vein thrombosis or for unilateral renal vein thrombosis in a solitary functioning kidney. Long-term low-molecular-weight heparin may be preferred for renal vein thrombosis associated with a renal cell carcinoma. The optimal duration of systemic anticoagulation is unknown, but anticoagulation can be discontinued in patients whose membranous nephropathy goes into remission.

PROGNOSIS

Systemic anticoagulation is generally successful in preventing further thromboembolic events with an acceptable rate of bleeding complications, particularly if anti-platelet therapy is not used concurrently. Renal prognosis depends largely on the cause of the renal vein thrombosis and whether that cause resolves, persists, or recurs.[22]

GENERAL REFERENCES

For the General References and other additional features, please visit Elsevier eBooks+ at https://ebooks.health.elsevier.com.

Grade A References

A1. Piaggio D, Bracale U, Pecchia L, et al. Endovascular treatment versus medical therapy for hypertensive patients with renal artery stenosis: an updated systematic review. *Ann Vasc Surg.* 2019;61:445-454.

A2. Raman G, Adam GP, Halladay CW, et al. Comparative effectiveness of management strategies for renal artery stenosis: an updated systematic review. *Ann Intern Med.* 2016;165:635-649.

111 NEPHROLITHIASIS

DAVID A. BUSHINSKY

Kidney stones are composed of crystals in a protein matrix. Most crystals contain calcium, which is generally complexed with oxalate, phosphate, or both, whereas other stones are composed of uric acid, magnesium ammonium phosphate (struvite), or cystine, alone or in combination. Kidney stones form when the saturation of their components exceeds the solubility of the solid phase in urine.

EPIDEMIOLOGY

The annual incidence of kidney stones in industrialized nations exceeds 1 per 1000 persons, with a lifetime risk of about 10% in women and about 15% in men. The incidence of stone formation peaks in the fourth and fifth decades, and prevalence increases with age until approximately 70 years in men and 60 years in women. In the United States, the prevalence of nephrolithiasis has increased from 3% in the late 1970s to more than 5%, an increase that is likely due to changes to diet and lifestyle, as well as more accurate diagnosis.[1] The estimated yearly economic cost of kidney stones exceeds $5 billion in the United States.

In the United States, Whites are more likely to develop renal stones than are other ethnic groups. Stones are more common in hot, dry climates, perhaps because greater fluid loss through the skin and respiratory epithelium leads to more concentrated urine. Many occupations make it inconvenient to utilize a restroom, and these individuals often avoid fluids in an effort to avoid urination, thereby leading to excretion of concentrated urine. Insufficient rehydration among people who engage in physical activity and have large insensible losses also leads to concentrated urine.

Obesity is correlated with the risk for kidney stone formation. Individuals weighing more than 220 pounds or having a body mass index greater than 30 are significantly more likely to form stones than are individuals who weigh less than 150 pounds or have a body mass index between 21 and 22.9.

The types of stones vary around the world,[2] but in the United States, the majority of stones are calcium oxalate and/or calcium phosphate (>80%), and less than 10% are pure uric acid stones. By comparison, about 70% of stones in the Mediterranean and Middle East are composed of uric acid. Magnesium ammonium phosphate (struvite) stones account for 1 to 25% of stones, whereas cystine stones comprise 1 to 2% of stones.[3]

PATHOBIOLOGY

Human bone is composed of calcium and phosphate, principally in the form of apatite. Once humans reach their adult height and their skeleton is fully mineralized, the net amount of calcium that is absorbed by nonpregnant individuals must be excreted in the urine. Similarly absorbed phosphate that is not needed for bone mineralization or cell growth must be excreted. Oxalate is an end product of metabolism, and it too must be excreted in the urine. The need for water conservation by terrestrial humans often leads to excretion of these ions in relatively scant amounts of urine, thereby promoting increased saturation with respect to the solid phases of calcium oxalate and/or calcium phosphate. Increasing saturation drives the formation of the solid crystal phase and is expressed as the ratio of calcium oxalate (or phosphate) ion activity to its solubility. At ratios of greater than 1, termed supersaturation, a solid phase can form, whereas the substances remain in solution at ratios less than 1. When urine is supersaturated, ions can bond to form the more stable, solid phase, which is termed *nucleation*. Homogeneous nucleation refers to the bonding of similar ions into crystals. The more common and thermodynamically favored heterogeneous nucleation occurs when crystals grow on dissimilar crystals or substances as cellular debris in the urine. Although humans produce inhibitors of stone formation, such as osteopontin and Tamm-Horsfall protein, supersaturation can overwhelm this inhibition, and a solid phase will form.

Calcium Stones

About 70 to 80% of kidney stones contain calcium, which is often complexed with oxalate or phosphate. Calcium-containing kidney stones are most often caused by excessive excretion of calcium (hypercalciuria), oxalate (hyperoxaluria), or urate (hyperuricosuria) or insufficient excretion of citrate (hypocitraturia).[4]

Calcium-containing stone formation has a strong genetic component.[5] Idiopathic hypercalciuria is thought to be a polygenic disorder in which a generalized dysregulation of calcium transport in the kidney, intestine, and bone leads to increased urinary calcium. A number of single-nucleotide polymorphisms, in genes coding for the calcium-sensing receptor, the vitamin D receptor, and osteopontin, and others, have been associated with calcium nephrolithiasis. Overall, 14 monogenic mutations account for 15% of nephrolithiasis/nephrocalcinosis, and genetic factors appear to explain about 20 to 35% of the interindividual variation in excretion of ions critical to stone formation.

Urinary oxalate is derived from endogenous metabolism of glyoxylate and ascorbic acid or from dietary sources, such as cocoa, nuts, tea, and certain leafy green vegetables such as spinach. The three main causes of hyperoxaluria are excessive oxalate ingestion *(dietary oxaluria)*, excessive intestinal absorption of oxalate *(enteric oxaluria)* that is paradoxically observed in malabsorptive gastrointestinal disorders, and excessive endogenous oxalate production seen in certain hepatic enzyme deficiencies (*primary hyperoxaluria;* Chapter 189). Additionally, ethylene glycol, a common automobile antifreeze, is metabolized to oxalate and can cause excessive urinary oxalate excretion in conjunction with severe metabolic acidosis and renal failure (Chapter 96).

Enteric oxaluria results in elevated urinary oxalate levels (60 to 100 mg/day).[6] In gastrointestinal malabsorptive conditions such as Crohn disease (Chapter 127), celiac sprue (Chapter 126), jejunoileal bypass (Chapter 201), and chronic pancreatitis (Chapter 130), malabsorbed fatty acids bind dietary calcium, thereby leaving oxalate free to pass into the colon, where it is more likely to be absorbed owing to the presence of bile acids; this excess oxalate is then subsequently filtered by the glomerulus and excreted in the urine. Intestinal bacteria also can influence oxalate levels by degrading it, preventing its absorption, or even stimulating its secretion from the circulation into the intestine.

Primary hyperoxaluria (Chapter 189) results from defects in hepatic enzymes in the liver glyoxylate pathway; the results are substantial endogenous oxalate production and a marked elevation of urinary oxalate (80 to 300 mg/day).[7] Oxalate deposits in numerous organs, including the heart, bone marrow, muscle, and renal parenchyma, where they lead to renal failure, cardiomyopathy, and bone marrow suppression at an early age. In type 1 primary hyperoxaluria, which accounts for about 80% of cases, the hepatic enzyme alanine glyoxylate aminotransferase, which converts glyoxylate to glycine, is deficient because of one of a large number of mutations in the *AGXT* gene. With deficient alanine glyoxylate aminotransferase, the glyoxylate is converted to oxalate. In the milder type 2 primary hyperoxaluria, which represents approximately 10% of cases, patients lack D-glycerate reductase and glyoxylate reductase owing to mutations in the *GRHPR* gene. Type 3 primary hyperoxaluria, which accounts for about 5% of cases, is a result of mutations in the *HOGA1* gene that catalyzes the cleavage of 4-hydroxy-2-oxoglutarate to pyruvate and glyoxylate.

Nephrolithiasis and nephrocalcinosis can also result from a variety of monogenic disorders, such as Dent disease (X-linked recessive nephrolithiasis; Chapter 113), McCune-Albright syndrome (Chapters 212 and 229), osteogenesis imperfecta type 1 (Chapter 239), and congenital lactase deficiency (Chapter 126).

Citrate inhibits stone formation by combining with calcium to form a soluble complex that reduces the availability of calcium to bind with oxalate or phosphate. The principal risk factor for hypocitraturia is a high protein intake. Men often have lower urinary citrate concentrations than women. Distal renal tubular acidosis (Chapter 104) promotes the formation of calcium phosphate stones owing to bone demineralization and an alkaline tubular pH.

Calcium oxalate kidney stones form on calcium phosphate deposits, termed Randall plaques, which are located in the renal papillae. Randall plaque formation is positively correlated with urine calcium excretion and negatively correlated with urine volume and pH. These calcium phosphate crystals, in the form of apatite, originate around the thin loop of Henle and then extend into the interstitium without eroding into the tubular lumen or damaging the tubular cells. The crystals move toward the urinary space, where they form Randall plaques, which are visible on cystoscopy and also may be seen as medullary calcifications on computed tomography (CT). In the presence of urine that is supersaturated with respect to calcium oxalate, these ions may form a crystal that increases in size to several millimeters or even a centimeter. The stone can break off from the Randall plaque and then migrate to, irritate, and possibly obstruct the ureter.

Uric Acid Stones

The incidence of uric acid stones appears to be rising in the United States in parallel with the increase in obesity, which leads to renal insulin resistance and a very low urine pH.[8] Over 5 times as much uric acid is soluble in a urine with a pH of 6.5 compared with a pH of 5.3. Diarrhea and diets high in animal protein can contribute to an acidic urinary pH. Most patients with uric acid stones have a reduced urine pH, and some have low urine volumes or elevated urinary uric acid levels. Uric acid stone formers have greater body weight and a higher incidence of insulin resistance and type 2 diabetes mellitus. Insulin resistance also leads to impaired urinary ammonium excretion, thereby resulting in the excretion of more hydrogen ions as titratable acids and lower urine pH, which reduces the solubility of ammonium.

Hyperuricosuria may be seen in patients who ingest large quantities of dietary purine, such as organ meats, shellfish, certain fish (e.g., anchovies, sardines, herring, and mackerel), meat extracts (e.g., bouillon and consommé), and protein. Hyperuricemic disorders, including gout (Chapter 252), myeloproliferative disorders, tumor lysis syndrome, and certain inborn errors of metabolism, can also contribute to an increased urinary uric acid. Medications such as salicylates and probenecid can be hyperuricosuric.

Struvite Stones

Struvite stones, sometimes called *triple phosphate stones, magnesium ammonium phosphate stones,* and *infection stones,* comprise only about 10 to 25% of all stones but constitute the majority of staghorn calculi, which are large stones that extend beyond a single renal calyx.[9] Struvite stones are far more common in women than in men, in large part owing to women's increased susceptibility to upper urinary tract infections (Chapter 263). Similarly, any patient with urinary stasis, such as patients with neurogenic bladders, indwelling urinary catheters, or spinal cord lesions, is susceptible to struvite stones.

Struvite stones form only in the presence of both increased production of ammonium and an alkaline urine ($pH \geq 7$), which occur only with urease-producing bacteria. *Proteus mirabilis* (Chapter 281) is a common urease-producing bacterium, but other gram-negative and gram-positive bacteria, such as *Klebsiella* spp. and *Staphylococcus epidermidis,* as well as *Mycoplasma* spp. (Chapter 293) and yeast species, have been implicated in urease production. By comparison, *Escherichia coli* does not produce urease.

Cystine Stones

Cystinuria (Chapter 113), which is an autosomal dominant disorder with incomplete penetrance or an autosomal recessive disorder caused by mutations of the *SLC3A1* gene or the *SLC7A9* gene, results in decreased renal tubular reabsorption and excessive urinary excretion of the dibasic amino acids cystine, ornithine, lysine, and arginine.[10] The resulting urinary excretion of cystine

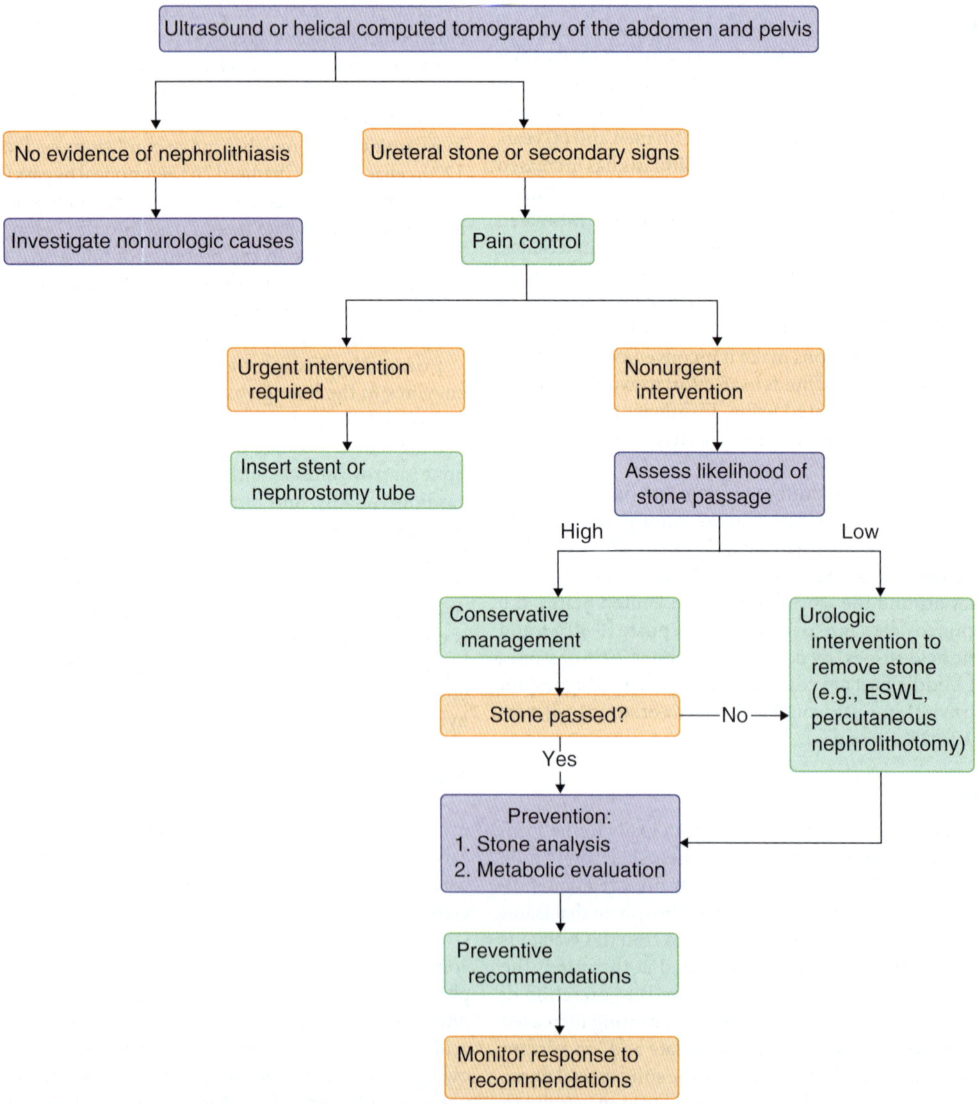

FIGURE 111-1. Algorithm for evaluation of suspected renal colic. ESWL = extracorporeal shock wave lithotripsy. (From Curhan GC. Nephrolithiasis. In: Goldman L, Schafer AI, eds. *Goldman's Cecil Textbook of Medicine.* 24th ed. Philadelphia: Elsevier Saunders; 2012.)

in the typical volume of urine exceeds its solubility of about 250 mg/L and enables stone formation. Although normal people excrete about 30 to 50 mg of cystine per day, heterozygotes for cystinuria excrete about 400 mg/day, and homozygotes often excrete about 600 mg/day. Thus, homozygotes must continually excrete more than 2 L of urine each day to avoid stone formation. Cystinuria is unrelated to the much more severe disorder *cystinosis* (Chapter 113), which results in extensive intracellular cystine accumulation.

CLINICAL MANIFESTATIONS

Patients with kidney stones often present with pain and/or hematuria, and less often present with urinary tract infections (Chapter 263) or acute kidney injury (Chapter 106), either owing to bilateral obstruction or unilateral obstruction in a single functioning kidney (Fig. 111-1). Patients often complain of severe ureteral colic. The pain is of abrupt onset and can intensify into severe, excruciating flank pain. The pain may migrate anteriorly along the abdomen and inferiorly to the groin, testicles, or labia majora as the stone moves down the ureter toward the ureterovesical junction. The pain resolves only after the stone passes or is removed. Microscopic or gross hematuria is common, and patients occasionally present with painless hematuria (see Fig. 100-3). The finding of a stone on radiographic examination does not preclude another cause. Conversely, even large calculi may be asymptomatic and be discovered during the investigation of unrelated symptoms. Obstruction caused by calculi may also be painless, and nephrolithiasis should always be considered in the differential diagnosis of unexplained acute or chronic kidney disease (Chapters 106 and 116).

DIAGNOSIS

The physical examination can provide clues to the diagnosis of kidney stones but is not diagnostic. Some patients have demonstrable flank tenderness, and a rare patient with hyperuricemia will have tophi (Chapter 252). However, the physical examination is most helpful for not showing other potential causes of pain. The suspicion of a kidney stone generally obligates radiographic evaluation. Radiographic studies can be deferred, however, in patients in whom the clinical diagnosis is clear, who have no evidence of infection, who are able to eat and drink, and who can be managed on oral analgesics.

Ultrasonography is an easy and rapid way to detect possible urinary obstruction without exposing the patient to ionizing radiation. Ultrasound can detect clinically significant renal calculi, with about an 85% sensitivity for detecting the ureteral stones that cause acute symptoms. Among emergency department patients with suspected nephrolithiasis, those who undergo ultrasonography have a lower cumulative radiation exposure than those randomized to CT without any significant differences in high-risk diagnoses, serious adverse events, pain scores, or subsequent rehospitalizations or emergency department visits.[A1] A helical CT scan or a low radiation CT scan without radiographic contrast can detect kidney stones with both a sensitivity and a specificity exceeding 95% (Fig. 111-2).[11] Based on the density of the stone, it also can often differentiate a calcium-containing stone from a cystine or uric acid stone. An added benefit is that helical CT is often helpful in determining the cause of nonstone abdominal pain (Chapter 119). In certain situations, such as in human immunodeficiency virus (HIV)–infected patients thought to have stones induced by a protease inhibitor, a helical CT scan with contrast is often required because the stones are not radiopaque and do not obstruct the ureter.

Approximately 90% of kidney stones are radiopaque and may be detected on a simple abdominal radiograph. Unfortunately, however, the stone is often obscured by stool, vertebrae, or abdominal gas, so the sensitivity of a plain abdominal radiograph is about 55%, and its specificity is only about 75%. Uric acid stones are radiolucent and cannot be detected radiographically without contrast.

Intravenous pyelography has a sensitivity of about 75% and a specificity of more than 90% for detecting renal calculi. Intravenous pyelography is also useful for identifying structural abnormalities of the urinary tract, such as a medullary sponge kidney (Chapter 112), that predisposes to stone formation. However, an intravenous pyelogram often does not detect nonobstructing radiolucent stones because they do not create a filling defect. An intravenous pyelogram exposes the patient to more radiation than a plain radiograph but less than a CT scan. It also carries the risk of radiographic contrast material, which is greater in individuals with underlying renal compromise. With the widespread availability of ultrasonography and helical CT scans, an intravenous pyelogram is rarely indicated.

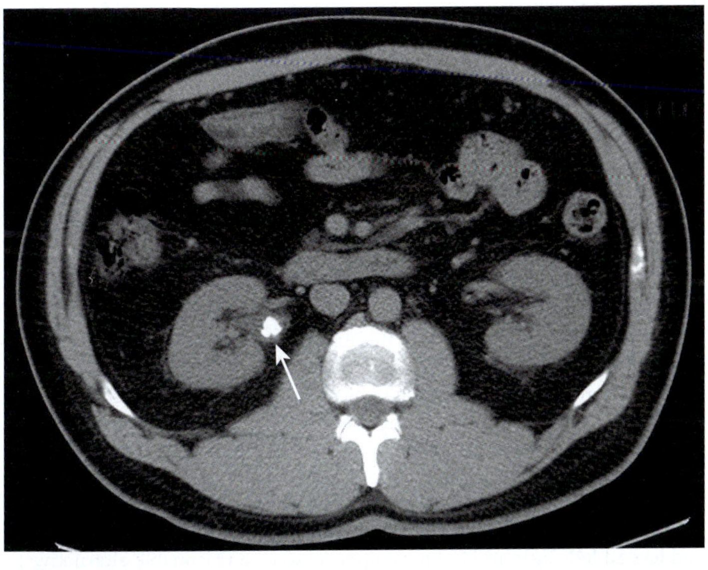

FIGURE 111-2. High-resolution helical computed tomographic (CT) scan of the upper part of the abdomen demonstrating a stone in the right renal pelvis (*arrow*). There is no hydronephrosis. (From Curhan GC. Clinical crossroads: a 44-year-old woman with kidney stones. *JAMA*. 2005;293:1107-1114.)

TREATMENT

Medical Therapy

Because the pain of renal colic can be excruciating, pain control is critical after the definitive diagnosis has been made. If nausea and vomiting prevent the use of oral medication, parenteral medication is typically required. Nonsteroidal anti-inflammatory drugs (NSAIDs; Table 26-4) are as or more effective compared with opiates for renal colic and are preferred because they have fewer side effects.[A2,A3] An intravenous or intramuscular option is ketorolac (15 to 30 mg), and an oral option is ibuprofen (200 to 400 mg/dose every 4 to 6 hours with a maximum daily dose of 1.2 g) in patients who can tolerate oral medication. Because NSAIDs can cause acute kidney injury, especially in patients who are dehydrated or have pre-existing kidney injury, adequate hydration (e.g., normal saline at 75 to 150 mL/hour) is essential, but neither high-volume fluid therapy nor diuretics promote the passage of the stone. If necessary, oral oxycodone (5 to 15 mg every 4 to 6 hours as needed) may be added to ibuprofen for outpatient pain control. The dose and frequency of administration of oxycodone should be reduced in patients who have renal impairment.

Medical Expulsive Therapy

Kidney stones 5 mm or smaller have about a 70% probability of passing spontaneously, whereas stones between 5 and 7 mm have a 60% chance, stones 7 to 9 mm have a 48% chance, and stones 9 mm or larger have a 25% chance of passing spontaneously. Stones located more distally in the ureter are more likely to pass spontaneously. Medical expulsive therapy may be cautiously attempted with ureteral stones smaller than 10 mm diameter for 4 to 6 weeks if pain is controlled, kidney function is normal, and there is no evidence of urinary tract infection or significant obstruction.[12] The patient must be followed closely, generally with repeat ultrasound examinations every week or 2 weeks.

Expulsive therapy can reduce ureteral spasm and increase spontaneous passage rates by about 50%. Meta-analyses demonstrate an overall benefit for the α-blocker tamsulosin (0.4 mg orally daily),[A4,A5] which appears to promote the passage of the stone more quickly and effectively than the calcium-channel blocker nifedipine (nifedipine XL 30 mg daily or twice daily). Other options include a phosphodiesterase type 5 inhibitor (e.g., tadalafil 10 mg/day for 10 days) or a selective α_{1a} receptor blocker (e.g., silodosin 4 mg/day). Silodosin appears more effective than tamsulosin for promoting the passage of large, distal ureteral stones.[A6]

Initial Surgical Treatment

Stones that cause obstruction, infection, acute kidney injury, or intractable pain must be removed expeditiously. In general, larger and more proximal stones are less likely to pass spontaneously, even with medical expulsive therapy, and are often an indicator for earlier intervention. Approximately 15% of all kidney stones require an intervention to remove them. For example, removal of small, asymptomatic kidney stones at the time of surgery to remove a ureteral or contralateral stone reduces the rate of relapse.[A7]

The approach to stone removal depends on its size, location, and composition, as well as on urinary tract anatomy. The major options for ureteral stone removal include percutaneous nephrolithotomy, extracorporeal shock wave lithotripsy, and ureteroscopy; open surgical extraction is rarely required. Percutaneous nephrolithotomy involves the passage of a flexible scope through the kidney and into the urinary space. Extracorporeal shock wave lithotripsy focuses external sound waves onto the kidney stone, thereby causing it to fragment into smaller stones that can more easily be passed spontaneously. Ureteroscopy involves the passage of a ureteroscope into the ureter with removal or laser fragmentation of the stone. Meta-analyses suggest that ureteral stones should be treated with ureteroscopy or shock wave lithotripsy rather than percutaneous nephrolithotomy and that percutaneous nephrolithotomy is the treatment of choice for lower pole renal stones and the majority of large kidney stones (≥15 mm),[A8] because it results in longer stone-free rates and a lower need for retreatment, even though it is associated with more complications, usually minor, and a longer hospitalization compared with shock wave lithotripsy.

Medical Evaluation

After an initial stone episode, the recurrence rate in nontreated patients is estimated to be about 25% at 3 to 5 years and about 50% at 5 to 10 years. As a result, every patient who forms an initial stone should undergo evaluation with the goal of preventing recurrent stones. The history should focus on uncovering factors that predispose to stone formation. All stones should be analyzed to assist in defining the underlying metabolic abnormality and to guide therapy.[13]

A careful dietary history, including an estimate of fluid intake, is essential. Many stone formers are erroneously instructed to eliminate all calcium from their diet, a practice that not only increases stone formation but also may induce bone demineralization. Sodium intake should be estimated because sodium excretion obligates calcium excretion, thereby potentially leading to urinary supersaturation. Excessive animal protein intake increases metabolic acid production, which increases bone demineralization and calciuria.

Hypercalcemic disorders—including malignancy (Chapter 227), hyperparathyroidism (Chapter 227), and sarcoidosis (Chapter 83)—often result in hypercalciuria, increased urinary supersaturation, and calcium stone formation. Malabsorptive gastrointestinal disorders, such as Crohn disease (Chapter 127) and celiac disease (Chapter 126), or weight reduction surgery (Chapter 201), such as ileal resection or jejunoileal bypass, will often result in calcium oxalate stone formation from increased oxalate absorption and excretion as well as volume depletion.

Medications that can cause calcium stone formation include loop diuretics, which increase urinary calcium excretion, as well as salicylates and probenecid, which increase urinary uric acid excretion. Various medications that can themselves precipitate into stones include intravenous acyclovir, high-dose sulfadiazine, triamterene, and the antiretroviral agents indinavir and nelfinavir. Other medications that inhibit renal tubular carbonic anhydrase activity, such as acetazolamide and topiramate, can lead to metabolic acidosis, bone resorption, hypercalciuria, lower urinary citrate excretion, and higher urinary pH, all of which promote the formation of calcium phosphate stones.

The number and frequency of stones formed, the patient's age at the time of the first stone, the size of the stone, and an analysis of the composition of the stone are also important clues. Stones that develop at a young age suggest a genetic disorder, such as primary hyperoxaluria or cystinuria. Large staghorn calculi in elderly patients are consistent with struvite stones. A stone's response to intervention is also helpful: cystine stones do not fragment well with lithotripsy, and stones that recur frequently in a single kidney suggest a unilateral anatomic abnormality.

Basic laboratory testing should include levels of serum electrolytes (sodium, potassium, chloride, and bicarbonate), creatinine, calcium, phosphorus, uric acid, 25-hydroxyvitamin D, and thyroid-stimulating hormone. If the serum calcium is above and the serum phosphorus is below the midrange of normal, a serum parathyroid hormone level should be obtained.

An elevated urine specific gravity suggests inadequate fluid intake. Hematuria may indicate irritation to the urothelial lining by a stone. Characteristic crystals (see Fig. 100-10) are more common than in nonstone formers. The presence of hexagonal crystals (see Fig. 100-9) mandates that cystinuria be excluded. Patients with struvite stones generally have an elevated urine pH (>7.4) owing to the splitting of urea into ammonia and bicarbonate, whereas a low urinary pH (<5.5) raises the suspicion of uric acid stones. An elevated urine pH combined with bacteriuria (Chapter 263) suggests struvite stones. Because urease production may stimulate struvite stone formation despite low bacterial colony counts, the laboratory must identify all bacteria and determine antibiotic sensitivities even with low colony counts. If no bacteria are isolated, cultures for *Ureaplasma urealyticum* should be requested. The combination of an elevated urinary pH (6.5 to 7.2) with a low serum potassium and serum bicarbonate level strongly suggests distal renal tubular acidosis (Chapter 104).

In patients with recurrent stones and/or high-risk characteristics for recurrence, a 24-hour urine collection can determine the levels of calcium, oxalate, citrate, sodium, urate, phosphorus, and creatinine, as well as the calculation of supersaturation with respect to calcium oxalate, calcium phosphate, and uric acid (Table 111-1). Increased ion excretion of the components of a stone leads to increased rates of forming recurrent stones. An elevated supersaturation should lead the clinician to determine the individual components of the urine that are causing the increased supersaturation, and efforts can then be made to rectify these abnormalities. Cystine should also be measured at least once in every stone former to exclude cystinuria and regularly in patients who form cystine stones. Multivitamins should be discontinued about 5 days before the collection to prevent any antioxidant effect on the urine sample.

TABLE 111-1 OPTIMAL 24-HOUR URINE VALUES IN PATIENTS WITH NEPHROLITHIASIS

PARAMETER	VALUE
Volume	>2-2.5 L
pH	>5.5 and <7.0 (24-hr specimen not required)
Calcium	<250 mg
Oxalate	<40 mg
Sodium	<2000 mg
Uric acid	<750 mg
Phosphorus	<1100 mg
Citrate	>320 mg
Supersaturation with respect to calcium oxalate	<5
Supersaturation with respect to calcium phosphate	0.5-2
Supersaturation with respect to uric acid	0-1

Urine creatinine should be measured to ensure the adequacy of collection and should be >15 mg/kg in men and >10 mg/kg in women. Supersaturation is the ratio of the ion activity product and its solubility product.

PREVENTING RECURRENT STONES

Preventive treatment (Fig. 111-3) emphasizes advising the patient to increase oral fluid intake to produce a urine volume greater than 2 L per day, an oral intake that will reduce recurrent stone formation by about 50%.[A9-A10]

Calcium Stones

Because urine calcium excretion is directly correlated with urine sodium excretion, decreasing sodium intake will decrease urine calcium excretion and reduce supersaturation.[14] Patients with calcium stones should limit daily sodium intake to no more than 2 g per day and reduce animal protein intake to 0.8 to 1.0 g/kg per day.

The recommended calcium intake for a 19- to 50-year-old man or woman is 1000 mg of elemental calcium per day, and a number of studies demonstrate decreased formation of calcium stones when people consume diets adequate in calcium, presumably because appropriate calcium intake is needed for intestinal binding of dietary oxalate to prevent its absorption. Dairy products are preferred over calcium supplements because clinical studies indicate that women taking supplemental vitamin D and calcium have a significant increase in stone formation.

Patients with persistent hypercalciuria often benefit from longer-acting thiazide diuretics (e.g., chlorthalidone 12.5 to 25 mg/day), which directly lower urinary calcium and reduce recurrent stone formation by about 50%.[A11] However, a short-acting thiazide diuretic given once daily does not reduce symptomatic recurrences.[A12] Thiazides are effective only if patients restrict dietary sodium. In patients with hypercholesterolemia or hyperglycemia, indapamide (1.25 to 5 mg/day) can be used because it has less effect on these parameters. If patients develop hypokalemia, dietary potassium intake should be increased, or a potassium supplement can be administered. Allopurinol should be prescribed as for gout (300 mg daily; see Chapter 252). Potassium citrate (10 to 40 mEq/day) will increase urinary citrate excretion, bind urinary calcium, and further decrease recurrent stone formation.[A13] Potassium citrate is available as a wax-matrix tablet. A 24-hour urine collection can be repeated in a month or two to assess the response to therapy. Sodium-glucose cotransporter-2 (SGLT2) inhibitors appear to reduce the risk of nephrolithiasis by 50%[A14] but are not currently recommended for routine prophylactic use.

Patients with diet-related hyperoxaluria should be instructed to limit or avoid foods with high oxalate content such as cocoa, nuts, tea, and green leafy vegetables such as spinach. Because dietary calcium and oxalate bind in the gut, patients should consume these foods with calcium-containing foods. For enteric hyperoxaluria, treatment is first directed at the underlying disorder and then at instituting therapy for the cause of the steatorrhea (Chapter 126). Dietary oxalate should be restricted, and dietary calcium and oxalate should be ingested at the same meal. A diet that is low in fat; that is high in fruits, vegetables, and low-fat dairy products; that is rich in grains, fish, poultry, beans, seeds, and nuts; and that contains fewer sweets and less added sugar and red meat appears to be a reasonable alternative to a low-oxalate diet. Additional fluid intake and potassium citrate are often beneficial. Reloxaliase, which is an oral nonabsorbable oxalate-degrading enzyme,[15] is currently in clinical trials.

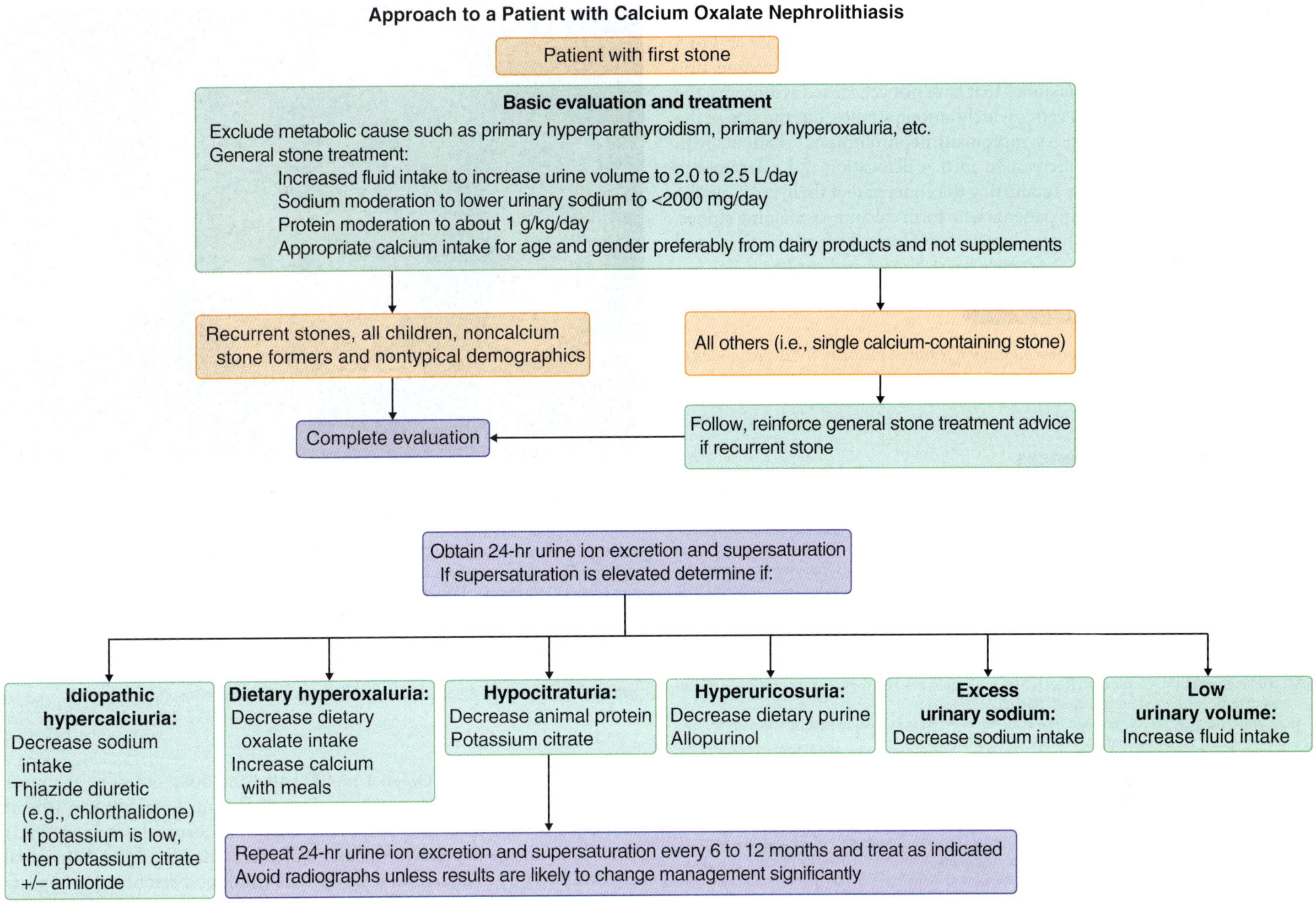

FIGURE 111-3. Approach to a patient with calcium oxalate nephrolithiasis.

In some patients with type 1 primary hyperoxaluria, pyridoxine (vitamin B_6) can increase enzyme activity and reduce oxalate production. These patients should also be treated with measures that reduce the precipitation of calcium oxalate, such as ample fluid intake and potassium citrate (10 to 40 mEq/day). Lumasiran, which is a small interfering RNA that decreases the levels of glycolate oxidase thereby resulting in less production of oxalate, reduces urinary oxalate levels by approximately 50% and reduces plasma oxalate levels into the normal range in patients who have type 1 primary hyperoxaluria.[A15] Lumasiran has the potential to eliminate the clinical manifestations, such as renal failure, of type 1 primary hyperoxaluria and to prevent the need for curative liver transplantation. All patients with type 1 primary hyperoxaluria should be seen by specialists and be considered for treatment with this therapy.

Calcium stones may be found in patients with hyperuricosuria. These patients often excrete excess amounts of urinary uric acid but normal amounts of urinary calcium and oxalate. Compared with patients with pure uric acid stones, they generally have a higher urinary pH (about 5.5). The mechanism by which uric acid promotes calcium stone formation is unclear. Therapy generally consists of dietary purine restriction, increased fluid intake, and the addition of allopurinol (300 mg daily) if necessary.

If moderation of dietary protein is not successful in patients with hypocitraturia, oral potassium citrate is given (10 to 40 mEq/day). Serum levels of potassium and bicarbonate must be closely monitored, especially in patients with chronic kidney disease.

Uric Acid Stones

Uric acid stones are radiolucent and are thus most often visualized with CT. Therapy for patients with uric acid stones begins with nonspecific measures such as increasing fluid intake, a low purine diet, and lowering animal protein intake to increase urinary pH. Ideally, the urinary pH should be elevated to approximately 6.5 to 7.0, a level that not only prevents new stone formation but also can dissolve existing uric acid stones without promoting calcium phosphate deposition. Potassium citrate (10 to 40 mEq/day) may be required to raise the urinary pH sufficiently. If all else fails, the carbonic anhydrase inhibitor acetazolamide (250 to 500 mg/day) may be initiated to raise urine pH. Because concomitant hyperuricemia may be present, allopurinol (100 to 300 mg daily) may be indicated to lower the serum uric acid level.

Struvite Stones

Struvite stones rapidly grow to a large size and may promptly recur if not completely removed. Therapy requires complete surgical stone removal coupled with appropriate long-term antibiotics (Chapter 263), selected on the basis of cultures of stone fragments retrieved from surgery. Antibiotics should be continued at full doses until the urine is sterile and then continued at a lower dose. Monthly surveillance cultures should be performed until the urine remains sterile for 3 consecutive months. Antibiotics can then be discontinued with monthly surveillance urine cultures for another year.

Cystine Stones

Cystine kidney stones, which usually develop by the second or third decade of life, are radiopaque and may appear as staghorn calculi or multiple stones. The disease should be suspected in any patient with an early onset of stones, frequently recurrent nephrolithiasis, and a family history of the disease. Although the presence of the classic hexagonal cystine crystals in the urine (see Fig. 100-9 in Chapter 100) may suggest the diagnosis, anyone suspected of the disorder should have a quantitative cystine measurement on a 24-hour urine sample.[16]

The goal of treatment is to lower the urinary cystine concentration below the limits of solubility.[17] Patients are advised to drink sufficient quantities of water to maintain excreted cystine in solution. Patients should moderate intake of sodium and animal protein foods, which contain large amounts of methionine, which is a precursor of cystine. Because cystine is more soluble at a higher pH, urinary alkalinization with potassium citrate (10 to 40 mEq/day) can be used to maintain a urinary pH $\geq$ 7.0. Chelating agents reduce the free cystine concentration by forming more soluble compounds and should be prescribed by a specialist owing to their high incidence of side effects.

PROGNOSIS

The recurrence rate of calcium oxalate nephrolithiasis is about 25% at 3 to 5 years and about 50% at 5 to 10 years, and the rate is higher for cystine, uric acid, and struvite stones.[18] For stones that have not yet caused symptoms, the risk of developing symptoms varies widely among studies, but the size of the stone is not predictive of future symptomatic nephrolithiasis.[19] Patients with kidney stones often have an increase in aortic calcification and a decrease in bone mineral density, thereby supporting the concept that there is dysregulation in calcium homeostasis in patients who form calcium-containing stones. Patients with nephrolithiasis have a higher risk of losing kidney function[20] and also have an increased risk for coronary heart disease and stroke.

GENERAL REFERENCES

For the General References and other additional features, please visit Elsevier eBooks+ at https://ebooks.health.elsevier.com.

Grade A References

A1. Wang RC, Fahimi J, Dillon D, et al. Effect of an ultrasound-first clinical decision tool in emergency department patients with suspected nephrolithiasis: a randomized trial. *Am J Emerg Med.* 2022;60:164-170.
A2. Pathan SA, Mitra B, Straney LD, et al. Delivering safe and effective analgesia for management of renal colic in the emergency department: a double-blind, multigroup, randomised controlled trial. *Lancet.* 2016;387:1999-2007.
A3. Pathan SA, Mitra B, Cameron PA. A systematic review and meta-analysis comparing the efficacy of nonsteroidal anti-inflammatory drugs, opioids, and paracetamol in the treatment of acute renal colic. *Eur Urol.* 2018;73:583-595.
A4. Hollingsworth JM, Canales BK, Rogers MA, et al. Alpha blockers for treatment of ureteric stones: systematic review and meta-analysis. *BMJ.* 2016;355:1-11.
A5. Campschroer T, Zhu X, Vernooij RW, et al. Alpha-blockers as medical expulsive therapy for ureteral stones. *Cochrane Database Syst Rev.* 2018;4:CD008509.
A6. Liu XJ, Wen JG, Wan YD, et al. Role of silodosin as medical expulsive therapy in ureteral calculi: a meta-analysis of randomized controlled trials. *Urolithiasis.* 2018;46:212-218.
A7. Sorensen MD, Harper JD, Borofsky MS, et al. Removal of small, asymptomatic kidney stones and incidence of relapse. *N Engl J Med.* 2022;387:506-513.
A8. Tsai SH, Chung HJ, Tseng PT, et al. Comparison of the efficacy and safety of shockwave lithotripsy, retrograde intrarenal surgery, percutaneous nephrolithotomy, and minimally invasive percutaneous nephrolithotomy for lower-pole renal stones: a systematic review and network meta-analysis. *Medicine (Baltimore).* 2020;99:e19403.
A9. Bao Y, Tu X, Wei Q. Water for preventing urinary stones. *Cochrane Database Syst Rev.* 2020;2:CD004292.
A10. Wang Z, Zhang Y, Wei W. Effect of dietary treatment and fluid intake on the prevention of recurrent calcium stones and changes in urine composition: a meta-analysis and systematic review. *PLoS One.* 2021;16:e0250257.
A11. Li DF, Gao YL, Liu HC, et al. Use of thiazide diuretics for the prevention of recurrent kidney calculi: a systematic review and meta-analysis. *J Transl Med.* 2020;18:106.
A12. Dhayat NA, Bonny O, Roth B, et al. Hydrochlorothiazide and prevention of kidney-stone recurrence. *N Engl J Med.* 2023;388:781-791.
A13. Phillips R, Hanchanale VS, Myatt A, et al. Citrate salts for preventing and treating calcium containing kidney stones in adults. *Cochrane Database Syst Rev.* 2015;10:CD010057.
A14. Balasubramanian P, Wanner C, Ferreira JP, et al. Empagliflozin and decreased risk of nephrolithiasis: a potential new role for SGLT2 inhibition? *J Clin Endocrinol Metab.* 2022;107:e3003-e3007.
A15. Garrelfs SF, Frishberg Y, Hulton SA, et al. Lumasiran, an RNAi therapeutic for primary hyperoxaluria type 1. *N Engl J Med.* 2021;384:1216-1226.

112 CYSTIC KIDNEY DISEASES

M. AMIN ARNAOUT

DEFINITION AND EPIDEMIOLOGY

The term *cystic kidney diseases* refers to a heterogeneous group of hereditary and acquired disorders characterized by the presence of unilateral or bilateral renal cysts.[1] When acquired singly or in small numbers and in the absence of any other pathology, renal cysts are termed *simple cysts*, which are present in approximately 50% of individuals older than 40 years, are usually not loculated, and tend to bulge out from the renal surface (Fig. 112-1). The polycystic kidney diseases (PKDs), by comparison, constitute a clinically important group of genetically mediated disorders characterized by prominent, expanding, typically bilateral renal cysts. PKDs are classified as dominant, recessive, or X-linked, based on their pattern of inheritance. Autosomal dominant PKD, with a prevalence rate between 1 in 400 and 1 in 2000,[2] is among the most common monogenic diseases in humans and accounts for about 8 to 10% of all end-stage renal disease in the United States. Autosomal dominant PKD develops in an age-dependent manner and affects mainly adults. Autosomal recessive PKD, by contrast, is a relatively rare childhood disorder that appears in 1 in every 6000 to 50,000 live births. Renal cysts are also seen in several other rare hereditary kidney diseases and in several syndromic PKDs (Table 112-1). Collectively, the hereditary PKDs generally affect both sexes and all races equally and cost more than $1 billion annually to manage in the United States alone. *Acquired cystic kidney disease* refers to the multiple bilateral renal cysts that occur in 90% of patients who have received renal replacement therapy for 8 years or longer. Acquired cystic kidney disease is associated with increased rates of renal cell carcinoma.

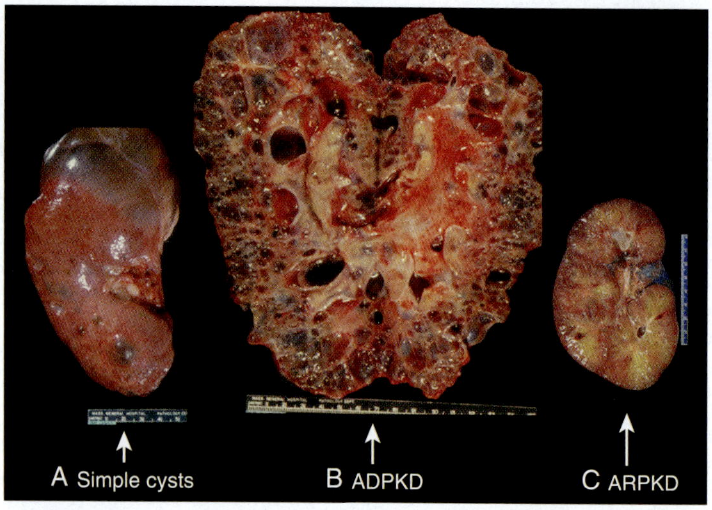

FIGURE 112-1. **Gross pathology of selected cystic kidney diseases. A, Photograph of a kidney with multiple simple cysts. The cysts bulge out from the surface of a normal-sized kidney. B, Sagittal cross section of a kidney from an adult with autosomal dominant polycystic kidney disease (ADPKD). Multiple macroscopic cysts have resulted in an enlarged but still reniform kidney (note the evidence of prior hemorrhage within some of the cysts). (Courtesy Dr. Robert Colvin, Massachusetts General Hospital.) C, Sagittal cross section of a kidney segment from a patient with autosomal recessive polycystic kidney disease (ARPKD). It shows multiple, small, slit-like radially oriented cysts (ranging from 0.2 cm up to 1.8 cm in greatest dimension) that replace the entire cortex and medulla and are arranged perpendicular to the external surface. Patchy foci of hemorrhage are also present. (Courtesy Dr. Alyaa Al-Ibraheemi, Boston Children's Hospital.)**

AUTOSOMAL DOMINANT POLYCYSTIC KIDNEY DISEASE

PATHOBIOLOGY

Autosomal dominant PKD is a systemic disorder characterized by cyst formation in multiple organs, including the kidneys, other ductal organs, and the cardiovascular system. Renal cysts originate as outpouchings of tubules and may arise from any portion of the nephron, with up to 1% of nephrons involved. The outpouchings expand and eventually separate from the parent tubules, yielding cysts (Fig. 112-2). Cyst growth is caused by proliferation of the cyst lining cells and by abnormal fluid accumulation that results when chloride-driven fluid secretion outpaces absorption. Cyst expansion and fibrosis (induced by cystic epithelium-derived chemokines, cytokines, and growth factors that attract macrophages and fibroblasts) cause compression and obstruction of noncystic normal tubules, thereby resulting in upstream tubular dilation. The kidneys become massively enlarged, and kidney function progressively declines.

Genetics

Heterogeneous mutations in *PKD1* and *PKD2* cause ADPKD and account for approximately 80% and 15% of the cases, respectively. Mutations in *GANAB*, *DNAJB11*,[3] and *ALG9*, which code for endoplasmic reticulum enzymes involved in the protein biosynthetic pathway, account for fewer than 1% of cases. Carriers of loss-of-function mutations in *GANAB*, which encodes GIIα, have mild autosomal dominant PKD and variable degrees of polycystic liver disease. Carriers of inactivating mutations in *DNAJB11*, which encodes the chaperon protein ERdj3, have a phenotypic hybrid of autosomal dominant PKD and autosomal dominant tubulointerstitial kidney disease (TKD), characterized

TABLE 112-1 COMPARISON OF CLINICAL FEATURES OF CYSTIC KIDNEY DISEASES

DISEASE	INHERITANCE	FREQUENCY	GENE PRODUCT	AGE OF ONSET	CYST ORIGIN	RENOMEGALY	CAUSE OF ESRD	OTHER MANIFESTATIONS
Simple cysts	No	50% in persons age 40 yr and older	None*	Adulthood	Anywhere (usually cortical)	No	No	None
ACKD	No	90% of ESRD patients at 8 yr	None*	Years after onset of ESRD	Proximal and distal tubules	Rarely	No	None
ADPKD	AD	1 : 400-1000	Polycystin-1(PC1); Polycystin-2 (PC2); GIIα; ERdj3; ALG9	20s and 30s	Anywhere (including Bowman capsule)	Yes No (for ERdi3, ALG9)	Yes (for PC1, PC2, or ERdj3) No (for GIIα or ALG9)	Primarily in PKD1/PKD2-disease: liver cysts, cerebral aneurysms, hypertension, mitral valve prolapse, kidney stones, urinary tract infections
ARPKD	AR	1 : 10,000-40,000	Fibrocystin/polyductin; DZIP1L	First year of life	Distal nephron, collecting duct	Yes	Yes	Hepatic fibrosis Hypertension Pulmonary hypoplasia
NPH	AR	1 : 80,000	Nephrocystins (NPH1–20) MAPKBP1	Childhood or adolescence	Loop of Henle, distal convoluted tubule	No	Yes	Retinal degeneration Neurologic, skeletal, hepatic, and cardiac malformations
ADTKD-UMOD	AD	Rare	Uromodulin	Adolescence	Cortico-medullary	No	Yes	Gout
ADTKD-MUC1	AD	Rare	Mucin-1	Adolescence	Cortico-medullary	No	Yes	Gout (less prevalent and later onset)
ADTKD-REN	AD	Rare	Renin	Childhood	Cortico-medullary	No	Yes	Anemia Early-onset gout Hyperkalemia Mild hypotension
ADTKD-SEC61A1	AD	Rare	α1 subunit of Sec61 translocon	Childhood	Glomerular	No	Yes	Anemia Recurrent infections Early-onset gout Developmental defects Cognitive impairment
ADTKD-HNF1B	AD; spontaneous	Rare	HNF1β	Childhood or adulthood	Cortico-medullary	Rarely	Variable	Early-onset diabetes and pancreatic hypoplasia Hypomagnesemia Hyperthyroidism Liver function abnormalities Gout Renal and urogenital anomalies Intellectual disability Risk of renal cell carcinoma
MSK	No; AD	1 : 5000-20,000	None*	Adulthood	Medullary collecting duct	No	No	Kidney stones
Bardet-Biedl syndrome	AR	1 : 65,000-160,000	BBS 1-21	Childhood	Renal calyces	Rarely	Yes	Syndactyly and polydactyly Obesity Retinal dystrophy Male hypogenitalism Hypertension Intellectual disability
Oral-facial-digital syndrome-1	XD	1 : 250,000	OFD1 protein	Childhood or adulthood	Renal glomeruli	Rarely	Yes	Malformation of the face, oral cavity, and digits Liver cysts Intellectual disability
HIPKD	AR	Rare	Phosphomannomutase 2	Childhood	Renal glomeruli	Yes	Yes	Hypoglycemic seizures Occasional liver cysts ARPKD-like phenotype
Tuberous sclerosis	AD	1 : 10,000	Hamartin (TSC1), tuberin (TSC2)	Childhood	Loop of Henle, distal convoluted tubule	Rarely	Rarely	Renal cell carcinoma Tubers Seizures Angiomyolipomas Hypertension
VHL syndrome	AD	1 : 40,000	VHL protein	20s	Cortical nephrons	Rarely	Rarely	Retinal angioma CNS hemangioblastoma Renal cell carcinoma Pheochromocytoma

*No known genetic susceptibility.

ACKD = acquired cystic kidney disease; AD = autosomal dominant; ADPKD = autosomal dominant polycystic kidney disease; ADTKD = autosomal dominant tubulointerstitial kidney disease; ALG9 = α-1,2-mannosyltransferase; AR = autosomal recessive; ARPKD = autosomal recessive polycystic kidney disease; CNS = central nervous system; DZIP1L = DAZ interacting protein 1-like; ERdj3 = ER DnaJ homologue glycoprotein encoded by DnaJ homolog subfamily B member 11; ESRD = end-stage renal disease; GIIα = glucosidase II alpha subunit; HIPKD = PKD with hyperinsulinemic hypoglycemia; HNF1β = hepatocyte nuclear factor 1 β; MSK = medullary sponge kidney; MUC1 = mucin-1; NPH = nephronophthisis; REN = renin; UMOD = uromodulin; VHL = von Hippel-Lindau; XD = X-linked dominant.

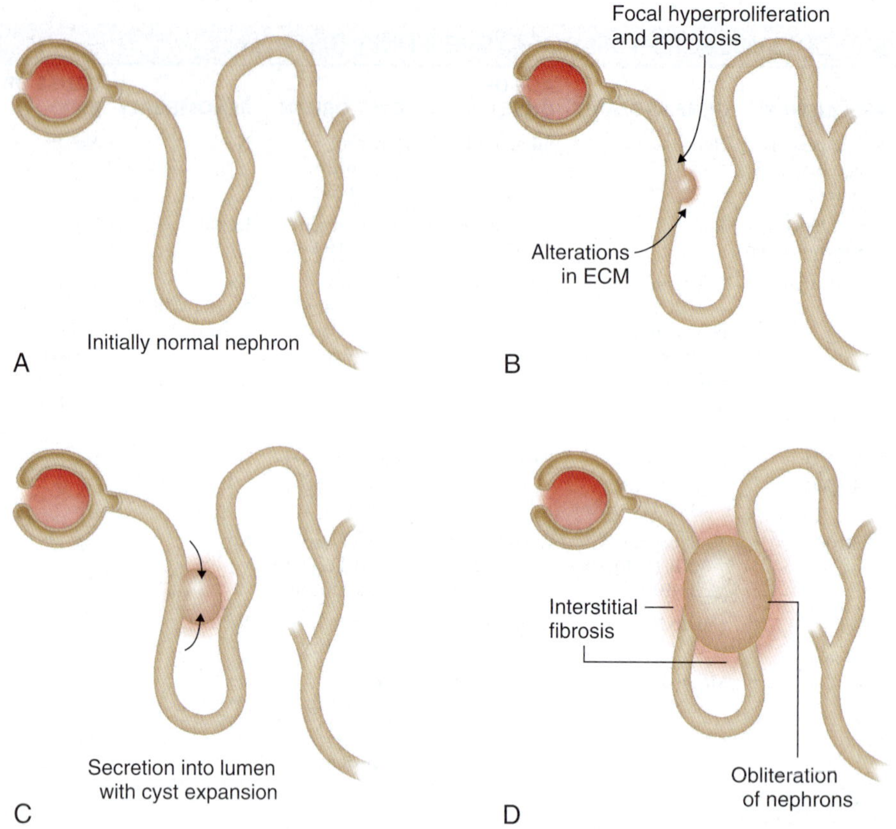

FIGURE 112-2. A to D, Steps involved in cyst formation in autosomal dominant polycystic kidney disease. Note that this process occurs hundreds or thousands of times during the natural history of the disease. ECM = extracellular matrix.

by normal-sized cystic kidneys, liver cysts, and progressive interstitial fibrosi that lead to late-onset end-stage renal disease and is reminiscent of autosomal dominant TKD-UMOD (defective proteostasis caused by *DNAJB11* variants might affect uromodulin trafficking as well). Carriers of inactivating mutations in *ALG9*, which encodes alpha-1,2-mannosyltransferase, develop both kidney and liver cysts, but they have milder disease than typical autosomal dominant PKD. In *GANAB-*, *DNAJB11-* and *ALG9*-associated ADPKD, cystogenesis appears to be driven by variable defects in the folding and maturation of PC1. In a minority of autosomal dominant PKD cases, no demonstrable mutations are found in these genes, thereby suggesting that additional genes may be involved.[4]

PKD1 is 54 kb long and is located on chromosome 16p13.3, adjacent to the tuberous sclerosis 2 (*TSC2*) gene. *PKD1* has 46 exons, generates a 14-kb transcript, and encodes a 4302-residue protein called polycystin-1 (PC1), the first described member of an expanding polycystin protein family. The 5′ region of human *PKD1* (to exon 33) is replicated on the same chromosome, resulting in approximately six copies of *PKD1*-like pseudogenes, which must be distinguished from the *PKD1* gene in direct mutational analysis. Most mutations in *PKD1* are inactivating truncation mutations or affect protein biogenesis, trafficking, or stability. To date, over 2300 mutations have been identified throughout the gene (http://pkdb.mayo.edu/) but especially in the 3′ half. Loss of function mutations and mutations in the 5′ half of the gene are associated with more severe disease, with only about 20% of patients retaining adequate renal function at 60 years of age (compared with about 40% of those with 3′ mutations).

The 68-kb *PKD2* gene is located on chromosome 4q13-23, transcribes 15 exons, and generates a 5-kb transcript, which encodes a protein of 968 residues called polycystin-2 (PC2). To date, 278 heterogeneous mutations in *PKD2* have been identified. The greater number of cysts that occur at an early age in *PKD1* compared with *PKD2* disease is likely a result of a higher frequency of mutations in the longer *PKD1* coding region and the presence of six *PKD1*-like pseudogenes that may be involved in recombination-based gene conversion and rearrangements.

Because renal cysts develop from approximately 1% of nephrons, somatic inactivation of the normal *PKD1* or *PKD2* allele (somatic second hit model) has been proposed as the main mechanism of cyst initiation. Alternatively, the *PKD1* or *PKD2* haploinsufficiency state may produce wide stochastic fluctuations in levels of the normal gene product and may reduce it to below a critical disease-causing threshold in the absence of a somatic second hit (haploinsufficiency model). The genomic instability associated with the *PKD1* or *PKD2* haploid state may increase the likelihood of somatic second hits, which contribute to disease progression by providing cysts with a growth or survival advantage.

There are wide variations in the onset and severity of autosomal dominant PKD even among affected members of the same family. This variability could arise from variable frequency and timing of the somatic inactivation of the respective normal allele. Variability in disease onset and severity can also result from bilineal inheritance of *PKD1* and *PKD2* mutant alleles or by inheritance of hypomorphic or incompletely penetrant variants of either gene. Mosaicism in a parent in whom a mutation has arisen de novo could result in one sibling having the disease while another is disease free despite sharing the identical inherited haplotype at the *PKD* locus. Digenic inheritance of mutant *PKD1, PKHD1, TSC2,* or *HNF1B* alleles can result in ADPKD in infancy. Other modifier loci beyond the known disease genes as well as nongenetic risk factors (e.g., smoking, caffeine, acute kidney injury, and male sex hormones) may also modulate the formation of renal cysts.

Gene Products

PKD1 encodes PC1, which consists of a large 11-pass receptor-like glycoprotein with a relatively short cytoplasmic carboxyl terminus (E-Fig. 112-1). The PC1 ectodomain contains multiple functional motifs, which are also present in cell adhesion receptors, thereby suggesting a role in cell-cell or cell-matrix interactions or both. PC2, which is encoded by *PKD2*, is a 6-pass atypical transient receptor potential-type channel with cytoplasmic amino- and carboxy-termini. Its six-transmembrane segment exhibits homology to the carboxyl terminal six-transmembrane segment of PC1. PC1 binding to PC2 and the cleavage of PC1 at the G protein–coupled receptor proteolytic site (resulting in N-terminal and C-terminal fragments that remain tethered) are necessary for their normal folding and export from the endoplasmic reticulum to the Golgi apparatus and subsequently to the surface of the cell. Emerging evidence suggests that the primary function of the PC1/PC2 complex is in primary cilia that are ubiquitously expressed on cell surfaces. The PC1/PC2 complex transitions from the Golgi apparatus via polycystin-bearing vesicles to the transition fibers and then undergoes facilitated trafficking to enter the cilium.[5]

PC1 and PC2 are widely expressed with overlapping non-identical distributions in tissues. PC1 expression is highest during kidney development and progressively declines thereafter, becoming mainly limited to the collecting duct in the normal adult kidney, although it can be upregulated in response to renal injury. By comparison, renal expression of PC2 is maintained throughout development and predominates in the medullary thick ascending limb and distal cortical tubules in the normal adult kidney. Disruption of the PC1/PC2 complex in primary cilia appears to be critical to the genesis of the PKD phenotype, but the precise function the PC1/PC2 complex plays in primary cilia remains obscure.

Experimental studies have suggested that developing renal tubules with high proliferative indices are more sensitive to the reduction in PC1 or PC2 levels, with disease severity radically altered depending on the time of gene inactivation. Maintenance of higher proliferative indices in the distal nephron epithelium relative to that in the proximal nephron may explain the predominance of cysts in the distal nephron in adult human autosomal dominant PKD.

CLINICAL MANIFESTATIONS

Autosomal dominant PKD has a highly variable presentation, even within families. The clinical features of *PKD2*-associated autosomal dominant PKD are indistinguishable from those of *PKD1*-associated disease. However, *PKD2* disease is milder, with an older average age of onset—about 75 years versus 55 years for *PKD1*-associated disease—owing to the development of fewer cysts at an early age rather than to a slower cyst growth rate.

Despite an estimated 100% penetrance by age 90 years, only half the individuals with heterozygous mutations in *PKD1* or *PKD2* are ever diagnosed clinically with autosomal dominant PKD. Of these, the majority present in the third or fourth decade of life with symptoms referable to renal cystic disease. However, autosomal dominant PKD can develop at any age, including infancy, and it can have a nonrenal presentation. Renomegaly may predominate the clinical picture, with abdominal distention, discomfort, or pain; however, renomegaly also can be discovered incidentally on physical examination or after radiographic studies of the abdomen.

Nocturia, one of the earliest signs of abnormal renal function in autosomal dominant PKD, reflects the early impairment in the ability to concentrate urine owing to disruption of renal architecture by the cysts. Hematuria is typical, but proteinuria is less prominent than in many other renal diseases. Cyst hemorrhage and sometimes rupture, which can occur spontaneously or after trauma, present as sharp pain and hematuria. Recurrent cyst infection (Chapter 263), usually by common urinary tract-infecting organisms, is characterized by flank or abdominal pain, fever, rigors, leukocytosis, and occasionally sepsis. Kidney stones (Chapter 111) occur in 20 to 36% of patients, with uric acid stones slightly more common than calcium oxalate stones; predisposing factors include urinary stasis, defective trapping of urea in the medulla, low urine pH, hypocitraturia, hyperoxaluria, hypercalciuria, and hypomagnesuria. Anemia features less prominently than in other renal diseases, probably because of the relatively well-preserved secretion of erythropoietin.

Cardiovascular disease, which is common in autosomal dominant PKD, manifests as biventricular diastolic dysfunction even in young patients with normal blood pressure and renal function, thoracic and abdominal aortic aneurysms, and cervicocephalic and coronary aneurysms. Arterial hypertension is present in approximately 70% of cases before renal dysfunction is detected. Development of hypertension at a young age is associated with a four-fold increased risk of end-stage renal disease and increased cardiovascular morbidity. The risk for preeclampsia is also higher than in the general population.

Intracranial aneurysm occurs in 4 to 8% of asymptomatic autosomal dominant PKD patients, but the incidence is higher in patients with a family history of nonruptured (10% risk) or ruptured intracranial aneurysm (20% risk; Chapter 377). Autosomal dominant PKD-associated aneurysms tend to rupture at a smaller size and in younger individuals—on average, 10 years younger than among the general population. Although usually clinically silent, intact cerebral aneurysms can present with focal neurologic symptoms and headaches. By contrast, aneurysms that rupture lead to subarachnoid hemorrhage (Chapter 377) and have dramatic presentations that include severe headaches, seizures, altered sensorium, and death. Aortic and coronary artery aneurysms are also more prevalent in patients with autosomal dominant PKD, and the frequency of aortic insufficiency is increased.

Although almost never severe enough to cause end-stage liver disease, age-dependent hepatic cysts occur in 30 to 80% of patients with autosomal dominant PKD and can lead to signs and symptoms of mass effect, infection, hemorrhage, and rupture.[6] Estrogen intake and multiparity in women are risk factors for developing larger and more symptomatic liver cysts. The cysts that occasionally form in other organs, such as the pancreas, spleen, brain, ovaries, epididymis, and prostate, are usually asymptomatic. Sperm abnormalities and defective motility may occur but rarely cause male infertility. Bronchiectasis (Chapter 78) is three-fold more common, inguinal hernias may be more prevalent, and colonic diverticulosis and diverticulitis are more common in end-stage renal disease patients with autosomal dominant PKD.

DIAGNOSIS

Renomegaly, typically presenting in the third or fourth decade of life with a positive family history and common extrarenal manifestations, such as hypertension, are useful findings in making a presumptive diagnosis of autosomal dominant PKD. In these cases, renal ultrasonography is frequently diagnostic. Because only about 75% of individuals give a family history of autosomal dominant PKD, ultrasound screening of asymptomatic parents or grandparents may be required to uncover diagnostically relevant silent autosomal dominant PKD.[7]

A diagnosis of autosomal dominant PKD can be made in an asymptomatic individual by ultrasonography (Fig. 112-3A). To account for the common age-dependent appearance of simple cysts, autosomal dominant PKD is diagnosed if at least three renal cysts (distributed in one or both kidneys) are present in individuals 15 to 29 years old (sensitivity, 0.82; specificity, 1.0) or 30 to 39 years old (sensitivity, 0.96; specificity, 1.0), if at least two renal cysts are present in each kidney in individuals 40 to 59 years old (sensitivity, 1.0; specificity, 0.99), or if at least four renal cysts are detected in each kidney in individuals 60 years of age or older (sensitivity, 1.0; specificity, 1.0). Fewer than two renal cysts in an individual from an autosomal dominant PKD family with an unknown genotype age 40 years or older or the absence of renal cysts in such an individual age 30 to 39 years is sufficient to exclude the disease, with negative predictive values of 100% and 99.3%, respectively. A negative ultrasound result is less accurate in excluding disease in individuals younger than 30

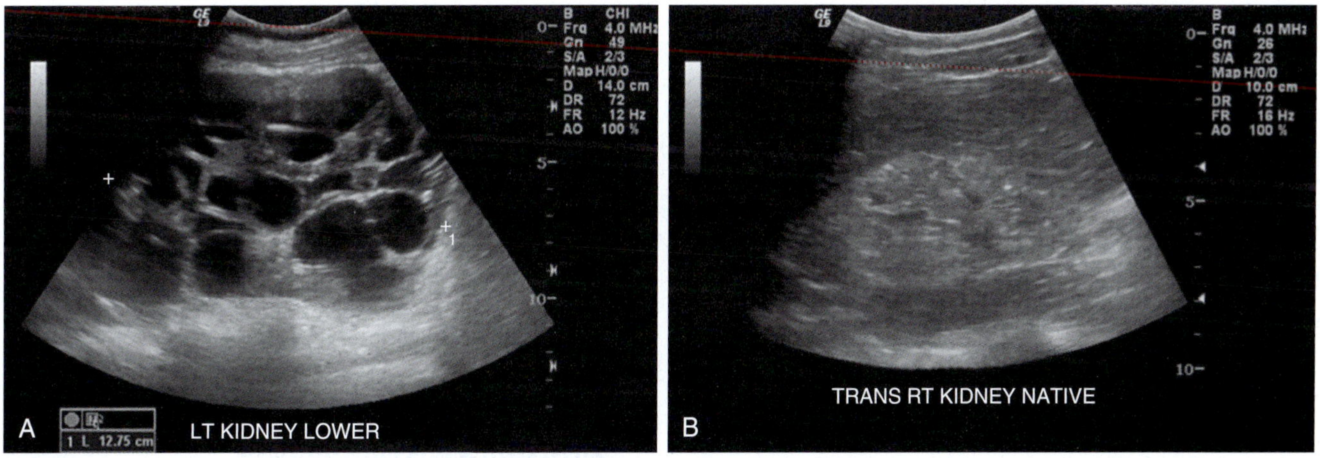

FIGURE 112-3. A, Ultrasound image of a kidney from a patient with autosomal dominant polycystic kidney disease. B, Ultrasound image of a kidney from a patient with autosomal recessive polycystic kidney disease. (Courtesy Dr. Javier M. Romero and Jennifer A. McDowell, Massachusetts General Hospital.)

years, so computed tomography (CT) or magnetic resonance imaging (MRI) is recommended. When a young relative is being considered as a potential kidney donor to a family member with end-stage autosomal dominant PKD, contrast-enhanced, three-dimensional CT or magnetic resonance angiography is required because these tests can detect 3-mm cysts compared with ultrasonography's ability to detect 10-mm cysts.

Cerebral aneurysms are increasingly being detected with MRI in autosomal dominant PKD patients. Four-vessel cerebral angiography remains the gold standard and is often used for surgical planning.

DNA-based diagnosis of autosomal dominant PKD by means of direct sequencing is commercially available and detects mutations in more than 90% of affected individuals. Whole-genome sequencing may have a much higher sensitivity and specificity for the diagnosis because it is better at distinguishing the *PKD1* gene from six similar pseudogenes.[8] It also can detect mosaicism, which accounts for about 10% of cases otherwise missed by genetic testing.[9] Testing is recommended when imaging study results are equivocal, in a young transplant donor from an autosomal dominant PKD family when imaging study results are negative, or to facilitate preimplantation genetic diagnosis.[10]

Monitoring Progressive Renal Disease

Despite ongoing renal cyst expansion, the glomerular filtration rate (GFR) and the serum creatinine level are generally maintained within the normal range in autosomal dominant PKD patients until the fourth to sixth decade of life. These markers are therefore insensitive for monitoring disease progression, especially in young patients. Reduced renal blood flow is the most sensitive prognostic indicator of renal progression. Estimating height-adjusted total kidney volume from measurements of kidney length, width, and thickness using MRI, CT, or ultrasonography can reliably monitor disease progression in the early stages of autosomal dominant PKD when the GFR is still in the normal range, and each 100-mL increment of height-adjusted total kidney volume increases the odds of reaching stage 3 chronic kidney disease by about 1.5-fold. Although gadolinium-enhanced MRI provides excellent detail of kidney structures, MRI without gadolinium is recommended to monitor kidney volume, especially in autosomal dominant PKD patients with a reduced GFR, because of concern about nephrogenic systemic fibrosis (Chapter 246) and further impairment of renal function associated with its use. Height-adjusted total kidney volume progressively increases in most patients who have autosomal dominant PKD but at widely differing rates, ranging from less than 1% to more than 10% annually. Renal function declines as the kidneys enlarge,[11] and patients who have rapidly progressive autosomal dominant PKD are most likely to benefit from treatment.[12]

PREVENTION AND TREATMENT

Management strategies are aimed at monitoring for complications of autosomal dominant PKD and treating them, as well as providing genetic counseling.[13] Frequent monitoring and effective treatment of hypertension (Chapter 64; see Tables 64-7 and 64-9) are essential because hypertensive patients have a greater annual increase in kidney volume, as well as a higher prevalence of left ventricular hypertrophy, ischemic heart disease, and stroke, compared with normotensive patients. The goals of blood pressure control are the same as for other patients with renal disease, including the attainment of a symptom-free blood pressure of 120/80 mm Hg or less. Angiotensin-converting enzyme inhibitors or angiotensin receptor blockers are the first-line antihypertensive drugs in autosomal dominant PKD. Hypertensive autosomal dominant PKD patients who are young (15 to 49 years), have stage 1 or 2 cystic kidney disease, and do not have diabetes mellitus or significant cardiovascular comorbidities may benefit from blood pressures of 95/60 to 110/75 mm Hg, a level associated with a slower increase in total kidney volume, a greater decline in left-ventricular-mass index, and a greater reduction in urinary albumin excretion, but not a delay in the reduction in the glomerular filtration rate. Dietary salt restriction also may be beneficial in the management of autosomal dominant PKD.

Oral tolvaptan (45 to 90 mg in the morning and 15 to 30 mg in the afternoon as tolerated) slows the increase in total kidney volume and the decline in kidney function in patients with normal creatinine clearance and in patients with moderate-to-advanced kidney disease.[A1,14,15] It can also reduce kidney pain.[A2] The small but significant clinical effect may be the result of reduced cell proliferation, direct intrarenal hemodynamic effects, or both. Tolvaptan induces a four-fold increased risk of hepatocellular injury, so liver function testing before initiation and at specific intervals (at 2 and 4 weeks, then monthly for 18 months, then every 3 months thereafter) is required in all patients with autosomal dominant PKD.[16] Overall, nearly 25% of patients do not tolerate tolvaptan, and it is not routinely used in children.

Treatment of urinary tract infection (Chapter 263) and prevention of nephrolithiasis (Chapter 111) are the same as in the general population and include standard antimicrobial therapy and increased fluid intake, respectively. Renal and hepatic cyst infections are optimally treated with lipophilic antibiotics that possess cyst-penetrating capabilities, including ciprofloxacin, trimethoprim, clindamycin, and vancomycin. Blood or urine cultures and sensitivities are used to guide the choice of antibiotic therapy.

Cyst hemorrhage and rupture, with resultant pain and hematuria, are usually managed conservatively with rest and analgesics; nonsteroidal anti-inflammatory drugs (NSAIDs) are avoided owing to their antiplatelet action and potential renal toxicity. Alternatives include acetaminophen 500 mg up to every 4 hours for mild to moderate pain, nonopiates such as tramadol 50 mg up to every 4 hours for moderate to severe pain, and the addition of an oral or transdermal opioid (see Table 26-6 in Chapter 26) as needed. Patients with enlarged kidneys should be advised to avoid playing contact sports, and those with massively enlarged kidneys should refrain from wearing belts and seatbelts. Some patients with unusually painful cysts respond to cyst fluid aspiration, cyst deroofing, or ethanol-induced sclerosis.

Nephrectomy is rarely indicated before the onset of end-stage renal disease. Renal replacement therapies, including renal transplantation (Chapter 117), are at least as effective as in other causes of end-stage renal disease.[17]

The massive cystic enlargement of the liver commonly seen by midlife in women with autosomal dominant PKD makes it prudent to avoid estrogen intake and repeated pregnancies. Partial hepatectomy has been successful in improving the quality of life in patients with massive liver enlargement, but liver transplantation is the only curative therapy.[18]

Magnetic resonance angiography screening is not routinely recommended for asymptomatic patients without a family history of cerebral aneurysm or subarachnoid hemorrhage, but it is recommended for patients with a positive personal or family history and for patients who experience a new onset of severe headache or central nervous system symptoms or signs. It also may be considered in those with high-risk occupations, such as airline pilots, and for patients with incapacitating anxiety. The risk of a patient with a positive family history developing a new aneurysm after an initially negative magnetic resonance angiography result is 2.6% at a mean follow-up period of 9.8 years, so rescreening every 5 to 10 years in such cases may be appropriate, especially in patients with early-onset hypertension or a history of heavy smoking. Asymptomatic patients with positive family history of cerebral aneurysms and positive magnetic resonance angiography results should be followed closely with a neurosurgeon and monitored by annual magnetic resonance angiography screening. The decision to perform surgical clipping or endovascular embolization should take into consideration the age of the patient, the size of the aneurysm and its location, and a previous history of cerebral bleeding (Chapter 377).

Patients should be advised that their children have a 50% probability of inheriting a disease-causing germline mutation. DNA-based diagnostics are most useful in identifying the germline mutation prenatally or preimplantation. As DNA-based diagnostics become more widely available and less expensive and as promising new treatment options are developed, genetic counseling will become an increasingly important component of prevention.

Experimental Therapies

Current therapeutic efforts are targeting increased cell proliferation of cystic epithelium and abnormal fluid secretion into cysts (E-Fig. 112-2).[19] The metabolically stable somatostatin analogue octreotide (long-acting release at a dose of 40 mg every 28 days)[20] can slow the expansion of renal cysts but does not slow the decline in renal function and also is associated with substantial side effects.[A3] Indirect inhibition of mTOR via activation of AMPK with metformin (E-Fig. 112-2) has shown promise in a phase II trial.[A4] Bosutinib, an oral dual Src/Bcr-Abl tyrosine kinase inhibitor, can reduce the rate of kidney enlargement but has not been shown to slow the decline in glomerular filtration.[A5] A trial evaluating the value of tesevatinib, which is a multi-kinase inhibitor, on the progression of height-adjusted total kidney volume in autosomal dominant PKD is ongoing.

PROGNOSIS

The rate of progression of renal disease is highest in men with poorly controlled hypertension, an early age at diagnosis, mutations (particularly truncations) in *PKD1*, and higher initial height-adjusted total kidney volume.[21] Higher salt intake but not higher protein intake is associated with more rapidly progressive disease.[22] Kidney cysts develop earlier in *PKD1* than in *PKD2* disease, but the rate of expansion is similar, indicating that the basic difference in phenotype is in cyst initiation, not expansion. Whereas the presence of one affected family member who developed end-stage renal disease by age 60 years is highly predictive of PKD1 disease (positive predictive value, 100%; sensitivity, 75%), the development of end-stage renal disease after age 70 years in a family member is highly predictive of PKD2 disease (positive predictive value, 95%; sensitivity, 75%). Approximately 5% of all autosomal dominant PKD patients with cerebral aneurysms die from aneurysmal rupture.

AUTOSOMAL RECESSIVE POLYCYSTIC KIDNEY DISEASE

DEFINITION AND EPIDEMIOLOGY

Autosomal recessive PKD is a multisystem childhood disorder characterized by severe and early PKD dominated by dilation of the kidney collecting ducts, systemic hypertension, biliary ductal plate dysgenesis in neonates, and portal tract fibrosis in older children.[23]

PATHOBIOLOGY

Autosomal recessive PKD is mainly caused by heterogeneous mutations in *PKHD1* (polycystic kidney and hepatic disease 1) and rarely by mutations in *DZIP1L*. Located on chromosome 6q21, *PKHD1* has 67 exons and spans a genomic region of approximately 470 kb, the longest open reading frame of which is 12,222 base pairs long. *PKHD1* encodes a unique type I membrane protein, fibrocystin/polyductin, comprising 4074 amino acids, with a large extracellular segment that contains multiple IPT/TIG (*Ig*-like, *P*lexins, *T*ranscription factors) domains, a PA14 domain, a PbH1 (*P*arallel β-*h*elix repeat) domain, 2 G8 domains, a cleavage site, and a short cytoplasmic carboxyl terminus that includes a cilia targeting signal. The precise physiologic function of fibrocystin/polyductin in collecting duct and biliary duct epithelium is not clear, but its domains are known to mediate cell motility and invasion (IPT domains), extracellular protein and carbohydrate binding, and catalytic processing (PA14, PbH1, and G8 domains). Alternatively spliced transcripts of *PKHD1* encode a membrane protein with variable extracellular domains, as well as forms lacking the transmembrane segment. Biallellic truncating mutations in *PKHD1* are associated with perinatal renal disease, whereas patients with biallelic missense mutations may present later because some functional protein is produced.

Fibrocystin is predominantly expressed in the cortical and medullary collecting ducts, the thick ascending limbs of Henle and bile ducts. It is also found to a lesser degree in the pancreas, liver, and lungs, which are also affected in autosomal recessive PKD. Fibrocystin interacts with PC2 within the PC1/PC2 complex, where loss of fibrocystin downregulates PC2. Fibrocystin–PC2 interactions may regulate function of the ciliary PC1/PC2 complex.

Located on chromosome 3q22, 1-q23 *DZIP1L* encodes DZIP1L, which is widely expressed and is localized primarily to the centrioles and distal end of basal bodies. The localization of PC1 and PC2 to the ciliary membrane is compromised in DZIP1L-mutant cells, thereby suggesting that DZIP1L is required for regulating the integrity of the transition zone.

CLINICAL MANIFESTATIONS

Although autosomal recessive PKD can present as renal cysts discovered radiographically either antenatally or during adulthood, it usually manifests as bilateral abdominal masses and renal insufficiency in infancy. It carries a 30% mortality rate owing to severe pulmonary hypoplasia; oligohydramnios, presumably linked to in utero renal disease, likely accounts for the pulmonary hypoplasia. Hypertension is almost universal, typically develops before renal impairment is apparent, and probably accelerates the decline in renal function. Findings related to renal tubular dysfunction may be present and include polyuria, enuresis, hyponatremia, and hyperchloremic metabolic acidosis. Cystic complications related to infection and rupture also occur, although hematuria is an infrequent finding.

Hepatic fibrosis, secondary to dilation of the intrahepatic and extrahepatic bile ducts, manifests as recurrent ascending cholangitis (Chapter 141) and portal hypertension with splenomegaly and esophageal varices. Pancreatic fibrosis is rarely a clinical concern.

DIAGNOSIS

The demonstration by abdominal ultrasonography (see Fig. 112-3B) or CT of symmetrically enlarged polycystic kidneys that retain their reniform shape (owing to uniform microcystic dilation of the distal tubules and collecting ducts) and hepatic fibrosis is sufficient to diagnose autosomal recessive PKD. In contrast to autosomal dominant PKD cysts, autosomal recessive PKD cysts tend to retain their connections with the originating nephron.

Aside from an occasional affected sibling, a family history is often not elicited. Distinguishing autosomal recessive PKD from autosomal dominant PKD, especially in patients presenting in childhood or adulthood, may require a liver biopsy to document otherwise undetectable hepatic fibrosis. Gene-based diagnostics in autosomal recessive PKD are helpful in making a firm diagnosis,[24] especially in patients with late-onset disease, and they are useful in preimplantation and prenatal diagnosis. Mutations in *DZIP1L* is considerably rarer than mutations in *PKHD1*, perhaps in part owing to the larger size of *PKHD1*.

TREATMENT AND PREVENTION

In the absence of specific therapy for autosomal recessive PKD, management goals focus on early detection and on treatment of the complications of hypertension, urinary tract or cyst infection, end-stage renal disease, and portal hypertension. Kidney transplantation may be necessary in late childhood in patients with autosomal recessive PKD who present with renal disease perinatally. Treatment of portal hypertension may require liver transplantation or portosystemic shunting (Chapter 140). Treatment of hypertension begins with ACE inhibitors and angiotensin receptor blockers (see Tables 64-7 and 64-9 in Chapter 64), which are generally effective. As in all children with end-stage renal disease, attention to nutrition and renal osteodystrophy is paramount (Chapter 116). With improving sensitivity of gene-based diagnostics, prenatal counseling will play a more active role in prevention.

PROGNOSIS

For patients with autosomal recessive PKD, the highest mortality rates occur during the first year of life. Males and females are equally affected. Approximately 50 to 80% of patients who survive this period live past 15 years of age. End-stage renal disease with macroscopic cysts, interstitial fibrosis, and shrunken kidneys can take up to 20 years to develop; but in rare instances, it never occurs.

NEPHRONOPHTHISIS

DEFINITION AND EPIDEMIOLOGY

Nephronophthisis is the most common genetic cause of end-stage renal disease in childhood and adolescence, during which it accounts for 5 to 15% of cases of end-stage renal disease. It is an autosomal recessive kidney disorder caused by mutations in a number of genes that encode nephronophthisis proteins (nephrocystins), which are expressed in the centrosome and basal body of primary cilia, with some also localizing to adherens junctions or focal adhesions in epithelia.[25] Homozygotic and compound heterozygotic mutations in at least 20 known genes (*NPH1* through *NPH20* and *MAPKBP1*) account for about 30% of cases. Infantile, juvenile, and adolescent variants have been described based on the median age of onset of ESRD. Infantile nephronophthisis is characterized by mutations in the *NPH2* gene. The juvenile form is the most common and is caused by mutations in *NPH1*. The adolescent form is caused by mutations in *NPH3*. Mutations in *MAPKBP1*, which encodes MAPKABP1, a microtubule-binding protein, are a rare cause of late-onset cilia-independent nephronophthisis.

Nephronophthisis is characterized pathologically by renal interstitial fibrosis, tubular atrophy with basement membrane thickening and disruption, and renal cysts and diverticula that are largely restricted to the loops of Henle and distal tubules at the corticomedullary junctions. Kidney size is generally normal or reduced, except in the rare infantile variant that leads to end-stage renal disease by 3 years of age. Expression of *NPH* genes at extrarenal sites accounts for the associated retinal, neural, liver, and skeletal abnormalities. Each of the *NPH* genes is associated with a somewhat different phenotype, although some share common phenotypes, explained by protein-protein interactions between two or more nephrocystins. Cerebello-ocular-renal syndromes associated with nephronophthisis can sometimes include early-onset retinitis pigmentosa when the syndrome is caused by mutations in *NPH5* and *NPH6*.

CLINICAL MANIFESTATIONS

Presenting symptoms include polyuria, growth failure, and anemia. Polyuria occurs early, owing to reduced urinary concentrating ability and to salt wasting. A decreased growth rate is related to chronic dehydration, and growth failure and anemia occur with the onset of end-stage renal disease. Blood pressure is normal, and edema is absent before the onset of renal failure. Hematuria and proteinuria are absent or minimal. Patients with mutations in specific *NPH* genes may also present with eye defects, oculomotor apraxia, congenital amaurosis, retinitis pigmentosa, neural anomalies, cerebellar ataxia, seizures, liver fibrosis, skeletal defects, scoliosis, cleft palate, and situs inversus.

DIAGNOSIS

The diagnosis relies on clinical suspicion of the disorder in a pediatric or adolescent patient who presents with end-stage renal disease and extrarenal manifestations such as abnormal eye movements, intellectual disability, and polydactyly. Differential diagnosis includes renal dysplasia, early-onset autosomal dominant PKD, urinary tract obstruction, autosomal dominant TKD, and autosomal recessive PKD. Abdominal ultrasonography, MRI (without gadolinium), electroretinography, and full neurologic and ophthalmologic evaluations should assess the patient's renal, liver, retinal, and neurologic status. Renal ultrasonography showing loss of corticomedullary differentiation, increased parenchymal echogenicity, and occasionally small medullary or corticomedullary cysts in normal-sized or moderately small kidneys is highly suggestive of juvenile nephronophthisis in a child with severe uremia. Genetic testing may be required for a conclusive diagnosis. A renal biopsy showing evidence of chronic tubulointerstitial nephritis may be necessary to confirm the diagnosis if genetic testing is not available.

TREATMENT AND PREVENTION

Treatment is largely supportive, focusing on the progressive renal failure and the need for dialysis and transplantation. Prenatal genetic testing in families with a genetic diagnosis of nephronophthisis is feasible. DNA-based diagnostics are most useful in identifying the germline mutation prenatally or preimplantation.

AUTOSOMAL DOMINANT TUBULOINTERSTITIAL KIDNEY DISEASE (MEDULLARY CYSTIC KIDNEY DISEASE)

Autosomal dominant tubulointerstitial kidney disease is a group of genetic disorders characterized by an autosomal dominant inheritance, medullary cysts, and slowly progressive loss of kidney function beginning in the teenage years.[26] It shares a number of histologic features with nephronophthisis, including tubular basement membrane disintegration, tubular cyst formation, and tubulointerstitial inflammation and fibrosis.

Mutations in one of five genes—*UMOD/MCKD2, MUC1/MCKD1, REN, SEC61A1* and *HNF1B*—cause autosomal dominant tubulointerstitial kidney disease. *UMOD* on chromosome 16p12 encodes an 85-kD nonciliary protein, uromodulin, which is expressed on the luminal side of renal epithelium in the thick ascending limb of Henle loop and early distal convoluted tubules. Uromodulin kidney disease (also known as familial juvenile hyperuricemic nephropathy type 1, uromodulin storage disease, and glomerulocystic kidney disease) is the most common subtype, accounting for the majority of cases. Recent data indicate that *UMOD* mutations in uromodulin are encountered in 2 to 3% adults with chronic kidney disease. The mutations impair trafficking of furosemide-sensitive Na-K-2Cl transporter to the apical membrane of the thick ascending limb, thereby causing mild sodium wasting and volume contraction, with a secondary increase in proximal tubule urate reabsorption and hyperuricemia. Intracellular accumulation of the mutant protein causes tubular cell death. Affected patients do not have an increased incidence of urinary tract infections or renal calculi.

MUC1 on chromosome 1q21 encodes mucin-1, a transmembrane protein expressed in the distal nephron, the gastrointestinal and respiratory tracts, and skin, with no known function. The autosomal dominant TKP-MUC1 phenotype, which is limited to the kidneys, accounts for approximately 30% of autosomal dominant tubulointerstitial kidney disease. Gout and hyperuricemia occur late, secondary to loss of kidney function.

Mutations in *REN*, which encodes renin on chromosome 1q32.1, are rarer causes of autosomal dominant tubulointerstitial kidney disease. The clinical and laboratory manifestations resemble other low renin states. Anemia, caused by decreased levels of angiotensin II (a positive regulator of erythropoiesis), precedes the development of chronic kidney disease. Hyperuricemia develops early, likely owing to relative hypotension and increased proximal absorption of uric acid. Accumulation of the abnormal renin leads to tubular cell death and chronic kidney disease.

HNF1B nephropathy results from mutations in the gene encoding the widely expressed transcription factor hepatocyte nuclear factor-1-beta. *HNF1B* is located on chromosome 17q12 and mediates the development of a variety of tissues, including the kidney, liver, pancreas, and genital tract. This cystic renal disease may be accompanied by variable renal and extra renal manifestations (see Table 112-1). Renal function may be normal or may decline to end-stage renal disease. Neither mutation type nor position correlates with severity of disease.

DIAGNOSIS

Corticomedullary cysts, which are present in most adult patients with autosomal dominant tubulointerstitial kidney disease, cannot always be recognized on ultrasonography or computed tomography because they tend to be very small. A presumptive diagnosis is based on a strong family history and a bland urinary sediment with minimal proteinuria. Mutational analysis is necessary to make a definitive diagnosis.

TREATMENT

Except for the treatment of hyperuricemia and gout, when present (Chapter 252), the management of pancreatic insufficiency (in autosomal dominant tubulointerstitial kidney disease—HNF1B) and of low blood pressure and hyperkalemia (in autosomal dominant tubulointerstitial kidney disease—REN) is similar to that of patients with nephronophthisis.

MEDULLARY SPONGE KIDNEY

Medullary sponge kidney, a rare disorder of unknown pathogenesis, is characterized by congenitally acquired inner medullary and papillary collecting duct dilations, hypercalciuria, and a mild defect in urinary concentration and acidification secondary to tubular dysfunction.[27] Medullary sponge kidney is usually nonhereditary, but autosomal dominant inheritance has been described in several families.

Patients present with microscopic or gross hematuria and recurrent kidney stones, usually by the second or third decade of life. Medullary sponge kidney also may be an incidental finding on an intravenous pyelogram that shows the characteristic pooling of contrast material within the cystic collecting ducts. Differential diagnosis includes other causes of medullary nephrocalcinosis such as hyperparathyroidism, renal tubular acidosis type I, hypervitaminosis D, milk-alkali syndrome, and sarcoidosis.

TREATMENT AND PROGNOSIS

Basic treatment is aimed at controlling stone formation by stabilizing urinary pH. End-stage renal disease is uncommon, and long-term prognosis is excellent.

OTHER INHERITED CYSTIC SYNDROMES

TUBEROUS SCLEROSIS AND VON HIPPEL-LINDAU SYNDROME

Autosomal dominant renal cyst formation is seen in tuberous sclerosis and von Hippel-Lindau syndrome (Chapter 385). In tuberous sclerosis, cyst formation is commonly associated with hypertension; this disorder can resemble autosomal dominant PKD and is associated with about a 5% incidence of renal cell carcinoma. In von Hippel-Lindau syndrome, cyst formation can also lead to features of autosomal dominant PKD; more importantly, the syndrome is associated with a 25% incidence of renal cell carcinoma.

TREATMENT

Treatment is discussed in Chapter 385.

RARE CHILDHOOD SYNDROMES

Bardet-Biedl syndrome is an autosomal recessive disorder characterized by vision loss, obesity, hypertension, delayed development of motor skills, behavioral problems, and dystrophy of the hands, kidneys, and male genitals. Mutations in at least 21 genes involved in maintenance and function of cilia have been identified. About 45% of cases result from mutations in *BBS1* or *BBS10*, but in about 25% of cases, the defective gene remains to be identified. Calyceal cysts and calyceal clubbing predominate the renal lesion and are best diagnosed by intravenous urography rather than ultrasonography. Renal impairment is frequent and is an important cause of death.

Oral-facial-digital syndrome is a rare neurodevelopmental ciliopathy characterized by malformations of the brain, face, oral cavity, and digits. It is inherited in an X-linked dominant pattern and is caused by defects in the *OFD1* gene, which encodes OFD1 protein expressed in the centrosome and basal body of primary cilia but has an undetermined function. Renal (primarily glomerular) cysts are found in as many as 50% of patients, all females; males carrying the mutation die in utero. End-stage renal disease has been reported in affected girls and women ranging in age from 11 to 72 years.

Polycystic kidney disease with hyperinsulinemic hypoglycemia, is caused by biallelic mutations in *PMM2*, which encodes phosphomannomutase 2, an isomerase involved in synthesis of dolichol-P-oligosaccharides. Hyperinsulinemic hypoglycemic polycystic kidney disease presents in early childhood with hypoglycemic seizures owing to altered insulin secretion, enlarged glomerulocystic kidneys and occasional liver cysts. The severity of cystic kidney disease is variable, with few patients progressing to end-stage renal disease.[28]

TREATMENT

Control of blood pressure (Chapter 64) is important. For hyperinsulinemic hypoglycemic polycystic kidney disease, chronic diazoxide therapy can treat the hypoglycemia. No specific treatments are currently available for these conditions, and the affected children should be managed at specialized centers.

ACQUIRED CYSTIC KIDNEY DISEASE

Acquired cystic kidney disease is largely confined to the end-stage renal disease population on dialysis (Chapter 117). Cysts arise from proximal and distal tubule dilations in small end-stage kidneys regardless of cause, mode of dialysis, or presence of a functioning kidney transplant. Identifiable risk factors include duration of end-stage renal disease, older age, male sex, Black race, and chronic hypokalemia.

CLINICAL MANIFESTATIONS AND DIAGNOSIS

Acquired cystic kidney disease is usually asymptomatic, but it occasionally leads to enlarged kidneys with associated abdominal discomfort and pain. Cyst hemorrhage, which is more common than cyst infection, presents with flank pain, anemia, or hematuria. The most significant complication of acquired cystic kidney disease is malignant conversion of cysts into renal cell carcinoma (Chapter 182). Carcinomas commonly present as hematuria and are 2 to 200 times more common in patients with acquired cystic kidney disease than in the general dialysis population.

Acquired cystic kidney disease is diagnosed by ultrasonography or computed tomography (CT), demonstrating multiple and bilateral renal cysts in a patient with preexisting chronic renal failure or end-stage renal disease. In contrast to autosomal dominant or recessive PKD, the kidneys are usually not enlarged, and there is no family history of PKD. Renal CT or MRI is preferable to detect cysts in small kidneys and to assess for malignant conversion.

TREATMENT AND PREVENTION

No strategies are available to prevent the appearance or delay the expansion of renal cysts in patients on hemodialysis, but cysts may stabilize or regress after successful renal transplantation. New or frank hematuria raises the concern of renal cell carcinoma (Chapter 182), which should be assessed using ultrasonography and contrast-enhanced CT. Any evidence of septa formation, solid material, or contrast enhancement within a cyst is suspicious for carcinoma and warrants consideration of nephrectomy.

PROGNOSIS

Asymptomatic acquired cystic kidney disease does not affect survival. The incidence of renal cell carcinoma in patients with acquired cystic kidney disease is approximately 0.18% per year. Although metastasis is less common at the time of diagnosis in patients with acquired cystic kidney disease than in other patients with renal cell carcinoma, the 5-year mortality rates are higher, likely related to the almost invariable coexistence of end-stage renal disease.

GENERAL REFERENCES

For the General References and other additional features, please visit Elsevier eBooks+ at https://ebooks.health.elsevier.com.

Grade A References

A1. Lu J, Xu W, Gong L, et al. Efficacy and safety of tolvaptan versus placebo in the treatment of patients with autosomal dominant polycystic kidney disease: a meta-analysis. *Int Urol Nephrol.* 2022;55:631-640.

A2. Casteleijn NF, Blais JD, Chapman AB, et al. Tolvaptan and kidney pain in patients with autosomal dominant polycystic kidney disease: secondary analysis from a randomized controlled trial. *Am J Kidney Dis.* 2017;69:210-219.

A3. Griffiths J, Mills MT, Ong AC. Long-acting somatostatin analogue treatments in autosomal dominant polycystic kidney disease and polycystic liver disease: a systematic review and meta-analysis. *BMJ Open.* 2020;10:e032620.

A4. Perrone RD, Abebe KZ, et al. Primary results of the randomized trial of metformin administration in polycystic kidney disease (TAME PKD). *Kidney Int.* 2021;100:684-696.

A5. Tesar V, Ciechanowski K, Pei Y, et al. Bosutinib versus placebo for autosomal dominant polycystic kidney disease. *J Am Soc Nephrol.* 2017;28:3404-3413.

113

HEREDITARY NEPHROPATHIES AND DEVELOPMENTAL RENAL/URINARY ABNORMALITIES

LISA M. GUAY-WOODFORD

HEREDITARY NEPHROPATHIES

The proximal tubule is responsible for reclaiming most of the filtered glucose, amino acids, uric acid, phosphate, bicarbonate, and low-molecular-weight proteins. The loop of Henle and the distal nephron reabsorb approximately 30% of the filtered sodium chloride and 50% of the filtered divalent cations. The collecting duct, under the regulatory control of aldosterone, fine-tunes sodium reabsorption and secretes hydrogen and potassium ions. In the terminal collecting duct, antidiuretic hormone regulates water reabsorption and urinary concentration.

Inherited renal tubular disorders are a group of conditions in which the normal renal tubular reabsorption of ions, organic solutes, and water (Chapter 102) is disrupted because of defects in single genes.[1] These defects can be categorized by the nephron segment affected (Table 113-1).

DISORDERS OF PROXIMAL TUBULE FUNCTION

CYSTINURIA

Cystinuria is characterized by defective proximal tubular reabsorption of cystine and dibasic amino acids, thereby resulting in increased excretion of cystine and the risk of forming cystine-containing urinary stones (Chapter 111).[2] This autosomal recessive trait has an estimated prevalence of 1 in 7000 individuals. Two cystinuria genes have been identified: *SLC3A1,* which encodes the heavy subunit, rBAT; and *SLC7A9,* which encodes the light subunit, $b^{O,+AT}$. Several large studies indicate that mutations in *SLC3A1* are more common than mutations in *SLC7A9*. Mutations in *SLC3A1* cause cystinuria type A, mutations in *SLC7A9* cause cystinuria type B, and mutations in both genes cause mixed genotype cystinuria.

CLINICAL MANIFESTATIONS AND DIAGNOSIS

Although the severity of the disease is similar in all types of cystinurias, the clinical presentation can be quite variable, and the onset of disease may occur from infancy to the seventh decade of life. Cystine stones are radiopaque and often form the nidus for secondary calcium oxalate stones. Symptoms include renal colic, which may be associated with urinary tract obstruction and/or infection. Affected children can be identified by elevated urinary cystine levels, but testing must be performed after tubular transport has fully matured (at age 2 years). Genetic testing is available, but not mandatory for diagnosis, which can be established by stone analysis and/or quantitative 24-hour urine analysis.

TREATMENT

Conservative therapy with hydration (target specific gravity <1.005), reduced intake of sodium (children 1 to 1.5 mEq/day; adults 100 mEq/day), reduced intake of dietary methionine, and urinary alkalinization is sufficient for many patients with cystinuria. However, recurrent stones may cause renal damage, so such patients should be treated with thiol-containing agents such as D-penicillamine (pediatric dose, 20 to 30 mg/kg/day in four divided doses; adult dose, 0.5 to 1.2 g/day in four divided doses) or tiopronin (pediatric dose, 15 to 40 mg/kg/day in three divided doses; adult dose 800 to 1500 mg/day divided in three doses). Therapy should maintain the unbound urinary cystine concentration below 250 mg/L.

CYSTINOSIS

Cystinosis is the most common inherited cause of renal Fanconi syndrome. It also affects the eyes, muscles, central nervous system, lungs, and various endocrine organs. This autosomal recessive disorder is caused by mutations in the gene *CTNS,* which encodes cystinosin, a lysosomal cystine transporter. Defects in this transporter lead to the accumulation of intralysosomal cystine crystals and widespread cellular destruction.

TABLE 113-1 HEREDITARY NEPHROPATHIES BY NEPHRON SEGMENT

NEPHRON SEGMENT	DISORDER	INHERITANCE	MAJOR RENAL FEATURES
PROXIMAL TUBULE			
	Renal glycosuria	AR	Isolated glycosuria
	Proximal renal tubular acidosis	AR	Hyperchloremic, hypokalemic, metabolic acidosis
	Carbonic anhydrase II deficiency	AR	Mixed proximal and distal renal tubular acidosis
	Hartnup disease	AR	Neutral aminoaciduria
	Lysinuric protein intolerance	AR	Protein intolerance, basic aminoaciduria
	Cystinuria	AR	Type A: Urinary calculi Type B: Urinary calculi
	Cystinosis	AR	Infantile: Renal Fanconi syndrome Late-onset: Renal Fanconi syndrome Non-nephropathic: Renal Fanconi syndrome
	Hypophosphatemic rickets	X-linked AD AR	Renal phosphate wasting, hypophosphatemia Renal phosphate wasting, hypophosphatemia Renal phosphate wasting, hypophosphatemia
	Dent disease	X-linked	Dent disease 1: Nephrocalcinosis, urinary calculi; low-molecular-weight proteinuria Dent disease 2: Nephrocalcinosis, urinary calculi; low-molecular-weight proteinuria
	Lowe syndrome	X-linked	Renal Fanconi syndrome
	Hereditary fructose intolerance	AR	Renal Fanconi syndrome
	Tyrosinemia, type I	AR	Renal Fanconi syndrome
	Wilson disease	AR	Renal Fanconi syndrome
	Fanconi-Bickel syndrome	AR	Renal Fanconi syndrome with hepatorenal glycogenosis
	Renal hypouricemia	AR	Hypouricemia, nephrolithiasis, and exercise-induced acute renal failure
LOOP OF HENLE			
	Bartter syndrome	AR AD	Type 1: Hypokalemic, hypochloremic metabolic alkalosis Type 2: Hypokalemic, hypochloremic metabolic alkalosis Type 3: Hypokalemic, hypochloremic metabolic alkalosis Type 4: Hypokalemic, hypochloremic metabolic alkalosis Type 5: Hypokalemic, hypochloremic metabolic alkalosis
DISTAL TUBULE			
	Gitelman syndrome	AR	Hypokalemic, hypochloremic, metabolic alkalosis
	Familial hypomagnesemia with hypercalciuria	AR	Severe renal magnesium and calcium wasting
	Isolated hypomagnesemia	AD	Renal magnesium wasting
	SeSAME syndrome (EAST syndrome)	AR	Hypokalemia, metabolic alkalosis, and hypomagnesemia
COLLECTING DUCT			
	Liddle syndrome	AD	Low renin hypertension
	Glucocorticoid-remediable hyperaldosteronism	AD	Low renin hypertension
	Apparent mineralocorticoid excess	AR	Low renin hypertension
	Pseudohypoaldosteronism, type 1	AR AD	AR: Hyponatremic, hypokalemic, metabolic acidosis AD: Hyponatremic, hypokalemic, metabolic acidosis
	Pseudohypoaldosteronism, type 2 (Gordon syndrome)	AD	Low renin hypertension with hyperkalemia
	Distal renal tubular acidosis	AR AD	AR: Hyperchloremic, hypokalemic, metabolic acidosis AD: Hyperchloremic, hypokalemic, metabolic acidosis
	Carbonic anhydrase II deficiency	AR	Mixed proximal and distal renal tubular acidosis
	Nephrogenic diabetes insipidus	X-linked AR and AD	X-linked: Urinary concentrating defect AR and AD: Urinary concentrating defect

AD = autosomal dominant; AR = autosomal recessive; SeSAME = seizures, sensorineural deafness, ataxia, intellectual disability (mental retardation), and electrolyte imbalances.

CLINICAL MANIFESTATIONS AND DIAGNOSIS

Three clinical presentations have been described. The most severe is infantile (classic) cystinosis, which manifests in the first year of life with renal tubular acidosis, impaired growth, and evidence of renal Fanconi syndrome, including aminoaciduria, glucosuria, phosphaturia, and low-molecular-weight proteinuria.

In untreated patients, progressive renal damage results in end-stage kidney disease by 10 years of age. A less severe, late-onset (juvenile or intermediate) form causes renal dysfunction in adolescence and involves cystine deposits in the cornea. The mildest form, an ocular, non-nephropathic form, features photophobia but no renal issues.

TREATMENT AND PROGNOSIS

The mainstay of therapy is oral cysteamine (dose: 60 to 90 mg/kg/day or 1.35 to 1.90 g/m^2/day, divided every 6 hours), which is an aminothiol that can lower intracellular cystine content by 90%.[3] In well-treated patients, cysteamine delays renal functional decline, enhances growth, prevents hypothyroidism, and lowers muscle cystine content. Therefore, early diagnosis and prompt, proper treatment are critical for preventing or significantly delaying the complications of cystinosis. Twice-daily dosing with delayed-release cysteamine bitartrate (at approximately 70% of the patient's usual dose) is as efficacious as cysteamine for reducing white blood cell cystine levels in patients with nephropathic cystinosis.

DENT DISEASE

Dent disease is an X-linked recessive renal tubular disorder characterized by low-molecular-weight proteinuria, hypercalciuria with nephrocalcinosis, and progressive renal failure. Low-molecular-weight proteinuria is the most consistent clinical feature, but there is wide variability in other manifestations of proximal tubular dysfunction. Atypical presentations have been reported, including amino aciduria, glycosuria, uricosuria/hypouricemia, kaliuresis/hypokalemia, and phosphaturia/hypophosphatemia. In two thirds of patients, the disease is caused by mutations in the *CLCN5* gene (Dent-1). A smaller proportion of patients (15 to 20%) have mutations in *OCRL* (Dent-2), the gene associated with Lowe oculocerebrorenal syndrome.

TREATMENT AND PROGNOSIS

No specific treatment is available, so treatment is designed to reduce nephrolithiasis and nephrocalcinosis with thiazide diuretics and often potassium citrate (see Chapter 111). End-stage kidney disease occurs at a median age of 40 years.[4]

DISORDERS OF LOOP OF HENLE AND DISTAL TUBULE FUNCTION

THE BARTTER-GITELMAN DISORDERS

The Bartter-Gitelman syndromes are a group of disorders that are characterized by markedly reduced salt transport in the thick ascending limb of Henle (Bartter syndrome) or in the distal convoluted tubule (Gitelman syndrome).[5]

Bartter syndrome is an autosomal recessive disorder that is caused by mutations in one of five genes—*SLC12A2,* encoding the sodium-potassium-chloride cotransporter NKCC2; *KCNJ1,* encoding the ROMK1 potassium ion channel; *CLCNKB,* encoding the ClC-Kb basolateral chloride ion channel; *BSND,* encoding barttin, a regulatory subunit required for basolateral chloride channel targeting to the membrane; and *MAGED,* encoding the melanoma antigen D2 (MAGE-D2). Defects in these genes cause Bartter syndrome types I, II, III, IV, and V, respectively. All five syndromes are characterized by disrupted salt transport in the thick ascending limb. In addition, severe gain-in-function mutations in *CASR,* the gene encoding the extracellular calcium ion–sensing receptor CaSR, can cause a Bartter-like phenotype (referred to as the Bartter-like subform of familial hypocalcemia) that is distinguished from the others by autosomal dominant transmission and associated hypocalcemic hypercalciuria. Most patients with Gitelman syndrome have defects in *SLC12A3,* the gene that encodes the sodium-chloride cotransporter NCCT. However, a minority of patients with the Gitelman phenotype have mutations in *CLCNKB.*

CLINICAL MANIFESTATIONS AND DIAGNOSIS

Individuals with Bartter syndrome exhibit renal salt wasting, lowered blood pressure, polyuria, hypokalemic metabolic alkalosis,[6] and hypercalciuria with a variable risk of nephrocalcinosis. Bartter syndrome mimics the effects of long-term furosemide treatment (E-Fig. 113-1). In comparison, individuals with Gitelman syndrome have a disorder resembling the effects of long-term thiazide administration: milder renal salt wasting, normal blood pressure, hypokalemic metabolic alkalosis, hypomagnesemia, and hypocalciuria. Clinical differences between Bartter and Gitelman syndromes relate to the severity of salt wasting, whereas phenotypic differences among Bartter types I through V correlate with the specific physiologic roles played by the individual transporters or channels in the kidney and other organs.

Genetic testing can confirm these diagnoses by detecting the specific mutation. However, it is not usually required in clinical practice.

TREATMENT

The mainstay of treatment includes replacing salt and water losses and providing potassium supplementation to maintain serum levels greater than 3 mEq/dL.[7] For patients with perinatal (types I, II, IV, V) Bartter syndrome, nonsteroidal anti-inflammatory drugs (e.g., indomethacin 2 to 4 mg/kg/day in two to four divided doses) may be beneficial. In patients with Gitelman syndrome and some patients with Bartter syndrome type III, oral magnesium supplementation may be required to maintain serum levels above 1.2 mg/dL. In patients who have Gitelman syndrome with persistent symptomatic hypokalemia despite therapeutic adherence or who have unacceptable side effects, treatment with potassium-sparing diuretics (e.g., amiloride 10-20 mg/day), a selective aldosterone antagonist (eplerenone 150 mg/day), or a combination of these agents may be effective.

DISORDERS OF COLLECTING DUCT FUNCTION

LIDDLE SYNDROME (PSEUDOALDOSTERONISM)

Liddle syndrome is an autosomal dominant form of salt-sensitive hypertension (Chapter 64) caused by mutations in the β or γ subunit of the epithelial sodium channel, which is expressed at the apical surface of collecting duct cells and plays a critical role in maintaining salt balance and blood pressure.[6] Both the β and γ subunits regulate the channel activity of the α subunit. Mutations in either of these regulatory subunits result in increased epithelial sodium channel activity and Liddle syndrome. Severe hypertension typically manifests in childhood, with features of hypokalemic metabolic alkalosis that resemble primary aldosteronism. However, the secretion of renin and aldosterone is suppressed in this disorder.

TREATMENT

The clinical abnormalities can be ameliorated by a low-salt diet plus a potassium-sparing diuretic (e.g., amiloride 5 to 20 mg/day or triamterene 100 to 200 mg twice daily), which acts as an antagonist of the epithelial sodium channel. Spironolactone is not useful because genetic alterations in the regulatory subunits disrupt mineralocorticoid regulation of the channel.

DISTAL RENAL TUBULAR ACIDOSIS

Distal renal tubular acidosis results from failure of the collecting duct α-intercalated cells to excrete fixed acids (see Fig. 104-1 in Chapter 104). Both autosomal dominant and autosomal recessive forms of distal renal tubular acidosis have been described. Mutations in the *CA2* gene encoding carbonic anhydrase II or the *SLC4A1* gene encoding the chloride-bicarbonate exchanger AE1 cause autosomal dominant distal renal tubular acidosis and are rarely associated with recessive forms of the disease. Mutations in genes encoding subunits of the vacuolar hydrogen–adenosine triphosphatase (V-type H^+-ATPase) proton pump are the primary causes of autosomal recessive distal renal tubular acidosis. V-type ATPases are ubiquitous, multisubunit protein complexes that mediate the ATP-dependent transport of protons. In the kidney, V-type ATPases are the major proton-secreting pumps in the distal nephron and are involved in net proton secretion (bicarbonate generation) or proton reabsorption (net bicarbonate secretion). Defects in two genes, *ATP6V1B1* and *ATP6V0A4,* which encode subunits of the H^+-ATPase, cause distal renal tubular acidosis with or without associated sensorineural deafness.

CLINICAL MANIFESTATIONS AND DIAGNOSIS

Clinical consequences include hypokalemic, hyperchloremic metabolic acidosis; impaired growth; hypercalciuria; hypocitraturia; nephrocalcinosis; nephrolithiasis; rickets in children; and osteomalacia in adults. Classic distal renal tubular acidosis can be distinguished from other metabolic acidoses by an inappropriately high urine pH (>5.5), diminished net acid excretion, positive urinary anion gap, and low urinary ammonium concentration (Table 113-2).[8]

TREATMENT

Treatment with alkali supplementation as citrate salts (1 to 2 mEq/kg/day in adults and 3 to 6 mEq/kg/day in children) corrects the metabolic acidosis as well as the hypocitraturia, thereby preventing nephrolithiasis.[9] In contrast to proximal renal tubular acidosis, urinary potassium wasting can be ameliorated with alkali therapy alone.

DEVELOPMENT OF THE KIDNEY AND URINARY TRACT

The human kidney and urogenital tract develop from three principal embryonic structures: the metanephric mesenchyme, the mesonephric (wolffian) duct, and the cloaca (Fig. 113-1). At 4 to 5 weeks of gestation, the ureteric bud originates as a diverticulum of the mesonephric duct. Reciprocal interactions between the branching ureteric bud and the metanephric mesenchyme induce kidney development, with the metanephros undergoing an epithelial transformation to form the glomeruli and the proximal and distal tubules. The ureteric bud branches give rise to the collecting ducts, the renal pelvis, the ureter, and the bladder trigone. Approximately 60% of the nephron mass is formed in the second half of gestation, and the number of nephrons in the normal human kidney varies widely from about 250,000 to over 2 million.

Concurrent with the initial nephrogenic events, the urorectal fold divides the cloaca into the urogenital sinus and the future rectum. The mesonephric duct develops into the trigone of the urinary bladder, which is the posterior part of the bladder wall. Between 5 and 6 weeks of gestation, the second genital duct (müllerian duct) appears and runs in parallel with the wolffian duct. In males, the müllerian duct subsequently regresses, and the wolffian duct proceeds to form the epididymis, the vas deferens, the seminal vesicle, and the ejaculatory duct. In females, the wolffian duct regresses, and the müllerian ducts fuse to form the ureterovaginal primordium, which merges with the urogenital sinus and eventually gives rise to the uterus, the oviducts, and the proximal vagina. The remnants of the allantois form the urachus, a fibrous cord that connects the bladder to the umbilicus.

ABNORMALITIES OF THE URINARY TRACT

Congenital abnormalities of the kidney and urinary tract encompass a diverse set of structural malformations that result from defects in the developing urinary system.[10] These abnormalities occur in 3 to 11% of the population and account for approximately 50% of all congenital abnormalities.[11] Although 10 to 20% of cases are attributable to single gene mutations or genomic disorders, the majority of sporadic cases appear to involve complex interactions of multiple genetic variants and environmental factors.[12,13]

The most common malformation (~20%) is ureteropelvic junction obstruction. Renal parenchymal anomalies include agenesis, hypoplasia, dysplasia, malrotation, and ectopia. Pelviureteral abnormalities include megaureter, ectopic ureter, horseshoe kidney, duplex collecting system, and vesicoureteral reflux. Abnormalities of posterior urethral valves can occur concurrently. Prenatal ultrasonographic surveillance has substantially improved detection and prompt initiation of treatment, but these disorders remain important causes of infant mortality, as well as morbidity in older children and adults, including progression to renal failure.

RENAL AGENESIS

Renal agenesis reflects a complete failure of nephrogenesis. Unilateral agenesis can occur as an isolated abnormality or as a component of syndromic disorders, such as Turner syndrome (Chapter 214). As an isolated entity, the complete absence of one kidney occurs in 1 in 1000 to 1500 individuals. The incidence is higher in males and occurs somewhat more frequently on the left side; in about half the patients, the ipsilateral ureter and hemitrigone are also absent. The remaining kidney is usually enlarged owing to compensatory hypertrophy, but it may be ectopic or malrotated. Vesicoureteral reflux is observed on the contralateral side in about 30% of patients.

Renal agenesis is commonly associated with genital anomalies, thereby suggesting that it represents a developmental field defect. In females, absence of the ipsilateral oviduct and malformation of the uterus and vagina result from maldevelopment of the müllerian duct, whereas in males, wolffian duct–derived structures, such as the vas deferens and the seminal vesicles, are often absent. Other associated anomalies can involve the cardiovascular system (30%), musculoskeletal system (14%), and adrenal gland (10%). Unilateral renal agenesis is found in 30% of patients with the VACTERL syndrome, an association of vertebral, anal, cardiac, trachea-esophageal, renal, and limb defects.

Bilateral renal agenesis has an estimated incidence of 1 in 4000 births and is associated with the Potter sequence, which includes pulmonary hypoplasia, a characteristic facies, and deformities of the spine and limbs. At birth, these neonates have a critical degree of pulmonary hypoplasia that is incompatible with survival. The familial association of unilateral and bilateral renal agenesis, renal dysplasia, and congenital hydronephrosis occurs in hereditary renal adysplasia syndrome (Online Mendelian Inheritance in Man entry 191830), a rare autosomal dominant disorder with variable penetrance.

RENAL HYPOPLASIA

The term *renal hypoplasia* describes small kidneys with normally differentiated nephrons that are reduced in number. *Oligomeganephronia* describes a form of bilateral renal hypoplasia with a marked reduction in nephron number and associated hypertrophy of individual glomeruli and tubules. This abnormality occurs sporadically as an isolated developmental defect that must be differentiated from acquired renal atrophy and the genetic disorders nephronophthisis and autosomal dominant tubulointerstitial kidney disease (formerly known as medullary cystic kidney disease). Renal function declines slowly, with progression to end-stage kidney failure in the second to third decade of life.

RENAL DYSPLASIA

Renal dysplasia, which can be associated with various abnormalities of kidney size, results from abnormal metanephric differentiation that causes anomalous and/or incompletely differentiated renal elements. Small dysplastic kidneys are commonly referred to as *aplastic*. Large dysplastic kidneys are often cystic; the most extreme type is referred to as *multicystic dysplastic kidney*.

Unilateral dysplasia may be asymptomatic well into adult life. Small aplastic and large multicystic dysplastic kidneys are nonfunctioning and can be distinguished from renal agenesis by imaging studies. The ipsilateral ureter is typically atretic. Contralateral malformations, including obstruction and vesicoureteral reflux, are common. Unilateral multicystic kidneys involute over time and often disappear. Unilateral aplasia and multicystic dysplasia may be manifestations of the hereditary renal adysplasia syndrome. Bilateral multicystic dysplastic kidneys are incompatible with neonatal survival.

TABLE 113-2 FEATURES OF THE INHERITED RENAL TUBULAR ACIDOSES

DISORDER	RENAL TRANSPORT DEFECT	MINIMAL URINE pH DURING ACIDOSIS	ALKALI SUPPLEMENTATION	UAG DURING ACIDOSIS
Proximal renal tubular acidosis	↓ Proximal bicarbonate reabsorption	<5.5	Children: 10-15 mEq HCO_3^-/kg/day	0 or +
Carbonic anhydrase II deficiency	↓ Proximal bicarbonate reabsorption and ↓ distal acidification	Variable	Variable	0 or +
Distal renal tubular acidosis	↓ Distal acidification	>5.5	Adults: 1-2 mEq HCO_3^-/kg/day Children: 3-6 mEq HCO_3^-/kg/day	+ +

HCO_3^- = bicarbonate; UAG = urinary anion gap = $[Na^+] + [K^+] - [Cl^-]$. In renal tubular acidosis, the UAG is usually 0 or positive. By comparison, the UAG is negative in metabolic acidosis associated with diarrheal illness.

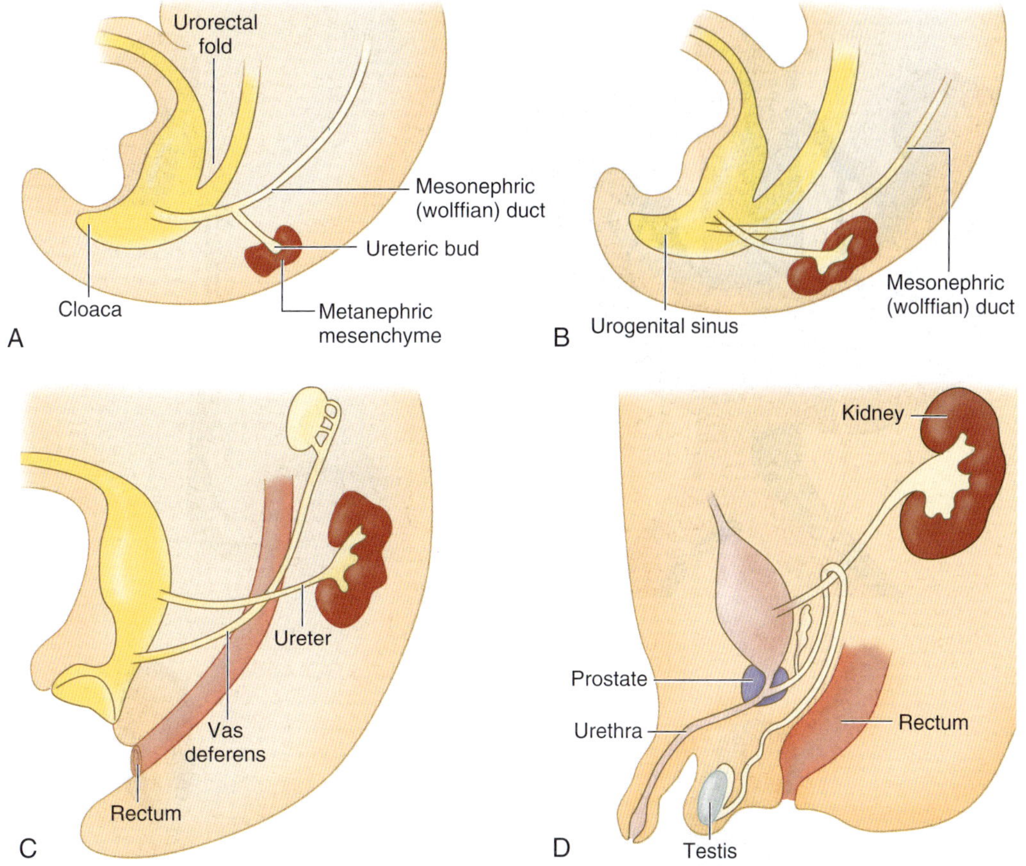

FIGURE 113-1. Key events in the development of the male urinary tract. In the 4-week embryo, the ureteric bud emerges from the wolffian duct (**A**). Reciprocal interactions between the branching ureteric bud and the metanephric mesenchyme induce kidney development. Concurrently, the cloaca is divided by the urorectal fold into the urogenital sinus and the future rectum (**B**). In the 8-week male embryo, the wolffian duct begins to give rise to the epididymis, the seminal vesicles, and the caudal part of the vas deferens (**C**). By 9 weeks, axial growth of the fetal spine prompts the developing kidney to ascend from the pelvis to its final lumbar position. The external genitalia develop between 8 and 16 weeks, and testicular descent begins in month 7 of gestation (**D**).

RENAL AND URETERAL STRUCTURAL ABNORMALITIES

RENAL MALROTATION AND ECTOPIA

Metanephric kidney development begins caudally. By 9 weeks of gestation, the kidney has ascended to its normal level (L1-L3), and the renal pelvis has rotated 90 degrees toward the midline. Anomalies of ascent and/or failure of rotation are common. Bilateral renal ectopia is often associated with kidney fusion. The most common fusion anomaly is the horseshoe kidney, which occurs in 1 in 500 newborns with a 2 : 1 male predominance. Renal ascent is prevented by the root of the inferior mesenteric artery (Fig. 113-2A). Crossed renal ectopia can occur with or without fusion. Supernumerary (extra) kidneys are typically ectopic and vary in location. Although almost one third of patients with renal ectopia remain asymptomatic, the associated malrotation of the renal pelvis increases the risk of hydronephrosis, infection, and stone formation.

PELVIURETERAL ABNORMALITIES

Obstruction of the ureteropelvic junction impedes the flow of urine from the renal pelvis into the ureter. It is one of the most frequently occurring urinary tract anomalies in infants, occurring in 1 in 1000 live births with male predominance. In congenital obstruction of the ureteropelvic junction, urologic anomalies in the contralateral system are common, including renal agenesis, renal dysplasia, multicystic dysplasia, and vesicoureteral reflux. Ureteropelvic junction obstruction may occur in adults secondary to external compression, kinking, or stenosis of the proximal ureter. Surgical intervention is indicated if there is associated renal function impairment, pyelonephritis, stones, or pain.

Hydrocalyx or *hydrocalycosis* refers to dilation of a major calyx that can result from intrinsic obstruction, such as in infundibular stenosis, or in the context of extrinsic compression of the pelvis, caused by a vessel or a parapelvic cyst. In comparison, *megacalycosis* represents a nonobstructive, dysplastic lesion found primarily in males, in which the calyces are dilated and usually increased in number. Associated renal medullary hypoplasia causes malformation of the renal papillae.

Calyceal diverticula are cystic structures connected by a narrow channel to an adjacent minor calyx. In imaging studies, these diverticula typically fill with contrast material, which distinguishes them from renal parenchymal cysts.

Partial duplication of the renal pelvis and ureter is a common anomaly that occurs more frequently in females, is typically unilateral, and is clinically insignificant.

URETERIC ANOMALIES

Ectopic ureters usually reflect complete ureteric and renal duplication. Approximately 10% are bilateral. The ectopic ureter typically drains the dysplastic upper pole of a duplex kidney and inserts below the normal vesicoureteral junction into the lower trigone of the bladder or the proximal urethra. Ectopic ureters occur more frequently in females, and the insertion sites can include the vagina and the vulva, with resulting incontinence. An ectopic ureter is often associated with a ureterocele, which is a cystic dilation of the terminal ureter (see Fig. 113-2B). In children, ureteroceles can be associated with urinary tract infection and obstruction of the bladder neck or even of the contralateral ureter. In adults, the clinical presentation usually involves associated infection, ureteric stones, or both.

A *megaureter*, or grossly dilated ureter, has multiple potential causes, including intrinsic ureteric obstruction by a stone, bladder outflow obstruction, vesicoureteral reflux, and external compression of the distal ureter. In contrast, primary megaureter results from a functional obstruction of the distal ureter caused by an aperistaltic segment (see Fig. 113-2C).

VESICOURETERAL REFLUX

In the normal urinary tract, urinary reflux from the bladder into the ureters is prevented by a functional valve-like mechanism at the vesicoureteral junction. The competence of this valve is dependent on several critical factors, such as the intramural length of the ureter, the position of the ureteric orifice in the bladder, and the integrity of the bladder wall musculature.

Primary vesicoureteral reflux results from incompetence of the vesicoureteral junction owing to the shortened length of the ureter's submucosal segment

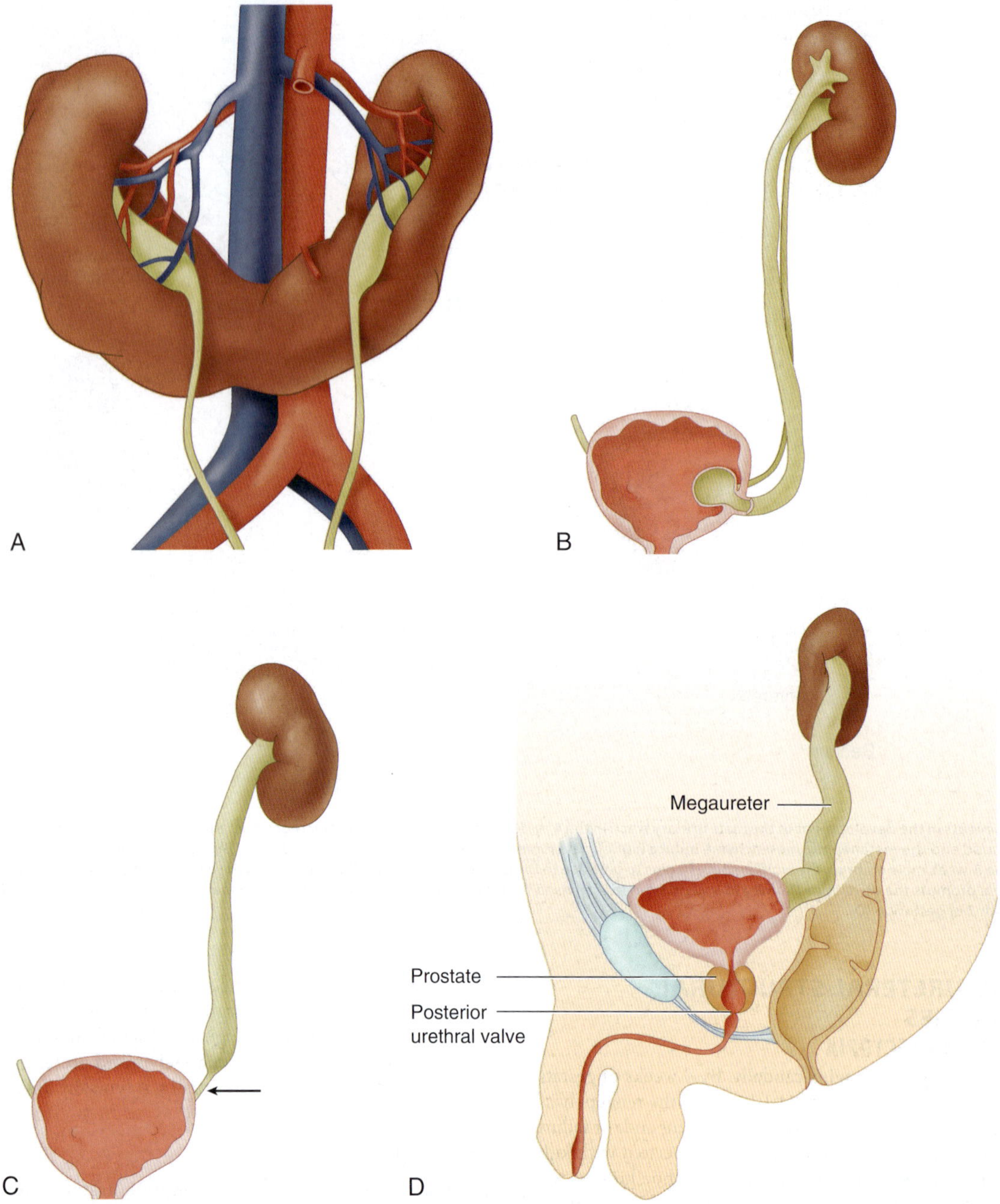

FIGURE 113-2. **Developmental abnormalities of the urinary tract. A, Horseshoe kidney. B, Ectopic ureter associated with a ureterocele. C, Megaureter with the aperistaltic segment *(arrow)*. D, Bladder outlet obstruction caused by posterior urethral valves.**

and the lateral, ectopic position of its orifice. It is estimated to occur in 1 to 2% in children. Familial clustering of vesicoureteral reflux suggests that genetic factors contribute to the pathogenesis, but each implicated gene accounts for only a small number of affected patients.[14]

As the intramural ureter lengthens with age, primary vesicoureteral reflux tends to remit or disappear. Vesicoureteral reflux can also occur secondary to obstructive maldevelopment of the lower urinary tract in children, such as in triad syndrome and posterior urethral valves, or secondary to masses that obstruct the bladder or urethra (in adults). In both primary and secondary vesicoureteral reflux, intrarenal reflux can lead to the development of reflux nephropathy, a tubulointerstitial lesion (Chapter 108) associated with gross scarring at the renal poles. In addition, the development of a glomerular lesion consistent with focal and segmental glomerulosclerosis (Chapter 107) can cause proteinuria, hypertension, and progressive loss of renal function.

Primary vesicoureteral reflux is diagnosed in about 30 to 40% of children who have imaging studies after urinary tract infections (Chapter 263). Frequent urinary tract infection, higher grades of vesicoureteral reflux, and the presence of bladder and bowel dysfunction are risk factors for renal cortical scarring, and the rates of spontaneous resolution of reflux and of endoscopic surgical success depend upon bladder and bowel dysfunction.

TREATMENT

For children with grade I through IV vesicoureteral reflux, antimicrobial prophylaxis does not decrease the risk of renal scarring,[A1] which occurs significantly more frequently in kidneys with grade IV reflux than in kidneys with low-grade or no reflux. For most patients, conservative management is preferred, using an individualized, risk-based approach under expert supervision. One endoscopic injection of a dextranomer/hyaluronic acid copolymer provides an efficient and safe long-term treatment in about 80% of treated patients with advanced vesicoureteral reflux,[15,16] but surgery has a higher cure rate.[A2] Further studies are needed to determine whether this minimally invasive approach should replace traditional surgical correction as the first-line therapy in many patients.

LOWER URINARY TRACT ABNORMALITIES

TRIAD SYNDROME (PRUNE-BELLY SYNDROME, EAGLE-BARRETT SYNDROME)

Triad syndrome, also referred to as prune-belly syndrome or Eagle-Barrett syndrome, involves a constellation of anomalies including congenital absence or deficiency of the abdominal wall musculature, gross ureteral dilation, bladder wall thickening, prostatic hypoplasia, and bilateral undescended testes (cryptorchidism). The full syndrome is expressed only in males, and surviving individuals are typically infertile. Patients with an incomplete syndrome can have anomalies of the abdominal wall musculature, bladder, and upper urinary tract; 3 to 5% of these patients are females. Although the specific molecular causes have yet to be defined, defects in mesenchymal development appear to cause poor prostate and bladder differentiation, ureteral smooth muscle aplasia with consequent ureteral aperistalsis, and varying degrees of renal dysplasia. Patients with triad syndrome have associated anorectal malformations, musculoskeletal anomalies, and, rarely, cardiac anomalies. In the immediate postnatal period, prognosis depends on the severity of extra-genitourinary defects. Long-term outcome correlates with the degree of renal dysplasia and the success of urodynamic management.

BLADDER ABNORMALITIES

Bladder exstrophy results from a midline closure defect involving the lower anterior abdominal wall, the bladder, and the external genitalia. These abnormalities have been attributed to a primary defect in the differentiation of the cloacal membrane, but the precise molecular events remain unclear. Variants in genes involved the morphogenesis of the urinary tract are linked to the pathogenesis of bladder exstrophy.[17] In severe cases, bladder exstrophy may be associated with imperforate anus and rectal atresia. Clinical studies suggest a correlation between the success of bladder reconstruction and long-term preservation of renal function.

In adults, neuropathic or neurogenic bladder (Chapter 115) has numerous etiologic contributors, including central nervous system trauma, stroke, disorders such as Parkinson disease, spinal trauma, multiple sclerosis, and peripheral nerve damage caused by trauma or surgery. In children, myelomeningocele (spina bifida) is the most common cause of neurogenic bladder dysfunction. Other forms of myelodysplasia, such as spinal dysraphism (spina bifida occulta) and sacral agenesis, are less common causes.

TREATMENT

Treatment focuses on the management of incontinence (Chapter 115) and the prevention and treatment of urinary tract infections (Chapter 263).

POSTERIOR URETHRAL VALVES

In male infants, posterior urethral valves are the most common cause of bladder outflow obstruction, with resulting bilateral hydronephrosis and megaureters. However, among all infants with hydronephrosis, only 10% have posterior urethral valves. The urethral obstruction results from defective reabsorption of mucosal folds in the posterior urethra, just distal to the verumontanum of the prostatic urethra. As a result, dilation of the proximal urethra, bladder wall hypertrophy and trabeculation, associated vesicoureteral reflux, and varying degrees of renal dysplasia are present (see Fig. 113-2D). Surgical management strategies are dictated by the age of the child and the degree of associated renal insufficiency. Survival and long-term renal outcome depend on the severity of the associated renal dysplasia.

GENERAL REFERENCES

For the General References and other additional features, please visit Elsevier eBooks+ at https://ebooks.health.elsevier.com.

Grade A References

A1. Mattoo TK, Chesney RW, Greenfield SP, et al. Renal scarring in the randomized intervention for children with vesicoureteral reflux (RIVUR) trial. *Clin J Am Soc Nephrol.* 2016;11:54-61.

A2. Salih EM, Eldamanhory H, Selmy GI, et al. Comparison of subureteral endoscopic injection of dextranomer/hyaluronic acid and Lich-Gregoir ureteral reimplantation in the treatment of pediatric primary vesicoureteral reflux: a prospective randomized study. *J Laparoendosc Adv Surg Tech A.* 2021;31:719-723.

114 BENIGN PROSTATIC HYPERPLASIA AND PROSTATITIS

STEVEN A. KAPLAN

BENIGN PROSTATIC HYPERPLASIA

DEFINITION

The prostate gland is composed of four zones: peripheral, central, transitional, and stroma. It can also be divided by lobes: anterior, posterior, lateral, and median (Fig. 114-1).

A normal prostate volume in young men is about 20 mL (where 1 mL is equivalent to 1 gram), but it increases from an average of about 24 mL to 38 mL between ages 50 to 80 years. In benign prostatic hyperplasia (BPH), the calculated volume exceeds 30 mL, but the degree of prostatic enlargement that causes symptoms is highly variable.

EPIDEMIOLOGY

Age is the major risk factor for BPH. A histologic diagnosis of BPH will develop in approximately 50% of men older than 50 years of age and 90% of men in their 80s. Of these men, approximately 50% will develop notable lower urinary tract symptoms, which increase in prevalence in a linear fashion between the ages of 40 and 80 years. With increasing worldwide longevity, BPH has become a major global challenge.[1]

PATHOBIOLOGY

As the bladder fills with urine, it normally is able to maintain a low intravesical pressure via sympathetic nerve stimulation despite the increasing volume. However, an enlarged prostate may cause lower urinary tract symptoms by directly obstructing the flow of urine or by increasing the muscle tone of the prostate. Men with bladder outlet obstruction due to BPH often have overactive bladder detrusor function, thereby resulting in urinary retention. In addition, changes in the vascularity of the prostate or the urinary bladder can contribute to the development of symptoms. The growth of the prostate gland is dependent on androgens and androgen receptors, and it is reduced by 5α-reductase inhibitors that block the conversion of testosterone to dihydrotestosterone.[2]

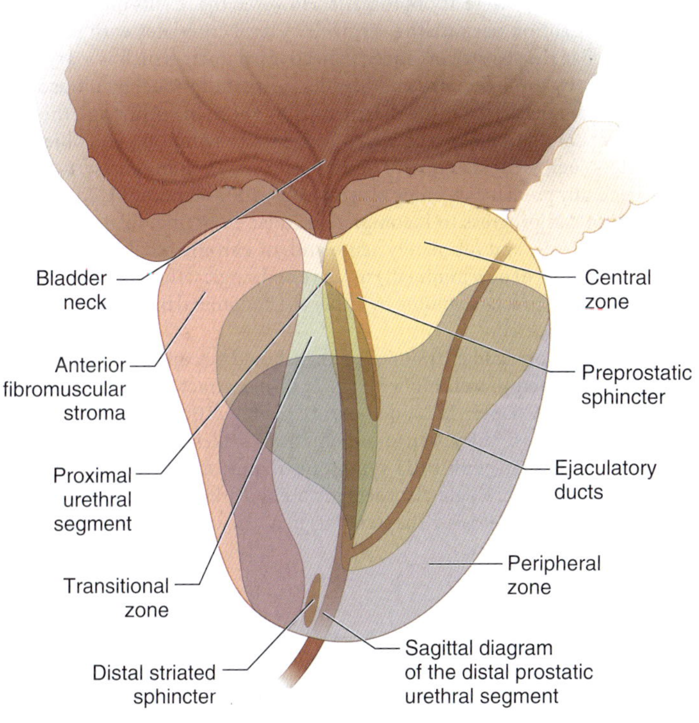

FIGURE 114-1. Anatomy of the prostate.

Enlargement typically is a combination of stromal hypertrophy and glandular hyperplasia, mostly in the central zone. BPH is a histologic diagnosis defined by the proliferation of smooth muscle and epithelial cells within the prostatic transition zone.

CLINICAL MANIFESTATIONS

Benign prostatic hyperplasia can lead to lower urinary tract symptoms, which can have a significant negative impact on quality of life. The presence of lower urinary tract symptoms is often indicative of bladder outlet obstruction secondary to BPH. Symptoms may significantly impair health-related quality of life and are classified as voiding (i.e., hesitancy, weak stream, straining, and prolonged voiding), storage (i.e., frequency, urgency, nocturia, urge incontinence, and voiding of small volumes), or postmicturition (i.e., postvoid dribble, incomplete emptying).[3] Most patients who have lower urinary tract symptoms present with a combination of these symptoms. The symptoms of overactive bladder (Chapter 115) and lower urinary tract symptoms secondary to BPH often overlap.

DIAGNOSIS

Assessment should begin with a medical history and review of the patient's medications. The medical history should include any causes that may lead to bladder dysfunction, such as cerebrovascular disease, previous surgical procedures, and a history of prostatic disease. Diuretics and over-the-counter preparations, such as nasal decongestants and antihistamines, may exacerbate the patient's urinary symptoms. Furthermore, dietary factors such as water, caffeine, alcohol, and artificial sweeteners can be important contributors to the overall clinical manifestations of symptoms because they serve as direct bladder irritants and diuretics. Urinary symptoms should be assessed in a standardized fashion with validated instruments such as the International Prostate Symptom Score (IPSS) (Fig. 114-2) and observed over time.

Abdominal examination should be performed to identify the presence of a palpable bladder, which could be a sign of urinary retention. The physical examination should include a prostate examination to evaluate its size and the possible presence of nodules. The digital rectal examination gives only an approximate estimate of size because only the posterior half is palpated. A focused neurologic examination is also important to assess a patient's mental status, ambulatory status, lower extremity neuromuscular function, and anal sphincter tone.

Laboratory Findings

Urinalysis should be performed to screen for hematuria and urinary tract infection (Chapter 263). A serum prostate-specific antigen (PSA) level should be measured because it can detect asymptomatic prostate cancer (Chapter 186) that may require treatment even in men who would not be candidates for treatment if they were asymptomatic. However, the results must be interpreted with caution because the serum PSA level correlates with prostatic volume even in the absence of cancer. Objective parameters such as maximum urinary flow by uroflowmetry and bladder postvoid residual by ultrasound should also be measured if the diagnosis is in question.[4] Although there is not a direct correlation between lower urinary tract symptoms and objective parameters such as prostate size or flow rate, prostate volume and serum PSA levels generally predict worsening of symptoms. Long-standing bladder outlet obstruction can progress to incomplete bladder emptying, bilateral hydroureteronephrosis, and ultimately acute and/or chronic renal insufficiency. Given the myriad of new minimally invasive and surgical therapeutic options, measurement of prostate volume by either the abdominal or transrectal route should be considered.

Other causes of bladder dysfunction that should be considered during the assessment of men presenting with lower urinary tract symptoms include bladder cancer (Chapter 182), diabetes (Chapter 210), urethral strictures, and bladder stones. The absence of hematuria makes bladder cancer very unlikely, but patients with BPH symptoms require cystoscopy if they also have hematuria. Neurologic disorders including Parkinson disease (Chapter 378) and multiple sclerosis (Chapter 380) may also cause lower urinary tract symptoms in men.

TREATMENT

The treatment of BPH aims to improve subjective symptoms and quality of life as well as to prevent progression of the disease.[5] Over time, treatment has evolved away from surgical therapy and largely to medical therapy.[6,7]

Men who are mildly symptomatic, defined as a score of 7 or less on the IPSS questionnaire, can be observed (Fig. 114-3). Lifestyle changes that may improve symptoms include fluid restriction, timed voiding, and double voiding. Patients who have moderate symptoms, defined as 8 to 19 points on the IPSS, and who are not seriously bothered by their symptoms may also be observed with periodic reassessment to monitor whether urinary retention, refractory hematuria, infections, or other complications develop. Men with more substantial symptoms should be treated medically.[8]

Medications

α-Adrenergic antagonists, which decrease bladder outlet resistance by relaxing urethral smooth muscle and possibly striated sphincter tone, are considered the first-line treatment of male lower urinary tract symptoms[A1] (Table 114-1). Their side effects include orthostatic hypotension, sexual dysfunction, and dizziness. All medications in this class should be discontinued before cataract surgery for fear of floppy-iris syndrome.

The 5α-reductase inhibitors dutasteride and finasteride are also effective for the treatment of BPH, with evidence suggesting that dutasteride is preferred.[A2] These agents reduce prostate size by suppressing testosterone and dihydrotestosterone production. As a result, these agents reduce the number of episodes of acute urinary retention and decrease the need for surgical treatment of BPH, and they are particularly helpful for the treatment of patients with higher prostate volumes. Side effects of these medications include erectile dysfunction, reduced libido, and decreased ejaculate volume.

The phosphodiesterase type 5 inhibitor tadalafil also improves lower urinary tract symptoms and IPSS scores secondary to BPH.[A3] However, tadalafil is not as efficacious as α-adrenergic antagonists or 5α-reductase inhibitors for improving maximal urinary flow.

Antimuscarinic agents, which target the muscarinic cholinergic receptors in the bladder to reduce overactivity that occurs as a result of changes in detrusor function, are safe and efficacious for the treatment of BPH. Options include tolterodine, solifenacin, and fesoterodine.

Another class of agents used to treat overactive bladder symptoms are β_3-agonists such as mirabegron and vibegron. Mirabegron and vibegron stimulate β_3-receptors, thereby causing smooth muscle relaxation in the bladder.[A4]

Combination drug therapy is an option when single-drug therapy is insufficient. Data suggest that the best combination is adding a 5α-reductase inhibitor to an α-adrenergic blocker,[A5] although the combination of an α-adrenergic blocker and a phosphodiesterase 5 inhibitor is also efficacious.[A6,A7] Similarly, the combination of tamsulosin, dutasteride, and an antimuscarinic agent or A β_3-agonists (see Table 114-1) can improve overactive bladder symptoms that have responded inadequately to tamsulosin alone.[A8] Saw palmetto, the most commonly used phytotherapeutic agent, does not improve urinary parameters during a treatment period of 12 months in randomized trials and is not recommended even as add-on therapy.

Surgical Treatments

Many minimally invasive treatment options are available for BPH.[9,10] Prostatic urethral lift delivers permanent transprostatic implants through a cystoscope to open the prostatic parenchyma mechanically. This treatment is limited to patients with a prostate smaller than 80 g and without significant middle lobe hypertrophy, in whom it is as good as or better than surgical prostatectomy.[A9] Transurethral radiofrequency-induced water therapy induces a delayed coagulation necrosis of prostatic tissue, thereby resulting in a decrease in prostate volume.[A10] The advantages of these procedures (i.e., lower risks for retrograde ejaculation, strictures, hematuria, and blood transfusions) must be balanced against increased risks for dysuria, urinary retention, recurrent symptoms, and the need for retreatment compared with transurethral resection of the prostate.[A11]

Electrosurgically based transurethral resection of the prostate, either via a monopolar or bipolar approach, is the "gold standard" in endoscopic treatment of symptomatic BPH. Because of improvements in medical therapy and minimally invasive options, the number of transurethral resection of the prostate procedures performed in the United States has declined, although it still remains the most commonly performed urologic procedure.

Bipolar transurethral resection of the prostate uses bipolar instead of monopolar electrocautery and saline as an irrigant. This procedure resects large amounts of prostatic tissue from the transitional zone and central zone but decreases complications, such as hyponatremia and perioperative bleeding requiring transfusion. For patients with very large prostate glands (i.e., 80 g and larger), transurethral resection of the prostate procedures may require prolonged operative times, and an open surgical approach may be necessary for adequate debulking of the obstructing prostatic tissue.

Other surgical technologies include various laser vaporization techniques[A12] or microwave therapy.[A13] Laser technologies can be effective alternatives to electrosurgical approaches, although their long-term durability remains to be defined. Prostatic artery embolization is another possible treatment, though data on its efficacy and safety are limited.[A14]

	Not at all	Less than 1 time in 5	Less than half the time	About half the time	More than half the time	Almost always
1. Over the past month or so, how often have you had a sensation of not emptying your bladder completely after you finished urinating?	0 ☐	1 ☐	2 ☐	3 ☐	4 ☐	5 ☐
2. Over the past month or so, how often have you had to urinate again less than two hours after you finished urinating?	0 ☐	1 ☐	2 ☐	3 ☐	4 ☐	5 ☐
3. Over the past month or so, how often have you found you stopped and started again several times when you urinated?	0 ☐	1 ☐	2 ☐	3 ☐	4 ☐	5 ☐
4. Over the past month or so, how often have you found it difficult to postpone urination?	0 ☐	1 ☐	2 ☐	3 ☐	4 ☐	5 ☐
5. Over the past month or so, how often have you had a weak urinary stream?	0 ☐	1 ☐	2 ☐	3 ☐	4 ☐	5 ☐
6. Over the past month or so, how often have you had to push or strain to begin urination?	0 ☐	1 ☐	2 ☐	3 ☐	4 ☐	5 ☐

7. Over the past month, how many times did you most typically get up to urinate from the time you went to bed at night until the time you got up in the morning?

0 ☐ none	1 ☐ 1 time	2 ☐ 2 times	3 ☐ 3 times	4 ☐ 4 times	5 ☐ 5 or more times

Total IPSS Score = sum of questions 1–7 = ______

Quality of life due to urinary symptoms

If you were to spend the rest of your life with your urinary condition just the way it is now, how would you feel about that?

Delighted	Pleased	Mostly satisfied	Mixed—about equally satisfied and dissatisfied	Mostly dissatisfied	Unhappy	Terrible
0 ☐	1 ☐	2 ☐	3 ☐	4 ☐	5 ☐	6 ☐

FIGURE 114-2. **International Prostate Symptom Score (IPSS). The seven symptom questions constitute a scale initially developed by the American Urological Association. The eighth question about quality of life is scored separately. (From Barry MJ, Fowler FJ Jr, O'Leary MP, et al. The American Urological Association symptom index for benign prostatic hyperplasia: the Measurement Committee of the American Urological Association. *J Urol*. 1992;148:1549.)**

PROGNOSIS

Over time, the symptoms of BPH often increase and require medications or a procedure. Recurrent episodes of prostatitis can exacerbate symptoms. Patients should be counseled about the likelihood of progression, the natural history of lower urinary tract symptoms (including the risk for urinary tract infections [Chapter 263]) related to BPH, and the treatment options that can be offered.

PROSTATITIS

EPIDEMIOLOGY AND PATHOBIOLOGY

Prostatitis is usually a clinical diagnosis based on signs and symptoms that occur as a result of inflammation of the prostate gland. The overall prevalence of prostatitis is approximately 8%, and it affects men of a wide age range. Swelling or inflammation of the prostate gland, which may be due to various causes, can have a significant impact on quality of life. The current classification system defines the various types of prostatitis on the basis of whether it is acute or chronic, associated with infection, or associated with pelvic pain (Table 114-2).

The causative organisms of acute bacterial prostatitis are usually similar to those that cause other common genitourinary infections (Chapter 263) and include *Escherichia coli* and *Enterococcus* spp. About 60% of patients with chronic bacterial prostatitis have evidence of ongoing infection based on polymerase chain reaction (PCR) testing of their expressed prostatic secretions, with *Chlamydia trachomatis, Ureaplasma urealyticum, Mycoplasma genitalium*, and *Mycoplasma hominis* the most common organisms detected. The pathogenesis of chronic prostatitis/chronic pelvic pain syndrome, however, remains unclear.

CLINICAL MANIFESTATIONS

Acute bacterial prostatitis (type I) is characterized by acute infection of the prostate gland. Presenting symptoms include pelvic, perineal, penile, or ejaculatory pain as well as irritative or obstructive voiding symptoms and sexual dysfunction. Patients with severe infections can present with fever and chills and can become septic (Chapter 94). Type II prostatitis is characterized by recurrent or relapsing infection caused by the same organism. These patients tend to be less sick during each episode and usually present with voiding symptoms and pain.

Type III prostatitis is characterized by pelvic discomfort or pain for more than 3 of the 6 months before evaluation. Type III patients have repeatedly negative urine cultures. Classification into type IIIa or IIIb is contingent on the presence of leukocytes in semen, post–prostate massage urine, or prostatic secretions. Patients with type IV prostatitis do not experience any symptoms of prostatitis. Leukocytes or inflammatory cells are found in prostate tissue, semen, or expressed prostatic secretions.

DIAGNOSIS

The diagnosis of prostatitis requires a careful history, physical examination, and examination of the urine. The physician must ask pertinent questions about voiding history, sexual history, symptoms, pain, neurologic disorders, and prior pelvic surgery. The National Institutes of Health Chronic Prostatitis Symptom Index (NIH-CPSI), which is a standardized tool for the evaluation and assessment of prostatitis, consists of nine parts that outline three major areas of prostatitis: pain, urinary symptoms, and quality of life (Fig. 114-4). The NIH-CPSI is not specifically for making the diagnosis of prostatitis, but it is very useful for longitudinally monitoring changes in symptoms over time after a diagnosis of prostatitis has been established. The physical examination should include an abdominal, external genital, perineal, and digital rectal examination. Attention should be placed on identifying pelvic wall discomfort, structural abnormalities, or prostatic pain on digital rectal examination.

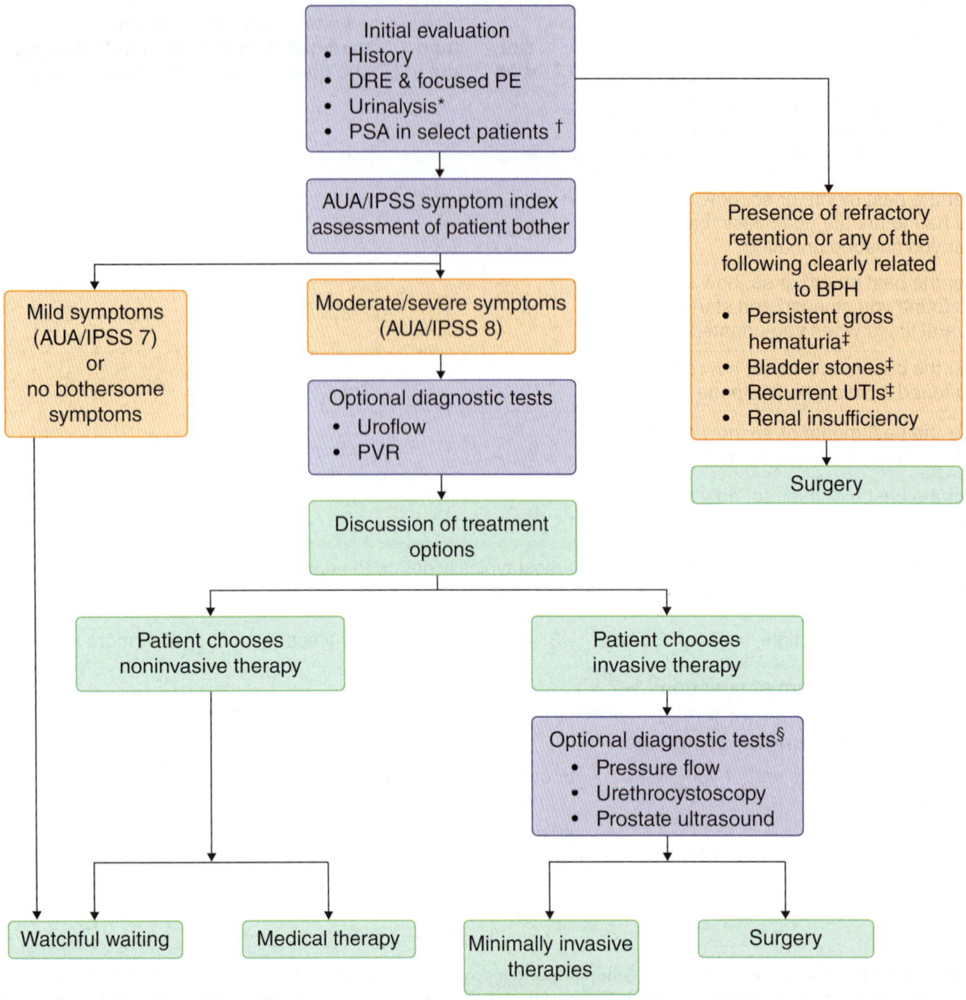

FIGURE 114-3. **Algorithm of management of benign prostatic hyperplasia (BPH).** *In patients with clinically significant prostatic bleeding, a course of a 5 alpha-reductase inhibitor may be used. If bleeding persists, tissue ablative surgery is indicated. †Patients with at least a 10-year life expectancy for whom knowledge of the presence of prostate cancer would change management or patients for whom the PSA measurement may change the management of voiding symptoms. ‡After exhausting other therapeutic options. §Some diagnostic tests are used in predicting response to therapy. Pressure-flow studies are most useful in men prior to surgery. AUA = American Urological Association; DRE = digital rectal exam; IPSS = International Prostate Symptom Score; PE = physical exam; PSA = prostate-specific antigen; PVR = postvoid residual urine; UTI = urinary tract infection. (©2003 American Urological Association Educations and Research, Inc.)

TABLE 114-1 ORAL MEDICATIONS AND RECOMMENDED DAILY DOSES FOR MALE LOWER URINARY TRACT SYMPTOMS

α-BLOCKERS	5α-REDUCTASE INHIBITORS	α-BLOCKER AND 5α-REDUCTASE INHIBITOR	ANTIMUSCARINICS	PHOSPHODIESTERASE TYPE 5 INHIBITORS	β_3-ADRENERGIC RECEPTOR ACTIVATOR
Alfuzosin 10 mg	Dutasteride 0.5 mg	Dutasteride and tamsulosin 0.5/0.4 mg	Darifenacin 7.5, 15 mg	Tadalafil 5 mg	Mirabegron 25, 50 mg
Doxazosin 1-8 mg	Finasteride 5 mg		Fesoterodine 4, 8 mg	Sildenafil and vardenafil not FDA approved for BPH	Vibegron 75 mg
Tamsulosin 0.4 mg			Oxybutynin 5, 10, 15 mg		
Terazosin 1-10 mg			Oxybutynin XL 5, 10, 15 ER mg		
Silodosin 4, 8 mg			Tolterodine 1, 2 mg Tolterodine LA 2, 4 ER mg Trospium 20, 60 mg Solifenacin 5, 10 mg		

BPH = benign prostatic hypertrophy; ER = extended-release; FDA = U.S. Food and Drug Administration; LA = long acting; XL = extended release.

TABLE 114-2 CLASSIFICATION OF PROSTATITIS

	CATEGORIES			
	I	II	III	IV
Term	Acute bacterial prostatitis	Chronic bacterial prostatitis	Chronic prostatitis/chronic pelvic pain syndrome (CP/CPPS) IIIa. Inflammatory CPPS IIIb. Noninflammatory CPPS	Asymptomatic inflammatory prostatitis
Characteristics	Acute infection of prostate gland	Recurrent or relapsing infection caused by the same organism; not acute	90% of cases of chronic prostatitis are presumed to be nonbacterial; diagnosis of exclusion Characteristic symptoms Discomfort or pain in pelvic region for more than 3 months within the past 6 months Pelvic, perineal, penile, or ejaculatory pain; irritative or obstructive voiding symptoms, sexual dysfunction No documented recurrent urinary tract infections; repeated negative cultures Classification into IIIa or IIIb determined by presence of leukocytes in semen, post–prostate massage urine, or prostatic secretion	No symptoms of prostatitis Leukocytes or inflammatory cells present in prostate tissue, semen, or expressed prostatic secretions

Laboratory Evaluation

Urinalysis and urine culture should be performed for every patient. Historically, the four-specimen test was recommended, with specimens obtained from the initial voided bladder urine, midstream voided bladder urine, expressed prostatic secretions obtained during prostate massage, and voided bladder urine collected after prostate massage. Leukocytes in the third specimen suggest the diagnosis of prostatitis. Leukocytes without bacteria suggest inflammation consistent with nonbacterial prostatitis. However, this four-step approach is rarely used today because it has not proved to be useful as a diagnostic tool or for directing treatment. It has been replaced by either a semen culture or a midstream urine culture and by examination of a voided urine specimen after prostate massage.

Urodynamic methods offer valuable insight for patients experiencing predominantly voiding symptoms. Other conditions, such as prostatic obstruction, primary bladder neck obstruction, dysfunctional voiding, urethral obstruction, and detrusor-sphincter dyssynergia, may be defined with the help of postvoid residual, pressure-flow urodynamics, or videourodynamics. These conditions, in comparison to prostatitis, have many effective treatment options.

Measurement of a postvoid residual urine volume by ultrasound can be used to assess incomplete emptying because urinary retention can be a risk factor for recurrent infections.[11] Low maximum urine flow rates suggest bladder outlet obstruction, decreased detrusor contractility, or both as an alternative explanation for lower urinary tract symptoms and poor flow. However, for those who fail to respond to treatment, PCR analysis of semen to evaluate for possible fastidious organisms (e.g., *C. trachomatis, U. urealyticum, Mycoplasma* species, and *Neisseria gonorrhoeae*) may be useful for the evaluation of chronic prostatitis. Cultures of urethral swabs may be used to evaluate patients with potentially undiagnosed sexually transmitted diseases (Chapter 264). Other diagnostic tests include semen analysis and culture, which are useful for patients with complaints of abnormal-smelling semen or infertility.

Cystoscopy is an adjunct to urodynamics in the evaluation of chronic prostatitis/chronic pelvic pain syndrome, especially before any surgical intervention. Cystoscopy is also performed for evaluation of hematuria or abnormal cytology findings because prostate cancer (Chapter 186) or bladder cancer (Chapter 182) can cause symptoms similar to chronic pelvic pain syndrome.

PSA testing should be ordered on the basis of prostate cancer screening (Chapter 186) but has no specific role in evaluation of prostatitis symptoms. Acute prostatitis can increase the serum level of PSA, but it usually returns to normal levels with appropriate antibiotics within 1 to 3 months. PSA can be elevated and even can wax and wane in patients with chronic prostatitis/chronic pelvic pain syndrome. Patients with chronic prostatitis have a less well-defined decrease in PSA after a course of antibiotics. Anywhere from one third to two thirds of men undergoing prostate biopsy have chronic inflammation, but the correlation with symptoms of prostatitis is unclear.

Transrectal ultrasound can identify a prostatic abscess and is generally recommended for patients who have recurrent prostatitis or who do not respond to treatment. The potential utility of pelvic computed xerographic scanning and transrectal magnetic resonance imaging is unclear.

TREATMENT

Acute Bacterial Prostatitis

Oral or intravenous antibiotics are usually effective for curing acute prostatitis, and progression to chronic bacterial prostatitis is uncommon.[12] Typical first-course antibiotics include oral fluoroquinolones (e.g., levofloxacin 500 mg once daily or ofloxacin 300 mg twice daily) and sulfonamides (e.g., trimethoprim/sulfamethoxazole 160 mg/800 mg twice daily) for 6 weeks. Patients who are unable to tolerate oral medications and patients with signs of sepsis may require broad-spectrum intravenous antibiotics (e.g., ampicillin 2 g every 6 hours plus gentamicin 1.5 mg/kg every 8 hours until afebrile) followed by 6 weeks of oral therapy as before. A prostatic abscess may require interventional therapy.[13]

Chronic Bacterial Prostatitis

Antibiotic therapy is the mainstay of treatment for chronic bacterial prostatitis.[14] Antibiotics with good lipid solubility, good enteric bacterial coverage, and a high pK_a have the best prostatic penetration. These antibiotics include quinolones, sulfa-based preparations, macrolides, tetracyclines, and aminoglycosides. The fluoroquinolones (e.g., ciprofloxacin 500 mg twice daily, levofloxacin 500 mg once daily, or ofloxacin 300 mg twice daily) have equivalent success rates in patients with chronic bacterial prostatitis and are generally the first-line treatment. In cases in which atypical bacteria, such as chlamydia, are suspected to be the cause of chronic bacterial prostatitis, better results may be achieved by macrolide antibiotics, such as azithromycin (500 mg twice daily). Most studies demonstrate effective treatment with 30 days of therapy, but some clinicians prescribe 6 weeks of therapy as for acute prostatitis because the recurrence rate is as high as 40% within a year. Delivery of antibiotics by intraprostatic injection or anal submucosal injection is rarely used.

Treatments for Chronic Prostatitis/Chronic Pelvic Pain Syndrome

The optimal regimen for the treatment of chronic prostatitis/chronic pelvic pain syndrome is not known, and the response to treatment is often disappointing.[15] Prolonged courses of antibiotics generally are not effective. One option is to perform PCR testing of expressed prostatic secretions and to use antibiotics only if the test result is positive. Current empirical therapy uses a combination of α-blockers, adrenergic antagonists, phosphodiesterase 5 inhibitors,[A15,A16] and anti-inflammatory agents (e.g., ibuprofen 400 mg three times daily or naproxen 200 mg twice daily). Neuroleptics, such as gabapentin, have been tried but appear to be no better than placebo and have side effects. The potential value of allopurinol is unclear. Many phytotherapies have been tried, but improvements have not been dramatic or consistent in various trials.

Conservative supportive therapies include warm sitz baths and special diets that avoid spicy foods, caffeine, alcohol, and other urinary irritants. Behavioral therapies and stress reduction can augment the efficacy of medications,[A17] and therapies that aim to improve relaxation and to re-educate pelvic floor muscle function can improve symptoms in highly stressed individuals with dysfunctional voiding. Options include biofeedback and bladder retraining. Unproven treatments include trigger point massage combined with relaxation and electromagnetic pelvic floor therapy, acupuncture, and percutaneous tibial nerve stimulation.[A18] Prostate massage can be combined with other therapies, but its efficacy has been variable.

PROGNOSIS

Most patients with type I prostatitis are effectively treated with oral or intravenous antibiotics, although some cases do not respond to treatment and

NIH-Chronic Prostatitis Symptom Index (NIH-CPSI)

Pain or Discomfort

1. In the last week, have you experienced any pain or discomfort in the following areas?

	Yes	No
a. Area between rectum and testicles (perineum)	☐1	☐0
b. Testicles	☐1	☐0
c. Tip of the penis (not related to urination)	☐1	☐0
d. Below your waist, in your pubic or bladder area	☐1	☐0

2. In the last week, have you experienced:

	Yes	No
a. Pain or burning during urination?	☐1	☐0
b. Pain or discomfort during or after sexual climax (ejaculation)?	☐1	☐0

3. How often have you had pain or discomfort in any of these areas over the last week?

☐ 0 Never
☐ 1 Rarely
☐ 2 Sometimes
☐ 3 Often
☐ 4 Usually
☐ 5 Always

4. Which number best describes your AVERAGE pain or discomfort on the days that you had it, over the last week?

☐ ☐ ☐ ☐ ☐ ☐ ☐ ☐ ☐ ☐ ☐
0 1 2 3 4 5 6 7 8 9 10
NO PAIN — PAIN AS BAD AS YOU CAN IMAGINE

Urination

5. How often have you had a sensation of not emptying your bladder completely after you finished urinating, over the last week?

☐ 0 Not at all
☐ 1 Less than 1 time in 5
☐ 2 Less than half the time
☐ 3 About half the time
☐ 4 More than half the time
☐ 5 Almost always

6. How often have you had to urinate again less than two hours after you finished urinating, over the last week?

☐ 0 Not at all
☐ 1 Less than 1 time in 5
☐ 2 Less than half the time
☐ 3 About half the time
☐ 4 More than half the time
☐ 5 Almost always

Impact of Symptoms

7. How much have your symptoms kept you from doing the kinds of things you would usually do, over the last week?

☐ 0 None
☐ 1 Only a little
☐ 2 Some
☐ 3 A lot

8. How much did you think about your symptoms, over the last week?

☐ 0 None
☐ 1 Only a little
☐ 2 Some
☐ 3 A lot

Quality of Life

9. If you were to spend the rest of your life with your symptoms just the way they have been during the last week, how would you feel about that?

☐ 0 Delighted
☐ 1 Pleased
☐ 2 Mostly satisfied
☐ 3 Mixed (about equally satisfied and dissatisfied)
☐ 4 Mostly dissatisfied
☐ 5 Unhappy
☐ 6 Terrible

Scoring the NIH-Chronic Prostatitis Symptom Index Domains

Pain: Total of items 1a, 1b, 1c,1d, 2a, 2b, 3, and 4 = ______

Urinary Symptoms: Total of items 5 and 6 = ______

Quality of Life Impact: Total of items 7, 8, and 9 = ______

FIGURE 114-4. National Institutes of Health (NIH) Chronic Prostatitis Symptom Index. (Modified from Litwin MS, McNaughton-Collins M, Fowler FJ Jr, et al. The National Institutes of Health chronic prostatitis symptom index: development and validation of a new outcome measure. Chronic Prostatitis Collaborative Research Network. *J Urol.* 1999;162:369-375.)

progress to type II prostatitis. The natural history of type II, type III, and type IV prostatitis remains undefined.

GENERAL REFERENCES

For the General References and other additional features, please visit Elsevier eBooks+ at https://ebooks.health.elsevier.com.

Grade A References

A1. Jung JH, Kim J, MacDonald R, et al. Silodosin for the treatment of lower urinary tract symptoms in men with benign prostatic hyperplasia. *Cochrane Database Syst Rev.* 2017;11:CD012615.

A2. Li Y, Ma J, Qin XH, et al. The efficacy and safety of dutasteride and finasteride in patients with benign prostatic hyperplasia: a systematic review and meta-analysis. *Transl Androl Urol.* 2022;11:313-324.

A3. Cui J, Cao D, Bai Y, et al. Efficacy and safety of 12-week monotherapy with once daily 5 mg tadalafil for lower urinary tract symptoms of benign prostatic hyperplasia: evidence-based analysis. *Front Med (Lausanne)*. 2021;8:744012.
A4. Sebastianelli A, Russo GI, Kaplan SA, et al. Systematic review and meta-analysis on the efficacy and tolerability of mirabegron for the treatment of storage lower urinary tract symptoms/overactive bladder: comparison with placebo and tolterodine. *Int J Urol*. 2018;25:196-205.
A5. Kang D, Hu C, Fu Y, et al. Combination of alpha-blocker and 5α-reductase inhibitor for treatment of benign prostatic hyperplasia. *Clin Invest Med*. 2017;40:E200-E210.
A6. Takeda M, Yokoyama O, Yoshida M, et al. Safety and efficacy of the combination of once-daily tadalafil and alpha-1 blocker in Japanese men with lower urinary tract symptoms suggestive of benign prostatic hyperplasia: a randomized, placebo-controlled, cross-over study. *Int J Urol*. 2017;24:539-547.
A7. Zhang J, Li X, Yang B, et al. Alpha-blockers with or without phosphodiesterase type 5 inhibitor for treatment of lower urinary tract symptoms secondary to benign prostatic hyperplasia: a systematic review and meta-analysis. *World J Urol*. 2019;37:143-153.
A8. Yamanishi T, Asakura H, Seki N, et al. Efficacy and safety of combination therapy with tamsulosin, dutasteride and imidafenacin for the management of overactive bladder symptoms associated with benign prostatic hyperplasia: a multicenter, randomized, open-label, controlled trial (DIrecT study). *Int J Urol*. 2017;24:525-531.
A9. Franco JVA, Jung JH, Imamura M, et al. Minimally invasive treatments for benign prostatic hyperplasia: a Cochrane network meta-analysis. *BJU Int*. 2022;130:142-156.
A10. McVary KT, Gittelman MC, Goldberg KA, et al. Final 5-year outcomes of the multicenter randomized sham-controlled trial of a water vapor thermal therapy for treatment of moderate to severe lower urinary tract symptoms secondary to benign prostatic hyperplasia. *J Urol*. 2021;206:715-724.
A11. Franco JV, Jung JH, Imamura M, et al. Minimally invasive treatments for lower urinary tract symptoms in men with benign prostatic hyperplasia: a network meta-analysis. *Cochrane Database Syst Rev*. 2021;7:CD013656.
A12. Wei HB, Guo BY, Tu YF, et al. Comparison of the efficacy and safety of transurethral laser versus open prostatectomy for patients with large-sized benign prostatic hyperplasia: a meta-analysis of comparative trials. *Investig Clin Urol*. 2022;63:262-272.
A13. Franco JV, Garegnani L, Escobar Liquitay CM, et al. Transurethral microwave thermotherapy for the treatment of lower urinary tract symptoms in men with benign prostatic hyperplasia. *Cochrane Database Syst Rev*. 2021;6:CD004135.
A14. Jung JH, McCutcheon KA, Borofsky M, et al. Prostatic arterial embolisation for men with benign prostatic hyperplasia: a Cochrane review. *BJU Int*. 2023;131:32-45.
A15. Franco JVA, Turk T, Jung JH, et al. Pharmacological interventions for treating chronic prostatitis/chronic pelvic pain syndrome: a Cochrane systematic review. *BJU Int*. 2020;125:490-496.
A16. Deng W, Du X, Zhou W, et al. Systematic review and meta-analysis: α-adrenergic receptor blockers in chronic prostatitis. *Ann Palliat Med*. 2021;10:9870-9878.
A17. Burgio KL, Kraus SR, Johnson TM Jr, et al. Effectiveness of combined behavioral and drug therapy for overactive bladder symptoms in men: a randomized clinical trial. *JAMA Intern Med*. 2020;180:411-419.
A18. Qin Z, Wu J, Tian J, et al. Network meta-analysis of the efficacy of acupuncture, alpha-blockers and antibiotics on chronic prostatitis/chronic pelvic pain syndrome. *Sci Rep*. 2016;6:1-11.

115 URINARY INCONTINENCE

NEIL M. RESNICK AND CATHERINE E. DUBEAU

DEFINITION

Urinary incontinence is the involuntary leakage of urine sufficient to be a health or social problem.

EPIDEMIOLOGY

More than twice as common in women than in men, the prevalence of incontinence increases with age, although at least some degree of urinary incontinence is reported by 11% of women aged 22 to 27 years.[1] Incontinence afflicts 15 to 30% of older adults living at home, one third of those in acute care settings, and more than half of those in nursing homes. Its estimated cost in the United States exceeded $83 billion in 2020, with out-of-pocket costs for patients of more than $500.

Urinary incontinence predisposes to perineal rashes, pressure ulcers, urinary tract infections, falls, and fractures, and it is associated with embarrassment, stigmatization, isolation, depression, anxiety, sexual dysfunction, and risk for institutionalization. Many seriously ill elderly consider it an outcome worse than death.

Despite its prevalence and adverse consequences, geriatric incontinence remains largely neglected, by patients and physicians alike. This neglect is unfortunate because its increased prevalence with age relates more to age-associated diseases and functional impairments than to age itself. Most important, incontinence is usually treatable and often curable at all ages, even in the frail, although the approach in older patients must be broader than that employed in younger patients.[2]

PATHOBIOLOGY

At any age, continence depends not only on the integrity of lower urinary tract function but also on the presence of adequate mentation, mobility, motivation, and manual dexterity. Although incontinence in younger patients is rarely associated with deficits in these domains, such deficits occur commonly in older patients and can cause or exacerbate incontinence or influence therapeutic approaches. Some data suggest that genomics[3] and the microbiome[4] may play a role in increasing susceptibility, particularly for urge incontinence.

With age, bladder capacity does not change, but bladder sensation and contractility decrease.[5] At the cellular level, detrusor smooth muscle develops a "dense band pattern" characterized by dense sarcolemmal bands with depleted caveolae. This depletion may mediate the age-related decline in bladder contractility. In addition, an incomplete disjunction pattern characterized by scattered protrusion junctions develops and may underlie the high prevalence of involuntary bladder contractions (detrusor overactivity) in older adults of both sexes. Bladder ischemia and/or inflammation likely also contribute.[6] Urethral length and sphincter strength decrease in women, whereas the prostate enlarges in most men and causes obstruction in about 50% of them. The postvoid residual volume in the bladder also increases in both sexes but normally to less than 100 mL. In addition, older persons often excrete most of their fluid intake at night, even in the absence of venous insufficiency, renal disease, heart failure, or prostatic obstruction. Because this shift in nocturnal fluid excretion is coupled with an age-associated increase in sleep disorders, most older adults have at least one episode of nocturia per night.

None of these age-related changes causes incontinence, but all predispose to it. This predisposition, combined with the increased likelihood that an older person will encounter an additional pathologic, physiologic, or pharmacologic insult, explains the increased prevalence of incontinence with age. Thus, the onset or exacerbation of incontinence in an older person is often due to precipitants that are outside the lower urinary tract and that are amenable to medical intervention.

Causes of Transient Incontinence

Incontinence is transient in up to one third of community-dwelling elderly individuals and in up to half of acutely hospitalized patients. Although most transient causes are outside the lower urinary tract (Table 115-1), three points warrant emphasis. First, the risk for transient incontinence is increased if, in addition to physiologic changes of the lower urinary tract, there also are pathologic changes. Anticholinergic agents are more likely to cause retention and overflow incontinence in individuals with a weak or obstructed bladder, whereas excess urine output is more likely to cause urge incontinence in individuals with detrusor overactivity or impaired mobility. Second, these transient causes may persist if left untreated and should not be dismissed merely because incontinence is long-standing. Third, identification of the most common cause is of little value because causes vary among individuals, and geriatric incontinence is rarely due to just one cause.

Causes of Established Incontinence Related to the Lower Urinary Tract

Detrusor Overactivity

Detrusor overactivity, also called involuntary bladder contraction or *overactive bladder*, generally causes *urge incontinence* and is the most common type of lower urinary tract dysfunction in incontinent elderly people, in whom it accounts for about two thirds of cases. Histologically, detrusor overactivity is associated with the complete disjunction pattern, with widening of the intercellular space, reduction of normal (intermediate) muscle cell junctions, and emergence of novel protrusion junctions and ultraclose abutments that connect cells together in chains. These connections may mediate a change in cell coupling from a mechanical to an electrical mechanism that results in involuntary bladder contraction. Other potential causes include ischemia, abnormalities in suburothelial myofibroblasts, and changes in central nervous system structural and functional control mechanisms.

At any age, detrusor overactivity is usually idiopathic, but it can be associated with a variety of other causes that may affect prognosis and management. Such conditions include cerebral disease, upper motor neuron lesions (Chapters 369 and 387), urethral obstruction, stress incontinence, bladder calculus, and bladder carcinoma (Chapter 182).

Stress Incontinence

Stress incontinence, which is the second most common cause of incontinence in older women and the dominant cause in middle-aged women, usually reflects

TABLE 115-1 CAUSES OF TRANSIENT INCONTINENCE: DIAPERS MNEMONIC

Delirium	Result of underlying illness or medication; incontinence is secondary and abates once the cause of delirium is corrected	
Infection—*symptomatic* UTI	Acute, symptomatic UTI may cause or worsen incontinence, but the far more common *asymptomatic* bacteriuria does not	
Atrophic urethritis/vaginitis	Characterized by vaginal erosions, telangiectasia, petechiae, and friability; may cause or contribute to incontinence	
Pharmaceuticals	*Drug type:*	*Potential effects on continence:*
	Sedative-hypnotics (e.g., long-acting benzodiazepines; alcohol)	Sedation, delirium, decreased mobility
	Anticholinergics (dicyclomine, disopyramide, sedating antihistamines, antipsychotics, tricyclic antidepressants, cyclobenzaprine, anti-Parkinson, antidepressants [not SSRIs])	Urinary retention, overflow incontinence, delirium, impaction; the antipsychotics also decrease mobility
	Opiates	Urinary retention, stool impaction, sedation, delirium
	α-Adrenergic antagonists	Relax sphincter; may induce stress incontinence in women
	α-Adrenergic agonists	Urinary retention in men (tighten sphincter, prostate)
	Calcium-channel blockers, especially the dihydropyridines	Nocturnal diuresis due to fluid retention
	"Loop" diuretics (thiazide-like agents only rarely cause it)	Polyuria, frequency, urgency
	NSAIDs	Nocturnal diuresis due to fluid retention
	Thiazolidinediones	Nocturnal diuresis due to fluid retention
	Some nociceptives (gabapentin, pregabalin)	Nocturnal diuresis due to fluid retention; sedation; delirium
	Dopamine receptor agonists (e.g., ropinirole, pramipexole)	Nocturnal diuresis due to fluid retention
	Angiotensin-converting enzyme inhibitors	Drug-induced cough leads to stress incontinence in women
	Vincristine	Urinary retention due to neuropathy
	Cholinesterase inhibitors	Urinary incontinence
Excess urine output	From large intake, diuretic agents (caffeinated beverages, alcohol), and metabolic disorders (hyperglycemia, hypercalcemia); nocturnal incontinence may result from obstructive sleep apnea or mobilization of peripheral edema (heart failure, venous insufficiency, side effects of medications)	
Restricted mobility	Often results from overlooked, correctable conditions such as arthritis, pain, foot problems, postprandial hypotension, or fear of falling	
Stool impaction	May cause both fecal and urinary incontinence that remit with disimpaction	

NSAIDs = nonsteroidal anti-inflammatory drugs; SSRI = selective serotonin reuptake inhibitor; UTI = urinary tract infection.
Adapted from Resnick NM, Tadic SD, Yalla SV. Geriatric incontinence and voiding dysfunction. In: Wein AJ, Novick AC, Partin AW, et al, eds. *Campbell-Walsh Urology*, 10th ed. St. Louis: Elsevier; 2012.

insufficient urethral support plus some degree of sphincter weakness. Obese women are more likely to progress to mixed incontinence over time.[7] Stress incontinence is rare in men but can result from sphincter damage following radical, but not transurethral, prostatectomy.

Urethral Obstruction

Urethral obstruction is the second most common cause of established incontinence in older men, although most obstructed men are not incontinent. When obstruction is associated with incontinence, it usually presents as urge incontinence owing to the associated detrusor overactivity; overflow incontinence is uncommon. Outlet obstruction is rare in women but may result from a bladder neck suspension or from urethral kinking associated with a large cystocele.

Detrusor Underactivity

Detrusor underactivity is usually idiopathic. When it causes incontinence, it is associated with overflow incontinence (<10% of incontinence).

Damaged Innervation

Damage to lower urinary tract innervation can cause several types of dysfunction. A brain lesion may cause detrusor overactivity. A spinal cord lesion (Chapters 175 and 369) above the sacral level can cause both detrusor overactivity and detrusor-sphincter dyssynergia, a condition in which the sphincter contracts rather than relaxes during detrusor contraction; the result can be severe outlet obstruction and hydronephrosis. A spinal cord lesion below the sacral level can cause detrusor underactivity, sphincter weakness, or both. Peripheral and autonomic nerve damage can cause still additional problems, such as decreased bladder emptying and sensation in postural tachycardia syndrome.[8] Thus, because *neurogenic bladder* is such a nonspecific term, it is preferable to refer to the specific dysfunction causing incontinence.

Causes of Incontinence Unrelated to the Lower Urinary Tract (Functional Incontinence)

"Functional" incontinence, which is often cited as a distinct type of geriatric incontinence and attributed to deficits of cognition and mobility, implies that urinary tract function is normal. However, normal urinary tract function is the exception, even in continent elderly people, and is rarely observed in incontinent elderly people. Moreover, incontinence is not inevitable, even with dementia or immobility. Among the most severely demented institutionalized residents, nearly 20% are continent; among those who can transfer from a bed to a chair, nearly half are continent. Functionally impaired individuals also are the most likely to suffer from factors that cause transient incontinence, and a diagnosis of functional incontinence may result in failure to detect these reversible causes. Finally, if functionally impaired individuals also have urethral obstruction or stress incontinence, they may benefit from targeted therapy. Nonetheless, functional impairment often contributes to incontinence, and addressing its causes and those of transient incontinence may ameliorate incontinence sufficiently to obviate the need for further investigation.

CLINICAL MANIFESTATIONS

The manifestations of transient incontinence depend on the underlying condition. Occasionally, patients present with incontinence that is more difficult to characterize clinically without further testing.

Detrusor Overactivity

Detrusor overactivity usually manifests as *urge incontinence*, characterized by leakage that follows the *abrupt* onset or intensification of a desire to void and the leakage of a moderate to large amount of urine. Urinary frequency (>8 voids/day) and nocturia are also frequently present. Some patients with detrusor overactivity may present with precipitant leakage without urgency symptoms.

Detrusor overactivity exists as two subsets in elderly people: one in which contractile function is preserved and one in which it is impaired. The latter condition, termed *detrusor hyperactivity with impaired contractility*, has several implications. First, because the bladder is weak, these patients may develop urinary retention, which can mimic that seen in patients with outlet obstruction and detrusor underactivity. Second, even in the absence of retention, detrusor hyperactivity with impaired contractility mimics other lower urinary tract causes of incontinence. For instance, if the involuntary detrusor contraction occurs coincident with a stress maneuver and if the weak contraction is not detected, detrusor hyperactivity with impaired contractility will be misdiagnosed as stress incontinence. Alternatively, because detrusor hyperactivity with impaired contractility may be associated with urinary urgency, frequency, weak flow rate, elevated residual urine (e.g., >150 mL), and bladder trabeculation, in men, it may mimic prostatic obstruction. Third, use of a bladder relaxant for detrusor hyperactivity with impaired contractility may result in urinary retention owing to bladder weakness, thereby requiring a lower dose or an alternative therapeutic approach.

Stress Incontinence and Mixed Incontinence

Stress incontinence is leakage that coincides *instantaneously* with both the onset and cessation of a cough or other cause of increased abdominal pressure; nocturnal leakage is rare. Some women report both urge and stress incontinence, termed *mixed incontinence*. To plan treatment, it is useful to determine which component is the most bothersome. In men with sphincter damage following radical prostatectomy, leakage resembles the intermittent drip of a leaky faucet.

DIAGNOSIS

Older persons in particular should be screened for incontinence. In addition to a targeted clinical evaluation (Table 115-2),[9,10] a bladder diary can provide diagnostic clues and guide therapy (E-Fig. 115-1). For example, incontinence occurring only between 8 AM and noon may be caused by a morning loop diuretic. Incontinence that occurs at night in a demented man with heart failure, but not during a 4-hour nap in his wheelchair, is likely due to nocturnal diuresis associated with his heart failure and not to dementia, impaired mobility, or prostatic obstruction. A woman with volume-dependent stress incontinence may leak only on the way to void after a full night's sleep, when her bladder contains more than 400 mL—more than it ever does during her continent waking hours.

Because urinary retention is difficult to detect by examination and can affect diagnosis and therapy, the postvoid residual volume usually should be determined, except in a middle-aged woman who desires only behavioral therapy for a classic presentation of stress incontinence.[11,12] Urodynamic testing is generally recommended only when diagnostic certainty is required or before nonroutine surgery (not required prior to most surgery for uncomplicated stress incontinence) or if there is evidence of a serious underlying cause of the incontinence, such as a brain or spinal cord lesion, or hydronephrosis. Urodynamic evaluation comprises a battery of tests designed to assess the lower urinary tract during the filling and voiding phases of micturition. The selection among tests depends on the clinical setting and question to be answered; for instance, measuring detrusor pressure and urine flow during voiding can determine whether urethral obstruction is present, whereas monitoring bladder and urethral pressures during the filling phase and with coughing may be helpful for patients with an atypical presentation of mixed incontinence.

TABLE 115-2 CLINICAL EVALUATION OF URINARY INCONTINENCE

HISTORY
Symptom type (urge, stress, overflow, or mixed)
Incontinence frequency, severity, and duration
Pattern (diurnal, nocturnal or both; also, e.g., after taking medications)
Precipitants
Associated symptoms (straining to void, incomplete emptying, dysuria, hematuria, suprapubic/perineal discomfort or numbness)
Alteration in bowel habit/sexual function (because of proximity to the bladder and shared innervation)
Other relevant factors (cancer, acute illness, neurologic disease, pelvic or lower urinary tract surgery/radiation therapy
Medications, including nonprescription agents (see Table 115-1)
PHYSICAL EXAMINATION
General examination to identify and/or assess relevant medical conditions (e.g., heart failure, peripheral edema)
Brief assessment of cognitive and physical function (e.g., MiniCog, Get Up and Go [see Chapters 361 and 371])
If stress incontinence is suspected, determine whether leakage *coincides* with the onset *and* cessation of a single, forceful cough
Palpate for bladder distention after voiding
Pelvic examination to detect atrophic vaginitis, lichen sclerosis, mass, prolapse (if beyond the vagina, there is increased risk for urinary retention)
Rectal examination for skin irritation, resting tone and voluntary control of anal sphincter, prostate nodule; fecal impaction (*note:* prostate size correlates poorly with presence of urethral obstruction)
Neurologic examination, especially mental status and elemental examination, including sacral reflexes and perineal sensation
INITIAL INVESTIGATION
Bladder diary (see E-Fig. 115-1)
Metabolic survey (electrolytes, calcium, glucose, and urea nitrogen as appropriate)
Measure postvoid residual volume, by portable ultrasound if available
Urinalysis to detect sterile hematuria or infection; culture if new-onset or worsening incontinence
Renal ultrasound to detect hydronephrosis in men whose postvoid residual volume urine exceeds about 200 mL
Urine cytology for patients with hematuria, pain, or unexplained new-onset or worsening incontinence
Uroflowmetry for men in whom urethral obstruction is suspected
Cystoscopy for patients with hematuria, suspicion of lower urinary tract pathology (e.g., bladder fistula, stone, or tumor; urethral diverticulum), or need for lower urinary tract surgery

Adapted from Resnick NM, Yalla SV. Management of urinary incontinence in the elderly. *N Engl J Med.* 1985;313:800-805.

TREATMENT

Optimal therapy requires a multifactorial approach (Table 115-3), including treatment of any associated causes, underlying medical conditions, functional impairments, fluid intake, and the urinary tract abnormality itself.[13] Treatment of the precipitants alone may be sufficient to restore continence, even if there is coexisting urinary tract dysfunction. For example, a flare of hip arthritis in a woman with age-related detrusor overactivity may decrease mobility sufficiently to convert her urinary urgency into incontinence. Treatment of the arthritis, rather than the involuntary detrusor contractions, will not only restore continence but also lessen pain and improve mobility. Because of their frequency, reversibility, and association with morbidity beyond incontinence, any transient causes (see Table 115-1) should be addressed first.

Although pads and diapers have a role, they remain an adjunct to more specific therapy. Urinary catheters should rarely be used for chronic incontinence because of the high risk of urinary tract infection (Chapter 263).

Lifestyle Interventions

Lifestyle interventions include education, self-monitoring with a bladder diary, adjustment of fluid and caffeine intake, weight loss for overweight women with stress incontinence, smoking cessation, and use of aids (e.g., a bedside urinal).[A1] Phone-based apps also show promise for the self-management of urge and mixed incontinence.[A2] Helpful online resources are available for patients.[14–16]

Behavioral Therapy

Behavioral therapy[17] includes pelvic muscle exercises and bladder retraining (progressively increasing voiding intervals, strategies to cope with urgency).[A3] For each option, group education is an effective alternative to individual instruction.[A4]

For stress incontinence, pelvic muscle exercises are effective but less so than surgery,[A5] and combining the two does not enhance efficacy.[A6] Acupuncture[A7] and pessaries[18] can also be effective.

For urge incontinence, behavioral therapy is as effective as pharmacotherapy. However, combining the two is more effective than either alone[A8] because neither therapy generally abolishes involuntary bladder contractions.

For institutionalized patients who are cognitively impaired but can state their name and are partly mobile, regular daytime reminders to void ("prompted voiding") have proved effective for daytime incontinence. Wet checks and protective garments are appropriate for the others.[A9]

Pharmacotherapy

Currently approved drugs have not proved effective for stress incontinence or overflow incontinence. For urge incontinence, several bladder relaxants are modestly and equally effective (Table 115-4), including in vulnerable older patients.[A10] All anticholinergic agents can cause dry mouth, constipation, and visual blurring, with some variation among agents. Their use can also be associated with short- and long-term cognitive impairment, although this complication appears to be very uncommon.[19] Nevertheless, each may be well tolerated, even in cognitively impaired elderly patients, when they are prescribed properly and cognitive status is monitored. Patients who are taking a cholinesterase inhibitor, which can cause incontinence, have three options: delay intervention because the incontinence will often subside, reconsider the benefits of continued cholinesterase treatment, or consider adding a non-anticholinergic agent.

The choice among these drugs may also depend on other considerations. For instance, immediate-release oxybutynin has the quickest onset of action, thereby making it an inexpensive and effective choice for patients who need control at predictable times. Other drugs, although more expensive, can be used less often and can be better tolerated for daily use.

The β_3-adrenergic agonists mirabegron[A11] and vibegron have efficacy similar to the anticholinergic agents and may be preferable when there is concern for anticholinergic or cognitive adverse effects. If needed, mirabegron also may be combined with an anticholinergic for improved efficacy. Desmopressin should be avoided in older persons due to the risk of severe hyponatremia.

Ultimately, the choice of medication should depend on ease of use, cost, and avoidance of adverse effects in an individual patient. Regardless of the drug selected, the key is to begin with a low dose and increase it slowly, realizing that full benefit may not apparent be for 2 to 3 months and that adverse effects may offset the benefit. With such titration, urge incontinence can be controlled in about one third of patients and substantially improved in another one third. Success rates are lower in patients with moderate-severe dementia.

For urinary incontinence in the setting of atrophic vaginitis, a 3- to 12-month course of topical estrogen can be useful, although oral estrogen can worsen incontinence.[A12]

Surgical Procedures

Stress Incontinence

For women with stress incontinence or stress-predominant mixed incontinence, surgery has proved effective and relatively durable at all ages. Periurethral bulking injection can help frail women or those with mild stress incontinence, but it does not generally restore continence.[20] However, urethral sling and mid-urethral tape suspension procedures can cure most women for at least 5 years. For women with more complex stress incontinence and women who have adequate cognitive and functional capacity, an artificial sphincter can be moderately effective, although experience is still limited.

Urge Incontinence

For urge incontinence, surgical intervention, including neuromodulation,[21] tibial nerve stimulation,[22] and injections of onabotulinum toxin,[A13] are third-line agents. Limited available data suggest that their efficacy may be only modestly better than the efficacy of pharmacotherapy and that older patients may not fare as well as younger ones. Older patients treated with onabotulinum toxin also are more likely to develop urinary retention and urinary tract infections.

Issues Specific to Men

Apart from atrophic vaginitis, the transient causes of incontinence in men are the same as in women. However, owing to the frequency of prostate enlargement, urinary retention occurs more often in the setting of conditions that suppress detrusor contractility (e.g., fecal impaction) or use of drugs such as anticholinergics, α-adrenergic agonists, and opiates. Urge incontinence is equally common in men as in women, but it may be associated with an obstructive prostate. Therapeutic considerations for incontinence related to prostatic hypertrophy include α-adrenergic agonists and 5-α reductase inhibitors, as well as prostate surgery (see Table 115-3, Fig. 114-3, and Table 114-1). Antimuscarinics and mirabegron (both used in combination with an α-blocker) are also helpful. Botulinum toxin may be useful as well, but it appears to be less effective than in women.[A14] Stress incontinence is rare in men unless they have undergone radical (not transurethral) prostatectomy for carcinoma.[23] In such cases, anti-incontinence surgery, such as a male sling operation or creation of an artificial urinary sphincter, is moderately successful[A15] but is usually reserved for incontinence that is moderate to severe and persists for more than a year in men who otherwise have a good prognosis. As in women, overflow incontinence is uncommon but, when present, in men it is more likely due to obstruction.

PREVENTION

Data suggest that group- or community-based education and behavioral modification programs may be helpful in older women. Weight loss can reduce the risk for stress incontinence.[24]

TABLE 115-3 STEPWISE APPROACH TO TREATMENT OF URINARY INCONTINENCE*

CONDITION	CLINICAL TYPE OF INCONTINENCE†	TREATMENT
Detrusor overactivity with normal contractility	Urge	1. Bladder retraining or prompted voiding regimens. 2. ± Bladder relaxant medication if needed and not contraindicated (see Table 115-4). If treatment fails, consider posterior tibial neurostimulation, sacral neuromodulation, or intradetrusor injection of onabotulinumtoxinA. 3. Indwelling catheterization alone is often unhelpful because detrusor spasms often increase, leading to leakage around the catheter. 4. In selected cases, induce urinary retention pharmacologically and add intermittent or indwelling catheterization.‡
Detrusor hyperactivity with impaired contractility	Urge§	1. If bladder empties adequately, behavioral methods (as above) ± bladder relaxant medication (low doses; especially feasible if sphincter incompetence coexists). 2. If residual urine >150 mL, augmented voiding techniques¶ or intermittent catheterization (± bladder relaxant medication). If neither is feasible, undergarment or indwelling catheter.‡ 3. In selected cases, induce urinary retention pharmacologically and add intermittent or indwelling catheterization.‡
Stress incontinence	Stress	1. Conservative methods (weight loss if obese; treatment of cough or atrophic vaginitis; physical maneuvers to prevent leakage [e.g., tighten pelvic muscles before cough, cross legs]; occasionally, use of tampon or pessary is helpful). 2. If leakage threshold ≥150 mL identified, adjust fluid excretion and voiding intervals appropriately. 3. Pelvic muscle exercises ± biofeedback/weighted intravaginal cones; must continue indefinitely. 4. Surgery (sling, artificial sphincter, periurethral bulking injections).
Urethral obstruction (see Chapter 114)	Urge/overflow‖	1. Conservative methods (including adjustment of fluid excretion, bladder retraining/prompted voiding) if hydronephrosis, recurrent symptomatic UTI, and hematuria have been excluded. 2. α-Adrenergic antagonist (α_{1a} specific may be better tolerated in patients with orthostatic hypotension). 3. Also consider adding a bladder relaxant if detrusor overactivity coexists, postvoid residual volume is small, and surgery is not desired/feasible; *monitor postvoid residual volume!* 4. 5-α Reductase inhibitor, if not contraindicated and the patient either prefers it or is not a surgical candidate; clinical benefit takes months. 5. Surgery (incision, prostatectomy) is an effective alternative before or after these steps.
Underactive detrusor	Overflow	1. Decompress for at least several days (the larger the postvoid residual volume, the longer should be the decompression [up to a month]) and then perform a voiding trial. 2. Exclude urethral obstruction if this has not already been done. 3. If cannot void or if postvoid residual volume remains large, try augmented voiding techniques¶ ± α-adrenergic antagonist but only if some voiding possible; bethanechol *rarely* useful. 4. If fails or voiding is not possible, intermittent or indwelling catheterization.‡

*These treatments should be initiated only after adequate toilet access has been ensured, contributing conditions have been treated (e.g., atrophic vaginitis, UTI, fecal impaction, heart failure), fluid management has been optimized, and unnecessary or exacerbating medications have been addressed. For additional details, see text.

†*Urge:* leakage in the absence of stress maneuvers and urinary retention, usually preceded by *abrupt* onset or intensification of the need to void; stress: leakage that coincides instantaneously with stress maneuvers, in the absence of urinary retention or detrusor contraction; overflow: frequent leakage of small amounts associated with urinary retention.

‡UTI prophylaxis can be used for recurrent symptomatic UTIs but only if catheter is not indwelling.

§May also mimic stress or overflow incontinence.

‖Also can cause postvoid "dribbling" alone, which is treated conservatively (e.g., by sitting to void and allowing more time, "double voiding," and in men by gently "milking" the urethra after voiding).

¶Augmented voiding techniques include Credé (application of suprapubic pressure) and Valsalva (straining) maneuvers and double voiding. They should be performed only after voiding has begun.

UTI = urinary tract infection.

Adapted and updated from Resnick NM. Voiding dysfunction and urinary incontinence. In: Beck JC, ed. *Geriatric Review Syllabus.* New York: American Geriatrics Society; 2011:141-154.

TABLE 115-4 BLADDER RELAXANT AGENTS FOR URGE INCONTINENCE

- Anticholinergic
  - Oxybutynin IR, 7.5-20 mg daily (2.5-5 mg three or four times daily; doses >2.5 mg four times daily can be problematic and rarely helpful); oxybutynin XL, 5-30 mg once daily; oxybutynin patch (3.9 mg/day) twice weekly; oxybutynin 10% gel (1 g topically once per day)
  - Tolterodine, 1-2 mg twice daily; tolterodine LA, 4 mg once daily
  - Darifenacin, 7.5-15 mg once daily
  - Solifenacin, 5-10 mg once daily
  - Trospium, 20 mg daily to twice daily; 60 mg (extended release) once daily
  - Fesoterodine, 4-8 mg once daily
- β_3-Adrenergic agonist
  - Mirabegron, 25-50 mg once daily
  - Vibegron 75 mg daily

PROGNOSIS

Incontinence is associated with sexual dysfunction and other adverse effects on quality of life.[25] Limited data suggest that incontinence progresses in about one third of patients and remits in about 10 to 15%, although it is unclear how much of the remission reflects intervention or improvement in functional or medical status.

GENERAL REFERENCES

For the General References and other additional features, please visit Elsevier eBooks+ at https://ebooks.health.elsevier.com.

Grade A References

A1. Kilpatrick KA, Paton P, Subbarayan S, et al. Non-pharmacological, non-surgical interventions for urinary incontinence in older persons: a systematic review of systematic reviews. The SENATOR project ONTOP series. *Maturitas*. 2020;133:42-48.

A2. Wadensten T, Nyström E, Nord A, et al. App-based self-management of urgency and mixed urinary incontinence in women: one-year follow-up. *Neurourol Urodyn*. 2022;41:945-954.

A3. Dumoulin C, Cacciari LP, Hay-Smith EJC. Pelvic floor muscle training versus no treatment, or inactive control treatments, for urinary incontinence in women. *Cochrane Database Syst Rev*. 2018;10:CD005654.

A4. Dumoulin C, Morin M, Danieli C, et al. Group-based vs individual pelvic floor muscle training to treat urinary incontinence in older women: a randomized clinical trial. *JAMA Intern Med*. 2020;180:1284-1293.

A5. Balk EM, Rofeberg VN, Adam GP, et al. Pharmacologic and nonpharmacologic treatments for urinary incontinence in women: a systematic review and network meta-analysis of clinical outcomes. *Ann Intern Med*. 2019;170:465-479.

A6. Sung VW, Borello-France D, Newman DK, et al. Effect of behavioral and pelvic floor muscle therapy combined with surgery vs surgery alone on incontinence symptoms among women with mixed urinary incontinence: the ESTEEM randomized clinical trial. *JAMA*. 2019;322:1066-1076.

A7. Liu Z, Liu Y, Xu H, et al. Effect of electroacupuncture on urinary leakage among women with stress urinary incontinence: a randomized clinical trial. *JAMA*. 2017;317:2493-2501.

A8. Burgio KL, Krause SR, Johnson TM, 2nd, et al. Effectiveness of combined behavioral and drug therapy for overactive bladder symptoms in men: a randomized controlled clinical trial. *JAMA Intern Med*. 2020;180:411-419.

A9. Roe B, Flanagan L, Maden M. Systematic review of systematic reviews for the management of urinary incontinence and promotion of continence using conservative behavioural approaches in older people in care homes. *J Adv Nurs*. 2015;71:1464-1483.

A10. Wagg A, Staskin D, Engel E, et al. Efficacy, safety, and tolerability of mirabegron in patients aged > 65yr with overactive bladder wet: a phase IV, double-blind, randomized, placebo-controlled study (PILLAR). *Eur Urol*. 2020;77:211-220.

A11. Drake MJ, Chapple C, Esen AA, et al. Efficacy and safety of mirabegron add-on therapy to solifenacin in incontinent overactive bladder patients with an inadequate response to initial 4-week solifenacin monotherapy: a randomised double-blind multicentre phase 3b study (BESIDE). *Eur Urol*. 2016;70:136-145.

A12. Rahn DD, Ward RM, Sanses TV, et al. Vaginal estrogen use in postmenopausal women with pelvic floor disorders: systematic review and practice guidelines. *Int Urogynecol J*. 2015;26:3-13.

A13. Ginsberg DA, Drake MJ, Kaufmann A, et al. Long-term treatment with onabotulinumtoxina results in consistent, durable improvements in health related quality of life in patients with overactive bladder. *J Urol*. 2017;198:897-904.

A14. De Nunzio C, Brucker N, Bschleipfer T, et al. Beyond antimuscarinics: a review of pharmacological and interventional options for overactive bladder management in men. *Eur Urol*. 2021;79:492-504.

A15. Abrams P, Constable LD, Cooper D, et al. Outcomes of a noninferiority randomised controlled trial of surgery for men with urodynamic stress incontinence after prostate surgery (MASTER). *Eur Urol*. 2021;79:812-823.

116 CHRONIC KIDNEY DISEASE

ANDREW S. LEVEY AND MARK J. SARNAK

Chronic kidney disease represents a heterogeneous group of disorders that become increasingly common as the population ages. Diabetes (Chapter 210), hypertension (Chapter 64), and autoimmune glomerular diseases (Chapter 107) are the most common causes of chronic kidney disease worldwide, but systemic infections, drug toxicity, and environmental exposures are important causes in selected populations. Irrespective of the cause, many kidney diseases follow a progressive course and cause complications in virtually every organ system. In patients in whom the rate of disease progression is fast or life expectancy is long, the disease may culminate in kidney failure that leads to uremia and death.

DEFINITION

Chronic kidney disease is defined as the presence of either a marker of kidney damage, such as more than 30 mg/day of albuminuria, or a glomerular filtration rate less than 60 mL/min/1.73 m^2 for 3 or more months.[1] The threshold value for albuminuria reflects a more than three-fold elevation above the normal value of 5 to 10 mg/day, whereas the threshold glomerular filtration rate reflects a more than 50% reduction below the normal value of approximately 125 mL/min/1.73 m^2. Irrespective of age, both of these abnormalities are associated with an increased risk of progressive kidney disease, altered metabolism and excretion of many drugs by the kidney, complications, and death (E-Fig. 116-1).[2]

EPIDEMIOLOGY

The prevalence of chronic kidney disease in U.S. adults is approximately 11.5% (Fig. 116-1), including approximately 4.7% of the population that has increased albuminuria with a glomerular filtration rate greater than 60 mL/min/1.73 m^2 (stages G1 and G2) and 6.8% of the population that has a glomerular filtration rate less than 60 mL/min/1.73 m^2 (stages G3 to G5). The glomerular filtration rate declines by an average rate of approximately 1 mL/min/1.73 m^2 per year after about age 40 years, but with a wide range among individuals. The cause of the decline with age is not well understood, but the decline may be due to senescence, kidney disease, or both. Irrespective of cause, 25% of individuals in the United States have a glomerular filtration rate less than 60 mL/min/1.73 m^2 by age 70 years and older.

In the United States, an estimated 800,000 or so individuals, equivalent to about 0.25% of the population, have kidney failure (stage G5) and require kidney replacement therapy with dialysis or transplantation (Chapter 117), and this prevalence has been rising by approximately 20,000 per year due to the growth and aging of the population.[3] The age-adjusted incidence of the initiation of kidney replacement therapy has been declining, however, perhaps related to better and earlier management. Unfortunately, the rising prevalence of obesity may increase incidence of kidney failure in future years because of the earlier onset of diabetes and hypertension.

The worldwide prevalence of kidney disease in adults and children is estimated to be about 9%, or about 700 million people.[4] About 30% of chronic kidney disease is attributed to diabetes. The annual mortality from chronic kidney disease is about 1.2 million owing to kidney failure itself and 1.4 million owing to an increased incidence of cardiovascular disease, thereby representing about 4.6% of total mortality and making it the twelfth leading worldwide cause of death. The disability-adjusted life years lost vary widely among regions of the world (E-Fig. 116-2). The risk for chronic kidney disease is associated with increased susceptibility (e.g., old age, family history, history of acute kidney disease, member of ethnic or racial minority in the United States, reduced nephron mass because of low birthweight or a prior partial or complete nephrectomy), or with exposure to conditions that cause chronic kidney disease, such as diabetes and hypertension [Table 116-1]). Chronic kidney disease is more common in older, male, Black, and Hispanic individuals in the United States.[5]

		Stages of Albuminuria (description and range)		
		A1	A2	A3
		normal to mildly increased	moderately increased	severely increased
		<30 mg/g <3 mg/mmol	30-299 mg/g 3-29 mg/mmol	≥300 mg/g ≥30 mg/mmol
Stages of the Glomerular Filtration Rate (mL/min/1.73m^2)	G1, normal or high, >90	56%	2%	0.4%
	G2, mildly decreased, 60-89	33%	2%	0.3%
	G3, mildly to moderately decreased, 45-59	4%	0.8%	0.2%
	G3b, moderately to severely decreased, 30-44	1.0%	0.4%	0.2%
	G4, severely decreased, 15-29	0.2%	0.1%	0.1%
	G5, kidney failure, <15	0%	0%	0.1%

FIGURE 116-1. Approximate percentage of the U.S. population by glomerular filtration rate and albuminuria. For population studies, chronic kidney disease is generally defined as albuminuria greater than 30 mg/day or a decreased glomerular filtration rate (<60 mL/min/1.73 m^2). The prevalence of chronic kidney disease in U.S. adults is 11.5%, which is the rounded sum of all shaded cells. Albuminuria stages A$_2$ and A$_3$ correspond to microalbuminuria and macroalbuminuria, respectively. Albuminuria stage A3 includes nephrotic-range albuminuria (greater than about 2000 mg/day). Albuminuria (in mg/day) equals albuminuria (in mg/g) if the urinary creatinine excretion equals 1.0 g/day. For albuminuria: 1.0 mg/g = 0.113 mg/mmol. GFR = glomerular filtration rate. Prognosis is color coded: white = low risk; yellow = moderately increased risk; orange = high risk; red = very high risk. (Modified from Kidney Disease: Improving Global Outcomes [KDIGO]. KDIGO 2012 clinical practice guideline for the evaluation and management of chronic kidney disease. *Kidney Int Suppl.* 2013;3:1-150 and based on data from the National Health and Nutrition Examination Survey [NHANES] 1999-2006.)

Causes of kidney disease are classified according to the site of pathologic findings (e.g., glomerular, tubulointerstitial, vascular, and cystic and congenital diseases that affect multiple sites), as well as the presence or absence of systemic disease affecting the kidney. Among older adults, diabetes and hypertension are the most common causes in Europe and North America, whereas congenital anomalies of the kidney and urinary tract (Chapter 113) and glomerular diseases (Chapter 107) are more common in children and young adults. Autoimmune glomerular diseases are also common in East Asia (Chapter 107). Chronic infections causing glomerular and interstitial diseases are more common in low- and middle-income nations. Tubulointerstitial diseases are known to be endemic in certain areas due to exposure to aristolochic acid, heavy metals, fine particulate matter, or extremes of heat and agricultural work (Chapter 108). An important risk factor in people of West African ancestry is inheritance of two of the G1 or G2 variants of *APOL1*, likely reflective of a selective advantage from resistance to *Trypanosoma brucei*,[6] which confers an approximately four-fold greater risk of kidney failure.

PATHOBIOLOGY

Irrespective of the initial mechanism, most kidney diseases progress through a final common pathway that culminates in pathologic features of glomerular, interstitial, and vascular sclerosis in which tubular atrophy coexists with glomerular and tubular hypertrophy and the formation of cysts. These pathologic changes result in a progressive increase in albuminuria and a decline in the glomerular filtration rate.

In health, proteinuria is minimal because of low permeability of the glomerular capillary wall to high-molecular-weight plasma proteins and the efficient receptor-mediated tubular reabsorption of filtered low-molecular-weight plasma proteins (Fig. 116-2).[7] The normal urine protein excretion rate and albumin excretion rate are generally less than 50 and 10 mg/day, respectively. Proteinuria can be classified by increased glomerular permeability to macromolecules (glomerular; Chapter 107), decreased tubular reabsorption of filtered proteins (tubular; Chapter 108) due to disorders of tubular epithelium; or increased filtered load of low-molecular-weight proteins, such as immunoglobulin light chains. Regardless of the cause, the presence of albumin and other macromolecules in glomerular filtrate may be associated with progressive tubular and interstitial damage, thereby contributing to the subsequent decline in glomerular filtration rate.

Large increases in albuminuria (greater than approximately 2.0 g/day, corresponding to proteinuria above approximately 3.5 g/day) can give rise to nephrotic syndrome (Chapter 107), with a decreased serum albumin level, edema, hypercholesterolemia, and hypercoagulability (Table 116-2). Loss of albumin in the urine lowers plasma oncotic pressure, thereby resulting in redistribution of plasma to the interstitial space, increased renal tubular reabsorption of sodium chloride and water, and retention of extracellular fluid (Chapter 107). Decreased oncotic pressure stimulates increased production of plasma proteins by the liver, including apolipoproteins, thereby leading to hyperlipidemia. The urinary loss of anticoagulant proteins (e.g., antithrombin,

TABLE 116-1 CAUSES OF CHRONIC KIDNEY DISEASE

	EXAMPLES OF SYSTEMIC DISEASES AFFECTING THE KIDNEY	EXAMPLES OF PRIMARY KIDNEY DISEASE (ABSENCE OF SYSTEMIC DISEASES AFFECTING THE KIDNEY)
Glomerular diseases (Chapter 107)	Diabetes (Chapter 210), obesity (Chapter 201), systemic autoimmune diseases (systemic lupus erythematosus [Chapter 245], antineutrophil cytoplasmic antibody–associated vasculitis, cryoglobulinemia, Henoch-Schonlein purpura [Chapter 249], Goodpasture syndrome), systemic infections (bacterial endocarditis or endovascular infection [Chapter 47], human immunodeficiency virus [Chapter 359], hepatitis B virus, hepatitis C virus [Chapter 135], schistosomiasis [Chapter 326]), drugs (vascular endothelial growth factor inhibitors, gold, penicillamine, pamidronate), neoplasia (light chain deposition disease, amyloidosis [Chapter 174])	Diffuse, focal, or crescentic proliferative glomerulonephritis (postinfectious, immunoglobulin A nephropathy, complement factor 3 glomerular nephritis, anti–glomerular basement membrane nephritis); focal and segmental glomerulosclerosis, membranous nephropathy, minimal change disease, inherited podocytopathies
Tubulointerstitial diseases (Chapter 108)	Systemic infections (*Legionella* [Chapter 290], leptospirosis, streptococci [Chapter 268]), autoimmune (acute interstitial nephritis, tubulointerstitial nephritis, and uveitis [Chapter 108], systemic lupus erythematosus [Chapter 245], Sjogren syndrome [Chapter 247], immunoglobulin G4 interstitial nephritis), sarcoidosis (Chapter 83), drugs (nonsteroidal anti-inflammatory drugs, iodinated contrast, calcineurin inhibitors, aminoglycoside antibiotics, β-lactam antibiotics, vancomycin, tenofovir, amphotericin, cis-platinum, ifosfamide), metabolic disorders (hyperuricemia due to tumor lysis, hypokalemia [Chapter 103], hypercalcemia [Chapter 227]), environmental toxins (heavy metals, aristolochic acid; Chapter 20), neoplasia (e.g., multiple myeloma; Chapter 173)	Urinary tract infections (bacteria, *Mycobacteria*, schistosomiasis), stones, obstruction, inherited tubulointerstitial diseases (autosomal dominant [medullary cystic disease], autosomal recessive [nephronophthisis])
Vascular diseases	Atherosclerosis (Chapter 65), hypertension (Chapter 64), ischemia (Chapter 110), cholesterol emboli (Chapter 66), thrombotic microangiopathy (hemolytic uremic syndrome [Chapter 158], thrombotic thrombocytopenic purpura [Chapter 158]), systemic sclerosis (Chapter 246)	Fibromuscular dysplasia, radiation
Cystic and congenital diseases	Polycystic kidney disease (Chapter 112), Alport syndrome, Fabry disease (Chapter 192)	Congenital anomalies of the kidney and urinary tract (CAKUT)

Genetic diseases are not considered separately because some diseases in each category are now recognized as having genetic determinants.
Adapted from Kidney Disease: Improving Global Outcomes (KDIGO). KDIGO 2012 clinical practice guideline for the evaluation and management of chronic kidney disease. *Kidney Int Suppl.* 2013;3:1-150.

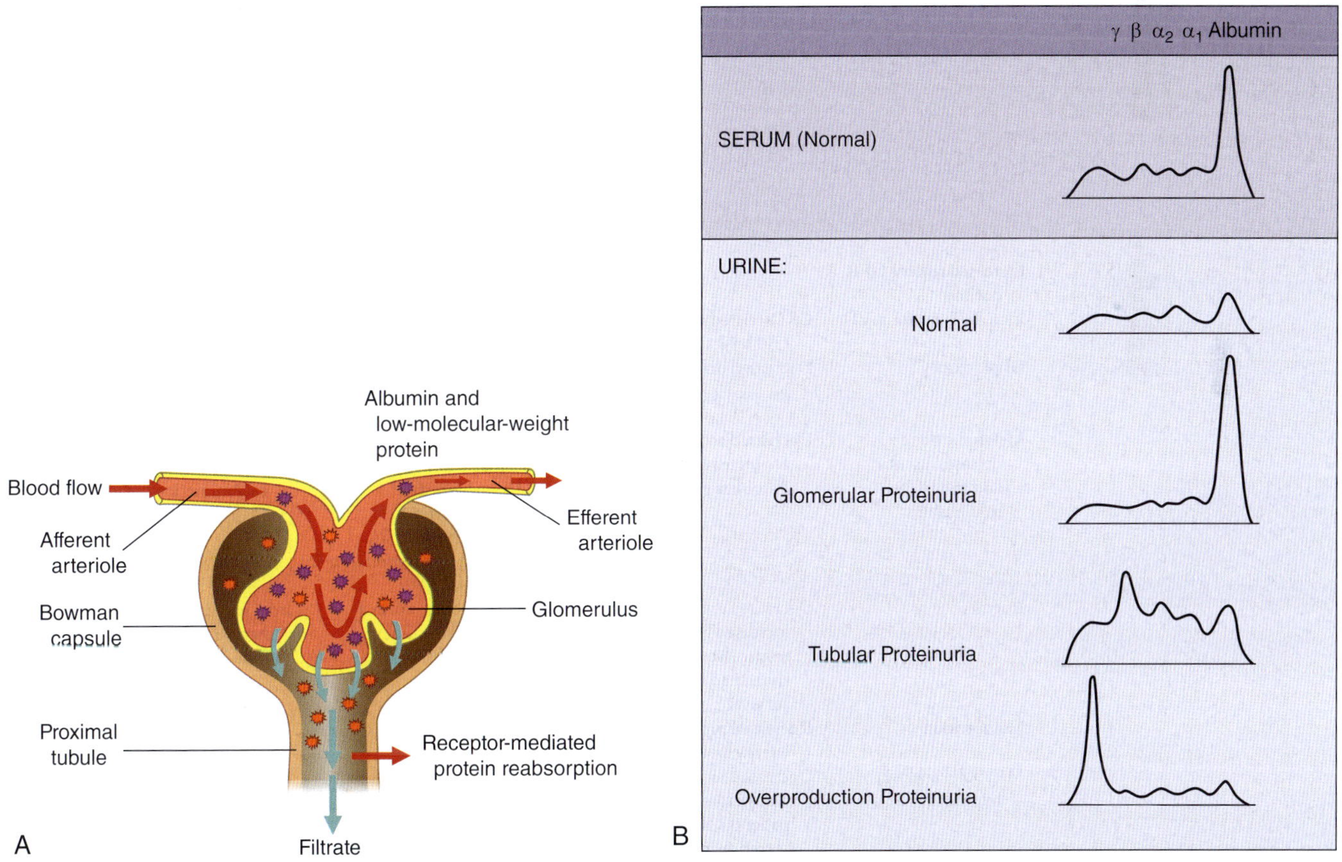

FIGURE 116-2. **Pathophysiology of proteinuria. A,** Glomerular filtration barrier to macromolecules (albumin) and tubular reabsorption of low-molecular-weight proteins. **B,** Normal serum protein electrophoresis and patterns of proteinuria. **A,** In health, proteinuria is minimal because of the low permeability of glomerular capillary wall to high-molecular-weight serum proteins, such as albumin (*purple symbols*, approximately 65,000 daltons) and gamma globulins (approximately 150,000 daltons), as well as the efficient receptor-mediated tubular reabsorption of filtered low-molecular-weight serum proteins, such as α-1, α-2, and β-globulins (e.g., β-2 microglobulin, cystatin C, β-trace protein, and immunoglobulin light chains; *orange symbols*, approximately 10,000 to 20,000 daltons). Other proteins in normal urine include proteins secreted by the tubule, such as uromodulin (the most abundant protein in normal urine and present in aggregates of up to several million daltons), and from the lower urinary and genital tracts. **B,** Normal serum protein electrophoresis showing separate peaks for albumin and globulins (α-1, α-2, β, and γ), according to molecular weight and charge (albumin is most anionic). Normal urine protein electrophoresis shows minimal amounts of all serum proteins. Glomerular proteinuria shows predominantly albumin; tubular proteinuria shows predominantly α-1, α-2, and β-globulins; and overproduction proteinuria shows light-chain immunoglobulins. These patterns can also be detected by measurement of urinary albumin and total protein, specific low-molecular-weight serum protein or light chains, and immunofixation. (From Stevens LA, Lafayette LA, Perrone RD, et al. Laboratory evaluation of kidney disease. In: RW Schrier, ed. *Diseases of the Kidney and Urinary Tract*. Philadelphia: Lippincott Williams & Wilkins; 2007:299-336.)

TABLE 116-2 CHRONIC KIDNEY DISEASE CLINICAL DISORDERS, MECHANISM, MANIFESTATIONS, AND MANAGEMENT (CLINICAL ACTION PLAN) BY GLOMERULAR FILTRATION RATE AND ALBUMINURIA STAGES

ALBUMINURIA STAGE	ALBUMIN EXCRETION RATE (mg/24 h) AND APPROXIMATELY EQUIVALENT ALBUMIN TO CREATININE RATIO (mg/g)*	DISORDER	MECHANISM	MANIFESTATIONS	MANAGEMENT (CLINICAL ACTION PLAN)*
A1	<30				Diagnose and treat the cause Treat comorbid conditions Evaluate for reversible CKD risk factors Start measures to slow CKD progression and reduce CVD risk (lifestyle and diet, blood pressure control, glycemic control in diabetes, lipid-lowering and antithrombotic therapy if indicated)
A2	30-299	Increased risk for GFR decline	Tubulointerstitial damage from uptake of filtered macromolecules	CKD progression	ACE inhibitors or angiotensin receptor blockers; SGLT2 inhibitors; mineralocorticoid-receptor antagonists and GLP1 agonists in diabetes
		Increased risk for CVD	Pro-inflammatory and prothrombotic state	Clinical CVD	
A3	≥300	Nephrotic syndrome if albumin to creatinine ratio above about 2000 or protein to creatinine ratio above about 3500	Low serum oncotic pressure; increased hepatic synthesis of lipoproteins; loss of serum anticoagulant proteins; kidney edema	Low serum albumin (<3.5 g/dL), edema, hyperlipidemia, DVT, acute GFR decline	Diuretics, statins, anticoagulants, albumin infusions as necessary for refractory edema or acute GFR decline

GFR STAGE	GFR (mL/min/1.73 m^2)	DISORDER	MECHANISM	MANIFESTATIONS	MANAGEMENT (CLINICAL ACTION PLAN)*
G1	>90				Diagnose and treat the cause Treat comorbid conditions Evaluate for reversible CKD risk factors Start measures to slow CKD progression and reduce CVD risk (lifestyle and diet, blood pressure control, glycemic control in diabetes, lipid-lowering and antithrombotic therapy if indicated)
G2	60-89				Estimate progression
G3a[†] G3b[†]	45-59 30-44	Increased risk for GFR decline			Consider alkali therapy, dietary protein restriction
		Increased risk for CVD	CKD-related nontraditional CVD risk factors	Hypertension, heart failure, myocardial ischemia, stroke	Consider intensifying CVD risk factor management
		Drug toxicity	Decreased drug excretion	Increased serum drug concentrations, side effects, drug-drug interactions	Adjust medication dosages as indicated
		Metabolic bone disease, vascular and soft tissue calcification	Decreased active vitamin D_3, increased PTH and fibroblast growth factor 23	High serum phosphorus, normal or low serum calcium, increased bone reabsorption (osteitis fibrosa cystica), decreased bone formation (osteomalacia)	Dietary phosphate restriction, phosphate-binding agents, calcitriol, calcimimetics
		Anemia	Decreased erythropoietin, increased hepcidin, relative iron deficiency, shortened red blood cell survival	Low hemoglobin, normal MCV, low reticulocyte count	Iron, erythropoietin-stimulating agents, hypoxia inducible factor stabilizers, red blood cell transfusions
		Malnutrition	Decreased protein and energy intake	Weight loss, low serum albumin	Referral to registered dietitian nutritionist, appropriate protein intake
		Metabolic acidosis, hyperkalemia	Decreased renin and aldosterone (in some patients), decreased acid secretion, decreased potassium secretion	Low serum bicarbonate, high or normal serum anion gap, high serum potassium	Alkali therapy, dietary potassium restriction, potassium-binding agents
		Sexual and reproductive disorders	Increased prolactin	Amenorrhea, menorrhagia, impotence, oligospermia, galactorrhea	
G4	15-29			Many of the disorders noted earlier (for example, hypertension, 75%; anemia, 30%; hyperphosphatemia, 20%)	Prepare for kidney replacement therapy (transplantation and/or dialysis) or comprehensive conservative treatment

TABLE 116-2 CHRONIC KIDNEY DISEASE CLINICAL DISORDERS, MECHANISM, MANIFESTATIONS, AND MANAGEMENT (CLINICAL ACTION PLAN) BY GLOMERULAR FILTRATION RATE AND ALBUMINURIA STAGES—cont'd

GFR STAGE	GFR (mL/min/1.73 m²)	DISORDER	MECHANISM	MANIFESTATIONS	MANAGEMENT (CLINICAL ACTION PLAN)*
G5	<15	Symptoms of uremia	Retention of toxic solutes	Fatigue, anorexia, nausea, vomiting, peripheral neuropathy, pruritus, serositis (pericardial and pleural effusions), encephalopathy, increased risk for infections, coagulopathy with gastrointestinal bleeding More of the disorders noted earlier (for example, hypertension, 75%; anemia, 50%; hyperphosphatemia, 30%)	If symptoms of uremia are present, start kidney replacement therapy or comprehensive conservative treatment Treat symptoms

*Clinical action plan is cumulative, meaning that the plan for later stages (lower GFR and higher albuminuria) includes the plan from earlier stages (higher GFR and lower albuminuria).
†There is wide variability in the level of GFR at which clinical manifestations occur. Manifestations can be detected by laboratory testing at stages G3a to G3b. Treatment is often deferred until stages G3b to G4.
ACEI = angiotensin-converting enzyme inhibitor; ARB = angiotensin II receptor blocker; CKD = chronic kidney disease; CVD = cardiovascular disease; DVT = deep vein thrombosis; GFR = glomerular filtration rate; GLP1 = glucagon-like peptide 1; MCV = mean corpuscular volume; MRA = mineralocorticoid receptor antagonist; PTH = parathyroid hormone; SGLT2 = sodium-glucose transport protein 2.

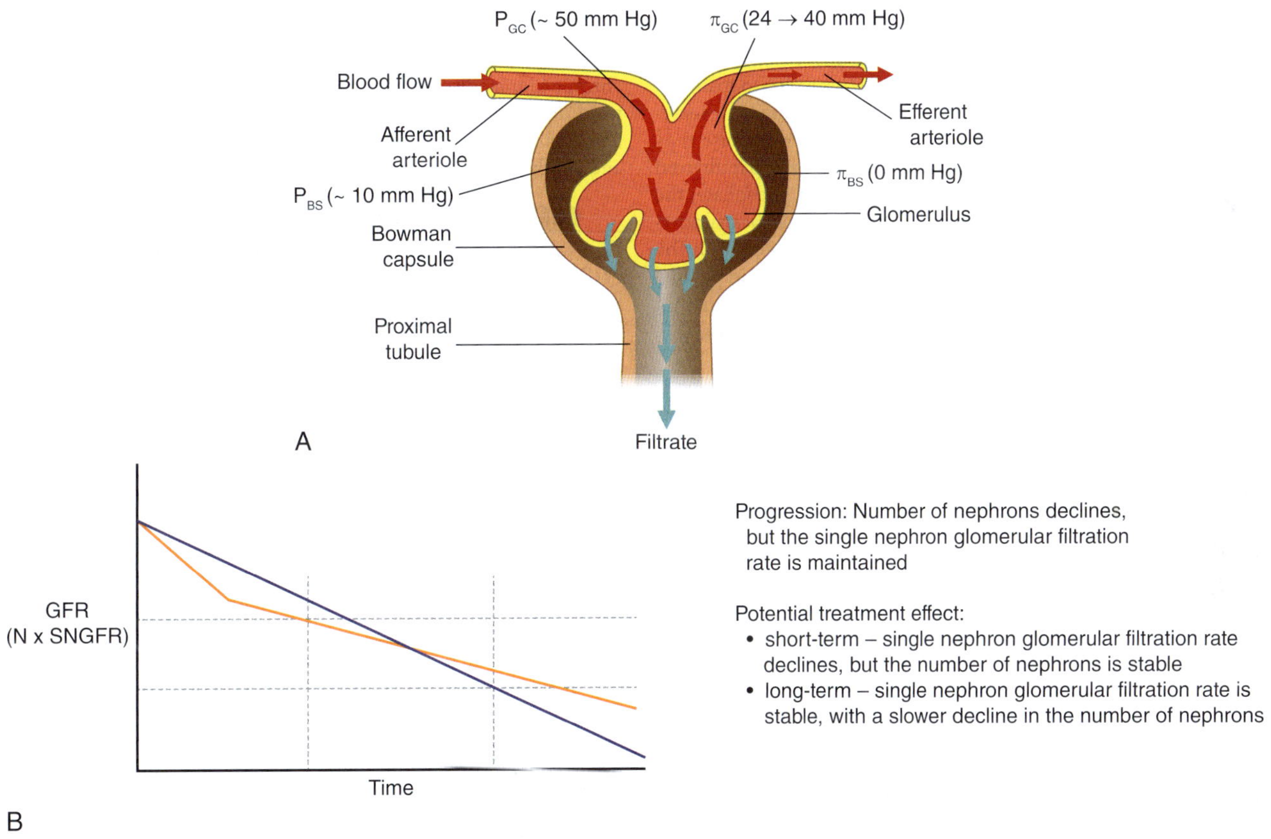

FIGURE 116-3. **Pathophysiology of decreased glomerular filtration rate. A,** Hemodynamic determinants of the single nephron glomerular filtration rate. **B,** Mechanism of interventions to slow glomerular filtration rate decline. **A,** In health, a high glomerular filtration rate reflects a high filtration pressure gradient across the glomerular capillary wall (the difference between the hydrostatic pressure gradient [the hydrostatic pressure in the glomerular capsule (P_{GC}) compared with the pressure in Bowman space (P_{BS})] and oncotic pressure gradients [the oncotic pressure in the glomerular capillary (π_{GC}) compared with the oncotic pressure in Bowman space (π_{BS})]) and the high ultrafiltration coefficient of the glomerular capillary wall (K_F, the product of surface area times hydraulic permeability). **B,** Glomerular filtration rate is the product of the number of nephrons times the average single nephron glomerular filtration rate. A decline in glomerular filtration reflects a loss of nephrons. Some therapies for chronic kidney disease reduce the single-nephron glomerular filtration rate but slow the loss of nephrons, thereby initially lowering the glomerular filtration rate (short-term effect) but subsequently slowing the rate of decline of glomerular filtration (long-term effect). GFR = glomerular filtration rate; SNGFR = single nephron GFR.

proteins S and C) and increased liver production of clotting factors and other procoagulant proteins results in hypercoagulability that can manifest as renal vein or deep vein thrombosis.[8] Decreased plasma volume and interstitial edema in the kidney may cause acute kidney injury. Smaller increases in albuminuria (30 to 2000 mg/day, A2 to A3, subnephrotic range) may parallel endothelial damage in other organs and be associated with pro-inflammatory or prothrombotic signals that increase the risk of cardiovascular disease and other complications of chronic kidney disease.

In health, the normal glomerular filtration rate is approximately 125 mL/min/1.73 m² in young adults owing to a high filtration pressure gradient (the difference between hydrostatic and oncotic pressure gradients) across the glomerular capillary wall and its high ultrafiltration coefficient (the product of surface area times hydraulic permeability) (Fig. 116-3). In principle, the glomerular filtration rate is the product of the nephron number (approximately 1 million per kidney) times the mean single-nephron glomerular filtration rate. A decreased glomerular filtration rate is often caused by a decreased number of nephrons and increased nephron glomerular filtration rate per remnant nephron (single nephron hyperfiltration). This hyperfiltration is caused by the combined effect of glomerular hypertrophy and increased filtration pressure from decreased glomerular capillary resistance, with greater reduction in afferent than efferent resistance. These changes may be considered adaptive because the increase in the single nephron glomerular filtration rate enables continued excretion of solutes despite a decreased number of nephrons, but it is also maladaptive because the increased pressure may damage remnant nephrons, thereby leading to progressive loss of nephrons and a further decline in the glomerular filtration rate. The number of nephrons may also be reduced in premature and low-birthweight infants, thereby leading to subsequent higher risk for the development of chronic kidney disease.[9] Numerous other mechanisms, with or without hyperfiltration and proteinuria, may contribute to the progression of kidney disease.

Therapies targeted to the glomerular adaptations can lower filtration pressure either by increasing afferent resistance or by decreasing efferent resistance and inducing an initially faster glomerular filtration rate decline (short-term or acute effect) followed by a subsequent slowing in the rate of decline in glomerular filtration (long-term or chronic effect), presumably by slowing of the loss of nephrons (Fig. 116-3B). Albuminuria is also generally reduced by such therapies.

The uremic syndrome, which occurs at a glomerular filtration rate below 15 mL/min/1.73m^2 (stage G5, kidney failure), is characterized by retention of solutes that are normally excreted by the kidney (e.g., urea, creatinine, phosphorus, hydrogen ion, potassium, sodium, chloride, unmeasured anions, low-molecular-weight proteins, lipids, and carbohydrates; see Table 116-2). The increased concentration of retained solutes can be directly toxic to cells, such as cells of the neuromuscular and immune systems. In addition, the retention of solutes may also stimulate regulatory systems to try to maintain their net excretion by decreasing their reabsorption or increasing their secretion. However, these tubular adaptations may be maladaptive because they have adverse consequences in other organ systems. For example, parathyroid hormone (PTH) is increased in response to the retention of phosphate; the result is reabsorption of bone and the potential for tertiary hyperparathyroidism if the hyperparathyroidism becomes autonomous (Chapter 227). The kidney's endocrine and metabolic functions also tend to decline in parallel with decreased excretory function; examples include decreased production of erythropoietin and 1,25-dihydroxycholecalciferol (activated vitamin D_3), as well as decreased urinary production of ammonia.

With smaller decreases in glomerular filtration rate, the retention of solutes is less marked but still may cause complications (see Table 116-2). For example, most patients with chronic kidney disease have hypertension, often with onset at stages G1 to G2, due to a combination of increased extracellular fluid volume from the retention of sodium chloride and increased systemic vascular resistance from a deficiency in nitric oxide and a failure to suppress the sympathetic nervous system and the renin-angiotensin system.

Increased PTH and deficiency of active vitamin D_3 are among the earliest complications of decreased glomerular filtration rate, generally occurring at stage G3a. The metabolic bone disease of chronic kidney disease includes renal osteodystrophy as well as vascular and soft tissue calcification. Renal osteodystrophy is characterized by a combination of bone lesions from increased secretion of PTH (osteitis fibrosa cystica) and a deficiency of active vitamin D_3 (osteomalacia).

The anemia of chronic kidney disease (Chapter 144) is hypoproliferative and normochromic, largely due to a deficiency in erythropoietin, the accumulation of hepcidin, and relative iron deficiency. However, the survival of red cells is also diminished. Anemia generally first appears at stage G3a to G3b but is usually mild (hemoglobin >10 g/dL) until stage G4.

Muscle and fat wasting is primarily due to decreased intake of protein and energy owing to anorexia, although gastrointestinal symptoms (nausea, vomiting, and diarrhea) may contribute at stage G5. Micronutrient deficiencies may also occur. Other causes of muscle and fat wasting may include the accumulation of leptin, ghrelin deficiency, inflammation, and metabolic acidosis. Malnutrition may also be a side effect of dietary restrictions.

Metabolic acidosis (Chapter 104) in chronic kidney disease is caused by retention of hydrogen ion owing to decreased tubular secretion. The most common cause (uremic acidosis) is the decreased production of ammonia owing to decreased nephron mass at stages G3b to G5. A concomitant elevation in the anion gap occurs at stage G4 to G5 owing to the reduced filtration of unmeasured anions. Nevertheless, an acid urine pH is preserved, and the serum bicarbonate level usually stabilizes between 12 and 18 mEq/L because of buffering of retained hydrogen ions in bone. Causes of metabolic acidosis in chronic kidney disease at stage G1 to G2 include impaired acidification (e.g., distal renal tubular acidosis, nonacid urinary pH , usually with hypokalemia), impaired bicarbonate reabsorption (proximal renal tubular acidosis, alkaline urine pH during the generation phase but acid urine pH in the steady-state phase, usually with hypokalemia), and hyporeninemic hypoaldosteronism (type 4 renal tubular acidosis, acid urine pH, usually with hyperkalemia).

Hyperkalemia (Chapter 103), which generally begins at stages G3b to G4, is usually caused by the retention of potassium owing to a combination of excessive dietary intake, decreased filtered load, and decreased tubular secretion. Potassium retention directly stimulates the secretion of aldosterone by the adrenal zona glomerulosa, thereby leading to increased tubular secretion of potassium. The inhibition of the renin-angiotensin system leads to impaired secretion of aldosterone and to type 4 renal tubular acidosis with resulting hyperkalemia. Causes of hyperkalemia without potassium retention include a transcellular shift of potassium from intracellular to extracellular fluid (for example, due to metabolic acidosis, hyperglycemia, or β-adrenergic blockade) or cell lysis.

As the glomerular filtration rate falls, prolactin is retained. Elevated prolactin levels contribute to disturbances in the hypothalamic-pituitary axis and can cause sexual and reproductive disorders at stage G3b to G4. The toxicity of numerous retained solutes leads to peripheral neuropathy, uremic encephalopathy, and an increased risk of infections at stage G5.

Chronic kidney disease is a risk factor for cardiovascular disease, including atherosclerosis (e.g., coronary ischemia and myocardial infarction, cerebral ischemia and stroke, and aortic and peripheral vascular disease), left ventricular hypertrophy, and heart failure. In addition to the increased prevalence of traditional risk factors (e.g., older age, male sex, diabetes, hypertension, hyperlipidemia, obesity, smoking, and physical inactivity) in patients with chronic kidney disease, chronic kidney disease itself also appears to be a risk factor for left ventricular hypertrophy and cardiovascular disease, due in part to increased levels of fibroblast growth factor 23 as well as to pro-inflammatory and prothrombotic states.

CLINICAL MANIFESTATIONS

Clinical manifestations depend on the degree of albuminuria and the severity of the reduction in the glomerular filtration rate (see Table 116-2).[10] Chronic kidney disease is usually silent in its early stages. The earliest manifestation may be the new onset or worsening of hypertension, abnormalities on a urinalysis, electrolyte or acid-base abnormalities, or the development of edema. Often symptoms are nonspecific, such as fatigue or lassitude.

Albuminuria generally indicates glomerular damage and is the earliest marker of kidney damage in conditions such as diabetes, hypertension, and obesity. Subnephrotic-range albuminuria (30 to 2000 mg/day, stages A2 to A3) has few clinical manifestations but is associated with increased risk of cardiovascular disease, anemia, infections, and cognitive impairment. Nephrotic syndrome can cause severe edema, deep vein thrombosis or pulmonary embolism, or acute kidney injury.

A decreased glomerular filtration rate may lead to the accumulation of drugs that are excreted by the kidney, with an increased risk for side effects owing to toxicity and drug-drug interactions. Side effects can also occur due to increased renal toxicity of radiographic contrast agents that contain iodine and the systemic toxicity of gadolinium (Chapter 246). Superimposed acute kidney injury (Chapter 106) is common due to side effects of drugs used to treat chronic kidney disease, cardiovascular disease, and other frequently occurring comorbid conditions.

Many clinical manifestations of decreased glomerular filtration rate may occur at stages G3b to G4. Renal osteodystrophy may cause pathologic fractures and soft tissue masses. Hyperphosphatemia may elevate the calcium-phosphate concentration product in excess of its solubility in extracellular fluid, causing soft tissue and vascular calcification, leading to noncompliant large arteries, left ventricular hypertrophy, heart failure, and, rarely, necrosis of skin and underlying soft tissue owing to ischemia (calciphylaxis). Anemia may cause weakness and contribute to heart failure. Muscle and fat wasting may cause weight loss, often superimposed on preexisting obesity. At stage G3b, the serum anion gap may be in the normal range (normal anion gap metabolic acidosis). At stage G4 to G5, the serum anion gap is usually increased due to retention of inorganic anions (phosphates and sulfates), and high anion gap metabolic acidosis appears. Consequences of chronic metabolic acidosis in chronic kidney disease include osteopenia due to dissolution of calcium salts, as well as muscle wasting and faster progression of kidney disease. Mild hyperkalemia (serum potassium 5.0 to 5.5 mEq/L; Chapter 103) is common, especially in patients treated with drugs that inhibit the renin-angiotensin-aldosterone system. Moderate hyperkalemia (serum potassium 5.5 to 6.5 mEq/L) is more common at stage G3b, and severe hyperkalemia (serum potassium >6.5 mEq/L) is seen with more advanced chronic kidney disease. Sexual and reproductive disorders may include amenorrhea, menorrhagia, impotence, oligospermia, or galactorrhea.

Kidney failure (glomerular filtration rate <15 mL/min 1.73 m^2, stage G5) can give rise to signs of uremia. The uremic syndrome includes hypertension, extracellular fluid overload, metabolic bone disease, anemia, malnutrition, peripheral neuropathy, pruritus, gastrointestinal symptoms, pericarditis (Chapter 62), encephalopathy, and an increased risk for infections.

DIAGNOSIS

Patients with possible chronic kidney disease should be evaluated systematically (Table 116-3) to define whether they meet the diagnostic criteria (Table 116-4), based on the degree of their albuminuria (>30 mg/day), the decline in their glomerular filtration rate (<60 mL/min 1.73 m^2), and the chronicity of these changes (3 or more months) (Table 116-5). In patients who are determined to have chronic kidney disease, the disease should be classified according to its severity, based on the degree of albuminuria and the glomerular filtration rate (see Fig. 116-1 and see Table 116-2), as well as on its cause (see Table 116-1).

TABLE 116-3 GUIDE FOR THE DETECTION, EVALUATION, AND MANAGEMENT OF CHRONIC KIDNEY DISEASE

1. **Recognition of increased risk of chronic kidney disease**	• Increased susceptibility to chronic kidney disease • Exposure to conditions that cause chronic kidney disease
2. **Testing for chronic kidney disease**	• Measure serum creatinine to estimate glomerular filtration rate • Measure urinary albumin • Assess other markers of kidney damage that are specific to the risk (urine sediment, imaging abnormalities, renal tubular syndromes, kidney biopsy) • Perform confirmatory tests (if indicated)
3. **Detection of chronic kidney disease**	• Duration >3 months (documented or inferred) • Markers of kidney damage • Glomerular filtration rate <60 mL/min per 1.73 m^2 (estimated or measured)
4. **Evaluation of clinical diagnosis for implementation of cause-specific therapy**	• Diabetic kidney disease (type 1 or 2) • Nondiabetic kidney disease (glomerular disease other than diabetic glomerulosclerosis, vascular diseases, tubulointerstitial diseases, cystic or congenital diseases) • Kidney disease in kidney transplant recipients
5. **Assessment of stage for implementation of stage-based cause-independent therapy**	• Albuminuria stages • Glomerular filtration rate stages
6. **Prognosis (risk assessment with detection, evaluation, and management tailored to patient's risk)**	• Predictive instruments using level of albuminuria and glomerular filtration rate plus other factors specific for the outcome (kidney failure, kidney disease progression, acute kidney injury, chronic kidney disease, cardiovascular disease and other complications, mortality)

Modified from Levey AS, Coresh J. Chronic kidney disease. *Lancet*. 2012;379:165-180.

TABLE 116-4 CRITERIA FOR CHRONIC KIDNEY DISEASE (ANY OF THE FOLLOWING PRESENT FOR >3 MONTHS)

Markers of kidney damage (one or more)	Albuminuria (albumin excretion rate ≥30 mg/24 hr; albumin to creatinine ratio ≥30 mg/g; albumin to creatinine ratio stages A2-A3) Urine sediment abnormalities Imaging abnormalities Electrolyte and other abnormalities due to tubular disorders Pathologic abnormalities History of kidney transplantation
Decreased GFR	Glomerular filtration rate <60 mL/min/1.73 m^2 (glomerular filtration rate stages G3a-G5)

From Kidney Disease: Improving Global Outcomes (KDIGO). KDIGO 2012 clinical practice guideline for the evaluation and management of chronic kidney disease. *Kidney Int Suppl*. 2013;3:1-150.

Evaluation of Duration

Evaluation of duration of the kidney disease distinguishes chronic kidney disease (>3 months) from acute kidney injury (Chapter 106).[11] The duration can be documented either by review of past medical records or inferred from specific findings. For example, oliguria or a decreased glomerular filtration rate in the setting of acute illness suggests acute kidney injury. Small kidneys on imaging studies or chronic illness signifies chronic kidney disease. Many kidney diseases can cause either acute or chronic disease, but acute tubular necrosis, the most common cause of acute kidney injury, does not have a chronic phase, and diabetic kidney disease, the most common cause of chronic kidney disease, does not have an acute phase.

Evaluation of Markers of Kidney Damage

Albuminuria signifies increased glomerular permeability, and a large quantity of albuminuria generally signifies a glomerular disease. The albumin excretion rate in a timed urine sample is the gold standard for assessing albuminuria, but an albumin to creatinine ratio in an untimed "spot" urine sample is recommended as the initial test because of its specificity and convenience.[12] As a rough guide, an albumin excretion rate of less than 30 mg/day corresponds approximately to a protein excretion rate of less than 150 mg/day and a dipstick protein reading of negative to trace positive. An albumin excretion rate of greater than 300 mg/day corresponds approximately to a protein excretion rate greater than 500 mg/day and a dipstick that is 1+ positive or greater. Renal tubular disorders may cause abnormalities of serum and urine electrolytes as well as urine pH, glucose, amino acids, and low-molecular-weight proteins in the absence of other markers of kidney damage or a decreased glomerular filtration rate. The evaluation of these disorders usually requires referral to specialists.

Evaluation of the urine sediment can be helpful to determine whether hematuria or pyuria reflect kidney damage (Chapter 101). Dysmorphic red blood cells (RBCs) indicate a glomerular disease (Chapter 107), RBC casts suggest a proliferative glomerulonephritis (Chapter 107), and white blood cell casts suggest pyelonephritis (Chapter 263) or tubulointerstitial nephritis (Chapter 108). Oval fat bodies and fatty casts are found in diseases with proteinuria. Renal tubular epithelial cells and casts may be seen in any parenchymal kidney disease; in the absence of hematuria and proteinuria, such cells may indicate acute tubular necrosis.

Ultrasound is generally the first imaging modality because it is noninvasive, does not require contrast, and has high sensitivity for detecting hydronephrosis, cortical scarring, masses (Chapters 182 and 186), stones (Chapter 111), polycystic kidney disease (Chapter 112), and large or small kidneys. CT and MRI with contrast or diagnostic angiography may be necessary for further delineation of the kidney structures, and percutaneous antegrade or cystoscopic retrograde procedures may be necessary to evaluate the renal collecting system.

Pathologic abnormalities are the gold standard for kidney damage, but biopsy of the kidney is an invasive procedure that is generally reserved for evaluation of markers of kidney damage or decreased glomerular filtration rate when knowledge of the pathologic findings will affect treatment. The main complication of percutaneous biopsy is bleeding, which occurs more frequently in patients who have hypertension, a lower glomerular filtration rate, and biopsy of native as compared with transplanted kidneys.

Evaluation of the Glomerular Filtration Rate

Approximately 90% of clinical laboratories in the United States report an estimated glomerular filtration rate (eGFR) whenever a serum creatinine is measured. Equations to estimate the eGFR use serum concentrations of creatinine and cystatin (Table 116-6), which are endogenous filtration markers that vary inversely with the glomerular filtration rate, plus demographic variables (e.g., with age, with or without sex, and without race), which serve as surrogates for factors other than the glomerular filtration rate that influence their serum concentrations.[13,14] Factors other than glomerular filtration rate that influence the serum creatinine concentration include its generation by muscle and diet, tubular secretion, and extrarenal elimination by intestinal bacteria. Unfortunately, the eGFR lacks precision; in populations with no systematic bias, only 80 to 90% of eGFR calculations are within 30% of the measured glomerular filtration rate. Systematic underestimation of the measured glomerular filtration rate can be observed in individuals who have a large muscle mass, who eat large amounts of meat, who take creatine supplements, or who are treated with medications that inhibit the tubular secretion of creatinine (e.g., trimethoprim, fenofibrate,

TABLE 116-5 EVALUATION OF CHRONIC KIDNEY DISEASE

Duration >3 mo on the basis of documentation or inference. Duration is necessary to distinguish chronic kidney disease from acute kidney injury

- Clinical assessment can indicate duration
  - Review of previous laboratory data
  - Acute illness or oliguria suggests acute kidney injury
  - Chronic illness or small kidneys indicate chronic kidney disease
- Documentation of duration is not usually available in epidemiologic studies

Kidney damage as defined by structural abnormalities or functional abnormalities other than decreased glomerular filtration rate. Markers of kidney damage may suggest cause of disease

Albuminuria as a marker of kidney damage. Increased glomerular permeability, urine albumin to creatinine ratio >30 mg/g

- The normal urinary albumin to creatinine ratio in young adults is ≤10 mg/g. Urine albumin to creatinine ratio stages 10-29, 30-300, and >300 mg are high-normal, high, and very high, respectively
- Threshold value of 30 mg/g roughly corresponds to urine dipstick values of trace or 1+, dependent on urine concentration
- High urinary albumin to creatinine ratio can be confirmed by urine albumin excretion in a timed urine collection

Abnormalities in urinary sediment as markers of kidney damage

- Dysmorphic red blood cells in glomerular disease
- Red blood cell casts in proliferative glomerulonephritis
- White blood cell casts in pyelonephritis or interstitial nephritis
- Oval fat bodies or fatty casts in diseases with proteinuria
- Granular casts and renal tubular epithelial cells in many parenchymal diseases (nonspecific)

Imaging abnormalities as markers of kidney damage (ultrasound, computed tomography, and magnetic resonance imaging with or without contrast, isotope scans, angiography)

- Hydronephrosis due to obstruction
- Cortical scarring due to infarcts, pyelonephritis, or vesicoureteral reflux
- Polycystic kidney disease
- Kidney stones
- Renal artery stenosis
- Renal masses or enlarged kidneys due to infiltrative diseases
- Small and echogenic kidneys (common in late stages of chronic kidney disease because of many parenchymal diseases)

Renal tubular syndromes as markers of kidney damage

- Renal tubular acidosis
- Nephrogenic diabetes insipidus
- Bartter and Gittelman syndromes
- Fanconi syndrome
- Cystinuria
- Familial hypomagnesemia with hypercalciuria and nephrocalcinosis

Pathologic abnormalities as markers of kidney damage

- Glomerular diseases
- Vascular diseases
- Tubulointerstitial diseases
- Cystic diseases
- Congenital diseases

Glomerular filtration rate (GFR) <60 mL/min per 1.73 m^2

- Glomerular filtration rate is the best overall index of kidney function in health and disease
- Normal glomerular filtration rate in young adults is about 125 mL/min per 1.73 m^2; glomerular filtration rate <15 mL/min per 1.73 m^2 is defined as kidney failure
- Glomerular filtration rate may be assessed by measurement of clearances of exogenous filtration markers (measured glomerular filtration rate) or estimated from serum concentrations of endogenous filtration markers (estimated glomerular filtration rate)
- Estimated glomerular filtration rate using serum creatinine is the first step in glomerular filtration rate evaluation
  - Non–glomerular filtration rate determinants of serum creatinine include generation by muscle or diet, tubular secretion, and extrarenal elimination by gastrointestinal tract bacterial creatininase
  - In populations with acute illness or chronic comorbid illness, estimated glomerular filtration rate from creatinine may have systematic error (bias) compared to measured glomerular filtration rate
  - In populations in which estimated glomerular filtration rate from creatinine does not have bias, estimated glomerular filtration rate from creatinine lacks precision: only 80-90% of estimated glomerular filtration rates are within 30% of measured glomerular filtration rate
- Confirmatory tests for decreased estimated glomerular filtration rate from creatinine include estimated glomerular filtration rate using serum cystatin C or the combination of serum creatinine and cystatin C; measured creatinine clearance; or measured glomerular filtration rate using inulin, iothalamate, iohexol, ethylene-diamine tetracetic acid, or diethylene triamine pentaacetic acid

Cause of chronic kidney disease. Classification of cause is based on

- Site of documented or presumed pathologic abnormalities
- Presence or absence of systemic disease affecting the kidneys

Modified from Levey AS, Coresh J. Chronic kidney disease. *Lancet*. 2012;379:165-180.

ritonavir, cobicistat, dolutegravir, and other antiviral agents) or inhibit bacterial creatininase (broad-spectrum antibiotics). In contrast, systematic overestimation of the measured glomerular filtration rate can be observed in individuals who have muscle wasting, eat a vegetarian or low-protein diet, or have large losses of creatinine-containing extravascular fluid, such as when pleural or peritoneal effusions are continuously drained and replaced with intravenous fluids. Cystatin C is an alternative filtration marker that is recommended as a confirmatory test to estimate the glomerular filtration rate. Serum cystatin C is not affected by muscle mass, diet, or tubular secretion, but it is affected by smoking, obesity, inflammation, thyroid hormones, and glucorticosteroids, independent of glomerular filtration rate. The estimation of glomerular filtration rate by cystatin C is not more accurate than a

TABLE 116-6 EQUATIONS FOR ESTIMATING THE GLOMERULAR FILTRATION RATE

Using the serum creatinine level only $142 \times \min(Scr/k,1)^{\alpha} \times \max(Scr/k,1)^{-1.200} \times 0.9938^{age} \times 1.012$ [if female] where Scr is serum creatinine, k is 0.7 for females and 0.9 males, α is −0.241 for females and −0.302 for males, min indicates the minimum of Scr/k or 1, max indicates the maximum of Scr/k or 1
Using the serum cystatin level only $133 \times \min(Scys/0.8,1)^{-0.499} \times \max(Scys/0.8,1)^{-1.328} \times 9962^{age} \times 0.932$ [if female] where Scys is serum cystatin C
Using both the serum creatinine and serum cystatin level $135 \times \min(Scr/k,1)^{\alpha} \times \max(Scr/k,1)^{-0.544} \times \min(Scys/0.8,1)^{-0.323} \times \max(Scys/0.8,1)^{-0.778} \times 0.9961^{age} \times 0.963$ [if female] where Scr is serum creatinine, Scys is serum cystatin C, k is 0.7 for females and 0.9 males, α is −0.219 for females and −0.144 for males, min indicates the minimum of Scr/k or 1, max indicates the maximum of Scr/k or 1

From National Kidney Foundation calculator: https://kidney.org/professionals/kdoqi/gfr_calculator.

glomerular filtration rate estimated by creatinine, but together they are more accurate than either alone.

Evaluation of Cause

For evaluation of cause, the classification can be simplified into diabetic (Chapter 109) versus nondiabetic diseases of native kidneys and diseases in kidney transplant recipients (Chapter 117). In general, further diagnostic testing should be guided by the likelihood of detecting a treatable disease (Chapter 100).

Diabetic kidney disease is the most common cause of kidney disease in adults in high-income nations, and the clinical features of diabetic glomerulosclerosis can be easily recognized without specialized diagnostic tests (Chapter 109). Slowly worsening albuminuria, hypertension, and a progressive decline in glomerular filtration rate are typical, whereas hematuria, pyuria, and imaging abnormalities are usually absent.

Among the nondiabetic kidney diseases, hypertensive nephrosclerosis (Chapter 64) is the most common. It has no distinct markers, but increased albuminuria can occur before or after the onset of a decreased glomerular filtration rate. Hypertensive retinopathy (Fig. 391-24) and left ventricular hypertrophy are common, whereas hematuria, pyuria, and imaging abnormalities are typically absent. However, hypertension is a common complication of other kidney diseases, and an abnormal urine sediment or a family history of early onset of kidney disease suggests another primary cause of the kidney disease. Many cases of presumed hypertensive nephrosclerosis in individuals of West African descent may be associated with *APOL1* pathogenic variants (Chapter 107).

TREATMENT

General Principles

Management, which is based on the cause of chronic kidney disease and its stage, should begin as soon as the disease is detected. Cause-specific therapy that is directed at factors that cause chronic kidney disease may induce remission and slow progression. Stage-based therapies, which are directed by the level of albuminuria and the glomerular filtration rate, aim to slow the progression and prevent complications of chronic kidney disease, irrespective of the cause (see Table 116-2). Stage-based recommendations are cumulative, so recommendations for late stages include recommendations for early stages. Although many common problems can be managed with existing guidelines by non-nephrologists, specialty nephrology referral is recommended for patients with an uncertain diagnosis, an albumin to creatinine ratio greater than 300 mg/g (stage A3), a glomerular filtration rate less than 30 mL/min/1.73 m^2 (stage G4 to G5), or complications that are difficult to manage.

Cause-Specific Treatment for Chronic Kidney Disease

Glycemic control (Chapter 210) can retard the development of diabetic glomerulosclerosis, and blood pressure control (Chapter 64) can retard the development of hypertensive nephrosclerosis. However, no specific treatment can reverse either disease. For patients who have diabetic kidney disease, the recommended HbA_{1c} target is similar as for patients who have diabetes without kidney disease, although less strict targets may be appropriate for patients with comorbid conditions. Specific treatments (see Table 116-1) are available for many other causes of nondiabetic kidney disease, including glomerular diseases (Chapter 107) and the withdrawal of exposure to toxic drugs (Chapter 106).

Stage-Based Treatment Independent of Cause

Therapies to slow the progression of chronic kidney disease and reduce cardiovascular risk in patients with chronic kidney disease are the mainstays of treatment for most patients. Patients must avoid drugs that are toxic to the kidneys and reduce the dosage of drugs that are excreted by the kidney

Lifestyle and Diet Recommendations

As in the general population, a healthy eating pattern, physical activity, and tobacco cessation are recommended to reduce the risk of cardiovascular disease. A healthy eating pattern accounts for all foods and beverages within an appropriate calorie level and limits saturated fats and trans fats, added sugars, and sodium. A Mediterranean-type diet (Fig. 13-1) may improve lipid profiles, and a DASH-sodium diet (Table 13-4) may lower blood pressure and reduce the production of acid.[15] Dietary sodium restriction (<2.0 g/day) is recommended for patients who have hypertension. The recommended dietary allowance for protein for the general population is approximately 0.8 g/kg/day, which is far below the average protein intake in high-income nations. Some guidelines recommend a dietary protein intake of 0.6 to 0.8 g/kg/day at stage G3 to G5 because of its favorable effect on ameliorating solute retention and the potential to slow the progression of chronic kidney disease. Maintenance of a total energy intake of 25 to 35 kcal/kg/day while consuming a low-protein diet is recommended to avoid protein-calorie malnutrition. Involvement of a registered dietitian nutritionist is essential.

Blood Pressure Control

A systolic blood pressure less than 130 mm Hg is key, and a systolic blood pressure less than 120 mm Hg (using standardized office-based measurements) is recommended by some guidelines.[16] Caution is advised because a lower blood pressure goal may initially be associated with an increased risk of reducing the glomerular filtration rate, especially in older patients with comorbid conditions. Renin-angiotensin-aldosterone system inhibition with an ACE inhibitor or an angiotensin receptor blocker (Tables 64-7 and 64-9) is recommended for patients with albuminuria with or without diabetes to reduce albuminuria and slow the decline in the glomerular filtration rate,[A1] with diuretics[A2] and calcium channel antagonists as additional agents and calcium channel antagonists as the third agent (Chapter 64). Nonsteroidal mineralocorticoid receptor antagonists (e.g., finerenone 20 mg once daily if the glomerular filtration rate is greater than 60 mL/min/1.73m^2 and 10 mg once daily if it is 25 to 59 mL/mm/1.73m^2) are also effective in patients with diabetes and albuminuria.[A3,A4]

Sodium Glucose Transport Protein 2 (SGLT2) Inhibition and Glucagon-like Peptide 1 Agonists

SGLT2 inhibitors reduce sodium glucose cotransport in the proximal tubule, thereby resulting in natriuresis, weight loss, and lower blood pressure. Treatment with these medications[17] reduces albuminuria, slows the decline of the glomerular filtration rate, and reduces the risk for kidney failure and cardiovascular disease in patients who have albuminuria with diabetic (Chapter 109) or nondiabetic kidney disease.[A5-A7] These agents (e.g., canagliflozin 100 mg daily, dapagliflozin 5 mg daily, and empagliflozin 10 mg daily) recommended for patients with albuminuria who have type 2 diabetes (Chapter 109) or who do not have diabetes, but they are not approved for use in patients who have type 1 diabetes. Glucagon-like peptide-1 agonists also reduce albuminuria and slow the decline in glomerular filtration rate in patients with type 2 diabetes and albuminuria.[18]

Lipid-Lowering Therapy and Antithrombotic Agents

Patients with chronic kidney disease are at increased risk of cardiovascular disease (Chapter 40). A healthy diet (Chapters 13 and 201), statins (Chapter 190), and other therapies are recommended to reduce low-density lipoprotein (LDL) cholesterol levels and thereby reduce this risk.[19] When clinically indicated, antithrombotic agents appear to have similar efficacy as in patients who do not have chronic kidney disease; however, the risk of hemorrhagic side effects is higher in patients with chronic kidney disease, and the dose of antithrombotic agents often must be adjusted (Chapter 70). In contrast to their cardiovascular benefit, neither lipid-lowering therapy nor antithrombotic agents appear to have a beneficial effect on the progression of the kidney disease itself.

Treatment of Complications of Albuminuria

Diuretics are generally needed to control edema due to nephrotic syndrome (Chapter 107). In refractory cases, albumin infusion can be administered at the same time.[20] ACE inhibitors and angiotensin receptor blockers (Table 64-7) are useful to reduce albuminuria, but they may cause hypotension and hyperkalemia. Anticoagulants can be used to prevent or treat deep vein thrombosis (Chapter 68) and renal vein thrombosis (Chapter 110).

Treatment of Complications of a Decreased Glomerular Filtration Rate

Exogenous alkali can prevent and treat metabolic acidosis due to chronic kidney disease. It also can slow the decline in the glomerular filtration rate in patients with or without metabolic acidosis and in diabetic and nondiabetic kidney disease.[A8] A reasonable starting dose is sodium bicarbonate at 650 mg twice daily, titrated to a target serum bicarbonate of approximately 22 to 24 mEq/L.

Extracellular fluid volume retention may be a potential risk of therapy with sodium bicarbonate.

Mild hyperkalemia (potassium level 5 to 5.5 mEq/L) generally requires no treatment other than education to avoid foods with large concentrations of potassium. Levels higher than 5.5 mEq/L generally require treatment[21] (Chapter 103). Urgent therapy for higher levels may include calcium gluconate to prevent cardiac arrhythmias; insulin, glucose, and bicarbonate to shift potassium from extracellular to intracellular fluid; loop diuretics, potassium-binding agents, and dialysis to remove potassium from the body; and treatment of reversible causes of hyperkalemia. If there are no reversible disorders, prevention includes dietary potassium restriction (<2 g/day) and potassium-binding agents (Chapter 103).

Metabolic bone disease is treated with phosphate-binding agents to maintain a normal serum phosphorus level (Chapter 105) and with activated vitamin D_3 (e.g., calcitriol starting at 0.25 µg to 0.5 µg orally every day or every other day depending on the glomerular filtration rate and the PTH level) or its analogues. In dialysis patients, calcimimetics (e.g., cinacalcet starting at 30 mg orally daily) should be used to suppress PTH. Subtotal parathyroidectomy is required in refractory cases of tertiary hyperparathyroidism (Chapter 207).

Treatment of symptomatic anemia includes iron repletion if indicated, erythropoiesis-stimulating agents, and red cell transfusions. To stimulate erythropoiesis, erythropoiesis-stimulating agents (e.g., darbepoetin alpha starting at 0.45 µg/kg every 4 weeks) are generally begun when the hemoglobin level is less than 9 g/dL in patients who have symptoms of anemia, who are likely to need red cell transfusions, and in whom the goal is to reduce the risk of alloimmunization or other transfusion-related risks (Chapter 162). Erythropoiesis-stimulating agents are associated with an increased risk of deep vein thrombosis and cardiovascular disease, so they are generally reserved for patients with stages G4 to G5 chronic kidney disease and are used to raise the hemoglobin level only to 10 to 11 g/dL because higher levels are associated with more cardiovascular complications. Hypoxia-inducible factor-stabilizing agents also are effective for raising the hemoglobin level[A9,A10] but are not currently approved in the United States for patients who are not being treated by dialysis because of safety concerns.

Kidney Replacement Therapy and End-of-Life Care

Kidney failure (glomerular filtration rate <15 mL/min/1.73 m^2), which is the end stage of chronic kidney disease, is treated for as long as possible with comprehensive conservative care, which is management of clinical disorders and symptoms of uremia to maintain quality of life without dialysis. When such care is no longer adequate for controlling symptoms and signs, kidney replacement therapy (Chapter 117) is required. Dialysis is effective in resolving the most severe symptoms and signs, but it is associated with many complications and often does not result in full resolution of symptoms and signs. Since both quality of life and survival are limited with dialysis, especially for older patients, kidney transplantation is preferred, whenever possible, to resolve symptoms and extend life. Unfortunately, it is not available to all patients.

End-of-life care (Chapter 3) refers to maintaining comfort at the end of life in patients treated by transplantation, dialysis, or comprehensive conservative care. A shared decision model is recommended for implementation of these modalities of therapy, and planning should begin well in advance of the onset of uremic symptoms.

PREVENTION

Primary prevention of chronic kidney disease refers to the prevention and treatment of risk factors for chronic kidney disease, including diabetes, hypertension, cardiovascular disease, and other associated systemic disorders, as well as reducing exposure to drugs and environmental toxins that cause kidney disease. Adoption of public health guidelines for a healthy lifestyle and diet can lower the prevalence of hypertension, diabetes, obesity, and cardiovascular disease. Secondary prevention to slow the progression of kidney disease relies upon early detection, such as evaluating albuminuria to assess kidney damage and the serum creatinine level to estimate the glomerular filtration rate, in patients who have hypertension, diabetes, cardiovascular disease, and other systemic diseases associated with an increased risk for chronic kidney disease.[22] Failure to assess markers of kidney damage delays the detection of chronic kidney disease and the ability to implement measures to slow its progression. Detection of albuminuria or other markers of kidney damage enables implementation of measures to slow progression before glomerular filtration rate declines, thereby potentially increasing the interval until the onset of kidney failure (E-Fig. 116-3). Tertiary prevention in chronic kidney disease refers to kidney replacement therapy for kidney failure to prevent complications and death.

PROGNOSIS

The prognosis in chronic kidney disease depends primarily on the cause of disease, the level of albuminuria and glomerular filtration rate, and the availability of treatment. Kidney disease often progresses even after the diseases that initially caused it are no longer active. Explanations include systemic hypertension, proteinuria, increased glomerular capillary pressure with increased glomerular filtration, and accumulation of nephrotoxins.

Risk stratification is an important consideration for the detection, evaluation, and management of chronic kidney disease. The Kidney Failure Risk Equation (https://ckdpcrisk.org/kidneyfailurerisk/) predicts the 2-year and 5-year risk of kidney failure with replacement therapy in people with glomerular filtration rate less than 60 mL/min/1.73 m^2 using four variables (age, sex, glomerular filtration rate, and albumin to creatinine ratio) or eight variables (the same four variables plus serum albumin, bicarbonate, calcium, and phosphorus). The Timing of Clinical Outcomes in CKD with Severely Decreased GFR instrument (https://ckdpcrisk.org/lowgfrevents/) predicts the 2-year and 4-year risk of kidney failure with replacement therapy, cardiovascular disease, and death in people with glomerular filtration rate less than 30 mL/min/1.73 m^2 from 10 variables (age, sex, race, glomerular filtration rate, albumin to creatinine ratio, systolic blood pressure, body mass index, presence or absence of diabetes, history of smoking, and history of cardiovascular disease).[23]

GENERAL REFERENCES

For the General References and other additional features, please visit Elsevier eBooks+ at https://ebooks.health.elsevier.com.

Grade A References

A1. Bhandari S, Mehta S, Khwaja A, et al. Renin-angiotensin system inhibition in advanced chronic kidney disease. *N Engl J Med*. 2022;387:2021-2032.
A2. Agarwal R, Sinha AD, Cramer AE, et al. Chlorthalidone for hypertension in advanced chronic kidney disease. *N Engl J Med*. 2021;385:2507-2519.
A3. Bakris GL, Agarwal R, Anker SD, et al. Effect of finerenone on chronic kidney disease outcomes in type 2 diabetes. *N Engl J Med*. 2020;383:2219-2229.
A4. Pitt B, Filippatos G, Agarwal R, et al. Cardiovascular events with finerenone in kidney disease and type 2 diabetes. *N Engl J Med*. 2021;385:2252-2263.
A5. Heerspink HJL, Stefánsson BV, Correa-Rotter R, et al. Dapagliflozin in patients with chronic kidney disease (DAPA-CKD). *N Engl J Med*. 2020;383:1436-1446.
A6. Heerspink HJL, Sjöström CD, Jongs N, et al. Effects of dapagliflozin on mortality in patients with chronic kidney disease: a pre-specified analysis from the DAPA-CKD randomized controlled trial. *Eur Heart J*. 2021;42:1216-1227.
A7. The EMPA-KIDNEY Collaborative Group, Herrington WG, Staplin N, et al. Empagliflozin in patients with chronic kidney disease. *N Engl J Med*. 2023;288:117-127.
A8. Hutlin S, Hood C, Campbell KL, et al. A systematic review and meta-analysis on effects of bicarbonate therapy on kidney outcomes. *Kidney Int Rep*. 2020;6:695-705.
A9. Chertow GM, Pergola PE, Farag YMK, et al. Vadadustat in patients with anemia and non-dialysis-dependent CKD. *N Engl J Med*. 2021;384:1589-1600.
A10. Singh AK, Carroll K, McMurray JJV, et al. Daprodustat for the treatment of anemia in patients not undergoing dialysis. *N Engl J Med*. 2021;385:2313-2324.

117 TREATMENT OF IRREVERSIBLE RENAL FAILURE

DAVID COHEN AND ANTHONY MICHAEL VALERI

Chronic kidney disease (Chapter 116) tends to progress over time as glomerular capillary hypertension leads to glomerular hyperfiltration, which in turn precipitates progressive injury, glomerulosclerosis, tubulointerstitial fibrosis, and progressive loss of nephrons, regardless of the original insult. Irreversible and advanced end-stage renal disease requires renal replacement therapy, which can be broadly categorized as hemodialysis, peritoneal dialysis, and renal transplantation. In the United States, about 800,000 people receive some form of renal replacement therapy; approximately 480,000 people receive in-center hemodialysis, 16,000 people receive home hemodialysis, 65,000 people are on peritoneal dialysis, and 245,000 have a functioning kidney transplant. Approximately 180,000 people develop end-stage renal disease every year.[1]

Renal replacement therapy must be initiated when fluid and electrolyte derangements, particularly hyperkalemia, acidosis, or volume overload, can no longer be adequately controlled with dietary modifications and medications (Chapter 116) or if uremic symptoms, such as anorexia, nausea, vomiting, gastritis pericarditis, or encephalopathy, develop (Table 117-1). Renal replacement therapy typically is required when the estimated glomerular filtration rate (eGFR) is below 10 mL/minute, although it may be needed at an eGFR of 10 to 15 mL/minute when comorbid conditions, particularly heart failure, make medical management even more challenging and difficult. In one small randomized trial of critically ill patients with stage 2 acute kidney injury (defined as a serum creatinine level ≥2 times baseline or urinary output <0.5 mL/kg/hour for ≥12 hours and a plasma neutrophil gelatinase-associated lipocalin level >150 ng/mL), early initiation of renal replacement therapy reduced 90-day mortality compared with delayed initiation.[A1] However, larger randomized trials of intensive care unit patients with stage 3 acute kidney injury showed no reduction in mortality, and patients whose dialysis was delayed tended to have earlier diuresis, fewer adverse events, and a shorter duration of renal replacement therapy.[A2,A3] The routine initiation of dialysis (creatinine level 7.5 mg/dL) is no better than standard dialysis beginning at a creatinine level of approximately 10 mg/dL.[A4] Furthermore, intensive dialytic renal support therapy is no better than standard dialytic therapy, and intermittent hemodialysis and continuous renal replacement therapy lead to similar clinical outcomes in acute renal failure. It also is important to verify that the prescribed dialysis is received and that standardized measures are achieved. Some patients—especially patients in an increased catabolic state, trauma patients, and patients receiving glucocorticoids—may require dialysis more than three times per week to achieve adequate therapy. Neither furosemide nor low-dose dopamine improves outcome, even though low-dose dopamine may temporarily improve metrics of renal physiology.

Hemodialysis relies on diffusion across a semipermeable artificial membrane, whereas peritoneal dialysis brings the blood and the dialysate solution in contact across a natural biologic membrane. The diffusion of solutes along their respective concentration gradients across a semipermeable membrane removes nitrogenous waste products and corrects imbalances of potassium, calcium, magnesium, phosphorus, and acid. In addition, plasma water filters across the membrane and, by convection, drags solutes across the membrane in approximately the same concentration as in the plasma water. The electrolyte concentrations in the dialysate solution are not necessarily physiologic but are intentionally varied with respect to their potassium, calcium, magnesium, and bicarbonate concentrations to favor correction of the plasma toward a more normal physiologic state. For example, a typical dialysate solution might use a potassium concentration of 2 mEq/L and a bicarbonate concentration of 35 mEq/L to enable correction of hyperkalemia and uremic metabolic acidosis. Convection across the dialysis membrane is driven by either a hydrostatic pressure gradient applied across the membrane (hemodialysis) or an oncotic pressure gradient using high-dextrose concentrations or a large, poorly absorbed carbohydrate polymer in the dialysate solution (peritoneal dialysis) for the removal and filtration of excess salt and water from the body.

DIALYSIS

HEMODIALYSIS

Conventional hemodialysis is typically provided at an outpatient dialysis unit where patients are treated three times per week for 3 or 4 hours per session. The measures used for determining the adequacy of treatment are based on urea clearance (as a surrogate marker molecule for the generation and clearance of small-molecular-weight nitrogenous waste products, <500 daltons). The simplest measure is the urea reduction ratio, which is the percentage fall in the blood urea nitrogen level with each dialysis session, with a goal of 65% or greater, or a single pool normalized urea clearance based on the single pool variable volume urea kinetic model (*spKt/V*) of 1.2 or greater on a thrice-weekly dialysis schedule. More precise measurements can fine-tune the dialysis in an individual patient. A more intensive protocol for increased urea clearance with a 40% increase in the *spKt/V* from 1.32 to 1.53 on a thrice-weekly schedule does not improve survival, perhaps because it increases the likelihood of hypotension during dialysis. More frequent hemodialysis, whether as in-center hemodialysis or nocturnal home hemodialysis six times per week, improves outcomes such as kidney-specific measures of quality of life, blood pressure, regression of left ventricular hypertrophy, and serum phosphorus levels, but it did not reduce mortality at 12 months, although longer follow-up (median of 3.6 years) showed a 46% reduction in mortality.[A5]

Patients on hemodialysis are exposed to a large volume of dialysate solution (typically 36 to 48 L/hour during dialysis) and must be protected against even small quantities of impurities, such as trace minerals, bacteria, and bacterial endotoxins, in the dialysis solution. To this end, dialysate solutions are prepared from concentrates diluted with water prepared by reverse osmosis systems or deionizer tanks to remove undesired trace cations and anions and then filtered through small micron-sized pore filters to remove bacteria and their byproducts. Exposure to low levels of bacteria and bacterial byproducts may contribute to the chronic inflammation seen in some patients on hemodialysis.

In critically ill patients who are hemodynamically unstable, one alternative is continuous venovenous hemofiltration, which requires central venous access (double-lumen catheter) and blood flows between 150 and 300 mL/minute. Plasma water under pressure passes across one side of a highly permeable membrane, thereby allowing both water and solutes up to about 60 kD to be removed. In contrast to hemodialysis, urea, creatinine, and phosphate are cleared at similar rates (convective clearance) during hemofiltration, but with improved clearance of larger molecular weight solute ("middle molecules"). The filtrate is discarded, and the fluid lost is partially replaced with a solution containing the major crystalloid components of the plasma at physiologic levels. However, there is no evidence from randomized trials that continuous venovenous hemofiltration offers a survival advantage compared with intermittent hemodialysis in patients with acute renal failure.

New modes of hemodialysis, used predominantly outside the United States, have sought to take advantage of convection to increase the clearance of middle molecules by using high-flux dialysis membranes and ultrafiltration rates of more than 20 L of fluid per dialysis session. In a large randomized trial, this approach, termed high-efficiency postdilution online hemofiltration, reduced all-cause mortality by 30%.

Uremic toxins are classified as low molecular weight (<500 daltons), middle molecular weight (500-60,000) protein-derived metabolites/solutes, and protein-bound solutes. Conventional hemodialysis is most efficient at the removal of low-molecular-weight uremic solutes (<500 daltons). One method to increase the removal of larger-molecular-weight uremic solutes ("middle molecules" in the 500 to 5000 dalton range) is by extending the time on dialysis to permit greater diffusion of these molecules across the dialysis membrane. However, the benefits of this approach remain unclear. Another method of increasing the clearance of middle-molecular-weight uremic solutes is by the use of membranes with larger pore sizes (referred to as medium cutoff dialyzers), which are able to achieve clearances comparable to or, for molecules at the higher end of this range, superior to hemodiafiltration with standard dialyzers. The concern, however, is the filtration and loss of albumin and the long-term implications in terms of overall nutritional status.[A6-A8]

The most common complications during hemodialysis are vascular access problems, hypotension, muscle cramps, nausea, vomiting, headache, and chest pain. Excessive fluid removal is the most frequent cause of hypotension, but persistent hypotension may be caused by sepsis (Chapter 94), myocardial ischemia (Chapter 57), pericardial tamponade (Chapter 62), arrhythmias (Chapters 49 to 53), and active bleeding. A rare complication is an air embolus (Chapter 68), which is manifested with agitation, cough, dyspnea, and chest pain. The patient should be given 100% oxygen and positioned with the left side down (Duran position) in Trendelenburg, or flat and supine, in an attempt to trap air in the right ventricle.

TABLE 117-1 INDICATIONS FOR DIALYSIS IN CHRONIC KIDNEY DISEASE

Uremic encephalopathy or neuropathy
Pericarditis or pleuritis
Bleeding attributable to uremia
Fluid overload refractory to diuretics
Hypertension poorly responsive to medication
Persistent hyperkalemia, metabolic acidosis, hypercalcemia, hypocalcemia, or hyperphosphatemia refractory to medical therapy
Malnutrition or weight loss
Persistent nausea and vomiting

From Tolkoff-Rubin N. Treatment of irreversible renal failure. In: Goldman L, Schafer AI, eds. *Goldman's Cecil Medicine*. 24th ed. Philadelphia: Elsevier Saunders; 2012.

PERITONEAL DIALYSIS

Peritoneal dialysis,[2] which is an alternative mode of renal replacement therapy, is usually performed at home by the patient or the patient's family. A peritoneal dialysis catheter is implanted through a surgically created tunnel in the abdominal wall and inserted into the peritoneal cavity. The catheter's tip in the pelvis is used to instill a dialysis solution into the peritoneal cavity and then to drain the solution from it. Peritoneal dialysis uses the peritoneal membrane, which consists of the visceral peritoneum, the interstitial tissues, and the mesenteric capillaries, as the filter across which the diffusion of solutes and convection of plasma water occur. Different forms include continuous ambulatory peritoneal dialysis, which is typically performed with 1.5- to 3-L exchanges of peritoneal dialysis solution instilled in the abdomen through a Tenckhoff catheter four times per day; automated peritoneal dialysis, which is performed with a cycler machine at night cycling 1.5 to 3 L of peritoneal dialysis fluid into and out of the abdomen four or five times overnight; and continuous cyclic peritoneal dialysis, a hybrid of continuous ambulatory peritoneal dialysis and automated peritoneal dialysis that uses cycler therapy at night combined with one or two manual exchanges during the day. *Kt/V* urea is the total volume clearance of urea (*Kt*) normalized to the urea space, *V*, which is approximately equal to total body water. For patients who are treated with peritoneal dialysis, residual renal function is often important for ensuring adequate clearance of uremic toxins. For such patients, residual renal function is measured periodically by a 24-hour urine collection. Then the amount of clearance of urea is also measured from the fluid drained from the patient's abdominal cavity after a dialysate exchange to be sure that total urea clearance, from the dialysate plus residual renal function, meets the minimal clearance that is recommended for the patient.

Clearance of small solutes is a key predictor of survival in patients undergoing peritoneal dialysis, and residual renal function also plays a critical role. Current guidelines advocate a minimal target *Kt/V* urea of at least 1.7 per week. Every effort should be made to maintain residual renal function as long as possible by avoiding nephrotoxins such as nonsteroidal anti-inflammatory drugs, iodinated contrast agents, and aminoglycosides. As residual renal function diminishes over time, the peritoneal dialysis prescription needs to be adjusted accordingly.

MEDICAL ISSUES

Renal replacement therapy is concerned not only with adequate dialytic clearance of nitrogenous waste products, the restoration of acid-base and electrolyte balance, and the control of salt and water balance but also with preserving adequate access sites for dialysis, nutrition, and the management of anemia, bone diseases, and cardiovascular risk.

Access Issues

The optimal dialysis access for hemodialysis is a native vein arteriovenous fistula, which can be created by the surgical anastomosis of the radial artery to the cephalic vein or of the brachial artery to either the brachiocephalic or the basilic vein. If a patient's veins are inadequate, a synthetic graft can be placed between the radial, brachial, or axillary artery and the brachiocephalic, basilic, or axillary vein as an alternative. Most commonly, these grafts are made from a synthetic polymer, expanded polytetrafluoroethylene. Less frequently, urgent temporary access can be obtained with a dual-lumen central venous dialysis catheter that is inserted into the internal jugular (preferable) or subclavian vein (right preferred to left). Dialysis access requires periodic Doppler monitoring to detect stenoses that can lead to reduced or even inadequate blood flow, thereby resulting in inadequate urea clearance and, if untreated, thrombosis. These stenoses can be treated by percutaneous transluminal angioplasty, with drug-coated balloons preferable to standard angioplasty,[A9] although stenting is sometimes required to maintain adequate luminal patency.

Nutrition

Adequate nutrition is important for optimizing outcome with renal replacement therapy, and rates of hospitalization are reduced when patients ingest at least 1 g/kg/day of protein. Another marker of nutritional status is the serum albumin level, which generally serves as a reasonable predictor of outcomes with renal replacement therapy.

Anemia

Anemia in end-stage renal disease is due to the reduced production of erythropoietin by the diseased kidneys, a shortened half-life of red blood cells, and the potential loss of red blood cells in the extracorporeal dialysis circuit and the gastrointestinal tract (related to intermittent anticoagulation for the hemodialysis procedure). Erythropoietic stimulating agents should aim to avoid transfusion by maintaining the hemoglobin level generally above 9 g/dL but not higher than 11 g/dL because higher levels are associated with more cardiovascular complications. Patients who have relative or absolute iron deficiency, as evidenced by a transferrin saturation below 20 to 25% or a serum ferritin level below 200, are often relatively resistant to erythropoietic stimulating agents and can benefit from the concurrent administration of a 1-g course (during 8 to 10 dialysis sessions) of intravenous iron (iron sucrose, ferric gluconate, ferumoxytol, or ferric carboxymaltose).[A10]

Unlike the original class of erythropoietic stimulating agents, which were erythropoietin or modified forms of it, a new class of agents (e.g., roxadustat, vadadustat, and daprodustat) inhibits the metabolism and degradation of the α subunit of hypoxia-inducible factor.[A11–A13] This factor stimulates the production of erythropoietin from the kidney and liver and also enhances the mobilization and utilization of iron from stores in the reticuloendothelial system by suppressing the production of hepcidin in the liver. Daprodustat is the first of these drugs to be approved by the U.S. Food and Drug Administration for the treatment of anemia in end-stage renal disease patients on dialysis.

Metabolic Bone Disease

Metabolic bone disease and phosphorus imbalance are common in end-stage renal disease. Clinical manifestations of renal osteodystrophy (Chapter 116) can range from adynamic bone disease to osteomalacia (Chapter 226) to secondary hyperparathyroidism (Chapter 227) and osteitis fibrosa cystica. The goals of therapy are to achieve a serum phosphorus level within or close to the normal physiologic range, typically about 2.5 to 5.5 g/dL; a corrected calcium (0.8 × [4 − Serum albumin level] + Serum calcium level])–phosphorus product less than 55; and an intact parathyroid hormone level within two to nine times the upper limit of normal.[3] Management includes the restriction of dietary phosphate to 750 to 1000 mg/day of elemental phosphorus; the use of phosphate binders (calcium carbonate or acetate, sevelamer carbonate, lanthanum carbonate, or potentially other cationic agents, magnesium or ferric ion) with meals to bind phosphate in the intestines and to reduce its absorption; the use of activated forms of vitamin D (e.g., calcitriol [0.5 to 4 μg IV or 0.5 to 1 μg PO], paricalcitol [1 to 15 μg IV or PO], or doxercalciferol [1 to 6 μg IV or 5 to 20 μg PO] at each hemodialysis session) to stimulate the parathyroid cells to suppress parathyroid hormone secretion; and cinacalcet (30 to 180 mg daily) to reduce secondary hyperparathyroidism significantly by nearly 70%, even though it does not provide a survival benefit over activated vitamin D therapy alone. Etelcalcetide, which is an intravenous calcimimetic, that is, administered during dialysis sessions, appears to be an equally effective alternative to daily oral cinacalcet.[A14]

Hyperphosphatemia can also lead to pruritus, which occurs in about 50% of patients. If moderate-to-severe pruritus persists, however, intravenous difelikefalin (0.5 μg/kg three times per week) can significantly reduce itching and improve itch-related quality of life.[A15] Reducing the serum phosphorus level is the key treatment.

Cardiovascular Disease

Cardiovascular disease is the leading cause of morbidity and mortality in patients on dialysis. The mainstay of blood pressure control in renal replacement therapy is to achieve the lowest tolerated postdialysis weight to facilitate blood pressure control and enhance the body's sensitivity to antihypertensive agents. The general approach to antihypertensive medication therapy is similar to the approach for other patients, with the exception that diuretics are not helpful (see Tables 64-7 and 64-9). The ideal or goal interdialytic blood pressure for the patient with end-stage renal disease is probably 125 to 145 mm Hg systolic.

Dialysis-dependent chronic kidney disease is an indicator for the same type of aspirin therapy and β-adrenergic blockade used in survivors of a myocardial infarction (Chapters 57 and 58). Statin therapy (Chapter 190) is often recommended, but statins are not of proven benefit for reducing major cardiovascular events or overall mortality in dialysis patients despite clinically relevant reductions in low-density lipoprotein cholesterol levels. The addition of spironolactone (25 mg daily) can reduce the risk of a cardiovascular or cerebrovascular event by about 50%. Control of diabetes (Chapter 210) is important, but mortality in hemodialysis patients is not increased until the hemoglobin A_{1c} level is 8.5% or higher. In patients with chronic kidney disease and stable moderate or severe coronary disease, an initial invasive coronary strategy is no better than a conservative guideline-based strategy.[A16,A17]

Amyloidosis

Dialysis-associated amyloidosis (Chapter 174), typically seen in patients who have been on dialysis for more than 10 to 12 years, is caused by the deposition of end-products of β_2-microglobulin catabolism as amyloid fibrils. The clinical syndrome includes carpal tunnel syndrome (Chapter 388), arthropathy, and autonomic neuropathy (Chapter 386).

Infection

Infection is the second leading cause of morbidity and mortality in dialysis patients. For example, patients on hemodialysis account for about 8% of all patients who develop bacterial endocarditis (Chapter 61), with *S. aureus* and enterococcal endocarditis being equally common.[4]

In hemodialysis, vascular access sites are the primary sources of bacteria and account for about 75% of all cases of bacteremia. In a patient with possible catheter-related bacteremia, blood culture specimens should be obtained both from the catheter and from a peripheral vein. Most vascular access infections are caused by staphylococcal organisms (Chapter 267) and should be treated empirically with vancomycin (15 to 20 mg/kg or approximately 1 g) at the end of each dialysis session, adjusted to blood levels, unless another organism is cultured. In patients with systemic sepsis (Chapter 94) with hemodynamic instability, the line should be pulled promptly and reinserted only after blood cultures are negative for at least 48 hours and the patient has defervesced. Interim dialysis can use an alternative access site, such as a temporary non-tunneled catheter. A prolonged course of antibiotic therapy (4 to 8 weeks) is recommended for bacteremia or fungemia that persists after the catheter is removed or in patients with evidence of endocarditis (Chapter 61), septic arthritis (Chapter 251), osteomyelitis (Chapter 251), epidural abscess (Chapter 381), or other metastatic infection.

With peritoneal dialysis, infection is the most frequent reason that the catheter must be removed and therapy discontinued. Infection is suspected by erythema, tenderness, induration, or purulent or bloody drainage. Peritonitis must be suspected in patients with abdominal pain and cloudy dialysate; the physical examination usually shows abdominal tenderness, often with rebound. The peritoneal fluid white blood cell count is typically above 100/μL with a predominance of neutrophils, although lymphocytes may predominate with fungal or mycobacterial infections. Polymicrobial infections should raise the possibility of a perforated diverticulum (Chapter 128), ruptured appendix (Chapter 128), ischemic bowel (Chapter 129), incarcerated hernia (Chapter 128), pancreatitis (Chapter 130), or gynecologic conditions (Chapters 184, and 219) and should prompt an emergent abdominal computed tomography scan. *Staphylococcus epidermidis* (Chapter 267) is the most common cause of peritonitis, but *Pseudomonas* species (Chapter 282) account for 5 to 8% of cases. Recommended initial empirical treatment is intraperitoneal, unless there is evidence of bacteremia or hematogenous spread of the infection. Options include vancomycin (15 to 30 mg/kg in one exchange every 5 to 7 days as guided by serum levels) or a cephalosporin (e.g., cefazolin, 15 to 20 mg/kg in one exchange daily) together with intravenous or intraperitoneal administration of a third-generation cephalosporin with antipseudomonal activity (e.g., ceftazidime, 1 to 1.5 g in one exchange daily) or gentamicin (0.6 mg/kg in one exchange daily) for at least 2 weeks.

Staphylococcus aureus (Chapter 267) is the most common organism for exit site and tunnel infections. Treatment options include empirical oral penicillinase-resistant penicillins (e.g., dicloxacillin, 250 to 500 mg twice daily), fluoroquinolones (e.g., ciprofloxacin, 250 mg twice daily or 500 mg daily), trimethoprim-sulfamethoxazole (e.g., 80 mg/400 mg twice daily or 160 mg/800 mg daily), and cephalosporins (e.g., cephalexin, 500 mg two to three times per day). Vancomycin should be avoided as first-line therapy except for methicillin-resistant *S. aureus*. Mupirocin nasal ointment applied to the exit site twice daily for 5 days every 4 weeks significantly reduces the incidence of *S. aureus* exit site infections.

PROGNOSIS

The prognosis of patients with end-stage renal disease on chronic dialysis depends on their age and other comorbid conditions, especially diabetes. On average, the 5-year survival rate is about 40 to 50% and is similar for hemodialysis and peritoneal dialysis. Survival rates are markedly lower than for the age-matched U.S. population (Table 117-2). The leading cause of death is arrhythmic cardiac arrest, but about 15% of deaths are related to withdrawal of dialysis.

RENAL TRANSPLANTATION

For appropriate patients, renal transplantation continues to be the best treatment for advanced chronic kidney disease. The success of renal transplantation has increased dramatically during the past several decades owing to improved surgical technique, improved medical care, and safer and more effective immunosuppressive medications. Although transplant recipients do not have a normal life expectancy, current 5-year survival rates are nearly twice as high as for similar patients who remain on dialysis or on the transplant waiting list. Several long-held axioms have been proved false, most notably the need for long-term steroid therapy, the impossibility of transplantation in the face of antidonor human leukocyte antigen (HLA) antibodies (positive crossmatch), the inability to transplant ABO-incompatible donor-recipient pairs, and the inability to create long-term tolerance. Despite this remarkable progress, the number of patients on the waiting list far exceeds the number of available kidneys, and the long-term survival rates for kidneys and patients remain disappointing.

EPIDEMIOLOGY

Over 26,000 total renal transplants, including combined kidney-pancreas, kidney-liver, and kidney-heart, are performed annually in the United States. The most common disease leading to renal transplantation is diabetic nephrosclerosis (Chapter 109), followed by hypertensive nephrosclerosis (Chapter 110) and other forms of glomerulonephritis (Chapter 107). Kidney transplant recipients vary in age from infants to older than 80 years, with the majority being between 35 and 64 years of age. About 65% of the kidneys transplanted

TABLE 117-2 EXPECTED REMAINING YEARS OF LIFE IN PREVALENT PATIENTS WITH END-STAGE RENAL DISEASE AND IN THE GENERAL POPULATION, BY AGE, SEX, AND END-STAGE RENAL DISEASE TREATMENT MODALITY

	END-STAGE RENAL DISEASE PATIENTS, 2020					
	DIALYSIS		*TRANSPLANT*		*GENERAL U.S. POPULATION*	
AGE	**FEMALE**	**MALE**	**FEMALE**	**MALE**	**FEMALE**	**MALE**
40-44	8.9	9.4	26.7	24.4	39.6	35.3
45-49	7.7	8.2	23.0	20.8	35.0	30.9
50-54	6.8	7.0	19.6	17.4	30.6	26.8
55-59	5.9	6.0	16.5	14.5	26.3	22.8
60-64	5.1	5.0	13.6	11.9	22.2	19.1
65-69	4.4	4.2	10.9	9.7	18.2	15.7
70-74	3.7	3.6	8.7	7.7	14.5	12.4
75-79	3.3	3.0	6.9*	6.0*	11.1	9.4
80-84	2.8	2.6			8.1	6.9
85+	2.4	2.1			3.8	3.3

*For patients age 75+ years.

Table shows the expected remaining lifetime, in years, for the 2020 prevalent end-stage renal population and the general U.S. population. The table illustrates the markedly foreshortened projected lifespan for patients with end-stage renal disease relative to those without. In individuals aged 40-44 years, for example, there is a >25-year projected lifespan difference between men receiving dialysis (expectancy 9.4 years) and men in the general population (expectancy 35.3 years); the difference was >30 years for women receiving dialysis.

Data Source: USRDS ESRD database. 2022 Annual Data Report, End Stage Renal Disease Chapter 6, Table 6-1, https://usrds-adr.niddk.nih.gov/2022, and National Vital Statistics Report Volume 71, 2022. United States Life Tables 2020, Tables 2,3.

in the United States are from deceased donors, with the other 35% from living donors, who include both living genetically related family members and genetically unrelated donors, most often spouses or friends. The number of deceased kidney donors has increased in recent years, in part due to the opioid epidemic, whereas the number of living donors has remained relatively constant, as has the number of patients on the active transplant waitlist. Currently, the number of patients on the active waitlist is three times larger than the supply of kidneys; and, as a result, the median waiting time for a patient listed for kidney transplantation exceeds 4 years. Fewer than 50% of candidates on the waitlist are transplanted within 5 years of listing, and approximately one third either die or are removed from the waitlist without having received a transplant. Due to improved survival and reduced costs of kidney transplantation compared with dialysis, the U.S, government has recently taken initiatives to encourage increased rates of transplantation for patients with end-stage renal disease.[5]

Renal Transplant Success Rates

For deceased donor kidney transplants, the overall 1-year success rate is approximately 93%, and the 10-year success rate is approximately 50%. For recipients of live donor kidney transplants, the overall 1-year success rate is more than 97%, and the 10-year success rate is 65%.

KIDNEY DONATION

Potential *living kidney donors* undergo a thorough evaluation to ensure that age-adjusted renal function is normal, that the surgical risk of donor nephrectomy is acceptably low, and that there are no medical conditions that would increase the risk of future renal disease in the donor. In addition, all donors are screened for transmissible infections or malignant neoplasms.

Potential donors must be capable of understanding the risks and benefits of live kidney donation, cannot be coerced into donating, and cannot condition the donation on the receipt of money or other valuable goods. Federal law prohibits the buying and selling of organs. Although recent data suggest that live kidney donors have a 3.5- to 5.3-fold higher risk for developing end-stage renal disease compared with healthy non-donors during the 10 years after donation, the absolute risk remains less than 1%.[6] Gestational hypertension or preeclampsia also is more likely in kidney donors than in matched nondonors.

Potential recipients who have a willing and medically and psychosocially suitable live donor, but who either have preformed antidonor HLA antibodies or are blood group incompatible with their potential donor, can receive successful transplants by desensitization protocols that involve intravenous immune globulin and plasmapheresis to reduce the level of antidonor HLA antibodies or isoagglutinins. Despite remarkable short-term success, the high incidence of antibody-mediated rejection has made long-term success rates somewhat disappointing, at about 60 to 70% at 5 years. However, data indicate that patients who receive kidney transplants from HLA-incompatible live donors still realize a substantial survival benefit compared with similar patients who wait for compatible transplants from deceased donors or who remain on the waitlist. An increasingly popular alternative to desensitization is kidney-paired donation. In this scenario, two recipients, each with an incompatible live donor who is compatible with the other recipient, exchange donors, thereby creating two immunologically compatible donor-recipient pairs. Over 1000 annual paired donation transplants in the United States now account for approximately 15% of all living-donor transplants. In some situations, more complicated exchanges may involve multiple donor-recipient pairs.

The majority of deceased donors are brain dead, as a result of head trauma (Chapter 368), cerebrovascular catastrophe (Chapter 377), or anoxia (Chapter 50), but continue to maintain a normal circulation. The Uniform Anatomical Gift Act of 1968 and subsequent revisions equate brain death with death (Chapter 2) and permit organ donation after a declaration of brain death, provided there is consent from the family of the deceased. Events surrounding brain death and organ procurement may result in acute kidney injury, and renal biopsies are frequently performed before implantation to assess kidney quality and potential longevity.

The shortage of available donor organs continues to plague the field of clinical transplantation. Attempts to increase the number of donor organs have included the use of lower quality kidneys, such as kidneys from older donors or donors with a history of diabetes mellitus or hypertension. Deceased donor kidneys are now rated on a continuous grading system—the Kidney Donor Profile Index (KDPI). Characteristics used to calculate the KDPI include the donor's age, height and weight, serum creatinine, history of hypertension, history of diabetes, hepatitis C status, whether the donation was after a cardiac death, and the cause of death. Lower KDPI values—higher quality kidneys—are associated with a lower inherent estimated risk of kidney failure (longer anticipated function after transplantation), whereas transplantation of kidneys with higher KDPI values will result in shorter estimated allograft survival times. This prognosis allows for better informed decision making on the part of both patients and physicians. Developing algorithms to facilitate the optimal use of suboptimal kidneys will continue to be a challenge. Protocols have also been developed to allow organ recovery from deceased donors after cessation of cardiac function (donation after cardiac death [DCD] donors). These kidneys function as well as those recovered by traditional donation after brain death.

Initiatives to increase the deceased donor pool include kidney transplantation from a human immunodeficiency virus (HIV)-positive donor to an HIV-infected recipient. With the availability of curative treatment for hepatitis C (Chapter 135), infected donor kidneys can now be used for hepatitis C-negative recipients, who then receive antiviral therapy immediately after transplantation.[7,8]

WHO IS A CANDIDATE FOR RENAL TRANSPLANTATION?

All patients with advanced chronic kidney disease must be informed about the option of transplantation. Candidates must undergo an age and gender appropriate comprehensive medical and psychosocial evaluation to determine their suitability. The major elements of the evaluation include an assessment of cardiovascular risk,[9,10] urologic suitability, cancer screening, risk of infection, and overall frailty. Because cardiovascular disease is common in end-stage renal disease patients, cardiovascular testing is often undertaken in patients older than 50 years and in patients with a history of diabetes (Chapter 401). In general, contraindications to transplant include active uncontrolled infection, cancer not amenable to treatment, advanced untreatable cardiac disease, cirrhosis, advanced chronic lung disease, inability to follow the post-transplant medical regimen owing to psychosocial reasons, and poor perioperative risk. For otherwise suitable patients with advanced liver, lung, cardiac disease, combined liver-kidney, lung-kidney, or heart-kidney transplantation may be an appropriate option. Despite consensus guidelines, the criteria for listing a candidate for transplant vary among transplant centers.[11]

ALLOCATION

The national systems in the U.S. (the United Network for Organ Sharing) and in virtually every country oversee the distribution of deceased donor kidneys. Given the imbalance between demand and supply, this allocation system attempts to balance equity and utility. Some prioritization is given to patients who are likely to have the best allograft survival, but all suitable candidates have a chance to receive a kidney.

The national system for the allocation of deceased donor organs in the United States is divided into 58 donor service areas, each with an organ procurement organization responsible for procuring and allocating deceased donor organs. The distribution of these organs is first local, then regional, and finally national if no local compatible recipient exists. Waiting time for active listing can begin from the date a patient first starts dialysis, or when their eGFR is <20 mL/minute. The current allocation system largely prioritizes waitlisted candidates with longest waiting time as first in line for the next available compatible kidney within their blood group. Each waitlisted patient receives an Estimated Post-Transplant Survival (EPTS) score based on four factors: time on dialysis, current diagnosis of diabetes, prior solid organ transplants, and age. Patients with low EPTS scores (longer predicted post-transplant survival) are prioritized to receive donor organs with longer anticipated function, beginning the practice of longevity matching in kidney allocation. Special consideration is given to children who are waitlisted prior to age 18 years, patients with high levels of anti-HLA antibodies (for whom compatible donors are difficult to find), patients receiving combined (heart-kidney, liver-kidney, or lung-kidney) transplants, and patients for whom a potential donor has a high degree of HLA matching.[12]

IMMUNOSUPPRESSION

Notwithstanding several reports of successful medication-free long-term renal allograft survival in small numbers of carefully selected patients undergoing complicated conditioning regimens, long-term immunosuppression remains obligatory in virtually all patients to achieve long-term renal allograft survival. The principal drivers of the immune response to an organ allograft and the principal obstacle to organ acceptance are the HLA antigens (Chapter 38). HLA-identical siblings enjoy the best long-term survival rates, and increasing degrees of HLA antigen *mis*match continue to be associated with inferior long-term outcomes (Chapter 38).

Immunosuppressive treatment can be divided into three phases: induction, maintenance, and antirejection (Table 117-3). Induction immunosuppression consists of antilymphocyte antibodies given within the first week immediately after transplantation. Maintenance immunosuppression refers to those medications given daily as long as the allograft is functioning. Antirejection therapy is given to treat episodes of acute or chronic rejection.

For about two thirds of patients, the standard maintenance therapy for the long-term prevention of renal allograft rejection is a three-drug regimen: a calcineurin inhibitor, a purine synthesis inhibitor, and a corticosteroid—tacrolimus, mycophenolate, and prednisone. In the approximately one third of patients with a low-to-moderate risk of rejection, corticosteroids can be safely withdrawn within the first week after transplantation,[A18] and a dual-therapy regimen of mycophenolate and tacrolimus is continued. Outcomes appear to be similar with either regimen. In a randomized trial, however, substituting belatacept (a costimulation blocker) for cyclosporine reduced the 7-year risk of death from graft failure more than 40% and resulted in significantly improved allograft function without an increase in any adverse events, despite a higher number of early acute rejection episodes.[A19]

Induction therapy consists of polyclonal or monoclonal antilymphocyte antibodies administered in the first week after transplantation. Approximately 80% of kidney transplant recipients are in centers that administer induction therapy, the majority with rabbit-derived polyclonal antilymphocyte serum (usually 6 mg/kg total dose) and the others with either basiliximab (20 mg, day 0 and day 4) or alemtuzumab (30-mg single dose). The goals of induction therapy include a reduction in the number of acute rejection episodes in the first several weeks or months after transplantation, a long-term reduction in the overall number of acute rejection episodes, and a resulting improvement in long-term success rates. The addition of cell-based biologic products (regulatory T cells, dendritic cells, or macrophages) is an experimental approach under investigation, with the goal of permitting a reduction in long-term immunosuppression, without any compromise in results (Chapter 38).[13]

REJECTION AND ITS TREATMENT

Despite the availability of more effective and safer immunosuppressive medications, rejection remains an ever-present threat, and a significant proportion of allograft failures are ultimately caused by immune-mediated injury. Classically, there are three types of rejection: hyperacute, acute, and chronic. Histological definitions of acute and chronic rejection are based on criteria (Banff Classification) established and periodically updated by a working group of pathologists and clinicians. Most recently, the category of chronic T-cell mediated rejection has been recognized, and criteria for its diagnosis have been outlined.[14]

Hyperacute rejection occurs when a kidney is transplanted into a recipient who is presensitized to the donor. The recipient's circulating preformed antidonor antibodies may target HLA antigens, blood group (ABO) antigens, or endothelial cell antigens expressed on the donor kidney. The result is immediate endothelial injury and irreversible thrombosis of the transplant. Because of the prescreening of all donor-recipient pairs for the presence of such antidonor antibodies, hyperacute rejection occurs in less than 1% of all renal transplants.

Acute rejection is characterized clinically by an increase in the serum creatinine level over days to weeks, often in the absence of symptoms. On pathologic examination, acute rejection is most frequently "cellular" and characterized by T-lymphocyte infiltration of the tubules, interstitium, and of the vascular structures in more severe rejection. Acute rejection now occurs in only 10 to 15% of transplant patients during the first post-transplantation year and about another 10% in the second year. The majority of acute rejections occur in the first 3 to 6 months after transplantation and are clinically mild, treatable, and reversible. Other causes of allograft dysfunction (e.g., hemodynamic factors such as hypotension and volume depletion, urinary tract obstruction, drug-induced nephrotoxicity, and BK polyomavirus nephropathy) must be excluded. Percutaneous biopsy of the allograft is required to establish the diagnosis with certainty, to determine the type and severity of the rejection, and to guide therapeutic decisions. Acute cellular rejection should be treated immediately, either with high-dose intravenous corticosteroid therapy for milder forms or with polyclonal antilymphocyte sera for steroid-resistant or more severe acute rejection episodes. Such treatment is usually effective at resolving the episode.

Between 10 and 20% of patients have acute antibody-mediated rejection injury, due either to preformed antidonor antibodies or to the development of de novo donor specific antibodies. A hallmark of acute antibody-mediated rejection is the deposition of C4d, a metabolite of a complement component C4, in the peritubular capillaries, accompanied by inflammatory cells in the peritubular capillaries. This antibody-mediated rejection may occur alone or in combination with cellular rejection. Early antibody-mediated rejection is much more common in patients with a prior history of exposure to alloantigen through transfusion, pregnancy, or prior transplantation. The development of sensitive reagents for detection of circulating antidonor antibodies has greatly facilitated the diagnosis of antibody-mediated rejection. Treatment is more problematic, and patients frequently receive plasmapheresis to remove antidonor antibodies, high dose corticosteroids, and/or polyclonal antilymphocyte globulin, as well as various regimens of intravenous immune globulin. Although

TABLE 117-3 IMMUNOSUPPRESSIVE MEDICATIONS USED IN RENAL TRANSPLANTATION

CLASS	DRUGS	HOW USED	MECHANISM OF ACTION	MAJOR ADVERSE EFFECTS
Steroids	Prednisone, methylprednisolone	Induction, maintenance, antirejection	Multiple sites, anti-inflammatory; inhibit production of multiple cytokines	Poor wound healing, weight gain, diabetes, acne, hypertension, cushingoid appearance
Calcineurin inhibitors	Tacrolimus and cyclosporine	Maintenance	Inhibit calcineurin, prevent interleukin-2 production	Nephrotoxicity, hypertension, diabetes mellitus
Purine synthesis inhibitors	Azathioprine	Maintenance	Metabolized to 6-mercaptopurine	Anemia, leukopenia, thrombocytopenia
	Mycophenolic acid	Maintenance	Inhibits purine synthesis by the inhibition of inosine monophosphate dehydrogenase, specific for the purine de novo pathway on which lymphocytes depend	Anemia, leukopenia, thrombocytopenia; teratogenic
mTOR inhibitors	Sirolimus, everolimus	Maintenance	Inhibit mTOR (mammalian target of rapamycin), block lymphocyte response to growth factors	Poor wound healing, proteinuria, hyperlipidemia
Costimulation blockade	Belatacept	Maintenance	Human recombinant fusion protein combining the extracellular portion of cytotoxic T lymphocyte–associated antigen-4 (CTLA-4) with the Fc fragment of human IgG; this binds to the CTLA-4 receptor, preventing engagement of CTLA-4 on the T cell, preventing costimulation	Central nervous system post-transplantation lymphoproliferative disease
T cell–depleting antibodies	Thymoglobulin	Induction, antirejection	Rabbit-derived polyclonal antilymphocyte serum (multiple targets)	Infusion reaction, leukopenia, thrombocytopenia
	Alemtuzumab	Induction	Anti-CDS2	
Anti-IL2R monoclonal antibodies	Basiliximab	Induction	Block interleukin-2 receptor (IL2R)	Rare infusion reaction

Ig = immunoglobulin.

this treatment is often effective in reversing acute antibody-mediated rejection, successful elimination of antidonor antibody and prevention of alloantibody resynthesis are much more difficult. Chronic antibody-mediated rejection frequently follows an episode of acute antibody-mediated rejection.

Chronic rejection is characterized by a slow decline in allograft function, generally during a period of months to years, and frequently accompanied by proteinuria. Although it can occur in the absence of documented episodes of acute rejection and after many years of stable allograft function, early acute rejection is a major risk factor for later chronic rejection and allograft failure. The development of donor-specific anti-HLA antibodies appears to be a strong risk factor for subsequent allograft failure. Antibodies targeting non-HLA loci are also likely to play an important role.[15,16] Anti-HLA antibodies are detectable in a high percentage of cases of chronic allograft dysfunction.[17] Biopsy may show evidence of T cell–induced injury, antibody-induced injury with deposits of C4d, transplant glomerulopathy, or a combination of these findings. In many patients with long-term deterioration of allograft function, however, the only findings are interstitial fibrosis and tubular atrophy, often accompanied by arteriolar hyalinosis, without clear-cut evidence as to the cause. Unfortunately, no treatment has been proved to be effective for chronic T cell or chronic antibody-mediated rejection, which are common causes of long-term allograft failure.

OTHER COMPLICATIONS OF RENAL TRANSPLANTATION

Immunosuppression in renal transplant recipients is associated with a number of adverse effects, the most important of which are infection, malignant neoplasia, and nephrotoxicity.

Infection

Infections occurring in the first few weeks after transplantation are generally nosocomial (Chapter 260), donor derived, present in the recipient at the time of transplantation, or a result of complications of the surgical procedure, such as wound, catheter-associated, or urinary tract infections (Chapter 263) (Fig. 117-1). Next is a period of 5 to 6 months during which opportunistic infection or reactivation of latent infection, such as cytomegalovirus (CMV) infection (Chapter 347) or Epstein-Barr virus (EBV) infection (Chapter 348), is most likely to occur. Later in the course, when the doses of immunosuppressive medication are decreased, community-acquired infections are most common. This timeline is partly a function of infection prophylaxis, given to all renal transplant recipients to minimize infectious complications during periods of highest risk, including perioperative antibiotics to prevent wound and urinary tract infection (Chapter 263), trimethoprim-sulfamethoxazole to prevent *Pneumocystis jiroveci* pneumonia (Chapter 313), oral nystatin or clotrimazole to prevent oral candidiasis (Chapter 310), and oral valganciclovir (see Table 328-4) to prevent CMV disease (Chapter 347). Urinary tract infections (Chapter 263) are the most frequent bacterial infections that lead to hospitalizations in kidney transplant recipients, and the most common organism is *Escherichia coli*.

Up to 30% of patients develop active infection with the BK polyomavirus (Chapter 341), which is trophic for the urinary epithelia. In 5 to 10% of patients, this infection leads to tubulitis and interstitial nephritis, which may result in significant allograft injury. Histologically, BK polyomavirus nephritis is often difficult to distinguish from acute rejection without the use of a special SV40 stain that identifies the large T antigen of BK virus. Approximately 80 to 90% of the general population has serologic evidence of exposure to BK polyomavirus, so infection in the renal transplant recipient may be due to reactivation, superinfection, or primary infection. Interestingly, BK nephropathy is very rare in equally immunosuppressed recipients of other organ transplants. The most important noninvasive indicator of possible BK viral nephropathy is BK viremia, which can be documented in about 10 to 20% of renal transplant recipients. It is presently estimated that 5 to 10% of all renal transplant recipients develop BK virus–induced nephritis and allograft dysfunction, which leads to allograft failure in about half of these patients. Monitoring for BK viremia or viruria is strongly recommended, especially in the first year post-transplant. BK viremia and BK viral nephropathy should be treated initially with a reduction in immunosuppression. No effective antiviral therapy exists for patients who do not respond to lowered immunosuppression.

CMV infection (Chapter 347) continues to be a major cause of morbidity in renal transplant recipients. CMV is widely distributed in the general population, with seroprevalence rates from 40 to 90%, so infections may be due to reactivation, superinfection, or primary infection. CMV disease may be limited to fever and malaise, but frequently causes significant morbidity and even mortality after infecting the gastrointestinal tract, lungs, or liver. Most transplant centers use oral valganciclovir (see Table 328-4) for CMV prophylaxis for 7 months or more after transplantation for all patients at risk, especially seronegative

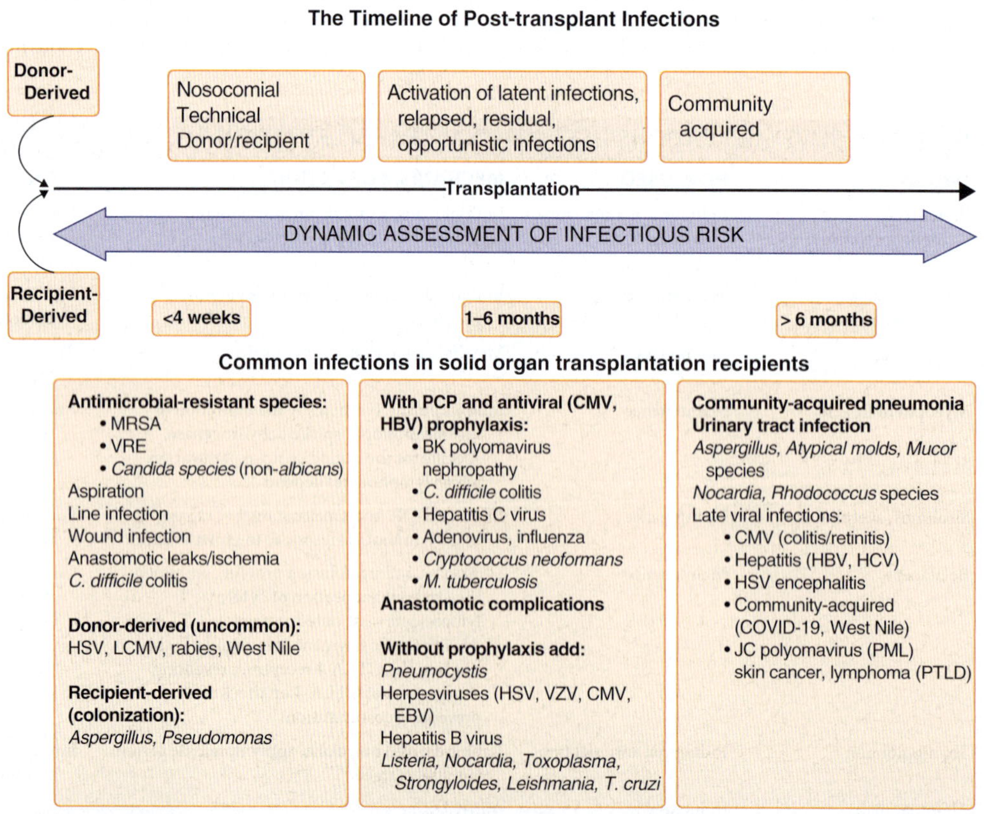

FIGURE 117-1. **Timeline of post-transplantation infections.** CMV = cytomegalovirus; COVID-19 = coronavirus disease 2019; EBV = Epstein-Barr virus; HBV = hepatitis B virus; HCV = hepatitis C virus; HSV = herpes simplex virus; LCMV = lymphocytic choriomeningitis virus; MRSA = methicillin-resistant *Staphylococcus aureus;* PCP = *Pneumocystis* pneumonia; PML = progressive multifocal leukoencephalopathy; PTLD = post-transplantation lymphoproliferative disease; VRE = vancomycin-resistant enterococci; VZV = varicella-zoster virus. (From Fishman JA. Introduction: infection in solid organ transplant recipients. *Am J Transplant*. 2009;9[Suppl 4]:S3-S6.)

recipients who receive transplants from seropositive donors. Another alternative is frequent post-transplantation monitoring, with treatment reserved for patients who develop viremia. Regardless of the initial strategy, approximately 10% of patients have later viral activation and require additional treatment. Antiviral therapy (Chapters 328) is usually highly effective.

EBV infection (Chapter 348) also may represent a primary infection, reactivation, or superinfection. EBV may cause a mononucleosis-like syndrome, but the more serious concern in renal transplant patients is a form of lymphoma termed post-transplantation lymphoproliferative disease (Chapters 171 and 348).

Renal transplant patients who are infected with severe acute respiratory syndrome coronavirus-2 have a higher mortality (15 to 30%) than the general population.[18] There is no agreed-upon protocol for the safe reduction of immunosuppression that will protect the allograft while mitigating the course of the infection. Vaccination against coronavirus disease 2019 (COVID-19) appears effective and protective against severe disease, albeit less so than in the non-immunosuppressed population.[19]

Malignant Neoplasia

Renal transplant patients develop some malignant neoplasms at higher rates than in the general population.[20] These malignancies include post-transplantation lymphoproliferative disorder related to EBV, Kaposi sarcoma (Chapter 359) caused by human herpesvirus 8 (Chapter 345), and cervical (Chapter 184) and anal (Chapter 131) carcinomas caused by human papillomavirus (Chapter 344). Post-transplantation lymphoproliferative disease most commonly involves the renal allograft, but it may involve any organ, including the gastrointestinal tract, lung, and central nervous system. Treatment usually involves a reduction in immunosuppression and chemotherapy (Chapter 171). Long-term patient survival rates approach 75%.

The relative risks of many common solid carcinomas are also elevated about two-fold, but with the exception of nonmelanoma skin cancers, the absolute risks remain low. Lifetime risk of nonmelanoma skin cancers (Chapter 188) may be as high as 70%. Annual skin screening and the attentive use of ultraviolet-blocking skin creams are strongly recommended. Otherwise, transplant recipients should follow the same standard screening guidelines as the general population for breast (Chapter 183), colon (Chapter 179), prostate (Chapter 186), and lung (Chapter 177) cancer. Whether immunosuppression should be reduced in patients who develop malignant neoplasms other than post-transplantation lymphoproliferative disease is unknown.

Calcineurin Inhibitor–Induced Nephrotoxicity

Calcineurin inhibitors (cyclosporine and tacrolimus; Chapter 28), which are arguably the most effective antirejection medications used in kidney transplantation, ironically cause a chronic, usually mild and stable, impairment of GFR in virtually all patients who receive them. Superimposed, acute reversible cyclosporine or tacrolimus nephrotoxicity may occur in patients who experience sudden elevations in drug blood levels. These acute episodes usually resolve when the dose of cyclosporine or tacrolimus is reduced. Of greater concern is long-term, irreversible calcineurin inhibitor–induced nephrotoxicity, which can cause allograft failure. This diagnosis is often difficult to make because there are few if any absolutely specific histologic biopsy findings. As a result, careful monitoring of blood calcineurin inhibitor levels is essential to avoid supratherapeutic levels (risking nephrotoxicity and infection) or subtherapeutic levels (risking rejection).

New-Onset Diabetes

By 36 months after transplantation, 30 to 40% of patients develop glucose intolerance or frank diabetes, which may be caused by corticosteroids, tacrolimus, and, to a lesser extent, cyclosporine. Treatment is as for diabetes in the general population (Chapter 210), with appropriate adjustment in the dose of insulin and oral agents for renal function. Patients who develop diabetes have poorer outcomes, including higher rates of cardiovascular events, graft failure, and death. Sodium glucose cotransporter 2 (SGLT2) inhibitors may be safe and appropriate treatment options for transplant patients, perhaps even for patients without diabetes mellitus.[A20]

MANAGEMENT OF THE PATIENT AFTER RENAL TRANSPLANTATION

In the initial few months after transplantation, patients are generally seen weekly. The interval then typically expands to once monthly for the remainder of the first year and every 2 to 6 months thereafter. Routine testing includes measurement of blood pressure, renal function, calcineurin inhibitor blood levels, lipid levels, glucose levels, BK polyomavirus assays, and proteinuria. Polymerase chain reaction analysis for CMV or EBV is indicated in selected patients. Monitoring for metabolic bone disease is also recommended, by parathyroid hormone and vitamin D levels as well as by bone densitometry. Influenza and pneumococcal vaccinations are strongly recommended for renal transplant recipients, but live vaccines are contraindicated (Chapter 15).

PROGNOSIS

Five-year kidney allograft survival is approximately 90% for recipients of living donor kidneys and 75% for recipients of deceased donor kidneys. Ten-year survival rates are approximately 70% and 45 to 50%, respectively.[21] Allograft failure with return to dialysis or retransplantation accounts for about 50% of long-term allograft failures.[22] Progressive loss of function in the long-term renal allograft is most commonly the result of chronic rejection but also may be due to nonimmunologic causes, such as calcineurin inhibitor nephrotoxicity, hypertension, diabetes, or recurrent glomerular disease (Table 117-4). A standardized evaluation (Table 117-5) can help establish the cause.

The importance of immunologic (or alloantigen-dependent) factors is illustrated by the fact that death-censored living donor transplants between HLA-identical siblings have a 94% 10-year graft survival, compared with 81% for parental or other less well-matched living donor kidneys and 40 to 50% overall for cadaveric kidney recipients.[23] Deceased donor kidneys with zero or one HLA-A, B, or DR mismatches have a higher success rate (close to 65% at 10 years) than do deceased donor kidneys with two or more antigen mismatches, which have 15 to 30% lower absolute survival rates.

Factors unrelated to anti-allograft immunity are also associated with reduced long-term success rates. These include hypertension, a kidney from an older (>50 years) donor, hyperlipidemia, diabetes mellitus, calcineurin inhibitor nephrotoxicity, recurrent glomerular disease, and a maladaptive response to hemodynamic injury, which is caused by elevated glomerular flow and pressure. Chronic calcineurin inhibitor toxicity leads to end-stage renal disease in at least 5 to 10% of recipients of nonrenal transplants and is likely to have at least a comparable long-term impact in renal transplant patients. Virtually all primary glomerular diseases (Chapter 107), including focal segmental glomerulosclerosis, membranous nephropathy, membranoproliferative glomerulonephritis, and immunoglobulin A (IgA) nephropathy, can recur after transplantation. Recurrent glomerulonephritis is a common cause of proteinuria and nephrotic syndrome after transplantation and may be responsible for up to 10% of all graft failures. For example, graft failure is significantly higher in patients with membranoproliferative glomerulonephritis, focal segmental glomerulosclerosis, membranous nephropathy, and IgA nephropathy compared with adult polycystic kidney disease. Renal biopsy is required to establish the diagnosis in a long-term renal allograft with deteriorating function or proteinuria and to distinguish immune-related from non–immune-related causes. Whether noninvasive biomarkers of actual or impending allograft injury (e.g., circulating donor-derived cell-free DNA or gene expression panels in peripheral blood or urine) will substitute for renal biopsy, in at least some

TABLE 117-4 COMMON CAUSES OF RENAL ALLOGRAFT DYSFUNCTION

Volume depletion: Nausea, vomiting, diarrhea, poor fluid intake, hemorrhage
Medication induced: Diuretics, antihypertensive medications, nonsteroidal anti-inflammatory drugs, calcineurin inhibitors, angiotensin-converting enzyme inhibitors
Urinary tract obstruction: Bladder outlet obstruction, ureteral obstruction
Transplant renal artery stenosis
Infection: Bacteremia, urinary tract infection
Rejection: Cell mediated, antibody mediated

TABLE 117-5 EVALUATION OF RENAL ALLOGRAFT DYSFUNCTION

History: Fluid intake and loss, medication changes, fever
Physical examination: Blood pressure, pulse rate, temperature, weight, edema, allograft tenderness or swelling
Laboratory tests: Serum creatinine level, BK virus detection by polymerase chain reaction analysis of urine or blood, calcineurin inhibitor levels, antidonor antibody testing, urine protein analysis, urine and blood cultures
Doppler ultrasound to assess for possible urinary tract obstruction or transplant renal artery stenosis
Renal biopsy

situations, is an area of active investigation. In the other 50% of failures, a patient dies with a functioning allograft. The most common cause of death in these patients is cardiovascular, due to the high prevalence of diabetes, hypertension, and hyperlipidemia, as well as the high burden of preexisting cardiovascular disease in transplant candidates. Although there are no specific guidelines for the prevention, monitoring, or management of cardiovascular disease after renal transplantation, standard risk factor reduction guidelines are generally considered applicable, including the use of statins (Chapter 190), and antihypertensive medications, to meet blood pressure targets (Chapter 64). The other leading causes of long-term death in renal transplant recipients are infection, sepsis, and malignant disease, all of which are complications of long-term immunosuppression.

GENERAL REFERENCES

For the General References and other additional features, please visit Elsevier eBooks+ at https://ebooks.health.elsevier.com.

Grade A References

A1. Zarbock A, Kellum JA, Schmidt C, et al. Effect of early vs delayed initiation of renal replacement therapy on mortality in critically ill patients with acute kidney injury: the ELAIN randomized clinical trial. *JAMA.* 2016;315:2190-2199.

A2. Gaudry S, Hajage D, Schortgen F, et al. Initiation strategies for renal-replacement therapy in the intensive care unit. *N Engl J Med.* 2016;375:122-133.

A3. Bagshaw SM, Wald R, Adhikari NKJ, et al. Timing of initiation of renal-replacement therapy in acute kidney injury. *N Engl J Med.* 2020;383:240-251.

A4. Gaudry S, Hajage D, Benichou N, et al. Delayed versus early initiation of renal replacement therapy for severe acute kidney injury: a systematic review and individual patient data meta-analysis of randomised clinical trials. *Lancet.* 2020;395:1506-1515.

A5. Chertow GM, Levin NW, Beck GJ, et al. Long-term effects of frequent in-center hemodialysis. *J Am Soc Nephrol.* 2016;27:1830-1836.

A6. Hull KL, March DS, Churchward DR, et al. The effect of extended-hours hemodialysis on outcomes: a systematic review and meta-analysis. *Hemodial Int.* 2020;24:133-147.

A7. Kirsch AH, Lyko R, Nilsson LG, et al. Performance of hemodialysis with novel medium cut-off dialyzers. *Nephrol Dial Transplant.* 2017;32:165-172.

A8. Weiner DE, Falzon L, Skoufos L, et al. Efficacy and safety of expanded hemodialysis with the Theranova 400 Dialyzer: a randomized controlled trial. *CJASN.* 2020;15:1310-1319.

A9. Lookstein RA, Haruguchi H, Ouriel K, et al. Drug-coated balloons for dysfunctional dialysis arteriovenous fistulas. *N Engl J Med.* 2020;383:733-742.

A10. Macdougall IC, White C, Anker SD, et al. Intravenous iron in patients undergoing maintenance hemodialysis. *N Engl J Med.* 2019;380:447-458.

A11. Chen N, Hao C, Liu B-C, et al. Roxadustat treatment for anemia in patients undergoing long-term dialysis. *N Engl J Med.* 2019;381:1011-1022.

A12. Eckardt K-U, Agarwal R, Aswad A, et al. Safety and efficacy of vadadustat for anemia in patients undergoing dialysis. *New Engl J Med.* 2021;384:1601-1612.

A13. Singh AK, Carroll K, Perkovic V, et al. Daprodustat for the treatment of anemia in patients undergoing dialysis. *N Engl J Med.* 2021;385:2325-2335.

A14. Block GA, Bushinsky DA, Cheng S, et al. Effect of etelcalcetide vs cinacalcet on serum parathyroid hormone in patients receiving hemodialysis with secondary hyperparathyroidism: a randomized clinical trial. *JAMA.* 2017;317:156-164.

A15. Fishbane S, Jamal A, Munera C, et al. A phase 3 trial of difelikefalin in hemodialysis patients with pruritus. *N Engl J Med.* 2020;382:222-232.

A16. Spertus JA, Jones PG, Maron DJ, et al. Health status after invasive or conservative care in coronary and advanced kidney disease. *N Engl J Med.* 2020;382:1619-1628.

A17. Bangalore S, Maron DJ, O'Brien SM, et al. Management of coronary disease in patients with advanced kidney disease. *N Engl J Med.* 2020;382:1608-1618.

A18. Woodle ES, Gill JS, Clark S, et al. Early corticosteroid cessation vs long-term corticosteroid therapy in kidney transplant recipients: long-term outcomes of a randomized clinical trial. *JAMA Surg.* 2021;156:307-314.

A19. Vincenti F, Rostaing L, Grinyo J, et al. Belatacept and long-term outcomes in kidney transplantation. *N Engl J Med.* 2016;374:333-343.

A20. Halden TAS, Kvitne KE, Midtvedt K, et al. Efficacy and safety of empagliflozin in renal transplant recipients with posttransplant diabetes mellitus. *Diabetes Care.* 2019;42:1067-1074.

XIII

GASTROINTESTINAL DISEASES

118

APPROACH TO THE PATIENT WITH GASTROINTESTINAL DISEASE

KENNETH R. MCQUAID

The luminal gastrointestinal (GI) tract (esophagus, stomach, duodenum, small and large intestine, and anus) and pancreas are responsible for digestion, for the absorption of nutrients and fluids, and for the temporary storage and excretion of undigested waste. The GI tract has an epithelial lining with an enormous surface area that provides nutrient absorption and serves as a barrier to microorganisms. In addition, the GI tract has a large innate and adaptive immune system that interfaces with luminal food antigens, host proteins, commensal and pathogenic bacteria, and parasites and must decide which antigens to tolerate and which require immune activation.[1] The GI tract also contains an extensive enteric endocrine system that regulates food intake, weight control, and glucose homeostasis as well as secretions from the stomach, intestine, and pancreas. Finally, it has an enteric nervous system that is integrated with the autonomic and central nervous systems to control gastric emptying, intestinal motility, and defecation.[2]

Numerous diseases within and outside the GI tract may alter normal function by causing structural damage (erosion, ulceration, perforation, stenosis, or obstruction), bleeding, inflammation, abnormal absorption or secretion of nutrients and electrolytes, or abnormal motility. Despite its anatomic and physiologic complexity, the GI system has only a limited repertoire of symptoms and signs to express conditions that may be either serious or clinically insignificant: abdominal pain, heartburn, regurgitation, dysphagia, odynophagia, dyspepsia, nausea and vomiting, gas and bloating, weight loss, diarrhea, constipation, overt or occult GI tract bleeding, and incontinence.

GENERAL APPROACH TO PATIENTS WITH GASTROINTESTINAL SIGNS AND SYMPTOMS

An appropriate history and physical evaluation usually can narrow the differential diagnosis of GI complaints. A specific diagnosis can almost always be established thereafter by the judicious use of laboratory, endoscopic, or imaging studies (Table 118-1). Not surprisingly, the site of the abdominal pain has a significant correlation with the organ involved.[3]

CLINICAL HISTORY

The clinician should elicit the nature of the complaint, including its acuity, severity, location, radiation, duration, pattern (steady vs. colicky; abrupt vs. gradual onset), and relationship to food, meals, and bowel movements. Symptoms that arise from the GI tract are almost always improved or worsened by eating or by bowel movements. For symptoms of recent onset, it is important to elicit recent dietary intake, a medication history, potential exposure to enteric infections, coronavirus disease 2019 (COVID-19), or sexually transmitted infections (Chapter 264), and recent travel. It is also useful to establish whether there are signs or symptoms that suggest a systemic illness, including fever, weight loss, arthralgias, fatigue, weakness, and rash.

Most nonsurgical GI diseases are manifested with mild to moderate symptoms that develop gradually and do not require immediate attention. Acute symptoms that require urgent assessment are severe abdominal pain and overt GI bleeding (Chapter 121) that is manifested by hematemesis, melena, or large-volume hematochezia. Severe or dramatic abdominal pain that develops acutely during minutes to hours requires urgent evaluation to determine whether surgical intervention is required. Severe vomiting or diarrhea with signs of dehydration also warrants urgent attention.

Mild to moderate chronic or intermittent symptoms that have been present for a long period can be evaluated in a deliberate fashion. A substantial proportion of chronic GI complaints has no obvious organic or biochemical basis and ultimately is classified as *functional* GI disorders (Chapter 123). Complaints that have been ongoing for years rarely are attributable to readily remedied structural disorders. In patients with chronic GI symptoms, it is important to elicit and to address the current reason for seeking evaluation, which may include concern for underlying serious illness (especially cancer), a change in the character or severity of symptoms, life stressors, and depression. Asking the patient what he or she thinks or fears may provide insights into the proportion of the complaint attributable to these amplifying issues, regardless of whether the problem is functional or structural in origin.

A dietary history (Chapter 198) should be obtained. For acute symptoms of nausea, vomiting, diarrhea, or abdominal pain, intake during the previous 24 to 48 hours should be reviewed for clues to a food-borne illness, including possible exposure to a contaminated food or water source and similar symptoms in other people (Chapter 262). Possible exposure to COVID-19 during the previous 10 days should be assessed.[4] For chronic or intermittent complaints, a recall of meals and types of foods eaten during the previous 1 to 2 days provides insight into eating habits and the amounts and types of fruits and vegetables, whole grains, fiber, protein, fat, and dairy products ingested. A relationship between specific foods and symptoms may be found. For example, dairy products (lactose intolerance), whole grains, legumes or cruciferous vegetables, or fatty meals (malabsorption) may cause pain, flatulence, or diarrhea, and a low-fiber diet may cause chronic constipation. Recent and long-term changes in body weight should be elicited. Involuntary loss of more than 5% of body weight during the prior 12 months is worrisome for serious disease and significant malnutrition (Chapter 197).

The number and consistency of bowel movements should be elicited, and any change in bowel habits must be explored. Signs of acute GI bleeding (melena or hematochezia) or inflammatory colitis (blood, mucus, or pus) should be elicited. Improvement in symptoms after passage of flatus or a bowel movement suggests a disorder of the colon or anorectum.

PAST MEDICAL HISTORY

The past medical history should be reviewed for conditions that may cause acute or chronic GI symptoms, including endocrine disorders such as diabetes (Chapter 210) and thyroid dysfunction (Chapter 207), cardiovascular diseases such as heart failure (Chapter 45) and peripheral vascular disease (Chapter 65), chronic liver disease and portal hypertension (Chapter 139), neurologic conditions such as Parkinson disease (Chapter 378) and neuromuscular disorders (Chapter 366), and rheumatologic and collagen vascular disorders (Chapter 236). In addition to their impact on GI tract function, the severity of these conditions must be considered in weighing the risks of diagnostic studies, especially endoscopy. Patients with symptomatic or advanced respiratory insufficiency (Chapter 90), sleep apnea (Chapter 374), valvular heart disease (Chapter 60), coronary artery disease (Chapter 39), heart failure (Chapter 45), cirrhosis (Chapter 139), cerebrovascular disease (Chapter 375), neuromuscular disease (Chapter 390), or dementia (Chapter 371) have an increased risk of sedation-related complications during endoscopy.

A list of prescription and nonprescription medications, vitamins, minerals, and other nutritional supplements should be obtained, paying particular attention to any that were recently initiated or changed. Herbal supplements (Chapter 30) are commonly used but are seldom reported without direct questioning. Medications are potential causes of odynophagia, dyspepsia, nausea or vomiting, abdominal pain, diarrhea, and constipation. The use of antiplatelet agents and anticoagulants should be determined. The risks of stopping versus continuing these medications must be weighed in patients who have acute or chronic GI bleeding or in whom a therapeutic procedure is to be performed.

SOCIAL HISTORY

The patient's personal relationships, employment history, quality of life, alcohol intake (Chapter 364), and smoking (Chapter 363) history should be determined. It can be very informative to observe both verbal and nonverbal interactions between the patient and a partner or caregiver during an interview. Alcohol may cause heartburn, dyspepsia, nausea, diarrhea, or chronic liver disease. Many patients are reluctant to disclose the full extent of their alcohol intake on direct questioning; therefore, in addition to asking how often they imbibe (days/week and drinks/day), it may be revealing to inquire about their preferred beverage and how it is purchased (location, volume, and frequency). Cigarette smoking is associated with an increased risk of heartburn, peptic ulcer disease, Crohn disease, and GI malignant neoplasms.

Clinicians should inquire about the degree to which GI symptoms are disrupting a patient's life. GI illness may affect dietary and bowel habits, sleep, and sense of vitality. Concerns about dietary intolerances, inability to eat, inability to have comfortable bowel movements, uncontrolled diarrhea or gas, fecal urgency, or fecal incontinence may affect a patient's social life, personal and sexual relationships, employment, and sense of optimism.

The social history should also be reviewed for recent stressors that may precipitate or exacerbate GI symptoms, including marital or interpersonal discord, personal or family illness, bereavement, financial pressures, job loss, and change in employment. To elicit such information, it may be helpful to tell patients that stress worsens many conditions and to inquire whether they believe stress may be contributing to their problem.

For elderly, disabled, or marginally housed patients, it is important to elicit how they obtain and prepare their meals and how they access toilet facilities. For patients undergoing GI procedures, it is important to determine whether they have mental, physical, or social barriers that would make it difficult to comply with preprocedural instructions (including bowel preparation) and whether they have an able-bodied adult who can accompany them to the procedure and observe them at home, if necessary, afterward.

FAMILY HISTORY

The family history should be reviewed for GI disorders with a heritable component, especially celiac disease (Chapter 126), inflammatory bowel diseases (Chapter 127), and neoplasms of the GI, gynecologic, and genitourinary tracts.

PHYSICAL EXAMINATION

Nonabdominal Examination

The nonabdominal examination should assess nutritional status (Chapter 198) and any signs of systemic conditions that may cause GI symptoms or that must be considered in weighing the risks and benefits of further testing, especially endoscopy. Vital signs should be obtained in all patients. Low-grade fever (<100.5° F) is common in inflammatory conditions, including gastroenteritis, inflammatory bowel disease, appendicitis, cholecystitis, and diverticulitis. High fever (>102° F) suggests sepsis, pelvic or intra-abdominal infections (e.g., cholangitis, pelvic inflammatory disease, pyelonephritis), or peritonitis. Hemodynamic instability (hypotension or tachycardia) suggests intravascular depletion due to poor oral intake, acute GI or intra-abdominal bleeding, severe diarrhea, or peritonitis. A body mass index of less than 18 suggests malnourishment.

A general survey should be performed to assess for signs of weight loss (fat and muscle wasting), malnutrition (dry or thin skin, hair loss, edema, anasarca), and vitamin deficiencies (pellagra, scurvy). Skin lesions may provide clues to systemic conditions such as liver disease (jaundice, spider telangiectasias, palmar erythema), inflammatory bowel disease (erythema nodosum, pyoderma gangrenosum), celiac disease (dermatitis herpetiformis), vasculitis, and rare GI malignant neoplasms, polyposis syndromes, and pancreatic endocrine tumors (Chapters 178, 179, and 213). An oral examination looks for mucocutaneous candidiasis (which may reflect immunosuppression), ulcerations (which may reflect inflammatory bowel disease, vasculitis, viral infection, or vitamin deficiencies), and glossitis or angular cheilitis (which may reflect vitamin deficiencies). With the exception of supraclavicular lymph nodes, peripheral lymph nodes are uninvolved with GI diseases but should be examined when systemic infection or advanced malignant disease is suspected (Chapter 154). Examination of the lungs and cardiovascular system should focus on evidence of conditions that might increase the risk of moderate sedation in the event that endoscopy is required (respiratory insufficiency, heart failure) and of conditions that increase the risk of intestinal ischemia (atrial fibrillation, valvular heart disease, peripheral vascular disease) (Chapter 129). The extremities should be evaluated for edema and peripheral pulses. Finally, a brief neurologic assessment should be performed to screen for intracranial mass lesions or other neurologic disorders that may be manifested with GI symptoms.

Abdominal Examination

The abdominal examination begins with a visual inspection of the abdomen and inguinal region for scars (due to prior surgeries or trauma), asymmetry (suggesting a mass or organomegaly), distention (due to obesity, ascites, or intestinal ileus or obstruction), prominent periumbilical veins (suggesting portal hypertension), or hernias (umbilical, ventral, inguinal). The examination proceeds with auscultation followed by percussion, and it ends with light and deep palpation.

In patients *without* abdominal pain, auscultation of bowel sounds to assess intestinal motility has limited usefulness and may be omitted. Percussion may be performed before or in conjunction with light and deep palpation. Initial cursory light percussion across the upper, mid, and lower abdomen is useful to denote areas of dullness and tympany as well as to elicit unanticipated areas of pain or tenderness before palpation. More extensive percussion provides limited but useful information about the size of the liver and spleen, gastric or intestinal distention, bladder distention, and ascites (Chapters 132 and 139). Gentle, light palpation promotes abdominal relaxation and allows the detection of muscle resistance (guarding), abdominal tenderness, and superficial masses of the abdominal wall or abdomen. Deeper palpation of the abdominal organs (liver, spleen, kidneys, aorta) and abdominal cavity may detect enlargement or abnormal masses. Superficial or deep masses should be assessed for size, location, mobility, content (solid, liquid, or air), and the presence or absence of tenderness. The consistency of a patient's response to palpation with and without distraction is particularly useful in those with suspected chronic functional abdominal discomfort. Superficial masses include hernias, lymph nodes, subcutaneous abscesses, lipomas, and hematomas. Neoplasms (liver, gallbladder, pancreas, stomach, intestine, kidney), abscesses (appendicitis, diverticulitis, Crohn disease), or aortic aneurysms may represent deep abdominal masses.

Examination of the right upper quadrant should assess the liver size, contour, texture, and tenderness. Liver size is crudely estimated by percussion of the upper and lower borders of liver dullness in the midclavicular line. Liver contour and tenderness are best assessed during held inspiration by deep palpation along the costal margin. Examination of the left upper quadrant is useful to detect splenomegaly (Chapter 154), although a normal-sized or even an enlarged spleen often cannot be detected. Percussion in the left upper quadrant near the tenth rib (posterior to the midaxillary line) may detect splenic dullness that is distinct from gastric or colonic tympany. The tip of an enlarged spleen may be palpated during inspiration if the examiner supports the left costal margin with the left hand while palpating below the costal margin with the right hand. Ascites should be suspected in a patient with a protuberant abdomen and bulging flanks. To screen for ascites, percussion of the flanks should be performed to assess the level of dullness. If the level of flank dullness appears to be increased, the most sensitive test for ascites is to check for "shifting" dullness when the patient rolls from the supine to the lateral position.

Digital Rectal and Pelvic Examinations

The digital rectal examination is intrusive and uncomfortable and should be performed only when necessary, such as in patients with perianal or rectal symptoms, incontinence, difficult defecation, suspected inflammatory bowel disease, and acute abdominal pain. The digital examination, with or without fecal occult blood testing, is not a useful screening test for colorectal cancer (Chapter 179). However, in patients with acute or chronic GI bleeding (Chapter 121), it is a rapid means of assessing the stool for color and occult blood. The perianal area should be visually inspected for rashes, soilage (suggesting incontinence or fistula), fistulas, fissures, skin tags, external hemorrhoids, and prolapsed internal hemorrhoids (Chapter 131). After gentle digital insertion, the anal canal should be assessed for resting tone and voluntary squeeze. The distal rectal vault should be swept circumferentially to palpate for mass lesions, tenderness, or fluctuance.

LABORATORY STUDIES

Blood Tests

Blood tests routinely obtained in the evaluation of patients with GI symptoms include a complete blood count, liver tests (Chapter 133), serum chemistries, and, in selected cases, pancreatic enzymes and markers of inflammation. GI causes of anemia include acute or chronic GI blood loss, inflammatory bowel disease, nutrient malabsorption (folate, iron, or vitamin B_{12}), and chronic liver disease. Microcytosis suggests iron deficiency due to chronic GI blood loss or malabsorption. Macrocytosis may be attributable to folate or B_{12} malabsorption, medications (e.g., immunomodulators used for inflammatory bowel disease), or chronic liver disease. An elevated platelet count suggests chronic inflammation (e.g., inflammatory bowel disease) or GI blood loss with compensatory marrow production. A low platelet count may be attributable to portal hypertension with splenic sequestration. Low serum albumin may be caused by chronic GI disorders that result in weight loss, nutrient malabsorption, chronic inflammation, loss of protein across abnormal GI mucosa (i.e., protein-losing enteropathy), or decreased hepatic synthesis (e.g., chronic liver disease). Abnormal liver test results may be due to acute or chronic liver diseases, disorders of the pancreas or biliary tract, and medications (Chapter 133). Serum amylase and lipase are obtained to screen for pancreatitis (Chapter 130) in patients with acute abdominal pain. Increased levels of inflammatory markers, such as an elevated erythrocyte sedimentation rate and C-reactive protein, are nonspecific but useful in the management of patients with inflammatory bowel disease (Chapter 127).

Serum ferritin reflects total body iron and may be decreased in patients with chronic GI blood loss or intestinal malabsorption (e.g., celiac disease). Deficiencies in the fat-soluble vitamins (A, D, E, K) (Chapter 126) may reflect disorders of malabsorption that result in steatorrhea. The serum international

TABLE 118-1 APPROACH TO COMMON GASTROINTESTINAL SYMPTOMS AND SIGNS

	ABDOMINAL PAIN	GI BLEEDING	DIARRHEA	STEATORRHEA	CONSTIPATION
History (ascertain the following)	Duration: acute vs. chronic Onset: sudden vs. 1-2 hr vs. gradual Character: visceral (vague or dull, steady or cramping, diffuse) or parietal (severe, well localized, worse with movement) Location: upper, middle, or lower; radiation Associated symptoms: vomiting, hematemesis, diarrhea, hematochezia, melena, constipation, obstipation, jaundice Previous episodes Other diseases	Acute vs. chronic (duration); intermittent vs. continuous; quantity; hematemesis, melena, or hematochezia; associated pain and location; symptoms of anemia (e.g., dyspnea, chest pain, lightheadedness); medication use (especially aspirin, NSAIDs, anticoagulants); previous episodes; risk factors for chronic liver disease (alcohol, hepatitis)	Acute (<2 wk) vs. chronic (duration); fever, weight loss, or abdominal pain; stool character: number per 24 hr, watery or bloody, large vs. small volume, change in volume with eating, greasy; dietary history (especially lactose); history of IBD, pancreatic disease, intestinal surgery, DM; recent change in medications or antibiotic use; community outbreak or similar symptoms in family members; potential exposure to contaminated food; elderly immunosuppressed host; risk of HIV or sexually transmitted disease; COVID-19 exposure	Duration; weight loss; stool number, consistency (greasy), presence of blood; abdominal pain; flatulence; history of excessive alcohol, chronic liver disease, pancreatitis, intestinal dysmotility, surgery, DM; history of easy bruising, night blindness, bone pain, osteoporosis, dermatitis herpetiformis	Acute vs. chronic (duration); age; number of stools per week; difficulty with defecation (straining, incomplete evacuation, digital manipulation); bloating or discomfort; blood on stools, weight loss; dietary fiber and fluid intake; chronic illness (DM, neuromuscular, endocrine); abdominal surgeries; medications, impaired mobility
Physical findings (evaluate for the following)	Fever, HR, BP Appearance: calm, restless, motionless Inspect: skin, distention, hernias Bowel sounds: present, absent, roaring Percussion and palpation: organomegaly, mass (abscess), focal tenderness, guarding Peritoneal signs: sharp pain with cough, shaking, percussion, light palpation	HR, BP, orthostatic findings; abdominal pain present or absent; signs of chronic liver disease and portal hypertension (which may indicate varices); jaundice, spider angiomas, hepatosplenomegaly; ascites; examine nasogastric aspirate for blood ("coffee grounds" vs. bright red); examine stool for blood (Hemoccult) and color (melena, maroon, or bright red)	HR, BP, orthostatic findings; fever; wasting; presence of abdominal tenderness or mass; perianal disease; extraintestinal symptoms of IBD (e.g., oral ulcers, arthritis, erythema nodosum)	Wasting, presence or absence of abdominal mass or tenderness; rash (vitamin deficiencies) or excessive bruising (vitamin K deficiency); jaundice or signs of chronic liver disease	Assess mobility and chronic medical conditions; abdominal distention; palpable stool within bowel in left lower quadrant; rectal examination—impacted stool, anal fissure, rectal prolapse, pelvic floor descent with straining, rectocele
Laboratory tests	CBC, BUN, Cr, glucose, amylase, lipase, liver tests (ALT, AST, bilirubin, alkaline phosphatase), albumin, INR, U/A, urine β-HCG; nasal swab for COVID-19	CBC, BUN, Cr, liver tests, INR, type and cross	CBC, BUN, Cr, glucose, electrolytes, liver tests, albumin, C-reactive protein Selected cases: consider serum chromogranin A, VIP, calcitonin, gastrin, glucagon, urinary 5-HIAA; stool for culture, ova, parasites or multiplex PCR tests; nasal swab for COVID-19; consider fecal weight, fat, elastase, calprotectin, electrolytes, laxative screen	CBC, glucose, liver tests, albumin, electrolytes, celiac disease antibody (IgA anti-tTG or EMA or IgG DGP, if IgA deficiency); assessment of vitamin and mineral absorption (A, D) and INR (K is fat soluble), folate, iron, calcium, phosphate, B_{12}; stool for fecal elastase and qualitative fat; stool for quantitative fecal fat; breath test for bacterial overgrowth	CBC, Chem-7, calcium, magnesium, phosphate, TFTs; selected patients with severe constipation may undergo anal manometry with balloon expulsion,
Endoscopy	EGD, colonoscopy	EGD, colonoscopy, enteroscopy, wireless capsule study	Colonoscopy (including ileal inspection) with biopsies; EGD with duodenal biopsies; wireless capsule study	EGD with duodenal biopsies	Colonoscopy if recent change in bowel habits
Imaging	CT scan or ultrasound; MR or CT enterography; angiography	CT angiography, angiography	Small bowel enterography: CT, MRI, (Crohn disease); somatostatin receptor scintigraphy	CT of the abdomen (pancreatic calcifications; biliary dilation)	Usually not necessary; colonic transit studies; MRI or barium defecography

5-HIAA = 5-hydroxyindoleacetic acid; ALT = alanine transaminase; AST = aspartate transaminase; BP = blood pressure; BUN = blood urea nitrogen; CBC = complete blood count; CNS = central nervous system; COPD = chronic obstructive pulmonary disease; COVID-19 = coronavirus disease 2019; Cr = creatinine; CT = computed tomography; DGP=deamidated gliadin peptide; DM = diabetes mellitus; EGD = esophagogastroduodenoscopy; EMA=endomysial antibody; ESR = erythrocyte sedimentation rate; GERD = gastroesophageal reflux disease; GI = gastrointestinal; HbA_{1C} = hemoglobin A_{1C}; HCG = human chorionic gonadotropin; HIV = human immunodeficiency virus; HR = heart rate; IBD = inflammatory bowel disease; INR = international normalized ratio; KCl = potassium chloride; MRI = magnetic resonance imaging; NSAIDs = nonsteroidal anti-inflammatory drugs; RBC = red blood cell; TFTs = thyroid function tests; tTG = tissue transglutaminase; U/A = urinalysis; VIP = vasoactive intestinal polypeptide.

Modified from Proctor DD. Approach to the patient with gastrointestinal disease. In: Goldman L, Ausiello D, eds. *Cecil Textbook of Medicine,* 23rd ed. Philadelphia: Saunders-Elsevier; 2008.

NAUSEA AND VOMITING	DYSPHAGIA	ODYNOPHAGIA	HEARTBURN AND REGURGITATION	ANOREXIA	WEIGHT LOSS
Nausea with or without emesis; acute vs. chronic (duration); intermittent vs. constant; presence or absence of severe abdominal pain, comorbid illnesses, especially peptic ulcer, endocrine (DM), cardiac, psychiatric; medications; history of excessive alcohol; COVID-19 exposure	Oropharyngeal vs. esophageal dysphagia; solids vs. liquids; acute vs. chronic (duration); intermittent vs. progressive; GERD symptoms present or absent; weight loss; history of food impactions, allergies, atopic conditions, skin changes, cold hands (Raynaud phenomenon)	Duration of pain with swallowing; underlying immunosuppression (e.g., HIV infection, DM); caustic ingestion; use of medications that cause topical injury (especially NSAIDs, KCl, bisphosphonates, iron, antibiotics, zidovudine)	Duration of symptoms; location; relation to meals or specific foods; nocturnal symptoms; dysphagia or chest pain; extraesophageal manifestations: cough, hoarseness, asthma	Acute vs. chronic (duration); association with different foods; psychiatric disease (e.g., depression, dementia); chronic or undiagnosed medical conditions (e.g., DM, thyroid or adrenal disease, COPD, advanced heart failure, renal insufficiency, malignant disease, HIV infection); medication use	Acute vs. chronic (duration); age; total amount (>5% is significant); intentional vs. unintentional; appetite increased or decreased; rapid vs. gradual; change in physical activity; documented vs. undocumented; fever or sweats; anorexia, nausea, vomiting; diarrhea, steatorrhea, blood in stool; abdominal pain; history or symptoms of chronic medical, neurologic, or psychiatric illness; medications; alcohol and substance abuse
Acute with severe abdominal pain: evaluate for GI obstruction, pancreatitis, mesenteric ischemia, biliary colic, appendicitis, or other conditions causing peritonitis Acute without abdominal pain: evaluate for pregnancy, medications, food poisoning, infectious gastroenteritis, COVID-19, hepatitis, CNS disease, postoperative ileus Chronic: evaluate for medications, chronic gastric outlet obstruction (due to ulcer disease or malignant disease), impaired GI motility (gastroparesis), other chronic medical conditions, intracranial disorders, psychiatric disease (bulimia)	Usually normal; examine oropharynx and neck for lymphadenopathy and masses; evaluate the skin for sclerodermatous changes	Usually normal; evaluate oropharynx for thrush, herpetic lesions, caustic injury; general examination for signs of underlying immunosuppression	Usually normal, unless extraesophageal manifestations are present	Wasting; fever; signs of bulimia (e.g., loss of tooth enamel, knuckle ulcerations and calluses); abdominal masses; enlarged lymph nodes	Wasting; malnutrition; poor dentition or poorly fitting dentures; thyromegaly; COPD or heart failure; abdominal masses; enlarged lymph nodes; pelvic masses in women; diabetic neuropathy; signs of depression, dementia, or bulimia
β-HCG, CBC, serum electrolytes, BUN, Cr, glucose, HbA_{1c}, liver tests, albumin, TFTs, cortisol	CBC; eosinophilia or elevated IgE in some patients with eosinophilic esophagitis	CBC, HIV test, fasting glucose	Usually normal	CBC, Chem-7, liver tests, albumin, HIV test, TFTs	CBC, Chem-7, HbA_{1c}, TFTs, liver tests, C-reactive protein or ESR, calcium, phosphate, albumin, HIV test, morning cortisol
EGD to exclude gastric outlet obstruction	EGD with biopsies or dilation, esophageal motility study	EGD with biopsies	EGD (to detect erosive esophagitis or Barrett esophagus); ambulatory pH/impedance probe	Directed at detecting underlying disease (e.g., if a GI cause is suspected, EGD or colonoscopy with biopsies may be helpful)	Directed at detecting underlying disease (e.g., if a GI cause is suspected, EGD or colonoscopy with biopsies may be helpful)
CT of the abdomen; if chronic, also consider head CT, gastric emptying study, CT or MR enterography	Esophagogram (barium swallow) will show stricture, Schatzki ring, mass	Usually not necessary	Usually not necessary	Directed at detecting underlying disease (e.g., if a GI cause is suspected, abdominal CT may be helpful)	Directed at detecting underlying disease (e.g., chest or abdominal CT may be helpful)

normalized ratio may be elevated in patients with cholestasis because of malabsorption of vitamin K or in patients with chronic liver disease because of decreased hepatic synthetic function. Serum B_{12} may be decreased in patients with autoimmune gastritis (pernicious anemia), gastric bypass surgery, or malabsorption because of small bowel bacterial overgrowth or disease of the terminal ileum (e.g., Crohn disease).

Specialized laboratory tests that may be useful for the diagnosis of specific diseases include stool *Helicobacter pylori* antigen in patients with duodenal ulcer disease or dyspepsia, antibodies to tissue transglutaminase immunoglobulin A (IgA) or deamidated gluten peptide (IgG) in celiac disease, and CA19-9 in pancreaticobiliary malignant disease.

Stool Examination

Fecal occult blood testing is useful to evaluate iron deficiency anemia and acute or chronic GI blood loss. In patients with acute diarrhea, assessment for infectious agents is indicated if diarrhea is bloody, severe, associated with severe abdominal pain or fever, or if the patient is immunocompromised. In most clinical settings, molecular testing of stool specimens is now preferred for initial screening of a panel of bacteria (including *Clostridioides difficile*), viruses, and parasites, with results available within 1 to 5 hours.[5,6] Stool specimens also may be submitted for leukocyte or lactoferrin testing, culture for routine bacterial pathogens (e.g., *Salmonella, Campylobacter, Shigella*), and, in selected patients, testing for *C. difficile, Escherichia. coli 0157:H7*, Shiga toxin, and parasites (*Giardia, Entamoeba histolytica*). To distinguish among the causes of chronic diarrhea (Chapter 126), stool samples may be sent for assessment of electrolytes, leukocytes (microscopy, calprotectin, or lactoferrin), elastase, and fecal fat.

ENDOSCOPY AND RADIOLOGY

Endoscopy (Chapter 120) and radiographic studies (Chapter 119) play a major role in the evaluation and management of many GI disorders. Esophageal manometry and esophageal pH and impedance monitoring can be useful for the evaluation of heartburn, reflux, and other esophageal symptoms (Chapter 124). Anorectal manometry may be useful in some patients with fecal incontinence and defecatory dysfunction (Chapter 131). Breath tests are commonly used to diagnose *H. pylori* infection (a urease breath test; Chapter 125), lactose intolerance, and small bowel bacterial overgrowth (a hydrogen and methane breath test with lactulose or glucose; Chapter 126).

The diagnosis of a functional GI disorder is made after organic disorders have been excluded by clinical evaluation and limited, directed diagnostic testing. "Overtesting" should be avoided. Thereafter, the emphasis should switch from finding a "cause" of the symptoms to implementing successful coping and adaptive behaviours.

ABDOMINAL PAIN

Abdominal pain, which is a frequent complaint among outpatients in the office setting and emergency department, may be benign and self-limited or the presenting symptom of severe, life-threatening disease. Chronic abdominal pain that has been present for months or years in the absence of other organic illness is almost always functional in origin and does not require urgent evaluation. By contrast, most patients with severe acute abdominal pain require a thorough but emergent evaluation, which may quickly reveal an acute surgical illness (Chapter 128).

PATHOBIOLOGY

Stimulation of hollow abdominal viscera is mediated by splanchnic afferent fibers within the muscle wall, visceral peritoneum, and mesentery that are sensitive to distention and contraction. Visceral afferent nerves are loosely organized, innervate several organs, and enter the spinal cord at several levels. Thus, visceral pain is vague or dull in character and diffuse; patients attempting to localize the pain often move their entire hand over the upper, middle, or lower abdomen. Most visceral pain is steady, but cramping, intermittent pain or "colic" results from peristaltic contractions caused by partial or complete obstruction of the small intestine, ureter, or uterine tubes. In contrast to visceral innervation, a dense network of nerve fibers that follow a spinal T6 to L1 somatic distribution innervates the parietal peritoneum. Pain fibers of the parietal peritoneum are stimulated by stretch or distention of the abdominal cavity or retroperitoneum; direct irritation from infection, pus, or secretions (e.g., caused by a ruptured viscus); or inflammation caused by contact between the parietal peritoneum and an adjacent inflamed organ (e.g., appendicitis). Parietal pain is sharp, well characterized, and localized by the patient to a precise location on the abdomen, often by pointing with one finger.

The GI viscera (liver, biliary system, pancreas, and GI tract) arise during embryologic development from midline structures that have bilateral innervation. Thus, GI visceral pain is typically localized to the abdominal midline.

ACUTE ABDOMINAL PAIN

CLINICAL MANIFESTATIONS

History

The history should determine the time course, character, and location and radiation pattern of the pain (Table 118-2). Severe abdominal pain that begins

TABLE 118-2 TYPICAL MANIFESTATIONS OF KEY CAUSES OF ACUTE AND CHRONIC ABDOMINAL PAIN

CONDITION	LOCATION	QUALITY	ONSET	AGGRAVATING OR RELIEVING FACTORS	ASSOCIATED SYMPTOMS OR SIGNS	DIAGNOSTIC STUDIES
Peptic ulcer disease (Chapter 125)	Epigastric, occasionally RUQ, rarely LUQ	Dyspepsia: mild to moderate aching discomfort, pain, burning, gnawing, postprandial fullness	Days	Variable relief with antacids; may be relieved by, worsened by, or unrelated to meals	Recurrent; associated factors (e.g., *Helicobacter pylori*, aspirin, NSAIDs)	Anemia, upper endoscopy, *H. pylori* testing
Acute pancreatitis (Chapter 130)	Epigastric, radiates to midback (occasionally RUQ or LUQ)	Diffuse, steady, stabbing, penetrating	1-2 hr	Aggravated by food; better when lying still and with narcotics	Severe nausea and vomiting; reduced or absent bowel sounds; associated factors (e.g., alcohol, gallstones)	Elevated amylase and lipase, CT
Acute cholecystitis (Chapter 141)	Epigastric, then moves to RUQ; may radiate to right scapula	Gradual, steady increase, moderate to severe	Hours	May follow a fatty meal; better with narcotics and surgery	Nausea, some vomiting, fever	Elevated WBC count, US or CT
Acute appendicitis (Chapter 128)	Periumbilical, then moves to RLQ	Vague initially; gradual, steady increase to intense, localized, pain	Hours	Unprovoked; better with narcotics and surgery	Anorexia, nausea, obstipation; occasional vomiting, fever late	Elevated WBC count, US or CT
Diverticulitis (Chapter 128)	LLQ or suprapubic	Moderate to severe, steady or cramping, sharp or aching, localized	Hours to days	Unprovoked; better with narcotics and antibiotics or surgery	Anorexia, nausea, distention, constipation or loose stools; partial relief with passage of flatus or BM; fever late	Elevated WBC count, CT
Ruptured viscus and peritonitis (Chapter 128)	Diffuse	Intense	Minutes to hours	Worse with cough or movement; better when lying still or with narcotics or surgery	Fever, anorexia, nausea, vomiting; lack of bowel sounds; tenderness with percussion, light touch, rebound; guarding and rigidity (late); loath to move	Elevated WBC count, CT

TABLE 118-2 TYPICAL MANIFESTATIONS OF KEY CAUSES OF ACUTE AND CHRONIC ABDOMINAL PAIN—cont'd

CONDITION	LOCATION	QUALITY	ONSET	AGGRAVATING OR RELIEVING FACTORS	ASSOCIATED SYMPTOMS OR SIGNS	DIAGNOSTIC STUDIES
Intestinal ischemia (Chapter 129)	Small intestine—periumbilical; proximal (right) colon—periumbilical or RLQ; distal colon—LLQ	Severe, stabbing pain out of proportion to physical findings	Minutes	Chronic ischemia—occurs after eating; acute ischemia—usually unprovoked; better with narcotics, thrombus dissolution, stenting, surgical resection	Nausea, bloody diarrhea; associated factors (e.g., hypotension, cardiac arrhythmias)	Elevated WBC count, CT or MR with angiography, or colonoscopy (colonic ischemia)
Strangulated hernia (Chapter 128)	Localized	Sharp, localized, intense; crampy or steady	Minutes to hours	Previous hernia history; unprovoked; better with narcotics and decompression, including surgery	Anorexia, nausea, vomiting, no stool or flatus passage if obstruction; bowel sounds variable—hyperactive early if obstruction present, but absent bowel sounds late, especially with peritonitis	Elevated WBC count, CT, US
Small or large bowel obstruction (Chapter 128)	Small intestine—periumbilical; proximal (right) colon—periumbilical or right abdomen; distal (left) colon—LLQ	Early—diffuse, colicky, crampy; late—steady and better localized	Hours to days	Aggravated by food; better with narcotics, NGT decompression, or surgery	Distention, anorexia, nausea, vomiting; no stool or flatus passage; small intestine—increased hyperperistaltic (rushes) bowel sounds (early) or quiet abdomen (late); large intestine—bowel sounds variable; associated factors (e.g., hernia, previous surgery)	CT
Abdominal abscess (Chapter 128)	Located over the abscess, usually LLQ or RLQ	Insidious, intense, constant	Days	May be aggravated by movement; better with abscess drainage	Fever, anorexia, nausea, abdominal mass	Elevated WBC count, CT
Acute hepatitis (Chapter 134)	RUQ	Dull or intense; localized	Days	Worse with deep inspiration	Jaundice, anorexia, nausea; liver enlarged and tender to palpation; associated factors (e.g., alcohol, infection)	Abnormal liver test results
GERD (Chapter 124)	Substernal or epigastric	Burning, gnawing	Days to years	Provoked by large or fatty meals or recumbency; relief with antacids	Recurrent; may have regurgitation, dysphagia, or extraesophageal manifestations (e.g., asthma, chronic cough, laryngitis)	Upper endoscopy (usually normal), ambulatory pH/impedance probe
Nonulcer (functional) dyspepsia (Chapter 123)	Epigastric	Mild to moderate discomfort, pain, burning, gnawing, postprandial fullness	Years	May be worsened by meals; cannot be reliably distinguished from ulcer disease by history alone	Other symptoms of functional disorders (IBS, fibromyalgia, pelvic pain)	Normal EGD
IBS (Chapter 123)	Variable; usually lower abdomen	Vague, crampy, sense of urgency	Years	Pain may be precipitated by dietary factors or stress; associated with change in bowel characteristics (e.g., frequency, form, difficulty with passage); relieved with stool passage	Bloating and abdominal distention	Normal sigmoidoscopy, colonoscopy, and CT, but these are usually not necessary for diagnosis
Chronic pancreatitis (Chapter 130)	Epigastric or periumbilical, radiates to midback	Intense, localized	Days to years	Aggravated by food; better with narcotics	Anorexia, nausea, vomiting; associated factors (e.g., alcohol); DM (with advanced disease)	Amylase and lipase may be normal; CT may show calcifications, dilated pancreatic duct, pseudocyst; increased fecal fat and decreased fecal elastase if pancreatic insufficiency
Inflammatory or infectious enterocolitis (Chapters 128 and 262)	Small intestine—periumbilical; large intestine—right or left side of the abdomen over the colon; rectum—tenesmus	Crampy	Hours to days	Better with stool passage and treatment of underlying cause	Nausea, vomiting, bloody diarrhea; associated factors (e.g., infectious—food transmission; IBD—prolonged duration, family history)	Stool studies for culture, colonoscopy with biopsies

CT = computed tomography; DM = diabetes mellitus; EGD = esophagogastroduodenoscopy; GERD = gastroesophageal reflux disease; IBS = irritable bowel syndrome; LLQ = left lower quadrant; LUQ = left upper quadrant; MR = magnetic resonance; NGT = nasogastric tube; NSAIDs = nonsteroidal anti-inflammatory drugs; RLQ = right lower quadrant; RUQ = right upper quadrant; US = ultrasound; WBC = white blood cell count.

suddenly during seconds to minutes indicates a catastrophic event, such as esophageal rupture, perforated peptic ulcer or viscus, ruptured ectopic pregnancy, ruptured aortic aneurysm, acute mesenteric ischemia, or myocardial infarction. Pain that progresses within 1 to 2 hours is consistent with a rapidly progressive inflammatory disorder (e.g., cholecystitis, appendicitis, pancreatitis), acute obstruction of a viscus (small intestinal obstruction, which is often related to adhesions from prior intraperitoneal surgery[7]; ureteral colic), or organ ischemia caused by a strangulated blood supply (volvulus, strangulated hernia, ovarian torsion). Pain that is less severe and develops during several hours is more commonly caused by a medical rather than a surgical condition, including upper GI disorders (dyspepsia), intestinal disorders (gastroenteritis, inflammatory bowel disease), liver disorders (hepatitis, abscess), urinary disorders (cystitis, pyelonephritis), and gynecologic infections; however, the slow evolution of surgical disorders such as cholecystitis (Chapter 141), appendicitis or diverticulitis (Chapter 128), and intra-abdominal abscesses must not be overlooked.

The character of the pain provides important information about whether the symptoms are due to visceral stimulation or parietal stimulation (peritonitis). Patients with peritonitis may report severe localized pain or irritation with activities or maneuvers that stretch or move the parietal peritoneum, such as walking, moving in bed, and coughing; as a result, they tend to lie quietly to avoid painful stimulation. By contrast, patients with visceral pain may move or walk restlessly or attempt a bowel movement in an effort to relieve their symptoms.

The location of pain in the upper, middle, or lower abdomen is a crude but important indicator of the diagnosis (Fig. 118-1). Visceral pain arising from the foregut (esophagus, stomach, proximal duodenum, bile duct, gallbladder, pancreas) most often is manifested in the epigastrium. Pain derived from the midgut (small intestine, appendix, ascending colon, proximal transverse colon) occurs in a periumbilical location. Pain derived from the hindgut (distal transverse colon, left colon, rectum) localizes to the lower midline between the umbilicus and symphysis pubis. Paired intra-abdominal organs such as the kidneys, ureters, ovaries, and fallopian tubes have unilateral innervation that localizes pain to the side of the involved organ. As some surgical conditions progress, the character and location of the pain shift from a visceral to a parietal pain pattern. Thus, early cholecystitis (Chapter 141) may be manifested with vague midline epigastric pain that progresses to sharp right upper quadrant pain as localized peritoneal irritation develops. Likewise, appendicitis (Chapter 128) commonly begins with vague, diffuse periumbilical pain that evolves to sharp, well-localized right lower quadrant pain as peritonitis ensues.

Anorexia, vomiting, diarrhea, distention, and constipation are commonly seen with abdominal pain caused by both medical and surgical disorders. Although nonspecific, the *absence* of any of these symptoms is evidence against an emergent surgical or medical disorder because severe illness usually leads to reflex stimulation or inhibition of gastric and intestinal peristalsis. Vomiting is common in medical and surgical disorders involving the upper GI tract, including acute gastroenteritis, pancreatitis, gastric and small intestinal obstruction, and biliary tract disease. Pain that precedes the onset of vomiting is typical of surgical conditions, whereas the reverse is true of medical conditions (e.g., food poisoning, gastroenteritis). Abdominal pain with prominent diarrhea is most commonly caused by a medical condition (e.g., gastroenteritis, inflammatory bowel disease). Although constipation alone is a nonspecific complaint, the absence of stool passage and flatus is consistent with complete bowel obstruction or paralytic ileus.

Jaundice accompanying acute abdominal pain virtually always indicates a hepatobiliary disorder (Chapter 133), including obstruction of the biliary duct (choledocholithiasis, pancreatic carcinoma, cholangiocarcinoma), complications of acute cholecystitis, acute hepatitis (viral, ischemic), and hepatic malignant neoplasms. The possibility of cholangitis should be considered and excluded in all patients with acute abdominal pain and jaundice, especially if the patient has fever, chills, hypotension, altered mental status, or leukocytosis. Hematemesis with upper abdominal pain suggests a Mallory-Weiss tear, alcoholic gastritis, or peptic ulcer disease. Hematochezia with abdominal pain is most commonly caused by medical conditions such as infectious gastroenteritis or inflammatory bowel disease, but it also may be caused by ischemic colitis or mesenteric ischemia. Gross hematuria may be due to cystitis (Chapter 263) or a ureteral stone (Chapter 111). Abdominal pain with weight loss may be due to inflammatory bowel disease, chronic mesenteric ischemia, or advanced GI malignant neoplasms. In women, a missed menstrual period, adnexal pain, spotting, or cramping may suggest pregnancy, ectopic pregnancy, or spontaneous abortion. Acute pain between cycles may be caused by ovarian follicles or ruptured corpus luteum cysts. Pelvic pain with fever, chills, or cervical discharge suggests pelvic inflammatory disease.

The past medical history and review of systems can provide clues about systemic and extra-abdominal conditions that may be manifested with abdominal pain. Acute coronary syndromes (Chapter 57), heart failure (Chapter 45),

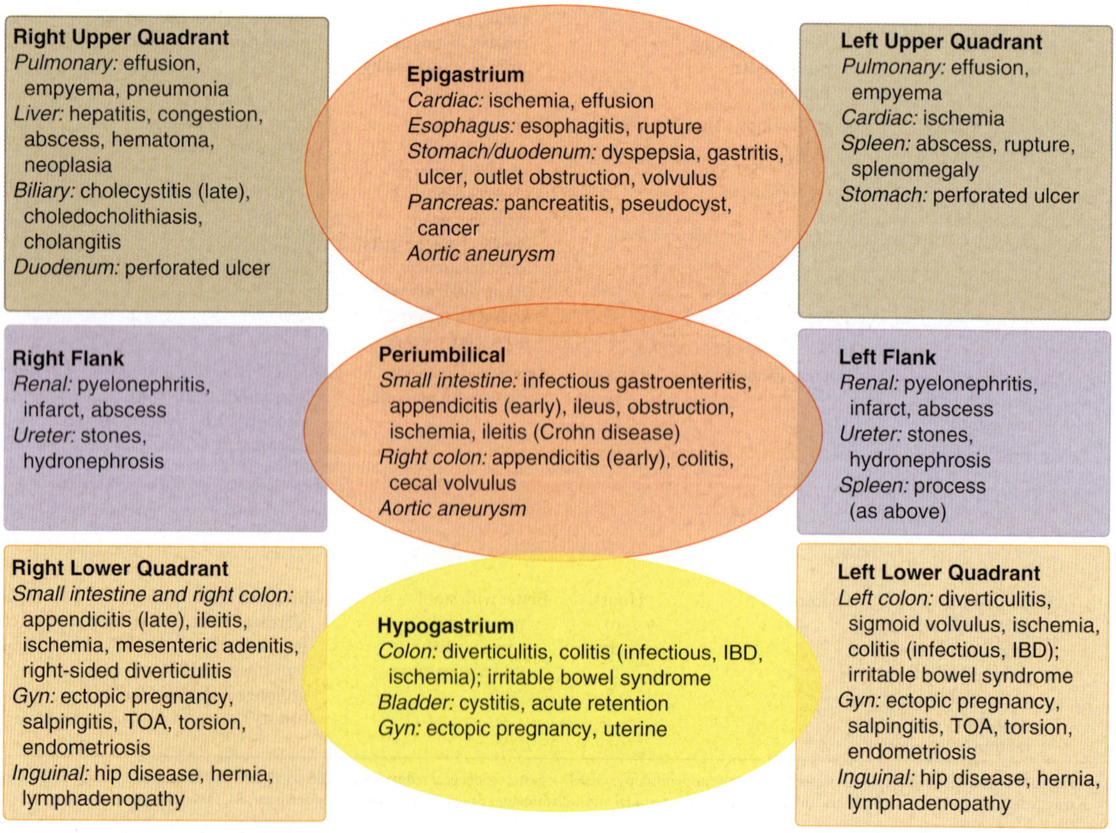

FIGURE 118-1. Differential diagnosis of abdominal pain by its initial location. Gyn = gynecologic; IBD = inflammatory bowel disease; TOA = tubo-ovarian abscess.

pneumonia (Chapter 85), or empyema may cause dyspepsia, epigastric or right or left upper quadrant pain, nausea, and vomiting. Metabolic conditions such as uremia (Chapter 116), diabetes with hyperglycemia or ketoacidosis (Chapter 210), hypercalcemia (Chapter 227), or acute adrenocortical insufficiency (Chapter 208) may cause pain, nausea, vomiting, and diarrhea. Acute intermittent porphyria (Chapter 194) and familial Mediterranean fever (Chapter 254) may cause recurrent episodes of severe pain and peritonitis that may be misdiagnosed, leading to unnecessary surgeries. Other causes of acute abdominal pain include narcotic withdrawal (Chapter 365), insect or reptile bites (Chapter 98), and lead or arsenic poisoning (Chapter 20).

Physical Examination

The physical examination must identify life-threatening illnesses that require urgent surgical evaluation. Nevertheless, the examination must be orderly, careful, and complete. If the examiner immediately palpates the site of maximal pain, the patient is unlikely to relax and to cooperate for the remainder of the examination.

First, the patient should be observed and the abdomen inspected. Most patients remain calm, cooperative, and freely capable of moving during the examination. Patients who are writhing or restless may have pain due to visceral distention (e.g., renal colic, intestinal obstruction), whereas patients who lie motionless may have peritonitis. Gentle shaking of the bed or having the patient cough may elicit sharp, well-localized pain in patients with parietal but not with visceral pain. Auscultation should be performed before percussion or palpation so that intestinal activity is undisturbed. An abdomen that is quiet except for infrequent squeaks or tinkles suggests peritonitis or ileus. Loud peristaltic rushes that occur in synchrony with abdominal pain suggest small bowel obstruction. Light percussion across the upper, middle, and lower abdomen can determine any site of focal tenderness suggestive of peritonitis. Light palpation should be performed with one or two fingers (not the whole hand), beginning away from where the patient localizes the pain and gradually moving to the site of pain. Thereafter, gentle, deeper palpation of the entire abdomen is performed gradually, including the region of tenderness. An attempt should be made to palpate for an abdominal aortic aneurysm (Chapter 63). Examination also should include the inguinal and femoral canals, umbilicus, and surgical scars for evidence of incarcerating hernias. The presence of focal tenderness indicates parietal peritoneal irritation. Voluntary or involuntary tightening of the muscle wall ("guarding") may occur during palpation. With gentle, steady compression of the abdomen with one hand, voluntary guarding usually subsides, allowing the examination to proceed. Persistent involuntary guarding indicates peritonitis with reflex muscle wall contraction. Testing for "rebound tenderness" in patients with suspected peritonitis is not recommended because it causes significant pain and is usually not necessary to establish the diagnosis. When the presentation strongly suggests a nonserious GI disorder but the patient has significant tenderness with palpation, it is useful to use the stethoscope ostensibly to listen for bowel sounds but actually to reproduce the pressure of palpation. A significant discrepancy in the tenderness elicited by the stethoscope and by digital palpation may be seen in patients who are anxious, have functional complaints, or are seeking secondary gain. A digital rectal examination should be performed in most patients with acute abdominal pain to evaluate for tenderness or fluctuance that suggests a perirectal abscess and to assess the stool for signs of overt or occult blood. Women with lower abdominal pain should have a pelvic examination by a skilled examiner to evaluate for gynecologic disease. Some specific and dramatic findings point to particular diagnoses (Table 118-3).

TABLE 118-3 PHYSICAL SIGNS IN PATIENTS WITH ACUTE ABDOMINAL PAIN

SIGN	DESCRIPTION	DIAGNOSIS
Murphy sign	Cessation of inspiration during right upper quadrant examination	Acute cholecystitis
McBurney sign	Tenderness located midway between anterior superior iliac spine and umbilicus	Acute appendicitis
Cullen sign	Periumbilical bluish discoloration	Retroperitoneal hemorrhage Pancreatic hemorrhage Ruptured abdominal aortic aneurysm
Grey Turner sign	Bluish discoloration of flanks	Retroperitoneal hemorrhage Pancreatic hemorrhage Ruptured abdominal aortic aneurysm
Kehr sign	Severe left shoulder pain	Splenic rupture Ectopic pregnancy rupture
Obturator sign	Pain with flexed right hip rotation	Appendicitis
Psoas sign	Pain with straight leg raising against resistance (right side)	Appendicitis

Special Populations

Increased diligence is required in the evaluation of patients in whom abdominal signs and symptoms may be minimal until the disease process is far advanced. Such patients include the elderly (Chapter 24) and patients who have dementia (Chapter 371), psychiatric disturbances (Chapter 362), or spinal cord injuries. An admitting diagnosis of "altered mental status," "failure to thrive," "obstipation," or "fever of unknown origin" may stem from serious intra-abdominal conditions. Disorders that may be overlooked in the elderly include bowel perforation, bowel obstruction, cholecystitis, diverticulitis, volvulus, mesenteric ischemia, and abdominal aortic aneurysm. In patients with chronic liver disease, the presence of ascites may mask the signs and symptoms of serious surgical conditions such as cholecystitis, appendicitis, and diverticulitis. Even in the presence of perforation, signs of peritonitis may be lacking because the ascites fluid separates the visceral peritoneum and parietal peritoneum. Likewise, immunocompromised populations, who are at risk for infectious, drug-related, and iatrogenic complications, may manifest few physical findings or laboratory abnormalities. Owing to the limitations of the clinical evaluation in these vulnerable populations, there should be a low threshold for the use of abdominal imaging.

Abdominal Pain Developing in the Hospital

When pain develops as a new problem in a hospitalized patient, it is usually caused by a limited number of conditions. Postprocedural complications may cause perforation, infection, or bleeding (intraperitoneal, retroperitoneal, or within solid organs). Shunting of splanchnic blood flow in severely ill medical or surgical patients may cause stress gastritis, nonocclusive mesenteric ischemia, or acalculous cholecystitis. Adynamic ileus or acute colonic pseudo-obstruction is common in critically ill or postoperative patients and is manifested as diffuse abdominal pain and distention. *C. difficile* (Chapter 271) colitis is a common cause of pain, diarrhea, and distention, especially in patients receiving antibiotics. Constipation (Chapter 122), which is a common problem in hospitalized patients, may go unnoticed until pain and distention develop. Finally, many medications can cause dyspepsia and abdominal pain.

DIAGNOSIS

Patients with acute abdominal pain should have a complete blood count with differential; leukocytosis is present in most acute surgical conditions (Fig. 118-2). A pregnancy test is required in women of childbearing age. Serum levels of electrolytes, glucose, blood urea nitrogen, and creatinine assess hydration, acid-base status, and renal function. Liver chemistries and pancreatic enzymes should be obtained in most patients, but especially in those with upper abdominal pain, jaundice, or vomiting. An elevation in aspartate or alanine aminotransferase levels may reflect choledocholithiasis with acute biliary obstruction (Chapter 141), acute gallstone pancreatitis (Chapter 130), or a hepatocellular process (Chapter 134). Painful jaundice with a significant rise in the alkaline phosphatase level usually reflects cholestasis caused by extrahepatic biliary obstruction (Chapter 141). Amylase and lipase levels are elevated in most patients with acute pancreatitis, but minor amylase elevations also occur with a perforated viscus or mesenteric ischemia (Chapter 129). Urinalysis may demonstrate pyuria, hematuria, or bacteriuria due to ureteral calculi (Chapter 111) or urinary tract infection (Chapter 263).

Imaging

Ultrasound is preferred in suspected pregnancy and to evaluate for other acute gynecologic disorders, such as tubo-ovarian abscess, ruptured corpus luteum cyst, or ovarian torsion; it is also preferred for the initial evaluation of suspected acute cholecystitis (Chapter 141) and ureteral stones with hydronephrosis and for the bedside evaluation of unstable patients. In most other settings, abdominal computed tomography (CT) with oral and intravenous administration of contrast material (when possible) is preferred and can provide

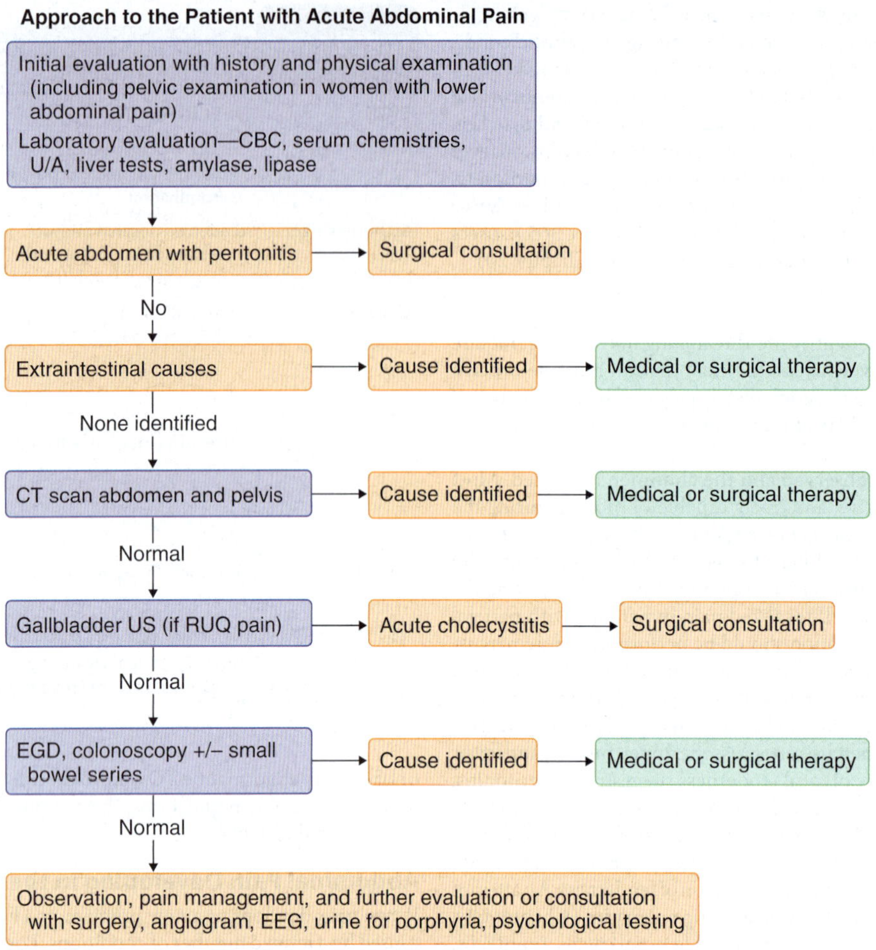

FIGURE 118-2. **Approach to the patient with acute abdominal pain.** CBC = complete blood count; CT = computed tomography; EEG = electroencephalography; EGD = esophagogastroduodenoscopy; RUQ = right upper quadrant; U/A = urinalysis; US = ultrasonography.

a definitive diagnosis in up to 90% of patients with acute severe abdominal pain[A1] (Chapter 119). Abdominal CT may be falsely negative early in the course of acute pancreatitis, mesenteric ischemia, cholecystitis, appendicitis,[8] and diverticulitis, especially if it is performed without contrast enhancement.

TREATMENT

Once the diagnosis is clear, treatment of the underlying condition is initiated. For uncomplicated acute appendicitis diagnosed by CT scan, antibiotics are an alternative to urgent surgery,[A2] but they are associated with a 25 to 30% rate of readmission or surgery in the next year. As a result, the international consensus is generally for urgent surgery.[9] In patients with diverticulitis, antibiotics are the usual first-line therapy (Chapter 128).[10] In patients with nonspecific acute abdominal pain and no clear diagnosis, early laparoscopy is useful for diagnosis, but outcomes such as complication rates, readmission rates, and length of hospitalization are no better than with a strategy of active observation.

CHRONIC ABDOMINAL PAIN

Chronic or recurrent abdominal pain that has been present for months to years may be caused by structural (organic) disease, but the majority of patients have a functional disorder such as irritable bowel syndrome (Chapter 123). Common organic causes of chronic abdominal pain include medications with GI side effects, peptic ulcer disease (Chapter 125), inflammatory bowel disease (Chapter 127), chronic pancreatitis (Chapter 130), biliary tract disease (Chapter 141), GI cancers (Chapters 178 and 179), and endometriosis (Chapter 218). The clinician should attempt to distinguish patients with symptoms or signs of organic disease, in whom further diagnostic investigation is warranted, from those with probable functional disease (Fig. 118-3). Although functional disorders occur in all age groups, the symptoms usually begin before the age of 40 years. "Alarm" features that suggest a structural disorder and are inconsistent with a functional disorder are fever, severe pain, significant weight loss, jaundice, progressive dysphagia, recurrent vomiting, nocturnal pain or diarrhea, and stools that are bloody or positive for fecal occult blood. Laboratory study findings should be normal with functional disorders; therefore, an unrevealing evaluation for anemia; leukocytosis; and levels of iron, albumin, C-reactive protein, and vitamins A, D, or B_{12} argues against structural or organic disease.

In patients younger than 50 years with a suspected functional disorder and no alarm features (e.g., family history of colon cancer or inflammatory bowel disease or abnormalities on screening blood tests), further testing should be minimized, and the emphasis should be shifted to managing symptoms, coping, and making lifestyle changes (Chapter 123). In patients who may have organic disease, testing often includes a combination of upper GI endoscopy, colonoscopy, and ultrasound or CT imaging.

GAS AND BLOATING

BELCHING

Belching (eructation), which is the involuntary or voluntary release of gas from the esophagus or stomach, commonly occurs during or after a meal. Virtually all belching is caused by swallowed air, which may be increased by eating quickly, drinking carbonated beverages, chewing gum, and smoking. Gas also may be produced within the stomach by antacids, especially sodium bicarbonate, which rapidly neutralize gastric acid and release carbon dioxide. Belching seldom reflects serious GI dysfunction but may be increased in patients with gastroesophageal reflux (Chapter 124), functional dyspepsia (Chapter 123), or gastroparesis (Chapter 122). Chronic, excessive, repetitive supragastric belching is a functional disorder caused by transient ingestion of air into the esophagus (caused by subconscious diaphragmatic contraction and upper esophageal sphincter relaxation) and its subsequent expulsion; it is treated with behavioral modification.

FLATUS

Flatus, or "gas," is a normal byproduct of digestion. Otherwise healthy adults pass flatus 10 to 20 times daily and excrete up to 1500 mL. Thus, it is difficult to distinguish patients with abnormal or excessive gas production from those with only a heightened awareness of or sensitivity to normal production. Increased flatulence with diarrhea may be symptomatic of disorders of malabsorption,

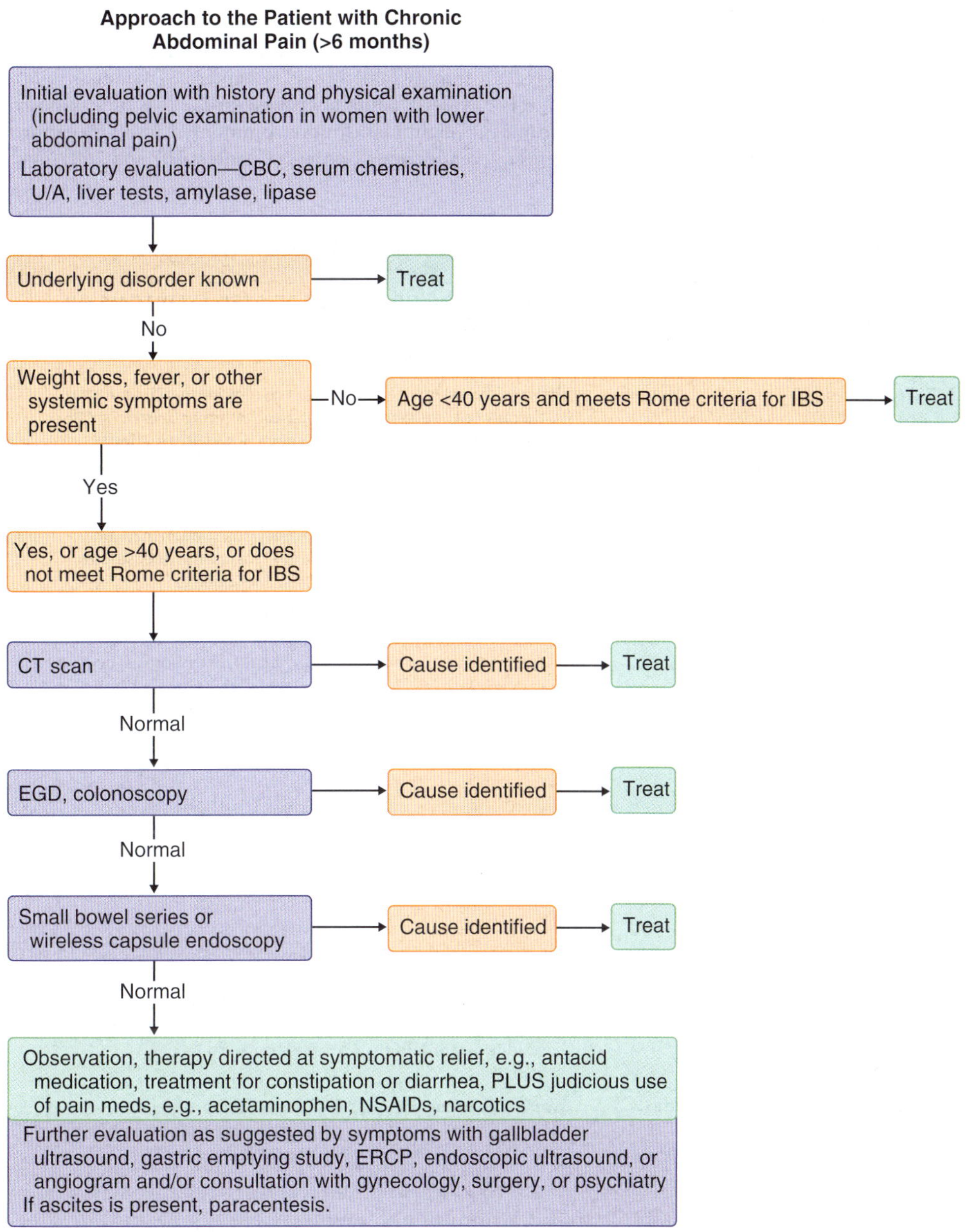

FIGURE 118-3. **Approach to the patient with chronic abdominal pain.** CBC = complete blood count; CT = computed tomography; EGD = esophagogastroduodenoscopy; ERCP = endoscopic retrograde cholangiopancreatography; IBS = irritable bowel syndrome; NSAIDs = nonsteroidal anti-inflammatory drugs; U/A = urinalysis.

including celiac disease (Chapter 126), pancreatic insufficiency (Chapter 130), and small intestinal bacterial overgrowth (Chapter 126).

In normal adults, flatus is derived from two sources: swallowed air and colonic bacterial fermentation of FODMAPs (fermentable oligosaccharides, disaccharides, and monosaccharides and polyols), which are short-chain carbohydrates that may be incompletely absorbed in the small intestine and result in the colonic production of carbon dioxide or methane. FODMAPs include lactose (dairy products), fructose, fructans, polyols, and galacto-oligosaccharides. Fructose is present in fruit, especially apples and pears, and is a major component of corn syrups that are widely used as sweeteners. Polyols include sorbitol, which is a natural sugar in stone fruit (peaches, apricots, plums, prunes) and a common added sweetener in sugar-free candies, as well as trehalose, which is present in mushrooms. Fructans and oligosaccharides are plentiful in cruciferous vegetables (cabbage, broccoli, cauliflower, Brussels sprouts, turnips, rutabagas), garlic, onions, legumes (beans, soy, lentils, peas), pasta, and whole grains.[11]

BLOATING AND DISTENTION

Bloating and distention are common complaints among patients with functional GI disorders (Chapter 123).[12] As chronic, isolated symptoms, they are almost never caused by serious structural disease. Functional bloating may be caused by heightened sensitivity to minor increases in intestinal gas or impaired transit of gas, even though the total volume of intestinal gas is within normal limits. The acute onset of distention in conjunction with alarm symptoms such as cramping pain, weight loss, nausea, vomiting, obstipation, or diarrhea warrants further evaluation for disorders that cause intestinal obstruction (Chapter 128) or malabsorption (Chapter 126).

TREATMENT

Patients with long-standing flatulence in the absence of other symptoms or signs of GI disease can be treated conservatively. Avoidance of carbonated beverages, chewing gum, sorbitol- and fructose-containing sweeteners, and gas-producing vegetables improves symptoms in most patients.[A3] Lactase deficiency may be confirmed by a lactose breath test. Underlying GI illness is suggested by the recent onset of flatulence with other symptoms of organic disease, including weight loss, abdominal pain, diarrhea, distention, and abnormal laboratory studies (Chapter 126). A positive fecal fat analysis confirms malabsorption and merits further investigation (see Table 126-6). Suspected small bowel bacterial overgrowth may be confirmed by carbohydrate breath tests[A4] or treated empirically with antibiotics.

Rifaximin (550 mg three times daily for 2 weeks) is effective for functional bloating, pain and loose or watery stool, but dietary and behavioral changes and reassurance may also be useful.[A5] Although some clinical studies suggest benefit with probiotics, the overall data are inconclusive.[13] In one randomized trial of patients with irritable bowel syndrome with predominant bloating, fecal transplantation improved bloating, pain, and flatulence.[A6]

INVOLUNTARY WEIGHT LOSS

The unintentional loss of more than 5% of baseline weight within a 12-month period is frequently due to a serious underlying medical or psychiatric illness.[14] Weight loss is seldom the sole presenting sign of medical disorders, but it is often revealed during the clinical evaluation of other complaints. Chronic weight loss in the elderly is commonly caused by depression; dementia; difficulty with chewing or swallowing; malignant disease; medications; alcoholism; or physical and social limitations to procuring, preparing, and eating meals (Table 118-4) (Chapter 23). Gradual, mild weight loss occurs in some elderly patients because of the loss of lean body mass. In young patients, weight loss is more commonly caused by eating disorders (Chapter 200), endocrine disorders (Chapters 207 and 208), or chronic GI conditions such

TABLE 118-4 CAUSES OF INVOLUNTARY WEIGHT LOSS

CONDITION	QUALITY	DURATION	AGGRAVATING OR RELIEVING FACTORS	ASSOCIATED SYMPTOMS OR SIGNS	DIAGNOSTIC STUDIES
WEIGHT LOSS SECONDARY TO GASTROINTESTINAL CAUSES					
GI, pancreatic, or hepatobiliary malignant disease (Chapters 178-181)	Progressive, fast	Months	Better with cancer therapy (e.g., surgery, XRT, chemotherapy)	Dysphagia (esophageal); anorexia, nausea, vomiting (gastric, small or large bowel obstruction); visible or occult blood in stool; altered bowel habits; jaundice or hepatomegaly (biliary obstruction, hepatic tumor, metastatic disease); iron deficiency anemia	CBC, FOBT, ferritin, CEA, CA19-9, AFP, EGD, colonoscopy, abdominal CT, PET
Malabsorption (Chapter 126) (poor absorption of nutrients due to pancreatic insufficiency, small intestinal mucosal disorders, or bacterial overgrowth)	Progressive, slow	Months to years	Diarrhea or steatorrhea, excessive flatulence; worse with eating and resolves with NPO status	Usually associated with increased appetite; may have anemia (iron, B_{12}, folate), osteoporosis, or osteomalacia (vitamin D, calcium, phosphorus); easy bruising (vitamin K), night blindness (vitamin A)	Stool for fecal fat (qualitative or quantitative); fecal elastase; vitamins A and D and INR; calcium, ferritin, B_{12}, albumin; celiac disease antibodies (e.g., IgA anti-tTG, or antiendomysial antibodies, IgG deamidated gliadin peptide); EGD with small bowel biopsy; breath test for bacterial overgrowth
Inflammatory bowel disease (especially Crohn disease) (Chapter 127)	Progressive, slow	Months	Eating causes pain, cramps, increased diarrhea and urgency; improved by low-residue diet or NPO status	Bloody stools, abdominal cramps and pain, perianal disease, extraintestinal manifestations (e.g., oral ulcers, uveitis, erythema nodosum, arthralgias)	CBC, albumin, ESR, CRP, fecal calprotectin, colonoscopy with biopsies, CT or MR enterography, wireless capsule study
GI motility disorders (Chapter 122)	Intermittent, slow	Years	Worse with eating	Nausea, vomiting, distention, diarrhea, or constipation may be present	EGD and colonoscopy, gastric emptying study, CT or MR enterography, surgical full-thickness intestinal biopsies
Cirrhosis (Chapter 139)	Muscle wasting with edema, so weight may increase	Months to years	Worse with salt or fluid intake	Ascites, peripheral edema	Liver biopsy
Chronic intestinal ischemia (Chapter 129)	Progressive	Months to years	Worse with eating	Afraid to eat; postprandial abdominal pain, nausea; associated atherosclerotic disease	CT or MR angiography
WEIGHT LOSS SECONDARY TO NONGASTROINTESTINAL CAUSES					
Poor or inadequate calorie intake due to social factors (Chapter 197)	Intermittent or progressive, acute (hospitalized) or chronic	Days to months to years	Common in elderly, teenagers; exacerbated by poor dentition or poorly fitting dentures	Will eat if food is made available	Review dietary log and how food is obtained and prepared
Medications	Intermittent or progressive	Months	Worse with medication; resolves with discontinuation of offending drug	Anorexia, nausea, vomiting	Review alcohol, recreational drugs, and prescription medications (stimulants, antidepressants, metformin, glucagon-like peptide-1 analogs, dopamine, anticholinergics, cardiovascular agents)
Non-GI malignant disease	Progressive	Months	Better with cancer therapy (e.g., surgery, XRT, chemotherapy)	Anorexia, nausea, vomiting; pain; metastatic disease	Calcium, cortisol; CT for underlying disease, PET
Endocrine disorders: DM, hyperthyroidism, adrenal insufficiency (Chapters 207, 208,and 210)	DM—appetite increased or decreased, early satiety; hyperthyroidism—increased appetite	Months to years	Worse with disease chronicity	DM: gastroparesis, neuropathy, retinopathy, nephropathy Adrenal insufficiency: nausea, vomiting, diarrhea, abdominal pain	Serum glucose, Hgb A_{1c}, TFT, cortisol

TABLE 118-4 CAUSES OF INVOLUNTARY WEIGHT LOSS—cont'd

CONDITION	QUALITY	DURATION	AGGRAVATING OR RELIEVING FACTORS	ASSOCIATED SYMPTOMS OR SIGNS	DIAGNOSTIC STUDIES
Chronic infections, including HIV and TB (Chapters 299 and 359)	Progressive, fast	Months	Better with directed therapy, megestrol acetate (Megace)	Nausea, anorexia, other infections	HIV test, PPD, cultures, biopsies if necessary
Systemic inflammatory disorders	Progressive, moderate	Months to years	Better with directed therapy, megestrol acetate (Megace)	Arthritis, rash, vasculitis	ANA, RF, ESR, CRP
Chronic renal failure (Chapter 116)	Progressive, slow; edema may increase weight	Months to years	Better with dialysis, megestrol acetate (Megace)	Nausea, anorexia, weight gain	BUN, Cr, 24-hr creatinine clearance
Advanced COPD or heart failure (Chapters 45 and 76)	Progressive, slow	Months to years	Better with oxygen and specific treatment	Fatigue, dyspnea, edema, wasting	Pulmonary function testing or two-dimensional echocardiography
Psychiatric illness: depression, manic-depressive illness (Chapter 362)	Progressive, slow	Months to years	Depression common in elderly; flat affect; manic phase associated with hyperactivity and decreased intake	Psychological testing	
Psychogenic eating disorders—anorexia nervosa, bulimia (Chapter 200)	Intermittent or progressive	Months to years	Worse with stressors	Refusal to eat, loss of tooth enamel, calluses and healing ulcerations of hand	Psychiatric testing
Substance abuse (alcohol, opiates, CNS stimulants)	Intermittent or progressive	Months	Resolves with discontinuation	Anorexia, nausea, vomiting	Careful interview; patients may deny or minimize

AFP = α-fetoprotein; ANA = antinuclear antibody; BUN = blood urea nitrogen; CBC = complete blood count; CEA = carcinoembryonic antigen; CNS = central nervous system; COPD = chronic obstructive pulmonary disease; Cr = creatinine; CRP = C-reactive protein; CT = computed tomography; DM = diabetes mellitus; EGD = esophagogastroduodenoscopy; ESR = erythrocyte sedimentation rate; FOBT = fecal occult blood test; GI = gastrointestinal; Hgb = hemoglobin; HIV = human immunodeficiency virus; INR = international normalized ratio; MR = magnetic resonance; NPO = nothing orally; PET = positron emission tomography; PPD = purified protein derivative; RF = rheumatoid factor; TB = tuberculosis; TFT = thyroid function test; tTG = tissue transglutaminase; XRT = x-ray therapy.
Modified from Proctor DD. Approach to the patient with gastrointestinal disease. In: Goldman L, Ausiello D, eds. *Cecil Textbook of Medicine*, 23rd ed. Philadelphia: Saunders-Elsevier; 2008.

as inflammatory bowel disease (Chapter 127) or celiac disease (Chapter 126). In chronic medical conditions, involuntary weight loss is usually caused by a combination of decreased appetite (anorexia) and varying degrees of cachexia; examples include advanced malignant disease, chronic infections (human immunodeficiency virus [HIV], tuberculosis), heart failure, chronic kidney or liver disease, end-stage lung disease, and adrenal insufficiency. Weight loss that occurs in the presence of normal or increased appetite suggests increased metabolism and energy expenditure caused by endocrine disorders, such as poorly controlled diabetes (Chapter 210) or hyperthyroidism (Chapter 207), or GI disorders that result in food malabsorption (Chapter 126). Chronic GI disorders that cause progressive narrowing or obstruction of the esophagus (cancer, achalasia), stomach (cancer, peptic ulcer disease with gastric outlet obstruction), small intestine (Crohn disease), or arterial circulation (chronic mesenteric ischemia) may cause weight loss as a result of dysphagia, vomiting, or postprandial pain that limits the ability to ingest sufficient calories.

DIAGNOSIS

The cause of weight loss (see Table 118-4) is usually evident from the history, physical examination, and routine laboratory studies, including complete blood count, electrolytes, liver chemistries, thyroid-stimulating hormone, urinalysis, and, when appropriate, HIV serology (Fig. 118-4). A chest radiograph should be obtained in patients who smoke, have any respiratory symptoms, or are older than 40 years. In one large study, patients with involuntary weight loss had a two- to three-fold increased risk of a new cancer diagnosis within the next 2 years, but the absolute rate of such a diagnosis was only 2.2%.[15]

Signs of dehydration or severe malnutrition may require an assessment for nutritional deficiencies (Chapter 197) and nutritional support (Chapter 198). Other symptoms and signs necessitate consideration of additional diagnostic testing. Weight loss with increased appetite merits an assessment of thyroid function (Chapter 207), glucose intolerance (Chapter 210), and malabsorption (Chapter 126). Suspected malabsorption may be confirmed by a positive fecal fat analysis. GI symptoms suggesting obstruction or occult GI malignant disease can be evaluated with upper GI endoscopy, upper GI radiographic series, colonoscopy, or abdominal CT. Psychiatric evaluation may be warranted in patients with signs of depression, early dementia, or eating disorders. In up to 25% of patients, no cause of weight loss is found.[16]

NAUSEA AND VOMITING

Nausea is an unpleasant feeling of the impending need to vomit. *Vomiting* is the forceful oral expulsion of gastric contents as a result of retrograde contraction of the duodenum and antrum with compression of the thoracoabdominal musculature. Nausea and vomiting may be caused by a number of GI and non-GI disorders, but they are best categorized according to chronicity and the presence of abdominal pain. The acute onset of vomiting *with* severe abdominal pain suggests a serious illness potentially requiring surgical intervention, including GI obstruction (Chapter 128), mesenteric ischemia (Chapter 129), pancreatitis (Chapter 130), biliary colic (Chapter 141), and conditions causing peritonitis (Chapter 128), such as appendicitis or a perforated viscus. Acute vomiting *without* abdominal pain is most commonly caused by pregnancy (Chapter 221), myocardial infarction (Chapter 58), medications (including chemotherapy), migraine headache (Chapter 367), food poisoning (Chapter 262), infectious gastroenteritis (Chapter 262), hepatitis (Chapters 134 and 135), upper GI bleeding, postoperative ileus, motion sickness (Chapter 396), vestibular neuritis (Chapter 396), or acute central nervous system disease. Gastrointestinal symptoms (nausea, vomiting, or watery diarrhea) are present in up to 10% of patients who are infected with severe acute respiratory syndrome coronavirus 2 (SARS-CoV-2; Chapter 336) and may precede respiratory symptoms. Chronic or recurrent nausea and vomiting *with* abdominal pain are commonly caused by GI disorders that result in the partial or intermittent obstruction of the stomach or small intestine and conditions that result in chronic intestinal pseudo-obstruction (Chapter 122). Chronic nausea and vomiting *without* abdominal pain may be due to disorders that impair gastric emptying or small intestine motility and non-GI causes, including medications, cannabinoids,[17] pregnancy, intracerebral disorders, cardiac disease, endocrine disease, labyrinth disorders, psychiatric disease (including bulimia), gastroparesis, cyclical vomiting syndrome, and functional disorders. Vomiting of undigested food eaten hours earlier suggests gastric obstruction or gastroparesis. Abdominal distention or feculent emesis suggests obstruction of the small intestine.

DIAGNOSIS

Most cases of acute vomiting without abdominal pain are self-limited and require no evaluation (Fig. 118-5). Medication-related symptoms and pregnancy should be excluded. With severe vomiting, serum electrolyte values

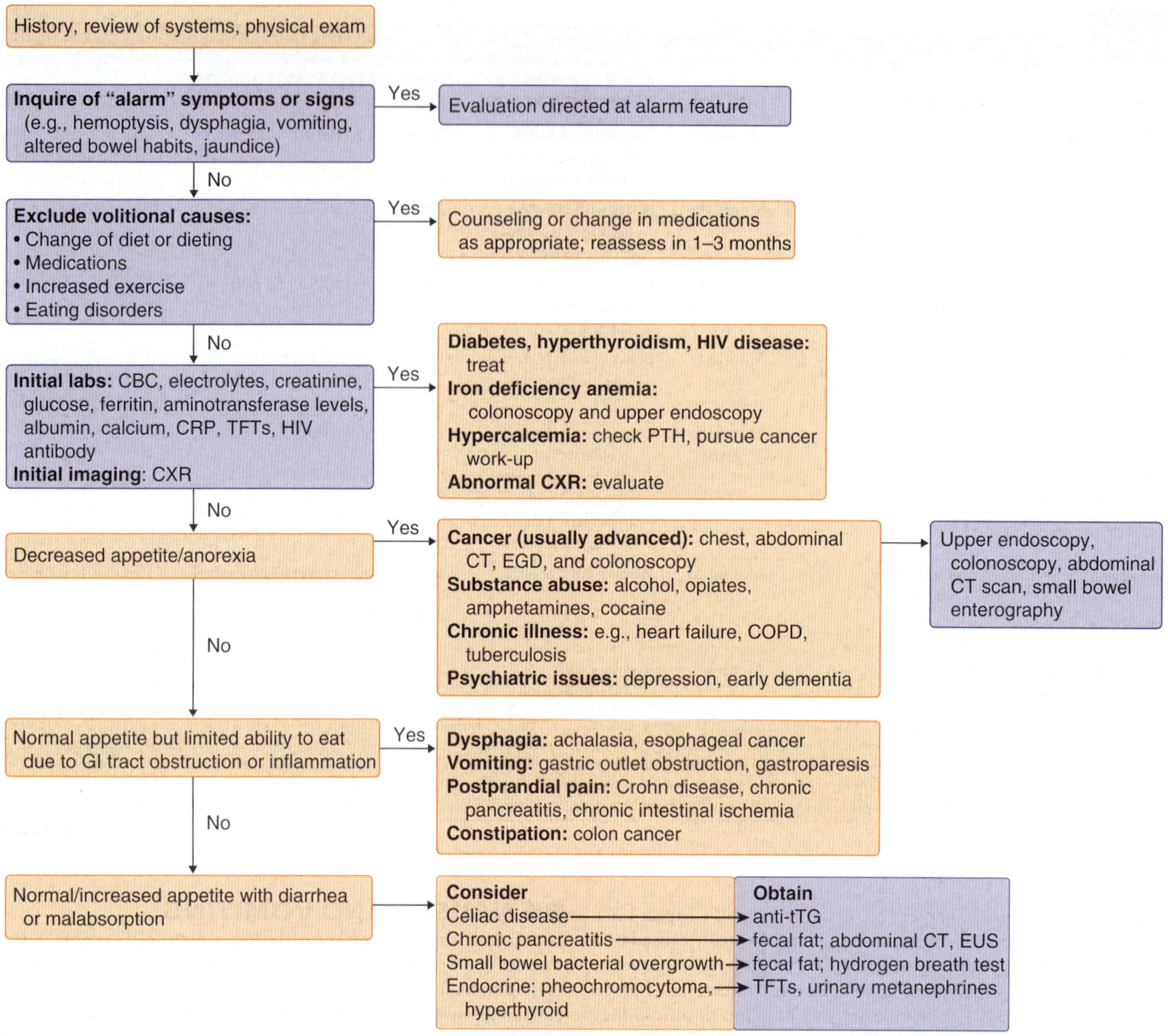

FIGURE 118-4. Approach to the patient with unintentional weight loss of more than 5%. CBC = complete blood count; COPD = chronic obstructive pulmonary disease; CRP = C-reactive protein; CT = computed tomography; CXR = chest radiograph; EGD = esophagogastroduodenoscopy; EUS = endoscopic ultrasound; GI = gastrointestinal; HIV = human immunodeficiency virus; PTH = parathyroid hormone; TFTs = thyroid function tests; tTG = tissue transglutaminase.

should be obtained. Hyperglycemia may cause acute gastroparesis. Increased liver chemistries or pancreatic enzymes suggest hepatobiliary or pancreatic disease. In patients with acute abdominal pain and vomiting, abdominal plain radiography or CT is performed to look for evidence of GI obstruction, a perforated viscus, or pancreaticobiliary disease. In patients with chronic vomiting of uncertain cause, the goal is to distinguish structural GI disorders, GI motility disorders, and non-GI disorders. Esophagogastroduodenoscopy, enterography, abdominal cross-sectional imaging, GI motility studies, and head CT or magnetic resonance imaging may be indicated.

TREATMENT

The approach to the medical treatment of nausea and vomiting depends on the cause (Table 118-5). Patients who are receiving moderately emetogenic chemotherapy are frequently managed with a 5-HT_3 receptor antagonist[18] and dexamethasone; a neurokinin-1 receptor antagonist[19] or olanzapine[A7] can be added for highly emetogenic regimens.[20] For patients with mildly emetogenic regimens or vomiting from other causes, treatment with single or combinations of anticholinergic agents, dopamine receptor antagonists, 5-HT_3 receptor antagonists,[A8] or cannabinoids[A9] usually provide symptomatic relief.[21] For refractory vomiting due to gastroparesis, gastric electrical stimulation[A10] or peroral endoscopic pyloromyotomy[22] may be considered.

CONSTIPTION

Constipation (Chapter 122), which is the most common digestive symptom, occurs in 15% of the population. Constipation may refer to fewer than three bowel movements per week; hard or lumpy stools; or difficulty during defecation, characterized by straining, a sensation of obstruction or incomplete evacuation, or the need to engage in manual manipulations to promote evacuation. Constipation may be caused by systemic conditions that slow colonic transit, including neuromuscular disease, endocrine disorders, and electrolyte abnormalities, or by lesions that obstruct the passage of stool through the distal colon or anorectum, such as neoplasms, strictures, prolapse, and aganglionosis (Hirschsprung disease).[23] Opioid-induced constipation is increasingly common owing to the opioid epidemic.

TREATMENT

Most patients do not have an apparent cause and are deemed to have chronic idiopathic constipation owing to colonic inertia, dyssynergic defecation, or functional disorders (e.g., irritable bowel syndrome). Most patients can be successfully treated with adequate fluids, fiber supplements, osmotic agents (polyethylene glycol), and/or nonprescription stimulant laxatives (e.g., once-daily bisacodyl, 5 to 10 mg, or senna, 17.6 to 34.4 mg).[A11] Management of chronic refractory constipation may require linaclotide (72 to 290 μg daily), plecanatide (3 mg daily), lubiprostone (24 μg twice daily), or prucalopride (1 to 2 mg daily; see Table 122-3), whereas patients with dyssynergia may respond to biofeedback.[24] For opioid-induced constipation, a combination of an osmotic and stimulant laxative is recommended as initial treatment. Patients who have an inadequate response may benefit from the addition of a peripherally acting μ-opioid receptor antagonist (e.g., naloxone, naloxegol, or naldemedine) or the serotonin-4 receptor agonist prucalopride (1 to 2 mg daily; Table 122-3).[A12]

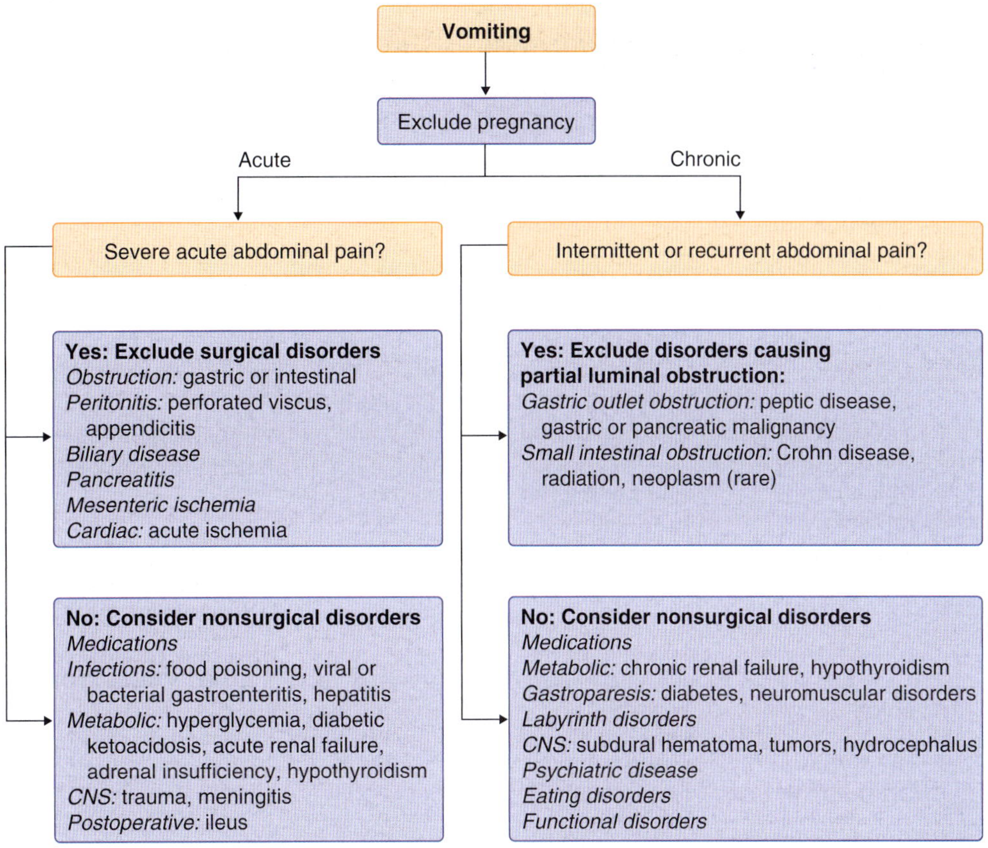

FIGURE 118-5. **Approach to the patient with vomiting.** CNS = central nervous system.

TABLE 118-5 MEDICAL TREATMENT OF NAUSEA AND VOMITING

DRUG	USUAL INDICATIONS	USUAL DOSE (RANGE)	ROUTE	COMMENTS
ANTICHOLINERGIC-ANTIHISTAMINE AGENTS	Most commonly: GIDz, motion sickness, vertigo			Side effects: sedation, dizziness, delirium, blurred vision, glaucoma, bronchospasm, tachycardia, urinary retention Avoid concomitant alcohol or CNS depressants; use with caution in elderly patients
Scopolamine patch	MS	1.5 mg/72 hr	Patch	
Dimenhydrinate	MS	50 mg (50-100 mg) q4-6h	PO, IM, IV	Maximum 400 mg/24 hr
Cyclizine	MS, GIDz	50 mg q8h	PO, IM	Maximum 200 mg/24 hr
Meclizine	MS, V	25-50 mg q24h	PO	
Diphenhydramine	GIDz	25-50 mg q6h 50-100 mg q6h	PO, IV IM	
Promethazine	GIDz, PONV, MS	25 mg (12.5-25 mg) q6-12h 25 mg (12.5-50 mg) q4-6h	PO, PR IV, IM	Phenothiazine derivative, but lacks significant antidopaminergic effects Avoid perivascular extravasation or subcutaneous injection(severe tissue necrosis)
Trimethobenzamide	GIDz, PONV	200 mg q6-8h	IM	
DOPAMINE RECEPTOR ANTAGONISTS	Most commonly: acute, nonsurgical gastrointestinal disorders (viral gastroenteritis), PONV, CTX			Side effects: neuromuscular (extrapyramidal) symptoms—agitation, restlessness, involuntary movements, dystonia, torticollis, laryngospasm, Parkinson-like features
Prochlorperazine	GIDz, PONV, CTX with low-emetic risk	5-10 mg q6-8h 25 mg q12h	PO, IV, IM PR	Maximum dose 20-40 mg/24 hr; avoid subcutaneous injection (irritation)
Metoclopramide	GIDz Mildly emetogenic CTX	10 mg (10-20 mg) q6-8h 1-2 mg/kg before and 2 hr after CTX	PO, IV, IM IV	Modest efficacy at these doses High doses infrequently used owing to availability of safer, more effective CTX regimens; use with diphenhydramine to reduce adverse side effects
Droperidol	PONV	2.5 mg (1.25-5 mg) preinduction and q4-6h as needed	IV, IM	May cause QTc prolongation and torsades de pointes; use is restricted to patients who fail to respond to other agents

TABLE 118-5 MEDICAL TREATMENT OF NAUSEA AND VOMITING—cont'd

DRUG	USUAL INDICATIONS	USUAL DOSE (RANGE)	ROUTE	COMMENTS
Olanzapine	Highly emetogenic CTX: used in combination with 2-3 other antiemetic agents	10 mg q24h on days 1-4	PO	Antipsychotic that blocks dopamine D2 and serotonin 5HT-2 receptors; side effects include sedation and hyperglycemia
CORTICOSTEROIDS				
Dexamethasone	PONV CTX	4-8 mg once preinduction 8-20 mg on day 1; 8 mg on days 2-4	PO, IV PO, IV	Most beneficial when used with other agents (e.g., 5-HT_3 RA, neurokinin-1 RA)
BENZODIAZEPINES				Used to reduce anxiety and anticipatory vomiting
Lorazepam	CTX	1-2 mg q4-6h	PO, IV	
CANNABINOIDS				May stimulate appetite; adverse side effects (sedation, dizziness, dysphoria, dry mouth) limit use
Dronabinol	GIDz, CTX	5-10 mg q6-8h	PO	
Nabilone	GIDz, CTX	1-2 mg q12h	PO	
5-HT_3 RECEPTOR ANTAGONISTS	PONV, CTX			All except palonosetron may cause QTc prolongation (dose-dependent) with risk of cardiac arrhythmias PONV prevention: give IV immediately before anesthesia induction Prevention of CTX-induced vomiting: give single dose 30 min (IV) to 1 hr (PO) before CTX
Ondansetron	PONV CTX, RadTx	4 mg once 4-8 mg 8 mg once	IV PO IV	
Granisetron	CTX, RadTx	1 mg twice daily 1 mg once	PO IV	
Dolasetron	CTX, PONV	100 mg once daily	PO only	
Palonosetron	CTX PONV	0.25 mg once 0.5 mg 0.075 mg	IV PO, 1-3 days IV	Second generation antagonist with higher affinity for 5-HT3 receptors and longer half-life; does not cause QTc prolongation
NEUROKININ-1 RECEPTOR ANTAGONISTS	Highly emetogenic CTX			Used exclusively in combination with a 5-HT_3 RA or dexamethasone
Aprepitant		125 mg on day 1; 80 mg on days 2-3	PO	
Rolapitant		180 mg 1-2 hr before CTX	PO	
Fosaprepitant		150 mg on day 1	IV	Aprepitant 80 mg PO on days 2-3
Netupitant 300 mg/ palonosetron 0.5 mg combination		1 capsule 1 hr before CTX	PO	
ANTIEMETIC REGIMENS FOR CHEMOTHERAPY				
Mildly emetogenic CTX	Option 1 Option 2 Option 3	Dexamethasone 8 mg Dopamine receptor antagonist 5-HT_3 RA	IV or PO	One dose only One dose only One dose only
Moderately emetogenic CTX		Day 1: 5-HT_3 RA plus dexamethasone 8 mg with or without neurokinin-1 RA	IV or PO	Days 2-3: continue oral 5-HT_3 RA and/or dexamethasone 8 mg to reduce delayed emesis
Highly emetogenic CTX		Day 1: 5-HT_3 RA plus dexamethasone 12 mg plus neurokinin-1 RA plus olanzapine	IV or PO	Days 2-4: olanzapine and dexamethasone 8 mg PO daily; if aprepitant given on day 1, continue 80 mg PO days 2-4. Regimens may vary.

5-HT_3 = serotonin or 5-hydroxytryptamine$_3$; CNS = central nervous system; CTX = chemotherapy; GIDz = acute, nonsurgical gastrointestinal disorders associated with nausea and vomiting (e.g., viral gastroenteritis); IM = intramuscularly; IV = intravenously; MS = motion sickness; PO = orally; PONV = postoperative nausea and vomiting; PR = per rectum; RA = receptor antagonist; RadTx = radiation therapy–induced nausea and vomiting; V = vertigo.

Modified from Proctor DD. Approach to the patient with gastrointestinal disease. In: Goldman L, Ausiello D, eds. *Cecil Textbook of Medicine*, 23rd ed. Philadelphia: Saunders-Elsevier; 2008.

GASTROINTESTINAL BLEEDING

GI bleeding (Chapter 121) may be acute and clinically apparent (overt) or chronic, slow, and clinically inapparent (occult). The location of acute GI bleeding is described as either upper or lower, according to whether the source is proximal or distal to the ligament of Treitz (distal duodenum). Upper GI bleeding, which is three times more common than lower GI bleeding, is manifested by bloody emesis (hematemesis), coffee ground emesis, and, in most cases, black stools (melena). Common causes of significant bleeding are peptic ulcer disease, esophageal varices, Mallory-Weiss tears, erosive gastritis or esophagitis, and vascular ectasias.[25] Major lower GI bleeding is manifested by large-volume maroon or bright red bloody stools (hematochezia). Although 80 to 90% of patients with hematochezia have a lower source of bleeding, massive upper GI bleeding also may cause hematochezia. Approximately 95% of major lower GI bleeding arises from the colon and 5% from the small intestine. Lower GI bleeding is increased in patients older than

50 years, in whom diverticulosis accounts for 60% of cases; the remainder are due to ischemia, neoplasms, ulcers, vascular ectasias, or hemorrhoids. In patients younger than 50 years, bleeding is more commonly attributable to inflammatory bowel disease, hemorrhoids, or infectious colitis, but the incidence of colonic neoplasia is increasing in patients ages 40 to 50 years.[26]

Occult GI bleeding refers to GI blood loss that is small in volume and not apparent to the patient but is detectable by tests for fecal occult blood. Chronic occult bleeding may result in iron deficiency anemia.[27] Both upper endoscopy and colonoscopy should be performed to look for a source of occult bleeding, most commonly gastroesophageal or colonic neoplasia, erosive esophagitis or gastritis, ulcer disease, or vascular ectasia. In patients with recurrent iron deficiency and occult blood loss in whom no source is found on upper and lower endoscopy, video capsule endoscopy, CT enterography, or enteroscopy is performed to look for a small bowel source (vascular ectasia, ulcer, or neoplasm)

FECAL INCONTINENCE

Fecal incontinence (Chapter 131) is dependent on a number of factors, including a solid or semisolid stool, a compliant and distensible rectal reservoir, the ability to sense rectal fullness, an intact internal anal sphincter (an involuntary muscle innervated by the enteric nervous system), an intact external anal sphincter and puborectalis (voluntary muscles innervated by the pudendal nerve), and the mental and physical ability to reach a toilet facility when needed.[28] Minor incontinence, which occurs in 10% of people older than 70 years, is characterized by the inability to control flatus or by the seepage of fecal matter that results in soiling of the perianal area and undergarments. It tends to be intermittent, occurring after bowel movements; when coughing, lifting, or passing flatus; or when stools are loose. Major incontinence is characterized by the partial or complete inability to control bowel movements reliably, resulting in gross, involuntary loss of feces and the need to wear a diaper. It occurs in less than 1% of the population and is virtually always caused by a central nervous system disorder that results in diminished awareness of bowel needs, neuropathy, or damage to the anal sphincters.

OTHER GASTROINTESTINAL COMPLAINTS

Heartburn, esophageal regurgitation, dysphagia,[29] odynophagia, and noncardiac chest pain suggest esophageal disease (Chapter 124). *Dyspepsia*, which refers to bothersome, intermittent, mild to moderate upper abdominal or epigastric symptoms (burning, pain, early satiation, postprandial fullness) can be caused by peptic ulcer disease (Chapter 125) or esophageal disease (Chapter 124), or it can be functional in origin (Chapter 123).[30] An orderly diagnostic approach (Fig. 118-6) can help distinguish among the various causes, avoid unnecessary testing, and minimize symptoms.

Diarrhea, which is defined pathophysiologically as an increase in stool weight to more than 200 g/day, can be caused by malabsorption of osmotically active substances or by increased intestinal secretion of electrolytes and water. In clinical practice, however, stool weight is seldom quantified, and the term *diarrhea* refers to an increase in stool liquidity or frequency (more than three bowel movements per day). Acute and chronic diarrhea (Chapter 126) should be distinguished because the evaluation and treatment are different. In young adults with chronic diarrhea, the leading causes are irritable bowel syndrome (Chapter 123), inflammatory bowel disease (Chapter 127), microscopic colitis (Chapter 126), bile acid diarrhea,[31] malabsorption, drugs, food additives, and diabetes (Chapter 210).

GENERAL REFERENCES

For the General References and other additional features, please visit Elsevier eBooks+ at https://ebooks.health.elsevier.com.

Grade A References

A1. Hajibandeh S, Loutfi M, Hajibandeh S, et al. Routine versus selective computed tomography in non-traumatic acute abdominal pain: meta-analysis of randomised trials. *Langenbecks Arch Surg*. 2020;405:283-291.

A2. de Almeida Leite RM, Seo DJ, Gomez-Eslava B, et al. Nonoperative vs operative management of uncomplicated acute appendicitis: a systematic review and meta-analysis. *JAMA Surg*. 2022;157:828-834.

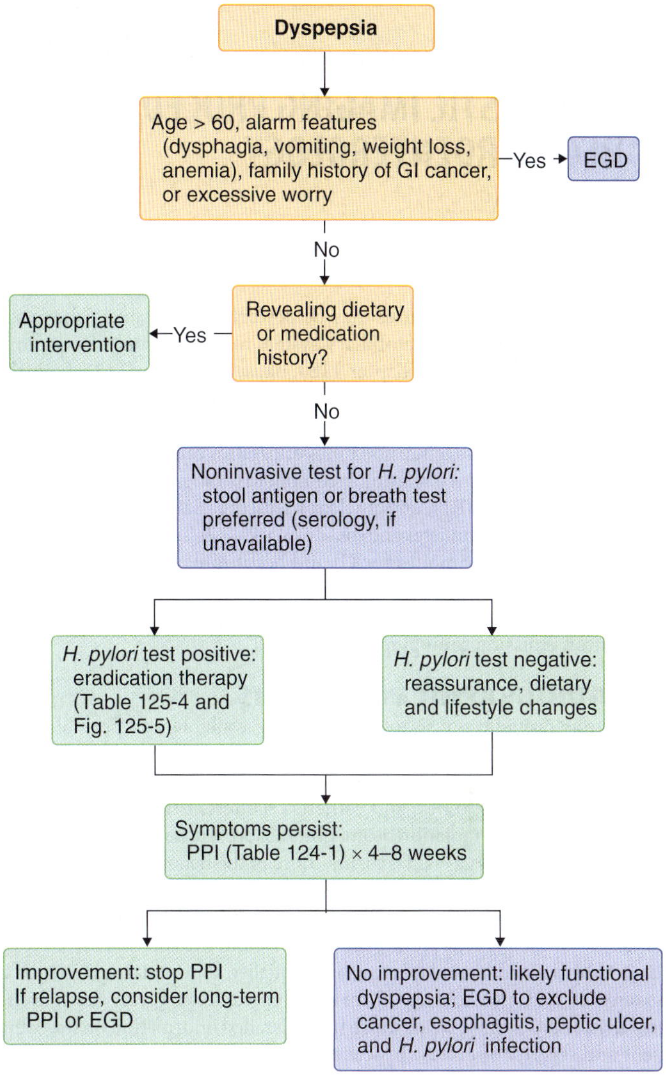

FIGURE 118-6. Approach to the patient with dyspepsia. EGD = esophagogastroduodenoscopy; GI = gastrointestinal; PPI = proton pump inhibitor.

A3. Zhang Y, Feng L, Wang X, et al. Low fermentable oligosaccharides, disaccharides, monosaccharides, and polyols diet compared with traditional dietary advice for diarrhea-predominant irritable bowel syndrome: a parallel-group, randomized controlled trial with analysis of clinical and microbiological factors associated with patient outcomes. *Am J Clin Nutr*. 2021;113:1531-1545.

A4. Hammer HF, Fox MR, Keller J, et al. European guideline on indications, performance, and clinical impact of hydrogen and methane breath tests in adult and pediatric patients: European Association for Gastroenterology, Endoscopy and Nutrition, European Society of Neurogastroenterology and Motility, and European Society for Paediatric Gastroenterology, Hepatology and Nutrition consensus. *United European Gastroenterol J*. 2022;10:15-40.

A5. Black CJ, Staudacher HM, Ford AC. Efficacy of a low FODMAP diet in irritable bowel syndrome: systematic review and network meta-analysis. *Gut*. 2022;71:1117-1126.

A6. Holvoet T, Joossens M, Vazquez-Castellanos JF, et al. Fecal microbiota transplantation reduces symptoms in some patients with irritable bowel syndrome with predominant abdominal bloating: short- and long-term results from a placebo-controlled randomized trial. *Gastroenterology*. 2021;160:145-157.

A7. Hashimoto H, Abe M, Tokuyama O, et al. Olanzapine 5 mg plus standard antiemetic therapy for the prevention of chemotherapy-induced nausea and vomiting (J-FORCE): a multicentre, randomised, double-blind, placebo-controlled, phase 3 trial. *Lancet Oncol*. 2020;21:242-249.

A8. Weibel S, Schaefer MS, Raj D, et al. Drugs for preventing postoperative nausea and vomiting after general anesthesia: an abridged Cochrane network meta-analysis. *Anaesthesia*. 2021;76:962-973.

A9. Chow R, Valdez C, Chow N, et al. Oral cannabinoid for the prophylaxis of chemotherapy-induced nausea and vomiting—a systematic review and meta-analysis. *Support Care Canc*. 2020;28:2095-2103.

A10. Ducrotte P, Coffin B, Bonaz B, et al. Gastric electrical stimulation reduces refractory vomiting in a randomized crossover trial. *Gastroenterology*. 2020;158:506-514.

A11. Rao SS, Brenner DM. Efficacy and safety of over-the-counter therapies for chronic constipation: an updated systematic review. *Am J Gastroenterol*. 2021;116:1156-1181.

A12. Vijayvargiya P, Camilleri M, Vijayvargiya P, et al. Systematic review with meta-analysis: efficacy and safety of treatments for opioid-induced constipation. *Aliment Pharmacol Ther*. 2020;52:37-53.

119

DIAGNOSTIC IMAGING PROCEDURES IN GASTROENTEROLOGY

LAURA R. CARUCCI

A variety of imaging procedures may be performed to evaluate the gastrointestinal (GI) tract and hepatobiliary system for a spectrum of symptoms, including abdominal pain (Chapter 118), nausea (Chapter 118), vomiting, heartburn (Chapter 123), diarrhea (Chapter 126), constipation (Chapter 122), bloating, GI bleeding (Chapter 121), weight loss (Chapter 118), or abnormal laboratory test results. Imaging modalities utilized for these procedures include radiography, fluoroscopy, ultrasound, computed tomography (CT), magnetic resonance imaging (MRI), and nuclear medicine. Each modality provides varying utility with advantages and disadvantages.[1,2] In addition, these modalities offer advanced techniques for GI and hepatobiliary imaging, including CT and MR enterography, CT colonography (virtual colonoscopy), MR cholangiopancreatography (MRCP), MR elastography, CT and MR angiography, and positron emission tomography (PET)/CT.

RADIOGRAPHIC PLAIN FILMS

Radiography provides quick, low-cost, readily available, and portable evaluation of the abdomen and pelvis. Abdominal radiographs may be ordered to evaluate acute abdominal pain and to assess for obstruction, ileus, perforation, post-surgical changes, tubes, and catheters. Different tissue types absorb a varying amount of the radiation beam. Bone absorbs more of the beam and will appear white, whereas gas will transmit more of the beam to the detector and appear black. Radiographs therefore can be utilized to evaluate the bowel gas pattern, calcifications, radiopaque foreign bodies, and the osseous structures, and they may also provide some information about the soft tissues. Although radiography is a readily available first-line modality, abdominal radiographs are less sensitive and specific than CT for many processes involving the abdomen and pelvis, and CT can provide much more detailed information on the overall extent and severity of disease processes.

Abdominal radiographs show the distribution of bowel gas and caliber of bowel. A combination of supine and upright or decubitus radiographs is preferred over supine imaging alone and can provide more detail about potential bowel obstruction or extraluminal air. The pattern of bowel gas and air-fluid levels can help distinguish between entities such as small bowel obstruction (Fig. 119-1), colonic obstruction, volvulus, or ileus. In addition to bowel gas, radiographs may reveal gas in atypical or unexpected locations, including pneumoperitoneum (Fig. 119-2), pneumatosis (Fig. 119-3), pneumobilia, portal venous gas, retroperitoneal gas, subcutaneous emphysema, gas in an abscess, or gas in the gallbladder.

Pneumoperitoneum may be recognized on supine radiographs by the appearance of gas on both sides of the bowel wall (Rigler sign); linear, angulated, or triangular areas of lucency; gas in the most non-dependent portion of the abdomen in the midline, under the central tendon of the diaphragm; or outlining spaces and structures such as the falciform ligament (see Fig. 119-2). An upright or decubitus radiograph increases the sensitivity for detecting free air. With optimal patient positioning and technique, as little as 1 to 2 mL of free air can been seen on abdominal radiography. However, pneumoperitoneum may be identified in only 50% of patients with documented visceral perforation because of technical limitations, including poor image quality, suboptimal field of view, and exclusion of the uppermost peritoneal cavity on the image. CT is the most accurate and sensitive diagnostic modality for detecting pneumoperitoneum.

Abdominal radiographs are also useful to evaluate radiopaque foci such as calcifications (gallstones, renal stones, fecoliths), foreign bodies (ingested or inserted foreign bodies, ballistic fragments), surgical devices (bariatric lap band) (Fig. 119-4), drains, tubes, and retained surgical material (sponge, lap pads, needles). Radiography can localize radiopaque intra-abdominal foreign bodies with a sensitivity of 90% and specificity of 100%.

FLUOROSCOPY

Fluoroscopy studies use contrast agents that may be swallowed, injected, or instilled into the GI tract in conjunction with radiographic images. Fluoroscopy studies are relatively quick, inexpensive, minimally or noninvasive, and widely available. Typical GI fluoroscopy procedures that may be performed include modified barium swallow, esophagram, upper GI series, upper GI series with small bowel follow-through, contrast enema, colostomy enema, and defecography.

Contrast agents utilized include water-soluble iodinated contrast material, barium, and air. Water-soluble contrast is preferred for possible leaks,

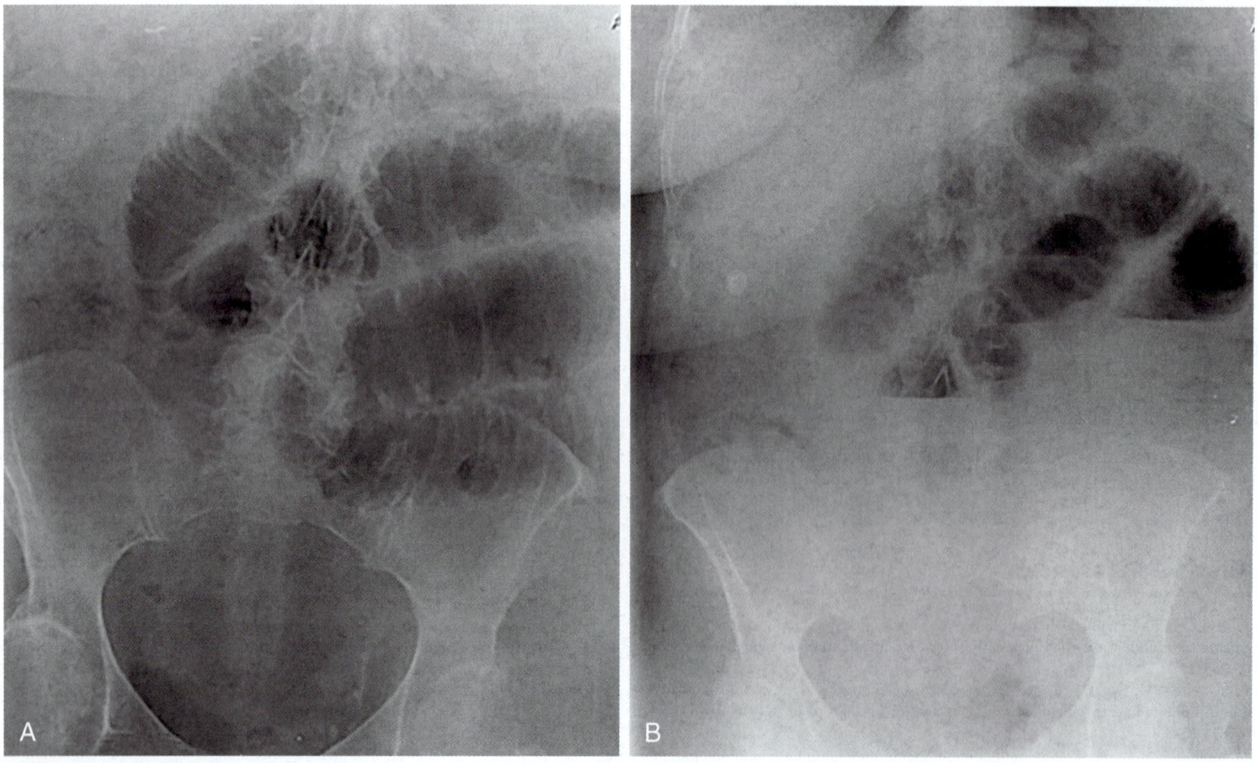

FIGURE 119-1. **Small bowel obstruction.** Supine (A) and upright (B) radiographs of the abdomen show dilated gas-filled loops of small bowel with a small amount of gas in the colon. The colon is not dilated. Small bowel air-fluid levels are noted on the upright radiograph. The findings are consistent with small bowel obstruction.

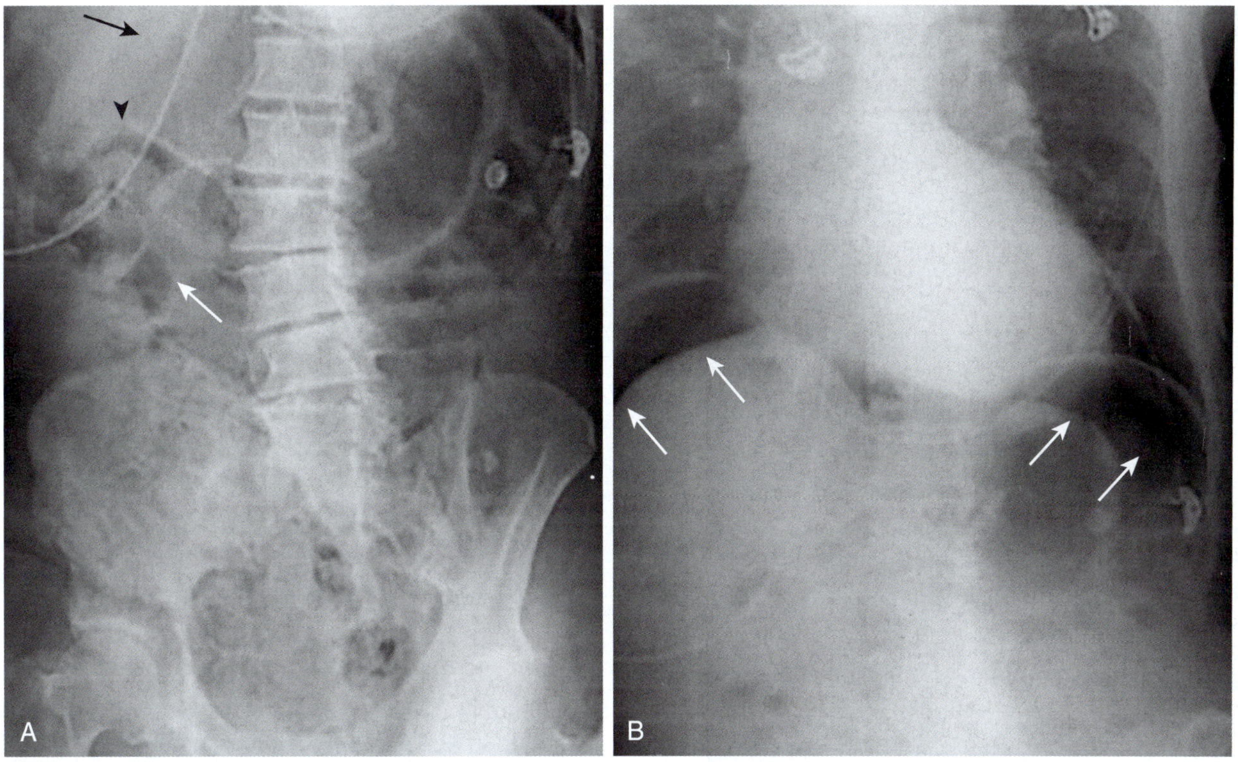

FIGURE 119-2. **Pneumoperitoneum. A,** A supine radiograph of the abdomen shows pneumoperitoneum. There is increased lucency throughout the upper abdomen (*black arrow*) with angulated gas in the right upper quadrant (*arrowhead*), and both sides of the bowel wall are visible (Rigler sign) (*white arrow*). **B,** An upright radiograph confirms a large amount of free air layering under the diaphragm (*arrows*).

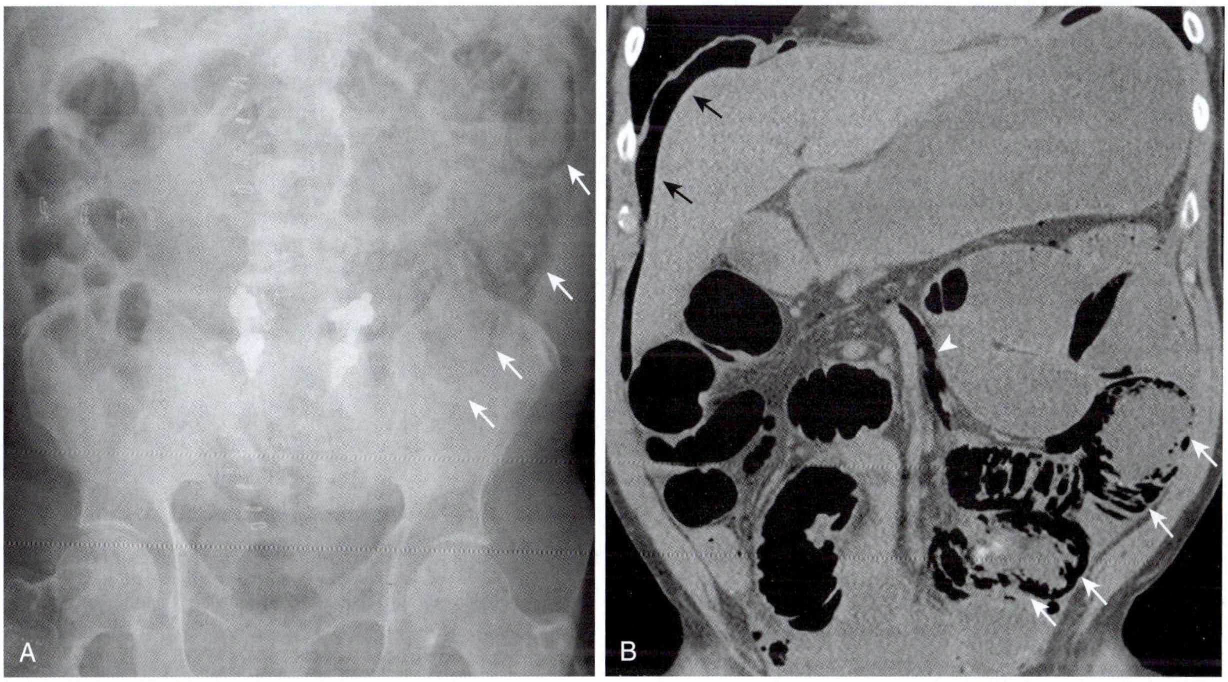

FIGURE 119-3. **Pneumatosis. A,** A supine radiograph of the abdomen shows dilated small bowel loops with lucency in the bowel wall due to pneumatosis (*arrows*). Also note skin staples and hardware in the lumbar spine. Pneumatosis is much more readily visible on the coronal computed tomographic (CT) image without intravenous contrast (*white arrows*). **B,** Also seen on the CT is associated mesenteric venous gas (*arrowhead*) and free air (*black arrows*).

perforations, suspected impacted foreign bodies, and following trauma, surgery, or instrumentation. Barium is preferred otherwise.

Double contrast techniques, which utilize barium in conjunction with air to distend the lumen, are best for mucosal detail (Fig. 119-5). Single contrast techniques are used for debilitated or postoperative patients and to evaluate for leaks (Fig. 119-6).

GI fluoroscopy studies evaluate the bowel lumen but provide limited information about surrounding structures other than secondary findings, such as mass effect and displacement. Fluoroscopy studies provide anatomic, structural, mucosal, and functional information about the bowel. In particular, fluoroscopy studies may detect congenital anomalies, infectious or inflammatory conditions (including inflammatory bowel disease; Chapter 127), filling defects (polyps, masses) (see Fig. 119-5), outpouchings (e.g., ulcers [Chapter 125], diverticula [Chapter 128]), extravasation (leak) (see Fig. 119-6), fistulae, and obstruction (e.g., mass, stricture, adhesive disease, intussusception). Also, fluoroscopic studies are ideally suited to evaluate post-surgical anatomy and complications

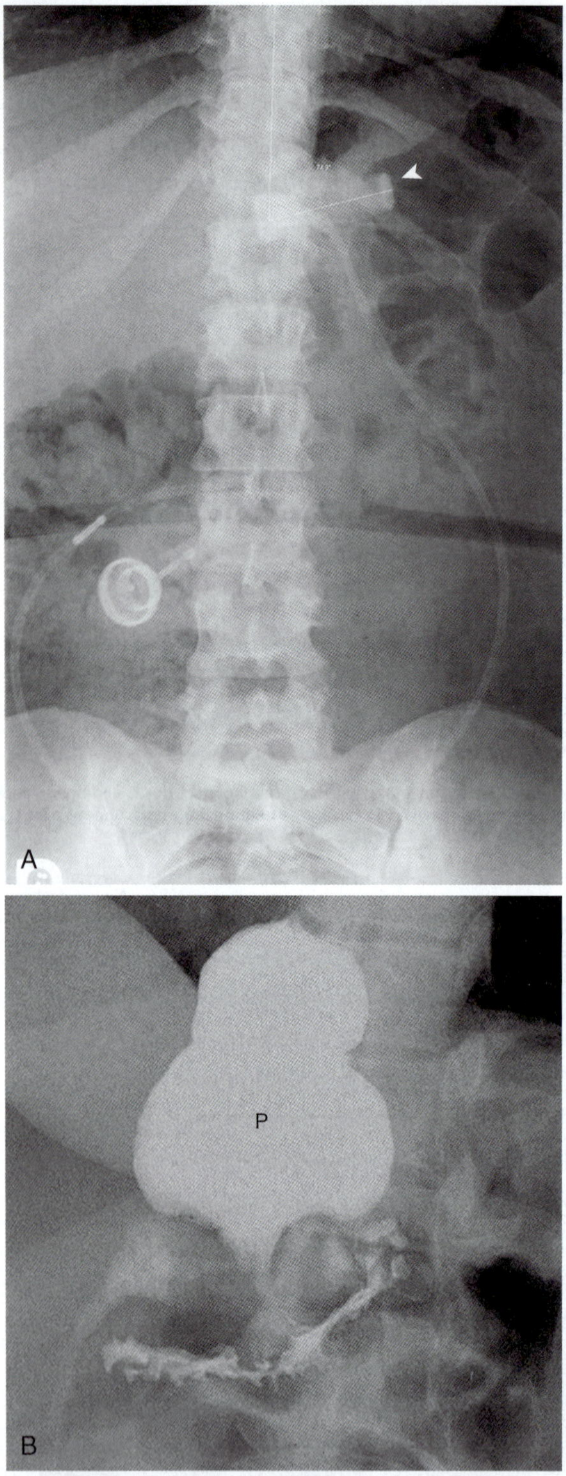

FIGURE 119-4. Gastric band bariatric surgery: band slippage with fundic herniation. **A,** A supine radiograph of the abdomen shows a gastric band device. The radiograph allows for evaluation of the surgical components, including the band itself (*arrowhead*), the connecting tubing, and the injectable reservoir. The inflatable band around the proximal stomach is too inferiorly located and horizontal in position (*arrowhead*). **B,** An upper gastrointestinal fluoroscopic spot image shows a dilated gastric pouch (*P*) above the band, with partial obstruction owing to band slippage with fundic herniation.

(see Fig. 119-4). Although CT is a high-yield study for diagnosis of small bowel obstruction and its cause, upper GI series with small bowel follow-through can further evaluate the cause and degree of obstruction and provide useful information about bowel transit time. Fluoroscopy can also be used for interventions, including feeding tube and drainage catheter placement and repositioning. For patients with inflammatory bowel disease, however, CT and MR enterography are now much more commonly performed than is a fluoroscopic small bowel follow-through. Similarly, CT colonography is more often performed than a double contrast barium enema to screen for colorectal cancer.

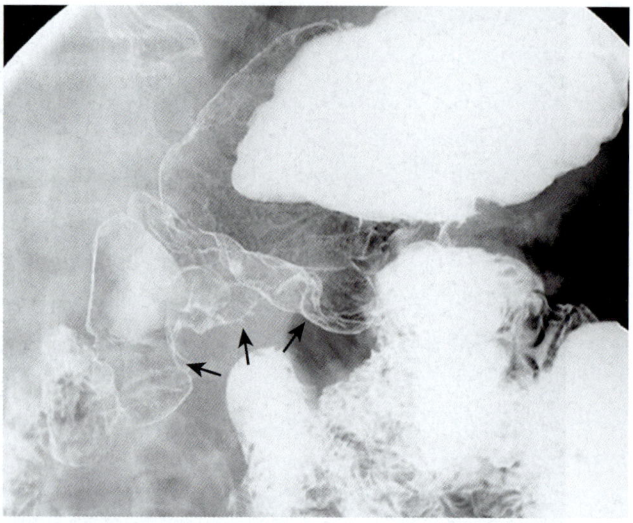

FIGURE 119-5. Gastric cancer. A double contrast upper gastrointestinal fluoroscopic spot image shows a lobulated mass along the greater curvature of the gastric body (*arrows*), consistent with a primary gastric neoplasm.

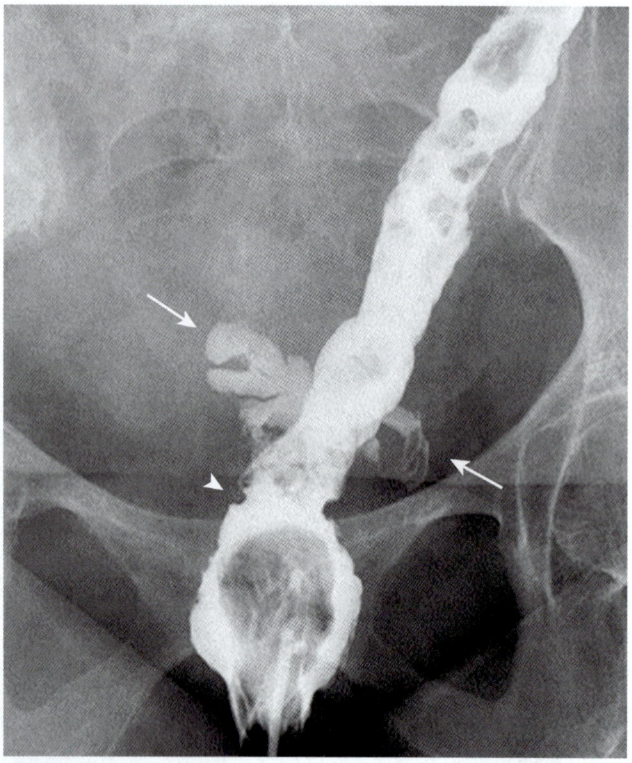

FIGURE 119-6. Colorectal anastomotic leak. A single contrast enema utilizing water-soluble contrast shows a colorectal anastomosis (*arrowhead*) as well as a large collection of amorphous extraluminal contrast (*arrows*) owing to anastomotic leak.

Fluoroscopy, which allows for real-time imaging and observing changes over time, can be used to evaluate the swallowing mechanism, esophageal motility and reflux, and bowel transit time. For example, an esophagram can assess for a spectrum of structural and mucosal abnormalities (including ulcer, stricture, mass, and hiatal hernia), evaluate esophageal motility, and detect gastroesophageal reflux and its complications (Fig. 119-7).[3] Modified barium swallow studies and esophagrams constitute a larger percentage of fluoroscopy studies now performed,[4] because the pharynx and esophagus are not as readily evaluated with cross sectional techniques.[5] Modified barium swallow can evaluate the swallowing mechanism, assess for aspiration using various consistencies and compensatory maneuvers, and determine potential strategies to improve swallowing function[6]; it is particularly useful in patients who have neurologic and musculoskeletal conditions, trauma, recurrent upper respiratory infections, and aspiration pneumonia.

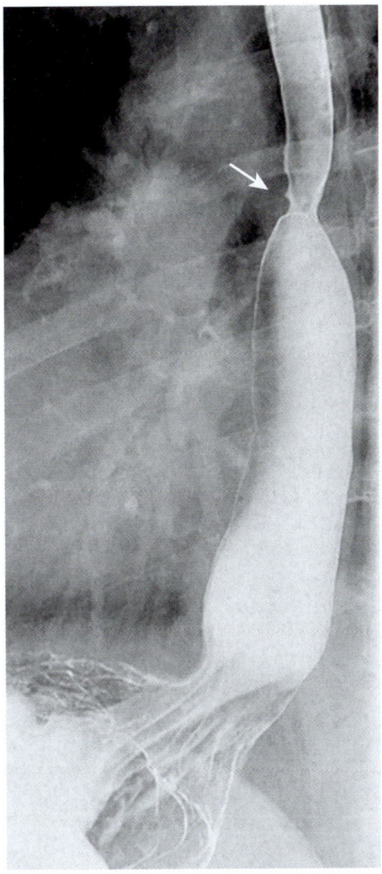

FIGURE 119-7. **Barrett esophagus.** A fluoroscopic spot image from an esophagram shows a patulous gastroesophageal junction; marked spontaneous gastroesophageal reflux was also seen at fluoroscopy. A focal stricture with mild associated irregularity in the mid to upper thoracic esophagus (*arrow*) is due to Barrett esophagus.

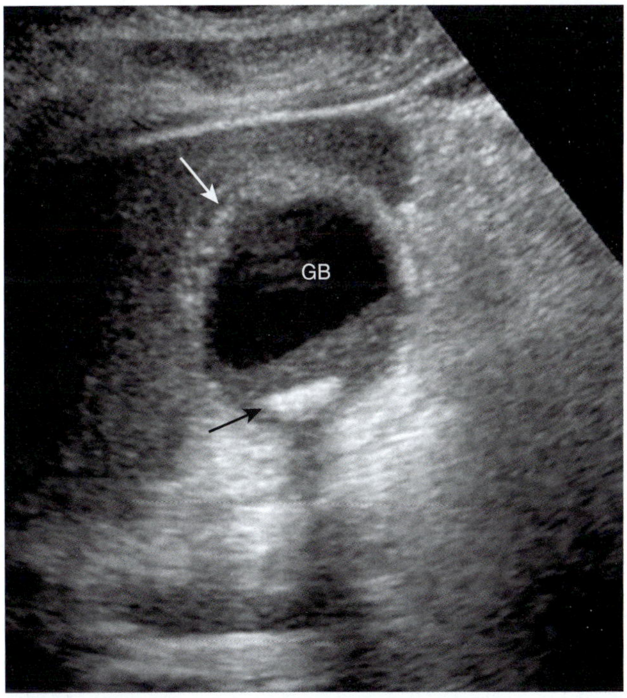

FIGURE 119-8. **Cholelithiasis and acute cholecystitis.** Ultrasound of the gallbladder (*GB*) shows echogenic, shadowing stones (*black arrow*) surrounded by layering sludge. Also noted is gallbladder wall thickening (*white arrow*) with trace adjacent fluid. A sonographic Murphy sign was also noted upon scanning.

ULTRASOUND

Abdominal ultrasound provides real-time imaging that utilizes high-frequency sound waves emitted by a transducer or probe, most often placed on the skin surface. Sound waves bounce back to the transducer to varying degrees based on the type of tissue, thereby creating images of the solid organs and vasculature of the abdomen. Ultrasound is noninvasive, portable, and does not utilize ionizing radiation or iodinated contrast material. These characteristics make ultrasound an excellent first test to evaluate patients who have suspected disease or abnormalities of the liver, gallbladder, biliary tree, spleen, pancreas, kidneys, and the abdominal cavity, as well as the inferior vena cava, aorta, and portal vein. Ultrasound may also be performed utilizing transvaginal, transrectal, or endoscopic probes, and it may be utilized for image-guided biopsy and intervention.

However, images are acquired only where the probe is placed, and ultrasound is therefore operator dependent. Also, it may be difficult to evaluate the entire contents of the abdomen owing to a large body habitus, the patient's positioning, artifact from skin dressings, and artifact from bowel gas. Ultrasound waves are blocked by bowel gas, thereby often limiting evaluation of the common bile duct and pancreas. As a result, more detailed evaluation often requires CT or other modalities.

A liver Doppler examination provides more detailed information about the hepatic vasculature and can evaluate vascular patency, direction of flow, and vascular waveforms. Doppler ultrasound techniques can also be used to diagnose vascular thrombosis (Chapter 129), varices (Chapter 139), cavernous transformation of the portal vein, aneurysms, and vascular anomalies (Chapter 129).

Ultrasound is well suited to evaluate the gallbladder (Chapter 141) and right upper quadrant pain.[7] Sound waves travel through fluid, thereby making ultrasound an ideal modality to evaluate the gallbladder. The normal gallbladder is fluid-filled, transmits sound, and appears hypoechoic (dark) on ultrasound. Gallstones appear echogenic (bright) and result in "acoustic shadowing" as the sound waves fail to propagate through stones (Fig. 119-8). Ultrasound is the method of choice for the diagnosis of gallstones with high sensitivity and accuracy (>95%), and ultrasound can differentiate cholelithiasis from sludge, polyps, or masses. In the setting of acute cholecystitis, ultrasound may reveal gallstones, gallbladder wall thickening, adjacent fluid, gallbladder distension (see Fig. 119-8), and a sonographic Murphy sign (focal tenderness corresponding to a sonographically localized gallbladder). Biliary ductal dilation may be recognized, but the cause may not be revealed if the common duct and pancreas are obscured by bowel gas. MR or CT may be performed to evaluate for the etiology of biliary obstruction (i.e., pancreatic mass, choledocholithiasis).

Ultrasound is useful to assess for diffuse hepatic processes, and it can evaluate the liver's size, morphology, and echotexture. In cirrhosis (Chapter 139), the liver appears echogenic, heterogeneous, and nodular in contour (Fig. 119-9).[8] Ultrasound can also identify findings of portal hypertension, including splenomegaly, ascites, and collateral vessels. Ultrasound can detect focal solid organ lesions and can readily determine a cystic or solid nature of a lesion. Doppler techniques can be utilized to determine the lesion's vascularity (see Fig. 119-9). CT and MR are superior to ultrasound overall to characterize liver lesions (i.e., benign lesions, primary tumor, metastasis), but contrast-enhanced ultrasound can assist in characterizing a liver lesion sonographically. Ultrasound following intravenous (IV) injection of a contrast agent, consisting of gas within microbubbles, can show enhancement of the lesions.

COMPUTED TOMOGRAPHY

CT, which uses x-ray technology, can image the entire contents of the abdomen and pelvis within only a few minutes, while providing excellent anatomic detail. Images can be reconstructed in multiple planes, and 3D images can also be generated. Abdominopelvic CT, which allows for evaluation of the bowel as well as solid organs, mesentery, peritoneum, and vasculature, is often performed with iodinated intravenous contrast to provide more detailed evaluation of abdominal contents. Oral contrast may be administered as well to help evaluate the bowel. Contrast may also be administered rectally or injected into the bladder, a fistula, or a drainage catheter prior to imaging.

CT of the abdomen and pelvis is ideally suited to evaluate patients who present with an acute abdomen (Chapters 118 and 128), because CT can detect even minimal pneumoperitoneum and can evaluate the entirety of the bowel and abdominal vasculature. Free air, pneumatosis, abscesses, and signs of infection, including peritonitis, are more readily visualized on CT than with radiography (see Fig. 119-3). CT also can evaluate for bowel processes, including appendicitis (Chapter 128 and Figs 128-3 and 128-4),[9] diverticulitis (Chapter 128 and Fig 128-6; Fig. 119-10),[10] volvulus, intussusception (Fig. 119-11), infectious and inflammatory conditions (including inflammatory bowel disease; Chapter 127), ischemia (Chapter 129),[11] trauma, perforation,

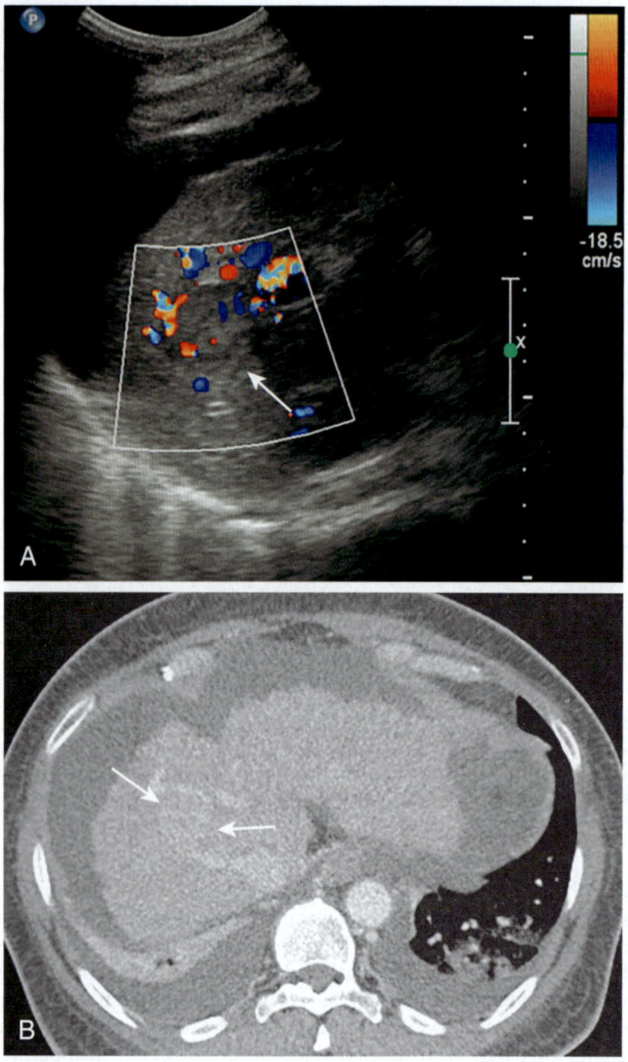

FIGURE 119-9. **Cirrhosis with hepatocellular carcinoma. A,** Abdominal ultrasound using color Doppler technique shows a small, nodular, echogenic, and heterogeneous liver due to cirrhosis. A focal mass is noted with internal vascularity seen with color Doppler (*arrow*). There is perihepatic fluid. **B,** Contrast-enhanced axial computed tomographic image in the same patient shows a nodular, cirrhotic liver; ascites; and a corresponding enhancing liver lesion (*arrows*) consistent with hepatocellular carcinoma.

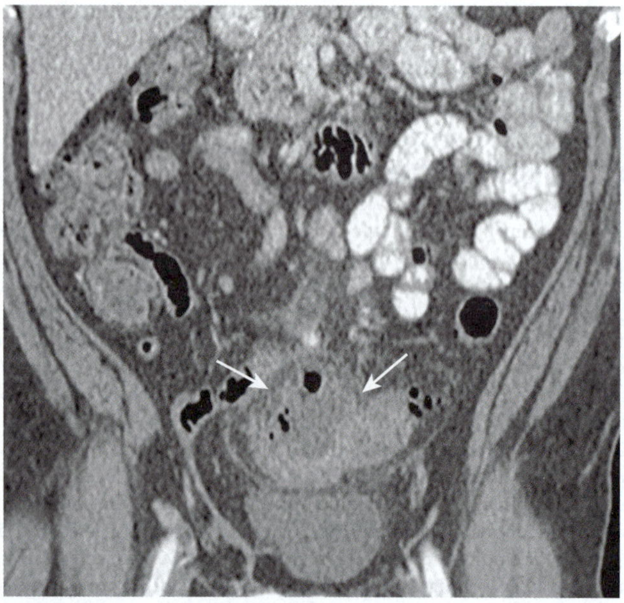

FIGURE 119-10. **Acute sigmoid diverticulitis with abscess.** A coronal contrast-enhanced computed tomographic image reveals diverticulosis in the sigmoid colon. There is focal sigmoid colon wall thickening with adjacent inflammatory change and an abscess (*arrows*) along the sigmoid colon due to diverticulitis.

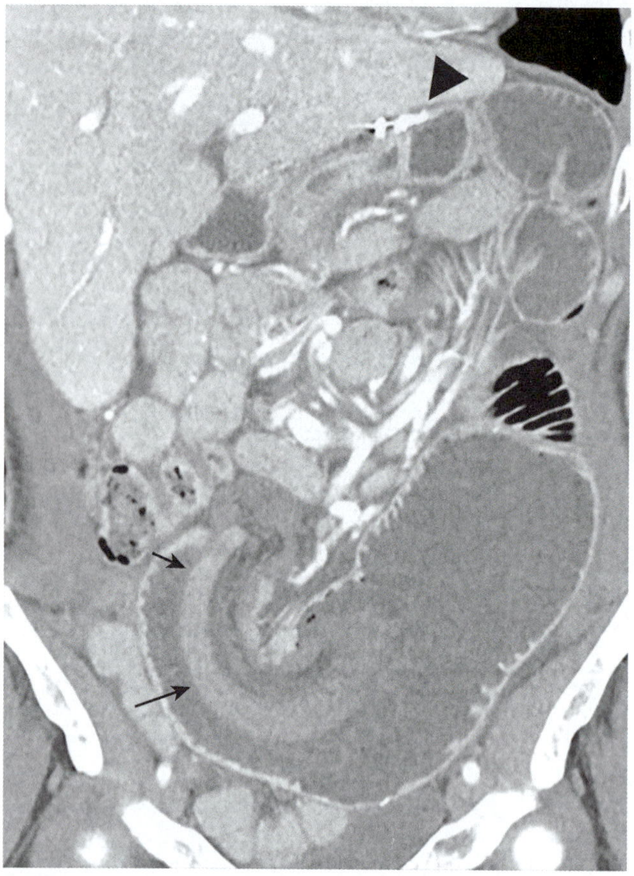

FIGURE 119-11. **Small bowel obstruction due to intussusception following Roux-en-Y gastric bypass.** A coronal contrast-enhanced CT image shows markedly dilated small bowel consistent with obstruction and due to intussusception (*arrows*) at the jejunojejunal anastomosis in a patient status post Roux-en-Y gastric bypass. Note clips near the gastrojejunal anastomosis (*arrowhead*).

fistulas, bowel obstruction, and intrinsic or extrinsic masses. CT also allows for diagnosis of relatively benign entities that may mimic more severe pathology by presenting with an acute abdomen, such as epiploic appendagitis and omental infarction.

CT can detect diffuse processes involving the liver, including cirrhosis, along with its possible associated findings and complications, such as splenomegaly, ascites, collateral vessels, or hepatocellular neoplasm (see Fig. 119-9). Diffuse pancreatic processes, such as pancreatitis (Chapter 130) and its associated complications (such as ascites, fluid collections, vascular thromboses, and pseudoaneurysms), also are well characterized with CT. CT is better than ultrasound for detailing whether a lesion is likely benign or malignant (i.e., hepatic hemangioma, cyst, primary tumor, or metastasis).

Ultrasound, which is more sensitive than CT for the detection of cholelithiasis, should be the first-line procedure for the evaluation of the gallbladder itself. However, CT allows for visualization of the entire biliary tree and the underlying cause of biliary obstruction (i.e., pancreatic mass), but MR is more sensitive for the detection of choledocholithiasis.

In addition to bowel and solid organs, the mesentery and peritoneum are also included in their entirety on CT, thereby allowing for diagnosis of mesenteric masses, tumor implants, adenopathy, hematoma, abscesses, ascites, peritonitis, and carcinomatosis. CT can assess for disease spread throughout the abdomen and pelvis. CT with IV contrast also allows for evaluation of the mesenteric and hepatic vasculature (Fig. 119-12), aorta, inferior vena cava, and any potential collateral vessels. CT is often utilized to diagnose and stage primary tumors in the abdomen and pelvis and to assess for metastases to lymph nodes, solid organs, the peritoneum, and bone (Fig. 119-13). CT is also utilized to evaluate the therapeutic response of tumors.

CT angiography is useful to diagnose atherosclerotic disease, arterial thrombosis, embolic disease, vasculitis, aneurysms, dissections, vascular encasement by tumor, mesenteric ischemia, or GI bleeding. Slight protocol and image timing modifications allow for more optimal evaluation of these processes, and noninvasive CT angiography has largely replaced conventional angiography for many indications.

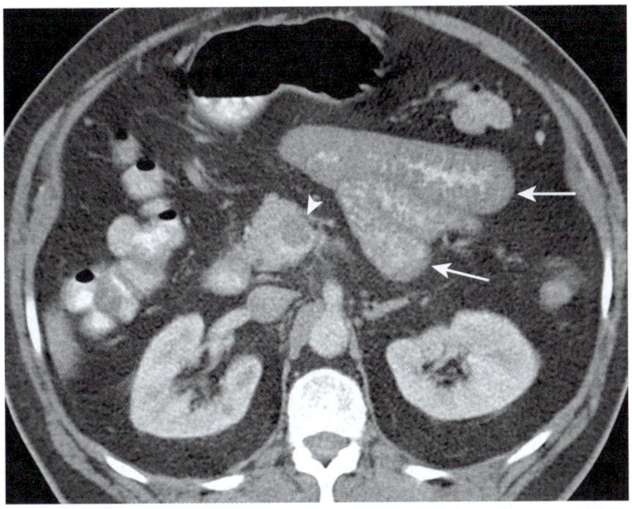

FIGURE 119-12. **Superior mesenteric vein (SMV) thrombosis.** An axial computed tomographic image with intravenous contrast shows a filling defect in the SMV consistent with thrombus (*arrowhead*). Associated jejunal wall thickening (*arrows*) is due to ischemic changes.

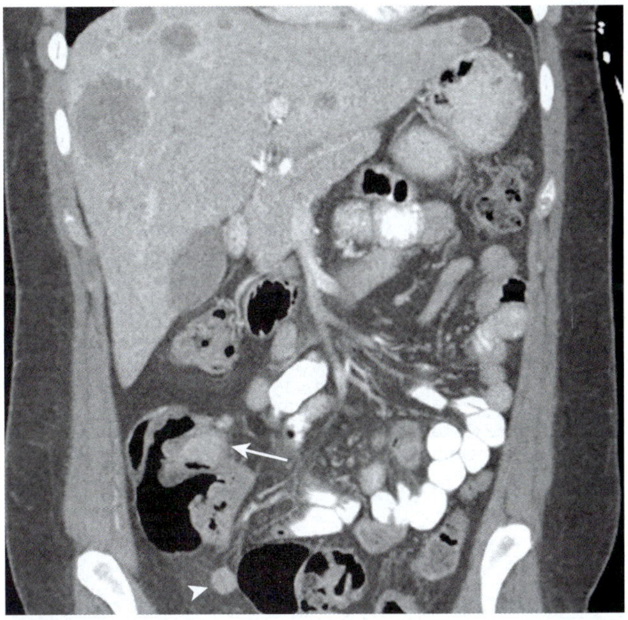

FIGURE 119-13. **Metastatic neuroendocrine tumor.** A coronal contrast-enhanced computed tomographic image shows an enhancing mass along the ileocecal valve (*arrow*) consistent with a primary neuroendocrine tumor. Multiple hepatic metastases are noted as well as a peritoneal tumor implant in the right lower quadrant (*arrowhead*).

CT enterography is a CT study optimized to evaluate the small bowel. Neutral oral contrast is administered to distend the bowel, and IV contrast is given to evaluate the bowel wall and its enhancement pattern. CT enterography can identify areas of bowel involvement and active inflammation in inflammatory bowel disease, as well as assess for complications such as strictures, fistulas, abscess, and obstruction. CT enterography can also evaluate for possible small bowel masses and determine a cause for low-grade, intermittent, or chronic small bowel obstruction.

CT colonography, or virtual colonoscopy, is a low-radiation-dose, noninvasive, safe, and effective screening examination for colorectal cancer. CT colonography can detect pre-cancerous polyps before cancer develops.[12] The entire colon is evaluated without the need for the patient to be sedated. 2D and 3D display techniques are utilized to "fly-through" the inside of the colon (Fig. 119-14). CT colonography is now widely accepted as an alternative to conventional colonoscopy for screening for colorectal cancer.[13]

MAGNETIC RESONANCE IMAGING

MRI, which utilizes a strong magnetic field to generate high-resolution images that can be acquired in any plane, provides excellent soft tissue detail, thereby allowing for better characterization of focal lesions as compared with CT. As with CT, MRI can image the entire abdominal contents. MRI allows for many imaging options, and studies are typically tailored for a specific provided indication. However, MRI requires much longer time for image acquisition and therefore may lead to problems with claustrophobia as well as respiratory or motion artifact. The strong magnetic field necessary for MRI also leads to artifacts, safety issues, and certain contraindications, largely related to implanted devices (infusion pumps, vascular clips, implants, certain pacemakers).

MRI can evaluate diffuse processes involving a solid organ, such as the liver, and associated findings. MRI allows for detection and characterization of focal lesions even better than CT. For example, MRI can differentiate focal liver lesions based on their tissue properties, including cysts, biliary hamartomas, hemangiomas, focal nodular hyperplasia, hepatocellular carcinomas (Chapter 181), and metastases (Fig. 119-15). Intravenous gadolinium-based contrast media aid in the characterization of lesions and vascular involvement (Fig. 119-16). The characterization of liver lesions in particular may be further improved with hepatocyte-specific gadolinium contrast agents that are taken up by the liver and excreted in bile, thereby allowing for the differentiation of lesions such as focal nodular hyperplasia versus metastasis. MRI may also be used to diagnose and stage tumors, such as rectal cancer; MRI can localize the

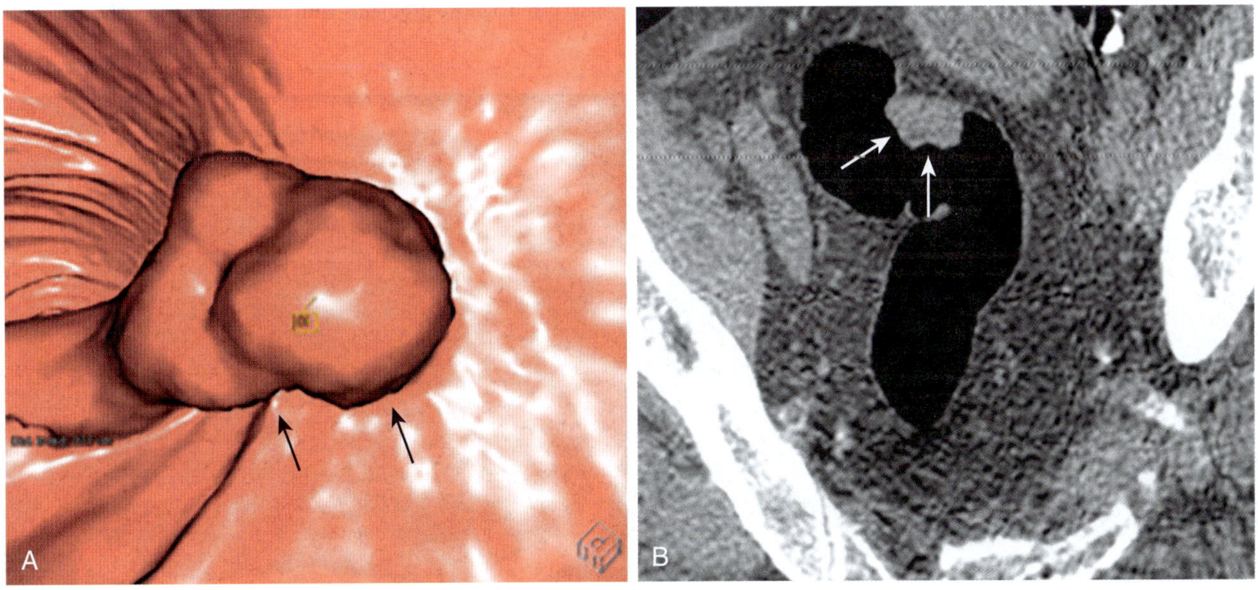

FIGURE 119-14. **Polypoid lesion in the sigmoid colon on screening computed tomographic colonography. A,** 3D intraluminal fly-though and (**B**) 2D axial computed tomographic image show a 2.5-cm lobulated polypoid lesion in the sigmoid colon (*arrows*).

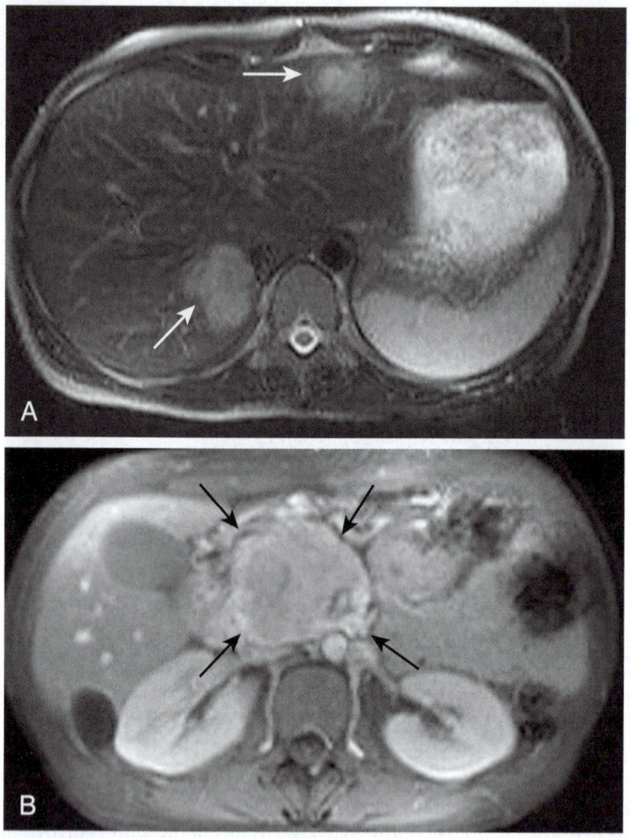

FIGURE 119-15. Pancreatic neuroendocrine tumor with liver metastases. A, Axial T2-weighted magnetic resonance (MR) image shows two moderately bright lesions in the liver (*arrows*). Heterogenous enhancement was seen following contrast (not shown). Imaging features are consistent with hepatic metastatic disease. **B,** Axial post contrast T1 fat-suppressed MR image in the abdomen more inferiorly shows a large heterogenous mass in the proximal pancreas (*arrows*) consistent with pancreatic neuroendocrine tumor.

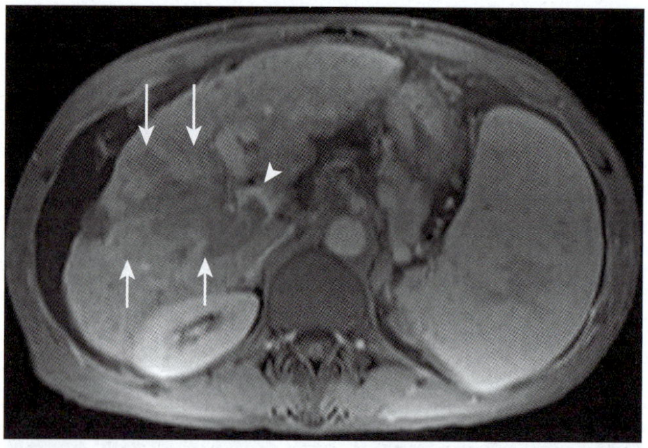

FIGURE 119-16. Hepatocellular carcinoma with tumor thrombus in the main portal vein. Axial post contrast T1 fat-suppressed MR image of the abdomen shows cirrhosis with ascites and splenomegaly. There is a large ill-defined mass in the right lobe (*arrows*) consistent with hepatocellular carcinoma. There is extent into the main portal vein with tumor thrombus (*arrowhead*).

tumor, evaluate the extent of tumor in the rectal wall, and assess for involvement of surrounding lymph nodes and other structures.

MRI allows for quantitative evaluation in the liver. MRI can be used to detect and quantify hepatic fat (hepatic steatosis) (Fig. 119-17) and hepatic iron deposition (hemosiderosis, hemochromatosis; Chapter 196).[14] In addition, MR elastography is a noninvasive technique to evaluate for liver stiffness and therefore estimate and stage fibrosis in patients with liver disease.[15]

MRI can identify biliary obstruction and determine its cause, including choledocholithiasis and pancreatic masses (Fig. 119-18). MR cholangiopancreatography (MRCP), which is a noninvasive method to evaluate the biliary and pancreatic ducts, has replaced endoscopic retrograde cholangiopancreatography for many diagnostic indications. MRCP sequences are optimized to show fluid, such as in the biliary tree and pancreatic duct. This technique is useful to diagnose biliary stones (Fig. 119-19), strictures, cholangitis, masses, variant anatomy, and the relationship of masses to the ducts.

MR angiography may be especially useful in patients who cannot undergo CT angiography because of renal insufficiency or allergy to iodinated contrast agents. MR enterography can evaluate disease activity and response to therapy in patients with inflammatory bowel disease, as well as associated complications, such as stricture (Fig. 119-20), fistula, obstruction, and abscesses. As with CT enterography, neutral oral contrast and IV contrast are administered to determine the bowel wall enhancement pattern. MRI allows for a more detailed evaluation of bowel wall thickening and can determine the presence of edema or fibrosis in the bowel wall. Since it has no ionizing radiation, MR enterography is especially useful in younger patients who have inflammatory bowel disease and who will need multiple examinations over time.

NUCLEAR MEDICINE

Functional nuclear medicine studies for GI processes include gastric emptying and hepatobiliary scintigraphy. A gastric emptying study can diagnose gastroparesis and delayed gastric emptying (Chapter 122). A small meal tagged with radioactive material is ingested and images are obtained over the stomach over time to determine how the stomach empties. Hepatobiliary scintigraphy (cholescintigraphy, hepatobiliary iminodiacetic acid [HIDA] scan) can diagnose problems with hepatic function, the bile ducts, and the

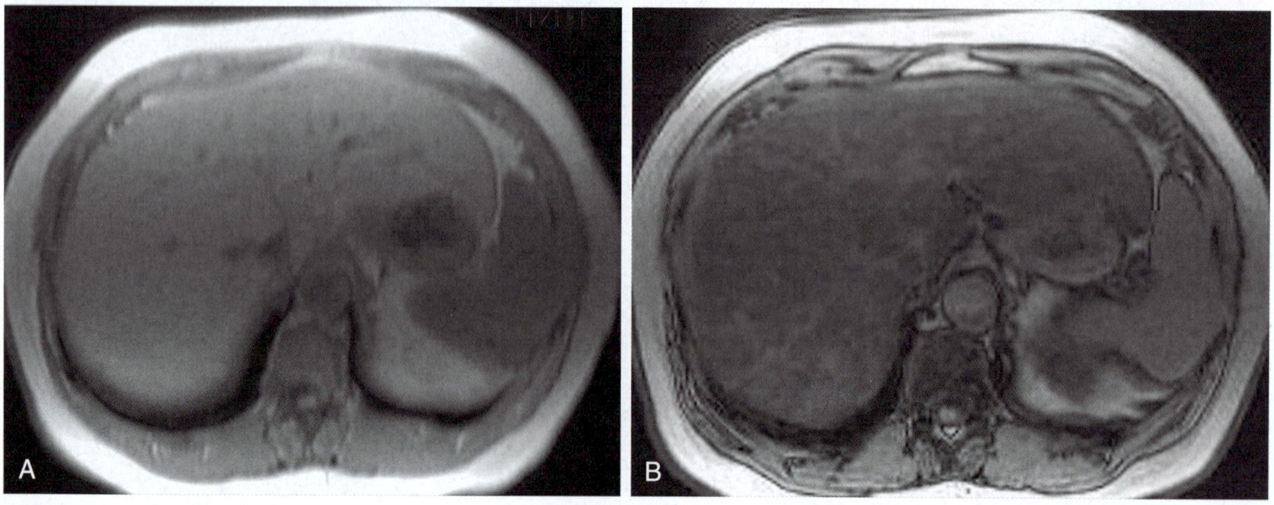

FIGURE 119-17. Hepatic steatosis with chemical shift imaging. Axial T1 in-phase **(A)** and out-of-phase **(B)** magnetic resonance images show pronounced loss of signal intensity throughout the liver on out-of-phase images as compared with in-phase images (the liver is darker) due to diffuse hepatic steatosis.

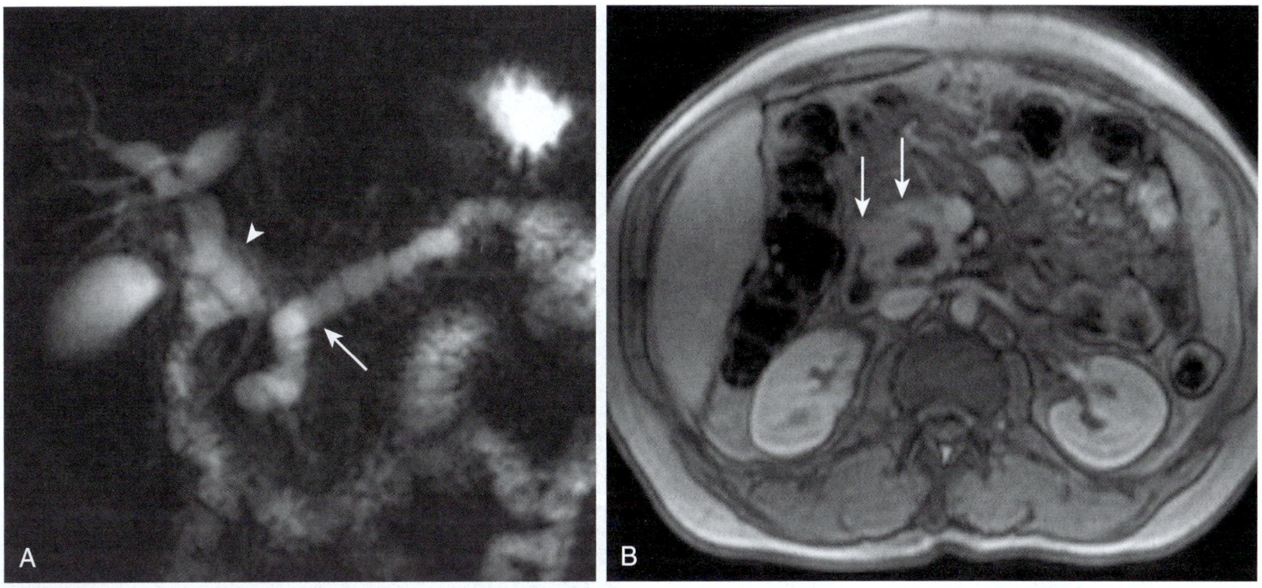

FIGURE 119-18. Biliary and pancreatic ductal dilatation due to pancreatic head cancer. A, Coronal thick slab T2-weighted magnetic resonance cholangiopancreatography image shows a double duct sign with biliary (*arrowhead*) and pancreatic (*arrow*) ductal dilatation with abrupt transition in the proximal pancreas. There is an indwelling biliary stent. **B,** Axial post contrast T1 fat-suppressed magnetic resonance image shows a mass in the pancreatic head (*arrows*) consistent with primary pancreatic cancer.

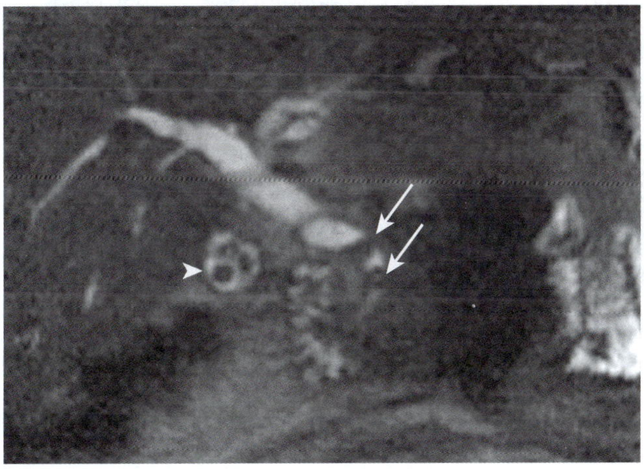

FIGURE 119-19. Choledocholithiasis. Coronal T2-weighted magnetic resonance cholangiopancreatography image shows biliary ductal dilatation with two filling defects in the common duct (*arrows*) consistent with choledocholithiasis. Also note stones in the gallbladder (*arrowhead*).

gallbladder (Chapter 141). A radiolabeled agent is injected intravenously, taken up by the liver, excreted in bile, and subsequently enters the small bowel. Images over time show how well the gallbladder empties and can be used to diagnose acute cholecystitis, acalculous cholecystitis, biliary obstruction, bile leaks or fistulas, and congenital biliary anomalies. This study may be especially useful following an indeterminant ultrasound for possible acute cholecystitis.

GI bleeding scintigraphy is a noninvasive means to diagnose and localize a site of active GI bleeding (Chapter 121), with a reported sensitivity of 93% and specificity of 95%. This study, which is most often performed with 99mTc-tagged red blood cells, can detect active bleeding into the bowel lumen at a rate as low as 0.1 mL/min. This study also allows for imaging over several hours, so it may be especially beneficial in the setting of intermittent bleeding.

Nuclear medicine studies are also useful to diagnose and stage tumors. A ^{111}In-labeled octreotide study (Octreoscan) can be used to visualize tumors bearing somatostatin receptors, because octreotide is a somatostatin analog. This approach is especially useful for diagnosis, staging, and follow-up of neuroendocrine tumors (gastrinoma, insulinoma, and glucagonoma; Chapter 213), carcinoid tumors, paragangliomas, and pancreatic islet cell tumors (Chapter 211).

Positron emission tomography with ^{18}F-labeled fluorodeoxyglucose (^{18}F-FDG PET) is a powerful imaging tool for evaluating many cancers and provides functional information about cancer cells. ^{18}F-FDG, a glucose analog, accumulates

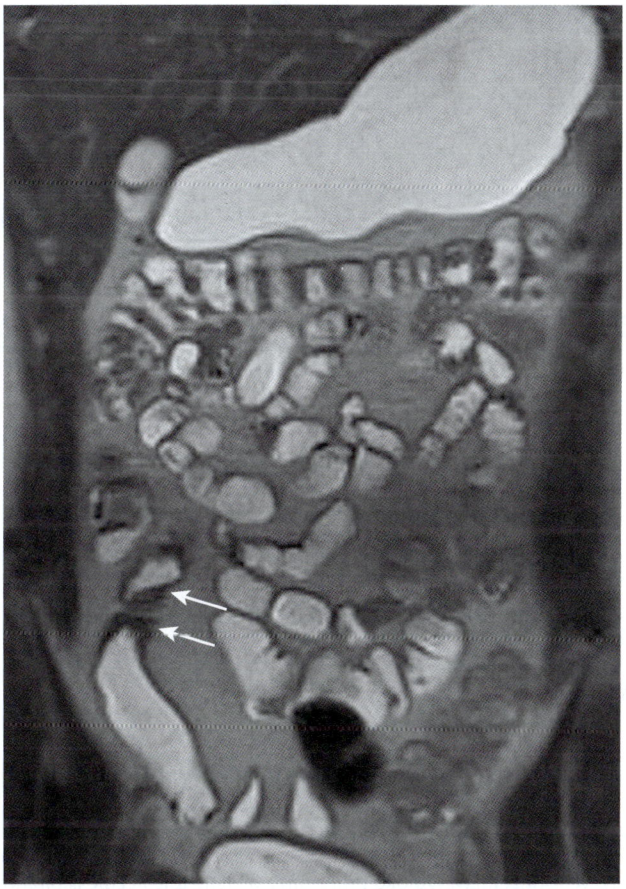

FIGURE 119-20. Crohn disease on magnetic resonance (MR) enterography. A coronal T2-weighted MR image shows Crohn involvement of the distal ileum with wall thickening and associated fibrofatty proliferation of the mesentery. There is a mild stricture (*arrows*) with mild proximal dilatation.

in malignant tissues because malignant cells have an elevated rate of glycolytic activity as compared with normal surrounding cells. Malignant cells therefore exhibit increased uptake of ^{18}F-FDG on imaging. ^{18}F-FDG PET used in conjunction with CT (i.e., PET/CT) can provide biologic, functional, and anatomic information, and areas of increased uptake can be correlated with accompanying CT images (Fig. 119-21). This approach can be used to diagnose and stage tumors, to search for metastatic disease, and to assess for residual or

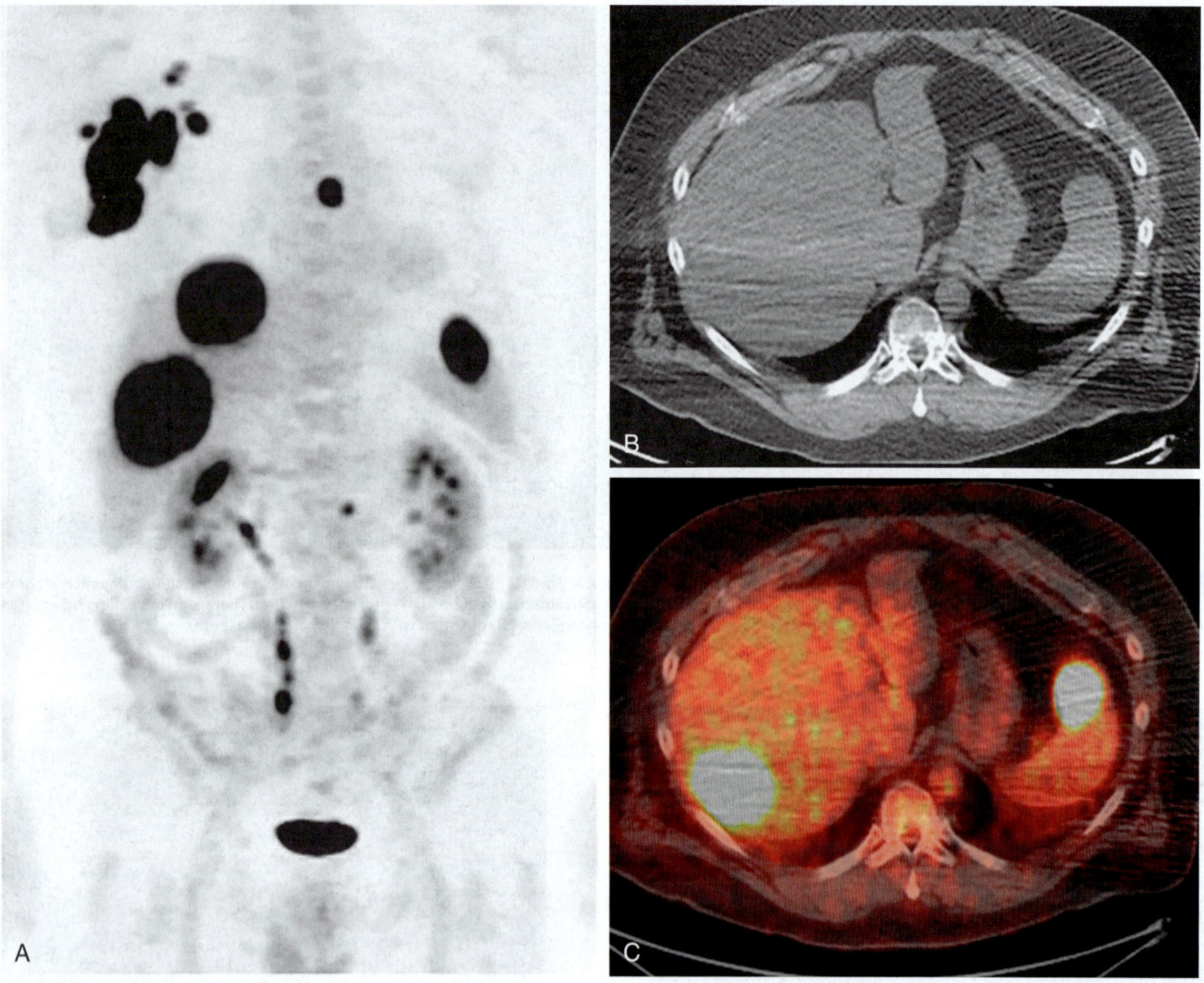

FIGURE 119-21. **Metastatic disease on positron emission tomography/computed tomography (PET/CT). A,** Coronal PET image shows increased uptake in right axillary lymphadenopathy and mediastinal lymphadenopathy as well as liver and spleen involvement. **B,** Lesions in the liver and spleen are barely perceptible on the axial noncontrast CT image. **C,** These lesions are much more conspicuous on the fused axial PET/CT image.

recurrent tumor after treatment. Because PET provides metabolic information, it is superior to CT alone to distinguish active tumor from treated scar. PET/MR, which utilizes high-resolution MR images in conjunction with PET, is a promising new technology with similar attributes but is currently much less readily available than PET/CT.

INTERVENTIONAL PROCEDURES

A variety of interventional procedures (Chapter 120) may be performed in the GI tract and hepatobiliary system using fluoroscopy, ultrasound, or CT guidance. In some cases, a combination of modalities may allow for the safest procedure. MR guidance is much less common because of the longer time needed to acquire images and special considerations owing to the magnetic field.

Interventional image-guided procedures include fine needle aspiration or core biopsy of a mass, drainage of an abscess, placement of a percutaneous cholecystostomy tube, biliary drainage and intervention, paracentesis, and placement of a feeding tube. CT- or ultrasound-guided tumor ablation (including cryoablation, thermal ablation, and alcohol ablation) may be performed for liver tumors (Chapter 181), and is especially useful for unresectable tumors and in patients who are poor surgical candidates.

Vascular interventional procedures include treatment of aneurysms or pseudoaneurysms (such as from pancreatitis), diagnosis and treatment of GI bleeding, placement of a transjugular intrahepatic portosystemic shunt (Chapter 139), and chemoembolization. Chemoembolization may be used to treat primary or metastatic liver lesions (Chapter 181). Chemotherapeutic agents are injected directly into the artery that supplies a tumor, and the artery is then embolized, thereby trapping the medications in the area of the tumor and allowing for treatment with higher chemotherapeutic doses but less systemic toxicity.

GENERAL REFERENCES

For the General References and other additional features, please visit Elsevier eBooks+ at https://ebooks.health.elsevier.com.

120 GASTROINTESTINAL ENDOSCOPY

KENNETH K. WANG

The three major applications of gastrointestinal (GI) endoscopy in medicine include: diagnostic applications to define the source of gastrointestinal bleeding, to stage gastrointestinal cancers, and to obtain samples for histology or culture; therapeutic applications, such as providing hemostasis, resecting lesions, remodeling of the GI tract to manage obesity and to create passages, either between lumens or to fluid collections; and combined modality procedures with interventional radiology or surgery. In current practice, GI endoscopy has evolved from being primarily a straightforward diagnostic endoscopic technique for the colon and upper GI lumen to being a more versatile diagnostic and now therapeutic technique.

In the United States, endoscopy in healthy individuals is typically performed under deep sedation with propofol, but conscious sedation with midazolam and fentanyl is an alternative in straight-forward procedures (Chapter 400). In appropriate patients who desire to drive soon after the procedure or who cannot be accompanied by a family member or friend, the procedure can be performed without sedation.

Ideally, patients should discontinue anticoagulants and antiplatelet agents long enough before the procedure to reverse their effects (Chapter 70) and restart them in consultation with the specialists who recommended them (Table 120-1).[1] Bridging anticoagulation (Fig. 399-3) generally increases the risk of periprocedural bleeding without reducing the risk of thromboembolism[A1] and should be considered only in patients who are at very high risk of thromboembolism.[2]

Each procedure has specific indications but also carries risks (Table 120-2).

DIAGNOSTIC ENDOSCOPY

UPPER GI ENDOSCOPY

Upper endoscopy consists of examination of a portion of the posterior pharynx including the epiglottis, upper esophageal sphincter area, larynx, and vallecula.

TABLE 120-1 ANTITHROMBOTIC THERAPY FOR ELECTIVE ENDOSCOPY

Thrombotic Risk Low to High	ENDOSCOPIC RISK OF BLEEDING	
	LOW*	HIGH†
	Continue anticoagulant	Discontinue warfarin, then restart warfarin on same day of procedure Delay reinitiating DOAC until adequate hemostasis is achieved
	Continue antiplatelet agent	Continue aspirin and discontinue $P2Y_{12}$ inhibitors for at least 5 days and switch to aspirin (or continue aspirin if on dual therapy)
		If high risk for thrombosis,‡ strongly consider bridge therapy with LMWH (e.g., enoxaparin, 1.5 mg/kg q24h or 1.0 mg/kg q12h) until oral anticoagulant is again effective Delay reinitiating DOACs until adequate hemostasis is achieved

*Diagnostic upper gastrointestinal endoscopy, colonoscopy, or flexible sigmoidoscopy, including mucosal biopsy; endoscopic retrograde cholangiopancreatography; capsule endoscopy; enteral stent deployment (controversial); endoscopic ultrasound without fine-needle aspiration; argon plasma coagulation; Barrett ablation.

†Polypectomy, biliary or pancreatic sphincterotomy, treatment of varices, percutaneous endoscopic gastrostomy or jejunostomy, therapeutic balloon-assisted enteroscopy, endoscopic ultrasound with fine-needle aspiration, endoscopic hemostasis, tumor ablation, cystogastrostomy, ampullary resection, endoscopic mucosal resection, endoscopic submucosal dissection, pneumatic or bougie dilation.

‡Any mitral valve prosthesis, any caged-ball or tilting disc aortic valve prosthesis, recent (within 6 months) cerebrovascular accident or transient ischemic attack, recent (within 3 months) venous thromboembolism, severe thrombophilia (deficiency of protein C, protein S, or antithrombin; antiphospholipid antibodies).

DOAC = direct-acting oral anticoagulant; LMWH = low-molecular-weight heparin.

Adapted from ASGE Standards of Practice Committee, Acosta RD, Abraham, NS, et al. The management of antithrombotic agents for patients undergoing GI endoscopy. *Gastrointest Endosc.* 2016;83:3-16.

The entire esophagus and stomach are visualized. The duodenal bulb as well as the first and second portions of the duodenum are part of the standard examination.

INSTRUMENT

Flexible endoscopes are equipped with a high-resolution video chip at the end of a flexible tube and two fiberoptic light bundles. The endoscope has a water channel for irrigation of the camera lenses and a suction channel that can remove liquids and doubles as an instrument channel through which a variety of accessories (e.g., biopsy forceps to obtain tissue, brushes to obtain cytologic specimens, snares to remove polyps, or bipolar probes to cauterize bleeding vessels) can be passed.

PREPARATION

All upper endoscopic procedures require fasting for at least 6 hours prior to the procedure to permit adequate visualization. Patients who are receiving a per oral endoscopic myotomy for achalasia should be on clear liquids for 2 days prior to the procedure. Broad spectrum antibiotics (e.g., cefazolin 2 g intravenously preprocedure) are routinely given due to the stasis and bacterial overgrowth in the esophagus. Chronic medications can be taken orally the morning of the procedure, with minimum oral fluids to help pass the pills.

In patients who have a history of aspiration or cognitive impairment, preprocedural tracheal intubation may be advisable to protect the airway. Preprocedural intubation also is often required to prevent aspiration of blood in patients who have an active upper GI bleed, especially patients who are known to have cirrhosis and portal hypertension, because they will not be fully alert after the procedure. Patients with gastroparesis or with gastric or esophageal obstruction should also be considered for airway protection because of the likelihood of retained food.

INDICATIONS

A common indication for upper GI endoscopy is to determine the presence of a GI disease such as ulcers or esophagitis and/or and to explain a symptom (Table 120-3).

THE PROCEDURE

Unless the patient is intubated, the procedure is performed with the patient in the left lateral position to decrease the chance of aspiration. The esophagus is inspected, especially for esophagitis and varices, and then the stomach is inspected for gastric varices, ulcers, evidence of intestinal metaplasia or gastritis, and neoplasms (Fig. 120-1). Retroflexion is necessary in the fundus of the stomach to visualize the gastric cardia as well as the incisura, which is one of the most likely sites for intestinal metaplasia. The endoscope then is passed down to the second portion of the duodenum. The standard endoscope visualizes the papilla of Vater in only about 50% of cases because it is on the side wall of the duodenum and not within the field of view.

Adjuncts to Standard Endoscopy

Contrast agents that can increase the visibility of flat neoplasms include Lugol solution, which is diluted and sprayed on the surface of the squamous esophagus to help diagnose squamous neoplasia. The normal squamous mucosa takes up the iodine and appears brown, whereas neoplastic areas with either cancer or dysplasia will not take up the iodine and appear as unstained tissue that should be biopsied or resected depending on the degree of suspicion. A widely used alternative is narrow-band imaging, which uses blue light to illuminate the mucosa and highlight its features, particularly the small mucosal capillary patterns that become distorted in dysplastic tissue. In the stomach, a mixture of acetic acid and indigo carmine can detect gastric carcinoma and also enhance its borders to guide en bloc removal. Despite their utility, however, dyes are not popular in Western countries because of the difficulties in application and the contamination they create in the endoscope. Nonetheless, in high-risk patients, such as those with Lynch syndrome (Chapter 179), contrast agents can enhance detection of small early gastric cancers. Other tools to aid in the diagnosis of premalignant disease include devices such as confocal laser endomicroscopy that can magnify the views of the mucosa and assess the leakiness of the microvascular system, but this approach is infrequently used clinically in part because it requires administration of intravenous fluorescein. Volume laser endomicroscopy, which is a version of optical coherence tomography, has the potential to scan large areas of tissue at high resolution without contrast agents and is commercially available for scanning the esophagus.

TABLE 120-2 COMPLICATIONS OF ENDOSCOPY

ENDOSCOPIC COMPLICATION	INCIDENCE (%)	SPECIFIC PROPHYLAXIS
GENERAL COMPLICATIONS		
Complications related primarily to sedation (cardiovascular and postprocedure respiratory depression, aspiration)	0.6-0.7	Airway protection with massive upper gastrointestinal bleeding Preprocedure medical evaluation, intraprocedure and postprocedure monitoring Anesthesiology consultation for high-risk patients
Perforation	0.1-0.3 (upper endoscopy) 0.14-0.25 (colonoscopy)	None (except careful technique, possible benefit to "underwater" technique)
Bleeding	0.3 (upper endoscopy) 0.7-2.5 (polypectomy)	Carefully balance risk and benefits Discontinue or reduce anticoagulant use before high-risk procedures
Bacteremia and infection complications (endocarditis, bacterial ascites)	<0.1	Antibiotics for patients at risk for endocarditis (patients with artificial valves, pulmonary-systemic shunts, previous history of endocarditis), with synthetic vascular grafts, and with bacterial ascites (cirrhotics)
Death	0.6 (upper endoscopy) 0.2 (colonoscopy)	
COMPLICATIONS ASSOCIATED WITH SPECIALIZED PROCEDURES		
Pancreatitis (ERCP)	3-20	Rectal indomethacin
Cholangitis (ERCP)	0.1-2	Preprocedure antibiotics
Wound infections (PEG)	3-4	Preprocedure antibiotics

ERCP = endoscopic retrograde cholangiopancreatography; PEG = percutaneous endoscopic gastrostomy.
From Pasricha PJ. Gastrointestinal endoscopy. In: Goldman L, Schafer AI, eds. *Goldman-Cecil Medicine*, 26th ed. Philadelphia: Elsevier; 2020:834-840.

TABLE 120-3 INDICATIONS FOR UPPER GI ENDOSCOPY

- Dyspepsia unresponsive to medical therapy
- Development of alarm symptoms including dysphagia, odynophagia, weight loss
- Persistent symptoms of reflux despite medical therapy
- Surveillance for upper GI malignancy
- Bleeding thought to be due to upper GI source or occult GI bleeding

GI = gastrointestinal.

ENDOSCOPIC ULTRASONOGRAPHY

Endoscopic ultrasonography combines an endoscope with an ultrasound array at its tip to visualize anatomy in three dimensions. Pulse doppler signals can assess blood flow, and elastography can assess tissue characteristics.

INSTRUMENT

A circular array instrument is best for mapping out the visceral surface of the esophagus and duodenum, whereas a linear array ultrasound endoscope is used for needle aspiration and biopsy because it can use Doppler ultrasound to ensure that the needle bypasses vascular structures and can observe the needle throughout its entire passage into a lymph node or organ.

PREPARATION

The preparation for an upper GI endoscopic ultrasound is similar to endoscopy. Coagulation parameters should be normalized before endoscopic ultrasonography, fine-needle aspiration, or biopsy may be performed. Deep sedation is generally used because of the length of the procedure.

INDICATIONS

The most common indications for endoscopic ultrasound are to stage esophageal, gastric, pancreatic, and biliary cancers by determining their depth, degree of circumferential involvement, and overall size.[3,4] Fine-needle biopsy is indicated for lesions that require more knowledge of tissue architecture (e.g., lymphoma) or type of infiltration (e.g., autoimmune pancreatitis). Ultrasound can guide fine-needle aspiration of lymph nodes or metastases to solid organs, especially in the liver. It can also be an adjunctive test to stage pulmonary cancer when lymph nodes are not accessible from the bronchi. Other indications include defining a lesion's vascularity, measuring portal pressure, or assessing and treating arterial vessels that feed bleeding lesions such as ulcers.

PROCEDURE

The echoendoscope is passed into the esophagus like a routine endoscope. However, the transducer portion of the endoscope is rigid and is of greater diameter than an endoscope, so passage can be more difficult in the presence of mechanical obstructions, such as an esophageal diverticulum or bone spurs in the cervical spine. Scanning begins in the posterior pharynx, where structures such as the thyroid gland and carotid arteries are very apparent. The aortic arch, aortic-pulmonic window, descending aorta, left atrium, and pulmonary vessels can be examined. Generally, examinations follow the aorta into the abdomen, where visualization of the gastro-hepatic ligament, superior mesenteric artery, and celiac axis provides landmarks in the abdomen. The celiac axis gives rise to the splenic artery and allows visualization of the body and tail of the pancreas. The left lobe of the liver is easily scanned, as is the gallbladder. From the duodenum, the portal vessel, biliary tree, and pancreatic head can be visualized, and ultrasound can be used to guide biopsy of a pancreatic mass (Fig. 120-2). Any lesions such as lymph nodes can be sampled with the linear echoendoscope. Some lesions that appear obvious on computed tomographic (CT) scanning may be invisible to ultrasound, but small lesions around the pancreas are generally better visualized on endoscopic ultrasound. Biopsies and aspirates can be routinely performed.

Under ultrasound guidance, therapeutic stents can be placed across the gastric wall into the gallbladder to decompress an inflamed gallbladder[5] or into the jejunum to bypass an obstruction caused by pancreatic cancer. Vascular access with endoscopic ultrasound can measure portal pressures, embolize arterial bleeding sites that cannot be approached by interventional radiology, and define feeder vessels for bleeding ulcers.

ENDOSCOPIC RETROGRADE CHOLANGIOPANCREATOGRAPHY (ERCP)

Endoscopic retrograde cholangiopancreatography (ERCP) can examine the biliary tree and pancreatic ducts. ERCP commonly includes fluoroscopy to visualize the dye infused within the pancreatic or biliary system, so all patients should be appropriate candidates for exposure to contrast agents and radiation.

INSTRUMENT

The typical side viewing endoscope has a rigid tip very similar in length to the echoendoscope, with the same issues regarding passage into the esophagus. The therapeutic duodenoscope is about 125 cm long with a 4.2-mm working channel that allows for passage of accessories such as the cholangioscope. The channel also has a lever that permits the user to angle a catheter into the ampulla of Vater.

PREPARATION

Patients should be fasting as for routine upper GI endoscopy. The instrument visualizes at 90 degrees to the axis of the endoscope and has no forward viewing capacity, so the esophagus must be known to be free of diverticula, strictures, or tumors. In preparation for the injection of dye and for the interventional procedure, coagulation status must be determined and normalized if possible. If the risk of precipitating pancreatitis is high (i.e., younger patient age, female

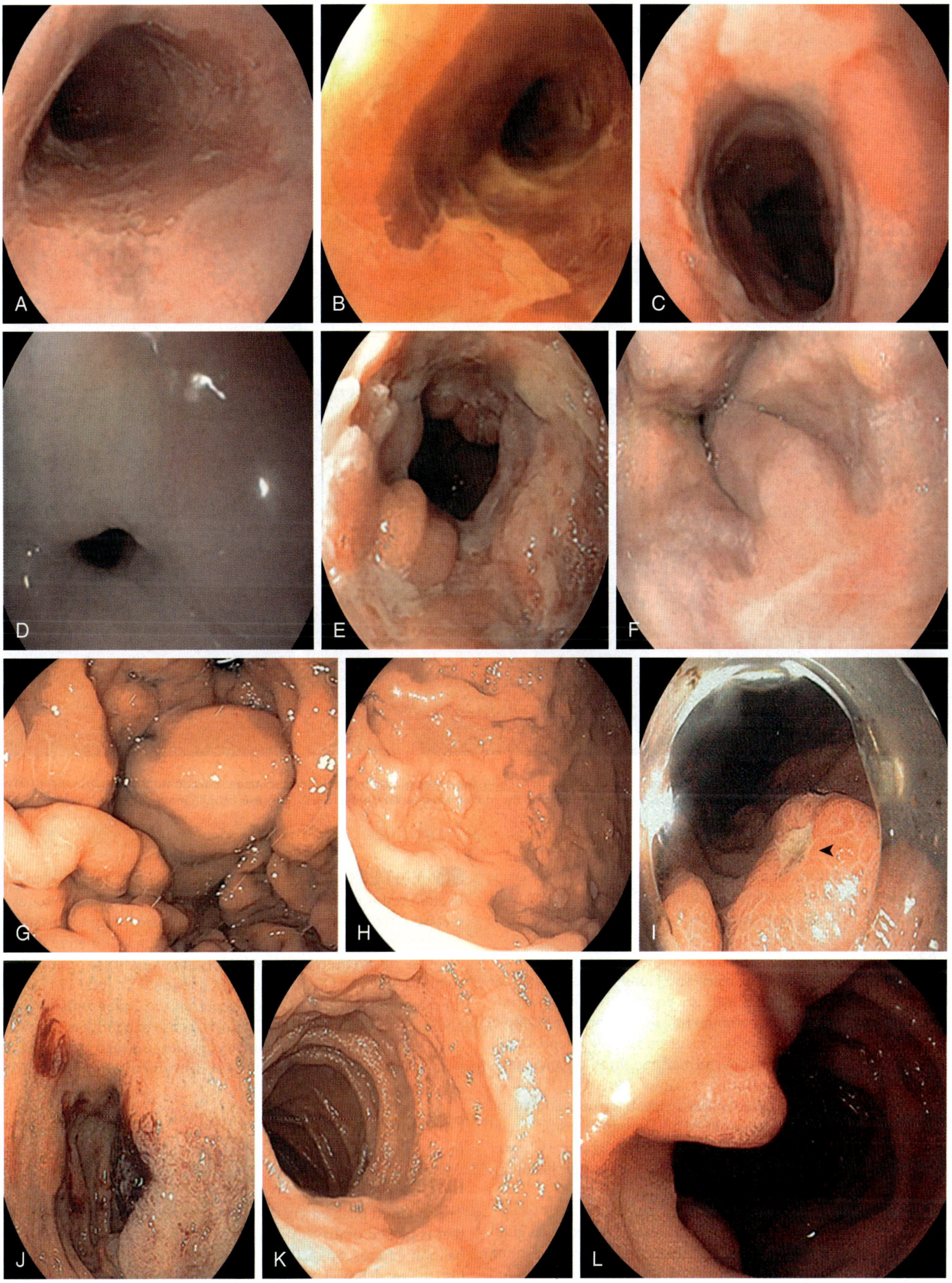

FIGURE 120-1. Endoscopic images of abnormalities that can be observed in the upper gastrointestinal tract. A, Barrett esophagus with areas of salmon colored mucosa indicative of esophageal intestinal metaplasia. **B,** After Lugol solution has been applied to the esophageal mucosa, areas of whitish appearing mucosa that do not take up iodine suggest dysplasia. **C,** Streaks of inflammation consistent with relatively severe erosive esophagitis. **D,** Esophageal stricture with narrowing of the esophageal lumen but no evidence of inflammation. **E,** Excavating distal esophageal cancer. **F,** Submucosal esophageal varices near the gastroesophageal junction without evidence of recent bleeding. **G,** Rugal folds in the stomach, with the expanded fold in the center of the figure representing a gastric varix. **H,** Hyperplastic polyp, which is common in patients who are taking proton pump inhibitors and generally are benign, in the center of the field. **I,** Ulcer (*black arrow*) elevated in the body of the stomach. **J,** Duodenal ulcer in the bulb of the duodenum. **K,** Adenoma (the center of the image) in the duodenum, where adenomatous polyps can be found, although benign Brunner glands are often found in the duodenal bulb. **L,** Normal ampulla of Vater.

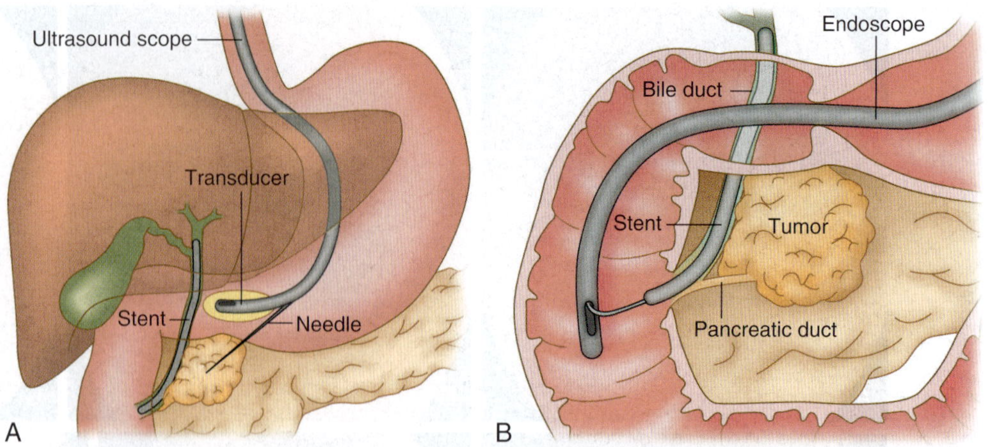

FIGURE 120-2. Biopsy of a pancreatic mass guided by endoscopic ultrasonography (A) and the placement of a stent into a malignant bile duct stricture with endoscopic retrograde cholangiopancreatography (B). (From Brugge WR, Van Dam J: Pancreatic and biliary endoscopy. *N Engl J Med.* 1999;341:1808-1816. Copyright ©1999 Massachusetts Medical Society. All rights reserved.)

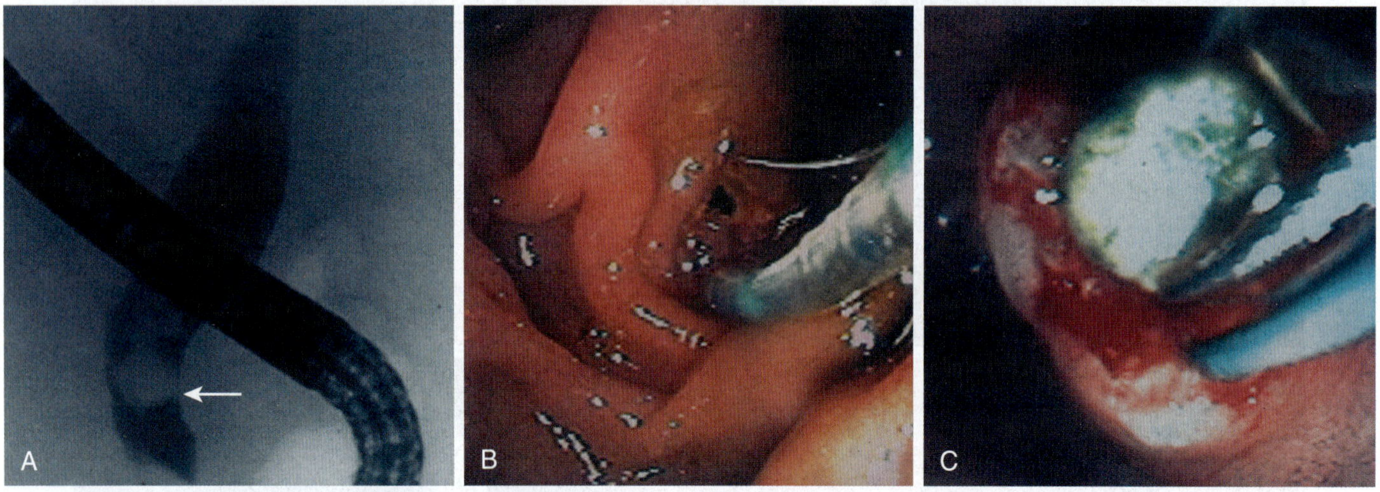

FIGURE 120-3. Biliary sphincterotomy and stone removal from the bile duct. A, Endoscopic retrograde cholangiographic image showing stones (*arrow*) in the distal common bile duct. B, Endoscopic image of a sphincterotome in the bile duct with the wire cutting the roof of the ampulla (sphincter). C, A stone is being removed from the bile duct by an endoscopically passed basket. (Courtesy of Pankaj Jay Pasricha, MD.)

gender, sphincter of Oddi dysfunction, previous pancreatitis, abnormal serum bilirubin), pre-procedural prophylaxis with a sulindac (100 mg) enema can decrease the risk of ERCP-induced pancreatitis.[A2]

INDICATIONS

ERCP is usually performed to evaluate obstructive jaundice, pancreatitis, or a pancreatic mass when other imaging tests are equivocal or demonstrate lesions that require therapy, such as a common bile duct stone. For example, suspected choledocholithiasis warrants ERCP for diagnosis and potential treatment (Fig. 120-3). ERCP also is often performed for chronic pancreatitis and ampullary polyps. In acute pancreatitis (Chapter 130), ERCP is often delayed until inflammation has subsided unless suspected pancreatic ductal disruption necessitates stenting. Indeterminate biliary or pancreatic ductal strictures found on magnetic resonance cholangiopancreatography (Chapter 119) may require brushings and biopsies on ERCP to define their histology.

PROCEDURE

The endoscope is typically introduced in a blind fashion using manual guidance. When the instrument passes into the second portion of the duodenum, the ampulla of Vader can be identified. The pancreatic duct is usually found directly perpendicular to the mucosa, whereas the common bile duct is much more angulated. In patients who have a pancreas divisum, the minor papilla, which is usually found at the first portion of duodenum, may need to be cannulated to access the main pancreatic duct. Once the appropriate duct is identified on fluoroscopy with contrast or with the use of a guidewire through the endoscope, accessories can be introduced for therapeutic (e.g., to extract a stone or to place a stent to bypass a stenosis or tumor) or diagnostic (e.g., to obtain tissue from an indeterminate stricture or mass) purposes. Small caliber endoscopes can be passed through a therapeutic duodenoscope (larger operating channel required) to visualize the pancreatic or biliary ducts and take small biopsies or cytologic specimens from any suspicious lesions.[6]

ENTEROSCOPY

In standard upper GI endoscopy, visualization usually extends only to the second portion of the duodenum. The easiest way to visualize the entire duodenum and a significant distance (about a half meter) into the jejunum is to use push enteroscopy, which is generally performed with a pediatric colonoscope. Most occult bleeding GI lesions (Chapter 121) are visible using this technique. Other accessories permit the endoscopist to extract foreign bodies, take specimens for diagnosis, perform a polypectomy, place a stent, dilate strictures, and even treat bleeding lesions such as telangiectasias. If the lesion is beyond the reach of these instruments, more technically difficult procedures can be employed.

PREPARATION

Preparation is as for upper GI endoscopy.

INSTRUMENT

The standard push enteroscope is usually a dedicated pediatric colonoscope that is passed orally through the stomach and into the small bowel. Single balloon enteroscopy with an overtube allows the enteroscope to be guided into the small bowel. Single balloon procedures can examine altered anatomy, such as in patients who have had bariatric surgery with a Roux-Y anastomosis.

To traverse the full jejunum, a double balloon system, with balloons on both an overtube and on the distal end of the endoscope, can be inflated and deflated to plicate the small bowel onto the shaft of the endoscope. By collapsing the small bowel onto its sheath, the endoscope can be slowly manipulated through the entire small bowel. A motorized spiral enteroscopy[7] device with an overtube that corkscrews the intestine over the tube is an emerging alternative to using a balloon to pull the intestine over the overtube. An endoscopic tattoo can be placed at the furthest distal extent of the antegrade enteroscopy, so that a colonoscopic examination from below can advance through the ileocecal valve and then to the tattoo, thereby confirming that the entire small bowel has been investigated.

INDICATIONS

The indications for enteroscopy are usually related to occult gastrointestinal bleeding (Chapter 121) or further definition of a lesion visualized on small bowel imaging. It can be used to define extent of disease, such as in celiac sprue (Chapter 126) or inflammatory bowel disease (Chapter 127), if needed. Therapeutic uses include aid in placing jejunal feeding tubes, dilating strictures, aid in performing ERCP in cases of altered anatomy such as after bowel bypass, and removal of small intestinal polyps.

PROCEDURE

Patients are positioned in the left lateral position to reduce the risk of aspiration. The advancement of this device requires fluoroscopy to confirm the location of the enteroscope when lesions are found. In addition, treatment options are limited given the long length (200 cm) of the instrument. The instrument is valuable in the diagnosis of conditions that have eluded other techniques, such blood loss in the small intestine (Chapter 121), small intestinal masses (Chapter 179), and inflammatory and malabsorptive conditions of the intestines (Chapter 126).

COLONOSCOPY

Colonoscopy is used for diagnostic and therapeutic purposes from the rectum to the ileocecal valve. Use of a colonoscope requires familiarity with the anatomy of the colon and the tendency of the colon to twist and form loops in the sigmoid and transverse colon, thereby causing difficulty in advancing the instrument unless these loops can be reduced. The colon's haustral folds also can make visualization more difficult.

INSTRUMENT

A standard adult colonoscope is about 168 cm in length and has a larger channel for suction and passage of accessories compared with an upper GI endoscope. However, the diameter of the colonoscope is also larger and the insertion tube is more flexible to allow retroflexion at various critical points in the colon, such as in the cecum or in the rectum. The diameter of the colonoscope can identify significant colonic strictures because it will be unable to pass through them.

PREPARATION

A good colonic preparation, which is essential for a complete examination,[8] often is the most unpleasant part of the procedure, and patients will be more adherent if they are strongly encouraged to take the preparations as directed.[A3] Common high-volume preparations use a nonabsorbable osmotic agent (polyethylene glycol) mixed with water and drunk by the patient in a split-dose fashion (half the evening prior to the procedure and the other half the morning of the procedure). This split-dose method is better tolerated and more effective in clearing stool than are single-dose regimens.[A4] Refrigerating the solution is often beneficial in decreasing its taste, and sucking on lemon wedges or ice cubes also can blunt its flavor. Some patients find that drinking the solution through a straw also can decrease its unpleasant taste. Finally, chewing gum before drinking a glass of the solution also makes the preparation more palatable. Although patients often rely on the color of the effluent and the absence of solid stool as indicators of adequate preparation, patients should continue to take the complete bowel preparation until the entire preparation is consumed to ensure an adequate colonic preparation. In patients who are at risk of a poor preparation (e.g., patients who have had poor preparations in the past, nonambulatory or hospitalized patients, and patients who are unable to consume the full preparation, such as patients with diabetic gastroparesis), it also may be necessary to begin a liquid diet 24 to 36 hours before the scheduled colonoscopy and increase the amount of solution to avoid solid foods in the GI tract and to ensure adequate colonic cleansing. The consequences of inadequate preparation include the need to repeat the preparation for another procedure, the inability to detect significant lesions in the colon, and an increased risk of adverse events such as perforation or bleeding.

INDICATIONS

Colonoscopy is most commonly performed to screen for colon cancer (Chapter 179). It is also indicated to evaluate possible lower GI bleeding (Chapter 121) from conditions such as a tumor or polyp (Chapter 179), inflammatory bowel diseases (Chapter 127), diverticular disease (Chapter 128), or a mucosal telangiectasia (Figs. 120-4 and 120-5).

PROCEDURE

The procedure typically begins with the patient on the left lateral position, which generally allows easier passage into the sigmoid colon. The patient may be switched to the supine position once the splenic flexure is reached, particularly when using water immersion, which is better tolerated and very useful when removing polyps, rather than carbon dioxide insufflation, which is often uncomfortable and can produce nausea and bloating postprocedure. The water immersion technique instills warm water into the colon to distend it.

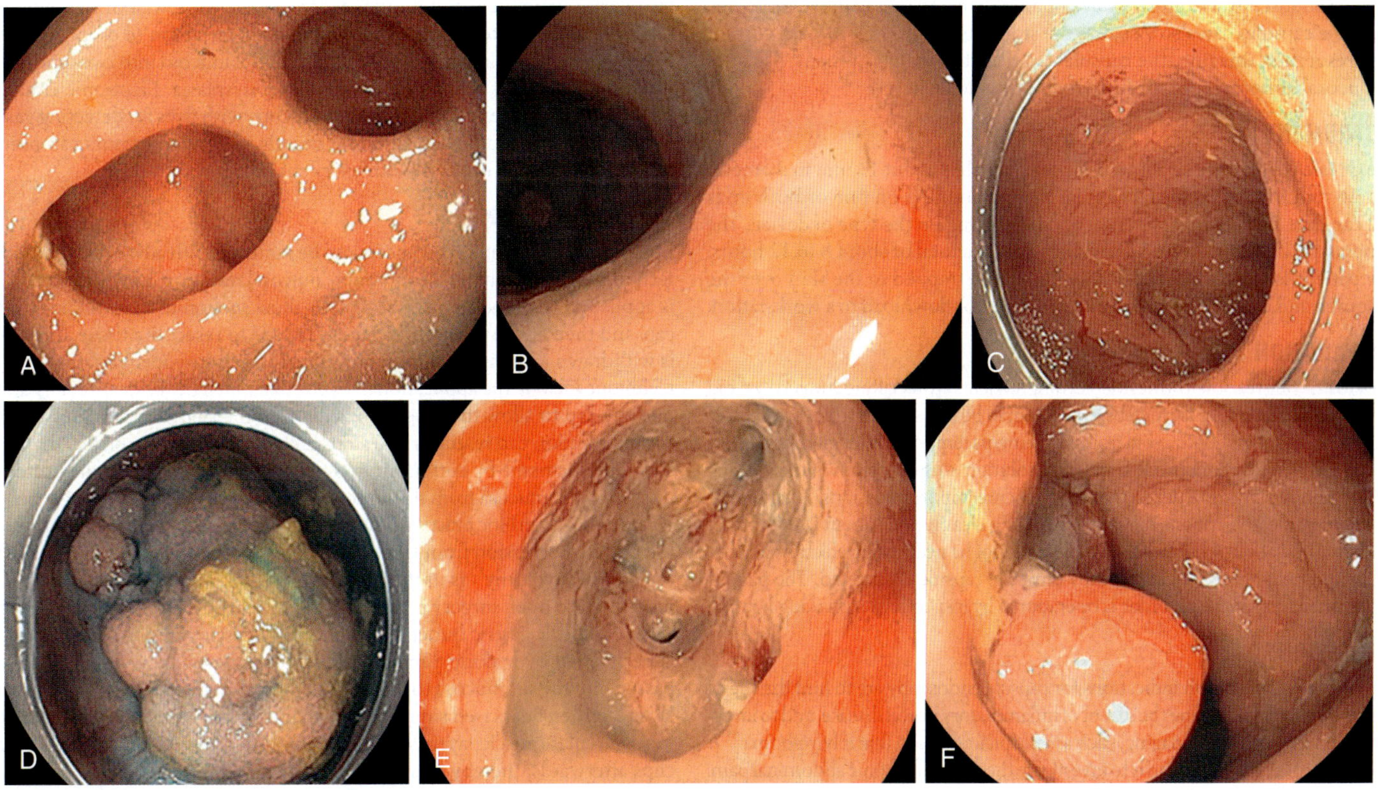

FIGURE 120-4. **Images of colonic pathology. A,** Large mouthed colonic diverticula, which are normal findings particularly in older patients. **B,** Colonic ulcer often found in the context of inflammatory bowel disease, most commonly Crohn disease. **C,** Chronic ulcerative colitis, with small pseudopolyps indicative of chronic disease. **D,** Large colonic polyp, likely an adenoma; despite its size this polyp can usually be removed endoscopically. **E,** Ulcerated colon with a fistula at the base. Colonic ulcers can fistulize to bladder, vagina, small bowel, and stomach depending on location of the fistula. **F,** Ulcerated polyp with polypoid edges, suspicious for malignant transformation.

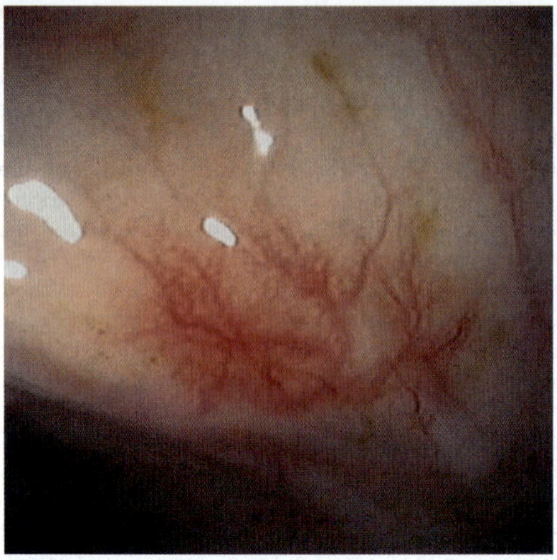

FIGURE 120-5. **Mucosal telangiectasia (arteriovenous malformation) in the colon.** The patient presented with hematochezia. The lesion was subsequently cauterized endoscopically. (Courtesy of Pankaj Jay Pasricha, MD.)

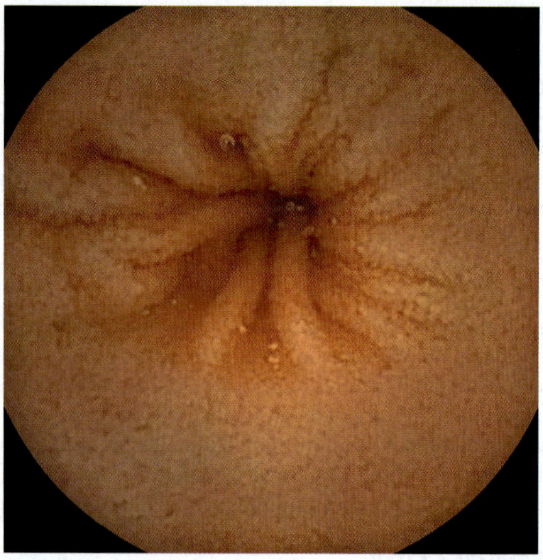

FIGURE 120-6. **Typical normal-appearing small bowel on capsule endoscopy.** Although resolution is far less than standard endoscopy, villi can easily be appreciated on the capsule images.

The hypotonic nature of the fluid allows water to infiltrate the mucosa, thereby making removal of colon polyps easier. Examination of the cecum and right side of the colon is generally better on withdrawal with the patient supine.

Since polyps are often found and removed, patients must have their anticoagulants and antiplatelet medications stopped in sufficient time to ensure adequate hemostasis.[9] Removal techniques using small wire snares are routine, but specialized snares can grasp even flat polyps, and combination devices can inject fluid underneath the polyps to aid in safe removal by providing a cushion underneath the lesion. Water immersion polypectomy likewise can facilitate mucosa swelling with hypotonic fluid without the need for an injection. If a colonoscopy is being performed to evaluate gastrointestinal bleeding, however, polypectomy will often be deferred because postprocedural bleeding could easily be confused with bleeding from the original hemorrhagic site.[10]

CAPSULE ENDOSCOPY

Capsule endoscopy was initially developed to detect lesions in the small bowel. Steerable capsules can also visualize the stomach and the colon. With current high-resolution imaging, the capsule can detect bleeding sites and flag sites of mucosal abnormalities for further endoscopic review.

INSTRUMENT

The device is literally a swallowed capsule, which is about 11 mm in diameter and 26 mm in length, with a camera that is mounted on one or both ends and can take 2 to 18 images per second depending on the type of device. The cameras are battery powered and can image for a total of about 8 to 12 hours. The patient is connected to an antenna that is strapped to the skin over the abdomen and can receive and store the images for download to a workstation.

PREPARATION

Prior to imaging the small bowel for bleeding, patients are usually requested to avoid eating foods that might leave debris in the small bowel, such as fruit or vegetable seeds. Patients also should avoid iron supplements temporarily. Beginning the day before the procedure, a bowel preparation solution is usually given in the evening to help remove any food debris that may obscure important lesions. After ingesting the capsule, the patient may start ingesting clear liquids about 2 hours later and light food about 4 hours later. Patients cannot be near strong electromagnetic fields (e.g., magnetic resonance scan) until the capsule is excreted. The patient also should be sure the recorder is operational by inspecting its blinking light.

INDICATIONS

The three most common indications for capsule endoscopy are to find the site of obscure bleeding, to define the extent of inflammatory bowel disease, and to investigate a finding on other imaging, such as a suspicious lesion that is lymphoma.[11] A more controversial indication is to investigate the cause of chronic abdominal pain.

PROCEDURE

The patient returns the recorder, which can be downloaded and reviewed by an appropriately trained physician. The artificial intelligence in the software will identify areas of suspicious lesions, which are tagged for review. Areas of potential bleeding are also indicated. The physician can then review all images for potential sources of bleeding or areas of abnormality that may indicate bleeding such as ulceration (Fig. 120-6). Since images are not reviewed until after the capsule has passed, current devices cannot be used therapeutically; however, new generations of steerable capsules under magnetic control may be equipped with potential therapies, such as hemostatic sprays that could be released when a suspicious area is identified.

ADVANCED ENDOSCOPY

ADVANCED IMAGING

With the use of in vivo dyes such as fluorescein, even capillary blood flow can be visualized. The glandular structure and the microenvironment of early neoplastic lesions can be visualized using confocal laser endomicroscopy via a standard endoscope, via endoscopic ultrasound-guided fine-needle aspiration into cystic structures, or a duodenoscope to view the wall of the bile duct. Optical coherence tomography can visualize 7 linear cm of esophagus with one scan, thereby allowing reconstruction of the mucosa into two- and three-dimensional images that assess the extent of dysplasia. Electronic enhancement methods are replacing chromoendoscopy with dyes for detecting gastric neoplasia. The visualization of blood vessels in luminal tumors can predict the depth of tumor invasion with excellent accuracy.

TISSUE RESECTION

Most large polyps and early cancers can be removed with advanced endoscopic techniques. One example is endoscopic mucosal resection, by which a small cap is applied to the tip of the endoscope to allow suction to draw tissue into the cap, and then a wire snare with cautery is used to resect the tissue. The tissue is withdrawn into the cap and removed via the endoscope. Variations of this technique include the application of bands that pinch the tissue after it is drawn into the cap to allow the easier application of the snare. Endoscopic submucosal dissection can resect large lesions en bloc, thereby completely removing all neoplastic tissue by cutting around the area of neoplasia and then carefully dissecting the mucosa from the underlying muscle layer. For Barrett esophagus (Chapter 124), en bloc mucosal resection followed by ablation therapy can reduce the risk of progression from low-grade dysplasia to higher grade dysplasia.[A5,A6]

Per-oral myotomy[12] is useful for treating achalasia, with outcomes at least equivalent to open surgery in appropriate patients.[A7] It is also useful for some cases of pyloric gastric outlet obstruction and gastroparesis.[13] This technique is performed by making a mucosal incision to permit the endoscope to be passed into the submucosa to tunnel along the muscularis propria. The muscle layer can then be incised similar to a Heller myotomy, except usually only the inner circular muscle layer is cut. The tunnel can be sealed with hemostatic clips afterwards, thereby permitting easier closure.

In the colon, routine cautery of tissue surrounding a resected polyp can be performed using the avulsion technique, which entails grasping tissue with a small forceps that can apply electrocautery to the edges of the resection. This technique decreases the risk of recurrent polyps.

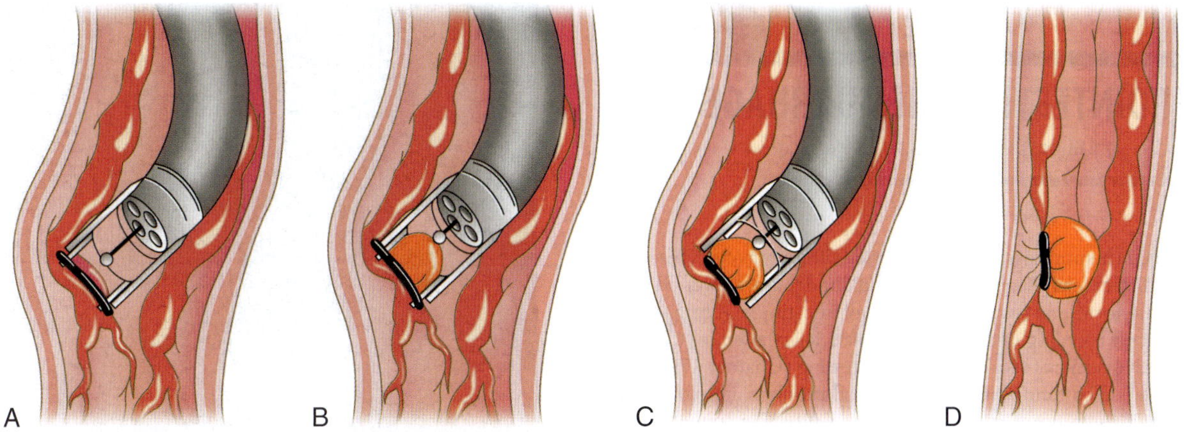

FIGURE 120-7. **Endoscopic variceal ligation technique. A,** The endoscope, with attached ligating device, is brought into contact with a varix just above the gastroesophageal junction. **B,** Suction is applied, drawing the varix-containing mucosa into the dead space created at the end of the endoscope by the ligating device. **C,** The tripwire is pulled, releasing the band around the aspirated tissue. **D,** Completed ligation. (From Pasricha PJ. Gastrointestinal endoscopy. In: Goldman L, Schafer AI, eds. *Goldman-Cecil Medicine,* 26th ed. Philadelphia: Elsevier; 2020:834-840.)

ESOPHAGEAL VARICES

Patients with portal hypertension commonly undergo an endoscopy to exclude possible esophageal or gastric varices (Chapter 139). Prophylactic treatment is recommended in patients who have bled previously, when large esophageal varices are present, and when the endoscopy shows variceal stigmata such as pseudoaneurysms or fibrin clots that are consistent with prior bleeding. Active variceal bleeding can be difficult to treat endoscopically because the bleeding areas may not be visible. Temporizing measures to include using a tube that can tamponade the bleeding by occluding the vessels at the gastroesophageal junction with a balloon. If this approach is unsuccessful, the esophageal balloon can then be inflated to tamponade the esophageal varices. Once bleeding is controlled, variceal banding (Fig. 120-7) can be performed to occlude the varices. Bleeding gastric varices are usually best managed by carefully injecting cyanoacrylate glue, which produces clotting within the vessel.

REMODELING ORGANS

Endoscopic devices to create a fundoplication for controlling gastroesophageal reflux disease (Chapter 124)[14] are useful only in selected cases because repair of the diaphragmatic hernia also is required in patients who have hernias that are large enough to require a procedure to control reflux.[A8] In bariatric procedures, the stomach can be plicated endoscopically, similar to a surgical gastric sleeve procedure but without removal of gastric tissue.[15] Other endoscopic procedures for weight loss include the short-term (less than 6 months) placement of gastric balloons that cause early satiety and moderate weight loss.[A9] Malabsorption can be produced either by bypassing the duodenum with a stent or by ablating the duodenal mucosa.[16]

CREATING ANASTOMOSES

The endoscopic creation of a percutaneous opening into the lumen of the GI tract can provide access for feeding into the stomach (percutaneous endoscopic gastrostomy) or jejunum (in patients at high risk for aspiration) in patients who require long-term nutrition (Chapter 198). The creation of an anastomosis between the bile duct and the stomach, using endoscopic ultrasound-guided placement of a stent under fluoroscopy, can decompress biliary obstruction in patients who have pancreatic or distal biliary cancers (Chapters 180 and 181). Placing a stent to bypass a duodenal obstruction caused by a pancreatic tumor is another palliative option.[17] However, these internal anastomoses usually provide only short-term palliation because of evolving anatomy as the tumor progresses.

REPAIR OF SURGICAL COMPLICATIONS

Endoscopic techniques can repair anastomotic leaks, drain abscesses around luminal surfaces, complete surgical resection of tumors that have positive neoplastic margins, and restore luminal integrity in areas of postoperative stenosis. For stenosis caused by surgical ischemia, temporary stenting with fully covered metal can provide short-term relief, but restenosis often occurs when the stent is removed because long-term stent deployment leads to erosion of the stent and the potential for perforation and bleeding. Drainage of abscesses can be achieved by endoscopic ultrasound-guided placement of lumen-apposing metal stents into the abscess and then cleaning out the abscess with the endoscope;[18] as the abscess drains away, the stents can eventually be removed. Sponges with low vacuum can be placed in the lumen of abscesses around the esophagus to help clear them.

COMBINED PROCEDURES

In rendezvous procedures, an interventional radiologist advances wires into the biliary system to help the endoscopist identify the location of a hidden papilla or pass a stricture that cannot be passed using wires inserted proximally via the papilla. In severe esophageal strictures, a gastrostomy can be performed, and then an endoscope can be placed into the stomach, where it is then advanced proximally toward the mouth to rendezvous with an endoscope passed by a gastroenterologist from the throat.[19] Using cutting tools, a lumen can be constructed between the two endoscopes. Full thickness resections of the gastrointestinal tract are often both more efficient and safer for the patient when performed as combined procedures by an endoscopist and surgeon, with the closure of the defect performed laparoscopically.

GENERAL REFERENCES

For the General References and other additional features, please visit Elsevier eBooks+ at https://ebooks.health.elsevier.com.

Grade A References

A1. Kuo HC, Liu FL, Chen JT, et al. Thromboembolic and bleeding risk of periprocedural bridging anticoagulation: a systematic review and meta-analysis. *Clin Cardiol.* 2020;43:441-449.

A2. Kang X, Guo X, Chen Z, et al. The incidence and severity of post-ERCP pancreatitis in patients receiving standard administration of NSAIDs: a systematic review and meta-analysis. *J Gastrointest Surg.* 2022;26:2380-2389.

A3. Guo X, Yang Z, Zhao L, et al. Enhanced instructions improve the quality of bowel preparation for colonoscopy: a meta-analysis of randomized controlled trials. *Gastrointest Endosc.* 2017;85:90-97.e6.

A4. Radaelli F, Paggi S, Hassan C, et al. Split-dose preparation for colonoscopy increases adenoma detection rate: a randomised controlled trial in an organised screening programme. *Gut.* 2017;66:270-277.

A5. Qumseya BJ, Wani S, Gendy S, et al. Disease progression in Barrett's low-grade dysplasia with radiofrequency ablation compared with surveillance: systematic review and meta-analysis. *Am J Gastroenterol.* 2017;112:849-865.

A6. Pouw RE, Klaver E, Phoa KN, et al. Radiofrequency ablation for low-grade dysplasia in Barrett's esophagus: long-term outcome of a randomized trial. *Gastrointest Endosc.* 2020;92:569-574.

A7. Mundre P, Black CJ, Mohammed N, et al. Efficacy of surgical or endoscopic treatment of idiopathic achalasia: a systematic review and network meta-analysis. *Lancet Gastroenterol Hepatol.* 2021;6:30-38.

A8. Xie P, Yan J, Ye L, et al. Efficacy of different endoscopic treatments in patients with gastroesophageal reflux disease: a systematic review and network meta-analysis. *Surgl Endosc.* 2021;35:1500-1510.

A9. Loo JH, Lim YH, Seah HL, et al. Intragastric balloon as bridging therapy prior to bariatric surgery for patients with severe obesity (BMI $\geq$ 50 kg/m^2): a systematic review and meta-analysis. *Obes Surg.* 2022;32:489-502.

121

GASTROINTESTINAL HEMORRHAGE

THOMAS O. KOVACS AND DENNIS M. JENSEN

Gastrointestinal (GI) hemorrhage can be manifested clinically as overt bleeding from the upper GI tract (esophagus, stomach, and duodenum), lower GI tract (colon), or obscure locations (usually in the small intestine).[1] Alternatively, it can occur as occult bleeding detected by iron deficiency anemia (Chapter 145) or by a positive result of fecal occult blood testing (Chapter 179).

GI hemorrhage is a common worldwide clinical problem and continues to be associated with significant morbidity and mortality. The annual hospitalization rate for upper GI bleeding is now estimated to be about 300,000 hospitalizations per year in the United States. Lower GI bleeding occurs less frequently, at about 20% of the rate of upper GI bleeding, but increases substantially with age and may occur more frequently than upper GI bleeding in the elderly. Overall, for patients hospitalized for GI bleeding, 40% occurs in the upper GI tract, 25% in the lower GI tract, and 35% in an undefined location. Mortality rates from upper GI hemorrhage are high, varying from 3.5 to 7% in the United States.

UPPER GASTROINTESTINAL BLEEDING

CLINICAL MANIFESTATIONS

Upper GI bleeding occurs proximal to the ligament of Treitz. Patients with upper GI bleeding usually present with hematemesis (vomiting blood or coffee-ground material) or melena (black, tarry stool). In large series, about 50% of patients have hematemesis and melena, about 30% have hematemesis alone, and about 20% have only melena. On occasion, however, hematochezia (passage per rectum of red blood or clots) may be the only manifestation of a bleeding ulcer, and about 15% of all patients who present with hematochezia have an upper GI source. Peptic ulcer disease (Fig. 121-1) is the most common cause of acute upper GI hemorrhage, accounting for about 40% of cases. Other common causes are esophageal and gastric varices and erosive esophagitis. Variceal bleeding, which occurs in the setting of portal hypertension, is discussed in Chapter 139. Other conditions, such as Mallory-Weiss tears (Fig. 121-2; Chapter 124), angiodysplasia, watermelon stomach, tumors, and Dieulafoy lesion, occur less frequently than peptic ulcer (Table 121-1). The mortality from nonulcer bleeding is comparable to that from ulcer hemorrhage in high-risk patients, so all causes of upper GI hemorrhage contribute to the morbidity and cost of care associated with it.

DIAGNOSIS

Initial assessment includes a medical history, vital signs, physical examination (including digital rectal examination), and laboratory evaluation. Patients should be asked questions that can help determine the diagnostic possibilities for the bleeding source. For example, peptic ulcer bleeding (Chapter 125) should be suspected in patients taking daily aspirin or nonsteroidal anti-inflammatory drugs (NSAIDs). For patients with known or suspected liver disease, bleeding related to portal hypertension (such as varices or portal hypertensive gastropathy; Chapter 139) should be strongly considered. Heavy alcohol intake or vomiting should suggest a Mallory-Weiss tear (Chapter 124). A feeding tube or a chronic nasogastric tube and a history of gastroesophageal reflux disease raise the suspicion for severe erosive esophagitis (Chapter 124).

The physician should check the vital signs with attention to signs of hypovolemia, such as hypotension, tachycardia, and orthostasis. The patient's skin should be examined for petechiae (see Fig. 158-2), purpura (see Fig. 406-10), spider angiomas, and palmar erythema (see Fig. 132-2), and the abdomen should be assessed for ascites (see Fig. 132-4), hepatomegaly, or splenomegaly, which may indicate portal hypertension. Tenderness or a mass may indicate an intra-abdominal tumor.

Routine placement of a nasogastric or orogastric tube is not recommended for patients with upper GI hemorrhage. Such a tube may, however, potentially be useful in selected patients to localize bleeding to the upper GI tract in patients with hematochezia, hemodynamic instability, and absence of overt

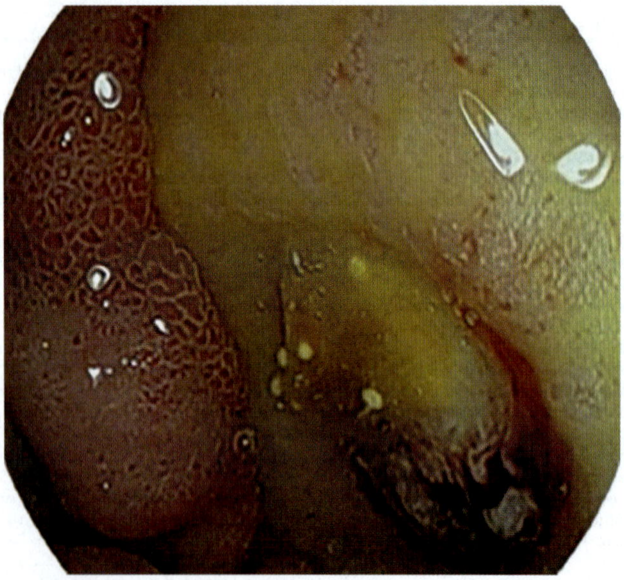

FIGURE 121-1. Large duodenal ulcer with a bleeding visible vessel.

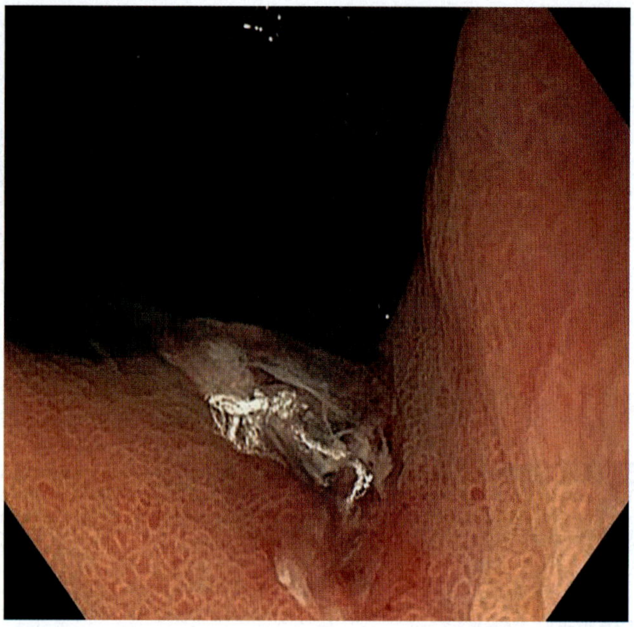

FIGURE 121-2. Mallory-Weiss tear with an overlying clot at the gastroesophageal junction.

TABLE 121-1 CAUSES OF SEVERE UPPER GASTROINTESTINAL (GI) BLEEDING IN ONE LARGE CENTER

DIAGNOSIS	%
Peptic ulcer (gastric or duodenal)	38
Gastric or esophageal varices	16
Erosive esophagitis	13
Upper GI tumors	7
Upper GI angiomas*	6
Mallory-Weiss tear	4
Gastric or duodenal erosions	4
Dieulafoy lesion	2
Other†	2
No upper GI cause found‡	8

*Upper GI angiomas include single or multiple angiectasia, watermelon stomach, and Osler-Weber-Rendu telangiectasia.
†Other lesions were surgical anastomoses, Cameron ulcers, aortoenteric fistulas, and hemobilia.
‡No cause found in esophagus, stomach, or duodenum, but 2% had mouth, nose, or pharyngeal bleeding sites.

signs of upper GI bleeding; help clear gastric blood for better endoscopic visualization; and minimize the risk of aspiration.

Peripheral blood should be sent for standard hematology, chemistry, liver, and coagulation studies as well as for typing and crossmatching for packed red blood cells (Chapter 162). Hemoglobin concentration and hematocrit may not accurately reflect blood loss because equilibration with extravascular fluid requires 24 to 72 hours. A low platelet count suggests chronic liver disease, dilution, drug reaction, or a hematologic disorder. In upper GI bleeding, the blood urea nitrogen level typically increases to a greater extent than the creatinine level owing to increased intestinal absorption of urea after the breakdown of blood proteins. However, this phenomenon can be misleading in the setting of renal insufficiency or rapid transit of blood. An elevated international normalized ratio can be observed in chronic liver disease and in patients who are taking warfarin.

TREATMENT

Acute Management

Resuscitation efforts should be initiated simultaneously with assessment in the emergency department and continue during the hospitalization.[2] Large-bore (14- or 16-gauge) intravenous catheters are recommended, with normal saline infused as fast as necessary to maintain hemodynamic stability. A restrictive transfusion strategy (red blood cell transfusions given only at hemoglobin level <7 g/dL, with a post-transfusion target of 7 to 9 g/dL) is better than a liberal strategy for reducing 45-day mortality and further bleeding in patients with acute upper GI hemorrhage.[3] These results can be generalized to patients with non-exsanguinating upper GI bleeding[A1] but not to patients who are hypotensive due to severe hemorrhage or have associated cardiovascular disease, in whom a hemoglobin target of 9 to 10 g/dL is recommended.[4] Guidelines also advocate platelet transfusion for patients with active bleeding and a low platelet count (<50,000/μL), but there is no benefit from platelet transfusions in patients who are on antiplatelet agents but have normal platelet levels. For patients who develop upper GI hemorrhage while taking anticoagulants, such as a vitamin K antagonist or a direct-acting oral anticoagulant, it is reasonable to proceed to upper endoscopy before correcting the medication effects. To prevent aspiration, which can cause considerable morbidity and mortality, endotracheal intubation should be considered in patients with active hematemesis or altered mental status.

Nonvariceal Hemorrhage

Endoscopic Therapy

Endoscopy can identify the site of bleeding and provide therapeutic hemostasis in most patients.[5] Patients with evidence of active bleeding (hematemesis, red blood by nasogastric lavage, or hemodynamic instability) should undergo emergency endoscopy as soon as possible (within 12 hours) after medical resuscitation. An intravenous prokinetic agent (either erythromycin 250 mg or metoclopramide 10 mg) 30 to 60 minutes before endoscopy may help move blood out of the stomach and into the small intestine, thereby improving endoscopic visualization. In other patients, endoscopy between 6 and 24 hours after presentation appears to be as safe and effective as emergent endoscopy.[A2,A3]

In addition to localization of the bleeding source, endoscopic evaluation can provide prognostic information and stratify the risk of rebleeding on the basis of the presence or absence of stigmata of recent hemorrhage (Table 121-2).[6] In addition to endoscopic stigmata, other clinical and laboratory factors that predict a poor prognosis include older age, bleeding onset in the hospital, medical comorbidities (especially hepatic, renal, and malignant disease), shock, coagulopathy, fresh blood in the nasogastric lavage, and the need for multiple blood transfusions. Risk stratification using clinical scoring systems, such as the Glasgow-Blatchford score (Table 121-3), may also identify patients at very low risk (score = 0 to 1) of rebleeding or mortality and thereby allow safe, early discharge from the emergency department with outpatient follow-up.

The goal of endoscopic therapy is to stop acute bleeding and to reduce the risk of recurrent bleeding. Most endoscopic therapies were designed for peptic ulcer hemorrhage, but they can be used for other causes of nonvariceal upper GI bleeding, in which underlying arteries are the source of bleeding. Available treatments include injection (epinephrine or sclerosants such as absolute ethanol), thermal coagulation (with multipolar/bipolar or heater probe), and mechanical compression (hemostatic clips). Injection therapy is effective, safe, and inexpensive, but it is sometimes inadequate for definitive hemostasis when it is used alone. When epinephrine injection is combined with either thermal coagulation or hemoclips, hemostasis is achieved in more than 95% of patients with active bleeding, and rebleeding rates are decreased by more than 50%. A device with a larger, over-the-scope clip may be useful for re-treating patients who rebleed after initial hemostasis.[A4,A5]

Endoscopic therapy is reserved for lesions that have high-risk stigmata for rebleeding (e.g., active arterial bleeding, nonbleeding visible vessel, or adherent clot) or moderate-risk stigmata, such as oozing, bleeding without associated clot, or nonbleeding visible vessel.[7] It is not warranted for low-risk stigmata (clean-based ulcer or flat pigmented spot, unless arterial blood flow is underneath the flat spot), which have the lowest risk of rebleeding (Fig. 121-3). Some causes of upper GI bleeding, such as gastric or duodenal erosions and neoplasms, generally are not amenable to endoscopic treatment and require appropriate medical or surgical therapy.

Recurrent bleeding after endoscopic treatment directly increases mortality, raises transfusion requirements, and prolongs hospitalization. Independent

TABLE 121-2 ENDOSCOPIC STIGMATA OF RECENT HEMORRHAGE FOR PEPTIC ULCER BLEEDS

STIGMATA	PREVALENCE (%)	RISK OF REBLEEDING ON MEDICAL TREATMENT (%)	REBLEED RISK AFTER ENDOSCOPIC HEMOSTASIS (%)*
Active spurting bleeding	12	80-90	15-30
Non-bleeding visible vessel	22	40-50	15-30
Adherent clot	10	30-35	15-20
Oozing bleeding without other stigmata	14	10-20	0-5
Flat spot with underlying arterial blood flow	5	10-20	0-5
Flat spot without underlying blood flow	5	<5	–†
Clean ulcer base	32	3	–†

*Reduction in bleeding risk is with the administration of a proton pump inhibitor after successful endoscopic hemostasis.

†Endoscopic hemostasis is not recommended for clean-based ulcers or flat spots without underlying blood flow.

From Kovacs TOG, Jensen DM. Endoscopic therapy for severe ulcer bleeding gastrointestinal. *Endosc Clin N Am.* 2011;21:681-696 and Jensen DM, Kovacs TOG, Ohning GV, et al. Doppler endoscopic probe monitoring of blood flow improves risk stratification and outcomes of patients with severe non-variceal upper gastrointestinal hemorrhage. *Gastroenterology.* 2017;152:1310-1318.

TABLE 121-3 GLASGOW-BLATCHFORD SCORE

ADMISSION RISK MARKER	SCORE
Blood urea (mg/dL)	
18.2-22.3	2
22.4-27.9	3
28.0-69.9	4
≥70	6
Hemoglobin (g/dL)	
Men	
12-13	1
10-11.9	3
<10	6
Women	
10-12	1
<10	6
Systolic blood pressure (mm Hg)	
100-109	1
90-99	2
<90	3
Pulse ≥100/min	1
History and comorbidities	
Melena	1
Syncope	2
Hepatic disease*	2
Cardiac failure†	2

*Known history or clinical and laboratory findings of chronic or acute hepatic disease.

†Known history or clinical and echocardiographic findings of cardiac failure.

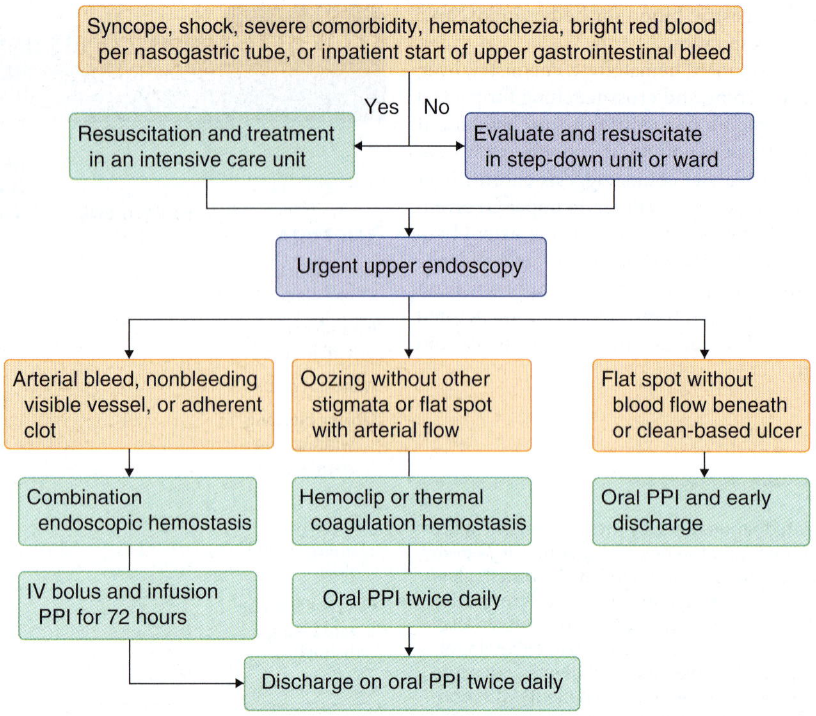

FIGURE 121-3. **Management algorithm for nonvariceal upper gastrointestinal hemorrhage.** IV = intravenous; PPI = proton pump inhibitor.

predictors of recurrent hemorrhage after successful endoscopic therapy include hemodynamic instability, comorbid illness, posterior duodenal location, and large ulcer size. Patients with these high-risk ulcer features may benefit from more aggressive posthemostasis triage and management.

Use of a Doppler endoscopic probe to detect blood flow underneath stigmata of a recent nonvariceal upper GI hemorrhage provides a more objective way to stratify the risk of patients with ulcer hemorrhage as well as a safe and effective method to improve outcomes. Persistence of a positive Doppler signal after endoscopic treatment correlates with rebleeding, and Doppler probe–guided endoscopic hemostasis significantly reduces 30-day rebleeding rates compared with standard, visually guided hemostasis.[A6] Patients who have residual arterial blood flow after endoscopic hemostasis have significantly higher rebleeding rates than do patients in whom arterial blood flow is successfully obliterated.

Medical Therapy

The most common cause of upper GI bleeding is peptic ulcer disease, and the most common cause of peptic ulcer disease in developed countries is NSAID use. Aspirin and other NSAIDs should be discontinued in patients with bleeding peptic ulcers, unless there is a contraindication to do so (e.g., secondary prophylaxis for stroke). Patients with documented *Helicobacter pylori* infection should be treated with combination antibiotics and a proton pump inhibitor (Chapter 125). After documentation of *H. pylori* eradication, maintenance antisecretory treatment is not needed unless the patient also requires NSAIDs or anticoagulation therapy.

Proton pump inhibitors (see Table 124-1) are the mainstay of medical therapy for hemostasis and healing of peptic lesions. Acid suppression can promote platelet aggregation and clot formation as well as reduce the risk of rebleeding. High-dose intravenous proton pump inhibitors (bolus followed by continuous infusion [e.g., pantoprazole 80 mg followed by 8 mg/hour for 72 hours]) after successful endoscopic hemostasis reduce rebleeding rates and mortality in patients with high-risk stigmata of recent hemorrhage. For patients with high-risk stigmata, either this same regimen or intermittent high-dose proton pump inhibitor therapy may be equally effective.[8] Patients with low-risk or no stigmata can be treated with an oral proton pump inhibitor (e.g., esomeprazole or pantoprazole 40 mg twice daily) and considered for early discharge. Pre-endoscopic proton pump inhibitor treatment is controversial since it does not alter clinical outcomes, but it may downstage the severity of the stigmata of recent hemorrhage and decrease the need for endoscopic intervention. Therefore, in patients with suspected ulcer bleeding, proton pump inhibitors given as an intravenous bolus may be used while waiting for the endoscopy, but this therapy cannot substitute for endoscopy and should not delay it.

The optimal management approach for patients who develop peptic ulcer–related GI bleeding while receiving antiplatelet or anticoagulant therapy is controversial, but rapid reversal of antithrombotic treatments is generally important (Chapter 70).[9] In patients who have a bleeding peptic ulcer while receiving low-dose aspirin therapy followed by successful endoscopic hemostasis and high-dose intravenous proton pump inhibitor therapy, the incidence of recurrent ulcer bleeding at 30 days is twice as high (10% vs. 5%) in patients who continue low-dose aspirin compared with those who did not. However, patients who continue low-dose aspirin have a significantly lower mortality rate compared with the placebo group because of lower rates of cardiovascular and cerebrovascular complications. Current recommendations[10] suggest that patients with upper GI hemorrhage who need secondary cardiovascular prophylaxis should resume low-dose aspirin treatment as soon as the cardiovascular risks outweigh the gastrointestinal risks, usually within 7 days, while continuing proton pump inhibitors (e.g., esomeprazole or pantoprazole 40 mg daily). Such a policy increases the risk of recurrent bleeding by about 65% but also decreases the risk of thromboembolism by about 65% and all-cause mortality by about 50%.[11] Among the direct-acting oral anticoagulants, apixaban (Chapter 70) may be associated with the lowest risk of major GI bleeding.[12]

Patients with idiopathic (non–*H. pylori*, non-NSAID) peptic ulcers should receive long-term acid suppression therapy. For this purpose, limited data suggest that proton pump inhibitors and histamine 2 receptor antagonists are about equally effective, although the former may be slightly better.[A7]

Variceal Bleeding

The treatment of variceal bleeding is discussed in Chapter 139.

LOWER GASTROINTESTINAL BLEEDING

DEFINITION AND EPIDEMIOLOGY

Lower GI hemorrhage generally refers to bleeding from the colon and anorectum. Severe lower GI bleeding occurs with an annual incidence of 20 per 100,000 population, much less frequently than upper GI bleeding. Patients are usually older and present with painless hematochezia, typically without orthostasis. If orthostasis is present, a brisk upper GI bleed, which occurs in 15 to 20% of cases of severe hematochezia, should be considered. The most common cause of severe colorectal hemorrhage is from diverticulosis (Chapter 128). Other frequent causes include internal hemorrhoids (Chapter 131), ischemic colitis (Chapter 129), rectal ulcer (Chapter 131), and delayed bleeding from postpolypectomy ulcers at a median of 8 days (range, 5 hours to 17 days) after the procedure (Table 121-4). In most patients, the bleeding stops and does not recur. The overall mortality rate from lower GI bleeding is 2 to 4%.

DIAGNOSIS

Patients with hematochezia should have a careful history, physical examination, and laboratory evaluation, analogous to the evaluation for upper GI bleeding.[13] The history may help in the differential diagnosis. A history of diverticulosis (see Figs. 128-5 and 128-6) may raise the suspicion for a diverticular bleed (Chapter 128). Abdominal cramping followed by bloody diarrhea suggests ischemic colitis (see Fig. 129-2). A recent polypectomy makes a postpolypectomy bleed more likely.

After medical resuscitation, most patients will need to undergo colonoscopy, although a flexible sigmoidoscopy or anoscopy may be an alternative in cases in which it is highly likely that the bleeding source is from the anorectum or distal colon (Fig. 121-4). Colonoscopy is critical for identifying a luminal source of bleeding as well as for potential hemostasis of amenable lesions.[14] Urgent colonoscopy within 12 hours of admission improves diagnostic yield but has not been shown to reduce either the rate of rebleeding or transfusion requirements.[A8] To cleanse the colon adequately and to visualize the colonic mucosa, a bowel purge with 6 L or more of a polyethylene glycol solution should be administered before the procedure. Colonoscopic treatment (Fig. 121-4) of focal bleeding sources with stigmata of hemorrhage (Fig. 121-5) uses the same methods (epinephrine and either thermocoagulation or hemoclips) as for upper GI bleeding. In addition, coagulation of angiectasias and bleeding biopsy sites is feasible during colonoscopy.[15]

If colonoscopy does not reveal the source of bleeding, an upper endoscopic evaluation should be performed. If both are negative, capsule endoscopy (Chapter 120), if it is locally available, may be the preferred way to look for a small intestinal source of bleeding. Alternatively, if bleeding persists or is too rapid for a colonoscopy to be performed, a tagged red blood cell nuclear scan or angiography may be performed to localize the bleeding. The red blood cell scan can help localize bleeding if it occurs at a rate of at least 0.1 mL/minute. However, a positive scan localizes bleeding to a general region of the abdomen but not to a specific anatomic site. CT angiography, which can detect bleeding rates of 0.3 to 0.5 mL/minute, is a more useful imaging test to identify the anatomic source of hemorrhage. Angiography has the advantage that it can treat the bleeding source with embolization of the bleeding vessel. However, it requires a faster bleeding rate (at least 0.5 mL/minute). These imaging studies cannot identify nonbleeding stigmata and usually do not yield an etiologic diagnosis.

TABLE 121-4 MOST COMMON COLONIC SOURCES OF SEVERE HEMATOCHEZIA IN A SERIES OF 486 CASES (EXPRESSED AS PERCENTAGE OF COLONIC SOURCES)*

Diverticulosis	32%
Internal hemorrhoids	13%
Ischemic colitis	12%
Rectal ulcers	8%
Colonic angiodysplasia, angiectasia, angiomas, or radiation proctopathy	7%
Ulcerative colitis, Crohn disease, other colitis	6%
Postpolypectomy ulcer	5%
Other lower gastrointestinal tract sources	6%

*Less common causes include surgical anastomotic ulcers or sutures, nonsteroidal anti-inflammatory agent colopathy, metastases, portal hypertensive colopathy, lymphoma, and endometriosis.

TREATMENT

Surgical management rarely is needed for hemostasis of lower GI bleeding because most bleeding is either self-limited or easily managed with medical or endoscopic therapy.[16] The main indications for surgery are malignant lesions (Chapters 131 and 179), diffusely bleeding lesions that fail to respond to medical therapy (such as ischemia; Chapter 129), and recurrent diverticular hemorrhage (Chapter 128). If the bleeding source can be localized preoperatively to a particular area of the colon, a segmental resection can be performed rather than a subtotal colectomy. In patients who have lower GI bleeding while on aspirin, the continuation of aspirin is associated with higher risk of recurrent lower GI bleeding but a lower risk of serious cardiovascular events and death.[17] Patients who develop GI bleeding while on antithrombotic medications for atherosclerotic conditions (e.g., coronary, peripheral vascular, or cerebrovascular artery disease) have a 20-fold increase in the likelihood of a new gastrointestinal cancer[18] and require the same aggressive evaluation as patients who bleed without using such medication.

OBSCURE AND OCCULT GASTROINTESTINAL BLEEDING

DEFINITION AND EPIDEMIOLOGY

Obscure GI bleeding is persistent or recurrent bleeding, despite negative initial GI evaluation—including upper endoscopy, push enteroscopy (which reaches farther into the small intestine), and colonoscopy, as well as radiologic evaluation of the small intestine, such as small bowel follow-through or CT or MR

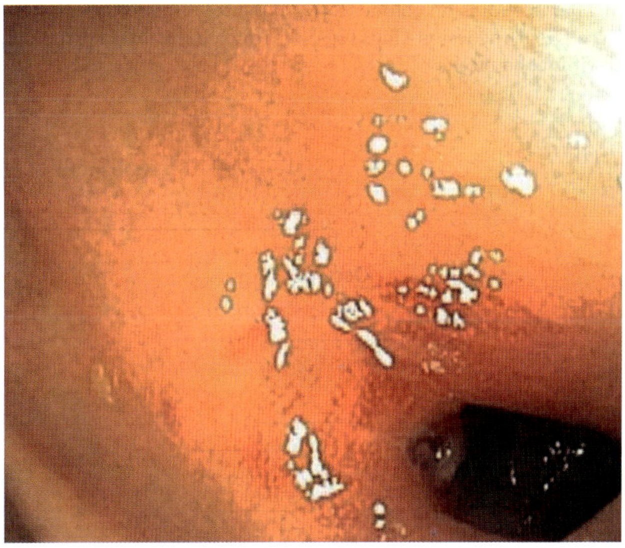

FIGURE 121-5. Colon diverticulum with a visible vessel.

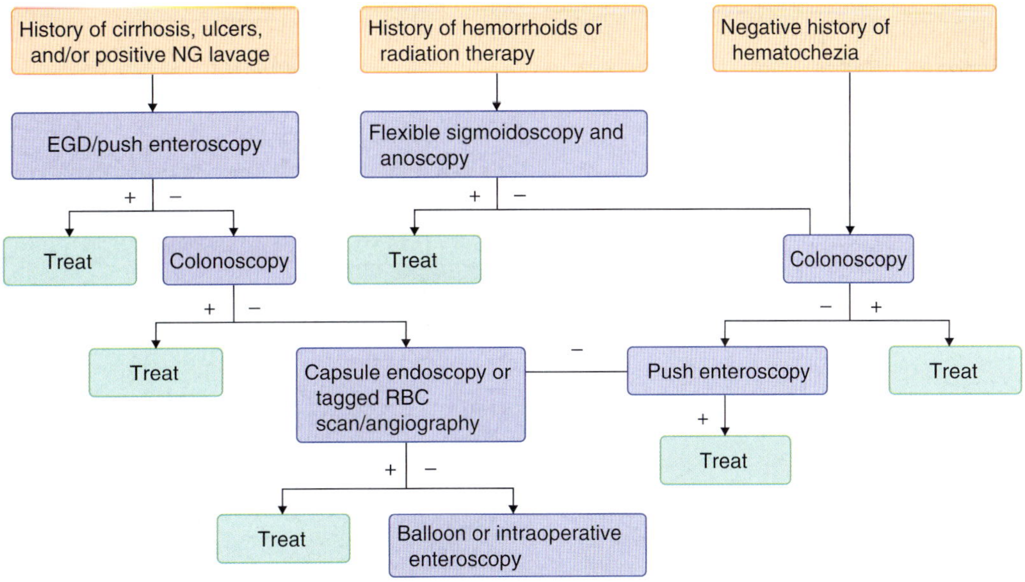

FIGURE 121-4. Management algorithm for severe hematochezia. EGD = esophagogastroduodenoscopy; NG = nasogastric; RBC = red blood cell; + = diagnostic findings; – = no diagnostic findings.

TABLE 121-5 SMALL INTESTINAL LESIONS FOUND IN 488 PATIENTS DURING DOUBLE-BALLOON ENTEROSCOPY FOR OBSCURE GASTROINTESTINAL BLEEDING

LESION	FREQUENCY (RANGE)
None	40% (0-57)
Angiectasias	31% (6-55)
Ulcerations	13% (2-35)
Malignancy	8% (3-26)
Other	6% (2-22)

enterography.[19] Obscure GI bleeding can be classified as either overt (melena, maroon stool, or hematochezia) or occult bleeding (positive result of fecal occult blood testing, usually in the setting of iron deficiency anemia).

In most large series of hospitalized patients, 5% of overt GI bleeding cases are considered to be obscure, and 75% of these patients have bleeding from the small intestine that is beyond the reach of an upper endoscope or colonoscope. Angiectasias (see Fig. 120-5) are the most common source of small intestinal bleeding, followed by ulcers and tumors (Table 121-5). Other causes for obscure GI bleeding include lesions that are within reach of standard endoscopes but that were not recognized as the bleeding site (e.g., a large hiatal hernia with lesions known as Cameron ulcers on endoscopy or internal hemorrhoids on colonoscopy) and intermittently bleeding lesions such as a Dieulafoy lesion (Fig. 121-5),[20] which is an aberrant submucosal vessel without an ulcer.

Iron deficiency (Chapter 145) has a prevalence of 2 to 5% among adult men and postmenopausal women. It can occur from overt or occult blood loss (e.g., GI tract lesions, menorrhagia), iron malabsorption (celiac disease, atrophic gastritis), and red blood cell destruction (hemolysis). It should be suspected in patients with low mean corpuscular volume, low ferritin level, or low transferrin saturation.

DIAGNOSIS

The approaches to overt and occult obscure GI bleeding are similar (Fig. 121-6). In the case of recurrent overt bleeding, upper endoscopy, push enteroscopy, and colonoscopy should be repeated, with the type of bleeding dictating which endoscopic procedure to do first. Colonoscopy with anoscopy should be done first if there is hematochezia. If there is melena, a push small bowel enteroscopy should be performed. If the first procedure is unremarkable, evaluation should be undertaken from the opposite end. If the second test result is negative, capsule endoscopy should be performed (Chapter 120).[21] If bleeding from the small intestine is seen on capsule endoscopy, further attempts to diagnose and to treat the bleeding should be performed with either deep enteroscopy (using a balloon overtube to slide much farther along into the small intestine) or intraoperative enteroscopy. All of these long enteroscopes facilitate diagnosis and hemostasis. If the capsule endoscopy is negative and rapid rebleeding recurs, a tagged red blood cell scan or angiography may be used to localize the bleeding site and assist with subsequent intraoperative enteroscopy.

For occult GI bleeding, colonoscopy should be performed first because fecal occult blood testing was designed to screen for colorectal cancer (Chapter 179). Upper endoscopy and push enteroscopy should follow if the colonoscopy is unremarkable. Afterward, the algorithm is the same as for overt bleeding; however, if the capsule endoscopy is negative, efforts should be focused toward providing supportive care rather than further evaluation.

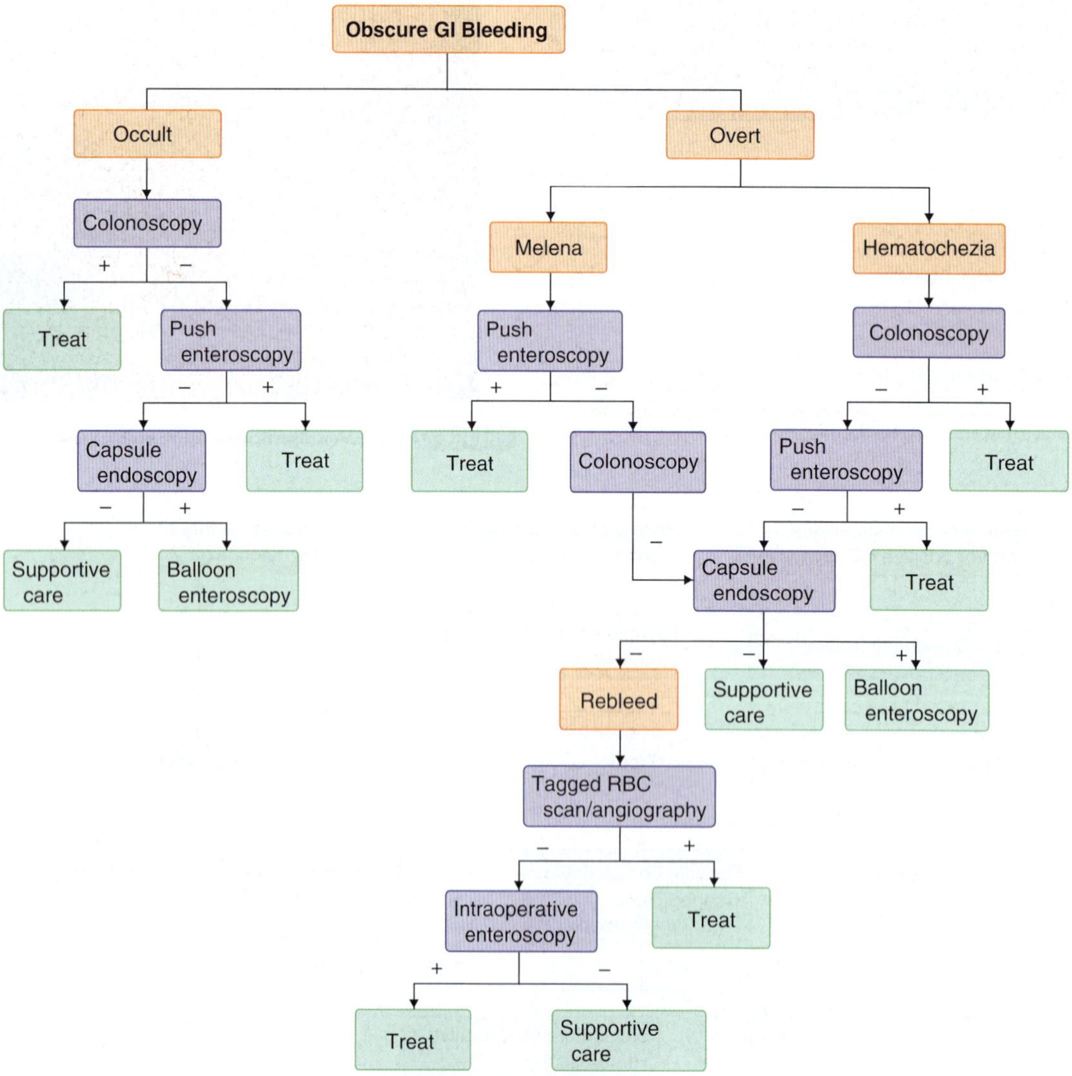

FIGURE 121-6. Management algorithm for obscure gastrointestinal bleeding. GI = gastrointestinal; RBC = red blood cell; + = diagnostic findings; – = no diagnostic findings.

Iron Deficiency Anemia

GI evaluation of iron deficiency anemia (Chapter 145) is indicated in adult men, regardless of age, and postmenopausal women. Women who have not reached menopause may warrant a GI evaluation after obvious or potential causes of iron deficiency and blood loss, such as chronic menorrhagia, have been excluded. Colonoscopy should be performed first, followed by upper endoscopy and push enteroscopy if the colonoscopy is negative.[22] Duodenal biopsy specimens should be taken to look for evidence of celiac disease (Chapter 126). In the absence of other potential sources of iron deficiency anemia, *H. pylori* should be treated, if present, because *H. pylori* infection decreases iron absorption and may produce microerosions that bleed. If all three of these endoscopic procedures are unrevealing, capsule endoscopy should be performed. If the capsule study is negative, investigation into non-GI causes of iron deficiency (Chapter 145) may be pursued.

GENERAL REFERENCES

For the General References and other additional features, please visit Elsevier eBooks+ at https://ebooks.health.elsevier.com.

Grade A References

A1. Odutayo A, Desborough MJR, Trivella M, et al. Restrictive versus liberal blood transfusion for gastrointestinal bleeding: a systematic review and meta-analysis of randomized controlled trials. *Lancet Gastroenterol Hepatol.* 2017;2:354-360.
A2. Lau JYW, Yu Y, Tang RSY, et al. Timing of endoscopy for acute upper gastrointestinal bleeding. *N Engl J Med.* 2020;382:1299-1308.
A3. Merola E, Michielan A, de Pretis G. Optimal timing of endoscopy for acute upper gastrointestinal bleeding: a systematic review and meta-analysis. *Intern Emerg Med.* 2021;16:1331-1340.
A4. Jensen DM, Kovacs T, Ghassemi KA, et al. Randomized controlled trial of over-the-scope clip as initial treatment of severe nonvariceal upper gastrointestinal bleeding. *Clin Gastroenterol Hepatol.* 2021;19:2315-2323.e2.
A5. Meier B, Wannhoff A, Denzer U, et al. Over-the-scope-clips versus standard treatment in high-risk patients with acute non-variceal upper gastrointestinal bleeding: a randomised controlled trial (STING-2). *Gut.* 2022;71:1251-1258.
A6. Jensen DM, Kovacs TOG, Ohning GV, et al. Doppler endoscopic probe monitoring of blood flow improves risk stratification and outcomes of patients with severe nonvariceal upper gastrointestinal hemorrhage. *Gastroenterology.* 2017;152:1310-1318.
A7. Wong GLH, Lau LHS, Ching JYL, et al. Prevention of recurrent idiopathic gastroduodenal ulcer bleeding: a double-blind, randomized trial. *Gut.* 2020;69:652-657.
A8. Niikura R, Nagata N, Yamada A, et al. Efficacy and safety of early vs elective colonoscopy for acute lower gastrointestinal bleeding. *Gastroenterology.* 2020;158:168-175.

122 DISORDERS OF GASTROINTESTINAL MOTILITY

MICHAEL CAMILLERI

DEFINITION

Motility disorders result from impaired control of the neuromuscular apparatus of the gastrointestinal tract. Associated symptoms include recurrent or chronic nausea, vomiting, bloating, abdominal discomfort, and constipation or diarrhea in the absence of intestinal obstruction.

PATHOBIOLOGY

Normal Physiology

Neuroenteric Control

Motor function of the gastrointestinal tract depends on the contraction of smooth muscle cells and their integration and modulation by enteric and extrinsic nerves as well as pacemaker cells, such as the interstitial cells of Cajal. Extrinsic neural control consists of cranial and sacral parasympathetic nerves (excitatory to nonsphincteric muscle) and the thoracolumbar sympathetic supply (excitatory to sphincters, inhibitory to nonsphincteric muscle). The vagus nerve innervates from the stomach to the right colon. Parasympathetic innervation of the distal colon arises from sacral segments S2 to S4. Sympathetic fibers to proximal and mid-gut and to the colon arise from the intermediolateral column of the spinal cord (T5 to T10 and T11 to L3, respectively). The prevertebral ganglia integrate afferent impulses from the gut and mediate reflex control of abdominal viscera.

The enteric nervous system, which is capable of autonomous control of the gut, comprises about 100 million neurons organized in ganglionated plexuses. The larger myenteric or Auerbach plexus, between the longitudinal and circular muscle layers, is responsible for motility, and the submucosal or Meissner plexus controls absorption, secretion, and mucosal blood flow. The enteric nervous system also plays an important role in visceral afferent function.

Pacemaker cells, which coordinate muscle contraction and sense distortion, serve as intermediaries between the enteric nerves and the smooth muscle cells. Electrical control activity spreads through interneurons in the contiguous segments of the gut via neurochemical activation by transmitters that may be excitatory (e.g., acetylcholine, substance P) or inhibitory (e.g., nitric oxide, somatostatin).

Gastric and Small Bowel Motility

The motor functions of the stomach and small intestine are characterized by distinct patterns of motor activity in the fasting and postprandial periods (E-Fig. 122-1). The fasting period is characterized by a cyclic motor phenomenon, the interdigestive migrating motor complex. In healthy individuals, one cycle of this complex is completed every 60 to 90 minutes. The complex has three phases: quiescence (phase I), intermittent pressure activity (phase II), and an activity front (phase III) during which the stomach and small intestine contract at their highest frequencies (3 per minute in the stomach, 12 per minute in the duodenum, 8 per minute in the ileum). Another characteristic motor pattern in the distal small intestine is prolonged propagated contraction, which empties residue from the ileum into the colon in bolus transfers.

In response to the ingestion of food, the proximal stomach accommodates the food by a vagally mediated reduction in tone, thereby facilitating the ingestion of food without an increase in pressure. Liquids empty from the stomach in an exponential manner, and the rate of emptying varies with calorie content and viscosity. The half-emptying time for non-nutrient liquids in healthy individuals is usually less than 20 minutes. Solids are retained selectively in the stomach, where they undergo acid and peptic digestion as well as "churning" or trituration by high liquid shearing forces in the antrum. Digestible food particles are emptied after their size is reduced by trituration to less than 2 mm. Gastric emptying of solids is characterized by an initial lag period followed by a linear post-lag emptying phase. Secretion of hormones that mediate the motor and digestive process (e.g., gastrin for acid secretion; cholecystokinin for gallbladder contraction and bile and pancreatic secretion; and insulin, glucagon, and incretins such as glucagon-like peptide 1 for glucose regulation) is integrated with the arrival of food or chyme at different levels of the gut to ensure optimal digestion and signal satiation.

The small intestine transports solids and liquids at approximately the same rate. As a result of the lag phase for the transport of solids from the stomach, liquids typically arrive in the colon before solids. Chyme moves from ileum to colon intermittently in boluses propelled by contractions. In the postprandial period, the interdigestive migrating motor complex is replaced by an irregular pattern of contractile activity that persists for about 1 hour for each 200 kcal ingested.

Vomiting is characterized by a stereotypic sequence of motor events, including contractions of the stomach, abdominal muscles, and diaphragm. This sequence is followed immediately in the proximal small bowel by a propagated, rhythmic contractile response similar to the migrating motor complex.

Colonic Motility

The normal colon displays short-duration (phasic) contractions and a background contractility or tone. Nonpropagated phasic contractions segment the colon and facilitate mixing, retention of residue, and formation of solid stool. High-amplitude propagated contractions, which exceed 75 mm Hg, propagate over a distance of at least 15 cm at a propagation velocity of 0.15 to 2.2 cm/second and contribute to the movement of feces in the colon. In health, these contractions occur on average five or six times per day, most often postprandially and between 6 am and 2 pm.

Colonic transit is slow most of the time but rapid at other times. Residue may be retained for prolonged periods in the ascending and transverse colon; alternatively, a mass movement may deliver the contents to the sigmoid colon in seconds. Feeding stimulates movement of colonic content (a gastrocolonic response). In health, the average mouth-to-cecum transit time is about 6 hours, and transit times through the right colon, left colon, and sigmoid colon are about 12 hours each. Decreased calorie intake slows colonic transit, whereas

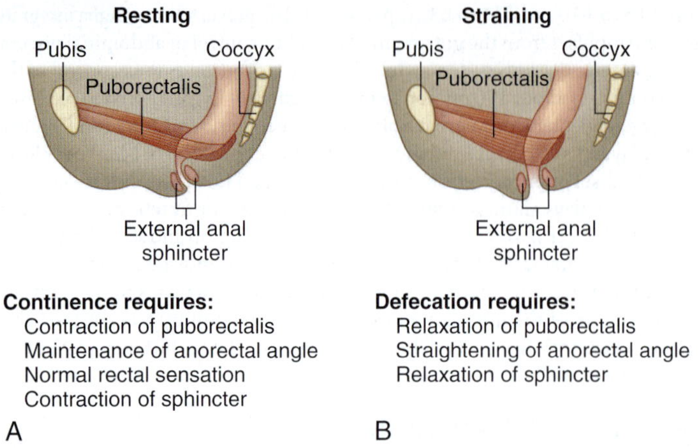

FIGURE 122-1. Pelvic floor and anorectal functions during continence and defecation. Sagittal view through the pelvis in the resting (A) and straining (B) postures. Coordinated functions of pelvic floor (puborectalis) and anal sphincter are essential for continence and defecation.

meals greater than 500 kcal, especially if fat-rich, stimulate colonic motility and propulsion. Outlet obstruction in patients with pelvic floor dysfunction or voluntary suppression of defecation often slow colonic transit and decrease the motor response to feeding.

Fluid reabsorption influences gastrointestinal transit. Approximately 9 L of fluid enters the gut from oral intake and endogenous secretions. The small intestine delivers about 1.5 L of fluid to the colon, where most is reabsorbed, leaving a maximum of 200 mL of water excreted in normal stool. Up to 3 L of fluid can be reabsorbed by the colon over 24 hours, unless the ileocolonic flow rate or colonic motility overwhelm the colon's capacity or reabsorption.

Defecation and Continence

Normal defecation requires a series of coordinated actions of the colon, rectum, pelvic floor, and anal sphincter muscles (Fig. 122-1). Distention of the rectum results in the relaxation of the internal anal sphincter (rectoanal inhibitory reflex) and simultaneous contraction of the external anal sphincter to maintain continence. The anal transition zone can sense the difference between solid or liquid stool and gas.

TABLE 122-1 CLASSIFICATION OF GASTROPARESIS AND PSEUDO-OBSTRUCTION

TYPE	NEUROPATHIC	MYOPATHIC
Infiltrative	Progressive systemic sclerosis Amyloidosis	Progressive systemic sclerosis Amyloidosis Systemic lupus erythematosus Ehlers-Danlos syndrome Dermatomyositis
Familial	Familial visceral neuropathies	Familial visceral myopathies Metabolic myopathies
Idiopathic	Idiopathic intestinal pseudo-obstruction	Sporadic hollow visceral myopathy
Neurologic	Porphyria Heavy metal poisoning Brain stem tumor Parkinson disease Multiple sclerosis Spinal cord transection	Myotonia Other dystrophies
Infectious	Chagas disease Cytomegalovirus Norwalk virus Epstein-Barr virus	
Drug induced	Tricyclic antidepressants Narcotic agents Anticholinergic agents Antihypertensives Dopaminergic agents Vincristine Laxatives	
Paraneoplastic	Small cell lung cancer Carcinoid syndrome	
Postsurgical/Injury	Postvagotomy with or without pyloroplasty or gastric resection Spinal cord injury	
Endocrine	Diabetes mellitus Hypothyroidism or hyperthyroidism Hypoparathyroidism	

DISEASES OF SLOW TRANSIT THROUGH THE STOMACH AND SMALL BOWEL

PATHOBIOLOGY

Gastrointestinal motility disturbances (Table 122-1) result from disorders of the extrinsic nervous system, enteric nervous system, intestinal pacemakers or smooth muscle. Neuropathic patterns are characterized by normal amplitude but incoordinated contractions, whereas myopathies are characterized by low-amplitude contractions (average <40 mm Hg in the antrum and <10 mm Hg in the small bowel).

Genetic defects that result in congenital dysmotility include abnormalities of *RET*, the gene that encodes the tyrosine kinase receptor, and abnormalities in the endothelin B system. Neural crest cells migrate from the vagal and sacral crest to the developing gut and, over time, colonize the entire developing alimentary canal and its appendages. Endothelin B serves to retard maturation of migrating neural crest cells, thus facilitating colonization of the entire gut with nerve cells.

EXTRINSIC NEUROPATHIC DISORDERS

Extrinsic neuropathic processes include vagotomy, trauma, Parkinson disease (Chapter 378), diabetes (Chapter 210), amyloidosis (Chapter 174), a paraneoplastic syndrome usually associated with small cell carcinoma of the lung (Chapter 177), and effect of medications, such as α_2-adrenergic agonists, glucagon-like peptide 1 analogues, opiates, and anticholinergics, on neural control.

Damage to the autonomic nerves may lead to motor, secretory, and sensory disturbances, most frequently resulting in constipation. Fasting colonic motility and tone remain normal, but a reduced left colon response to feeding as well as decreased rectal tone and sensitivity may lead to colorectal dilation and fecal impaction.

ENTERIC AND INTRINSIC NEUROPATHIC DISORDERS

Disorders of the enteric nervous system or interstitial cells of Cajal are usually the result of an infectious (e.g., viral), degenerative, immune, or inflammatory process associated with infiltration of the myenteric plexus with inflammatory cells.

SMOOTH MUSCLE DISORDERS

Disturbances of smooth muscle may result in significant disorders of gastric emptying and of transit through the small bowel and colon. Motility disturbances may be the result of metabolic disorders, such as hypothyroidism (Chapter 207) and hyperparathyroidism (Chapter 227), but these patients more commonly present with constipation. Scleroderma may result in focal or general dilation, wide-mouthed diverticula, and delayed transit in the stomach, small bowel, and colon. The amplitude of contractions is reduced, and bacterial overgrowth may result in steatorrhea or pneumatosis intestinalis. Mitochondrial neurogastrointestinal encephalomyopathy is an autosomal recessive condition that may be manifested with hepatic failure in neonates, seizures or diarrhea in infants, and hepatic failure or chronic intestinal pseudo-obstruction in adults.

CLINICAL MANIFESTATIONS

The clinical features of gastroparesis[1,2] and chronic intestinal pseudo-obstruction[3] are similar and include nausea, vomiting, early satiety, abdominal discomfort, distention, bloating, and anorexia. Severe cases, which occur mostly in patients with disorders of smooth muscle, may be accompanied by dilation, weight loss, depletion of mineral and vitamin stores. Diarrhea and constipation indicate that the motility disorder extends beyond the stomach. Vomiting may result in aspiration pneumonia (Chapter 82) or Mallory-Weiss esophageal tears (Chapters 121 and 124), and patients with a generalized motility disorder may have abnormal swallowing or delayed colonic transit.

A careful family and medication history is essential. Review of systems may reveal an underlying collagen vascular disease (e.g., scleroderma) or disturbances of extrinsic autonomic neural control, including orthostatic dizziness, difficulties with erection or ejaculation, recurrent urinary tract infections, dry mouth, dry eyes, dry vagina, difficulties with visual accommodation in bright lights, and absence of sweating.

On physical examination, a succussion splash indicates stasis, typically in the stomach. The hands and mouth may reveal signs of Raynaud phenomenon or scleroderma (Chapter 246). Testing of pupillary responses (to light and accommodation), external ocular movements, blood pressure in the lying and standing positions, and general features of a peripheral neuropathy can identify patients with an associated neurologic disturbance (e.g., diabetic neuropathy) or mitochondrial cytopathies (see under the Smooth Muscle Disorders section in this chapter).

The differential diagnosis includes mechanical obstruction, functional gastrointestinal disorders, anorexia nervosa, and the rumination syndrome. The rumination syndrome is a relatively common, underdiagnosed condition that is manifested with early (0 to 30 minutes) postprandial, effortless regurgitation of undigested food after virtually every meal.

DIAGNOSIS

Diagnosis requires documentation of delayed gastric emptying of a digestible solid meal. The clinician should assess the acuity of symptoms and the patient's state of hydration and nutrition. The goals of the evaluation are to determine what regions of the digestive tract are malfunctioning and whether the symptoms are due to a neuropathy or a myopathy (Fig. 122-2). Key steps include the following:

1. *Suspect and exclude mechanical obstruction* by upper gastrointestinal endoscopy and small bowel imaging studies, including a small bowel follow-through, computed tomographic enterography, and magnetic resonance enteroclysis. Capsule endoscopy should be avoided because of the potential risk of retention of the capsule. These studies rarely identify the cause, however, except for systemic sclerosis and mitochondrial cytopathy, which are characterized by megaduodenum, multiple small bowel diverticula, and pneumatosis intestinalis.
2. *Assess gastric and small bowel motility.* After mechanical obstruction and alternative diagnoses such as Crohn disease (Chapter 127) have been excluded, a transit profile of the stomach should be performed using a radiolabeled solid meal followed by scintigraphy at 0, 1, 2, 3, 4, and 6 hours, or a stable isotope breath test. Delayed gastric emptying is associated with symptoms of gastroparesis.[4] If the underlying cause of the motility disturbance is known, it is usually unnecessary to pursue further diagnostic testing. If the cause is unclear, gastroduodenal manometry by use of a multilumen tube with sensors in the distal stomach and proximal small intestine can differentiate a neuropathic process (normal-amplitude contractions but abnormal patterns of contractility) from a myopathic process (low-amplitude contractions in the affected segments, typically <10 mm Hg in the small intestine). A wireless motility capsule also can assess contraction amplitude if the intestine is not dilated to more than 5 cm. Manometry may also identify pylorospasm, which may respond to per-oral endoscopic myotomy.
3. *Identify the pathogenesis* (see Table 122-1). Other tests for neuropathic causes assess autonomic dysfunction (Chapter 389), autoantibodies associated with paraneoplastic syndromes, and brain stem function. In patients with a myopathic disorder of unclear cause, the evaluation should consider amyloidosis (immunoglobulin electrophoresis, fat aspirate, or rectal biopsy; Chapter 174), systemic sclerosis (topoisomerase I; Chapter 246), and thyroid disease (Chapter 207). In appropriate settings, porphyria (Chapter 194) and Chagas disease (Chapter 318) may need to be excluded. Diabetes mellitus (Chapter 210) is associated with gastroparesis, pylorospasm, intestinal pseudo-obstruction, diarrhea, constipation, and fecal incontinence.[5] In refractory cases, genetic testing or full-thickness biopsy of the small intestine (E-Fig. 122-2) may be required to identify metabolic muscle disorders and mitochondrial cytopathies (Chapter 389).
4. *Identify complications of the motility disorder, including bacterial overgrowth, dehydration, and malnutrition.* In patients presenting with diarrhea, it is important to assess nutritional status and to exclude bacterial overgrowth by culture of small bowel aspirates or glucose-hydrogen breath test (Chapter 126). Bacterial overgrowth is relatively uncommon in neuropathic disorders but is found more often in myopathic conditions, such as scleroderma, that are associated more often with dilation or low-amplitude contractions. An empirical trial of antibiotics (see later) often is used instead of formal testing.

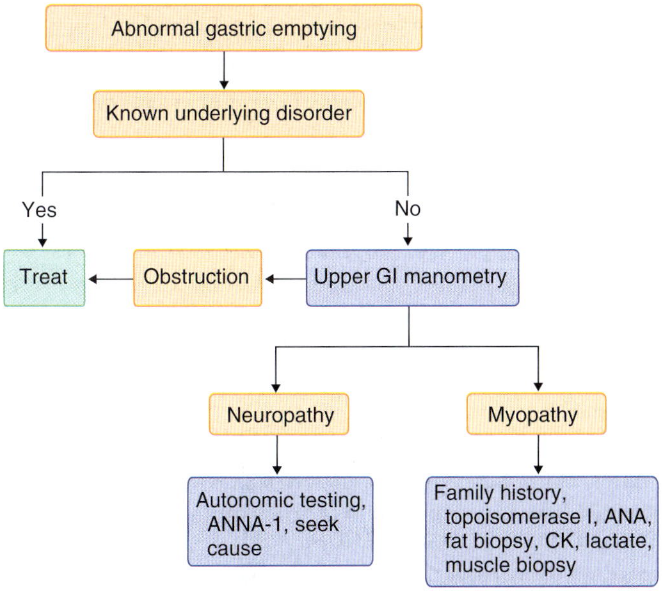

FIGURE 122-2. Flow diagram outlines steps in diagnosis of idiopathic gastroparesis and intestinal pseudo-obstruction. ANA = antinuclear antibody; ANNA-1 = type 1 antineuronal nuclear antibody; CK = creatine kinase; GI = gastrointestinal.

TREATMENT

Rehydration, electrolyte repletion, and nutritional supplementation are particularly important during acute exacerbations of gastroparesis and chronic intestinal pseudo-obstruction. Initial nutritional measures include small solid particle meals (blenderized solids) or low-fiber liquid food supplements with the addition of iron, folate, calcium, and vitamins D, K, and B_{12} at the usually recommended daily levels. In patients with more severe symptoms, enteral or parenteral supplementation may be required.[6] If it is anticipated that enteral supplementation may be needed for more than 3 months, a jejunostomy feeding tube is recommended. These tubes may be placed with the aid of endoscopy. Gastrostomy tubes should be avoided in patients with gastroparesis except for venting purposes.

Medical Therapy

Prokinetic Agents

Medications often can enhance gastric emptying and improve symptoms in patients with neuromuscular motility disorders.[A1] Tradipitant (an experimental antagonist of tachykinin receptor 1 given orally at 85 mg twice daily) can significantly reduce nausea and vomiting in patients with diabetic or idiopathic gastroparesis.[A2] Aprepitant (125 mg/day for 4 weeks) also appears to be efficacious for gastroparesis and related disorders.[A3]

Erythromycin, a macrolide antibiotic that stimulates motilin receptors at higher doses (250 to 500 mg) and cholinergic mechanisms at lower doses (40 to 80 mg) accelerates gastric emptying in gastroparesis. Erythromycin is most effective when it is used intravenously (3 mg/kg every 8 hours by slow infusion) during acute exacerbations of gastroparesis. Efficacy wanes over 14 days because of tachyphylaxis. Pyridostigmine (30 to 60 mg every 6 hours tablet or liquid formulation) is also sometimes used. In patients who do not respond to other treatments, metoclopramide (a dopamine antagonist with mild prokinetic and antiemetic properties) can be useful for up to 3 months as a rapid oral disintegrating tablet, intranasal spray, elixir, or parenteral preparation. It should be taken orally (15 to 30 minutes before meals and at bedtime). Usual doses are 5 to 10 mg four times daily, but patients may experience side effects (changes in affect, anxiety) at relatively low doses (even 30 to 40 mg/day).

Domperidone (10 to 20 mg, three times per day before meals) is another dopamine antagonist available through an investigational drug application to the U.S. Food and Drug Administration and local Institutional Review Board. Its efficacy appears similar to metoclopramide, with lower risk of involuntary movements. Domperidone-induced cardiac arrhythmias may occur in patients with specific polymorphisms in the cytochrome P-450 3A4 gene, which encodes the enzyme that metabolizes domperidone (Chapter 25). Genetic screening is not recommended in any guidelines.

Experimental medications for gastroparesis include relamorelin, an agonist of ghrelin receptor (given subcutaneously once or twice daily), which can speed gastric emptying and improve the symptoms of gastroparesis in diabetic patients,[A4] and felcisetrag, an intravenous 5-HT4 receptor agonist, which accelerates gastric emptying in idiopathic and diabetic gastroparesis.[A5]

Antiemetic Agents

Antiemetics (Table 118-5), including diphenhydramine (25 mg orally up to two times per day for up to 3 months) and promethazine (orally or by suppository, 25 mg up to two times per day) can treat nausea and vomiting in patients with gastroparesis and intestinal pseudo-obstruction. The serotonin 5-HT$_3$ antagonists (e.g., ondansetron, 4 or 8 mg tablet or oral dissolution tablet; or granisetron which is available as a transdermal patch) also may be used.

Other Approaches

Octreotide (50 µg subcutaneously at bedtime), a cyclized analogue of somatostatin, induces small intestinal activity that mimics phase III of the interdigestive migrating motor complex. It actually retards gastric emptying and small bowel transit. Octreotide may be used before sleep to sweep residue toward the colon and to avoid bacterial overgrowth.

Antibiotic therapy, typically using different antibiotics for 7 to 10 days each month in an attempt to avoid bacterial resistance, is indicated in patients with documented, symptomatic bacterial overgrowth. Common antibiotics include doxycycline (50 to 100 mg twice daily), metronidazole (250 mg three times daily), and double-strength trimethoprim-sulfamethoxazole (two tablets twice daily). Use of antibiotics in patients with diarrhea and fat malabsorption secondary to bacterial overgrowth results in significant symptomatic relief.

Surgical and Endoscopic Therapy

Surgical decompression is rarely necessary in patients with chronic pseudo-obstruction. Venting enterostomy (jejunostomy) is effective, however, in relieving abdominal distention and bloating and in reducing the frequency with which nasogastric intubations and hospitalizations are required for acute exacerbations compared with the period before vent placement. Access to the small intestine by enterostomy also provides a means to deliver nutrients and should be considered in patients with intermittent symptoms. Surgical treatment should be considered whenever the motility disorder is localized to a resectable portion of the gut: completion gastrectomy for patients with post–gastric surgical stasis syndrome, and colectomy with ileorectostomy for intractable constipation associated with chronic colonic pseudo-obstruction.

Gastric electrical stimulation may improve symptoms in some patients with severe gastroparesis.[A6] Botulinum injection of the pylorus, followed if successful by gastric per-oral endoscopic myotomy or pyloric surgery, is a promising therapy for troublesome cases.[7]

Small bowel transplantation currently is limited to patients who have intestinal failure and reversible liver disease induced by total parenteral nutrition or who have life-threatening or recurrent catheter-related sepsis. Isolated transplantation of the small intestine is associated with higher graft and patient survival and fewer complications related to rejection and infection.

DISEASES OF RAPID TRANSIT THROUGH STOMACH AND SMALL BOWEL

DUMPING SYNDROME AND ACCELERATED GASTRIC EMPTYING

Dumping syndrome and accelerated gastric emptying typically follow truncal vagotomy and gastric drainage procedures (Chapter 125), fundoplication for gastric esophageal reflux disease (Chapter 124), or bariatric procedures such as sleeve gastrectomy or Roux-en-Y gastric bypass. A high calorie (usually carbohydrate) content of the liquid phase of the meal evokes a rapid insulin response with secondary hypoglycemia.

The management of dumping syndrome and accelerated gastric emptying emphasizes dietary maneuvers, such as avoidance of high-nutrient liquid drinks and possibly addition of guar gum or pectin to retard gastric emptying of liquids. Pharmacologic treatment with octreotide, 25 to 100 µg subcutaneously before meals, retards intestinal transit and inhibits the hormonal responses that lead to hypoglycemia.

RAPID TRANSIT DYSMOTILITY OF THE SMALL BOWEL

Rapid transit of material through the small bowel may occur in postvagotomy diarrhea (Chapter 126), short bowel syndrome (Chapter 126), diabetic diarrhea (Chapter 126), and carcinoid diarrhea (Chapter 213) and result in significant losses of fluid and electrolytes. Ileal resection or disease and idiopathic bile acid malabsorption may induce colonic secretion and secondary diarrhea. Accelerated transit may be confirmed by scintigraphic studies.

Treatment goals are to restore hydration and nutrition and to slow small bowel transit by avoiding hyperosmolar drinks and replacing with iso-osmolar or hypo-osmolar oral rehydration solutions. The fat content in the diet should be reduced to approximately 50 g/day to avoid delivery of unabsorbed fat to the colon. All electrolyte and nutritional deficiencies of calcium, magnesium, potassium, and water-soluble and fat-soluble vitamins should be corrected. In patients with less than 1 m of residual small bowel, it may be impossible to maintain fluid and electrolyte homeostasis without parenteral support. In patients with a longer residual intestinal segment, oral nutrition, pharmacotherapy, and supplements are almost always effective.

The opioid agent loperamide (2 to 4 mg 30 minutes before meals and at bedtime for a total dose of 16 mg/day) suppresses the motor response to feeding and improves symptoms. Bile acid binding, such as with cholestyramine (4 g three times daily) or colesevelam (1.875 g twice daily), is indicated for patients with suspected or proven bile acid malabsorption.[8] Clonidine (0.1 mg daily as oral tablet or dermal patch) or a 5-HT_3 antagonist (e.g., ondansetron, 4 to 8 mg three times daily) is used rarely in addition to loperamide. Octreotide (50 µg subcutaneously three times daily, 5 minutes before meals) may be used in patients for whom the oral agents are ineffective or poorly tolerated.

COLONIC MOTILITY DISORDERS

Constipation

EPIDEMIOLOGY

Constipation is a common clinical problem, reported by about 20% of the population, and 40% of Americans report needing to strain excessively to pass their bowel movements.[9]

PATHOBIOLOGY

In functional constipation, transit is normal, and there is no evacuation disorder. These patients may have pain in association with constipation, and there is overlap with constipation-predominant irritable bowel syndrome (Chapter 123). In patients with acquired slow-transit constipation, unassociated with colonic dilation, the number of interstitial cells of Cajal in the different layers of the colon is reduced compared with controls.

Idiopathic megarectum and megacolon can be either congenital or acquired; an enteric nervous system defect is suspected. In megacolon, the dilated segment shows normal phasic contractility but decreased colonic tone, with smooth muscle hypertrophy and fibrosis of the muscularis mucosa, circular muscle, and longitudinal muscle layers.

Acquired defects in the enteric nervous system may result in constipation in Chagas disease (Chapter 318), which is caused by infection with *Trypanosoma cruzi* and results in the destruction of myenteric neurons.

DIAGNOSIS

It is essential to distinguish an evacuation disorder, also called functional outlet obstruction (Table 122-2), from constipation resulting from slow transit or other causes.[10] In a tertiary center, about 25% of patients presenting with constipation have impaired evacuation, and the remainder have constipation associated with either normal transit (also called functional constipation) or delayed colonic transit (also called slow-transit constipation). Characterization of constipated patients without rectal evacuation disorders (Fig. 122-3) relies on the measurement of transit with radiopaque markers or scintigraphy.

TABLE 122-2 CLINICAL CLUES SUGGESTIVE OF AN EVACUATION DISORDER

HISTORY
Prolonged straining to expel stool
Taking up unusual postures on the toilet to facilitate stool expulsion
Support of perineum or digitation of rectum or vagina to facilitate rectal emptying
Inability to expel enema fluid
Constipation after subtotal colectomy for constipation
RECTAL EXAMINATION (WITH PATIENT IN LEFT LATERAL POSITION)
Inspection
Anus "pulled" forward during attempts to simulate strain during defecation
Anal verge descends <1 cm or >4 cm during attempts to simulate strain during defecation
Perineum balloons down during straining, and rectal mucosa prolapses through anus
Palpation
High anal sphincter tone at rest precludes easy entry of examining finger (in absence of painful perianal condition, e.g., anal fissure)
Anal sphincter pressure during voluntary squeeze is minimally higher than tone at rest
Perineum descends <1 cm or >4 cm during attempts to simulate strain during defecation
Puborectalis muscle palpable through posterior rectal wall is tender
Palpable mucosal prolapse during straining
"Defect" in anterior wall of the rectum, suggestive of rectocele
ANORECTAL MANOMETRY AND BALLOON EXPULSION (WITH PATIENT IN LEFT LATERAL POSITION)
Average anal sphincter resting tone >80 cm H_2O or squeeze pressure >240 cm H_2O
Failure of balloon expulsion despite addition of 200 g weight
ABDOMINO-PELVIC RADIOGRAPH
Rectal gas area >9 cm^2

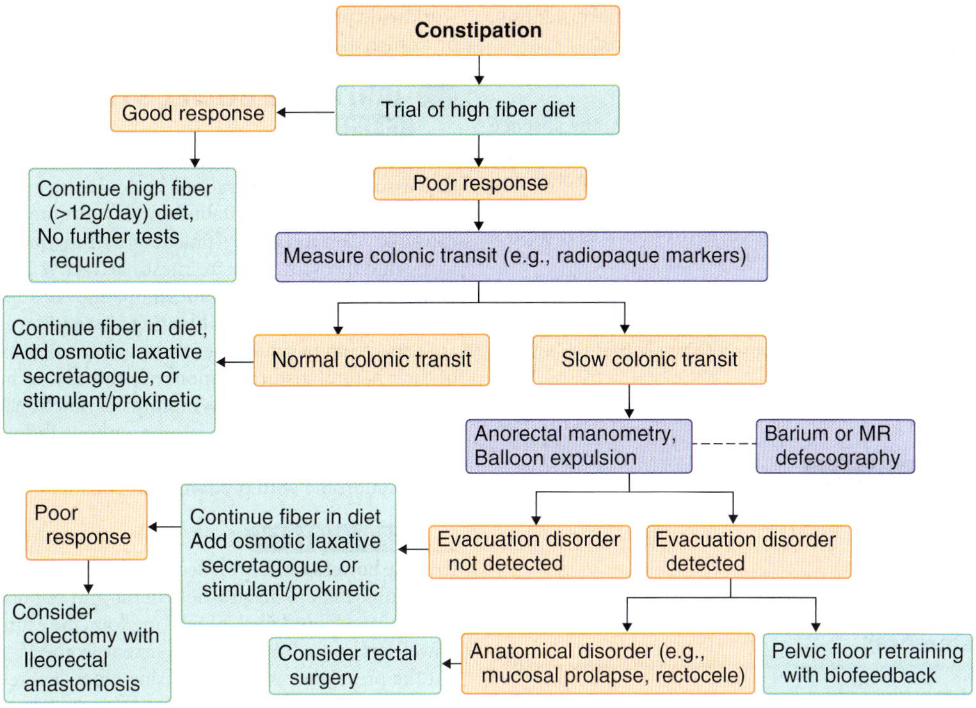

FIGURE 122-3. Algorithm in the management of constipation.

TREATMENT

The average daily fiber intake is around 12 g/day. In patients with normal-transit constipation, 20 to 30 g/day is effective to relieve constipation. In patients with slow-transit constipation, drug-induced constipation, or evacuation disorders, however, supplementation of 30 g of fiber per day does not result in any improvement in constipation. A second step is to add an osmotic laxative, such as a magnesium salt[A7] or polyethylene glycol solution, to enhance the retention of fluid within the lumen by osmotic forces, to increase fluidity, and to facilitate aboral transport of colonic contents. If these measures do not suffice, a prokinetic or stimulant agent,[11] such as bisacodyl (5 to 10 mg every 1 to 2 days) may be added (Table 122-3).[A8]

In more difficult-to-treat cases, prucalopride (1 to 2 mg daily) accelerates colonic transit and is beneficial in chronic constipation.[A9] Other pharmacologic approaches include lubiprostone (24 µg twice daily); linaclotide (72 µg, 145 µg, or 290 µg daily), or plecanatide (3 mg). These drugs as well as naloxegol (a peripheral µ-opioid antagonist at 12.5 or 25 mg daily), methylnaltrexone (0.15 mg/kg subcutaneously every other day for 2 weeks or 450 mg/day orally), naldemedine (0.2 mg daily), and the combination of oxycodone with naloxone (the latter displaces oxycodone from µ-opioid receptors in the gut) are effective in patients with opiate-induced constipation as a complication of advanced illness or noncancer pain.[A10]

When these approaches do not work, the patient should be reassessed to exclude an evacuation disorder (Chapter 131). For evacuation disorders, a biofeedback treatment program with muscle relaxation of the anal sphincters and pelvic floor results in a 70% or greater cure rate for the constipation.

Surgical Therapy

In patients whose constipation is not associated with an evacuation disorder and does not respond to aggressive medical therapies (including combinations described earlier), laparoscopic colectomy with ileorectostomy is effective in relieving constipation.

TABLE 122-3 TREATMENTS FOR CHRONIC CONSTIPATION

IDIOPATHIC CONSTIPATION
Bulk Agents
Psyllium (10 g daily), methylcellulose, calcium polycarbophil, wheat dextrin
Nonabsorbed Substances
PEG 3350 (17 g daily)
Lactulose (20 g daily)
Magnesium hydroxide (1 g daily)
Stimulants
Bisacodyl (5-10 mg daily)
Senna (8.6 mg, 2 to 4 tabs daily)
Prucalopride (1-2 mg daily)
Secretory Drugs
Lubiprostone (24 µg twice daily)*
Linaclotide (72 µg, 145 µg, or 290 µg daily)
Plecanatide (3 mg daily)
OPIOID-INDUCED CONSTIPATION
Opioid Receptor Antagonists
Naloxegol (12.5-25 mg daily)
Naloxone/oxycodone (20 mg/40 mg)
Methylnaltrexone (0.15 mg/kg subcutaneously every other day for 2 weeks or 450 mg orally per day)
Naldemedine (0.2 mg daily)

*Also indicated for opioid-induced constipation.
PEG 3350 = polyethylene glycol-electrolyte.
Adapted from Wald A. Constipation: advances in diagnosis and treatment. *JAMA.* 2016;315:185-191.

HIRSCHSPRUNG DISEASE

DEFINITION

Hirschsprung disease occurs in 1 in 5000 live births. It is characterized by a localized segment of narrowing of the distal colon as a result of failure of local development of intrinsic nerves in the myenteric plexus.[12]

PATHOBIOLOGY

A relative deficiency of *KIT*-positive interstitial cells of Cajal has been reported in Hirschsprung disease and chronic intestinal pseudo-obstruction. The majority of familial and sporadic Hirschsprung disease is associated with *RET* oncogene mutations, but mutations in *EDNRB, GDNF*, and *EDN3* have been reported as well. Hirschsprung disease is well characterized histologically by the absence of ganglion cells in the myenteric and submucosal plexus and the presence of hypertrophied nerve trunks in the space normally occupied by the ganglion cells. In the muscle layers of the colon involved with Hirschsprung disease, deficiency of nerve growth factor receptors also contributes to the dysfunction. The narrowing and failure of relaxation in the aganglionic segment are thought to be due to the lack of neurons containing nitric oxide synthase.

CLINICAL MANIFESTATIONS

Hirschsprung disease is usually diagnosed at birth because of failure to pass meconium or the presence of megacolon, although it may be identified in childhood as a result of fecal retention, constipation, or abdominal distention. Onset of symptoms or diagnosis after the age of 10 years is rare.

DIAGNOSIS

Diagnosis is based on the typical focal narrowing of the colon, the absence of the rectoanal inhibitory reflex (relaxation of anal sphincter pressure at rest during distention of a balloon in the rectum depends on natural preservation and maturation of intrinsic nerves in the distal bowel), and a deep rectal biopsy specimen showing absence of submucosal neurons with hypertrophied nerve trunks.

TREATMENT

Treatment involves excision of the affected bowel segment or a pull-through procedure by which normal bowel is anastomosed to the cuff of the lower rectum, just above the anal sphincters.

GENERAL REFERENCES

For the General References and other additional features, please visit Elsevier eBooks+ at https://ebooks.health.elsevier.com.

Grade A References

A1. Vijayvargiya P, Camilleri M, Chedid V, et al. Effects of promotility agents on gastric emptying and symptoms: a systematic review and meta-analysis. *Gastroenterology*. 2019;156:1650-1660.

A2. Carlin JL, Liberman VR, Dahal A, et al. Efficacy and safety of tradipitant in patients with diabetic and idiopathic gastroparesis in a randomized, placebo-controlled trial. *Gastroenterology*. 2021;160:76-87.e4.

A3. Pasricha PJ, Yates KP, Sarosiek I, et al. Aprepitant has mixed effects on nausea and reduces other symptoms in patients with gastroparesis and related disorders. *Gastroenterology*. 2018;154:65-76.

A4. Camilleri M, McCallum RW, Tack J, et al. Efficacy and safety of relamorelin in diabetics with symptoms of gastroparesis: a randomized, placebo-controlled study. *Gastroenterology*. 2017;153:1240-1250.

A5. Chedid V, Brandler J, Arndt K, et al. Randomised study: effects of the 5 HT4 receptor agonist felcisetrag versus placebo on gut transit in patients with gastroparesis. *Aliment Pharmacol Ther*. 2021;53:1010-1020.

A6. Ducrotte P, Coffin B, Bonaz B, et al. Gastric electrical stimulation reduces refractory vomiting in a randomized crossover trial. *Gastroenterology*. 2020;158:506-514.e2.

A7. Morishita D, Tomita T, Mori S, et al. Senna versus magnesium oxide for the treatment of chronic constipation: a randomized, placebo-controlled trial. *Am J Gastroenterol*. 2021;116:152-161.

A8. Rao SSC, Brenner DM. Efficacy and safety of over-the-counter therapies for chronic constipation: an updated systematic review. *Am J Gastroenterol*. 2021;116:1156-1181.

A9. Luthra P, Camilleri M, Burr NE, et al. Efficacy of drugs in chronic idiopathic constipation: a systematic review and network meta-analysis. *Lancet Gastroenterol Hepatol*. 2019;4:831-844.

A10. Vijayvargiya P, Camilleri M, Vijayvargiya P, et al. Systematic review with meta-analysis: efficacy and safety of treatments for opioid-induced constipation. *Aliment Pharmacol Ther*. 2020;52:37-53.

123 IRRITABLE BOWEL AND FUNCTIONAL UPPER GASTROINTESTINAL SYNDROMES

LIN CHANG

Functional gastrointestinal disorders are a spectrum of chronic gastrointestinal disorders that are characterized by specific symptoms depending on the region that is involved.[1] Functional gastrointestinal disorders have been traditionally known to be syndromes without a structural or biochemical basis to explain their clinical features. However, alterations in the bidirectional communication between the brain and the gut are increasingly being implicated in their motility disturbances, visceral hypersensitivity, altered mucosal and immune function, altered gut microbiota, and altered central nervous system (CNS) processing, all of which may vary among individuals or even in the same individual over time. As a result, these conditions are now referred to as disorders of gut-brain interaction.

The most current and widely used classification system is the Rome IV diagnostic criteria, which has defined a number of functional gastrointestinal disorders, by far the most common of which are irritable bowel syndrome, functional dyspepsia, and functional heartburn. Based on these criteria, the worldwide prevalence of functional gastrointestinal disorders is estimated to be as high as 40%.[2]

IRRITABLE BOWEL SYNDROME

DEFINITION

Irritable bowel syndrome is characterized by chronic or recurrent abdominal pain associated with alterations in stool form and/or frequency (i.e., diarrhea and/or constipation). Irritable bowel syndrome, which is frequently diagnosed in primary care and referral practices, is a functional bowel disorder attributable to the middle or lower gastrointestinal tract. It also includes functional constipation (also known as chronic idiopathic constipation), functional diarrhea, and functional abdominal bloating/distention. Functional bowel disorders are a spectrum of syndromes that can transition to another over time because of their natural history, response to therapy, or both. For example, a patient may initially present with symptoms of functional constipation, such as hard and infrequent stools and straining without abdominal pain, but later develop abdominal pain associated with constipation and meet criteria for irritable bowel syndrome with predominant constipation.

EPIDEMIOLOGY

Irritable bowel syndrome is seen worldwide, but its prevalence varies based on geographic region, diagnostic criteria, and population studied. In the United States, Canada, and the United Kingdom, the estimated prevalence of irritable bowel syndrome based on the current Rome IV diagnostic criteria is 4.6%,[3] but the prevalence was higher using older, less restrictive criteria. In a global epidemiology study in 33 countries on six continents, the worldwide prevalence of irritable bowel syndrome was 4.1% based upon Rome IV criteria, but it was more common in women (5.2%) than in men (2.9%).[4] Using predominantly a physician's diagnosis of irritable bowel syndrome, the estimated incidence is about 38 per 10,000 person-years.

The three main subtypes of irritable bowel syndrome are based upon the usual stool form (i.e., irritable bowel syndrome with predominant constipation, irritable bowel syndrome with predominant diarrhea, and irritable bowel syndrome with mixed bowel habits). Patients who have irritable bowel syndrome but whose stool form pattern does not meet criteria for one of these three bowel habit subtypes is defined as having irritable bowel syndrome unclassified. Using Rome IV criteria, irritable bowel syndrome with predominant diarrhea and irritable bowel syndrome with mixed bowel habits each accounted for 35 to 40% of irritable bowel patients, irritable bowel syndrome with predominant constipation accounted for about 25%, and less than 5% were irritable bowel syndrome unclassified. However, the subtypes of irritable syndrome can transition over time in the same patient.

Up to 50% of individuals with symptoms of irritable bowel syndrome do not seek health care, but functional bowel disorders are nevertheless estimated to generate about 4.4 million annual physician visits.[5] When they do seek health care, patients with irritable bowel syndrome are more likely to have diagnostic tests and abdominal or pelvic surgeries compared with other patients, although many of these interventions are neither necessary nor recommended by professional society guidelines. Health care–seeking about irritable bowel syndrome symptoms is associated with older age, a higher level of concern about bowel function, bloating, and a greater impact on social activities. Patients with irritable bowel syndrome also have increased health care visits and costs associated with nongastrointestinal symptoms as well as a significant comorbidity from other somatic and psychological disorders. In addition to increased direct medical expenses, irritable bowel syndrome is associated with absenteeism from work and impaired work productivity.

PATHOBIOLOGY

Irritable bowel syndrome is a multifactorial disorder that results from a dysregulation of gut-brain interactions, thereby resulting in alterations of intestinal motility, visceral perception, autonomic nervous system function, stress responsiveness, mucosal and immune function, gut microbiota, and CNS modulation of viscerosensory input. Risk factors that increase the risk of developing irritable bowel syndrome and of triggering symptomatic flares include genetic predisposition, environmental factors (e.g., adverse childhood experiences and infectious gastroenteritis), food, and stress.

Familial and Genetic Factors

Irritable bowel syndrome clusters in families, and the odds of having affected relatives are 1.75-fold to 2.75-fold higher than among relatives of unaffected persons. However, compelling evidence shows that environmental factors also influence the presence of irritable bowel syndrome, potentially to a greater degree than genetic heritability.

Large genome-wide association studies have found that polymorphisms on chromosome 9q31.2 are significantly more common in women but not men with irritable bowel syndrome compared with controls. Another large study found six independent susceptibility loci. Four of these six loci also have been associated with mood and anxiety disorders and/or genes expressed in the nervous system, thereby suggesting a key role for neuronal pathways within the brain-gut axis.

About 2 to 3% of patients with irritable bowel syndrome have rare genetic variants that may result in a functional abnormality at the level of the gastrointestinal tract.[6] These variants include functional polymorphisms of the voltage-gated channel $Na_v1.5$ (*SCN5A*) causing a channelopathy and potentially a loss of function in voltage dependence or mechanosensitivity and sucrase-isomaltase gene variants indicative of reduced levels of a disaccharide enzyme that may protect against chronic diarrhea. Other associations include a homozygous short allele of the serotonin transporter gene (*5-HTTLPR*) and polymorphisms in the genes that encode for serotonin type 3 receptors. However, all these findings must be interpreted cautiously until treatment studies validate their causality.

Postinfection Irritable Bowel Syndrome

The strongest risk factor for irritable bowel syndrome, especially irritable bowel syndrome with predominant diarrhea, is an acute gastrointestinal infection, which increases the risk of irritable bowel syndrome at 12 months by about four-fold regardless of whether the infection was bacterial, protozoal/parasitic, or viral in nature.[7] The risk is especially increased in individuals who are younger, female, or have a history of gastroesophageal reflux disease, dyspepsia, more severe diarrheal illness, anxiety, or depression.

Stressful Life Events

An important risk factor for the development and exacerbations of irritable bowel syndrome is stressful life events.[8] Implicated stressful life events include physical, sexual, or emotional/verbal abuse; history of severe illness; death or mental illness of a parent; incarceration of an individual in the household; and exposure to wartime conditions.

Increased Visceral Perception

The perception of gut stimuli is influenced by the integrated activity and communication among the gut lumen, mucosa, submucosa, enteric nervous system, and CNS.[9,10] Stimuli within the gut (e.g., contractile activity, distension) are detected and transmitted via primary afferent nerves that project to the dorsal horn of the spinal cord, with neurons located in the dorsal root ganglia. This sensory input ascends along the dorsal column and then to the contralateral ventroposterolateral nucleus of the thalamus, brainstem nuclei, and cortical regions. Visceral stimuli are assessed by the salience network and insula, which assess the importance of these signals and whether they are perceived as normal gut sensations, abdominal discomfort, or pain. The two main brain output systems to the gut are the autonomic nervous system and descending pain modulatory pathways. The autonomic nervous system regulates and modulates gut motility, immune responses, and sensation, whereas the pain facilitatory and inhibitory pathways regulate pain sensitivity at the level of the spinal cord's dorsal neurons, which receive afferent visceral input.

Increased perception of visceral stimuli and symptoms of irritable bowel syndrome develop from either greater sensitivity of visceral afferent pathways (peripheral sensitization) or central amplification of visceral afferent input at the level of the brain and spinal cord (central sensitization). Peripheral sensitization of sensory nerves occurs when nerves are activated by mediators released from immune and/or epithelial cells, such as occurs in inflammation or infection.

Patients with irritable bowel syndrome have overall lowered thresholds for pain or discomfort when exposed to rectal or colonic balloon distension (i.e., visceral hypersensitivity) compared with healthy individuals. However, this hypersensitivity typically is seen only in a subset of patients with irritable bowel syndrome and only modestly correlates with the severity of their symptoms.

Altered CNS Processing and Modulation

Multimodal brain imaging studies have demonstrated both structural and functional alterations in task-related brain networks in patients with irritable bowel syndrome. Neuroimaging findings associated with irritable bowel syndrome include greater volume and cortical thickness of the sensorimotor cortex that correlates with the severity of symptoms; alterations in resting state functional connectivity of the anterior insula and amygdala; greater engagement of the salience detection and emotional arousal networks in response to rectal balloon distension; decreased corticolimbic inhibitory feedback; and increased activation of the central autonomic network that regulates autonomic nervous system response. These findings support the role of the CNS and brain-gut interactions in irritable bowel syndrome pathophysiology.

Gut Transit and Motility

Alterations in small intestinal and colonic motility in irritable bowel syndrome include increased colonic motility during fasting, in the postprandial state, and with psychological or physical stressors. A subset of patients with irritable bowel syndrome with predominant diarrhea have a more rapid intestinal transit time that can be induced by psychological and physical stress. About 50% of patients with irritable bowel syndrome with predominant diarrhea have accelerated colon transit times.

Peripheral Gastrointestinal Factors

The gut is composed of a network of cells and mediators that affect gastrointestinal function and contribute to the symptoms of irritable bowel syndrome. This peripheral gut network can communicate with the brain via multiple routes, including neural, endocrine, and inflammatory pathways. The brain-to-gut communication is mainly mediated via the autonomic nervous system pathways to the gut.

Patients with irritable bowel syndrome have an increase in colonic mucosal nerves that express substance P, transient receptor potential vanilloid type 1 cannabinoid, and protease-activated receptors. Some patients with irritable bowel syndrome have altered mucosal barrier function and decreased expression of tight junction proteins in the jejunum and colon. Increased permeability has been associated with greater severity of abdominal pain, visceral hyperalgesia, and altered bowel habits. Immune activation involving mast cells and T lymphocytes may mediate dysfunction of the intestinal barrier, abnormalities in motility, and visceral pain in irritable bowel syndromes.

Increased immune activation has been demonstrated in the colonic mucosa of patients with irritable bowel syndromes, including increased numbers of mast cells adjacent to sensory neurons in the colonic mucosa. Mast cells release mediators such as histamine that may activate afferent nerves and result in peripheral sensitization and increased abdominal pain. Disruption of the mucosal barrier associated with changes in expression of tight junction proteins in response to food allergens suggests that patients with irritable bowel syndrome have nonclassical food allergies that may contribute to postprandial symptoms.

The fecal microbiota of patients with irritable bowel syndrome often shows an abundance of Enterobacteriaceae, family Lactobacillaceae, and genus *Bacteroides*, as well as decreased amount of Clostridiales I, genus *Faecalibacterium*, and genus *Bifidobacterium*.[11] These findings have biologic plausibility because the microbes that are increased in irritable bowel syndrome produce organic acids (e.g., lactic acid), reduce mucosal glycoproteins, or contain pathogenic bacteria. The microbes that are decreased in irritable bowel syndrome produce butyrate, which is an energy source for epithelial cells, have anti-inflammatory effects, and are thought to maintain gut health. About 25% patients with irritable bowel syndrome have bile acid diarrhea.

Dysregulated Stress Responsiveness

Growing evidence supports that irritable bowel syndrome is a stress-sensitive disorder. The stress of the hypothalamic-pituitary-adrenal axis is dysregulated in response to experimental stress or hormone challenge in patients with irritable bowel syndrome compared with healthy controls. This stress can increase visceral sensitivity, gut motility and permeability, and immune responses.

CLINICAL MANIFESTATIONS

The hallmark feature of irritable bowel syndrome is chronic or recurrent pain that is associated with diarrhea, constipation, or both.[12] Postprandial symptoms, which are reported by about two thirds of patients, include abdominal pain, bloating, and flatulence. Meal-related symptoms are often triggered by larger meals, foods rich in carbohydrates or fats, coffee, alcohol, and spicy foods.

Women with irritable bowel syndrome are more likely to have constipation and less likely to have diarrhea compared with men. Symptoms can worsen just prior to menses, when estrogen and progesterone levels decline. Irritable bowel syndrome is also more commonly diagnosed in patients under age 50 years.

Extraintestinal symptoms and conditions that may coexist with irritable bowel syndrome include temporomandibular joint disorder, interstitial cystitis/painful bladder syndrome, dysmenorrhea (Chapter 218), migraine headaches (Chapter 367), fibromyalgia (Chapter 253), chronic fatigue syndrome (Chapter 253), anxiety (Chapter 362), depression (Chapter 362), and somatization. Patients with irritable bowel syndrome also are more likely to report subjective sleep disturbances (Chapter 374), especially when they have more severe gastrointestinal symptoms.

In about one third of patients, irritable bowel syndrome can coexist with other functional gastrointestinal disorders, such as functional dyspepsia and functional heartburn.[13] Most patients note a decreased quality of life because of gastrointestinal symptoms, abdominal pain, and psychological stress. For example, patients often report difficulty concentrating; feeling self-conscious; and having a fear of leaving the house, traveling, or being in places without bathrooms.

DIAGNOSIS

Symptom-Based Criteria

A systematic approach with limited diagnostic testing typically is sufficient to make the diagnosis of irritable bowel syndrome (Fig. 123-1), using the symptom-based Rome IV criteria (Table 123-1).[14] The Rome criteria also can classify irritable bowel syndrome into subtypes based on the most frequent

TABLE 123-1 DIAGNOSTIC CRITERIA FOR IRRITABLE BOWEL SYNDROME

1. Symptoms:
   A. Recurrent abdominal pain (at least 1 day per week, on average, in the last 3 months) with symptoms for at least 6 months and associated with two or more of the following:
      - Related to defecation
      - Associated with a change in frequency of stool
      - Associated with a change in form (appearance) of stool

   B. Symptoms that cumulatively support the diagnosis of irritable bowel syndrome:
      - Abnormal stool frequency: ≤3 bowel movements per week or >3 bowel movements per day
      - Abnormal stool form: lumpy/hard stool or loose/watery stool
      - Defecation straining
      - Urgency
      - Feeling of incomplete bowel movement
      - Passing mucus
      - Bloating or feeling of abdominal distention
2. Absence of alarm symptoms, such as:
   - New-onset symptoms at age ≥50 years
   - Unintentional weight loss
   - Hematochezia or melena not related to hemorrhoids
   - Nocturnal diarrhea
   - Anemia
   - Palpable abdominal mass or lymphadenopathy
   - Family history of colorectal cancer, inflammatory bowel disease, or celiac disease

Adapted from Mearin F, Lacy BE, Chang L, et al. Bowel disorders. *Gastroenterology*. 2016;150:1393-1407 and Mayer EA. Functional gastrointestinal disorders: irritable bowel syndrome, dyspepsia, esophageal chest pain, and heartburn. In: Goldman L, Schafer A, eds. *Goldman-Cecil Medicine*, 26th ed. Philadelphia: Elsevier; 2020:852-859.

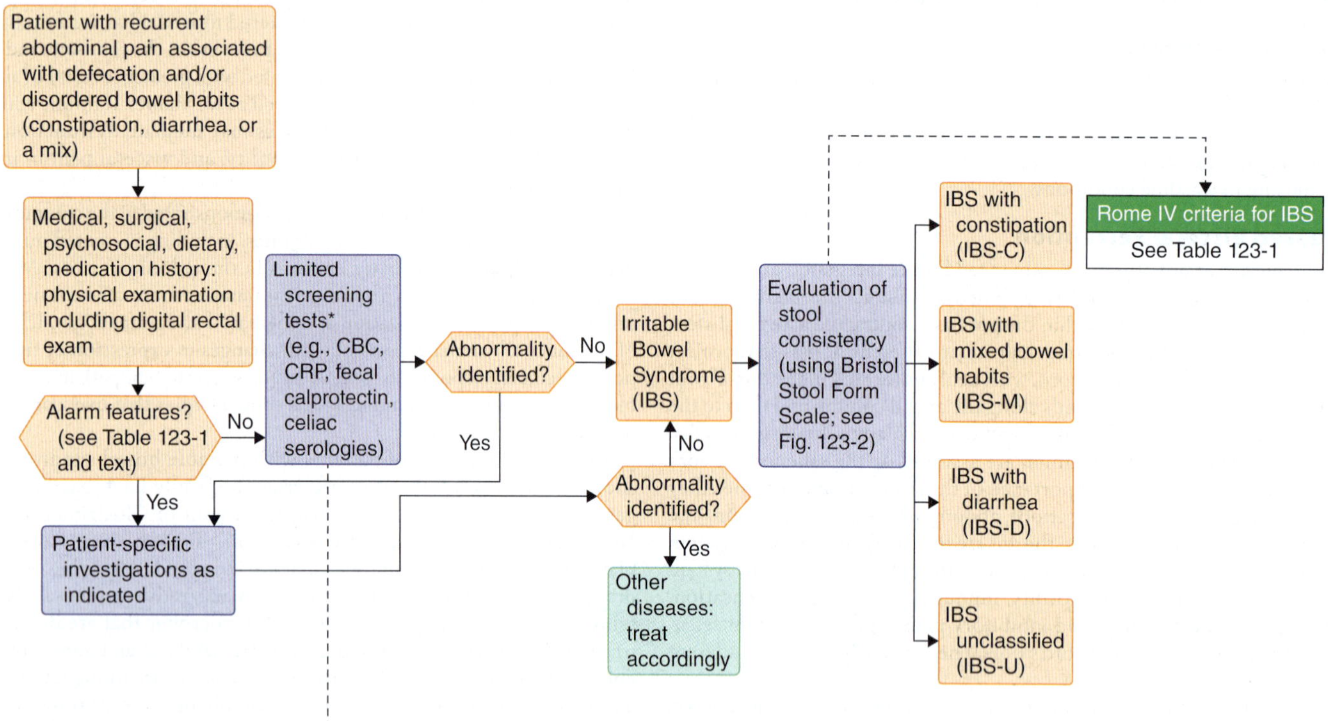

*Limited screening tests

Recommended	IBS population	Not recommended
Positive diagnostic strategy vs. diagnosis of exclusion	All IBS	Routine stool testing
Celiac serologies	IBS-D	Routine colonoscopy <45 yrs
Fecal calprotectin/lactoferrin	IBS-D	Food allergy or insensitivities testing
C-reactive protein	IBS-D	Lactulose or glucose hydrogen breath testing
Bile acid diarrhea testing	IBS-D where bile acid diarrhea is suspected	
Giardia stool antigen	IBS-D if giardia is endemic	
Anorectal physiology testing	IBS with suspected pelvic floor dysfunction and/or refractory constipation	

FIGURE 123-1. Diagnostic algorithm for irritable bowel syndrome. The recommendations for limited diagnostic testing are summarized from society guidelines. Rome IV diagnostic criteria for irritable bowel syndrome shown. CBC = complete blood count; CRP = C-reactive protein; IBS = irritable bowel syndrome. (From Chang L. How to Approach a Patient with Difficult to Treat IBS. Invited review, Gastroenterology, Mentoring, Education and Training section. *Gastroenterology* 2021;161[4]:1092-1098.)

stool form (Fig. 123-2) at a time when the patient is not taking medications to treat diarrhea or constipation.

The differential diagnosis for symptoms consistent with irritable bowel syndrome includes celiac disease (Chapter 126), inflammatory bowel disease (i.e., ulcerative colitis and Crohn disease; Chapter 127), microscopic or collagenous colitis (Chapter 126), colon cancer (Chapter 127), bile acid diarrhea (Chapter 126), and food intolerances. Alarm features or "red flags" that suggest these alternative diagnoses include the new onset of symptoms after age 50 years; rectal bleeding; weight loss; iron deficiency anemia; nocturnal diarrhea; and a family history of colon cancer, inflammatory bowel disease, or celiac disease. The presence of an alarm feature should prompt a targeted diagnostic evaluation of the clinical symptoms. However, testing often does not reveal another cause of the patient's symptoms, and many patients with red flag symptoms are ultimately diagnosed with irritable bowel syndrome.

Diagnostic Testing

Since irritable bowel syndrome is a diagnosis of exclusion, diagnostic testing (Fig. 123-1; Table 123-2) is targeted to exclude other potential causes of the patient's symptoms.[15] Guidelines recommend a serum IgA anti-tissue transglutaminase to assess for celiac disease, with a duodenal biopsy if the serologic test is positive. Since IgA deficiency is not uncommon in the general population, however, this test can be falsely negative and should be combined with a total IgA level. In

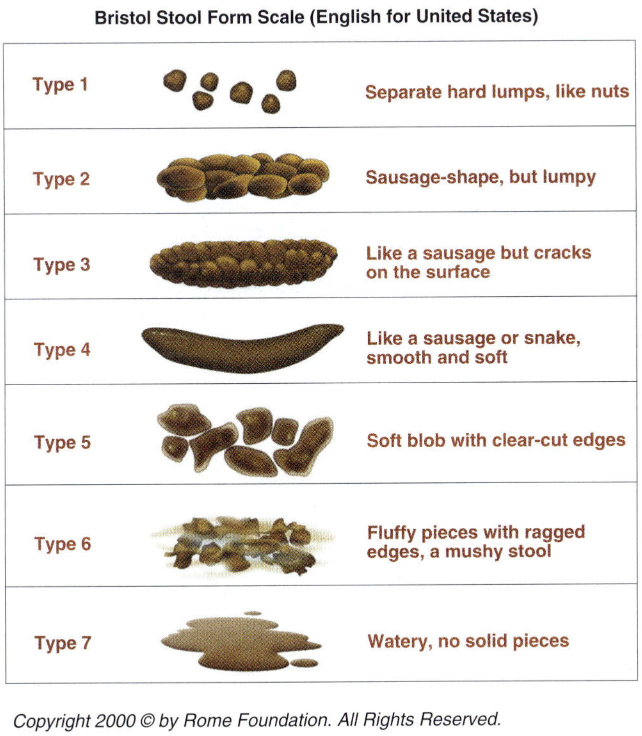

FIGURE 123-2. The Bristol Stool Form Scale. (Distributed with the kind permission of The Rome Foundation.)

TABLE 123-2 DIAGNOSTIC TESTING IN THE EVALUATION OF SUSPECTED IRRITABLE BOWEL SYNDROME

1. Generally recommended tests
Complete blood count
C-reactive protein
Fecal calprotectin/lactoferrin
Celiac serologies (IgA anti-tissue transglutaminase level and IgA level)
Colonoscopy in new-onset irritable bowel syndrome symptoms at age ≥50 years
Stool *Giardia* test (antigen or PCR) in endemic areas
Stool testing for bacteria and parasites if a relevant travel history
2. Tests generally NOT recommended
Colonoscopy if age <50 years without alarm features
Stool studies for infection without a history of travel to high-risk regions
Food allergy or intolerance testing
Lactose or glucose hydrogen breath tests

Ig = immunoglobulin; PCR = polymerase chain reaction.

IgA-deficient patients, a serum IgG anti-tissue transglutaminase level and/or an IgG deaminated gliadin peptide level should be used to screen for celiac disease.

Most guidelines do not recommend a routine colonoscopy in patients who are under the age of 45 to 50 years without alarm features.[16] If a colonoscopy is performed, random colon biopsies should be taken in patients with diarrheal symptoms to examine for microscopic or collagenous colitis.

TREATMENT

Overall Approach

A prompt and clear diagnosis can facilitate appropriate treatment in a timely manner. The patient's acceptance of the diagnosis, ability to recognize fluctuating symptom patterns, and knowledge regarding how to prevent flares and treat symptoms when they arise aids in an increased perceived sense of control over them. Providing educational resources validates irritable bowel syndrome as a real condition and empowers patients to learn how to manage their symptoms.

Treatment should consider the most bothersome symptoms, the severity of symptoms, the impact of symptoms on quality of life, the presence of comorbid conditions, psychological impact, prior treatment history, and the patient's preferences.[17–19] A clinician-patient relationship founded on effective communication is of utmost importance in providing effective care and improving patient outcomes.[20]

Mild symptoms of irritable bowel syndrome have little or no impact on the patient's quality of life and may require nothing more than a positive diagnosis of irritable bowel syndrome, education, reassurance, dietary advice, and over-the-counter medications. Moderate symptoms that affect daily activities commonly also require pharmacotherapy. Severe symptoms, which have a significant impact on quality of life, coexist with psychological distress or extraintestinal symptoms, or have failed to respond to prior treatments, require an integrated approach, usually with both pharmacologic and behavioral treatment.[21] Strategies to prevent flares include avoidance of dietary triggers and stressors that can exacerbate symptoms. For irritable bowel syndrome with predominant diarrhea (Fig. 123-2) and irritable bowel syndrome with predominant constipation (Fig. 123-3), treatments typically focus on interventions to normalize bowel habits and reduce abdominal pain.

Therapies for Multiple Types of Irritable Bowel Syndrome

Diet

Dietary treatment is a first-line treatment for irritable bowel syndrome. A 1- to 2-week food and symptom diary can help determine if symptoms are triggered by specific foods that should be avoided.[22] A diet that is low in fermentable oligosaccharides, disaccharides, monosaccharides, and polyols (FODMAPs) can improve global irritable bowel symptoms, especially in patients with predominant diarrhea, and also can reduce abdominal pain, abdominal bloating, and abnormal bowel habits.[A1,A2] This diet is best explained and supervised by a trained dietitian, who can also guide the gradual reintroduction of foods if the strict elimination diet is succesful. By comparison, a gluten-free diet is of less clear benefit, though it may be tried in patients in whom gluten products consistently exacerbate symptoms.

Soluble Fiber

Fiber supplementation (up to 25 to 35 g of psyllium fiber daily) can be beneficial, especially in patients who have predominant constipation, and can be tried in other patients as well. However, fiber may cause abdominal discomfort and gas, so lower doses should be used initially, followed by a gradual increase.[A3] Guidelines specifically recommend soluble (e.g., psyllium) but not insoluble fiber (e.g., wheat bran). Although psyllium is less likely to improve overall symptoms compared with medications, it is also less likely to cause adverse events.

Medications

Medications can help relieve the spasms, constipation, diarrhea, and pain of irritable bowel syndrome (Table 123-3).[23]

Antispasmodics and Peppermint Oil

Antispasmodic agents, which exert their potential benefits via a direct effect on intestinal smooth muscle or via anticholinergic or antimuscarinic properties, are generally efficacious for improving symptoms of irritable bowel syndrome.[24] The most common adverse events are dry mouth, dizziness, and blurred vision. Peppermint oil also is useful to relieve abdominal pain and global symptoms of irritable bowel syndrome.

Probiotics

Combination probiotic products can reduce global symptoms of irritable bowel syndrome by about 20%,[25] but data from randomized trials are mixed and so are the recommendations of various professional societies. Probiotics may be most useful in patients who have persistent bloating.

Central Brain-Gut Neuromodulators

Centrally acting brain-gut neuromodulators can be used to treat irritable bowel symptoms and not necessarily anxiety or depression. These agents, which

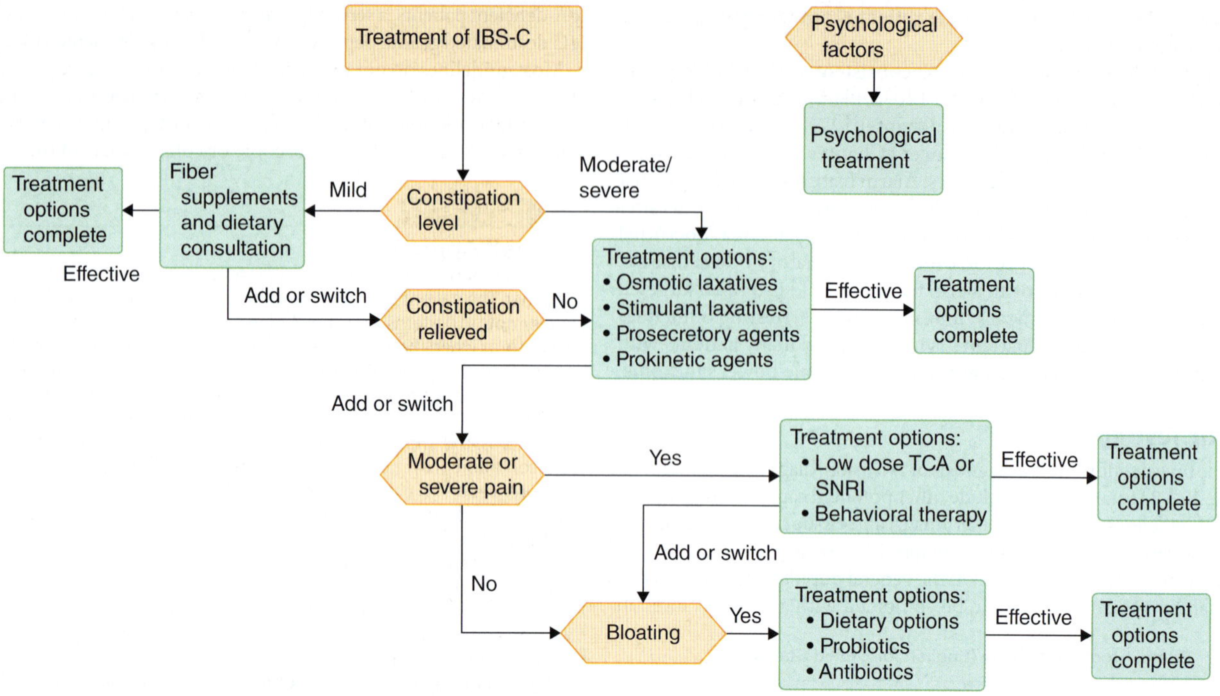

FIGURE 123-3. Treatment algorithm for irritable bowel syndrome with constipation predominance (IBS-C). SNRI = serotonin-norepinephrine reuptake inhibitor; TCA = tricyclic antidepressants. (Adapted with permission obtained from the Rome Foundation.)

TABLE 123-3 EVIDENCE-BASED ORAL TREATMENTS FOR IRRITABLE BOWEL SYNDROME

SYMPTOMS AND MEDICATION	DOSE	COMMON OR SERIOUS SIDE EFFECTS
PAIN AND SPASM		
Antispasmodics		
Peppermint oil	1 to 2 capsules three times daily or as needed	Heartburn, nausea, vomiting
Hyoscyamine	0.125 mg three to four times daily or as needed	Dry mouth, blurred vision, dizziness, constipation
Dicyclomine	10 mg three to four times daily or as needed	Dry mouth, blurred vision, dizziness
Central Neuromodulators		
Amitriptyline (TCA)	10 to 25 mg at bedtime, can increase gradually up to 100 mg at bedtime	Sedation, dry mouth, constipation
Desipramine (TCA)	10 to 25 mg at bedtime, can increase gradually up to 100 mg at bedtime	Dry mouth, dizziness
Nortriptyline (TCA)	10 to 25 mg at bedtime, can increase gradually up to 100 mg at bedtime	
Citalopram (SSRI)	5 to 20 mg daily	Sexual dysfunction, headache, nausea, sedation, insomnia, dizziness, sweating, withdrawal symptoms
Fluoxetine (SSRI)	20 to 40 mg daily	
Paroxetine (SSRI)	10 to 50 mg daily	
Sertraline (SSRI)	25 to 150 mg daily	
CONSTIPATION		
Laxatives and Secretory Modulators		
Polyethylene glycol 3350	17 g in 125 mL water daily	Nausea, bloating
Lactulose	10 g daily, can increase to 20 to 40 g daily	Diarrhea, bloating, cramping
Lubiprostone	8 μg twice daily	Nausea, diarrhea, headache, abdominal pain and discomfort
Linaclotide	290 μg daily	Diarrhea, abdominal pain, flatulence
Plecanatide	3 mg daily	Diarrhea, flatulence
Tenapanor	50 mg twice daily	Diarrhea, abdominal distension, flatulence
Prokinetic		
Tegaserod (5-HT4 agonist)	6 mg twice daily in women under age 65 years without a history of cardiovascular ischemic events	Diarrhea, headache, nausea, flatulence
DIARRHEA		
Opioid Receptor Agents		
Loperamide	2 mg, can increase up to 4 mg four times daily	Constipation
Eluxadoline	75 to 100 mg twice daily	Constipation, nausea, sphincter of Oddi dysfunction, pancreatitis
5HT3 Antagonists		
Alosetron	0.5 to 1.0 mg twice daily	Constipation, ischemic colitis (rare)

TABLE 123-3 EVIDENCE-BASED TREATMENTS FOR IRRITABLE BOWEL SYNDROME—cont'd

SYMPTOMS AND MEDICATION	DOSE	COMMON OR SERIOUS SIDE EFFECTS
Bile Acid Sequestrants		
Bile acid sequestrants (cholestyramine, colesevelam)	Cholestyramine: start at 2 to 4 g/day and titrate up to 24 g/day to response Colesevelam: two 625-mg tablets twice daily Colestipol: 1 g twice daily, can increase by 1 g/day every other day up to 16 g daily depending on response	Abdominal cramps, constipation
BLOATING		
Antibiotics		
Rifaximin	550 mg three times daily for 14 days	Abdominal pain, nausea
Probiotics		
Bifidobacterium infantis 35624	1 capsule per day	None
Activia	1 container twice daily	None

SSRI = selective serotonin reuptake inhibitor; TCA = tricyclic antidepressant.

Adapted from Mayer EA. Functional gastrointestinal disorders: irritable bowel syndrome, dyspepsia, esophageal chest pain, and heartburn. In: Goldman L, Schafer A, eds. *Goldman-Cecil Medicine*, 26th ed. Philadelphia: Elsevier; 2020:852-859.

include tricyclic antidepressants, selective serotonin reuptake inhibitors, and serotonin-norepinephrine reuptake inhibitors (see Table 362-5), may decrease pain perception by modulating the CNS processing of visceral stimuli, enhancing descending pain inhibitory pathways, decreasing the firing of primary sensory afferent nerves, altering gastrointestinal transit, and treating comorbid psychological symptoms.

Pooled data suggest that tricyclic antidepressants (Table 362-5) can improve global symptoms of irritable bowel syndrome in about 35% of patients[A4] and may be especially useful for abdominal pain. Preferred formulations are desipramine or nortriptyline (10 to 25 mg at bedtime), which are less likely to cause sedation, constipation, and dry mouth.

Selective serotonin reuptake inhibitors appear to have a similar efficacy for improving global symptoms, with fewer side effects than tricyclic antidepressants, but they do not seem to be as efficacious for reducing abdominal pain. Serotonin-norepinephrine reuptake inhibitors also can reduce chronic pain, particularly in patients who cannot tolerate or take tricyclic antidepressants.

Pharmacotherapy for Irritable Bowel Syndrome with Predominant Constipation (See Fig.123-2)

Medications should be used in patients who have at least moderately severe symptoms despite dietary interventions and over-the-counter remedies.[26] Medications generally should be tried sequentially for 8 to 12 weeks since their maximal effects for reducing abdominal pain, discomfort, and bloating can require at least 6 to 8 weeks of therapy. Combination therapy has not been evaluated in randomized clinical trials but can be used in clinical practice if patients have a partial response to a single treatment.

Over-the-Counter Laxatives

Osmotic laxatives, such as polyethylene glycol, are commonly used, over-the-counter, relatively inexpensive agents that are safe and well tolerated in patients with irritable bowel syndrome with predominant constipation. Polyethylene glycol is efficacious for improving the frequency and form of stools but not for reducing abdominal pain or global symptoms. Side effects include abdominal pain, diarrhea, nausea, and flatulence, all of which occur in a dose-dependent manner.

Lubiprostone

Lubiprostone (8 μg twice daily), which is a peripherally acting chloride channel activator that increases intestinal chloride secretion, can improve symptoms of constipation, stool consistency, straining, abdominal pain, bloating, and discomfort in patients with irritable bowel syndrome with predominant constipation.[A5,A6] The most common side effects of lubiprostone are nausea, which may be reduced by taking the drug with meals, and diarrhea.

Linaclotide and Plecanatide

Linaclotide and plecanatide are minimally absorbed peptides that activate guanylate cyclase C receptors on the luminal side of the intestinal epithelium, increase levels of cyclic guanosine monophosphate, and result in enhanced luminal secretion of chloride and bicarbonate. Linaclotide also may decrease firing of visceral sensory nerves, thereby reducing abdominal pain. Linaclotide (290 μg daily) can reduce abdominal pain and increase spontaneous bowel movements.[A7] Plecanatide (3 mg daily) has similar benefits.[A8] The most common side effect of both of these agents is diarrhea, which may remit if lower doses are used.

Tenapanor

Tenapanor is a minimally absorbed, small molecule inhibitor of the gastrointestinal sodium/hydrogen exchanger isoform 3, which is a transporter that is involved in the reabsorption of sodium and water. Tenapanor (50 mg twice daily) is effective for treating constipation and abdominal pain,[A9] with diarrhea as its most common adverse event.

Pharmacologic Therapies for Irritable Bowel Syndrome with Predominant Diarrhea (See Fig. 123-4)

μ-Opioid Receptor Agonists

Loperamide, which is a peripheral opioid agonist, is efficacious in reducing the frequency of stools in patients who have irritable bowel syndrome with predominant diarrhea, but it does not improve global irritable bowel syndrome symptoms or abdominal pain.[27] Because of the lack of effect on global symptoms, loperamide is a first-line treatment predominately for patients with mild abdominal pain.

Eluxadoline (starting at 100 mg twice daily but reducing the dose to 75 mg twice daily if the higher dose is not tolerated) is a μ- and a κ-opioid receptor agonist and a δ-opioid receptor antagonist that is efficacious for reducing diarrhea and abdominal pain in patients with irritable bowel syndrome with predominant diarrhea.[A10] Contraindications include mild or moderate hepatic impairment, the lack of a gallbladder, known or suspected biliary duct obstruction, pancreatic disease, sphincter of Oddi dysfunction, and alcohol use disorder. The most common side effects are nausea and constipation.

Rifaximin

Rifaximin is a broad-spectrum, minimally absorbed antibiotic that is approved for the treatment of irritable bowel syndrome with diarrhea at a dose of 550 mg three times daily for 14 days.[A11] Subsequent retreatment with up to three courses of rifaximin can also be effective. Rifaximin is generally well tolerated, but the most common side effects are nausea and abdominal pain.

Alosetron

Alosetron is a 5-HT_3 receptor antagonist that influences the brain-gut axis to slow gastrointestinal transit and reduce visceral hypersensitivity. Because alosetron can cause ischemic colitis (rate of 1.1 per 1000 patient years) and serious complications of constipation (0.66 per 1000 patient years), it is available in the United States only under a risk evaluation and mitigation strategy under expert oversight for women with severe irritable bowel syndrome with predominant diarrhea who have failed traditional treatment.

Bile Acid Sequestrants

Some patients with irritable bowel syndrome with predominant diarrhea are thought to have bile acid diarrhea (Chapter 141), which can be confirmed by fecal bile acid levels. If confirmed, bile acid diarrhea can be treated with a bile acid sequestrant (see Table 123-3), but an empiric trial of a bile acid sequestrant also may be considered.

Psychological Interventions

Psychological therapies that reduce stress-sensitive symptoms of irritable bowel syndrome include standard and minimal contact cognitive-behavioral therapy, gut-directed hypnotherapy, relaxation training/therapy, psychotherapy, mindfulness meditation, stress management, and training in emotional awareness and expression.[A12] Cognitive-behavioral therapy aims to reduce maladaptive

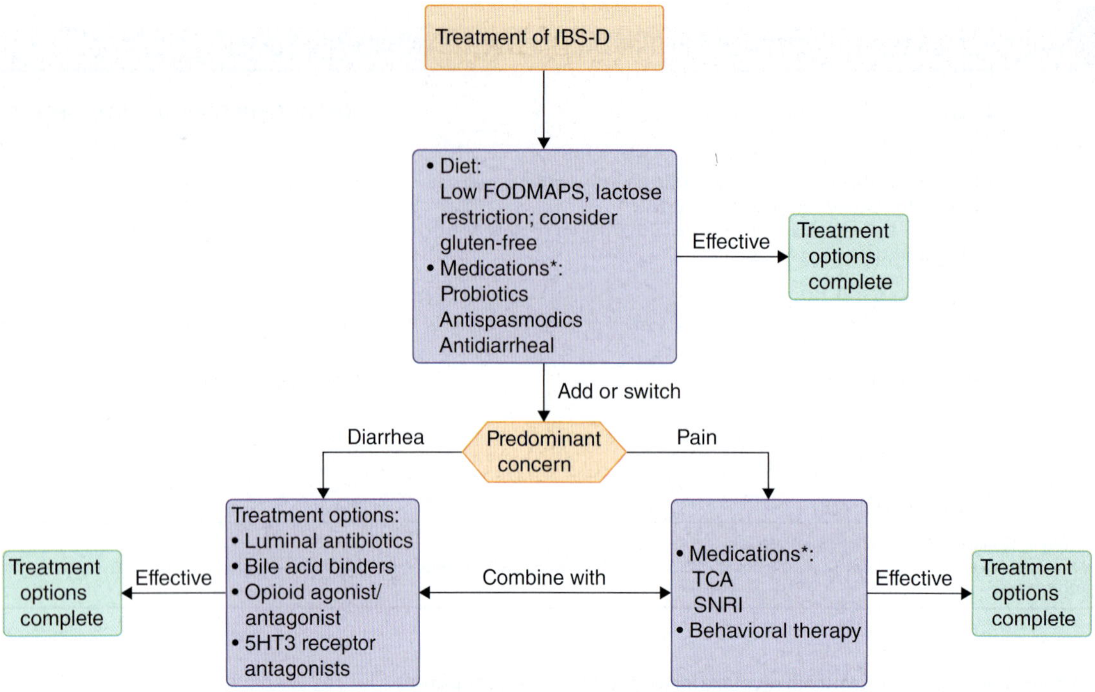

FIGURE 123-4. **Treatment algorithm for irritable bowel syndrome with diarrhea predominance (IBS-D). *See Table 123-3. FODMAPS = fermentable oligosaccharides, disaccharides, monosaccharides, and polyols; SNRI = serotonin-norepinephrine reuptake inhibitor; TCA = tricyclic antidepressants. (Adapted with permission from the Rome Foundation.)**

thoughts that can influence behaviors and emotional responses, thereby exacerbating physical symptoms. Gut-directed hypnotherapy focuses on relaxation and repeated suggestions focused on improving gut-brain communication and on reinterpretating visceral signals arising from the gut during routine activities such as digestion as being natural, comfortable, and unimportant. For patients with persistent bothersome symptoms despite standard care, an integrated care model of physicians working synergistically with dietitians, health psychologists, and even pelvic floor therapists, in person or using Internet-based programs, can improve quality of life.[28] Compared with usual care and education, psychological therapies are associated with about a 30% reduction of the symptoms of irritable bowel syndrome and are recommended for selected patients who understand the role of brain-gut behavioral therapy for irritable bowel syndrome, have the time and motivation to make behavioral changes, and experience avoidance and significant distress regarding symptoms and/or respond poorly to other therapies (see Figs. 123-2 and 123-3).

TABLE 123-4 ROME IV DIAGNOSTIC CRITERIA FOR FUNCTIONAL DYSPEPSIA*

1. One or more of the following bothersome symptoms:
    - Postprandial fullness
    - Early satiation
    - Epigastric pain
    - Epigastric burning

and

2. No evidence of structural disease (including at upper endoscopy) that is likely to explain the symptoms

*The criteria must be fulfilled for the last 3 months with onset of symptoms at least 6 months before diagnosis.

Adapted from Stanghellini V, Chan FK, Hasler WL, et al. Gastroduodenal disorders. *Gastroenterology*. 2016;150:1380-1392.

PROGNOSIS

About 30 to 45% of patients with irritable bowel syndrome have persistent symptoms for up to 12 years. Psychological symptoms, particularly anxiety and a negative perception of stressful life events, are associated with persistent symptoms. Other risk factors for persistent symptoms include female gender, younger age, and prior anxiety or depression.

FUNCTIONAL DYSPEPSIA

DEFINITION AND EPIDEMIOLOGY

Functional dyspepsia is the most common functional gastrointestinal disorder, with a prevalence of about 7%. The Rome IV diagnostic criteria for functional dyspepsia comprises bothersome (i.e., impacts usual activities) postprandial fullness, early satiety, epigastric pain, and/or epigastric burning in the absence of structural disease to explain these symptoms (Table 123-4). Heartburn, which is excluded from the definition of functional dyspepsia, may nevertheless coexist with it. Epigastric pain syndrome and postprandial distress syndrome are the two subtypes of functional dyspepsia (Table 123-5). Epigastric pain syndrome is characterized as bothersome epigastric pain or burning on one or more days per week in the past 3 months. Postprandial distress syndrome is defined as bothersome early satiety or postprandial fullness on 3 or more days per week in the previous 3 months. Almost two thirds of patients with functional dyspepsia have postprandial distress syndrome, over 15% have epigastric pain syndrome, and the remainder have symptoms that overlap both postprandial distress syndrome and epigastric pain syndrome.

Risk factors for functional dyspepsia include female sex, smoking, use of nonsteroidal anti-inflammatory drugs, acute gastroenteritis, psychological disorders (particularly anxiety), and *Helicobacter pylori* infection (Chapter 125).[29] Eradication of *H. pylori* has a statistically significant but unfortunately small likelihood of relieving symptoms of functional dyspepsia. If a patient who has symptoms of functional dyspepsia also has *H. pylori* infection and if eradication of *H. pylori* resolves these symptoms, the patient is classified as having *H. pylori* gastritis and not functional dyspepsia.

PATHOBIOLOGY

The pathobiology of functional dyspepsia includes delayed or rapid gastric emptying, visceral hypersensitivity, and impaired gastric accommodation, as well as gastric and duodenal hypersensitivity to distention, acid, low-grade inflammation (e.g., eosinophilia), mucosal permeability, and food antigens. About 30% of patients with functional dyspepsia have delayed gastric emptying time, which prompts the ongoing debate as to whether these patients should be diagnosed as having functional dyspepsia with delayed gastric emptying or as having gastroparesis (Chapter 122). However, symptoms other than severe nausea do not correlate well with gastric emptying time.[30]

CLINICAL MANIFESTATIONS AND DIAGNOSIS

The initial diagnostic evaluation of functional dyspepsia is based on the assessment of symptoms and alarm features (Fig. 123-5).[31] The presence of alarm features (Table 123-6) warrants an upper endoscopy to exclude conditions such as gastric cancer (Chapter 178) or serious esophageal disease (Chapter 124) as well as to perform a biopsy to detect *H. pylori*. If alarm features are absent and the patient is younger than age 60 years (or under age 55 years in regions with a high prevalence of gastric cancer), endoscopy is not required, but noninvasive testing for *H. pylori* (e.g., a stool antigen test [Table 125-3; Fig. 125-5]) is indicated.

TABLE 123-5 ROME IV DIAGNOSTIC CRITERIA FOR SUBGROUPS OF PATIENTS WITH FUNCTIONAL DYSPEPSIA*

POSTPRANDIAL DISTRESS SYNDROME

One or both of the following bothersome symptoms at least 3 days per week:
1. Postprandial fullness (severe enough to impact usual activities)
2. Early satiation

Supportive Criteria

1. Postprandial epigastric pain or burning, epigastric bloating, excessive belching, and nausea can also be present.
2. Vomiting warrants consideration for another diagnosis.
3. Heartburn is not a dyspeptic symptom but may often coexist.
4. Symptoms that are relieved by evacuation of feces or gas should generally not be considered as part of dyspepsia.

EPIGASTRIC PAIN SYNDROME

Must include at least one of the following bothersome symptoms at least 1 day a week:
1. Epigastric pain (i.e., severe enough to impact on usual activities)
2. Epigastric burning (i.e., severe enough to impact on usual activities)

Supportive Criteria

1. Pain may be induced by ingestion of a meal, relieved by ingestion of a meal, or may occur while fasting.
2. Postprandial epigastric bloating, belching, and nausea can also be present.
3. Persistent vomiting likely suggests another disorder.
4. Heartburn is not a dyspeptic symptom but may often coexist.
5. The pain does not fulfill biliary pain criteria.
6. Symptoms that are relieved by evacuation of feces or gas generally should not be considered as part of dyspepsia.

*The criteria must be fulfilled for the last 3 months with symptom onset at least 6 months before diagnosis.

Adapted from Stanghellini V, Chan FK, Hasler WL, et al. Gastroduodenal disorders. *Gastroenterology*. 2016;150:1380-1392.

TABLE 123-6 ALARM SYMPTOMS ASSOCIATED WITH AN UNDERLYING UPPER GASTROINTESTINAL MALIGNANCY

Unintentional weight loss
New-onset dyspepsia after age 55 years
Dysphagia
Persistent vomiting
Any overt gastrointestinal bleeding, hematemesis, or melena
Family history of esophageal or gastric cancer
Iron deficiency anemia
Palpable abdominal mass or lymph node

From Mayer EA. Functional gastrointestinal disorders: irritable bowel syndrome, dyspepsia, esophageal chest pain, and heartburn. In: Goldman L, Schafer A, eds. *Goldman-Cecil Medicine*, 26th ed. Philadelphia: Elsevier; 2020:852-859.

TREATMENT

If *H. pylori* is not detected, empiric therapy with a proton pump inhibitor (see Table 124-1) is typically recommended.[A13] If symptoms persist, additional treatment is based on the subtype of functional dyspepsia. In patients with postprandial distress syndrome, buspirone (10 mg three times daily) and mirtazapine (15 mg at bedtime) have demonstrated efficacy. Tricyclic antidepressants (see Table 362-5) can relieve symptoms compared with placebo, particularly in patients who have abdominal pain and a normal gastric emptying time.

PROGNOSIS

The long-term prognosis for functional dyspepsia is favorable in the majority of patients, and life expectancy is similar to that of the general population.

FUNCTIONAL HEARTBURN

Functional heartburn is retrosternal burning discomfort or pain that radiates retrosternally, is unresponsive to optimal antisecretory therapy, and is not

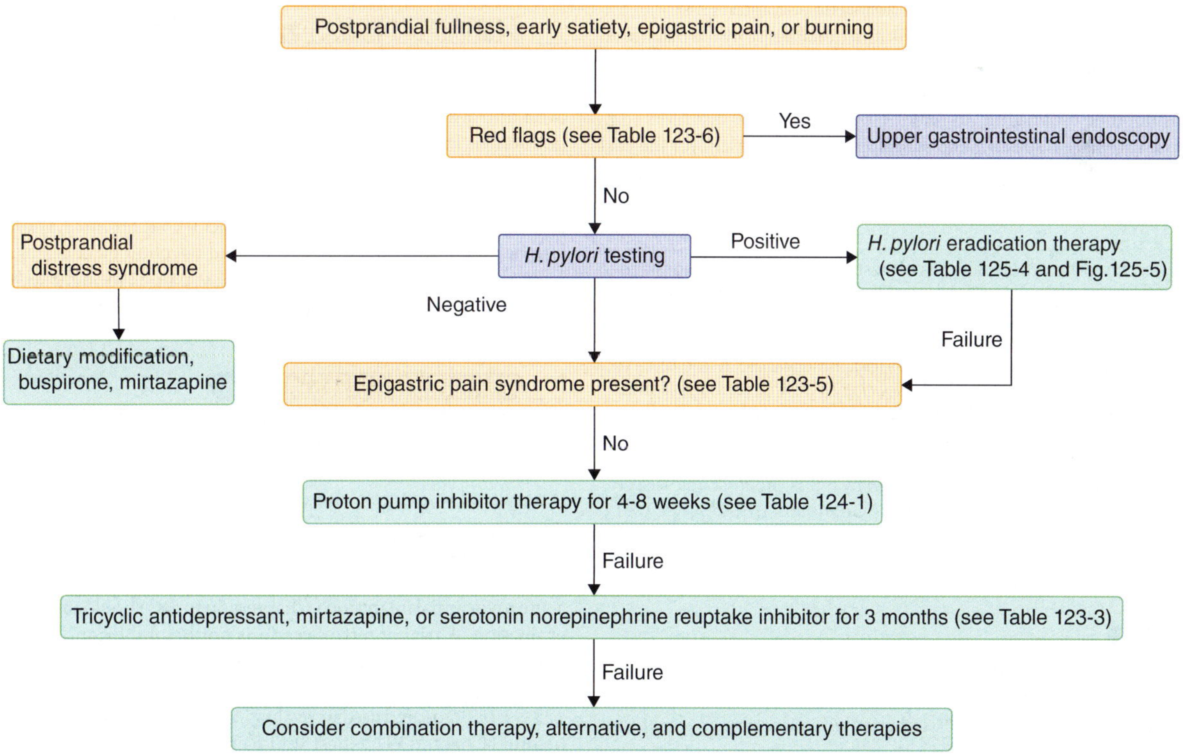

FIGURE 123-5. Algorithm for functional dyspepsia. A recommended approach to patients who present with epigastric pain, postprandial fullness, and early satiety, who meet the Rome IV diagnostic criteria for functional dyspepsia (see Table 123-4), and who lack any alarm features (see Table 123-6). In the setting of treatment failure, the physician should re-evaluate all clinical and laboratory findings to determine whether further diagnostic testing might be beneficial to assess the patients for alternative causes of the symptoms. (From Mayer EA. Functional gastrointestinal disorders: irritable bowel syndrome, dyspepsia, esophageal chest pain, and heartburn. In: Goldman L, Schafer AI, eds. *Goldman-Cecil Medicine*, 26th ed. Philadelphia: Elsevier; 2020:852-859.)

accompanied by gastroesophageal reflux disease or esophageal mucosal, motility, or structural abnormalities to explain the symptoms. Even if some gastroesophageal reflux is detected, symptoms are not correlated with it. Although patients may have some degree of epigastric discomfort, the chest symptoms predominate.

EPIDEMIOLOGY

Functional heartburn is very common. The global prevalence of functional heartburn is about 1%, but it is approximately 25% in patients whose heartburn responds to a proton pump inhibitor and 50% in patients whose heartburn does not respond to a proton pump inhibitor. The presence of coexistent irritable bowel syndrome is a strong predictor of functional heartburn.

PATHOBIOLOGY

The pathobiology of functional heartburn is likely related to visceral hypersensitivity to antral and esophageal distention, altered esophageal motility in the absence of a clinically detectable motility disorder, and psychological factors.

CLINICAL MANIFESTATIONS

Patients with functional heartburn, which unlike dyspepsia is felt in the chest rather than the abdomen, complain of typical heartburn symptoms that usually are triggered by food intake and psychosocial stress but are refractory to acid-suppressive therapy with proton pump inhibitors. By definition, they also have negative endoscopic and acid monitoring evaluations of the esophagus.

DIAGNOSIS

An endoscopy with biopsies is performed in patients whose heartburn symptoms do not respond to an adequate trial of empirical proton pump inhibitor therapy in order to exclude other esophageal or gastric diseases, such as eosinophilic esophagitis, pill-induced esophagitis, stricture, Barrett esophagus, and malignancy (Chapter 124). If endoscopy is normal, ambulatory pH monitoring alone or with impedence should be conducted without acid suppression in patients who do not have proven gastroesophageal reflux and with acid suppression in patients who have proven gastroesophageal reflux. If esophageal acid (pH <4) exposure time is less than 4% of the time of a complete study, high-resolution esophageal manometry should be performed to exclude a major esophageal motility disorder such as achalasia (Chapter 124).

Based on the Rome IV criteria (Table 123-7), functional heartburn is diagnosed if heartburn is present at least twice per week with all of the following criteria: no relief of symptoms with optimal antisecretory therapy; absence of gastroesophageal reflux, eosinophilic esophagitis, or major esophageal motor disorders (e.g., achalasia, diffuse esophageal spasm); and symptoms that are present for the past 3 months with an onset of symptoms at least 6 months prior to the diagnosis.

TABLE 123-7 ROME IV DIAGNOSTIC CRITERIA FOR FUNCTIONAL HEARTBURN

Must include all of the following:
- Burning retrosternal discomfort or pain
- No relief of symptoms despite optimal antisecretory therapy
- Absence of evidence that gastroesophageal reflux (abnormal acid exposure and symptoms) or eosinophilic esophagitis is the cause of symptoms
- Absence of major esophageal motor disorders (e.g., achalasia/esophagogastric junction outflow obstruction, diffuse esophageal spasm, jackhammer esophagus, absent peristalsis)

*The criteria must be fulfilled for the last 3 months with the onset of symptoms at least 6 months before diagnosis, with a frequency of at least twice per week.

Aziz Q, Fass R, Gyawali CP, et al. Functional esophageal disorders. *Gastroenterology*. 2016;150:1368-1379.

TREATMENT

Treatment of functional heartburn consists of lifestyle modifications, pharmacotherapy with neuromodulators, and behavioral therapy.[32] Lifestyle modifications include identifying and managing triggers such as foods, stress, or physical activities that precipitate symptoms. Antisecretory medications such as standard- or double-dose proton pump inhibitors (e.g., omeprazole 20 mg once to twice daily; see Table 124-1) can be helpful, especially if gastroesophageal reflux coexists.[33] Low doses of tricyclic antidepressants (e.g., imipramine; starting at 10 to 20 mg at bedtime) or selective serotonin reuptake inhibitors (e.g., fluoxetine 10 to 20 mg daily) are considered the mainstay of treatment for functional heartburn. For truly refractory heartburn caused by reflux, laparoscopic Nissen fundoplication is better than continued medical treatment (see Chapter 124). Cognitive-behavioral therapy may be helpful. Acupuncture and esophageal-directed hypnotherapy (Chapter 30) are reserved for refractory cases.

PROGNOSIS

The prognosis and long-term natural history of functional heartburn are not completely known. Up to two thirds of patients continue to have heartburn over 2 years of follow-up, whereas about 20% experience a reduction in symptoms.

FUNCTIONAL CHEST PAIN OF LIKELY ESOPHAGEAL ORIGIN

DEFINITION

Functional chest pain of presumed esophageal origin (Table 123-8) is a chronic midline chest pain that is not explained by cardiac causes, gastroesophageal reflux, or esophageal motility disorders (Chapters 39 and 124).

TABLE 123-8 ROME IV DIAGNOSTIC CRITERIA FOR FUNCTIONAL CHEST PAIN OF PRESUMED ESOPHAGEAL ORIGIN*

Must include all of the following:
- Retrosternal chest pain or discomfort; cardiac causes should be excluded
- Absence of associated esophageal symptoms, such as heartburn and dysphagia
- Absence of evidence that gastroesophageal reflux or eosinophilic esophagitis are the cause of the symptoms
- Absence of major esophageal motor disorders (e.g., achalasia/esophageal-gastric outflow obstruction, diffuse esophageal spasm, jackhammer esophagus, absent peristalsis)

*The criteria must be fulfilled for the last 3 months with the onset of symptoms at least 6 months before diagnosis, with a frequency of at least once a week.

From Mayer EA. Functional gastrointestinal disorders: irritable bowel syndrome, dyspepsia, esophageal chest pain, and heartburn. In: Goldman L, Schafer A, eds. *Goldman-Cecil Medicine*, 26th ed. Philadelphia: Elsevier; 2020:852-859.

EPIDEMIOLOGY AND PATHOBIOLOGY

Functional chest pain has a prevalence rate as high as 25% and is a leading cause of acute chest pain (see Table 39-2), especially in younger patients. Men and women are equally affected, and it is more commonly reported in younger individuals, perhaps because repeated reassurance decreases the complaint in other individuals. Nevertheless, many patients undergo repeated and unnecessary diagnostic cardiac evaluations. Patients with functional chest pain often have anxiety or panic attacks (Chapter 362), thereby suggesting a link between functional chest pain and psychological issues.

The pathobiology of esophageal chest pain is thought to be similar to that of functional heartburn. In addition, however, increased esophageal muscle contraction has been implicated.

CLINICAL MANIFESTATIONS

Functional chest pain is often indistinguishable from the pain of acute myocardial ischemia or myocardial infarction (Chapters 57 and 58). Although the pain is typically substernal, it can radiate to the arm and neck. The pain is unrelated to exercise and can persist for hours.

DIAGNOSIS

Patients who present with chest pain (see Table 39-2) suspicious for angina or acute myocardial infarction (Chapters 56 to 58) should undergo prompt cardiac evaluation. A trial of nitroglycerin is not helpful diagnostically because it can relieve esophageal spasm as well as myocardial ischemia. If the cardiac evaluation is negative, other causes of functional chest pain should be evaluated (Table 123-9), but repeated cardiac evaluations for recurrent symptoms usually are not helpful (Chapter 39). Chest wall pain, tenderness on palpation, or changes in pain with movement usually are musculoskeletal in origin (Chapter 39).

An association with certain foods or concurrent heartburn or dyspepsia can sometimes differentiate between acid-induced versus non–acid-related causes. In patients with alarm symptoms (see Table 123-6), such as weight loss, progressive dysphagia, or anemia, upper endoscopy is required. Testing for esophageal motility disorders (Chapter 124) is useful for severe or recurrent symptoms.

TABLE 123-9 DIFFERENTIAL DIAGNOSIS OF FUNCTIONAL CHEST PAIN

ORGANIC ESOPHAGEAL CAUSES
Gastroesophageal reflux disease
Achalasia
Virus- or pill-induced esophagitis
Eosinophilic esophagitis
NONGASTROINTESTINAL CAUSES
Cardiac chest pain
Chest wall pain
Pulmonary disease
Panic attack

From Mayer EA. Functional gastrointestinal disorders: irritable bowel syndrome, dyspepsia, esophageal chest pain, and heartburn. In: Goldman L, Schafer A, eds. *Goldman-Cecil Medicine,* 26th ed. Philadelphia: Elsevier; 2020:852-859.

TREATMENT

Many patients with functional chest pain have atypical gastroesophageal reflux disorder (Chapter 124) and benefit from a therapeutic trial with a proton pump inhibitor (e.g., omeprazole 20 mg daily). The optimal duration of treatment is unclear, but an attempt should be made to discontinue proton pump inhibitors after several months of successful therapy. If the patient's response is equivocal, 24-hour pH testing can be considered (Chapter 124). In patients who do not respond to a proton pump inhibitor, testing for esophageal motility disorders (Chapter 124) should be performed to look for conditions such as high-amplitude contractions, diffuse esophageal spasm, or achalasia. Fears regarding possible cardiac disease must be addresseed explicitly, and patients must be reassured by the negative results of the cardiac evaluation.

Low-dose tricyclic antidepressants (e.g., amitriptyline, imipramine, or desipramine 10 to 50 mg at bedtime) may be useful. For persistent symptoms, cognitive-behavioral therapy or mindfulness-based stress reduction may be beneficial.

PROGNOSIS

Functional chest pain has a benign prognosis, although many patients may request repeated cardiac evaluations if symptoms persist and diminish quality of life.

GENERAL REFERENCES

For the General References and other additional features, please visit Elsevier eBooks+ at https://ebooks.health.elsevier.com.

Grade A References

A1. Black CJ, Staudacher HM, Ford AC. Efficacy of a low FODMAP diet in irritable bowel syndrome: systematic review and network meta-analysis. *Gut.* 2022;71:1117-1126.

A2. Carbone F, Van den Houte K, Besard L, et al. Diet or medication in primary care patients with IBS: the DOMINO study - a randomised trial supported by the Belgian Health Care Knowledge Centre (KCE Trials Programme) and the Rome Foundation Research Institute. *Gut.* 2022;71:2226-2232.

A3. Black CJ, Yuan Y, Selinger CP, et al. Efficacy of soluble fibre, antispasmodic drugs, and gut–brain neuromodulators in irritable bowel syndrome: a systematic review and network meta-analysis. *Lancet Gastroenterol Hepatol.* 2020;5:117-131.

A4. Ford AC, Lacy BE, Harris LA, et al. Effect of antidepressants and psychological therapies in irritable bowel syndrome: an updated systematic review and meta-analysis. *Am J Gastroenterol.* 2019;114:21-39.

A5. Black CJ, Burr NE, Quigley EMM, et al. Efficacy of secretagogues in patients with irritable bowel syndrome with constipation: systematic review and network meta-analysis. *Gastroenterology.* 2018;155:1753-1763.

A6. Nelson AD, Black CJ, Houghton LA, et al. Systematic review and network meta-analysis: efficacy of licensed drugs for abdominal bloating in irritable bowel syndrome with constipation. *Aliment Pharmacol Ther.* 2021;54:98-108.

A7. Atluri DK, Chandar AK, Bharucha AE, et al. Effect of linaclotide in irritable bowel syndrome with constipation (IBS-C): a systematic review and meta-analysis. *Neurogastroenterol Motil.* 2014;26:499-509.

A8. Shah ED, Kim HM, Schoenfeld P. Efficacy and tolerability of guanylate cyclase-C agonists for irritable bowel syndrome with constipation and chronic idiopathic constipation: a systematic review and meta-analysis. *Am J Gastroenterol.* 2018;11:329-338.

A9. Chey WD, Lembo AJ, Yang Y, et al. Efficacy of tenapanor in treating patients with irritable bowel syndrome with constipation: a 26-week, placebo-controlled phase 3 trial (T3MPO-2). *Am J Gastroenterol.* 2021;116:1294-1303.

A10. Lembo AJ, Lacy BE, Zuckerman MJ, et al. Eluxadoline for irritable bowel syndrome with diarrhea. *N Engl J Med.* 2016;374:242-253.

A11. Lembo A, Pimentel M, Rao SS, et al. Repeat treatment with rifaximin is safe and effective in patients with diarrhea-predominant irritable bowel syndrome. *Gastroenterology.* 2016;151:1113-1121.

A12. Black CJ, Thakur ER, Houghton LA, et al. Efficacy of psychological therapies for irritable bowel syndrome: systematic review and network meta-analysis. *Gut.* 2020;69:1441-1451.

A13. Ford AC, Tsipotis E, Yuan Y, et al. Efficacy of *Helicobacter pylori* eradication therapy for functional dyspepsia: updated systematic review and meta-analysis. *Gut.* 2022;71:1967-1975.

124 DISEASES OF THE ESOPHAGUS

GARY W. FALK AND DAVID A. KATZKA

NORMAL ANATOMY AND PHYSIOLOGY

The esophagus, which averages about 27 cm in length, is a hollow muscular tube consisting of the mucosa, submucosa, and muscularis layers, with the notable absence of a serosal layer. The mucosa is a stratified squamous nonkeratinized epithelium that transitions to a columnar epithelium at the gastroesophageal junction. The muscular layer of the esophagus is composed of striated muscle in the upper one third and smooth muscle in the lower two thirds. These muscular components are arranged as an inner circular and an outer longitudinal layer. Located between the circular and longitudinal muscle layers is Auerbach (myenteric) plexus, whereas Meissner plexus is located within the submucosa and innervates the muscularis mucosae. The esophagus is bound by an upper esophageal sphincter proximally and the lower esophageal sphincter distally. The upper esophageal sphincter contains functional contributions from the inferior pharyngeal constrictor proximally and the cricopharyngeus distally. By contrast, the lower esophageal sphincter is anatomically and histologically indistinguishable from the lower esophagus. Blood supply for the cervical portion is derived from branches of the inferior thyroid artery. The intrathoracic segment of the esophagus receives its blood supply from bronchial arteries and direct branches from the aorta, and the left gastric and the inferior phrenic arteries supply the abdominal portion of the esophagus. Venous drainage follows the arterial supply in the cervical and abdominal portions, whereas the thoracic esophagus drains into the azygous and hemiazygos system. Likewise, the lymphatic drainage of the esophagus is segmental, with the cervical portion draining into deep cervical lymph nodes, the thoracic portion into the superior and posterior mediastinal lymph nodes, and the abdominal portion into the gastric and celiac lymph nodes.

The motor functions of the esophagus are to transport a food bolus from the oropharynx into the stomach and then to keep food from returning to the esophagus after it has entered the stomach. The upper esophageal sphincter and the proximal third of the esophagus compose the first portion of the esophagus. The upper esophageal sphincter is approximately 2 to 4 cm in length. The recurrent laryngeal nerve inferiorly and a pharyngeal plexus superiorly supply the upper esophageal sphincter. The muscle layers close the esophageal lumen and shorten the esophagus to facilitate forward transport through the proximal esophagus. After food traverses the proximal esophagus, it moves into the distal two thirds of the esophagus, where peristalsis is achieved by sequential muscular contraction mediated through an interplay of inhibitory and excitatory neurotransmitters. Peristalsis may be primary, that is, initiated by a swallow, or secondary, that is, stimulated by refluxed gastric contents. Although local mechanisms control most esophageal motor function, vagal input is important in the distal esophagus, where smooth muscle myopathies and autonomic neuropathies can cause dysfunction. The distal esophagus is separated from the stomach by the lower esophageal sphincter, which is 4 to 5 cm in length and is functionally distinct because it maintains a tonic high-pressure zone. This sphincter relaxes nearly completely upon swallowing to allow the passage of food and then regains its tone to provide a barrier against reflux. It also relaxes transiently during normal functions, such as belching and vomiting. The vagus nerve, acetylcholine, and nitric oxide influence tone, but the lower esophageal sphincter tone is influenced by the crural diaphragm as the esophagus traverses the diaphragmatic hiatus.

Esophageal Functional Testing

Options for esophageal functional testing include barium esophagography, high-resolution esophageal manometry, and esophageal impedance testing. Barium esophagography (Chapter 119) reveals both anatomic and physiologic information about luminal lesions, such as malignancies, ulceration, diverticula, hiatal hernia, and strictures; intramural lesions, such as leiomyomas; and extrinsic lesions, such as occur from vascular (aorta, right atrium, subclavian artery) impingement or solid lesions (pulmonary malignancy, adenopathy) that compress the esophagus. Radiography is also an excellent tool for studying motility patterns, such as peristalsis with either liquid or solid contrast material, while precisely visualizing how the esophagus handles a bolus rather than by implying function from pressure or impedance changes.

High-resolution esophageal manometry measures pressure changes generated by esophageal wall contraction and changes in tone using multiple sensors that simultaneously measure pressure from the pharynx to the lower esophageal sphincter.[1] Esophageal impedance testing detects the movement of an intraluminal bolus by measuring conductance between catheter-based electrodes based on the substance that is in contact with each electrode. Air, which is a poor conductor of electric current, will yield high impedance, whereas swallowed or refluxed liquids, which are excellent conductors of electricity, will generate a low impedance signal. From these measurements, the direction and velocity of the transport of air and bolus can help assess peristaltic function and the reflux of acid and nonacid gastric contents. Impedance can also reflect site-specific esophageal mucosal permeability, thereby providing further insight into mucosal integrity and disease in inflammatory or metaplastic conditions.

A functional luminal imaging probe is a balloon-based device that measures pressures in response to controlled volumetric distentions. When used in the esophagus, it can measure the compliance of the esophageal wall and lower esophageal sphincter, as well as esophageal body motility. This procedure is increasingly being used to evaluate disorders such as eosinophilic esophagitis, achalasia, obstruction of the esophagogastric junction outlet, and unexplained dysphagia.

Symptoms of Esophageal Disease

The most common symptom of esophageal disease is heartburn, which is defined as a sensation of substernal burning. Chest pain without typical heartburn may occur in a variety of esophageal disorders, including gastroesophageal reflux and motor disorders such as in achalasia. However, esophageal pain and even heartburn can be indistinguishable from cardiac angina (Chapter 39), so care must be taken when a patient at risk for coronary artery disease complains of heartburn for the first time.

Dysphagia, or difficulty swallowing, is another cardinal symptom of esophageal disease. Dysphagia with only solid food tends to occur with structural lesions, which cause esophageal constriction, whereas dysphagia with both liquids and solids occurs more often with motility disorders. Patients with oropharyngeal dysphagia will commonly complain of a feeling of food "sticking" in the throat or the inability to propel the bolus from the mouth to the pharynx; they may also complain of the need for multiple swallowing motions to clear the bolus. Since the cranial nerves that generally control the initial phases of swallowing are responsible for other functions as well, symptoms that may be associated with oropharyngeal dysphagia include drooling, dysarthria (due to tongue dysfunction), nasal regurgitation (due to failure to seal off the nasal passage), or coughing and aspiration (due to failure to elevate and cover the laryngeal vestibule). Dysphagia that results from abnormalities in the body of the esophagus may be referred to the chest or the neck, so the location of dysphagia does not predict the location of the disease. Dysphagia may also lead to a variety of behavioral accommodations, including maneuvers such as slow eating, food aversion, avoidance of hard solid food, and drinking of large amounts of liquids with solid meals.

Regurgitation, which is another typical esophageal symptom, may be described as the feeling of food coming up into the chest or, more dramatically, into the mouth. When regurgitation occurs early in the meal, it suggests a proximal lesion. Regurgitation later in the meal suggests a motility abnormality such as achalasia.

Food impaction is an extreme esophageal symptom. When impaction occurs in the oropharynx, it may lead to tracheal impaction or compression. With more distal esophageal lesions, impaction may occur any time during the meal, almost always from a mechanical cause. Patients experience the sudden onset of chest pain and the sensation of food sticking, typically after solids such as meats, raw vegetables, and sticky rice. With complete impaction, patients who cannot handle secretions because of the obstructing bolus are at risk for aspiration, esophageal rupture, and perforation.

GASTROESOPHAGEAL REFLUX DISEASE

DEFINITION

Gastroesophageal reflux disease (GERD) develops when the reflux of stomach contents into the esophagus causes troublesome symptoms or complications.

EPIDEMIOLOGY

It is estimated that GERD, defined as at least weekly heartburn or acid regurgitation, has a prevalence ranging from 10 to 20% in the Western world and less than 5% in Asia. In the United States, estimates are that as many as 44% of people may have had GERD symptoms and 30% have had such symptoms in the prior week. The prevalence also tends to be higher in North America than Europe and higher in northern Europe than in southern Europe. Risk factors for developing GERD include obesity, particularly central obesity, and possibly increasing age. A genetic component may also play a role because GERD is more common in patients with a positive family history and in monozygotic twins than in dizygotic twins.

PATHOBIOLOGY

The esophagus is protected from the harmful effects of refluxed gastric contents by the antireflux barrier at the gastroesophageal junction, by esophageal clearance mechanisms, and by epithelial defensive factors. The antireflux barrier consists of the lower esophageal sphincter, crural diaphragm, phrenoesophageal ligament, and angle of His, which causes an oblique entrance of the esophagus into the stomach. The attachment of the lower esophageal sphincter to the crural diaphragm results in increased pressure during inspiration and when intra-abdominal pressure increases. Disruption of normal defense mechanisms leads to pathologic amounts of reflux.

Reflux of gastric contents from the stomach into the esophagus occurs in healthy individuals, but refluxed gastric contents are normally cleared in a two-step process: volume clearance by peristaltic function and neutralization of small amounts of residual acid by weakly alkaline swallowed saliva. In normal healthy individuals, physiologic reflux occurs primarily when the lower esophageal sphincter transiently relaxes in the absence of a swallow because of a vagally mediated reflex that is stimulated by gastric distention. In GERD patients, transient relaxation of the lower esophageal sphincter or a low resting lower esophageal sphincter pressure can result in regurgitation, especially when intra-abdominal pressure is increased. In some patients, a primary increase in intra-abdominal pressure overcomes normal lower esophageal sphincter pressure. These patients may have a rumination and/or supragastric belching variant of gastroesophageal reflux.[2]

A hiatal hernia, which results in axial and vertical spatial separation between the augmenting effects of the crural diaphragm and the lower esophageal sphincter, predisposes to reflux events by widening the opening of the gastroesophageal junction and decreasing the pressure of the lower esophageal sphincter. The result is an increased exposure of the esophagus to acid and gastric contents, with increased reflux events during transient physiologic relaxation of the lower esophageal sphincter and/or increased gastric pressure. Hernias also act as a reservoir for gastric contents when normal esophageal clearance mechanisms result in trapping of fluids in the hernia sac. These contents can reflux into the esophagus when the lower esophageal sphincter relaxes during subsequent swallowing.

Normal individuals also have an unbuffered acid pocket in the gastric cardia, which escapes the buffering effects of a meal in the postprandial period. This region is a source of postprandial reflux and may explain the chronic inflammation often seen in the cardia and distal esophagus. In reflux patients, the acid pocket is more common and longer in length than in normal individuals. Displacement of the acid pocket into a hiatal hernia also appears to increase acidic reflux in patients with GERD.

Increased intra-abdominal fat associated with obesity increases intragastric pressure, which increases the gastroesophageal pressure gradient and the frequency of transient lower esophageal sphincter relaxation, thereby predisposing gastric contents to migrate into the esophagus. In addition, obesity enhances the spatial separation of the crural diaphragm and the lower esophageal sphincter, thereby predisposing obese individuals to a hiatal hernia. The metabolic syndrome (Chapter 210) that is associated with obesity also may have an independent effect in promoting esophageal injury in GERD.

The normal defense mechanisms based on peristalsis and saliva also can be impaired. Peristaltic dysfunction is associated with an increasing severity of esophagitis, and ineffective peristaltic clearance may occur when the amplitude of esophageal contractions is less than 20 mm Hg. Saliva production may be impaired by a variety of mechanisms, such as smoking and Sjögren syndrome (Chapter 247).

The esophageal mucosa contains several lines of defense. A pre-epithelial barrier constitutes a small unstirred water layer combined with bicarbonate from swallowed saliva and from the secretions of submucosal glands. A second epithelial defense is composed of cell membranes and tight intercellular junctions, cellular and intercellular buffers, and cell membrane ion transporters. The postepithelial line of defense is composed of the blood supply to the esophagus. Acid and acidified pepsin in the refluxate are the key factors that damage the intercellular junctions, increase intracellular permeability, and dilate intercellular spaces. If sufficient quantities of refluxate diffuse into the intercellular spaces, cellular damage may occur. Signs and symptoms of GERD occur when defective epithelium comes into contact with refluxed acid, pepsin, or other noxious gastric contents. In addition to the direct noxious effects of refluxed acid, pepsin, and bile, refluxed gastric juice stimulates esophageal epithelial cells to secrete chemokines that attract inflammatory cells into the esophagus, thereby damaging the esophageal mucosa.

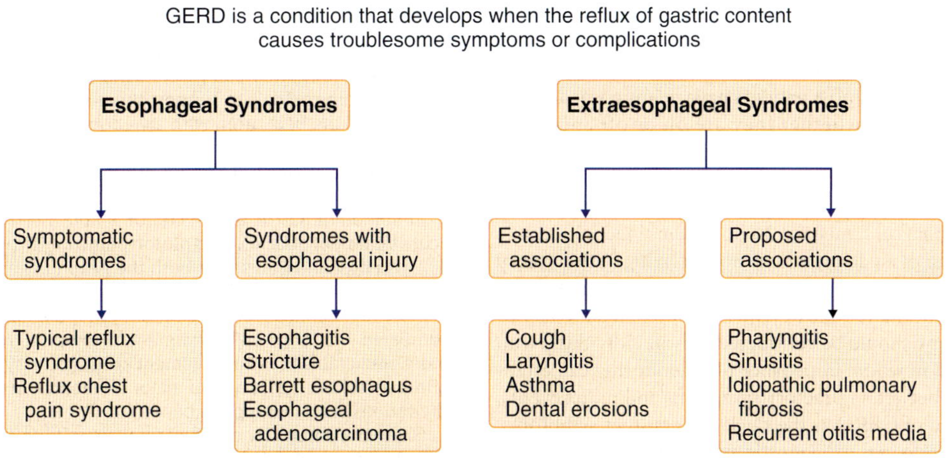

FIGURE 124-1. **Montreal classification of gastroesophageal reflux disease (GERD).** (From Vakil N, van Zanten S, Kahrilas P, et al. The Montreal definition and classification of gastroesophageal reflux disease: a global evidence-based consensus. *Am J Gastroenterol*. 2006;101:1900-1920.)

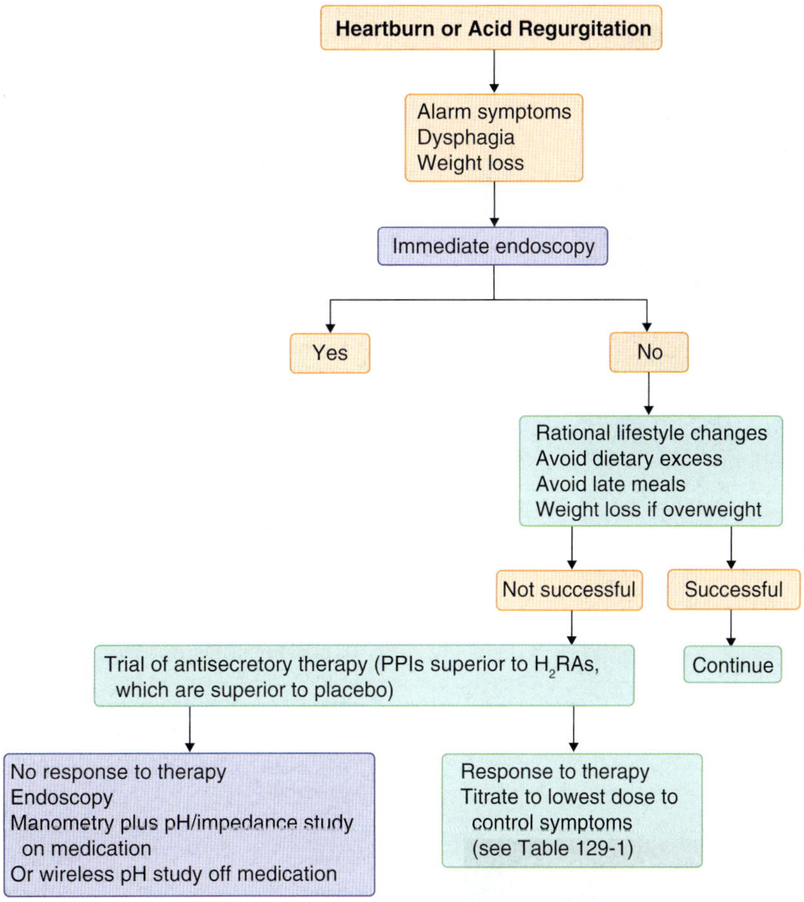

FIGURE 124-2. **Algorithm for the management of heartburn or regurgitation symptoms.** Surgery is indicated only for patients who are intolerant of antisecretory therapy or who have ongoing symptoms, especially regurgitation if reflux is well documented. H_2RA = histamine-2 receptor antagonist; PPI = proton pump inhibitor. (Based on Kahrilas PJ, Shaheen NJ, Vaezi MF. American Gastroenterological Association Institute technical review on the management of gastroesophageal reflux disease. *Gastroenterology*. 2008;135:1392-1413.)

CLINICAL MANIFESTATIONS

The classic symptoms of GERD are heartburn and acid regurgitation; atypical symptoms include chest pain, dysphagia, and odynophagia. Extraesophageal manifestations of reflux disease can include cough (Chapter 71), laryngitis (Chapter 397), asthma (Chapter 75), and dental erosions, but these symptoms are more easily attributable to GERD if accompanied by classic signs and symptoms of reflux disease and by objective testing that demonstrates increased reflux (Fig. 124-1). Other proposed associations that do not reliably respond to acid suppression and hence are not clearly related to GERD include pharyngitis, sinusitis, otitis media, throat clearing, and idiopathic pulmonary fibrosis.

When excessive gastric contents overwhelm the mucosal protective factors in the esophagus, esophagitis may be manifest as erosions or ulceration of the esophagus and may also lead to fibrosis with stricturing, columnar metaplasia (Barrett esophagus), or esophageal adenocarcinoma (Chapter 178). However, approximately two thirds of individuals with reflux symptoms have no evidence of esophageal damage by endoscopy.

DIAGNOSIS

When GERD is associated with typical signs and symptoms, such as heartburn or acid regurgitation, that are responsive to antisecretory therapy, no diagnostic evaluation is warranted,[3] except perhaps in patients who have high-risk characteristics for Barrett esophagus, such as smoking, older age, and absence of *H. pylori* infection.[4] However, recommendations on screening vary, and the cost-effectiveness of screening is uncertain.[5]

Diagnostic endoscopy is warranted in individuals who fail to respond to 4 to 8 weeks of therapy or have alarm symptoms or signs such as dysphagia, weight loss (Fig. 118-4), anemia, gastrointestinal bleeding, or persistent heartburn (Fig. 124-2). Endoscopy permits the detection of erosive esophagitis and complications such as a peptic stricture (Fig. 124-3) and Barrett esophagus (Fig. 124-4); mucosal biopsy, which is crucial in these settings, also excludes conditions that can mimic GERD, such as eosinophilic esophagitis. However, most patients have no mucosal damage seen on endoscopy, regardless of whether they are on or off antisecretory therapy.

Esophageal manometry is useful to exclude achalasia in patients with suggestive symptoms. Esophageal reflux testing may be performed using 48- to 96-hour devices attached to the esophageal lumen, or 24-hour combined impedance and pH monitoring.[6] Testing of a patient who is not receiving antisecretory therapy can document abnormal esophageal acid exposure and establish the relationship between symptoms and reflux events. Testing of a patient who is on acid-suppression therapy should be considered only in individuals who have established GERD and in whom impedance pH monitoring can establish the relationship, if any, between refractory symptoms and reflux events, thereby permitting exclusion of GERD as the cause of persistent symptoms. Barium radiography has no role in the diagnostic evaluation of patients with uncomplicated reflux disease.

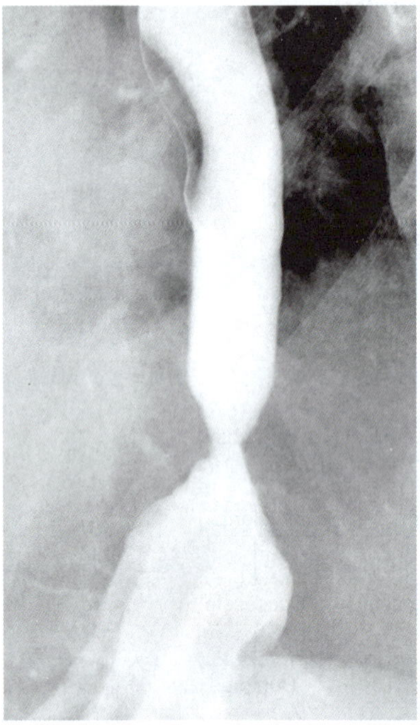

FIGURE 124-3. **Barium radiograph of a peptic stricture.** (Courtesy Marc Levine, MD.)

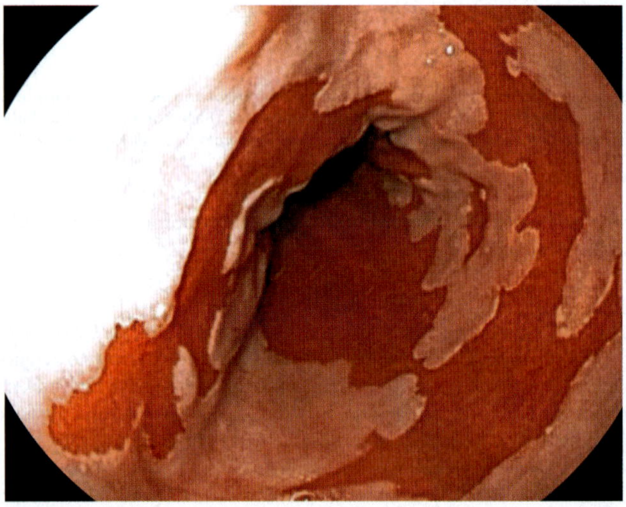

FIGURE 124-4. **Endoscopic appearance of Barrett esophagus. Note the white-appearing normal squamous mucosa displaced above the true end of the esophagus. The intervening mucosa appears salmon pink.**

TREATMENT

Although avoidance of foods or beverages that may provoke symptoms, such as alcohol, coffee, spicy foods, and late meals, makes physiologic sense, data from clinical trials to support these maneuvers are lacking. Elevation of the head of the bed, often with a wedge device, for patients with nocturnal regurgitation or heartburn also is logical. Given the association of obesity and GERD symptoms, weight loss should be part of any treatment program for obese patients.

Inhibition of gastric acid secretion (Table 124-1) is the cornerstone of the acute treatment of GERD,[7] and proton pump inhibitors are superior to histamine (H_2)–receptor antagonists for both the healing of esophagitis and the control of symptoms. For example, twice-daily proton pump inhibitor therapy results in more rapid endoscopic healing but not more rapid resolution of symptoms compared with once-daily treatment.[A1] However, the healing of esophagitis is more predictable than improvement in heartburn symptoms, even with proton pump inhibitors. There are no major differences in treatment efficacy among the various proton pump inhibitors.

Given the chronicity of reflux symptoms, long-term maintenance therapy with proton pump inhibitors is typically required, especially for patients with erosive esophagitis. Dosing should be titrated to the lowest dose necessary to control symptoms. Data to support the use of proton pump inhibitors in the management of extraesophageal GERD syndromes are weak, although selected patients, usually those with accompanying symptoms of classic heartburn and acid regurgitation, may benefit. The safety profile of proton pump inhibitors is excellent, but short-term adverse events such as headaches and diarrhea may occur. Long-term use of proton pump inhibitors has been associated with a variety of adverse consequences (vitamin B_{12} deficiency, *Clostridioides difficile* infection, community-acquired pneumonia, hip fracture, metabolic bone disease, diabetes mellitus, and small intestinal bacterial overgrowth), but the magnitude of any such risks is low enough that they do not offset their benefit.[8]

Although proton pump inhibitors are superior to H_2-receptor antagonists for long-term maintenance therapy as well as for short-term relief, H_2-receptor antagonists are superior to placebo and are useful in patients who cannot tolerate proton pump inhibitors. No high-quality data exist to support the common practice of using metoclopramide as either monotherapy or an adjunct to acid suppression therapy; furthermore, its potential adverse effects argue against the use of this drug in any GERD patients. In patients

TABLE 124-1 DRUG THERAPY FOR ESOPHAGEAL DISORDERS

AGENT	DOSE
ANTACIDS: LIQUID (TO BUFFER ACID AND INCREASE LESP)	
For example, Mylanta II/Maalox TC (acid-neutralizing capacity, 25 mEq/5 mL)*	15 mL qid 1 hr after meals and at bedtime or as needed
GAVISCON (TO DECREASE REFLUX VIA A VISCOUS MECHANICAL BARRIER AND BUFFER ACID)	
$Al(OH)_3$, $NaHCO_3$, Mg trisilicate, alginic acid	2-4 tablets qid and at bedtime or as needed
H_2-RECEPTOR ANTAGONISTS (TO DECREASE ACID SECRETION)	
Cimetidine	400 mg bid or 200 mg qid
Ranitidine	150 mg bid-qid or 10 mL qid; maintenance dose, 150 mg bid or 10 mL bid
Famotidine	20-40 mg bid or 2.5-5 mL bid
Nizatidine	150 mg bid
PROTON PUMP INHIBITORS (TO DECREASE ACID SECRETION AND GASTRIC VOLUME)†	
Omeprazole	20-40 mg/day; maintenance dose, 20 mg/day
Lansoprazole	15-30 mg/day; maintenance dose, 15 mg/day
Pantoprazole	40 mg/day; maintenance dose, 40 mg/day
Rabeprazole	20 mg/day; maintenance dose, 10-20 mg/day
Esomeprazole	20-40 mg/day; maintenance dose, 20 mg/day
Dexlansoprazole	30-60 mg/day; maintenance dose, 30 mg/day

*Patients with reflux are not generally hypersecretors of gastric acid, so the therapeutic doses of antacids are based on their capacity to buffer (normal) basal acid secretion rates of approximately 1 to 7 mEq/hr (mean, 2 mEq/hr) and peak meal-stimulated acid secretion rates of about 10 to 60 mEq/hr (mean, 30 mEq/hr).

†High-dose therapy is a twice-daily administration of the usually daily dose.

$Al(OH)_3$ = aluminum hydroxide; bid = twice daily; H_2 = histamine; LESP = lower esophageal sphincter pressure; Mg = magnesium; $NaHCO_3$ = sodium bicarbonate; qid = four times daily.

who have persistent symptoms despite proton pump inhibitor therapy, prolonged wireless monitoring off of proton pump therapy can identify patients whose symptoms are not acid-related and who can safely discontinue acid-suppression therapy.[A2]

If, however, patients have documented esophagitis, are intolerant of proton pump inhibitors or unresponsive to them, or regurgitate large volumes, an antireflux procedure should be considered.[9] Newer minimally invasive options in carefully selected patients (including full-thickness plication, various approaches to augment of the lower esophageal sphincter, and transoral incisionless fundoplication) can normalize esophageal acid exposure in about 50% of patients.

Antireflux surgery is an option for patients who have documented esophagitis, who are intolerant of proton pump inhibitors or unresponsive to them, or who regurgitate large volumes. Laparoscopic antireflux surgery is equivalent to continued proton pump inhibitor therapy for the healing of esophagitis and for the treatment of chronic GERD in patients who initially respond to proton pump inhibitors. In patients with persistent regurgitation despite proton pump inhibitor therapy, however, laparoscopic surgery is better than continued medical therapy for relieving symptoms,[A3,A4] even though about 15 to 20% of patients have recurrent symptoms severe enough to warrant another procedure. Surgery also has a number of serious complications that may affect quality of life, including dysphagia, vagal nerve injury, gas bloat syndrome, and diarrhea.

PROGNOSIS

Patients with GERD generally do well with conservative antireflux measures and proton pump inhibitor therapy. When surgery is required, the outcome is usually excellent.

PEPTIC STRICTURES

Esophageal strictures are a well-recognized complication of GERD, especially in older patients with long-standing reflux symptoms, but population-based studies suggest that the incidence of new and recurrent strictures is declining. Peptic strictures are thought to be a consequence of severe inflammation, which leads to fibrosis, scarring, esophageal shortening, and loss of compliance of the lumen.

CLINICAL MANIFESTATIONS AND DIAGNOSIS

Symptoms are typically dysphagia to solids with or without antecedent symptoms of heartburn or acid regurgitation. Strictures may be diagnosed by barium radiography or with upper endoscopy, but barium esophagograms (see Fig. 124-3) have a higher sensitivity for detecting subtle lesions, especially if performed with a solid challenge such as a barium-impregnated pill. However, peptic strictures must be distinguished from a wide variety of other causes of luminal narrowing, including pills, prior nasogastric tube intubation, neoplasia, infection, radiation, surgical anastomosis, some systemic diseases, caustic substances, eosinophilic esophagitis, lichen planus, and extrinsic compression. As a result, endoscopic biopsy and cytology are critical for distinguishing benign from malignant causes of strictures.

TREATMENT

Endoscopic dilation, which remains the cornerstone of therapy, should be done gradually to achieve a luminal diameter that is sufficiently large to relieve symptoms—typically a diameter of 13 mm or greater. After dilation is accomplished, patients should receive chronic proton pump inhibitor therapy (see Table 124-1). For recalcitrant peptic strictures, injection of triamcinolone into the stricture is superior to sham injection in patients who receive balloon dilation and post-procedure proton pump inhibitors.

PROGNOSIS

Endoscopic dilation will usually alleviate symptoms, but repetitive dilation is required in a significant minority of patients.

BARRETT ESOPHAGUS

Barrett esophagus, which is an acquired condition that results from severe esophageal mucosal injury, is a metaplastic change in the lining of the distal tubular esophagus, where the normal squamous epithelium is replaced by a columnar epithelium. Barrett esophagus would be of little importance if not for its well-recognized association with adenocarcinoma of the esophagus (Chapter 178). However, the risk for cancer in an individual patient with Barrett esophagus is low.

EPIDEMIOLOGY

Barrett esophagus is found in approximately 5 to 15% of patients who undergo endoscopy for symptoms of GERD.[10] Population-based studies suggest that the prevalence of Barrett esophagus is approximately 1.3 to 1.6%, but about 45% of affected patients do not have reflux symptoms. Barrett esophagus is predominantly a disease of middle-aged White men, but about 25% of patients are women or are younger than 50 years. The prevalence of Barrett esophagus increases until a plateau is reached between the seventh and ninth decades. Risk factors include frequent and long-standing reflux episodes, smoking, male sex, older age, and central male pattern obesity.

PATHOBIOLOGY

Barrett esophagus results from severe esophageal mucosal injury. Patients who develop Barrett esophagus typically have more esophageal acid and bile exposure, the former based on 24-hour pH monitoring, and almost always have a hiatal hernia, which is typically longer and associated with larger defects than in patients without Barrett esophagus. However, why some patients with GERD develop Barrett esophagus whereas others do not remains unclear, as does the cell of origin of columnar metaplasia. Candidates include dedifferentiation of squamous epithelium into columnar epithelium or stimulation of stem cells from either the basal layer of the esophageal epithelium, the esophageal submucosal glands, gastric cardia, residual embryonal stem cells at the gastroesophageal junction, or the bone marrow. The transcription factor CDX2, which can be induced by both acid and bile salts, appears to play a role in promoting the development of the columnar epithelium in the distal esophagus and gastroesophageal junction.[11] A small subset of patients may have an inherited predisposition to Barrett esophagus, although the genetics of the disease are incompletely understood.

CLINICAL MANIFESTATIONS

The development of reflux symptoms at an earlier age, an increased duration of reflux symptoms, an increased severity of nocturnal reflux symptoms, and prior complications of GERD such as esophagitis, ulceration, stricture, and bleeding may raise the likelihood of Barrett esophagus. Nevertheless, patients with Barrett esophagus are difficult to distinguish clinically from patients whose GERD is uncomplicated by a columnar-lined esophagus. Patients with Barrett esophagus may paradoxically have impaired sensitivity to esophageal acid perfusion and even lack symptoms of GERD.

DIAGNOSIS

Endoscopically, Barrett esophagus is characterized by displacement of the squamocolumnar junction so that it is now proximal to the gastroesophageal junction, which is defined by the proximal margin of gastric folds (see Fig. 124-4). The diagnosis of Barrett esophagus is established if the squamocolumnar junction is displaced 1 cm or more proximal to the gastroesophageal junction and if intestinal metaplasia, which is characterized in part by acid mucin-containing goblet cells, is detected by biopsy.[12]

The precise junction of the stomach and the esophagus may be difficult to determine endoscopically owing to the presence of a hiatal hernia, inflammation, and the dynamic nature of the gastroesophageal junction. If the squamocolumnar junction is above the level of the esophagogastric junction, as defined by the proximal margin of the gastric folds, biopsy specimens should be obtained for confirmation of columnar metaplasia.

Intestinal or columnar metaplasia may be seen in the cardia of normal individuals as well as in persons with chronic reflux disease, and the prevalence of intestinal metaplasia at a normal-appearing gastroesophageal junction varies from 5 to 36%. Dysplasia and an increased risk for carcinoma have been reported in patients who have intestinal metaplasia of the gastroesophageal junction or cardia, but the magnitude of that risk appears to be far less than that of Barrett esophagus and surveillance is not warranted.

Another potential approach to diagnosis is the cytosponge-trefoil factor 3, which is a non-endoscopic cell collection device coupled with an immunohistochemical biomarker. This small mesh sponge within a soluble gelatin capsule is attached to a string. The patient swallows the capsule, which is then retrieved about 5 minutes later. The mesh slightly abrades the esophageal mucosa, thereby collecting cells for analysis. In one randomized trial, this approach significantly increased the early diagnosis of Barrett esophagus.[A5]

TREATMENT

Patients who are diagnosed with Barrett esophagus require surveillance endoscopy at regular intervals (Fig. 124-5). They characteristically worry about cancer risk, which they may overestimate, face higher life insurance premiums, and may receive conflicting information on how best to treat their condition.

Proton pump inhibitors (see Table 124-1), which are the cornerstone of medical therapy for Barrett esophagus, consistently relieve symptoms and heal esophagitis. However, proton pump inhibitors, even at high doses, do not provide clear regression of Barrett histology, perhaps because alleviation of reflux symptoms is not necessarily equivalent to normalization of esophageal acid exposure. In fact, abnormal acid exposure persists in approximately 25% of Barrett esophagus patients despite twice-daily proton pump inhibitors. The precise importance of complete control of esophageal acid exposure in patients with Barrett esophagus remains unknown, but the combination of high-dose proton pump inhibitor therapy plus aspirin (300 to 325mg daily) can reduce the progression to high-grade dysplasia, adenocarcinoma, or death in patients with Barrett metaplasia.[A6] Antireflux surgery effectively alleviates GERD symptoms, and the indications for surgery are the same as those for patients with GERD without Barrett esophagus. Surgery should not, however, be viewed as a better cancer prevention tool.

Current practice guidelines, based on observational data, recommend endoscopic surveillance of patients with documented Barrett esophagus in an attempt to detect dysplasia and cancer at an early and potentially curable stage.[12] Before entering into a surveillance program, patients should be advised about risks and benefits, including the limitations of surveillance endoscopy as well as the importance of adhering to appropriate surveillance intervals. Other considerations include age, likelihood of survival over the next 5 years, and ability to tolerate either endoscopic or surgical interventions for early esophageal adenocarcinoma.

Systematic four-quadrant biopsies should be obtained at 2-cm intervals along the entire length of the Barrett segment after inflammation related to GERD is controlled with antisecretory therapy. Mucosal abnormalities, especially in the setting of high-grade dysplasia, should be resected endoscopically.

Surveillance intervals, determined by the presence and grade of dysplasia, are based on a limited understanding of the biology of esophageal adenocarcinoma. Surveillance for patients without dysplasia should occur every 3 to 5 years after an initial negative examination. If low-grade dysplasia is found, the diagnosis should first be confirmed by an expert gastrointestinal pathologist because of the marked interobserver variability in the interpretation of these biopsies. If confirmed, aggressive proton pump inhibitor therapy (see Table 124-1) is recommended to decrease inflammation and regeneration, which may make pathologic interpretation difficult. A repeat endoscopy should then be performed within 6 months of the initial diagnosis. If low-grade dysplasia is again confirmed, options include continued surveillance at 6- to 12-month intervals or radio frequency ablation, but ablation significantly reduces the risk for progression to high-grade dysplasia or to adenocarcinoma over the next 3 years.[A7]

If high-grade dysplasia is found, an experienced gastrointestinal pathologist should confirm the diagnosis. For patients with confirmed high-grade dysplasia, endoscopic ablation therapy with radio frequency ablation, endoscopic mucosal resection, or a combination is now recommended instead of surgery or continued surveillance.[13] For high-grade dysplasia patients with any visible abnormality, endoscopic mucosal resection is recommended for optimal diagnosis and staging. Surgery with esophagectomy is reserved only for patients who fail to respond to endoscopic ablation therapy or if the cancer is beyond stage T1a (intramucosal cancer).

PROGNOSIS

The risk that a patient with Barrett esophagus will develop esophageal adenocarcinoma is now estimated to be approximately 0.1 to 0.3% annually. With appropriate surveillance,[14] most patients with Barrett esophagus will never develop esophageal adenocarcinoma and will die of other causes.

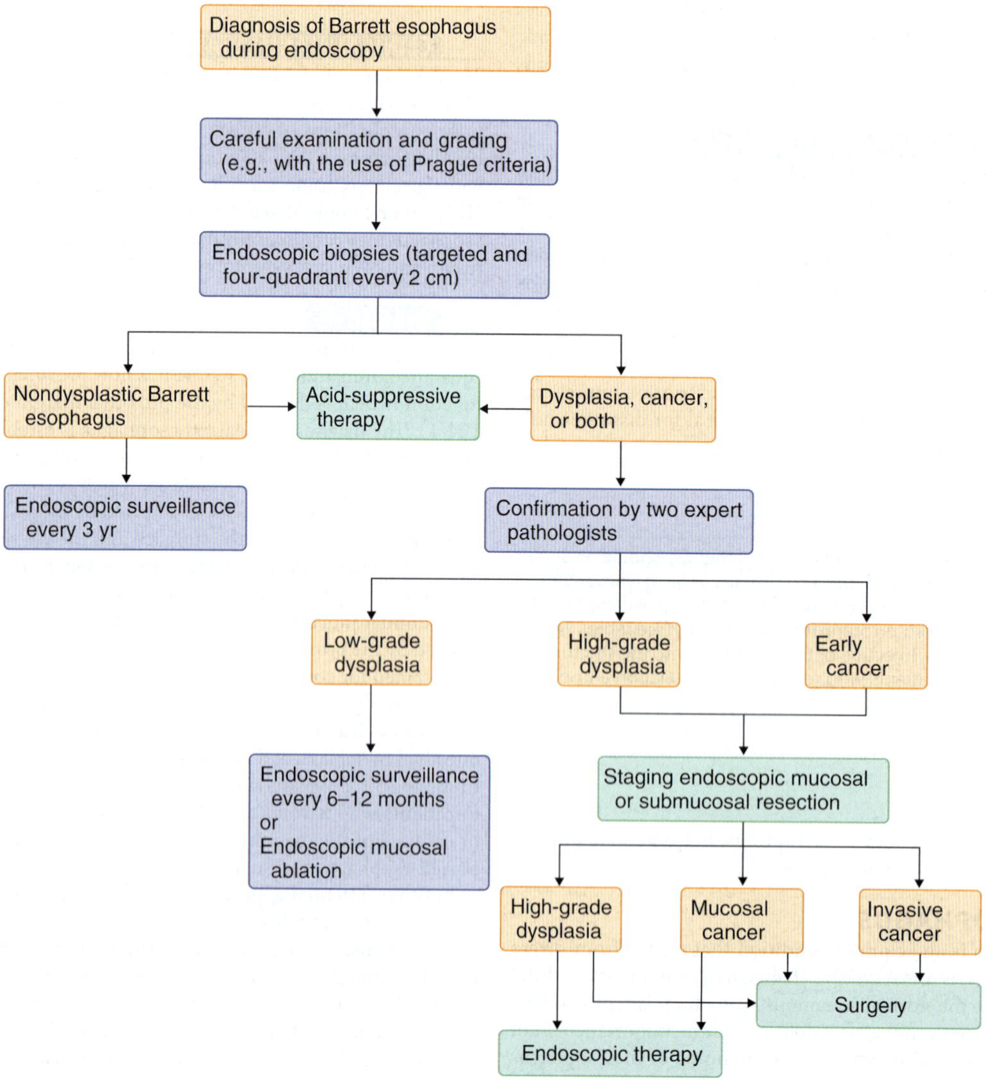

FIGURE 124-5. Proposed treatment algorithm for patients with Barrett esophagus. (From Sharma P. Barrett's esophagus. *N Engl J Med.* 2009;361:2548-2556.)

ESOPHAGITIS

EOSINOPHILIC ESOPHAGITIS

Eosinophilic esophagitis is probably caused by an aberrant immune or antigenic response to food and aeroallergens that trigger chronic inflammation with dense eosinophilia in the esophageal mucosa. The disease is most common in children, adolescents, and young adults, but middle-aged adults are often affected as well. The estimated prevalence is about 0.5 to 1 case per 1000 population. Patients often have a personal and family history of other allergic disorders. A genetic predisposition is suggested by abnormal gene profiles in almost 50% of children with this disorder.

CLINICAL MANIFESTATIONS AND DIAGNOSIS

Children present with failure to thrive, nausea, vomiting, abdominal pain, and dyspeptic symptoms, whereas adults present with solid food dysphagia, food impaction, or chest pain. Boerhaave syndrome (see later) may also occur with this disease. Diagnosis is made by classic findings on endoscopy, such as linear furrowing, white exudates, and multiple rings (Fig. 124-6), accompanied by biopsies demonstrating eosinophilic infiltration (Table 124-2) in the absence of other conditions that can cause esophageal eosinophilia, such as GERD, achalasia, vasculitis, hypereosinophilic syndrome, Crohn disease, Ehlers-Danlos syndrome, graft versus host disease, infections, and drug hypersensitivity. The severity of the condition and its response to therapy can be assessed by both endoscopic and histologic criteria.[15]

TREATMENT AND PROGNOSIS

Treatment options for eosinophilic esophagitis include food elimination diets,[A8] proton pump inhibitors (see Table 124-1), and topical steroids.[16-18] Many patients may benefit from an empiric one, two, four- (or six-) food elimination diet that eliminates cow's milk protein (casein), soy, wheat, eggs, peanut/tree nuts, and seafood. An elemental diet also may be prescribed for severe disease. A formal allergy evaluation (Chapter 230) is required only in individuals with accompanying atopic diseases. Topical steroids (e.g., swallowed fluticasone, 880 μg twice daily; budesonide orodispersible tablets, 0.5 mg twice daily; or budesonide suspension, 1 mg twice daily) can safely sustain remission in 75% of patients, whereas up to 95% of patients may relapse when treatment is stopped.[A9,A10] Dupilumab (300 mg subcutaneously weekly for 12 weeks) is a useful option.[A11,19]

Most patients do well after an initial course of treatment. However, relapse is typical once therapy is discontinued, and chronic therapy is often needed, especially for those with prior complications such as food impaction, strictures, or a narrow-caliber esophagus.

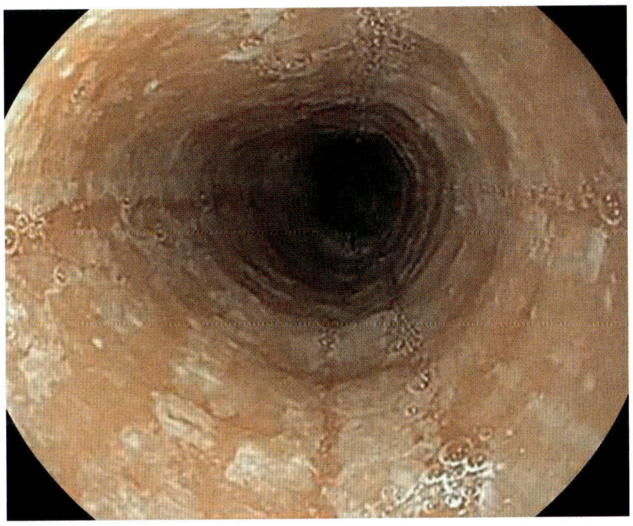

FIGURE 124-6. Endoscopic corrugated (ringed) appearance of esophagus in eosinophilic esophagitis.

TABLE 124-2 GUIDELINES FOR THE DIAGNOSIS OF EOSINOPHILIC ESOPHAGITIS

- Characteristic demographic and endoscopic findings
- Clinical symptoms of esophageal dysfunction
- *At least* 15 eosinophils in 1 high-power biopsy field
- Exclusion of other causes of esophageal eosinophilia

PILL-INDUCED ESOPHAGITIS

Pills (Table 124-3) can induce esophageal injury by producing a caustic acid solution (e.g., ascorbic acid and ferrous sulfate), producing a caustic alkaline solution (e.g., alendronate, button batteries), placing a hyperosmolar solution in contact with the esophageal mucosa (e.g., potassium chloride), or causing direct drug toxicity to the esophageal mucosa (e.g., tetracycline). Because prolonged contact is an essential part of the injury, predisposing factors for pill-induced injury include anatomic barriers, such as a stricture, a prominent aortic arch that compresses the esophagus, or improper ingestion of the pill because of inadequate fluid or improper positioning (i.e., lying down directly after taking the pill). The most common medications are tetracycline and its derivatives, but other commonly implicated medications include nonsteroidal anti-inflammatory drugs, bisphosphonates, ferrous sulfate, quinidine, and potassium chloride.

Patients usually complain of the acute onset of severe odynophagia. Radiographic or endoscopic findings may range from discrete ulceration to diffuse esophagitis. Treatment is generally supportive with discontinuation of the medication until the injury resolves. Although acid suppression is commonly recommended, there is no proof that this approach is beneficial. Patients should be given careful instructions to avoid lying down immediately after ingesting medication and to drink adequate fluids to prevent injury. Rarely, pill-induced injury may lead to strictures and even fistulas.

CAUSTIC INJURY

Potentially devastating caustic esophageal injuries may be caused by highly alkaline solutions, such as sodium hydroxide, or highly acidic solutions, such as sulfuric acid. The most common products that contain these substances are drain cleaners and industrial strength cleaners, but other corrosive substances include hair relaxers, oven and toilet bowl cleaners, and button batteries. Patients require emergent endoscopy to determine the degree of injury,

TABLE 124-3 MEDICATIONS COMMONLY ASSOCIATED WITH ESOPHAGITIS OR ESOPHAGEAL INJURY

ANTIBIOTICS
Tetracycline Doxycycline Clindamycin Penicillin Rifampin Cloxacillin
ANTIVIRAL AGENTS
Zalcitabine Zidovudine Nelfinavir
BISPHOSPHONATES
Alendronate Etidronate Pamidronate
CHEMOTHERAPEUTIC AGENTS
Dactinomycin Bleomycin Cytarabine Daunorubicin 5-Fluorouracil Methotrexate Vincristine Crizotinib
NONSTEROIDAL ANTI-INFLAMMATORY DRUGS
Aspirin Naproxen Ibuprofen
OTHER MEDICATIONS
Quinidine Potassium chloride Ferrous sulfate Ascorbic acid Multivitamins Theophylline

which helps predict long-term prognosis. No clear evidence supports routine steroids or antibiotics. Many patients will have lifelong disease marked by chronic strictures that require frequent dilation and even esophageal reconstruction. In patients with a severe initial injury, the risk for esophageal cancer is significantly increased.

ESOPHAGEAL MOTOR DISORDERS

OROPHARYNGEAL DYSFUNCTION

The cricopharyngeus and inferior pharyngeal constrictor are composed of striated muscle and innervated by upper motor neurons, the brain stem, and the cerebral cortex. Both primary myopathic and neuropathic disorders can result in dysfunction. The most common neurologic cause of oropharyngeal dysphagia is a cerebrovascular accident (Chapter 376). Other neuropathic disorders that may also affect function include myasthenia gravis (Chapter 390), brain stem tumors (Chapter 175), amyotrophic lateral sclerosis (Chapter 387), Parkinson disease (Chapter 378), Alzheimer disease (Chapter 371), post-polio syndrome (Chapter 349), Guillain-Barré syndrome (Chapter 388), and botulism (Chapter 271). Myogenic disorders that cause dysfunction include paraneoplastic antibody-mediated syndromes (Chapter 164), thyroid disease (Chapter 207), primary myopathies (Chapter 389) such as dermatomyositis and inclusion body myositis and drugs that cause myopathy such as statins and amiodarone.

Patients with oropharyngeal abnormalities experience dysphagia, often accompanied by postprandial coughing, hoarseness, and aspiration pneumonia. Treatment focuses on the underlying myopathic or neurologic cause and swallowing therapy, but prognosis is often poor owing to limited treatment options.

ACHALASIA

Achalasia, which is the prototypic esophageal motility disorder,[20] is characterized by insufficient relaxation of the lower esophageal sphincter accompanied by loss of esophageal peristalsis.

EPIDEMIOLOGY AND PATHOBIOLOGY

Achalasia can occur in patients of almost any age, from infants to nonagenarians, but it most commonly presents between 30 and 60 years of age. The prevalence is 10 per 100,000 in the United States, with all races affected and an equal distribution in men and women. The pathophysiology of achalasia most likely reflects an antibody-mediated autoimmune myenteric plexopathy in the lower esophageal sphincter and a generalized neuropathy in the esophageal body. The triggering event is unclear, but a viral cause is suggested. Injury to the lower esophageal sphincter neurons leads to a relative selective deficiency of nitric oxide. With this loss of the main functional inhibitory neurotransmitter, the sphincter loses its ability to relax. The neurochemical process that leads to aperistalsis is unclear.

CLINICAL MANIFESTATIONS AND DIAGNOSIS

The cardinal symptoms of achalasia are dysphagia to both liquids and solids, regurgitation, and chest pain. Some patients may have more subtle symptoms, including heartburn, presumably caused by esophageal stasis of acidic food content, weight loss, and aspiration pneumonia; in these settings, diagnosis is often delayed.

The diagnosis of achalasia relies on esophageal manometry and barium radiography. The classic radiographic appearance is esophageal dilation, stasis of contrast material, and a "bird's beak" appearance to the lower esophageal sphincter (Fig. 124-7). Manometry demonstrates high residual pressures of the lower esophageal sphincter and either simultaneous contractions or complete absence of peristaltic contractions (E-Fig. 124-1). Whether classification systems based on manometric findings can predict response is being studied. Endoscopy is recommended to exclude secondary causes of achalasia, such as gastroesophageal junctional cancer. Occasionally, patients present with a massively dilated esophagus and marked food retention. Radiographically, these patients develop a "sigmoid" esophagus with a radiographic picture similar to a sigmoid colon.

Achalasia may represent a paraneoplastic presentation of some malignancies, particularly small cell lung cancer (Chapter 177); in these patients, the tumor produces an antineuronal antibody (anti-Hu) that mediates the autoimmune lower esophageal sphincter plexopathy and produces a syndrome identical to primary achalasia. Some tumors, such as proximal gastric cancer, may also metastasize to or directly extend into the lower esophageal sphincter and produce an achalasia-like picture, possibly owing to extrinsic compression or tumor infiltration.

TREATMENT

Treatment options to decrease the functional obstruction at the level of the lower esophageal sphincter include the intrasphincteric injection of botulinum toxin, pneumatic dilation, surgical myotomy, and peroral endoscopic myotomy. Injection of botulinum toxin during endoscopy reduces symptoms and improves esophageal emptying in up to 90% of patients. Because symptoms typically recur within 6 to 24 months, this treatment is best for patients who are not candidates for more definitive therapies or to confirm the diagnosis of achalasia when clinical, radiographic, and manometric criteria are not conclusive.

In pneumatic dilation, a 30- to 40-mm pneumatic balloon is placed fluoroscopically to straddle the lower esophageal sphincter; the balloon is then inflated to tear the muscle fibers of the lower esophageal sphincter. In general, one pneumatic dilation will achieve 5 years of symptomatic remission in 70% of patients, and three dilations will succeed in 90% of patients. The downside of this procedure is the risk for perforation, which occurs in less than 1% of patients in experienced hands.

The third approach is a Heller myotomy, which is now typically performed laparoscopically. This long myotomy starts at least 2 cm below the lower esophageal sphincter and extends for about 6 cm upward past the sphincter; a loose fundoplication is performed to prevent gastroesophageal reflux. The 5-year success rate approaches 90%. Randomized controlled trials suggest that either pneumatic dilation or Heller myotomy will provide comparable clinical results over 2 years.[A12]

Peroral endoscopic myotomy is an alternative to laparoscopic myotomy. Results at 2 years are equal to or better than for pneumatic dilation[A13,A14] or laparoscopic Heller myotomy, and long-term follow-up data are encouraging; however, reflux is observed in approximately 50% of patients. As a result, patients should be aware of this issue when selecting between the endoscopic and laparoscopic approaches and should undergo endoscopy at 6 to 12 months after peroral endoscopic myotomy.[21]

In patients with massive dilation, esophageal dysfunction may warrant total esophagectomy because of life-threatening symptoms such as continued weight loss, recurrent aspiration pneumonia, or tracheal compression. In patients with underlying paraneoplastic malignancy, treatment of the tumor may be helpful, and botulinum toxin has been tried with anecdotal success.

PROGNOSIS

No treatment approach is curative, and all are palliative. Recurrent symptoms may be related to an incomplete myotomy, herniation or unwrapping of the fundoplication, esophageal strictures, Barrett esophagus, or just the natural history of the disease. Achalasia patients also may be predisposed to squamous cell carcinoma of the esophagus, although current evidence does not support cancer screening.

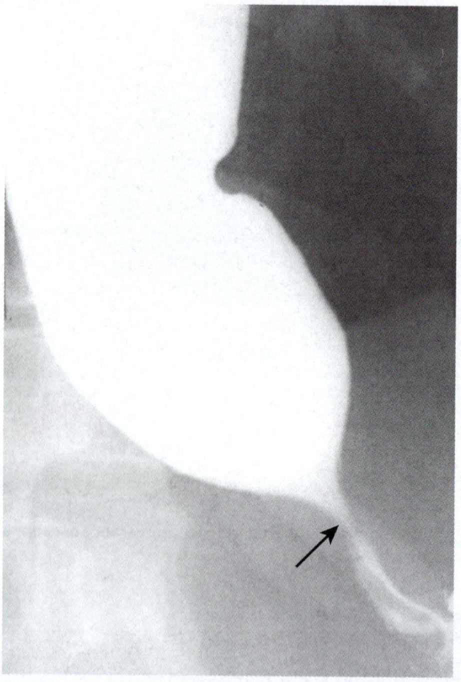

FIGURE 124-7. **Esophagogram of a patient with idiopathic achalasia. Note the dilated esophagus and distal tapering result in a "bird's beak" deformity in the area of the lower esophageal sphincter *(arrow)*.** (Courtesy Marc Levine, MD.)

DIFFUSE ESOPHAGEAL SPASM

Diffuse esophageal spasm is found in fewer than 5% of patients who undergo manometry for symptoms of chest pain, dysphagia, or both. The pathophysiology of diffuse esophageal spasm is not well understood, but a deficiency of nitric oxide in the esophageal body may lead to a loss of control of esophageal peristalsis, high pressures, and rapid velocity contractions.

CLINICAL MANIFESTATIONS AND DIAGNOSIS

Classically, patients have symptoms of intermittent chest pain (Chapter 123), dysphagia, or both. On endoscopic ultrasound, patients may demonstrate thickening of the circular and longitudinal muscle layers. Diffuse esophageal spasm is defined manometrically by premature rapid contractions in at least 20% of all swallows, accompanied by normal peristalsis.[22] Radiographically, diffuse esophageal spasm is characterized by a "corkscrew" esophagus with multiple simultaneous contractions that obliterate the lumen (Fig. 124-8).

TREATMENT AND PROGNOSIS

Treatment of these patients is challenging, and clinical trials have not demonstrated efficacy of any therapy. Empirical therapy may be tried with agents that relax smooth muscle or augment the nitric oxide content, such as hyoscyamine (0.125 mg sublingually), calcium-channel antagonists (nifedipine, 10 mg sublingually), nitroglycerin (0.3 mg sublingually), and sildenafil (50 mg orally). Injection of botulinum toxin into the esophageal body has had equivocal results. Antidepressants, particularly low-dose tricyclics (e.g., imipramine, 10 to 50 mg before bedtime), have had some success. For patients with dysphagia, sphincter options include botulinum toxin injection and pneumatic dilation, but surgery is not indicated unless there is evidence of achalasia. Early results of peroral endoscopic myotomy are encouraging. In general, these disorders can be difficult to manage but are not life-threatening.

OTHER MOTILITY DISORDERS

Jackhammer esophagus and hypertensive peristalsis are recently described manometric diagnoses that formerly were called nutcracker esophagus. Both are characterized by high-amplitude peristaltic contractions and are of uncertain clinical significance. Antisecretory therapy with proton pump inhibitors (see Table 124-1) is often warranted.

Isolated incomplete relaxation of the lower esophageal sphincter, also known as esophagogastric junction outflow obstruction, may represent a variant of achalasia and should be treated as such in patients with dysphagia and supportive findings or functional imaging or impedance planimetry. This entity also may be seen with structural and vascular abnormalities in the vicinity of the gastroesophageal junction. Patients with manometric findings of low-amplitude contractions, failed contractions, or contractions with large breaks have weak peristalsis, which is commonly seen in patients with severe underlying GERD.

STRUCTURAL ABNORMALITIES

CRICOPHARYNGEAL BARS

A cricopharyngeal bar diagnosed by a prominent impression of the cricopharyngeus, reflects an inability to relax the upper esophageal sphincter maximally during the flow of barium, with a sustained decrease in compliance. The decrease in cross-sectional area of the upper esophageal sphincter is likely caused by fibrosis. This condition may be asymptomatic or accompanied by symptoms of oropharyngeal dysphagia to solids. Treatment of symptomatic patients is either large-caliber dilation or surgical or endoscopic myotomy; the clinical results are generally excellent.

ESOPHAGEAL DIVERTICULA

Esophageal diverticula are encountered in fewer than 1% of upper gastrointestinal radiographic studies and account for less than 5% of cases of dysphagia. Esophageal diverticula may occur in one of three locations: above the upper esophageal sphincter, in the mid-esophagus, and just above the lower esophageal sphincter.

Zenker diverticulum is a pouch that protrudes posteriorly above the upper esophageal sphincter (Fig. 124-9). This protrusion occurs through a triangular region known as Killian triangle, which is bordered above by fibers of the inferior constrictor muscle and below by the cricopharyngeal muscle. It is thought to be caused by increased hypopharyngeal pressure that results from decreased compliance and impaired opening of the upper esophageal sphincter. Small diverticula may be asymptomatic, but increasing size is associated with globus, dysphagia to solids or liquids, regurgitation of undigested food, halitosis, and aspiration. Although no treatment is needed for asymptomatic patients, open or endoscopic surgery is indicated when symptoms occur. Prognosis after surgery is excellent.

Mid-esophageal diverticula, which are focal outpouchings of the middle of the esophagus, are thought to be related to an underlying abnormality of esophageal motility. Past tuberculosis may result in such diverticula. Symptoms typically include dysphagia with or without regurgitation, and diagnosis is usually made with barium contrast radiography. Surgical diverticulectomy with myotomy or endoscopic myotomy is reserved for patients with symptoms.

Epiphrenic diverticula are herniations of mucosa and submucosa through the muscular layers of the distal 10 cm of the esophagus. They are most commonly caused by functional lower esophageal sphincter obstruction, owing to

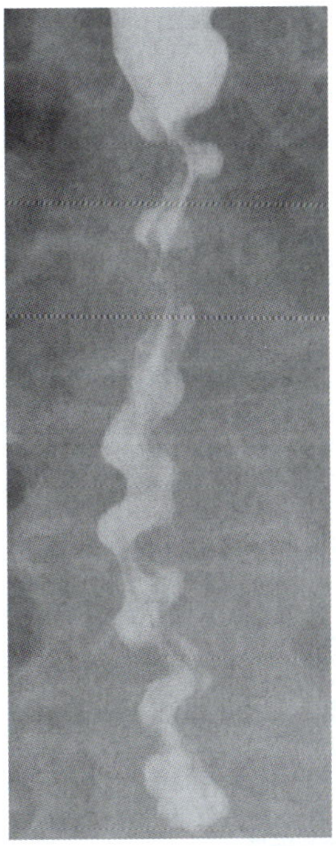

FIGURE 124-8. Barium esophagogram showing a "corkscrew" esophagus in a patient with diffuse esophageal spasm. The patient had dysphagia, chest pain, and normal endoscopic findings. (Image courtesy of Marc Levine, MD.)

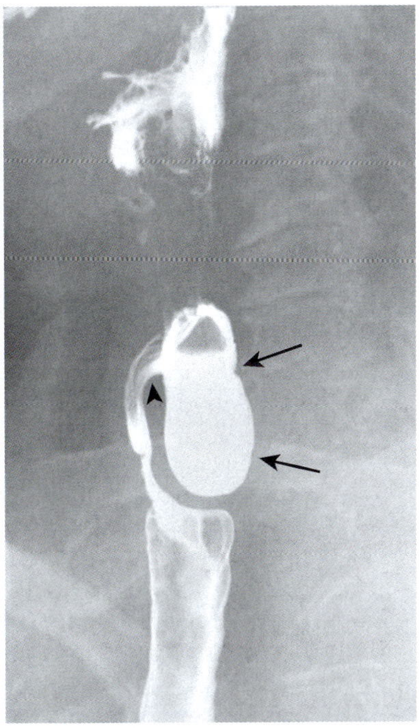

FIGURE 124-9. Barium radiograph of Zenker diverticulum *(arrows)* and cricopharyngeus *(arrowhead)*. (Courtesy Marc Levine, MD.)

underlying motility abnormalities such as achalasia or diffuse esophageal spasm, but also may be associated with mechanical obstruction, owing to a leiomyoma, prior surgery, stenosis, stricture tumor, or web. Epiphrenic diverticula may be asymptomatic or cause dysphagia, regurgitation, odynophagia, chest pain, heartburn, or aspiration. Diagnosis is typically made by barium radiography (Fig. 124-10), but endoscopy is recommended to exclude a structural cause of obstruction, and esophageal manometry is recommended to evaluate for underlying motility abnormalities. No therapy is warranted in asymptomatic patients, but symptomatic patients generally do well with surgical diverticulectomy, repair of the defect in the esophageal wall, and relief of the underlying obstruction, usually with a myotomy and partial fundoplication.

RINGS AND WEBS

Esophageal rings are concentric areas of narrowing, usually in the distal esophagus. *Schatzki ring* (Fig. 124-11) is a thin, fixed, circumferential membrane-like narrowing at the gastroesophageal junction, typically at the proximal border of a hiatal hernia. The cause may be congenital, secondary to a pleat of redundant mucosa, or related to gastroesophageal reflux. Symptoms typically occur if the ring results in a lumen that is 13 mm or less in diameter. Classic symptoms are intermittent dysphagia to solids or impaction of solid food. Diagnosis is best accomplished with barium radiography, especially for rings larger than 13 mm in diameter, which may be missed at the time of endoscopy. Treatment involves use of large-caliber dilators at least 18 mm in diameter. Long-term therapy with proton pump inhibitors (see Table 124-1) may prevent relapses. Most patients relapse after a single dilation.

Muscular rings, which are located several centimeters above the squamocolumnar junction, are composed of mucosa, submucosa, and muscle. Barium radiography and endoscopy reveal a focal constriction of variable diameter. Optimal therapy is unclear. Dilation leads to only partial or temporary relief. Other treatment modalities include injection of botulinum toxin and anticholinergic agents.

Esophageal webs are thin, eccentric, membranous areas of narrowing that may be found anywhere in the esophagus but most commonly are in the proximal region (Fig. 124-12). The pathogenesis of webs is unknown, but they are associated with a number of systemic diseases, including bullous skin disorders, chronic graft-versus-host disease, and iron deficiency anemia.

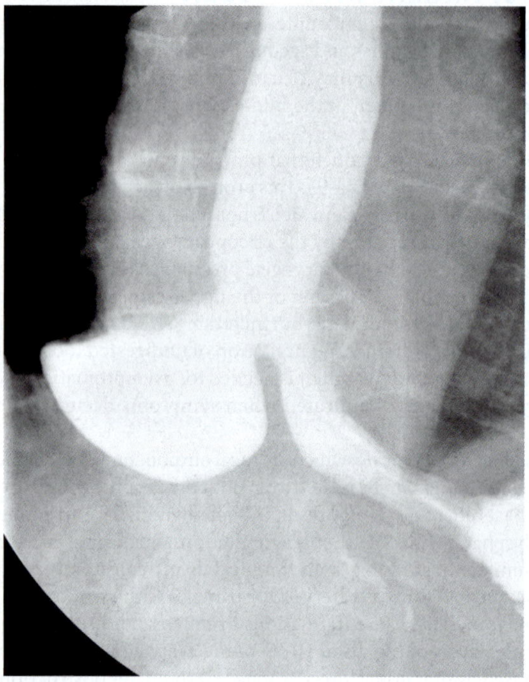

FIGURE 124-10. Barium radiograph of an esophageal epiphrenic diverticulum. (Courtesy Marc Levine, MD.)

HIATAL HERNIA

A hiatal hernia involves herniation of elements of the abdominal cavity through the diaphragmatic hiatus. A sliding, or type I, hernia, in which the gastroesophageal junction is displaced above the diaphragmatic hiatus, is the most common type. Type I hiatal hernias typically are not associated with symptoms or are associated with heartburn or acid regurgitation. Treatment is the same as for GERD.

In a type II, or true, paraesophageal hernia, which is uncommon, the gastroesophageal junction is in its normal location, but the fundus and parts of the greater curvature of the stomach herniate into the mediastinum alongside the esophagus. With type III or mixed paraesophageal hernia, the gastroesophageal junction and a large part of the stomach herniate into the mediastinum. Both types of paraesophageal hernias present with symptoms of postprandial distress, such as epigastric pain, chest pain, substernal fullness, shortness of breath, nausea, or vomiting. Iron deficiency anemia may be seen with large hiatal hernias in which at least one third of the stomach is in the chest; linear gastric erosions at the top of gastric folds at the level of the diaphragm have been implicated as a cause of chronic blood loss. Asymptomatic paraesophageal hernias do not require surgery. Symptomatic paraesophageal hernias warrant surgical therapy because of the risk for strangulation, bleeding, perforation, or obstruction.

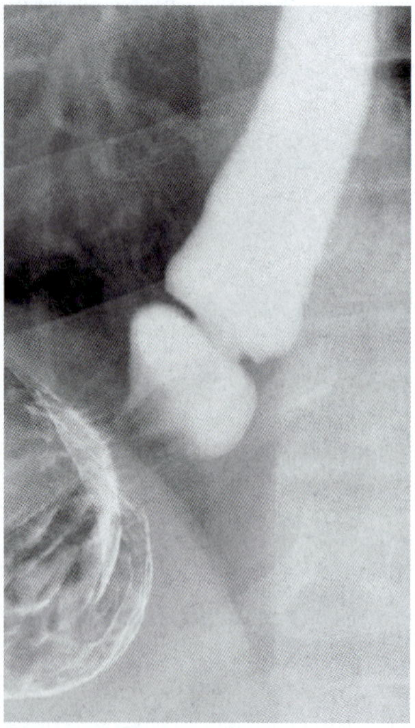

FIGURE 124-11. Barium radiograph of Schatzki ring. (Courtesy Marc Levine, MD.)

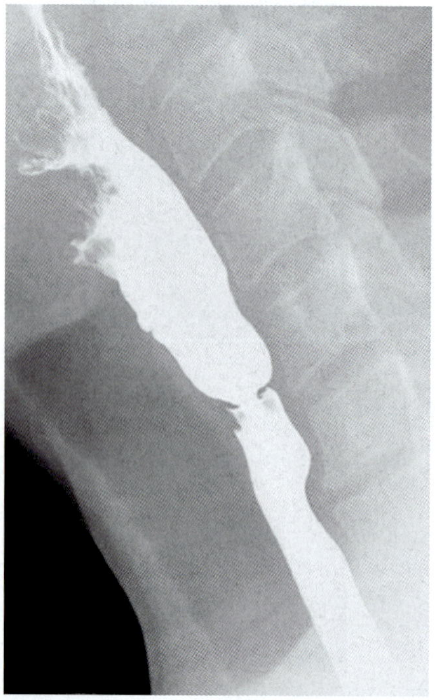

FIGURE 124-12. Barium radiograph of an esophageal web. (Courtesy of Marc Levine, MD.)

THE ESOPHAGUS IN SYSTEMIC DISEASES

SCLERODERMA

Up to 90% of patients with scleroderma (Chapter 246) have esophageal involvement, thereby making it the most common gastrointestinal abnormality in the disease.[23] The classic manometric and radiologic findings are aperistalsis of the distal two thirds of the esophagus and hypotensive or patulous lower esophageal sphincter on manometry or radiography, respectively. Only one third of scleroderma patients have these classic findings. These findings result initially because of neuropathy and later because of the myopathy. The main clinical manifestation is severe gastroesophageal reflux. Delayed gastric emptying may also occur. Marked esophageal stasis may also lead to *Candida* esophagitis. A patulous (on radiography) or hypotensive (on manometry) lower esophageal sphincter strongly supports the diagnosis. Proton pump inhibitor therapy (see Table 124-1) is the cornerstone of treatment. Lifestyle changes, including small frequent meals and avoiding nighttime meals, may reduce the gastric symptoms. Antireflux surgery can exacerbate dysphagia by creating a functional high-pressure zone in the distal esophagus and is thus usually contraindicated. Unfortunately, many patients suffer from chronic GERD and are at risk for developing Barrett esophagus and recurrent strictures.

AMYLOIDOSIS

Amyloidosis (Chapter 174) may lead to smooth muscle and autonomic nervous system dysfunction that involves the esophagus in a pattern similar to scleroderma. Patients will have both dysphagia and severe reflux because of esophageal aperistalsis and a hypotensive lower esophageal sphincter. Dysphagia may result not only from the motility changes but also from diffuse esophageal rigidity and loss of compliance owing to amyloid infiltration of the esophageal wall. Rarely, an achalasia-like pattern may develop. No treatment improves the esophageal manifestations of amyloidosis, other than treatment for the underlying disease and high-dose proton pump inhibitors given twice daily.

OTHER SYSTEMIC DISEASES

Dermatomyositis (Chapter 248) principally involves the striated muscle of the oropharynx and proximal esophagus, but sometimes the distal esophagus may lose normal peristaltic function. Symptoms can be oropharyngeal or esophageal depending on the site of greatest muscular involvement. Dysphagia may be an early presenting symptom of dermatomyositis, and the esophagus may be involved in 10 to 50% of patients. Treatment is directed at the generalized myositis because there are no specific treatments for the esophagus. Swallowing therapy may sometimes be helpful. Return of swallowing commonly lags behind recovery of other striated muscle symptoms.

Esophageal involvement in *systemic lupus erythematosus* (Chapter 245) is not as prominent as in scleroderma, dermatomyositis, or mixed connective tissue disease. Dysphagia occurs in fewer than 15% of patients and may be caused by decreased salivation from secondary Sjögren syndrome or reduced esophageal peristalsis. Other causes of esophageal symptoms in patients with systemic lupus erythematosus include GERD, esophageal ulcers, esophageal infection, and medication-induced esophagitis. *Behçet disease* (Chapter 249) causes esophageal ulcers in less than 15% of affected patients. Ulcers are typically located in the middle third of the esophagus and are often associated with ulcers in the stomach, ileum, or colon. Rare esophageal lesions include strictures, varices, and fistulas connecting with the trachea. These complications can be severe and debilitating.

Esophageal involvement in *Crohn disease* (Chapter 127) is uncommon but has been described in up to 1 to 2% of patients. Occasionally, isolated esophageal disease may occur. Ulceration is the most common manifestation, but strictures, fissures, esophagobronchial fistulas, mediastinal abscesses, and aphthoid lesions have been described. Patients typically complain of dysphagia and odynophagia. Treatment and prognosis are as for the underlying Crohn disease.

In the *Ehlers-Danlos syndrome* (Chapter 239), hiatal hernias are common, and structural esophageal defects such as giant epiphrenic diverticula, megaesophagus, and spontaneous esophageal rupture may also be seen.

SKIN DISORDERS THAT INVOLVE THE ESOPHAGUS

Lichen planus (Chapter 405) often involves the esophagus. Patients generally present in the fourth to seventh decade of life. Histologically, the lesions in up to 25 to 50% of patients show a characteristic lymphohistiocytic inflammatory infiltrate and apoptotic basal keratinocytes known as Civatte bodies. Lesions classically occur on the buccal mucosa and the tongue, but the disease may also involve other areas of the oral cavity and the esophagus, conjunctiva, nose, larynx, stomach, bladder, and anus. Most patients are asymptomatic or have only minor symptoms, but patients with severe esophageal lichen planus often develop strictures and may present with dysphagia, odynophagia, and weight loss. Strictures are typically proximal but may be variable in length and location, sometimes involving most of the esophageal body. Patients may present with esophageal lichen planus in the absence of extraesophageal disease. Endoscopic findings, which can be subtle and nonspecific, include peeling mucosa, hyperemic focal abnormalities, and submucosal plaque or papules. High-dose systemic steroids, starting with at least 40 mg prednisone and then tapering over 1 to 2 months, are often successful, but relapse is common when steroids are tapered. Topical steroids, tacrolimus, and methotrexate also have been tried. Dilation and intralesional steroids can alleviate the symptoms associated with strictures, but symptoms frequently recur in less than a year and necessitate repeat dilations. The esophageal lesions of lichen planus may have malignancy potential.

Pemphigus vulgaris (Chapter 406) patients who experience acute flares may have upper gastrointestinal symptoms (dysphagia, odynophagia, or retrosternal burning) in 80% of cases and biopsy-proven esophageal pemphigus lesions in nearly 50% of cases. Pemphigus vulgaris may rarely be isolated to the esophagus. Paraneoplastic pemphigus (Chapter 406), most commonly reported with lymphoreticular disease, also may involve the esophagus. Like lesions on the skin, esophageal lesions may be flaccid blisters or erosions, but they may also appear as red longitudinal lines along the entire esophagus. Like cutaneous and oral pemphigus, esophageal pemphigus is generally treated with corticosteroids.

In *mucous membrane pemphigoid* (cicatricial pemphigoid; Chapter 406), the esophagus is the most common site of gastrointestinal involvement, but esophageal disease occurs in less than 15% of patients. The esophageal disease can present as long as 10 years after disease onset and may be the only presentation of the disease. Patients complain of dysphagia and odynophagia. Imaging typically shows erosions, strictures, bullae, or webs. Treatment generally is as for the skin disease.

In *dystrophic epidermolysis bullosa* (Chapter 406), approximately 70 to 95% of patients develop esophageal stenosis or strictures. Strictures are especially common in children with recessive dystrophic epidermolysis bullosa, whereas fewer than 10% of patients with dominant dystrophic epidermolysis bullosa develop strictures by age 50 years.

ESOPHAGEAL INFECTIONS

HERPES SIMPLEX VIRUS

Herpes simplex virus (HSV; Chapter 345) esophagitis, which is usually caused by HSV-1, is a well-recognized disease in immunocompromised patients but may also occur in immunocompetent hosts. HSV typically presents as severe odynophagia. Endoscopy and radiology characteristically demonstrate multiple ulcers and friable mucosa, predominantly involving the distal esophagus. Mucosal biopsies demonstrate typical intranuclear inclusion bodies. Depending on the severity of the esophageal disease and the underlying health of the patient, treatment options may include intravenous acyclovir, 5 mg/kg every 8 hours for 7 days, or oral acyclovir, 400 mg five times daily for 7 days, combined with symptomatic treatment.

CANDIDIASIS

Esophageal candidiasis is common in patients with human immunodeficiency virus (HIV) infection or with impaired cellular immunity owing to hematologic malignancies, immunosuppressive therapy, or diabetes mellitus.[24] Esophageal candidiasis is also seen in immunocompetent patients who are taking corticosteroids and in individuals with marked esophageal stasis, such as patients with advanced achalasia or scleroderma. Esophageal candidiasis characteristically presents with symptoms of odynophagia, dysphagia, and chest pain. Endoscopy demonstrates scattered or coalescent yellow-white mucosal plaques (Fig. 124-13). Given the high prevalence of esophageal candidiasis in HIV patients, some recommend treating symptomatic HIV patients empirically and reserving endoscopy for refractory symptoms. Mild oropharyngeal candidiasis may be treated with topical clotrimazole (10 mg troche five times daily for 7 to 14 days) or nystatin (600,000 units four times daily for 7 to 10 days), whereas oral fluconazole (100 mg daily for 7 to 14 days) is needed for moderate to severe oropharyngeal and esophageal candidiasis.[25] Intravenous fluconazole and amphotericin B deoxycholate (Chapter 307) are appropriate options for severe esophageal candidiasis and toxemia or for patients who cannot tolerate oral therapy.

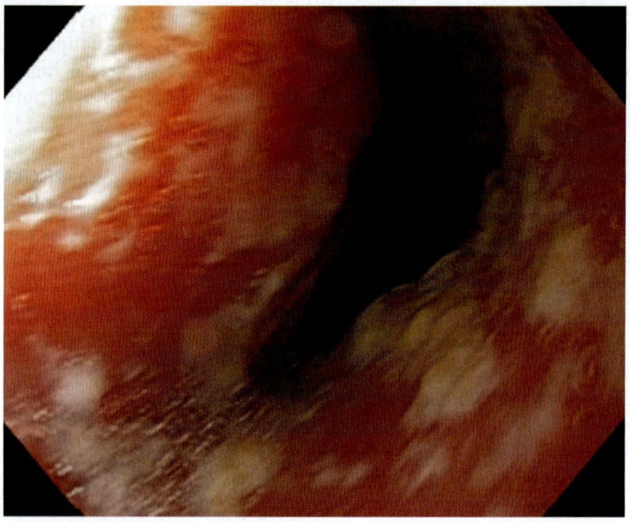

FIGURE 124-13. *Candida* esophagitis.

CYTOMEGALOVIRUS

Cytomegalovirus (CMV; Chapter 347) infection of the esophagus is almost exclusively found in immunocompromised patients. Patients infected with the HIV virus with low CD4 counts are most commonly affected, but CMV also occurs in transplant recipients on immunosuppressive therapy and in immunosuppressed patients with malignancy. Patients typically have severe odynophagia with evidence of radiographic or endoscopic esophageal ulcers. Treatment is usually with intravenous ganciclovir (5 mg/kg once or twice daily for 10 to 14 days) or foscarnet (90 mg/kg every 8 to 12 hours until healing occurs).

BACTERIAL ESOPHAGITIS

Bacterial infection of the esophagus is uncommon but can occur in immunosuppressed patients, typically those with neutropenia and malignancy. Patients present with chest pain or odynophagia, or both, and endoscopy reveals extensive erosions, usually in the distal esophagus. Biopsy and Gram stain reveal acute and chronic inflammation and bacteria, commonly gram-positive organisms, especially viridans-group streptococci, *Staphylococcus aureus*, *Staphylococcus epidermidis*, and *Bacillus* species. Treatment is with the appropriate antibiotics administered parenterally.

HUMAN PAPILLOMAVIRUS

Esophageal infections with human papillomavirus (HPV; Chapter 344) are typically asymptomatic. HPV lesions are most frequently found in the mid to distal esophagus as erythematous macules, white plaque, nodules, or exuberant frondlike lesions. The diagnosis is made by histologic demonstration of koilocytosis (an atypical nucleus surrounded by a ring), giant cells, or immunohistochemical stains. Treatment is usually not necessary, although large lesions may require endoscopic removal. Other treatments, such as interferon, bleomycin, and etoposide, have yielded varying results. HPV infection is a risk factor for esophageal squamous cell carcinoma (Chapter 178), but the value of endoscopic surveillance is not known.

MISCELLANEOUS ESOPHAGEAL CONDITIONS

Esophageal Emergencies

BOERHAAVE SYNDROME

Boerhaave syndrome, or spontaneous rupture of the esophagus, is a transmural full-thickness tear of the esophageal wall. A sudden rise in intraesophageal pressure during forceful vomiting is the cause in most cases. The tear is most commonly in the lower third of the esophagus, 2 to 3 cm proximal to the gastroesophageal junction.

CLINICAL MANIFESTATIONS AND DIAGNOSIS

The classic presentation is vomiting, lower thoracic pain, and subcutaneous emphysema. Other findings may include pleural effusions, especially left-sided, tachypnea, abdominal rigidity, fever, and hypotension. Because the condition is rare and classic antecedent vomiting is not always reported, rupture is often recognized only after the development of mediastinitis.

The chest radiograph may demonstrate mediastinal widening, a unilateral pleural effusion, hydropneumothorax, and pneumomediastinum. The esophagram, typically with a water-soluble agent, reveals extravasation, although false-negative results may be encountered. Computed tomography (CT) scanning with an oral contrast agent, which is perhaps the best diagnostic option, typically demonstrates air in the mediastinum.

MALLORY-WEISS TEAR

A Mallory-Weiss tear (see Fig. 124-2) is a mucosal tear, often at the gastroesophageal junction, usually caused by severe vomiting or retching. The syndrome is more common in alcoholic patients. In about 85% of patients, it is associated with acute upper gastrointestinal bleeding, which requires transfusion in about 70% of patients and urgent intervention in about 10% of cases. Mortality is about 5%, similar to the mortality in severe bleeding ulcers. Most tears heal spontaneously within about 48 hours.

IATROGENIC PERFORATION

Esophageal perforation may occur as a result of a variety of iatrogenic causes, including endoscopy, dilation, endosonography, or surgery, as well as with foreign body ingestion. Typical symptoms include chest pain with or without abdominal pain, subcutaneous emphysema, and fever. Diagnosis may be made immediately at the time of endoscopy or radiography. Chest radiographs may show pneumomediastinum, subcutaneous emphysema, hydrothorax, or hydropneumothorax. A Gastrografin swallow may show a leak, and chest CT may show mediastinal air. Acute perforations are life-threatening emergencies that warrant immediate closure before contamination of the mediastinum. For acute perforation caused by endoscopy, endoscopic clips or stents are an option. Conservative therapy also is an option for well-contained perforations with minimal mediastinal, pleural, or peritoneal contamination and no obvious signs of sepsis. Prognosis is generally good if the perforation is recognized and treated early, preferably within 12 to 24 hours.

TREATMENT AND PROGNOSIS

Successful therapy depends on early recognition and the underlying condition of the patient. The classic approach is operative repair in conjunction with broad-spectrum antibiotics and nutritional support, especially if the diagnosis is made within the first 24 hours. Aggressive conservative therapy with percutaneous drains, broad-spectrum parenteral antibiotics, and nutrition also has been successful. In selected individuals, endoscopic insertion of self-expanding covered metallic stents or over the scope clips, with or without pleural drainage as needed, is an option. The mortality rate can be as high as 100% without treatment.

FOREIGN BODIES

Impaction of food or foreign bodies is a common gastrointestinal emergency. Meat impaction is most commonly seen in adults, but other foreign objects that also may be ingested accidentally or by design include batteries, coins, and bones. Many patients have an underlying esophageal abnormality, such as Schatzki ring, stricture, eosinophilic esophagitis, tumor, or achalasia. The clinical presentation includes dysphagia, odynophagia, foreign body sensation, chest pain, excessive salivation, and difficulty handling secretions. Immediate endoscopic extraction or gentle advancing of the bolus with concomitant airway protection is recommended because prolonged impaction may result in penetration into the esophageal wall followed by perforation and mediastinitis.

ESOPHAGEAL VARICES

Esophageal varices are described in Chapter 139.

ESOPHAGEAL FISTULA

Tracheoesophageal fistulas may arise from a variety of different causes, including trauma, infectious esophagitis, necrosis after prolonged endotracheal intubation, esophageal cancer, and radiation therapy. Patients are often critically ill and may not tolerate surgery. Metallic stents are a treatment option.

Atrial-esophageal fistulas are a rare complication after radio frequency ablation (Chapter 54) for atrial fibrillation. The clinical presentation is nonspecific and includes features such as dysphagia, fever, leukocytosis, bacteremia, massive intestinal bleeding, and septic shock. Diagnosis requires a high index of suspicion and is aided by a chest CT scan. Surgery is required; the prognosis is excellent with early recognition and treatment but can be dire if treatment is delayed.

CONGENITAL ABNORMALITIES

ESOPHAGEAL ATRESIA AND TRACHEOESOPHAGEAL FISTULA

Children with congenital esophageal anomalies commonly survive into adulthood after successful surgery. As adults, these patients typically have gastroesophageal reflux that warrants proton pump inhibitor therapy. Strictures at prior surgical anastomoses are common, and patients may require periodic endoscopic dilation. Eosinophilic esophagitis may also occur.

HETEROTOPIC GASTRIC MUCOSA (INLET PATCH)

Inlet patches, which are areas of gastric columnar epithelium, are present in up to 4.5% of adults and are usually found incidentally at the time of routine endoscopy. Typically, a red columnar patch varying in size from a few millimeters to a few centimeters is seen just below the cricopharyngeus. Inlet patches can be associated with hoarseness, sore throat, and globus sensation. Strictures, ulcers, and rare malignant transformation also have been described. Treatment options include proton pump inhibitors (see Table 124-1) and endoscopic ablation.

OTHER CONGENITAL ESOPHAGEAL DISORDERS

Duplication cysts, which may be located anywhere in the esophagus, may be in continuity with or separate from the esophageal lumen. Symptoms, which may present initially in adulthood, include dysphagia owing to luminal compression, chest pain, and regurgitation. Treatment is surgical.

Dysphagia lusoria is caused by an aberrant right subclavian artery that originates from the right aortic arch and causes partial compression of the esophagus as it crosses over to the left side. Patients may complain of dysphagia. This condition is most commonly detected incidentally during barium radiography, where it is visualized as a crossing diagonal impression at the junction of the proximal and middle thirds of the esophagus. Surgery is rarely indicated because of the complexity of the operation and the difficulty in establishing a clear relationship between the radiographic findings and symptoms.

GENERAL REFERENCES

For the General References and other additional features, please visit Elsevier eBooks+ at https://ebooks.health.elsevier.com.

Grade A References

A1. Zhang H, Yang Z, Ni Z, et al. A meta-analysis and systematic review of the efficacy of twice daily PPIs versus once daily for treatment of gastroesophageal reflux disease. *Gastroenterol Res Pract.* 2017;2017:9865963.

A2. Yadlapati R, Masihi M, Gyawali CP, et al. Ambulatory reflux monitoring guides proton pump inhibitor discontinuation in patients with gastroesophageal reflux symptoms: a clinical trial. *Gastroenterology.* 2021;160:174-182.

A3. Richter JE, Kumar A, Lipka S, et al. Efficacy of laparoscopic Nissen fundoplication vs transoral incisionless fundoplication or proton pump inhibitors in patients with gastroesophageal reflux disease: a systematic review and network meta-analysis. *Gastroenterology.* 2018;154:1298-1308.

A4. Spechler SJ, Hunter JM, Jones KM, et al. Randomized trial of medical versus surgical treatment for refractory heartburn. *N Engl J Med.* 2019;381:1513-1523.

A5. Fitzgerald RC, di Pietro M, O'Donovan M, et al. Cytosponge-trefoil factor 3 versus usual care to identify Barrett's oesophagus in a primary care setting: a multicentre, pragmatic, randomised controlled trial. *Lancet.* 2020;396:333-344.

A6. Jankowski JAZ, de Caestecker J, Love SB, et al. Esomeprazole and aspirin in Barrett's oesophagus (AspECT): a randomised factorial trial. *Lancet.* 2018;392:400-408.

A7. Qumseya BJ, Wani S, Gendy S, et al. Disease progression in Barrett's low-grade dysplasia with radiofrequency ablation compared with surveillance: systematic review and meta-analysis. *Am J Gastroenterol.* 2017;112:849-865.

A8. Mayerhofer C, Kavallar AM, Aldrian D, et al. Efficacy of elimination diets in eosinophilic esophagitis: a systematic review and meta-analysis. *Clin Gastroenterol Hepatol.* 2023;S1542-3565(23)00078-2. [Epub ahead of print.]

A9. Dellon ES, Lucendo AJ, Schlag C, et al. Fluticasone propionate orally disintegrating tablet (APT-1011) for eosinophilic esophagitis: randomized controlled trial. *Clin Gastroenterol Hepatol.* 2022;20:2485-2494.

A10. Straumann A, Lucendo AJ, Miehlke S, et al. Budesonide orodispersible tablets maintain remission in a randomized, placebo-controlled trial of patients with eosinophilic esophagitis. *Gastroenterology.* 2020;159:1672-1685.

A11. Dellon ES, Rothenberg ME, Collins MH, et al. Dupilumab in adults and adolescents with eosinophilic esophagitis. *N Engl J Med.* 2022;387:2317-2330.

A12. Baniya R, Upadhaya S, Khan J, et al. Laparoscopic esophageal myotomy versus pneumatic dilation in the treatment of idiopathic achalasia: a meta-analysis of randomized controlled trials. *Clin Exp Gastroenterol.* 2017;10:241-248.

A13. Ponds FA, Fockens P, Lei A, et al. Effect of peroral endoscopic myotomy vs pneumatic dilation on symptom severity and treatment outcomes among treatment-naive patients with achalasia: a randomized clinical trial. *JAMA.* 2019;322:134-144.

A14. Werner YB, Hakanson B, Martinek J, et al. Endoscopic or surgical myotomy in patients with idiopathic achalasia. *N Engl J Med.* 2019;381:2219-2229.

125 ACID PEPTIC DISEASE

ERNST J. KUIPERS

Acid peptic diseases can involve the esophagus (Chapter 124), the stomach, and the duodenum. Dyspeptic symptoms also can occur in patients who have no endoscopic abnormalities, in whom it is termed *nonulcer dyspepsia* (Chapter 123).

DEFINITIONS

Gastric and duodenal ulcers usually occur in an area of inflamed mucosa. This inflammation, termed *gastritis, duodenitis*, or *bulbitis*, can be recognized by endoscopic signs of edema and erythema of the mucosa, but microscopic evaluation of endoscopic biopsy specimens is required for a definitive diagnosis of mucosal inflammation.

Gastritis is categorized by endoscopic and histologic criteria, with granulocytes predominating in active gastritis and mononuclear cells in chronic gastritis. Gastritis is classified further by the segment of the involved stomach: antral-predominant gastritis, corpus-predominant gastritis, or pangastritis. Finally, the absence or presence of premalignant stages of damage to the mucosa as a result of long-standing inflammation defines the categories of nonatrophic and atrophic gastritis, respectively. High-definition endoscopy, when combined with magnification and image enhancement, allows adequate visualization of features of gastritis, atrophy, and intestinal metaplasia. Gastritis features include antral nodularity, absence of connecting venules, and enlarged gastric folds. Sometimes, the mucosa has a typical miniature cobblestone appearance, termed *nodular gastritis* (a finding particularly in children colonized by *Helicobacter pylori*), or grossly enlarged folds without evidence of cancer, termed *hypertrophic gastritis*. Disappearance of gastric folds and enhanced mucosal vasculature are findings of *atrophic gastritis*. Atrophy may be accompanied by *intestinal metaplasia*, which appears as gray-white patches (white-light endoscopy) or light-blue lines ("light-blue crests") on the mucosal surface (narrow-band imaging).

A *peptic ulcer* is a mucosal defect at least 0.5 cm in diameter that penetrates the muscularis mucosae. Smaller mucosal defects are called *erosions* (Fig. 125-1). Gastric ulcers are subdivided into proximal ulcers, located in the body of the stomach, and distal ulcers, located in the antrum and angulus of the stomach. Gastric ulcers are located mainly along the lesser curvature, in particular at the transitional zone of corpus- to antral-type mucosa. This transitional zone is often in the area of the angulus but may shift proximally. Duodenal ulcers usually are located on the anterior or posterior wall of the duodenal bulb (Fig. 125-2) or occasionally at both sites ("kissing" ulcers). Lesions distal

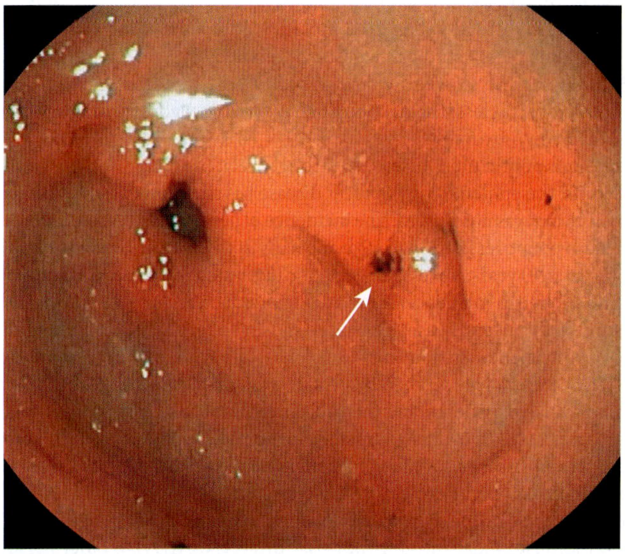

FIGURE 125-1. Endoscopic view of uncomplicated erosive gastritis. The erosion appears as a small, superficial mucosal break with a black base (*arrow*).

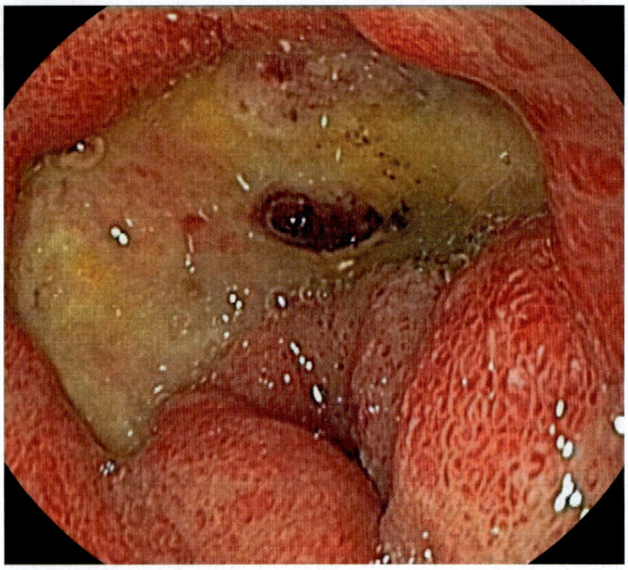

FIGURE 125-2. **Endoscopic view of an ulcer at the anterior wall of the duodenal bulb. The ulcer has a clean base, with a visible vessel appearing as a dark red protruding spot close to the lower ulcer rim. The surrounding mucosa is inflamed and swollen.**

to the duodenal bulb are termed *postbulbar ulcers*. Patients who previously underwent a distal gastric resection (Billroth I or II procedure) or a gastric bypass (Chapter 201) can develop ulceration at the anastomosis (*anastomotic* or *marginal ulcer*). However, ulcers occurring after Billroth II resection are located predominantly in the jejunal mucosa at the junction between the afferent and efferent loops. Other peptic ulcers can occur at sites of metaplastic or heterotopic gastric mucosa, for example, in Meckel diverticulum, the rectum, or Barrett esophagus. Patients with a large hiatal hernia can develop gastric ulceration, known as *Cameron ulcers*, at the herniation. *Dieulafoy ulcers*, which are small mucosal defects over an intramural arteriole, can lead to severe bleeding. Although these lesions can occur throughout the gastrointestinal tract, two thirds occur in the stomach.

EPIDEMIOLOGY

The worldwide prevalence of gastritis reflects the prevalence of *H. pylori*. Colonization with this bacterium is virtually always associated with chronic active gastritis, which persists as long as an individual remains colonized and only slowly disappears 6 to 24 months after bacterial eradication. An estimated 4.4 billion people worldwide are colonized with *H. pylori*.[1] Colonization usually occurs in the first decade of life and then remains lifelong. In developing countries, high colonization rates result in a high prevalence of *H. pylori* gastritis (often ≥75%) in all age groups, including children. In Western countries, the colonization pressure in children has decreased markedly in recent decades, thereby leading to a birth-cohort phenomenon for the prevalence of *H. pylori* gastritis—currently less than 20% in young adults but 40 to 60% in elderly persons. Some recent studies suggest that this decrease in *H. pylori* prevalence in children may be slowed by factors such as the increasing use of daycare facilities. Nevertheless, the decline of *H. pylori* in developed country populations has been inexorable.

Although peptic ulcer disease is strongly related to *H. pylori* gastritis and duodenitis, the epidemiology of ulcer disease has shown secular variation even when *H. pylori* was ubiquitous. The incidence of peptic ulcer disease rose steeply in Western countries in the late 19th and early 20th centuries and has decreased over the past 40 years; nevertheless, peptic ulceration remains a common disorder. The decline in incidence, associated with a decrease in hospital admissions and surgery for ulcer disease, is believed mostly to reflect the decreasing prevalence of gastric colonization with *H. pylori*. It also results from the widespread application of eradication therapy, which strongly reduced recurrent ulcers in *H. pylori*–positive patients, and the widespread use of acid-suppressive medications. Nevertheless, hospital admissions for complications of ulcers and mortality from ulcer disease have shown a far less marked decline in both the United States and other countries because the reduction in *H. pylori*–associated ulcers in younger persons has been partly counterbalanced by an increase in ulcers related to nonsteroidal anti-inflammatory drugs (NSAIDs) in older persons.

In Western countries, duodenal ulcers occur more frequently than gastric ulcers. The predominant age at which duodenal ulcers occur is between 20 and 50 years, whereas gastric ulcers most commonly occur in patients older than 40 years. The incidence of gastroduodenal ulcer disease is approximately 1 to 2 per 1000 inhabitants per year. Although the prevalence of *H. pylori* colonization is nearly identical in males and females, two thirds of patients with ulcers are male. More than 50% of patients have a recurrent ulcer within 12 months of healing in the absence of treatment. Maintenance acid-suppressive therapy reduces this recurrence rate, but only therapeutic measures that remove the underlying cause of the ulcer can prevent most ulcer recurrences.

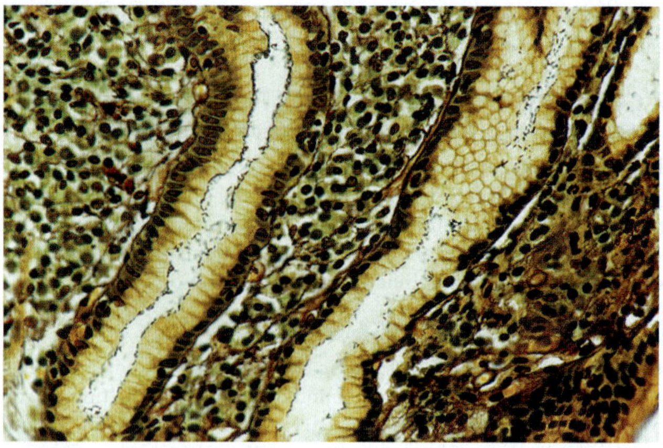

FIGURE 125-3. **Gastric mucosa colonized with *Helicobacter pylori* appearing as curved bacilli on the mucosal surface.**

PATHOBIOLOGY

Helicobacter pylori

Most peptic ulcers are associated with colonization with *H. pylori* (Fig. 125-3).[2] However, most persons who are *H. pylori* positive do not have any specific complaints, nor do they develop ulcer disease. The estimated risk for the development of ulcer disease during persistent *H. pylori* colonization is 5 to 15%—that is, three-fold to eight-fold higher than the risk in patients who are *H. pylori* negative. The risk for the development of an ulcer in the presence of *H. pylori* is determined by a combination of host- and bacteria-related factors. Host factors include immune response, smoking, and stress. Genome-wide association studies have identified a relationship between polymorphisms in the toll-like receptor gene and the interleukin-1β gene with the prevalence of *H. pylori*. This relationship may in part explain the variation in risk for *H. pylori* colonization and thus the risk for *H. pylori*–associated disease, including peptic ulcer. Bacterial factors that enhance mucosal inflammation and increase the risk for ulcer include a high production of the *VacA* product, which reflects the presence of the s1m1 genotype; a high level of cytokine induction, owing to the presence of genes in the *cag* pathogenicity island; and enhanced adherence to the gastric epithelium as a result of bacterial expression of *babA* and *oipA*.

Nonsteroidal Anti-inflammatory Drugs and Aspirin

The other common cause of gastroduodenal ulcer disease is the use of NSAIDs. At least 2 to 4% of the population in many countries use acetylsalicylic acid, acetic acid derivatives (diclofenac, indomethacin, sulindac), or propionic acid derivatives (ibuprofen, ketoprofen, naproxen) on a daily basis. The risk for ulcer disease is dose and duration dependent. Within 14 days after the start of such treatment, about 5% of patients develop erosions or ulcers. In patients who continue therapy for 4 weeks or longer, this proportion increases to 10%, but many are clinically silent. The concomitant presence of *H. pylori* infection increases the incidence of NSAID-related ulcers.

The risk for an ulcer during NSAID use is higher in patients who are older than 60 years; patients with a previous ulcer; patients who use corticosteroids, selective serotonin reuptake inhibitors, or aldosterone antagonists; and patients with major comorbid diseases. In patients who use anticoagulants, such as warfarin and new oral anticoagulants (thrombin and factor Xa inhibitors), or who have severe comorbid disease, an NSAID-induced ulcer is more likely to lead to life-threatening gastroduodenal hemorrhage.

On the basis of their activities, NSAIDs are divided into cyclooxygenase 1 (COX1) and COX2 inhibitors (Chapter 26). The COX1 enzyme is involved in the production of prostaglandins, which play a role in normal cell regulation. The COX2 enzyme, which is also involved in the production of prostaglandins, is induced by inflammatory responses. Most NSAIDs have a nonselective

COX inhibitory effect; selective COX2 inhibitors are associated with fewer gastroduodenal ulcers, but their use has been limited because of their adverse coronary effects (Chapter 26). The strong association between NSAIDs and ulcer disease and the risk for recurrence of ulcers with their continued use require that patients with ulcers be thoroughly assessed for any use of NSAIDs.

Helicobacter pylori–Negative, Non-NSAID Ulcer Disease

In most series, *H. pylori* and NSAID use account for 80 to 95% of cases of ulcer disease. The remaining cases are often referred to as *idiopathic* or *H. pylori–negative, non-NSAID* acid peptic disease. The proportion of ulcer disease that is idiopathic is increasing throughout the world as the prevalence of *H. pylori* decreases. Further, it is likely that some ulcers in *H. pylori*–positive patients were not caused by *H. pylori*. Consistent with this notion is the fact that some *H. pylori*–positive patients develop recurrent ulcers after successful bacterial eradication, so presumably their ulcer disease was idiopathic. It is not known whether the increase in idiopathic ulcer disease is simply proportional to the decrease in *H. pylori*–associated ulcers or whether it reflects a true increase in the incidence of idiopathic ulcers.

In patients with idiopathic ulcer disease, specific clues to the underlying cause are often provided by the medical history, including comorbidity and drug use; the endoscopic appearance of the ulcer; and the histologic features of the ulcer's margins and surroundings. In most cases, these initial data can be used to direct further diagnostic studies (Table 125-1).

Malignant Ulcer Disease

Gastroduodenal ulcers can result from underlying malignancies. In the stomach, such tumors are related to gastric adenocarcinoma and, rarely, to mucosa-associated lymphoid tissue (MALT) lymphomas (Chapter 178). Malignant ulcers in the duodenum may result from primary duodenal carcinomas or from penetrating pancreatic cancers. Duodenal cancers have an association with polyposis syndromes, especially familial adenomatous polyposis and, to a much lesser extent, *MUTYH*-associated polyposis and Peutz-Jeghers syndrome (Chapter 179). In both the stomach and the duodenum, ulcer disease also may be caused by metastatic tumors, including cancers of the breast, colon, thyroid, or kidney, or by melanoma, disseminated lymphoma, or Kaposi sarcoma. Malignant ulcers are characteristically irregular in shape with heaped borders, but they also may be flat or depressed. Current high-resolution and magnification endoscopes allow visualization of the altered mucosal structure surrounding an ulcer, including changes in the microvascular pattern. Primary gastric adenocarcinomas often occur in mucosal areas with atrophic and intestinal metaplastic changes. For a definite diagnosis of malignancy, multiple biopsy specimens are needed, usually from the ulcer margins.

Systemic Inflammatory Disorders

A few gastroduodenal ulcers are caused by systemic inflammatory diseases, in particular, Crohn disease (Chapter 127). Patients with Crohn disease affecting

TABLE 125-1 DIFFERENTIAL DIAGNOSIS OF PEPTIC ULCER DISEASE

ORIGIN	CONDITION	FREQUENCY*	DIAGNOSTIC TEST	FINDINGS
Microbes	*Helicobacter pylori*	Very common	*H. pylori* tests Histology	Bacteria, enzymes, antigens, antibodies Gastritis
	Helicobacter heilmannii	Rare	Histology	Spiral bacteria, gastritis
	Treponema pallidum	Very rare	Serology	Antibodies
	Mycobacterial infection	Very rare	Histology, immune response testing, chest radiograph	Acid-fast bacteria, granuloma, immune response, pulmonary infiltrate
	Cytomegalovirus, herpes simplex virus type 1, Epstein-Barr virus	Rare	Histology, serology	Virus inclusions, antibodies
Drug use	NSAIDs, aspirin	Very common	History, urine test	NSAID use
	Bisphosphonates	Rare	History	Bisphosphonate use
	Corticosteroids	Rare	History	Corticosteroid use, comorbidity
	Amphetamines, cocaine	Rare	History, drug testing	Drug use
	Anticoagulants, coagulopathy	Rare	Endoscopy	Ulcer after intramural bleed
	Immune checkpoint inhibitors	Rare	Endoscopy	Ulceration
	Calcium polystyrene sulfonate	Rare	Endoscopy	Ulceration
Malignancy	Gastric cancer	Common	Histology	Malignancy
	Duodenal cancer	Rare	Histology, CT	Malignancy
	Pancreatic cancer	Common	Histology, CT	Malignancy
	Mucosa-associated lymphoid tissue lymphoma	Rare	Histology	Malignancy
	Metastatic cancer	Rare	Histology	Malignancy
	Gastric sarcoma	Very rare	Histology	Malignancy
Gastritis syndromes	Eosinophilic gastritis	Rare	Histology	Eosinophilic infiltration
	Lymphocytic gastritis	Rare	Histology, celiac disease screening	Lymphocytic infiltration, villous atrophy
Hyperacidity syndromes	Zollinger-Ellison syndrome	Rare	Serum gastrin, secretin test	Extreme hypergastrinemia, positive secretin test
	Antral G-cell hyperfunction	Very rare	Serum gastrin, secretin test	Moderate hypergastrinemia, negative secretin test
	Retained gastric antrum	Very rare	Medical history, gastrin	Billroth II resection, hypergastrinemia
	Systemic mastocytosis	Very rare	Histology of affected sites	Mast cell infiltration
	Chronic myelogenous leukemia	Very rare	Leukemia evaluation	Leukemia
Ischemia	Mesenteric vascular occlusion	Common	Angiography	Vascular disease
	Polycythemia vera	Rare	Blood counts	Polycythemia
Specific ulcer types	Cameron ulcer	Common	Endoscopy	Ulcer in large hiatal hernia
	Marginal ulcer	Common	Endoscopy	Ulcer at anastomosis
	Dieulafoy ulcer	Common	Endoscopy	Singular bleeding focus with minimal mucosal disruption
Systemic inflammation	Crohn disease	Common	Histology, ileocolonoscopy	Inflammation, granulomas
	Vasculitides	Rare	Histology, systemic evaluation	Vasculitis, signs of systemic disease
	Gastric amyloidosis	Very rare	Histology	Amyloid deposition
Other conditions	Stress ulcer	Fairly common in patients in intensive care units	Endoscopy	—
	Radiation therapy, chemotherapy	Rare	Endoscopy, history	—

*Frequency as a cause of gastroduodenal ulcer disease.
CT = computed tomography; NSAID = nonsteroidal anti-inflammatory drug.

the proximal gastrointestinal tract often have multiple ulcers characterized by irregular longitudinal shapes. Ulcers in the duodenum occur on top of Kerckring folds. Patients with gastroduodenal ulcers from Crohn disease do not invariably have evidence of disease elsewhere in the digestive tract, nor do blood tests always suggest an active inflammatory bowel disorder. The demonstration of ulcerative inflammation elsewhere in the digestive tract, in particular in the terminal ileum and colon, strongly supports the diagnosis of Crohn disease, as do noncaseating granulomas on biopsy specimens. However, the absence of granulomas does not exclude Crohn disease, and these lesions are not specific for Crohn disease; they also are associated with *H. pylori* gastritis and other conditions, particularly sarcoidosis (Chapter 83). Sarcoidosis can also lead to gastroduodenal ulcer disease.

Other inflammatory disorders that can cause gastritis or gastroduodenal ulcers include various forms of vasculitis affecting the mesenteric system, in particular, Behçet disease (Chapter 249), Henoch-Schönlein purpura (Chapter 249), Takayasu arteritis (Chapters 63 and 249), polyarteritis nodosa (Chapter 249), systemic lupus erythematosus (Chapter 245), Churg-Strauss syndrome (Chapter 249), and granulomatosis with polyangiitis (Chapter 249). Lymphocytic gastroduodenitis, which is strongly associated with celiac disease (Chapter 126), may lead to duodenal ulceration and subsequent stenotic web formation. Ulcer disease also may occur in patients with polycythemia vera (Chapter 152), possibly in relation to reduced mucosal blood flow. Vasculitis underlying ulcer disease should be considered in patients with chronic or recurrent ulceration in whom other causes have been excluded. Lymphocytic phlebitis, which is a rare vasculitic inflammatory disorder that affects the mesenteric veins, may cause gastric ulcers. Systemic amyloidosis (Chapter 174) affecting the stomach wall may lead to gastric ulcers. Rare cases of duodenal ulceration have been described in the presence of annular pancreas or congenital bands obstructing the descending duodenum.

Hypergastrinemic Syndromes

Peptic ulcers can result from chronic gastric hyperacidity related to hypergastrinemia. The most important hypergastrinemic disorder is Zollinger-Ellison syndrome (Chapter 213), a condition of marked hyperacidity leading to severe peptic ulcer disease caused by a gastrin-producing endocrine tumor. These patients usually have multiple bulbar and postbulbar duodenal ulcers that are resistant to conventional acid-suppressive therapy. The diagnosis can be confirmed by the presence of a high fasting serum gastrin level (often, but not always, ≥10-fold increased and >1000 pg/mL). Similar gastrin levels are sometimes seen in patients treated for chronic ulcer disease with high-dose proton pump inhibitors. For clarification, secretin testing can be performed: in patients with Zollinger-Ellison syndrome, the injection of secretin (1 U/kg) increases serum gastrin levels by more than 50%, or 120 pg/mL or greater, in persons with fasting gastrin levels less than 10-fold above normal. Imaging techniques, such as computed tomography (CT), magnetic resonance imaging, isotope scanning, endoscopic ultrasonography, videocapsule endoscopy, and balloon-assisted enteroscopy, may be used to detect the primary tumor, which is often located in either the pancreas or the proximal small bowel. In some patients, Zollinger-Ellison syndrome occurs as part of the multiple endocrine neoplasia syndrome (Chapter 212), particularly in association with hyperparathyroidism. Other hypergastrinemic hyperacidity syndromes are retained gastric antrum syndrome (see later) and antral G-cell hyperfunction. In the latter, fasting serum gastrin levels are only modestly increased and do not rise after the injection of secretin, but they respond in an exaggerated way to meals, thereby leading to hyperacidity. When the condition occurs in an *H. pylori*–positive patient, bacterial eradication therapy may be curative. However, some patients with G-cell hyperfunction are *H. pylori* negative.

Ischemia

Stenosis or occlusion of the celiac trunk or the superior mesenteric artery (Chapter 129) also can lead to ulceration in the mucosa of the proximal digestive tract (Fig. 125-4). These ulcers typically occur in elderly patients who have known severe atherosclerosis or risk factors for it, but they can also occur in younger subjects with mesenteric obstruction due to other causes, as well as in patients with marked chronic heart failure. Ischemic ulcers tend to heal slowly and to recur. Pallor of the mucosa, consistent with decreased mucosal blood flow, may be noted at endoscopy. Upper mesenteric ischemia is often associated with upper abdominal pain, which can be elicited by a meal or by physical activity. These symptoms may cause patients to decrease their food intake, leading to weight loss before their clinical presentation. The prevalence of upper mesenteric ischemia with secondary ulcer disease is unknown, in part owing to its variable presentation, often with a history of gradual symptoms; the lack of standardized and reliable diagnostic tests; and clinicians' unfamiliarity with the condition.[3] Diagnostic evaluation includes a duplex ultrasound scan for vascular flow and conventional or CT angiography of the affected arteries. Gastroduodenal mucosal perfusion can be functionally measured by means of tonometry and by directly measuring mucosal oxygen saturation during endoscopy; however, these tests are not widely available.

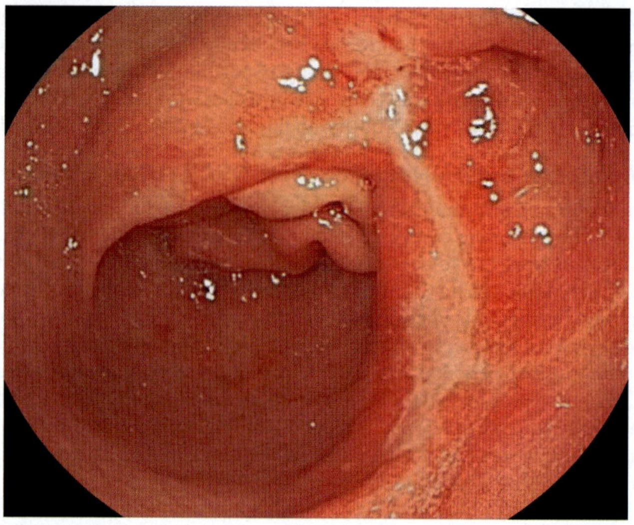

FIGURE 125-4. Endoscopic view of an irregular gastric ulcer at the posterior wall and smaller curvature in a patient with chronic mesenteric ischemia due to subtotal stenosis of the celiac trunk.

Stress Ulcers

Patients with severe medical conditions, such as major trauma, sepsis, extensive burns, head injury, or multiorgan failure, can develop stress ulcers in the stomach or duodenum. Major risk factors for stress ulceration in severely ill patients include mechanical ventilation, coagulopathy, and hypotension, but factors such as hepatic and renal failure and the use of ulcerogenic medications may contribute. Stress ulcers occur independently of *H. pylori* colonization. Ulcers associated with head injury are known as Cushing ulcers, and ulcers associated with extensive burns are known as Curling ulcers. Stress ulcers were once common in patients in intensive care units, but improvements in overall management, including respiratory and hemodynamic care, acid inhibition, and emphasis on adequate feeding, have reduced the incidence of these ulcers, which currently affect 1 to 2% of these patients. Stress ulcers may be asymptomatic, but they can also cause complications, especially bleeding.

Other Factors

Cameron Ulcer

Patients with large hiatal hernias (Chapter 124) may present with proximal gastric ulcers, termed *Cameron ulcers*, at the level of the hiatus, where the stomach is compressed. These ulcers are usually asymptomatic but may cause occult or overt bleeding. During upper gastrointestinal endoscopy, patients with large hiatal hernias and iron deficiency anemia should be carefully examined in normal and retroverted positions for the presence of Cameron ulcers.

Anastomotic or Marginal Ulceration

Patients who have undergone partial gastrectomy sometimes develop recurrent ulcers, often located at the anastomosis or within the jejunum immediately opposite the anastomosis. Ischemia and chronic inflammation, in particular resulting from biliary reflux, may cause such ulcers. If biopsies exclude cancer, treatment includes acid suppression and *H. pylori* eradication, if needed. Anastomotic ulcers after bariatric gastric surgery appear to be related to local ischemia. They have no clear correlation with *H. pylori*, and preoperative *H. pylori* eradication does not appear to reduce the incidence of such ulcers. However, proton pump inhibitor therapy may reduce their incidence. Peptic ulcer disease can also be associated with the retained gastric antrum syndrome when the antrum is not completely excised from the detached duodenum during partial gastrectomy surgery. Because it then lacks exposure to acid and therefore is not physiologically downregulated, it continues to secrete gastrin despite normal or even high acid levels. Marginal ulcers can also occur after bariatric Roux-en-Y gastric bypass surgery.

Other Microbial Organisms

Colonization with *Helicobacter heilmannii* (formerly known as *Gastrospirillum hominis*), which is probably a zoonotic organism, is associated with mild gastritis and sometimes with transient ulcer disease. Ulcer disease also may be infectious, resulting from secondary syphilis (Chapter 295), mycobacterial infection (Chapter 299), infection with herpes simplex virus type 1 (Chapter 371), varicella-zoster virus (Chapter 346), cytomegalovirus infection (Chapter 347), or Epstein-Barr virus (Chapter 348).

Alcohol

Short-term heavy alcohol use or long-term moderate to heavy alcohol use can lead to signs of acute and chronic gastritis. No evidence indicates that this type of gastritis is associated with a significant risk for peptic ulceration, although alcohol use increases the risk for bleeding in patients with peptic ulcer disease.

Hyperhistaminic Syndromes

Similar to the hypergastrinemic syndromes, persistent elevation of histamine can lead to hyperacidity as a result of the chronic stimulation of parietal cells. Elevated histamine levels are observed in two rare syndromes. *Systemic mastocytosis* (Chapter 235) is characterized by a proliferation of mast cells in the bone marrow, skin, liver, spleen, and gastrointestinal tract, often associated with both spontaneous and trigger-induced (e.g., alcohol) release of histamine and other vasoactive substances. Patients with systemic mastocytosis often have gastrointestinal symptoms, including pain, diarrhea, and blood loss. Ulceration results from chronic gastric acid hypersecretion. Clues to the diagnosis include symptoms of pruritus, urticaria, or rash. The bone marrow and affected organ mast cell infiltrates carry a specific *C-kit* mutation and express CD2 and CD25. Histamine hypersecretion leading to peptic ulcer disease also can occur in *chronic myelogenous leukemia* (Chapter 170) with basophilia.

Other Drugs

Oral bisphosphonates, used widely for osteoporosis (Chapter 225), may induce gastric erosions and ulcerations in an estimated 3 to 10% of treated patients. The risk for ulcer disease may be synergistically increased by NSAID use but is probably independent of *H. pylori* colonization. Although corticosteroid treatment can be complicated by peptic ulcer disease, the relative risk is only slightly increased, except in patients with serious comorbid diseases, patients using long-term or high-dose therapy, or patients with prior ulcers. Other patients who use corticosteroids are not at serious risk for ulcer disease and therefore do not require measures to prevent ulcers. Similarly, the use of aldosterone antagonists is also associated with an increased risk for peptic ulcer and ulcer bleeding, likely related to impaired mucosal healing.

Persons who use amphetamines and crack cocaine (Chapter 365) frequently develop ulcer disease, often with perforation, possibly as a result of vascular insufficiency. Chemotherapy, particularly when given selectively as a high-dose intra-arterial infusion in the celiac system, can be complicated by ulcer disease. Patients on anticoagulant therapy and those with other coagulopathies may rarely develop intramural hematoma of the gastrointestinal tract. Depending on the location, these hematomas may cause obstruction, but they can also leave large ulcers when they rupture into the lumen. Radiation therapy of the upper abdomen is sometimes complicated by chronic ischemic ulceration, especially as a late complication.

CLINICAL MANIFESTATIONS

The clinical manifestations of acid peptic disease (Table 125-2) do not always predict the various morphologic presentations found at endoscopy. Indeed, a silent ulcer may be recognized only when it presents abruptly with a complication, most commonly hemorrhage or perforation, or it may be discovered incidentally when a diagnostic test is performed for other reasons. Nevertheless, the typical presentation of acid peptic disease is recurrent episodes of pain. The pain is almost invariably located in the epigastrium and may radiate to the back or, less commonly, to the thorax or other regions of the abdomen (see Table 125-2). Some patients describe the pain as burning or piercing, whereas others describe it as an uncomfortable feeling of emptiness of the stomach, referred to as *painful hunger*. Indeed, the pain may improve with the ingestion of food, only to return in the postprandial period. The timing of the pain in relation to meals and to the soothing effects of food is nonspecific, however, and may also occur in patients with functional dyspepsia without ulcer. Nocturnal epigastric pain that awakens a patient several hours after a late meal is more likely to represent ulcer pain.

TABLE 125-2 KEY SYMPTOMS AND SIGNS OF PEPTIC ULCER

UNCOMPLICATED ULCER
No symptoms ("silent ulcer" in up to 40% of cases)
Epigastric pain
Pain may radiate to the back, thorax, other parts of the abdomen (cephalad most likely, caudad least likely)
Pain may be nocturnal (most specific), "painful hunger" relieved by food, or continuous (least specific)
Nausea
Vomiting
Heartburn (mimics or associated with gastroesophageal reflux)
COMPLICATED ULCER
Severe abdominal pain
Shock
Abdominal boardlike rigidity (and rebound and other signs of peritoneal irritation)
Free intraperitoneal air
Hemorrhage
Hematemesis and/or melena
Hemodynamic changes, anemia
Previous history of ulcer symptoms (80%)
Gastric outlet obstruction
Satiation, inability to ingest food, eructation
Nausea, vomiting (and related disturbances)
Weight loss

Aside from the pain during symptomatic episodes, patients may complain of retrosternal burning (heartburn) or acidic regurgitation into the throat, symptoms that reflect associated gastroesophageal reflux (Chapter 124), which is aggravated by hyperacidity or delayed gastric emptying. Nausea and vomiting may also occur but are nonspecific. The presence of significant diarrhea should raise the possibility of Zollinger-Ellison syndrome (Chapter 213), but diarrhea also may result from the intensive use of magnesium-containing antacids. In untreated patients, symptoms tend to be intermittent, with flares of daily pain lasting 2 to 8 weeks, separated by prolonged asymptomatic intervals. During periods of remission, patients may feel well and may be able to eat even heavy or spicy meals without apparent discomfort.

Physical Examination

The physical examination is usually unrevealing. If significant bleeding has occurred (Chapter 121), the patient may present with pallor and may be hypovolemic (Chapter 92). It is always useful to inquire about the characteristics of the stool because ulcer-related bleeding may manifest not only obviously in the form of hematemesis but also insidiously as melena (black feces). In the case of massive ulcer bleeding with the rapid bowel passage of blood, patients may also present with red rectal blood loss. When a patient has acute perforation, severe epigastric and abdominal pain usually develops, and the patient appears distressed. Characteristically, intense contracture of the abdominal muscles is apparent on palpation, together with rebound tenderness and other signs of peritoneal irritation. With large amounts of intra-abdominal air, percussion may reveal hypertympany over the liver.

DIAGNOSIS

In a patient who presents with symptoms consistent with ulcer disease, the diagnostic evaluation should proceed along two different but complementary paths: confirmation of the anatomic abnormality and investigation of its cause (Table 125-3). In most patients, it is advisable to follow both diagnostic paths simultaneously, but sometimes it is reasonable to skip the anatomic verification as a cost-saving strategy and proceed to management based on probable cause.

Anatomic Diagnosis

Upper gastrointestinal endoscopy (Chapter 120) is the primary investigative tool in patients suspected of having acid peptic disease. This technique can detect erosive gastritis (see Fig. 125-1) or an ulcer in the gastric wall or duodenal bulb (see Fig. 125-2). Because of the high prevalence and the spontaneous improvement of dyspeptic symptoms, endoscopy generally should not be performed immediately; rather, its use should be restricted to patients with persistent or recurrent symptoms. However, immediate endoscopy is indicated in patients with alarm symptoms such as weight loss, dysphagia, anorexia, considerable vomiting, anemia, or signs of occult or overt bleeding.

TABLE 125-3 DIAGNOSTIC PATHS AND TOOLS IN ULCER DISEASE

PATH 1: MORPHOLOGIC DIAGNOSIS
Gastroduodenoscopy Barium contrast (inferior alternative) Endoscopic ultrasound (selected cases only) Computed tomography (useful in selected cases)
PATH 2: ETIOLOGIC DIAGNOSIS
***Helicobacter pylori* Testing**
Histologic examination of gastric mucosa with appropriate stains Serum antibodies Stool antigen test Carbon-13 urea breath test
Ulcer Associated with Nonsteroidal Anti-inflammatory Drug Use
History of drug ingestion Decreased platelet aggregation Molecular identification of drugs, pro-drugs, metabolites (complex, expensive)
Acid Hypersecretory Syndromes
Serum gastrin elevation Gastrin provocative tests (intravenous secretin, meal) Gastric analysis (acid titration)

Endoscopy, which is the gold standard for diagnosis, is both highly sensitive and highly specific for the detection of ulcer disease. The most common locations for a peptic ulcer are the stomach and duodenal bulb, but peptic ulcers sometimes occur in the esophagus, the small bowel, and a Meckel diverticulum lined with heterotopic gastric mucosa. Endoscopic ultrasound may detect an unsuspected submucosal component or enlarged lymph nodes, such as may occur in gastric neoplasia, especially lymphoma and linitis plastica (Chapter 178). Ulcers in the dorsal wall of the duodenal bulb, especially at the transition from the bulb to the postbulbar descending portion of the duodenum, are most difficult to visualize. They sometimes require a side-viewing endoscope, particularly when endoscopic treatment is needed. Other regions where gastroduodenal ulcers can be easily missed are the cardia and the gastric angulus. Dieulafoy lesions may be difficult to diagnose because of their small mucosal defects and intermittent bleeding. Some patients require more than one endoscopy, preferably during acute bleeding, to localize the lesion. Endoscopy is also useful for ascertaining the presence of concomitant disorders, including esophagitis and duodenitis, or complications, such as bleeding or a visible vessel (see Fig. 125-2); obtaining biopsy specimens for histologic examination and to assess for *H. pylori* (see Fig. 125-3); and performing therapeutic interventions.

In rare cases, such as stenosis that blocks the advancing endoscope, conventional barium contrast radiographs (Chapter 119) are indicated. Additional investigations by endosonography or CT are needed when underlying malignant disease is suspected. The endoscopist should obtain biopsy samples from all gastric ulcers, especially those with a suspicious appearance, to exclude potential malignant disease. Because duodenal ulcers are less likely to be malignant, biopsies are usually not required unless malignancy is specifically suspected.

Etiologic Diagnosis

Diagnosis must focus on establishing the cause of the ulcer. The first step is to determine whether *H. pylori* or NSAID use is present because these are the major risk factors for peptic ulcers and can be contributing factors in ulcers with other precipitating causes.

Testing for *Helicobacter pylori*

In populations with high *H. pylori* prevalence, nearly all patients with peptic ulcer disease are positive for *H. pylori*, so diagnostic testing has little value except when antimicrobial susceptibility testing is needed. The prevalence of *H. pylori* remains high in immigrants from developing countries, where most people become *H. pylori* positive in youth. In Western countries, approximately 50% of individuals who are older than 65 years are colonized with *H. pylori*, but the prevalence is less than 20% in those younger than 30 years. In these younger persons, the proportion of patients with ulcers who are *H. pylori* negative is higher than in older patients, making diagnostic testing for *H. pylori*, followed by targeted therapy in those who are positive for the bacterium, more attractive than empirical therapy.

The presence of *H. pylori* can be ascertained by four possible approaches: gastric biopsies, serum, stool, or breath test.[4] The first method, *gastric mucosal biopsies*, is the standard procedure when diagnostic endoscopy is initially performed. Routine hematoxylin and eosin staining is sensitive and specific for *H. pylori*. However, the accuracy of this technique may be affected by sampling error, improper orientation of the specimen, and recent therapy with proton pump inhibitors or antibiotics. The presence of *H. pylori* in gastric mucosal biopsies also can be assessed by rapid urease testing, which has a high positive predictive value, although false-negative tests occur in patients using proton pump inhibitors or antibiotics and in patients with marked atrophic gastritis and intestinal metaplasia. Finally, biopsies can be cultured for *H. pylori* when it is important to assess antimicrobial resistance in patients with recurrent disease after previous antibiotic treatment.

A second option is *serology*, which is simple, inexpensive, and accurate, although its predictive value is lower in areas where the prevalence of *H. pylori* is low. Serology is not helpful to verify whether *H. pylori* has been eradicated with antibiotics because it may take more than 6 months or even 1 to 2 years for *H. pylori* antibodies to decrease to undetectable levels.

A third option is a *stool H. pylori antigen test*, which is similar in accuracy to standardized serologic testing. Finally, the *carbon-13* or *carbon-14 urea breath test*, which relies on the detection of *H. pylori* urease activity, is a noninvasive and relatively simple test, but it is more expensive than stool or blood testing. Although the test usually becomes negative as soon as *H. pylori* treatment is begun, a minimum interval of 6 to 8 weeks after therapy has ended is recommended to reduce false-negative results.

Nonsteroidal Anti-inflammatory Drugs

NSAIDs are usually established as the putative cause of an ulcer based on information obtained from the patient. Assessment of NSAID use in an individual patient presenting with ulcer disease can be difficult both because NSAID use is common and often intermittent and because many different NSAIDs are widely available over the counter in most countries. NSAID use is usually evaluated by detailed medical history, focusing not only on current and recent drug use, and especially over-the-counter treatments, but also on symptoms of pain, including musculoskeletal complaints. Further information from family members, family practitioners, and pharmacists is sometimes helpful. If surreptitious use of NSAIDs is suspected, direct serum and urine testing for aspirin and NSAID derivatives is feasible, or aspirin use can be assessed indirectly by a platelet adherence assay; however, these tests are not commonly used in clinical practice.

Hypersecretory Syndromes

Hypersecretory syndromes not related to *H. pylori* or NSAIDs are rare causes of ulcer disease and are diagnosed by special tests (see Table 125-3). Zollinger-Ellison syndrome should be strongly considered in patients with multiple ulcers, particularly in atypical locations such as distal to the duodenal bulb, and when diarrhea is present because these findings are uncommon in *H. pylori*–related peptic ulcer disease. Hypergastrinemic syndromes (e.g., Zollinger-Ellison syndrome, antral G-cell hyperplasia) are best diagnosed by a determination of serum gastrin levels, both basal and after stimulation with intravenous secretin (gastrinoma detection) or a test meal (antral G-cell hyperplasia detection). When detected early, gastrinomas may be resectable (Chapter 213).

Gastric analysis, by quantified aspiration of gastric juice through a nasogastric tube (both basal and after stimulation with subcutaneous pentagastrin), is indicated in only two rare circumstances: patients with elevated serum gastrin levels suggestive of Zollinger-Ellison syndrome or antral G-cell hyperplasia but with equivocal responses to standard gastric provocative tests, and patients with indirect signs of gastric hypersecretion (e.g., enlarged folds and abundant clear fluid at endoscopy), normal gastrin levels, and negative provocative gastrin tests but who may still be hypersecretors, such as patients with recurrent ulcer disease despite a prior vagotomy with or without antrectomy. A basal acid output greater than 15 mEq/hour or greater than 5 mEq/hour in a postoperative patient is considered a positive test result.

The diagnosis of Zollinger-Ellison syndrome is best confirmed by gastric analysis showing a basal acid output greater than 15 mEq/hour in conjunction with a fasting serum gastrin level exceeding 1000 pg/mL in the presence of gastric pH less than 2. To bypass the cumbersome gastric analysis, a gastric pH determination showing a fasting pH of 2 or less is adequate. For serum gastrin levels in the range of 100 to 1000 pg/mL and intragastric pH>2, an increase in the serum gastrin to more than 200 pg/mL after a secretin stimulation test is suggestive of the diagnosis. An elevated serum gastrin level alone is not sufficient to diagnose Zollinger-Ellison syndrome because serum gastrin levels tend to increase over time with atrophic gastritis and also can be markedly increased in patients receiving proton pump inhibitor therapy.

Other Causes

In patients in whom a gastroduodenal ulcer cannot be ascribed to colonization with *H. pylori*, use of NSAIDs, or a hypersecretory syndrome, the establishment of a definite etiologic diagnosis may require a more thorough evaluation, starting with a medical history that focuses on the use of other ulcerogenic agents and the presence of symptoms that could suggest an underlying systemic disease. The next step is to evaluate biopsy samples from ulcer borders and from the antrum, corpus, and duodenum. The ulcer specimens may reveal overt or suspicious signs of malignancy, in particular adenocarcinoma (Chapter 178) or lymphoma. In these cases, further diagnostic evaluation should include staging of the malignancy. Alternatively, the biopsies may provide evidence of other infectious conditions, specific types of gastritis, celiac disease, ischemia, amyloidosis, or a systemic inflammatory condition. These data can be combined with clues provided by the endoscopic evaluation, including the character and location of the ulcer, signs of ischemia, and signs of inflammation at other locations. Further evaluation should focus on the presence of systemic disorders and may include a chest radiograph, angiography, colonoscopy, and abdominal CT.

Differential Diagnosis

The differential diagnosis of ulcer-like symptoms includes many disorders of the upper abdominal organs, including malignant diseases of the stomach (Chapter 178), duodenum (Chapter 179), pancreas (Chapter 180), or bile ducts (Chapter 181). The differential diagnosis of upper abdominal symptoms also includes liver and gallstone disease (Chapter 141), pancreatitis (Chapter 130), and motility disorders (Chapter 122). In many patients with upper abdominal dyspeptic complaints, no underlying cause can be identified. In this "nonulcer" or functional dyspepsia group, complaints characteristic of gastroesophageal reflux, ulcer symptoms, or dysmotility symptoms may be prominent. Some patients (generally 5%) benefit from eradication of *H. pylori*, with a slow decrease of dyspeptic complaints over 12 to 24 months, but functional dyspepsia is not a proven or widely accepted indication for treatment of *H. pylori*. If such treatment is considered, both the patient and the physician should be prepared for persistent symptoms despite eradication of *H. pylori* and potentially for the emergence of antimicrobial-resistant *H. pylori*, which may result in a spiral of multiple courses of therapy in an attempt to remove resistant organisms.

Diagnostic Scenarios: Acute or Initial Clinical Presentation

Younger (≤45 years old) patients without alarm symptoms or signs such as anemia, rapid weight loss, or other evidence of serious disease do not necessarily require endoscopy, and malignant gastric disease is unlikely. When a physician is treating a patient who lives in an area of the world with a relatively high prevalence of *H. pylori* infection (>10% of the population is positive), a test-and-treat approach can begin with an *H. pylori* stool antigen determination, urea breath test, or *H. pylori* serologic examination. However, although commonly practiced, the test-and-treat approach has never been documented to improve outcomes, except in the setting of endoscopically confirmed peptic ulcer disease. If the *H. pylori* test is positive, the patient can be treated with the appropriate *H. pylori* eradication drugs (see later) and observed for 4 to 6 weeks. If a patient with dyspeptic symptoms is taking an NSAID, either orally or parenterally, the first therapeutic approach is to discontinue these drugs and to prescribe a proton pump inhibitor for 4 to 6 weeks. In patients who test negative for *H. pylori* and who are not taking NSAIDs or who do not improve after these drugs are discontinued, endoscopy is indicated to determine whether an ulcer is present.

Conversely, gastroenterologists more commonly proceed directly to endoscopy. If no abnormalities are apparent or the endoscopic study shows only "gastritis" without an overt ulcer, a biopsy should be obtained to ascertain by histologic examination or urease testing whether *H. pylori* is present. If *H. pylori* is present, then eradication treatment may be pursued. However, the efficacy of *H. pylori* eradication for the relief of functional dyspeptic symptoms is only about 6 to 12% greater than with placebo,[A1] and eradication therapy increases the risk for reflux-related symptoms (Chapter 124), especially in Asian patients.

If endoscopic examination reveals an ulcer, its location determines the subsequent approach. An ulcer in the duodenal bulb has only a remote chance of representing a malignant lesion and need not routinely be examined by biopsy. By contrast, biopsy is mandatory for a gastric ulcerative lesion identified at endoscopy because malignant gastric disease may present with similar clinical manifestations and may resemble benign ulcer disease morphologically. Even if histologic assessment does not identify a malignant process, repeat endoscopy is recommended about 1 month after therapy to verify complete healing and for biopsy of the scar.

TREATMENT

Helicobacter pylori–Associated Ulcers

H. pylori–associated ulcers often heal spontaneously, but acid-suppressive therapy accelerates healing and ameliorates symptoms. Four weeks of acid-suppressive therapy heals 70 to 80% of ulcers, and this number increases to more than 90% after 8 weeks of therapy. If *H. pylori* colonization persists, however, ulcers recur in 50 to 90% of patients within 12 to 24 months; this rate can be reduced to 20 to 30% with maintenance acid suppression and to less than 5% with *H. pylori* eradication.[A2] Eradication treatment is therefore mandatory (Table 125-4).[5,6] The success of eradication treatment strongly depends on therapy adherence and antimicrobial resistance.[7,8] Resistance of *H. pylori* to metronidazole varies between 20 and 80% throughout the world. Clarithromycin resistance is increasing and ranges between 10 and 50% in many regions owing to the widespread use of macrolides to treat upper respiratory infections. Resistance to amoxicillin and tetracycline is rare and is not usually relevant in clinical practice. Levofloxacin resistance was very rare a decade ago, but it now ranges between 10 and 50% in many regions of the world. Because of this worldwide increase in prevalence of antimicrobial resistance, *H. pylori* eradication regimens continue to evolve.

The conventional regimen is empiric "triple" therapy for 14 days.[9,10] This treatment remains a standard regimen for regions and populations with a clarithromycin resistance below 15%, such as in Northern Europe and North America. Triple therapy combines a proton pump inhibitor or potassium-competitive acid blocker (vonoprazan 20 mg twice daily)[A3] with two antibiotics, usually combinations of amoxicillin, a nitroimidazole, and clarithromycin, with the latter sometimes being replaced by levofloxacin.[A4] Double-dose proton pump inhibitor therapy (dose equivalent to omeprazole 40 mg twice daily) also increases eradication rates by approximately 10% and is preferred. For patients in whom such therapy fails, a 14-day course of quadruple therapy (see later) eradicates *H. pylori* in an additional 80% of patients (Fig. 125-5). Adding probiotic capsules to standard triple therapy appears to hasten the resolution of symptoms and increase the eradication of *H. pylori*.[A5]

Because of the increased prevalence of antimicrobial resistance, initial empiric "quadruple" therapies[A6] or susceptibility-guided antibiotic treatment[A7] are increasingly being recommended over initial empiric "triple therapy" because of their better first-line efficacy. Bismuth-based quadruple therapy consists of a proton pump inhibitor, a bismuth compound, and two antibiotics, usually tetracycline and a nitroimidazole (see Table 125-4). This regimen leads to eradication in about 85 to 90% of patients. Non–bismuth-based quadruple therapies consist of a proton pump inhibitor plus three antibiotics, usually given for 14 days (see Table 125-4). The three forms of non–bismuth-based quadruple therapy (sequential, hybrid, and concomitant therapy) differ in their antibiotic dosing schedule. Sequential therapy consists of a proton pump inhibitor with amoxicillin, usually given for 5 days, followed by a proton pump inhibitor with clarithromycin and a nitroimidazole for another 5 days. Ten-day sequential therapy is equally effective as 14-day triple therapy.[A8] Hybrid therapy starts with the same 5-day combination of a proton pump inhibitor with amoxicillin and then continues the amoxicillin for the next 5 days together with clarithromycin and metronidazole. Concomitant therapy, which gives these same drugs all together for 14 days, is the most effective, in particular when given for 14 days with a proton pump inhibitor in a dose of 40 mg twice daily.

Continuation of acid-suppressive therapy after antibiotic treatment is needed only when symptoms persist or in cases of complicated ulcer disease until eradication of *H. pylori* has been confirmed. Ascertainment of therapeutic efficacy must be delayed at least 1 month after the end of treatment to prevent false-negative results related to the organism's temporary suppression but not eradication. When repeat endoscopy is needed (e.g., a gastric ulcer requires repeated histologic examination to exclude underlying malignancy), repeat screening for *H. pylori* can be performed using gastric biopsy specimens for histologic examination, culture, or urease testing. If no clinical indication exists for repeat endoscopy, *H. pylori* status can be determined by a carbon-13 urea breath test, stool *H. pylori* antigen, or repeated serology. Serologic determination is based on a more than 40 to 50% decrease in immunoglobulin G antibody levels in the first 6 months after treatment compared with pretreatment levels in that patient; ideally, the (frozen) pretreatment and post-treatment specimens should be examined simultaneously by the same laboratory using the same assay.

After successful *H. pylori* eradication, the risk for recurrent infection in most populations is less than 1% per year. In a minority of patients, ulcers recur either owing to reinfection or in the presence of another ulcerogenic factor, particularly NSAID use. Quinolone-based quadruple therapy (including bismuth) for 10 or more days is an excellent second-line therapy for patients who do not respond to initial therapy.[11]

Disease Related to Nonsteroidal Anti-inflammatory Drug Use

In patients who are diagnosed with acid peptic disease while they are taking NSAIDs or aspirin, the first step is to stop such therapy. Acid suppression with a proton pump inhibitor (in doses similar to those used for *H. pylori*) leads

TABLE 125-4 OVERVIEW OF ORAL ANTIBIOTICS USED FOR *HELICOBACTER PYLORI* ERADICATION

DRUG CLASS	DRUG	TRIPLE THERAPY* DOSE	BISMUTH-BASED QUADRUPLE THERAPY† DOSE	NON–BISMUTH-BASED QUADRUPLE THERAPY‡ DOSE
Acid suppression	Proton pump inhibitor	40 mg bid[§]	20-40 mg bid[§]	20-40 mg bid[§]
	Potassium competitive acid blocker	20 mg bid[††]	20 mg bid[††]	20 mg bid[††]
Standard antimicrobials	Bismuth compound[‖]		2 tablets bid	
	Amoxicillin	1 g bid	1 g bid	1 g bid
	Metronidazole[¶]	500 mg bid	500 mg tid	500 mg bid
	Clarithromycin	500 mg bid		500 mg bid
	Tetracycline		500 mg qid	
Salvage antimicrobials	Levofloxacin**	500 mg qd	500 mg od	500 mg qd
	Rifabutin	150 mg bid	150 mg bid	
	Furazolidone	100 mg bid	100 mg bid	
	Doxycycline		100 mg bid	100 mg bid
	Nitazoxanide		500 mg bid	500 mg bid

*Triple therapy consists of a proton pump inhibitor or bismuth compound, together with two of the listed antibiotics, usually given for 7 to 14 days.

†Bismuth-based quadruple therapy consists of a proton pump inhibitor plus the combination of a bismuth compound and two antibiotics, usually given for 7 to 14 days.

‡Non-bismuth-based quadruple therapy consists of a proton pump inhibitor, plus three antibiotics usually given for 10 days and sometimes extended to 14 days. The three forms of non–bismuth-based quadruple therapy differ in their antibiotic dosing schedules: (1) sequential therapy gives amoxicillin for the first half of the course and then metronidazole and clarithromycin for the second half; (2) hybrid therapy starts with amoxicillin for the first half and then continues the second half with amoxicillin, clarithromycin, and metronidazole; (3) concomitant therapy combines all three antibiotics throughout the usual 10- to 14-day therapy. Other combinations of antibiotics are occasionally used.

§Proton pump inhibitor dose equivalent to omeprazole 20 to 40 mg bid. (See Table 124-1 for doses of other proton pump inhibitors.)

‖Bismuth subsalicylate or subcitrate.

¶An alternative is tinidazole 500 mg bid.

**Alternatives are moxifloxacin 400 mg qid and sitafloxacin 100 mg bid.

††Equivalent to vonoprazan 20 mg bid.

bid = twice daily; qd = daily.

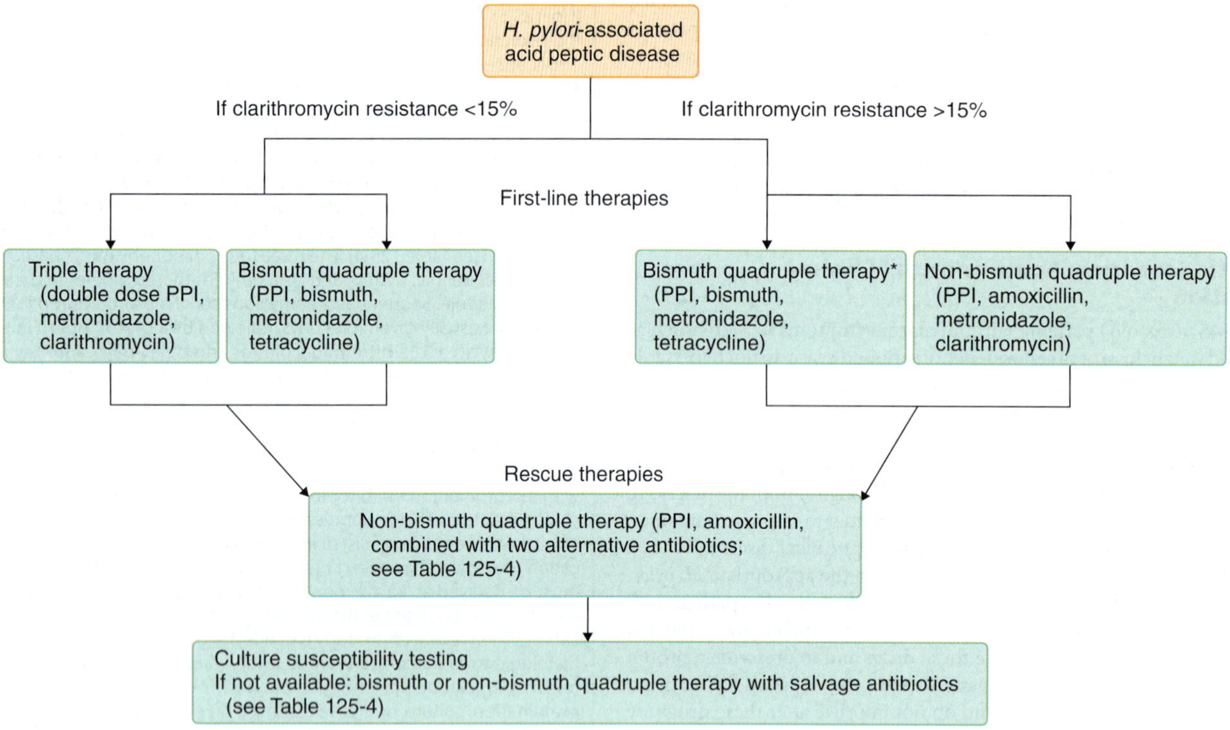

FIGURE 125-5. **Management of *H. pylori*–associated acid peptic disease.** See text and Table 125-4 for duration of therapy. PPI = proton pump inhibitor. *Preferred therapy if clarithromycin resistance >15%.

to healing of 85% of NSAID-induced gastric ulcers and more than 90% of duodenal ulcers within 8 weeks of therapy, whereas acid suppression with a histamine-2 (H_2)-receptor blocker, equivalent to ranitidine 300 mg twice daily (see Table 125-1), heals approximately 70% of ulcers within 8 weeks. The mucosal-protective drug misoprostol (200 mg four times daily) has a similar effect to the H_2 blockers. Treatment must be continued for at least 8 weeks, and maintenance therapy is needed in patients who continue to take NSAIDs. Gastric ulcers, larger lesions, and recurrent lesions heal more slowly.

Ulcer occurrence during NSAID therapy suggests a causal relationship, but patients should also be tested for *H. pylori*. In patients who are *H. pylori* positive, eradication therapy should be considered because there are no clear clinical parameters distinguishing between these etiologic factors.

Idiopathic Ulcer Disease

Patients with idiopathic ulcer disease despite a thorough assessment for underlying causes are treated primarily with an acid suppressant, usually a proton pump inhibitor, because they are at considerable risk for recurrent ulcer disease. After the underlying cause is identified and adequately treated, acid-suppressive therapy can be withdrawn if there are no additional risk factors for ulcer disease, such as NSAID therapy or *H. pylori* infection. If the cause of the idiopathic ulceration is not clarified and there is doubt about the adequacy of the diagnostic testing for *H. pylori*, empirical eradication therapy can be considered, especially when there is histologic evidence of chronic active gastritis without further explanation. If related to unidentified *H. pylori*, gastritis should slowly disappear after successful eradication therapy.

PREVENTION

Primary Prevention

A test-and-treat strategy for *H. pylori* colonization is sometimes considered for patients with dyspeptic symptoms, but there is no specific way to prevent *H. pylori*–associated ulcer disease. By contrast, primary prevention of NSAID-associated ulcer disease is widely advocated for patients at high risk because of a prior ulcer, severe concomitant disease, or use of warfarin or high-dose corticosteroids as well as for critically ill patients in intensive care units. H_2 blockers (at a dose equivalent to ranitidine 300 mg twice daily; Table 124-1) partially prevent duodenal ulcer disease during NSAID therapy but have no effect on preventing gastric ulcers unless a higher dose (equivalent to famotidine 40 mg twice daily) is given. Proton pump inhibitors[A9] (at a dose equivalent to omeprazole 20 mg once daily; Table 124-1) and misoprostol (in doses varying between 400 and 800 mg/day) partially protect against both gastric and duodenal ulcers during NSAID use. Misoprostol and proton pump inhibitors are equally effective, but adherence with therapy is lower with misoprostol owing to its side effects. Patients should be advised of the importance of adherence because less than 80% adherence to gastroprotection is associated with a more than two-fold increased risk for ulcer disease compared with those who are fully adherent. During low-dose aspirin therapy, primary prevention of ulcers is advocated for the same risk groups, using a proton pump inhibitor or an H_2-receptor antagonist.[A10] *H. pylori* eradication also can reduce aspirin-associated peptic ulcer bleeding.[A11] For the prevention of stress ulcers in patients in intensive care units,[12] proton pump inhibitors and histamine-2 receptor blockers are approximately equally effective, but some data suggest that proton pump inhibitors may be preferred.[A12]

Secondary Prevention

Secondary prevention of *H. pylori*–associated ulcer disease is mandatory and consists of successful bacterial eradication. Testing to ascertain *H. pylori* status after eradication therapy is indicated in patients with prior complicated ulcer disease or with persistent or recurrent symptoms after therapy, as well as in patients who fail to complete the therapeutic course.

Secondary prevention of NSAID-related ulcer disease is preferentially achieved by the withdrawal of NSAIDs. In patients who must continue taking NSAIDs, a change to a selective COX2 inhibitor[A13] in combination with a proton pump inhibitor at a dose equivalent to esomeprazole 20 mg twice daily is advocated, especially for patients with complicated ulcer disease. This combination is associated with a lower risk for secondary peptic ulcer complications than treatment with a COX2 inhibitor alone.

Secondary prevention of recurrent ulcers in patients who use aspirin may depend on *H. pylori* status. In *H. pylori*–positive patients, *H. pylori* eradication is as effective as a proton pump inhibitor for the prevention of recurrent ulcers. *H. pylori*–negative patients require additional acid-suppressive therapy at a dose equivalent to esomeprazole 20 mg twice daily.[A14] Secondary prevention of idiopathic ulcer disease consists primarily of maintenance therapy with a proton pump inhibitor and treatment of the underlying condition. When there is doubt about the accuracy of the diagnostic assessment for *H. pylori*, an empirical course of eradication treatment can be considered.

Complications

Hemorrhage

Hemorrhage (Chapter 121), which is the most common complication of peptic ulcer disease, occurs in about one in six patients with ulcers over the course of their ulcer activity. Ulcers caused by NSAIDs account for a larger proportion of these hemorrhages. Peptic ulcer is thus the most common cause of nonvariceal upper gastrointestinal bleeding, accounting for 40 to 60% of cases in most populations. Bleeding is associated with a 5 to 15% risk for rebleeding and up to a 10% risk for mortality. Hemorrhage may occur along a continuum from a serious acute event associated with hemodynamic shock and high mortality to slow or intermittent blood loss leading to chronic anemia. Approximately 80% of patients with bleeding ulcers describe a prior history of symptomatic disease, and about 20 to 30% have suffered a previous hemorrhage. Assessment of the magnitude of bleeding is of paramount importance in determining the need for transfusion and subsequent management (Table 125-5). Initial hematocrit levels may be misleading and are likely to

TABLE 125-5 PARAMETERS OF THE ROCKALL, BLATCHFORD, AND AIMS65 SCORING SYSTEMS FOR UPPER GASTROINTESTINAL BLEEDING*

		ROCKALL SYSTEM†		*BLATCHFORD SYSTEM*‡		*AIMS65*§	
SCORING CATEGORIES	**SCORING PARAMETERS**	**PARAMETER**	**SCORE**	**PARAMETER**	**SCORE**	**PARAMETER**	**SCORE**
Age	Age (yr)	60-79	1	N/A	—	>65	1
		≥80	2				
Clinical status	Systolic blood pressure	<100	2	100-109	1	≤90	1
				90-99	2		
				<90	3		
	Pulse	>100	1	>100	1	N/A	—
	Melena	N/A	—	Present	1	N/A	—
	Syncope	N/A	—	Present	1	N/A	—
	Altered mental status	N/A	—	N/A	—	Present	1
	Comorbidities	Any major comorbidity	2	Hepatic disease	2	N/A	—
		Renal or liver failure, or disseminated malignancy	3	Cardiac failure	2		
Laboratory parameters	Blood urea, mmol/L	N/A	—	6.5-7.9	2	N/A	—
				8.0-9.9	3		
				10-24.9	4		
				>25.0	6		
	Hemoglobin, g/dL	N/A	—	Men: 12.0-13.0	1	N/A	—
				Women: 10.0-12.0	1		
				Men: 10.0-12.0	3		
				Men and women: <10.0	6		
	INR	N/A	—	N/A	—	>1.5	1
	Albumin	N/A	—	N/A	—	<3.0 g/dL	1
Endoscopy	Endoscopic diagnosis	No focus, or Mallory-Weiss tear	0	N/A	—	N/A	—
		Upper GI malignancy	2				
		All other diagnoses	1				
	Endoscopic SRH	None/dark spot only	0	N/A	—	N/A	—
		Blood/clot/vessel	2				

*The Blatchford (Stanley AJ, Ashley D, Dalton HR, et al. Outpatient management of patients with low-risk upper-gastrointestinal haemorrhage: multicentre validation and prospective evaluation. *Lancet.* 2009;373:42-47) and AIMS65 (Saltzman JR, Tabak YP, Hyett BH, et al. A simple risk score accurately predicts in-hospital mortality, length of stay, and cost in acute upper GI bleeding. *Gastrointest Endosc.* 2011;74:1215-1224) systems are pre-endoscopy scoring systems; the Rockall system (Rockall TA, Logan RF, Devlin HB, et al. Risk assessment after acute upper gastrointestinal haemorrhage. *Gut.* 1996;38:316-321) has a pre- and post-endoscopy component. The Blatchford system is a tool to select patients for early discharge and later endoscopy during office hours. The Rockall score can help to assess the risk for rebleeding and mortality. The AIMS65 predicts mortality.

†Scores before and after endoscopy. Low risk defined as scores of ≤2, high risk defined as scores ≥6.

‡Low risk defined as score of 0.

§Low risk defined as score of ≤1, high risk as score of ≥2.

GI = gastrointestinal; INR = international normalized ratio; N/A = not applicable; SRH = stigmata of recent hemorrhage.

fall because of hemodilution. Rapid bleeding is usually apparent on the basis of clinical signs (pallor, systolic blood pressure ≤100 mm Hg, pulse ≥100 beats/minute); immediate fluid resuscitation is indicated to prevent circulatory collapse. Transfusion is needed in patients with marked anemia. Restrictive transfusion using a hemoglobin threshold of 70 to 80 g/L is associated with fewer transfusions and lower risks for rebleeding and mortality.[A15] Mortality is particularly related to complications of the bleed, such as aspiration, and exacerbation of underlying disease, such as pulmonary, cardiovascular, renal, and hepatic disease. On rare occasions, patients may actually bleed to death, especially when a larger artery is affected, such as when an ulcer in the posterior wall of the duodenal bulb perforates the gastroduodenal artery. The stopping of such bleeding is therefore a medical emergency.[13]

Initial treatment aims at hemodynamic stabilization. Endoscopy is the mainstay of therapy and should be performed emergently or within 24 hours of presentation in high-risk cases, especially patients who are hemodynamically unstable, require transfusion, or have more severe comorbidities.[14] Endoscopy can be performed to ascertain the origin of the bleeding and, if necessary, provide therapy to stop the bleed and reduce the risk for rebleeding.

The appearance of the ulcer determines the need for endoscopic treatment and the risk for rebleeding (Table 125-6) and mortality. "Clean base" ulcers and those with flat and pigmented spots carry a low risk for rebleeding and do not require endoscopic treatment. In contrast, ulcers with active bleeding or stigmata of recent bleeding, in particular a visible vessel or adherent clot, require treatment to stop the bleed and reduce the otherwise high risk for recurrence.

Endoscopic therapy may lead to a three-fold reduction in episodes of recurrent bleeding and in the need for surgical intervention, as well as a 40% reduction in mortality. Treatment modalities include injection therapy with epinephrine or a sclerosant, thermocoagulation, and mechanical pressure by means of clips. Thermocoagulation can be performed by direct contact, such as with a heater probe, or by a noncontact method, such as argon plasma coagulation. The efficacy of these methods is generally comparable, except that epinephrine injection alone is inferior to the other modalities but can be useful when combined with any of the others. If an adherent clot is found, an attempt should be made to remove it by water flushing or snaring to allow an assessment of the underlying ulcer base and the treatment of any underlying visible vessels to reduce the risk for rebleeding.

Pre-endoscopy administration of intravenous proton pump inhibitor therapy (at a dose equivalent to a bolus of 80 mg esomeprazole, followed by a continuous infusion of 8 mg/hour until endoscopy) reduces bleeding and the need for emergent endoscopic treatment, but it has no effect on the need for transfusion or the occurrence of rebleeding or death. For patients with active bleeding or stigmata of recent bleeding, endoscopic treatment should be followed by an intravenous proton pump inhibitor given as a bolus at a dose equivalent to 80 mg esomeprazole over 30 minutes, followed by a continuous infusion at a dose equivalent to esomeprazole 8 mg/hour for 72 hours to reduce rebleeding and the need for further intervention. Intermittent oral or intravenous therapy at 6- to 12-hour intervals in a cumulative daily dose equivalent to 80 to 160 mg esomeprazole may be equally effective, although more evidence is needed in patients from Western countries. Other therapies, including tranexamic acid, vasopressin, somatostatin, and octreotide, should be considered experimental (Chapter 121). Second-look endoscopy is not routinely indicated but can be considered in very high-risk cases, particularly when there is doubt about the adequacy of initial visualization or treatment.

About 70 to 80% of rebleeds occur within the first 3 days and generally should be managed by repeat endoscopy. If endoscopy fails to stop the bleed or prevent further rebleeding, surgery and interventional radiology are equivalent options. Surgery includes stitching of the ulcer and occlusion of the feeding artery, usually the gastroduodenal artery. Interventional radiology uses angiography to insert coils in the culprit vessel at the site of the bleed. Single-center observational experience suggests that each of these methods is equally effective in the hands of experienced clinicians, and the choice depends on local availability and expertise.

The risk for a fatal outcome of an upper gastrointestinal hemorrhage can be estimated based on five clinical and endoscopic parameters (see Table 125-5). In several studies, mortality in patients with a bleeding peptic ulcer was less than 2% among those with a score of 2 points or less, 10% in those with 3 to 5 points, and up to 46% in those with 6 points or more. Management of patients who recover after a peptic ulcer hemorrhage is similar to the treatment of patients with uncomplicated ulcers. Eradication of *H. pylori* provides excellent protection against both recurrence and rebleeding of *H. pylori*–related ulcers. NSAID-induced ulcers are preferentially managed by the withdrawal of NSAIDs or, if this is not feasible, by the combination of a COX2 inhibitor and a proton pump inhibitor at a dose equivalent to esomeprazole 20 mg twice daily. In patients with a history of ulcer bleeding and concomitant cardiovascular disease requiring antiplatelet therapy, the combination of low-dose aspirin and a proton pump inhibitor at a dose equivalent to esomeprazole 20 mg twice daily is associated with a lower risk for complicated ulcer than is clopidogrel monotherapy. If a patient who requires antiplatelet therapy presents with a bleeding ulcer, antiplatelet therapy should be continued or restarted as soon as possible if the risk for a cardiovascular event outweighs the risk for recurrent bleeding.

Perforation

Perforation may manifest as an acute event, whereby gastric contents spill into the peritoneal cavity, or more insidiously as the ulcer slowly penetrates into surrounding tissues. Acute free perforation typically causes abrupt and severe abdominal pain associated with abdominal muscular spasm that produces boardlike rigidity of the abdomen and other manifestations of peritoneal irritation. Secondary hemodynamic shock is common. The clinical diagnosis can be confirmed in approximately 80% of patients by a plain chest radiograph with the patient standing (Fig. 125-6); a CT scan can be obtained if doubt persists. Leukocytosis and elevated C-reactive protein levels develop rapidly, and mild hyperamylasemia may occur. Treatment begins by correcting hemodynamic, fluid, and electrolyte imbalances. Nasogastric suction is helpful, and prophylactic antibiotics (e.g., amoxicillin-clavulanic acid 1 g every 8 hours intravenously) are usually administered. Unless a specific contraindication exists, emergency surgery is usually indicated,[15] although more conservative approaches are sometimes appropriate. Given the success in achieving the long-term cure of ulcer disease through the eradication of *H. pylori* and the

TABLE 125-6 ENDOSCOPY RESULTS IN PATIENTS WITH BLEEDING ULCERS

ENDOSCOPY RESULT	ULCER CHARACTERISTICS*	RISK FOR RECURRENT BLEEDING (%)
Active bleeding	Arterial bleeding	80-90
	Oozing bleeding	10-30
Stigmata of recent bleeding	Nonbleeding visible vessel	50-60
	Adherent clot	25-35
	Flat pigmented spot	0-8
No signs of bleeding	Clean ulcer base	0-12

*The ulcer characteristics determine the risk for recurrent bleeding during follow-up.

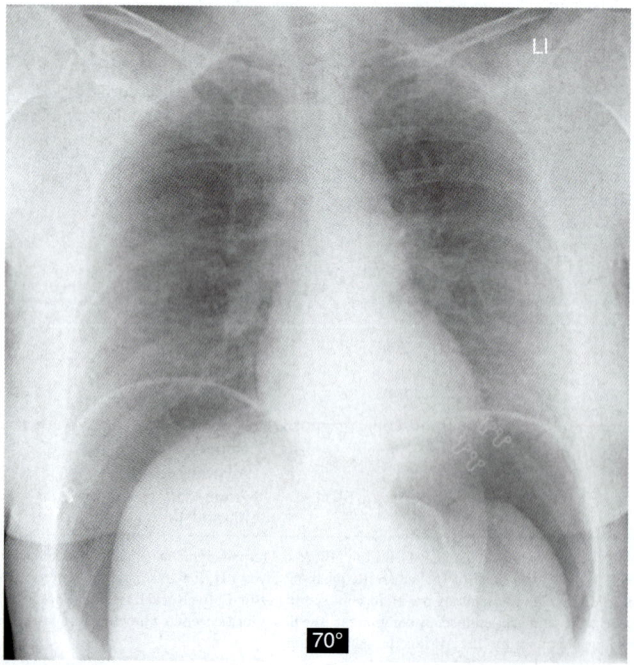

FIGURE 125-6. **Plain chest radiograph in an upright patient with a perforated ulcer. The radiograph shows free air under the diaphragm.**

withdrawal of NSAIDs, suturing of the perforated ulcer may be adequate, permitting the patient to avoid a more radical vagotomy with or without gastric resection.

Intractability

Intractability is a term strictly applied to an ulcer that persists even after intensive and prolonged proton pump inhibitor therapy. Symptoms may or may not be present. These rare cases may result from poor compliance with recommended treatment, surreptitious use of ulcerogenic drugs, or other diseases (e.g., Crohn disease, ischemia, infection with bacteria other than *H. pylori*, viral infection). If these issues are recognized and these diagnoses are pursued, further complications and interventions such as surgical vagotomy and pyloroplasty can almost always be avoided.

Acid peptic disease related to alcohol or bisphosphonates should be addressed by discontinuing the precipitating agent. Treatment of Zollinger-Ellison syndrome requires high-dose proton pump inhibitors and/or surgery (Chapter 213). Rare ulcers caused by Crohn disease (Chapter 127), vasculitis (Chapter 249), sarcoidosis (Chapter 83), polycythemia vera (Chapter 152), amyloidosis (Chapter 174), and other rare disorders should be addressed by treating the underlying condition. Stress ulcers and Cameron ulcers are treated by potent acid-suppressive therapy (e.g., omeprazole 20 mg twice daily).

Stenosis

Gastric outlet obstruction is now a rare complication of ulcer disease because of the early detection and treatment of most ulcers. Most patients who develop clinically relevant gastric outlet obstruction have had an ulcer in the duodenal bulb and/or pyloric channel. Edema and inflammation play an important role, and occasionally a patient with active disease presents with symptoms of outlet obstruction as manifested by nausea, vomiting, and gastric stasis without a tight, chronic stenosis. Management therefore involves three key steps. The first is nasogastric tube aspiration and gastric lavage to clear the stomach of retained debris, followed by early endoscopy. This step facilitates an accurate diagnosis. Nasogastric suction may need to be maintained for several days if vomiting resumes when the tube is clamped. The second step consists of intense antisecretory therapy using intravenous proton pump inhibitors in a dose equivalent to a bolus of 80 mg esomeprazole over 30 minutes, followed by a continuous infusion of 8 mg/hour. Finally, the cause of the ulcer needs to be addressed, usually by eradicating *H. pylori* and withdrawing NSAIDs. If the initial treatment resolves the clinical situation and the patient can resume eating, it is often not necessary to undertake further treatment of the outlet stenosis; however, tight, fibrous scarring may require endoscopic balloon dilation or surgery.

PROGNOSIS

Most peptic ulcers heal spontaneously within weeks to months. However, if the underlying condition is not adequately treated, a large proportion of ulcers recur. Both initial and recurrent ulcers can give rise to complications. The four major complications are intractability, perforation, hemorrhage, and stenosis. Each distinct situation requires specific management approaches. Patients with complicated ulcer disease are at particular risk for recurrent complications and need careful assessment for secondary prevention. In patients who take long-term acid suppressive therapy, especially with proton pump inhibitors, the risks for community-acquired pneumonia and vitamin B_{12} deficiency (Chapters 150 and 199) are increased but overall mortality is not.[16] The treatment of *H. pylori* infection appears to reduce the risk of gastric cancer.[17,A16]

GENERAL REFERENCES

For the General References and other additional features, please visit Elsevier eBooks+ at https://ebooks.health.elsevier.com.

Grade A References

A1. Ford AC, Tsipotis E, Yuan Y, et al. Efficacy of *Helicobacter pylori* eradication therapy for functional dyspepsia: updated systematic review and meta-analysis. *Gut.* 2022. [Epub ahead of print.]
A2. Ford AC, Gurusamy KS, Delaney B, et al. Eradication therapy for peptic ulcer disease in Helicobacter pylori-positive people. *Cochrane Database Syst Rev.* 2016;4:CD003840.
A3. Shinozaki S, Kobayashi Y, Osawa H, et al. Effectiveness and safety of vonoprazan versus proton pump inhibitors for second-line Helicobacter pylori eradication therapy: systematic review and meta-analysis. *Digestion.* 2021;102:319-325.
A4. Rokkas T, Gisbert JP, Malfertheiner P, et al. Comparative effectiveness of multiple different first-line treatment regimens for *Helicobacter pylori* infection: a network meta-analysis. *Gastroenterology.* 2021;161:495-507.
A5. Yu M, Zhang R, Ni P, et al. Efficacy of *Lactobacillus*-supplemented triple therapy for *H. pylori* eradication: a meta-analysis of randomized clinical trials. *PloS One.* 2019;14:e0223309.
A6. Liou JM, Fang YJ, Chen CC, et al. Concomitant, bismuth quadruple, and 14-day triple therapy in the first-line treatment of Helicobacter pylori: a multicentre, open-label, randomised trial. *Lancet.* 2016;388:2355-2365.
A7. Gingold-Belfer R, Niv Y, Schmilovitz-Weiss H, et al. Susceptibility-guided versus empirical treatment for *Helicobacter pylori* infection: a systematic review and meta-analysis. *J Gastroenterol Hepatol.* 2021;36:2649-2658.
A8. Nyssen OP, McNicholl AG, Megraud F, et al. Sequential versus standard triple first-line therapy for Helicobacter pylori eradication. *Cochrane Database Syst Rev.* 2016;6:CD009034.
A9. Yang M, He M, Zhao M, et al. Proton pump inhibitors for preventing non-steroidal anti-inflammatory drug induced gastrointestinal toxicity: a systematic review. *Curr Med Res Opin.* 2017;33:973-980.
A10. Chan FK, Kyaw M, Tanigawa T, et al. Similar efficacy of proton-pump inhibitors vs H2-receptor antagonists in reducing risk of upper gastrointestinal bleeding or ulcers in high-risk users of low-dose aspirin. *Gastroenterology.* 2017;152:105-110.
A11. Hawkey C, Avery A, Coupland CAC, et al. Helicobacter pylori eradication for primary prevention of peptic ulcer bleeding in older patients prescribed aspirin in primary care (HEAT): a randomised, double-blind, placebo-controlled trial. *Lancet.* 2022;400:1597-1606.
A12. Alhazzani W, Alshamsi F, Belley-Cote E, et al. Efficacy and safety of stress ulcer prophylaxis in critically ill patients: a network meta-analysis of randomized trials. *Intensive Care Med.* 2018;44:1-11.
A13. Chan FKL, Ching JYL, Tse YK, et al. Gastrointestinal safety of celecoxib versus naproxen in patients with cardiothrombotic diseases and arthritis after upper gastrointestinal bleeding (CONCERN): an industry-independent, double-blind, double-dummy, randomised trial. *Lancet.* 2017;389:2375-2382.
A14. Scally B, Emberson JR, Spata E, et al. Effects of gastroprotectant drugs for the prevention and treatment of peptic ulcer disease and its complications: a meta-analysis of randomised trials. *Lancet Gastroenterol Hepatol.* 2018;3:231-241.
A15. Odutayo A, Desborough MJ, Trivella M, et al. Restrictive versus liberal blood transfusion for gastrointestinal bleeding: a systematic review and meta-analysis of randomised controlled trials. *Lancet Gastroenterol Hepatol.* 2017;2:354-360.
A16. Ford AC, Yuan Y, Forman D, et al. Helicobacter pylori eradication for the prevention of gastric neoplasia. *Cochrane Database Syst Rev.* 2020;7:CD005583.

126 APPROACH TO THE PATIENT WITH DIARRHEA AND MALABSORPTION

CAROL E. SEMRAD

DEFINITIONS

Normal stool frequency ranges from three times per week to three times per day. As a symptom, diarrhea can be described as a decrease in stool consistency (increased fluidity), stools that cause urgency or abdominal discomfort, or an increase in the frequency of stool. Consistency is defined as the ratio of fecal water to the water-holding capacity of fecal insoluble solids, which are composed of bacterial mass and dietary fiber. Because it is difficult to measure stool consistency and because stool is predominantly (60 to 85%) water, stool weight becomes a reasonable surrogate of consistency.

As a sign, diarrhea is defined by the weight or volume of stool measured over a 24- to 72-hour period. Daily stool weights of children and adults are less than 200 g, and greater stool weights are an objective definition of diarrhea; however, this definition misses 20% of diarrheal symptoms in patients who have loose stools that are less than this daily weight.

Acute diarrheas persist for less than 2 to 3 weeks or, rarely, 6 to 8 weeks. The most common cause of acute diarrhea is infection. Chronic diarrheal conditions persist for at least 4 weeks and, more typically, 6 to 8 weeks or longer. The four mechanisms of diarrhea are osmotic, secretory, exudative, and altered motility. Because many diarrheal diseases are due to more than one of these mechanisms, it is clinically useful to categorize diarrhea as malabsorptive (fatty), watery, and inflammatory.

EPIDEMIOLOGY

Diarrhea is a leading cause of mortality worldwide and is particularly problematic for elderly people and for children younger than 5 years of age in developing nations. Infectious diarrheal conditions cause approximately 445,000 worldwide childhood deaths annually, despite the improved use of oral rehydration solutions, zinc, and vitamin A supplements. Rotavirus infection (Chapter 350) is the most common cause of fatal childhood diarrhea, but the introduction of the oral monovalent rotavirus vaccine has significantly decreased its mortality rate in both developing and developed nations.

In the United States, norovirus has surpassed rotavirus as the leading cause of gastroenteritis requiring medical care. Approximately 48 million Americans suffer from food-borne illness each year, including about 128,000 annual hospitalizations and 3000 deaths, most in elderly people. The major pathogens that cause diarrhea result in an estimated $17.6 billion in annual health care costs and days lost from work.

PATHOBIOLOGY

Fluid and Electrolyte Transport

Whether a hypotonic meal, such as a steak and water, or a hypertonic meal, such as milk and a doughnut, is consumed, the volume of the meal is augmented by gastric, pancreatic, biliary, and duodenal secretions. The permeable duodenum then renders the meal approximately isotonic with an electrolyte content similar to that of plasma by the time it reaches the proximal jejunum. As the intestinal slurry moves toward the colon, the Na^+ concentration in the luminal fluid remains constant, but Cl^- is reduced to 60 to 70 mmol/L, and bicarbonate (HCO_3^-) is increased to a similar concentration as the result of Cl^- and HCO_3^- transport mechanisms in the enterocyte and HCO_3^- secretion in the ileum (E-Fig. 126-1A and B). In the colon, K^+ is secreted, and the Na^+ transport mechanism of the colonocyte, together with the low epithelial permeability, extracts Na^+ and fluid from the stool. As a result, the Na^+ content of stool decreases to 30 to 40 mmol/L; K^+ increases from 5 to 10 mmol/L in the small bowel to 75 to 90 mmol/L; and poorly absorbed divalent cations, such as Mg^{2+} and Ca^{2+}, are concentrated in stool to values of 5 to 100 mmol/L. The anion concentrations in the colon change drastically because bacterial degradation of carbohydrate (i.e., unabsorbed starches, sugars, and fiber) creates short-chain fatty acids that attain concentrations of 80 to 180 mmol/L; at colonic pH, organic anions, such as acetate, propionate, and butyrate, are present. In the setting of carbohydrate malabsorption, the generation of high concentrations of these short-chain fatty acids may decrease stool pH to 4 or lower. The osmolality of the stool is approximately that of plasma (280 to 300 mOsm/kg H_2O) when it is passed.

At the cellular level, Na^+ transport by the epithelium from lumen to blood (by Na^+-coupled sugar and amino acid transport in the small intestine, by Na^+/H^+ exchange proteins in the small intestine and proximal colon, and by aldosterone-regulated Na^+ channels [ENaC] in the distal colon) creates a favorable osmotic gradient for absorption (see E-Fig. 126-1A and C). Chloride transport by the epithelium from blood to lumen (by cystic fibrosis transmembrane conductance regulator [CFTR] and the calcium-activated chloride channel in the small intestine and colon) creates an osmotic gradient for secretion (see E-Fig. 126-1B). Normally, the intestine is in a net absorptive state, regulated by extrinsic adrenergic nerves and proabsorptive neuropeptides and hormones (see E-Fig. 126-1D). Stimulation of secretion by neurotransmitters, hormones, and inflammatory mediators (Table 126-1) can offset this balance. A heterozygous missense mutation (c.2519 G→T) in GUCY2C on chromosome 12 causes familial diarrhea by increasing GC-C signaling.

Diarrhea is due primarily to alterations of intestinal fluid and electrolyte transport and less to smooth muscle function. Each 24 hours, 8 to 10 L of fluid enters the duodenum. The diet supplies 2 L of this fluid; the remainder comes from salivary, gastric, hepatic, pancreatic, and intestinal secretions. The small intestine normally absorbs 8 to 9 L (80%) of this fluid and presents 1.5 L to the colon for absorption. Of the remaining fluid, the colon absorbs all but approximately 100 mL. Diarrhea can result from increased secretion by the small intestine or the colon if the maximal daily absorptive capacity of the colon (4 L) is exceeded. Alternatively, if the colon is diseased so that it cannot absorb even the 1.5 L normally presented to it by the small intestine, diarrhea results.

Watery diarrheas may be due to osmotic, secretory, or inflammatory mechanisms. With ingestion of a poorly absorbed (e.g., Mg^{2+}) or unabsorbable (polyethylene glycol, lactulose, or, in lactase-deficient individuals, lactose) solute, the osmotic force of the solute pulls water and secondarily sodium and chloride ions into the intestinal lumen. A considerable proportion of the osmolality of stool results from the nonabsorbed solute. This gap between stool osmolality and the sum of the electrolytes in the stool causes osmotic diarrhea.

Active chloride secretion or inhibited sodium absorption, which also creates an osmotic gradient favorable for the movement of fluids from blood to lumen, explains the pathophysiology of the secretory diarrheas. Agents that increase enterocyte cyclic adenosine monophosphate (cAMP) (e.g., cholera toxin, prostaglandins), cyclic guanosine monophosphate (cGMP) (e.g., *Escherichia coli* stable toxin), or intracellular ionized calcium (Ca^{2+}) (e.g., acetylcholine) (see Table 126-1) inhibit non-nutrient Na^+ absorption and stimulate Cl^- secretion (see Table 126-1 and E-Fig. 126-1B and D).

TABLE 126-1 STIMULI OF INTESTINAL SECRETION

AGENT	INTRACELLULAR MEDIATOR	RELATED DIARRHEAL ILLNESS
Cholera, *Escherichia coli* heat labile toxin, *Salmonella, Yersinia*	cAMP	Travelers, endemic
E. coli heat stable toxin	cGMP	Travelers, endemic
Rotatoxin (NSP4)	?	Viral gastroenteritis
Serotonin, PAF	Ca	Inflammatory, allergic
PG, leukotrienes	cAMP, Ca	Invasive enteric bacteria,* inflammatory bowel diseases
PG	cAMP	Villous adenoma
Histamine	Ca	Intestinal allergies, mastocytosis, scombroid poisoning
VIP	cAMP	VIPoma, ganglioneuromas
5-HT, substance P, bradykinin	Ca	Malignant carcinoid
Calcitonin	?	Medullary carcinoma thyroid
Acetylcholine	Ca	Insecticides, nerve gas poisoning, cholinergic drugs
Ricinoleic acid	cAMP, Ca	Laxative abuse†
Caffeine	cAMP	Coffee, sodas, tea

5-HT = 5-hydroxytryptamine; Ca = calcium; cAMP = cyclic adenosine monophosphate; cGMP = cyclic guanosine monophosphate; PAF = platelet-activating factor; PG = prostaglandin; VIP = vasoactive intestinal peptide.

Shigella spp, Clostridioides difficile, enteroinvasive, Escherichia coli, Vibrio parahaemolyticus, Clostridium perfringens.

†Also phenolphthalein, anthraquinone, bisacodyl, dioctyl sodium sulfosuccinate, and senna.

Inflammatory diarrhea, which may be watery or bloody, are characterized by enterocyte damage, villus atrophy, and crypt hyperplasia. The damaged enterocyte membrane of the small intestine has decreased disaccharidase and peptide hydrolase activity, reduced or absent Na^+-coupled sugar or amino acid transport mechanisms, and reduced or absent sodium chloride absorptive transporters. Conversely, the hyperplastic crypt cells maintain their ability to secrete Cl^- (and perhaps HCO_3^-). If the inflammation is severe, immune-mediated vascular damage or ulceration allows blood, pus, and protein to leak (exudate) from capillaries and lymphatics and contribute to the diarrhea. Activation of lymphocytes, phagocytes, and fibroblasts releases various inflammatory mediators that induce intestinal chloride secretion (see E-Fig. 126-1D). Interleukin-1 (IL-1) and tumor necrosis factor (TNF), which also are released into the blood, cause fever, anorexia, and malaise.

ACUTE DIARRHEA

CLINICAL MANIFESTATIONS

Approximately 80% of acute diarrheas are due to infections with viruses, bacteria, and parasites. The remainder are due to medications that have an osmotic force, stimulate intestinal fluid secretion, damage the intestinal epithelium, or contain poorly absorbable or nonabsorbable sugars (e.g., sorbitol), or less commonly fecal impaction, pelvic inflammation (e.g., acute appendicitis [Chapter 128]), or intestinal ischemia (Chapter 129).

Food-Borne and Water-Borne Infectious Diarrhea

Most infectious diarrheas are acquired through fecal-oral transmission from water, food, or person-to-person contact (Table 126-2). Patients with infectious diarrhea often complain of nausea, vomiting, and abdominal cramps that are associated with watery, malabsorptive, or bloody diarrhea and fever (dysentery). As documented using polymerase chain reaction (PCR) methods of diagnosis, most outbreaks of nonbacterial acute gastroenteritis in the United States and other countries are caused by noroviruses (Norwalk agent; Chapter 350). Rotavirus (Chapter 350) predominantly causes diarrhea in infants, usually in the winter months, but also may cause nonseasonal acute diarrhea in adults, particularly in elderly people.[1] Mechanisms for diarrhea include decreased fluid absorption due to destruction of villus enterocytes and stimulation of fluid secretion by NSP4 rotatoxin and viral activation of the enteric nervous system. Ebola virus *(Filoviridae)* infects endothelial cells, macrophages, and dendritic cells. The mechanism for the massive watery diarrhea is not known.

TABLE 126-2 EPIDEMIOLOGY OF ACUTE INFECTIOUS DIARRHEA AND INFECTIOUS FOOD-BORNE ILLNESS

VEHICLE	CLASSIC PATHOGENS
Water (including foods washed in such water)	*Vibrio cholerae*, norovirus (Norwalk agent), *Giardia*, *Cryptosporidium*
Food	*Salmonella, Campylobacter, Shigella* spp
Poultry	Enterohemorrhagic *Escherichia coli*
Beef, unpasteurized fruit juice	Tapeworm
Pork	*V. cholerae, Vibrio parahaemolyticus*, and *Vibrio vulnificus; Salmonella* and *Shigella* spp; hepatitis A and B viruses;
Seafood and shellfish (including raw sushi and gefilte fish)	tapeworm; anisakiasis
Cheese, milk	*Listeria* spp
Eggs	*Salmonella* spp
Mayonnaise-containing foods and cream pies	Staphylococcal and clostridial food poisonings
Fried rice	*Bacillus cereus*
Fresh berries	*Cyclospora* spp
Canned vegetables or fruits	*Clostridium* spp
Sprouts	Enterohemorrhagic *E. coli, Salmonella* spp
Animal-to-person (pets and livestock) contact	*Salmonella, Campylobacter, Cryptosporidium*, enterohemorrhagic *E. coli*, and *Giardia* spp
Person-to-person (including sexual) contact	All enteric bacteria, viruses, and parasites
Daycare center	*Shigella, Campylobacter, Cryptosporidium*, and *Giardia* spp; viruses; *Clostridioides difficile*
Hospitalization, antibiotics, or chemotherapy	*C. difficile*
Swimming pool	*Giardia* and *Cryptosporidium* spp
Foreign travel	*E. coli* of various types; *Salmonella, Shigella, Campylobacter, Giardia*, and *Cryptosporidium* spp; *Entamoeba histolytica*

spp = species.
Modified from Powell DW. Approach to the patient with diarrhea. In : Yamada T, Alpers DH, Owyang C, et al, eds. *Textbook of Gastroenterology*, 3rd ed. Philadelphia: Lippincott-Raven; 1999.

The incidence of food-borne bacterial diseases in the United States decreased significantly during the coronavirus disease 2019 (COVID-19) pandemic, in large part because of less international travel but also likely because of increased hand-washing, closure of some child care centers, and decreased restaurant dining.[2] Incidence is highest for *Campylobacter jejuni* (Chapter 279), followed by *Salmonella* (Chapter 284) and *E. coli* O157:H7 (Chapter 280), and less commonly *Shigella* (Chapter 285), *Yersinia, Vibrio* (Chapter 278), *Cyclospora* (Chapter 324), and listeria (Chapter 272). *Vibrio* infection is predominantly due to the consumption of raw shellfish. Outbreaks of *E. coli* O157:H7 have been associated with petting zoos, uncooked ground beef, and green leafy vegetables. These bacteria most often invade the distal small bowel and colon, where they multiply intracellularly and damage the epithelium. Diarrhea is due to the stimulation of intestinal secretion by inflammatory mediators, decreased absorption across the damaged epithelium, and exudation of protein into the lumen. *Shigella* spp and enterohemorrhagic *E. coli* produce a similar toxin, the "Shiga toxin," which is cytotoxic to intestinal epithelial cells and causes inflammation, cell damage, and diarrhea with blood and pus.

Outbreaks of *Cryptosporidium* (Chapter 321) have been reported in water parks. This parasite causes diarrhea by adhering and fusing to the epithelial cell membrane in the small bowel, thereby causing cell damage. Organisms that are specific for seafood include *Vibrio parahaemolyticus* (Chapter 278), which causes either watery or bloody diarrhea, and *Vibrio vulnificus*, which causes watery diarrhea and, especially in patients with liver disease, a fatal septicemia. Ingestion of meat contaminated by anthrax (Chapter 272) causes fever, diffuse abdominal pain, and bloody stool or vomitus. Anthrax invades the intestinal mucosa; the organism, or anthrax toxin, causes inflammation, ulceration, and necrosis.

In addition to enteric infections, certain systemic infections (e.g., viral hepatitis [Chapter 134], listeriosis [Chapter 272], legionellosis [Chapter 290]), mycoplasma, and emerging infections (e.g., Hanta virus [Chapter 351], severe acute respiratory syndrome coronavirus 2 [SARS-CoV-2; Chapter 336], avian influenza [Chapter 332]) may cause or manifest with substantial diarrhea.

Environmental and Food Poisonings

Food poisoning refers to the accumulation of toxin in food owing to the growth of toxin-producing organisms, most commonly *Staphylococcus aureus* (Chapter 267), *Bacillus cereus, Clostridium perfringens* (Chapter 271), and *Clostridium botulinum* (Chapter 271). Diarrhea is usually of rapid onset, as early as 4 hours after ingestion, and is often associated with vomiting. Natural toxins also are responsible for mushroom *(Amanita)* poisoning (Chapter 96), which can also cause acute liver and kidney failure.

Environmental poisonings may be caused by heavy metals (arsenic from rat poison, gold, lead, mercury) that impair cell energy production. Arsenic (Chapter 20) also induces cardiovascular collapse at high doses. Insecticide (organophosphates and carbamates) poisoning occurs most commonly in field workers or from the ingestion of contaminated herbs or teas (Chapter 96); diarrhea, excessive saliva, and pulmonary secretions are caused by acetylcholine-stimulated chloride secretion in intestine and other epithelia. Patients often have associated vomiting and abdominal cramps.

Seafood is a common source of food poisoning, particularly fin fish and bivalve shellfish. Most of these toxins cause varying combinations of gastrointestinal (nausea, vomiting, diarrhea) and neurologic (tingling and burning around the mouth, facial flushing, sweating, headache, palpitations, and dizziness) symptoms within hours of seafood ingestion (Chapter 98). Similar symptoms are reported in patients with scombroid poisoning, which is caused by ingestion of decaying flesh of blood fish (tuna, mahi-mahi, marlin, or mackerel) that release large amounts of histamine (Chapter 98).

Marine dinoflagellates (algae) produce toxins that can cause paralytic shellfish poisoning, diarrhetic shellfish poisoning, and ciguatera (Chapter 98). Sporadic outbreaks of diarrhetic shellfish poisoning "red tides" occur when bivalve mollusks ingest dinoflagellates that produce saxitoxins (voltage-sensitive sodium-channel blocker) and okadaic acid (a lipid-soluble toxin that inhibits serine and threonine protein phosphatases 1 and 2A). Ingestion of contaminated mollusks by humans results in diarrhea and neurologic symptoms. Saxitoxins cause predominantly neurologic symptoms (paralytic, neurotoxic, or amnestic shellfish poisonings) and okadaic acid gastrointestinal symptoms (diarrhetic shellfish poisoning).

Food-chain passage of another dinoflagellate spp *(Gambierdiscus toxicus)* to fin fish (mackerel, amberjack, snapper, grouper, or barracuda) results in the accumulation of ciguatoxin (Chapter 98) that causes a seafood poisoning called ciguatera. Ciguatoxin activates voltage-sensitive sodium channels and causes neurologic and gastrointestinal symptoms. Fish from the Albemarle-Pamlico estuary (eastern United States) ingest toxic dinoflagellates that cause *Pfiesteria piscicida* poisoning. The dinoflagellate toxins cause nausea, vomiting, abdominal pain, diarrhea, and neurologic symptoms such as fatigue, myalgias, pruritus, circumoral paresthesias, reversal of hot and cold sensation, psychiatric abnormalities, and memory loss. The neurologic symptoms may persist for months to years. Puffer fish poisoning by tetrodotoxin, a voltage-sensitive sodium-channel blocker produced by the fish, causes neurologic symptoms, respiratory paralysis, and death.

Traveler's Diarrhea

North American travelers to developing countries and travelers on airplanes and cruise ships are at high risk for acute infectious diarrhea. Common causes of traveler's diarrhea (Chapter 265) include norovirus, enterotoxic or enteroaggregative *E. coli, Shigella*, and giardiasis.[3] *E. coli* heat-stable toxin binds to guanylate cyclase in the enterocyte brush-border membrane, where it results in elevation of intracellular cGMP. *E. coli* heat-labile toxin, similar to cholera toxin, binds to the monosialoganglioside GM_1 in the brush-border membrane, thereby resulting in the activation of adenylate cyclase and the elevation of intracellular cAMP. cAMP and cGMP stimulate intestinal chloride secretion and inhibit the nutrient-independent absorption of sodium and chloride. Sodium-glucose absorption is not affected, hence the basis for oral rehydration therapy. Cholera toxin permanently binds to adenylate cyclase until the natural turnover of the intestinal epithelium in 5 to 7 days, thereby resulting in persistent secretion and severe diarrhea. DNA sequencing to detect genome sequences of *Vibrio cholerae* isolates suggests human introduction as the cause of recent outbreaks. Of the annual average of six cases of cholera reported in the United States, most are associated with travel.

Antibiotic-Associated Diarrhea

Antibiotics are a common cause of hospital-acquired diarrhea that occurs in approximately 20% of patients receiving broad-spectrum antibiotics, with approximately 30% of cases caused by *Clostridioides difficile* (Chapter 271). Strains that produce increased levels of toxins A and B and a binary toxin have emerged. These strains are associated with an increase in the incidence and severity of *C. difficile* infections, including fulminant *C. difficile* colitis that can lead to colectomy or even death. The A and B toxins produced by *C. difficile* can cause diarrhea. In animal models, IL-8, substance P, and leukotriene B_4 were found to mediate toxin A–stimulated intestinal fluid secretion. *C. difficile* can cause severe diarrhea, pseudomembranous colitis, or toxic megacolon.

Nosocomial Hospital Diarrhea

Diarrhea is the most common nosocomial illness among hospitalized patients and residents in long-term care facilities. Common causes include antibiotic-associated diarrhea, *C. difficile* infection, medications, fecal impaction, tube feeding, and underlying illness. Magnesium-containing laxatives, antacids, and lactulose cause osmotic diarrheas. Bisacodyl laxatives cause secretory diarrhea. Liquid formulations of medications cause diarrhea (elixir diarrhea) because of the high content of sorbitol or other nonabsorbable sugars (e.g., mannitol) used to sweeten the elixir; patients prescribed liquid medications through feeding tubes may receive more than 20 g of sorbitol daily. An important but poorly understood cause of diarrhea is enteral (tube) feeding (Chapter 198), particularly in critically ill patients, who often develop diarrhea. Dysmotility, increased intestinal permeability, and low sodium content in enteral formulas may be contributing factors.

Patients in mental health institutions and nursing homes have a high incidence of nosocomial infectious diarrhea (e.g., *C. difficile* and less commonly *Shigella, Salmonella,* hemorrhagic *E. coli, Giardia, Entamoeba histolytica*). Infectious diarrhea, 50% or more of which is caused by *C. difficile,* is also common in acute care hospitals. Severe *C. difficile* infection also has been reported among peripartum women. If outside foods are not brought to hospitalized patients, the likelihood of a nosocomial infection caused by *Salmonella* or *Shigella* is extremely rare. Immunosuppressed patients are also susceptible to nosocomial viral infections (rotavirus, norovirus, adenovirus, and coxsackievirus).

Cancer Treatment and Medication-Related Diarrhea

Abdominal or whole-body radiation virtually always causes an increased frequency of bowel movements that are often watery. Cancer chemotherapy with amsacrine, azacitidine, cytarabine, dactinomycin, daunorubicin, doxorubicin, floxuridine, 5-fluorouracil, 6-mercaptopurine, methotrexate, plicamycin, IL-2, and resveratrol may cause mild to moderate diarrhea. Irinotecan (CPT-11) or oxaliplatin and the combination of 5-fluorouracil plus leucovorin are frequent causes of severe watery diarrhea.

Immune checkpoint inhibitors of cytotoxic T-lymphocyte antigen (CTLA-4) and programmed death ligand PD-(L) cause diarrhea in up to 40% of patients. Colitis with or without enteritis is the cause. Evaluation of patients with significant diarrhea (>4 stools over baseline) includes exclusion of infection, measurement of fecal calprotectin or lactoferrin, and/or endoscopic biopsies.[4] If unrecognized and untreated, this form of severe colitis can be fatal.

Olmesartan, an angiotensin II receptor antagonist (ARB), causes severe diarrhea as a result of a sprue-like enteropathy. Angiotensin-converting enzyme (ACE) inhibitors may cause abdominal pain and diarrhea resulting from visceral angioedema. Colchicine, neomycin, methotrexate, and *para*-aminosalicylic acid damage the enterocyte membrane. Cholestyramine, colestipol, and colesevelam bind bile salts and can result in malabsorptive diarrhea, especially in patients who have had an ileal resection. Gold therapy causes intestinal inflammation and diarrhea.

Daycare Diarrhea

More than 7 million children in the United States attend daycare, where diarrhea is extremely common, and secondary infection of family members occurs in 10 to 20% of cases. Most outbreaks of diarrhea are due to rotavirus or norovirus; less common causes are *Shigella* (Chapter 285), *Giardia* (Chapter 322), and *Cryptosporidium* (Chapter 321).

Runner's Diarrhea

Diarrhea occurs in 10 to 25% of individuals who exercise vigorously, especially women marathon runners and triathletes. Some athletes have associated abdominal cramps, urgency, nausea, or vomiting. The pathophysiology of runner's diarrhea is unknown. Release of intestinal secretogogues, especially prostaglandins, hormones, or ischemia, may be involved.

DIAGNOSIS

Acute watery diarrhea may be due to infections, food toxins, or medications, or the acute diarrhea may signal the onset of a chronic disease (Fig. 126-1; see Tables 126-1 and 126-2). Multiplex PCR testing on stool is a rapid and sensitive method to detect bacterial, viral, and parasitic pathogens (Chapter 262), but it does not distinguish particles from live organisms or provide antibiotic sensitivity. The diagnostic approach in patients with fever and watery or bloody diarrhea should focus on multiplex PCR testing of stool for pathogens.[5] A positive result requires a culture for antimicrobial sensitivity and contact tracing. A test for *Vibrio* is needed in those who recently traveled to a cholera-endemic area.

Routine stool testing is not indicated when diarrhea occurs after 3 to 5 days of hospitalization, except in patients with neutropenia, human immunodeficiency virus (HIV) infection, or signs of enteric infection. In patients with more than three watery stools daily, particularly patients who have recently used antibiotics, been hospitalized, or are peripartum, a two-test approach is recommended for the diagnosis of *C. difficile* infection (Chapter 271). A positive stool PCR or glutamate dehydrogenase test is followed by an enzyme-based immunoassay for toxins to help distinguish true infection from a carrier state.[6]

Organisms that cause diarrhea but are not routinely cultured by clinical microbiology laboratories include *Yersinia* (Chapter 288), *Plesiomonas,* enterohemorrhagic *E. coli* serotype O157:H7 (Chapter 280), *Aeromonas, Cyclospora,* microsporidia, and noncholera *Vibrio* (Chapter 278). Parasites such as *Giardia* (Chapter 322), *Cryptosporidium* (Chapter 321), and *Strongyloides* (Chapter 327) can be difficult to detect in stool but may be diagnosed by stool antigen testing or intestinal biopsy (Chapter 262).

TREATMENT

Goals for the treatment of diarrhea include fluid replacement, antidiarrheal agents, nutritional support, and antimicrobial therapy when indicated. Because death in patients with acute diarrhea is caused by dehydration, the first task is to assess the degree of dehydration and to replace fluid and electrolyte deficits.

Fluid Replacement

Severely dehydrated patients should be treated with intravenous lactated Ringer solution or saline solution, with additional potassium and bicarbonate as needed. Oral rehydration solutions, which are used extensively to replace diarrheal fluid and electrolyte losses, are effective because they contain sodium, sugars, and, often, amino acids that use nutrient-dependent sodium uptake transporters. In alert patients with mild to moderate dehydration, oral rehydration solution is equally effective as intravenous hydration in repairing fluid and electrolyte losses. Oral rehydration solutions can be given to infants and children in volumes of 50 to 100 mL/kg over 4 to 6 hours; adults may need to drink 1000 mL/hour. Reduced-osmolarity solutions (Na^{2+} 75 mmol/L, osmolarity 245 mmol/L versus Na^{2+} 90 mmol/L, osmolarity 311 mmol/L in standard solutions) are better tolerated and effective in noncholera diarrhea but may cause hyponatremia in patients with high-volume diarrhea, particularly children. Glucose-based solutions, although effective in rehydrating the patient, may worsen the diarrhea. In contrast to glucose-based solutions, polymeric rice-based solutions decrease diarrhea in cholera victims; rice is digested to many glucose monomers that aid in the absorption of intestinal secretions. These solutions may not decrease stool output in acute diarrhea, but they will effectively rehydrate the patient despite continued diarrhea. After rehydration has been accomplished, oral rehydration solutions are given at rates equaling stool loss plus insensible losses until the diarrhea ceases.

Reducing Diarrhea

Bismuth subsalicylate (Pepto-Bismol, 525 mg orally every 30 minutes to 1 hour for five doses, may repeat on day 2) is safe and efficacious in bacterial infectious diarrhea. Opiates and anticholinergic drugs are not recommended for invasive bacterial infectious diarrhea because these drugs paralyze intestinal motility and predispose to increased colonization, invasion, and prolonged excretion of infectious organisms. The opiate loperamide is safe in acute or traveler's diarrhea, provided that it is not given to patients with dysentery (high fever, with blood or pus in the stool), and especially when administered concomitantly with effective antibiotics. A combination of loperamide (2 mg orally four times daily)

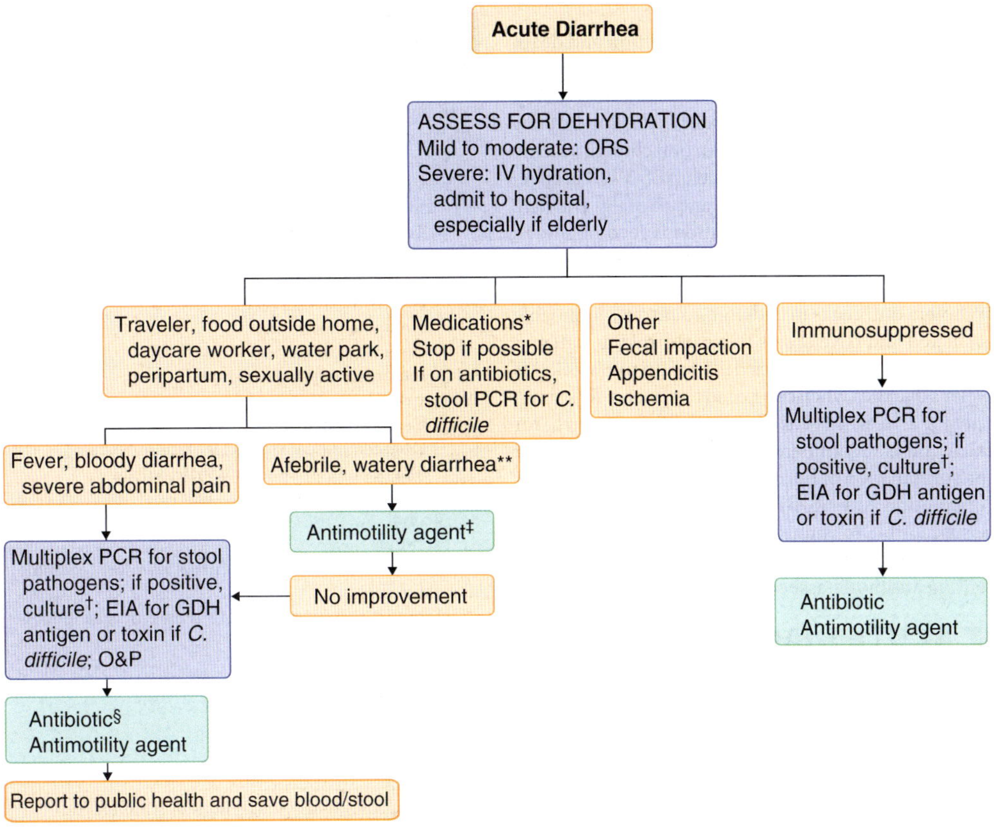

FIGURE 126-1. **Approach to the diagnosis of acute diarrhea.** *More than 700 medications cause diarrhea, including caffeine, protease inhibitors, immune checkpoint inhibitors, thyroid preparations, metformin, mycophenolate mofetil, sirolimus, cholinergic drugs, colchicine, selective serotonin reuptake inhibitors, proton pump inhibitors, histamine-2 blockers, 5-ASA derivatives, angiotensin-converting enzyme inhibitors and receptor blockers, bisacodyl, senna, aloe, anthraquinones, and magnesium- or phosphorus-containing medications. †Specifically request culture for *Yersinia, Plesiomonas, Vibrio,* enterohemorrhagic *Escherichia coli* serotype O157:H7, and *Aeromonas* if suspected. ***Vibrio* testing if travel to cholera-endemic area. ‡If high suspicion for *Clostridioides difficile* or invasive bacterial infection, wait for PCR studies before starting. Racecadotril has antisecretory effects without paralyzing intestinal motility and can be used if available. §Not recommended for patients with bloody diarrhea due to *E. coli* O157:H7. EIA = enzyme-based immunoassays; GDH = glutamate dehydrogenase; IV = intravenous; O&P = ova and parasites; ORS = oral rehydration solution; PCR = polymerase chain reaction.

plus simethicone (125 mg orally four times daily) may reduce the abdominal cramps and duration of traveler's diarrhea. Racecadotril (100 mg orally three times daily in adults, 1.5 mg/kg of body weight orally three times daily in children), an intestinal enkephalinase inhibitor that is antisecretory but does not paralyze intestinal motility, is effective in the treatment of acute diarrhea in children and adults. The diarrhea associated with enteral nutrition (Chapter 198) often can be managed with pectin (4 g/kg body weight daily) or, if there are no contraindications, with loperamide (2 mg orally four times daily for 3 to 7 days, maximal dose 16 mg daily), and diarrhea is not a reason to stop tube feeding unless stool volumes exceed 1 L/day.

Anxiolytics (e.g., diazepam 2 mg orally two to four times daily) and antiemetics (e.g., promethazine 12.5 to 25 mg orally once or twice daily) that decrease sensory perception may make symptoms more tolerable and are safe. Some foods or food-derived substances (green bananas, pectins [amylase-resistant starch], zinc) lessen the amount or duration of diarrhea in children. Unabsorbed amylase-resistant starches are metabolized in the colon to short-chain fatty acids that enhance fluid absorption. Zinc supplementation (20 mg of elemental zinc orally once daily) is effective in preventing recurrences of diarrhea in malnourished children; copper deficiency is a potential complication of prolonged zinc therapy. Probiotics are not beneficial in children with acute diarrhea,[A1] but large randomized trials have not been reported in adults.

Antibiotics

While the clinician is awaiting stool culture results to guide specific therapy (Chapter 266), the fluoroquinolones (e.g., ciprofloxacin, 500 mg orally twice daily for 1 to 3 days, or levofloxacin, 500 mg orally daily for 1 to 3 days) are the treatment of choice when antibiotics are indicated (see Fig. 126-1). Trimethoprim-sulfamethoxazole (1 double-strength tablet orally twice daily for 5 days or 2 single-strength tablets orally twice a day for 5 days) is second-line therapy. If the symptom complex suggests *Campylobacter* infection, azithromycin (500 mg/day orally for 3 days) should be added. Regardless of the cause of infectious diarrhea, patients should be treated with antibiotics if they are immunosuppressed; have valvular, vascular, or orthopedic prostheses; have congenital hemolytic anemias (especially if salmonellosis is involved); or are extremely young or old.

Certain infectious diarrheas should be treated with antibiotics, including those associated with shigellosis (Chapter 285), cholera (Chapter 278), pseudomembranous enterocolitis (Chapter 271), parasitic infestations (Chapter 321 to 323), and sexually transmitted diseases (Chapter 264). Treatment of *E. coli* serotype O157:H7 infection is not recommended at present because current antibiotics do not appear to be helpful and the incidence of complications (hemolytic-uremic syndrome) may be greater after antibiotic therapy. Antibiotics are not effective for viral diarrhea or cryptosporidiosis.

For traveler's diarrhea, ciprofloxacin (500 mg orally twice daily for 3 days) is an effective treatment. The nonabsorbable antibiotic rifaximin (200 mg taken orally three times daily or 400 mg twice daily for 3 days) is safe and effective for treatment of traveler's diarrhea in Mexico, but it may not be effective against *Campylobacter* and *Shigella* infections.

Fluoroquinolone-resistant and trimethoprim-sulfamethoxazole–resistant strains of *Shigella, E. coli, Salmonella, Campylobacter*, and *C. difficile* have emerged. Azithromycin (500 mg orally on day 1 and 250 mg/day orally for 4 days) may be an effective alternative treatment for resistant strains of *Shigella* and *Campylobacter* and for traveler's diarrhea acquired in Mexico.

If *C. difficile* is suspected on an epidemiologic basis, fidaxomicin (200 mg orally twice a day for 10 days) is superior to vancomycin (125mg orally four times daily for 10 days)[A2] to prevent of recurrent infection. Other antibiotics and gastric acid suppressants, which are risk factors for recurrent infection, should be discontinued if possible.[7] In patients with recurrent *C. difficile* infection or a high risk for recurrence, immunotherapy with bezlotoxumab (a monoclonal antibody against *C. difficile* toxin B, given as a one-time dose of 10 mg/kg intravenously [IV] infused over 1 hour) decreases recurrence rates.[A3] Fecal microbiota transplantation is more effective than vancomycin for the treatment of recurrences, with resolution rates of 90% compared with 30% for vancomycin.[A4] Non–*C. difficile* antibiotic-induced diarrhea is generally mild and self-limited, and it usually clears spontaneously or in response to cholestyramine therapy (4 g orally four times daily for 2 weeks).

Treatment for chemotherapy-induced and radiation-induced mild to moderate diarrhea includes loperamide (2 mg orally four times daily) and nonsteroidal anti-inflammatory drugs (NSAIDs) (e.g., naproxen, 250 to 500 mg orally twice daily). Octreotide may be an effective treatment in those with severe diarrhea in doses up to 700 µg/day subcutaneously (SQ). Treatment of diarrhea due to checkpoint inhibitor enterocolitis includes discontinuing the offending agent and starting systemic glucocorticoids (the equivalent of 0.5 to 2 mg/kg prednisone given orally or intravenously), with a 4- to 6-week taper. If no response is seen in 72 hours or the response is incomplete after 1 week, infliximab (5 mg/kg) or vedolizumab (300 mg) should be given intravenously at weeks 0, 2, and 6.

PREVENTION

Rotavirus vaccination (Chapter 350) reduces the risk for infection and death and generally results in milder symptoms among those infected. Travelers to high-risk countries (Central America and parts of Latin America, Africa, Asia, the Middle East) should avoid ingestion of tap water and ice and of raw meat, raw seafood, and raw vegetables (Chapter 265). An oral cholera vaccine against recombinant toxin B subunit and killed whole-cell (rBS-WC) is effective in preventing infection from the O1 El Tor strain and partially effective against enterotoxigenic *E. coli* strains. Cholera vaccination is recommended for relief workers and health professionals who work in endemic countries and for individuals who are immunocompromised or have chronic illnesses or hypochlorhydria. To stop cholera outbreaks in endemic countries, vulnerable communities must be vaccinated and have access to clean drinking water.

Bismuth subsalicylate (525 mg orally four times daily for up to 3 weeks) is effective in preventing traveler's diarrhea when compared to placebo. Rifaximin (200 to 1100 mg/day orally for 2 weeks) is effective for reducing the risk for traveler's diarrhea in Mexico and is recommended for those at high risk for health complications.[A5] The combination of rifaximin plus loperamide is better than either one alone. Loperamide and NSAIDs are taken prophylactically by many runners who are susceptible to runner's diarrhea, but it is not clear whether they are effective. Oral probiotics (e.g., lactobacilli and bifidobacteria) are not effective for preventing antibiotic-associated acute diarrhea.

PERSISTENT ACUTE DIARRHEA

Persistent diarrhea for more than 2 weeks develops in about 3% of individuals who travel to developing countries. Common causes include parasitic infections (e.g., *Giardia* [Chapter 322], *Cryptosporidium* [Chapter 321]) and bacterial infections (e.g., enteroaggregative *E. coli* [Chapter 280], *Shigella* [Chapter 285], and *Salmonella* [Chapter 284]). The evaluation should include culture for bacterial pathogens and methods for detecting bacterial, viral, and protozoal infections (e.g., multiplex PCR) as well as microscopy for protozoal infections. Antimicrobial therapy can be empirically given to patients who have recently returned from the developing world but should preferably be given based on the results of laboratory testing.

CHRONIC DIARRHEA

An estimated 5% of the U.S. population suffers from chronic diarrhea, and approximately 40% of these individuals are older than 60 years of age. The causes of chronic diarrhea include persistent infectious or inflammatory diarrheas, malabsorptive syndromes, and watery diarrheas (Table 126-3).

CLINICAL MANIFESTATIONS

Patients with malabsorption (Table 126-4) can present with a variety of gastrointestinal or extraintestinal manifestations (Table 126-5). Significant malabsorption of fat and carbohydrate usually causes chronic diarrhea, abdominal cramps, gas, bloating, and weight loss. Steatorrhea (fat in the stool) manifests as oily, foul-smelling stools that are difficult to flush down the toilet. Stools may be large and bulky (e.g., pancreatic insufficiency) or watery (e.g., bacterial overgrowth, mucosal diseases). Individuals with malabsorption also can present with manifestations of vitamin and mineral deficiencies. Dyspnea can be caused by anemia from iron, copper, folate, or vitamin B_{12} deficiency. Manifestations of calcium, magnesium, or vitamin D malabsorption include paresthesias and tetany resulting from hypocalcemia or hypomagnesemia and bone pain from osteomalacia or osteoporosis-related fractures. Paresthesias and ataxia are manifestations of cobalamin and vitamin E deficiency. Alternatively, neuropathy may be due to malnutrition or copper deficiency. Dermatitis herpetiformis (Chapter 406) is a blistering, burning, itchy rash on the extensor surfaces and buttocks that is associated with celiac disease.

Inflammatory diarrheas may manifest with fever and abdominal pain or with edema to suggest chronic protein loss. Patients may have multiple, low-volume, bloody stools with tenesmus to suggest proctitis or have severe diarrhea as a result of graft-versus-host disease (GVHD) or celiac disease. Systemic manifestations of inflammatory bowel disease include polymigratory arthritis, sacroiliitis, erythema nodosum, pyoderma gangrenosum, leukocytoclastic angiitis, uveitis, and oral aphthous ulcers.

DIAGNOSIS

A detailed history and physical examination lead to a diagnosis in 25 to 50% of patients with chronic diarrheas (see Table 126-1 and Fig. 126-2). In young adults with chronic diarrhea, the leading causes are irritable bowel syndrome, inflammatory bowel disease, microscopic colitis, bile acid diarrhea, malabsorption, drugs, food additives, thyroid disease, and diabetes mellitus. The addition

TABLE 126-3 CAUSES OF CHRONIC DIARRHEA

Persistent infectious diarrheas (see Table 126-2)
Brainerd diarrhea
Malabsorptive syndromes (see Tables 126-4 and 126-6)
Common causes
Celiac disease
Infection (*Giardia lamblia*, HIV/AIDS-related)
Tropical sprue
Crohn disease
Radiation enteritis
Gastric bypass surgery
Dumping syndrome
Chronic pancreatitis
Intestinal bacterial overgrowth
Watery diarrhea
Osmotic diarrhea
Disaccharidase deficiencies (lactase, sucrase)
Magnesium, sodium phosphate, sulfate
Sorbitol, fructose
Alcohol
Factitious
Functional watery diarrhea (irritable bowel syndrome)
Pure secretory
Hormone-secreting tumors (VIPoma, neuroendocrine, gastrinoma, medullary thyroid cancer)
Systemic mastocytosis
Villous adenoma
Idiopathic
Inflammatory diarrheas
Inflammatory bowel disease
Eosinophilic gastroenteritis
Microscopic colitis (collagenous or lymphocytic)
Food allergy

AIDS = acquired immunodeficiency syndrome; HIV = human immunodeficiency virus; VIP = vasoactive intestinal peptide.

TABLE 126-4 CAUSES OF MALABSORPTION

MECHANISM OF MALABSORPTION	CONDITIONS
Impaired mixing	Partial/total gastrectomy Gastric bypass surgery
Impaired lipolysis	Chronic pancreatitis Pancreatic cancer Congenital lipase or colipase deficiency Gastrinoma
Impaired micelle formation	Severe liver disease Bacterial overgrowth Crohn disease Ileal resection Gastrinoma
Impaired mucosal absorption	Lactase deficiency Abetalipoproteinemia Giardiasis Celiac disease Tropical sprue Agammaglobulinemia Amyloidosis AIDS-related Radiation enteritis Graft-versus-host disease Whipple disease Eosinophilic gastroenteritis Drugs Lymphoma Autoimmune enteritis Short-bowel syndrome
Impaired nutrient delivery	Congenital lymphangiectasia Lymphoma Tuberculosis Constrictive pericarditis Severe congestive heart failure
Unknown	Hypoparathyroidism Adrenal insufficiency Hyperthyroidism Carcinoid syndrome

AIDS = acquired immunodeficiency syndrome.

TABLE 126-5 CLINICAL CONSEQUENCES OF MALABSORPTION OF NUTRIENTS, WATER, AND ELECTROLYTES

NUTRIENT MALABSORBED	CLINICAL MANIFESTATION
Protein	Wasting, edema
Carbohydrate and fat	Diarrhea, abdominal cramps and bloating, weight loss, growth retardation
Fluid and electrolytes	Diarrhea, dehydration
Iron	Anemia, cheilosis, angular stomatitis
Calcium and vitamin D	Bone pain, fractures, tetany
Magnesium	Paresthesias, tetany
Vitamin B_{12} and folate	Anemia, glossitis, cheilosis, paresthesias, ataxia (vitamin B_{12} only)
Vitamin E	Paresthesias, ataxia, retinopathy
Vitamin A	Night blindness, xerophthalmia, hyperkeratosis, diarrhea
Vitamin K	Ecchymoses
Riboflavin	Angular stomatitis, cheilosis
Zinc	Dermatitis, hypogeusia, diarrhea
Selenium	Cardiomyopathy
Essential fatty acids	Dermatitis
Copper	Anemia, mental deterioration, neuropathy

of stool culture and examination for ova and parasites, determination of stool fat, and flexible sigmoidoscopy or colonoscopy with biopsy raises the diagnostic rate to approximately 75%. The remaining 25% of patients with chronic diarrhea may need extensive testing and perhaps hospitalization to make a diagnosis.

A history of 10 to 20 daily bowel movements that do not respond to fasting suggests secretory diarrhea (Fig. 126-3).[8] A history of peptic ulcer should suggest gastrinoma (Chapter 213) or systemic mastocytosis (Chapter 235). Physical examination is helpful only if the thyromegaly of medullary carcinoma (Chapter 207), the cutaneous flushing of the neuroendocrine tumors and systemic mastocytosis, the dermatographism of systemic mastocytosis, or the migratory necrolytic erythema of glucagonoma (Chapter 213) is evident. Autonomic dysfunction (e.g., postural hypotension, impotence, gustatory sweating) is almost invariably present in diabetic diarrhea.

Evaluation for malabsorption begins with a careful elicitation of bowel habits and a description of the stool; weight loss; travel; food or milk tolerance; underlying gastrointestinal, pancreatic, or liver diseases; abdominal surgery; radiation or chemotherapy treatments; family history; and drug and alcohol use.

Blood Tests

Blood measurements (see Fig. 126-2) of iron, folate, vitamin B_{12}, prothrombin time (vitamin K), and other fat-soluble vitamins (A, E, and D) help evaluate malabsorption. Specific antibody tests should be sent when celiac disease is suspected (see later). Peripheral blood findings of leukocytosis, eosinophilia, elevated erythrocyte sedimentation rate or C-reactive protein, hypoalbuminemia, or low total serum protein suggest an inflammatory diarrhea, whose hallmark is the presence of blood, either overt or occult, and leukocytes or calprotectin (a nondegradable leukocyte protein) in the stool.

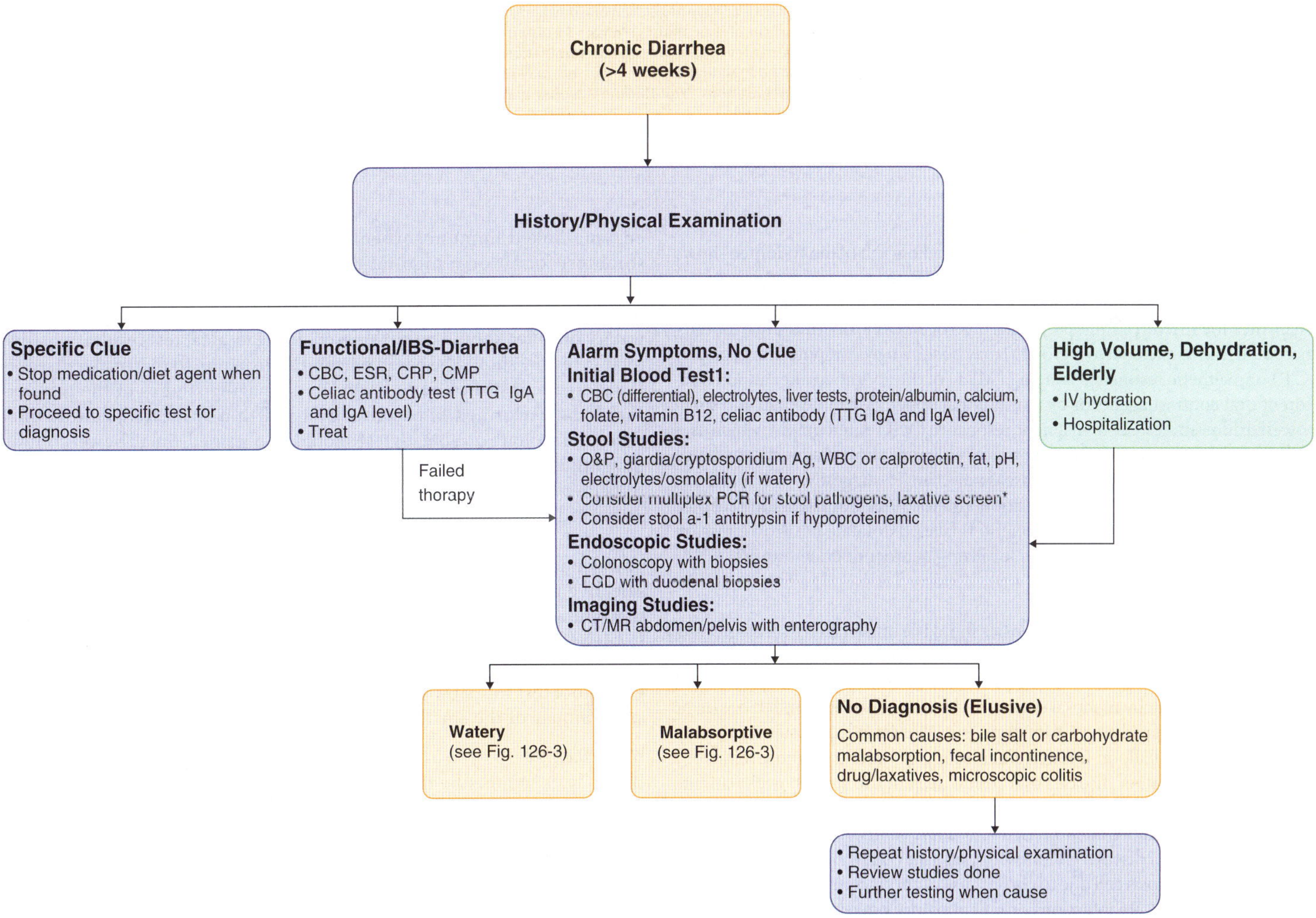

FIGURE 126-2. **Initial approach to chronic diarrhea.** *Perform multiplex PCR for stool pathogens in those who are immunosuppressed; perform laxative screen if laxative abuse is suspected. Ag = antigen; CBC = complete blood count; CMP = comprehensive metabolic panel; CRP = C-reactive protein; CT = computed tomography; EGD = esophagogastroduodenoscopy; EIA = enzyme-based immunoassay; ESR = erythrocyte sedimentation rate; IgA = immunoglobulin A; IV = intravenous; MR = magnetic resonance; O&P = ova and parasites; PCR = polymerase chain reaction; TTG = tissue transglutaminase; WBC = white blood cells.

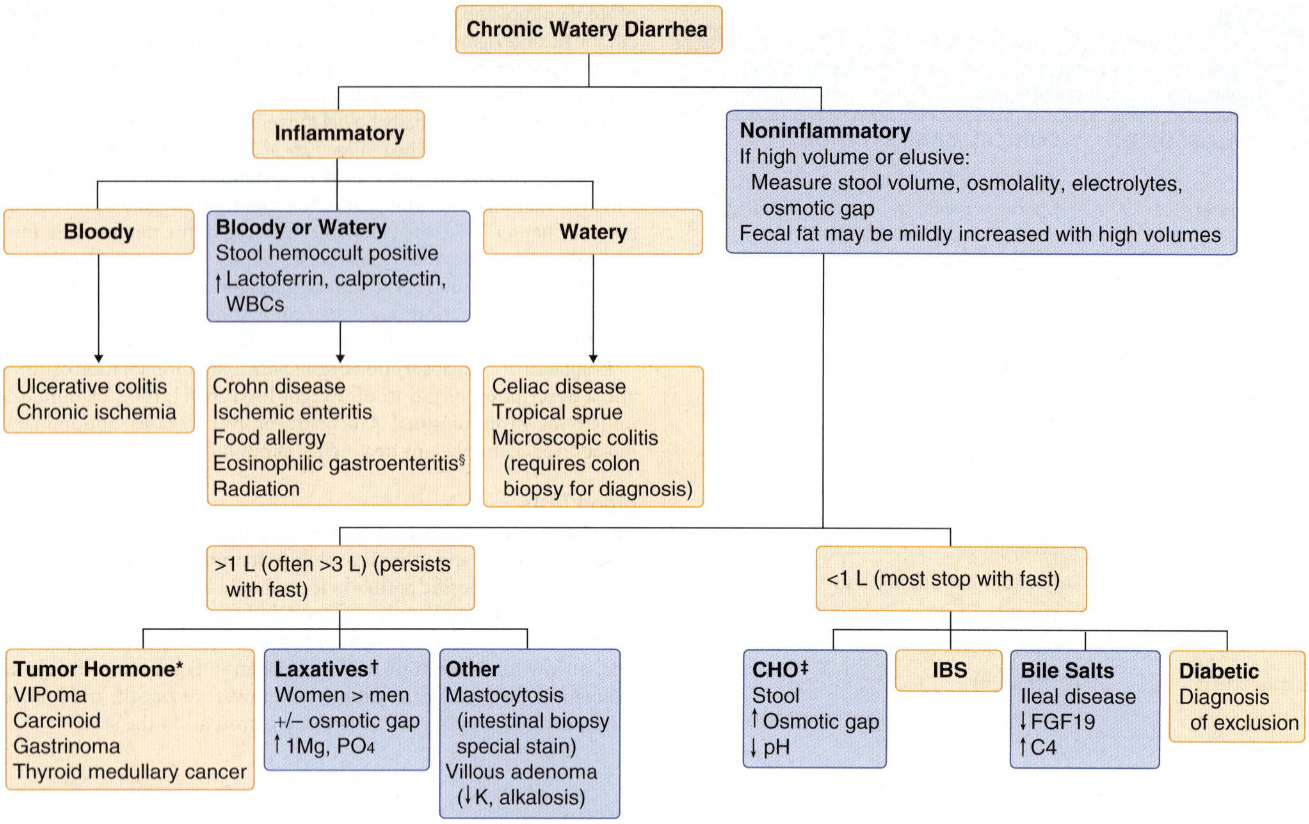

FIGURE 126-3. **Approach to the evaluation of watery diarrhea.** Many diarrheas have more than one mechanism (i.e., osmotic, secretory, inflammatory). Other causes include medications, postsurgical (vagotomy, Nissan wrap, cholecystectomy), hyperthyroidism, and alcohol. *VIPoma: >3 L output daily "pancreatic cholera," elevated VIP level. Carcinoid: elevated urine 5-hydroxyindole acetic acid, positive OctreoScan. Gastrinoma: elevated gastrin level, positive secretin stimulation test, diarrhea due to high volume of acid secretion. Thyroid medullary cancer: elevated calcitonin level. †Stool volume may be high or low volume depending on dose ingested, may respond to fasting. ‡Carbohydrate malabsorption (CHO) may be due to lactase deficiency, dietary fructose, sorbitol in diabetic candies or liquid medications. §Full-thickness biopsy may be needed for diagnosis. C4 = 7α-hydroxy-4-cholesten-3-one; FGF = fibroblast growth factor; IBS = irritable bowel syndrome; WBCs = white blood cells.

Imaging

Malabsorption may be suggested if a flat plate radiograph of the abdomen shows pancreatic calcification (Chapter 119). Some diseases (e.g., previous gastric surgery, gastrocolic fistulas, blind loops from previous intestinal anastomoses, small intestine strictures, multiple jejunal diverticula, abnormal intestinal motility that could lead to bacterial overgrowth) may be shown by computed tomography (CT) or magnetic resonance imaging (MRI) of the abdomen after administration of oral contrast agents or by a traditional upper gastrointestinal and small bowel barium studies. CT or magnetic resonance (MR) enterography, which uses oral neutral contrast to enhance the bowel wall, may show diagnostic evidence of advanced inflammatory bowel disease or changes suggestive of lymphoma, eosinophilic gastroenteritis, or radiation enterocolitis. Somatostatin receptor scintigraphy with gallium-68 or copper-64–labeled dotatate positron emission tomography (PET) scan is useful in localizing neuroendocrine tumors.

Endoscopy and Biopsy

Upper endoscopy with duodenal biopsies should be undertaken if serologic tests for celiac disease are positive or diagnostic clues suggest small bowel mucosal malabsorption (Chapter 120). Some patients with celiac disease may have mild inflammation or patchy mucosal disease and require duodenal bulb biopsies or enteroscopy with jejunal biopsies for diagnosis. Wireless video capsule endoscopy (Chapter 120) and balloon-assisted enteroscopy are used to diagnose refractory celiac disease and other diseases that reside deep in the small bowel. Patients with severe watery or elusive diarrhea should have a colonoscopy to the terminal ileum to assess for villous adenomas, microscopic colitis, mastocytosis, or early inflammatory bowel disease. Colonoscopy also may show brown pigmentation suggestive of melanosis coli due to chronic use of anthracene laxatives. Terminal ileal ulcers may indicate infectious or inflammatory bowel disease.

Other Laboratory Tests

Malabsorption

If chronic diarrhea is the presenting symptom, a stool examination for ova and parasites and a PCR test for *Giardia* or stool antigen-capture enzyme-linked immunosorbent assay (ELISA) should be obtained. A stool test for fat on a high-fat diet (70 to 100 g/day) is the best available screening test for malabsorption (Table 126-6). If the fecal fat test result is negative, selective carbohydrate malabsorption or other causes of watery diarrhea should be considered. If the fecal fat test result is positive, further testing should be based on clinical suspicion for particular diseases. If pancreatic insufficiency is suspected, imaging studies of the pancreas should be performed. If bacterial overgrowth is suspected, culture of an intestinal aspirate or a breath test should be obtained. Small bowel contrast imaging is useful in detecting structural abnormalities that predispose to bacterial overgrowth (Table 126-7). If proximal mucosal damage is suspected, multiple duodenal biopsies should be obtained. If there are no clues, CT or MR enterography may help to detect middle and distal small bowel mucosal diseases. Some individuals with celiac disease present with selective nutrient deficiencies without diarrhea. In these cases, a tissue transglutaminase (tTG) immunoglobulin A (IgA) antibody test and total IgA level should be performed. In patients hospitalized for severe diarrhea or malnutrition, a more streamlined evaluation usually includes a multiplex PCR stool test for pathogens; stool fat test; an abdominal imaging study; and a biopsy of the small intestine and colon.

Watery Diarrhea

Breath tests to measure the respiratory excretion of H_2 and methane after administration of carbohydrates can assess carbohydrate malabsorption or bacterial overgrowth (see Table 126-6).

The diagnosis of rare neuroendocrine tumors, such as carcinoids, gastrinoma, VIPoma, medullary carcinoma of the thyroid, glucagonoma, somatostatinoma, and systemic mastocytosis, is made by showing elevated blood levels of serotonin, chromogranin A, or urinary 5-hydroxyindoleacetic acid and serum levels for gastrin, vasoactive intestinal peptide, calcitonin, glucagon, somatostatin, histamine, or prostaglandins (Chapter 213). Somatostatin receptor scintigraphy and PET dotatate scanning are useful in the diagnosis and evaluation of neurodendocrine tumors (Chapter 213).

TABLE 126-6 TESTS FOR THE EVALUATION OF MALABSORPTION*

TEST	COMMENTS
GENERAL TESTS OF ABSORPTION	
Quantitative stool fat test	Gold standard test of fat malabsorption. Requires ingestion of a high-fat diet (70-100 g) for 2 days before and during the collection. Stool is collected for 2-3 days. Normally, <7 g/24 hr is excreted on a high-fat diet. Borderline abnormalities of 8-14 g/24 hr may be seen in secretory or osmotic diarrheas that are not caused by malabsorption. There are false-negative findings if fat intake is inadequate. False-positive results can occur if the nonabsorbable fat olestra is ingested or mineral oil laxatives or rectal suppositories (e.g., cocoa butter) are given to the patient before stool collection.
Qualitative stool fat test	The nuclear magnetic resonance method determines the percentage of fat in the stool (normal, <20%). The test depends on an adequate fat intake (100 g/day). There is high sensitivity (90%) and specificity (90%) with fat malabsorption of >10 g/24 hr. Sensitivity drops with stool fat in the range of 6-10 g/24 hr.
Hydrogen breath test	Most useful in the diagnosis of lactase deficiency. An oral dose of lactose (25 g) is administered after measurement of basal breath H_2 levels. The sole source of H_2 in the mammal is bacterial fermentation; unabsorbed lactose makes its way to colonic bacteria, resulting in excess breath H_2. A *late peak* within 3-6 hr of >20 ppm of exhaled H_2 after lactose ingestion suggests lactose malabsorption. Absorption of other carbohydrates (e.g., sucrose, glucose, fructose) also can be tested.
SPECIFIC TESTS FOR MALABSORPTION	
Tests for Pancreatic Function	
Secretin stimulation test	The gold standard test of pancreatic function. Requires duodenal intubation with a double-lumen tube and collection of pancreatic juice in response to intravenous secretin. Allows measurement of bicarbonate (HCO_3^-) and pancreatic enzymes. A sensitive test of pancreatic function, but labor intensive and invasive.
Secretin-enhanced MRCP	Noninvasive test for the detection of exocrine dysfunction in early chronic pancreatitis. The signal intensity ratio of pancreas to spleen has a significant positive correlation with the pancreatic fluid bicarbonate level as measured by the ductal secretin test. A ratio of 1 : 2 has a 77% sensitivity and 83% specificity for diagnosing pancreatic exocrine dysfunction, and it also has a strong correlation with histopathology of non-calcific chronic pancreatitis.
Fecal elastase-1 test	Stool test for pancreatic function. Equal sensitivity to the secretin stimulation test for the diagnosis of moderate to severe pancreatic insufficiency. Unreliable with mild insufficiency. False-positive results occur with increased stool volume and intestinal mucosal diseases.
Tests for Bacterial Overgrowth	
Quantitative culture of small intestinal aspirate	Gold standard test for bacterial overgrowth. Greater than 10^3 colony-forming units (CFU)/mL in the jejunum suggests bacterial overgrowth. Requires special anaerobic sample collection, rapid anaerobic and aerobic plating, and care to avoid oropharyngeal contamination. False-negative results occur with focal jejunal diverticula and when overgrowth is distal to the site aspirated.
Hydrogen breath test	The 50-g glucose breath test has a sensitivity of 90% for growth of 10^5 colonic-type bacteria in the small intestine. If bacterial overgrowth is present, increased H_2 is excreted in the breath. An early hydrogen level (<90 min) of >20 ppm suggests bacterial overgrowth. Specificity is increased when performed with simultaneous nuclear scintigraphy to define transit time to the cecum. False-positive results occur in patients with rapid transit. False-negative results occur with non–hydrogen-producing organisms. Concomitant measurement of breath methane improves test sensitivity.
Tests for Mucosal Disease	
Small bowel biopsy	Obtained for a specific diagnosis when there is a high index of suspicion for small intestinal disease. Several biopsy specimens (4-5) must be obtained to maximize the diagnostic yield. Distal duodenal biopsy specimens are usually adequate for diagnosis, but occasionally duodenal bulb biopsies or enteroscopy with jejunal biopsy specimens is necessary. Small intestinal biopsy provides a specific diagnosis in some diseases (e.g., intestinal infection, Whipple disease, abetalipoproteinemia, agammaglobulinemia, lymphangiectasia, lymphoma, amyloidosis). In other conditions, such as celiac disease and tropical sprue, the biopsy specimens show characteristic findings, but the diagnosis is made by positive celiac serology or improvement after specific treatment.
Test of Ileal Function	
^{75}SeHCAT test	This is a test of bile acid absorption. Seven days after ingestion of radiolabeled synthetic selenium–homocholic acid conjugated with taurine (^{75}SeHCAT), whole-body retention is measured by a gamma-counting device. The result is expressed as a fraction of baseline ingestion. Retention values of <10% are abnormal and indicate bile acid malabsorption with a sensitivity of 80-90% and specificity of 70-100%. The radiation dose is equivalent to that of a plain chest x-ray. Liver disease and bacterial overgrowth may give false results. Not approved for use in the United States.

*Not all these tests are readily available. A strong suspicion for any disease warrants forgoing an extensive work-up and obtaining the test with highest diagnostic yield. In some cases, empirical treatment, such as removing lactose from the diet of an otherwise healthy individual with lactose intolerance, is warranted without any testing.
MRCP = magnetic resonance cholangiopancreatography.

Inflammatory Diarrhea

Stool occult blood, white blood cells, and calprotectin are helpful tests for bowel inflammation. Video capsule endoscopy of the small bowel may detect ulcerations deep in the small bowel not reachable by standard upper or lower endoscopy and not detected with conventional radiologic imaging. However, the risk for capsule retention in the small bowel is high in patients with Crohn disease or heavy NSAID use, particularly when there is a history of obstructive symptoms. The most sensitive test for protein-losing enteropathy is measurement of intestinal protein loss by 24-hour stool excretion or clearance of α_1-antitrypsin.

Stool Examination in Elusive Diarrhea

An important adjunct to diagnosing the cause of diarrhea is to examine the stool. The greasy, bulky stool of steatorrhea and the bloody stool of gut inflammation are distinctive. Stool collections (see Table 126-6) can be analyzed for weight, volume, fat, electrolytes (Na^+, K^+, Cl^-), osmolality, pH, and a laxative screen (SO_4^{2-}, PO_4^{2-}, Mg^{2+}). Stool or urine can be analyzed for emetine (a component of ipecac), bisacodyl, castor oil, or anthraquinone.

Carbohydrate malabsorption lowers stool pH because of colonic fermentation of carbohydrate to short-chain fatty acids. Stool pH less than 5.3 usually means pure carbohydrate malabsorption, whereas in the generalized malabsorptive diseases, stool pH is greater than 5.6 and usually greater than 6.0.

The normal stool osmotic gap, which is the difference between stool osmolality (or 290 mOsm) and twice the stool Na^+ and K^+ concentrations, is 50 to 125. In secretory diarrheas, the colon's capacity for adjusting electrolyte concentrations is overwhelmed, the stool osmotic gap is less than 50, and stool electrolytes more nearly resemble plasma electrolytes (Na^+ concentrations are usually >90 mmol/L, K^+ concentrations usually <10 mmol/L), except for higher HCO_3^- concentrations (usually >50 mmol/L). In osmotic diarrhea, the

TABLE 126-7 ABNORMALITIES CONDUCIVE TO BACTERIAL OVERGROWTH

STRUCTURAL
Blind intestinal loops
End or side-to-side intestinal anastomoses
Ileocecal valve resection
Duodenal and jejunal diverticula
Strictures (Crohn disease, radiation enteritis)
Adhesions (postsurgical)
Gastrojejunocolic fistulas
MOTOR
Scleroderma
Diabetes mellitus
Idiopathic pseudo-obstruction
HYPOCHLORHYDRIA
Atrophic gastritis
Proton pump inhibitors
MISCELLANEOUS
Immunodeficiency states
Pancreatitis
Cirrhosis
Chronic renal failure

presence of uncharged solute or unmeasured cation in the colonic lumen draws in water, depresses stool Na^+ (usually <60 mmol/L) and K^+ concentrations, and results in a stool osmotic gap greater than 125. Stools with Na^+ concentrations between 60 and 90 mmol/L and calculated osmotic gaps between 50 and 100 can result from either secretory or malabsorptive abnormalities. Patients with Mg^{2+}-induced diarrhea may be diagnosed by fecal Mg^{2+} values of more than 50 mmol/L. Sodium anion–induced diarrheas (Na_2SO_4, Na_2PO_4) mimic secretory diarrhea because the stool Na^+ content is high (>90 mmol/L) and there is no osmotic gap; this diarrhea may be diagnosed by determining stool Cl^- concentration because these anions displace stool Cl^-, resulting in a depressed stool Cl^- value (usually <20 mmol/L). A low stool osmolality suggests contamination of stool with dilute urine or water in the case of factitious diarrhea.

SPECIFIC CAUSES OF CHRONIC DIARRHEA

PROLONGED, PERSISTENT INFECTIOUS DIARRHEAS

Prolonged infectious diarrheas (>2 weeks) may be due to persistent or recurrent infections. These diarrheas occur most commonly in children exposed to unsafe drinking water in developing countries, patients who have acquired immunodeficiency syndrome (AIDS) or are immunosuppressed for other reasons, and recent travelers. Recurrent or prolonged infectious diarrhea may lead to severe malnutrition and death (mortality rate, 50%). Treatment for children includes nutrition support with supplemental vitamin A (200,000 IU orally twice yearly) and zinc (20 mg elemental orally daily for 14 days). Severe disease may require total parenteral nutrition.

In patients with AIDS, protracted diarrhea may be caused by treatable agents such as *E. histolytica, Giardia*, or *Strongyloides* or by organisms such as *Cryptosporidium, Isospora belli*, and microsporidia that are difficult to treat or untreatable. The most effective treatment is retroviral therapy to improve the immune system (Chapter 357).

In travelers returning from developing countries who have infectious diarrhea that persists for longer than 3 to 4 weeks, stool should be examined for culture and for ova and parasites. In patients with a recent history of antibiotic use, stool also should be sent for *C. difficile* toxin or PCR. Any specific organisms that are identified should be treated. If treatment with trimethoprim-sulfamethoxazole or a fluoroquinolone has been unsuccessful, tetracycline (250 mg orally four times daily for 7 to 10 days), doxycycline (100 mg orally two times a day for 7 to 10 days), or metronidazole (250 mg orally three times daily for 7 to 10 days) can be tried. After documented infectious diarrhea, 25% of patients experience pain, bloating, urgency, a sense of incomplete evacuation, and loose stools for 6 months or longer; some of these patients have celiac disease, so screening (see later) is warranted in this setting. When no other cause is found, these patients are deemed to have postinfectious irritable bowel syndrome.

Sporadic outbreaks of severe, prolonged diarrhea, often greater than 1 year in duration, occasionally have been reported. This form of prolonged diarrhea is called *Brainerd diarrhea*. The organism has yet to be identified. The diarrhea is difficult to treat; cholestyramine (4 g orally three times daily) may be helpful.

MALABSORPTIVE SYNDROMES

Malabsorption is caused by many different diseases, drugs (e.g., the lipase inhibitor orlistat; Chapter 201), and nutritional products (the nonabsorbable fat olestra) that impair intraluminal digestion, mucosal absorption, or delivery of the nutrient to the systemic circulation (E-Fig. 126-2; see Table 126-4). Dietary fat is the nutrient most difficult to absorb. Fatty stools (steatorrhea) are the hallmark of malabsorption; a stool test for fat is the best screening test. Malabsorption does not always cause diarrhea. Clinical signs of vitamin or mineral deficiencies may occur in the absence of diarrhea. A careful focused history is crucial in guiding further testing to confirm the suspicion of malabsorption and to make a specific diagnosis (Fig. 126-4). The goals of treatment are to correct or treat the underlying disease and replenish losses of water, electrolytes, and nutrients.

CONDITIONS THAT IMPAIR INTRALUMINAL DIGESTION

Most digestion and absorption of nutrients occur in the small intestine (see E-Fig. 126-2). Carbohydrates and most dietary proteins are water soluble and readily digested by pancreatic enzymes. Pancreatic proteases (trypsinogen, chymotrypsinogen, procarboxypeptidases) are secreted from acinar cells in inactive forms. The cleavage of trypsinogen to trypsin by the duodenal brush-border peptidase enteropeptidase (enterokinase) allows trypsin to cleave the remaining trypsinogen and other proteases to their active form.

Most dietary lipids (long-chain triglycerides, cholesterol, and fat-soluble vitamins) are water insoluble and must undergo lipolysis and incorporation into mixed micelles before they can be absorbed across the intestinal mucosa. Pancreatic lipase, in the presence of its cofactor, colipase, cleaves long-chain triglycerides into fatty acids and monoglycerides. The products of lipolysis interact with bile salts and phospholipids to form mixed micelles, which also incorporate cholesterol and fat-soluble vitamins (D, A, K, and E) in their hydrophobic centers. Bicarbonate secreted from pancreatic duct cells is physiologically important to neutralize gastric acid because pancreatic enzyme activity and bile salt micelle formation are optimum at a luminal pH of 6 to 8.

IMPAIRED MIXING

Surgical alterations, such as partial gastrectomy with gastrojejunostomy (Billroth II anastomosis) or gastrointestinal bypass surgeries for obesity, result in the release of biliary and pancreatic secretions into the intestine at a site remote from the site of entry of gastric contents. This imbalance can result in impaired lipolysis and impaired micelle formation, with subsequent fat malabsorption. Bypass of the duodenum also impairs absorption of iron, folate, and calcium. Rapid transit through the jejunum contributes to the malabsorption of nutrients. Individuals with these conditions also have surgical anastomoses that predispose to bacterial overgrowth.

DUMPING SYNDROME

After esophageal (distal esophagectomy, myotomy for achalasia), gastric (gastrectomy, non–pylorus-sparing Whipple surgery, gastrojejunostomy, Nissan wrap, and hiatal hernia repair), and bariatric (Roux-en-Y gastric bypass) surgeries, the unregulated delivery of concentrated sugars and food into the duodenum and jejunum results in altered insulin regulation, maldigestion, osmotic movement of fluid into the intestinal lumen, and rapid transit such that intestinal contact time is insufficient for absorption of nutrients. Glucagon-like peptide-1 (GLP-1) plays a key role in the pathophysiologic response of hyperinsulinemic hypoglycemia following the ingestion of concentrated sweets.[9] Patients may present with severe diarrhea, malabsorption, abdominal cramping, gas, and weight loss. Some patients have associated sweatiness, dizziness, and altered cognition because of postprandial hypoglycemia. Diagnosis is made by characteristic symptoms and a mixed meal tolerance test or continuous glucose monitoring for hypoglycemia.

Treatment is with a diet that is low in concentrated sugars divided into six small meals. Administration of pectin (15 g with each meal) may slow gastric emptying in patients who have a stomach. In patients who are refractory to dietary measures, a short-acting somatostatin analogue (e.g., octreotide, 25

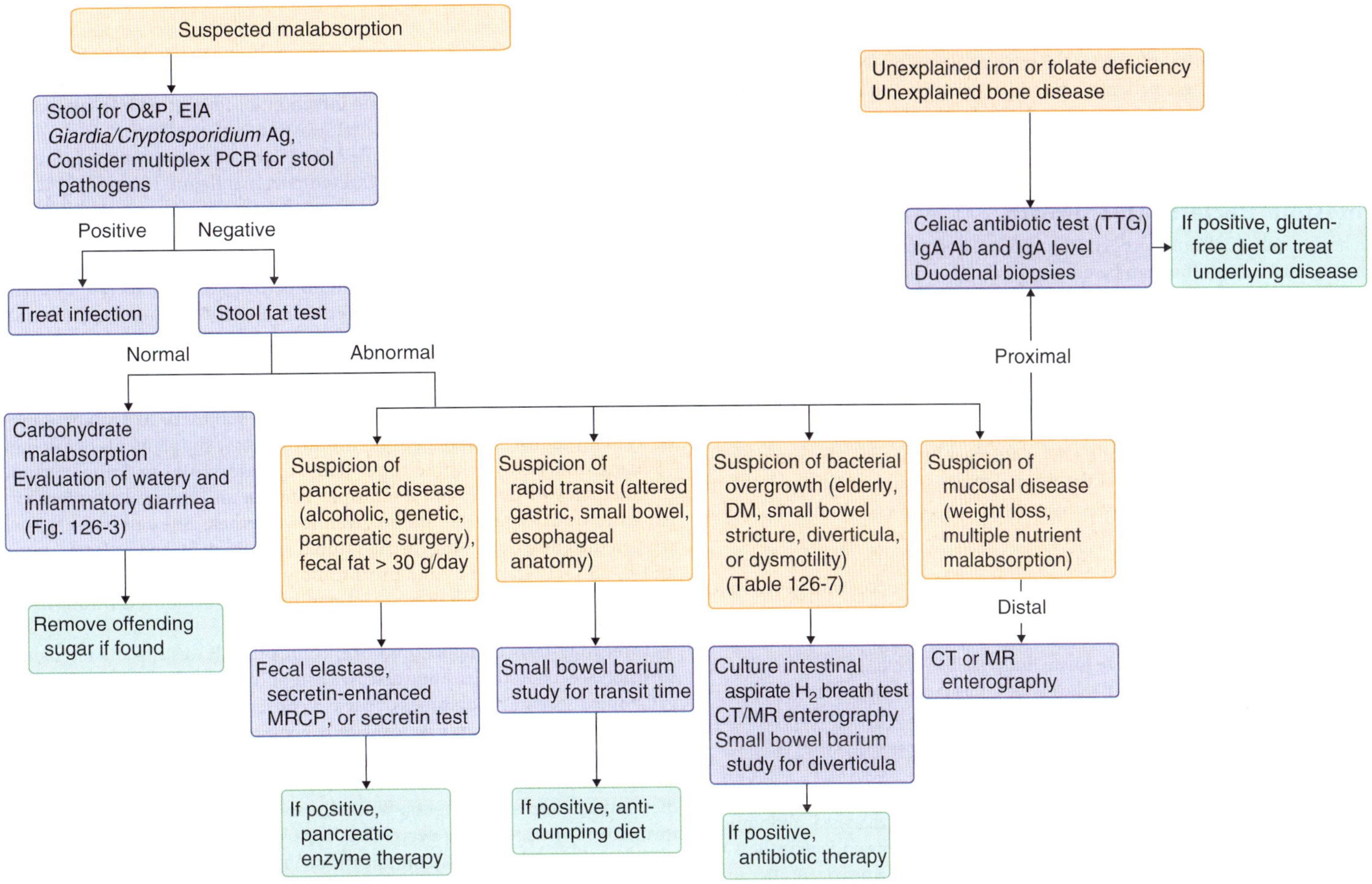

FIGURE 126-4. **Approach to the diagnosis of malabsorption.** Ab = antibody; Ag = antigen; CT = computed tomography; DM = diabetes mellitus; EIA = enzyme immunoassay; Ig = immunoglobulin; MR = magnetic resonance; MRCP = magnetic resonance cholangiopancreatography; O&P = ova and parasites; PCR = polymerase chain reaction; TTG = tissue transglutaminase.

to 200 μg SQ three times daily) or the better tolerated intramuscular preparation (10 to 20 mg monthly) improves dumping symptoms. In patients with predominant reactive hypoglycemia 1 to 3 hours after a meal (late dumping), an α-glycosidase hydrolase inhibitor (e.g., acarbose, 50 to 100 mg orally three times daily) that blocks carbohydrate absorption in the small bowel may be beneficial. Continuous jejunal tube feeding is also effective. GLP-1 receptor agonists also are a promising therapy for patients with symptomatic hypoglycemia.

IMPAIRED LIPOLYSIS

A deficiency in pancreatic lipase may be caused by the congenital absence of pancreatic lipase or by destruction of the pancreatic gland as a result of alcohol-related pancreatitis, cystic fibrosis, or pancreatic cancer. Pancreatic lipase also can be denatured by excess secretion of gastric acid (e.g., gastrinoma; Chapter 213). In such cases, lipase denaturation can be offset by treatment with a high-dose proton pump inhibitor (e.g., omeprazole 60 mg/day orally) to block acid secretion.

CHRONIC PANCREATITIS

Chronic pancreatitis (Chapter 130) is the most common cause of pancreatic insufficiency and impaired lipolysis. In the United States, chronic pancreatitis most commonly results from alcohol use disorder; in contrast, tropical (nutritional) pancreatitis is most common worldwide. Malabsorption of fat does not occur until more than 90% of the pancreas is destroyed.

CLINICAL MANIFESTATIONS

Individuals with pancreatic causes of malabsorption typically present with bulky, fat-laden stools (usually >30 g of fat daily), abdominal pain, and diabetes, although some present with diabetes in the absence of gastrointestinal symptoms. Stools usually are not watery because undigested triglycerides form large emulsion droplets with little osmotic force and, in contrast to fatty acids, do not stimulate water and electrolyte secretion in the colon. Deficiency of fat-soluble vitamins is seen only rarely, presumably because gastric and residual pancreatic lipase generates enough fatty acids for some micelle formation. In severe disease, subclinical protein malabsorption, manifested by the presence of undigested meat fibers in the stool, and subclinical carbohydrate malabsorption, manifested by gas-filled, floating stools, can occur. Weight loss, when it occurs, is most often caused by decreased oral intake to avoid abdominal pain or diarrhea and less commonly by malabsorption. Pancreatic enzyme replacement and analgesics are the mainstays of treatment for chronic pancreatitis (see Table 130-5 in Chapter 130).

DIAGNOSIS

Between 30 and 40% of individuals with alcohol-related chronic pancreatitis have calcifications on abdominal radiographs. A qualitative or quantitative test for fecal fat is positive in individuals whose pancreas is more than 90% destroyed. Noninvasive tests of pancreatic function are not sensitive enough to detect mild to moderate insufficiency, so secretin-enhanced magnetic resonance cholangiopancreatography (MRCP) or the endoscopic secretin stimulation test is preferred (see Table 126-6) if it can be obtained.

IMPAIRED MICELLE FORMATION

Bile salt concentrations in the intestinal lumen can fall to less than the critical concentration (2 to 3 mmol/L) needed for micelle formation because of decreased bile salt synthesis (severe liver disease), decreased bile salt delivery (cholestasis), or removal of luminal bile salts (bacterial overgrowth, terminal ileal disease or resection, cholestyramine therapy, acid hypersecretion). Fat malabsorption resulting from impaired micelle formation is generally not as severe as malabsorption resulting from pancreatic lipase deficiency, presumably because fatty acids and monoglycerides can form lamellar structures, which to a certain extent can be absorbed. Malabsorption of fat-soluble vitamins (D, A, K, and E) may be marked, however, because micelle formation is required for their absorption.

Decreased Bile Salt Synthesis and Delivery

Malabsorption can occur in individuals with cholestatic liver disease or bile duct obstruction, as well as in occasional patients who have undergone prior cholecystectomy.[10] The clinical consequences of malabsorption are seen most often in women with primary biliary cirrhosis because of the prolonged nature of the illness. Although these individuals can present with steatorrhea, osteoporosis or, less commonly, osteomalacia is the most common presentation. The cause of bone disease in these patients is poorly understood and often is not related to vitamin D deficiency. Bone disease is treated with calcium supplements (and vitamin D if a deficiency is documented), weight-bearing exercise, and a bisphosphonate (e.g., alendronate, 10 mg/day orally or 70 mg orally once weekly).

Intestinal Bacterial Overgrowth

In health, only small numbers of lactobacilli, enterococci, gram-positive aerobes, or facultative anaerobes can be cultured from the upper small bowel lumen. Motility and acid are the most important factors in keeping the number of bacteria in the upper small bowel low. Any condition that produces local stasis or recirculation of colonic luminal contents allows development of a predominantly "colonic" flora (coliforms and anaerobes, such as *Bacteroides* and *Clostridium*) in the small intestine (see Table 126-7).[11] Anaerobic bacteria cause impaired micelle formation by releasing cholylamidases, which deconjugate bile salts. The unconjugated bile salts, with their higher pK_a, are more likely to be in the protonated form at the normal upper small intestinal pH of 6 to 7 and can be absorbed passively. As a result, the concentration of bile salts decreases in the intestinal lumen and can fall to less than the critical micellar concentration, causing malabsorption of fats and fat-soluble vitamins. Vitamin B_{12} deficiency and carbohydrate malabsorption also can occur with generalized bacterial overgrowth. Anaerobic bacteria ingest vitamin B_{12} and release proteases that degrade brush-border disaccharidases. Although anaerobic bacteria use vitamin B_{12}, they synthesize folate. Individuals with bacterial overgrowth may have low serum vitamin B_{12} levels but normal or high folate levels; this helps distinguish bacterial overgrowth from tropical sprue, in which vitamin B_{12} and folate levels are usually low because of decreased mucosal uptake.

CLINICAL MANIFESTATIONS

Individuals with bacterial overgrowth can present with diarrhea, abdominal cramps, gas and bloating, anorexia, weight loss, and signs and symptoms of vitamin B_{12} and fat-soluble vitamin deficiency. Watery diarrhea occurs because of the osmotic load of unabsorbed carbohydrates and stimulation of colonic secretion by unabsorbed fatty acids.

DIAGNOSIS

The diagnosis of bacterial overgrowth should be considered in elderly people and in individuals with predisposing underlying disorders (see Table 126-7).[12] Bacterial overgrowth may be associated with the irritable bowel syndrome. The identification of greater than 10^3 CFU/mL in a culture of small intestinal aspirate is the gold standard in diagnosis but is not readily available. Noninvasive options, which have a wide range of sensitivities and specificities compared with those of intestinal culture, are the carbohydrate substrate-based glucose hydrogen and methane breath tests (see Table 126-6). In individuals with low vitamin B_{12} levels, a Schilling test before and after antibiotic therapy can be diagnostic if available (Chapter 150).

TREATMENT

The goals of treatment are to correct the structural or motility defect, if possible; to eradicate offending bacteria; and to provide nutritional support.[13] Acid-reducing agents should be stopped, if possible. Treatment with antibiotics should be based on culture results whenever possible; otherwise, empirical treatment is given. Rifaximin (400 mg orally three times daily) is effective,[A6] but less so in individuals with an excluded (blind) intestinal loop. Tetracycline (250 to 500 mg orally four times daily), doxycycline (100 mg orally two times daily), or a broad-spectrum antibiotic against aerobes and enteric anaerobes (ciprofloxacin, 500 mg orally twice daily; amoxicillin-clavulanic acid, 250 to 500 mg orally three times daily; cephalexin, 250 mg orally four times daily with metronidazole, 250 mg orally three times daily) should be given for 14 days. In patients with small bowel dysmotility, prokinetic agents such as prucalopride (2 to 4 mg orally once daily), metoclopramide (10 mg orally four times daily) or erythromycin (250 to 500 mg orally four times daily) can be tried. Octreotide (50 μg subcutaneously every day) may improve motility and reduce bacterial overgrowth in individuals with scleroderma. If the structural abnormality or motility disturbance cannot be corrected, the patient is at risk for malnutrition and deficiencies of vitamin B_{12} and fat-soluble vitamins. Cyclic treatment (1 to 3 weeks of every 4 to 6 weeks) with rotating antibiotics may be required in these patients to prevent recurrent bouts of bacterial overgrowth. If supplemental calories are needed, medium-chain triglycerides should be given because they do not depend on micelle formation for their absorption. Monthly treatment with vitamin B_{12} should be considered, along with supplemental vitamins D, A, K, and E and calcium.

ILEAL DISEASE

Disease of the terminal ileum is most commonly due to Crohn disease, which also may lead to ileal resection, but it also can be caused by radiation enteritis, tropical sprue, tuberculosis, *Yersinia* infection, or idiopathic bile salt malabsorption. These diseases cause bile salt wasting in the colon.

The clinical consequences of bile salt malabsorption are related directly to the length of the diseased or resected terminal ileum. In an adult, if less than 100 cm of ileum is diseased or resected, watery diarrhea results because of stimulation of colonic fluid secretion by unabsorbed bile salts. Bile acid diarrhea responds to cholestyramine (2 to 4 g taken at breakfast, lunch, and dinner).[14] If more than 100 cm of ileum is diseased or resected, bile salt losses (>3 g/day) in the colon exceed the capacity for increased bile salt synthesis in the liver, the bile salt pool shrinks, and micelle formation is impaired. As a result, steatorrhea ensues, and fatty acid–induced intestinal secretion synergizes with the bile acid–induced secretion to cause diarrhea. Treatment is with a low-fat diet, vitamin B_{12} (300 to 1000 μg subcutaneously or intramuscularly once every month), dietary supplements of calcium (500 mg orally two or three times daily, monitor 24-hour urine calcium for adequacy of dose), and a multiple vitamin and mineral supplement. An antimotility agent should be given for diarrhea. Bile salt binders may worsen diarrhea. Screening for fat-soluble vitamin deficiencies (vitamins A and E, 25-OH vitamin D, and prothrombin time) and bone disease (bone densitometry, serum calcium, intact parathyroid hormone, 24-hour urine for calcium) should be done.

Three long-term complications of chronic bile salt wasting and fat malabsorption are renal stones, bone disease (osteoporosis and osteomalacia), and gallstones. Oxalate renal stones occur as a consequence of excess free oxalate absorption in the colon. Free oxalate is generated when unabsorbed fatty acids bind luminal calcium, which is then unavailable for binding oxalate. Renal oxalate stones sometimes can be avoided with a low-fat, low-oxalate diet and calcium supplements. Bone disease is caused by impaired micelle formation with a resulting decrease in absorption of vitamin D; year-round sun exposure reduces this complication. Vitamin D (50,000 U orally one to three times per week) and calcium supplements (500 mg orally two to three times daily) should be given to susceptible individuals, but vitamin D levels and serum and urinary calcium must be monitored for response to treatment because excess vitamin D can be toxic. The mechanism of gallstone formation in these individuals is unclear; pigmented gallstones are most common.

CONDITIONS THAT IMPAIR MUCOSAL ABSORPTION

PATHOBIOLOGY

Nutrients are absorbed along the entire length of the small intestine, with the exception of iron and folate, which are absorbed in the duodenum and proximal jejunum, and bile salts and cobalamin (vitamin B_{12}), which are absorbed in the distal ileum. The efficiency of nutrient uptake at the mucosa is influenced by the number of villus absorptive cells, the presence of functional hydrolases and specific nutrient transport proteins on the brush-border membrane, and transit time. Transit time determines the contact time of luminal contents with the brush-border membrane and influences the efficiency of nutrient uptake across the mucosa.

Mucosal malabsorption can be caused by specific (usually congenital) brush-border enzyme or nutrient transporter deficiencies or by generalized diseases that damage the small intestinal mucosa or result in surgical resection or bypass of the small intestine. The nutrients malabsorbed in these general malabsorptive diseases depend on the site of intestinal injury (proximal, distal, or diffuse) and the severity of damage. The main mechanism of malabsorption in these conditions is a decrease in surface area available for absorption. Some conditions (infection, celiac disease, tropical sprue, food allergies, and GVHD) are characterized by intestinal inflammation and villus flattening; others are characterized by ulceration (ulcerative jejunitis, NSAIDs, Crohn disease), infiltration (amyloidosis), or ischemia (radiation enteritis, mesenteric ischemia).

Long-chain fatty acids are transported across the microvillus membrane of villus epithelial cells by CD36 and the fatty acid transport protein FATP4. The bile salts from mixed micelles remain in the intestinal lumen and are absorbed in the distal ileum by sodium-dependent cotransport. Oligosaccharides and larger oligopeptides (products of pancreatic enzyme digestion), sucrose, and lactose are hydrolyzed further by enzymes present in the brush-border membrane of villus epithelial cells before they are absorbed. Although only sugar monomers (glucose, galactose, fructose) can be taken up at the apical epithelial cell membrane, dipeptides and tripeptides are readily taken into the cell.

Water-soluble vitamins are readily absorbed throughout the small intestine. Fat-soluble vitamins, minerals, and cobalamin are more difficult to absorb because of the requirement for micelle formation (vitamins D, A, K, and E), a divalent charge (magnesium, calcium, iron), or selected sites of uptake in the intestine (iron, cobalamin). Calcium is absorbed best in the proximal small intestine by a vitamin D–dependent calcium channel (TRPV6). Magnesium is absorbed in the small intestine by members of the transient receptor potential family (TRPM6 and TRPM7). Mutations in TRPM6 have been identified in the rare disorder hereditary hypomagnesemia. Ferrous iron is transported into intestinal epithelial cells by a proton-coupled metal-ion transporter (DMT1 or Nramp2) that has specificity for Fe^{2+} and other divalent cations (Mn^{2+}, Co^{2+}, Cd^{2+}, Cu^{2+}, Ni^{2+}, and Pb^{2+}). The reduced form of copper (Cu^{1+}) is absorbed by the copper transporter 1 (CTR1). Zinc (Zn^{2+}) is predominantly absorbed by the Srt-, Irt-like protein ZIP4. The absorption of calcium and nonheme iron is enhanced by solubilization with hydrochloric acid. Intraluminal compounds such as oxalate, phytate, and long-chain fatty acids bind to calcium and magnesium, decreasing their absorption. Individuals with severe mucosal disease or short-bowel syndrome with high fecal fluid outputs lose magnesium and zinc from endogenous secretions.

Folates (Chapters 150 and 199) are both taken in the diet and produced by bacteria in the colon. Dietary folates are reduced to their monoglutamate form in the lumen of the proximal intestine and absorbed predominantly by a proton-coupled folate transporter. Deficiency can be caused by poor intake or malabsorption secondary to intestinal disease or drugs.

The cobalamins (Chapters 150 and 199) are abundant in foods containing animal proteins (e.g., meat, seafood, eggs, milk). Dietary cobalamin is released from food in the stomach by acid-peptic digestion and binds to haptocorrin at gastric pH. Pancreatic enzymes degrade haptocorrin, thereby freeing cobalamin to bind to gastric intrinsic factor, which that is secreted from parietal cells. The intrinsic factor–cobalamin complex then travels to the distal ileum and binds to the cubam complex (cubulin and amnionless). Once transported into ileal enterocytes, intrinsic factor is degraded; cobalamin binds to transcobalamin II and is transported in the blood stream to target tissues. Various mutations in the factors required for these processes can cause hereditary juvenile cobalamin deficiency. Cobalamin (vitamin B_{12}) deficiency in industrialized countries is rarely due to poor dietary intake but rather reflects the inability to absorb cobalamin. This inability may be caused by a lack of intrinsic factor, consumption of cobalamin by overgrowth of anaerobic bacteria in the small bowel lumen, ileal disease or resection, or defective transcobalamin II. Large amounts of cobalamin are present in the liver (2 to 5 mg), and cobalamin is reabsorbed from bile through the enterohepatic circulation, thereby limiting daily losses to less than 1 μg. It usually takes 10 to 12 years for cobalamin deficiency to develop after it is eliminated from the diet, but deficiency can occur more rapidly (2 to 5 years) with malabsorptive syndromes. If lack of gastric acid causes food-cobalamin malabsorption, treatment with oral cyanocobalamin supplementation (Chapter 150) is curative.

LACTASE DEFICIENCY

EPIDEMIOLOGY

Acquired lactase deficiency is the most common cause of selective carbohydrate malabsorption. Most individuals, except those of northern European descent, begin to lose lactase activity by the age of 2 years. The prevalence of lactase deficiency is highest (85 to 100%) in persons of Asian, African, and Native American descent.

PATHOBIOLOGY

The persistence or nonpersistence of lactase activity is associated with a single nucleotide polymorphism C/T_{-13910} that is found upstream of the lactase gene on chromosome 2q21-22. Hypolactasia is associated with the C/C_{-13910} genotype in diverse ethnic groups. The mechanism by which this variant downregulates the lactase gene is not known, but functional studies suggest genotype-dependent alterations in levels of messenger RNA.

CLINICAL MANIFESTATIONS

Adults with lactase deficiency typically complain of gas, bloating, and diarrhea after the ingestion of milk or dairy products but do not lose weight. Unabsorbed lactose is osmotically active, drawing water followed by ions into the intestinal lumen.[15] On reaching the colon, bacteria metabolize lactose to short-chain fatty acids, carbon dioxide, and hydrogen gas. Short-chain fatty acids are transported with sodium into colonic epithelial cells, facilitating the reabsorption of fluid in the colon. If the colonic capacity for the reabsorption of short-chain fatty acids is exceeded, an osmotic diarrhea results (see later discussion of carbohydrate malabsorption in watery diarrhea).

DIAGNOSIS

The diagnosis of acquired lactase deficiency can be made by empirical treatment with a lactose-free diet, which results in resolution of symptoms; by the hydrogen breath test after oral administration of lactose; or by genetic testing. Many intestinal diseases cause secondary reversible lactase deficiency, including viral gastroenteritis, celiac disease, giardiasis, and bacterial overgrowth.

CELIAC DISEASE

DEFINITION AND EPIDEMIOLOGY

Celiac disease is a chronic inflammatory condition of the small intestine precipitated by the ingestion of wheat, rye, and barley in individuals with certain genetic predispositions.[16] The prevalence in general populations worldwide is approximately 1%. High-risk groups for celiac disease include first-degree relatives and individuals with type 1 diabetes mellitus, autoimmune thyroid disease, autoimmune liver disease, and Down, Turner, or Williams syndromes. Approximately 5% of patients diagnosed with diarrhea-predominant irritable bowel syndrome or with microscopic (lymphocytic) colitis have celiac disease.

PATHOBIOLOGY

Environmental and genetic factors are important in the development of celiac disease, with data suggesting a relationship with prior reovirus infection.[17] Approximately 10% of first-degree relatives of affected individuals are found to have celiac disease. Predisposition has been mapped to the human leukocyte antigen (HLA)-D region on chromosome 6. More than 90% of northern Europeans with celiac disease have the DQ2 heterodimer encoded by alleles DQA1*0501 and DQB1*0201, compared with 20 to 30% of controls. A smaller celiac group carries HLA-DQ8. Many non-HLA alleles identified in genome-wide association studies account for a small portion of genetic risk. Most such genes are involved in adaptive and innate immune responses. Overlap variants have been identified in diabetes, rheumatoid arthritis, and Crohn disease.

The alcohol-soluble protein fraction of wheat gluten, the gliadins, and similar prolamins in rye and barley trigger intestinal inflammation in susceptible individuals. Oat grains, which have prolamins rich in glutamine but not proline, are rarely toxic. Gliadins and similar prolamins with high proline content are relatively resistant to digestion by human proteases. Many gliadin and prolamin peptides have been identified that stimulate HLA-DQ2– and HLA-DQ8–restricted intestinal T-cell clones from individuals with celiac disease. In blood lymphocyte comprehensive screen assays, three immunodominant prolamin peptides have been identified from wheat, barley, and rye in DQ2 celiac individuals; dominant peptides differ in those with DQ8. The DQ2 protein expressed on antigen-presenting cells has positively charged binding pockets; tTG (the autoantigen recognized by endomysial antibody) may enhance intestinal inflammation by deamidation of select glutamine residues in gliadin and similar prolamins to negatively charged glutamic acid. In the deamidated form, most gliadin peptides have a higher binding affinity for DQ2 and are more potent stimulants of gluten-sensitized T cells. Villous atrophy may be caused by inflammation that is triggered by γ-interferon released from DQ2- or DQ8-restricted CD4 T cells in the lamina propria. Intraepithelial lymphocytes also directly kill intestinal epithelial cells under the influence of IL-15 released from stressed enterocytes.

CLINICAL MANIFESTATIONS

Celiac disease usually manifests early in life, at approximately 2 years of age (after wheat has been introduced into the diet), or later in the second to fourth decades of life, but it can occur at any age. It may first manifest clinically after abdominal surgery or an episode of infectious diarrhea.

Adults with celiac disease in the United States often present with anemia or osteoporosis without diarrhea and no or mild other gastrointestinal symptoms. Other extraintestinal manifestations of celiac disease include rash (dermatitis herpetiformis), neurologic disorders (peripheral neuropathy, ataxia, epilepsy), psychiatric disorders (depression, paranoia), reproductive disorders (infertility, spontaneous abortion), short stature, dental enamel hypoplasia, chronic hepatitis, and pancreatitis.

A minority of patients present with severe diarrhea, weight loss or growth retardation, and the clinical manifestations of vitamin and mineral deficiencies.

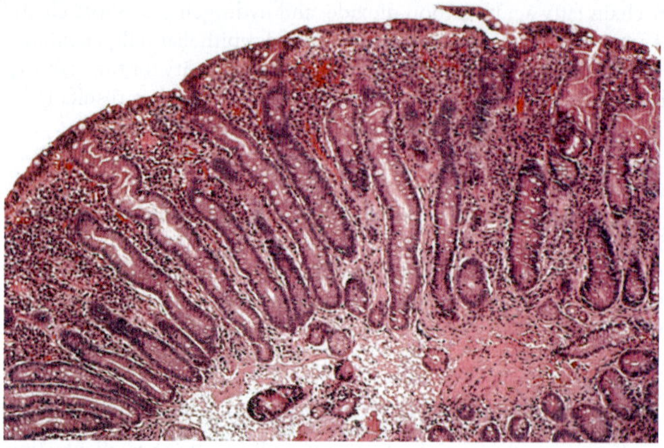

FIGURE 126-5. **Intestinal biopsy appearance of flattened villi, hyperplastic crypts, and increased intraepithelial lymphocytes.** (Courtesy John Hart, MD.)

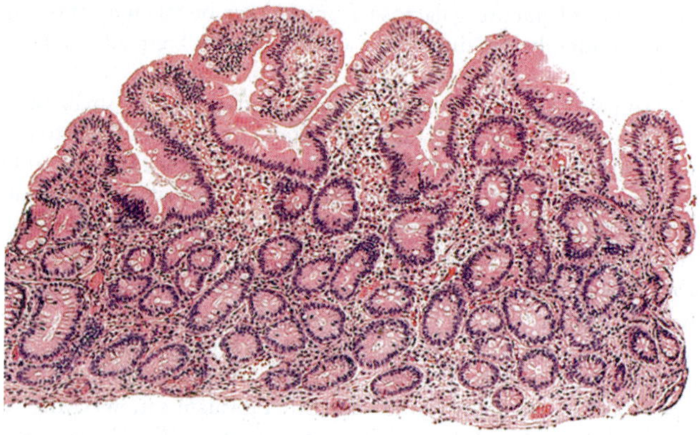

FIGURE 126-6. **Regeneration of villi after initiation of a gluten-free diet.** (Courtesy of John Hart, MD.)

Cobalamin deficiency is more common (10% of patients) than previously thought and usually corrects itself on a gluten-free diet. Symptomatic individuals require supplementation of vitamin B_{12}. Diarrhea is caused by many mechanisms, including a decreased surface area for water and electrolyte absorption, the osmotic effect of unabsorbed luminal nutrients, an increased surface area for chloride secretion (crypt hyperplasia), and the stimulation of intestinal fluid secretion by inflammatory mediators and unabsorbed fatty acids. Some individuals have impaired pancreatic enzyme secretion caused by decreased mucosal cholecystokinin release or bacterial overgrowth that may contribute to diarrhea. Individuals with nonceliac gluten sensitivity have wheat-related intestinal and extraintestinal symptoms similar to those of celiac disease but lack intestinal inflammation or celiac serologic markers. Fermentable oligosaccharides, disaccharides, monosaccharides, and polyols (FODMAPs) and gluten or nongluten wheat proteins (amylase trypsin inhibitors) may be the offending agents.

DIAGNOSIS

Routine screening for celiac disease is not recommended. In individuals who have subtle symptoms or in symptomatic high-risk groups, however, screening with anti-tTG IgA antibody testing is a cost-effective strategy.[18] High titer (>10-fold) of the anti-tTG IgA antibody is virtually diagnostic of celiac disease. EMA IgA antibodies, detected by indirect immunofluorescence, are highly sensitive (90%) and specific (95 to 99%) for active celiac disease in skilled laboratory testing. An ELISA test to detect antibodies against tTG has equal sensitivity to the EMA test but is less specific at lower titers. The anti-deamidated gliadin (a biotinylated synthetic γ-gliadin peptide with glutamic acid substituted for glutamine), antibody immunofluorometric assay has an inferior sensitivity and specificity compared with the anti-tTG IgA antibody.

Patients with mild disease may have negative antibody study results.[19] Anti-tTG, gliadin peptide, and EMA IgA antibodies tests are negative in individuals with selective IgA deficiency (present in up to 3% of individuals with celiac disease). In these patients, the anti-deamidated gliadin IgG antibody, which has a sensitivity and specificity close to that of the tTG IgA antibody, is helpful in diagnosis. In equivocal cases (negative serologic findings and equivocal biopsy result or positive serologic findings and normal biopsy result), HLA genotyping is useful to exclude the diagnosis of celiac disease in persons who lack the *DQ2* or *DQ8* gene.

The diagnosis of celiac disease can be confirmed by characteristic abnormalities seen on duodenal biopsies and improving when a gluten-free diet is instituted (Figs. 126-5 and 126-6). Mucosal flattening may be observed endoscopically as scalloped or reduced duodenal folds. Characteristic features found on intestinal biopsy include blunted or absent villi (villous atrophy), crypt hyperplasia, increased intraepithelial lymphocytes, and infiltration of the lamina propria with plasma cells and lymphocytes. In some individuals, the only abnormal biopsy finding is increased intraepithelial lymphocytes. However, individuals who have a TTG IgA antibody titer greater than 10-fold positive has a high enough predictive value for an abnormal duodenal biopsy characteristic of celiac disease that no biopsy is needed in this subset of individuals.[20,21] The decision to forgo biopsy for diagnosis should be under the guidance of a gastroenterologist.

TREATMENT

Treatment consists of a lifelong gluten-free diet. Wheat, rye, and barley grains should be excluded from the diet. Rice and corn grains are tolerated. Oats (if not contaminated by wheat grain) are tolerated by most. Early referral to a registered dietitian knowledgeable in the gluten-free diet and to a reputable celiac support group or website is crucial in maintaining dietary adherence. Owing to secondary lactase deficiency, a lactose-free diet should be recommended until symptoms improve.

In a preliminary trial, inhibition of transglutaminase-2 attenuated gluten-mediated mucosal damage and tended to improve symptoms[A7] Other therapies under study include exogenous oral enzymes that degrade gluten peptides, tight junction regulators, IL-15 inhibitors, and immune therapies to promote oral gluten tolerance.

Bone densitometry should be performed on individuals diagnosed with celiac disease who are older than 30 years of age because up to 70% have osteopenia or osteoporosis. Patients with diarrhea and weight loss should be screened for vitamin and mineral deficiencies. Documented deficiencies of vitamins and minerals should be replenished (Table 126-8), and women of childbearing age should take folic acid supplements. Bone mass often improves on a gluten-free diet alone. Patients with vitamin D or calcium deficiency should receive supplements (Chapter 199), with the dose monitored by 25-OH vitamin D levels and a 24-hour urine test for calcium. Celiac disease is associated with an increased risk for hospitalization with influenza and pneumococcal infection, so vaccination against both is recommended.

Most patients with seronegative villous atrophy do not have celiac disease. Most such patients have villous atrophy due to another cause or will have spontaneous improvement despite continuing to ingest gluten.

PROGNOSIS

Of patients with celiac disease treated with a gluten-free diet, 90% experience symptomatic improvement within 2 weeks. The most common cause of a poor dietary response is continued ingestion of gluten. Other possibilities include a missed intestinal infection (see later), an alternative diagnosis (e.g., ARB use particularly in elderly patients with a sprue-like enteropathy but negative celiac serologic findings, agammaglobulinemia [diagnosed by hypogammaglobulinemia and lack of plasma cells on small bowel biopsy], autoimmune enteritis [diagnosed by a positive anti-enterocyte antibody and crypt apoptosis or loss of goblet cells on small bowel biopsy]), bacterial overgrowth, pancreatic insufficiency, microscopic colitis, or other food allergies (cow's milk, soy protein). Between 4 and 40% of patients with celiac disease with symptomatic improvement have incomplete histologic recovery on a gluten-free diet; in such patients, a stricter diet may further improve symptoms and histology. A small percentage of patients with severe symptoms and enteropathy do not improve despite a strict gluten-free diet. In such patients, repeat intestinal biopsy with special lymphocyte marker studies is indicated. Some patients will have collagen deposition beneath the surface epithelium (collagenous sprue) or a polyclonal population of intraepithelial lymphocytes (refractory celiac disease type I). Others will have ulcerative jejunitis or a monoclonal population of intraepithelial T cells with an aberrant phenotype or clonal T-cell receptor-γ gene rearrangements (refractory celiac disease type II), which are predictive of enteropathy-associated T-cell lymphoma (Chapter 171) that portends a poor prognosis. Video capsule endoscopy and device-assisted enteroscopy may be helpful in establishing these diagnoses. Patients

TABLE 126-8 VITAMIN AND MINERAL DOSES USED IN THE TREATMENT OF MALABSORPTION

VITAMIN	ORAL DOSE	PARENTERAL DOSE
Vitamin A*	Water-soluble A, 25,000 U/day†	
Vitamin E	Water-soluble E, 400-800 U/day†	
Vitamin D‡	25,000-50,000 U/day	
Vitamin K	5 mg/day	
Folic acid	1 mg/day	
Calcium§	1500-2000 mg elemental calcium/day Calcium citrate, 500 mg calcium/tablet† Calcium carbonate, 500 mg calcium/tablet†	
Magnesium	Liquid magnesium gluconate†	2 mL of a 50% solution (8 mEq), total dose, in both buttocks IM
	1-3 tbsp (12-36 mEq magnesium) in 1-2 L of ORS or sports drink sipped throughout the day Magnesium chloride hexahydrate† 100-600 mg elemental magnesium/day	
Zinc	Zinc gluconate† 20-50 mg elemental zinc/day‖	
Iron	150-300 mg elemental iron/day Polysaccharide-iron complex†	Iron sucrose¶ Sodium ferric gluconate complex¶
	Iron sulfate or gluconate	Iron dextran (as calculated for anemia) (IV or IM¶; Chapter 145)
B-complex vitamins	1 megadose tablet/day	
Vitamin B_{12}	2 mg/day	1 mg IM or SQ/mo**
Copper	Copper sulfate 2-3 mg/day	1-2 mg IV/day

*Monitor serum vitamin A level to avoid toxicity, especially in patients with hypertriglyceridemia.
†Form best absorbed or with least side effects.
‡Monitor serum calcium and 25-OH vitamin D levels to avoid toxicity.
§Monitor 24-hr urine calcium to assess adequacy of dose.
‖If intestinal output is high, additional zinc should be given. Monitor for copper deficiency with high doses.
¶Parenteral therapy should be given in a supervised outpatient setting because of the risk for fatal reactions. Decreased risk for fatal reactions when compared with iron dextran.
**For vitamin B_{12} deficiency, 1 mg IM or SQ twice per week for 4 wk, then once per month.
IM = intramuscular; IV = intravenous; ORS = oral rehydration solution; SQ = subcutaneous.

with collagenous sprue, autoimmune enteritis, or refractory celiac disease type I often respond to prednisone (20 to 40 mg/day orally) or budesonide (9 mg opened capsule orally daily).

Patients with celiac disease have a higher likelihood of having other autoimmune conditions, such as type 1 diabetes, thyroiditis, rheumatoid arthritis, inflammatory bowel disease, systemic lupus erythematosus, Sjögren syndrome, primary biliary cirrhosis, autoimmune hepatitis, vitiligo, and pancreatitis. Interestingly, approximately one third of patients with idiopathic sporadic ataxia have transglutaminase-6 antibodies, consistent with gluten-induced disease.

Individuals with celiac disease have a 15 to 35% increased risk of mortality.[22] They also are at increased risk for cancer, particularly T cell lymphoma (Chapter 171) and small bowel carcinoma[23] (Chapter 171), with highest risks in the first year of after diagnosis and in patients over age 60 years. T-cell lymphoma is rare and should be suspected in individuals who have abdominal pain, recurrence of symptoms after initial response to a gluten-free diet, or refractory celiac disease.

TROPICAL SPRUE

Tropical sprue is an inflammatory disease of the small intestine associated with the overgrowth of predominantly coliform bacteria. It occurs in residents or travelers to India, Southeast Asia, Puerto Rico, and parts of the Caribbean. With the expansion of tourism and the global economy, this may be an underrecognized cause of enteropathy or mistaken for celiac disease. Individuals classically present with diarrhea and megaloblastic anemia secondary to vitamin B_{12} and folate deficiency, but some have anemia only. Intestinal biopsy characteristically shows subtotal and patchy villous atrophy in the proximal and distal small intestine, which may be caused by the effect of bacterial toxins on gut structure or by the secondary effects of vitamin B_{12} deficiency on the gut (megaloblastic gut). Diagnosis is based on history, documentation of vitamin B_{12} and/or folate deficiency, and the presence of an abnormal small intestinal biopsy report. Treatment is a prolonged course of tetracycline (250 mg orally four times daily) or doxycycline (100 mg orally two times daily), folic acid (5 mg/day orally), and, with coexistent deficiency, vitamin B_{12} injections (1000 µg weekly) until symptoms resolve. Relapse or reinfection occurs in 20%, mainly in natives of the tropics.

GIARDIA LAMBLIA

Giardia lamblia infection (Chapter 322), the most common protozoal infection in the United States, can cause malabsorption in individuals infected with many trophozoites, especially the immunocompromised or IgA-deficient hosts. Malabsorption occurs when many organisms cover the epithelium and cause mucosal inflammation, which results in villous flattening and a decrease in absorptive surface area. Stool for ova and parasites at this stage of infection is often negative because of the attachment of organisms in the proximal small intestine. Diagnosis can be made by PCR, stool antigen-capture ELISA test, or duodenal biopsy.

HUMAN IMMUNODEFICIENCY VIRUS

Diarrhea, malabsorption, and wasting are common in individuals with AIDS but are seen less frequently with improved antiretroviral therapy (Chapter 359). In patients who are receiving highly active antiretroviral therapy, diarrhea is more likely to be due to protease inhibitors than to enteric infection.

Malabsorption is usually due to infection with cryptosporidia, *Mycobacterium avium-intracellulare* complex, *I. belli*, or microsporidia. *AIDS enteropathy* (a term used if no organism is identified) also can cause malabsorption. Mechanisms of malabsorption and diarrhea include villous atrophy, increased intestinal permeability, rapid small bowel transit (in patients with protozoal infection), and ultrastructural damage of enterocytes (in AIDS enteropathy). Among individuals with AIDS and diarrhea, results of fecal fat absorption are frequently abnormal. Serum albumin, vitamin B_{12}, and zinc levels are often low. Vitamin B_{12} deficiency is caused mainly by ileal disease, but low intrinsic factor and decreased transcobalamin II may be contributing factors. Management of malabsorption should focus on restoring the immune system by treating the underlying HIV infection with antiviral therapy. If possible, the offending organism should be treated with antibiotics. If the organism cannot be eradicated, chronic diarrhea and malabsorption result; treatment in these cases consists of antimotility agents and a lactose-free, low-fat diet. Pancreatic enzyme replacement therapy can be tried in HIV-infected individuals who are taking highly active antiretroviral therapy or nucleoside analogues and who have fat malabsorption of obscure origin. If supplemental calories are needed, liquid oral supplements that are predigested and high in medium-chain triglycerides (semi-elemental) are tolerated best. Vitamin and mineral deficiencies should be screened for and treated.

WHIPPLE DISEASE

Whipple disease (Chapter 305), which is a rare cause of malabsorption, manifests with gastrointestinal complaints in association with systemic symptoms, such as fever, joint pain, or neurologic manifestations.[24] Approximately one third of patients have cardiac involvement, most commonly culture-negative endocarditis. Occasionally, individuals present with ocular or neurologic disease without gastrointestinal symptoms. The gram-positive actinomycete, *Tropheryma whippelii*, can be detected by PCR of duodenal biopsy specimens, gastric juice, saliva, urine,[25] or stool. Small intestinal biopsy shows villous blunting and infiltration of the lamina propria with large macrophages that stain positive with the periodic acid–Schiff method and are filled with the organism. It is important to distinguish these macrophages from macrophages infected with *M. avium-intracellulare* complex (Chapter 300), which stain positive on acid-fast staining and are found in individuals with AIDS. Treatment is with a prolonged course of broad-spectrum antibiotics (e.g., ceftriaxone 2 g/day IV or meropenem 1 g IV three times daily; then trimethoprim 160 mg and sulfamethoxazole 800 mg orally two times daily for 1 year or trimethoprim 160 mg and sulfamethoxazole 800 mg orally two times daily for 1 year). Relapses occur, but initial treatment with parenteral ceftriaxone or meropenem appears to be associated with a low relapse rate.

GRAFT-VERSUS-HOST DISEASE

Diarrhea occurs frequently after allogeneic hematopoietic stem cell transplantation (Chapter 163). Immediately after transplantation, diarrhea is caused by the toxic effects of cytoreductive therapy on the intestinal epithelium. From 20 to 100 days after transplantation, diarrhea is usually due to GVHD or infection. Patients with GVHD present clinically with a skin rash, hepatic cholestasis, buccal mucositis, anorexia, nausea, vomiting, abdominal cramps, and diarrhea. The diagnosis of GVHD in the gastrointestinal tract can be made on biopsy of the stomach, small intestine, or colon. In mild cases, the mucosa appears normal on inspection at endoscopy, but apoptosis of gastric gland or crypt cells can be found on biopsy. In severe cases, denudation of the intestinal epithelium results in diarrhea and malabsorption and often requires parenteral nutritional support. Octreotide (50 to 250 μg SQ three times daily) may be helpful in controlling voluminous diarrhea. Treatment of acute GVHD is with steroids (or antithymocyte globulin or ruxolitinib for steroid-refractory disease) combined with parenteral nutritional support until intestinal function returns.

SHORT-BOWEL SYNDROME

Malabsorption caused by small bowel resection or surgical bypass is called the short-bowel syndrome. The most common causes in the United States are massive resection of the jejunum, owing to strangulated bowel, volvulus, or ischemia (mesenteric or after intra-abdominal surgery), and jejunal exclusion, owing to gastric bypass surgery. Short-bowel syndrome resulting from Crohn disease and radiation enteritis now is less common because of improved medical and radiation therapies. The severity of malabsorption depends on the site and extent of resection; the capacity for adaptive hyperplasia, dilation, and elongation; and the function of the residual bowel. Mechanisms of malabsorption after small bowel resection include a decreased absorptive surface area, decreased luminal bile salt concentration, rapid transit, and bacterial overgrowth. Limited jejunal resection is tolerated best because bile salt and vitamin B_{12} absorption remain normal. Ileal resection is less well tolerated because of the consequences of bile salt wasting and the limited capacity of the jejunum to undergo adaptive hyperplasia. Adaptive hyperplasia in residual small bowel after resection depends on nutrients, endogenous secretions (pancreatic and biliary juice), local factors (trefoil peptides, prostaglandins, polyamines), growth hormone and growth factors (epidermal growth factor [EGF], insulin-like growth factor-1 [IGF1], transforming growth factor-α [TGF-α], IL-11). The glucagon-like peptide-2 (GLP2) produced in L cells in the terminal ileum and colon is a potent stimulant of adaptive hyperplasia in the jejunum in response to a meal. Using intestinal stem cell technology, epithelial organoids have been successfully grown in culture systems, but bowel regeneration has not yet been accomplished.

When less than 100 cm of jejunum remains, the colon takes on an important role in caloric salvage and fluid reabsorption. Malabsorbed carbohydrates are digested by colonic bacteria to short-chain fatty acids, which are absorbed in the colon.

TREATMENT

In patients who have a colon, parenteral nutrition may be avoided using a diet rich in complex carbohydrates, oral rehydration solution, an acid-reducing agent, and an antimotility agent (loperamide 2 to 8 mg orally up to four times a day; diphenoxylate and atropine 1 to 2 tablets orally up to four times a day; codeine 15 to 60 mg orally up to four times a day).[26] In comparison, individuals with fewer than 100 cm of jejunum and no colon have high jejunostomy outputs and often require intravenous fluids or parenteral nutrition to survive. These individuals waste sodium, chloride, bicarbonate, magnesium, zinc, and water in their ostomy effluent. Dietary modifications should include a high-salt, nutrient-rich diet given in small meals. An oral rehydration solution with a sodium concentration 75 to 90 mmol/L is absorbed best. Oral vitamin and mineral doses higher than the usual U.S. recommended daily allowances are required (see Table 126-8). Vitamin B_{12} should be given parenterally (500 to 1000 μg intramuscularly or subcutaneously every month). Magnesium deficiencies are often difficult to replenish with oral magnesium because of its osmotic effect in the intestinal lumen. A liquid magnesium preparation added to an oral rehydration solution and sipped throughout the day may minimize magnesium-induced fluid losses. Potent antimotility agents, such as tincture of opium (0.3 to 1 mL orally four times daily) or liquid morphine 20 mg/mL (1 mL orally four times daily), often are needed to slow transit and maximize contact time for nutrient absorption. High-volume jejunostomy outputs can be lessened by inhibiting endogenous secretions with a proton pump inhibitor (e.g., omeprazole, 40 mg orally one time daily, or lansoprazole, 30 mg orally one time daily) and, in severe cases (>3 L/day output), octreotide (100 to 250 μg subcutaneously three times daily; if effective, convert to an equivalent long-acting monthly dosage). The benefit of octreotide may be offset by its potential to inhibit intestinal adaptation and impair pancreatic enzyme secretion with doses greater than 300 μg/day.

In the most severe cases, supplemental calories must be provided by nocturnal tube feeding or parenteral nutrition. Treatment with growth hormone (0.1 mg/kg/day SQ) with or without glutamine (30 g/day orally) for 4 weeks may reduce parenteral nutrition requirements in patients who have had massive intestinal resections. Teduglutide (0.05 mg/kg/day SQ), a glucagon-like peptide-2 analogue that stimulates adaptive hyperplasia in remnant intestine after resection, improves absorption, and reduces parenteral nutrition requirements. Small bowel transplantation should be considered for individuals who require parenteral nutrition to survive and then develop progressive liver disease or venous access problems. Bioengineering of intestine using organoids and scaffolding systems is a promising future therapy.[27]

PROGNOSIS

Long-term complications include bone disease, renal stones (oxalate stones if the colon is present, urate stones with a jejunostomy), gallstones, bacterial overgrowth, fat-soluble vitamin deficiencies, essential fatty acid deficiency, and D-lactic acidosis.

CONDITIONS THAT IMPAIR NUTRIENT DELIVERY TO THE SYSTEMIC CIRCULATION

Insoluble lipids (present in chylomicrons) are exocytosed across the basolateral membrane of epithelial cells into the intestinal lymphatics. From there, they enter the mesenteric lymphatics and the general circulation through the thoracic duct. Sugar monomers, amino acids, and medium-chain fatty acids are transported across the basolateral membrane of intestinal epithelial cells into capillaries and into the portal circulation. Sugar monomers are transported across the basolateral membrane by the facilitative glucose transporter isoform (GLUT2) and amino acids by facilitative amino acid carriers (see E-Fig. 126-1C).

IMPAIRED LYMPHATIC DRAINAGE

Diseases that cause intestinal lymphatic obstruction, such as primary congenital lymphangiectasia (malunion of intestinal lymphatics), and diseases that result in secondary lymphangiectasia (lymphoma, tuberculosis, Kaposi sarcoma, retroperitoneal fibrosis, constrictive pericarditis, severe heart failure) result in fat malabsorption. The increased pressure in the intestinal lymphatics leads to leakage and sometimes rupture of lymph into the intestinal lumen, with the loss of lipids, γ-globulins, albumin, and lymphocytes. The diagnosis of lymphangiectasia can be made by intestinal biopsy, but the specific cause may be more difficult to identify. Individuals with lymphangiectasia malabsorb fat and fat-soluble vitamins and have protein loss into the intestinal lumen. The most common presentation is hypoproteinemic edema. Nutritional management includes a high protein and low-fat diet and supplementation with medium-chain triglycerides, which are absorbed directly into the portal circulation. Fat-soluble vitamins should be given if deficiencies develop.

CONGENITAL MALABSORPTION AND DIARRHEA

A number of congenital disorders, mostly autosomal recessive, alter nutrient digestion, epithelial cell transport, or villus epithelial architecture. These disorders usually present within the first few weeks of life and may become targets for stem cell therapy.

Mutations in sugar disaccharidases include lactase (rare), sucrose-isomaltase, maltase-glucoamylase, and trehalase (digests trehalose in mushrooms) deficiencies. These disorders are characterized by osmotic diarrhea when the offending sugar is introduced into the diet. Diagnosis is made by a low stool pH (owing to conversion of malabsorbed sugar to short-chain fatty acids by colonic bacteria), reduced enzyme activity on duodenal biopsy, and genetic testing. The treatment is to feed alternative sources of carbohydrates. Congenital enterokinase (enteropeptidase) deficiency due to missense mutations in the gene causes severe protein malabsorption owing to the inability to activate trypsinogen and other pancreatic proteases in the intestinal lumen. Treatment is with supplemental pancreatic enzymes.

Defects in epithelial transport proteins include congenital glucose-galactose malabsorption (mutation in the *SGLT1* gene) that results in severe carbohydrate malabsorption. Congenital chloride and sodium diarrheas are rare autosomal recessive disorders caused by mutations in the epithelial Cl^-/HCO_3^- (SLC26A) and the Na^+/H^+ exchanger (SCL9A3, GUCY2C), respectively. These disorders cause maternal polyhydramnios and fluid-filled bowel loops in utero as well as severe diarrhea at birth. Diagnosis in the newborn is made by high stool chloride levels and metabolic alkalosis in congenital chloride diarrhea, high stool sodium levels and metabolic acidosis in congenital sodium diarrhea, and genetic testing.

Abetalipoproteinemia is due to defects in chylomicron formation and exocytosis at the basolateral membrane of intestinal epithelial cells that are necessary for the delivery of lipids to the systemic circulation. Mutations in the microsomal triglyceride transfer protein (MTP), apolipoprotein B gene, and SAR1B (triggers coat protein of vesicles in the endoplasmic reticulum) result in chylomicron retention in epithelial cells. Children with this disorder have fat malabsorption and the consequences of vitamin E deficiency (retinopathy and spinocerebellar degeneration). Biochemical tests show low plasma levels of apoprotein B, triglyceride, and cholesterol. Membrane lipid abnormalities result in red blood cell acanthosis (burr cells). Intestinal biopsy, which is diagnostic, is characterized by engorgement of epithelial cells with lipid droplets. Treatment is with a low-fat diet containing medium-chain triglycerides and high doses of fat-soluble vitamins, especially vitamin E.

Homozygous loss-of-function mutations in the gene encoding CD55 (decreased decay-accelerating factor with hyperactivation of complement) cause protein-losing enteropathy, often accompanied by primary intestinal lymphangiectasia, edema due to hypoproteinemia, and malabsorption. Affected individuals often may have recurrent infections and angiopathic thromboembolic disease (CHAPLE syndrome).

Defects in villus epithelial cell structure presents at birth with severe malabsorption. Microvillus inclusion disease is due to defects in intraepithelial cellular protein transport and epithelial polarization. Mutations have been identified in myosin type 5 motor protein (*MYO5B*) and syntaxin-3 (*STX3*) genes. Tufting enteropathy is characterized by disorganized enterocytes at villus tips (tufts). Mutations have been identified in EpCAM and SPINK2 to suggest disorders in tight junction formation. Most infants with these disorders require parenteral nutrition or small bowel transplantation for survival.

WATERY DIARRHEA

Watery diarrhea may be due to osmotic, secretory, inflammatory, or often combined mechanisms (see Fig. 126-3).

INGESTION OF NONABSORBABLE OR POORLY ABSORBABLE SOLUTES

MAGNESIUM AND SODIUM PHOSPHATE AND SULFATE DIARRHEAS

Magnesium, phosphate, and sulfate are poorly absorbed minerals. Individuals who ingest significant amounts of magnesium-based antacids or high-potency multimineral and multivitamin supplements or those who surreptitiously ingest magnesium-containing laxatives or nonabsorbable anion laxatives, such as Na_2PO_4 (neutral phosphate) or Na_2SO_4 (Glauber or Carlsbad salt), may develop osmotically induced, watery diarrhea that may be high volume.

SORBITOL AND FRUCTOSE DIARRHEA

Dietetic food, chewing gum, candies, and medication elixirs that are sweetened with sorbitol, which is an unabsorbable carbohydrate, can cause diarrhea. Excessive consumption of pears, prunes, peaches, and apple juice, which also contain sorbitol and fructose, a poorly absorbable sugar, can result in diarrhea. Most soft drinks are now sweetened with fructose-containing corn syrup and may be a cause of diarrhea when ingested in high concentrations.

RAPID INTESTINAL TRANSIT

A small amount of carbohydrate in the diet is unabsorbed by the normal small intestine. Diets that are high in carbohydrate and low in fat may allow rapid gastric emptying and rapid small intestinal motility, thereby leading to carbohydrate malabsorption and osmotic diarrhea. Rapid transit time also occurs in thyrotoxicosis (Chapter 207). Because of the production of H_2 and carbon dioxide gas by colonic bacteria, abdominal gas and cramping may be the predominant symptoms.

BILE ACID DIARRHEA

Ileal malabsorption of bile salts results in the stimulation of colonic fluid secretion and watery diarrhea. Three types of bile acid malabsorption induce diarrhea. Type 1 results when severe disease (e.g., Crohn disease), resection, or bypass of the distal ileum allows bile salts to escape absorption (see earlier). Type 2 may be congenital: rarely owing to a defect in the intestinal sodium bile acid transporter but more commonly owing to increased bile salt production (associated with decreased levels of fibroblast growth factor 19 [FGF19], an intestinal fibroblast growth factor that normally downregulates bile salt synthesis in the liver, and increased levels of 7-α-hydroxy-4-cholesten-3-one [7αC4], which is a marker of bile acid synthesis, in blood). The result is increased bile salt production that overwhelms reabsorption in the ileum. Type 3 is caused by various conditions, including prior cholecystectomy, celiac disease, pancreatic insufficiency, microscopic colitis, bacterial overgrowth, gastric surgery, or vagotomy. Postulated mechanisms include a bile salt storage problem, increased production, decreased recycling, or saturation of absorption.

Primary (type 2) bile acid diarrhea is now thought to account for up to 30% of cases of functional or irritable bowel syndrome with chronic diarrhea (Chapter 123).[28] The diagnosis is made by selenium homocholic acid taurine (^{75}SeHCAT) testing (see Table 126-6), a 48-hour stool collection for bile acids on a high-fat diet, or fasting blood tests that measure FGF19 and C4 levels.

TREATMENT

Diarrhea due to types 1 and 2 often responds to cholestyramine (2 to 4 g orally two to four times daily), colestipol (5 g orally two or three times daily), or the more potent and better tolerated bile salt binder colesevelam (625-mg tablet orally two to six times daily). Obeticholic acid (25 mg orally daily), a farnesoid X receptor agonist that stimulates FGF19 production, may lessen the frequency of bile acid diarrhea but may cause pruritis.[29] Fat-soluble vitamin deficiency is a potential risk with chronic use of bile salt binders. Although many patients with type 3 respond to cholestyramine or colesevelam, some do not. In these patients, motility-altering drugs such as opiates (e.g., loperamide, 2 to 4 mg orally two to four times daily) and anticholinergics (e.g., hyoscyamine sulfate, 0.125 to 0.250 mg orally two to four times daily) may be of benefit.

TRUE SECRETORY DIARRHEAS

High-volume secretory diarrheas (see Fig. 126-3) can be caused by hormones or cytokines that are secreted by rare endocrine tumors, including carcinoid tumors (Chapter 213), gastrinomas (Chapter 213), VIPomas of the pancreas (Chapter 213), and medullary carcinoma of the thyroid (Chapter 207). Diarrhea is also seen in 60 to 80% of patients with systemic mastocytosis (Chapter 235). Diarrhea resulting from gastrinoma is distinct in that it is caused by high volumes of hydrochloric acid secretion that overwhelm the reabsorptive capacity of the colon and by maldigestion of fat owing to pH inactivation of pancreatic lipase and precipitation of bile salts.

VILLOUS ADENOMAS

Large (4 to 18 cm) villous adenomas, particularly in the rectum or occasionally the sigmoid colon, may cause secretory diarrhea of 500 to 3000 mL/24 hours characterized by hypokalemia, chloride-rich stool, and metabolic alkalosis. Increased numbers of goblet cells and increased prostaglandin E_2 are responsible for the diarrhea. Chloride wasting in the stool and metabolic alkalosis are also found in congenital chloridorrhea, which is caused by a defect in the intestinal Cl^-/HCO_3^- transporter. The metabolic alkalosis distinguishes these two diarrheas from most other diarrheas that cause metabolic acidosis. A villous adenoma is usually diagnosed by colonoscopy. The prostaglandin antagonist indomethacin (25 to 100 mg/day orally) reduces the diarrhea in some patients; resection is curative.

DIABETES MELLITUS–RELATED DIARRHEA

Constipation is more common than diarrhea in patients with diabetes (Chapter 210). High-volume, watery diarrhea, often with nocturnal incontinence, occurs in 20% of patients with poorly controlled type 1 diabetes. These patients usually have concomitant neuropathy, nephropathy, and retinopathy. The diarrhea may be due to several causes, including celiac disease, anal incontinence, bacterial overgrowth related to dysmotility, medications (metformin, acarbose), and autonomic neuropathy. If no specific cause is found, clonidine (initial dose 0.1 mg orally twice daily and titrated slowly to a maximal dose of 0.5 to 0.6 mg orally twice daily) may be helpful. Patients with neuropathy frequently have impaired anal sphincter function, and high-dose loperamide (4 mg orally four times daily) may improve the incontinence.

ALCOHOL-RELATED DIARRHEA

Diarrhea related to alcohol ingestion (Chapter 364) may be due to rapid intestinal transit, decreased bile and pancreatic secretion, nutritional deficiencies such as folate or vitamin B_{12}, or alcohol-related enteric neuropathy. Diarrhea may be acute with binge drinking, or it may be chronic and watery and persist for days or weeks. The diarrhea slowly resolves with abstinence from alcohol, proper nutrition, and the repletion of vitamin deficiencies.

FACTITIOUS DIARRHEA

Approximately 30% of patients referred to tertiary centers have chronic diarrhea from laxative abuse. The diarrhea is usually severe and watery, often with nocturnal symptoms. Some patients may have abdominal pain, weight loss, nausea, vomiting, hypokalemic myopathy, and acidosis. Stool volumes range from 300 to 3000 mL/day depending on the dose of laxative ingested. In the United States, bisacodyl is the most common cause. Other culprits include anthraquinone (senna, cascara, aloe, rhubarb) or osmotic laxatives (neutral phosphate, Epsom salts, and magnesium citrate). Some patients abuse other agents that cause diarrhea, such as the diuretics furosemide and ethacrynic acid.

More than 90% of laxative abusers are women who have underlying eating disorders such as anorexia nervosa or bulimia (Chapter 200) or middle-aged women who have complicated medical histories and who often work in health care. In patients with unexplained diarrhea, laxative screening of stool and urine (see later) should be performed to exclude this syndrome before an extensive medical evaluation is performed for other causes of chronic diarrhea.

CHRONIC IDIOPATHIC SECRETORY DIARRHEA

In a small subset of patients with secretory diarrhea, no cause is found despite an extensive evaluation. These cases are labeled as chronic idiopathic secretory diarrhea. In most patients, the diarrhea resolves within 6 to 24 months, which suggests a possible postinfectious or Brainerd diarrhea. If no diagnosis is found after thorough testing and a search for surreptitious laxative abuse, a therapeutic trial with bile salt–binding drugs (e.g., cholestyramine, 4 g orally before meals three times daily, or the more potent colesevelam, 625-mg tablet two to six times daily) or opiates (e.g., loperamide, 2 mg orally four times daily, maximal dose 16 mg daily) is warranted.

INFLAMMATORY DIARRHEAS

Diarrhea resulting from inflammation is characterized by watery or bloody stools, fecal leukocytes, and loss of protein in the stool (see Fig. 126-3).

INFLAMMATORY BOWEL DISEASE

See Chapter 127.

EOSINOPHILIC GASTROENTERITIS

Eosinophilic gastroenteritis is an increasingly recognized condition of unknown etiology characterized by infiltration of eosinophils in the mucosa, muscle, or serosal layers of the gastrointestinal tract.[30] Mast cells play a role in the pathogenesis. Approximately 50% of patients have atopic histories. Infestation with nematodes (Chapter 327) must be excluded before this diagnosis is made. Diarrhea occurs in 30 to 60% of patients with mucosal disease. Patients with involvement of the muscle layer often present with abdominal pain, nausea, and vomiting indicative of gastric outlet or intestinal obstruction. Peripheral eosinophilia is present in about 70% of patients. The disease may involve the entire gastrointestinal tract from esophagus to anus, or it may be isolated to a segment. With diffuse involvement, patients may have steatorrhea, protein-losing enteropathy, and blood loss.

Management includes an elimination diet or an elemental diet. Budesonide (9 mg orally daily) or prednisone (0.5 to 1 mg/kg orally daily) is highly effective, but relapses are common when corticosteroids are tapered. Lirentelimab, a monoclonal antibody against siglec-8 (sialic acid-binding immunoglobulin-like lectin 8 expressed on eosinophils and mast cells) is a promising therapy that significantly decreases tissue eosinophil counts and improves clinical symptoms.[A8]

MICROSCOPIC (COLLAGENOUS AND LYMPHOCYTIC) COLITIS

These two conditions, collectively known as *microscopic colitis,* may or may not be the same disease or variants of the same disease.[31] Lymphocytic colitis is equally prevalent in men and women, whereas collagenous colitis occurs 10 times more often in middle-aged or elderly women. These conditions may be associated with autoimmune disease or with NSAID use. There is an increased prevalence (5%) of microscopic colitis among individuals with celiac disease. These diseases may be categorized as either inflammatory or secretory diarrheas. An epidemiologic relationship to medications such as NSAIDs, proton pump inhibitors, selective serotonin reuptake inhibitors, and smoking has been reported, and increased luminal prostaglandin levels may cause the diarrhea. Enteric infections, food hypersensitivity, and intraluminal bile have been proposed as triggers for prostaglandin release from lymphocytes.

Antidiarrheal agents such as loperamide (2 mg orally four times daily) are the mainstay of therapy for mild diarrhea, which usually has a benign and self-limited course. Budesonide (4.5 to 9 mg orally daily) is the most effective therapy.[A9] In patients who do not tolerate or respond to it, an alternative is bismuth subsalicylate therapy (8 chewable 262-mg tablets orally daily). Patients with refractory disease may require corticosteroids (e.g., prednisone, 40 mg/day orally), a trial of azathioprine, or anti–TNF-α antibodies.

FOOD ALLERGY AND HYPERSENSITIVITY

Food allergies or sensitivities, especially to cow's milk and egg protein, are a well-established cause of enterocolitis in children, with an estimated frequency of 5%. Symptoms of abdominal cramps, diarrhea, and sometimes vomiting occur shortly after ingestion of the allergen (Chapter 233). Food hypersensitivity reactions are reported in 20 to 25% of adults and can lead to anxiety and disordered eating.[32] The role of food allergy in causing diarrhea in adults is less clear owing to the lack of a reliable diagnostic test. Allergy testing correlates poorly with intestinal allergy. The most common food allergens are milk, soy, eggs, seafood, nuts, and wheat. Sequential elimination diets can be diagnostic and therapeutic.

RADIATION ENTERITIS

Patients who receive pelvic radiation for malignancies of the female urogenital tract, gastrointestinal tract, or the male prostate may develop chronic radiation enterocolitis[33] 6 to 24 months after total doses of radiation greater than 40 to 60 Gy (Chapters 18 and 128), but symptoms can develop as late as 20 years after treatment. Early abnormalities include an increase in inflammatory mediators, an increase in cholinergic stimulation of intestinal tissue, and endothelial cell apoptosis that precedes epithelial cell apoptosis. The last finding suggests that vascular injury is the primary event. Diarrhea may be caused by bile acid malabsorption if the ileum is damaged, by bacterial overgrowth if radiation causes small intestinal strictures or bypass, or by radiation-induced chronic inflammation of the small intestine and colon. Rapid transit also may contribute to malabsorption and diarrhea.

TREATMENT

Treatment is often unsatisfactory. Anti-inflammatory drugs (mesalamine, corticosteroids) and antibiotics have been tried with little success. Cholestyramine (4 g orally three times daily) and NSAIDs (e.g., naproxen, 250 to 500 mg orally twice daily) may help, as may opiates (loperamide, 2 mg orally four times daily, or loperamide-*N*-oxide, 3 mg orally two times daily). Hyperbaric oxygen therapy may be useful for refractory disease. Surgery carries a high morbidity.

PROTEIN-LOSING GASTROENTEROPATHY

Severe protein loss through the gastrointestinal tract can be caused by mucosal diseases such as lymphangiectasia, lymphatic obstruction, bacterial or parasitic infection, gastritis (Chapter 125), gastric cancer, collagenous colitis, inflammatory bowel disease (Chapter 127), celiac disease, sarcoidosis (Chapter 83), lymphoma (Chapter 171), tuberculosis (Chapter 299), Ménétrier disease (Chapter 178), eosinophilic gastroenteritis, and food allergies. A variety of extraintestinal diseases, including systemic lupus erythematosus (Chapter 245), heart failure (Chapter 45), and constrictive pericarditis (Chapter 62), also can be causative. Patients with systemic lupus erythematosus (Chapter 245) may present with protein-losing enteropathy as the only manifestation of their disease.

The typical clinical presentation is hypoproteinemia with edema. Diarrhea is a frequent symptom but not always present. Depending on the cause, patients may have lymphocytopenia (from lymphatic obstruction), steatorrhea, and fat-soluble vitamin deficiencies (especially with primary intestinal lymphangiectasia or celiac disease).

Evaluation includes exclusion of renal, liver, heart disease as a cause followed by testing for suspected gastrointestinal mucosal diseases. MRI may play a role in detecting intestinal/mesenteric edema and lymphatic dilation. The α1-antitrypsin clearance test is useful for diagnosis and to evaluate the magnitude of protein loss.[34] Treatment focuses on the underlying disease.

MISCELLANEOUS DISEASES

Although acute mesenteric arterial or venous thrombosis manifests as an acute bloody diarrhea, chronic mesenteric vascular ischemia (Chapter 129) may manifest as watery diarrhea. Gastrointestinal tuberculosis (Chapter 299) and histoplasmosis (Chapter 308) manifest as diarrhea that may be either bloody or watery, as do certain immunologic diseases, such as Behçet syndrome and Churg-Strauss syndrome. All of these diseases may be misdiagnosed as inflammatory bowel disease

(Chapter 127). Neutropenic enterocolitis, an ileocolitis that occurs in patients with neutropenia and leukemia, sometimes is caused by *C. difficile* infection.

TREATMENT

Antidiarrheal agents are of two types: those used for mild to moderate diarrheas and those used for severe secretory diarrheas. A major shortcoming of opiates, the most commonly prescribed antidiarrheal agents, is that they have no antisecretory effect. Rather, they act by decreasing intestinal motility, thereby allowing longer contact time with the mucosa for improved fluid absorption. The exception is racecadotril, an enkephalinase inhibitor, that blocks intestinal fluid secretion without affecting motility.

Bulk-forming agents (psyllium, 7 g in 8 oz water orally up to five times daily and methylcellulose, 3 to 6 tablets twice daily with 300 mL of water) act by binding water and increasing the consistency of stool. Pectin has been shown to have proabsorptive activity. These agents may be useful in patients with fecal incontinence. Bismuth subsalicylates (524 mg orally every hour up to eight doses daily) have mild antisecretory and antimotility effects and are effective and safe in mild diarrheas.

The opiates may be symptomatically useful in mild to moderate diarrhea. Deodorized tincture of opium, codeine, and diphenoxylate with atropine largely have been supplanted by loperamide. Loperamide does not pass the blood-brain barrier and has a high first-pass metabolism in the liver; it has a high therapeutic-to-toxic ratio and is essentially devoid of addiction potential. It is safe in adults, even in total doses of 24 mg/day. The usual dose is 2 to 4 mg two to four times daily. Opiates may be harmful in patients with severe diarrhea because large volumes of fluid may pool in the intestinal lumen (third space), and stool output is no longer a reliable gauge for replacing fluid losses. The antimotility effects are a problem in infectious diarrhea because stasis may enhance bacterial invasion and delay clearance of microorganisms from the bowel. Opiates and anticholinergics also are dangerous in severe inflammatory bowel disease or severe *C. difficile* infection, where they may precipitate megacolon.

Antidiarrheal agents that are used for the treatment of severe secretory and inflammatory diarrheas generally have profiles with more serious side effects. The somatostatin analogue octreotide (initial dose, 100 to 600 µg subcutaneously in two to four divided doses daily; maximal dose, 1500 µg daily) lessens diarrhea in the carcinoid syndrome and in neuroendocrine tumors because it inhibits hormone secretion by the tumor. It is also effective in the treatment of dumping syndrome and chemotherapy-related diarrheas. Long-acting octreotide (20 to 30 mg intramuscularly every month) is available for once-a-month dosing. Octreotide can suppress pancreatic enzyme secretion and make diarrhea worse; it also may be of only limited usefulness in short-bowel syndrome and AIDS diarrhea. Crofelemer (125 mg orally twice daily), a chloride channel inhibitor extracted from the bark latex of the South American tree *Croton lechleri*, improves HIV-related chronic diarrhea. Agents such as phenothiazine and calcium-channel blockers have mild antisecretory effects, but side effects limit their use. Clonidine (initial dose, 0.1 mg orally twice daily, titrated slowly to a maximal dose of 0.5 to 0.6 mg twice daily) is most useful in opiate withdrawal diarrhea and is sometimes useful in diabetic diarrhea; postural hypotension may limit its use, particularly in patients with diabetes. Alosetron (0.5 mg orally twice daily for 4 weeks, maximal dose 1 mg orally twice daily) may be justified for severe diarrhea-predominant irritable bowel syndrome; associations with ischemic colitis and severe constipation have limited its use. Indomethacin (250 to 500 mg orally twice daily), a cyclooxygenase blocker that inhibits prostaglandin production, is useful in the treatment of diarrheas caused by acute radiation, AIDS, or villous adenomas of the rectum or colon; occasionally, it may be useful in neuroendocrine tumors and food allergy. For eosinophilic gastroenteritis, corticosteroids (prednisone, 20 to 40 mg/day orally for 7 to 10 days) are the mainstay of therapy. Lirentelimab, a monoclonal antibody against siglec-8, depletes eosinophils, inhibits mast cell activation, and is a promising new therapy. Food elimination diets are not usually effective. Treatment of inflammatory bowel disease is described in Chapter 127.

GENERAL REFERENCES

For the General References and other additional features, please visit Elsevier eBooks+ at https://ebooks.health.elsevier.com.

Grade A References

A1. Vassilopoulou L, Spyromitrou-Xioufi P, Ladomenou F. Effectiveness of probiotics and synbiotics in reducing duration of acute infectious diarrhea in pediatric patients in developed countries: a systematic review and meta-analysis. *Eur J Pediatr*. 2021;180:2907-2920.
A2. Okumura H, Fukushima A, Taieb V, et al. Fidaxomicin compared with vancomycin and metronidazole for the treatment of *Clostridioides (Clostridium) difficile* infection: a network meta-analysis. *J Infect Chemother*. 2020;26:43-50.
A3. Wilcox MH, Gerding DN, Poxton IR, et al. Bezlotoxumab for prevention of recurrent *Clostridium difficile* infection. *N Engl J Med*. 2017;376:305-317.
A4. Dembrovszky F, Gede N, Szakács Z, et al. Fecal microbiota transplantation may be the best option in treating multiple *Clostridioides difficile* infection: a network meta-analysis. *Infect Dis Ther*. 2021;10:201-211.
A5. Fan H, Gao L, Yin Z, et al. Probiotics and rifaximin for the prevention of travelers' diarrhea: a systematic review and network meta-analysis. *Medicine (Baltimore)*. 2022;101:e30921.
A6. Gatta L, Scarpignato C. Systematic review with meta-analysis: rifaximin is effective and safe for the treatment of small intestine bacterial overgrowth. *Aliment Pharmacol Ther*. 2017;45:604-616.
A7. Schuppan D, Mäki M, Lundin KEA, et al. A randomized trial of a transglutaminase 2 inhibitor for celiac disease. *N Engl J Med*. 2021;385:35-45.
A8. Dellon ES, Peterson KA, Murray JA, et al. Anti-siglec-8 antibody for eosinophilic gastritis and duodenitis. *N Engl J Med*. 2020;383:1624-1634.
A9. Münch A, Bohr J, Miehlke S, et al. Low-dose budesonide for maintenance of clinical remission in collagenous colitis: a randomised, placebo-controlled, 12-month trial. *Gut*. 2016;65:47-56.

127 INFLAMMATORY BOWEL DISEASE

GARY R. LICHTENSTEIN

DEFINITION

Inflammatory bowel disease refers to two chronic idiopathic inflammatory disorders: ulcerative colitis and Crohn disease. Characteristic clinical, endoscopic, and histologic features are critical for the diagnosis of these disorders, but no single individual finding is absolutely diagnostic for one disease or the other. Mucosal ulceration in Crohn disease may be transmural and may occur anywhere in the gastrointestinal tract, most commonly in the distal ileum and proximal colon. The hallmark of ulcerative colitis is continuous ulceration starting in the rectum and limited to the colon. Approximately 10% of patients with inflammatory bowel disease have what is called "inflammatory bowel disease-undetermined," a term used when Crohn colitis cannot be distinguished from ulcerative colitis.

EPIDEMIOLOGY

Inflammatory bowel disease occurs worldwide, but the highest incidence is found in North America, the United Kingdom, and northern Europe. Data suggest an increasing incidence and prevalence over time and in different regions around the world, although ulcerative colitis remains slightly more prevalent than Crohn disease. The incidence of ulcerative colitis in North America is estimated to be about 19 per 100,000 person-years and 24 per 100,000 person-years in Europe, with a prevalence of approximately 280 per 100,000 persons in North America and up to 500 per 100,000 persons in Europe. The incidence of Crohn disease in North America is estimated to be about 20 per 100,000 person-years and 13 per 100,000 person-years in Europe, with a prevalence of approximately 320 per 100,000 person-years in North America and in Europe.[1]

Crohn disease and ulcerative colitis may occur at any age, but both have their peak incidence in the second to fourth decade, with a second peak in the seventh decade. The female-to-male ratio for both ulcerative colitis and Crohn disease suggests no gender preference.

Crohn disease and ulcerative colitis are complex polygenic disorders, for which having a family history of inflammatory bowel disease is a risk factor. Crohn disease and ulcerative colitis occur in all ethnic and socioeconomic groups, but their incidence is highest in White and Jewish people of Eastern European (Ashkenazi) descent. In North America and the United Kingdom, however, the incidence of Crohn disease in African Americans and African Caribbeans appears to be approaching that of Whites. Studies of migrants from certain developing countries in South Asia to the United Kingdom suggest an increased prevalence of inflammatory bowel disease in subsequent generations, presumably because of environmental influences.

Cigarette smoking is associated with a worse prognosis in patients with Crohn disease but an improved course in ulcerative colitis. Nonsteroidal anti-inflammatory drugs (NSAIDs) appear to be associated with new onset of inflammatory bowel disease and with exacerbations of disease. Appendectomy for an inflammatory indication has been suggested as protective against the development of ulcerative colitis. Diet does not clearly affect the course of inflammatory bowel disease.

PATHOBIOLOGY

Although the trigger for inflammatory bowel disease is not known, three major pathways likely activate the disease: a genetic predisposition, immune dysregulation, and an environmental trigger.[2] A possible explanation is that the inability of the innate immune system to clear microbial antigens, combined with increased intestinal epithelial permeability to antigens, eventually leads to an overactive adaptive immune response.[3]

Genetics

Of patients with inflammatory bowel disease, 5 to 20% have another family member with inflammatory bowel disease. First-degree relatives have a 10- to 15-fold increased risk for developing inflammatory bowel disease. The concordance rate of developing Crohn disease in identical twins, siblings, and first-degree relatives is 50%, 0 to 3%, and 5 to 10%, respectively. Ulcerative colitis follows similar genetic patterns but with slightly lower risk rates. Twenty percent of patients with a positive family history of inflammatory bowel disease will have discordant disease type: one family member with Crohn disease and another with ulcerative colitis.

More than 200 gene susceptibility loci have been linked to inflammatory bowel disease, with at least 30 specific for Crohn disease and more than 20 specific for ulcerative colitis.[4] *NOD2/CARD15*, which is located on chromosome 16 (16q12) and expressed in intestinal epithelial Paneth cells, macrophages, and dendritic cells, is involved in the expression of an intracellular receptor that senses muramyl dipeptide, which is a peptidoglycan component of gram-positive bacteria. Activation of *NOD2* leads to activation of nuclear factor κ-B (NF-κB), which mediates transcription of numerous proinflammatory cytokines. A mutation in the leucine-rich domain of the NOD2 protein, which interacts with bacterial lipopolysaccharide, leads to failure in activation of NF-κB and is associated with the development of Crohn disease.

The *ATG16L1* gene on chromosome 2 and the *IRGM* gene on chromosome 5 also have been associated with increased susceptibility to Crohn disease. Both are members of a family of genes involved in autophagy, an autonomous process that involves the maintenance of cellular homeostasis and organelle turnover, as well as the processing of intracellular pathogens, the subsequent presentation of antigens, and the regulation of cell signaling. Toll-like receptor-4 gene polymorphisms are associated with both Crohn disease and ulcerative colitis. Polymorphisms of the interleukin-23 (IL-23) receptor gene are associated with ulcerative colitis and a varied risk for Crohn disease. The presence of an adenylate cyclase 7 (*ADCY7*) missense mutation leads to an excessive inflammatory response that predisposes to ulcerative colitis. Human leukocyte antigen (HLA) class II polymorphisms, especially in HLA-DR molecules, may confer increased risk for ulcerative colitis and possibly Crohn as well. The *OCTN1* gene (located on chromosome 5q31) and the *DLG5* gene (located on chromosome 10) are associated with Crohn disease. *DLG5* encodes a scaffolding protein that is important for maintaining epithelial integrity in various organs, whereas *OCTN1* encodes for an ion channel that regulates cell-to-cell signaling in the intestinal epithelium.

Inflammatory bowel disease also has been associated with Turner syndrome (Chapter 214), glycogen storage type Ib (Chapter 191), and the Hermansky-Pudlak syndrome (triad of albinism, platelet aggregation defect, and accumulation of ceroid-like pigment in tissue) (Chapter 159). Inflammatory bowel disease also is associated with various diseases that have known genetic predisposition, including ankylosing spondylitis (Chapter 244), psoriasis (Chapter 405), atopy (Chapter 230), eczema (Chapter 405), celiac sprue (Chapter 126), cystic fibrosis (Chapter 77), primary sclerosing cholangitis (Chapter 141), multiple sclerosis (Chapter 380), autoimmune thyroid disease (Chapter 207), autoimmune hemolytic anemia (Chapter 146), primary biliary cirrhosis (Chapter 141), myasthenia gravis (Chapter 390), and Cogan syndrome (Chapter 249).

PATHOPHYSIOLOGY

Microbes likely play a part in the development of inflammatory bowel disease. In several animal models of colitis, colitis does not develop in a sterile environment but can be induced after the introduction of commensal bacteria. For instance, helminth infection protects mice with *Nod2* mutations, which otherwise make them susceptible to Crohn disease, by inhibiting colonization by an inflammatory *Bacteroides* species. *Debaryomyces hansenii* (also known as *Candida famata*) has recently been implicated as a fungus that is found in Crohn disease tissue and can lead to dysregulated healing.[5]

Diverting the fecal stream away from active mucosal inflammation, such as in an ileostomy, also helps alleviate inflammation in Crohn disease. Crohn disease and ulcerative colitis preferentially occur in the terminal ileum and colon, which contain the highest concentration of bacteria, on the order of approximately 10^{12} organisms per gram of luminal contents. Antibiotics, particularly antibiotics with broad-spectrum anaerobic coverage, are helpful in the treatment of Crohn disease. More recently, several genetic polymorphisms associated with sensing the intestinal microbial environment and triggering an immune response have been linked to inflammatory bowel disease.

Both Crohn disease and ulcerative colitis are products of a dysregulated innate immune system that triggers T cells and a humoral response. T_H17 cells, which are activated in Crohn disease and ulcerative colitis, are stimulated by IL-23, which is produced by antigen-presenting cells.

Western-type diets (which are typically high in protein, fat, salt, sugar, other additives, and preservatives but low in fruit, vegetables, and fiber) are associated with almost a two-fold increased risk of developing inflammatory bowel disease.[6] Such foods and additives may disrupt the gut microbiota and propagate of immune activation.

Pathology

Crohn Disease

As a result of a dysregulated immune system, patients with Crohn disease develop aphthous ulcers, which are superficial mucosal ulcers. As the disease progresses, the ulceration becomes deeper, transmural, and discrete; it may form a serpiginous pattern and may occur anywhere from the mouth to the anus in a noncontinuous pattern. The most common location for ulceration is the ileocecal region. In some patients, chronic disease leads to the formation of fibrotic strictures, and approximately 30% of patients may develop fistulas in the course of their disease.

In early Crohn disease, the histopathologic findings are characterized by an acute inflammatory infiltrate in the lamina propria, with cryptitis, and crypt abscesses. Later in the disease process, the crypt architecture becomes distorted, with a lymphocytic infiltrate and a resulting branching and shortening of the crypts. Noncaseating granulomas, which may be found in up to 15% of endoscopic biopsy specimens and up to 70% of surgical specimens, are not unique to Crohn disease but help confirm the diagnosis when other classic features are present.

Surgical specimens also may show transmural intestinal wall inflammation and fat creeping on the serosal surface.

Ulcerative Colitis

In mild ulcerative colitis, the mucosa is granular, hyperemic, and edematous in appearance. As the disease becomes more severe, the mucosa ulcerates, and the ulcers may extend into the lamina propria. Ulcerative colitis starts in the rectum and may extend proximally in a continuous pattern, but it affects only the colon. Pseudopolyps may form owing to epithelial regeneration after recurrent acute attacks. With chronic disease, the colonic mucosa may lose the normal fold pattern, the colon may shorten, and the colon may appear narrowed.

In early ulcerative colitis, the histopathologic findings are characterized by epithelial necrosis, an acute inflammatory infiltrate in the lamina propria, with cryptitis and crypt abscesses. In chronic disease, a predominant lymphocytic infiltrate and distortion of crypt architecture are seen.

CLINICAL MANIFESTATIONS

Symptoms of inflammatory bowel disease are varied and may be a consequence of the location of the disease, the duration of disease, and any anatomic complications of the disease, such as strictures and fistulas in Crohn disease (Table 127-1).

TABLE 127-1 CLINICAL CHARACTERISTICS OF CROHN DISEASE AND ULCERATIVE COLITIS

CHARACTERISTICS	CROHN DISEASE	ULCERATIVE COLITIS
Peak age of onset (years of age)	15-30, 2nd peak in the 7th decade	20-40, 2nd smaller peak beyond the 7th decade
Sex distribution (F/M)	1.2/1	1/1
Potential sites of gastrointestinal involvement	Esophagus to anus	Colon
Skipped areas of involvement	+	–
Transmural inflammation	+	–
Type of ulceration	Usually discrete	Continuous
Fistula	+	–
Stricture	+	–
Perianal disease (fissure, skin tags)	+	–

Symptoms

Crohn Disease

The terminal ileum is affected in about 70% of patients with Crohn disease. Primary ileal disease occurs in 30% of patients, whereas ileocolonic disease occurs in 40%. Symptoms may include abdominal pain, typically in the right lower quadrant, diarrhea, hematochezia, and fatigue. With more severe disease, fever and weight loss may be present. Some patients may present with obstructive symptoms, such as abdominal pain, abdominal distention, and nausea.[7]

Only approximately 5% of patients develop Crohn disease in the upper gastrointestinal tract, and esophageal Crohn disease occurs in fewer than 2% of patients. Subjects with upper gastrointestinal Crohn disease may present with dysphagia, odynophagia, chest pain, or heartburn. Gastroduodenal disease occurs in 0.5 to 4% of patients and commonly occurs along with distal disease. Symptoms may include upper abdominal pain. Isolated jejunal disease is rare; if the jejunum is involved, there is also distal small bowel involvement. Up to 30% of patients have perianal disease (Chapter 131) that may include the development of fistulas, abscesses, fissures, and skin tags. Symptoms of perianal disease include pain and discharge. Fever may be present if there is an abscess.

Fistulae, which are internal tracts that connect one organ to another (e.g. rectovaginal, enterovesicular, perianal) or to the skin surface (e.g., anus to skin), can occur anywhere in the gastrointestinal tract and develop in 20 to 40% of Crohn patients. Penetrating Crohn disease also may cause intra-abdominal and perianal abscesses owing to a fistula with a blind end or intestinal perforation. External fistulas, which present with symptoms of fluid discharge from the cutaneous opening, can be enterocutaneous or perianal. Internal fistulas can be enteroenteric, rectovaginal, or enterocolonic. Patients may present with persistent abdominal pain and fever with an abscess in this location.

Ulcerative Colitis

As with Crohn disease, symptoms and signs of ulcerative colitis depend on the extent and severity of disease. At the time of diagnosis, 14 to 37% of patients have pancolitis, 36 to 41% have disease extending beyond the rectum, and 44 to 49% have proctosigmoiditis. Symptoms include hematochezia, diarrhea, tenesmus, production of excessive mucus, urgency to defecate, and abdominal pain. In the setting of proctitis or proctosigmoiditis, patients may have constipation with difficulty defecating. With more extensive and severe colonic involvement, patients also may have weight loss and fever. They also may have nausea and vomiting because of abdominal pain, fatigue because of anemia, and peripheral edema as a consequence of hypoalbuminemia.

Physical Examination

Signs on physical examination are representative of the type of disease as well as its location and severity. Oral ulcers may be present in Crohn disease. The location of abdominal tenderness usually reflects the location of intestinal involvement. In Crohn disease, abdominal tenderness is classically in the right lower quadrant and may include fullness or a mass depending on the severity of inflammation. Peritoneal signs may occur when penetrating Crohn disease causes intestinal perforation. Rectal examination may reveal skin tags, hemorrhoids, fissure, and fistulae. Additionally, the finding of a rectal stricture maybe a sign of current or past Crohn involvement.

Extraintestinal Manifestations

Arthropathy, the most common extraintestinal manifestation (Table 127-2), affects up to 10 to 20% of subjects. Peripheral arthralgias, arthritis, ankylosing spondylitis (Chapter 244), and sacroiliitis may exacerbate with gastrointestinal symptoms. Dermatologic disorders, such as erythema nodosum (in 10 to 15% of patients; see Fig. 407-24) and pyoderma gangrenosum (in 1 to 2% of patients; Chapter 240), develop in up to 15% of patients. Ocular disorders, especially uveitis and episcleritis (Chapter 391), may occur in 5 to 15% of patients with irritable bowel disease. Patients with inflammatory bowel disease also have up to a 10% risk for renal calculi, especially calcium oxalate stones (Chapter 111), in the setting of fat malabsorption with Crohn disease in the small bowel. Uric acid stones can occur in the setting of severe volume depletion. Patients with inflammatory bowel disease, especially patients with ulcerative colitis, are at increased risk for primary sclerosing cholangitis—2 to 7.5% of patients develop this disorder, and 70 to 80% of patients with this disorder have underlying inflammatory bowel disease (Chapter 141).

Extraintestinal Complications

Patients with inflammatory bowel disease are susceptible to extraintestinal complications from the disease itself or medications used to treat disease.

TABLE 127-2 EXTRAINTESTINAL COMPLICATIONS OF INFLAMMATORY BOWEL DISEASE

COMPLICATIONS	CROHN DISEASE	ULCERATIVE COLITIS
Ocular disorders (uveitis, episcleritis)	+	+
Arthropathy	+	+
Oral ulcers	+	–
Skin disorders (pyoderma gangrenosum, erythema nodosum)	+	+
Nephrolithiasis	+	+
Primary sclerosing cholangitis	+	+
Bone disorders (osteoporosis, osteomalacia)	+	–
Thromboembolic disease	+	+
B_{12} deficiency	+	–

These complications include osteoporosis, osteomalacia, arthritic complications, thromboembolic events, pulmonary disease,[7] and renal, dermatologic, and neurologic complications. Osteoporosis occurs in approximately 15% of patients, and steroid therapy (Chapter 28) is the major risk factor; avascular necrosis of the hip and septic arthritis are unusual complications of steroids or other immunosuppressive therapies. Cheilitis may be a result of iron deficiency anemia (Chapter 145). Patients with inflammatory bowel disease are at an increased risk for thromboembolic disease, especially in the setting of active intestinal disease, even when compared with other autoimmune diseases such as rheumatoid arthritis and celiac disease. Secondary amyloidosis with renal involvement can be a consequence of chronic inflammation. Asthma is the most common pulmonary disorder observed in association with Crohn disease. Patients also are at risk for optic neuritis and multiple sclerosis (Chapter 380), as well as for peripheral neuropathy (Chapter 388) from vitamin B_{12} deficiency, which may occur as a result of poor absorption owing to active small bowel disease, surgical resection, or small intestinal bacterial overgrowth.

DIAGNOSIS

When diarrhea (Chapter 126) is the predominant symptom, the initial evaluation should include a thorough medical history, testing for infectious colitis (Chapter 126), and screening for endocrine-metabolic disorders such as hyperthyroidism (Chapter 207) and hypocalcemia (Chapter 227). Infections with organisms such as *Salmonella* (Chapter 284), *Shigella* (Chapter 285), *Amoeba* (Chapter 323), *Giardia* (Chapter 322), *Escherichia coli* O157:H7 (Chapter 280), and *Campylobacter* (Chapter 279) can be accompanied by bloody diarrhea, abdominal cramps, and an endoscopic mucosal appearance identical to that of ulcerative colitis. Stool studies are needed to diagnose or exclude these infections. If hematochezia and abdominal pain are the predominant symptoms, the differential diagnosis is broad (Table 127-3).

Diagnostic Evaluation

Endoscopic Evaluation

In a patient with symptoms suggestive of inflammatory bowel disease and no evidence for an infection to explain the symptoms, endoscopic evaluation is essential. Colonoscopy is the initial endoscopic test for patients who present with lower gastrointestinal symptoms such as diarrhea and hematochezia, except in the presence of acute severe peritoneal symptoms. Colonoscopy up to and including the terminal ileum is important if there is a potential diagnosis of inflammatory bowel disease. Small bowel imaging (such as small bowel follow-through or computed tomography [CT] enterography, or magnetic resonance imaging [MRI] enterography) also may be needed to determine whether there is small bowel disease or to determine the distribution of disease. Capsule endoscopy is useful if all other endoscopic and radiologic testing is nondiagnostic, but Crohn disease of the small bowel is still suspected. Findings on capsule endoscopy should be followed by endoscopy to obtain biopsies. Capsule endoscopy should not be performed if Crohn disease is complicated by a known small bowel stricture. If it is uncertain whether a stricture is present, a patency capsule can be used initially to discern if it passes.

TABLE 127-3 DIFFERENTIAL DIAGNOSIS OF ILEITIS AND COLITIS

INFECTIONS	**MEDICATIONS/TOXINS**
Bacterial	Nonsteroidal anti-inflammatory drugs
Aeromonas	Pancreatic enzyme supplements—fibrosing colopathy
Campylobacter jejuni	Phosphosoda bowel preparations
Chlamydia (proctitis)	Radiation
Clostridioides difficile	**INFLAMMATORY**
Mycobacterium tuberculosis	Appendicitis
Salmonella	Diverticular disease
Shigella	Eosinophilic gastroenteritis
Enterohemorrhagic *Escherichia coli*	Nongranulomatous ulcerative jejunoileitis (celiac disease)
Yersinia	**NEOPLASIA**
Viral	Carcinoid
Cytomegalovirus	Carcinoma primary or metastatic
Herpes simplex virus (proctitis)	Lymphoma
Human immunodeficiency virus	Mycosis fungoides
Fungal	Malignant histiocytosis
Histoplasma capsulatum	**MISCELLANEOUS**
Parasitic	Amyloidosis
Entamoeba histolytica	Sarcoidosis
Helminths	Endometriosis
VASCULAR	Tubo-ovarian abscesses
Collagen Vascular Disease	
Behçet disease	
Churg-Strauss syndrome	
Henoch-Schönlein purpura	
Systemic lupus erythematosus	
Polyarteritis nodosa	
Ischemia	

Modified from Aberra FN, Lichtenstein GR. Crohn disease. In: Talley NJ, Kane SV, Wallace MD, eds. *Practical Gastroenterology and Hepatology: Small and Large Intestine*. Wiley-Blackwell; 2010:225-235.

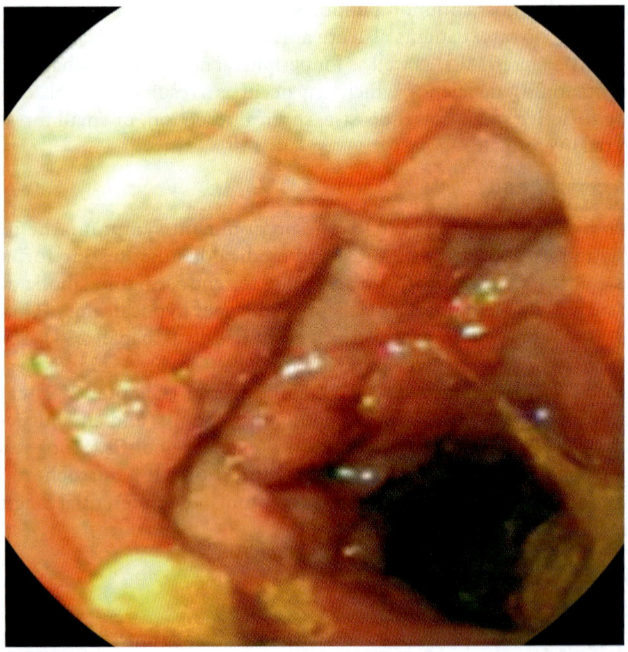

FIGURE 127-1. Endoscopic appearance of Crohn disease with cobblestoning.

Crohn Disease

Early endoscopic findings in Crohn disease include superficial small mucosal ulcers, also called aphthous ulcers. As the severity of Crohn disease progresses, the ulcerations become deeper and may become round, linear, or serpiginous. Intersecting longitudinal and transverse ulcers cause a cobblestone mucosal appearance, with "stone" areas representing normal mucosa (Fig. 127-1). Areas of ulceration, which are typically interspersed with normal "skip" areas, may occur anywhere from the esophagus to anus but are most common in the ileocecal region. Isolated colonic disease occurs in 25% of patients, and 60% will have rectal involvement, thereby making it at times difficult to differentiate from ulcerative colitis.

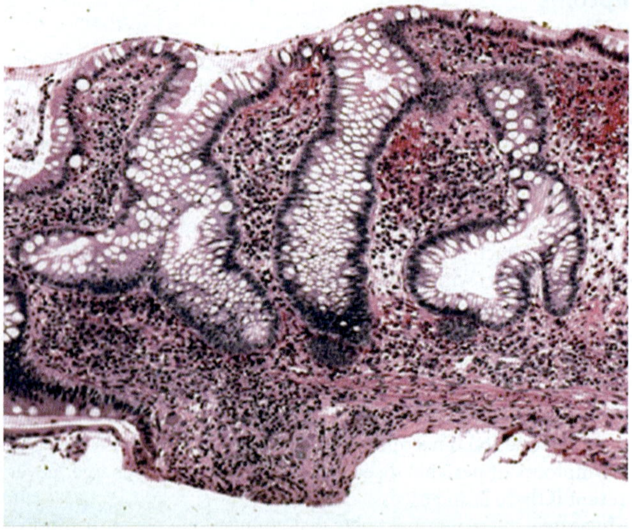

FIGURE 127-2. **In ulcerative colitis, histopathology from colonic biopsies reveals features of crypt distortion and lymphocytic infiltration in the mucosa.** (Modified from AGA Institute Slides 2010.)

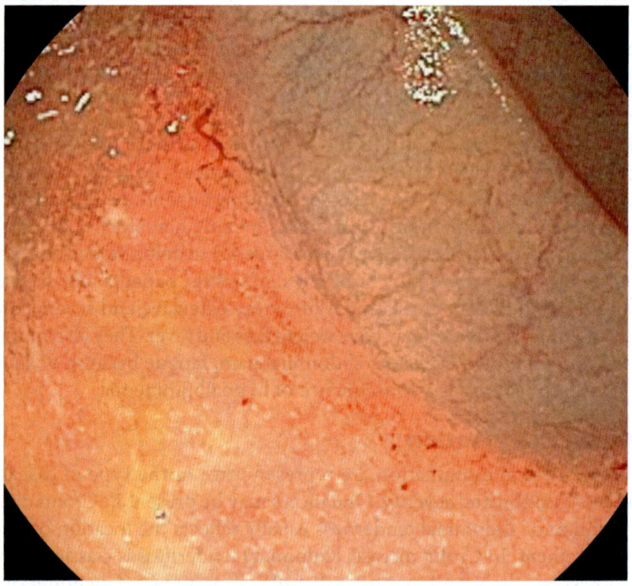

FIGURE 127-3. **Endoscopic appearance of ulcerative colitis.**

The diagnosis of inflammatory bowel disease is contingent upon accurate histopathologic results, so biopsy of the affected area(s) is key. Findings of an inflammatory infiltrate in the lamina propria and distortion of the crypt architecture support the diagnosis (Fig. 127-2). The diagnosis of Crohn disease may be made by histopathologic examination alone if noncaseating granulomas are seen, but granulomas are rarely found on endoscopic biopsies. The diagnosis of Crohn disease is usually based on a combination of information gleaned from histopathologic findings, colonoscopy, and small bowel imaging. A skip pattern of ulceration, ulceration in the small bowel or upper gastrointestinal tract, or the presence of fistulas support the diagnosis of Crohn disease. Colonic and small bowel ulceration occur in several other disorders, including infections that may not be detected by routine stool studies (such as enterohemorrhagic *E. coli*), vascular disorders, immune-related enterocolitis, neoplasia, diverticulitis, radiation, and medications such as NSAIDs (see Table 127-3).

Ulcerative Colitis

The diagnosis of ulcerative colitis is based on endoscopic findings (Video 127-1) and histopathology.[8] Early in the disease process, patients develop diffuse mucosal erythema with loss of the normal mucosal vascular pattern. In mild disease, the mucosa may have a granular and edematous appearance. As the disease becomes more severe, the mucosa becomes more friable, bleeds easily when the mucosa is touched, and may eventually ulcerate (Fig. 127-3). Endoscopic findings, which start in the rectum and may extend proximally in a continuous pattern, affect only the colon. The term "backwash ileitis" describes a spillover effect from ulcerative colitis and should not be construed as actual involvement of the terminal ileum by ulcerative colitis. Pseudopolyps may form owing to epithelial regeneration after recurrent attacks in patients with long-standing disease. The presence of pseudopolyps is thought to be a marker of more severe disease. With chronic disease, the colonic mucosa may lose its normal fold pattern, and the colon may shorten and appear narrowed. Careful endoscopic observation—including the observed vascular pattern, bleeding, and ulceration—can assess the severity of ulcerative colitis and monitor its response to treatment.

Features such as crypt distortion, continuous mucosal inflammation starting from the rectum, absence of granulomas, and absence of small bowel disease are consistent with ulcerative colitis. Early in the disease process, chronic inflammatory findings, such as crypt distortion, may not be present, and the diagnosis may be more difficult to establish.

Radiology

Radiologic imaging is vital and almost always should be obtained when inflammatory bowel disease, particularly Crohn disease, is suspected. CT enterography and magnetic resonance imaging (MRI) enterography have supplanted barium studies (such as an upper gastrointestinal series, small bowel follow-through, and barium enema) to diagnose the extent, severity, and type of disease (strictures and fistulas) of Crohn disease. CT and MRI enterography are also useful for the detection of abdominal abscesses and perineal abscesses.

Laboratory Findings

Anemia may result from chronic disease, blood loss, or nutritional deficiencies of iron, folate, or vitamin B_{12}. A modestly elevated leukocyte count is indicative of active disease, but a marked elevation suggests an abscess or another suppurative complication. The erythrocyte sedimentation rate and C-reactive protein are nonspecific serum inflammatory markers that are commonly used to monitor the activity of disease. Fecal calprotectin levels tend to be elevated in active disease and lower when patients are in remission.[9] Hypoalbuminemia is an indication of malnutrition and is common with active disease. Ileal disease or resection of more than 100 cm of distal ileum results in a diminished serum vitamin B_{12} level because of malabsorption.

Serologic Markers

Serologic markers are supportive but may not be used independently to diagnose inflammatory bowel disease. Anti–*Saccharomyces cerevisiae* antibodies (ASCA), which are antibodies to yeast, are present in 40 to 70% of patients with Crohn disease and in less than 15% of patients with ulcerative colitis. The combination of elevated ASCA immunoglobulin A (IgA) and IgG titers is highly specific for Crohn disease, ranging from 89 to 100%. Perinuclear antineutrophil cytoplasmic antibodies (pANCA) are present in 20% of Crohn patients, primarily in colon-predominant disease, and in 55% of patients with ulcerative colitis. ASCA-positive and pANCA-negative disease are associated with a sensitivity of 55% and specificity of 93% for Crohn disease. The antimicrobial antibodies anti-I2 (Crohn disease–related protein from *Pseudomonas fluorescens*), anti-Cbir1 (flagellin-like antigen), and anti-OmpC (*E. coli* outer membrane porin C) are also associated with Crohn disease.

TREATMENT

The aim of medical therapy is to reduce inflammation and subsequently induce and maintain clinical remission while simultaneously healing the mucosa. Medications used to treat inflammatory bowel disease include the categories of 5-aminosalicylate (5-ASA), antibiotics, corticosteroids, immunomodulators (azathioprine, mercaptopurine, methotrexate, and ozanimod), and biologics (infliximab, adalimumab, certolizumab pegol, golimumab, vedolizumab, natalizumab, and ustekinumab; Table 127-4). The specific medical therapy selected[10] is based on the location, extent (nonpenetrating and nonstricturing, stricturing, and penetrating and fistulizing disease), severity of disease, and future prognosis. Patients with high-risk disease (high potential for future surgery or complications such as fistula and abscess) or high disease activity are considered candidates for biologic therapy.[11] Supportive medical therapy, such as antidiarrheal and antispasmodic medications, also may be used. In patients over age 60 years, who represent about 15% of newly diagnosed cases, the risk-benefit ratio of more aggressive therapies may be less favorable.[12]

Categories of Medical Therapy

5-Aminosalicylate

5-ASA, which acts as a topical anti-inflammatory within the lumen of the intestine, is used to treat mild to moderate ulcerative colitis and as maintenance therapy for patients in remission.[A1,A2] Sulfasalazine is the combination of a sulfapyridine with 5-ASA; 5-ASA is responsible for the anti-inflammatory property of this drug, whereas sulfapyridine is the carrier that allows 5-ASA to be delivered to the colon. Other oral formulations of 5-ASA allow it to be delivered to the intestine by different mechanisms. Mesalamine is released in the intestine based on a pH delivery model, whereas sulfasalazine, olsalazine, and balsalazide are released in the intestine by bacterial cleavage of a covalent bond between 5-ASA and a prodrug. For rectal and sigmoid disease, 5-ASA suppository and enema preparations are also effective for induction and maintenance of remission in patients with ulcerative colitis. Adverse events associated with 5-ASAs are uncommon but may include nausea, dyspepsia, hair loss, headache, pancreatitis, worsening diarrhea, and hypersensitivity reactions.

Corticosteroids

Corticosteroids are primarily used to treat flares of ulcerative colitis and Crohn disease. Oral formulations may be used for mild to moderate disease, whereas systemic corticosteroids are used for moderate to severe disease.

Enteric-coated budesonide, a pH-dependent ileal release formulation, is an oral corticosteroid with high topical activity and low systemic bioavailability (10%). Enteric-coated budesonide is indicated for treatment of active mild to moderate ileocecal Crohn disease. Budesonide MMX is released in the colon and is available for treatment of mild to moderately active ulcerative colitis. Budesonide foam is administered rectally with an applicator in the colon for mild to moderately active ulcerative colitis limited to the rectum and sigmoid colon. Oral corticosteroids such as prednisone and methylprednisolone are used for moderate to severe disease, starting at doses ranging from 40 to 60 mg/day for 1 to 2 weeks, then typically tapered over a period of 8 to 12 weeks. Intravenous methylprednisolone is used for severe disease, with dosing ranging from 40 to 60 mg/day. When symptoms are controlled, systemic corticosteroids are not recommended because of their substantial side effects and their lack of efficacy for maintaining remission (Chapter 28).

Immunomodulation

In patients who remain symptomatic despite 5-ASA therapy or who have moderate to severe Crohn disease[A3] or ulcerative colitis,[A4] immunomodulators can provide substantial benefit.[13]

Janus-Kinase Inhibition

Tofacitinib (an oral, nonselective inhibitor of the Janus kinase family) has a more rapid onset of activity for moderate to severe ulcerative colitis[A5] at 10 mg orally twice daily for at least 8 weeks, then 5 or 10 mg twice daily with the medication discontinued if an adequate therapeutic benefit is not achieved by 16 weeks. Side effects include activation of nonsystemic herpes zoster, an abnormal lipid profile, thrombosis, and the potential risk of lymphoma.

Upadacitinib (an oral, selective inhibitor of the Janus kinase family) has a rapid onset of activity and is approved for the treatment of moderate to severely active ulcerative colitis.[A6] The induction dose (45 mg once daily for 8 weeks) should be followed by a maintenance dose (usually 15 mg once daily, but 30 mg once daily can be considered for patients who have refractory, severe, or extensive disease), but dosing should be at the lowest effective dose in the individual patient. Upadacitinib should be discontinued if adequate therapeutic response is not achieved with the 30 mg dosage.

Anti–Tumor Necrosis Factor-α Agents

Monoclonal antibody therapy directed against tumor necrosis factor-α (anti–TNF-α) include infliximab (which is a chimeric mouse-human IgG1 monoclonal antibody that is infused intravenously), adalimumab and golimumab (which are fully human IgG1 antibodies that are self-administered subcutaneously), and certolizumab pegol (which is a chimeric pegylated Fab fragment IgG-4 to TNF-α administered subcutaneously). Infliximab is effective against moderate to severe Crohn disease, fistulizing Crohn disease, and moderate to severe ulcerative colitis that has failed to respond to conventional therapy, as well as in patients who have ulcerative colitis with high-risk prognostic indicators. Adalimumab and certolizumab pegol are effective for moderate to severe Crohn disease that has failed to respond to conventional therapy, and adalimumab and golimumab are useful for moderate to severe ulcerative colitis that has failed to respond to conventional therapy or have high active disease with high-risk prognostic indicators.

In patients with early Crohn disease, timely use and escalation of anti–TNF-α treatment based on symptoms and biomarkers (e.g., a fecal calprotectin ≥250 μg/g of stool, a C-reactive protein level ≥5 mg/L, a Crohn Disease Activity Index ≥150 [E-Table 127-1], or prednisone use in the previous week) results in better clinical and endoscopic outcomes than does symptom-driven decisions alone. Before anti-TNF therapy is considered, however, risk versus benefit needs to be assessed in each individual patient, given the potential risks, including infection and malignancy.

Other Biologics

Natalizumab (a humanized IgG4 monoclonal antibody, against the α_4 subunit of $\alpha_4\beta_1$ and $\alpha_4\beta_7$ integrins expressed on all leukocytes except neutrophils) is useful for treatment of moderate to severe Crohn disease that is refractory to other therapies, but strict guidelines must be followed because of its associated risk for progressive multifocal leukoencephalopathy (Chapter 341). Another small adhesion molecule, vedolizumab (see Table 127-4) is used in patients who have

TABLE 127-4 MEDICAL THERAPIES FOR INFLAMMATORY BOWEL DISEASE

DRUG	DOSE	RELEASE SITE
5-AMINOSALICYLATES		
Sulfasalazine (Azulfidine)	2-6 g PO/day	Colon
Mesalamine (Asacol, Lialda, Apriso)	2.4-4.8 g PO/day	Distal ileum, colon
Olsalazine (Dipentum)	1-3 g PO/day	Colon
Balsalazide (Colazal)	6.25 g PO/day	Colon
Mesalamine (Pentasa)	2-4 g PO/day	Duodenum, jejunum, ileum, colon
Mesalamine (Rowasa), enema, suppository	4 g/day (enema) 1 g/day (suppository)	Rectum/sigmoid Rectum
Mesalamine (Canasa), suppository	1 g/day (suppository)	Rectum
CORTICOSTEROIDS		
Budesonide (Entocort EC)	Induction: 9 mg PO daily Maintenance: 6 mg PO daily	Small intestine
Budesonide (MMX, UCERIS)	Induction 9 mg PO daily	Colon
Budesonide (UCERIS foam)	2 mg budesonide per metered dose 1 metered dose administered twice daily for 2 weeks followed by 1 metered dose administered once daily for 4 weeks	Colon
Prednisone	0.25-0.75 mg/kg PO daily	Systemic
Methylprednisolone	40-60 mg IV daily	Systemic
IMMUNOMODULATORS		
Upadacitinib	45 mg PO once daily for 8 weeks then 15 mg PO a day further for at least 8 weeks. A maintenance dose of 30 mg PO once daily can be considered for patients who have refractory, severe, or extensive disease. Upadacitinib should be discontinued if an adequate therapeutic response is not achieved with the 30 mg dose	
Tofacitinib	10 mg PO twice daily for 8 weeks then 5 to 10 mg PO twice daily for 8 weeks further then 10 mg twice daily for at least 8 weeks; followed by 5 or 10 mg twice daily, depending on therapeutic response	Systemic
6-Mercaptopurine	1.5 mg PO/kg/day	Systemic
Azathioprine	2.5 mg PO/kg/day	Systemic
Methotrexate	Induction: 25 mg SQ weekly for 4 months Maintenance: 15-25 mg SQ weekly	Systemic
Cyclosporine	2-4 mg/kg/day IV	Systemic
Ozanimod	1 mg PO daily	Systemic
BIOLOGICS		
Infliximab	Induction: 5 mg/kg IV weeks 0, 2, 6 Maintenance: 5-10 mg/kg IV every 8 weeks	Systemic
Adalimumab	Induction: 160 mg SQ week 0, 80 mg week 2 Maintenance: 40 mg SQ every other week	Systemic
Golimumab	Induction: 200 mg SQ week 0 and 100 mg week 2 Maintenance: 100 mg SQ every 4 weeks	Systemic
Certolizumab pegol	Induction: 400 mg SQ weeks 0, 2, 4 Maintenance: 400 mg SQ every 4 weeks	Systemic
Natalizumab	300 mg IV every 4 weeks	Systemic
Vedolizumab	Induction: 300 mg IV at 0, 2, and 6 weeks Maintenance: 300 mg IV every 8 weeks	Systemic
Ustekinumab	Induction: intravenous: Up to 55 kg: 260 mg; greater than 55 kg to 85 kg: 390 mg; greater than 85 kg: 520 mg Maintenance: 90 mg SQ every 8 weeks	
Risankizumab	Induction: 600 mg IV at 0, 4, and 8 weeks Maintenance: 180 mg or 360 mg SQ at week 12 and every 8 weeks thereafter	

IV = intravenously; PO = orally; SQ = subcutaneously.

moderate to severe ulcerative colitis and adult patients with moderate to severe Crohn disease when one or more standard therapies (corticosteroids, immunomodulators, or TNF blocker medications) have not provided an adequate response. Ustekinumab (a monoclonal antibody to the p40 subunit of interleukin-12 and interleukin-23), used as intravenous induction therapy followed by subcutaneous maintenance therapy, can induce and maintain clinical remission in patients with moderately to severely active ulcerative colitis.[A7] Risankizumab (a monoclonal antibody to the p19 subunit of interleukin-23) given as an intravenous induction followed by subcutaneous maintenance therapy (see Table 127-4) can induce and maintain clinical remission in patients with moderately to severely active Crohn disease.[A8,A9] Ozanimod (an oral sphingosine phosphate agonist that reduces lymphocytes at 1 mg orally daily) has rapid onset of action and can induce and maintain remission in patients with moderate to severe ulcerative colitis.[A10]

Other Immunomodulators

The use of azathioprine, 6-mercaptopurine, and methotrexate has fallen out of favor as primary therapy for patients with ulcerative colitis and Crohn disease, because of the superior efficacies and safety profiles of biologic and other agents. These immunomodulators have a slow onset of action, often requiring several months of administration before their benefits are achieved, so they are used principally for maintenance of remission.

Azathioprine, the prodrug of 6-mercaptopurine, typically is prescribed at a dose of 2 to 3 mg/kg/day; the equivalent dose of 6-mercaptopurine is 1.5 mg/kg/day. Side effects include allergic reactions, pancreatitis, myelosuppression, nausea, infections, hepatotoxicity, and malignancy, especially lymphoma. The white blood cell count and liver chemistries must be monitored routinely. Methotrexate, which is a folic acid antagonist, is given as 25 mg intramuscularly or subcutaneously once per week for 16 weeks for active Crohn disease and 15 mg to 25 mg intramuscularly or subcutaneously once per week for maintaining remission. In addition to its use as primary therapy for Crohn disease, methotrexate has been used in conjunction with other biologic agents to reduce immunogenicity.

Antibiotics

The exact mechanism for the beneficial effect of broad-spectrum antibiotics in the treatment of inflammatory bowel disease is not known. Potential mechanisms include eliminating small intestinal bacterial overgrowth, eradicating a bacterially mediated antigenic trigger by altering the intestinal microbiome, and potential immunosuppressive properties (e.g., metronidazole). The primary role of antibiotics is in Crohn disease, where metronidazole (10 to 20 mg/kg/day for 4 to 8 weeks), ciprofloxacin (500 mg orally [PO] twice daily for 4 to 8 weeks), or both are primary inductive therapies for perianal fistulae. Antibiotics are not used as primary therapy for ulcerative colitis or luminal Crohn disease because they do not induce mucosal healing.

Crohn Disease Medical Therapy

Mild to Moderate Crohn Disease

Sulfasalazine (3 to 6 g/day) is superior to placebo for treating active symptoms of ileocolonic and colonic Crohn disease, with response rates ranging from 45 to 55% for mild to moderate disease.[14] However, sulfasalazine is not clearly effective for small bowel disease alone (Fig. 127-4) and has not been demonstrated to heal the colonic or ileal mucosa. For mild to moderate Crohn disease involving the distal small intestine or proximal colon, enteric-coated budesonide (9 mg/day) provides approximately a 70% response rate after 8 weeks and is significantly more effective than mesalamine (4 g/day) for distal ileal and right colonic disease. Early combined immunosuppression with an anti–TNF-α antagonist and an antimetabolite is more effective than conventional management and more effective than either agent as monotherapy.

Upper gastrointestinal Crohn disease (jejunal, duodenal, gastric, and esophageal) is uncommon, and few clinical trials are available to assess therapies for this location. Because local therapies such as 5-ASAs and budesonide are not released in these locations, systemic immunosuppressants (azathioprine, mercaptopurine, methotrexate, infliximab, adalimumab, and certolizumab pegol, natalizumab, vedolizumab, risankizumab, and ustekinumab; see Table 127-4 for doses) are the mainstays of therapy.[15] In the absence of comparative trials, initial therapy might include the use of anti-TNF therapy alone on in combination with an antimetabolite (6-mercaptopurine, azathioprine, or methotrexate), ustekinumab, risankizumab, or vedolizumab.

Moderate to Severe Crohn Disease

Patients with moderate to severe disease are often initially treated with systemic corticosteroids, but corticosteroids should not be used as maintenance therapy. Biologics can be used initially as therapy for patients with high-risk disease or severe disease activity.[16,17] A meta-analysis suggests that either adalimumab, infliximab plus azathioprine, or ustekinumab are the three most effective therapies for induction and maintenance of remission of Crohn disease.[A11] For example, infliximab (5 mg/kg at 0, 2, and 6 weeks and then every 8 weeks) alone or infliximab plus azathioprine (2.5 mg/kg/day) is more effective than azathioprine alone, and initial combined therapy (corticosteroids, daily azathioprine, and infliximab) is preferable to reserving it only for patients who do not respond to corticosteroids plus azathioprine or who have aggressive disease. However, the benefit of using these medications as combination therapy versus individual monotherapy must be assessed in the context of the potential risk of long-term use.

Of patients with Crohn disease who are treated for at least 1 year with infliximab and azathioprine, approximately 50% will experience a relapse within 1 year after discontinuation of infliximab. Given the significant escalated risk for lymphoma in patients under the age 35 years, especially in men, methotrexate is often used in place of azathioprine or 6-mercaptopurin in this patient population. Patients who do not respond to conventional therapy, including an anti-TNF agent (e.g., adalimumab or certolizumab pegol), may be considered for vedolizumab, ustekinumab, or natalizumab (see Table 127-4 for dosing).

For severe Crohn disease, patients should be hospitalized, given nothing by mouth, rehydrated with intravenous fluids, and administered parenteral corticosteroids. Patients who respond to parenteral corticosteroids should be switched to high-dose oral corticosteroids (prednisone, 40 to 60 mg/day), with the dose of prednisone gradually reduced. Patients who have severe Crohn disease and who do not respond to parenteral corticosteroids within 3 to 5 days should be considered for either infliximab or surgery. A course of total parenteral nutrition (Chapter 198) may be useful as adjunctive therapy.

Fistulizing Crohn Disease

Fistulas (Chapter 131) occur in one third of patients with Crohn disease, and perianal fistulas represent the most common location. Asymptomatic internal fistulas rarely require therapy. A concomitant abscess, which may occur in the setting of a fistula, must be excluded before initiating immunosuppressive therapy. Surgery may be required. Medical treatment depends on the location and associated complications.

High-output enterocutaneous fistulas in the setting of proximal small bowel involvement can lead to outputs of more than 500 mL/day and can cause severe volume depletion. Initial management requires volume repletion. In the postoperative setting, a fistulous opening is usually in the area of a wound, and it is imperative to protect the healing skin from infection caused by the drainage

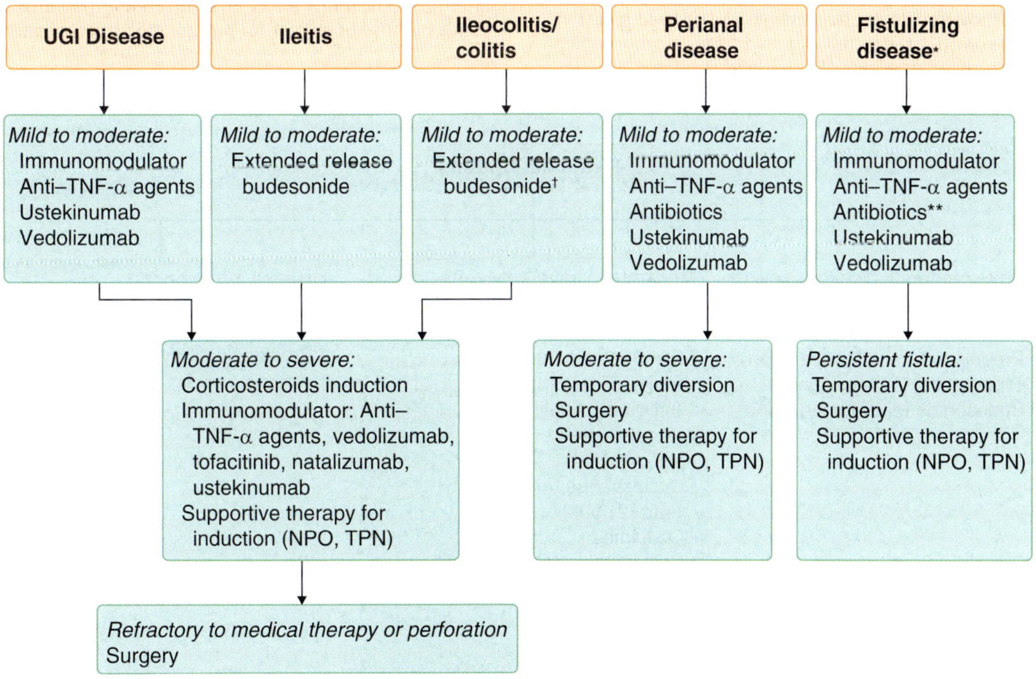

FIGURE 127-4. Crohn disease treatment algorithm. *Abscess should be excluded before initiating medical therapy. †Proximal colon disease involvement. **Perianal location. NPO = nothing by mouth; TNF-α = tumor necrosis factor-α; TPN = total parenteral nutrition; UGI = upper gastrointestinal.

from either an ostomy bag or a catheter used for a high-output fistula. High-output fistulas will rarely close spontaneously and typically will require surgical closure. Low-output fistulas are usually treated initially with anti–TNF-α therapy (e.g., infliximab, adalimumab, or certolizumab; see Table 127-4 for dosing).

Perianal fistulas are classified into simple and complex (Chapter 131). A simple fistula is located below the dentate line (i.e., most of the anal sphincter) and has one track. A complex fistula passes through the intersphincteric (high location), transsphincteric, or suprasphincteric region and may have multiple tracks. Simple fistulas respond well to medical therapy, initially with metronidazole (10 to 20 mg/kg/day PO for 4 to 8 weeks) and/or ciprofloxacin (500 mg PO twice daily for 4 to 8 weeks), but patients will also require additional treatment of the fistula and of any coexisting mucosal disease under expert supervision. Anti–TNF-α agents, ustekinumab, and vedolizumab (see Table 127-4 for dosing) are the first-line medical therapy. Patients with fistulas without rectal mucosal Crohn disease may respond well to fistulotomy, whereas patients with mucosal involvement may benefit from seton placement rather than fistulotomy. Complex fistulas usually require a combination of surgical and medical therapy. In the setting of intractable disease, colonic or ileal diversion may allow for rectal and perianal healing; in severe cases, proctocolectomy may be necessary.

For Crohn disease–related rectovaginal fistulas, medical therapy with anti–TNF-α agents (see Table 127-4 for dosing) or even azathioprine or 6-mercaptopurine is usually considered before surgery. Surgical therapy, such as fistulotomy and mucosal advancement flap surgery, may be considered.

Enterovesicular or colovesicular fistulas may be treated with antimetabolite therapy or anti–TNF-α agents, or both, but recurrent urinary tract infection is an indication for surgery. Surgery usually involves resection of involved bowel and closure of the bladder defect.

Asymptomatic internal fistulas, such as enteroenteric fistulas, do not require surgical intervention, but treatment with an anti-TNF agent (see Table 127-4 for dosing) or perhaps azathioprine or 6-mercaptopurine and/or a biologic agent may be considered. Internal fistulas, such as cologastric and coloduodenal, may cause substantial symptoms because of bypass of part of the intestine. If medical management fails or if an abscess forms, surgery is recommended.

Medical Management of Ulcerative Colitis

The decision guiding which therapy is appropriate for a specific patient with ulcerative colitis is dependent upon several factors, including anatomic distribution of disease; severity of disease activity; and risk (prognosis) of disease (Figure 127-5).[18] When focusing on anatomic distribution of ulcerative colitis as a guide to therapies, several options exist, including suppositories, retention enemas, topical foam, oral therapy, and parenteral therapy. Suppositories are effective to treat proctitis in the distal 20 cm of the colon. Topical foam and enemas are effective for distal and left-sided colitis. Oral therapy and parenteral therapy are effective for all locations of disease.[19]

Proctitis

For active ulcerative proctitis, topical 5-ASA (enema and suppository) in combination with oral treatment is superior to oral treatment alone.[20] Topical 5-ASA is superior to topical corticosteroids for treatment of active ulcerative proctitis; rectal 5-ASA therapy produces a faster response when given with oral 5-ASA. Corticosteroid enemas, suppositories, or foam[A12] also can be used if 5-ASA fails. 5-ASA or corticosteroid retention enemas can be used for active disease up to the splenic flexure (i.e., the rectum, sigmoid colon, and descending colon). Another approach to proctitis or distal colitis is an oral aminosalicylate, although a response may not be evident for 3 to 4 weeks. Additionally, once-a-day extended-release budesonide (budesonide MMX) and topical budesonide foam[A13] are effective for mild to moderately active ulcerative proctosigmoiditis, with fewer steroid-related side effects than conventional corticosteroids.

Extensive Colitis, Mild to Moderate

In patients with mild to moderate activity ulcerative colitis extending proximal to the splenic flexure, the initial drug of choice is an oral 5-ASA; efficacy increases with increasing doses. Even with more extensive disease, supplementation of oral 5-ASA with 5-ASA enemas or suppositories may help reduce the symptoms of fecal urgency that result from rectal involvement, and budesonide MMX provides incremental benefit. In patients with more than five or six bowel movements per day, in patients in whom a more rapid response is desired, or in patients who have not responded to 3 to 4 weeks of 5-ASA, the treatment of choice is oral corticosteroids. Patients with severe diarrhea, systemic symptoms, or significant amounts of blood in their stool should be started on prednisone 40 mg/day; most patients respond to oral corticosteroids within a few days. After the symptoms are controlled, prednisone can be tapered gradually by 5 mg every 1 to 2 weeks. Patients who respond to oral prednisone and can be fully withdrawn from it should be maintained on 5-ASA.

Severe Colitis

If patients with severe ulcerative colitis do not begin to respond to corticosteroids at the equivalent dose of methylprednisolone 60 mg IV within 3 to 5 days or do not completely respond within 7 to 10 days, options include colectomy, infliximab, or cyclosporine[21] (see Table 127-4 for dosing). Tofacitinib (10 mg twice daily) also can improve symptoms and maintain remission in patients with moderate to severe active ulcerative colitis.[22] Ozanimod (1 mg orally daily) also is effective in this situation for inducing and maintaining remission.

For patients whose disease flares whenever the corticosteroids are withdrawn or their corticosteroid dose is lowered, temptation to continue high-dose corticosteroid must be avoided. If the patient requires a substantial dose (>15 mg/day of prednisone) for more than 4 months, a trial of a biologic agent (infliximab, adalimumab, golimumab, vedolizumab, or ustekinumab) or an immunomodulator (azathioprine, mercaptopurine, ozanimod, tofacitinib, or upadacitinib) should be considered for maintenance of remission.[A14-A16] All those agents are efficacious, but vedolizumab may be the most efficacious and safe option.[A17] The choice among these agents requires expert guidance and consideration of the presence or absence of extraintestinal manifestations, the severity of the disease, the presence or absence of other comorbid conditions, the patient's preferences, and insurance coverage. Attempts should be made to reduce the steroid dose, and the goal of treatment is complete steroid withdrawal.

Fecal microbial transplantation is an experimental approach to the treatment of ulcerative colitis. Data so far are promising but inconclusive.[23]

Acute Flare

The most common indication for hospitalization in patients with ulcerative colitis is intractable diarrhea, although blood loss is also common. Patients with severely active ulcerative colitis should be evaluated for toxic megacolon by abdominal radiography or CT. Antidiarrheal medications and anticholinergic medications are contraindicated in patients with severe ulcerative colitis because of the risk for precipitating toxic megacolon. The mainstays of

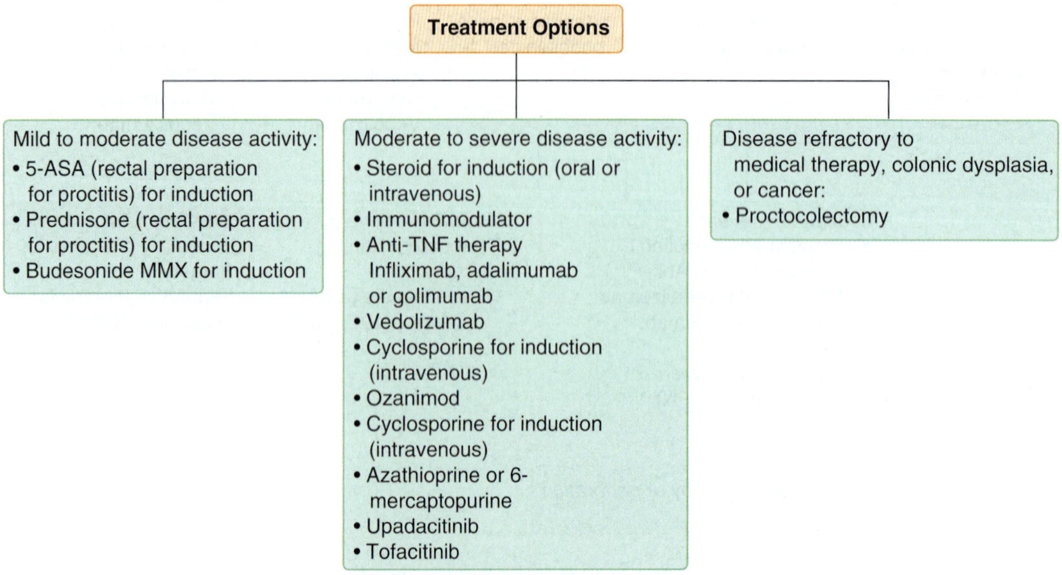

FIGURE 127-5. Ulcerative colitis treatment algorithm. 5-ASA = 5-aminosalicylic acid; MMX = multi-matrix system; TNF = tumor necrosis factor.

therapy for severe ulcerative colitis are rehydration with intravenous fluids and intravenous corticosteroids (hydrocortisone, 300 mg/day; prednisolone, 60 to 80 mg/day; or methylprednisolone, 40 to 60 mg/day). Total parenteral nutrition (Chapter 198) may be necessary in patients with malnutrition. Patients with peritoneal signs or signs of systemic infection should be treated with parenteral antibiotics (Chapter 128). Patients who do not respond in 3 to 5 days should be considered for either colectomy, a trial of intravenous cyclosporines, or a trial of infliximab (see Table 127-4 for dosing).

Maintenance Therapy

Aminosalicylates reduce recurrent disease in patients with ulcerative colitis, and essentially all patients should receive maintenance therapy with a 5-ASA preparation. However, the utility of 5-ASA preparations in patients who are using biologic agents is less well established, and data suggest that once a patient initiates a biologic, aminosalicylates do not add clinical benefit and can be discontinued. Corticosteroids are not effective as maintenance therapy and should not be used in this way. Azathioprine, 6-mercaptopurine, tofacitinib, upadacitinib, ozanimod, infliximab, adalimumab (160 mg at week 0, 80 mg at week 2, and then 40 mg every other week), ustekinumab, and golimumab (see Table 127-4 for dosing) are effective for maintenance therapy in patients whose ulcerative colitis is not controlled by 5-ASA.

Surgical Therapy

Crohn Disease

Since surgical resection does not cure Crohn disease and recurrences are likely after resection, the approach should be conservative in terms of the amount of bowel resected. Failure of medical management is a common cause for resection in patients with Crohn disease, but complications (e.g., obstruction, fistula, and abscess) are often the indications for resection. Overall, the overall 1-, 5-, and 10-year risks of surgery in patients with Crohn disease are about 12%, 18%, and 26%.

For Crohn disease of the small bowel, the most common surgical procedure is segmental resection for obstruction or fistula; the incidence of a recurrence severe enough to require repeat surgery after ileal or ileocolic resection is approximately 25% after 10 years and 35% after 15 years in the absence of biologic therapies. For patients with extensive colonic disease that includes the rectum, the procedure of choice is total proctocolectomy with a Brooke (end) ileostomy. Total colectomy with ileal pouch anal anastomosis is not appropriate in Crohn colitis because recurrent disease in the ileal segment of the new pouch would require a repeat operation and loss of a long segment of ileum. Anti-TNF monotherapy (e.g., infliximab, adalimumab, or certolizumab; see Table 127-4 for dosing) appears to be the most effective strategy for postoperative prophylaxis for Crohn disease,[A18] but ustekinumab and vedolizumab (see Table 127-4 for dosing) also may be effective.

Ulcerative Colitis

For ulcerative colitis, colectomy is a curative procedure. Emergency colectomy may be required in patients with toxic megacolon or a severe fulminant attack without toxic megacolon. Fortunately better medical therapy has substantially reduced the need for colectomy for refractory disease to about 3% at one year, 7% after 5 years, at 10% after 10 years.[24] The decision for or against colectomy and among types of surgery requires expert consultation. The standard operation for ulcerative colitis is proctocolectomy and a Brooke ileostomy, but creating a pouch from the terminal 30 cm of ileum and pulling the distal end of the pouch through the anal canal can preserve anal function and avoid an ileostomy. Ileoanal anastomosis is sometimes complicated by inflammation in the ileal pouch (termed *pouchitis*), which can be treated with antibiotics (typically, metronidazole, 500 mg three times daily or 20 mg/kg/day, or ciprofloxacin, 500 mg twice daily for 2 weeks). The risk for malignancy (see later) also can be an indication for colectomy.

Complications

Crohn Disease

Abscesses

Abscesses, which are common complications in Crohn disease, result from extension of a mucosal fissure or ulcer through the intestinal wall and into extraintestinal tissue. Leakage of intestinal contents through a fissure into the peritoneal cavity results in an abscess. Abscesses occur in 15 to 20% of patients with Crohn disease, especially in the terminal ileum. The typical clinical manifestation of an intra-abdominal abscess is fever, abdominal pain, abdominal tenderness, and leukocytosis. A CT scan is the preferred modality to diagnose intra-abdominal abscess. Broad-spectrum antibiotic therapy, including anaerobic coverage, is indicated. Percutaneous drainage of abscesses in patients with Crohn disease may improve the clinical picture but does not provide adequate therapy because of persistent communication between the abscess cavity and the intestinal lumen. Resection of the involved intestine is usually required for definitive therapy.

Obstruction

Obstruction is a common complication of Crohn disease, particularly in the small intestine, and is a leading indication for surgery. In Crohn disease, mucosal thickening from acute inflammation, muscular hyperplasia and scarring as a result of previous inflammation, or adhesions may cause small bowel obstruction. Obstruction also may occur because of impaction of a bolus of fibrous food in a stable, long-standing stricture. Cramping abdominal pain and diarrhea, which worsen after meals and resolve with fasting, suggest obstruction. Strictures may be evaluated by CT enterography, MRI enterography, oral contrast studies, barium enema, or colonoscopy, depending on the anatomic location. Corticosteroids (e.g., methylprednisolone, 40 to 60 mg/day IV, or hydrocortisone, 200 to 300 mg/day IV for 5 to 14 days) are useful if acute inflammation is an important component of the obstructive process, but not if the obstruction is caused by fibrosis. A common error in the management of Crohn disease is inappropriate treatment with long courses of corticosteroids in patients who have obstructive symptoms from fixed anatomic lesions. If the obstruction does not resolve with nasogastric suction and corticosteroids, surgery is necessary.[25]

Perianal Disease

Perianal disease is a potentially disabling complication of Crohn disease. Ulcerations in the anal canal may coalesce and result in fistula formation (Chapter 131). The fistulous openings are most commonly found in the perianal skin but can occur in the groin, vulva, or scrotum. Fistulas are accompanied by drainage of serous or purulent material. If the fistula does not drain freely, there is local accumulation of pus (perianal abscess) with redness, pain, and induration. The pain of a perianal abscess is exacerbated by local pressure that may result from defecation, sitting, or walking. The typical physical manifestation of an abscess is redness with tenderness on digital examination; fluctuance also may be present. Persistent severe perianal Crohn disease can result in destruction of the anal sphincter and subsequent fecal incontinence. Adequate evaluation of perianal disease generally requires endoscopic examination under anesthesia. Cross-sectional CT or MRI can define the presence and extent of perianal abscesses. The goals of therapy for perianal disease are relief of local symptoms and preservation of the sphincter. Limited disease can be approached with sitz baths and metronidazole, but most cases also require adequate external drainage. Infliximab, adalimumab, certolizumab pegol, ustekinumab, vedolizumab, azathioprine, or 6-mercaptopurine (see Table 127-4 for dosing) may be useful in healing perianal disease, but the disease may reactivate when the drug is stopped. Allogeneic, expanded, adipose-derived stem cells are an experimental treatment for complex perianal fistulas in patients whose Crohn disease does not respond to conventional or biologic treatments or both.

Ulcerative Colitis

One of the most significant complications of ulcerative colitis is toxic megacolon, which is dilation of the colon to a diameter greater than 6 cm associated with worsening of the patient's clinical condition and the development of fever, tachycardia, and leukocytosis. Physical examination may reveal postural hypotension, abdominal tenderness over the distribution of the colon, and absent or hypoactive bowel sounds. Agents that reduce gastrointestinal motility, such as antispasmodics and antidiarrheal agents, have the potential to initiate or exacerbate toxic megacolon. Medical therapy is designed to reduce the likelihood of perforation and return the colon to normal motor activity as rapidly as possible. The patient is given nothing by mouth, and nasogastric suction is begun. Intravenous fluids should be administered to replete water and electrolyte abnormalities, broad-spectrum antibiotics (e.g., ampicillin-sulbactam, given as 1 g ampicillin plus 0.5 g sulbactam, 1.5 to 3 g every 6 hours for 5 to 14 days; levofloxacin, 500 mg/day IV, plus metronidazole, 500 mg IV or PO twice daily; cefazolin, 500 mg IV three times daily, plus metronidazole, 500 mg IV or PO twice daily; or trimethoprim-sulfamethoxazole, 8 to 10 mg/kg/day IV or PO in two to four divided doses, plus metronidazole, 500 mg IV or PO twice daily for approximately 7 days or until symptomatic improvement) are given in anticipation of possible peritonitis as a result of perforation, and parenteral corticosteroids are administered at a dose equivalent to more than 40 to 60 mg of prednisone per day. Signs of improvement include a decrease in abdominal girth and the return of bowel sounds. Deterioration is marked by the development of rebound tenderness, increasing abdominal girth, and cardiovascular collapse. If the patient does not begin to show signs of clinical improvement during the first 24 to 48 hours of medical therapy, the risk for perforation increases markedly, and surgical colectomy is indicated.

Follow-Up

Colon Cancer, Dysplasia, and Colonoscopic Surveillance

The risk for colorectal cancer (Chapter 179) is increased beginning after 8 years of disease and continues to increase in subsequent years.[26] The incidence of colorectal adenocarcinoma is 60 to 100% higher in persons with inflammatory bowel disease than in the general population but has been decreasing over time, likely at least in part because of advances in modern therapies. Patients with extensive ulcerative colitis have a markedly increased risk for colon cancer, patients with left-sided disease have an intermediate risk, and patients with long-standing ulcerative colitis are at risk for colorectal cancer even if their symptoms have been relatively mild or even quiescent for 10 to 15 years.

Colon cancers may be submucosal and may be missed at colonoscopy. Colon cancer in patients with ulcerative colitis is most commonly associated with dysplastic changes in the mucosa, often at multiple sites in the colon. Although recent data have demonstrated that most dysplasia is visible, not all dysplasia can be identified by visual inspection, so microscopic examination of biopsy specimens is required.

In patients with long-standing ulcerative colitis, current practice guidelines recommend colonoscopy with surveillance using chromoendoscopy or narrow band imaging, with biopsies of abnormal lesions or random colon biopsies, beginning 8 years after the onset of disease and repeated every 1 to 2 years.[27] If the specimens show dysplasia and if a discrete polypoid lesion with well-defined borders cannot be identified, colectomy is recommended.[28]

The risk for colon cancer in patients with Crohn colitis is similar to the risk in patients with a similar extent of ulcerative colitis. Surveillance colonoscopy is also recommended in patients with Crohn colitis.

Pregnancy

Fertility in women with inflammatory bowel disease usually is normal or only minimally impaired, and the incidence of prematurity, stillbirth, and developmental defects in the offspring of women with inflammatory bowel disease, except fetal complications may be somewhat more likely when the mother's disease is clinically active, regardless of drug therapy. Previous proctocolectomy or the presence of an ileostomy is not an impediment to successful completion of a pregnancy, but women who have had ileal pouch anal anastomosis surgery with a total proctocolectomy have markedly reduced fertility.

If a woman's disease is inactive at the time of conception, it is likely that it will remain inactive during the course of the pregnancy. Ulcerative colitis that is active at the time of conception tends to worsen. In patients with active Crohn disease at the time of conception, the degree of activity remains the same in two thirds of women; of the other one third, some improve clinically and others deteriorate.

Sulfasalazine does not harm the fetus, but pregnant women have an increased requirement for folic acid and sulfasalazine interferes with folate absorption by competitively inhibiting the jejunal enzyme folate conjugase. Therefore, women who are taking sulfasalazine and who are pregnant or considering pregnancy should receive folate supplementation (1 mg twice daily) to ensure that the fetus receives adequate amounts for normal development. The use of corticosteroids by pregnant women with inflammatory bowel disease is associated with an increased rate of premature rupture of the membranes and a higher rate of cleft lip. In general, it appears that the risk to the pregnancy of treatment with sulfasalazine or corticosteroids is less than the risk in allowing disease activity to go untreated.

Most of the data on the teratogenicity of azathioprine and 6-mercaptopurine in pregnancy are derived from the transplant literature and involve higher doses than are commonly used for inflammatory bowel disease. Reported fetal effects in the transplant population include congenital malformations, immunosuppression, prematurity, and growth retardation. The risks of these medications in the inflammatory bowel disease population are not completely known, given that only a small number of such patients have been formally studied.

Infliximab, adalimumab, golimumab, certolizumab pegol, vedolizumab, and ustekinumab are considered to be safe during pregnancy, but the risks of these agents are not completely known, because only a relatively small number of patients have been formally studied. To date, data are inadequate to assess fetal risk and guide therapy with ozanimod upadacitinib, and tofacitinib during pregnancy.

PROGNOSIS

Ulcerative Colitis

Recurrent flares and remissions characterize typical ulcerative colitis. A rapidly progressive initial attack results in serious complications in approximately 10% of patients. Complete recovery after a single attack may occur in another 10% of patients. Some patients may actually have had an acute undetected infection rather than true ulcerative colitis. The probability that a patient with clinically inactive disease will remain in remission the following year is 80 to 90%. By comparison, patients with clinically active disease have a 70% probability of relapse during the following year.

Patients who present with ulcerative proctitis have the best overall prognosis, and only approximately 5% of patients with proctitis will require colectomy over a lifetime. Severe complications are very uncommon, but the disease will extend more proximally in the colon in up to 50% of patients. Ulcerative colitis–related mortality has decreased substantially since the introduction of corticosteroids, and recent studies suggest that long-term survival rates for patients with ulcerative colitis are similar to those of the general population.

Crohn Disease

The manifestations of Crohn disease can wax and wane. A patient with clinically active Crohn disease has a 70 to 80% chance of having active disease in the subsequent year, whereas 80% of patients in remission will remain so over the following year. Over the course of a 4-year period, approximately 25% of patients will have persistently active disease after diagnosis, 25% will remain in remission, and 50% will have a fluctuating course with years of remission and years with clinically active disease. Approximately 75 to 80% of all patients with luminal and fistulizing Crohn disease will require surgical intervention for their disease, with approximately 50% of them requiring surgery within 6 months of diagnosis. The rate for a second surgery for luminal Crohn disease ranges from 25 to 38% within 5 years, and 40 to 70% will need reoperation by 15 years.

Patients with Crohn disease have an increased mortality rate, approximately 1.3 to 1.5 times higher than the general population, unrelated to whether they have small intestine or large intestine involvement, or both. This excess mortality, which is most notable in the first few years after diagnosis, is most commonly related to complications of Crohn disease (e.g., colorectal cancer, shock, volume depletion, protein-calorie malnutrition, and anemia). Whether aggressive use of immunomodulators and biologic therapy will alter the natural course of disease is unknown.

GENERAL REFERENCES

For the General References and other additional features, please visit Elsevier eBooks+ at https://ebooks.health.elsevier.com.

Grade A References

A1. Wang Y, Parker CE, Feagan BG, et al. Oral 5-aminosalicylic acid for maintenance of remission in ulcerative colitis. *Cochrane Database Syst Rev.* 2016;5:CD000544.

A2. Wang Y, Parker CE, Bhanji T, et al. Oral 5-aminosalicylic acid for induction of remission in ulcerative colitis. *Cochrane Database Syst Rev.* 2016;4:CD000543.

A3. Barberio B, Gracie DJ, Black CJ, et al. Efficacy of biological therapies and small molecules in induction and maintenance of remission in luminal Crohn's disease: systematic review and network meta-analysis. *Gut.* 2022;72:264-274.

A4. Burr NE, Gracie DJ, Black CJ, et al. Efficacy of biological therapies and small molecules in moderate to severe ulcerative colitis: systematic review and network meta-analysis. *Gut.* 2022;71:1976-1987.

A5. Sandborn WJ, Su C, Sands BE, et al. Tofacitinib as induction and maintenance therapy for ulcerative colitis. *N Engl J Med.* 2017;376:1723-1736.

A6. Danese S, Vermeire S, Zhou W, et al. Upadacitinib as induction and maintenance therapy for moderately to severely active ulcerative colitis: results from three phase 3, multicentre, double-blind, randomised trials. *Lancet.* 2022;399:2113-2128.

A7. Sands BE, Sandborn WJ, Panaccione R, et al. Ustekinumab as induction and maintenance therapy for ulcerative colitis. *N Engl J Med.* 2019;381:1201-1214.

A8. Ferrante M, Panaccione R, Baert F, et al. Risankizumab as maintenance therapy for moderately to severely active Crohn's disease: results from the multicentre, randomised, double-blind, placebo-controlled, withdrawal phase 3 FORTIFY maintenance trial. *Lancet.* 2022;399:2031-2046.

A9. D'Haens G, Panaccione R, Baert F, et al. Risankizumab as induction therapy for Crohn's disease: results from the phase 3 ADVANCE and MOTIVATE induction trials. *Lancet.* 2022;399:2015-2030.

A10. Sandborn WJ, Feagan BG, D'Haens G, et al. Ozanimod as induction and maintenance therapy for ulcerative colitis. *N Engl J Med.* 2021;385:1280-1291.

A11. Singh S, Murad MH, Fumery M, et al. Comparative efficacy and safety of biologic therapies for moderate-to-severe Crohn's disease: a systematic review and network meta-analysis. *Lancet Gastroenterol Hepatol.* 2021;6:1002-1014.

A12. Sandborn WJ, Bosworth B, Zakko S, et al. Budesonide foam induces remission in patients with mild to moderate ulcerative proctitis and ulcerative proctosigmoiditis. *Gastroenterology.* 2015;148:740-750.

A13. Sandborn WJ, Bosworth B, Zakko S, et al. Budesonide foam induces remission in patients with mild to moderate ulcerative proctitis and ulcerative proctosigmoiditis. *Gastroenterology.* 2015;148:740-750.

A14. Archer R, Tappenden P, Ren S, et al. Infliximab, adalimumab and golimumab for treating moderately to severely active ulcerative colitis after the failure of conventional therapy (including a review of TA140 and TA262): clinical effectiveness systematic review and economic model. *Health Technol Assess.* 2016;20:1-326.

A15. Sands BE, Peyrin-Biroulet L, Loftus EV Jr, et al. Vedolizumab versus adalimumab for moderate-to-severe ulcerative colitis. *N Engl J Med.* 2019;381:1215-1226.

A16. Sands BE, Sandborn WJ, Panaccione R, et al. Ustekinumab as induction and maintenance therapy for ulcerative colitis. *N Engl J Med.* 2019;381:1201-1214.

A17. Lasa JS, Olivera PA, Danese S, et al. Efficacy and safety of biologics and small molecule drugs for patients with moderate-to-severe ulcerative colitis: a systematic review and network meta-analysis. *Lancet Gastroenterol Hepatol.* 2022;7:161-170.

A18. Singh S, Garg SK, Pardi DS, et al. Comparative efficacy of pharmacologic interventions in preventing relapse of Crohn's disease after surgery: a systematic review and network meta-analysis. *Gastroenterology.* 2015;148:64-76.

128

INFLAMMATORY AND ANATOMIC DISEASES OF THE INTESTINE, PERITONEUM, MESENTERY, AND OMENTUM

JOHN F. KUEMMERLE

CONGENITAL STRUCTURAL ABNORMALITIES

MECKEL DIVERTICULUM

Meckel diverticulum, which is the most common congenital anomaly of the gastrointestinal (GI) tract, is present in 2 to 3% of the population and is more common in men. Meckel diverticulum occurs when the omphalomesenteric or vitelline duct connecting the fetal yolk sac to the primordial gut fails to close during development. Located on the antimesenteric border, the Meckel diverticulum is commonly found within about 100 cm of the ileocecal valve and typically is 1 to 10 cm in size. Heterotopic tissue is found in about 50% of Meckel diverticula, most commonly gastric or pancreatic tissue but usually not both. The presence of heterotopic tissue correlates with the development of symptomatic complications, with a lifetime risk of about 6%.

CLINICAL MANIFESTATIONS

The complications from a Meckel diverticulum include lower GI bleeding, obstruction, diverticulitis, and perforation.[1] Bleeding can occur when the production of acid from heterotopic gastric mucosa causes ileal ulcerations. Obstruction can result from volvulus around the diverticulum, intussusception of the diverticulum into the intestine, or herniation of the diverticulum and adjacent intestine. Inguinal, femoral, and umbilical hernias all can occur. Repeated and chronic inflammation at the neck of the diverticulum and nearby ileum also can lead to intestinal fibrosis and bowel obstruction. The most common complications are intestinal bleeding in children and obstruction in adults.

DIAGNOSIS

The diagnosis of a Meckel diverticulum can be challenging. Radionuclide imaging with sodium pertechnetate (^{99m}Tn) can be used in cases of bleeding because both normal and heterotopic gastric mucosa take up the tracer (Fig. 128-1). This test has high sensitivity and specificity in children but higher rates of false-positive and false-negative tests in adults. Crohn disease (Chapter 127) and other ileal inflammatory diseases can yield false-positive results. Radiographic imaging with a barium small bowel follow-through typically is not helpful because the diverticulum does not fill with barium contrast. Enteroclysis increases the yield of barium imaging by increasing the pressure and filling of the diverticulum. Angiography can visualize the vestigial vitelline artery that arises from the superior mesenteric artery or a superior mesenteric artery branch that directly feeds the diverticulum or adjacent ileum. Both small bowel capsule endoscopy (Chapter 120) and double-balloon enteroscopy can identify a Meckel diverticulum during the evaluation of obscure bleeding.

TREATMENT AND PROGNOSIS

The management of bleeding, obstruction, or perforation that occurs in association with a Meckel diverticulum is open or laparoscopic surgical resection of the diverticulum and possibly of adjacent ulcerated and bleeding ileum. The surgical resection of a Meckel diverticulum incidentally identified at the time of surgery for another condition is controversial given the low lifetime risk of complications but can be considered in young men, patients with large diverticula, or patients with suspected heterotopic tissue. After identification and treatment, the prognosis is excellent because the Meckel diverticulum is removed, and the risk of complications is eliminated.

INTESTINAL ATRESIA AND STENOSIS, MALROTATION, GASTROSCHISIS, AND OMPHALOCELE

The congenital disorders of intestinal atresia and stenosis, malrotation, gastroschisis, and omphalocele disorders usually present early in infancy and childhood, but sometimes the diagnosis of stenosis or malrotation may

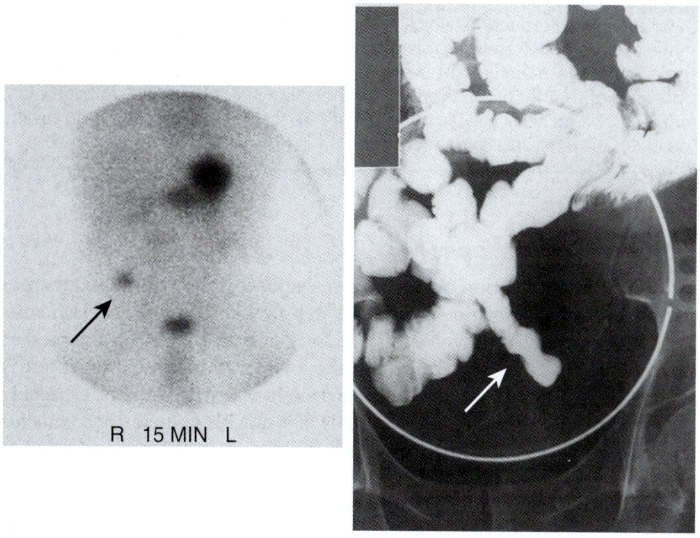

FIGURE 128-1. **Meckel diverticulum. Nuclear medicine imaging with ^{99m}Tn pertechnetate scan shows tracer uptake in a Meckel diverticulum (*arrow* in left panel) and in the stomach and bladder. Barium radiography in the same patient also shows the Meckel diverticulum (*arrow* in right panel).**

be made in adulthood. With the exception of pyloric stenosis, significant long-term morbidity and mortality are associated with these anomalies even after surgical correction. Patients with malrotation or gastroschisis typically present with complications of their surgery, including adhesions, bowel obstruction, or abdominal wall hernias. Patients with intestinal atresia and resulting short gut syndrome also have significant morbidity and mortality related to intestinal failure and the need for long-term total parenteral nutrition.

ACQUIRED STRUCTURAL DISORDERS

VOLVULUS

Intestinal volvulus, which is pathologic twisting of the intestine around the mesentery, can result in obstruction of the proximal bowel. Because the mesentery is involved, possible complications include vascular compromise, bowel necrosis, bowel perforation, and peritonitis. The most susceptible regions for volvulus are the sigmoid colon, cecum, and occasionally the transverse colon, with an estimated annual incidence of two to six cases per 100,000. Sigmoid volvulus is most common in men, with a peak age in the 80s, whereas cecal volvulus is more common in women, who typically present in their 60s. Elderly institutionalized individuals are at the highest risk. Small bowel volvulus is uncommonly observed in U.S. adults but can result from preexisting anomalies such as malrotation or congenital bands of Ladd.

CLINICAL MANIFESTATIONS

Volvulus can present with symptoms and signs of acute bowel obstruction, including pain that may be out of proportion to physical findings. Nausea and vomiting are usually present. The presentation also can be more insidious or intermittent with constipation, laxative use, and a previously recognized dilated colon. Physical findings include abdominal distention, tympanic percussion, rebound, guarding, and rigidity. Escalating pain and tenderness can indicate colonic ischemia and perforation.

DIAGNOSIS

The diagnosis of colonic volvulus can be made using abdominal radiographs, which demonstrate a distended colon, loss of haustrations, and a typical "bent inner tube" sign with the apex in the right upper quadrant of the abdomen (Fig. 128-2A) or the "omega" sign (Fig. 128-2B). In cases of a cecal volvulus, the dilated cecum is observed in the epigastrium or in the left upper quadrant. A water-soluble contrast-enhanced radiograph can identify the point of obstruction due to volvulus.

TREATMENT AND PROGNOSIS

Patients with colonic volvulus should have nothing per oral cavity (NPO) with nasogastric (NG) tube decompression and receive appropriate fluid volume resuscitation. In the absence of complete obstruction or signs of ischemia or perforation, patients with a sigmoid volvulus can undergo emergent colonoscopy and attempted reduction, which is successful in up to 75% of cases.[2] Surgical intervention is indicated for volvulus involving the cecum, transverse colon, or small intestine, as well as after colonoscopic reduction of a sigmoid volvulus because of the risk of recurrence. The mortality rate is about 9% for sigmoid volvulus, 7% for cecal volvulus, and about 17% for combined sigmoid and cecal volvulus or transverse colon volvulus.

INTUSSUSCEPTION

Intestinal intussusception occurs when a segment of bowel invaginates into the adjacent distal intestine and results in bowel obstruction and ischemia. Intussusception usually involves just the small intestine, but it can also present as small intestinal intussusception into the colon. Although intussusception is a common cause of small bowel obstruction in pediatric patients, especially after rotavirus vaccination (Chapter 350), it is rare in adults and accounts for only about 5% of small bowel obstruction. The cause of intussusception is infrequently identified in children, but a cause can be identified in about 90% of adult cases. Typical precipitating causes in adults include small intestinal polyps, benign tumors (including leiomyomas and neurofibromas), malignant tumors, inflammatory bowel disease (Chapter 127), postoperative adhesions, Meckel diverticulum, and feeding tubes.[3]

CLINICAL MANIFESTATIONS

Most patients present with symptoms of partial bowel obstruction, including pain, nausea, and vomiting, and some patients have diarrhea with occult or overt bleeding. The clinical picture can be confusing when the patient has intermittent symptoms from a spontaneously resolved event. A mass may be palpable on examination. Passage of "currant jelly" stools is characteristic of intussusception, especially in children.

DIAGNOSIS

The diagnosis of intussusception is usually made using computed tomography (CT), which reveals a characteristic alternating high- and low-attenuation target-like or sausage-shaped lesion that represents the invaginated intestinal segments. However, because of the confusing presentation of intussusception in adults, a combination of plain radiographs, upper GI series, and barium enema frequently is required for an adequate evaluation.

TREATMENT AND PROGNOSIS

Colonic intussusceptions are treated surgically in adults because of the high likelihood that a colonic malignancy is the causative lesion. For small intestinal intussusception, a randomized trial showed that hydrostatic reduction is superior to pneumatic reduction in children.[A1] This approach has been tried in adults in whom no other significant causative lesion is present. However, adults with small intestinal intussusception frequently have an underlying pathologic cause, so their treatment consists primarily of surgical intervention and bowel resection, which not only resolves the obstruction but also provides a diagnosis of the causative lesion. If the predisposing cause can be diagnosed and corrected, the prognosis is good, and recurrence rates are low. If the underlying cause is not fully correctable such as with neurofibromatosis (Chapter 385) or adhesions, intussusceptions may recur.

HERNIAS

Anatomically, hernias comprise a herniated viscus, the hernial sac (internal wall of the hernia lined by peritoneum), and the hernial ring. Whereas an external hernia occurs when the viscus lies outside the abdomen, an internal hernia occurs when the viscus lies in an abnormal location within the abdominal cavity. Secondary hernias can occur at previous sites of incision or injury. Incisional, inguinal, and umbilical hernias comprise 90% of all hernias. Hernias are common and occur in about 5% of the population within their lifetimes. For inguinal hernias alone, the lifetime cumulative incidence is estimated to be 43% in men and 6% in women. By comparison, femoral, umbilical, and incisional hernias occur twice as often in women.

CLINICAL MANIFESTATIONS, DIAGNOSIS, AND TREATMENT OF SPECIFIC HERNIAS

Epigastric hernias

Epigastric hernias occur at sites of congenital weakness in the midline between the xiphoid and umbilicus along the linea alba. Small epigastric hernias may be asymptomatic or difficult to identify. Larger epigastric hernias can present as nodules, sometimes with tenderness. Multiple hernias may be present. Diagnosis is made by physical examination complemented by ultrasound or CT imaging. They can be repaired surgically if symptomatic or if complications are present.

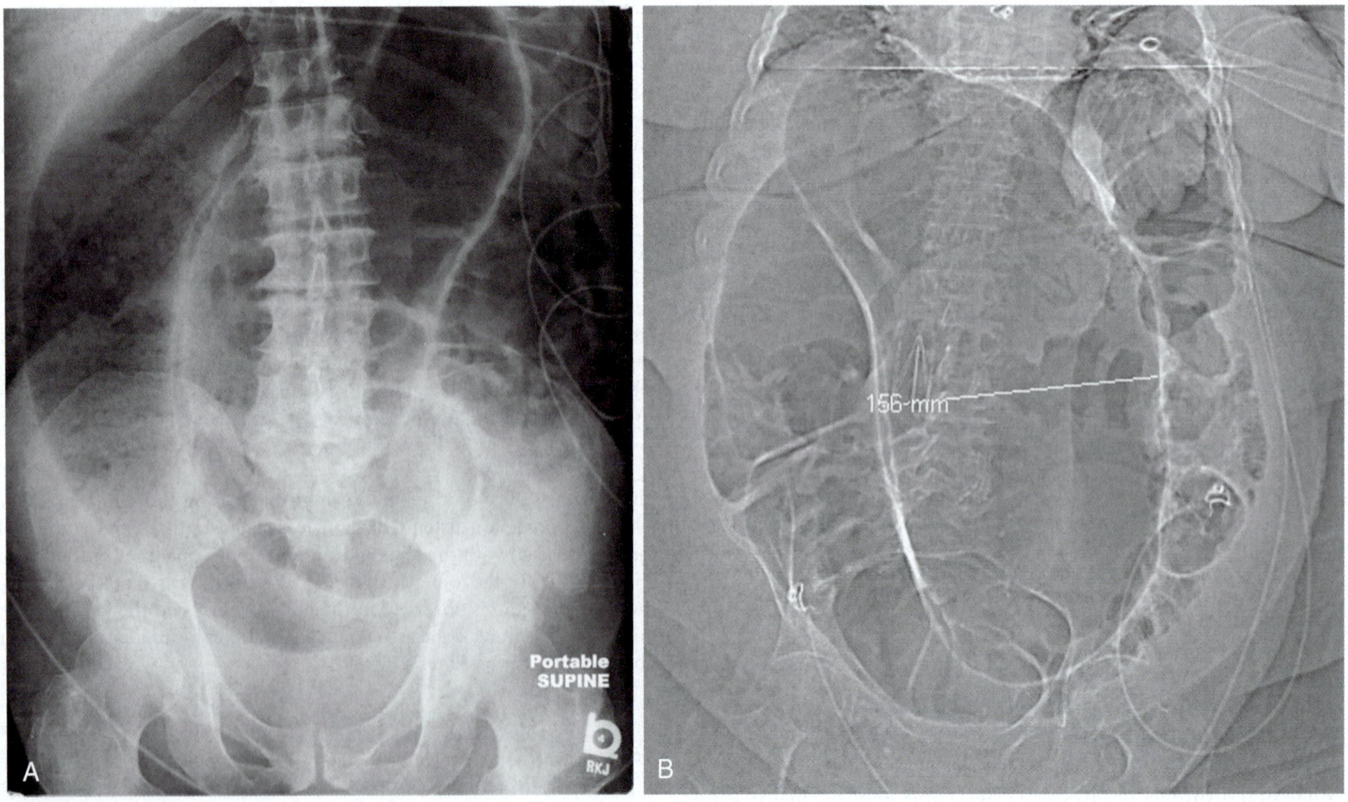

FIGURE 128-2. Sigmoid volvulus. Plain abdominal radiograph shows the presence of a sigmoid volvulus. **A,** "Bent inner tube" sign. **B,** "Omega" or "coffee bean" sign.

Umbilical hernias

Umbilical hernias occur in association with obesity, in multiparous women, and in patients with ascites. They present as a protuberant mass palpable at the umbilicus. Incarceration of small bowel or omentum is common, and strangulation occurs in about one third of umbilical hernias. Umbilical hernias can be repaired surgically, with mesh repair preferable to suture repair,[A2] if they are symptomatic or associated with complications, but ascites should be controlled for the hernia repair to succeed.

Groin hernias

Groin hernias present with bulging in this region, particularly with Valsalva maneuvers. Whereas direct inguinal hernias occur at the site of weakness at the base of the Hesselbach triangle, indirect inguinal hernias occur lateral to the Hesselbach triangle. Both direct and indirect inguinal hernias are above the inguinal ligament. Femoral hernias occur below the inguinal ligament in the femoral canal. Pain is typically mild, but more severe pain or colicky abdominal pain suggests incarceration or strangulation. Palpation can reveal the presence of a groin hernia that increases in size with standing or increased intra-abdominal pressure, such as a Valsalva maneuver, but palpation may be difficult in obese patients. In unclear cases, CT imaging can be helpful. The differential diagnosis of an inguinal bulge also includes adenopathy, lipoma or other tumors, testicular torsion of an undescended testicle, and abscess. Femoral hernias should be repaired when first diagnosed because of their risk for strangulation. Because the presence of strangulation can reliably be made only at surgery, more severe symptoms warrant early surgical intervention.

Watchful waiting is an acceptable option for men with minimally symptomatic inguinal hernias, although the majority of men will ultimately be referred for surgery, primarily because of pain, within 10 years.[4] The treatment of symptomatic groin hernias is surgical, now usually by open mesh-based techniques or laparoscopic repair, with mesh techniques probably providing slightly better long-term results.[A3] Open repair can be performed under local anesthesia, whereas laparoscopic repair, which generally results in less postoperative pain and an earlier return to normal activities, requires general anesthesia and carries a small risk of major intra-abdominal injury.[5]

Pelvic hernias

Pelvic hernias occur through a weakened pelvic floor and are six-fold more common in women, especially with advancing age. The most common form is an obturator hernia, but less common forms include a sciatic hernia through the sciatic foramen or perineal hernias through the pelvic floor musculature. Most obturator hernias present with acute bowel obstruction. A tender mass may be palpable near the obturator canal on rectal or vaginal examination. Inner thigh pain on internal rotation of the hip may be present in 50% of patients. Diagnosis can be aided using CT imaging. The treatment is surgical.

Incisional hernias

Incisional hernias can develop after 1 to 4% of laparotomy incisions. Incisional hernias may cause chronic abdominal discomfort, especially with maneuvers that increase intra-abdominal pressure. Repair is usually performed with prosthetic mesh, which appears to provide better outcomes than suture repair[6] and is also useful for prophylaxis against a future incisional hernia at the time of a midline laparotomy.[A4]

More rare hernias include lumbar hernias (which are more common in men and after surgery for trauma), Spigelian hernias occurring through the linea semilunaris in elderly patients, and internal hernias that occur when an intraperitoneal organ protrudes into a separate compartment within the abdomen. Some hernias occur in surgically created defects or because of congenital defects (e.g., paraduodenal, pericecal, or foramen of Winslow). Up to 15% of internal hernias occur through mesenteric or omental defects. Most patients present with intermittent symptoms of pain and bowel obstruction or strangulation. Radiologic studies can be of variable assistance. The differential diagnosis should include volvulus, adhesions, and tumors. The diagnosis can be made using barium studies and CT imaging. Surgery is needed to reduce the herniated viscus and close any defect.

INFLAMMATION OF THE INTESTINE AND COLON

APPENDICITIS

Appendicitis, which is the most common intra-abdominal pathology that requires emergency surgery, affects about 1 per 1000 adults annually worldwide.[7] The lifetime prevalence of appendicitis is 8.7% in men and 6.9% in woman. Lifetime rates of appendectomy are higher, 12% in men and 23% in women, because the diagnosis may be difficult to confirm noninvasively and because of the practice of operating on patients in whom the condition is highly suspected.[8] About one third of patients have luminal obstruction of the vermiform appendix, most commonly caused by an appendicolith but also occasionally by lymphoid hyperplasia or tumors, including carcinoid tumors (Chapter 213). Gangrenous appendicitis is almost always associated with luminal obstruction.

CLINICAL MANIFESTATIONS AND DIAGNOSIS

The differential diagnosis of appendicitis is extensive (Table 128-1). Current guidelines for diagnosis include characteristic history and physical findings of abdominal pain; localized tenderness; or other signs of acute appendicitis, including increased right lower quadrant pain with cough, pain with flexion and internal rotation of the hip, pain with passive extension of the right hip, and increased right lower quadrant pain during palpation of the left lower quadrant. Laboratory evidence of inflammation includes leukocytosis, greater than 10,000/μL but usually less than 18,000/μL unless perforation has occurred, with left shift, and elevated markers such as the C-reactive protein or procalcitonin level. The use of a standardized approach, the Adult Appendicitis Score (Table 128-2),[9] can reduce unnecessary imaging and hospital admissions.[A5] However, none of these tests are accurate enough to make or exclude the diagnosis of appendicitis in patients with an intermediate probability score. The preferred diagnostic test is multidetector CT, preferably using a low-dose, 2 mSv CT, which has a sensitivity and specificity of at least 94%[A6] and perhaps higher and can also detect perforation (Figs. 128-3 and 128-4). Nonenhanced CT is nearly as good as contrast-enhanced CT for diagnosing acute appendicitis,[10] while limiting exposure to iodinated contrast and its potential adverse effects in patients for whom it is a concern. A point-of-care ultrasound is helpful if positive, but a negative test does not exclude the diagnosis. Even expert ultrasonography is less sensitive and specific, 83% and 93%, respectively than CT, but it is useful when CT is contraindicated, such as in pregnant women or a suspected ectopic pregnancy. Magnetic resonance imaging is no better than CT but is an accurate option for pregnant women.[11]

TREATMENT AND PROGNOSIS

When acute appendicitis is suspected, emergent surgical consultation and appendectomy are indicated. Laparoscopic appendectomy is preferred over open appendectomy because of lower rates of postoperative complications and a more rapid return to normal eating and activity, except open appendectomy is preferred in patients with evidence of perforation.[A7] Preoperative antibiotics (e.g., cefotetan, 2 g intravenously, or cefoxitin, 2 g intravenously followed by three postoperative doses or ticarcillin–clavulanic acid) reduce infectious complications in otherwise uncomplicated appendicitis. Because perforation of the appendix increases the risk of mortality from 0.0002% to 3% and increases the morbidity rate from 3% to 47%, the traditional approach is that a negative laparotomy is an acceptable trade-off to missing true appendicitis.

A nonoperative approach using antibiotics to treat uncomplicated appendicitis[12] can reduce routine surgical morbidity but at the expense of more than

TABLE 128-1 DIFFERENTIAL DIAGNOSIS OF ACUTE APPENDICITIS

SURGICAL CAUSES
Intestinal obstruction
Intussusception
Acute cholecystitis (Chapter 141)
Mesenteric adenitis (especially from adenoviral infection; Chapter 333)
Meckel diverticulitis
Right-sided colonic diverticulitis
UROLOGIC CAUSES
Right nephrolithiasis (Chapter 111)
Right pyelonephritis (Chapter 263)
GYNECOLOGIC CAUSES
Ectopic or tubal pregnancy
Ruptured or torsed ovarian cyst
Right-sided salpingitis or tubo-ovarian abscess (Chapter 264)
MEDICAL CAUSES
Yersinia (Chapter 288) or *Campylobacter* (Chapter 279) enterocolitis
Crohn ileitis (Chapter 127)
Pneumonia (Chapter 85)
Diabetic ketoacidosis (Chapter 210)
Herpetic neuralgia (especially right 10th and 11th nerves; Chapter 346)
Porphyria (Chapter 194)
Tuberculous colitis (Chapter 299)

TABLE 128-2 ADULT APPENDICITIS SCORE

	VARIABLE	VALUE
Symptoms and findings	RLQ pain	2
	Pain relocation	2
	RLQ tenderness	
	Woman age 16-49 years	1
	All others	3
	Guarding	
	Mild	2
	Moderate or severe	3
Laboratory	Leukocytosis (WBC/μL)	
	≥7,200 and <10,900	1
	≥10,900 and <14,900	2
	≥14,000	3
	Proportion of neutrophils (%)	
	≥62 and <75	2
	≥75 and <83	3
	≥83	4
	CRP (mg/L) and symptoms <24 h	
	≥4 and <11	2
	≥11 and <25	3
	≥25 and <83	5
	≥83	1
	CRP (mg/L) and symptoms >24 h	
	≥12 and <53	2
	≥53 and <152	2
	≥152	1
Total score	≤10 low probability	
	11-15 intermediate probability	
	≥16 high probability	

CRP = C-reactive protein; RLQ = right lower quadrant; WBC = white blood cell count. Online calculator: http://www.appendicitisscore.com/.
From Sammalkorpi HE, Mentula P, Leppäniemi A. A new adult appendicitis score improves diagnostic accuracy of acute appendicitis—a prospective study. *BMC Gastroenterol.* 2014;14:114.

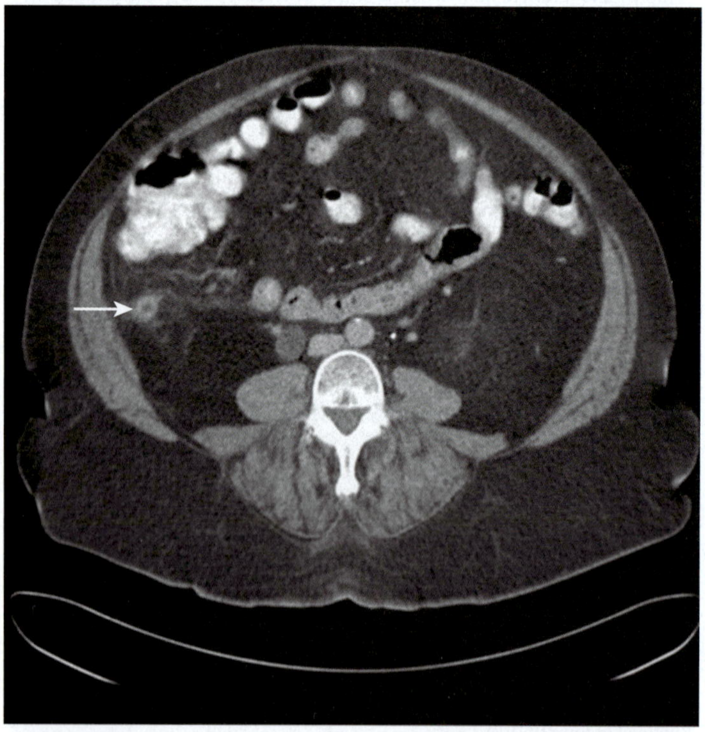

FIGURE 128-3. **Appendicitis.** A computed tomography scan shows an inflamed appendix with a diameter greater than 1 cm (*arrow*) consistent with acute, uncomplicated appendicitis.

a two-fold increase in complications, including about a 2% risk of rupture, a 1% risk of gangrenous appendicitis, and a 25 to 30% need for readmission or surgery within 3 to 12 months.[A8,A9] If antibiotics are chosen for uncomplicated appendicitis, 2 days of intravenous ertapenem (1 g daily) followed by 5 days of oral levofloxacin (500 mg daily) and metronidazole (500 mg three times daily) is slightly better than 7 days of oral moxifloxacin (400 mg daily).[A10]

The benefits of surgery are most notable in patients with an appendicolith. In the United States, the professional consensus tends to favor surgical appendectomy, except in patients who have had prior surgical complications, but informed decision making is recommended because many patients may prefer a nonoperative approach.[12]

For a perforated appendix with abscess formation, immediate appendectomy yields similar results to a strategy of percutaneous ultrasound- or CT-guided drainage, intravenous (IV) antibiotics, and laparoscopic appendectomy about 10 weeks later. In the setting of perforation, once-daily dosing with ceftriaxone and metronidazole for 7 to 10 days is as good as triple-dose therapy.

Complications develop in more than 15% of patients, with an overall mortality rate of about 3% in patients with perforated appendicitis. Complications are uncommon in surgically treated nonperforated appendicitis. Patients who have appendectomies for suspected but not confirmed appendicitis have a prognosis that depends on whether they had an underlying disease, such as Crohn disease (Chapter 127) or carcinoid tumor (Chapter 213). In adults over age 40 years, the risk of developing a right-sided colon cancer may be increased by as much as 10-fold,[13] so careful follow-up is warranted.

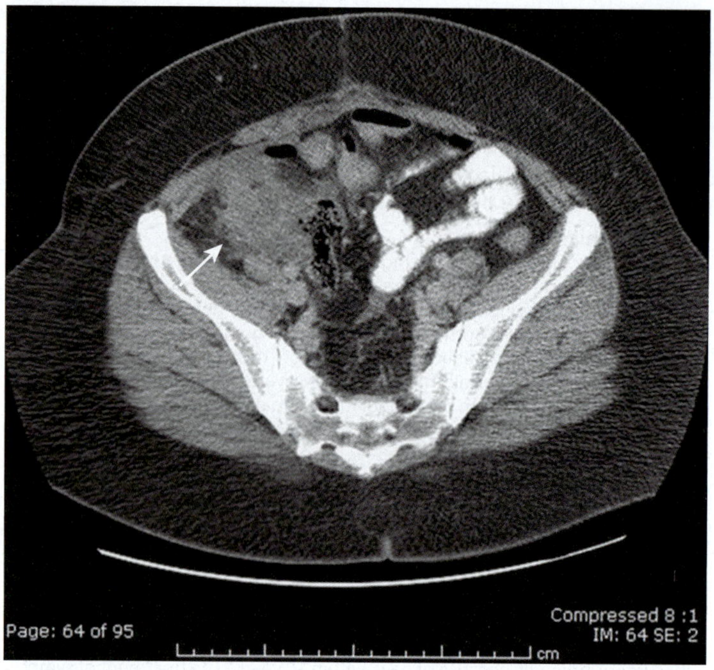

FIGURE 128-4. **Appendicitis.** A computed tomography scan shows appendicitis complicated by perforation with abscess formation (*arrow*). (Courtesy of Charlene Prather, MD.)

DIVERTICULITIS OF THE COLON

Colonic diverticula are technically pseudodiverticula. They form when the colonic mucosa and submucosa herniate through the muscularis propria of the colon. A spectrum of problems can result from diverticulosis, including diverticulitis, which is an infected diverticulum, or diverticular bleeding, which is manifested as acute lower GI bleeding (Chapter 121).[14] Diverticular disease (Fig. 128-5 and E-Fig. 128-1) affects about 10% of middle-aged adults and increases in prevalence up to about 80% in elderly adults. Acute diverticulitis is now more common than acute appendicitis in the emergency departments of developed countries.[14]

Colonic diverticula form at the site where the nutrient artery, the vasa recta, penetrates the muscularis propria. Diverticulosis in Western populations is most common in the left colon and has been thought to be associated with the low-fiber content of the typical Western diet, although recent epidemiologic studies cast doubt on this hypothesis. Diverticulosis can occur anywhere in the colon, however, and it is more commonly observed in the right colon in Asian populations.

The lifetime risk of diverticulitis is up to 25%. Diverticulitis is thought to occur when impacted material in the diverticulum compresses the blood supply, thereby resulting in a microperforation. Diverticulitis can be complicated further by free perforation, abscess, or fistula formation.

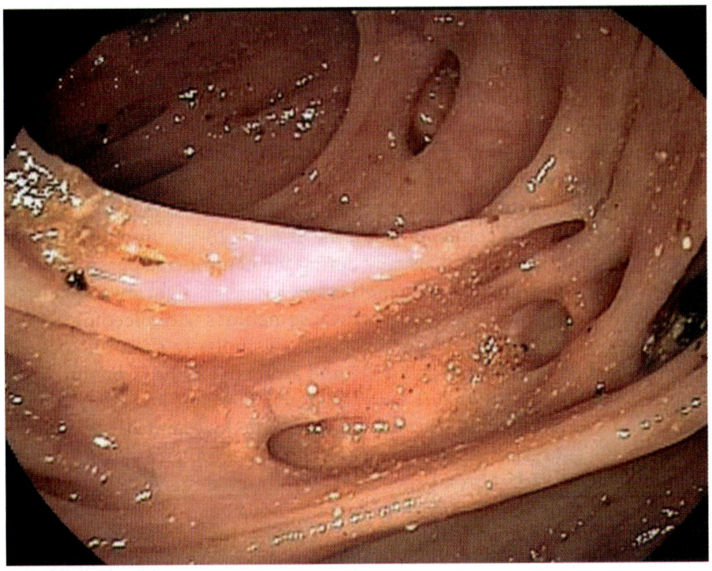

FIGURE 128-5. Sigmoid diverticulosis. The colonoscopic appearance of sigmoid diverticulosis coli.

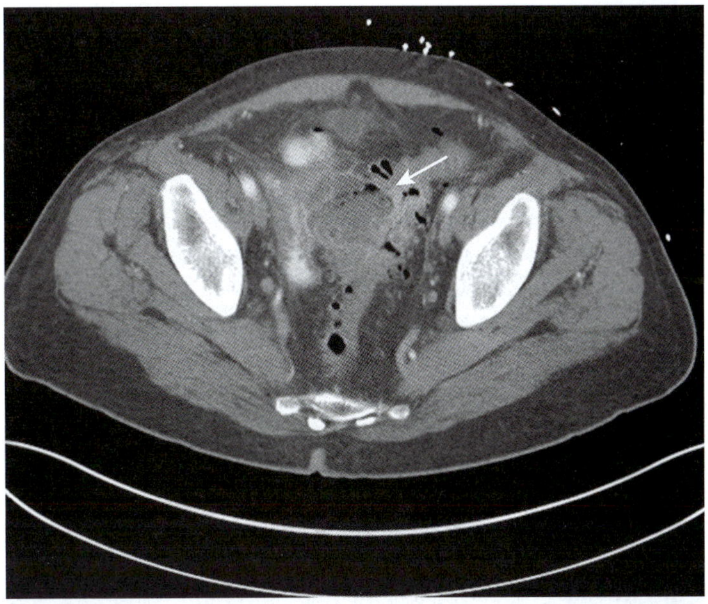

FIGURE 128-6. Diverticulitis. A computed tomography scan shows acute diverticulitis with perforation. An abscess (*arrow*) is seen presenting as a fluid and air-filled collection.

CLINICAL MANIFESTATIONS

The majority of patients with colonic diverticulosis are asymptomatic. Patients with diverticulitis commonly present with localized pain, fever, and anorexia. The pain may radiate to the back, flank, or suprapubic region. Nausea and vomiting, constipation or diarrhea, or urinary symptoms may be variably present. Physical examination typically reveals left lower quadrant tenderness, sometimes with localized guarding or a palpable mass. Rebound tenderness or peritoneal signs should suggest the presence of free perforation. Visible diverticular bleeding is rare in the setting of acute diverticulitis. Leukocytosis is present. When the acutely inflamed diverticulum is adjacent to the bladder, sterile pyuria may be found.

DIAGNOSIS

The clinical suspicion of acute diverticulitis is correct in only about 40 to 56% of cases, so the diagnosis must be confirmed in the appropriate setting by leukocytosis plus an ultrasound examination or a CT scan showing diverticulosis coli with localized inflammation of the colonic wall and pericolic fat at the site of acute diverticulitis.[15,16] A CT scan also can demonstrate free perforation, abscess, or fistula formation (Fig. 128-6). Because of the increased risk of perforation, invasive testing such as barium enema or colonoscopy is contraindicated when a diagnosis of acute diverticulitis is being entertained. The differential diagnosis of acute diverticulitis includes inflammatory bowel disease (Chapter 127), gastroenteritis, appendicitis, and colon cancer (Chapter 179) with perforation.

TREATMENT

Perforated diverticulitis with rupture of fecal material into the full peritoneum is a life-threatening surgical emergency. For diverticulitis with purulent but nonfecal peritonitis, randomized trials comparing laparoscopic peritoneal lavage with surgical resection have shown essentially no difference in outcomes.[A11] For diverticulitis with focal abscess formation, treatment is percutaneous CT-guided drainage and subsequent surgery, usually laparoscopic, typically after 6 weeks.[17]

Uncomplicated acute diverticulitis is usually treated with antibiotics, but antibiotics have limited benefit.[A12] A 7- to 10-day course of oral antibiotics (e.g., amoxicillin–clavulanate[18] [500 mg/125 mg] alone or ciprofloxacin [750 mg twice daily] plus metronidazole [500 mg four times daily]), perhaps after a single IV dose of antibiotics, is as effective and safe as hospitalization for IV antibiotics.[19] Patients who can tolerate clear liquids can be treated in the outpatient setting with gradual advancement of their diet. Patients who are unable to tolerate eating should be admitted to the hospital for IV fluids and antibiotics (e.g., levofloxacin 750 mg daily and metronidazole 500 mg every 6 hours or piperacillin–tazobactam 3.375 g every 6 hours). For diverticular and other intra-abdominal infections that have had adequate surgical treatment, fixed-duration antibiotic therapy of approximately 4 days provides similar outcomes to longer courses until after the resolution of physiologic abnormalities (about 8 days).

Although the risks associated with one episode of uncomplicated diverticulitis are low, with a mortality rate that is less than 1%, complicated diverticulitis, defined as diverticulitis with abscess, fistula formation, free perforation, or obstruction, is associated with increased inpatient morbidity in up to 25% of cases and has a mortality rate as high as 5%. Furthermore, these risks increase with a second episode of complicated diverticulitis. Elective segmental colectomy typically has been recommended to patients after two to three episodes of complicated diverticulitis and in young patients even after a first episode. However, recent evidence suggests that the risk of complicated diverticulitis after recovery from uncomplicated diverticulitis is only about 5% and is actually lower, not higher, after subsequent episodes of uncomplicated diverticulitis. However, prophylactic elective surgery is probably preferable in patients who have either three or more episodes of acute diverticulitis within 2 years or have persistent abdominal complaints for more than 3 months after a confirmed episode of left-sided diverticulitis.[A13–A15]

Acute diverticulitis can be complicated by colitis or late stricture formation. About 40% of patients with complicated diverticulitis have significant morbidity, and their mortality rate is about 6%, but it is only about 2% in patients without perforation. There is no convincing evidence that a high-fiber diet prevents recurrent diverticular disease or that nuts or any particular foods should be favored or avoided.

OTHER INTESTINAL INFLAMMATORY CONDITIONS

SMALL INTESTINAL ULCERS

Most primary idiopathic ulcers are found in the mid- to distal ileum, where they can be solitary or multiple. A careful history is necessary to exclude other precipitating causes of small intestinal ulcers, including drug exposure and other systemic diseases (Table 128-3). Pathologically, these ulcers can be differentiated from Crohn disease or chronic ulcerative jejunoileitis by the absence of granulomas. Barium contrast studies including enteroclysis can make the diagnosis, and CT or magnetic resonance enterography also can be helpful. In the absence of bowel obstruction, video capsule endoscopy is often the preferred test. Therapy with anti-inflammatory or immunosuppressive medications has not proven helpful. Therapy is typically directed to complications, including perforation and obstruction, with segmental surgical resection. However, the risk of ulcer recurrence is high.

Drug-induced ulcerations are common and can result from nonsteroidal anti-inflammatory drugs (NSAIDs), potassium chloride preparations, vasoactive medications, antimetabolites, and cocaine. Video capsule endoscopy can make the diagnosis (Fig. 128-7). NSAID-induced injury is similar to Crohn disease, with transmural injury and the risk of stricture formation. Treatment is aimed at avoiding the offending agent, if possible. A recent randomized trial demonstrated that adding a proton pump inhibitor to a non-selective NSAID actually increased the short-term risk of drug-induced small bowel injury.[A16]

A variety of systemic conditions also can manifest with small intestinal ulcerations. Patients with Crohn disease (Chapter 127) can have ulcers of

TABLE 128-3 CAUSES OF SMALL INTESTINAL ULCERS

CATEGORY	CAUSES
Acidic	Meckel diverticulum, Zollinger-Ellison syndrome
Drug-induced	Potassium chloride, NSAID, antimetabolite
Idiopathic	Primary ulcer, Behçet disease
Infectious	Tuberculosis, typhoid, *Yersinia*, *Strongyloides* superinfection
Inflammatory	Crohn disease, SLE, chronic jejunoileitis
Metabolic	Uremia
Neoplastic	Malignant histiocytosis, lymphoma, adenocarcinoma
Radiation	Radiation enteritis
Vascular	Mesenteric vascular insufficiency, vasculitis, arteritis

NSAID = nonsteroidal anti-inflammatory drug; SLE = systemic lupus erythematosus.

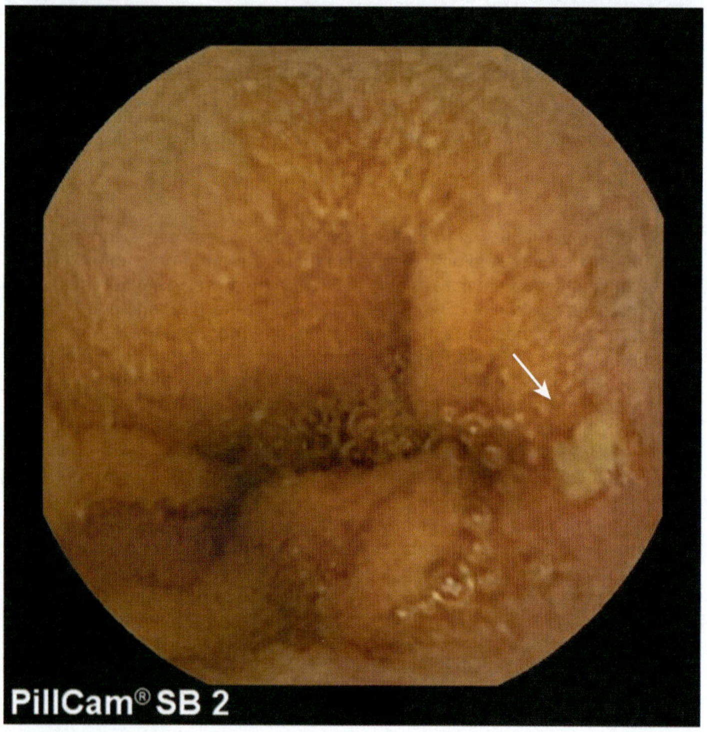

FIGURE 128-7. **Nonsteroidal anti-inflammatory drug (NSAID)–induced enteropathy.** The wireless capsule endoscopy appearance of a jejunal ulceration (*arrow*) caused by NSAID use.

any portion of the GI tract. Systemic lupus erythematosus (Chapter 245), rheumatoid arthritis (Chapter 243), scleroderma (Chapter 246), polyarteritis nodosa (Chapter 249), and Henoch-Schönlein purpura (Chapter 249) can present with small intestinal ulcerations that are thought to be secondary to microthrombosis and vasculitis. Mesenteric vasculitis presents as nausea, vomiting, fever, and GI bleeding.

Behçet disease (Chapter 249) is a systemic process that causes intestinal ulcers, typically in the ileocecal region, in fewer than 1% of cases. Although symptoms are similar to those of Crohn disease, pathologically Behçet disease-related ulcers are deep and do not have surrounding inflammation or granulomas. The optimal treatment of this disease has yet to be delineated. Patients frequently are treated with immunomodulators (Chapter 249), and surgery is reserved for ulcer-related complications.

Sarcoidosis (Chapter 83) uncommonly involves the intestine. Its presentation is similar to Crohn disease, with small and large intestinal ulceration and noncaseating granulomas. Patients commonly have nausea, vomiting, diarrhea, abdominal pain, and protein-losing enteropathy. Treatment is targeted to controlling the systemic disease.

Mycobacterium tuberculosis (Chapter 299) typically involves the distal ileum and cecum. A waxing and waning course can mimic the symptoms and location commonly seen in Crohn disease. The diagnosis is suspected based on a history of exposure, particularly in endemic regions, and confirmed by colonoscopy with biopsy, stains, and culture. Treatment is as for disseminated tuberculosis (Chapter 299).

Histoplasma capsulatum (Chapter 308) presents with ulcerations and polypoid masses that mimic tumors, typically in an immunocompromised patient. Patients present with diarrhea, bleeding, and obstruction. The granulomas seen on biopsy must be differentiated from Crohn disease, tuberculosis, and sarcoidosis. Treatment involves managing the systemic infection.

Neutropenic enterocolitis, or typhlitis (E-Fig. 128-2),[20] is an inflammation of the intestine or colon, usually during the neutropenic phase 10 to 14 days after high-dose induction chemotherapy. It involves right lower quadrant abdominal pain, distention, and diarrhea, sometimes with bleeding. These findings in themselves are nonspecific and are similar to *Clostridioides difficile*–associated colitis (Chapter 271) and ischemic colitis (Chapter 129). Diagnosis is based on typical CT scan findings of thickened bowel wall; bowel distention, especially of the cecum; and associated inflammatory changes. Treatment is conservative, with bowel rest and decompression when bowel dilation is present, and broad-spectrum antibiotics. Leukocyte-stimulating agents are often used to reverse the neutropenia (Chapter 153). Treatment of bleeding is supportive with transfusions and correction of any coagulopathy. Surgery is indicated in the setting of intractable bleeding or perforation. The symptoms resolve rapidly with resolution of neutropenia.

VISCERAL ANGIOEDEMA

Visceral angioedema can be idiopathic, or it can be a complication of hereditary and acquired C1 esterase inhibitor deficiency (Chapter 232), hypocomplementemia, drugs (especially angiotensin-converting enzyme inhibitors), or foods. Patients with GI angioedema commonly present with abdominal pain and distention, nausea, vomiting, and diarrhea. Some patients also have evidence of mucous membrane swelling, hives, wheezing, or dyspnea. On CT scan, thickened, fluid-filled loops of small bowel and ascites also may be seen. Symptoms commonly occur episodically, persist for 1 to 3 days and may recur periodically. The diagnosis is established by discontinuing the implicated drug or food, low serum levels of C4, low C1 esterase quantitative levels, or reduced C1 esterase functional activity. C1 esterase inhibitor deficiency can be treated successfully with C1 inhibitor therapy (Chapter 232).

RADIATION ENTERITIS

Radiation injury[21] can occur in the small or large intestine as a result of therapy for gynecologic, urologic, rectal, or retroperitoneal tumors. Acute injury, which can occur during the course of treatment, is associated with nausea, diarrhea, and abdominal or rectal discomfort. The risk is related to radiation dose. Chronic injury typically presents 6 months to 2 years after treatment and presents with progressive bowel obstruction owing to continued inflammation and fibrosis. Patients with radiation proctitis present with rectal pain, bleeding, and occasionally diarrhea.

Acute radiation injury is usually self-limited to the period of treatment, but up to 5% of patients can progress to chronic radiation injury to the small intestine, and up to 15% of patients experience chronic radiation proctitis. Radiation enteritis and stricture formation can be seen on barium radiographs or CT scans. The characteristic neovascularization pattern of telangiectasias from radiation proctitis is seen on endoscopy.

One-third to one-half of patients develop bleeding, which can be minor and intermittent or more substantial. Whereas patients who do not require transfusion have a 70% chance of remission, patients with chronic radiation enteritis who need transfusion have a low rate of remission (20%) and have subsequent high morbidity and even mortality rates. Radiation proctitis can be difficult to treat.

Two therapies, endoscopic argon plasma coagulation and rectal formalin infusion, were demonstrated to have similar efficacy in a recent RCT.[A17] Surgery for intestinal radiation enteritis, which can be required in up to one third of patients with strictures or bleeding, is associated with a high complication rate and should be avoided if possible.

PERITONEAL DISORDERS

PERITONITIS

Peritonitis, which is a local or generalized inflammation that involves the visceral and parietal peritoneum, can occur as a primary or secondary process. Primary peritonitis in adults is the spontaneous infection of ascites in a patient with cirrhosis (Chapter 139) in the absence of an overt intra-abdominal source. The use of acid-suppressive therapy appears to increase the risk of developing spontaneous bacterial peritonitis three-fold in hospitalized patients with cirrhosis.

Secondary peritonitis develops when disease or injury to the intestine results in bacterial contamination from a perforated viscus (e.g., peptic ulcer disease, appendicitis, diverticulitis, penetrating trauma, or iatrogenic), from iatrogenic causes (e.g., peritoneal dialysis or surgical contamination), from granulomatous disease (e.g., tuberculosis or fungal infections), or from chemical or aseptic exposures (e.g., bile, urine, or radiographic barium).

CLINICAL MANIFESTATIONS AND DIAGNOSIS

Abdominal pain is the hallmark of peritonitis. It can be sudden in onset in the setting of a perforated viscus or more insidious in nature in the setting of granulomatous or chemical causes. Patients with peritonitis typically lie supine with flexed knees and exhibit shallow breathing. Physical examination reveals a distended abdomen with tenderness to palpation, localized or generalized guarding, and rigidity. Associated symptoms include fever, nausea, vomiting, and leukocytosis with a left shift. Some patients with bacterial peritonitis rapidly develop septic shock (Chapter 94).

Granulomatous peritonitis has a more insidious presentation, and 70% of patients have symptoms for 4 months before diagnosis. Systemic symptoms include fever, malaise, anorexia, and weight loss. The abdomen is diffusely tender. Leukocytosis can be absent.

Patients with tuberculous peritonitis (Chapter 299) often have a positive skin test result or infiltrates on their chest radiograph. The peritoneal fluid typically has a high protein level (<3 g/dL), a low glucose (<30 mg/dL), and elevated leukocytes (<250 cells/μL); fluid stains and cultures are unhelpful, but polymerase chain reaction (PCR)–based tests can be diagnostic. The laparoscopic appearance of tuberculous peritonitis is characteristic, with fibrous masses from the parietal peritoneum and granulomas.

Plain abdominal radiographs may show evidence of paralytic ileus, and free air under the diaphragm on upright views confirms the presence of a perforated viscus. CT scan is more sensitive, 70 to 100%, than plain radiographs for detecting free air and may also demonstrate the underlying cause (Fig. 128-8). CT/positron emission tomography can be useful for distinguishing tuberculous peritonitis from peritoneal carcinomatosis.[22]

In young patients, appendicitis and a perforated duodenal ulcer (Chapter 125) are common causes. In older patients, perforated diverticula and cancer (Chapter 179) are more common. In women of child-bearing age, tubal pregnancy and a ruptured tubo-ovarian abscess must be considered (Chapters 264 and 275). Secondary peritonitis is usually caused by a mixed flora of bacteria, including *Escherichia coli, Streptococcus faecalis, Pseudomonas aeruginosa, Klebsiella mirabilis, Bacteroides fragilis, Clostridium* spp, and anaerobic streptococci.

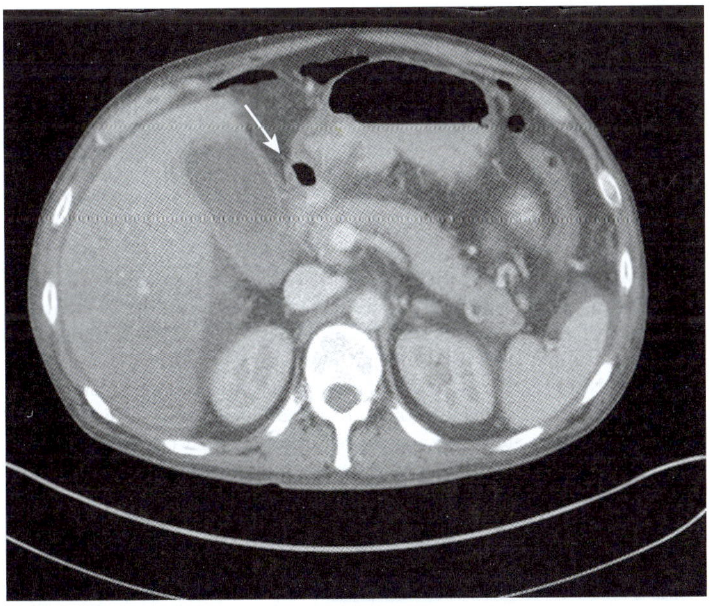

FIGURE 128-8. **Peritonitis.** A computed tomography scan in a patient with peritonitis showing a thickened duodenal wall from a perforated duodenal ulcer (*arrow*) found at the time of surgical exploration.

TREATMENT AND PROGNOSIS

Treatment of acute suppurative peritonitis relies on prompt adequate resuscitation with IV fluids and broad-spectrum IV antibiotics. Treatment regimens include: piperacillin–tazobactam, 3.375 g every 6 hours; ampicillin–sulbactam, 3.0 g every 6 hours; ciprofloxacin, 500 mg every 12 hours, and metronidazole, 1 g every 12 hours; levofloxacin, 750 mg every 24 hours; cefepime, 2 g every 12 hours, and metronidazole, 1 g every 12 hours; or imipenem–cilastatin sodium, 500 mg every 6 hours.[A18] Early diagnosis and surgical intervention for acute peritonitis from perforated viscus is critical. The mainstay of treatment for tuberculous peritonitis is at least 6 months of a multidrug regimen (Chapter 299).

Chemical aseptic peritonitis can be complicated by secondary bacterial infection. Treatment is similar to that of acute suppurative peritonitis, with intervention to control the source of peritoneal contamination.

The outcome of peritonitis depends on its cause as well as the rapidity of treatment. The mortality rate can be as low as 15% in patients who have correctable causes, such as a perforated appendix, and who do not develop multiorgan failure before treatment but as high as 50% for postoperative infective peritonitis.

PERITONITIS AS A COMPLICATION OF CHRONIC AMBULATORY PERITONEAL DIALYSIS

The most common complication of chronic ambulatory peritoneal dialysis is infectious peritonitis from bacterial contamination (Chapter 117), which commonly results from poor technique. In contrast to polymicrobial acute suppurative peritonitis, peritonitis complicating chronic ambulatory peritoneal dialysis is typically monomicrobial with gram-positive cocci in the majority of cases and gram-negative species in the remainder of cases. Fungal peritonitis is rare. Symptoms can be milder than in other forms of peritonitis, with patients often presenting with diffuse abdominal pain, low-grade fever, and leukocytosis. The exchange fluid is characteristically turbid and may be the only sign of infection. The diagnosis is based on these physical findings, turbid dialysate with less than 100 leukocytes/μL, and a positive dialysate culture that determines the microbe involved. Treatment is with intraperitoneal antibiotics. The dialysis catheter should be removed in the setting of an inadequate response to therapy, fungal or tuberculous peritonitis, or concomitant skin infection. The risk of peritonitis can be reduced by the judicious use of prophylactic intravenous vancomycin and oral nystatin or fluconazole.[A19]

ADHESIONS

Peritoneal adhesions, which are the most commonly observed cause of bowel obstruction,[23] can occur at any time after a laparotomy,[24] with rates about one-third lower with laparoscopic as compared with open surgery.[25] Adhesions are also the most common cause of small bowel obstruction in patients who have not had prior abdominal surgery.[26] Patients who have had intra-abdominal infection, ischemia, and peritonitis are at increased risk. Patients present with complete or incomplete bowel obstruction, which is usually manifested as colicky abdominal pain, nausea, and vomiting (including feculent vomiting), abdominal distention, and an absence of flatus or stooling. Bowel obstruction can be diagnosed on plain radiographs or CT scan from the presence of dilated bowel and air-fluid levels, with decompressed bowel distal to the site of obstruction (Fig. 128-9). Treatment of bowel obstructions is with NG tube decompression and fluid resuscitation. A nonoperative approach can be attempted in cases of partial bowel obstruction or in patients who have had numerous prior laparotomies, which make surgical exploration more complicated. However, urgent laparotomy for lysis of adhesions must be performed before bowel ischemia develops. In patients with chronic abdominal pain, surgical exploration for the intent of lysing adhesions without clear evidence of obstructing adhesions should be avoided. Patients who develop postoperative adhesions can progress to bowel obstruction and develop recurrent adhesions despite surgical lysis of the adhesions.

PERITONEAL CARCINOMATOSIS AND MALIGNANT ASCITES

Peritoneal carcinomatosis results when malignancy spreads throughout the peritoneal cavity and eventually encases the viscera. The cause can be primary tumors of the peritoneal cavity (e.g., mesothelioma and sarcoma), dissemination of an intra-abdominal malignancy (e.g., gastric, colon, pancreatic, ovarian, or neuroendocrine tumors), lymphomas, metastatic spread from extra-abdominal malignancy (e.g., breast, lung, or melanoma), and pseudomyxoma peritonei (a rare condition with gelatinous peritoneal implants from mucinous neoplasms of the appendix or ovary).

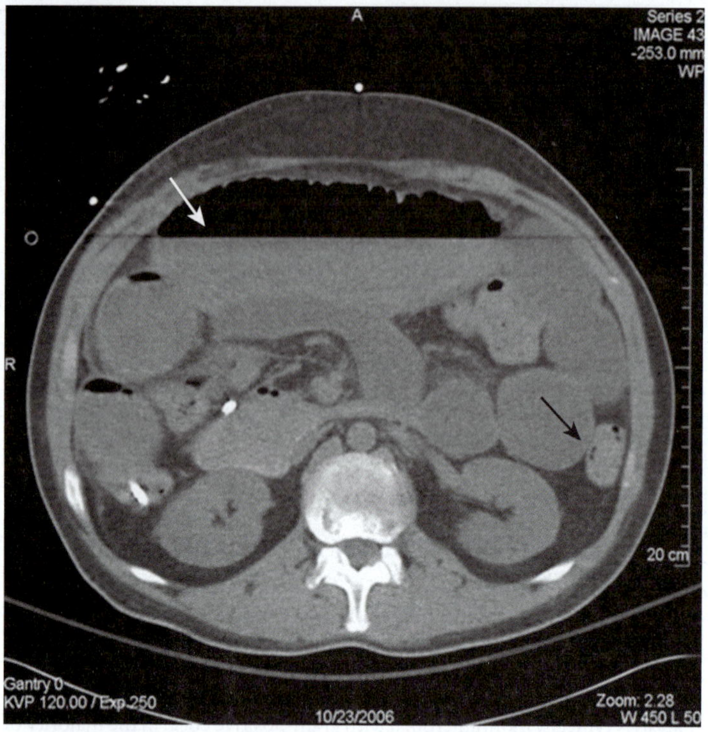

FIGURE 128-9. Small bowel obstruction. A computed tomography scan shows dilated, fluid-filled small bowel (*white arrow*) and a nondilated colon (*black arrow*) in a patient with a small bowel obstruction from adhesions found at the time of surgical exploration.

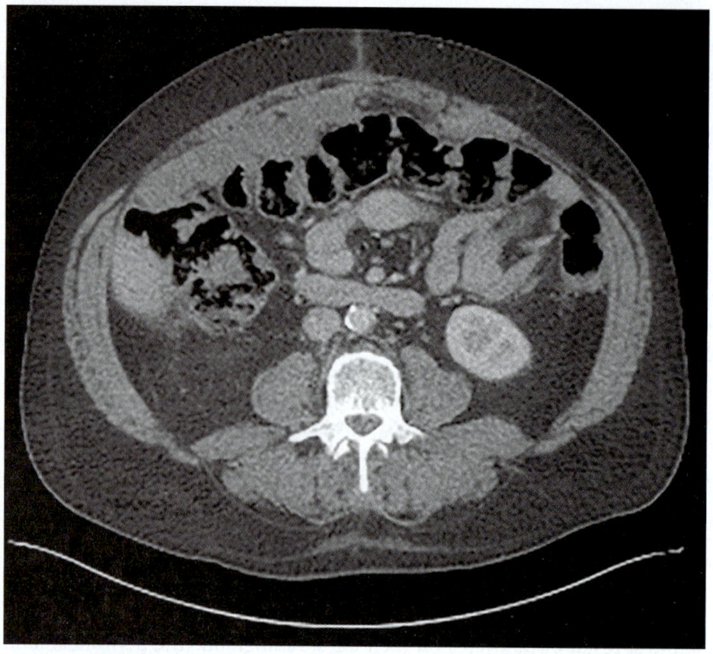

FIGURE 128-10. Carcinomatosis. A computed tomography scan shows peritoneal carcinomatosis in a patient with colon cancer.

CLINICAL MANIFESTATIONS AND DIAGNOSIS

The presentation of peritoneal carcinomatosis is nonspecific, with complaints of abdominal pain, anorexia, nausea, vomiting, malaise, and weight loss. Ascites is the most common physical finding. Malignant ascites is rare, accounting for less than 10% of cases of ascites.

Although ultrasound examination may document ascites, CT is preferred to identify carcinomatosis and the origin of the underlying cause (Fig. 128-10). Diagnostic paracentesis can be performed to obtain cell count and differential, culture, and cytologic examination. A serum to ascites albumin ratio of less than 1.1 mg/dL suggests malignant ascites, but the differential diagnosis also includes pancreatic ascites (Chapter 130), nephrotic syndrome (Chapter 107), and peritoneal tuberculosis. Laparoscopy can disclose the typical tumor implant stubbing the peritoneum. Biopsy and appropriate stains can verify the presence of mesothelioma (Chapters 86 and 177) by detecting hyaluronic acid on Alcian stain in a specimen that has a negative carcinoembryonic antigen stain and no mucin on a periodic acid–Schiff stain. By contrast, carcinomas have no hyaluronic acid but show mucin and have a positive carcinoembryonic antigen stain.

TREATMENT AND PROGNOSIS

Treatment is typically palliative owing to the late presentation of disease. Malignant ascites responds poorly to diuretic therapies, and repeated therapeutic paracentesis may be needed. Recent data suggest some benefit from cytoreductive surgery and hyperthermic intraperitoneal chemotherapy.

DISEASES OF THE MESENTERY AND OMENTUM

The differential diagnosis of mesenteric and omental disorders include a variety of rare disorders, including inflammation, cysts, and tumors that can be benign or malignant (Table 128-4).

Mesenteric panniculitis presents in middle or later age with a slight male predilection. Symptoms typically include nonspecific abdominal pain, weight loss, nausea, vomiting, and low-grade fever, but patients occasionally can present with an acute abdomen. A palpable mass is felt in the majority of patients. The diagnosis can be confirmed by CT scan. Lesions should be biopsied to exclude malignancy but generally are not amenable to complete resection. Significant improvement in the symptoms of this generally self-limited process has been reported with progesterone, corticosteroids, azathioprine, or cyclophosphamide, but evidence to recommend their general use is lacking.

TABLE 128-4 MESENTERIC DISEASES

PRIMARY INFLAMMATORY DISEASE
Panniculitis
Retractile mesenteritis
CYSTS
Developmental
Traumatic
Neoplastic
Infectious
TUMORS
Benign tumors
Lipoma
Leiomyoma
Hemangioma
Malignant tumors
Liposarcoma
Leiomyosarcoma
Rhabdomyosarcoma
Metastatic tumor
Mesenteric fibromatosis

Mesenteric and omental cysts and solid tumors are rare disorders. Patients present with a constellation of nonspecific symptoms. They can be identified with CT scan. Surgical resection will provide the definitive diagnosis and determine whether a benign or malignant condition is present.

Mesenteric fibromatosis (desmoid tumors) is a rare noninflammatory condition that may be associated with familial adenomatosis polyposis (Chapter 179). Fibromatoses are locally aggressive tumors that may present as stable or rapidly growing intra-abdominal masses. They have a high rate of recurrence after incomplete surgical resection, in patients with multicentric disease, or if precipitated by surgical trauma itself.

GENERAL REFERENCES

For the General References and other additional features, please visit Elsevier eBooks+ at https://ebooks.health.elsevier.com.

Grade A References

A1. Xie X, Wu Y, Wang Q, et al. A randomized trial of pneumatic reduction versus hydrostatic reduction for intussusception in pediatric patients. *J Pediatr Surg*. 2018;53:1464-1468.
A2. Kaufmann R, Halm JA, Eker HH, et al. Mesh versus suture repair of umbilical hernia in adults: a randomised, double-blind, controlled, multicentre trial. *Lancet*. 2018;391:860-869.
A3. Lockhart K, Dunn D, Teo S, et al. Mesh versus non-mesh for inguinal and femoral hernia repair. *Cochrane Database Syst Rev*. 2018;9:CD011517.
A4. Jairam AP, Timmermans L, Eker HH, et al. Prevention of incisional hernia with prophylactic onlay and sublay mesh reinforcement versus primary suture only in midline laparotomies (PRIMA): 2-year follow-up of a multicentre, double-blind, randomised controlled trial. *Lancet*. 2017;390:567-576.
A5. Andersson M, Kolodziej B, Andersson RE. Randomized clinical trial of Appendicitis Inflammatory Response score-based management of patients with suspected appendicitis. *Br J Surg*. 2017;104:1451-1461.
A6. LOCAT Group. Low-dose CT for the diagnosis of appendicitis in adolescents and young adults (LOCAT): a pragmatic, multicentre, randomised controlled non-inferiority trial. *Lancet Gastroenterol Hepatol*. 2017;2:793-804.
A7. Talha A, El-Haddad H, Ghazal AE, et al. Laparoscopic versus open appendectomy for perforated appendicitis in adults: randomized clinical trial. *Surg Endosc*. 2020;34:907-914.
A8. CODA Collaborative, Davidson GH, Flum DR, et al. Antibiotics versus appendectomy for acute appendicitis—longer-term outcomes. *N Engl J Med*. 2021;385:2395-2397.
A9. Flum DR, Davidson GH, Monsell SE, et al. A randomized trial comparing antibiotics with appendectomy for appendicitis. *N Engl J Med*. 2020;383:1907-1919.
A10. Sippola S, Haijanen J, Gronroos, et al. Effect of oral moxifloxacin vs intravenous ertapenem plus oral levofloxacin for treatment of uncomplicated acute appendicitis: the APPAC II randomized clinical trial. *JAMA*. 2021;325:353-362.
A11. Azhar N, Johanssen A, Sundström T, et al. Laparoscopic lavage vs primary resection for acute perforated diverticulitis: long-term outcomes from the Scandinavian diverticulitis (SCANDIV) randomized clinical trial. *JAMA Surg*. 2021;156:121-127.
A12. Araya-Quezada C, Torres-Bavestrello L, Gómez-Barbieri G, et al. Antibiotics for acute uncomplicated diverticulitis in hospitalized patients. *Medwave*. 2021;21:e8140.
A13. van de Wall BJ, Stam MA, Draaisma WA, et al. Surgery versus conservative management for recurrent and ongoing left-sided diverticulitis (DIRECT trial): an open-label, multicentre, randomised controlled trial. *Lancet Gastroenterol Hepatol*. 2017;2:13-22.
A14. Bolkenstein HE, Consten ECJ, van der Palen J, et al. Long-term outcome of surgery versus conservative management for recurrent and ongoing complaints after an episode of diverticulitis: 5-year follow-up results of a multicenter randomized controlled trial (DIRECT-Trial). *Ann Surg*. 2019;269:612-620.
A15. Santos A, Mentula P, Pinta T, et al. Comparing laparoscopic elective sigmoid resection with conservative treatment in improving quality of life of patients with diverticulitis: the laparoscopic elective sigmoid resection following diverticulitis (LASER) randomized clinical trial. *JAMA Surg*. 2021;156:129-136.
A16. Washio E, Esaki M, Maehata Y, et al. Proton pump inhibitors increase incidence of nonsteroidal anti-inflammatory drug-induced small bowel injury: a randomized, placebo-controlled trial. *Clin Gastroenterol Hepatol*. 2016;14:809-815.
A17. Furtado FS, Furtado GB, Oliviera AT, et al. Endorectal formalin instillation or argon plasma coagulation for hemorrhagic radiation proctopathy therapy: a prospective and randomized clinical trial. *Gastrointest Endosc*. 2021;93:1393-1400.
A18. Sawyer RG, Claridge JA, Nathens AB, et al. Trial of short-course antimicrobial therapy for intraabdominal infection. *N Engl J Med*. 2015;372:1996-2005.
A19. Campbell D, Mudge DW, Craig JC, et al. Antimicrobial agents for preventing peritonitis in peritoneal dialysis patients. *Cochrane Database Syst Rev*. 2017;4:CD004679.

129 VASCULAR DISEASES OF THE GASTROINTESTINAL TRACT

CHARLES J. KAHI

INTESTINAL ISCHEMIA

Intestinal ischemia can be caused by a variety of disorders that result in decreased blood supply to the bowel. The injury itself, as well as its presentation, management, and outcome, vary depending on acuity, the splanchnic vessel(s) affected, the presence or absence of collateral circulation, the segment and the length of bowel involved, and whether the arterial or venous circulation is compromised. Recognition and appropriate management are crucial to improve patients' outcomes.[1]

EPIDEMIOLOGY

About 1 in 1000 hospital admissions is related to intestinal ischemia. Intestinal ischemia can be occlusive or nonocclusive, and can also be classified as acute or chronic, arterial or venous, and small bowel or colonic ischemia. Risk factors for intestinal ischemia include older age and conditions that predispose to arterial disease (e.g., atherosclerosis, fibromuscular dysplasia, abdominal aortic aneurysm, trauma, vasculitis), embolism (e.g., cardiac arrhythmias, cardioversion, heart failure, cardiomegaly, dyskinesia, valvular heart disease, recent myocardial infarction, cardiac catheterization, intracardiac thrombus, atheromatous cholesterol embolism), low-flow states (e.g., sepsis, dialysis, reduced cardiac output, vasoconstrictive drugs), or pathologic thromboses (hypercoagulable and hyperviscosity states, portal hypertension, trauma, malignancy, inflammation). Intestinal arterial and venous thrombosis have also been seen as complications of severe acute respiratory syndrome coronavirus 2 (Chapter 336).[2]

PATHOBIOLOGY

Blood flow to the digestive system is largely supplied by the celiac axis, superior mesenteric artery, and inferior mesenteric artery. The celiac axis gives rise to the left gastric artery, common hepatic artery, and splenic artery. These arteries and their branches (gastroduodenal, right gastroepiploic, and anterior superior pancreaticoduodenal) supply portions of the esophagus (also supplied from the aorta, right intercostal, bronchial, inferior thyroid, short gastric, and left phrenic arteries), stomach, duodenum, pancreas, and liver. The superior mesenteric artery supplies the majority of the small intestine and right colon via the inferior (anterior and posterior) pancreaticoduodenal arteries, the middle colic, right colic, and ileocolic arteries. The inferior mesenteric artery supplies the left colon via the left colic artery and proximal rectum via the superior rectal artery. The distal rectum receives its arterial supply from the internal iliac artery. Collateral vessels connect the three major systems: the superior and inferior mesenteric arteries can communicate through the marginal artery of Drummond, which runs along the mesenteric border, the meandering mesenteric artery (arc of Riolan) at the base of the mesentery, and the central anastomotic artery. The celiac axis and superior mesenteric artery are connected via the pancreaticoduodenal arcade (formed from the superior pancreaticoduodenal branch of the celiac axis and inferior pancreaticoduodenal branch of the superior mesenteric artery), the arc of Barkow, and the arc of Buhler. Collateral vessels vary from person to person, but in general, the stomach, duodenum, and rectum have extensive collaterals and are thus more resistant to ischemic events. Conversely, the splenic flexure and descending colon have more limited collaterals, thereby creating "watershed" areas that are more vulnerable to ischemia during low blood flow states.

Blood flow to the intestine is regulated by the sympathetic nervous system, angiotensin II, vasopressin, and prostaglandins. Under normal conditions, intestinal blood flow accounts for nearly 10% of cardiac output, and it may increase to 25% in the postprandial state. The bowel can withstand a 75% reduction of blood flow for up to 12 hours, whether due to arterial, venous, occlusive, or nonocclusive causes. This adaptability is because only a fraction of mesenteric capillaries are open under normal circumstances, and the bowel responds to reduced blood flow by increasing capillary flow and the efficiency of oxygen extraction. However, prolonged and severe reduction in blood flow can result in generalized mesenteric vasoconstriction, which diminishes flow through collaterals, thereby leading to potentially irreversible ischemia even if the underlying cause is corrected. Diminished delivery of oxygen and nutrients to the bowel results in ischemic injury; reperfusion after an ischemic episode can also injure the bowel. These insults are mediated by oxygen radicals, reduced endothelial synthesis of nitric oxide, and an enhanced cellular inflammatory response. In early stages, the damage involves the bowel mucosa, but it may progress to transmural necrosis.

ACUTE MESENTERIC ISCHEMIA

Acute mesenteric ischemia of the small bowel is considered a medical emergency, and delays in identification and management can result in death within a short period of time. Acute mesenteric ischemia should be distinguished from colonic ischemia, which has a generally better prognosis. Categories of acute mesenteric ischemia include superior mesenteric artery embolus or thrombosis, nonocclusive mesenteric ischemia, focal segmental ischemia, and mesenteric venous thrombosis.

CLINICAL MANIFESTATIONS

A high index of suspicion is critical so the diagnosis can be made before the intestine suffers irreversible damage. A cardinal symptom is abdominal pain, which is typically out of proportion to the amount of abdominal tenderness elicited on physical examination.[3] The pain can be periumbilical or ill-defined. In general, acute mesenteric ischemia should be considered in older patients who develop rapid-onset abdominal pain in the context of a cardiac arrhythmia, heart failure, a recent myocardial infarction, a retrograde aortic catheterization, or hypotension. It should also be suspected in younger patients who have hypercoagulable states (Chapter 67) or who use vasoactive substances (Chapter 365) and who have persistent and unexplained abdominal pain. Other features at presentation may include fever, nausea and vomiting, diarrhea, and abdominal distention. In elderly patients, the presenting symptoms may be nonspecific, such as an altered mental state.

The pattern and rapidity of the onset of symptoms can offer clues to the etiology. Patients with an embolism can present with abrupt abdominal pain and forceful bowel movements, whereas a more indolent onset and course are generally seen in mesenteric venous thrombosis. In nonocclusive mesenteric ischemia, pain may be absent or not a dominant feature. Occult gastrointestinal bleeding is common in acute mesenteric ischemia, but overt bleeding is not (in contrast to colonic ischemia); its occurrence is usually a late and ominous development, which suggests intestinal infarction. If acute mesenteric ischemia progresses, abdominal findings may become more apparent and include tenderness, distention, and peritoneal signs.

DIAGNOSIS

Laboratory findings may initially be normal and generally lack sufficient reliability for early diagnosis.[4] D-dimer is a sensitive early marker, but it has high false-positive rates. Leukocytosis (>15,000/mL with a neutrophilic shift) and elevations in levels of serum amylase, phosphate, lactate dehydrogenase, creatine kinase, aminotransferases, and lactate may be seen, but these are usually associated with later-stage disease and lack sufficient sensitivity and specificity. Novel serologic markers are actively being studied but have not yet entered routine practice.

Plain radiographs are usually unrevealing in early acute mesenteric ischemia. With progression of the ischemic injury, abnormalities may include ileus, thumbprinting (due to submucosal hemorrhage), pneumatosis linearis, or portal venous gas. Although these findings are nonspecific, their presence correlates with a worse prognosis, and plain radiographs are useful to exclude other conditions. Doppler ultrasonography is generally not recommended because it only allows evaluation of the proximal aspects of the celiac axis and superior mesenteric artery, and it is not reliable in the assessment of nonocclusive mesenteric ischemia. Computed tomography (CT) scans of the abdomen and pelvis may be normal in early acute mesenteric ischemia or may reveal bowel wall thickening, submucosal hemorrhage, mesenteric venous thrombosis, mesenteric stranding, pneumatosis, or portal venous gas in more advanced cases (Fig. 129-1).

Standard contrasted CT is most useful for the diagnosis of mesenteric venous thrombosis, but it is generally less helpful for diagnosing acute mesenteric ischemia, especially in its early stages. CT angiography is the diagnostic imaging modality of choice,[5] with a sensitivity and specificity of about 95%, while also allowing concomitant evaluation of other abdominal structures. CT angiography should be performed without oral contrast owing to the risk of obscuring the mesenteric vessels and delaying diagnosis. Magnetic resonance (MR) angiography also has high diagnostic accuracy and may be preferred for patients who are hypersensitive to iodinated contrast dye, but it is less readily available and more time-consuming to obtain than CT angiography. Although CT angiography and MR angiography perform well for occlusive acute mesenteric ischemia, they are both less reliable for nonocclusive mesenteric ischemia. The gold standard for the diagnosis and specific classification of acute mesenteric ischemia is selective mesenteric angiography, which also has therapeutic applications for the delivery of medications or the placement of a stent. However, given its wide availability and ease of performance, CT angiography has largely replaced conventional angiography for the primary diagnosis of acute mesenteric ischemia.

PROGNOSIS

Untreated acute mesenteric ischemia resulting in intestinal infarction is associated with a mortality rate of over 70%, but prompt diagnosis and treatment significantly improve outcomes. Two-year survival rates are nearly 90% using intensive multidisciplinary and multimodal approaches.

TREATMENT

Arterial acute mesenteric ischemia involving the small bowel is associated with high mortality (greater than 70% if there is intestinal infarction). Prompt diagnosis and management are essential,[6] and patients benefit from a multidisciplinary approach (Fig. 129-2).

Initial management for all patients should include intravascular volume resuscitation, broad-spectrum antibiotics with gram-negative and anaerobic coverage to prevent sepsis secondary to bacterial translocation from the gut (e.g., a third-generation cephalosporin or fluoroquinolone plus metronidazole and piperacillin-tazobactam; see Table 266-4), and attention to any underlying precipitating factors such as heart failure (Chapter 46) or cardiac arrhythmias (Chapters 52 and 53). The presence of peritoneal signs or of imaging findings suggestive of transmural intestinal necrosis should prompt urgent exploratory laparotomy. If feasible, preoperative angiography is useful because it can help tailor the surgical approach and is associated with significantly lower postoperative morbidity and mortality, particularly for occlusive acute mesenteric ischemia. Depending on the subtype of mesenteric ischemia and severity of the patient's condition, surgery may include embolectomy, thrombectomy, resection of necrotic bowel, and vascular bypass.[7] Papaverine (60-mg bolus followed by 30 to 60 mg/hr continuous infusion for 12 to 48 hours) is a phosphodiesterase inhibitor that is used pre- and postoperatively for occlusive acute mesenteric ischemia (superior mesenteric artery embolism and superior mesenteric artery thrombosis) and as a primary treatment modality for nonocclusive mesenteric ischemia to minimize splanchnic vasoconstriction and decrease the risk of reperfusion injury. Other vasodilators such as alprostadil (20-µg bolus followed by 60 to 80 µg/24 hr infusion until clinical improvement) can also be used.[8] Options for selected patients with occlusive acute mesenteric ischemia who do not require surgery include thrombolysis and endovascular stent placement. Long-term care involves addressing underlying predisposing factors (e.g., smoking cessation, lipid-lowering therapy), lifelong therapy with aspirin in patients who undergo surgery, and dual antiplatelet therapy (usually with aspirin plus clopidogrel) in patients who undergo endovascular intervention (Chapter 59).

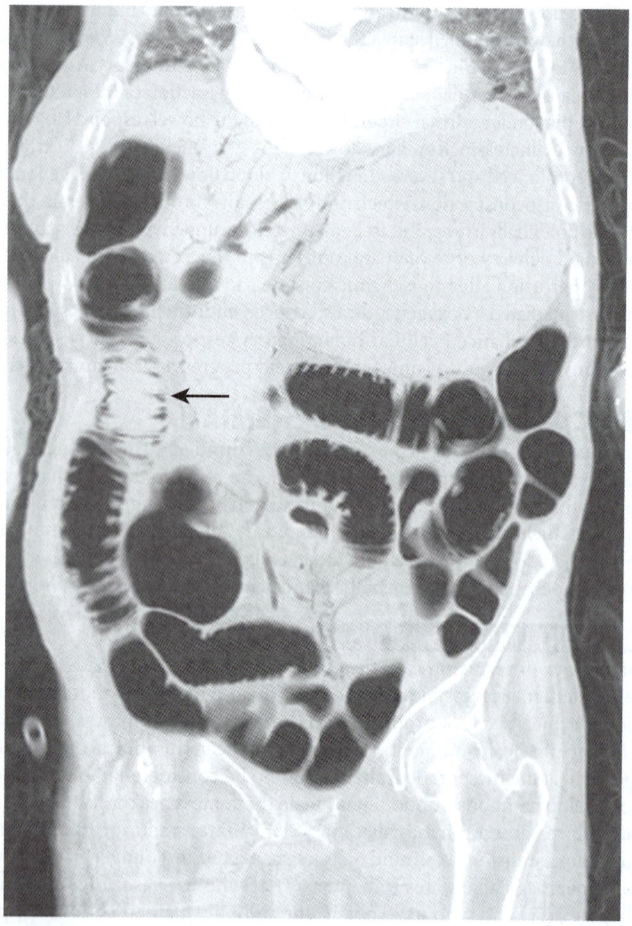

FIGURE 129-1. **Pneumatosis *(arrow)* and intrahepatic portal venous gas in a patient with cardiac arrhythmias and small intestinal ischemia.** (From Gore RM, Yaghmai V, Thakrar KH, et al. Imaging in intestinal ischemic disorders. *Radiol Clin North Am.* 2008;46:845-875.)

SPECIFIC ACUTE MESENTERIC ISCHEMIA SYNDROMES

Superior Mesenteric Artery Thrombosis

Superior mesenteric artery thrombosis, also referred to as acute mesenteric arterial occlusive disease, is estimated to account for more than 50% of cases of acute mesenteric ischemia. It can occur in the context of preexisting symptomatic chronic mesenteric ischemia (see later) in 20 to 50% of cases. These patients typically report preexisting postprandial abdominal pain, weight loss, and sitophobia (fear of eating). Atherosclerotic disease involving other vascular beds (coronary, carotid, peripheral arterial) is common, and risk factors overlap with those of atherosclerosis in general (age, smoking, hypertension, diabetes, hyperlipidemia). The most common site of thrombosis is just distal to the origin of the superior mesenteric artery. The diagnosis can be established by CT angiography or MR angiography, although selective mesenteric catheter angiography is often used to direct and administer therapy. Papaverine (e.g., a 60-mg bolus followed by 30 to 60 mg/hr continuous infusion for 12 to 48 hours) or another vasodilator such as alprostadil (20- µg bolus followed by 60 to 80 µg/24 hr infusion until clinical improvement) is administered into the superior mesenteric artery to

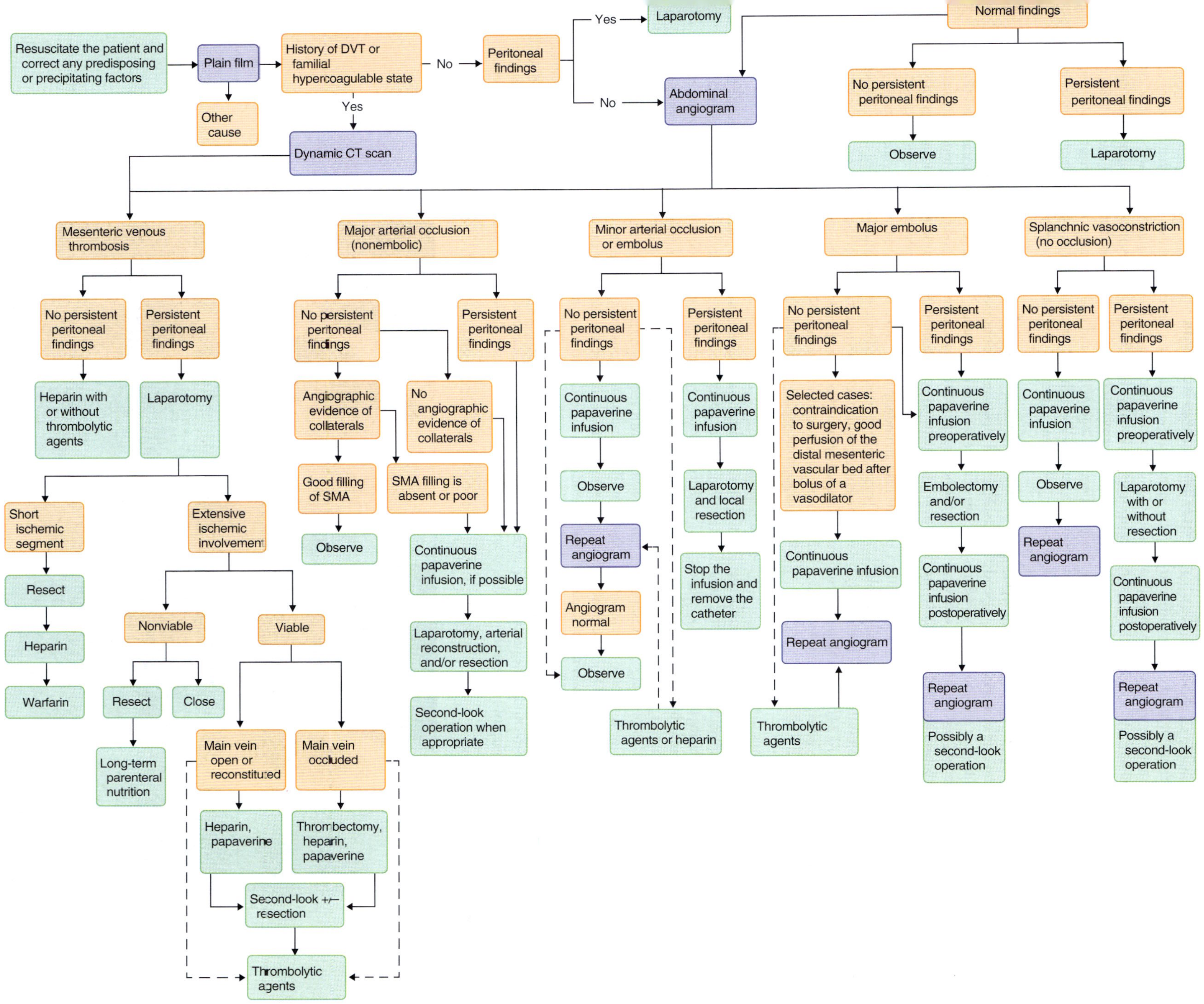

FIGURE 129-2. Algorithm for managing patients with suspected acute mesenteric ischemia: diagnosis and management. Solid lines indicate an accepted management plan; dashed lines indicate an alternative management plan. CT = computed tomography; DVT = deep vein thrombosis; SMA = superior mesenteric artery. (From American Gastroenterological Association Medical Position Statement: guidelines on intestinal ischemia. *Gastroenterology*. 2000;118:951-953 [corrected algorithm in *Gastroenterology*. 2000;119:281].)

alleviate reflex splanchnic vasoconstriction. Thrombolytic therapy (using tissue plasminogen activator infused at a rate of 0.5 to 1 mg/hr), with or without angioplasty and endovascular stenting, is an option in selected cases; however, most patients require surgical thrombectomy and bypass grafting.

Superior Mesenteric Artery Embolism

Superior mesenteric artery embolism is responsible for about 30% of cases of acute mesenteric ischemia. It usually results from left atrial or left ventricular mural thrombi (due to atrial fibrillation, for example), which tend to lodge just distal to the origin of the superior mesenteric artery (E-Fig. 129-1). Selected patients with minor emboli (distal to the ileocolic artery take-off) or with incomplete occlusion may be candidates for thrombolytic therapy with tissue plasminogen activator, administered via a catheter inserted in the vicinity of the embolus, to lyse clot material and alleviate abdominal pain. Emboli that occur proximal to the take-off of the ileocolic artery are termed major, and such patients usually require laparotomy, as do patients with peritoneal signs. Surgical interventions, including embolectomy and bowel resection, depend on operative findings. Some patients will require a second-look surgery within 24 hours to reassess the viability of the small bowel and the adequacy of resection. Vasodilators such as papaverine or alprostadil are used similarly to the management of superior mesenteric artery thrombosis. Patients with superior mesenteric artery embolism may benefit from systemic anticoagulation with unfractionated heparin to prevent clot propagation and further distal embolization, although this benefit must be balanced against the risk of hemorrhage. If surgery is performed, anticoagulation is resumed 24 hours postoperatively. Patients with atrial fibrillation and embolic events generally require long-term anticoagulation (Chapter 52).

Nonocclusive Mesenteric Ischemia

Nonocclusive mesenteric ischemia is the cause of up to 20% of cases of acute mesenteric ischemia. The syndrome results from splanchnic vasoconstriction, which initially occurs as a protective mechanism during low arterial blood flow to the intestine, such as seen in patients with cardiac arrhythmias, heart failure, myocardial infarction, shock, sepsis, burns, pancreatitis, hemorrhage, dialysis, and vasospasm due to vasoactive substances (e.g., cocaine, digoxin, vasopressin, amphetamines). In patients with nonocclusive mesenteric ischemia, the splanchnic vasoconstriction persists despite correction of the precipitating event, thereby leading to bowel ischemia. Abdominal pain may not be a major hallmark and is sometimes overshadowed by other clinical features, such as cardiovascular instability. Given the underlying pathophysiology, the standard of care for nonocclusive mesenteric ischemia is correction of the precipitating event(s), diagnosis by selective mesenteric angiography, and treatment with a continuous infusion of a vasodilator (see earlier) into the superior mesenteric artery to reverse splanchnic vasoconstriction. The infusion is continued until angiography (generally repeated daily) demonstrates that the vasoconstriction is resolved (Figs. 129-3A and 129-3B). Surgical exploration with resection of necrotic bowel is indicated in the presence of peritoneal signs.

Focal Segmental Ischemia

Focal segmental ischemia has a better prognosis than other forms of acute mesenteric ischemia because the length of involved bowel and the extent of necrosis are usually more limited. Causes include atheromatous emboli (Chapter 66), vasculitis (see later), strangulated hernias (Chapter 128), radiation therapy (Chapter 18), and oral contraceptives (Chapter 220). Some patients may develop a chronic enteritis with strictures that can mimic Crohn disease. Treatment is surgical resection of the involved bowel.

Mesenteric Venous Thrombosis

Splanchnic[9] and mesenteric venous thromboses, which account for nearly 10% of cases of acute mesenteric ischemia, have acute and subacute forms that are distinguished based on the duration since the onset of symptoms. Patients with subacute mesenteric venous thrombosis may present with fluctuating symptoms (abdominal pain, nausea, distention, diarrhea) persisting weeks to months. Many patients have an underlying inherited or acquired hypercoagulable state (Table 129-1) or portal hypertension, but some have no identifiable cause. The superior mesenteric vein, often with involvement of the portal and splenic veins, is most frequently thrombosed, and the inferior mesenteric vein is rarely affected. Presenting symptoms in acute thrombosis are similar to those of the arterial forms of acute mesenteric ischemia, notably pain out of proportion to physical examination findings. Gastrointestinal bleeding, if present, usually indicates bowel infarction.

CT with IV contrast has greater than 90% accuracy for the diagnosis of mesenteric venous thrombosis and is the modality of choice given its availability and ease of performance. Findings may include thickening and enhancement of the bowel wall, distention, hazy mesentery, indistinct bowel wall margins, new ascites, and enlargement of the superior mesenteric vein with an intraluminal thrombus. MR venography has very high diagnostic accuracy but is less readily available, more time-consuming, and more costly. Selective mesenteric angiography can help establish the diagnosis and guide therapy (Fig. 129-4) but is generally not needed when standard CT is diagnostic.

Therapy follows similar principles as for arterial acute mesenteric ischemia: fluid resuscitation, antibiotics with gram-negative and anaerobic coverage (e.g., a third-generation cephalosporin or fluoroquinolone plus metronidazole and piperacillin-tazobactam; see Table 266-4), avoidance of vasoconstrictors,

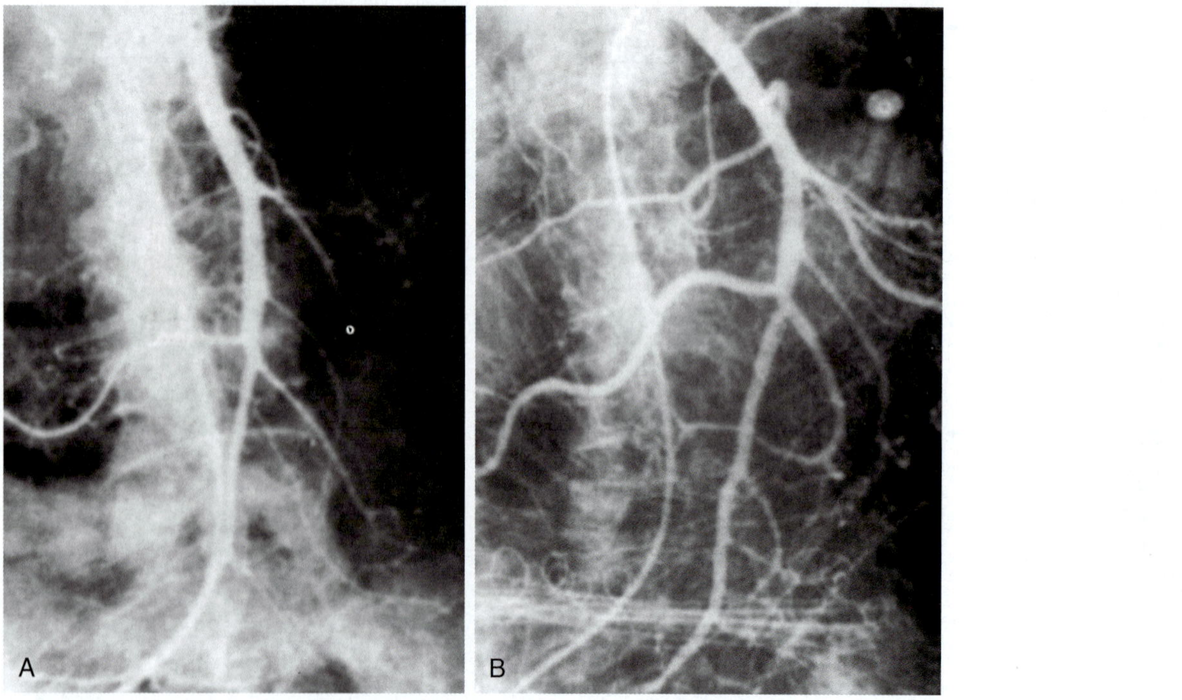

FIGURE 129-3. Selected films from superior mesenteric angiography. A, Diffuse vasoconstriction characteristic of nonocclusive mesenteric ischemia. B, Intra-arterial infusion of papaverine (30 to 60 mg/hr) resulted in vasodilation.

TABLE 129-1 CONDITIONS ASSOCIATED WITH MESENTERIC VENOUS THROMBOSIS

PROTHROMBOTIC STATES (See Chapter 67)
Antithrombin deficiency
Protein C deficiency
Protein S deficiency
Factor V Leiden
Prothrombin gene G20210A mutation
Antiphospholipid antibodies
Hyperhomocysteinemia
Oral contraceptives
Pregnancy
Neoplasms
INTRA-ABDOMINAL INFLAMMATION AND SEPSIS
Peritonitis
Pancreatitis
Diverticulitis
Inflammatory bowel disease
Appendicitis
Cholecystitis
HEMATOLOGIC DISORDERS
Paroxysmal nocturnal hemoglobinuria
Polycythemia vera
Essential thrombocythemia
Sickle cell disease
LIVER CIRRHOSIS
Portal hypertension
Variceal sclerotherapy
OTHERS
Abdominal surgery
Blunt abdominal trauma

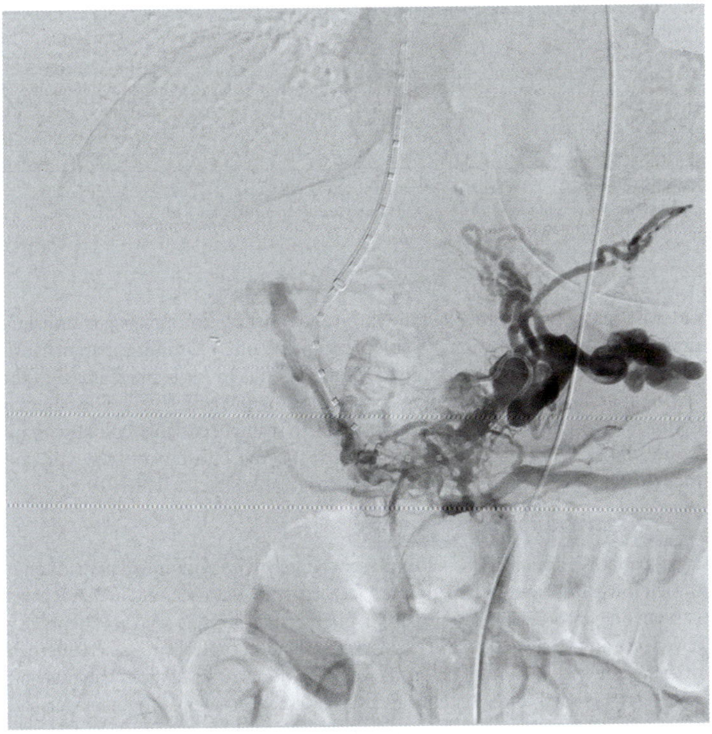

FIGURE 129-4. Selective mesenteric angiogram of a patient with superior mesenteric venous thrombosis and extrahepatic portal vein thrombosis.

and systemic anticoagulation with heparin (Table 68-6).[10] The presence of peritoneal signs or other findings suspicious for bowel infarction require laparotomy with or without bowel resection and infusion of a vasodilator. Selected patients may benefit from thrombolytic therapy. Patients with mesenteric venous thrombosis and an underlying hypercoagulable state should receive lifelong anticoagulation therapy with warfarin or a direct-acting oral

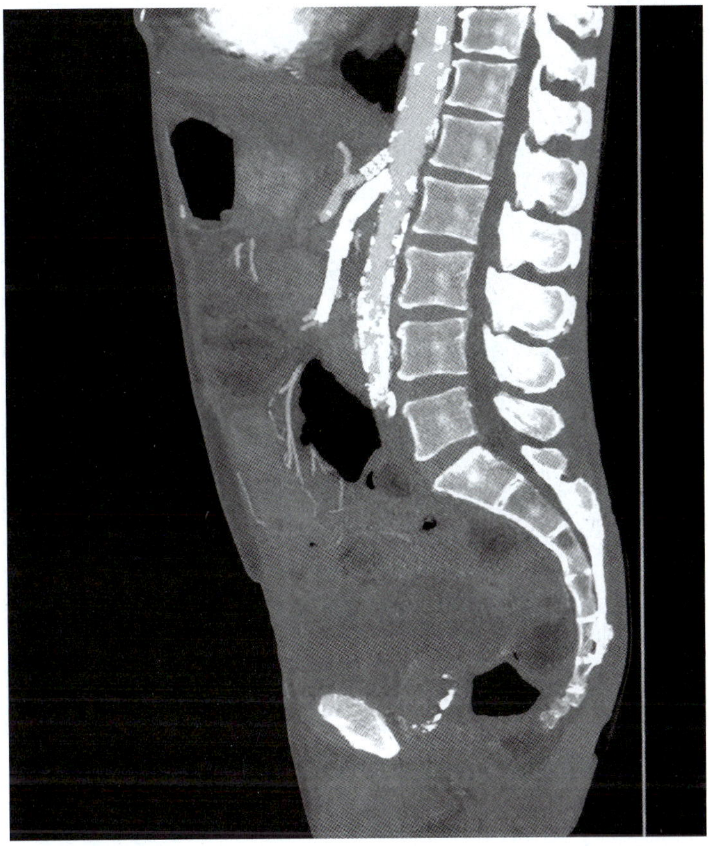

FIGURE 129-5. Computed tomographic angiography of a patient who had chronic mesenteric ischemia and who was treated with endovascular stenting of the celiac axis and superior mesenteric artery. Note the extensive atherosclerotic disease.

anticoagulant (Table 70-6);[11] otherwise, a 3- to 6-month course of anticoagulation is thought to be adequate. The prognosis of mesenteric venous thrombosis is generally better than that of the arterial variants of acute mesenteric ischemia.

Chronic mesenteric venous thrombosis is distinct from the acute and subacute forms; patients may present with gastrointestinal bleeding from esophageal or gastric varices owing to portal or splenic vein thrombosis in the absence of symptoms at the time of the initial thrombotic event. Treatment is aimed at controlling hemorrhage and underlying portal hypertension.

CHRONIC MESENTERIC ISCHEMIA

Chronic mesenteric ischemia, which is almost always caused by atherosclerotic disease of the mesenteric vessels, generally involves the origins of at least two of the three major mesenteric arteries (celiac axis, superior mesenteric artery, inferior mesenteric artery) (Fig. 129-5). The risk factors are the same as for atherosclerosis (Chapter 40), including age, smoking, hypertension, diabetes, and hyperlipidemia, and many patients have atherosclerotic disease involving other vascular beds.

CLINICAL MANIFESTATIONS

A hallmark symptom is postprandial pain in the upper or mid-abdomen, starting within 30 minutes after eating, increasing in severity, and gradually subsiding over a few hours. Weight loss may occur as a result of sitophobia; other symptoms include nausea, vomiting, bloating, diarrhea, and constipation. The syndrome may progress with time, and episodes of pain may become more prolonged and unrelated to eating, indicative of worsening vascular narrowing and increased risk of acute thrombosis. The occurrence of sudden severe pain in a patient with known or suspected chronic mesenteric ischemia implies a superimposed acute thrombotic event. Uncommon associations are unexplained gastroduodenal ulcerations that do not heal with acid suppression, small bowel biopsy findings of villous atrophy, and delayed gastric emptying. Physical findings in patients with advanced disease may include cachexia or an abdominal bruit.

DIAGNOSIS

The diagnosis of chronic mesenteric ischemia may be challenging: the prevalence of atherosclerosis is high in older patients, and abdominal pain may not

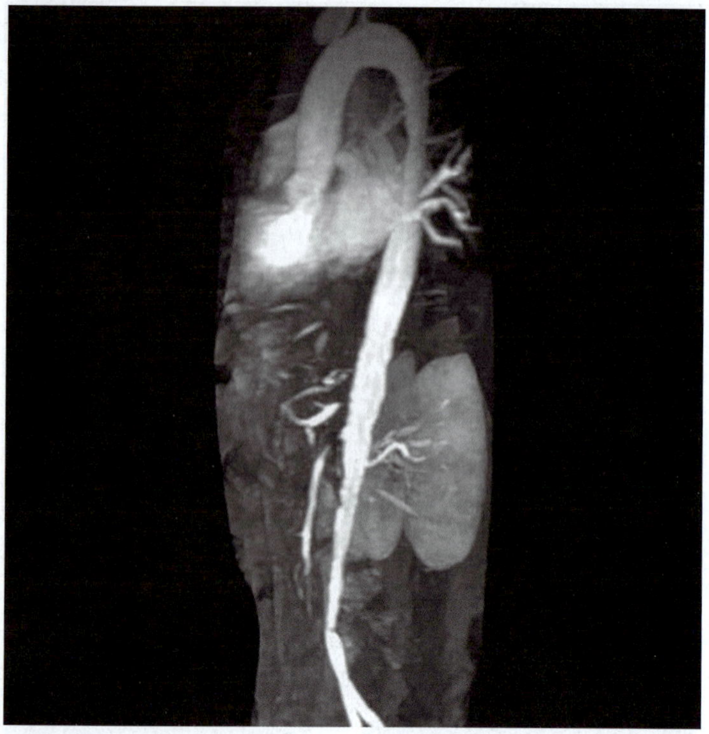

FIGURE 129-6. Magnetic resonance angiography in a patient with chronic mesenteric ischemia. This image shows severe stenosis at the origins of the celiac axis and the superior mesenteric artery. (Courtesy Thomas Casciani, MD.)

necessarily be due to mesenteric vascular occlusive disease. Available imaging modalities, such as CT angiography, can reveal stenoses in the mesenteric vessels but cannot ascertain whether ischemia is present. Doppler ultrasonography can screen for stenoses in the proximal aspects of the celiac axis and superior mesenteric artery; increased flow velocities of at least 200 cm/sec (celiac axis) and 275 cm/sec (superior mesenteric artery) are associated with a stenosis of at least 70%. Both CT angiography and MR angiography (Fig. 129-6 and Video 129-1) are useful for detecting arterial stenoses, but neither is sensitive enough to exclude chronic mesenteric ischemia when the pretest probability is high. Gastric tonometry exercise testing, which measures the gastric-arterial Pco_2 gradient (an increase after exercise is indicative of ischemia), has shown promise for diagnosing ischemia but is not widely available. Selective mesenteric angiography remains a cornerstone of the evaluation, because the diagnosis requires the presence of clinical symptoms, occlusion of at least two of the three major mesenteric vessels, and exclusion of other potential causes of postprandial abdominal pain (e.g., cancer, gastroparesis, volvulus, bowel obstruction, pancreatobiliary disease, paraesophageal hernias).

TREATMENT

In patients who have symptoms consistent with chronic mesenteric ischemia, have appropriate angiographic findings, and have no other potential causes, revascularization is indicated. Mesenteric angioplasty with or without stent placement is the treatment of choice, with open surgery reserved for selected younger patients and patients who are not suitable for endovascular repair,[12,13] and is associated with shorter hospital stay and lower morbidity. However, surgery is more effective long-term because it is associated with better long-term patency rates and a lower risk of recurrent symptoms.

TABLE 129-2 CONDITIONS AND MEDICATIONS ASSOCIATED WITH COLON ISCHEMIA

CARDIOVASCULAR
Atherosclerosis
Atrial fibrillation
Cerebrovascular disease
Congestive heart failure
Ischemic heart disease
Hypertension
Hypotension
Peripheral vascular disease
Shock
PULMONARY
Chronic obstructive pulmonary disease
GASTROINTESTINAL
Constipation
Diarrhea
Irritable bowel syndrome
OTHER MEDICAL CONDITIONS
Diabetes
Rheumatologic disorders
SURGERY
Abdominal surgery
Cardiovascular (including aortic) surgery
Ileostomy
Laparoscopy
MEDICATIONS AND DRUGS
Constipation-inducing medications
Immunomodulators (antitumor necrosis factor-α, interferon)
Illicit drugs (amphetamines, cocaine)
Antibiotics
Appetite suppressants
Chemotherapeutic agents (including taxanes)
Decongestants (including pseudoephedrine)
Diuretics
Ergot alkaloids
Hormonal therapies (including oral contraceptives)
Laxatives
Psychotropics
Serotoninergics (including alosetron)

Adapted from Brandt LJ, Feuerstadt P, Longstreth GF, et al. ACG clinical guideline: epidemiology, risk factors, patterns of presentation, diagnosis, and management of colon ischemia (CI). *Am J Gastroenterol.* 2015;110:18-44.

COLON ISCHEMIA

Colon ischemia is the most common ischemic syndrome of the bowel. It is diagnosed in about 10 to 20% of patients who present to the hospital with lower gastrointestinal bleeding, and its incidence is estimated at about 16 per 100,000 person-years in the general population. Colon ischemia is also referred to as "ischemic colitis"; however, an inflammatory phase is not consistently found, so the preferred term is colon ischemia. Colon ischemia encompasses a spectrum of injury, including reversible colopathy (most common, about 50%), transient colitis, chronic colitis, stricture, gangrene, and fulminant universal colitis. Most cases occur in older patients (>60 years old), in whom the most common cause is transient nonocclusive hypoperfusion of a colonic segment, often without apparent cause. Although older patients are prone to colon ischemia in "watershed areas" of the colon (splenic flexure-descending colon), a segmental pattern of involvement is common, most often involving the left colon. In younger patients, colon ischemia is more likely to be caused by the use of vasoactive substances (e.g., cocaine, methamphetamines), vasculitis, or hypercoagulable states (Table 129-2).

CLINICAL MANIFESTATIONS

Most patients with colon ischemia present acutely with abdominal pain, often in the left lower quadrant, associated with fecal urgency, diarrhea, and hematochezia. Passage of maroon stool may also occur, but bleeding is rarely severe. Patients may have fever and tachycardia. The physical examination typically reveals tenderness over the affected portion of colon, as well as abdominal distention. Patients with isolated right-sided colon ischemia tend to have more severe pain, which overshadows bleeding. As with acute mesenteric ischemia, the presence of peritoneal signs mandates prompt surgical consultation. About 25% of cases of colon ischemia are isolated right-side colon ischemia, which can complicate low-flow states such as hypotension and sepsis, chronic kidney disease, and hemodialysis, presumably secondary to intravascular fluid shifts.

DIAGNOSIS

No single test can conclusively diagnose colon ischemia, but the diagnosis can be established with judicious use of diagnostic modalities in the appropriate clinical context.[14] The differential diagnosis includes inflammatory bowel disease (ulcerative colitis and Crohn disease; Chapter 127), infectious colitis

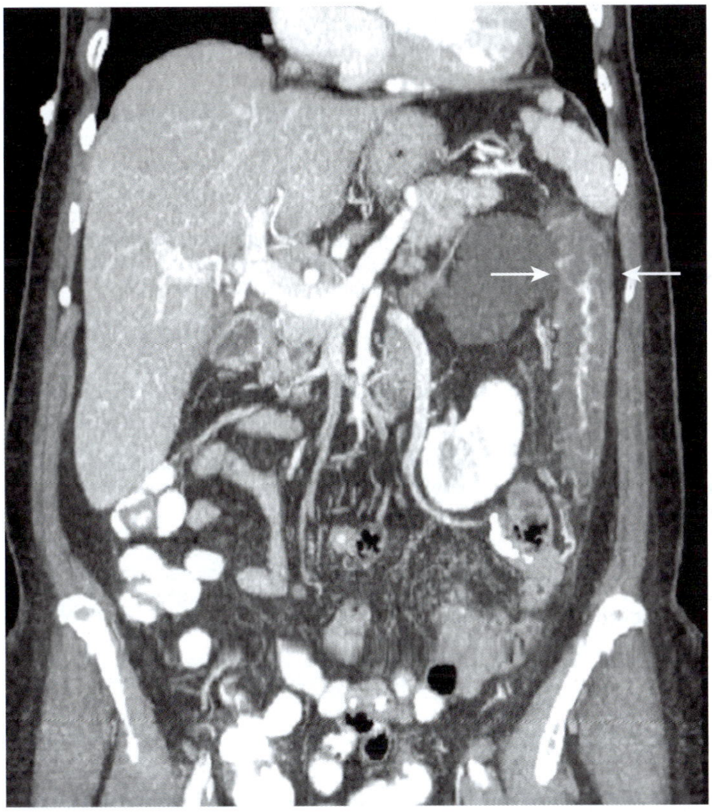

FIGURE 129-7. **Colon ischemia. There is mural thickening (*arrows*) of the proximal descending colon and submucosal edema. (From Gore RM, Yaghmai V, Thakrar KH, et al. Imaging in intestinal ischemic disorders. *Radiol Clin North Am.* 2008;46:845-875.)**

(Chapter 126), and mechanical obstruction due to colorectal cancer (Chapter 179), fecal impaction, or stricture.

Laboratory findings may be normal, but the presence of leukocytosis and elevated blood levels of urea nitrogen and lactate are indicative of a more severe course. Plain radiographs may be normal or show thumbprinting. A CT scan with IV contrast, which is useful to exclude other diagnostic possibilities and to assess the severity and distribution of the ischemic process, may show segmental colonic edema and inflammation with or without pericolonic inflammatory stranding (Fig. 129-7); however, these findings are nonspecific and can also be seen in inflammatory bowel disease, infectious colitis, and diverticulitis. Colonoscopy is the best test to diagnose colon ischemia, because it allows direct visualization of the mucosal biopsy and assessment of the distribution and severity of the disease process. Most colonoscopic findings are nonspecific (erythema, edema, segmental patchy ulcerations, subepithelial hemorrhages), but the presence of a "single stripe sign" (E-Fig. 129-2) in the left colon is a reliable indicator of colon ischemia. Visceral angiography is typically not required. However, patients with isolated right-sided colon ischemia tend to have a more aggressive course. This is because the superior mesenteric artery supplies blood to the right side of the colon and most of the small intestine, so ischemia confined to the right colon may be a sentinel event for ischemia involving the small intestine (E-Fig. 129-3).

Unlike patients with left-sided colon ischemia, those with isolated right-sided colon ischemia should undergo CT angiography or traditional angiography to evaluate the mesenteric circulation for possible occlusion of the superior mesenteric artery.

TREATMENT

Colon ischemia is usually self-limited, and symptoms generally resolve within 2 to 3 days with supportive care: volume replacement, bowel rest, correction of conditions leading to hypoperfusion such as systemic hypotension, avoidance of vasoconstrictive medications, and broad-spectrum antibiotics (e.g., third-generation cephalosporin or fluoroquinolone plus metronidazole, and piperacillin-tazobactam; see Table 266-4) with gram-negative and anaerobic coverage, especially in patients with severe colon ischemia (Fig. 129-8). Surgery is reserved for patients with signs and symptoms of gangrene, perforation, or massive bleeding.[15] Patients with persistent symptoms have a higher incidence of complications, including gangrene, perforation, segmental colitis, and stricture. Strictures, which can form over weeks to months, may require surgical resection.

VASCULITIS

Vasculitis (Chapter 249) can involve the gastrointestinal tract, usually in association with systemic involvement. The gastrointestinal manifestations, which depend on the size of the vessels involved, include abdominal pain, nausea or vomiting, diarrhea, and overt bleeding. The ischemic process is typically due to immune complex deposition that leads to the activation of complement and resulting inflammation, which may then lead to focal segmental ischemia. Treatment usually requires immunosuppressive medications (Chapter 28) or surgical resection in selected situations.

LARGE VESSEL VASCULITIS

Takayasu disease and *giant cell arteritis* (Chapter 63) rarely involve the mesenteric circulation. Takayasu arteritis most often affects young women of Asian background and has been associated with ulcerative colitis and Crohn disease (Chapter 127).

MEDIUM VESSEL VASCULITIS

Polyarteritis nodosa (Chapter 249) is the most common underlying diagnosis in vasculitis involving the gastrointestinal tract. The disease is characterized by segmental microaneurysms, which occur more frequently in the small bowel than in the colon. The gallbladder, spleen, liver, and pancreas may be involved. The syndrome may be associated with chronic hepatitis B infection (Chapter 135). Abdominal pain is the most common symptom, but gastrointestinal bleeding and perforation have also been reported.

Infantile febrile mucocutaneous lymph node syndrome (Kawasaki disease; Chapter 249) is a necrotizing vasculitis that can affect young children and cause abdominal pain, ileus, obstruction, and perforation.

Malignant atrophic papulosis (Degos disease) is a rare occlusive vascular disease affecting mainly the skin and intestine. Spontaneous perforation may occur owing to ischemia, and the disease has a poor prognosis.

SMALL VESSEL VASCULITIS

Systemic lupus erythematosus (Chapter 245) is associated with a variety of gastrointestinal manifestations.[16] Lupus vasculitis involving the mesenteric vessels may present with a clinical syndrome of focal segmental ischemia or chronic mesenteric ischemia, but some patients develop significant gastrointestinal bleeding. Lupus mesenteric vasculitis requires prompt recognition and immunosuppressive management.

Antineutrophil cytoplasmic antibody (ANCA)–associated vasculitis includes granulomatosis with polyangiitis, microscopic polyangiitis, and eosinophilic granulomatosis with polyangiitis (Churg-Strauss syndrome; Chapter 249). Gastrointestinal tract involvement is variable, with abdominal pain and bleeding the most common symptoms.

Henoch-Schönlein purpura (Chapter 249) typically presents in children with palpable purpura, arthritis, and abdominal pain. The cause is deposition of immunoglobulin A immune complexes in blood vessel walls. Gastrointestinal involvement is common and usually manifested by pain and bleeding owing to mucosal and submucosal hemorrhages.

Hypersensitivity vasculitis rarely involves the splanchnic vessels and is associated with a variety of drugs, chemicals, and infections.

Behçet disease (Chapter 249) is characterized by oral and genital ulcers. Both large-vessel and small-vessel vasculitis may occur. Gastrointestinal manifestations include abdominal pain, diarrhea, overt bleeding, and perforation due to deep ulcerations. The ileocecal area is most commonly involved.[17]

For each of these conditions, treatment is aimed at the underlying vasculitis.

VASCULAR ANOMALIES AND DISORDERS

Vascular anomalies of the gastrointestinal tract are common, especially with older age. *Angioectasia* (also referred to as vascular ectasia) is a general term that refers to the process whereby a blood vessel is lengthened or dilated. *Angiodysplasia* has often been used interchangeably with angioectasia. *Telangiectasia* is similar, but the term is usually used in the context of systemic disorders, such as hereditary hemorrhagic telangiectasia and scleroderma. *Arteriovenous malformation* is a congenital lesion, whereas *angioma* is a vascular neoplasm that can be benign (hemangioma) or malignant (angiosarcoma).

ANGIOECTASIA

Angioectasia is the most common vascular abnormality of the gastrointestinal tract, and its prevalence increases with age. Angioectasias consist

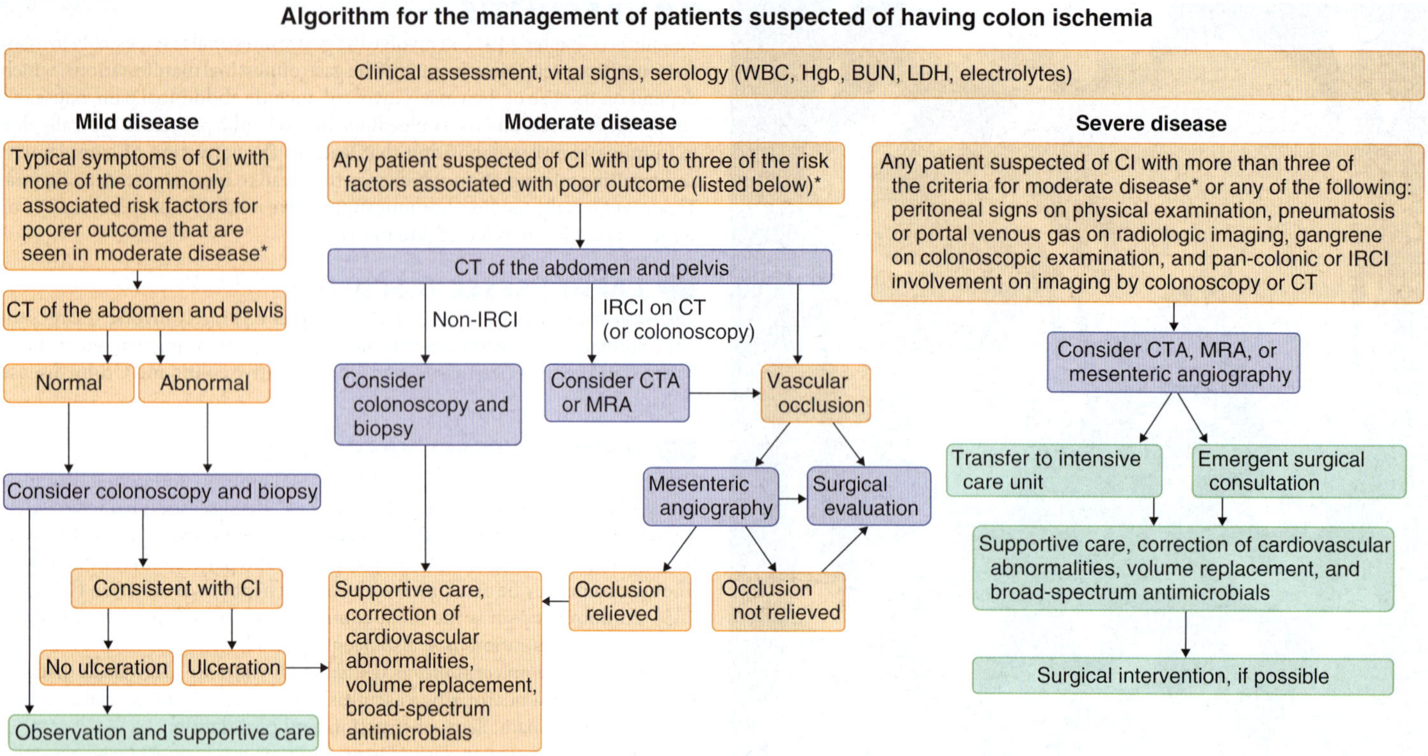

FIGURE 129-8. **Colon ischemia algorithm.** Diagnosis and treatment of colon ischemia (CI) based upon disease severity. *Risk factors associated with poor outcome: male gender, hypotension (systolic blood pressure <90 mm Hg), tachycardia (HR >100 beats per min), abdominal pain without rectal bleeding, BUN >20 mg/dL, Hgb <12 g/dL, LDH >350 U/l, serum sodium <136 mEq/L(mmol/L), WBC >15 × 10^9/cmm. BUN = blood urea nitrogen; CT = computed tomography; CTA = computed tomography angiography; Hgb = hemoglobin; IRCI = isolated right-colon ischemia; LDH = lactate dehydrogenase; MRA = magnetic resonance angiography; MRI = magnetic resonance imaging; WBC = white blood cell count. (From Brandt LJ, Feuerstadt P, Longstreth GF, et al. ACG clinical guideline: epidemiology, risk factors, patterns of presentation, diagnosis, and management of colon ischemia [CI]. *Am J Gastroenterol.* 2015;110:18-44.)

of thin-walled, distorted mucosal and submucosal arterioles, venules, and capillaries. Angioectasias are most frequently located in the cecum and ascending colon, can be single or multiple, and can sometimes be found concomitantly in the small intestine and stomach. Associations include systemic sclerosis (Chapter 246), chronic renal failure (Chapter 116), von Willebrand disease (Chapter 159), aortic stenosis (Chapter 60), and left ventricular assist devices (Chapter 93).

CLINICAL MANIFESTATIONS

Most angioectasias are asymptomatic and found incidentally during endoscopy. However, some may cause painless bleeding, which can be occult or overt (hematochezia, melena, hematemesis).[18] The bleeding is typically recurrent and mild, but about 15% of patients develop massive bleeding.

DIAGNOSIS

The diagnosis is most often established at endoscopy, either incidentally or during investigations for anemia or gastrointestinal bleeding (Fig. 129-9). The lesions may be difficult to discern in patients who are hypovolemic or have received meperidine for sedation; in the latter situation, naloxone can be considered to reverse the opioid effect and improve visualization. Small bowel angioectasias beyond the reach of endoscopes require videocapsule endoscopy[19] or small bowel balloon-assisted enteroscopy for diagnosis and treatment (Chapter 121).

TREATMENT

Incidental angioectasias found at endoscopy or colonoscopy in asymptomatic individuals do not require intervention. Endoscopic modalities, which can effectively control hemorrhage from angioectasias, include bipolar electrocoagulation, argon plasma coagulation (E-Figs. 129-4A and 129-4B), and application of hemoclips. Rebleeding occurs in some patients and requires repeat intervention. When endoscopic hemostasis is not feasible owing to active bleeding or inaccessible lesion location, visceral angiography can be diagnostic and therapeutic by allowing embolization of the bleeding lesion. Thalidomide (25 mg orally 4 times daily) has antiangiogenic properties and has been reported to be effective in some patients with refractory bleeding from intestinal angioectasias. Other pharmacologic options include octreotide (50 to 100 µg subcutaneously twice a day) and bevacizumab (5 mg/kg every 2 weeks for a total of six infusions).

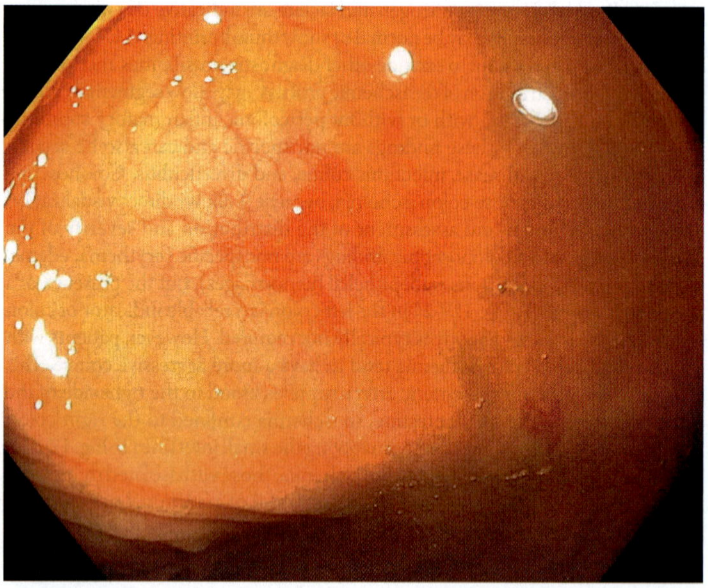

FIGURE 129-9. **Colonic angioectasia.**

DIEULAFOY LESION

Dieulafoy lesion is a persistently large submucosal artery with an overlying mucosal defect. This lesion is most often found in the proximal portion of the stomach within 6 cm of the gastroesophageal junction, but it has also been reported in the esophagus, small intestine, colon, and rectum. Clinical manifestations include overt bleeding (Chapter 121), which can be brisk, massive, and recurrent (Fig. 129-10). In some patients, diagnosis may be delayed because the vascular protuberance can be subtle and difficult to visualize at endoscopy.

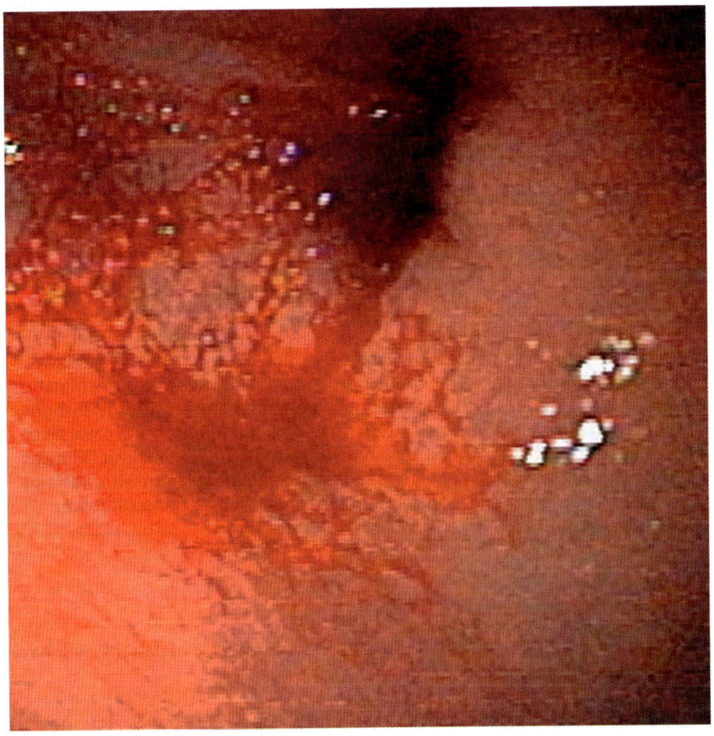

FIGURE 129-10. Brisk bleeding from a Dieulafoy lesion in the stomach of a patient with melena.

Endoscopic treatment is usually effective.[20] Options include injection, electrocoagulation, argon plasma coagulation, band ligation, and hemoclip application.

HEREDITARY HEMORRHAGIC TELANGIECTASIA

Hereditary hemorrhagic telangiectasia, also known as Osler-Weber-Rendu disease (Chapter 159), is an inherited autosomal dominant disorder. Patients typically have visible telangiectasias on their lips and mucous membranes, as well as telangiectasias in their gastrointestinal tract and other organs. The spectrum of symptoms varies with age: affected children tend to have frequent epistaxis, whereas overt recurrent gastrointestinal bleeding predominates in older age groups. Telangiectasias on the lips (see Fig. 159-3), buccal mucosa, and tongue are highly suggestive. Most patients have recurrent melena (sometimes compounded by swallowed blood from epistaxis), and some patients become transfusion-dependent. Diagnosis is based on clinical criteria (epistaxis, telangiectasias, visceral lesions, hereditary hemorrhagic telangiectasia in a first-degree relative) and can be confirmed by testing for mutations in the endoglin and activin receptor-like kinase-1 genes. Endoscopic therapy is the mainstay of management, particularly for actively bleeding lesions.

OTHER ECTASIAS

Patients with *Turner syndrome* (Chapter 217), *scleroderma* (Chapter 246), and *CREST syndrome* (Chapter 246) may also have gastrointestinal tract telangiectasias. In patients with portal hypertension (Chapter 139), vascular ectasias can involve venules and capillaries in the stomach (*congestive gastropathy*), in the small bowel (*congestive enteropathy*), and in the colon (*congestive colopathy*). In the stomach, ectasia and thrombosis can result in so-called watermelon stomach (gastric antral vascular ectasia), in which erythematous streaks, similar to the stripes on a watermelon, are visible by endoscopy in the antrum and radiate toward the pylorus and even the gastric cardia. Occult bleeding is common, and melena can occur. If iron replacement alone is not adequate, argon plasma coagulation is the treatment of choice.

AORTOENTERIC FISTULAS

After abdominal aortic aneurysm surgery (Chapter 63), an *aortoenteric fistula* can develop, often because of infection of the graft. Fistulas typically communicate with the third or fourth portion of the duodenum and can occur several years after surgery. Massive and even fatal gastrointestinal bleeding may result. When gastrointestinal bleeding develops in patients who have had prior abdominal aortic surgery, the evaluation must include urgent upper endoscopy to exclude another definitive source of the bleeding. CT aids the diagnosis, which should be suspected in the appropriate clinical context. If no alternative bleeding source can be definitively found, explorative surgery is indicated.

An *atrioesophageal fistula* may be caused by thermal damage to the heart or esophagus. Examples of precipitating events include radiofrequency ablation procedures for arrhythmias (Chapter 54) or for Barrett esophagus (Chapter 124).

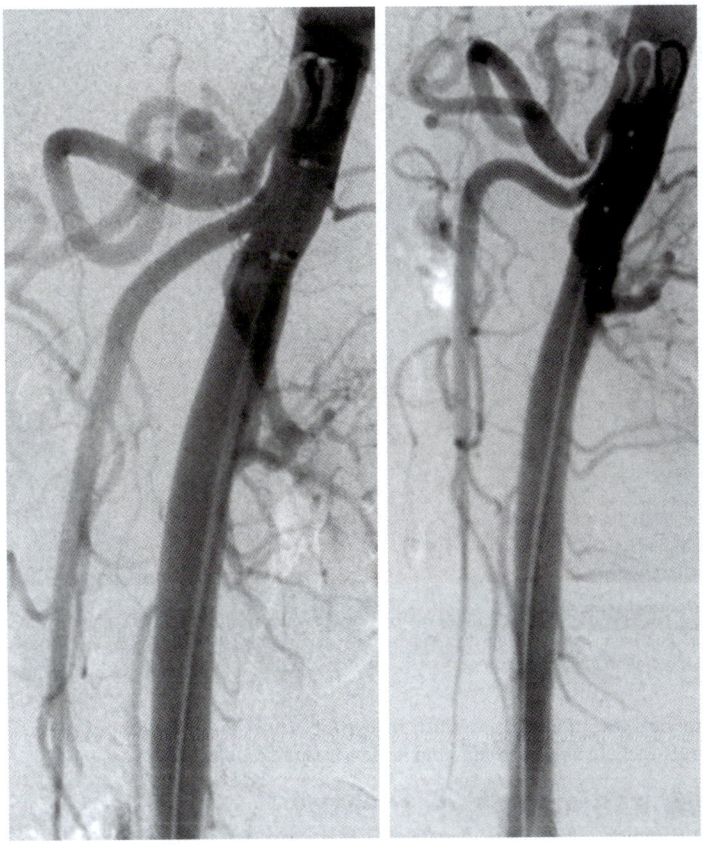

FIGURE 129-11. Celiac artery compression syndrome is caused by a low-lying median arcuate ligament, which results in compression of the celiac artery. This phenomenon is accentuated during expiration. (Courtesy Himanshu Shah, MD.)

CELIAC ARTERY COMPRESSION SYNDROME

Celiac artery compression syndrome, also known as median arcuate ligament syndrome, is a rare and poorly understood pseudo-ischemic syndrome. Most patients are young and otherwise healthy. Postprandial upper abdominal pain and diarrhea may be caused by extrinsic compression of the celiac axis by the median arcuate ligament of the diaphragm or by pressure on the celiac ganglion itself. Sitophobia can result in considerable weight loss, and some patients have an epigastric bruit that intensifies with expiration. Visceral angiography supports the diagnosis (Fig. 129-11), although asymptomatic patients also can have a localized bruit and even celiac axis compression on angiography. Surgical therapy is an option if patients have otherwise unexplained symptoms that are consistent with the syndrome.

SUPERIOR MESENTERIC ARTERY SYNDROME

Superior mesenteric artery syndrome refers to impingement of the duodenum by the superior mesenteric artery owing to narrowing of the angle between the superior mesenteric artery and aorta. The resulting mechanical obstruction can cause rapid weight loss because gastric outlet obstruction results in abdominal pain and postprandial vomiting. Imaging typically shows evidence of obstruction in the third portion of the duodenum, with a cutoff and proximal dilation. Treatment of the underlying condition (adequate nutrition and weight gain) can be curative, but surgery is sometimes needed.

HEMANGIOMAS

Hemangiomas are uncommon, usually benign vascular tumors that can be found throughout the gastrointestinal tract, often in the rectum or colon. They may be single or multiple and can be classified as cavernous, capillary, or mixed. Cavernous rectal hemangiomas tend to be large and bleed profusely, but colonic hemangiomas may cause slow, occult bleeding. Small hemangiomas can be treated endoscopically, but large or multiple lesions may require

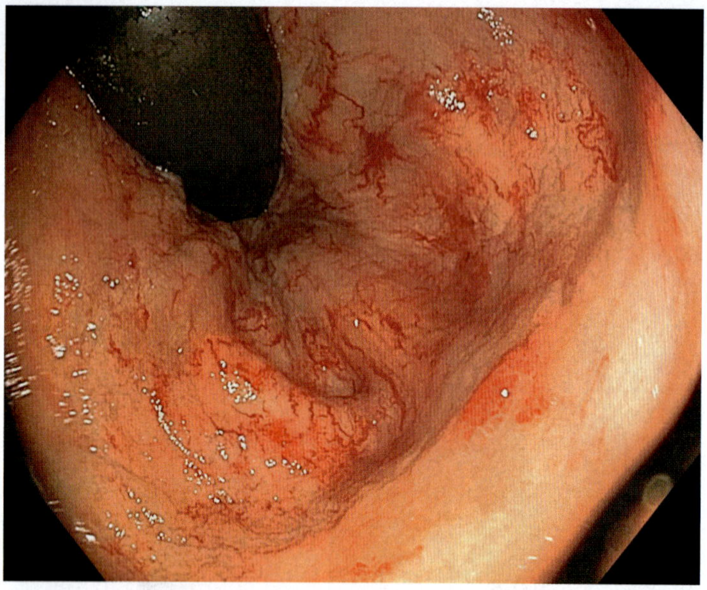

FIGURE 129-12. Radiation proctopathy. Retroflexed view of the rectum showing multiple large and serpiginous vascular ectasias in a patient with hematochezia and history of radiation for prostate cancer.

surgical resection. Rare vascular malignant neoplasms of the gastrointestinal tract include *angiosarcomas* and *hemangioendotheliomas*.

RADIATION PROCTOPATHY

A common radiation-mediated injury to the gastrointestinal tract is radiation proctopathy (Chapter 128), typically in patients treated for prostate cancer. Patients with acute radiation proctopathy (within 6 weeks of therapy) can present with tenesmus and diarrhea, whereas those with chronic radiation proctopathy (onset 6 to 24 months after therapy) can have significant hematochezia owing to radiation-associated vascular ectasias. Endoscopy reveals mucosal fibrosis and a proliferation of vascular ectasias, which are the source of bleeding (Fig. 129-12). Argon plasma coagulation is usually an effective treatment for bleeding.

HEPATIC AND SPLENIC VASCULAR DISEASE

Abnormalities of the hepatic and splenic arteries and veins affect fewer than 1 person per 2000.

BUDD-CHIARI SYNDROME

Budd-Chiari syndrome can be the result of any process that interferes with the normal outflow of blood through the hepatic vein, such as constrictive pericarditis (Chapter 62) and veno-occlusive disease (Chapter 136). The most common cause is thrombosis of one, two, or all three of the major hepatic veins, with or without extension of thrombus and even occlusion into the inferior vena cava.[21] More than 50% of cases of Budd-Chiari syndrome are related to a hypercoagulable state (Chapter 67), such as a factor V (Leiden) gene mutation, antiphospholipid antibody syndrome, protein C deficiency, protein S deficiency, antithrombin III deficiency, a chronic myeloproliferative disorder (e.g., polycythemia vera [Chapter 152], essential thrombocythemia [Chapter 152], myeloid metaplasia [Chapter 152]), paroxysmal nocturnal hemoglobinuria, or other hypercoagulable state conditions (Chapter 67). Other causes include malignancies (direct compression or invasion of hepatic veins), infections (liver abscess), pregnancy, inflammatory disorders (e.g., sarcoidosis, inflammatory bowel disease, connective tissue disease), membranous obstruction (webs) of the inferior vena cava, or spontaneous thrombosis, owing to a hypercoagulable state (Chapter 67).

CLINICAL MANIFESTATIONS

Budd-Chiari syndrome usually progresses insidiously over weeks to months as patients develop hepatomegaly, upper abdominal pain, and ascites. Rare patients may present acutely with encephalopathy, jaundice, ascites, and liver failure.

DIAGNOSIS

Most patients have only mild to moderate nonspecific elevations in serum aspartate and alanine aminotransferase levels. *JAK2* mutation analysis may detect a chronic myeloproliferative disorder. Screening for factor V (Leiden); antiphospholipid antibodies; and deficiencies in protein C, protein S, and antithrombin III is appropriate if the cause is not clear. Doppler ultrasound of the liver is the initial diagnostic test of choice[22]; contrast CT scanning or MR angiography can detect the absence of hepatic venous flow or venous thrombosis (or both). The diagnosis can be confirmed by hepatic venography (see Fig. 129-7), which also can guide therapy.

TREATMENT

Therapy includes diagnosis and treatment of underlying conditions, anticoagulation (intravenous heparin; see Table 68-6 in Chapter 68) to prevent the propagation of thrombi, and treatment of the ascites (e.g., diuretics; Chapter 139). Most patients require interventional radiologic procedures, such as angioplasty, stenting, or transjugular intrahepatic portosystemic shunts, to restore hepatic venous flow.[23] If endovascular procedures are not successful, a surgical shunt can drain the portal and/or mesenteric veins into the inferior vena cava. Liver transplantation (Chapter 140) should be considered for fulminant liver failure or cirrhosis, or both. Most patients require lifelong anticoagulation with warfarin or a newer oral anticoagulant (Chapter 70), even after liver transplantation.

PROGNOSIS

The 5-year survival rate is more than 80%, but about 50% of patients will have a major bleed, often related to invasive therapy.

PORTAL VEIN THROMBOSIS

The most common causes of acute portal vein thrombosis are cirrhosis, hypercoagulable states, intra-abdominal malignancy, inflammatory disorders (e.g., pancreatitis, Crohn disease), and medical procedures (e.g., splenectomy, cholecystectomy, gastrectomy, liver transplantation, transjugular intrahepatic portosystemic shunt). As with Budd-Chiari syndrome, many patients have a *JAK2* mutation.

CLINICAL MANIFESTATIONS AND DIAGNOSIS

Clinical manifestations include portal hypertension with variceal bleeding and ascites (Chapter 139).[24] Abdominal pain may indicate intestinal ischemia as the thrombus extends into the superior mesenteric vein. Fever, chills, and liver tenderness suggest pylephlebitis, which can result in systemic sepsis. The diagnosis is usually established by Doppler ultrasound or by CT or MR angiography.

TREATMENT

Anticoagulation with warfarin (Tables 70-2 and 70-4) to an international normalized ratio (INR) of 2 to 3 or enoxaparin (1 mg/kg subcutaneously twice a day) is recommended for at least 3 months and should be continued chronically in patients who have persistent risk factors for thrombosis or whose thrombus extends into the mesenteric veins.[25] Pylephlebitis usually requires intravenous parenteral antibiotics (e.g., piperacillin/tazobactam, ticarcillin/clavulanate, carbapenem, or a third-generation cephalosporin plus metronidazole; see Chapter 266). Parenteral antibiotics are typically given for about 2 weeks, and total treatment duration is at least 6 weeks, with the choice of antibiotics guided by blood culture results.

In patients who have cirrhosis complicated by acute or chronic portal vein thrombosis, endoscopy is recommended to diagnose and treat esophageal varices (Chapter 120).

Patients with *chronic* portal vein thrombosis can be asymptomatic but often have portal hypertension and hypersplenism. A biliary cholangiopathy may cause jaundice that requires biliary stenting. After varices are treated, noncirrhotic patients benefit from rivaroxaban (15 mg daily) if they do not have major risk factors for thrombosis[A1] and may benefit from chronic warfarin anticoagulation (Chapter 68) if they have ongoing risk factors for thrombosis. Transjugular intrahepatic portosystemic shunting is more effective than endoscopic band ligation plus propranolol to prevent future variceal bleeding in such patients (Chapter 139).[A2]

PROGNOSIS

Mortality rates in treated patients are less than 10%.

SPLENIC VEIN THROMBOSIS

Splenic vein thrombosis is usually caused by a tumor (e.g., pancreatic cancer), pancreatitis, or trauma. Isolated gastric varices and splenomegaly often develop. Liver function and portal pressure are normal. Doppler ultrasound, MR, and

CT can help make the diagnosis. In symptomatic patients, splenectomy is the treatment of choice.

HEPATIC AND SPLENIC ARTERIAL DISEASE

Nonocclusive hepatic arterial disease (*ischemic hepatitis*) develops if the arterial blood supply to the liver is inadequate, usually as a result of severe or sustained shock (Chapter 92), hypotension, volume depletion, or sepsis. Aminotransferase levels typically rise acutely to greater than 1000 U/L and return to their baseline by about 40 to 60% per day after restoration of adequate hepatic arterial blood.

Hepatic artery thrombosis is extremely rare except after liver transplantation (Chapter 140), where it can present with abnormal liver function tests, bile duct injury (e.g., biliary stricture, cholangitis, liver abscess), or liver failure. Doppler ultrasound and angiography will confirm the diagnosis. Patients often require biliary stenting with drainage of any abscesses, followed by surgical reconstruction of the hepatic artery or repeat liver transplantation.

Splenic or hepatic artery aneurysms are usually caused by atherosclerosis, vasculitis, trauma, portal hypertension, pancreatitis, infection, or pregnancy. Clinical manifestations can include abdominal pain and intra-abdominal hemorrhage. Hepatic artery aneurysms can cause hemobilia. The diagnosis is established by angiography. Symptomatic aneurysms (generally 1 cm or larger in the hepatic artery and 2 cm or larger in the splenic artery) require surgery. When a splenic artery aneurysm is discovered during pregnancy, the high likelihood of bleeding is an indication for treatment, usually by interventional radiology.

Fistulas from the hepatic artery to the portal vein are rarely seen in hereditary hemorrhagic telangiectasia or as a result of trauma or malignancy. The resultant portal hypertension may cause abdominal pain, ascites, and gastrointestinal bleeding. Involvement of the hepatic artery may lead to biliary strictures and hepatobiliary infection. Radiographic embolization, surgery, or liver transplantation may be required.

MISCELLANEOUS VASCULAR DISORDERS

Blue rubber bleb nevus syndrome is characterized by purple-blue cutaneous venous malformations, which can affect the gastrointestinal tract, most commonly the small intestine. Gastrointestinal bleeding may occur, but endoscopic therapy is usually contraindicated because the lesions can involve the full thickness of the bowel. Surgical resection is usually needed.

In *Klippel-Trenaunay* syndrome, port-wine-colored cutaneous hemangiomas, hemihypertrophy, and varicose veins are seen. The *Parkes Weber* form includes arteriovenous fistulas; gastrointestinal involvement is uncommon.

In *Ehlers-Danlos syndrome type IV* (Chapter 239), small bowel ischemia and perforation as well as arterial rupture may develop. Patients with *pseudoxanthoma elasticum type I* (Chapter 239) are at risk for gastrointestinal or intraperitoneal hemorrhage, as are patients with *visceral arterial aneurysms* that result from atherosclerosis, fibrodysplasia, vasculitis, trauma, portal hypertension, pancreatitis, or pregnancy.

Thromboangiitis obliterans (Berger disease; Chapter 66) typically affects young men who smoke cigarettes. Mesenteric involvement is uncommon and usually manifested by distal occlusions of the mesenteric circulation.

Malignant atrophic papulosis (Degos disease) is a rare occlusive vascular disease affecting mainly the skin and intestine. Spontaneous perforation may occur owing to ischemia, and the disease has a poor prognosis.

GENERAL REFERENCES

For the General References and other additional features, please visit Elsevier eBooks+ at https://ebooks.health.elsevier.com.

Grade A References

A1. Plessier A, Goria O, Cervoni JP, et al. Rivaroxaban prophylaxis in noncirrhotic portal vein thrombosis. *NEJM Evid.* 2022;1.

A2. Lv Y, Qi X, He C, et al. Covered TIPS versus endoscopic band ligation plus propranolol for the prevention of variceal rebleeding in cirrhotic patients with portal vein thrombosis: a randomised controlled trial. *Gut.* 2018;67:2156-2168.

130 PANCREATITIS

CHRIS E. FORSMARK

ACUTE PANCREATITIS

DEFINITION

Acute pancreatitis is a discrete episode of cellular injury and inflammation in the pancreas, usually with symptoms of abdominal pain, nausea, and vomiting. It is accompanied by elevations in serum levels of amylase or lipase and/or radiographic evidence of pancreatic inflammation, edema, or necrosis. Although the pancreas can recover normal function and appearance after an episode, recovery may not be complete, especially if the necrosis is substantial. In patients with recurrent episodes, there can be a shift from acute inflammation, necrosis, and apoptosis to chronic inflammation and fibrosis that are characteristic of chronic pancreatitis. Acute and chronic pancreatitis are on a continuum, and it may be difficult to differentiate acute relapsing pancreatitis from evolving chronic pancreatitis.

EPIDEMIOLOGY

The incidence of acute pancreatitis in the United States is around 40 cases per 100,000 population, with about 300,000 hospital admissions annually, thereby making acute pancreatitis one of the most common gastrointestinal discharge diagnoses in U.S. hospitals. The cost of caring for these patients is about $4 to $6 billion annually. The incidence of acute pancreatitis is increasing in the United States and many other countries,[1] owing to more frequent use of diagnostic tests and to an increasing prevalence of gallstones and other risk factors in the setting of the obesity epidemic.

PATHOBIOLOGY

Acute pancreatitis is caused by premature activation of digestive enzymes within pancreatic acinar cells. Increased intracellular calcium and the activation of trypsinogen to trypsin appear to be the critical initial steps, with trypsin then activating other proteases within the gland.[2] These activated enzymes produce cell injury and necrosis. Necrosis can involve the pancreas as well as surrounding fat and structures, thereby leading to fluid extravasation into the surrounding retroperitoneal spaces ("third space" losses). Necrosis sufficient to be visible on a contrast-enhanced computed tomographic (CT) scan is termed acute necrotizing pancreatitis and distinguished from the milder interstitial pancreatitis, in which necrosis is not visible on a CT scan. In addition to the pancreatic damage, the release of pro-inflammatory cytokines and activated digestive enzymes into the systemic circulation can produce a systemic inflammatory response syndrome and organ system failure, including hypotension, renal failure, and acute respiratory distress syndrome (Chapter 90). Gallstones (Chapter 141) and alcohol (Chapter 364) together account for around two thirds of all cases of acute pancreatitis, but causes vary by age and sex, and the cause is unknown in a significant proportion of cases (Table 130-1).

Gallstones (Chapter 141)

Passage of a gallstone through the ampulla of Vater with transient obstruction of the pancreatic duct is the initiating event for gallstone pancreatitis. Only about 5% of all patients with gallstones develop pancreatitis, and patients with smaller gallstones ($\leq$5 mm), which can pass the cystic duct and reach the ampulla, are at highest risk. Microlithiasis, defined as tiny gallstones and/or biliary sludge that are not easily visible on routine imaging, is often the cause in patients initially labeled as having acute idiopathic pancreatitis.

Alcohol (Chapter 364)

More than 5 years of alcohol intake averaging more than 5 to 8 drinks daily is usually required before pancreatitis develops, but most people with this level of intake do not develop pancreatitis.[3] A variety of cofactors have been proposed, including a high-fat diet, genetic variability in detoxifying enzymes, coexistent genetic mutations, and cigarette smoking. The evidence is strongest for smoking. By the time patients have a first clinical episode of acute alcoholic pancreatitis, most already have evidence of underlying chronic pancreatitis.

TABLE 130-1 CAUSES OF ACUTE PANCREATITIS

ETIOLOGY	EXAMPLES
Gallstones	Gallstones (Chapter 141) Microlithiasis
Drugs and toxins	Ethyl and methyl alcohol (Chapters 364 and 96) Tobacco (Chapter 363) Azathioprine, 6-mercaptopurine, pentamidine, didanosine, sulfonamides, thiazides, aminosalicylates, valproic acid, and others Scorpion venom (Chapter 98) Organophosphate insecticides (Chapter 96)
Metabolic	Hypertriglyeridemia (Chapter 190) Hypercalcemia (Chapter 227)
Trauma	Post-ERCP (Chapter 120) Blunt or penetrating trauma Postoperative
Obstruction of the pancreatic duct	Benign pancreatic duct stricture Benign ampullary stricture (e.g., celiac disease, Crohn disease, diverticulum) Ampullary adenoma or adenocarcinoma (Chapter 181) Pancreatic ductal adenocarcinoma (Chapter 180) Intraductal papillary mucinous neoplasm (Chapter 180)
Infections	Cytomegalovirus (Chapter 347), mumps (Chapter 340), rubella (Chapter 339), Coxsackie B (Chapter 349), *Candida* (Chapter 310), histoplasmosis (Chapter 308), *Ascaris* (Chapter 327)
Genetics	*PRSS1* mutations *CFTR* mutation *SPINK1* mutation Other mutations
Autoimmune pancreatitis	Type 1 Type 2
Idiopathic pancreatitis	

ERCP = endoscopic retrograde cholangiopancreatography.

The peak of alcoholic pancreatitis is in ages of 20 to 50, and it is more common in men. The mechanism of alcoholic pancreatic injury involves a mixture of direct toxicity, oxidative stress, and alterations in pancreatic enzyme secretion.

Drugs, Toxins, and Metabolic Factors

Drug-induced pancreatitis is a rare and generally idiosyncratic event. Although many drugs have been implicated, the evidence is most compelling for 6-mercaptopurine and azathioprine (up to a 4% attack rate), as well as for valproic acid (the leading cause in an analysis of over 1000 cases of drug-induced acute pancreatitis).[4] Other agents include L-asparaginase, didanosine, pentamidine, valproic acid, furosemide, mesalamine, ciprofloxacin, prednisone, olanzapine, sulfonamides, and aminosalicylates. Toxins that may cause acute pancreatitis include methyl alcohol, organophosphate insecticides, and venom from certain scorpions.

Levels of serum triglycerides above 500 mg/dL, and usually greater than 1000 mg/dL, can cause acute pancreatitis, but the mechanism is not known.[5] The risk appears to be higher in overweight persons.[6] Hypercalcemia is an exceedingly rare cause of acute pancreatitis.

Trauma

Iatrogenic trauma to the pancreas and pancreatic duct during performance of an endoscopic retrograde cholangiopancreatography (ERCP; Chapter 120) can cause pancreatitis, with the risk averaging less than 5% for patients with simple common bile duct stones or malignancy but up to 20% in some high-risk subgroups.

Penetrating and blunt trauma, ranging from a contusion to severe crush injury and even transection of the gland, can cause pancreatitis. Acute presentation is the rule, but some patients with milder injury may present in a subacute or chronic fashion. Ischemic injury to the gland can occur after surgical procedures, especially cardiopulmonary bypass, and cause severe pancreatitis.

Obstruction of the Pancreatic Duct

Obstruction of the pancreatic duct by a pancreatic ductal adenocarcinoma (Chapter 180), an ampullary adenoma or carcinoma, or an intraductal papillary mucinous neoplasm can cause acute pancreatitis. The diagnosis of pancreatic duct obstruction is usually established with magnetic resonance imaging (MRI) with magnetic resonance cholangiopancreatography (MRCP) or with endoscopic ultrasound. Benign strictures of the pancreatic duct at the ampulla of Vater may be caused by celiac disease (Chapter 126), duodenal Crohn disease (Chapter 127), and periampullary diverticulum. Current evidence does not support the role of sphincter of Oddi dysfunction as a cause of acute pancreatitis. Studies of pancreas divisum as a potential cause of acute pancreatitis are ongoing.

Infections

Ascaris lumbricoides (Chapter 327) may cause pancreatitis by obstructing the pancreatic duct as the worms migrate through the ampulla of Vater. Viruses that may infect the pancreatic acinar cells directly and may cause pancreatitis include cytomegalovirus (Chapter 347), Coxsackie B virus (Chapter 349), adenovirus (Chapter 349), and mumps virus (Chapter 340).

Autoimmune Pancreatitis

Two forms of autoimmune pancreatitis have been identified.[7] The most common presentation is obstructive jaundice that mimics pancreatic adenocarcinoma or chronic pancreatitis. These are discussed under "Chronic Pancreatitis."

Genetics

Mutations in the cationic trypsinogen gene (*PRSS1*), which have been identified in families with hereditary pancreatitis, are more commonly seen in association with chronic pancreatitis but can present early in the course as acute pancreatitis. Many additional mutations and polymorphisms are associated with both acute and chronic pancreatitis. These affected genes include the cystic fibrosis conductance regulator (*CFTR*), serine protease inhibitor kazal type 1 (*SPINK1*), chymotrypsin C, calcium-sensing receptor, carboxy ethyl lipase, claudins, and others.

CLINICAL MANIFESTATIONS

Abdominal pain, nausea, and vomiting are the hallmark symptoms of acute pancreatitis. The abdominal pain is usually in the epigastric region and often radiates to the back. The pain is steady, reaches its maximum intensity over 30 to 60 minutes, and persists for days. These characteristic symptoms may be masked in patients who present with delirium, multiple organ system failure, or coma.

The physical examination usually reveals tachycardia. Hypotension, tachypnea, dyspnea, and low-grade fever are observed in more severe cases. Confusion, delirium, and, rarely, even coma may be present. The abdomen is often distended with diminished bowel sounds. Tenderness to palpation of the abdomen, which may be epigastric or more diffuse, is typical, whereas rebound and guarding are unusual. Dullness to percussion in the lower lung fields may be noted owing to pleural effusion. Rare physical findings include ecchymoses of the flank (Grey-Turner sign) or umbilicus (Cullen sign), which occur when fluid and blood track into these spaces from the retroperitoneum. Jaundice may be present if there is biliary obstruction by a stone. The presence of systemic inflammatory response syndrome (Chapter 94) is predictive of more severe pancreatitis. Tachycardia, dyspnea, tachypnea, orthostatic hypotension, pleural effusion, oxygen desaturation, or shock signals more substantial third-space losses, a higher likelihood of a variety of complications, and a worse prognosis. More severe pancreatitis is characterized by more substantial pancreatic and peripancreatic necrosis, more peripancreatic fluid collections, and more dysfunction of extrapancreatic organs.

DIAGNOSIS

The diagnosis of acute pancreatitis is suggested by clinical features and confirmed by laboratory and imaging studies that exclude other serious intra-abdominal conditions and help define the severity and most likely cause of the pancreatitis.[8]

The diagnosis of acute pancreatitis requires at least two of the following three criteria: abdominal pain consistent with pancreatitis, serum amylase or lipase of at least three times the upper limit of normal, or imaging findings consistent with acute pancreatitis on imaging (contrast CT, MRI, or ultrasound). Patients with mild pancreatitis have no local (pancreatic fluid collection or necrosis) or systemic complications (organ failure complications), patients with moderate pancreatitis have local complications and/or transient organ system failure that persists for less than 48 hours, and patients with severe pancreatitis have organ failure that persists for more than 48 hours.

Laboratory Tests

Amylase and Lipase

Most patients with acute pancreatitis have elevations in serum levels of amylase or lipase within a few hours of the onset of symptoms. Lipase is generally preferred over amylase as a diagnostic test because of its superior specificity. Although elevation to more than three times the upper limit of normal is the recommended cutoff for diagnosing acute pancreatitis, up to 25% of cases may not reach this threshold. Lipase levels tend to remain elevated longer than amylase levels, but both decline gradually over several days. Elevations more than three times the upper limit of normal are most specific for acute pancreatitis. Amylase and lipase levels may be normal in patients with acute pancreatitis, particularly if the measurement is delayed for several days after the onset of symptoms, and marked hypertriglyceridemia can interfere with their accurate measurement. Both enzymes are cleared by the kidney, and renal failure can falsely raise the level of these enzymes up to five times the upper limit of normal in the absence of pancreatitis.

Amylase and lipase levels also can be elevated in a variety of other conditions that may mimic acute pancreatitis, including intestinal ischemia and infarction (Chapter 129), bowel obstruction (Chapter 128), cholecystitis (Chapter 141), and choledocholithiasis (Chapter 141). In addition, amylase levels may be elevated from ectopic pregnancy, acute salpingitis, and a variety of extra-abdominal conditions such as parotitis (Chapter 340), lung cancer (Chapter 177), and head trauma (Chapter 368).

In some patients, only the amylase level or the lipase level may be elevated. Serial measurements of amylase or lipase in patients with established acute pancreatitis are not useful in clinical decision making. In patients with recurrent attacks of pancreatitis, the peak level of amylase or lipase tends to diminish progressively.

Other Laboratory Tests

In severe pancreatitis, leukocytosis, azotemia, and hemoconcentration may be seen. Failure of the blood urea nitrogen (BUN) level or hematocrit to normalize with fluid resuscitation is associated with more substantial third-space losses and a worse prognosis. Hyperglycemia, hypocalcemia, and mild hypertriglyceridemia also can develop. Elevations in alanine aminotransferase levels more than three times the upper limit of normal are most suggestive of gallstones, although any significant elevation in liver chemistries should raise the possibility of gallstone pancreatitis (Chapter 141).

Determining Etiology

To identify the cause of acute pancreatitis, the history should focus on alcohol and tobacco use, previous biliary colic, drug history, family history, and recent trauma. Because gallstones are the leading cause of acute pancreatitis, accounting for about 40% of cases, all patients should have an abdominal ultrasound examination to look for gallstones. Gallstone pancreatitis should be suspected if stones or a dilated bile duct is seen on imaging studies or if abnormal liver chemistries are present.

A careful history, often with corroboration from family members, will help diagnose alcoholic pancreatitis, which accounts for about 20% of cases, as well as medication- or toxin-induced pancreatitis and traumatic pancreatitis. Serum chemistries will help identify unusual cases caused by severe (>1000 mg/dL) hypertriglyceridemia.

If these initial approaches are unrevealing, MRI with MRCP or endoscopic ultrasound (EUS) can detect small gallstones, microlithiasis, or underlying premalignant or malignant causes (particularly in patients over age 40 years).[9] More specialized investigations, such as genetic testing, are usually reserved for patients who have had multiple attacks of unexplained pancreatitis.

Of the 25% of patients who do not have an identified cause after a basic initial evaluation, microlithiasis is the most common underlying explanation. With additional evaluation and testing, only about 10% of patients are ultimately labeled as having truly idiopathic pancreatitis. Idiopathic pancreatitis is more common in women, and especially elderly women, than in men.

Imaging Studies

Imaging studies are used not only in establishing the diagnosis but also in determining the cause and prognosis. In most patients, both ultrasound and CT are used in a complementary fashion.

Abdominal ultrasonography can confirm the presence of acute pancreatitis by documenting pancreatic enlargement, edema, or associated peripancreatic fluid collections. Visualization of the pancreas may be limited owing to body habitus or overlying intestinal gas. In patients with gallstone pancreatitis, ultrasonography is more accurate than CT in identifying gallstones in the gallbladder or a dilated common bile duct.

CT is more accurate than ultrasonography in confirming the diagnosis of acute pancreatitis and in documenting the presence of pancreatic necrosis and peripancreatic fluid collections. CT is also particularly helpful in excluding intra-abdominal conditions that can mimic acute pancreatitis. Pancreatic parenchyma that opacifies on CT with intravenous contrast is still viable, whereas parenchyma that does not enhance is necrotic (Fig. 130-1). The extent of pancreatic necrosis has prognostic importance but is generally not clearly visible on CT until at least 3 days after presentation. CT scans are not routinely required in all patients with acute pancreatitis but should be performed when the diagnosis is not clear and in patients who have a first attack, severe disease, systemic complications, or disease that is slow to improve.

MRI is equivalent to CT in its ability to document acute pancreatitis, identify necrosis, and diagnose or exclude other diseases that could mimic acute pancreatitis. In addition, MRCP is much better than CT for identifying gallstones. In critically ill patients, MRI is more difficult than CT to perform.

ERCP and endoscopic ultrasonography are important in both diagnosis and therapy of acute pancreatitis. Endoscopic ultrasonography, which is primarily used to establish the cause when the initial evaluation is unrevealing, is particularly accurate in identifying underlying malignancy, premalignant lesions such as ampullary adenoma, and small gallstones or microlithiasis. ERCP is not used for diagnosis, but it can be very useful for therapeutic purposes.

Determining Severity

Severe pancreatitis is characterized by organ system failure and by local pancreatic complications such as necrosis, fluid collections, or pseudocysts.[10] Organ failure can be single or multiple, early- or late-onset, and progressive, persistent, or transient. In severe acute pancreatitis, renal failure, pulmonary failure, and circulatory failure most commonly occur as part of the systemic inflammatory response.

During the acute attack, poorly demarcated fluid collections around the pancreas track into various retroperitoneal and peritoneal spaces. Much of this inflammatory fluid will resolve, but some will form into a more rounded and circumscribed fluid collection, called a pseudocyst (Fig. 130-2). Similarly, areas of pancreatic and peripancreatic necrosis will eventually develop a surrounding wall and begin to soften and liquefy, thereby becoming "walled-off pancreatic necrosis." For both fluid and necrosis, this process usually takes several weeks. It is important to distinguish pseudocysts from walled-off pancreatic necrosis; they appear similar on a CT scan but are easily distinguishable on MRI or endoscopic ultrasonography, because necrotic collections contain both solid and liquid material. Greater degrees or amounts of necrosis generally correlate with a higher risk of an adverse outcome, particularly if infection develops in the devitalized necrotic tissue. Although many patients with pancreatic

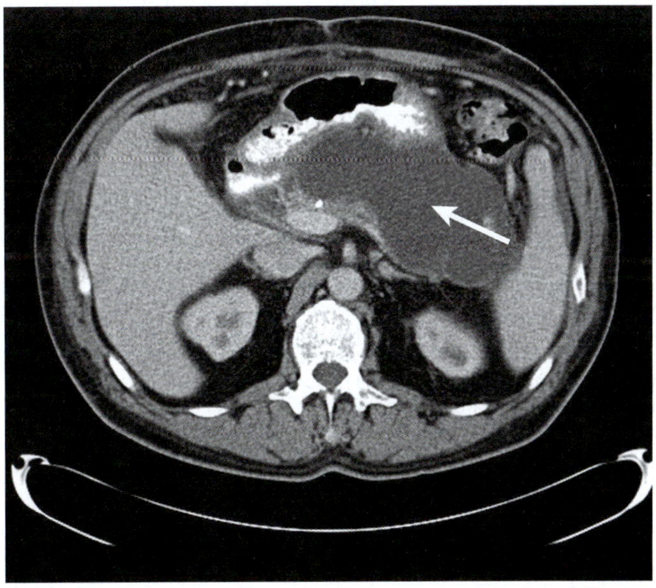

FIGURE 130-1. A computed tomographic scan demonstrating a large area of pancreas that does not enhance with intravenous contrast (*arrow*), consistent with pancreatic necrosis.

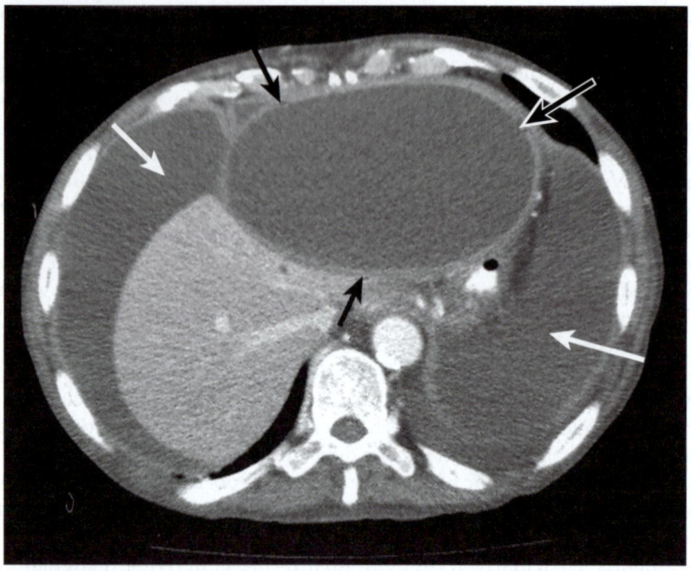

FIGURE 130-2. A large pseudocyst is seen (*black arrows*). In addition, ascites surrounding the liver (*white arrows*) is noted due to a leak from the pseudocyst (pancreatic ascites).

necrosis may not develop organ system failure, organ system failure is quite rare in the absence of pancreatic necrosis.

Risk Stratification

A number of clinical features identify patients at higher risk, including patients who are older, obese, or have more serious or more numerous comorbid conditions. Obesity in particular dramatically increases the risk of more severe pancreatitis. Additional clinical features that can be predictive include the presence of the systemic inflammatory response syndrome, particularly if it persists for more than 48 hours, and laboratory features consistent with intravascular volume depletion (elevated hematocrit or BUN). In addition to this qualitative estimate of prognosis, a number of multiple-factor scoring systems have been developed in an attempt to help guide clinicians in gauging prognosis, but there is no evidence that these complex multiple-factor scoring systems are superior to experienced clinical judgment.

TREATMENT

General Supportive Care

The majority of patients will recover within several days, but it is usually not possible to identify these patients at the time of admission.

All patients should initially be given nothing by mouth (NPO). Pain control often requires parenteral narcotics, and hydromorphone (in divided doses of 1 to 2 mg IV every 4 to 6 hours initially, with titration as needed) is generally preferred.

However, nonsteroidal anti-inflammatory agents (NSAIDs) may be as successful as narcotics by 24 hours.[A1] Patients with significant third-space loss, often augmented by prior poor oral intake or fluid losses through vomiting, will have evidence of intravascular fluid depletion. Even in mild pancreatitis, fluid losses may be substantial. Appropriate fluid resuscitation (Chapter 92) is recommended in all practice guidelines.[11] Moderate fluid resuscitation (1.5 mL/kg/hour of lactated Ringer solution in all patients, preceded by a 10 mL/kg bolus only if the patient is hypovolemic), with reassessments and adjustments at 12, 24, 48, and 72 hours[A2] to correct blood pressure and pulse, to reduce the hematocrit and BUN to normal, and to ensure a urine output of at least 0.5 mL/kg/hour, is preferred. More aggressive infusion of fluid worsens outcomes, primarily by increasing the risk of respiratory failure owing to fluid overload but also by increasing the risk of organ system failure, heart failure, and an abdominal compartment syndrome. To avoid these potential adverse effects, fluid therapy must be guided by whether the patient has the physiologic reserve to handle it.

Treatment of nausea and vomiting may be needed, and 5-HT3 antagonists (Table 118-5) are generally preferred. Nasogastric suction is rarely needed.

Patients with mild or moderate pancreatitis can be fed when they feel able to tolerate it, even before enzyme levels are completely normalized or pain is entirely absent. Beginning oral feeding within 48 hours after hospitalization is as safe as starting later and also reduces hospital length of stay. There is no need to begin with a clear liquid diet: feeding can be initiated with a low-fat solid diet as the first meal.

TABLE 130-2 COMPLICATIONS OF ACUTE PANCREATITIS

COMPLICATION	EXAMPLES
Systemic complications	Hypotension and shock Adult respiratory distress syndrome Acute renal failure Disseminated intravascular coagulation Hypocalcemia Hypertriglyceridemia Hyperglycemia Encephalopathy and coma
Gastrointestinal bleeding	Stress ulceration Pseudoaneurysm
Local (pancreatic) complications	Acute peripancreatic fluid collection Pseudocyst (infected and sterile) Acute necrotic collection Walled-off pancreatic necrosis (infected and sterile) Duodenal and biliary obstruction

In patients with more severe pancreatitis (based upon early organ system failure, substantial third-space fluid losses, or comorbid conditions), admission to an intermediate care unit or intensive care unit (ICU) is appropriate. Careful monitoring for progressive organ system failure, metabolic complications, and fluid status is critical in these patients. In patients with severe pancreatitis, enteral nutrition (oral or tube feeding) is safer and less expensive than total parenteral nutrition, which should be utilized exceedingly rarely. Patients who appear to have sufficiently severe disease that they might not be able to eat for 5 to 7 days can be considered for tube feeding. Alternatively, waiting for up to 5 days to see if patients with severe acute pancreatitis can eat is reasonable, with tube feeding reserved for those who are unable to eat after 5 days.[12] In patients given tube feeding, there is no difference if the tube is nasogastric, nasoduodenal, or nasojejunal. In addition, there is no evidence that elemental or semi-elemental formulas are better than standard polymeric formulas.

Treatment of Complications

Most patients who develop acute gallstone pancreatitis have already passed the offending stone into the duodenum, but patients with a persistent or multiple stones are at higher risk of developing cholangitis and (possibly) more severe pancreatitis. Current practice guidelines recommend urgent ERCP in patients whose gallstone pancreatitis is complicated by evidence of cholangitis (e.g., fever, jaundice, right upper quadrant pain) and early ERCP for patients with evidence of a persistent bile duct stone (e.g., visible persistent stone on imaging study, jaundice, persistently dilated bile duct, or worsening liver chemistries at 48 hours after admission). In patients who have severe pancreatitis, as evidenced by early and progressive organ system failure but who do not have cholangitis, early ERCP is not better than conservative care.[A3]

The systemic complications (Table 130-2) that develop in patients with severe acute pancreatitis include some that are similar to those commonly encountered in other ICU patients (e.g., ventilator-associated pneumonia, line sepsis) as well as the specific metabolic complications of severe pancreatitis[13] Hyperglycemia is common and may contribute to higher rates of infections. In severe acute pancreatitis, ionized calcium levels are usually normal, but hypocalcemia is common owing to a diminished serum albumin level; treatment is not needed in the absence of signs of hypocalcemia, such as tetany or a Chvostek sign (Chapter 227). Mild hypertriglyceridemia is common, but underlying hypertriglyceridemia does not cause acute pancreatitis unless triglyceride levels surpass 1000 mg/dL. Triglyceride levels drop promptly when the patient is made NPO.

Infections in patients with acute pancreatitis include urinary tract infections, pneumonia, line infections, and *Clostridioides difficile*. High-quality nursing care, antibiotic stewardship, and careful attention to catheters and lines can minimize these infections. In addition, patients with necrotizing pancreatitis may develop infected pancreatic necrosis. Although infected necrosis has a substantial impact on prognosis, prophylactic antibiotics are not beneficial for patients with sterile necrosis. Infected necrosis typically occurs 2 to 3 weeks into the illness and is heralded by fever, leukocytosis, and worsening abdominal pain. The responsible organisms are usually gram-negative rods and other gut flora, but *Staphylococcus aureus* is an important agent as well. If infected necrosis is suspected, a contrast CT scan should be obtained. The finding of gas in the necrotic collection is a specific but not sensitive sign of infected necrosis. A CT-directed fine-needle aspiration of the necrotic area can be obtained for culture and Gram stain but is not required in patients in whom clinical features, such as fever, leukocytosis, and worsening abdominal pain, are strongly suggestive of infected pancreatic necrosis. Antibiotics with deferred surgery if needed is as good as immediate surgical drainage for infected necrotizing pancreatitis.[A4] Antibiotics with appropriate penetration into necrosis (e.g., imepenem/cilastatin 500 mg IV/q 8 hours, meropenem 500 mg IV/q 8 hours, metronidazole 500 mg

IV/q 8 hours plus ciprofloxacin 400 mg IV/q 8 hours, or ceftazidime 500 mg IV/q 8 hours; see Table 266-4 in Chapter 266) should be initiated if infection is suspected or documented, and the specific regimen can be tailored to the organism if known. Intravenous antibiotics should be continued for several weeks to allow the necrotic material to demarcate fully, begin to liquefy, and become encapsulated. If patients become septic, it is reasonable to place a percutaneous drain into the collection to stabilize the patient. When this walled-off necrosis is sufficiently liquefied to allow less invasive approaches, therapy can include percutaneous, endoscopic, or minimally invasive surgical therapy.[14] Endoscopic transgastric necrosectomy is generally preferred, although minimally invasive surgical approaches are also effective.[A5-A7] Open surgical drainage should be avoided.

Fluid collections around the pancreas (acute peripancreatic fluid collections) are common in acute pancreatitis and do not require any specific therapy. Most will resolve spontaneously, but some will mature into an encapsulated pseudocyst. It is important to distinguish a pseudocyst (usually outside the confines of the pancreas and filled with fluid) from an area of necrosis (usually inside the confines of the pancreas and a mixture of solid and liquid material). Therapy also is not needed for asymptomatic pseudocysts, even if they are large, but therapy is indicated for pseudocysts that cause abdominal pain, obstruct a surrounding hollow viscus, or are associated with infection or bleeding. A pseudocyst can be treated successfully using endoscopic, percutaneous, or minimally invasive surgical techniques, and the choice among these approaches can be determined by local expertise and anatomic location.

Bleeding may complicate a pseudocyst, and bleeding into the cyst may reach the intestine through the pancreatic duct. In some patients, bleeding into the pseudocyst may be caused by a pseudoaneurysm of a nearby visceral artery; this type of bleeding may be massive. Unexplained gastrointestinal bleeding or a sudden, unexplained drop in the hematocrit in a patient with pancreatitis or a pseudocyst should prompt an emergent contrast CT scan, followed by embolization if a pseudoaneurysm is identified.

Treatment to Prevent Relapsing Pancreatitis

Preventing relapse requires a clear knowledge of the precipitating cause. Abstinence from alcohol and tobacco should be strongly encouraged, including referral to appropriate resources. Cholecystectomy prevents subsequent attacks of gallstone pancreatitis and should be accomplished within the index hospitalization.[A8] In patients with presumed "idiopathic" acute pancreatitis, an empiric cholecystectomy can be considered, provided that alternative causes have been excluded,[15] because many of these patients have gallstones as the etiology.[A9] In patients who have gallstone pancreatitis but who are not surgical candidates, endoscopic biliary sphincterotomy provides reasonable protection from subsequent attacks. Control of serum lipids prevents subsequent attacks of hypertriglceridemic pancreatitis. Therapy of lesions that obstruct the pancreatic duct, such as strictures and ampullary adenomas, may also prevent relapse.

The risk of post-ERCP pancreatitis is reduced with careful patient selection, the use of peri-procedural NSAID suppositories, by aggressive intravenous hydration, or by the placement of small-caliber temporary pancreatic duct stents.[A10]

PROGNOSIS

More than 80% of all patients with acute pancreatitis recover promptly without developing severe pancreatitis, but up to 30% may ultimately develop diabetes or exocrine pancreatic insufficiency. Mortality is usually from progressive multiple organ system failure, either from the acute pancreatitis itself or from hospital-acquired infections, including infection of pancreatic fluid collections or necrotic pancreatic tissue. Early organ failure (within 24 hours of admission), multiple organ system failure, and persistent or progressive (present beyond 48 hours after admission) organ failure are associated with prolonged hospitalization, ICU admission, need for surgery, and death. Overall mortality is about 2%, but it can approach 30% in patients with more severe comorbid conditions (and particularly obesity) and in patients who develop pancreatic necrosis, infection, or organ system failure. Although high-quality ICU care reduces mortality, no specific therapy is currently proven to reduce these risks.

For patients with acute alcoholic pancreatitis, long-term mortality is about four-fold higher than in the general population, mostly owing to alcohol-related conditions. Acute pancreatitis due to hypertriglyceridemia also has an adverse prognosis. For other causes, long-term mortality is minimally elevated compared with the general population.

CHRONIC PANCREATITIS

DEFINITION

Chronic pancreatitis is a syndrome associated with a wide spectrum of predisposing risk factors and environmental triggers. Chronic pancreatitis usually evolves after episodes of recurrent acute pancreatitis, and the transition between acute and chronic pancreatitis may be difficult to identify. Common features include abdominal pain, exocrine and/or endocrine insufficiency, and imaging evidence of pancreatic atrophy, calcification, or dilated pancreatic duct.[16] The progression of chronic pancreatitis is variable, but it often culminates in irreversible and widespread pancreatic fibrosis with chronic inflammation and damage to nerves, ducts, acini, and islets.

EPIDEMIOLOGY

The prevalence of symptomatic chronic pancreatitis in Western countries is about 40 to 70 per 100,000 persons, with an estimated incidence of 5 to 8 cases/100,000. In the United States, chronic pancreatitis accounts for about 125,000 outpatient visits and 25,000 hospitalizations annually. Interestingly, the prevalence of histologic evidence of chronic pancreatitis in autopsy studies approaches 5%, indicating that many people develop some pancreatic damage as a consequence of normal aging, other diseases (e.g., diabetes), or exposure to toxins (such as smoking or consumption of alcohol) but do not develop any symptoms or signs of chronic pancreatitis during life.

PATHOBIOLOGY

Multiple genetic polymorphisms and mutations can predispose to chronic pancreatitis, and various environmental and immunologic triggers can initiate the disease.[17] Episodes of acute inflammation, whether clinical or subclinical, eventually change the inflammatory milieu of the pancreas, with a shift to chronic inflammation, cell injury, cell death, the activation of pancreatic stellate cells, and the progression to fibrosis. This process becomes self-sustaining and produces the characteristic histologic damage.

The mechanisms of pain of chronic pancreatitis are complex. Damage to pancreatic nociceptive nerves and neuroimmune interaction driven by the chronic inflammatory state is the primary cause of pain, but the chronic pain can eventually produce visceral, spinal cord, and central hyperalgesia.

Alcohol and Tobacco

Alcohol causes about 50% of all cases of chronic pancreatitis in the United States. The risk is dose dependent, but it usually requires sustained ingestion of alcohol of 4 to 5 drinks daily over more than 5 years. The majority of people (95%) who consume this much alcohol do not develop chronic pancreatitis, pointing to important cofactors such as genetic risk factors and cigarette smoking. Smoking increases the risk of chronic pancreatitis by two- to three-fold, with a dose-dependent effect. Smoking is estimated to account for 25% of the attributable risk of chronic pancreatitis, and continued smoking after diagnosis accelerates the course of the disease. These risks also appear to be synergistic, such that the combination of alcohol and tobacco is more than an additive effect.

Genetic

Hereditary pancreatitis is an autosomal dominant disease characterized by early onset of acute and chronic pancreatitis, the development of exocrine and endocrine pancreatic insufficiency, and a high risk of pancreatic adenocarcinoma (Chapter 180). Mutations in the *PRSS1* gene in these families appear to cause a gain in function in which the mutant trypsinogen, once activated to trypsin, is difficult to inactivate. This trypsin, if present in an amount that overwhelms normal protective mechanisms, can activate other pancreatic enzymes and lead to pancreatic damage and eventually to chronic pancreatitis. One of the protective mechanisms is a trypsin inhibitor called the *SPINK1* protein. Loss-of-function mutations in *SPINK1* predispose to chronic pancreatitis. Major mutations in the *CFTR* lead to cystic fibrosis (Chapter 77), which may be associated with chronic pancreatitis and pancreatic atrophy, depending upon the location of the mutation. Certain mutations in *CFTR* predispose to chronic pancreatitis, without causing the sinopulmonary features of classic cystic fibrosis. A number of additional genetic polymorphisms in the calcium-sensing receptor, chymotrypsin C, carboxyethyl lipase, claudins, and others are also associated with chronic pancreatitis. With the exception of *PRSS1*, these polymorphisms predispose to chronic pancreatitis and may function as modifying genes but are not sufficient to cause chronic pancreatitis.

Pancreatic Duct Obstruction

Chronic obstruction of the pancreatic duct by benign, premalignant, and malignant conditions can cause chronic pancreatitis to develop in the gland upstream from the obstruction. Examples include duodenal diseases causing obstruction at the ampulla (celiac disease, Crohn disease, ampullary adenoma or carcinoma) and benign (after severe pancreatitis, pancreatic surgery, or abdominal trauma) and malignant pancreatic duct strictures (pancreatic ductal adenocarcinoma, intraductal papillary mucinous neoplasms).

Other Causes

Autoimmune pancreatitis is a disease that most often presents as a masslike lesion in the pancreas with obstructive jaundice, mimicking cancer, but it also may present as chronic pancreatitis and rarely as acute pancreatitis.[18] Because cancer is more common than autoimmune pancreatitis, it must be excluded (usually with endoscopic ultrasonography). Type 1 autoimmune pancreatitis is characterized by diffuse swelling of the pancreas, elevation of the serum IgG4 level, and involvement of other organs, especially with biliary strictures, salivary gland inflammation, retroperitoneal fibrosis, and renal lesions. Histologically, these organs are infiltrated by chronic inflammatory cells, especially plasma cells bearing IgG4 on their surface, as is part of the spectrum of IgG4-related disease.[19] Type 2 autoimmune pancreatitis, which affects only the pancreas and is not associated with elevations in IgG4, may have potential overlap with autoimmune cholangitis.

Although most chronic pancreatitis follows multiple episodes of acute pancreatitis, a single severe acute attack that causes substantial pancreatic necrosis can cause a ductal stricture or destroy enough gland to produce exocrine and endocrine insufficiency. Other diseases that cause repeated attacks of pancreatitis can lead to chronic pancreatitis. For example, hypertriglyceridemia causes recurrent acute pancreatitis that leads to chronic pancreatitis.

CLINICAL MANIFESTATIONS

Abdominal pain is the most common symptom and is responsible for the greatest negative impact on quality of life. The pain may be episodic or constant, and it is generally present in the epigastrium with radiation to the back.[20] Some patients will present initially with an episode of acute pancreatitis and thereafter develop evidence of chronic pancreatitis, but others will have obvious chronic pancreatitis at their first presentation. If pain is episodic, the patient may be labeled as having acute pancreatitis or an acute flare of chronic pancreatitis. When pain is severe, nausea and vomiting may occur. Pain may worsen, improve, or remain stable over time. Up to 5% of patients do not have pain and instead present with exocrine (steatorrhea, weight loss) or endocrine (diabetes mellitus) pancreatic insufficiency. The disease tends to be progressive over time, even if the original cause (e.g., alcohol) is removed. The pain also may become self-perpetuating even if therapy is successful.

DIAGNOSIS

The diagnosis may be suspected based on the clinical features but should be confirmed by tests that identify structural damage to the pancreas or derangements in pancreatic function (Table 130-3).[21] Serum levels of amylase or lipase are not useful for diagnosing chronic pancreatitis. Serum trypsinogen (also called trypsin) is abnormally low in patients with chronic pancreatitis that is advanced enough to cause steatorrhea but is often normal in patients with less advanced disease. Serum glucose levels will be elevated in patients with endocrine insufficiency.

Chronic pancreatitis is a slowly progressive disease in which visible damage to the gland (e.g., on a CT scan) and functional failure (e.g., steatorrhea or diabetes mellitus) may not be apparent for years. All diagnostic tests are most accurate when the disease is far advanced, and all are far less accurate in the early stages of disease.

TABLE 130-3 DIAGNOSTIC TESTS FOR CHRONIC PANCREATITIS*

STRUCTURAL	FUNCTIONAL
Biopsy	Hormonal (secretin) test
Endoscopic ultrasonography	Fecal elastase
Magnetic resonance imaging with magnetic resonance cholangiopancreatography, with or without secretin infusion	Serum trypsin level
Computed tomography	Fecal fat
Endoscopic retrograde cholangiopancreatography	Blood glucose level
Ultrasonography	
Plain abdominal radiography	

*Listed in approximate order of decreasing sensitivity.

From a practical perspective, the diagnosis is established in most patients by CT or MRI.[22] The diagnostic challenge lies with patients who present with a severe pain syndrome suggestive of chronic pancreatitis but who have a normal or minimally abnormal CT or MRI. In these patients, MRI with secretin-MRCP or endoscopic ultrasonography is the best choice, unless a secretin-based pancreatic function test is available. ERCP should not be used for diagnostic purposes alone.

In about 20% of patients, no clear cause of chronic pancreatitis is identified, and this may be more common in women. Some patients may have underlying genetic mutations, and others may be surreptitiously using alcohol and/or tobacco. Two general forms of idiopathic chronic pancreatitis are observed. In the first, pain is the predominant feature, and the onset of disease is in young adulthood. In the second, the onset is in middle age, and exocrine and endocrine insufficiency, rather than abdominal pain, are the major clinical manifestations. As more genetic polymorphisms are identified, the relative prevalence of idiopathic pancreatitis is shrinking.

Tests of Pancreatic Structure

Plain abdominal radiographs may demonstrate diffuse or focal pancreatic calcification in patients with advanced chronic pancreatitis). Although specific for chronic pancreatitis, these findings are detected only after years of disease.

Abdominal ultrasound is of limited utility because overlying gas often limits the ability to visualize the pancreas. An abnormal pancreatic duct, pancreatic calcifications, gland atrophy, or changes in echotexture are seen in about 60% of patients.

CT is the most widely used diagnostic test for chronic pancreatitis, and high-quality images can be obtained of the pancreas and pancreatic duct. Characteristic findings include a dilated pancreatic duct, ductal or parenchymal calcifications, and atrophy (Fig. 130-3). These structural changes take years to develop, so CT is not as accurate in early or less advanced disease. Like CT, MRI allows detailed images of the pancreas, and the addition of MRCP allows even better assessment of pancreatic duct morphology. Secretin can be administered at the time of MRCP to allow better visualization of the pancreatic duct. MRI with secretin-MRCP is more sensitive for detecting the early changes of chronic pancreatitis than is CT.

Endoscopic ultrasonography allows very detailed images of the pancreatic parenchyma and duct (Fig. 130-4). Normal endoscopic ultrasonography essentially excludes chronic pancreatitis, whereas very abnormal endoscopic ultrasonography is highly consistent with chronic pancreatitis. ERCP provides the most detailed images of the pancreatic duct, as well as the opportunity to provide therapy (see later). Changes in the duct include dilation, irregularity, ductal stones, and strictures (Fig. 130-5). However,

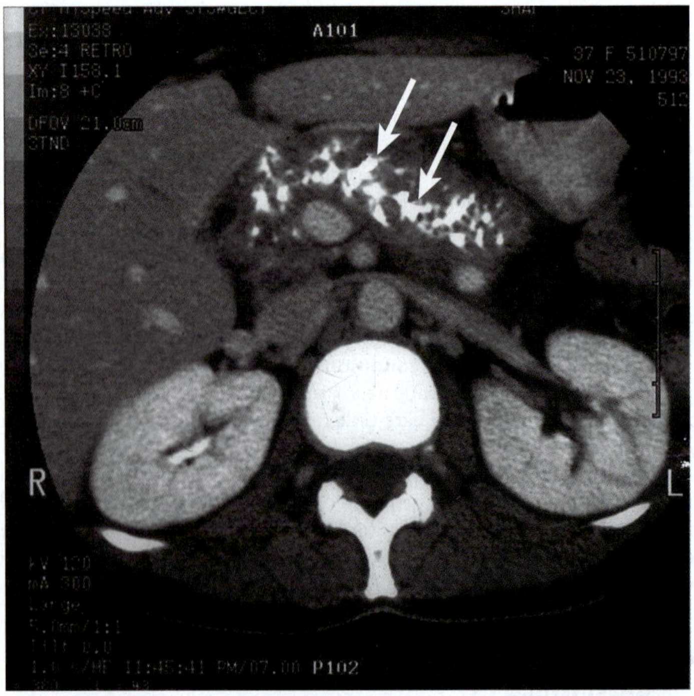

FIGURE 130-3. A computed tomographic scan demonstrating diffuse pancreatic calcification in a patient with long-standing chronic pancreatitis (*arrows*).

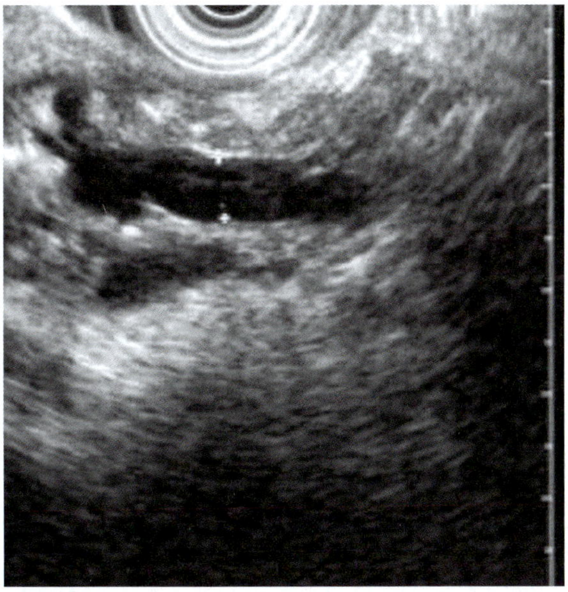

FIGURE 130-4. An endoscopic ultrasound in a patient with chronic pancreatitis, demonstrating a dilated pancreatic duct (*marks on margin of main duct*).

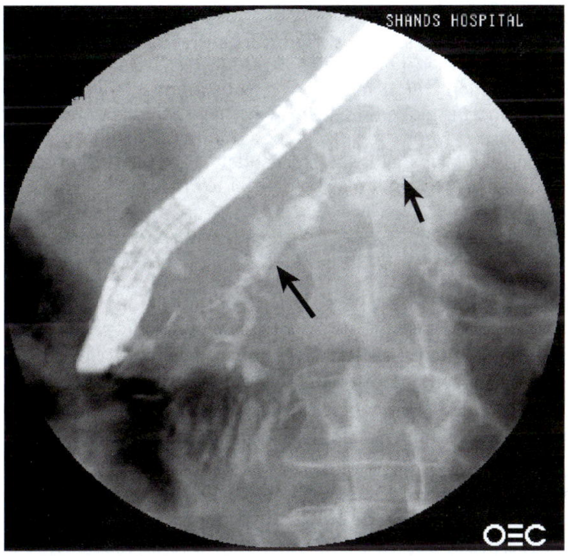

FIGURE 130-5. An endoscopic retrograde cholangiopancreatography demonstrating a very irregular pancreatic duct with areas of dilation and stricturing in a patient with chronic pancreatitis (*arrows*).

ERCP carries a risk of causing pancreatitis, so it should be utilized only when therapy is planned.

Tests of Pancreatic Function

Quantification of fat in stool during a 72-hour collection while on a high-fat diet can be used to document steatorrhea but is rarely performed. Qualitative analysis of fat with Sudan staining of a stool specimen has poor sensitivity and specificity. Fecal levels of pancreatic elastase are diminished to less than 200 μg/g in patients with exocrine pancreatic insufficiency. The test can be performed while patients are taking pancreatic enzyme therapy.

For a direct pancreatic function test, a tube or endoscope is passed into the duodenum, where pancreatic secretions are collected and analyzed for bicarbonate concentration, after a supraphysiologic dose of secretin is administered. A normal study is defined by at least one of the samples having a bicarbonate concentration of 80 mEq/L or more. The test becomes abnormal earlier in the disease process than any other test, so it is best suited to diagnose chronic pancreatitis earlier in its clinical course. However, the test is not widely available or used.

TREATMENT

Medical therapy starts with vigorous attempts to assist patients in stopping alcohol and tobacco, if applicable.

Treatment of Pain

Many patients will require analgesics. It is appropriate to start with the less potent agents first (such as NSAIDs or tramadol 50 to 100 mg every 6 hours). In most patients, it is helpful to add an adjunctive agent such as a gabapentoid (e.g., pregabalin starting at 75 mg two times daily), a tricyclic antidepressant (e.g., amitriptyline starting at 50 mg at night or nortriptyline starting at 10 mg at night), a selective serotonin reuptake inhibitor, or a combined serotonin and norepinephrine uptake inhibitor at the usual starting dose (Table 362-5).[23] Combinations of these adjunctive agents are also utilized. Antioxidants (mixtures of selenium, vitamins E and C, β-carotene, and methionine) may also have some beneficial effect on pain in selected patients with preexisting deficiencies.

Sudden worsening of pain should lead to a search for specifically treatable complications, including pseudocyst, obstruction of a surrounding hollow organ (e.g., duodenum or bile duct), or superimposed carcinoma. A good-quality CT or MRI is usually sufficient to exclude these possibilities. These imaging tests may also help in choosing appropriate therapy. Patients with a dilated duct (generally >5 mm) are the best candidates for endoscopic and surgical therapy for pain. Patients without ductal dilation are not suitable for most endoscopic and surgical therapy and must rely instead on medical therapy (Table 130-4). Unfortunately, pain often persists despite therapy. A celiac plexus block using bupivacaine can be performed relatively easily and safely, but substantial relief of pain is unpredictable and at best is achieved for only weeks.

Other Medical Therapy

Pancreatic enzyme therapy is commonly used to treat exocrine insufficiency and occasionally to treat pain, although evidence is lacking on its effectiveness for

TABLE 130-4 TREATMENT FOR PAIN

Medical therapy	Analgesics and adjunctive agents • Tramadol 50 mg, 1-2 three times daily • Pregabalin, starting at 75 mg two times daily • Gabapentin, starting at 100 mg at night • Amitryptiline, starting at 50 mg at night • Nortriptyline, starting at 10 mg at night • SSRIs (e.g., citalopram, fluoxetine, sertraline, paroxetine) at recommended starting dose (see Table 362-5) Antioxidants • Typical mixture containing vitamin C (1000 mg), vitamin E (300 IU), selenium (500 μg), methionine (2 g), and β-carotene (10,000 IU) total daily dose
Nerve block	Endoscopic ultrasonography–guided nerve block
Endoscopic therapy	Stent Stone removal, lithotripsy
Surgical therapy	Pancreaticojejunostomy (modified Puestow operation) Partial pancreatic resection (Whipple operation, duodenum preserving pancreatic head resection, others) Total pancreatectomy with islet-cell auto-transplantation

CT = computed tomography; SSRI = selective serotonin reuptake inhibitor.

TABLE 130-5 ENZYME THERAPY FOR EXOCRINE PANCREATIC INSUFFICIENCY

PRODUCT	FORMULATION	LIPASE CONTENT/CAPSULE OR PILL*
Zenpep	Enteric-coated porcine	3000; 5000; 10,000; 15,000; 20,000; 25,000; 40,000
Creon	Enteric-coated porcine	3000; 6000; 12,000; 24,000; 36,000
Pancreaze	Enteric-coated porcine	4200; 10,500; 16,800; 21,000; 37,000
Pertzye	Enteric-coated porcine with bicarbonate	4000; 8000; 16,000; 24,000
Viokace	Non–enteric-coated porcine tablet†	10,440; 20,880

*In USP units.
†Must be co-administered with an H_2 blocker (e.g., famotidine 20 mg twice daily) or a proton pump inhibitor (e.g., omeprazole 20 mg/day).

pain. Autoimmune pancreatitis responds promptly to steroid therapy (usually 40 mg of prednisone daily for 4 weeks, with a taper of 5 mg/week over the next 7 weeks), but relapse commonly occurs, particularly in patients with biliary obstruction. Continuing prednisone at a low daily dose (e.g., 5 to 7.5 mg for 3 years),[A11] or the use of alternative agents (e.g., azathioprine or rituximab, under the direction of a specialist), may be required to maintain remission.

Endoscopic Therapy and Lithotripsy

ERCP can be used to dilate strictures and place stents across the stricture. Ductal stones, if they are not too large and are not impacted, may also be removed. Larger stones usually require lithotripsy to reduce the stone to fragments that are manageable. ERCP is most useful in patients who have a dominant obstruction in the pancreatic head with upstream ductal dilation. Such ERCP therapy is technically successful in more than 80% of carefully selected patients, and pain relief may be seen in 70 to 80% of patients, although treatment usually requires several endoscopic procedures.[24]

Surgical Therapy

Surgery also generally requires a dilated pancreatic duct and is somewhat more effective and more durable than is endoscopic therapy.[A12] Surgery can involve decompression of the pancreatic duct, resection of the pancreas, or a combination of the two. The most commonly performed procedure, the modified Puestow procedure, involves a longitudinal incision of the pancreatic duct from the body of the pancreas to as close to the duodenum as possible, and this duct is overlaid with a defunctionalized small intestinal limb to drain it. At the time of surgery, ductal strictures can be incised and ductal stones can be removed. The procedure is relatively simple in patients with a dilated pancreatic duct (>5 mm). Pain relief in the short term is good (>80%), with about 50% obtaining long-term relief of pain. Alternative surgical procedures for pain include partial resection of the pancreas, typically the head of the gland. These operations, which include the classic pancreatico-duodenectomy (Whipple operation), as well as several variations of a duodenum-preserving pancreatic head resection, provide equal short-term pain relief[A13] and better long-term pain relief than a modified Puestow but perhaps with higher morbidity. Some evidence suggests surgery earlier in the clinical course is more effective.[A14] Total pancreatectomy, usually coupled with auto-transplantation of harvested islet cells, is currently considered a therapy of last resort in adults.

Exocrine Insufficiency

Steatorrhea and maldigestion do not occur until approximately 90% of pancreatic enzyme secretion is lost, usually after at least 5 to 10 years of disease. Patients may note weight loss and oily stools but often do not complain of diarrhea.[25] Patients with chronic pancreatitis and exocrine insufficiency maldigest fat, protein, and carbohydrates, but fat maldigestion is usually most severe (including fat-soluble vitamins, particularly vitamin D). The diagnosis of exocrine insufficiency is usually suggested by symptoms of oily or floating stools and weight loss. A formal 72-hour stool fat analysis is the most accurate method to document steatorrhea and to gauge effectiveness of therapy but is rarely done. Instead, the clinical features and a fecal elastase lower than 200 μg/g stool, coupled with an appropriate response to enzyme replacement therapy, is the best substitute for 72-hour fecal fat testing.

Pancreatic enzyme replacement therapy (Table 130-5) can normalize fat and fat-soluble vitamin absorption, maintain normal nutrition and weight, and prevent complications such as osteoporosis.[A15] Both enteric-coated capsules and non–enteric-coated tablets are available. Enzymes are identified by the lipase content of the pill or capsule, although they all contain proteases and amylase as well. The goal of enzyme therapy is to provide at least 10% of normal pancreatic output with each meal (90,000 USP units of lipase/meal). Since most patients are still producing some enzymes (including gastric lipase), it may not be necessary to prescribe the full dosage of 90,000 USP units with each meal; 40,000 to 50,000 is a reasonable starting point.

If non–enteric-coated preparations are selected, cotreatment with an H_2-blocker (e.g., famotidine 20 mg twice daily or equivalent) or proton pump inhibitor (e.g., omeprazole 20 mg daily or equivalent) is required to prevent acid denaturation of lipase; such cotreatment is not needed with enteric-coated preparations. Enzymes should be taken during the meal. Supplementation with vitamin D (400 to 1000 IU daily) and calcium (1.0 to 1.5 g daily) is appropriate because of the risks of osteoporosis (Chapter 225) and osteopenia. Measurement of fat-soluble vitamin levels and periodic bone mineral density testing are recommended. The success of enzyme therapy is generally defined as weight gain, reduction or absence of visible oil in the stool, and correction of fat-soluble vitamin levels. Failure of enzyme therapy is most often due to an inadequate dose. Increasing the dose up to the full 90,000 USP units during meals and encouraging compliance is appropriate as a first step. No generic products are available in the United States, so cost may be a major cause of noncompliance. Some patients may not respond owing to the presence of a second disease that also causes malabsorption, such as small intestinal bacterial overgrowth.

Endocrine Insufficiency

Similar to exocrine insufficiency, diabetes mellitus (Chapter 210) is a very late complication of chronic pancreatitis, occurring years or decades after the onset of disease. In contrast to type 1 diabetes mellitus, destruction of the entire islet, which has been termed type 3C diabetes mellitus, reduces secretion of both insulin and glucagon.[26] The absence of glucagon increases the risk that overly aggressive insulin therapy may lead to hypoglycemia. In most patients, therefore, insulin treatment is not aimed at exceedingly tight glucose control. Unfortunately, these patients are at similar risk for microvascular complications as are all other patients with diabetes.

Pancreatic Pseudocyst

Pancreatic pseudocysts, when they are discovered in patients with chronic pancreatitis, are generally mature and have a visible capsule surrounding them. As in acute pancreatitis, benign pseudocysts in chronic pancreatitis do not require therapy if they are not producing symptoms and are not infected. However, some cystic structures in and around the pancreas are cystic neoplasms (Chapter 180), not pseudocysts. Symptomatic pseudocysts require drainage, whereas neoplasms require resection. Features that suggest a cystic neoplasm include a cyst with a thick or nodular wall, a cyst with multiple internal septations, or a cyst occurring in a patient who does not have a history of pancreatitis. Any combination of these features should lead to further investigation, generally with endoscopic ultrasonography and aspiration.

Symptomatic pseudocysts can be treated with endoscopic, percutaneous, or surgical therapy with equal efficacy. In most centers, endoscopic ultrasonography-guided drainage is becoming first-line therapy with excellent short- and long-term results. Complications of pseudocysts include infection, bleeding (discussed earlier), and rupture. Pseudocysts may leak into the peritoneal compartment (pancreatic ascites) or track into the chest (pancreatic pleural effusion). Patients usually present with abdominal distension or dyspnea, rather than abdominal pain. Amylase level in the fluid is usually greater than 4000 U/L. Endoscopic therapy with stent placement across the connection between pseudocyst and pancreatic duct is highly effective in this situation.

Malignancy

Chronic pancreatitis is a strong risk factor for pancreatic ductal adenocarcinoma (Chapter 180), with a lifetime risk of about 4%, which is 8- to 16-fold above the general population.[27] *KRAS* mutations may be found in chronic pancreatitis. The risk of cancer is higher in patients who have hereditary pancreatitis and who also smoke, in whom the risk may be as high as 40%. Other genetic causes and smoking also increase the risk of secondary pancreatic malignancy, as may type 3C diabetes mellitus. It may be difficult to visualize cancer in an already diseased pancreas.

PREVENTION

Currently, there are no reliable methods to prevent chronic pancreatitis. Patients at risk for chronic pancreatitis, such as members of families with hereditary pancreatitis or patients with strong genetic predispositions, should avoid alcohol and tobacco. Similarly, patients with established chronic pancreatitis should avoid these agents, which hasten the progression of the disease.

PROGNOSIS

With prolonged follow-up of 10 to 20 years, the majority of patients will develop exocrine or endocrine insufficiency. Overall mortality is increased three- to six-fold compared with age-matched controls. Patients who are older, smoke, or have alcohol as the cause are at highest risk of mortality. Overall, 10-year survival approximates 70%, and 20-year survival is about 45%. Death is usually not due to pancreatitis itself but rather to malignancy, postoperative complications, and complications of alcohol (Chapter 364) or tobacco (Chapter 363).

GENERAL REFERENCES

For the General References and other additional features, please visit Elsevier eBooks+ at https://ebooks.health.elsevier.com.

Grade A References

A1. Thavanesan N, White S, Lee S, et al. Analgesia in the initial management of acute pancreatitis: a systematic review and meta-analysis of randomised controlled trials. *World J Surg.* 2022;46:878-890.

A2. de-Madaria E, Buxbaum JL, Maisonneuve P, et al. Aggressive or moderate fluid resuscitation in acute pancreatitis. *N Engl J Med.* 2022;387:989-1000.

A3. Schepers NJ, Hallensleben NDL, Besselink MG, et al. Urgent endoscopic retrograde cholangiopancreatography with sphincterotomy versus conservative treatment in predicted severe acute gallstone pancreatitis (APEC): a multicentre randomised controlled trial. *Lancet.* 2020;396:167-176.

A4. Boxhoorn L, van Dijk SM, van Grinsven J, et al. Immediate versus postponed intervention for infected necrotizing pancreatitis. *N Engl J Med.* 2021;385:1372-1381.

A5. Bang JY, Arnoletti JP, Holt BA, et al. An endoscopic transluminal approach, compared with minimally invasive surgery, reduces complications and costs for patients with necrotizing pancreatitis. *Gastroenterology.* 2019;156:1027-1040.

A6. van Brunschot S, van Grinsven J, van Santvoort HC, et al. Endoscopic or surgical step-up approach for infected necrotising pancreatitis: a multicentre randomised trial. *Lancet*. 2018;391:51-58.
A7. Hollemans RA, Bakker OJ, Boermeester MA, et al. Superiority of step-up approach vs open necrosectomy in long-term follow-up of patients with necrotizing pancreatitis. *Gastroenterology*. 2019;156:1016-1026.
A8. Moody N, Adiamah A, Yanni F, Gomez D. Meta-analysis of randomized clinical trials of early *versus* delayed cholecystectomy for mild gallstone pancreatitis. *Br J Surg*. 2019;106:1442-1451.
A9. Räty S, Pulkkinen J, Nordback I, et al. Can laparoscopic cholecystectomy prevent recurrent idiopathic acute pancreatitis? A prospective randomized multicenter trial. *Ann Surg*. 2015;262:736-741.
A10. Akshintala VS, Sperner Weiland CJ, Bhullar FA, et al. Non-steroidal anti-inflamamtory drugs, intravenous fluids, pancreatic stents, or their combinations for the prevention of post-endoscopic retrograde choloangiopancreatography pancreatitis: a systematic review and network meta-analysis. *Lancet Gastroenterol Hepatol*. 2021;S2468-1253.
A11. Masamune A, Nishimori I, Kikuta K, et al. Randomised controlled trial of long-term maintenance corticosteroid therapy in patients with autoimmune pancreatitis. *Gut*. 2017;66:487-494.
A12. Ahmed Ali U, Pahlplatz JM, Nealon WH, et al. Endoscopic or surgical intervention for painful obstructive chronic pancreatitis. *Cochrane Database Syst Rev*. 2015;3:CD007884.
A13. Diener MK, Huttner FJ, Kieser M, et al. Partial pancreatoduodenectomy versus duodenum-preserving pancreatic head resection in chronic pancreatitis: the multicentre, randomised, controlled, double-blind ChroPac trial. *Lancet*. 2017;390:1027-1037.
A14. Issa Y, Kempeneers MA, Bruno MJ, et al. Effect of early surgery vs endoscopy-first approach on pain in patients with chronic pancreatitis: the ESCAPE randomized clinical trial. *JAMA*. 2020;323:237-247.
A15. de la Iglesia-García D, Huang W, Szatmary P, et al. Efficacy of pancreatic enzyme replacement therapy in chronic pancreatitis: systematic review and meta-analysis. *Gut*. 2017;66:1354-1355.

131 DISEASES OF THE RECTUM AND ANUS

ROBERT D. MADOFF AND GENEVIEVE B. MELTON

ANATOMY

The Rectum

The rectum and anal canal make up the final portion of the hindgut. In general, the colon transitions distally to the rectum at the level of the sacral promontory, where the taeniae coli splay to form a continuous longitudinal muscle layer and then extends approximately 12 to 18 cm distally. The peritoneum covers the upper two thirds of the rectum anteriorly and is usually more limited laterally. The rectum and its mesentery are surrounded posteriorly by endopelvic fascia, and this anatomic package contains the relevant lymphovascular structures that should be removed intact during rectal cancer surgery. The rectum also has two or three curves within its lumen created by submucosal folds called the valves of Houston. The second valve is often used as a rough guideline for the intraperitoneal cavity anteriorly.

Blood supply to the rectum originates from the inferior mesenteric artery proximally and internal iliac arteries distally. The inferior mesenteric artery terminates as the superior rectal artery, which supplies the rectum and the upper one third of the anal canal. Additionally, internal iliac arteries give off the middle rectal arteries and the inferior rectal arteries (inferior via the internal pudendal artery) to supply the distal rectum and anal canal. The proximal rectum drains predominantly into the superior rectal venous plexus and then to the inferior mesenteric vein and portal venous system. By contrast, the caudal rectum and anal canal drain mainly into the systemic venous circulation through the inferior and middle rectal veins into the internal iliac veins and inferior vena cava. Generally, the lymphatic drainage of the rectum follows the arterial supply, so the lymphatic spread of rectal tumors is to the inferior mesenteric and internal iliac lymph nodes. As a result of the rectum's dual blood supply and drainage, pulmonary metastatic spread occurs earlier and more often with rectal cancers than with colon cancers. Innervation to the rectum involves both the sympathetic and parasympathetic plexus. The sympathetic nerves arise from the first three lumbar segments of the spinal cord, whereas the parasympathetic nerve supply originates from the caudal three sacral nerve roots.

The Anal Canal

The anal canal, which begins at the level of the *levator ani* muscle and extends to the anal verge opening, is about 2.5 to 5 cm in length and is surrounded by the internal and external anal sphincter muscles. The anorectal junction, which can be easily appreciated on digital rectal examination, is the point where the rectum angulates posteriorly from the axis of the anal canal. The internal anal sphincter, which is responsible for about 70% of the resting anal tone, is an extension of the inner circular smooth muscle layer of the rectum. The external sphincter muscle comprises skeletal muscle and is under voluntary control. The dentate line is located about 2 cm proximal to the anal verge (anal opening). Hemorrhoids are classified as internal versus external according to their relative location proximal or distal to the dentate line.

The mucosal lining changes histologically along the course of the anal canal. Superiorly, the anal canal consists of columnar epithelium that mirrors the rectum. Approximately 1 to 2 cm above the level of the dentate line is a transitional zone, where columnar, cuboidal, transitional, and squamous epithelia cells are found. This admixture of cells constitutes the derivation of the term "basaloid" as it relates to anal canal cancers and marks the proximal boundary for anal cancer surveillance. Distal to this line, the squamous epithelium extends to the anal verge and perianal skin, eventually adding glandular and hair follicles that resemble skin elsewhere on the body. Infected anal glands are a frequent cause of perianal abscess and fistula. Below the dentate line, lymphatic drainage generally goes to the inguinal nodes. The external anal sphincter is innervated by fibers from S4 and the internal pudendal nerve. Somatic sensation of the anal canal comes from the inferior rectal nerve via the pudendal nerve. This somatic sensation ceases 1 to 2 cm above the dentate line, which explains why some procedures such as hemorrhoid ligation can be performed in the office without anesthesia.

SPECIFIC ANORECTAL CONDITIONS

Hemorrhoids

EPIDEMIOLOGY AND PATHOBIOLOGY

An estimated 15 million or more individuals, about 5 to 12% of adults, in the United States experience symptoms related to hemorrhoids each year, and these individuals generate over 4 million annual office visits. However, the true incidence and prevalence of hemorrhoids are unknown because several anorectal conditions that are commonly attributed to "hemorrhoids" are actually caused by other conditions.

Despite a commonly held notion that hemorrhoids are always abnormal, they actually are normal structures that are identifiable even in the fetus. Hemorrhoids are vascular cushions that consist of connective tissue, smooth muscle, and both arterioles and veins. Functionally, they likely aid with overall fecal continence by serving as a malleable gasket that improves the seal of the anal canal.

Hemorrhoids are *not* rectal varices, which are distinct vascular entities that can develop in the setting of portal hypertension. *Hemorrhoidal disease* is a more appropriate term to describe the pathologic state with hemorrhoids that generates symptoms. The hemorrhoidal arteriolar component explains why hemorrhoidal bleeding is typically bright red in color and can be copious in quantity. Causative factors that can provoke hemorrhoidal symptoms include constipation, diarrhea, older age, pregnancy, and prolonged straining with defecation. Over time, repeated stretching of the anal canal damages the supporting tissue and results in downward displacement of the vascular cushions. Although none of these precipitating factors has been established rigorously, each can cause either increased abdominal pressure or obstruction of venous return, thereby leading to engorgement and enlargement of the vascular cushions.

CLINICAL MANIFESTATIONS AND DIAGNOSIS

The most common symptom of internal hemorrhoids is bright red bleeding. This bleeding is typically painless and is most often seen on the toilet tissue or in the toilet bowl. The quantity of blood is variable, but patients may occasionally describe blood dripping or squirting into the toilet bowl. Passage of dark blood or blood mixed in the stool suggests a more proximal source. Internal hemorrhoids are classified based on the symptoms they cause. As internal hemorrhoids enlarge, they are also associated with redundant rectal mucosa that protrudes from the anus with defecation. Early hemorrhoids bleed but do not prolapse (grade 1). Initial protrusion reduces spontaneously (grade 2); more advanced protrusion requires digital reduction (grade 3) and, at its most advanced form, becomes irreducible (grade 4) (Fig. 131-1). Internal hemorrhoids are insensate and do not themselves result in pruritus, but they can cause itching owing to associated perianal soiling or mucus deposition caused by mucosal prolapse. Additionally, patients may complain of anal discomfort or pressure, mucus discharge, extra tissue at the verge (i.e., mucosal prolapse), or a sensation of incomplete evacuation.

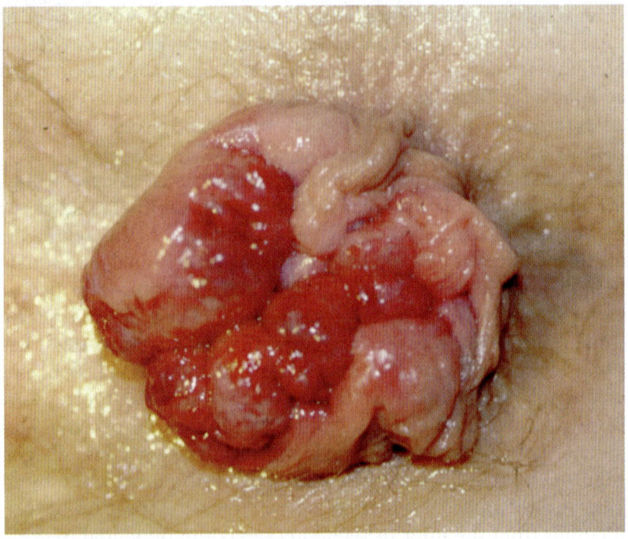

FIGURE 131-1. Grade 4 nonreducible internal and external hemorrhoids.

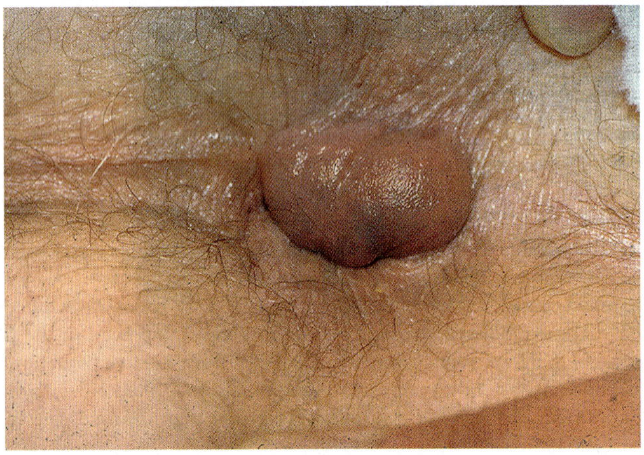

FIGURE 131-2. Thrombosed external hemorrhoid.

Individuals with anorectal symptoms frequently present complaining of "hemorrhoids" or are even referred from other physicians with a diagnosis of hemorrhoids. Although hemorrhoids may be present, they are often not the source of the underlying complaint. Therefore, it is always incorrect—and sometimes dangerous—for the physician to apply this diagnosis without completing an adequate evaluation. Fortunately, the initial evaluation is simple, and the correct diagnosis is often suspected based on history alone and confirmed by a limited visual and endoscopic examination. Internal hemorrhoids are best visualized with a slotted anoscope.

Rectal bleeding should never be attributed to hemorrhoids alone, even if hemorrhoids are visible; at a minimum, flexible sigmoidoscopy is required to exclude more proximal pathology. For more concerning symptoms or high-risk patients (e.g., personal or family history of colorectal cancer, persistent bleeding despite adequate treatment, unscreened individuals over age 45 years), a full evaluation of the large intestine should be performed by colonoscopy. The rising incidence of colon and rectal cancers (Chapter 179) in individuals under age 45 years serves to emphasize the point that unexplained rectal symptoms require thorough evaluation at all ages and should not simply be attributed to "hemorrhoids."

External hemorrhoids are usually asymptomatic and should be differentiated from perianal skin tags, which may cause difficulties with perianal hygiene, particularly when they are large or elongated. External hemorrhoids become symptomatic when they thrombose, thereby causing acute-onset pain and swelling (Fig. 131-2). Thrombosed external hemorrhoids, which are usually diagnosed by simple inspection of the anus, appear as an external lump, covered by anoderm and skin, with the underlying thrombosis giving it a purple appearance. Occasional patients who present with extensive, circumferential thrombosis require urgent surgical consultation.

TABLE 131-1 INTERNAL HEMORRHOIDS: GRADING AND MANAGEMENT

GRADE	SYMPTOMS AND SIGNS	MANAGEMENT
1	Bleeding No prolapse	Dietary modifications* Rubber band ligation Infrared coagulation Injection sclerotherapy
2	Prolapse with spontaneous reduction Bleeding, seepage	Rubber band ligation Infrared coagulation Dietary modifications* Injection sclerotherapy Doppler hemorrhoidal artery ligation
3	Prolapse requiring digital reduction Bleeding, seepage	Surgical hemorrhoidectomy Rubber band ligation Dietary modifications* Doppler hemorrhoidal artery ligation
4	Prolapsed, cannot be reduced Strangulated	Surgical hemorrhoidectomy Urgent hemorrhoidectomy

*Dietary modifications include increasing the consumption of fiber, bran, or psyllium and water. Dietary modifications are always appropriate for the management of hemorrhoids and to prevent recurrence after banding or surgery (or both).

TREATMENT

Grade 1 hemorrhoids often respond to dietary manipulation alone: increased dietary fiber, addition of a fiber supplement, and increased water intake (Table 131-1).[1,2] The goal, which may not be readily achievable, is approximately 25 to 30 g of fiber and 8 glasses of water daily. Patients often require a dietary fiber supplement to reach the recommended fiber intake. Patient education should also include maintaining proper bowel habits, including limiting time on the commode and avoiding straining with defecation.

More advanced hemorrhoids require specific therapy, which is almost always office-based. The most popular and simplest technique is rubber band ligation, whereby a tiny rubber band (internal diameter approximately 1 mm) is placed around some of the redundant rectal mucosa and prolapsing hemorrhoid well above the dentate line. The banded tissue sloughs in 7 to 14 days, an event occasionally heralded by rectal bleeding, which can be significant in rare cases. The result of surgery is a pexy effect for the prolapsing hemorrhoid and ligation of part of the blood flow to the hemorrhoid pile. Recovery is relatively straightforward for most patients. Banding can be repeated at 3- to 4-week intervals until bleeding and protrusion are controlled. Bands placed too close to the dentate line cause immediate severe pain and must be removed promptly. Patients who are at high risk of bleeding because of intrinsic coagulopathies or treatment with anticoagulant agents should not undergo rubber band ligation, unless these agents can be discontinued prior to the procedure, owing to the increased risk of postprocedure bleeding. Alternative office therapies for moderate internal hemorrhoids include injection sclerotherapy and infrared coagulation. Thrombosed external hemorrhoids that are early in their course (up to 72 hours since onset), have not responded to conservative therapy, or have thrombosed repeatedly also can be treated by excision in the office under local anesthesia or, if required because of size and location, may require excision in the operating room.

Operative hemorrhoidectomy is needed in only a minority of patients with advanced disease. Indications for hemorrhoidectomy include irreducible prolapse, a substantial external component, and failure of more conservative therapies. The most common approach is an excisional hemorrhoidectomy, which is generally performed on an outpatient basis. Excisional hemorrhoidectomy can also be performed using a coagulation device that seals the tissue, with comparable results and potentially less recurrence (weak evidence).[A1] An alternative approach is Doppler-guided hemorrhoidal artery ligation, after which recurrence rates of 3 to 60% have been reported. Recurrent hemorrhoids are less frequent after hemorrhoidal artery ligation than after a single rubber band ligation,[A2] but hemorrhoidal artery ligation typically must be performed in the operating room and is associated with more pain. Stapled hemorrhoidopexy, which entails resecting a ring of rectal mucosa proximal to the internal hemorrhoids using a circular stapling device, has mostly fallen out of favor because of its higher recurrence rate and a small but worrisome risk of significant complications, such as chronic pain, rectovaginal fistula, and staple line bleeding.

PERIANAL ABSCESS

EPIDEMIOLOGY AND PATHOBIOLOGY

Several superficial and deep spaces around the rectum and anal canal normally contain loose areolar tissue that can serve as potential spaces for perianal infections. Perianal abscess is a common condition, but its incidence is not well documented. Approximately 80% of perianal abscesses are caused by infection of the anal glands that track toward the skin, whereas other causes include simple skin infections, trauma, inflammatory bowel disease, anorectal surgery, malignancy, and immunosuppression.

CLINICAL MANIFESTATIONS AND DIAGNOSIS

Patients most commonly present with complaints of perianal pain and swelling with or without antecedent events such as trauma. In most cases, a local area of erythema, tenderness, and fluctuance can be appreciated on physical examination. However, these findings are often absent in abscesses in certain locations, including intersphincteric abscesses in the plane between the internal and external sphincter muscles, as well as in supralevator and deep ischiorectal locations. These abscesses should still be suspected based on a history of increasing pain and fever, as well as focal perianal tenderness on the physical examination.

As with all acutely painful anal conditions, digital examination should generally be avoided. Likewise, office instrumentation with an anoscope or proctoscope is contraindicated because these examinations cause substantial pain and typically yield little, if any, diagnostic information. When the cause of the acute pain cannot be determined in the office, prompt examination under anesthesia should be performed. Adjunctive computed tomographic (CT) scanning, magnetic resonance imaging (MRI), or endorectal ultrasound can provide valuable information, particularly in settings of occult, recurrent, or complex disease.

TREATMENT

Treatment for perianal abscess is prompt incision and drainage, which usually can be performed in the office.[3] Large or deep (e.g., postanal or horseshoe) abscesses are best evaluated in the operating room with proper sedation. Antibiotics do not adequately penetrate abscess cavities, and extension of a local infection can lead to sepsis and complex long-term problems. Therefore, antibiotic therapy is inadequate and should never be given in an attempt to avoid or delay incision and drainage. After incision and drainage, antibiotics (e.g., 7 days of oral metronidazole 500 mg every 8 hours and ciprofloxacin 500 mg every 12 hours in addition to standard care) may reduce the rate of subsequent fistula formation.[A3] Antibiotics are especially recommended in immunocompromised patients (e.g., patients with poorly controlled HIV or diabetes mellitus, transplant recipients, and patients undergoing chemotherapy), patients with extensive cellulitis or severe systemic symptoms, and patients at high risk for endovascular infection (e.g., patients with cardiac shunts or prosthetic valves). In patients who fail to improve following incision and drainage, prompt surgical reevaluation is warranted because the problem is likely to be a residual abscess that requires further drainage.

ANAL FISTULA

EPIDEMIOLOGY

An anal fistula, which represents the chronic form of a perianal abscess in which the tract from the infected anal gland to the abscess cavity does not adequately heal, can occur in 30 to 50% of patients following a perianal abscess.[4] This usually manifests as one or more chronic tracts from the anal canal to the perianal skin. The incidence of anal fistula is about 8.6 per 100,000. Fistulae are two to three times more common in men than in women.

PATHOBIOLOGY

After a perianal abscess is drained, the internal opening—the site at the dentate line where the infected gland originated—can remain patent, thereby leaving a source for recurrent infection as well as a tract from the internal anal gland to the abscess cavity and its drainage site. Multiple or atypical anal fistulae should always raise the diagnostic suspicion of Crohn disease, which can occasionally be isolated to the perianal area.

Anal fistulae are characterized by their relationship to the sphincter complex. The simplest and most common (approximately 70%) fistula is intersphincteric—located in the plane between the internal and external sphincter muscles. Transsphincteric fistulas (about 20 to 25%), which traverse both the internal and external sphincter muscles, are classified either as low fistulae, which traverse only the distal external sphincter, or high fistulae, which traverse the more proximal portions of the external sphincter. Suprasphincteric fistulae originate at the dentate line and loop over the entire sphincter complex. Extrasphincteric fistulae have internal openings remote from the dentate line; most originate from a pelvic abscess caused by a ruptured appendix (Chapter 128), diverticulitis (Chapter 128), or Crohn disease (Chapter 127).[5] A horseshoe fistula, which has external openings with associated tracts on both sides of the midsagittal plane, most commonly has a single internal opening in the posterior midline.

CLINICAL MANIFESTATIONS AND DIAGNOSIS

Anal fistulae sometimes present as recurrent abscesses in the same location as the original one or as persistent and sometimes intermittent purulent drainage from an abscess site that has failed to heal completely. Patients may often think the area has healed for several weeks or longer prior to experiencing the same feeling of a "boil" forming in the identical area, spontaneously rupturing, and relieving their symptoms.

The diagnosis of an anal fistula is established by history and by visualization of an external opening in the perianal skin. A fibrous fistula tract can sometimes be palpated along the course of the fistula from the skin toward the anal canal. An internal opening is occasionally visible on anoscopy, but a visible internal opening is not necessary to identify a fistula and to make a presumptive diagnosis.

TREATMENT

Treatment of anal fistulae is surgical. Most fistulae are cured by being laid open via a fistulotomy to eliminate the original source of infection at the internal opening. The fistula tract can then heal by secondary intention. However, this approach divides sphincter muscle and puts the patient at risk for impaired fecal continence in proportion to the quantity of muscle involved. In general, intersphincteric and low transsphincteric fistulae can be safely laid open if the patient has normal baseline continence and no underlying predisposing factors for diarrhea (e.g., colitis) or recurrent fistulae (e.g., Crohn disease). Because the anterior sphincter mechanism is relatively short and subject to injury following vaginal delivery, fistulotomy for anterior fistulae in women must be undertaken only after careful consideration.

When a high or complex fistula is identified, the first step is often placement of a seton, a suture, or other material (now commonly a Silastic vessel loop) that is passed though the fistula tract, out the anus, and secured to itself. The seton guarantees that the external fistula opening will not heal over, so a recurrent abscess is much less likely to supervene. After being left in for several weeks, the tract often scars around the seton and becomes fibrotic. Treatment options to eliminate the internal opening include endorectal advancement flap repair and ligation of the intersphincteric fistula tract. Because Crohn disease–associated fistulae tend to be multiple and recurrent, fistulotomy is avoided, except for the most superficial fistulae. In general, patients with Crohn disease are best served by placement of long-term draining setons and medical therapy for their underlying disease (Fig. 131-3).

PROGNOSIS

After appropriate surgery, about 85% of anal fistules are healed at 6 years.

ANAL FISSURE

EPIDEMIOLOGY

Anal fissures can occur at any age but most frequently affect young adults. Men and women are equally affected.

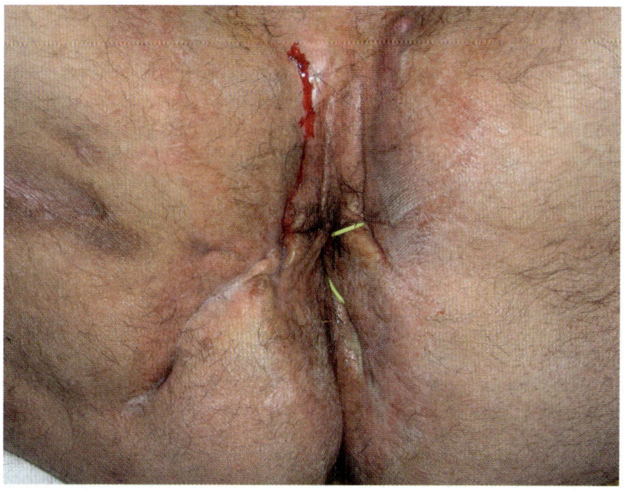

FIGURE 131-3. Crohn disease fistulae. Silastic setons in place with several additional draining tracts and evidence of prior surgery.

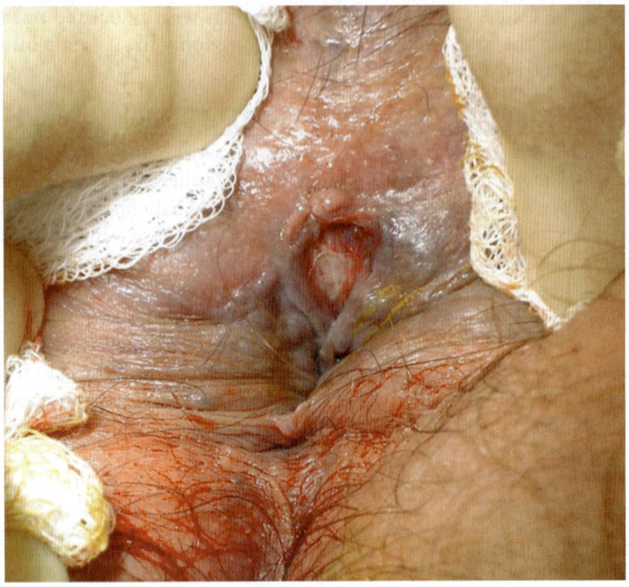

FIGURE 131-4. **Anal fissure.** This longitudinal tear occurs just inside the anal margin.

PATHOBIOLOGY

An anal fissure, which is a longitudinal tear typically with ulceration in the anoderm, occurs just inside the anal margin (Fig. 131-4). The underlying pathophysiology of anal fissures is hypertonia of the internal anal sphincter. Typical anal fissures occur at the midline; most commonly they occur posteriorly, but about 15% are found anteriorly or both anteriorly and posteriorly. "Off-the-midline" fissures may represent a routine fissure, but they generally require examination under anesthesia with culture, biopsy, and pathologic evaluation to exclude other causes such as anal cancer, Crohn disease, syphilis, HIV, leukemia, or tuberculosis.

CLINICAL MANIFESTATIONS AND DIAGNOSIS

Patients with anal fissures generally present with pain during and after bowel movements. Fissures are sometimes precipitated by a bout of constipation or a period of excessive diarrhea, but no specific precipitating event is usually noted. Patients typically describe severe anal pain that may persist for hours or even continue until exacerbation by the next bowel movement. There is sometimes an association with minor bright red bleeding, most commonly seen in small quantities that streak the stool or the toilet tissue. Whereas an acute anal fissure appears as a superficial split in the perianal skin and anoderm, chronic anal fissures, defined by their presence for at least 6 to 8 weeks, are often associated with a "sentinel" skin tag (so-called because its presence should suggest the presence of an underlying fissure) or a hypertrophied anal papilla located just proximal to the fissure at the dentate line, as well as more extensive tearing and ulceration. Well-established fissures may have fibrotic margins with "rolled edges" of the anoderm and visible internal anal sphincter fibers at their base.

Most fissures can be readily observed on physical examination by applying opposing traction to the buttocks. In general, no further examination is performed at that time when a classic anal fissure is identified. Digital and endoscopic examination typically should be delayed until the patient has healed to avoid causing pain. However, patients should be advised that they will require subsequent examination, which may include anoscopy or colonoscopy to exclude other anorectal or more proximal pathology.

TREATMENT

In addition to treating any instigating bowel abnormalities (e.g., constipation or diarrhea), most therapies for anal fissures are directed at the underlying hypertonia of the internal anal sphincter.[6] Approximately 40% of fissures heal with fiber supplementation and increased fluid intake alone, including the great majority of acute fissures. Patients are also advised to take warm sitz baths for symptomatic relief, especially following bowel movements.

Two pharmacologic approaches can augment diet and sitz baths: topical sphincter relaxants and botulinum toxin injection. Topical nitroglycerine (0.2 to 0.8%) or a topical calcium-channel blocker such as diltiazem gel (2%) applied externally around the anal orifice two to four times daily reduces sphincter tone and often leads to healing. Both drugs have similar efficacy, but nitroglycerine has the disadvantage of causing headaches, lightheadedness, or syncope owing to systemic vasodilation in approximately 25% of patients. Botulinum toxin injection into the internal anal sphincter appears to promote healing with recurrence rates similar to topical treatments. Overall, these more conservative approaches unfortunately are only marginally better than placebo for healing chronic fissures, and recurrent fissures occur in approximately 50% of patients.

For patients who fail medical therapy or who are simply too subjectively miserable to pursue pharmacologic treatment, lateral internal sphincterotomy is an appropriate and generally safe approach that is easily performed under monitored local anesthesia in an outpatient setting.[A4] Recovery after lateral internal sphincterotomy is rapid, and fissure healing is expected in more than 90% of cases. Sphincterotomy as first-line therapy provides higher healing rates, fewer relapses, and fewer side effects than topical nitroglycerine, with fewer symptoms, greater satisfaction, and no difference in continence at long-term follow-up. However, a small percentage of patients who undergo sphincterotomy develop minor seepage or even actual incontinence. Therefore, the sphincterotomy should be "tailored" to adjust the amount of internal anal sphincter according to the size of the fissure and the patient's overall amount of internal anal sphincter to maintain sufficient sphincter muscle. When such patients have refractory fissures, a trial of botulinum toxin injection, potentially in conjunction with a topical sphincter relaxant, is often a good alternative. A new experimental treatment is the injection of recently collected autologous adipose tissue, which has been reported to heal up to 55% of perianal fistulas in patients with Crohn disease.[7]

PRURITUS ANI

EPIDEMIOLOGY

The reported incidence of pruritus ani ranges from 1 to 5% in the general population, though it is likely much higher. Men are more commonly affected than women (4 : 1), and this condition is most common in the fourth through the sixth decades of life. Primary or idiopathic pruritus is responsible for 50 to 90% of all cases of pruritus ani.

CLINICAL MANIFESTATIONS AND DIAGNOSIS

Pruritus ani, or perianal itching, is a very common symptom but is not a disease in and of itself. The most common cause is likely inadequate perianal hygiene, often exacerbated by scratching, which leads to excoriation of the skin, further inflammation, and worsening pruritus.[8] Secondary causes include dermatologic, infectious, systemic, and lower gastrointestinal disease, as well as local irritants. Some of these sources include prolapsing hemorrhoids, anal fistulas, and anal incontinence, as well as specific dermatologic conditions such as contact dermatitis, psoriasis, lichen sclerosis, squamous intraepithelial neoplasia (formerly called Bowen disease), and perianal Paget disease (intraepidermal adenocarcinoma).

Diagnosis is typically based on a history of intractable itching despite trials of several over-the-counter medications and physical examination to exclude an obvious inciting source. The severity of the condition can be classified as stage 0—normal skin; stage 1—red and inflamed skin; stage 2—lichenified skin; and stage 3—lichenified skin as well as coarse ridges and often ulcerations.

TREATMENT

A therapeutic trial of symptomatic empiric management is effective in more than 90% of patients. Options include improved hygiene, avoidance of potential contact allergens (e.g., soaps and over-the-counter topical treatments), and use of either talc to absorb excess moisture or a barrier cream such as zinc oxide.[9] Mechanical scratching will perpetuate the cycle of inflammation and must be strictly avoided. Some patients benefit from the avoidance of certain foods, including caffeinated beverages, alcohol, milk, chocolate, and tomatoes. Mild topical steroids such as 1% hydrocortisone are sometimes helpful, but stronger steroid preparations are frequently counterproductive and should be avoided when they are not indicated for a specific dermatologic diagnosis. The placement of a small fluff of absorbent cotton at the anal verge can help to wick away moisture and collect any drainage before it can be in prolonged contact with the skin. Other adjuncts include drying the perianal skin with a hairdryer after bathing and replacing toilet paper with nondetergent, nondeodorant, nonalcoholic hypoallergenic wipes. Skin biopsies and dermatologic consultation should be obtained when a primary dermatologic condition is suspected or when the perianal irritation fails to heal with conservative therapy.

FECAL INCONTINENCE

EPIDEMIOLOGY AND PATHOBIOLOGY

Involuntary loss of stool or flatus is a relatively common problem that, when severe, can be socially isolating and debilitating. About 2% of individuals in the United States report incontinence symptoms, but the prevalence is more common in women and the elderly, and it also is substantially higher in patients who visit primary care providers and gastroenterologists. Almost half of U.S. nursing home patients suffer from fecal incontinence. Factors such as embarrassment, denial, and the degree of symptoms hinder a determination of true prevalence. Patients presenting with fecal incontinence often have concomitant urinary incontinence (Chapter 115), and up to 25% of women with fecal incontinence have at least one associated pelvic floor disorder.

Normal continence involves the coordinated interaction between multiple different neuronal pathways and the pelvic and perineal structures. In addition, several factors including bowel motility, stool consistency, evacuation efficiency, mental status, and sphincter integrity all play a role in normal regulation.[10] Sphincter disruption related to vaginal delivery is a common cause that often affects young women; many incontinent women who present later in life have an underlying sphincter injury for which they can no longer compensate. Other causes of incontinence include fecal impaction, surgical or traumatic sphincter injury, rectal prolapse, neurologic disorders (e.g., diabetic neuropathy, stroke, multiple sclerosis, brain or spinal cord injury), chronic diarrheal states, dementia, impaired mobility, and poor access to toilet facilities.

CLINICAL MANIFESTATIONS AND DIAGNOSIS

Because fecal incontinence is a symptom and not a disease, the diagnosis is based on history alone. Specific evaluation of the incontinent patient can include anal manometry, anal ultrasound, pudendal nerve testing, and defecography. Anal endoscopic ultrasonography, which is generally a helpful test, accurately depicts sphincter anatomy and reliably identifies sphincter defects. Some patients with fecal incontinence may have concomitant disorders such as impaired evacuation, pelvic prolapse, or urinary incontinence; urogynecologic evaluation should be performed when appropriate.

TREATMENT

Mild incontinence is often treated successfully by the addition of a fiber supplement to make stools less liquid and the use of an antimotility agent, such as loperamide 2 to 4 mg up to four times daily, to treat diarrhea. Biofeedback also is sometimes successful.

For individuals with significant sphincter disruptions, surgical repair (sphincteroplasty) usually leads to substantial improvement (Fig. 131-5). Unfortunately, this improvement tends to wane over time, so sacral nerve modulation, which requires placement of an electrical lead into the S3 sacral foramen and implantation of an electrical stimulator, is usually a better option. Sacral nerve modulation is highly effective for fecal incontinence,[11] with about 40% of patients regaining continence and another 45% noting improvement at 36 months.

For patients without a sphincter defect, sacral nerve modulation is one option, but another option is transanal submucosal injection of dextranomer in stabilized hyaluronic acid. These injections add bulk to the perianal tissues, thereby allowing the perianal tissues to coapt together. As a result, injection therapy is most effective in patients who have a small amount of leakage and not loss of full bowel movements. After two treatments of four injections each, reported fecal incontinence decreases by about 50%, but many patients require repeat injections. This treatment should not be used in patients who are immunosuppressed or who have had prior radiation therapy, rectal prolapse, or inflammatory bowel disease.

For patients with severe refractory incontinence, creation of a colostomy should be strongly considered. Initial reluctance notwithstanding, most patients regain control of their bowel function and report a substantially improved quality of life.

RECTAL PROLAPSE

EPIDEMIOLOGY AND PATHOBIOLOGY

Rectal prolapse is a full-thickness protrusion of the rectum beyond the anal sphincter. It occurs in about 1% of adults over age 65 years, and about 90% of cases are in women. Prolapse is caused by an internal rectal intussusception that eventually becomes more severe and then progresses so that the full thickness of the rectal wall protrudes externally. Risk factors include multiparity, a history of pelvic surgery, higher body mass index, chronic diarrhea or constipation with significant straining, connective tissue disorders, and neurologic diseases. Uncorrected prolapse also frequently leads to fecal incontinence by mechanically stretching the sphincter complex and causing a stretch injury to the pudendal nerves, with frank loss of fecal material when the rectal mucosa prolapses externally.

CLINICAL MANIFESTATIONS AND DIAGNOSIS

The main clinical manifestation of rectal prolapse is the protruding rectal mass (Fig. 131-6). The protrusion most commonly occurs with bowel movements, but with time it may occur with coughing or sneezing, and eventually it can occur spontaneously. Approximately 75% of patients have at least minor complaints of fecal incontinence, whereas complaints of "constipation,"

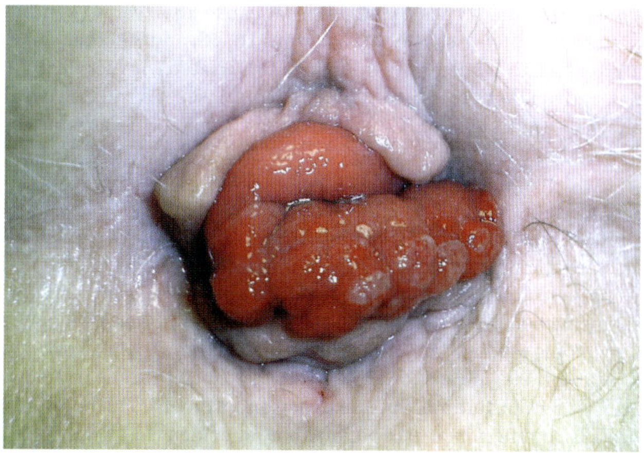

FIGURE 131-6. **Rectal mucosal prolapse. The main clinical manifestation of rectal prolapse is the protruding rectal mass.**

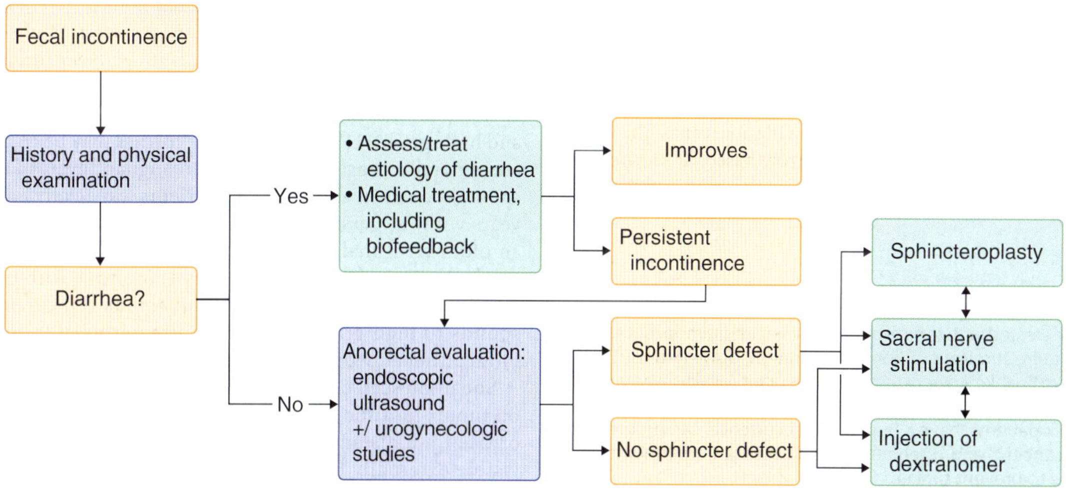

FIGURE 131-5. **Algorithm for fecal incontinence.** (Adapted from Madoff RD, Parker SC, Varma MG, et al. Fecal incontinence in adults. *Lancet*. 2004;364:621-632.)

which are often caused by unsuccessful attempts to evacuate the intussuscepting rectum, occur in 15 to 65%. Other associated symptoms include chronic mucus discharge, pelvic discomfort, and minor bleeding. Patients can also rarely present with an incarcerated or strangulated prolapse that mandates urgent intervention.

The diagnosis of rectal prolapse is confirmed on physical examination. Full-thickness prolapse, which is characterized by concentric mucosal folds of the rectum, must be differentiated from circumferential mucosal prolapse, which is characterized by radial folds alone. The prolapse is often best demonstrated by having the patient strain on a commode. Ancillary studies do not routinely alter management, but colonoscopy should be performed to help exclude other pathology. Defecography is also helpful to diagnose internal rectal intussusception and associated pelvic floor abnormalities, such as rectocele and enterocele.

TREATMENT

Nonoperative measures will not correct rectal prolapse, so conservative measures should be considered only in patients who have very minor and minimally symptomatic prolapse or who are poor surgical candidates. A ventral rectopexy with mesh (either biologic or nonabsorbable), which involves mobilizing the rectum anteriorly, suturing the mesh to the anterior rectal wall, and then fixing the mesh to the sacrum, is the procedure of choice. This operation, which can be performed laparoscopically or robotically, can help to correct rectoceles and is associated with less postoperative constipation and recurrence than prior surgical alternatives.[A5]

HUMAN PAPILLOMAVIRUS

EPIDEMIOLOGY AND PATHOBIOLOGY

Human papillomavirus (HPV), which is the most common sexually transmitted infection, is a cause of anal dysplasia and cancer. The approximately 40 HPV subtypes that can cause anogenital infections are divided into low-risk types (e.g., types 6 and 11) that cause anal warts (condyloma acuminata) and high-risk types (e.g., types 16, 18, and 33) that can cause anal dysplasia and cancer. HPV infection is associated with cervical, vulvar, vaginal, and penile cancers, and some patients have HPV-related dysplasia or cancer in multiple sites. Over 90% of anal cancers are attributable to HPV infection.

The incidence of anal cancer has been steadily increasing, from 0.6 per 100,000 in 1973 to 1.0 per 100,000 in 2001 and 2.0 per 100,000 in 2018. In the United States alone, an estimated 9090 individuals develop anal cancer annually, and approximately 1400 will die from it.[12] These epidemiologic trends have been attributed to a particularly rapid increase in anal cancers among men who have sex with men, especially men infected with HIV. Anal HPV, including the high-risk serotypes, is highly prevalent in at-risk populations (sex workers, intravenous drug users, transplant recipients, men who have sex with men, and HIV-positive men and women). Furthermore, anal dysplasia is common in at-risk populations, as evidenced by the 30 to 50% prevalence of high-grade anal dysplasia among HIV-positive men who have sex with men seen in specialty clinics in New York and San Francisco. Other associated risk factors for both dysplasia and anal cancer include a history of other HPV-related genital dysplasia or malignancy (cervical, vaginal, or vulvar), prior sexually acquired diseases, anoreceptive intercourse, multiple sexual partners, and cigarette smoking.

ANAL WARTS

CLINICAL MANIFESTATION AND DIAGNOSIS

Anal warts can occur in the perianal skin and within the anal canal. The lesions are raised, epithelialized (when external), and narrow based. Their spectrum of appearances can range from scattered individual warts to a confluent mass of warts (Fig. 131-7).

TREATMENT

External warts can be treated with topical podophyllin or imiquimod, but extensive warts usually require surgical excision or fulguration. Untreated warts can rarely progress to form Bushke-Löwenstein tumors—giant, locally invasive condyloma acuminata that frequently contain in situ or invasive cancer. Anal warts, especially in high-risk patients, have a high risk of recurrence, can progress to dysplasia and anal cancer,[13] and often require multiple local treatments and ongoing surveillance to prevent cancer.

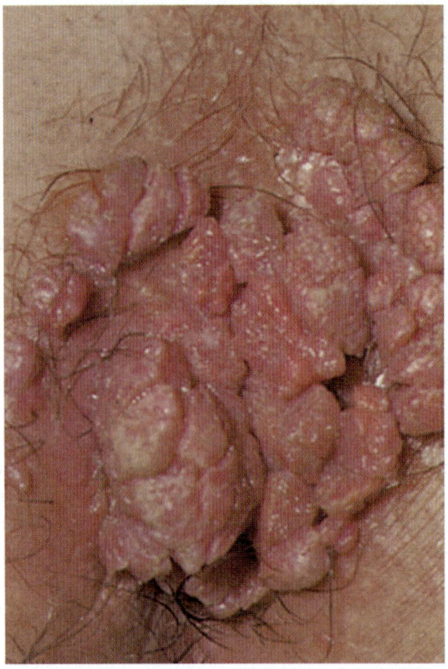

FIGURE 131-7. Anal condyloma. These can occur as individual warts or as a confluent mass.

ANAL CANCER

Anal cancer is almost always a manifestation of HPV infection (Chapter 344), especially HPV 16 and 18.[14] Other significant but less common anal cancers include adenocarcinoma, melanoma, and Paget disease.

Anal cancer is a common problem in the HIV-positive population, especially in men who have sex with men. In the United States, anal cancer is nearly 20 times more common in HIV-positive individuals than in the uninfected population. However, the incidence has been declining by 7% per year since 2008, presumably because of more effective antiretroviral therapy. Other independent risk factors include low nadir CD4 counts, alcohol use, and smoking.

CLINICAL MANIFESTATIONS AND DIAGNOSIS

The most common symptoms of anal cancer are bleeding, pain, and a palpable mass. The cancer may be seen externally as an ulcerated mass or may be palpated within the anal canal. Anal dysplastic lesions may appear as anal warts or as flat, pigmented lesions, or they may be invisible to the naked eye. They are best visualized using anal microscopy after topical application of 3 to 5% acetic acid (see later). Biopsy is necessary to make the diagnosis.[15]

Thorough palpation of the inguinal lymph nodes is important to detect the presence of any clinically relevant adenopathy, but proper staging for anal canal malignancies requires a chest, abdominal, and pelvic CT scan. Pelvic MRI is useful to assess the size and depth of the lesion as well as the presence and location of any involved regional lymph nodes.

The great majority of anal cancers are variants of squamous cell carcinoma. The terms *anal dysplasia, anal intraepithelial neoplasia*, and *squamous intraepithelial lesion* differ slightly but have often been used interchangeably. Squamous intraepithelial lesions are divided into low-grade (LSIL) and high-grade (HSIL) groups; the former may be transient, but the latter are generally considered to be premalignant even though they may clear spontaneously in about 20% of patients, especially patients below age 45 years without persistent HPV16.[16] Anal intraepithelial neoplasia (AIN), an older term that is being supplanted by the squamous intraepithelial terminology, is divided into grades 1, 2, and 3, with grades 2 and 3 being classified as high-grade lesions. Squamous cell carcinoma in situ corresponds to high-grade squamous intraepithelial lesion and grade 3 anal intraepithelial neoplasia.

Squamous cell carcinoma of the anus is divided into two groups based on tumor location: cancers of the anal margin (extending from the anal orifice for a distance up to 5 cm) and cancers of the anal canal. Tumors visible externally but extending into the anal canal are considered anal canal lesions.

TREATMENT

Management of the patient with anal dysplasia is controversial. Many authorities advocate a screening and treatment approach based on that used for cervical cancer (Chapter 184), which is another HPV-associated disease. High-risk individuals are screened with anal Papanicolaou smears, and high-definition anal microscopy (analogous to colposcopy of the cervix) is performed when abnormal cytology is detected. Using this technique, dysplastic lesions can be identified and focally ablated[A6] or treated with topical imiquimod or 5-fluorouracil. Reported complete response rates vary significantly (≈30 to 80%), and side effects (pain, irritation, and ulceration) may require withdrawal of therapy. More extensive dysplasia requires microscopy-directed targeted ablation in the operating room.

Chemoradiotherapy is standard first-line treatment for squamous cell cancer of the anal canal. Current radiation protocols most frequently use 45-Gy external beam radiation therapy in 25 fractions, with a boost to the primary tumor and involved inguinal nodes to a total dose of 54 to 59 Gy. Standard chemotherapy utilizes 5-fluorouracil (1000 mg/m^2 per 24 hours, continuous infusion for 96 hours, starting on days 1 and 29) in combination with mitomycin C (most commonly 10 mg/m^2 intravenous bolus on days 1 and 29). Abdominoperineal resection with permanent colostomy is reserved for tumors that fail to respond to chemoradiation and those that recur. Similarly, groin dissection is performed only when involved inguinal nodes fail chemoradiation.

Early squamous cell cancers of the anal margin can be locally excised if a satisfactory margin can be obtained without injuring the anal sphincter and if there is no evidence of nodal spread. More advanced anal margin tumors are treated with chemoradiotherapy as described for anal canal tumors. Combined chemoradiation therapy is the primary treatment for most squamous cell carcinomas of the anal canal.

PREVENTION

In addition to its proven efficacy in the prevention of cervical neoplasia in women, HPV vaccination appears to be effective in preventing external genital lesions and intraepithelial neoplasm in HIV-uninfected men. The use of an HPV vaccine may reduce anal intraepithelial neoplasm in men who have sex with men, but it does not appear to benefit HIV-infected men.[A7]

Routine HPV vaccination is recommended at age 11 to 12 years, but it can be administered starting at age 9 years in both males and females (Chapter 15).[17] A catch-up vaccination is recommended in previously unvaccinated females between ages 13 and 26 years and in males between ages 13 and 21 years and in individuals who did not complete the vaccine series. For males 22 to 26 years, catch-up HPV vaccination is recommended in men who have sex with men and in immunocompromised men (including HIV-infected males).

OTHER SEXUALLY TRANSMITTED ANORECTAL DISEASES

A number of sexually transmitted diseases (Chapter 264) of the anorectum occur most frequently in individuals who practice anoreceptive intercourse. Common causative agents include *Treponema pallidum* (Chapter 295), *Neisseria gonorrhoeae* (Chapter 275), *Chlamydia trachomatis* (Chapter 294), herpes simplex (Chapter 345), and HIV (Chapter 353). Other sexually transmitted pathogens are *Shigella* (Chapter 285), *Campylobacter jejuni* (Chapter 279), *Haemophilus ducreyi* (Chapter 276), *Calymmatobacterium granulomatis* (Chapter 292), *Entamoeba histolytica* (Chapter 323), *Giardia lamblia* (Chapter 322), and *Isospora belli* (Chapter 324).

The widely variable presentations range from asymptomatic to anal pain, pruritus, discharge, fever, cramps, and bloody diarrhea. Clinical suspicion followed by appropriate and specific testing is necessary to make the correct diagnosis, and clinicians should consider the possibility of simultaneous infections. Treatment addresses the specific infection.

GENERAL REFERENCES

For the General References and other additional features, please visit Elsevier eBooks+ at https://ebooks.health.elsevier.com.

Grade A References

A1. Aibuedefe B, Kling SM, Philp MM, et al. An update on surgical treatment of hemorrhoidal disease: a systematic review and meta analysis. *Int J Colorectal Dis*. 2021;36:2041-2049.
A2. Brown SR, Tiernan JP, Watson AJM, et al. Haemorrhoidal artery ligation versus rubber band ligation for the management of symptomatic second-degree and third-degree haemorrhoids (HubBLe): a multicentre, open-label, randomised controlled trial. *Lancet*. 2016;388:356-364.
A3. Ghahramani L, Minaie MR, Arasteh P, et al. Antibiotic therapy for prevention of fistula in-ano after incision and drainage of simple perianal abscess: a randomized single blind clinical trial. *Surgery*. 2017;162:1017-1025.
A4. Emile SH, Khan SM, Adejumo A, et al. Ligation of intersphincteric fistula tract (LIFT) in treatment of anal fistula: an updated systematic review, meta-analysis, and meta-regression of the predictors of failure. *Surgery*. 2020;167:484-492.
A5. Lobb HS, Kearsey CC, Ahmed S, et al. Suture rectopexy versus ventral mesh rectopexy for complete full-thickness rectal prolapse and intussusception: systematic review and meta-analysis. *BJS Open*. 2021;5:zraa037.
A6. Palefsky JM, Lee JY, Jay N, et al. Treatment of anal high-grade squamous intraepithelial lesions to prevent anal cancer. *N Engl J Med*. 2022;386:2273-2282.
A7. Wilkin TJ, Chen H, Cespedes MS, et al. A randomized, placebo-controlled trial of the quadrivalent human papillomavirus vaccine in human immunodeficiency virus-infected adults aged 27 years or older: AIDS Clinical Trials Group Protocol A5298. *Clin Infect Dis*. 2018;67:1339-1346.

XIV

DISEASES OF THE LIVER AND BILIARY SYSTEM

132 APPROACH TO THE PATIENT WITH LIVER DISEASE

PAUL MARTIN

The liver serves multiple key functions, including metabolism of the products of ingested food, production of amino acids to form proteins, detoxification of ingested drugs, conversion of nitrogenous substances from the gut into urea, formation of clotting factors, metabolism of bilirubin, processing of lipids absorbed from the intestine, and excretion of its products as bile. The liver also stores glycogen, which is a source of glucose, and helps contain infections by removing bacteria from the blood stream. These diverse functions reflect the activities of hepatocytes, bile duct cells called cholangiocytes, Kupffer cells, endothelial cells, and portal fibroblasts.

The liver has a dual blood supply: 70% is delivered by the portal vein, which drains the intestine, and the remainder is delivered by the hepatic artery. After arrival in the liver, nutrient-rich portal blood passes along the hepatic sinusoids in close contact with lining hepatocytes before draining into the hepatic vein. The hepatocytes detoxify, metabolize, and synthesize the products of digestion. Bilirubin, which is produced by breakdown of red cells and other hemoproteins by reticuloendothelial cells predominantly in the liver and spleen, is transported to the hepatocytes, bound to albumin, and solubilized by them for biliary excretion.

Liver disease causes loss of hepatocellular capacity, with diminished detoxification, excretory, and synthetic functions. Hepatocyte dysfunction results in impaired production of clotting factors, albumin, and other proteins, as well as reduced endogenous formation of lipids. Hepatocyte injury from a variety of causes, including viruses, alcohol, autoimmune disorders, and drug hepatotoxicity, is accompanied by leakage of cellular enzymes into the systemic circulation (Chapter 133). Coagulopathy, decreased serum albumin, and hyperbilirubinemia are observed with more profound hepatocellular injury. Portal hypertension occurs because of disruption of the low-pressure intrahepatic blood flow from the portal to the systemic venous circulation owing to hepatic fibrosis. Consequences of portal hypertension include accumulation of abdominal ascites and the development of portal-systemic venous collaterals with portal-systemic shunting, with formation of varices and development of hepatic encephalopathy. Vascular disorders, including portal vein thrombosis, can result in portal hypertension in the absence of parenchymal liver disease.

The diversity of the liver's functions, its complicated blood supply, and its intimate relationship with the biliary tree contribute to the divergent manifestations of liver disease. The initial complaint often reflects whether the cause is diffuse, such as acute viral hepatitis with widespread hepatocyte injury that manifests as malaise or fatigue, or whether the cause is discrete, such as when biliary obstruction from a gallstone in the common bile duct manifests as severe abdominal pain. Patients may present with multiple complaints, such as nausea and anorexia owing to hepatocellular disease accompanied by right upper quadrant discomfort due to stretching of the hepatic capsule by parenchymal cell edema and inflammation. Patients with more advanced liver disease, such as decompensated cirrhosis (Chapter 139), may have substantial hepatocellular dysfunction with jaundice and coagulopathy in addition to portal hypertension with ascites and bleeding esophageal varices. Many patients who present with hepatic symptoms or signs may have extrahepatic disease; for example, a tender, enlarged liver may be caused by a systemic disorder, such as heart failure with hepatic congestion, rather than a primary hepatic disorder. In patients with cirrhosis, the initial presentation of previously unrecognized liver disease may be a major complication such as variceal hemorrhage, which in turn can precipitate hepatic encephalopathy and other features of frank hepatic decompensation.

HISTORY

Patients with liver disorders come to medical attention for a variety of reasons,[1] ranging from the incidental discovery of abnormal liver chemistries[2] to decompensated cirrhosis. Many complaints related to liver disease, such as fatigue, are nonspecific; unless liver disease is considered in the differential diagnosis, recognition of the hepatic origin of these complaints may be delayed.

In clinical practice, a frequent manifestation of asymptomatic liver disease is discovery of abnormal liver biochemistries during a life insurance application, annual physical examination, or attempt to donate blood. It is important to inquire about occasions when liver biochemistries may have been obtained to determine whether hepatic dysfunction is long-standing or more recent. In a patient with hepatic dysfunction, inquiry should be made about the presence of malaise, anorexia, fatigue, and weight change. Jaundice (Chapter 133) is a dramatic manifestation of possible liver disease. A patient may first notice lighter-colored stools or dark urine rather than scleral icterus. The absence of these latter changes suggests that unconjugated hyperbilirubinemia is due to hemolysis rather than intrinsic liver disease. Not infrequently, a patient may be unaware of jaundice until it is noted by others.

Abdominal pain (Chapter 118) related to liver disease can have a variety of explanations. Symptomatic gallstones (Chapter 141) can present with the abrupt onset of severe epigastric or right upper quadrant discomfort, often after a large meal and frequently associated with nausea and vomiting. The pain is often steady rather than colicky and can radiate widely, including to the chest and back. A patient may not be able to achieve a position that lessens the pain, which may last several hours. More persistent pain, particularly if associated with weight loss and jaundice, raises concern about malignant bile duct obstruction. Pain is also common in parenchymal liver disease in the absence of biliary tract disease. Many patients with chronic hepatocellular disorders, such as chronic hepatitis C (Chapter 135) or nonalcoholic fatty liver disease (NAFLD) (Chapter 138), complain of vague right upper quadrant discomfort that has no particular relieving or aggravating factors. Abdominal pain, which can be severe, is also frequent in acute viral hepatitis (Chapter 134), as well as with the hepatic congestion that results from back pressure in heart failure or hepatic vein occlusion, as in Budd-Chiari syndrome (Chapter 129).

Fatigue, anorexia, and malaise can be present in both acute and chronic liver disease. In acute liver disorders such as acute viral hepatitis (Chapter 134), drug-induced liver disease (Chapter 136), or an acute manifestation of autoimmune hepatitis (Chapter 135), patients may report profound fatigue, nausea, and malaise with decreased appetite and substantial associated weight loss. Distaste for cigarettes is said to be characteristic of acute viral hepatitis. Fatigue is also prominent in chronic liver disease such as chronic hepatitis C (Chapter 135). Pruritus is a prominent feature of cholestatic disorders, such as primary biliary cirrhosis, sclerosing cholangitis, or cholestatic drug reactions, particularly when patients are frankly icteric; however, pruritus also occurs in chronic parenchymal liver disease, most notably chronic hepatitis C, and in acute viral hepatitis. Easy bruising in patients with liver disease reflects coagulopathy and/or thrombocytopenia.

Fever in a patient with hepatic dysfunction is experienced in the prodrome of acute hepatitis A, as well as in alcoholic hepatitis and drug-induced liver disease. In a patient with suspected biliary obstruction, fever suggests complicating bacterial cholangitis or acute cholecystitis. Ascites is most frequently a manifestation of cirrhosis and portal hypertension in a patient with liver disease. Patients note increasing abdominal girth, which may be preceded by ankle edema. Weight gain owing to fluid retention may be masked by concomitant loss of muscle mass. The onset of ascites in the absence of a history of liver disease suggests a vascular event, such as hepatic vein occlusion (Chapter 129), or a nonhepatic cause of ascites, such as nephrotic syndrome or heart failure. Accumulation of ascites in a patient with liver disease may be subtle, with a slowly increasing waist circumference, or it may be more rapid, such as in a cirrhotic patient who receives fluid resuscitation after gastrointestinal bleeding. Although ascites in a patient with liver disease implies the presence of cirrhosis, ascites also can complicate severe acute liver disease, including alcoholic hepatitis and viral hepatitis, in which it suggests a poor prognosis.

Hepatic encephalopathy (Chapter 139), which is a neuropsychiatric disorder in patients with liver disease, can range from subtle cognitive impairment to deep coma.[3] Early symptoms include a disturbed sleep pattern with nocturnal insomnia and daytime somnolence. More advanced encephalopathy can result in impairment of memory, confusion, and difficulty completing routine tasks. However, new-onset confusion or coma in a patient with liver disease should not be presumed to reflect hepatic encephalopathy unless other explanations, such as sedative overdose or subdural hematoma, have been excluded. Important precipitants of hepatic encephalopathy in a cirrhotic patient include gastrointestinal bleeding, bacterial infection (e.g., spontaneous bacterial peritonitis), electrolyte imbalance, and renal insufficiency, all of which need to be excluded during the initial clinical evaluation. In a patient with acute liver failure, coma as a consequence of cerebral edema may be impossible to distinguish from advanced hepatic encephalopathy unless the increased intracranial pressure results in papilledema.

Gastrointestinal hemorrhage resulting from bleeding varices is usually profuse and often abrupt in onset. It typically presents with hematemesis or melena (Chapter 121), and frequently coexisting postural hypotension or presyncope indicates major blood loss. The increased protein load in the gut can precipitate hepatic encephalopathy. Nonvariceal causes of gastrointestinal bleeding in a patient with liver disease include portal gastropathy (Chapter 121).

RISK FACTORS FOR LIVER DISEASE

An important aspect of the history is identification of possible risk factors for liver disease. The history should include directed questioning about alcohol consumption, including frequency and pattern (Chapter 364). The age of initial alcohol use and whether consumption has increased with age should be ascertained. Family members also should be asked about their perception of the patient's alcohol use and whether it has resulted in difficulties in personal relationships or work performance. Other clues to alcohol abuse are a history of convictions for driving under the influence of alcohol, motor vehicle accidents, and physical symptoms of alcohol dependence (Chapter 364). More circumspect questioning may be required to elicit a history of recreational drug use. Not infrequently, a patient with suspected viral hepatitis admits to smoking marijuana or snorting cocaine but does not acknowledge intravenous drug use. With the increasing frequency of nonalcoholic fatty liver disease as a cause of hepatic dysfunction (Chapter 138), comorbid conditions such as diabetes mellitus, hyperlipidemia, sleep apnea, and weight gain should be noted.

Medication use, whether prescription or over-the-counter, must be assessed because drug-induced liver disease is an important cause of apparently cryptogenic hepatic dysfunction and is not limited to therapeutic drugs (Chapter 136).[4] Increasingly, herbal and "natural" products (Chapter 30) are ingested for a variety of maladies, and patients may fail to disclose their use because they do not perceive these agents to have side effects or may sense that the physician does not endorse their use. As with alcohol, it is important to quantify the amount of medication ingested and over what period. The social history should include details about recent travel and contact with individuals with viral hepatitis through intimate, household, or occupational contact. It is also important to ask about vigorous physical activity that can result in elevated aminotransferase levels of nonhepatic origin.

ASSESSING DURATION OF LIVER DISEASE

The differential diagnosis in a patient with liver disease is determined to a large extent by the presentation, such as jaundice or ascites. In many patients, however, the timing of more subtle findings such as elevated aminotransferases is difficult to determine. Prior blood test results should be retrieved to determine whether hepatic dysfunction is long-standing or more recent. Hepatic dysfunction of less than 6 months' duration is regarded as acute and is frequently self-limited, whereas abnormalities that persist for more than 6 months are unlikely to resolve spontaneously. If the patient has had a cholecystectomy, it is important to determine the indication. Incidental gallstones are sometimes assumed to be the cause of abnormal liver chemistries in a patient with parenchymal liver disease and can lead to an unnecessary cholecystectomy. Thrombocytopenia owing to portal hypertension in a patient with unrecognized cirrhosis may have been investigated in the past without a firm conclusion being reached.

REVIEW OF OTHER ORGAN SYSTEMS

While focusing on liver-related symptoms, it is important not to overlook other diagnostic clues, associated disorders, and complications. Sicca symptoms, including dry eyes and mouth, are common in primary biliary cholangitis (Chapter 141); florid features of scleroderma and CREST syndrome (Chapter 246) are other associations. Dyspnea in a patient with hepatic dysfunction may reflect cardiac failure with hepatic congestion (Chapter 45). Other explanations include hepatopulmonary syndrome (Chapter 139), with the characteristic complaint of platypnea-dyspnea (often with chest tightness) that is worse in the upright position owing to aggravation of the ventilation-perfusion mismatch because of intrapulmonary shunting. A hydrothorax in decompensated cirrhosis can cause dyspnea, as can emphysema in patients with liver disease caused by α_1-antitrypsin deficiency. A history of premature menopause is common in middle-aged women with cirrhosis, as is decreased libido and sexual potency in cirrhotic men. Arthralgias are often reported in viral hepatitis, and hemochromatosis (Chapter 196) may manifest with involvement of the proximal interphalangeal joints or chondrocalcinosis of the knees; increased skin pigmentation and diabetes mellitus are other features of this disorder. Accelerated osteopenia occurs in many liver diseases, including primary cirrhosis, primary sclerosing cholangitis, and alcoholic cirrhosis; osteopenia may be aggravated by corticosteroid use in autoimmune hepatitis. Alcoholic peripheral neuropathy (Chapter 384) can manifest with pain and paresthesias. Tremor and inattentiveness in a younger patient with hepatic dysfunction suggest Wilson disease (Chapter 195). Diarrhea and rectal bleeding in a patient with cholestatic liver disease suggest associated inflammatory bowel disease (Chapter 127).

FAMILY HISTORY

The family history should include an inquiry not only about relatives with liver disease but also associated extrahepatic conditions. Hereditary hepatic conditions (see later), such as Wilson disease and hemochromatosis, may occur in several members of a sibship. In α_1-antitrypsin deficiency, some family members may experience predominantly emphysema rather than cirrhosis. Similarly, renal failure in a family member of a patient with hepatic cysts suggests adult polycystic disease (Chapter 112). A family history of inflammatory bowel disease may be a clue to primary sclerosing cholangitis in a patient with cholestatic liver chemistries. The history in patients with suspected alcoholic liver disease may reveal other family members with alcoholism.

PHYSICAL EXAMINATION

GENERAL CONDITION

In a patient with suspected liver disease, it is crucial to resist the temptation to palpate the abdomen immediately, thus potentially ignoring other important diagnostic clues. Apart from seeking icterus, the initial observation should note whether muscle wasting, cutaneous stigmata of liver disease, abdominal distention, and peripheral edema are present. The vital signs may reflect the hyperdynamic circulation characteristic of cirrhosis, with a resting tachycardia, wide pulse pressure, and low blood pressure resulting from peripheral vasodilation. Fetor hepaticus, which is described as a musty smell, may be detected when a cirrhotic patient exhales and must be distinguished from more frequent halitosis caused by poor dental hygiene.

MUCOCUTANEOUS FINDINGS

Icterus (Fig. 132-1) is best confirmed by examination of the sclera or, if necessary, under the tongue, where elastin tissue retains bilirubin. Grayish skin discoloration in hemochromatosis may be most evident in the skin folds in the groin or axilla. Acanthosis nigricans can be observed in nonalcoholic fatty liver disease (Chapter 138). A Kayser-Fleischer ring (see Fig. 195-2), caused by the deposition of copper in the Descemet membrane, is a brownish circle around the periphery of the iris and may require slit lamp examination to detect; it always should be sought in a patient with suspected Wilson disease (Chapter 195). Poor dentition is characteristic in alcoholic or drug-abusing individuals, and excessive dental caries may result from decreased saliva production in sicca syndrome. Parotid gland swelling is occasionally observed in alcoholic patients. Central cyanosis and clubbing are found in the hepatopulmonary syndrome. Temporal muscle wasting and "paper money" facial skin, owing to atrophy with telangiectasia, are signs of advanced liver disease. Xanthelasma from lipid deposits may be observed on the eyelids and skin around the orbits in patients with cholestatic liver disease. Spider nevi on the face and thorax are not pathognomonic of liver disease, especially in women, but they are suggestive if more than a few are present. Palmar erythema (Fig. 132-2) may be normal in women but suggests liver disease in men. Dupuytren contracture (see Fig. 138-1), the retraction of the palmar fascia with subsequent contracture of the palms and fingers, can be a sign of alcoholic liver disease, although it

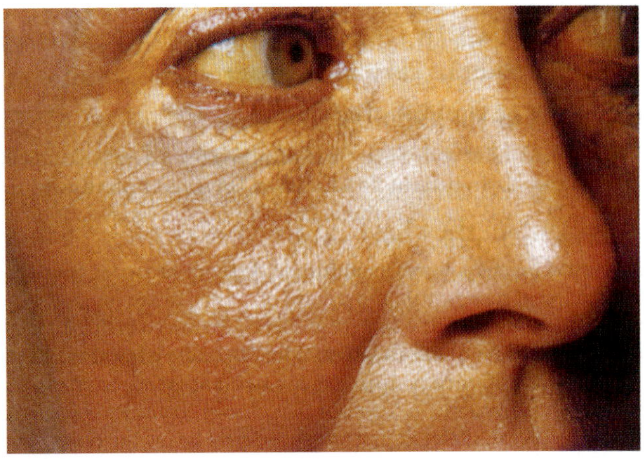

FIGURE 132-1. Scleral icterus.

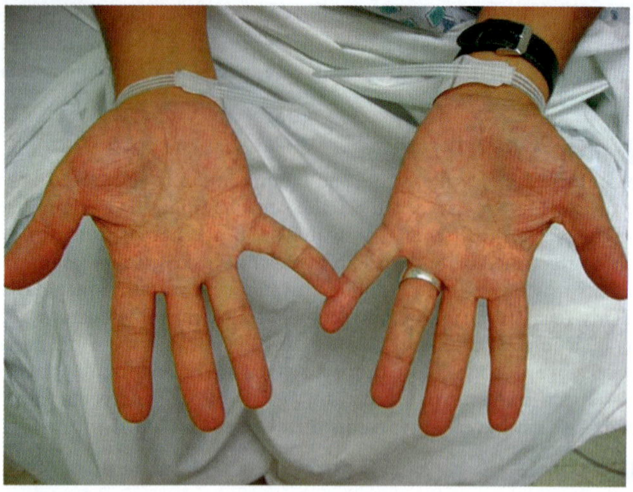

FIGURE 132-2. Palmar erythema.

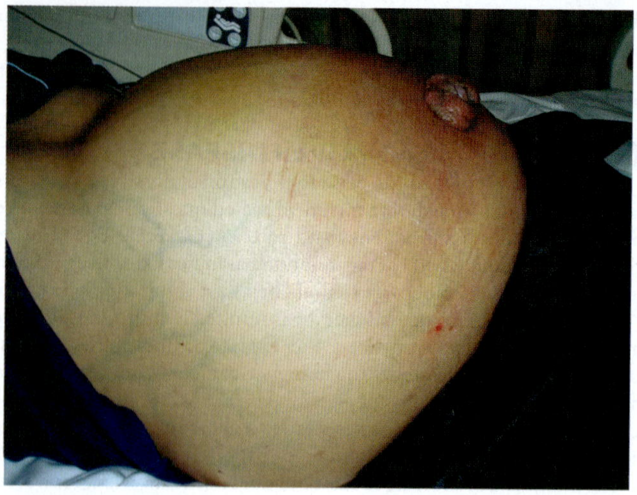

FIGURE 132-4. Ascites.

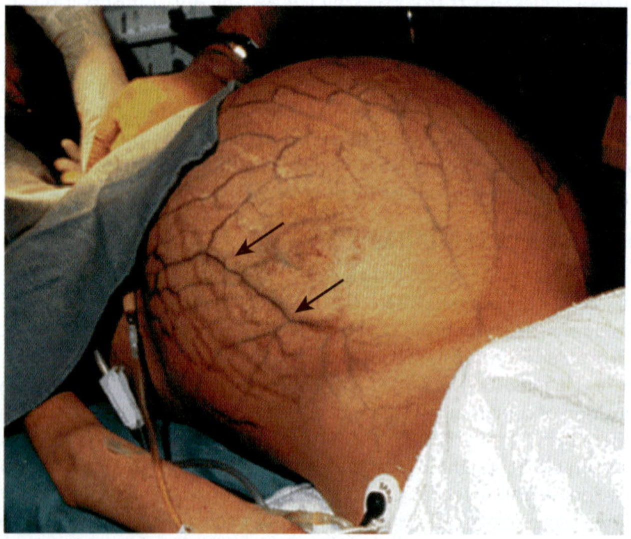

FIGURE 132-3. **Caput medusae.** Photograph shows caput medusae accentuated by a large amount of ascites in a patient being prepared for liver transplantation. An extensive plexus of veins is seen emanating from the umbilical region and radiating across the anterior abdominal wall. Note the large vein coursing inferiorly along the right flank (*arrows*). This is the superficial epigastric vein, which drains into the external iliac vein. (From Henseler KP, Pozniak MA, Le FT, et al. Three-dimensional CT angiography of spontaneous portosystemic shunts. *Radiographics*. 2001;21:691-704.)

is also described in patients with epilepsy or diabetes mellitus, as well as in individuals who have work-related contractures. Petechiae and ecchymoses reflect impaired production of clotting factors and hypersplenism in advanced liver disease. Patches of white discoloration on the nails may be present in advanced liver disease. Scratch marks from pruritus may be observed on the trunk and extremities of patients with cholestatic liver disease. Sparing of the center of the back can lead to a less pigmented butterfly-shaped area because patients cannot reach that area with their fingernails.

EXAMINATION OF THE ABDOMEN

Abdominal distention with ascites and dilation of collateral veins owing to portal hypertension represent florid signs of advanced liver disease. Caput medusae (Fig. 132-3) in the periumbilical area implies recanalization of the umbilical vein with portal hypertension.

Abdominal percussion may confirm the presence of ascites (Fig. 132-4). Shifting dullness results from movement of ascites to the most dependent portion of the abdomen. The subject should be examined in the supine position, with percussion of the abdomen from the midline toward the right or left flank. A change from a tympanic sound to a dull sound signifies a change from air to fluid, and the location of that change identifies the surface of the fluid pool. Next, the examiner should percuss below the point at which dullness is elicited and ask the subject to turn toward the examiner. With the subject on his or her side, the examiner percusses again at the same point where tympany converted to dullness. If that spot is now tympanic, shifting dullness has been detected as a result of movement of the air-fluid boundary; this finding supports the presence of ascites. This maneuver should be performed sequentially on each side for confirmation. A fluid wave can be felt by placing the medial border of one hand on the abdomen and tapping the right or left lateral abdominal walls; the resulting wave is felt by the first hand. Scrotal edema and abdominal wall hernias are often present in patients with long-standing ascites. Abdominal tenderness in a patient with ascites suggests peritonitis (e.g., spontaneous bacterial peritonitis or the result of a perforated viscus). However, it is important to note that abdominal tenderness is frequently absent in spontaneous bacterial peritonitis.

The liver is dull to percussion. Percussion of the right upper quadrant can determine the liver span, normally 6 to 12 cm in the midclavicular line. The liver span may be diminished in a patient with cirrhosis, whereas hepatomegaly (Fig. 132-5) is detected in hepatic congestion resulting from heart failure, nonalcoholic fatty liver disease, and cholestatic forms of cirrhosis. The liver is best examined with the patient in the supine position, arms parallel to the side of the body and knees bent to relax the abdominal muscles. Palpation should begin in the right lower quadrant of the abdomen and move upward toward the rib cage so that the liver edge is felt on the way up. A normal liver edge is smooth and sometimes slightly tender when palpated. In general, a liver edge that is felt up to 2 cm below the right costal margin is considered normal, but a normal-sized liver can be displaced downward by other abnormalities, such as emphysema. In thin subjects, the liver edge may be felt on deep inspiration, even if it is normal in size.

The liver can feel hard and irregular, as in cirrhosis, or slightly tender, enlarged, and smooth, as in acute viral hepatitis, alcoholic hepatitis, or hepatic congestion, as occurs with right heart failure. The liver can extend across the midline, and the left lobe can be felt in the epigastrium. When the location of the edge of the liver is unclear, the scratch test may be more accurate than palpation.[A1] The bell of the stethoscope is placed on the right upper quadrant over the rib cage while scratching the surface of the abdominal wall from the mid-abdomen toward the liver; the sound of the scratch is amplified in an area under which the liver lies. In the presence of ascites, the liver edge may be detected by exerting quick pressure with the fingertips below the rib cage.

A palpable gallbladder suggests obstruction of the biliary system, whereas tenderness elicited by palpation during inspiration (the Murphy sign) suggests acute cholecystitis. Marked hepatic tenderness with hepatomegaly is observed in patients with a hepatic abscess (Chapter 137).

Splenomegaly (Chapter 154) is suggested by dullness to percussion between the 9th and 11th ribs in the left midaxillary line. A palpable spleen tip implies portal hypertension in a patient with chronic liver disease, although an enlarged spleen also can be detected in acute viral hepatitis and infiltrative disorders that involve both the liver and the spleen (see Table 154-5). Rectal examination is obligatory if gastrointestinal bleeding is suspected because of melena, anemia, or unexplained hepatic encephalopathy.

COMPLETE PHYSICAL EXAMINATION

The presence of rales and elevation of the jugular venous pressure suggest heart failure or pericardial disease as a cause of hepatic congestion.[5] Loss of secondary sexual characteristics in liver disease is reflected by a loss of axillary and

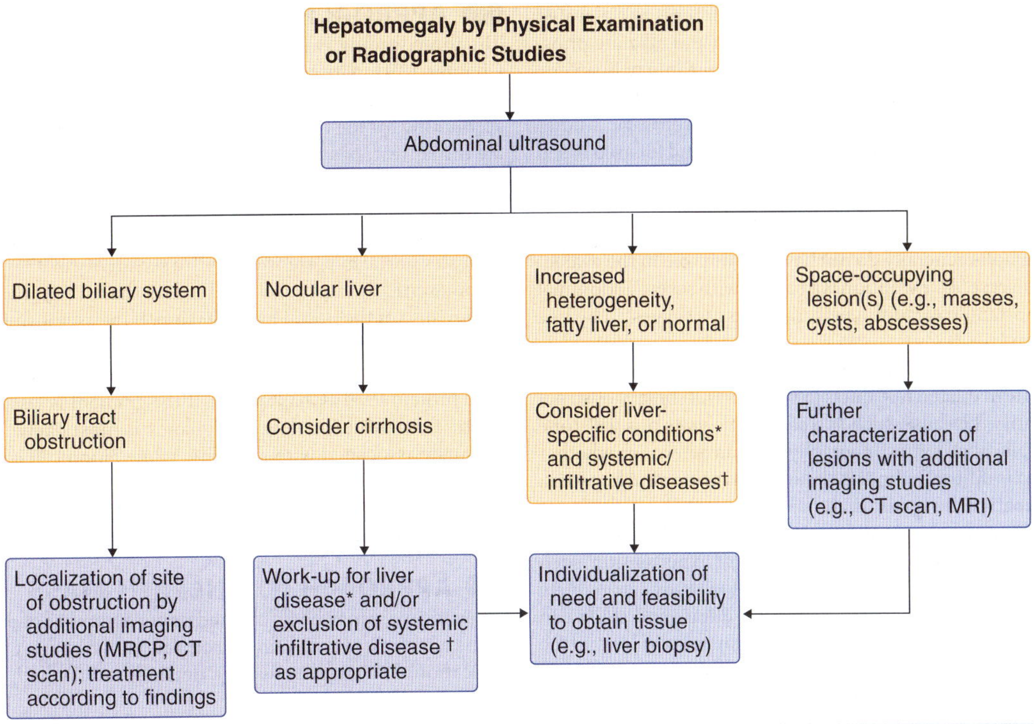

FIGURE 132-5. Diagnostic approach to hepatomegaly. *Conditions to be excluded include viral hepatitis, alcohol- and drug-induced liver disease, steatohepatitis, autoimmune liver diseases, and metabolic disorders, including hemochromatosis, Wilson disease, and α_1-antitrypsin deficiency. †Systemic and infiltrative diseases include amyloidosis, lymphoma, sarcoidosis, and infectious processes such as disseminated tuberculosis and fungemia. CT = computed tomography; MRCP = magnetic resonance cholangiopancreatography; MRI = magnetic resonance imaging.

TABLE 132-1 APPROACH TO COMMON HEPATIC COMPLAINTS

PRESENTATION	COMMON SYMPTOMS	COMMON PHYSICAL SIGNS	DIAGNOSTIC STUDIES	COMMON DIAGNOSES
Ascites	Abdominal distention and pain, ankle edema	Flank dullness Shifting dullness Fluid wave	Ultrasound with Doppler Diagnostic paracentesis Urinalysis	Cirrhosis Budd-Chiari syndrome Heart failure Nephrotic syndrome
Hepatic encephalopathy	Sleep disorientation, confusion, coma	Asterixis Altered mentation Fetor hepaticus	Serum ammonia Blood cultures Stool Hemoccult Serum creatinine and electrolytes	Decompensated cirrhosis Acute liver failure Other metabolic encephalopathies (renal, respiratory)
Hepatic mass	None or abdominal pain	Hepatic bruit or rub	α-Fetoprotein Ultrasound CT scan MRI Biopsy	Benign lesions: Hemangioma, adenoma, focal nodular hyperplasia Malignant lesions: Hepatocellular carcinoma, cholangiocarcinoma, metastases
Abdominal pain	Nausea, vomiting, fever	Right upper quadrant tenderness Palpable gallbladder Murphy sign	Ultrasound HIDA scan Paracentesis for ascites if present	Biliary colic Acute cholecystitis Hepatic congestion Hepatic metastases

CT = computed tomography; HIDA = hepatobiliary iminodiacetic acid; MRI = magnetic resonance imaging.

pubic hair, as well as feminization of body habitus in a male patient. Testicular atrophy also may be present. Peripheral edema is common in decompensated cirrhosis and may occur before ascites is obvious.

Neuropsychiatric alterations can include subtle changes in personality or more overt hepatic encephalopathy. Constructional apraxia (e.g., inability to draw a five-pointed star or to write legibly) in a fully conscious patient is a typical finding in hepatic encephalopathy. Asterixis, which is characterized by a series of extensor and flexor wrist movements, can be elicited by having the patient extend the arms, with dorsiflexion of the wrists, while separating the fingers for at least 15 seconds. Tremors (Chapter 379) are nonspecific but are also common in advanced cirrhosis.

DIAGNOSTIC STUDIES (TABLE 132-1)

LABORATORY STUDIES

The initial evaluation of liver disease involves a battery of blood tests, which can assess hepatic necroinflammation (serum aminotransferases), cholestatic biliary tract dysfunction (alkaline phosphatase, γ-glutamyl transpeptidase), excretory function (bilirubin), and synthetic function (coagulation factors, albumin) (Chapter 133). In hepatocellular dysfunction caused by viral hepatitis (Chapter 134), aminotransferase levels are elevated, with the serum alanine aminotransferase (ALT) level higher than the aspartate aminotransferase (AST) level. In alcoholic hepatitis (Chapter 138), AST elevation exceeds that of ALT. In patients with biliary obstruction or cholestatic liver diseases (Chapter 141), such as primary biliary cirrhosis or a cholestatic drug reaction, bilirubin and generally alkaline phosphatase levels are elevated. Impairment of synthetic function leads to a decreased serum albumin level over days to weeks. The prothrombin time, expressed as the international normalized ratio (INR), is a more sensitive test of hepatic synthetic function and becomes prolonged within several hours after a major hepatic insult. Portal hypertension owing to advanced hepatic fibrosis or cirrhosis results in a decreased platelet count resulting from hypersplenism. Although these general patterns of liver dysfunction are helpful in the initial evaluation of liver disease, they are nonspecific. For example, a patient with a predominantly hepatocellular process and elevated aminotransferase levels may also have elevated bilirubin and alkaline phosphatase levels as well as a low serum albumin level if liver injury is severe. Nevertheless, initial blood tests should identify the predominant pattern of abnormality and direct further diagnostic evaluation with serologic studies and abdominal imaging, which should be carefully selected and focused based upon the initial clinical evaluation.

ABDOMINAL IMAGING

Plain abdominal radiographs generally do not have a major role in the evaluation of suspected liver disease. An exception is a patient with severe abdominal pain, in whom it is important to exclude a perforated viscus suggested by free air under the diaphragm.

Ultrasonography should be the initial investigation in patients with obstructive jaundice. It can confirm dilated bile ducts in patients with biliary obstruction and often can identify the cause, such as a pancreatic mass or a gallstone lodged in the common bile duct. Ultrasonography also can determine whether the hepatic parenchyma is diffusely abnormal, such as in acute viral hepatitis; it can identify bright hepatic echo texture in nonalcoholic fatty liver disease or a coarsened echo texture in cirrhosis. In addition to confirming the presence of ascites, ultrasonography can identify other signs of portal hypertension, such as splenomegaly or intra-abdominal varices. A Doppler flow study can evaluate blood flow through the portal and hepatic vessels. An ultrasound study can identify hepatic masses and distinguish a cystic mass from a solid lesion (see later). Computed tomography (CT) and magnetic resonance imaging (MRI) add greater detail to the assessment of the hepatic vasculature, hepatic masses, and hepatic vascular structures. For the evaluation of focal liver lesions, the sensitivities of ultrasonography, contrast, CT, and MRI are similar. MRI can obtain a detailed cholangiogram, thereby avoiding a more invasive endoscopic retrograde cholangiopancreatography in many patients with suspected bile duct obstruction or disease (Chapters 119 and 120).

Transient elastography assesses hepatic fibrosis by measuring liver stiffness based on the propagation of shear waves in liver tissue, and it has largely replaced liver biopsy for this purpose.[6] In addition to measuring liver stiffness, transient elastography, often combined with standard ultrasonography, can assess the degree of attenuation by fat and thereby can also estimate hepatic steatosis. Magnetic resonance–based elastography may be preferred in the presence of ascites or obesity.[7] A low stiffness score and a normal platelet count can identify patients who are at low risk for variceal bleeding.[8]

MEASUREMENT OF TRANSJUGULAR PRESSURE

Transjugular pressure measurements are indicated in patients who have atypical presentations of portal hypertension (e.g., when it is unclear whether liver disease is the cause) or occasionally to assess whether portal hypertension is severe enough to warrant prophylaxis against variceal hemorrhage (Chapter 139). A catheter is advanced under fluoroscopy into the hepatic vein, and the free hepatic venous pressure is measured. The catheter is then advanced further until it becomes "wedged" in a small hepatic vein venule. A small balloon occludes the venule, and the wedged hepatic vein pressure, which reflects hepatic sinusoidal pressure, is obtained. The portal pressure gradient, which is derived by subtracting the free pressure measurement from the wedged pressure measurement, is normally less than 5 mm Hg. Varices form at a gradient greater than 10 mm Hg, whereas ascites and variceal hemorrhage occur only when the gradient is greater than 12 mm Hg. A transjugular approach also increases the safety of liver biopsy in the presence of ascites, coagulopathy, or thrombocytopenia when standard percutaneous liver biopsy is hazardous.

LIVER BIOPSY

Although liver biopsy had been the definitive test to assess the severity of hepatic inflammation and fibrosis in diffuse hepatocellular disease, its use has diminished in large part due to the availability of transient elastography. Nevertheless, it retains an important role in the diagnosis of autoimmune hepatitis (Chapter 135), drug hepatotoxicity (Chapter 136), and small duct primary sclerosing cholangitis (Chapter 141).[9] However, because of its potential complications, such as intra-abdominal bleeding, biopsy is recommended only when less invasive testing does not yield a definitive diagnosis or prognosis or when additional information,[10] such as quantitative determination of hepatic copper in Wilson disease or hepatic iron in hemochromatosis, is necessary for definitive diagnosis (see later). Liver biopsy under radiographic guidance is also indicated if a hepatic mass cannot be characterized as benign or malignant by noninvasive means.[11]

APPROACH TO NEW-ONSET ASCITES

The three leading causes of ascites in the United States are cirrhosis (85%; Chapter 139), peritoneal malignancy (7%), and heart failure (3%; Chapter 46), with nephrotic syndrome (Chapter 107) and tuberculosis (Chapter 299) accounting for the remainder. Diagnostic paracentesis, which is the appropriate initial test, has a low complication rate, including ascitic fluid leak (in about 5% of patients with cirrhosis) and bleeding or infection (less than 2% of patients). A serum-ascites albumin gradient (defined as serum albumin concentration minus ascitic albumin concentration) level of 1.1 g/dL or greater indicates portal hypertension, with a sensitivity of 97% and specificity of 90%. If the ascitic fluid protein level is less than 2.5 g/dL, cirrhosis is the most likely cause of the portal hypertension. If the ascitic fluid protein level is more than 2.5 g/dL, heart failure is the likely cause of the portal hypertension (see Table 139-3), and the diagnosis can be confirmed by an elevated brain natriuretic protein level (Chapter 45). If the gradient is less than 1.1 g/dL and the ascitic fluid protein is low, malignancy is most likely. Malignant ascites also is usually associated with an ascitic white blood cell count greater than 500/μL. Spontaneous bacterial peritonitis (Chapter 128) is diagnosed based on an ascitic neutrophil count above 250 cells/μL or more if secondary causes of peritonitis can be excluded.

APPROACH TO A HEPATIC MASS

A hepatic mass may be discovered under a number of different circumstances and is often an incidental finding on abdominal imaging performed for another indication. The initial evaluation depends upon whether the mass is cystic or solid (Fig. 132-6).[12]

HEPATIC CYSTS

Most hepatic cysts are benign and incidental. Simple hepatic cysts are typically solitary and asymptomatic, although larger cysts may cause abdominal discomfort. Ultrasonography, which is usually diagnostic, shows an anechoic fluid-filled space, an imperceptible wall, and posterior acoustic enhancement (Fig. 132-7A and B). Worrisome features, including the presence of symptoms or increasing size, require exclusion of a cystadenoma. On ultrasound a cystadenoma is hypoechoic with irregular walls and septations. Hepatic resection is indicated because malignant transformation can occur.

Multiple hepatic cysts may suggest the presence of autosomal dominant adult polycystic disease.[13] Polycystic liver disease can occur in conjunction with polycystic kidney disease (Chapter 112) or without it. Isolated polycystic liver disease is associated with mutations in the *PRCKSCH* gene, which encodes the glucosidase 2 subunit β enzyme, and in Sec63, which is part of a large protein complex involved in protein translocation in the endoplasmic reticulum, but many other genetic mutations have also been described.[14] Adult polycystic liver disease typically is asymptomatic, although some patients note dull right upper quadrant pain, fullness, sense of a mass, and increasing abdominal girth. Rupture of a cyst, hemorrhage into a cyst, infection of a cyst, or torsion of a cyst may cause severe pain. Physical examination may include hepatomegaly, cachexia due to weight loss, and ascites. As cysts increase in number and size with age, they may become palpable. On ultrasound, multiple fluid-filled cysts are present without internal echoes unless bleeding or infection has occurred. Treatment with long-acting somatostatin analogues (e.g., lanreotide 120 mg subcutaneously every 4 weeks) can modestly reduce the volumes of liver cysts.[A2] Interventions indicated for symptoms include aspiration or resection. Polycystic liver disease usually does not result in clinical hepatic impairment, and prognosis depends on the severity of any concurrent polycystic renal disease. In some cases, however, large, symptomatic, or bleeding cysts may raise the consideration of liver transplantation,[15] often with combined kidney transplantation (Chapter 117) for associated renal cysts and kidney failure.

Caroli disease, which is a rare congenital abnormality with cystic dilation of the intrahepatic biliary tree, can be associated with cholangitis and biliary stones.[16] Many patients ultimately develop cholangiocarcinoma (Chapter 141). Magnetic resonance cholangiopancreatography demonstrates intrahepatic dilations with normal ducts in between and a normal common bile duct. Endoscopic treatment is indicated for cholangitis, although resection or liver transplantation may ultimately be required.

SOLID HEPATIC MASS

Most solid hepatic masses are asymptomatic, but some patients may have vague right upper quadrant discomfort. The abrupt onset of more severe pain suggests a complication, such as hemorrhage or rupture. The approach to a solid hepatic mass (Fig. 132-8) is influenced by the presence or absence of underlying chronic liver disease, such as chronic viral hepatitis, as well as

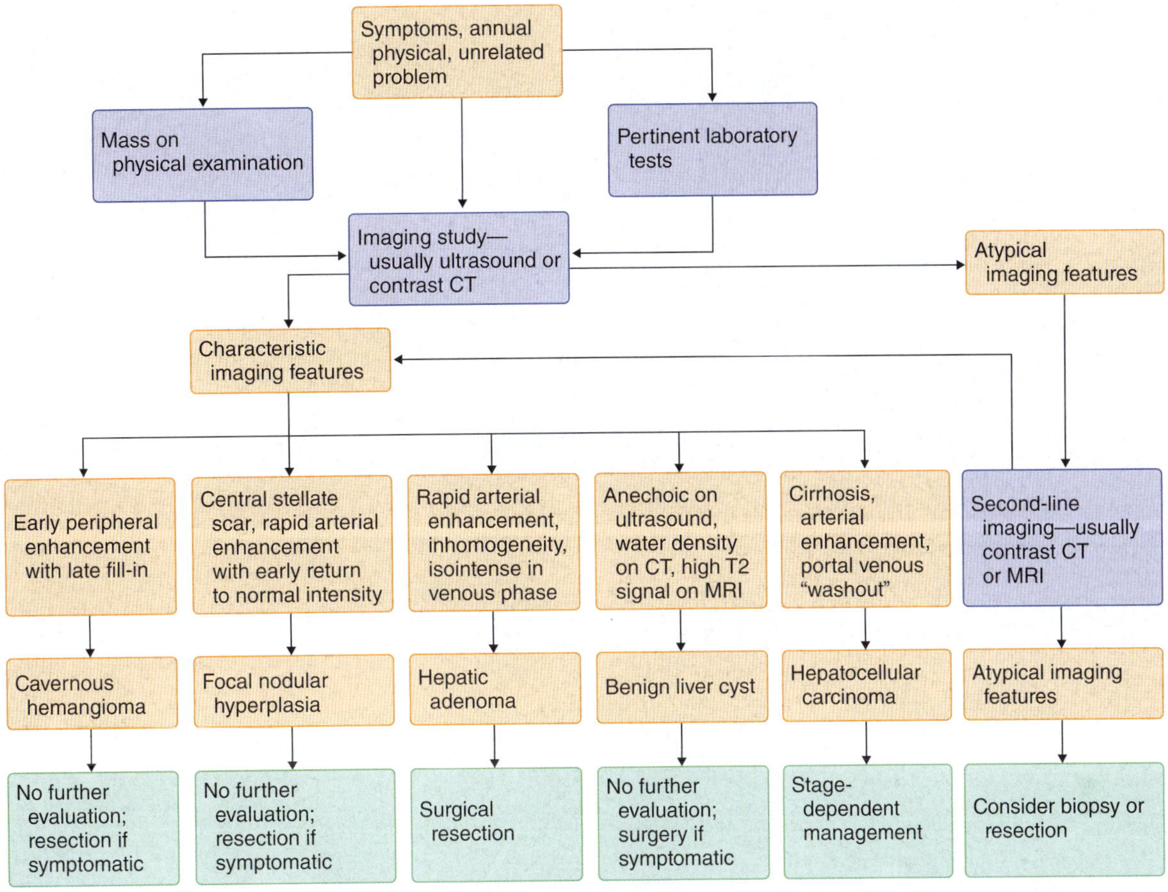

FIGURE 132-6. **Approach to evaluating the patient with a mass lesion in the liver.** This flowchart shows an algorithm for evaluating and managing common liver mass lesions. CT = computed tomography; MRI = magnetic resonance imaging. (From Roberts LR. Liver and biliary tract tumors. In: Goldman L, Schafer AI, eds. *Goldman's Cecil Medicine*, 24th ed. Philadelphia: Saunders; 2012.)

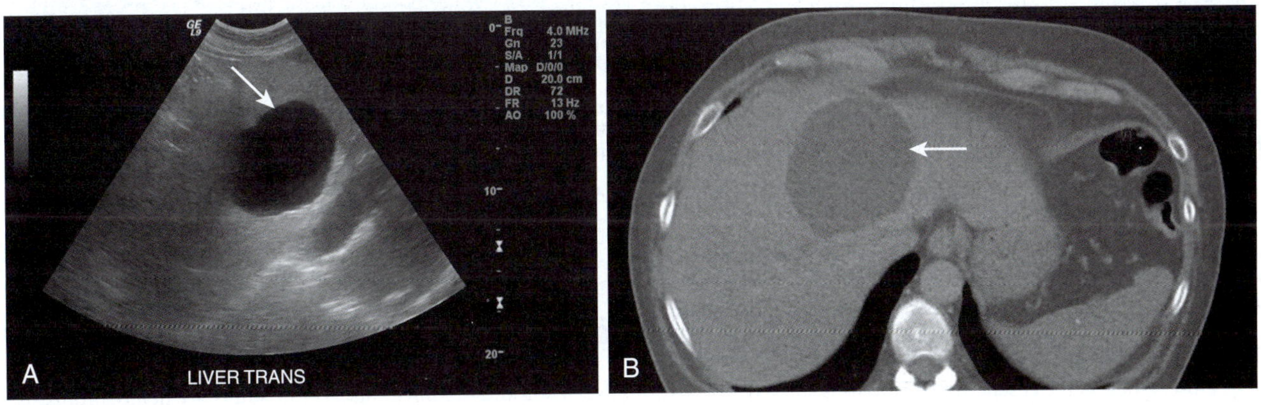

FIGURE 132-7. **Simple hepatic cyst. A,** Ultrasound demonstrates clear contents and an imperceptible wall (*arrow*). **B,** On a computed tomographic scan, a simple hepatic cyst is characterized by the lack of septation and an imperceptible wall (*arrow*). (Courtesy of Dr. B. Madrazo.)

whether an extrahepatic malignancy with hepatic metastases is a consideration. If chronic liver disease is present, a solid mass must be assumed to represent primary hepatocellular carcinoma (Chapter 181) until proven otherwise. By comparison, a solid lesion in the absence of underlying liver disease is more likely to be benign and incidental. Benign hepatic adenomas are commonly discovered in young to middle-aged women and are not associated with hepatic dysfunction. With modern contrast studies, it is usually possible to make a confident radiologic diagnosis about the nature of a solid hepatic mass. Important examples include the initial peripheral filling and retention of contrast dye by a hemangioma (see Fig. 132-8A, B, and C), the rapid arterial filling of a hepatocellular carcinoma with subsequent "washout" of contrast during the portal venous phase (see Fig. 181-4), or the central scar typical of focal nodular hyperplasia (see Fig. 132-8D). If a benign etiology cannot be adequately determined noninvasively, then biopsy may be necessary.

Hepatic hemangiomas are the most common benign solid hepatic mass. On ultrasound, the lesion is hyperechoic, with a typical hypervascular appearance on contrast-enhanced abdominal CT or MRI. Generally, no intervention is required unless there is a clear association with abdominal symptoms, increasing size, or a complication such as rupture.

Hepatic adenomas (Chapter 181) are benign epithelial hepatic tumors associated with the use of oral contraceptives with a higher estrogen content. On ultrasound, adenomas are hyperechoic, reflective of their fat content, but become anechoic if hemorrhage has occurred. Contrast CT and MRI show arterial enhancement and varying signal intensity reflecting steatosis and hemorrhage, if present. Biopsy may be needed for diagnosis. Potential complications of adenomas, especially if greater than 5 cm, include spontaneous hemorrhage and rupture. Malignant transformation is more common in men and in adenomas with a β-catenin exon 3 mutation. Such patients and patients

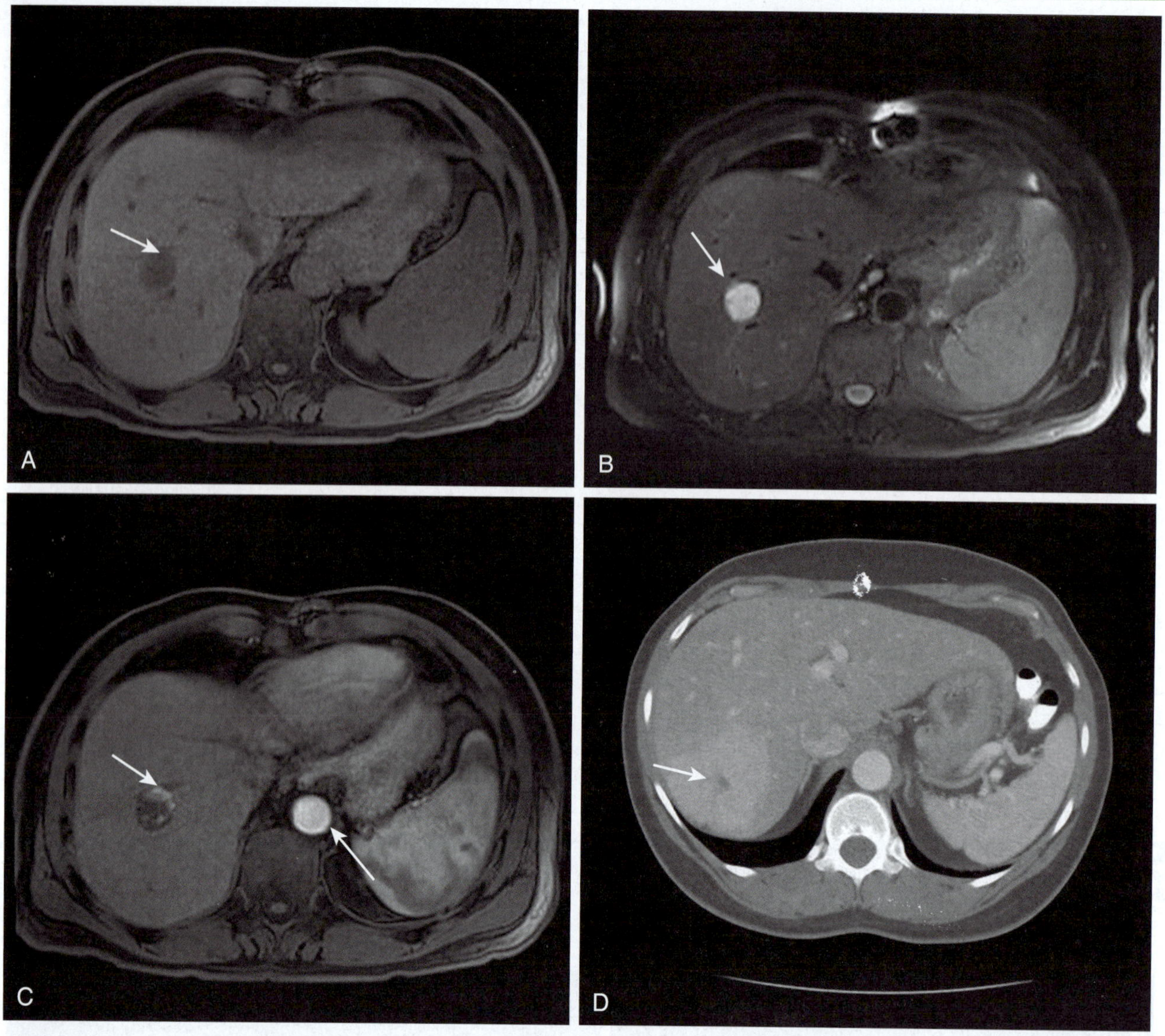

FIGURE 132-8. **Solid hepatic mass. A,** Hemangioma seen as a solid mass (*arrow*) on the T1 phase of a magnetic resonance (MR) imaging scan. **B,** Hemangioma on MR T2 image is characterized by a high signal density (*arrow*). **C,** A hemangioma fills slowly (*shorter arrow*) from the periphery after intravenous contrast is administered (*longer arrow*). **D,** Focal nodular hyperplasia is characterized by a central scar (*arrow*) in the late venous phase of a contrast computed tomographic scan. (Courtesy of Dr. B. Madrazo.)

with adenomas greater than 5 cm should undergo prophylactic hepatic resection.[17] Discontinuation of oral contraceptives may lead to a decrease in size.

Focal nodular hyperplasia, which is a benign lesion characterized by a central scar, is thought to represent a hyperplastic response due to a vascular malformation. Identification of the scar by ultrasound, CT, or MRI is diagnostic (see Fig. 132-8D). Observation in the absence of symptoms is advised.

Multiple regenerative 1- to 3-mm nodules clustered around the portal triads characterize nodular regenerative hyperplasia. It is associated with a variety of systemic disorders, predominantly autoimmune, including rheumatoid arthritis, systemic lupus erythematosus, and polymyalgia rheumatica; neoplastic such as myeloproliferative syndromes; and medications, including thiopurines. Symptoms, if present, reflect associated portal hypertension. Diagnosis is by biopsy, which shows hypertrophied hepatocytes clustered around the center of the nodules with peripheral atrophy. Management is directed to the associated portal hypertension (Chapter 139).

Hepatocellular carcinoma (Chapter 181) is a frequent complication of cirrhosis of any cause as well as chronic hepatitis B infection even in the absence of cirrhosis. Patients usually will have evidence of cirrhosis with hepatic dysfunction. Because surveillance for hepatocellular carcinoma is now recommended in individuals at risk, this tumor is increasingly identified when asymptomatic and potentially curable. On ultrasound, hepatocellular carcinoma appears solid. Owing to its predominantly arterial blood supply compared with that of normal hepatic parenchyma, intravenous contrast is rapidly taken up by a hepatic cellular carcinoma and then "washes out" on CT scan or MR imaging (see Fig. 181-4). Serum α-fetoprotein is elevated in approximately 60% of cases. Therapeutic options depend on the tumor's size and severity of associated liver disease.

APPROACH TO THE PATIENT WITH INHERITED LIVER DISEASE

The major inherited liver diseases in adults are hemochromatosis, Wilson disease, cystic fibrosis, and α_1-antitrypsin deficiency. These disorders may be suspected by their extrahepatic manifestations or may be detected during evaluation of unexplained hepatic dysfunction.

Hereditary hemochromatosis (Chapter 196), which is the most common inherited liver disorder, is most frequently due to mutations in the *HFE* gene (located on chromosome 6p22.2), typically at C282Y and H63D. Approximately 1 in 250 individuals of Northern European descent are homozygous for C282Y, the major *HFE* mutation, although only a minority develop phenotypic manifestations.[18] Liver blood test abnormalities, if present, are nonspecific. Definitive diagnosis is confirmed by detection of C282Y homozygote or compound heterozygote (C282Y/H63D). MRI or CT scan can confirm excessive hepatic iron. Liver biopsy is unnecessary for diagnosis but is advised for a serum ferritin greater than 1000 µg/L because the patient is likely to be cirrhotic. Iron accumulates in hepatocytes, but not in Kupffer cells, in a periportal to pericentral gradient (Fig. 132-9). By comparison, secondary iron overload accumulates in Kupffer cells in conditions such as ineffective erythropoiesis. Quantitative iron measurement in liver tissue, calculated as the µmol of iron/g dry weight liver/age, can confirm the diagnosis. Treatment of hemochromatosis is by phlebotomy (Chapter 196).

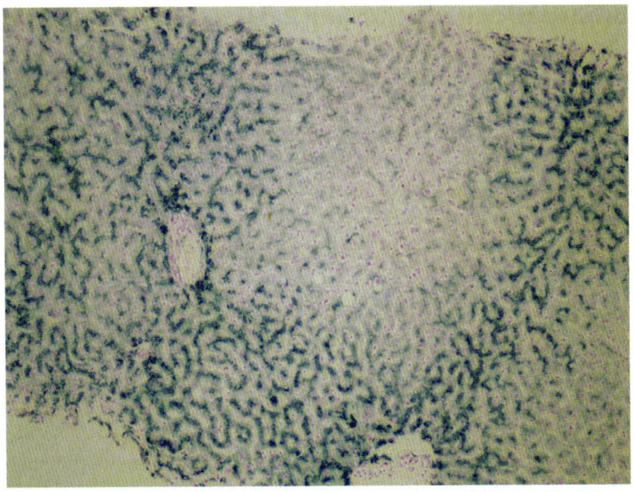

FIGURE 132-9. **Liver biopsy in hemochromatosis (Prussian blue stain for iron).** Iron deposition is found in a periportal distribution, predominantly in parenchymal cells (hepatocytes). (From Bacon BR. Inherited and metabolic disorders of the liver. In: Goldman L, Schafer AI, eds. *Goldman's Cecil Medicine*, 24th ed. Philadelphia: Saunders; 2012.)

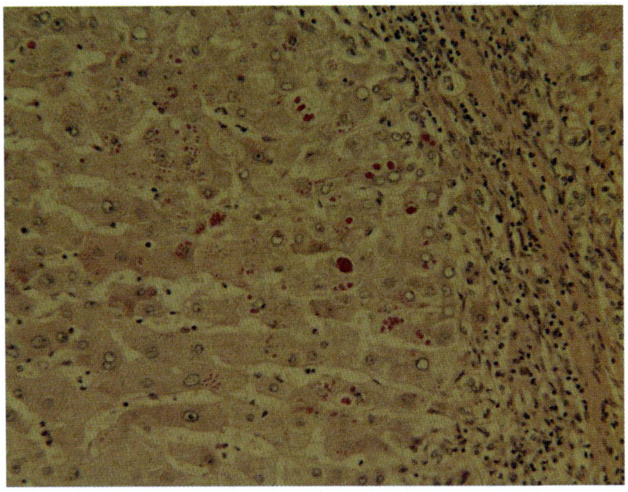

FIGURE 132-10. **Liver biopsy in α_1-antitrypsin deficiency.** On a periodic acid–Schiff, diastase-resistant stain, α_1-antitrypsin globules, with a characteristic magenta color, are found at the periphery of the lobule. (From Bacon BR. Inherited and metabolic disorders of the liver. In: Goldman L, Schafer AI, eds. *Goldman's Cecil Medicine*, 24th ed. Philadelphia: Saunders; 2012.)

α_1-Antitrypsin deficiency, which results from inherited mutations in this serine protease inhibitor, prevents its export from hepatocytes, where its accumulation causes liver inflammation, fibrosis, and cirrhosis.[19] Deficiency of circulating α_1-antitrypsin results in panlobular emphysema (Chapter 76) even in nonsmokers. The disease is most frequent in persons of European ancestry. Inheritance is autosomal recessive with codominant inheritance because each allele provides 50% of circulating α_1-antitrypsin. A large number of alleles have been identified in the proteinase inhibitor (Pi) gene, with MM associated with normal circulating α_1-antitrypsin levels and the most common abnormal alleles, S and Z, associated with reduced levels. PiZZ homozygotes, who have the most severe α_1-antitrypsin deficiency, have only 15% of normal circulating levels and are prone to liver and lung disease. Liver disease has a bimodal distribution, with neonatal hepatitis and cholestatic jaundice manifesting in early life and cirrhosis in adulthood. Only approximately one third of adults with the PiZZ phenotype develop cirrhosis, thereby implying that other cofactors are involved in disease progression. For example, Pi*Z heterozygosity, found in 2.4% of Whites, increases the risk of cirrhosis secondary to either alcoholic or nonalcoholic fatty liver disease (Chapter 139) by about six-fold.[20] Other phenotypes with α_1-antitrypsin deficiency (e.g., PiMZ or PiSZ) increase the risk for liver disease, whereas null variants have lung but not liver disease. The condition may be suspected as the result of a low α_1-1 globulin level on protein electrophoresis, and the diagnosis can be confirmed by demonstration of a low serum α_1-antitrypsin level followed by Pi testing to determine the phenotype. Liver function test abnormalities are generally nonspecific, although the albumin level can be low and the INR prolonged if cirrhosis is present. Liver biopsy, which shows the extent of fibrosis, is characterized by periodic acid–Schiff (PAS)-positive, diastase-resistant globules in the periphery of the lobule (Fig. 132-10). Weekly intravenous α_1-antitrypsin protein concentrate infusions, which are approved by the U.S. Food and Drug Administration, might prevent progression of lung disease by restoring serum and alveolar α_1-antitrypsin levels. Fazirsiran, which is an RNA interference therapeutic, is an experimental approach to improving liver enzyme abnormalities.[21]

Wilson disease (Chapter 195) is excessive copper accumulation in liver and extrahepatic tissues owing to an inherited disorder in copper transport from hepatocytes to bile. Hepatic manifestations include chronic hepatitis and cirrhosis, most typically appearing by the fourth decade of life, although they can manifest later. A characteristic finding in a fulminant manifestation of Wilson disease is hemolysis with an abnormally low alkaline phosphatase level, jaundice, and coagulopathy. More typically, patients have elevated aminotransferase levels without hemolysis at presentation. Diagnosis usually is based on an elevated 24-hour urinary copper level and low serum ceruloplasmin levels, but in unclear cases the quantification of increased hepatic copper content by biopsy is definitive.[22] Copper chelation prevents disease progression.

Cystic fibrosis (Chapter 77) is usually dominated by pulmonary complications, but liver disease is an important cause of morbidity and mortality in adults.[23] In patients with elevated alkaline phosphatase and bilirubin levels, biliary cirrhosis (Chapter 141) can develop owing to abnormal bile viscosity. Whether new therapies for cystic fibrosis lung disease will improve liver disease is unknown. Ursodeoxycholic acid may improve biochemical test results but has no clear benefit on outcome. Liver transplantation (Chapter 140) may be necessary for decompensated cirrhosis.

GENERAL REFERENCES

For the General References and other additional features, please visit Elsevier eBooks+ at https://ebooks.health.elsevier.com.

Grade A References

A1. Huelsen A, Fischer J, Hegarty J, et al. The scratch test for identifying the lower liver edge is at least as accurate as percussion and is significantly more effective for young trainees-a randomised comparative trial. *N Z Med J*. 2016;129:53-63.

A2. Griffiths J, Mills MT, Ong AC. Long-acting somatostatin analogue treatments in autosomal dominant polycystic kidney disease and polycystic liver disease: a systematic review and meta-analysis. *BMJ Open*. 2020;10:e032620.

133 APPROACH TO THE PATIENT WITH JAUNDICE OR ABNORMAL LIVER TESTS

KEVIN M. KORENBLAT

JAUNDICE AND HYPERBILIRUBINEMIA

DEFINITION

Jaundice, from the French *jaune* ("yellow"), is the yellow-orange discoloration of the skin, conjunctivae, and mucous membranes that results from an elevated plasma bilirubin level. Mild hyperbilirubinemia may be clinically undetectable, but jaundice becomes evident at plasma bilirubin greater than 3 to 4 mg/dL, depending on the patient's skin pigmentation, the conditions of observation, and the bilirubin fraction that is elevated. Hyperbilirubinemia may result from increased bilirubin production or inherited or acquired defects in the metabolism of hepatic bilirubin.

PATHOBIOLOGY

Bilirubin Metabolism

Bilirubin Production

Bilirubin is the degradation product of the heme moiety of hemoproteins, a class of proteins involved in the transport or metabolism of oxygen (E-Fig. 133-1). Normal adults produce approximately 4 mg of bilirubin per kilogram of body weight per day. Between 70 and 90% of bilirubin is derived from the hemoglobin in erythrocytes, which are sequestered and destroyed by the mononuclear phagocytic cells of the reticuloendothelial system, principally in the spleen, liver, and bone marrow. The remainder is from the turnover of nonhemoglobin hemoproteins, such as myoglobin, the P-450 cytochromes, catalase, and peroxidase, principally in the liver. Ineffective erythropoiesis, which is the premature destruction of newly formed erythrocytes in the bone marrow, contributes a minor fraction. Bilirubin is more than just a byproduct of a degradatory pathway; it has antioxidant and immune modulating properties, and it is a ligand for cellular receptors.[1]

The two-step conversion of heme to bilirubin begins with the opening of the heme molecule at its α bridge carbon by the microsomal enzyme *heme oxygenase*, a process that results in the formation of equimolar quantities of carbon monoxide and the green tetrapyrrole biliverdin. This nontoxic, water-soluble pigment is the main excretory product of heme in birds, reptiles, and amphibians. However, biliverdin cannot cross the placenta. Accordingly, its reduction to bilirubin in mammals by a second enzyme, *biliverdin reductase*, allows its transplacental removal from the fetus into the maternal circulation, from which it can be excreted by the maternal liver. The unconjugated bilirubin produced in the periphery is transported in plasma to the liver. Because of its insolubility in aqueous media, it is kept in solution by tight but reversible binding to albumin. A number of compounds, including salicylates, sulfonamides, furosemide, and radiographic contrast agents, can competitively displace bilirubin from its binding sites on albumin, a phenomenon that is of little clinical significance except in neonates, in whom the resulting increased concentration of unbound bilirubin raises the risk for kernicterus.

Disposition of Bilirubin by the Liver

Excretion of bilirubin from the body is a major function of the liver (see E-Fig. 133-1), where the specialized microanatomy enhances the extraction of protein-bound compounds from the circulation. Hepatic translocation of bilirubin from blood to bile involves four distinct steps: (1) uptake of unconjugated bilirubin, principally by facilitated transport and, to a lesser extent, diffusion; (2) intracellular binding, mainly to various cytosolic proteins of the glutathione-*S*-transferase family; (3) conversion in the endoplasmic reticulum of unconjugated bilirubin to bilirubin monoglucuronides and diglucuronides by a specific uridine 5′-diphospho-glucuronosyltransferase (UDP-glucuronosyltransferase) isoform designated UGT1A1, encoded by the *UGT1* gene complex; and (4) transfer of bilirubin monoglucuronides and diglucuronides into bile by a canalicular membrane adenosine triphosphate (ATP)–dependent transporter designated multidrug resistance–associated protein 2 (MRP2) and also known as canalicular multispecific organic anion transporter (cMOAT) or ATP-binding cassette sub-family C member 2 (ABCC2). MRP2 is encoded by the gene *ABCC2*, a member of the ATP-binding cassette (ABC) transporter superfamily of genes. Conjugated bilirubin is secreted also across the hepatocyte sinusoidal membrane by multidrug resistance–associated protein 3 (MRP3), particularly when the transport capacity of MRP2 is exceeded. MRP2 and MRP3 share a 48% amino acid identity.

Conjugation of unconjugated bilirubin to bilirubin monoglucuronides and diglucuronides is a critical process that greatly increases the aqueous solubility of bilirubin, thereby enhancing its elimination from the body while simultaneously reducing its ability to diffuse across biologic membranes, including the blood-brain barrier. In newborn infants, a decreased capacity to conjugate bilirubin leads to unconjugated hyperbilirubinemia (physiologic jaundice of the newborn). If severe, this hyperbilirubinemia may then lead to kernicterus. Phototherapy by exposure to light in the blue spectrum (390 to 470 nm) converts bilirubin to water-soluble photoisomers that are readily excreted in bile, thereby protecting the central nervous system from bilirubin toxicity. Gilbert syndrome and Crigler-Najjar syndrome types 1 and 2, which result from genetic defects in bilirubin conjugation, are characterized by unconjugated hyperbilirubinemia; by contrast, Dubin-Johnson syndrome, which results from inheritable defects in MRP2, is characterized by conjugated or mixed hyperbilirubinemia. Loss of function of the membrane organic ion transport proteins OATP1B1 and OATP1B3 causes Rotor syndrome, also a conjugated or mixed hyperbilirubinemia.

Enterohepatic Circulation and Excretion of Bilirubin

Normal human bile contains an average of less than 5% unconjugated bilirubin, 7% bilirubin monoconjugates, and 90% bilirubin diconjugates. Following canalicular secretion, conjugated bilirubin passes down the gastrointestinal tract without reabsorption by either the gallbladder or intestinal mucosa. Although some bilirubin reaches the feces, most is converted to urobilinogen and to related compounds by bacteria within the ileum and colon. Urobilinogen is reabsorbed and returns to the liver through the portal circulation, where it is re-excreted into bile. This process of enterohepatic recirculation occurs with urobilinogen, bile salts, and some medications. Any urobilinogen not taken up by the liver reaches the systemic circulation, from which it is cleared by the kidneys. Normal urine urobilinogen excretion is 4 mg/day or less. Hemolysis increases the load of bilirubin entering the gut and therefore the amount of urobilinogen formed and reabsorbed. Liver disease decreases hepatic extraction of bilirubin; as a result, plasma urobilinogen levels rise and more urobilinogen is excreted in the urine. Cholestasis, bile duct obstruction, or antibiotics that reduce or eliminate the bacterial conversion of bilirubin to urobilinogen decrease the formation and urinary excretion of urobilinogen.

Unconjugated bilirubin ordinarily does not reach the gut except in neonates or, by ill-defined alternative pathways, in the presence of severe unconjugated hyperbilirubinemia (e.g., Crigler-Najjar type 1). In these circumstances, unconjugated bilirubin is reabsorbed from the gut, thereby amplifying the hyperbilirubinemia.

Measurement of Bilirubin in Plasma

The total plasma bilirubin concentration in normal adults is less than 1 to 1.5 mg/dL. Modern analytic techniques show that normal plasma contains principally unconjugated bilirubin, with only a trace of conjugated bilirubin. Clinical laboratories quantify plasma bilirubin by a reaction in which bilirubin is cleaved by a diazo reagent under acidic conditions to form azobilirubin that is quantitated spectrophotometrically. Bilirubin conjugates react rapidly ("prompt" or "direct"-reacting bilirubin). Unconjugated bilirubin reacts slowly because the site of attack by the diazo reagent is protected by internal hydrogen bonding. Measurement of the total plasma bilirubin concentration requires addition of an agent, such as a detergent, to solubilize the unconjugated bilirubin.

The "indirect"-reacting bilirubin is calculated by subtracting the direct-reacting bilirubin from the total. Although physicians traditionally equate the direct-reacting fraction of bilirubin in plasma with conjugated bilirubin and the indirect fraction with unconjugated bilirubin, this approach is, at best, an approximation. The unqualified interpretation of direct and indirect fractions as reflecting conjugated and unconjugated bilirubin, respectively, may lead to diagnostic errors, particularly in the diagnosis of hereditary hyperbilirubinemias. In common practice, 10 to 20% of the bilirubin in normal plasma gives a prompt (direct) diazo reaction even though more than 95% of total bilirubin in normal plasma is unconjugated. Thus, at virtually any total bilirubin concentration, a direct-reacting fraction of less than 15% of the total bilirubin can be considered as essentially all unconjugated.

When the direct-reacting fraction is greater than 15%, a simple dipstick test for bilirubinuria may clarify the situation. Unconjugated bilirubin is not excreted in urine regardless of the height of its plasma concentration because its binding to albumin is too tight for effective glomerular filtration and it is not secreted by the tubules. In comparison, conjugated bilirubin in the blood under conditions of parenchymal liver disease or bile duct obstruction is loosely bound to albumin and readily filtered at the level of the glomerulus. Even modest degrees of conjugated hyperbilirubinemia result in bilirubinuria, which is *always* a pathologic finding. With prolonged conjugated hyperbilirubinemia, some of the conjugated bilirubin binds *covalently* to albumin and produces what is designated the delta (δ)-bilirubin fraction. Although δ-bilirubin gives a direct diazo reaction, it is not filterable by the glomerulus and does not appear in the urine; it disappears slowly from the plasma, with the 14- to 21-day half-life of the albumin to which it is bound. δ-Bilirubin can account for the slow rate at which a mixed or predominantly conjugated (direct) hyperbilirubinemia resolves as hepatitis improves or biliary obstruction is relieved. Although δ-bilirubin is not easily measured, its presence can be inferred when an elevated direct-reacting bilirubin persists after bilirubinuria resolves.

Transcutaneous bilirubinometry is an alternative method for measuring bilirubin in infants with neonatal jaundice. The method is based on the measurement of the light reflected from the percutaneous transmission of visible light and can be used to screen newborns.

Bilirubin Kinetics

The plasma unconjugated bilirubin concentration ([UCB]) is determined by a balance between the bilirubin production rate (BRP) and hepatic bilirubin clearance (C_{BR}) according to the relationship:

$$[UCB] \approx BRP/C_{BR}$$

C_{BR} is analogous to the creatinine clearance test of kidney function; it is a measure of the rate at which bilirubin is extracted from plasma, and it is a true quantitative test of liver function. This equation indicates that [UCB] is directly proportional with increases in BRP and inversely proportional with C_{BR}, thereby providing a basis for classifying unconjugated hyperbilirubinemias according to their pathogenesis.

Increased Bilirubin Production

An increased production of bilirubin can be caused by hemolysis, an accelerated destruction of transfused erythrocytes, resorption of hematomas, or ineffective erythropoiesis owing to lead poisoning, megaloblastic anemia related to deficiency of either folic acid or vitamin B_{12}, sideroblastic anemia, congenital erythropoietic porphyria, or myeloproliferative or myelodysplastic diseases. In these settings, other liver tests are typically normal and the hyperbilirubinemia is modest, rarely exceeding 4 mg/dL; higher values imply concomitant hepatic dysfunction. However, after brisk blood transfusion or resorption of massive hematomas caused by trauma, the increased bilirubin load may be transiently sufficient to lead to observable jaundice. The causes of hemolysis are numerous (Chapters 146 and 147). Besides specific blood disorders, mild hemolysis accompanies many acquired diseases. In the setting of systemic disease, which may include a degree of hepatic dysfunction, hemolysis may produce a component of conjugated hyperbilirubinemia in addition to an elevated unconjugated bilirubin concentration. Prolonged hemolysis may lead to the formation of pigmented gallstones that contain calcium salts of bilirubin.

Decreased Hepatic Bilirubin Clearance

Decreased Bilirubin Uptake

Bilirubin uptake by hepatocytes involves both facilitated transport and passive diffusion. Decreased bilirubin uptake is believed to explain the initial increase in unconjugated bilirubin associated with rifampin use.

Impaired Bilirubin Conjugation

The most frequent cause of decreased bilirubin clearance is a decrease in bilirubin conjugating activity. Bilirubin conjugation with glucuronic acid is catalyzed principally by a UDP-glucuronosyltransferase, which is designated UGT1A1 and encoded by the *UGT1* gene complex. The *UGT1A1* gene is assembled by alternative splicing of a bilirubin-specific variant of exon 1, designated exon A_1, with four common exons (exons 2 to 5) that encode the shared carboxyl terminal end of all *UGT1*-encoded proteins. Its promoter region normally contains an $A(TA)_6TAA$ TATA box–like construct.

APPROACH TO THE PATIENT WITH HYPERBILIRUBINEMIA

Hyperbilirubinemia and jaundice may result from isolated disorders of bilirubin metabolism, liver disease, or obstruction of the biliary tract. Jaundice represents the most visible sign of hepatobiliary disease of many causes (Table 133-1).

GENETIC DISORDERS OF BILIRUBIN CONJUGATION

The hereditary hyperbilirubinemias (Table 133-2) are a group of five syndromes in which hyperbilirubinemia occurs as an isolated biochemical abnormality, without evidence of liver disease.

CRIGLER-NAJJAR AND GILBERT SYNDROMES

Crigler-Najjar syndrome types 1 and 2 and Gilbert syndrome are hereditary forms of unconjugated hyperbilirubinemia that have been known for more than two decades to result principally from mutations in *UGT1A1*. In Crigler-Najjar type 1, essentially no functional enzyme activity is present; in Crigler-Najjar type 2, enzymatic activity can be as much as 10% of normal; and in Gilbert syndrome, the enzymatic activity is 10 to 33% of normal levels. The resulting bilirubin concentrations are 18 to 45, 6 to 25, and 1.5 to 4 mg/dL, respectively (Table 133-2). Because total UGT1A1 enzymatic activity must be less than 50% of normal to produce unconjugated hyperbilirubinemia, phenotypic expression of mutations in this enzyme requires either homozygosity or double heterozygosity, and each of these disorders is inherited in an autosomal recessive pattern. Individuals of Black or White ancestry with Gilbert syndrome are typically homozygous for an $A(TA)_7TAA$ promoter mutation; this polymorphism is designated *UGT1A1*28*. Structural mutations in exon 1 of *UGT1A1* causing modest reductions in enzymatic activity have been reported in some Japanese patients with Gilbert syndrome. To date, at least 130 different mutations in *UGT1A1* associated with hereditary hyperbilirubinemia have been identified, including ones linked to Crigler-Najjar type 1 and type 2. Other studies in patients with unconjugated hyperbilirubinemia have also identified mutations and polymorphism in multiple additional regions of *UGT1A*, including its promoter region, in the solute carrier protein SCLO1B1, and in the enzymes heme oxygenase and biliverdin reductase A that influence serum bilirubin concentrations.

Crigler-Najjar Syndrome Type 1

Crigler-Najjar type 1 is characterized by a striking unconjugated hyperbilirubinemia that appears in the neonatal period, persists for life, and is unresponsive to phenobarbital.[2] Most patients (type 1A) exhibit defects in the glucuronide conjugation of a spectrum of substrates in addition to bilirubin as the result of homozygous or compound heterozygous mutations in one of the common exons (2 to 5) of the *UGT1* complex. In a smaller subset (type 1B), a mutation in the bilirubin-specific exon A1 limits the defect to bilirubin conjugation. Fifty-nine structurally diverse *UGT1A1* mutations can cause Crigler-Najjar type 1; their common feature is that they all encode proteins with absent or, at most, traces of enzymatic activity.

Before the availability of phototherapy, most patients with Crigler-Najjar type 1 died of bilirubin encephalopathy (kernicterus) in infancy or early childhood. Optimal treatment for a neurologically intact patient includes approximately 12 hours/day of phototherapy from birth throughout childhood, perhaps supplemented by exchange transfusion in the neonatal period; use of oral calcium phosphates to bind bilirubin isomers generated by phototherapy and, thereby, disrupt enterohepatic circulation; and early liver transplantation, before the onset of brain damage. Plasmapheresis can temporarily control abrupt increases in bilirubin.

Crigler-Najjar Syndrome Type 2

Bilirubin concentrations are typically lower in Crigler-Najjar type 2, and plasma bilirubin levels can be reduced to 3 to 5 mg/dL by phenobarbital. At least 48 different mutations of *UGT1A1* have been associated with Crigler-Najjar type 2; all encode a bilirubin-UDP-glucuronosyltransferase with markedly reduced but detectable enzymatic activity. Although much less common in Crigler-Najjar type 2, kernicterus has occurred at all ages, typically associated with factors that temporarily raise the plasma bilirubin concentration above baseline (e.g., fasting, intercurrent illness). For this reason, phenobarbital therapy is often recommended; a single bedtime dose usually maintains clinically safe plasma bilirubin concentrations.

Gilbert Syndrome

Gilbert syndrome is the most common form of the hereditary hyperbilirubinemias.[3] The most common polymorphism is the homozygous $A(TA)_7TAA$ promoter polymorphism designated as the UGT1A1*28 allele. Approximate allelic frequencies are 42%, 30%, and 10% in Black, White, and Asian populations, respectively. In Asian populations, polymorphisms in coding regions are more common than the *28 allele. The high prevalence of Gilbert syndrome often explains the frequency of mild unconjugated hyperbilirubinemia in liver transplant recipients and why population-level studies of bilirubin levels tend to skew toward higher levels. Plasma bilirubin concentrations are most often less than 3 mg/dL, although both higher and lower values are frequent, with increases of two-fold to three-fold commonly occurring with fasting and intercurrent illness. The phenotypic distinction between mild Gilbert syndrome and a normal state is often blurred. Phenobarbital's ability to induce hepatic enzyme activity normalizes both the bilirubin concentration and C_{BR}. Oxidative drug metabolism and the disposition of many, but not all, xenobiotics that are metabolized by glucuronidation appear to be normal in Gilbert syndrome. A critical exception is the antitumor agent irinotecan (CPT-11), whose active metabolite (SN-38) is glucuronidated specifically by UGT1A1. In patients with Gilbert syndrome, irinotecan can cause intractable diarrhea, myelosuppression, and other serious toxicities. The estrogen modulator raloxifene is also a substrate for UGT1A1, and the presence of the homozygous *28 allele results in a two-fold higher exposure to the medication and a greater increase

TABLE 133-1 DIFFERENTIAL DIAGNOSIS OF HYPERBILIRUBINEMIA AND JAUNDICE

DISORDERS OF BILIRUBIN METABOLISM WITHOUT LIVER DISEASE

- Unconjugated Hyperbilirubinemia
  - Increased bilirubin production
    - *Examples:* Hemolysis, ineffective erythropoiesis, blood transfusion, resorption of hematomas
  - Decreased hepatocellular uptake
    - *Examples:* Drugs (e.g., rifampin)
  - Decreased conjugation
    - *Examples:* Gilbert and Crigler-Najjar syndromes, physiologic jaundice of the newborn, breast milk jaundice, HIV protease inhibitors
- Conjugated or Mixed Hyperbilirubinemia
  - Decreased canalicular transport: Dubin-Johnson syndrome
  - Decreased reuptake of bilirubin conjugates: Rotor syndrome

LIVER DISEASE

- Acute or Chronic Hepatocellular Dysfunction
  - Acute or subacute hepatocellular injury
    - *Examples:* Viral hepatitis A, B, C, E; hepatotoxins (e.g., ethanol, acetaminophen, mushroom [*Amanita phalloides*] poisoning); drugs (e.g., isoniazid, diclofenac); metabolic diseases (e.g., Wilson disease, Reye syndrome); pregnancy-related (e.g., acute fatty liver of pregnancy, HELLP); hepatic ischemia (e.g., shock)
  - Chronic hepatocellular disease
    - *Examples:* Hepatitis B, B and D, C, and E; hepatotoxins (e.g., organic solvents, vitamin A); nonalcoholic and alcoholic fatty liver disease; autoimmune hepatitis; metabolic disease (Wilson disease, hemochromatosis, α_1-antitrypsin deficiency)
- Hepatic Disorders with Cholestasis
  - Familial cholestatic disorders
    - Single gene disorders
      - *Examples:* Benign recurrent intrahepatic cholestasis; progressive familial intrahepatic cholestasis; Navajo neurohepatopathy syndrome; North American Indian cholestasis
  - Diffuse infiltrative disorders
    - Familial cholestatic disorders of unknown pathogenesis
      - *Examples:* Aagenaes syndrome
    - *Examples:* Granulomatous diseases (e.g., bacterial, mycobacterial, fungal, rickettsial, and trepenomal infections, sarcoidosis, lymphoma), medications (e.g., phenytoin, carbamazepine), amyloidosis, infiltrative malignancies, extramedullary hematopoiesis
  - Inflammation of intrahepatic bile ductules and/or portal tracts
    - *Examples:* Primary biliary cholangitis, liver allograft rejection, graft-versus-host disease
  - Miscellaneous conditions
    - *Examples:* Uncommon presentations of viral or alcoholic hepatitis, intrahepatic cholestasis of pregnancy, contraceptive jaundice, estrogens, anabolic steroids, postoperative cholestasis, cholestasis of sepsis, total parenteral nutrition, drug-induced liver injury (amoxicillin-clavulanate)

BILE DUCT OBSTRUCTION

- Choledocholithiasis
- Diseases of the Bile Ducts
  - Inflammation, infection
    - *Examples:* Primary sclerosing cholangitis, AIDS cholangiopathy, hepatic artery thrombosis, hepatic arterial infusion pump chemotherapy, postsurgical biliary strictures
  - Neoplasms (e.g., cholangiocarcinoma)
- Extrinsic Compression of the Biliary Tree
  - Neoplasms
    - *Examples:* Pancreatic carcinoma, metastatic lymphadenopathy, hepatoma
  - Pancreatitis with or without pseudocyst formation
  - Vascular enlargement (e.g., aneurysm, cavernous transformation of portal vein)

AIDS = acquired immunodeficiency syndrome; HELLP = hemolysis, elevated liver enzymes, and low platelets; HIV = human immunodeficiency syndrome.

in bone density. Although Gilbert syndrome has no association with disease, occasional reports have suggested an association of the UGT1A1*28 allele with a decreased risk for cardiovascular and inflammatory diseases, an association that has been attributed to the vasodilatory and antioxidant effects of bilirubin and heme oxygenase.[4]

UNCONJUGATED HYPERBILIRUBIN IN THE NEWBORN PERIOD

Most neonates develop mild, physiologic jaundice from unconjugated hyperbilirubinemia between days 2 and 5 after birth because of hepatic immaturity and low UGT1A1 levels. Neonates can also experience early and late-onset jaundice from breast milk from two processes. Early onset jaundice occurs within 1 to 3 days of life and is attributed to the reduced calorie intake associated with breastfeeding. Late-onset jaundice occurs within 4 to 5 days of birth and can arise from the inhibition of bilirubin conjugation by the progestational steroid $3\alpha,20\beta$-pregnanediol and certain fatty acids present in breast milk. Peak bilirubin levels are typically less than 5 to 10 mg/dL, and levels return to normal within 2 weeks as mechanisms fostering bilirubin disposition mature. Prematurity, with or without hemolysis, is associated with higher bilirubin levels that may require phototherapy.

CONJUGATED OR MIXED HYPERBILIRUBINEMIA

Two phenotypically similar but mechanistically distinct inherited disorders, Dubin-Johnson syndrome and Rotor syndrome, are characterized by conjugated or mixed hyperbilirubinemia with normal values for other standard liver tests (see Table 133-2). Dubin-Johnson syndrome results from any of several mutations in the *ABCC2* gene that encodes MRP2, and Rotor syndrome is associated with mutations in *SLCO1B1* and *SLCO1B3*. Serum bilirubin levels tend to be modestly elevated (2 to 5 mg/dL), and aminotransferase levels tend to be normal.

In both Dubin-Johnson and Rotor syndromes, liver function is normal. The syndromes can be distinguished from other conditions and from one another by analysis of urine porphyrin excretion. In Dubin-Johnson syndrome, total urine coproporphyrin levels are normal, but coproporphyrin I constitutes 80% of the total; typically coproporphyrin III is 75% of the total.[5] In Rotor syndrome, total coproporphyrin levels are elevated two- to five-fold.

LIVER AND BILIARY TRACT DISEASE

Jaundice is a common sign of generalized hepatobiliary dysfunction, both acute and chronic. Icteric hepatobiliary disease is readily distinguished from the isolated disorders of bilirubin metabolism because the increase in plasma bilirubin concentration occurs in association with other markers of hepatobiliary disease (Fig. 133-1).

Liver diseases can be categorized as those in which the primary injury results from inflammation and hepatocellular necrosis, inhibition of bile flow (cholestasis), or a combination of the two. The cholestatic disorders can be further subdivided into those resulting from mechanical obstruction of the bile duct flow and those from intrahepatic cholestasis, from a multitude of conditions that include several familial cholestatic syndromes; infiltrative disorders, inflammatory or neoplastic conditions; and drug-induced liver injury (see Table 133-1).

TABLE 133-2 PRINCIPAL FEATURES OF THE HEREDITARY DISORDERS OF BILIRUBIN METABOLISM

FEATURE	CRIGLER-NAJJAR SYNDROME TYPE 1	CRIGLER-NAJJAR SYNDROME TYPE 2	GILBERT SYNDROME	DUBIN-JOHNSON SYNDROME	ROTOR SYNDROME
Incidence	Very rare	Rare	Up to 12% of population	Rare	Rare
Total serum bilirubin (mg/dL)	18-45 (usually >20), unconjugated	6-25 (usually ≤20), unconjugated	Typically ≤4 in absence of fasting or overt hemolysis; mostly unconjugated	Typically 2-5, less often ≤25; approximately 60% direct reacting	Usually 3-7, occasionally ≤20; approximately 60% direct reacting
Defect(s) in bilirubin metabolism*	Bilirubin UGT1A1 conjugating activity markedly reduced: trace to absent	Bilirubin UGT1A1 conjugating activity reduced: ≤10% of normal	Complex haplotype Bilirubin UGT1A1 conjugating activity typically reduced to 10-33% of normal; reduced bilirubin uptake in some cases; mild hemolysis in up to 50% of patients	Impaired canalicular secretion of conjugated bilirubin owing to MRP2 mutation	Impaired hepatic secretion or storage of conjugated bilirubin owing to impaired reuptake of bilirubin conjugates resulting from simultaneous OATP1B1 and OATP1B3 mutations
Routine liver tests	Normal	Normal	Normal	Normal	Normal
Serum bile acids	Normal	Normal	Normal	Usually normal	Normal
Pharmacologic responses/ special features	No response to phenobarbital	Phenobarbital reduces bilirubin by ≤75%	Phenobarbital reduces bilirubin, often to normal	Increased bilirubin concentration with estrogens; diagnostic urine coproporphyrin isomer pattern (total is normal, with isomer I increased to ≥80% of total)	Characteristic urine coproporphyrin excretion pattern (total is increased ≤2.5-fold in ≈65% of cases but isomer I always <80% of total)
Major clinical features	Kernicterus in infancy if untreated; may occur later despite therapy	Rare late-onset kernicterus with fasting	None	Occasional hepatosplenomegaly	None
Hepatic morphology/ histology	Normal	Normal	Normal; occasionally increased lipofuscin pigment	Liver grossly black; coarse, dark centrilobular pigment	Normal
Bile bilirubin fractions†	>90% unconjugated	Largest fraction (mean 57%) monoconjugates	Mainly diconjugates but monoconjugates are increased (mean 23%)	Mixed conjugates, reported increase in diconjugates	Increased conjugates
Inheritance (all autosomal)	Recessive	Recessive	Promoter mutation is recessive; missense mutation often dominant	Recessive; rare kindred appears dominant	Recessive
Diagnosis	Clinical and laboratory findings, lack of response to phenobarbital	Clinical and laboratory findings, response to phenobarbital	Clinical and laboratory findings; promoter genotyping; liver biopsy rarely necessary	Clinical and laboratory findings; liver biopsy unnecessary if coproporphyrin studies available	Clinical and laboratory findings; urine coproporphyrin analysis
Treatment	Phototherapy or tin protoporphyrin as short-term therapy; liver transplantation definitive	Consider phenobarbital if baseline bilirubin ≥8 mg/dL	None necessary	Avoid estrogens; no other therapy necessary	No treatment necessary

*UGT1A1 = bilirubin specific isoform of the UGT1 family of uridine diphosphate glucuronosyltransferases.
†Bilirubin in normal bile: <5% unconjugated bilirubin, with an average of 7% bilirubin monoconjugates and 90% bilirubin diconjugates.

FAMILIAL CHOLESTASIS SYNDROMES

Bile secretion, which is essential both for the elimination of metabolic wastes and for the solubilization and subsequent absorption of specific nutrients, is a complex, energy-dependent process in which three genes encoding ABC (ATP binding cassette) transporters (*ATP8B1*, *ABCB11*, and *ABCB4*) play critical roles. Cholestatic disorders of childhood (E-Table 133-1) can be caused by a wide range of developmental, heritable, and acquired conditions. Congenital disorders of bile duct development include extrahepatic biliary atresia, progressive familial intrahepatic cholestasis,[6] and Alagille syndrome.[7]

Signs and symptoms associated with progressive familial intrahepatic cholestasis 1 include stunted growth, diarrhea, jaundice, and pruritus.[8] The pruritus from cholestatic disorders can be treated by interruption of the enterohepatic circulation by blockade of the apical bile salt transporter in the ileum.[9] Odevixibat (40 mcg/kg orally once daily) is indicated for the treatment of pruritus in patients 3 months of age and older with progressive familial intrahepatic cholestasis, and maralixibat (190 mcg/kg orally daily for 7 days, then 380 mcg/kg daily, as tolerated) is indicated for treatment of cholestatic pruritus in patients 1 year of age or older with Alagille syndrome.[A1] Treatment can also include reduction of bile acids by partial biliary external diversion, in which bile from the gallbladder is drained by a jejunal conduit externally.

Benign recurrent intrahepatic cholestasis is a rare, autosomal recessive disorder characterized by recurrent attacks of sometimes disabling malaise, pruritus, and jaundice, beginning in childhood or adulthood and varying in duration from weeks to months. Intervals between attacks may vary from months to years, and care is directed at managing the symptoms of fatigue and pruritus. Some cases are associated with progressive hepatic fibrosis.

ACQUIRED CONJUGATION DEFECTS

A modest reduction in bilirubin conjugating capacity occurs in advanced hepatitis or cirrhosis (Chapter 139). In these settings, however, conjugation is better preserved than canalicular excretion. Pharmacologic and

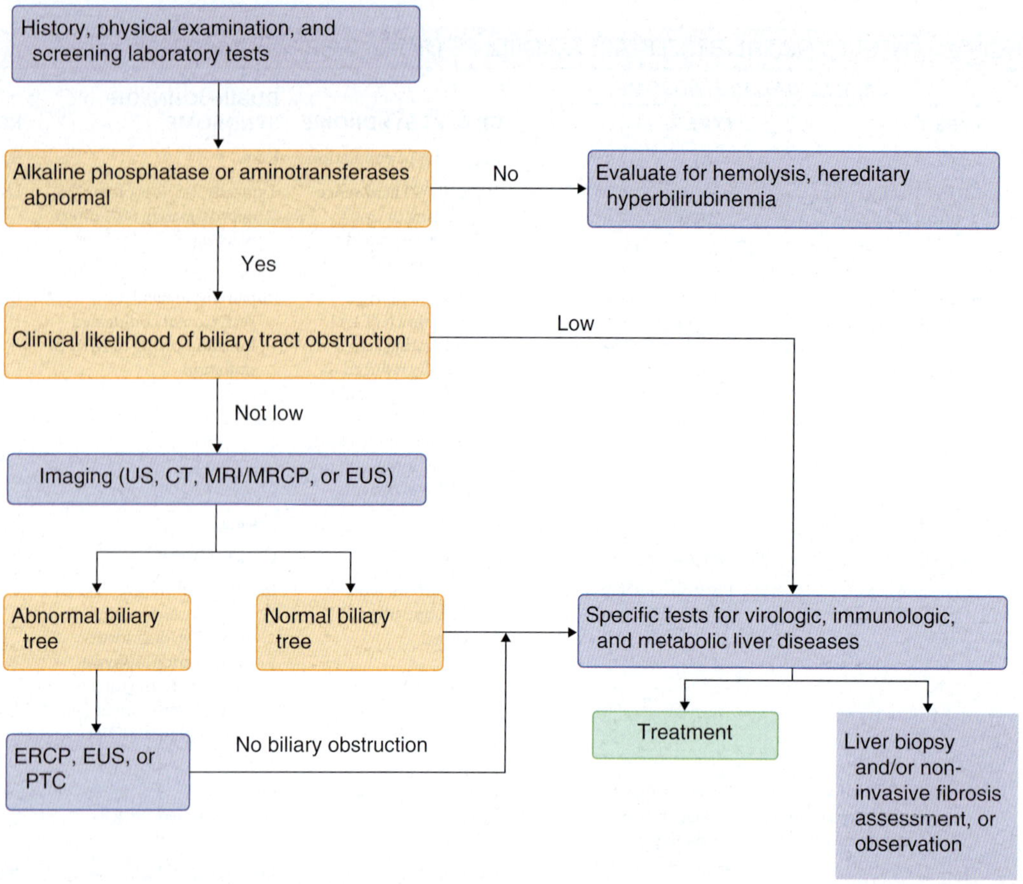

FIGURE 133-1. **Diagnostic algorithm for the evaluation of hyperbilirubinemia and other liver test abnormalities and signs and symptoms suggestive of liver disease.** CT = computed tomography; ERCP = endoscopic retrograde cholangiopancreatography; EUS = endoscopic ultrasound; MRCP = magnetic resonance cholangiopancreatography; MRI = magnetic resonance imaging; PTC = percutaneous transhepatic cholangiogram; US = ultrasound. (Modified from Lidofsky SD, Scharschmidt BF. Jaundice. In: Feldman M, Scharschmidt BF, Sleisenger MH, eds. *Gastrointestinal and Liver Disease*. 6th ed. Philadelphia: WB Saunders; 1998:227.)

metabolic perturbations may lead to acquired reductions in bilirubin conjugation. Medications known to inhibit UGT1A1 function include the human immunodeficiency virus (HIV) protease inhibitors (indinavir and atazanavir) and sorafenib, which is a multikinase inhibitor. Various other drugs (e.g., pregnanediol and the antibiotics chloramphenicol and gentamicin) also may cause unconjugated hyperbilirubinemia by inhibiting UGT1A1. In all settings in which UGT1A1 inhibitors cause unconjugated hyperbilirubinemia, the presence of Gilbert syndrome amplifies the hyperbilirubinemia.

JAUNDICE IN PREGNANCY

Jaundice in pregnancy (Chapter 221) includes any liver disease that occurs during pregnancy.[10] Conditions unique to pregnancy include elevation of aminotransferase and bilirubin levels during the first trimester with hyperemesis gravidarum. Intrahepatic cholestasis of pregnancy, which occurs during the second and third trimesters, is associated with intrauterine demise and resolves spontaneously after delivery. Mutations and sequence variations in genes encoding biliary transporters, especially *ABCB4* and *ABCB11*, have been reported in some but not all cases. Acute fatty liver or HELLP (*h*emolysis, *e*levated *l*iver enzymes, and *l*ow *p*latelets) syndrome occurs in association with preeclampsia in the third trimester. Acute fatty liver may resemble fulminant hepatic failure, with early delivery a prerequisite to maternal recovery.

POSTOPERATIVE JAUNDICE

This multifactorial syndrome can be caused by increased bilirubin production (e.g., breakdown of transfused erythrocytes, resorption of hematomas), decreased hepatic bilirubin clearance (e.g., bacteremia, endotoxemia, parenteral nutrition, perioperative hypoxia), or both. Postoperative hyperbilirubinemia (Chapter 401) is often accompanied by a several-fold increase in levels of alkaline phosphatase, GGT, or both. Aminotransferase levels are, at most, minimally elevated, and synthetic function is typically normal. The differential diagnosis includes biliary obstruction (Chapter 141) or hepatocellular injury related to shock, medication-induced liver injury (Chapter 136), or viral hepatitis (Chapters 134 and 135). The resolution of postoperative jaundice tends to parallel the overall postoperative course.

DIAGNOSIS

Accurate diagnosis and the distinction between acute and chronic disease often depend on appropriate selection and interpretation of laboratory and imaging studies. Tests used in initial evaluation of liver disease fall into two categories: tests that indicate injury, most commonly the aminotransferase levels, and tests that measure, or at least reflect, actual function. The results of laboratory testing can be informative for the magnitude of their deviation from the reference range, or as binary data to distinguish normal from abnormal. Serial determinations often can be helpful to assess the course of disease or the outcome of an intervention.

Serum Enzyme Tests

The levels of hepatic enzymes found in plasma are a measure of hepatocyte turnover or injury. Enzymes released during normal hepatocyte turnover are believed to be the basis for normal circulating levels. Cell injury and cell death activate phospholipases that create holes in the plasma membrane, thereby increasing the release of intracellular contents.

Aminotransferases

The aminotransferases catalyze transfer of the α-amino group of aspartate (aspartate aminotransferase [AST]) or alanine (alanine aminotransferase [ALT]) to the α-keto group of α-ketoglutarate, with pyridoxal phosphate (vitamin B_6) as a cofactor. Laboratory methods that assay aminotransferase activity require supplementation with vitamin B_6 to avoid falsely decreased activity in subjects who are vitamin B_6 deficient.

Normal serum levels, which are established locally from samples obtained from normal populations, may vary appreciably in different populations but are typically 40 IU/L or less (see Appendix). Deviations from the reference ranges should be expressed as multiples of the upper limits of the reference range.

Values >20 times the upper limit of normal can occur with acute hepatocyte injury from shock, viral infection, or immune- or medication-induced injury. ALT is a purely cytosolic enzyme. Distinct isoforms of AST are present in cytosol and mitochondria, and AST is also found on the plasma membrane. Expression of the mitochondrial isoform and its physiologic export from the hepatocyte are upregulated by ethanol.

Circulating levels of AST and ALT are elevated in most hepatic diseases,[11] and the degree of aminotransferase activity found in plasma roughly reflects the current activity of the disease process. There are, however, exceptions, and aminotransferases can both underestimate and overestimate the degree of hepatic injury. In alcohol-related hepatitis (Chapter 138), aminotransferase levels greater than 10 times the upper limit of normal are uncommon, and levels exceeding this threshold may suggest an additional cause of organ injury. In nonalcoholic fatty liver disease (Chapter 138), normal values for ALT may be found in an appreciable fraction of patients with steatohepatitis, fibrosis, or even cirrhosis. By contrast, conditions as diverse as papillary stenosis, transient choledocholithiasis (Chapter 141), and some forms of acute viral hepatitis (Chapter 134) manifest minimal histologic changes despite aminotransferase levels in excess of 10 times the upper limit of normal. Conversely, aminotransferase levels may decline during the course of massive hepatic necrosis because liver injury is so extensive that little enzyme activity remains. In rare circumstances, antibodies to AST result in an antibody-enzyme complex called a macroenzyme that has a delayed clearance from the circulation.

Aminotransferase levels are useful in several distinct ways. First, they provide a relatively specific screening test for hepatobiliary disease, including the diagnosis of previously unsuspected chronic hepatitis B or C. Although AST levels may be increased with diseases of other organs (notably myocardial and skeletal muscle), the source of increased aminotransferase activity can often be elucidated by consideration of the clinical context in which it arises. Aminotransferase levels are also used to monitor the activity of an acute or chronic parenchymal liver disease and its response to therapy.

Aminotransferase levels also can be elevated in patients with severe systemic disease. For example, aminotransferase levels may be elevated in over 90% of patients hospitalized with coronavirus 2019 (COVID-2019; Chapter 336) infection,[12] in whom they appear to indicate hepatic injury.

Aminotransferase levels may provide diagnostic clues. In most liver diseases, the ratio of AST to ALT is usually 1 or less; however, ratios are typically 2 or higher in alcoholic fatty liver and alcoholic hepatitis (Chapter 138) as a reflection of increased synthesis and secretion of mitochondrial AST into plasma and selective loss of ALT activity because of the pyridoxine deficiency commonly seen in alcoholism. An elevated AST/ALT ratio also occurs in acute liver failure from Wilson disease (Chapter 195).

Alkaline Phosphatases

Alkaline phosphatases are widely distributed enzymes (e.g., liver, bile ducts, intestine, bone, kidney, placenta, and leukocytes) that catalyze the release of orthophosphate from ester substrates at an alkaline pH. The normal activity level in adult serum is dependent on the patient's age and sex, as well as the method of measurement.[13] Two widely used current methods have upper limits of normal in adults of 85 and 110 IU/L (see Appendix). Serum levels higher than the reference range are normal in children and in pregnancy. Bone alkaline phosphatase participates in the deposition of hydroxyapatite in osteoid. In other sites, including the liver, its phosphatase activity may facilitate movement of molecules across cell membranes. Serum alkaline phosphatase activity principally reflects the contribution of hepatic and bone isoforms; the intestinal form may account for 20 to 60% of the total after a fatty meal, and blood groups B and O are associated with sustained increases. There is a substantial placental contribution to the alkaline phosphatase level late in pregnancy; the Regan isozyme, a variant that appears identical to the placental form, is associated with hepatocellular cancer (Chapter 181), lung cancer (Chapter 177), and other neoplasms.

Elevations in the serum alkaline phosphatase in cholestatic hepatobiliary disease result from two distinct mechanisms: increased synthesis and secretion of the enzyme and solubilization from the apical (canalicular) surface of hepatocytes and the luminal surface of biliary epithelial cells by the increased local concentrations of bile acids that occur with cholestasis. The first step in the evaluation of alkaline phosphatase is to elucidate the source of the elevation. The placenta, bone, and intestine are non-hepatobiliary sources, and increases in activity can be seen in pregnancy and disorders of increased bone turnover, including Paget disease (Chapter 228), osteomalacia (Chapter 226), and osseous metastatic disease. When the source of the alkaline phosphatase is inapparent from the clinical history, elevation of the gamma-glutamyl transferase (GGT) or 5'-nucleotidase (5'-NT) make a hepatobiliary source likely. The interpretation of a normal GGT is more complicated; although the GGT can be normal in non-hepatobiliary disorders, it is also typically normal in intrahepatic cholestasis of pregnancy, and in some familial cholestatic disorders. With a serum half-life of approximately 1 week, serum alkaline phosphatase levels may remain elevated for days to weeks after resolution of biliary obstruction. This delay may be especially misleading when accompanied by prolonged direct-reacting hyperbilirubinemia owing to delayed clearance of delta bilirubin.

Modest increases in serum alkaline phosphatase (<3 times the upper limit of normal) occur in many hepatic parenchymal disorders, including hepatitis and cirrhosis. Greater increases (3 to 10 times the upper limit of normal) usually indicate obstruction of bile flow. Although the highest levels usually reflect obstruction of the common bile duct, elevations also can occur with obstruction of intrahepatic bile ducts from infiltrative conditions that arise from granulomatous processes (sarcoidosis [Chapter 83], mycobacterial infection [Chapters 299 and 300]), malignancy (lymphoma, cholangiocarcinoma, or metastatic cancer), or amyloidosis (Chapter 174).

Other Hepatic Enzymes

5'-nucleotidase (5'-NT) is a plasma membrane enzyme that cleaves orthophosphate from the 5' position on the pentose sugar of adenosine or inosine phosphate. Leucine aminopeptidase (LAP) is a ubiquitous cellular peptidase. The serum levels of both usually increase in cholestasis. Accordingly, their major use is to confirm whether an elevated alkaline phosphatase is of hepatobiliary origin. Both enzymes may be increased in the later stages of a healthy pregnancy.

Gamma-glutamyl transpeptidase (GGT) is present in many tissues. Its serum activity increases in hepatobiliary disease but also in neuromuscular diseases, pancreatic disease (even in the absence of biliary obstruction), pulmonary disease, and during the ingestion of ethanol and other inducers of microsomal enzymes. Nevertheless, because serum GGT levels are usually normal in bone disease, the enzyme may be helpful in confirming the hepatic origin of alkaline phosphatase. Lactate dehydrogenase levels are often elevated in hepatic ischemia and other conditions that result in hepatic necrosis.

Tests Based on Clearance of Metabolites and Drugs

A major function of the liver is to remove various metabolites and toxins from the blood. In liver disease, clearance of such molecules may be impaired because of loss of parenchymal cells, diminished bile secretion, biliary obstruction, decreased cellular uptake or metabolism, or reduced or heterogeneous hepatic blood flow. Serum levels of metabolites produced at a relatively constant rate (e.g., bilirubin) can be particularly useful indicators of liver function.

Bilirubin

The differential diagnosis of hyperbilirubinemia (see earlier) includes generalized liver disease, inherited disorders of bilirubin metabolism (e.g., Gilbert, Crigler-Najjar, Dubin-Johnson, and Rotor syndromes), and nonhepatic conditions (e.g., hemolysis). Higher bilirubin levels correlate with a poorer prognosis in most forms of chronic liver disease.

Ammonia

Ammonia, a byproduct of amino acid metabolism, is removed from blood by the liver, converted to urea in the Krebs-Henseleit cycle, and excreted by the kidneys. In the setting of portosystemic shunting or severe hepatic dysfunction, ammonia levels rise. Measurements of blood ammonia are typically used to confirm a diagnosis of hepatic encephalopathy (Chapter 139); however, they do not strongly correlate with the severity of the encephalopathy (Chapter 139). The correlations may be improved if the measurement is made rapidly on an iced arterial blood sample. Elevated ammonia levels also occur when ammonia production is increased by intestinal flora, by the kidney (in response to metabolic alkalosis or hypokalemia), or in rare genetic diseases that affect the pathway of urea synthesis.[14]

Tests Reflecting Hepatic Synthetic Function

Coagulation Tests

Prothrombin Time

The prothrombin time (PT) reflects the plasma concentrations of both extrinsic and common pathway factors, that is, factors VII, X, and V; prothrombin; and fibrinogen. A prolonged PT most often results from vitamin

K deficiency, liver disease, or the therapeutic use of warfarin-like anticoagulants. Vitamin K, a fat-soluble vitamin, is found in many foods and is also synthesized by gut bacteria (Chapter 161). Vitamin K deficiency can be caused by poor dietary intake and malabsorptive states, including the fat malabsorption that results from cholestasis, and with antibiotic suppression of gut flora, particularly in patients who receive inadequate vitamin K replacement.

The half-lives of clotting factors are typically less than 1 day. Factor VII, which has the shortest half-life, is usually the earliest and most severely depressed during periods of defective hepatic synthesis. Because the PT is dependent on factor VII, it responds rapidly with changes in hepatic synthetic function; it is useful for following the course of acute liver diseases, in which a significant or growing prolongation of the PT may indicate a poor prognosis (Chapters 139 and 140). An abnormal PT that is due solely to vitamin K deficiency usually becomes normal within 24 to 48 hours after parenteral repletion; however, if decreased synthesis of clotting factors reflects hepatocyte dysfunction, there may be little or no response to vitamin K.

Although the prolongation of PT with liver disease is generally accepted as indicative of defective clotting factor synthesis, the synthesis of both procoagulant and anticoagulant proteins is disturbed in liver disease. The physiologic consequences of this rebalancing of coagulation may preserve the coagulation response. Prolongation of the PT may also reflect an acquired dysfibrinogenemia or spur cell hemolytic anemia, both of which can occur in decompensated cirrhosis (Chapter 139).

Albumin

Albumin is produced solely by the liver. Its plasma concentration reflects a balance between its synthetic rate of approximately 100 to 200 mg/kg/day and plasma half-life of approximately 21 days. The synthetic rate is affected by the patient's nutritional state, thyroid and glucocorticoid hormone levels, plasma colloid osmotic pressure, exposure to hepatotoxins (e.g., alcohol), and presence of systemic disorders, liver disease, or both. Many conditions increase albumin losses and shorten its plasma half-life, including nephrotic syndrome (Chapter 107), protein-losing enteropathy (Chapter 126), severe burns (Chapter 97), exfoliative dermatitis, and major gastrointestinal bleeding (Chapter 121). Hypoalbuminemia in cirrhosis indicates diminished hepatic synthetic function.

Hematologic Tests in Liver Disease

In moderate to severe acute liver diseases, varying degrees of cytopenias can be seen with all three cell lineages. The most common finding is thrombocytopenia from hypersplenism, which can be a surrogate marker of portal hypertension. Anemia may reflect low-grade hemolysis or marrow depression. Bone marrow suppression may be caused by ethanol or drugs, and aplastic anemia has an uncommon but recognized association with acute viral hepatitis. Zieve syndrome (spur cell hemolytic anemia and hypertriglyceridemia) is a rare but well-characterized complication of severe alcoholic liver disease (Chapter 138). Modest leukopenia, often with atypical lymphocytes, also may be present. Chronic liver disease, especially if cholestatic, may be accompanied by target cells, erythrocytes with an expanded cell membrane that reflects abnormalities in serum lipids.

APPROACH TO THE PATIENT WITH JAUNDICE OR ABNORMAL LIVER TESTS

History, Physical Examination, and Initial Laboratory Studies

Patients with liver disease may present with jaundice or other signs or symptoms, or the disease may be detected in the asymptomatic patient by the finding of abnormal liver tests during a routine evaluation. Regardless of how the patient comes to medical attention, the diagnostic approach (see Fig. 133-1) begins with a careful history, physical examination, and screening laboratory studies (measurement of total and direct bilirubin, ALT, AST, alkaline phosphatase levels, and PT) to formulate an initial differential diagnosis.[15,16] The ability to distinguish between liver disease and biliary tract obstruction is the major goal of the initial evaluation (Table 133-3).

Historic details relevant to the assessment of liver disease include quantification of alcohol consumption, use of medications including complementary and alternative supplements, injection drug use, prior hepatobiliary surgery, and a family history of liver disease. Physical evidence of cirrhosis (e.g., spider angiomas, gynecomastia, ascites, splenomegaly) supports the diagnosis of chronic parenchymal disease. Laboratory testing should help to distinguish primary hepatocellular injury from a cholestatic or mixed pattern. Hepatic synthetic function and signs of portal hypertension (thrombocytopenia) should be assessed. Serologic testing can further elucidate the causes of liver disease. It is also important to recognize that laboratory patterns alone commonly are not sufficient to make or exclude a diagnosis.

TABLE 133-3 OBSTRUCTIVE JAUNDICE VERSUS CHOLESTATIC LIVER DISEASE

FEATURE	SUGGESTS OBSTRUCTIVE JAUNDICE	SUGGESTS PARENCHYMAL LIVER DISEASE
History	Abdominal pain Fever, rigors Prior biliary surgery Acholic stools	Anorexia, malaise, myalgias, suggestive of viral prodrome Known infectious exposure Use of injection drugs or intranasal cocaine Exposure to known hepatotoxin Family history of jaundice
Physical examination	High fever Abdominal tenderness Palpable abdominal mass	Ascites Other stigmata of liver disease (e.g., prominent abdominal veins, gynecomastia, spider angiomata, asterixis, encephalopathy, Kayser-Fleischer rings)
Laboratory studies	Elevated alkaline phosphatase level with varying degrees of hyperbilirubinemia Prothrombin time that is normal or normalizes with vitamin K administration	Elevated aminotransferase levels Prolonged prothrombin time that does not correct with vitamin K administration Blood tests indicative of specific liver disease

Imaging Studies

If extrahepatic obstruction is suspected, its site and nature can be determined in virtually all patients. A reasonable initial step is the use of a noninvasive imaging study such as ultrasonography or magnetic resonance cholangiopancreatography (MRCP) to determine whether the intrahepatic or extrahepatic biliary system, or both, are dilated, thereby implying mechanical obstruction. Because of its lesser expense, portability, and convenience, ultrasound is often the procedure of choice for the diagnosis of cholelithiasis (Chapters 132 and 141). Biliary obstruction may be less apparent in cirrhosis, and mild biliary dilation without obstruction is common after cholecystectomy.

The biliary tree can be examined by endoscopic retrograde cholangiopancreatography (ERCP; Chapter 120) or percutaneous transhepatic cholangiography. Endoscopic ultrasound (EUS) (Chapter 120) is a complementary approach that permits internal ultrasonographic analysis of the pancreas, extrahepatic bile ducts, and regional lymph nodes and blood vessels. EUS combined with fine needle aspiration permits tissue sampling of abnormalities in areas such as the bile ducts and pancreas that typically have been difficult to sample percutaneously.

Selection of Imaging Tests

Liver ultrasound is an ideal screening test to evaluate the liver architecture, assess for surface nodularity and parenchymal mass lesions, and exclude biliary obstruction. Ultrasound is relatively inexpensive in comparison to other imaging modalities, is widely available, and avoids ionizing radiation. The identification of mass lesions on ultrasound will commonly prompt further cross-sectional imaging with either computed tomography or magnetic resonance imaging. If imaging reveals evidence of biliary obstruction or if obstruction is still considered likely despite imaging findings, cholangiography by ERCP or PTC, both of which offer therapeutic and diagnostic capabilities, may be an appropriate choice. In patients with an intermediate probability of obstruction, MRCP is a reasonable study. Individual radiology units have different levels of expertise for these procedures, and the local radiology staff may be quite helpful in recommending the best procedure for a given patient.

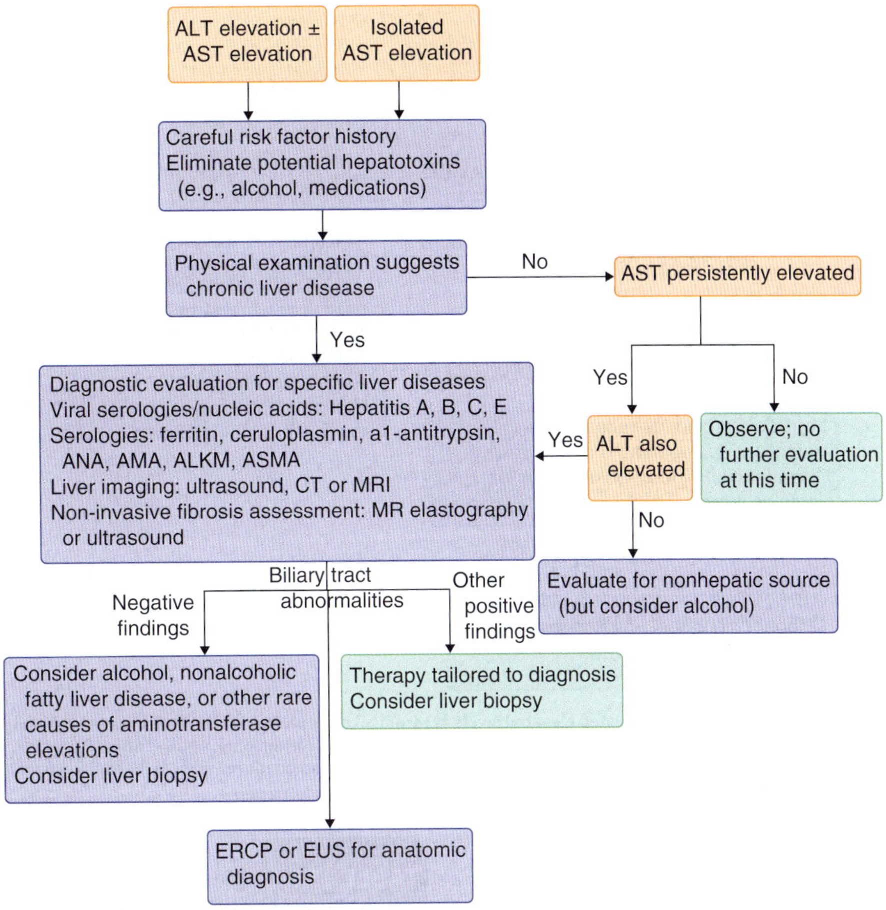

FIGURE 133-2. **Approach to the evaluation of isolated elevated levels of serum alanine aminotransferase (*ALT*), aspartate aminotransferase (*AST*), or both in the asymptomatic patient.** ALKM = anti–liver/kidney microsomal antibody; ANA = antinuclear antibody; AMA = antimitochondrial antibody; ASMA = anti–smooth muscle antibody; CT = computed tomography; ERCP = endoscopic retrograde cholangiopancreatography; EUS = endoscopic ultrasound; MR = magnetic resonance; MRI = magnetic resonance imaging.

Asymptomatic Aminotransferase Abnormalities

Epidemiologic data suggest that up to 25% of asymptomatic adult Americans have a mild to moderate elevation of aminotransferase levels. The incidental discovery of such abnormalities is currently the most frequent means by which liver disease is first recognized. Whereas up to one third of such patients have no elevation on subsequent testing, others may prove to have any of the common forms of liver disease including chronic viral hepatitis (Chapter 135) and nonalcoholic fatty liver disease (Chapter 138). Persistent elevations of liver test levels should prompt careful clinical evaluation (Fig. 133-2), including laboratory testing of aminotransferase levels and hepatic synthetic function. Serologic studies for viral, autoimmune, and metabolic conditions can provide further insights into diagnosis. When appropriate, changes in aminotransferase levels observed in response to weight loss, the withdrawal of medications, or alcohol sobriety can be very helpful. The evaluation can be further aided by elastography to assess for hepatic fibrosis or liver biopsy when tissue characterization is necessary for a diagnosis (Chapter 132).

Alkaline Phosphatase Elevation

A careful history identifies patients at risk for intrahepatic cholestasis related to drugs or toxins (Chapter 136). The presence of hilar adenopathy or arthritis may implicate sarcoidosis (Chapter 83), although hepatic sarcoidosis can be present without extrahepatic disease. Many patients with isolated elevation of the alkaline phosphatase level have nonhepatic causes, such as pregnancy or bone disease. The origin of an elevated alkaline phosphatase can be determined by fractionation into its constituent fractions (Fig. 133-3). A hepatic source is highly likely if the serum GGT is also abnormal.

Imaging of the liver and biliary tree is necessary when the alkaline phosphatase is of hepatobiliary origin. The diagnostic approach typically begins with liver ultrasound, but MRCP may be an appropriate first choice in, for example, individuals who have inflammatory bowel disease (Chapter 127), in which the probability of primary sclerosing cholangitis (Chapter 141) is increased. Serologic studies should include an antimitochondrial antibody; a positive result suggests primary biliary cholangitis. Other less common (and nonexhaustive) causes of cholestatic liver test include amyloidosis (Chapter 174), tuberculosis (Chapter 299), fungal infections, extramedullary hematopoiesis, Langerhans cell histiocytosis (Chapter 155), infiltrative neoplasms, and sepsis.

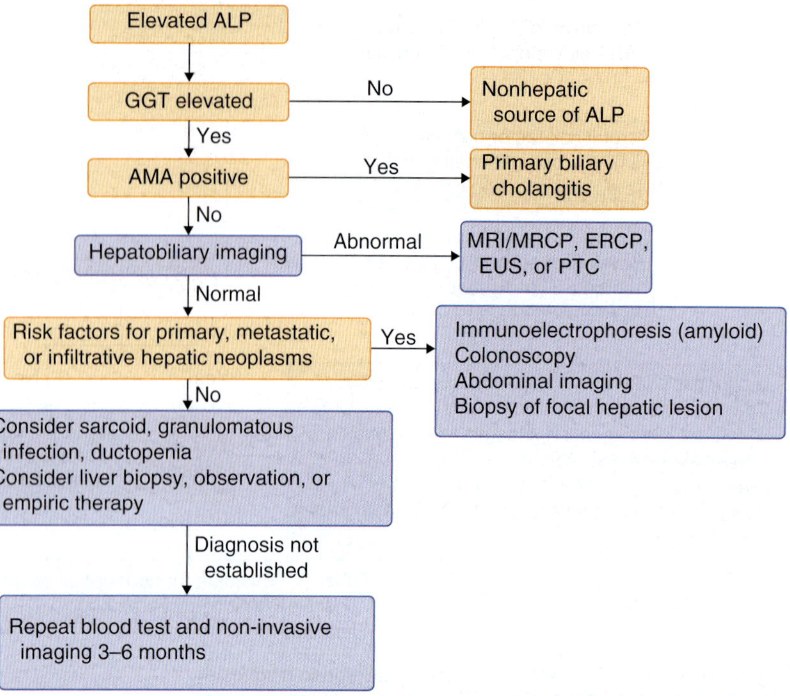

FIGURE 133-3. **Approach to the asymptomatic patient with isolated elevated levels of serum alkaline phosphatase (*ALP*).** In cases with a high index of suspicion of biliary tract disease (e.g., sclerosing cholangitis), cholangiography may be warranted even in the face of normal ultrasound imaging. AMA = antimitochondrial antibody; ERCP = endoscopic retrograde cholangiopancreatography; EUS = endoscopic ultrasound; GGT = γ-glutamyl transpeptidase; MRCP = magnetic resonance cholangiopancreatography; MRI = magnetic resonance imaging; PTC = percutaneous transhepatic cholangiogram; US = ultrasonography.

GENERAL REFERENCES

For the General References and other additional features, please visit Elsevier eBooks+ at https://ebooks.health.elsevier.com.

Grade A Reference

A1. Gonzales E, Hardikar W, Stormon M, et al. Efficacy and safety of maralixibat treatment in patients with Alagille syndrome and cholestatic pruritus (ICONIC): a randomised phase 2 study. *Lancet*. 2021;398:1581-1592.

134 ACUTE VIRAL HEPATITIS

JEAN-MICHEL PAWLOTSKY

Infection with a hepatotropic virus causes an acute episode of liver inflammation, referred to as *acute hepatitis*, which can lead to either spontaneous clearance of the infectious agent or its persistence, which in turn leads to chronic infection for a subset of these viruses. Five hepatitis viruses are responsible for the vast majority of acute hepatitis cases (Table 134-1):[1] hepatitis A virus (HAV); hepatitis B virus (HBV); hepatitis C virus (HCV); hepatitis D, or delta, virus (HDV), which is a defective viroid using the hepatitis B surface antigen (HBsAg) as its envelope; and hepatitis E virus (HEV).[2] Other viruses may cause acute inflammatory liver disease, including members of the Herpesviridae family such as human cytomegalovirus, Epstein-Barr virus, and herpes simplex virus. In one study from Spain, the most common causes of acute viral hepatitis cases were: 28% hepatitis B, 18% hepatitis C, 14% hepatitis A, and 14% Epstein-Barr virus (Chapter 348),[3] but severe acute respiratory syndrome coronavirus 2 (SARS-CoV-2) infection also is often accompanied by acute hepatitis. Adenovirus infection has led to outbreaks of hepatitis in children. It is unclear to what extent other viruses, such as parvovirus B19 or human herpesvirus 6, can also cause acute hepatitis. Patients who present with an acute viral hepatitis syndrome but negative virologic tests are referred to as having non–A-to-E hepatitis, perhaps attributable to hepatotropic viruses that have yet to be identified. The worldwide incidence of acute viral hepatitis is decreasing because of global improvements in hygiene and the development and use of efficient vaccines against HBV, to a lesser extent against HAV, and perhaps in the future, HEV.

TABLE 134-1 VIRUSES RESPONSIBLE FOR ACUTE VIRAL HEPATITIS AND LIKELIHOOD OF CHRONIC EVOLUTION

VIRUS	EVOLUTION TO CHRONIC VIRAL HEPATITIS
Hepatitis A virus	Never
Hepatitis B virus	>90% (perinatal acquisition) to <1% (adult infection)
Hepatitis C virus	50-80%
Hepatitis D or delta virus	2% (coinfection) to 90% (superinfection)
Hepatitis E virus	Occasionally in immunosuppressed patients
Other viruses Human cytomegalovirus Epstein-Barr virus Herpes simplex virus Human herpesvirus 6 Parvovirus B19 SARS-CoV-2	May establish chronic infection (except SARS-CoV-2), not associated with chronic hepatitis

GENERAL FEATURES OF ACUTE VIRAL HEPATITIS

PATHOBIOLOGY

Acute viral hepatitis is characterized by acute necroinflammation of the liver. Because none of the hepatotropic viruses is cytopathic, liver injury is mediated by a strong cytotoxic T cell–mediated reaction against infected hepatocytes that express viral antigens at their surface. Pro-inflammatory cytokines, natural killer cells, and antibody-dependent cellular cytotoxicity also appear to play a role in liver necroinflammation. Successful immune elimination may lead to viral clearance, which may or may not be associated with lifelong immunity, depending on the infecting agent. The immune reaction is sometimes so potent that the patient develops subfulminant or even fulminant hepatitis that requires liver transplantation (Chapter 140). In some patients—the proportion varies, according to the virus responsible for acute hepatitis—the immune response fails and chronic infection is established (Chapter 135).

CLINICAL MANIFESTATIONS

After infection, there is an incubation period from a few days to a few weeks, depending upon the causative agent (Fig. 134-1). This incubation period is generally characterized by nonspecific symptoms, including fatigue, nausea, loss of appetite, flulike symptoms, and/or right upper quadrant pain (Table 134-2). The incubation period is often characterized by leukopenia and relative lymphocytosis. Immune-mediated symptoms, including rash, hives, arthralgias, angioneurotic edema, and fever, are observed in 10 to 20% of patients during the preicteric phase.

During the acute stage of the disease, symptoms may vary widely, from asymptomatic to subicteric, icteric or severe, and fulminant. The icteric form, which is not frequent, is characterized by fatigue, anorexia, nausea, dysgeusia, jaundice, dark urine, light-colored stool, and weight loss. Physical examination reveals jaundice and hepatic tenderness. Hepatomegaly and splenomegaly may be present. On laboratory testing, acute viral hepatitis is characterized by elevated total and direct serum bilirubin levels and aminotransferase levels that are often greater than 10 times the upper limit of normal. Cholestatic acute hepatitis is associated frequently with prolonged and fluctuating jaundice and pruritus. After 1 to 3 weeks, on average, both clinical and laboratory signs progressively improve and return to normal. Some patients, however, may experience a relapse before definitive resolution.

Signs of hepatic failure (Chapter 140), including changes in personality, aggressive behavior, sleeping disorders, and hepatic encephalopathy, characterize fulminant forms of acute viral hepatitis. Coma can supervene rapidly, and widespread hemorrhage may develop.

DIAGNOSIS

The diagnosis of acute hepatitis is suspected based on elevated serum aminotransferase levels, which are generally more than 10 times the upper limit

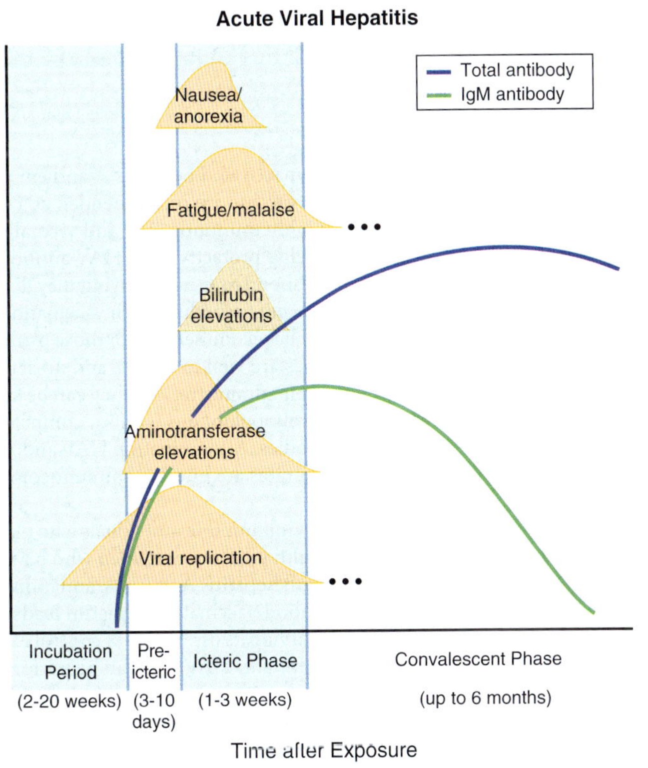

FIGURE 134-1. **Typical course of acute viral hepatitis. IgM = immunoglobulin M.**

of normal (Table 134-3). Total and direct bilirubin levels are elevated if the acute hepatitis is subicteric or icteric. Alkaline phosphatase levels may be elevated in cases of cholestatic hepatitis.

Serologic and eventually molecular testing identifies the causal agent. Liver biopsy or a non-invasive assessment of liver inflammation and fibrosis are generally not required. All cases of acute hepatitis should be reported to the local, state, or national health department as soon as possible after diagnosis.

TREATMENT

In addition to virus-specific therapy for HBV and HCV,[4] patients with acute viral hepatitis should avoid alcohol consumption and acetaminophen. Sexual contact should be avoided if the partner is not protected (i.e., not HBV vaccinated). Patients with subfulminant or fulminant hepatitis should be supported in an intensive care unit setting and evaluated for possible liver transplantation (Chapter 140).

TABLE 134-2 COMMON CLINICAL MANIFESTATIONS OF ACUTE VIRAL HEPATITIS

PHASES OF INFECTION	DURATION*	MANIFESTATIONS*
Incubation	2-20 weeks	Virus detectable in blood Aminotransferase and bilirubin levels normal No antibody detectable
Preicteric	3-10 days	Nonspecific symptoms: fatigue, anorexia, nausea, vague right upper quadrant pain Viral titers peak Aminotransferase levels begin to rise Immune complex-mediated hypersensitivity reaction (≈10-20% of cases) with rash, hives, arthralgias, fever
Icteric	1-3 weeks	Jaundice appears; dark urine and light stools seen Nonspecific symptoms worsen Weight loss, dysgeusia, pruritus may occur Hepatosplenomegaly may develop Aminotransferase levels typically >10 times normal Antibodies appear Viral titers decline Rare extrahepatic manifestations (aseptic meningitis, encephalitis, seizures, ascending flaccid paralysis, nephrotic syndrome, seronegative arthritis)
Recovery	Up to 6 months	Symptoms resolve gradually Antibody levels rise Aminotransferase and bilirubin levels normalize
Chronic	After 6 months	See Chapter 135

*Varies by virus.

TABLE 134-3 LABORATORY TESTING FOR SUSPECTED ACUTE VIRAL HEPATITIS

GENERAL EVALUATION
Alanine aminotransferase Aspartate aminotransferase Alkaline phosphatase International normalized ratio (INR)
FIRST-LINE DIAGNOSTIC TESTS
Anti-HAV IgM HBsAg, anti-HBc IgM Anti-HCV antibodies HCV RNA Anti-HEV IgM
SECOND-LINE DIAGNOSTIC TESTS
Anti-HAV IgM present: none advised HBsAg and anti-HBc IgM present: HDV antigen, anti-HDV antibodies HCV RNA present with or without anti-HCV antibodies: none advised Anti-HEV IgM present: none advised No virologic marker: See Fig. 134-3

HAV = hepatitis A virus; HBc = hepatitis B core; HBsAg = hepatitis B surface antigen; HBV = hepatitis B virus; HCV = hepatitis C virus; HDV = hepatitis D virus; HEV = hepatitis E virus; IgM = immunoglobulin M.

PROGNOSIS

Prognosis depends on the degree of prolongation of the prothrombin time, as well as the degree of elevation of the bilirubin and lactate levels. A factor V level less than 40% or any signs of encephalopathy are indications for hospitalization. Death is extremely rare and occurs only in fulminant cases. Other signs of poor prognosis are persistently worsening jaundice, ascites, and an acute decrease in the size of the liver. Serum aminotransferase levels and viral genome levels have no prognostic value.

HEPATITIS A

DEFINITION

The Pathogen

HAV is a member of the Picornaviridae family, genus *Hepatovirus*. The hepatitis A viral particle is a 27-nm nonenveloped icosahedral nucleocapsid that expresses the hepatitis A antigen and contains a positive-stranded RNA genome approximately 7.5 kb long. Three different HAV genotypes have been described in humans (genotypes I, II, and III, further divided into subtypes A and B), with genotype I predominating worldwide. Other genotypes have been isolated in nonhuman primates. It is currently unclear to what extent different genotypes are associated with distinct clinical courses of infection.

EPIDEMIOLOGY

HAV infection has a worldwide distribution, and infections can be sporadic or occur in epidemic outbreak. The incidence of acute cases and the seroprevalence vary according to the hygiene, sanitation, housing, and socioeconomic standards of a given region, with a seroprevalence as low as approximately 13% in Sweden but up to 100% in many countries with poor sanitary conditions and hygienic practices. In developing countries, infection generally occurs at a young age and most of the population has been exposed and is protected after age 10 years. In countries with good sanitary and hygienic conditions, however, infection can occur at any age, and the prevalence of exposed, immune subjects slowly increases with age. In the United States, according to the Centers for Disease Control and Prevention, the incidence of acute hepatitis A declined from 12.0 cases per 100,000 individuals in 1995 to 0.5 cases per 100,000 individuals by 2012, but has subsequently increased to 3.8 cases per 100,000 individuals in 2018 owing to widespread outbreaks among persons reporting drug use and homelessness.

HAV is generally transmitted via the fecal-oral route, most often directly from person to person or through the ingestion of fecally contaminated food[5] or water. Transmission by blood transfusion has been reported, and isolated cases of apparent perinatal transmission have been described. High-risk groups for acute hepatitis A include travelers to developing countries, children in day care centers and their parents, men who have sex with men, injection drug users, homeless persons, patients who receive plasma products for hemophilia, and persons in institutions.[6]

PATHOBIOLOGY

The genome serves as a messenger RNA and contains a single open reading frame that encodes both structural and non-structural viral proteins. After attachment to a specific receptor at the surface of hepatocytes, the virus penetrates into cells and is uncoated. Subsequent events occurring exclusively in the cytoplasm include translation of the single open reading frame into a polyprotein that is later processed to generate the mature viral proteins; replication in a membrane-bound replication complex that generates new viral genomes, which are subsequently used for viral protein production and viral particle assembly; and packaging of newly formed genomes into new particles that are exported out of the cells. The virus is secreted into bile and, to a lesser extent, serum.

CLINICAL MANIFESTATIONS

Typically, the incubation period is 15 to 45 days (see Table 134-2). In most cases, acute infection takes a mild and unrecognized course. The incidence of symptomatic, icteric cases increases with the age at infection.[7] Acute hepatitis A in adults may require hospitalization in up to 13% of cases; prolonged courses of 6 to 9 months have been reported in 10% of adult patients with a diagnosis of acute hepatitis A. Hepatitis A is the most common cause of relapsing cholestatic hepatitis.

DIAGNOSIS

The diagnosis of acute hepatitis A is based on the detection of anti-HAV immunoglobulin M (IgM) in serum by enzyme immunoassay. IgM serum levels peak during the second month of infection (Fig. 134-2). HAV RNA can be transiently detected in stool and other body fluids by polymerase chain reaction (PCR) 3 to 10 days before the onset of illness and for 1 to 2 weeks thereafter; however, HAV RNA testing is not necessary. When the infection resolves, anti-HAV IgM disappears after 4 to 12 months, but anti-HAV IgG persists for life and confers definitive and durable protection against infection.

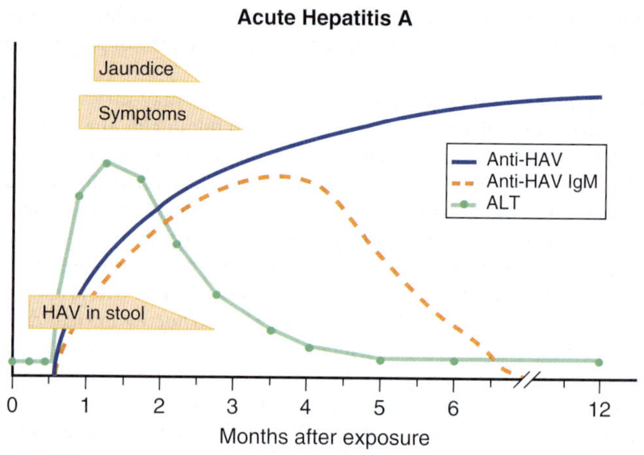

FIGURE 134-2. Serologic course of acute hepatitis A. ALT = alanine aminotransferase; HAV = hepatitis A virus; IgM = immunoglobulin M.

TREATMENT

Because HAV infection is self-limited, no specific antiviral treatment is required. In severe cases, patients may need to be hospitalized. If liver function is deteriorating, patients may need to be assessed for liver transplantation, which is the only therapeutic option for acute liver failure (Chapter 140).

PREVENTION

HAV vaccines (Chapter 15) consist of inactivated hepatitis A antigen purified from cell culture. Two doses of the vaccine are recommended at a 6- to 18-month interval. All vaccines are highly immunogenic, and virtually all healthy persons who are vaccinated develop protective anti-HAV antibodies. Patients with chronic liver disease also respond to vaccination but may display lower anti-HAV titers. An accelerated vaccine schedule, with vaccination on days 0, 7, and 21, is also effective and may be recommended for those planning to travel to endemic areas. HAV vaccines are well tolerated, and no serious adverse events have been linked with their administration; they can be safely administered with other vaccines or immunoglobulins without compromising the development of protective antibodies. A combination HAV and HBV vaccine is also available. Seroconversion rates are lower in immunocompromised individuals.

HAV vaccination is recommended for nonimmune individuals who plan to travel to endemic countries, medical health professionals, men who have sex with men, persons who are in contact with hepatitis A patients, and individuals with chronic liver diseases. A childhood vaccination program leads to a significant decline in HAV infection, justifying its use as part of control efforts in endemic countries. Serologic testing for anti-HAV IgG can be performed before vaccination in adults born in endemic countries and in individuals older than 50 years born in industrialized areas; persons with detectable IgG are protected and should not be vaccinated. For postexposure prophylaxis, both HAV vaccination and immunoglobulin are about 98% effective, with vaccination having the advantage of preventing secondary cases. HAV vaccine and immunoglobulin commonly are used together in this setting.

Long-term follow-up studies after complete HAV vaccination show that anti-HAV IgG titers sharply decline during the first year after vaccination but remain detectable in almost all individuals for at least 10 years. Protective anti-HAV antibody titers persist for at least 27 years after the successful vaccination of children and young adults.

PROGNOSIS

Acute hepatitis A infection generally resolves without complications in 3 to 4 weeks and never evolves to chronic infection. Prolonged elevation of serum aminotransferase levels has been reported. Relapses a few weeks after the acute case also have been observed. Prolonged courses may occur in children and immunosuppressed individuals.

Cholestatic hepatitis A is unusual and has a good prognosis, with full recovery within a few weeks. Fulminant hepatitis A is rare, occurring in less than 0.1% of cases, but its incidence and mortality increase with the patient's age at acquisition. In the United States, 4% of all cases of fulminant hepatitis are caused by HAV infection. Overall, mortality of acute hepatitis A is 1.8% in patients older than 50 years. In patients with chronic hepatitis B, superinfection with HAV is associated with a 6- to 23-fold higher morbidity and mortality.

ACUTE HEPATITIS B

DEFINITION

The Pathogen

HBV is a member of the Hepadnaviridae family, genus *Hepadnavirus*. The infectious virion, the Dane particle, is 42 to 47 nm in diameter. It possesses an envelope and a capsid or core that contains the partially double-stranded, circular DNA genome and the HBV polymerase. The HBV genome is the smallest known human virus genome, with approximately 3000 nucleotides.

EPIDEMIOLOGY

Two billion individuals worldwide have been in contact with HBV, and approximately 300 million individuals have chronic infection. In the United States, approximately 0.3% of the population is chronically infected. Although the worldwide incidence of chronic HBV infection is decreasing as a result of prevention and vaccination, the absolute prevalence of chronically infected individuals has increased as a result of the increase in the world population. HBV virions are produced and circulate in very high amounts in HBV-infected individuals, who are highly contagious. Four principal routes of transmission are responsible for acute HBV infections: (1) sexual transmission, which is the principal route in industrialized areas; (2) perinatal mother-to-infant transmission, which is associated with a very high (>90%) rate of chronic infection and is the principal cause of HBV transmission in Asia; (3) horizontal transmission through nonsexual interindividual contact, which is frequent at a young age in Africa and is associated with evolution to chronicity in approximately 15% of cases; and (4) percutaneous transmission by blood and blood products, unsafe medical or surgical materials, or injection drug use.

In industrialized countries, groups at high risk for HBV infection include individuals born in areas where HBV is endemic, including immigrants and adopted children; individuals who were not vaccinated as infants and whose parents were born in regions where HBV is endemic; household and sexual contacts of HBsAg-positive individuals; persons who have ever injected drugs; persons with multiple sexual partners or a history of sexually transmitted disease; men who have sex with men; inmates of correctional facilities; patients infected with HCV or HIV; patients undergoing renal dialysis; recipients of blood or blood products before 1987; and health care workers.[8]

PATHOBIOLOGY

The HBV genome contains four overlapping open reading frames that encode a number of structural and non-structural viral proteins. The pre-S/S gene encodes the three surface proteins—small (S), middle (M), and large (L)—that express HBsAg. The pre-C/C gene encodes the core protein, that expresses the hepatitis B core (HBc) antigen, and the hepatitis B e (HBe) protein, a secreted non-structural protein that plays a role in immune tolerance to HBV replication. The P gene encodes the HBV polymerase, whose two motifs—a reverse transcriptase motif and an RNAse H motif—code for two enzymes involved in HBV replication. Finally, the X gene encodes the X protein, which is a transactivator involved in HBV replication that bears oncogenic properties. The blood of infected patients contains not only infectious viruses but also a large excess of empty, non-infectious HBV envelopes.

The complex HBV life cycle involves multiple steps: fixation to the sodium taurocholate cotransporting polypeptide, which is the main HBV receptor molecule at the surface of hepatocytes; internalization; fusion and release of the nucleocapsid containing the HBV DNA genome and the associated HBV polymerase molecule in the cell cytoplasm; transport into the nucleus, where decapsidation occurs and the DNA genome molecule is released; transformation of the viral genome by the viral polymerase into a covalently closed circular DNA, which is the episomal form responsible for persistence of the HBV genome in the nucleus of infected hepatocytes; generation of messenger RNAs and viral protein synthesis; generation of a pregenomic RNA, which serves as a template for reverse transcription that generates the long DNA strand; degradation of the pregenomic RNA by the RNAse H activity of the viral polymerase; DNA-dependent DNA polymerase activity of the reverse transcriptase motif, which synthesizes the short complementary DNA strand in newly formed nucleocapsids; and, finally, budding into the endoplasmic reticulum, maturation, and export of newly formed virions.

Ten HBV genotypes (A through J), which differ by approximately 8% of their genomic nucleotide sequence, have different geographic distributions and may be associated with different clinical outcomes. Genotype A predominates in Northern and Western Europe, whereas genotype D is the most frequent genotype in the Mediterranean area and in Eastern Europe. In non-Asian populations in the United States, genotype A predominates in men who have sex with men, whereas genotype D is the most frequent in intravenous drug users. In Asia and in Asian immigrants living in industrialized countries, genotypes B and C predominate. Genotype C has been associated with a higher incidence of severe liver disease and hepatocellular carcinoma compared with genotype B in Asia, perhaps because this genotype spread earlier than the others.

CLINICAL MANIFESTATIONS

Typically, the incubation period is 30-150 days. Jaundice has been reported in up to one third of adult patients with acute hepatitis B, but most cases are unrecognized. Among symptomatic patients (see Table 134-2), the manifestations are similar to those of other causes of acute viral hepatitis.

DIAGNOSIS

Four markers should be sought for the diagnosis of acute hepatitis B: HBsAg, total anti-HBc antibodies, anti-HBc IgM, and anti-HBs antibodies (Table 134-4). Acute hepatitis B is characterized by the simultaneous presence of both HBsAg and anti-HBc IgM (Fig. 134-3). Total anti-HBc antibodies are also present, whereas anti-HBs antibodies are not. During the convalescence phase, patients lose HBsAg before the appearance of anti-HBs antibodies; they have isolated anti-HBc antibodies, and the diagnosis is based on the presence of anti-HBc IgM. Recovery is characterized by the appearance of anti-HBs antibodies. The presence of both total anti-HBc and anti-HBs antibodies characterizes recovery from acute hepatitis B. Anti-HBc IgG remains at high levels for the patient's lifetime, whereas anti-HBs antibody titers may fluctuate and sometimes become undetectable after several years. Quantitative HBsAg assessment may be useful during the course of acute hepatitis B because if the HBsAg level does not rapidly decrease, the patient is at risk for chronic evolution. Patients who remain positive for HBV DNA or HBeAg 6 weeks after the onset of symptoms are likely to develop chronic infection.

TREATMENT

Acute HBV infection usually does not require antiviral therapy, and most patients spontaneously clear the infection. Overall, antiviral therapy does not reduce 1-year mortality.[A1] However, antiviral therapy with a nucleoside or a nucleotide analogue (currently entecavir [0.5mg daily] or tenofovir [tenofovir disoproxil fumarate, 245 mg daily, or tenofovir alafenamide, 25 mg daily] until the signs of severity regress) is recommended in patients with severe acute hepatitis B, characterized by a coagulopathy or persistent symptoms or marked jaundice for more than 4 weeks, to prevent progression to acute liver failure and avoid subsequent liver transplantation or death.[9] Treatment should be initiated before signs of acute liver failure are present. Antiviral therapy does not cause hepatitis B to become a chronic infection.

PREVENTION

Because not everyone has been vaccinated, individuals who are aware that they are infected with HBV should take steps to avoid transmitting the infection to others. This is accomplished by ensuring that their sexual contacts and household members are vaccinated; using barrier protection during sexual intercourse; not sharing instruments such as toothbrushes, razors, and combs; cleaning blood spills with detergent or bleach; and not donating blood, organs, or sperm.

TABLE 134-4 SEROLOGIC PROFILES OBSERVED IN DIFFERENT PHASES OF ACUTE, SELF-RESOLVING HEPATITIS B

PHASE OF INFECTION	HBsAg	ANTI-HBc IgM	TOTAL ANTI-HBc ANTIBODIES	ANTI-HBs ANTIBODIES
Incubation	+	+/−	+/−	−
Acute hepatitis	+	+	+	−
Convalescence	−	+	+	−
Recovery	−	−	+	+

HBc = hepatitis B core; HBs = hepatitis B surface; HBsAg = hepatitis B surface antigen; IgM = immunoglobulin M.

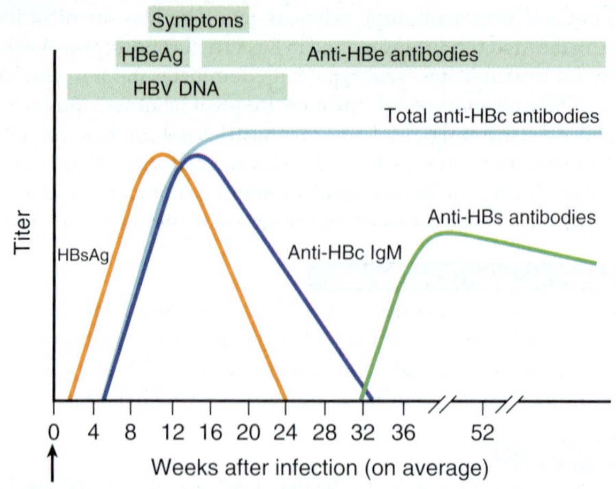

FIGURE 134-3. **Kinetics of hepatitis B virus (HBV) markers during acute self-resolving hepatitis B.** The *arrow* indicates infection. HBc = hepatitis B core; HBeAg = hepatitis B e antigen; HBs = hepatitis B surface; HBsAg = hepatitis B surface antigen; IgM = immunoglobulin M.

Prevention of HBV infection is based on vaccination. Universal infant vaccination programs have been initiated in many countries. High-risk individuals (e.g., health care workers, dialysis patients, family members and sexual partners of HBV carriers, pregnant women, and men who have sex with men) should be screened for HBV infection by HBsAg and anti-HBs antibody testing, and seronegative persons should be vaccinated.[10]

Vaccination consists of the administration of recombinant HBsAg in three injections at 0, 1, and 6 months in adults. A lower dose is given at the same time points in newborns, children, and adolescents. Adults on dialysis require four injections at months 0, 1, 2, and 6. HBV vaccination elicits a potent neutralizing response, characterized by the presence of isolated anti-HBs antibodies at high titers. A titer greater than 10 IU/L is considered protective. The seroconversion rate is higher than 90% in healthy individuals. HBV vaccines are well tolerated. Injection site reactions within 1 to 3 days, as well as mild general reactions, are common and transient. Post-vaccination testing for anti-HBs antibodies to document seroconversion is not routinely recommended. However, persons who remain at risk for HBV infection, such as infants of HBsAg-positive mothers, health care workers, dialysis patients, and sexual partners of HBV carriers, should be tested to determine their response to vaccination.

Of vaccinated persons, 3 to 10% respond poorly or do not respond, especially smokers, obese patients, and elderly individuals. Non-responders should receive another full course of vaccination, often with an increased dose. Other options include intradermal application and the co-administration of adjuvants and cytokines. One third to two thirds of vaccinated individuals lose their anti-HBs antibodies after 10 to 15 years. It is unclear whether these persons are still protected. Thus, persons at risk should receive booster immunization if anti-HBs antibodies have been lost.

When nonimmune persons or vaccinated individuals with an anti-HBs titer below 10 IU/L have contact with HBV-contaminated materials (e.g., needles) or have sexual intercourse with an HBV-infected person, active-passive immunization (i.e., infusion of hepatitis B immunoglobulin) plus active immunization (vaccination) is recommended within 48 hours after exposure. Vaccination alone is sufficient in persons with anti-HBs antibody titers between 10 to 100 IU/L, and no action is required if the anti-HBs titer is above 100 IU/L.

Tenofovir disoproxil fumarate (245 mg orally per day from 24 to 28 weeks of gestation until up to 12 weeks after delivery) can substantially reduce mother-to-child transmission of HBV in mothers with high viral loads (>200,000 IU/mL) or high HBsAg levels (>10,000 IU/mL).[A2] However, this long-standing practice may not be required in settings in which the baby is ensured to be given HBV immune globulin at birth as well as HBV vaccine at birth and at months 1, 2, 4, and 6.[A3]

Infants born to HBsAg-positive mothers must receive hepatitis B immunoglobulin and be vaccinated within 12 hours of birth; this regimen reduces the rate of vertical HBV transmission from 95% to less than 5%. Cesarean section is not needed if active-passive immunization is to be performed. Mothers of vaccinated infants can breast-feed, and breast-feeding is not contraindicated on tenofovir treatment.

PROGNOSIS

Fulminant hepatitis is more frequent in acute HBV infection than in other types of acute viral hepatitis, with an incidence of approximately 0.1%. Factors associated with adverse outcomes of acute hepatitis B include advanced age, female sex, and perhaps some strains of virus. Whether infection with a precore mutant strain is associated with more severe or fulminant disease is still debated.

Among patients infected at birth, the rate of spontaneous recovery after an acute HBV infection is less than 5%, whereas adult infections spontaneously resolve in 95 to 99% of cases. Spontaneous resolution confers lifelong immunity, which is usually characterized by the presence of both anti-HBs antibodies and anti-HBc antibodies. Anti-HBs antibodies may become undetectable several years after resolution, but patients rapidly produce protective antibodies if they are re-exposed to HBV.

ACUTE HEPATITIS C

DEFINITION

The Pathogen

HCV is a member of the Flaviviridae family, genus *Hepacivirus*. The genome is a single-stranded, positive, linear RNA molecule whose 5′ end contains an internal ribosome entry site involved in polyprotein translation; the genome also includes one single open reading frame and a short 3′ noncoding region involved in replication. The genome is contained in a protein capsid or core, which itself is surrounded by a lipid bilayer envelope into which two inserted viral glycoproteins mediate viral entry into target cells.

EPIDEMIOLOGY

HCV is present in all continents, and an estimated 58 million individuals are chronically infected, with about 1.5 million new infections occurring each year. In industrialized countries, the incidence of HCV infection has declined considerably owing to blood screening and measures to prevent viral infections in people who inject drugs. However, approximately 50,000 new cases of acute hepatitis C have been estimated to occur annually in the United States according to the Centers for Disease Control and Prevention, mostly in intravenous drug users. HCV incidence and prevalence are higher in developing areas of the world, where the main route of HCV infection is unsafe medical or surgical procedures; only approximately 50% of blood products are screened for anti-HCV antibodies in these countries, and approximately 40% of all injections are given with reused equipment. Egypt's estimated 7% prevalence in people 19 to 65 years is the highest worldwide, owing to unsafe injection campaigns for the treatment of schistosomiasis in the 1950s to 1960s and subsequent person-to-person transmission. Although the incidence of acute hepatitis C has declined in Egypt during the past 15 years, a substantial number of cases of acute hepatitis are still caused by HCV.

HCV is transmitted almost exclusively by infected blood. Preventive screening with highly sensitive enzyme immunoassays and, in many settings, nucleic acid testing has virtually eliminated the risk for post-transfusion HCV infection (theoretical risk: <1 in 2 million donations in the United States, 1 in 34 million donations in France). As a result, the principal route for HCV transmission in industrialized countries is now drug injection, which is responsible for 60 to 80% of new cases. The incidence of HCV infection in people who inject drugs is as high as 39 per 100 person years. In this context, imprisonment is an important risk factor for acquiring HCV infection in industrialized countries.

Nosocomial transmission through the use of improperly decontaminated materials or the contaminated hands or gloves of health care workers is responsible for a substantial number of new infections worldwide. HCV also can be transmitted by tattooing, piercing, or acupuncture if standard precautions are not implemented. Although HCV can be acquired after accidental needlestick exposure, the risk for infection is low (<1%), and health care workers have only a slightly higher prevalence of HCV than the general population. HCV can be transmitted to household members who share instruments such as scissors, razors, and combs. Sexual transmission is unusual, but outbreaks of acute hepatitis have been reported in communities of men who have high-risk sex with men. The risk for mother-to-infant transmission of HCV is less than 5% and is generally related to exposure to the mother's blood in the perinatal period. Cesarean sections are not recommended, and breast-feeding is not contraindicated (except in the presence of cutaneous nipple lesions). Factors possibly associated with high transmission rates include the level of HCV viremia and maternal intravenous drug use. In 10 to 30% of cases, no apparent risk factor for HCV infection is identifiable, suggesting other potential sources of community-acquired hepatitis C.

PATHOBIOLOGY

Entry of HCV into cells is mediated by several receptor molecules, including glycosaminoglycans, CD81, scavenger receptor B1, claudin-1, and occludin. Entry is followed by fusion. Decapsidation of viral nucleocapsids liberates free genomic RNAs into the cell cytoplasm, where they serve, together with newly synthesized RNAs, as messenger RNAs for synthesis of the HCV polyprotein. The post-translational processing of the HCV polyprotein results in the generation of 10 proteins, including 3 structural proteins (the core protein and the two envelope glycoproteins) and 7 non-structural proteins. HCV replication takes place in the replication complex (or "membranous web") that associates viral proteins, cellular components, and nascent RNA strands. It is catalyzed by the RNA-dependent RNA polymerase. Viral particle formation is initiated by the interaction of the core protein with genomic RNA. Newly produced virus particles leave the host cell via constitutive secretory pathways.

Phylogenetic analyses of HCV strains isolated in various regions of the world have identified eight main HCV genotypes, designated 1 through 8 (with genotypes 1 to 6 being the most prevalent worldwide). These HCV types comprise a large number of subtypes, identified by lowercase letters (1a, 1b, etc.). The genotypes' nucleotide sequences differ by 31 to 34%, and their amino acid sequences differ by approximately 30%; in contrast, the subtypes' nucleotide sequences differ by between 20 and 23%, with marked differences in particular genomic regions. The high prevalence and diversity of HCV genotype 3 and 6 strains in Asia and of genotype 1, 2, 4, and 5 strains in Africa suggest that these types and subtypes emerged and diversified in these regions. In industrialized countries, a small number of HCV genotypes, including 1a, 1b, 2a, 2b, 2c, 3a, and 4a, have been introduced and spread rapidly among exposed populations. Subtypes 1a and 1b predominate all over the world. The most common genotypes in the United States are 1a and 1b (≈75%), 2a, 2b and 3a (15% to 20%), and 4, 5, and 6 (below 5%). Genotype 3a is more prevalent in Western Europe, where it accounts for up to 35% of cases, especially among people who inject drugs. Genotype 4 is highly prevalent in the Middle East and Africa. Its incidence and prevalence are increasing in people who inject drugs in industrialized countries. Genotype 5 is rare outside South Africa, and genotype 6 is rare outside Southeast Asia. Genotype 7 was identified in Central Africa and genotype 8 in Punjab, India. Infections with different genotypes do not differ in terms of the clinical manifestations, progression, or disease severity.

CLINICAL MANIFESTATIONS

HCV RNA becomes detectable in the serum 3 to 7 days after exposure. HCV core antigen becomes detectable 1 to 3 days later. HCV RNA and HCV core antigen levels rise rapidly during the first weeks, followed by serum aminotransferase levels 2 to 8 weeks after exposure. Anti-HCV antibodies arise late in the course of acute hepatitis C and may not be present at the onset of symptoms and serum aminotransferase elevation.

After an incubation period that ranges from 15 to 120 days, acute hepatitis C usually remains asymptomatic and is undiagnosed. Nonspecific symptoms such as fatigue, low-grade fever, myalgias, nausea, vomiting, or itching may be present. Jaundice occurs in only 20 to 30% of patients, usually 2 to 12 weeks after infection. Serum aminotransferase levels commonly exceed 10 times the upper limit of normal in the acute stage, even in the absence of symptoms. Patients who are coinfected with human immunodeficiency virus have more severe acute symptoms.[11] Fulminant hepatitis C has been reported but appears to be exceptional in the absence of another chronic underlying liver disease.

DIAGNOSIS

When acute hepatitis C is suspected, patients should be tested for both anti-HCV antibodies by enzyme immunoassay and HCV RNA with a sensitive molecular biology technique. HCV core antigen detection by means of rapid enzyme immunoassay can be used as an alternative to HCV RNA detection.[12] Four marker profiles can be observed, based on the presence or absence of either marker (Table 134-5). The presence of HCV RNA in the absence of anti-HCV antibodies is strongly indicative of acute HCV infection, which will be confirmed by seroconversion (i.e., the appearance of anti-HCV antibodies) a few days to weeks later. Acutely infected patients can have both HCV RNA and anti-HCV antibodies at the time of diagnosis; in this case, it is difficult to distinguish acute hepatitis C from an acute exacerbation of chronic hepatitis C or acute hepatitis of another cause in a patient with chronic hepatitis C.

Acute hepatitis C is very unlikely if both anti-HCV antibodies and HCV RNA are absent or if anti-HCV antibodies are present without HCV RNA (Fig. 134-4). Patients in the latter group should be retested in a few weeks, however, because HCV RNA may be temporarily undetectable owing to transient, partial control of viral replication before the infection becomes chronic (Fig. 134-5). Apart from such cases, the presence of anti-HCV antibodies in the absence of HCV RNA is generally seen in patients who have recovered from a past HCV infection. Nevertheless, this pattern cannot be differentiated from a false-positive enzyme immunoassay result, the exact prevalence of which is unknown.

TABLE 134-5 PATTERNS OF HEPATITIS C VIRUS (HCV) MARKERS AND THEIR SIGNIFICANCE DURING ACUTE HEPATITIS C

ANTI-HCV ANTIBODIES	HCV RNA	DIAGNOSIS
−	−	Not acute hepatitis C
−	+	Acute hepatitis C
+	−	Probably not acute hepatitis C (retest in a few weeks)
+	+	Difficult to differentiate acute from chronic hepatitis C

HCV = hepatitis C virus.

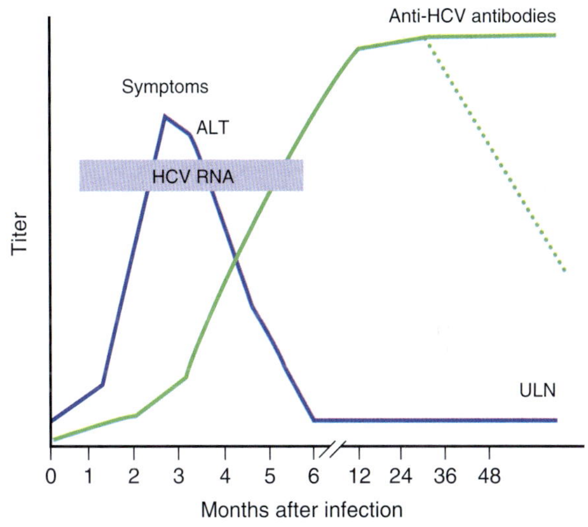

FIGURE 134-4. **Kinetics of hepatitis C virus (HCV) markers during acute self-resolving hepatitis C.** ALT = alanine aminotransferase; ULN = upper limit of normal.

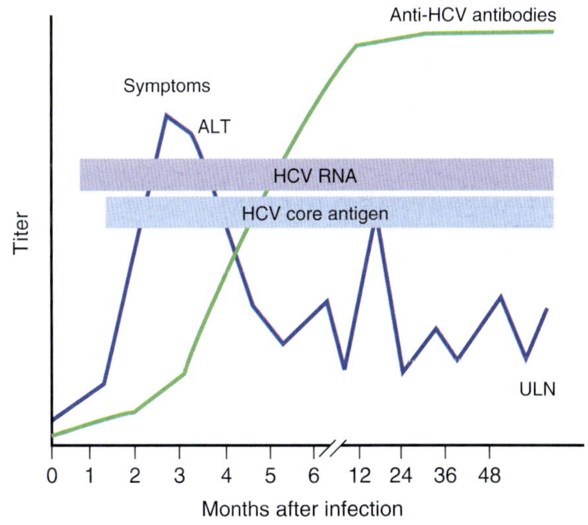

FIGURE 134-5. **Kinetics of hepatitis C virus (HCV) markers during acute hepatitis C that evolves toward chronic infection.** ALT = alanine aminotransferase; ULN = upper limit of normal.

TREATMENT

Treatment of acute hepatitis C should be considered not only because it prevents chronic HCV infection, which can lead to serious clinical sequelae, but also because HCV viremia is associated with a risk for transmitting HCV to other persons, especially in high-risk groups. Although 20 to 50% of patients will spontaneously clear the virus without treatment, immediate treatment is cost-effective and recommended[13] because it provides higher rates of viral clearance, mostly because asymptomatic patients tend to be less adherent with the close follow-up needed to monitor them for the institution of appropriately timed delayed therapy.[14]

Patients with acute hepatitis C should be treated with an all-oral combination of pan-genotypic, direct-acting antiviral drugs for 8 weeks. Options include the fixed-dose, once daily combination of sofosbuvir (400 mg) and velpatasvir (100 mg) or the fixed-dose combination (3 pills in the morning) of glecaprevir (100 mg) and pibrentasvir (40 mg) (see Table 134-5).[15,16] The cure of HCV infection should be assessed by HCV RNA disappearance from serum or plasma at 12 and 24 weeks post-treatment, because late relapses have been reported.

After accidental needlestick exposure, neither immunoglobulin nor post-exposure prophylaxis is recommended. Patients should be monitored with HCV RNA and aminotransferase level testing at baseline, week 2, and 4 and 6 months after exposure. Patients who have documented infection should be treated as described earlier.

PREVENTION

Prevention of HCV transmission is based on standard precautions such as screening of blood and blood products by an enzyme immunoassay for anti-HCV antibodies and/or nucleic acid testing for HCV RNA, application of standard medical and surgical hygiene procedures, and safe use of syringes and materials for drug preparation in people who inject drugs. One-time screening is also recommended for all individuals over age 18 years.[17] Needle exchange programs and education regarding the risks of drug use (including intranasal cocaine) and the risk for transmission from shared injection equipment are important. These interventions combined with effective treatment of chronic hepatitis (Chapter 135) will substantially reduce the risk of acute hepatitis C in the future.[18]

No prophylactic vaccine is or will soon be available against HCV.

PROGNOSIS

Approximately 50 to 80% of patients are unable to clear HCV spontaneously and develop chronic infection. Spontaneous recovery is more frequent if infection is acquired at birth (≈50%) and if acute hepatitis is symptomatic. It is unclear whether the genotype influences recovery rates. Other factors associated with better rates of spontaneous recovery include female sex, early decline of HCV RNA levels, and high aminotransferase or bilirubin levels. Patients who spontaneously recover may retain detectable anti-HCV antibodies for years to decades, but they are not protected against HCV reinfection.

ACUTE HEPATITIS D (DELTA)

DEFINITION

The Pathogen

HDV, which is a satellite of HBV, can be transmitted only to patients who are acutely or chronically infected with HBV. Its single, negative-strand, circular RNA genome of approximately 1700 nucleotides folds in native conditions into a nearly complementary rodlike structure that contains a ribozyme. The HDV genome encodes one single structural protein, the hepatitis D (HD) protein, which expresses HDAg. The 36-nm infectious HDV virion comprises the HD protein and the genome, both enclosed within an HBsAg-expressing coat derived from empty HBV envelopes.

EPIDEMIOLOGY

Pooled data suggest that about 5% of chronic HBV carriers, or approximately 15 million individuals worldwide, are also infected with HDV.[19] The prevalence of HDV infection in HBV-infected patients varies according to the geographic area because it is transmitted primarily through parenteral exposure. As a result, its prevalence in Western countries is 20-fold higher on average in HBsAg-positive individuals who inject drugs than in non–drug users. By comparison, the prevalence of HDV has decreased substantially in southern Europe, probably owing to universal HBV vaccination programs, improvement in hygiene and living conditions, and implementation of standard precautions to prevent HIV infection. The incidence of HDV is increasing in Russia, Eastern Europe, Japan, and India.

PATHOBIOLOGY

HDV uses host RNA polymerase II for its replication, following the rolling circle model. Within cells, HDV RNA is associated with multiple copies of the HD protein to form a ribonucleoprotein complex. This complex is exported by the HBV envelope, which contains the three HBV envelope proteins, into the Golgi apparatus before being secreted.[20]

HDV has eight genotypes (HDV-1 to HDV-8), which differ from one another by at least 20% of their nucleotide sequences. HDV genotypes can be segregated into 2 to 4 sub-genotypes, which differ from one another by at least 10% of their nucleotide sequences. HDV-1 is the most prevalent HDV genotype worldwide, whereas other genotypes have regional geographic distributions.

CLINICAL MANIFESTATIONS

HDV can be acquired at the same time as HBV (coinfection) or by a chronic HBsAg carrier (superinfection). Coinfection is characterized by one or two episodes of acute hepatitis, depending on the respective amounts of HBV and HDV present in the inoculum; acute hepatitis can range from mild to fulminant. In contrast, when chronic HBV carriers are superinfected by HDV, acute hepatitis D is generally severe, often fulminant, and generally becomes chronic.

DIAGNOSIS

Three markers of HDV infection are total anti-HD antibodies, anti-HD IgM, and HDV RNA; the latter can be detected and quantified by real-time PCR. All HBsAg-positive patients should be tested, and the diagnosis of HDV infection is based on the presence of anti-HD antibodies. Chronic HBV carriers with risk factors for HDV superinfection should be tested regularly.

In patients with a self-resolving HBV-HDV coinfection, HDV RNA and anti-HD IgM are only transiently present and are often missed. Anti-HBc IgM indicates concomitant acute HBV infection.

In HDV superinfection of a chronic HBsAg carrier, no anti-HBc IgM is present. HDV RNA is found in serum or plasma before and during the acute episode, whereas both total anti-HD antibodies and anti-HD IgM are present during the acute phase. Anti-HD antibodies and sometimes anti-HD IgM remain at high levels if the disease becomes chronic.

TREATMENT

No treatments are of proven benefit for acute hepatitis D, although several are being actively investigated.[21]

If, however, patients are coinfected with hepatitis B, then treatment of the hepatitis B should be pursued.

PREVENTION

The most effective means of preventing HDV infection is HBV vaccination, because individuals who are protected against HBV cannot be infected with HDV. In chronic HBsAg carriers, standard hygiene and behavioral precautions should be practiced to avoid superinfection with HDV.

PROGNOSIS

In patients who are acutely coinfected with HBV and HDV, only approximately 2% become chronic HDV carriers. In contrast, when HDV infection is acquired by chronic HBV carriers, approximately 90% also become chronic carriers of HDV, and the risk of developing cirrhosis is increased four-fold.[22]

ACUTE HEPATITIS E

DEFINITION

The Pathogen

HEV is a member of the genus *Orthohepevirus* in the Hepeviridae family. HEV is a small, nonenveloped virus. Its genome is a positive sense, single-stranded RNA molecule. Eight HEV genotypes (1 to 8) have been described: genotypes 1 and 2 appear to be strictly human, whereas genotypes 3 to 8 appear to be of animal origin but can also infect humans.

PATHOBIOLOGY AND EPIDEMIOLOGY

HEV transmission is principally fecal-oral. HEV is endemic in most developing areas of the world, where acute infections are sporadic or occur during large epidemics related to the contamination of drinking water. Seroprevalence data suggest that one third of the world's population has been infected with HEV.[23] Every year, an estimated 20 million HEV infections worldwide lead to an estimated 3.3 million symptomatic cases of hepatitis E.

Genotype 1 has been found principally in Asia and North Africa, whereas genotype 2 has been isolated in cases from Central America and Western Africa. No animal reservoir is known for these genotypes, and transmission appears to be linked to the contamination of food or drinking water. In industrialized countries, HEV genotypes 1 and 2 are not present. HEV genotypes 3 and 4 are endemic in various wild and domestic animal species, and zoonotic transmission appears to be the main route of transmission in Europe, the United States, and Asia. Diagnosed cases of acute hepatitis E have increased constantly in Western Europe and North America in recent years, and high HEV seroprevalence has been described in special at-risk populations, such as butchers or farmers. Transmission may be favored by the consumption of uncooked meat and direct contact with infected animals. It is now thought to be the most common cause of acute viral hepatitis worldwide. Additionally, acute HEV may be observed in immunocompromised patients.

CLINICAL MANIFESTATIONS

The incubation period is 3 to 8 weeks. HEV infection causes only mild, nonspecific symptoms in the majority of cases, especially if the infection is acquired early in life. Immunocompetent individuals clear the virus spontaneously. The peak of viremia occurs early during infection, whereas the peak of aminotransferase activity is reached approximately 6 weeks after infection. Severe disease is more frequent in pregnant women and in patients with underlying chronic liver disease, who may rarely progress to fulminant hepatic failure. Some patients with Guillain-Barré syndrome (Chapter 388) have had a preceding acute hepatitis E infection. Chronic infections have been reported in immunosuppressed patients, especially recipients of organ transplants.

DIAGNOSIS

Patients with acute hepatitis should be tested for hepatitis E. Diagnosis of acute hepatitis E is based on the detection of anti-HEV IgM antibodies, which appear within 6 weeks and persist for 3 to 12 months. No assays are yet approved by the U.S. Food and Drug Administration. HEV RNA also can be detected in feces, serum, or plasma, where its presence is transient. Anti-HEV IgG generally persists for life after acute infection.

TREATMENT

Treatment of acute hepatitis E is not recommended because the vast majority of patients recover spontaneously.[24] Severe and fulminant cases should be referred to specialized units, where ribavirin monotherapy can be successful.

PREVENTION

Improving public hygiene and eating well-cooked meat are the best defenses against hepatitis E. Travelers to areas of the world where hygiene standards are low, particularly pregnant women, should be cautioned about drinking the water and eating uncooked food. A prophylactic vaccine based on recombinant HEV proteins has been approved in China, but is not yet available elsewhere. Its efficacy remains 87% at 4.5 years.[A4] Other HEV vaccines are in the developmental phase.

PROGNOSIS

Acute cases can be severe in elderly patients, and fulminant cases are frequent among pregnant women who are infected during large-scale waterborne epidemics. Overall case fatality rates range from zero to 10%, and less than 1% of fatal cases of acute hepatitis in the United States are attributed to hepatitis E. HEV genotypes 3 and 4 are less virulent than genotypes 1 and 2. Sporadic cases in industrialized areas are generally benign. HEV does not commonly evolve into chronic infection, but immunosuppressed patients can become chronic carriers.

OTHER TYPES OF ACUTE VIRAL HEPATITIS

Infection by members of the Herpesviridae family, such as cytomegalovirus (Chapter 347), Epstein-Barr virus (Chapter 348),[25] and herpes simplex virus (Chapter 345), should be considered in the differential diagnosis of unclear episodes of elevated liver enzymes in the absence of markers of acute hepatitis virus infection, especially in immunocompromised individuals. For instance, cytomegalovirus infection can be associated with graft loss after liver transplantation (Chapter 140). Parvovirus B19 (Chapter 342) may persist in the liver and worsen liver disease in patients with chronic hepatitis B and perhaps in patients with chronic HCV infection. Human herpesvirus 6 variant A has been linked with syncytial giant-cell hepatitis. Transient anicteric elevations of aminotransferase levels are often observed in patients with SARS-CoV-2 infection. Human adenovirus infection (Chapter 333) has caused outbreaks of acute hepatitis in children.[26]

NON-A-TO-E HEPATITIS

Rare patients develop acute hepatitis of presumed viral cause but have no markers of known hepatitis viruses. Some of these cases may be due to variants of known hepatitis viruses, in particular HBV, that are not detected by the usual serologic and molecular methods. However, the existence of other, unknown hepatotropic viruses cannot be excluded.

GENERAL REFERENCES

For the General References and other additional features, please visit Elsevier eBooks+ at https://ebooks.health.elsevier.com.

Grade A References

A1. Mantzoukis K, Rodríguez-Perálvarez M, Buzzetti E, et al. Pharmacological interventions for acute hepatitis B infection: an attempted network meta-analysis. *Cochrane Database Syst Rev.* 2017. CD011645.

A2. Pan CQ, Duan Z, Dai E, et al. Tenofovir to prevent hepatitis B transmission in mothers with high viral load. *N Engl J Med.* 2016;374:2324-2334.

A3. Jourdain G, Ngo-Giang-Huong N, Harrison L, et al. Tenofovir versus placebo to prevent perinatal transmission of hepatitis B. *N Engl J Med.* 2018;378:911-923.

A4. Zhang J, Zhang XF, Huang SJ, et al. Long-term efficacy of a hepatitis E vaccine. *N Engl J Med.* 2015;372:914-922.

135 CHRONIC VIRAL AND AUTOIMMUNE HEPATITIS

JEAN-MICHEL PAWLOTSKY

DEFINITION

Chronic hepatitis is defined by chronic necroinflammation of the liver and may be due to various causes, including hepatotropic viruses (Chapter 134), autoimmunity, alcohol (Chapter 138), metabolic disorders (Chapter 132), and other less common factors. Chronic infection by hepatitis viruses is by far the main cause of chronic hepatitis worldwide, with nearly 300 million individuals chronically infected with hepatitis B virus (HBV) and nearly 60 million individuals infected with hepatitis C virus (HCV). Chronic viral hepatitis B and C are the leading causes of cirrhosis (Chapter 139) and hepatocellular carcinoma (Chapter 181) worldwide and account for more than 1 million deaths per year.[1] Chronic HBV infection can be associated with infection by hepatitis D virus (HDV). Hepatitis A virus does not cause chronic hepatitis. Hepatitis E virus (HEV) generally does not cause chronic hepatitis, except in immunosuppressed patients.

CLINICAL MANIFESTATIONS

The clinical symptoms of chronic viral and autoimmune hepatitis are typically nonspecific, and many patients have no symptoms. Fatigue, sleep disorders, and right upper quadrant pain may be present. Often the diagnosis is made when liver test abnormalities are identified by blood testing during a routine health evaluation or assessment for an unrelated problem or at the time of voluntary blood donation. More advanced symptoms include poor appetite, nausea, weight loss, muscle weakness, itching, dark urine, and jaundice. Patients can progress to full-blown cirrhosis (Chapter 139), with its typical clinical manifestations. If cirrhosis is present, weakness, weight loss, abdominal swelling, edema, bruisability, gastrointestinal bleeding, and hepatic encephalopathy with mental confusion may arise. Other findings may include spider angiomas, palmar erythema (see Fig. 132-2), ascites (see Fig. 132-4), edema, and skin excoriations.

DIAGNOSIS

Levels of alanine aminotransferase (ALT) and aspartate aminotransferase (AST) are usually elevated (generally two to five times the upper limit of normal), but they can remain within the normal range for long periods of time in patients with chronic viral hepatitis B or C. The ALT level is generally higher than the AST level. Both can reach 10 to 25 times the upper limit of normal during acute exacerbations. Biologic tests can establish the etiologic diagnosis (Table 135-1).

Alkaline phosphatase and γ-glutamyl transpeptidase levels are usually minimally elevated unless cirrhosis is present. Serum bilirubin and albumin levels and the prothrombin time are normal unless the patient has advanced cirrhosis. Serum immunoglobulin levels are mildly elevated or normal in chronic viral hepatitis but may be very elevated in autoimmune hepatitis. Results that suggest the presence of advanced fibrosis are a platelet count below 160,000, AST levels higher than ALT levels, elevation in serum bilirubin, decrease in serum albumin, prolongation of the prothrombin time, elevation in α-fetoprotein levels, and presence of high globulin levels.

Liver ultrasound can determine the texture and size of the liver and spleen, exclude hepatic masses, and assess the gallbladder, intrahepatic bile ducts, and portal venous flow. Computed tomography and magnetic resonance imaging of the liver are helpful if a mass or other abnormality is found by ultrasound.

Liver biopsy has been critical for diagnosis and to determine the severity of disease. Hepatocellular necrosis is typically eosinophilic degeneration or ballooning degeneration throughout the parenchyma, greater in the periportal area, spotty, or piecemeal. Fibrosis also typically begins in the periportal regions and can link adjacent portal areas or portal and central areas (bridging fibrosis), distort the hepatic architecture, and lead to cirrhosis and portal hypertension. The histologic grade of chronic hepatitis can be determined by combining scores for periportal necrosis and inflammation, lobular necrosis and inflammation, and portal inflammation.

Recently, noninvasive physical methods (such as hepatic transient elastography or acoustic radiation force impulse imaging) and serologic markers have proved accurate for the assessment of mild fibrosis and cirrhosis, without requiring liver biopsy, in patients with chronic hepatitis B and C. However, these tests are less accurate for distinguishing moderate or advanced fibrosis, and their results may be influenced by ongoing liver inflammation, so liver biopsy remains the reference method in chronic hepatitis of nonviral causes. For example, liver biopsy can help exclude other causes of chronic hepatitis, including alcoholic liver disease, fatty liver and steatohepatitis (Chapter 138), drug-induced liver disease (Chapter 136), sclerosing cholangitis (Chapter 141), iron overload (Chapter 196), and veno-occlusive disease (Chapter 129), each of which can coexist with viral or autoimmune hepatitis.

TREATMENT AND PROGNOSIS

Chronic HBV infection is not curable, but it usually can be controlled by appropriate antiviral drugs. HCV infection is curable, and more than 95% of treated patients are cured. Autoimmune hepatitis responds to immunosuppression with corticosteroids and azathioprine.

TABLE 135-1 ETIOLOGIC DIAGNOSIS OF CHRONIC HEPATITIS

DIAGNOSIS	SCREENING TESTS	CONFIRMATORY TESTS
Chronic hepatitis B	HBsAg	HBV DNA
Chronic hepatitis C	Anti-HCV antibodies	HCV RNA
Chronic hepatitis D	Anti-HDV antibodies	HDV RNA
Autoimmune hepatitis	Auto-antibodies (ANA; anti-SMA; anti-LKM1; anti-LC1; anti-SLA/LP)	Exclusion of other causes and patterns of clinical disease
Drug-induced liver disease	History	Rechallenge, if necessary, if considered safe
Wilson disease	Ceruloplasmin	Urine copper concentration
Cryptogenic hepatitis	Exclusion of other causes	

ANA = antinuclear antibody; anti-LC1 = anti–liver cytosol type 1; anti-LKM1 = anti–liver-kidney microsomal 1 antibody; anti-SLA/LP = anti–soluble liver antigen/liver pancreas antibodies; anti-SMA = anti–smooth muscle actin; HBsAg = hepatitis B surface antigen; HBV = hepatitis B virus; HCV = hepatitis C virus; HDV = hepatitis D virus.

CHRONIC HEPATITIS B

EPIDEMIOLOGY

Approximately 300 million individuals, or 4% of the world's population, are carriers of chronic HBV.[2] Two billion individuals, or one human being in three, have been in contact with the virus. In North America, Western and Northern Europe, and Australia, less than 2% of the population are chronic hepatitis B surface antigen (HBsAg) carriers. In the United States, the prevalence is approximately 0.3%, so approximately 860,000 Americans are infected. In Eastern Europe, South America, the Mediterranean basin, and the Indian subcontinent, the prevalence of chronic HBsAg carriage is between 2 and 8%. Highly endemic areas, with a rate of chronic HBsAg carriage exceeding 8%, include China, Southeast Asia, sub-Saharan Africa, and the native populations of the Far North of America.

HBV is the main cause of primary liver cancer (hepatocellular carcinoma; Chapter 181) worldwide, with approximately 350,000 new cases attributable to HBV every year. Hepatocellular carcinoma is more likely in the presence of underlying cirrhosis, but HBV has oncogenic properties of its own, and hepatocellular carcinoma can occur in noncirrhotic HBV patients.

PATHOBIOLOGY

HBV is not a cytopathic virus. Rather, liver injury in chronic hepatitis B is a consequence of the local immune response at the immune elimination phase. In particular, liver injury is related to cytotoxic T cells that recognize and kill infected hepatocytes that express HBV antigens at their surface and to the local production of cytokines. Chronic inflammation triggers fibrogenesis through the activation of hepatic stellate cells. The hepatitis B X protein may also directly activate fibrogenesis. As a result, many patients with chronic hepatitis B have progressive fibrosis, which may evolve into cirrhosis.

The rate of chronicity after an acute HBV infection is more than 95% among infants infected at birth. This risk diminishes as the age at acquisition increases, and it is less than 5% in individuals infected as adults. Chronic HBV infection is defined by HBsAg carriage that persists for more than 6 months after the acute episode. Chronic HBsAg carriage typically evolves through three phases: immune tolerant, immune elimination, and inactive.

The immune tolerant phase is generally short if the infection occurred during adulthood, but it persists for years to decades in patients infected at birth or during early childhood. At the immune tolerant stage, the immune response of the host "tolerates" HBV infection and does not cause liver inflammation or hepatocyte destruction. The immune tolerant phase is characterized by the presence of hepatitis B e antigen (HBeAg), very high levels of HBV DNA in blood, normal serum or plasma aminotransferase levels, and no or minimal inflammatory activity on liver biopsy. However, these patients have detectable immune responses against HBV antigens, their liver histology is not strictly normal, and they display a high level of HBV DNA integration and clonal hepatocyte expansion, indicating that hepatocarcinogenesis is already underway.

The immune elimination phase is characterized by an active immune response that causes necroinflammatory lesions and triggers hepatic fibrogenesis and progressive fibrosis. ALT and AST levels are increased, but HBV DNA levels are lower than during the immune tolerant phase and frequently fluctuate. The immune elimination phase has a variable duration, ranging from a few weeks to several decades. HBeAg, when present, defines HBeAg-positive chronic hepatitis B. HBeAg can be cleared and replaced by anti-HBe antibodies, defined as HBe seroconversion. HBe seroconversion may lead to the persistence of HBV replication and chronic inflammation, defined as HBeAg-negative chronic hepatitis B, or to the inactive HBsAg carrier state. Patients with HBeAg-positive chronic hepatitis B are infected with a wild-type virus and are able to secrete the HBe protein. Patients with HBeAg-negative chronic hepatitis B are infected with so-called precore mutant viruses, which cannot produce the HBe protein because they have a stop codon in the pre-C gene, or with core promoter mutant viruses, which produce considerably lower amounts of HBe protein. Because of the prevalence of the HBV genotype D in Euro-Mediterranean and African countries, HBeAg-negative/anti–HBe-positive chronic hepatitis B is seven to nine times more frequent than HBeAg-positive disease in those locations.

The inactive HBsAg carriage phase is the result of successful immune elimination leading to HBe seroconversion. ALT and AST levels are normal, HBV DNA is undetectable or at very low levels, and patients without preexisting cirrhosis have normal liver histology.

CLINICAL MANIFESTATIONS

Patients with chronic hepatitis B are generally asymptomatic. The most common symptom is fatigue, but sleep disorders, difficulty concentrating, and upper

TABLE 135-2 VIROLOGIC MARKER PROFILES IN PATIENTS WITH CHRONIC HEPATITIS B VIRUS INFECTION

	HBsAg	ANTI-HBs Ab	HBeAg	ANTI-HBe Ab	ANTI-HBc Ab IgM	ANTI-HBc Ab TOTAL	HBV DNA
Chronic hepatitis							
HBeAg-positive	+	–	+	–	–*	+	≥2 × 10^4 IU/mL
HBeAg-negative	+	–	–	+	–*	+	≥2 × 10^3 IU/mL
Inactive carrier	+	–	–	+	–	+	<2 × 10^3 IU/mL
Reactivation	+	–	+/–	+/–	+/–	+	≥2 × 10^3 IU/mL

*Anti-HBc IgM can be detected at low titers.
Ab = antibodies; Ag = antigen; HBc = hepatitis B core; HBe = hepatitis B e; HBs = hepatitis B surface; HBV = hepatitis B virus; IgM = immunoglobulin M.

right quadrant pain are often observed. Chronic hepatitis B is characterized biologically by elevated aminotransferase levels, and ALT levels can fluctuate substantially during the immune elimination phase. Moderate cholestasis, with mildly elevated alkaline phosphatase and γ-glutamyl transpeptidase levels, also can be present, especially in patients with cirrhosis.

HBeAg-negative chronic hepatitis B is generally more severe than the HBeAg-positive variety. The incidence of spontaneous HBe seroconversion among HBeAg-positive patients is 8 to 12% per year when they are in the immune elimination phase; HBe seroconversion often follows a transient ALT flare. Some of these patients evolve toward inactive HBsAg carriage, whereas others switch into an HBeAg-negative form of chronic hepatitis B, with elevated ALT levels and an HBV DNA level greater than 2000 IU/mL.

The annual incidence of cirrhosis varies from 2 to 10% in patients with chronic HBV infection, with a cumulative incidence of approximately 20% at 5 years. The risk for cirrhosis is two- to four-fold higher in HBeAg-negative patients compared with HBeAg-positive ones. The annual incidence of hepatocellular carcinoma in patients with chronic hepatitis B varies from 1% in patients without cirrhosis to 2 to 8% in cirrhotic patients, with the higher rates occurring in older patients. Patients with cirrhosis (Chapter 139), hepatocellular carcinoma (Chapter 181), or both have the typical signs associated with these conditions. Rarely, chronic HBV infection is associated with extrahepatic manifestations, including glomerulonephritis (Chapter 107), most often in children, and polyarteritis nodosa (Chapter 249), mostly in adults.

DIAGNOSIS

Serologic markers used to diagnose chronic hepatitis B (Table 135-2) include HBsAg, anti-HBs antibodies, total anti–hepatitis B core (HBc) antibodies and anti-HBc immunoglobulin M (IgM), HBeAg, and anti-HBe antibodies. Molecular markers include HBV DNA; real-time polymerase chain reaction (PCR)–based or transcription-mediated amplification (TMA)–based assays are the best way to detect and quantify HBV DNA.[3]

Chronic HBV infection is defined by the persistence of HBsAg in the serum for more than 6 months after the acute episode. The majority of subjects with isolated anti-HBc antibodies are not viremic. However, some individuals who test positive for anti-HBc antibodies, but not for HBsAg or anti-HBs antibodies, may be viremic; in these cases, some viruses' amino acid substitutions in the HBsAg sequence make HBsAg undetectable with current enzyme immunoassays. Other individuals may have such low-level HBV replication in their livers that HBV DNA is not detectable in blood ("occult" hepatitis B). Screening is recommended periodically in high-risk individuals and once (together with HCV and HIV testing) in all adults.[A1]

Serum or plasma ALT and HBV DNA levels are important markers of severity and prognosis. The assessment of severity, including the grade of necroinflammation and the stage of fibrosis, has traditionally been based on the liver biopsy (Fig. 135-1), but serologic markers, transient elastography, or acoustic radiation force impulse imaging have replaced liver biopsy in the pretreatment assessment of the severity of chronic hepatitis B in most patients.

PREVENTION AND TREATMENT

Patients with chronic hepatitis B should be vaccinated against hepatitis A virus, abstain from alcohol, and avoid immunosuppressive therapies unless absolutely necessary. HBV-infected patients who require corticosteroids, rituximab, or other chemotherapy for other conditions should receive entecavir 0.5 mg/day, tenofovir disoproxil fumarate 245 mg/day, or tenofovir alafenamide 25 mg/day during therapy and for 12 months after its cessation as prophylaxis against reactivation of hepatitis B.

The goals of chronic hepatitis B therapy are to suppress HBV replication, reduce the histologic activity of chronic hepatitis, and lessen the risk for cirrhosis and hepatocellular carcinoma.[4,5] HBV infection cannot be completely eradicated because of the persistence of covalently closed circular DNA (cccDNA) in the nucleus of infected hepatocytes. As a result, therapy attempts to reduce HBV DNA levels as much as possible—ideally, below the limit of detection of real-time PCR or TMA assays (10 to 15 IU/mL)—to ensure a degree of viral suppression that will lead to biochemical remission, histologic improvement, and prevention of complications.

Two different types of drugs for the treatment of chronic hepatitis B are pegylated interferon-α (IFN-α) and nucleoside/nucleotide analogues. Pegylated IFN-α2a, administered subcutaneously at a dose of 180 μg/week for 48 weeks, improves various markers of HBV infection in both HBeAg-positive (Table 135-3) and HBeAg-negative (Table 135-4) patients. The most frequent side effects of IFN-α are flulike symptoms after the injections, fatigue, anorexia, weight loss, and alopecia. The most concerning side effects are neutropenia, thrombocytopenia, anxiety, irritability, depression, and suicidal ideation.

Nucleoside analogues (e.g., entecavir) require triple phosphorylation to be active, whereas nucleotide analogues (e.g., tenofovir) need only two phosphorylations to be active. These drugs are given orally (PO) once daily at the following dosages: 0.5 mg for entecavir, 245 mg for tenofovir administered as the pro-drug tenofovir disoproxil fumarate, or 25 mg for tenofovir administered as the prodrug tenofovir alafenamide. All have short-term benefits on various markers of HBV infection in HBeAg-positive (see Table 135-3) and HBeAg-negative (see Table 135-4) patients. Entecavir and tenofovir are used because they are the most potent inhibitors of HBV replication,[A2,A3] and they are the least likely to select for resistant HBV variants. These drugs are generally well tolerated. Renal impairment and decreases in mineral bone density are rarely seen with tenofovir disoproxil fumarate; these side effects are not observed with tenofovir alafenamide because the active compound is concentrated in the liver.

Patients should be considered for treatment when their HBV DNA levels are greater than 2000 IU/mL and/or their serum ALT levels are abnormal if noninvasive assessment or liver biopsy shows moderate to severe active necroinflammation, fibrosis, or both. Patients with an HBV DNA level above 20,000 IU/mL and ALT above 2 times the upper limit of normal should be treated regardless of the degree of fibrosis. Indications for treatment must also consider the patient's age and health status, as well as the availability of antiviral agents in individual countries. Patients in the immune tolerant phase and those with mild hepatitis on liver biopsy or noninvasive markers should not be treated, but follow-up ALT levels and HBV DNA assays are mandatory. Patients with compensated cirrhosis and detectable HBV DNA should be treated even if their ALT levels are normal, their HBV DNA levels are below 2000 IU/mL, or both. Patients with decompensated cirrhosis require urgent antiviral treatment.

Two treatment strategies can be considered: a 48-week course of pegylated IFN-α or long-term oral treatment with nucleoside/nucleotide analogues. Their combined use does not seem to improve the rate of sustained virologic response after treatment.

Pegylated IFN-α can provide a sustained virologic response, defined as a sustained HBe seroconversion (clearance of HBeAg, which is replaced by anti-HBe antibodies) and an HBV DNA level that remains below 2000 IU/mL after a 48-week course of treatment; an ALT flare can be observed at the time of HBeAg loss in patients in whom treatment is successful. Pegylated IFN-α treatment can be considered as an initial treatment option in patients with mild to moderate HBeAg-positive or -negative chronic hepatitis B. Practically, it should be reserved for patients with the best chance of a sustained virologic response off treatment—HBeAg-positive patients with high baseline ALT levels (more than three times the upper limit of normal) and HBV DNA levels below 2 × 10^6 IU/mL. Pegylated IFN-α therapy is contraindicated in patients with advanced cirrhosis and in immunosuppressed patients. Patients infected with HBV genotypes A and B generally respond better to IFN-α therapy than do patients infected with genotypes C and D, but the predictive value of the HBV genotype for an individual patient is weak. Patients who fail to achieve a sustained virologic response after a single course of pegylated IFN-α are candidates for nucleoside/nucleotide analogue therapy.

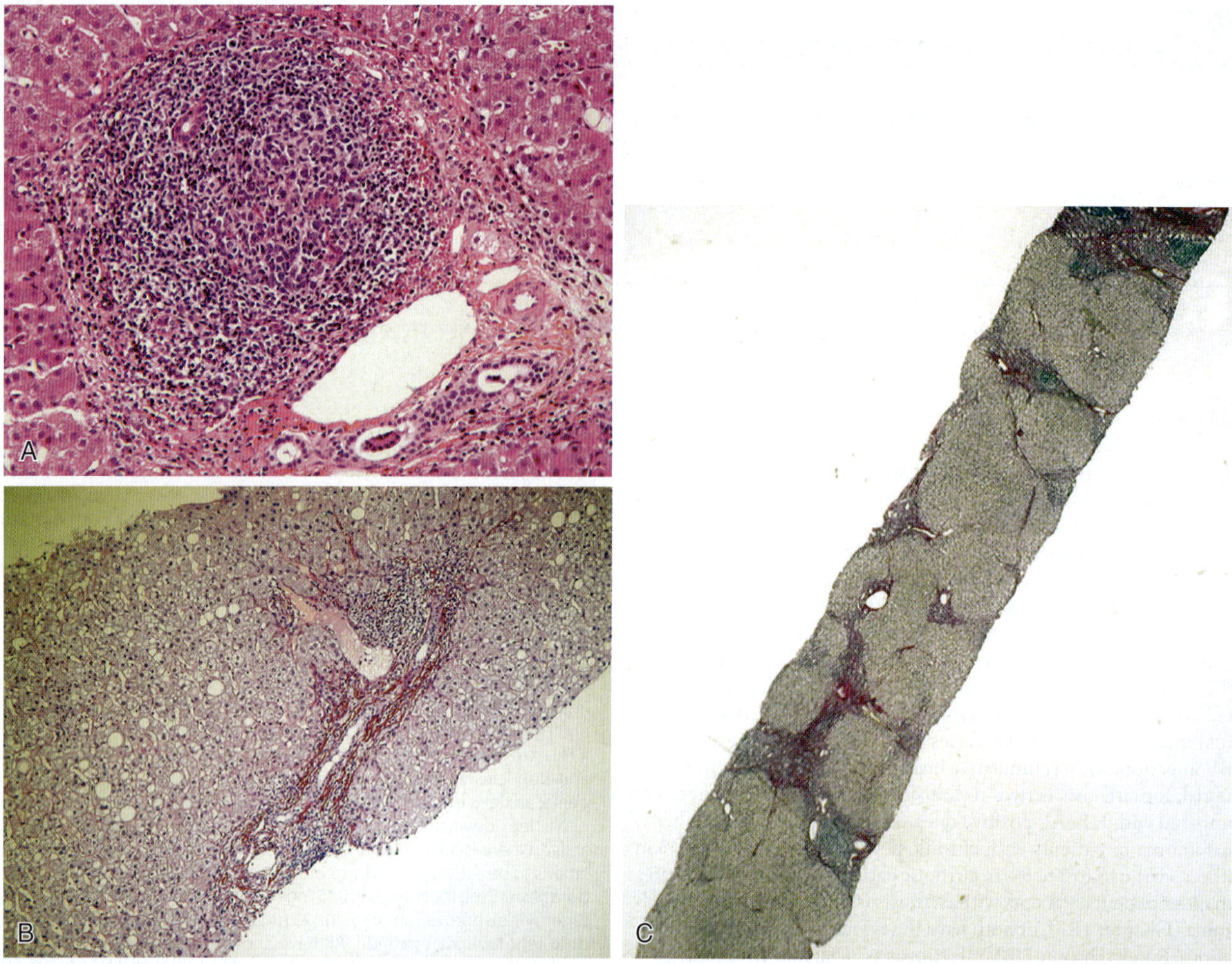

FIGURE 135-1. **Liver biopsies in patients with chronic hepatitis C. A,** Lymphoid nodule with germinal center; minimal interface hepatitis (hematein-eosin, magnification 200×). **B,** Mild fibrosis, Metavir score F1 (picrosirius-hemalun, magnification 100×). **C,** Extensive fibrosis, Metavir score F3 (picrosirius-hemalun, magnification 20×). (Courtesy Prof. Elie-Serge Zafrani, Department of Pathology, Henri Mondor Hospital, Créteil, France.)

Long-term treatment with nucleoside/nucleotide analogues is indicated in the majority of patients with chronic hepatitis B. Tenofovir (available as tenofovir disoproxil fumarate or liver-targeted tenofovir alafenamide) or entecavir, which are the most potent drugs with an optimal resistance profile, are recommended as first-line monotherapies. Entecavir or tenofovir alafenamide should be selected over tenofovir disoproxil fumarate in patients >60 years old, patients with bone disease (chronic steroid use or use of other medications that worsen bone density, history of fragility fracture, osteoporosis) and patients with renal alteration (eGFR <60 mL/min/1.73 m^2, albuminuria >30 mg/24 hour or moderate dipstick proteinuria, low phosphate <2.5 mg/dL, dialysis). HBV DNA should be suppressed to undetectable levels (<10 to 15 IU/mL) with a sensitive real-time PCR-based or TMA-based assay. If the HBV DNA level is reduced but still detectable in a compliant patient, the other agent may be added; however, the long-term safety of combined tenofovir and entecavir is unknown. When HBeAg-positive patients seroconvert to anti-HBe antibody-positive or HBeAg-negative patients lose their HBsAg (with or without anti-HBs seroconversion), treatment should be continued for at least an additional 12 months. In all other cases, treatment should be continued for life and adherence is particularly important.

Virologic breakthroughs—defined by a subsequent increase of the HBV DNA level of 1 log or more above the nadir level—in patients receiving entecavir or tenofovir are exclusively a result of nonadherence. Virologic breakthrough is generally followed a few weeks later by a biochemical breakthrough in which a previously normal ALT level rises above normal. In a patient who develops resistance to any nucleoside/nucleotide analogue other than entecavir or tenofovir, switching to tenofovir (either tenofovir disoproxil fumarate or tenofovir alafenamide) and possibly adding entecavir are the only efficient strategies, although the long-term safety of the combination of tenofovir and entecavir is not known. In patients with lamivudine, telbivudine, or entecavir resistance, treatment should be switched to tenofovir. Patients who have resistance to adefovir should be switched to tenofovir, and entecavir should be added if HBV DNA plateaus. Patients with multidrug resistance should receive the combination of tenofovir and entecavir. The combination of tenofovir and emtricitabine, a nucleoside analogue similar to lamivudine, in a single tablet (approved for HIV but not for HBV therapy) is also a valid option in cases of resistance to any of these drugs.

In patients with cirrhosis, nucleoside/nucleotide analogue therapy is the only option. In patients with decompensated disease, efficient antiviral treatment with entecavir or tenofovir most often stabilizes the patient's condition and can also delay or obviate the need for liver transplantation. If transplantation is needed, post-transplant administration of anti-HBV immunoglobulins in combination with entecavir or tenofovir prevents recurrent HBV in the vast majority of cases. Patients with a low risk of recurrence can discontinue anti-HBV immunoglobulins but should continue monoprophylaxis with entecavir or tenofovir.

PROGNOSIS

Every year, approximately 0.5% of inactive HBsAg carriers spontaneously lose HBsAg, and most of them acquire anti-HBs antibodies. Reactivations are possible in inactive HBV carriers, especially if they become immunosuppressed, such as when they are treated for other conditions with corticosteroids, rituximab, or other chemotherapeutic agents. HBV reactivations often evolve into a subfulminant or fulminant form.

The risk of cirrhosis (Chapter 139) in chronic hepatitis B is 2 to 10% per year, and it is significantly associated with a higher HBV DNA level, older age, alcohol consumption, coinfection with other hepatotropic viruses, and coinfection with human immunodeficiency virus (HIV). The cumulative incidence of liver decompensation is about 15 to 20% at 5 years in patients with compensated cirrhosis. The complications of cirrhosis, including hepatocellular carcinoma, are among the main causes of mortality in HBV-infected patients, and the annual incidence of death is about 3 to 4%. In patients who are treated with long-term entecavir/tenofovir, however, 8-year survival is now similar to the general population.[6] The likelihood of developing hepatocellular carcinoma (Chapter 181) is approximately 1% per year in patients without cirrhosis and

TABLE 135-3 RESULTS OF MAJOR STUDIES FOR THE TREATMENT OF HBeAg-POSITIVE CHRONIC HEPATITIS B AT 6 MONTHS FOLLOWING 48 OR 52 WEEKS OF PEGYLATED IFN-α (PEGIFN-α) AND AT 48 OR 52 WEEKS OF NUCLEOSIDE/NUCLEOTIDE ANALOGUE THERAPY

		PegIFN-α	*NUCLEOSIDE/NUCLEOTIDE ANALOGUE*		
	PLACEBO/CONTROL GROUPS	*PegIFN-α2a* 180 µg ONCE WEEKLY	ENTECAVIR 0.5 mg DAILY	TENOFOVIR DISOPROXIL FUMARATE 245 mg DAILY	TENOFOVIR ALAFENAMIDE 25 mg DAILY
HBe seroconversion	4-6%	32%	21%	21%	10%
HBV DNA <60-80 IU/mL	0-17%*	14%	67%	76%	64%‡
ALT normalization†	7-24%	41%	68%	68%	72%
HBsAg loss	0-1%	3%	2%	3%	1%

*HBV DNA levels were assessed with various molecular assays, with different lower limits of detection.
†The definition of ALT normalization varied among different trials.
‡The lower limit of HBV DNA detection/quantification was different across studies (<29 IU/mL for tenofovir alafenamide studies).
Ag = antigen; ALT = alanine aminotransferase; HBe = hepatitis B e; HBs = hepatitis B surface; HBV = hepatitis B virus; IFN = interferon.
Modified from: EASL 2017 clinical practice guidelines on the management of hepatitis B virus infection. *J Hepatol.* 2017;67:370-398.

TABLE 135-4 RESULTS OF MAJOR STUDIES FOR THE TREATMENT OF HBeAg-NEGATIVE CHRONIC HEPATITIS B AT 6 MONTHS FOLLOWING 48 WEEKS OF PEGYLATED IFN-α (PEGIFN-α) AND AT 48 OR 52 WEEKS OF NUCLEOSIDE/NUCLEOTIDE ANALOGUE THERAPY

		PegIFN-α	*NUCLEOSIDE/NUCLEOTIDE ANALOGUE*		
	PLACEBO/CONTROL GROUPS	PegIFN-α2a 180 µg ONCE WEEKLY	ENTECAVIR 0.5 mg DAILY	TENOFOVIR DISOPROXIL FUMARATE 245 mg DAILY	TENOFOVIR ALAFENAMIDE 25 mg DAILY
HBV DNA <60-80 IU/mL	0-20%*	19%	90%	93%	94%‡
ALT normalization†	10-29%	59%	78%	76%	83%
HBsAg loss	0%	4%	0%	0%	0%

*HBV DNA levels were assessed with various molecular assays, with different lower limits of detection.
†The definition of ALT normalization varied among different trials.
‡The lower limit of HBV DNA detection/quantification was different across studies (<29 IU/mL for tenofovir alafenamide studies).
Ag = antigen; ALT = alanine aminotransferase; HBe = hepatitis B e; HBs = hepatitis B surface; HBV = hepatitis B virus; IFN = interferon.
Modified from: EASL 2017 clinical practice guidelines on the management of hepatitis B virus infection. *J Hepatol.* 2017;67:370-398.

2 to 8% per year in patients with cirrhosis, and it is significantly associated with a higher HBV DNA level, male sex, old age, a family history of hepatocellular carcinoma, reversion from anti-HBe–positive to HBeAg-positive, and coinfection with other hepatotropic viruses. HBV carriers who have cirrhosis or who are at risk for hepatocellular carcinoma should be screened every 6 to 12 months with an ultrasound examination and an α-fetoprotein level.

Liver histology, including necroinflammation and fibrosis, improves in patients who have chronic hepatitis B, who are on long-term nucleoside/nucleotide analogue therapy, and who maintain low/undetectable HBV DNA levels. In addition, the risks of developing cirrhosis, of decompensation of cirrhosis, and of hepatocellular carcinoma are significantly reduced but not eliminated as compared with untreated patients, especially patients who already have cirrhosis or have a family history of hepatocellular carcinoma.

CHRONIC HEPATITIS C

EPIDEMIOLOGY

HCV, which is present on all continents, is estimated to cause chronic infection in approximately 58 million individuals. The prevalence of chronic HCV infection, which varies geographically, is estimated to be about 0.7% in the United States (affecting 2.4 million individuals), 0.5% in the Americas overall, 1.3% in Europe, 0.5% in Southeast Asia, 0.9% in Africa, and 0.5% in the Western Pacific region. The highest prevalence is in Egypt (9% overall, but up to 40% in certain rural areas), where infection was initially spread by intramuscular injections for schistosomiasis during treatment campaigns several decades ago. Hepatitis C virus still causes more deaths in the United States than does HIV, largely because most cases remain undiagnosed, and it causes approximately 290,000 deaths per year worldwide.

PATHOBIOLOGY

Acute HCV infection evolves into chronic infection in 50 to 80% of cases depending on the age at acquisition (children versus adults, respectively). Even patients who spontaneously recover and maintain detectable anti-HCV antibodies are not protected against reinfection. Persistence of infection is related to a qualitatively and quantitatively altered CD4+ T-helper cell and cytotoxic T lymphocyte response that fails to eradicate infection. The plasticity of the viral genomes is responsible for the coexistence of closely related but genetically different viral populations in equilibrium in the patient's replicative environment. This genetic diversity allows continuously generated variant viral populations to be selected by timely changes in the replicative environment.

Chronic HCV infection is responsible for necroinflammatory lesions of varying severity, sometimes associated with steatosis, which is the accumulation of triglycerides in hepatocytes. HCV is not a cytopathic virus. Liver injury in chronic hepatitis C is related to the action of immune effectors that recognize and kill infected hepatocytes that express HCV antigens at their surface and the local production of various cytokines and chemokines. Chronic inflammation triggers fibrogenesis through the activation of hepatic stellate cells. Fibrosis progresses at nonlinear rates that are generally faster in older patients, in males, and in the presence of chronic alcohol intake, viral coinfections, or immunosuppression. The severity of chronic hepatitis is independent of the HCV RNA level and of the HCV genotype. This chronic inflammation and progression of fibrosis predispose patients to cirrhosis (Chapter 139), which is present in approximately 20% of HCV-infected patients, and hepatocellular carcinoma (Chapter 181), which occurs at an incidence rate of 1 to 5% per year in patients with cirrhosis.

CLINICAL MANIFESTATIONS

Acute hepatitis C (Chapter 134) is most often asymptomatic and therefore undiagnosed. The most common symptom associated with chronic HCV infection is fatigue, but it may remain inapparent for years. ALT levels are usually moderately elevated and fluctuate, but they can remain normal for weeks to months despite active hepatitis on liver biopsy. Moderate cholestasis can be present in patients with cirrhosis. Patients with cirrhosis (Chapter 139), hepatocellular carcinoma (Chapter 181), or both have the typical signs associated with these conditions.

HCV is the main cause of type II and type III mixed cryoglobulinemia (Chapter 173). Low levels of circulating cryoglobulins, which contain HCV RNA, anti-HCV antibodies, rheumatoid factor, and low levels of complement, can be found in 50 to 70% of cases, whereas elevated rheumatoid factor (Chapter 243) is found in 70% of cases. Fewer than 1% of HCV-infected patients develop symptoms of cryoglobulinemic vasculitis (Chapter 249), including fatigue, myalgias, arthralgias, rash (purpura, hives, leukocytoclastic vasculitis), neuropathy, and membranoproliferative glomerulonephritis.[7] Cryoglobulinemia can be severe and lead to end-stage renal disease or severe neuropathies, and long-term cryoglobulinemia has been linked to non–Hodgkin B-cell lymphomas (Chapter 171).

Low titers of antinuclear and anti–smooth muscle antibodies can be found in HCV-infected patients, but they do not have any clinical significance. HCV has been reported to trigger the symptoms of porphyria cutanea tarda (Chapter 194), and an association with lichen planus (Chapter 405) has been suggested.

DIAGNOSIS

Chronic HCV infection is defined by the persistence of HCV RNA for more than 6 months. Chronic hepatitis C is diagnosed by the simultaneous presence of anti-HCV antibodies and HCV RNA (or HCV core antigen where available). Detectable HCV replication in the absence of anti-HCV antibodies is observed almost exclusively in patients who are profoundly immunosuppressed, on hemodialysis, or agammaglobulinemic.

The strategy for HCV screening varies in different areas according to the local prevalence. In the United States, screening for HCV is recommended once between the ages of 18 and 79 years for everyone. HCV screening is based upon detecting anti-HCV antibodies in a centralized laboratory. However, tests performed at the patient's care site, such as rapid diagnostic tests using fingerstick whole blood or saliva (or fingerstick whole blood sampled on dried blood spots), can improve access to screening and linkage to care. Confirmation of infection is based upon the detection of HCV RNA by a molecular method, or alternatively, HCV core antigen by enzyme immunoassay. Reflex testing (HCV RNA confirmation on the same sample as was used to detect anti-HCV antibody) is recommended to improve linkage-to-care. The level of HCV replication does not correlate with the severity of liver disease or with the risk for progression to cirrhosis or hepatocellular carcinoma.

Determination of the HCV genotype is no longer recommended. Laboratory testing often reveals high levels of monoclonal rheumatoid factor and cryoglobulins.

TREATMENT

Chronic HCV infection is curable by antiviral therapy. The goal of therapy is to achieve a sustained virologic response, defined by undetectable HCV RNA at 12 weeks (possibly 24 weeks) after the end of therapy using a sensitive HCV RNA assay with a lower limit of detection of 10 to 20 IU/mL. Sustained virologic response corresponds to a definitive cure of infection.

All treatment-naïve and previously treated patients with chronic HCV infection should be treated without delay, regardless of the severity of liver disease or extra-hepatic manifestations, except in highly unusual situations in which they have contraindications to available oral anti-HCV drugs. Noninvasive assessment of liver fibrosis prior to therapy is required to identify patients who have advanced fibrosis and cirrhosis and who therefore will need post-treatment follow-up for the possible development of hepatocellular carcinoma. Careful assessment of drug-drug interactions is also required prior to initiating therapy (www.hep-druginteractions.org).

Treatment regimens are based on combinations of orally administered antiviral drugs (Chapter 328) that have pan-genotypic antiviral properties (i.e., are active against all known HCV genotypes and subtypes). These combinations provide a sustained virologic response and cure infection in more than 95% of patients. Current anti-HCV drugs belong to three classes, including nucleotide analogues (sofosbuvir), protease inhibitors (glecaprevir, voxilaprevir), and NS5A inhibitors (daclatasvir, velpatasvir, pibrentasvir). These medications, which are available as standalone drugs (sofosbuvir, daclatasvir) or as one-pill fixed-dose combinations of two or three drugs (sofosbuvir/velpatasvir, glecaprevir/pibrentasvir, sofosbuvir/velpatasvir/voxilaprevir), are safe and well-tolerated, with headache and fatigue as the most frequently reported side effects. Generic formulations of HCV drugs are available in low- and middle-income countries and can be used, provided that quality controls are met and guaranteed by the provider.

Due to their virologic efficacy, ease of use, safety, and tolerability, pan-genotypic combination regimens must be used to treat chronic hepatitis C. Treatment is guided by the presence of compensated or decompensated cirrhosis, and prior exposure to oral anti-HCV drugs. Patients infected with HCV can be treated with one of four regimens[8-10] (Table 135-5): the fixed-dose combination of sofosbuvir and velpatasvir[A4-A6]; the fixed-dose combination of glecaprevir and pibrentasvir[A7-A12]; the fixed-dose triple combination of sofosbuvir, velpatasvir, and voxilaprevir[A13]; and the combination of sofosbuvir with the fixed-dose combination of glecaprevir and pibrentasvir. In settings where these combinations are not available or not affordable, the pan-genotypic combination of sofosbuvir and daclatasvir, often available as generic drugs, can also be used with a high probability of sustained virologic response.

Sofosbuvir/velpatasvir should be administered for 12 weeks in patients with chronic hepatitis C without cirrhosis or with compensated cirrhosis. Glecaprevir/pibrentasvir should be administered for 8 weeks in patients without cirrhosis and in patients with compensated cirrhosis who are treatment-naïve, and for 12 weeks in patients with compensated cirrhosis who failed a previous treatment with pegylated interferon α and/or sofosbuvir plus ribavirin.

For patients who do not have a sustained virologic response after treatment with oral anti-HCV drug regimens, retreatment with the triple combination of sofosbuvir, velpatasvir, and voxilaprevir for 12 weeks provides a high rate of sustained virologic response.[A14] In very difficult-to-cure patients (patients who failed twice or more to achieve a sustained virologic response after a combination regimen including a protease and/or an NS5A inhibitor), the triple combination of sofosbuvir, velpatasvir, and voxilaprevir, or the triple combination of sofosbuvir and glecaprevir/pibrentasvir for 12 weeks with weight-based ribavirin (1000 or 1200mg in patients <75 kg or ≥75 kg, respectively) should be administered, and/or treatment duration can be prolonged to 16 to 24 weeks.

Because the risk of advanced liver disease is significantly increased in patients with other coexisting causes of liver disease, patients with chronic hepatitis C should abstain from alcohol and, unless there are other contraindications, should be vaccinated for hepatitis A and B (Chapter 15).

Patients Coinfected with HIV

Patients with coexisting HIV infection should be considered like non-HIV coinfected patients in terms of treatment indications and virologic response to therapy. The only difference to take into account is potential drug-drug interactions with antiretroviral drugs.[A15,A16]

Patients with Decompensated Cirrhosis or Recurrent HCV after Liver Transplantation

In patients who have decompensated cirrhosis or a history of decompensation, protease inhibitors are contraindicated, so these patients should be treated with the combination of sofosbuvir and velpatasvir plus weight-based ribavirin (1000 mg for patients <75 kg, 1200 mg for patients ≥75 kg). When ribavirin cannot be used because of contraindications (anemia, significant coronary or cerebrovascular disease, or renal insufficiency) or poor tolerance, 24 weeks of treatment without ribavirin is recommended. Because ribavirin is teratogenic, it is essential that adequate contraception be practiced during therapy and for at least 6 months thereafter in both men and women.

For patients who have decompensated cirrhosis with an indication for liver transplantation (Chapter 140), those with a Model for End-Stage Liver Disease (MELD; Table 139-2) score below approximately 20 are likely to benefit from curing HCV prior to transplantation. In patients with more severe liver disease (MELD score >20), transplant followed by treatment of graft reinfection with sofosbuvir and velpatasvir or with glecaprevir and pibrentasvir is recommended.

PROGNOSIS

Spontaneous HCV clearance in patients with chronic hepatitis C is exceptional. The HCV RNA level has no prognostic value in chronic hepatitis C. An estimated 20% of patients with chronic hepatitis C develop cirrhosis (Chapter 139) after an average of 20 years of progression in the absence of therapy. Cirrhosis remains compensated for many years in the vast majority of patients, but decompensation occurs at an annual rate of 2 to 5% in cirrhotic patients. After a first decompensation, the mortality rate related to portal hypertension, hepatocellular insufficiency, and hepatocellular carcinoma is 10% per year, with a 50% survival rate at 5 years. The risk for death increases with advancing age, male gender, and the severity of cirrhosis.

Hepatocellular carcinoma (Chapter 181) is rare in patients with chronic hepatitis C without cirrhosis. In patients with cirrhosis, the incidence of hepatocellular carcinoma is 2 to 4% per year, most often in patients with compensated cirrhosis. HCV has become the most common cause of hepatocellular carcinoma in most industrialized countries.

After successful anti-HCV therapy, the risk of hepatocellular carcinoma is eliminated for patients who do not have cirrhosis or other causes of liver disease. The risk is considerably reduced but not eliminated in patients with cirrhosis, especially in the presence of other causes of liver disease. Late relapses in patients who have achieved a sustained virologic response are most often reinfections in individuals with high-risk practices.

CHRONIC HEPATITIS D

EPIDEMIOLOGY

HDV infection occurs only in HBsAg carriers. Only approximately 2% of patients acutely coinfected with HDV and HBV develop chronic hepatitis D. In chronic HBV carriers superinfected by HDV, however, 90% of patients become chronic HDV carriers. Overall, 4.5% of chronic HBsAg carriers, or about 12 million individuals, are chronically infected with HDV.

CLINICAL MANIFESTATIONS

Chronic hepatitis D is generally severe, with more than 80% of patients developing cirrhosis. Compared with patients who have chronic hepatitis B alone, patients with chronic infection with both HBV and HDV are three times as likely to develop hepatocellular carcinoma and twice as likely to die.

DIAGNOSIS

Markers of HDV infection should be sought at least once in every chronic HBsAg carrier. Total anti-HD antibodies remain at high levels in chronic HDV infection, and HDV RNA is present. Although all chronic HDV carriers also are chronic HBsAg carriers, chronic HDV carriers generally have low or undetectable HBV DNA levels because HDV inhibits HBV replication.

PREVENTION

Chronic HDV infection is best prevented by HBV vaccination, because individuals who are protected against HBV cannot be infected with HDV. In chronic HBsAg carriers, standard hygiene and behavioral precautions should be practiced to avoid superinfection with HDV. Once acute HDV infection occurs, no secondary prevention strategy is successful.

TREATMENT

Pegylated IFN-α2a (180 μg once weekly) for 48 weeks can provide a virologic response rate that is approximately 50% on treatment,[11] but only about 25% of patients have undetectable HDV RNA 24 weeks after the end of treatment. Longer treatment duration may increase the virologic response rates.

Bulevirtide, an HDV entry inhibitor (2 mg once daily by subcutaneous injection as monotherapy or coadministered with a nucleoside or a nucleotide analogue for treatment of underlying HBV infection),[A17] also suppresses HDV. The optimal treatment duration is unknown, and treatment should be continued as long as associated with clinical benefit. Whether HDV-infected patients might benefit from the combination of bulevirtide and pegylated IFN-α2a remains to be determined.

TABLE 135-5 ANTIVIRAL REGIMENS FOR CHRONIC HEPATITIS C INFECTION

TREATED POPULATION	CIRRHOSIS STATUS	PRIOR TREATMENT EXPERIENCE	SOFOSBUVIR/VELPATASVIR: ONE TABLET CONTAINING 400 mg OF SOFOSBUVIR AND 100 mg OF VELPATASVIR ONCE DAILY	GLECAPREVIR/PIBRENTASVIR: THREE TABLETS CONTAINING 100 mg OF GLECAPREVIR AND 40 mg OF PIBRENTASVIR ONCE DAILY WITH FOOD	SOFOSBUVIR/VELPATASVIR/VOXILAPREVIR: ONE TABLET CONTAINING 400 mg OF SOFOSBUVIR, 100 mg OF VELPATASVIR AND 100 mg OF VOXILAPREVIR ONCE DAILY	SOFOSBUVIR +GLECAPREVIR/PIBRENTASVIR: ONE TABLET CONTAINING 400 mg OF SOFOSBUVIR PLUS THREE TABLETS CONTAINING 100 mg OF GLECAPREVIR AND 40 mg OF PIBRENTASVIR ONCE DAILY WITH FOOD	SOFOSBUVIR + DACLATASVIR*: ONE TABLET CONTAINING 400 mg OF SOFOSBUVIR PLUS ONE TABLET CONTAINING 60 mg OF DACLATASVIR ONCE DAILY
Treatment-naïve or treatment-experienced (pegylated interferon-alpha and/or sofosbuvir plus ribavirin)	No cirrhosis	Treatment-naïve	12 weeks	8 weeks	No	No	12 weeks
		Treatment-experienced	12 weeks	8 weeks	No	No	12 weeks
	Compensated cirrhosis	Treatment-naïve	12 weeks	8 weeks	No	No	12 weeks
		Treatment-experienced	12 weeks	12 weeks	No	No	12 weeks
Failure to achieve a sustained virologic response after oral direct-acting antiviral drug treatment	No cirrhosis	First failure of oral direct-acting antiviral drugs	No	No	12 weeks	No	24 weeks with ribavirin[†]
		Very difficult-to-cure patients (patients who failed twice or more to achieve a sustained virologic response after a combination regimen including a protease and/or an NS5A inhibitor)	No	No	12, 16, or 24 weeks ± ribavirin[†]	12, 16, or 24 weeks ± ribavirin[†]	24 weeks with ribavirin[†]
	Compensated cirrhosis	First failure of oral direct acting antiviral drugs	No	No	12 weeks	No	24 weeks with ribavirin[†]
		Very difficult-to-cure patients (patients who failed twice or more to achieve a sustained virologic response after a combination regimen including a protease and/or an NS5A inhibitor)	No	No	12, 16, or 24 weeks ± ribavirin[†]	12, 16, or 24 weeks ± ribavirin[†]	24 weeks with ribavirin[†]

TABLE 135-5 ANTIVIRAL REGIMENS FOR CHRONIC HEPATITIS C INFECTION—cont'd

TREATED POPULATION	CIRRHOSIS STATUS	PRIOR TREATMENT EXPERIENCE	SOFOSBUVIR/ VELPATASVIR ONE TABLET CONTAINING 400 mg OF SOFOSBUVIR AND 100 mg OF VELPATASVIR ONCE DAILY	GLECAPREVIR/ PIBRENTASVIR THREE TABLETS CONTAINING 100 mg OF GLECAPREVIR AND 40 mg OF PIBRENTASVIR ONCE DAILY WITH FOOD	SOFOSBUVIR/ VELPATASVIR/ VOXILAPREVIR ONE TABLET CONTAINING 400 mg OF SOFOSBUVIR, 100 mg OF VELPATASVIR AND 100 mg OF VOXILAPREVIR ONCE DAILY	SOFOSBUVIR +GLECAPREVIR/ PIBRENTASVIR ONE TABLET CONTAINING 400 mg OF SOFOSBUVIR PLUS THREE TABLETS CONTAINING 100 mg OF GLECAPREVIR AND 40 mg OF PIBRENTASVIR ONCE DAILY WITH FOOD	SOFOSBUVIR + DACLATASVIR* ONE TABLET CONTAINING 400 mg OF SOFOSBUVIR PLUS ONE TABLET CONTAINING 60 mg OF DACLATASVIR ONCE DAILY
Decompensated cirrhosis	Decompensated cirrhosis	Treatment-naïve	12 weeks with ribavirin† or 24 weeks if ribavirin contraindications	No	No	No	12 weeks with ribavirin† or 24 weeks if ribavirin contraindications
		Treatment-experienced (any treatment received)	12 weeks with ribavirin† or 24 weeks if ribavirin contraindications	No	No	No	12 weeks with ribavirin† or 24 weeks if ribavirin contraindications
Recurrent hepatitis C after liver transplant	No cirrhosis	Treatment-naïve	12 weeks	12 weeks	No	No	12 weeks
		Pretransplant treatment-experienced	12 weeks	12 weeks	No	No	12 weeks
	Compensated cirrhosis	Treatment-naïve	12 weeks	12 weeks	No	No	12 weeks
		Pretransplant treatment-experienced (any treatment received	12 weeks	12 weeks	No	No	12 weeks
	Decompensated cirrhosis	Treatment-naïve	12 weeks with ribavirin† or 24 weeks if ribavirin contraindications	No	No	No	12 weeks with ribavirin† or 24 weeks if ribavirin contraindications
		Pretransplant treatment-experienced (any treatment received)	12 weeks with ribavirin† or 24 weeks if ribavirin contraindications	No	No	No	12 weeks with ribavirin† or 24 weeks if ribavirin contraindications

*In settings where the other combinations are not available or not affordable, where they are often available as generic drugs.
†Ribavirin should be administered at the dose of 1000 or 1200 mg in patients <75 kg or ≥75 kg, respectively.

CHRONIC HEPATITIS E

HEV infection is usually an acute self-limiting disease, but in developed countries it causes chronic infection with rapidly progressive cirrhosis in organ transplant recipients, patients with hematologic malignancies that require chemotherapy, and immunosuppressed HIV-infected individuals, either from a latent virus reactivated by immunosuppression or from a virus transmitted at the time of transplantation. Almost all cases of chronic infection have been in immunosuppressed patients. About one in 3000 blood donors in England are HEV-RNA–positive, even though they are usually seronegative despite their viremia, and can transmit the infection to more than 40% of the recipients of their blood products.

CLINICAL MANIFESTATIONS AND DIAGNOSIS

Diagnosis of acute hepatitis E is based on the detection of anti-HEV IgM antibodies. HEV RNA also can be detected in blood or feces, where its presence is transient. Immunosuppressed patients, such as solid organ transplant recipients, with chronic hepatitis E harbor repeatedly positive anti-HEV antibodies and HEV RNA in blood.

TREATMENT AND PREVENTION

There is no validated treatment of chronic HEV infection.[12] In the transplant setting, reduction in the levels of immunosuppression lead to viral clearance in 30% of cases. Ribavirin (600 mg/day) is associated with about an 80% sustained virologic response rate and is considered first-line treatment.[13] Pegylated interferon-α also can be effective. Reducing the level of immunosuppression can result in viral clearance in approximately one third of patients. A vaccine to prevent HEV infection has been developed and is licensed in China but is not yet available elsewhere.

AUTOIMMUNE HEPATITIS

Autoimmune hepatitis is a chronic inflammatory liver disorder characterized by the presence of autoantibodies in serum, high levels of serum immunoglobulins, and a frequent association with other autoimmune diseases.

EPIDEMIOLOGY AND PATHOBIOLOGY

Autoimmune hepatitis typically manifests between the ages of 15 and 25 years or between the ages of 45 and 60 years, and it is more common in women. The incidence rate is approximately 1.7 per 100,000 population per year. Along with primary biliary cirrhosis (Chapter 141) and primary sclerosing cholangitis (Chapter 141), autoimmune hepatitis is one of the three major autoimmune liver diseases.

Autoimmune hepatitis is believed to be caused by autoimmune reactions against normal hepatocytes in genetically predisposed persons or persons exposed to unidentified triggers of an autoimmune process against liver antigens. Associations are seen with the human leukocyte antigen (HLA) class I B8 and class II DR3 and DR52a loci. In Asians, autoimmune hepatitis is associated with HLA DR4.

CLINICAL MANIFESTATIONS AND DIAGNOSIS

Autoimmune hepatitis tends to be more severe at its onset than chronic hepatitis B or C, and it progresses to end-stage liver disease if not treated with immunosuppression.[14] Although it is occasionally detected by elevated serum aminotransferase levels on a routine health evaluation, most patients present with fatigue and jaundice.[15] Elevations of bilirubin or alkaline phosphatase indicate more severe or advanced disease. Patients typically have marked elevations in serum γ-globulin, specifically immunoglobulin G, as well as autoantibodies directed at non–organ-specific cellular constituents.

Type 1 autoimmune hepatitis (approximately 90% of cases) is characterized by titers of 1:80 or higher (>1:20 in children) of antinuclear, anti–smooth muscle, anti-actin, and/or anti–soluble liver antigen/liver pancreas antibodies. Type 2 autoimmune hepatitis is characterized by similar elevations of anti–liver-kidney microsomal 1 antibodies and/or anti–liver cytosol 1 antibodies, without antinuclear or anti–smooth muscle antibodies. However, auto-antibodies are not detected in 20 to 35% of cases.

Liver biopsy shows features that are typical of all chronic types of hepatitis, except plasma cell infiltrates. Noninvasive physical markers, such as transient elastography, magnetic resonance elastography, or acoustic radiation force impulse imaging, correlate strongly with the histologic stage of fibrosis, but their accuracy may be impaired by inflammation at the time of diagnosis and during the first months of treatment.

The differential diagnosis of autoimmune hepatitis includes drug-induced liver injury (Chapter 136). Sustained biochemical resolution after glucocorticoid withdrawal reinforces the diagnosis of a self-limited drug-induced liver injury, whereas recrudescence of laboratory abnormalities is consistent with autoimmune hepatitis.

TREATMENT

The clinical symptoms and liver test abnormalities of autoimmune hepatitis generally respond promptly to prednisone.[16,17] Induction therapy should be based on 0.5 to 1.0 mg/kg/day prednisone or prednisolone. If the initial response is good, azathioprine should be added gradually, up to 1.0 to 2.0 mg/kg/day, starting 2 weeks after steroid initiation, while the steroid dose is gradually tapered.[18] In patients without cirrhosis and or acute severe autoimmune hepatitis, budesonide (3 mg three times daily, reduced to twice daily following remission), can be used instead of prednisone/prednisolone in combination with azathioprine. The dose of immunosuppression should be individualized to achieve and maintain normal ALT and immunoglobulin G levels.

In cases of treatment failure, incomplete response, or intolerance to first-line agents, either mycofenolate mofetil (20 mg/kg/day initially, increased to a maximum of 3 g/day) or tacrolimus (1 to 8 mg/day) chronically can achieve and maintain biochemical remission.[19] Infliximab or rituximab are possible alternative therapies after first-line and second-line regimens have failed. After 3 years or more of remission, therapy can be carefully withdrawn, but severe and even fatal flares can occur weeks to months later.

PROGNOSIS

The prognosis is generally related to the histologic stage of the disease. Patients who initially respond to therapy may do well for many years. Patients who progress to end-stage liver disease requre liver transplantation (Chapter 140).[20]

CRYPTOGENIC CHRONIC LIVER DISEASE

Cryptogenic chronic liver disease refers to chronic hepatitis or cirrhosis of unknown cause after excluding hepatitis B, C, D, and E; autoimmune hepatitis; steatohepatitis (Chapter 138); alcoholic liver disease (Chapter 138); drug-induced hepatitis (Chapter 136); and inherited and metabolic liver diseases (Chapter 132). Tests to exclude these conditions include serum levels of α_1-antitrypsin, iron, and ceruloplasmin and, if necessary, urine and liver copper concentrations. In its later stages, nonalcoholic steatohepatitis may be associated with little or no fat.

GENERAL REFERENCES

For the General References and other additional features, please visit Elsevier eBooks+ at https://ebooks.health.elsevier.com.

Grade A References

A1. Chou R, Blazina I, Bougatsos C, et al. Screening for hepatitis B virus infection in nonpregnant adolescents and adults: updated evidence report and systematic review for the US Preventive Services Task Force. *JAMA*. 2020;324:2423-2436.

A2. Hsu YC, Chen CY, Chang IW, et al. Once-daily tenofovir disoproxil fumarate in treatment-naïve Taiwanese patients with chronic hepatitis B and minimally raised alanine aminotransferase (TORCH-B): a multicentre, double-blind, placebo-controlled, parallel-group, randomised trial. *Lancet*. 2021;21:823-833.

A3. Chan HL, Fung S, Seto WK, et al. Tenofovir alafenamide versus tenofovir disoproxil fumarate for the treatment of HBeAg-positive chronic hepatitis B virus infection: a randomised, double-blind, phase 3, non-inferiority trial. *Lancet Gastroenterol Hepatol*. 2016;1:185-195.

A4. Feld JJ, Jacobson IM, Hezode C, et al. Sofosbuvir and velpatasvir for HCV genotype 1, 2, 4, 5, and 6 infection. *N Engl J Med*. 2015;373:2599-2607.

A5. Curry MP, O'Leary JG, Bzowej N, et al. Sofosbuvir and velpatasvir for HCV in patients with decompensated cirrhosis. *N Engl J Med*. 2015;373:2618-2628.

A6. Foster GR, Afdhal N, Roberts SK, et al. Sofosbuvir and velpatasvir for HCV genotype 2 and 3 infection. *N Engl J Med*. 2015;373:2608-2617.

A7. Zeuzem S, Foster GR, Wang S, et al. Glecaprevir-pibrentasvir for 8 or 12 weeks in HCV genotype 1 or 3 infection. *N Engl J Med*. 2018;378:354-369.

A8. Kwo P, Poordad F, Asatryan A, et al. Glecaprevir and pibrentasvir yield high response rates in patients with HCV genotype 1-6 without cirrhosis. *J Hepatol*. 2017;67:263-271.

A9. Asselah T, Kowdley KV, Zadeikis N, et al. Efficacy of glecaprevir/pibrentasvir for 8 or 12 weeks in patients with hepatitis C virus genotype 2, 4, 5, or 6 infection without cirrhosis. *Clin Gastroenterol Hepatol*. 2018;16:417-426.

A10. Forns X, Lee SS, Valdes J, et al. Glecaprevir plus pibrentasvir for chronic hepatitis C virus genotype 1, 2, 4, 5, or 6 infection in adults with compensated cirrhosis (EXPEDITION-1): a single-arm, open-label, multicentre phase 3 trial. *Lancet Infect Dis*. 2017;17:1062-1068.

A11. Wyles D, Poordad F, Wang S, et al. Glecaprevir/pibrentasvir for hepatitis C virus genotype 3 patients with cirrhosis and/or prior treatment experience: a partially randomized phase 3 clinical trial. *Hepatology*. 2018;67:514-523.

A12. Brown RS , Jr, Buti M, Rodrigues L, et al. Glecaprevir/pibrentasvir for 8 weeks in treatment-naïve patients with chronic HCV genotypes 1-6 and compensated cirrhosis: the EXPEDITION-8 trial. *J Hepatol*. 2020;72:441-449.

A13. Jacobson IM, Lawitz E, Gane EJ, et al. Efficacy of 8 weeks of sofosbuvir, velpatasvir, and voxilaprevir in patients with chronic HCV infection: 2 phase 3 randomized trials. *Gastroenterology*. 2017;153:113-122.

A14. Bourliere M, Gordon SC, Flamm SL, et al. Sofosbuvir, velpatasvir, and voxilaprevir for previously treated HCV infection. *N Engl J Med*. 2017;376:2134-2146.

A15. Wyles D, Brau N, Kottilil S, et al. Sofosbuvir and velpatasvir for the treatment of hepatitis C virus in patients coinfected with human immunodeficiency virus type 1: an open-label phase 3 study. *Clin Infect Dis*. 2017;65:6-12.

A16. Rockstroh JK, Lacombe K, Viani RM, et al. Efficacy and safety of glecaprevir/pibrentasvir in patients coinfected with hepatitis C virus and human immunodeficiency virus type 1: the EXPEDITION-2 study. *Clin Infect Dis*. 2018;67:1010-1017.

A17. Wedemeyer H, Aleman S, Brunetto M, et al. Efficacy and safety of bulevirtide monotherapy given at 2 mg or 10 mg dose level once daily for treatment of chronic hepatitis delta: week 48 primary end point result from a phase 3 randomized, multicenter, parallel design study. *J Hepatol*. 2022;77:S4.

136 DRUG-INDUCED LIVER INJURY

PAUL B. WATKINS

DEFINITION

Drug-induced liver injury can be caused by drugs or by druglike substances, including herbal products. Because some drugs can cause minor abnormalities of liver chemistries that are of no health concern, drug-induced liver injury is defined in terms of threshold values for liver chemistries (Table 136-1).[1] The clinical presentation of drug-induced liver injury can be predominantly hepatocellular, cholestatic, or a mixture of each, as defined by the ratio of the serum alanine aminotransferase (ALT) level to the alkaline phosphatase level. A hepatocellular presentation primarily reflects death of hepatocytes with release of their contents, including ALT and aspartate aminotransferase (AST), into circulation, whereas a cholestatic presentation reflects injury to the bile ductular epithelium (cholangiocytes) or to processes that selectively affect the liver's ability to make and secrete bile. A mixed injury reflects a combination of these processes. Since no tests can definitively confirm most cases, the diagnosis is often one of exclusion.[2]

EPIDEMIOLOGY

Drug-induced liver injury is a rare event considering the very large number of different drugs used by patients. Estimated rates are fewer than 20 drug-induced liver injuries per 100,000 person-years in Western countries[3] but higher in mainland China. However, due to challenges in diagnosing drug-induced liver injury and incomplete reporting, the true incidence may be 10 times higher. Antimicrobial agents are the major class of implicated drugs in Western countries, whereas herbal medications are the most frequently reported cause in Asian countries.

In U.S. tertiary medical centers, about 10% of cases of severe acute hepatitis may be caused by drug-induced liver injury. Acetaminophen is the dominant cause of acute and fatal drug-induced liver injury. About 10 to 15% of cases are related to dietary and herbal supplements.

PATHOBIOLOGY

The liver is particularly susceptible to drug-induced injury because it sees the highest concentration of drugs after oral administration and because it is the major site for the metabolism of drugs, thereby resulting in a high concentration of potentially toxic drug metabolites. Drugs that cause liver injury can be divided into three categories: direct/intrinsic toxins, which cause liver injury that is clearly dose-related and generally occurs within days of dosing; idiosyncratic toxins, for which the relationship between the dose and liver injury is complex, and liver injury typically occurs suddenly after weeks to months of chronic treatment; and indirect toxicity, in which liver injury occurs as a side effect of the drug's desired therapeutic actions (typically immune suppressants that activate viral hepatitis or immune checkpoint inhibitors that result in a liver-directed T-cell response) (Table 136-2).[4] Acetaminophen (paracetamol) is the most important direct/intrinsic drug that causes liver injury, not only because it is a frequent cause of liver failure but also because an antidote (N-acetyl cysteine) is effective if given soon after ingestion of an overdose. Idiosyncratic drug-induced liver injury generally reflects an adaptive immune attack on the liver.

If drugs are not directly excreted as unchanged in the urine, the liver is the major site where they are metabolized. Most drugs are lipophilic and are transformed in the liver from nonpolar compounds into more hydrophilic metabolites via oxidative pathways mediated by the cytochromes P-450 (CYPs), often followed by conjugation to polar ligands so they can be excreted in the urine or bile. Other important metabolic pathways for some drugs may include acetylating enzymes, glutathione-*S*-transferase, and alcohol dehydrogenase.

TABLE 136-1 INTERNATIONAL CONSENSUS CRITERIA FOR DRUG-INDUCED LIVERY INJURY

A. Drug-induced liver injury is defined by any of the following peak serum values (assuming a healthy liver prior to the event):
   - Serum alanine aminotransferase level 5 or more times the upper limit of normal
   - Serum alkaline phosphatase level 2 or more times the upper limit of normal in the absence of bone pathology
   - Serum alanine aminotransferase level 3 or more times the upper limit of normal and total serum bilirubin level 2 or more times the upper limit of normal in the absence of hemolysis or Gilbert syndrome

B. The clinical pattern of drug-induced liver injury is defined by the R-value, which is calculated as the alanine aminotransferase : alkaline phosphatase ratio, where each is expressed in terms of the upper limit of normal when the patient first meets the criteria for drug-induced liver injury:
   - Hepatocellular drug injury if $R \geq 5.0$
   - Mixed drug injury if $R > 2.0$ to < 5.0
   - Cholestatic drug injury if $R \leq 2.0$

Drug-Induced liver Injury (DILI): Current status and future directions for drug development and post-market settings. A consensus by a CIOMS Working Group 2020. Council for International Organizations of Medical Sciences; 2020. Available at https://cioms.ch/publications/product/drug-induced-liver-injury/.

DIRECT/INTRINSIC HEPATOTOXICITY

PATHOBIOLOGY

In cases of direct/intrinsic hepatotoxicity, the parent drug or, more usually, a toxic (or "reactive") metabolite formed by the metabolism of the parent drug, directly causes injury and death to liver cells. Virtually every user will develop this liver toxicity if they receive a high enough dose, but the threshold dose that causes toxicity can vary substantially among individuals.

Acetaminophen

The most important drug that causes direct hepatotoxicity is acetaminophen (also called paracetamol), which accounts for over 50% of cases of acute liver failure in the United States, Europe, and Australia. After a person consumes a therapeutic dose of acetaminophen, the majority of the drug undergoes glucuronidation or sulfation, thereby resulting in harmless metabolites that are rapidly excreted in urine (E-Fig. 136-1). Less than 10% of acetaminophen is normally converted to the potentially toxic metabolite, N-acetyl-p-benzoquinone imine (NAPQI). Therapeutic doses of acetaminophen are generally safe because NAPQI is rapidly detoxified through conjugation to glutathione. However, when a healthy person consumes a very large dose of acetaminophen (typically more than 12 grams as a single dose), the sulfation pathway can become saturated, thereby resulting in a greater fraction of this larger dose being converted to NAPQI. The excess NAPQI results in an increase in covalent binding to cellular proteins, particularly in mitochondria. This protein binding activates a subsequent series of signaling pathways that involve c-Jun N terminal kinase and can lead to the death of hepatocytes. The time taken to activate these pathways presumably accounts for the typical 24-hour latency between consumption of a toxic dose of acetaminophen and onset of elevated liver chemistries. Patient-specific factors that can significantly reduce the dose threshold for acetaminophen toxicity include poor nutrition and fasting (which can deplete the substrate for glucuronidation), as well as excessive ethanol intake (which can induce CYP2E1; see E-Fig. 136-1). Patients with cirrhosis (Chapter 139) may also be more susceptible, thereby leading to the current recommendation not to exceed 2 g in 24 hours in this population.

Other Direct Liver Toxins

Other drugs that cause liver toxicity by direct mechanisms include cocaine, aspirin, nicotinic acid, many anticancer drugs, and pyrrolizidine alkaloids that are contained in some plant products (Table 136-3). For *Amanita* poisoning (Chapter 96) after ingestion of the mushrooms *Amanita phalloides* (death cap) or *Amanita virosa* (deadly agaric), the dose-dependent toxic effect on the liver is attributed to amatoxin, an ingredient of the mushrooms that enhances the toxic effect by its enterohepatic recirculation characteristics; the toxic effect is exerted on each cycle of the recirculation through the liver.[5]

Statin drugs (Chapter 190) can cause dose-dependent, asymptomatic elevations in serum ALT in 1 to 4% of treated individuals, but clinically significant liver injury is quite rare, and progression to liver failure is almost unheard of. Hence, no patient should be denied statin treatment over liver safety concerns.

CLINICAL MANIFESTATIONS

Acetaminophen

After a single and usually intentional overdose of acetaminophen, the clinical presentation has four potential stages (E-Fig. 136-2).[6] The first stage includes up to 24 hours after the ingestion, during which symptoms may include nausea, vomiting, and abdominal discomfort. The second stage, which marks the

TABLE 136-2 TYPICAL FEATURES OF DRUG-INDUCED LIVER INJURY

	DIRECT/INTRINSIC	IDIOSYNCRATIC	INDIRECT
Implicated drugs	Acetaminophen is major cause (see Table 136-3)	Many drugs, especially antibiotics and herbal products (see Table 136-4)	Immune modulators, including checkpoint inhibitors
Dose-related	Yes	Less likely at doses <50 mg/day	No
Latency	1 to several days	1-3 months	1-6 months
Genetic predisposition	Variants in phase 1 or phase 2 metabolism	HLA risk alleles	Unknown
Pathogenesis	Reactive metabolites	Adaptive immune attack on the liver	Viral cytolysis or an adaptive immune attack on the liver
Pathophysiology	Reactive metabolites damage organelles and initiate death-signaling pathways	Cytotoxic T cells kill liver cells	Activation of viral infection or reduced immune tolerance
Pathology	Pericentral necrosis with little inflammation	Panacinar inflammation and cell death	Variable

TABLE 136-3 DRUGS AND TOXINS THAT CAUSE DOSE-RELATED INJURY

DRUG OR TOXIN
Acetaminophen
Alcohol
Amiodarone
Cocaine
Cyclophosphamide
Cyclosporine
Methotrexate
Niacin
Nonsteroidal anti-inflammatory drugs (principally bromfenac, phenylbutazone)
Oral estrogens or androgens
Tetracyclines
Toxins (yellow phosphorus, carbon tetrachloride, *Amanita* toxin, bacterial toxins)
Zidovudine

initial elevation of liver chemistries, typically starts about 24 hours after the ingestion when the patient may feel entirely well. Serum AST and ALT levels rise rapidly to very high levels, initially with AST levels typically higher than ALT levels. Elevations in the serum bilirubin level and international normalized ratio (INR) reflect significant loss of liver function. The third stage, which is marked by the peaking of serum ALT and AST, typically occurs 3 to 4 days after the ingestion. If the injury is severe, the serum bilirubin level and INR will continue to increase, and the patient may develop fulminant hepatic failure, often accompanied by kidney failure. The fourth stage is recovery with return of all liver chemistries and the INR to normal over 2 weeks. Because death of liver cells ceases after the first several days after ingestion, the serum enzymes fall at the rate of their half-lives (ALT about 2 days, AST about 1 day).

Other Direct Liver Toxins

Other direct liver toxins cause hepatic steatosis and lactic acidosis, which typically present with fatigue, nausea, and weight loss within the first month of starting treatment with the culprit drug. Drugs implicated in causing this type of liver injury include intravenous tetracycline and d-nucleosidase drugs, including zidovudine (AZT). Liver chemistries may be only minimally elevated, and liver histology reveals microvesicular steatosis similar to that observed when aspirin causes Reye syndrome. Chronic treatment with several drugs (e.g., tamoxifen or methotrexate) can cause fatty liver without lactic acidosis, often in the setting of obesity or type 2 diabetes. Acute alcoholic injury also results in fatty liver (Chapter 138).

Bland cholestasis occurs in healthy young men who consume androgen-containing supplements to build muscle bulk (see E-Fig. 136-2D).[7] Long-term use of estrogens, especially in high doses, is associated with benign liver adenomas, and long-term use of androgen-containing supplements can cause liver cancer.

Sinusoidal obstruction syndrome (previously termed veno-occlusive disease), which can be acute or subacute forms of this phenotype, presents with abdominal pain and weight gain owing to the rapid accumulation of ascites. Offending drugs are generally chemotherapeutic agents, typically alkylating agents such as cyclophosphamide.

DIAGNOSIS

In an otherwise healthy person, sudden development of extremely high (more than 50 times the upper limit of normal) ALT and AST values, followed by resolution at the half-lives of these enzymes, is almost pathognomonic for acetaminophen overdose.[8] Nevertheless, the diagnosis of acetaminophen drug-induced liver injury can be challenging during the first stage, when it is based on the history of the amount ingested and the timing of the ingestion. Since some patients may not admit to having taken an overdose and liver chemistries will generally not be abnormal during the first stage, measurement of an acetaminophen blood level is key to diagnosis. For other causes of direct liver injury, the diagnosis is based on exposure to a known toxin.

Rare exposures to other liver toxins (Table 136-3), such as poisonous mushrooms or industrial solvents, also can present with a clinical picture similar to acetaminophen poisoning. The diagnosis is based on evidence of exposure since there is no definitive diagnostic test.

TREATMENT

N-acetyl cysteine, which repletes liver stores of glutathione, is a very effective treatment for acetaminophen overdose,[A1] especially if administered during stage 1. Intravenous dosing can begin with 140 mg/kg in 300 mL of 5% dextrose given over 1 hour, followed by a dose of 70 mg/kg in 5% dextrose given over a 1-hour period every 4 hours for 48 hours. Alternatively, a loading dose of 140 mg/kg can be given orally, followed by 70 mg/kg every 4 hours for 17 doses (72 hours), with subsequent dosing dependent on the predicted and measured toxic levels of acetaminophen as a function of time since a single overdose (https://www.mdcalc.com/acetaminophen-overdose-nac-dosing#next-steps). Critically ill patients require intensive care. Liver transplantation (Chapter 140) is often required for fulminant hepatic failure.

For other direct liver injuries, no specific treatments are available. Care is supportive, with liver transplantation often required for liver failure.

PREVENTION

Patients who have accidentally overdosed should be advised to read the labels on all analgesics, cold, and sleep remedies to keep total acetaminophen dosing within the recommended range. Patients who have intentionally overdosed require psychiatric consultation (Chapter 362).

PROGNOSIS

The prognosis is excellent if NAC is administered within stage 1. If serial assessments of acetaminophen levels indicate that the half-life is longer than 5.5 hours, progressive liver injury is likely.

IDIOSYNCRATIC HEPATOTOXICITY

EPIDEMIOLOGY

Idiosyncratic drug-induced liver injury is a rare but potentially serious event that occurs during recommended dosing of the implicated drug at a frequency less than 1 : 1000 treated patients. Although idiosyncratic hepatotoxicity is not generally dose-related, it is less likely to occur when the daily dose of drug is less than 50 mg per day and can occasionally occur when the daily dose is increased after prolonged treatment (>1 year) at a lower dose. The most common drugs that cause idiosyncratic drug-induced liver injury are antimicrobial agents (e.g., fluoroquinolones) and herbal and dietary supplements (Table 136-4). Herbal supplements dominate in China[9] and other parts of Asia, and the incidence of drug-induced liver injury related to dietary and herbal supplements is increasing in the United States as well.[10] The risk appears to increase with factors such as older age and alcohol use (Table 136-5).

PATHOBIOLOGY

Idiosyncratic drug-induced liver injury often results from a cytotoxic T-cell response to drug-induced neoantigen(s) presented on the surface of liver cells. This response typically occurs because of covalent binding of a drug metabolite to an endogenous liver protein, thereby resulting in altered peptide fragments presented by class 1 HLA molecules.[11] However, creation of a novel antigen alone is not thought to be sufficient to initiate an immune attack on the liver (E-Fig. 136-3).[17] A number of genetic variants, particularly HLA alleles (Table 136-6), increase the susceptibility to idiosyncratic hepatotoxicity[13]. Due to the rarity of idiosyncratic drug-induced liver injury, however, the vast majority of patients treated with these drugs do not get drug-induced liver injury even if they carry the corresponding risk allele. Genetic variants in CYP isoenzymes likely also partially explain a predisposition to drug-induced liver injury. In addition, a polymorphism in the *PTPN22* gene, which is believed to influence T-cell activation, also is associated with about a 50% increased risk for drug-induced liver injury.

The usual response to an initial adaptive immune attack on the liver due to a drug is spontaneous resolution, even with continued exposure to the offending drug, because of immune tolerance mechanisms. The typical latency reflects, at least in part, the time needed to complete the multiple sequential steps involved (E-Fig. 136-3). Once the injury is initiated, it may progress for days or rarely weeks after discontinuing the offending drug. In some cases (see E-Fig. 136-2, panel B), the adaptive immune attack can occur within days after starting treatment, presumably as a reflection of a sufficient pre-existing

TABLE 136-4 MOST COMMON CAUSES OF IDIOSYNCRATIC DRUG-INDUCED LIVER INJURY

TYPE OF MEDICATION	%	SPECIFIC DRUGS*	%
Antimicrobials	32	Amoxicillin-clavulanate	8
Herbal and dietary supplements	12	Isoniazid	4
Cardiovascular agents	7	Nitrofurantoin	4
Central nervous system agents	7	Sulfamethoxazole/trimethoprim	3
Antineoplastic agents	4	Minocycline	2
Analgesics	3	Cefazolin	2
Immunomodulatory drugs	2	Azithromycin	2
Endocrine drugs	2	Ciprofloxacin	1
Rheumatologic treatments	1	Levofloxacin	1
Gastrointestinal agents	1	Diclofenac	1

*Excludes herbal and dietary supplements.

Adapted from Chalasani N, Bonkovsky HL, Fontana R, et al. Features and outcomes of 899 patients with drug-induced liver injury: the DILIN Prospective Study. *Gastroenterology*. 2015;148:1340-1352.

TABLE 136-5 FACTORS THAT MAY PREDISPOSE TO IDIOSYNCRATIC DRUG-INDUCED LIVER INJURY

Elderly age
Alcohol use
Female gender
Renal disease
Foods such as grapefruit that interfere with the metabolism of some drugs
Concomitant drugs
Genetic factors

TABLE 136-6 HLA ALLELES ASSOCIATED WITH RISK FOR IDIOSYNCRATIC DRUG-INDUCED LIVER INJURY DUE TO CERTAIN DRUGS

DRUG	HLA ALLELE	ODDS RATIO OF INCREASED RISK
Amoxicillin/clavulanic acid	A*02:01	2.3
	DRB1*15:01	2.8
Fenofibrate	A*33:01	59
Flucloxacillin	B*57:01	81
Flupirtine	DRB1*16:01-DQB1*05:02	19
Green tea extract	B*35:01	12
Lumiracoxib	DRB1*15:01-DQB1*06:02	5.0
Minocycline	B*35:02	30
Sulfamethoxazole/ trimethoprim	B*14:01	9.2
Terbinafine	A*33:01	41
Ticlopidine	A*33:01	163
Ximelagatran	DRB1*07:01-DQA1*02:01	4.4

population of appropriately primed T cells prior to starting treatment with the implicated drug, perhaps due to prior treatment with the same drug, or prior exposure to a structurally similar viral antigen.

CLINICAL MANIFESTATIONS

About 50% of cases present within 30 days of starting the drug, and about 80% of cases present within 90 days (see E-Fig. 136-2, panel B).[14] Occurrences beyond 1 year of treatment are very rare and usually occur with drugs that are not taken continuously, such as minocycline for acne or nitrofurantoin for urinary tract infections.

Different drugs can cause different types of liver reactions (Table 136-7), but clinically the damage presents as a hepatocellular, cholestatic, or mixed injury. Most cases of drug-induced liver injury are hepatocellular reactions, which account for 60% of cases and are characterized by elevated levels of AST and ALT. Cholestatic reactions[15] can be caused by trimethoprim-sulfamethoxazole, captopril, and body-building dietary supplements that contain androgenic compounds. Nodular regenerative hyperplasia manifests with fatigue, weight loss, ascites, and other complications of portal hypertension, usually after at least 6 months of continuous treatment with the offending drug. Drugs implicated as causing this phenotype include azathioprine, mercaptopurine, and thioguanine.

TABLE 136-7 IDIOSYNCRATIC TOXIN AND DRUG REACTIONS

REACTION TYPE	SOME IMPLICATED DRUGS OR TOXINS
Hepatocellular	Carbamazepine, fluoroquinolones, cyclosporine, herbs, methimazole, isoniazid, lovastatin, nefazodone, trazodone, venlafaxine
Cholestatic or mixed	Anabolic steroids, captopril, carbamazepine, chlorpromazine, estrogen, erythromycin, amoxicillin/clavulanate
Fibrosis	Methotrexate, excess vitamin A
Granulomatous	Allopurinol, diltiazem, nitrofurantoin, sulfa drugs, quinidine
Autoimmune	Nitrofurantoin, minocycline
Immunoallergic	Halothane, phenytoin, sulfamethoxazole
Steatohepatitis	Amiodarone, perhexiline maleate, tamoxifen

DIAGNOSIS

The most commonly used tool to aid in the diagnosis of drug-induced liver injury is the Roussel Uclaf Causality Assessment Method (RUCAM; Table 136-8; https://www.ncbi.nlm.nih.gov/books/NBK548272/), which considers answers to a series of questions such as time to detection of drug-induced liver injury from start of treatment, rate of resolution after stopping treatment, and whether the drug is known to cause hepatotoxicity. The sum of the points (>8 = highly probable, 6 to 8 = probable, 3 to 5 = possible, 1 to 2 = unlikely, 0 = excluded) after completing the exercise corresponds to scales of confidence on a causal link.

The RUCAM instrument does not consider the characteristic clinical presentations (or signatures) of the drugs that cause idiosyncratic reactions (see Table 136-4 and https://www.ncbi.nlm.nih.gov/books/NBK548473/). However, one drug can have more than one "signature," and many drugs have similar signatures.

A liver biopsy is generally not necessary to make the diagnosis of idiosyncratic drug-induced liver injury but is generally recommended when other potentially treatable diseases that have characteristic histology are being considered, such as autoimmune hepatitis (Chapter 135). For drugs for which specific genetic polymorphisms (see Table 136-6) increase risk, genetic testing may occasionally be helpful, particularly if the patient is being treated with multiple potential culprit drugs.

TREATMENT

Other than stopping treatment with the offending drug, no specific treatments are usually recommended for idiosyncratic drug-induced liver injury.[16,17] Drug-induced liver injury due to valproate, which presents with elevated blood levels of ammonia and altered mental status, may respond to treatment with carnitine (loading dose of 100 mg/kg intravenously [6 g maximum] over 30 minutes followed by maintenance doses of 15 mg/kg every 4 hours over 10 to 30 minutes). Oral administration of cholestyramine (8 g orally 3 times daily for 11 days) can hasten removal of some lipophilic drugs with long half-lives (e.g., leflunomide). Nevertheless, corticosteroids (typically starting with the equivalent of 40 mg prednisone daily with subsequent titration and tapering according to the patient's response) are often administered if the drug-induced liver injury mimics autoimmune hepatitis (Chapter 135) or if the liver injury is progressing towards liver failure, especially if clinical signs of hypersensitivity (fever, rash, and peripheral eosinophilia) are present.[18]

TABLE 136-8 SCORING SYSTEM TO ASSESS CAUSALITY OF HEPATOCELLULAR REACTIONS

FACTOR	SCORE*
TEMPORAL RELATIONSHIP OF START OF DRUG TO START OF ILLNESS	
Initial treatment: 5-90 days; subsequent treatment course: 1-15 days	+2
Initial treatment: <5 or >90 days; subsequent treatment course: >15 days	+1
From cessation of drug: ≤15 days[†]	+1
COURSE	
ALT decreases ≥50% from peak within 8 days	+3
ALT decreases ≥50% from peak within 30 days	+2
If the drug is continued, inconclusive	0
RISK FACTORS	
Alcohol[‡]	+1
No alcohol[‡]	0
Age ≥ 55 yr	+1
Age < 55 yr	0
CONCOMITANT DRUG	
Concomitant drug with suggestive time of onset	−1
Concomitant drug known to be a hepatotoxin with suggestive time of onset	−2
Concomitant drug with further evidence of involvement (rechallenge)	−3
NUMBER OF NONDRUG CAUSES	
Hepatitis A, B, or C; biliary obstruction; alcoholism (AST ≥ 2 × ALT); recent hypotension; and CMV, EBV, and HSV infections all excluded	+2
4-5 causes excluded	+1
<4 causes excluded	−2
Nondrug cause highly probable	−3
PREVIOUS INFORMATION ON HEPATOTOXICITY OF DRUG IN QUESTION	
Package insert mentions	+2
Published case reports but not on package label	+1
Reaction unknown	0
RECHALLENGE	
Positive (ALT doubles with drug alone)[§]	+2
Compatible (ALT doubles, compounding features)[§]	+1
Negative (increase in ALT but ≤2 × ULN)[§]	−2
Not done	0

*Causality is highly probable (score >8), probable (score 6-8), possible (score 3-5), unlikely (score 1-2), or excluded (score ≤0).
[†]For cholestatic reactions, ≤30 days.
[‡]For cholestatic reactions, alcohol, or pregnancy.
[§]For cholestatic reactions, substitute alkaline phosphatase (or total bilirubin) for ALT.
ALT = alanine aminotransferase; AST = aspartate aminotransferase; CMV = cytomegalovirus; EBV = Epstein-Barr virus; HSV = herpes simplex virus; ULN = upper limit of normal.
Modified from Danan G, Benichou C. Causality assessment of adverse reactions to drugs. I. A novel method based on the conclusions of international consensus meetings: application to drug-induced liver injuries. *J Clin Epidemiol.* 1993;46:1323-1330; and Benichou C, Danan G, Flahault A. Causality assessment of adverse reactions to drugs. II. An original model for validation of drug causality assessment methods: case reports with positive rechallenge. *J Clin Epidemiol.* 1993;46:1331-1336.

PREVENTION

Patients who have a suspected drug-induced liver injury should have this fact prominently noted in the medical record and should not receive that drug again. To capture an idiosyncratic drug-induced liver injury early in its course and prior to the onset of jaundice, patients taking some drugs (e.g., antibiotic treatment for more than 2 weeks and many anticancer drugs, including kinase inhibitors, azathioprine, and most antiseizure drugs) should be routinely monitored with liver chemistries during the first 3 to 6 months of treatment, although the value of routine liver test monitoring has not been conclusively established by randomized trials.

PROGNOSIS

The vast majority of patients with drug-induced liver injury will recover after discontinuing treatment with the offending drug, but up to 20% will still have biochemical evidence of drug-induced liver injury at 6 months. Patients who develop hepatocellular jaundice have a greater than 10% chance of developing liver failure, regardless of the causative drug. The number of liver transplantations (Chapter 140) for liver failure caused by herbal products continues to rise.[19]

INDIRECT HEPATOTOXICITY

Indirect drug-induced liver injury refers to liver injuries that result as a consequence of the desired therapeutic actions of the drug. This phenomenon is a quite common form of drug-induced liver injury that is increasing as more immune modulatory medications enter the marketplace.

Examples of indirect drug-induced liver injury include flaring of preexisting viral hepatitis due to immune suppression that may result from treatment with corticosteroids and some monoclonal antibodies (e.g., daclizumab and anti–tumor necrosis factor alpha agents).[20] The other major type of indirect hepatotoxicity results from drugs that increase immune responses to cancer, such as checkpoint inhibitors[21] (which remove immune tolerance and spark an adaptive immune attack on the liver and other organs). Liver cell stress and neoantigen presentation must also be present for the reduction in immune tolerance to cause liver injury (E-Fig. 136-3), and concomitant treatment with a drug that can cause liver injury increases the risk.

CLINICAL MANIFESTATIONS AND DIAGNOSIS

Indirect hepatotoxicity is usually hepatocellular or mixed. It typically arises within 3 months after the start of therapy but can appear later. Many cases are anicteric and asymptomatic; sometimes, however, the hepatitis can worsen and rarely become life-threatening if untreated.

Indirect hepatotoxicity is typically detected by routine monitoring of liver chemistries during therapy with the offending agent. Reactivation of viral hepatitis is detected by serum viral counts.

TREATMENT AND PROGNOSIS

Reactivation viral hepatitis may require antiviral treatment (Chapter 134). Liver injury due to checkpoint inhibitors appears to respond to corticosteroids (e.g., 40 mg of prednisone daily, with subsequent titration and tapering according to the patient's response).

Concomitant treatment with drugs well-recognized to be hepatotoxic should be avoided. Full recovery is expected with timely recognition and appropriate treatment.

GENERAL REFERENCES

For the General References and other additional features, please visit Elsevier eBooks+ at https://ebooks.health.elsevier.com.

Grade A Reference

A1. Chiew AL, Gluud C, Brok J, et al. Interventions for paracetamol (acetaminophen) overdose. *Cochrane Database Syst Rev.* 2018;2:CD003328.

137 BACTERIAL, PARASITIC, FUNGAL, AND GRANULOMATOUS LIVER DISEASES

K. RAJENDER REDDY

INFECTIONS OF THE LIVER

Infections of the liver can be due to a variety of pathogens, including bacteria, fungi, amebae, protozoa, helminths, spirochetes, and rickettsiae.[1] The manifestations of these infections are protean; some are generic to all infections, whereas others are specific to particular infections. The epidemiology can vary and depend upon the geographic region of the world. In endemic areas, *Entamoeba histolytica* (Chapter 323) is a key consideration in the differential diagnosis of a liver abscess (Table 137-1).

BACTERIAL INFECTIONS

PYOGENIC LIVER ABSCESS

DEFINITION

Pyogenic liver abscess is a focal collection of purulent bacterial material and necroinflammatory debris. It can be solitary or multiple and can be caused by one or more aerobic and/or anaerobic bacteria.

EPIDEMIOLOGY

Pyogenic liver abscess has an estimated global incidence of approximately 1.1 to 2.3 per 100,000 person-years, whereas in the United States the incidence is reported to be approximately 3.6 per 100,000 and has been rising. The risk is about three-fold higher in patients with diabetes.[2] Biliary obstruction, caused by a malignancy or benign disease, accounts for 50 to 60% of pyogenic liver abscesses, whereas portal pyemia, due to appendicitis or other intra-abdominal infections (e.g., diverticulitis), accounts for about 20% of cases.[3] Studies from Asia, where *Klebsiella pneumoniae* is the primary etiologic source of pyogenic liver abscess,[4] have proposed a correlation with underlying colorectal neoplasms, some of which are evident at the time of diagnosis but also with a five- to eight-fold higher risk of newly diagnosed colorectal cancers in the 3 years after diagnosis. However, it is yet to be determined whether these findings can be extrapolated to other regions of the world.

PATHOBIOLOGY

Bacteria can enter the liver via the portal system from infections in areas drained by the mesenteric system into the portal system, such as appendicitis. Other mechanisms for pyogenic liver abscess include bacterial cholangitis owing to benign or malignant obstruction and infection of the liver from a systemic bacteremia, such as an infection of the oral cavity. Pyogenic liver abscess can also be caused by blunt or penetrating trauma, including such unusual causes as the ingestion of a toothpick or fish bone that can cause an intestinal perforation, fistula to the liver, and subsequent abscess formation. Liver abscesses can occur in a transplanted graft owing to vascular compromise caused by hepatic artery thrombosis and ischemic bile duct strictures.

Multiple organisms can cause pyogenic liver abscess. The most common organism, *Klebsiella pneumoniae* (Chapter 281) often is associated with biliary tract disease. Other aerobes include *Escherichia coli*, group D streptococci, β-hemolytic streptococci, and *Staphylococcus aureus*. Anaerobic infection is often seen with colonic disease. Less common causes of liver abscesses include *Actinomyces, Nocardia asteroides, Yersinia pseudotuberculosis* and *Yersinia enterocolitica, Listeria monocytogenes, Campylobacter jejuni, Legionella pneumophila, Mycobacterium tuberculosis, Salmonella typhi* or *Salmonella paratyphi, Candida albicans*, and *Bartonella henselae*. Most often, the organism recovered from an abscess cavity is single, but multiple organisms can be isolated in as many as a third of patients. Bacteria may not be isolated from the abscess because of prior antibiotic therapy or the failure to perform proper anaerobic cultures.

CLINICAL MANIFESTATIONS

The signs and symptoms associated with a liver abscess typically include fever, right upper quadrant abdominal pain, chills, nausea, vomiting, weight loss, and jaundice. The presentation can be acute or indolent. An associated bacteremia is seen in approximately 50% of the patients, and about 15% of patients may develop septic shock. About 10% of patients develop metastatic infections in other sites.

DIAGNOSIS

Appropriate diagnosis requires a high degree of clinical suspicion, and diagnosis is sometimes delayed. Usually, however, the diagnosis is made promptly with the wide availability of the various radiologic modalities. The two common causes of liver abscesses are pyogenic and amebic abscesses, and it is important to make a distinction because the prognosis and management differ.[5] Amebic abscesses can infrequently become secondarily infected with other bacteria.

The diagnosis of an abscess is based on a constellation of clinical, bacteriologic, and radiologic features.[6] Ultrasonography and computed tomography (CT) scanning are the most common radiologic modalities to diagnose an abscess cavity reliably,[7] either as single or multiple lesions (Fig. 137-1A and B). CT is the preferred diagnostic modality to detect an abscess, with sensitivity of more than 90%. Any concurrent biliary obstruction also can be diagnosed by these imaging modalities. Approximately 50% of patients have multiple abscesses. On CT the lesion is seen as a fluid collection with irregular borders and cavity wall edema. One drawback to this imaging modality is that no specific features differentiate a pyogenic abscess from other infectious causes (i.e., amebic or fungal). Another drawback is that a very early stage abscess may not be well formed and may have characteristics more suggestive of a solid mass. On noninvasive imaging studies, it is critical to distinguish an abscess from a tumor or a simple cyst. Various events, such as bleeding into a cyst, calcification, necrosis, and bleeding into a tumor, may confuse the distinction. A finding of smaller (<2 cm) peripheral lesions that surround a central abscess (the cluster sign) can help exclude a hepatic neoplasm. Calcification suggests

TABLE 137-1 FEATURES OF BACTERIAL AND AMEBIC ABSCESSES

	DEMOGRAPHICS	RISK FACTORS	SYMPTOMS	LABORATORY FINDINGS	RADIOGRAPHIC FEATURES	DIAGNOSIS	TREATMENT
Bacterial liver abscess	50-70 years old Male = female	Recent bacterial infection, biliary obstruction, diabetes mellitus	Fevers, chills, malaise, anorexia, diarrhea, cough, pleuritic chest pain, RUQ pain	Leukocytosis, anemia, elevated alkaline phosphatase and bilirubin, low albumin, positive blood cultures (50%)	Multifocal (50%), usually right lobe, irregular margins	Aspirate (70-80% positive)	Percutaneous drainage and antibiotics
Amebic liver abscess	18-50 years old Male > female	Alcohol intake, HLA-DR3, oral and anal sex, contaminated enema apparatus, travel to or living in an endemic area	Fever, RUQ pain, hepatic tenderness, anorexia, weight loss, uncommon to have colitis	Leukocytosis, no eosinophilia, mild anemia, elevated alkaline phosphatase, elevated ESR, positive serology	Single abscess (80%), usually right lobe, wall enhancement seen on CT scan with IV contrast	Aspirate (trophozoites rarely seen) can rule out superimposed bacterial infection, positive serology and risk factors	Metronidazole and iodoquinol

CT = computed tomography; ESR = erythrocyte sedimentation rate; HLA = human leukocyte antigen; IV = intravenous; RUQ = right upper quadrant.

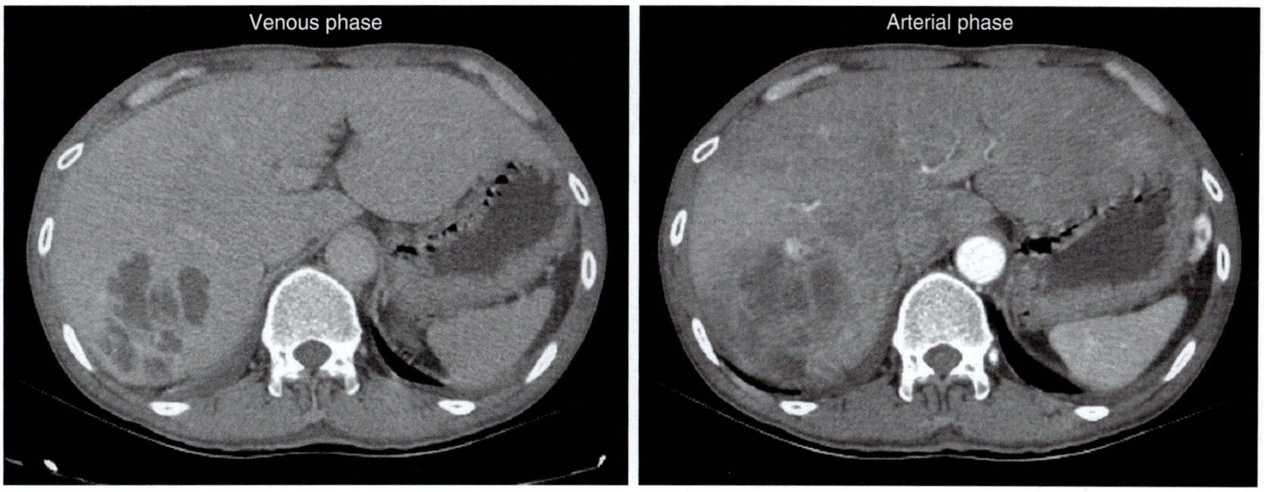

FIGURE 137-1. A and B, Computed tomographic scans of pyogenic liver abscess. (Courtesy Dr. Chalermrat Bunchorntavakul, Bangkok, Thailand.)

bleeding into a tumor, but it also can be seen in the wall of an echinococcal cyst. Nonspecific radiologic features, including elevation of the right hemidiaphragm, right lower lung lobe atelectasis, and right pleural effusion, are seen in up to 30% of patients with pyogenic liver abscesses. Magnetic resonance imaging and tagged white blood scans add little to the diagnosis of a liver abscess.

Microbial cultures are essential. In addition to blood cultures, the abscess cavity should be aspirated percutaneously, with either ultrasound or CT guidance, and the aspirate should be cultured for aerobic and anaerobic organisms as well as examined for amebae if there is any suspicion of an amebic abscess. Blood cultures are positive in only approximately 50% of cases. In approximately 15 to 20% of cases, multiple organisms are identified in the abscess cavity, but 20 to 50% of cases may have negative cultures despite appropriate culture techniques.

TREATMENT

Immediate broad-spectrum antibiotic coverage and the prompt identification and treatment of the source of the infection are essential for successful outcomes.[8] As soon as the causative bacterium is identified, the antibiotic regimen can be tailored appropriately. Recommendations should be guided by the culture and by prevailing bacterial resistance patterns. Monotherapy with a β-lactam or β-lactamase inhibitor such as ampicillin-sulbactam (3 g intravenously [IV] every 6 hours) or piperacillin-tazobactam (3.375 or 4.5 g IV every 6 hours) or ticarcillin-clavulanate (3.1 g IV every 6 hours) can be used, or a third-generation cephalosporin such as ceftriaxone (1 g IV daily or 2 g IV every 12 hours for central nervous system infections) *plus* metronidazole (500 mg IV every 8 hours) can be considered. Alternate regimens for consideration include a fluoroquinolone (such as ciprofloxacin 400 mg IV every 12 hours or levofloxacin 500 or 750 mg IV daily) *plus* metronidazole (500 mg IV every 8 hours) and monotherapy with a carbapenem such as imipenem-cilastatin (500 mg IV every 6 hours), meropenem (1 g IV every 8 hours), doripenem (500 mg IV every 8 hours), or ertapenem (1 g IV daily). The duration of therapy is partly based on the response to therapy. An average of 4 to 6 weeks of antibiotic therapy is reasonable, and the last 2 to 4 weeks of the antibiotic regimen can be administered orally. For documented *Klebsiella pneumoniae* liver abscess treated with 5 to 7 days of intravenous antibiotics, an additional 28 days of oral ciprofloxacin is as good as an additional 28 days of intravenous ceftriaxone.[A1] Abscesses that are difficult to drain or are slow to demonstrate radiographic resolution require longer courses of therapy. Importantly, radiologic abnormalities resolve more slowly than clinical and biochemical features, so the latter should be used as a guide for tailoring the therapeutic regimen.

Antibiotics alone can sometimes successfully resolve small, multiple pyogenic abscesses, but most patients (≥70%) will require drainage of the abscesses. Percutaneous drainage is recommended, with subsequent management dictated by the size and number of abscesses. Abscesses of up to 5cm in diameter can be managed with a single aspiration. Larger abscesses are probably better managed with catheter drainage[A2,A3] until the output is less than approximately 20 to 25mL per day, at which time the catheter can be removed. Endoscopic ultrasound-guided drainage is an option if the abscess cannot be accessed percutaneously.[9] Surgical drainage is seldom required because of the advancements in percutaneous drainage and is reserved for loculated abscesses and abscesses that do not respond to percutaneous drainage and antibiotics. Biliary obstruction is treated with endoscopic retrograde cholangiopancreatography or transhepatic cholangiography (Chapter 141) with accompanying biliary drainage. For pyogenic abscesses in transplanted livers, management and proper biliary drainage may be difficult to achieve because of the diffuse nature of the biliary strictures.

PROGNOSIS

Abscesses smaller than 10 cm can take up to 16 weeks to resolve, whereas abscesses larger than 10 cm may take an average of an additional 6 weeks to resolve. Mortality from pyogenic liver abscess is associated with older age and with comorbidities such as cirrhosis, diabetes, chronic renal failure, and malignancy. Jaundice is an ominous sign. In developed countries the mortality rate ranges from 2 to 12%.

NON-ABSCESS HEPATIC BACTERIAL INFECTIONS

Bacterial infections of the liver can also cause more diffuse infections without frank abscess formation. Implicated organisms include *Listeria monocytogenes* (Chapter 272), *Yersinia enterocolitica* (Chapter 288), *Salmonella typhi* and *Salmonella paratyphi* (Chapter 284), *Legionella* (Chapter 290), *Ehrlichia* (Chapter 302), and gonococci (Chapter 275). There are no specific features associated with these infections, and these organisms do not necessarily cause abscesses. Patients with chronic liver disease are especially at risk for *Listeria* infection. Patients with active enteric *Yersinia* infection can have secondary liver involvement with or without liver abscesses. Disseminated gonococcal infections (Chapter 275) can cause a perihepatitis (Fitz-Hugh-Curtis syndrome), which can be manifested with right upper quadrant pain and tenderness.

Systemic bacteremia can cause a variety of hepatobiliary abnormalities, which may range from elevated aminotransferase and alkaline phosphatase levels (Chapter 133) to the cholestasis of sepsis with the development of jaundice. Several organisms can disrupt normal liver function after entering the blood stream, the most common of which are *E. coli*, *Klebsiella* spp, *Streptococcus pneumoniae*, and *S. aureus*. Typically, in patients suffering from jaundice, sources of bacteremia include pneumonia, urinary tract infection, and soft tissue infection, although organisms may originate from a range of other sites. The hepatic biochemical abnormalities associated with bacteremia may be related to factors such as hemodynamic instability and liver hypoperfusion, as well as to the infection. Associated renal failure, a blood transfusion–derived bilirubin load, and drugs may complicate the picture. The course of cholestasis may be prolonged for several days to a few weeks, but it typically resolves with resolution of the systemic infection. There is no specific treatment for the cholestasis related to a systemic infection, but it is important to rule out drug-induced cholestasis that may evolve as a consequence of one or more of the antibiotics.

FUNGAL DISEASES OF THE LIVER

Except for hepatosplenic candidiasis, clinically significant fungal diseases of the liver are unusual. Typically, other fungal infections will also be manifested as liver granulomas but will not show the high, swinging pyrexia that is characteristic of hepatosplenic candidiasis. Tissue cultures are required to confirm a diagnosis.

HEPATOSPLENIC CANDIDIASIS

EPIDEMIOLOGY AND PATHOBIOLOGY

Hepatosplenic candidiasis typically is caused by *Candida albicans*, but other species, including *C. tropicalis*, *C. parapsilosis*, *C. glabrata*, and *C. krusei*, have occasionally been reported. It occurs as part of disseminated candidiasis (Chapter 310), most commonly in patients with solid organ or hematopoietic stem cell transplants or acute leukemia, but rarely in patients with lymphoma,

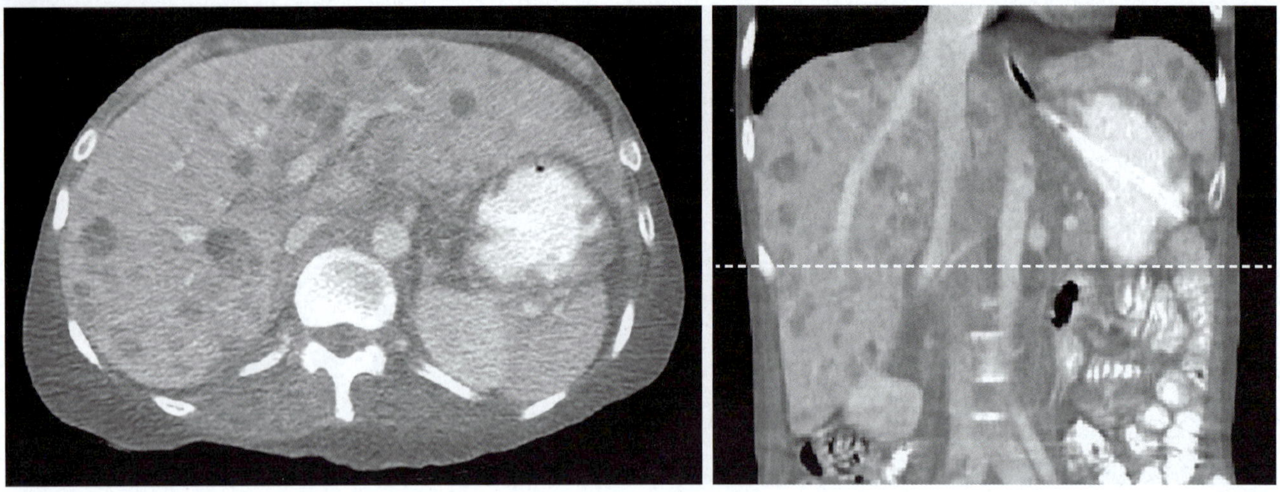

FIGURE 137-2. Multiple filling defects in the liver and spleen in a patient with hepatic and splenic candidiasis. (Courtesy of Dr. Sirina Ekpanyapong, Bangkok, Thailand.)

aplastic anemia, and sarcoma. With the current widespread use of prophylactic antifungal agents early in the course of the disease in patients with acute leukemia, hepatosplenic candidiasis develops in only 1 to 2% of patients, more commonly with acute lymphoblastic leukemia than with acute myeloid leukemia. Hepatosplenic candidiasis presumably results from translocation of *Candida* species from the gastrointestinal tract into the blood stream as a result of prolonged neutropenia and a breach in mucosal integrity.

CLINICAL MANIFESTATIONS AND DIAGNOSIS

Hepatosplenic candidiasis (Fig. 137-2) is manifested by persistent and high spiking fevers in a patient who was previously neutropenic and has now returned to a normal neutrophil count.[10] Right upper quadrant pain, nausea, vomiting, and anorexia may accompany fever.

Patients typically have elevated levels of alkaline phosphatase and less commonly of aminotransferases, bilirubin, and leukocytes. CT, which is the imaging modality of choice, classically shows multiple lucencies representing microabscesses in the liver, spleen, and kidneys. If the CT scan is nondiagnostic but clinical suspicion remains high, magnetic resonance imaging should be performed. A definitive diagnosis is usually made on a liver biopsy specimen that shows multiple granulomas and may show yeast and hyphal forms with special stains. However, biopsy often will not show evidence of infection, especially in cases in which antifungal therapy has been used. Although biopsy is the only means to establish a definitive diagnosis, it often is not required because the clinical, laboratory, and radiographic manifestations of the disease are almost always sufficient to establish a specific diagnosis.

TREATMENT AND PROGNOSIS

The mainstay of therapy is antifungal therapy. In clinically stable patients, oral fluconazole (400 mg orally, daily) can be used. In acutely ill patients a lipid formulation of amphotericin B (3 to 5 mg/kg IV daily) or an echinocandin for several weeks is recommended. The echinocandin options include caspofungin (70 mg loading dose then 50 mg IV daily), anidulafungin (200 mg loading dose then 100 mg IV daily), or micafungin (100 mg IV daily). After several weeks of such therapy, patients can be transitioned to oral fluconazole at 400 mg daily or to voriconazole (6 mg/kg IV q12 hours for first 24 hours, then 3 to 4 mg/kg IV q12 hours or 200 mg orally q12 hours) or posaconazole (IV: 300 mg IV 9 to 12 hours on day 1, then 300 mg IV daily or 300 mg orally 9 to 12 hours on day 1, then 300 mg orally daily) in fluconazole-resistant isolates. Treatment should continue until the lesions resolve on follow-up CT scans, typically within 6 months of treatment. Patients receiving chemotherapy or stem cell transplants are at a higher risk for developing hepatosplenic candidiasis; for this reason, patients who have a history of hepatosplenic candidiasis should be treated prophylactically with fluconazole (400 mg orally, daily) to prevent relapse.

PROGNOSIS

With prolonged treatment with antifungal agents, there has been good success at treating hepatosplenic candidiasis.

OTHER FUNGAL DISEASES

Several additional fungal infections affect the liver, although rarely. *Coccidioides immitis* is often asymptomatic but may lead to fungal hepatitis characterized by increased alkaline phosphatase and the development of hepatic granulomas. Hepatic *Cryptococcus neoformans* infection is rare but has a higher prevalence in patients with acquired immunodeficiency syndrome (AIDS), in whom it typically causes hepatomegaly. In the non–human immunodeficiency virus (HIV)–infected patient, disseminated cryptococcosis less frequently can result in focal granulomatous hepatitis, which may clinically mimic viral hepatitis, or can be manifested as obstructive jaundice secondary to sclerosing cholangitis. *Histoplasma capsulatum* infects individuals who inhale the fungus, but most cases are subclinical. In symptomatic hepatic histoplasmosis, two thirds of patients will present with hepatomegaly, with some showing splenic enlargement as well. On histologic examination, histoplasmosis can cause multiple granulomas diffusely distributed throughout the liver, although a more common finding is portal lymphohistiocytic infiltrate. *Paracoccidioides brasiliensis* most commonly infects adult men, and autopsy series have shown hepatic involvement in up to 50% of patients who die of this infection. Some individuals may present with hepatomegaly or jaundice, although the latter is found in less than 6% of patients. Aminotransferase levels are often elevated in the early stages of the disease; changes in alkaline phosphatase or bilirubin levels tend to occur in the later stages. Biopsy may reveal lesions ranging from small granulomas to diffuse infiltration of yeast forms and fibrosis, often with bile duct involvement. In all of these examples, fungal cultures are necessary to establish a definitive diagnosis.

PARASITIC, PROTOZOAL, AND HELMINTHIC INFECTIONS OF THE LIVER

AMEBIC LIVER ABSCESS

EPIDEMIOLOGY

Entamoeba histolytica is found throughout the world where the barriers between human feces and food and water are inadequate. After malaria, it is the second leading cause of death from parasitic diseases worldwide, accounting for an estimated 40,000 to 100,000 deaths annually. In the United States, most cases of amebiasis arise in immigrants from endemic areas and people living in states that border Mexico.[11] Travelers to endemic areas are also at risk; ingestion of amebic cysts and colonization of the gastrointestinal tract can occur years before the development of a liver abscess. Amebic liver abscesses mainly affect men between the ages of 18 and 50 years but are also more common in postmenopausal women, thereby suggesting a hormonal protective effect. Other risk factors include alcohol intake, human leukocyte antigen (HLA)-DR3, oral and anal sex, and contaminated enema apparatuses.

PATHOBIOLOGY

Entamoeba histolytica has a simple life cycle consisting of the cyst (infectious form) and trophozoite (the motile stage associated with disease); it infects only humans and some nonhuman primates. Cysts are ingested and mature into trophozoites in the intestinal lumen. The development of amebic colitis is not essential for liver abscess formation. *E. histolytica* trophozoites penetrate through the mucosa and submucosal tissues and enter the portal circulation. *E. histolytica* blocks intrahepatic portal venules. When the trophozoites reach the liver, they create their unique abscesses, which are well-circumscribed regions of dead hepatocytes, liquefied cells, and cellular debris that are surrounded by a rim of connective tissue, a few inflammatory cells, and amebic trophozoites. The adjacent liver parenchyma is unaffected. Given the small numbers of amebae relative to the size of the abscess, it is suggested that *E. histolytica* can cause hepatocyte death without direct contact.

CLINICAL MANIFESTATIONS

Patients can present with amebic liver abscesses months to years after traveling to an endemic area, so a detailed travel history is essential for the diagnosis. The disease should be suspected in patients with an appropriate travel history, fever, right upper quadrant pain, and substantial hepatic tenderness. Jaundice is extremely uncommon. Symptoms are usually acute (<10 days in duration) but can be chronic, with anorexia and weight loss. Patients with acute disease tend to have multifocal disease, whereas patients with a more indolent course tend to have a solitary lesion. Laboratory data tend to demonstrate a leukocytosis without eosinophilia, mild anemia, an elevated alkaline phosphatase level, and a high erythrocyte sedimentation rate.

DIAGNOSIS

Although some individuals with amebic liver abscesses have concurrent amebic colitis, the majority of patients have no bowel symptoms; hence, the results of stool microscopy for *E. histolytica* trophozoites and cysts are usually negative. The diagnosis relies on identification of space-occupying lesions in the liver and a positive amebic serology.[12] Both ultrasound and CT scan are very sensitive (Fig. 137-3), but neither provides absolute specificity for amebic liver abscesses. Serologic testing is highly sensitive (>94%) and specific (>95%). False-negative test results can be obtained within the first 7 to 10 days of infection, but repeat testing will usually be positive. Polymerase chain reaction testing of the abscess aspirate has proved valuable for making the diagnosis in returning travelers. Aspiration of the lesion may be necessary to exclude a primary or secondary bacterial infection.

TREATMENT AND PROGNOSIS

Metronidazole (500 to 750 mg orally three times daily) is usually the first-line treatment. Clinical improvement is often seen within 72 to 96 hours, but treatment should be continued for 7 to 10 days. Tinidazole at 2g daily for 5 days is especially effective and may be better tolerated, in part because of its shorter treatment regimen.[A4] Alternatives include ornidazole (0.5g twice daily for 5 to 10 days) and nitazoxanide (500mg twice daily for 10 days).[A5] Drainage is not necessary, even for large abscesses of 5 to 10cm,[13] except in patients who do not respond within 5 days. The abscess usually will shrink by about 50% within a week, but the mean time to complete radiologic resolution is 3 to 9 months. Repeated imaging in a clinically improving patient may lead to unwarranted concern and unnecessary treatment.

Treatment must also address the removal of all of the cysts from the intestinal lumen in patients with evidence of intraluminal infection. A recommended treatment is iodoquinol (650 mg orally three times a day for 20 days) to prevent continued colonization and possible recurrence of the liver abscess. Alternative regimens for treating intraluminal infection include paromomycin (25 to 30 mg/kg per day orally in three divided doses for 7 days) or diloxanide furoate (500 mg orally three times day for 10 days). The overall mortality rate from amebic abscess is 1 to 3%, whereas it is less than 1% if diagnosed and treated early.

OTHER PROTOZOAL LIVER DISEASES

In addition to *E. histolytica*, other protozoal diseases that affect the liver include *Cryptosporidium* (Chapter 321), *Toxoplasma gondii* (Chapter 320), *Leishmania* (Chapter 319), *Plasmodium* (Chapter 316), and *Babesia microti* (Chapter 324) (Table 137-2).

HELMINTH INFECTIONS

Echinococcosis and Hydatid Cyst Disease

EPIDEMIOLOGY AND PATHOBIOLOGY

Human cystic echinococcosis (Chapter 325) is a zoonosis caused by the larval cestode *Echinococcus granulosus*. It is often referred to as hydatid cyst disease because of the watery cysts that characterize the infection.

The disease remains endemic in sheep-raising areas of the world, including Africa, the Mediterranean region of Europe, the Middle East, Asia, South America, Australia, and New Zealand. Dogs are the definitive hosts for *E. granulosus*, and sheep are the major intermediate hosts, although yaks, goats, and camels are other relevant intermediate hosts. Humans are only accidental hosts when they ingest food or water that is fecally contaminated with eggs. Human contact with sheepdogs, which are in frequent contact with livestock, is a major risk for infection.

The disease cycle begins when an adult tapeworm infects the intestinal tract of the definitive host (dogs usually). The adult tapeworm then produces eggs, which are expelled in the host's feces. Intermediate hosts become infected by ingesting the eggs of the parasite in fecally contaminated food. Inside the intermediate host, the eggs hatch and release tiny hooked embryos (called oncospheres), which travel in the blood stream and eventually lodge in the liver, lungs, or kidneys, where they develop into hydatid cysts. Inside these cysts grow thousands of tapeworm larvae, the next stage in the life cycle of the parasite.

CLINICAL MANIFESTATIONS

The initial infection is asymptomatic, but an enlarging hydatid liver cyst can cause abdominal pain, nausea, hepatomegaly, or a palpable mass. Patients may describe symptoms of mild upper right quadrant pain, urticarial rash, and episodes of pruritus. If the cyst ruptures, serious complications can develop. Cysts that perforate into the peritoneum can lead to the development of extrahepatic cysts and may induce an allergic reaction leading to an increase of eosinophils in the blood, pruritic urticaria, and systemic anaphylaxis. In most cases, however, cysts rupture into bile ducts, which can result in cholestatic jaundice, cholangitis, or biliary pain.

DIAGNOSIS

On ultrasound or CT scans (Fig. 137-4), the hydatid cysts are often large with a flaky appearance that is referred to as hydatid sand.[14] CT imaging also may show multiple daughter cysts or a fluid density cyst with peripheral focal areas of calcification.[15] Fluid is of variable density depending on the amount of proteinaceous debris.

Hydatid cysts of liver can be diagnosed by a serologic assay, the Weinberg reaction, but it can be falsely negative in up to 38% of cases. An enzyme-linked immunosorbent assay may be more sensitive. Eosinophilia is not a feature unless the cyst ruptures; in fact, there usually are no changes in blood chemistries.

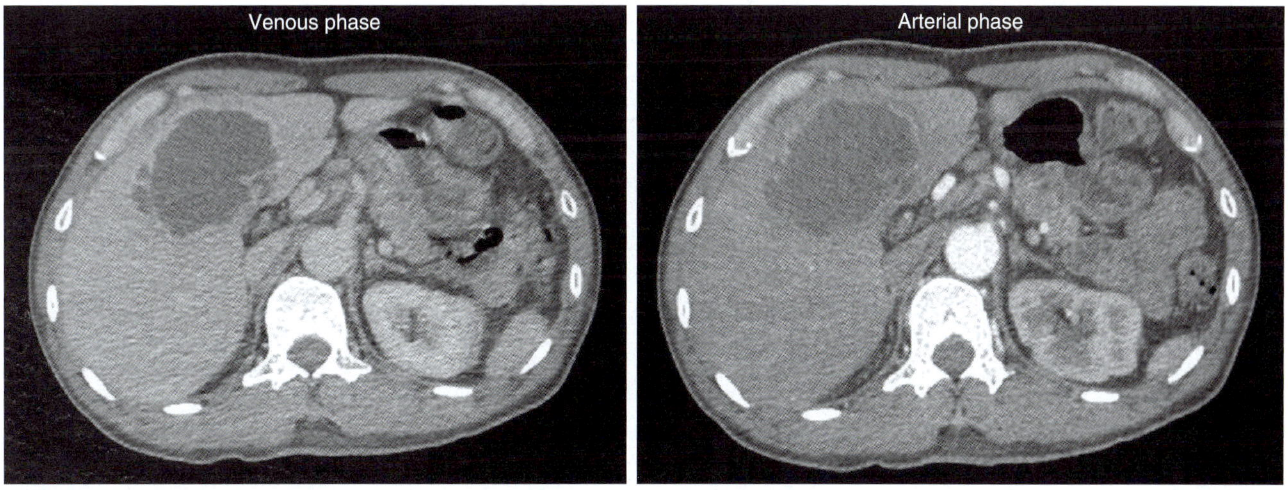

FIGURE 137-3. **Computed tomographic scan of an amebic liver abscess.** (Courtesy Dr. Chalermrat Bunchorntavakul, Bangkok, Thailand.)

TABLE 137-2 PARASITIC INFECTIONS INVOLVING THE LIVER

	CHARACTERISTICS	ENDEMIC AREAS	RISK FACTORS AND ENDEMIC AREAS	MAJOR HEPATIC MANIFESTATIONS	SYMPTOMS AND SIGNS	LABORATORY FINDINGS	RADIOGRAPHIC FEATURES	DIAGNOSIS	TREATMENT
MAJOR PROTOZOA									
Entamoeba histolytica	Ingested cysts develop into invasive trophozoites that colonize the colon and occasionally spread to the liver by the portal blood	Mexico, regions of Central and South America, India, and regions of Africa	Male gender, alcohol intake, HLA-DR3, oral and anal sex, and contaminated enema apparatuses	Amebic liver abscesses develop as a tissue response to trophozoite invasion with acute and chronic manifestations (see text)	Fever, RUQ pain, and substantial hepatic tenderness	Leukocytosis without eosinophilia, mild anemia, elevated serum AP, and high ESR	US, CT, and MRI can detect abscess but cannot always differentiate amebic from pyogenic. On CT or MRI, amebic abscess sometimes appears "cold" with bright rim	Imaging, serology, stool antigen test (microscopic evaluation of stool has a poor yield)	Metronidazole (500-750 mg PO tid × 7-10 days) *or* tinidazole (2 g daily × 5 days); Iodoquinol (650 mg PO tid × 20 days) *or* paromomycin (25-30 mg/kg PO daily in three divided doses × 7 days) *or* diloxanide furoate (500 mg PO tid × 10 days), also needed to eradicate intestinal colonization
OTHER PROTOZOA									
Cryptosporidium spp and microsporidia	Ingested cysts develop into trophozoites in intestinal mucosa	Worldwide distribution	AIDS	Biliary tract infection with obstruction and cholangitis	See Chapter 321	See Chapter 321	See Chapter 321	See Chapter 321	See Chapter 321
Toxoplasma gondii	Ingestion of oocysts in contaminated soil or water or in infected meat; systemic spread of tachyzoites in the circulation	Worldwide distribution	Consumption of undercooked meat, contact with soil, and travel outside the United States, Europe, or Canada	Immunocompetent: asymptomatic or hepatomegaly and mild LFT elevations Immunocompromised: occasional overt hepatitis	See Chapter 320	See Chapter 320	See Chapter 320	See Chapter 320	See Chapter 320
Leishmania spp	Sand fly bite transmits promastigotes; proliferation in the reticuloendothelial system	Worldwide distribution	Children age 10 and younger and immunocompromised adults Contact with sand flies	Hepatosplenomegaly months to years after infection	See Chapter 319	See Chapter 319	See Chapter 319	See Chapter 319	See Chapter 319
Plasmodium spp	Mosquito (*Anopheles*) bite transmits sporozoites	Multiple regions throughout the world	Exposure to anopheline mosquito bites	Proliferation in hepatocytes causes hepatomegaly, enzyme elevations, and jaundice	See Chapter 316	See Chapter 316	See Chapter 316	See Chapter 316	See Chapter 316
Babesia microti	Tick bite transmits the agent, which parasitizes erythrocytes	Europe	Asplenia is a risk for fatal hepatic failure, especially bovine babesiosis	Mild liver enzyme elevations	See Chapter 324	See Chapter 324	See Chapter 324	See Chapter 324	See Chapter 324
MAJOR HELMINTHS									
Schistosoma spp	Cercaria in fresh water penetrate the skin, travel by the circulation to portal vein radicals	*S. mansoni* found in South America, Africa, and Middle East *S. japonicum* found in Far East (mostly China and Philippines)	Contact with fresh water containing cercaria of schistosomes	Progressive presinusoidal blood flow obstruction, periportal fibrosis, portal hypertension, varices, ascites, splenomegaly	Initial infection presents as itching; later presentations include fever, diarrhea, chills, headaches, or hives Hematemesis from ruptured gastroesophageal varices	Eosinophilia and splenomegaly Seroconversion occurs within 4-6 weeks	Extensive calcification with typical "turtle-back" appearance along portal tracts	Rectal biopsy, liver biopsy, microscopic examination of stool	Praziquantel (single dose of 40 mg/kg for *S. haematobium*, *S. mansoni*, or *S. intercalatum* infections; two divided doses of 60 mg/kg for *S. japonicum* or *S. mekongi* infections) with a second dose 6-12 weeks later if necessary

Echinococcus granulosus	Eggs of small (3-7 mm) tapeworms in stool of canid hosts; ingested eggs produce larval oncospheres that migrate to the liver and form cysts in sheep, humans, and other intermediate hosts	Worldwide distribution, found especially in sheep-raising areas (Africa, the Mediterranean region of Europe, the Middle East, Asia, South America, Australia, and New Zealand)	Ingestion of food or water fecally contaminated with eggs and human contact with sheepdogs	Initial infection asymptomatic Liver cysts increase in diameter by 1-5 cm yearly and cause variable abdominal pain, hepatomegaly, and variable eosinophilia Occasional cyst rupture, secondary bacterial infection	Enlarged hydatid cyst can cause abdominal pain, nausea, hepatomegaly, or a palpable mass Mild RUQ pain, urticaria, and episodes of pruritus	Positive Weinberg reaction (false-negative reaction in 38% of cases) or ELISA analysis Eosinophilia seen in ruptured cysts	On US or CT, cysts appear flaky, sometimes showing daughter cysts or peripheral focal calcification; fluid is of variable density	Imaging, Weinberg reaction, or ELISA	Albendazole (15 mg/kg/day, divided into two doses, up to maximum 400 mg, PO bid × 1-3 months; up to 6 months if necessary); cysts without daughter cysts can be drained percutaneously; complicated cysts, including those communicating with the biliary tree, often require surgical treatment
Echinococcus multilocularis	Eggs of small tapeworms in stool of foxes; ingested eggs produce oncospheres in the liver of rodents, humans, and other intermediate hosts	Endemic in Northern hemisphere	Human exposure increasing with growing fox populations	Metacestodes colonize the liver as a tumor-like mass of small vesicles	See Chapter 325	See Chapter 325	See Chapter 325	See Chapter 325	See Chapter 325
Fasciola spp	Leaf-shaped flukes up to 13 × 30 mm derived from ingested cysts; the fluke excysts in the duodenum, migrates directly across the bowel wall into the peritoneal cavity, and burrows directly into the liver (or occasionally out to the skin)	Worldwide distribution	Consumption of freshwater or aquatic plants contaminated by colonized livestock	Adult flukes live in the common and hepatic bile ducts, causing obstruction that leads to thickening of the ducts, dilation, and fibrosis of the proximal biliary tree	Acute: fever, abdominal pain, eosinophilia Chronic: symptomatic biliary obstruction, variable eosinophilia	Serologic tests include hemagglutination, complement fixation, ELISA, and counterimmunoelectrophoresis. Anemia, leukocytosis, eosinophilia, elevated AP, and hypergammaglobulinemia are often seen	CT is most useful: liver shows hypodense nodules or tortuous tracks; thickening of the liver capsule, subcapsular hematoma, and parenchymal calcification may also be seen	Serology, stool examination	Triclabendazole, 10 mg/kg PO once or twice
Opisthorchis spp and *Clonorchis sinensis*	Flukes of 8-25 mm derived from ingested cysts; the fluke excysts in the duodenum and migrates into the bile ducts	*Opisthorchis* spp: Southeast Asia, central and eastern Europe (particularly Siberia) *C. sinensis:* China, Japan, Vietnam, and Korea	Consumption of raw, pickled, dried, smoked, or salted freshwater fish or crayfish originating from East Asia or, in the case of *Opisthorchis felineus,* Russia and Eastern Europe	Acute: typically asymptomatic Chronic: abdominal pain, fever, anorexia, tender hepatomegaly, sometimes eosinophilia Late sequelae: intermittent biliary obstruction, cholelithiasis, cholecystitis, cholangitis, secondary bacterial abscesses, cholangiocarcinoma	Chronic infection presents as dyspepsia, abdominal pain, diarrhea, nausea, vomiting, anorexia, weight loss, fevers, hepatomegaly, and urticaria Acute presentation includes serum sickness, intrahepatic pigment stones, and facial edema Other rare complications are cholangitis, pancreatitis, and obstructive jaundice	Anemia, leukocytosis, eosinophilia, elevated AP, and hypergammaglobulinemia	US may detect flukes in biliary tree CT shows small hypodense nodules	Serology and stool examination	Praziquantel, 25 mg/kg/day PO tid × 2 days

TABLE 137-2 PARASITIC INFECTIONS INVOLVING THE LIVER—cont'd

	CHARACTERISTICS	ENDEMIC AREAS	RISK FACTORS AND ENDEMIC AREAS	MAJOR HEPATIC MANIFESTATIONS	SYMPTOMS AND SIGNS	LABORATORY FINDINGS	RADIOGRAPHIC FEATURES	DIAGNOSIS	TREATMENT
Toxocara spp	Nematode infection disseminates to cause visceral larva migrans after ingestion of soil contaminated with dog or cat feces	Highest prevalence in southeastern United States	Consumption of food contaminated with soil containing eggs; distributed throughout the United States	Often an asymptomatic cause of eosinophilia (exclude *Trichinella, Strongyloides,* filaria, hookworm, schistosomiasis) Hepatomegaly is common, but nonhepatic manifestations dominate the clinical picture	See Chapter 327	See Chapter 327	See Chapter 327	See Chapter 327	See Chapter 327
OTHER HELMINTHS									
Ascaris lumbricoides	Ingested eggs develop into larvae that migrate to the lungs and are coughed and swallowed; develop into roundworms 15-30 mm long in the small intestine	Global distribution with higher prevalence in Africa, South America, India, and the Far East; 20% of the world's population is colonized	Consumption of fecally contaminated food or water, particularly in young children	Colonization is typically asymptomatic with eosinophilia Biliary migration of worms can cause symptomatic biliary obstruction, cholangitis, cholecystitis, and secondary bacterial liver abscess	Sensitized patients during pulmonary phase present with asthma-like symptoms, hemoptysis, chest pain, and cyanosis Urticaria and other allergic reactions sometimes seen Patients in intestinal phase show cognitive and nutritional impairment with abdominal pain, hepatomegaly, cholangitis, and obstructive jaundice	Leukocytosis with eosinophilia Hyperbilirubinemia occasionally seen	Movement of the worms within the biliary tree can sometimes be observed A "bull's-eye" appearance can be seen on cross-sectional imaging	Stool examination, imaging, and ERCP (Video 137-1)	Albendazole, 400 mg PO once
Capillaria hepatica	Ingested eggs develop into larvae in the intestinal mucosa; larvae migrate to the liver by portal blood flow and develop into short-lived roundworms	Human infection is rare	Consumption of food contaminated with rodent feces	Fever, eosinophilia, and hepatomegaly; subsequent foci of liver fibrosis, granulomas, and calcification in involved areas	Persistent fever, eosinophilia, and hepatomegaly most common Splenomegaly, anorexia, nausea, vomiting, night sweats, and altered bowel habits also seen	Anemia, eosinophilia, moderately elevated liver enzymes, increased ESR, and hypergammaglobulinemia	US shows nonspecific hyperechoic areas in the portal spaces	Stool and liver biopsy	Mebendazole, 200 mg PO bid × 20 days
Strongyloides stercoralis	Ingested eggs develop into 1.5- to 2.5-mm nematodes that invade the hepatic vasculature, lymphatics, and biliary tract	Tropical and subtropical areas including southeast United States and southern and eastern Europe	Consumption of food contaminated with soil containing eggs, infection with HTLV-1, and immunocompromised individuals	Hepatic disease in the setting of immunosuppression: jaundice, abdominal pain; eosinophilia is uncommon	Recurrent urticaria, abdominal pain, diarrhea, and cough; mild jaundice and hepatomegaly in the absence of splenomegaly	Eosinophilia and hypoalbuminemia Patients may have elevated liver enzymes	Imaging studies not used in diagnosis	Serology and stool examination	Ivermectin (single dose, 200 µg/kg orally × 1-2 days) or Albendazole (400 mg PO bid × 7 days)

AIDS = acquired immunodeficiency syndrome; AP = alkaline phosphatase; bid = twice daily; CT = computed tomography; ELISA = enzyme-linked immunosorbent assay; ERCP = endoscopic retrograde cholangiopancreatography; ESR = erythrocyte sedimentation rate; HLA = human leukocyte antigen; HTLV = human T-cell lymphotropic virus; LFT = liver function test; MRI = magnetic resonance imaging; PO = orally; RUQ = right upper quadrant; spp = species; tid = three times daily; US = ultrasonography.

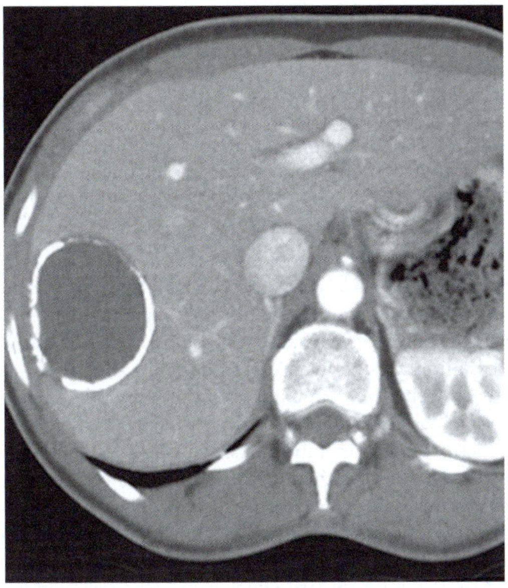

FIGURE 137-4. Computed tomographic scan of a hepatic echinococcal cyst. (Courtesy Dr. Chalermrat Bunchorntavakul, Bangkok, Thailand.)

TREATMENT AND PROGNOSIS

Uncomplicated, asymptomatic, inactive cysts can be observed without treatment.[16] Otherwise, however, drug therapy includes the antiparasitic agent albendazole (15 mg/kg/day, divided into two doses, to a maximum 400 mg orally twice daily) for 1 to 3 months, although a 6-month duration has also been used.[17] However, treatment with albendazole alone is not effective, so drainage is essential to the effective treatment of hydatid cysts. Cysts without daughter cysts can be drained percutaneously. Percutaneous drainage consisting of puncture and aspiration, followed by injection and reaspiration of a scolicidal solution is better than needle aspiration[A6] and has fewer side effects than open drainage, provided that patients receive concomitant antihelminthic therapy, such as albendazole starting 1 week before surgery and continuing 4 weeks postoperatively to minimize risk of secondary echinococcosis in the event of spillage. Chlorhexidine, hydrogen peroxide, 80% alcohol, or 0.5% cetrimide are preferred scolicidal agents rather than hypertonic saline or formalin.

Complicated cysts, however, typically require surgery. For example, if the cyst communicates with the biliary tree, injection of scolicidal agents carries an almost universal risk of secondary sclerosing cholangitis and is contraindicated. In such cases, the cyst must be treated surgically, either by cystectomy or hepatic resection.

The prognosis is generally good, with complete cure expected after successful percutaneous or surgical treatment. However, spillage occurs in 2 to 25% of cases, depending on the location of the cyst and the surgeon's experience. The operative mortality rate varies from 0.5 to 4% for the same reasons.

Schistosomiasis

EPIDEMIOLOGY AND PATHOBIOLOGY

Schistosomiasis is an infection of trematodes. *Schistosoma* (Chapter 326) cause periportal fibrosis and liver cirrhosis owing to deposition of eggs in the small portal venules.[18] *S. mansoni* and *S. japonicum* lead to liver disease. Infection with *S. mansoni* is found in parts of South America, Africa, and the Middle East. Infection with *S. japonicum* is found in the Far East, mostly China and the Philippines. Although primary infection does not occur in the United States, 5% of the world's population (200 million people) may be infected, thereby making it a major international health concern and highly prevalent in immigrants.

Humans become infected after contact with water that contains the infective stage (cercaria) of *schistosomes*. After penetration of the skin, the larvae migrate to the lungs and then to the venules of the mesentery, urinary bladder, or ureters. They release eggs in the venules of the mesentery, and the eggs enter the liver through the portal vein, where they become lodged in the terminal branches of the portal venules. The lodged eggs cause a granulomatous inflammation, and the lesions heal by periportal fibrosis. *S. japonicum* is more virulent than *S. mansoni* because its infections produce 10 times more eggs. Hepatic fibrosis may be independent of parasite burden related primarily to the host's inflammatory response.[19]

CLINICAL MANIFESTATIONS

Initial infection is manifested as itching that is caused by skin penetration by larvae. Several weeks later, patients may complain of fever, diarrhea, chills, headaches, or hives. At this time, patients will have eosinophilia. During the next 5 to 15 years, periportal liver fibrosis develops and leads to presinusoidal portal hypertension, splenomegaly (Chapter 154), and gastroesophageal varices (Chapter 124). With *S. japonicum*, however, the progression can be much more rapid, with little interval between the acute and chronic disease. Hepatic function is generally well preserved, and patients generally present with hematemesis from ruptured gastroesophageal varices.

DIAGNOSIS

Schistosomal eggs typically have lateral or terminal spines and are easy to detect on microscopic examination of feces or on a rectal biopsy specimen. Seroconversion occurs within 4 to 8 weeks of infection but cannot distinguish active infection from a history of exposure. Newer, more sensitive and specific molecular and immunodiagnostic techniques (including polymerase chain reaction–enzyme-linked immunosorbent assay systems) for detection of schistosome DNA in feces or serum and plasma have the potential to diagnose schistosomiasis in all stages of clinical disease, not only when the adult worms are producing eggs. Imaging may show extensive calcification with the typical "turtle-back" appearance along the portal tracts reflecting the clustered, calcified eggs along the portal triads. Ultrasound can assess the degree of periportal fibrosis.[20,21] Liver biopsy may demonstrate an egg of *S. mansoni* along with intense granulomatous change in the portal tract (E-Fig. 137-1).

TREATMENT AND PROGNOSIS

Praziquantel (a single dose of 40 mg/kg for *S. haematobium, S. mansoni*, or *S. intercalatum* infections; two divided doses of 60 mg/kg for *S. japonicum* or *S. mekongi* infections), which is the preferred treatment, is effective in 70 to 100% of cases. However, a second dose can be given 6 to 12 weeks later, particularly in patients with eosinophilia, high antibody titers, or persistent symptoms. Despite treatment, 5 to 20% of patients develop significant hepatic fibrosis. Treatment of portal hypertension may be necessary. The mortality is 0.05% with heavy *S. mansoni* infection and 1.8% for severe *S. japonicum* infection. Bleeding from esophageal varices is the most serious complication. Chronic infection can lead to hepatocellular carcinoma.

GRANULOMATOUS DISEASES OF THE LIVER

Granulomas, which are found in up to 15% of liver biopsies, can be an incidental finding or may represent a wide array of liver diseases (Table 137-3). A granuloma is an accumulation of epithelioid cells, including transformed macrophages, mononuclear cells, and other inflammatory cells. Granulomas may have associated necrosis (caseating), as in tuberculosis (Chapter 299), or may be non-necrotizing (noncaseating), as in sarcoidosis (Chapter 83). In addition, fibrin-ring granulomas are characterized by a vacuole encircled by a ring of fibrinoid necrosis and surrounded by lymphocytes and histiocytes, as seen in Q fever.

An incidental granuloma requires minimal further evaluation. Tuberculosis should be excluded. Sarcoidosis also should be considered because it is the most common cause of granulomas in the United States. An antimitochondrial antibody should be obtained to exclude primary biliary cirrhosis (Chapter 139). The use of potentially causative drugs should be stopped (see Table 137-3).

SARCOIDOSIS

Sarcoidosis (Chapter 83), which is the most frequently identified cause of hepatic granuloma in the United States, affects all racial and ethnic groups and occurs at all ages. In patients with sarcoidosis, the liver is the third most commonly involved organ, after the lymph nodes and lung; approximately 20 to 30% of patients with sarcoidosis have noncaseating granulomas on liver biopsy.[22] The classic granuloma is found mainly in the portal triads, with a cluster of large epithelioid cells and often with multinucleated giant cells.

CLINICAL MANIFESTATIONS AND DIAGNOSIS

Hepatic involvement of sarcoidosis is often subclinical, and only a minority of patients will present with pruritus, fever, abdominal pain, hepatomegaly,

TABLE 137-3 CAUSES OF GRANULOMATOUS LIVER DISEASE

DIAGNOSIS	SPECIAL AND UNIQUE FEATURES
Sarcoidosis	Evidence of pulmonary sarcoidosis, granulomas found on biopsy of other organs, elevated ACE level
Bacterial infections	
Mycobacterium tuberculosis	Caseating granulomas on biopsy, positive PPD response or interferon-gamma release assay, active pulmonary tuberculosis
Other mycobacteria (*M. avium-intracellulare, M. leprae, M. mucogenicum, M. bovis*)	HIV, exposure history
Other bacteria (brucellosis, listeriosis, melioidosis, tularemia, yersiniosis, Bartonellosis, Q fever, syphilis, psittacosis)	Fever, exposure history
Viral infections (cytomegalovirus, Epstein-Barr virus, hepatitis C, hepatitis B, hepatitis A)	Serology for acute or recent exposure
Fungal infections (histoplasmosis, coccidioidomycosis, blastomycosis, nocardiosis, candidiasis)	Fever, immunocompromised
Parasitic infections (schistosomiasis, *Ascaris lumbricoides*, toxoplasmosis, visceral leishmaniasis)	Travel to endemic regions, positive serologic testing
Primary biliary cirrhosis	Female sex, positive AMA, elevated IgM
Malignant diseases (Hodgkin disease, non-Hodgkin lymphoma, renal cell carcinoma)	Evidence of malignant disease in kidney or bone marrow
Drug reactions (allopurinol, chlorpropamide, phenylbutazone, sulfonamides, carbamazepine, glyburide, quinidine, quinine, diltiazem, hydralazine, rosiglitazone, phenytoin, methyldopa, procainamide, amoxicillin-clavulanic acid, mebendazole, mesalamine, acetaminophen, pyrazinamide, halothane, isoniazid, norfloxacin)	Exposure history
Toxins (beryllium, copper sulfate, Thorotrast)	Previous exposure history
Miscellaneous (talc, Crohn disease, granulomatosis with polyangiitis [formerly Wegener granulomatosis], post-jejunoileal bypass, mineral oil lipogranulomas, hepatic allograft rejection, chronic granulomatous disease)	History of IV drug use, history of liver transplantation, diarrhea

ACE = angiotensin-converting enzyme; AMA = antimitochondrial antibody; HIV = human immunodeficiency virus; IgM = immunoglobulin M; IV = intravenous; PPD = purified protein derivative.

cholestatic jaundice, or portal hypertension.[23] In some patients, the granulomatous injury and destruction of the interlobular bile ducts eventually cause ductopenia and a histologic picture similar to primary biliary cirrhosis (Chapter 141). In other patients, damage to the large bile ducts may lead to a syndrome that mimics primary sclerosing cholangitis (Chapter 141). Other patients may present with focal liver lesions suggestive of malignant neoplasm.

Patients typically have a marked elevation of the serum alkaline phosphatase level. Angiotensin-converting enzyme (ACE) levels also are characteristically elevated but may not be helpful in differentiating sarcoidosis from other chronic liver diseases, such as primary biliary cirrhosis, in which it also may be elevated. The presence of noncaseating granulomas in a patient with clinically suspected sarcoidosis generally establishes the diagnosis. However, granulomas do not correlate with liver function test results or duration of disease.

TREATMENT AND PROGNOSIS

In general, hepatic sarcoidosis does not need to be treated except in patients with other indications for treatment (Chapter 83). Corticosteroids improve liver function test results but do not alleviate portal hypertension, and serial biopsies often show little improvement. Other therapies used in uncontrolled studies include ursodeoxycholic acid, methotrexate, and azathioprine.[24] Sarcoidosis that leads to portal hypertension and fibrosis may ultimately require liver transplantation (Chapter 140), although sarcoidosis may recur in the new organ.

OTHER GRANULOMATOUS LIVER DISEASES

In addition to sarcoidosis, another major cause of granulomatous liver disease is tuberculosis (Chapter 299). Miliary tuberculosis, caused by *Mycobacterium tuberculosis*, commonly results in hepatic granulomas, and patients present with hepatomegaly, abnormal liver function test results, or both. A biopsy revealing caseating granulomas along with a positive PPD (purified protein derivative) response and active pulmonary tuberculosis can help in establishing a diagnosis. Other mycobacteria are also known to cause granulomatous liver disease including *M. avium intracellulare*, *M. genavense*, and *M. scrofulaceum* (Chapter 300).

Other causes of granulomatous liver disease include zoonotic infections such as cat-scratch disease (Chapter 291), Q fever (Chapter 302), and brucellosis (Chapter 286). Cat-scratch disease, which primarily affects children, is caused by *Bartonella henselae*, with cats serving as the main reservoir for the organism. Patients typically present with lymphadenopathy associated with persistent pyrexia of unknown origin, abdominal pain, and weight loss. *B. henselae* can be identified by a Warthin-Starry stain or an imaging study may demonstrate scattered defects in the liver. Q fever is caused by the intracellular gram-negative rickettsial organism *Coxiella burnetii*. Most infections are asymptomatic, but may have self-limited influenza-like symptoms, pneumonia, and hepatitis. A liver biopsy may demonstrate fibrin-ring granulomas (doughnut shaped) in the background of nonspecific reactive hepatitis and steatosis. Brucellosis, which is not common in the United States, is caused by at least four species of *Brucella: B. abortus, B. suis, B. melitensis,* and *B. canis.* The disease is manifested as recurrent high fevers, drenching sweats, malaise, arthralgia, fatigue, abdominal pain, anorexia, and headaches. Patients often have hepatomegaly. Hepatic biochemical abnormalities are nonspecific and show elevated serum levels of aminotransferases and alkaline phosphatase. The granulomas formed by this infection are typically smaller than those caused by sarcoidosis or tuberculosis, and a definitive diagnosis can be established by serologic testing.

It is important to keep in mind that hepatic granulomas are formed naturally as a consequence of the immune response, so they may be seen in infections with hepatic involvement. Many of the diseases noted above can manifest as granulomatous liver disease (see Table 137-3): listeriosis (Chapter 272), yersiniosis (Chapter 288), candidiasis (Chapter 310), histoplasmosis (Chapter 308), coccidioidomycosis (Chapter 308), and schistosomiasis (Chapter 326). Viral infections (e.g., cytomegalovirus, hepatitis A, hepatitis B, and hepatitis C), primary biliary cirrhosis (Chapter 139), malignancies, and certain drug reactions (Chapter 136) have all been etiologically linked to granulomatous liver disease.

GENERAL REFERENCES

For the General References and other additional features, please visit Elsevier eBooks+ at https://ebooks.health.elsevier.com.

Grade A References

A1. Molton JS, Chan M, Kalimuddin S, et al. Oral vs intravenous antibiotics for patients with Klebsiella pneumoniae liver abscess: a randomized, controlled noninferiority study. *Clin Infect Dis.* 2020;71:952-959.

A2. Ahmed M, Alam J, Hussain S, et al. Prospective randomized comparative study of percutaneous catheter drainage and percutaneous needle aspiration in the treatment of liver abscess. *ANZ J Surg.* 2021;91:E86-E90.

A3. Al-Sayaghi KM, Alhujaily M, Zaky MK, et al. Percutaneous needle aspiration versus catheter drainage in the management of liver abscess: an updated systematic review and meta-analysis. *ANZ J Surg.* 2022. [Epub ahead of print.].

A4. Pandey S, Gupta GK, Wanjari SJ, et al. Comparative study of tinidazole versus metronidazole in treatment of amebic liver abscess: a randomized control trial. *Indian J Gastroenterol.* 2018;37:196-201.

A5. Goel V, Jain A, Sharma G, et al. Evaluating the efficacy of nitazoxanide in uncomplicated amebic liver abscess. *Indian J Gastroenterol.* 2021;40:272-280.

A6. Akhan O, Erdoğan E, Ciftci TT, et al. Comparison of the long-term results of puncture, aspiration, injection and re-aspiration (PAIR) and catheterization techniques for the percutaneous treatment of CE1 and CE3a liver hydatid cysts: a prospective randomized trial. *Cardiovasc Intervent Radiol.* 2020;43:1034-1040.

138 ALCOHOLIC AND NONALCOHOLIC STEATOHEPATITIS

NAGA P. CHALASANI AND JACQUELYN MAHER

Alcohol-associated liver disease and nonalcoholic fatty liver disease (NAFLD), which represent two of the most common forms of liver disease, can lead to cirrhosis, liver cancer, liver failure, and death. Although these two conditions have different risk factors and natural histories, in both conditions (Table 138-1) the hepatocytes are characterized by macrovesicular steatosis, which is the accumulation of triglycerides as one large cytoplasmic globule that displaces the nucleus. In microvesicular steatosis, cytoplasmic accumulation of fat occurs as multiple small globules with a central (intact) nucleus.

ALCOHOL-ASSOCIATED LIVER DISEASE

DEFINITION

Excessive alcohol consumption (Chapter 364) causes alcohol-associated liver disease and can significantly worsen other liver disorders, such as viral hepatitis (Chapter 135) and hemochromatosis (Chapter 196). Although most individuals who consume alcohol do not consume it excessively and do not develop any physical or social consequences, some alcoholics consume sufficient alcohol and, presumably because of other predisposing factors, develop alcohol-associated liver disease. Alcohol-associated liver disease is a spectrum of chronic liver diseases ranging from alcoholic fatty liver to acute alcoholic hepatitis and cirrhosis.

Alcohol-associated fatty liver disease will develop in nearly 90% of individuals who consume alcohol heavily (on average, >6 drinks per day), but only a subset of individuals develop the severe conditions of alcoholic hepatitis and alcohol-associated cirrhosis. Genetic predisposition and environmental factors are likely to play a role in the pathogenesis of acute alcoholic hepatitis and alcohol-associated cirrhosis, but such factors have not been well defined. Nearly 50% of the patients with alcoholic hepatitis have preexisting cirrhosis (Chapter 139), and individuals who do not yet have cirrhosis are at high risk for its development, especially if they continue to consume alcohol.

EPIDEMIOLOGY

The true prevalence of alcoholic liver disease is not known, but nearly 1% of North American adults are thought to have alcohol-associated liver disease. Among individuals with alcohol use disorder, the prevalence of alcohol-associated liver disease is about 12%.[1] Even these figures are considered underestimates, however, because milder forms of alcohol-associated liver disease are not associated with symptoms and often are unrecognized. Alcohol-associated liver disease accounts for about 50% of deaths from cirrhosis and 40 to 45% of all deaths from liver disease. Over the last decade, alcohol-associated liver disease was the primary cause of almost one third of liver transplants (Chapter 140) in the United States, thereby replacing hepatitis C virus infection as the leading cause of liver transplantation in the United States. Based on an increase in the frequency of alcohol consumption, especially high-risk drinking, the incidence of alcoholic liver disease in the U.S. population is likely to increase significantly in the future.

PATHOBIOLOGY

The mechanisms underlying alcoholic liver injury can be broadly categorized into those caused by the effects of alcohol directly on hepatocytes and those caused by the effects mediated by Kupffer cells. The hepatocyte-specific mechanisms include the altered redox state induced by alcohol and aldehyde dehydrogenase reactions; the oxidative stress and lipid peroxidation caused by the induction of CYP2E1 enzymes and the mitochondrial electron transfer system; the effects of alcohol upon the nuclear transcription factors AMP kinase and SREBP-1c; protein adduct formation; and altered methionine and folate metabolism with resulting stress on the endoplasmic reticulum. Chronic alcohol consumption increases gut permeability, and the resulting portal endotoxemia activates Kupffer cells. Activated Kupffer cells release a number of proinflammatory mediators. These include tumor necrosis factor-α (TNF-α); transforming growth factor-β1; interleukins 1, 6, 8, and 10; and platelet-derived growth factor. TNF-α has a plethora of biologic effects and causes hepatocyte apoptosis, whereas transforming growth factor-β1 and platelet-derived growth factor play important roles in stellate cell activation, collagen production, and hepatic fibrosis.

Of the known risk factors for the development of alcohol-associated liver disease (Table 138-2), the amount of alcohol consumed is the single most important. For unclear reasons, only 30 to 35% of individuals with heavy and long-term drinking develop alcoholic hepatitis, and fewer than 20% develop cirrhosis. Women are at higher risk; for example, the risk of alcoholic cirrhosis increases after 10 years of alcohol consumption at quantities of more than 60 to 80 g/day in men, whereas in women, it can develop at quantities of only more than 20 g/day. Moreover, the peak incidence of alcohol-associated liver disease in women is approximately a decade earlier than in men. The type of alcoholic beverage consumed may not be as critical, but "spirits" and beer may be more hepatotoxic than wine. Hispanics and American Indians may be predisposed to more significant alcoholic liver injury. Both obesity and protein-calorie malnutrition, in which micronutrients and antioxidant capacity are diminished, also are important predispositions.

Polymorphisms in genes associated with lipid metabolism (*PNPLA3* and *HSD17B13*), alcohol metabolism (alcohol and aldehyde dehydrogenases and cytochrome P-450 enzymes), and dysregulated cytokine production (e.g., *TNF*) may influence susceptibility to alcohol-related liver injury. Candidate genes impacting alcohol-related cirrhosis include *PNPLA3, HSD17B13 TM6SF2*, and *MBOAT7, MARC1*, and *HNRNPUL1*.[2] In patients with other forms of chronic liver disease (e.g., viral hepatitis B or C), concomitant alcohol consumption significantly aggravates liver injury.

CLINICAL MANIFESTATIONS

Patients with alcohol-associated liver disease may have signs and symptoms from underlying alcoholism as well as those caused by liver disease. Stigmata of chronic alcoholism include palmar erythema (see Fig. 132-2), spider nevi, bilateral gynecomastia, testicular atrophy, bilateral parotid enlargement, and Dupuytren contractures (Fig. 138-1). The clinical features of liver disease will depend on the stage of alcohol-associated liver disease, that is, whether a patient has fatty liver or more advanced liver disease, such as alcoholic hepatitis and cirrhosis.

Patients with alcohol-associated fatty liver disease are generally asymptomatic, but some patients may have anorexia, fatigue, right upper quadrant discomfort, and tender hepatomegaly. These patients also may have biochemical

TABLE 138-1 COMMON CAUSES OF MACROVESICULAR AND MICROVESICULAR STEATOSIS

MACROVESICULAR STEATOSIS	MICROVESICULAR STEATOSIS
Obesity, type 2 diabetes, metabolic syndrome, and dyslipidemia (nonalcoholic fatty liver disease)	Reye syndrome
Excessive alcohol consumption	Medications (valproate, antiretroviral medicines, intravenous tetracycline)
Hepatitis C (genotype 3)	Heat stroke
Wilson disease	Acute fatty liver of pregnancy
Lipodystrophy starvation	HELLP syndrome
Jejunoileal bypass	Inborn errors of metabolism (lecithin–cholesterol acyltransferase deficiency, cholesterol ester storage disease, Wolman disease)
Parenteral nutrition	
Medications (amiodarone, methotrexate, tamoxifen, corticosteroids, antipsychotics)	

HELLP = *h*emolysis, *e*levated *l*iver enzymes, and *l*ow *p*latelets.

TABLE 138-2 RISK FACTORS FOR ALCOHOL-ASSOCIATED LIVER DISEASE AND NONALCOHOLIC FATTY LIVER DISEASE (NAFLD)

ALCOHOL-ASSOCIATED LIVER DISEASE	NAFLD
MAJOR	**MAJOR**
Amount and duration of alcohol consumption	Obesity
Female gender	Type 2 diabetes
Genetic factors	Dyslipidemia
Protein-calorie malnutrition	Metabolic syndrome
MINOR	**MINOR**
Type of beverage	Polycystic ovary syndrome
Binge drinking	Hypothyroidism
Obesity	Obstructive sleep apnea
Hispanic ethnicity	Hypopituitarism
	Hypogonadism

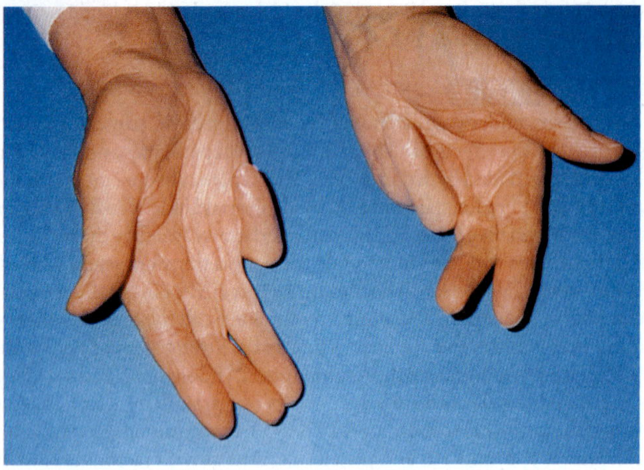

FIGURE 138-1. **Dupuytren contracture.** (From Gudmundsson KG, Jonsson T, Arngrimsson R. Guillaume Dupuytren and finger contractures. *Lancet*. 2003;362:165-168.)

evidence of alcoholism and alcohol-associated liver disease with macrocytosis as well as elevated levels of aspartate aminotransferase (AST) and γ-glutamyl transpeptidase. Patients with alcohol-associated fatty liver typically do not have jaundice, ascites, or splenomegaly.

Patients with alcoholic hepatitis may have a more dramatic presentation with severe malaise, fatigue, anorexia, fever, evidence of protein-calorie malnutrition, and features of decompensated liver disease, including jaundice, coagulopathy, ascites, and encephalopathy. However, these classic features are not universally present. Physical examination invariably shows at least some features of chronic alcoholism, and jaundice (see Fig. 132-1), ascites (see Fig. 132-4), and splenomegaly are common. The laboratory examination findings are typically abnormal. Common hematologic abnormalities include leukocytosis with neutrophil predominance, macrocytic anemia (Chapter 150), thrombocytopenia (Chapter 158), and prolonged prothrombin time. Liver biochemistries (Chapter 133) are abnormal with an elevated AST and ratio of AST to alanine aminotransferase (ALT), alkaline phosphatase, γ-glutamyl transpeptidase, and total bilirubin but decreased levels of serum albumin. The AST rarely exceeds 300 IU/L. Serum electrolyte abnormalities, including hypokalemia (Chapter 103), hypomagnesemia (Chapter 105), hypocalcemia (Chapter 227), and hypophosphatemia (Chapter 105), are frequent. Patients with alcoholic cirrhosis have the same clinical features that are common to other types of cirrhosis (Chapter 139) but also with striking features of underlying chronic alcoholism, including gynecomastia in males and significant muscle wasting.

DIAGNOSIS

The diagnosis of alcohol-associated liver disease strongly depends on the history of excessive alcohol consumption and the presence of liver disease.[3,4] Although laboratory abnormalities are not specific for alcohol-associated liver disease, they can be suggestive in the context of excessive alcohol consumption. An AST/ALT ratio of greater than 2 is typical in alcohol-associated liver disease, and ALT values greater than 150 to 200 IU/L are very rare in alcohol-associated liver disease. Serology testing for coexisting chronic viral hepatitis (Chapter 135) is critical. Diagnostic dilemmas arise when a patient denies excessive alcohol consumption in the face of clinical features that are suggestive of alcohol-associated liver disease. Interviewing family members about specific alcohol consumption may be helpful in the accurate ascertainment of alcohol consumption. Serum and urinary levels of ethyl glucuronide and ethyl sulfate are sensitive and specific markers of recent alcohol consumption, but they are not commonly measured in clinical practice. Hepatic imaging by ultrasound, computed tomography, or magnetic resonance imaging will show changes consistent with hepatic steatosis or more advanced forms of liver disease, such as cirrhosis and portal hypertension. Imaging is also important to exclude other forms of liver disease, including malignant disease and biliary obstruction. Imaging findings suggestive of alcohol-associated liver disease include an enlarged caudate lobe, greater visualization of the right posterior hepatic notch, and focal fat sparing or geographic fat distribution.

Because specific treatments for heavy alcohol drinking and alcohol-associated hepatitis may be harmful in patients with other liver diseases, it is important to exclude other predominant or coexisting liver diseases, including chronic viral hepatitis (Chapter 135) and drug-induced liver injury, especially from acetaminophen (Chapter 136), by history, blood tests, and biopsy if needed. Hyperferritinemia generally reflects an acute phase reactant, rather than an iron overload disorder, so it usually will return to normal when the acute liver injury resolves.

Liver biopsy is the key to distinguishing alcohol-associated liver disease from other entities, characterizing the nature of the liver disease, and determining whether a patient has fatty liver or more advanced alcoholic hepatitis. Histologic features of alcohol-associated fatty liver include macrovesicular steatosis that is predominantly centrilobular (zone 3) in nature. In alcoholic hepatitis, the biopsy is more striking and reveals macrovesicular steatosis, lobular neutrophilic infiltration, Mallory hyaline, ballooning degeneration of the hepatocytes, and perivenular fibrosis. In general, patients with alcoholic hepatitis also have histologic evidence of chronic liver injury in the form of more advanced fibrosis (periportal or bridging fibrosis or cirrhosis).

TREATMENT

Total abstinence, which is the most important treatment measure, is mandatory for the improvement of the clinical and histologic features of alcohol-associated liver disease. Its benefits are unequivocal, even in patients with severe decompensation. However, long-term abstinence is difficult to achieve, so a multidisciplinary approach with counseling and medications that promote abstinence should be considered. Disulfiram is not commonly used because of its poor tolerability and hepatotoxicity. Opioid antagonists, such as naltrexone (50 mg/day for up to 6 months or even longer), nalmefene (20 mg/day as maintenance), and acamprosate (333-mg tablets, two tablets three times each day for 1 year), can help promote abstinence when they are used as part of a multidisciplinary approach.

Alcohol-associated fatty liver disease requires no specific treatment other than abstinence. Patients with alcoholic hepatitis, however, have increased short- and long-term mortality and should be considered for therapeutic interventions in addition to mandatory abstinence.[5,6] If a patient's clinical manifestations and/or liver biopsy findings are consistent with alcoholic hepatitis and there is no evidence of other inflammatory liver diseases, such as hepatitis C (Chapter 135), prednisolone (40 mg/day for 4 weeks) should be given to carefully selected patients[7] with severe alcoholic hepatitis who have a score higher than 32 on the Maddrey discriminant function (4.6 × [patient's prothrombin time − control prothrombin time] + total bilirubin level) and encephalopathy but do not have gastrointestinal bleeding or systemic infection. Studies have suggested that a Model for End-Stage Liver Disease (MELD) score (see Table 139-2) higher than 21 can substitute for the Maddrey score to guide the use of prednisolone. Such therapy appears to reduce mortality at 1 month,[A1] but probably not thereafter.[A2] Adding intravenous *N*-acetylcysteine (on day 1 at a dose of 150, 50, and 100 mg/kg of body weight in 250, 500, and 1000 mL of 5% glucose solution during a period of 30 minutes, 4 hours, and 16 hours, respectively; and on days 2 through 5, 100 mg/kg/day in 1000 mL of 5% glucose solution) to prednisolone appears to be superior to prednisolone alone in terms of a significantly lower mortality at 1 month and a somewhat but not significantly lower mortality at 6 months.[A3] Pentoxifylline is not of incremental value when added to corticosteroids.[A4] A variety of newer agents are currently in clinical trials.[8]

All patients with alcoholic hepatitis and alcoholic cirrhosis should be assessed and treated for protein-calorie malnutrition and micronutrient deficiency. Hospitalized patients with severe decompensation should be considered for enteral nutrition (Chapter 198).

Complications such as ascites, spontaneous bacterial peritonitis, encephalopathy, variceal bleeding, hepatorenal syndrome, osteoporosis, and hepatopulmonary syndrome may occur in patients with decompensated alcoholic cirrhosis and must be managed carefully (Chapter 139). Liver transplantation is a reasonable option in patients with decompensated alcoholic cirrhosis, and observational data suggest that early liver transplantation can improve survival in patients with severe, medically refractory alcoholic hepatitis. Although 6 months of abstinence and strong social support are generally required for eligibility (Chapter 140),[9] liver transplantation can be performed with good outcomes in severely ill but highly selected patients with acute alcoholic hepatitis before completing 6 months of abstinence. Patients with alcoholic cirrhosis, especially males, are at risk for hepatocellular carcinoma (Chapter 181) and should be screened with semiannual liver imaging and serum α-fetoprotein levels. They also may be at risk for extrahepatic malignant disease, notably head and neck, lung, and esophageal cancer. For Dupuytren contracture, injection of collagenase *Clostridium histolyticum* can reduce the severity and improve the range of motion significantly.

PROGNOSIS

Alcoholic fatty liver is generally reversible with total abstinence for a few months. The survival of patients with alcoholic hepatitis has improved over the last decade, but about 20% of patients die within 6 months after presentation, and patients with biopsy-documented alcohol-associated liver disease have a five-fold increased risk of death compared with that of the general population.[10]

Predictors of poor outcome include the severity of disease as quantified by approaches such as the MELD score (Chapters 139 and 140), the severity of fibrosis and the neutrophilic infiltration on liver biopsy, and continued alcohol use. Some data also suggest a poorer prognosis in patients who are homozygous for the rs738409:G variant in the *PNPLA3* gene.

NONALCOHOLIC FATTY LIVER DISEASE

DEFINITIONS

On histologic examination, NAFLD resembles alcohol-associated liver disease, but it occurs in individuals without significant alcohol consumption. Average alcohol consumption of more than two drinks per day in men and more than one drink per day in women generally is not consistent with a diagnosis of NAFLD. In addition, the definition of NAFLD excludes patients with a history of exposure to steatogenic medications, such as amiodarone, methotrexate, or tamoxifen.

NAFLD encompasses a spectrum of abnormal liver histologic features, ranging from simple steatosis to nonalcoholic steatohepatitis (NASH) and cirrhosis. In simple steatosis, liver histology reveals macrovesicular steatosis without ballooning degeneration of hepatocytes or liver fibrosis. NASH, which is a more advanced form of NAFLD, is histologically characterized by macrovesicular steatosis, ballooning degeneration of the hepatocytes, and sinusoidal fibrosis.

EPIDEMIOLOGY

NAFLD is one of the most common causes of elevated liver enzymes and chronic liver disease in the Western world. Its incidence in adults and children is rising rapidly because of the ongoing epidemics of obesity (Chapter 201), type 2 diabetes mellitus (Chapter 210), and metabolic syndrome. Its prevalence is high in certain populations of patients; for example, nearly 80% of patients with type 2 diabetes and 90% of morbidly obese individuals have imaging evidence of NAFLD, but it also can occur in about 7% of non-obese individuals in the United States and over 15% of non-obese Asians. Nearly one third of adults in westernized countries are estimated to have NAFLD,[11] and about 5% of adults may have NASH.[12] These percentages compare reasonably well with other data suggesting that the prevalence of cirrhosis from NAFLD is about 2%. Hispanics and Whites are at higher risk for NAFLD, whereas its prevalence is intriguingly low in African Americans.

PATHOBIOLOGY

The major risk factors for NAFLD include obesity, type 2 diabetes mellitus (Chapter 210), metabolic syndrome, and dyslipidemia. Other comorbidities associated with NAFLD include polycystic ovary syndrome (Chapter 217), hypothyroidism (Chapter 207), hypopituitarism (Chapter 205), hypogonadism (Chapter 216), and sleep apnea (Chapter 374).

Two fundamental but related defects in NAFLD are insulin resistance/hyperinsulinemia and excessive levels of circulating nonesterified fatty acids, which are released from adipose tissue and taken up by hepatocytes.[13] An excessive influx of nonesterified fatty acids into hepatocytes results in macrovesicular steatosis, which is predominantly centrilobular in location.

In addition, patients with NAFLD have increased de novo lipogenesis in the liver. Although patients with NAFLD robustly esterify free fatty acids into neutral triglycerides, free fatty acids that remain unesterified within hepatocytes are considered the primary mediators of cell injury (lipotoxicity). In the background of hepatic steatosis, factors that promote cell injury, inflammation, and fibrosis include oxidative stress, endoplasmic reticulum stress, apoptosis, adipocytokines, and stellate cell activation. The sources of oxidative stress include mitochondria and microsomes. Adipocytokines that play an important role in the pathogenesis of NAFLD include adiponectin and TNF-α. It is unclear why some patients with NAFLD exhibit NASH, whereas other patients with a comparable risk factor profile have only simple steatosis. There is a consistent and significant relationship between *PNPLA3* genetic polymorphisms and the severity of steatosis and other histologic features of NAFLD. Other polymorphisms that correlate positively with NAFLD are formed in *GCKR, TM6SF2*, and *MBOAT7*. Conversely, a polymorphism in *HSD17B13* offers protection against NAFLD and its severity.

CLINICAL MANIFESTATIONS

NAFLD is often asymptomatic but may rarely cause fatigue and right upper quadrant pain. Physical examination may reveal hepatomegaly, palmar erythema (see Fig. 132-2), and spider nevi. If liver disease is advanced, the features of liver failure, such as ascites, encephalopathy, and abdominal collateral vessels, are present. Simple steatosis is benign with a minimal risk of cirrhosis, whereas NASH is progressive and can lead to cirrhosis (Chapter 139) and liver failure (Chapter 140). In up to 20% of patients with NASH, liver histologic features will worsen and cirrhosis will develop during a 10- to 15-year period. Severe obesity, advancing age, and diabetes are thought to be risk factors for disease progression. Progressive disease during the early phase can be identified by a repeat liver biopsy or by noninvasive imaging tests, such as vibration-controlled transient elastography or magnetic resonance elastography. In later stages, however, the signs and symptoms of portal hypertension (e.g., abdominal collateral vessels and low platelet count) indicate the development of cirrhosis. Patients with NASH-induced cirrhosis are at risk for development of hepatocellular carcinoma (Chapter 181). Patients with NAFLD have several metabolic risks that predispose them to atherosclerosis, and coronary artery disease is the most common cause of death in patients with NAFLD.

DIAGNOSIS

NAFLD is generally suspected when aminotransferase levels are asymptomatically elevated in an individual with metabolic risk factors (obesity, diabetes, or the metabolic syndrome) or when liver imaging (ultrasound, computed tomography, or magnetic resonance imaging) obtained for another reason shows fatty infiltration (Fig. 138-2).[14] The diagnosis of NAFLD requires that there is no history of previous or ongoing significant alcohol consumption, no exposure to steatogenic medications, and no evidence of other causes of liver disease, such as viral hepatitis B or C. Elevated levels of aminotransferases, although common, are not required for the diagnosis of NAFLD. In contrast to alcohol-associated liver disease, ALT levels are higher than AST levels, but they rarely exceed 250 IU/L. In general, AST and ALT levels do not have diagnostic or prognostic significance. Mild hyperferritinemia is common and should not be confused with hereditary hemochromatosis (Chapter 196). Similarly, low-grade autoantibody (antinuclear antibody, anti–smooth muscle antibody) positivity is not uncommon and should not be confused with autoimmune liver disease (Chapter 135). Because steatosis is common in patients with Wilson disease (Chapter 195), serum ceruloplasmin levels should be obtained as part of the diagnostic evaluation in individuals who are younger than age 45 years.

Fatty liver on ultrasonography has a positive predictive value of only 77% and a negative predictive value of only 67% compared with liver biopsy. Abdominal magnetic resonance imaging is more accurate, but its high cost limits its usefulness in routine practice. Because neither of these imaging tests can differentiate simple steatosis from NASH or identify cirrhosis until hepatic fibrosis has caused nodular liver or overt portal hypertension, liver biopsy is required to establish the presence of NASH or cirrhosis. Common indications for a percutaneous liver biopsy in patients with NAFLD include persistently high aminotransferase levels, inability to exclude a competing or a coexisting cause (e.g., iron overload or autoimmune liver disease), and clinical suspicion of NASH and advanced fibrosis. In patients with NASH, liver histology shows steatosis, inflammation, ballooning, and fibrosis (Fig. 138-3).[15] However, liver histology alone cannot reliably distinguish NASH

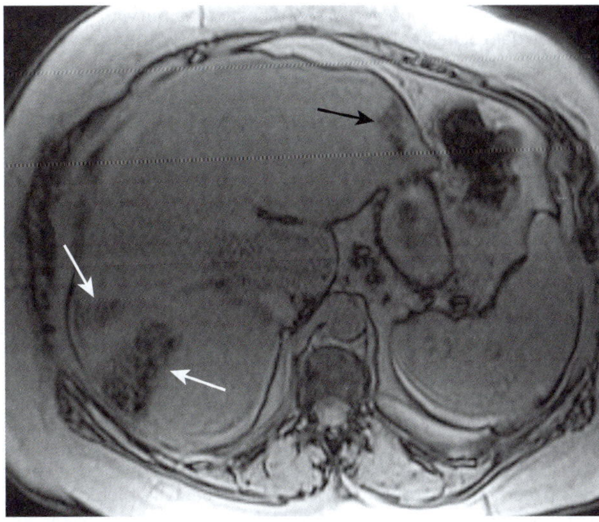

FIGURE 138-2. Magnetic resonance image of chronic liver disease due to nonalcoholic fatty liver disease. Out-of-phase T1-weighted images show focal fat infiltration of varying shapes in right lobe *(white arrows)* and left lobe *(black arrow)*. (Courtesy Professor Kumar Sandrasegaran, Indiana University School of Medicine, Indianapolis, Ind.)

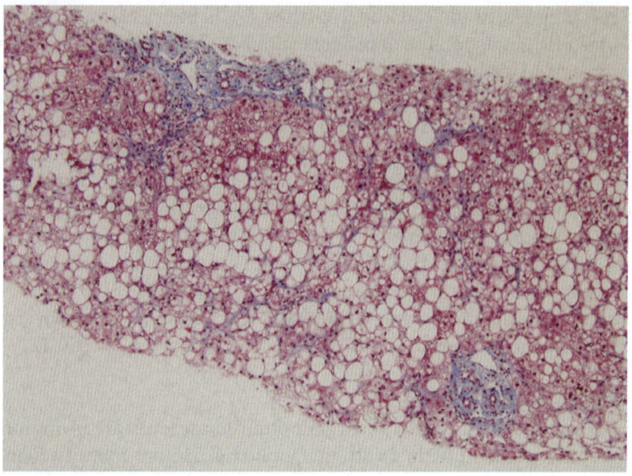

FIGURE 138-3. **Liver biopsy specimen showing nonalcoholic steatohepatitis with increased fat and with early cirrhosis.** (Courtesy of the NASH Clinical Research network.)

from alcoholic hepatitis because these two entities have remarkably similar microscopic features. Vibration controlled transient elastography, which now can be performed as a point-of-care test, can provide an estimate of liver fibrosis in NAFLD in clinical practice.

TREATMENT

Lifestyle modification with dietary restriction and regular exercise is the first choice of treatment for NAFLD.[16,17] Weight reduction, a low refined-sugar diet, and increased physical activity reduce liver fat, improve glucose control and insulin sensitivity, and improve histopathologic features.[A5,A6] It is generally recommended that patients with NAFLD lose 10% of their body weight in a gradual fashion, but this goal is difficult to achieve. If resources are available, a multidisciplinary approach with behavioral therapy, dietary advice, and monitoring by a professional nutritionist and an exercise expert is more successful than a prescriptive approach (Chapter 201). Weight loss via bariatric surgery in obese patients (Chapter 201) has been reported to resolve liver biopsy finding in about 80% of patients, with a progressive reduction in fibrosis.[18]

Pharmacotherapy options[19–21] include vitamin E (800 IU of α-tocopherol administered daily for 2 years), which can significantly improve liver enzymes and histologic findings in NASH and NAFLD.[A7] Statins (e.g., atorvastatin 20 mg daily) with or without vitamins C and E can improve liver test results and reduce subsequent NAFLD.[A8] Liraglutide (a glucagon-like peptide-1 agonist at 1.8 mg daily subcutaneously) can safely lead to a histologic resolution of NASH.[A9,A10] Semaglutide (subcutaneously daily at 0.4 mg for 72 weeks) also has been highly effective in resolving steatohepatitis but does not significantly improve fibrosis in individuals with NASH and clinically significant fibrosis.[A11] Lanifibranor (a peroxisome proliferator-activated receptor agonist at 1200 mg daily) can improve the inflammatory components of NASH and may reduce fibrosis.[A12]

Thiazolidinedione insulin sensitizers (pioglitazone and rosiglitazone) improve steatosis, inflammation, ballooning, and perhaps fibrosis, but with the side effect of an average gain of nearly 10 pounds.[A13] Unfortunately, the weight gain that is common with thiazolidinediones may offset the histologic benefits that they offer.

Supplemental omega-3 polyunsaturated fatty acids have shown promise in small controlled trials.[A14] Treatment with pentoxifylline (400 mg three times daily) may improve liver enzymes and liver histologic findings in individuals with NASH.

Obeticholic acid (an FXR agonist) has shown some histologic efficiency,[A15] but longer-term studies are awaited. An engineered fibroblast growth factor 19 (FGF19) administered over 12 weeks has shown dramatic improvement in hepatic fat in a proof-of-concept study in adults with NASH.[A16,A17] Inhibition of dihydroceramide desaturase 1 is a potential target for treating hepatic steatosis.[22] Another potential agent is resmetirom, a selective thyroid hormone receptor-β agonist (80 mg orally twice daily).[A18]

Patients with NAFLD often have dyslipidemia that puts them at excessive risk for coronary artery disease; their dyslipidemia (Chapter 190) should be treated aggressively with statins and other lipid-lowering agents, which can be safely administered to patients with NAFLD and NASH. In morbidly obese individuals with NASH and other significant metabolic comorbidities, foregut bariatric surgery can lead to significant improvement in hepatic histologic features,[A19] but the physician must exclude the presence of portal hypertension before offering this type of surgery. Carefully selected patients with decompensated cirrhosis due to NASH can be treated with liver transplantation (Chapter 140), but recurrence during the post-transplantation period is common.[23]

PREVENTION

The measures to prevent NAFLD include maintaining optimal body weight, exercising regularly, and treating any associated metabolic comorbidities such as diabetes and dyslipidemia. Avoidance of saturated fat, high fructose intake, and alcohol consumption may reduce the development of NAFLD.

PROGNOSIS

Steatosis alone is generally benign, whereas steatohepatitis is often progressive. Liver fibrosis on biopsy is also independently associated with long-term liver failure and mortality.[24,25] One third of NAFLD patients may have remission within 7 years, mostly depending on modest weight reduction. Otherwise, however, data are sparse regarding the risk and risk factors for the progression of NAFLD and NASH to cirrhosis and liver failure.

Because NAFLD often coexists with one or more components of the metabolic syndrome, its presence reflects guarded long-term overall prognosis. The long-term complications in patients with simple steatosis generally result from cardiovascular disease and atherosclerosis, not from liver failure (Chapter 140).[26]

Patients with NASH also are at risk for liver failure and liver cancer (Chapter 181),[27] in addition to their significantly increased risk of cardiovascular disease. For example, among patients with NASH on their initial biopsy, one third or more develop progressive fibrosis during a mean follow-up interval of about 5 years. Older age, diabetes, and ballooning and fibrosis on liver biopsy are important predictors of progression. In the United States, NAFLD is now second only to alcohol-associated liver disease as a cause of being listed for liver transplantation.

GENERAL REFERENCES

For the General References and other additional features, please visit Elsevier eBooks+ at https://ebooks.health.elsevier.com.

Grade A References

A1. Lee YS, Kim HJ, Kim JH, et al. Treatment of severe alcoholic hepatitis with corticosteroid, pentoxifylline, or dual therapy: a systematic review and meta-analysis. *J Clin Gastroenterol.* 2017;51:364-377.

A2. Pavlov CS, Varganova DL, Casazza G, et al. Glucocorticosteroids for people with alcoholic hepatitis. *Cochrane Database Syst Rev.* 2017;11:CD001511.

A3. Singh S, Murad MH, Chandar AK, et al. Comparative effectiveness of pharmacological interventions for severe alcoholic hepatitis: a systematic review and network meta-analysis. *Gastroenterology.* 2015;149:958-970.

A4. Louvet A, Thursz MR, Kim DJ, et al. Corticosteroids reduce risk of death within 28 days for patients with severe alcoholic hepatitis, compared with pentoxifylline or placebo—a meta-analysis of individual data from controlled trials. *Gastroenterology.* 2018;155:458-468.

A5. Kenneally S, Sier JH, Moore JB. Efficacy of dietary and physical activity intervention in non-alcoholic fatty liver disease: a systematic review. *BMJ Open Gastroenterol.* 2017;4:1-12.

A6. Schwimmer JB, Ugalde-Nicalo P, Welsh JA, et al. Effect of a low free sugar diet vs usual diet on nonalcoholic fatty liver disease in adolescent boys: a randomized clinical trial. *JAMA.* 2019;321:256-265.

A7. Sato K, Gosho M, Yamamoto T, et al. Vitamin E has a beneficial effect on nonalcoholic fatty liver disease: a meta-analysis of randomized controlled trials. *Nutrition.* 2015;31:923-930.

A8. Pastori D, Polimeni L, Baratta F, et al. The efficacy and safety of statins for the treatment of non-alcoholic fatty liver disease. *Dig Liver Dis.* 2015;47:4-11.

A9. Armstrong MJ, Gaunt P, Aithal GP, et al. Liraglutide safety and efficacy in patients with non-alcoholic steatohepatitis (LEAN): a multicentre, double-blind, randomised, placebo-controlled phase 2 study. *Lancet.* 2016;387:679-690.

A10. Dong Y, Lv Q, Li S, et al. Efficacy and safety of glucagon-like peptide-1 receptor agonists in non-alcoholic fatty liver disease: a systematic review and meta-analysis. *Clin Res Hepatol Gastroenterol.* 2017;41:284-295.

A11. Newsome PN, Buchholtz K, Cusi K, et al. A placebo-controlled trial of subcutaneous semaglutide in nonalcoholic steatohepatitis. *N Engl J Med.* 2021;384:1113-1124.

A12. Francque SM, Bedossa P, Ratziu V, et al. A randomized, controlled trial of the pan-PPAR agonist lanifibranor in NASH. *N Engl J Med.* 2021;385:1547-1558.

A13. He L, Liu X, Wang L, et al. Thiazolidinediones for nonalcoholic steatohepatitis: a meta-analysis of randomized clinical trials. *Medicine (Baltimore).* 2016;95:1-9.

A14. He XX, Wu XL, Chen RP, et al. Effectiveness of omega-3 polyunsaturated fatty acids in non-alcoholic fatty liver disease: a meta-analysis of randomized controlled trials. *PLoS ONE.* 2016;11:1-22.

A15. Younossi ZM, Ratziu V, Loomba R, et al. Obeticholic acid for the treatment of non-alcoholic steatohepatitis: interim analysis from a multicentre, randomised, placebo-controlled phase 3 trial. *Lancet.* 2019;394:2184-2196.

A16. Harrison SA, Neff G, Guy CD, et al. Efficacy and safety of aldafermin, an engineered FGF19 analog, in a randomized, double-blind, placebo-controlled trial of patients with nonalcoholic steatohepatitis. *Gastroenterology.* 2021;160:219-231.

A17. Sanyal A, Charles ED, Neuschwander-Tetri BA, et al. Pegbelfermin (BMS-986036), a PEGylated fibroblast growth factor 21 analogue, in patients with non-alcoholic steatohepatitis: a randomised, double-blind, placebo-controlled, phase 2a trial. *Lancet.* 2019;392:2705-2717.

A18. Harrison SA, Bashir MR, Guy CD, et al. Resmetirom (MGL-3196) for the treatment of non-alcoholic steatohepatitis: a multicentre, randomised, double-blind, placebo-controlled, phase 2 trial. *Lancet.* 2019;394:2012-2024.

A19. Lassailly G, Caiazzo R, Ntandja-Wandji L-C, et al. Bariatric surgery provides long-term resolution of non-alcoholic steatohepatitis and regression of fibrosis. *Gastroenterology.* 2020;159:1290-1301.

139

CIRRHOSIS AND ITS SEQUELAE

GUADALUPE GARCIA-TSAO

DEFINITION

Cirrhosis, which can be the final stage of any chronic liver disease, is a diffuse process characterized by fibrosis and conversion of normal architecture to structurally abnormal nodules (Fig. 139-1). These "regenerative" nodules lack normal lobular organization and are surrounded by fibrous tissue. The process involves the whole liver and generally is considered irreversible. Although cirrhosis is histologically an "all-or-nothing" diagnosis, it can be classified clinically by its status as compensated or decompensated. Decompensated cirrhosis is defined by the presence of ascites, variceal bleeding, encephalopathy, or jaundice, which are complications that result from the main consequences of cirrhosis: portal hypertension and liver insufficiency.

EPIDEMIOLOGY

Because many patients with cirrhosis are asymptomatic until decompensation occurs, it is difficult to assess the real prevalence and incidence of cirrhosis in the general population. The prevalence of chronic liver disease or cirrhosis worldwide is estimated to be 100 (range, 25 to 400) per 100,000 subjects, but it varies widely by country and by geographic region.

Cirrhosis is an important cause of morbidity and mortality worldwide and in the United States. According to the latest Global Burden of Diseases study, cirrhosis annually causes more than 1.32 million deaths worldwide and about 45,000 deaths in the United States, making it the 11th leading cause of death overall.[1] Importantly, chronic liver disease and cirrhosis mainly affect individuals between 25 and 64 years of age. As chronic liver disease affects people in their most productive years of life, it has a significant impact on the economy as a result of premature death, illness, and disability.

Any chronic liver disease can lead to cirrhosis (Table 139-1). The main causes of cirrhosis in Western and industrialized countries are alcohol-related (Chapter 138) and nonalcoholic steatohepatitis (Chapter 138),[2,3] whereas viral hepatitis B (Chapter 135) is the primary cause in China and other Asian countries. Hepatitis C (Chapter 135) was the most common cause of cirrhosis in the United States until effective antiviral therapy became available. Other causes of cirrhosis include autoimmune liver diseases, such as primary biliary cholangitis (Chapter 135), primary sclerosing cholangitis (Chapter 135), autoimmune hepatitis (Chapter 135), and metabolic diseases such as hemochromatosis (Chapter 196) and Wilson disease (Chapter 195). Heterozygous carriage of the alpha1-antitrypsin Pi*Z variant, which is present in up to 10% of persons of European descent, increases the risk of liver cirrhosis in patients with liver disease or alcohol abuse (Chapter 138). When all potential causes have been investigated and excluded, cirrhosis is considered "cryptogenic." Many cases of cryptogenic cirrhosis are now thought to be due to nonalcoholic steatohepatitis (Chapter 138).

PATHOBIOLOGY

Liver Fibrosis and Cirrhosis

The key pathogenic feature underlying liver fibrosis and cirrhosis is activation of hepatic stellate cells. Hepatic stellate cells, which are known as *Ito cells* or *perisinusoidal cells*, are located in the space of Disse between hepatocytes and sinusoidal endothelial cells. Normally, hepatic stellate cells are quiescent and serve as the main storage site for retinoids (vitamin A). In response to injury, hepatic stellate cells become activated, as a result of which they lose their vitamin A, proliferate, develop a prominent rough endoplasmic reticulum, and secrete extracellular matrix (collagen types I and III, sulfated proteoglycans, and glycoproteins). In addition, they become contractile myofibroblasts.

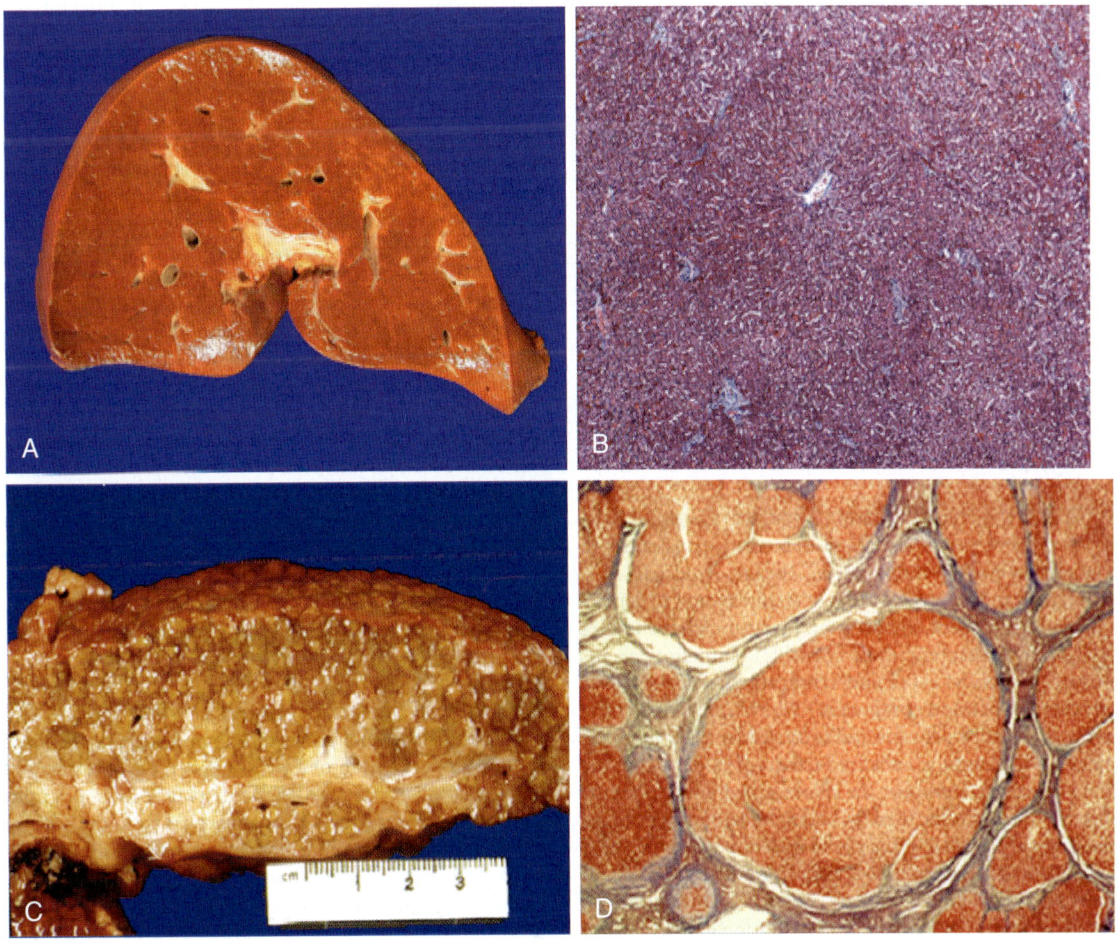

FIGURE 139-1. Gross and microscopic images of a normal and cirrhotic liver. A, Gross image of a normal liver with a smooth surface and homogeneous texture. **B,** On microscopic examination, liver sinusoids are organized, and vascular structures are normally distributed. **C,** Gross image of a cirrhotic liver. The liver has an orange-tawny color with an irregular surface and a nodular texture. **D,** On microscopic examination, the architecture is disorganized, and there are regenerative nodules surrounded by fibrous tissue.

TABLE 139-1 CAUSES OF CIRRHOSIS

MAIN FACTORS CAUSING CIRRHOSIS
Alcoholic liver disease
Nonalcoholic fatty liver disease
Chronic hepatitis B
OTHER CAUSES OF CIRRHOSIS (<2% OF ALL CASES)
Chronic hepatitis C
Cholestatic and autoimmune liver diseases
Primary biliary cirrhosis
Primary sclerosing cholangitis
Autoimmune hepatitis
Intrahepatic or extrahepatic biliary obstruction
Mechanical obstruction
Biliary atresia
Cystic fibrosis
Metabolic disorders
Hemochromatosis
Wilson disease
α_1-Antitrypsin deficiency
Glycogen storage diseases
Abetalipoproteinemia
Porphyria
Hepatic venous outflow obstruction
Budd-Chiari syndrome
Veno-occlusive disease
Right-sided heart failure
Drugs and toxins
Intestinal bypass
Indian childhood cirrhosis

A number of genetic polymorphisms have been associated with a higher risk of cirrhosis related to alcohol or obesity,[4] but their clinical utility remains unclear.

Unlike other capillaries, normal hepatic sinusoids lack a basement membrane. The sinusoidal endothelial cells themselves contain large fenestrae (100 to 200 nm in diameter) that permit the passage of large molecules with molecular masses up to 250,000 daltons. Collagen deposition in the space of Disse, as occurs in cirrhosis, leads to defenestration of the sinusoidal endothelial cells ("capillarization" of the sinusoids), thereby altering exchange between plasma and hepatocytes and resulting in a decreased sinusoidal diameter that is further exacerbated by the contraction of stellate cells.

Complications of Cirrhosis

The two main consequences of cirrhosis are portal hypertension, with the accompanying hyperdynamic circulatory state, and liver insufficiency (Fig. 139-2). The development of varices and ascites is a direct consequence of portal hypertension and the hyperdynamic circulatory state, whereas jaundice occurs as a result of an inability of the liver to excrete bilirubin (i.e., liver insufficiency). Encephalopathy is the result of both portal hypertension and liver insufficiency. Ascites, in turn, can become complicated by infection, which is called *spontaneous bacterial peritonitis*, and by functional renal failure, which is called *hepatorenal syndrome*.

Portal Hypertension and the Hyperdynamic Circulatory State

In cirrhosis, portal hypertension results from both an increase in resistance to portal flow and an increase in portal venous inflow.[5] The initial mechanism is increased sinusoidal vascular resistance (Fig. 139-3) secondary to (1) deposition of fibrous tissue and subsequent compression by regenerative nodules (fixed component), which could theoretically be amenable to antifibrotic agents and could be ameliorated by resolving the underlying etiologic process, and (2) active vasoconstriction (functional component), which is amenable to the action of vasodilators such as nitroprusside and is caused by a deficiency in intrahepatic nitric oxide (NO), as well as enhanced activity of vasoconstrictors.

Early in the portal hypertensive process, the spleen grows and sequesters platelets and other formed blood cells, thereby leading to hypersplenism. In addition, vessels that normally drain into the portal system, such as the coronary vein, reverse their flow and shunt blood away from the portal system to the systemic circulation. These portosystemic collaterals are insufficient to decompress the portal venous system and offer additional resistance to portal flow. As collaterals develop, an increase in portal blood inflow, which results from splanchnic vasodilation, maintains the portal hypertensive state. Splanchnic arteriolar vasodilation is, in turn, secondary to increased production

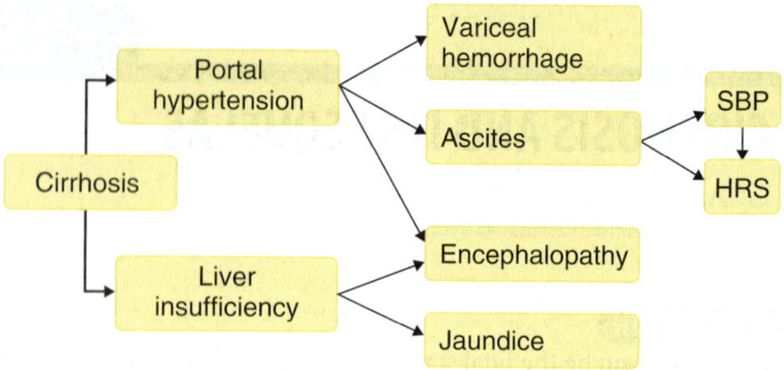

FIGURE 139-2. **Complications of cirrhosis result from portal hypertension or liver insufficiency.** Varices and variceal hemorrhage are a direct consequence of portal hypertension. Ascites results from sinusoidal portal hypertension and can be complicated by infection (spontaneous bacterial peritonitis [SBP]) or renal dysfunction (hepatorenal syndrome [HRS]). Hepatic encephalopathy results from portosystemic shunting (i.e., portal hypertension) and liver insufficiency. Jaundice results solely from liver insufficiency.

of NO. Thus, the paradox in portal hypertension is that a deficiency of NO in the intrahepatic vasculature leads to vasoconstriction and increased resistance, whereas overproduction of NO in the extrahepatic circulation leads to vasodilation and increased portal flow.

In addition to splanchnic vasodilation, there is systemic vasodilation, which by causing a decreased *effective* arterial blood volume leads to activation of neurohumoral systems (renin-angiotensin-aldosterone system), retention of sodium, expansion of plasma volume, and development of a hyperdynamic circulatory state. This hyperdynamic circulatory state maintains portal hypertension, thereby leading to the formation and growth of varices, and plays an important role in the development of all other complications of cirrhosis.

Varices and Variceal Hemorrhage

The complication of cirrhosis that results most directly from portal hypertension is the development of portal-systemic collaterals, the most relevant of which are those that form through dilation of the coronary and gastric veins and constitute gastroesophageal varices. The initial formation of esophageal collaterals depends on a threshold portal pressure, clinically established by a hepatic venous pressure gradient of 10 to 12 mm Hg, below which varices do not develop.

Development of a hyperdynamic circulatory state leads to further dilation and growth of varices and eventually to their rupture and variceal hemorrhage, one of the most dreaded complications of portal hypertension. Tension in a varix determines variceal rupture and is directly proportional to variceal diameter and intravariceal pressure and inversely proportional to variceal wall thickness.

Ascites and Hepatorenal Syndrome

Ascites, which is the accumulation of intraperitoneal fluid, in cirrhosis is secondary to sinusoidal hypertension and retention of sodium. Cirrhosis leads to sinusoidal hypertension by blocking hepatic venous outflow both anatomically by fibrosis and regenerative nodules and functionally by increased postsinusoidal vascular tone. Similar to the formation of esophageal varices, a threshold hepatic venous pressure gradient of 12 mm Hg is needed for the formation of ascites. In addition, retention of sodium replenishes the intravascular volume and allows the continuous formation of ascites. Retention of sodium results from vasodilation that is mostly due to an increase in the production of NO. With progression of cirrhosis and portal hypertension, vasodilation is more pronounced, thereby leading to further activation of the renin-angiotensin-aldosterone and sympathetic nervous systems and resulting in further sodium retention (refractory ascites), water retention (hyponatremia), and renal vasoconstriction (hepatorenal syndrome).[6]

Spontaneous Bacterial Peritonitis

Spontaneous bacterial peritonitis, an infection of ascitic fluid, occurs in the absence of perforation of a hollow viscus or an intra-abdominal inflammatory focus, such as an abscess, acute pancreatitis, or cholecystitis. Bacterial translocation, or the migration of bacteria from the intestinal lumen to mesenteric lymph nodes and other extraintestinal sites, is the main mechanism implicated in spontaneous bacterial peritonitis. Impaired local and systemic immune defenses are a major element in promoting bacterial translocation and, together with shunting of blood away from the hepatic Kupffer cells through portosystemic collaterals, allow a transient bacteremia to become more prolonged, thereby colonizing ascitic fluid. Spontaneous bacterial peritonitis occurs in patients with reduced ascites defense mechanisms, such as a low

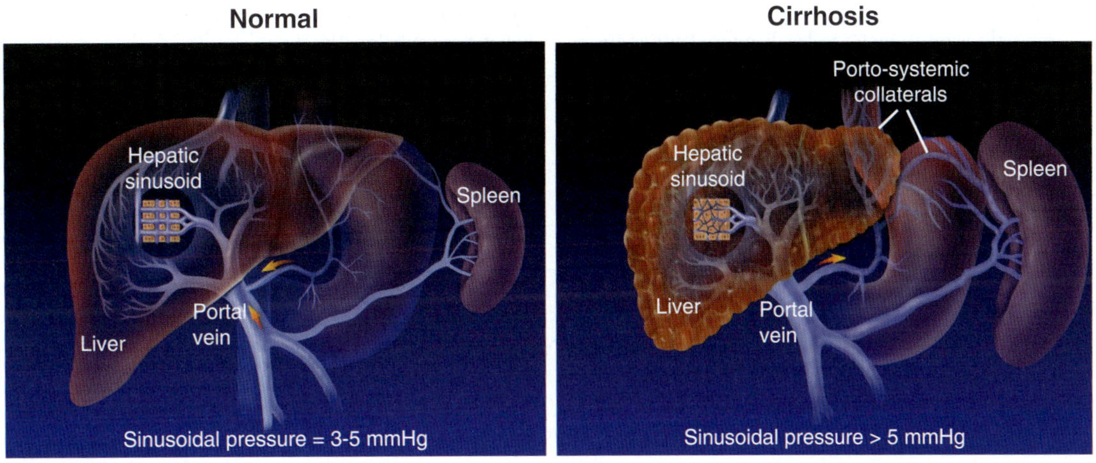

FIGURE 139-3. **Hepatic sinusoidal pressure is increased in cirrhosis.** In the normal liver (*left*), the intrahepatic vasculature is compliant, and the hepatic venous pressure gradient, which is a measure of sinusoidal pressure, is 5 mm Hg or lower. In the cirrhotic liver (*right*), the sinusoidal architecture is distorted by regenerative nodules and fibrosis that lead to increased intrahepatic resistance, portal hypertension, splenomegaly, and portosystemic collaterals; the hepatic venous pressure gradient is above 5 mm Hg. Complications of cirrhosis develop after the gradient increases above 10 to 12 mm Hg.

complement level in ascitic fluid. Another factor that promotes bacterial translocation in cirrhosis is intestinal bacterial overgrowth attributed to a decrease in small bowel motility and intestinal transit time. Infections, particularly from gram-negative bacteria, can precipitate renal dysfunction through worsening of the hyperdynamic circulatory state.

Encephalopathy

Hepatic encephalopathy is brain dysfunction caused by liver insufficiency, portosystemic shunting, or both.[7] Ammonia, a toxin normally removed by the liver, plays a key role in its pathogenesis. In cirrhosis, ammonia accumulates in the systemic circulation because of shunting of blood through portosystemic collaterals and decreased liver metabolism (i.e., liver insufficiency). The presence of large amounts of ammonia in the brain damages supporting brain cells or astrocytes and leads to structural changes characteristic of hepatic encephalopathy (Alzheimer type II astrocytosis). Ammonia results in upregulation of astrocytic peripheral-type benzodiazepine receptors, the most potent stimulants of neurosteroid production. Neurosteroids are the major modulators of γ-aminobutyric acid, which results in cortical depression and hepatic encephalopathy. Other toxins, such as manganese, also accumulate in the brain, particularly the globus pallidus, where they lead to impaired motor function. Other yet-to-be-elucidated toxins may also be involved in the pathogenesis of encephalopathy.

Jaundice

Jaundice (Chapter 133) in cirrhosis results from the inability of the liver to excrete bilirubin and is therefore the result of liver insufficiency. However, in cholestatic diseases leading to cirrhosis (e.g., primary biliary cirrhosis, primary sclerosing cholangitis, vanishing bile duct syndrome), jaundice is more likely due to biliary damage than to liver insufficiency. Other indicators of liver insufficiency, such as the presence of encephalopathy or prolongation of the international normalized ratio, help determine the most likely contributor to hyperbilirubinemia (Chapter 133).

Cardiopulmonary Complications

The hyperdynamic circulatory state eventually results in high-output heart failure with decreased peripheral utilization of oxygen, a complication that has been referred to as *cirrhotic cardiomyopathy*. Vasodilation at the level of the pulmonary circulation leads to arterial hypoxemia, the hallmark of hepatopulmonary syndrome. Normal pulmonary capillaries are 8 µm in diameter, and red blood cells (slightly less than 8 µm) pass through them one cell at a time, thereby facilitating oxygenation. In *hepatopulmonary syndrome*, the pulmonary capillaries are dilated up to 500 µm, so passage of red cells through the pulmonary capillaries may be many cells thick. As a result, a large number of red cells are not oxygenated, which causes the equivalent of a right-to-left shunt.

Conversely, *portopulmonary hypertension*[8] occurs when the pulmonary bed is exposed to vasoconstrictive substances that may be produced in the splanchnic circulation and bypass metabolism by the liver; the initial result is reversible pulmonary hypertension. However, because these factors result in endothelial proliferation, vasoconstriction, in situ thrombosis, and obliteration of vessels, irreversible pulmonary hypertension ensues.

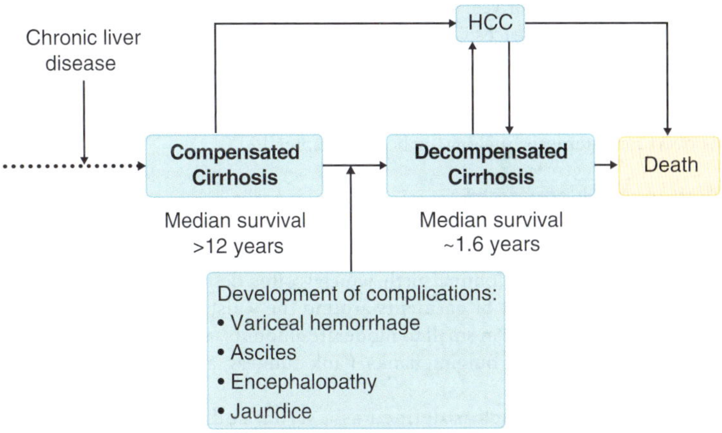

FIGURE 139-4. **Natural history of cirrhosis.** Any chronic liver disease will lead to cirrhosis. Initially, cirrhosis will be compensated (median survival, >12 years), but once complications (ascites, variceal hemorrhage, encephalopathy, jaundice) develop, it becomes decompensated (median survival, 1.6 years). Hepatocellular carcinoma (HCC) can develop at any stage and precipitate decompensation and death.

CLINICAL MANIFESTATIONS

The clinical manifestations of cirrhosis range widely, depending on the stage of cirrhosis, from an asymptomatic patient with no signs of chronic liver disease to a patient who is confused and jaundiced with severe muscle wasting and ascites. The natural history of cirrhosis is characterized by an initial phase, termed *compensated* cirrhosis, followed by a rapidly progressive phase marked by the development of complications of portal hypertension or liver dysfunction (or both), termed *decompensated* cirrhosis (Fig. 139-4).[9] In the compensated phase, liver synthetic function is mostly normal, and portal pressure, although increased, is below the threshold level required for the development of varices or ascites. As the disease progresses, portal pressure increases and liver function worsens, thereby resulting in the development of ascites, portal hypertensive gastrointestinal bleeding, encephalopathy, and jaundice.[10] The development of any of these clinically detectable complications marks the transition from a compensated to a decompensated phase. Progression to death may be accelerated by the development of other complications, such as recurrent gastrointestinal bleeding, renal impairment (refractory ascites, hepatorenal syndrome), hepatopulmonary syndrome, and sepsis (spontaneous bacterial peritonitis). The development of hepatocellular carcinoma (Chapter 181) may accelerate the course of the disease at any stage (see Fig. 139-4). Transition from a compensated to a decompensated stage occurs at a rate of approximately 5 to 7% per year. The median time to decompensation, or the time at which half the patients with compensated cirrhosis will become decompensated, is about 6 years.

Compensated Cirrhosis

In this stage, cirrhosis is mostly asymptomatic and is diagnosed either during the evaluation of chronic liver disease or fortuitously during routine physical examination, biochemical testing, imaging for other reasons, endoscopy showing gastroesophageal varices, or abdominal surgery in which a nodular liver is detected. Nonspecific fatigue, weight loss, decreased muscle mass, decreased libido, or sleep disturbances may be the only complaints. About 40% of patients with compensated cirrhosis have esophageal varices. Nonbleeding gastroesophageal varices are asymptomatic, and their presence (without bleeding) does not denote decompensation.

Decompensated Cirrhosis

At this stage, there are signs of decompensation: ascites, variceal hemorrhage, jaundice, hepatic encephalopathy, or any combination of these findings. Ascites, which is the most frequent sign of decompensation, is present in 80% of patients with decompensated cirrhosis.

Variceal Hemorrhage

Gastroesophageal varices are present in approximately 50% of patients with newly diagnosed cirrhosis. The prevalence of varices correlates with the severity of liver disease and ranges from 40% in Child A cirrhotic patients (Table 139-2) to 85% in Child C cirrhotic patients.

Both the development of varices and the growth of small varices occur at a rate of 7 to 8% per year. The incidence of a first variceal hemorrhage in patients with small varices is about 5% per year, whereas medium and large varices bleed at a rate of approximately 15% per year. Large varices, severe liver disease, and red wale markings on varices are independent predictors of variceal hemorrhage. Bleeding from gastroesophageal varices can be manifested as overt hematemesis, melena, or both (Chapter 121).

Ascites and Hyponatremia

Ascites is the most common cause of decompensation in cirrhosis and occurs at a rate of 7 to 10% per year. The most frequent symptoms associated with ascites are increased abdominal girth, which is often described by the patient as tightness of the belt or garments around the waist, and recent weight gain. When it is present in small to moderate amounts, ascites can be identified on examination by bulging flanks, flank dullness, and shifting dullness (Chapter 132).

Hyponatremia, which is defined as a serum sodium concentration <130 mEq/L (Chapter 102), is present in about 25% of patients with cirrhosis and ascites. However, patients with cirrhosis do not usually have the neurologic manifestations of hyponatremia, presumably because it typically develops gradually. Nevertheless, hyponatremia is a marker of the severity of cirrhosis and is associated with poorer quality of life and the development of hepatic encephalopathy.

Hepatorenal syndrome is a type of prerenal kidney injury that occurs in patients with cirrhosis and ascites.[11] It represents the extreme of the spectrum of abnormalities that lead to cirrhotic ascites and is the result of maximal peripheral vasodilation, as well as maximal activation of hormones that cause the retention of sodium and water and intense vasoconstriction of the renal arteries. Hepatorenal syndrome is divided into two types based on clinical characteristics and prognosis. Type 1 hepatorenal syndrome (now called hepatorenal syndrome–acute kidney injury) is rapidly progressive *acute* kidney injury in which the rise in serum creatinine concentration occurs within a 2-week period. Type 2 hepatorenal syndrome (now called hepatorenal syndrome–non-acute kidney injury) is more slowly progressive and associated with ascites that is refractory to diuretics. Patients with hepatorenal syndrome usually have tense ascites that responds poorly to diuretics, but no specific symptoms or signs typify this entity.

Spontaneous Bacterial Peritonitis

About one third of patients with cirrhosis are admitted for bacterial infection or acquire a bacterial infection during hospitalization, the most common being spontaneous bacterial peritonitis. The two most important predictors of the development of bacterial infection are the severity of liver disease and admission for gastrointestinal hemorrhage. The most frequent clinical manifestations of spontaneous bacterial peritonitis are fever, jaundice, and abdominal pain. On physical examination, there is typically abdominal tenderness, with or without rebound tenderness, or ileus (or both). However, up to one third of patients with spontaneous bacterial peritonitis initially may have no abdominal symptoms or symptoms of infection[12] and may present instead with encephalopathy, acute kidney injury, or evidence of shock.

Hepatic Encephalopathy

Hepatic encephalopathy, which is the neuropsychiatric manifestation of cirrhosis, occurs at a rate of approximately 2 to 3% per year. Hepatic encephalopathy associated with cirrhosis is of gradual onset and rarely fatal. It is manifested as a wide spectrum of neurologic and psychiatric abnormalities ranging from subclinical alterations to coma. Clinically, it is characterized by alterations in consciousness and behavior ranging from inversion of the sleep-wake pattern and forgetfulness (grade 1); to confusion, bizarre behavior, and disorientation (grade 2); to lethargy and profound disorientation (grade 3); to coma (grade 4). On physical examination, early stages may demonstrate only a distal tremor, but the hallmark of overt hepatic encephalopathy is the presence of asterixis. In addition, patients with hepatic encephalopathy may have sweet-smelling breath, a characteristic termed *fetor hepaticus*.

Pulmonary Complications

Hepatopulmonary syndrome is associated with exertional dyspnea, which can lead to extreme debilitation. Clubbing of the fingers, cyanosis, and vascular spiders may be seen on physical examination. Hepatopulmonary syndrome is present in approximately 5 to 10% of patients awaiting liver transplantation.

Portopulmonary hypertension is manifested as exertional dyspnea, syncope, and chest pain.[13] On examination, an accentuated second sound and right ventricular heave are prominent (Chapter 69).

TABLE 139-2 THE TWO MOST COMMONLY USED SCORING SYSTEMS IN CIRRHOSIS

1. CHILD-TURCOTTE-PUGH (CTP) SCORE (RANGE, 5-15)

	POINTS ASCRIBED		
Parameters	**1**	**2**	**3**
Ascites	None	Grade 1-2 (or easy to treat)	Grade 3-4 (or refractory)
Hepatic encephalopathy	None	Grade 1-2 (or induced by a precipitant)	Grade 3-4 (or spontaneous)
Bilirubin (mg/dL)	<2	2-3	>3
Albumin (g/dL)	>3.5	2.8-3.5	<2.8
Prothrombin time (seconds > control) or INR	<4 <1.7	4-6 1.7-2.3	>6 >2.3

CTP classification: Child A: score of 5-6; Child B: score of 7-9; Child C: score of 10-15

2. MODEL OF END-STAGE LIVER DISEASE (MELD) SCORE (RANGE, 6-40)

$[0.957 \times \text{LN (creatinine in mg/dL)} + 0.378 \times \text{LN (bilirubin in mg/dL)} + 1.12 \times \text{LN (INR)} + 0.643] \times 10$

MELD-Na is calculated first by determining the traditional MELD ($MELD_{(0)}$); if the initial $MELD_{(i)}$ score is 12 or greater, the score is adjusted by incorporating the serum sodium value

$$[MELD_{(0)} + 1.32 \times (137\text{-Na}) - [0.033 \times MELD(i) \times (137\text{-Na})]$$

INR = international normalized ratio; LN = natural logarithm.

DIAGNOSIS

The diagnosis of cirrhosis should be considered in any patient with chronic liver disease. In asymptomatic patients with *compensated cirrhosis*, typical signs of cirrhosis may not be present, and the physical examination and laboratory test findings may be entirely normal. The diagnosis may often require histologic confirmation by liver biopsy, which is the "gold standard" for the diagnosis of cirrhosis. However, liver biopsy is an invasive procedure subject to sampling error, and the presence of cirrhosis can often be confirmed noninvasively by a combination of serum biomarkers, imaging techniques, and measurements of liver stiffness.

Physical Examination

On physical examination, stigmata of cirrhosis consist of muscle atrophy, mainly involving the bitemporal muscle regions and the thenar and hypothenar eminences; spider angiomas, mostly on the trunk, face, and upper limbs; and palmar erythema involving the thenar and the hypothenar eminences and the tips of the fingers. Although muscle atrophy is a marker of liver insufficiency, spider angiomas and palmar erythema are markers of vasodilation and a hyperdynamic circulation. Men may have hair loss on the chest and abdomen, gynecomastia, and testicular atrophy. Petechiae and ecchymoses may be present as a result of thrombocytopenia or a prolonged prothrombin time. Dupuytren contracture, which is a thickening of the palmar fascia, occurs mostly in alcoholic cirrhosis. A pathognomonic feature of cirrhosis is the finding on abdominal examination of a small right liver lobe, with a span of less than 7 cm on percussion, and a palpable left lobe that is nodular with increased consistency. Splenomegaly may also be present and is indicative of portal hypertension. Collateral circulation on the abdominal wall (caput medusae) may also develop as a consequence of portal hypertension. Absence of any of these physical findings does not exclude cirrhosis.

Laboratory Tests

Laboratory test results suggestive of cirrhosis include even subtle abnormalities in serum levels of albumin or bilirubin or elevation of the international normalized ratio. The most sensitive and specific laboratory finding suggestive of cirrhosis in the setting of chronic liver disease is a low platelet count (<150,000/μL), which occurs as a result of portal hypertension and hypersplenism. Other serum markers that are often abnormal include levels of aspartate aminotransferase, γ-glutamyl transpeptidase, hyaluronic acid, α_2-macroglobulin, haptoglobin, tissue metalloproteinase inhibitor 1, and apolipoprotein A. Combinations of these tests have been used to predict the presence of cirrhosis, but they are not as accurate as imaging studies.

Imaging Studies

Confirmatory imaging tests include computed tomography, ultrasound, and magnetic resonance imaging. Findings consistent with cirrhosis include a nodular contour of the liver, a small liver with or without hypertrophy of the left or caudate lobe, splenomegaly, and, in particular, identification of intra-abdominal collateral vessels indicative of portal hypertension (Fig. 139-5). With increasing fibrosis, the liver becomes stiff, and this stiffness can be measured by ultrasound (transient elastography, acoustic radiation force impulse imaging), or magnetic resonance imaging. Measurement of liver stiffness, a new noninvasive technique, appears to be useful in the diagnosis of cirrhosis and in excluding its presence. These tests are becoming more widely available, and typical findings on any of these imaging studies, together with a compatible clinical picture, are indicative of the presence of cirrhosis. A liver biopsy then would not be required unless the degree of inflammation or other features require investigation.

In *decompensated cirrhosis*, detection of ascites, variceal bleeding, or encephalopathy in the setting of chronic liver disease essentially establishes the diagnosis of cirrhosis, so a liver biopsy is not necessary to establish the diagnosis. Patients with decompensated cirrhosis often exhibit malnutrition, more severe muscle wasting, more numerous vascular spiders, and hypotension and tachycardia as a result of the hyperdynamic circulatory state.

Portal Pressure Measurements

Direct measurements of portal pressure involve catheterization of the portal vein, are cumbersome, and may be associated with complications. Hepatic vein catheterization with measurement of wedged and free pressure is the simplest, safest, most reproducible, and most widely used method to indirectly measure portal pressure. Portal pressure measurements are expressed as the hepatic venous pressure gradient: the gradient between wedged hepatic venous pressure, which is a measure of sinusoidal pressure, and free hepatic or inferior vena cava pressure, which is used as an internal zero reference point. In a patient with clinical evidence of portal hypertension (e.g., varices), the hepatic venous pressure gradient is useful in the differential diagnosis of the cause of portal hypertension: it will be normal (3 to 5 mm Hg) in prehepatic causes of portal hypertension, such as portal vein thrombosis, and in intrahepatic but presinusoidal causes, such as schistosomiasis (Chapter 326); but it will be abnormal (≥6 mm Hg) in sinusoidal causes of portal hypertension, such as cirrhosis, and in postsinusoidal causes, such as veno-occlusive disease. In patients with compensated viral or alcoholic cirrhosis, a hepatic venous pressure gradient of 10 mm Hg or greater ("clinically significant" portal hypertension) predicts the development of decompensation, and its reduction with pharmacologic therapy predicts a favorable outcome in patients with cirrhosis. In patients with variceal hemorrhage, a hepatic venous pressure gradient of more than 20 mm Hg predicts recurrent variceal hemorrhage and may portend death. Measurements of liver stiffness correlate with hepatic venous pressure measurements and can help stratify patients with compensated cirrhosis, regardless of etiology, into those with and without clinically significant portal hypertension.

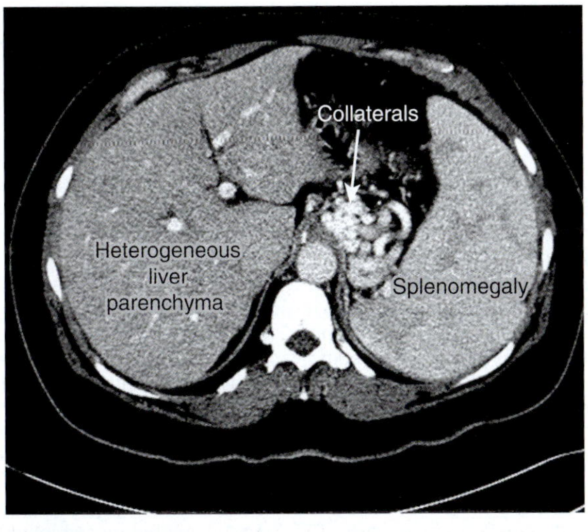

FIGURE 139-5. Computed tomography in a patient with compensated cirrhosis. The liver parenchyma is heterogeneous, there is splenomegaly, and, importantly, there are portosystemic collaterals.

Complications of Cirrhosis

Varices and Variceal Hemorrhage

Upper gastrointestinal endoscopy (Chapter 120) remains the main method for diagnosis of varices and variceal hemorrhage. Varices are classified as small (straight, minimally elevated veins above the esophageal mucosal surface), medium (tortuous veins occupying less than one third of the esophageal lumen), or large (occupying more than one third of the esophageal lumen). The diagnosis of variceal hemorrhage is made when diagnostic esophagogastroduodenoscopy shows one of the following: active bleeding from a varix, a "white nipple" overlying a varix, clots overlying a varix, or varices with no other potential source of bleeding.

Ascites

The most common cause of ascites is cirrhosis, which accounts for 80% of cases. Peritoneal malignant disease (e.g., peritoneal metastases from gastrointestinal tumors or ovarian cancer), heart failure (Chapter 45), and peritoneal tuberculosis (Chapter 299) together account for another 15% of cases. The initial, most cost-effective, and least invasive method to confirm the presence of ascites is abdominal ultrasonography.

Diagnostic paracentesis is a safe procedure that should be performed in every patient with new-onset ascites, even in those with coagulopathy. Ultrasound guidance should be used in patients in whom percussion cannot locate the ascites or in whom a first paracentesis attempt does not yield fluid. The fluid in a patient with new-onset ascites should always be evaluated for albumin (with simultaneous estimation of serum albumin), total protein, and polymorphonuclear (PMN) blood cell count, and bacteriologic cultures and cytology should be performed. The PMN cell count and bacteriologic culture are useful to exclude infection (either spontaneous or secondary bacterial peritonitis), and cytologic evaluation is needed if peritoneal carcinomatosis is suspected. Depending on the clinical setting, additional tests can be performed on the fluid: glucose and lactate dehydrogenase levels (if secondary bacterial peritonitis is suspected), smear and culture for acid-fast bacilli (if peritoneal tuberculosis is suspected), and amylase level (if pancreatic ascites is suspected).

The serum-ascites albumin gradient and ascites protein levels are useful in the differential diagnosis of ascites (Table 139-3). The serum-ascites albumin gradient correlates with sinusoidal pressure and will therefore be elevated (>1.1 g/dL) in patients in whom the source of ascites is the hepatic sinusoid (e.g., cirrhosis or cardiac ascites). Protein levels in ascitic fluid are an indirect marker of the integrity of the hepatic sinusoids: normal sinusoids are permeable structures that "leak" protein, whereas sinusoids in cirrhosis are "capillarized" and do not leak as much protein. The three main causes of ascites—cirrhosis, peritoneal malignant disease or tuberculosis, and heart failure—can easily be distinguished by combining the results of both the serum-ascites albumin gradient and ascites total protein content. Cirrhotic ascites typically has a high serum-ascites albumin gradient and low protein, cardiac ascites has a high serum-ascites albumin gradient and high protein, and ascites secondary to peritoneal malignant disease typically has a low serum-ascites albumin gradient and high protein. A high serum B-type natriuretic peptide has a high diagnostic accuracy in the diagnosis of ascites due to heart failure.

TABLE 139-3 USING THE SERUM-ASCITES ALBUMIN GRADIENT AND THE ASCITES TOTAL PROTEIN LEVEL TO DIAGNOSE THE CAUSE OF ASCITES

CONDITION	SERUM-ASCITES ALBUMIN GRADIENT*	ASCITES TOTAL PROTEIN LEVEL†
Cirrhosis	High	Low
Malignant ascites	Low	High
Cardiac ascites	High	High

*High is more than 1.1 g/dL; low is less than 1.1 g/dL.
†High is more than 2.5 g/dL; low is less than 2.5 g/dL.

Hepatorenal Syndrome

Hepatorenal syndrome is a diagnosis of exclusion, but patients typically have ascites that is unresponsive to diuretics, and most have hyponatremia. The differential diagnosis of acute kidney injury in cirrhosis includes conditions that worsen vasodilation, such as sepsis, the use of vasodilators, and large-volume paracentesis not accompanied by albumin infusion; conditions that decrease effective arterial blood volume, such as gastrointestinal hemorrhage, overdiuresis, or diarrhea (often induced by overdoses of lactulose); conditions that induce renal vasoconstriction, such as nonsteroidal anti-inflammatory drugs; and nephrotoxic insults, such as from aminoglycosides. As a result, the diagnosis of hepatorenal syndrome can only be made after diuretics have been discontinued, any condition that leads to worsening of the hemodynamic status of the cirrhotic patient has been excluded or treated, and intravascular volume has been expanded with albumin.

Spontaneous Bacterial Peritonitis

A high index of suspicion and early diagnosis are key in the management of spontaneous bacterial peritonitis. Diagnostic paracentesis should be performed in any patient with symptoms or signs of spontaneous bacterial peritonitis, including unexplained encephalopathy and renal dysfunction. Because spontaneous bacterial peritonitis is often asymptomatic and frequently community acquired, diagnostic paracentesis should be performed when any patient with cirrhosis is admitted to the hospital, regardless of the cause for admission.

The diagnosis of spontaneous bacterial peritonitis is established by an ascitic fluid PMN count >250/μL. Bacteria can be isolated from ascitic fluid in only 40 to 50% of cases, even with sensitive methods such as inoculation directly into a blood culture bottle. Spontaneous bacterial peritonitis is mostly a non-bacterial infection, usually with a gram-negative enteric organism. However, the widespread use of antibiotic prophylaxis in cirrhosis has led to an increased prevalence of infections with multidrug-resistant organisms. Anaerobes and fungi very rarely cause spontaneous bacterial peritonitis; their presence, as well as a polymicrobial infection, should raise suspicion of secondary bacterial peritonitis.

Hepatic Encephalopathy

The diagnosis of overt hepatic encephalopathy is mainly clinical and based on a history and physical examination that shows alterations in consciousness and behavior as well as the presence of asterixis. Ammonia levels are unreliable, and there is poor correlation between the grade of hepatic encephalopathy and ammonia blood levels. High levels (>150 μmol/L) are, however, indicative of hepatic encephalopathy and can be useful in the evaluation of a patient with neurocognitive disturbances of unknown origin. Psychometric tests and an electroencephalogram, which typically shows generalized slow waves and the presence of triphasic waves, are commonly used in research but are not generally used for clinical diagnosis. Minimal or subclinical hepatic encephalopathy, which is present in up to 80% of patients with cirrhosis, is diagnosed solely on the basis of abnormal results of psychometric and neuropsychological tests of attention (e.g., number connection test, digit symbol test) and psychomotor function (e.g., grooved pegboard). Screening of patients with cirrhosis for minimal hepatic encephalopathy is not widely recommended because diagnostic tests are not standardized and the benefits of treatment are uncertain.

Hepatopulmonary Syndrome and Portopulmonary Hypertension

The diagnostic criteria for hepatopulmonary syndrome are arterial hypoxemia with a Pa_{O_2} of less than 80 mm Hg or an alveolar arterial oxygen gradient of greater than 15 mm Hg, along with evidence of pulmonary vascular shunting on contrast echocardiography (Chapter 43) or a ^{99m}Tc-labeled macroaggregated albumin scan demonstrating abnormal shunting of radioactivity to the brain. Portopulmonary hypertension is diagnosed by the presence of mean pulmonary arterial pressure higher than 25 mm Hg on right-sided heart catheterization, provided pulmonary capillary wedge pressure is less than 15 mm Hg.

TREATMENT

Treatment of cirrhosis should ideally be aimed at interruption or reversal of fibrosis. Although antifibrotic drugs have not been shown to reverse fibrosis consistently or to improve outcomes in patients with cirrhosis, eradication of the hepatitis C or the hepatitis B virus has been associated with regression of fibrosis. Treatment of compensated cirrhosis is currently directed at preventing the development of decompensation by (1) treating the underlying liver disease (e.g., antiviral therapy for hepatitis C or B) to reduce fibrosis and to prevent decompensation; (2) avoiding factors that could worsen liver disease, such as alcohol, hepatotoxic drugs, and superimposed viral infections; (3) lowering portal pressure by the use of nonselective β-adrenergic blockers (e.g., carvedilol, propranolol) that have been shown to prevent variceal hemorrhage and decompensation in patients with compensated cirrhosis; and (4) screening for hepatocellular carcinoma (so it can be treated at an earlier stage) (Fig. 139-6).[14] Treatment of decompensated cirrhosis focuses on specific decompensating events and the option of liver transplantation. Increasingly, data reveal that different therapies for the same complication may be applicable to patients with different risk profiles, mainly based on severity of the disease (see Table 139-2).

Varices and Variceal Bleeding

Reducing portal pressure decreases the risk for the development of varices and variceal hemorrhage, as well as the risk for ascites and death. Nonselective β-adrenergic blockers (propranolol, nadolol) reduce portal pressure by producing splanchnic vasoconstriction and decreasing portal venous inflow. In patients with cirrhosis and medium or large varices that have never bled, nonselective β-blockers significantly reduce the risk for first variceal hemorrhage.[A1] In patients who have compensated cirrhosis with no or small varices, nonselective β-blockers significantly reduce the risk of decompensation.[A2] Carvedilol (a nonselective β-blocker with vasodilating properties) is more effective than other β-blockers for lowering portal pressure[A3] and also reduces decompensation and death in patients who have compensated cirrhosis with significant portal hypertension.[A4] Therefore, carvedilol at a dose of 3.125 to 12.5 mg/day is now recommended to prevent decompensation.[15] In patients who cannot tolerate or have contraindications to nonselective β-blockers, endoscopic variceal ligation (see Fig. 125-3), a therapy that aims to obliterate varices by placing rubber rings on variceal columns, is at least as useful as traditional nonselective β-blockers to prevent a first variceal hemorrhage but will not prevent ascites. Ligation has no effect on portal pressure and can lead to hemorrhage from ligation-induced ulcers. Among patients who have cirrhosis, screening endoscopy should be repeated every 2 to 3 years in patients with no varices, every 1 to 2 years in patients with small varices, and sooner in patients with decompensated disease so that ligation can be instituted before the varices grow in size and bleed.

Patients with cirrhosis and variceal hemorrhage require resuscitation in an intensive care unit. However, over-transfusion should be avoided because it can precipitate rebleeding. Hemoglobin values should be maintained at about 8 g/dL. Prophylactic antibiotics should be used in this setting not only to prevent bacterial infections but also to decrease rebleeding and death. The recommended antibiotic is ceftriaxone at a dose of 1 g/day for 5 to 7 days.

The most effective specific therapy for the control of active variceal hemorrhage is the combination of a vasoconstrictor with endoscopic therapy. Safe vasoconstrictors include terlipressin, somatostatin, and the somatostatin analogues octreotide and vapreotide; they can be initiated at admission to the hospital and continued for 2 to 5 days. The vasoconstrictor currently available in the United States is octreotide, which is used as a 50-μg intravenous bolus followed by an infusion at 50 μg/hour. The preferred endoscopic therapy to control variceal hemorrhage is esophageal variceal ligation.[A5] In cases in which bleeding continues despite vasoconstrictors and ligation, an esophageal stent appears to be more effective as a bridge to a more definitive therapy and is safer than balloon tamponade, although it may not reduce mortality.[A6]

The transjugular intrahepatic portosystemic shunt (TIPS) is generally recommended for patients who fail to respond to standard therapy (Fig. 139-7). In patients at high risk of failure, Child C (score 10 to 13) patients and Child B patients who have actively bleeding varices at endoscopy, preemptive TIPS placement (24 to 48 hours after admission) is associated with a reduced failure rate and a significant improvement in survival. Therefore, preemptive "early" TIPS should be considered in high-risk subpopulations of patients with variceal hemorrhage.[A7–A9] Even though patients with cirrhosis and coagulopathy (prolonged international normalized ratio or decreased platelet count) have a higher risk of not responding to hemostasis for variceal hemorrhage or bleeding from procedures (ligation, paracentesis, TIPS, surgery), neither recombinant factor VII nor eltrombopag has proved beneficial in randomized trials, and neither is recommended.

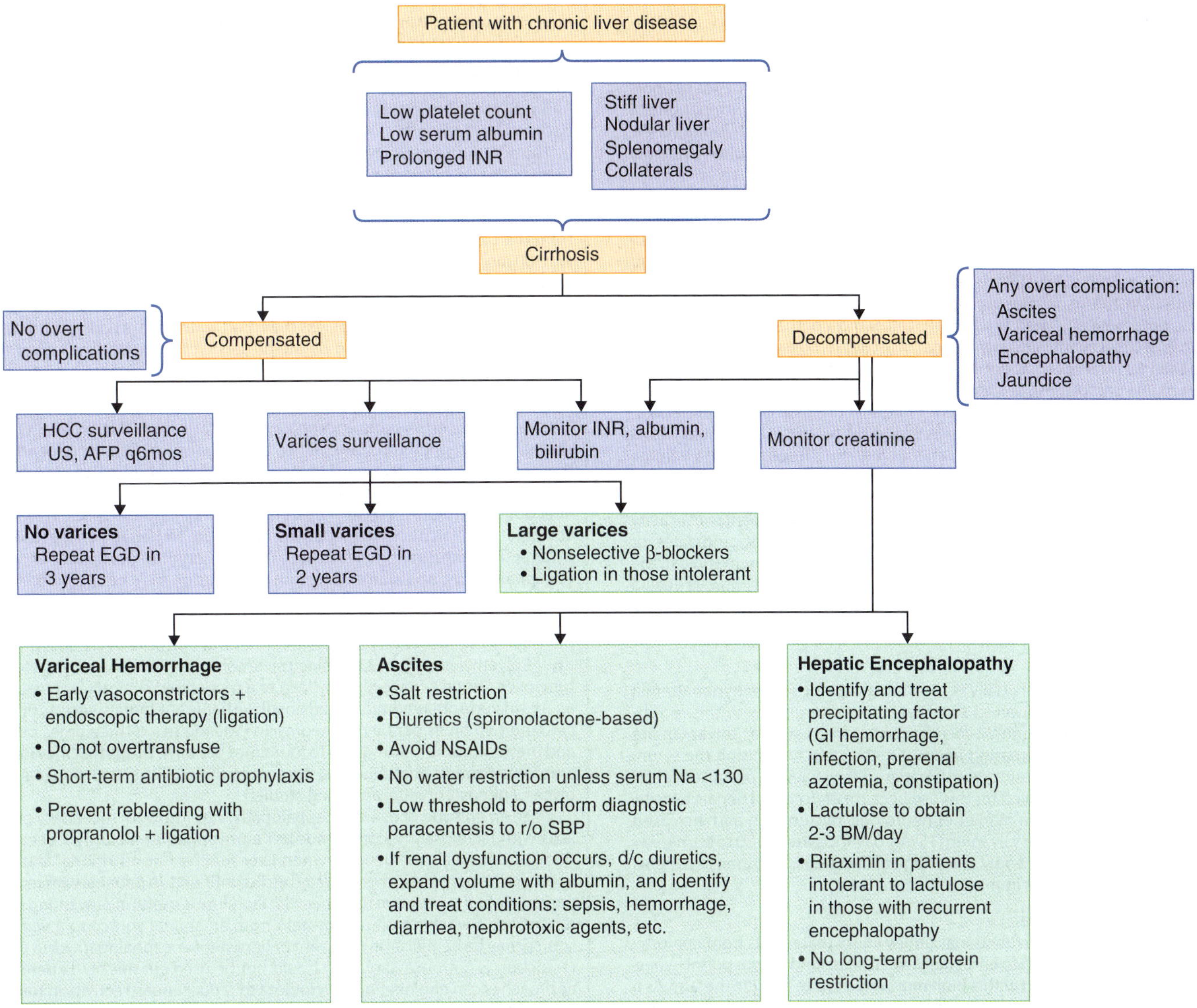

FIGURE 139-6. **Summary of the management of compensated and decompensated cirrhosis.** AFP = α-fetoprotein; BM = bowel movement; d/c = discontinue; EGD = esophagogastroduodenoscopy; GI = gastrointestinal; HCC = hepatocellular carcinoma; INR = international normalized ratio; Na = sodium; NSAIDs = nonsteroidal anti-inflammatory drugs; r/o = rule out; SBP = spontaneous bacterial peritonitis; US = ultrasound.

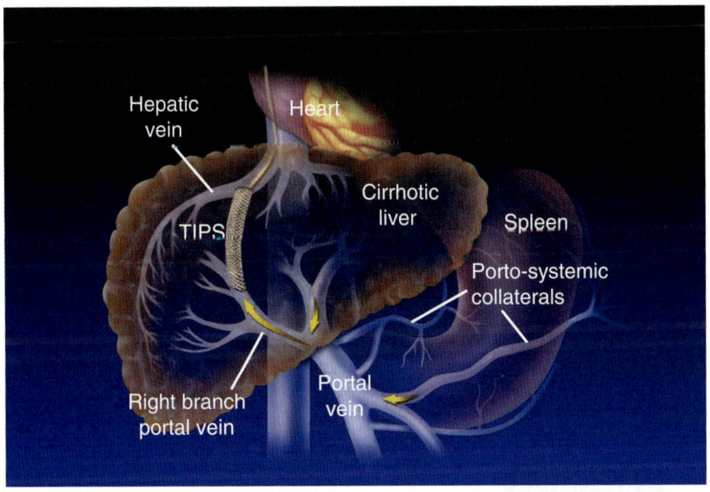

FIGURE 139-7. **Transjugular intrahepatic portosystemic shunt (TIPS).** This shunt is performed by interventional radiologists and consists of an expandable metal stent (most often coated with polytetrafluoroethylene) that connects a branch of the portal vein (high-pressure vein) to a branch of the hepatic vein (low-pressure vein). The shunt decompresses the portal system and portosystemic collaterals, and therefore it is used in the treatment of selected patients with cirrhosis and variceal hemorrhage. The shunt also decompresses the hepatic sinusoids and therefore is also used in the treatment of refractory ascites.

After control of hemorrhage, the 1-year recurrence of hemorrhage without treatment is high, at about 60%. Therefore, therapy to prevent rebleeding should be instituted before the patient is discharged. The recommended therapy is a combination of nonselective β-blockers (propranolol or nadolol) and endoscopic variceal ligation.[A10] The dose of β-blockers should be the maximum dose that is tolerated, and endoscopic variceal ligation should be repeated every 2 to 4 weeks until the varices are obliterated. Patients who had TIPS placed during the episode of acute variceal hemorrhage do not require β-blockers or ligation but do require periodic Doppler examination of the shunt to assess its patency.

Shunt therapy, either surgical or through radiologic placement of a TIPS, should be used in patients whose variceal bleeding has persisted or recurred despite combined pharmacologic and endoscopic therapy. Both types of shunts are equally effective, and the choice will depend on local expertise. Although the uncovered TIPS frequently occludes, polytetrafluoroethylene-covered stents are associated with lower occlusion rates and lower rates of hepatic encephalopathy. In a randomized trial, covered stents were more effective than β-blockers in preventing variceal rebleeding in patients with cirrhosis, but they produced slightly more adverse events without increasing survival time or quality of life.[A11]

Ascites

Salt restriction and diuretics constitute the mainstay of management of ascites.[16] Dietary sodium intake should be restricted to 2 g/day. A more restrictive diet is not recommended and may compromise nutritional status.

Spironolactone, which is more effective than loop diuretics, should be started at a dose of 100 mg/day (once a day in the morning). The dose should be adjusted every 3 to 4 days to a maximal effective dose of 400 mg/day. Furosemide, at an escalated dose from 40 to 160 mg/day, can be started concurrently with spironolactone if ascites is tense or added subsequently if weight loss is inadequate or if hyperkalemia develops with spironolactone alone. The goal is weight loss of 1 kg in the first week and 2 kg/week subsequently. However, diuretics should be reduced if the rate of weight loss is more than 0.5 kg/day in patients without peripheral edema or more than 1 kg/day in patients with peripheral edema. Side effects of diuretic therapy include hypovolemic hyponatremia, hyperkalemia, renal dysfunction, encephalopathy, and, with spironolactone, painful gynecomastia.

In the acute setting, albumin infusion alone appears to be of no benefit and can increase the risk of pulmonary edema.[A12] However, the addition of long-term human albumin (40 g twice weekly for 2 weeks, then 40 g weekly) to spironolactone and furosemide can significantly reduce recurrent ascites[A13] and improve 18-month survival.[A14]

In the 10 to 20% of patients with ascites who are refractory to diuretics, large-volume paracentesis, aimed at removal of all or most of the fluid, plus albumin at a dose of 6 to 8 g intravenously per liter of ascites removed, particularly when more than 5L is removed at once, is a reasonable approach. The frequency of large-volume paracentesis is dictated by the rapidity at which the ascites reaccumulates. TIPS with uncovered stents is more effective than large-volume paracentesis plus albumin in preventing recurrent ascites but is associated with a higher rate of encephalopathy. In patients requiring frequent large-volume paracentesis (more than twice per month), a polytetrafluoroethylene-covered TIPS can improve survival.[A15] A peritoneovenous shunt, with use of a subcutaneously placed silicone tube that transfers ascites from the peritoneal cavity to the systemic circulation, can be used in patients who are not candidates for TIPS or liver transplantation. Automated flow pumps to move ascitic fluid to the bladder can reduce the need for large-volume paracentesis and improve quality of life in patients with medically untreatable ascites, but they require surgical placement and are at risk for infection.[A16]

Hyponatremia

Fluid restriction to 1.5 liters daily is recommended for severe hyponatremia (serum sodium concentration <130 mEq/L), but adherence with this recommendation is poor. Although V2-receptor antagonists such as tolvaptan are sometimes effective at increasing free water excretion and raising the serum sodium level in hyponatremic cirrhotic patients, they have no overall effect on survival and are not approved for this use because of potential hepatotoxicity. Because hyponatremia is a marker of neurologic dysfunction and increased mortality, short-term use of tolvaptan (15 mg/day, increased to 30 to 60 mg/day if needed) may be indicated only as a bridge to liver transplantation in patients in whom transplantation is imminent (Chapter 140).

Hepatorenal Syndrome

Hepatorenal syndrome is a functional kidney injury that results from hemodynamic abnormalities owing to end-stage liver disease and severe portal hypertension, and it is associated with a high mortality despite specific therapy. As a result, documented hepatorenal syndrome in the absence of prerenal azotemia or acute tubular necrosis represents a priority for transplantation (Chapter 140). Specific therapies for hepatorenal syndrome that have been used to "bridge" a patient to transplantation include vasoconstrictors (terlipressin, norepinephrine, octreotide plus midodrine) plus albumin, TIPS, and extracorporeal albumin dialysis, which is an experimental hemofiltration dialysis method that uses an albumin dialysate. The largest experience is with the use of terlipressin, which at a dose of 0.5 to 2.0 mg intravenously every 4 to 6 hours leads to a higher reversal rate of hepatorenal syndrome compared with placebo.[A17] However, terlipressin can also cause adverse effects, such as respiratory failure, and must be used with caution.

Spontaneous Bacterial Peritonitis

Empirical antibiotic therapy with an intravenous third-generation cephalosporin (e.g., cefotaxime 2 g intravenously every 12 hours or ceftriaxone 2 g intravenously every 24 hours) should be initiated as soon as the diagnosis is established and before culture results are available; the minimal duration of therapy should be 5 days. Response to recommended empirical antibiotics is significantly lower in patients with health care–associated infections (i.e., infections that occur in patients who have been in a health care facility within the prior 3 months) and particularly low in nosocomial infections (i.e., infections that occur >48 hours after hospitalization) because more infections are caused by multidrug-resistant organisms. In these settings, broader-spectrum antibiotics (e.g., vancomycin-tazobactam, imipenem, ertapenem [Chapter 94]) should be given initially and then modified after culture results and antibiotic sensitivities are obtained. Aminoglycosides should be avoided because of the high incidence of renal toxicity in cirrhotic patients.

Repeated diagnostic paracentesis should be performed 2 days after antibiotics are started, by which time the number of PMN neutrophils in ascitic fluid should have decreased by more than 25% from baseline. Lack of response should prompt further investigations to exclude secondary peritonitis. The renal dysfunction associated with spontaneous bacterial peritonitis can be prevented by the intravenous administration of albumin, particularly in patients who have any evidence of renal dysfunction (blood urea nitrogen >30 mg/dL or creatinine >1 mg/dL, or both) or serum bilirubin concentration higher than 4 mg/dL at the time of diagnosis. Albumin at a dose of 1.5 g per kilogram of body weight at diagnosis, repeated on the third day at an intravenous dose of 1 g per kilogram of body weight, can reduce the risk of renal failure and acute mortality. However, this dosing is empirical, should not exceed 100 g per dose, and does not reduce 3-month mortality in cirrhotic patients with infections other than spontaneous bacterial peritonitis.[A18]

The administration of nonabsorbable (or poorly absorbable) antibiotics can prevent the development of spontaneous bacterial peritonitis and other infections in cirrhosis by selectively eliminating gram-negative organisms in the gut.[17] However, norfloxacin, which was used for this purpose, was withdrawn from the U.S. market in 2014. Reasonable alternatives include oral ciprofloxacin 500 mg every day or rifaximin 600 mg twice daily.[18] Long-term antibiotic prophylaxis may be justified only in two groups: patients who have recovered from a previous episode of spontaneous bacterial peritonitis and patients who have an ascites protein level of less than 1 g/L with advanced liver and circulatory dysfunction as evidenced by the presence of jaundice, hyponatremia, or renal dysfunction.

Hepatic Encephalopathy

Treatment of overt hepatic encephalopathy starts by exclusion of alternative causes of altered mental status. Once the diagnosis of hepatic encephalopathy has been made, treatment involves identifying and treating the precipitating factor and reducing the ammonia level. Precipitating factors include infections, overdiuresis, gastrointestinal bleeding, high oral protein load, and constipation. Narcotics and sedatives contribute to hepatic encephalopathy by directly depressing brain function. TIPS is a common precipitant of hepatic encephalopathy, and shunt reduction or occlusion may be required. Among agents aimed at decreasing ammonia production in the gut, lactulose (15 to 30 mL orally twice daily adjusted to obtain two or three soft bowel movements per day) is the first choice for the treatment of episodic overt encephalopathy.[19] Polyethylene glycol 3350-electrolyte solution (4 L orally or by nasogastric tube over 4 hours), however, may lead to a more rapid clinical response. Other agents include orally administered nonabsorbable antibiotics, such as rifaximin (550 mg two times per day),[A19] neomycin (500 mg to 1 g three times per day), and metronidazole (250 mg two to four times per day). Drugs that may increase ammonia fixation in the liver, such as L-ornithine-L-aspartate, benzoate, and glycerol phenylbutyrate, are being studied.

Once an episode of overt encephalopathy has resolved, secondary prophylaxis with lactulose is recommended. If a precipitating factor has been identified and is well controlled or when liver function or nutritional status has improved, prophylactic therapy may be discontinued. In patients with recurrent encephalopathy, rifaximin together with lactulose is useful in preventing further recurrence. Switching dietary protein from an animal source to a vegetable source may be beneficial in recurrent or persistent encephalopathy, but protein restriction is not necessary and should not be used chronically. Experimental approaches can engineer gut microbiota to reduce urease activity in mice, but whether this approach can be extended to humans is unknown.

Pulmonary Complications

Hepatopulmonary syndrome rarely resolves spontaneously, and medical therapy is disappointing.[20] TIPS is not generally recommended. The only viable treatment is liver transplantation (Chapter 140).

By comparison, liver transplantation is indicated only in a subset of patients with portopulmonary hypertension. In fact, a mean pulmonary arterial pressure higher than 45 mm Hg is an absolute contraindication to liver transplantation. The use of vasodilators should be considered in these patients (Chapter 69).

Surgical Therapy

Liver Transplantation

Orthotopic liver transplantation (Chapter 140), which is the definitive therapy for cirrhosis, is indicated when the risk for dying of liver disease is greater than the risk for dying of transplantation, as determined by a Child-Pugh score of 7 or higher (see Table 139-2) or a Model for End-Stage Liver Disease (MELD) score of 15 or higher. MELD and MELD-Na (see Table 139-2), which estimate the risk for 3-month mortality, are used to determine the priority for liver transplantation. The number of available deceased donor organs is lower than the number of patients awaiting liver transplantation; as a result, 15 to 20% of patients awaiting liver transplantation in the United States die before an organ becomes available.

PREVENTION

Treatment of the underlying liver disease, before the development of cirrhosis, is a primary prevention strategy. Because the major causes of cirrhosis are related to lifestyle choices such as injection drug use (Chapter 365), alcohol consumption (Chapter 364), obesity, and unprotected sex, primary prevention programs that focus on encouraging alcohol abstinence, reducing high-risk behavior for hepatitis virus infection, weight reduction, and vaccination for hepatitis B are even better prevention strategies.

PROGNOSIS

The outcome of cirrhosis depends on the patient's stage. Patients with compensated cirrhosis die of liver disease only after transition to a decompensated stage. The 10-year survival rate of patients who remain in a compensated stage is approximately 90%, whereas their likelihood of decompensation is 50% at 10 years. Inception cohort studies of patients with compensated cirrhosis show a median survival of all patients, including those in whom decompensation develops over time, of about 10 years. Overall, the median survival after decompensation is about 2 years.[21] Survival is even lower in patients with refractory ascites, hyponatremia, or recurrent variceal hemorrhage and is lowest in patients who are hospitalized with an acute decompensating event, in whom 28-day mortality is about 30% and correlates with the number of organ failures present. Hepatocellular carcinoma develops at a fairly constant rate of 3% per year and is associated with a worse outcome at whatever stage it develops.

Predictors of survival are somewhat different in compensated and decompensated patients. Parameters of portal hypertension (varices, splenomegaly, platelet count, γ-globulin) assume greater importance in compensated patients, whereas renal dysfunction, hemorrhage, and hepatocellular carcinoma are important predictive factors in patients with decompensated cirrhosis. In clinical practice, the Child-Pugh score is applicable to all cirrhotic patients, and the MELD score is used in decompensated patients to determine priority for liver transplantation (see Table 139-2).

GENERAL REFERENCES

For the General References and other additional features, please visit Elsevier eBooks+ at https://ebooks.health.elsevier.com.

Grade A References

A1. Kerbert AJC, Chiang FWT, van der Werf M. Hemodynamic response to primary prophylactic therapy with nonselective β-blockers is related to a reduction of first variceal bleeding risk in liver cirrhosis: a meta-analysis. *Eur J Gastroenterol Hepatol.* 2017;29:380-387.

A2. Villanueva C, Albillos A, Joan Genescà J, et al. β blockers to prevent decompensation of cirrhosis in patients with clinically significant portal hypertension (PREDESCI): a randomised, double-blind, placebo-controlled, multicentre trial. *Lancet.* 2019;393:1597-1608.

A3. Zacharias AP, Jeyaraj R, Hobolth L, et al. Carvedilol versus traditional, non-selective beta-blockers for adults with cirrhosis and gastroesophageal varices. *Cochrane Database Syst Rev.* 2018;10:CD11510.

A4. Villanueva C, Torres F, Kumar Sarin S, et al. Carvedilol reduces the risk of decompensation and mortality in patients with compensated cirrhosis in a competing-risk meta-analysis. *J Hepatol.* 2022;77:1014-1025.

A5. Roberts D, Best LM, Freeman SC, et al. Treatment for bleeding oesophageal varices in people with decompensated liver cirrhosis: a network meta-analysis. *Cochrane Database Syst Rev.* 2021;4:CD013155.

A6. Escorsell A, Pavel O, Cardenas A, et al. Esophageal balloon tamponade versus esophageal stent in controlling acute refractory variceal bleeding: a multicenter randomized, controlled trial. *Hepatology.* 2016;63:1957-1967.

A7. Nicoară-Farcău O, Han G, Rudler M, et al. Effects of early placement of transjugular portosystemic shunts in patients with high-risk acute variceal bleeding: a meta-analysis of individual patient data. *Gastroenterology.* 2021;160:193-205.

A8. Plaz Torres MC, Best LM, Freeman SC, et al. Secondary prevention of variceal bleeding in adults with previous oesophageal variceal bleeding due to decompensated liver cirrhosis: a network meta-analysis. *Cochrane Database Syst Rev.* 2021;3:CD013122.

A9. Nicoară-Farcău O, Han G, Rudler M, et al. Effects of early placement of transjugular portosystemic shunts in patients with high risk acute variceal bleeding: a meta-analysis of individual patient data. *Gastroenterology.* 2021;160:193-205.

A10. Albillos A, Zamora J, Martinez J, et al. Stratifying risk in the prevention of recurrent variceal hemorrhage: results of an individual patient meta-analysis. *Hepatology.* 2017;66:1219-1231.

A11. Holster IL, Tjwa ET, Moelker A, et al. Covered transjugular intrahepatic portosystemic shunt versus endoscopic therapy + beta-blocker for prevention of variceal rebleeding. *Hepatology.* 2016;63:581-589.

A12. China L, Freemantle N, Forrest E, et al. A randomized trial of albumin infusions in hospitalized patients with cirrhosis. *N Eng J Med.* 2021;384:808-817.

A13. Sandi BB, Leão GS, de Mattos AA, et al. Long-term albumin administration in patients with cirrhosis and ascites: a meta-analysis of randomized controlled trials. *J Gastroenterol Hepatol.* 2021;36:609-617.

A14. Caraceni P, Riggio O, Angeli P, et al. Long-term albumin administration in decompensated cirrhosis (ANSWER): an open-label randomised trial. *Lancet.* 2018;391:2417-2429.

A15. Bureau C, Thabut D, Oberti F, et al. Transjugular intrahepatic portosystemic shunts with covered stents increase transplant-free survival of patients with cirrhosis and recurrent ascites. *Gastroenterology.* 2017;152:157-163.

A16. Bureau C, Adebayo D, Chalret de Rieu M, et al. Alfapump® system vs. large volume paracentesis for refractory ascites: a multicenter randomized controlled study. *J Hepatol.* 2017;67:940-949.

A17. Wong F, Pappas SC, Curry MP, et al. Terlipressin plus albumin for the treatment of type 1 hepatorenal syndrome. *N Engl J Med.* 2021;384:818-828.

A18. Thévenot T, Bureau C, Oberti F, et al. Effect of albumin in cirrhotic patients with infection other than spontaneous bacterial peritonitis. A randomized trial. *J Hepatol.* 2015;62:822-830.

A19. Bureau C, Thabut D, Jezequel C, et al. The use of rifaximin in the prevention of overt hepatic encephalopathy after transjugular intrahepatic portosystemic shunt: a randomized controlled trial. *Ann Intern Med.* 2021;174:633-640.

140 LIVER FAILURE AND TRANSPLANTATION

ROBERT J. FONTANA

LIVER FAILURE

EPIDEMIOLOGY AND PATHOBIOLOGY

Acute liver failure, which is a rare disorder seen in 2000 to 3000 U.S. patients each year, is defined as a severe acute liver injury that precipitates the sudden onset of encephalopathy and coagulopathy (international normalized ratio [INR] > 1.5).[1] By definition, acute liver failure results from an insult within the prior 6 months. Acute-on-chronic liver failure is defined when liver injury of longer duration worsens and causes liver failure or other complications of portal hypertension.[2]

Nearly 50% of all cases of acute liver failure are caused by acetaminophen hepatotoxicity (Chapters 96 and 136), whereas idiosyncratic drug-induced liver injury (Chapter 136), autoimmune hepatitis (Chapter 135), acute hepatitis B (Chapter 134), and shock liver (Chapter 92) account for more than a quarter of cases.[3]

Acute-on-chronic liver failure can sometimes be precipitated by the same acute insults that cause acute liver failure. More commonly, however, acute-on-chronic liver failure occurs when cirrhosis (Chapter 139) decompensates because of a comparatively minor insult superimposed on serious but compensated underlying liver disease, or when ongoing alcoholic liver disease (Chapter 138), fatty liver disease (Chapter 138), or a metabolic liver disease (e.g., hemochromatosis [Chapter 196] or Wilson disease [Chapter 195]) causes severe progressive injury.

Liver failure results in loss of the liver's ability to synthesize coagulation factors and metabolize ammonia. The rapid loss of hepatocytes results in a massive release of cytokines, thereby leading to tissue hypoxia and lactic acidosis. The encephalopathy of acute liver failure is mediated by cerebral edema, not by the portosystemic shunting and portal hypertension of cirrhosis (Chapter 139).

CLINICAL MANIFESTATIONS AND DIAGNOSIS

The clinical manifestations of liver failure are the same as the manifestations of severe cirrhosis (Chapter 139). Hepatic encephalopathy and coagulopathy are the dominant features, but ascites, hepatorenal syndrome, hepatopulmonary syndrome, and portopulmonary hypertension typically occur. Variceal bleeding is more common in acute-on-chronic liver failure.

Patients with acute liver failure typically have the rapid onset of the encephalopathy and coagulopathy (INR > 1.5), but the onset can be slower in patients who have acute-on-chronic liver failure.[4] The severity of acute liver failure and the adequacy of tissue perfusion (e.g., serum pH and lactate level) can be assessed by measuring blood levels of markers that are synthesized by the liver (e.g., the INR, factor V level, and serum albumen level) or processed by the liver (e.g., serum arterial ammonia level and bilirubin level) and then monitoring them serially. Because factor V is the coagulation factor with the shortest half-life, it is the most sensitive biomarker to detect trends over time. The patient's grade of encephalopathy should be assessed on a scale of 1 (subtle, minimal change in consciousness), 2 (disoriented, inappropriate), 3 (somnolent but arousable), or 4 (comatose).

TREATMENT

Patients who have acute liver failure should be stabilized in an intensive care unit, where any neurologic, respiratory, hemodynamic, infectious, and renal complications should be addressed.[5] *N*-acetylcysteine (a 140 mg/kg loading dose followed by 70 mg/kg every 4 hours) should be administered immediately to all patients with suspected acetaminophen hepatotoxicity (Chapter 136). Based on limited data that raise the possibility of its potential benefit, N-acetylcysteine is also commonly recommended in acute liver failure caused by idiosyncratic drug-induced liver injury, hepatitis B, and autoimmune hepatitis, as well as acute liver failure of indeterminate cause, especially in patients who have grade 1 or 2 encephalopathy.[6]

Removal of the offending agent for idiosyncratic drug-induced liver injury (Chapter 136), nucleos(t)ide analogues for acute hepatitis B (Chapter 134), acyclovir for herpes simplex virus (Chapter 345), copper chelation and plasmapheresis for Wilson disease (Chapter 195), corticosteroids for autoimmune hepatitis (Chapter 135), delivery of the infant for pregnancy-related liver disease (Chapter 221), and a continuous heparin infusion for Budd-Chiari syndrome (Chapter 129) should be implemented.

The management of varices and variceal bleeding, ascites, hyponatremia, hepatorenal syndrome, and the hepatopulmonary syndrome is as recommended for cirrhosis. Although coagulopathy is inherent to acute liver failure, routine transfusions of plasma and platelets are not recommended because the excess volume can exacerbate cerebral and pulmonary edema without significant benefit.

To prevent intracranial hypertension, the head of the bed should be elevated above 30 degrees from horizontal, and efforts should be taken to minimize movement and Valsalva maneuvers. All sedative and psychotropic drugs should be avoided because of their delayed clearance. For acute kidney injury, continuous renal replacement therapy is preferred over hemodialysis and may help improve outcomes by reducing systemic ammonia levels.[7] When patients develop grade 3 encephalopathy, their respiratory status should be carefully monitored so that they can be electively intubated with a target PCO_2 of 28 to 30 mm Hg to facilitate intracerebral vasoconstriction.[8]

Invasive intracranial pressure (ICP) monitoring using intraparenchymal devices should be considered to guide medical therapy in nonresponsive patients with grade 3 or 4 encephalopathy because other signs of worsening neurologic function (e.g., posturing, dilated pupils, abnormalities on a brain computed tomographic scan) are frequently not present. Placement of an ICP monitor carries a 10 to 20% risk of intracranial bleeding, so all patients should receive desmopressin (20 μg) plus individualized doses of recombinant factor VIIa, fresh frozen plasma, or plasma factor concentrate under expert supervision to lower the risk of hemorrhage to less than 5%.[9] Surges in ICP that reduce cerebral perfusion pressure may be treated with an intravenous bolus of hypertonic saline (1 to 4 mL/kg of 3 to 10% saline over 30 minutes) or mannitol (0.5 to 1 mg/kg IV), with concomitant monitoring of serum sodium and osmolarity levels. Pentobarbital (100 to 150 mg bolus followed by 1 to 3 mg/kg/hour) can be used in patients who have refractory cerebral edema. Moderate hypothermia to 32° to 33° C via external cooling blankets may be helpful, but data are currently insufficient to recommend its routine use.

Serious bacterial infections are documented in about 80% of patients with acute liver failure, including fungal infections in about 20%. Any fever requires comprehensive evaluation (Chapters 259 and 260), with a low threshold for starting empirical broad-spectrum antibiotics while awaiting culture results if patients suffer from clinical deterioration.

PROGNOSIS

The likelihood of spontaneous recovery from acute liver failure without liver transplant can be estimated by knowing its cause, the initial severity of hepatic encephalopathy, the need for vasopressor or ventilatory support, and the laboratory parameters (e.g., the INR and bilirubin level) and vital organ function over time. Acute liver failure that is pregnancy-related or caused by acetaminophen, ischemia, or hepatitis A has a higher rate of spontaneous liver recovery (50 to 70%) compared with other causes of acute liver failure (20 to 50%). Hypophosphatemia is suggestive of liver regeneration and is a positive prognostic sign.

Patients who have a predicted transplant-free survival of less than 80% (see https://appadvice.com/app/acute-liver-failure-prognostic) should be considered for early transfer to a liver transplant center for further evaluation. Even if patients initially are at lower risk, however, they may require emergency liver transplantation if they exhibit no signs of liver recovery and regeneration, despite disease-specific interventions and general supportive care. Qualifying patients should be placed on the liver transplant waiting list with the highest priority, known as status 1A. With emergency surgery, patients in acute liver failure can achieve a 2-year survival as high as 92% with excellent neurologic and clinical outcomes. However, only 30% of listed patients who have acute liver failure undergo transplantation because of either spontaneous improvement or the development of a contraindication to liver transplantation. As a result, acute liver failure accounts only for 3 to 5% of annual liver transplants in the United States.

When patients with decompensated cirrhosis (Chapter 139) develop acute-on-chronic liver failure with variceal hemorrhage, ascites, and/or hepatic encephalopathy, they should be referred for evaluation for a liver transplant because of their increased risk of short-term mortality.[10,11,12] Adult patients with compensated cirrhosis have a median survival of 12 years and typically do not require referral for a possible liver transplant unless they have a Sodium-Model for End-Stage Liver Disease (Na-MELD) score above 15 (see Table 139-2), progressive protein calorie malnutrition, or severe clinical symptoms (e.g., muscle wasting, severe pruritus, recurrent encephalopathy, ascites, or gastrointestinal bleeding) that will improve with liver transplant. Patients who have the hepatopulmonary syndrome or portopulmonary hypertension (Chapter 139) may qualify for a higher priority on the waiting list via Na-MELD exception scores.

LIVER TRANSPLANTATION

Liver transplantation is a life-saving therapy for selected patients who have severe acute or chronic liver failure, as well as patients who have certain genetic, metabolic, and intrahepatic neoplastic disorders. In the United States, over 150 liver transplant centers perform nearly 9000 liver transplants annually. Deceased donors account for about 95% of transplanted livers, whereas about 5% are from living donors (Fig. 140-1).[13] At any given time, approximately 13,000 patients are on the liver transplant waiting list. The size of the deceased organ donor pool has gradually increased owing to the use of livers from deceased donors who are elderly or have hepatic steatosis, chronic hepatitis C, or prior hepatitis B infection. Nevertheless, the pre-transplant mortality rate for patients on the waiting list remains 7 to 12 deaths per 100 waiting list-years. By comparison, the 1- and 5-year recipient survival rates are now about 93 and 82%, respectively (Fig. 140-2).

INDICATIONS FOR LIVER TRANSPLANTATION

Chronic alcohol-related liver disease (Chapter 138), is now the most common underlying indication for liver transplant (Fig. 140-3) because of the success of antiviral therapies for treating chronic hepatitis C (Chapter 135). Nonalcoholic fatty liver disease (Chapter 138) is another increasing indication for liver transplant because of the obesity epidemic in the United States and other developed and even developing countries (Chapter 201).

Acute or Acute-on-Chronic Liver Failure

Liver transplantation is reserved for patients who have acute or acute-on-chronic liver failure with a high 90-day risk of death, as well as patients who

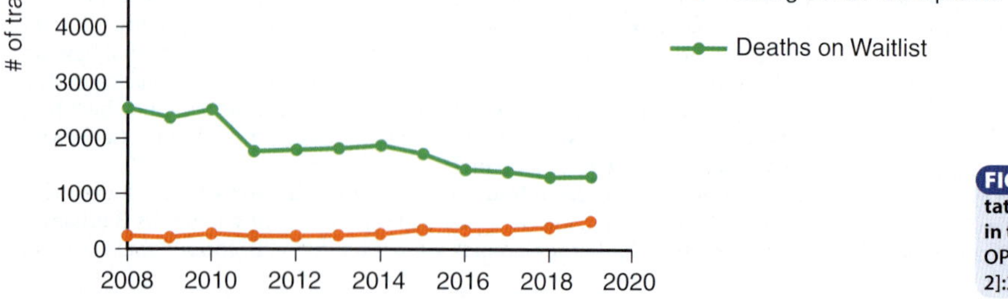

FIGURE 140-1. **Annual number of patients undergoing liver transplantation, living donor liver transplantation, and dying on the waiting list in the United States.** (Based on data from Kwon AJ, Kim WR, Lake JR, et al. OPTN/SRTR 2019 annual data report: river. *Am J Transplant.* 2021;21[Suppl 2]:208-315. Courtesy of Jason Pan, MD.)

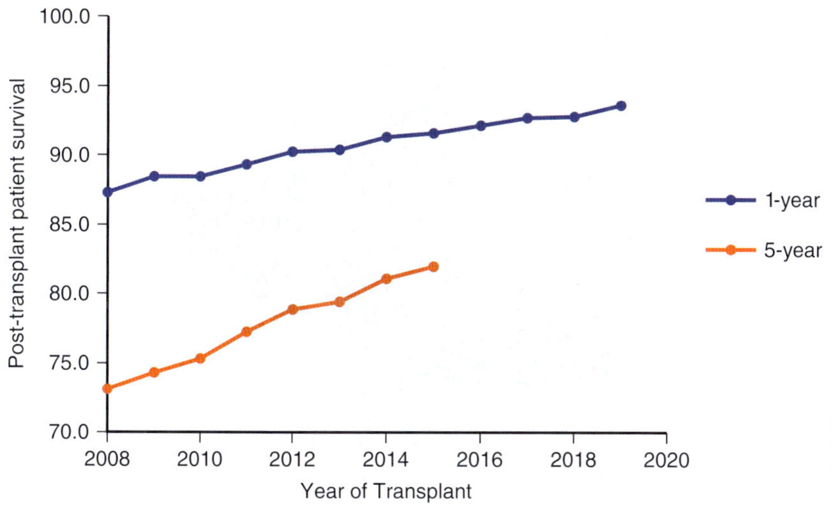

FIGURE 140-2. **The 1- and 5-year adult liver transplant patient survival rates in the United States.** (Based on data from Kwon AJ, Kim WR, Lake JR, et al. OPTN/SRTR 2019 annual data report: river. *Am J Transplant.* 2021;21[Suppl 2]:208-315. Courtesy of Jason Pan, MD.)

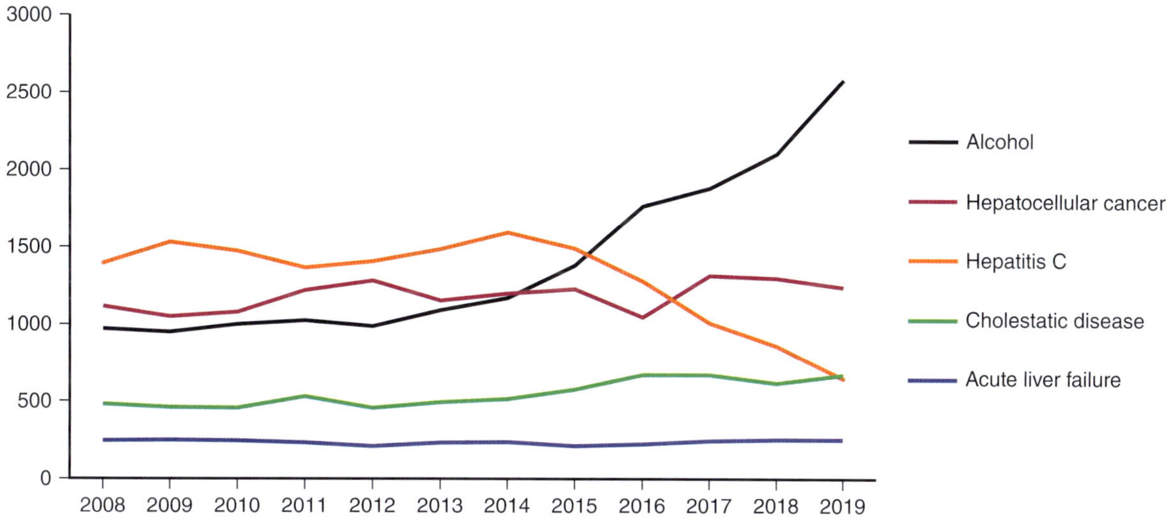

FIGURE 140-3. **Leading indications for adult liver transplantation in the United States** (Based on data from Kwong AJ, Kim WR, Lake JR, et al. OPTN/SRTR 2019 annual data report: liver. *Am J Transplant.* 2021;21[Suppl 2]:208-315. Courtesy of Jason Pan, MD.)

have metabolic, genetic, and neoplastic diseases that may be cured with liver transplantation.[14] When a patient with progressive cirrhosis experiences hepatic decompensation (e.g., ascites, variceal hemorrhage, portal vein thromboses, hepatic encephalopathy), progressive protein calorie malnutrition, or deteriorating laboratory indices, the patient should be referred for liver transplant evaluation. Most patients who have cirrhosis and a Na-MELD score of 15 or higher (Table 139-2) are likely to have a survival benefit with transplantation. Patients who have unique qualifying complications of portal hypertension (e.g., hepatopulmonary syndrome or refractory hepatic hydrothorax) may also receive high priority.[15]

Hepatobiliary Cancer

Hepatocellular carcinoma is the primary indication for 10 to 20% of adult liver transplants in the United States. To qualify for transplant independently of their Na-MELD score, patients must have: no evidence of extrahepatic disease or vascular invasion; one lesion that is less than 5 cm in size, or two or three lesions, each less than 3 cm in size; and a serum α-fetoprotein level less than 1000 ng/mL. Hepatocellular carcinoma patients who meet these criteria have a 5-year post-transplant survival approaching 80%.[16] If locoregional therapy, radiation, or chemoembolization (Chapter 181) reduces the size of the tumor(s), patients who do not meet these criteria may be downstaged, become eligible for transplantation, and do as well as patients who met transplantation criteria without downstaging.

Selected patients with locally advanced perihilar cholangiocarcinoma may also qualify for transplantation, regardless of their Na-MELD score if they have unresectable disease or have underlying liver disease that would make them poor candidates for resection surgery. Before transplantation, such patients should receive neoadjuvant chemotherapy and radiation (Chapter 181) and then undergo operative staging to ensure that they have no lymphatic, intrahepatic, or extrahepatic metastases. In eligible patients, the 5-year recurrence-free survival with neoadjuvant therapy and liver transplant is about 65%. Other uncommon indications for liver transplantation include hemangioendotheliomas and metastatic neuroendocrine and carcinoid tumors to the liver (Chapter 213).

Metabolic Disorders

Inborn errors of metabolism, such as primary hyperoxaluria, urea cycle disorders, and organic acidemias (Chapter 189) do not cause parenchymal liver disease or fibrosis.[17] However, liver transplantation can correct the enzymatic defects by lowering ammonia levels in urea cycle disorders and organic acidemia, lowering oxalate levels in primary hyperoxaluria, and providing normal protein in patients with familial amyloid polyneuropathy (Chapter 174). Liver transplantation also can prevent progression of systemic manifestations of these diseases but does not typically reverse preexisting systemic clinical manifestations, such as the intellectual deficits in the urea cycle disorders and organic acidemias or advanced neurologic symptoms and cardiac disease in familial amyloidosis or in patients with Wilson disease.

SELECTION FOR TRANSPLANTATION

Liver transplant candidates should be carefully evaluated by a multidisciplinary team to ensure that they have severe enough disease to warrant transplantation but also will be able to tolerate the surgery and associated immunosuppression with a favorable 5-year outcome. The presence of severe cardiopulmonary disease, active use of illicit substances or alcohol, frailty, and nonadherence with medical care are contraindications to transplantation (Table 140-1). A patient's eligibility for transplantation may vary over time and should be reassessed

TABLE 140-1 CONTRAINDICATIONS TO LIVER TRANSPLANTATION

Relapsing illicit substance or alcohol use
Inadequate social support
Severe or untreated psychiatric disease or behavioral concerns
Severe cardiopulmonary disease
Active extrahepatic malignancy
Uncontrolled sepsis or other severe infections
Active HIV infection with AIDS-defining illness
Irreversible neurologic disease
Anatomic anomalies or extensive vascular thromboses that are prohibitive to transplant
Severe malnutrition and frailty

AIDS = acquired immunodeficiency syndrome; HIV = human immunodeficiency virus.

whenever they undergo a clinical change, hospitalization, or a decompensating liver-related event.

Preoperative Medical Assessment

The pre-transplant evaluation process initially involves confirming the cause of the liver disease and determining whether any treatment other than transplantation may be effective. Then an assessment of the patient's severity of disease, operative risk, and nutritional and functional status is undertaken. Patients should complete age- and gender-appropriate cancer screenings (e.g., head and neck examination, skin examination, colonoscopy, mammography, pelvic examination, prostate-specific antigen determination). Blood typing is needed to ensure proper matching with potential donors, but matching by human leukocyte antigen (HLA) type is not required.

Liver transplantation surgery places significant stress on the heart and lungs, so patients with heart failure, inadequately treated coronary artery disease, severe valvular disease, or moderate to severe pulmonary hypertension are frequently excluded from consideration. All transplant candidates should have an electrocardiogram, a transthoracic echocardiogram with Doppler and bubble study to exclude intrapulmonary shunting, and a chest radiograph to screen for cardiopulmonary disease. Patients at risk for coronary artery disease should undergo formal cardiac stress testing with follow-up coronary angiography as indicated (Chapters 44 and 56).[18] Patients who have smoked or have underlying lung disease should undergo pulmonary function tests (Chapter 73) and pulse oximetry. Patients who have stage IV or V chronic kidney disease (Chapter 116) or who have been on hemodialysis for more than 90 days may be considered for combined liver and kidney transplantation.

Because of the need for lifelong immunosuppression, recipients of liver transplants are at risk for both bacterial and opportunistic infections. A careful dental examination is important to exclude an oral source of chronic infection. Latent pathogens such as tuberculosis (Chapter 299), Epstein-Barr virus (Chapter 348), cytomegalovirus (Chapter 347), toxoplasma (Chapter 320), and hepatitis B (Chapter 135) may reactivate in the setting of immunosuppression, so patient's prior exposure must be assessed before transplantation to plan for proper prophylaxis. Vaccinations against hepatitis A, hepatitis B, influenza, pneumococcus, herpes zoster, and COVID-19 infection (Chapter 15) are recommended before transplantation whenever possible. Patients with well-controlled human immunodeficiency virus (HIV) on stable antiretroviral therapy (Chapter 357) may undergo liver transplantation at specialized centers with good outcomes. However, patients with uncontrolled HIV infection or acquired immunodeficiency syndrome are excluded from liver transplantation because their outcomes are poor.

Patients who have severe malnutrition (Chapter 198), frailty (Chapter 24), morbid obesity (Chapter 201), or are older than age 70 years must be carefully assessed on an individual basis because they are at higher risk for postoperative complications and poor allograft function. Preoperative contrast-enhanced computed tomographic (CT) or magnetic resonance (MR) imaging of the liver is recommended in most centers for surgical planning and to evaluate for portal vein thromboses and atherosclerosis of the major vessels.

Preoperative Psychosocial Assessment

Successful liver transplantation requires long-term adherence to medication regimens, laboratory monitoring, and outpatient follow-up, as well as continued lifelong abstinence from alcohol, tobacco, and other illicit substances. Poor adherence may arise from a lack of motivation, poor social support, inability to maintain insurance coverage, and severe or untreated psychiatric conditions or substance use disorders. Long-term (≥6 months) preoperative abstinence from alcohol is desirable, in part to determine whether liver function may improve, but is not as predictive of the likelihood of recidivism as are factors such as social isolation, underlying psychiatric conditions, and family support. For example, selected patients with severe alcoholic hepatitis and a first episode of hepatic decompensation that is refractory to corticosteroids may do well after emergent liver transplantation combined with intensive post-transplantation treatment of the alcohol use disorder.[19]

A multidisciplinary team that involves hepatologists, social workers, psychiatrists, and psychologists may best identify and address any potential barriers to transplantation. In addition, liver transplantation candidates are typically screened with periodic toxicology testing, such as a serum phosphatidylethanol level, urine toxicology, urine ethyl glucuronide, and urine cotinine levels. Formal pre-transplantation education instructs patients, their families, and caregivers about the process of transplantation and the need for lifelong abstinence from illicit substances and compliance with medical treatments.

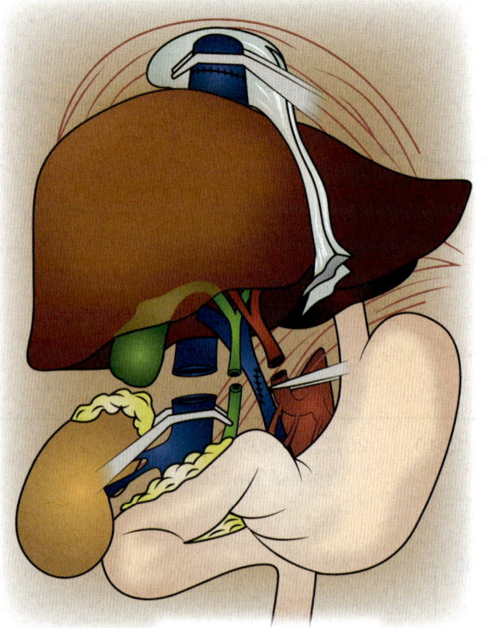

FIGURE 140-4. The four major anastomoses created during a standard liver transplant operation. The recipient's main portal vein is typically sewn to the donor's portal vein in an end-to-end manner. The venous outflow can be created via direct insertion of the individual hepatic veins onto the recipient vena cava or via a side-to-side cavocavostomy. Hepatic artery blood flow is established via an end-to-end arterial anastomosis. (From Karp SJ, Alexopoulous S. Liver transplantation. In: Townsend CM Jr, Beauchamp RD, Evers BM, et al, eds. *Sabiston Textbook of Surgery,* 21st ed. St. Louis, MO: Elsevier; 2022: 614-626.)

Listing for Liver Transplantation

Once an adult patient is medically, psychosocially, and financially approved to be added to the liver transplant waiting list, their priority is determined by their calculated Na-MELD score (Table 139-2), which is correlated with the likelihood of dying in the next 3 months without liver transplantation. The minimal Na-MELD score required to be listed for liver transplantation varies by center, but the usual requirement is a score of at least 15 points or evidence of complications of portal hypertension or progressive protein calorie malnutrition. Once on the list, organs are generally offered to ABO-identical or compatible patients who have the highest laboratory Na-MELD score, but critically ill adults may be upgraded to a higher priority if they are in an intensive care unit with fulminant liver failure, have acutely decompensated Wilson disease, or have acute failure of a previously transplanted liver.[20]

THE TRANSPLANTATION PROCEDURE

Liver transplant surgery entails three phases that requires 3 vascular and 1 biliary anastomoses: removal of the native liver, the anhepatic state, and engraftment (Fig. 140-4). Significant intra-operative bleeding typically requires large volumes of blood products and procoagulants.

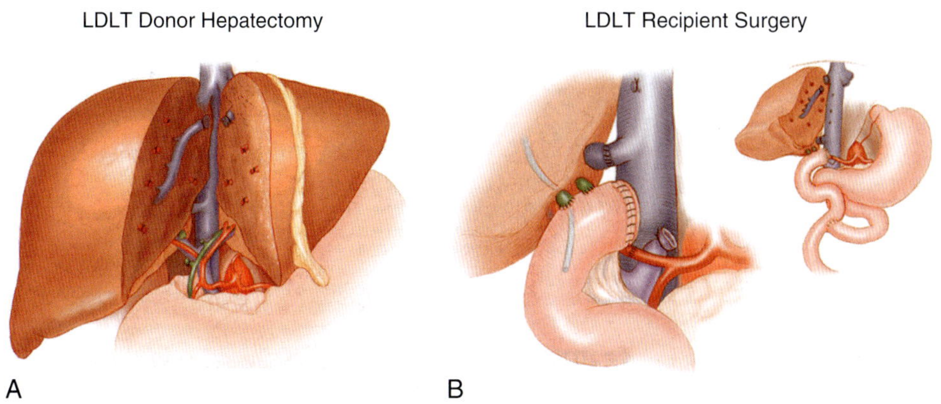

FIGURE 140-5. **Living related donor hepatectomy (A) and orthotopic implantation of the right lobe graft (B).** LDLT = living donor liver transplantation. (From Everson GT. Hepatic failure and liver transplantation. In: Goldman L, Schafer AI, eds. *Goldman-Cecil Medicine,* 26th ed. Philadelphia: Elsevier; 2020:998-1004.)

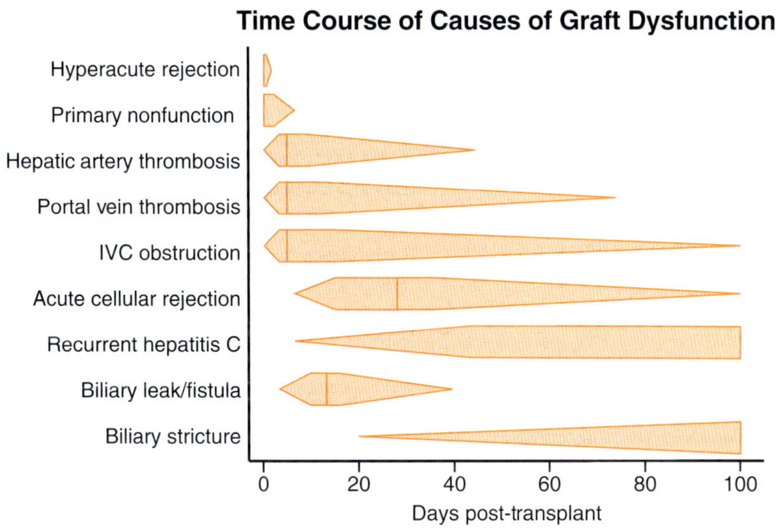

FIGURE 140-6. **Time course of causes of graft dysfunction.** Hyperacute rejection is rare (ABO incompatibility) but occurs in the first few hours to days. Primary nonfunction, vascular thrombosis, and biliary leaks are early events, and acute rejection episodes occur after the first 7 days. Recurrent hepatitis C may begin early but typically is manifested after the first 2 or 3 weeks after transplantation. Biliary strictures evolve more slowly and tend to be later events. IVC = inferior vena cava. (From Everson GT. Hepatic failure and liver transplantation. In: Goldman L, Schafer AI, eds. *Goldman-Cecil Medicine,* 26th ed. Philadelphia: Elsevier; 2020:998-1004.)

In the United States, approximately 95% of adult liver transplants use organs from deceased donors. Most deceased donor livers are procured from individuals who have experienced brain death due to head trauma, intracranial bleeding, or prolonged anoxia. However, about 8% are from critically ill patients who do not meet criteria for brain death (Chapter 373) but who may still qualify to be a liver donor after controlled withdrawal of life support. Livers from these latter donors have a higher risk of complications, such as ischemic cholangiopathy and primary non-function, because of prolonged warm ischemia following withdrawal of life-support. Cold ischemia time, which is the time between removal of the organ from the donor and implantation into the recipient, typically ranges from 4 to 8 hours. Advanced techniques for hypothermic[A1] and for normothermic[A2,21] perfusion can maintain the integrity of the graft during cold ischemia and may help expand the donor pool. Due to concerns of excessive travel time, livers from deceased donors over age 70 years or whose livers were harvested after cardiac death are offered to local liver transplantation programs.

Living donor liver transplantation can expedite liver transplantation and improve survival. Living donor liver transplantation is generally reserved for outpatients who have cirrhosis, liver tumors, or metabolic defects and who are not of high enough priority to qualify for a cadaveric liver (Fig. 140-5).[22] A portion of the larger right liver lobe (segments 5 to 8, which weigh 600 to 1000 grams) is typically used in an adult-to-adult transplantation (see Fig. 140-5).

POST-TRANSPLANTATION COMPLICATIONS AND CARE

Early post-transplantation complications (Fig. 140-6) related to the surgery include intra-abdominal bleeding, primary nonfunction of the graft, small-for-size syndrome, hepatic artery thrombosis, and bile leaks.[23,24] Subacute complications, which occur 1 to 3 months after surgery, include strictures of the biliary anastomosis, acute cellular rejection, and opportunistic infections. Late complications beyond 1 year include post-transplant lymphoproliferative disorder (Chapter 348), de novo malignancy, and recurrence of the original liver disease. Cardiovascular disease and malignancy are the leading causes of death after 1 year.

Surgical Complications

Primary nonfunction of the graft is the most serious perioperative complications but fortunately occurs in only 2 to 4% of recipients. Primary nonfunction is characterized by high aminotransferase levels, an elevated INR, lactic acidosis, and renal failure. Patients with primary nonfunction within 7 days of transplantation are highest priority for another transplant.

Hepatic artery thrombosis, which develops in less than 5% of patients and typically manifests with high levels of aminotransferases, coagulopathy, acidosis, or bile leaks early on and cholangiopathy later, can be diagnosed by liver ultrasound with Doppler. If surgical or radiologic interventions are not possible or successful, patients with hepatic artery thrombosis within 7 days after transplantation are highest priority for re-transplantation.

Biliary complications, such as bile leaks, biliary anastomotic strictures, and ischemic cholangiopathy, occur in 20 to 30% of recipients. Bile leaks tend to occur within days of the transplant. Ischemic cholangiopathy typically results in multiple, diffuse intrahepatic strictures that present clinically at 1 to 6 months after transplantation and may require percutaneous transhepatic cholangiography or re-transplantation for definitive management.

Infectious Complications

In the days after surgery, patients are prone to wound and surgical site infections, ventilator-associated pneumonia, catheter-associated bloodstream infections, and infections of non-anatomic fluid collections that arose during surgery (e.g., biloma, hematoma). In the first month after transplantation, high levels of immunosuppression raise the risk of infection with opportunistic pathogens (Fig. 140-7). Patients are typically prescribed trimethoprim-sulfamethoxazole[25] (usually one double strength tablet three times a week) to prevent *Pneumocystis* infections (see Table 313-2) and oral antifungal agents (e.g., fluconazole 100 mg per day) for 3 to 6 months after transplantation. The risk for cytomegalovirus is highest when the donor is anti-cytomegalovirus

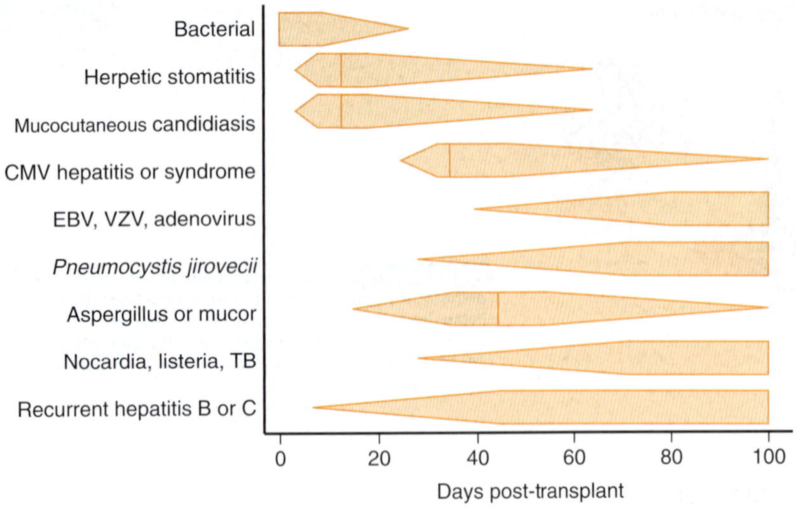

FIGURE 140-7. **Time course for infectious complications.** Bacterial and mucocutaneous viral or candidal infections occur early, and most of the others occur after the first 2 or 3 weeks after transplantation. CMV = cytomegalovirus (Chapter 347); EBV = Epstein-Barr virus (Chapter 348); TB = tuberculosis (Chapter 299); VZV = varicella-zoster virus (Chapter 346). (From Everson GT. Hepatic failure and liver transplantation. In: Goldman L, Schafer AI, eds. *Goldman-Cecil Medicine*, 26th ed. Philadelphia: Elsevier; 2020:998-1004.)

TABLE 140-2 ORAL IMMUNOSUPPRESSION MEDICATIONS

DRUG	DOSE	MONITORING	ADVERSE EFFECTS
CALCINEURIN INHIBITORS			
Cyclosporine	100-200 mg bid	Trough blood level 50 to 200 ng/mL	Nephrotoxicity Neurotoxicity
Tacrolimus	1-2 mg bid	Trough blood level 4 to 10 ng/mL	Hypertension Diabetes mellitus
mTOR INHIBITORS			
Sirolimus	1-3 mg daily	Trough blood level 4 to 12 ng/mL	Leukopenia, neutropenia
Everolimus	1-2 mg bid	Trough blood level 3 to 10 ng/mL	Thrombocytopenia Hyperlipidemia Vascular thrombosis Poor wound healing Mouth ulcers Pneumonitis
ANTIMETABOLITES			
Azathioprine	50-200 mg daily	CBC with platelets Chemistry panel including liver enzymes	Neutropenia Thrombocytopenia Anemia Hepatotoxicity, pancreatitis
Mycophenolate mofetil	500-1000 mg bid	CBC with platelets	Neutropenia GI disturbance Teratogen
CORTICOSTEROIDS			
Prednisone	5-20 mg daily	Clinical	Hypertension Diabetes/metabolic syndrome Osteoporosis Impaired healing

bid = twice daily; CBC = complete blood count; GI = gastrointestinal; mTOR = mammalian target of rapamycin.

IgG positive and the recipient is anti-cytomegalovirus IgG negative; in this situation, antiviral prophylaxis with valganciclovir (900 mg per day) is recommended. Beyond 6 months, patients remain at-risk for community-acquired bacterial and viral infections. When patients with hepatitis B infection undergo liver transplantation, post-transplantation oral nucleoside analogues (such as entecavir or tenofovir, see Chapter 135) are required to suppress viral replication along with hepatitis B immunoglobulins in selected individuals based on their virological profile at the time of transplantation. Recipients with detectable hepatitis C RNA can usually be cleared of infection with a 12-week course of pangenotypic, combination oral direct-acting antiviral agents (see Table 135-5).

Immunosuppression and Rejection

Immunosuppressive medications and associated prophylactic agents are generally managed by the patient's liver transplant team, but all clinicians should be familiar with the general approach and common toxicities (Table 140-2).[26] The initial immunosuppression for adult liver transplant recipients typically consists of high-dose intraoperative corticosteroids followed by tacrolimus, mycophenolate mofetil, and a steroid taper over 3 to 6 months. As early as 6 to 12 months after liver transplantation, healthy and uncomplicated liver transplant recipients may be tapered to a single calcineurin inhibitor (e.g., cyclosporine or tacrolimus).[A3] Some patients are also treated with mammalian target of rapamycin (mTOR) inhibitors (sirolimus or everolimus) combined with a low-dose calcineurin inhibitor in an effort to minimize nephrotoxicity. The target trough level of the calcineurin inhibitors and mTORs can generally be reduced over time if the patient has stable allograft function and evidence of immunologic tolerance.

Because calcineurin inhibitors and mTOR inhibitors are metabolized by cytochrome P-450 3A4/5, commonly used antifungal agents (e.g., azoles, caspofungin), some antibiotics (e.g., macrolides), non-dihydropyridine calcium-channel blockers, amiodarone, and other agents that are also metabolized by CYP3A4 must be carefully dosed and monitored to be sure that their blood levels do not increase or result in dangerous levels of immunosuppressants. Conversely, St. John's wort, rifampin, and some anticonvulsants (e.g., carbamazepine, phenytoin) can induce P-450 levels and reduce blood levels of immunosuppressive agents.

Acute T-cell–mediated rejection of the liver is most common during the first 10 days, and over 50% of cases of acute rejection occur in the first 90 days. Acute rejection should be suspected whenever the patient has unexplained allograft dysfunction or elevations in liver biochemistries.[27,28] The gold standard for the diagnosis is liver biopsy, which demonstrates variable degrees of portal inflammation, bile duct injury, and vascular endothelial inflammation (E-Fig. 140-1). The majority of patients with acute rejection will respond to a short course of intravenous corticosteroids and an increased dose of their maintenance immunosuppression under expert care. Repeated episodes of acute rejection can also lead to chronic ductopenic rejection, which is associated with obliteration of the bile ducts. Affected patients are slower to improve and may merit consideration for re-transplantation.

Antibody-mediated rejection may arise in a small proportion of recipients due to the development of donor-specific antibodies. In such cases, an increase in immunosuppression and/or plasmapheresis or IV immunoglobulin may be required under expert care.

Post-transplant lymphoproliferative disorders typically present in the first 12 to 18 months, but they can develop in up to 5% of recipients over their lifetimes. Post-transplant lymphoproliferative disorders usually occur when a patient has uncontrolled replication of Epstein-Barr virus (Chapter 348) because they are overly immunosuppressed. The diagnosis is confirmed by biopsy of a suspicious lymph node, solid organ, or bone marrow. About 50% of patients respond to a 25 to 50% reduction in immunosuppression within 1 month. Second- and third-line treatments include antiviral agents, rituximab, and chemoradiation therapy (see Chapter 348).

Long-Term Management

Beyond the first year, recipients of liver transplants are at increased risk for accelerated atherosclerosis, obesity, chronic kidney disease, and malignancy compared with age and gender-matched controls. Cardiovascular disease risk factors (e.g., hypertension [Chapter 64], hyperlipidemia [Chapter 190], diabetes [Chapter 210], obesity [Chapter 201]) should be aggressively managed with medications and diet. Patients who are on long-term immunosuppression should undergo screening and surveillance for cancer, including annual skin examinations by a dermatologist due to the high incidence of squamous cell and basal cell carcinomas (Chapter 188). Metabolic bone disease and vitamin D deficiency are frequent, so patients should receive oral calcium, vitamin D, and bisphosphonates (Chapter 225) to reduce the risk of bone fractures. Recurrent liver disease includes primary sclerosing cholangitis (Chapter 141), primary biliary cholangitis (Chapter 141), fatty liver disease (Chapter 138), and autoimmune hepatitis (Chapter 135).

Vaccination against herpes zoster reactivation, influenzae, pneumococcus, and COVID-19 are recommended in all recipients of liver transplants (Chapter 15). However, live virus vaccines should be avoided.

GENERAL REFERENCES

For the General References and other additional features, please visit Elsevier eBooks+ at https://ebooks.health.elsevier.com.

Grade A References

A1. Van Rijn R, Schurink IJ, de Vries Y, et al. Hypothermic machine perfusion in liver transplantation: a randomized trial. *N Engl J Med*. 2021;384:1391-1401.

A2. Markmann JF, Abouljoud MS, Ghobrial M, et al. Impact of portable normothermic blood-based machine perfusion on outcomes of liver transplant: the OCS Liver PROTECT randomized clinical trial. *JAMA Surg*. 2022;157:189-198.

A3. Fairfield C, Penninga L, Powell J, et al. Glucocorticosteroid-free versus glucocorticosteroid-containing immunosuppression for liver transplanted patients. *Cochrane Database Syst Rev*. 2018;4:CD007606.

141

DISEASES OF THE GALLBLADDER AND BILE DUCTS

EVAN L. FOGEL AND STUART SHERMAN

GALLBLADDER

Gallstones

EPIDEMIOLOGY

Gallstone disease is one of the most common and costly digestive diseases, with an estimated annual direct cost of $15 billion in the United States. Newly diagnosed gallstone disease occurs in more than 1 million people annually in the United States, and more than 750,000 cholecystectomies are now performed annually. The prevalence of gallstones is about 10 to 15% in American and European adults, with women affected about twice as often as men. Cholesterol gallstones are uncommon in individuals younger than 20 years, but a sharp increase is noted with each decade up to approximately the age of 70 years, particularly in women. About 20% of women and 10% of men have gallstones by 60 years of age. Together, approximately 12% of Americans, or 36 million men and women, harbor gallstones.

In the United States, the prevalence of stones is highest in Mexican American women (26%), followed by White women (17%) and African American women (14%). The prevalence of gallstones is extremely high in Native Americans, especially in women. In Chileans and Bolivians of Indian ancestry, gallstones are also common, and gallstone-associated cancer is the most common gastrointestinal cancer in these countries.

Environmental factors and genetic predisposition are likely to play an interactive role in gallstone formation. Pregnancy may contribute to the predominance of cholesterol stones in younger women because it is associated with progesterone-induced impaired gallbladder emptying and estrogen-mediated increased cholesterol saturation of bile. The prevalence of gallbladder stones in nulliparous women is approximately one tenth of that noted in multiparous women (1.3 vs. 13%). Exogenous estrogen administration in the form of hormone replacement therapy and oral contraceptives is also associated with stone formation. Other medications, including somatostatin analogues, ceftriaxone, and clofibrate, have been associated also with an increased incidence of gallbladder stones.

Obesity is a major risk factor for the development of cholesterol stones. Obese individuals have an increase in biliary cholesterol secretion relative to bile acid and lecithin secretion, thereby resulting in bile supersaturation. However, rapid weight loss is also associated with an increased risk for gallstones. Diminished ileal absorption of bile acids, due to surgical resection or bypass or to active inflammation (e.g., Crohn disease), may also lead to an increased likelihood of gallstones. Adherence to a modified Mediterranean diet (Fig. 13-1) or Dietary Approaches to Stop Hypertension (DASH) diet (Table 13-4) is associated with lower risk of symptomatic gallstone disease.[1]

PATHOBIOLOGY

Gallstone Formation

Gallstones represent a failure to maintain certain biliary solutes, primarily cholesterol and calcium salts, in a solubilized state. Gallstones are classified by their cholesterol content as either cholesterol or pigment stones. Pigment stones are further classified as either black or brown. Most cholesterol stones contain calcium salts in their core, and pure cholesterol gallstones are uncommon (10%). In most American populations, 70 to 80% of gallstones are cholesterol,[2] and black pigment stones account for most of the remaining 20 to 30%. Potential genetic susceptibility loci for gallstone disease include a common variant (p.D19H) of the hepatic and intestinal cholesterol transporter ABCG5/G8 and loss-of-function mutations in the ABCB4 transporter.[3]

In normal bile, cholesterol is soluble in the form of mixed micelles with optimal concentration of bile salts and phospholipids. With disproportionate concentrations, bile becomes supersaturated, and the excess cholesterol precipitates as monohydrate crystals. These crystals become embedded in gallbladder mucin gel with bilirubinate to form biliary sludge, which may eventually aggregate into a gallbladder stone.

Black pigment stones make up a small proportion of gallstones. These stones consist of polymerized calcium bilirubinate, precipitated as a result of exceeding the solubility of calcium and unconjugated bilirubin. In addition to increasing age, the formation of black pigment stones is more common in individuals who have conditions that create an excessive amount of unconjugated bilirubin (e.g., chronic hemolysis in hemoglobinopathies, cirrhosis, ineffective erythropoiesis), who are being fed by total parenteral nutrition (Chapter 198), or who have ileal diseases. Black pigment stones are typically tarry, are usually not associated with infected bile, and are located almost exclusively in the gallbladder.

By contrast, brown pigment stones are coarse in texture and are primarily formed in the bile duct as a result of bacterial infection that releases β-glucuronidase to hydrolyze glucuronic acid from bilirubin. Phospholipid hydrolysis also increases, thereby leading to precipitation of calcium, bilirubin, and free fatty acids and also resulting in the formation of brown pigment stones. Brown pigment stones account for 30 to 90% of gallstones in Asian populations, may also occur throughout the entire biliary tree, and are frequently associated with pyogenic cholangiohepatitis.

Gallbladder contractility is impaired in some patients with gallstones. Although gallbladder dysfunction can be the consequence of gallstone disease or of excessive cholesterol infiltration into the gallbladder's smooth muscle, evidence suggests that gallbladder stasis itself can lead to gallbladder stone formation. A normal gallbladder ejects 10 to 20% of its contents into the duodenum in response to enteric nervous stimulation. The presence of postprandial intestinal fat further increases gallbladder contractility, which is mediated by the enteric nervous system and cholecystokinin. Gallbladder stasis is frequently evident in patients with risk factors for forming gallstones, including obesity, pregnancy, rapid weight loss, and prolonged fasting (Table 141-1). Somatostatin analogues may predispose to gallstone formation by decreasing gallbladder emptying. Furthermore, gallbladder dysmotility is an independent risk factor for recurrent gallstones in patients who have been treated with extracorporeal shock wave lithotripsy.

Acute Calculous Cholecystitis

The most common complication of gallstone disease is acute cholecystitis, which occurs in 15 to 20% of symptomatic patients. Acute cholecystitis results when a stone becomes lodged at the gallbladder–cystic duct junction, where it impairs gallbladder outflow and drainage. The extent of inflammation and the progression of acute cholecystitis are related to the duration and degree of obstruction. In the most severe cases, this process can lead to ischemia and necrosis of the gallbladder wall. More often, the stone spontaneously dislodges, and the inflammation gradually resolves. Acute cholecystitis is primarily an inflammatory rather than an infectious process, but about 50% of patients with acute cholecystitis have secondary bacteriobilia, most commonly with *Escherichia coli*.

CLINICAL MANIFESTATIONS

The clinical spectrum of cholelithiasis ranges from the asymptomatic state to fatal complications. Among patients with asymptomatic gallstones, approximate annual risks are 1% for biliary pain, 0.3% for acute cholecystitis, 0.2% for symptomatic choledocholithiasis, and 0.04 to 1.5% for gallstone pancreatitis. However, these low individual percentages represent a huge population-wide number of symptomatic patients, given the frequency of gallstones. Overall, about 1 to 2% of asymptomatic individuals with gallstones develop serious symptoms or complications each year related to their gallstones.

The majority of gallstones are asymptomatic and are discovered on imaging studies performed for other indications. In such individuals, the gallbladder fills and empties normally, and the gallstones remain in the gallbladder and do not obstruct the cystic duct. Over time, however, asymptomatic gallstones can become symptomatic and be manifested as biliary colic due to impaction of a gallstone at the neck of the gallbladder or cystic duct. Although the pain is commonly termed biliary colic, the majority of patients actually note constant pain due to obstruction of the cystic duct and a progressive increase in gallbladder wall tension, rather than the paroxysmal pain of typical colic. The pain usually is located in the right upper quadrant or epigastrium and frequently radiates to the back and right scapula. Although biliary colic classically occurs after fatty meals, an association with meals is present in only 50% of patients, and the pain often develops more than 1 hour after eating. The duration of pain is typically 1 to 5 hours, but it may persist up to 24 hours. Pain persisting beyond 24 hours suggests that acute inflammation or cholecystitis is present. Episodes of biliary colic are usually less frequent than one episode per week. Other symptoms, such as nausea and vomiting, accompany each episode in 60 to 70% of cases. Bloating and belching are also present in 50% of patients. Fever and jaundice occur much less frequently with simple biliary colic. Although some patients with gallstones have continuous pain, predominantly in the back or the left upper quadrant, rather than episodic pain, alternative causes should be considered in such patients.

Acute Calculous Cholecystitis

Patients with acute cholecystitis typically present with right upper quadrant pain similar to biliary colic.[3] In acute cholecystitis, however, the pain is usually unremitting, may last several days, and is often associated with nausea, emesis, anorexia, and fever. On physical examination, patients usually have a low-grade fever, with localized right upper quadrant tenderness and guarding. The presence of a Murphy sign, an inspiratory arrest during deep palpation of the right upper quadrant, is the classic physical finding of acute cholecystitis. A palpable right upper quadrant mass is appreciated in one third of patients and usually represents omentum that has migrated to the area around the gallbladder in response to the inflammation. Mild jaundice (bilirubin level <6 mg/dL) may be present. Significant jaundice is rare with acute cholecystitis but when present suggests the presence of common bile duct stones, cholangitis, or obstruction of the common hepatic duct by severe pericholecystic inflammation because of the impaction of a large stone in the Hartmann pouch, which mechanically obstructs the bile duct (i.e., Mirizzi syndrome; Fig. 141-1). Mirizzi syndrome, which occurs in about 0.1% of patients with gallstones and 0.7 to 4% of patients after cholecystectomy, may lead to chronic inflammation, compression of the bile duct associated with clinical jaundice (Mirizzi type A), necrosis, and fibrosis. Ultimately, a cholecystocholedochal fistula may occur (Mirizzi type B). High fever suggests ascending cholangitis, often with bacterial infection (Fig. 141-2). Acute cholecystitis may coexist with choledocholithiasis or its complications of acute cholangitis and gallstone pancreatitis.

DIAGNOSIS

Transabdominal ultrasound is the radiologic procedure of choice to identify gallstones (Fig. 141-3). Because the ultrasound waves cannot penetrate the stones, acoustic shadowing is seen posterior to the stones, thereby facilitating diagnosis. Free-floating gallbladder stones will also move to a dependent position when the patient is repositioned during scanning. If both of these features are present, the positive predictive value of ultrasound approaches 100%. Nonshadowing echoes alone, however, may be caused by gallbladder polyps. Gallstones may be missed because of a lack of contrasting bile around the stones, as may occur with an impacted cystic duct stone or when the gallbladder is filled with stones. Small gallstones may not cast an acoustic shadow. An ileus with increased abdominal gas, as can occur with acute cholecystitis or pancreatitis (Chapter 130), may limit visualization of the gallbladder. Overall, the false-negative rate of ultrasound for detection of gallstones is less than 5% but may increase to 15% with acute cholecystitis. Ultrasound may also demonstrate dilation of the intrahepatic and extrahepatic bile ducts. Dilated ducts may signify obstruction due to stones in the common bile duct, distal strictures, or malignant obstruction (Chapters 180 and 181).

TABLE 141-1 RISK FACTORS ASSOCIATED WITH GALLSTONE FORMATION

NONMODIFIABLE FACTORS	MODIFIABLE FACTORS
Increasing age	Pregnancy and parity
Female gender	Obesity
Ethnicity	Low-fiber, high-calorie diet
Genetics, family history	Prolonged fasting
	Medications: clofibrate, estrogens, octreotide
	Low-level physical activity
	Rapid weight loss
	Hypertriglyceridemia, low high-density lipoprotein
	Metabolic syndrome
	Gallbladder stasis
	Terminal ileal disease or resection
	Total parenteral nutrition, fasting state

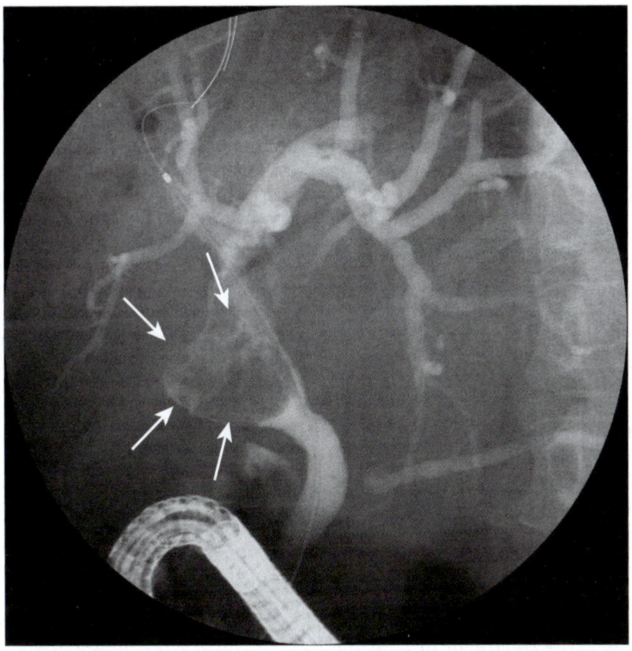

FIGURE 141-1. A bile duct stricture is seen at endoscopic retrograde cholangiopancreatography, representing Mirizzi syndrome (type A), with a large stone *(arrows)* in the proximal cystic duct, causing extrinsic compression of the bile duct.

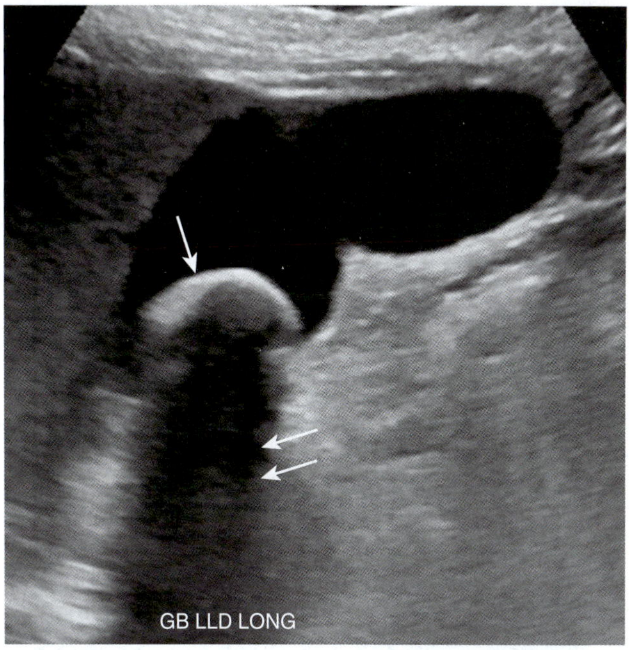

FIGURE 141-3. Ultrasound image of the long axis of the gallbladder. The image shows a dependent gallstone *(single arrow)* and acoustic shadow *(double arrows)*.

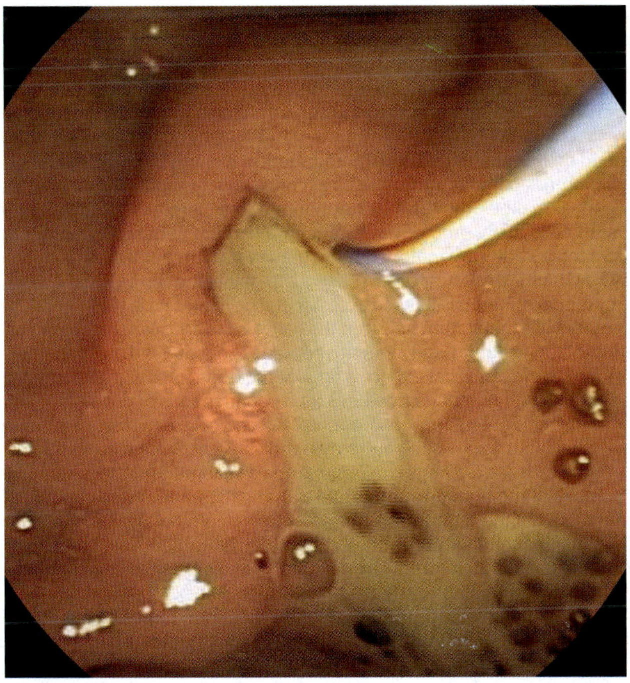

FIGURE 141-2. Endoscopic image of pus exiting the biliary orifice in this patient who presented with ascending cholangitis secondary to choledocholithiasis (note several small stones in duodenum).

Ultrasound has a sensitivity and specificity of 85% and 95%, respectively, for the diagnosis of acute cholecystitis. In addition to the presence of gallstones, findings suggestive of acute cholecystitis include thickening of the gallbladder wall (>4 mm) and the presence of pericholecystic fluid. Focal tenderness directly over the gallbladder (sonographic Murphy sign) also is suggestive of acute cholecystitis.

Cholescintigraphy provides a noninvasive, anatomic, and functional evaluation of the liver, gallbladder, bile duct, and duodenum, although it has generally been superseded by ultrasound for this purpose, except in certain situations, such as identification of a suspected occult bile leak after cholecystectomy or a functional gallbladder disorder (see later). In this procedure, technetium 99 m (^{99m}Tc)–labelled iminodiacetic acid derivatives are injected intravenously, taken up by the liver, and excreted into the bile. These hepatobiliary iminodiacetic acid (HIDA) scans provide functional information about the liver's ability to excrete radiolabelled substances into a nonobstructed biliary tree. The tracer should be taken up by the liver, gallbladder, common bile duct, and duodenum within 1 hour. Nonvisualization of the gallbladder 1 hour after the injection of the radioisotope with filling of the bile duct and duodenum indicates an obstructed cystic duct and in the acute clinical setting is highly sensitive (95%) and specific (95%) for acute cholecystitis, although false-positive results are often seen in the setting of gallbladder stasis (e.g., critically ill patients, total parenteral nutrition). Slow uptake of the tracer by the liver suggests hepatic parenchymal disease. Filling of the gallbladder and bile duct with delayed or absent filling of the intestine may suggest an obstruction at the level of the major papilla.

Abdominal computed tomography (CT) is less sensitive than ultrasound for the diagnosis of gallstones and is primarily indicated for the diagnosis of complications of gallstone disease, such as acute cholecystitis, choledocholithiasis, pancreatitis, and gallbladder cancer. By comparison, *plain abdominal radiographs* are of little value in the evaluation of gallbladder disease because only 15% of gallstones contain sufficient calcium to appear radiopaque. Plain films can be useful, however, for the diagnosis of other causes of acute abdominal pain (e.g., perforated viscus, bowel obstruction). Rarely, abdominal films may show a calcified gallbladder wall (Fig. 141-4) in chronic cholecystitis or findings such as pneumobilia or gallstone-associated ileus in acute cholecystitis.

A CT scan also is frequently performed to evaluate an acutely ill patient with abdominal pain. The CT scan can detect gallstones, gallbladder wall thickening, pericholecystic fluid and edema, and air in the gallbladder or gallbladder wall (emphysematous cholecystitis), but it is generally much less sensitive than ultrasonography for finding these conditions.

Magnetic resonance imaging is highly sensitive for the diagnosis of both gallstones and common duct stones, but stones smaller than 3 mm may be missed. Endoscopic ultrasound provides excellent imaging of the gallbladder and biliary tree but is rarely the primary imaging modality for detection of a gallbladder stone. Endoscopic collection of bile for crystal analysis may serve as a surrogate for microlithiasis not seen on transabdominal ultrasound.

With cholecystitis, laboratory evaluation can show a mild leukocytosis, with a white blood cell count of 12,000 to 15,000 cells/μL. However, many patients have a normal white blood cell count. Leukocytosis greater than 20,000 cells/μL should suggest further complications of cholecystitis, such as gangrene, perforation, or cholangitis. Mild elevations in serum bilirubin, alkaline phosphatase, aminotransferase, and amylase levels may also be seen with acute cholecystitis.

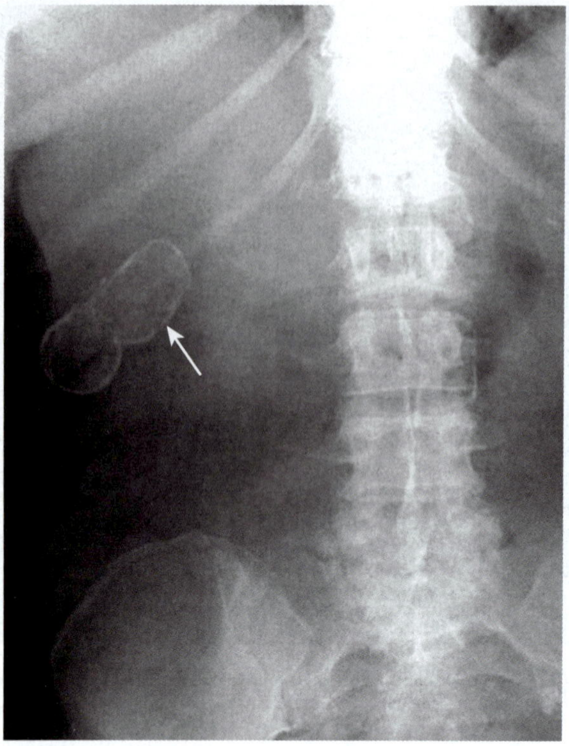

FIGURE 141-4. Plain abdominal radiograph illustrating a porcelain gallbladder. Note the calcified gallbladder wall.

TREATMENT

The treatment approach to gallstones depends on symptoms, complications, and whether there are stones in the common bile duct (Fig. 141-5).

Silent Gallstones

The longer that stones remain silent, the less likely they are to cause symptoms. In one large series, 20% of patients with initially silent gallstones developed events (8% uncomplicated, 12% complicated) at a median of 17 years. Risks were higher in women and in patients with multiple stones or a stone larger than 10 mm. Almost all patients will develop symptomatic disease before developing one of the serious complications of gallstones. Therefore, prophylactic cholecystectomy is not generally indicated in patients with asymptomatic gallstones.

In select groups of patients, however, prophylactic cholecystectomy should be considered, even when gallbladder stones are absent. A porcelain gallbladder with a calcified gallbladder wall is associated with a 5% or higher risk for malignant transformation, high enough to justify cholecystectomy. Patients with a long common channel between the bile and pancreatic ducts (i.e., anomalous pancreaticobiliary duct junction; see later) also are at significant risk for gallbladder cancer and should undergo prophylactic cholecystectomy. Acute cholecystitis is a potentially life-threatening condition in immunosuppressed patients, so prophylactic cholecystectomy is generally recommended before or at the time of major organ transplantation. Data also support cholecystectomy in patients undergoing bariatric weight loss surgery even in the absence of gallstones because of their nearly 30% risk for developing gallstones and requiring cholecystectomy during rapid weight loss in the first year after surgery. Prophylactic cholecystectomy adds minimal morbidity and mortality risks to most bariatric operations[4] and is clearly indicated in patients with gallstones. Some patients with silent gallbladder stones may also benefit from prophylactic cholecystectomy. In patients with sickle cell disease (Chapter 149), for example, cholecystitis can precipitate a crisis with substantial operative risks. Large gallstones (>3 cm) are more frequently associated with acute cholecystitis and gallbladder carcinoma. Because gallbladders containing stones that are larger than 3 cm in diameter have a 10-fold greater risk for developing malignancy than do those containing stones that are smaller than 1 cm, prophylactic cholecystectomy may also be indicated in these patients.

Symptomatic Gallstones in Outpatients

Although initial conservative management followed by elective surgery is reasonable in patients with mild symptoms,[A1] early surgery within 24 hours is generally preferred for patients with uncomplicated biliary colic. If patients do not have severe pain that lasts for >15 minutes, is located in the epigastrium or right upper quadrant, radiates to the back, and responds to simple analgesics, a conservative strategy of delaying surgery may be a reasonable alternative.[A2]

Day surgery is as safe and effective as an overnight stay.[A3] More than 95% of cholecystectomies are performed laparoscopically, with about 3% of elective procedures converted to an open procedure in the operating room. Contraindications to laparoscopic surgery include significant bleeding and Child class C cirrhosis (Chapter 139). Some patients with severe chronic obstructive pulmonary disease or heart failure may not tolerate the pneumoperitoneum required for laparoscopic surgery, and the prior upper abdominal surgery may increase the difficulty of or preclude laparoscopic cholecystectomy. Serious complications of laparoscopic cholecystectomy are rare, with a reported incidence of 0.6 to 1.5% for any bile duct leaks and 0.3 to 0.6% for a major bile duct injury. Although these risks are higher than for open surgery, the overall mortality rate (<0.3%) is lower for laparoscopic surgery, and the postoperative recovery is much easier. Outcomes for laparoscopic cholecystectomy are comparable among low- and high-volume centers. Robotic-assisted cholecystectomy appears to be as effective as laparoscopic cholecystectomy but is associated with a significant increase in complications and costs.[5]

Inpatient Acute Calculous Cholecystitis

In patients with an acute attack of cholecystitis warranting hospital admission, medical stabilization with intravenous fluids as needed, broad-spectrum antibiotics (e.g., piperacillin-tazobactam 3.375 g every 6 hours; or ceftriaxone 1 to 2 g once daily, plus metronidazole 500 mg every 6 hours; or levofloxacin, 500 mg once daily, plus metronidazole) and parenteral analgesics are indicated (see Table 26-4 in Chapter 26). The duration of antibiotic therapy is tailored to clinical improvement.

Early laparoscopic cholecystectomy within 2 days of the onset of symptoms is the treatment of choice for acute cholecystitis unless there are contraindications.[A4] Such surgery significantly reduces morbidity,[6] length of hospital stay,[A5] and time to return to work compared with open surgery. However, the conversion rate to an open procedure is about 25% compared with a rate of about 3% for elective laparoscopic surgery. If the bilirubin level is less than 4 mg/dL with no signs of cholangitis (i.e., intermediate risk for the presence of a bile duct stone), initial cholecystectomy with intraoperative cholangiography results in a shorter length of stay and fewer bile duct investigations compared with sequential common duct endoscopic assessment followed by subsequent surgery, without increasing morbidity. Laparoscopic fenestrating or reconstituting subtotal cholecystectomy is a safe "bailout" procedure in difficult operative situations.[7] Reconstituting subtotal cholecystectomy, which retains a small remnant gallbladder, may have better outcomes, but these techniques depend on intraoperative findings and surgical expertise.[A6]

In high-risk patients whose medical conditions preclude cholecystectomy, endoscopic gallbladder drainage is preferred over percutaneous cholecystostomy so as to allow prompt gallbladder drainage.[A7,A8] In expert hands, endoscopic retrograde cholangiopancreatography (ERCP)–guided stent drainage may be possible if contrast and a subsequent guidewire can be passed through the cystic duct, thereby allowing access to the gallbladder via the major papilla. Placement of a metal stent between the gallbladder and alimentary tract using endoscopic ultrasound is an alternative that does not depend on a patent cystic duct. Both techniques have success rates higher than 90%, with improved pain scores and lower reintervention rates than percutaneous drainage.[8]

If such drainage and appropriate antibiotics do not lead to clear improvement within 24 hours, however, laparotomy is indicated because failure to improve after percutaneous drainage is usually caused by gangrene of the gallbladder or perforation. If cholecystostomy is successful and the acute episode resolves, the patient can electively undergo either cholecystectomy or percutaneous stone extraction and removal of the cholecystostomy tube. Ideal timing of cholecystectomy after cholecystostomy is uncertain,[9,10] and nearly two thirds of patients may not proceed to cholecystectomy within the same calendar year.

Nonsurgical options for the treatment of gallstone disease are rarely used today because of their limited efficacy and the widespread application of laparoscopic cholecystectomy. Oral dissolution therapy (e.g., ursodeoxycholic acid, 15 mg/kg/day) may be considered in patients who have cholesterol gallstones, but it completely dissolves stones in only 40% of patients, and stones recur in up to 50% of patients within 5 years after therapy is stopped. Lifelong therapy, therefore, may be necessary. The direct infusion of organic solvents (methyl *tert*-butyl ether) into the gallbladder also is efficacious only for cholesterol gallstones, and the recurrence rate is similar to that of oral dissolution therapy. Extracorporeal shock wave lithotripsy can be considered for a single radiopaque stone that is 0.5 to 2 cm in diameter, regardless of its type, but only a small percentage of symptomatic patients fit these criteria. As a result, this therapy is limited to an extremely select group of patients.

PREVENTION

Moderate physical activity and dietary management (high fiber intake, avoidance of saturated fatty acids) may lower the risk for gallstone disease. Daily administration of cholecystokinin (3.5 μg) in patients receiving prolonged total parenteral nutrition may prevent formation of gallbladder sludge. Oral ursodeoxycholic acid (15 mg/kg/day) is beneficial to prevent gallstone disease during rapid weight loss and in patients who need long-term somatostatin

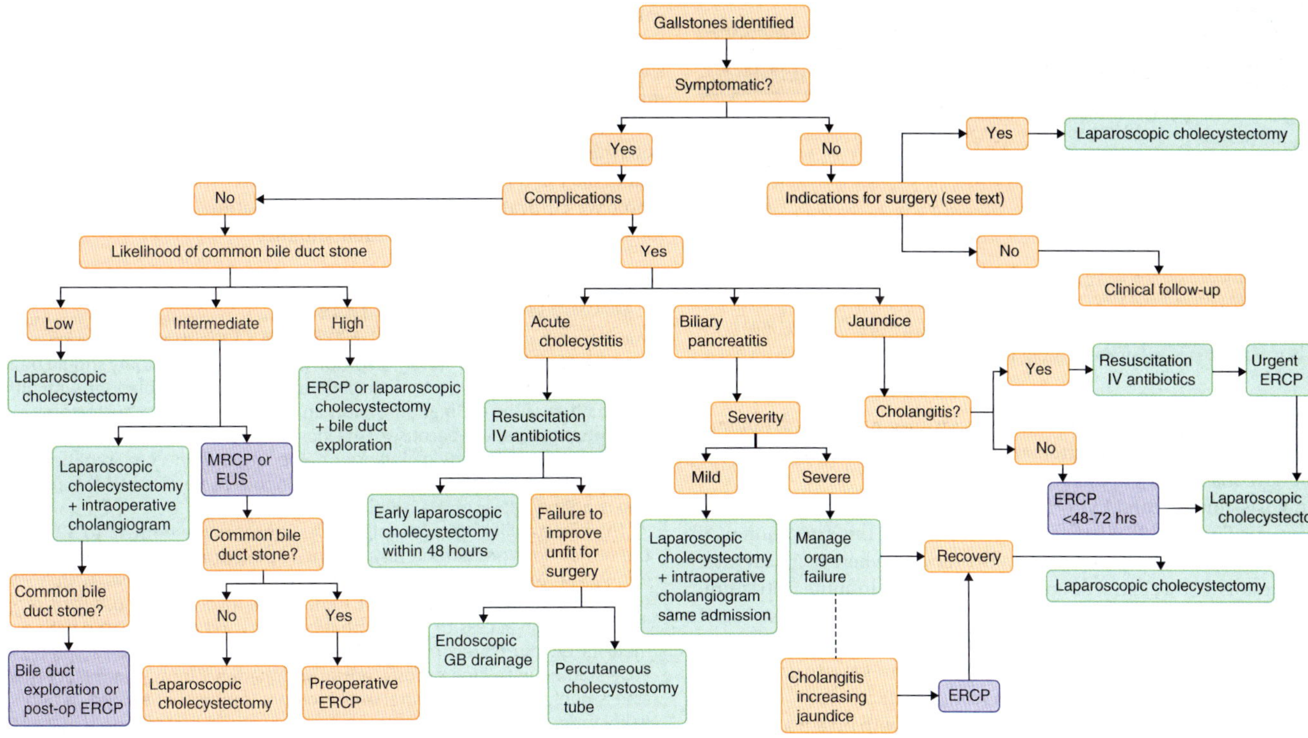

FIGURE 141-5. **Algorithm for the treatment of gallstones.** ERCP = endoscopic retrograde cholangiopancreatography; EUS = endoscopic ultrasound; GB = gallbladder; IV = intravenous; MRCP = magnetic resonance cholangiopancreatography.

therapy. For secondary prevention (i.e., in patients with gallstones already present), there are insufficient data to support the use of any medical therapy.

Complications of Acute Calculous Cholecystitis

Several complications of acute cholecystitis include empyema of the gallbladder, emphysematous cholecystitis, and gangrene leading to gallbladder perforation. Each of these complications can be associated with significant morbidity and mortality and therefore requires prompt surgical intervention. In 1 to 2% of patients with acute cholecystitis, the gallbladder will perforate into an adjacent hollow viscus, thereby creating a cholecystenteric fistula; the duodenum (79%) and the hepatic flexure of the colon (17%) are the most common sites. The episode of acute cholecystitis generally resolves as the gallbladder spontaneously decompresses after the fistula forms. If a large gallstone passes from the gallbladder into the small intestine, a mechanical bowel obstruction, termed gallstone ileus, may result. Gallstone ileus occurs in 10 to 15% of patients with a cholecystenteric fistula. Patients with gallstone ileus present with signs and symptoms of intestinal obstruction—nausea, vomiting, and abdominal pain. Abdominal films will demonstrate small bowel distention and air-fluid levels and may give additional clues to the source of the obstruction (pneumobilia or a calcified gallstone distant from the gallbladder). The initial management of gallstone ileus includes relieving the obstruction. Most frequently, this goal can be achieved by removing the gallstone through an enterotomy, although endoscopic retrieval of the offending stone can be done, depending on where the stone is located.

Acute Acalculous Cholecystitis

Acute acalculous cholecystitis, which accounts for 5 to 10% of all cases of acute cholecystitis, usually occurs in critically ill patients after trauma, burns, long-term parenteral nutrition, and major nonbiliary operations (e.g., abdominal aneurysm repair, cardiopulmonary bypass). The cause of acute acalculous cholecystitis remains unclear, although gallbladder stasis with increased bacterial colonization and ischemia have been implicated.

The symptoms and signs of acute acalculous cholecystitis are similar to those of acute calculous cholecystitis, with right upper quadrant pain and tenderness, fever, and leukocytosis. The disease often has a more fulminant course than acute calculous cholecystitis and more frequently progresses to gangrene, empyema, or perforation. Except for the absence of gallstones, ultrasound and CT findings are similar to those of calculous cholecystitis, including gallbladder wall thickening and pericholecystic fluid. On cholescintigraphy, the gallbladder does not fill; however, the false-positive rate (absent gallbladder filling without acute acalculous cholecystitis) may be as high as 40%.

Emergency cholecystectomy is recommended if the diagnosis is established or even if clinical suspicion is high because the risk for gangrene, perforation, or empyema exceeds 50%. Cholecystectomy rather than cholecystostomy is usually required, but percutaneous cholecystostomy or endoscopic gallbladder stenting is recommended in patients unable to undergo surgery. The mortality rate for acute acalculous cholecystitis can be as high as 40%, mostly because of the concomitant illnesses in patients who develop this disease.

FUNCTIONAL GALLBLADDER DISORDER

Some patients present with typical symptoms of biliary colic but do not have any evidence of gallstones on ultrasound examination. If further investigations such as liver chemistries, amylase and lipase levels, CT scan, and even upper gastrointestinal endoscopy are unremarkable, the diagnosis of a functional gallbladder disorder should be considered. The pathobiology is poorly understood, but one possibility is that the obesity epidemic has increased the population-wide accumulation of fat in the gallbladder wall—cholecystosteatosis—thereby decreasing the gallbladder's ability to empty. Some patients may have intermittent gallbladder outlet obstruction due to cystic duct spasm, poor coordination between the contraction of the gallbladder and the sphincter of Oddi, or dysmotility of the gallbladder. In a cholecystokinin-stimulated ^{99m}Tc-HIDA scan, cholecystokinin is infused intravenously after the gallbladder has filled with the ^{99m}Tc-labeled radionuclide, and a gallbladder ejection fraction is calculated 20 minutes later. An ejection fraction of less than 35% at 20 minutes is considered abnormal, and most of these patients have histopathologic evidence of chronic cholecystitis, although a low gallbladder ejection fraction is not specific for a functional gallbladder disorder (Table 141-2). The efficacy of laparoscopic cholecystectomy is controversial in this setting, but the Society of American Gastrointestinal and Endoscopic Surgeons recommends it. The percentage of patients undergoing cholecystectomy for functional gallbladder disorder in the United States during the past 15 years has increased from less than 5% to more than 20% of patients having the gallbladder removed. Additionally, patients who have symptoms of typical biliary colic and a markedly high gallbladder ejection fraction (i.e., gallbladder hyperkinesia) may also benefit from cholecystectomy, even though they do not have gallstones.[A9]

TUMORS OF THE GALLBLADDER

Benign

Cholesterol polyps are not true neoplasms but rather are cholesterol-filled projections of gallbladder mucosa that protrude into the lumen. These polyps account for approximately 50% of all polypoid gallbladder lesions, are usually

TABLE 141-2 SETTINGS IN WHICH A LOW GALLBLADDER EJECTION FRACTION MAY BE IDENTIFIED

Functional gallbladder disorder (chronic acalculous cholecystitis)
Cystic duct obstruction
Sphincter of Oddi dysfunction
Asymptomatic, healthy individuals
Diabetes
Pregnancy
Cirrhosis
Obesity
Celiac disease
Medications (narcotic analgesics, calcium-channel antagonists, oral contraceptive agents, benzodiazepines, histamine-2 receptor antagonists)

smaller than 1 cm, are typically found incidentally on imaging studies as nonmobile filling defects, are usually asymptomatic unless associated with gallstones, and do not have malignant potential.

Adenomyosis consists of a hypertrophic gallbladder muscle layer with mucosal diverticula called Rokitansky-Aschoff sinuses. This condition may affect the gallbladder locally, particularly in the fundus, where it appears as a hemispheric lesion with a central dimple; segmentally, as an annular stricture; or diffusely, when it involves the entire gallbladder wall. The cause is not entirely clear but may be secondary to a gallbladder motility disorder. Isolated adenomyosis can cause biliary-type symptoms and can progress to gallbladder cancer, so prophylactic cholecystectomy is recommended.

Gallbladder adenomas are benign epithelial tumors with malignant potential. Adenomas usually are manifested as solitary, nonmobile filling defects on ultrasound. Polyps smaller than 0.5 cm, regardless of total polyp number, can be observed with serial imaging studies, namely ultrasound, every 12 months. Larger polyps, however, may harbor a carcinoma in situ, and cholecystectomy is recommended for polyps larger than 1 cm and for any patients older than 50 years with biliary symptoms.

Malignancy

Gallbladder cancer is the most common biliary tract malignant neoplasm and fifth most common gastrointestinal cancer overall, with approximately 7000 new cases diagnosed annually in the United States (2.5 cases/100,000 population). The usual age at onset is the sixth or seventh decade, with a female-to-male ratio of 3 : 1. Gallbladder cancer is more common in Native Americans, Mexicans, Alaskans, and American Hispanics, as well as in residents of Israel, Chile, and northern Japan.

Perhaps because of chronic inflammation, gallbladder cancer is strongly associated with gallstones, which are identified in more than 90% of patients with gallbladder carcinoma. Conversely, only 1% of patients with gallstones develop gallbladder carcinoma. Choledochal cysts are associated with an increased risk for malignant neoplasms throughout the biliary tree, including the gallbladder, perhaps because of increased stasis, chronic inflammation, and infection. In patients with choledochal cysts, excision of extrahepatic cysts is recommended to avoid biliary tract cancer. By comparison, biliary sphincterotomy alone may be adequate for a type III extrahepatic cyst.

About 90% of gallbladder cancers are adenocarcinomas (90% scirrhous, 5% papillary, 5% colloid). The remaining tumors are anaplastic or squamous cell cancers. Gallbladder cancers spread by local extension and direct invasion of adjacent structures, including the common hepatic duct, liver, duodenum, and colon. Lymphatic drainage is to adjacent lymph nodes, and disseminated disease is to the liver and the peritoneal surface.

Most patients (80%) present with abdominal pain of less than 1 month in duration, which may be difficult to distinguish from symptoms of biliary colic or acute cholecystitis. Nausea and vomiting (50%) and weight loss (40%) are often present, and jaundice (30%) is a poor prognostic sign that typically signifies porta hepatis involvement with tumor. Up to 20% of gallbladder cancers are found at cholecystectomy performed for gallstones, whereas incidental cancers are found at 1% of cholecystectomies.

Diagnosis may be difficult preoperatively because laboratory test results may be normal or nonspecific even when advanced disease is manifested by hypoalbuminemia and anemia. There is no reliable tumor marker. Liver test results are abnormal when the tumor or periportal lymphadenopathy is associated with biliary obstruction. Ultrasonography has a sensitivity of 75 to 80% for detection of gallbladder cancer, with findings ranging from a complex luminal mass to gallbladder wall thickening, polypoid mass, or gallstones. Doppler ultrasound has a sensitivity and specificity of about 80% for the diagnosis of gallbladder cancer. Detection of color flow within a lesion supports the diagnosis, but its absence does not exclude malignancy.[11] CT or magnetic resonance cross-sectional imaging can assess the extent of disease, including regional and distant metastases. Endoscopic ultrasound may aid in determining the extent of local invasion and nodal involvement, but it rarely is necessary in the preoperative evaluation. ERCP is indicated only in patients who have clinical evidence of biliary obstruction and are being considered for stent placement to palliate their jaundice.

PREVENTION AND TREATMENT

Patients with gallstones larger than 3 cm have a 10-fold increased risk for development of gallbladder cancer, so prophylactic cholecystectomy should be considered even in an asymptomatic patient. A porcelain gallbladder, with diffuse calcification of the gallbladder wall, is an indication for cholecystectomy in the asymptomatic patient because of the increased risk for cancer. Cholecystectomy also is indicated for any gallbladder polyp larger than 1 cm, in patients with choledochal cysts other than type III, in anomalous pancreaticobiliary union, and in adenomyosis of the gallbladder.

The resectability rates for gallbladder cancer range from 15 to 30%. When the tumor does not extend beyond the lamina propria layer of the gallbladder wall (T1a), simple cholecystectomy alone may be curative, with a 5-year survival rate approaching 100%.[12] Tumors that involve the muscularis propria (T1b) may gain access to the lymphatic system and be associated with occult metastases. Current recommendations for pT1b cancers involve complete operative staging with laparoscopy, portal lymphadenectomy, cystic duct margin assessment, and partial central liver excision. Tumors that extend through the gallbladder wall (stage II/III) require a more extensive resection (cholecystectomy, partial central hepatectomy, lymph node dissection). Stage II tumors (no invasion beyond the gallbladder serosa) may have up to a 60 to 80% 5-year survival rate, whereas stage III tumors have a 25% 5-year survival rate. Median survival with unresectable (stage IV) disease is typically less than 6 months. Radiation therapy has not been shown to be effective, whereas chemotherapy regimens in unresectable disease (typically similar to regimens for pancreatic cancer [Chapter 180]) are associated with response rates of approximately 20%. Capecitabine (1250 mg/m^2 twice daily on days 1 to 14 of a 21-day cycle, for eight cycles) appears to improve overall survival in patients with resected cancer when used as adjuvant therapy,[A10] while second-line FOLFOX (folinic acid, fluorouracil, and oxaliplatin) chemotherapy leads to a clinically meaningful increase in 6- and 12-month overall survival rates after progression on cisplatin and gemcitabine.[A11] Molecular-targeted therapies may be helpful in a subset of patients.[13] Because of the late presentation of this disease and spread of tumor at diagnosis, the overall 5-year survival is less than 10%.

BILE DUCTS

Bile Duct Stones

PATHOBIOLOGY

Bile duct stones, or choledocholithiasis, can be classified as either primary or secondary. Primary duct stones develop de novo within the bile ducts, whereas secondary stones develop in the gallbladder and subsequently pass into the bile duct. In the Western world, more than 85% of all bile duct stones are secondary. Primary duct stones typically occur in conditions associated with bile stasis (e.g., benign biliary strictures, sclerosing cholangitis, choledochal cysts, periampullary diverticula), which promotes bacterial overgrowth with subsequent bilirubin deconjugation and the breakdown of biliary lipids, thereby resulting in the formation of brown pigment stones.

CLINICAL MANIFESTATIONS

Bile duct stones are discovered incidentally in 5 to 12% of patients during the evaluation of gallbladder stones and suspected cholecystitis. It is difficult to determine whether the existing bile duct stones are asymptomatic in patients who present with biliary pain alone because pain can originate from either the gallbladder stones or bile duct stones. More than 50% of patients with retained bile duct stones experience recurrent symptoms during a follow-up period of 6 months to 13 years, and 25% of cases develop serious complications.

Common clinical symptoms and signs of bile duct stones include epigastric or right upper quadrant pain, fever, and jaundice (referred to as the Charcot triad). Pain can be mild or severe, and severe episodes must be differentiated from other potentially life-threatening events. Occasional patients may present with painless jaundice and weight loss mimicking pancreaticobiliary malignant disease (Chapter 180).

DIAGNOSIS

Patients with cholangitis, with or without associated pancreatitis (Chapter 130), typically have elevated serum aminotransferase levels. The serum bilirubin level usually is less than 15 mg/dL with choledocholithiasis because most bile duct stones cause intermittent, incomplete biliary obstruction. In unusual cases, the serum aminotransferase levels can be profoundly elevated (up to 2000 IU/L), mimicking acute viral hepatitis.

Although ultrasound is the most common initial test for patients with suspected gallbladder stones, it has a low sensitivity rate (25 to 60%) for detection of bile duct stones, in part because the bile duct may not be dilated in acute obstruction. CT scan may demonstrate calcified bile duct stones (Fig. 141-6), but its sensitivity for this purpose is generally little better. CT is useful, however, for identifying other potential causes of biliary obstruction (e.g., mass lesion) and local complications, such as a liver abscess (Chapter 137). Magnetic resonance cholangiopancreatography (MRCP) and endoscopic ultrasound can detect bile duct stones with an accuracy comparable to that of ERCP (Fig. 141-7). Because of potential procedure-related risks, ERCP is now reserved for patients with confirmed or a high suspicion of biliary disease who are likely to require therapeutic intervention.

TREATMENT

Given the potential serious complications of bile duct stones (i.e., cholangitis, pancreatitis),[14] specific therapy is generally required regardless of symptoms. About 85 to 90% of bile duct stones can be removed at ERCP by standard balloon dilation and basket extraction after biliary endoscopic sphincterotomy, with a complication rate, including pancreatitis, bleeding, cholangitis, cholecystitis, and perforation, of less than 10%. Data are conflicting on whether asymptomatic patients are at increased risk for post-ERCP pancreatitis compared with patients who have symptomatic bile duct stones.[15–17] Endoscopic biliary orifice dilation without sphincterotomy may reduce some acute complications but increases the risk for pancreatitis and may lead to more subsequent procedures.[18]

The 10 to 15% of bile duct stones that cannot be removed by standard ERCP are generally larger than 1.5 cm, impacted, or located above a stricture.[19] Alternative therapies include the use of large-diameter dilation balloons (12 to 18 mm)[A12] and fragmentation by mechanical or electrohydraulic lithotripsy. Whenever stones cannot be completely removed endoscopically, biliary stents should be placed to ensure adequate biliary drainage and to prevent recurrent symptoms while awaiting further therapy. Long-term biliary stenting can also be used in patients with severe comorbid medical conditions that preclude surgery or repeated endoscopic interventions.

Ideally, patients with concomitant gallbladder and bile duct stones would be best treated with a single laparoscopic cholecystectomy and bile duct exploration, which is preferable to ERCP followed by cholecystectomy.[A13] However, only a minority of surgeons can successfully perform laparoscopic bile duct exploration, so open common bile duct exploration is generally performed if endoscopic and laparoscopic approaches are unsuccessful. A novel combined laparoendoscopic rendezvous procedure, where ERCP is facilitated by transcystic wire passage into the bile duct and duodenum at the time of cholecystectomy, is equivalent to the two-stage procedures in terms of ductal stone clearance, with less pancreatitis, lower morbidity, and shorter hospital stay despite a longer procedural time.[A14]

Complications of Bile Duct Stones

Cholangitis is a potentially life-threatening disease that results from bacterial infection of obstructed bile. Systemic toxicity occurs when intraductal pressure is sufficiently elevated to cause reflux of bacteria or endotoxin into the blood. About 80 to 90% of cases of acute cholangitis is caused by choledocholithiasis, with the remaining cases caused by a benign biliary stricture (e.g., primary sclerosing cholangitis, chronic pancreatitis, postoperative bile duct injury, or narrowing at an anastomosis) or by malignant biliary obstruction, typically after previous endoscopic instrumentation and stent placement. In certain parts of the world, parasitic biliary obstruction (e.g., *Ascaris*; Chapter 327) may be manifested with cholangitis. The most common bacteria are gram-negative bacilli and *Streptococcus* spp, but *Enterococcus* species are frequently seen in patients with occluded biliary stents. Prompt antibiotic therapy (e.g., intravenous ceftriaxone 1 to 2 g once daily; ampicillin-sulbactam 1.5 to 3 g every 6 hours; piperacillin-tazobactam 3.375 g every 6 hours; ciprofloxacin 400 mg twice daily; or levofloxacin 500 mg orally once daily) is critical and usually can permit conservative management with endoscopic biliary decompression within 24 to 48 hours.[A15] However, urgent decompression is indicated if improvement is not seen within a few hours. The advantages of ERCP are that it can delineate the cause of obstruction, obtain bile for culture, and rapidly decompress the biliary tree definitively by removing the stone or temporarily by placing a stent without removing the stone. Routine stenting is not indicated after successful stone removal unless the adequacy of biliary drainage is uncertain.

Acute gallstone pancreatitis accounts for up to 50% of cases of acute pancreatitis in Western countries (Chapter 130). Most patients quickly respond to conservative therapy, but some develop severe pancreatitis. Although early ERCP with biliary sphincterotomy and stone removal (Fig. 141-8) would appear to be an attractive therapeutic option, early ERCP does not reduce mortality or complications except in patients with biliary obstruction or clear evidence of cholangitis.[A16] After recovery from an episode of biliary pancreatitis, laparoscopic cholecystectomy with intraoperative cholangiography is recommended to prevent further episodes, preferably during the same hospital admission.[A17] If a common bile duct stone is found at intraoperative cholangiography, laparoscopic or open common bile duct exploration and stone removal can be accomplished with high success rates in experienced hands, or postoperative ERCP can remove any retained stones.[A18]

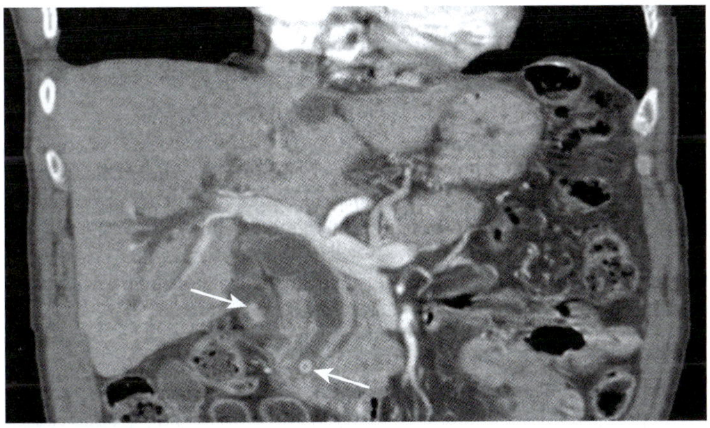

FIGURE 141-6. Computed tomography scan demonstrating calcified gallstones and a distal bile duct stone.

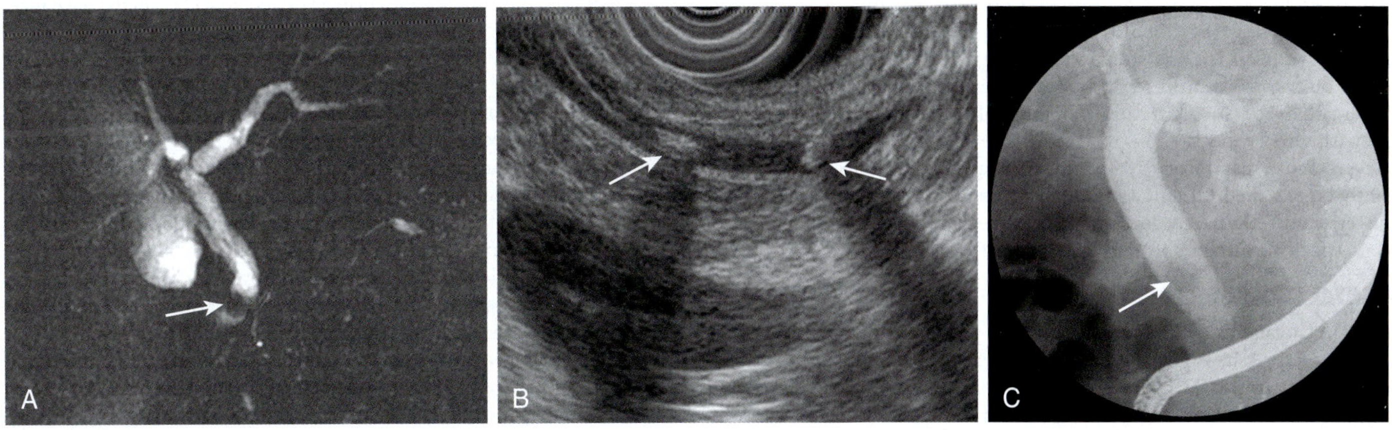

FIGURE 141-7. Common bile duct stones seen at magnetic resonance cholangiopancreatography (A), endoscopic ultrasound (B), and endoscopic retrograde cholangiopancreatography (C).

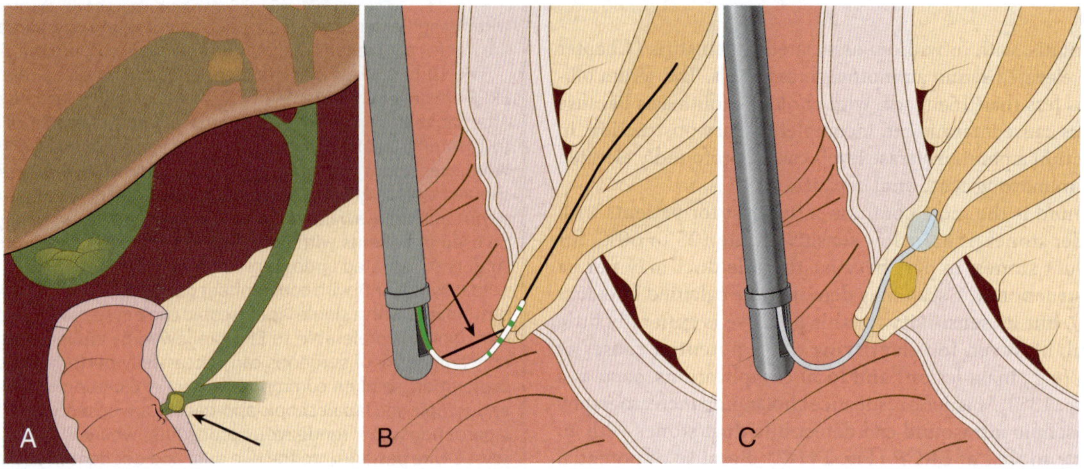

FIGURE 141-8. A, A stone that is impacted in the distal bile duct is causing biliary pancreatitis, with gallbladder stones also seen. B, Performance of biliary sphincterotomy. C, Subsequent stone removal by balloon sweep.

PREVENTION

Up to 25% of patients may have recurrent bile duct stones, with or without a gallbladder, but it remains uncertain what proportion of these recurrent stones are in fact overlooked residual stones from a prior event. A dilated extrahepatic bile duct (≥13 mm) and periampullary diverticula are risk factors for recurrent stones, perhaps by increasing biliary stasis. Identification and treatment of biliary strictures, papillary stenosis, and gallstones in patients with gallbladder in situ are essential for preventing recurrent stones. Unfortunately, no preventive therapy has been proved effective, although ursodeoxycholic acid (15 mg/kg/day) appears to reduce the risk for gallstones during weight loss.

BENIGN BILIARY STRICTURES

Postoperative extrahepatic bile duct strictures occur after 0.25 to 1% of cholecystectomies. Most of these lesions are manifested as abnormal liver test results, obstructive jaundice, and cholangitis within 2 to 3 months postoperatively, although the presentation can be delayed. The cholangiogram commonly shows a short, smooth narrowing near the cystic duct stump with proximal duct dilation (Fig. 141-9). Strictures typically must be redilated, and stents are exchanged at 3- to 4-month intervals for 8 to 12 months until the stricture is nearly as open as the downstream bile duct. About 80% of patients will have a good result. Covered self-expandable metal stents are as good as multiple plastic stents for resolving strictures, with fewer ERCP procedures needed to achieve resolution.[A19] However, some patients will ultimately require a bilioenteric bypass. Strictures more than 2 cm in length, strictures with clips placed securely across the duct, or strictures associated with resected segments of duct require surgical intervention.

Intrapancreatic common bile duct strictures, which may occur in 3 to 46% of patients with chronic pancreatitis, can lead to secondary biliary cirrhosis or recurrent cholangitis. With the complication of cholangitis or jaundice, intervention is clearly indicated, typically with ERCP and stent placement. In the absence of cholangitis or jaundice, either surgical repair or endoscopic biliary decompression with multiple plastic stents (Fig. 141-10) has traditionally been recommended when the alkaline phosphatase level is consistently more than twice the upper limit of normal during a 6-month period of observation. Biliary strictures that complicate liver transplantation (Chapter 140) are usually treated similarly with good results.

Severe acute respiratory syndrome coronavirus 2 (SARS-CoV-2) frequently targets the liver, but a rapidly progressive cholangiopathy has also been reported.[20] The pathogenesis of this disorder remains poorly understood, and no specific treatment options are currently available.

ORIENTAL CHOLANGIOHEPATITIS

Recurrent cholangitis with hepatolithiasis has a prevalence of more than 10% in parts of East Asia, especially in Taiwan, owing to infection with *Ascaris lumbricoides* (Chapter 327) and *Clonorchis sinensis* (Chapter 326). This condition results in local strictures and dilation of the intrahepatic biliary tree. Biliary stasis and subsequent bacterial infection cause brown stones to form. Most patients have recurrent cholangitis, but cholangiocarcinoma can also ensue. Ultrasound or CT can establish the diagnosis. Treatment includes intravenous fluids and antibiotics. Endoscopic stone removal is usually the preferred treatment, but localized surgical resection targeted to the cultured organisms may be necessary.

PRIMARY SCLEROSING CHOLANGITIS

DEFINITION

Primary sclerosing cholangitis is a chronic cholestatic disease characterized by fibrosing inflammation of segments of the intrahepatic and extrahepatic bile ducts.[21] It results in progressive narrowing of the duct lumen and ultimately may be manifested with recurrent episodes of ascending cholangitis or, alternatively, may progress to secondary biliary cirrhosis and its associated complications. Cholangiocarcinoma (Chapter 181) is a dreaded complication with a reported incidence of 25 to 40% at autopsy or liver transplantation.

EPIDEMIOLOGY

The true prevalence of primary sclerosing cholangitis is unknown, but current estimates are 0.2 to 8.5 per 100,000 in the U.S. population. Its prevalence is much higher in populations in which inflammatory bowel disease (Chapter 127) is more common. Affected men outnumber women in a 2 : 1 ratio, with the mean age at diagnosis of 32 to 40 years. However, primary sclerosing cholangitis has been reported in infants, children, and the elderly.

PATHOBIOLOGY

The cause of primary sclerosing cholangitis and the mechanisms responsible for its progression are unknown. However, autoimmune and genetic causes are supported by its frequent association with inflammatory bowel disease and the increased prevalence of the HLA B8, DR3 haplotype. Evidence from both fecal- and mucosa-associated microbial studies suggests that patients with primary sclerosing cholangitis harbour an abnormal enteric microbiome. About two thirds of patients with primary sclerosing cholangitis have ulcerative colitis or Crohn colitis, and it is rarely associated with Crohn disease that is limited to the small bowel. However, only 1 to 13% of patients with colitis are diagnosed with primary sclerosing cholangitis during their lifetime. First-degree relatives of patients with primary sclerosing cholangitis have a 9- to 39-fold increased risk for development of the disease.

On pathologic examination, involved segments of bile ducts in strictured areas show diffuse thickening with a mononuclear inflammatory cell infiltrate. The most characteristic biopsy features are bile duct proliferation, periductal fibrosis, periductal inflammation, and loss of bile ducts. Obliterative cholangitis with a chronic inflammatory cell infiltrate and periductular "onion ring" fibrosis is strongly associated with primary sclerosing cholangitis but is infrequently observed in biopsy specimens. Given the patchy nature of the disease and possible lack of significant intrahepatic involvement, however, the histologic appearance of primary sclerosing cholangitis is variable and may resemble extrahepatic biliary obstruction, chronic active hepatitis, or, rarely, primary biliary cirrhosis.

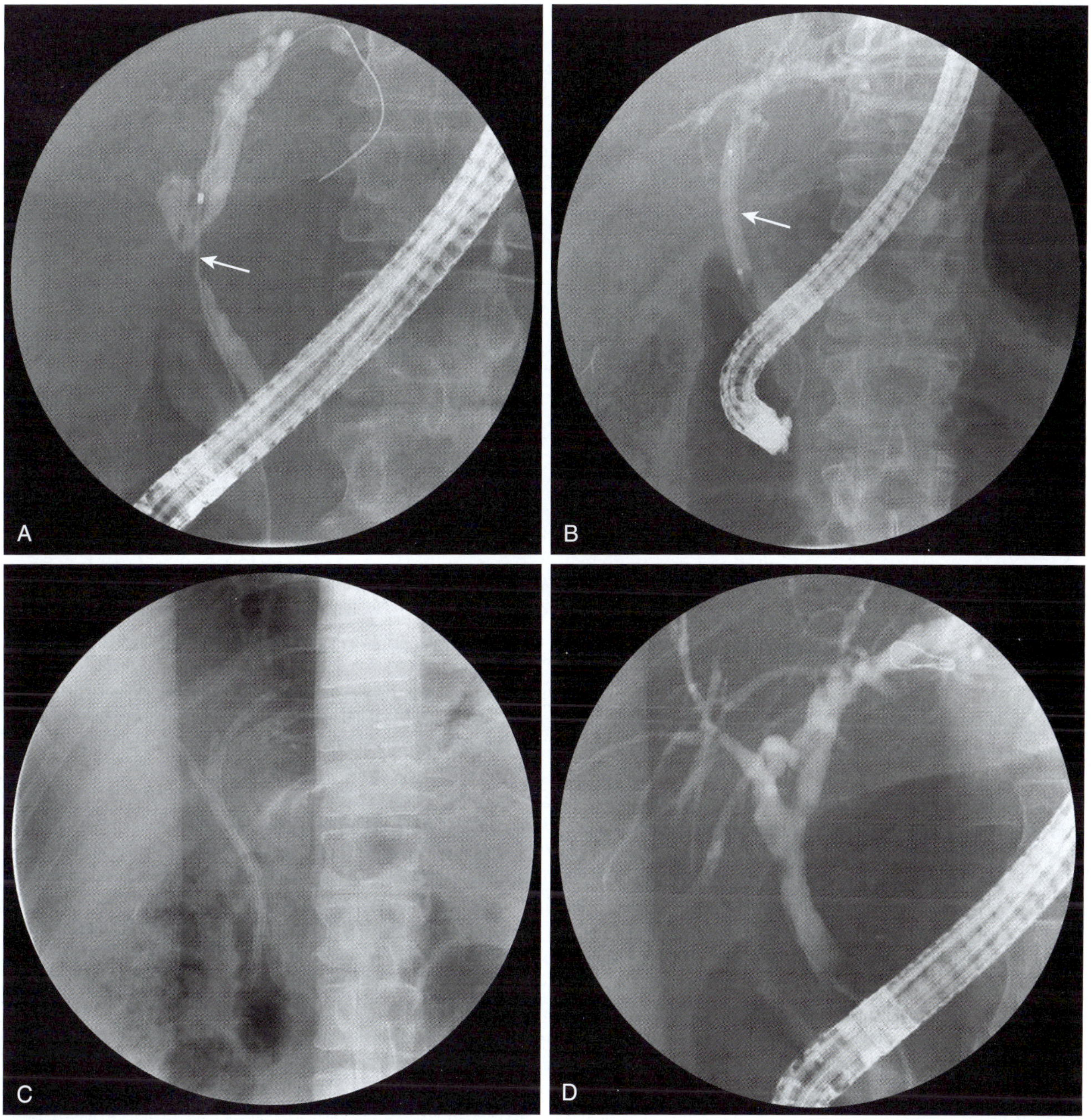

FIGURE 141-9. Endoscopic retrograde cholangiopancreatography images obtained from a patient who presented with painless jaundice 8 months after cholecystectomy. **A,** Benign common hepatic duct stricture. **B,** Balloon dilation of the stricture. **C,** Multiple stents placed. **D,** Resolution of stricture after a 1-year stenting interval.

CLINICAL MANIFESTATIONS

Most patients with primary sclerosing cholangitis are asymptomatic at presentation and are identified after investigation of an elevated alkaline phosphatase level (Chapter 133).[22] Overall, about 90% of patients have an elevated alkaline phosphatase level, with or without mildly elevated serum aminotransferase levels. Fatigue, anorexia, malaise, and weight loss are common but may erroneously be attributed to a patient's inflammatory bowel disease. Patients may exhibit signs or symptoms of cholestatic liver disease, including pruritus, upper abdominal pain, and fever. The serum bilirubin concentration is elevated in only about 40% of patients at presentation. Some patients have anemia, hypoalbuminemia, or hypergammaglobulinemia, and a prolonged international normalized ratio suggests biliary obstruction or synthetic dysfunction. Nearly 90% of patients will have a positive perinuclear antineutrophilic cytoplasmic antibody, but this antibody is also nonspecific and may be found in both ulcerative colitis (Chapter 127) and autoimmune hepatitis (Chapter 135). Antinuclear or anti–smooth muscle antibodies are found in 25% of patients but are not specific, and a positive antimitochondrial antibody suggests primary biliary cholangitis as the diagnosis.

DIAGNOSIS

Cholangiography is necessary to establish the diagnosis of primary sclerosing cholangitis (Fig. 141-11).[23] MRCP generally is the test of choice, but ERCP may be indicated if MRCP is inconclusive, particularly when the disease is confined to small intrahepatic ducts. The role of biopsy remains uncertain owing to the segmental nature of the disease and the overlap of the histologic features with other disease states. Diffuse multifocal strictures are usually short, with intervening normal or dilated segments that give a beaded appearance. Other frequent findings on cholangiography include pseudodiverticula, mural irregularities, and biliary stones and sludge. Secondary causes of sclerosing cholangitis include obstruction (postoperative, autoimmune cholangiopathy, choledocholithiasis, and recurrent pyogenic cholangitis), ischemic (hepatic artery instillation of the chemotherapeutic agent 5-fluorouracil, radiation, and paroxysmal nocturnal hemoglobinuria), and neoplastic (cholangiocarcinoma, hepatocellular carcinoma, lymphoma, and metastasis).

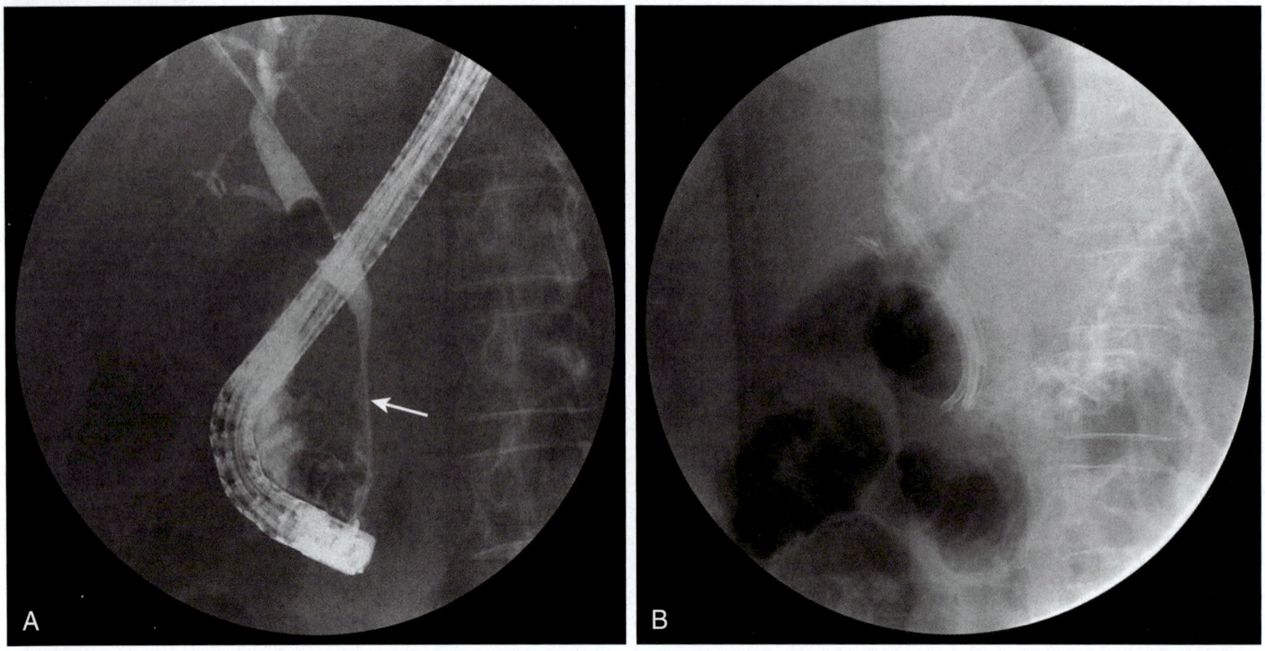

FIGURE 141-10. **Endoscopic retrograde cholangiopancreatography images obtained from a patient with a history of alcohol abuse who presented with pruritus and was found to have a markedly elevated alkaline phosphatase level. A,** A smooth distal bile duct stricture is seen (*arrow*). **B,** Four stents have been placed through the stricture.

TREATMENT

The chronic cholestasis of primary sclerosing cholangitis can be treated with cholestyramine (4 to 8 g/day), ursodeoxycholic acid (15 mg/kg/day), rifampicin (300 to 600 mg/day), or phenobarbital (30 to 120 mg/day) with modest success. Obeticholic acid, which is a potent farnesoid X receptor agonist approved for the treatment of primary biliary cholangitis (at 5 to 10 mg once daily), reduces the serum alkaline phosphatase level in patients with primary sclerosing cholangitis, although its effects on disease progression are not known.[A20] Another experimental farnesoid X receptor agonist, cilofexor, has shown promise in patients who have large-duct primary sclerosing cholangitis.[A21] Fat-soluble vitamin deficiencies (Chapter 199) must be corrected. The prevalence of osteoporosis (Chapter 225) in primary sclerosing cholangitis is between 4 and 10%, so bone densitometry should be performed at diagnosis and every 2 to 3 years thereafter. Supplementation with oral vitamin D and calcium seems prudent, even in the absence of symptomatic deficiency. Treatment with bisphosphonates (Chapter 225) is reserved for patients with confirmed osteoporosis. Unfortunately, no medical treatment slows the progression of disease; ursodeoxycholic acid, D-penicillamine, corticosteroids, cyclosporine, methotrexate, and colchicine have all been shown to be ineffective for improving survival or delaying the time to liver transplantation. Whether repeated endoscopic treatment to maintain bile duct patency can improve outcomes is unknown, although patients with a dominant stricture may benefit.[24] Furthermore, short-term stents are not superior to balloon dilatation and are associated with a significantly higher occurrence of treatment-related adverse events (e.g., cholangitis, pancreatitis).[25]

Liver transplantation (Chapter 140) is the only potentially curative therapy. The 1-year and 5-year survival rates typically are in the 90% and 80% range, respectively. Primary sclerosing cholangitis may recur in the transplanted organ in 15 to 20% of patients.

PROGNOSIS

The natural history of primary sclerosing cholangitis is variable and incompletely understood. Asymptomatic patients have a much better prognosis than symptomatic patients, with 10-year actuarial survival rates of 80% and 50%, respectively. In symptomatic patients, the median time of survival until death or liver transplantation is 9 years, compared with 12 to 18 years for all patients with primary sclerosing cholangitis, regardless of symptoms. An elevated serum bilirubin level and hepatomegaly appear to correlate with a poor prognosis, whereas cholangiographic appearance, the presence or absence of inflammatory bowel disease, and the patient's age do not. Cholangiocarcinoma (Chapter 181) is a dreaded complication of primary sclerosing cholangitis, and the risk appears to be greatest in patients with long-standing ulcerative colitis and cirrhosis.

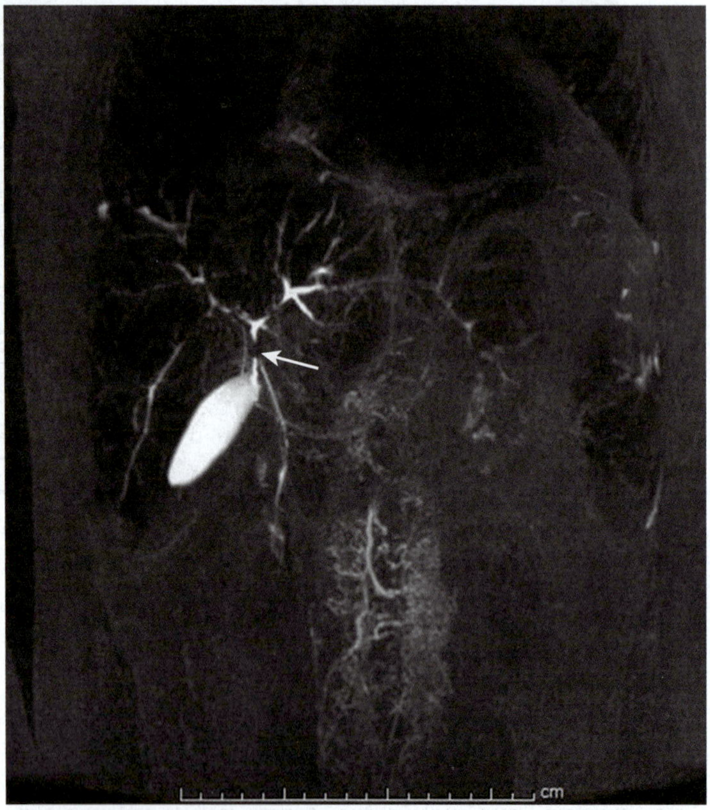

FIGURE 141-11. **Magnetic resonance cholangiopancreatography demonstrating the typical cholangiographic features of primary sclerosing cholangitis.** Note the narrowed segment of the common bile duct (*arrow*) as well as the diffuse strictures and dilated segments of several intrahepatic bile ducts, giving the classic "beaded" appearance.

CHOLEDOCHAL CYSTS AND ANOMALOUS PANCREATICOBILIARY DUCT JUNCTION

Choledochal cysts are uncommon anomalies of the biliary tree that are manifested as cystic dilation of the intrahepatic or extrahepatic ducts (or both). The incidence is 1 in 100,000 to 150,000 births in Western populations and 1 in 1000 in Asian populations. There is a 3 : 1 to 4 : 1 female-to-male preponderance.

TABLE 141-3 CLASSIFICATION OF CHOLEDOCHAL CYSTS

TYPES	DESCRIPTION	PROPORTION OF CHOLEDOCHAL CYSTS
I	Segmental or diffuse fusiform dilation of the bile duct	50-80%
II	Choledochal diverticulum	2%
III	Dilation of the intraduodenal portion of the bile duct	1.4-5%
IVa	Multiple intrahepatic and extrahepatic cysts	15-35%
IVb	Multiple extrahepatic cysts	
V (Caroli disease)	Single or multiple dilations of the intrahepatic ducts	20%
VI	Dilatation of the cystic duct between the neck of the gallbladder and the common hepatic duct	Rare

These cysts (E-Fig. 141-1) usually involve only the extrahepatic biliary tree, but they can present as extrapancreatic bile duct diverticula, involve only the intraduodenal part of the common bile duct, or present as multiple intrahepatic and extrahepatic cysts (Table 141-3). An anomalous pancreaticobiliary duct junction (E-Fig. 141-2) is frequently associated with choledochal cysts but may be found in isolation, especially in Asian populations.

Patients with choledochoceles commonly have biliary colic, cholangitis, jaundice, or unexplained pancreatitis. Bile reflux may also result in acute pancreatitis or predispose to biliary cancers.

Cholangiography, preferably by ERCP, is the diagnostic "gold standard," although MRCP can also delineate the anatomy noninvasively. Because of the increased risk for development of biliary tract cancers, cyst resection (including cholecystectomy) is the generally recommended treatment, although it does not eliminate the risk entirely.[26]

BILIARY FISTULA

A biliary fistula represents an injury to the bile duct, most commonly seen as a complication of cholecystectomy, common bile duct exploration, or inadvertent operative injury of the bile duct or as a consequence of a local infection. Rarely, biliary fistulas result from long-standing untreated biliary tract disease. With more widespread use of laparoscopic cholecystectomy, the incidence of bile duct injury, including biliary fistula, has increased, but it remains less than 0.5% in most published series.

Postoperative bile duct leaks are usually manifested within a week after surgery, with patients presenting with abdominal pain (90%), tenderness (80%), fever (75%), nausea and vomiting (50%), and jaundice (40%). Clinically detectable ascites is rare. Biochemical testing is usually nonspecific, with variable elevations in serum liver test values and the white blood cell count.

Patients with suspected biliary fistulas often undergo abdominal ultrasonography or CT to look for evidence of a biloma as well as a hepatobiliary scan to diagnose the leak. However, ERCP is the most sensitive test to detect a biliary fistula. Treatment options for biliary leaks include percutaneously or endoscopically placed biliary drains or stents and surgical drainage and repair of the leak.

VANISHING BILE DUCT SYNDROMES

The vanishing bile duct syndrome is characterized by a paucity of intrahepatic bile ducts, an elevated alkaline phosphatase level, and cholestasis. Causes include primary biliary cholangitis, primary sclerosing cholangitis, autoimmune hepatitis (Chapter 135), graft-versus-host disease, chronic liver transplant rejection (Chapter 140), ischemia, intrahepatic chemotherapy, drug toxicity (e.g., ampicillin, amoxicillin, flucloxacillin, erythromycin, tetracycline, doxycycline, cotrimoxazole), human immunodeficiency virus (HIV) infection (Chapter 359), sarcoidosis (Chapter 83), and histiocytosis. Ursodeoxycholic acid (15 mg/kg/day) can increase bile flow, but the condition inexorably progresses to biliary cirrhosis, which ultimately requires liver transplantation.

PRIMARY BILIARY CHOLANGITIS

Primary biliary cholangitis, previously known as primary biliary cirrhosis, is an obliterative autoimmune cholangiopathy that involves the small and medium-sized bile ducts and that slowly progresses during a decade or so. As the ducts are obliterated, patients develop cholestasis, fibrosis, and, ultimately, liver failure.[27]

EPIDEMIOLOGY

About 95% of patients with primary biliary cholangitis are women, and the peak age at onset is between 20 and 60 years. The incidence of the disease may be increasing. In the United States, the estimated annual incidence is about 4.5 per 100,000 per year for women and 0.7 for men. Because of the limited life expectancy of affected patients, the age- and gender-adjusted prevalence of primary biliary cholangitis is about 65 per 100,000 in women and about 12 per 100,000 in men.

PATHOBIOLOGY

Although the mechanism of progressive destruction of the small interlobular ducts is unknown, primary biliary cholangitis is considered to be an autoimmune disorder. Genome-wide studies show an association with HLA, interleukin-12A, and interleukin-12RB2 variants, suggesting that interleukin-12 signaling might be important. The disease progresses slowly and can eventually lead to biliary cirrhosis, portal hypertension, and liver failure. The classic histologic finding is noncaseating granulomas and paucity of bile ducts in the portal tracts.

CLINICAL MANIFESTATIONS

The most common symptoms are fatigue (50%), which can be debilitating and is unrelated to the degree of underlying liver disease, and pruritus (30%), but about 50% of patients are asymptomatic at the time of diagnosis. Many patients are initially seen by dermatologists for pruritus, which may be first noticed in pregnancy but persists after delivery.

Autoimmune syndromes associated with primary biliary cholangitis include autoimmune thyroid dysfunction (Chapter 207), Sjögren syndrome (Chapter 247), Raynaud phenomenon (Chapter 246), and celiac disease (Chapter 126). Vitamin D malabsorption can also lead to metabolic bone disease (Chapters 225 and 226).[28]

DIAGNOSIS

The first clue to primary biliary cholangitis is an elevated serum alkaline phosphatase level, which should be confirmed by an elevated γ-glutamyl transpeptidase level (Chapter 133). The antimitochondrial antibody level has a sensitivity and specificity of more than 95% when the titer is higher than 1 : 40, and it may be positive even before there is any clinical or biochemical evidence of the disease. By comparison, the bilirubin level often is not elevated until later in the course of the disease, with most of the elevation typically due to an elevation in conjugated bilirubin. Total immunoglobulins are generally normal, but immunoglobulin M levels can be elevated.

An ultrasound examination of the biliary tree is critical to confirm the absence of extrahepatic disease. A liver biopsy is occasionally needed to confirm the diagnosis, particularly in antimitochondrial antibody–negative patients, and to stage the disease.

TREATMENT

Ursodeoxycholic acid therapy (12 to 15 mg/kg/day) improves serum bilirubin, alkaline phosphatase, and cholesterol levels and has a variable effect on pruritus.[29] Unfortunately, it does not relieve fatigue, reduce mortality, or delay the need for liver transplantation. In patients who do not respond to ursodeoxycholic acid, obeticholic acid in a daily dose of 10 mg can significantly reduce alanine aminotransferase, alkaline phosphatase, and γ-glutamyl transpeptidase levels, but its effect on clinical outcomes such as liver failure and the need for liver transplantation is unknown.[A22] Bezafibrate therapy also improves liver chemistry test results and pruritus[A23] but has not been shown to reduce liver-related mortality or overall mortality. Saroglitazar, a peroxisome proliferator–activated receptor agonist, may also lead to improved alkaline phosphatase levels in patients who are resistant to or intolerant of ursodeoxycholic acid.[30]

There is no definite benefit from steroids, colchicine, azathioprine, or methotrexate. Bisphosphonates (Chapter 225) are commonly prescribed for the accompanying metabolic bone disease, but their benefit is uncertain. Liver transplantation (Chapter 140) is indicated for refractory disease. The post-transplantation prognosis is excellent, with 2-year and 5-year survival rates of 80% and 70%, respectively. However, studies suggest an 8 to 40% recurrence in the transplanted liver.

PROGNOSIS

Up to two thirds of asymptomatic patients become symptomatic within 2 to 4 years. Significant bridging fibrosis or cirrhosis on biopsy carries a worse prognosis. Prognosis is also influenced by the serum bilirubin and albumin levels, the international normalized ratio, older age, and the presence of peripheral edema. Liver failure develops in about 25% of patients within 10 years after diagnosis, and median survival after diagnosis is 12 to 15 years.

BILE DUCT TUMORS

BENIGN

Benign bile duct tumors are exceedingly rare compared with malignant tumors and are much less common than benign gallbladder tumors. They can be divided into three histologic types (papillomas, adenomas, cystadenomas), may be solitary or multiple, and often are found incidentally during the evaluation of bile duct dilation or intraductal filling defects. Patients may be asymptomatic or have symptoms of biliary obstruction. Treatment typically consists of surgical bile duct resection with hepaticojejunostomy reconstruction. Even benign tumors tend to recur after excision, and some undergo malignant change.

CHOLANGIOCARCINOMA

Cholangiocarcinoma is discussed in Chapter 181.

AMPULLARY TUMORS

Benign ampullary lesions seen on endoscopic or radiologic studies include heterotopic gastric mucosa, a lipoma, or an impacted common bile duct stone. Primary tumors of the ampulla of Vater can be premalignant or malignant, but the overwhelming majority (>95%) are either adenomas or adenocarcinomas. The prevalence of ampullary adenomas has been estimated to be 0.04 to 0.12% in autopsy series, but the prevalence is higher in patients with hereditary polyposis syndromes (Chapter 179), in which ampullary adenomas occur in up to 80% of individuals and progress to malignancy in 4%.

Malignant ampullary lesions are most commonly adenocarcinomas, although metastatic breast cancer, renal cell cancers, and melanomas also have been identified. Carcinoid tumors (Chapter 213) and other neuroendocrine tumors are rare. Ampullary adenomas probably follow an adenoma-to-carcinoma sequence similar to colorectal adenocarcinoma (Chapter 179), with a 25 to 85% risk for transformation to carcinoma.

Patients with ampullary lesions may present with biliary colic, obstructive jaundice, pancreatitis, or nonspecific upper abdominal pain, with or without fluctuating serum liver test results, malaise, and anorexia. However, ampullary lesions are often found incidentally on cross-sectional imaging or during upper endoscopy performed for a different indication.

For ampullary adenomas, options include observation with surveillance biopsies and attempts to resect the lesion completely through endoscopy or surgery. Surveillance of an ampullary adenoma in the setting of familial adenomatous polyposis is reasonable if the lesion is small (<1 cm) and asymptomatic, but resection is preferred if advanced histology (e.g., villous features, dysplasia) is identified. Surgical resection has been the standard for ampullary tumors. Treatment modalities include pancreatoduodenectomy, which has a high rate of morbid and even fatal complications, and transduodenal excision, which is associated with high recurrence rates. The 5-year survival rates after pancreaticoduodenectomy range from 64 to 80% for patients with node-negative disease and from 17 to 50% for node-positive disease. Limited data exist regarding adjuvant therapy, the benefits of which are uncertain. A common practice is to treat these patients in a manner similar to patients with resected pancreatic adenocarcinomas (Chapter 180). Patients who present with unresectable disease tend to receive combination gemcitabine (1000 mg/m^2) plus cisplatin (25 mg/m^2) chemotherapy, each administered on days 1 and 8, every 3 weeks for eight cycles. Palliative biliary stenting can be performed in individuals who have a short life expectancy.

In patients with small, localized, and clearly benign ampullary adenomas, endoscopic resection represents an alternative to surgical therapy in appropriately selected patients (E-Fig. 141-3). Whether endoscopic resection is effective for larger or higher-risk adenomas is uncertain. Furthermore, recurrence rates after endoscopic papillectomy approach 20%, thereby emphasizing the need for careful follow-up endoscopic surveillance.

SPHINCTER OF ODDI DYSFUNCTION

Sphincter of Oddi dysfunction is a benign, noncalculous obstruction to the flow of bile or pancreatic juice through the pancreaticobiliary junction. It may be manifested clinically by pain, pancreatitis (Chapter 130), abnormal liver test results, or abnormal pancreatic enzymes. Post-cholecystectomy pain resembling the patient's preoperative biliary colic occurs in at least 10 to 20% of patients.

Evaluation of patients with suspected sphincter of Oddi dysfunction includes standard serum liver chemistries, serum amylase and lipase levels, and an abdominal ultrasound examination or CT scan. The specimens for serum enzyme studies should be drawn during bouts of pain, if possible. Mild elevations (less than two times the upper limits of normal) are frequent in sphincter of Oddi dysfunction, whereas greater abnormalities are more suggestive of stones, tumors, and parenchymal liver disease. The findings on CT and abdominal ultrasound studies are usually normal, but abnormal liver or pancreatic enzymes or a dilated bile duct or pancreatic duct may occasionally be found. ERCP and sphincter of Oddi manometry may be considered in patients who have objective evidence of pancreatic or biliary disease (abnormal liver or pancreatic enzymes or a dilated bile or pancreatic duct) or clinically significant or disabling symptoms and in whom definitive sphincter ablation is planned if abnormal sphincter function is found. In patients without objective evidence of pancreatic or biliary disease, ERCP and manometry are no longer recommended.[A24]

Medical therapy with nonspecific antispasmodics (e.g., dicyclomine 10 to 20 mg every 6 hours; hyoscyamine 0.375 mg every 12 hours) or smooth muscle relaxants (e.g., nifedipine 60 mg daily) for a 1-month trial should be considered in patients with pancreaticobiliary-type pain (with or without abnormal liver enzyme, amylase, or lipase levels) or a dilated bile or pancreatic duct. If patients do not respond satisfactorily, ERCP and endoscopic sphincterotomy can improve pain in 55 to 95% of patients with abnormal findings on laboratory testing or abdominal imaging. Alternatively, only about 25% of patients without objective evidence of pancreatic or biliary disease improve after sphincterotomy.

GENERAL REFERENCES

For the General References and other additional features, please visit Elsevier eBooks+ at https://ebooks.health.elsevier.com.

Grade A References

A1. Loozen CS, Oor JE, van Ramshorst B, et al. Conservative treatment of acute cholecystitis: a systematic review and pooled analysis. *Surg Endosc.* 2017;31:504-515.

A2. van Dijk AH, Wennmacker SZ, de Reuver PR, et al. Restrictive strategy versus usual care for cholecystectomy in patients with gallstones and abdominal pain (SECURE): a multicentre, randomised, parallel-arm, non-inferiority trial. *Lancet.* 2019;393:2322-2330.

A3. Tang H, Dong A, Van L. Day surgery versus overnight stay laparoscopic cholecystectomy: a systematic review and meta-analysis. *Dig Liv Dis.* 2015;47:556-561.

A4. Zafar S, Obirieze A, Adesibikan B, et al. Optimal time for early laparoscopic cholecystectomy for acute cholecystitis. *JAMA Surg.* 2015;150:129-136.

A5. Roulin D, Saadi A, Di Mare L, et al. Early versus delayed cholecystectomy for acute cholecystitis, are the 72 hours still the rule? *Ann Surg.* 2016;264:717-722.

A6. Koo JGA, Chan YH, Shelat VG. Laparoscopic subtotal cholecystectomy: comparison of reconstituting and fenestrating techniques. *Surg Endosc.* 2021;35:1014-1024.

A7. Ahmed O, Rogers AC, Bolger JC, et al. Meta-analysis of outcomes of endoscopic ultrasound-guided gallbladder drainage versus percutaneous cholecystostomy for the management of acute cholecystitis. *Surg Endosc.* 2018;32:1627-1635.

A8. Teoh AYB, Kitano M, Itoi T, et al. Endosonography-guided gallbladder drainage versus percutaneous cholecystostomy in very high-risk surgical patients with acute cholecystitis: an international randomised multicentre controlled superiority trial (DRAC 1). *Gut.* 2020;69:1085-1091.

A9. Eltyeb HA, Al-Leswas D, Abdalla MO, Wayman J. Systematic review and meta-analyses of cholecystectomy as a treatment of biliary hyperkinesia. *Clin J Gastro.* 2021;14:1308-1317.

A10. Primrose JN, Fox RP, Palmer DH, et al. Capecitabine compared with observation in resected biliary tract cancer (BILCAP): a randomised, controlled, multicentre, phase 3 study. *Lancet Oncol.* 2019;20:663-673.

A11. Lamarca A, Palmer DH, Wasan HS, et al. Second-line FOLFOX chemotherapy versus active symptom control for advanced biliary tract cancer (ABC-06): a phase 3, open-label, randomised, controlled trial. *Lancet Oncol.* 2021;22:690-701.

A12. Facciorusso A, Gkolfakis P, Ramai D, et al. Endoscopic treatment of large bile duct stones: a systematic review and network meta-analysis. *Clin Gastroenterol Hepatol.* 2023;21:33-44.e9.

A13. Pan L, Chen M, Ji L, et al. The safety and efficacy of laparoscopic common bile duct exploration combined with cholecystectomy for the management of cholecystocholedocholithiasis: an up-to-date meta-analysis. *Ann Surg.* 2018;268:247-253.

A14. Lin Y, Su Y, Yan J, et al. Laparoendoscopic rendezvous versus ERCP followed by laparoscopic cholecystectomy in the management of cholecystocholedocholithiasis: a systemic review and meta-analysis. *Surg Endosc.* 2020;34:4214-4224.

A15. Iqbal U, Khara HS, Hu Y, et al. Emergent versus urgent ERCP in acute cholangitis: a systematic review and meta-analysis. *Gastrointest Endosc.* 2020;91:753-760.

A16. Schepers NJ, Hallensleben NDL, Besselink MG, et al. Urgent endoscopic retrograde cholangiopancreatography with sphincterotomy versus conservative treatment in predicted severe acute gallstone pancreatitis (APEC): a multicentre randomised controlled trial. *Lancet.* 2020;396:167-176.

A17. Moody N, Adiamah A, Yanni F, et al. Meta-analysis of randomized clinical trials of early versus delayed cholecystectomy for mild gallstone pancreatitis. *Br J Surg.* 2019;106:1442-1451.

A18. Gao YC, Chen J, Qin Q, et al. Efficacy and safety of laparoscopic bile duct exploration versus endoscopic sphincterotomy for concomitant gallstones and common bile duct stones: a meta-analysis of randomized controlled trials. *Medicine (Baltimore).* 2017;96:1-10.

A19. Ramchandani M, Lakhtakia S, Costamagna G, et al. Fully covered self-expanding metal stent vs multiple plastic stents to treat benign biliary strictures secondary to chronic pancreatitis: a multicenter randomized trial. *Gastroenterology*. 2021;161:185-195.
A20. Kowdley KV, Vuppalanchi R, Levy C, et al. A randomized, placebo-controlled, phase II study of obeticholic acid for primary sclerosing cholangitis. *J Hepatol*. 2020;73:94-101.
A21. Trauner M, Gulamhusein A, Hameed B, et al. The nonsteroidal farnesoid X receptor agonist Cilofexor (GS-9674) improves markers of cholestasis and liver injury in patients with primary sclerosing cholangitis. *Hepatology*. 2019;70:788-801.
A22. Nevens F, Andreone P, Mazzella G, et al. A placebo-controlled trial of obeticholic acid in primary biliary cholangitis. *N Engl J Med*. 2016;375:631-643.
A23. Corpechot C, Chazouilléres O, Rousseau A, et al. A placebo-controlled trial of bezafibrate in primary biliary cholangitis. *N Engl J Med*. 2018;378:2171-2181.
A24. Cotton PB, Pauls Q, Keith J, et al. The EPISOD study: long-term outcomes. *Gastrointest Endosc*. 2018;87:205-210.

XV

HEMATOLOGIC DISEASES

142 HEMATOPOIESIS AND HEMATOPOIETIC GROWTH FACTORS

KENNETH KAUSHANSKY

Hematopoiesis is the process by which bone marrow stem cells develop into all of the cell types present in the blood (erythrocytes, neutrophils, eosinophils, basophils, monocytes, platelets, T lymphocytes, B lymphocytes, and natural killer cells) (Fig. 142-1). The regulation of the numbers of each cell type is carefully controlled by paracrine and endocrine hematopoietic growth factors, which exert antiapoptotic, proliferative, and differentiative effects on hematopoietic stem, progenitor, and maturing blood cells. Many of these glycoproteins are now produced by recombinant DNA technology and have been among the most successful therapeutics in modern medicine.

HEMATOPOIETIC STEM AND PROGENITOR CELLS

Hematopoietic stem cells comprise 1 in 10^5 to 10^6 marrow cells and are not morphologically distinguishable from other progenitors or small lymphocytes but can be purified to homogeneity using physical characteristics and combinations of monoclonal antibodies (including $CD34^+$) to cell surface proteins. The two critical characteristics of a hematopoietic stem cell are its ability to differentiate into all blood cell types and to self-renew. The decision to self-renew or differentiate is a stochastic process, at the stem cell stage and at the subsequent multipotent or unipotent stages of differentiation, that can be influenced by a number of cell extrinsic (growth factors and stromal proteins) and cell intrinsic (transcription factors) molecules. Hematopoietic stem cells reside in specialized microenvironments (niches) within the bone marrow. The complex and diverse stromal cell populations that comprise the critical perivascular stem cell niche include endothelial cells, CXCL12 abundant reticular [CAR] cells, nestin+ mesenchymal stem cells, and megakaryocytes and provide signals that support stem cell maintenance, self-renewal, and long-term multilineage repopulation ability.[1]

Clonal hematopoiesis with somatic mutations, which can be detected by DNA sequencing, is more common with advancing age (currently referred to as clonal hematopoiesis of undetermined potential [CHIP]),[2] and is associated with higher risks of hematologic cancer and all-cause mortality.[3] Some genes that are mutated in patients with myeloid cancers are frequently mutated in apparently healthy persons; these mutations may represent characteristic early events in the development of hematologic cancers[4] and are associated with increased risk of atherosclerotic cardiovascular disease.[5] Interestingly, the concordance of clonal hematopoiesis among twins is limited, thereby suggesting in utero or subsequent environmental influences.[6] Evidence based on recapitulating the genetic changes in patients with CHIP in engineered mice strongly suggests that dysregulated inflammation in the affected monocytes/macrophages is responsible for the excess cardiovascular and cerebrovascular disease seen in such patients.[7,8]

HEMATOPOIETIC CELL EXPANSION: HEMATOPOIETIC GROWTH FACTORS

A large number of transcription factors regulate stem cell number and differentiation state. Several molecular switches have been identified that determine hematopoietic cell fate.

Equally important to hematopoiesis is a group of hematopoietic growth factors that share structural homology and bind to nonredundant type I transmembrane proteins belonging to the cytokine receptor family. Many of these proteins are the physiologic regulators of a specific lineage of blood cells (e.g., erythropoietin, granulocyte colony-stimulating factor, thrombopoietin); others appear to represent redundant hematopoietic growth-promoting activities of molecules essential for other biologic functions (e.g., interleukin-3 [IL-3], interleukin-11 [IL-11], granulocyte-macrophage colony-stimulating factor).

Erythropoietin is produced predominantly by the kidneys and to a lesser extent in the liver and acts on marrow erythroid progenitors to enhance their survival, proliferation, and differentiation. Levels of erythropoietin are inversely related to hemoglobin concentrations in the blood, sensed as renal oxygen tension. In the presence of tissue (renal) hypoxia, the transcription factor hypoxia-induced factor (HIF) 1α is stabilized against proteasome-mediated

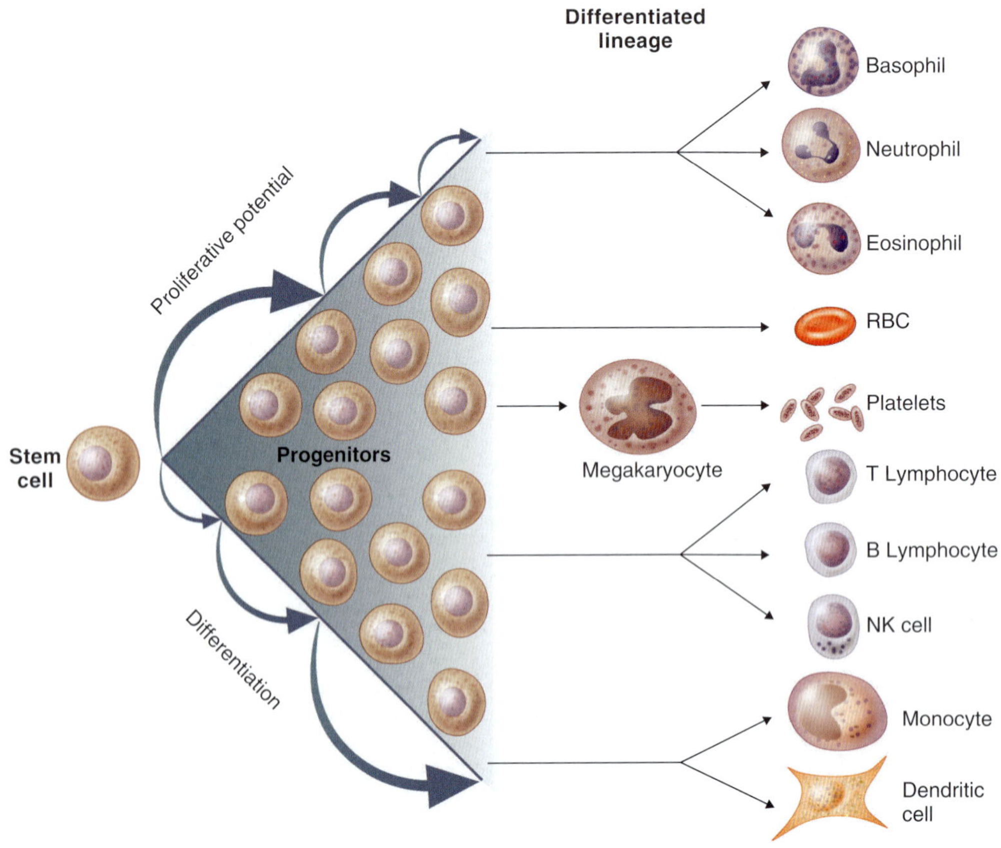

FIGURE 142-1. **Hierarchical model of lymphohematopoiesis.** NK = natural killer; RBC = red blood cell.

destruction and drives erythropoietin transcription by binding to a critical hypoxia responsive element located in the 3′ untranslated region of the gene. Genetic elimination of erythropoietin or its receptor results in embryonic lethality, establishing that although other cytokines can influence erythropoiesis, red blood cell production is absolutely dependent on the hormone.

Granulocyte colony-stimulating factor stimulates the production of neutrophils from their marrow progenitors (Fig. 142-2). Levels of the hormone are also inversely related to neutrophil numbers but are regulated primarily by inflammatory stimuli, including tumor necrosis factor-α (TNF-α) and IL-1α acting on endothelial cells, fibroblasts, and macrophages. Similar to the action of erythropoietin on erythroid progenitors, granulocyte colony-stimulating factor acts to enhance the survival, proliferation, and differentiation of neutrophil progenitors.[9] In addition, the cytokine acts to functionally activate the mature cells it helps to produce. Genetic elimination of granulocyte colony-stimulating factor or its receptor in mice reduces neutrophil levels to 25% of normal, the only hormone known to exert this great an impact on granulopoiesis.

Thrombopoietin, the primary regulator of platelet production, is produced in the liver and by marrow stromal cells. Plasma levels of the hormone are normally inversely related to platelet mass and are regulated by the level of senescent platelet uptake, mediated by the hepatocyte Ashwell-Morrell receptor; inflammation, mediated by IL-6; removal of thrombopoietin by circulating platelets; and by transcriptional feedback inhibition of the thrombopoietin gene in marrow stromal cells by platelet granule proteins. Similar to erythropoietin and granulocyte colony-stimulating factor, thrombopoietin stimulates the survival, proliferation, and differentiation of its corresponding lineage, megakaryocytes and their precursors, and primes mature platelets to respond to platelet activation agonists.[10] But unlike the other two cytokines, thrombopoietin also has important, nonredundant effects on the hematopoietic stem cell, which has important implications for leukemogenesis. Genetic elimination of thrombopoietin or its receptor in mice or congenital nonsense or missense mutations in the gene for the thrombopoietin receptor in humans results in platelet levels approximately 10% of normal and a reduction in stem cells, eventuating in aplastic anemia in children by 1 to 2 years of age.

Chemokines and other cytokines also regulate hematopoiesis. The chemokine ligands CXCR2 and CXCL4 affect the survival and self-renewal of hematopoietic stem cells,[11] as does interferon signaling, the effects of which vary with the type of interferon but can play an important role during inflammation.[12] Additional cytokine-receptor systems are essential for one or more aspects of hematopoiesis and mature blood cell function and include IL-7, critical for all types of lymphocyte production; IL-5, the primary regulator of eosinophil production; IL-4, responsible for immunoglobulin class switching in B lymphocytes; IL-15, essential for normal natural killer cell differentiation; and IL-2, a lymphocyte activation cytokine.

Although the effects of these hematopoietic cytokines are clear, a number of lines of evidence suggest that they may exert additional effects outside of blood cell production. For example, both erythropoietin and the leukocyte colony-stimulating factors (GM-CSF and G-CSF) have been found to protect neurons against damage in experimental models of traumatic and ischemic brain injury.[13,14] Although holding much promise, initial clinical trials of erythropoietic stimulating agents in such settings have not yet proven clear efficacy.[15]

The molecular mechanisms by which the hematopoietic growth factors affect blood cell survival, proliferation, and differentiation are becoming increasingly well understood. Binding of cognate ligand to each of the hematopoietic cytokine receptors results in activation of one or more tyrosine kinases, either tethered cytoplasmic kinases of the Janus (JAK) family for the hematopoietic cytokine receptor family or the intrinsic kinase of the cytokines that use the receptor tyrosine kinase class of receptors (stem cell factor, Flt3 ligand, and macrophage colony-stimulating factor). After activation, these kinases phosphorylate tyrosine residues within the cytoplasmic domains of each receptor, providing docking sites for cytoplasmic signaling intermediates possessing Src homology (SH)2 domains. Among the best characterized SH2 domain-containing proteins that bind to hematopoietic receptors are nascent transcription factors, such as the signal transducers and activators of transcription (STAT) proteins; adapter proteins, including Grb2, Gab1, tensin2, and SHC; phosphatases, for example, SHP1 and SHP2; and the regulatory subunit (p85) of phosphoinositol-3-kinase (PI3K). When bound to one or more of the newly induced phosphotyrosine residues of the cytokine receptor or receptor tyrosine kinase, these secondary molecules are phosphorylated, either by JAK or other kinases, making them competent to bind additional molecules (e.g., the adapters that ultimately activate Ras, and p85 PI3K that binds its kinase [p110] subunit) or are activated as transcription factors (e.g., STATs). The downstream effector molecules then activated include a number of kinases, transporter molecules, and transcription factors, ultimately leading to hematopoietic cell survival, proliferation, and differentiation.

CLINICAL USES OF HEMATOPOIETIC CELLS AND GROWTH FACTORS

The clinical development of erythropoietin and related compounds (erythropoietic stimulating agents), granulocyte colony-stimulating factor, and thrombopoietin receptor agonists represent some of the very best examples of harnessing recombinant DNA technology for therapeutic benefit. Patients with renal failure, widespread inflammation, or bone marrow replacement and those undergoing chemotherapy for cancer all experience variable degrees of anemia that is often very debilitating. Administration of erythropoietic stimulating agents (ESAs) almost invariably results in a rapid reticulocyte response and correction of the anemia. Most patients undergo an enhanced sense of well-being as the blood hemoglobin concentration rises to 10 g/dL. Clinical trials have demonstrated the efficacy of these agents in patients with renal failure and with cancer, although recent analyses call into question the safety of these agents in some settings.[A1] For example, patients receiving higher levels of the drug for anemia secondary to kidney failure progressed to requiring dialysis more frequently and experienced increased cardiovascular events, such as myocardial infarction and stroke, than patients on low levels of the hormone sufficient to maintain their blood Hgb at 10 g/dL or lower. The only patients who regularly demonstrate a poor response are individuals with severe inflammation. Overall, erythropoietic stimulating agents are safe and effective drugs for patients with anemia caused by a wide range of conditions, but their use and dose must be carefully considered.

Many patients undergoing cytotoxic therapy for cancer experience severe neutropenia and are thus at substantial risk for life-threatening infection. Clinical trials of recombinant granulocyte colony-stimulating factor in patients undergoing aggressive chemotherapy for leukemia and solid tumors resulted in the Food and Drug Administration (FDA) approval of the drug for use in patients undergoing chemotherapy of intensity sufficient to produce severe neutropenia (Chapter 153). The use of the drug and its numerous biosimilars

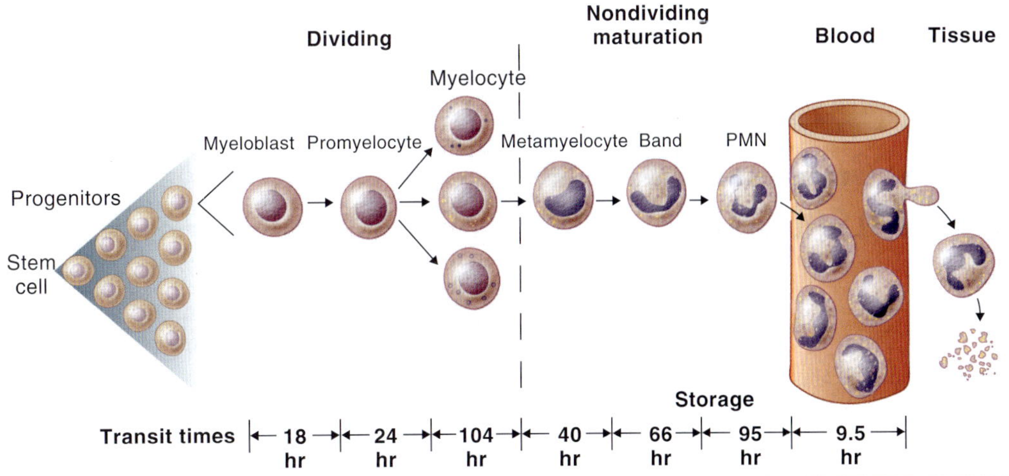

FIGURE 142-2. **Neutrophil production system.** PMN = polymorphonuclear leukocyte.

is associated with the more rapid return of neutrophils to safe levels if administered soon after the inciting chemotherapy is completed, but not at the nadir of neutrophil production, and results in lower risk of severe infections. However, the use of granulocyte colony-stimulating factor has not enhanced survival in patients with any tumor type. And similar to the use of erythropoietin in patients with cancer, the administration of granulocyte colony-stimulating factor to some patients receiving cytotoxic chemotherapy for cancer (e.g., breast cancer) has been associated with a statistically significant increase in cancer recurrence, although this finding is controversial.

Thrombopoietin was cloned and characterized in 1994 and was quickly advanced to clinical trials following the model of granulocyte colony-stimulating factor use in patients undergoing cancer chemotherapy. Initial results with the intact hormone and a truncated version that included only the receptor-binding domain were mixed, and use of the truncated form of the drug, administration to healthy volunteer donors to improve platelet apheresis yields, resulted in a significant number of subjects developing antidrug antibodies that cross-reacted with their native thrombopoietin, resulting in severe thrombocytopenia. This experience caused manufacturers of thrombopoietin to cease clinical trials. Instead, several small molecules that bind to and stimulate the thrombopoietin receptor and stimulate thrombopoiesis have been developed for clinical use.[A2,A3] Two such drugs approved by the FDA for use in patients with severe immune thrombocytopenia include a peptibody that contains four copies of a thrombopoietin receptor–binding peptide grafted onto an immunoglobulin scaffold and a small organic molecule that is orally bioavailable and binds to a spatially distinct site on the thrombopoietin receptor. The use of each drug results in a high rate of platelet responses into the normal range in patients with severe immune thrombocytopenia (Chapter 158) who were refractory to conventional therapies. It was initially thought that although thrombopoietin receptor agonists would stimulate platelet production in excess of immune destruction, they would not alter the pathophysiology of immune thrombocytopenia purpura (ITP), and hence be required for very long periods of time. However, a growing number of patients who have extremely refractory ITP have been reported no longer to require a thrombopoietin receptor agonist after a variable number of months of therapy, thereby suggesting that these drugs might be able to alter the immune response in such patients. In addition to the treatment of patients with ITP, thrombopoietin receptor agonists have been approved for use in patients with thrombocytopenia secondary to interferon treatment of hepatitis C viral infection and for patients with aplastic anemia. Additional clinical indications are being tested.

GENERAL REFERENCES

For the General References and other additional features, please visit Elsevier eBooks+ at https://ebooks.health.elsevier.com.

Grade A References

A1. Amato L, Addis A, Saulle R, et al. Comparative efficacy and safety in ESA biosimilars vs. originators in adults with chronic kidney disease: a systematic review and meta-analysis. *J Nephrol.* 2018;31:321-332.

A2. Kuter DJ, Tarantino MD, Lawrence T. Clinical overview and practical considerations for optimizing romiplostim therapy in patients with immune thrombocytopenia. *Blood Rev.* 2021;49:100811.

A3. Bussel J, Kulasekararaj A, Cooper N, et al. Mechanisms and therapeutic prospects of thrombopoietin receptor agonists. *Semin Hematol.* 2019;56:262-278.

143

THE PERIPHERAL BLOOD SMEAR

BARBARA J. BAIN

With the development of sophisticated automated instruments to count and characterize blood cells, Romanowsky (Wright-Giemsa or May-Grünwald-Giemsa)–stained peripheral blood smears are now performed on only a minority of blood specimens received in a hematology laboratory. Nevertheless, the blood smear remains important for a number of reasons: it can (1) verify the result of an automated instrument, (2) provide an immediate specific diagnosis, or (3) indicate a narrow range of diagnostic possibilities, permitting focused rather than indiscriminate investigation.[1-3] A blood film can provide a rapid diagnosis in cases in which speed is crucial, such as in acute promyelocytic leukemia, thrombotic thrombocytopenic purpura, Burkitt lymphoma, and certain infections.[4] It also can aid in the rapid diagnosis of malaria (Chapter 316)[5] and babesiosis (Chapter 324).[6] Sometimes a smear reveals an error in an automated blood count[7] or provides unexpected information that is of value in patient management.[8]

Usually, blood smears are initially interpreted by a laboratory scientist. In some countries, it is customary for clinicians to examine the blood smears of their own patients because the clinician has the final responsibility for integrating all information and making a diagnosis. However, the interpretation of a blood smear can be difficult, and a trained laboratory hematologist or hematopathologist often has a major role in interpreting smears that may have been initially examined by a laboratory scientist.[9] Digital microscopy permits a preliminary assessment and is a practical option for expert evaluation and triage of peripheral blood smears in locations where experienced staff are not available on site.[10]

It is crucial that, when requesting a blood count, the clinician provides all the essential information needed to interpret the count and any associated smear. Regardless of whether the clinician examines the blood film, he or she must be able to interpret the written report issued by the laboratory. To do so, the clinician must be familiar with the terms generally used by laboratory staff and the possible significance of the abnormalities described. The most important of these terms are illustrated in Figs. 143-1 through 143-20.

REASONS FOR PERFORMING A BLOOD SMEAR

A blood smear may be requested by a clinician or initiated by a laboratory scientist or a laboratory hematologist. Clinical findings that should lead a clinician to request a blood smear are summarized in Table 143-1.

Laboratory scientists and physicians may initiate a blood smear that has not been requested by the clinician if the clinical details indicate the possibility of a significant hematologic abnormality. However, they are also likely to evaluate a blood smear in response to abnormalities revealed by an automated instrument. These abnormalities may be quantitative or qualitative. Quantitative abnormalities that require evaluation include anemia, polycythemia, macrocytosis, microcytosis, neutrophilia, lymphocytosis, eosinophilia, thrombocytopenia, and thrombocytosis.

Modern automated instruments are able to "flag" the presence of qualitative abnormalities that require a blood film to be examined for confirmation of the abnormality or for further elucidation. "Flags" are generated in response to the electrical impedance or the light scattering characteristics of individual cells. Some instruments are dependent on cytochemical reactions of cells or on the cells' ability to polarize light. Most instruments can indicate the

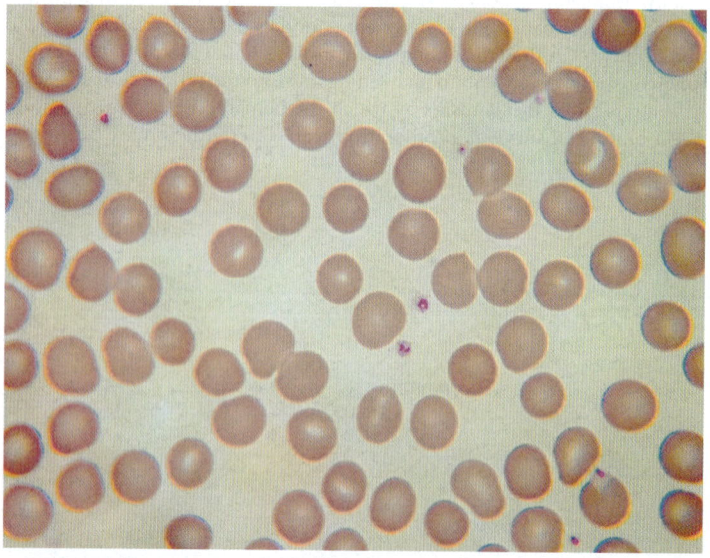

FIGURE 143-1. Normal peripheral blood smear. These normal red cells are described as *normocytic* (i.e., of normal size) and *normochromic* (i.e., their staining characteristics are normal). Normal erythrocytes are biconcave discs, causing them to have an area of central pallor that does not exceed one third the diameter of the cell. There are also scattered normal platelets (×1000).

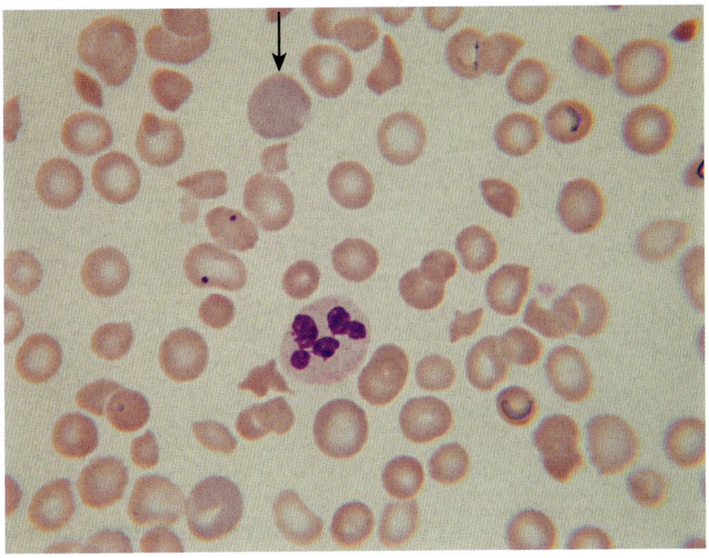

FIGURE 143-2. **Smear showing multiple abnormalities.** There is *anisocytosis*, defined as an increased variation in cell size; *poikilocytosis*, defined as an increased variation in cell shape; and *polychromasia*, defined as the presence of erythrocytes with a blue tinge to their cytoplasm—indicating a young cell recently released from the bone marrow in which the polychromasia is due to the presence of RNA. *Polychromatic cells* are erythrocytes with a blue tinge; because polychromatic cells are larger than normal mature erythrocytes, they are known as *polychromatic macrocytes* (*arrow*). The film also shows two cells containing bluish purple *Howell-Jolly bodies;* these inclusions are nuclear remnants (×1000).

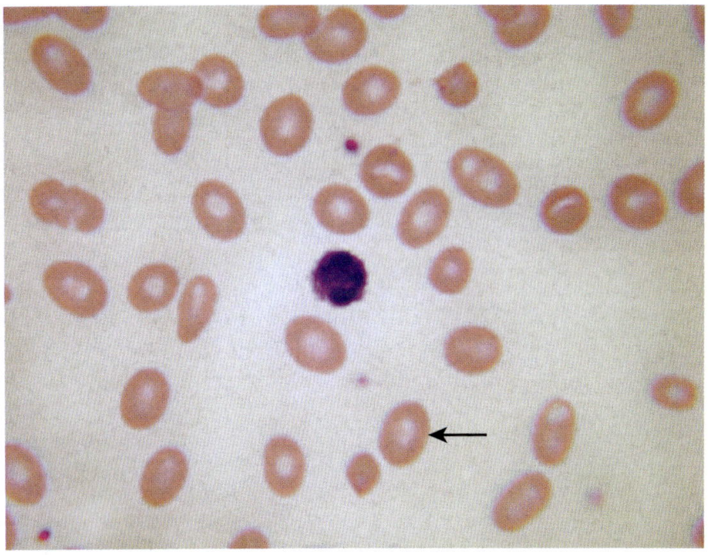

FIGURE 143-4. **Macrocytic anemia.** A *macrocyte* is recognized on a blood film as a cell with a diameter that is considerably greater than that of the nucleus of a small lymphocyte. In addition, this smear shows *oval macrocytes* (also known as *macro-ovalocytes*), defined as cells that are larger than normal and oval in shape (*arrow*). They are of considerable diagnostic importance, being characteristic of megaloblastic anemia and Southeast Asian ovalocytosis; they can also be seen in dyserythropoiesis (×1000).

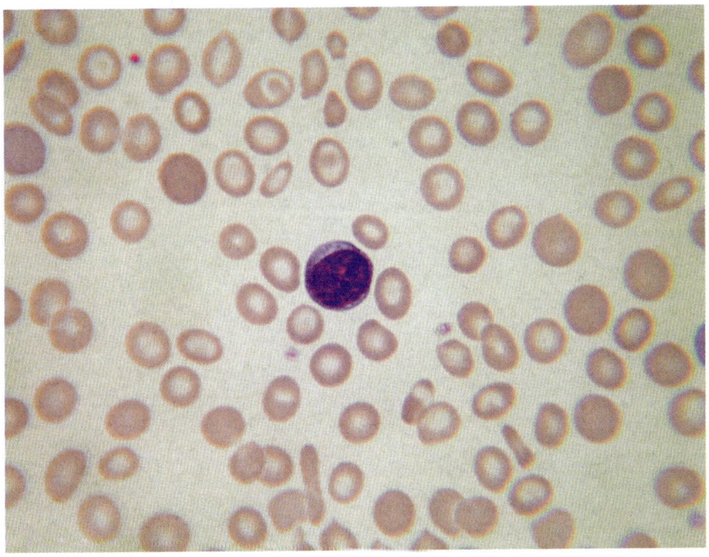

FIGURE 143-3. **Microcytic red cells from a case of thalassemia minor (β-thalassemia heterozygosity).** In a blood smear, a *microcyte* can be defined as a cell with a diameter less than that of the nucleus of a normal small lymphocyte (generally 7 to 8 μm). There are also some cells showing *hypochromia*, an area of central pallor that is larger than one third of the diameter of the red cell. In addition, there are two *target cells*, with a hemoglobinized area in the center of the area of pallor (×1000).

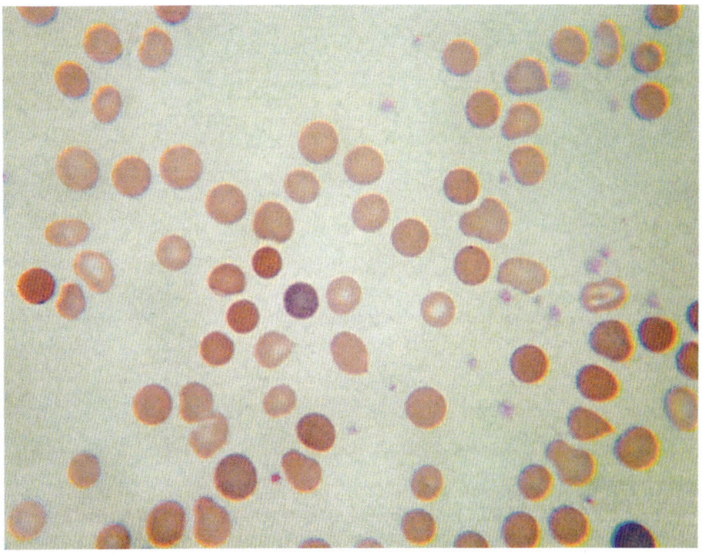

FIGURE 143-5. **Hereditary spherocytosis.** A *spherocyte* is a red cell that lacks central pallor because of its spherical shape. In hereditary spherocytosis, there are usually cells in which the central pallor is reduced rather than absent, and they are intermediate in shape between a spherocyte and a *discocyte*, which is an erythrocyte with the normal shape of a biconcave disc (×1000).

possibility of the presence of blast cells, reactive or other atypical lymphocytes, granulocyte precursors, or nucleated red blood cells. Some instruments can enumerate nucleated red blood cells. Instruments using a cytochemical reaction for peroxidase to help identify neutrophils, eosinophils, and monocytes may flag the appearance of large, unstained (i.e., peroxidase-negative) cells; such cells may indicate a harmless inherited peroxidase deficiency, but sometimes such cells are lymphoma cells, reactive lymphocytes, or leukemic blast cells. Instruments often flag the possibility of an erroneous platelet count, such as when there is an overlap in size between platelets and red cells or when light-scattering characteristics suggest the presence of platelet aggregates (a potential cause of pseudothrombocytopenia). A reported increase in basophil count should generally also be regarded as a flag because it often represents a pseudobasophilia, resulting from the presence of leukemia or lymphoma cells. Some instruments alert the instrument operator to the possible presence of malaria parasites.

International consensus guidelines indicate which automated instrument results require blood smear review. Whether a review is needed is determined in part by whether that specimen is the first one obtained from that patient and whether there has been a significant change from a previously validated result (referred to as a *delta check*). Laboratory computers can be programmed to indicate when a result meets the criteria for smear review.

Automated red cell measurements can, to some extent, replace examination of the blood film.[11] An increased red cell distribution width indicates the presence of anisocytosis. A decreased mean cell volume is usually a reliable indicator of microcytosis. A reduction in the mean cell hemoglobin concentration indicates hypochromia (for most instruments, however, this measurement is less sensitive than the human eye in the detection of hypochromia). An increased mean cell volume usually indicates macrocytosis, but examination of a smear is necessary both to confirm that the result is not an artifact and to elucidate the cause. Some instruments can measure the hemoglobin concentration in individual cells and thus flag the presence of hyperdense cells; however, a blood film is still necessary to distinguish spherocytes from irregularly contracted

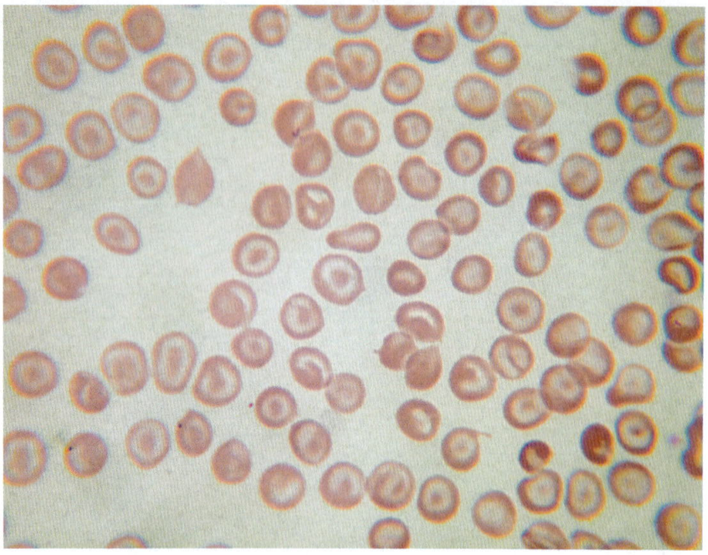

FIGURE 143-6. **Target cells.** A *target cell* is an erythrocyte with a hemoglobinized area in the middle of the normal area of central pallor (×1000).

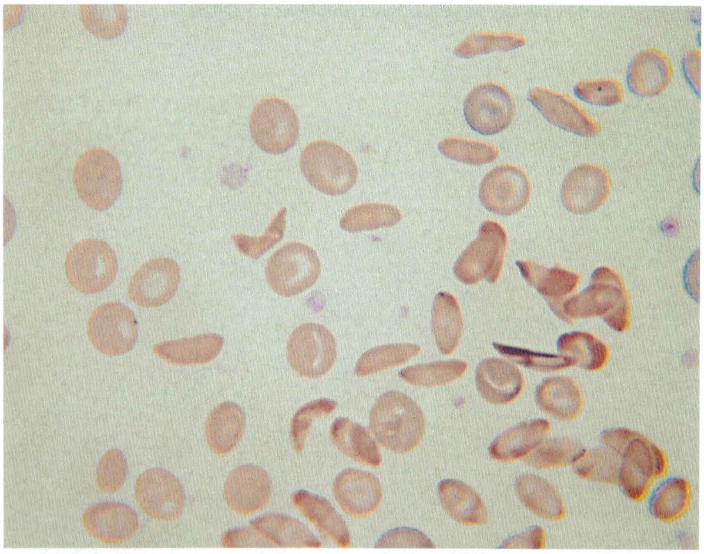

FIGURE 143-7. **Sickle cells.** A *sickle cell* is a cell with a sickle or crescent shape resulting from the polymerization of hemoglobin S. These cells are seen in sickle cell anemia (homozygosity for hemoglobin S) as well as in compound heterozygous states such as sickle cell/hemoglobin C disease and sickle cell/β-thalassemia, which also lead to sickle cell disease. This smear also shows target cells and boat-shaped cells with a lesser degree of polymerization of hemoglobin S than in a classic sickle cell (×1000).

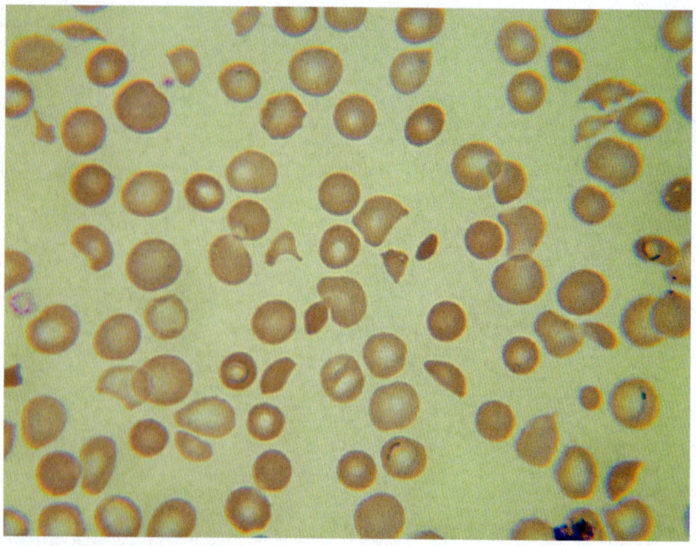

FIGURE 143-8. **Red cell fragmentation.** *Red cell fragments* or *schistocytes* are defined as fragments of erythrocytes. In addition to small angular fragments, there may be *microspherocytes*, cells of reduced size and spherical in form (also known as *spheroschistocytes*), and *keratocytes*, cells with two or four hornlike projections. Keratocytes can result from removal of a Heinz body, as well as from red cell fragmentation. Some schistocytes are referred to as *helmet cells* because of their typical shape. Schistocytes are seen in microangiopathic hemolytic anemias and in mechanical hemolysis (×1000).

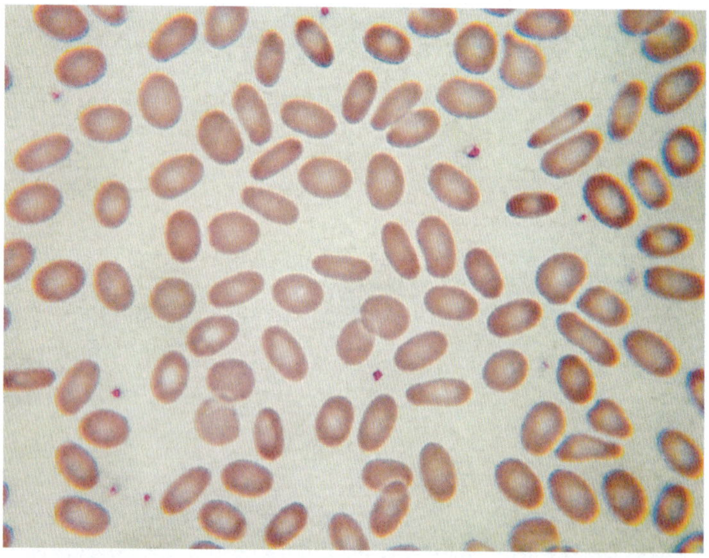

FIGURE 143-9. **Hereditary elliptocytosis.** An *elliptocyte* is an elliptical red cell. When seen in the numbers present in this smear, they are indicative of hereditary elliptocytosis; smaller numbers are seen in other conditions such as iron deficiency anemia, in which they are sometimes referred to as *pencil cells* (×1000).

cells, sickle cells, and other cells that have an increased hemoglobin concentration. Most instruments produce a histogram of the size distribution of red cells, and some do the same for the distribution of hemoglobin concentration; either of these graphic representations may show dimorphic red cells (i.e., two populations of cells).

THE BLOOD SMEAR IN THE DIFFERENTIAL DIAGNOSIS OF ANEMIA

MICROCYTIC ANEMIAS

In microcytic anemias (Chapter 145), the automated count is of considerable importance and may permit a distinction between iron deficiency and thalassemia heterozygosity. In iron deficiency, there is initially a normocytic normochromic anemia; only when the deficiency becomes more severe is there microcytosis. Conversely, in β-thalassemia heterozygosity, there is usually a normal or near-normal hemoglobin concentration, but the red blood cell count is increased, and there is marked microcytosis (low mean cell volume) together with a parallel reduction in mean cell hemoglobin. The blood film provides supplementary information that can favor one diagnosis or the other. Iron deficiency is more likely to be associated with hypochromia and elliptocytes ("pencil cells"), whereas in β-thalassemia heterozygosity, there is microcytosis, hypochromia is less marked, and there are more likely to be target cells and basophilic stippling. Individuals with α-thalassemia involving the deletion of two α genes (−α/−α) or (− −/α α) have red cell indices similar to those of β-thalassemia heterozygosity; in this case, the blood film usually does not provide any additional diagnostically useful information, although individuals with nondeletional α-thalassemia due to hemoglobin Constant Spring have prominent basophilic stippling. When there is deletion of a single α gene, the blood count is either less abnormal or normal, and the blood smear does not provide any extra diagnostically useful information. The blood smear is, however, a useful supplement to the blood count in suggesting a diagnosis of hemoglobin H disease (Chapter 148). The blood count shows anemia, marked microcytosis (low mean cell

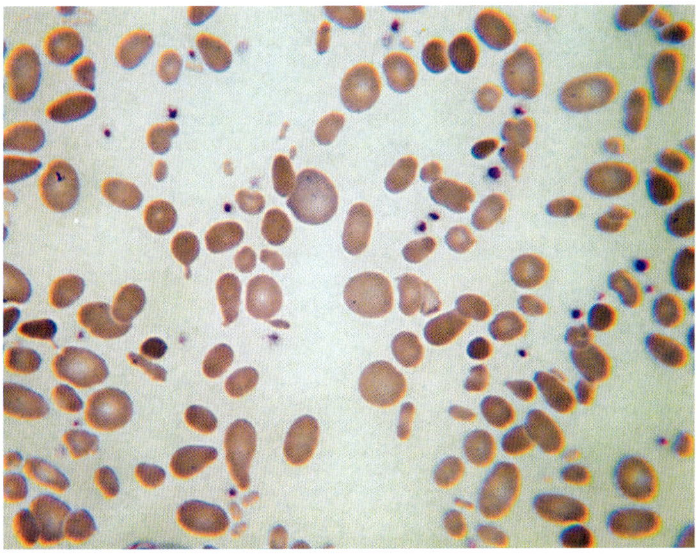

FIGURE 143-10. **Hereditary pyropoikilocytosis.** This smear shows striking poikilocytosis, including elliptocytes, microspherocytes and other fragments, as well as teardrop cells. Hereditary pyropoikilocytosis is a congenital condition, similar to hereditary elliptocytosis, which usually results from the inheritance of two different mutated genes, one from each parent, and is characterized by a severe hemolytic anemia (×1000).

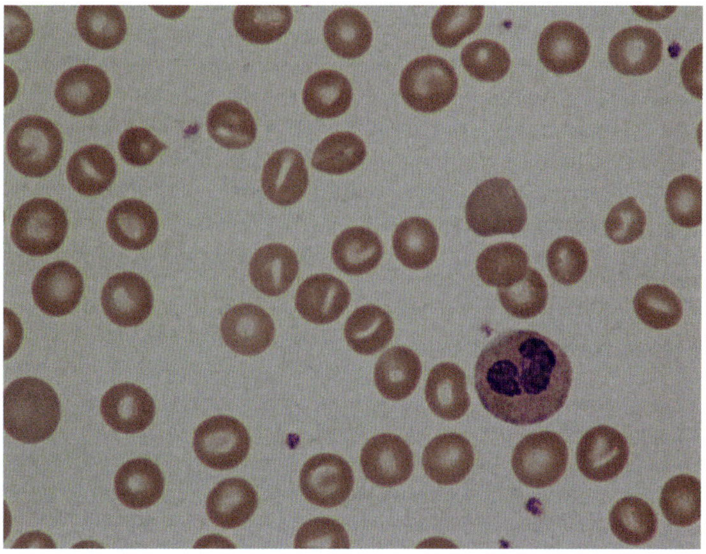

FIGURE 143-12. **Stomatocytosis.** A *stomatocyte* is a cell that appears to have a central mouth-shaped or slitlike stoma. Among the less common causes are hereditary stomatocytosis and phytosterolemia (also known as sitosterolemia). Alcohol and hydroxycarbamide (hydroxyurea) therapy are more common causes (×1000).

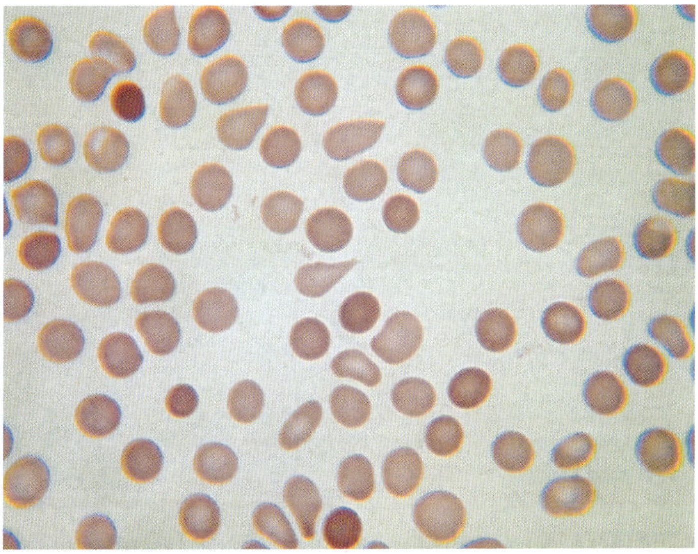

FIGURE 143-11. **Teardrop poikilocytes.** *Teardrop poikilocytes*, or *dacrocytes*, are teardrop-shaped red cells; they are characteristic of primary myelofibrosis but are also seen in myelofibrosis following other myeloproliferative neoplasms or secondary to bone marrow infiltration and in megaloblastic anemia (×1000).

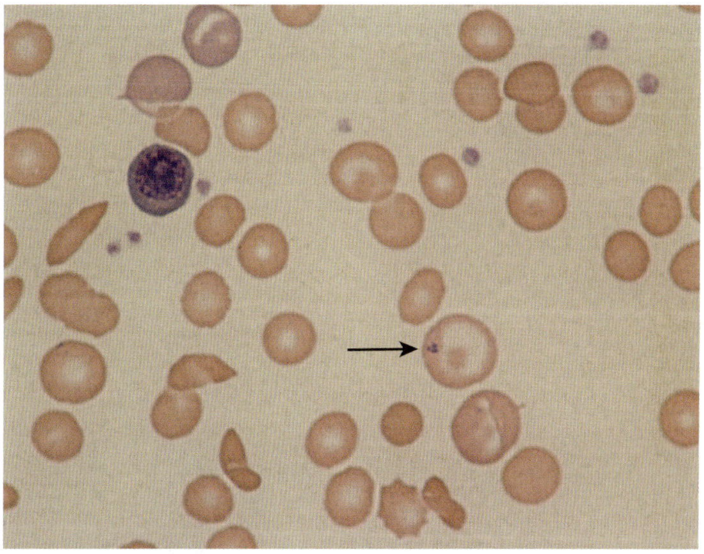

FIGURE 143-13. **A cluster of Pappenheimer bodies within a target cell in sickle cell anemia.** A *Pappenheimer body* is an iron-containing red cell inclusion. It is smaller and more angular than a Howell-Jolly body and stains navy blue rather than purple. Pappenheimer bodies are seen following splenectomy, in other hyposplenic states, and in sideroblastic anemias. The smear also shows boat-shaped cells, a nucleated red blood cell, polychromatic macrocytes, and a polychromatic stomatocyte (×1000). A Perls stain confirms the iron content in a Pappenheimer body.

volume and mean cell hemoglobin), and usually a reduction in the mean cell hemoglobin concentration. The smear usually shows marked poikilocytosis in addition to microcytosis, and there may be polychromasia, correlating with an elevated reticulocyte count. Iron deficiency anemia should also be distinguished from anemia of chronic disease. The blood counts may be quite similar in the two conditions, but microcytosis is less common in anemia of chronic disease, and the smear often shows features of inflammation, such as increased rouleaux formation, background staining (as a result of increased plasma proteins), and sometimes neutrophilia. Other rare microcytic anemias that must be distinguished from iron deficiency include congenital sideroblastic anemia (Chapter 145) and lead poisoning. In congenital sideroblastic anemia, the film is dimorphic, with one population of hypochromic microcytes and another of normochromic normocytic cells. In lead poisoning, the presence of basophilic stippling and polychromasia in a patient with microcytosis can suggest the diagnosis. Sometimes a blood film provides the first clue that apparent microcytosis is actually the result of red cell fragmentation.

MACROCYTIC ANEMIAS

A blood film can be important in distinguishing true macrocytosis from factitious macrocytosis as a result of the presence of red cell agglutinates (see Fig. 143-16). Diagnostic features that can suggest the cause of macrocytosis are shown in Table 143-2.

A smear is particularly important in evaluating the possibility of a megaloblastic anemia (Chapter 150) (Figs. 143-4 and 143-21). Sometimes assays of vitamin B_{12} and folate are normal despite a deficiency, and only the blood film features suggest the true diagnosis and indicate the need for further investigation.

NORMOCYTIC NORMOCHROMIC ANEMIA

A blood smear is only occasionally useful in determining the cause of a normocytic normochromic anemia. Signs of inflammation may be present in

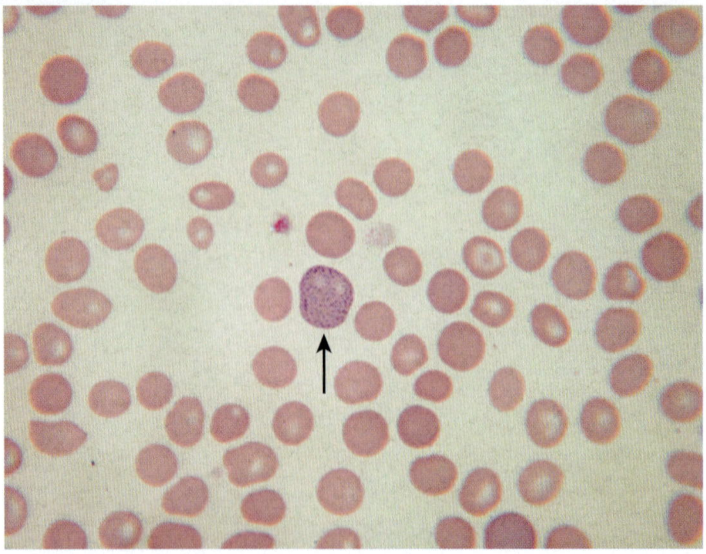

FIGURE 143-14. **Basophilic stippling.** *Basophilic stippling*, also known as punctate basophilia, means that there are fine (as in this case) or coarse purplish blue dots dispersed through the red cell (*arrow*). They are a very nonspecific feature occurring in thalassemia trait, lead poisoning, pyrimidine 5′-nucleotidase deficiency, and dyserythropoiesis in general (×1000).

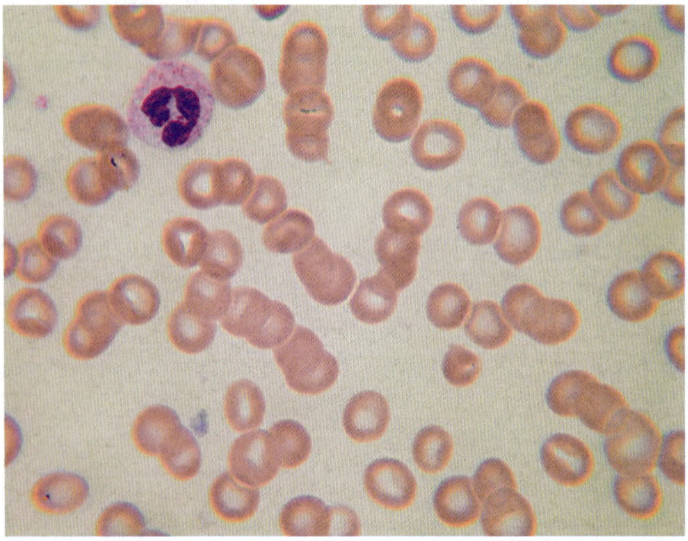

FIGURE 143-15. **Rouleaux formation.** *Rouleaux* are stacks of red cells, often compared to stacks of coins. Rouleaux formation results from an increase of high-molecular-weight globulins in the plasma, either as a reactive change or as a result of secretion of a paraprotein in a plasma cell neoplasm (×1000).

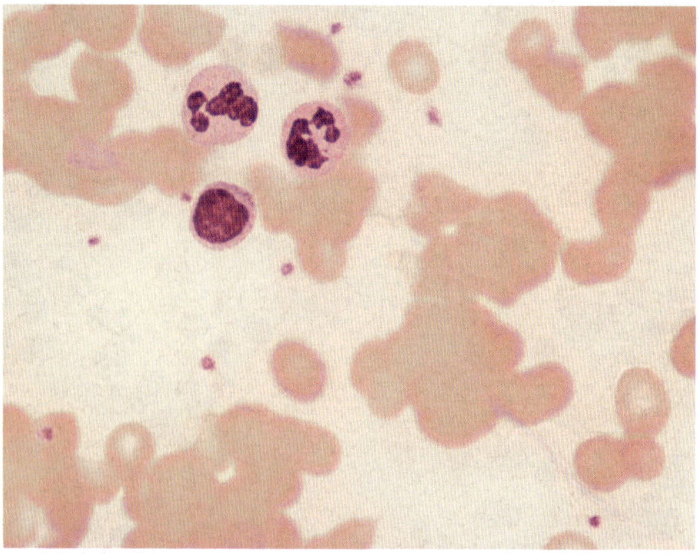

FIGURE 143-16. **Red cell agglutination.** *Red cell agglutinates* are irregular aggregates of red cells, often seen in *Mycoplasma pneumoniae* infection; other infections, such as infectious mononucleosis; and in chronic cold hemagglutinin disease (×1000).

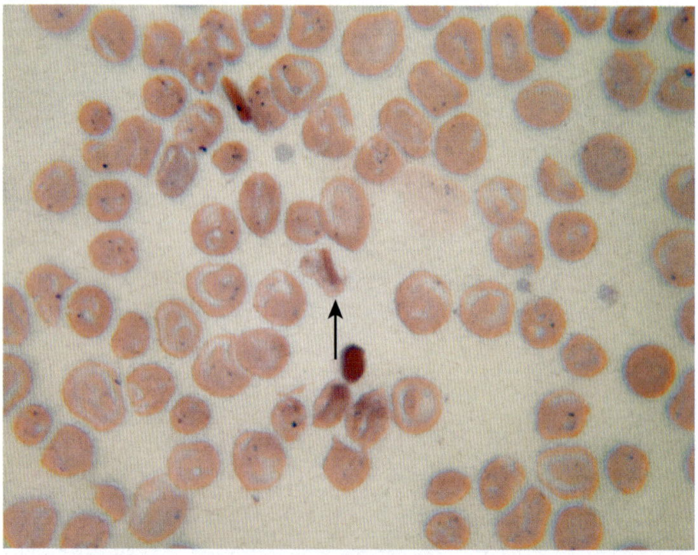

FIGURE 143-17. **Homozygous hemoglobin C or hemoglobin C disease.** Three *hemoglobin C crystals* are present, one indicated by an *arrow*. Hemoglobin C crystals are usually six-sided, with a long axis having parallel edges. In addition to hemoglobin C disease, these crystals can also be seen in sickle cell/hemoglobin C compound heterozygosity and in hemoglobin C/β^0 thalassemia (×1000).

anemia of chronic disease. Rouleaux formation and increased background staining can also indicate multiple myeloma. Polychromasia suggests the possibility of young red cells as a result of recent blood loss or hemolysis. Small numbers of acanthocytes may indicate hypothyroidism or anorexia nervosa. Dysplastic features, such as hypogranular or pseudo-Pelger neutrophils, suggest a myelodysplastic syndrome.

HEMOLYTIC ANEMIAS

The possibility of hemolysis is suggested by the presence of polychromasia and macrocytosis. Specific causes of hemolysis are suggested by the presence of various poikilocytes, as shown in Table 143-3.

The distinction between spherocytes and irregularly contracted cells is important; both are dense cells with absent central pallor, but the differential diagnosis is quite different. Recognition of the features of oxidant damage is important in diagnosing glucose-6-phosphate dehydrogenase (G6PD) deficiency because sometimes an assay for G6PD performed during an acute hemolytic episode is normal (Chapter 147). In addition to irregularly contracted cells, there may be ghost cells, hemi-ghost cells ("blister cells"), and even Heinz bodies protruding from the red cells and confirmed on a Heinz body preparation. The observation of these features is an indication to repeat the assay when the acute hemolytic episode is over.

ASSESSMENT OF THROMBOCYTOPENIA, THROMBOCYTOSIS, AND PLATELET MORPHOLOGY

A blood smear is essential to validate the count whenever an automated count shows thrombocytopenia (e.g., a count $<60 \times 10^9$/L) (Chapter 158). This should be done quickly before patient management is altered, such as by postponing surgery or initiating further diagnostic workup. A platelet transfusion should never be given for an unexpected thrombocytopenia without microscopic confirmation of the count. A factitiously low platelet count is often the result of in vitro platelet aggregation (Chapter 157) and is occasionally the result of platelet satellitism (platelets surrounding neutrophils, generally seen in samples anticoagulated with EDTA), and possibly also with platelet phagocytosis. To detect aggregates reliably, the edges and the tail of the smear

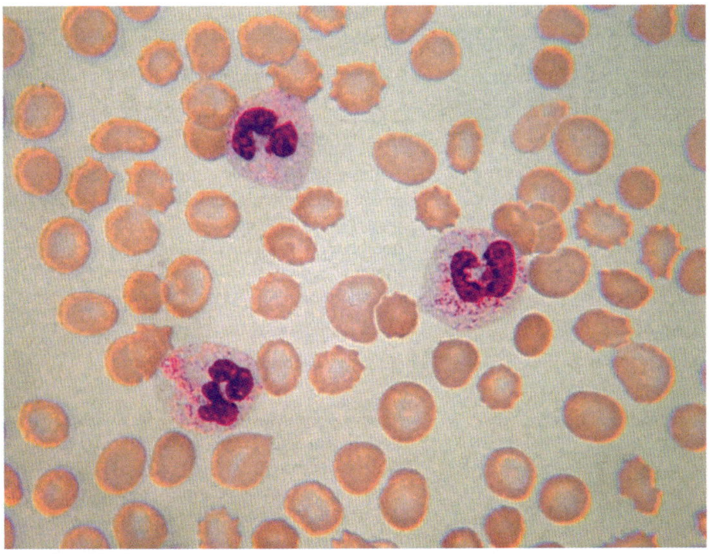

FIGURE 143-18. **Toxic granulation.** *Toxic granulation* refers to heavy staining of azurophilic granules of neutrophils. When accompanied by neutrophil vacuolation, it is often indicative of infection, but toxic granulation can also result from inflammation, tissue damage, administration of granulocyte colony-stimulating factor, and normal pregnancy. Rarely it results from chronic neutrophilic leukemia or a leukemoid reaction to multiple myeloma (×1000).

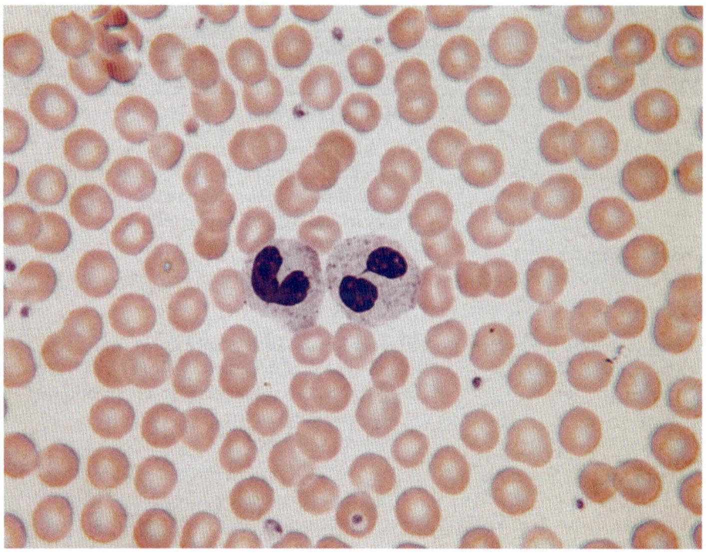

FIGURE 143-20. **Pelger-Huët anomaly.** A *Pelger-Huët anomaly* is a cytologic abnormality of neutrophils in which there is hypolobulation of nuclei and increased chromatin clumping. Nuclei may have a shape resembling a peanut or a pince-nez, as in the example shown. The Pelger-Huët anomaly is inherited, but similar pseudo-Pelger neutrophils are seen in myelodysplastic syndromes, in which the neutrophils may also be hypogranular (×1000). They can also be seen as an acquired reversible phenomenon in response to specific drugs, including tacrolimus and mycophenolate mofetil.

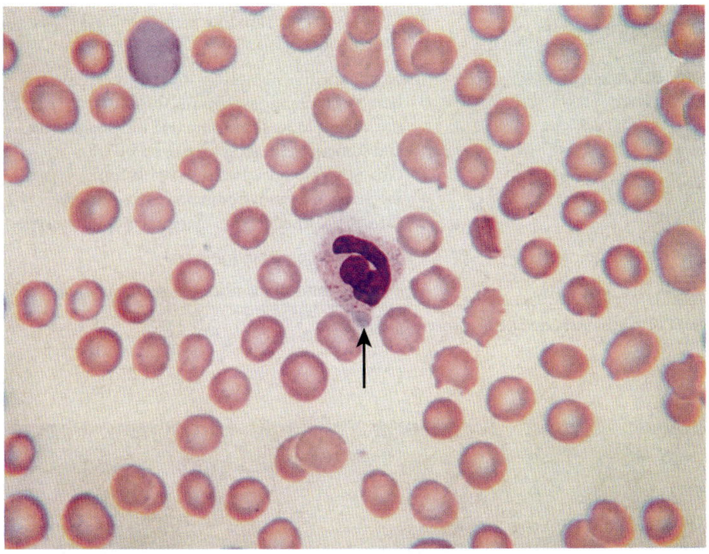

FIGURE 143-19. **Döhle body.** A *Döhle body* (*arrow*) is a pale blue-gray amorphous inclusion near the cell membrane of a neutrophil. Döhle bodies can result from infection and inflammation. Similar but different inclusions (larger and more angular) are seen in the May-Hegglin anomaly (MYH9-related disorder) (×1000).

TABLE 143-1 CLINICAL FEATURES SUGGESTING THE NEED FOR A BLOOD SMEAR

CLINICAL FEATURE	REASON TO PERFORM A BLOOD SMEAR
Lymphadenopathy or splenomegaly	May be indicative of infectious mononucleosis or another reactive condition or of leukemia or lymphoma
Clinically evident anemia	Helps in the differential diagnosis
Bruising or bleeding tendency, including unexplained retinal hemorrhages	May confirm thrombocytopenia or show morphologically abnormal platelets (which may have defective function); sometimes shows acute leukemia or other condition causing bone marrow failure
Acute kidney injury	Hemolytic-uremic syndrome and thrombotic thrombocytopenic purpura should be confirmed or excluded
Jaundice and hypertension in a pregnant woman	May show schistocytes, supporting a diagnosis of HELLP syndrome
Bone pain	May indicate multiple myeloma, bone marrow infiltration, or sickle cell disease
Unexplained chest or abdominal pain or acute splenic enlargement in a child	Possible sickle cell disease
Unexplained hyperbilirubinemia	Assessment of possible hemolysis

HELLP = hemolysis, elevated liver enzymes, low platelets.

should be examined. The presence of fibrin strands also suggests the activation of coagulation and an erroneous platelet count.

If a low platelet count is confirmed, the film may give clues to the cause (Chapter 158).[12] Giant platelets (Figs. 143-22 and 143-23) occur in a number of inherited thrombocytopenias, including Bernard-Soulier syndrome and MYH9-related disorders (the May-Hegglin anomaly and related conditions).[13] Small platelets are less common but are a feature of Wiskott-Aldrich syndrome. Agranular platelets occur in gray platelet syndrome, and platelets with a reduced number of larger-than-normal granules are seen in Jacobsen/Paris-Trousseau syndrome. The presence of May-Hegglin inclusions (Döhle-like bodies; see Fig. 143-19) in neutrophils indicates that the cause of the thrombocytopenia is a mutation in *MYH9*. In acquired thrombocytopenias, increased platelet turnover is often accompanied by the presence of large platelets, whereas bone marrow failure is associated with platelets of normal size. It is important to look for red cell fragments to confirm or exclude a diagnosis of thrombotic thrombocytopenic purpura and atypical hemolytic-uremic syndrome in any patient with the apparent recent onset of thrombocytopenia; because platelet transfusions are usually contraindicated in these conditions, the smear should be examined before platelet transfusion is contemplated. Occasionally the smear reveals clinically unsuspected malaria. The smear of any patient with the apparent recent onset of severe thrombocytopenia should be examined carefully for evidence of acute promyelocytic leukemia; the leukemic cells may be infrequent in the circulating blood. Hemorrhagic manifestations and a low platelet count can also be indicative of meningococcal septicemia; in some patients, organisms are seen in the blood smear and the diagnosis is confirmed; in other patients, only marked toxic changes in neutrophils are detected.

Thrombocytosis should also be confirmed on a smear. Factitiously elevated counts may be the result of the presence of red cell fragments (in

TABLE 143-2 USEFUL FEATURES FOR DETERMINING THE CAUSE OF MACROCYTIC ANEMIA

CAUSE	SMEAR FEATURES
Megaloblastic anemia (vitamin B_{12} or folic acid deficiency)	Oval macrocytes, teardrop poikilocytes, hypersegmented neutrophils; when severe, marked anisocytosis and poikilocytosis, which may include red cell fragments
Ethanol excess	Target cells and stomatocytes; anisocytosis and poikilocytosis less than in megaloblastic anemia
Liver disease	Target cells, stomatocytes
Myelodysplastic syndromes, including sideroblastic anemias	Other dysplastic features such as hypogranular and hypolobulated neutrophils; if erythropoiesis is sideroblastic, a population of hypochromic microcytic cells and Pappenheimer bodies
Chronic hemolytic anemia	Polychromasia; characteristic poikilocytes sometimes present (e.g., irregularly contracted cells if there is an unstable hemoglobin)

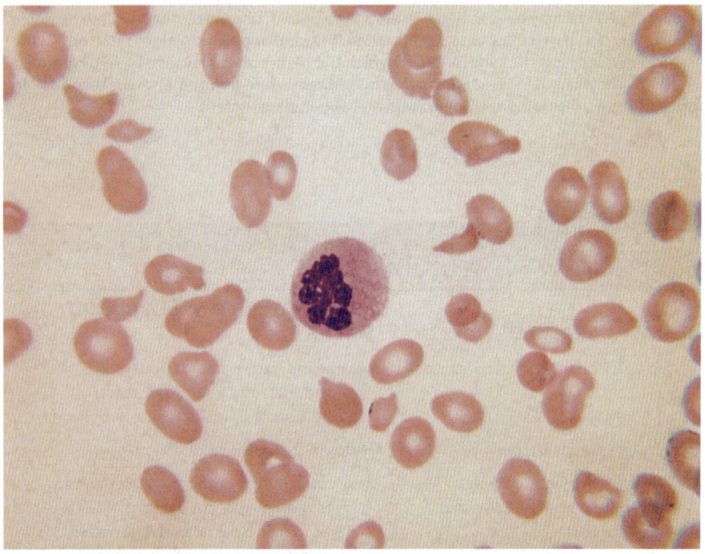

FIGURE 143-21. Hypersegmented neutrophils. A *hypersegmented neutrophil* is one in which the nucleus has more than five lobes, as in this example from an individual with megaloblastic anemia. Neutrophil hypersegmentation is also said to be present if there are increased numbers of neutrophils with five lobes or if the median lobe count is increased. Hypersegmented neutrophils should be distinguished from macropolycytes, in which an increased lobe count results from a doubled content of DNA (×1000).

microangiopathic or mechanical hemolytic anemia, burns, or accidental in vitro heating of the blood sample), white cell fragments (in acute leukemia and, less often, in lymphoma), cryoglobulin precipitates, or microorganisms (particularly *Candida* species). If the count is confirmed, the blood smear may be useful to indicate a likely cause (e.g., features of hyposplenism or the presence of basophilia in a myeloproliferative disorder).

It is sometimes necessary to examine a smear to confirm that an apparently normal platelet count is valid. This should always be done in patients with acute leukemia and an elevated white cell count; the presence of white cell fragments of a similar size to platelets can suggest that the platelet count is at a safe level when it is in fact dangerously low. Counting the ratio of platelets to other particles of similar size permits the count to be corrected. Any unexpectedly normal count should be confirmed; for example, the sudden rise of the automated platelet count in a patient being treated for a hematologic neoplasm may be the result of fungi that have colonized an indwelling intravenous line and are being shed into the blood stream.

LEUKOCYTOSIS AND LEUKOPENIA

The finding of leukocytosis is not necessarily an indication for a blood smear (Chapter 153). For example, this finding would be expected in a patient with infection or following surgery or trauma, in which case smear confirmation is not required. However, unexpected leukocytosis requires examination of a smear.

TABLE 143-3 BLOOD SMEAR FEATURES SUGGESTING A SPECIFIC CAUSE OF INHERITED OR ACQUIRED HEMOLYTIC ANEMIA

BLOOD SMEAR FEATURES	CONDITIONS SUGGESTED
Spherocytes	Hereditary spherocytosis, autoimmune hemolytic anemia, alloimmune hemolytic anemia (e.g., hemolytic disease of the newborn, delayed hemolytic transfusion reaction), drug-induced immune hemolytic anemia, *Clostridium perfringens* sepsis
Elliptocytes	Hereditary elliptocytosis
Oval macrocytes plus stomatocytes	Southeast Asian ovalocytosis
Irregularly contracted cells	Glucose-6-phosphate dehydrogenase deficiency, oxidant damage from chemicals or drugs in individuals with normal red cell enzymes (e.g., dapsone administration), liver failure due to Wilson disease (release of copper from liver), unstable hemoglobin, hemoglobin C homozygosity
Sickle cells and boat-shaped cells	Sickle cell disease (e.g., sickle cell anemia or compound heterozygous states such as S/C, S/D-Punjab, S/O-Arab, S/β-thalassemia)
Target cells	Hemoglobin C homozygosity, other hemoglobinopathies, hereditary xerocytosis
Stomatocytes	Hereditary stomatocytosis, phytosterolemia
Acanthocytes	Liver failure (spur cell hemolytic anemia)
Basophilic stippling	Lead poisoning, pyrimidine 5′-nucleotidase deficiency
Red cell fragments (schistocytes)	Microangiopathic hemolytic anemia (including hemolytic-uremic syndrome, thrombotic thrombocytopenic purpura, HELLP syndrome, and sometimes hemolysis associated with disseminated intravascular coagulation), mechanical hemolytic anemia (e.g., defective cardiac prosthetic valve, march hemoglobinuria)
Erythrophagocytosis	Paroxysmal cold hemoglobinuria
Red cell agglutinates	Acute or chronic cold antibody-induced hemolysis

HELLP = hemolysis, elevated liver enzymes, low platelets.

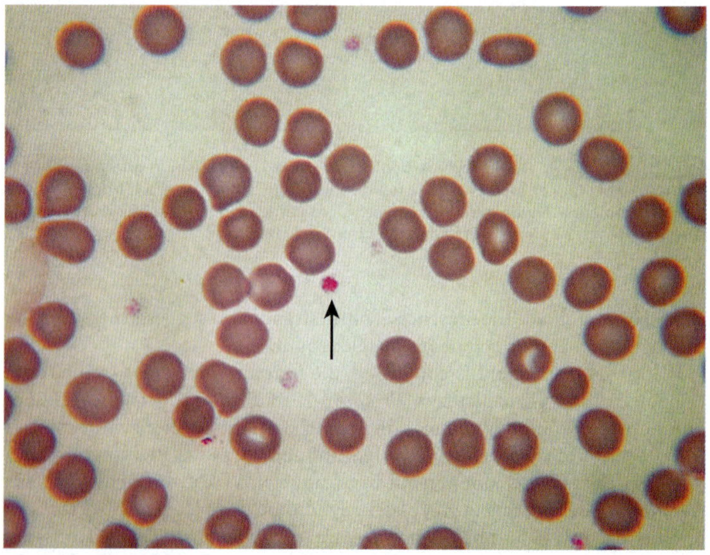

FIGURE 143-22. Normal-sized platelet *(arrow)*. Platelets have central granules, although this is not apparent in this photomicrograph (×1000).

Artifactual white count elevation is unusual but can occur as a result of cryoglobulinemia, hyperlipidemia, or the presence of *Candida* species. Distinguishing reactive changes from leukemia on the basis of morphology is usually straightforward for neutrophil leukocytosis but more difficult for lymphocytosis. In

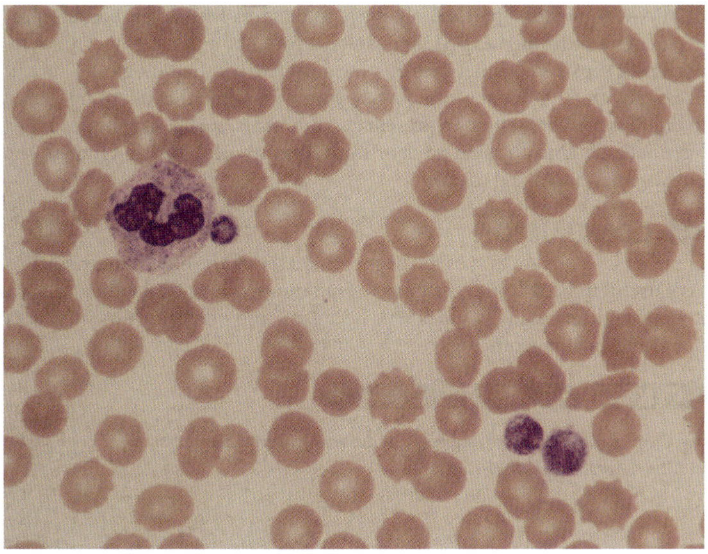

FIGURE 143-23. Giant platelets. Giant platelets are as large as or larger than normal red cells. Giant platelets can indicate increased platelet turnover or an inherited or acquired defect in thrombopoiesis (×1000).

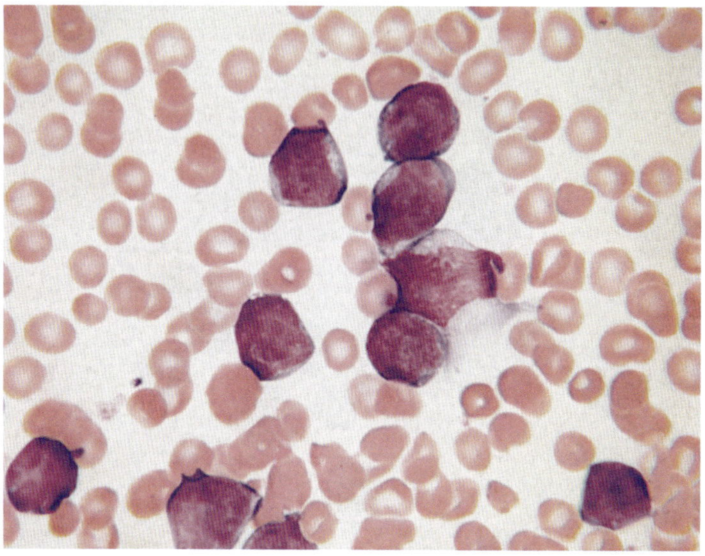

FIGURE 143-24. Acute lymphoblastic leukemia. Numerous agranular blast cells with a high nuclear-to-cytoplasmic ratio are present. Platelets are decreased in number (×1000).

reactive leukocytosis, there is usually toxic granulation, and Döhle bodies may be present (see Figs. 143-18 and 143-19). Vacuolation is particularly characteristic of bacterial infection, and there may be some degranulation of neutrophils. The hematologist should be aware of the changes induced by granulocyte colony-stimulating factor so that they are not confused with a response to infection. Granulocyte colony-stimulating factor can cause toxic granulation, Döhle bodies, vacuolation, and the presence of macropolycytes (giant neutrophils) and circulating neutrophil precursors. The changes typical of leukemia are discussed later.

Leukopenia (Chapter 153) usually requires a film for confirmation and elucidation. The exception is when it is expected in a given clinical context, such as when a patient has had recent chemotherapy. Rarely, an apparent leukopenia is artifactual, owing to the aggregation of neutrophils mediated by an autoantibody or resulting from infection-induced changes in adhesion molecules of the leukocyte surface membrane.

With some automated instruments, it is necessary to confirm that reported neutropenia is real. If the automated count is based on peroxidase cytochemistry, the presence of an inherited deficiency will lead to an apparent neutropenia associated with an increase of large, unstained (i.e., peroxidase-negative) cells. The scatter plot is characteristic, but because the same features could be due to acute leukemia with neutropenia and circulating blast cells, a smear is needed for confirmation.

LEUKEMIAS AND LYMPHOMAS

The blood smear is critical in the diagnosis of leukemias and lymphomas. The lymphoblasts of acute lymphoblastic leukemia are usually medium-sized agranular cells with relatively scanty cytoplasm (Fig. 143-24), whereas in acute myeloid leukemia, blast cells are generally larger, with more plentiful cytoplasm that may contain granules or Auer rods (Fig. 143-25). Myeloid blast cells vary in appearance according to whether they are myeloblasts or monoblasts. Myeloblasts are usually medium sized and may have plentiful granules, scanty granules, or no visible granules; they may contain Auer rods or, rarely, giant granules. Monoblasts are much larger cells with plentiful cytoplasm containing few granules and, very rarely, Auer rods. Megakaryoblasts are present in some patients and are sometimes cytologically distinctive because of their tendency to form cytoplasmic blebs or develop platelet-type granules.

Chronic myeloid leukemia has a very characteristic blood smear (Fig. 143-26) in which the most numerous cells are myelocytes and mature neutrophils. Eosinophils and basophils are also present. Dysplastic features are generally absent. In atypical Philadelphia chromosome–negative chronic myeloid leukemia, monocytosis is more frequent and dysplastic features are present. Chronic myelomonocytic leukemia is characterized by increased monocytes, some of them immature, with inconspicuous dysplastic features and infrequent granulocyte precursors. Chronic neutrophilic leukemia and a neutrophilic leukemoid reaction to a plasma cell neoplasm have similar hematologic features and need to be distinguished by supplementary tests, including analysis for a *CSF3R* mutation.[14]

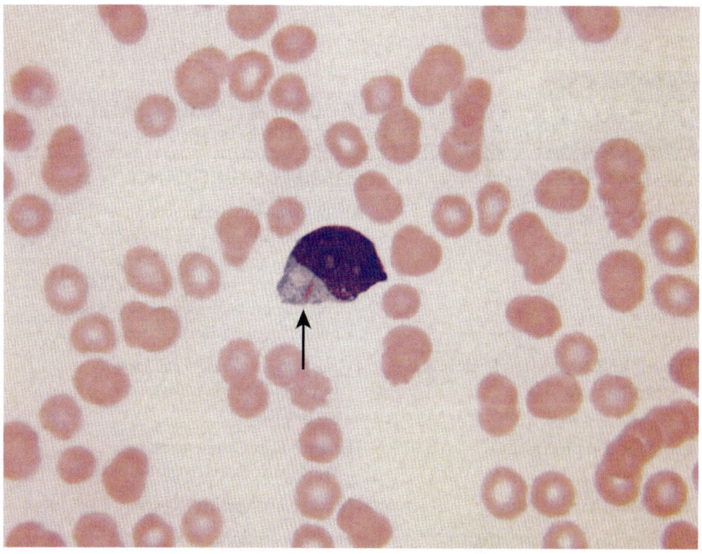

FIGURE 143-25. Auer rod. An Auer rod (*arrow*) is a rod-shaped inclusion in the cytoplasm of cells of myeloid lineage formed by the crystallization of azurophilic granule constituents. Auer rods are seen only in acute myeloid leukemia and high-grade myelodysplastic syndromes. They are usually seen in blast cells but are occasionally found in maturing cells (×1000).

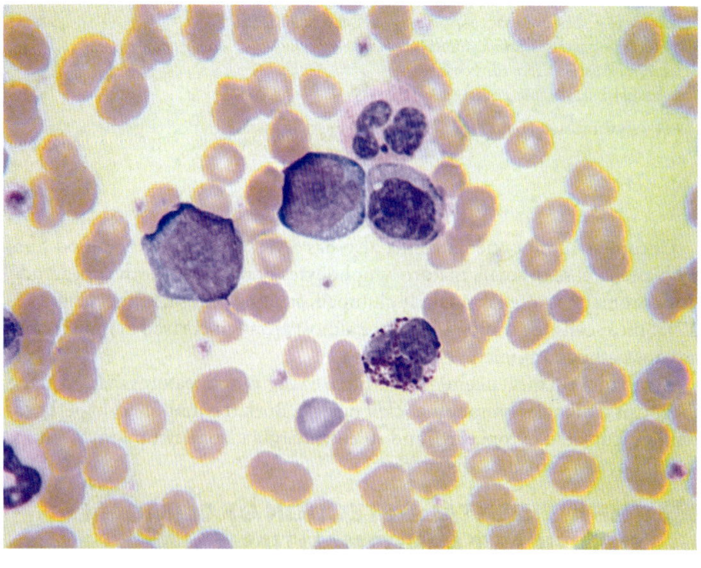

FIGURE 143-26. Chronic myeloid leukemia. In this view there are myeloblasts, a myelocyte, a basophil, and a segmented neutrophil (×1000).

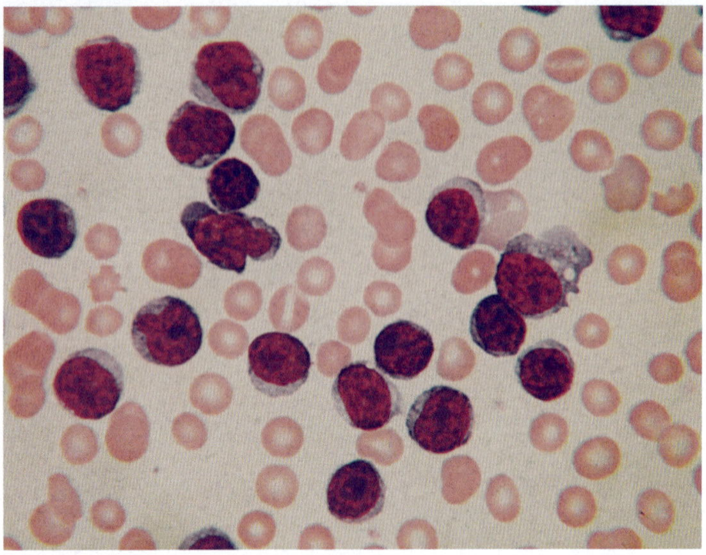

FIGURE 143-27. **Chronic lymphocytic leukemia.** There are large numbers of rather monotonous, mature small lymphocytes with chromatin clumping. Smear cells (or smudge cells), reflecting the mechanical fragility of the cells, are characteristic but are not seen in this photomicrograph (×1000).

TABLE 143-4 INCIDENTAL BUT CLINICALLY RELEVANT BLOOD SMEAR OBSERVATIONS

OBSERVATION	POSSIBLE SIGNIFICANCE
Acanthocytes	Abetalipoproteinemia, neuroacanthocytosis (includes choreoacanthocytosis, McLeod phenotype, Huntington-like disease 2, and pantothenate-kinase–associated neurodegeneration)
Howell-Jolly bodies, target cells, and acanthocytes	Hyposplenism (congenital, previous splenectomy, celiac disease, amyloidosis)
Cryoglobulin precipitates	Hepatitis C, multiple myeloma, Waldenström macroglobulinemia
Vacuolated lymphocytes	Inherited metabolic disorders
Parasites (e.g., malaria parasites, *Babesia*, microfilaria, trypanosomes, *Leishmania*)	Parasitic infection
Fungi (*Candida* spp, *Histoplasma capsulatum, Talaromyces marneffei, Cryptococcus neoformans, Malassezia furfur*)	Disseminated fungal infection or, in the case of *Candida*, colonization of an indwelling intravenous line
Bacteria (e.g., pneumococcus, meningococcus, *Capnocytophaga canimorsus, Borrelia, Ehrlichia, Anaplasma, Yersinia pestis*)	Bacterial infection
Leukoerythroblastic blood film	Bone marrow infiltration (e.g., metastatic malignancy)

Chronic lymphocytic leukemia also has a very characteristic blood film, with an increase of small, mature lymphocytes of rather uniform appearance. The chromatin is often irregularly clumped, creating a mosaic effect (Fig. 143-27). Smear cells (or smudge cells) are almost always increased in number but are not pathognomonic.

Lymphoma in the leukemic phase often has cytologic features that aid in the diagnosis. Follicular lymphoma (cleft nuclei), Burkitt lymphoma (hyperbasophilic vacuolated cytoplasm), and splenic marginal zone lymphoma (villous lymphocytes) can all be distinctive.

THE INCIDENTAL DETECTION OF CLINICALLY SIGNIFICANT ABNORMALITIES

Sometimes the examination of a blood film reveals unexpected but clinically significant information. Examples are given in Table 143-4. Detection of microorganisms is particularly likely in patients with acquired immunodeficiency syndrome (AIDS), hyposplenic patients, and patients with overwhelming sepsis, but sometimes they are detected in immunologically normal patients with only trivial symptoms. It should be noted that microorganisms in blood smears sometimes represent contaminants, particularly if specimens have been obtained by skin prick or from the umbilical cord and if there has been a delay in making the film.

CONCLUSION

Despite major advances in other diagnostic methods, the blood smear remains very useful in hematologic diagnosis. Sometimes it is critical either because it yields a diagnosis very quickly or because it provides information that is not available in any other way.

GENERAL REFERENCES

For the General References and other additional features, please visit Elsevier eBooks+ at https://ebooks.health.elsevier.com.

144

APPROACH TO THE ANEMIAS

ROBERT T. MEANS, JR.

Anemia is defined as a significant reduction in the volume of erythrocytes, or red blood cells, in the body. The red blood cell is an anucleate biconcave disc, approximately 8 μm in diameter, composed of various enzymes and chemicals surrounded by a lipid bilayer. The major component of the red blood cell is hemoglobin. A normal red blood cell contains 30 to 40 pg of hemoglobin. Hemoglobin is a highly specialized molecule, optimally enabled to deliver oxygen from the lungs through the circulation to the peripheral tissues and to remove carbon dioxide from the peripheral tissues and return it to the lungs for expiration. The red blood cell is generated in the bone marrow from erythroid precursors (Chapter 142) and survives approximately 120 days in the circulation before its clearance by the reticuloendothelial system.

The direct measurement of the red cell mass is a complex process; therefore, surrogate measures are used to define anemia in the clinical setting. The most common measures are the blood hemoglobin concentration and the hematocrit. The red blood cell count per microliter is also reported in routine hematologic analysis but is rarely used to define anemia. The hematocrit derives its name from the graduated tube in which blood was centrifuged for analysis. The percentage of the blood column represented by red cells compressed by centrifugation (also called packed cell volume) is the quantity physically represented by the hematocrit. Hematocrit values determined by centrifugation-based techniques are used mainly in limited-resource environments where electronic cell counting is not available. In laboratories where complete blood counts are performed using electronic cell counting methods, the hematocrit is a calculated value reflecting the product of the red blood cell count and the mean corpuscular volume of the red cells, both of which are measured directly. Because the hemoglobin concentration is directly measured rather than calculated, many physicians prefer to use the measurement of hemoglobin in the definition of anemia.

PATHOBIOLOGY

Anemia and Oxygen Delivery

The function of hemoglobin is to deliver oxygen to tissues. Oxygen delivery is a function of blood flow, blood hemoglobin content as reflected by hemoglobin concentration, and the gradient between arterial and venous oxygen content (Fick equation). The effect of anemia on blood hemoglobin content is readily apparent, and it also has a role in the other elements of the Fick equation.

In severe anemia associated with blood volume loss or in severe anemia with preserved blood volume, heart rate typically increases, and blood flow is

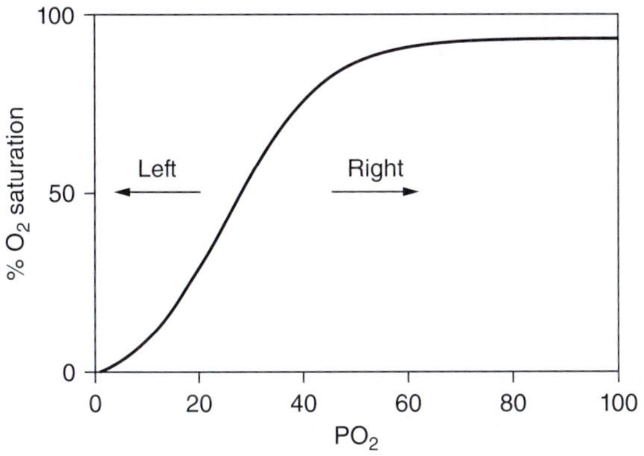

FIGURE 144-1. Oxyhemoglobin dissociation curve. Directions of right and left shift indicated. The curve plots the percentages of hemoglobin in its saturated (oxygen-laden) form on the vertical axis as a function of ambient oxygen tension on the horizontal axis. A rightward shift of the curve indicates a decreased affinity of hemoglobin for oxygen, making it easier for hemoglobin to release its oxygen to supply hypoxic tissue through which the blood passes.

shunted from the periphery to critical organs such as the brain, liver, kidneys, and coronary circulation to preserve oxygen delivery.

The arterial/venous oxygen gradient is also affected by anemia. When the oxyhemoglobin dissociation curve is shifted to the right, the oxygen affinity of hemoglobin is decreased—it requires a higher partial pressure of oxygen to attain a given level of hemoglobin saturation, and oxygen is more readily released to the tissues (Fig. 144-1). In anemia, the principal cause of a right shift is increased intracellular 2,3 diphosphoglycerate (DPG, also called 2,3 bisphosphoglycerate), a product of red cell metabolism. A right shift can also be induced by hyperthermia, hypercapnia, or acidosis. The opposite conditions can produce a left shift, resulting in oxygen being held more tightly by hemoglobin (high affinity).

Methemoglobin

Hemoglobin is composed of two α-globin chains and two β-globin chains, each of which has a covalently bound iron-containing porphyrin ring. Movement of the iron atom in relation to the plane of the porphyrin ring results in changes in the oxygen affinity of hemoglobin. Iron in normal hemoglobin is in the reduced ferrous state (Fe^{2+}). When hemoglobin iron becomes oxidized to the ferric state (Fe^{3+}), it is no longer able to bind oxygen and is called methemoglobin. Under normal circumstances, red cells contain a cytochrome b_5-based enzymatic system that rapidly reduces methemoglobin iron back to the ferrous state.

Methemoglobinemia occurs when this system fails. It may be a congenital condition, or it may be the result of exposure to toxic agents, perhaps in association with a subclinical cytochrome b_5 deficiency (Table 144-1). There are also mutations in globin genes that result in variant hemoglobins (M-hemoglobin) in which iron stabilizes in the ferric state.

Patients with methemoglobin concentrations greater than 10% show cyanosis (bluish discoloration of the skin) with normal oxygen saturation on arterial blood gas. Pulse oximetry may be inaccurate in methemoglobinemia. Arterial blood in methemoglobinemia is a chocolate brown color that does not become red with oxygen exposure. However, addition of potassium cyanate (KCN) to the blood sample will cause the blood to become red with methemoglobinemia but not with M-hemoglobins. Most blood gas machines, particularly in hospitals, can quantify methemoglobin.

Congenital methemoglobinemia patients typically do well even with methemoglobin concentrations of 30 to 40% because of adaptation and primarily have the cosmetic or social problem of cyanosis. Ascorbic acid (vitamin C) may be helpful, or methylene blue can be used. In contrast, acute methemoglobinemia from toxic exposure can be life threatening. Lethargy or headache can occur at methemoglobin levels around 20%. Above 40%, confusion, altered consciousness, and dyspnea can be noted. At concentrations above 50 to 60%, coma and death may occur. The treatment for acute methemoglobinemia is methylene blue 1 to 2 mg/kg, although higher doses up to 6 to 7 mg/kg can be required. M-hemoglobins do not require treatment.

Regulation of Red Cell Production

The primary regulator of red cell production is the effectiveness of oxygen delivery. This critical need may explain why hemoglobin concentration or hematocrit are controlled in a relatively narrow normal range as compared to the white blood count or platelet count, where the upper limit of normal may

TABLE 144-1 CAUSES OF METHEMOGLOBINEMIA

CONGENITAL*
Cytochrome b_5 reductase deficiency
Type I: erythrocyte enzyme deficiency only
Type II: generalized enzyme deficiency (persistent neurologic features)
ACQUIRED
Local Anesthetics
Benzocaine
Lidocaine
Procaine
Phenazopyridine (Pyridium)
Anti-infectives
Dapsone
Nitrofurantoin
Primaquine
Sulfonamides
Nitrates/Nitrites
Amyl nitrate
Isobutyl nitrite
Nitroglycerin
Other Medications
Acetaminophen
Rasburicase
Zopiclone
Other Compounds
Aniline dyes
Henna (2-hydroxy-1,4-napthoquinone)
Phenylhydroxylamine

*Congenital M-hemoglobins clinically and functionally resemble methemoglobins but are biochemically and genetically distinct.

be two or three times the lower limit of normal. The mediator that translates peripheral oxygen need to red cell production is the hormone erythropoietin. After birth, the predominant physiologic site of erythropoietin production is the kidney, although the liver retains some limited capacity for erythropoietin production. Neoplasms arising from liver, kidney, or other tissues may secrete erythropoietin in an unregulated manner. Anemia results in decreased oxygen tension in the renal cortex, thereby inducing the transcription factor HIF (hypoxia-inducible factor), which in turn upregulates erythropoietin production. Erythropoietin binds to specific receptors on erythroid progenitors in the marrow leading to increased red cell production. When correction of anemia normalizes the oxygen tension in the renal cortex, erythropoietin production falls back to basal levels. Ambient hypoxia, or underoxygenation of the blood by a right-to-left cardiopulmonary shunt, also leads to the production of erythropoietin. This hypoxia causes the erythrocytosis seen in dwellers at high altitudes and in individuals with uncorrected cyanotic heart disease.

Although an adequate supply of other factors such as iron, vitamin B_{12}, or folate is required for red cell production, polycythemia does not occur in the absence of an increased erythropoietin stimulus. Red cell production has feedback regulation of iron availability through the erythroferrone/hepcidin/ferroportin axis (Chapter 145).

CLINICAL MANIFESTATIONS

Symptoms

In general, the symptoms of anemia are nonspecific and highly dependent on the patient's general physical condition or other comorbid illnesses. Anemia of rapid onset, as may be seen with massive acute hemolysis or with acute blood loss, is more likely to be symptomatic than anemia from red cell underproduction or from slow gastrointestinal blood loss. In both of these cases, the total blood volume is preserved, and there is time for the cardiovascular system to accommodate to the changes in hematocrit. Preservation of blood volume and cardiovascular accommodation are likely the reasons that patients with slow-onset anemias such as B_{12} deficiency are traditionally reported to become symptomatic at much lower hemoglobin concentrations or hematocrits than patients with iron deficiency anemia from blood loss. A person with coronary artery disease or chronic obstructive lung disease is more likely to become symptomatic than an anemic individual without those disorders who has the same hemoglobin concentration.

Common symptoms in anemia include fatigue but typically not dyspnea. Palpitations or a sense of the heart racing or pounding may occur, representing a more rapid heart rate and increased ejection fraction in order to maintain oxygen delivery. Symptomatology in anemia syndromes that develop as a consequence of some other disease (such as the anemia of inflammation in association with rheumatoid arthritis) will most likely be dominated by the symptoms of the associated disease. Pica, the desire to eat nonnutritive substances such as ice, is very specific to iron deficiency. Restless leg syndrome may also be a manifestation of iron deficiency.

Physical Findings

Pallor may occur in patients with anemia but may be difficult to appreciate in patients seen for the first time due to the widespread differences in skin pigmentation among healthy individuals, but its presence in mucous membranes obviates that variable. Pallor can also occur in other conditions associated with shunting of blood away from the periphery to the critical organs. In the assessment of anemia, pallor of the conjunctival mucosa or of the creases in the palm are more specific than pallor in other sites. Pallor of the conjunctival mucosa generally indicates a hemoglobin concentration less than 9 g/dL, and failure of the palmar creases to become more prominent when the extended fingers are pushed down, thereby extending the palm, generally indicates a hemoglobin no higher than 7 to 8 g/dL. Tachycardia and a systolic ejection murmur may develop as a result of anemia and cardiovascular accommodation to it. Peripheral edema, which may be occasionally seen with moderately severe anemia, may reflect a combination of high-output heart failure and loss of oncotic pressure associated with fewer blood cells. On rare occasions, retinal hemorrhages may be seen on fundoscopic examination in severe anemia. All of these vascular and cardiac manifestations of anemia will resolve with correction of anemia.

DIAGNOSIS

Medical History

The initiating step of any evaluation for anemia is demonstration by hemoglobin concentration or hematocrit that the patient is anemic (see Tables 144-2 and 144-3). A number of elements in the history and physical examination can guide the subsequent laboratory evaluation (Tables 144-4 and 144-5). Duration of anemia assists in distinguishing congenital from chronic or acute causes. Because iron deficiency is the most common etiology of anemia in clinical medicine, dietary history (vegetarian or vegan) and a history of blood loss should always be pursued. In women, this questioning should also include asking about the number of previous pregnancies and whether iron supplementation was used during pregnancy. Every child delivered at term represents an investment of 800 mg of maternal iron (Chapter 145). Persistent jaundice suggests active hemolysis, and episodic jaundice is frequently observed in individuals with congenital hemolytic anemias, whether they result from metabolic defects such as glucose-6-phosphate dehydrogenase (G6PD) deficiency or from red cell membrane defects such as hereditary spherocytosis. A history of cholelithiasis in early adulthood is suggestive of congenital hemolytic disorders. A history of chronic inflammatory disorders raises the possibility of the anemia of inflammation (Chapter 145). A history of petechiae or easy bruising or a history of recurrent infection raises the possibility of a hematopoietic disorder not limited to the erythroid lineage. A family history of a specific diagnosis, such as sickle cell anemia or thalassemia, is obviously helpful. Similarly, a history of family members with episodes of jaundice following minor illnesses suggests a congenital hemolytic anemia. In contrast, a history of a similar disorder in the mother, aunts, and sisters of a female patient with suspected iron deficiency is not particularly helpful in the diagnosis of anemia.

Physical Examination

Certain physical findings may help guide the evaluation of anemia by providing clues to specific syndromes, underlying disorders, or bleeding (Table 144-5). Evidence of bleeding mandates evaluation for iron deficiency. Petechiae, purpura, or thrush suggests abnormalities of the platelets or white cells and raises the possibility of a generalized marrow disorder not limited to the erythroid lineage. Frontal bossing (prominence of the forehead due to expansion of red marrow in the skull) is seen in congenital hemolytic anemias but can be a normal variant; in general, adults with hemolytic anemia and this physical finding have had their diagnosis defined earlier in life. The neurologic findings of B_{12} deficiency generally require a more thorough examination than is part of the routine physical examination (Chapter 150).

Complete Blood Counts

The usual complete blood count provided by automated cell counters includes a variety of directly measured and calculated parameters, which at a minimum include the white blood cell count, the red blood cell count, the hemoglobin concentration and hematocrit, the platelet count, and the red cell indices described later. Many automated counters also provide a differential white blood count and a semiquantitative description of red cell abnormalities. Decreased counts of white blood cells and platelets are discussed in Chapters 153 and 158, respectively. Typical values are shown in Table 144-2. Clinicians should become familiar with the normal values specific to the laboratories they use.

The hemoglobin, hematocrit, and red cell counts are all concentrations, which means that a change in the plasma volume can elevate them or decrease them relative to the actual total body red cell mass. An example of an anemia associated with a normal or slightly increased red cell mass occurs in the second trimester of normal pregnancy. In contrast, an elevated hemoglobin concentration or hematocrit with a normal or decreased total body red cell mass can be seen in dehydration or the capillary leak syndrome

Red cells can also be described by parameters called red cell indices, which are routinely calculated by most electronic cell counters. These include the mean corpuscular volume (MCV), the mean corpuscular hemoglobin (MCH),

TABLE 144-2 NORMAL RED BLOOD CELL MEASUREMENTS

MEASUREMENT	NORMAL RANGE
Hemoglobin concentration	12-16 g/dL Female 13.5-17.5 g/dL Male
Hematocrit	36-48% Female 40-52% Male
Red blood cell (RBC) count	4.0-5.4 × 10^6/μL Female 4.5-6.0 × 10^6/μL Male
Mean corpuscular volume (MCV)	81-99 fL
Mean corpuscular hemoglobin (MCH)	30-34 pg
Mean corpuscular hemoglobin concentration (MCHC)	30-36 g/dL
RBC size distribution width (RDW)	
RDW-CV	12-15%
RDW-SD	37-47 fL
Reticulocyte percentage*	0.5-1.5%
Absolute reticulocyte count	20,000-100,000/μL
Reticulocyte production index	0.5-2.5%

*The same normal range applies to corrected reticulocyte counts.
RDW-CV = RDW-coefficient of variation; RDW-SD = RDW-standard deviation.

TABLE 144-3 DEFINITION OF RED CELL INDICES AND RETICULOCYTE PARAMETERS

$$\text{Mean corpuscular volume (MCV)} = \frac{\text{Hematocrit}}{\text{Red blood cell count}}$$

$$\text{Mean corpuscular hemoglobin (MCH)} = \frac{\text{Hemoglobin concentration}}{\text{Red blood cell count}}$$

Mean corpuscular hemoglobin concentration (MCHC)

$$= \frac{\text{MCH}}{\text{MCV}} \text{ or } \frac{\text{Hemoglobin concentration}}{\text{Hematocrit}}$$

Absolute reticulocyte count = Reticulocyte percentage × Red blood cell count

$$\text{Corrected reticulocyte count (hematocrit)} = \text{Reticulocyte percentage} \times \frac{\text{Hematocrit}}{42}$$

Corrected reticulocyte count (hemoglobin) =

$$\text{Reticulocyte percentage} \times \frac{\text{Hemoglobin concentration}}{15}$$

$$\text{Reticulocyte production index (RPI)} = \frac{\text{Corrected reticulocyte count (hematocrit)}}{\text{Maturation factor}}$$

HEMATOCRIT RANGE	MATURATION FACTOR
36-45%	1.0
26-35%	1.5
16-25%	2.0
Less than 16%	2.5

TABLE 144-4 MEDICAL HISTORY IN THE APPROACH TO ANEMIA

GENERAL
Duration (lifelong; chronic; intermittent; acute)
Previous blood transfusion
Family history of anemia
CLUES TO IRON DEFICIENCY/BLOOD LOSS
Change in bowel habits (melena, hematochezia, diarrhea)
Other bleeding
Surgical procedures
Pica (ice)
Restless leg symptoms
CLUES TO HEMOLYSIS
Jaundice (episodic, sustained, family history)
Hemoglobinuria
Cholelithiasis/cholecystectomy in early adulthood
CLUES TO SYSTEMIC HEMATOLOGIC DISEASE
Purpura/petechiae
Recurrent infections, including oral candidiasis
CLUES TO SYSTEMIC DISORDERS ASSOCIATED WITH ANEMIA
Rheumatologic/collagen vascular disease (anemia of inflammation)
Renal disease (anemia of chronic kidney disease)
Infections (recent or chronic, anemia of inflammation)
Endocrinopathy (anemia associated with endocrine deficiency)
Malignancy (anemia of inflammation)
Weight loss (anemia of inflammation; also nonspecific)

TABLE 144-5 PHYSICAL EXAMINATION FINDINGS IN THE APPROACH TO ANEMIA

FACTORS THAT MAY CAUSE OVER- OR UNDERESTIMATION OF THE DEGREE OF ANEMIA
Edema/anasarca
Other signs of congestive heart failure
Orthostatic hypotension/poor skin turgor
CLUES TO IRON DEFICIENCY/BLOOD LOSS
Heme-positive stool
Telangiectasias
CLUES TO HEMOLYSIS
Jaundice
Splenomegaly
Right upper quadrant abdominal tenderness
Frontal bossing (hemoglobinopathy/thalassemia)
CLUES TO B_{12}/FOLATE DEFICIENCY
Glossitis
Decreased vibratory sensation/proprioception
CLUES TO SYSTEMIC HEMATOLOGIC DISEASE
Purpura/petechiae
Oral thrush
Splenomegaly
Lymphadenopathy

and the mean corpuscular hemoglobin concentration (MCHC) (Table 144-3). Another parameter automatically calculated by most electronic cell counters is the red cell distribution width (RDW), which represents either the coefficient of variation of the distribution curve of red cell sizes (RDW-CV) or the standard deviation of the red cell distribution width curve (RDW-SD) and is a marker of red cell anisocytosis (variation in size).

Red blood cell parameter determinations (Table 144-2) will vary between laboratories depending upon the equipment used and on the population serving as the basis for the normal range. For example, the normal red cell values among patients living at high altitude are higher than those in normal subjects at sea level due to lower ambient oxygen tension driving higher erythropoietin production. Normal values are different between newborns, children, and adults and between men and women after puberty. The difference in normal hemoglobin concentration, hematocrit, and red cell count between adult men and women is attributed to the action of testosterone in sensitizing erythroid progenitors to erythropoietin.

Reticulocyte Count

Red cells newly released from the bone marrow that have shed their nuclei but still contain some nuclear material in the cytoplasm are called reticulocytes. Reticulocytes were traditionally measured through supravital staining on fresh smears, but now are most frequently measured by flow cytometry technology incorporated into electronic blood counters. On the routine Wright-Giemsa–stained peripheral blood smear, reticulocytes are slightly larger than red cells, have little or no central pallor, and have a more grayish (polychromatic) tinge to the cytoplasm. The reticulocyte activity in a particular specimen can be expressed in a variety of ways (Table 144-3). All are based on the principle that the reticulocyte response of the marrow to anemia varies with the degree of anemia. The uncorrected reticulocyte count, sometimes called the reticulocyte percentage, represents the percentage of red blood cells that are reticulocytes. However, an uncorrected reticulocyte count of 2% would be entirely normal in a person with a hematocrit of 42% or hemoglobin concentration of 14 g/dL but would be grossly inadequate in a person with a hematocrit of 20% or hemoglobin concentration of 7 g/dL. The other reticulocyte parameters represent an effort to adjust this uncorrected value for the degree of anemia. The simplest and most common adjustment is to express the reticulocyte count as the absolute reticulocyte count, which is the reticulocyte percentage multiplied by the red blood cell count. The most complex is the reticulocyte production index (RPI), which corrects the reticulocyte count for the degree of anemia and then adjusts by a factor that compensates for the release of less mature reticulocytes into the circulation under circumstances of more severe anemia.

Reticulocyte counts are helpful in the initial approach to anemia in distinguishing anemias due to underproduction of red cells from those associated with adequate or increased production but shortened survival in the circulation. During treatment of anemia, increases in the reticulocyte count can predict response to therapy prior to increments in the hemoglobin concentration or hematocrit. Alternately, failure of the reticulocyte count to increase at the expected time can predict failure of current therapy and dictate a change of approach.

Blood Smear Examination

Even in the era of more sophisticated electronic hematologic analysis, including ability of device software to provide descriptions of red cells, value remains in the examination of peripheral blood smear (Chapter 143) by a physician familiar with the clinical situation of the patient. In congenital hemolytic anemias, the morphologic changes characteristic of red cell membrane abnormalities may be seen (spherocytes, elliptocytes, etc.). The "bite" and "blister" red cells found in hereditary defects of red cell oxidative metabolism are unlikely to be appreciated except by direct examination by a clinician. Sideroblastic anemia is characterized as a microcytic anemia (see later) but is frequently associated with a normal MCV because the sideroblastic clone is not large enough to alter the average red cell size. The finding of a dimorphic red cell population is a significant clue to this disorder but may also be seen in partially treated iron deficiency. Macroovalocytes and hypersegmented neutrophils are highly suggestive of B_{12} deficiency.

Bone Marrow Examination

Bone marrow aspiration and biopsy are required for the diagnosis of many primary marrow disorders giving rise to anemia. In general, it is most likely to be indicated in underproduction anemias rather than in those associated with an appropriate or increased reticulocyte response. However, paroxysmal nocturnal hemoglobinuria (PNH), which can include elements of both hemolysis and marrow failure, is an exception. Disorders that require bone marrow examination for diagnosis at the present time are aplastic anemia and pure red cell aplasia, myelodysplastic syndromes, and anemias associated with marrow replacement (lymphoma, leukemia, myelofibrosis, myeloma, or metastatic cancer). Marrow examination is rarely required for assessment of iron status, given the availability of other diagnostic tools (Chapter 145). Bone marrow examination for the diagnosis of anemia should include both aspiration and biopsy and routinely include Prussian blue staining for evaluation of iron stores and possible detection of ringed sideroblasts. Flow cytometry to phenotype myeloid or lymphoid/plasma cell populations should also be performed, as should standard cytogenetics, when suspecting a clonal disorder. If there is suspicion on clinical grounds of a specific disease associated with a molecular abnormality, polymerase chain reaction (PCR) or fluorescence in situ hybridization (FISH) testing for that abnormality should be performed. Molecular studies for parvovirus in cases of possible pure red cell aplasia can be performed on peripheral blood. A more recent discovery is that clonal abnormalities of hematopoiesis can be identified on peripheral blood molecular testing, particularly in the elderly (Chapter 142).[1] It is possible that such testing may obviate the need for bone marrow examination in certain selected populations.[2]

TABLE 144-6 INITIAL ASSESSMENT OF ANEMIA

INPATIENT/HOSPITAL-BASED CLINIC SETTING*
History and physical examination
Complete blood counts with indices
Reticulocyte count
Peripheral blood smear review
AMBULATORY CLINIC SETTING
History and physical examination
Complete blood counts with indices
Reticulocyte count
Peripheral blood smear review (if/when possible)
Iron assessment for iron deficiency anemia/anemia of inflammation
Serum iron concentration
Serum total iron binding capacity and serum percent transferrin saturation
Serum ferritin concentration

*This approach would also apply in an ambulatory setting with in-office laboratory capacity.

Initial Laboratory Approach to Anemia

The traditional approach to the evaluation of anemia has been to obtain a complete blood count with indices and reticulocyte count, categorize the anemia on that basis, and then proceed with specific testing indicated by reticulocyte count and MCV, informed by the findings on history and physical examination and review of the blood smear. This is an appropriate and intellectually valid approach at any time, but particularly in the inpatient or hospital-based clinic settings. In the ambulatory practice environment for many internists, third-party payers may mandate that laboratory studies be sent to outside reference laboratories. The consequence of such policies is that blood count and reticulocyte count results may not be available on the day of the visit, and personal review of the blood smear may be challenging. In such a practice environment, it is reasonable to include an assessment of iron status in the initial laboratory evaluation of anemia. Iron deficiency anemia and the anemia of inflammation (also called anemia of chronic disease)[3] can both be diagnosed by these tests and are the two most common etiologies of anemia (Chapter 145). Although iron deficiency anemia is more likely to be microcytic and anemia of inflammation is more likely to be normocytic, both of these syndromes can be either microcytic or normocytic; therefore, it is likely that iron testing will be needed in nearly all circumstances not associated with an elevated reticulocyte response. This approach is outlined in Table 144-6.

ANEMIAS ASSOCIATED WITH INCREASED RETICULOCYTE PRODUCTION

Anemia associated with increased reticulocyte production after adjustment for anemia suggests the presence of either blood loss or hemolysis (Fig. 144-2). In certain situations, bleeding or hemolysis may not be associated with an appropriate reticulocyte response; these situations typically indicate some concurrent restriction on red cell production such as iron or folate deficiency.

ANEMIA DUE TO BLOOD LOSS

The symptoms of acute blood loss are dependent on the rapidity and volume of blood loss and secondarily on the site of blood loss. They are heavily influenced by effects of hypovolemia. Hypovolemia and loss of the oxygen-carrying capacity of red cells may impair oxygen delivery to tissues.

In the initial setting of acute blood loss, plasma and red cells are depleted in their same relative ratio. The result of this is that the hemoglobin concentration and hematocrit do not change acutely. As the intravascular volume is expanded, either rapidly with exogenous intravenous colloid or crystalloid in the setting of trauma, or more slowly by endogenous redistribution of plasma from the extravascular space, the hematocrit and hemoglobin concentration will begin to move downward over hours to days to reveal the true extent of loss of circulating red cell mass. In this setting, therefore, the degree of blood loss is initially underestimated by the blood counts. Further complicating the situation in the case of acute trauma is cytokine activation and the "coagulopathy of trauma." For this reason, trauma transfusion protocols have been developed in which packed red blood cells, fresh frozen plasma, and platelet concentrate are administered in specific ratios in order to return as quickly as possible to the physiologic state.[4]

Clinical findings vary with the volume and site of blood loss. Bleeding into the gastrointestinal tract can lead to hematemesis, melena, and/or hematochezia, depending on the location and rate of bleeding. The serum blood urea nitrogen (BUN) concentration will rise out of proportion to the creatinine level even with relatively modest gastrointestinal bleeding due to the breakdown and absorption of hemoglobin protein. When a patient has a large hematoma, whether intracavitary or between tissue planes, hyperbilirubinemia and occasionally clinically apparent jaundice, as well as some rise in BUN, may occur as the extravascular hemoglobin breaks down. Bleeding may be associated with reactive thrombocytosis and occasionally leukocytosis.

The management of massive blood loss is by transfusion (Chapter 162) and correction of the cause of bleeding. In smaller-volume acute blood loss, where the hemoglobin concentration comes to equilibrium at a point that does not impair oxygen delivery in that specific patient, patients may be allowed to recover on their own, mobilizing their own iron stores. When there is concern about adequate iron stores, iron replacement can be given.

Chronic blood loss is rarely at a level that produces acute volume shifts and the dramatic symptomatology of acute blood loss. The reticulocyte count remains appropriately elevated until iron becomes depleted by its utilization for increased erythropoiesis, at which time the reticulocyte response decreases and the hemoglobin concentration and hematocrit begin to drift downward. The decline in MCV begins shortly after the hemoglobin concentration and hematocrit fall below the normal range.

ANEMIA DUE TO HEMOLYSIS

Hemolysis (Chapters 146 to 149) indicates a reduction in the survival of red cells in the circulation from increased red cell destruction. Some reduction in red cell survival is an element in many hematologic syndromes, including the anemia observed with chronic kidney disease, the anemia seen with inflammation, and the anemia seen with liver disease (distinct from spur cell anemia). Microangiopathic hemolytic morphology is occasionally seen in disseminated intravascular coagulation.

Certain laboratory studies raise suspicion of a hemolytic anemia and some confirm it (Table 144-7). These are not specific to any etiology of hemolytic anemia. The distinction between extravascular hemolysis (which includes hemolysis in the spleen) and intravascular hemolysis is helpful in understanding these disorders at the pathophysiologic level. However, it is not absolute in terms of diagnostic testing. While the haptoglobin tends to become lower in intravascular hemolysis, it is generally decreased in extravascular hemolysis also. Hemoglobinemia and hemoglobinuria are specific for intravascular hemolysis.

The causes of hemolysis (Table 144-8) can be grouped using a classification that separates etiologies that are (1) entirely external to the red cell (e.g., immunologic, mechanical, or toxic processes); (2) defects that are intrinsic to the red cell membrane (e.g., hereditary spherocytosis or spur cell anemia), and (3) processes primarily related to red cell metabolism or to abnormalities of hemoglobin. The enzymatic defects producing hemolysis are typically related to oxidative metabolism and particularly to oxidative stress, such as that induced by medications.

The approach to the diagnosis of the various classes of hemolytic anemia syndromes (Fig. 144-2) begins with the examination of the peripheral smear. Identification of the characteristic microangiopathic changes of thrombotic thrombocytopenic purpura immediately provides direction to life-saving therapy. Similarly, congenital defects in the intrinsic proteins of the red cell membrane produce specific morphologic features, which can lead rapidly to a confirmable diagnosis. If the morphology on the peripheral blood smear is normal or shows only a small number of spherocytes, then evaluation for an immunologic etiology of hemolysis should be pursued. In general, autoimmune hemolytic anemia is associated with an abnormal direct antiglobulin (Coombs) test. In individuals with a previous transfusion history or a history of pregnancy in which fetal-maternal transfusion may have occurred, the possibility of other immune hemolytic mechanisms arises, and an antibody screen (also called the indirect antiglobulin test) should be ordered. If negative, metabolic or toxic causes of hemolysis should be considered.

Sustained hemolysis of any etiology creates an increased demand for folic acid, and it is reasonable to supplement individuals with chronic hemolysis with folate (1 mg/day). In countries that do not routinely fortify food with folic acid, a higher level of supplementation may be needed. During pregnancy, when folate demands are increased, a higher level of supplementation than the recommended 0.8 mg/day is reasonable for individuals with chronic hemolysis. Hemolysis that is primarily extravascular is generally not associated with increased iron demands, because the hemoglobin iron from the hemolyzed red cells is recycled in the reticuloendothelial system. In intravascular hemolysis, the haptoglobin/hemopexin system for recycling heme iron is readily overwhelmed and iron supplementation may be necessary.

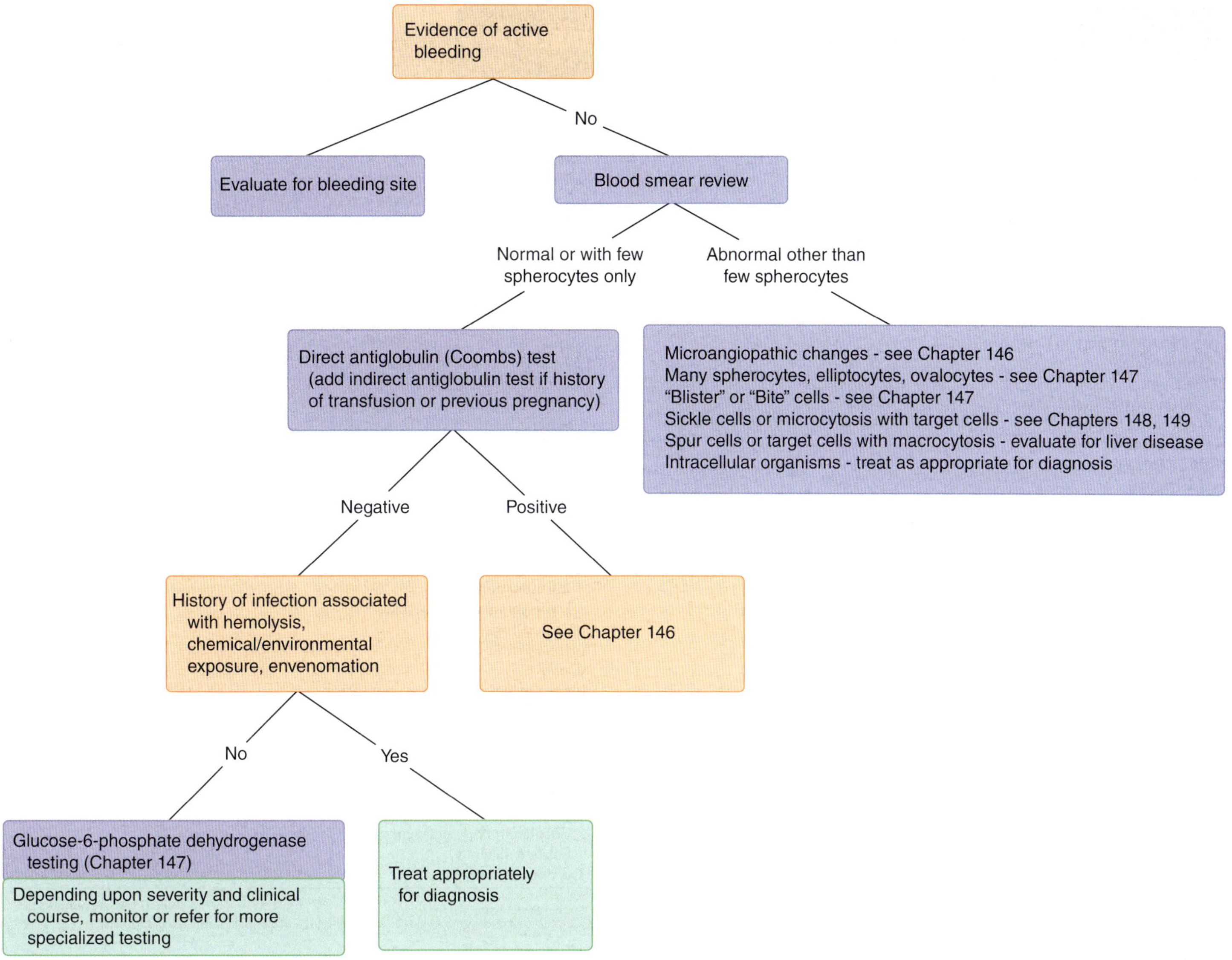

FIGURE 144-2. **Approach to the workup of hemolysis, beginning with examination of the peripheral blood smear.** (See Chapter 143.)

TABLE 144-7 GENERAL LABORATORY FINDINGS IN HEMOLYTIC ANEMIA

FINDINGS SUGGESTIVE OF HEMOLYSIS
Peripheral blood smear
Polychromasia
Abnormal red cell morphology
Elevated reticulocyte count (adjusted for anemia)
Elevated serum bilirubin (indirect/unconjugated)
Elevated serum lactate dehydrogenase
Slightly elevated serum aspartate aminotransferase
FINDINGS CONFIRMATORY OF HEMOLYSIS
Decreased serum haptoglobin (lower in intravascular hemolysis)
Increased plasma hemoglobin
Increased urobilinogen
Hemoglobinuria (intravascular hemolysis)
Hemosiderinuria (intravascular hemolysis; chronic or recurrent)

ANEMIAS ASSOCIATED WITH INADEQUATE RETICULOCYTE RESPONSE (UNDERPRODUCTION ANEMIAS)

The vast majority of anemias seen in adults are associated with decreased red cell production. A useful approach to the evaluation of these anemias is to classify them by MCV as microcytic, normocytic, or macrocytic (Table 144-9 and Fig. 144-3). A limitation to this approach is that the MCV used in defining this model was based on examination of the blood smear and not necessarily on the measured MCV value provided by the electronic cell counter. The dimorphic population of microcytic and normocytic red cells seen in sideroblastic anemia has already been mentioned. In the presence of concurrent inflammation or of elevated serum immunoglobulin (whether polyclonal or monoclonal), stacking of red cells ("rouleaux formation") as they pass through the aperture of the counter may artifactually elevate the measured MCV.

MICROCYTIC ANEMIAS

Microcytic anemias (Chapter 145) share the common pathogenesis of defective cellular hemoglobin synthesis. These defects may be at the globin level, as in the hemoglobinopathies and thalassemia, or may affect synthesis of the heme moiety. Lead poisoning suppresses ferrochelatase, interfering with synthesis of the heme porphyrin ring. Anemia of inflammation (anemia of chronic disease) is typically normocytic but may be associated with a slight reduction in MCV. In general, an MCV less than 75 fL would not be seen in the anemia of inflammation. The lowest MCVs will be seen in the hemoglobinopathies and thalassemias. A normal RDW in microcytic anemia is more likely to represent a hemoglobinopathy or thalassemia rather than iron deficiency.

MACROCYTIC ANEMIAS

Macrocytic anemias (Chapters 150, 151, and 167) represent a variety of diagnoses and pathophysiologic mechanisms. Inflammation or hypergammaglobulinemia can produce a laboratory artifact resulting in an elevated reported MCV. The elevated MCV in reticulocytosis is not an artifact because reticulocytes are larger than mature red cells. Liver disease or alcohol use are frequently associated with a mildly macrocytic anemia due to changes in red cell membrane lipids. Although the anemia of hypothyroidism is most commonly associated with a normal MCV, macrocytosis is

TABLE 144-8 ETIOLOGIES OF HEMOLYTIC ANEMIA

EXTERNAL TO RED BLOOD CELL
Hypersplenism
Immunologic
Autoimmune
Alloimmune
Microangiopathic
Thrombotic microangiopathy
Thrombotic thrombocytopenic purpura
Hemolytic uremic syndrome (typical/atypical)
Mechanical fragmentation
Valvular heart disease (native and prosthetic)
Foot-strike hemolysis (march hemoglobinuria)
Malignant hypertension
Giant hemangioma/Kasabach-Merritt
Thermal injury
Infections
Malaria (blackwater fever)
Clostridial sepsis
Babesiosis
Toxic/Metabolic
Chemical
Arsine
Copper
Lead
Venoms
Snake bite
Spider bite (brown recluse)
MEMBRANE DEFECT
Acquired
Paroxysmal nocturnal hemoglobinuria
Spur cell anemia
Congenital
Red cell membrane protein defect
Hereditary spherocytosis, similar disorders
INTERNAL DEFECT
Hemoglobinopathy
Sickle hemoglobin syndromes
Other hemoglobinopathy syndromes
Thalassemia syndromes
Red cell metabolic abnormalities
Glucose-6-phosphate dehydrogenase deficiency, similar disorders
Hypophosphatemia (acquired)

TABLE 144-9 CLASSIFICATION OF ANEMIA BY MEAN CORPUSCULAR VOLUME (MCV)

MICROCYTIC: DEFECTS IN CELLULAR HEMOGLOBIN SYNTHESIS
Iron deficiency anemia
Hemoglobinopathy*
Thalassemia
Sideroblastic anemia (congenital)
Anemia of inflammation (some cases)
Lead poisoning
NORMOCYTIC
Iron deficiency anemia (early)
Sickle cell anemia—homozygous or sickle cell trait
Anemia of inflammation (most cases)
Unexplained anemia of the elderly
Anemia of chronic kidney disease
Physiologic anemia of pregnancy
Anemia of endocrine deficiency
Hypothyroidism—most cases
Adrenal insufficiency
Androgen deficiency
Myelodysplastic syndrome
Marrow replacement
Pure red cell aplasia
Aplastic anemia (many cases)
MACROCYTIC
Laboratory artifacts
Inflammation
Hypergammaglobulinemia
Reticulocytosis
Anemia of liver disease
Alcohol
Anemia of hypothyroidism (some cases)
Copper deficiency
Primary marrow failure
Diamond Blackfan anemia
Myelodysplastic syndrome (including acquired sideroblastic anemia)
Aplastic anemia (some cases)
Megaloblastic anemia
Cobalamin (B_{12}) deficiency
Folate deficiency
Hydroxyurea therapy

*Homozygous sickle cell anemia (SS), sickle cell trait (AS), and hemoglobin C trait are normocytic. Compound heterozygote sickle cell syndromes like sickle-thalassemia are microcytic.

sometimes reported, and it is frequently classified as a macrocytic anemia. The syndromes outlined earlier are usually associated with an MCV less than 105 to 115 fL.

Other macrocytic anemias result from impaired DNA synthesis. These disorders include the classic megaloblastic anemias from cobalamin (B_{12}) and folate deficiency as well as primary marrow failure disorders such as the myelodysplastic syndromes and Diamond Blackfan anemia. These causes of anemia are frequently associated with abnormalities of other cell lineages. The myelosuppressive agent hydroxyurea also produces striking macrocytosis as part of its expected effect. In primary marrow failure disorders, the MCV is typically less than 110 fL. Megaloblastic anemia may be associated with extremely elevated MCV: as the MCV rises above 115 fL, the likelihood of cobalamin or folate deficiency increases. Hydroxyurea can produce elevated MCV in a similar range. Copper deficiency may be confused with cobalamin deficiency because it also is associated with neurologic findings, but the MCV is typically less than 110 fL.

NORMOCYTIC ANEMIAS

Normocytic anemias also represent a mixed group of disorders. In some cases, they are caused by a primary marrow failure state, as in pure red cell aplasia or aplastic anemia. In most other circumstances, they represent anemia associated with another systemic disorder.[5]

Iron deficiency anemia in its early stages, like the anemia of acute blood loss, is associated with a normal MCV. After iron stores are depleted, a process of iron-depleted erythropoiesis begins. As the red cells produced under these conditions become a larger proportion of the total red cell population, the MCV begins to decline. The anemia of inflammation[6] (Chapter 145) is likely the most common normocytic anemia syndrome after acute blood loss or early iron deficiency.

Myelodysplastic syndromes and other primary bone marrow failure disorders can be normocytic in many cases. Pure red cell aplasia presents as an isolated normochromic normocytic anemia with striking reticulocytopenia. In patients with isolated anemia and a reticulocyte count of 0.1% or less or an absolute reticulocyte count less than 10,000/μL, a bone marrow examination should be performed to evaluate for this diagnosis.

SPECIFIC ANEMIA SYNDROMES

ANEMIA OF CHRONIC KIDNEY DISEASE

Anemia is almost invariable in significant renal insufficiency, beginning when the estimated glomerular filtration rate (eGFR) falls below 45 mL/min/1.73 m^2 body surface area. Anemia is a less frequent complication of polycystic kidney disease because of secretion of erythropoietin by the cysts.

The major pathogenetic factor in the anemia of chronic kidney disease is erythropoietin deficiency. The use of recombinant erythropoietin (erythropoiesis-stimulating agents) has substantially mitigated this problem, although even in the erythropoietin era 48% of predialysis patients and 28% of hemodialysis patients have hematocrit values <30%. Other mechanisms contributing to the anemia of kidney disease are suppression of the erythroid progenitor response to anemia and shortened red cell survival. Shortened red cell survival has a number of proposed mechanisms, including decreased ability to regulate cellular oxidative stress, effects of toxic metabolites accumulated in uremia, and membrane lipid peroxidation.

Red cells are normocytic and normochromic. Echinocytes ("burr cells") are sometimes present. The reticulocyte count is decreased for the degree of anemia. Erythropoietin concentrations are generally not helpful in making a diagnosis because the usual feedback relationship between hemoglobin concentration/hematocrit and erythropoietin secretion is lost. eGFR <45 mL/min/

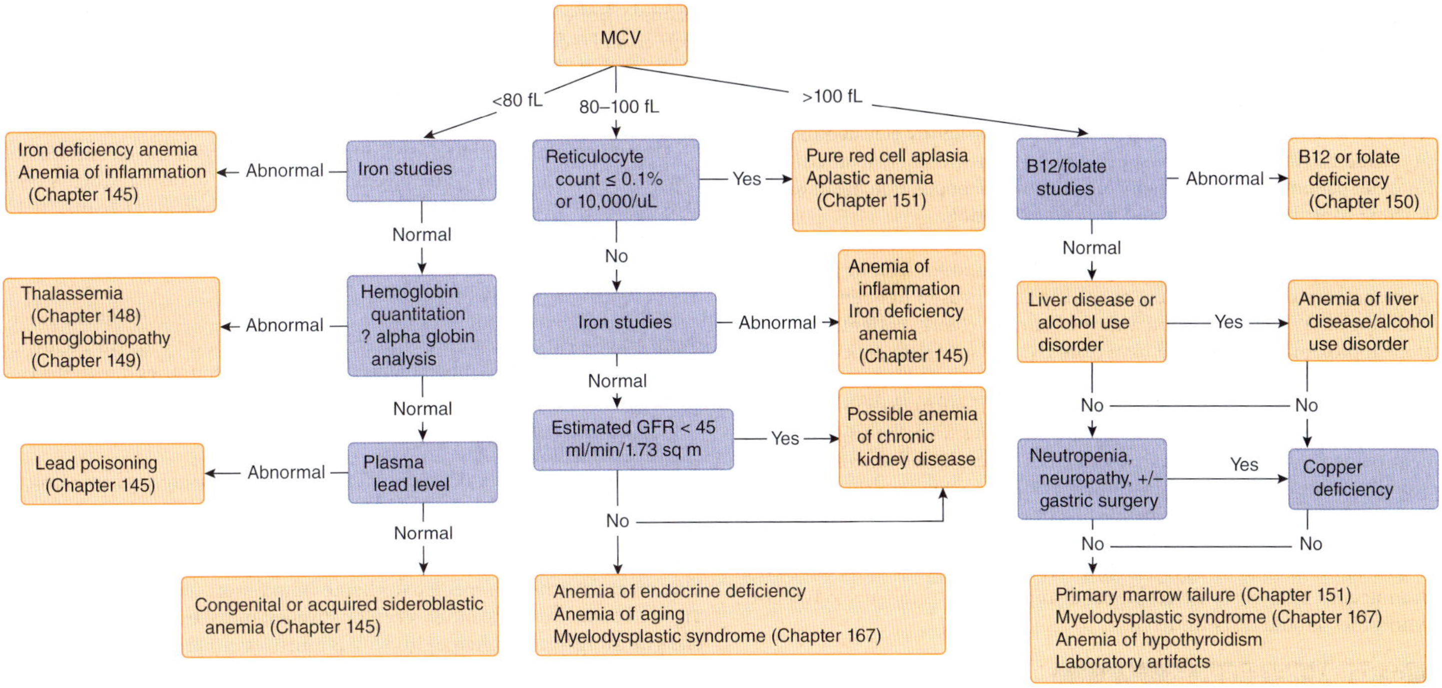

FIGURE 144-3. Approach to anemia based on the mean corpuscular volume (MCV). GFR = glomerular filtration rate.

1.73 m^2 surface area is the principal "permissive" condition for anemia of chronic kidney disease.

TREATMENT

The anemia of chronic kidney disease (Chapter 116 and 117) is treated with recombinant erythropoietin or an erythropoietin analog aiming for a hemoglobin level of 9 to 11 g/dL.[A1,A2] Daprodustat, which is an oral inhibitor of hypoxia-inducible factor prolyl hydroxylase and which stimulates erythropoiesis and regulates iron metabolism, is approved by the U.S. Food and Drug Administration (FDA) for patients who are on dialysis.[A3] To avoid the adverse complications of overcorrection or even just correction to normal with erythropoiesis-stimulating agents (such as seizures, accelerated hypertension, or thrombosis), treatment is not started until the hemoglobin concentration is less than 9 g/dL, and is suspended when the hemoglobin target of 9 to 11 g/dL is reached.[7] Iron supplementation should be considered when the transferrin saturation is less than 30% or serum ferritin concentration is less than 500 ng/mL. Hepcidin effects impair iron absorption in renal failure,[8] and intravenous iron is more effective for supplementation than is oral iron.[9] Resistance to erythropoietin therapy most commonly reflects iron deficiency or concurrent inflammation; folate deficiency may also contribute to erythropoietin resistance.

ANEMIA OF LIVER DISEASE

The majority of patients with chronic liver disease are mildly anemic.[10] Total blood volume in cirrhosis and other chronic liver diseases is typically increased 10 to 15%, but may be expanded as much as 30%. Dilution of the red cell mass by expanded plasma volume is a major element in the anemia of liver disease.

The hemoglobin concentration is typically 10 to 12 g/dL in cirrhosis. Red cells are generally macrocytic with an average MCV of 107 fL. Chronic alcohol abuse or even binges of alcohol consumption without established liver disease also cause mild macrocytosis, although the MCV remains generally less than 105 fL. Although alcohol abusers are at increased risk for dietary folate deficiency, folate deficiency typically is not the cause of these changes. Target cells may be present. Target cells in liver disease have an increased diameter that distinguishes them from the microcytic target cells of hemoglobinopathies or thalassemia. The reticulocyte count is generally near the appropriate level for the degree of anemia. Marked reticulocytosis may be seen with spur cell anemia or when recovering from heavy acute alcohol ingestion.

The major pathogenetic factor in the anemia of liver disease is shortened red cell survival. Many mechanisms contribute, with abnormalities in the lipid composition of the red cell membrane likely the most important. Splenic sequestration or abnormalities of oxidative metabolism may also contribute. Other factors that may contribute include suppression of erythroid progenitors by alcohol, dietary folate deficiency, or gastrointestinal blood loss and possible iron deficiency. Spur cell anemia, a morphologically distinctive consequence of abnormal red cell lipid composition in liver disease, may be associated with striking reticulocytosis. Greater than 5% spur cells in the red cell population is associated with decreased survival in liver disease.

Specific treatment of uncomplicated anemia of liver disease is not required, beyond encouraging good nutrition and alcohol abstinence. Patients should be evaluated for concurrent blood loss and iron or folate deficiency.

ANEMIA OF ENDOCRINE DEFICIENCY

Anemia in endocrine deficiencies such as hypothyroidism and adrenal or androgen insufficiency is "adaptive" in a sense, since it reflects an adjustment to downregulated basal metabolism. The degree of anemia is typically mild to moderate and of itself rarely causes symptomatology. These diagnoses should be considered after more significant etiologies of anemia such as iron deficiency or renal insufficiency have been ruled out. Less than one-third of cases of anemia in hypothyroidism are macrocytic; otherwise, anemia in endocrine deficiency is normocytic. Anemia in adrenal insufficiency may be masked by volume contraction. Anemia may be the only finding in androgen deficiency. Treatment of the underlying deficiency corrects the anemia of endocrine deficiency.

PHYSIOLOGIC ANEMIA OF PREGNANCY

A decrease in the hemoglobin concentration is a normal feature of pregnancy. Beginning around the seventh week of pregnancy, the red cell mass begins to expand up to 15 to 25% above prepregnancy baseline. At roughly the same time, the plasma volume begins to expand disproportionately, ultimately reaching 40 to 50% above baseline during weeks 16 to 24.[11] This dilutional anemia with increased red cell mass is referred to as "physiologic anemia of pregnancy." Normocytic anemia with a hemoglobin concentration greater than 11 g/dL in the late first trimester or 10 g/dL in the second and third trimesters of an uncomplicated pregnancy can be attributed to the physiologic anemia of pregnancy without further testing. Lower hemoglobin concentrations or microcytic or macrocytic anemia require evaluation. The mostly likely contributors to anemia in pregnancy are iron deficiency or folate deficiency, demand for both of which is increased during pregnancy. In the absence of a preexisting deficiency or an increased demand induced by hemolysis, the 0.8-mg daily folate dose recommended for neural tube defect prophylaxis is sufficient to avoid folate deficiency during pregnancy in countries where food fortification with folate is standard. Higher doses may be required in other circumstances.[A4] Although routine iron supplementation during pregnancy is generally not recommended in guidelines, it is quite common in the United States; such patients have a lower likelihood of developing iron deficiency in pregnancy or postpartum.

ANEMIA OF AGING

The frequency of anemia in both men and women increases after the age of 50. By age 65, roughly 10% of men and women are anemic. The prevalence of anemia is three- to four-fold increased in African Americans over 65 compared to persons of White European ancestry but only slightly elevated in Latino populations. However, gender-specific mean hemoglobin/hematocrit values for older patients are nearly identical to the overall population mean values.[12] Anemia contributes to frailty and morbidity in aging.

The increased frequency of anemia with aging in part reflects age-related declines in renal function, gastric acidity (required for iron or B_{12} absorption), and testosterone in men, as well as an increased frequency of other pathology.[13] When large populations of anemic elderly patients are evaluated, approximately one third have iron, B_{12}, and/or folate deficiency (with iron deficiency predominant); one third have anemia of inflammation and/or anemia of chronic kidney disease (with anemia of inflammation three times more frequent); and one third have other etiologies, with the largest component being normocytic anemia described as "unexplained anemia of aging." Studies of this entity suggest that it is a cytokine/hepcidin-driven analog of the anemia of inflammation/anemia of chronic disease. Specific treatment is not required. In elderly individuals with persistent unexplained anemia and abnormalities in other lineages or mild macrocytosis, bone marrow examination or molecular analysis to detect clonal disorders such as the myelodysplastic syndromes should be considered.

GENERAL REFERENCES

For the General References and other additional features, please visit Elsevier eBooks+ at https://ebooks.health.elsevier.com.

Grade A References

A1. Hayashi T, Maruyama S, Nangaku M, et al. Darbepoetin Alfa in patients with advanced CKD without diabetes: randomized, controlled trial. *Clin J Am Soc Nephrol.* 2020;15:608-615.

A2. Mohamed MMG, Oyenuga M, Shaikh S, et al. Hypoxia inducible factor-prolyl hydroxylase inhibitors in anemic patients with non-dialysis dependent chronic kidney disease: a meta-analysis of randomized clinical trials. *Int Urol Nephrol.* 2023;55:167-171.

A3. Singh AK, Cizman B, Carroll K, et al. Efficacy and safety of daprodustat for treatment of anemia of chronic kidney disease in incident dialysis patients: a randomized clinical trial. *JAMA Intern Med.* 2022;182:592-602.

A4. Obeid R, Schon C, Wilhelm M, et al. The effectiveness of daily supplementation with 400 or 800 microg/day folate in reaching protective red blood folate concentrations in non-pregnant women: a randomized trial. *Eur J Nutr.* 2018;57:1771-1780.

145 MICROCYTIC AND HYPOCHROMIC ANEMIAS

THOMAS G. DELOUGHERY

IRON DEFICIENCY

DEFINITION

Iron deficiency occurs when the body iron stores are insufficient to support iron metabolism. Iron deficiency can occur without anemia; in this setting, the lack of iron in tissues leads to fatigue, alopecia, and other symptoms. Further depletion of iron stores, however, will lead to a progressive microcytic anemia. In functional iron deficiency, iron stores are adequate, but the affected individual is unable to mobilize them to support erythropoiesis.

EPIDEMIOLOGY

In the United States, the prevalence of iron deficiency is about 1 to 2% in men but is much higher in women. Women are at greater risk for developing iron deficiency due to obligate iron losses through menstruation, with an average loss of 35 mL of blood and 16 mg of iron per menstrual period. Iron requirements in women average 1 to 3 mg per day, with higher needs for women with heavier menses. Dietary iron intake is often inadequate to maintain iron balance.[1] For example, bone marrow stores may be absent in 25% of healthy college-age women and reduced in another 33%. The average pregnancy requires 900 mg of iron stores, with requirements rising to 6 mg/day at the end of the third trimester. Furthermore, approximately 15% of women lose over 500 mL of blood at delivery, thereby adding further stress on iron stores.[2]

After menstrual blood loss, gastrointestinal bleeding is the second leading cause of iron deficiency. Some bleeding is acute, but gastrointestinal lesions also can cause gradual blood loss over long periods of time (Chapter 121). Gastrointestinal cancer, especially colon cancer but also gastric cancer, is found in up to 10% of older patients with iron deficiency anemia. Ulcers and gastritis are common nonmalignant causes of blood loss.

Iron deficiency is also seen more commonly in the elderly likely due to dietary factors in combination with chronic health conditions. The incidence of iron deficiency also is much higher in developing countries due to the lack of bioavailable dietary sources of iron.

PATHOBIOLOGY

Iron is found in a variety of foods. Meat is the richest source of heme iron, in which iron is in the ferrous form (Fe^{2+}). Iron from nonheme sources is largely in the ferric form (Fe^{3+}), which is reduced by stomach acid to the ferrous form (Fig. 145-1). In the jejunum, two receptors on the mucosal cells absorb iron. One receptor, which is specific for heme-bound iron, absorbs 30 to 40% of ingested heme iron. The other receptor, divalent metal transporter (DMT1), takes up inorganic (nonheme) iron but is much less efficient, thereby explaining the superior absorption of heme iron compared with inorganic iron. Iron is exported from the enterocyte via the transmembrane protein ferroportin (SCL40A1). Iron is subsequently delivered to plasma transferrin, which can carry up to two iron molecules and is the main transport molecule for iron. Transferrin delivers iron to the marrow, where it binds to the transferrin receptor on the red cell membrane.[3] This complex of transferrin-receptor is internalized into the cell by endocytosis. The lower pH of the endosome results in release of iron from the complex. The iron-less complex recycles to the cell surface, transferrin is released, and the cycle restarts. In a growing red cell, about 80,000 transferrin molecules bind on and off every second. Excess iron is taken to the liver, where it is stored. Ferritin, which is the storage protein for iron, consists of 24 ferritin subunits that create a shell that can store up to 4500 iron molecules. In dying red cells, iron contained in hemoglobin is reprocessed by binding to ferritin in macrophages, and it is then transferred to transferrin for recycling, either into newly developing red cells or to storage in the liver. This iron cycle is extremely efficient and loses less than 5% of iron contained in the total red cell mass.

The key protein of iron metabolism, hepcidin, controls iron absorption and the release of iron from its stores.[4] Hepcidin binds to ferroprotein, thereby leading to its degradation. When hepcidin degrades ferroprotein, iron cannot be released from the enterocyte or hepatocytes, thereby leading to both a lack of iron absorption and a halt in iron release to developing red cells. Hepcidin synthesis is upregulated not only by iron but also by inflammation. Hypoxia reduces levels of hepcidin, whereas erythropoiesis and iron deficiency increase levels of hepcidin. Rare mutations in proteins of iron absorption can lead to severe iron deficiency, but these conditions most commonly present in childhood.

The two major causes of iron deficiency are blood loss and reduced absorption of iron. Blood loss, most commonly from gynecologic or gastrointestinal sources, is the predominant cause for iron deficiency. The other mechanisms for iron deficiency are issues with the absorption of iron and the influence of iron-poor diets (Table 145-2). For example, the increasing avoidance of dietary meat is leading to an increase in iron deficiency because nonheme iron can be inadequate to maintain iron stores, especially in women. Lactovegetarians are at even higher risk.[5]

Gastrointestinal Causes

Any source of gastrointestinal bleeding (Chapter 121) can cause iron deficiency, but some gastrointestinal diseases have additional adverse effects on iron balance. For example, *Helicobacter pylori* infections can result in iron deficiency because of bleeding from ulcers (Chapter 125), but infection also results in achlorhydria, which impairs the ability to convert iron from its ferric to its ferrous form and thereby decreases the absorption of iron. *Heliobacter pylori* infections may also lead to autoimmune gastritis, which leads to iron deficiency in its early stages and to B_{12} deficiency in its later stages.

Obese patients are often iron deficient, with about 8% of obese patients having elevated hepcidin levels as a marker of reduced iron absorption. After bariatric surgery, the prevalence of iron deficiency can be as high as 50%,

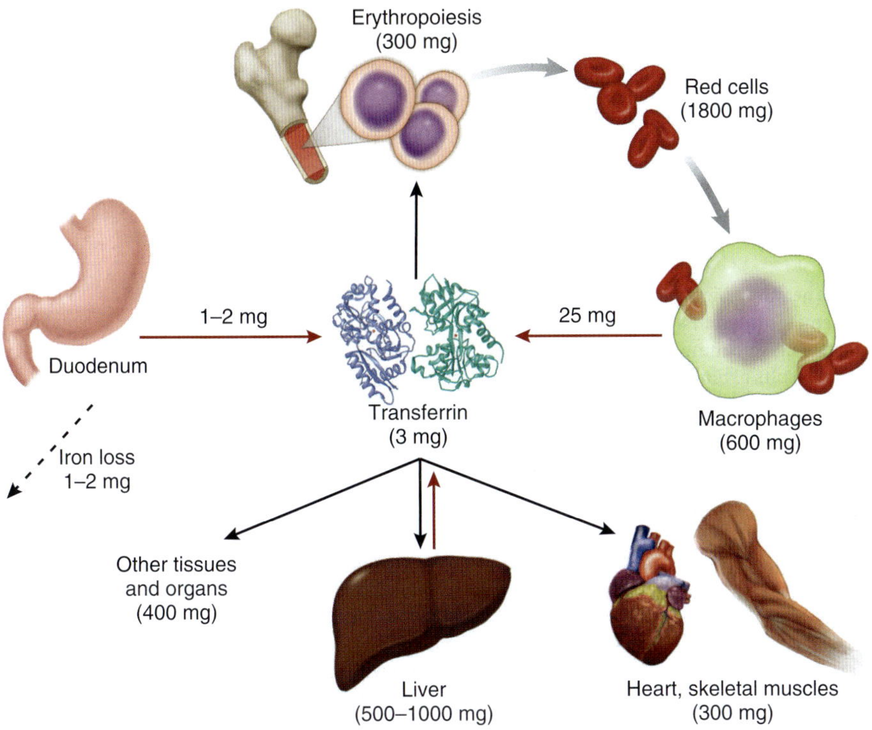

FIGURE 145-1. **Iron distribution in the body.** Schematic representation of iron distribution in the body. The iron carrier transferrin transports iron to all organs. The average content of iron in different tissues/organs for an adult male is shown in parentheses. Most iron is consumed for hemoglobin synthesis in red blood cells. Iron recycling from macrophages, which clear senescent red cells by phagocytosis, provides most usable iron. Duodenal iron absorption is limited to 1 to 2 mg daily and corresponds to the daily physiologic loss. (From Camaschella C. Microcytic and hypochromic anemias. In: Goldman L, Schafer AI, eds. *Goldman-Cecil Medicine*. 26th ed. Philadelphia: Elsevier; 2020:1035-1040.)

TABLE 145-1 MICROCYTIC HYPOCHROMIC ANEMIA

Iron deficiency
See Table 145-2
Anemia of inflammation – blocked delivery of iron to the developing red cell
Thalassemia – disruption of hemoglobin protein synthesis
Sideroblastic anemia – disruption of heme synthesis
Congenital
ALAS2 mutations
SLC25A38 mutations
GLRX5 mutations
Acquired
Myelodysplastic syndromes
Drugs/toxins
Ethanol
Isoniazid
Linezolid
Pyrazinamide
Copper deficiency

TABLE 145-2 CAUSES OF IRON DEFICIENCY

Menstrual losses
Pregnancy and delivery
Gastrointestinal causes
Cancer
Gastritis
Helicobacter pylori
Atrophic gastritis
Ulcers
Bariatric surgery
Celiac disease (even with gluten-free diet)
Hookworm and other parasites
Inflammatory bowel disease
Meckel diverticulum
Vascular malformations
Diet
Drugs
Aspirin
Nonsteroidal anti-inflammatory agents
Proton pump inhibitors
Hematuria
Athletes undergoing intense training
Obesity
Inherited defects in iron metabolism

with the prevalence increasing every subsequent year after surgery. Since the main site of gastrointestinal iron absorption is the duodenum, surgeries that bypass this part of the bowel are associated with a higher incidence of iron deficiency. For example, the risk is higher for more complex surgeries, such as the Roux-en-Y, than sleeve gastrectomy.[6]

Athletes are at risk for iron deficiency, with gastrointestinal blood loss as the major cause. Furthermore, exercise-induced hemolysis, caused by foot striking and perhaps also by intense muscle contractions, can lead to urinary losses of iron. Decreased iron absorption may also contribute because levels of hepcidin are often elevated in athletes due to training-induced inflammation.

Patients who have inflammatory bowel disease (Chapter 127) have a high prevalence of iron deficiency because bowel inflammation results in reduced absorption of iron as well as gastrointestinal blood loss. In addition, the marked inflammatory state leads to a rise in hepcidin levels, thereby blocking iron absorption. Celiac disease (Chapter 126) can also be accompanied by severe iron deficiency, owing to reduced absorption of iron, gastrointestinal blood loss, and increased hepcidin levels. Even when on a gluten-free diet, patients may not be able to absorb enough iron to avoid long-term iron deficiency.[7]

Both aspirin and nonsteroidal anti-inflammatory agents can lead to iron deficiency through overt bleeding from ulcers and/or increased subtle gastrointestinal blood loss. For example, a daily aspirin increases blood loss from 0.8 mL/day to 5.0 mL/day. Protein pump inhibitors reduce stomach acid, hinder the conversion of ferric to ferrous iron, and can lead to iron deficiency. This risk of iron deficiency is less with H_2-blockers.

Parasitic infections are a common cause of gastrointestinal blood loss in developing countries. Hookworm infections (Chapter 327) are classically associated with iron deficiency, with each worm capable of ingesting 0.5 mL of blood a day. Other parasites associated with iron deficiency are whipworm (Chapter 327) and schistosomiasis (Chapter 326).

Other Causes

Another source of blood loss is the genitourinary system. Bladder or renal lesions that result in chronic hematuria can lead to iron deficiency over time. In women, a frequent source of excess menstruation is dysfunctional uterine bleeding and fibroids (Chapter 184). In chronic hemolytic disorders (Chapters 146 and 147), ongoing hemoglobinuria can rarely result in iron deficiency.

Patients who have heart failure (Chapter 45) have an increased prevalence of both overt and functional iron deficiency, with rates of true iron deficiency as high as 13 to 42% and an even higher percentage having functional iron deficiency. In patients who are on renal dialysis (Chapter 117), blood loss with dialysis and the use of erythropoiesis-stimulating agents lead to depletion of iron stores. The effective use of erythropoiesis-stimulating agents requires efficient mobilization of stored iron, but this process can be blunted by the inflammation of renal disease.

CLINICAL MANIFESTATIONS

Because iron deficiency anemia often slowly worsens, otherwise healthy patients may tolerate marked anemia. As a result, iron deficiency anemia is often first suggested based on a complete blood count ordered for routing screening. Iron deficiency anemia is usually suspected or diagnosed from results of blood tests pointing to microcytic anemia, low serum iron, and low ferritin.[8]

Iron deficiency can lead to symptoms due to both the lack of iron itself and the resultant anemia. The most common and disabling symptom of iron deficiency anemia is fatigue, which can occur with even modest reductions in iron stores. Older patients with underlying comorbid conditions typically develop dyspnea and may even develop new onset or worsening angina.

A common complaint in iron-deficient women is hair loss, with increased loss reported in women with ferritins under 100 ng/dL. The pattern most associated with iron deficiency is diffuse nonscarring scalp alopecia (Chapter 409). Another common symptom of iron deficiency is cold intolerance, perhaps because iron is important for the effectiveness of thyroid hormone. Restless leg syndrome (Chapter 374), in which patients have leg cramps, unpleasant leg sensations, and the need to move the legs at night, is also a symptom of low iron stores.[9] Some patients report increased bruising and/or generalized pruritus. In advanced iron deficiency, patients may develop glossitis, angular stomatitis, brittle or spoon nails (koilonychia), or dysphagia due to esophageal webs (Plummer-Vinson syndrome).

Pica, which is an unusual craving for eating ice or clay, is a common symptom in patients with iron deficiency. While this overall condition is not specific for iron deficiency, the preference for eating ice may be both sensitive and specific for the condition.

DIAGNOSIS

The serum ferritin level correlates with body iron stores in healthy patients and is the most reliable and cost-effective test to diagnose iron deficiency. Since ferritin is an acute phase reactant, an iron-replete patient may have a very high ferritin level, but it is rare for an iron-deficient patient to have a ferritin level over 100 ng/mL. A ferritin level of less than 15 ng/mL is very specific for iron deficiency, but iron deficiency cannot be excluded in older patients or in patients who have inflammatory conditions unless the ferritin level is greater than 100 ng/mL. Ferritin values under 50 ng/mL should be considered abnormal in a symptomatic patient.

The anemia of iron deficiency is classically a microcytic anemia (Table 145-1) without reticulocytosis (Fig. 145-2), but these findings are neither sensitive nor specific (Table 145-3) since thalassemia and the anemia of inflammation (Chapter 144) can also lead to microcytosis. A low red cell mean corpuscular volume is generally a late finding seen with severe iron deficiency, but concurrent medical issues such as liver disease, folate deficiency, or B_{12} deficiency (Chapter 144) may blunt or obscure the decrease in red cell size.

A serum iron level is not effective as a diagnostic test since it is low in the anemia of inflammation, can be falsely elevated with oral iron intake in iron-deficient patients, and varies markedly from day to day. An elevated total iron binding capacity (TIBC) is specific for iron deficiency, but its sensitivity is low because it is reduced by inflammation, aging, and poor nutrition. Iron saturation percentages are also unreliable because they depend on both the TIBC and serum iron level, so saturation is also low in the anemia of chronic disease. Serum levels of soluble transferrin receptor are increased in iron deficiency, and levels also can be increased in any condition associated with increased red cell mass, such as in hemolytic anemias. The gold standard for iron deficiency is the bone marrow iron stain, but this invasive and expensive procedure is rarely, if ever, indicated.

Determining the Underlying Cause

A priority in care of the patient with iron deficiency is determining the cause. Given that the body has no natural mechanisms for eliminating iron, blood loss must always be assumed.[10] Testing of the stool for blood can identify patients with blood loss; however, most stool tests require 10 mL or more of daily blood loss to be positive, and losses less than 10 mL/day can still lead to iron deficiency. Because of this limitation, any man with unexplained iron deficiency or any iron-deficient woman over age 40 years should undergo both upper and lower gastrointestinal endoscopy to evaluate for occult blood loss (see Fig. 121-6). In problematic cases, capsule endoscopy may be required (Chapter 121).[11] Premenopausal women over age 40 years should also undergo testing, as should any person with gastrointestinal symptoms, family history of colon cancer, weight loss, or blood in the stool. A thorough menstrual history should be also obtained. A urinalysis is important, although occult hematuria is rarely persistent enough to lead to iron deficiency.

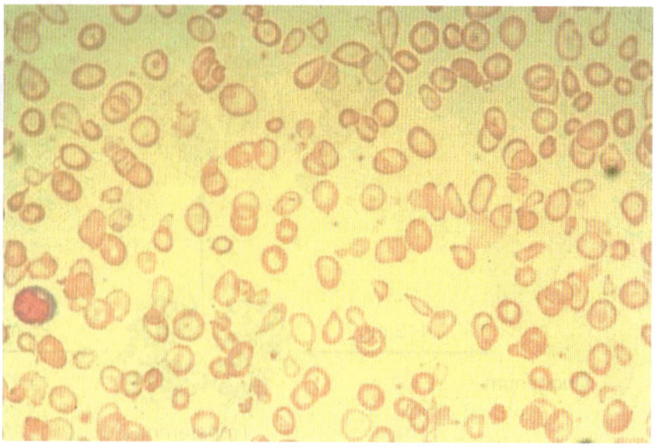

FIGURE 145-2. Microcytic hypochromic blood smear.

Differential Diagnosis

Iron deficiency anemia must be distinguished from α- or ß-thalassemia, in which serum iron and serum ferritin levels are normal or high. A low serum iron level with a high ferritin level is typical of the anemia of chronic inflammation, in which serum hepcidin levels are normal or high, and inflammatory markers such as the erythrocyte sedimentation rate and the C-reactive protein level are usually elevated. Sideroblastic anemia is associated with iron overload and an increased ferritin level; it can be confirmed by finding ringed sideroblasts on bone marrow smears.

TREATMENT

Repletion of iron can ameliorate symptoms of iron deficiency and restore a normal red blood cell mass. Eating a diet higher in bioavailable iron can help treat iron deficiency[A1] and can maintain iron stores, but even the best diet alone is usually inadequate to replete iron stores. Meat is the food that is richest in iron due to its heme iron. Cooking with iron skillets can also increase dietary iron, but the amount of iron enrichment is variable.

Oral Iron Supplementation

Ferrous sulfate (325 mg once daily) is effective for patients without conditions that preclude oral therapy. However, lower doses (15 to 20 mg of elemental iron daily) can be as effective and are better tolerated with fewer gastrointestinal side effects.[12]

Multiple oral iron preparations exist (Table 145-4), and no one compound appears to be superior to another.[A2] If ferrous sulfate is not tolerated, then ferrous gluconate, which has less elemental iron per tablet, can be tried.

The iron supplement is best taken on an empty stomach or with meat protein (cow, pork, and fish) to increase its absorption. Vitamin C may also increase the absorption of iron, whereas concomitant calcium and fiber can decrease its absorption. Tea, which is a potent inhibitor of iron absorption, can reduce absorption by 90%. Coffee also decreases iron absorption by about 60%.

With oral supplementation, the reticulocyte count should rise within 1 week, and hemoglobin concentration should start rising by the second week of therapy. Iron should be continued until iron stores are replete, with a goal ferritin level of 50 to 100 ng/dL.

Gastrointestinal side effects of oral iron are common, with 30 to 50% of patients reporting symptoms that may be related to esophageal erosions and gastritis. The side effects of stomach pain and constipation can hinder compliance. Taking a smaller dose of elemental iron and even decreasing to every other day can maintain effectiveness[A3] while reducing these symptoms. In patients whose iron deficiency does not respond to oral iron, adherence to and tolerability of oral iron should be assessed. Conditions to consider include celiac disease (Chapter 126), autoimmune gastritis (Chapter 125), *Helicobacter pylori* infections, persistent menorrhagia, and ongoing gastrointestinal losses.

TABLE 145-3 DIAGNOSIS OF IRON DEFICIENCY

TEST	IRON DEFICIENCY	ANEMIA OF CHRONIC INFLAMMATION	IRON DEFICIENCY AND INFLAMMATION	SIDEROBLASTIC ANEMIA
Serum iron	Decreased	Decreased	Decreased	Often increased
Mean corpuscular volume	Decreased/Normal	Decreased/Normal	Decreased/Normal	Normal
Total iron-binding capacity	Increased	Decreased	Decreased/Normal	Normal
Saturation (%)	Decreased (usually <16%)	Decreased (usually <30%)	Decreased (usually <20%)	Increased (usually >45%)
Ferritin (μg/L)	Decreased (usually <15 ng/mL)	Increased (usually >200 ng/mL)	Decreased (usually <100 ng/mL)	Increased (usually >200 ng/mL)

TABLE 145-4 COMMONLY PREPARED IRON PREPARATIONS

AGENT	TYPICAL SINGLE DOSE
ORAL	
Ferrous sulfate	325 mg (65 mg elemental iron)
Ferrous gluconate	325 mg (35 mg elemental iron)
Iron bisglycinate	25 mg elemental iron
INTRAVENOUS	
Ferric carboxymaltose	750-1000 mg
Ferric derisomaltose	1000 mg
Ferumoxytol	510-1020 mg
Low molecular weight iron dextran	1000 mg

Intravenous Iron Therapy

Parenteral iron should be used in any iron-deficient patient who is not responding to or cannot tolerate oral iron. If the hemoglobin concentration has not responded within 2 weeks, it is unlikely the patient will respond to oral iron. In patients who have ongoing bleeding, the iron loss may be too great for oral iron to overcome. Bowel issues, such as surgical resection or inflammatory bowel disease, can also lead to resistance to oral iron. *H. pylori* infection and celiac disease lead to impaired absorption of iron. Patients with known absorption problems, such as history of bowel surgery or bariatric procedures, should preferentially receive intravenous iron. In pregnancy, intravenous iron has been shown to be superior to oral iron.[A4]

Replacement iron formulations include low molecular weight iron dextran (given as a 1000 mg single replacement dose over one hour), ferumoxytol (given as 510 mg over 15 minutes, repeated once in 3 to 8 days), ferric carboxymaltose (given as two 750 mg doses a week apart), and ferric derisomaltose (up to 1000 mg over 20 minutes). Patients who need a magnetic resonance imaging scan must inform their doctors if they received ferumoxytol because it can function as a contrast agent. With iron carboxymaltose, about 75% of recipients experience a fall in the serum phosphorus level to less than 2.0 mg/dL,[A5] and symptomatic hypophosphatemia can occur.

All intravenous iron preparations contain carbohydrates that bind the elemental iron to prevent reactions. Nevertheless, a disadvantage of intravenous iron is an infusion reaction, which is not a true allergic reaction but rather is related to the activation of complement by the labile free iron (complement activation-related pseudoallergy). Since these reactions are not allergic in nature, administering a test dose is not helpful. Rates of mild reactions are about 1 in 200, and rates of major reactions are about 1 in 200,000. Reactions that require hospitalization are very rare but can be seen with any iron product.[13] Iron infusion should be administered under the supervision of experienced clinicians who are skilled and equipped to deal with infusion reactions. All patients should be observed for 30 minutes after the infusion. Diphenhydramine premedication should be avoided because it can worsen symptoms.

In general, the infusion is stopped for mild reactions and then resumed at a slower rate once symptoms resolve. For more severe reactions, fluids (e.g., 500 mL of normal saline) and corticosteroids (e.g., 150 to 500 mg of hydrocortisone) are helpful. If patients do not respond or develop anaphylaxis (Chapter 233), they should also be treated with epinephrine intravenously (1 mL or a 1/10,000 solution) or intramuscularly (0.3 to 0.5 mL of a 1/1000 solution), oxygen, and more fluids; such patients should be transferred to an acute care setting.

Formulas that calculate the total iron deficit tend to be unreliable, so the most pragmatic approach is to use a 1000-mg replacement dose. Patients with severe iron deficiency anemia may have deficits that exceed 1 g, so a ferritin level should be checked 2 to 4 weeks after an infusion. If the ferritin is not higher than 50 ng/dL at that time, another iron dose should be given. After a patient receives intravenous iron, the ferritin should be checked every 3 to 4 months; if it falls below 50 ng/dL, the iron infusion should be repeated. Patients with ongoing gastrointestinal bleeding should have the ferritin level checked more often and may require frequent infusions.

Oral iron supplementation in iron-deficient but not anemic women (serum ferritin measurements under 50 ng/mL) improves fatigue. In patients who have heart failure, repletion of deficient iron stores can improve cardiac function and quality of life, and also to reduce hospitalization.[A6–A8] In such patients, intravenous iron replacement appears to be superior to oral replacement.[A9] In patients who have restless leg syndrome (Chapter 374) with abnormal ferritin levels, iron replacement can markedly reduce symptoms.[A10] In patients who are on hemodialysis, proactive iron treatment is preferred over reactive treatment.[A11]

PREVENTION

The recommended dietary iron intake is 8 mg/day for adults and postmenopausal women, 18 mg for premenopausal women, and 27 mg/day during pregnancy. Meats are rich in heme iron, and iron in meat is much more effectively absorbed. Nonmeat sources of iron contain less bioavailable iron, and it is difficult to ingest large enough amounts to meet iron requirements.

PROGNOSIS

The prognosis of iron deficiency is excellent once stores are replete. Some patients, especially those who have had bariatric surgery or inflammatory bowel disease, may require chronic iron infusions.

ANEMIA OF CHRONIC DISEASE (ANEMIA OF INFLAMMATION)

Any type of illness can be accompanied by an anemia that is due to direct results of the inflammatory state. Although this type of anemia especially accompanies cancer and severe infections, it is increasingly recognized as a complication of conditions such as heart failure[14] and chronic pulmonary disease.[15]

PATHOBIOLOGY

Inflammation leads to anemia by several different mechanisms.[16] Inflammatory cytokines such as interleukin (IL)-6 increase the levels of serum hepcidin, which blocks the absorption of iron. The impaired release of iron from its stores results in iron-restricted erythropoiesis. Normally, ferroportin allows export of iron from enterocytes, macrophages, and hepatocytes. However, hepcidin binds to and leads to the degradation of ferroportin, which blocks the export of iron to the blood and to developing red cells. These cytokines also suppress the production of erythropoietin, so serum erythropoietin levels will be lower than predicted for a given degree of anemia. In addition, the half-life of the red cell is shorter.

CLINICAL MANIFESTATIONS AND DIAGNOSIS

The degree of anemia varies with the degree of inflammation. Most patients will have hemoglobin concentrations in the 8 to 10 g/dL range, but concentrations can be as low as 7 g/dL. The anemia of inflammation can be microcytic, owing to the impaired delivery of iron to the developing erythrocyte, but it is rare to be less than 70 fL. The anemia can further add to the symptomatic burden of the underlying disorder.

The diagnosis is typically made by excluding other causes for the anemia (e.g., nutritional deficiencies of iron, folate, or vitamin B_{12}, multiple myeloma in older patients, bone marrow disorders) and documenting the presence of adequate iron stores (serum ferritin > 100 ng/dL). Serum levels of erythropoietin are lower than would be expected for the degree of anemia. Due to iron sequestration, the iron saturation percentage is decreased.

TREATMENT

The most effective therapy of anemia of chronic disease is treatment of the underlying disorder. Unless the patient is frankly iron deficient, patients do not benefit from either oral or intravenous iron unless they are also receiving an indicated erythropoiesis-stimulating agent. Such agents are commonly prescribed in chronic kidney disease (Chapters 116 and 117) and sometimes prescribed in cancer patients who are undergoing chemotherapy, but they are not generally used for other causes. In the future, the use of hepcidin antagonists may be of benefit.

SIDEROBLASTIC ANEMIA

The rarest cause of microcytic anemia are the sideroblastic anemias. By definition, ringed sideroblasts must be seen on bone marrow examination. Ringed sideroblasts are abnormal red cell precursors in which aggregates of iron surround the nucleus due to disruption of the synthesis of heme.[17]

Sideroblastic anemia can be acquired or inherited.[18] The most common inherited form is X-linked sideroblastic anemia due to mutations in the *ALAS2* gene. The enzyme product of this gene controls the first step in the synthesis of heme, so mutations lead to disruption of its synthesis. Rarer autosomal recessive forms include mutations in *SLC25A38*, which is needed to import the amino acid glycine that is required for the synthesis of heme, and glutaredoxin 5, which impairs *ALAS2* gene translation.

Acquired forms of sideroblastic anemia can be due to myelodysplastic syndromes (Chapter 167) or to drugs or toxins that interfere with the synthesis of heme. Implicated drugs include ethanol, isoniazid, pyrazinamide, and linezolid. Copper deficiency, either because of inadequate dietary intake or overabundant ingestion of zinc, can lead to ringed sideroblasts.[19]

CLINICAL MANIFESTATIONS AND DIAGNOSIS

Given the number of entities that can lead to sideroblastic anemia, presentations can vary. Younger patients presenting with inherited sideroblastic anemia will present with microcytic anemia. In acquired forms, red cells can range from microcytic to macrocytic, but the blood smear will show a population of microcytic red cells. In copper deficiency, patients often have neurologic manifestations such as myelopathy.

Diagnosis is made by a bone marrow examination that shows ringed sideroblasts (Fig. 145-3). Precise diagnosis can be made by use of molecular diagnostic techniques once drugs and toxins have been excluded.

TREATMENT AND PROGNOSIS

Treatment of inherited sideroblastic anemia is supportive with transfusion and management of the subsequent iron overload, although some patients will respond to high-dose vitamin B6 (pyridoxine) or to a stem cell transplant.[20] For acquired forms, discontinuation of the toxic agent is crucial and, as in the case of alcohol-induced sideroblastosis (Chapter 364), may lead to rapid resolution with adequate nutrition. For myelodysplastic syndrome (Chapter 167), treatment of the underlying marrow disease is indicated.

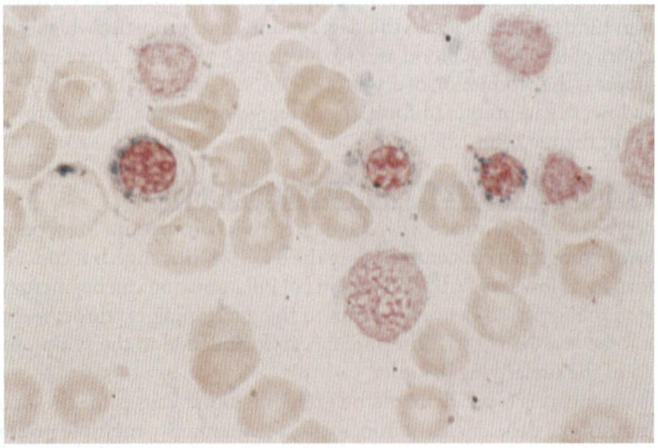

FIGURE 145-3. **Ringed sideroblasts.** Prussian blue iron stain of the bone marrow shows ringed sideroblasts, which are erythroblasts with perinuclear rings of iron-laden mitochondria. (From Camaschella C. Microcytic and hypochromic anemias. In: Goldman L, Schafer AI, eds. *Goldman-Cecil Medicine*. 26th ed. Philadelphia: Elsevier; 2020:1035-1040.)

GENERAL REFERENCES

For the General References and other additional features, please visit Elsevier eBooks+ at https://ebooks.health.elsevier.com.

Grade A References

A1. Skolmowska D, Glabska D, Kolota A, et al. Effectiveness of dietary interventions to treat iron-deficiency anemia in women: a systematic review of randomized controlled trial. *Nutrients*. 2022;14:2724.
A2. Gamad N, Saha PK, Sharma P, et al. A randomized controlled trial comparing the efficacy, tolerability, and cost of oral iron preparations in iron-deficiency anemia in pregnancy. *J Obstet Gynaecol Res*. 2021;47:3828-3841.
A3. Kaundal R, Bhatia P, Jain A, et al. Randomized controlled trial of twice-daily versus alternate-day oral iron therapy in the treatment of iron-deficiency anemia. *Ann Hematol*. 2020;99:57-63.
A4. Govindappagari S, Burwick RM. Treatment of iron deficiency anemia in pregnancy with intravenous versus oral iron: systematic review and meta-analysis. *Am J Perinatol*. 2019;36:366-376.
A5. Wolf M, Rubin J, Achebe M, et al. Effects of iron isomaltoside vs ferric carboxymaltose on hypophosphatemia in iron-deficiency anemia: two randomized clinical trials. *JAMA*. 2020;323:432-443.
A6. Jankowska EA, Kirwan BA, Kosiborod M, et al. The effect of intravenous ferric carboxymaltose on health-related quality of life in iron-deficient patients with acute heart failure: the results of the AFFIRM-AHF study. *Eur Heart J*. 2021;42:3011-3020.
A7. Van Veldhussen DJ, Ponikowski P, van der Meer P, et al. Effect of ferric carboxymaltose on exercise capacity in patients with chronic heart failure and iron deficiency. *Circulation*. 2017;136:1374-1383.
A8. Ponikowski P, Kirwan BA, Anker SD, et al. Ferric carboxymaltose for iron deficiency at discharge after acute heart failure: a multicentre, double-blind, randomised, controlled trial. *Lancet*. 2020;396:1895-1904.
A9. Mei Z, Chen J, Luo S, et al. Comparative efficacy of intravenous and oral iron supplements for the treatment of iron deficiency in patients with heart failure: a network meta-analysis of randomized controlled trials. *Pharmacol Res*. 2022;182:106345.
A10. Bae H, Cho YW, Kim KT, et al. Randomized, placebo-controlled trial of ferric carboxymaltose in restless legs syndrome patients with iron deficiency anemia. *Sleep Med*. 2021;84:179-186.
A11. Macdougall IC, White C, Anker SD, et al. Intravenous iron in pateints undergoing maintenance hemodialysis. *N Engl J Med*. 2019;380:447-458.

146

AUTOIMMUNE AND INTRAVASCULAR HEMOLYTIC ANEMIAS

MARC MICHEL

DEFINITION

Hemolytic anemia is defined as an anemia due to a shortened lifespan of mature red blood cells (RBCs) in the peripheral blood. According to the cause, hemolysis and accelerated destruction of RBCs can take place within the vasculature (intravascular hemolysis) and/or in the liver or spleen (extravascular hemolysis). Hemolytic anemia can be the consequence of an intrinsic (intracorpuscular) and often genetically determined defect of the red cell membrane or a red cell constituent (hemoglobin structure or enzyme machinery). Alternatively, hemolytic anemia can result from an extrinsic (extracorpuscular) and typically acquired abnormality that attacks the RBC's membrane (immune, infectious, toxic) (Table 146-1).

Autoimmune hemolytic anemia is a rare acquired autoimmune disease in which autoantibodies directed toward autologous red cell membrane antigens lead to their accelerated destruction.[1] The diagnosis of autoimmune hemolytic anemia is thus based on the presence of a positive direct antiglobulin (Coombs) test and on the absence of any other hereditary or acquired cause of hemolysis.[2] In autoimmune hemolytic anemia, hemolysis is mainly extravascular, but some features of concomitant intravascular hemolysis may be present at onset. In addition to autoimmune hemolytic anemia, other causes of immune-mediated hemolytic anemias that are not mediated by autoantibodies may occur, including some drug-induced hemolytic anemias or post-transfusional hemolytic reactions due to the presence of alloantibodies or to other more complex mechanisms. Paroxysmal nocturnal hemoglobinuria (PNH) is a rare and potentially life-threatening acquired clonal blood disorder with protean manifestations in which RBCs are abnormally vulnerable to activation of complement. The resulting chronic intravascular hemolysis is the hallmark of the classic hemolytic form of the disease, with the release of free hemoglobin contributing to many of its clinical manifestations.

TABLE 146-1 MAIN CAUSES OF HEMOLYTIC ANEMIAS

INTRACORPUSCULAR	EXTRACORPUSCULAR
DISORDERS OF THE RBC MEMBRANE	**IMMUNOLOGIC**
Inherited	• Autoimmune HA
• Hereditary spherocytosis	• Alloimmunization
• Hereditary elliptocytosis	• Delayed hemolytic transfusion reaction
• Hereditary stomatocytosis	• Drug-induced HA
Acquired	**MECHANICAL**
• Paroxysmal nocturnal hemoglobinuria	• Thrombotic thrombocytopenic purpura
HEMOGLOBINOPATHY	• Atypical or typical hemolytic-uremic syndrome
Qualitative defect in hemoglobin	• Other microangiopathies
• Sickle cell disease	• HELLP syndrome
• Unstable hemoglobins	• Prosthetic heart valve dysfunction (valve hemolysis)
Quantitative defect in hemoglobin	• Acanthocytosis
• β-Thalassemia	**INFECTIOUS**
• α-Thalassemia	• Malaria
RBC ENZYME ABNORMALITY	• Babesiosis, *Clostridium perfringens*, gram-positive bacteria
• G6PD deficiency	**TOXIC**
• Pyruvate kinase deficiency	• Exogenous: thermal burns; industrial copper, lead poisoning, spider bite, snake bite, mushrooms ingestion.
• Others: pyrimidine 5′ nucleotidase deficiency	• Endogenous: Wilson disease (copper overload)
	• Drug related

G6PD = glucose-6-phosphate dehydrogenase; HA = hemolytic anemia; HELLP = hemolysis, elevated liver, low platelets; RBC = red blood cell.

IMMUNE HEMOLYTIC ANEMIAS

Autoimmune Hemolytic Anemia

EPIDEMIOLOGY

Autoimmune hemolytic anemia can affect both children (mainly before the age of 5 years) and adults, and its estimated overall (not age-adjusted) annual incidence is 2.4 per 100,000 individuals.[3] In children, males tend to be more frequently affected; the female : male sex ratio is 1.5:2 in adults. Median age at onset is 58 years in adults, with more than two thirds of the patients age 40 years and above. This age distribution may be related to the increased frequency of lymphoproliferative malignancies in the elderly, with an age-related increase in secondary autoimmune hemolytic anemia due to lymphoma.

The estimated annual incidence of cold-agglutinin disease, which is a rare form of autoimmune hemolytic anemia, is 0.18/100,000. The median age at diagnosis is 67 years,[4,5] with a female prevalence.

Most cases of autoimmune hemolytic anemias occur sporadically but may be sometimes associated, mostly in children, with an underlying hereditary primary immunodeficiency. Autoimmune hemolytic anemia usually occurs as an isolated immune cytopenia but can sometimes be associated, either concomitantly or sequentially, with immune thrombocytopenia (ITP, Chapter 158) and/or autoimmune neutropenia in the setting of Evans syndrome. Among autoimmune hemolytic anemias, the so-called warm autoimmune hemolytic anemia (see Diagnosis and Classification) accounts for 70 to 80% of all cases and almost 90% of the cases in children. Paroxysmal cold hemoglobinuria is a very uncommon subtype of autoimmune hemolytic anemia seen almost exclusively in children. Autoimmune hemolytic anemia can be primary (or idiopathic) or associated with an underlying disease or condition (secondary autoimmune hemolytic anemia).

PATHOBIOLOGY

The pathogenesis of autoimmune hemolytic anemia is a complex multistep process involving not only the autoantibodies but also various effectors of the immune system, including the complement system and macrophages, as well as B and T lymphocytes.[6] Whereas the mechanisms leading to hemolysis are partially elucidated (antibody-dependent cell-mediated cytotoxicity and complement dependent cytotoxicity being primarily involved), the mechanisms leading to the breakdown of self-tolerance are far from fully understood and are mainly extrapolated from mouse models.

Immunoglobulin G (IgG) anti–red cell autoantibodies mediate the destruction of RBCs outside the circulating blood (extravascular hemolysis). In contrast, when lytic components of the complement system participate in the process, the destruction of red cells usually occurs directly within the circulation (intravascular hemolysis) and/or in the liver.[7]

In warm autoimmune hemolytic anemia, the autoantibody targeting RBCs is mainly of the IgG_1 isotype. It is able to bind to macrophage Fc gamma receptor; therefore, extravascular hemolysis takes place mainly in the reticuloendothelial system of the spleen. Autoantigens on RBC membranes targeted by autoantibody are, by decreasing frequency, (1) peptides from the Rhesus system (in approximately one third of cases); (2) band 3 protein; and (3) glycophorin A, an RBC membrane glycoprotein. In other cases, the antibodies have specificity for antigens in the Kell or Duffy blood group system and very rarely for ABO antigens. In less than 10% of the cases of warm autoimmune hemolytic anemia, no specificity can be found. In contrast to warm autoimmune hemolytic anemia, cold agglutinins are IgM autoantibodies that react at cold temperatures with polysaccharides on the red cell surface and mainly with i and I antigens and less commonly with the Pr glycoprotein and sialylated polysaccharides. Cold agglutinins associated with *Mycoplasma pneumoniae* infection have an anti-I specificity, whereas those related to infectious mononucleosis have anti-i specificity. More recently, infection with the severe acute respiratory syndrome virus coronavirus-2 (SARS-CoV2), whose protein spike shares some homology with ankyrin 3, has also been recognized as a viral trigger of autoimmune hemolytic anemia. In cold agglutinin disease, the cold agglutinins are almost always anti-I monoclonal IgM antibodies with a VH4-34 heavy chain, a heavy chain shape of the antigen-binding surface that favors attachment to polysaccharides.

DIAGNOSIS

Clinical Symptoms

The clinical symptoms of autoimmune hemolytic anemia are those of anemia (e.g., unusual fatigue, exertional dyspnea, tachycardia) and/or those due to active hemolysis (jaundice with or without dark urine, especially when there is intravascular hemolysis). In patients with high-affinity cold agglutinins, exposure to cold can also precipitate episodes of acrocyanosis by inducing massive agglutination of RBCs in the capillary circulation of the hands, feet, or even nose tip and ears. Mild splenomegaly may be present especially in warm autoimmune hemolytic anemia, whereas splenomegaly is uncommon in cold agglutinin disease unless there is an underlying B-cell lymphoma.

General Laboratory Tests

Elevated serum levels of indirect bilirubin and lactate dehydrogenase (LDH) and decreased serum haptoglobin are the usual, albeit nonspecific, features of hemolytic anemia. Laboratory signs of intravascular destruction of RBCs (hemoglobinemia, hemoglobinuria, and hemosiderinuria) are unusual in the setting of autoimmune hemolytic anemia. Once hemolytic anemia has been recognized, the diagnosis of autoimmune hemolytic anemia is usually relatively easy and based first on the identification of anti-RBC autoantibody by means of the direct antiglobulin (Coombs) test, and then on the exclusion of other causes of hemolytic anemia. A careful examination of the peripheral blood smear is essential, keeping in mind that an increase in the number of spherocytes (particularly microspherocytes) can be observed in approximately 30 to 40% of cases of autoimmune hemolytic anemias (Chapter 147).[8]

The Direct Antiglobulin (Coombs) Test

The direct antiglobulin (Coombs) test reveals antibody-coated RBCs central to the diagnosis of autoimmune hemolytic anemia. The indirect antiglobulin (Coombs) test evaluates the presence of incomplete antibodies in the patient's serum. As presently used, the standard antiglobulin reagent contains antibodies to test for the presence of all four classes of IgG and components of complement (usually C3 and C4) on standard gel tubes.

A positive direct antiglobulin test requires cautious interpretation when there are no other features of autoimmune hemolytic anemia. False-positive test results are not unusual. The reported incidence of positive antiglobulin (Coombs) tests in normal blood donors and the general populations of hospitalized patients varies widely—from 1 in 100 to 1 in 15,000. Differences in the technique used to perform the test account for this variation. The usual reason for a false-positive direct antiglobulin test is nonspecific, low-avidity adherence of serum IgG to red cells whereas some patients with systemic lupus erythematosus or B-cell lymphoid malignancies may produce true anti-RBC auto-antibodies without active hemolysis. False-negative direct antiglobulin tests in true autoimmune hemolytic anemia are rare (~5% of all autoimmune hemolytic anemias) and are usually due to low-affinity autoantibodies that spontaneously elute from the red cell surfaces in vitro, or to IgA antibodies, or to amounts of erythrocyte-coating antibodies that are below the limit of detection by the antiglobulin test. The diagnosis of direct antiglobulin test–negative autoimmune hemolytic anemia can be considered only after the exclusion of other potential causes of hereditary and acquired hemolytic anemia.

Classification of Autoimmune Hemolytic Anemia: Warm versus Cold Autoimmune Hemolytic Anemia

Once the diagnosis of autoimmune hemolytic anemia is established, classification of the type of autoimmune hemolytic anemia involved is essential.[9] According to the direct antiglobulin test pattern and the optimal temperature at which the autoantibody reacts with human RBCs, autoimmune hemolytic anemias (warm and cold) are typically subdivided into four major subtypes: warm autoimmune hemolytic anemia; cold autoimmune hemolytic anemia (including chronic cold agglutinin disease); mixed-type autoimmune hemolytic anemia; and the exceptional paroxysmal cold hemoglobinuria.[10] The great majority of cold-reactive autoantibodies are called "cold agglutinins;" cold hemolysins are much less common. A small proportion (~5%) of patients may exhibit both cold-reactive and warm-reactive autoantibodies, indicating a mixed autoimmune hemolytic anemia type. The distinction between cold autoimmune hemolytic anemia and warm autoimmune hemolytic anemia is very important because the mechanisms of RBC injury, the primary site of hemolysis, and the therapeutic approaches are different. Table 146-2 summarizes the main features of the different types of autoimmune hemolytic anemia.

In warm autoimmune hemolytic anemias, which represent 70 to 80% of all autoimmune hemolytic anemias in adults, the direct antiglobulin test pattern is either solely IgG-positive or IgG plus C_3–positive. Autoantibodies are mainly of the IgG_1 isotype, and they bind and react optimally with RBCs at a temperature of 37° C (range, 35 to 40° C). In warm autoimmune hemolytic anemia, the hemolysis is mainly extravascular and occurs predominantly in the spleen. On the other hand, in autoimmune hemolytic anemia, due to cold autoantibodies, which account for 15 to 20% of AIHAs, the usual direct antiglobulin test pattern is IgG-negative and C3-positive, and circulating cold agglutinins are detectable in the serum at a significant titer (i.e., >1/64). Cold antibodies are almost exclusively of IgM isotype, which are able to activate the classical complement pathway but are seldom found fixed on the RBC membrane in vitro as they are rapidly eluted ex vivo before the test can be performed. Cold antibodies typically react with RBCs at temperatures below 30° C (optimum, 4° C) and lead to various degrees of extravascular hemolysis, predominantly in the liver rather than the spleen. In rare cases of AIHAs (~5 to 10%) known as mixed-type AIHAs, autoantibodies (mostly of IgM isotype) can react with RBCs within a wide range of temperature (thermal amplitude from 4 to 37° C). Last, paroxysmal cold hemoglobinuria is a very uncommon AIHA subtype seen almost exclusively in children; it is due to an IgG hemolysin reacting with autologous RBCs at low temperatures (2 to 10° C) that can be detected only by means of the Donath Landsteiner test, a test available only in few referral laboratories. In addition to these four distinct subtypes of AIHAs, drug-induced hemolytic anemias must be regarded as a distinct entity (see Drug-Induced Hemolytic Anemia). Besides the distinction between warm autoimmune hemolytic anemia and cold autoimmune hemolytic anemia; autoimmune hemolytic anemias are also classified as primary (or idiopathic) or secondary, depending on the presence or absence of an underlying disease or condition promoting immune dysregulation. On average, 50 to 60% of warm autoimmune hemolytic anemias are secondary (see Table 146-3 for associated conditions) and, therefore, a minimal workup must be performed at the time of diagnosis in every patient to search for an underlying disease or condition (Table 146-4). It is important to emphasize that a presumably primary form of warm autoimmune hemolytic anemia can precede by many years the finding of a non-Hodgkin lymphoma; therefore, patients with warm autoimmune hemolytic anemia must be followed beyond remission.

Regarding autoimmune hemolytic anemias due to cold autoantibodies, in children and young adults, these are mainly secondary to either bacterial (*M. pneumoniae* infection) or viral (Ebstein-Barr virus or cytomegalovirus) infection, whereas in adults aged over 50, although rare, chronic cold agglutinin disease is by far the main cause of cold autoimmune hemolytic anemia. Although cold agglutinin disease has long been considered as a primary (i.e., idiopathic) form of autoimmune hemolytic anemia, it is now recognized that about 90% of cases of cold agglutinin disease are associated with a monoclonal

TABLE 146-2 MAIN CHARACTERISTICS OF VARIOUS TYPES OF AUTOIMMUNE HEMOLYTIC ANEMIA

AUTOIMMUNE HEMOLYTIC ANEMIA TYPE	EPIDEMIOLOGY/ TYPE OF HEMOLYSIS	RATE OF SECONDARY AUTOIMMUNE HEMOLYTIC ANEMIA	AUTOANTIBODY ISOTYPE	OPTIMAL TEMPERATURE	DIRECT ANTIGLOBULIN TEST PATTERN	ELUATE	AUTOANTIBODY SPECIFICITY (TARGETED ANTIGENS)
Warm autoimmune hemolytic anemia	~70-80% of all autoimmune hemolytic anemia Adult > children (mean age 3 years), mostly EV hemolysis, subacute onset (rarely abrupt with associated IV hemolysis)	~50% of the cases (see Table 146-3)	IgG >> IgA, IgM	37° C	IgG ± C_3	IgG	Antigens of the Rh system, band 3, glycophorin, A
Cold agglutinin syndrome	~20-30% of all autoimmune hemolytic anemia cases in adults Age >50 years EV ± IV hemolysis	Mainly secondary monoclonal IgM kappa gammopathy in 90% of the cases ± features of definite clonal B-cell lymphoproliferative disorder	IgM >>> IgA or IgG Cold agglutinins titer >1/500	4° C	C_3	negative	I antigen > i >> Pr
Cold transient autoimmune hemolytic anemia	Children, young adults IV hemolysis	Infections (*Mycoplasma pneumoniae*, Ebstein-Barr virus, etc.)	Polyclonal IgM Cold agglutinins titer ≥1/64	4° C	C_3	negative	I > i antigens
Paroxysmal cold hemoglobinuria	Children (rare), exceptional in adults Acute IV hemolysis	Infections (*Mycoplasma pneumoniae* virus)	IgG (Donath-Landsteiner hemolysin)	>30° C	C_3	negative	P + c antigens (biphasic hemolysins)
Mixed-type autoimmune hemolytic anemia	Adult Mainly EV hemolysis	Mainly B-cell lymphoma	IgG, IgM ± AF ~ 1/500	Wide range (4°-37° C)	IgG ± C_3	IgG	Polyreactivity

EV = extravascular; Ig = immunoglobulin G; IV = intravascular.

TABLE 146-3 MAIN DISORDERS OR CONDITIONS ASSOCIATED WITH WARM AUTOIMMUNE HEMOLYTIC ANEMIA

Hematologic disorders and lymphoproliferative diseases:
- Chronic lymphoid leukemia,* acute lymphoblastic leukemia,† LGL leukemia
- B-cell lymphoma,* Hodgkin lymphoma
- Angioimmunoblastic T-cell lymphoma
- Castleman disease
- Myelodysplasias, myelofibrosis

Solid tumors: thymoma/ovarian dermoid cyst/carcinoma

Autoimmune and inflammatory diseases
- Systemic lupus erythematosus, antiphospholipid syndrome
- Rheumatoid arthritis
- Ulcerative colitis, pernicious anemia/thyroiditis
- Myasthenia gravis
- Autoimmune hepatitis, giant cell hepatitis*
- Sarcoidosis
- Eosinophilic fasciitis

Infections:
- Virus: Epstein-Barr virus,* hepatitis C, cytomegalovirus, SARS-CoV-2
- Bacteria: tuberculosis/brucellosis/syphilis/babesiosis

Drugs

Primary immunodeficiencies
- Common variable immunodeficiency
- Hyper-IgM syndrome,† ALPS†
- CTLA4† or LRBA deficiency†
- IPEX syndrome,† APECED syndrome†

Others
- Pregnancy
- Postallogenic bone marrow transplantation or liver or small bowel transplant*
- Rosai-Dorfman disease

*Diseases that can also be associated with cold autoimmune hemolytic anemia.
†Seen almost exclusively in childhood.
ALPS = autoimmune lymphoproliferative syndrome; APECED = autoimmune polyendocrinopathy-candidiasis-ectodermal dystrophy; CTLA4 = cytotoxic T lymphocyte–associated protein 4; IgM = immunoglobulin M; IPEX = immune dysregulation, polyendocrinopathy, enteropathy X-linked syndrome; LGL = large granular lymphocytes; LRBA = lipopolysaccharide-responsive and beige-like anchor protein; SARS-CoV-2 = severe acute respiratory syndrome coronavirus 2.

TABLE 146-4 RECOMMENDED WORKUP IN WARM AUTOIMMUNE HEMOLYTIC ANEMIA

1. Antinuclear antibodies (± anti-DNA antibodies if ANA-positive)
2. Anticardiolipin antibodies and lupus anticoagulant*
3. Serum protein electrophoresis and immunoelectrophoresis
4. Immunophenotyping of peripheral lymphocytes (flow cytometry)
5. CT scan of the chest, abdomen, and pelvis (in the absence of obvious SLE of APS)
6. Bone marrow biopsy: recommended in the presence of hypogammaglobulinemia and/or monoclonal gammopathy and/or abnormal lymphadenopathy on the CT imaging

*Especially in case of a previous episode of venous and/or arterial thrombosis or in case of recurrent miscarriage in women and systematically before splenectomy.
ANA = antinuclear antibodies; APS = antiphospholipid syndrome; CT = computed tomography; SLE = systemic lupus erythematosus.

IgM kappa and with other features of indolent clonal B cell lymphoproliferative disorder. As a result, it must be distinguished from Waldenström macroglobulinemia (Chapter 173) or lymphoplasmacytic lymphoma in the bone marrow (Chapter 171). Hemolytic anemia is seldom very severe in the setting of cold agglutinin disease, and it is classically exacerbated by exposure to cold or infections.

DRUG-INDUCED IMMUNE HEMOLYTIC ANEMIA

There are several mechanisms by which a drug can induce hemolytic anemia, and true drug-induced autoimmune hemolytic anemias are rare. Many drugs or drug metabolites have the potential to elicit antidrug antibodies. Drugs that form covalent bonds with proteins in the red cell membrane can bind antidrug antibodies to the red cell surface, thereby causing a positive direct antiglobulin test and, in some cases, initiating antibody-mediated destruction of red cells. Other drugs, such as the cephalosporins, can bind to red cell membranes and take up IgG nonspecifically from plasma. In these cases, there is no antidrug antibody. The diagnosis of drug-induced immune-mediated hemolytic anemia should be considered if the patient has a history of taking a suspected medication, there is acute complement-mediated hemolysis, only complement components are detectable on the red cell surface, or the patient's serum reacts with red cells in the presence of the suspected drug. Some drugs can induce true autoantibodies against red cells. Fludarabine, a purine nucleoside analogue used in the treatment of chronic lymphocytic leukemia, and monoclonal antibodies against tumor necrosis factor-α (infliximab and adalimumab), T cells (alemtuzumab), α4 integrin (natalizumab), and interleukin-2 receptor (daclizumab) also have this property, the cause of which is unknown. Notably, there is no definitive way of distinguishing drug-induced autoimmune hemolytic anemia from primary autoimmune hemolytic anemia. Immune checkpoint inhibitors, mostly anti-PD1 agents but also to a lesser extent anti-PDL1 and anti-CTLA4 monoclonal antibodies, which are currently used worldwide to treat various cancers, have become an important and increasing cause of drug-induced autoimmune hemolytic anemias.

TREATMENT

Supportive Care and Transfusion

Regardless the type of autoimmune hemolytic anemia, folic acid supplementation (5 to 10 mg/day) is warranted in patients with active autoimmune hemolytic anemia and increased erythropoiesis to prevent its depletion, which may be misinterpreted as a treatment failure. RBC transfusions are also indicated in patients with disabling symptoms of anemia and/or a significant underlying cardiovascular disorder (e.g., coronary artery disease or heart failure). Although younger patients may tolerate a stable hemoglobin level as low as 6 g/dL, maintaining a hemoglobin level of at least 8 g/dL is usually recommended in patients with major comorbidities. It is important for the managing physician to understand that no patient with symptomatic autoimmune hemolytic anemia should be denied blood transfusions because of an "incompatible crossmatch." The blood bank should be informed of the patient's status. Indeed, the patient's positive direct antiglobulin test almost always interferes with compatibility testing, so the role of the blood bank is to provide packed red cells that are the least incompatible ones in regard to the specificity of the patient's autoantibody. Close communication and cooperation between the clinician and the specialist in transfusion medicine are therefore essential for reducing the risks associated with transfusion in patients with autoimmune hemolytic anemia. Because transfused RBCs can be destroyed by the patient's autoantibodies, rapid transfusion of large volumes of RBCs must be avoided because they can have serious consequences. This risk is increased if the patient also has alloantibodies induced by previous transfusions or pregnancy. Units of packed RBCs should therefore not be administered at a rate that exceeds 1 mL/kg/hour. In cold autoimmune hemolytic anemia and cold agglutinin disease, prewarmed (at a temperature close to 37° C) packed RBCs are recommended. Plasma exchange is sometimes used for patients with life-threatening autoimmune hemolytic anemia, but there is no robust evidence supporting its efficacy and safety in the literature.

In transfusion-dependent patients with inadequate reticulocytosis, the transient off-label use of an erythropoiesis-stimulating agent by specialists may provide a 70% response rate for increasing the hemoglobin level and avoiding a transfusion.[11] Plasma exchanges can be temporarily helpful in cases of severe hemolysis and/or in preparation for surgery (e.g., cardiac surgery) that requires cold exposure.[12]

Treatment of Transient (Acute) Cold Autoimmune Hemolytic Anemias

In cases of transient cold autoimmune hemolytic anemias induced by an infection, the onset is usually abrupt, and the degree of anemia may be profound and sometimes life-threatening, requiring transfusion of prewarmed packed RBCs, which must not be postponed (Fig. 146-1). In addition to supportive care, the use of antibiotics is justified in case of pneumonia due to *M. pneumoniae*. A short course of corticosteroids can sometimes be considered in case of severe cold autoimmune hemolytic anemia secondary to a viral infection (Epstein-Barr virus) in order to reduce the duration of anemia, but this practice is neither consensual nor evidence-based.

Management of Chronic Cold Agglutinin Disease

The management of cold agglutinin disease has long been only supportive and symptomatic (see Fig. 146-1). Avoidance of exposure to cold is still the mainstay in management of cold agglutinin disease, especially to avoid cold-induced circulatory symptoms, but this measure is often not sufficient to avoid episodes of hemolysis. In cases of infections and other acute phase reactions, the levels of both C3 and C4 increase due to their enhanced production, resulting in exacerbation of complement-dependent cytotoxicity directed toward autologous RBCs and increased hemolysis. Consequently, prompt treatment of febrile infections or other illnesses as well as the prevention of infection by influenza and/or pneumococcal vaccines are strongly recommended in patients

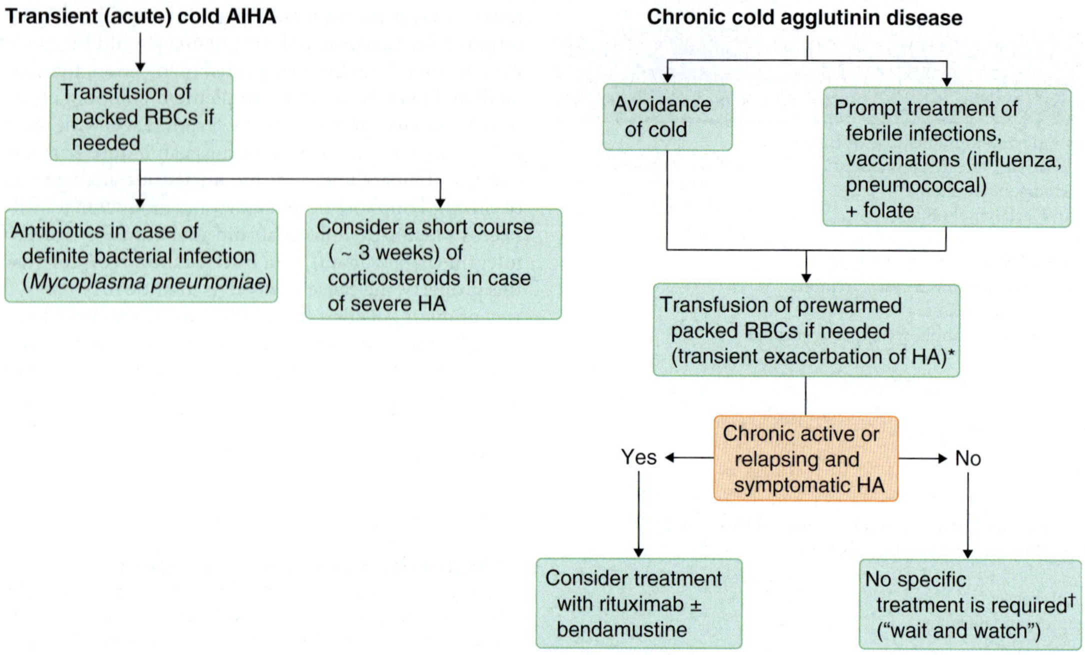

FIGURE 146-1. **Proposed algorithm for the management of cold autoimmune hemolytic anemias (AIHAs). *The transient use of erythropoiesis-stimulating agents can be considered off-label, †unless the underlying B cell–clonal lymphoproliferative disorder requires specific management. HA = hemolytic anemia; RBCs = red blood cells.**

with cold agglutinin disease. In case of exacerbation of hemolysis and severe anemia, transfusion of prewarmed packed RBCs must be considered because patients with cold agglutinin disease are often elderly with significant comorbid conditions. Whereas cold agglutinin disease is usually considered a relatively indolent and slowly progressive lymphoproliferative disorder with a relatively good prognosis, transfusion dependency may be observed in some patients with recurrent episodes of active hemolysis.

For patients with active or relapsing symptomatic episodes of cold hemolytic anemia that warrants treatment, rituximab either alone or in combination with bendamustine[A1] offers the best response rate (up to 75% response), but the toxicity of bendamustine and the increased risk of severe infection is a limitation for frail elderly patients. Another potential option for patients who require transfusions is sutimlimab,[13] which is a selective upstream inhibitor of the classical complement pathway (given at 45 to 60 mg/kg intravenously weekly for 4 weeks, then every 2 weeks).[A2] Some responses also have been reported in smaller studies with bortezomib plus dexamethasone or with ibrutinib.

In transfusion-dependent patients with normal or only slightly elevated reticulocyte counts, the transient use of an erythropoiesis-stimulating agent off-label may be useful as a transfusion-sparing strategy. Plasma exchange can be temporarily helpful in cases of severe hemolysis and/or in preparation for surgery requiring cold exposure such as lung-heart surgery.

Management of Primary Warm Autoimmune Hemolytic Anemias

First-Line Treatment: Corticosteroids

Primary warm autoimmune hemolytic anemias usually have a chronic course, and except for the few patients with mild compensated hemolysis with a normal or almost normal hemoglobin level, treatment is usually needed (Fig. 146-2). In contrast to cold agglutinin disease, corticosteroids are the cornerstone of therapy in warm autoimmune hemolytic anemias and should be given as first-line treatment. Intravenous immunoglobulin (IVIG) has only little efficacy in warm autoimmune hemolytic anemias and should be considered (at 2 g/kg over 2 days) only as potential rescue therapy for severe, transfusion-dependent autoimmune hemolytic anemia in the absence of response to corticosteroids. The corticosteroid regimen is usually based on oral prednisone or prednisolone at an initial daily dose of 1 to 2 mg/kg daily. By analogy with other autoimmune diseases, the use of intravenous methylprednisolone at a dose of 250 to 1000 mg/day for 1 to 3 days may be considered in patients with profound anemia, although no clinical trials supporting its superior efficacy are available. The starting dose of oral prednisone is usually maintained for 3 to 4 weeks and then tapered progressively if at least a partial response is achieved. There is no consensus concerning the total duration of treatment, but because the likelihood of early relapse is high when the treatment is prematurely stopped, corticosteroids should be maintained for at least 3 months after a complete response is achieved (defined by normalization of hemoglobin with no evidence of active hemolysis). Except for children, the use of alternate-day prednisone before stopping the treatment is not recommended. The efficacy of corticosteroids can take a few days to 2 weeks, so blood transfusions may be necessary at autoimmune hemolytic anemia onset, especially in case of severe anemia in young children or elderly adults for maintaining a "safe" hemoglobin level. After 2 to 3 weeks of treatment with corticosteroids, a clinically significant response is observed in 80 to 85% of the cases. Except for the few patients who are truly refractory to corticosteroids, the major issue that clinicians have to deal with when treating patients with warm autoimmune hemolytic anemia is that approximately 50 to 60% of them are found to be dependent on corticosteroids to suppress hemolysis. Thus, flares of relapses of warm autoimmune hemolytic anemia may occur either within weeks after withdrawal of corticosteroids or even on treatment when the dose of daily prednisone is decreased below a threshold, which is usually between 10 to 15 mg daily, a dose that is associated with several long-term adverse effects. Overall, only one third of patients can be considered to be in complete remission off-treatment 1 year after the onset of disease.

Second-Line Treatment

Rituximab

The efficacy of rituximab, the chimeric monoclonal antibody that targets the CD20 antigen on B lymphocytes, was first shown in refractory warm autoimmune hemolytic anemia in children with a response rate reaching up to 100% in some studies. In adults, rituximab was also shown to have significant efficacy in primary warm autoimmune hemolytic anemias in randomized trials, with a 75% overall response rate at 1 year.[A3,A4] The usual dose is 375 mg/m^2 by intravenous infusion once a week for 4 weeks, but other regimens such as fixed doses of 1000 mg 2 weeks apart as in rheumatoid arthritis can be used. Safety is usually good, although late-onset neutropenia and opportunistic infections such as *Pneumocystis jiroveci* pneumonia may rarely occur, so primary prophylaxis (Table 146-4) with trimethoprim-sulfamethoxazole (160 mg/800 mg) three times per week (Chapter 313) is wise when patients with autoimmune hemolytic anemia treated are with rituximab. Taken together, the data from the literature clearly support, whenever possible, the use of rituximab (off-label) as an early second-line treatment and before splenectomy for patients with warm autoimmune hemolytic anemia who have had no or little response to corticosteroids and for elderly patients with comorbidities such as diabetes who are at high risk for developing corticosteroid-induced side effects. When rituximab is administered before splenectomy, vaccination against *Streptococcus pneumoniae, Haemophilus influenzae* type B, and/or *Neisseria meningitidis* should be administered whenever possible 2 weeks before rituximab because splenectomy may be required thereafter (see Chapter 154 for specific recommendations).

Splenectomy

Splenectomy has long been the preferred second-line option for primary warm autoimmune hemolytic anemias. The rate of sustained response after splenectomy is approximately 60 to 70%, but clear predicting factors for response are still lacking. The perioperative risk of laparoscopic splenectomy is low and acceptable, with a mortality rate of less than 1%. The most feared complications, even after the laparoscopic procedure, remain the rare but unpredictable risk of overwhelming sepsis and the risk of postoperative thromboembolic complications, especially in the splanchnic veins. Perioperative low-molecular-weight heparin is therefore recommended in patients who have warm autoimmune hemolytic anemia and who undergo splenectomy and especially in those who also have positive antiphospholipid antibodies. The best time for splenectomy

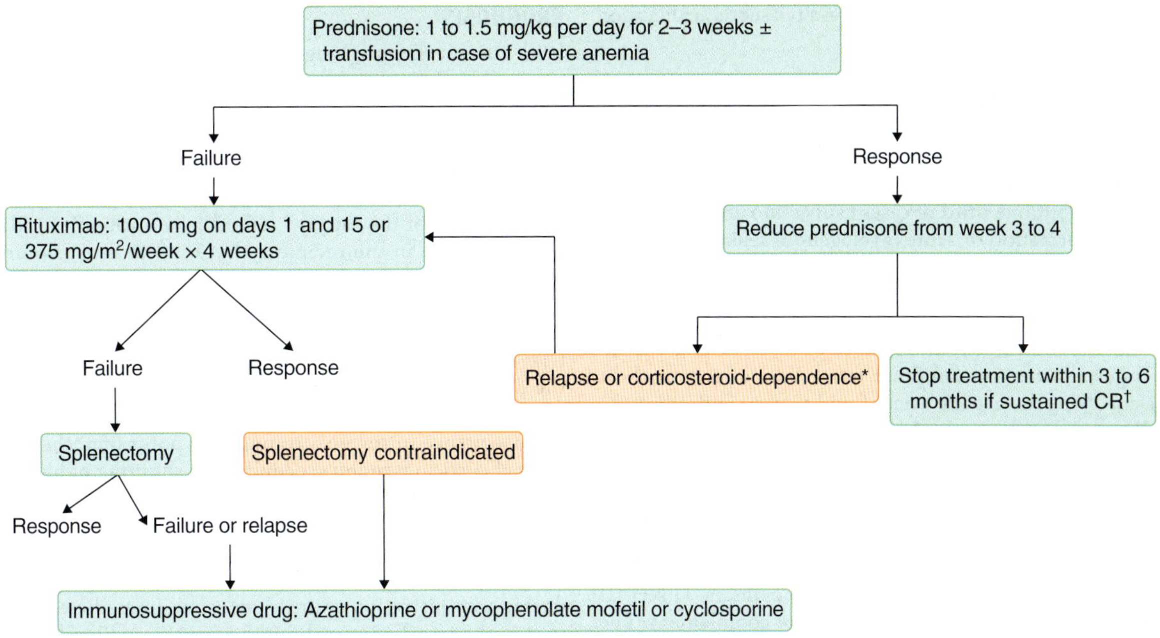

FIGURE 146-2. **Proposed algorithm for the treatment of primary warm-reactive autoimmune hemolytic anemia in adults.** *Need to maintain daily prednisone at more than 10 mg to maintain at least a partial remission (i.e., hemoglobin level ≥10 g/dL with at least a 2-g increase from baseline). †Complete remission (CR) = hemoglobin level >12 g/dL without hemolysis.

is controversial now that alternatives such as rituximab are available at least in some countries. In children aged less than 5 to 7 years, this procedure should be avoided or delayed as long as possible. In adults, it must be considered early in the course of the disease in patients who have failed to respond to both corticosteroids (or need high and unacceptable doses to maintain at least a partial remission) and rituximab.

Danazol

In patients dependent on corticosteroids, the use of danazol, an attenuated androgen analogue, at 400 to 800 mg/day can be helpful as a corticosteroid-sparing strategy in adults requiring a dose of daily prednisone greater than 15 mg to maintain a remission. However, because of its common androgenic side effects, its use is usually limited in female patients, and its potential liver toxicity makes long-term use difficult also in men.

Other Treatment Lines

Immunosuppressive and Cytotoxic Agents

In patients with refractory warm autoimmune hemolytic anemia in whom splenectomy and rituximab have failed or in patients those who are reluctant to undergo splenectomy or are not suitable candidates for splenectomy, the management is mainly based on experience and mostly retrospective data in the literature, as opposed to controlled, prospective, comparison trials. The efficacy of azathioprine, cyclophosphamide, and to a lesser extent cyclosporine and mycophenolate mofetil has been reported in small case series. The choice depends on the efficacy/safety ratio individualized for each patient. These drugs should be reserved for patients who have failed to respond to rituximab and to splenectomy or are not suitable candidates for splenectomy. For multirefractory patients, promising results have been reported with the combination of bortezomib and dexamethasone under expert supervision.

PAROXYSMAL NOCTURNAL HEMOGLOBINURIA

DEFINITION

Paroxysmal nocturnal hemoglobinuria (PNH) is a rare and potentially life-threatening clonal blood disorder with protean manifestations caused by an acquired somatic mutation in the phosphatidylinositol glycan (*PIG-A*) gene. In pluripotent hematopoietic stem cells, the mutation in *PIG-A* leads to a deficiency of glycosylphosphatidylinositol (GPI) anchors and GPI-anchored proteins, including the complement regulatory proteins CD55 and CD59 normally expressed on the surface of RBCs. PNH RBCs are therefore highly vulnerable to activation of complement on their surfaces (especially in case of fever, acidosis, or hypoxia) and the formation of the membrane attack complex (Chapter 37). The resulting chronic intravascular hemolysis is the hallmark of the classic hemolytic form of the disease, and the release of free hemoglobin contributes to most of its clinical manifestations (dysphagia, recurrent abdominal pain, erectile dysfunction).

EPIDEMIOLOGY

PNH can occur at any age but is most common between 10 and 50 years. The mean age at diagnosis is about 34 years (median age is about 40), and the female : male ratio is close to 1. Median survival after diagnosis is approximately 20 years. It is a rare disorder with an estimated prevalence in the population of about one per million in the population. There is no sex preference, and a family history of PNH is highly unusual.

PATHOBIOLOGY

PNH is due to a somatic mutation that causes a defect in the red cell membrane. The disease begins in a single hematopoietic stem cell when the *PIG-A* gene on the short arm of the active X chromosome acquires a mutation. The *PIG-A* gene encodes PIG-A, an enzyme that is essential for the synthesis of GPI. The location of *PIG-A* on the X chromosome allows a single mutation in the gene to affect GPI synthesis. This lipid normally forms a peptide link with the C-terminal amino acid of numerous proteins, anchoring them to the red cell membrane. Molecular genetic studies indicate that the PNH clone upregulates genes that make the PNH clone resistant to apoptosis and immune attack. The mutation in a hematopoietic stem cell affects *PIG-A* in blood cells of all lineages. Almost 150 different mutations of *PIG-A* have been identified. Most of them inactivate *PIG-A* and cause total loss of GPI in the descendants of the carrier stem cell. Red cells with complete deficiency of GPI are termed *PNH III erythrocytes*, and those with partial deficiency are called *PNH II erythrocytes*. The coexistence of PNH III and PNH II red cells in the same patient indicates the presence of two mutant clones. A small number of hematopoietic stem cells in normal people bear the *PIG-A* mutation; they have no proliferative advantage and persist in small numbers. In normal blood, the frequency of *PIG-A*–deficient cells is about 1 in 50,000 red cells. In contrast to those with PNH, however, the deficient cells in normal subjects arise from committed hematopoietic cells. The presence of *PIG-A*–deficient cells in normal subjects suggests that PNH involves not only the *PIG-A* mutation but also a second step, perhaps a mutation, that allows expansion of the mutated clone.

Functional Consequences of Deficiency of GPI

The membrane inhibitor of reactive hemolysis (CD59, or protectin) and CD55, an inhibitor of C3 convertase, are two of the many proteins that GPI normally anchors to the red cell. They prevent polymerization of C9, the final step in assembly of the membrane attack complex that begins with cleavage of C5 to C5b. Deficiencies of CD59 and CD55 allow unimpeded assembly of the membrane attack complex on the erythrocyte surface, thereby initiating intravascular hemolysis. A variety of nonspecific factors, such as a reduction in the pH of blood, can activate complement. The morning hemoglobinuria that occurs in some cases of PNH is probably the result of subtle acidification of blood during sleep.

CLINICAL MANIFESTATIONS

Classically, some patients with PNH arise in the morning and pass dark urine. The typical paroxysms of hemoglobinuria occur on a background of chronic, low-grade intravascular hemolysis that causes constant hemosiderinuria in PNH. About one third of cases evolve into aplastic anemia (Chapter 151). Transformation to acute myelogenous leukemia is a rare event. Abdominal pain, dysphagia, and erectile dysfunction are additional clinical features. The basis of these symptoms is probably scavenging by free plasma hemoglobin of endogenous nitric oxide, a regulator of vasomotor and smooth muscle tone. In about one third of cases, venous thrombosis occurs in unusual sites and can cause intra-abdominal splanchnic vein thrombosis involving the hepatic veins (Budd-Chiari syndrome), the portal veins, or less frequently cerebral vein thrombosis (Chapter 140). Splenomegaly is uncommon; hepatomegaly and ascites point to the complication of intra-abdominal venous thrombosis. Hemosiderinuria is the result of chronic intravascular hemolysis. Subtle or overt signs of bone marrow damage (leukopenia and thrombocytopenia) are frequent. The extent of red cell destruction in PNH depends on the number of PNH red cells in blood, the level of GPI on the red cell membrane (PNH III cells are devoid of GPI), and the surface activation of complement. The anemia is often aggravated by iron deficiency caused by chronic urinary iron loss in the form of hemosiderinuria. A direct antiglobulin test–negative hemolytic anemia associated with iron deficiency should raise the suspicion of PNH. The basis of the tendency to develop venous thrombosis is unclear. Hypercoagulability caused by the release of prothrombotic materials in red cell and platelet membranes (which are also abnormal in PNH) and impaired fibrinolysis have been implicated. Nitric oxide scavenging by free plasma hemoglobin may also damage endothelial cells and cause aggregation of platelets.

DIAGNOSIS

The diagnosis of PNH is suspected in case of an acquired and Coombs-negative intravascular hemolytic anemia and can be established by flow cytometry demonstrating a deficiency of GpI-linked proteins (CD24/CD57 and CD14) on both neutrophils and monocytes, as well as CD59 on RBCs. Another reagent with utility in flow cytometry is aerolysin, a bacterial protein that binds to the GPI anchor. Data strongly suggest that the fluorescent aerolysin variant (FLAER) is the best and most reliable reagent to study GPI-linked antigens on leukocytes, helpful for diagnosing PNH.

The clone size in PNH is usually correlated with the degree of intravascular hemolysis.

TREATMENT

Eculizumab, a humanized monoclonal antibody against C5, reduces the signs of intravascular hemolysis, the requirement for transfusions, and the incidence of thrombosis in PNH.[A5] In PNH, it is usually given at a dose of 600 mg every week for 4 weeks, followed 1 week later by a 900-mg dose, and then at 900 mg every other week.[14,15] Complement blockade is not always complete. Before being treated with eculizumab, every patient should be vaccinated against *Meningococcus A, B,* and *C* and, in many countries, a long-term prophylaxis with oral penicillin is also strongly recommended. Beyond transfusion-dependent hemolytic anemia, the occurrence of disease-related venous thrombosis is also a strong indication for eculizumab in the setting of PNH in combination with anticoagulation. Ravulizumab (given as a single weight-based loading dose of 2400 to 3000 mg followed by 3000 to 3600 mg every 8 weeks starting 2 weeks later) is another complement inhibitor that also binds to C5, has a much longer terminal half-life compared with eculizumab, and can provide equivalent results.[A6,A7] Crovalimab is a subcutaneous C5 inhibitor that may prove useful, especially in patients who are resistant to eculizumab and ravulizumab.[16] Subcutaneous pegcetacoplan (1080 mg subcutaneously twice weekly), which targets complement protein C3 rather than C5, can inhibit extravascular as well as intravascular hemolysis and may provide even better disease control than the C5 inhibitors.[A8] Combined inhibition of both C3 and C5 under expert supervision may become an option in persistent cases.[17] Hematopoietic stem cell transplantation is curative but is reserved for patients who have some pancytopenia that does not respond to complement therapy.

PROGNOSIS

With current therapy, long-term survival is expected. However, progression to bone marrow failure (Chapter 151) is associated with a poorer prognosis.

HEMOLYTIC TRANSFUSION REACTIONS

The cause of hemolytic transfusion reactions (Chapter 162) is intravascular lysis of the donor's red cells by antibodies (alloantibodies or isoantibodies) in the recipient that bind to one or more blood group antigens on the transfused cells. The recipient's isoantibodies can be natural anti-A or anti-B antibodies, or they can be induced by previous transfusions or pregnancy. Whether IgM or IgG, the isoantibodies trigger the assembly of lytic complement components on the surface of the donor's red cells. The rapid formation of large amounts of C3a and C5a fragments causes hypotension and bronchospasm. Renal failure is a consequence of severe, prolonged hypotension; the main renal lesion is renal cortical ischemia secondary to shunting of blood away from the kidneys. Hemoglobin itself is not nephrotoxic. The signs and symptoms of a hemolytic transfusion reaction are nonspecific and include fever, back pain, urticaria, dyspnea, hypotension, and evidence of disseminated intravascular coagulation. These nonspecific signs appear and worsen during administration of the transfusion. Immediate steps must be taken to stop the transfusion, submit the transfused blood and a sample of the patient's blood to the blood bank, and order tests of plasma and urine for free hemoglobin. Hydration is key to prevent renal failure. Intravenous fluid, usually normal saline, should be started at once and be combined with a diuretic (usually furosemide) in amounts needed to sustain a urine flow rate of at least 100 mL/hour. Patients with sickle cell disease (Chapter 149) are at high risk of delayed hemolytic transfusion reaction, a complication that can be life-threatening and require prompt management (Chapter 162).[18]

OTHER CAUSES OF INTRAVASCULAR HEMOLYSIS

Conditions in which vascular abnormalities (e.g., valve hemolysis), toxins (e.g., venomous snake bites), infections (e.g., malaria, babesiosis, clostridial sepsis), or drugs damage RBCs, cause them to lose pieces of membrane, and ultimately fragment into free hemoglobin-releasing particles should be considered in the differential diagnosis of intravascular hemolysis (Tables 146-2 and 146-3). Most of these conditions are readily apparent from the history and physical examination. Treatment focuses on the underlying cause of the hemolysis.

GENERAL REFERENCES

For the General References and other additional features, please visit Elsevier eBooks+ at https://ebooks.health.elsevier.com.

Grade A References

A1. Berentsen S, Randen U, Oksman M, et al. Bendamustine plus rituximab for chronic cold agglutinin disease: results of a Nordic prospective multicenter trial. *Blood.* 2017;130:537-554.

A2. Röth A, Berentsen S, Barcellini W, et al. Sutimlimab in patients with cold agglutinin disease: results of the randomized placebo-controlled phase 3 CADENZA trial. *Blood.* 2022;140:980-991.

A3. Michel M, Terriou L, Roudot-Thoraval F, et al. A randomized and double-blind controlled trial evaluating the safety and efficacy of rituximab for warm auto-immune hemolytic anemia in adults (the RAIHA study). *Am J Hematol.* 2017;92:23-27.

A4. Liu AP, Cheuk DK. Disease-modifying treatments for primary autoimmune haemolytic anaemia. *Cochrane Database Syst Rev.* 2021;3:CD012493.

A5. Zhou S, Dong X, Chen C, et al. Efficacy and safety of eculizumab for paroxysmal nocturnal hemoglobinuria: a systematic review and meta-analysis. *J Pediatr Hematol Oncol.* 2021;43:203-210.

A6. Lee JW, Sicre de Fontbrune F, Wong Lee Lee L, et al. Ravulizumab (ALXN1210) vs eculizumab in adult patients with PNH naïve to complement inhibitors: the 301 study. *Blood.* 2019;133:530-539.

A7. Kulasekararaj AG, Hill A, Langemeijer S, et al. One-year outcomes from a phase 3 randomized trial of ravulizumab in adults with paroxysmal nocturnal hemoglobinuria who received prior eculizumab. *Eur J Haematol.* 2021;106:389-397.

A8. Hillmen P, Szer J, Wietz I, et al. Pegcetacoplan versus eculizumab in paroxysmal nocturnal hemoglobinuria. *N Engl J Med.* 2021;384:1028-1037.

147

HEMOLYTIC ANEMIAS: RED BLOOD CELL MEMBRANE AND METABOLIC DEFECTS

PATRICK G. GALLAGHER

The mature erythrocyte differs from all other cells in the body. Lacking a nucleus, DNA, RNA, and ribosomes, it cannot synthesize RNA, DNA, or protein. It does not divide, it has no mitochondria, it cannot perform the Krebs cycle, and it lacks an electron transport system for oxidative phosphorylation. After enucleation, the reticulocyte, the precursor of the mature erythrocyte, leaves the marrow and enters the circulation equipped with a full complement of enzymes, transporters, signaling molecules, and all other proteins necessary to perform the essential functions of the red blood cell (RBC) during its lifespan.

The erythrocyte membrane accounts for only about 1% of the total weight of an RBC, yet it plays a critical role in the maintenance of normal RBC homeostasis through a number of mechanisms. These include retention of vital compounds and removal of metabolic waste, regulation of erythrocyte metabolism and pH, and import of iron required for hemoglobin (Hb) synthesis during erythropoiesis. The membrane maintains a slippery exterior so that erythrocytes do not aggregate or adhere to endothelial cells. The membrane skeleton, a network of proteins on the inner surface of the RBC, provides the strength and flexibility needed to maintain the normal shape and deformability of the erythrocyte.

The principal functions of erythrocyte metabolism in the mature erythrocyte include maintenance of adequate supplies of adenosine triphosphate (ATP), production of reducing substances to act as antioxidants, and control of oxygen affinity of Hb by production of adequate amounts of 2,3-diphosphoglycerate (2,3-DPG). Because the mature erythrocyte has lost its ability to perform oxidative phosphorylation, its energy is supplied by anaerobic glycolysis though the Embden-Meyerhof pathway, by oxidative glycolysis through the hexose monophosphate shunt, and through nucleotide salvage pathways.

THE ERYTHROCYTE MEMBRANE

NORMAL FUNCTION

Composed of a lipid bilayer and an underlying cortical membrane skeleton (Fig. 147-1), the membrane provides the erythrocyte the deformability and stability required to withstand its travels through the circulation. In one circulatory cycle throughout the body, an erythrocyte is subjected to high shear stress in the arterial system, dramatic size and shape changes in the microcirculation with capillary diameters as small as 7.5 μm, and marked fluctuations in tonicity, pH, and Po_2.[1]

Membrane Lipids

Red blood cell membrane lipids are asymmetrically distributed across the bilayer membrane, reflecting a steady state involving a constant exchange of phospholipids between the two bilayer hemileaflets. Glycolipids and cholesterol are intercalated between the phospholipids in the bilayer with their long axes perpendicular to the bilayer plane. Glycolipids, located in the external half of the bilayer with their carbohydrate moieties extending into the aqueous phase, carry several important RBC antigens and serve other significant functions. Phospholipids are asymmetrically organized; choline phospholipids, phosphatidylcholine, and sphingomyelin are primarily in the outer half of the bilayer, whereas amino phospholipids, phosphatidylethanolamine, and phosphatidylserine (PS) are in the inner half of the bilayer. In pathologic states such as thalassemia, sickle cell disease, and diabetes, loss of phospholipid asymmetry with externalization of PS leads to activation of blood clotting through conversion of prothrombin to thrombin and facilitates macrophage attachment to erythrocytes, marking them for destruction. Mature erythrocytes are unable to synthesize fatty acids, phospholipids, or cholesterol de novo and depend on lipid exchange and fatty acid acylation as mechanisms for phospholipid repair and renewal.

Membrane Proteins

Membrane proteins are classified as either *integral*, penetrating or crossing the lipid bilayer and interacting with the hydrophobic lipid core, or *peripheral*, interacting with integral proteins or lipids at the membrane surface but not penetrating into the bilayer core. Integral membrane proteins include the glycophorins, Rh proteins, Kell and Duffy antigens, and transport proteins such as band 3 (AE1, anion exchanger 1, SLC4A1), Na^+,K^+-ATPase, Ca^{2+}-ATPase, and Mg^{2+}-ATPase. Numerous membrane receptors and antigens are present on integral membrane proteins. Peripheral membrane proteins are on the cytoplasmic membrane face and include enzymes such as glyceraldehyde-3-phosphate dehydrogenase and the structural proteins of the spectrin-actin–based membrane skeleton.

Integral Membrane Proteins

Band 3, the major integral protein of the RBC, has two primary functions: ion transport and maintenance of protein–protein interactions. Band 3 mediates chloride–bicarbonate exchange and provides a binding site for glycolytic enzymes, Hb, and the skeletal proteins ankyrin, protein 4.1, and protein 4.2.

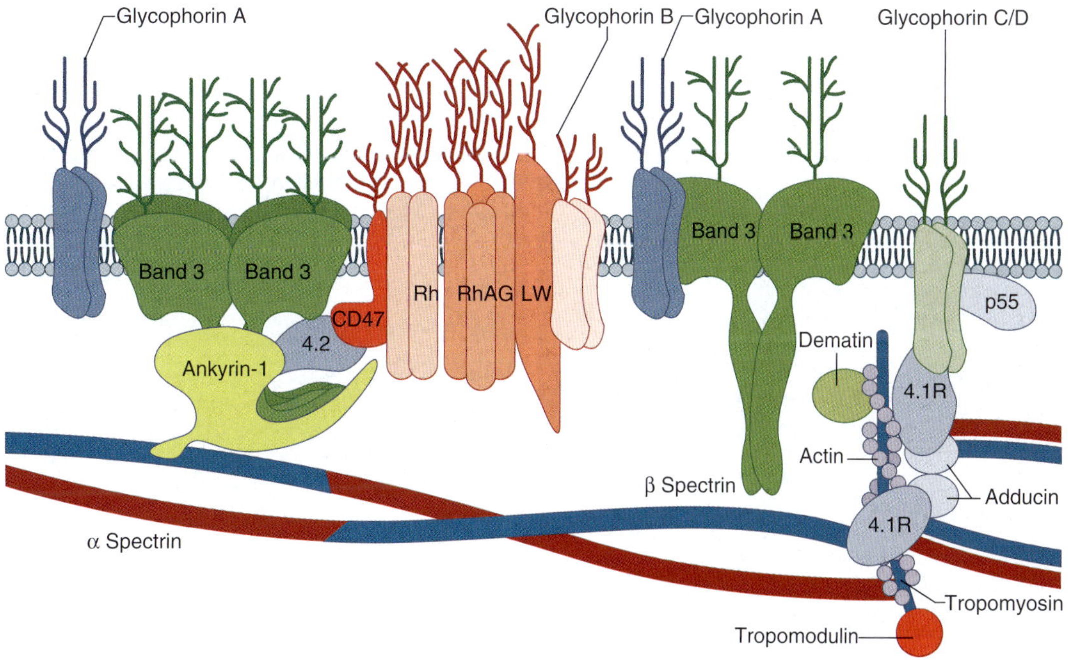

FIGURE 147-1. The erythrocyte membrane. A model of the major proteins of the erythrocyte membrane is shown: α and β spectrin, ankyrin, band 3 (the anion exchanger), 4.1 (protein 4.1) and 4.2 (protein 4.2), actin, and glycophorin. LW = Landsteiner Wiener glycoprotein; Rh = Rhesus polypeptide; RhAG = Rh-associated glycoprotein. (From Perrotta S, Gallagher PG, Mohandas N. Hereditary spherocytosis. *Lancet*. 2008;372:1411-1426.)

A single *N*-glycan chain attached to an asparagine in the membrane spanning domain of band 3 is composed of *N*-acetyl-d-lactosamine units arranged in an unbranched, linear fashion in fetal erythrocytes (i antigen) and in a branched fashion in adult cells (I antigen).

The glycophorins are the next most abundant family of integral membrane proteins. They provide most of the negative surface charge required by RBCs to avoid sticking to each other and to the vascular wall. They are involved in transmembrane signaling and carry receptors for *Plasmodium falciparum*, a number of viruses and bacteria, and several blood group antigens.

Peripheral Membrane Proteins

Spectrin is the major component of the membrane skeleton. It is composed of two subunits, α and β spectrin, that are structurally related but functionally distinct. Spectrin is highly flexible and assumes a variety of conformations, an unusual property that may be critical for normal membrane pliancy. The spectrin-based membrane skeleton is linked to the plasma membrane through the actin–protein 4.1 junctional complex; through spectrin–ankyrin interactions; and through binding of a multiprotein complex containing Rh proteins, Rh-associated glycoproteins, CD47, LW, glycophorin B, and protein 4.2 to ankyrin. Protein 4.1, a protein necessary for normal membrane stability, interacts with spectrin, actin, and other proteins of the RBC membrane. Ankyrin serves as the primary linkage protein for the high-affinity binding of spectrin to the inner membrane through interactions with the cytoplasmic domain of band 3. Protein 4.2 is a peripheral membrane protein that helps link the skeleton to the lipid bilayer through interactions with ankyrin and band 3.

Erythrocyte membrane disorders result from alterations in the quantity or quality (or both) of individual proteins and their dynamic interactions with each other. Disruption of the vertical protein–protein interactions of the membrane, that is, the spectrin-ankyrin–band 3 linkage or the band 3–protein 4.2 interaction, leads to uncoupling of the membrane skeleton from the lipid bilayer. This leads to membrane instability with loss of lipids and some integral membrane proteins, resulting in loss of membrane surface area and the phenotype of spherocytosis. Disruption of the horizontal interactions of membrane skeleton proteins, including perturbation of spectrin self-association or junctional complex protein–protein interactions, leads to membrane instability, altered membrane deformability and mechanical properties, and the phenotype of elliptocytosis.

Erythrocyte membrane disorders also result from abnormal cation permeability or disturbed erythrocyte hydration (see later section on "Hereditary Stomatocytosis Syndromes.")

DISORDERS OF THE ERYTHROCYTE MEMBRANE

Hemolytic anemias caused by defects in the erythrocyte membrane comprise an important group of hereditary anemias. Hereditary spherocytosis, hereditary elliptocytosis, and hereditary pyropoikilocytosis are the most common disorders among this group.[2] Detailed clinical studies carried out years ago have now been complemented by biochemical and genetic studies, providing a better understanding of the pathogenesis of these disorders as well as the normal biology of the erythrocyte membrane.

HEREDITARY SPHEROCYTOSIS

DEFINITION

Hereditary spherocytosis is a group of disorders characterized by spherical erythrocytes on the peripheral blood smear (Fig. 147-2A). Clinical, laboratory, and genetic heterogeneity characterize this group of disorders.

EPIDEMIOLOGY

Hereditary spherocytosis affects approximately one in 2000 to 4000 individuals of northern European ancestry.[3] Found worldwide, it is much more common in Whites than individuals of African ancestry.

PATHOBIOLOGY

The primary defect in hereditary spherocytosis is the loss of erythrocyte membrane surface area caused by defects in erythrocyte membrane proteins,

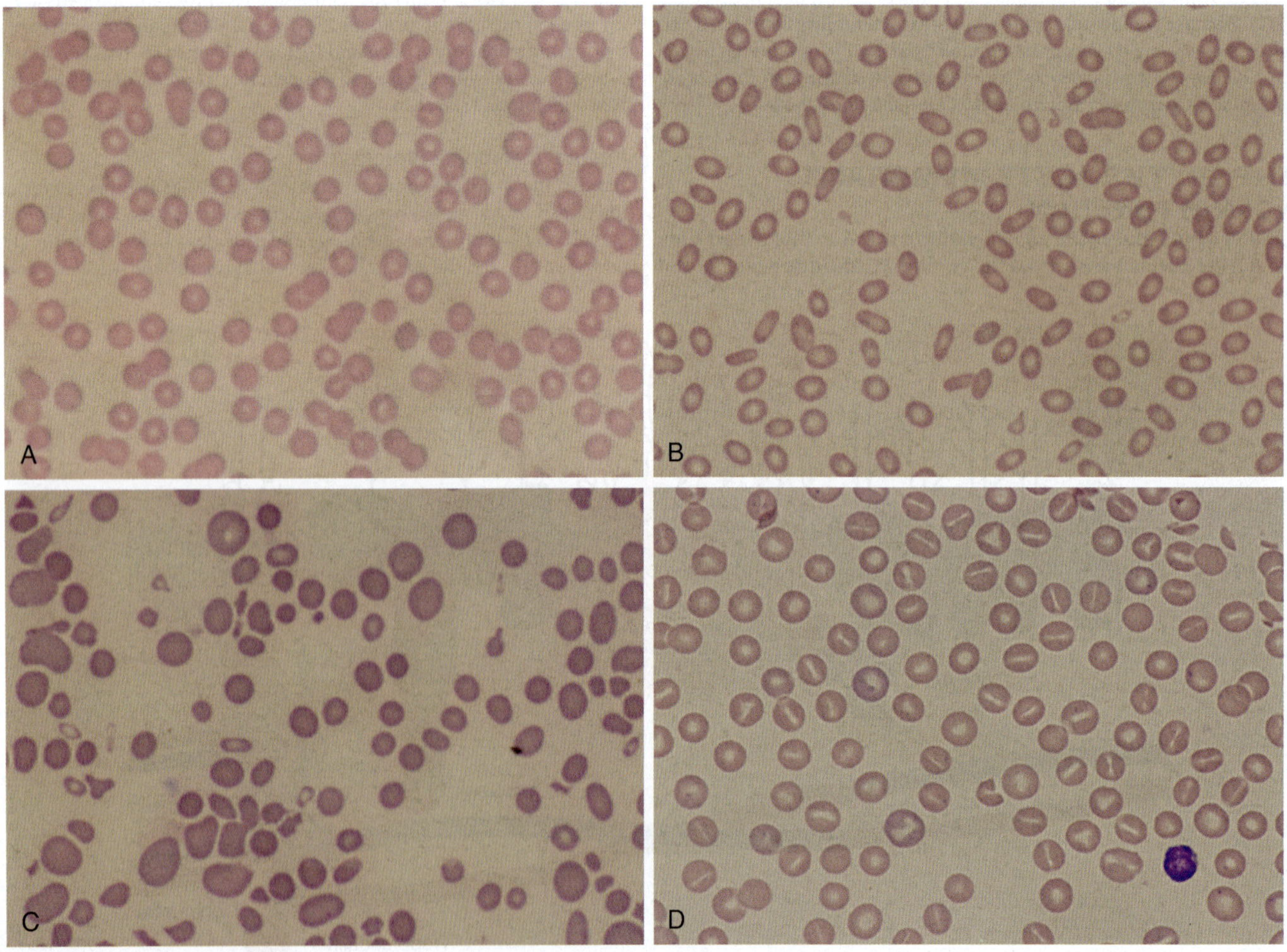

FIGURE 147-2. Peripheral blood smears in disorders of erythrocyte shape. A, Hereditary spherocytosis. Characteristic small spherocytes lacking central pallor are seen. B, Hereditary elliptocytosis. Smooth, cigar-shaped elliptocytes are seen. C, Hereditary pyropoikilocytosis. Pronounced microcytosis, poikilocytosis, fragmentation of erythrocytes, and elliptocytes are seen. D, Hereditary stomatocytosis.

including α spectrin, β spectrin, ankyrin, band 3, and protein 4.2. Qualitative or quantitative defects of one or more of these membrane proteins lead to membrane instability, which, in turn, leads to membrane loss. In approximately two thirds of hereditary spherocytosis patients, inheritance is autosomal dominant. In the remaining patients, inheritance is nondominant owing to either a de novo mutation or autosomal recessive inheritance. Cases with autosomal recessive inheritance are caused by defects in either α spectrin or protein 4.2. Rare cases of homozygous hereditary spherocytosis have been reported, resulting in fetal death or severe hemolytic anemia. In most cases, hereditary spherocytosis mutations are "private," that is, each individual has a unique mutation, implying that there is no selective evolutionary advantage to hereditary spherocytosis.

The spleen plays a critical, albeit secondary, role in the pathophysiology of hereditary spherocytosis. Splenic destruction of poorly deformable spherocytes is the primary cause of hemolysis experienced by hereditary spherocytosis patients. Abnormal erythrocytes are trapped in the splenic microcirculation and ingested by phagocytes. Moreover, the splenic environment is hostile to erythrocytes, with low pH, low glucose, and low ATP concentrations and high local concentrations of toxic free radicals produced by adjacent phagocytes, all contributing to membrane damage.

CLINICAL MANIFESTATIONS

The clinical manifestations of the spherocytosis syndromes vary widely[4] and are determined by the density and deformability of the abnormal red cells.[5] The classic triad of hereditary spherocytosis is anemia, jaundice, and splenomegaly. Rarely, patients may have severe hemolytic anemia presenting in utero or shortly after birth and continuing through the first year of life. These patients may require multiple blood transfusions, and in some cases, splenectomy in infancy. Many patients with hereditary spherocytosis escape detection throughout childhood. In these patients, the diagnosis of hereditary spherocytosis is not made until they are being evaluated for unrelated disorders later in life or when complications related to anemia or chronic hemolysis occur. Although the lifespan of an erythrocyte in these patients may be shortened to only 20 to 30 days, they adequately compensate for their hemolysis with increased bone marrow erythropoiesis.

Chronic hemolysis leads to the formation of bilirubinate gallstones (Chapter 141), the most frequently reported complication in patients with hereditary spherocytosis. Although gallstones have been observed in early childhood, most appear in adolescents and young adults.

Other complications of hereditary spherocytosis include aplastic, hemolytic, and megaloblastic crises. Aplastic crises occur after virally-induced bone marrow suppression and present with anemia, jaundice, fever, and vomiting. The most common etiologic agent in these cases is parvovirus B19 (Chapter 342). Hemolytic crises, usually associated with viral illnesses and occurring before 6 years of age, are generally mild and present with jaundice, increased spleen size, and a decrease in hematocrit. Megaloblastic crises occur in hereditary spherocytosis patients with increased folate demands, such as the pregnant patient, growing children, or patients recovering from an aplastic crisis.

Uncommon manifestations of hereditary spherocytosis include skin ulceration, gout, chronic leg dermatitis, cardiomyopathy, spinal cord dysfunction, movement disorders, and extramedullary erythropoiesis. In patients with untreated severe hereditary spherocytosis, poor growth and findings attributable to extramedullary hematopoiesis, such as hand and skull deformities, may be observed.

DIAGNOSIS

Patients with hereditary spherocytosis may present at any age, usually with anemia, hyperbilirubinemia, or an abnormal blood smear. In evaluating a patient with suspected hereditary spherocytosis, particular attention should be paid to the family history, including questions about anemia, jaundice, gallstones, and splenectomy. The initial laboratory investigation should include a complete blood count with a peripheral smear, reticulocyte count, direct antiglobulin test (Coombs test), and serum bilirubin. When the peripheral smear or family history is suggestive of hereditary spherocytosis, flow cytometric analysis of eosin-5-maleimide–labelled erythrocytes (EMA binding) or an incubated osmotic fragility test (discussed later) should be obtained. Rarely, additional, specialized testing is required to confirm the diagnosis.

Overall, laboratory findings in hereditary spherocytosis are heterogeneous. Erythrocyte morphology (Chapter 143) is distinctive but not diagnostic (Fig. 147-2A). Typical hereditary spherocytosis patients have blood smears with easily identifiable spherocytes lacking central pallor. Some patients present with only a few spherocytes on peripheral smear, but others present with numerous small, dense spherocytes and bizarre erythrocyte morphology. Specific morphologic findings have been identified in patients with certain membrane protein defects such as pincered erythrocytes (band 3) or spherocytic acanthocytes (β spectrin). When examining a peripheral blood smear in a case of suspected spherocytosis, it is important to have a high-quality smear with the erythrocytes well separated and some cells with central pallor in the field of examination because spherocytes are a common artifact on peripheral blood smears. Other disorders with spherocytes on peripheral blood smear are listed in Table 147-1.

TABLE 147-1 DISORDERS WITH SPHEROCYTES ON PERIPHERAL BLOOD FILM

Hereditary spherocytosis
Autoimmune hemolytic anemia
Thermal injuries
Microangiopathic and macroangiopathic hemolytic anemias
Hepatic disease
Clostridial septicemia
Transfusion reactions with hemolysis
Poisoning with certain snake, spider, and *Hymenoptera* venoms
Severe hypophosphatemia
Heinz body anemias
ABO incompatibility (neonates)

The mean corpuscular hemoglobin concentration (MCHC) is increased (between 34.5 and 38) in patients with hereditary spherocytosis owing to relative cellular dehydration. The mean corpuscular volume (MCV) is usually normal or slightly decreased. Many cell counters provide a histogram of MCHCs claimed to be accurate enough to identify nearly all patients with hereditary spherocytosis.

In a normal erythrocyte, a redundancy of cell membrane gives the cell its characteristic discoid shape and provides it abundant surface area. In spherocytes, there is a decrease in surface area relative to cell volume, resulting in their abnormal shape. This change is reflected in the increased osmotic fragility found in these cells. Osmotic fragility is tested by adding increasingly hypotonic concentrations of saline to RBCs. Normal erythrocytes are able to increase their volume by swelling, but spherocytes, which are already at maximal volume for surface area, burst at higher saline concentrations than normal. Approximately one fourth of hereditary spherocytosis individuals will have a normal osmotic fragility on freshly drawn RBCs, with the osmotic fragility curve approximating the number of spherocytes seen on peripheral smear. However, after incubation at 37° C for 24 hours, hereditary spherocytosis RBCs lose membrane surface area more readily than normal because their membranes have become leaky and unstable. Thus, incubation accentuates the defect in hereditary spherocytosis erythrocytes and brings out the defect on osmotic fragility, making incubated osmotic fragility the standard test in diagnosing hereditary spherocytosis (Fig. 147-3, *bottom panel*). When the spleen is present, a subpopulation of very fragile erythrocytes that have been conditioned by the spleen form the tail of the osmotic fragility curve. This tail disappears after splenectomy. The osmotic fragility test suffers from poor sensitivity, with as many as 20% of mild cases of hereditary spherocytosis missed after incubation. It is unreliable in patients who have small numbers of spherocytes and in patients who have been recently transfused. It is abnormal in other conditions in which spherocytes are present.

Eosin-5-maleimide (EMA) binding is a flow cytometry–based test used in the diagnosis of hereditary spherocytosis.[6] EMA is a fluorescent dye that binds to band 3 and Rh-related proteins in the erythrocyte membrane. In hereditary spherocytosis, the mean fluorescence of EMA-stained erythrocytes is lower compared with control because of the reduction of band 3 and related proteins, typically decreased to approximately 65% of normal (Fig. 147-3, *top panel*). Although primary defects of band 3 protein are seen in only about 25% of hereditary spherocytosis patients, decreased fluorescence intensity is also observed in the erythrocyte membranes of hereditary spherocytosis patients with defects in other membrane proteins such as ankyrin and spectrin. This is thought to be attributable to transmission of long-range effects of mutant protein defects across the membrane lattice, ultimately influencing the amount of EMA binding to band 3. EMA binding has good sensitivity and specificity and is simple and rapidly performed.[7]

Specialized testing is available for studying difficult cases or cases in which additional information is desired. Useful tests for these purposes include structural and functional studies of erythrocyte membrane proteins, such as protein

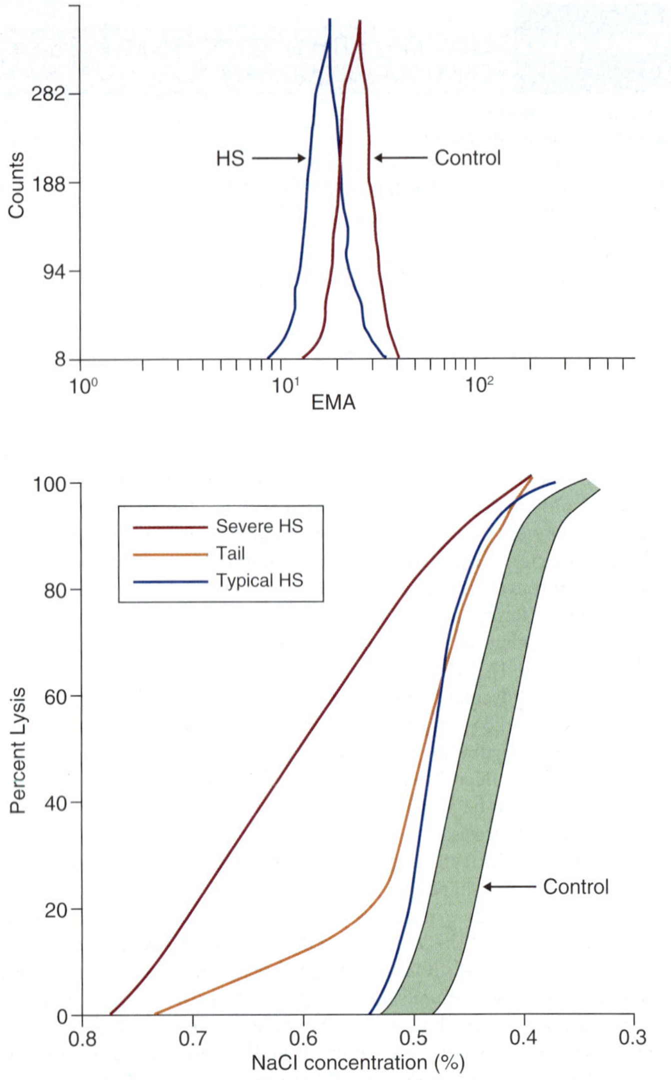

FIGURE 147-3. Testing in hereditary spherocytosis. *Top panel*, Eosin-5-maleimide (EMA) binding. Histogram of fluorescence of EMA-labeled erythrocytes from a normal control and a patient with typical hereditary spherocytosis. Decreased fluorescence is observed from hereditary spherocytosis (HS) erythrocytes. *Bottom panel*, Osmotic fragility curves in hereditary spherocytosis. The *shaded region* is the normal range. Results representative of both typical and severe spherocytosis are shown. A tail, representing fragile erythrocytes conditioned by the spleen, is common in spherocytosis patients prior to splenectomy. (From Gallagher PG. Abnormalities of the erythrocyte membrane. *Pediatr Clin North Am* 2013;60:1349-1352.)

quantitation, limited tryptic digestion of spectrin, spectrin, and ion transport. Membrane deformability may be examined using an ektacytometer.

Genetic diagnosis of hereditary spherocytosis has become widely available and the associated costs continue to decrease. The precise role of molecular diagnosis is evolving. Next-generation sequencing panels could become a cost-effective approach to molecular diagnosis of hereditary hemolytic anemia, especially when the family history is uninformative or when routine laboratory testing fails to identify the causative hemolytic process.[8] In difficult cases, such as when there is transfusion dependence, genetic testing may be diagnostic. Some experts recommend genetic testing to verify the diagnosis prior to splenectomy.

Other laboratory manifestations in hereditary spherocytosis are manifestations of ongoing hemolysis. Increased serum bilirubin, increased lactate dehydrogenase, increased urinary and fecal urobilinogen, and decreased serum haptoglobin reflect increased erythrocyte destruction. Because of the high risk for gallstones, routine interval ultrasonography to detect gallstones is recommended even if patients are asymptomatic.

After diagnosing a patient with hereditary spherocytosis, family members should be examined for presence of the disease. This can be of great epidemiologic importance, particularly for very old and very young patients. Prenatal diagnosis of hereditary spherocytosis has been made in a few cases, but this is rarely necessary.

TREATMENT AND PROGNOSIS

Splenic sequestration and destruction is the primary determinant of erythrocyte survival in hereditary spherocytosis patients. Splenectomy cures or alleviates anemia in most patients, reducing or eliminating the need for transfusions. The risk for cholelithiasis is also decreased to nearly background levels. After splenectomy, spherocytes remain in the peripheral blood, but their lifespan becomes near normal.

In the past, splenectomy was routinely performed in all patients with hereditary spherocytosis.[9] However, the risk of overwhelming post-splenectomy infection; the emergence of penicillin-resistant pneumococci; and the growing recognition of the increased risk of post-splenectomy cardiovascular disease (particularly thrombosis, pulmonary hypertension, and increased risk of atherosclerosis) have led to reevaluation of the role of splenectomy in the treatment of hereditary spherocytosis (Chapter 154).[10,11] In addition, with growing globalization, the important role of the spleen in protection of individuals living in or traveling to geographic regions where parasitic diseases such as malaria or babesiosis occur have reemerged. When splenectomy is considered, health care providers, the patient, and family members must review and weigh the benefits of splenectomy against the immediate and long-term risks of the procedure. Considering the risks and benefits, a reasonable approach is to splenectomize all patients with severe spherocytosis and all patients who have significant signs or symptoms of anemia, including growth failure, skeletal changes, leg ulcers, and extramedullary hematopoietic tumors. Other candidates for splenectomy are older patients who have hereditary spherocytosis and also have vascular compromise of vital organs. Whether patients with moderate hereditary spherocytosis and compensated, asymptomatic anemia should undergo splenectomy is controversial.

When splenectomy is indicated, laparoscopic splenectomy has become the method of choice. This technique results in less postoperative discomfort, a quicker return to preoperative diet and activities, shorter hospitalization, decreased costs, and smaller scars. Even massive spleens can be removed laparoscopically because the spleen is placed in a large bag, diced intraoperatively, and eliminated through suction catheters. Partial splenectomy was initially advocated for infants and young children with significant anemia associated with erythrocyte membrane disorders to allow for palliation of hemolysis and anemia while maintaining some residual splenic immune function. This procedure is now being suggested by some for most hereditary spherocytosis patients.[12] Guidelines, which reflect changes in current opinion about surgical management, include (1) preference for a laparoscopic approach, (2) performance of splenectomy ideally after the age of 6 years, (3) no indication for extended thrombosis prophylaxis after splenectomy for hereditary spherocytosis, and (4) avoidance of splenectomy in patients with some forms of hereditary stomatocytosis because of an increased risk of venous thromboembolism.

Before splenectomy (Chapter 154), patients should be immunized with vaccines against pneumococcus, *Haemophilus influenzae* type B, and meningococcus. Post-splenectomy care includes counseling of patients (or parents) to seek prompt medical care in case of febrile illness, to seek medical care after dog or cat bites, and to receive prophylaxis if traveling to malaria-endemic areas. Use of routine antibiotics after splenectomy for prevention of pneumococcal sepsis is controversial and data are lacking to indicate or refute their prescription. Many providers prescribe daily oral penicillin prophylaxis, 250 to 500 mg twice a day, for 2 or more years post-splenectomy. Before splenectomy and post-splenectomy if hemolysis does not abate, hereditary spherocytosis patients should take folic acid (1 mg/day orally) to prevent folate deficiency.

HEREDITARY ELLIPTOCYTOSIS AND RELATED DISORDERS

DEFINITION

Hereditary elliptocytosis is characterized by the presence of elliptical or oval cigar-shaped erythrocytes on peripheral blood smears of affected individuals (see Fig. 147-2B).

EPIDEMIOLOGY

Hereditary elliptocytosis has been estimated to occur in approximately one in 2000 to 4000 individuals. The true incidence of hereditary elliptocytosis is unknown because its clinical severity is heterogeneous, and many patients are asymptomatic. It is common in African Americans and people of Mediterranean ancestry, presumably because elliptocytes confer some resistance to malaria. In parts of Africa, the incidence of hereditary elliptocytosis approaches one in 100.

PATHOBIOLOGY

The principal defect in hereditary elliptocytosis is mechanical weakness or fragility of the erythrocyte membrane skeleton. Qualitative and quantitative defects in a number of RBC membrane proteins have been described in hereditary elliptocytosis, including α spectrin, β spectrin, protein 4.1, and glycophorin C. Most defects occur in spectrin, the principal structural protein of the erythrocyte membrane skeleton. αβ Spectrin heterodimers self-associate into tetramers and higher order oligomers that are critical for erythrocyte membrane stability as well as erythrocyte shape and function. Most spectrin defects in hereditary elliptocytosis impair the ability of spectrin dimers to self-associate into tetramers and oligomers, thereby disrupting the membrane skeleton. Structural and functional defects of protein 4.1 appear to disrupt the spectrin–actin contact in the membrane skeleton. Glycophorin C variants are also deficient in protein 4.1. The precise pathobiology of how elliptocytes are formed in these syndromes is unclear.

Genetically, hereditary elliptocytosis is heterogeneous with multiple genetic loci. A wide variety of mutations have been described in the α spectrin, β spectrin, protein 4.1, and glycophorin C genes, including point mutations, gene deletions and insertions, and messenger RNA processing defects. Several mutations have been identified in a number of individuals of the same genetic background, suggesting a "founder effect" for these mutants, which supports the hypothesis that there has been genetic selection for elliptocytosis because these RBCs confer some resistance to malaria. Most cases of hereditary elliptocytosis are inherited in an autosomal dominant pattern, with rare cases of de novo mutations.

CLINICAL MANIFESTATIONS

The clinical presentation of hereditary elliptocytosis is heterogeneous, ranging from asymptomatic carriers to patients with severe, life-threatening anemia. Most patients with hereditary elliptocytosis are asymptomatic and are diagnosed incidentally during testing for unrelated conditions. Asymptomatic carriers have been identified who possess the same molecular defect as an affected hereditary elliptocytosis relative but who have normal peripheral blood smears. The erythrocyte lifespan is decreased in only about 10% of patients. This subset of patients with hereditary elliptocytosis and decreased erythrocyte lifespan experience hemolysis, anemia, splenomegaly, and intermittent jaundice. Many of these patients have parents with typical hereditary elliptocytosis and thus are homozygotes or compound heterozygotes for defects inherited from each of the parents. Symptoms may vary among members of the same family; indeed, they may vary in the same individual at different times.

HEREDITARY PYROPOIKILOCYTOSIS

Hereditary pyropoikilocytosis is a rare cause of anemia with distinctive erythrocyte morphology on peripheral blood smear (see Fig. 147-2C) and has a picture similar to that seen in patients with severe burns. Patients typically present in infancy with severe anemia and peripheral blood smear findings of elliptocytosis, poikilocytosis, pyknocytosis, and fragmentation. Microspherocytosis is common, and the MCV is usually very low (50 to 70 fL). Most patients are of African ancestry. At least one third of hereditary pyropoikilocytosis patients have a parent or sibling with typical hereditary elliptocytosis, as they share common mutations in the self-association site of spectrin. Patients with hereditary pyropoikilocytosis tend to experience severe hemolysis and anemia in infancy that gradually improves, evolving toward typical hereditary elliptocytosis later in life.

DIAGNOSIS

Cigar-shaped elliptocytes on peripheral blood smear are the hallmark of hereditary elliptocytosis (see Fig. 147-2B). These normochromic, normocytic elliptocytes vary in number from a few to 100%. The likelihood of hemolysis does not correlate with the number of elliptocytes present. Ovalocytes, spherocytes, stomatocytes, and fragmented cells may also be seen. In some cases, pyknocytes may be prominent. Elliptocytes may be seen in association with other disorders, including megaloblastic anemias, hypochromic microcytic anemias (iron deficiency anemia and thalassemia), myelodysplastic syndromes, and myelofibrosis; however, elliptocytes generally make up fewer than one third of RBCs in these conditions. History and additional laboratory testing usually clarify the diagnosis of these disorders. In typical cases, the incubated osmotic fragility is normal, but in severe hereditary elliptocytosis and hereditary pyropoikilocytosis, incubated osmotic fragility is increased, and EMA binding is decreased.

Other laboratory findings in hereditary elliptocytosis are similar to those found in other hemolytic anemias and are nonspecific markers of increased erythrocyte production and destruction. The reticulocyte count generally is less than 5% but may be higher when hemolysis is severe.

Similar to hereditary spherocytosis, specialized laboratory procedures are available to study the erythrocyte membranes of hereditary elliptocytosis and hereditary pyropoikilocytosis patients. These studies are not routinely required to make the diagnosis of hereditary elliptocytosis or hereditary pyropoikilocytosis, but they may be helpful in studying problematic cases and in elucidating the underlying molecular defects.

TREATMENT

Therapy is rarely needed in patients with hereditary elliptocytosis. In rare cases, occasional RBC transfusions may be required. In cases of severe hereditary elliptocytosis and hereditary pyropoikilocytosis, splenectomy has been palliative because the spleen is the site of erythrocyte sequestration and destruction. Many practitioners think that the same indications for splenectomy in hereditary spherocytosis should be applied to patients with symptomatic hereditary elliptocytosis or hereditary pyropoikilocytosis. Post-splenectomy patients with hereditary elliptocytosis or hereditary pyropoikilocytosis experience increased hematocrits, decreased reticulocyte counts, and improvement in clinical symptoms. Similar post-splenectomy guidelines as outlined for hereditary spherocytosis should be followed.

Patients should be followed for signs of decompensation during acute illnesses. Interval ultrasonography to detect gallstones should be performed. In patients with significant hemolysis, folate (1 mg/day orally) should be administered daily.

HEREDITARY STOMATOCYTOSIS SYNDROMES

Red blood cell hydration is primarily determined by the intracellular concentration of monovalent cations. A net increase in sodium and potassium ions causes water to enter, forming *stomatocytes* (see Fig. 147-2D) or *hydrocytes*, but a net loss of sodium and potassium produces dehydrated RBCs, or *xerocytes*. Numerous descriptions of congenital or familial hemolytic anemias associated with abnormal cation permeability and, in some cases, disturbed RBC hydration have been reported.[13] These span the range from severe hydrocytosis to severe xerocytosis. In many cases, the molecular bases of this group of disorders are unknown. An unusual characteristic of the stomatocytosis syndromes is a predisposition to thrombosis after splenectomy. Acquired stomatocytosis has been associated with acute alcoholism and hepatobiliary disease, vinca alkaloid administration, neoplasms, and cardiovascular disease. Stomatocytosis is also sometimes observed as a processing artifact.

Overhydrated Hereditary Stomatocytosis (Hydrocytosis)

This group of disorders is characterized by stomatocytes, erythrocytes with a mouth-shaped (stoma) area of central pallor on peripheral blood smear (see Fig. 147-2D), severe hemolysis, macrocytosis (110-150 fL), elevated erythrocyte sodium concentration, reduced potassium concentration, and increased total Na^+ and K^+ content. The excess cations expand cell water, producing large, osmotically fragile cells with low MCHCs (24 to 30%). The clinical severity of overhydrated hereditary stomatocytosis is variable; some patients experience hemolysis and anemia, but others are asymptomatic. Missense mutations in the Rh-associated glycoprotein (*RHAG*) and in band 3 (*SLC4A1*) have been identified in discrete subsets of hydrocytosis patients.

Dehydrated Hereditary Stomatocytosis (Xerocytosis)

Blood smears from patients with dehydrated hereditary stomatocytosis exhibit contracted and spiculated RBCs, dessicytes, a variable number of stomatocytes, and target cells. Most patients have nearly normal erythrocyte morphology, with only a few target cells and an occasional echinocyte or stomatocyte. The MCV (95-115 fL) and MCHC are increased, and the osmotic fragility is reduced (i.e., resistance to osmotic lysis). The characteristic biochemical abnormality is a decreased potassium concentration and total monovalent cation content. Dominantly inherited mutations in PIEZO1 are found in most xerocytosis patients. PIEZO proteins are the recently identified pore-forming subunits of channels that mediate mechanotransduction in mammalian cells. In erythrocytes, PIEZO1 carries the Er blood group antigens.[14] Association of PIEZO variants with changes in erythrocyte hydration suggest that these proteins play an important role in erythrocyte volume homeostasis. A few hereditary xerocytosis patients have been found to have mutations in the Gardos channel, encoded by *KCNN4*, important in the pathogenesis of erythrocyte dehydration in sickle cell disease.

Intermediate Syndromes and Hereditary Stomatocytosis Variants

Hydrocytosis and xerocytosis represent the extremes of a broad spectrum of RBC permeability defects. In fact, families with features of both conditions have been reported. Some patients with severe permeability defects have little or no hemolysis. The proportion of stomatocytes and the degree of sodium influx do not correlate with each other, and neither correlates with the amount of hemolysis or anemia.

ERYTHROCYTE METABOLISM

NORMAL METABOLISM

The primary functions of the erythrocyte, gas transport and exchange, are maintained without a net change in energy state. However, several critical functions of the erythrocyte depend on the production and expenditure of energy. As erythrocytes age, glucose utilization and ATP levels fall, leading to decreased membrane deformability and, ultimately, a shortened lifespan. Lower potassium levels, higher sodium levels, and decreased membrane lipids are also seen in ATP-deficient, aging erythrocytes.

Erythrocytes do not undergo oxidative phosphorylation and do not store glycogen; thus, they must constantly catabolize glucose from the blood stream through the Embden-Meyerhof pathway and the hexose monophosphate shunt as a source of energy (Fig. 147-4). Erythrocytes incorporate glucose from the plasma through facilitated transfer, with erythrocyte glucose levels rapidly equilibrating with changes in blood glucose levels. Glucose is the preferred carbohydrate of the RBC, but fructose and mannose are metabolized almost as readily. Inside the erythrocyte, glucose is converted to glucose-6-phosphate or to fructose by sorbitol. Glucose-6-phosphate follows one of three pathways: (1) most (≈90%) enters the Embden-Meyerhof pathway, where it is converted into lactate, pyruvate, and ATP; (2) some (≈5 to 10%) enters the hexose monophosphate shunt to produce reduced intermediates and ribulose 5-phosphate, the latter of which eventually enters the Embden-Meyerhof pathway; and (3) a tiny fraction (<1%) is converted to glucose-1-phosphate and then to glycogen.

Embden-Meyerhof Pathway

The Embden-Meyerhof pathway of glycolysis is the primary source of ATP, 2,3-DPG and nicotinamide adenine dinucleotide, reduced form (NADH) in erythrocytes (see Fig. 147-4). Most of the energy generated by erythrocytes is through the Embden-Meyerhof pathway followed by storage as high-energy phosphates such as ATP or as reducing energy in the form of glutathione or pyridine nucleotides (NADH and nicotinamide adenine dinucleotide phosphate, reduced form [NADPH]). This pathway metabolizes about 90% of erythrocyte glucose with the catabolism of 1 mole of glucose yielding 2 moles of ATP and 2 moles of lactate. Two moles of ATP per mole of metabolized glucose seems insignificant compared with the Krebs cycle of intermediary metabolism, in which 1 mole of glucose metabolized produces 38 moles of ATP. However, this ATP production is adequate to renew 150 to 200% of the total RBC ATP every hour.

The Embden-Meyerhof pathway is also the primary source of NADH, a necessary cofactor for NADH methemoglobin reductase, which maintains heme iron in the reduced state. Without this reaction, heme iron would be oxidized to methemoglobin, which is not a functional oxygen transporter.

Finally, the Rapoport-Luebering shunt of the Embden-Meyerhof pathway (see Fig. 147-4) produces 2,3-DPG, a compound found in high concentrations in erythrocytes but in low concentrations in other cells. After it is formed, under physiologic conditions of pH and solute concentrations, 2,3-DPG binds reversibly to tetramers of deoxyhemoglobin with greater affinity than it does to oxyhemoglobin. By binding to deoxyhemoglobin, it allosterically upregulates the release of the remaining oxygen bound to the Hb, enhancing the ability of erythrocytes to release oxygen near tissues that need it most.

Hexose Monophosphate Shunt (Pentose Phosphate Pathway)

In the hexose monophosphate shunt (see Fig. 147-4), glucose-6-phosphate undergoes oxidation followed by a series of reactions to yield

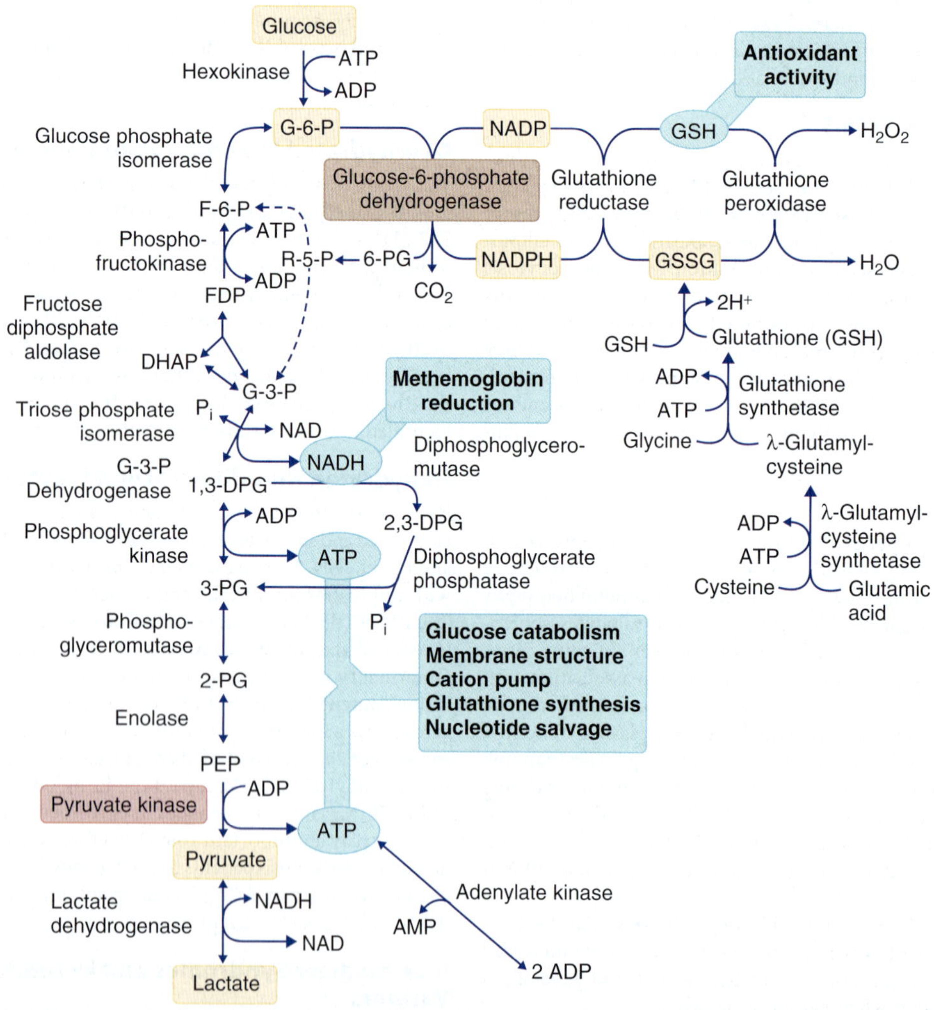

FIGURE 147-4. Pathways of energy metabolism in the erythrocyte. Glucose-6-phosphate may be degraded anaerobically to lactate through the Embden-Meyerhof pathway or oxidatively through the hexose monophosphate shunt. Pentose phosphates (R-5-P) can reenter anaerobic glycolysis as fructose-6-phosphate (F-6-P) and glyceraldehyde-3-phosphate (G-3-P) after conversion by enzymes of the terminal pentose phosphate pathway or as a product of adenosine or inosine degradation. 2,3-Diphosphoglycerate (2,3-DPG) may be generated instead of adenosine triphosphate (ATP) through diversion of triose through the Rapoport-Luebering shunt. Glutathione may be synthesized directly from constituent amino acids; its cycling from oxidized (GSSG) to reduced forms (GSH) depends on reduced pyridine cofactor (NADPH) generation. ADP = adenosine diphosphate; DHAP = dihydroxyacetone phosphate; FDP = fructose-1,6-diphosphate; NAD = nicotinamide adenine dinucleotide; NADP = nicotinamide adenine dinucleotide phosphate; NADPH = nicotinamide adenine dinucleotide phosphate, reduced form; PEP = polyestradiol phosphate.

fructose-6-phosphate and glyceraldehyde-3-phosphate, intermediates in the glycolytic pathway. The hexose monophosphate shunt is the primary source of erythrocyte NADPH, with 2 moles of NADPH produced for each mole of glucose metabolized. NADPH is required for the reduction of oxidized glutathione and some protein sulfhydryl groups.

Mature erythrocytes synthesize large amounts of reduced glutathione. Glutathione protects erythrocytes from oxidants, including hydrogen peroxide (H_2O_2), superoxide anions (O_2^-), and hydroxyl radicals (OH), which are produced as byproducts of the oxidation of heme by oxygen. Oxidants are also produced by activated phagocytes (e.g., during infection) and by erythrocytes after exposure to certain agents. When oxidants accumulate, they damage cellular proteins and lipids. Detoxification of H_2O_2 is significantly enhanced by glutathione peroxidase. Glutathione is converted to oxidized glutathione and to mixed disulfides with protein thiols. Glutathione levels are restored by glutathione reductase. In this process, NADPH is oxidized to nicotinamide adenine dinucleotide phosphate (NADP), which stimulates the hexose monophosphate shunt to regenerate NADPH. After oxidant stress, hypoxia, or acidosis, erythrocytes can increase the amount of glucose metabolized through the hexose monophosphate shunt up to 10- to 20-fold to generate increased amounts of reduced glutathione. The tight coupling of glutathione metabolism with the hexose monophosphate shunt protects the mature erythrocyte from oxidative stress.

DISORDERS OF ERYTHROCYTE METABOLISM

Congenital nonspherocytic hemolytic anemia traditionally includes erythrocyte disorders not due to defects of the RBC membrane or hemoglobin, immune-mediated disease, or other diseases such as paroxysmal nocturnal hemoglobinuria. Congenital nonspherocytic hemolytic anemia is a heterogeneous group of disorders associated with various metabolic abnormalities of the erythrocytes, including enzymopathies of glucose, glutathione, and nucleotide metabolism. Similar to the membrane disorders, clinical, biochemical, and genetic heterogeneity are typical within the enzymopathies. Hemolysis may develop as a result of either enzyme or antioxidant deficiency or dysfunction (e.g., abnormal substrate or cofactor binding), altered activation or inhibition characteristics, or decreased stability or specific activity.

Peripheral blood smears in congenital nonspherocytic hemolytic anemia, with the exception of pyrimidine 5′-nucleotidase deficiency, are unremarkable. Osmotic fragility of fresh erythrocytes is normal. Response to splenectomy is variable. Inheritance is heterogeneous. A thorough family history is important and may be of assistance in determining the diagnosis. Manifestations of the metabolic defect are usually confined to the erythrocyte but may occasionally involve nonerythroid cells.

Definitive diagnosis of metabolic abnormalities of the erythrocyte depends on qualitative or quantitative assays of specific enzyme activity or identification of the specific genetic mutation by DNA analysis. Results of enzyme assays should be interpreted with caution because they only sample surviving RBCs in the peripheral blood and the metabolic milieu of these cells is not necessarily comparable to cells already hemolyzed; in vitro enzyme assay conditions may not accurately reflect the in vivo environment; transfusions before the assay may obscure the underlying metabolic defect; and leukocyte contamination may lead to spurious results. Finally, average enzyme activity may not accurately reflect activity in subpopulations of erythrocytes. This is particularly true when there is reticulocytosis, which may yield artificially elevated mean enzyme activity owing to higher enzyme levels found in reticulocytes.

DISORDERS OF THE EMBDEN-MEYERHOF PATHWAY

Defects of the Embden-Meyerhof pathway are inherited in an autosomal recessive fashion, and usually hemolysis is seen only in homozygotes or compound heterozygotes. Heterozygotes, whose erythrocytes contain less than normal amounts of mutant enzyme, are clinically normal. An exception is phosphoglycerate kinase deficiency, an X-linked disorder with hemolysis found only in males. In this group of disorders, hemolysis is chronic, is not typically influenced by drugs or other inciting agents, and is attributed to insufficient levels of erythrocyte ATP. Splenomegaly from trapping of mutant erythrocytes is common. The hostile splenic environment contributes to the shortened erythrocyte lifespan. When performing specific diagnostic enzyme assays, measurement of glycolytic intermediates may assist in diagnosis because concentrations of intermediates are increased upstream of a defect and decreased downstream of a defect.

Pyruvate Kinase Deficiency

Pyruvate kinase deficiency accounts for approximately 90% of inherited defects of the Embden-Meyerhof pathway and is the second most common inherited erythrocyte enzymopathy associated with anemia after glucose-6-phosphate dehydrogenase (G6PD) deficiency (see later). Pyruvate kinase deficiency is found worldwide, but it is most common in individuals of northern European descent.

PATHOBIOLOGY

Pyruvate kinase catalyzes the conversion of phosphoenolpyruvate (PEP) to pyruvate, generating ATP. Deficient or defective pyruvate kinase leads to decreased levels of erythrocyte ATP, disturbing many cellular processes such as signaling and maintenance of water and ion content, leading to energy failure and dehydration. Upstream catabolites accumulate in the erythrocyte, including 2,3-DPG, which shifts the oxygen dissociation curve to the right, enhancing tissue oxygenation and ameliorating some of the physiologic effects of anemia. Early pyruvate kinase-deficient reticulocytes retain the ability to use oxidative phosphorylation to produce ATP, bypassing their defect. This ability is lost as reticulocytes mature and is markedly dampened in the hypoxic environment of the spleen.

Pyruvate kinase deficiency is inherited in an autosomal recessive manner. Affected individuals are homozygous or compound heterozygotes for pyruvate kinase defects. Heterozygotes are clinically normal or exhibit very minimal hemolysis. Mutation studies reveal a wide range of variants, with a few mutations enriched in certain populations.[15]

CLINICAL MANIFESTATIONS

Clinical manifestations in pyruvate kinase deficiency are heterogeneous, ranging from asymptomatic to transfusion-dependent hemolytic anemia.[16] More severely affected patients present in infancy or early childhood with anemia, jaundice, and splenomegaly. Occasionally, patients may escape detection until later in life when complications related to anemia and chronic hemolysis occur such as cholelithiasis or aplastic crisis or when the diagnosis is made during evaluation of the patient for another condition.

DIAGNOSIS

The peripheral blood smear demonstrates normocytic, normochromic erythrocytes, sometimes with spiculations (Fig. 147-5A). Poikilocytes and acanthocytes may also be seen. Reticulocytosis is common. Osmotic fragility of fresh erythrocytes is usually normal. Occasional patients exhibit a population of osmotically fragile cells after incubation.

NADH fluorescence is a commonly used screening test for pyruvate kinase deficiency. PEP and NADH are mixed with the patient's blood, incubated, and spotted on filter paper, and fluorescence is measured. Direct enzyme assay, which uses PEP as substrate for pyruvate kinase, performed on leukocyte-free hemolysate, is the gold standard for the diagnosis of pyruvate kinase deficiency. This detects all but the few rare patients with dysfunctional, thermolabile enzyme variants without enzyme deficiency. Leukocytes must be carefully depleted from the samples because they contain more than 300 times the pyruvate kinase activity of erythrocytes. Genetic diagnosis for pyruvate kinase deficiency is now widely available. Molecular diagnosis is particularly helpful in patients after transfusion, when prenatal diagnosis is desired, and when sample shipping and preparation precludes direct enzyme assay. To ascertain the diagnosis most accurately using molecular techniques, study of parental DNA is required, unless the patient is homozygous for a deleterious mutation, to determine if the variants detected are in *cis* or *trans* for precise diagnosis.

TREATMENT

Most patients require expectant management, with only rare transfusions, such as during an aplastic episode.[17] Mitapivat, an oral, small-molecule allosteric activator of pyruvate kinase in red cells,[18] can increase the hemoglobin level in adults with pyruvate kinase deficiency and a missense *PKLR* mutation.[A1] In severe cases, patients may be transfusion dependent. In these cases, splenectomy typically lessens hemolysis and ameliorates the anemia. After splenectomy, some patients develop marked reticulocytosis, up to 50 to 70%. This paradoxical reticulocytosis is attributed to increased reticulocyte survival after removal of the hostile splenic environment.

Other Disorders of the Embden-Meyerhof Pathway

Other abnormalities of the Embden-Meyerhof pathway have been described. Hexokinase deficiency is quite uncommon, with great phenotypic variability in reported cases. Severely affected patients have had anemia beginning in infancy and may require blood transfusions. Glucose phosphate isomerase (GPI) deficiency is the third most common hemolytic enzymopathy. GPI deficiency

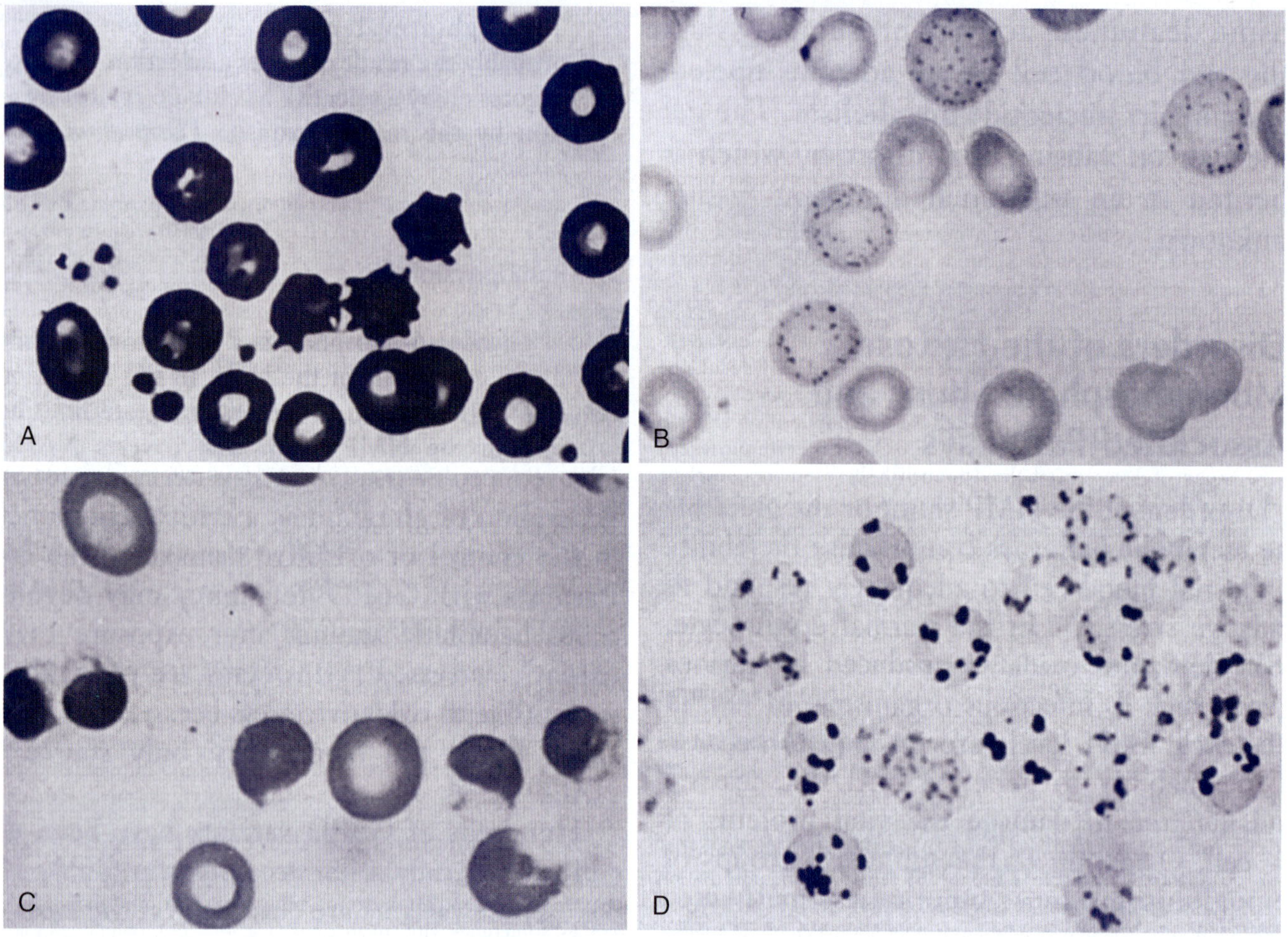

FIGURE 147-5. **Peripheral blood smears in erythrocyte enzymopathies. A,** Pyruvate kinase deficiency. **B,** Pyrimidine 5′-nucleotidase deficiency. **C,** Glucose-6-phosphate dehydrogenase (G6PD) deficiency. **D,** Heinz bodies in G6PD deficiency. (**B** from Paglia DE. Disorders of erythrocyte glycolysis and nucleotide metabolism. In: Handin RI, Lux SE, Stossel TP, eds. *Blood: Principles and Practice of Hematology*. Philadelphia: JB Lippincott; 1995:1877-1896.)

usually presents in infancy or early childhood with moderate to severe hemolytic anemia. Rare cases of GPI deficiency may also be complicated by neurologic symptomatology. Phosphofructokinase deficiency may involve erythrocytes, muscle, or both. The presentation is usually in adolescence with exertional myopathy. Hemolytic anemia has been described in isolated cases of 2,3-bisphosphoglycerate mutase deficiency and phosphoglycerate kinase deficiency.

DISORDERS OF NUCLEOTIDE METABOLISM

Mature erythrocytes lack the ability to synthesize purine and pyrimidine nucleotides de novo. However, they are able to form some nucleotides through salvage pathways.

Pyrimidine 5′-Nucleotidase Deficiency

Pyrimidine 5′-nucleotidase degrades the pyrimidine nucleotides of RNA to cytidine and uridine, which can diffuse out of the cell. When pyrimidine 5′-nucleotidase is deficient, nondiffusible, partially degraded RNAs accumulate, leading to the marked basophilic stippling characteristic of pyrimidine 5′-nucleotidase-deficient erythrocytes (see Fig. 147-5B). These accumulated pyrimidine nucleotides inhibit the transport of oxidized glutathione out of RBCs, leading to high levels of erythrocyte glutathione. Clinically, the patient has mild to moderate hemolytic anemia and splenomegaly. The cause of the hemolysis remains cryptic. Typically, splenectomy does not ameliorate the hemolysis and anemia.

DISORDERS OF THE HEXOSE MONOPHOSPHATE SHUNT (PENTOSE PHOSPHATE PATHWAY) AND ASSOCIATED PATHWAYS

Disorders of the hexose monophosphate shunt or of the glutathione metabolic pathways (see Fig. 147-4) compromise the ability of the RBC to respond adequately to oxidative stress. In normal erythrocytes, glutathione detoxifies oxidants produced by various agents and infection. In G6PD-deficient erythrocytes, because of the inability to generate NADPH, glutathione levels are inadequate, leaving the cell susceptible to oxidant stress. Oxidation of Hb sulfhydryl groups leads to the production of methemoglobin and intracellular Hb precipitates called *Heinz bodies.* Heinz bodies (see Fig. 147-5D), usually visualized on peripheral blood smears with supravital stains such as methyl violet, attach to and damage the erythrocyte membrane. They induce clustering of immunoglobulins and band 3 protein, marking the erythrocyte for opsonization by phagocytes and eventual removal from the circulation. Heinz bodies are "pitted" from circulating cells by the spleen and are commonly seen on smears of patients after splenectomy. "Bite cells," erythrocytes with localized invaginations, possibly at the site of Heinz body injury or removal, are seen during acute hemolytic episodes (Chapter 143). In addition to damage from Heinz body formation, glutathione-deficient erythrocytes undergo peroxidation of membrane phospholipids and oxidative cross-linking of spectrin, decreasing membrane deformability and further promoting splenic trapping.

Glucose-6-Phosphate Dehydrogenase Deficiency

G6PD deficiency is the most common inherited disorder of erythrocyte metabolism, affecting more than 400 million people worldwide.[19,20] The high prevalence of G6PD deficiency is thought to be attributable to genetic selection because G6PD-deficient erythrocytes have a selective advantage against invasion by the malaria parasite *Plasmodium falciparum*.

EPIDEMIOLOGY AND PATHOBIOLOGY

G6PD is the initial and rate-limiting step in the hexose monophosphate shunt (see Fig. 147-4), which converts NADP into NADPH. NADPH is required for the generation of glutathione, a critical constituent in the prevention of oxidative damage to the cell. G6PD-deficient patients may develop acute hemolytic anemia after exposure to oxidative stress. Although G6PD is a ubiquitous enzyme, erythroid cells are particularly susceptible to oxidative stress because the hexose monophosphate shunt is their only source of NADPH.

Hundreds of G6PD variants have been described, but only a few are common. Variants are classified on the basis of biochemical characteristics, electrophoretic mobility, ability to use substrate analogue, Km for NADP and G6PD, pH

TABLE 147-2 FEATURES OF G6PD VARIANTS

VARIANT	GENOTYPE	ENZYME ACTIVITY (% OF NORMAL)	ENZYME THERMAL STABILITY	ACTIVITY (K_{CAT} S^{-1})	ENZYME CATALYTIC CLASSIFICATION	WHO CLINICAL DISTRIBUTION
G6PD B	None	100	Normal	275	IV	Worldwide
G6PD A+	Val68Met	85	Normal	247	IV	Africa
G6PD A-	Val68Met, Asn126AsP	10-23	Low	137	III	Africa
G6PD Mahidol	Gly163Ser	0.6	Normal	207	II	Southeast Asia
G6PD Mediterranean	Ser188Phe	<5	Low	98	II	Middle East, Southcentral Asia
G6PD Canton	Arg463Leu	4	Slight decrease	123	II	North Vietnam and South China

From Luzzatto L, Ally M, Notaro R. Glucose-6-phosphate dehydrogenase deficiency. *Blood*. 2020;136:1225-1240.

activity profile, and thermal stability. The normal enzyme, Gd^{B}, is present in 99% of White Americans and 70% of African Americans. A normal variant, Gd^{A+}, found in 20% of African Americans, has a faster electrophoretic mobility than Gd^{B}. Gd^{A-}, the most common variant associated with hemolysis, is found in about 10% of African Americans and in many Africans. Gd^{A-} has decreased catalytic ability compared with Gd^{A+}. Gd^{Med}, the second most common variant associated with hemolysis, is common in the Mediterranean area, in India, and in Southeast Asia, with a prevalence of up to 5 to 50%. Gd^{Med} exhibits markedly decreased catalytic activity. Gd^{Canton}, a variant common in Asian populations, produces a clinical syndrome similar to Gd^{A-}. Features of several G6PD variants are shown in Table 147-2.

Gd^{B} activity decreases as normal cells age, with a half-life of approximately 60 days. Despite very low levels of or no active G6PD, older erythrocytes maintain the ability to produce NADPH and maintain a glutathione response to oxidative stress. The Gd^{A-} variant has a half-life of only 13 days, so young cells have a normal amount of enzyme activity, but older RBCs are grossly deficient. Because of this heterogeneity in G6PD levels, individuals with the Gd^{A-} variant experience only limited hemolysis after oxidant exposure.

More than 100 mutations in the *G6PD* gene, localized to Xq28, have been described. Most mutations are amino acid substitutions that influence enzyme kinetics, stability, or both, with a few rare deletions and splicing mutations described. Because it is X-linked, G6PD deficiency primarily affects males. Males have only one G6PD allele and express only one G6PD type. Females can express one or two G6PD types. The Lyon hypothesis specifies that only one X chromosome is active in any given cell; thus, any given cell in a heterozygous female is either normal or deficient. In females who are heterozygous for G6PD deficiency, average G6PD activity may be normal or mildly, moderately, or severely reduced, depending on the degree of lyonization. G6PD-deficient erythrocytes in heterozygous females are susceptible to the same oxidant stress as G6PD-deficient cells in males, but, typically, the overall degree of hemolysis is less because there is a smaller population of vulnerable cells.

CLINICAL MANIFESTATIONS

G6PD deficiency is divided into five classes based on clinical severity and degree of enzyme deficiency. Class I is characterized by congenital nonspherocytic hemolytic anemia without precipitating cause and severe G6PD deficiency. Class II is characterized by intermittent hemolysis and severe G6PD deficiency. Class III is characterized by hemolysis after oxidant stress and mild G6PD deficiency. Class II and III together represent more than 90% of G6PD variants. Classes IV and V are clinically asymptomatic. The most clinically significant syndromes of G6PD deficiency are acute hemolytic anemia; neonatal jaundice; and rarely, congenital nonspherocytic hemolytic anemia.

Acute hemolytic anemia is the most dramatic clinical presentation of G6PD deficiency with acute intravascular hemolysis after exposure to an oxidative stress. Oxidative stresses include ingestion of certain drugs such as primaquine or sulfa-containing compounds, exposure to naphthalene (mothballs), ingestion of fava beans, or infection, the latter being the most common cause of hemolysis. Table 147-3 lists drugs that should be avoided in G6PD-deficient patients. Presenting symptoms include irritability, fever, nausea, abdominal pain, and diarrhea within 48 hours of oxidant exposure. Hemoglobinuria, jaundice, and anemia ensue. The spleen and liver may be enlarged and tender. Cases with severe anemia may precipitate congestive heart failure. Laboratory findings include a normochromic, normocytic anemia with anisocytosis and reticulocytosis. Poikilocytes and bite cells may be seen. Heinz bodies, a classic finding in G6PD deficiency, may be seen but are an inconsistent finding because these damaged cells are rapidly cleared from the circulation in the spleen. Additional laboratory findings may include hemoglobinuria and the presence of free Hb in the blood.

TABLE 147-3 AGENTS TO BE AVOIDED BY GLUCOSE-6-PHOSPHATE DEHYDROGENASE–DEFICIENT PATIENTS*

ANTIMALARIALS

Primaquine (people with the African A^{-} variant may take it at reduced dosage, under surveillance)
Pamaquine
Chloroquine (may be used under surveillance when required for prophylaxis or treatment of malaria)

SULFONAMIDES AND SULFONES

Sulfanilamide
Sulfapyridine
Sulfadimidine
Sulfacetamide (Albucid)
Acetyl sulfisoxazole (Gantrisin)
Salicylazosulfapyridine (Salazopyrin)
Dapsone
Sulfoxone
Glucosulfone sodium (Promin)
Sulfamethoxazole-trimethoprim (Bactrim, Septra)

OTHER ANTIBACTERIAL COMPOUNDS

Nitrofurans—nitrofurantoin, furazolidone, nitrofurazone
[Nalidixic acid]
Chloramphenicol
p-Aminosalicylic acid

ANALGESICS

Acetylsalicylic acid (aspirin): moderate doses can be used
Acetophenetidin (Phenacetin)
Safe alternative: Paracetamol

ANTHELMINTICS

β-Naphthol
Stibophen
Niridazole

MISCELLANEOUS

Vitamin K analogues (1 mg of menaphthone can be given to babies)
Naphthalene (moth balls)
Probenecid
Dimercaprol (BAL)
Methylene blue
Arsine†
Phenylhydrazine†
Acetylphenylhydrazine†
Toluidine blue
Mepacrine

*Drugs in bold print should be avoided by people with all forms of glucose-6-phosphate dehydrogenase (G6PD) deficiency. Drugs in normal print should be avoided, in addition, by G6PD-deficient people of Mediterranean, Middle Eastern, and Asian origin. Items in normal print and within square brackets apply only to people with the African A^{-} variant.

†These drugs or chemicals may cause hemolysis in normal people if given in large doses. Many other drugs may produce hemolysis in certain individuals.

Another clinically significant syndrome of G6PD deficiency is neonatal jaundice. Jaundice is seldom present at birth, with the peak incidence of onset between days 2 and 3 of life. The severity of hyperbilirubinemia is variable. It may be severe, resulting in kernicterus or even death. In most cases, however, hyperbilirubinemia is adequately treated with phototherapy. In neonatal jaundice, it is important to note that the anemia is very rarely severe. The etiology of neonatal jaundice remains controversial. Neonatal jaundice is increased in G6PD-deficient infants who also carry a polymorphism of the uridine diphosphoglucuronyl transferase (*UDPGT1*) gene associated with Gilbert syndrome.

Chronic nonspherocytic hemolytic anemia is associated with uncommon variants of G6PD deficiency, usually mutant enzymes unable to maintain basal NADPH production. Presentation may be in the neonatal period when neonatal jaundice is accompanied by anemia in a male. The degree of chronic anemia in congenital nonspherocytic hemolytic anemia caused by G6PD deficiency has been variable. Some patients have compensated hemolysis, but others require intermittent transfusions. Transfusion dependence occurs in the most severe cases.

G6PD deficiency, which suppresses the antioxidant system, has been suggested to worsen severity of COVID-19 infection which activates pro-oxidant responses. This association was not identified in a genome-wide association study of patients with severe COVID-19.[21] This possible association needs to be further explored in clinical trials.

DIAGNOSIS

The G6PD reaction (glucose-6-phosphate + $NADP^+ \rightarrow$ 6-phosphogluconolactone + NADPH + H^+) reduces $NADP^+$ to NADPH. Formation of NADPH and NADH can be observed directly because they fluoresce in the visible spectrum when illuminated with long-wave ultraviolet light. Based on this observation, several simple screening tests performed using inexpensive long-wave ultraviolet light have been devised, and rapid testing has a very high sensitivity. However, these tests are semiquantitative, categorizing a sample as normal or deficient. They are unreliable after an acute hemolytic episode and do not typically detect female heterozygotes. Positive screening test results should be confirmed by spectrophotometric assay or DNA studies because of the risk of false-positive results.

Definitive assay of the enzyme depends on direct spectrophotometric measurement of NADPH production. Although more sensitive than screening tests, this still requires 20 to 30% G6PD-deficient cells to obtain an abnormal result. Sensitivity can be increased by comparing the level of G6PD deficiency with levels of other age-dependent erythrocyte enzymes, especially when testing is temporally in close proximity to an acute hemolytic episode. The cyanide-ascorbate test measures the ability of erythrocytes to prevent the oxidation of Hb by ascorbate. Using intact erythrocytes, as few as 10 to 15% deficient cells can be detected, making this test useful for detecting female heterozygotes and males after a hemolytic episode. This test also detects other perturbations of the hexose monophosphate shunt or glutathione metabolism. Genetic testing can be performed in difficult cases or when a molecular diagnosis is desired.[22]

TREATMENT

The best treatment for an individual with acute hemolytic anemia is careful prescription of medications and avoidance of inciting agents (see Table 147-3).[23,24] Outside of acute hemolytic episodes, these patients do not require any special therapy. Acute hemolytic anemia episodes are managed with particular attention to hematologic, cardiopulmonary, and renal complications of hemolysis. Management of neonatal jaundice does not differ from that recommended for other causes of neonatal hyperbilirubinemia. In congenital nonspherocytic hemolytic anemia, management is expectant. Exposure to oxidant stresses should be avoided. Blood transfusions may be necessary during acute hemolytic episodes. In severe cases of congenital nonspherocytic hemolytic anemia, splenectomy may ameliorate the anemia.

DISORDERS OF GLUTATHIONE METABOLISM

Defects of glutathione metabolism may be associated with hemolysis. Erythrocytes from patients lacking glutathione synthetase or γ-glutamylcysteine synthetase, enzymes involved in glutathione synthesis, have very low levels of glutathione. Clinically, these disorders resemble G6PD deficiency. There is mild to moderate chronic hemolytic anemia with increased susceptibility to oxidant stress.

GENERAL REFERENCES

For the General References and other additional features, please visit Elsevier eBooks+ at https://ebooks.health.elsevier.com.

Grade A Reference

A1. Al-Samkari H, Galactéros F, Glenthøj A, et al. Mitapivat versus placebo for pyruvate kinase deficiency. *N Engl J Med*. 2022;386:1432-1442.

148

THE THALASSEMIAS

MARIA DOMENICA CAPPELLINI

DEFINITION

The thalassemias, or more comprehensively the thalassemia syndromes, are a heterogeneous group of inherited hemolytic anemias characterized by deficient or absent production of one of the globin chains of hemoglobin. This deficiency leads to an imbalance in the synthesis of globin chains, an imbalance that is the hallmark of all the thalassemia syndromes.

EPIDEMIOLOGY

Taken together, the thalassemias are the most common recessive single-gene disorders in the world, with approximately 270 million or more people carrying one recessive gene. Each year, more than 40,000 children are born with one of the thalassemia syndromes, and about half of these individuals will become transfusion dependent. The extremely high frequency of the hemoglobin disorders compared with other monogenic diseases reflects natural selection mediated by the relative resistance of carriers against *Plasmodium falciparum* malaria (Chapter 316). Other factors that may be involved include the widespread practice of consanguineous marriage, increased maternal age in poorer countries, gene drift, and founder effects. For these reasons, the thalassemias are most frequent in southeastern and southern Asia,[1] in the Middle East, in the Mediterranean countries, and in northern and central Africa. However, as the result of recent mass migrations from the Middle East, Africa, and South East Asia, thalassemias are now encountered worldwide.

PATHOBIOLOGY

Normal adult red cells contain 97% adult hemoglobin (HbA: $\alpha_2\beta_2$), with approximately 2.5% of the minor component HbA_2 ($\alpha_2\delta_2$) and a small amount of fetal hemoglobin (HbF: $\alpha_2\gamma_2$). Because the stable tetramer $\alpha_2\beta_2$ is the major component of hemoglobin after birth, the two main forms of thalassemia are α-thalassemias and β-thalassemias. Because β-chain synthesis is fully activated only after birth, it follows that β-thalassemias are not expressed as a disease in intrauterine life; rather, they are manifested as γ-chain synthesis declines during the first year of life. In contrast, because α chains are shared by both fetal and adult hemoglobin, α-thalassemias are manifested in both fetal and adult life.

The thalassemia syndromes can be classified based on their genetics, clinical phenotypes, and transfusion requirements (Table 148-1).[2] Patients with transfusion-dependent β-thalassemia (β-thalassemia major or severe HbE–β-thalassemia) require lifelong, regular transfusions for survival, whereas patients with non–transfusion-dependent β-thalassemia (β-thalassemia intermedia or mild to moderate HbE–β-thalassemia) require no transfusions, occasional transfusions because of specific circumstances (e.g., pregnancy, surgery, or acute infection), or frequent transfusions but for a limited period (e.g., to support a growth spurt during childhood or manage a clinical complication).[3]

Genetics

Six different types of globin chains (α, β, γ, δ, ε, ζ) are found in normal human hemoglobin at different stages of development. In the very early embryo, hemoglobin synthesis is restricted to the yolk sac and the production of hemoglobins Gower 1 ($\zeta_2\varepsilon_2$), Gower 2 ($\alpha_2\varepsilon_2$), and Portland ($\zeta_2\gamma_2$). Subsequently, at about

TABLE 148-1 GENETIC AND CLINICAL CLASSIFICATIONS OF THE THALASSEMIAS

	GENETIC	CLINICAL	TRANSFUSION REQUIREMENT
α-Thalassemias	α^0	α-Minor	No transfusion
	α^+	HbH disease	Occasional transfusions
	Deletion (−α)	Hydrops fetalis	
	Nondeletion (α^T)		NA
β-Thalassemias	β^0	β-Minor	No transfusions
	β^+	Thalassemia intermedia	Occasional transfusions
	Variant with high HbA_2	Thalassemia major	Regular transfusions
	Normal HbA_2		
	Silent		
	Dominant		
	Unlinked to β-gene cluster		
δβ-Thalassemias	$(\delta\beta)^0$	δβ-Minor	Occasional transfusions
	$(\delta\beta)^+$	Thalassemia intermedia	
	$(^A\gamma\delta\beta)^0$		
HPFH	Deletion	Silent increase in HbF	No transfusions
	Nondeletion		
	Unlinked to β-gene cluster		

HbA = adult hemoglobin; HbF = fetal hemoglobin; HbH = hemoglobin H; HPFH = hereditary persistence of fetal hemoglobin.

8 weeks of gestation, the fetal liver takes over, synthesizing predominantly HbF ($\alpha_2\gamma_2$) and a small amount (<10%) of HbA. Between about 18 weeks and birth, the bone marrow progressively replaces the liver as the major site of red cell production; this shift is accompanied in the later stages of gestation by a reciprocal switch in production of HbA rather than HbF, so that HbF production drops to less than 2% by the end of the first year of life.

The globin genes are encoded in separate gene clusters. The α cluster (ζ,α_2,α_1) lies at the telomere of chromosome 16, whereas the β cluster ($\varepsilon,{}^G\gamma$ and ${}^A\gamma,\delta,\beta$) lies at chromosome 11p15.5. In both clusters, the genes are aligned 5′ to 3′ in the order in which they are expressed during development. Both sets of genes are under the regulation of enhancer-like elements (hypersensitive site [HS]–40 for α cluster and locus control region for β cluster) that lie some distance away at the 5′ end of the cluster. Deletion of these enhancer elements results in inactivation of any related globin gene. There are two α genes/alleles (α_2 and α_1) that differ by a few nucleotides in intron 2 and the 3′ untranslated region but nevertheless produce identical protein products. The output of the α_2 gene exceeds that of the α_1 gene by two- to three-fold.

The region around a DNase1 hypersensitive site at 40 kilobases (kb) upstream of the ζ-globin gene (HS-40) is the major regulator of α-globin gene expression. The β cluster contains a single pseudo-β gene, whereas the β cluster enhancer consists of five elements marked by erythroid-specific DNase1 hypersensitive sites lying 6 to 20 kb upstream of the ε-globin gene, with each element containing several binding sites for erythroid-specific and other transcription factors. All together, these elements are known as the locus control region, and each element contributes to the overall locus control region activity. In addition, there is an erythroid-specific hypersensitive site approximately 20 kb downstream of the β-globin gene; when the cluster is activated, the upstream and downstream hypersensitive sites are brought into proximity with the gene promoters to activate their transcription.

The individual globin genes share many general features; for example, each consists of three coding sequence exons separated by two introns in identical position but of variable length for a total length of approximately 1500 nucleotides. This structure has been highly conserved throughout evolution. The upstream regions flanking the first exon contain a number of sequence motifs that are necessary for specifying correct transcriptional initiation. A TATA box is found at 30 base pairs upstream of the initiation site together with one or more CCAAT sites at 70 base pairs upstream. The gene promoters also contain a CACCC or CCGCCC box that binds erythroid Krüppel-like factor (EKLF) 1, and some have binding sites for erythroid transcription factor GATA-1. In model systems, mutations introduced into such sequences lead to reduction in the level of transcription.

All the thalassemias have a similar pattern of inheritance; in most cases, the gene defects are transmitted in a mendelian autosomal recessive fashion. Thus, the severe, symptomatic varieties usually result from the interaction of more than one genetic determinant, for example, compound heterozygosity or homozygosity. The inheritance of α-thalassemia is more complicated because it involves the products of the linked pairs of α genes (αα) (see Clinical Manifestations).

Molecular Basis of Thalassemias

The α- and β-thalassemias are divided into disorders in which no chains are produced from the affected chromosomes (α^0 and β^0) and disorders in which the output of the chains is reduced (α^+ and β^+). For the α-thalassemias, the most common molecular defects are deletions of one or both α genes, which are designated −α and − −, respectively. The single α gene is thought to have arisen by crossover between two misaligned α genes on the homologous chromosome that can give rise to chromosomes with either single (−α) or triplicated (ααα) α-globin genes. To date, more than 40 different deletions that involve both α genes, resulting from illegitimate or nonhomologous recombination, have been reported. The lengths of deletion vary from 5.2 to more than 40 kb; the most common are those from Southeast Asia, the Mediterranean, and the Philippines, designated $--^{SEA}$, $--^{MED}$, and $--^{FIL}$, respectively. Nondeletion types of α-thalassemia (α^α) are much less common than the deletion forms; in most cases, they result from single oligonucleotide mutations in regions where the α gene sequence is critical for normal expression. Because expression of the α_2 gene is two to three times greater than that of the α_1 gene, it is not surprising that most of the nondeletion mutants predominantly affect expression of the α_2 gene. The mutations may affect the initiation codon or splicing signals, cause frame shifts, or introduce premature stop codons. At least five single-nucleotide variants affect the natural termination codon (TAA) of the α_2-globin gene. Among these, hemoglobin Constant Spring ($\alpha^{cs}\alpha$) is the most common and extensively studied. Finally, there are several α-globin variants that are so unstable that they undergo rapid, post-synthetic degradation. In such situations, β chains remain in excess within the red cell, and the patient carriers of these α-chain variants, by definition, have α-thalassemia. To date, 17 unstable α variants have been shown to produce the phenotype of α-thalassemia to a greater or lesser extent.

Like the α-thalassemias, the β-thalassemias are classified as β^0 (in which no β-globin is produced) and β^+ (in which some but less than normal β-globin is produced). In some cases, the defects in β-chain production are so mild that they are designated β^{++}. So far, more than 400 different thalassemic mutations of the β-globin gene have been reported; most are point mutations within the gene or its immediate flanking sequence. A few β-thalassemia mutations that segregate independently of the β-globin gene cluster have been described, presumably involving *trans*-acting regulatory factors. The distribution of alleles is highly variable from one population to another; but within each population, only a few alleles are common. The nondeletion forms of β-thalassemia account for most β-thalassemia alleles. An updated list of mutations (including transcriptional mutations, RNA processing mutations, and mutations affecting translation) is accessible at the Globin Gene Server website (http://globin.cse.psu.edu).

Simple deletions of the β-globin gene are rare, ranging in size from 290 base pairs to more than 60 kb. The 619–base pair deletion at the 3′ end of the β gene is relatively common among Sind and Punjabi populations in India and Pakistan. The remaining deletions are restricted to single families, are necessarily β^0-thalassemias, and interestingly are associated with unusually high levels of HbA_2 in heterozygotes. Large deletions that affect the entire β-globin gene cluster $(\varepsilon\gamma\gamma\delta\beta)^0$ are rare and restricted to single families. Finally, some highly unstable β-chain variants may be manifested as a dominant form of β-thalassemia.

The δβ-thalassemias and hereditary persistence of fetal hemoglobin are the result of deletions affecting various parts of the β-globin locus. These deletions are partially compensated by an increased expression of the γ genes that raises the level of HbF. The length of deletion accounts for different forms of δβ-thalassemia, including both ${}^G\gamma$ and ${}^A\gamma$ genes or only ${}^A\gamma$, and varies from 9 to 100 kb. Hemoglobin Lepore is a hybrid of δ and β chains resulting from a crossover between the two misaligned genes; this hemoglobin is synthesized inefficiently and gives rise to a form of δβ-thalassemia. Deletions of δ and β genes are also the molecular basis for many forms of hereditary persistence of fetal hemoglobin that, usually have higher levels of compensatory HbF production than the δβ-thalassemias. Hereditary persistence of fetal hemoglobin[4] also can be caused by point mutations in the promoter region upstream from the transcription start site in either the ${}^G\gamma$ or ${}^A\gamma$ genes that alter the binding of one or more transcription factors. Genetic studies have identified three major quantitative trait loci that account for 20 to 50% of the common variation in

HbF levels in patients with β-thalassemia and sickle cell disease as well as in healthy adults.

CLINICAL MANIFESTATIONS

The clinical manifestations (phenotype expression) of thalassemia syndromes are extremely variable and depend on the degree of globin chain imbalance.[5]

α-Thalassemias

There are two major classes of α-thalassemias: α^0, in which both α genes are inactivated (− −/); and α^+, in which only one of the pair is defective because of α gene deletion or mutation (−α or $\alpha\alpha^T$). The clinical spectrum of α-thalassemias correlates well with the number of the affected α genes, that is, from normal to the loss of all four genes.

The α-thalassemias are common in areas where β-thalassemias are also found at a high frequency. Thus, the coinheritance of α- and β-thalassemia trait may occur and even ameliorate the hematologic parameters. In families in which α- and β-thalassemias are present, genotyping is essential. The unstable mutant Hb^{CT} causes a severe reduction in α_2-globin expression from the affected chromosome; therefore, the carriers and particularly the homozygotes have a more severe phenotype than α-thalassemia minor but not as severe as most cases of HbH disease.

α-Thalassemia Minor

The inheritance of a normal allele (αα) with one of the α^+ or α^0 alleles most frequently results in α-thalassemia minor (− −/αα; −α/αα; $-\alpha^T/\alpha\alpha$; $\alpha^T\alpha/-\alpha$;−α/−α). In general, carriers of such genotypes have lower levels of total hemoglobin, mean corpuscular volume, and mean cell hemoglobin but higher red blood cell counts than normal. The greatest differences are seen in mean cell hemoglobin, which is usually less than 26 pg. The peripheral blood smear shows various degrees of hypochromia with some target cells and occasional poikilocytes (Chapter 143). In carriers of α^0-thalassemia (− −/αα), it is possible to generate a few red cell HbH inclusions (β_4). The carriers of nondeletional forms ($\alpha\alpha^T/\alpha\alpha$) show slightly more marked hematologic changes than those for deletional forms. The hemoglobin constitution of adult carriers of α^+- or α^0-thalassemia is indistinguishable from normal but has slightly lower levels of HbA_2. Traces of hemoglobin Bart (γ_4) in the neonatal period are detectable in a large proportion of neonates with α-thalassemia, and they decline during the first 6 months after birth.

Hemoglobin H Disease

HbH disease most frequently results from the co-presence of α^+- and α^0- thalassemia, and not surprisingly most patients originate from the populations of southeastern Asia, the Mediterranean, and the Middle East. HbH disease is a diagnosis attributed to subjects older than 6 months having a sufficient globin imbalance to produce detectable levels of HbH (>1 to 2%) in their peripheral blood together with inclusion bodies (β_4 tetramers) in their red cells on peripheral smear. The clinical phenotypes encompass a wide spectrum from mild clinical manifestations to thalassemia intermedia and are included in the so-called non–transfusion-dependent thalassemias. The predominant features of HbH disease are a hypochromic, microcytic anemia with jaundice, and hepatosplenomegaly. Because the main mechanism of the anemia is hemolysis rather than dyserythropoiesis, only a few patients have clinical evidence of an expanded erythron. The most common complication of HbH disease is the development of hypersplenism due to severe splenomegaly (Chapter 154). Other complications include gallstones, leg ulcers, increased risk for infection, folic acid deficiency, and increased risk for venous thrombosis mainly after splenectomy. Hemoglobin levels range in different series from 3 to 12 g/dL, with fluctuations that may occur after exposure to an oxidant drug, infection, or transient aplasia possibly due to intercurrent viral infection. Rarely, patients with HbH disease require regular blood transfusions. The anemia is associated with reticulocytosis and typical thalassemic changes of the red cell indices. The relative amount of HbH varies from 1 to 40%. The values of HbA_2 are always reduced. The peripheral blood film shows hypochromia with variable anisopoikilocytosis, target cells, and basophilic stippling. The characteristic feature of HbH disease is that it is always possible to generate multiple inclusions in the red cells after incubation with brilliant cresyl blue. The bone marrow shows marked erythroid hyperplasia.

Hydrops Fetalis

The most severe form of α-thalassemia is hydrops fetalis, in which all four α-globin genes are deleted (genotype − −/− −). Because α-globin chains are absent during gestation, hemoglobin Bart (γ_4) becomes the dominant hemoglobin. Because of its high oxygen affinity, hemoglobin Bart is unable to deliver oxygen to tissues, and the intrauterine consequences are progressive severe anemia, severe ineffective erythropoiesis with marked extramedullary erythropoiesis, massive organomegaly, heart failure, severe hypoalbuminemia, and edema. The hemoglobin levels range from 3 to 20 g/dL; the peripheral blood film is characterized by marked anisopoikilocytosis, large hypochromic macrocytes, and many nucleated red cells. The hemoglobin consists almost entirely of hemoglobin Bart (80 to 90%), with some remaining HbH and Portland. Mothers of these infants often have a history of previous neonatal deaths. Without medical care, women carrying these fetuses may have delivery and postpartum complications (e.g., retained placenta, eclampsia, sepsis) (Chapter 221).

Several reports describe α-thalassemia in association with intellectual disability (so-called ATR-16 syndrome). These conditions are mainly due to large deletions (one or two megabases) of the tip of chromosome 16, including the α-globin gene cluster. However, several cases have no deletions or other apparent abnormalities of the α-globin gene cluster. It has been shown that these patients with a peculiar phenotype characterized by severe mental retardation, dysmorphic facies, genital abnormalities, and α-thalassemia have a disorder that maps to the X chromosome (ATR-X syndrome).

β-Thalassemias

The β-thalassemias, which include a considerably heterogeneous group of disorders of hemoglobin synthesis, are characterized by a reduced output of the β chains of adult hemoglobin.[6] The clinical classification includes thalassemia major (transfusion dependent), thalassemia intermedia (of intermediate severity, non–transfusion dependent), and thalassemia minor (asymptomatic) (Fig. 148-1 and see Table 148-1). The severity of the clinical manifestations correlates well with the degree of imbalance of globin chains. Depending on the β-globin gene defects and their interaction, the production of β-globin chains is quantitatively reduced to different degrees, whereas the synthesis of α-globin continues as normal. The result is an accumulation of excess unmatched α-globin chains in the erythroid precursors. The free α-globin chains, which are not able to form stable tetramers, precipitate in the erythroid precursors where they form inclusion bodies that damage the red cell membrane, thereby causing premature destruction of erythroid precursors in the bone marrow (ineffective erythropoiesis). Ineffective erythropoiesis leads to a sequence of events responsible for bone marrow expansion, anemia, hemolysis, splenomegaly, and increased iron absorption. Any factor that reduces the degree of chain imbalance and the magnitude of α-chain excess, such as coinheritance of α-thalassemia or an innate ability to increase fetal hemoglobin, will ameliorate the clinical expression of the disease (Fig. 148-2).[7]

β-Thalassemia Minor

Thalassemia minor is the heterozygous state of β-thalassemia. Subjects with thalassemia minor are "carriers" of a single β-globin gene defect, and they are usually asymptomatic except for a mild microcytic anemia. The carriers are usually identified incidentally[8] during an intercurrent illness, in the course of a family study, or as part of a population survey. Carriers of β-thalassemia may have a triplicated α-gene allele: its coinheritance may cause a mild thalassemia intermedia phenotype due to the excess of α chains production.

The anemia is mild, microcytic, and hypochromic, and it is usually associated with a diagnostic elevation (>3.5%) in the level of HbA_2. However, coincidental iron deficiency can lower elevated HbA_2 levels to the normal range. Carriers of β-thalassemia with normal HbA_2 also have been observed in settings in which an individual with mild thalassemia intermedia was found to have one parent with typical β-thalassemia minor with elevated HbA_2, whereas the other showed either minimal or no hematologic abnormalities and normal HbA_2. Subjects with normal HbA_2 are usually carriers of silent β^{++} mutations (β^{++}). The blood smear shows characteristic microcytosis and hypochromia, with some variation in size and shape of the red cells. The presence of target cells is variable. The hematologic features are remarkably similar among different ethnic groups.

β-Thalassemia Intermedia

Thalassemia intermedia, which is a non–transfusion-dependent thalassemia disorder, describes patients with anemia, splenomegaly, and a wide spectrum of clinical severity without the full manifestations found in thalassemia major.[9] Mildly affected patients, who are almost completely asymptomatic until adult life, experience only mild anemia and spontaneously maintain hemoglobin levels between 7 and 10 g/dL. Patients with more severe thalassemia intermedia

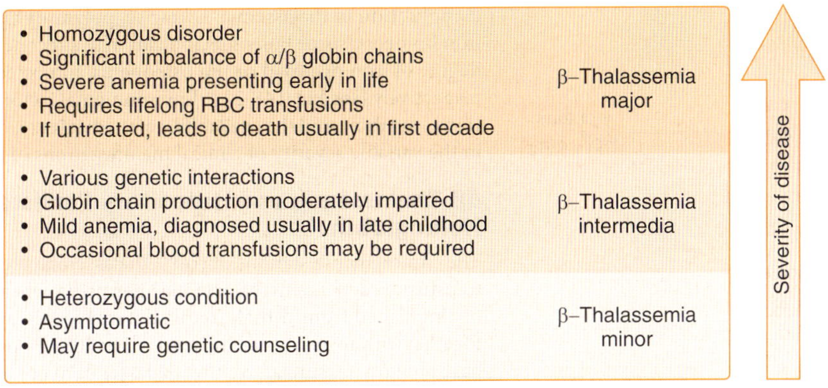

A

	Thalassemia major more likely	Thalassemia intermedia more likely
Clinical		
Presentation (years)	< 2	> 2
Hb levels (g/dL)	< 7	7–10
Liver/spleen enlargement	Severe	Moderate to severe
Hematologic		
HbF (%)	> 50	10–50 (may be up to 100%)
HbA2 (%)	> 3.5	< 4
Genetic		
Parents	Both carriers of high HbA2 β-thalassemia	One or both atypical carriers: high HbF β-thalassemia, borderline HbA2
Molecular		
Type of β-chain mutation	Severe	Mild/silent
Coinheritance of α-thalassemia	No/rare	Yes
Hereditary persistence of fetal hemoglobin	No	Yes
δβ-thalassemia	No	Yes
Gγ XmnI polymorphism	No	Yes

B

FIGURE 148-1. **A, Clinical classification of β-thalassemias, from β-thalassemia minor to β-thalassemia major, according to the disease severity. β-Thalassemia minor subjects are asymptomatic, whereas at the severe extreme, β-thalassemia major patients are transfusion dependent. In between is a wide spectrum of clinical phenotypes labeled thalassemia intermedia because of different genetic interactions characterized by moderate to severe transfusion-independent anemia. B, Tentative criteria to differentiate thalassemia major from thalassemia intermedia at presentation. HbA = adult hemoglobin; HbF = fetal hemoglobin; RBC = red blood cell.**

generally present between the ages of 2 and 6 years; although they are able to survive without regular transfusion therapy, growth and development can be retarded. Most thalassemia intermedia patients are homozygotes or compound heterozygotes for mild to moderate β-gene mutations ($\beta^+/\beta^+;\beta^0/\beta^+$); less commonly, only a single β-globin gene is affected. Because the clinical severity of the disease is dictated by the different extent of globin chain imbalance, at least three different mechanisms may promote the mild clinical characteristics of thalassemia intermedia compared with thalassemia major: inheritance of mild or silent β-gene mutations; coinheritance of determinants associated with increased γ-chain production, which contributes to neutralizing the large proportion of unbound α chains; and coinheritance of α-thalassemia, which reduces the synthesis of α chains, thereby reducing the α/non-α chain imbalance.

Three main factors are responsible for the clinical sequelae in patients with thalassemia intermedia: degree of ineffective erythropoiesis, chronic anemia, and iron overload.[10] The ineffective erythropoiesis primarily depends on the underlying molecular defects and is due to precipitation of free α chains in erythroid precursors in the bone marrow, where they cause membrane damage and premature cell death. The degree of ineffective erythropoiesis is the primary determinant of the anemia of thalassemia intermedia; peripheral hemolysis of mature, circulating red cells, and an overall reduction in hemoglobin synthesis are secondary. Hemolysis and damaged red cells that expose negatively charged membrane phosphatidyl-serine residues have been linked to the development of a hypercoagulable state and increased risk for pulmonary hypertension (Chapter 69) in patients with thalassemia intermedia.

Chronic anemia and chronic ineffective erythropoiesis lead to an inappropriate increase in gastrointestinal iron absorption, thereby resulting in iron overload even in the absence of blood transfusion. The mechanism is a reduced expression of hepcidin, a hepatic peptide that plays a central role in iron homeostasis (Chapter 196). Moreover, the growth and differentiation factor 15 (GDF15), which is secreted by erythroid precursors and overexpressed in the presence of ineffective erythropoiesis, may suppress the synthesis of hepcidin. Erythroferrone, secreted by erythroblasts, may also play a role in hepcidin regulation. Taken together, ineffective erythropoiesis (leading to increased GDF15) and chronic anemia/hypoxia result in hepcidin suppression, increased dietary iron absorption from the gut, and increased release of recycled iron from the reticuloendothelial system, thereby leading to an iron overload situation similar to that observed in patients with hereditary hemochromatosis syndromes (which also are characterized by impaired hepcidin production; Chapter 196).

As a consequence of these pathophysiologic processes, several complications are seen in patients with thalassemia intermedia but not with thalassemia major, especially in non-splenectomized patients. Cholelithiasis is much more common in thalassemia intermedia than in thalassemia major because of ineffective erythropoiesis and peripheral hemolysis. Extramedullary hematopoiesis, as a compensatory mechanism, leads to the formation of erythropoietic tissue masses that primarily involve the spleen, liver, lymph nodes, and vertebrae. These masses may cause neurologic problems, such as spinal cord compression (sometimes causing paraplegia) and intrathoracic masses. Leg ulcers that are rare in well-transfused patients with thalassemia major are common in adult patients with thalassemia intermedia. Thrombotic risk is definitely increased in patients with thalassemia intermedia, especially after splenectomy. Although stroke is rare in thalassemia intermedia, asymptomatic brain damage, including ischemia,

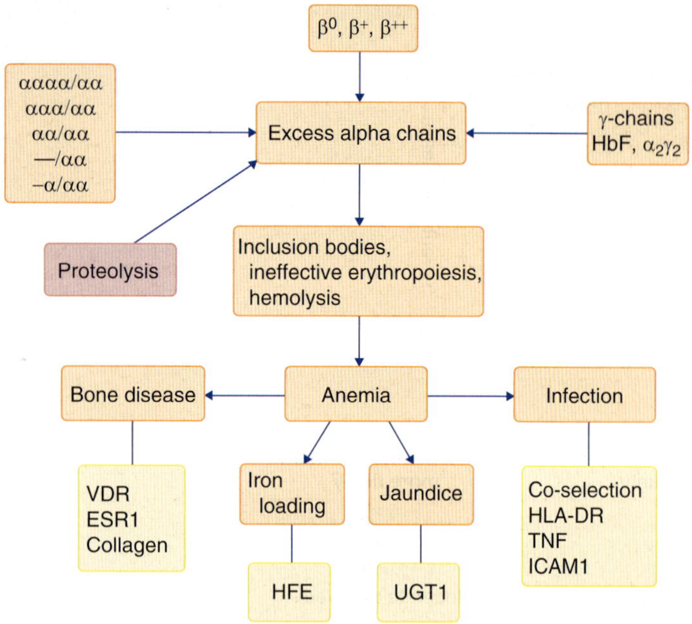

FIGURE 148-2. **Pathophysiology of β-thalassemias and modifiers of globin chain imbalance.** The severity of ineffective erythropoiesis is dependent on the degree of excess free α chains that result primarily from three different mechanisms: (1) inheritance of severe, mild, or silent β-chain mutations; (2) coinheritance of determinants associated with increased γ-chain production; and (3) coinheritance of α-thalassemia. A phenotype of thalassemia intermedia may result from the increased production of α-globin chains by a triplicated (ααα) or quadruplicated (αααα) α genotype associated with β heterozygosity. Inheritance of polymorphisms or mutations of genes involved in bone, iron, and bilirubin metabolism as well as in infection may contribute to modify the clinical course of the disease. ESR1 = estrogen receptor 1; HbF = fetal hemoglobin; HFE = hereditary hemochromatosis gene; HLA = human leukocyte antigen; ICAM1 = intercellular adhesion molecule 1; TNF = tumor necrosis factor; UGT1 = UDP-glucose : glycoprotein glucosyltransferase 1; VDR = vitamin D receptor.

has been documented by magnetic resonance imaging (MRI) and computed tomography. Pulmonary hypertension (Chapter 69) is prevalent in thalassemia intermedia patients (approximately 60%) and is thought to be the primary cause of heart failure in this patient population. Liver disease due to viral infection is less frequent than in thalassemia major; however, abnormal liver enzymes are frequently observed in patients with thalassemia intermedia, primarily because of hepatocyte damage resulting from iron overload. In some of the oldest patients with thalassemia intermedia, long-term overload has resulted in cirrhosis (Chapter 139) and hepatocellular carcinoma (Chapter 181), similar to what may be found in hereditary hemochromatosis (Chapter 196).

β-Thalassemia Major

The major forms of β-thalassemia (still sometimes called Cooley anemia) are disorders in which life can be sustained only by regular blood transfusions. This condition usually results from the homozygous state or from the compound heterozygous state for severe β-gene mutations (β^0). The typical forms of thalassemia major become manifested during the first year of life, during which γ chains are switched off but not replaced by β-chain synthesis. Left untreated, these infants are incapable of maintaining a hemoglobin level above 5 g/dL, show marked bone deformities and growth retardation, and are considered as "transfusion-dependent thalassemia patients." They develop the "thalassemic" facies due to frontal bossing of the skull and protrusion of the jaws and cheekbones. The magnitude of the increase in erythropoiesis may result in extramedullary masses arising usually from the sternum and ribs. Progressive hepatosplenomegaly, which is a constant finding, leads to pancytopenia. The early childhood of the untreated or inadequately treated thalassemia major patients is interspersed with various complications, including recurrent infections, spontaneous fractures, gallstones, and leg ulcers.[11]

Heart failure in thalassemia major is multifactorial but is thought to be principally related to chronic anemia and the toxic effects of iron overload in the myocardium (Chapters 47 and 196). Liver disease is due to iron overload (Chapter 196), but other genetic modifiers may affect the outcome of complications in different ways. For example, the presence of a polymorphic variant in the UGT1A1 promoter responsible for Gilbert syndrome (Chapter 133) may increase the predisposition to cholelithiasis, which is already a common complication in thalassemia. Likewise, polymorphisms in genes involved in iron homeostasis or bone metabolism may affect negatively or positively the degree of iron overload or the osteopenia and osteoporosis (Chapter 225), respectively (see Fig. 148-2).[12] Environmental factors, including social conditions, nutrition, and the availability of medical care, have also been implicated in the variable severity of clinical manifestations of thalassemia major.

δβ-Thalassemia and Hereditary Persistence of Fetal Hemoglobin

The clinical manifestations of $(\delta\beta)^0$-thalassemias are similar to those of non–transfusion-dependent thalassemia intermedia, whereas the heterozygotes are distinguished from β-thalassemia heterozygotes by normal levels of HbA_2 together with an increased HbF level of 5 to 20%. Homozygotes for Hb_{Lepore} may have phenotypes similar to either thalassemia major or thalassemia intermedia. Subjects affected by deletion or nondeletion forms of hereditary persistence of fetal hemoglobin are usually asymptomatic.

Any of the β-thalassemia defects may be coinherited with β-chain variants (HbS, HbC, HbE) and cause a clinically relevant β-thalassemia phenotype of different severity. These variants further illustrate that β-thalassemia syndromes have a wide clinical spectrum and that specific therapeutic approaches may completely change the clinical course and the natural history of these disorders (Fig. 148-3).

Hemoglobin E and Hemoglobin E Thalassemias

Hemoglobin E (HbE) is caused by a substitution of glutamic acid by lysine at codon 26 of the β-globin gene. It is a common mutation, especially in the Indian subcontinent and Southeast Asia and among people who have emigrated from those regions. The frequency of HbE approaches 60% in many regions of Thailand, Laos, and Cambodia. HbE results in reduced synthesis of the β-E chain and therefore has the phenotype of a mild form of β-thalassemia. HbE trait has little clinical significance; it may be associated with slight microcytosis without anemia, but it could be mistaken for iron deficiency without appropriate laboratory testing. Homozygous HbEE individuals have mild anemia and microcytosis, occasional splenomegaly, and peripheral blood smears showing red cell changes similar to those seen in thalassemia trait, including target cells. In this condition, hepcidin is suppressed, thereby leading to iron accumulation—even in the absence of blood transfusions and certainly worsened by them.

HbE interacts with different forms of α-thalassemia to produce a wide variety of clinical disorders.[13] Its coinheritance with β-thalassemia, a condition called HbE/β-thalassemia, is the most common severe form of β-thalassemia in Asia and globally represents about 50% of the clinically severe β-thalassemias.

DIAGNOSIS

The diagnosis of thalassemia may be required in a patient with an appropriate, suggestive clinical picture or for the identification of a heterozygote subject as part of a family study or population screening program. The general approach is common to any form of thalassemia, regardless of presentation (Fig. 148-4). The primary evaluation is based on the red cell indices by electronic cell counter and the red cell morphology on a well-stained blood film. Individuals with mean corpuscular volume below 80 fL and mean corpuscular hemoglobin below 27 pg with normal iron parameters require further investigation. The red blood cell number is usually higher than normal. In the presence of anemia with thalassemic red cell changes, the next step is the evaluation of hemoglobin fractions (HbA, HbA_2, HbF, or hemoglobin variants) by electrophoresis on cellulose acetate at alkaline pH or, even better, by high-performance liquid chromatography that enables the precise measurement of HbA_2, HbF, and HbA and the provisional identification of a large number of hemoglobin variants, including HbE. An HbA_2 level above 3.5% associated with hypochromic microcytic red cells is diagnostic of β-thalassemia minor. HbA_2 values between 3.2 and 3.5% (borderline) should be interpreted with care because they could be due to interaction of more than one thalassemic defect (α and β), a silent β mutation, or concomitant iron deficiency. If iron deficiency is present, it should be corrected and the HbA_2 estimation repeated. The majority of individuals with thalassemic red cell indices with normal or low HbA_2 and normal HbF will be α^0-thalassemia carriers or α^+-thalassemia homozygotes. Carriers of α^0-thalassemia may have a few red cells with HbH inclusions. Microcytosis with low or normal HbA_2 levels with elevated HbF (2 to 20%) indicates heterozygosity for δβ-thalassemia. Patients with hereditary persistence of fetal hemoglobin usually have normal red blood cell indices but increased levels of HbF with different intercellular distribution (homogeneous or

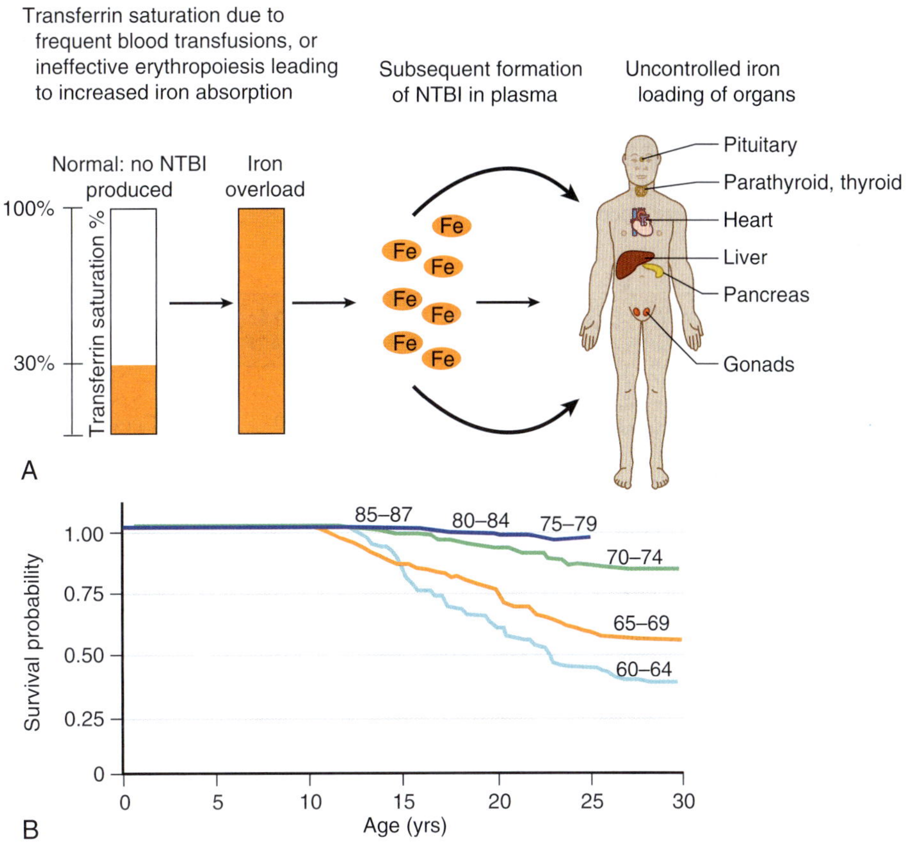

FIGURE 148-3. A, Transfusion iron overload and specific organ loading. B, Survival of Italian thalassemia major patients by cohort of birth. NTBI = non–transferrin-bound iron.

pancellular with the exception of heterocellular hereditary persistence of fetal hemoglobin) compared with δβ-thalassemia (uneven or heterocellular).

The definitive diagnosis of the thalassemia syndromes involves the identification of the underlying mutations by polymerase chain reaction (PCR) restriction enzyme analysis, PCR allele-specific oligonucleotides, gap PCR, and direct sequencing that at present is probably the easiest and most reliable method. For deletion forms of α-thalassemia, the multiplex ligation-dependent probe amplification is a recently introduced, useful method.

TREATMENT AND PROGNOSIS

Life expectancy is normal in patients with β-thalassemia minor. Other patients affected by different forms of thalassemia develop a variety of complications mainly due to iron overload, which requires monitoring to direct iron chelation therapy. The most notable are heart failure and iron overload in the liver.

Medical Treatment

Thalassemia Minor

No specific treatment is required for α- or β-thalassemia heterozygotes (carriers, thalassemia minor), but they should receive appropriate genetic counseling. During pregnancy, thalassemia-carrying women may become more anemic, so they should be observed carefully, mainly during the second and third trimesters, and supported with folic acid. When true iron deficiency is associated with thalassemia traits, iron supplementation should be provided, and levels of transferrin saturation and ferritin should be monitored.

Hemoglobin H Disease

HbH patients in general have higher hemoglobin levels (8 to 9 g/dL) and do not need regular blood transfusion. Supplementation with folic acid (2 to 5 mg/day) is generally recommended, especially in pediatric patients. The major complications in HbH disease are hemolytic crises that may occur during or after acute infections; in such cases, immediate intervention, including blood transfusions and treatment for infections, should be promptly administered. Prognosis generally depends on the degree of transfusion-dependency and iron overload.

Thalassemia Intermedia and Major

The clinical management of thalassemia intermedia and thalassemia major remains challenging. Prolongation of life, now well into the third or fourth decade, is accompanied by several complications, partly due to the underlying disorder and partly as a consequence of the treatment with blood transfusions and iron overload.

Patients with thalassemia intermedia generally experience puberty late, but they have normal sexual development and are usually fertile. Women with thalassemia intermedia may have successful pregnancies, although complications may occur during pregnancy. Overall prognosis generally depends on the degree of transfusion-dependency and iron overload.

In untreated β-thalassemia major, the mortality rate is high around puberty. However, children who are well transfused to maintain a hemoglobin level above 9 g/dL have relatively normal growth and development, and if they are adequately transfused and are fully adherent with iron chelation therapy (see Iron Overload) can enter puberty and become sexually mature. Unfortunately the current adult population of thalassemia major patients often suffers from now-avoidable side effects of long-term treatment, including transfusion-associated infections (particularly hepatitis B and hepatitis C infection [Chapters 134 and 135] and, in some populations, HIV infection [Chapter 355]), as well as end-organ damage (liver, heart, endocrine glands) due to unsatisfactory long-term iron chelation. The main causes of death in adult thalassemia major patients still remain cardiac complications, mainly in poorly chelated patients, although liver cirrhosis is also increasing because of the prolongation of life.

The supportive treatment of thalassemia major patients, best provided by a team of experts, includes regular transfusion therapy and iron chelation. The optimal transfusion regimen involves regular blood transfusions, usually administered every 2 to 5 weeks, to maintain the pretransfusion hemoglobin levels above 9 to 10.5 g/dL. The decision to initiate lifelong transfusion therapy should be based on a definitive diagnosis of severe thalassemia, taking into account the molecular defects, the severity of anemia on repeated measurement, the level of ineffective erythropoiesis, and the clinical criteria (such as failure to thrive or bone changes). It is advisable that thalassemia major patients receive leukoreduced packed red cells to minimize transfusion reactions and the transmission of pathogens. Adverse reactions to red blood cell transfusions may occur during or after transfusion and can be hemolytic and nonhemolytic. Transfusion-related acute lung injury is rare but severe and must be immediately managed (Chapter 162).

Many patients with thalassemia major commonly require splenectomy because of hypersplenism, but optimal management may delay or even obviate the need for splenectomy. Splenectomy should be considered only for patients whose annual blood consumption increases progressively and is responsible for significant increases in iron stores despite good chelation therapy or in the presence of symptoms due to splenic enlargement or hypersplenism. The major complication of splenectomy is severe and sometimes overwhelming infection (Chapter 154). Because removal of the spleen may reduce the primary immune response to encapsulated organisms, it is advisable to delay splenectomy until patients are at

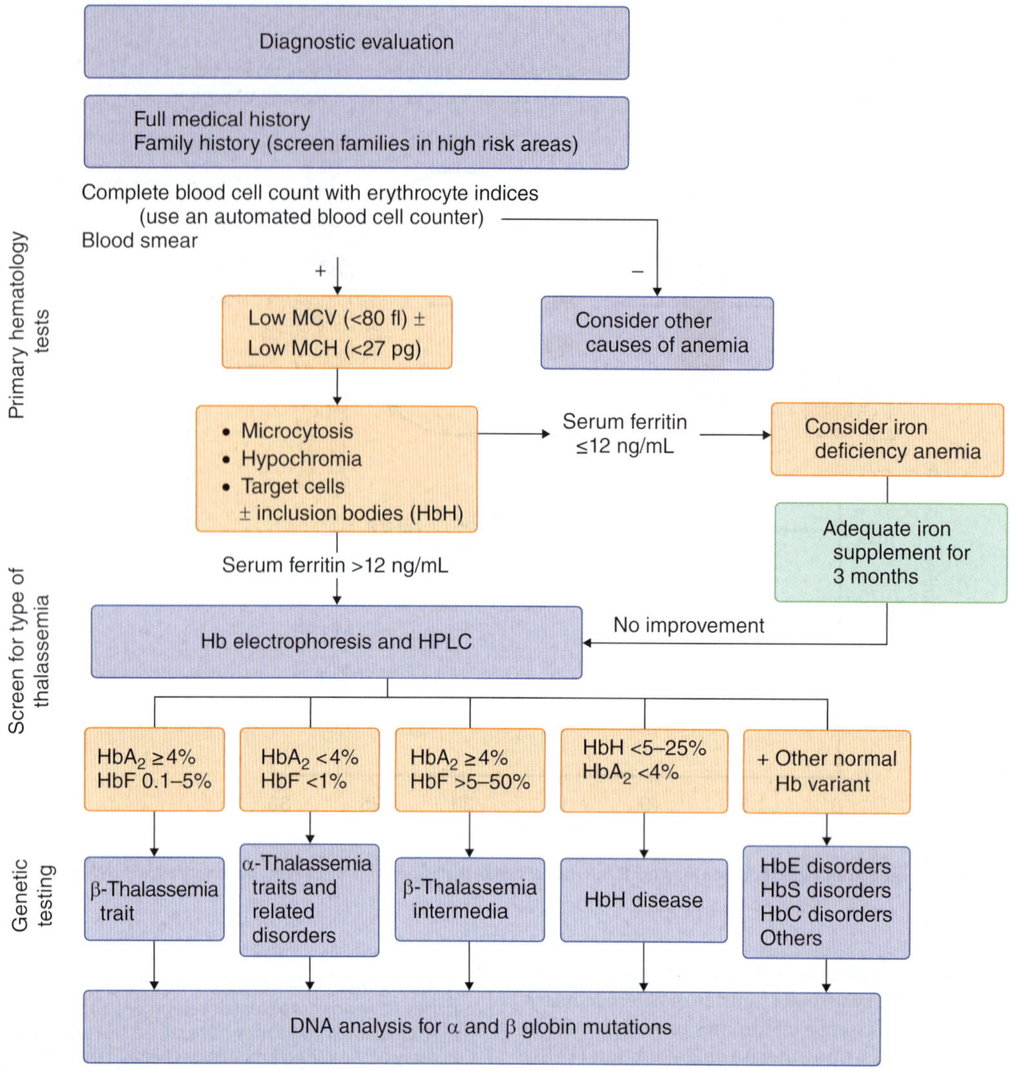

FIGURE 148-4. **Diagnostic approach to suspected thalassemia.** Hb = hemoglobin; HPLC = high-performance liquid chromatography; MCH = mean corpuscular hemoglobin; MCV = mean corpuscular volume.

least 5 years old. The mortality rate for overwhelming infection after splenectomy in patients with thalassemia is approximately 50% despite intensive supportive care. Therefore, it is mandatory to adopt preventive measures including immunoprophylaxis (vaccination against *Streptococcus pneumoniae,* pneumococcus, and meningococcus) (Chapter 154), chemoprophylaxis, and education of the parent and patient to recognize and to report febrile illnesses. After splenectomy, patients with thalassemia also have an increased risk of thrombosis.

The management of non–transfusion-dependent thalassemia intermedia is more complicated because of the wide heterogeneity of phenotypes. However, increasing evidence supports the benefit of preventive transfusion therapy to decrease the incidence of complications rather than reserving transfusion for when complications develop. The initiation of iron chelation therapy in patients with thalassemia intermedia depends not only on the amount of excess iron but also on the rate of iron accumulation, the duration of exposure to excess iron, and various other factors in individual patients.

Increasing Red Cell Release

Two new molecules, sotatercept[14] and luspatercept,[15] which are activin-type IIA and IIB receptor fusion proteins, can increase the release of mature erythrocytes into the circulation by acting mainly on late-stage erythropoiesis. Luspatercept (a recombinant fusion protein that binds to select transforming growth factor β superfamily ligands, given subcutaneously at a dose of 1.00 to 1.25 mg/kg every 3 weeks) is approved for adults with transfusion-dependent β-thalassemia, in whom it can reduce the transfusion burden by at least 33%, with analogous reductions in serum ferritin levels and no clinically meaningful changes in liver or myocardial iron concentrations.[A1]

Stimulation of Hemoglobin F Synthesis

An alternative treatment of β-thalassemia consists of the pharmacologic stimulation of HbF synthesis. In humans, hemoglobin switch from HbF to HbA occurs in the period around birth as a result of γ- to β-globin gene switching. A number of pharmacologic agents able to reactivate HbF synthesis have been identified, including hypomethylating agents, histone deacetylase inhibitors, and hydroxyurea. Whereas the effect of these pharmacologic treatments (particularly hydroxyurea) in sickle cell disease is clear (Chapter 149), their benefit on the clinical course of β-thalassemia is presently limited, perhaps because of the higher level of HbF required in β-thalassemia to achieve clinical results compared with those observed in sickle cell disease.

The reduction of α-globin expression may provide an equally plausible approach to ameliorating clinically severe forms of β-thalassemia, especially in patients with hemoglobin E β-thalassemia, who comprise about 50% of all patients born each year with severe β-thalassemia.

Experimental Therapies

Gene therapy (Chapter 34) using a lentivirus vector[16] or genome editing through CRISPR/Cas9 technology[17] is a potentially useful approach for increasing fetal hemoglobin production in patients who have thalassemia syndromes. Ongoing clinical trials are assessing efficacy in patients with transfusion-dependent β-thalassemia. New molecules with the potential ability to correct ineffective erythropoiesis or to generate iron-restricted erythropoiesis are in phase 2 clinical trials.

Iron Overload

Iron overload, which is an inevitable and serious complication of long-term blood transfusion therapy and hyperabsorption of dietary iron, requires adequate treatment to prevent early death, mainly from iron-induced cardiac disease.[18] The principal methods of determining body iron levels (Chapter 196) are measurements of the serum ferritin level and assessment of liver iron concentration from biopsy tissue or, as an alternative noninvasive method, by R2 MRI. High serum ferritin levels (>2500 μg/L) and high liver iron concentration (>15 g/dry weight) indicate high risk for significant morbidity and mortality. A cut-off of 800 μg/L ferritin and more than 7 g/dry weight liver iron concentration have been associated with high risk for morbidity in thalassemia intermedia and other forms of non–transfusion-dependent thalassemias.

Cardiac iron can be measured by a T2* MRI procedure that allows estimation of the cardiac iron load. MRI T2* values below 10 milliseconds are always associated with severe iron load and high risk for heart failure within 1 year. MRI T2* values above 20 milliseconds are considered normal, meaning no iron in the heart. Echocardiography also may be useful to evaluate functional changes.

For other organs, including liver disease, endocrinopathies, lung disease, thrombophilia, and bone disease, the diagnostic approaches are similar to those used in hemochromatosis (Chapter 196).

The oral iron chelator deferasirox is effective and safe in removing excess iron from different organs, including the heart[A2,A3] and is the first-line treatment in most countries.[19] The dose should be individualized according to age, history of adherence with previous chelation, and other factors. Monitoring and adjustment of iron chelation by repeated measurements of ferritin, calculation of iron intake by transfusions, and, whenever possible, measurement of cardiac and liver iron at least once by MRI are mandatory.

Prior to the availability of oral agents, the standard chelation therapy was deferoxamine, given for 10 to 24 hours daily as a slow, continuous, subcutaneous infusion 5 to 7 days per week. Unfortunately, adherence with the rigorous regimen of daily subcutaneous infusions is a serious limiting factor, and life expectancy in nonadherent patients is not different from that of untreated patients. The combination of deferasirox plus deferoxamine can further reduce iron overload compared with deferasirox alone.[A4]

Another oral iron chelator, deferiprone (75 to 100 mg/kg/day), may be more effective than deferoxamine in protecting the heart from the accumulation of iron.[A5] However, its use is restricted to U.S. patients who are unable to use deferoxamine or patients with an unsatisfactory response to deferoxamine, as judged by serum ferritin levels and by liver iron concentrations. A potential benefit of combined deferoxamine and deferiprone therapy has been observed, and this combination should be considered for patients with high levels of heart iron or cardiac dysfunction.

In patients with thalassemia major and cardiac siderosis, amlodipine added to chelation therapy reduces cardiac iron more effectively than chelation therapy alone,[A6,A7] but larger studies will be required to inform the evaluations. The use of proton pump inhibitors may further reduce serum ferritin levels.[A8]

Hydrops Fetalis

Infants with hydrops fetalis syndrome almost always die either in utero (30 to 40 weeks' gestation) or soon after birth, but some infants with hemoglobin Bart hydrops fetalis can survive with in utero blood transfusions and premature delivery by caesarean section. However, subsequent development is abnormal, and survivors require regular blood transfusions after birth.

Bone Marrow Transplantation

Allogeneic hematopoietic cell transplantation (Chapter 163) in thalassemia syndromes has been increasingly successful during the past two decades, mainly in β-thalassemia major.[20] Predictors of poor transplant outcome are hepatomegaly, history of irregular chelation, and hepatic fibrosis. Patients are categorized into three risk classes. Class 1 patients have none of these adverse risk factors, class 2 patients have one or two adverse risk factors, and class 3 patients have all three. The probabilities of thalassemia-free survival for patients younger than age 17 years at the time of hematopoietic cell transplantation from a human leukocyte antigen (HLA)-identical relative were 87% and 85%, respectively, in patients belonging to class 1 and class 2 and much lower in young patients in class 3. The progressive adjustment of conditioning regimens in class 3 patients and in adults (>17 years old) has significantly reduced the incidence of transplant-related mortality in patients in class 3. Only 25 to 30% of patients with diseases potentially curable by hematopoietic cell transplantation have a suitable HLA-compatible sibling. Bone marrow transplantation from unrelated donors increases significantly the incidence of acute and chronic graft-versus-host disease, particularly in thalassemia. A study from the Eurocord cooperative group reported the outcome of 33 patients with class 1 and class 2 thalassemia who received cord blood hematopoietic stem cells from an HLA-identical sibling; no patient died of transplant-related complications, suggesting that related cord blood hematopoietic cell transplantation is a safe procedure for thalassemia patients.

UNSTABLE HEMOGLOBINOPATHIES

More than 80 rare mutant hemoglobins have been reported to cause hemolytic anemia by either amino acid replacements or deletions that significantly lower the solubility of hemoglobin. These mutant hemoglobins thereby form intracellular precipitates that can be detected as so-called Heinz bodies when the blood smear is exposed to a supravital stain. Structural abnormalities include mutations that weaken the linkage between heme and globin, disrupt secondary (α-helical) structure, or introduce a charged or polar side group into the hydrophobic interior of the globin subunit.

This disorder, sometimes called congenital Heinz body hemolytic anemia, is inherited in an autosomal dominant manner. Severely affected individuals have jaundice, splenomegaly, and, on occasion, dark brown urine due to the release of heme and aberrant conversion to dipyroles. The instability of a few of these globin mutants is so extreme that they cannot be detected by routine laboratory methods. The result is a thalassemia phenotype with microcytosis and ineffective erythropoiesis. Like individuals with glucose-6-phosphate dehydrogenase deficiency (Chapter 147), patients with unstable hemoglobin mutants often lack clinical symptoms and signs of hemolysis until they develop an infection or are exposed to an oxidant drug.

The diagnosis can be established by a combination of a positive Heinz body preparation and either abnormal hemoglobin electrophoresis or demonstration of a precipitate after exposure of a hemolysate to heat or isopropanol. Some clinics have access to a reference laboratory that can identify the specific mutation by α- and β-globin DNA sequencing.

Most individuals with this disorder do not require treatment, but some are symptomatic from severe anemia. Splenectomy generally results in a significant increase in red cell mass. However, the fraction of Heinz body–positive red cells increases markedly after splenectomy, and these patients are at significant risk for development of pulmonary hypertension and cor pulmonale.

GENERAL REFERENCES

For the General References and other additional features, please visit Elsevier eBooks+ at https://ebooks.health.elsevier.com.

Grade A References

A1. Cappellini MD, Viprakasit V, Taher AT, et al. A phase 3 trial of luspatercept in patients with transfusion-dependent β-thalassemia. *N Engl J Med*. 2020;382:1219-1231.

A2. Bollig C, Schell LK, Rücker G, et al. Deferasirox for managing iron overload in people with thalassaemia. *Cochrane Database Syst Rev*. 2017;8:CD007476.

A3. Dou H, Qin Y, Chen G, et al. Effectiveness and safety of deferasirox in thalassemia with iron overload: a meta-analysis. *Acta Haematol*. 2019;141:32-42.

A4. Eghbali A, Shokri P, Afzal RR, et al. A 1-year randomized trial of deferasirox alone versus deferasirox and deferoxamine combination for the treatment of iron overload in thalassemia major. *Transfus Apher Sci*. 2019;58:429-433.

A5. Elalfy MS, Adly A, Awad H, et al. Safety and efficacy of early start of iron chelation therapy with deferiprone in young children newly diagnosed with transfusion-dependent thalassemia: a randomized controlled trial. *Am J Hematol*. 2018;93:262-268.

A6. Sadaf A, Hasan B, Das JK, et al. Calcium channel blockers for preventing cardiomyopathy due to iron overload in people with transfusion-dependent beta thalassaemia. *Cochrane Database Syst Rev*. 2018;7:CD011626.

A7. Gupta V, Kumar I, Raj V, et al. Comparison of the effects of calcium channel blockers plus iron chelation therapy versus chelation therapy only on iron overload in children and young adults with transfusion-dependent thalassemia: a randomized double-blind placebo-controlled trial. *Pediatr Blood Cancer*. 2022;69:e29564.

A8. Eghbali A, Khalilpour A, Taherahmadi H, et al. Pantoprazole reduces serum ferritin in patients with thalassemia major and intermedia: a randomized, controlled study. *Therapie*. 2019;74:507-512.

149

SICKLE CELL DISEASE AND OTHER HEMOGLOBINOPATHIES

JO HOWARD

SICKLE CELL DISEASE

DEFINITION

Sickle cell disease is caused by a mutation in the β-globin gene. The resulting clinical syndromes are characterized by chronic hemolytic anemias and can be complicated by vaso-occlusion and vasculopathy that can cause widespread acute and chronic organ damage as well as premature mortality.

EPIDEMIOLOGY

The sickle mutation became prominent several thousands of years ago in Sub-Saharan African and Arab-Indian populations. Its persistence was due to a selective advantage in areas where falciparum malaria was endemic, with sickle trait carriers estimated to have approximately 90% protection against severe malaria infection. The carrier frequency is now highest in West and Central Africa (up to 50%), in Arab populations in the Middle East, and in some populations in India (Fig. 149-1). Forced movement of African populations during the slave trade and, more recently, migration because of war and economic pressures have led to increasing numbers of carriers and affected individuals in the Americas, the Caribbean, Europe, and worldwide.

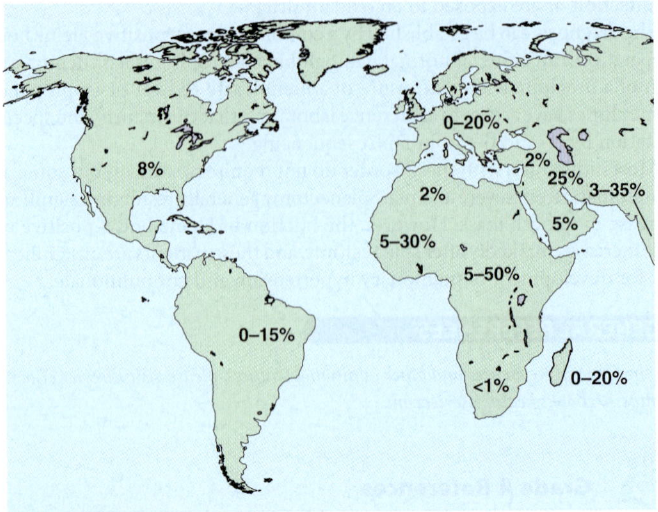

FIGURE 149-1. Worldwide prevalence of the sickle cell trait. Shown are the percentages of individuals with sickle cell trait in regions of the world where the hemoglobin S (HbS) gene is often present. In each geographic area, the prevalence of sickle cell trait can vary markedly according to racial or ethnic group, by historical migration patterns, and even from village to village. Not shown is the high concentration of the HbS gene in areas of Europe, such as London, Manchester, and Paris, where migrants from Africa or Afro-Caribbean populations have settled.

The prevalence of sickle cell disease and sickle trait varies across the world, but more than 75% of the estimated 300,000 to 400,000 births affected annually with sickle cell anemia (HbSS) occur in Sub-Saharan Africa, with these numbers predicted to increase.[1]

PATHOBIOLOGY

Globin, which is the protein portion of hemoglobin, has an iron-containing porphyrin heme ring that allows the molecule to transport oxygen efficiently. Mutations that cause changes in the amino acid sequence of the globin polypeptide can cause clinically significant diseases, including sickle cell disease, that collectively are termed hemoglobinopathies. Sickle hemoglobin (HbS:$\alpha_2\beta_2^s$), which is caused by an adenine (A) to thymidine (T) substitution (GAG to GTG) in codon 6 of the β-globin gene (HBB), results in a valine residue (Glu6Val) instead of the normal glutamic acid residue (Fig. 149-2). Homozygous sickle cell disease (HbSS) is an autosomal recessive condition, so each offspring of two sickle cell carrier parents has a 25% chance of being affected (Fig. 149-3AI).

HbS polymerizes when it becomes deoxygenated, and this polymerization distorts the shape of red cells into the characteristic sickle shape (Fig. 149-3Aii) and leads to red cell damage, hemolysis, and vaso-occlusion. The deoxygenation of red cells occurs in the circulation as they cross the capillary bed; but as they return to the lungs, oxygen uptake occurs, and the polymers deaggregate. This sickling–desickling cycle is repeated as the red cell recirculates, but if the passage of red cells is delayed, cell sickling, membrane damage, and vaso-occlusion occur before transit through the microvasculature is complete. The formation of polymers (and the severity of sickling) may be increased by a higher intracellular hemoglobin concentration, low pH, and raised temperature and can be decreased by the presence of other intracellular hemoglobins, such as fetal hemoglobin (HbF).

The polymerization of sickle hemoglobin leads to red cell damage by several mechanisms that result in red cell destruction (hemolysis) and vaso-occlusion.[2] Most hemolysis is extravascular because it occurs when macrophages

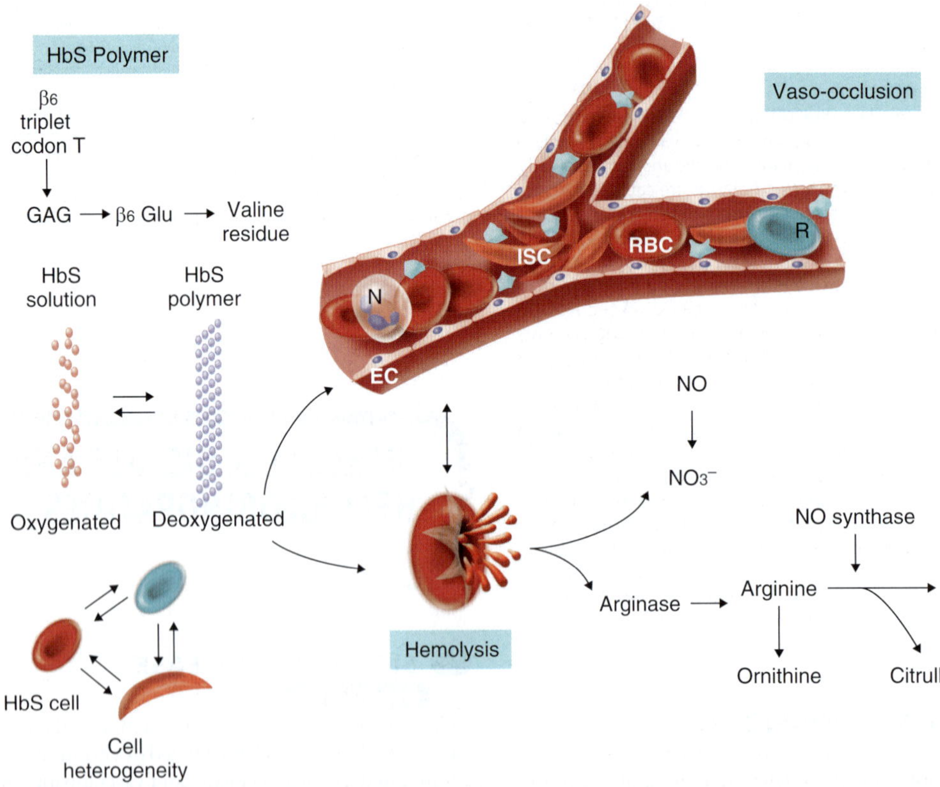

FIGURE 149-2. Pathophysiology of sickle cell disease. An adenine (A) to thymidine (T) transversion (A6T) at codon 6 in the β-hemoglobin gene on chromosome 11 (*HBB*) leads to the substitution of a glutamic acid codon by a valine codon. β6 valine allows the hemoglobin S (HbS) molecule ($\alpha_2\beta_2^S$) to polymerize when it is deoxygenated. DeoxyHbS polymer injures the erythrocyte and leads to a heterogeneous population of sickle cells with damaged membrane cytoskeleton, reduced cation and water content, and altered distribution of membrane lipids. In the vasculature, sickle cells interact with endothelium and other blood cells to cause vaso-occlusion. Some damaged erythrocytes hemolyze intravascularly, thereby releasing heme into the plasma to scavenge nitric oxide (NO) and to reduce hemoglobin to methemoglobin and nitrate. NO, by binding soluble guanylate cyclase, converts cyclic guanosine triphosphate to guanosine monophosphate, thereby relaxing vascular smooth muscle and causing vasodilation. A state of reduced endothelial NO bioavailability in sickle cell disease impairs the homeostatic vascular functions of NO, such as inhibition of platelet activation and aggregation and transcriptional repression of genes transcribing cell adhesion molecules. Hemoglobin, heme, and heme iron catalyze the production of oxygen radicals and protein nitration, potentially further limiting NO bioavailability and activating endothelium. Lysed erythrocytes also liberate arginase, which destroys L-arginine, the substrate for NO production, providing another mechanism for endothelial NO deficiency. The normal balance of vasoconstriction versus vasodilation is therefore skewed toward vasoconstriction as well as endothelial activation and proliferation. EC = epithelial cell; ISC = irreversibly sickled cell; N = neutrophil; R = reticulocyte; RBC = red blood cell.

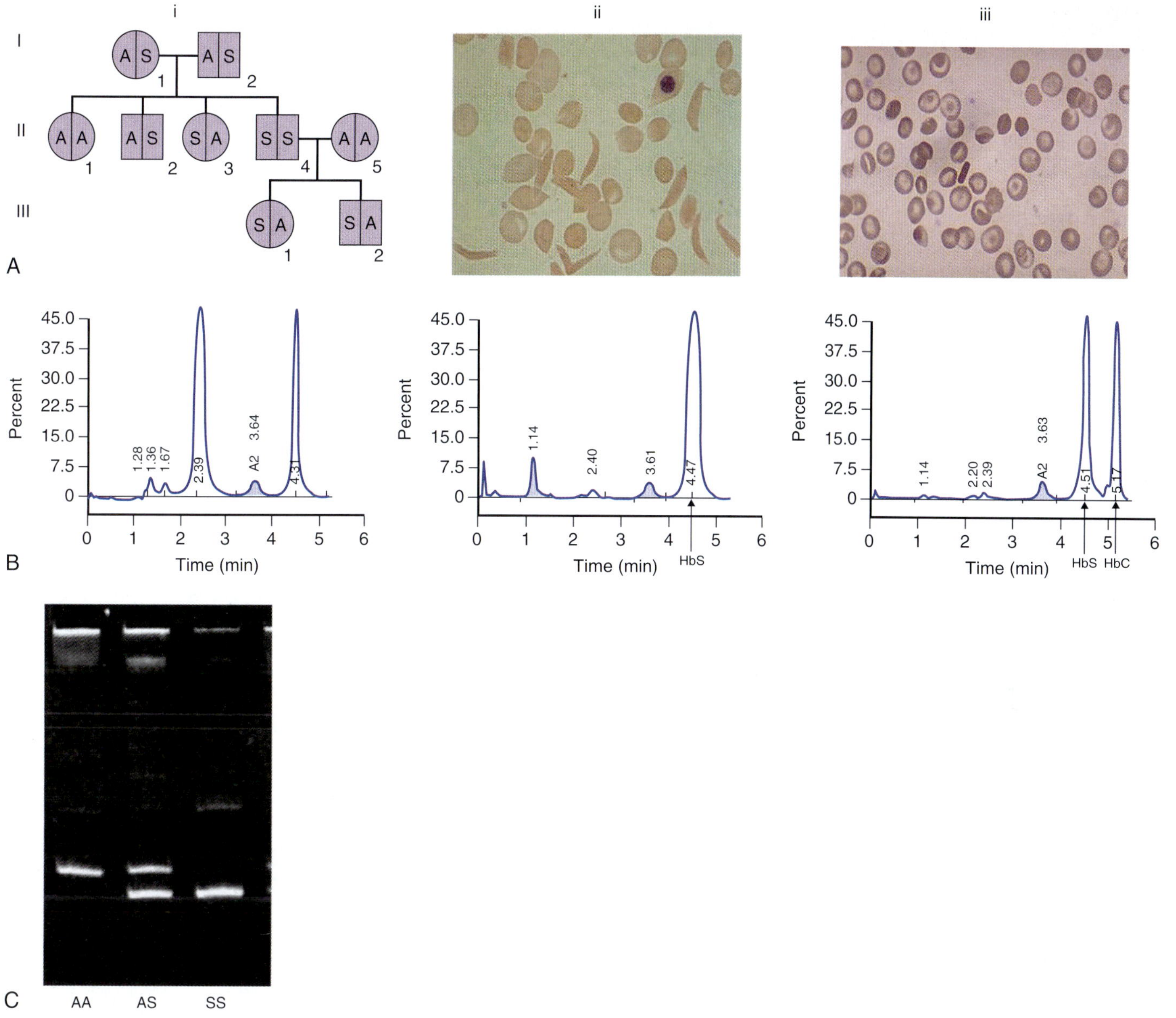

FIGURE 149-3. **Diagnosis of sickle cell disease. A, A prototypical family structure in which both parents (I) have sickle cell trait and each offspring (II) has a 25% chance of having sickle cell anemia (SS). Each child of an affected parent (III) will have sickle cell trait (SA) if the other parent has a normal hemoglobin (AA) genotype. The blood films *(center* and *right)* are from patients with sickle cell anemia and hemoglobin SC (HbSC) disease, respectively. Note the irreversibly sickled cells in the former and the hemoglobin C (HbC) crystal and target cells in the latter. B, High-performance liquid chromatography profiles from patients with sickle cell trait *(left)*, sickle cell anemia *(center)*, and HbSC disease *(right)*. C, Amplification-refractory mutation system–based separation of the β-globin genes from a normal subject (AA), a carrier of sickle cell trait (AS), and a patient with sickle cell anemia (SS).**

recognize damaged sickle erythrocytes, thereby resulting in erythrophagocytosis. Intravascular hemolysis liberates hemoglobin into the circulation, where it binds to, and thereby depletes, free plasma haptoglobin and scavenges nitric oxide (NO). In addition, these sickled red cells adhere to activated vascular endothelial cells, thereby promoting inflammation as well as leukocyte and platelet adherence to endothelium. These interactions with endothelium lead to vascular obstruction, tissue ischemia, and then vaso-occlusion. Endothelial cells respond to biologic modifiers that are generated during these vaso-occlusive episodes and the resulting inflammation. The initiation of vaso-occlusion is complex, and mechanisms include the following:

- Cellular damage from adhesive interactions among sickle cells, leucocytes, endothelial cells, and platelets and involving cell adherence molecules such as P selectin, which is expressed on endothelial cells and platelets when they are activated. Leukocytes are then captured on the endothelium.
- Adherent sickle cells and shear stresses that release reactive oxidant species express endothelin and disturb NO balance.
- Reperfusion injury, which can activate endothelial cells and stimulate inflammation.
- Reticulocytes, which are prematurely released from the bone marrow and have adhesive ligands that augment interactions between erythrocytes and endothelial cells.

Hemoglobin variants that have the β-globin gene Glu6Val substitution (HbS) are prone to polymerization. Accumulation of these HbS polymers within sickled erythrocytes causes cellular injury, thereby leading to the clinical syndrome of sickle cell disease. In homozygous sickle cell disease (HbSS) or coinheritance of HbS and β^0-thalassemia (HbSβ^0-thalassemia), the cells contain HbS and no HbA and have the greatest clinical severity (sickle cell anemia). The coinheritance of HbS with other hemoglobin variants (e.g., HbC, HbE, HbSβ^+-thalassemia, HbSD^{Punjab}, HbSO^{Arab}) are also associated with sickling disorders of varying severity (Table 149-1). Although most of the more than 1000 hemoglobin mutations are clinically insignificant, others can occasionally affect the stability and function of hemoglobin and cause hemolytic anemia, disordered oxygen transport, or methemoglobinemia (Chapter 144).

CLINICAL MANIFESTATIONS

Sickle Cell Trait (Sickle Cell Carrier; HbAS)

Approximately 18 to 25% of the population of Sub-Saharan Africa are sickle cell carriers and have what is termed sickle cell trait. Carriers are protected against intracellular sickling because the red cells contain a predominance of HbA compared with HbS (usually 35 to 40% HbS) and because the HbA inhibits hemoglobin polymerization, except under extreme conditions (prolonged

TABLE 149-1 GENETIC AND LABORATORY FEATURES OF COMMON SICKLE HEMOGLOBINOPATHIES*

GENOTYPE	GENETICS	PREVALENCE AMONG AFRICAN AMERICANS†	HEMATOCRIT (%)	MCV (fL)	HbS (%)	HbA_2 (%)	HbF (%)	SEVERITY‡
Sickle cell anemia (HbSS)	Homozygous HbS	1 : 600	18-28	85-95	>85	2-3	2-15	4
HbSS-α-thalassemia	Homozygous HbS α^+-thalassemia	30% of HbSS patients	25-33	70-85	>85	4-6	2-15	4
HbSC disease (HbSC)	Compound heterozygous HbS, HbC	1 : 800	28-40	70-85	50	2-3	1-8	2
HbS-β^0-thalassemia (HbS-β^0-Thal)	Compound heterozygous HbS, β^0-thalassemia	1 : 1600	20-30	65-75	>85	4-6	5-15	4
HbS-β^+-thalassemia (HbS-β^+-Thal)	Compound heterozygous HbS, β^+-thalassemia	1 : 1600	30-40	60-70	70-95	4-6	2-10	1-3
HbSE disease (HbSE)	Compound heterozygous HbS, HbE	Rare§	30-45	70-80	60	2-3	1	1-2
HbS-HPFH	Compound heterozygous HbS and gene deletion HPFH	Rare	38-45	70-80	70	2	20-30	0
Sickle cell trait (HbAS)¶	Heterozygous HbS	1 : 12	38-50	80-90	35-40	2-3	<1	0
Normal (HbAA)	Homozygous HbA	—	38-50	80-90	0	2-3	<1	—

*Many other abnormal globin genes can be found as compound heterozygotes with the HbS gene. The most common of these are α-thalassemia, HbD, HbO (Arabia), HbG (Philadelphia), HPFH, Hb Hope, and Hb Lepore. Average ranges of laboratory values are shown, but these can vary according to the patient's age.

†These figures differ by the prevalence of the involved genes in the population studied. In West and Central Africa, where the disease is most common, approximately 2% of all newborns have sickle cell disease. The prevalence of the HbC trait in African Americans is 3%, and that of the β-thalassemia trait is 1%. About 30% of African Americans carry an α-thalassemia gene, which can alter the phenotype of sickle cell disease by causing microcytosis, reduced cell density, and less hemolysis.

‡Severity of disease compared with sickle cell anemia, clinically the most severe genotype. This is a qualitative ranking of the clinical severity of each genotype; within each genotype, there is great clinical heterogeneity.

§Although this combination is still a rare genotype, the rising Asian population in the United States (HbE is a Southeastern Asian gene) will make it more frequent with time. With few cases reported compared with the other genotypes, the phenotype of HbSE disease is not totally defined. It may resemble HbS-β^+-thalassemia, with symptoms appearing mainly in adults.

¶Sickle cell trait should not be classified as a form of sickle cell disease. About 8% of African Americans are carriers of HbS. Carriers are hematologically normal with a normal life expectancy. The few abnormalities traceable to the presence of HbS, besides the renal lesions, include a four-fold increased risk for pulmonary embolism, an increased risk for splenic infarction at high altitude, and a higher risk for dying during the course of exertional heat illness.

Hb = hemoglobin; HbF = fetal hemoglobin; HPFH = hereditary persistence of HbF; MCV = mean corpuscular volume.

hypoxia, acidosis, or dehydration). The carrier state is not generally regarded as harmful; carriers have a normal life expectancy but may experience clinical complications.[3]

Limited epidemiologic studies of individuals with sickle cell trait suggest an increased risk for extreme exercise- and physical exertion–related injury, broadly including exertional rhabdomyolysis, heat-associated collapse, and unexplained sudden death.[4,5] Sickle cell trait can likewise be a cause of death during training and competition in athletes.

Renal abnormalities are among the most common manifestations of sickle cell trait, including hematuria and impaired urinary concentrating ability, and can lead to albuminuria and chronic kidney disease. Individuals with sickle cell trait are at increased risk for venous thromboembolism, specifically pulmonary embolism.[6]

Sickle Cell Disease

Sickle cell disease has remarkably variable clinical manifestations. An individual patient can have almost all known complications, whereas others may have virtually no complications but nevertheless die suddenly. Some individuals have severe complications but do not demonstrate other manifestations. Thus, the phenotypic variability of sickle cell disease is striking despite being a prototypical "single-gene" mendelian disorder. Specific sickle cell genotypes have differing severity, with HbSS and HbSβ^0-thalassemia following a similarly severe disease course, whereas HbSC, HBSβ^+-thalassemia (and the other genotypes) tend to have a milder disease phenotype. However, some patients with HbSS may have infrequent pain episodes and few complications, whereas some patients with HbSC may experience frequent severe pain crises. Factors causing this phenotypic variability include coinheritance of disease-modifying genes, including HbF and α-thalassemia, as well as variations in genes that affect inflammation, nitric oxide biology, oxidant injury, cell-cell interactions, vasoregulation, coagulation, and hemostasis.

Multiorgan Disease and Variation with Age

Although sickle cell disease is most commonly associated with anemia and repeated pain episodes, the pathophysiologic process can affect all organs in the body (Table 149-2). Acute complications include an increased risk for infection, stroke, and chest complications. Chronic complications include chronic lung disease, chronic renal failure, pulmonary hypertension, and ophthalmologic complications.

TABLE 149-2 ACUTE AND CHRONIC COMPLICATIONS OF SICKLE CELL DISEASE

SYSTEM	ACUTE COMPLICATIONS	CHRONIC COMPLICATIONS
Neurologic	Acute ischemic stroke Acute hemorrhagic stroke Venous sinus thrombosis	Silent cerebral ischemia Vasculopathy (moyamoya disease) Headache Cognitive dysfunction
Cardiorespiratory	Acute chest syndrome	Pulmonary hypertension Asthma Chronic sickle lung disease Sleep-disordered breathing Myocardial impairment
Renal	Acute renal failure Hematuria Urinary tract infection	Enuresis Proteinuria Chronic renal failure
Urologic	Priapism	Erectile dysfunction
Orthopedic	Osteomyelitis	Avascular necrosis
Ophthalmologic	Vitreous hemorrhage Retinal detachment Retinal artery occlusion	Retinopathy
Others	Acute splenic sequestration Acute hepatic sequestration Gallstone disease (biliary colic, cholecystitis)	Chronic splenomegaly Splenic dysfunction Sickle hepatopathy Leg ulceration

Complications typically vary with age. Dactylitis (pain crisis affecting hands and feet) is often the first symptom seen in young children when the levels of

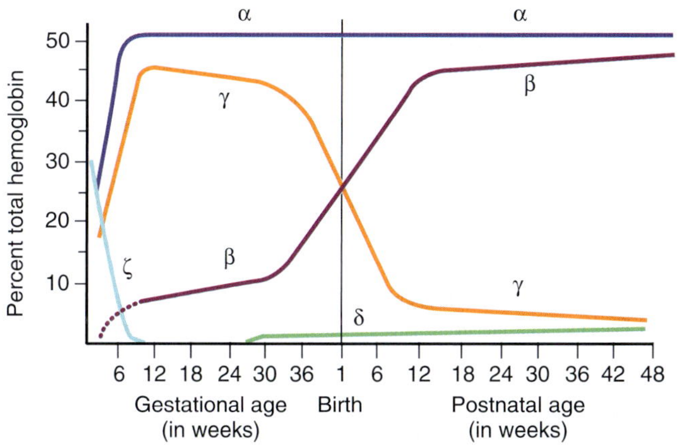

FIGURE 149-4. **Human globin genes.** Expression of globin genes during development. The α chains are expressed throughout gestation and adult life, the fetal γ-globin chains are expressed predominantly in utero, and the β-globin and δ-globin genes are expressed mainly postnatally. This switching of gene expression patterns accounts for the different hemoglobins present in the embryo, fetus, and adult. This phenomenon also accounts for the observation that disorders of α-globin can affect both fetus and adult, whereas β-globin chain diseases usually are not clinically apparent in the first months of life, when fetal hemoglobin levels are still high.

HbS increase between 6 and 12 months of age as hemoglobin switches from HbF to HbS (Fig. 149-4). Splenic dysfunction, which occurs early in life, increases susceptibility to infection and results in high rates of infective deaths in the absence of antibiotic prophylaxis and vaccination. Splenic sequestration is most common in affected individuals who are younger than age 5 years before the development of splenic infarction, although it may occur later in persons with milder disease phenotypes. Before the introduction of transcranial Doppler screening and primary stroke prevention (see later), stroke was most common in young children and in older adults; the risk is now markedly less in children but not in adults.

Most chronic organ damage does not become clinically significant until adulthood, but invariably organ damage will begin in early childhood. For example, although evidence of renal dysfunction (e.g., hyposthenuria and microalbuminuria) occurs in early childhood, end-stage renal failure is uncommon before late adulthood. Similarly, acute chest syndrome, asthma, and sleep-disordered breathing are all common in children, but severe chronic lung disease becomes apparent in adulthood. Pulmonary hypertension, retinopathy, leg ulcers, and avascular necrosis are all uncommon in childhood but much more common in adults. With an increasing life expectancy, sickle cell disease has now evolved into a debilitating disorder with substantial morbidity resulting from ongoing sickle cell vasculopathy and multiorgan damage.[7] Patients should be offered the option of curative therapies as their best option for improved long-term survival and quality of life.

Pain

Acute Pain

Acute pain episodes (vaso-occlusive crises) are the hallmark of sickle cell disease, occur with unpredictable frequency, may be triggered by infection, dehydration, or stress, or may occur with no precipitant. Pain crises are the most common reason for hospital admission in patients with sickle cell disease, but pain is also experienced frequently in the community and can have a significant impact on quality of life. Almost 30% of adults with sickle cell disease have pain on more than 95% of days, and only about 15% have pain on fewer than 5% of days. Overall, patients experience pain on about 50% of days but use health care on fewer than 5% of days.

Young children typically experience pain in the fingers and toes (dactylitis), but older children and adults tend to experience pain in the arms, legs, and trunk. Examination of the affected area is usually normal, but swelling and acute tenderness may be evident. No diagnostic tests exist for sickle crisis, so diagnosis is usually based on the patient's history. An individual patient will usually describe the pain as typical for sickle cell disease, and atypical pain requires further investigation to look for alternative causes.

Chronic Pain

Chronic pain refers to pain that persists for more than 3 months. In patients with sickle cell disease, chronic pain may be due to an identifiable underlying cause, most commonly avascular necrosis. However, some patients experience severe daily pain with no clear stimulus, perhaps because of central sensitivity syndromes that are associated with an increased sensitivity to painful and nonpainful stimuli and are precipitated and reinforced by repeated painful and stressful stimuli.

Anemia

Patients with HbSS/HbSβ^0-thalassemia usually have a baseline hemoglobin of 6 to 9 g/dL, whereas patients with HbSC and HbSβ^+-thalassemia will have a higher baseline hemoglobin of 8 to 12 g/dL. Patients usually tolerate this degree of anemia, although some patients experience significant fatigue. Anemia, sometimes associated with renal dysfunction, often worsens in older adulthood.

Acute anemia (a decrease in hemoglobin of >2 g/dL) may be associated with worsening symptoms of fatigue and breathlessness, and intervention with transfusion may be required. Causes of acute anemia include worsening hemolysis, parvovirus (erythrovirus) B19 infection (potentially causing pure red cell aplasia or hypoplasia), splenic sequestration, folate deficiency, and any cause of anemia seen in non–sickle cell disease patients. Parvovirus B19 (Chapter 342), which causes slapped-cheek syndrome in children, usually manifests as an acute viral illness with profound anemia and reticulocytopenia. Splenic sequestration is most common in young children before splenic infarction and is characterized by anemia and splenic enlargement.

Neurologic Complications

Acute Ischemic Stroke

In untreated children and adults with sickle cell disease, strokes occur in approximately 10% of patients by age 20 years and 25% by age 40 years. Cerebral vasculopathy is the most common cause in children, but adults also have comorbid conditions such as diabetes, hypertension, and atrial fibrillation. Acute ischemic stroke can also occur in the context of acute pain crisis or acute anemia. The typical features of acute ischemic stroke (Chapter 376) include hemiparesis, facial droop, or dysphasia, but patients may present with loss of consciousness or behavioral change.

Acute Hemorrhagic Stroke

Patients with sickle cell disease also are at increased risk for intracerebral, intraventricular, subdural, and subarachnoid hemorrhage (Chapter 377), often related to the underlying cerebral vasculopathy. The prevalence of both moyamoya (a rare, chronic occlusive cerebrovascular disease characterized by progressive stenosis of the intracranial terminal carotid arteries with an abnormal vascular network at the base of the brain) and cerebral aneurysms are increased in this group of patients. Presentation with headache and decreased consciousness is more common than with focal neurologic signs.

Silent Cerebral Infarction and Other Neurologic Complications

MRI of patients with sickle cell disease frequently shows small ischemic lesions that are not associated with neurologic deficits. These silent cerebral infarcts increase with increasing age and are associated with cognitive impairment, including a reduction in IQ. MRI screening of children may identify affected individuals at an early age. Venous sinus thrombosis, posterior reversible encephalopathy syndrome, and headaches are also more common in patients with sickle cell disease.

Cardiorespiratory Complications

Acute Chest Syndrome

Acute chest syndrome is an acute illness characterized by fever and/or respiratory symptoms accompanied by a new pulmonary infiltrate on chest radiograph. Patients may present to the hospital with acute chest syndrome, or it may develop 1 to 3 days after admission for an acute pain crisis. Etiologies include infection (bacterial or viral), fat embolism, and pulmonary infarction (Chapter 68). Severity is variable, but it may result in severe hypoxia, respiratory failure, and death.

Pulmonary Hypertension

Pulmonary hypertension, with a mean pulmonary artery pressure of 25 mm Hg or greater, is reported in 6 to 11% of adults with sickle cell disease and is associated with increased mortality. Pathogenesis is multifactorial and includes left-sided heart disease, chronic lung disease, chronic thromboembolic disease, and intravascular hemolysis. *N*-terminal pro–brain natriuretic peptide (BNP) levels are typically elevated, and echocardiography is the best noninvasive test.

Chronic Lung Disease and Sleep-Disordered Breathing

About 20% of children with sickle cell disease have asthma, which may be caused by increased pulmonary capillary blood flow or by the chronic inflammation of the lungs. The prevalence of asthma is not increased in adults with sickle cell disease, but about 70% of adults with sickle cell disease develop restrictive lung defects, which can be associated with daytime hypoxia, chest pain, and progressive restrictive lung defects and fibrosis on high-resolution CT scanning. Sleep-disordered breathing (Chapter 374), with nocturnal hypoxia and obstructive sleep apnea, is seen in up to 40% of children and 60% of adults with sickle cell disease.

Renal and Urologic Complications

Renal complications are seen in up to 60% of patients with sickle cell disease, commencing in early childhood and progressing with increasing age. A distal renal tubule–concentrating defect, which is an early manifestation of renal damage, results in hyposthenuria (an inability to concentrate urine), nocturnal enuresis, and a predisposition to dehydration. An increased glomerular filtration rate (GFR), owing to anemia and high cardiac output, leads to glomerular hypertrophy and damage and then to microalbuminuria, which is seen in 20% of children and 60% of adults with sickle cell disease and can progress to unselective proteinuria and even nephrotic syndrome (Chapter 107).

Hematuria, which is also common in sickle cell disease as well as in sickle cell trait (see earlier), can be due to renal papillary necrosis. This syndrome can be painful and profuse. Renal medullary carcinoma is a highly aggressive malignancy that predominantly afflicts young adults and adolescents with sickle cell hemoglobinopathies.

Acute kidney injury (Chapter 106) occurs in 2 to 10% of patients who are admitted with acute painful crisis and can be precipitated by dehydration, sepsis, and drugs. Cortical ischemia, perhaps due to sickling in the low-flow low-oxygen cortical areas of the kidney, also can contribute to tubular interstitial disease (Chapter 108). Progressive renal dysfunction can result in end-stage kidney disease, with a requirement for dialysis or renal transplantation.

Priapism

Priapism is a persistent, prolonged, and painful penile erection unrelated to sexual stimulation. Priapism is common in men and boys with sickle cell disease and may occur as short, intermittent, self-limited episodes (stuttering priapism) or as severe acute episodes lasting for more than an hour (fulminant priapism). Acute priapism may be preceded by stuttering priapism and can result in long-term erectile dysfunction.

Infection

Sickle cell patients experience increased morbidity and mortality from infection, in part due to functional asplenia or hyposplenia (Chapter 154), and also due to increased rates of gram-negative sepsis. Hyposplenia develops from infancy and leads to a deficiency in response to encapsulated bacteria and hence increased risk for invasive infection with organisms such as *Streptococcus pneumoniae* (Chapter 268), *Neisseria meningitides* (Chapter 274), and *Haemophilus influenzae* type b (Chapter 277). Patients with sickle cell disease are more likely to have adverse outcomes from coronavirus disease 2019 (COVID-19) infection (Chapter 336).[8]

DIAGNOSIS

Routine Blood Tests

The usual steady-state hemoglobin level is 5 to 10 g/dL in HbSS and is higher in the milder phenotypes. The anemia in HbSS is typically normochromic and normocytic, but microcytosis is often seen in HbSC disease, and marked microcytosis and hypochromia are seen in HbSβ-thalassemia. Most affected individuals have reticulocytosis and evidence of hemolysis with a raised bilirubin and lactate dehydrogenase (LDH). The blood film in HbSS will show numerous sickle cells, polychromasia, and features of hyposplenism (in adults). In addition, hypochromia is also prominent in HbSβ-thalassemia. In HbSC disease, target cells, densely staining contracted boat-shaped red cells, and HbC crystals may be seen with less sickled cells and polychromasia than in HbSS (see Figs. 149-3Aii and 149-3Aiii).

Analysis of Hemoglobin Type

High-pressure liquid chromatography (HPLC) is now the most common method of hemoglobin analysis. Variant hemoglobins are identified by their elution time from an ion exchange column and can be quantified. HPLC is quick, is reliable, and allows high throughput of samples (see Fig. 149-3B). Confirmatory testing should be performed with alternative techniques. These include the following:

- The sickle solubility test will detect sickling of hemoglobin in solution by treatment with a reducing agent. It is specific for sickle hemoglobin but does not differentiate among HbAS, HbSS, and other compound heterozygotes of sickle cell hemoglobin.
- Hemoglobin electrophoresis was the first method used to demonstrate hemoglobin variants but is time-consuming and labor-intensive.
- DNA sequence analysis identifies the specific globin gene mutation (see Fig. 149-3C).
- Tandem mass spectrometry identifies the specific amino acid change in the globin chain.

Screening

Screening for sickle cell trait is currently required in some branches of the U.S. Armed Forces because of an increased risk from complications of extreme exercise. Antenatal screening aims to identify couples at high risk for an affected pregnancy to enable counseling and prenatal diagnosis (via chorionic villus sampling or amniocentesis) early enough to allow reproductive choice. Preconceptual screening provides couples with information about the risks of an affected birth before conception and allows them to consider the option of preimplantation diagnosis.

TREATMENT AND PREVENTION

General Measures

Sickle cell disease is a chronic disease for which good nutrition and a high fluid intake should be encouraged. Patients and their families should be educated about acute complications and should be taught how to palpate the spleen, how to manage simple pain crises, and when to go to the emergency department. Regular outpatient clinic visits will ensure appropriate screening for chronic disease complications (including screening for stroke risk) and early intervention.[9] The increased production of red blood cells, combined with inadequate nutrition, leads to accelerated consumption of folic acid; supplementary folic acid is typically recommended, although patients with a good dietary intake may not require it. There are significant psychosocial implications of chronic illness, and patients and their families should be offered psychological and social support if needed. The transition from pediatric to adult care is a time of heightened vulnerability and should be managed in a structured way.

Management of Complications

Pain

Mild acute pain episodes can be managed at home with simple analgesia (acetaminophen, nonsteroidal anti-inflammatory drugs; Table 26-4), fluids, and rest, but more severe pain crises may need hospital admission for strong opiate analgesia (Table 26-6). Patients and their families should be made aware of situations when they should be seen in the hospital (Table 149-3).

Inpatients typically require parenteral analgesic. Patients often find patient-controlled analgesic devices beneficial, and the use of patient-controlled analgesic may reduce total opiate intake. Patients being treated with opiates should be monitored for respiratory depression and excessive sedation and should be offered adjuvant therapy to manage opiate side effects (emesis [Table 118-5], constipation [Table 122-3], and pruritus [Table 403-10]). Doses of opiate pain relief should be titrated down as soon as pain settles.

Patients with acute pain episodes should be monitored for the development of other complications, particularly acute chest syndrome, which typically begins 24 to 72 hours after the onset of an acute pain crisis and is more common in patients who have chest and back pain. Early incentive spirometry may reduce the subsequent incidence of acute chest syndrome, and regular monitoring of oxygen saturations will allow early identification of those with worsening hypoxia, which can be a precursor to acute chest syndrome. Patients with recurrent acute pain crisis should be offered hydroxyurea therapy.

TABLE 149-3 SYMPTOMS THAT SHOULD PROMPT HOSPITAL ADMISSION: "RED FLAG" EVENTS

- Severe pain not settling with usual analgesia
- Atypical pain
- Temperature >38° C
- Chest pain
- Shortness of breath
- Neurologic symptoms (e.g., weakness of a limb or facial droop, diminished level of consciousness)
- Pain associated with unusually severe headaches
- Severe lethargy
- Priapism
- Severe jaundice

Chronic pain can be difficult to treat and worsened by opiate therapy. Referral to chronic pain services is often helpful (Chapter 26).

Infection and Infection Prophylaxis

Vaccination for pneumococcus, meningococcus, and *Haemophilus* (Chapter 15) decreases the risk for early mortality and morbidity from invasive bacterial disease, but vaccine-resistant serotypes can still cause serious infections. Infections, especially with encapsulated organisms, require prompt antibiotic treatment.

Stroke

For patients with suspected strokes, urgent magnetic resonance imaging (MRI) or MR angiography can confirm and localize the stroke, although computed tomography (CT) may be used in emergency situations to exclude acute hemorrhagic stroke. Xanthochromia in cerebrospinal fluid can confirm a subarachnoid hemorrhage.

After initial management with hydration and oxygenation, urgent exchange transfusion should be performed to minimize ischemic damage and improve perfusion of the brain. If there is marked anemia (hemoglobin <6 g/dL), simple transfusions may be given to achieve a post-transfusion hemoglobin concentration of about 10 g/dL and HbS percentage of less than 30%, but initial exchange transfusion may prevent recurrent stroke more effectively than initial simple transfusion.[10] In adults with sickle cell disease, thrombolysis appears to be safe in the absence of hemorrhagic transformation.[11]

For an acute hemorrhagic stroke, treatment should be on a specialized neurosurgery unit and should generally be similar to treatment of patients without sickle cell disease. However, exchange transfusion therapy should be considered before neurosurgical intervention.

The risk for recurrent stroke is high, and transfusion therapy seems to be more effective than hydroxyurea in preventing recurrent stroke. Patients should be offered long-term blood transfusion to maintain HbS percentage of less than 30%, most effectively by repeated automated or manual exchange transfusions, although the optimal duration of such therapy is uncertain.[A1] Surgical revascularization may be indicated for patients with recurrent acute ischemic stroke or progressive vasculopathy.

Children who have silent cerebral infarction may benefit from educational or medical intervention. Chronic transfusion therapy may be of benefit, particularly in patients who have abnormal transcranial Doppler studies.

On transcranial Doppler screening in children, a raised time-averaged mean of maximal velocity is associated with an increased risk of stroke. In such children, a blood transfusion strategy to maintain HbS% at less than 30% can reduce the risk of stroke by 90%. As a result, transcranial Doppler scanning is now routine in children ages 2 to 16 years. Stopping transfusions after 3 years leads to an increased risk of recurrent stroke, whereas changing to hydroxyurea therapy after 1 year of transfusions is as effective as continuing with transfusion.[A2]

Cardiorespiratory

Initial treatment of the acute chest syndrome is supportive with pain relief, antibiotics, and oxygen therapy, but more severe presentations may require treatment with simple or exchange transfusion and/or noninvasive or invasive respiratory support.[12] Patients with severe or recurrent acute chest syndrome should be offered treatment with hydroxyurea.

Patients with catheterization-proved pulmonary hypertension should be offered sickle cell disease–modifying therapy or specific therapy for pulmonary hypertension (see Fig. 69-6) under the guidance of an expert. For sleep-disordered breathing (Chapter 374), treatment with nocturnal oxygen or noninvasive respiratory support may be required.

Renal and Urologic Disease

Hematuria may require blood transfusion and occasionally interventional radiology or surgery. Hematuria in patients older than age 40 years, particularly if painless, always should be evaluated by a urologist.

Proteinuria is associated with progression of chronic kidney disease, so patients should be offered screening for proteinuria (with albumin-creatinine or protein-creatinine ratio). Early intervention with angiotensin-converting enzyme inhibitors or angiotensin receptor blockers is indicated in patients who have significant proteinuria (protein-creatinine ratio >50 mg/mmol). Renal function should be monitored regularly to allow optimization of the treatment of hypertension and proteinuria and thereby slow progression.

Priapism

Young men with sickle cell disease should be educated about priapism and encouraged to come to the emergency department for episodes that persist for more than 1 hour. Initial conservative management includes pain relief, fluids, gentle exercise and urination, and oral α-adrenergic agents (etilefrine). If the priapism fails to resolve, a urologist should be contacted to perform penile aspiration, which can be combined with the injection of α-adrenergic agents into the corpus cavernosa. The procedure will often cause detumescence; if not, further surgical intervention will be needed. Transfusion therapy may be helpful to support surgery and possibly to relieve persistent priapism. Treatment of stuttering priapism should be considered for symptomatic relief and with the aim of preventing future episodes of fulminant priapism. Oral α-adrenergic agents and antiandrogens should be considered under guidance of an expert urologist, and phosphodiesterase type 5 (PDE5) inhibitors also may be considered.

Management of Pregnancy

Although most women with sickle cell disease should expect to have successful pregnancies and healthy babies, these pregnancies are associated with an increased rate of maternal and fetal morbidity and mortality. Complications include increased sickle complications (pain, chest complications), pregnancy complications (infection, raised blood pressure), and high rates of premature birth and fetal growth restriction. Women should be counseled about the risks of pregnancy during their routine outpatient appointments, and preconceptual care should include partner screening, review of medications, and evaluation of chronic complications that may affect the pregnancy. When pregnant, women should be enrolled into multidisciplinary antenatal care with an obstetrician who has experience in sickle cell disease and a hematologist. Caregivers should consider prescribing daily low-dose aspirin (e.g., 81 mg daily) for prevention of preeclampsia (Chapter 221). Patients should be followed regularly throughout pregnancy with blood pressure, urinalysis, and ultrasound monitoring. Prophylactic transfusion is not recommended for all pregnancies but may reduce the risk for pain crisis, chest complications, and fetal complications. If there are no obstetric complications, the pregnancy should be allowed to continue to term, anticipating spontaneous labor and normal delivery. Women with sickle cell disease are at increased risk for venous thrombosis (Chapter 68), and their risk should be assessed using appropriate tools and the need for thromboprophylaxis considered (Chapter 221).[13]

Management of Surgery

General anesthesia is associated with increased risk for complications, in particular, increased pain crises and acute chest crises. These complications can be reduced with careful preoperative care (hydration, oxygenation) and consideration of preoperative blood transfusion. In low- to moderate-risk surgery in patients with non-HbSS genotypes, transfusion may not be needed. Simple transfusion aiming for a hemoglobin concentration of more than 9 g/dL is as effective as exchange transfusion for low- and moderate-risk surgery, but high-risk surgery (cardiac or neurosurgery) requires preoperative exchange transfusion.[14]

Disease-Modifying Therapies

Hydroxyurea

Hydroxyurea increases HbF levels and reduces cellular adhesion and hemolysis. Randomized controlled trials in various settings have shown that hydroxyurea reduces acute pain episodes, chest crises, and rates of hospitalization in adults and children with sickle cell anemia with few side effects regardless of the severity of symptoms.[A3] Dose-escalation protocols (up to 30 mg/kg/day) are superior to fixed-dose protocols (at 20 mg/kg/day).[A4] In addition, hydroxyurea reduces the risk of stroke in patients who have elevated transcranial Doppler studies. Adherence to hydroxyurea clearly reduces emergency visits and hospitalizations.[15] Hydroxyurea should be offered to all infants, children, and adolescents with sickle cell anemia, irrespective of severity, and to adults with recurrent pain episodes, severe or recurrent acute chest syndrome, and symptomatic anemia.

Hydroxyurea is well tolerated. Its main side effect is myelosuppression, and regular blood monitoring is required while on the drug. Because of suggestive evidence regarding teratogenicity and effects on spermatogenesis, hydroxyurea should be avoided in patients who are trying to conceive.

Anemia and Blood Transfusion

Red cell transfusion is used both to treat the acute complications of sickle cell disease and as long-term disease-modifying therapy. Patients who have chronic anemia may need intervention with hydroxyurea, transfusions, or erythropoiesis-stimulating agents. Acute anemia typically requires blood transfusion, aiming for a return to the patients' baseline hemoglobin concentration.

Acute indications for transfusion include acute anemia, acute chest syndrome, stroke, and multiorgan failure. Transfusion is not indicated for the treatment of simple acute pain crises. Long-term transfusion is indicated for primary and secondary stroke prevention and for the prevention of recurrent pain episodes or recurrent acute chest syndrome if there has not been a response to hydroxyurea therapy.

Blood can be administered as a simple or "top-up" transfusion to increase hemoglobin levels and improve oxygen-carrying capacity or as an exchange transfusion (manual or automated). Exchange transfusion allows a more marked reduction of HbS compared with HbA and is more likely to reduce vaso-occlusion.[16] In view of the increased risk for alloimmunization and delayed hemolytic transfusion reactions in patients with sickle cell disease, blood should be ABO Rh (CcDEe) and Kell compatible, and blood should be antigen-negative for clinically significant antibodies that are currently or have previously been detected (Chapter 162).

Long-term or frequent intermittent transfusion can result in iron overload and iron deposition in the liver and other organs. The patient should be monitored with ferritin and liver iron quantification by MRI, and iron chelation therapy should be instigated if the patient is iron-loaded (see Chapter 196). Both deferasirox and desferrioxamine are effective and licensed for use in sickle cell disease. Deferiprone is not currently licensed for use in sickle cell disease but is also effective.

TABLE 149-4 NEW MEDICATIONS FOR TREATMENT OF SICKLE CELL DISEASE

DRUG NAME	MODE OF ACTION	DOSE	LICENSED INDICATIONS (UNITED STATES)
L-Glutamine	Antioxidant	5 g-15 g orally, twice daily based on body weight	Reduction of acute complications in sickle cell disease in adults and pediatric patients 5 years and older
Crizanlizumab	Anti-P selectin	5 mg/kg IV infusion over 30 min on Week 0, 2, and every 4 weeks thereafter	Reduction in the frequency of vaso-occlusive crises in adults and pediatric patients 16 years and older with sickle cell disease
Voxelotor	HbS polymerization inhibitor	1500 mg orally, daily	The treatment of sickle cell disease in adults and pediatric patients 12 years and older

HbS = hemoglobin S; IV = intravenous.

Other Disease Modifying Therapies (Table 149-4)

L-Glutamine, an antioxidant, can reduce the rate of vaso-occlusive pain crises and hospital admissions.[A5] Crizanlizumab, an anti-P selectin agent, reduces the frequency of vaso-occlusive cries and increases the median time to first and second crisis.[A6] Both drugs are useful to reduce the frequency of vaso-occlusive pain events in patients who have frequent pain crises. Voxelotor, which is a hemoglobin modifier that inhibits the polymerization of hemoglobin and reduces hemolysis, raises hemoglobin by 1.0 g/dL in over 50% of recipients without adverse events.[A7]

Other promising agents currently in development for the acute or long-term treatment of sickle cell disease act through different mechanisms. Examples include drugs targeting HbS polymerization (e.g., pyruvate kinase activators),[17] histone deacetylase inhibitors, and drugs targeting inflammation (e.g., interleukin 1-beta [IL-1b] blockade). A randomized trial of canakinumab, which is an IL-1b blocker, did not show a pre-specified reduction in pain but did show reduction in markers of inflammation, sickle cell disease–related adverse events, and hospitalization rates.[A8]

Curative Therapies

Stem Cell Therapy

Successful hematopoietic stem cell transplantation (Chapter 163) is a potentially curative option for sickle cell disease. When performed in young patients, hematopoietic stem cell transplantation from human leukocyte antigen (HLA)–matched siblings results in excellent overall survival and event-free survival.[18] The utility of this approach is limited because only about 10 to 20% of sickle cell disease patients will have HLA-identical siblings available as donors. Hematopoietic stem cell transplantation from alternative donors (particularly haplo-identical transplants) have shown good outcomes in small studies but are associated with increased morbidity and mortality. There is increasing evidence of the efficacy of reduced-intensity conditioning approaches in adults, associated with reduced adverse effects.[19]

Gene Therapy

Gene therapy (Chapter 34), which is another potentially curative option for sickle cell disease, involves manipulation of hematopoietic stem cells to correct or circumvent the sickle mutation followed by autologous transplantation of the manipulated cells. Clinical trials using lentiviral vectors to add modified antisickling β-globin variants have showed sustained production of the modified β-globin with reduced hemolysis and resolution of severe vaso-occlusive events.[20] Gene-editing techniques using CRISPR/Cas9 technology to encourage production of fetal hemoglobin (HbF) also can be effective, with persistence of high levels of HbF and elimination of vaso-occlusive pain crises for at least 1 year.[21]

PROGNOSIS

In resource-rich countries with universal neonatal screening, antibiotic prophylaxis, improved supportive care, and successful research trials, most children with sickle cell disease reach adulthood. In the United States, nearly 95% of persons with sickle cell disease reach age 18 years. Nevertheless, adults with sickle cell disease still have a high burden of pain and comorbidity, and the median age of death is 43 years.[22] The extent to which newer drugs will impact chronic organ damage, quality of life, and longevity is unclear. In Sub-Saharan Africa, by contrast, where almost 80% of the projected 306,000 newborns worldwide with sickle cell disease are born, mortality remains 50 to 90% before age 5 years.

OTHER HEMOGLOBINOPATHIES

Hemoglobin C trait is a benign condition in which lysine replaces glutamic acid at the same sixth position on the hemoglobin beta chain where valine causes the sickle cell mutation. Homozygous HbC disease is associated with a mild hemolytic anemia and splenomegaly. HbC disease is characterized by a peripheral smear with a large population of target cells (see Fig. 149-3Aiii), with some red cells containing crystals. Individuals with HbC disease generally do not have clinical sickle crises or other complications. HbS/HbC disease occurs in about 1 per 1100 Black Americans. Patients who have HbS/HbC disease tend to have a clinical syndrome intermediate in severity between homozygous hemoglobin C disease and homozygous sickle cell anemia. Treatments, when needed, are similar to those for sickle cell anemia.

Hemoglobin E and the HbE thalassemias are discussed in Chapter 143.

Other than HbS, HbC, and HbE, most hemoglobinopathies do not cause clinical abnormalities. Among those that may have some clinical complications are some of the unstable hemoglobin variants, in which the mutant hemoglobin tends to precipitate intracellularly and causes a so-called Heinz body hemolytic anemia. These conditions are covered in the section on "Unstable Hemoglobinopathies" in Chapter 143. Another group of hemoglobinopathies are globin chain mutations that cause increased binding of oxygen by the abnormal hemoglobin, that is, the high-oxygen-affinity hemoglobin variants. These individuals generally have a secondary erythrocytosis as a compensatory response to their relative ineffectiveness in releasing O_2 to tissues. High-oxygen-affinity hemoglobinopathies are best diagnosed by formal study of the patient's oxyhemoglobin dissociation curve and P-50 values, which can be obtained with a commercially available instrument such as the Hemox-Analyzer, which measures in vitro deoxygenation of the sample using nitrogen gas and simultaneously determines oxygen tension with a Clarke electrode. Estimations of the P-50 by blood gas analyzers on venous blood are more convenient but have not been well validated in the screening of hemoglobin variants with high oxygen affinity. Despite their polycythemia, these patients do not have the other diagnostic characteristics of polycythemia vera (Chapter 152).

GENERAL REFERENCES

For the General References and other additional features, please visit Elsevier eBooks+ at https://ebooks.health.elsevier.com.

Grade A References

A1. Estcourt LJ, Kohli R, Hopewell S, et al. Blood transfusion for preventing primary and secondary stroke in people with sickle cell disease. *Cochrane Database Syst Rev.* 2020;7:CD003146.

A2. Ware RE, Davis BR, Schultz WH, et al. Hydroxycarbamide versus chronic transfusion for maintenance of transcranial Doppler flow velocities in children with sickle cell anaemia—TCD with transfusions changing to hydroxyurea (TWiTCH): a multicentre, open-label, phase 3, non-inferiority trial. *Lancet.* 2016;387:661-670.

A3. Tshilolo L, Tomlinson G, Williams TN, et al. Hydroxyurea for children with sickle cell anemia in Sub-Saharan Africa. *N Engl J Med.* 2019;380:121-131.

A4. John CC, Opoka RO, Latham TS, et al. Hydroxyurea dose escalation for sickle cell anemia in sub-Saharan Africa. *N Engl J Med.* 2020;382:2524-2533.

A5. Niihara Y, Miller ST, Kanter J, et al. A phase 3 trial of l-glutamine in sickle cell disease. *N Engl J Med.* 2018;379:226-235.

A6. Ataga KI, Kutlar A, Kanter J, et al. Crizanlizumab for the prevention of pain crises in sickle cell disease. *N Engl J Med.* 2017;376:429-439.

A7. Vichinsky E, Hoppe CC, Ataga KI, et al. A phase 3 randomized trial of voxelotor in sickle cell disease. *N Engl J Med.* 2019;381:509-519.

A8. Rees D, Kilinc Y, Unal S, et al. A randomized placebo-controlled double-blind trial of canakinumab in children and young adults with sickle cell anemia. *Blood.* 2022;139:2642-2652.

150

MEGALOBLASTIC ANEMIAS

SALLY P. STABLER

DEFINITION

Megaloblastic anemia is defined as an anemia or pancytopenia resulting from failure of DNA synthesis and imbalance of maturation between the nucleus and the cellular cytoplasm resulting in large cells subject to maturation arrest and early destruction. Large, macrocytic, red blood cells are also seen in conditions other than megaloblastic anemia (Table 150-1). In practical terms, however, many of the causes of macrocytic red blood cells overlap with those of full-blown megaloblastic anemias. The most frequent causes of severe megaloblastic anemia are deficiencies of cobalamin (vitamin B_{12}) and folate, two vitamins with interrelated roles in the synthesis of thymidine and purines for DNA synthesis[1,2] (Table 150-2).

EPIDEMIOLOGY

Cobalamin Deficiency

Cobalamin is synthesized only by microorganisms, and humans obtain the vitamin through ingestion of animal-source foods because plants do not utilize cobalamin.[3] There are many populations in the world that do not consume adequate cobalamin-containing food due to scarcity and expense of animal-source food or belief systems against the use of such foods. Recommended daily allowances in the United States have been set at 2.4 μg/day, which is readily achieved with an omnivorous diet containing meat, dairy, eggs, fish, or shellfish. Lactovegetarians are at high risk for dietary deficiency,[4] and foods targeted to vegetarian populations in high-resource countries can be supplemented with cobalamin.[5] The fetus and breast-feeding infant obtain cobalamin from the mother, and thus requirements are increased to 2.6 μg for pregnancy and 2.8 μg for lactating women. The breast milk of cobalamin-deficient women has low concentrations of the vitamin and their infants can have severe developmental and growth impairment. An efficient enterohepatic circulation of cobalamin prevents loss of the vitamin so that individuals on deficient or marginal diets will take years to become deficient if the gastrointestinal tract is functioning.[6]

Cobalamin is a trace component of food-bound proteins in the diet, and most causes of severe deficiency relate to the inability to absorb the vitamin. The failure of secretion of gastric intrinsic factor due to an autoimmune disease of the gastric mucosa is known as pernicious anemia and results in life-threatening anemia, pancytopenia, or myeloneuropathy unless treated.[7] Surgery or disease of the stomach, pancreas, or ileum also will cause deficiency.[8] The normal processes of cobalamin absorption are shown in Fig. 150-1.

The incidence of pernicious anemia is reported to range from 1 to 50 per 100,000 persons per year, depending on the criteria used for diagnosis. The prevalence has been described as 50 to 4000 cases per 100,000 persons, again depending on diagnostic criteria. Pernicious anemia becomes more common with age, and the highest prevalence occurs in persons of African or European ancestry with lower incidence and prevalence in East Asians.[9] Mild atrophic gastritis with protein-bound cobalamin malabsorption occurs in up to 20% of older adults, particularly Whites. Dietary cobalamin deficiency is population dependent, but can range from 30 to 50% in areas of South America, Africa, and India.

TABLE 150-1 CAUSES OF MACROCYTOSIS

NONMEGALOBLASTIC DISORDERS
Reticulocytosis
Alcohol abuse/heavy use
Chronic liver disease
Thyroid disorders (hypothyroidism)
Chronic lung disease with hypoxemia
Cold agglutinins and paraproteinemias
Hyperglycemia
Primary bone marrow disorders (e.g., myelodysplasia)
MEGALOBLASTIC ANEMIAS (SEE TABLE 150-2)
Cobalamin (vitamin B_{12}) deficiency
Folate deficiency
Other megaloblastic anemias

Folate Deficiency

In contrast to cobalamin, folates are abundant in foods of plant origin and are also found in dairy and organ meats. Folates are susceptible to loss in cooking, particularly if the cooking water is discarded and not incorporated into the dish. Populations with limited access to or distaste for vegetables, legumes, or fruits may have folate deficiency. Alcohol and some other drugs interfere with folate absorption or promote excretion and are major causes of folate deficiency seen clinically. Folates are absorbed mainly in the upper small

TABLE 150-2 CAUSES OF MEGALOBLASTIC ANEMIA

COBALAMIN (VITAMIN B_{12}) DEFICIENCY
Lack of intrinsic factor
Pernicious anemia (type A gastritis)
Gastrectomy, gastric bypass
Congenital defect in gastric intrinsic factor
Food cobalamin malabsorption
Atrophic gastritis (type B gastritis)
Gastric or achlorhydria
Exocrine pancreatic dysfunction
Disorders of the distal ileum
Surgical resection of distal 1-2 ft.
Inflammatory bowel disease
Surgical reconstruction—ileal conduit or cystoplasty
Congenital defects of cubam receptor (Imerslund-Gräsbeck syndrome)
Usurpation of intestinal cobalamin
Tropical sprue, bacterial overgrowth, blind loops
Parasitic infection—*Diphyllobothrium latum* and *Giardia lamblia*
Nutritional cobalamin deficiency
Breast-fed infant of a deficient mother
Diet lacking animal source food, such as vegan, lacto-ovo vegetarian, or impoverished low-meat diet
Drug-induced cobalamin deficiency
Nitrous oxide abuse or anesthesia in a cobalamin-deficient patient
Metformin, histamine blocking or proton pump inhibitor drugs
Inborn errors of cobalamin metabolism
Transport—transcobalamin deficiency
Cellular metabolism—mutations that cause combined methylmalonic acidemia and homocystinuria (CblC-J)
FOLATE DEFICIENCY
Nutritional folate deficiency
Lack of fresh fruit, green leafy vegetables, legumes, organ meats
Anorexia nervosa and other eating disorders
Alcohol abuse combined with poor nutrition
Folate malabsorption
Celiac or tropical sprue
Crohn disease and other small intestinal diseases
Increased demand or loss
Pregnancy
Hemolytic anemias
Proliferative skin diseases
Leukemias
Hemodialysis
Drug-caused folate deficiency
Antifolates—methotrexate, pemetrexed, pralatrexate, pyrimethamine, sulfasalazine, trimethoprim
Anticonvulsants—phenytoin, carbamazepine, valproic acid
Methylation-requiring drugs—L-Dopa, high-dose niacin, α-lipoic acid
Inborn errors of folate metabolism
MTHFD1 deficiency
PCFT (*SLC46A1*) mutation
MEGALOBLASTIC ANEMIA NOT DUE TO COBALAMIN OR FOLATE DEFICIENCY
Inborn errors
Thiamine responsive megaloblastic anemia (*SLC19A2* mutation)
Hereditary orotic aciduria
Lesch-Nyhan syndrome
Drugs affecting DNA synthesis
Cancer chemotherapy—hydroxyurea, azathioprine, others
Antiretrovirals—zidovudine, stavudine
Tyrosine kinase inhibitors—imatinib, sunitinib, others

CblC-J = cobalamin C, D, E, F, G, and J (defects); MTHFD1 = methylenetetrahydrofolate dehydrogenase 1; PCFT = proton-coupled folate transporter.

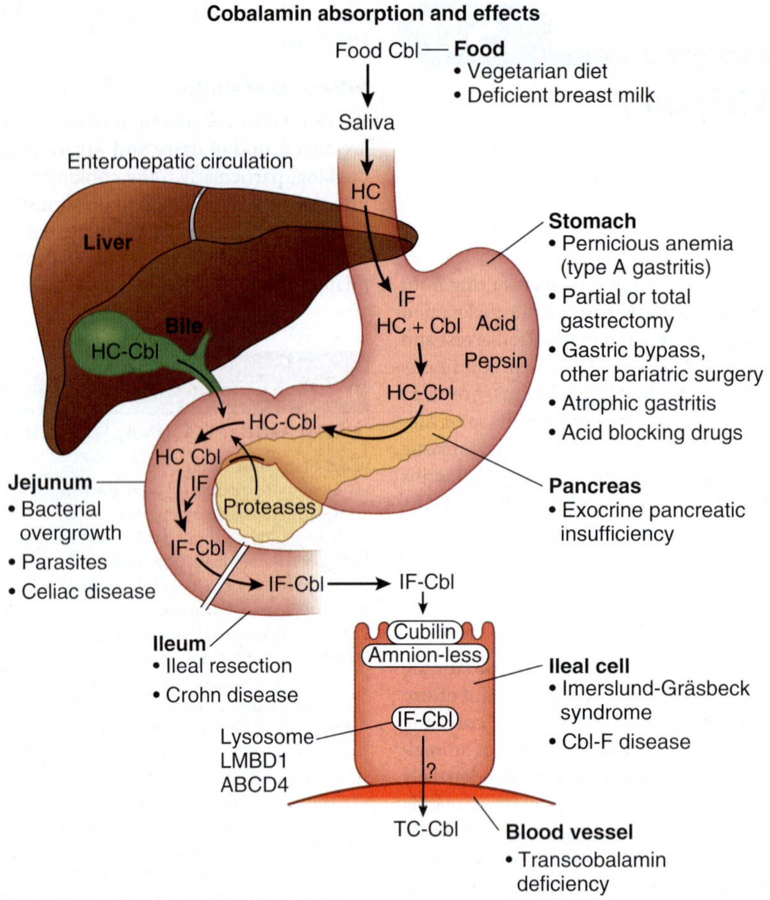

FIGURE 150-1. **The normal processes of cobalamin (Cbl) absorption and associated defects are shown.** ABCD4 = ATP binding cassette subfamily D member 4 (defect); Cbl = cobalamin; Cbl-F = cobalamin F (defect); HC = haptocorrin (also called R-protein or R-factor); IF = intrinsic factor; LMBD1 = probable lysosomal cobalamin transporter (defect); TC = transcobalamin. (Adapted from Stabler SP. Megaloblastic anemias: pernicious anemia and folate deficiency. In: Young NS, Green SL, High KA, eds. *Clinical Hematology*, Philadelphia: Mosby Elsevier; 2006:242-251.)

intestine; thus, diseases such as celiac or tropical sprue, bacterial overgrowth, or inflammatory bowel diseases are complicated by clinical folate deficiency. Many countries including the United States, Canada, Chile, Costa Rica, and South Africa have fortified grain products with folic acid. This has virtually eliminated folate deficiency except in those persons with impaired absorption or high alcohol intake. Countries without fortification may have a significant folate-deficient population depending on customary dietary food patterns which in resource-poor countries provide less than 50% of recommended folate intake.[10,11]

A recommended daily allowance for folate in the United States is 400 µg for adult men and nonpregnant women. The requirement has been increased to 600 µg for pregnant women and 500 µg for lactating women. Food folates are polyglutamated and are less bioavailable than the synthetic folic acid used to fortify food and supplements, which has made estimation of total folate intake more difficult in fortified populations.

PATHOBIOLOGY

Cobalamin

Cobalamin is necessary for only two enzymatic reactions in higher animals. In one reaction methyl-cobalamin is a cofactor for the enzyme methionine synthase, which uses methyl-tetrahydrofolate (methyl-THF) to methylate homocysteine to form methionine. Methionine can be activated to S-adenosylmethionine, which is the methyl donor for many reactions including the important synthesis of creatine, lipids, neurotransmitters, DNA methylation, and many other compounds. The demethylated folate product, THF, is the precursor for the other folate coenzymes. One coenzyme, 5, 10-methyleneTHF, participates in the formation of thymidine from dUMP by thymidylate synthase. Thymidine is critical for DNA synthesis and the accumulation of uracil is harmful; if incorporated into DNA it can cause prolongation of the cell cycle, chromosomal damage, and maturation arrest. Apoptosis may occur due to the impaired DNA repair with cell fragmentation and resulting cell death.

The buildup of methyl-THF, which cannot be converted to THF due to the decrease in methionine synthase activity, is referred to as the "methylfolate trap." This build-up causes a secondary state of folate deficiency in the cobalamin-deficient patient. Methyl-THF is not a good substrate for polyglutamation and therefore it diffuses out of cells and will be lost in the urine. The impairment in methionine synthase activity is the primary cause for the indistinguishable megaloblastic anemia seen with either cobalamin or folate deficiency. When methionine synthase activity is impaired, serum homocysteine levels increase (Chapter 193).

The second cobalamin-dependent reaction uses adenosyl-cobalamin to convert a product of propionic acid metabolism, L-methylmalonyl-CoA, to succinyl-CoA by the enzyme L-methylmalonyl-CoA mutase. When the mutase is blocked by deficiency of adenosyl-cobalamin, the methylmalonyl-CoA is hydrolyzed to methylmalonic acid, a compound with unknown metabolic fate. Elevated methylmalonic acid has been shown to be a sensitive indicator of impaired mutase activity and thus of cobalamin deficiency in many experimental cellular or animal models as well as in human patients.[12] There are no roles for folate metabolism in this pathway.

Cobalamin Absorption

The cobalamin in unfortified food consists of the coenzyme forms bound to the two enzymes. Because there are only trace amounts of cobalamin (average 4 to 6 µg in omnivorous diets) there is a multistep process involving binding proteins and receptors to provide for absorption of the vitamin. The normal processes of absorption are shown in Fig. 150-1 and reviewed elsewhere in detail. Food is mixed with saliva and digested in the stomach where pepsin and gastric acid release cobalamin from the food protein allowing it to bind to haptocorrin (HC), also called R-protein or R-factor, a glycoprotein present in saliva. The HC-cobalamin complex moves to the duodenum where it is joined by HC-cobalamin recycled from bile. Pancreatic proteases with bicarbonate digest the HC releasing cobalamin to be bound by intrinsic factor (IF), which had been secreted by the gastric parietal cells. IF binding is specific for true cobalamin and does not bind the cobalamin analogues found widely in the environment. The IF-cobalamin complex travels to the distal ileum where it is bound by the cubam receptor, a complex of cubilin and amnionless. The IF-cobalamin complex is internalized in lysosomes and two specific exporters (products of the LMBD1 and ABCD4 genes) are required to export it into the cytoplasm. Eventually cobalamin is bound to transcobalamin (TC), which is the physiologic delivery protein. A specific transcobalamin receptor (CD 320) facilitates cellular uptake wherein the TC is degraded by lysosomes and the cobalamin becomes available for intracellular processes. There are many intracellular transporters and enzymes responsible for the eventual appearance of the coenzyme forms of methyl-cobalamin on methionine synthase and adenosyl-cobalamin on L-methylmalonyl-Co-A mutase. The study of congenital defects in these enzymes, which are designated Cbl A-Cbl J, has elucidated much of this complicated metabolism. Some of these disorders are included in Table 150-2.

Cobalamin Transport

About 80% of total cobalamin in blood is bound to HC and only 10 to 20% to the delivery protein, TC. TC is known to be the most important carrier because inborn errors in TC lead to infantile megaloblastic anemia and severe disability. In contrast, deficiencies of HC are moderately common and do not appear to result in disease. HC binds analogues of cobalamin that are abundant in the human colon, foods, and the environment and may have a role in sequestering the analogues to facilitate their excretion. HC is present in white blood cells such as granulocytes. HC-cobalamin is taken up by the asialoglycoprotein receptors in the liver, which may facilitate the removal of analogues by secretion into the bile. There are problems in interpreting total cobalamin values because the cobalamin bound to TC is a small part of the circulating total, as discussed in the section on Diagnosis.

Malabsorption of Cobalamin as a Cause of Deficiency

Pernicious Anemia

Pernicious anemia was recognized many decades before cobalamin was identified because of the histamine-fast achlorhydria found in some patients with fatal progressive macrocytic pancytopenia. It is misnamed because it is a gastric disease, and many patients may not even have anemia. Pernicious anemia is due to a chronic inflammatory attack on the mucosa of the fundus and body of the stomach in which there are inflammatory infiltrates and an immune response to gastric H/K ATPase in the parietal cells. With atrophy of the gastric mucosa there is loss of the gastric parietal cells which produce IF in addition to stomach acid. This type A gastritis takes many years to develop and initially may cause iron deficiency anemia before the lesion is severe enough to result in the loss of IF.

Patients may produce anti-intrinsic factor antibodies, which can also block absorption of cobalamin. The cobalamin secreted into bile is lost in pernicious anemia because there is no IF in the duodenum to bind the cobalamin. Thus, instead of the usual normal loss of about 1 μg of cobalamin per day there may be 5 to 9 μg lost, greatly shortening the time to develop deficiency.

Helicobacter pylori is another cause of chronic gastritis, although it mostly affects the antrum of the stomach (Type B gastritis). Whether *H. pylori* plays a role in the progression of pernicious anemia and cobalamin deficiency is still undefined.

Pernicious anemia is found in association with other autoimmune disorders such as endocrinopathies like autoimmune thyroid disease, type I diabetes mellitus, and vitiligo. Relatives of patients with pernicious anemia may have the full spectrum of autoimmune diseases. The relationship between Graves disease and pernicious anemia is especially strong with about a quarter of the patients having both illnesses. It is important that women with autoimmune thyroid disease have adequate cobalamin status prior to pregnancy and throughout lactation.

Protein-Bound Cobalamin Malabsorption

Less severe forms of gastric atrophy appear in older adults, most frequently in those of European ancestry, wherein a loss of pepsin and gastric acid prevents the total release of cobalamin[13] from protein binding in food. Stomach acid–blocking medications may also impair the absorption of protein-bound cobalamin. The actual risk is uncertain because these medications are used frequently in an aging population that also has age-related gastric atrophy. Patients with gastric atrophy may be identified by serum markers as discussed in the Diagnosis section.

Cobalamin Malabsorption Due to Surgery

Total gastrectomy invariably results in severe cobalamin deficiency due to the loss of IF after 1 to 5 years depending on the underlying status of cobalamin stores. Bariatric surgery such as the Roux-en-Y gastric bypass and sleeve gastrectomy cause the food-cobalamin stream to be separated from the cells secreting IF because the stomach is bypassed. The cubam receptor is present in the distal 1 to 2 feet of ileum, so its loss due to inflammatory bowel disease or the surgical use of distal ileum to create an ileal conduit diversion or ileal cystoplasty causes cobalamin deficiency.

Other Causes of Malabsorption

Exocrine pancreatic dysfunction may cause failure of digestion of HC and release of cobalamin for binding by IF. Bacterial overgrowth as seen in tropical sprue has been shown to cause both cobalamin and folate deficiency. Infestation with a freshwater fish tapeworm, *Diphyllobothrium latum*, is an uncommon cause of usurpation of cobalamin in the duodenum. *Giardia lamblia* is a more common protozoal intestinal infection that may cause decreased cobalamin absorption.

Congenital Malabsorption of Cobalamin

Abnormal gastric IF (GIF) manifests as megaloblastic anemia in infancy or childhood, depending on the underlying cobalamin status at birth. Much more common disorders include mutations in the cubam receptor which have been found in either the cubilin or amnionless protein. This was initially described in Scandinavia and was given the name Imerslund-Gräsbeck disease, but it is particularly common in the Middle East. It is not known whether heterozygotes for these mutations might be more predisposed to nutritionally or atrophic gastritis-induced cobalamin deficiency.

Cobalamin Deficiency Due to Drugs

Many studies have reported on the effects of metformin on cobalamin status. Although it does appear to decrease serum cobalamin levels and may cause malabsorption in the ileum, it is not known whether it can induce full-blown megaloblastic anemia. The anesthetic agent nitrous oxide is a definite cause of cobalamin deficiency, usually manifesting as myeloneuropathy. The gas inactivates methionine-synthase and increases excretion of cobalamin, therefore repeated use induces a severe deficiency. Prolonged continuous use will cause bone marrow aplasia in about 10 days. Persons at risk are often employed in dental or medical offices where nitrous oxide is available or abuse nitrous oxide–containing whipping cream dispensers. There are also reports of a subacute neurologic progression of cobalamin deficiency occurring in patients with unrecognized pernicious anemia after only one episode of nitrous oxide anesthesia, symptoms occurring over days to weeks.[14] Often neurologic damage is permanent despite adequate replacement with cobalamin.

Folate

Folate Metabolism

The role of methyl-THF as a cofactor for methionine synthase was described above. However, there are other folate coenzymes that function as cofactors for many enzymes involved in amino acid metabolism, purine synthesis, methylation reactions, one carbon metabolism, and regulatory functions. Inhibition of these reactions due to folate deficiency can cause decreased cellular growth and proliferation, which is exploited in the use of antifolates for cancer chemotherapy. One cellular form, 5,10-methyleneTHF, is at a branch point to be used by thymidylate synthase to produce the thymidine necessary for DNA synthesis, or is reduced irreversibly by 5,10-methylenetetrahydrofolate reductase (MTHFR) to methyl-THF. As discussed above, methyl-THF must be converted by cobalamin-dependent methionine synthase before the folate can be used in other reactions. A common polymorphism in MTHFR (C677T), known as the thermolabile mutation, renders the enzyme somewhat less efficient and results in higher homocysteine and lower folate levels when folate intake is low. The prevalence of the polymorphism is quite variable, ranging from less than 1% in Africans to 30% in Mediterranean, Mexican, and northern Chinese populations. Its association with risk for various human disorders has been extensively studied but not clearly defined. The polymorphism changes the proportions of folate coenzyme forms, decreasing methyl-THF, and thus circulating folate levels. The increase in homocysteine levels and decrease in folate levels is most apparent in populations on low or marginal folate intakes.

Folate Absorption and Transport

Natural food folates are polyglutamated and must be hydrolyzed by an upper small intestinal brush border enzyme, folylpolyglutamate hydrolase. Folate monoglutamate is transported into the cells by a surface protein–coupled folate transporter (PCFT). Folic acid (nonreduced folate), a stable form, is used in supplements and fortified grains and has a bioavailability of about 90%. Folic acid is reduced to THF and then methylated and released into the plasma. The reduced folate carrier (RFC, solute carrier family, SLC19A1) transports folates into and out of the cell. Absorbed folates in the portal circulation are taken up in the liver, polyglutamated, and retained or released into the circulation or bile. Circulating folates are bound to proteins, particularly albumin. Red blood cells accumulate folates during erythropoiesis, and thus the red cell folate level may more constantly reflect long-term folate status than serum folate. Concentrations of folates in CSF are three-fold higher than in blood, and the choroid plexus has abundant receptors for uptake and transport.

Causes of Nutritional Folate Deficiency

Nutritional folate deficiency occurs in the areas of the world that do not currently have folate food fortification. The foods containing the highest amount of naturally occurring folate are dark green leafy vegetables, beans and other legumes, nuts, orange juice, and liver or other organ meats. Potatoes, many fruits, and eggs have moderate amounts of folate but dairy items and muscle meat are much lower in folate. In high-resource countries, cereals, snack bars, sport drinks, and other foods promoted for health and exercise are often fortified with folic acid. Natural food folate intake has been estimated to be roughly 200 μg/day with an extra 200 μg in nonsupplement users from the added folic acid in fortified grains in persons in the United States. Total folate in supplement users was much higher, between 700 to 1000 μg per day. Low serum folate was found in approximately 15% in surveys of the U.S. population prior to the food folate fortification program. Nutritional folate deficiency is common in areas of the world with limited opportunity for consumption of fresh vegetable foods and is particularly a problem for women of childbearing age who require increased quantities to prevent folate deficiency–associated pregnancy complications. Folate-deficient diets are often deficient in other nutrients such as vitamin C, iron, and other vitamins and minerals.

Malabsorption of Folate

The serum folate level decreases within 3 weeks of severe folate malnutrition or malabsorption and megaloblastic bone marrow changes occur after 15 to 20 weeks. Folate malabsorption occurs in diseases of the upper small intestine and is rarely seen after gastrectomy or with Roux-en-Y gastric bypass. Celiac disease, which causes villous atrophy of the small intestine, causes folate deficiency in up to half of the patients. Tropical sprue, a cause of chronic diarrhea and progressive small intestinal villous atrophy, also causes folate deficiency with or without cobalamin deficiency. Inflammatory bowel disease, particularly Crohn disease, causes folate deficiency in addition to iron and vitamin B_{12} deficiency.

Conditions with Increased Folate Requirements

Diseases in which there is increased cellular proliferation may result in folate depletion. This includes skin diseases such as psoriasis and chronic hemolytic anemias, particularly sickle cell disease. Folates and other water-soluble vitamins are lost during renal hemodialysis.

Alcohol and Folate Deficiency

Alcohol abuse is the most common cause of folate deficiency manifesting megaloblastic anemia. Even well-nourished alcoholics may have macrocytosis and elevated homocysteine values, often when serum folate and hemoglobin are still normal. Alcohol-induced impairment of folate metabolism is exacerbated by poor nutrition. Megaloblastic anemia due to alcohol-associated folate deficiency still occurs despite the food folate fortification program in the United States. Folate-deficient alcoholics have been shown to have impaired intestinal absorption of folate, oxidative destruction of folates, impaired hepatic uptake, reduced storage, and enhanced renal excretion. Effects on the enzymes of methionine metabolism, particularly methionine synthase, are likely due to the toxic metabolites of ethanol. It may be difficult to recognize megaloblastic anemia in alcoholics because their frequently coexisting iron deficiency due to gastrointestinal bleeding may mask macrocytosis. In addition, alcohol induces sideroblastic anemia, an iron utilization defect, which can also mask macrocytosis. Nonalcohol related causes of cirrhosis can cause macrocytosis due to membrane abnormalities in the red cells, even with adequate folates.

Drugs That Cause Folate Deficiency

There are many drugs that interfere with folate metabolism (Table 150-2). The anticonvulsants, particularly carbamazepine, phenytoin, valproate, and phenobarbital have all been shown to cause macrocytosis, folate depletion, and hyperhomocysteinemia. Folic acid supplements improve folate status without preventing the antiseizure efficacy. There are many antifolates in common use, being exploited for their inhibitory effect on cellular proliferation such as methotrexate, pemetrexed, and pralatrexate used in cancer chemotherapy and in rheumatic diseases. It is interesting that the beneficial effect of methotrexate in rheumatoid arthritis is not counteracted by providing supplemental folic acid. Some antibiotics such as trimethoprim, pyrimethamine, and some sulfa derivatives are antifolates. Sulfasalazine used for inflammatory bowel disease will also cause folate depletion. Functional folate deficiency can be induced by drugs that require methylation for metabolism by depleting the normal stores of methyl groups. Drugs such as L-dopa, high-dose niacin, and an over-the-counter agent, α-lipoic acid, all raise homocysteine.

Inborn Errors of Folate Metabolism

There are two inborn errors of folate that present as megaloblastic anemia: methylenetetrahydrofolate dehydrogenase deficiency (MTHFD1) and hereditary folate malabsorption due to mutations in the protein-coupled folate transporter (PCFT). MTHFD1 deficiency has been found in six infants and children with megaloblastic anemia, immunodeficiency, or inflammatory conditions and hyperhomocysteinemia. Treatment with high doses of folic acid or folinic acid were beneficial in several of the patients. It is not yet known whether this disorder will be found in adult medicine.

Severe deficiencies of MTHFR (not the common thermolabile polymorphism) cause hyperhomocysteinemia with low methionine, but **not** megaloblastic anemia. These patients may present with thrombotic complications of hyperhomocysteinemia (Chapter 67) and neurologic deficits (Chapter 384). Treatment with betaine and folic acid greatly improves the prognosis.

CLINICAL MANIFESTATIONS

Definition of Macrocytosis

The best definition of macrocytosis is red blood cell mean cell volume (MCV) that is higher than the expected value for any individual patient. Clinicians who rely on laboratory reported ranges such as 80 to 100 fL will make errors in diagnosis because the MCV is affected by ethnicity and age. For instance, 30% of persons with African ancestry in the United States have one deleted α hemoglobin subunit and their median MCV is about 84 fL. It would take much longer for these individuals to increase the MCV to greater than 100 fL than someone whose normal MCV was 92 fL. Persons with β-thalassemia trait, hemoglobin E, and iron deficiency will also not usually have an increase in MCV to more than 100 fL despite the coexistence of severe megaloblastic anemia. Individuals with a combination of microcytic red cell indices and megaloblastosis may have oval macrocytes visible on the peripheral blood smear and a high red cell distribution width (RDW).

The causes of macrocytosis are shown in Table 150-1. As indicated, macrocytosis is not equivalent to megaloblastosis: there are many causes of macrocytic peripheral red blood cell indices that are not associated with a megaloblastic state. Reticulocytes, newly released red cells that are less than 24 hours old, are at their largest size and decrease as they age over 120 days in the circulation. Thus, reticulocytosis will increase the MCV, in many cases to over 100 fL. A rise in MCV may be the first sign of autoimmune hemolytic anemia and is also commonly found in patients with fragmentation anemia, sickle cell anemia, or with hemolysis due to infectious agents. Macrocytosis can be seen in patients who are post-splenectomy or have liver disease of any type, especially with associated alcoholism. Severe portal hypertension causes macrocytosis with thrombocytopenia and leukopenia mimicking a true megaloblastic anemia when examining only the peripheral blood smear. Chronic lung disease, particularly with associated hypoxia-induced polycythemia, is frequently macrocytic. Hypothyroidism and severe hyperglycemia also cause macrocytosis. The primary bone marrow disorders such as aplastic anemia, pure red cell aplasia, myelodysplastic syndrome, idiopathic myelofibrosis, and multiple myeloma may cause striking macrocytosis, with or without associated cytopenias. Cold agglutinins and paraproteinemias cause red cell clumping, which may lead to rouleau formation that can cause an erroneously high MCV. Drugs with effects on DNA synthesis, such as antiretrovirals, chemotherapy agents, and antifolates, cause macrocytosis.

Complications of Megaloblastic Anemias

Examples of peripheral blood smears and bone marrow aspirate and biopsy in megaloblastic anemia are shown in Fig. 150-2A-D (also see Chapter 143). The hallmark of megaloblastic pathology in the marrow is that cells are large ("megalo") and their nuclei have not matured ("blastic"); thus there are oval macrocytes and occasionally even a megaloblastic nucleated red blood cell detected on the peripheral blood smear. Other red blood cells are misshapen and fragmented and can be mistaken for schistocytes as seen in fragmentation anemias. There may be thrombocytopenia and leukopenia when

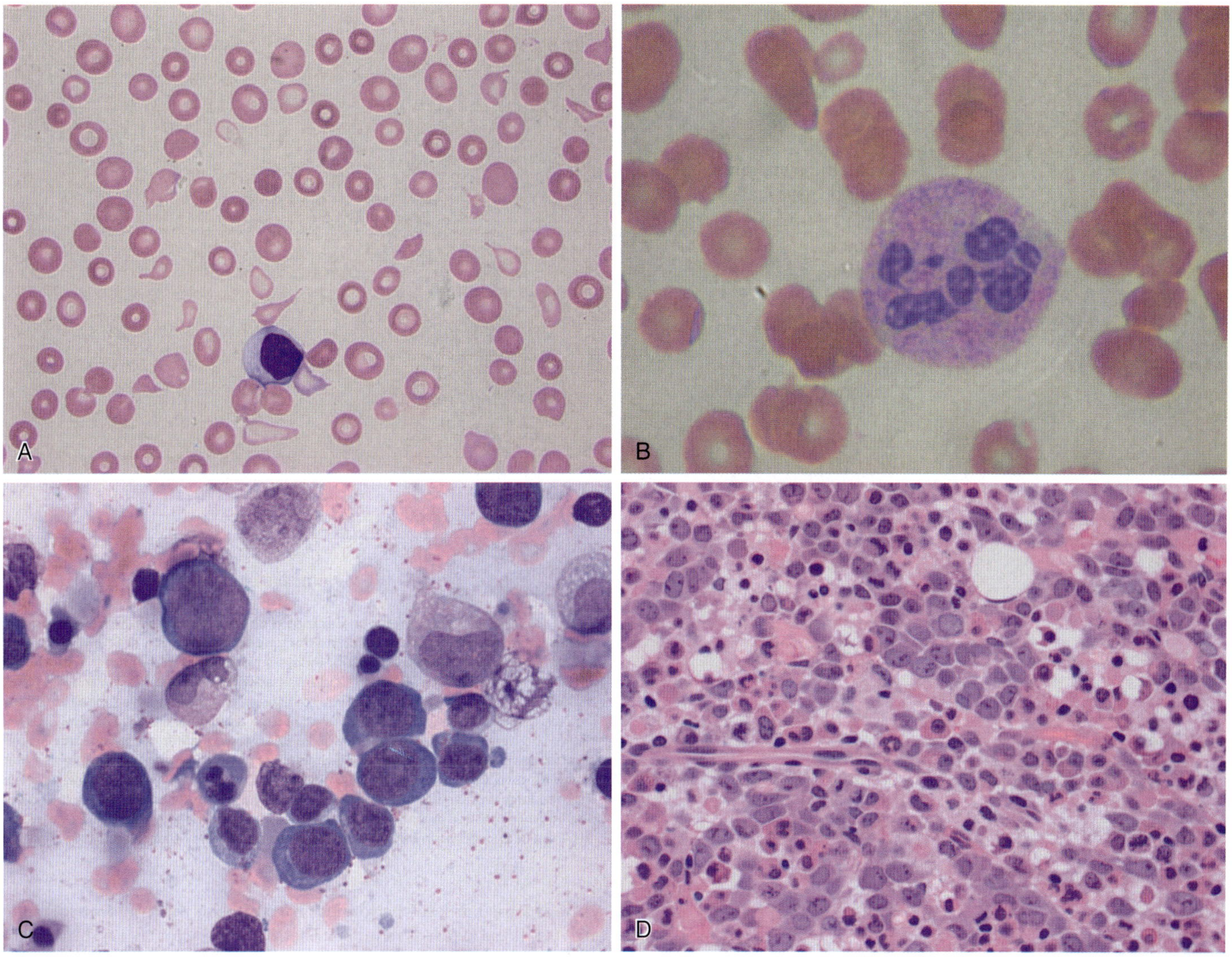

FIGURE 150-2. **Photomicrographs of peripheral smear, bone marrow aspirate, and biopsy are shown. A,** Oval macrocytes and fragmented red blood cells are present in a smear from a patient with severe cobalamin deficiency and thalassemia trait, demonstrating an extreme range in size and shape of the red blood cells. **B,** Hypersegmented neutrophil. **C,** A group of megaloblastic red cell precursors all with an open lacy chromatin pattern is shown from a bone marrow aspirate. Red cell dysplasia and giant metamyelocytes are also present. **D,** The bone marrow biopsy shows hypercellularity with a predominance of large erythroblasts and many mitotic figures, all potentially confused with acute leukemia. The erythroid hyperplasia in the bone marrow of a patient with megaloblastic anemia is due to "ineffective erythropoiesis." (Photomicrographs: 2B courtesy of John W. Ryder, MD, Department of Pathology, University of Colorado School of Medicine; 2 A, C, and D courtesy of Zenggang Pan, MD, PhD, Department of Pathology, University of Colorado School of Medicine.)

anemia becomes severe. Hypersegmented granulocytes are present. The presence of one 6-lobed or five 5-lobed granulocytes per 100 cells is considered abnormal. Some red blood cells may show basophilic stippling. A megaloblastic blood smear with oval macrocytes and fragmented red blood cells with thrombocytopenia has frequently been mistaken for microangiopathic hemolytic anemia such as thrombotic thrombocytopenia, as documented by case reports. Reticulocytopenia in megaloblastic anemias differentiates these microangiopathic-appearing red cells in the peripheral smear from hemolytic anemias. The bone marrow biopsy and aspirate smear is hypercellular with a decreased myeloid : erythroid ratio. There is delayed maturation of erythroblasts, which to the inexperienced observer may even suggest a diagnosis of acute leukemia because they are large cells with open chromatin and blue cytoplasm. The normal process of shrinking and condensing of the nucleus during erythropoiesis is impaired so that the chromatin pattern remains open and lacy (i.e., "megaloblastic"). Although nuclear maturation is delayed, cytoplasmic maturation (e.g., hemoglobinization of the cytoplasm) proceeds unimpaired, leading to the morphologic phenomenon of "nuclear cytoplasmic dissociation." These red cell precursors have poor survival within the bone marrow and pathologic abnormalities suggestive of cellular dysplasia with nuclear fragments in the red cells are present. The cellular apoptosis causes intramedullary hemolysis or "ineffective erythropoiesis." Maturation of white cell precursors is delayed, producing giant metamyelocytes and bands. Flow cytometry of the bone marrow demonstrates left shifts in erythroblasts and white cell precursors which again could lead the unwary to diagnose acute leukemia. Cytogenetic studies may show chromosomal fragmentation and in some cases even clonal abnormalities which correct with vitamin replacement and resolution of megaloblastic anemia.

Intramedullary hemolysis causes indirect hyperbilirubinemia, low serum haptoglobin, and sometimes extreme values for lactate dehydrogenase. The presence of markers of hemolysis and fragmented cells on a peripheral blood smear accompanied by a normal instead of low reticulocyte count can mimic hemolytic anemia. Furthermore, defects of cobalamin metabolism, such as a cobalamin-C mutation, can present with the hemolytic-uremic syndrome.

Other tissues that have rapid cellular turnover may become likewise megaloblastic. This abnormality is particularly common in the gastrointestinal tract, where it sometimes causes malabsorption. Cells of the uterine cervix can become megaloblastic and appear dysplastic. Impairment of spermatogenesis can cause infertility. Atrophy and glossitis of the tongue mucosa may occur. Some individuals may have areas of skin hyperpigmentation.

Neurologic Abnormalities Due to Cobalamin Deficiency

Cobalamin is necessary for the development and initial myelination and maintenance of the spinal cord and brain. Demyelination can be demonstrated on imaging in both brain and spinal cord as depicted schematically in Fig. 150-3. Cobalamin-deficient infants may have delay or failure in normal myelination which occurs during the first year of life. The demyelinating lesion, often termed "subacute combined degeneration," begins with symptoms of symmetric paresthesia, usually in the lower extremities but sometimes involving

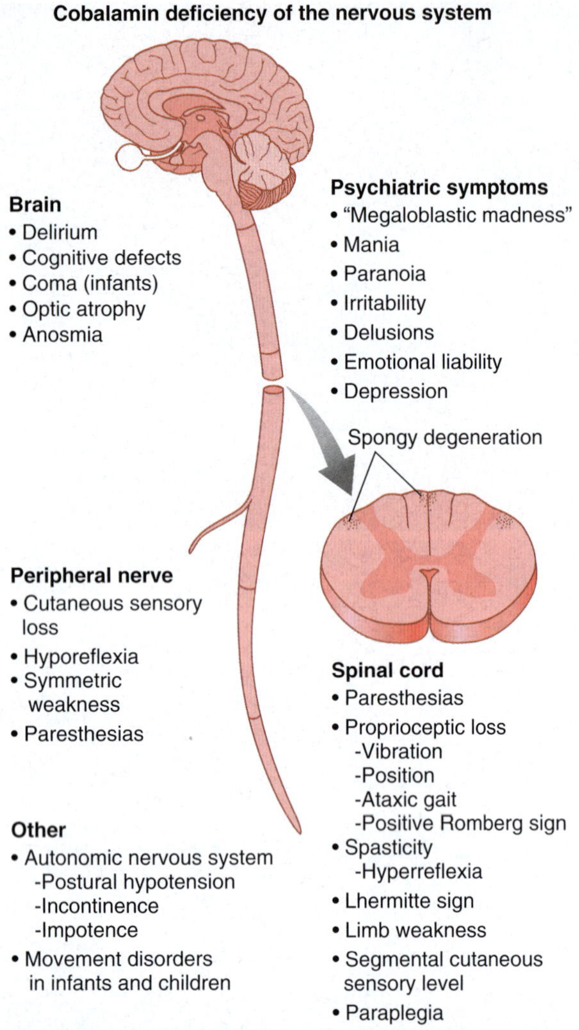

FIGURE 150-3. The myriad symptoms and signs of cobalamin deficiency of the nervous system are shown. These range from paresthesias without objective signs to severe motor loss, even quadriplegia. The spongy degeneration shown in the cross-section depiction of the spinal cord may be seen on magnetic resonance imaging as increased signal intensity on T2 weighted images often described as an inverted "V" sign. Also see Chapter 388. (Adapted from Stabler SP. Megaloblastic anemias: pernicious anemia and folate deficiency. In: Young NS, Green SL, High KA, eds. *Clinical Hematology*, Philadelphia: Mosby Elsevier; 2006:242-251.)

the hands first. There is early impairment of proprioception ending with loss of vibration and position sense manifesting as ataxic gait. Other common signs and symptoms are shown in Fig. 150-3. As the severity of the spinal lesions increases weakness develops, with spasticity and hyperreflexia, and eventually patients may develop a segmental cutaneous sensory level and even paraplegia. Altered mental status occasionally occurs particularly with irritability, delusions, paranoia, lability, even mania called "megaloblastic madness" in the past.

The underlying biochemical lesions causing the neurologic disease are still unknown, although changes in lipids, growth factors, cytokines, or methylation status of proteins have all been studied. There is a strong inverse relationship between the severity of the neurologic abnormalities and the hematologic abnormalities. Therefore, the coexistence of anemia is helpful in a patient with a compatible neurologic disorder in suggesting cobalamin deficiency but is not required. Patients with a normal hemoglobin level and a neurologic presentation have similar metabolic abnormalities as do patients with anemia (Fig. 150-4). There is also an inverse relationship between the duration of neurologic abnormalities prior to diagnosis and the completeness of correction after adequate cobalamin replacement, so early diagnosis is imperative (see Chapter 384).

DIAGNOSIS

Cobalamin and Folate Biochemical Assays

Measurement of the serum cobalamin or folate level has been a time-honored method of screening. Original tests have been replaced today with automated

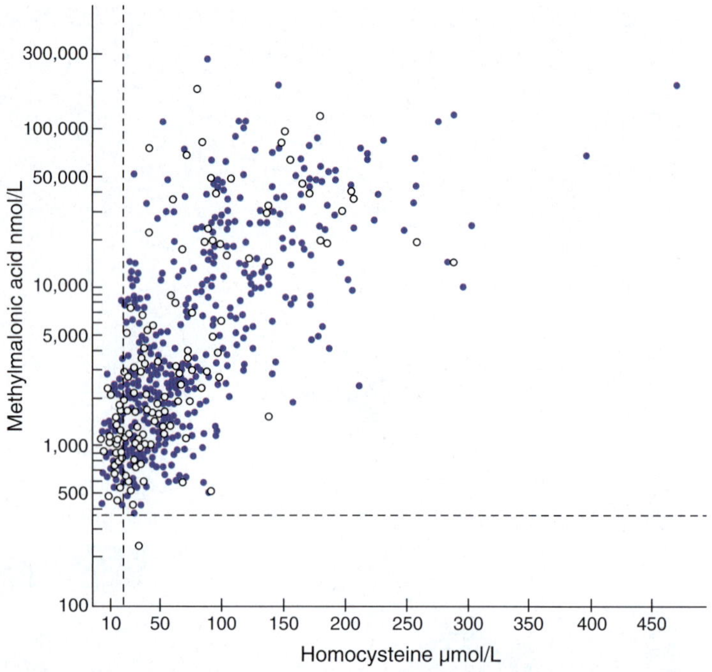

FIGURE 150-4. Serum methylmalonic acid plotted against serum homocysteine in patients with clinically ascertained and documented cobalamin deficiency. The serum methylmalonic acid plotted against homocysteine in about 500 patients with clinically ascertained cobalamin deficiency. Patients had either megaloblastic anemia (closed circles), which in most cases was proven to respond to cobalamin treatment, or a neurologic syndrome compatible with that found in cobalamin deficiency. Those shown as open circles had hematocrit values over 38%. Values were equal for methylmalonic acid and homocysteine whether the patients had anemia or mainly neurologic abnormalities. Methylmalonic acid was greater than 1000 nmol/L in 90% of these clinically proven patients. Hatched lines represent methylmalonic acid 376 nmol/L and homocysteine 21.3 µmol/L. (Previously published in Stabler S. Vitamin B12. In: Erdman, Jr. JW, McDonald IA, Zeisel SH, eds. *Present Knowledge in Nutrition*. 10th ed. Ames, IA: Wiley-Blackwell; 2012.)

assays of cobalamin levels performed on instruments with platforms for multiple analytes. These methods rely on purified intrinsic factor (IF) as the cobalamin binder, often using chemiluminescent microparticle immunoassays for detection. It has been reported that denaturation of anti-IF antibodies present in samples from patients with pernicious anemia can be incomplete, and thus normal to even high values of cobalamin are reported falsely. In general, the values reported from these automated methods are higher than with the historical assays, which complicates comparison of reference ranges. Extremely low values of serum cobalamin (<70 pg/mL) usually reflect deficiency associated with clinical abnormalities that will improve with treatment, but such patients are rare. There is a large equivocal range (100 to 300 pg/mL) in which further testing with metabolites is needed to distinguish between false-positive low and true-positive low or low normal values.

A low serum folate (<3 ng/mL) is clinically significant when found in food folate fortified countries such as the United States. Most authorities have, however, raised the lower limit of the reference range to 5 to 6 ng/mL, values that overlap with the median in populations without fortification. Red blood cell folate should be a good marker of longer-term folate status but the methodology of measuring folate in the presence of the red cell protein matrix has led to poor reproducibility, and the assay cannot be recommended for routine clinical use outside of research investigations.

An assay of the amount of cobalamin bound to transcobalamin, holo-transcobalamin (Holo-TC or "active B_{12}"), is available in Europe and Canada but not yet FDA-approved in the United States. Anti-intrinsic factor antibodies, which are present in pernicious anemia, do not affect this assay, but a polymorphism in the TC gene prevents measurement using this method. Holo-TC increases after oral intake of a large amount of cobalamin and thus is being developed as a test for absorption.

Methylmalonic Acid and Homocysteine Markers of Deficiency

Excess methylmalonic acid is produced when L-methylmalonyl-Co-A mutase is blocked by cobalamin deficiency. Therefore, elevated serum or urine methylmalonic acid has been proven to be a very sensitive indicator of cobalamin status. Patients who have low cobalamin values but normal serum methylmalonic acid do not respond to treatment and have false-positive low cobalamin levels. The methylmalonic acid value is the first test to become abnormal in infrequently treated patients with proven pernicious anemia. The methylmalonic value decreases immediately after treatment, normalizing within days to weeks. Thus, methylmalonic acid must be assayed prior to treatment. A common clinical error is to treat a patient who likely has a false-positive low cobalamin level and when anemia or the clinical symptoms do not respond, to proceed with assaying methylmalonic acid. After treatment, serum methylmalonic acid normalizes or decreases into the high normal range in seniors (<400 nmol/L) and others with mild renal insufficiency.

Methylmalonic acid values increase above the reference range in renal insufficiency but are usually less than 1000 nmol/L even in patients on renal dialysis. A related metabolite, 2-methylcitric acid, is measured with methylmalonic acid by some commercial testing laboratories and, if higher than the simultaneous methylmalonic acid value, will diagnose renal insufficiency rather than vitamin deficiency. Methylmalonic acid is a product of propionic acid metabolism; thus gut bacterial overgrowth can cause higher values sometimes responsive to antibiotics. A polymorphism in HIBCH, an enzyme in valine catabolism, may cause a mild increase in methylmalonic acid.

Patients with severe inborn errors of cobalamin metabolism rarely normalize methylmalonic acid, even with very intensive parenteral treatment. Such individuals are occasionally detected in adult medicine practices and should be referred to a metabolic center.

Homocysteine

Homocysteine levels increase when either cobalamin or folate deficiency impairs the activity of methionine synthase and cannot be used to distinguish between cobalamin or folate deficiency, because serum homocysteine levels are elevated in 95% of clinically proven folate-deficient individuals. When patients with elevated serum homocysteine levels are treated with the wrong vitamin, the homocysteine level does not decrease. Elevated homocysteine responds to treatment with the correct vitamin very rapidly, often within hours; thus, as in the case of methylmalonic acid, it must be measured prior to any treatment. Even nutritious hospital food may correct elevated homocysteine. Adding vitamins to intravenous fluids for suspected alcoholic patients in the emergency department will correct serum folate levels, and if homocysteine is not assayed rapidly it too will have fallen, yet the patient will still have unexplained megaloblastic anemia. There is a strong relationship between folate intake and homocysteine values in populations that are cobalamin replete. U.S. population serum homocysteine values fell by several μmol/L after folate food fortification. Renal failure increases homocysteine by unclear mechanisms because homocysteine is not dependent on urinary clearance, although the kidney is rich in homocysteine-metabolizing enzymes. Homocysteine can be elevated in hypothyroidism, severe pyridoxine deficiency, and in the presence of antifolate drugs.

If cobalamin is measured because of vague complaints of fatigue and nonspecific neurologic or psychiatric symptoms, most values lower than 200 pg/mL will be false-positive low. The sensitivity of a low cobalamin value (<200 pg/mL) is about 60%.

The sensitivity of a serum methylmalonic acid value higher than 400 nmol/L is about 98% for clinical deficiency, but its specificity for clinical abnormalities is much less because serum methylmalonic acid rises quickly in response to cobalamin depletion. It may be mildly abnormal in patients with other causes of anemia or neurologic syndromes, as seen frequently in seniors or vegetarians. Patients with modest elevations of methylmalonic acid (<700 nmol/L) may not have any clinical syndrome attributable to cobalamin deficiency.

Diagnosis of Pernicious Anemia

Blocking anti-intrinsic factor antibodies are found in 50 to 70% of patients. Anti–parietal cell antibodies are found in a higher percentage (90%) but are less specific because they are found in other autoimmune diseases and forms of gastritis. Demonstration of histamine-fast achlorhydria is rarely performed but is very specific for pernicious anemia. The gastric antrum is spared in pernicious anemia, and the gastrin-producing cells may become hyperplastic. Elevated fasting serum gastrin is suggestive of pernicious anemia. Another marker of the gastric mucosa is pepsinogen-1, which is low in pernicious anemia. These markers, however, are affected by the widespread use of proton pump inhibitor medications. At least a week after a cobalamin injection should elapse before testing for anti-intrinsic factor antibodies.

Endoscopy with gastric biopsy is the best method of diagnosing atrophic gastritis, and some experts recommend that patients with pernicious anemia have at least one screening endoscopy because they are at greater risk for carcinoid tumors and adenocarcinoma of the stomach. This approach would be mandatory for patients who have symptoms consistent with gastric neoplasm or coexisting iron deficiency.

A radio-labeled cobalamin absorption test known as the Schilling test is no longer available. A test using the increase in holo-TC values after three doses of unlabeled oral cobalamin is being investigated and may prove to be a good substitute.

Folate Malabsorption

There are no specific tests for folate malabsorption. The presence of a disease of the upper small intestine such as celiac disease, tropical sprue, or Crohn disease will point to folate malabsorption. Folate deficiency is often associated with iron and multiple other nutrient deficiencies in contrast to cobalamin deficiency due to pernicious anemia.

TREATMENT

Cobalamin Deficiency

The primary goals of treatment of cobalamin deficiency are to restore the normal tissue content of cobalamin (between 2 to 5 mg in an adult human) and prevent relapse. Parenteral administration of either cyano- or hydroxy-cobalamin is rapidly effective. Common treatment regimens in severely symptomatic patients would be daily intramuscular or subcutaneous injection of 1 mg (1000 μg) for 7 days or every other day for 2 weeks, followed by weekly injections for 8 weeks, then monthly. Less symptomatic patients could be loaded with biweekly or weekly doses for 8 weeks followed by monthly administration. Hydroxy-cobalamin is retained better than cyano-cobalamin and after loading can be given at 2- to 4-month intervals instead of monthly. About 150 μg is retained after an injection of 1 mg, which is why it is necessary to provide multiple injections during the loading treatment phase to achieve the replacement of 2 to 5 mg. However, a single 10,000 μg dose can correct pernicious anemia for at least 3 months.[15] Methylmalonic acid remains elevated in about 20% of pernicious anemia patients injected monthly with cyano-cobalamin, which will normalize with a shorter time interval between injections. There is no toxicity upper limit for cobalamin, and patients may claim that their well-being is enhanced by injections as frequent as every 2 to 3 weeks.

A small percentage (0.5 to 2%) of a high dose of oral cobalamin is absorbed by mass action in the upper intestinal tract without IF or an intact ileum. Randomized trials comparing parenteral and high oral doses (1000 to 2000 μg/day) have shown equivalent clinical correction, rise in serum cobalamin, and normalization of elevated methylmalonic[A1,A2] acid and homocysteine levels.[16] Patients with severe abnormalities should receive at least 2000 μg/day initially, so they absorb 20 to 40 μg/day. High-dose cobalamin tablets containing 500 μg to 2.5 mg dosages are available without prescription in the United States. Physician error is one of the leading causes of discontinuation of treatment in pernicious anemia. Patients should be taught to start self-directed treatment with high-dose oral tablets if denied medical follow-up for cobalamin deficiency. High-dose preparations may be less available in other parts of the world. There are also preparations designed for intranasal or sublingual use, which have been less studied in patients with true pernicious anemia. Patients and providers may have preferences as to cost, convenience, compliance, and comfort relating to injected versus oral treatment.[17]

The alternative cobalamin forms methyl- and adenosyl-cobalamin are also available for replacement but are unstable, converting to the aquo(hydroxy) form on exposure to light. There is no advantage in using these expensive alternatives because they will undergo the same metabolic conversions as does cyano- or hydroxyl-cobalamin. Treatment of neuropathic pain with methyl-cobalamin may be an exception.[18]

Treatment of Dietary Deficiency

Patients with dietary deficiency should be loaded with high dose oral or parenteral cobalamin to replete tissue stores (2 to 5 mg). This is crucial for vegetarian women contemplating pregnancy, especially from countries with high prevalence of cobalamin deficiency. The amount of cobalamin in maternal vitamins is too low to replete stores quickly; IF-mediated absorption is limited to 2 to 5 μg per day, so it would take an entire pregnancy to replace 1 to 2 mg, and the infant could be born deficient. The breast-feeding mother should also be loaded to normal stores because her breast milk will be deficient if only small supplements are used. The cobalamin-replete vegetarian can supplement smaller quantities such as in multivitamin tablets (i.e., 3 to 9 μg/day). Persons who avoid animal-source foods are often also deficient in iron and many other vitamins. There is a large literature on methods to improve growth and development of children in resource-poor countries with combinations of protein, iron, folic acid, cobalamin, and other nutrients.

Recommendations for Treatment of Seniors

The incidence of both true pernicious anemia and atrophic gastritis increase with age. The high usage of metformin and stomach acid–blocking drugs is also more prevalent with age, which compounds the potential malabsorption of cobalamin. Elevated methylmalonic acid, which corrects with cobalamin treatment, is very prevalent (up to 40%) in studies of the oldest old. Theoretically, smaller doses of cobalamin should be effective in patients who still have some residual IF, but studies in seniors have shown that at least 500 μg/day is necessary to correct most individuals with elevated methylmalonic acid. The Food and Nutrition Board recommended that seniors take an unspecified dose of cobalamin daily. It seems prudent to recommend a supplement of at least 1000 μg/day for individuals at risk for malabsorption. Many clinical trials of cobalamin and folate replacement in correcting diseases of aging such as cognitive impairment[A3,19,20] or osteoporosis have been disappointing. A possible exception is a trial of cobalamin in improving nerve conduction in seniors.

Treatment of Folate Deficiency

Because either cobalamin or folate deficiency causes megaloblastic anemia and elevated homocysteine levels, it is important to distinguish which vitamin is deficient or to treat potential deficiency of both. If serum methylmalonic acid is elevated then there is at least cobalamin deficiency (Table 150-3). This consideration is particularly important in countries with food folate fortification where almost all elevated homocysteine is due to cobalamin deficiency and not folate deficiency. Pharmacologic doses of folic acid (i.e., 1 mg daily) can partially correct megaloblastic anemia in cobalamin-deficient anemia, which has been termed "masking of pernicious anemia." Unfortunately, if neurologic lesions are present they will continue to progress and may become irreversible if a cobalamin-deficient patient is treated with only folate. Over-the-counter folic acid supplements are topped at 800 μg in the United States to prevent inadvertent use by patients with pernicious anemia. Prescription doses of 1 to 5 mg daily of oral folic acid are acceptable treatments for replacement. Patients who have ongoing alcoholism, gut malabsorption, hemolytic anemia, or other unknown pathology should remain on replacement indefinitely. Folic acid 1 mg daily can also be given to patients taking methotrexate for rheumatologic disease, or to patients taking niacin or L-dopa to prevent hyperhomocysteinemia. Pretreatment with folic acid and cobalamin is used with the multitargeted antifolate chemotherapy agents. There is no advantage to treating with methyl-THF over folic acid.

Treatment of Hyperhomocysteinemia

Severe hyperhomocysteinemia (homocysteine >50 μmol/L) is a prothrombotic condition whether due to classical homocystinuria, other inborn errors of metabolism, or vitamin deficiency (Chapter 193). There are many case reports of thrombosis as the presenting complaint in pernicious anemia. The association of hyperhomocysteinemia with vascular disease and thrombosis prompted many large trials of folic acid or combination B vitamin (high-dose cobalamin, vitamin B_6, plus folate) therapy in vascular disease, but the trials have not been successful or have been even harmful,[A4] except for a decrease the incidence of stroke in folate-deficient populations.[21] For example, a randomized trial of antihypertensive medication with or without folic acid, 800 μg daily, in China demonstrated a hazard ratio of 0.79 for decreased risk of stroke,[A5] and a trial of high-dose combination cobalamin, folic acid, and vitamin B_6 in high-altitude soldiers in India decreased thrombotic events by 54%.[A6] Beneficial effects of folic acid or combination B vitamin treatment are easier to prove in populations that are not already eating folate fortified food. Trials in patients with renal failure, especially on dialysis, have not shown benefit in homocysteine lowering and perhaps harm in diabetic kidney disease.

Any patient with extreme hyperhomocysteinemia (>100 μmol/L) should be investigated thoroughly with assay of methylmalonic acid and methionine and a documented response to treatment after replacement. Patients with milder types of pyridoxine-responsive classic homocystinuria may present in adulthood with thrombotic disease, although not with megaloblastic anemia. All patients with nonresponsive hyperhomocysteinemia should be referred to a metabolic center.

TABLE 150-3 USING METABOLITES TO DIAGNOSE COBALAMIN AND FOLATE DEFICIENCY

If methylmalonic acid is elevated >400 nmol/L, consider cobalamin deficiency
If homocysteine is elevated >14 μmol/L, then consider either cobalamin or folate or both deficiencies
Pretreatment metabolite testing will distinguish between true-positive and false-positive low cobalamin values
Metabolite testing is prudent in severe anemia/pancytopenia or demyelinating central nervous system disease regardless of vitamin levels

PREVENTION

Severe consequences of cobalamin deficiency can be prevented by investigating those patients at highest risk, which includes patients with autoimmune thyroid disease, vitiligo, history of gastrointestinal surgery, and family histories of pernicious anemia and autoimmunity. The tragedy of the cobalamin-deficient breast-fed infant should be completely avoidable if attention is paid to the prepregnancy cobalamin status of women who are at risk for deficiency especially with Graves or other autoimmune thyroid disease, vitiligo, status post bariatric or other gastrointestinal surgery, inflammatory bowel disease, and those who avoid animal-source foods. Women who limit animal-source food and immigrants from countries with known cobalamin deficiency should be proven to be cobalamin replete prior to pregnancy. Newborn screening programs using tandem mass spectrometry have revealed that there are as many infants with nutritional cobalamin deficiency as with the inborn errors of cobalamin metabolism. It is possible that prompt treatment of these infants will prevent the worst of the growth failure and neurodevelopmental abnormalities seen when they are discovered later.[22]

The widespread cobalamin and other micronutrient deficiencies in resource-poor areas of the world and in populations who shun animal-source foods is a difficult problem. Increasing meat, dairy, and other animal foods is an expensive approach for populations eating mostly plant-based proteins. Some fermented plant foods such as enset, tempeh, and algae derivatives do contain cobalamin although the concentrations are likely variable. Innovative approaches such as supplementing toothpaste have been tested and could potentially be useful.[A7] Another approach such as fortifying tea bags in India with both cobalamin and folic acid might be useful.

Prevention of Folate Deficiency

Folate food fortification, which has been adopted by many countries, can effectively raise folate levels.[A8] The programs were designed to increase folate status in women to prevent neural tube defects. Neural tube defects have decreased by 25 to 50% depending on the preexisting folate status of the population. Despite food fortification, women of childbearing age in the United States are recommended to take supplements of 400 μg of folic acid daily. Prenatal vitamins are fortified with folic acid at 1 mg/day and are recommended prior to conception and throughout gestation and breast-feeding. Folic acid supplements of 1 mg daily should be given to patients with inflammatory bowel disease, celiac disease, on methotrexate or older anticonvulsants, and to those with chronic hemolytic anemias. Dietary folate deficiency can be corrected by adding green leafy vegetables, legumes, fruits, and organ meats to the diet.

PROGNOSIS

Megaloblastic Anemia

Megaloblastic anemia due to cobalamin or folate deficiency should correct completely with the appropriate vitamin so long as there are no comorbidities. There is an increase in reticulocyte count within 5 days, and the hemoglobin normalizes by 1 to 2 months. Some patients can produce a unit of blood per week with replacement. Thrombocytopenia and leukopenia also correct within the first 2 weeks. Iron deficiency will manifest as a blunting of the hemoglobin response, a fall in MCV into the microcytic range, and a decrease in serum ferritin and iron saturation. The anemia of chronic renal failure may coexist in seniors with cobalamin deficiency and could be treated if appropriate with erythropoiesis-stimulating agents (Chapter 116). Patients with intestinal diseases may need combination cobalamin and folic acid treatment.

The most likely diagnosis in a failure of vitamin treatment is that of an incorrect diagnosis due to a false-positive low vitamin level. There may be cobalamin deficiency with coexisting myelodysplastic syndrome or other bone marrow disease. Folate-deficient alcoholics often have multifactorial anemia and a prolonged period of abstinence with folic acid treatment may be required, especially if the bone marrow is sideroblastic.

Correction of glossitis and other megaloblastic abnormalities in the intestinal tract may manifest as positive weight gain in malnourished patients.

Recurrent macrocytosis or anemia during adequate cobalamin replacement may suggest associated autoimmune disease, particularly thyroid disorders or autoimmune hemolytic anemia. Recurrent iron deficiency due to malabsorption from achlorhydria could be a continuing problem, especially pertinent in patients who have undergone bariatric surgery.

Cobalamin Deficiency of the Central Nervous System

The demyelinating nervous system pathology is not always reversible with cobalamin treatment (Chapter 384). The duration of and severity of symptoms before treatment is inversely correlated with the extent of correction of the abnormalities. Paresthesias and behavioral changes are the quickest and most likely to correct. Spinal cord lesions that have progressed to severe sensory loss and motor weakness usually do not correct fully. The cobalamin-deficient infant often has residual impairments and permanent disability. There is an occasional patient who develops paresthesias in the first few days after cobalamin replacement, which will resolve with further treatment.

It is important to document elevated methylmalonic acid or homocysteine in a patient who presents without megaloblastic anemia because there is a significant probability of a false-positive low cobalamin level in such patients. Lack of improvement or progression of neurologic symptoms and signs when cobalamin has been adequately replaced is proof that there is another cause for the symptoms. Diseases such as spinal stenosis or multiple sclerosis will not respond to cobalamin replacement, and delay in diagnosis during futile cobalamin therapy may harm the patient.

GENERAL REFERENCES

For the General References and other additional features, please visit Elsevier eBooks+ at https://ebooks.health.elsevier.com.

Grade A References

A1. Wang H, Li L, Qin LL, et al. Oral vitamin B_{12} versus intramuscular vitamin B_{12} for vitamin B_{12} deficiency. *Cochrane Database Syst Rev*. 2018;3:CD004655.

A2. Sanz-Cuesta T, Escortell-Mayor E, Cura-Gonzalez I, et al. Oral versus intramuscular administration of vitamin B12 for vitamin B12 deficiency in primary care: a pragmatic, randomised, non-inferiority clinical trial (OB12). *BMJ Open*. 2020;10:e033687.

A3. Markun S, Gravestock I, Jäger L, et al. Effects of vitamin B12 supplementation on cognitive function, depressive symptoms, and fatigue: a systematic review, meta-analysis, and meta-regression. *Nutrients*. 2021;13:923.

A4. Li Y, Huang T, Zheng Y, et al. Folic acid supplementation and the risk of cardiovascular diseases: a meta-analysis of randomized controlled trials. *J Am Heart Assoc*. 2016;5:e003768.

A5. Huo Y, Li J, Qin X, et al. Efficacy of folic acid therapy in primary prevention of stroke among adults with hypertension in China: the CSPPT randomized clinical trial. *JAMA*. 2015;313:1325-1335.

A6. Kotwal J, Kotwal A, Bhalla S, et al. Effectiveness of homocysteine lowering vitamins in prevention of thrombotic tendency at high altitude area: a randomized field trial. *Thromb Res*. 2015;136:758-762.

A7. Siebert AK, Obeid R, Weder S, et al. Vitamin B-12-fortified toothpaste improves vitamin status in vegans: a 12-wk randomized placebo-controlled study. *Am J Clin Nutr*. 2017;105:618-625.

A8. Centeno Tablante E, Pachón H, Guetterman HM, et al. Fortification of wheat and maize flour with folic acid for population health outcomes. *Cochrane Database Syst Rev*. 2019;7:CD012150.

151

APLASTIC ANEMIA AND RELATED BONE MARROW FAILURE STATES

AMY E. DEZERN AND ROBERT A. BRODSKY

IDIOPATHIC APLASTIC ANEMIA

DEFINITION

Idiopathic aplastic anemia is a hematopoietic stem cell disorder associated with markedly reduced marrow cellularity and markedly decreased hematopoiesis. The decreased hematopoiesis may disproportionately affect fewer lineages in early stages, but aplastic anemia is ultimately associated with trilineage hypoplasia.

EPIDEMIOLOGY

Aplastic anemia can be inherited or acquired. The majority of cases of acquired aplastic anemia are idiopathic, but causative conditions include viral infections and medications (Table 151-1).

Aplastic anemia is chiefly a disease of children and younger adults, with a second peak in incidence observed in patients age 60 years and older. Aplastic anemia is rare in Western Europe and the United States (fewer than two cases per million population per year). The incidence of aplastic anemia is higher in Asia at five to six cases per million population per year. The higher incidence in Asian countries has been linked to environmental factors such as chemicals or infections more than genetic factors. Both males and females are equally affected.

TABLE 151-1 PRIMARY AND SECONDARY CAUSES OF ACQUIRED APLASTIC ANEMIA

PRIMARY	
	Idiopathic aplastic anemia
	Pregnancy-associated aplastic anemia
	Classical paroxysmal nocturnal hemoglobinuria syndrome (Chapter 146)
SECONDARY	
	Drug associated (see E-Table 151-1)
	Iatrogenic/cytotoxic
	Radiation-associated
	Viruses (Epstein-Barr virus, cytomegalovirus, hepatitis A, B, or C))
	Autoimmune (autoimmune hepatitis and pancytopenia of autoimmune disease)

PATHOBIOLOGY

Acquired aplastic anemia is believed to be the result of an autoimmune attack directed at hematopoietic progenitor cells (Chapter 142). The immune attack is primarily directed by cytotoxic T cells that target hematopoietic stem cells and cause apoptosis, thereby leading to hematopoietic failure.[1,2]

Aplastic anemia is most often associated with normal cytogenetics. An abnormal karyotype in a patient with a hypocellular marrow is more consistent with a diagnosis of myelodysplastic syndrome (Chapter 167), although chromosomal abnormalities such as trisomy 8 or deletion 13q may still be consistent with an aplastic anemia diagnosis.

Acquired aplastic anemia generally lacks germline mutations, whereas inherited forms are driven by a germline mutation.[3] About 60 to 70% of idiopathic aplastic anemia patients demonstrate acquired clonality at the time of diagnosis on sensitive next-generation sequencing and array-based karyotyping using comparative genomic hybridization. The clones often remain despite therapies other than hematopoietic stem cell transplant and are frequently the source of relapse and/or progression.

CLINICAL MANIFESTATIONS

At initial presentation, many patients with aplastic anemia manifest symptoms of anemia, including fatigue, weakness, pallor, and headaches. Severe thrombocytopenia (Chapter 158) causes petechiae of the skin and mucous membranes, epistaxis, and/or gum bleeding. Fever and infections can also be seen in the presence of neutropenia (Chapter 153). However, some patients are identified earlier in the course of disease because of cytopenias found on routine laboratory testing before they have any symptoms or signs of the disease.

DIAGNOSIS

The diagnosis of aplastic anemia requires either a bone marrow with <25% of the normal cellularity or bone marrow with <50% normal cellularity in which less than 30% of the cells are hematopoietic. Cellularity is often profoundly decreased (<10%; Fig. 151-1), but small islands of hematopoiesis can be seen. The marrow aspirates in aplastic anemia do not show overt dysplastic changes, and blastic forms are not increased. The peripheral blood in aplastic anemia shows pancytopenia with a relative lymphocytosis, but is otherwise unremarkable.

Idiopathic aplastic anemia is a diagnosis of exclusion, and no single test can consistently distinguish aplastic anemia from other causes of bone marrow failure. However, extensive historical questions, findings on the physical examination, and laboratory diagnostics can help determine the cause of bone marrow failure (Table 151-2). Congenital forms must be excluded, especially in younger patients, prior to making a diagnosis of acquired aplastic anemia.[4] Aplastic anemia must be differentiated from hypoplastic myelodysplastic syndrome (Chapter 167), in which the mutational spectrum overlaps with aplastic anemia, as well as from inherited bone marrow failure disorders for which the phenotypic presentations might be indiscernible.

Aplastic anemia is further classified by the severity of the depression of peripheral blood counts. *Severe aplastic anemia* is defined by depression of blood counts involving at least two hematopoietic lineages (i.e., absolute reticulocyte count <60,000/μL, absolute neutrophil count <500/μL, or a platelet count <2000/μL) and bone marrow hypocellularity (<30%, excluding lymphocytes). *Very severe aplastic anemia* has an absolute neutrophil count of <200/μL, whereas *moderate aplastic anemia* is characterized by depression of blood counts not fulfilling the definition of severe disease (Table 151-3).

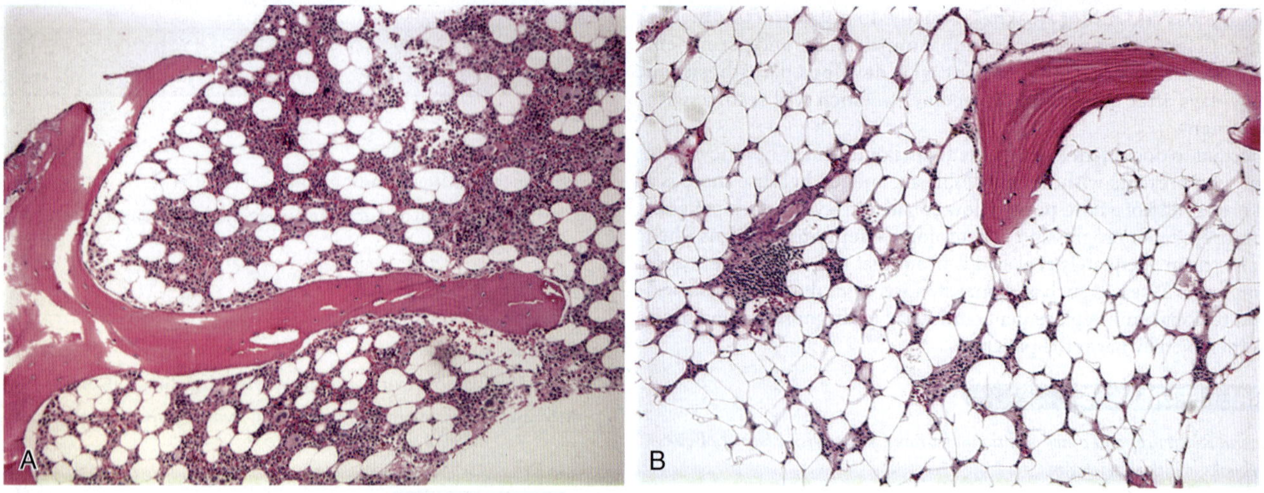

FIGURE 151-1. Two bone marrow biopsy samples from different patients. **A,** This specimen, from a normal individual, shows an abundance of hematopoietic cells, including myeloid and erythroid precursors and normal-appearing megakaryocytes. **B,** A specimen from a patient with severe aplastic anemia shows few detectable hematopoietic cells, and those that can be seen (one small nest) are lymphocytes. Some lymphoid cells are usually detectable and probably play an important pathophysiologic role in many cases of acquired idiopathic aplastic anemia, a disorder that is most often immunologically mediated. (Courtesy Dr. Ken Gatter, Oregon Health and Science University.)

TREATMENT

Definitive treatment with either immunosuppressive therapy or allogeneic hematopoietic stem cell transplantation (Chapter 163) is necessary for patients with severe or very severe aplastic anemia, but no standard of care exists for moderate aplastic anemia. Younger age (typically age <40 years) and the presence of a matched sibling donor favor the use of allogeneic hematopoietic stem cell transplantation, whereas older age (age >40 years) and absence of a matched sibling donor typically favor the use of immunosuppressive therapy. However, hematopoietic stem cell transplantation from haploidentical or unrelated donors is increasingly being used as front-line therapy for children and younger adults.

Hematopoietic Stem Cell Transplantation (HSCT)

Adolescents and young adults who meet criteria for severe disease and who have an HLA-matched sibling donor should proceed directly to hematopoietic stem cell transplantation (Chapter 163).[5] Predictors of survival following hematopoietic stem cell transplantation include matched sibling donor, recipient age <16 years, early transplant within 12 weeks of diagnosis, and a non-radiation conditioning regimen. Compared with standard immunosuppressive therapy, hematopoietic stem cell transplantation markedly reduces the risk of relapse and mitigates the risk for the later development of sequelae such as myelodysplasia, acute myeloid leukemia, or classical paroxysmal nocturnal hemoglobinuria. With increasingly good results with haploidentical[6] as well as unrelated donor hematopoietic stem cell transplantation, more patients are receiving hematopoietic stem cell transplantation for aplastic anemia (Fig. 151-2).

Immunosuppressive Therapy

Immunosuppressive therapy is often first-line therapy for adolescents and young adults who have severe aplastic anemia and who lack matched sibling donors as well as for medically fit adults (over age 40 years). Immunosuppressive therapy typically uses a combination of anti-thymocyte globulin (ATG), cyclosporine (12 to 15 mg/kg in divided doses twice daily), and eltrombopag[7] (a thrombopoetin-receptor agonist at 150 mg daily) in adults. Of the two ATG preparations commonly used in clinical practice, horse ATG (40 mg/kg/day for 4 days) appears to be superior in the front-line treatment of severe aplastic anemia.[A1] Eltrombopag increases response rates by about 20% compared with ATG and cyclosporine alone.[A2] Corticosteroids are also administered during the first 2 weeks under expert oversight to prevent serum sickness.

General Care

Supportive long-term care is imperative for patients who have aplastic anemia. Placement of a central venous catheter should be strongly considered for all patients given the frequency of phlebotomy, transfusions, and administration of therapeutic medications. Patients who have severe cytopenias require frequent and sometimes urgent blood product support. Blood products should be irradiated (to prevent transfusion-associated graft-versus-host disease) and leukocyte-reduced (to prevent alloimmunization and reduce the incidence of cytomegalovirus infections; see Chapter 162).

Fungal and bacterial infections are a major cause of death in patients with severe aplastic anemia, but an active fungal infection should not delay more definitive therapy such as immunosuppressive therapy or hematopoietic stem cell transplantation. Approaches to prophylactic antibiotic therapy vary among institutions, but adding prophylactic granulocyte colony stimulating factor to immunosuppressive therapy is not of incremental value.[A3]

Aplastic Anemia During Pregnancy

Aplastic anemia can rarely present during pregnancy. Spontaneous remission can occur in 25 to 30% of patients, often upon birth or termination of the pregnancy. Pregnant patients can be followed with stringent supportive care, or cyclosporine may be considered. Complications appear to be more likely in pregnant patients who have low platelet counts and associated paroxysmal nocturnal hemoglobinuria (Chapter 146).

PROGNOSIS

The hematopoietic response rate after immunosuppressive therapy is about 70 to 80%, and the probability of survival at 5 years ranges from 60 to 85%. Patients who are treated with horse ATG plus cyclosporine can have about a 60% overall survival at 15 years, but failure-free survival (survival without relapse or secondary clonal disease beyond 10 years) after immunosuppressive therapy is less than 50%. Survival outcomes continue to improve for alternative donor hematopoietic stem cell transplantation, and haploidentical transplantation with post-transplant cyclophosphamide represents a potential cure in patients who have severe aplastic anemia.

PAROXYSMAL NOCTURNAL HEMOGLOBINURIA

Paroxysmal nocturnal hemoglobinuria is a rare clonal disorder in which the activation of complement causes hemolytic anemia and sometimes bone marrow failure. A clone of paroxysmal nocturnal hemoglobinuria cells is seen in at least 50% of patients who have true aplastic anemia. Classical paroxysmal nocturnal hemoglobinuria is discussed in Chapter 146.

LARGE GRANULAR LYMPHOCYTE LEUKEMIA

DEFINITION AND EPIDEMIOLOGY

Large granular lymphocyte leukemia is a clonal lymphoid disorder characterized by a peripheral lymphocytosis of cytotoxic T-lymphocytes with concomitant cytopenias. Although an increase in the number of large granular lymphocytes can be associated with other entities, such as aplastic anemia or myelodysplastic syndrome, large granular lymphocyte leukemia is a distinct clinical entity.

Males and females are equally affected. The median age at diagnosis is 60 years, with very rare occurrence in younger children. The estimated incidence of large granular lymphocyte leukemia in the United States is 1 in 10,000,000 individuals. Large granular lymphocyte leukemia is associated with myelodysplastic syndrome (Chapter 167) in about 10% of cases.

PATHOBIOLOGY

The exact mechanism underlying the development of large granular lymphocyte leukemia is not fully understood. The leading hypothesis is the acquisition

TABLE 151-2 STANDARD EVALUATION OF A PATIENT WITH SUSPECTED APLASTIC ANEMIA TO ENCOMPASS RISK OF INHERITED DISORDERS

EVALUATION	PURPOSE
HISTORY AND PHYSICAL EXAMINATION	
Hematologic: Long-standing cytopenia(s) or macrocytosis Unexplained cytopenia(s) or macrocytosis, aplastic anemia, myelodysplastic syndrome, acute myeloid leukemia in one or more close relative(s)	Could suggest inherited bone marrow failure disorder due to identification of cytopenias at early age
Developmental: Short stature, physical anomalies (especially thumb or radial ray, cardiac, or renal)	Fanconi anemia or dyskeratosis congenita or thrombocytopenia-absent radius syndrome
Immunologic/Infectious Disease: Severe, recurrent, or atypical infections (e.g., mycobacterial, viral, fungal)	Could suggest GATA2 deficiency
Dermatologic: Gray hair prior to 25 Leukoplakia or nail dysplasia Reticulated skin pigmentation, café au lait macules	Could suggest dyskeratosis congenita or another short telomere syndrome
Pulmonary: Pulmonary fibrosis and/or early onset emphysema, pulmonary alveolar proteinosis, fungal or mycobacterial infection	Could suggest dyskeratosis congenita, another short telomere syndrome, or GATA2 deficiency
Abdominal: Pancreatic insufficiency, liver fibrosis, renal anomaly or malplacement	Could suggest dyskeratosis congenita, another short telomere syndrome, or Diamond Blackfan anemia
Oncologic: Head, neck, or anogenital squamous cell carcinoma, or early onset gastrointestinal cancer or multiple cancers in patient or close relatives	Could suggest short telomere syndrome
LABORATORY TESTING	
Complete blood count with differential and blood smear review	Assess severity of cytopenias and consider alternative etiologies
Reticulocyte count	Assess marrow response to anemia and use to assess the severity of aplastic anemia
Hemoglobin F%	Elevated levels may indicate an inherited bone marrow failure disorder
Levels of vitamin B_{12}, folate, copper, zinc, ferritin	Exclude vitamin or mineral deficiencies as cause or contributor to cytopenias
Serologies for hepatitis A/B/C, Epstein-Barr virus, parvovirus, and cytomegalovirus	Rule out infectious disease contributors to cytopenias and identify co-management needs during treatment and transplant
LDH, haptoglobin	Exclude a hemolytic component to anemia
Paroxysmal nocturnal hemoglobin clone	Assess presence or absence of GPI-anchored protein expression; presence suggests acquired rather than inherited disease
Antinuclear antibodies (plus anti-double-stranded DNA if positive)	Assess for systemic lupus erythematosus
Quantification of immunoglobulins A, G, M	Assess for additional immune deficits
Flow cytometry to assess numbers of B lymphocytes, T lymphocytes, and natural killer cells	Assess for additional immune deficits
Telomere length measurement of peripheral blood lymphocytes by fluorescence in situ hybridization	If telomere length <1st percentile, patient may have a short telomere syndrome and be at risk of increased transplant-related toxicity with standard preparative regimens
Chromosome breakage analysis on peripheral blood	If test is positive and consistent with a diagnosis of Fanconi anemia, Fanconi anemia–specific regimen should be utilized and patient is at increased risk of transplant-related toxicity.
Bone marrow aspirate and biopsy	Assess cellularity, iron stores, and reticulin fibrosis; exclude other marrow pathologies
Conventional karyotyping	Examine chromosomes in a sample of cells to identify genetic (acquired or inherited) problems as the cause of cytopenias
HLA typing	Determine HLA profile for stem cell donor search
Myeloid malignancy gene sequencing from peripheral blood or bone marrow	Evaluate for mutations in genes recurrently mutated in aplastic anemia (e.g., *PIGA, BCOR, BCORL1*) and/or myelodysplastic syndrome (e.g., epigenetic mutations, *TP53*).
Inherited bone marrow failure gene panel sequencing	Evaluate for multiple inherited bone marrow failure disorders (see E-Table 151-2) at once. Universal testing of young patients is also warranted.
Erythrocyte adenosine deaminase	Screen for Diamond Blackfan anemia

GPI = glycosylphosphatidylinositol; HIV = human immunodeficiency virus; HLA = human leukocyte antigen; LDH = lactase dehydrogenase.
Modified from DeZern AE, Churpek JE. Approach to the diagnosis of aplastic anemia. *Blood Adv.* 2021;5:2660-2671.

abnormalities in pathways that enhance survival, since normal large granulocytic lymphocytes undergo faster apoptosis whereas neoplastic lymphocytes appear to undergo reduced apoptosis. Mutations in *STAT3* are increased in patients with large granular lymphocyte leukemia, but these mutations are also detected when aplastic anemia, myelodysplastic syndrome, or pure red cell aplasia is associated with large granular lymphocytes.

CLINICAL MANIFESTATIONS

Patients most commonly present with asymptomatic neutropenia (Chapter 153) with or without concomitant anemia on routine laboratory evaluation, but some patients present with symptoms related to cytopenias. Large granular lymphocyte leukemia is also the most common cause of pure red cell aplasia in adults. Splenomegaly (Chapter 154), which is a common finding on physical

TABLE 151-3 CAMITTA CRITERIA FOR CLASSIFICATION OF APLASTIC ANEMIA

PERIPHERAL BLOOD CYTOPENIAS	NON-SEVERE (MODERATE) APLASTIC ANEMIA*	SEVERE APLASTIC ANEMIA†	VERY SEVERE APLASTIC ANEMIA‡
Bone marrow cellularity	<25%	<25%	<25%
Absolute neutrophil count		<500/μL	<200/μL
Platelet count		<20,000/μL	
Reticulocyte count		<1.0% corrected or <60,000/μL	

*Not meeting criteria for severe disease.
†Any 2 of 3.
‡Meets criteria for severe disease plus a lower absolute neutrophil count (<200/μL).

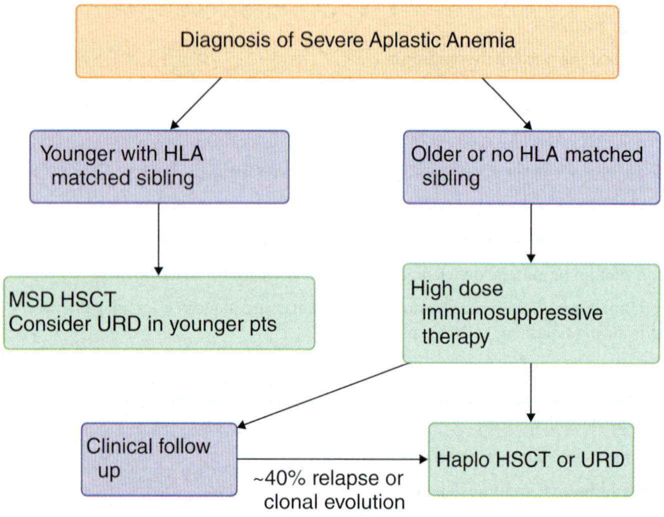

FIGURE 151-2. **Therapeutic considerations for severe aplastic anemia.** Haplo = haplo-identical; HLA = human leukocyte antigen; HSCT = hematopoietic stem cell transplantation; MSD = matched sibling donor; URD = unrelated living donor.

examination, is seen in 25 to 50% of cases and is classically associated with rheumatoid arthritis (Chapter 243) in males.

DIAGNOSIS

No single laboratory test is diagnostic of large granular lymphocyte leukemia. In the appropriate clinical context, however, a combination of histomorphology and flow cytometry with molecular diagnostic studies are sufficient for diagnosis.[8]

The peripheral blood often shows neutropenia with a relative lymphocytosis. Large granulocytic lymphocytes with relatively abundant pale cytoplasm, scattered eosinophilic granules, mature chromatin, and smooth nuclear borders (Fig. 151-3) are best seen in the peripheral blood rather than in a bone marrow sample.

However, large granulocytic lymphocytes can be increased not only in true large granular lymphocyte leukemia but also in reactive conditions, other non-neoplastic bone marrow failure conditions, and neoplastic hematologic malignancies. Distinguishing true large granular lymphocyte leukemia from these conditions can be challenging. Large granulocytic lymphocytes also are often transiently increased in patients with viral infections and can even be increased in individuals with normal white blood cell counts. By comparison, cytotoxic T-lymphocytes are elevated for more than 6 months in the peripheral blood, and the increase is not attributable to any other cause. As a result, flow cytometry is critical for diagnosis and will reveal an immunophenotypic profile that is indicative of an activated cytotoxic T cell (e.g., $CD3^+$, T cell receptor [TCR]-$\alpha\beta^+$, $CD57^+$, $CD4^-$, $CD5^{dim}$, $CD8^+$, $CD16^+$, $CD27^-$, $CD28^-$). Demonstration of clonal T-cell gene rearrangements is also an important part of the diagnostic evaluation.

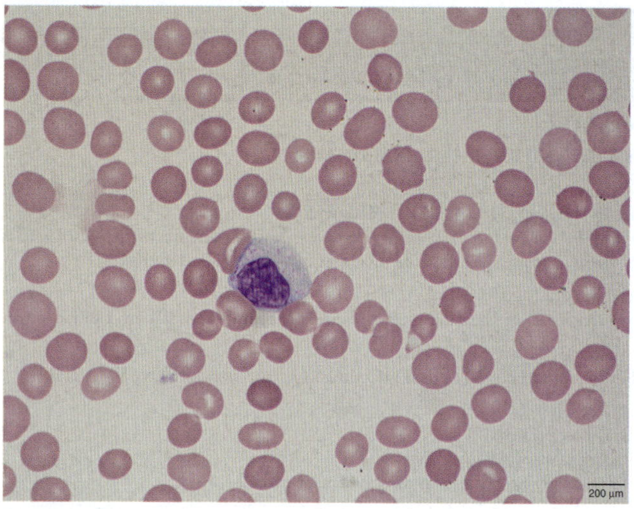

FIGURE 151-3. **Large granular lymphocyte.** (Courtesy of Rena Xian, MD, PhD.)

TREATMENT

Asymptomatic patients are best observed with routine blood counts and clinical follow-up, but treatment is indicated if patients are symptomatic because of severe cytopenias, recurrent infections, constitutional symptoms, or problematic splenomegaly (Chapter 154). Therapies commonly used under expert supervision include methotrexate, cyclophosphamide, cyclosporine, and alemtuzumab.[9] Patients often receive multiple sequential therapies because the disease often relapses.

When large granular lymphocyte leukemia is associated with the myelodysplastic syndrome (Chapter 167), it should be considered a paraneoplastic phenomenon; treatment should focus on the underlying myelodysplastic syndrome. The opposite is true with large granular lymphocyte leukemia–associated pure red cell aplasia, which often is more immune-responsive than pure red cell aplasia from other causes.

PROGNOSIS

Most cases of large granular lymphocyte leukemia follow a chronic course. Prognosis varies depending on the response to immunosuppressive therapy, as well as any underlying conditions, such as the myelodysplastic syndrome.

PURE RED CELL APLASIA

Pure red cell aplasia is a syndrome characterized by a severe normochromic, normocytic anemia (Chapter 144); reticulocytopenia; and the absence of erythroblasts from an otherwise normal bone marrow. Pure red cell aplasia is classified by the clinical course (acute or chronic) and underlying etiology (idiopathic or secondary).

PATHOBIOLOGY

Although pure red cell aplasia has numerous causes, the underlying etiology is thought to be immune-mediated.[10] Pure red cell aplasia may represent a primary hematologic disorder in the absence of any other disease or may develop secondary to parvovirus infection (Chapter 342), human immunodeficiency virus infection, a collagen vascular disease, leukemia, lymphoma, thymoma, solid tumors, treatment with recombinant human erythropoietin or other drugs, ABO-incompatible hematopoietic stem cell transplantation, and pregnancy.

CLINICAL MANIFESTATIONS

The acquired form of pure red cell aplasia presents either as an acute self-limited disease, predominantly seen in children, or as a chronic illness that is more frequently seen in adults. In adults, pure red cell aplasia presents as isolated anemia with normal (or slightly low) white blood cell and platelet counts. Large granular lymphocytes may be increased.

DIAGNOSIS

Evaluation for the possible causes of pure red cell aplasia includes assessing for a history of drug use, toxin exposure, or infections; abnormalities in liver and kidney function; immunologic examination for auto-antibodies; virologic studies to detect parvovirus B19 DNA, especially in patients with immunodeficiency and/or hemolytic anemia; and computed tomographic scanning to assess for a thymoma. Peripheral-blood flow cytometry should also be performed to quantify the concentration of large granulocytic lymphocytes.

However, the diagnosis of pure red cell aplasia requires a bone marrow biopsy and is often a diagnosis of exclusion. Bone marrow biopsies show normal to hypocellular marrow with absent or nearly absent erythroid precursors. Colony formation assays specifically for burst forming unit-erythroid may be informative. Increased colony formation assay growth is often seen in pure red cell aplasia, in keeping with the immune-mediated nature of this disorder, and higher growth correlates with a positive response to immunosuppressive therapy.

TREATMENT

During the initial evaluation, red cell transfusions can be given as necessary. Since about 10% of patients who have primary idiopathic pure red cell aplasia will have self-limited disease, other treatments can be delayed for about 1 month while watching for signs of recovery of erythropoiesis.

Immunosuppression is the mainstay of therapy for persistent pure red cell aplasia.[11] Corticosteroids (e.g., prednisone 20 to 60 mg) produce about a 75% response rate, but relapse occurs in up to 80% of patients when the dosage is tapered during the 24 months after remission. Cyclosporine under expert oversight yields an overall response rate of about 65%, but many patients do not remain in remission when cyclosporine is discontinued. Cyclophosphamide can provide an overall response rate of 40 to 60% after approximately 11 to 12 weeks of treatment.

For secondary pure red cell aplasias, removal of the inciting factor is critical. Pure red cell aplasia that is secondary to parvovirus B19 can be treated with intravenous immunoglobulin under expert oversight. About 25 to 30% of causes of thymoma-associated pure red cell aplasia show a hematologic response after surgical resection.

PROGNOSIS

Depending on the cause, the course can be acute and self-limiting or chronic with rare spontaneous remissions. In patients who have spontaneous remissions, no specific therapy is required other than transfusion for symptomatic anemia and cessation of possible offending drugs. For acquired chronic pure red cell aplasia, remissions can be attained with treatment, but the aplasia commonly recurs when therapy is discontinued.

INHERITED BONE MARROW FAILURE SYNDROMES

The inherited bone marrow failure syndromes are heterogeneous disorders in which at least one clinically significant cytopenia is present.[12] Many of the inherited bone marrow failure syndromes are associated with characteristic physical findings as well as notably increased risks of both solid and hematologic neoplasms.

FANCONI ANEMIA

Fanconi anemia is a genetic disorder that manifests as developmental abnormalities, progressive bone marrow failure, and an increased risk of developing both hematologic malignancies and carcinomas of the head, neck, and anogenital region at a relatively young age. The vast majority of families with Fanconi anemia exhibit autosomal recessive inheritance, but about 2% of cases are X-linked recessive. Fanconi anemia has an incidence of about 1/200,000 to 400,000 in most populations, but the incidence is higher in Ashkenazi Jews (about 1/30,000) and Afrikaners from South Africa (about 1/22,000). Most patients are diagnosed in the first decade of life, though some cases with milder phenotypes present later in life. Abnormalities in at least 23 genes that participate in a common DNA repair pathway called the Fanconi anemia pathway can result in defective DNA repair, which, in turn, leads to an increased mutation rate and oncogenesis.

CLINICAL MANIFESTATIONS AND DIAGNOSIS

Fanconi anemia is a very heterogeneous disease, with different mutations associated with different patterns of disease and severity. On physical examination, patients with Fanconi anemia show heterogeneous but characteristic physical findings, including café au lait spots, abnormalities of the thumbs, malformation of the ears and eyes, small stature, hypogonadism, and abnormalities of the gastrointestinal, genitourinary, cardiopulmonary, and central nervous systems. Patients typically present with an unusual macrocytosis and then later develop pancytopenia, thrombocytopenia, and ultimately bone marrow failure. Diagnosis is based on chromosomal fragility in blood lymphocytes, especially after exposure to alkylating agents, diepoxybutane, or mitomycin C.[13] Skin fibroblasts are often required for conclusive diagnosis.

TREATMENT

Approximately 50% of patients with Fanconi anemia initially respond to androgens under expert supervision, but androgen therapy has significant side effects such as liver toxicity, acne, and behavioral anomalies. Allogeneic hematopoietic stem cell transplantation provides a potential cure.

PROGNOSIS

Patients with low blood counts or cytogenetic abnormalities in the marrow have a relatively poor prognosis. By age 25 years, approximately 10% of patients develop acute leukemia (Chapter 168) and approximately 5% develop myelodysplastic syndrome. Even after a successful hematopoietic stem cell transplantation, patients remain at an increased risk of developing solid tumors[14] and should be regularly monitored.

DYSKERATOSIS CONGENITA AND SHORT TELOMERE SYNDROMES

Telomeres, which are tandem TTAGGG repeats at the ends of eukaryotic chromosomes, protect the integrity of the genetic material. Telomeres decrease in length with cell division. When the telomeres become too short, the resulting genomic instability allows for an increased rate of mutations and predisposes to oncogenesis. Nine proteins are currently known to participate in the maintenance of telomeres, and approximately 60% of patients with dyskeratosis congenita have a mutation in one of these genes.

The inheritance of dyskeratosis congenita may be autosomal dominant, autosomal recessive, or X-linked, and some patients also have de novo germline mutations. The median age at diagnosis is at about 15 years (range 0 to 75), and males are disproportionately affected, with a male:female ratio of approximately 3:1.

CLINICAL MANIFESTATIONS AND DIAGNOSIS

Dyskeratosis congenita is most often associated with a triad of characteristic skin and nail changes, bone marrow failure, and a predisposition for the development of cancers, particularly squamous cell carcinomas of the head and neck and anogenital region. Additional clinical findings may include premature graying, pulmonary fibrosis, short stature, immune deficiencies, avascular necrosis of the femur or humerus, and liver cirrhosis. Short telomere syndromes encompass a broader spectrum of disorders with both marrow failure and other systemic manifestations.[15]

The bone marrow is initially cellular, but all three lineages demonstrate gradual aplasia. Patients may progress to develop myelodysplastic syndrome or acute myeloid leukemia. Verification of shortened telomeres in white blood cells evaluated by flow cytometry with fluorescent in situ hybridization can confirm the diagnosis.

TREATMENT AND PROGNOSIS

Allogeneic hematopoietic stem cell transplantation, which is the only curative option, should be offered if the platelet count is 3000/μl , the absolute neutrophil count is <1000/μL, and the hemoglobin concentration is <8 g/dL. Without successful transplant, mean survival is 30 years, with most deaths related to infections, bleeding, and malignancy.[16]

DIAMOND–BLACKFAN ANEMIA

Diamond-Blackfan anemia is a rare congenital hypoplastic anemia that usually presents early in infancy. In familial cases, the pattern of inheritance is generally autosomal dominant, but a significant number of cases represent new mutations.

Diamond-Blackfan anemia is a ribosomopathy, and approximately 50% of patients carry known mutations that result in defective ribosomal function, especially mutations in the large or small subunit gene *RPS19*. The clinical disease is caused by insufficient production of a particular ribosomal protein (haploinsufficiency).

CLINICAL MANIFESTATIONS AND DIAGNOSIS

Very young patients present with anemia and reticulocytopenia, with an increase in mean corpuscular volume, hemoglobin F, and red cell adenosine deaminase. The hematologic findings are often accompanied by facial deformities (characterized by a short nose with a broad nasal bridge, widely spaced eyes, and thick upper lip), triphalangeal thumbs, microcephaly, congenital cataracts, and genitourinary and cardiac defects.

The bone marrow shows a selective loss of erythroid precursors. The myeloid lineage shows a full range of maturation, and megakaryocytes are normal in number and morphology. The finding of an elevated adenosine deaminase level in the serum is strongly suggestive of this disease, and the genetic diagnosis usually can be made with a Diamond-Blackfan anemia panel.

TREATMENT AND PROGNOSIS

Up to 80% of patients respond to corticosteroids (e.g., prednisone starting at 2 mg/kg/day, followed by a 0.5 mg/kg/day maximum maintenance dose).[17] Patients who do not respond within a month are considered steroid-refractory and require RBC transfusion support. Hematopoietic stem cell transplantation improves red cell production but does not protect against the development of the myelodysplastic syndrome or acute myeloid leukemia; as a result, matched unrelated hematopoietic stem cell transplantation is best reserved for steroid-refractory patients who require regular transfusions.

The outcomes of Diamond-Blackfan anemia are usually excellent, in particular for patients younger than age 10 years. However, Diamond-Blackfan patients have a marked increased risk for colon cancer, and all patients should be referred to a gastroenterologist for appropriate screening at around age 20 years.

OTHER MARROW FAILURE DISORDERS

Other extremely rare marrow failure disorders that can be seen, especially in children, typically require specific genetic panels or whole exome sequencing by an expert hematologist. Examples include mutations in *SAMD9* (sterile alpha motif domain protein 9) and *SAMD9L* (its paralogue SAMD9-like), sideroblastic anemia (Chapter 145), monosomy 7 predisposition syndromes, thrombocytopenia-absent radii syndrome, Pearson syndrome, and MonoMac (*GATA2*) syndrome.[18]

GENERAL REFERENCES

For the General References and other additional features, please visit Elsevier eBooks+ at https://ebooks.health.elsevier.com.

Grade A References

A1. Yang N, Chen J, Zhang H, et al. Horse versus rabbit antithymocyte globulin in immunosuppressive therapy of treatment-naive aplastic anemia: a systematic review and meta-analysis. *Ann Hematol.* 2017;96:2031-2043.

A2. Peffault de Latour R, Kulasekararaj A, Iacobelli S, et al. Eltrombopag added to immunosuppression in severe aplastic anemia. *N Engl J Med.* 2022;386:11-23.

A3. Tichelli A, Peffault de Latour R, Passweg J, et al. Long-term outcome of a randomized controlled study in patients with newly diagnosed severe aplastic anemia treated with antithymocyte globulin and cyclosporine, with or without granulocyte colony-stimulating factor: a severe aplastic anemia working party trial from the European group of blood and marrow transplantation. *Haematologica.* 2020;105:1223-1231.

152 POLYCYTHEMIA VERA, ESSENTIAL THROMBOCYTHEMIA, AND PRIMARY MYELOFIBROSIS

JASON GOTLIB

DEFINITION

In the 2022 International Consensus Classification, the major category of myeloproliferative neoplasms comprises seven diseases (Table 152-1), including polycythemia vera, essential thrombocythemia, and primary myelofibrosis.[1]

TABLE 152-1 2022 INTERNATIONAL CONSENSUS CLASSIFICATION OF MYELOPROLIFERATIVE NEOPLASMS

DISEASE
Chronic myeloid leukemia
Chronic neutrophilic leukemia
Polycythemia vera
Primary myelofibrosis
Prefibrotic/early primary myelofibrosis
Overt primary myelofibrosis
Essential thrombocythemia
Chronic eosinophilic leukemia, not otherwise specified
Myeloproliferative neoplasm, unclassifiable

The umbrella term "*BCR::ABL1*-negative myeloproliferative neoplasms" is used to distinguish these disorders from chronic myeloid leukemia (CML), which is also included in the myeloproliferative neoplasm category and molecularly defined by the *BCR::ABL1* fusion oncogene. (CML is discussed in Chapter 170.) Polycythemia vera, essential thrombocythemia, and myelofibrosis are chronic myeloid stem cell disorders characterized by excessive production of terminally differentiated cells and variable potential to evolve into acute myeloid leukemia (AML), also referred to as blast-phase myeloproliferative neoplasm. Although these neoplasms exist along a continuous disease spectrum, they each exhibit heterogeneous molecular, biologic, and clinical features that translate into unique natural histories.

EPIDEMIOLOGY

According to a meta-analysis of 34 studies, the combined annual incidence rates (IRs) for polycythemia vera, essential thrombocythemia, and primary myelofibrosis were 0.84, 1.03, and 0.47 per 100,000, respectively. Data from 2001 to 2012 found that the age-adjusted IRs were highest for polycythemia vera (10.9 per 1 million person-years) and essential thrombocythemia (IR = 9.6), and relatively lower for primary myelofibrosis (IR = 3.1). The median ages at diagnosis ranged from 65 to 70 years for the three myeloproliferative neoplasms. Excluding essential thrombocythemia, which predominates among females especially younger than 60 years of age, polycythemia vera and primary myelofibrosis are more commonly diagnosed in males. For all three myeloproliferative neoplasms, IRs are significantly lower among Hispanic Whites, Asian-Pacific Islanders, and Blacks compared to non-Hispanic Whites. Based on data from two large U.S. health plans spanning 2008 to 2010, prevalence rates ranged from 44 to 57 per 100,000 individuals for polycythemia vera, 38 to 57 per 100,000 for essential thrombocythemia, and 0.3 to 5.7 per 100,000 for myelofibrosis.

Risk factors associated with the development of myeloproliferative neoplasms require further study but have included Jewish descent, autoimmune conditions (e.g., Crohn disease), and male-predominant occupations including agricultural or other rural-sector workers with potential exposure to benzene or petroleum. The individual genetic background can influence the propensity for developing a myeloproliferative neoplasm. A five- to seven-fold increased risk of myeloproliferative neoplasm development was identified in first-degree relatives of patients with a myeloproliferative neoplasm.

PATHOBIOLOGY

A point mutation at base pair 1849 (G→T) in the *JAK2* gene results in substitution of the normal valine to phenylalanine in codon 617 (V617F) of exon 14. The somatic V617F mutation has been identified as a highly recurrent mutation in polycythemia vera, essential thrombocythemia, and primary myelofibrosis.[2,3] The mutation affects the autoinhibitory pseudokinase domain of *JAK2*, relieving inhibition of JAK2 kinase activity, and resulting in constitutive JAK-STAT signaling (Fig. 152-1). *JAK2* V617F is found in ≈95 to 98% of polycythemia vera patients and 50 to 60% of essential thrombocythemia and primary myelofibrosis patients; other myeloid neoplasms rarely exhibit *JAK2* mutations. Small in-frame insertions and deletions in exon 12 of the *JAK2* gene (e.g., codons 530 to 540 s) are restricted to ≈2% of polycythemia vera patients who are negative for the V617F mutation (Fig. 152-2).

The *JAK2* V617F mutation arises in a multipotent hematopoietic progenitor or hematopoietic stem cell. It is identified in all cells derived from the myeloid lineage but can also be found in B and NK cells and, more rarely, in

T cells. It has been identified in endothelial cells of the spleen and of splanchnic veins in patients with myelofibrosis or patients with a myeloproliferative neoplasm and the Budd-Chiari syndrome. *JAK2* V617F can evolve from a heterozygous to homozygous state due to uniparental disomy (copy-neutral loss of heterozygosity) involving the short arm of chromosome 9 (9p loss of heterozygosity) where the *JAK2* gene is located. The *JAK2* V617F variant allele frequency in granulocytes from myeloproliferative neoplasm patients can vary widely. The variant allele frequency is usually low (e.g., below 50%) in essential thrombocythemia and higher in polycythemia vera and primary myelofibrosis (frequently over 50%, attributable to loss of heterozygosity). Similarly, very high variant allele frequencies are commonly observed in myelofibrosis that evolves from polycythemia vera (post-polycythemia vera myelofibrosis) or myelofibrosis that evolves from essential thrombocythemia (post-essential thrombocythemia myelofibrosis).

Activating mutations in the gene encoding the thrombopoietin receptor *MPL* (most commonly *MPL* W515 L/K) are found in less than 5% of patients with essential thrombocythemia and up to 10% of individuals with myelofibrosis (see Fig. 152-2). These mutations in exon 10 (including the rare S505N variant) occur in the juxtamembrane, intracytosolic portion and stabilize the receptor in an active dimeric configuration. Mutations in exon 9 of the calreticulin (*CALR*) gene have been found in the overwhelming majority of nonmutated *JAK2/MPL* patients and account for 20 to 35% of all patients with essential thrombocythemia and myelofibrosis (see Fig. 152-2). Although more than 50 types of mutations have been described, *CALR* variants fall into two predominant subtypes: type 1 (52 base-pair deletion), which is more common in patients with myelofibrosis, and type 2 (5 base-pair insertion) mutations, which is more prevalent in essential thrombocythemia. All exon 9 mutations result in a +1 frameshift in the coding sequence, resulting in a modified carboxy terminus which lacks a KDEL motif responsible for preventing secretion of the protein from the endoplasmic reticulum (ER). The mutant CALR C-terminus also acquires a greater positive charge that leads to loss of multiple calcium-binding sites. Recent investigations have uncovered that mutant CALR binds to the extracellular domain of the thrombopoietin receptor, MPL (Chapter 142), resulting in activation of the JAK-STAT axis. The positive charge of the mutant CALR C-terminus and the protein's lectin activity are required to mediate this neomorphic oncogenic activity.[4] These findings highlight a new paradigm of a mutated ER chaperone protein activating a cytokine receptor, leading to cellular transformation.

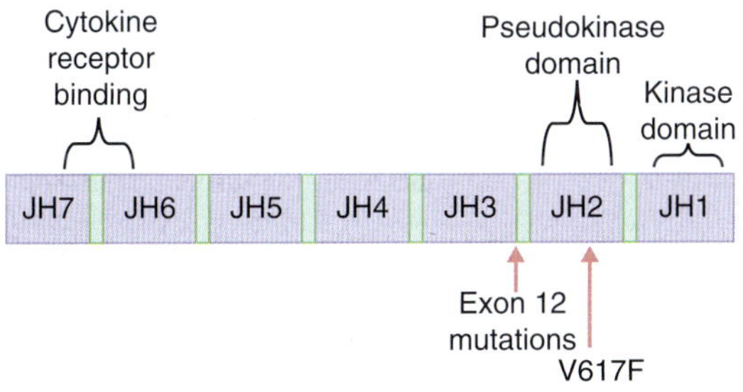

FIGURE 152-1. **Exon 12 and *JAK2* V617F gene mutations.** Scheme of the *JAK2* gene showing the positions of the V617F (exon 14) and exon 12 mutations. (From Levine RL, Gilliland DG. Myeloproliferative disorders. *Blood.* 2008;112:2190-2198. Fig. 2.)

LNK (SH2B3) is a negative regulator of JAK2 and normally functions to inhibit downstream STAT activation. Mutations in *LNK* have been found in 1 to 2% of patients with essential thrombocythemia or myelofibrosis, and rarely in patients with idiopathic erythrocytosis or polycythemia vera. Secondary *LNK* mutations may also occur during disease progression in *JAK2*- or *CALR*-mutant patients.

Approximately 10% of patients with essential thrombocythemia or primary myelofibrosis do not exhibit the canonical *JAK2, MPL,* or *CALR* driver mutations (so-called "triple-negative" myeloproliferative neoplasm patients) (see Fig. 152-2). Some of these patients exhibit cytogenetic abnormalities without evidence for a driver mutation, but no evidence of clonal hematopoiesis can be found in other patients. Rare patients exhibit alternative *JAK2* or *MPL* mutations that are present in the germline, consistent with a hereditary thrombocytosis.

Additional Molecular Abnormalities

Exome sequencing of a large cohort of patients with myeloproliferative neoplasm revealed that the median number of mutations in both polycythemia vera and essential thrombocythemia was 6.5, compared with 13 in myelofibrosis, consistent with it being a more advanced, genetically heterogeneous disease (Table 152-2). Besides *JAK2, CALR,* and *MPL*, mutations are found in genes encoding epigenetic regulators (*TET2, DNMT3A, ASXL1, EZH2, IDH1,* and *IDH2*), components of the splicing machinery (*SF3B1, SRSF2, U2AF1*), signal transduction (*CBL, SH2B3 [LNK]*), and tumor suppressor function (*TP53*).[5] Although identified in chronic-phase myeloproliferative neoplasms, acquisition of *TP53* mutations is commonly associated with disease acceleration, including transformation of myelofibrosis to blast-phase disease.

Genotype-Phenotype Correlations

The high prevalence of the *JAK2* V617F mutation in three clinically distinct myeloproliferative neoplasms raises the question of which factors contribute to the phenotypic diversity among polycythemia vera, essential thrombocythemia, and primary myelofibrosis. Differences in mutant allele burden of *JAK2* V617F likely modulate phenotype. Murine retroviral transplant models resulting in high levels of *JAK2* V617F expression produced a polycythemia vera–like phenotype with marked erythrocytosis. In contrast, transgenic models with more physiologic levels of *JAK2* V617F expression resulted in phenotypes resembling essential thrombocythemia and primary myelofibrosis. These animal models corroborate findings in patients, in whom the frequency of the *JAK2* V617F variant allele tends to be the highest in polycythemia vera and primary myelofibrosis, with lower levels in essential thrombocythemia. For patients with essential thrombocythemia, positivity for *JAK2* V617F tends to confer a polycythemia vera–like phenotype, with higher hemoglobin and lower platelet counts than in *JAK2* V617F–negative essential thrombocythemia patients.

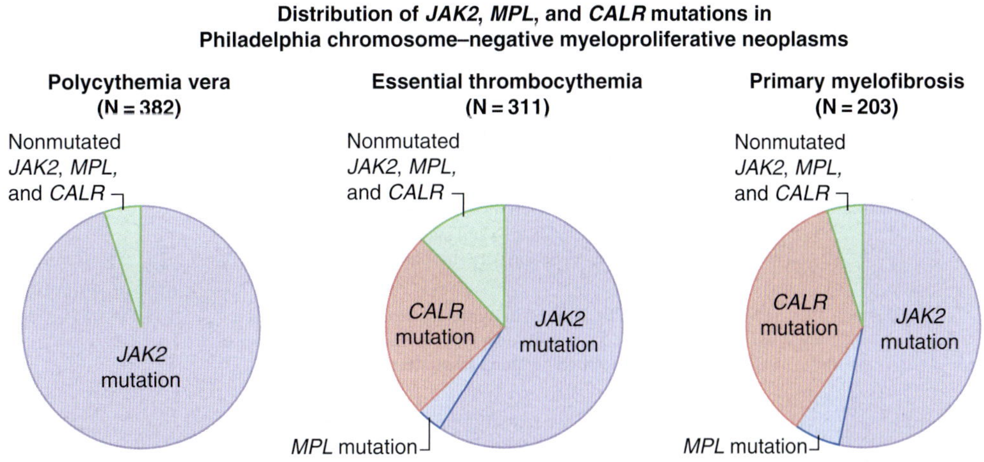

FIGURE 152-2. **Distribution of canonical *JAK2, MPL,* and *CALR* mutations in polycythemia vera, essential thrombocythemia, and primary myelofibrosis.** Relative distribution of *JAK2, CALR,* and *MPL* mutations in polycythemia vera, essential thrombocythemia, and primary myelofibrosis. All three mutations lead to constitutive activation of the Janus kinase/signal transducer and activator of transcription (JAK-SKAT) signaling axis. (From Klampfl T, Gisslinger H, Harutyunyan AS, et al. Somatic mutations of calreticulin in myeloproliferative neoplasms. *N Engl J Med.* 2013;369:2379-2390, Fig. 1a.)

TABLE 152-2 MUTATIONAL LANDSCAPE OF CHRONIC- AND BLAST-PHASE MYELOPROLIFERATIVE NEOPLASMS AND PROGNOSTIC RELEVANCE OF MOLECULAR ABNORMALITIES

MUTATION	CHROMOSOME LOCATION	FREQUENCY	PATHOGENETIC RELEVANCE	PROGNOSTIC ASSOCIATIONS
JAK2 (Janus kinase 2): *V617F*	9p24	PV: ≈96% ET: ≈55% PMF: ≈65%	Contributes to abnormal myeloproliferation and progenitor cell growth factor hypersensitivity	Intermediate prognosis and higher risk of thrombosis compared to patients with *CALR* mutation (PMF)
JAK2 exon 12 mutation	9p24	PV: ≈3%	Contributes to primarily erythroid myeloproliferation	Younger age, increased mean hemoglobin/hematocrit, and lower mean white blood cell and platelet counts at diagnosis compared to those with *JAK2* V617F-mutated PV. Both *JAK2* mutations are associated with similar rates of thrombosis, evolution to myelofibrosis or leukemia, and death in PV
CALR (Calreticulin): exon 9 deletions and insertions	19p13.2	PMF: ≈25% ET: ≈20% PV: 0%	Wild-type *CALR* is a multifunctional Ca^{2+} binding protein chaperone mostly localized in the endoplasmic reticulum	Improved survival compared to *JAK2* mutation and "triple-negative" PMF. Lower risk of thrombosis compared to *JAK2* mutation (ET, PMF) No difference in overall survival or myelofibrotic or leukemic transformation compared to *JAK2*-mutated ET *CALR* type 1/type 1-like with improved overall survival compared to *CALR* type 2/type 2-like and *JAK2* V617F mutation (PMF)
MPL (myeloproliferative leukemia virus oncogene): MPN-associated *MPL* mutations involve exon 10	1p34	ET: ~3% PMF: ~10%	Contributes to primarily megakaryocytic myeloproliferation	Intermediate prognosis and higher risk of thrombosis compared to patients with *CALR* mutation (PMF)
LNK, or *SH2B3* (a membrane-bound adaptor protein): MPN-associated mutations are monoallelic and involve exon 2	12q24.12	PV: rare ET: rare PMF: rare BP-MPN: ≈10%	Wild-type *LNK* is a negative regulator of JAK2 signaling	Inferior overall survival in ET
TET2 (TET oncogene family member 2): mutations involve several exons	4q24	PV: ≈16% ET: ≈5% PMF: ≈17% BP-MPN: ≈17%	TET proteins catalyze conversion of 5mC to 5hmC, which favors demethylated DNA. Both TET1 and TET2 display this catalytic activity. *IDH* and *TET2* mutations might share a common pathogenetic effect.	
ASXL1 (additional sex combs-like 1): exon 12 mutations	20q11.1	ET: ≈3% PMF: ≈13% BP-MPN: ≈18%	Wild-type *ASXL1* is needed for normal hematopoiesis and might be involved in coactivation of transcription factors and transcriptional repression	Independently associated with inferior overall survival and leukemia-free survival (PMF) Survival longest for *CALR* (+)/*ASXL1*(−) patients (median 10.4 years) and shortest in *CALR*(−)/*ASXL1*(+) patients (median 2.3 years). Intermediate survival (median 5.8 years) for *CALR*(+)/*ASXL1*(+) or *CALR*(−)/*ASXL1*(−) patients (PMF); worse overall and MF-free survival in PV
IDH1/*IDH2* (isocitrate dehydrogenase): exon 4 mutations	2q33.3/15q26.1	PV: ≈2% ET: ≈1% PMF: ≈4% BP-MPN: ≈20%	*IDH* mutations induce loss of activity for the conversion of isocitrate to 2-KG and gain in function in the conversion of 2-KG to 2-HG. 2-HG might be the mediator of impaired TET2 function in cells with mutant *IDH* expression	Independently associated with inferior leukemia-free survival (PMF); worse overall (*IDH1*) and leukemia-free survival (*IDH2*) in PV; inferior overall survival in ET (*IDH2*)
EZH2 (enhancer of zeste homolog 2): mutations involve several exons	7q36.1	PV: ≈3% PMF: ≈7% MDS: ≈6%	Wild-type *EZH2* is part of a histone methyltransferase (polycomb repressive complex 2 associated with H3 Lys-27 trimethylation). MPN-associated *EZH2* mutations might have a tumor suppressor activity, which contrasts with the gain-in-function activity for lymphoma-associated *EZH2* mutations	Independently associated with inferior overall survival (PMF); inferior overall and leukemia-free survival in ET
DNMT3A (DNA cytosine methyltransferase 3a): most frequent mutations affect amino acid R882	2p23	PV: ≈7% PMF: ≈7% BP-MPN: ≈14%	DNA methyl transferases are essential in establishing and maintaining DNA methylation patterns in mammals	
CBL (Casitas B-lineage lymphoma proto-oncogene): exon 8/9 mutations	11q23.3	PV: rare ET: rare MF: ≈6%	CBL is an E3 ubiquitin ligase that marks mutant kinases for degradation. Transforming activity requires loss of this function.	
IKZF1 (IKAROS family zinc finger 1): mostly deletions including intragenic	7p12	CP-MPN: rare BP-MPN: ≈19%	IKZF1 is a transcription regulator and putative tumor suppressor	
TP53 (tumor protein p53): exons 4 through 9	17p13.1	PMF: ≈4% BP-MPN ≈27%	A tumor suppressor protein that targets genes that regulate cell cycle arrest, apoptosis, and DNA repair	Associated with leukemic transformation (PMF and ET)

TABLE 152-2 MUTATIONAL LANDSCAPE OF CHRONIC- AND BLAST-PHASE MYELOPROLIFERATIVE NEOPLASMS AND PROGNOSTIC RELEVANCE OF MOLECULAR ABNORMALITIES—cont'd

MUTATION	CHROMOSOME LOCATION	FREQUENCY	PATHOGENETIC RELEVANCE	PROGNOSTIC ASSOCIATIONS
SF3B1 (splicing factor 3B subunit 1): mostly exons 14 and 15	2q33.1	PMF: ≈7%	SF3B1 is a component of the RNA spliceosome. *SF3B1* mutations are closely associated with ring sideroblasts.	Inferior overall and MF-free survival in ET
SRSF2 (serine/arginine-rich splicing factor 2): exon 2	17q25.1	PMF: ≈17%	SRSF2 is a component of the RNA spliceosome, whose dysfunction promotes defects in alternative splicing	Independently associated with inferior overall survival and leukemia-free survival (PMF); worse overall survival in PV, ET
U2AF1 (U2 small nuclear RNA auxiliary factor 1)	21q22.3	PMF: ≈16%	U2AF1 is a subunit of the U2 small nuclear ribonucleoprotein auxiliary factor involved in pre-mRNA processing	Independently associated with anemia (PMF); inferior overall survival with *U2AF1* Q157 compared to *U2AF1*-unmutated PMF; worse overall and MF-free survival in ET
Triple-negative (negative for *JAK2*, *MPL*, or *CALR* mutations)				Inferior leukemia-free survival compared to patients with *JAK2*- and/or *CALR*-mutated PMF. Inferior overall survival compared to patients with *CALR*-mutated PMF.

2-HG = 2-hydroxyglutarate; 2-KG = 2-ketoglutarate; 5hmC = 5-hydroxymethylcytosine; 5mC = 5-methylcytosine; BP-MPN = blast-phase MPN; CP-MPN= chronic-phase MPN; ET = essential thrombocythemia; MDS = myelodysplastic syndrome; MF includes both PMF and post-ET/PV myelofibrosis; MPN = myeloproliferative neoplasms; PMF = primary myelofibrosis; PV = polycythemia vera.

CLINICAL MANIFESTATIONS

Essential Thrombocythemia

Up to one half of patients may present with incidental thrombocytosis (defined as platelet count >450,000/μL) without symptoms. The frequency of vasomotor symptoms differs widely between series; such microvascular disturbances can manifest as headaches, lightheadedness, syncope, chest pain, visual disturbances (amaurosis fugax, scintillating scotomata, ophthalmic migraine), and erythromelalgia (Fig. 152-3) which manifests as burning pain of the hands or feet associated with erythema and warmth.[6] Incidence rates of arterial (e.g., cerebrovascular event, myocardial infarction, peripheral arterial disease) and venous (deep vein thrombosis, pulmonary embolism, superficial thrombophlebitis) thrombosis as well as hemorrhage also vary; however, rates of major thrombosis or bleeding are less than 10% at diagnosis and follow-up. Thrombosis of unusual sites such as the abdomen (e.g., mesenteric, portal, hepatic vein thrombosis [Budd-Chiari syndrome]) and central nervous system (e.g., cerebral venous sinus thrombosis; retinal vein or artery thrombosis) may also be observed. Differences in diagnostic criteria used for essential thrombocythemia as well as the potential for inclusion of patients with prefibrotic myelofibrosis may account for the variability in reported rates of splenomegaly (typically mild), which range from <10% to approximately 50% of patients.

In one study of 150 patients with essential thrombocythemia, the median platelet count ranged from 454,000 to 3,460,000/μL. There is no correlation between the degree of thrombocytosis and risk of thrombosis; however, patients with a platelet count higher than about 1.5 million/μL are at an increased risk for bleeding, attributable, in part, to acquired von Willebrand disease. Acquired von Willebrand disease is due to increased binding of large von Willebrand factor multimers, which are the most hemostatically effective components of the von Willebrand factor protein, to platelets and their removal from the plasma; the finding of decreased ristocetin cofactor activity (e.g., <30%) and loss of high-molecular-weight von Willebrand multimeric proteins on multimer analysis can help establish the diagnosis (Chapter 159).

Polycythemia Vera

Most patients with polycythemia vera are incidentally discovered to have an elevated hemoglobin (defined as hemoglobin >16.5 g/dL in men or >16.0 g/dL in women) and elevated hematocrit (defined as >49% in men or >48% in women). Increased blood hyperviscosity can lead to a constellation of physical examination findings, including hypertension, facial plethora, injection of the conjunctival small vessels and engorgement of the retinal veins on funduscopic examination, erythromelalgia (similar to essential thrombocythemia), splenomegaly (more frequent than hepatomegaly), and tophaceous gout.[7] Relatively common complaints include fatigue, aquagenic pruritus (itching following a warm bath or shower), headache, difficulty concentrating, lightheadedness/dizziness, and nondescript gastrointestinal symptoms such as epigastric discomfort and abdominal fullness/early satiety (E-Table 152-1). Neurologic symptoms, including tinnitus, paresthesias, and the aforementioned visual disturbances, are also encountered in polycythemia vera. In a large international

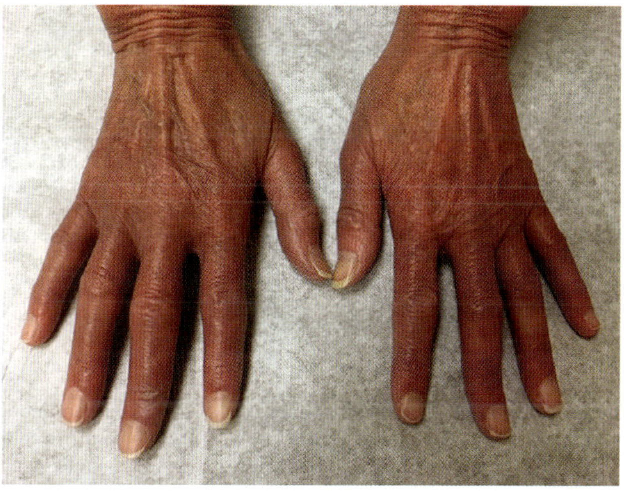

FIGURE 152-3. Erythromelalgia of the hands in a patient with polycythemia vera characterized by an exon 12 *JAK2* mutation.

study of patients with polycythemia vera, arterial thrombotic complication, venous thrombosis, or major hemorrhage were noted prior to or at the time of diagnosis in 16, 7, and 4% of patients, respectively.

Primary Myelofibrosis

The major clinical issues related to primary myelofibrosis include debilitating constitutional symptoms, splenomegaly, progressive cytopenias, potential for evolution to AML (15 to 20% of patients), and reduced survival. With advancing disease, the spleen can become massive in size (filling the left side of the abdomen and to the pelvic brim), resulting in abdominal pain (sometimes with referred left shoulder pain), early satiety, weight loss, and complications including splenic infarction.[8] Extramedullary hematopoiesis resulting in hepatomegaly is also common; complications of extramedullary hematopoiesis include portal hypertension, esophageal or gastric varices, and ascites. Myelofibrosis-associated anemia may be due to several causes, including ineffective hematopoiesis, splenic sequestration, gastrointestinal bleeding, autoimmune hemolytic anemia, or nutritional deficiencies (e.g., vitamin B_{12}). Extramedullary hematopoiesis may involve other sites besides the liver and spleen, such as the paravertebral space, lymph nodes, retroperitoneum, lungs or pleura, genitourinary organs, skin, and bowel. Pulmonary hypertension may be underdiagnosed in myelofibrosis and other myeloproliferative neoplasms and has been associated with increased symptoms (e.g., fatigue and dyspnea) and decreased survival. The incidence of arterial and venous thrombosis is similar to that of essential thrombocythemia.

TABLE 152-3 2022 INTERNATIONAL CONSENSUS CLASSIFICATION DIAGNOSTIC CRITERIA FOR POLYCYTHEMIA VERA, ESSENTIAL THROMBOCYTHEMIA, AND PRIMARY MYELOFIBROSIS

CRITERIA	POLYCYTHEMIA VERA[*]	ESSENTIAL THROMBOCYTHEMIA[†]	PRIMARY MYELOFIBROSIS[‡]
Major criteria	1. Elevated hemoglobin concentration (>16.5 g/dL in men; >16.0 g/dL in women) or elevated hematocrit (>49% in men; >48% in women) or increased red blood cell mass (>25% above mean normal predicted value) 2. Bone marrow biopsy showing age-adjusted hypercellularity with trilineage growth (panmyelosis), including prominent erythroid, granulocytic, and megakaryocytic proliferation with pleomorphic, mature megakaryocytes 3. Presence of *JAK2* V617F or *JAK2* exon 12 mutation	1. Platelet count ≥450,000/µL 2. Bone marrow biopsy showing proliferation mainly of the megakaryocytic lineage, with increased numbers of enlarged, mature megakaryocytes with hyperlobulated nuclei, no significant increase or left shift in neutrophil granulopoiesis or erythropoiesis; very rarely or minor (grade 1) increase in reticulin fibers 3. ICC criteria for *BCR::ABL1*-positive chronic myeloid leukemia, polycythemia vera, primary myelofibrosis, or other myeloid neoplasms are not met 4. *JAK2, CALR,* or *MPL* mutation	1. Megakaryocytic proliferation and atypia, without reticulin fibrosis grade >1, accompanied by increased age-adjusted bone marrow cellularity, granulocytic proliferation, and (often) decreased erythropoiesis (**PREFIBROTIC**)[§] 2. Megakaryocytic proliferation and atypia, accompanied by reticulin and/or collagen fibrosis grades 2 or 3 (**OVERT**)[‖] 3. ICC criteria for *BCR::ABL1*-positive chronic myeloid leukemia, polycythemia vera, essential thrombocythemia, myelodysplastic syndromes, or other myeloid neoplasms are not met 4. *JAK2* or *CALR* or *MPL* mutation, or presence of another clonal marker,[¶] or absence of reactive myelofibrosis[**]
Minor criteria	Subnormal erythropoietin level	Presence of a clonal marker[¶] or absence of reactive thrombocytosis	Presence of at least one of the following, confirmed on two separate determinations: • Anemia not attributed to a comorbid condition • Leukocytosis ≥11,000/µL • Palpable splenomegaly • LDH above the upper limit of normal • Leukoerythroblastosis (only in overt primary myelofibrosis)

[*]The diagnosis of polycythemia vera requires either all three major criteria or the first two major criteria plus the minor criteria. Major criterion 2 (bone marrow biopsy) may not be required in patients with sustained absolute erythrocytosis (hemoglobin concentration in men >18.5 g/dL or >16.5 g/dL in women and hematocrit values >55.5% in men and >49.5% in women) if the major criterion 3 and the minor criteria are present. However, initial myelofibrosis (present in as many as 20% of patients) can only be detected by bone marrow biopsy, and this finding may predict a more rapid progression to overt myelofibrosis (post–polycythemia vera myelofibrosis).

[†]The diagnosis of essential thrombocythemia requires that all major criteria or the first three major criteria plus the minor criteria are met.

[‡]The diagnosis of primary myelofibrosis requires that all three major criteria and at least one minor criterion are met.

[§]First major criterion definition for prefibrotic/early myelofibrosis only (not applicable to overt myelofibrosis).

[‖]First major criterion definition for overt myelofibrosis only (not applicable to prefibrotic/early myelofibrosis).

[¶]In the absence of any of the three major clonal mutations, a search for other mutations associated with myeloid neoplasms (e.g., *ASXL1, EZH2, TET2, IDH1, IDH2, SRSF2,* and *SF3B1* mutations) may be of help in determining the clonal nature of disease.

[**]Minor (grade 1) reticulin fibrosis secondary to infection, autoimmune disorder, or other chronic inflammatory conditions, hairy cell leukemia, or another lymphoid neoplasm, metastatic malignancy, or toxic (chronic) myelopathies.

ICC = International Consensus Classification; LDH = lactate dehydrogenase.

Patients with myelofibrosis exhibit the greatest symptom burden among the Philadelphia chromosome–negative myeloproliferative neoplasms. In addition to mechanical symptoms referable to splenomegaly, hypercatabolic signs and symptoms such as fatigue, night sweats, low-grade fevers, weight loss, pruritus, gout, and joint or bone pain (most commonly involving the lower extremities) tend to become more omnipresent and severe with disease evolution.

DIAGNOSIS

Diagnostic Criteria for Polycythemia Vera, Essential Thrombocythemia, and Primary Myelofibrosis

The International Consensus Classification uses a combination of histopathologic, laboratory, and molecular data to establish major and minor criteria for the diagnosis of polycythemia vera, essential thrombocythemia, and primary myelofibrosis (Table 152-3). To mitigate the risk of periprocedural bleeding, testing for acquired von Willebrand disease (Chapter 159) should be considered in patients who have elevated platelet counts (e.g., 1 to 1.5 million/µL) associated with major bruising or bleeding or in patients undergoing surgery or delivery of a pregnancy.

Other Causes of Erythrocytosis and Thrombocytosis

For patients presenting with an elevated hemoglobin, history taking should first try to determine whether a spurious erythrocytosis may be present due to hemoconcentration (seen in patients with volume depletion related to conditions such as burns, diarrhea, and diuretics). Family history is important for evaluating congenital forms of erythrocytosis, including causes associated with a decreased p50 (the oxygen tension at which hemoglobin is 50% saturated) such as a high-oxygen-affinity hemoglobin, 2,3-bisphosphoglycerate (2,3-BPG) deficiency, or methemoglobinemia (Chapter 144). Congenital forms of erythrocytosis associated with a normal p50 include mutations in the genes encoding *EPO*[9] or the *EPO* receptor and mutations of genes involved in the oxygen-sensing pathway (e.g., *VHL, HIF2A,* and *PHD2*) (Table 152-4). Erythrocytosis mutation panels are now commercially available to test for such variants.

In secondary types of acquired erythrocytosis (see Table 152-4), only red blood cells are increased, whereas in polycythemia vera, red blood cells, as well as the white blood count and platelet count, may be increased because only the latter is a pluripotent hematopoietic stem cell disorder. Molecular testing has greatly facilitated the evaluation of acquired forms of erythrocytosis; in this clinical context, identification of *JAK2* V617F (in 95 to 98% of patients with polycythemia vera) or an exon 12 *JAK2* mutation establishes the diagnosis of polycythemia vera. Iron deficiency and a subnormal EPO level (the latter is a minor diagnostic criterion) are common laboratory findings in polycythemia vera.

Similar to erythrocytosis, the evaluation of thrombocytosis is first directed to ruling out reactive causes, which are much more common than essential thrombocythemia (see Table 152-5). Hereditary forms of thrombocytosis are rare and may be related to germline mutations in the genes encoding thrombopoietin (*THPO*), gelsolin, or *MPL* and *JAK2*, which are distinct from the somatic *MPL* W515 L/K and *JAK2* V617F variants.

If essential thrombocythemia or primary myelofibrosis is suspected and molecular testing is negative for *JAK2* V617F, screening for *CALR* and/or *MPL* mutations is undertaken. Bone marrow examination with expert pathology interpretation is critical to distinguish between essential thrombocythemia (Fig. 152-4), prefibrotic myelofibrosis, and overt primary myelofibrosis (Fig. 152-5) and between clonal and reactive forms of myeloproliferation, particularly in cases where a clonal marker cannot be found (e.g., triple-negative patients). The peripheral blood smear may demonstrate large or giant platelets in all three myeloproliferative neoplasms. In primary myelofibrosis, variable degrees of leukoerythroblastosis may be observed, consisting of circulating immature granulocytes and nucleated and teardrop red blood cells (dacrocytes) (Chapter 143). Increased numbers of circulating $CD34^+$ cells can be detected in the blood, and their numbers increase with disease severity. The bone marrow reveals myeloid hyperplasia, clustered atypical megakaryocytes, and variable degrees of reticulin (or collagen) fibrosis (as well as osteosclerosis) depending on disease stage (see Fig. 152-5). Specific clinical and laboratory criteria have been codified for a diagnosis of post–polycythemia vera myelofibrosis

TABLE 152-4 DIFFERENTIAL DIAGNOSIS OF ERYTHROCYTOSIS

SPURIOUS ERYTHROCYTOSIS (also referred to as relative polycythemia, stress erythrocytosis, stress polycythemia, benign polycythemia, Gaisböck syndrome, and pseudopolycythemia)

A. Cases are characterized by an increased hematocrit and normal or decreased red blood cell (RBC) total mass resulting from a decreased plasma volume. Hemoconcentration can result from vomiting or diarrhea, burns, aggressive diuretic therapy, decreased fluid intake, diabetic ketoacidosis, and renal disease. Stress and hypertension can also be associated with a decreased plasma volume.

CONGENITAL ERYTHROCYTOSIS

A. Associated with reduced p50 (partial pressure of oxygen at which 50% of hemoglobin is saturated with oxygen)
  i. Mutant high-oxygen-affinity hemoglobinopathy
  ii. 2,3-Bisphosphoglycerate deficiency
  iii. Methemoglobinemia
B. Associated with normal p50
  i. *VHL* mutations (Chuvash polycythemia)
  ii. *PHD2* mutations
  iii. *HIF2A* mutations
  iv. *EPO* receptor mutations
  v. *EPO* gain-of-function mutation

ACQUIRED ERYTHROCYTOSIS

A. Primary (clonal): Polycythemia vera (associated with low EPO level)
B. Secondary (associated with normal to high EPO levels)
  i. Chronic hypoxia states
    (1) Chronic lung disease
    (2) Right-to-left cardiopulmonary shunts
    (3) High-altitude habitat
    (4) Tobacco use or carbon monoxide poisoning
    (5) Sleep apnea or hypoventilation syndrome
    (6) Renal artery stenosis
  ii. Hypoxia-independent
    (1) Use of androgens (e.g., testosterone; danazol)
    (2) Use of erythropoietin
    (3) Post–renal transplant
    (4) Anti-VEGF therapy
    (5) Erythropoietin-secreting tumors: hepatocellular carcinoma, renal cell carcinoma, (cerebellar) hemangioblastoma, uterine leiomyoma, meningioma, carcinoid tumor, metanephric adenoma, pheochromocytoma, parathyroid adenoma
    (6) POEMS

EPO = erythropoietin; POEMS = polyneuropathy, organomegaly, endocrinopathy, M protein, and skin (changes) syndrome; VEGF = vascular endothelial growth factor.

TABLE 152-5 DIFFERENTIAL DIAGNOSIS OF THROMBOCYTOSIS

PRIMARY (CLONAL)	SECONDARY (REACTIVE)
ESSENTIAL THROMBOCYTHEMIA	**INFECTION**
OTHER MYELOID NEOPLASMS	Acute bacterial/viral infections
Primary myelofibrosis	Chronic infections (e.g., tuberculosis)
Chronic myeloid leukemia	**NONMALIGNANT BLOOD CONDITIONS**
Del(5q) myelodysplastic syndrome	Iron deficiency anemia
Myelodysplastic/myeloproliferative neoplasms with ring sideroblasts and thrombocytosis (MDS)/MPN-RS-T	Acute blood loss
	Acute hemolytic anemia
	Rebound following use of chemotherapy
	Rebound following treatment of ITP
	Rebound from ETOH-related thrombocytopenia
	AUTOIMMUNE/INFLAMMATORY CONDITIONS
	Inflammatory bowel disease
	Vasculitides
	Rheumatoid arthritis
	Celiac disease
	MALIGNANCIES
	Lymphoma
	Metastatic cancer
	POEMS
	MEDICATIONS
	Thrombopoietin receptor agonists
	All-trans retinoic acid (ATRA)
	Interleukin-1β
	Vincristine
	Epinephrine
	Glucocorticoids
	TISSUE DAMAGE
	Severe trauma, burns
	Acute pancreatitis
	Myocardial infarction
	Postsurgical period (e.g., CABG)
	ALLERGIC REACTION
	EXERCISE

CABG = coronary artery bypass graft; ETOH = alcohol; ITP = immune (or idiopathic) thrombocytopenic purpura; MDS = myelodysplastic syndrome; POEMS = polyneuropathy, organomegaly, endocrinopathy, M protein, and skin (changes) syndrome.

and post–essential thrombocythemia myelofibrosis, including confirmation of a prior diagnosis of polycythemia vera or essential thrombocythemia and minimal thresholds of bone marrow fibrosis. Table 152-6 lists other causes of fibrosis involving the bone marrow.

TREATMENT

Essential Thrombocythemia and Polycythemia Vera

For patients with essential thrombocythemia and polycythemia vera, no therapy has been shown to alter the natural history of disease (e.g., transformation to post–polycythemia vera or post–essential thrombocythemia myelofibrosis, acute myeloid leukemia, or overall survival), and therapies are aimed at mitigating the risk of future vascular events and disease-related constitutional symptoms.[10] The therapeutic approaches to the two conditions have many similarities (Table 152-7).

Aspirin

Low-dose aspirin (100 mg daily), which is foundational to the treatment of polycythemia vera regardless of risk group, results in an approximately 60% reduction in the relative risk of the composite end point of nonfatal myocardial infarction, nonfatal stroke, or death from cardiovascular causes, without significantly increasing the risk of major bleeding.

In essential thrombocythemia, treatment decisions are based on the classification of patients into very low-, low-, intermediate-, and high-risk groups according to the revised International Prognostic Score for Essential Thrombocythemia (IPSET)–thrombosis risk stratification. For patients with very low-risk essential thrombocythemia (age ≤60 years, no *JAK2* mutation, no prior history of thrombosis), aspirin or observation alone may be considered. Pharmacologic data suggest an optimal aspirin regimen of 100 mg twice daily to maximize platelet inhibition without adverse effects.[A1] For a patient with low-risk essential thrombocythemia (age ≤60 years, with *JAK2* mutation, no prior history of thrombosis) or intermediate-risk essential thrombocythemia (age >60 years, no *JAK2* mutation, no prior history of thrombosis), only aspirin (81 mg daily) is recommended.

Cytoreductive Therapy

Cytoreductive therapy should be administered to patients who have high-risk essential thrombocythemia (history of thrombosis at any age or age >60 years with *JAK2* mutation), patients who have high-risk polycythemia vera, and patients who have lower-risk forms of essential thrombocythemia or polycythemia vera but who develop any signs or symptoms of new thrombosis, acquired von Willebrand disease, disease-related major bleeding, symptomatic progressive splenomegaly, progressive leukocytosis or thrombocytosis, worsening disease-related symptoms (pruritus, night sweats, fatigue), or vasomotor/microvascular disturbances (headaches, chest pain, erythromelalgia) refractory to aspirin.[11]

For polycythemia vera, intensive treatment to maintain a hematocrit target of less than 45% results in an almost four-fold reduction in the risk of cardiovascular death and major thrombosis compared with a hematocrit target of 45 to 50%. A lower hematocrit cutoff (42%) may be appropriate for females (attributed to their lower red blood cell mass compared with males) or for patients with progressive symptoms, but no randomized data are available to support this recommendation.

Hydroxyurea or pegylated interferons are generally considered front-line therapy, but interferons have become increasingly preferred in younger patients due to their ability to elicit high rates of hematologic remissions and molecular responses, without evidence of leukemogenicity.

Hydroxyurea

In high-risk essential thrombocythemia, hydroxyurea can reduce the risk of thrombosis from about 25% to about 5%. Hydroxyurea plus low-dose aspirin is at least as good as anagrelide plus low-dose aspirin and is recommended as first-line therapy for essential thrombocytopenia.[12] Initial and subsequent dosing of hydroxyurea is tailored to individual blood counts and tolerance. A typical starting dose is 500 to 1000 mg daily.

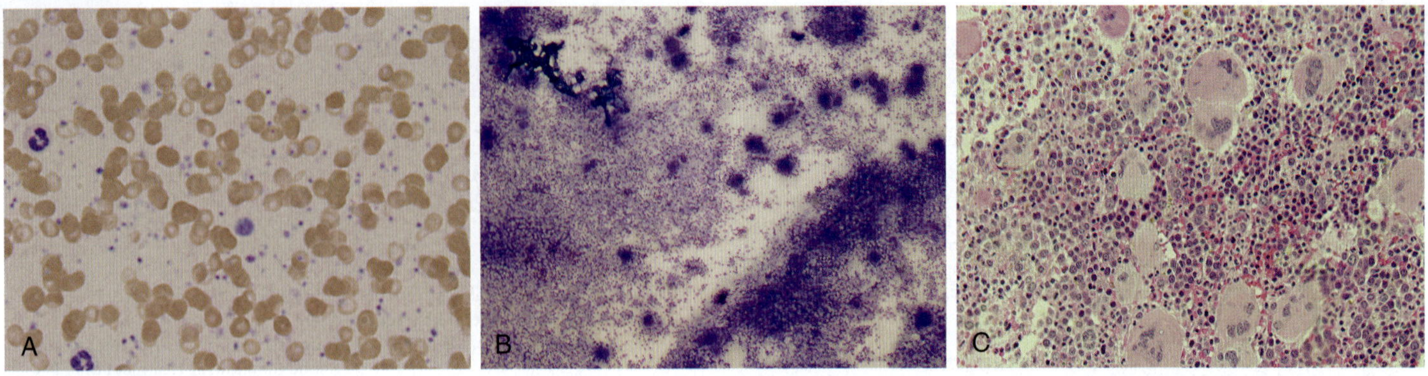

FIGURE 152-4. **Histopathology of essential thrombocythemia. A,** Peripheral blood demonstrating increased numbers of platelets, including large forms. Bone marrow aspirate (B) and core biopsy (C) revealing a marked increase in numbers of megakaryocytes.

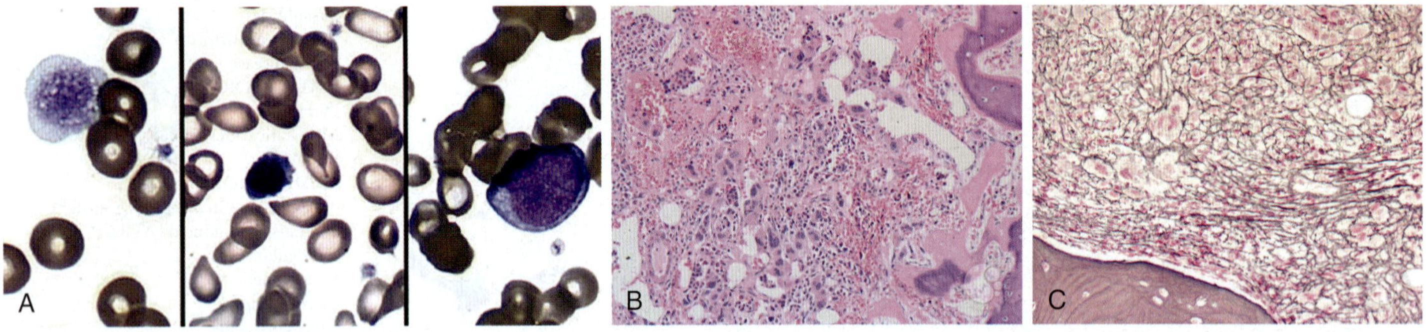

FIGURE 152-5. **Histopathology of primary myelofibrosis. A,** Leukoerythroblastic blood findings in primary myelofibrosis including a large platelet, teardrop red blood cells (dacrocytes), and a myeloblast. **B,** Core bone marrow biopsy showing megakaryocyte clustering with thick irregular bone trabeculae with osteomyelosclerosis (H&E stain × 100). **C,** Reticulin stain of bone marrow biopsy confirms extensive (grade MF-3) fibrosis. (*B and C,* Courtesy American Society of Hematology image bank, https://imagebank.hematology.org/.)

TABLE 152-6 CAUSES OF BONE MARROW FIBROSIS

MYELOID NEOPLASMS/DISORDERS
Primary myelofibrosis
Chronic myeloid leukemia
Myelodysplastic syndromes
Myelodysplastic/myeloproliferative neoplasms
Systemic mastocytosis
Chronic eosinophilic leukemias
Acute myeloid leukemias (including acute myelofibrosis/acute megakaryocytic leukemia)
Gray platelet syndrome
LYMPHOID NEOPLASMS
Hairy cell leukemia
Multiple myeloma
Lymphomas
HISTIOCYTIC AND DENDRITIC CELL NEOPLASMS
Langerhans cell histiocytosis
NONHEMATOLOGIC CONDITIONS
Autoimmune myelofibrosis
Connective tissue disorders
Chronic infections (e.g., tuberculosis)
Vitamin D deficiency (rickets)
Renal osteodystrophy
Pulmonary hypertension
Metastatic cancers (e.g., prostate, breast, gastric)

TABLE 152-7 RISK-BASED STRATIFICATION OF TREATMENT OPTIONS IN ESSENTIAL THROMBOCYTHEMIA AND POLYCYTHEMIA VERA

RISK GROUP*	ESSENTIAL THROMBOCYTHEMIA	POLYCYTHEMIA VERA
Very-low	Observation	N/A
Low	Low-dose aspirin	Low-dose aspirin + phlebotomy
Intermediate	Low-dose aspirin	N/A
High	Low-dose aspirin + cytoreduction Cytoreduction options: Hydroxyurea† or Interferons (based on patient-specific variables)‡ or Anagrelide	Low-dose aspirin + phlebotomy + cytoreduction Cytoreduction options: Hydroxyurea or Interferons (based on patient-specific variables)‡ Ruxolitinib for hydroxyurea-resistant or intolerant patients
	Manage cardiovascular risk factors; monitor for new thrombosis or bleeding; progressive disease-related signs and symptoms (e.g., splenomegaly, leukocytosis, thrombocytosis, pruritus, night sweats, fatigue)	

*Risk groups are defined in the text.
†For older patients, busulfan may be considered in patients not responding to or tolerating hydroxyurea
‡Interferon alfa-2b, peginterferon alfa-2a, or ropeginterferon alfa-2b (approved in the European Union and United States).
N/A = not applicable.

In polycythemia vera, the use of hydroxyurea plus phlebotomy as needed significantly reduces the risk of thrombosis compared with phlebotomy alone, probably without increasing the risk for leukemic transformation. As a result, hydroxyurea is a first-line cytoreductive therapy for polycythemia vera.[13]

Interferons

For patients with essential thrombocythemia or polycythemia vera, interferons (interferon alfa-2b, PEG-interferon alfa-2a, or PEG-interferon alfa-2b) are an alternative first-line treatment to hydroxyurea, particularly for younger patients or for pregnant women who need cytoreductive therapy (see Table 152-7). The addition of a polyethylene glycol (PEG) moiety to IFN-α results in a longer half-life, which translates into less frequent administration, more drug stability, less immunogenicity, and less toxicity and is favored by most practitioners. Nevertheless, depending on the study, PEG-interferons have resulted

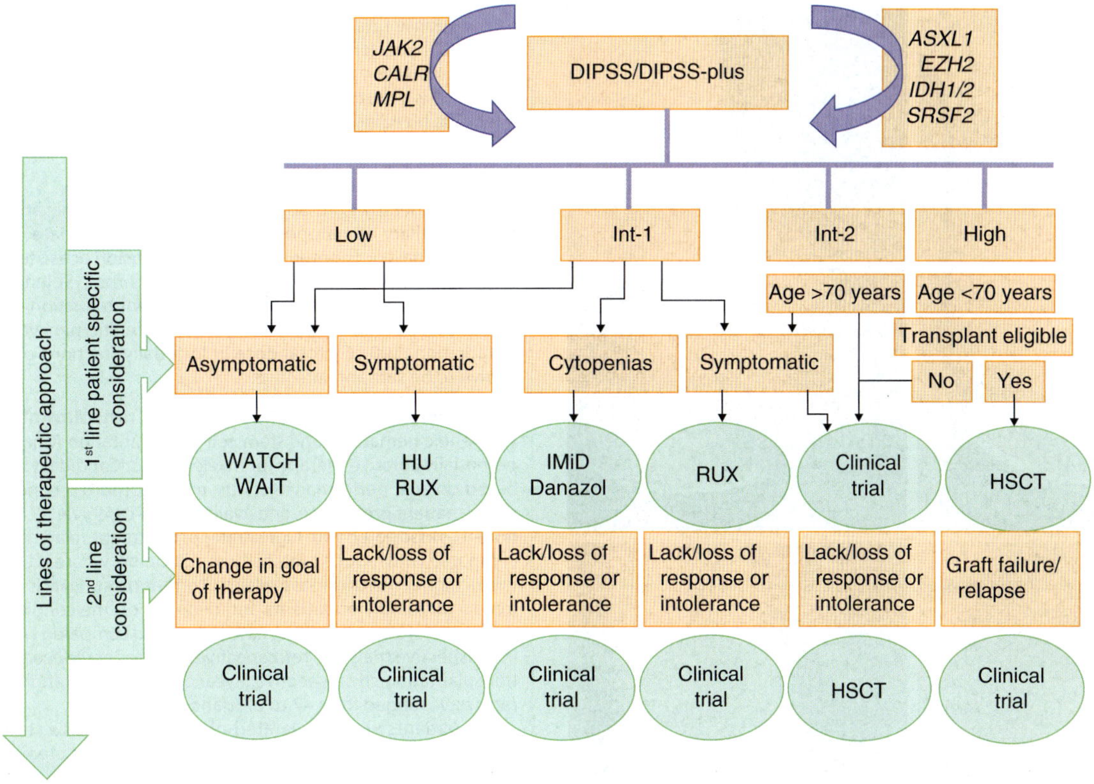

FIGURE 152-6. **Risk-based stratification for treatment decision making in myelofibrosis.** DIPSS = Dynamic International Prognostic Scoring System (see text under "Prognosis" for "Primary Myelofibrosis"); HSCT = hematopoietic stem cell transplant; HU = hydroxyurea; IMiD = immunomodulatory agents; Int = intermediate; RUX = ruxolitinib. (From Mascarenhas J. Looking forward: novel therapeutic approaches in chronic and advanced phases of myelofibrosis. *Hematology Am Soc Hematol Educ Program*. 2015;2015:329-339, Fig 3.)

in treatment discontinuation rates of 15 to 40%. Toxicities include myelosuppression, flulike symptoms (e.g., fatigue, myalgias/arthralgias), transaminitis, autoimmune phenomena, hypothyroidism, and depression.

Studies of PEG-interferon-alfa-2a in patients with polycythemia vera and essential thrombocythemia reveal complete hematologic remission rates of 75 to 95% and complete molecular remission of the *JAK2* V617F mutation in 17 to 24% of patients. The presence of *TET2, ASXL1, EZH2, DNMT3A*, and *IDH1/2* mutations is associated with failure to achieve a complete molecular remission.

In a randomized trial of pegylated IFN-alfa-2a compared with hydroxyurea in high-risk polycythemia vera and essential thrombocythemia, no significant differences were noted in response rates after 24 months.[A2] However, ropeginterferon-alfa-2b provides superior and durable hematologic and molecular response rates compared with hydroxyurea at 5 years.[A3] In low-risk polycythemia vera patients, ropeginterferon-alfa-2b can also increase the ability to maintain the hematocrit <45% in about 85% of patients compared with 60% of patients with phlebotomy alone (p = .0075).[A4]

Anagrelide

Anagrelide (starting at 1 mg twice daily and not to exceed 10 mg/day), which inhibits the maturation of megakaryocytes, can reduce the platelet count in essential thrombocythemia.[A5] However, it may be associated with more thrombotic and bleeding events than hydroxyurea.[A6] As a result, it is a second-line agent.

Ruxolitinib

Ruxolitinib, a *JAK1/JAK2* inhibitor (starting dose 10 mg twice daily), is useful in patients who have phlebotomy-dependent polycythemia vera with or without splenomegaly and an inadequate response to or intolerance of hydroxyurea. It can provide durable responses and improvement of disease-related symptoms, with generally good tolerability.[A7]

Other Agents

Busulfan is an alkylating agent that can be used as an alternative cytoreductive agent in older patients with polycythemia vera or essential thrombocythemia. Special care has to be given to adjusting the dose based on blood counts because prolonged severe myelosuppression/aplasia has been reported.

In polycythemia vera, iron deficiency and increased red blood cell production result in suppression of the master iron homeostasis hormone hepcidin, which in turn leads to increased iron availability for erythropoiesis. Clinical trials are now in progress evaluating whether hepcidin mimetics can reduce phlebotomy requirements in patients with polycythemia.[14]

Primary Myelofibrosis

The Dynamic International Prognostic Scoring System (DIPSS)-(Plus) risk stratification scheme is used to guide decision making regarding treatment options (Fig. 152-6), with clinical trials encouraged in all risk groups. Allogeneic hematopoietic stem cell transplantation is the only curative modality, and all other therapies are used with palliative intent. Transplant generally should be recommended for patients with intermediate-2 or high-risk disease, nontransplant therapy should be recommended for low-risk disease, and more individualized risk counseling is required for patients with intermediate-1 risk disease for which the risk-benefit ratio is less clear. In such individuals, low platelet counts and identification of potentially high molecular–risk mutations (e.g., *ASXL1*) may assist with decision making.

Individuals with asymptomatic low-risk primary myelofibrosis do not require treatment and are monitored regularly for symptoms and signs of disease progression.[15,16] Symptomatic patients with low- or intermediate-risk disease have demonstrated responses in splenomegaly and constitutional symptoms with ruxolitinib in nonrandomized studies. Although interferons can elicit hematologic responses, reduction of splenomegaly, and improvement of bone marrow histopathology in earlier stages of myelofibrosis, responses in more advanced forms of disease are modest.

Medical Therapy

Ruxolitinib, with dosing based on platelet count under expert supervision, is recommended to treat patients with intermediate- to high-risk primary, post–polycythemia vera myelofibrosis and post–essential thrombocytopenia myelofibrosis to mitigate symptomatic splenomegaly (Fig. 152-7) and disease-related symptoms. Ruxolitinib also is associated with about a 30% reduction in the risk of death. Therapy is generally continued until loss of response (e.g., worsening splenomegaly and/or symptoms or unacceptable toxicity).

The majority of patients treated with ruxolitinib do not experience significant reductions in *JAK2* V617F allele burden or bone marrow fibrosis. High-grade anemia and thrombocytopenia are common with ruxolitinib, usually improve after the first 8 to 12 weeks of therapy, and require careful dose adjustment to maximize efficacy while minimizing myelosuppression. Ruxolitinib is also associated with an increased risk of opportunistic infections, including herpes zoster, reactivation of hepatitis B virus, tuberculosis, and rare cases of progressive multifocal leukoencephalopathy.

JAK inhibitors are useful and reasonably well-tolerated.[17] The JAK2 inhibitor fedratinib (400 mg daily) is first- or second-line therapy for adult patients with intermediate-2 or high-risk primary or secondary (post–polycythemia vera or post–essential thrombocythemia) myelofibrosis and a baseline platelet count of ≥50,000 μL based on its ability to reduce splenic volume.[A8] However, it has a black box warning because of a potential increased risk of serious and fatal Wernicke encephalopathy. Thiamine levels must be checked in all patients prior to starting fedratinib and periodically during treatment.

Another *JAK1/JAK2* inhibitor, momelotinib (200 mg daily), is noninferior to ruxolitinib in reducing splenic volume,[A9] but is not as good for reducing the

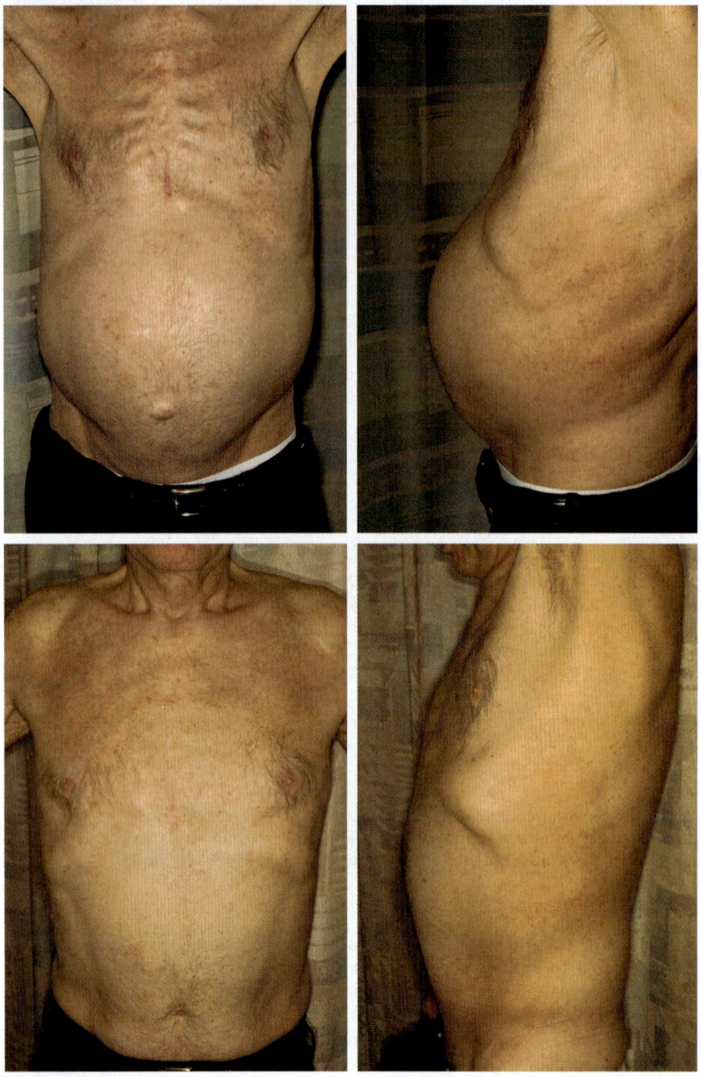

FIGURE 152-7. JAK inhibition in myelofibrosis. Marked reduction in massive splenomegaly after 2 months of JAK inhibitor therapy. (Photos courtesy Dr. Srdan Verstovsek, MD Anderson Cancer Center.)

symptomatic burden. In patients previously treated with ruxolitinib, momelotinib is not superior to best available therapy in reducing spleen volume.[A10] However, momelotinib may be useful to mitigate myelofibrosis-associated anemia by reducing hepcidin levels.

Pacritinib (200 mg twice daily)[A11,A12] is an oral multikinase inhibitor that targets JAK2 (as well as FLT3, CSF1R, and IRAK1) that can reduce splenic volume and improve symptoms, even in patients with severe baseline cytopenias. It is FDA-approved for myelofibrosis patients with a platelet count <50,000/μL.

Other drugs being evaluated as monotherapy or in combination with JAK inhibitors in the front- or second-line therapy include telomerase inhibitors (imetelstat), BET inhibitors (e.g., CPI-06010), BCL-2 inhibitors (e.g., navitoclax), lysine-specific demethylase 1 (LSD1) inhibitors (e.g., bomedemstat), MDM2 blockade (e.g., KRT-232), and various antifibrotic agents that target the bone marrow microenvironment.

Anemia is an unmet need not served (and often worsened) with ruxolitinib treatment. In addition to support with red blood cell transfusions, erythropoiesis-stimulating agents under expert supervision have exhibited responses in about one-third of patients with myelofibrosis. Androgens such as danazol (200 to 300 mg twice daily) can improve anemia in 20 to 30% of individuals, more commonly in non–transfusion-dependent patients. Prostate cancer screening and monitoring of liver function tests are recommended for patients receiving danazol. Luspatercept, which is an erythroid maturation agent that acts as an activin receptor type IIB fusion protein ligand trap that targets the transforming growth factor beta pathway, is currently under evaluation in myelofibrosis patients with anemia.

Splenectomy

The need for splenectomy has probably decreased since the availability of ruxolitinib. Nevertheless, patients who have symptomatic splenomegaly refractory to JAK inhibitors and hydroxyurea may respond to splenectomy, with about a 67% response rate for splenomegaly-related discomfort, a 50% response rate for portal hypertension, and a 23% response rate for transfusion-dependent anemia. However, surgical-related mortality is about 9%, and surgical-related morbidity is about 30%. Postsplenectomy complications (Chapter 154) include infection, bleeding, thrombosis, hepatomegaly, and extreme thrombocytosis or leukocytosis.

Radiation Therapy

Radiation therapy is an option for both hepatosplenic and nonhepatosplenic extramedullary hematopoiesis, which can be associated with complications such as spinal cord compression, pleural effusion or ascites, pulmonary hypertension, cardiac tamponade, and hydronephrosis. Splenic irradiation (100 to 500 cGy in 5 to 10 fractions) induces transient reduction in splenomegaly but can be associated with persistent, life-threatening pancytopenia. Lower doses of radiation (100 cGy total dose in four daily fractions of 25 cGy) have been shown to be safe and effective.

Allogeneic Hematopoietic Stem Cell Transplantation

Allogeneic hematopoietic stem cell transplantation (Chapter 163) is the only potentially curative therapy for myelofibrosis. Candidacy for transplantation is based on age, performance status, major comorbid conditions, psychosocial status, patient preference, and availability of caregiver(s). Myeloablative conditioning is associated with higher rates of treatment-related nonrelapse mortality compared with reduced-intensity conditioning, whereas the latter is associated with a higher risk of disease relapse. Long-term survival is observed in approximately 30 to 60% of patients and depends on the conditioning regimen and the source of stem cells (e.g., matched-sibling compared with unrelated donor). In prospective trials and retrospective analyses of reduced-intensity allogeneic transplantation, the respective 5-year overall survival and nonrelapse mortality rates have ranged from 47 to 67% and 16 to 24%.

For patients with accelerated-phase myelofibrosis (10 to 19% circulating blasts), reduced-intensity allogeneic hematopoietic stem cell transplantation can provide an estimated 5-year overall survival of 65% and a 5-year incidence of relapse of 30%.[18]

Special Situations

Pregnancy in the setting of polycythemia vera and essential thrombocythemia is a higher-risk clinical situation that warrants consultation with a high-risk obstetrician. Patients with essential thrombocythemia have an increased risk of first trimester pregnancy loss. The *JAK2* V617F mutation is an adverse prognostic factor for pregnancy outcome, and retrospective analyses have shown that low-dose aspirin is associated with a reduction in pregnancy complications, especially in patients with *JAK2*-mutated essential thrombocythemia. In low-risk pregnancy, low-dose aspirin is recommended throughout pregnancy, and low-molecular-weight heparin for 6 weeks postpartum; for high-risk pregnancy (previous microcirculatory disturbances, presence of two or more hereditary thrombophilic factors, severe complications in a previous pregnancy, age >35 years, and platelet count >1,000,000/μL), prophylactic low-molecular-weight heparin with low-dose aspirin is recommended throughout pregnancy and the postpartum period. Interferon is generally considered safe during pregnancy and is the preferred agent when cytoreduction is required and its benefits to the mother outweigh potential risks to the fetus. Hydroxyurea should be avoided, including during the breast-feeding period.

Given the thrombohemorrhagic diatheses observed in myeloproliferative neoplasms, optimization of blood counts (e.g., with phlebotomy or cytoreduction) is a high priority before elective surgery. Multidisciplinary collaboration with the surgical team is recommended to evaluate the type and duration of prophylactic antiplatelet or anticoagulation therapy needed in the perioperative setting, in conjunction with close surveillance of thromboembolism.

PROGNOSIS

Polycythemia Vera and Essential Thrombocythemia

Survival

In polycythemia vera, older age, leukocytosis, venous thrombosis, and abnormal karyotype adversely affect survival, with median survivals ranging from about 11 years to about 28 years. The cumulative incidence of transformation to leukemia is 2.3% at 10 years, 5.5% at 15 years, and 7.9% at 20 years. Resistance to hydroxyurea is associated with a 5.6-fold increase in the risk of death and a 6.8-fold increase in the risk of transformation to post–polycythemia vera myelofibrosis and AML.

In patients with essential thrombocythemia, age 60 years or older, leukocyte count of ≥11,000/μL, and prior thrombosis are associated with poorer survival. Based on weighted points assigned to these variables, patients were allocated to three risk categories: low (0 points; median survival not reached); intermediate (1 to 2 points; median survival 24.5 years); and high (3 to 4 points; median survival 13.8 years) (E-Table 152-2). The incidence of leukemic transformation is less than 5% in patients with essential thrombocythemia.

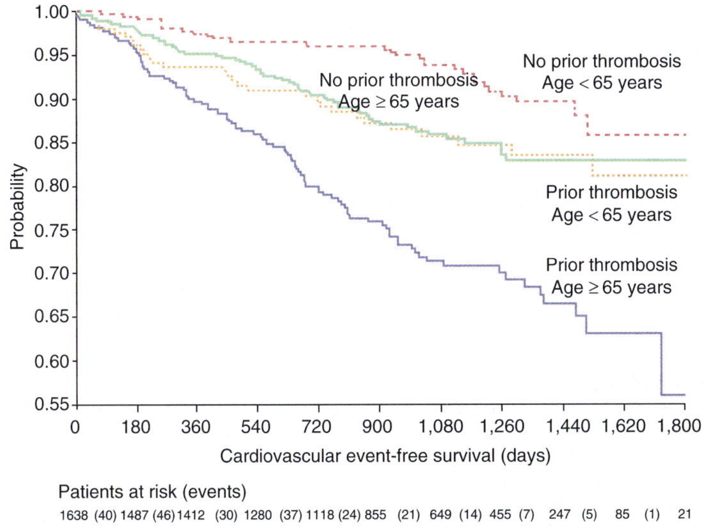

Risk group	# events/ 100 persons/year
Age <65 without prior thrombosis	2.5
Age ≥65 without prior thrombosis	4.9
Age <65 with prior thrombosis	5.0
Age ≥65 with prior thrombosis	10.9

FIGURE 152-8. **Cardiovascular event–free survival of 1638 patients with polycythemia vera according to age and history of thrombosis.**

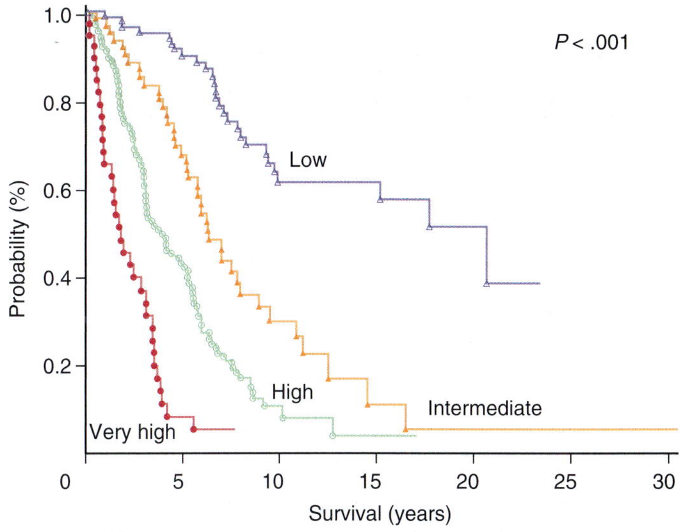

FIGURE 152-9. **Mutation-enhanced International Prognostic Score System 70-Plus: mutation-enhanced international prognostic score system for patients with primary myelofibrosis. Mayo training cohort. (Adapted from Guglielmelli P, Lasho TL, Rotunno G, et al. MIPSS70: mutation-enhanced international prognostic score system for transplantation-age patients with primary myelofibrosis. *J Clin Oncol.* 2018;36:310-318, Fig 1 and Table 3.)**

Thrombosis

Conventional assessment of thrombosis risk in essential thrombocythemia (and polycythemia vera) separates patients into low- and high-risk categories based on the absence or presence of either age older than 60 years or history of thrombosis (Fig. 152-8). Marked thrombocytosis (e.g., platelet count >1.5 million/µL) is associated with a higher risk of bleeding than thrombosis.

An international study of patients with essential thrombocythemia identified cardiovascular risk factors and *JAK2* V617F mutation status as additional independent risk factors that were used to validate a three-tiered prognostic model (IPSET-thrombosis) consisting of low-, intermediate-, and high-risk patients with respective thrombosis risks of 1.03%, 2.35%, and 3.56% of patients/year (see E-Table 152-2). IPSET-thrombosis outperformed the two-tiered (low-risk 0.95% of patients/year vs. high-risk 2.86% of patients/year) risk stratification in predicting future vascular events.

Subsequent analysis of IPSET-thrombosis revealed that among low-risk patients, thrombosis risk was significantly lower in patients with nonmutated *JAK2* in the absence of cardiovascular risk factors (0.44%) compared with when they are present (1.05%). In addition, the risk of thrombosis in the presence of the *JAK2* mutation without cardiovascular risk factors and in the presence of both *JAK2* mutation and cardiovascular risk factors were 1.59% and 2.57%, respectively. These observations led to the development of the revised IPSET-thrombosis scoring system, which has been independently validated and stratifies patients into four risk groups: very low risk (age ≤60 years, no prior history of thrombosis, and no *JAK2* mutation); low risk (age ≤60 years, no prior history of thrombosis, and having a *JAK2* mutation); intermediate risk (age >60 years, no prior history of thrombosis, and no *JAK2* mutation), and high risk (prior history of thrombosis and/or age >60 years with a *JAK2* mutation).

Primary Myelofibrosis

The Dynamic International Prognostic Scoring System (DIPSS)-Plus utilizes eight clinical and laboratory parameters to refine risk prognostication in patients with primary myelofibrosis: age >65 years, hemoglobin <10 g/dL, leukocyte count >25,000/µL, circulating blasts ≥1%, constitutional symptoms, unfavorable karyotype, red cell transfusion need, and platelet count <100,000/µL. Four risk categories were generated based on the number of adverse points: low risk (zero adverse points); intermediate-1 risk (1 adverse point); intermediate-2 risk (2 to 3 adverse points); and high risk (4 to 6 adverse points), with respective median survivals of 180, 80, 35, and 16 months. In a multivariate analysis, platelet count <100,000/µL and unfavorable cytogenetics were independent predictors of leukemia-free survival. The Mutation-enhanced International Prognostic Scoring System (MIPSS)-Plus prognostic scoring system integrates mutational data (absence of *CALR* type-1 mutation, presence of a high–molecular risk mutation [i.e., *ASXL1, EZH2, SRSF2, IDH1/2*], and presence of two or more high–molecular risk mutations) in addition to clinical and cytogenetic information to improve risk stratification in transplantation-eligible patients (Fig. 152-9).[19] The MIPSS70+ version 2.0 prognostic scoring system provides additional information about risk with the addition of a very high-risk cytogenetic category and the high-risk *U2AF1* Q157 mutation.

GENERAL REFERENCES

For the General References and other additional features, please visit Elsevier eBooks+ at https://ebooks.health.elsevier.com.

Grade A References

A1. Rocca B, Tosetto A, Betti S, et al. A randomized double-blind trial of 3 aspirin regimens to optimize antiplatelet therapy in essential thrombocythemia. *Blood.* 2020;136:171-182.
A2. Mascarenhas J, Kosiorek HE, Prchal JT, et al. A randomized, phase 3, trial of interferon-alfa versus hydroxyurea in polycythemia vera and essential thrombocythemia. *Blood.* 2022;139:2931-2941.
A3. Gisslinger H, Klade C, Georgiev P, et al. Ropeginterferon-2b versus standard therapy for polycythaemia vera (PROUD-PV and CONTINUATION-PV): a randomised, non-inferiority, phase 3 trial and its extension study. *Lancet Haematol.* 2020;7:e196-e208.
A4. Barbui T, Vannucchi AM, De Stefano V, et al. Ropeginterferon alfa-2b versus phlebotomy in low-risk patients with polycythemia vera (Low-PV study): a multicentre, randomized phase 2 trial. *Lancet Haematol.* 2021;8:e175-e184.
A5. Samuelson B, Chai-Adisaksopha C, Garcia D. Anagrelide compared with hydroxyurea in essential thrombocythemia: a meta-analysis. *J Thromb Thrombolysis.* 2015;40:474-479.
A6. Gotic M, Egyed M, Gercheva L, et al. Cardiovascular safety of anagrelide hydrochloride versus hydroxyurea in essential thrombocythaemia. *Cardiovasc Toxicol.* 2021;21:236-247.
A7. Passamonti, Palandri F, Saydam G, et al. Ruxolitinib versus best available therapy in inadequately controlled polycythaemia vera without splenomegaly (RESPONSE-2): 5-year follow up of a randomized, phase 3b study. *Lancet Haematol.* 2022;9:e480-e492.
A8. Pardanani A, Harrison C, Cortes JE, et al. Safety and efficacy of fedratinib in patients with primary or secondary myelofibrosis: a randomized clinical trial. *JAMA Oncol.* 2015;1:643-651.
A9. Mesa RA, Kidladjian JJ, Catalano JV, et al. SIMPLIFY-1: a phase III randomized trial of momelotinib versus ruxolitinib in janus kinase inhibitor-naïve patients with myelofibrosis. *J Clin Oncol.* 2017;35:3844-3850.
A10. Harrison CN, Vannucchi AM, Platzbecker U, et al. Momelotinib versus best available therapy in patients with myelofibrosis previously treated with ruxolitinib (SIMPLIFY 2): a randomised, open-label, phase 3 trial. *Lancet Haematol.* 2018;5:e73-e81.
A11. Mesa RA, Vannucchi AM, Mead A, et al. Pacritinib versus best available therapy for the treatment of myelofibrosis irrespective of baseline cytopenias (PERSIST-1): an international, randomised, phase 3 trial. *Lancet Haematol.* 2017;4:e225-e236.
A12. Mascarenhas J, Hoffman R, Talpaz M, et al. Pacritinib vs best available therapy, including ruxolitinib, in patients with myelofibrosis: a randomized clinical trial. *JAMA Oncol.* 2018;4:652-659.

153

LEUKOCYTOSIS AND LEUKOPENIA

NANCY BERLINER

The normal peripheral white blood cell count (WBC) ranges between 4500/µL and 10,000/µL, with a mean of 7500/µL, and is composed of neutrophils, lymphocytes, monocytes, basophils, and eosinophils. Because neutrophils usually represent about 60% of the peripheral WBC, derangement in the WBC usually reflects elevation or reduction in the absolute neutrophil count. Leukocytosis (an elevated WBC) and leukopenia (a depressed WBC) may be secondary to an underlying disease or exposure, or they may be manifestations of a primary hematologic disorder.

NORMAL NEUTROPHIL DYNAMICS

Neutrophils arise in the bone marrow from multipotent progenitor cells that also give rise to erythrocytes, megakaryocytes, eosinophils, basophils, and monocytes. Neutrophil precursors in the marrow mature over 6 to 10 days to form a storage pool of mature neutrophils (Fig. 153-1). Acetylation of C/EBPε, a member of the CCAAT/enhancer binding protein family of transcription factors, is required for secondary and tertiary granule formation and for terminal neutrophil differentiation. Together, the marrow populations make up about 95% of the body's total granulocyte mass (20% neutrophil precursors, 75% mature bands and neutrophils). The circulating neutrophil pool thus represents only the remaining approximately 5% of the body's total neutrophils, just over half of which at any given time are adherent to the vascular endothelium and pooled in the spleen, a phenomenon termed *margination*. Marginated neutrophils are poised for immediate release into the circulation during stress. The lifespan of neutrophils in the peripheral blood is up to 3 to 4 days. Once in the circulation, neutrophils subsequently migrate into tissues, where they can survive for 1 to 4 days. Changes in neutrophil number reflect these dynamics.

Neutrophilia can occur as the result of increased marrow production, increased release of neutrophils from the storage pool, or mobilization of neutrophils from the marginated pool. Neutropenia may be due to decreased marrow production, increased margination with or without sequestration by the spleen, or increased destruction of peripheral cells.

NEUTROPHILIA

Neutrophilia is usually reactive or secondary to an underlying inflammatory process such as infection, chronic inflammation, stress, drugs, nonhematologic malignancy, marrow stimulation (as in hemolysis or idiopathic thrombocytopenic purpura), or splenectomy. Primary causes of neutrophilia may be congenital, including hereditary neutrophilia, Down syndrome, and leukocyte adhesion deficiency, or they can be acquired, as in chronic myelogenous leukemia (CML) (Chapter 170) and other myeloproliferative neoplasms (Chapter 152) (Table 153-1).

EPIDEMIOLOGY AND PATHOBIOLOGY

Secondary Causes of Neutrophilia

Infection

Many acute bacterial infections can present with leukocytosis with a "left shift," referring to the circulation of more immature myeloid cells. This left shift most commonly is restricted to release of an increased number of band forms; however, in severe stress, one may also see circulating metamyelocytes and even earlier cells ("leukemoid reaction") (see Fig. 153-1) in the peripheral blood. Leukocytosis occurs within minutes to hours of infection owing to release of neutrophils from both the marrow and marginated pools. Examination of these neutrophils on peripheral smear may reveal evidence

TABLE 153-1 DIFFERENTIAL DIAGNOSIS OF NEUTROPHILIA

Primary hematologic etiologies
Congenital neutrophilia
Hereditary neutrophilia
Chronic idiopathic neutrophilia
Down syndrome
Leukocyte adhesion deficiency (LAD)
LAD-1
LAD-2
Acquired hematologic neoplasms
Myeloproliferative neoplasm
Chronic myelogenous leukemia
Polycythemia vera
Secondary to other disease entities
Infection
Acute via release from marginated and storage pools
Chronic via increased myelopoiesis (e.g., tuberculosis, fungal infection, chronic abscess, other chronic infections)
Chronic inflammation
Rheumatic disease: juvenile rheumatoid arthritis, rheumatoid arthritis, Still disease, and others
Inflammatory bowel disease
Granulomatous disease
Chronic hepatitis
Cigarette smoking
Stress
Myocardial infarction
Drug induced
Corticosteroids
β-Agonists
Lithium
Recombinant cytokine administration
Nonhematologic malignancy
Cytokine-secreting tumors (lung, tongue, kidney, urothelial tumors)
Marrow metastasis (myelophthisis)
Marrow stimulation
Hemolytic anemia, immune thrombocytopenia
Recovery from marrow suppression
Recombinant cytokine administration
Post-splenectomy

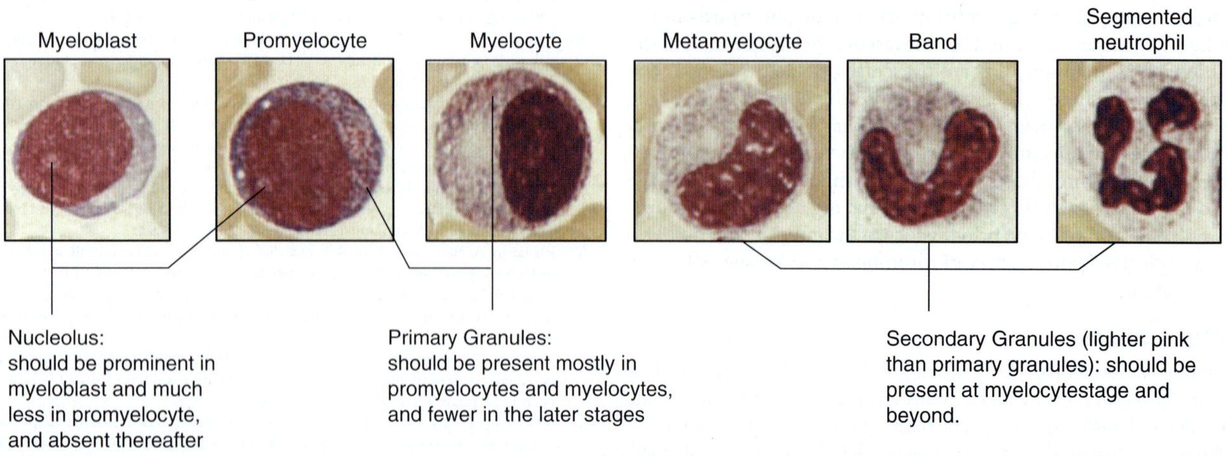

FIGURE 153-1. **Myeloid maturation in the bone marrow. Nucleoli are prominent in myeloblasts, much less frequent in promyelocytes, and absent in more mature forms. Primary granules are present in the cytoplasm of promyelocytes and myelocytes, and secondary granules predominate beyond the myelocyte stage.**

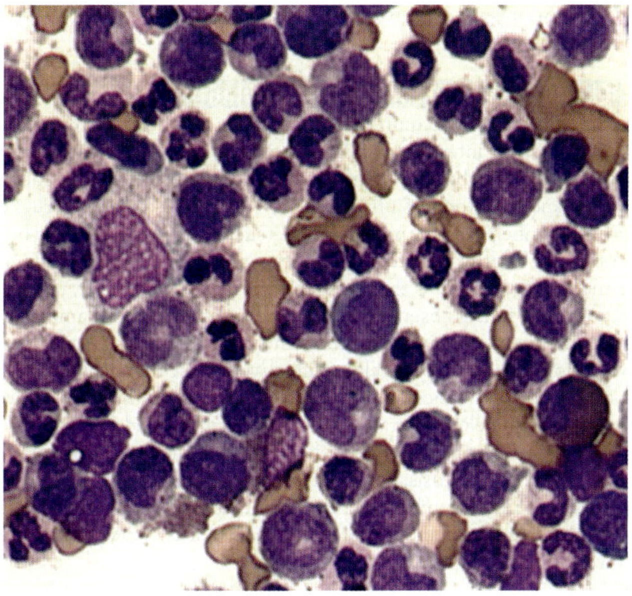

FIGURE 153-2. **Peripheral blood from a patient with leukemoid reaction.** From this smear, it would be impossible to distinguish a leukemoid reaction from chronic phase chronic myelogenous leukemia (Chapter 170). Distinction would depend on determination of the presence or absence of *BCR-ABL* fusion.

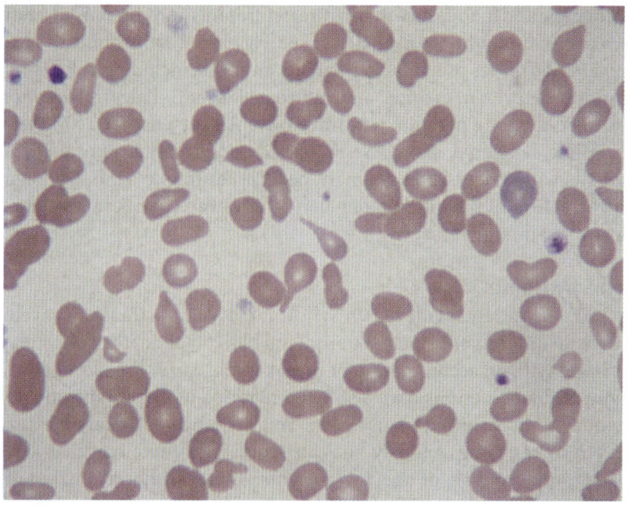

FIGURE 153-3. **Myelophthisic changes in erythrocyte morphology.** Note prominent teardrop forms. (From Rose M, Berliner N. Disorders of red blood cells. In: Andreoli TE, Benjamin IJ, Griggs RC, et al, eds. *Andreoli and Carpenter's Cecil Essentials of Medicine*, 8th ed. Philadelphia: Saunders; 2010:522, Fig. 49-2.)

of toxic granulation (see Fig. 143-18), Döhle bodies (see Fig. 143-19), and cytoplasmic vacuoles. Certain infections (e.g., *Clostridioides difficile* or tuberculosis in particular) are known to cause elevations in the WBC to greater than 30,000/μL in about one fourth of infected patients and may result in a *leukemoid reaction*,[1] defined as a WBC greater than 50,000/μL with a pronounced left shift (Fig. 153-2).

Chronic Inflammation

Leukocytosis due to chronic inflammation results from increased leukocyte (specifically neutrophil and monocyte) production as opposed to altered neutrophil distribution. Mature neutrophil pools become depleted with ongoing inflammation, and the marrow myeloid compartment expands to increase neutrophil production. Myriad cytokines, including tumor necrosis factor-α (TNF-α), granulocyte colony-stimulating factor (G-CSF), granulocyte-macrophage colony-stimulating factor (GM-CSF), macrophage inflammatory protein-1 (MIP-1), interleukin-1 (IL-1), IL-6, and IL-8, have been implicated in this marrow stimulation. Chronic inflammatory conditions that are commonly associated with leukocytosis and neutrophilia include juvenile rheumatoid arthritis, rheumatoid arthritis, Still disease, Crohn disease, ulcerative colitis, granulomatous infection, and chronic hepatitis. The WBC and neutrophil elevation in these cases is typically more modest than that seen in acute infection or inflammation.

Cigarette Smoking

Cigarette smoking can cause a neutrophilia in about 25 to 50% of chronic smokers and can persist for up to 5 years after smoking cessation. The mechanism of neutrophilia is unknown, although evidence suggests that cigarette smoke slows neutrophil apoptosis.

Stress

Within minutes of exercise, surgery, or stress, the number of circulating neutrophils increases, presumably because catecholamines stimulate the demargination of neutrophils. Some cases of stress-induced neutrophilia can be prevented by pretreatment with β-adrenergic antagonists (e.g., propranolol), thereby supporting the role of catecholamines in the demargination process. Exercise-induced neutrophilia, however, is not blocked by propranolol, thereby suggesting that it may instead be due to flow and mechanical perturbation of neutrophils in the lungs.

Myocardial Infarction

An elevated WBC has been described in the setting of acute myocardial infarction. The etiology of this leukocytosis is likely multifactorial and related, in part, to inflammation. Data suggest that individuals with higher white blood cell counts have poorer short- and long-term prognoses.

Drug Induced

The most well-known and widely used drugs associated with leukocytosis are corticosteroids. Other drugs that elevate the neutrophil count include β-agonists and lithium. Lithium causes neutrophilia by increasing the production of endogenous colony-stimulating factors (CSFs). G-CSF or GM-CSF treatment (Chapter 142) likewise causes neutrophilia, and although this is the desired effect, the neutrophilia can be quite pronounced.

Nonhematologic Malignancy

Leukocytosis can be seen in a number of nonhematologic malignancies. Some tumors (lung, head and neck, kidney, bladder) may secrete G-CSF as an ectopic hematopoietic growth factor. In cancer patients with hyperleukocytosis, genomic testing can discriminate myeloproliferative neoplasms from a paraneoplastic leukemoid reaction. Other tumors (lung, stomach, breast), when metastatic to the bone marrow, can cause a *leukoerythroblastic reaction*, characterized by left-shifted leukocytosis, thrombocytosis, and red cell abnormalities including nucleated and teardrop-shaped red blood cells (Fig. 153-3). The presence of nonhematopoietic entities invading the bone marrow (metastatic cancer, fibrosis, granulomatous disease) is termed *myelophthisis*.

Marrow Stimulation

Peripheral destruction of red cells and platelets, as seen with hemolytic anemia and idiopathic thrombocytopenic purpura, can result in stimulation of the bone marrow and a "spillover" leukocytosis. Recovery of cell counts following marrow suppression, as in the case of chemotherapy, can result in a rebound leukocytosis that may last several weeks.

Primary Causes of Neutrophilia

Hereditary Neutrophilia

Hereditary neutrophilia is an autosomal dominant genetic disease that is characterized by an elevated WBC in the 20,000 to 100,000/μL range with splenomegaly and widened diploe of the skull. The neutrophils function normally, and patients have no increased risk for bacterial infection or other sequelae. Hereditary neutrophilia can be caused by an autosomal dominant *GCSF3* gene mutation, which leads to constitutive activation of the G-CSF receptor.

Chronic Idiopathic Neutrophilia

Chronic idiopathic neutrophilia is a condition marked by leukocytosis in the 11,000 to 40,000/μL range with a normal bone marrow biopsy. In one series with a 20-year follow-up, patients with this condition had no medical sequelae from the elevated WBC.

Pelger-Huët Anomaly

Patients with the Pelger-Huët anomaly are often misdiagnosed as having a left-shifted WBC because many of their mature neutrophils are misinterpreted as band forms. Although these patients do not have leukocytosis, the Pelger-Huët anomaly often raises suspicion for an acute infection because of this apparent left shift. Pelger-Huët anomaly is due to a mutation in the lamin B receptor gene and manifests with mature neutrophils and condensed, clumped chromatin within a bilobed nucleus (see Fig. 143-20). A number of drugs can reversibly induce pseudo–Pelger-Huët anomaly, including colchicine, sulfonamides, ibuprofen, taxoids, and valproate. Pseudo–Pelger-Huët anomaly is also seen in some patients with myelodysplasia (Chapter 167). Vitamin B_{12} or folate deficiency can cause increased nuclear lobation of neutrophils in patients with Pelger-Huët anomaly, perhaps leading to a missed diagnosis. With correction of the vitamin deficiency, however, the aberrant neutrophil nuclear morphology returns.

Down Syndrome

Up to 10% of patients with Down syndrome develop a transient myeloproliferative disorder manifesting as peripheral blood leukocytosis with blasts in association with an accumulation of megakaryoblasts in the blood, liver, and marrow. Similar reactions have also been reported in phenotypically normal individuals with trisomy 21 mosaicism. Transient myeloproliferative disorder usually resolves spontaneously but can progress to acute megakaryoblastic leukemia in 23 to 30% of affected patients. This disorder is attributable to acquisition of mutations in the *GATA1* gene, which encodes a key transcription factor for hematopoietic regulation, leading to loss of normal GATA-1 expression and expression of a truncated GATA-1 protein. Evidence supports that these mutations are acquired during fetal life, and patients present in early infancy with transient myeloproliferative disorder. The pathogenesis of progression to acute megakaryoblastic leukemia presumably involves additional genetic and epigenetic events and is the focus of intense study.

Leukocyte Adhesion Deficiency

Patients with leukocyte adhesion deficiency also have persistent leukocytosis, defects in stimulus-dependent activation of neutrophils, recurrent infections, and delayed separation of the umbilical cord. Leukocyte adhesion deficiency is an abnormality of leukocyte adhesion reflecting the loss of surface adhesion molecules. Leukocyte adhesion deficiency-1 is due to absence or marked reduction in the common β chain of β2 integrins, resulting in loss of expression of leukocyte function–associated antigen 1 (LFA-1), the C3bi receptor, and GP150;95. This results in a failure to ingest and kill microbes opsonized by C3bi. In leukocyte adhesion deficiency-2, neutrophils lack sialyl Lewis X, the ligand for L-selectin expressed on endothelial cells. Neutrophils appear morphologically normal but are defective in chemotaxis, adherence, and phagocytosis.

Familial Cold Urticaria

Familial cold urticaria is marked by episodic fevers, leukocytosis, urticaria, rash, conjunctivitis, and muscle and skin tenderness with cold exposure. The rash is composed of infiltrating neutrophils. The syndrome appears to be related to decreased levels of C1-esterase inhibitor and is associated with mutations in the *CIAS1* gene on chromosome 1q.

Chronic Myelogenous Leukemia and Other Myeloproliferative Neoplasms

Chronic myelogenous leukemia (CML; Chapter 170), chronic neutrophilic leukemia, and the other myeloproliferative neoplasms (namely polycythemia vera and essential thrombocythemia; Chapter 152) are the principal acquired primary hematologic disorders associated with neutrophilia. CML on presentation should be distinguished from a leukemoid reaction. In contrast to a leukemoid reaction, CML is characterized by the presence of abnormalities of other blood cell lines ("panmyelosis") and by the presence of specific abnormalities. Therefore, the peripheral blood smear in CML (but not leukemoid reaction) demonstrates increased numbers in all cells of the neutrophilic series, classically with a greater proportion of myelocytes to metamyelocytes, and may display concomitant basophilia, eosinophilia, anemia, and thrombocytosis. Chronic neutrophilic leukemia, a rare myeloproliferative neoplasm, is characterized by hepatosplenomegaly and leukocytosis of at least 25,000/μL, with more than 80% of leukocytes being segmented neutrophil/band forms and less than 10% being immature granulocytes.[2] At least 50% of patients with chronic neutrophilic leukemia harbor mutations in the receptor for CSF-3 (*CSF3R; GCSFR*). Polycythemia vera and essential thrombocythemia, on the other hand, are notable for also having a marked increase in red cell mass and a marked thrombocytosis, respectively, which is often accompanied by leukocytosis.

Post-splenectomy

Patients develop leukocytosis following splenectomy, often long-standing, reflecting the loss of a major site of neutrophil margination. This is of no clinical importance, except insofar as it leads to unnecessary evaluation for other pathology.

CLINICAL MANIFESTATIONS AND DIAGNOSIS

As outlined previously, acquired leukocytosis is most commonly the result of acute or chronic infection or inflammation. When leukocytosis occurs in the absence of fever, aberrations in acute phase reactants, effusions, edema, or other signs and symptoms of inflammation, it may be secondary to drugs or an underlying nonhematologic malignancy. As such, leukocytosis should be seen as the sign of a healthy hematopoietic system responding to an outside stress. Bone marrow evaluation is therefore rarely indicated. However, persistence of leukocytosis in the absence of signs and symptoms of inflammation or infection, nonhematologic malignancy, and offending drugs should prompt an evaluation for a primary myeloproliferative disease or clonal hematologic neoplasm, particularly when there is evidence of a leukoerythroblastic reaction. CML and other myeloproliferative neoplasms can be ruled out by molecular diagnosis on the peripheral blood, as described in Chapter 170. In this setting of unexplained leukocytosis, bone marrow examination is indicated to evaluate for marrow infiltration by infection, tumor, or fibrosis and should include cultures for tuberculosis and fungal infection as well as cytogenetics and flow cytometry (Fig. 153-4).

LEUKOCYTOSIS DUE TO EXPANSION OF OTHER CELL LINES

Monocytosis and lymphocytosis can also elevate the WBC. Monocytosis, defined by an absolute monocyte count of greater than 500/μL, usually occurs in chronic inflammation resulting from infections (e.g., tuberculosis, syphilis, some viruses, and subacute bacterial endocarditis), autoimmune or granulomatous disease, and sarcoidosis.[3] Monocytosis can also be seen in malignancies, (e.g. preleukemic states, nonlymphocytic leukemia including acute myelomonocytic and monocytic leukemia, histiocytosis, Hodgkin disease, non-Hodgkin lymphoma, and various carcinomas).[4] Finally, monocytosis can be seen in the setting of chronic neutropenia, after splenectomy, and in the setting of recovery from marrow suppression (Table 153-2).

Lymphocytosis is defined by an absolute lymphocyte count of more than 5000/μL. The most common causes of lymphocytosis are viral infections such as Epstein-Barr virus (Chapter 348) and the hepatitis viruses (Chapter 134 and 135). Although most bacterial infections cause neutrophilia, pertussis and cat-scratch disease due to *Bartonella henselae* can cause lymphocytosis. Other infections that may cause a secondary lymphocytosis include toxoplasmosis and babesiosis. Hypersensitivity reactions due to drugs or serum sickness may also be associated with lymphocytosis.

Primary disorders causing lymphocytosis include chronic lymphocytic leukemia and monoclonal B-cell lymphocytosis (Table 153-3; see also Chapter 169). Low-count monoclonal B lymphocytosis can be detected in about 5% of adults over age 40 years and rarely progresses to chronic lymphocytic leukemia. By comparison, high-count monoclonal B lymphocytosis progresses to chronic lymphocytic leukemia at a rate of 1 to 2% per year.[5]

Eosinophilia (Chapter 156) is defined by an absolute eosinophil count of more than 400/μL.[6] Eosinophils proliferate under the influence of IL-5 and play a role in phagocytosis and modulating toxicity due to mast cell degranulation in hypersensitivity reactions. Eosinophilia is therefore most often seen in the setting of drug reactions, allergy, atopy, and asthma. A variety of infections, particularly parasitic infections and, to a lesser degree, fungal infections, can cause eosinophilia. Eosinophilia can also be the result of autoimmune and inflammatory conditions, as in eosinophilic granulomatosis with polyangiitis (formerly Churg-Strauss vasculitis). Atheroembolic disease and adrenal insufficiency may also cause eosinophilia. A number of cancers have been associated with polytypical expansion of eosinophils, including lymphomas and solid tumors. Clonal disorders of eosinophils have been observed in the setting of some leukemias. Finally, there is a heterogeneous group of disorders termed *hypereosinophilic syndromes* (Chapter 156). A *FIP1L1-PDGFRA* fusion gene has confirmed that some of these are primary clonal disorders of eosinophils; the clonality of other hypereosinophilic syndromes can be difficult to establish (see Table 156-1).

NEUTROPENIA

The risk for infection with neutropenia is highly dependent on the size of the neutrophil storage pool. Although neutropenia is defined by an absolute neutrophil count of less than 1500/μL, patients with neutrophil counts below this number have different risks and rates of infection depending on

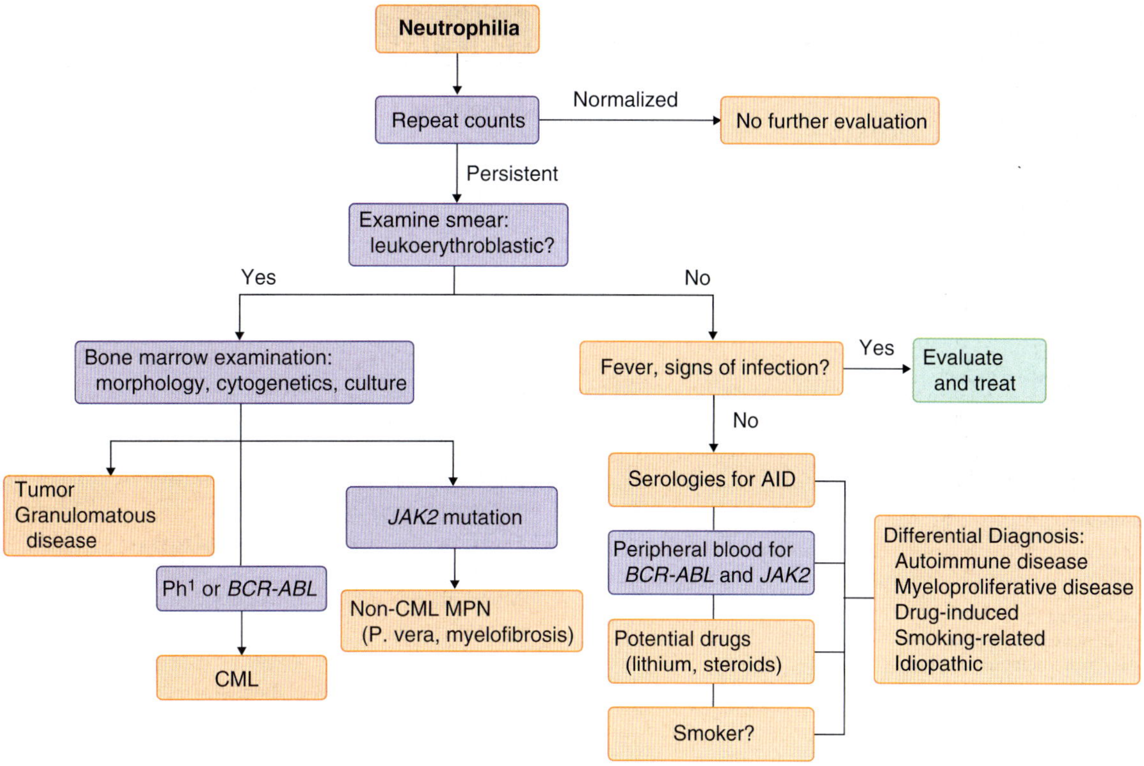

FIGURE 153-4. **Diagnostic approach to neutrophilia.** AID = autoimmune disease; CML = chronic myelogenous leukemia; ET = essential thrombocytopenia; MPN = myeloproliferative neoplasm; Ph^1 = Philadelphia chromosome; PV = P. vera.

TABLE 153-2 DIFFERENTIAL DIAGNOSIS OF MONOCYTOSIS

Infection
Granulomatous disease (tuberculosis, fungal disease)
Endocarditis
Syphilis
Autoimmune diseases
Lupus, rheumatoid arthritis
Giant cell arteritis
Vasculitis
Inflammatory bowel disease
Sarcoid
Malignancy
Primary hematologic malignancy
Chronic myelomonocytic leukemia
Acute myelomonocytic leukemia
Lymphoma
Solid tumors
Neutropenia
Associated with chronic neutropenia
Recovery form marrow suppression
Post-splenectomy

TABLE 153-3 DIFFERENTIAL DIAGNOSIS OF LYMPHOCYTOSIS

Infection
Viral infection
Epstein-Barr virus
Cytomegalovirus
Hepatitis
Bacterial infection
Pertussis
Bartonella
Tuberculosis
Syphilis
Rickettsia
Babesia
Hypersensitivity reactions
Serum sickness
Drug hypersensitivity
Primary hematologic disease
Chronic lymphocytic leukemia
Monoclonal B-cell lymphocytosis
Non-Hodgkin lymphoma

the cause of neutropenia. Patients who are neutropenic from chemotherapy, marrow failure, or marrow exhaustion experience infection at much higher rates than those with chronic neutropenic syndromes and immune-mediated neutropenia. Neutropenia may be congenital or acquired. The following sections first discuss congenital neutropenic disorders, the study of which has provided critical insights into normal myelopoiesis, and then the secondary causes of neutropenia (Table 153-4).

EPIDEMIOLOGY AND PATHOBIOLOGY

Primary Causes of Neutropenia

Normal Neutrophil Count for Duffy A-B- Individuals

The normal range of the neutrophil count is genetically determined and is variable. Several racial and ethnic groups have a relatively large proportion of individuals who are neutropenic by comparison to the published normal range, usually based on young, largely White individuals.[7] Single-nucleotide polymorphisms in the gene for the Duffy antigen receptor for chemokine are postulated to explain racial and ethnic differences in neutrophil counts. This polymorphism is seen among a variety of ethnic groups, including Blacks, Yemenite Jews, Falasha Jews, and African Bedouins.[8] Blood bank testing for Duffy A and B will demonstrate negativity for both antigens, thereby confirming this normal variant. An autosomal dominantly inherited condition called *benign familial neutropenia* is characterized by neutrophil counts in the 800 to 1400/µL range. Neither of these two forms of neutropenia is associated with *any* increased risk for infection.

Severe Congenital Neutropenia

Severe congenital neutropenia presents in the neonatal period with recurrent bacterial infections and neutrophil counts of less than 500/µL. Infections usually occur in the first months of life and often include omphalitis and perirectal abscesses. There is often an increase in monocytes and eosinophils. Bone marrow biopsy reveals a "maturation arrest" with an absence of mature neutrophil elements. Severe congenital neutropenia can follow autosomal

TABLE 153-4 DIFFERENTIAL DIAGNOSIS OF NEUTROPENIA

- Congenital neutropenia
  - Benign familial (constitutional) neutropenia
  - Duffy-null associated neutrophil count (DANC)
  - Severe congenital neutropenia
    - Autosomal dominant (*ELANE* mutation)
    - Autosomal recessive (Kostmann syndrome; *HAX2* mutation)
    - X-linked (*WASP* mutation)
    - Other rare defects (*G-CSFR* mutation, unknown)
  - Cyclic neutropenia
  - Shwachman-Diamond syndrome
  - Fanconi anemia
  - Dyskeratosis congenita
  - Glycogen storage disease type Ib
  - Myelokathexis
  - Chédiak-Higashi syndrome
  - Griscelli syndrome type II
  - Hermansky-Pudlak syndrome II
  - Barth syndrome
- Acquired neutropenia
  - Infection
  - Postinfection
  - Drug induced
  - Immune neutropenia
    - Primary immune neutropenia
    - Secondary to autoimmune disease
      - Rheumatoid arthritis
        - Felty syndrome
        - Large granular lymphocyte disease
      - Systemic lupus erythematosus
      - Granulomatosis with polyangiitis (formerly Wegener granulomatosis)
      - Hyperthyroidism
    - Pure white cell aplasia associated with thymoma
    - Large granular lymphocyte disease (independent of rheumatoid arthritis)
  - Primary bone marrow failure
    - Aplastic anemia
    - Myelodysplastic syndrome
    - Acute leukemia
  - Margination and hypersplenism
  - Vitamin and mineral deficiencies (including B_{12}, folate, copper)
  - Chronic idiopathic neutropenia in adults (CINA)

ELANE = neutrophil elastase gene; G-CSFR = granulocyte colony-stimulating factor receptor; WASP = Wiskott-Aldrich syndrome protein.

TABLE 153-5 CONGENITAL NEUTROPENIA SYNDROMES

SYNDROME	INHERITANCE PATTERN	GENE
SEVERE CONGENITAL NEUTROPENIA	Autosomal dominant	*ELANE* (~60%)
	Autosomal recessive	*HAX1* (~5%)
	X-linked	*WASP* (~5%)
	X-linked	*TAZ* (rare)
	Autosomal recessive	*G6PC3* (~2%)
	Autosomal dominant	*Gfi1* (rare)
	Autosomal dominant	*G-CSFR* (rare)
CYCLIC NEUTROPENIA	Autosomal dominant	*ELANE*
OTHER CONGENITAL SYNDROMES		
Shwachman-Diamond syndrome	X-Linked	*SBDS*
Fanconi anemia	Autosomal recessive	*FANCA-FANCO*
Dyskeratosis congenita	Variable	Telomerase and related genes
Glycogen storage disease type 1b	Autosomal recessive	*G-6-PT*
Myelokathexis	Autosomal dominant	*CXCR4*
Chédiak-Higashi syndrome	Autosomal recessive	*LYST*
Griscelli syndrome type 2	Autosomal recessive	*RAB27A*
Hermansky-Pudlak syndrome type 2	Autosomal recessive	*AP3B1*

ELANE = neutrophil elastase gene; *G6PC3* = glucose-6-phosphatase catalytic subunit 3 gene; G-6-PT = glucose-6-phosphatase translocase; *G-CSFR* = granulocyte colony-stimulating factor receptor gene; *LYST* = lysosomal trafficking regulatory gene; SBDS = Shwachman-Bodian-Diamond syndrome; *WASP* = Wiskott-Aldrich syndrome protein gene.

dominant and recessive and X-linked patterns of inheritance and is associated with mutations in a variety of genes (Table 153-5).[9]

Neutrophil elastase (ELANE) is a serine protease that is synthesized at high levels in the promyelocyte stage of neutrophil maturation and is packaged in primary granules. Though originally hypothesized to cause defective cellular trafficking and cytoplasmic accumulation leading to neutrophil apoptosis, newer evidence supports that ELANE mutations lead to accumulation of mutant elastase in the endoplasmic reticulum, with apoptosis resulting from activation of the unfolded protein response. Severe congenital neutropenia due to ELANE mutations is inherited in an autosomal dominant fashion.

Hax-1 is a mitochondrial protein with weak homology to bcl-2, and its absence results in mitochondrial-dependent apoptosis. Although all severe congenital neutropenia cases were originally referred to as Kostmann syndrome, that term is now reserved for this subgroup of autosomal recessive cases.

Wiskott-Aldrich syndrome protein regulates actin polymerization in hematopoietic cells, and deficiency of this protein results in the Wiskott-Aldrich syndrome, characterized by small platelets in low number, sinopulmonary infections, and eczema. Another phenotype of mutated Wiskott-Aldrich syndrome protein, however, is X-linked thrombocytopenia and neutropenia. Mutations in the glucose-6-phosphatase catalytic subunit 3 (*G6PC3*) are a more recently discovered cause of severe congenital neutropenia; homozygous loss of this metabolic enzyme also appears to lead to activation of the unfolded protein response and increased apoptosis of neutrophil precursors.

Severe congenital neutropenia was formerly a disease of infancy and early childhood because few, if any, patients survived to adulthood. However, G-CSF can raise neutrophil counts and prevent infection in most patients, thereby allowing most patients with severe congenital neutropenia to survive. Some patients require very high doses of G-CSF, but responses are seen in 80 to 90% of individuals. Increased survival led to the realization that severe congenital neutropenia predisposes to the development of myelodysplasia and acute myeloid leukemia (myelodysplasia/AML), with the development of myelodysplasia/AML at a rate of approximately 2% per year and a cumulative risk of about 20 to 30% over 10 years. Patients refractory to, or requiring very high doses of, G-CSF have a higher risk for leukemic transformation. The development of myelodysplasia/AML is often associated with the acquisition of a G-CSF receptor gene mutation. Considerable controversy exists concerning the role of lifelong G-CSF administration in the acquisition of other mutations and their contribution to malignant transformation in patients with severe congenital neutropenia (see Treatment later).

Two classes of G-CSF receptor mutations have been associated with severe congenital neutropenia and either hyper-responsiveness or hyporesponsiveness of the receptor. Initial studies aimed at demonstrating that severe congenital neutropenia was caused by mutation of the G-CSF or G-CSF receptor gene did not implicate such mutations in its pathogenesis. However, a small number of patients have been shown to have mutations in the G-CSF receptor gene that block ligand binding and produce a G-CSF–resistant form of severe congenital neutropenia. More important, however, the studies identified an acquired missense mutation that introduces a stop codon that leads to the deletion of the distal intracellular domain of the receptor known to be responsible for differentiation signaling. This mutation has been shown to cause hypersensitivity to G-CSF, suggesting that the mutation may play a role in the development of myelodysplasia/AML. However, whether this mutation in fact influences the development of myelodysplasia/AML and whether G-CSF increases the risk for developing the mutation remain subjects of significant controversy. Even in the presence of the G-CSF mutation, development of AML is associated with the acquisition of other myeloid leukemia–associated gene mutations.[10]

Cyclic Neutropenia

Cyclic neutropenia is defined by periods of neutropenia (≤200/μL) lasting 3 to 5 days and occurring at approximately 21-day intervals. Neutropenic periods may be marked by recurrent fevers, mouth sores, and infections of the skin, upper respiratory tract, and ears. Cyclic neutropenia can be dominantly inherited or sporadic, and it is associated with ELANE mutations in virtually all cases. Acquired cyclic neutropenia has been rarely associated with systemic diseases such as large granular lymphocytosis or T-cell lymphoma.

Other Congenital Syndromes with Associated Neutropenia

Several congenital disorders are associated with neutropenia.[11] These include Shwachman-Diamond syndrome, Fanconi anemia, dyskeratosis congenita, glycogen storage disease Ib, myelokathexis, Chédiak-Higashi syndrome, Griscelli syndrome II, and Hermansky-Pudlak syndrome II.

Shwachman-Diamond syndrome usually begins as an isolated neutropenia but progresses to marrow failure and is also associated with pancreatic dysfunction and skeletal abnormalities. The responsible gene, the Shwachman-Bodian-Diamond syndrome gene (*SBDS*), is involved in the regulation of ribosomal RNA. These patients carry an increased risk for leukemic transformation.

Fanconi anemia (Chapter 151) is due to mutations in genes involved in DNA repair, and as such, marrow failure develops later in these patients (median age, 7 years). Patients with Fanconi anemia often have concomitant short stature with upper limb anomalies and hyperpigmented café-au-lait spots, although about one third have no physical abnormalities. Screening is done by chromosomal fragility testing following exposure to diepoxybutane or mitomycin C and by direct assessment for known Fanconi gene mutations.

Dyskeratosis congenita (Chapter 151) is a syndrome of nail dystrophy, leukoplakia, and skin pigmentation abnormalities with associated neutropenia or aplastic anemia that typically does not present until the second decade of life. It is inherited in an autosomal dominant or recessive or X-linked fashion and is associated with mutations in genes involved in telomere maintenance. Dyskeratosis congenita is one of several diseases associated with telomere abnormalities, with wide-ranging manifestations including pulmonary fibrosis and hepatic cirrhosis as well as bone marrow failure.

Glycogen storage disease Ib (Chapter 191) is inherited as an autosomal recessive disorder characterized by intermittent neutropenia due to defects in the neutrophil respiratory burst with subsequent apoptosis of circulating neutrophils. Hepatomegaly and metabolic crises are also the hallmarks of this disease and are due to mutations in the gene for the glucose-6-phosphatase translocase enzyme.

The neutropenia of *myelokathexis* is due to retention of mature neutrophils in the bone marrow. During infection, however, patients with myelokathexis typically have a sudden rise in their neutrophils, making their clinical course relatively more benign. There is an association between this condition and hypogammaglobulinemia and warts: WHIM syndrome (*w*arts, *h*ypogammaglobulinemia, *i*mmunodeficiency, and *m*yelokathexis). Myelokathexis is caused by heterozygous mutations in the gene encoding chemokine receptor CXCR4.

Chédiak-Higashi syndrome, Griscelli syndrome II, and *Hermansky-Pudlak syndrome II* are all syndromes of albinism and neutropenia due to defects in vesicular trafficking. Chédiak-Higashi syndrome is due to mutations in a lysosomal trafficking regulatory gene (*LYST*) and is characterized by oculocutaneous albinism, bleeding, progressive neurologic disease, and increased susceptibility to hemophagocytic syndrome. Griscelli syndrome II, with nearly identical clinical manifestations as Chédiak-Higashi syndrome, is caused by mutations in the gene encoding the small guanosine triphosphatase RAB27A, which is involved in the release of myeloperoxidase from the primary granules of neutrophils. Hermansky-Pudlak syndrome II is due to mutations in the *AP3B1* gene, which encodes a part of a protein transport complex involved in vesicular trafficking and appears to be involved in the trafficking of neutrophil elastase. It is also marked by albinism, platelet abnormalities, and pulmonary fibrosis.

Barth syndrome is an X-linked autosomal recessive disorder characterized by neutropenia, cardiomyopathy, and growth retardation, with a high early childhood mortality from the associated heart disease. The causative mutation is in the *TAZ* gene, which encodes the tafazzin protein that is critical to remodeling cardiolipin in the mitochondrial membrane.

Secondary Causes of Neutropenia

Infection-Related Neutropenia

Several viral infections cause a transient neutropenia that typically resolves as the viremia abates. These include varicella, measles, rubella, hepatitis A and B, Epstein-Barr virus, influenza, parvovirus, and cytomegalovirus. The mechanisms are diverse and involve redistribution, decreased production, and immune destruction of neutrophils. Human immunodeficiency virus and acquired immunodeficiency syndrome also cause multifactorial leukopenia and neutropenia (Chapter 355). Patients often have splenomegaly and sequestration, but more commonly, the neutropenia reflects immune-mediated destruction. A myriad of atypical infections like *Mycobacterium tuberculosis*, ehrlichiosis, rickettsia, tularemia, brucellosis, and some staphylococcal infections can cause moderate neutropenia. Any infection leading to overwhelming sepsis can cause neutropenia, but this usually reflects consumption of marrow neutrophil reserves and is typically seen in newborns and elderly patients with limited marrow reserves. There is also increased margination of neutrophils during sepsis due to systemic activation of complement, exacerbating the neutropenia.

Drug-Induced Neutropenia and Neutropenia Due to Marrow Injury

Drug-induced neutropenia is the most common cause of neutropenia. Multiple drugs have been implicated in neutropenia and agranulocytosis, in both predictable and idiosyncratic patterns. Drug-induced neutropenias may reflect either suppression of marrow granulopoiesis or increased destruction of peripheral neutrophils. Many drugs cause direct dose-dependent marrow suppression, which is predictable and often mild. Others incite an idiosyncratic immune-mediated destruction that can present with profound agranulocytosis. Drug-induced neutropenia typically presents with a marked decline in neutrophils occurring after 1 to 2 weeks of exposure to the drug with recovery within 3 to 10 days of stopping the drug. However, atypical cases can present long after drug initiation, and others may be associated with a markedly delayed recovery (Fig. 153-5). Patients with drug-induced agranulocytosis may present with acute sepsis, leading to significant acute mortality. Recovery is often preceded by the appearance of monocytes and immature neutrophil forms. The more hypercellular the marrow is at diagnosis, the earlier marrow recovery may occur. Some common drugs known to cause neutropenia, in addition to antineoplastic, antiviral, and immunosuppressive agents, include clozapine;

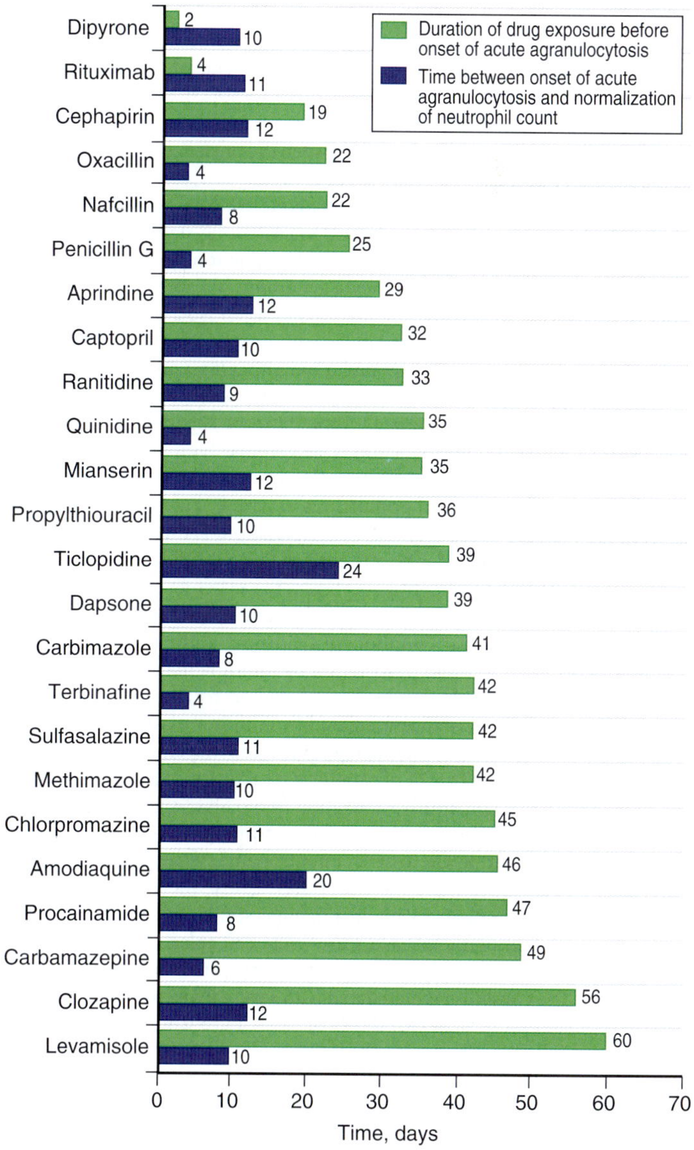

FIGURE 153-5. Median duration of treatment and neutropenia. Only drugs with more than three definite or probable reports of the time between onset of acute agranulocytosis and normalization of neutrophil count and the duration of treatment before onset of acute agranulocytosis were considered. (From Andersohn F, Konzen C, Garbe E. Systematic review: agranulocytosis induced by nonchemotherapy drugs. *Ann Intern Med*. 2007;146: 657-665.)

the antithyroidal thioamides including carbimazole, methimazole, and propylthiouracil; quinidine; procainamide; sulfasalazine; and levamisole, which is widely used as a cocaine adulterant and causes cocaine-associated neutropenia. Neutrophil recovery is speeded by G-CSF.

Radiation can induce marrow injury leading to acute or chronic marrow failure; in high doses, it is also a risk factor for the development of myelodysplasia and leukemia. These malignant hematopoietic diseases can themselves cause marrow failure because the malignant cells proliferate within the marrow and can also cause marrow fibrosis, both of which lead to cytopenias. These diseases are discussed in greater detail in Chapters 151 and 167, respectively. Likewise, metastatic carcinoma to the marrow can also cause marrow failure as the marrow becomes replaced by the metastatic cells.

Immune Neutropenia

Immune neutropenia can occur as an isolated phenomenon (primary immune neutropenia) or as a manifestation of an underlying systemic autoimmune disease (secondary immune neutropenia).[12] Primary autoimmune neutropenia is generally a disease of children, with a median age of onset of 6 to 12 months. Although infectious risk is increased, treatment is restricted to prophylactic antibiotics, with G-CSF reserved for acute infectious episodes. Ninety-five percent of patients undergo spontaneous remission within 2 years. Nearly all of these patients have antineutrophil antibodies directed against antigens derived from the FcγIIIb receptor; these antibodies mediate neutrophil destruction by either sequestration in the spleen or complement-mediated neutrophil lysis.

Secondary autoimmune neutropenia is a disease of adults and can be seen in association with hyperthyroidism, Wegener granulomatosis, rheumatoid arthritis, and systemic lupus erythematosus (SLE).[13] The role of antineutrophil antibodies in these patients is less clear. More than 50% of patients with SLE, for example, have antineutrophil antibodies, but many have normal neutrophil counts, and there is a poor correlation between the presence of the antibodies and neutrophil number.

Felty syndrome and *large granular lymphocyte syndrome* deserve separate mention. Felty syndrome occurs in association with long-standing rheumatoid arthritis (Chapter 243) and is characterized by splenomegaly and profound neutropenia. Large granular lymphocyte syndrome (Chapter 151) can occur either in the setting of rheumatoid arthritis or as an isolated phenomenon. Both Felty syndrome and large granular lymphocyte syndrome are associated with a proliferation of large granular lymphocytes, with a characteristic surface phenotype ($CD3^+$, $CD8^+$, $CD16^+$, and $CD57^+$). In rheumatoid arthritis, these two syndromes were originally thought to be separate diseases, with Felty syndrome being polyclonal and large granular lymphocyte syndrome representing a monoclonal proliferation. However, with increasing sensitivity of detection of monoclonal populations of lymphocytes, this distinction has become blurred. More than 90% of rheumatoid arthritis patients with either syndrome are human leukocyte antigen (HLA)-DR4-positive, leading to the postulate that the two entities represent the extremes of a single disease spectrum. This HLA restriction is not found among non–rheumatoid arthritis patients with large granular lymphocyte syndrome. Both syndromes cause immune-mediated neutrophil destruction by multiple mechanisms, including antineutrophil antibodies and cell-mediated destruction. Some patients may also have G-CSF resistance mediated by inhibitory G-CSF antibodies. The pathophysiology of large granular lymphocyte syndrome is incompletely understood. However, up to 50% of patients have activating mutations in Stat3, and all patients show constitutive activation of the Stat3 signaling pathway.

There are other rare forms of immune neutropenia. Isoimmune neonatal neutropenia is a moderate to severe neutropenia of the newborn due to transplacental passage of maternal antibodies against alleles inherited from the father, resulting in neutropenia in a manner similar to the development of anemia in Rh hemolytic disease. Pure white cell aplasia is a rare disease highlighted by a complete absence of myeloid precursors on bone marrow examination. The condition is associated with severe pyogenic infections and with thymoma in more than two thirds of cases. Pure white cell aplasia has also occurred following ibuprofen therapy.

Neutropenia Due to Increased Margination and Hypersplenism

Complement activation can result in both acute and chronic neutropenia as a result of increased margination of the circulating neutrophil pool. The increased neutrophil margination has been attributed to the fact that C5a renders neutrophils more adherent and prone to aggregation within the pulmonary vasculature and has been seen in patients suffering from burns and transfusion reactions. Complement activation may also lead to neutrophil destruction, as in paroxysmal nocturnal hemoglobinuria. Neutropenia can also reflect hypersplenism, although this is typically less common and less pronounced than the anemia and thrombocytopenia seen in patients with splenomegaly.

Neutropenia Due to Nutritional Deficiency

B_{12}, folate (Chapter 150), and copper deficiency are each associated with neutropenia. Copper deficiency is an underrecognized cause of neutropenia (usually seen with anemia), found especially in situations like total parenteral nutrition without copper supplementation, protein-losing enteropathies, celiac disease, gastric bypass surgery and postgastrectomy, malabsorption syndromes, and zinc toxicity. In addition to low serum copper and ceruloplasmin levels, distinct morphologic findings include hypogranularity and hypolobated nuclei (Pelger-Huet anomaly) on peripheral smear and cytoplasmic vacuolization of myeloid, as well as erythroid precursors and ringed sideroblasts.

Deficiencies in these vitamins and minerals result in ineffective myelopoiesis, maturation arrest, and megaloblastic changes with nuclear-cytoplasmic dyssynchrony. The characteristic finding in the setting of megaloblastic anemia is hypersegmentation of the neutrophil (Fig. 153-6).

Chronic Idiopathic Neutropenia

Chronic idiopathic neutropenia in adults is an acquired disorder characterized by prolonged neutropenia in the absence of any apparent underlying etiology. Chronic neutropenia is often an incidental finding on routine blood tests, making it impossible to know the duration of the neutropenia. Patients have no evidence of autoimmune disease, nutritional deficiency, or myelodysplasia. The syndrome is heterogeneous, with a wide range of neutrophil counts. A group of adults from Greece with chronic idiopathic neutropenia were found to have increased production of transforming growth factor-β (TGF-β), linked to a genetic polymorphism in the TGF-β locus, and consequent suppression of granulopoiesis by the bone marrow. These patients tend to have very mild neutropenia, with an absolute neutrophil count that is rarely less than 800. However, these patients should be distinguished from other adults with chronic idiopathic neutropenia, many of whom have an absolute neutrophil count below 200. The etiology of neutropenia in these patients is completely unknown, but the natural history of chronic idiopathic neutropenia in adults, even in the face of very low neutrophil counts, is generally benign. Most patients require no therapy, although those with very low counts may require G-CSF if they manifest severe infections. Some patients with recurrent infections or troublesome aphthous ulcers require chronic G-CSF treatment. These patients typically respond to low doses of G-CSF, and there is no increase in the development of myelodysplasia/AML.

CLINICAL MANIFESTATIONS AND DIAGNOSIS

Neutropenia is not usually associated with clinical signs and symptoms other than those of the underlying condition causing the low WBC. It becomes

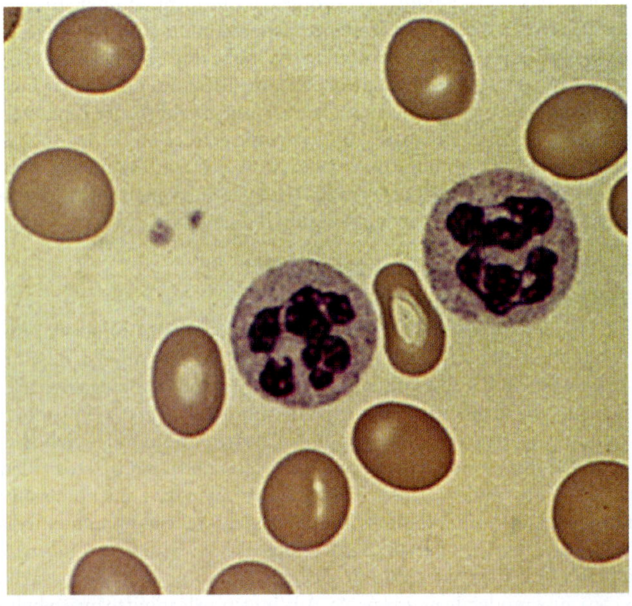

FIGURE 153-6. Peripheral blood with macrocytosis and hypersegmented neutrophils in megaloblastic anemia.

clinically evident, however, when it results in infection. Although patients with an absolute neutrophil count below 1000/μL have a slightly increased risk for infection, the risk increases substantially when the neutrophil count falls below 500/μL. With few neutrophils, the signs and symptoms of infection may be attenuated; pneumonia may be present with minimal infiltrate on chest radiograph, or a urinary tract infection may yield only a very mild pyuria. Therefore, fever in any neutropenic patient must be considered an emergency with prompt acquisition of cultures and rapid administration of empirical antibiotic therapy.

Because drug-induced neutropenia is the most common cause of acquired neutropenia, a careful inventory for drugs and toxins is warranted. Likewise, patients should be evaluated for potential precipitating malignant and inflammatory conditions. The time course of the neutropenia and infections can provide insight into the etiology (acute versus chronic, persistent versus cyclic, neonatal versus childhood versus adult onset). Attention should be paid to the skin, bones, appendages, and nails because abnormalities in these may point toward one of the congenital neutropenia syndromes. Evaluation of the complete blood count, peripheral blood smear, and vitamin B_{12} and folate levels should also be performed.

When the neutropenia is mild and associated with anemia and thrombocytopenia, the possibility of hypersplenism should be considered. Diagnosis can often be made by the finding of palpable splenomegaly. However, especially in obese patients, abdominal imaging may be used to evaluate spleen size. Abdominal ultrasound also allows the assessment of portal venous flow with Doppler studies. If splenic enlargement is confirmed, the etiology of the splenomegaly (Chapter 154) should be determined. The diagnosis of cyclic neutropenia formerly required demonstration of transient neutropenia through frequent blood counts over a course of 6 weeks but now can be established by sequencing of the elastase gene.

In other patients with chronic neutropenia without a history of infection, drug or toxin exposure, or B_{12} or folate deficiency, bone marrow examination should be performed to exclude myelodysplasia, with assessment of morphology, flow cytometry for the large granular lymphocyte syndrome, and cytogenetics. Once a normal marrow has been obtained, further bone marrow examination is not indicated in adults with chronic idiopathic neutropenia (Fig. 153-7).

TREATMENT

Management of the neutropenia patient is nuanced and depends on the etiology of the depressed count, its severity, and the presence or absence of fever.

Neutropenia After Chemotherapy

In *afebrile* adults with acquired neutropenia following chemotherapy, antibiotic prophylaxis with a quinolone (ciprofloxacin 500 mg orally twice a day, switched to 200 mg intravenously twice a day if the patient develops severe mucositis or intolerance to the oral formulation) or oral sulfamethoxazole/trimethoprim (1 double-strength tablet daily) can reduce all-cause mortality and is recommended along with antifungal prophylaxis (e.g., oral voriconazole 200 mg twice daily) in patients who are expected to have profound, protracted neutropenia (<100 neutrophils/μL for >7 days).[14] Trimethoprim-sulfamethoxazole is specifically recommended in patients at risk for *Pneumocystis jirovecii* pneumonia (Chapter 313), based on neutropenia in the setting of the equivalent of 20 mg or more of prednisone/day for 1 month or longer.

In afebrile neutropenia, the routine prophylactic administration of colony-stimulating factors does not appear to be beneficial,[A1] but many oncologic professional society guidelines recommend the use of prophylactic G-CSF in patients who are receiving chemotherapy and who have a 20% or greater risk for developing febrile neutropenia based on their age, comorbid illnesses, disease characteristics, and the myelotoxicity of the chemotherapy regimen. G-CSF is also recommended during hematopoietic stem cell transplantation (Chapter 163), for patients receiving chemotherapy for non-Hodgkin lymphoma (Chapter 171) or dose-dense chemotherapy, and for patients with a history of febrile neutropenia receiving further chemotherapy. In afebrile neutropenia, granulocyte transfusions may reduce the risk of infection but do not reduce mortality.[A2]

The approach to the patient with fever and neutropenia is discussed in detail in Chapter 260. Neutropenia with fever is a clinical emergency because patients are at risk for hemodynamic collapse and septic shock. Therefore, such patients should be evaluated thoroughly and cultured promptly, and empiric antibiotics should be administered within 30 to 60 minutes of presentation while awaiting culture results. The timely administration of antibiotics in neutropenic patients

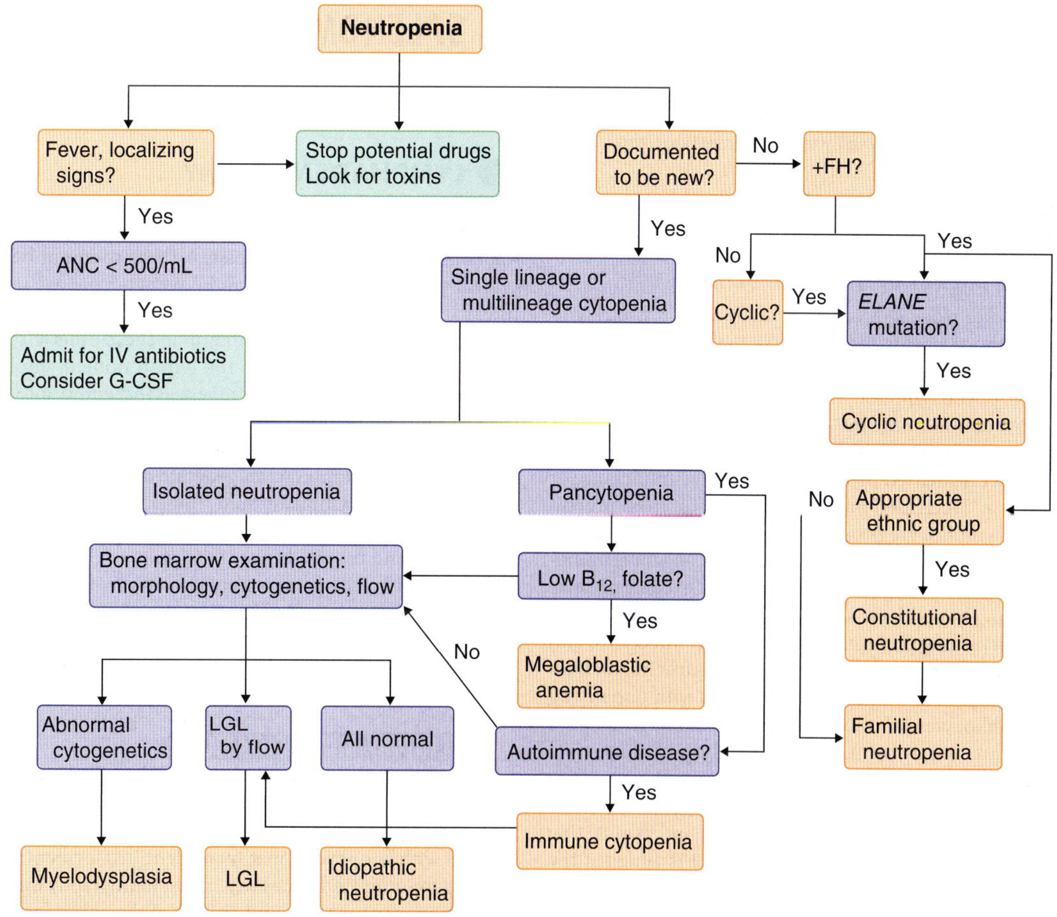

FIGURE 153-7. Diagnostic approach to neutropenia. ANC = absolute neutrophil count; *ELANE* = neutrophil elastase gene; FH = family history; G-CSF = granulocyte colony-stimulating factor; IV = intravenous; LGL = large granular lymphocyte syndrome.

at the onset of fever confers significant clinical benefit, with more rapid response and improved survival. The choice of treatment of patients with fever and neutropenia in the setting of cancer chemotherapy is based on the initial history and physical examination as well as a structured assessment of risk (Chapter 260).[15]

Other Neutropenias

Patients with immune neutropenia are typically treated with immunosuppressive therapy, including steroids, antithymocyte globulin, or cyclosporine, aimed primarily at treatment of the underlying autoimmune disease. Patients usually respond to G-CSF, although this treatment may induce a flare of joint symptoms in the setting of rheumatoid arthritis. Patients with the large granular lymphocyte syndrome often respond to low-dose methotrexate (10 mg/m^2 orally once a week), cyclosporine (100 to 600 mg or 2 to 10 mg/kg orally daily), or low-dose cyclophosphamide (50 to 100 mg orally daily).

Patients with *congenital neutropenia*, including idiopathic, severe congenital, or cyclic neutropenia, are usually successfully managed with G-CSF for years. With G-CSF, however, life expectancy has been extended into adulthood. Therapy is daily and chronic, given by subcutaneous injection, with doses varying by the type of neutropenia and the individual responsiveness to therapy. It is usually well tolerated, although accelerated bone loss has been observed. Growth and development appear unaffected. Patients with severe congenital neutropenia typically require the highest doses, whereas those with idiopathic neutropenia require the lowest.

In adults with *chronic idiopathic neutropenia*, G-CSF should be reserved for acute febrile episodes unless the patient has recurrent infections. Adults with chronic idiopathic neutropenia treated with G-CSF may experience significant side effects, including fever, gastrointestinal symptoms, and splenomegaly. Consequently, when adults with chronic idiopathic neutropenia require chronic G-CSF, it should be administered at the lowest dose necessary to prevent infections; it is usually sufficient to treat to maintain the absolute neutrophil count in the range of 300 to 500. Cyclic neutropenia is successfully treated with G-CSF and is not associated with an increased risk for leukemic transformation.

Pure white cell aplasia is immune mediated, and removal of the thymoma in thymoma-associated cases may not be sufficient for remission. Adjuvant therapy with cyclophosphamide, corticosteroids, cyclosporine, and intravenous immunoglobulin may be needed.

For patients with an inflammatory, infectious, or drug-induced neutropenia, the recommendation is to treat the underlying condition or stop the offending agent.

The use of antibiotics to prevent infection in other patients with chronic neutropenias has not been extensively studied but is typically not recommended and should be based on clinical context. There is no evidence that a low bacterial diet can prevent infection or mortality in neutropenic cancer patients.[A3]

Stem cell transplantation (Chapter 163) can be curative for a number of the congenital neutropenia and bone marrow failure syndromes, including Fanconi anemia. It is, however, not without risk and should therefore be reserved for patients with severe neutropenia complicated by recurrent infection definitively shown to be due to marrow failure.

LEUKOPENIA DUE TO DEFICIENCY OF OTHER CELL LINES

Lymphocyte production takes place in a variety of anatomic sites, and lymphocyte trafficking from those sites is bidirectional, making it difficult to understand lymphocyte dynamics in the same way that we do for neutrophils. Despite this, the peripheral lymphocyte count seems to be maintained in a narrow range at 2000 to 4000/μL, 20% of which are B cells and 70% of which are T cells. Lymphocytopenia is a total lymphocyte count of less than 1500/μL. It can reflect decreased production, defective trafficking, or increased loss or destruction. Decreased production can result from protein and calorie malnutrition; lymphocyte progenitor pool injury secondary to radiation, chemotherapy, or immunosuppressive agents; and congenital immunodeficiency states. Endogenous or exogenous glucocorticoid excess can cause lymphocytopenia by altering lymphocyte trafficking. This can also occur as the result of acute bacterial or fungal infections, certain viral infections, and granulomatous disease. Finally, many viruses cause direct destruction of lymphocytes, as do antilymphocyte antibodies seen in patients with underlying autoimmune diseases. Lymphocytes can also be lost from intestinal lymphatics in cases of protein-losing enteropathy, primary disease of the gut or intestinal lymphatics, or gut edema secondary to severe heart failure. Lymphocytopenia should prompt comprehensive assessment of the immune system, including lymphocyte subtyping, quantitative immunoglobulins, and skin testing to detect deficiencies of cell-mediated immunity. Treatment is aimed at the underlying disease, but intravenous immunoglobulin can be administered to patients with hypogammaglobulinemia, and transplantation can be performed in patients with severe deficiencies of cell-mediated immunity due to impaired lymphocyte production and function.

Monocytopenia, eosinopenia, and basophilopenia can accompany bone marrow failure syndromes or acute infection, malignancy, or severe injury and is thought to reflect elevations in glucocorticoids, prostaglandins, and epinephrine. These humoral factors have the greatest impact on eosinophils, and absence of eosinopenia in these settings should prompt suspicion for adrenal insufficiency, a primary myeloproliferative syndrome, parasitic infection, or primary hypereosinophilic syndrome. Monocytopenia is less frequent, probably owing to the diverse roles monocytes play in normal human physiology; prolonged and extreme monocytopenia may not be compatible with life.

GENERAL REFERENCES

For the General References and other additional features, please visit Elsevier eBooks+ at https://ebooks.health.elsevier.com.

Grade A References

A1. Skoetz N, Bohlius J, Engert A, et al. Prophylactic antibiotics or G(M)-CSF for the prevention of infections and improvement of survival in cancer patients receiving myelotoxic chemotherapy. *Cochrane Database Syst Rev*. 2015;12:CD007107.

A2. Estcourt LJ, Stanworth S, Doree C, et al. Granulocyte transfusions for preventing infections in people with neutropenia or neutrophil dysfunction. *Cochrane Database Syst Rev*. 2015;6:CD005341.

A3. van Dalen EC, Mank A, Leclercq E, et al. Low bacterial diet versus control diet to prevent infection in cancer patients treated with chemotherapy causing episodes of neutropenia. *Cochrane Database Syst Rev*. 2016;4:CD006247.

154

APPROACH TO THE PATIENT WITH LYMPHADENOPATHY OR SPLENOMEGALY

JANE N. WINTER

LYMPHADENOPATHY

Lymphadenopathy is very common in children and adolescents but is less common in adults. Lymph nodes are secondary lymphoid tissues located along the course of the lymphatic vessels. These round or bean-shaped structures typically measure less than 1 cm in diameter and are strategically situated to filter lymphatic fluid and to intercept microorganisms and other antigens. The hilus is the point of indentation in these otherwise round tissues where blood vessels enter and leave the lymph node. Lymphatic fluid enters the lymph node in afferent lymphatic vessels that empty into the subcapsular sinus, traverses the lymph node, and then leaves through a single efferent lymphatic at the hilus. Lymph nodes consist of B and T lymphocytes, macrophages, and dendritic cells that interact to generate an immune response to the antigens transported in the lymphatic fluid. These cells function together to generate the normal immune response by means of antigen processing, presentation, and recognition and the resulting proliferation of effector B and T lymphocytes.[1]

Lymph node enlargement generally results from cellular proliferation and expansion of lymph node components associated with the normal immune response to foreign antigens. Alternatively, it can be caused by infiltration of the lymph node by a neoplastic process or deposition of a foreign substance (e.g., in storage disease).

CLINICAL MANIFESTATIONS

Lymphadenopathy is usually noted incidentally by the patient on self-examination or is noted by a family member. Sometimes it is first detected by a physician on a physical examination. However, an increasing number of patients with lymphadenopathy are identified incidentally when they undergo imaging for unrelated issues (e.g., chest radiography for infectious symptoms; magnetic resonance imaging [MRI] of the spine for back pain related to a disc herniation). Occasionally an enlarged lymph node can become tender or become large enough to cause direct symptoms.

TABLE 154-1 TAKING A COMPLETE HISTORY IN THE ADULT PATIENT WITH LYMPHADENOPATHY

History of present illness
- Duration, recent changes
- Associated symptoms: fevers, drenching night sweats, shaking chills, weight loss, sore throat, arthritis or arthralgias, rash or skin lesions, pruritus, shortness of breath, chest pain
- Ill contacts, recent and remote travel, tick or insect bites

Past medical history
- Autoimmune disease, history of immunosuppressive therapy, history of infectious disease, history of recent vaccination

Family history
- Malignancy, especially hematologic malignancy, or infection
- Autoimmune disease

Social history
- Sexual activity—risk for HIV infection, other sexually transmitted diseases
- Occupation—exposure to toxins, livestock, pets
- Smoking or drinking

Medications: immunosuppressive agents, phenytoin, allopurinol, antibiotics

HIV = human immunodeficiency virus.

TABLE 154-2 CLUES TO THE CAUSE OF LYMPHADENOPATHY

Age
Symptoms
Localized versus generalized lymphadenopathy
Specific location/distribution
Tenderness, warmth, overlying erythema, mobility, pulsatile
Size

DIAGNOSIS

Lymph nodes that are larger than 1 cm are generally considered to be abnormal, although adenopathy in some locations is considered abnormal and worthy of investigation even when subcentimeter in size (supraclavicular, epitrochlear, or popliteal lymph nodes).

History and Physical Examination

A careful and complete history is the first and most important step in the evaluation of the patient with lymphadenopathy (Table 154-1). The age of the patient, recent travel history, possible infectious or toxic exposures through employment or hobbies, recent immunizations (e.g., COVID-19 vaccination is a frequent cause of unilateral axillary adenopathy),[2] current medications, and social, sexual, and family history may provide important clues to the cause (Table 154-2). A complete review of systems is required. Not only can the presence of symptoms be informative, but also their pattern, character, and duration (e.g., the high spiking fevers characteristic of Hodgkin lymphoma, known as Pel-Ebstein fevers) may suggest a cause. Similarly, particular symptoms such as pruritus suggest specific diagnoses (e.g., also Hodgkin lymphoma).

The physical examination must also be meticulous with attention not only to the distribution of the adenopathy but also to the presence of other physical findings (e.g., tonsillar enlargement in the patient with cervical adenopathy and Burkitt lymphoma [Chapter 171], parotid enlargement in Sjögren syndrome [Chapter 247], rash in T-cell lymphomas [Chapter 171], joint findings in autoimmune disorders, or a breast mass in the patient with axillary lymphadenopathy) (Table 154-3). Malignant lymph nodes are generally painless, whereas nodes that represent infection may be tender. Although exceptions occur, lymphadenopathy resulting from metastatic solid tumor is characteristically hard and may be fixed or matted, whereas lymphadenopathy representing hematologic malignancies is typically soft and may be mobile. Although borderline and slightly enlarged lymph nodes are commonly related to infectious causes, sizeable nodes are worrisome for malignancy and warrant prompt investigation. Often, no cause is identified, and careful follow-up is required.

Differential Diagnosis

The differential diagnosis of lymphadenopathy is vast. Whether lymphadenopathy is localized or generalized, its location, and the age of the patient all help to focus the investigation into its cause. Diffuse lymphadenopathy may occur in the setting of generalized infections, systemic disorders of the immune system, or widespread neoplasia (Table 154-4).

TABLE 154-3 EVALUATING THE PATIENT WITH LYMPHADENOPATHY

Complete physical examination with particular attention to:
- Tonsillar enlargement, evidence of superior vena cava syndrome
- Attention to all lymph node groups including epitrochlear, femoral
- Hepatosplenomegaly
- Rash
- Joints, deformities

Preliminary laboratory examination
- Complete blood count with differential, platelet count
- Sedimentation rate, testing for mononucleosis in the right setting

Imaging
- Chest radiograph (assess for mediastinal mass, hilar enlargement, infiltrate)
- Ultrasound for children up to age 14 years
- CT with intravenous contrast or contrast-enhanced MRI
- PET/CT not recommended unless diagnosis of lymphoma or other malignancy

Pathologic diagnosis
- Needle aspiration for investigation of infectious causes
- Core biopsy if excisional biopsy unsafe
- Excisional biopsy preferred especially if malignancy suspected

CT = computed tomography; MRI = magnetic resonance imaging; PET = positron emission tomography.

TABLE 154-4 DIFFERENTIAL DIAGNOSIS OF LYMPHADENOPATHY

CAUSES	EXAMPLES
Infectious	
Bacteria	Group A streptococcus, staphylococcal skin infections, syphilis, cat-scratch disease, *Chlamydia trachomatis*, typhoid fever, tuberculosis
Fungi	Histoplasmosis, blastomycosis, coccidioidomycosis
Parasites	Malaria, toxoplasmosis
Viruses	Infectious mononucleosis (Epstein-Barr virus), cytomegalovirus, HIV
Immune mediated	
Autoimmune disorders	Rheumatoid arthritis, systemic lupus erythematosus
Drug reactions	
Malignant	
Hematologic	Lymphoma, leukemia, myeloproliferative neoplasms
Solid tumors	Metastatic to lymph nodes
Unusual	
Storage disease	Gaucher disease, Niemann-Pick disease
Sarcoidosis	
Castleman disease	
Kawasaki vasculitis	
Kikuchi lymphadenitis	
Kimura disease	
Endocrinopathies	Addison disease
Sinus histiocytosis with massive lymphadenopathy (Rosai-Dorfman disease)	

HIV = human immunodeficiency virus.

Localized lymphadenopathy usually but not always results from a regional problem, such as infection or malignancy. The particular site may be informative. For example, recurrent sore throats and upper respiratory infections are regularly associated with tender submandibular and/or cervical adenopathy.[3] However, although cervical adenopathy in adults can be reactive hyperplasia from systemic infection, it is commonly caused by malignancies such as head and neck carcinomas, adenocarcinomas, small cell lung cancer, and lymphoma.[4] Epitrochlear or supraclavicular adenopathy is problematic in any adult or child, and it signifies likely disease. Inguinal adenopathy is common, often related to infection or trauma to the lower extremities, and often of little concern in the absence of other findings. Thoracic and mediastinal adenopathy may be caused by lung cancer (Chapter 177) but also by a variety of nonmalignant conditions including sarcoidosis (Chapter 83) and Castleman disease (Chapter 359) in addition to infection.[5]

Worldwide, infection by bacteria, mycobacteria, fungi, chlamydia, parasites, and viruses are the major causes of lymph node enlargement. Lymph node enlargement in the drainage region of any pyogenic infection is expected. Dramatic regional lymph node enlargement with fluctuant lymph nodes (i.e., buboes) is a hallmark of infection with the coccobacillus *Yersinia pestis* (Chapter 288), which causes bubonic plague. In cat-scratch fever, enlarged nodes close to the site of the flea bite carrying *Bartonella henselae* are common presenting signs (Chapter 291). Mediastinal lymphadenopathy may occur in inhalational anthrax (Chapter 272). Cervical adenopathy is commonly a manifestation of tuberculosis (Chapter 299). In contrast, diffuse adenopathy may represent a systemic infection with Epstein-Barr virus (i.e., infectious mononucleosis; Chapter 348), cytomegalovirus (Chapter 347), or human immunodeficiency virus (HIV; Chapter 359), or with the parasite *Toxoplasma gondii* (Chapter 320).

Autoimmune disorders may be associated with either localized or generalized lymphadenopathy. Lymph node enlargement in this setting is especially challenging given the increased frequency of malignant lymphoproliferative disorders in these patients. Biopsy (excisional when possible) and expert hematopathology consultation are required to exclude the possibility of lymphoma. Lymphadenopathy occurring as a result of a drug reaction is uncommon,[6] but it may be exceptionally difficult to distinguish histopathologically from malignant lymphoma. A wide range of drugs, including antiepileptics and antibiotics, have been reported to cause lymphadenopathy, but associated rash, eosinophilia, and liver function abnormalities are helpful in distinguishing a drug reaction (Chapter 234) from other causes.

Malignancy commonly manifests as lymphadenopathy. Enlarged lymph nodes (Fig. 154-1) may be involved or replaced by a hematologic malignancy such as Hodgkin (Chapter 172) or non-Hodgkin lymphoma (Chapter 171), or they may represent a site of metastasis from a solid tumor, most often occurring in the drainage area of the primary tumor.[7] For example, breast cancer (Chapter 183) is often accompanied by ipsilateral axillary nodal involvement and prostate cancer by iliac node involvement. Distant spread to the lymph nodes may also occur.

In addition to infectious, autoimmune, and malignant causes of lymphadenopathy, less common causes include storage diseases (as in Gaucher or Niemann-Pick disease; Chapter 192) or amyloidosis (Chapter 174; associated with a hematologic malignancy such as multiple myeloma or non-Hodgkin lymphoma, an inherited form of the disease, or with chronic inflammation). Sarcoidosis (Chapter 83) may manifest as enlarged lymph nodes, as can endocrinopathies such as thyroid disease (Chapter 207) or adrenal insufficiency (Chapter 208). Benign entities such as congenital lymphovascular malformations and branchial cleft cysts may present as a neck mass in a child.

Blood Testing

A routine complete blood count should be obtained. When signs and symptoms are consistent with an infectious cause, atypical lymphocytosis suggests Epstein-Barr virus infection, which can be confirmed by serology (Chapter 348).

Imaging

Imaging with computed tomography (CT) or MRI, with the latter preferred when radiation exposure is to be avoided such as during pregnancy, is the first step in the evaluation of worrisome palpable adenopathy in adults.[8] Ultrasonography is recommended as the preferred approach for children with cervical adenopathy and is also useful in adults for determining the size of the node and the possible presence of multiple nodes.[9,10] Clearly, borderline adenopathy or lymphadenopathy associated with symptoms or history suggestive of a benign origin (e.g., mononucleosis in a college student) does not merit immediate imaging and may be watched. Combined positron emission tomography (PET) and CT (PET/CT) should not be an initial test[11] but is very useful for staging and evaluation during and after treatment of patients who are diagnosed with a malignant lymphoma or a variety of solid tumors (Fig. 154-2).

Studies for infectious agents including cultures and special stains for infectious agents, immunophenotypic analysis by flow cytometry, and molecular studies complement morphology in making a diagnosis. In contrast, if head and neck cancer is in the differential diagnosis, the patient should have a complete ear, nose, and throat examination at the outset to avoid complicating subsequent surgery.

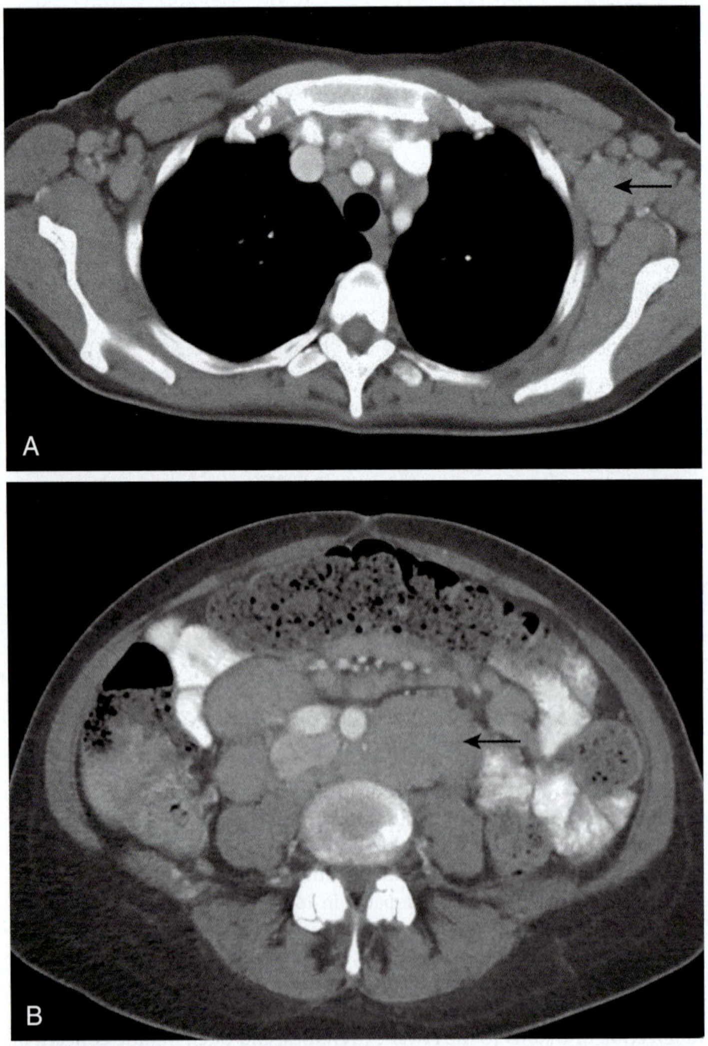

FIGURE 154-1. Axillary (A) and retroperitoneal lymph nodes (B) in a patient with follicular lymphoma. *Arrows* indicate examples of enlarged lymph nodes.

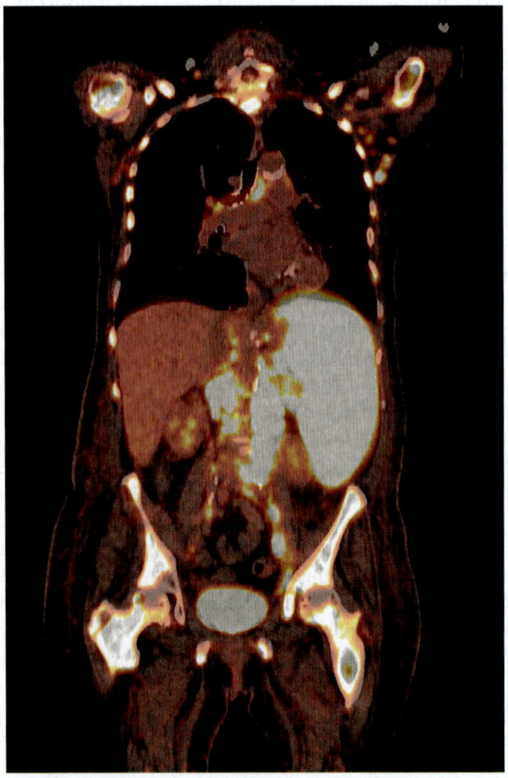

FIGURE 154-2. Fluorodeoxyglucose (FDG)-positron emission tomography (PET)/computed tomographic (CT) scan. The FDG-PET/CT scan demonstrates involvement of the spleen, lymph nodes, and bone in a patient with lymphoma.

Evaluation of a patient with incidentally noted lymphadenopathy on an imaging study poses a special challenge. For example, evaluation of the patient with incidentally noted intra-abdominal or pelvic adenopathy, like that of the patient with a new palpable mass, requires that the clinician integrate the clinical history and radiographic findings. A comparison of the radiologic findings to prior imaging studies can often eliminate concern if the findings are discovered to be long standing. Imaging findings considered worrisome by the American College of Radiology include (1) short axis diameter 1 cm or larger in the retroperitoneum; (2) abnormal architecture (round, indistinct hilum); (3) presence of enhancement (necrosis; hypervascularity); and (4) increased number of nodes defined as a cluster of three or more in a single nodal station or two or more in at least two regions. Biopsy should be considered if the nodes fall into any of these categories and there is clinical or laboratory evidence supporting the presence of a lymphoproliferative disorder. In many cases, the patient may be followed with repeat imaging in 3 to 6 months. If stable for 1 year, an abnormal lymph node or group of lymph nodes is most likely benign.

The location of the enlarged node(s), size, consistency, presence of generalized lymphadenopathy or hepatosplenomegaly, or associated symptoms are all helpful in developing an individualized approach. If nodes are large, 2 to 3 cm in size, and firm with associated symptoms, the risk for malignancy is high, and a diagnostic procedure should be performed expeditiously. A complete blood count with differential and examination of the peripheral smear along with a plain chest radiography may be helpful in sorting out which patient is best served by observation for what may be infectious mononucleosis or another infectious and uncomplicated process and who should proceed quickly to biopsy. A short course of antibiotics with close observation is often the preferred strategy with little risk if the patient is reliable and will return if the lump grows rather than regresses. Steroids should be avoided because they may mask the symptoms and cause shrinkage of the nodes in hematologic malignancies.

Biopsy

The decision to perform a biopsy of a lymph node depends on the clinical history and presentation as well as the ease with which a biopsy can be performed. For patients with symptoms, an early biopsy of a palpable lymph node may provide an answer to a puzzling case[12] but may add to the confusion if the biopsy result is not definitive. An excisional rather than a core biopsy is most likely to provide a definitive diagnosis,[13] but it is not practical in all cases. When no easily accessible peripheral nodes are available for biopsy, a core biopsy may be obtained by the interventional radiologists with the assistance of ultrasound or CT guidance. Fine-needle aspiration may be adequate to diagnose a solid tumor or infection but is insufficient for distinguishing malignant lymphoma from a reactive lymph node, and it is discouraged if lymphoma is in the differential diagnosis. An excisional biopsy remains the gold standard. Face-to-face discussion between the clinician and the pathologist is the most effective approach to determining a diagnosis, especially for the most challenging cases.

TREATMENT AND PROGNOSIS

The treatment of lymphadenopathy focuses on treatment of the underlying disease, which also determines prognosis. In some tumors, such as breast cancer (Chapter 183) and ovarian cancer (Chapter 184), removal of local lymph nodes is an important part of therapy.

SPLENOMEGALY

Splenomegaly is present in about 2% of adults in the United States, with no predilection by gender, age, or ethnicity. Causes include a wide variety of infections, primary liver disease, benign hematologic diseases, and malignancies.

The spleen is the largest lymphatic organ in the body, and some liken it to a very large lymph node. Similar to lymph nodes, the spleen has multiple and diverse functions, including its role as a filter removing defective red blood cells and infectious agents, its important role in immune response to blood-borne antigens, and a role in regulating blood volume.

Consistent with its multiple functions and its role as a massive filter, the spleen has an open circulation with three compartments: the white pulp, marginal zone, and red pulp. Blood enters the spleen through the splenic artery and its branches, filters through the splenic cords and periarterial lymphatic sheath, and is exposed in the white pulp to immunologically active cells including macrophages, B lymphocytes, and T lymphocytes. In the white pulp, microorganisms and foreign proteins are recognized, and an immune response to blood-borne antigens is initiated. In splenectomized individuals, the absence of this splenic function predisposes to certain infections, especially infections with encapsulated organisms such as *Streptococcus pneumoniae*.

Separating white pulp from red, the marginal zone acts as a transition zone. More than half the volume of the spleen is composed of splenic red pulp and consists primarily of erythrocytes along with macrophages, dendritic cells, and other white blood cells. Senescent or defective red blood cells are identified and destroyed in the red pulp. The process of hemolysis may be mechanical and/or immunologic as in autoimmune hemolytic anemia, in which the antibody-coated red blood cells are phagocytosed by macrophages. Perhaps less well appreciated, the spleen plays a role in regulating blood volume by means of a variety of mechanisms, including release of blood through splenic contraction and the splenorenal reflex that promotes retention of fluid and sodium by the kidneys during septic shock.

CLINICAL MANIFESTATIONS

Splenomegaly is commonly detected as an incidental finding on imaging performed for what appears to be an unrelated issue such as diverticulitis or nephrolithiasis. Given the obesity epidemic and the increasing reliance on testing rather than careful physical examination, it is uncommon for splenomegaly to be detected first on physical examination except as part of a careful evaluation of a patient who has a known predisposing condition.

Except with massive splenomegaly or acute obliteration of the splenic artery or vein, the patient is unlikely to have specific complaints related to splenomegaly itself. Pain in the left upper quadrant sometimes radiating to the left shoulder may be the first indication of a splenic infarct or an enlarged spleen. Rarely, the catastrophic signs and symptoms of splenic rupture are the first indications of splenomegaly. Unexplained weight loss related to early satiety caused by compression of the stomach by the enlarged spleen or unexplained cytopenias caused by hypersplenism may be the first indication of splenomegaly.

DIAGNOSIS

In contrast to lymphadenopathy, an enlarged spleen discovered on physical examination is nearly always abnormal and requires explanation. As with lymphadenopathy, the differential diagnosis of splenomegaly is wide ranging (Table 154-5), and the same principles hold. First, a careful history and physical examination, with attention to the age of the patient, the size of the spleen, and associated symptoms, will often but not always guide the investigation to the underlying cause. The majority of cases are due to infection, autoimmune disorders, or malignancies, but oftentimes no cause is identified, so careful follow-up is required.

TABLE 154-5 DIFFERENTIAL DIAGNOSIS OF SPLENOMEGALY

CAUSES	EXAMPLES
Infectious	
Bacteria	Endocarditis, brucellosis, syphilis, tuberculosis, Rocky Mountain spotted fever
Fungi	Histoplasmosis, toxoplasmosis
Parasites	Malaria, leishmaniasis
Viruses	Infectious mononucleosis (Epstein-Barr virus), HIV, cytomegalovirus
Immune mediated	
Autoimmune disorders	Rheumatoid arthritis, systemic lupus erythematosus, autoimmune hemolytic anemia
Drug reaction	Phenytoin
Malignant	
Hematologic	Lymphoma, leukemia, myeloproliferative neoplasm
Solid tumor	Metastatic to spleen
Congestive	Liver disease, portal vein thrombosis, congestive heart failure
Nonmalignant hematologic disorders	Hereditary spherocytosis, congenital or acquired hemolytic anemias, hemoglobinopathies, extramedullary hematopoiesis
Unusual	
Storage disease	Gaucher disease, Niemann-Pick disease
Sarcoidosis	
Cysts, pseudocysts	
Amyloidosis	

HIV = human immunodeficiency virus.

History

Similar to the approach to lymphadenopathy, a careful and complete history is the first and most important step in the evaluation of the patient with splenomegaly. The age of the patient, travel history, possible infectious or toxic exposures through employment or hobbies, recent immunizations, current medications, and social, sexual, and family history all may contribute important clues to the cause. A complete review of systems is required. A review of old records including imaging may provide evidence that splenomegaly is long-standing.

Physical Examination

Despite many approaches to palpating the spleen, a borderline or slightly enlarged spleen may be difficult to appreciate on examination. Positioning the patient in the right lateral decubitus position with knees slight flexed is a useful approach, especially for right-handed examiners. The examination should begin very low in the pelvis and work upwards to the left upper quadrant so as not to miss the edge of a massively enlarged spleen. Inspection and percussion combined with palpation provide the best chance of identifying the enlarged spleen. The patient should take deep breaths while checking for the tip of the spleen as it descends with deep inspiration. Splenomegaly is typically recorded as the number of centimeters the spleen descends below the left costal margin in the midclavicular line on deep inspiration. The physical examination in the patient with splenomegaly should be meticulous, including attention to the presence of lymphadenopathy, jaundice, tonsillar enlargement, joint effusions or swelling, and hepatomegaly.

Differential Diagnosis

The infectious causes of splenomegaly are myriad.[14,15] Geography and travel history are often important clues to an underlying infection. The most likely causes of splenomegaly in equatorial Africa or in a recent African immigrant are different from the causes in a North American urbanite. Bacterial infections commonly associated with splenomegaly include endocarditis (Chapter 61), brucellosis (Chapter 286), typhoid fever (Chapter 284), and rickettsial disorders such as Rocky Mountain spotted fever (Chapter 302). Mycobacterial infections including typical (Chapter 299) and atypical (Chapter 300) mycobacteria may manifest with splenomegaly, as can fungal infections such as histoplasmosis (Chapter 308). Among the parasitic disorders, malaria (Chapter 316) is nearly always accompanied by an enlarged spleen and should be high on the differential diagnosis list in the proper setting. Epstein-Barr virus (Chapter 348), which is the cause of infectious mononucleosis, is a common cause of splenomegaly that is usually self-limited. HIV (Chapter 359) may also be associated with splenomegaly, although often the causative agent is a coexisting infection with hepatitis C virus.

Autoimmune disorders such as rheumatoid arthritis (Chapter 243) and systemic lupus erythematosus (Chapter 245) are commonly associated with mild to moderate splenomegaly. Felty syndrome is characterized by splenomegaly, usually in the setting of long-standing rheumatoid arthritis, with associated neutropenia. Autoimmune hemolytic anemia (Chapter 146) is characterized by splenomegaly. Reactions to a variety of commonly prescribed drugs such as antibiotics may result in splenomegaly because of direct effects on the spleen, serum sickness (Chapter 36), or indirectly through effects on the liver.

Hematologic malignancies including myeloproliferative neoplasms frequently manifest with splenomegaly. Patients with lymphoproliferative disorders such as chronic lymphocytic leukemia (Chapter 169) or mantle cell lymphoma (Chapter 171) will in many cases have easily appreciated lymphadenopathy in addition to a palpable spleen. Isolated splenomegaly without associated lymphadenopathy is characteristic of hairy cell leukemia and myeloproliferative neoplasms such as primary myelofibrosis (Chapter 152).[16] Splenomegaly with weight loss related to compression of the stomach and early satiety may be the presenting complaint. Solid tumors may sometimes metastasize to the spleen and result in its enlargement, but this occurrence is unusual. Among solid tumors, malignant melanoma (Chapter 188) is the one most likely to be associated with splenic involvement, but even so, palpable splenomegaly is rare.

Congestive splenomegaly may occur as the result of chronic liver disease with portal hypertension (Chapter 139) or in the setting of splenic or portal vein thrombosis (Chapter 129). Disorders that result in excessive destruction of abnormal red blood cells such as hereditary spherocytosis (Chapter 147) or hemoglobinopathies are also associated with splenomegaly. Storage diseases such as Gaucher disease (Chapter 192), sarcoidosis (Chapter 83), amyloidosis (Chapter 174), thyrotoxicosis (Chapter 207), and hemophagocytic lymphohistiocytosis (Chapter 155) are among the other less common causes of splenomegaly.

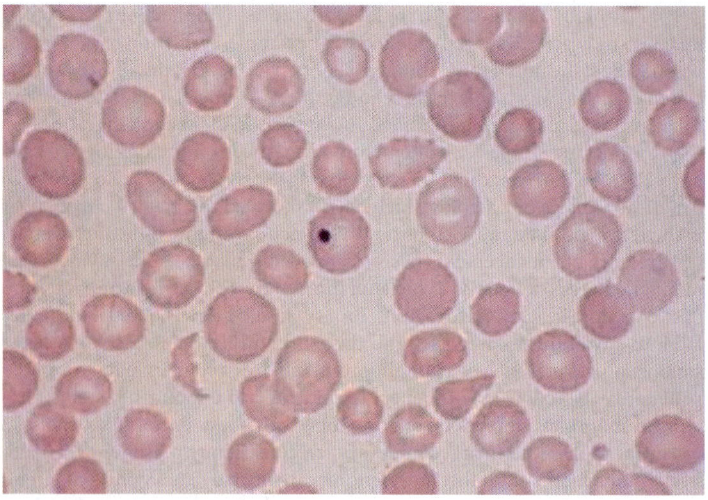

FIGURE 154-3. **Howell-Jolly body in an erythrocyte.** This finding is evidence of prior splenectomy or a nonfunctional spleen.

Laboratory Evaluation

Although the otherwise asymptomatic patient may be monitored, the symptomatic patient requires a diagnosis so that appropriate treatment may be initiated. Laboratory studies, especially the complete blood count and peripheral blood smear, are important tools in the investigation of the patient with splenomegaly. An enlarged spleen is frequently hyperfunctional ("hypersplenism") and sequesters red cells and platelets, thereby leading to anemia and thrombocytopenia. Leukopenia may also occur. In the presence of hypersplenism, examination of the peripheral smear (Chapter 143) in the patient with splenomegaly may show nucleated red blood cells and red cell abnormalities characteristic of chronic liver disease. The presence of abnormal lymphocytes (e.g., cells with projections as in hairy cell leukemia or with villous projections in splenic marginal zone lymphoma with villous lymphocytes) suggests the presence of a malignant leukemia or lymphoma. The presence of lymphoblasts points to acute lymphoblastic leukemia. In the absence of a functioning spleen, basophilic inclusions representing nuclear remnants, known as *Howell-Jolly bodies*, are seen in circulating red blood cells. The presence of Howell-Jolly bodies (Fig. 154-3) in peripheral blood indicates that the patient has either undergone splenectomy or has a nonfunctioning spleen, as in patients with sickle cell disease who have experienced repeated splenic infarcts.

Flow cytometric analysis can identify the abnormal cell population in many cases. A bone marrow aspirate and biopsy with immunohistochemistry, special stains, flow cytometric analysis, fluorescent in situ hybridization, cytogenetics, and additional molecular testing for particular mutations may be required for the complete evaluation of the patient with splenomegaly and a hematologic malignancy.

Elevated lactate dehydrogenase and uric acid levels are seen in lymphoid malignancies such as Burkitt lymphoma or other aggressive non-Hodgkin lymphomas, but also in myeloid malignancies. Examination of thick smears in patients suspected of malaria may show the offending parasite. Genetic testing may confirm a suspected diagnosis (e.g., in hemophagocytic lymphohistiocytosis).

Imaging

Not all palpable spleens are abnormal, especially in very thin individuals. The least invasive and most inexpensive approach to imaging the spleen is ultrasound, an approach that allows for sequential and accurate measurements. By ultrasound criteria, a spleen that is 13 cm or greater in length and more than 5 cm in thickness qualifies as enlarged.

In comparison with ultrasound, CT scans generally focus on the entire abdomen, not just the spleen, and provide important information that often provides an explanation for the splenomegaly. CT scans also will show

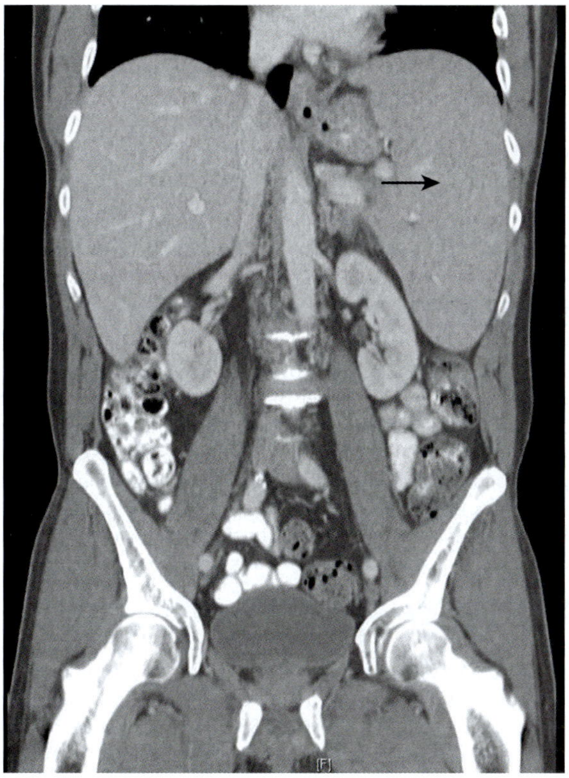

FIGURE 154-4. Splenomegaly (indicated by *arrow*) in a patient with hemophagocytic lymphohistiocytosis.

whether the spleen is diffusely enlarged or enlarged because of multiple nodules (Fig. 154-4). Fluorodeoxyglucose-PET does not distinguish among a variety of malignancies, infections, and other causes of splenomegaly, and it generally is not useful in the diagnostic evaluation of the patient with splenomegaly.

Biopsy

Because of the spleen's location and propensity to bleed, needle aspiration or core biopsy of the spleen is performed only at centers skilled and experienced in the procedure. If an extensive evaluation has not provided a likely explanation for splenomegaly and observation is judged to be imprudent, splenectomy may be performed laparoscopically or by laparotomy.[17,18] Because of the risk of surgical complications and long-term susceptibility to infection in splenectomized individuals, the relative risks and benefits of the procedure must be given serious consideration.[19] Once splenectomy is a possibility, immunization should proceed promptly in an attempt to reduce long-term risks. Appropriate vaccination before splenectomy and in asplenic individuals is of utmost importance (Table 154-6). Partial splenectomy is performed in some children with hereditary spherocytosis, splenic tumors, or splenic trauma in an attempt to reduce the long-term risk of sepsis.[20]

TABLE 154-6 RECOMMENDATIONS FOR PNEUMOCOCCAL, MENINGOCOCCAL, AND *HAEMOPHILUS INFLUENZAE* VACCINATION FOR ASPLENIC INDIVIDUALS

The following vaccines are used:	
Meningococcus	Quadrivalent meningococcal conjugate vaccine (Menveo) Meningococcal serogroup B vaccine (Trumenba or Bexsero)
Pneumococcus	23-valent pneumococcal vaccine (PPSV23, Pneumovax) 15-valent conjugate vaccine (PCV 15; Vaxneuvance); 20-valent conjugate vaccine (PCV 20; Prevnar 20)
Haemophilus influenzae	*H. influenza* type b (Hib) conjugate vaccine

GENERAL GUIDELINES

- Adults with functional asplenia (e.g., those with sickle cell disease) or those who require surgical splenectomy should be immunized with pneumococcal, meningococcal, and *H. influenza* vaccines
- If undergoing elective splenectomy, meningococcal, pneumococcal, and *H. influenzae* vaccines should be given at least 14 days before surgery. If not possible, they should be given after no less than 14 days after splenectomy
- Some recommend that the same vaccine combination be given again 8 weeks after the initial doses
- Multiple vaccines can be given at the same visit but injected at separate sites
- There is some variation in the specific recommendations listed below between guidelines from the U.S. Centers for Disease Control (CDC), the U.S. Advisory Committee on Immunization Practices, various institutions, and some European agencies

MENINGOCOCCAL VACCINES

- Quadrivalent meningococcal conjugate vaccines: two doses of Menveo or MenQuadfi, given 2 months apart *plus*
- Serogroup B meningococcal vaccines: either Trumenba (three doses at 0, 1-2, and 6 months apart) *or* Bexsero (two doses at least 1 month apart)
- Boost every 5 years with Menveo, Menactra, or MenQuadfi
- The two serogroup B vaccines are not interchangeable; the same vaccine product must be used for all doses in a series

PNEUMOCOCCAL VACCINES

- For before splenectomy: Prevnar 20 alone or Vaxneuvance followed by Pneumovax at least 8 weeks apart
- For functional asplenia: Prevnar 20 alone or Vaxneuvance followed by Pneumovax at least 8 weeks apart

***HAEMOPHILUS INFLUENZAE* VACCINE**

- Most adults are not at risk because they have already acquired specific antibodies against it through routine childhood vaccination or previous infection. However
- One dose of Hib vaccine can be given before splenectomy
- One dose of Hib vaccine can be given to functionally asplenic individuals

TREATMENT

If a likely cause, such as infectious mononucleosis or another infectious process, is identified and confirmed by testing, appropriate management should follow. The associated splenomegaly should resolve over time. Splenectomy may be indicated as part of the treatment of refractory immune thrombocytopenic purpura (Chapter 158) or inherited anemias such as hereditary spherocytosis (Chapter 147) or in cases of splenic abscess. Splenectomy also occasionally may be required for severe hypersplenism with cytopenias.

PROGNOSIS

Most incidentally identified splenic masses in asymptomatic patients will prove to be benign. When borderline in size, the significance of the incidentally noted spleen, like marginally enlarged lymph nodes, is unclear and requires follow-up. Follow-up imaging in short intervals (3 to 6 months) may establish a lesion to be unchanged and provide reassurance of its benign nature. Additional imaging modalities (e.g., MRI, PET/CT, and ultrasound) may be helpful in selecting appropriate patients for further investigation, including biopsy.

The patient without an obvious explanation for splenomegaly presents a difficult diagnostic challenge. Occult liver disease or an undiagnosed autoimmune process may emerge over time as an explanation for persistent splenomegaly in some of these patients.

Splenectomy or biopsy of focal splenic lesions may be the only diagnostic option in patients with persistent symptoms or progressive cytopenias. Splenectomy may have unintended consequences in patients with occult liver disease and portal hypertension and should be avoided in that setting. In the asymptomatic patient, close observation is often preferable to splenectomy.

GENERAL REFERENCES

For the General References and other additional features, please visit Elsevier eBooks+ at https://ebooks.health.elsevier.com.

155

HISTIOCYTOSES

BARRETT J. ROLLINS AND NANCY BERLINER

The histiocytoses comprise a family of diseases characterized by an accumulation of abnormal cells with features reminiscent of macrophages or dendritic cells. The term *histiocyte* refers to tissue macrophages that are the cell of origin for some histiocytoses. However, many of the other histiocytoses derive from nonmacrophage lineages or from hematopoietic stem cells.

The diagnostic category of histiocytosis embraces a number of heterogeneous but distinct clinical entities, some of which may co-occur in a single patient. Recent advances in molecular genetics provide the basis for a revised nosology that places histiocytic diseases into five groups (Table 155-1)[1,2]:

- L group. These include Langerhans cell histiocytoses and Erdheim-Chester disease because the occasional appearance of both diseases in the same patient suggests a common origin and because both diseases are characterized by somatic mutations in genes of the mitogen-activated protein kinase (MAPK) pathway. Indeterminate cell histiocytosis is also placed in the L group because it shares some characteristics with Langerhans cell histiocytosis.
- C group. These are non-Langerhans cell histiocytoses that involve the skin and/or mucosal surfaces. As in the L group, patients may present with mixtures of C group histiocytoses. They are subdivided into the xanthogranuloma and nonxanthogranuloma diseases. Some C group diseases also have a major systemic component, and mutations in MAPK pathway genes may be seen.
- M group. These are the malignant histiocytoses, which include primary malignancies such as malignant histiocytosis and secondary malignant histiocytoses that occur in the setting of leukemias, lymphomas, or other hematologic neoplasms. Mutations in MAPK pathway genes may occur in these diseases.
- R group. The paradigmatic member of this group is Rosai-Dorfman-Destombes disease, also known as sinus histiocytosis with massive lymphadenopathy. However, the R group also includes all of the other miscellaneous noncutaneous, non-Langerhans cell histiocytoses. Mutations in MAPK pathway genes may occur in these diseases.
- H group. This group contains the varieties of hemophagocytic lymphohistiocytosis and macrophage activation syndromes.

TABLE 155-1 CLASSIFICATION OF HISTIOCYTOSES AND MACROPHAGE/DENDRITIC CELL NEOPLASMS

L group	Langerhans cell histiocytosis (LCH) Indeterminate cell histiocytosis (ICH) Erdheim-Chester disease (ECD)
C group	Cutaneous non-Langerhans cell histiocytoses Xanthogranuloma (XG) family Juvenile xanthogranuloma (JXG) Adult xanthogranuloma (AXG) Solitary reticulohistiocytoma (SRH) Benign cephalic histiocytosis (BCH) Generalized disruptive histiocytosis (GEH) Progressive nodular histiocytosis (PNH) Xanthoma disseminatum (XD) Nonxanthogranuloma (non-XG) family Cutaneous Rosai-Dorfman-Destombes disease (RDD) Necrobiotic xanthogranuloma (NXG) Multicentric reticulohistiocytosis (MRH) Cutaneous non-Langerhans cell histiocytoses with major systemic involvement
R group	Familial Rosai-Dorfman-Destombes disease (RDD), also known as sinus histiocytosis with massive lymphadenopathy (SHML) Sporadic RDD Classical RDD Extranodal RDD RDD with neoplasia or immune disease Not otherwise classified
M group	Primary malignant histiocytoses Secondary malignant histiocytoses (associated with hematologic neoplasia) Subtypes: histiocytic, interdigitating, Langerhans, indeterminate
H group	Primary hemophagocytic lymphohistiocytosis (HLH) Secondary HLH HLH of unknown or uncertain origin

L GROUP

LANGERHANS CELL HISTIOCYTOSIS

EPIDEMIOLOGY

Langerhans cell histiocytosis occurs predominantly in children (median age, 3.8 years) but is also seen in adults.[3] Its overall incidence is 2.6 cases per million child years for all children younger than 14 years of age but with a strong trend toward a higher incidence in younger children. There is a slight excess of cases in male patients (1.2 : 1). The incidence of high-risk Langerhans cell histiocytosis is lower in Blacks than in Whites and higher in Hispanics than in non-Hispanics. The incidence in adults has been estimated at 1 to 2 cases per million. Pulmonary Langerhans cell histiocytosis, which occurs primarily in adults, is strongly associated with a smoking history.

PATHOBIOLOGY

The cardinal feature of Langerhans cell histiocytoses is an accumulation of abnormal histiocytes having abundant pale cytoplasm and a single kidney- or coffee bean–shaped nucleus (Fig. 155-1A). All pathologic Langerhans cells express the surface marker CD1a (Fig. 155-1B), and most express CD207, a mannose-binding lectin also known as Langerin. A majority of cells contain intracellular organelles called Birbeck granules, which can be detected by electron microscopy and are composed of CD207 molecules. The lesions are commonly accompanied by a robust inflammatory infiltrate the quality of which may vary depending on the clinical subtype (e.g., abundant eosinophils in eosinophilic granuloma of bone) (see Clinical Manifestations).

Langerhans cell histiocytosis is a neoplastic disease with clonal cells, most of which carry somatic activating mutations in genes that encode members of the MAPK pathway. Specifically, 50 to 60% have mutated *BRAF* (predominantly, but not exclusively, the mutation that encodes the oncogenic variant BRAF V600E), and 25 to 30% have activating mutations of *MAP2K1*. All cases show evidence for activation of extracellular signal-regulated kinase (ERK), the target of this kinase pathway, and the remaining 10 to 25% of cases without *BRAF* or *MAP2K1* mutations have mutations in other genes that activate the pathway, including *ARAF* and *RAS* family members, or translocations resulting in fusion proteins that activate *BRAF*.[4]

Historically, Langerhans cell histiocytosis was acknowledged to be a disease of histiocytes, but because the origin of Langerhans cell histiocytes was unknown, the disease was called histiocytosis X. Langerhans histiocytosis cells express CD1a and CD207 and have Birbeck granules, all of which are characteristic of normal Langerhans cells. However, the profile of genes expressed by Langerhans histiocytosis cells is closer to that of myeloid precursor cells than mature Langerhans cells. In addition, *BRAF* mutations can be detected in hematopoietic stem cells of patients whose Langerhans histiocytosis cells have *BRAF* mutations, a finding suggesting that Langerhans cell histiocytosis is more properly viewed as a myeloid neoplasm in which myeloid precursors may partially differentiate in a direction that allows them to acquire attributes that are also characteristic of Langerhans cells.

CLINICAL MANIFESTATIONS

Langerhans cell histiocytoses may occur at any age and involve any organ. However, the disease is more common in children, and the organs most frequently affected include the following:

- Bone (80% of cases). Skeletal lesions may be asymptomatic or may be associated with tenderness and swelling. The most common locations (in descending order of frequency) are skull, pelvis, femur, ribs, humerus, mandible, and spine, where they appear as punched-out lytic lesions without sclerosis on radiographs (Fig. 155-1C). Resorption of alveolar bone can lead to the appearance of so-called "floating teeth."
- Skin (33% of cases). The rash may be intensely petechial and include scaly and encrusted papules (Fig. 155-1D and E). When skin involvement is the presenting manifestation, the rash may be confused with seborrheic dermatitis and "cradle cap" in infants.
- Hypothalamus and pituitary stalk (25% of cases). Pituitary involvement can lead to diabetes insipidus, which was historically observed to occur in

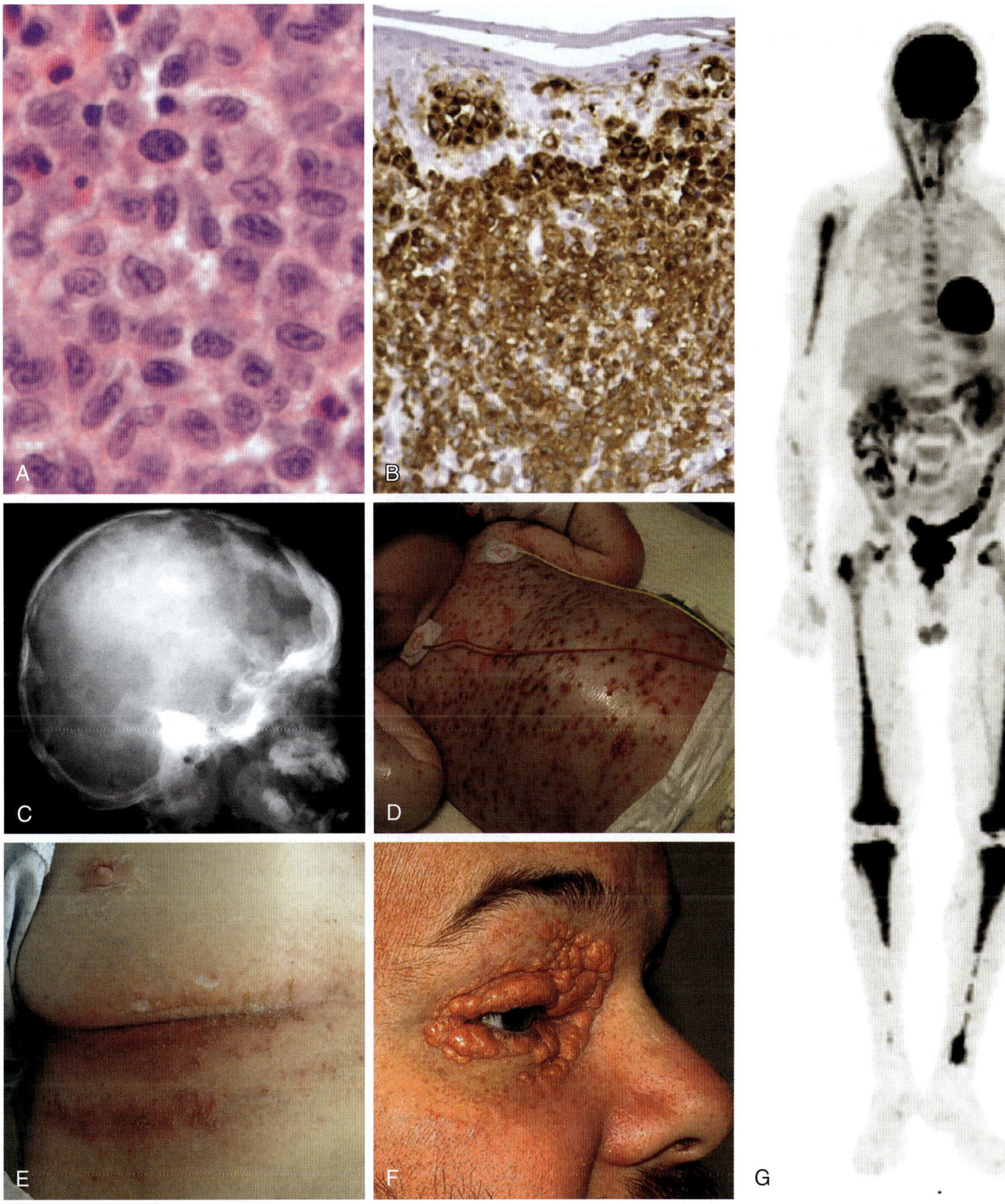

FIGURE 155-1. Histologic, radiographic, and cutaneous features of Langerhans cell histiocytosis (LCH) and Erdheim-Chester disease (ECD). A, Hematoxylin and eosin stain of a Langerhans cell histiocytosis bone lesion demonstrating the characteristic kidney- or coffee bean–shaped nuclei and abundant pink cytoplasm of Langerhans cell histiocytes (1000× magnification). **B,** CD1a immunostain of a Langerhans cell histiocytosis skin lesion showing uniformly stained Langerhans cell histiocytes infiltrating the upper dermis and focally involving the epidermis (200× magnification). **C,** Radiographic image showing lytic skull bone lesions in Langerhans cell histiocytosis. **D,** Cutaneous lesions in a child with multisystem Langerhans cell histiocytosis. **E,** Intertriginous lesion in an adult with cutaneous Langerhans cell histiocytosis. **F,** Periorbital xanthelasma in a patient with ECD. **G,** Fluorine-18–radiolabeled fluorodeoxyglucose positron emission tomographic (PET) scan of a patient with ECD showing bilateral and symmetrical abnormal signals in femora, tibiae, and humeri. (**A** and **B**, From Degar, BA, Fleming, MD, Rollins, BJ, Rodriguez-Galindo C. Histiocytoses. In: Orkin SH, Fisher DE, Ginsburg D, et al, eds. *Nathan and Oski's Hematology and Oncology of Infancy and Childhood*. 8th ed. Philadelphia: Elsevier Saunders; 2015:2104; **C** to **G**, From Emile J-F, Abla O, Fraitag S, et al. Revised classification of histiocytoses and neoplasms of the macrophage-dendritic cell lineages. *Blood*. 2016;127:2672-2781.)

25 to 50% of patients with Langerhans cell histiocytosis. With earlier diagnosis and effective chemotherapy, the contemporary incidence of diabetes insipidus has been reduced to 7 to 20%.

Involvement of the liver, spleen, bone marrow, or lungs occurs in 15% of cases; involvement of lymph nodes in 5 to 10%, and central nervous system (CNS; excluding pituitary) in 2 to 4%. Lung involvement is more frequent in adults than in children.

The clinical manifestations of Langerhans cell histiocytoses are extraordinarily diverse. However, some presentations were sufficiently stereotypic that they had been recognized as separate entities before the understanding that they are manifestations of the same disease. Importantly, the eponyms for these entities are no longer in use but are listed here to aid in understanding older literature:

- Hand-Schüller-Christian disease: triad of exophthalmos, diabetes insipidus, and bone lesions (especially cranial) in children; 15 to 40% of cases
- Letterer-Siwe disease (or Abt-Letterer-Siwe disease): multisystem disease involving skin, bone, lymph nodes, liver, and spleen in infants; poor prognosis
- Eosinophilic granuloma: bone only, often solitary; 60 to 80% of cases

TABLE 155-2 CLINICAL CLASSIFICATION OF LANGERHANS CELL HISTIOCYTOSIS*

CLINICAL GROUP	INVOLVED SYSTEM	INVOLVED ORGANS
1	Multisystem	Any risk organ†
2	Multisystem	≥2 organs *not including risk organs*
3	Single system • Multifocal‡ or special site§	≥2 lesions in one organ or in a special site§
—	Single system • Unifocal or localized	1 lesion in 1 organ

*Developed for the Langerhans Cell Histiocytosis-III (LCH-III) trial.
†Risk organs: bone marrow, liver, or spleen. (Lung is no longer classified as a risk organ.)
‡Multiple sites of involvement in a single organ system.
§Special sites confer increased risk of specific complications and include intracranial soft tissue extension or vertebral lesions with intraspinal soft tissue extension.

- Hashimoto-Pritzker disease (or congenital self-healing reticulohistiocytosis): self-limited skin involvement in newborns

The contemporary classification of Langerhans cell histiocytoses is based on clinical attributes that correlate with risk and therefore guide therapy. The two dimensions of risk are the number of organs involved (single system vs. multisystem disease) and the presence of disease in "risk organs" (defined as bone marrow, liver, or spleen; Table 155-2).

A late manifestation of Langerhans cell histiocytoses is neurodegeneration, which occurs in about 10% of surviving patients. Manifestations include ataxia, dysarthria, and dysmetria, along with neurocognitive decline and psychological difficulties. Magnetic resonance imaging (MRI) shows signal intensity changes in the cerebellar peduncles, basal ganglia, and pons. The clinical manifestations may wax and wane, but the disease is relentlessly progressive.

DIAGNOSIS

Because the clinical manifestations of Langerhans cell histiocytoses are nonspecific, clinicians must have a high index of suspicion in adult patients who present with a nonhealing seborrheic rash or solitary osteolytic lesion. In patients with diabetes insipidus, characteristic infiltration of the pituitary stalk may be seen on MRI. Pulmonary Langerhans cell histiocytoses should be considered in young smokers with dyspnea or a nonproductive cough whose plain chest radiographs show diffuse bilateral reticulonodular disease in the middle and upper lung zones. Computed tomography (CT) may show nodules or cysts.

Tissue analysis is mandatory. Histopathologic examination shows an infiltrate of histiocytic cells with pale cytoplasm and a single kidney- or coffee bean–shaped nucleus accompanied by varying numbers and types of inflammatory cells (see Fig. 155-1A). Eosinophils may be abundant. Definitive diagnosis requires a demonstration that the histiocytes stain for CD1a (see Fig. 155-1B). Positive staining for CD207 may further support the diagnosis of Langerhans cell histiocytosis. Electron microscopic examination for Birbeck granules has been supplanted by CD207 staining.

TREATMENT

Treatment strategies are evolving rapidly based on molecular testing, but decisions about specific therapies and their intensity have historically been driven by risk stratification. For example, patients with single system disease without organ dysfunction have an excellent prognosis and can be treated with local therapy (e.g., surgical curettage or radiation) or simply monitored and treated when symptomatic. More extensive disease requires systemic therapy, which typically begins with vinblastine and prednisone under expert supervision. Prolonging treatment in patients with multisystem disease decreases the risk of relapse from 54 to 37%. Thus, current standard of care for multisystem disease is vinblastine and prednisone induction followed by 12 months of continued therapy. Adding etoposide to the induction therapy may benefit patients with risk organ involvement.

Various approaches are available for relapsed or recurrent Langerhans cell histiocytosis, referred to historically as "reactivation," which occurs in 20 to 50% of patients. These patients can be placed into low-risk and high-risk categories. Low-risk patients are those who initially had low-risk multisystem Langerhans cell histiocytosis (i.e., no risk organ involvement or multifocal bone disease). Responses to a variety of second-line therapies have been documented, including 6-mercaptopurine and methotrexate, indomethacin, bisphosphonates, and nucleoside analogues such as cladribine, cytarabine, and clofarabine. High-risk patients are those who had risk organ involvement at presentation or showed a poor response to first-line treatment. Cladribine[5] and high-dose cytarabine may be effective in this setting, as is hematopoietic stem cell transplantation, but mortality is still significant.

The discovery of activating mutations in genes encoding MAPK pathway components has led to the use of rapidly advancing fibrosarcoma (RAF) and MAP kinase/ERK kinase 1 (MEK1) inhibitors, primarily in the relapsed setting.[6] In general, patients carrying sensitive mutations in *BRAF* or *MAP2K1*, including heavily pretreated patients, show remarkable responses to inhibitors of RAF (e.g., vemurafenib and dabrafenib), or MEK1 (e.g., cobimetinib, which has been approved by the FDA for use in patients with histiocytic neoplasms that do not carry the mutation encoding BRAF V600E). Optimal dosing has not yet been explored in a clinical trial, and treatment has generally been devised based on efficacy in other diseases. Most reports indicate that patients continue to respond to these inhibitors for as long as they are treated and have relapses when treatment is discontinued. Therefore, despite the remarkable efficacy of these agents, the roles that these inhibitors may play in curative or first-line treatment of Langerhans cell histiocytoses are currently unclear.

For adults with pulmonary Langerhans cell histiocytosis, smoking cessation is usually sufficient treatment. If not, these patients may be treated with corticosteroids. Patients with refractory cases may require lung transplantation.

PROGNOSIS

Outcomes in single system and low-risk disease are quite good. Overall survival for single system disease is more than 99%, with a relapse rate of 18%. In low-risk multisystem disease 5-year overall survival is 99% despite a 40 to 50% cumulative rate of relapse. Nonetheless, morbidities associated with the initial site of disease, especially orthopedic problems, may be long standing and significant. Patients with multisystem high-risk disease have an 84% 5-year overall survival with a 27% relapse rate in Langerhans cell histiocytosis-III. Failure to respond to initial therapy carries a dismal prognosis. Neurodegeneration may appear in up to 10% of patients several years after otherwise successful treatment and in the absence of active histiocytic disease. Sclerosing cholangitis (Chapter 141) may lead to long-term morbidity. The risk of developing leukemia or lymphoma is also higher than in the general population.[7]

ERDHEIM-CHESTER DISEASE

EPIDEMIOLOGY

Erdheim-Chester disease is extremely rare. Fewer than 1000 cases have been reported, and its precise incidence and prevalence are unknown. In contrast to Langerhans cell histiocytosis, Erdheim-Chester disease occurs primarily in adults between 40 and 70 years of age (mean age at diagnosis of 53 years),[8] although it may occur in children and infants. Male patients outnumber female patients by a ratio of nearly 3:1.

PATHOBIOLOGY

Histopathologic examination of lesions shows infiltration by foamy mononuclear histiocytes often accompanied by fibrosis and inflammation involving lymphocytes, neutrophils, or plasma cells. Occasional multinucleated giant cells may be observed. Because the histiocytes stain for CD68 and CD163, and not for CD1a, Erdheim-Chester disease histiocytes are thought to derive from the monocyte-macrophage lineage. Although these characteristics distinguish Erdheim-Chester disease from Langerhans cell histiocytosis, 20% of patients with Erdheim-Chester disease have concurrent Langerhans cell histiocytosis.

As in Langerhans cell histiocytosis, about 50% of patients with Erdheim-Chester disease have somatic mutations encoding BRAF V600E. Essentially all remaining patients have other genetic variants that activate the MAPK pathway, including mutations in *MAP2K1*, *ARAF*, *KRAS*, and *NRAS*, as well as gene fusions that activate *BRAF*, *ALK*, and *NTRK*. Mutations in *PIK3CA* have been observed and may co-occur with *BRAF* mutations.

CLINICAL MANIFESTATIONS

Histiocytic infiltration of bone occurs in nearly all patients, manifesting as symmetrical cortical sclerosis of diaphyseal and metaphyseal areas of long bones, often in the lower extremities (Fig. 155-1G). Patients may complain of mild juxta-articular pain but may also be asymptomatic in the presence of radiographic disease. Osteosclerosis of facial bones or other bones of the skull may also occur. CT or MRI may be necessary to detect lesions not seen on plain radiographs.

Cardiovascular involvement by fibrosis occurs in the majority of patients, may manifest as valvular abnormalities, conduction defects, or periaortic coating, and is one of the main causes of morbidity and mortality in Erdheim-Chester disease. Similar fibrosis may occur in the retroperitoneum, encircling the kidneys and leading to a progressive obstructive nephropathy. About 50% of patients with Erdheim-Chester disease have pulmonary disease involving the pleura, parenchyma, or both. About 40% of patients have CNS disease, including pituitary involvement leading to diabetes insipidus and mass lesions in various parts of the brain. CNS involvement portends a worse outcome. Cognitive impairment and behavioral changes may also occur in the absence of MRI-documented infiltration or masses, although they may be associated with gray matter volume loss. Cutaneous disease occurs in about 25% of patients and usually manifests as xanthelasma, most frequently involving the eyelids (Fig. 155-1F).

DIAGNOSIS

Diagnosis must be made by histologic examination of involved sites, preferably osteosclerotic bone. Because genetic analysis for mutations in MAPK pathway genes informs clinical care and because decalcification for histologic examination may preclude such analysis, sufficient material must be collected and processed separately for both histologic and genetic testing. Absence of CD1a or CD207 staining will distinguish Erdheim-Chester disease from Langerhans cell histiocytosis. However, 20% of patients with Erdheim-Chester disease have concurrent Langerhans cell histiocytosis. Clinical manifestations of Erdheim-Chester disease may be confused with those of Paget disease or POEMS (polyneuropathy, organomegaly, endocrinopathy, myeloma protein, and skin changes) syndrome (Chapter 173), but the histopathologic picture of these disorders is distinct. Juvenile xanthogranuloma is a histiocytic disease of the C group (see later), and its histopathologic features are very similar to those of Erdheim-Chester disease. However, juvenile xanthogranuloma typically occurs in young children and only rarely involves extracutaneous sites. When juvenile xanthogranuloma is disseminated, lesional cells may harbor activating mutations in genes of the MAPK pathway, which is reminiscent of Erdheim-Chester disease and places this form of juvenile xanthogranuloma in the L group.

When the tissue diagnosis of Erdheim-Chester disease is confirmed, the extent of disease should be determined. A full endocrine evaluation should be performed to assess pituitary involvement, and imaging studies should include long bones, skull, and pelvis, as well as CT or MRI evaluation of the brain, the full length of the aorta, and the retroperitoneum. These studies may reveal characteristic periaortic thickening ("coated" aorta) and retroperitoneal fibrosis ("hairy kidneys"). Fluorine-18–radiolabeled fluorodeoxyglucose uptake demonstrated by positron emission tomography has been reported to provide high specificity in the setting of osteosclerosis (Fig. 155-1G). The presence of cardiac conduction abnormalities should be evaluated by electrocardiography. Macrophage-like cells that stain for S100 and show emperipolesis may be seen histologically and could suggest a diagnosis of Rosai-Dorfman-Destombes disease, but the clinical presentation of Erdheim-Chester disease is distinct from that of Rosai-Dorfman-Destombes disease (see later).

TREATMENT

Because most cases of Erdheim-Chester disease are indolent, asymptomatic patients who have no CNS disease may be followed without treatment.[9] If patients have CNS disease or develop troublesome symptoms, systemic treatment is warranted. The nearly universal presence of mutations in genes encoding components of the MAPK pathway in this disorder has moved targeted therapies to the forefront. A basket trial of the RAF inhibitor vemurafenib, given to patients with a variety of diseases carrying a somatic mutation encoding BRAF V600E and including several cases of Erdheim-Chester disease, resulted in prolonged responses in 6 of 18 patients. Thus RAF inhibitors may be administered under expert supervision to patients whose disease carries activating mutations in *BRAF* or *ARAF*. Patients without these mutations may be treated with the MEK inhibitor cobimetinib which the FDA has approved for treating BRAF V600E-negative Erdheim-Chester disease.

If targeted therapies cannot be used, treatment with interferon (IFN) alfa (conventional or pegylated) is recommended because of a suggestion of survival benefit in a retrospective analysis. For patients in whom IFN treatment fails, cladribine or cyclophosphamide may produce responses. Glucocorticoids, interleukin-1 receptor (IL-1R) antagonists, and anti-TNF agents may also have activity. Radiotherapy may provide relief of local symptoms.

PROGNOSIS

Although therapies targeted against BRAF V600E or MEK1 produce impressive symptomatic and radiographic responses in most patients with Erdheim-Chester disease, the impact of these drugs on survival is currently unknown. In one small study of patients treated with IFN-alfa, 1- and 5-year overall survival rates were 93 and 41%, respectively, versus 86 and 28% in patients who did not receive interferon.

INDETERMINATE CELL HISTIOCYTOSIS

Indeterminate cell histiocytosis is an exceedingly rare disease that may manifest as a cutaneous eruption mimicking Langerhans cell histiocytosis, although some cases may involve lymph nodes only. It occurs in adults and may predominantly affect women, although no rigorous epidemiologic analyses have been performed. Histologic analysis of lesions shows a nonepidermotropic infiltration of histiocytes that may stain for CD1a, similar to Langerhans cell histiocytosis, but do not express CD207. One report describes a case with a somatic mutation encoding BRAF V600E and may support the notion that indeterminate cell histiocytosis is related to Langerhans cell histiocytosis. However, another report collected four cases, three of which showed the same *ETV3-NCOA2* gene fusion. Although the pathogenic relevance of this translocation is unknown, its recurrent appearance in indeterminate cell histiocytosis and its absence from Langerhans cell histiocytoses indicate that these are distinct entities.

C GROUP

These non-Langerhans cell histiocytoses are divided into those that are predominantly cutaneous versus those that have a significant systemic component. Each group is further divided into the xanthogranuloma and nonxanthogranuloma categories.

XANTHOGRANULOMA FAMILY

EPIDEMIOLOGY

This group comprises several diseases that are distinguished primarily on the basis of clinical presentation: patient age, anatomic site of involvement, and whether lesions are solitary, multiple, or disseminated. Juvenile xanthogranuloma is the most commonly occurring non-Langerhans cell histiocytosis. Although its published prevalence is 0.5% of pediatric tumors, the benign nature of juvenile xanthogranuloma likely leads to underreporting. A slight excess of cases in female patients has been observed (1.4:1).

PATHOBIOLOGY

Lesions contain a dermal infiltrate that includes histiocytes, occasional multinucleated giant cells that may have the features of Touton cells, and nonspecific inflammatory cells. Regressing lesions show replacement by fibrous tissue. Histiocytes stain for CD68, CD14, CD163, factor XIIIa, and fascin; S100 staining may be absent or variable, and the cells do not stain for CD1a or CD207.

Juvenile xanthogranuloma may occur in association with neurofibromatosis type 1, although the relationship between genetic abnormalities in NF1 and JXG is unknown. Mutations involving *NRAS, KRAS, BRAF, ARAF, MAP2K1*, and *MAPK1* have been reported, as well as activating RNF11/BRAF and MRC1/PDGFRB fusions. Mutations in *PIK3CD* have also been reported. To date, MAPK pathway mutations have been described only in disseminated and not cutaneous cases. Because of the phenotypic similarities between disseminated JXG and Erdheim-Chester disease, and because of the presence of mutations in MAPK genes in both, disseminated juvenile xanthogranuloma has been classified in the L group. Cutaneous juvenile xanthogranuloma remains in the C group.

CLINICAL MANIFESTATIONS

Juvenile xanthogranuloma is a benign disease in which a variable number of small (<2.0-cm) yellow-red skin nodules appear most commonly on the head, neck, or upper trunk, although they may occur anywhere. About 70% of lesions are solitary. Systemic disease occurs rarely and may involve liver, lung, spleen, lymph nodes, bone, and gastrointestinal tract. Both cutaneous and systemic lesions generally resolve spontaneously within a few months or years, with no clinically significant sequelae. Some cases of disseminated juvenile xanthogranuloma in newborns or juvenile xanthogranuloma producing symptoms may require treatment.

Xanthoma disseminatum is also in the xanthogranuloma family and manifests as a cutaneous eruption of brown papules or nodules on flexor and periorbital areas. It involves mucosal surfaces and has a significant visceral component. Xanthoma disseminatum primarily affects young adult men and has a chronic clinical course that may include diabetes insipidus.

DIAGNOSIS

The clinical appearance of cutaneous xanthogranuloma may be sufficiently characteristic that a diagnosis can be made by observation alone. Biopsy and immune staining may be required for ambiguous cases. Xanthogranuloma histiocytes stain for CD68, CD163, factor XIIIa, and fascin and do not stain for CD1a, CD207, and, generally, S100. Differential diagnosis includes the following: Langerhans cell histiocytosis, which can be distinguished by immune staining; papular xanthoma, the lesions of which contain more foam cells and fewer giant cells than xanthogranuloma; eruptive xanthoma, generally in hypertriglyceridemic adults; Spitz nevi; mastocytoma; and dermatofibroma.

TREATMENT

Patients with cutaneous juvenile xanthogranuloma may be observed without treatment. Patients with ocular involvement by juvenile xanthogranuloma or xanthoma disseminatum should be referred to an ophthalmologist for evaluation. Symptomatic visceral involvement may be treated, if necessary, with surgical excision, radiation therapy, or chemotherapy under expert supervision. Chemotherapeutic regimens used for Langerhans cell histiocytes may be effective in this setting.

PROGNOSIS

Cutaneous and visceral xanthogranuloma lesions spontaneously resolve, and the overall prognosis is excellent. Treatment outcomes for symptomatic visceral lesions are also good. Fatalities may occur rarely in infants with extensive hepatic involvement or CNS disease.

NONXANTHOGRANULOMA FAMILY

EPIDEMIOLOGY

Necrobiotic xanthogranuloma occurs in adults (average age of onset is in the sixth decade) and is accompanied by monoclonal gammopathy in 80% of patients.[10] There is no sex predilection. Multicentric reticulohistiocytosis is a disease of women in their 50s and 60s.[11] Rosai-Dorfman-Destombes disease may rarely be confined to the skin and in this manifestation should be considered a nonxanthogranuloma group C disease.

PATHOBIOLOGY

The pathobiology of necrobiotic xanthogranuloma is not understood, but its association with paraproteinemias has suggested that it may be a histiocytic reaction to the deposition of immunoglobulins. Histopathologic examination shows histiocytic xanthogranulomas with bands of necrosis in the dermis, accompanied by giant cells that may have a characteristic morphology for this disease. Lymphoid nodules and plasma cells may be seen.

One fourth of patients with multicentric reticulohistiocytosis have an underlying malignancy, thus raising the possibility that this is a paraneoplastic syndrome. However, no pathogenetic mechanism has been identified. Associated malignancies include breast and gastric cancers, as well as hematologic neoplasms.

CLINICAL MANIFESTATIONS

The cutaneous lesions of necrobiotic xanthogranuloma are discolored and indurated papules and nodules that may coalesce to form plaques, the centers of which may be atrophic. Periorbital areas are the most common site of involvement, but lesions may occur elsewhere on the face, trunk, arms, legs, and genitalia. The most common site of extracutaneous involvement is the eye and can manifest as uveitis or scleritis. Visceral involvement may also occur in a variety of sites but most commonly in the respiratory tract or cardiac structures.

The cutaneous lesions of multicentric reticulohistiocytosis are discolored papules that appear predominantly on the face, hands, forearms, and ears. The oral or nasal mucosa may also be involved. Periungual lesions may have a characteristic "coral bead" appearance. Patients with multicentric reticulohistiocytosis have a rapidly progressive destructive polyarthritis with systemic symptoms such as fever and weight loss.

DIAGNOSIS

Periorbital yellowish plaques with associated erythema and central atrophy or telangiectasias are highly suggestive of necrobiotic xanthogranuloma. Skin biopsy should be performed to confirm the diagnosis. Serum and urine electrophoresis should be performed to test for the presence of monoclonal gammopathy, and further hematologic work-up should be dictated by the results. Imaging of the chest, abdomen, and pelvis should be performed to assess visceral disease. The periorbital lesions of necrobiotic xanthogranuloma are distinguished from xanthelasmas or plane xanthomas by the former's larger size, induration, and erythema. Ocular involvement may be documented by conjunctival biopsy. Necrobiotic xanthogranuloma should also be distinguished from necrobiosis lipoidica, which occurs in patients with diabetes mellitus and has a histopathologic picture distinct from that of necrobiotic xanthogranuloma.

Histopathologic examination of multicentric reticulohistiocytosis shows frequent multinucleated giant cells and macrophages with eosinophilic cytoplasm. Multicentric reticulohistiocytosis may be reminiscent of fibroblastic rheumatism, although skin lesions in the latter are characterized histologically by fibrosis.

TREATMENT

Unlike xanthogranuloma, necrobiotic xanthogranuloma requires treatment because it does not spontaneously resolve and can produce disfiguring sequelae. No rigorous studies have identified an ideal treatment. Case reports suggest that alkylators such as chlorambucil or melphalan, with or without steroids, may be effective first-line therapy under expert supervision. Intravenous immunoglobulin has been used as second-line therapy, and lenalidomide has been used in patients with monoclonal gammopathy even in the absence of clinically documented multiple myeloma. Treatment of multicentric reticulohistiocytosis should be directed toward the underlying neoplasm if present.

PROGNOSIS

Scarring and ulceration may be common sequelae of cutaneous necrobiotic xanthogranuloma lesions. Patients with necrobiotic xanthogranuloma have an increased risk of developing hematologic malignancies and should be monitored. Treatment of the underlying neoplasm may not lead to resolution of multicentric reticulohistiocytosis.

R GROUP

The R group is composed primarily of the various manifestations of Rosai-Dorfman-Destombes disease, also known as sinus histiocytosis with massive lymphadenopathy.

EPIDEMIOLOGY

Sporadic Rosai-Dorfman-Destombes is a rare disease that occurs more commonly in children and young adults, with a peak incidence in the second and third decades. Overall prevalence is 5 per 100,000. The disease occurs more frequently in males and in individuals of African ancestry. Rosai-Dorfman-Destombes occurs in the lymph nodes of 20% of patients with H syndrome, which is associated with mutation in the *SLC29A3* gene. Nodal involvement also occurs in 41% of patients with autoimmune lymphoproliferative syndrome (ALPS) type Ia in which germline mutations affect *TNFRSF6*, which encodes Fas.

PATHOBIOLOGY

Nodal Rosai-Dorfman-Destombes is characterized by an accumulation in lymph node sinuses of large, polyclonal histiocytes with hypochromatic nuclei and pale cytoplasm, often showing emperipolesis (the presence of an intact cell within the cytoplasm of another cell). The histiocytes express macrophage markers, including S100, CD68, CD14, HLA-DR, and CD163, and do not express CD1a or CD207. Cortical regions of involved lymph nodes often have abundant plasma cells and activated B lymphocytes. Histiocytes may also accumulate in extranodal sites accompanied by plasma cells. The plasma cells are often immunoglobulin 4 (IgG4) positive. In some cases, histiocytes may harbor somatic mutations in MAPK pathway genes, *NRAS*, *KRAS*, *BRAF*, *ARAF*, and *MAP2K1*, suggesting that a subset of Rosai-Dorfman-Destombes disease may be associated with oncogenic driver mutations.

CLINICAL MANIFESTATIONS

Patients with nodal Rosai-Dorfman-Destombes present with nontender, massively enlarged cervical lymphadenopathy along with systemic inflammatory signs such as fever, leukocytosis, elevated erythrocyte sedimentation rate, and a polyclonal hypergammaglobulinemia. Nasal or tracheal obstruction may occur. Other involved nodal sites may include axilla, mediastinum, retroperitoneum, and inguinal regions. Extranodal involvement occurs in 43% of sporadic Rosai-Dorfman-Destombes cases, most commonly skin, nasal cavity, retro-orbital tissue, dura, bone, and soft tissue.

DIAGNOSIS

Diagnosis of Rosai-Dorfman-Destombes requires histopathologic examination of involved lymph nodes or extranodal tissues. The immunohistochemical staining pattern of the characteristic histiocytes is described earlier.

Rosai-Dorfman-Destombes disease can be distinguished from Langerhans cell histiocytosis by the absence of CD1a or CD207 staining. In cases of cutaneous involvement, differentiation from juvenile xanthogranuloma may be difficult. Intracranial Rosai-Dorfman-Destombes may have the radiographic appearance of meningioma, but characteristic cells may be seen in cerebrospinal fluid. Frequent IgG4-positive plasma cells in this disease may also raise a suspicion of IgG4-related disease (also known as hyper-IgG4 syndrome), although the clinical manifestations are distinct.

TREATMENT

Sporadic Rosai-Dorfman-Destombes disease generally has a favorable outcome and may resolve spontaneously over months to years. Symptomatic disease may be treated with corticosteroids, clofarabine, or radiation therapy under expert supervision. KRAS- or MEK-variant disease may respond to cobimetinib under expert oversight.[12]

PROGNOSIS

The prognosis of sporadic Rosai-Dorfman-Destombes is generally favorable.

M GROUP

The M group consists of malignant histiocytoses, which can be primary or can occur in association with other neoplasms.

EPIDEMIOLOGY

Malignant histiocytosis is rare, and its true incidence is unknown. It is a disease of adults, with a median age of diagnosis for the histiocytic sarcoma subtype in the mid-40s to mid-50s, and no sex imbalance. Secondary malignant histiocytosis may occur in the context of hematologic diseases such as acute lymphoblastic leukemia (but not acute myeloid leukemia), chronic lymphocytic leukemia, hairy cell leukemia, myelodysplastic syndrome, chronic myelomonocytic leukemia, follicular lymphoma, mediastinal germ cell tumors, and Langerhans cell histiocytosis.

PATHOBIOLOGY

Malignant histiocytosis cells are anaplastic and have frequent mitotic figures and atypical mitoses. Cells do not stain for epithelial markers such as keratins and epithelial membrane antigen (EMA), melanoma antigens such as melan-A and HMB45, B- and T-lymphocyte markers, and follicular dendritic cell markers. Malignant histiocytosis cells must express at least two of the histiocytic or dendritic cell markers CD68, CD163, CD4, or lysozyme and not express other histiocytosis markers such as S100, CD1a, or CD207. Malignant histiocytosis may manifest with various cellular phenotypes that are reminiscent of specific histiocytic cell types, and some pathologists have classified these as histiocytic, interdigitating dendritic cell, Langerhans cell, or indeterminate cell sarcomas. Recent recommendations suggest that the term *malignant histiocytosis* should be applied to the entire family of diseases and that the cellular phenotypes should be considered subtypes. In secondary malignant histiocytosis, clonal immunoglobulin rearrangements, translocations, or somatic mutations may appear both in the malignant histiocytosis cells and the cells of the underlying malignancy, a finding suggesting an evolutionary relationship between the two diseases.

CLINICAL MANIFESTATIONS

Patients may present with symptomatic mass lesions that can be accompanied by fever and weight loss. However, some lesions may be discovered incidentally through imaging studies. Disease may be unifocal or multifocal and can involve any organ, but malignant histiocytosis most commonly manifests in the intestinal tract, skin, or soft tissue. Malignant histiocytosis tumors generally progress rapidly.

DIAGNOSIS

Diagnosis depends on the presence of the histopathologic features described earlier. Other histiocytic or dendritic cell disorders such as Langerhans cell histiocytosis or hemophagocytic lymphohistiocytosis must be excluded. Malignant histiocytosis must also be distinguished from myeloid sarcomas, which are soft tissue collections of myeloid leukemia cells that are identical to leukemia cells in the circulation or bone marrow. Most challenging may be distinguishing the anaplastic cells of malignant histiocytosis from other aggressive malignancies such as diffuse large cell lymphoma, metastatic melanoma, and some metastatic carcinomas. Immunohistochemical staining patterns are useful to rule out these disorders.

TREATMENT

There is no standard of care for malignant histiocytosis. Depending on the sites of disease, effective approaches could include surgery, radiation therapy, or systemic chemotherapy, particularly regimens developed for aggressive lymphomas under expert supervision. A response to an RAF inhibitor in a histiocytic sarcoma carrying a BRAF V600E mutation has been reported, but this cannot be considered a standard therapeutic approach.

PROGNOSIS

A spectrum of outcomes can be seen in these patients, from spontaneous remission to recurrent and refractory disease. No markers have been described that reliably predict response to therapy.

H GROUP, INCLUDING HEMOPHAGOCYTIC LYMPHOHISTIOCYTOSIS

The H group comprises hemophagocytic lymphohistiocytosis, a disorder of immune hyperactivity that was originally described and characterized in infants and young children but is increasingly recognized as a disorder also seen in adults. In children, hemophagocytic lymphohistiocytosis is predominantly a congenital syndrome associated with homozygous genetic abnormalities that abolish the expression of key immune response genes necessary for normal T-cell and NK-cell responses (Chapter 231), although it may also be seen in association with certain infections and as a complication of systemic autoimmune disease. In adults, hemophagocytic lymphohistiocytosis is most commonly associated with lymphoid malignancy, but it also may be a complication of infection or autoimmune disease; in a subset of cases, no inciting abnormality can be found.[13]

EPIDEMIOLOGY

The estimated incidence of familial hemophagocytic lymphohistiocytosis is widely variable, reflecting both geographic variation and rate of successful detection. Estimates range from 1 to more than 200 in 300,000 births. Although it is a rare syndrome outside the pediatric population, the incidence of hemophagocytic lymphohistiocytosis in adults is impossible to estimate because it has been recognized as a syndrome occurring in adults only for the last 15 to 20 years. With increased recognition of the syndrome, it has become apparent that it is less rare than was previously appreciated. Hemophagocytic lymphohistiocytosis appears to be more common in China and Japan than it is in the West.

PATHOBIOLOGY

Hemophagocytic lymphohistiocytosis reflects an uncontrolled immune activation resulting from a failure of cytotoxic T-cell and NK-cell cytotoxicity. On recognition of antigen, these effector cells release perforin-containing cytolytic granules that contribute to lysis of the antigen-expressing target cell. Under normal conditions, target cell elimination limits antigen exposure, leading to downregulation of the immune response, termed *activation-induced cell death.* In familial hemophagocytic lymphohistiocytosis, however, homozygous null mutations in one of a series of genes involved in the synthesis, trafficking, and function of cytotoxic granules from cytotoxic immune cells, including *PRF1, UNC13D, STX11, STXBP2, RAB27A, LYST,* and *AP3B,* leads to inability to clear antigenic stimuli, thus causing a persistent and amplified immune response. The persistently activated cytotoxic T cells and NK cells release high levels of inflammatory cytokines, leading to macrophage activation, hemophagocytosis, and other manifestations of "cytokine storm." The inciting stimulus to the presentation of familial hemophagocytic lymphohistiocytosis is usually an infection, most frequently with Epstein-Barr virus (EBV). In children, secondary hemophagocytic lymphohistiocytosis may occur as a result of infection or autoimmune disease. In the setting of autoimmune disease, it is termed *macrophage activation syndrome.*

Hemophagocytic lymphohistiocytosis was nearly unrecognized as a disease that occurred in adults until the last 15 to 20 years. Since then it has become clear that, although rare, it is being increasingly diagnosed worldwide. It is not clear whether the increasing recognition of adult hemophagocytic lymphohistiocytosis reflects a higher incidence or greater ascertainment.

Most, if not all, adults with hemophagocytic lymphohistiocytosis are thought to have "secondary" or "acquired" hemophagocytic lymphohistiocytosis. The triggers of adult hemophagocytic lymphohistiocytosis include malignancy, infection, and systemic autoimmune disease. Malignancy (especially lymphoma) is the trigger for hemophagocytic lymphohistiocytosis in more than one half of adult patients. The mechanism of acquired hemophagocytic lymphohistiocytosis is much less well understood, although the pattern of immune hyperactivity and cytokine excess is similar.

With the increasing recognition of hemophagocytic lymphohistiocytosis in adults, significant attention has focused on polymorphisms and potential heterozygous mutations in the familial hemophagocytic lymphohistiocytosis genes that may predispose patients to acquire hemophagocytic lymphohistiocytosis in the presence of other triggers. In the original study examining the presence of genetic mutations in familial hemophagocytic lymphohistiocytosis genes in samples from adults suspected of having hemophagocytic lymphohistiocytosis, about 15% were found to have presumed hypomorphic alleles in the familial hemophagocytic lymphohistiocytosis genes. The most common mutation is in the perforin gene (*A92V*), and it is a polymorphism present in 5 to 8% of the general population. The effect of these mutations is unclear, although modeling suggests they may reduce the function of their cognate proteins, and some individuals have had detectable subtle abnormalities in NK-cell function. These mutations likely represent predisposing factors that are part of the pathogenesis of the disease in the setting of other triggers; however, the frequency of some of the mutations and their presence in asymptomatic family members suggest that they are not a driver of the disease.

CLINICAL MANIFESTATIONS

Familial hemophagocytic lymphohistiocytosis typically manifests in the first year of life, nearly always in the setting of infection, most commonly with Epstein-Barr virus. Children usually have prominent CNS symptoms, whereas this is much less frequent in adults. Adults may present with secondary hemophagocytic lymphohistiocytosis at any age. Patients frequently present with a fulminant picture of fever, cytopenias, and multiorgan failure, and they are often suspected of having septic shock. Because the inciting event in hemophagocytic lymphohistiocytosis is most commonly an infection, treatment of the infection may improve the patient's clinical status. However, recrudescence of symptoms is common because once hemophagocytic lymphohistiocytosis is triggered it is usually not self-limited without directed intervention. As delineated later in the diagnostic criteria for hemophagocytic lymphohistiocytosis, fever and cytopenias are often accompanied by splenomegaly, coagulopathy, dyslipidemia, liver function abnormalities, and elevated serum ferritin. Bone marrow aspiration frequently, although not always, demonstrates hemophagocytosis. Many of the clinical features of hemophagocytic lymphohistiocytosis are nonspecific, and diagnosis may be delayed. As discussed in the next section, the diagnosis, especially in adults, may be challenging.

DIAGNOSIS

The diagnostic criteria for hemophagocytic lymphohistiocytosis (Table 155-3) are based on pediatric hemophagocytic lymphohistiocytosis, but they generally perform well in diagnosing the disease in adults.[14] Other diagnostic algorithms have been designed with the intent of improving diagnostic accuracy, especially in adults, but they probably add little to the ability to diagnose hemophagocytic lymphohistiocytosis in adult patients, except perhaps at initial presentation or when some specialized tests such as the soluble IL-2 receptor (sIL2r or sCD25) are unavailable.

TABLE 155-3 DIAGNOSTIC CRITERIA FOR HEMOPHAGOCYTIC LYMPHOHISTIOCYTOSIS

Molecular diagnosis of familial disease
OR
At least 5 of the following 8 criteria:
Fever
Cytopenia of ≥2 lineages
Splenomegaly
Hypertriglyceridemia and/or hypofibrinogenemia
Ferritin >500 ng/mL
Soluble CD25/sIL2r >2400 U/mL
Hemophagocytosis in bone marrow, spleen, or lymph nodes
Low or absent NK-cell activity

NK = natural killer; sIL2r = soluble interleukin-2 receptor.

The first critical step in the diagnosis of hemophagocytic lymphohistiocytosis is to consider the diagnosis because until recently it was rarely entertained in adult patients. In considering the diagnosis, a thorough history should include details regarding recent infections, history of autoimmune disease, underlying malignancy, and underlying immune disorders. Testing should include complete blood count, full metabolic panel, triglycerides, fibrinogen, ferritin, and sIL2r where available. Thorough evaluation for bacterial, parasitic, mycobacterial, and fungal infection should be performed, as well as evaluation for viral infection to include both serology and viral titers for Epstein-Barr virus, cytomegalovirus, human immunodeficiency virus, influenza, hepatitis B and C, herpes simplex virus, varicella-zoster virus, parvovirus, adenovirus, and human herpesvirus-8. Patients should be evaluated for evidence of systemic autoimmune disease. Importantly, because lymphoma is a trigger of hemophagocytic lymphohistiocytosis in about half of adult patients, every effort should be made to find evidence for lymphoma. Patients should undergo marrow examination, and marrow samples should be sent for flow cytometry and T-cell gene rearrangement studies in addition to routine studies. When possible, full evaluation for lymphoma, including a positron emission tomographic (PET) scan, should be performed before initiation of therapy because therapy for hemophagocytic lymphohistiocytosis is likely to mask accompanying lymphoma and thereby impede its timely diagnosis.

Diagnosis of hemophagocytic lymphohistiocytosis requires demonstration of homozygous or compound heterozygous null mutations in familial hemophagocytic lymphohistiocytosis genes (seen in children) or fulfillment of five of eight criteria (see Table 155-3): fever, cytopenias, hypofibrinogenemia or hypertriglyceridemia, elevated ferritin, elevated soluble IL-2 receptor (sIL2r or sCD25), splenomegaly, hemophagocytosis in the bone marrow, and impaired NK-cell function. Because NK-cell function is highly variable outside of familial hemophagocytic lymphohistiocytosis and rarely tested, diagnosis in adults is usually made by satisfying five of the other seven criteria in Table 155-3.

Fever and cytopenias are universal findings in patients presenting with hemophagocytic lymphohistiocytosis. These signs are reflective of the exuberant secretion of inflammatory cytokines released by activated T and NK cells and macrophages, including IFN-γ, tumor necrosis factor-α, IL-2, IL-4, IL-6, and IL-10. Splenomegaly has been reported to occur in about half of adults with hemophagocytic lymphohistiocytosis, and its presence may reflect the duration of the illness before diagnosis. Hypertriglyceridemia and/or hypofibrinogenemia occur in at least 50% of adults with hemophagocytic lymphohistiocytosis. Elevated liver function test results, although not a criterion for the diagnosis, are seen in almost all patients.

Hyperferritinemia has often been considered the hallmark of hemophagocytic lymphohistiocytosis and macrophage activation syndrome. In children, a serum ferritin level higher than 10,000 mg/dL has been demonstrated to be more than 90% sensitive and specific for hemophagocytic lymphohistiocytosis. However, in adults, ferritin is less powerful for establishing the diagnosis. Survey of a database of patients for elevated ferritin revealed that even with ferritin levels higher than 50,000 mg/dL, fewer than 20% of patients will have hemophagocytic lymphohistiocytosis; conversely, among adults diagnosed with hemophagocytic lymphohistiocytosis, the ferritin level ranges from 600 mg/dL to more than 50,000 mg/dL. Therefore, the negative predictive value of a normal ferritin result is high, but it is not a discerning marker for hemophagocytic lymphohistiocytosis in adults. Because hyperferritinemia is a nonspecific consequence of macrophage activation, it is also elevated in other chronic inflammatory conditions, hemolytic anemia, and renal failure, all of which are more common in adults than in children.

The soluble form of the IL-2 receptor (sIL2r, sCD25) is also elevated in hemophagocytic lymphohistiocytosis. The IL-2 receptor is widely expressed by lymphocytes, monocytes, eosinophils, and NK cells; is cleaved by macrophage gelatinase (MMP9) to release the soluble form of the receptor; and is a marker of immune activation in many inflammatory disorders. Although it is elevated in nearly all, if not all, patients with hemophagocytic lymphohistiocytosis, it is not a readily available test. However, it can be an extremely valuable diagnostic marker. In particular, in adults, it is usually extremely elevated in lymphoma-associated hemophagocytic lymphohistiocytosis because the malignant lymphoma cells themselves express high levels of IL2r. The ratio of sIL2r to ferritin can help distinguish lymphoma-associated hemophagocytic lymphohistiocytosis from other forms of hemophagocytic lymphohistiocytosis in adults: the ratio is usually less than 1 in the absence of malignancy and greater than 2 in the setting of lymphoma-associated hemophagocytic lymphohistiocytosis.

Hemophagocytosis is often a prominent feature of hemophagocytic lymphohistiocytosis, but it is neither sensitive nor specific for the diagnosis. In adults, hemophagocytosis is often prominent, but many other diagnoses are associated with hemophagocytosis (e.g., acute viral infections and hemolytic anemias).

Evaluation for genetic mutations in familial hemophagocytic lymphohistiocytosis genes may be helpful in later management, but it is not urgent for the initial evaluation.

TREATMENT

Therapy of hemophagocytic lymphohistiocytosis is aimed at suppressing the abnormal immune response, usually through a combination of immunosuppressive and targeted anti–T-cell therapy (Fig. 155-2).[15] Because there have been no large trials of therapy for adult hemophagocytic lymphohistiocytosis, most adults are treated with the HLH-94 protocol, which was studied in a large prospective trial for pediatric hemophagocytic lymphohistiocytosis (Table 155-4). This therapy entails dexamethasone and etoposide with an 8-week induction course under expert supervision. Children with neurologic symptoms receive intrathecal methotrexate, but it is rarely necessary in adults. Following completion of the 8-week course, patients can be put on maintenance therapy with the addition of calcineurin inhibitors to intermittent dexamethasone and etoposide, usually as a bridge to stem cell transplantation. An alternative is the modified HLH-2004 protocol (Table 155-4). Patients with significant liver dysfunction can have initial dose reduction of etoposide with dose increases as function improves. Renal failure may also require dose reduction. Treatment should not usually be withheld for cytopenias, which often reflect disease activity rather than drug toxicity. However, adults often do not tolerate the initial bi-weekly dosing of etoposide, and it is usual to hold at least one of the initial four doses, or start immediately with weekly dosing.

TABLE 155-4 HLH-94 AND HLH-2004 PROTOCOLS FOR TREATMENT OF HEMOPHAGOCYTIC LYMPHOHISTIOCYTOSIS (HLH)

HLH-94 PROTOCOL
Initial Therapy for the First 8 Weeks:
Dexamethasone at 10 mg/m^2 orally per day weeks 1-2; 5 mg/m^2 per day weeks 3-4; 2.5 mg/m^2 per day weeks 5-6; 1.25 mg/m^2 per day week 7; taper during week 8
Etoposide at 150 mg/m^2 orally twice weekly for weeks 1-2; then once weekly
Intrathecal MTX (for children with neurologic symptoms only) at 12 mg per dose, given at weeks 3 and 4, with two additional doses at weeks 5 and 6 if progressive neurologic symptoms and/or abnormal CSF not improved after 2 weeks
Continuation Therapy/HSCT:
Dexamethasone at 10 mg/m^2 per day for 3 days, given every 2nd week
Etoposide 150 mg/m^2 × 1 in alternate weeks
Cyclosporine A beginning at week 9, dosing aimed at trough level of 200 μg/L
HLH-2004 PROTOCOL
Initial Therapy for the First 8 Weeks:
Same as HLH-94 Protocol, except (1) cyclosporine A beginning at day 1 and continuing into the Continuation phase. Recommend starting cyclosporine A at a daily dose of 6 mg/kg, with dosing aimed at trough level of 200 μg/L; and (2) adding prednisone to MTX for intrathecal injections (for children with neurologic symptoms only)
Continuation Therapy/HSCT as Soon as an Accepted Donor Is Identified

CSF = cerebrospinal fluid; MTX = methotrexate.

Modified from Bergsten E, Horne A, Aricó M, et al. Confirmed efficacy of etoposide and dexamethasone in HLH treatment: long-term results of the cooperative HLH-2004 study. *Blood*. 2017;130:2728-2738.

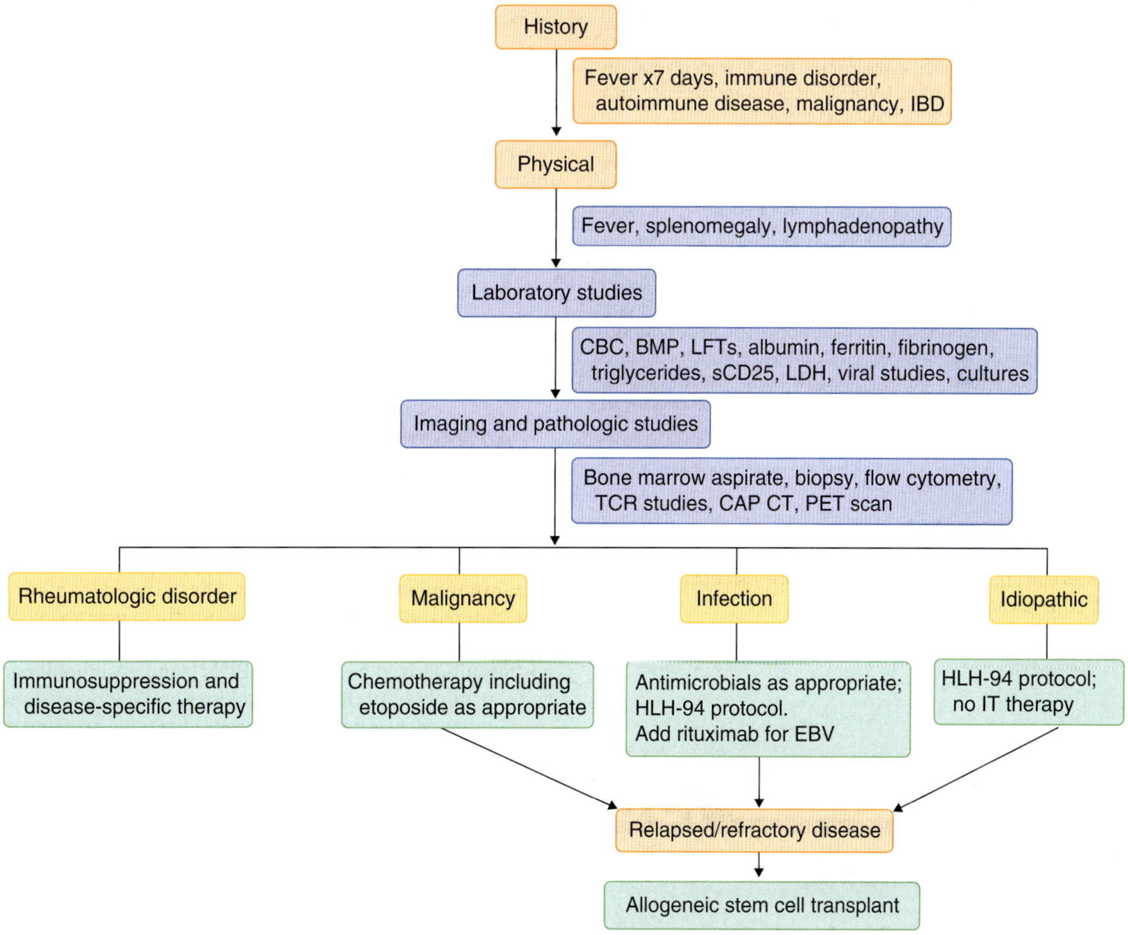

FIGURE 155-2. Approach to diagnosis and treatment of adult hemophagocytic lymphohistiocytosis (HLH). BMP = basic metabolic panel; CAP CT = chest, abdomen, pelvis computed tomography; CBC = complete blood count; EBV = Epstein-Barr virus; HLH-94 protocol (see text and grade A reference A2); IBD = inflammatory bowel disease; IT = immunotherapy; LDH = lactate dehydrogenase; LFTs = liver function tests; PET = positron emission tomography; sCD25 = soluble CD25; TCR = T-cell receptor.

Therapy is tailored to the underlying trigger for the syndrome. In patients with malignancy-associated hemophagocytic lymphohistiocytosis, treatment for the malignancy should be initiated immediately. Because most malignancy-associated hemophagocytic lymphohistiocytosis accompanies a lymphoma, therapy with an etoposide-containing regimen is recommended, and steroid therapy should be continued until the hemophagocytic lymphohistiocytosis has resolved. Epstein-Barr virus-related hemophagocytic lymphohistiocytosis is driven by viral infection of T lymphocytes, so treatment with the HLH-94 protocol should be administered without delay. In addition, rituximab is recommended to clear the B-cell reservoir of virus. Patients with no clear precipitating trigger ("idiopathic hemophagocytic lymphohistiocytosis") should receive the HLH-94 protocol with continued evaluation for underlying undiagnosed lymphoma or infection.

The one exception to the recommendation for cytotoxic therapy for adult hemophagocytic lymphohistiocytosis is for patients with macrophage activation syndrome. This subtype of hemophagocytic lymphohistiocytosis is often difficult to distinguish from an acute flare of the patient's underlying systemic autoimmune disease. Macrophage activation syndrome usually responds to intensification of immunosuppressive therapy for the primary disease and does not usually require cytotoxic therapy.

Patients who fail to respond to the HLH-94 protocol may receive salvage therapy with alemtuzumab, a monoclonal anti-CD52 antibody that destroys mature T cells, under expert supervision. This agent should be viewed as a bridge to stem cell transplant in eligible patients. In this setting, alemtuzumab has also been demonstrated to reduce the incidence of graft versus host disease (GVHD) after stem cell transplantation and is now incorporated into the conditioning regimen before stem cell transplantation for hemophagocytic lymphohistiocytosis.

The role of hematopoietic stem cell transplantation (HSCT) (Chapter 163) in hemophagocytic lymphohistiocytosis is evolving. Familial hemophagocytic lymphohistiocytosis is uniformly fatal without HSCT, but the necessity for other patients with HLH to undergo HSCT is less clear. In many children with infection-associated hemophagocytic lymphohistiocytosis, hemophagocytic lymphohistiocytosis resolves completely with HLH-94 therapy. The outcomes in adults are less clear, but adult patients who have refractory or relapsed disease or who have had life-threatening disease at presentation should be evaluated for transplantation. Patients must be in remission at the time of HSCT because patients with active hemophagocytic lymphohistiocytosis at the time of transplantation fare poorly and usually die of overwhelming GVHD. Outcomes are superior with reduced intensity conditioning. Successful HSCT is curative.

Novel therapies that may have an increasing role in the treatment of hemophagocytic lymphohistiocytosis include emapalumab and ruxolitinib. Emapalumab (1 mg/kg by intravenous infusion every 3-4 days, with dose increases up to 10 mg/kg based on clinical response and toxicity) is an FDA-approved antibody that targets IFN-γ and has been moderately effective for the treatment of refractory hemophagocytic lymphohistiocytosis in children.[16] It also may be useful for adults with hemophagocytic lymphohistiocytosis when combined with dexamethasone (5 to 10 mg/m^2) for the duration of treatment, although clinical studies in the adult population have not yet been performed. The Janus kinase 1/2 inhibitor ruxolitinib has been studied in early clinical trials and is not FDA approved for use in hemophagocytic lymphohistiocytosis, but it is a possible adjunct to therapy under expert supervision, especially in patients with intractable symptoms.

GENERAL REFERENCES

For the General References and other additional features, please visit Elsevier eBooks+ at https://ebooks.health.elsevier.com.

156 EOSINOPHILIC SYNDROMES

AMY D. KLION

DEFINITIONS

Eosinophils are terminally differentiated cells of the myeloid lineage that circulate in low numbers in the peripheral blood. Although normal ranges vary depending on the laboratory, blood eosinophilia is typically defined as an absolute eosinophil count of greater than 450/μL and hypereosinophilia as an absolute eosinophil count of 1500/μL or greater. Percentages of eosinophils in the total white blood count (WBC) can be misleading because they are affected by the relative numbers of neutrophils, which can be impacted by a number of factors (e.g., low neutrophil counts seen in certain racial/ethnic groups presumably due to polymorphisms in the Duffy antigen receptor [see Chapter 153] or the selective increase in neutrophils seen in response to glucocorticoids or bacterial infection). Tissue hypereosinophilia is loosely defined as extensive eosinophil infiltration in the opinion of the pathologist and may or may not be accompanied by blood eosinophilia. Consensus thresholds for tissue hypereosinophilia have not been defined, except for bone marrow eosinophilia (20% of nucleated cells) and eosinophilic esophagitis (≥15 eosinophils/high-power field).[1]

The hypereosinophilic syndrome can be defined by blood or tissue hypereosinophilia on at least two occasions with evidence of clinical manifestations attributable to the eosinophilia, regardless of the underlying etiology. This definition encompasses a number of clinical subtypes that differ in etiology and/or clinical manifestations and have prognostic and therapeutic implications (Table 156-1).[2] Hypereosinophilia or hypereosinophilic syndrome can be due to neoplastic or clonal proliferation of eosinophils (myeloid hypereosinophilia or hypereosinophilic syndrome), aberrant lymphocyte production of cytokines that promote eosinophilia (lymphoid hypereosinophilia or hypereosinophilic syndrome), inherited genetic abnormalities (familial hypereosinophilia or hypereosinophilic syndrome), or unknown causes (idiopathic hypereosinophilia or hypereosinophilic syndrome).[3,4] Overlap hypereosinophilic syndrome refers to eosinophilic disorders involving a single organ system, such as eosinophilic gastrointestinal disorders and eosinophilic fasciitis, or defined clinical entities, such as eosinophilic granulomatosis with polyangiitis (Chapter 249) or episodic angioedema and eosinophilia (Gleich syndrome), that overlap in clinical presentation with other subtypes of hypereosinophilic syndrome. Finally, secondary or associated hypereosinophilia or hypereosinophilic syndrome can complicate a wide variety of diseases and conditions, including helminth infection (Chapters 325 to 327), neoplasia, and drug hypersensitivity.

EPIDEMIOLOGY

Eosinophilia (absolute eosinophil count >450 eosinophils/μL) is common, occurring in 5 to 15% of the general population depending on the setting. The most frequent cause of mild to moderate eosinophilia worldwide is helminth infection, although atopic disease is the most likely culprit in industrialized settings. In contrast, hypereosinophilic syndrome (with the exception of some of the single-organ variants) is extremely rare, with an overall estimated prevalence of 0.3 to 6.3 per 100,000 in North America. The prevalence of eosinophilic esophagitis (Chapter 124) appears to be increasing, in keeping with an overall increase in the incidence of atopic disease, and has been estimated at 2.5 to 5 per 10,000 in the United States and Europe. Racial and ethnic differences have also been described.

PATHOBIOLOGY

Eosinophil Biology and Mediators of Tissue Damage

Eosinophils develop from pluripotent hematopoietic stem cells in the bone marrow (Chapter 142) under the influence of a complex array of transcription factors and cytokines, the most important of which is interleukin-5 (IL-5). Mature eosinophils are characterized by the presence of cytoplasmic granules that stain red with the acidic dye eosin. These granules contain four cationic proteins (major basic protein [MBP1], eosinophilic cationic protein [ECP], eosinophil-derived neurotoxin [EDN], and eosinophil peroxidase [EPO]) and a panoply of preformed cytokines and chemokines within a complex membranovesicular network. Release of granule proteins and mediators can occur in an indiscriminate way (through cytolysis or classic exocytosis) or selectively through a process called piecemeal degranulation.

Under homeostatic conditions, mature eosinophils are released into the blood, where they remain in the circulation for up to 36 hours before trafficking to the tissues. Data suggest that these "resident" eosinophils may play important regulatory roles in the maintenance of tissue integrity and cell-cell interactions. When eosinophils become activated, irrespective of the cause, they can cause tissue damage and other clinical manifestations through direct and indirect mechanisms. The latter include tissue deposition of cytotoxic eosinophil granule proteins and reactive oxygen intermediates, recruitment of inflammatory cells through the selective secretion of cytokines and chemokines, formation of lipid bodies with production of leukotrienes and other inflammatory mediators, and activation of mast cells, fibroblasts, and endothelial cells to promote fibrogenesis and thrombosis. Modulation of surface receptor expression and increased

TABLE 156-1 CLINICAL SUBTYPES OF HYPEREOSINOPHILIA/HYPEREOSINOPHILIC SYNDROMES

CLINICAL SUBTYPE	DEFINITION	EXAMPLES
Myeloid (clonal, neoplastic)	Presumed or proven primary neoplastic or clonal eosinophilia	*PDGFR*-associated myeloid neoplasms Chronic eosinophilic leukemia–not otherwise specified
Lymphocytic	Eosinophilia secondary to production of interleukin-5 or other eosinophil-promoting cytokines by aberrant and/or clonal lymphocytes	—
Familial	Hypereosinophilia in multiple generations	Autosomal dominant familial eosinophilia
Idiopathic	Unknown cause and exclusion of other clinical subtypes	—
Overlap	Clinically defined eosinophilic disorders, including those with single organ involvement, that overlap in clinical presentation with idiopathic or lymphocytic variant hypereosinophilic syndrome	Eosinophilic gastrointestinal disease Eosinophilic fasciitis Eosinophilic granulomatosis with polyangiitis Wells syndrome Episodic angioedema and eosinophilia
Secondary (associated)	Eosinophilia in the setting of a distinct diagnosis in which eosinophilia has been described in a subset of patients	See Table 156-2
Hypereosinophilia of unknown significance	Asymptomatic hypereosinophilia without evidence of end-organ manifestations or a primary myeloid etiology	—

PDGFR = platelet-derived growth factor receptor.

responsiveness to chemokines following activation also play important roles in eosinophil recruitment to the tissues and, ultimately, in disease pathogenesis.

Mutations

A number of recurrent genetic mutations have been described in clonal (neoplastic) eosinophilia.[5] The most common of these, an interstitial deletion in chromosome 4 leading to formation of the fusion gene *FIP1L1::PDGFRA*, likely causes eosinophil activation through a network of molecules including the IL-5 receptor, *JAK2*, and Lyn. The mechanisms of eosinophil activation in the setting of other mutations associated with clonal eosinophilia remain largely unexplored. Disease risk loci have been identified in a number of allergic disorders characterized by eosinophil accumulation and activation in tissues, including eosinophilic esophagitis.[6] Some of these, such as 5q22, encode genes known to be involved in eosinophil activation.

CLINICAL MANIFESTATIONS

The clinical manifestations of eosinophilia are very varied and include asymptomatic eosinophilia detected on a routine blood count, nonspecific symptoms such as fatigue and myalgia, and signs and symptoms related to eosinophilic tissue infiltration and/or complications of eosinophil-associated hypercoagulability. Although skin, pulmonary, and gastrointestinal manifestations are most frequent, any organ can be affected.[7] Moreover, there is considerable heterogeneity in the clinical manifestations within any given organ system. For instance, common presentations of eosinophilic skin involvement include intractable pruritus without rash, eczematous rash, urticaria, bullous lesions, and mucosal ulcerations. Although some clinical manifestations are more common in specific subtypes of hypereosinophilic syndrome (e.g., skin manifestations in lymphoid hypereosinophilic syndrome), there is considerable overlap in presentation among clinical subtypes. Moreover, the most serious clinical manifestations, such as endomyocardial fibrosis (Chapter 47)[8] and thromboembolism, can occur in any of the varied hypereosinophilic syndrome subtypes, including secondary or associated hypereosinophilic syndrome caused by untreated helminth infection or drug hypersensitivity.

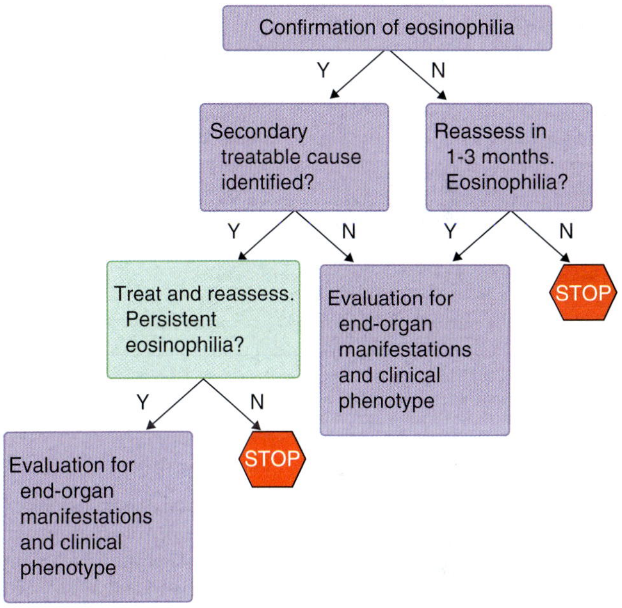

FIGURE 156-1. Initial approach to the clinically stable patient with unexplained eosinophilia. *Patients with idiopathic hypereosinophilia who are asymptomatic without end-organ manifestations are considered to have hypereosinophilia of undetermined significance (HEus).

DIAGNOSIS

Initial Diagnostic Evaluation

The first step in the diagnostic evaluation of the patient with eosinophilia is confirmation of the eosinophil count, while keeping in mind that fever, bacterial infection, and therapies, including glucocorticoids, that may be prescribed for other reasons can all suppress eosinophilia.[9] Once eosinophilia is confirmed, the next step is a search for secondary causes that require specific therapy directed at the underlying disorder (associated hypereosinophilic syndrome). If such a cause is identified, the patient should be treated and reassessed for resolution of the eosinophilia.

Differential Diagnosis

Patients with persistent eosinophilia and those without evidence of a clear secondary cause should undergo an initial evaluation aimed at the identification of end-organ involvement and classification by clinical subtype (Fig. 156-1). The diagnostic evaluation should be performed in a step-wise manner beginning with a careful history and physical examination, complete blood count with differential, and routine chemistries (including liver function tests and serum immunoglobulins). When possible, this evaluation should occur before institution of therapy because many diagnostic tests are affected by glucocorticoids and other therapies. However, treatment should not be delayed if life-threatening or disabling complications are present or imminent.

Although the differential diagnosis of eosinophilia is very broad, ranging from common allergic disorders to rare idiopathic hypereosinophilic syndromes, a careful history can substantially narrow the possibilities. Particular attention should be paid to medications and supplements, travel and exposures, risk factors for neoplasia, and prior medical history (especially asthma, atopic disease, and/or recurrent infections) because these may provide clues to secondary causes of eosinophilia, such as helminth infection, neoplasia, and immunodeficiency syndromes, that require therapy directed at the underlying cause rather than the eosinophilia itself (Table 156-2).[10] Whereas common allergic disorders, including asthma (Chapter 75) and atopic dermatitis (Chapter 405), can be associated with hypereosinophilia, especially in children, extremely high absolute eosinophil counts ($\geq$5000/µL) should prompt evaluation for another cause. A detailed review of systems should

TABLE 156-2 SELECTED SECONDARY CAUSES OF EOSINOPHILIA REQUIRING TREATMENT DIRECTED AT THE UNDERLYING CAUSE

CATEGORY	ETIOLOGIES	COMMENTS
Infection		
Helminthic	Varied	Most pronounced early in infection and with tissue invasive species
Protozoan	*Isospora belli* infection *Sarcocystis* infection	Other protozoan infections are not associated with eosinophilia
Ectoparasitic	Scabies Myiasis	Hypersensitivity reactions
Viral	HIV infection	Advanced disease
Bacterial	Chronic tuberculosis	Rare
Fungal	Coccidioidomycosis Cryptococcosis	Eosinophilia can complicate a wide variety of fungal infections
Neoplasia	Lymphoma	Hodgkin, non-Hodgkin
	Leukemia	Especially T-cell leukemias and pre-B cell ALL
	Carcinoma	Most commonly adenocarcinoma
Drug hypersensitivity	Varied	Prescription and nonprescription drugs, dietary supplements
Immunodeficiency	Varied	Hyper-IgE syndromes Omenn syndrome
Autoimmune and other immunologic disorders	Varied	Sarcoidosis Inflammatory bowel disease IgG4 disease Others
Other	Cholesterol embolism Hypoadrenalism Radiation Post-transplant status Cytokine therapy: IL-2, GM-CSF	—

ALL = acute lymphoblastic leukemia; GM-CSF = granulocyte-macrophage colony-stimulating factor; HIV = human immunodeficiency virus; IgE = immunoglobulin E; IgG4 = immunoglobulin G4; IL-2 = interleukin-2.

be obtained in all patients because the pattern of clinical manifestations can be suggestive of a particular diagnosis. For example, a history of aspirin sensitivity in an eosinophilic patient with worsening asthma and sinusitis is highly suggestive of aspirin-exacerbated respiratory disease (Chapters 75 and 394),[11] whereas symptoms of peripheral neuropathy in a similar patient should point to a diagnosis of eosinophilic granulomatosis with polyangiitis (Chapter 249).

It is extremely important to identify patients with primary myeloid disorders presenting as hypereosinophilic syndrome because these patients often have aggressive disease, and the approach to therapy is quite different from that of other eosinophilic disorders (see the Treatment section). Clinical and laboratory features suggestive of a primary myeloid disorder include dysplastic eosinophils and eosinophil precursors in the blood, anemia or erythrocytosis, thrombocytopenia, splenomegaly, and elevated serum levels of vitamin B_{12} and/or tryptase. Male gender should raise suspicion for *PDGFR*-associated myeloid neoplasms in this setting.

An initial screen for evidence of myeloid or lymphocytic variant hypereosinophilic syndrome should include serum vitamin B_{12} and tryptase levels, as well as immunophenotyping for T- and B-cell clonality by flow cytometry. Abnormal results, a peripheral eosinophil count of 5000/µL or greater, or other evidence suggestive of a hematologic malignancy (including lymphadenopathy, splenomegaly, or dysplastic or precursor cells on peripheral blood smear) should prompt a bone marrow aspirate and biopsy with standard cytogenetic analysis. Specific testing for recurrent molecular abnormalities associated with hypereosinophilic syndrome should be guided by the clinical features and, if suspected, should be included with the bone marrow examination, where their yield may be higher than in peripheral blood.[12] Although the recommended testing for end-organ damage depends on the clinical signs and symptoms, serum troponin levels, echocardiography, and pulmonary function tests should be performed in all patients to assess clinically evident or occult cardiopulmonary involvement such as endomyocardial fibrosis that can be suggested by echocardiographic abnormalities. Radiologic imaging of the chest, abdomen, and pelvis should also be considered in all patients to identify splenomegaly, lymphadenopathy, and clinically silent neoplastic or inflammatory disease.

TREATMENT

Initial Therapy

The most appropriate initial treatment for a patient with eosinophilia depends on its most likely cause, acuity, and accompanying severity of the clinical signs and symptoms. Glucocorticoids remain the first-line agent for most hypereosinophilic disorders, with four important exceptions: hypereosinophilic syndrome secondary to a treatable cause (associated hypereosinophilic syndrome), primary clonal or neoplastic hypereosinophilic syndrome with an identified mutation for which targeted therapy is available (i.e., imatinib-sensitive, *PDGFR* mutation–positive hypereosinophilic syndrome), eosinophilic gastrointestinal disease (which can sometimes be treated with dietary intervention alone), and patients with hypereosinophilia of unknown significance (who may not require therapy at all). The most appropriate dose of glucocorticoids for an individual patient has not been adequately studied, but the clinical subtype appears to be a useful predictor of systemic glucocorticoid response in hypereosinophilic syndrome.[13] Some eosinophilic disorders, including eosinophilic esophagitis (Chapter 124) and eosinophilic dermatitis, can be successfully managed with topical steroid therapy alone. If life-threatening or disabling complications, such as endomyocardial fibrosis, respiratory failure, or neurologic impairment, are present or imminent, high-dose glucocorticoid therapy (40 mg of prednisone or more daily under expert oversight) should be initiated without delay, even in the setting of associated hypereosinophilic syndrome, unless a treatable secondary cause is identified and is likely to respond rapidly to specific therapy. Ivermectin (200 µg/kg/day for 1 to 2 days) should be administered prior to glucocorticoid therapy in patients with potential exposure to *Strongyloides stercoralis* at any time during their life to prevent hyperinfection syndrome. The most appropriate second agent for treatment of glucocorticoid-refractory patients depends on the clinical subtype and most likely etiology of the eosinophilia, as discussed later.

Initial treatment of myeloid neoplasms that present as a hypereosinophilic syndrome should be guided by the molecular findings. Imatinib (100 mg orally daily; Chapter 170) is clearly the therapy of choice in *PDGFR* mutation–associated disease, with near 100% response rates reported in most series and the possibility of cure in some patients with long-term therapy.[14] Results with other targeted therapies, including *JAK* inhibitors, have been variable in patients with myeloid forms of hypereosinophilic syndrome to date, even in the presence of mutations in the corresponding gene. Consequently, glucocorticoids are often used initially with rapid addition of hydroxyurea or other second-line agents as needed under expert oversight. This approach is likely to change, however, as more experience is gained with targeted therapies.

Second-Line Agents

The selection of a second-line agent depends on a variety of factors, including the clinical subtype, physician's and patient's preference, and cost. Conventional agents used to treat glucocorticoid-resistant, *PDGFR* mutation–negative patients include hydroxyurea, interferon-α, methotrexate, and imatinib. Patients who are *PDGFR* mutation positive and who are intolerant of or resistant to imatinib should be treated with a second- or third-generation tyrosine kinase inhibitor with activity against *PDGFR*, with early consideration of hematopoietic stem cell transplant in nonresponders.

Targeted Therapies

The availability of therapeutic agents that specifically target eosinophils is rapidly changing the approach to the treatment of eosinophilic disorders. Three biologics that target eosinophils through the IL-5 axis, mepolizumab, reslizumab, and benralizumab, have been approved for the treatment of eosinophilic asthma based on randomized trials documenting reduction in asthma exacerbations with little or no toxicity (Chapter 75).[A1,A2] Mepolizumab (300 mg subcutaneously every 4 weeks) improves remission rates and length of remission in patients with treatment-refractory or relapsing eosinophilic granulomatosis with polyangiitis[A3,A4] and reduces disease flares in patients with steroid-responsive *PDGFRA*-negative hypereosinophilic syndrome.[A5] In phase II trials, benralizumab (30 mg subcutaneously every 4 weeks) reduced eosinophilia and improved clinical manifestations in patients with treatment-refractory hypereosinophilic syndrome,[A6] and a phase III study is ongoing. Although dupilumab (a monoclonal antibody to the IL-4 receptor) is approved by the U.S. Food and Drug Administration for the treatment of a number of eosinophilic disorders, including atopic dermatitis, asthma, and eosinophilic esophagitis,[A7] it has been associated with transient hypereosinophilia and, rarely, eosinophilic complications, so it should be used with caution in patients with elevated eosinophil counts.[15] Other novel agents currently in development for eosinophilic disorders, including biologics targeting eotaxin, lirentelimab (a monoclonal antibody to Siglec 8) and dexpramipexole, are likely to provide additional therapeutic options for the heterogeneous group of eosinophilic disorders.

PROGNOSIS

Although the prognosis of an individual patient with hypereosinophilic syndrome depends substantially on the clinical subtype, the severity of clinical manifestations at presentation, and treatment responsiveness, the overall prognosis has improved dramatically (>90% 5-year survival in most series) with advances in diagnostic tools and therapeutic approaches. The most clear-cut example has been the dramatic decrease in mortality in patients with clinical features consistent with an eosinophilic myeloid neoplasm (the majority of whom have *FIP1L1::PDGFRA*–associated disease) with imatinib therapy. In fact, mortality and morbidity in this group of patients (which were 30 to 50% at 5 years before the introduction of imatinib) are now almost entirely restricted to patients who present with irreversible cardiac or other life-threatening manifestations. Progression to lymphoma remains a concern in patients with the lymphocytic variant, particularly in patients with CD3-$CD4^+$ T-cell clones.

GENERAL REFERENCES

For the General References and other additional features, please visit Elsevier eBooks+ at https://ebooks.health.elsevier.com.

Grade A References

A1. Castro M, Zangrillia J, Wechsler ME, et al. Reslizumab for inadequately controlled asthma with elevated blood eosinophil counts: results from two multicenter, parallel, double-blind, randomised, placebo-controlled, phase 3 trials. *Lancet Respir Med.* 2015;3:355-366.

A2. FitzGerald JM, Bleeker ER, Nair P, et al. Benralizumab, an anti-interleukin-5 receptor α monoclonal antibody, as add-on treatment for patients with severe, uncontrolled, eosinophilic asthma (CALIMA): a randomised, double-blind, placebo-controlled phase 3 trial. *Lancet.* 2016;388:2128-2141.

A3. Wechsler ME, Akuthota P, Jayne D. Mepolizumab or placebo for eosinophilic granulomatosis with polyangiitis. *N Engl J Med.* 2017;376:1921-1932.

A4. Steinfeld J, Bradford ES, Brown J, et al. Evaluation of clinical benefit from treatment with mepolizumab for patients with eosinophilic granulomatosis with polyangiitis. *J Allergy Clin Immunol.* 2019;143:2170-2177.

A5. Roufosse F, Kahn JE, Rothenberg ME, et al. Efficacy and safety of mepolizumab in hypereosinophilic syndrome: a phase III, randomized, placebo-controlled trial. *J Allergy Clin Immunol.* 2020;146:1397-1405.

A6. Kuang FL, Legrand FA, Makiya M, et al. Benralizumab treatment for *PDGFRA*-negative hypereosinophilic syndromes. *N Engl J Med.* 2019;380:1336-1346.

A7. Dellon ES, Rothenberg ME, Collins MH, et al. Dupilumab in adults and adolescents with eosinophilic esophagitis. *N Engl J Med.* 2022;387:2317-2330.

157 APPROACH TO THE PATIENT WITH BLEEDING OR THROMBOSIS

ANDREW I. SCHAFER

MECHANISMS OF HEMOSTASIS AND THROMBOSIS

NORMAL HEMOSTASIS

The coagulation system is normally quiescent, and blood fluidity within blood vessels is maintained by the actions of a continuous monolayer of endothelial cells that line the intimal surface of the vasculature throughout the circulatory tree. At a site of vascular damage, the antithrombotic properties of endothelium are lost, and thrombogenic constituents of the subendothelial vessel wall become exposed to circulating blood. The result is rapid formation of a hemostatic clot that consists of platelets and fibrin and is localized to the area of vascular injury. Activation of platelets and formation of fibrin occur essentially simultaneously and interdependently to effect hemostasis. Subsequently, vascular repair is accomplished by thrombolysis and recanalization of the occluded site.[1]

Platelet activation at a site of vascular injury begins with the adhesion of platelets to the locally de-endothelialized intimal surface (i.e., platelet–vessel wall interaction). Platelet adhesion is mediated by von Willebrand factor, which sticks circulating platelets to the area of the damaged vessel wall by binding to its receptors located in platelet membrane glycoprotein Ib. The adherent platelets then undergo a "release reaction," during which they discharge constituents of their storage granules, including adenosine diphosphate (ADP), and simultaneously elaborate thromboxane A_2 from arachidonic acid through the aspirin-inhibitable cyclooxygenase reaction. ADP, thromboxane A_2, and other components of the release reaction act in concert to recruit and activate additional platelets from the circulation to the site of vascular injury. These activated platelets expose binding sites for fibrinogen by forming the surface membrane glycoprotein IIb/IIIa complex. In the process of platelet aggregation (platelet-platelet interactions), fibrinogen (or von Willebrand factor under conditions of high shear stress) mediates the final formation of an occlusive platelet plug.

Fibrin, which anchors the hemostatic platelet plug, is formed from soluble plasma fibrinogen by the action of the potent protease enzyme thrombin (Fig. 157-1). The fibrin mesh is stabilized by covalent cross-linking mediated by factor XIII. Thrombin is formed from its inactive (zymogen) plasma precursor, prothrombin, by the action of activated factor X (Xa) and its cofactor, factor Va. This sequence of reactions has classically been referred to as the *common pathway* of coagulation. Factor X can be activated by either the *tissue factor (extrinsic) pathway* or the *contact activation (intrinsic) pathway* of coagulation. The tissue factor pathway is now considered to be the major physiologic initiator of coagulation activation. It is triggered by the formation of the complex of tissue factor, which is exposed on the surfaces of activated vascular and blood cells, with activated factor VII (VIIa). The contact activation pathway involves a series (or cascade) of zymogen-protease reactions that are initiated by factor XII, high-molecular-weight kininogen, and prekallikrein. Activated factor XII (XIIa) converts factor XI to XIa, which in turn activates factor IX to IXa. Factor IXa is an enzyme that converts factor X to Xa, a reaction that requires factor VIIIa as a cofactor.

PHYSIOLOGIC ANTITHROMBOTIC MECHANISMS

Intact, normal endothelium promotes blood fluidity by inhibiting platelet activation. It likewise plays a crucial role in preventing fibrin accumulation.

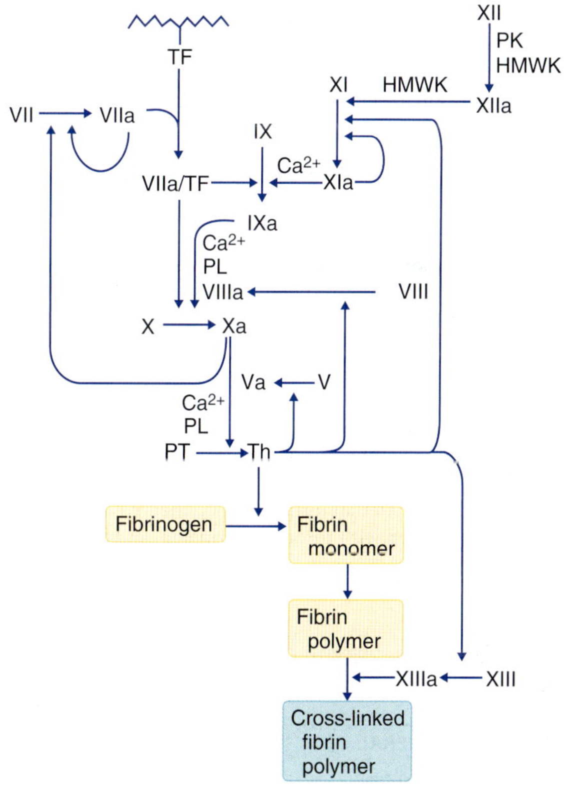

FIGURE 157-1. Coagulation cascade. This scheme emphasizes an understanding of (1) the importance of the tissue factor pathway in initiating clotting in vivo, (2) the interactions among pathways, and (3) the pivotal role of thrombin in sustaining the cascade by feedback activation of coagulation factors. HMWK = high-molecular-weight kininogen; PK = prekallikrein; PL = phospholipid; PT = prothrombin; TF = tissue factor; Th = thrombin. Roman numerals are coagulation factors (e.g., VII); when followed by a lowercase "a," they are the activated forms of those factors (e.g., VIIa). (From Schafer AI. Coagulation cascade: an overview. In: Loscalzo J, Schafer AI, eds. *Thrombosis and Hemorrhage*. Cambridge, MA: Blackwell Scientific Publications; 1994:3-12.)

Among the physiologic antithrombotic systems that produce this latter effect are (1) antithrombin III, (2) protein C and protein S, (3) tissue factor pathway inhibitor (TFPI), and (4) the fibrinolytic system. Antithrombin is the major protease inhibitor of the coagulation system: it inactivates thrombin and other activated coagulation factors. Heparin functions as an anticoagulant by binding to antithrombin and greatly accelerating these reactions. Heparin and heparin sulfate proteoglycans are naturally present on endothelial cells, so antithrombin inactivation of thrombin and other coagulation proteases most likely occurs physiologically on vascular surfaces rather than in fluid plasma. Activated protein C, with its cofactor protein S, functions as a natural anticoagulant by destroying factors Va and VIIIa, two essential cofactors of the coagulation cascade. Thrombin itself is the activator of protein C, and this reaction occurs rapidly only on the surfaces of intact vascular endothelial cells, where thrombin binds to the glycosaminoglycan thrombomodulin. TFPI is a plasma protease inhibitor that specifically quenches tissue factor–induced coagulation. Finally, what little fibrin can be produced, despite these potent physiologic antithrombotic mechanisms, is digested rapidly by the endogenous fibrinolytic system. Fibrinolysis is mediated by the protease plasmin, which is generated from plasminogen in plasma by the action of endothelium-derived plasminogen activators.

EVALUATION OF THE PATIENT WITH A POSSIBLE BLEEDING DISORDER

HISTORY AND PHYSICAL EXAMINATION

A thorough history is paramount in evaluating a patient for a possible systemic bleeding disorder. In addition to asking the patient about spontaneous bleeding episodes in the past, the responses to specific hemostatic challenges should be recorded. A bleeding tendency may be suspected if a patient previously experienced excessive hemorrhage after surgery or trauma, including common events such as circumcision, tonsillectomy, labor and delivery, menses, dental procedures, vaccinations, and injections. Conversely, a history of normal blood clotting after such specific challenges in the recent past is just as important to note. It may be a better test of the integrity of systemic hemostasis than any laboratory measurement can provide.

In a patient with a history of excessive or unexplained bleeding, the initial goal is to determine whether the cause is a systemic coagulopathy or localized anatomic or mechanical problem with a blood vessel. This situation is encountered most frequently in patients with excessive postoperative bleeding, which could be due to either local surgical trauma or a coagulation abnormality, or both. A history of prior bleeding suggests a coagulopathy, as does the finding of bleeding from multiple sites. However, this is not always the case. Even diffuse bleeding may arise from anatomic rather than hemostatic abnormalities, due to inherited or acquired primary vascular disorders rather than fluid-phase clotting abnormalities. Examples (Table 157-1) include Ehlers-Danlos syndrome; angiodysplasia; spontaneous, non-traumatic intracerebral hemorrhage caused by deep perforator arteriopathy or cerebral amyloid angiopathy; and recurrent mucosal hemorrhage in patients with hereditary hemorrhagic telangiectasia (Chapter 159). Conversely, a single episode of bleeding from an isolated site may be the initial manifestation of a systemic coagulopathy.

The history must include a survey of coexisting systemic diseases and drug ingestions that could affect hemostasis. Renal failure and the myeloproliferative neoplasms are associated with impaired platelet–vessel wall interactions and qualitative platelet abnormalities, connective tissue diseases and lymphomas are associated with thrombocytopenia, and liver disease causes a complex coagulopathy (Chapter 161). Ingestion of aspirin and other nonsteroidal anti-inflammatory drugs (NSAIDs) that cause nonselective inhibition of cyclooxygenase leads to platelet dysfunction; these drugs are often contained in over-the-counter preparations that patients may neglect to report without specific questioning. Other drugs, such as antibiotics, also may be associated with a bleeding tendency by causing abnormal platelet function or thrombocytopenia.[2] Finally, it is important to elicit a family history of bleeding problems. Although a positive history provides an important clue to a possible inherited coagulopathy, a negative history does not exclude a familial cause; for example, 20% of patients with classic hemophilia have a completely negative family history of bleeding.

Mild bleeding events are commonly reported by patients with and without subsequently laboratory-documented bleeding disorders, sometimes making it difficult for hematologists to define a "significant bleeding history." Using a web-based questionnaire, 25% of subjects in a healthy population reported epistaxis, 18% easy bruising (more commonly in women), 18% prolonged bleeding after dental extraction, and 47% of women heavy menstrual bleeding. Regarding the latter, in a study of 200 consecutive adolescents referred for heavy menstrual bleeding, a systemic bleeding disorder was diagnosed in 33%: low von Willebrand factor levels in 16%, von Willebrand disease in 11%, and qualitative platelet dysfunction in 4.5%.[3] More precise quantification of bleeding symptoms is being attempted by using "bleeding score" instruments such as the Vicenza bleeding score to help discriminate, in conjunction with laboratory testing, between healthy subjects and those with mild bleeding disorders.

Patterns of clinical bleeding, as revealed by the history and physical examination, may be characteristic of certain types of coagulopathy (Table 157-2). In general, patients with thrombocytopenia or qualitative platelet or vascular disorders present with bleeding from superficial sites in the skin and mucous membranes. These may involve petechiae, which are pinpoint cutaneous hemorrhages that appear particularly over dependent extremities (characteristic of severe thrombocytopenia), ecchymoses (common bruises), purpura, gastrointestinal and genitourinary tract bleeding, epistaxis, and hemoptysis. In these types of disorders, bleeding tends to occur spontaneously or immediately after trauma. In contrast, patients with inherited or acquired coagulation factor deficiencies, such as hemophilia, or those on anticoagulant therapy tend to bleed from deeper tissue sites (e.g., hemarthroses, deep hematomas, or retroperitoneal hemorrhage) and in a delayed manner after trauma.

LABORATORY TESTING

Screening Tests of Hemostasis

A few simple screening tests have traditionally been used in the initial evaluation of patients with a suspected coagulopathy: platelet count, bleeding time, prothrombin time (PT) (also reported as the INR), activated partial thromboplastin time (aPTT), and thrombin time (TT).[4] The North American Specialized Coagulation Laboratory Association (NASCOLA) has reported that most coagulation laboratories currently perform these tests as their "bleeding disorder panels."

Thrombocytopenia, reported by electronic particle counting, should be verified by examination of the peripheral smear. Pseudothrombocytopenia, a laboratory artifact of ex vivo platelet clumping, may be caused by the ethylenediaminetetraacetic acid (EDTA) anticoagulant used in tubes for blood cell counts, by other anticoagulants, or by nonphysiologic cold agglutinins acting at room temperature. It should be suspected whenever a very low platelet count is unexpectedly reported in a patient who does not exhibit any clinical

TABLE 157-1 CHARACTERISTIC PATTERNS OF BLEEDING IN SYSTEMIC DISORDERS OF HEMOSTASIS

TYPE OF DISORDER	SITES OF BLEEDING: GENERAL	SKIN	MUCOUS MEMBRANES	OTHER	ONSET OF BLEEDING	CLINICAL EXAMPLES
Platelet-vascular disorders	Superficial surfaces	Petechiae, ecchymoses	Common: oral, nasal, gastrointestinal, genitourinary	Rare	Spontaneous or immediately after trauma	Thrombocytopenia, functional platelet disorder, vascular fragility, disseminated intravascular coagulation, liver disease
Coagulation factor deficiency	Deep tissues	Hematomas	Rare	Common: joint, muscle, retroperitoneal	Delayed after trauma	Inherited coagulation factor deficiency, acquired inhibitor, anticoagulation, disseminated intravascular coagulation, liver disease

TABLE 157-2 FEATURES OF COAGULATION FACTOR DEFICIENCIES

DEFICIENCY	TYPICAL LABORATORY FINDINGS	APPROXIMATE PREVALENCE
Fibrinogen	Afibrinogenemia: TT ↑↑, aPTT ↑↑, PT ↑↑ Dysfibrinogenemia and hypofibrinogenemia: TT ↑, aPTT ↑, PT ↑↑	1 in 1 million
Prothrombin	TT normal, aPTT ↑, PT ↑	1 in 2 million
Factor V	TT normal, aPTT ↑, PT ↑	1 in 1 million
Combined factor V and VIII	TT normal, aPTT ↑, PT ↑	1 in 1 million
Factor VII	TT normal, aPTT normal, PT ↑	1 in 500,000
Factor X	TT normal, aPTT ↑, PT ↑	1 in 1 million
Factor XI	TT normal, aPTT ↑, PT normal	1 in 1 million
Factor XIII	TT, aPTT, and PT normal; specific assays required	1 in 2 million
Vitamin K–dependent coagulation factors	TT normal, aPTT ↑, PT ↑↑	<50 families reported

aPTT = activated partial thromboplastin time; PT = prothrombin time; TT = thrombin time.
Adapted from Palla R, Peyvandi F, Shapiro AD. Rare bleeding disorders: diagnosis and treatment. *Blood.* 2015;125:2052-2061.

bleeding. Pseudothrombocytopenia is indicated by the finding of platelet clumps on the peripheral smear, and the diagnosis is supported by the finding of simultaneously normal platelet counts in blood samples obtained by finger stick, in tubes containing other anticoagulants, or in a tube maintained at 37° C before platelet counting. Examination of the blood smear can also reveal clues to the cause of real thrombocytopenia, such as fragmented red blood cells in thrombotic thrombocytopenic purpura.

The bleeding time was a widely used clinical screening test for disorders of platelet–vessel wall interactions. It measures the time to cessation of bleeding after a standardized incision over the volar aspect of the forearm. However, the test is prone to problems related to quality control, reproducibility, sensitivity, and specificity. Therefore, because von Willebrand disease is the most common genetic cause of abnormal platelet–vessel wall interactions, most experts now recommend replacing the bleeding time with specific tests for von Willebrand disease (vWd screen) in the initial evaluation of patients with a suspected coagulopathy (Chapter 159). The entity of "low von Willebrand factor" activity (≥30 and ≤50 IU/dL), not meeting the diagnostic criteria of von Willebrand disease, has been associated with a bleeding tendency.[5] As an additional replacement for the bleeding time, especially when a functional (qualitative) abnormality of platelets is suspected by characteristic mucocutaneous bleeding or bruising, a global assay of platelet function can be appended to the panel of screening tests. This is most commonly a platelet function analyzer (PFA) closure time. The PFA and other platelet function studies (see later) must be performed after discontinuation of drugs that interfere with platelet function (e.g., aspirin and other NSAIDs).

The PT measures the integrity of the extrinsic and common pathways of coagulation (factors VII, X, and V; prothrombin; and fibrinogen) (Fig. 157-2). The aPTT measures the integrity of the intrinsic and common pathways of coagulation (high-molecular-weight kininogen; prekallikrein; factors XII, XI, IX, VIII, X, and V; prothrombin; and fibrinogen). The sensitivity of the PT and aPTT in detecting coagulation factor deficiencies may vary with the reagents used to perform these tests, and each laboratory must determine its own reference standards. It is important to note that the PT and aPTT are generally not sensitive enough to detect mild coagulation factor deficiencies, where the deficient factor level is >25%. For example, an individual with mild hemophilia (with factor VIII level of 35%) is likely to have a normal aPTT.[6] The TT is a screen for quantitative deficiencies and qualitative defects of plasma fibrinogen.

Follow-Up of Abnormal Screening Tests

Abnormalities in these screening tests of hemostasis may be pursued by more specialized tests to establish a specific diagnosis (Fig. 157-3).

An abnormal von Willebrand disease screen should be followed up with more specialized tests, including von Willebrand factor multimer analysis, to identify the type of von Willebrand disease involved. Abnormalities in the PFA closure time should be followed by more specialized light transmission aggregometry (LTA) of platelets using a panel of agonists (ADP, epinephrine, collagen, arachidonic acid, ristocetin) that induce characteristic changes in light transmission (or optical density) in stirred suspensions of freshly isolated platelets in plasma (PRP). LTA is still considered the "gold standard" for platelet function testing[7] (Chapter 159). In patients who have clinical bleeding problems, inherited disorders of platelet function are increasingly diagnosed by genomic testing.[8]

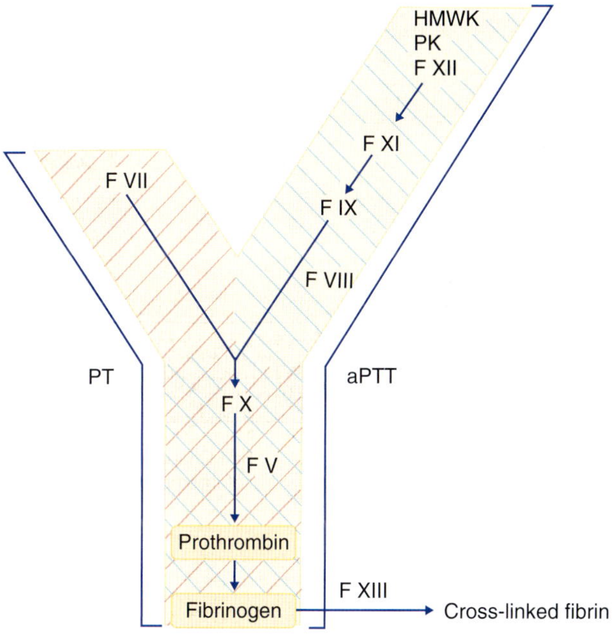

FIGURE 157-2. **Classic coagulation cascade.** The prothrombin time (PT) measures the integrity of the extrinsic and common pathways, whereas the activated partial thromboplastin time (aPTT) measures the integrity of the intrinsic and common pathways. Factor (F) XIII deficiency is not detected by PT or aPTT. HMWK = high-molecular-weight kininogen; PK = prekallikrein.

The finding of a prolonged PT and/or aPTT indicates either a deficiency of one or more coagulation factors or the presence of an inhibitor (Fig. 157-4), usually an antibody, directed at one or more components of the coagulation system. These two possibilities can be distinguished by performing a simple inhibitor screen, which involves a 1:1 mix of the patient's plasma and normal plasma. The premise of the test is that even if the patient's plasma is completely deficient (0% level) in a certain factor, mixing it 1:1 with normal plasma (100% level) should bring the concentration of that factor to 50% in the mixture; this is sufficient to correct the prolonged PT or aPTT. If correction occurs with the inhibitor screen, individual coagulation factor levels should be assayed for a specific deficiency state. If the 1:1 mix fails to correct the prolonged PT and/or aPTT, an inhibitor is likely to be present, and it is interfering with coagulation in vitro in both the patient's plasma and the normal plasma. Specific assays should then be performed to determine whether there is a true inhibitor against a coagulation factor (e.g., factor VIII antibody) or whether the inhibitor is a lupus anticoagulant. A prolonged TT, with or without prolongation of the PT and/or aPTT, suggests the presence of a quantitative deficiency or a qualitative defect of fibrinogen. These can then be distinguished by following up with simultaneously performed clottable (functional) and antigenic assays of fibrinogen: a disproportionately low clottable fibrinogen points to a functional fibrinogen abnormality (dysfibrinogenemia), whereas

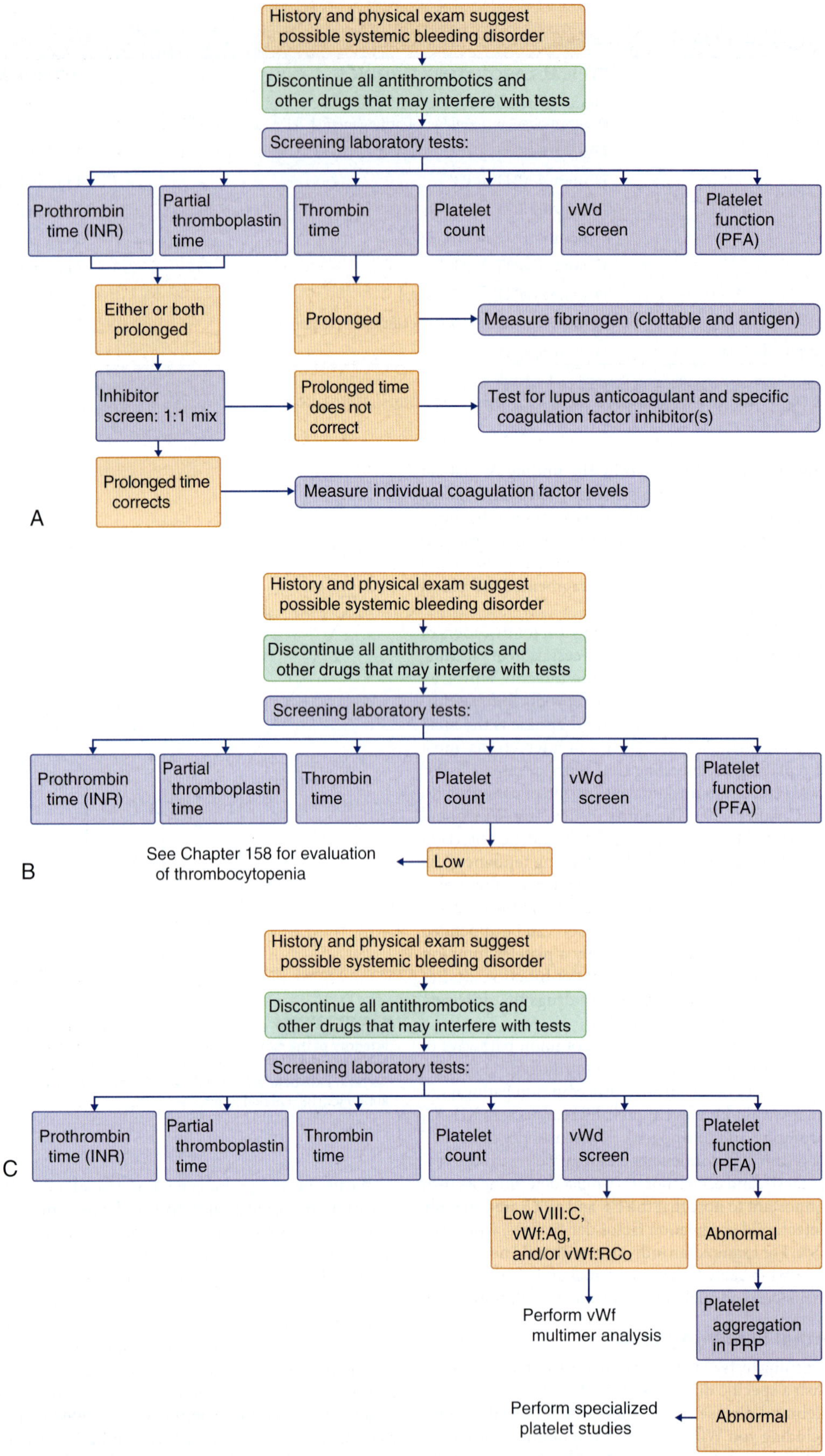

FIGURE 157-3. Algorithms for clinical and laboratory approach to the diagnosis of a patient with a suspected systemic bleeding disorder (coagulopathy). A to C, The critical importance of a thorough personal and family history and physical examination is emphasized before initiating a laboratory work-up. INR = international normalized ratio; PFA = platelet function analyzer; PRP = platelet-rich plasma; VIII:C = factor VIII coagulant activity; vWD = von Willebrand disease; vWf = von Willebrand factor; vWf:Ag = von Willebrand factor antigen; vWf:RCo = von Willebrand factor: ristocetin cofactor activity.

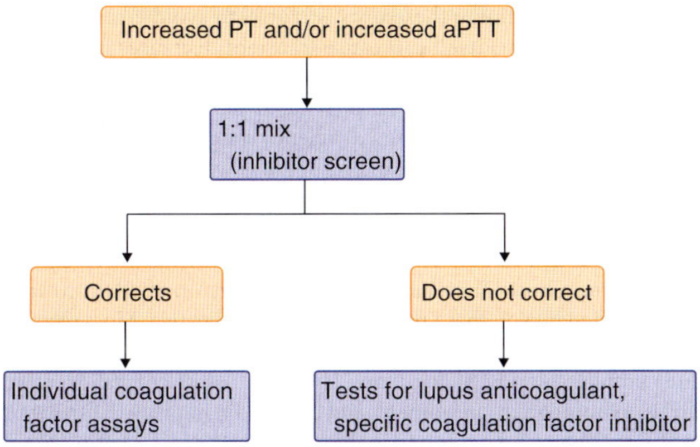

FIGURE 157-4. Approach to evaluating patients with prolonged prothrombin time (PT) or activated partial thromboplastin time (aPTT).

proportionately reduced levels of clottable and antigenic fibrinogen suggest a quantitative deficiency (hypofibrinogenemia or afibrinogenemia) (see Fig. 157-3A and Chapter 160).

Suspected Coagulopathy Despite Negative Screening Tests

Normal results for all these screening tests of hemostasis essentially usually exclude any clinically significant systemic coagulopathy. When all screening tests of coagulation are normal in a patient who is strongly suspected of having a systemic bleeding disorder, further testing might be necessary. Individual coagulation factor assays can reveal a mild factor deficiency even when the PT and aPTT are normal. Activated factor XIII catalyzes the covalent cross-linking of polymerized fibrin to solidify clot formation in vivo. However, the PT, aPTT, and thrombin time tests in vitro detect the formation of only fibrin that is not yet cross-linked (see Fig. 157-2). Therefore, since factor XIII deficiency (Chapter 160) is not detected by the PT and aPTT, specific testing for factor XIII activity is required.

Rare disorders of fibrinolysis also may be associated with normal screening tests, thereby necessitating more specialized tests when indicated (Chapter 161). Bleeding due to hyperfibrinolysis can be caused by increased levels of the fibrinolytic enzyme, plasmin. In turn, increased plasmin generation can be due to increased activators (tissue-plasminogen activator [tPA]), decreased plasmin substrate (hypoplasminogenemia), or decreased fibrinolytic inhibitors (α2-antiplasmin, plasminogen activator inhibitor-1 [PAI-1], or thrombin activatable fibrinolysis inhibitor [TAFI]). All of these proteins, as well as quantitative D-dimer levels, can be measured in clinical laboratories.[9]

Newer coagulation tests, known as global assays, have the potential to offer a more complete evaluation of a patient's overall clot-forming capability. These global assays, including thrombin generation tests and viscoelastic assays, have not yet advanced from experimental research to routine clinical practice.

Global Coagulation Laboratory and Point-of-Care Tests

Thrombin Generation Tests

Thrombin generation tests require separation of platelet-poor plasma (PPP) or platelet-rich plasma (PRP) from centrifuged whole blood. Thrombin generation in the patient's plasma can be then measured by comparing it to a calibrator of known thrombin activity, using automated fluorescence or chromogenic readouts. These tests measure primarily the coagulation arm of hemostasis and have been shown to be promising in evaluating thrombophilias in guiding antithrombotic therapy. The tests are limited at this time by their lack of validation as a clinical tool.

Clot Waveform Analysis

This test is based on the activated partial thromboplastin time (aPTT) assay, but with a prolonged light transmission readout that can monitor both the acceleration and deceleration of clotting, thereby reflecting the whole process of clot formation and clot lysis. It shows promise as a global test of disseminated intravascular coagulation (DIC) and for sensitive detection of mild coagulation factor deficiencies, but the method needs further validation and standardization.

Thromboelastography

Two types of semiautomated commercial devices available provide global assays of coagulation and fibrinolysis using point-of-care technology: the ROTEM (rotational thromboelastometry) analyzer and the thromboelastography analyzers. These tests are whole blood clotting tests in which a small aliquot of blood is rotated in a cuvette, and the strength, elasticity, and dissolution of the forming clot are measured with a torsion wire or by optical detection. The markedly increasing use of this technology is understandable; it is inherently attractive to have a bedside test that provides immediate, real-time, visualized monitoring and analysis of clot formation and lysis in whole blood incorporating the totality of the hemostatic system, including coagulation, fibrinolysis, and platelets.[10] A randomized trial of thromboelastography-guided blood component use in patients with cirrhosis and nonvariceal bleeding found that it leads to a significantly lower use of blood components than transfusions guided by INR and platelet count.[A1] However, systematic reviews have concluded at this time that most meaningful data on thromboelastography have come from their use in cardiac surgery involving cardiopulmonary bypass, where it has indeed reduced the need for transfusion of blood products.[A2] Randomized clinical trials have found that the use of thromboelastography-guided algorithms in place of traditional transfusion parameters in cirrhotic patients with severe coagulopathy (i.e., platelets <50,000 and/or INR >1.8) who are having active bleeding reduces the number of platelet, plasma, and cryoprecipitate transfusions.[A3] Its impact on producing other favorable clinical end points remains open to study.[11] For example, in two randomized trials, adding viscoelastography to routine coagulation studies did not improve overall outcomes after major trauma,[A4] and adding thromboelastography to such studies led to only a small reduction in blood loss from postpartum hemorrhage.[A5]

Other Point-of-Care Tests of Hemostasis

Other, more specialized but established point-of-care tests of hemostasis include the activated clotting time (ACT), which is used to monitor heparinization during extracorporeal circuits in cardiac bypass surgery and extracorporeal membrane oxygenation; handheld devices to measure the international normalized ratio (INR) for self-management at-home monitoring in patients taking vitamin K antagonists; and platelet function analyzers (i.e., the VerifyNow system), which measure platelet aggregation across fibrinogen-coated polystyrene beads in separate cartridges for assessment of resistance to antiplatelet drugs including aspirin, thienopyridines, and glycoprotein IIb-IIIa antagonists.

High-Throughput Sequencing

High-throughput sequencing can detect a molecular diagnosis in about 50% of all patients with a thrombotic, coagulation, platelet count, or platelet function disorder. In patients with otherwise unexplained bleeding disorders and normal hemostatic test results, it can find a molecular diagnosis in about 3% of patients.[12]

EVALUATION OF THE ASYMPTOMATIC PATIENT WITH ABNORMAL COAGULATION TESTS

In asymptomatic individuals who are discovered incidentally to have abnormalities in screening laboratory tests of hemostasis, the first critical question to ask is whether the findings are clinically relevant. Patients with inherited deficiencies of one of the contact activation coagulation factors (factor XII, high-molecular-weight kininogen, prekallikrein) characteristically have a markedly prolonged aPTT, yet they do not have a clinical bleeding tendency. Likewise, patients with lupus anticoagulants typically have prolongation of the aPTT and sometimes also the PT; they much more often have thrombotic rather than bleeding complications. In patients with heparin-induced thrombocytopenia, a marked decrease in the platelet count is sometimes associated with arterial and venous thrombosis rather than bleeding. It is crucial to view the clinical setting, history, physical examination, and screening laboratory tests as complementary facets of the approach to patients with suspected coagulopathies.

EVALUATION OF THE PREOPERATIVE PATIENT

Routine screening of all preoperative patients with a platelet count, bleeding time, PT, and aPTT is not only uninformative but also may be counterproductive if follow-up testing causes unnecessary expense and delays in surgery (Chapter 399). Preoperative bleeding time, PT, and aPTT do not predict surgical bleeding risk in patients who are not found to be at increased risk on clinical grounds, so a thorough clinical assessment should guide the need for these preoperative screening tests. Laboratory testing and possibly further specialized tests of coagulation are indicated for patients whose bleeding histories are suspicious for a hemostatic abnormality. Preoperative screening tests of coagulation are probably warranted for patients who cannot cooperate with an adequate clinical assessment and for those who will be undergoing procedures in which even minimal postoperative hemorrhage could be hazardous. Recent guidelines for preinterventional and preoperative hemostatic evaluation have likewise concluded that bleeding risk requires a detailed personal and family history of hemorrhagic events and physical examination; but individuals with a negative history and without conditions that may interfere with systemic hemostasis should not undergo coagulation testing.[13]

EVALUATION OF THE PATIENT WITH A POSSIBLE HYPERCOAGULABLE STATE

Most patients with venous thromboembolism (VTE) have an inherited basis for hypercoagulability (Chapter 67). Patients with inherited hypercoagulable states (or thrombophilia) typically present with an initial episode of VTE in early adulthood, but thrombotic manifestations may begin at any time from early childhood to old age. Patients usually have deep vein thrombosis of the lower extremities or pulmonary embolism, but other uncommon sites of venous thrombosis may be involved. Arterial thrombosis is not characteristically associated with inherited hypercoagulable states. Arterial thrombosis that occurs prematurely or in the absence of apparent risk factors should trigger a different line of investigation, possibly including evaluation for vasculitis, myeloproliferative neoplasms, hyperhomocysteinemia, antiphospholipid syndrome, and potential sources of systemic embolization.

The primary or hereditary hypercoagulable states (see Table 67-1) result from specific mutations or polymorphisms that lead to decreased levels of physiologic antithrombotic proteins or increased levels of procoagulant proteins. In contrast, the secondary or acquired hypercoagulable states are a heterogeneous group of disorders that predispose to thrombosis by complex mechanisms. VTE is often provoked by the combination of an underlying hypercoagulable genotype and an acquired prothrombotic, hypercoagulable state such as pregnancy, immobilization, or the postoperative state. Certain clinical characteristics suggest the presence of an inherited hypercoagulable state (Table 157-3). Patients with recurrent thrombosis should be tested for these disorders and, in most cases, committed to lifelong prophylactic anticoagulation. It is not clear whether it is essential to order these tests after a single episode of VTE. Counterintuitively, it has been found that most of the common inherited hypercoagulable states—which, to varying extents, clearly increase the risk for a *first* episode of VTE—are at best only weak predictors of *recurrent* VTE. It has been argued, therefore, that making a specific thrombophilia diagnosis after an initial episode of VTE will not influence the decision about the duration of prophylactic anticoagulation.[14] However, the increased risk for recurrent VTE with the more strongly prothrombotic mutations (e.g., antithrombin III, protein C or S deficiency), combined inherited thrombophilias, or antiphospholipid syndrome may necessitate long-term anticoagulation, and therefore their diagnosis after a first episode of VTE would in fact alter decisions about the duration of anticoagulation (see Fig. 67-1). Even if they are not maintained on long-term anticoagulation, patients with diagnosed primary hypercoagulable states should receive prophylactic anticoagulation during situations that pose a high risk for thrombosis, such as the peripartum period. There is no simple screening test for primary hypercoagulable states, and the timing of obtaining these tests is crucial to avoid erroneous diagnoses.[15] Acute thrombosis itself can cause transient decreases in the levels of antithrombin, protein C, and protein S. Heparin therapy can cause a decrease in plasma antithrombin activity. Warfarin therapy lowers the functional levels of protein C and protein S. Inherited deficiency states can be diagnosed spuriously under these conditions. Use of one of the newer anticoagulants can also interfere with laboratory tests, especially for lupus anticoagulant.

Patients who present with VTE have an increased risk for harboring an occult malignancy. This association is increased further in patients with recurrent and unprovoked thrombosis. There are conflicting opinions on whether an evaluation for occult malignancy in these patients must be exhaustive. Most recommend that evaluation can be limited to a thorough history, physical examination, routine complete blood cell count and chemistries, test of fecal occult blood, urinalysis, mammogram (in women), and chest radiograph, with further testing guided by any abnormalities found in this initial evaluation. Routine computed tomography scanning of the chest, abdomen, and pelvis is not indicated[A6] unless other testing suggests an abnormality[16] (see algorithm in Fig. 67-3).

In addition to classic deep vein thrombosis and pulmonary embolism, certain characteristic types of thrombosis may provide important clues to the cause and trigger a more directed evaluation. Migratory, superficial thrombophlebitis (Trousseau syndrome) or nonbacterial thrombotic endocarditis strongly suggests the presence of an occult malignancy (Chapter 67). Hepatic vein thrombosis (Budd-Chiari syndrome; Chapter 129) or portal vein thrombosis may indicate a myeloproliferative neoplasm (Chapter 152) or paroxysmal nocturnal hemoglobinuria (Chapter 146). Extensive inferior vena cava thrombosis may occur with renal cell carcinoma (Chapter 182). Warfarin-induced skin necrosis strongly suggests underlying protein C or protein S deficiency. Recurrent, spontaneous miscarriages are characteristic of the antiphospholipid syndrome (Chapter 160), although they are also associated with other thrombophilias.

GENERAL REFERENCES

For the General References and other additional features, please visit Elsevier eBooks+ at https://ebooks.health.elsevier.com.

Grade A References

A1. Kumar M, Ahmad J, Maiwall R, et al. Thromboelastography-guided blood component use in patients with cirrhosis with nonvariceal bleeding: a randomized, controlled trial. *Hepatology.* 2020;71:235-246.

A2. Wikkelsø A, Wetterslev J, Møller AM, et al. Thromboelastography (TEG) or rotational thromboelastometry (ROTEM) to monitor haemostatic treatment in bleeding patients: a systematic review and meta-analysis and trial sequential analysis. *Anaesthesia.* 2017;72:519-531.

A3. Rout G, Shalimar, Gunjan D, et al. Thromboelastography-guided blood product transfusion in cirrhosis patients with variceal bleeding: a randomized controlled trial. *J Clin Gastroenterol.* 2020;54:255-262.

A4. Baksaas-Aasen K, Gall LS, Stensballe J, et al. Viscoelastic haemostatic assay augmented protocols for major trauma haemorrhage (ITACTIC): a randomized, controlled trial. *Intensive Care Med.* 2021;47:49-59.

A5. Jokinen S, Kuitunen A, Uotila J, et al. Thromboelastometry-guided treatment algorithm in postpartum haemorrhage: a randomised, controlled pilot trial. *Br J Anaesth.* 2023;130:165-174.

A6. Carrier M, Lazo-Langner A, Shivakumar S, et al. Screening for occult cancer in unprovoked venous thromboembolism. *N Engl J Med.* 2015;373:697-704.

TABLE 157-3 CLINICAL CHARACTERISTICS OF PATIENTS WITH INHERITED HYPERCOAGULABLE STATES (THROMBOPHILIA)

Venous thromboembolism (>90% of cases)
Deep vein thrombosis or pulmonary embolism most common
Splanchnic or cerebral vein thrombosis rare but characteristic
Frequent family history of thrombosis
Typically autosomal dominant
First episode of thrombosis typically in young adulthood (<40 years)
Often apparently unprovoked (but an acquired thrombosis trigger is frequently identified with a careful history)
More common thrombophilias (factor V Leiden, prothrombin 20210 G→A) are associated with a lower thrombosis risk; rarer thrombophilias (antithrombin III, protein C, protein S deficiency) are associated with a higher thrombosis risk
Warfarin-induced skin necrosis or neonatal purpura fulminans with protein C or protein S deficiency (very rare)

158 THROMBOCYTOPENIA

CHARLES S. ABRAMS

DEFINITION

Thrombocytopenia is defined as a platelet count lower than the normal range, typically below 140,000/μL.

EPIDEMIOLOGY

With the widespread use of the routine complete blood count (CBC), asymptomatic individuals with incidentally discovered mild thrombocytopenia are being increasingly recognized. The clinical significance of mild thrombocytopenia (platelet counts between 100,000/μL and 150,000/μL) in the absence of other CBC abnormalities can be difficult to ascertain. Many, and perhaps most, of these individuals with mild chronic thrombocytopenia represent outliers of the normal distribution of platelet counts. However, others have thrombocytopenia that represents the early manifestation of an unrecognized disease.

After a decade, approximately 10% of patients with mild immune thrombocytopenia will develop ITP or another autoimmune disorder. However, approximately 90% of the subjects will continue to manifest borderline thrombocytopenia without developing another disorder during this period of time. It can be concluded that most individuals with isolated and asymptomatic chronic mild thrombocytopenia simply represent the lower end of the normal platelet count distribution. Consequently, international consensus groups have set the threshold for the diagnosis of ITP at a platelet count of less than 100,000/µL.

PATHOBIOLOGY

The causes of thrombocytopenia can be divided into three major categories: increased destruction of platelets, such as seen in immune-mediated causes; decreased production of platelets, usually due to an underlying bone marrow disorder; or sequestration of platelets within the spleen, as occurs in conditions that cause splenomegaly (hypersplenism).

Increased Platelet Destruction

In the absence of splenomegaly, the presence of increased megakaryocytes in an otherwise normal bone marrow implies that thrombocytopenia is due to increased platelet destruction. An acute drop in a patient's platelet count also implies that a peripheral destructive process is the likely cause. For example, a patient who develops abrupt thrombocytopenia during hospitalization most likely has a low platelet count caused by an infection or by the introduction of a new medication. Both nonimmune and immune processes can lead to a shortened platelet lifespan. Nonimmune reasons for the accelerated destruction of platelets include sepsis, disseminated intravascular coagulation (DIC), thrombotic thrombocytopenic purpura (TTP), hemolytic-uremic syndrome (HUS), preeclampsia or eclampsia, cardiopulmonary bypass, and giant cavernous hemangioma. Thrombocytopenia that occurs in these circumstances usually resolves with treatment of the underlying disorder, and platelet transfusions are rarely necessary. Thrombocytopenia due to TTP, HUS, or heparin-induced thrombocytopenia (HIT) is more characteristically associated with microvascular occlusion or thrombosis than with bleeding (Table 158-1).

Immune-mediated platelet destruction can result from drugs, alloimmune sensitization, or autoimmunity. Medications should always be considered as a possible cause of acute thrombocytopenia. The list of potential offending agents is long, but drugs with strong evidence of antibody-mediated platelet destruction include quinine, quinidine, sulfonamides (such as trimethoprim-sulfamethoxazole), β-lactam antibiotics (both penicillins and cephalosporins), vancomycin, procainamide, and gold salts. In addition to stopping the offending medication, platelet transfusions might be required for severe thrombocytopenia.

Decreased Platelet Production

Decreased platelet production occurs in primary diseases of the bone marrow, such as acute leukemia and aplastic anemia; myelophthisic processes in which bone marrow is affected by metastatic carcinoma, fibrosis, or other clonal hematopoietic disorders; following toxin-induced (such as chemotherapy or ethanol exposure) or radiation therapy–induced myelosuppression; and during infections with viruses such as HIV, cytomegalovirus (CMV), Epstein-Barr virus (EBV), and varicella. Thrombocytopenia also occurs when normal megakaryocyte proliferation is impaired by myelodysplasia.

Thrombocytopenia due to decreased platelet production is often accompanied by abnormalities of the white blood cells or red blood cells. This should be readily apparent by inspection of the CBC and review of the peripheral blood smear. When thrombocytopenia in this setting is accompanied by bleeding, the bleeding usually requires treatment by platelet transfusion. Additionally, when decreased platelet production is profound (less than 10,000/µL) and cannot be readily reversed, prophylactic platelet transfusion to prevent bleeding should be considered. However, as will be discussed in the following section, prophylactic platelet transfusion is problematic because of the short lifespan of platelets and the potential to develop alloantibodies that will limit the effectiveness of future platelet transfusions.

Platelet Sequestration

Approximately 30 to 40% of the circulating platelet mass is normally sequestered within the spleen. Enlargement of the spleen due to portal hypertension or infiltration is accompanied by expansion of the splenic platelet pool. Because hypersplenism by itself rarely causes a platelet count of less than 40,000/µL to 50,000/µL, bleeding due to thrombocytopenia from hypersplenism alone is unusual. In addition, if a patient with a large spleen has a platelet count of less than 40,000/µL, an additional etiology for the thrombocytopenia should be considered.

TABLE 158-1 DISORDERS THAT CAUSE BOTH THROMBOCYTOPENIA AND THROMBOSIS

Thrombotic thrombocytopenic purpura (TTP)
Hemolytic-uremic syndrome (HUS)
Heparin-induced thrombocytopenia (HIT)
Disseminated intravascular coagulation (DIC)
Paroxysmal nocturnal hemoglobinuria (PNH)
Vasculitis (such as systemic lupus erythematosus)
Antiphospholipid antibody syndrome

CLINICAL MANIFESTATIONS

In the absence of qualitative platelet defects (Chapter 159), excessive bleeding does not occur in thrombocytopenic patients following trauma or surgery unless the platelet count is lower than 75,000/µL. In otherwise hemostatically normal patients, spontaneous hemorrhage typically does not occur unless platelet counts are below 30,000/µL. Patients with platelet counts of less than 5000/µL to 10,000/µL are at a high risk for spontaneous, life-threatening hemorrhage. However, there is no absolute threshold for spontaneous bleeding due to thrombocytopenia. Bleeding may occur at higher counts when fever, sepsis, severe anemia, and other hemostatic defects are present, or when platelet function is impaired by medication. It is sometimes said that patients with wet purpura (mucocutaneous bleeding with blood blisters) are at particularly high risk for sudden catastrophic bleeding events. Therefore, it is critical that the physician consider the gamut of possibilities when diagnosing and managing a patient with a low platelet count.

DIAGNOSIS

Typically, the first step in diagnosing a patient with a low platelet count is to determine whether the thrombocytopenia is attributable to increased platelet destruction, decreased platelet production, or hypersplenism (Fig. 158-1). Since no single test can differentiate among the three possibilities, clinical evaluation is critical. A thorough history and physical examination, with attention to possible alternative explanations for thrombocytopenia, are mandatory. Particular attention should be paid to the duration of symptoms, which helps to determine whether the patient has acute or chronic thrombocytopenia. The clinician should also focus on the patient's recent exposure to new medications that might induce thrombocytopenia as a side effect.

Preliminary laboratory tests include a CBC with a differential, along with an examination of the peripheral blood smear (Chapter 143). Abnormalities in the number or morphology of the leukocytes or erythrocytes may indicate a systemic inflammatory disorder or a pathology within the bone marrow; fragmentation of red cells may suggest a microangiopathy such as thrombotic thrombocytopenic purpura (TTP), hemolytic-uremic syndrome (HUS), or disseminated intravascular coagulation (DIC). Clumping of the platelets on the peripheral blood smear may indicate that the patient has pseudothrombocytopenia (Chapter 157). This anomaly is usually due to an antibody that binds to and thereby agglutinates platelets only in the presence of hypocalcemia induced by ethylenediaminetetraacetic acid (EDTA) in the blood collection tube or when the blood sample is allowed to cool to room temperature. Repeating the platelet count in a blood sample that has been anticoagulated with heparin and kept warm until it is analyzed can help exclude this spurious diagnosis. Any additional testing to determine the cause of thrombocytopenia is based solely on the available clinical information derived from the history and examination of the patient. For example, testing for human immunodeficiency virus (HIV) would be prudent in a patient with risk factors. A bone marrow aspirate and biopsy are typically not required for a patient with thrombocytopenia who has an otherwise normal CBC and peripheral blood smear. However, a bone marrow aspirate and biopsy should be considered in older patients and in patients whose thrombocytopenia is progressive or in whom standard therapy has not been effective.

TREATMENT

For patients with decreased platelet production, the cornerstone of treatment is platelet transfusion (Chapter 162). For patients with other specific causes, however, platelet transfusions may or may not be a beneficial therapeutic option.

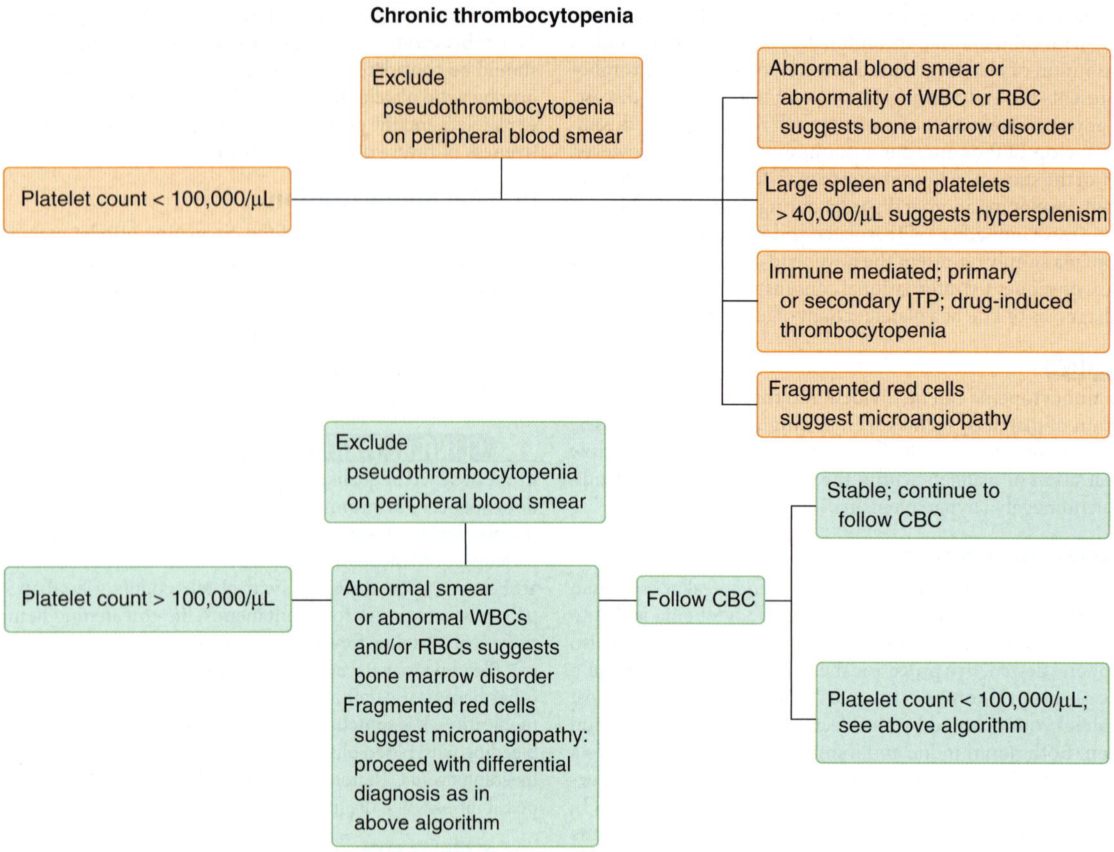

FIGURE 158-1. **Systematic approach to the evaluation of chronic thrombocytopenia.** CBC = complete blood count; ITP = immune (idiopathic) thrombocytopenic purpura; RBC = red blood cells; WBC = white blood cells.

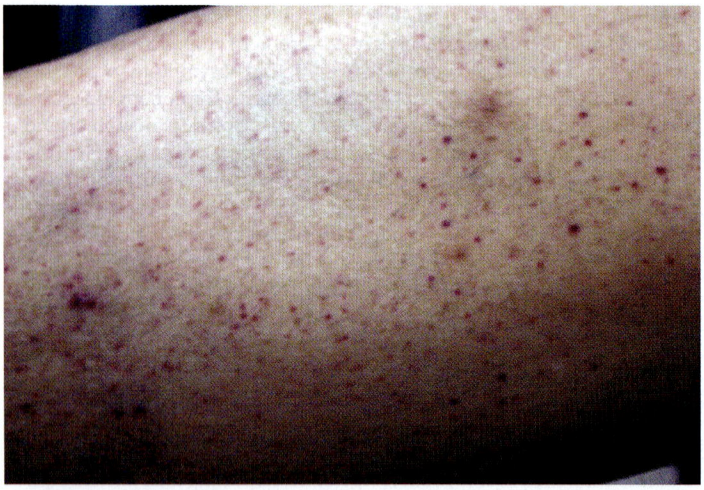

FIGURE 158-2. **Petechiae. Multiple pinpoint, nonblanching, erythematous macules found predominantly on skin of dependent extremities in patients with severe thrombocytopenia.**

Platelet Transfusions

Clinicians usually consider "wet" bleeding to be much more ominous than "dry" bleeding. Signs of wet bleeding include epistaxis, gingival bleeding, gastrointestinal bleeding, genitourinary bleeding, and bleeding around intravenous sites. Dry bleeding is defined as ecchymosis or petechiae (Fig. 158-2). Overt wet bleeding that is clearly due to thrombocytopenia is usually treated with platelet transfusion (Chapter 162). Prophylactic platelet transfusion for patients who are not bleeding is controversial. When making the decision whether to treat a nonbleeding patient with thrombocytopenia, the practitioner must consider the short lifespan of platelets (10 days), the 5- to 7-day shelf life of stored platelets, and the potential for the patient to develop transfusion-induced platelet alloantibodies. In patients undergoing treatment for acute leukemia, clinical trials have supported the practice of prophylactic platelet transfusions when the platelet count is below 5000/µL or 10,000/µL, rather than waiting until bleeding occurs in the severely thrombocytopenic patient.[1]

The indications for prophylactic platelet transfusions before interventional procedures are predominantly based on clinical experience and expert opinions, rather than on clinical trials. Current guidelines recommend platelet transfusion in patients with therapy-induced hypoproliferative thrombocytopenia and a platelet count of less than 10,000/µL. Prophylactic platelet transfusion is also indicated for patients having elective central venous catheter placement with a platelet count less than 20,000/µL and for patients having elective diagnostic lumbar puncture or major elective nonneuraxial surgery with a platelet count less than 50,000/µL (Table 158-2).[2] Platelet transfusions should continue for several days following procedures where the risk for bleeding or the complications resulting from bleeding are high. For extremely high-risk procedures that involve the nervous and ocular systems, the prophylactic platelet transfusions should be continued for at least 7 to 10 days.

A donated unit of blood contains approximately 50 billion platelets. Infusing this number of platelets into a patient should increase his or her platelet count by 20,000/µL divided by the patient's body surface area in square meters. Therefore, transfusion of one unit into an average-sized adult patient should increase the individual's platelet count by approximately 10,000/µL to 12,000/µL. Bags of platelets used for transfusions are typically obtained by pooling platelets derived from four to six blood donors. Therefore, a "unit" at one hospital may be derived from more donors than a "unit" obtained at another hospital.

Large quantities of platelets can be derived from a single donor by using apheresis technology (plateletpheresis) (Chapter 162). Because there is minimal loss of red blood cells with this technique, plateletpheresis allows one individual to donate very large numbers of platelets (equivalent to the number of platelets obtained from 6 units of donated blood). The risk for platelet alloimmunization is partially dependent on the number of individuals donating platelets to a patient. Therefore, single-donor plateletpheresis can minimize the risk of alloimmunization. To minimize exposure to blood products (Chapter 162), a strategy of low-dose (110 billion/m^2) transfusions requires more frequent platelet transfusions but ultimately results in fewer transfused platelets without the risk of bleeding complications compared with higher-dose transfusions in patients who require prophylactic platelet transfusion therapy for hypoproliferative thrombocytopenia.[3]

Several complications of platelet transfusion therapy must be kept in mind (also see Chapter 162). First, some patients can become alloimmunized against platelet antigens and can become refractory to future platelet transfusion therapy (discussed in detail later). Second, bacterial contamination of stored

TABLE 158-2 SUGGESTED MINIMUM PLATELET COUNTS BEFORE INVASIVE PROCEDURES

VERY HIGH-RISK PROCEDURES—75,000/μL TO 100,000/μL
Neurosurgery Ocular surgery (except cataract extraction) Thyroid surgery Prostatectomy
MODERATE-RISK PROCEDURES—50,000/μL
Liver biopsy Dental extraction Most surgical procedures
LOW-RISK PROCEDURES—30,000/μL
Endoscopy without biopsy Bronchoscopy without biopsy
VERY LOW-RISK PROCEDURES—NO PLATELET TRANSFUSIONS NECESSARY
Bone marrow biopsy Cataract extraction

platelets is a much more common complication than the infectious risk associated with red blood cell transfusions. Unlike red blood cells, which are stored frozen after being harvested from donated blood, platelets are sensitive to cool temperatures and therefore need to be stored at room temperature. This method of storage results in more bacterial overgrowth in the transfusion bags. Transfusion-associated bacterial sepsis is one of the most frequently reported causes of transfusion-induced mortality in the United States, and platelet transfusions are the most common blood products associated with sepsis. In contrast to the risk for bacterial infection, the risk for viral infection from platelet transfusions is no higher than it is for red blood cell transfusions. From a single unit of platelets, the risk for being exposed to HIV is less than 1 in 1.5 to 2 million, the risk for exposure to hepatitis B virus is less than 1 in 200,000, and the risk for exposure to hepatitis C virus is less than 1 in 1 to 2 million.

For thrombocytopenia caused by TTP or HIT, there is usually no indication for platelet transfusions because thrombosis occurs much more frequently than hemorrhage in these disorders. However, platelet transfusions may be considered under expert oversight for patients who have profound thrombocytopenia with life-threatening hemorrhage.

The Transfusion-Refractory Patient

Many patients do not have an optimal increase in their platelet count following transfusion. Although there are various definitions of platelet refractoriness, it is simplest to base this definition on the timing of platelet loss following transfusion. Patients who do not have the predicted rise in their platelet count (between 10,000/μL and 12,000/μL for every unit of donated platelets) should have their platelet count analyzed before their next platelet transfusion, 1 hour after that transfusion, and again 24 hours later. If their platelet count rises appropriately 1 hour after the transfusion but falls substantially 24 hours later, the patient has ongoing platelet consumption. This is often seen in patients with sepsis, DIC, severe active hemorrhage, or sometimes drug-mediated immune destruction of platelets. In these situations, the best therapy is to treat the underlying cause and to continue to support the patient with platelet transfusions as clinically indicated. Alternatively, some patients fail to have a significant increase in platelets even 1 hour after a transfusion. These patients may have hypersplenism, an autoantibody that eliminates not only endogenous platelets but also allogeneic donor platelets (as seen in patients with ITP or some patients with drug-mediated immune destruction of platelets), or alloantibodies that react with antigens on the transfused platelets.

Alloantibodies develop in approximately 20% of patients who are repeatedly exposed to platelet transfusions, and these patients present some of the most challenging management issues in transfusion medicine (Chapter 162). The alloantibodies may be directed against human leukocyte antigen (HLA) class I antigens (HLA-A and HLA-B) or against platelet-specific antigens present on the surface of the platelets. Because it appears that HLA class II antigens present on the surface of leukocytes are essential for the development of antibodies directed against HLA class I antigens, efforts to remove the contamination of leukocytes in platelet transfusion preparations can minimize alloantibody formation. Therefore, filters that trap leukocytes during transfusions are useful to prevent patients from becoming refractory to future platelet transfusions. After a patient develops alloantibodies against transfused platelets, the clinician and the blood bank should attempt to identify whether the alloantibody is directed against an HLA class I antigen or against a platelet-specific antigen. If the alloantibody can be identified, platelets derived from donors matched for an HLA class I antigen or the platelet-specific antigen can be used. Corticosteroids, intravenous immunoglobulin, splenectomy, and recombinant factor VIIa are probably of no value in maintaining hemostasis in platelet-refractory thrombocytopenic patients. Antifibrinolytic agents (e.g., ε-aminocaproic acid) under expert oversight might be helpful for patients with bleeding that is predominantly in the oral cavity or in the genitourinary tract. However, antifibrinolytic agents are contraindicated in patients with DIC (Chapter 161) because these agents can precipitate thrombotic events.

SPECIFIC CAUSES OF THROMBOCYTOPENIA

Drug-Induced Thrombocytopenia

PATHOBIOLOGY

Drug-induced thrombocytopenia is one of the most frequent causes of cytopenias evaluated by physicians.[4] Typically, drug-induced thrombocytopenia is the result of an immune reaction elicited by either the drug or by one of its metabolites. Sometimes the drug is simply deposited on the platelet surface, and antidrug antibodies lead to accelerated platelet clearance, primarily in the spleen. More frequently, the drug binds to a protein on the platelet surface and alters the conformation of the platelet protein in a way that is ultimately targeted by the immune system. In the absence of the drug or drug metabolites, this platelet neoantigen disappears, and the thrombocytopenia slowly resolves as new platelets are released from the bone marrow. Immune-mediated platelet destruction explains most drug-induced thrombocytopenias, but there are some exceptions. For example, chemotherapy and other bone marrow toxins can decrease platelet production and thereby induce thrombocytopenia by a mechanism independent of the immune system.

CLINICAL MANIFESTATIONS

The thrombocytopenia induced by medications can have a mild, moderate, or even severe course. Almost all types of drug-induced thrombocytopenia predispose the patient to the risk of hemorrhagic but not thrombotic complications. The notable exception to this rule is heparin-induced thrombocytopenia (discussed separately in the next section). A common difficult clinical situation occurs when an infected or otherwise critically ill patient develops abrupt thrombocytopenia. In this situation, it can be difficult to discern whether the thrombocytopenia is the result of the recent illness (such as a bacterial or viral infection) or its treatment (such as an antibiotic or another unrelated medication). It is also frequently challenging to discern drug-induced thrombocytopenia from ITP. For this distinction, the patient's medical history may be helpful. A gradually progressive thrombocytopenia over months to years is more consistent with ITP than with thrombocytopenia that is induced by a medication. Conversely, the rapid onset of thrombocytopenia following the initiation of a new medication indicates that the drug is the most likely culprit. The time between the initiation of the offending drug and the development of thrombocytopenia has not been well documented for most medications. However, thrombocytopenia typically begins days to a few weeks after the administration of most medications with this type of toxicity. Presumably, this lag time represents the period required for the patient to develop an immune response against the drug-platelet complex. Medications that have been taken safely for years before the onset of thrombocytopenia are unlikely to be the offending agents. In addition to an assessment of the patient's prescribed medications, a careful and comprehensive evaluation of the patient's over-the-counter medications is also necessary. Agents that contain quinine lead the list of often nonprescribed drugs that can induce life-threatening thrombocytopenia. Quinine is frequently contained in over-the-counter pills for leg cramps. Even the quinine in tonic water can induce severe thrombocytopenia ("gin and tonic purpura") when ingested by certain patients, since a drug-induced, immune-mediated thrombocytopenia usually is not related to the dose of the offending drug.

DIAGNOSIS

Some medications are much more likely to induce thrombocytopenia than others. Table 158-3 contains a partial list of drugs that frequently induce this type of toxicity. One particularly useful online database (www.ouhsc.edu/platelets/ditp.html) lists and periodically updates the level of evidence for specific drugs that may induce thrombocytopenia. With the exception of tests for HIT, laboratory tests for drug-induced thrombocytopenia do not have widespread applicability. Usually, drug-induced thrombocytopenia is proved

TABLE 158-3 DRUGS THAT ARE STRONGLY ASSOCIATED WITH THROMBOCYTOPENIA

ANTIBIOTICS AND ANTIVIRALS
Quinine, quinidine
Penicillin
Cephalosporin
Vancomycin
Trimethoprim-sulfamethoxazole
Sulfonamides, sulfonylureas
Linezolid
Valacyclovir
Ganciclovir
Indinavir
CARDIOVASCULAR MEDICATIONS
Abciximab
Tirofiban
Eptifibatide
Salicylates
Digoxin
Furosemide
MISCELLANEOUS
Cimetidine
Ranitidine
Famotidine
Valproate
Interferon
Oxaliplatin

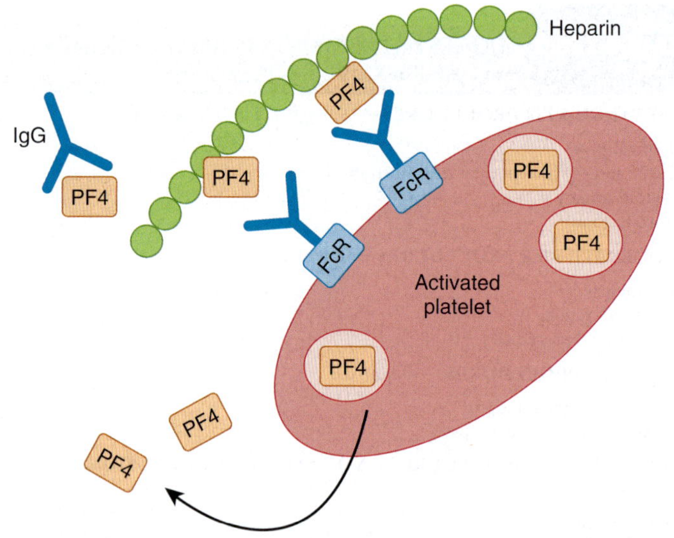

FIGURE 158-3. **Pathophysiology of heparin-induced thrombocytopenia.** Platelet factor 4 (PF4) is a protein that is stored in platelet granules and that is secreted from platelets upon their activation. Heparin can bind to PF4 and induce a conformational change within PF4 that in some patients produces an antibody-mediated immune response. Large complexes of immunoglobulin (Ig), heparin, and PF4 can accumulate on the platelet surface and stimulate the platelet when the Fc portion of the antibody interacts with the platelet's FcγRII receptor (FcR). Once activated, the platelets contribute to thrombosis. Additionally, the activated platelets secrete more PF4, which perpetuates the process.

only in retrospect, when the platelet count rises after the discontinuation of the suspected medication. Even then, the diagnosis is not conclusive unless thrombocytopenia recurs after rechallenging the patient with the offending drug (a practice that is almost never recommended).

TREATMENT

The best method for treating drug-induced thrombocytopenia is to stop all suspected offending medications.[5] Usually, no additional therapy is indicated. The thrombocytopenia typically begins to resolve without further intervention within days to a week of stopping the drug. The notable exceptions involve drugs with particularly long half-lives. Sulfonamides, quinine, and quinidine are notorious for inducing severe or even life-threatening thrombocytopenia. In patients with profound thrombocytopenia (<10,000/μL to 15,000/μL) or at a high risk for bleeding, platelet transfusions are indicated. When ITP cannot be confidently excluded and the thrombocytopenia is life-threatening, specific treatment for ITP can also be initiated (see later in this chapter).

HEPARIN-INDUCED THROMBOCYTOPENIA

EPIDEMIOLOGY

A special case of drug-induced immune-mediated thrombocytopenia associated with arterial and venous thrombosis, rather than bleeding, is heparin-induced thrombocytopenia (HIT).[6,7] It is seen in 2 to 5% of patients exposed to unfractionated heparin and in 0.7% of patients given low-molecular-weight heparin. HIT almost never occurs in patients who are exposed only to fondaparinux.

PATHOBIOLOGY

Platelets can secrete a protein called platelet factor 4 (PF4) that can bind to heparin. HIT is caused by an antibody that binds to this PF4-heparin complex (Fig. 158-3). Large complexes of antibodies directed against heparin-bound PF4 accumulate on the surface of platelets. At times, these anti-PF4 immunoglobulins bind to Fc receptors that are also present on the platelet surface, leading to activation of the platelet, release of more PF4, and a cycle of events that causes the stimulation of even more platelets. Ultimately, this also leads to the activation of the coagulation cascade, likely through exposure of tissue factor on the surface of activated macrophages. The activation of platelets and the clotting cascade results in the formation of both thrombi and thrombocytopenia.

CLINICAL MANIFESTATIONS AND DIAGNOSIS

Given the extensive use of heparin in hospitalized patients, HIT must always be considered when thrombocytopenia develops in this setting. However, patients with this syndrome often have multiple potential causes of thrombocytopenia, such as infections or other medications, so it is important to consider these other causes. Large retrospective studies of HIT have suggested that the onset of thrombocytopenia relative to the initiation of heparin therapy is useful in establishing or excluding this diagnosis. Immune-mediated HIT typically occurs 5 to 14 days after patients are given heparin by any route. HIT can even occur after subcutaneous injections of "minidose" heparin or following extremely low doses by heparin flush of intravenous lines. The 5- to 14-day lag between heparin exposure and the appearance of HIT is due to the time it takes for the immune response to generate the requisite antibodies against the heparin-PF4 complex. Some patients who have been exposed to heparin within the past several months may already have preexisting antibodies against the heparin-PF4 complex in their circulation. Therefore, when these patients are re-exposed to heparin, they may develop an acute onset of HIT even within the first day of the reinitiation of heparin. Whether or not pre-exposed to heparin, however, platelet-activating HIT antibodies are detectable at the onset of the HIT-related platelet count fall.

The unique timing of acute-onset HIT within hours of heparin re-exposure and the more typical development of HIT within 4 to 14 days of initial heparin exposure emphasize the importance of conducting a careful and critical history in establishing the diagnosis. HIT should be suspected in any patient who develops thrombocytopenia while on heparin therapy. Since the normal platelet count varies widely (140,000/μL to 450,000/μL), some patients may have a substantial decrease in their platelet count but still remain within the normal range. Therefore, a greater than 50% decrease in the platelet count of a patient on heparin should raise the suspicion of this syndrome. HIT should also be suspected in any patient who develops a thrombotic event while on heparin therapy. Some have used the 4 T scoring system to clinically assess the likelihood of HIT, as opposed to a different cause of thrombocytopenia. The 4 T score uses a combination of platelet count fall, timing of platelet count fall, coexisting occurrence of thrombosis, and other potential causes of thrombocytopenia to arrive at a clinical likelihood of HIT that is low probability, intermediate probability, or high probability.

Although antibodies against the heparin-PF4 complex are almost always present in patients with HIT, these antibodies are also frequently present in heparin-treated patients who do not have this disorder (i.e., those patients with neither thrombocytopenia nor thrombosis). There are two general categories of laboratory assays for the diagnosis of HIT: functional assays and immunologic assays (Table 158-4). Functional assays analyze whether the combination of heparin and the patient's plasma can induce normal platelets to aggregate or to secrete serotonin; these assays have very high specificity but relatively low sensitivity.[8] Immunologic assays test the patient's plasma for antibodies that bind to the heparin-PF4 complex; these assays have very high

TABLE 158-4 LABORATORY ASSAYS FOR HEPARIN-INDUCED THROMBOCYTOPENIA

ASSAY	SENSITIVITY (%)	SPECIFICITY (%)
Functional assay (e.g., serotonin release assay)	56-100%	>95%
PF4/heparin enzyme immunoassay (ELISA)	99%	30-70%

ELISA = enzyme-linked immunosorbent assay; PF4 = platelet factor 4.

sensitivity but lack specificity. Some studies show a good correlation between the amount of anti-PF4 antibodies present (such as determined by the optical density of an ELISA-based immunoassay) and the chance that the patient has clinically meaningful HIT. A *negative immunologic assay* is extremely useful in excluding this diagnosis, and a *positive functional assay* is useful in confirming the diagnosis of HIT. Several days may elapse before the test results are available. Therefore, in practice, these laboratory assays provide only confirmatory information. Urgent clinical decisions should *not* be deferred until such test results are available. The timing of the thrombocytopenia with respect to the heparin exposure and the degree of the platelet drop are the most important pieces of information needed by the physician when evaluating a patient suspected of having HIT.

Because platelets are consumed as they become activated, the clinical presentation of HIT is thrombocytopenia. However, it is unusual for the thrombocytopenia to actually cause bleeding in patients with HIT. Instead, HIT is a highly prothrombotic disorder. Both venous and arterial thromboses are common in HIT. Patients with HIT who do not have thrombosis on initial presentation still have a 20 to 30% chance of developing a thrombus within the next month. Nevertheless, the incidence of HIT-related clinical events is greatest immediately after diagnosis. More importantly, clinical studies report that the cessation of heparin alone frequently fails to prevent the development of new thrombotic events.

TREATMENT AND PREVENTION

If a patient is suspected of having HIT, all heparin should be stopped immediately. This includes subcutaneous injections of "minidose" heparin, heparin flushes of intravenous lines, and low-molecular-weight heparin; even heparin-coated intravenous catheters should be withdrawn. Alternative anticoagulation, such as the direct thrombin inhibitor argatroban, should be used (Chapter 70). Although not as well studied (nor FDA approved), both bivalirudin and fondaparinux appear to be viable alternatives. Accumulating evidence also suggests that the direct-acting oral anticoagulants (Table 70-6) can be used in patients with HIT,[9] using doses similar to what are used for the treatment of an acute venous thromboembolism but with a higher dose administered at the beginning of therapy (e.g., rivaroxaban 15 mg twice daily with food for 21 days then 20 mg with food once per day). Warfarin should not be used initially in cases of acute HIT because of its delayed therapeutic effect and its association with venous limb gangrene. However, when the platelet count has returned to a normal level as the acute episode of HIT starts to resolve, warfarin can be slowly introduced at a dose of 5 mg or less daily while an alternative anticoagulant such as argatroban is still being used. The warfarin dose can be gradually increased to achieve an international normalized ratio (INR) of 2 to 3. If the patient has had an acute thrombosis attributable to their HIT, they should be treated for a minimum of 3 months of anticoagulation. If the patient has thrombocytopenia but no thrombosis, anticoagulation is usually given for 4 to 6 weeks. Because patients rarely become profoundly thrombocytopenic as a result of HIT alone, platelet transfusions are typically not required and may actually precipitate thrombotic complications.

If low-molecular-weight heparin is used for prophylaxis instead of unfractionated heparin, the risk of HIT is much lower. However, low-molecular-weight heparins should never be used in the treatment of HIT because this drug can cross-react with the pathologic HIT antibodies.

CORONAVIRUS-2019

Coronavirus-2019 (COVID-19) infection (Chapters 335, 336, and 337) or vaccination against it can rarely result in immune thrombotic thrombocytopenia caused by platelet-activating antibodies against platelet factor 4.[10,11] The clinical manifestations are similar to autoimmune heparin-induced thrombocytopenia, with a predilection for venous thrombosis, pulmonary embolism, and cerebral venous sinus thrombosis.[12] The treatment is anticoagulation, but the precise best regimen is not currently known.

SEPSIS

Along with the exposure to certain drugs, bacterial and viral infections are among the most common causes of acute thrombocytopenia in hospitalized patients. Acute thrombocytopenia can be caused by the deposition of antibody-antigen complexes on the platelet surface through an "innocent bystander" phenomenon. These antibody-coated platelets are then cleared from the circulatory system by Fc receptor–expressing macrophages in the spleen. Thrombocytopenia associated with infections can also be due to DIC (as discussed in Chapter 161). It is notable that patients who are infected with severe acute respiratory syndrome coronavirus 2 (Chapter 334) usually have normal or elevated platelet counts despite having high D-dimer levels like patients with DIC. The treatment of sepsis-induced thrombocytopenia is directed at treating the underlying cause, along with the administration of platelet transfusions as clinically indicated.

IMMUNE THROMBOCYTOPENIC PURPURA

DEFINITION

ITP is an autoimmune disorder caused by circulating antiplatelet autoantibodies. An ITP-like picture can also be found in patients with autoimmune diseases, such as in systemic lupus erythematosus (Chapter 245); in low-grade lymphoproliferative disorders, such as chronic lymphocytic leukemia (Chapter 169); and in HIV infection (Chapter 359).

CLINICAL MANIFESTATIONS

ITP was classically thought to be a disease of young women. Although this description is appropriate for many individuals with this disorder, it is now appreciated that ITP can occur in patients of either sex and at any age. ITP is a chronic, recurring disorder in most adults, in stark contrast to pediatric patients, who usually suffer from acute ITP and much less frequently have chronic thrombocytopenia.

In contrast to patients with coagulation factor deficiencies who present with bleeding deep within their tissues, individuals with ITP (or other platelet disorders) typically have excessive mucocutaneous bleeding. Consequently, the clinician should inquire whether the patient has noticed epistaxis, gingival bleeding, easy bruising, hematuria, melena, or hematochezia. Female patients should also be asked about irregular or excessive vaginal bleeding. The physical examination should pay particular attention to signs of mucocutaneous bleeding. The patient should be thoroughly examined for petechiae (see Fig. 158-2) and ecchymosis as well as for evidence of hemorrhage within the conjunctiva, retina, and central nervous system.

DIAGNOSIS

In patients with ITP, the CBC is usually normal except for the thrombocytopenia, and their peripheral blood smear is remarkable only for a decreased number of platelets, some of which may be larger than normal. Splenomegaly is absent unless the ITP is due to an underlying disorder, such as lymphoma that is associated with splenomegaly. A bone marrow examination is usually not necessary in the absence of abnormalities other than thrombocytopenia on the CBC and peripheral blood smear. If performed, the bone marrow aspirate and biopsy of ITP patients typically show normal or increased numbers of megakaryocytes. However, the rest of their bone marrow is otherwise normal. These bone marrow findings are similar to what is observed in the bone marrows of patients who have other forms of destructive thrombocytopenia such as drug-induced thrombocytopenia. Antiplatelet antibody assays are neither sensitive nor specific and therefore should not be done. ITP must be distinguished from the rare syndrome of cyclic thrombocytopenia in which platelet counts spontaneously rebound, and bleeding, even at the nadir of the platelet count, tends to be mild.[13]

TREATMENT

First-Line Treatment

Initial management of ITP is guided by both symptoms and platelet count (Table 158-5).[14] Asymptomatic patients with platelet counts >30,000/μL can be followed without treatment.[15] If the patient is bleeding or has a platelet count <30,000/μL, either prednisone (1 mg/kg orally daily) or high-dose dexamethasone (4-day pulses of 40 mg intravenously per day every 28 days for several cycles) are both effective (Table 158-6), with a few trials showing better results with dexamethasone, and others (including the largest trial) showing no difference in long-term response rates.[A1] Oral prednisone has the advantage of allowing the dose to be titrated according to the platelet count. Although corticosteroids remain the first-line therapeutic modalities, mycophenolate mofetil under expert supervision is emerging as another first-line option.[A2]

TABLE 158-5 WHO SHOULD BE TREATED FOR IMMUNE THROMBOCYTOPENIC PURPURA (ITP)?

Guidelines for treatment of adult patients with ITP include the following recommendations:

1. Treatment should be administered to newly diagnosed patients if platelets are <30,000/μL.
2. First-line treatment should be a longer course of corticosteroids. IVIG should be used with corticosteroids when a more rapid increase in platelet count is required. Either IVIG or anti-D (where appropriate) should be used as first-line treatment if corticosteroids are contraindicated. If IVIG is used, the dose should be 1 g/kg once a day for 2 consecutive days.
3. Recommended second-line treatment in patients who are unresponsive to or relapse after the initial course of corticosteroids should be rituximab or a thrombopoietin receptor agonist. Splenectomy can be considered if treatment has been required for more than a year since it can produce lifelong responses in some patients.

IVIG = intravenous immunoglobulin.

TABLE 158-6 THERAPY FOR THE INITIAL MANAGEMENT OF IMMUNE THROMBOCYTOPENIC PURPURA

ORAL CORTICOSTEROIDS

The effect is dose dependent—approximately 80% of patients respond to 1 mg/kg/day. Toxicity also increases with the dose and duration of treatment, and side effects include glucose intolerance, immunosuppression, osteoporosis, and cataracts. Relapse is typical once therapy is tapered and discontinued. High-dose dexamethasone (40 mg/day for 4 days) has been reported to have a higher initial response rate and may be generally better tolerated than prednisone 1 mg/kg/day for 4 weeks followed by taper as initial first-line therapy.

INTRAVENOUS IMMUNOGLOBULIN

The effect is more rapid than daily prednisone. Administered at a dose of 1 g/kg/day for 2 consecutive days or 0.4 g/kg/day for 5 consecutive days. The response rates are approximately 80%, and the effects typically last 2 to 4 weeks. Toxicity includes headache, allergic reactions, and rarely, thrombosis.

ANTI-D IMMUNOGLOBULIN

It is administered at a dose of 50 to 75 μg/kg intravenously and should only be given to patients who have an Rh+ blood group. The response rates are dose dependent but can approach 75 to 80%. Hemolysis is a common toxicity but is usually mild. Rarely, hemolysis can be life threatening and can be associated with disseminated intravascular coagulation, renal failure, and end-organ infarction. It is generally ineffective in patients who have failed splenectomy.

TABLE 158-7 THERAPY FOR THE MANAGEMENT OF REFRACTORY IMMUNE THROMBOCYTOPENIC PURPURA

ORAL PREDNISONE

The effect is dose dependent and rapidly dissipates after discontinuation of the medication. Some patients can be maintained on a very low and tolerable daily dose (e.g., 5 mg). Long-term use is associated with infections, diabetes, osteoporosis, avascular necrosis, weight gain, and cataracts.

ORAL DEXAMETHASONE

This is administered at a dose of 40 mg/day for 4 consecutive days, repeated every 2 to 4 weeks for several months. Sustained response rates of 29 to 42% have been reported, although response rates are widely believed to be lower. Toxicity is similar to that of oral prednisone.

SPLENECTOMY

Durable (often lifelong) significant responses are seen in 65 to 70% of patients who undergo this procedure. More modest benefits are seen in another 10 to 15% of patients. There is no useful way to predict who will respond. Splenectomy is associated with surgical morbidity and some mortality (≈1-2%). Splenectomy produces lifelong immunosuppression to encapsulated and gram-positive organisms. Splenectomy is also associated with a small long-term risk of thrombosis.

RITUXIMAB

This is given at a dose of 375 mg/m^2/wk intravenously for a total of 4 weeks. Significant responses are seen in up to 60% of patients, and these responses typically last for months. Toxicity includes reactivation of hepatitis B, immunosuppression, and rarely, progressive multifocal leukoencephalopathy.

THROMBOPOIETIN RECEPTOR AGONISTS

These are administered daily (eltrombopag and avatrombopag) or weekly (romiplostim). An effect typically starts to be seen in 2 to 3 weeks and disappears shortly after the discontinuation of the medication. However, sustained, long-term effectiveness has been demonstrated while on the drug. Toxicity from long-term use is not well known but may include excessive thrombosis and bone marrow fibrosis.

Second-Line Treatment

Rituximab, a "humanized" murine monoclonal antibody against CD20 (a B-cell antigen), is widely used in patients who are unresponsive to first-line therapy. Complete response rates are seen in approximately 40% of patients, and meaningful response rate with platelet counts above 50,000/μL are seen in approximately 60% of patients. The combination of rituximab (375 mg/m^2 intravenously weekly for 4 weeks) plus dexamethasone (40 mg per day orally for 4 days) can induce higher response rates and longer time to relapse than dexamethasone alone.[16] However, the risk of grade 3 to 4 adverse events is increased when rituximab is combined with dexamethasone. Since the effect of rituximab usually requires 3 or more weeks, another therapy (such as corticosteroids) should be used initially if the patient is profoundly thrombocytopenic.

Peptides have been developed that bind to and activate the thrombopoietin (TPO) receptor; these agents are called TPO receptor agonists or thrombopoiesis stimulating agents. Because these recombinant drugs bear little structural similarity to native TPO, they do not trigger autoimmune anti-TPO antibodies. The FDA has approved two of these drugs, and several more are being used in other countries.

Romiplostim is a TPO receptor agonist composed of several copies of a receptor–binding peptide spliced into a recombinant antibody; it competes with endogenous TPO for binding to the TPO receptor and activates the receptor as would endogenous TPO.[A3] It is usually initiated at 2 to 3 μg/kg subcutaneously weekly, then slowly escalated to 10 μg/kg per week if needed. Eltrombopag[A4] and avatrombopag also activate the TPO receptor and improve thrombocytopenia and have the advantage of being administered orally. Eltrombopag is initiated at 50 mg orally daily (25 mg once daily in individuals with liver insufficiency or of East Asian ancestry), whereas avatrombopag is initiated at 20 mg orally per day. Subcutaneously administered romiplostim, orally administered eltrombopag, and orally administered avatrombopag are all capable of increasing platelet counts in approximately 70 to 90% of patients with ITP.[A5] Remarkably, these drugs can also increase the platelet counts of patients whose ITP is refractory to other treatment modalities, including splenectomy. However, adverse events, including bone marrow fibrosis and thromboembolism, have been reported. Unfortunately, these drugs' effects disappear soon after their discontinuation.

Fostamatinib, which is an oral inhibitor of Syk kinase (dosed at 100 mg twice daily, increasing to 150 mg twice daily if the platelet count remains below 50,000/mL after 4 weeks of therapy), can be useful in patients who have not responded to multiple other therapies.[A6] It results in a 40 to 45% initial response rate and 18% stable response rate with continuous therapy in previously treated patients with chronic immune thrombocytopenia. Side effects include diarrhea, nausea, hypertension, and neutropenia.[17]

Refractory ITP

Refractory patients may require immunosuppressive medications or splenectomy (Table 158-7). Immunosuppressive options include immunomodulating agents, such as intravenous immunoglobulin (IVIG), anti-Rh immunoglobulin (anti-D), cyclophosphamide, azathioprine, cyclosporine, mycophenolate mofetil, dapsone, interferon, and etanercept.[18]

Splenectomy can provide a durable complete response in approximately 66 to 70% of patients.[19,20] Approximately half of the remaining patients who do not have normal platelet counts following splenectomy achieve a partial response that is clinically meaningful. Unfortunately, 10 to 15% of patients derive no benefit from splenectomy. There is no test to predict whether a particular patient will respond to this treatment, although initial steroid responders and younger patients tend to have a better outcome. It should be noted that splenectomy is associated with small long-term risks of both infections and thrombosis (Chapter 154).

Patients who have ITP with severe thrombocytopenia (<5000/μL) or internal bleeding should be promptly treated with both high doses of pulse corticosteroids and IVIG. Platelet transfusions may be given concurrently with IVIG for critical bleeding.

THROMBOTIC THROMBOCYTOPENIC PURPURA

DEFINITION

Thrombotic thrombocytopenic purpura (TTP) is a consumptive thrombocytopenia associated with a mechanical hemolytic anemia.[21] The classic pentad of symptoms, which are thrombocytopenia, anemia, fever, neurologic problems, and renal abnormalities, are fully present in less than 10% of patients. Many patients today have only hemolytic anemia and thrombocytopenia. A good working definition for this diagnosis is thrombocytopenia along with a microangiopathic hemolytic anemia that is not associated with acute renal failure at presentation, disseminated intravascular coagulation, or another apparent cause. The poor specificity of the clinical features of this disease and the nonspecific laboratory abnormalities historically made TTP difficult to diagnose, but this has improved with the availability of ADAMTS13 testing. In the past, patients with untreated TTP had a mortality rate of 90% within 3 months. With modern therapy, patients with TTP have a mortality rate of approximately 10 to 20%.

PATHOBIOLOGY

Vascular endothelial cells normally secrete von Willebrand factor (vWF) (Chapter 159) that is composed of a large range of multimer sizes, including the so-called "ultralarge multimers." These latter forms bind to platelets very tightly even at low shear forces and therefore have the potential to create platelet aggregates in the circulation that might form microvascular occlusive thrombi, an undesirable result of vWF circulating with ultralarge multimers. However, a metalloproteinase identified as ADAMTS13 (*a d*isintegrin-like *a*nd *m*etalloprotease with *t*hrombo*s*pondin type 1 motif, member 13) is also normally present in blood and acts to cleave the ultralarge multimers of vWF, thereby preventing the formation of microvascular occlusions by platelet aggregates.[22] Most patients with adult-onset TTP have autoantibodies against ADAMTS13, thus causing an acquired deficiency of the enzyme and thereby permitting the circulation of thrombogenic ultralarge vWF multimers. Rare patients with inherited and recurrent TTP (Upshaw-Schulman syndrome) have a congenital deficiency of ADAMTS13.[23] Inherited or acquired ADAMTS13 deficiency causes the accumulation of ultralarge multimers of von Willebrand factor in plasma, which leads to platelet activation and the microvascular thrombosis that is characteristic of TTP (Fig. 158-4).

Characteristically, the thrombotic occlusions are in small terminal arterioles and capillaries and are composed mainly of platelets and von Willebrand factor within the damaged vascular lumen. In contrast to the pathology usually found in typical blood clots, the occlusions found in TTP patients contain very little fibrin and are referred to as hyaline thrombi.

Clinical assays of ADAMTS13 enzymatic activity are useful in diagnosing TTP. However, many patients can have a partial deficiency of ADAMTS13 without having TTP, so the absolute amount of deficiency is important. Levels of ADAMTS13 below 10% of normal are highly suggestive of TTP, while levels greater than 30% strongly argue against this diagnosis. Levels between 10 and 30% of normal are not very helpful.

Some patients reportedly developed TTP soon after taking an antiplatelet drug of the thienopyridine class. For example, clopidogrel can induce TTP, but the incidence is rare, about 1 in 250,000. Because the incidence of TTP in the general population is approximately 1 in 100,000, it is difficult to determine whether there is a significant risk for TTP in patients who are prescribed clopidogrel. The thienopyridine-derivative prasugrel has also been implicated in rarely causing TTP. Some patients have been diagnosed with TTP that was attributed to medications that directly injure the vascular endothelium (such as cyclosporine or tacrolimus). Most of these patients do not have TTP but have the related disorder HUS, discussed later in this chapter.

CLINICAL MANIFESTATIONS AND DIAGNOSIS

In TTP, patients can occasionally present with symptoms of excessive mucocutaneous bleeding, but they might also present with signs of a thrombotic event (including phlebitis, myocardial infarction, or stroke).[24] Abdominal pain is present in some patients, which is presumably due to intestinal ischemia. Signs of central nervous system disease, somnolence, and even coma can also be seen on presentation.

The two major hallmarks of TTP are microangiopathic hemolytic anemia and thrombocytopenia.[25] Microangiopathic hemolytic anemia is a non-immune-mediated hemolytic anemia caused by red cell fragmentation (Chapter 146). Patients with this disorder have typical laboratory findings of hemolytic anemia, including a high lactate dehydrogenase (LDH) level, elevated indirect bilirubin, low haptoglobin, and an increased reticulocyte count. Examination of the peripheral blood smear (Chapter 143) shows torn or fragmented red blood cells (schistocytes), and frequently also shows early red blood cell precursor cells (nucleated red blood cells). The thrombocytopenia may be mild if the disease is diagnosed at an early stage, but advanced cases of TTP can have platelet counts of less than 10,000/μL. Unlike most patients with typical thrombocytopenia, who tend to bleed excessively, patients with TTP have few hemorrhagic complications. Instead, they are markedly predisposed to thrombosis. In fact, a thrombotic complication in a thrombocytopenic patient is an important clue that TTP might be the cause of the thrombocytopenia (see Table 158-1). In the absence of plasmapheresis, TTP typically progresses and causes renal disease, neurologic symptoms, and fever. Since TTP now is often diagnosed in its early stages, patients usually only have microangiopathic hemolysis and thrombocytopenia.

TREATMENT

The prompt initiation of plasma exchange (plasmapheresis with plasma replacement) reduces the mortality rate associated with TTP from 90% to approximately 15%.[26] The mechanism of this benefit is partially due to the replacement of ADAMTS13. A randomized trial demonstrated that plasma exchange is more beneficial than plasma infusion for the treatment of TTP. This implies that some of the benefit of plasmapheresis is attributable to the removal of a pathologic substance from the patient's plasma. Assuming that the pathogenesis of most acquired forms of TTP is the antibody-mediated inhibition of ADAMTS13, plasma exchange has two benefits. First, it helps to remove the pathogenic antibody from the plasma. Second, the normal plasma infused into the patient during plasmapheresis repletes the deficiency of ADAMTS13.

Because patients with TTP can develop sudden thrombotic events (including stroke and myocardial infarction), and because patients can deteriorate quickly, it is prudent to initiate plasma exchange as rapidly as possible. Given the morbidity and mortality of untreated TTP, and given the relatively low risk of administering plasmapheresis, this therapy should be initiated even when

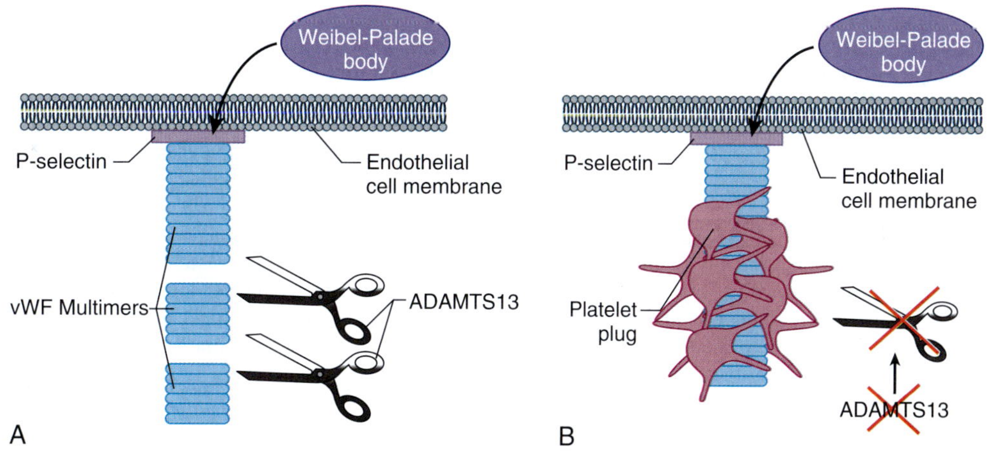

FIGURE 158-4. **Pathophysiology of thrombotic thrombocytopenia purpura (TTP). A, Von Willebrand factor (vWF) is synthesized in endothelial cells and stored in Weibel-Palade bodies. The vWF is assembled into ultralarge multimers that are cleaved after they are released into the blood stream by the protease ADAMTS13. The resultant smaller multimers of vWF only bind to platelets to participate in normal hemostasis. B, Most patients with TTP have severe deficiency of ADAMTS13 (less than 10% of normal). This results in the accumulation of ultralarge multimers of vWF within the circulation, which promote the excessive adhesion of platelets. The consequence is the formation of large plugs composed of vWF and platelets that can cause vascular occlusions.**

the diagnosis is not certain and without waiting for the results of ADAMTS13 testing. Plasmapheresis is not beneficial in children with Shiga toxin–induced HUS or in patients who develop HUS following their exposure to endothelium-toxic drugs, such as chemotherapy or calcineurin inhibitors (e.g., cyclosporine or tacrolimus).

Plasma exchange is administered to replace one entire plasma volume. An average-sized individual requires 20 to 30 units of fresh-frozen plasma for each plasmapheresis session. Therapy is usually administered daily, and patients are monitored for signs of improvement in their thrombocytopenia, hemolysis, neurologic symptoms, fever, and renal disease. Appropriate daily laboratory tests to monitor the patient are CBC, LDH, reticulocyte count, and creatinine. After the thrombocytopenia and hemolysis have been corrected for a few days, the daily plasmapheresis can either be discontinued or continued every other day for several more days. Most patients with TTP will start to respond within 3 to 5 days. A typical duration of therapy is 1 to 2 weeks, although some patients require treatment far beyond this usual time course.

A glucocorticoid is usually initiated at the start of treatment to decrease the production of anti-ADAMTS13 antibodies. Typically prednisone 1 mg/kg is administered daily, although some clinicians prefer to start with methylprednisolone 1000 mg daily for 3 days prior to starting prednisone.

Caplacizumab is an anti–von Willebrand factor, single-variable-domain immunoglobulin that inhibits the interaction between ultralarge von Willebrand factor multimers and platelets. Two randomized trials of patients with TTP showed that caplacizumab (10 mg subcutaneously daily) during plasma exchange and for 30 days afterward hastened resolution of the acute TTP episode and reduced the composite endpoint of TTP-related death, recurrent TTP, or a thromboembolic event.[A7,A8] Although caplacizumab can mildly shorten the number of days of plasma exchanges,[27] the very high cost of the drug has raised questions about its cost-effectiveness,[28] and suggests that it is best considered in patients who have neurologic or cardiac symptoms and in whom a very rapid response is needed to prevent impending catastrophic damage to these vital organs.

Additional immunosuppression with rituximab may be beneficial, but this drug does not decrease antibody production for weeks to months after its administration. If rituximab has any benefit in the treatment of TTP, it is probably only to minimize the incidence of late relapses.

Approximately one third to as many as one half of patients relapse after plasmapheresis is discontinued. These patients require a reinitiation of plasma exchange as well as administration of rituximab if this has not already been given.

Major complications of plasmapheresis do occur and are often attributable to the use of a central venous catheter. Hypotension, bacteremia, hemorrhage, and thrombosis are among the most common life-threatening complications of plasmapheresis therapy. Two specific complications deserve emphasis. First, patients taking an angiotensin-converting enzyme (ACE) inhibitor are susceptible to plasmapheresis-induced hypotension. This is due to these drugs' interference with bradykinin catabolism. Second, a patient who develops recurrent thrombocytopenia and a fever several days to a week into treatment may not be having an exacerbation of TTP, but rather may be developing central line–induced sepsis. Therefore, a vigorous investigation for infection should be initiated in patients who appear to be relapsing early.

HEMOLYTIC-UREMIC SYNDROME

DEFINITION

HUS is another cause of microangiopathic hemolytic anemia, and it may be difficult to distinguish from TTP.[29] When acute renal failure is predominant and there are no neurologic symptoms, many clinicians consider the syndrome to be HUS, not TTP. In contrast to TTP, HUS is not caused by a deficiency of ADAMTS13. Instead, HUS is probably caused by damage to endothelial cells leading to thrombosis in small blood vessels and fragmentation of red blood cells as they squeeze past the clots.

PATHOBIOLOGY AND CLINICAL MANIFESTATIONS

There are three major causes for HUS. The first, and most common, cause of HUS is a Shiga toxin–producing *E. coli* infection. This "typical" form of HUS occurs a few days after a bloody diarrhea syndrome induced by toxigenic *E. coli* (typically serotypes 157:H7 or O104:H4). The Shiga toxin binds to and damages glomerular endothelium, leading to localized thrombus formation, shearing of red cells, and kidney failure.

The next most common type of HUS is in patients who have inherited dysregulation of the alternative complement cascade (Chapter 37), now called complement-mediated (but formerly called atypical) HUS. The best-described genetic mutations cause a deficiency of factor H, which is a complement regulatory protease. HUS-inducing mutations in other components of complement regulation include those found in C3, factor B, CD46, and factor I. In complement-mediated HUS, complement is activated on endothelial cells. Frequently, an upper respiratory tract infection will precede the episode of microangiopathic hemolytic anemia. However, in contrast to typical HUS that is induced by an infection, the infection is only a trigger for complement-mediated HUS in a genetically susceptible host.

The least common variety of HUS is secondary HUS. This is usually caused by drugs or other medical conditions that directly or indirectly promote endothelial cell damage. Several drugs can also induce HUS by directly damaging the endothelial cells. These include calcineurin inhibitors, such as tacrolimus and cyclosporine; sometimes, lowering the dose of these drugs can reverse the microangiopathic hemolytic anemia. Cytotoxic drugs such as mitomycin C, cisplatin, and bleomycin can also induce HUS by directly damaging the endothelial cells. Secondary HUS can also be induced by a variety of autoimmune diseases, cancer, and pregnancy.

TREATMENT AND PREVENTION

Reducing the spread of Shiga toxin–producing *E. coli* is vital because antibiotics and antimotility drugs do not lower the risk for developing HUS symptoms. In contrast to TTP, there is little evidence that plasma exchange is beneficial in these cases. The clinical course and outcome of *E. coli* O104:H4–induced HUS are similar to infections with the more common O157:H7–induced HUS. Aggressive antibiotic therapy appears to be beneficial for reducing seizures and death. However, neither plasmapheresis nor glucocorticoids seem to be helpful for typical or secondary HUS. The infusion of plasma or plasmapheresis is uncertain in the treatment of the forms of HUS that are caused by the dysregulation of complement. Patients with complement-mediated HUS respond better to eculizumab or ravulizumab, which work by inhibiting the terminal complement cascade.

DISSEMINATED INTRAVASCULAR COAGULATION

Disseminated intravascular coagulation, which is a pathologic condition that depletes components of the coagulation system, including platelets, is discussed in detail in Chapter 161.

THROMBOCYTOPENIA DURING PREGNANCY

Thrombocytopenia occurs in approximately 10% of pregnant women.[30] It may be due to a normal variant of pregnancy (gestational thrombocytopenia), a pregnancy-specific condition (preeclampsia and HELLP [*h*emolysis, *el*evated *l*iver enzymes, and *l*ow *p*latelets]) syndrome, or a condition exacerbated by pregnancy (ITP, vasculitis, TTP). Thrombocytopenia occurs in approximately 7 to 10% of pregnancies, and about 75% of these cases are due to gestational thrombocytopenia, 15 to 20% are secondary to hypertensive disorders, 3 to 4% are due to an immune process, and the remaining 1 to 2% are rare constitutional thrombocytopenias, infections, and malignancies. The prognosis and treatment vary tremendously based on the underlying cause.

Gestational Thrombocytopenia

Gestational thrombocytopenia (incidental thrombocytopenia of pregnancy) is a mild, asymptomatic thrombocytopenia that typically occurs late in pregnancy. It occurs predominantly because of hemodilution from expanded plasma volume, although it is possible that there is also a component of increased platelet clearance. Gestational thrombocytopenia is not associated with fetal thrombocytopenia, and this form of maternal thrombocytopenia resolves spontaneously after delivery. Other than thrombocytopenia during previous pregnancies, women with gestational thrombocytopenia have no prior history of a low platelet count. This lack of previous thrombocytopenia helps to distinguish gestational thrombocytopenia from ITP. Additionally, in contrast to other causes of maternal thrombocytopenia, gestational thrombocytopenia does not occur before mid-second trimester, usually does not cause the platelet count to drop below 100,000/μL, and almost never causes a platelet count lower than 75,000/μL. Consequently, deviation from standard obstetric care is not required for a patient with gestational thrombocytopenia.

Preeclampsia

Preeclampsia causes proteinuria and hypertension during the later stages of pregnancy (Chapter 221). A minority of women with preeclampsia progress to have seizures; when this occurs, the syndrome is called *eclampsia*. Approximately 50% of women with preeclampsia have thrombocytopenia. Platelet counts are usually above 100,000/μL, and typically not less than 50,000/μL unless there is another coexisting reason. Some patients have an unusually severe form of preeclampsia called HELLP syndrome that is associated with a more significant thrombocytopenia, a microangiopathic hemolytic anemia, and markedly elevated liver function tests. Preeclampsia and HELLP syndrome are thought to result from a factor produced within the placenta because these syndromes usually resolve rapidly and spontaneously after delivery. However, the syndrome can also present postpartum. If these syndromes do not resolve spontaneously within 3 days, alternative diagnoses, such as ITP, TTP, or DIC should be considered. Consequently, immediate delivery of the child is recommended, if possible, because the microangiopathic process stops soon thereafter. If no improvement is seen by the third postpartum day and other causes, such as DIC, have been excluded, standard management for TTP, including plasma exchange, is recommended.

Immune Thrombocytopenia

ITP

Although a far less common cause of thrombocytopenia in a pregnant woman than gestational thrombocytopenia or preeclampsia, immune-mediated thrombocytopenia, particularly ITP, is the most common reason for a maternal platelet count less than 50,000/µL. Other than the magnitude of the thrombocytopenia, there is no laboratory test to differentiate ITP from gestational thrombocytopenia. Most patients with ITP or vasculitis during pregnancy have a history of thrombocytopenia before pregnancy. However, pregnancy can exacerbate or even unmask previously unrecognized autoimmune disorders like ITP. The antiplatelet IgG antibodies that cause ITP in the mother can cross the placenta and lead to thrombocytopenia in the fetus. Importantly, the platelet count in the unborn child does not correlate well with the platelet count of the mother, and attempts to sample fetal blood to monitor platelet counts are associated with significant risk.

Because most children born to women with ITP have a platelet count high enough for a successful delivery, the management of ITP focuses on keeping the maternal platelet count acceptable for the mother's safety. A platelet count above 30,000/µL is considered safe in the early stages of pregnancy and for vaginal delivery (although a platelet count above 80,000/µL is recommended for neuraxial anesthesia). A platelet count above 50,000/µL is acceptable for cesarean section. This can be managed by the use of oral glucocorticoids, and if necessary, by the administration of IVIG. Rituximab is not teratogenic but can cause prolonged lymphopenia in both the mother and the neonate. Although there are case reports of using romiplostim during pregnancy, the safety of thrombopoiesis-stimulating agents during pregnancy is not known. Splenectomy is rarely required and has a risk for inducing miscarriage when performed during the first trimester. This operation is also technically difficult during the later stages of pregnancy because of uterine enlargement.

TTP

The diagnosis of TTP during pregnancy can be difficult to make because many of the symptoms are identical to those of preeclampsia. If the symptoms develop during the early stages of pregnancy, when preeclampsia is unlikely, the diagnosis of TTP is more certain. The presence of hyperuricemia, hypoproteinemia, elevated liver transaminases, and direct bilirubin is more consistent with preeclampsia. The absence of elevated liver function abnormalities and the presence of a platelet count less than 20,000/µL or neurologic symptoms support the diagnosis of TTP. A very low (<10%) ADAMTS13 level also supports the diagnosis of TTP, but the results of this test might take some time.

POST-TRANSFUSION PURPURA AND NEONATAL ALLOIMMUNE THROMBOCYTOPENIA

Post-transfusion thrombocytopenia is due to the sensitization to platelet alloantigens, such as PlA1 (HPA-1a).[31] These alloimmune antibodies can cause profound thrombocytopenia approximately a week after a blood transfusion (post-transfusion purpura, or PTP). PTP is often induced by exposure to the small number of platelets that contaminate most red blood cell transfusions. It can be treated with IVIG or by plasma exchange. A similar alloimmune antibody produced by a pregnant woman can cause thrombocytopenia in her fetus (neonatal alloimmune thrombocytopenia, or NAIT). In this condition, the mother herself is not affected, but the neonate might have severe thrombocytopenia and bleeding. Neonatal alloimmune thrombocytopenia is treated with the transfusion of platelets derived from a PlA1-negative donor (most conveniently, the newborn's mother). Corticosteroids and IVIG have also been used.

VASCULITIS

Autoimmune diseases such as systemic lupus erythematosus (Chapter 245), rheumatoid arthritis (Chapter 243), and other forms of vasculitis can also cause thrombocytopenia. This cause is typically an ITP-like process that occurs in patients with a propensity for the development of autoantibodies. The treatment for these patients is immunosuppression, similar to the treatment for other patients with ITP. Some patients with active vasculitis and endothelial inflammation consume circulating platelets by promoting their adhesion to the damaged vessel wall. This creates a clinical picture that is difficult to distinguish from that of TTP without a tissue diagnosis that documents vasculitis or a very low (<10%) ADAMTS13 level. Because of the difficulty of discerning TTP from a flare-up of vasculitis, these patients are often treated with both plasma exchange and immunosuppression.

DILUTIONAL THROMBOCYTOPENIA

Thrombocytopenia does not typically occur after blood loss, possibly in part owing to the release of platelets from the splenic pool. Thrombocytopenia occasionally occurs after a massive hemorrhage. However, this is only when the hemorrhage is severe enough to necessitate the replacement of 1.5 to 2 times the total blood volume, which usually requires the transfusion of at least 15 to 20 units of packed red blood cells over a short period of time. Even in this circumstance, the thrombocytopenia is usually only mild to moderate. Therefore, the clinician should remain vigilant for another cause of the thrombocytopenia (such as DIC resulting from hemorrhage-induced hypotension and shock). When indicated, dilutional thrombocytopenia can be readily corrected with platelet transfusions.

CONGENITAL THROMBOCYTOPENIAS

Lifelong thrombocytopenia can be due to an inherited defect that affects platelet production or survival. Improved access to genetic testing has demonstrated that inherited thrombocytopenia is much more common than previously realized. Mutations in at least 32 genes can cause inherited thrombocytopenia. These disorders can be autosomal dominant (May-Hegglin anomaly and Sebastian syndrome), autosomal recessive (Bernard-Soulier disease, Fanconi anemia, gray platelet syndrome, thrombocytopenia with absent radius syndrome, and Paris Trousseau), or X-linked (Wiskott-Aldrich syndrome, GATA1-related, and FLNA-related). Many of these disorders are associated with other abnormalities in addition to thrombocytopenia such as kidney failure, cataracts, deafness, and predisposition to bone marrow failure or hematologic malignancies. A congenital cause of thrombocytopenia should be suspected in a patient who has long-standing moderate thrombocytopenia that was presumed to be treatment-refractory ITP. However, the majority of patients with chronic borderline thrombocytopenia and platelet counts greater than 100,000/µL continue to have stable platelet counts a decade later,[32] and many are likely to be outliers at the lower range of physiologic platelet counts.

GENERAL REFERENCES

For the General References and other additional features, please visit Elsevier eBooks+ at https://ebooks.health.elsevier.com.

Grade A References

A1. Mithoowani S, Gregory-Miller K, Goy J, et al. High-dose dexamethasone compared with prednisone for previously untreated primary immune thrombocytopenia: a systematic review and meta-analysis. *Lancet Haematol.* 2016;3:e489-e496.

A2. Bradbury CA, Pell J, Hill Q, et al. Mycophenolate mofetil for first-line treatment of immune thrombocytopenia. *N Engl J Med.* 2021;385:885-895.

A3. Yang R, Lin L, Yao H, et al. Therapeutic options for adult patients with previously treated immune thrombocytopenia: a systematic review and network meta-analysis. *Hematology.* 2019;24:290-299.

A4. Elgebaly AS, Ashal GE, Elfil M, et al. Tolerability and efficacy of eltrombopag in chronic immune thrombocytopenia: meta-analysis of randomized controlled trials. *Clin Appl Thromb Hemost.* 2017;23:928-937.

A5. Zhang J, Liang Y, Ai Y, et al. Eltrombopag versus romiplostim in treatment of adult patients with immune thrombocytopenia: a systematic review incorporating an indirect-comparison meta-analysis. *PLoS ONE.* 2018;13:e0198504.

A6. Bussel J, Arnold DM, Grossbard E, et al. Fostamatinib for the treatment of adult persistent and chronic immune thrombocytopenia: results of two phase 3, randomized, placebo-controlled trials. *Am J Hematol.* 2018;93:921-930.

A7. Peyvandi F, Scully M, Kremer Hovinga JA, et al. Caplacizumab for acquired thrombotic thrombocytopenic purpura. *N Engl J Med.* 2016;374:511-522.

A8. Scully M, Cataland SR, Peyvandi F, et al. Caplacizumab treatment for acquired thrombotic thrombocytopenic purpura. *N Engl J Med.* 2019;380:335-346.

159

VON WILLEBRAND DISEASE AND HEMORRHAGIC ABNORMALITIES OF PLATELET AND VASCULAR FUNCTION

JORGE DI PAOLA AND JAMES S. O'DONNELL

VON WILLEBRAND DISEASE

DEFINITION AND EPIDEMIOLOGY

Von Willebrand disease, which is the most common inherited bleeding disorder, is caused by quantitative or qualitative reductions in plasma von Willebrand factor (VWF). Significant bleeding symptoms due to reduced levels of von Willebrand factor are present in approximately 1 in 1000 individuals, with a prevalence that appears to be relatively consistent across different races and ethnicities. Importantly, however, population studies have demonstrated that not all people with reduced plasma levels of von Willebrand factor have clinically relevant bleeding, and the true prevalence of asymptomatic von Willebrand disease is less certain.

PATHOBIOLOGY

The human *VWF* gene consists of 52 exons and spans 178 kb on chromosome 12. Von Willebrand factor is a large multimeric plasma glycoprotein that plays two essential roles in normal hemostasis. First, it mediates platelet adhesion to exposed subendothelial tissues at sites of vascular injury. Second, von Willebrand factor acts as a carrier molecule for procoagulant factor VIII, thereby protecting it from premature proteolytic degradation and clearance. Von Willebrand factor and factor VIII circulate together in a noncovalent complex in normal plasma. In vivo, expression of von Willebrand factor is limited to endothelial cells and megakaryocytes. Von Willebrand factor that is synthesized within megakaryocytes is subsequently stored within the α-granules of their platelet progeny. This platelet von Willebrand factor accounts for 10 to 20% of the total amount that is present in normal platelet-rich plasma. In contrast, von Willebrand factor that is synthesized within endothelial cells is either released directly into the plasma through a constitutive secretory pathway or stored in dedicated organelles known as Weibel-Palade bodies. Consequently, under normal steady-state conditions, plasma von Willebrand factor is derived chiefly from endothelial cells. Regulated secretion of von Willebrand factor from its stores within Weibel-Palade bodies can be triggered by a variety of different secretagogues including histamine, thrombin, and desmopressin (DDAVP [1-desamino-8-D-arginine vasopressin]). Similarly, von Willebrand factor is secreted from α-granules following platelet activation.

Within endothelial cells, von Willebrand factor undergoes complex post-translational modification prior to its secretion into the plasma. In the endoplasmic reticulum, individual monomers of von Willebrand factor are assembled into dimers through the formation of C-terminal disulphide bonds. Subsequently, von Willebrand factor dimers form high-molecular-weight multimers in the Golgi after another round of N-terminal disulphide bond formation. As a result, von Willebrand factor circulates in the form of heterogeneous multimers that contain a variable number of subunits, ranging from a minimum of 2 to a maximum of 100. The largest multimers have molecular weights in excess of 20,000 Kd. Multimeric composition is a critical determinant of von Willebrand factor's functional activity. High-molecular-weight multimers bind both collagen and platelets with higher affinities, and they are more efficient in inducing platelet aggregation under high-shear conditions. In normal plasma, the multimeric composition of circulating von Willebrand factor is tightly regulated by a specific cleaving metalloprotease termed ADAMTS13 (a disintegrin and metalloproteinase with a thrombospondin type 1 motif, member 13).[1]

To facilitate platelet-plug formation at sites of vascular injury, von Willebrand factor also must be able to bind to exposed subendothelial collagen. Specific domains of von Willebrand factor interact with different types of collagen. For example, the A3 domain binds to collagen types I and III, whereas the principal binding site for types IV and VI collagen is located within the A1 domain.

In the normal population, plasma levels of von Willebrand factor typically vary between 50 to 150 IU/dL, and von Willebrand disease is classified into three distinct subtypes (Table 159-1). Type 1 von Willebrand disease is characterized by a partial quantitative deficiency in plasma levels of von Willebrand factor (<50 IU/dL) and accounts for the majority (about 75%) of cases. Type 2 von Willebrand disease includes patients who have qualitative disorders that impair one or more aspects of von Willebrand factor's normal functional activity. In these patients, the total amount of von Willebrand factor antigen (VWF:Ag) in the plasma may be normal or slightly reduced. In contrast, however, functional assays of von Willebrand factor are significantly reduced. Type 2 von Willebrand disease accounts for about 25% of cases and is further subdivided (type 2A, 2B, 2M, and 2N respectively) based upon the nature of the underlying qualitative defect of von Willebrand factor (Table 159-1). Type 3 von Willebrand disease is a rare (1 per million; about 1% of cases) and severe bleeding disorder characterized by near-complete deficiency in plasma von Willebrand factor.[2]

CLINICAL MANIFESTATIONS

Bleeding symptoms in patients with von Willebrand disease vary depending upon the residual levels of plasma VWF activity levels and the disease subtype. Patients typically present with mucocutaneous bleeding including epistaxis, gum bleeding, easy bruising, and bleeding from minor wounds. Recurrent gastrointestinal bleeding is a common presentation, particularly in patients with types 2 or 3 von Willebrand disease.[3]

Although von Willebrand disease is inherited in an autosomal manner, clinical disease is more prevalent in females because they face greater hemostatic challenges. For example, heavy menstrual bleeding occurs in up to 80% of women with von Willebrand disease and is often associated with iron deficiency (Chapter 145). Furthermore, undiagnosed von Willebrand disease is common (about 15% of cases) in women who present for investigation of

TABLE 159-1 CLASSIFICATION AND DIAGNOSIS OF VON WILLEBRAND DISEASE

TYPE VWD	DESCRIPTION	FVIII	RCo	VWF	RCo:VWF RATIO	MULTIMERS	SPECIAL TESTING
Normal range		50-150%	50-200%	50-200%	>0.7	Normal	
Type 1	Quantitative deficiency	↓ or N	<30%	<30%	>0.7	Normal distribution; decreased quantity	VWF propeptide:VWF ratio >0.6 in type 1 C; exon 28 DNA testing
Type 2A	Qualitative VWF defect	↓ or N	↓	N to ↓	<0.7	Loss of HMW forms	Exon 28 DNA testing
Type 2B	Qualitative gain of function; depletes HMW multimers	↓ or N	↓	N to ↓	<0.7	Loss of HMW forms	↑ RIPA low doses; exon 28 DNA testing
Type 2M	Qualitative defect	↓ or N	↓	N to ↓	<0.7	Normal	↓ CB
Type 2N	Qualitative defect only in FVIII binding	↓↓	N	N	>0.7	Normal	↓ VWF:FVIII binding study
Type 3	Near absence of VWF	↓↓	<3%	<3%	NA	None	
"Low VWF"	Borderline values	N	30-50%	30-50%	>0.7	Normal	

Typical or classical laboratory findings are described for each diagnosis. Expert interpretation is often required for patients without classical findings.
CB = collagen binding activity for VWF function; FVIII = factor VIII activity; HMW = high-molecular-weight; N = normal; Plt-VWD = platelet-type von Willebrand disease; RCo = ristocetin cofactor activity for VWF function; RIPA = ristocetin-induced platelet aggregation; VWF = von Willebrand factor antigen; ↑ = increased; ↓ = decreased value, with more arrows reflecting greater extent of decrease.
Data from Leebeek FWG, Eikenboom JCJ. Von Willebrand's disease. *N Engl J Med.* 2016;375:2067-80.

unexplained heavy menstrual bleeding. Significant bleeding can also occur in von Willebrand disease patients after hemostatic challenges, including dental extractions or surgical procedures.[4] Although plasma levels of von Willebrand factor progressively increase during pregnancy, women with von Willebrand disease have increased rates of both primary and secondary postpartum hemorrhage. Patients with type 3 von Willebrand disease have markedly reduced plasma factor VIII levels and present with recurrent spontaneous bleeding into joints. As in patients with severe hemophilia (Chapter 160), they can ultimately develop progressive arthropathy.

DIAGNOSIS

Clinical Assessment

A complete medical history and clinical examination are important in patients who undergo investigation for a possible bleeding tendency (Fig. 159-1). This history should include any family bleeding tendency or consanguinity, as well as a comprehensive list of current medications and health supplements. Clinical examination may demonstrate evidence of bleeding such as petechiae, ecchymosis, or hematomas. Signs of collagen vascular disorders (including skin laxity, joint hypermobility, joint dislocations, delayed wound healing) should be investigated. Any signs suggesting other inherited or acquired causes of bleeding disorders (e.g., senile purpura hereditary hemorrhagic telangiectasia, Cushing syndrome [Chapter 208], scurvy [Chapter 199], liver disease [Chapter 161], amyloidosis [Chapter 174], hypothyroidism [Chapter 207], paraproteinemia [Chapter 173], and myeloproliferative disorders) should be noted.

In clinical practice, the diagnosis of von Willebrand disease is based upon a bleeding phenotype combined with abnormal laboratory testing, sometimes aided by a family history. Investigation begins with an objective assessment of bleeding history (Fig. 159-1), which is best achieved using a standardized bleeding assessment tool (Table 159-2) to evaluate bleeding symptoms across different domains. Normal bleeding scores are less than 4 in males and less than 6 in females, so laboratory testing for von Willebrand disease and other bleeding disorders is indicated in males who score 4 or more or females who score 6 or more.[5]

Laboratory Evaluation

The prothrombin time (PT) and activated partial thromboplastin time (APTT) may be normal in patients with von Willebrand disease. Initial laboratory testing should also include measurement of plasma levels of von Willebrand factor antigen.[6] In view of the variability in plasma levels of von Willebrand factor, assays should be repeated on two separate occasions several weeks apart. Undetectable plasma levels of von Willebrand factor antigen (typically <3 IU/dL) are consistent with a diagnosis of type 3 von Willebrand disease, whereas partial quantitative deficiency (levels of 3 to 50 IU/dL) are diagnostic of type 1 von Willebrand disease (Fig. 159-1).[7] Since von Willebrand disease can be quantitative or qualitative in nature, laboratory testing must also include assessment of the various functional activities of von Willebrand factor (interactions with platelet GpIbα, collagen, and factor VIII). The von Willebrand factor ristocetin cofactor activity assay traditionally has been the gold standard test of von Willebrand factor function, but platelet-dependent von Willebrand factor activity is better measured by assays of von Willebrand factor glycoprotein 1b recombinant and von Willebrand factor glycoprotein 1b mutant. Commercial assays (typically containing types I and/or III collagen) can measure the binding of von Willebrand factor to collagen. Testing for the binding of von Willebrand factor to collagen types IV and VI has mainly been limited to research laboratories.

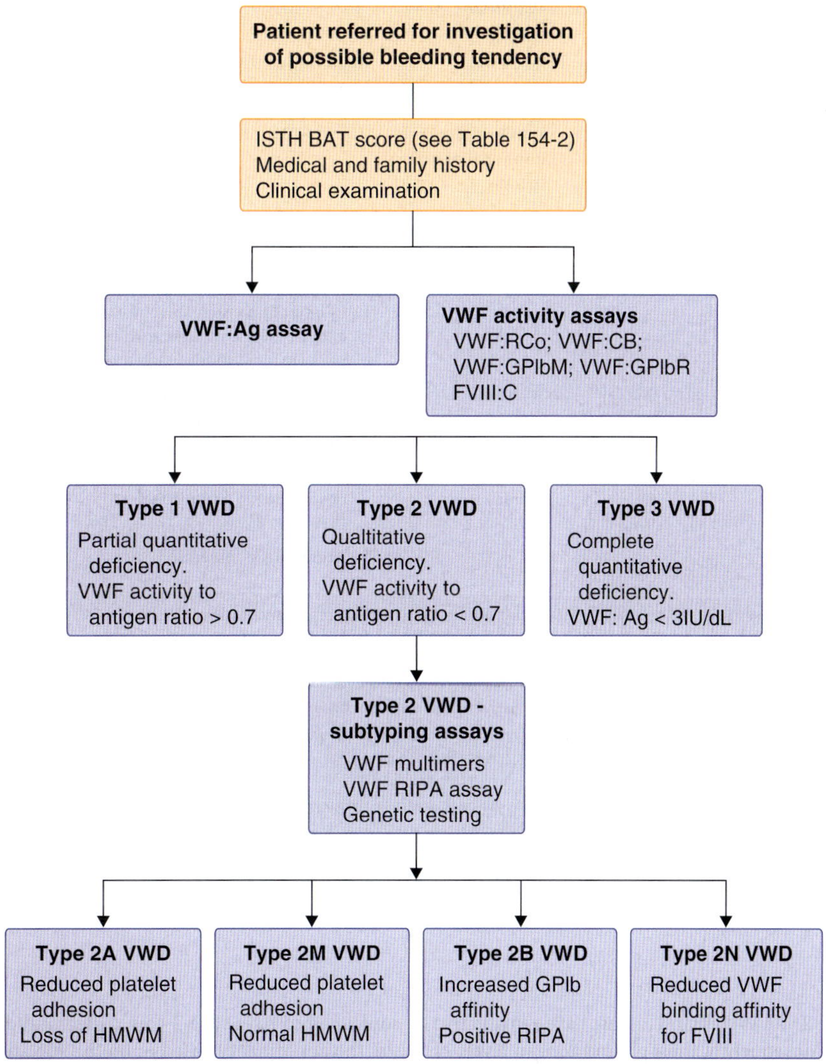

FIGURE 159-1. **Diagnostic algorithm for von Willebrand disease.** FVIII = factor VIII; FVIII:C = factor VIII procoagulant activity; HMWM = high-molecular-weight multimers; ISTH BAT = International Society on Thrombosis and Haemostasis Bleeding Assessment Tool; RIPA = ristocetin-induced platelet aggregation; VWD = von Willebrand disease; VWF = von Willebrand factor; VWF:Ag = von Willebrand factor antigen; VWF:CB = von Willebrand factor collagen binding; VWF:GPIbM = von Willebrand factor glycoprotein 1b mutant; VWF:GPIbR = von Willebrand factor glycoprotein 1b recombinant; VWF:RCo = von Willebrand factor ristocetin cofactor.

TABLE 159-2 INTERNATIONAL SOCIETY ON THROMBOSIS AND HAEMOSTASIS—SCIENTIFIC AND STANDARDIZATION COMMITTEE BLEEDING ASSESSMENT TOOL

	SCORE				
SYMPTOMS (UP TO THE TIME OF DIAGNOSIS)	**0***	**1***	**2**	**3**	**4**
Epistaxis	No/trivial	≥5/year or >10 minutes	Consultation only†	Packing or cauterization or antifibrinolytic	Blood transfusion or replacement therapy (use of hemostatic blood components and recombinant factor VIIa) or desmopressin
Cutaneous	No/trivial	For bruises 5 or more (>1 cm) in exposed areas	Consultation only†	Extensive	Spontaneous hematoma requiring blood transfusion
Bleeding from minor wounds	No/trivial	≥5/year or >10 minutes	Consultation only†	Surgical hemostasis	Blood transfusion, replacement therapy, or desmopressin
Oral cavity	No/trivial	Present	Consultation only†	Surgical hemostasis or antifibrinolytic	Blood transfusion, replacement therapy, or desmopressin
Gastrointestinal bleeding	No/trivial	Present and not associated with ulcer, portal hypertension, hemorrhoids, or angiodysplasia	Consultation only†	Surgical hemostasis or antifibrinolytic	Blood transfusion, replacement therapy, or desmopressin
Hematuria	No/trivial	Macroscopic	Consultation only†	Surgical hemostasis or iron therapy	Blood transfusion, replacement therapy, or desmopressin
Tooth extraction	No/trivial or never performed	Reported in ≤25% of all procedures, no intervention‡	Reported in ≥25% of all procedures, no intervention‡	Resuturing or packing	Blood transfusion, replacement therapy, or desmopressin
Surgery	No/trivial or never performed	Reported in ≤25% of all procedures, no intervention‡	Reported in ≥25% of all procedures, no intervention‡	Resuturing or packing	Blood transfusion, replacement therapy, or desmopressin
Menorrhagia	No/trivial	Consultation only† or Changing pads more frequently than every 2 hours or Clot and flooding	Time off work/school >2/year or Requiring antifibrinolytics or hormonal or iron therapy	Requiring combined treatment with antifibronlytics and hormonal therapy or present since menarche and >12 months	Acute menorrhagia requiring hospital admission and emergency treatment, requiring blood transfusion, replacement therapy, or desmopressin; or requiring dilatation and curettage or endometrial ablation or hysterectomy
Postpartum hemorrhage	No/trivial or no deliveries	Consultation only† or use of syntocin or lochia >6 weeks	Iron therapy or antifibrinolytics	Requiring blood transfusion, replacement therapy, or desmopressin; or requiring examination under anesthesia and/or the use of uterine balloon/package to tamponade the uterus	Any procedure requiring critical care or surgical intervention (e.g., hysterectomy, internal iliac artery legation, uterine artery embolization, uterine brace sutures)
Muscle hematomas	Never	Post-trauma, no therapy	Spontaneous, no therapy	Spontaneous or traumatic, requiring desmopressin or replacement therapy	Spontaneous or traumatic, requiring surgical intervention or blood transfusion
Hemarthrosis	Never	Post-trauma, no therapy	Spontaneous, no therapy	Spontaneous or traumatic, requiring desmopressin or replacement therapy	Spontaneous or traumatic, requiring surgical intervention or blood transfusion
Central nervous system bleeding	Never			Subdural, any intervention	Intracerebral, any intervention
Other bleeding§	No/trivial	Present	Consultation only†	Surgical hemostasis or antifibrinolytics	Blood transfusion, replacement therapy, or desmopressin
SCORE					

*Distinction between 0 and 1 is of critical importance. Score 1 means that the symptom is judged as present in the patient's history by the interviewer but does not qualify for a score 2 or more.

†Consultation only: the patient sought medical evaluation and was either referred to a specialist or offered detailed laboratory investigation.

‡Example: one extraction/surgery resulting in bleeding (100%): the score to be assigned is 2; two extractions/surgeries, one resulting in bleeding (50%): the score to be assigned is 2; three extractions/surgeries, one resulting in bleeding (33%): the score to be assigned is 2; four extractions/surgeries, one resulting in bleeding (25%): the score to be assigned is 1.

§Includes umbilical stump bleeding, cephalohematoma, cheek hematoma caused by sucking during breast/bottle feeding, conjunctival hemorrhage or excessive bleeding following circumcision or venipuncture. Their presence in infancy requires detailed investigation independently from the overall score.

From Rodeghiero F, Tosetto A, Abshire T, et al. ISTH/SSC bleeding assessment tool: a standardized questionnaire and a proposal for a new bleeding score for inherited bleeding disorders. *J Thromb Haemost.* 2010;8:2063-2065; Elbatarny M, Mollah S, Grabell J, et al. Normal range of bleeding scores for the ISTH-BAT adult aoject. *Haemophilia.* 2014;20:831-835; and isth-ssc_bleeding_assessment.pdf

By definition, patients with type 2 von Willebrand disease have a qualitative defect in von Willebrand factor. Consequently, their plasma antigen levels of von Willebrand factor are typically normal or only mildly reduced. However, a marked reduction in one or more aspects of the functional activity of von Willebrand factor results in an activity to antigen ratio below 0.7. In patients confirmed to have type 2 von Willebrand disease, the next step is to subclassify the abnormality based upon the specific nature of their qualitative defect using additional laboratory assays, including von Willebrand factor multimer analysis and the ristocetin-induced platelet aggregation assays (Fig. 159-1). Type 2A von Willebrand disease includes qualitative variants with reduced platelet adhesion and loss of high-molecular-weight multimers. In contrast, type 2M von Willebrand disease incorporates variants that have reduced platelet adhesion not caused by loss of high molecular multimers. Type 2B von Willebrand disease involves variants in which gain-of-function mutations lead to increased affinity for platelet GpIbα. Consequently, patients with type 2B von Willebrand disease can have fluctuating thrombocytopenia. Finally, type 2N von Willebrand disease is characterized by qualitative variants with decreased affinity for factor VIII.

Guidelines also recommend genetic testing for the diagnosis and subclassification of patients with type 2 von Willebrand disease, especially to distinguish type 2N from mild hemophilia A. Molecular analysis may also be useful for counseling and prenatal diagnosis in families with type 3 von Willebrand disease. In contrast, the utility of genetic testing in patients with type 1 von Willebrand disease remains unclear, because a variety of different sequence variants have been described spanning the *VWF* gene (https://databases.lovd.nl/shared/genes/VWF).

TREATMENT

Where possible, patients with von Willebrand disease should be managed in comprehensive referral centers with a multidisciplinary team that is experienced in treating patients who have bleeding disorders.[8] For elective procedures or bleeding complications, individualized treatment plans should be developed under expert oversight based on both patient- and procedure-related factors (Table 159-3). Patient-related factors to consider include the type of von Willebrand disease and the nadir levels of plasma von Willebrand factor antigen, von Willebrand factor activity, and factor VIII. Plasma levels of von Willebrand factor and factor VIII increase with aging in many patients with type 1 von Willebrand disease and may sometimes correct into the normal range, but even such levels may not result in a complete correction of the bleeding phenotype. Although the Bleeding Assessment Tool score can provide objective data on previous bleeding, it is less useful in patients who have had limited prior exposure to hemostatic challenges.

Tranexamic Acid

Tranexamic acid, which is a fibrinolytic inhibitor that is widely used in the treatment of von Willebrand disease, can be administered orally (typical dose 15 to 25 mg/kg three times daily) or intravenously (typical dose 15 mg/kg three times daily).[9] Even in high-risk populations (e.g., trauma, postpartum hemorrhage, major orthopedic surgery), tranexamic acid is associated with minimal thrombotic risk. However, tranexamic acid is usually avoided in patients with significant hematuria because it has been associated with clot retention and urinary obstruction.

DDAVP

DDAVP, which is a synthetic analog of L-arginine vasopressin, induces secretion of von Willebrand factor from Weibel-Palade body stores within endothelial cells and thereby can be used to elevate plasma levels of von Willebrand factor transiently. It can be administered intravenously (typical dose 0.3 μg/kg in 100 mL of normal saline infused over 20 minutes, maximum dose 25 to 30 μg) or can be given intranasally (300 μg total dose or 150 μg per nostril for persons >50 kg body weight). DDAVP is widely used in the treatment of type 1 von Willebrand disease and may also be useful in some patients with types 2A and 2M von Willebrand disease. However, it is generally avoided in type 2B von Willebrand disease, in which it can trigger significant thrombocytopenia, and it is not useful in patients with type 3 von Willebrand disease. Importantly, the increases in plasma levels of von Willebrand factor following DDAVP treatment vary significantly among individual patients with von Willebrand disease, so a DDAVP trial should be performed in each patient to define their individual response. Plasma levels of von Willebrand factor and factor VIII should be measured at 30 minutes and 4 hours post-DDAVP to assess both peak levels and the duration of the response. For acute bleeding or surgical procedures, DDAVP can be repeated every 12 to 24 hours, but tachyphylaxis can diminish the rise in the von Willebrand factor level following repeated treatments. DDAVP can cause fluid retention with secondary hyponatremia and seizures, so fluid restriction (1500 mL over 24 hours) is commonly instituted following DDAVP therapy. Plasma sodium levels should also be measured prior to any repeat dosing. DDAVP is generally avoided in elderly patients who have cardiovascular risk factors.

Plasma-Derived Concentrates of von Willebrand Factor

A number of different plasma-derived concentrates containing von Willebrand factor are licensed for use in patients whose von Willebrand disease fails to respond to DDAVP or who have contraindications to it.[10] In normal individuals, von Willebrand factor has a plasma half-life of approximately 12 to 16 hours, so treatment with DDAVP or plasma-derived von Willebrand factor concentrates can generally be administered once daily to prevent perioperative bleeding or to treat patients who present with acute bleeding. Current guidelines recommend that plasma activity levels of von Willebrand factor and factor VIII should be maintained at ≥50 IU/dL for at least 3 days after surgical procedures. Repeated infusions of factor VIII–containing von Willebrand factor concentrates have been associated with elevated levels of plasma factor VIII procoagulant activity and rare cases of thrombosis.

Recombinant von Willebrand Factor

Recombinant human von Willebrand factor (rVWF) concentrate, which differs from plasma-derived von Willebrand factor concentrates in that it is enriched in high-molecular-weight multimers and does not contain significant amounts of factor VIII, is highly effective.[A1] However, co-infusion of recombinant factor VIII may be necessary with the first dose of recombinant von Willebrand factor to ensure immediate hemostatic factor VIII levels are achieved. In the absence of concurrent recombinant factor VIII infusion, 6 hours may be required following the infusion of recombinant von Willebrand factor before plasma factor VIII procoagulant activity levels rise to above 40 IU/dL in patients with type 3 von Willebrand disease.

Platelet Transfusion

About 10 to 20% of von Willebrand factor is stored within platelet α-granules. Anecdotal reports suggest that platelet transfusion may be a useful adjunctive therapy in managing resistant bleeding in patients who have von Willebrand disease.

Von Willebrand Disease Management Strategies

Routine prophylaxis with von Willebrand factor usually is not required, except in patients who have severe disease or recurrent gastrointestinal bleeding.[11] Episodic treatment is key at the time of bleeding and prior to procedures that typically precipitate bleeding (Fig. 159-2). Prior to surgery, DDAVP or a von Willebrand factor concentrate should be infused.[12] Plasma von Willebrand factor activity and factor VIII procoagulant activity levels should then be assessed to ensure hemostatic levels have been achieved (≥ 50 IU/dL for minor procedures and ≈100 IU/dL for major surgery; Table 159-2). In addition, tranexamic acid should be commenced preoperatively and continued during the postoperative period. Following major surgery, trough levels of von Willebrand factor activity and factor VIII procoagulant activity levels should be repeated on a daily basis, with additional DDAVP or von Willebrand factor concentrate administered daily to maintain trough levels ≥50 IU/dL for at least 5 to 10 days (Table 159-2).[13,14]

TABLE 159-3 VON WILLEBRAND FACTOR REPLACEMENT GUIDELINES FOR BLEEDING/PROCEDURES

PROCEDURES/BLEEDING EVENTS DURATION	DOSING RECOMMENDATIONS
Major surgery: 7-14 days Cardiothoracic Cesarean section Craniotomy/Spinal cord Abdominal Prostatectomy	Initial dose: 40-60 RCo units/kg Maintenance doses: 20-40 RCo units/kg every 8-24 hr Monitor: FVIII and RCo trough and peak daily Targets: troughs >50%; peaks <200% RCo, <250% FVIII In responsive patients; may use desmopressin later in treatment
Minor surgery: 1-5 days Biopsies Complex dental extractions Gingival surgery Indwelling catheter placement Laparoscopies	Initial dose: 30-60 RCo units/kg Maintenance doses: 20-40 RCo units/kg every 12-48 hr Monitor: RCo and FVIII Targets: troughs >50%; peaks <200% RCo, <250% FVIII In responsive patients; may use desmopressin later in treatment Antifibrinolytic agent for 7-10 days is useful adjunct for dental procedures
Other procedures: one dose Cardiac catheterization Endoscopy with or without biopsies Liver biopsy Lacerations Simple dental extractions	Dose: 20-40 RCo units/kg Rare need for subsequent doses with multiple endoscopic biopsies Monitor: typically not done/required Desmopressin may suffice in very responsive patients Antifibrinolytic agent for 7-10 days useful adjunct for dental procedures

FVIII = factor VIII; RCo = ristocetin cofactor activity for von Willebrand factor function.
Adapted from Neff AT, Sidonio RF Jr. Management of VWD *Hematology Am Soc Educ Program*. 2014;1:536-541. From: Neff AT. Von Willebrand disease and hemorrhagic abnormalities of platelet and vascular function. In: Goldman L, Schafer AI. *Goldman-Cecil Medicine*. 26th ed. Elsevier; Philadelphia: 2020.

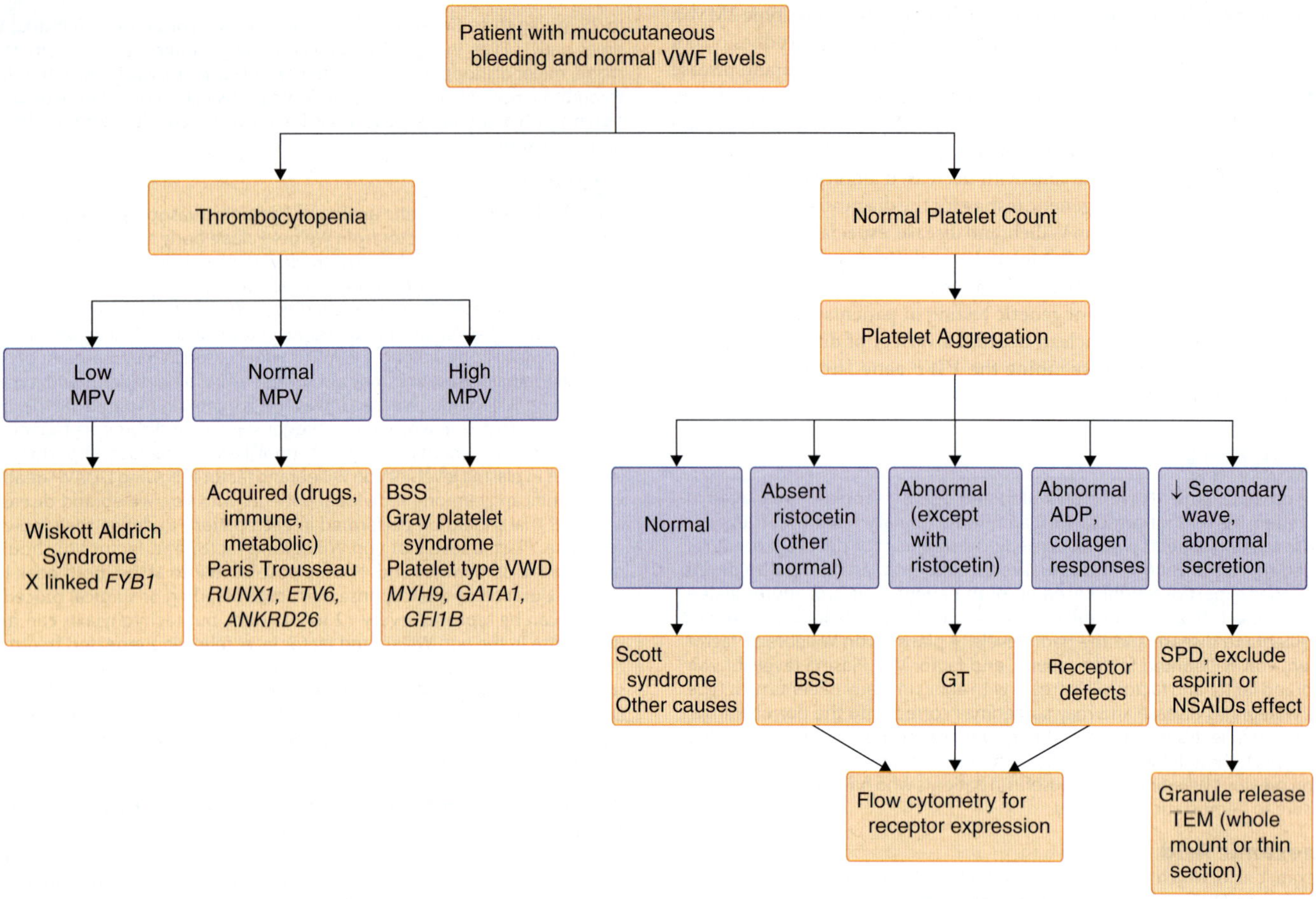

FIGURE 159-2. **Platelet disorder diagnostic algorithm.** ADP = adenosine diphosphate; BSS = Bernard-Soulier syndrome; GT = Glanzmann thrombasthenia; MPV = mean platelet volume; NSAIDs = nonsteroidal anti-inflammatory drugs; SPD = storage pool defect; TEM = transmission electron microscopy; VWD = von Willebrand disease.

PROGNOSIS

Some patients with type 1 and type 2 von Willebrand disease require specific treatment only around times of surgery, injury, or childbirth. However, other patients with severe type 1 and type 2 von Willebrand disease have recurrent lifelong bleeding issues that significantly impair their quality of life. Recurrent gastrointestinal bleeding often worsens with age, particularly in patients with type 2 VWD. Spontaneous joint bleeds can lead to progressive arthropathy in patients with type 3 VWD.

ACQUIRED VON WILLEBRAND SYNDROME

Acquired von Willebrand syndrome is an uncommon bleeding disorder that results from reduced plasma activity of von Willebrand factor in individuals who have no prior personal or family history of von Willebrand disease.[15] Acquired von Willebrand syndrome often occurs in association with underlying conditions, with 30 to 50% being associated with underlying lymphoproliferative disorders such as monoclonal gammopathy of undetermined significance (Chapter 173), multiple myeloma (Chapter 173), Waldenström macroglobulinemia (Chapter 173), non-Hodgkin lymphoma (Chapter 171), chronic lymphocytic leukemia (Chapter 168), and hairy cell leukemia (Chapter 168). Acquired von Willebrand syndrome has also been associated with a variety of other myeloproliferative disorders, autoimmune disorders, and malignancies. Mechanisms implicated in the pathogenesis of acquired von Willebrand syndrome include anti–von Willebrand factor antibodies that are associated with markedly enhanced clearance of von Willebrand factor. Cardiovascular disorders associated with pathological shear stress (e.g., aortic stenosis, extracorporeal membrane oxygenation, and left ventricular assist devices) can lead to loss of high-molecular-weight multimers due to enhanced proteolysis of von Willebrand factor by ADAMTS13.

TREATMENT

Management should focus primarily on treating any underlying conditions. Acute bleeding episodes can be difficult to manage and may be refractory to standard treatment options for von Willebrand disease. For example, although DDAVP and infusions of von Willebrand factor concentrate may cause an initial increase in levels of von Willebrand factor and factor VIII, these levels typically decline rapidly, so frequent monitoring is essential. Some patients with paraproteins may respond to intravenous immunoglobulin (IVIg), although responses in levels of von Willebrand factor and factor VIII may be delayed for several days. A combination of intravenous immunoglobulin and von Willebrand factor concentrate under expert supervision may be useful in managing elective procedures in some patients. Other treatment options include tranexamic acid, plasmapheresis, and recombinant factor VIIa.[16] Prognosis is generally determined by the prognosis of the underlying cause.

QUALITATIVE PLATELET DISORDERS

Inherited Platelet Bleeding Disorders

EPIDEMIOLOGY AND PATHOLOGY

Inherited disorders of platelet function are rare. These disorders include platelet receptor defects, platelet storage pool disorders, and a variety of other defects.

Each day, bone marrow megakaryocytes generate about 10^{11} anucleate platelets to maintain a platelet count of 150,000 to 450,000/μL. Platelets circulate in plasma and activate at sites of vascular injury to form a platelet clot. When the subendothelium is exposed due to injury, platelets bind to collagen, von Willebrand factor, and other extracellular matrix proteins via the von Willebrand factor receptor glycoprotein 1b/IX/V complex and collagen receptors such as $\alpha_2\beta_1$ and glycoprotein VI. This adhesion process triggers intracellular signaling events that lead to the activation of the fibrinogen receptor GPIIbIIIa, which is also known as integrin $\alpha_{2b}\beta_3$. The binding of fibrinogen leads to further signaling that causes platelets to change shape, granules to be released, and eventually the flipping of the membrane phospholipid layer to expose phosphatidyl serine, which provides docking sites for coagulation factors and ultimately supports the formation of a fibrin clot. In every step in the process, inherited platelet defects can compromise the performance and efficiency of these functions, thereby potentially leading to clinical bleeding.

CLINICAL MANIFESTATIONS

As with von Willebrand disease, bleeding associated with platelet disorders is often mucocutaneous (petechiae, purpura, ecchymoses, and hematomas), whereas joint or deep muscle bleeds are relatively uncommon. Affected women can have excessive menstrual bleeding (menorrhagia) and postpartum hemorrhage. Platelet dysfunction should also be suspected in the presence of increased bleeding following dental extraction, tonsillectomy, or other surgical procedures.

DIAGNOSIS

The bleeding assessment tool score used for von Willebrand disease is also useful in identifying patients with platelet function disorders, with a 99% probability if von Willebrand disease is excluded. A careful history may provide clues about whether the bleeding disorder is acquired or congenital, because platelet dysfunction may be related to other systemic disorders.

If studies for a plasma coagulation factor deficiency and von Willebrand disease are negative, functional platelet studies that should be performed at specialized centers include light transmission aggregometry, flow cytometry, and assays of platelet granule content and release (Fig. 159-2). Gene panels can test for inherited thrombocytopenias and disorders of platelet function in patients who have normal platelet counts, although the interpretation of such panels[17] can be challenging and they can miss large structural variants and deep intronic regions.[18]

TABLE 159-4 SOME COMMON AGENTS CAUSING ACQUIRED PLATELET DYSFUNCTION

TYPE OF AGENT	EXAMPLES
Antiplatelet agents	Aspirin, clopidogrel, prasugrel, ticagrelor, ticlopidine, abciximab, eptifibatide, tirofiban
Nonsteroidal anti-inflammatory agents	Ibuprofen, naproxen, indomethacin diclofenac, tolmetin, piroxicam
Selective serotonin reuptake inhibitors	Fluoxetine, paroxetine, sertraline
Plasma expanders	Dextrans, hydroxyethyl starch
Antihistamines	Chlorpheniramine, diphenhydramine
Foods and supplements	Vitamin E, fish oil, omega-3-fatty acids, alcohol, garlic, Chinese black tree fungus, ginger, cumin, turmeric, onion, cloves
Phosphodiesterase inhibitors	Cilostazol, dipyridamole, caffeine, theophylline, aminophylline, sildenafil

Data from Casari C, Bergmeier W. Acquired platelet disorders. *Thromb Res.* 2016;141(Suppl 2):S73-S75.

SPECIFIC QUALITATIVE PLATELET DISORDERS

Platelet Receptor Defects

The most commonly diagnosed receptor defects are Bernard-Soulier syndrome and Glanzmann thrombasthenia. Other platelet receptor defects associated with clinical bleeding include defects in the thromboxane, adenosine diphosphate, and collagen receptors, but these deficiencies are extremely rare and described in only a few families or cases.[19]

Bernard-Soulier Syndrome

Bernard-Soulier syndrome is an autosomal recessive disorder characterized by macrothrombocytopenia and caused by deficiency or dysfunction of GP1b/IX/V complex due to mutations in *GP1BA*, *GP1BB*, and *GP9*. In this disorder, platelets respond poorly to ristocetin in platelet aggregation studies but respond normally to other commonly used agonists, such as adenosine diphosphate (ADP), arachidonic acid, collagen, and epinephrine. The clinical presentation can be variable, but mucocutaneous bleeding is typically present. Flow cytometry usually confirms the absence of the receptor on the platelet surface, although some forms can present with a hypofunctional receptor expressed at lower levels than normal. The monoallelic form is much less severe and is associated with large platelets and somewhat low platelet counts; it can be diagnosed only by flow cytometry or genetic studies.

Glanzmann Thrombasthenia

Glanzmann thrombasthenia, which is also an autosomal recessive disorder of platelet aggregation, is caused by mutations in the genes *ITGA2B* and *ITGB3* that encode for the fibrinogen receptor GPIIbIIIa. Although the clinical presentation is also variable, bleeding tends to be severe since childhood. Patients exhibit normal platelet counts and normal platelet structure. Platelet light transmission aggregometry shows a normal response to ristocetin because the GPIb/IX/V complex is preserved, but responses to ADP, collagen, epinephrine, and arachidonic acid are very depressed or absent. The diagnosis of Glanzmann thrombasthenia can be confirmed by flow cytometry for the GPIIbIIIa receptor density and genetic testing. The complete absence of the receptor is defined as type 1, whereas moderate decreases to 10 to 20% of normal are defined as type 2.

Platelet Granule Defects

Disorders of platelet granules are rare. The most commonly diagnosed platelet function disorder is the platelet dense granule storage pool deficiency, which is usually diagnosed by a combination of mild bleeding, abnormal platelet aggregation (lack of secondary wave), and a decrease in the number of dense granules assessed by wet mount or thin section transmission electron microscopy. Bleeding is usually mild but can be more severe. In the autosomal recessive Hermansky-Pudlak syndrome, up to 10 different genes can have mutations that cause different subtypes. In this syndrome, which is accompanied by ocular albinism, platelets are normal in number and size, but the number of dense granules is severely decreased or even absent. Some patients with specific subtypes also develop severe pulmonary fibrosis, ophthalmologic complications, granulomatous colitis, and immune defects.

In Chédiak-Higashi syndrome (Chapters 153 and 231), a disorder of platelet dense granules is associated with oculocutaneous albinism, neutropenia, and severe immune deficiency. Patients also have large neutrophilic cytoplasmic inclusions and can develop life-threatening lymphohistiocytosis.

The autosomal recessive gray platelet syndrome is characterized by a complete absence of α-granules. This syndrome is caused by recessive loss of function mutations in *NBEAL2*. The platelets appear gray on a peripheral smear, and the diagnosis is confirmed by transmission electron microscopy. Although the bleeding diathesis is usually mild to moderate, the syndrome can be associated with splenomegaly and bone marrow fibrosis later in life. Other rare syndromes associated with abnormal α-granules are associated with mutations in *FLI1*, *GFI1B*, *STIM1*, and *GATA1*.

Other Inherited Platelet Function Disorders

Over 75 genes have been associated with inherited platelet disorders. These disorders are typically diagnosed on gene panels. Some of these disorders (e.g., mutations in *RUNX1*, *ETV6*, and *ANKRD26*) are associated with an increased risk of malignancies.

Acquired Platelet Dysfunction

The most common cause of acquired platelet dysfunction[20] is antiplatelet medications (Chapter 70), including aspirin, the thienopyridines (clopidogrel, prasugrel), nonthienopyridines P2Y12 inhibitors (ticagrelor, cangrelor), and the GPIIbIIIa inhibitors (tirofiban, eptifibatide, and abciximab). However, other drugs (Table 159-4) and dietary supplements can inhibit platelet function and result in easy bruising or bleeding.

Hematologic disorders such as paraproteinemias (Chapter 173), myeloproliferative neoplasms, and myelodysplastic syndrome (Chapter 167) can cause functional platelet disorders, sometimes accompanied by thrombocytopenia. Patients with end-stage renal disease (Chapter 116) or with liver failure (Chapter 140) often develop platelet dysfunction. Immune thrombocytopenic purpura also can be associated with platelet dysfunction owing to having antibodies against specific platelet receptors. Transient platelet dysfunction is seen during cardiac surgery with cardiopulmonary bypass.

TREATMENT

In most patients with congenital or acquired platelet disorders, transfusion of donor platelets is the recommended treatment. Unfortunately, patients who receive multiple platelet transfusions can become resistant because of immunity to platelet-specific or HLA-related antigens. In Glazmann thrombasthenia, alloimmunization can lead to a refractoriness to platelet transfusions; as a result, many experts prefer activated recombinant factor VIIa as the first line of treatment and reserve platelet transfusions for life-threatening bleeding.

DDAVP is effective in treating uremic bleeding and platelet dysfunction and may provide some benefit when individuals with a storage pool defect and Bernard-Soulier syndrome develop mild to moderate bleeding. Administration of DDAVP may cause fluid retention and hyponatremia, so precautions must be taken to prevent electrolyte imbalances.

Recombinant factor VIIa is useful in individuals with congenital and acquired disorders of platelet function, particularly in patients in whom platelet transfusion is ineffective. Recombinant factor VIIa increases the generation of thrombin at the site of damage to the vessel wall, thereby enhancing the recruitment of platelets. In individuals who have excessive mucocutaneous bleeding and in patients who are undergoing surgical procedures involving tissues of high fibrinolytic activity (e.g., nose, mouth, throat, and extraocular tissues), ε aminocaproic acid (5 g orally followed 1 hour later by 1 to 1.25 g/hour orally for 8 hours or until bleeding is controlled; maximum dose of 30 g/day), or tranexamic acid (15 to 25 mg/kg orally three times daily) can be useful.

HEREDITARY VASCULAR HEMORRHAGIC DISORDERS

HEREDITARY HEMORRHAGIC TELANGIECTASIA

Hereditary hemorrhagic telangiectasia, also known as Osler-Weber-Rendu syndrome, is an autosomal dominant disease with an estimated prevalence of approximately 1 in 5000. Hereditary hemorrhagic telangiectasia is characterized by vascular malformations involving the skin, nose, and gastrointestinal tract.

PATHOBIOLOGY

Sequence variations in a number of distinct genetic loci have been implicated in the pathogenesis of hereditary hemorrhagic telangiectasia. The affected genes encode proteins involved in regulating the signaling of the transforming growth factor (TGF-)β superfamily within endothelial cells.[21] A majority of patients (about 85%) have mutations of *ENG*, which encodes endoglin, or *ACVRL1*, which encodes activin receptor-like kinase (ALK1). Cumulatively, more than 500 different mutations of *ENG* or *ACVRL1* have been identified. Although all classical features can be seen in patients with either *ENG* (hereditary hemorrhagic telangiectasia type 1) or *ACVRL1* (hereditary hemorrhagic telangiectasia type 2) mutations, some genotype-phenotype correlations have been reported. For example, pulmonary and cerebral anterior venous malformations appear to be more common in type 1. Mutations affecting SMAD4 have also been described in a minority (2 to 3%) of patients and are associated with a concomitant precancerous state of juvenile polyposis.

CLINICAL MANIFESTATIONS

Vascular abnormalities are typically visible on the face and fingers (Fig. 159-3). Telangiectasia in the nose is associated with regular episodes of epistaxis that can be prolonged and severe in nature, and telangiectasia in the bowel can cause significant gastrointestinal bleeding (Chapter 121). As a result of recurrent bleeding, patients commonly have secondary iron-deficiency anemia (Chapter 145). The majority of patients with hereditary hemorrhagic telangiectasia also develop larger arteriovenous malformations within the brain, lungs, and liver. These malformations can contribute to pulmonary artery hypertension (Chapter 69), high-output heart failure (Chapter 45), and an increased risk for venous thrombosis.

DIAGNOSIS

Epistaxis and telangiectasias constitute the most common symptoms and signs of hereditary hemorrhagic telangiectasia and are part of standardized diagnostic criteria (Table 159-5). Telangiectasias and risk of gastrointestinal bleeding tend to become more apparent with aging, but the clinical diagnosis can be challenging in younger individuals, in whom genetic testing can be definitive.[22]

TABLE 159-5 DIAGNOSTIC CRITERIA FOR HEREDITARY HEMORRHAGIC TELANGIECTASIA

Recurrent spontaneous epistaxis
Multiple skin telangiectasias
Arteriovenous malformations (e.g., in lungs, brain, stomach, liver, intestines, spinal cord)
First-degree relative with the disease

Definitive disease = 3 or more criteria; possible disease = 2 criteria.

TREATMENT

Patients with epistaxis should use moisturizing topical therapies to humidify the nasal mucosa. Timolol gel (0.5 mL of 1% gel twice daily by syringe)[A2] and bevacizumab (7.5 mg/kg intravenously every 2 weeks)[A3] may be useful. Oral tranexamic acid (1 g three times daily) under expert guidance is effective, and local ablative therapies may be useful for significant epistaxis.[23] Patients with gastrointestinal bleeding require endoscopic evaluation (Chapter 120). Hemoglobin and ferritin levels should be closely monitored, and adequate iron replacement therapy must be given.

EHLERS-DANLOS SYNDROME

Ehlers-Danlos syndrome, which also can cause blood vessel rupture, is discussed in Chapter 239.

ACQUIRED VASCULAR HEMORRHAGIC DISORDERS

Patients with acquired vascular hemorrhagic disorders typically have no prior personal or family history of bleeding. Henoch-Schönlein purpura (Chapter 406) typically presents with a palpable lower extremity purpura, associated with arthralgias, abdominal pain, and renal injury. Scurvy (Chapter 199) typically presents with petechiae or bruising and with tiny perifollicular hemorrhages around corkscrew hairs. In senile purpura, diminished vascular support owing to aging and sun exposure result in easy bruising, especially on the dorsa of hands, forearms, and lower legs.

GENERAL REFERENCES

For the General References and other additional features, please visit Elsevier eBooks+ at https://ebooks.health.elsevier.com.

Grade A References

A1. Leebeek FWG, Peyvandi F, Escobar M, et al. Recombinant von Willebrand factor prophylaxis in patients with severe von Willebrand disease: phase 3 study results. *Blood*. 2022;140:89-98.
A2. Peterson AM, Lee JJ, Kallogjeri D, et al. Efficacy of timolol in a novel intranasal thermosensitive gel for hereditary hemorrhagic telangiectasia-associated epistaxis: a randomized clinical trial. *JAMA Otolaryngol Head Neck Surg*. 2020;146:1006-1014.
A3. Al-Samkari H, Kasthuri RS, Parambil JG, et al. An international, multicenter study of intravenous bevacizumab for bleeding in hereditary hemorrhagic telangiectasia: the InHIBIT-Bleed study. *Haematologica*. 2021;106:2161-2169.

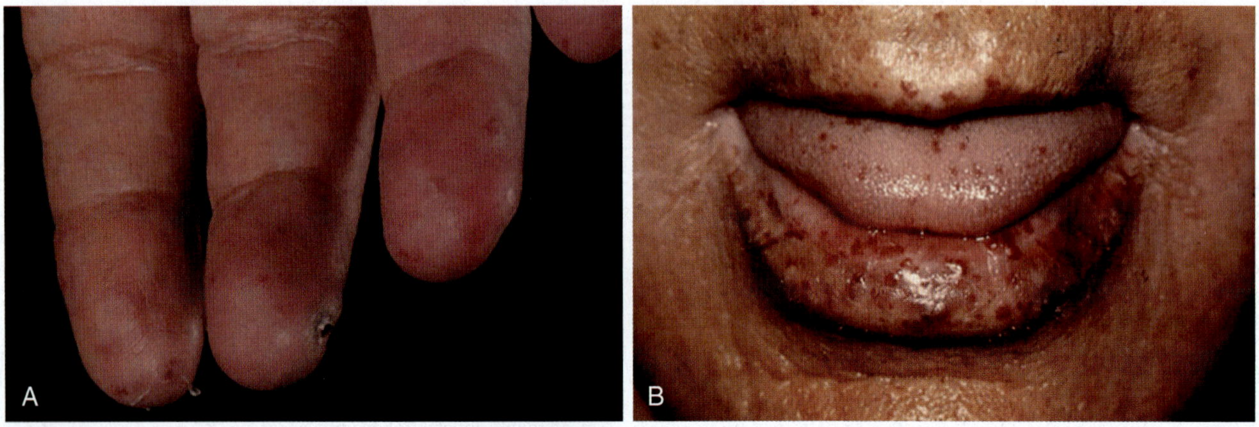

FIGURE 159-3. **Hereditary hemorrhagic telangiectasia (HHT).** Telangiectasias commonly occur on the fingers (A); face, lips, and tongue (B); and in other areas, including the nasal and gastrointestinal mucosa, and may develop in certain other internal organs. Skin or mucous membrane lesions typically blanch with pressure in contrast to petechiae, which do not. (A, Copyrighted and used with permission of the Mayo Foundation for Medical Education and Research, all rights reserved. B, Courtesy of Dr. Andrew Schafer.)

160

COAGULATION FACTOR DEFICIENCIES

MARGARET V. RAGNI

COAGULATION DEFICIENCIES

Severe coagulation deficiencies, or coagulopathies, are typically characterized by spontaneous or provoked bleeding, such as during surgery or trauma, and may result in life- or limb-threatening complications. By contrast, moderate and mild coagulopathies may remain clinically silent until they are detected coincidentally on routine laboratory screening tests (e.g., prothrombin time [PT], activated partial thromboplastin time [aPTT]), or when these tests are ordered to evaluate the cause of abnormal bleeding or bruising.

In general, coagulopathies may result from inadequate synthesis of coagulation factor proteins or from inhibition of activated factor proteins by acquired antibodies or anticoagulant medications. Qualitative defects, either congenital or acquired, may also result in bleeding.

Much of the morbidity of coagulopathies can be minimized or avoided altogether by prophylactic replacement of the deficient clotting factor proteins. In contrast to the lifelong clinical manifestations of hereditary or congenital coagulopathies, acquired deficiencies usually appear acutely in previously asymptomatic individuals; they may not be suspected and often remit spontaneously or after eradication of an inciting disease state or withdrawal of an offending medication. Acquired coagulation disorders may be associated with more severe bleeding than congenital disorders, in part because of the delay in diagnosis.

HEREDITARY HEMOPHILIAS

DEFINITION

Hemophilia A and hemophilia B are caused by deficiencies or defects in clotting factor VIII (antihemophilic factor) and factor IX (antihemophilic factor B, or Christmas factor), respectively.[1] A deficiency of either of these intrinsic coagulation pathway proteins results in inadequate formation of thrombin at sites of vascular injury.

EPIDEMIOLOGY

Hemophilia A and B are sex-linked recessive disorders estimated to occur in 1 in 5000 and 1 in 30,000 male births, respectively. The higher incidence of hemophilia A may be due to the greater amount of DNA at risk for mutation in the large factor VIII gene (186,000 base pairs) compared with the factor IX gene (34,000 base pairs). Hemophilia A and B are observed in all racial and ethnic groups, and more than 20,000 individuals are affected in the United States. A substantial proportion (30%) of hemophilia cases arise as new, spontaneous mutations. Overall, the hemophilias are much more common than the autosomal recessive coagulation disorders (see later), which often affect progeny from consanguineous relationships and require the inheritance of two defective alleles for the bleeding manifestations to become evident.

PATHOBIOLOGY

Genetics

As with other sex-linked recessive diseases, the genes for factor VIII and factor IX are located on the long arm of the X chromosome. Males with a defective allele on their single X chromosome transmit this gene to all their daughters, who are then obligate carriers, but to none of their sons. Because the offspring of female carriers inherit one affected X chromosome, half of their sons develop the coagulation disorder, and half of their daughters are obligate carriers. Female carriers may manifest bleeding symptoms, particularly postpartum bleeding, if the alleles on the X chromosome are unequally inactivated (lyonization), if the defective hemophilic allele is expressed in preference to the normal allele, and if plasma factor VIII levels are below 50%. Female hemophilia may arise as a result of mating between a hemophilic male and a female carrier (homozygous for the defective factor VIII or IX gene) or in carrier females who have the 45,XO karyotype (Turner syndrome) and are hemizygous for the defective hemophilia gene.

No single mutation is responsible for the hemophilias. Many missense and nonsense point mutations, deletions, and inversions have been described. Severe molecular defects predominate, with 40 to 50% of all cases of severe hemophilia A evolving from a unique inversion of intron 22 (the largest of the factor VIII introns). This inversion results from the recombination and translocation of DNA within intron 22 of the factor VIII gene, with areas of extragenic but homologous "nonfunctional" DNA located at a distance from intron 22. Other less common severe molecular defects include large gene deletions (5 to 10% of cases) and nonsense mutations (10 to 15% of cases). The encoded proteins resulting from these mutations are defective and do not express any factor VIII activity. Mild or moderate hemophilia A is commonly associated with point mutations and deletions. In contrast, factor IX mutations are more diverse, and severe hemophilia B is more likely caused by large deletions. Mutated clotting factor genes responsible for the hemophilias may also encode for the production of defective nonfunctional proteins that circulate in the plasma and are detected at normal quantitative levels by immunoassays but not by functional activity assays. A listing of the mutations that cause the hemophilias can be accessed via the Human Gene Mutation Database (www.hgmd.org).

CLINICAL MANIFESTATIONS

Hemophilia A and hemophilia B are clinically similar, with clinical severity corresponding inversely to the circulating levels of plasma coagulant factor VIII or IX activity. However, hemophilia A is associated with a higher frequency of bleeding, a greater need for factor replacement therapy, and more frequent hospitalizations, thereby suggesting greater clinical severity than in hemophilia B. Individuals with less than 1% of normal factor VIII or IX activity are classified as having "severe" disease, which is characterized by frequent spontaneous bleeding events in joints (hemarthrosis) and soft tissues and by profuse hemorrhage with trauma or surgery. Although spontaneous bleeding is uncommon in mild deficiencies (>5% normal activity), excess bleeding typically occurs with trauma or surgery. A moderate clinical course is associated with factor VIII or IX levels between 1 and 5%. Approximately 60% of all cases of hemophilia A are clinically severe, whereas only 20 to 45% of cases of hemophilia B are severe.

Severe hemophilia is typically suspected and diagnosed during infancy in the absence of a family history. Among newborns, intracranial hemorrhage is the leading cause of morbidity and mortality, with a cumulative incidence of about 4%. Intracranial hemorrhage does not appear to be related to the mode of delivery, although half of such hemorrhages occur in the newborn period. Circumcision within days after birth is accompanied by excessive bleeding in less than half of severely affected boys. The first spontaneous hemarthrosis in severely affected hemophilic boys usually occurs between 9 and 18 months of age, when ambulation begins. In moderately affected individuals, it generally does not occur until 2 to 5 years of age. The knees are the most prominent sites of spontaneous bleeds, followed by the elbows, ankles, shoulders, and hips; wrists are less commonly involved. Female carriers may also sustain joint bleeding and hemarthrosis, often unrecognized until years later, with sports and/or trauma.

Acute hemarthroses (Fig. 160-1) originate from the subsynovial venous plexus underlying the joint capsule and produce a tingling or burning sensation, followed by the onset of intense pain and swelling. On physical examination, the joint is swollen, hot, and tender to palpation, with erythema of the overlying skin. Joint mobility is compromised by pain and stiffness, and the joint is usually maintained in a flexed position.

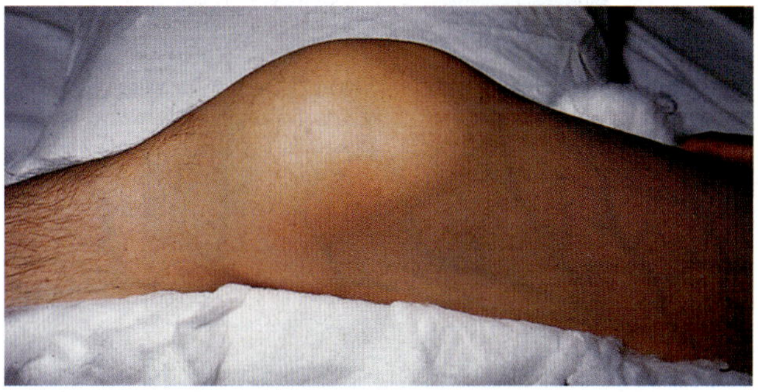

FIGURE 160-1. Acute hemarthrosis of the knee is a common complication of hemophilia. It may be confused with acute infection unless the patient's coagulation disorder is known, because the knee is hot, red, swollen, and painful. (From Forbes CD, Jackson WF. *Color Atlas and Text of Clinical Medicine*, 3rd ed. London: Mosby; 2003.)

Recurrent or untreated bleeds result in chronic synovial hypertrophy and, eventually, damage to the underlying cartilage, with subsequent subchondral bone cyst formation, bony erosion, and flexion contractures. Abnormal mechanical forces from weight bearing can produce subluxation, misalignment, loss of mobility, and permanent deformities of the lower extremities (Fig. 160-2). These changes are accompanied by chronic pain, swelling, arthritis, and disability. Plain radiographs and clinical examination of chronic hemarthroses often underestimate the extent of bone and joint damage; serial magnetic resonance imaging is the most sensitive technique to detect and monitor early and progressive disease, and early musculoskeletal ultrasound, performed in the office setting, may detect early joint disease even before symptoms occur.

Intramuscular hematomas account for about 30% of hemophilia-related bleeding events and are rarely life-threatening. Hematomas are usually precipitated by physical or iatrogenic trauma (e.g., after intramuscular injections) and may compromise sensory and motor function or arterial circulation if they entrap and compress vital structures in closed fascial compartments. The latter occurrence, termed *compartment syndrome*, presents with the rapid onset of swelling and severe pain in an extremity, unrelieved by factor infusion and standard analgesics, and is considered a medical emergency that may require fasciotomy to preserve tissue viability and provide pain relief. Retroperitoneal hematomas may be confused clinically with appendicitis or hip bleeds but should be suspected in a patient who is unable to stand erect due to the pain of muscle extension in the presence of hematoma. Immediate and aggressive treatment is required to prevent permanent anatomic deformity, such as flexion contracture, nerve damage, or pseudotumor formation (expanding hematomas that erode and destroy adjacent skeletal structures).

Bleeding from mucous membranes is not uncommon and when it involves the tongue or the retropharyngeal space, may threaten the airway. Gastrointestinal hemorrhage typically originates from anatomic lesions proximal to the ligament of Treitz and may be exacerbated by esophageal varices and/or thrombocytopenia secondary to cirrhosis and portal hypertension, or by the use of nonsteroidal anti-inflammatory drugs (NSAIDs) for the treatment of hemarthroses. Spontaneous bleeding in the genitourinary tract may arise from ureteral clots, renal stones, and/or less commonly, infection.

Intracranial bleeds occur in 10% of patients with a risk of 2% per year; they may be spontaneous or traumatic and are fatal in 30% of cases. Neuromuscular defects, seizure disorders, and intellectual deficits may ensue.

DIAGNOSIS

The diagnosis of hemophilia is suspected on the basis of a family and personal bleeding history and laboratory detection of prolongation of the aPTT (with normal PT). It is confirmed by significantly reduced plasma factor VIII or IX activity. As noted in Chapter 157, the aPTT is not a sufficiently sensitive screening test to be prolonged in mild hemophilia, where the factor VIII level is sometimes greater than 30% of normal. Severe hemophilia is usually recognized in infancy, with circumcision bleeding; by contrast, moderate or mild disease is recognized later in life after trauma or surgery. Hemophilia can be distinguished from von Willebrand disease (VWD; Chapter 159) by normal ristocetin cofactor and von Willebrand factor antigen levels. In type 2N VWD, the factor VIII level is significantly lower than ristocetin cofactor and von Willebrand factor antigen levels due to reduced factor VIII binding; this variant of VWD may require genotyping to distinguish it from hemophilia A. Other congenital intrinsic factor deficiencies (e.g., factor XI and XII) can be determined by coagulation factor–specific assays. Vitamin K deficiency (see later and Chapter 161) can be detected by the associated PT prolongation; deficiencies of factors II, VII, IX, and X; and resolution of the coagulation defect with vitamin K. The presence of heparin can be confirmed by correction of the aPTT after running the sample over a heparin absorption column. Failure of the aPTT to correct in a 1:1 mix with normal plasma suggests the presence of an inhibitor; specific inhibitors are associated with a single decreased factor level (usually factor VIII; see Alloantibody Inhibitors to Factors VIII and IX under Treatment), whereas blocking inhibitors cause nonspecific factor level changes associated with a positive hexagonal lipid assay (see Antiphospholipid Syndrome and Lupus Anticoagulant).

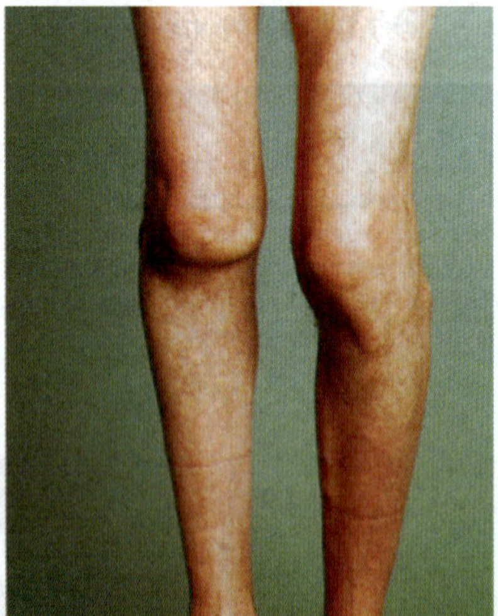

FIGURE 160-2. **Severe chronic arthritis in hemophilia.** The knee is the most commonly affected joint. Both knees are severely deranged in this patient. Note that the patient is unable to stand with both feet flat on the floor. (From Forbes CD, Jackson WF. *Color Atlas and Text of Clinical Medicine*, 3rd ed. London: Mosby; 2003.)

TREATMENT AND PREVENTION

General Care

Individuals with hemophilia cared for at hemophilia treatment centers have lower mortality and reduced costs of care compared with those receiving treatment elsewhere. The chronic care model practiced at hemophilia treatment centers emphasizes prevention to reduce joint disease and complications, optimization of factor dosing, counseling regarding safe sports, and the avoidance of aspirin and other drugs that inhibit platelet function, as well as management of surgical procedures and chronic transfusion-transmitted infections, including hepatitis C and HIV infection.

Treatment and Prevention of Bleeding

Replacement of Clotting Factors

Treatment and prevention of acute bleeding events in hemophilia A and B are based on replacement of the missing or deficient clotting factor protein to restore adequate hemostasis (Table 160-1). Use of factor on a prophylactic basis several times weekly to prevent bleeds can reduce or prevent joint bleeds and reduce joint arthropathy. All clotting factor concentrates available in the United States, whether plasma-derived or genetically engineered, are considered extremely safe; none has been implicated in the transmission of bloodborne viral pathogens or prions.

The goal of replacement therapy (see Table 160-1) is to achieve plasma factor VIII or IX activity levels that are sufficient to prevent spontaneous bleeds. As these events are individualized and vary by age, level of activity, and pharmacokinetics, the optimal level of treatment may vary among affected patients. In general, however, activity levels of 15% are sufficient to prevent spontaneous bleeding, whereas factor activity levels of 25 to 30% are recommended to treat minor spontaneous or traumatic bleeds (e.g., hemarthroses, persistent hematuria). At least 50% clotting factor activity levels are recommended for severe bleeds (e.g., major dental surgery, maintenance replacement therapy after major surgery or trauma), and 80 to 100% activity for any life-threatening or limb-threatening hemorrhagic event (e.g., major surgery, trauma). After major trauma or if visceral or intracranial bleeding is suspected, replacement therapy adequate to achieve 100% clotting factor activity should be administered immediately (within 5 to 10 minutes) *before* diagnostic procedures are initiated.

To calculate the initial dose of replacement factor, plasma factor VIII activity generally increases about 2% (0.02 IU/mL) for each unit of factor VIII administered per kilogram of body weight, and factor IX activity increases about 1% (0.01 IU/mL) for each unit of factor IX administered per kilogram of body weight. Therefore, a 70-kg individual with severe hemophilia A or B (factor VIII or IX activity <1% of normal) who requires replacement to 100% activity for major surgery should initially receive 3500 IU of factor VIII or 7000 IU of factor IX concentrate. The circulating half-lives of factors VIII and IX require subsequent dosing at half the initial dose every 8 to 12 hours for factor VIII and every 18 to 24 hours for factor IX, respectively. However, this empirical dosing should be individualized according to the patient's peak recovery and trough activity levels, using population pharmacokinetic modeling. The frequency of repeat dosing is also determined by the rapidity of pain relief, recovery of joint function, and resolution of active bleeding. Heterogeneity in the half-life of factor VIII concentrates is due to variability in clearance of von Willebrand factor.[2]

Replacement is usually maintained for at least 10 to 14 days after major surgery to allow proper wound healing and to avoid postoperative bleeding. In

TABLE 160-1 FDA-APPROVED COAGULATION PROTEINS AND REPLACEMENT THERAPIES AVAILABLE IN THE UNITED STATES

COAGULATION PROTEIN DEFICIENCY	INHERITANCE PATTERN	PREVALENCE	MINIMUM HEMOSTATIC LEVEL	REPLACEMENT SOURCES
Factor I (fibrinogen)			50-100 mg/dL	Cryoprecipitate, FFP, fibrinogen concentrate
Afibrinogenemia	Autosomal recessive	Rare (<300 families)		
Dysfibrinogenemia	Autosomal dominant or recessive	Rare (>300 variants)		
Factor II (prothrombin)	Autosomal dominant or recessive	Rare (25 kindreds)	30% of normal	FFP, factor IX complex concentrates
Factor V (labile factor)	Autosomal recessive	1 in 1 million births	25% of normal	FFP
Factor VII	Autosomal recessive	1 in 500,000 births	25% of normal	Recombinant factor VIIa (15-20 μg/kg), FFP, factor IX complex concentrates
Factor VIII (antihemophilic factor)	X-linked recessive	1 in 5000 male births	80-100% for surgery/life-threatening bleeds, 50% for serious bleeds, 25-30% for minor bleeds	Factor VIII concentrates (recombinant and recombinant extended-half-life factor VIII preferred)
Von Willebrand disease (also see Chapter 159)			>50% VWF antigen and ristocetin cofactor activity	DDAVP for mild to moderate disease (except type 2B; variable response in 2A); cryoprecipitate and FFP (not preferred, except in emergencies); plasma-derived factor VIII/VWF concentrate, viral attenuated, intermediate purity; recombinant VWF concentrate (the latter two proteins preferred for surgery, for disease unresponsive to DDAVP and for type 3)
Type 1 and 2 variants	Usually autosomal dominant	1% prevalence		
Type 3	Autosomal recessive	1 in 1 million births		
Factor IX (Christmas factor)	X-linked recessive	1 in 30,000 male births	25-50% of normal, depending on extent of bleeding, surgery	Factor IX concentrates (recombinant and recombinant extended half-life factor IX preferred); FFP not preferred except in dire emergencies
Factor X (Stuart-Prower factor)	Autosomal recessive	1 in 500,000 births	10-25% of normal	Plasma-derived factor X concentrate, FFP, or factor IX complex concentrates
Factor XI (hemophilia C)	Autosomal dominant; severe type is recessive	4% of Ashkenazi Jews; 1 in 1 million general population	20-40% of normal	FFP or factor XI concentrate
Factor XII (Hageman factor), prekallikrein, high-molecular-weight kininogen	Autosomal recessive	Not available	No treatment necessary	—
Factor XIII (fibrin stabilizing factor)	Autosomal recessive	1 in 3 million births	5% of normal	Recombinant FXIII concentrate, FFP, cryoprecipitate, or viral-attenuated factor XIII concentrate

DDAVP = desmopressin; FDA = U.S. Food and Drug Administration; FFP = fresh-frozen plasma; VWF = von Willebrand factor.

the management of bleeds or surgical procedures in patients with hemophilia, either repetitive bolus injections, as described earlier, or continuous infusion can be used for delivery of clotting factor replacement. The latter can provide constant levels of the deficient coagulation factor and can be cost-effective. Extended half-life recombinant factor VIII and IX[3] (including pegylated, albumin-fusion, nonacog alfa [factor IX], or Fc-fusion [Fc domain of immunoglobulin G_1, IgG_1]) are also available for prophylaxis or treatment, as they are safe and effective in reducing bleed frequency and prolong half-life 1.5- to 2-fold for factor VIII and 2.5- to 5.0-fold for factor IX. These agents have also been used successfully in surgery, but they are costly and may not be available at many hospitals. The typical dose frequency for extended half-life recombinant factor VIII is twice weekly at a dose of 50 to 65 IU/kg; for extended half-life recombinant factor IX, the dose is once every 1 to 2 weeks at a dose of 100 IU/kg.

Other Approaches to Augment Clotting

Nonfactor therapeutics given by subcutaneous administration also can be used as prophylaxis to prevent clinical bleeding. Emicizumab, which is the only such agent currently FDA-approved, is a bispecific monoclonal antibody that bridges activated factor IX and factor X to replace the function of missing activated factor VIII, whether due to a factor VIII inhibitor or factor VIII deficiency in hemophilia A. Emicizumab prophylaxis (1.5 mg/kg subcutaneously weekly or 3.0 mg/kg every 2 weeks, or 6.0 mg/kg every 4 weeks) is effective in reducing clinical bleeding in hemophilia A among patients of all ages, with or without inhibitors.[A1-A3] However, emicizumab is effective only for prevention but not for the treatment of acute bleeds. For acute treatment of bleeds or surgery in patients receiving emicizumab, factor replacement is required urgently. A novel intravenous factor VIII fusion protein, efanesoctocog alfa, in which recombinant factor VIIIFc is fused to von Willebrand factor, results in a four-fold increase in the half-life of factor VIII, thereby suggesting the possibility of weekly intravenous dosing.[4]

Hemarthroses

For hemarthroses, immediate or early replacement of the deficient clotting factor to normal hemostatic levels rapidly reverses the pain, whereas delayed treatment results in excess pain, morbidity, and joint damage. Optimal management once a bleed occurs includes rest, ice, (factor) concentrate, and elevation,[5] as well as protective mechanotherapy for balanced and incremental rehabilitation of injured tissues.[6]

The moderate or severe pain that accompanies acute hemarthroses responds to immediate analgesic relief. Narcotic analgesics, such as codeine or synthetic derivatives of codeine, are avoided because of their addictive potential, and early consultation with pain service physicians is recommended. Chronic acetaminophen analgesia, although helpful in low doses, may be associated with hepatic toxicity as higher doses are used, especially in patients with chronic hepatitis. For some patients compliant with prophylaxis, nonsteroidal anti-inflammatory drugs (NSAIDs; Table 26-4) may be used provided that bleeding does not occur. Aspirin (ASA) is generally contraindicated as it irreversibly inhibits platelet aggregation.

Over 75% of children and about 50% of adults engage in prophylaxis (preventive) factor infusions several times a week to maintain factor VIII or IX levels above 1% to prevent joint bleeds and the development of chronic hemophilic arthropathy. However, prophylaxis must be initiated before 4 years of age, the earlier the better, and in the absence of obesity to preserve joint motion.[7] For optimal outcomes, the patient and/or parent should be involved in decision making and the treatment plan.[8]

Although prophylaxis is the optimal strategy to prevent pain, reduced motion, and the disability of end-stage joint destruction, when prophylaxis has failed or was never initiated, surgery may be recommended. Synovectomy through open surgery or arthroscopy removes the inflamed tissue and may decrease pain and reduce recurrent bleeding, but usually only temporarily. Nonsurgical synovectomy (synoviorthesis), which involves the intra-articular administration of a radioisotope, may be considered in high-risk patients and for patients who have alloantibody inhibitors to factor VIII or IX (see later). Neither synovectomy nor synoviorthosis reverses joint damage, but both procedures may delay its progression. Non–weight-bearing exercises, such as swimming and isometrics, are important for periarticular muscle development and maintenance of joint stability for ambulation. Intractable pain and severe joint destruction secondary to repeated hemorrhage require prosthetic replacement. Chronic ankle pain responds best to open surgical or arthroscopic fixation and fusion (arthrodesis).

Genitourinary Bleeding

For genitourinary bleeding, clotting factor, fluid replacement, and, in children, a short course of steroids may be helpful to hasten resolution. However, genitourinary tract bleeding in patients with hemophilia may be worsened by the use of antifibrinolytic agents.

Alloantibody Inhibitors to Factors VIII and IX

Alloantibodies to infused factor VIII or, less frequently, to factor IX are usually detected in childhood after a median of 9 to 12 exposures to clotting factor. The prevalence of factor VIII alloantibodies among hemophilia A patients is 15 to 25%, whereas the prevalence of factor IX alloantibodies among hemophilia B patients is 1.5 to 3%.

Inhibitors are associated with hospitalization, cost, and early death. Inhibitors occur preferentially in patients who have a family history of inhibitors, patients who have large multidomain factor VIII and factor IX gene deletions, and in Black and Hispanic patients, but it is difficult to predict in whom inhibitors will develop. Among Black patients, gene sequence data suggest that mismatched factor VIII transfusions may account for the high risk of developing inhibitors. Nongenetic risk factors include early high-intensity or frequent daily exposure to factors to treat a bleed, trauma, or surgery. In previously untreated patients, the risk of developing inhibitors appears to be higher with recombinant than with plasma-derived factor.[A4]

Factor VIII–specific IgG1 antibodies appear first, followed by IgG3 and IgG4 antibodies. However, the appearance of factor VIII–specific IgG3 antibodies is always associated with the subsequent diagnosis of factor VIII inhibitors.[9]

The development of an alloantibody inhibitor is suspected when replacement therapy is ineffective in controlling bleeding symptoms. These antibodies completely neutralize clotting factor activity and prevent or reduce any increment in factor VIII or IX levels following bolus infusions of concentrate. Inhibitors are also associated with anaphylaxis and nephrotic syndrome.

Characterized as time and temperature dependent, inhibitors are quantitated in Bethesda units (BU). By definition, 1 BU is the amount of inhibitor that neutralizes 50% of the specific clotting factor activity in normal plasma. High responders, or patients with high-titer inhibitors (≥5 BU), mount an anamnestic antibody response to factor VIII clotting factor protein, usually within 5 to 7 days after subsequent exposure, and are no longer responsive to infused factor VIII. By contrast, low responders, or patients with low-titer inhibitors (<5 BU), do not manifest anamnesis, and such low-titer inhibitors can readily be overwhelmed by large amounts of human factor VIII or factor IX concentrate and can be successfully treated with three to four times the usual factor dose.

Management of patients with high-titer inhibitors[10] requires both assurance of hemostasis using bypass therapy and eradication of inhibitor formation (see Table 160-1). Bypass is typically accomplished with factor VIII inhibitor bypass activity (FEIBA; a plasma concentrate containing activated proenzymes of the prothrombin complex factors, prothrombin, and factors V11, IX and X). The usual treatment consists of one dose of FEIBA (75 IU/kg) or two doses of recombinant factor VIIa (90 to 270 μg/kg), although some patients may respond better to one agent than the other. Sequential use of FEIBA and recombinant factor VIIa (e.g., alternating every 6 hours) can improve hemostasis over single-agent treatment, but careful monitoring for thrombosis is necessary. The total dose of FEIBA should not exceed 20,000 IU in 24 hours.

Secondary prophylaxis in adults, with either recombinant factor VIIa, 90 μg/kg daily, 270 μg/kg daily, or FEIBA 85 IU/kg weekly, may significantly reduce bleeding rates as compared with on-demand treatment. Because neither agent is very effective alone and is limited by either total dose or dose frequency (VIIa must be given every 2 to 3 hours), these bypass agents may be alternated in selected patients (without cardiovascular risk, obesity, hypertension) every 3 hours for severe bleeds, surgery, or trauma. Alternatively, emicizumab prophylaxis (1.5 mg/kg subcutaneously weekly) may reduce bleeding events and improve quality of life compared with no prophylaxis in adults and children who have hemophilia A and have inhibitors.[A5,A6] By avoiding the need for factor VIII, inhibitor titers often decline.[11] Whether emicizumab and extended half-life agents such as recombinant factor VIIIFc will shorten the time to tolerance is currently uncertain. FEIBA should be avoided in patients who are receiving emicizumab because the combination increases the risk of thrombosis and thrombotic microangiopathy.

Eradication of inhibitors with immune tolerance induction is effective in about 75% of patients if initiated within 12 months of the detection of inhibitors. Immune tolerance induction regimens consist of daily factor concentrates (e.g., 200 IU/kg daily) to accomplish desensitization to infused factor. Immune tolerance induction is initiated as soon as the inhibitor is detected.[12] Maintenance of tolerance following induction usually, but not always, requires factor VIII or IX prophylaxis. Single or combination immunosuppressive agents (e.g., rituximab, mycophenolate, or cyclosporine) are variably effective. Other novel agents that promote thrombin generation by alternate pathways, including siRNA-antithrombin (fitusiran) and anti-TFPI, are in clinical trials to assess their safety and efficacy as potential bypass agents.[13] Preliminary data suggest bleeding frequency and factor use with these agents are reduced in inhibitor and noninhibitor patients.

Factor Concentrate–Transmitted Viral Infections

The prevalence of hepatitis C virus infection is about 90% in patients who were transfused from the late 1970s through the mid-1980s, and the prevalence of human immunodeficiency virus (HIV) infection is about 80% in patients who were transfused with factor VIII products and 50% in patients who were transfused with factor IX products from 1978 through the mid-1980s. Patients with HIV now can be controlled with highly active antiretroviral therapy (Chapter 357). Chronic hepatitis C infection (Chapter 135) remains the leading cause of death in hemophilia, in part because antiviral therapy does not prevent hepatocellular cancer in patients who have had long-standing chronic infection.

Ancillary and Other Therapies

Ancillary treatment strategies for the hemophilias include antifibrinolytic agents, such as ε-aminocaproic acid (50 mg/kg 3 to 4 times daily) or tranexamic acid (3 or 4 g orally daily in divided doses), to minimize mucous membrane bleeding, particularly in the oral cavity, and the application of fibrin glue to bleeding sites. Desmopressin (DDAVP) can be administered by nasal insufflation 30 minutes before a scheduled surgical procedure (one spray per nostril, to provide a total dose of 300 μg; or, in patients weighing less than 50 kg, 150 μg administered as a single spray). DDAVP may also be administered intravenously (dissolved in 50 mL normal saline) over 30 minutes at a dose of 0.3 μg/kg. DDAVP is especially useful in patients with mild hemophilia A because an adequate incremental rise in factor VIII activity can circumvent the use of clotting factor concentrates, and is generally available in most emergency department settings. Oral and intravenous fluid must be restricted to less than 1000 mL in any 24-hour period that DDAVP is administered whether to avoid hyponatremia and hyponatremic seizures. Other complications of DDAVP include facial flushing and tachyphylaxis (loss of response after three consecutive daily doses).

Gene Therapy for Hemophilia A and B

The hereditary hemophilias are model diseases for gene therapy[14] because they are caused by specific, well-defined gene mutations. A small, incremental rise in the synthesis of clotting factors can lead to substantially improved treatment and quality of life and inadvertent overexpression by successful gene transfer would not be detrimental.[15] Various adeno-associated (AAV) viral vectors carrying the Padua (FIX R338L) factor IX gain-of-function transgene in hemophilia B patients can achieve factor IX expression of 14 to 76% for up to 10 years.[16] In patients with severe hemophilia A, trials of AAV8-BDD-factor VIII and AAV5-BDD (B-domain deleted factor VIII)[17–19] have achieved factor VIII expression levels of 60% or higher for up to 3 years, but then waning to 20% or lower in some trials. These treatments resulted in a more than 90% reduction in annualized rate of bleeding events and use of factors in both hemophilia A and B. An immune response to the AAV capsid, associated with increases in liver aminotransferase levels, sometimes occurs but appears to be responsive to corticosteroids or possibly mycophenolate mofetil. Less immunogenic vectors, innovative delivery systems, and CRISPR gene editing are also being studied.

PREVENTION

Carrier Detection and Prenatal Diagnosis

Carrier detection and prenatal diagnosis have become technically feasible, very sensitive, and widely available. Noninvasive prenatal diagnosis by use of microfluidic digital PCR of maternal plasma DNA is based on the relative proportion of mutated versus normal alleles; it can detect an affected fetus as early as the eighth week of gestation. Because prenatal diagnosis requires the mother to have a known mutation, mothers are increasingly being tested in a nationwide hemophilia genotype program, MLOF (My Life, Our Future). However, at best only two thirds of carrier mothers will be identified because one third of new hemophilia cases arise as spontaneous mutations.

Early prenatal diagnosis is important to reduce intracranial bleeds in an infant with anticipated severe hemophilia by recommended caesarean delivery and to reduce circumcision-related bleeding by preventive factor treatment. Guidelines suggest caesarean section delivery be considered for any known male infants with severe hemophilia A. Vacuum extraction may increase cephalohematoma formation and is discouraged.

Early diagnosis is also important for the mother to reduce peripartum bleeding and advocate for genetic counseling regarding family planning. Next-generation sequencing, carrier testing, and prenatal diagnosis with genetic counseling are widely available in the United States through the network of federally funded hemophilia treatment centers. Fecundity rates remain high, and few confirmed carriers elect to terminate their pregnancies, even if an affected fetus is detected in utero. These decisions are influenced by the wide availability of safe and effective coagulation factor replacement concentrates and by the prospect of an eventual cure for the hemophilias through gene transfer or gene editing.

PROGNOSIS

The life expectancy of individuals with severe hemophilia is similar to that of the normal population. Although deaths from HIV and hepatitis C are declining, in part due to effective antiretroviral therapy for HIV (Chapter 357) and effective combination antiviral treatment for hepatitis C, patients with hemophilia and long-standing chronic hepatitis C infection prior to elective treatment still have a somewhat increased risk of hepatocellular carcinoma despite antiviral therapy.[20] Further, as patients with hemophilia live longer, malignancy and heart disease are becoming more common, and with them need for additional replacement during periods of chemotherapy-induced thrombocytopenia or antiplatelet therapy.[21] Among patients with alloantibody inhibitors, mortality rates are significantly higher than in other patients, so early diagnosis and early immune tolerance induction are recommended. Bleeding is also a leading cause of death, with a lifetime risk of intracranial hemorrhage of approximately 2 to 8%. Finally, the usual problems of aging are increasingly being recognized in those with hemophilia, including atherosclerosis, hypertension, hyperlipidemia, obesity, and diabetes. The impact of these conditions on the natural history of hemophilia, given several studies suggesting lower mortality from ischemic heart disease, remains to be seen.

ACQUIRED HEMOPHILIAS

EPIDEMIOLOGY AND PATHOBIOLOGY

Autoantibody inhibitors occur spontaneously in individuals with previously normal hemostasis. In contrast to alloantibody inhibitors in hemophilic men, which are directed against exogenous clotting factor, autoantibody inhibitors are directed against endogenous clotting factor, most commonly factor VIII. These autoantibodies typically arise in individuals with no past bleeding history, so the diagnosis may be missed until prolonged aPTT and aPTT mixed tests are obtained (Chapter 157). Although 50% of patients with autoantibody inhibitors have no obvious underlying cause, the other 50% are associated with autoimmune diseases, lymphoproliferative disorders, idiosyncratic drug reactions, pregnancy, and advanced age.

CLINICAL MANIFESTATIONS AND DIAGNOSIS

Massive hemorrhagic events, even more severe than in hemophilia patients with alloantibodies, and more commonly in soft tissues, may occur in those with autoantibodies because of a delay in diagnosis and treatment. The laboratory expression of autoantibodies is similar to that of alloantibodies, except that clotting factor activity is not completely neutralized. Residual clotting factor activities between 3 and 20% of normal are frequently observed in patients with autoantibodies.

TREATMENT

The same principles of replacement therapy for alloantibodies apply to these acquired autoantibody inhibitors.[22] The two goals of treatment are to stop the bleeding, assure hemostasis, and eradicate the inhibitor. For hemostasis, recombinant factor VIIa, activated prothrombin complex concentrate, or factor VIII bypass activity is commonly used, in similar doses used to achieve hemostasis with a success rate in over 90% of patients and thrombotic events in less than 5%. Emicizumab (3 mg/kg subcutaneously for 2 to 3 doses followed by 1.5 mg/kg every 3 weeks) can also be an effective prophylactic hemostatic therapy.[23]

Eradication of the inhibitor is significantly more successful (about 80%) in patients who are treated with corticosteroids (e.g., prednisone 1 mg/kg/day orally) and cyclophosphamide (150 mg/day orally or 500 to 750 mg/m^2 intravenous bolus every 3 to 4 weeks) than with corticosteroids alone (about 60%), with dose titration based on inhibitor levels and complicating cytopenias. Rituximab-based regimens (375 mg/m^2 intravenously weekly for 4 weeks) are also effective in about 60% of patients. High-dose intravenous immunoglobulin (IVIg)–based regimens under expert supervision may be effective in about 45% of patients. These agents are tapered and discontinued once the autoantibody has disappeared. The time to complete remission is about 5 weeks for corticosteroids plus cyclophosphamide, whereas rituximab-based regimens require twice as long to achieve remission.

PROGNOSIS

Patients with acquired hemophilia have a mortality rate of 15 to 25%, which is considerably higher than that observed with alloantibody factor VIII inhibitors. Survival in acquired hemophilia is influenced primarily by the achievement of a complete remission, age younger than 65 years at diagnosis, and any related diseases (malignancy vs. postpartum vs. others). Hemorrhagic complications are the primary cause of death, but about 15 to 20% of deaths are associated with sepsis, and about 70% of cases of sepsis arise as a complication of cyclophosphamide-induced neutropenia that may be avoided with future therapies.

VON WILLEBRAND DISEASE

The most common congenital bleeding disorder is von Willebrand disease, which is discussed in detail in Chapter 159.

FACTOR XI DEFICIENCY

EPIDEMIOLOGY

Factor XI deficiency has a prevalence of 1 in 1 million in the general population and 1 in 500 births in Ashkenazi Jewish families. The intrinsic pathway of coagulation of factor XI is the only contact-phase component that is associated with excessive bleeding complications when a deficiency exists.

PATHOBIOLOGY

Factor XI deficiency is predominantly an autosomal recessive trait, although some mutations may have a dominant transmission pattern. The factor XI gene (*FXI*) is located on chromosome 4, and the protein circulates as a homodimer, with each FXI monomer composed of four apple domains encoded by exons 3 through 10 and a protease domain encoded by exons 11 through 15. The Glu117 stop mutation in *FXI* is the most common cause of factor XI deficiency, due to poor secretion or stability of the truncated protein or decreased levels of messenger RNA. More than 170 mutations of *FXI* have been identified in factor XI–deficient patients (see www.factorxi.org), but close correlation between bleeding phenotype and genotype is lacking. Most mutations are missense or nonsense mutations and are located across all four apple domains and the serine protease region.

In Ashkenazi Jewish individuals, factor XI deficiency is common, with a heterozygote frequency of 8 to 10%; two predominant gene mutations occur with equal frequency and are designated type II (a stop codon in exon 5) and type III (a single base defect in exon 9). The most severe clinical disease is observed in patients who are homozygous for type II and who usually have less than 1% factor XI activity. Homozygous type III individuals also manifest severe symptoms, but typically less severe than those of type II patients; they have slightly higher factor XI levels of about 10 to 20%. Compound heterozygotes, type II/III, make up the bulk of factor XI–deficient patients; they have clinically mild disease, with factor XI levels between 30 and 50%.

In individuals of non-Ashkenazi Jewish ancestry, the mutations are more variable, although Cys128 stop has been described in several kindreds, and Cys38Arg has been found in several French Basque families. One third of patients who develop inhibitors are homozygous for Glu117 stop, which results in an absent *FXI*. Genotypic identification of affected patients is determined by measuring factor XI levels rather than by defining the specific gene defect.

CLINICAL MANIFESTATIONS

The clinical bleeding tendency in factor XI deficiency is less severe than that observed in severe hemophilia A or B and, in contrast to the hemophilias, does not correlate with the severity of the deficiency. Most individuals with less than 20% of normal factor XI activity experience excessive bleeding after trauma or surgery, but a few do not bleed. In contrast, bleeding has been observed in approximately 35 to 50% of mildly affected patients with factor XI levels between 20 and 50% of normal. Spontaneous hemorrhagic episodes, hemarthroses, and intramuscular and intracerebral bleeds are unusual; traumatic and surgical bleeds typically involve the mucous membranes. Patients undergoing tonsillectomy, prostatectomy, or dental extraction are at highest risk for bleeding unless replacement therapy is administered. Women may experience significant menorrhagia, and women with menorrhagia should be screened for both von Willebrand disease and factor XI deficiency. Patients with mild factor XI deficiency and coincident mild von Willebrand disease have an increased risk of bleeding.

DIAGNOSIS

Factor XI deficiency is diagnosed by a prolonged activated partial thromboplastic time (aPTt), normal prothrombin time (PT), and decreased factor XI activity ascertained in a specific quantitative clotting assay (normal range, 60 to 130%).

TREATMENT

Not all individuals with factor XI deficiency bleed, so it may be reasonable to monitor affected individuals with no treatment, especially if they have no family history of bleeding. For surgical or other major bleeding, fresh frozen plasma 15 to 20 mL/kg may be given, although potential complications include fluid overload and infection risk, which can be reduced with the use of pathogen-inactivated fresh frozen plasma,[24] if available. Use of factor XI concentrate, which is available in Europe but not the United States, may be complicated by thrombosis, which occurs in approximately 10% of patients, particularly in older individuals with preexisting cardiovascular disease or malignancy. Replacement dosing levels should not exceed 70% of factor XI activity. Repeat dosing with fresh frozen plasma or factor XI concentrate should take into consideration the long (60- to 80-hour) biologic half-life of factor XI in vivo.

The decision to treat heterozygotes with factor XI at levels greater than 20% is empirical and should be based on personal history of bleeding after trauma or surgery. There is no clear evidence that suggests any benefit of DDAVP. Because hemorrhagic complications originate most commonly from mucous membrane surfaces, antifibrinolytic agents such as ε-aminocaproic acid or tranexamic acid under expert supervision are frequently helpful as adjunctive therapy. In women with menorrhagia or postpartum hemorrhage, testing for von Willebrand disease is recommended because both diseases may be present, but testing should be postponed until 6 to 8 weeks after delivery to avoid hormone-induced increase in von Willebrand factor levels that may mask diagnosis.

Alloantibody inhibitors, which neutralize the hemostatic effects of exogenously administered factor XI replacement, can develop in patients with severe factor XI deficiency who have been exposed to plasma or factor XI concentrate. Recombinant factor VIIa can prevent bleeding during or after surgery in these patients.

DEFICIENCIES OF CONTACT ACTIVATION FACTORS

Although factor XI plays an important role in the activation of factor IX in the intrinsic pathway generation of thrombin, it is only one of the four components of the contact phase of coagulation (Chapter 157). Deficiencies in any of the other three factors (factor XII, prekallikrein, and high-molecular-weight kininogen) produce in vitro laboratory abnormalities. Even among those with severe factor XII deficiency (<1% activity), clinical bleeding does not occur. In fact, up to 8 to 10% with severe factor XII deficiency actually experience venous thromboembolic events, which are occasionally fatal. This finding has led to speculation that factor XII deficiency may lead to hypercoagulability through defective participation of the contact-phase proteins in the activation of fibrinolysis.

DIAGNOSIS

Deficiencies of each of these factors prolong the aPTT, often markedly, but it may normalize after prolonged incubation of the patient's plasma at 37° C with a negatively charged activator of the aPTT assay (i.e., kaolin or celite). Specific assays are also available to quantitate each of the contact factors.

TREATMENT

Deficiencies of the contact activation factors, however severe they are and however prolonged the associated aPTT may be, do not cause clinical bleeding problems, even in response to surgery or trauma. Therefore, no therapy is indicated for factor XII deficiency, prekallikrein deficiency, or high-molecular-weight kininogen deficiency. Routine anticoagulation regimens are used to treat thrombotic events.

FACTOR XIII (FIBRIN-STABILIZING FACTOR) DEFICIENCY

Factor XIII is a transglutaminase that is activated by thrombin and functions to cross-link fibrin to protect it from lysis by plasmin, the key enzyme of the fibrinolytic system. It is also involved in normal wound healing and tissue repair and seems to be crucial for maintaining a viable pregnancy. Homozygous severe deficiency states are rare and are inherited in an autosomal recessive manner, with a prevalence of 1 per 3 million births. Consanguinity is common. Most patients are deficient in the A-subunit (FXIII-A). Half of the molecular defects that account for A-subunit deficiency are missense mutations.

CLINICAL MANIFESTATIONS

Heterozygous carriers are usually asymptomatic, but homozygotes have life-long bleeding that typically starts shortly after birth with persistent bleeding around the umbilical stump. Intracranial bleeding events, usually precipitated by minimal trauma, occur commonly enough in infants (25%) to justify the initiation of a primary prophylaxis regimen of replacement therapy. Delayed bleeding after surgery and trauma is the hallmark of the disease. However, easy bruising, poor wound healing with defective scar formation and dehiscence, and hemarthroses are also characteristic. Spontaneous abortions are increased in severely affected women.

DIAGNOSIS

The diagnosis is usually suspected on clinical grounds, given that factor XIII deficiency is not detected by conventional screening coagulation tests (i.e., aPTT, PT). Most laboratories use a rapid screening assay that assesses the ability of a fibrin clot to remain intact with incubation in 5 mol/L of urea or 1% monochloroacetic acid. With factor XIII levels less than 1% of normal, the clot dissolves within 2 to 3 hours. However, the clot solubility tests are not standardized and have a low sensitivity.[25]

TREATMENT

Normal hemostasis is achieved with a factor XIII level of only 5% of normal. Replacement therapy for prophylaxis or the treatment of acute bleeds in factor XIII deficiency can be accomplished by administering plasma-derived factor XIII concentrate, which is pasteurized for viral safety, or fresh frozen plasma. Recombinant factor XIII is safe and effective in preventing bleeds in factor XIII–deficient patients. The dose is 10 to 20 U/kg intravenously given every 3 to 4 weeks. Acquired alloantibody inhibitors can develop in severely affected individuals. Autoantibodies also occur, usually in association with systemic lupus erythematosus.

DYSFIBRINOGENEMIA AND AFIBRINOGENEMIA

Approximately 300 abnormal fibrinogens have been described, but few cause hemostatic symptoms. Abnormal fibrinogens are rare, autosomally inherited proteins. Quantitative fibrinogen deficiencies (afibrinogenemia and hypofibrinogenemia) may result from mutations affecting fibrinogen synthesis or processing, whereas qualitative defects (dysfibrinogenemia) are caused by mutations that lead to abnormal polymerization, defective cross-linking, or defective assembly of the fibrinolytic system.

The prevalence of dysfibrinogenemia in patients with a history of thromboembolic episodes approaches 0.8%. A high prevalence of dysfibrinogenemia has been reported among patients with chronic thromboembolic hypertension, thereby implicating changes in the molecular structure of fibrin in the development of this disorder. Clinically insignificant dysfibrinogenemias may be acquired in association with hepatocellular carcinoma.

CLINICAL MANIFESTATIONS

More than 50% of the dysfibrinogenemias are asymptomatic, 25% are associated with a mild hemorrhagic tendency (commonly caused by defective release of fibrinopeptide A), and 20% predispose individuals to thrombosis (usually caused by impaired fibrinolysis; Chapter 67). Concurrent bleeding and thrombosis also may occur. Women experience a high incidence of pregnancy-related complications, such as spontaneous abortion and postpartum thromboembolic events. Thrombin times and reptilase times (plasma-based clotting times with the substitution of reptilase snake venom for thrombin) are not helpful in predicting whether an abnormal fibrinogen will be prothrombotic, prohemorrhagic, or asymptomatic. However, clinical history, fibrinopeptide release studies, and fibrin polymerization studies may be useful.

In contrast to the hepatic synthesis of a qualitatively abnormal protein in dysfibrinogenemia, congenital afibrinogenemia is an autosomal recessive disorder that causes markedly deficient production of the normal protein. Severe life-threatening hemorrhagic complications can occur at any site, beginning at birth with umbilical bleeding. Intracranial hemorrhage is a frequent cause of death. Poor wound healing is characteristic.

DIAGNOSIS

Abnormalities are usually detected incidentally when routine coagulation screening assays reveal decreased fibrinogen concentrations and prolonged thrombin clotting times. On further evaluation, discordance between functional and immunologic fibrinogen levels (>50 mg/dL more antigenic than functional) is observed; clotting times using snake venom (reptilase or ancrod) are variably prolonged.

Afibrinogenemia is usually detectable by specific functional or immunologic assays. Platelet dysfunction may accompany afibrinogenemia and exacerbate bleeding.

TREATMENT

Deficiencies of fibrinogen can be corrected by the administration of cryoprecipitate or a viral-attenuated (pasteurized), plasma-derived fibrinogen concentrate.[26] The target replacement goal is 100 mg/dL, and given a circulating biologic half-life of at least 96 hours, treatment every 3 to 4 days is adequate.

Thrombosis is a potential complication of treatment. Primary prophylaxis regimens may be useful in afibrinogenemia, with on-demand or prophylactic replacement for trauma or surgery. Fibrinogen replacement may reduce not only bleeding but also thrombosis. Individuals with thrombophilic manifestations should receive anticoagulation long-term, depending on risk-benefit assessment. Solvent/detergent plasma, which is a pooled human plasma that reduces allergic reactions and transfusion-related acute lung injury, or psoralen-treated fresh frozen plasma may be alternatives.

FACTOR V DEFICIENCY

Factor V is a component of the prothrombinase complex that assembles factors Va and Xa on the phospholipid membrane of the platelet for prothrombin (factor II) activation to thrombin.

CONGENITAL FACTOR V DEFICIENCY

Deficiency of factor V is a rare, autosomal recessive disorder (1 in 1 million births). The factor V Leiden protein, which is responsible for resistance to activated protein C and thrombophilia, does not affect factor V coagulant activity. The severity of plasma factor V deficiency correlates less well with the risk of clinical bleeding than does the factor V content in platelet α-granules. This observation illustrates the critical role of the platelet in promoting adequate hemostasis at bleeding sites and explains why transfusions of normal platelets may be preferred over fresh frozen plasma for the treatment of hemorrhagic episodes secondary to congenital or acquired factor V deficiency. Hemostasis can be maintained without correcting plasma factor V activity (>25% of normal). Recombinant factor VIIa has also been used off-label to treat bleeding in factor V deficiency.

COMBINED DEFICIENCIES OF FACTORS V AND VIII

Factors V and VIII are structurally homologous proteins, and combined deficiencies of these factors occur as an autosomal recessive disorder with a prevalence of 1 in 100,000 births among Jews of Sephardic origin. The disorder is believed to be caused by defective secretion due to mutations in export proteins in the endoplasmic reticulum of endothelial cells. The severity of bleeding is determined by the levels of these factors, which usually range from 5 to 30% of normal. Replacement therapy should be aimed at normalizing both clotting protein activities.

ACQUIRED FACTOR V DEFICIENCY

Acquired factor V deficiency has been described in individuals exposed to bovine factor V, which contaminates the thrombin preparations used topically to control bleeding during cardiovascular surgery. This abnormality probably represents the development of anti–bovine factor V antibodies that cross-react with the human factor V protein. Profuse bleeding accompanies this complication.

DEFICIENCIES OF VITAMIN K–DEPENDENT COAGULATION

DEFICIENCIES OF FACTORS II, VII, AND X

PATHOBIOLOGY AND CLINICAL MANIFESTATIONS

Congenital deficiencies of factors II (prothrombin), VII, and X are rare, autosomally inherited disorders. Heterozygotes (with factor levels approximately 20% of normal) are typically asymptomatic except in the immediate newborn period, when physiologic vitamin K deficiency exacerbates the underlying clotting factor deficiency. Homozygotes with clotting factor levels less than 10% of normal manifest variable symptoms. As with other coagulopathies, these deficiencies are usually suspected after neonatal umbilical stump bleeding. Thereafter, unless replacement or prophylactic therapy is provided, these patients are subject to mucosal bleeding from epistaxis, menorrhagia, and dental extractions; hemarthroses and intramuscular hematomas; and bleeding after surgery or trauma.

Acquired factor VII deficiency has been associated with Dubin-Johnson and Gilbert syndromes (Chapter 133). Acquired factor IX deficiency has been associated with Gaucher disease, because factor IX binds to glucocerebroside. Acquired factor X deficiency and amyloidosis are discussed later.

DIAGNOSIS

In the coagulation laboratory, factor VII deficiency is associated with a prolonged PT and a normal aPTT. This pattern localizes the deficiency to the extrinsic pathway. In contrast, deficiencies of factors II (prothrombin) and X prolong both the PT and the aPTT, with the defects localized to the common pathway of coagulation. A Russell viper venom–based clotting test can differentiate between these two deficiencies; as a direct activator of factor X, the assay is prolonged with factor X deficiency but not with factor II deficiency. Mixing patient plasma with normal plasma results in a correction of these assays, and specific clotting assays using plasma deficient in the coagulation protein to be studied can confirm the diagnosis.

TREATMENT

Replacement therapy is indicated for acute symptomatic bleeds and for prophylaxis before surgery. Plasma-derived factor X is available to treat bleeding in factor X deficiency. Alternatively, factor IX complex concentrates can be administered to achieve hemostatic levels of any of these vitamin K–dependent factors (25 to 30% of normal).

Bleeding complications caused by acquired IgG autoantibodies directed against any coagulation factor protein can be reversed rapidly, albeit temporarily, by extracorporeal immunoadsorption over a Sepharose-bound polyclonal antihuman IgG or staphylococcal A column, with concomitant replacement therapy and initiation of immunosuppression. Recombinant factor VIIa is increasingly used for surgery in patients with rare congenital coagulation deficiencies and Glanzmann thrombasthenia, but typically at lower doses than with hemophilia inhibitors—generally 10 to 15 μg/kg per dose for up to several days.

FACTOR DEFICIENCY IN AMYLOIDOSIS

Severe acquired deficiency of factor X, often accompanied by deficiencies of other vitamin K–dependent factors, occasionally occurs in individuals with systemic amyloidosis (Chapter 174). Because amyloid fibrils in the reticuloendothelial system bind endogenous and exogenous sources of factor X, replacement therapy with FFP or factor IX complex concentrates, even in large quantities, may not be sufficient. Recombinant factor VIIa concentrate has been used to reverse acute bleeding. Splenectomy may ameliorate recurrent bleeding complications.

OTHER ACQUIRED COAGULATION ABNORMALITIES

ANTIPHOSPHOLIPID SYNDROME AND LUPUS ANTICOAGULANT

EPIDEMIOLOGY

The antiphospholipid antibody syndrome is associated with recurrent thrombosis or recurrent pregnancy loss with autoantibodies directed against phospholipids. Antiphospholipid antibodies may include lupus anticoagulant, anticardiolipin antibody (CL), or anti-β2-glycoprotein-I (anti-β2-GPI). Thrombocytopenia is also a common finding in this prothrombotic disorder. Rarely, multiorgan failure may arise from widespread thrombosis, a syndrome called catastrophic antiphospholipid antibody syndrome.

PATHOBIOLOGY

The prothrombotic effects of antiphospholipid antibodies may derive from their ability to complex with β2-GPI in vivo (thereby negating their modulatory phospholipid-binding function) or through inhibition of protein C activation, interference with antithrombin III activity, and/or disruption of the annexin V shield, thereby preventing normal clot breakdown (fibrinolysis). Although complement and inflammation play a role in fetal loss in a murine model of antiphospholipid antibody syndrome, the pathogenic mechanism of pregnancy loss remains unclear. Although non–β2-GPI antibodies detected by CL enzyme-linked immunosorbent assay (ELISA) may play a role in early obstetric antiphospholipid antibody syndrome, and anti-β2-GPI antibodies with lupus anticoagulant activity play a role in late miscarriage, additional studies are needed to classify, understand, and manage this syndrome.

CLINICAL MANIFESTATIONS

Lupus anticoagulants prolong coagulation in in vitro assays but are not generally associated with clinical bleeding. Rarely, clinical bleeding may occur when antiphospholipid antibody antibodies interact with factor II (prothrombin), producing an acquired prothrombin (factor II) deficiency associated with accelerated clearance of lupus anticoagulant–prothrombin complexes from the circulation. Bleeding tendencies also may arise when the lupus anticoagulant targets platelet membranes and produces quantitative or qualitative platelet abnormalities. Other clinical findings in the antiphospholipid antibody syndrome include livedo reticularis, valvular heart lesions, and nephropathy. Clinically, although both arterial and venous thrombosis may occur in the antiphospholipid antibody syndrome, the most relevant is venous thrombosis and stroke in young adults. A diagnostic evaluation in those with arterial thrombosis should include transesophageal echocardiography to exclude a cardiac source for arterial clots. In obstetric patients, other causes of miscarriage should be excluded. A history of recurrent spontaneous abortion associated with antiphospholipid antibody syndrome is a risk factor for subsequent venous thromboembolism in the long term. Nonpregnant individuals with antiphospholipid antibody syndrome–associated thrombotic manifestations have a 50% risk of experiencing recurrent events over a 5-year period. Typically, recurrent thrombotic episodes occur in a pattern consistent with the initial findings (e.g., venous recurrence following an initial deep vein thrombosis).[27]

DIAGNOSIS

The diagnosis of antiphospholipid antibody syndrome is based on both clinical and laboratory criteria. Clinical criteria include arterial, venous, or small-vessel thrombosis in any tissue or organ and pregnancy morbidity.[28] The latter includes one or more pregnancy losses before 10 weeks' gestation; one or more pregnancy losses before 34 weeks due to eclampsia, preeclampsia, or placental insufficiency; or three or more spontaneous abortions before 10 weeks. Antiphospholipid antibody syndrome may be suspected in the setting of recurrent spontaneous miscarriages or pregnancy-related thromboembolic events, with the detection of cerebral arterial thromboses in young adults, in those with systemic lupus erythematosus (20 to 40%; Chapter 245) or other autoimmune diseases or lymphoproliferative malignancies, in those receiving psychotropic medications (e.g., chlorpromazine), or when incidental coagulation assays reveal aPTT prolongation.

Laboratory criteria for antiphospholipid antibody syndrome include the detection of one or more high-titer antiphospholipid antibodies (lupus anticoagulant, CL, anti-β2-GPI) on at least two occasions at least 12 weeks apart. Antiphospholipid antibodies can be detected by three assays: the lupus anticoagulant assay, the CL ELISA assay, and the β2-GPI ELISA assay. The lupus anticoagulant assay includes a screening test, based on a prolonged phospholipid-dependent clotting time; a mixing test that distinguishes the inhibitor (fails to correct in a 1 : 1 mix) from a deficiency state (corrects in a 1 : 1 mix); and a confirmatory test based on platelet neutralization to demonstrate that the inhibitor is phospholipid dependent (clotting time corrects) or a modified aPTT reagent based on the binding of hexagonal-phase phospholipids to lupus anticoagulants. The CL ELISA measures antibodies in dilute sera that bind to CL-coated plates, including those that bind to CL alone or bound to bovine β2-GPI and both IgG and IgM, but it may miss CL bound to human β2-GPI. The β2-GPI ELISA detects antibodies that bind to β2-GPI–coated irradiated plates, but it has reduced specificity owing to binding by nonpathogenic antibodies. Positivity in multiple assays is strongly associated with thrombosis and miscarriage. The risk of first thrombosis among asymptomatic individuals positive for lupus anticoagulants, CL, and β2-GPI antibodies, so-called triple-positive patients, is about 5% per year. Of the three assays, the β2-GPI ELISA is most strongly associated with thrombosis and early recurrent miscarriage; the lupus anticoagulant assay is associated with venous thrombosis, stroke, and late miscarriage. The greatest weight is given to a positive lupus anticoagulant test. From a practical standpoint, testing for all three antibodies at diagnosis is recommended to guide follow-up, because oral anticoagulants may interfere with the lupus anticoagulant test.

TREATMENT

Because of the high risk of recurrent thromboembolism, patients with the antiphospholipid antibody syndrome should receive antithrombotic therapy. The approach is based on achieving a balance between thrombosis risk and bleeding complications, especially in those with thrombocytopenia. Recommendations for patients who have the antiphospholipid antibody syndrome emphasize the use of unfractionated heparin or low-molecular-weight heparin (LMWH), with a 4- to 5-day overlap with warfarin, for acute venous thromboembolism, followed by long-term warfarin to a target international normalized ratio (INR) of 2.0 to 3.0. In individuals with thrombocytopenia, more frequent monitoring of the INR may be warranted to avoid bleeding complications. The direct oral anticoagulant rivaroxaban, although effective in prevention of venous thrombosis, is not as effective as warfarin for arterial thrombosis,[A7] so warfarin remains the treatment of choice in patients who have the antiphospholipid antibody syndrome. The duration of anticoagulation is based on a balance between the risks of bleeding compared with the risks of recurrent thrombosis.

For women with the antiphospholipid antibody syndrome and a prior pregnancy loss but no past thrombosis, the goal is to prevent recurrent pregnancy loss. Based on randomized trials, recommendations generally include low-dose aspirin (81 mg daily) in combination with prophylactic heparin or LMWH in the antepartum period.[29,30]

In the setting of bleeding or when the inherent risk of bleeding exceeds the risk of bleeding with treatment among patients with antiphospholipid antibody syndrome–associated thrombocytopenia and a platelet count below 20,000 to 30,000/μL, management is similar to that for idiopathic thrombocytopenic purpura (see Chapter 158). Case reports indicate that danazol, dapsone, aspirin, or chloroquine may be helpful adjuncts under expert supervision. In pregnant women with antiphospholipid antibody syndrome–associated thrombocytopenia, treatment is advised before epidural anesthesia or cesarean section. In the latter case, early delivery under cover of intravenous immunoglobulin is recommended.

Treatment of antiphospholipid antibody syndrome–associated bleeding is dependent on the site and severity of bleeding. For patients who are taking anticoagulant therapy, the anticoagulant should be withheld and an antidote (e.g., protamine or vitamin K) should be given. For thrombocytopenic bleeding, platelet transfusions should be administered, with red blood cell transfusions if necessary. If both thrombosis and bleeding occur, treatment should be directed at the component that is most life-threatening. In patients with a high bleeding risk, anticoagulants should be withheld or given at a lower dosage; patients with a high thrombotic risk despite thrombocytopenia should be anticoagulated and given agents to boost the platelet count.

In the life-threatening multisystem complication of catastrophic antiphospholipid syndrome, which is characterized by histopathologic evidence of small vessel thrombosis and dysfunction of multiple organs (e.g., lung, brain, heart, kidneys, skin, or gastrointestinal tract) over a short period of time, maximal anticoagulation, plasma exchange, and immunosuppressive therapy have been used under expert supervision. Eculizumab, an inhibitor of terminal complement, was effective in a patient with recurrent catastrophic antiphospholipid syndrome.

GENERAL REFERENCES

For the General References and other additional features, please visit Elsevier eBooks+ at https://ebooks.health.elsevier.com.

Grade A References

A1. Mahlangu J, Oldenburg J, Paz-Priel I, et al. Emicizumab prophylaxis in patients who have hemophilia A without inhibitors. *N Engl J Med.* 2018;379:811-822.

A2. Young G, Liesner R, Chang T, et al. A multicenter, open-label phase 3 study of emicizumab prophylaxis in children with hemophilia A with inhibitors. *Blood.* 2019;134:2127-2138.

A3. Callaghan MU, Negrier C, Paz-Priel I, et al. Long-term outcomes with emicizumab prophylaxis for hemophilia A with or without FVIII inhibitors from the HAVEN 1-4 studies. *Blood.* 2021;137:2231-2242.

A4. Peyvandi F, Mannucci PM, Garagiola I, et al. A randomized trial of factor VIII and neutralizing antibodies in hemophilia A. *N Engl J Med.* 2016;374:2054-2064.

A5. Oldenburg J, Mahlangu JN, Kim B, et al. Emicizumab prophylaxis in hemophilia A with inhibitors. *N Engl J Med.* 2017;377:809-818.

A6. Oldenburg J, Mahlangu JN, Bujan W, et al. The effect of emicizumab prophylaxis on health-related outcomes in persons with haemophilia A with inhibitors: HAVEN 1 Study. *Haemophilia.* 2019;25:33-44.

A7. Dufrost V, Wahl D, Zuily S. Direct oral anticoagulants in antiphospholipid syndrome: meta-analysis of randomized trials. *Autoimmun Rev.* 2021;20:102711.

161

DISSEMINATED INTRAVASCULAR COAGULATION AND BLEEDING IN LIVER FAILURE

ANDREW I. SCHAFER

DISSEMINATED INTRAVASCULAR COAGULATION

DEFINITION

Disseminated intravascular coagulation (DIC), also referred to as consumptive coagulopathy or defibrination, is caused by a wide variety of serious disorders (Table 161-1). In most patients, the underlying process dominates the clinical picture, but in some cases (e.g., occult malignant neoplasm, envenomation), DIC may be the initial or predominant manifestation of the disorder. DIC never occurs in isolation, without an inciting cause.

PATHOBIOLOGY

DIC is primarily a thrombotic process from a pathophysiologic perspective. However, its clinical manifestation may appear to be widespread hemorrhage in acute cases. The basic pathophysiologic mechanism (Fig. 161-1), regardless of cause, is entry into the circulation of procoagulant substances that trigger systemic activation of the coagulation system and platelets.[1] This results in disseminated deposition of fibrin-platelet thrombi within the microvasculature. In most cases, the procoagulant stimulus is tissue factor, a lipoprotein that is not normally exposed to blood. In DIC, tissue factor gains access to blood by tissue injury, its elaboration by malignant cells, or its expression on the surface of monocytes and endothelial cells by inflammatory mediators. Components of the inflammatory response and the coagulation system are reciprocally activated in some forms of DIC, such as sepsis. Tissue factor triggers generation of the coagulation protease thrombin, which induces fibrin formation and platelet activation. In some specific cases of DIC, procoagulants other than tissue factor (e.g., a cysteine protease or mucin in certain malignant neoplasms) and proteases other than thrombin (e.g., trypsin in pancreatitis, exogenous enzymes in envenomation) provide the procoagulant stimulus.

In acute, uncompensated DIC, coagulation factors are consumed at a rate in excess of the capacity of the liver to synthesize them, and platelets are consumed in excess of the capacity of bone marrow megakaryocytes to release them. The resulting laboratory manifestations under these circumstances are a prolonged prothrombin time (PT), a prolonged activated partial thromboplastin time (aPTT), and thrombocytopenia. Increased fibrin formation in DIC stimulates a heightened process of secondary fibrinolysis, in which plasminogen activators generate plasmin to digest fibrin (and fibrinogen) into fibrin(ogen) degradation products (FDPs). FDPs are potent circulating anticoagulants that further contribute to the bleeding manifestations of DIC. Intravascular fibrin deposition can cause fragmentation of red blood cells and lead to the appearance of schistocytes in blood smears (see Chapter 143); however, frank microangiopathic hemolytic anemia is unusual in DIC. Occlusive microvascular thrombosis in DIC can compromise the blood supply to some organs and lead to multiorgan failure, particularly when it is accompanied by systemic hemodynamic, inflammatory, and metabolic derangements.

TABLE 161-1 MAJOR CAUSES OF DISSEMINATED INTRAVASCULAR COAGULATION

INFECTIONS
Gram-negative bacterial sepsis
Other bacteria, fungi, viruses, Rocky Mountain spotted fever, malaria
IMMUNOLOGIC REACTIONS
Transfusion reactions (ABO incompatibility)
Organ transplant rejection
Hematopoietic stem cell transplantation
Chimeric antigen receptor (CAR) T-cell therapy
OBSTETRIC COMPLICATIONS
Amniotic fluid embolism
Retained dead fetus
Abruptio placentae
Toxemia, preeclampsia
Septic abortion
MALIGNANT NEOPLASMS
Pancreatic carcinoma
Adenocarcinomas
Acute promyelocytic leukemia
Other neoplasms
LIVER FAILURE
ACUTE PANCREATITIS
ENVENOMATION
RESPIRATORY DISTRESS SYNDROME
TRAUMA, SHOCK
Brain injury
Crush injury
Burns
Hypothermia or hyperthermia
Fat embolism
Hypoxia, ischemia
Surgery
VASCULAR DISORDERS
Giant hemangioma (Kasabach-Merritt syndrome)
Aortic aneurysm
Vascular tumors or malformations

Underlying Causes

DIC always has an underlying cause that must be identified and eliminated if the coagulopathy is to be managed successfully. The development of DIC in some of these disorders is associated with an unfavorable outcome. Infection is the most common cause of DIC. The syndrome is particularly associated with gram-negative or gram-positive sepsis (Chapter 94),[2] although it can be triggered by a variety of other bacterial, fungal, viral, rickettsial, and protozoal microorganisms. Severe acute respiratory syndrome coronavirus 2 (SARS-CoV-2) with coronavirus disease 2019 (COVID-19) infection (Chapter 336) can also be associated with a picture of DIC.[3]

The placenta and uterine contents are rich sources of tissue factor and other procoagulants that are normally excluded from the maternal circulation; a spectrum of clinical manifestations of DIC may accompany obstetric complications when this barrier is breached, especially in the third trimester. These syndromes range from acute, fulminant, and often fatal DIC in amniotic fluid embolism to chronic or subacute DIC with a retained dead fetus. Other obstetric problems associated with DIC include abruptio placentae, toxemia, and septic abortion.

Chronic forms of DIC are caused by a variety of malignant neoplasms, particularly acute myeloid leukemia,[4] pancreatic cancer (Chapter 180), and mucin-secreting adenocarcinomas of the gastrointestinal tract (Chapter 179), in which thrombotic rather than bleeding manifestations predominate. Treatment with all-*trans*-retinoic acid has greatly reduced the incidence of severe DIC in patients with acute promyelocytic leukemia (Chapter 168). Up to 50% of patients develop coagulopathy following chimeric antigen receptor (CAR) T-cell therapy, often in the form of DIC. Likewise, coagulopathy with features of DIC can develop with hematopoietic stem cell transplantation (Chapter 163). It is not known whether liver failure (see later) can cause DIC or whether its coexistence merely exacerbates intravascular coagulation because of impaired clearance of activated clotting factors, plasmin, and FDPs. Snake venom contains a variety of substances that can affect coagulation and endothelial permeability. Bites from rattlesnakes and other vipers can induce profound DIC by introduction of these exogenous toxins and release of endogenous tissue factor through tissue necrosis.

The likelihood and degree of DIC caused by trauma, surgery, and shock (Chapter 92) are related to the extent of tissue damage and the organs involved. The brain is a particularly rich source of tissue factor, so traumatic brain injury (Chapter 368) can precipitate acute DIC.[5] Large aortic aneurysms (Chapter 63), giant hemangiomas, and other vascular malformations can cause subclinical or clinical chronic DIC that is initiated locally within the abnormal vasculature but can spill into the systemic circulation.[6]

CLINICAL MANIFESTATIONS

The clinical manifestations of DIC are determined by the nature, intensity, and duration of the underlying stimulus. The coexistence of liver disease

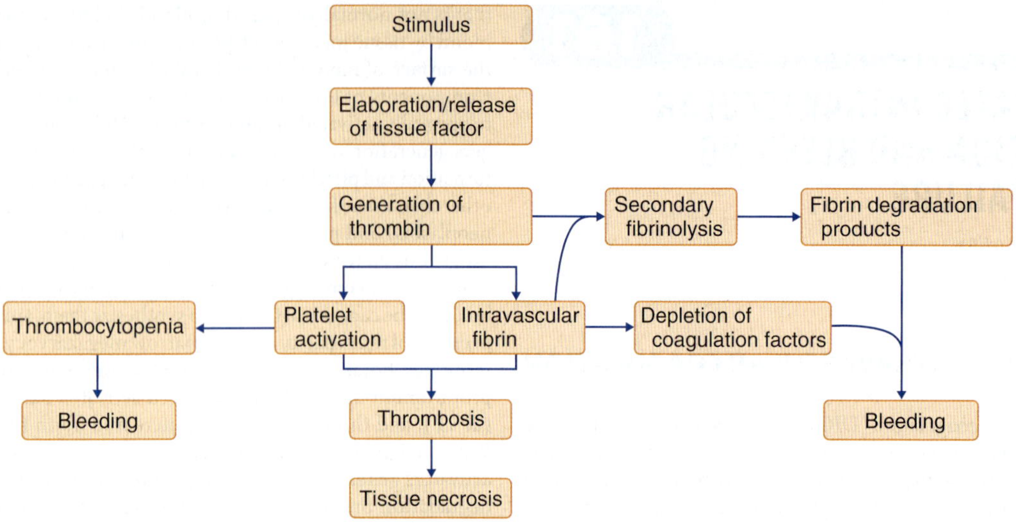

FIGURE 161-1. **Pathophysiologic process of bleeding, thrombosis, and ischemic manifestations in patients with disseminated intravascular coagulation.**

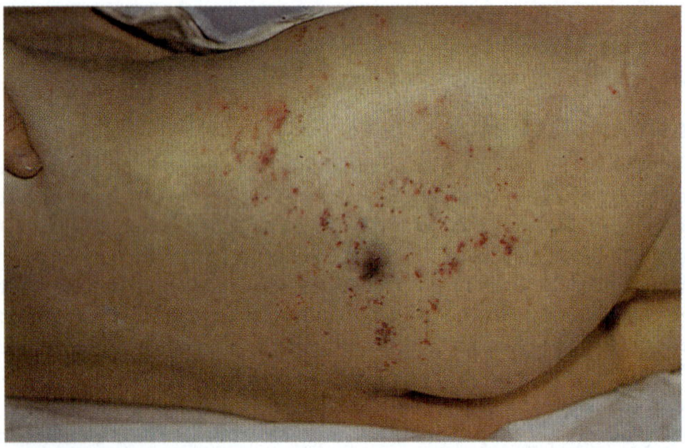

FIGURE 161-2. **Disseminated intravascular coagulation resulting from staphylococcal septicemia. Note the characteristic skin hemorrhage ranging from small purpuric lesions to larger ecchymoses. (From Forbes CD, Jackson WF. *Color Atlas and Text of Clinical Medicine*, 3rd ed. London: Mosby; 2003.)**

exacerbates DIC of any cause. Low-grade DIC is often asymptomatic and diagnosed only by laboratory abnormalities. Thrombotic complications of DIC occur most often with chronic underlying diseases, as exemplified by Trousseau syndrome in cancer (Chapter 67). The thrombotic phenotype of DIC, which occurs prototypically in association with solid tumor malignancies, can manifest as large vessel venous or arterial thrombosis, or as ischemic organ dysfunction due to microvascular thrombosis, or even as a thrombotic microangiopathy. DIC can present as acrocyanosis and gangrene of the digits in critically ill, hemodynamically compromised patients receiving vasopressors. Hemorrhagic necrosis of the skin (Fig. 161-2) and purpura fulminans may also be manifestations of DIC. Bleeding is the most common clinical finding in acute, uncompensated DIC. Bleeding can be limited to sites of intervention or anatomic abnormalities, but it tends to be generalized in more severe cases, including widespread ecchymoses and diffuse oozing from mucosal surfaces and orifices. In these cases, causes of which are exemplified by major trauma, abruptio placentae, or acute promyelocytic leukemia, the precipitating trigger is also a prothrombotic activation of the coagulation system but a fulminant, uncontrolled fibrinolytic response creates a bleeding or so-called fibrinolytic phenotype.

DIAGNOSIS

The laboratory diagnosis of fulminant acute DIC is not usually difficult.[7] Consumption and inhibition of the function of clotting factors cause prolongation of the PT, aPTT, and thrombin time. Consumption of platelets causes thrombocytopenia. Secondary fibrinolysis generates increased titers of FDPs, which can be measured by latex agglutination or D-dimer assays. Some schistocytes may be seen in the peripheral blood smear, but this finding is neither sensitive nor specific for DIC. Chronic or compensated forms of DIC are more difficult to diagnose, with highly variable patterns of abnormalities in "DIC screen" coagulation tests. Increased D-dimers and a prolonged PT are generally more sensitive measures than are abnormalities of the aPTT and platelet count. Overcompensated synthesis of consumed clotting factors and platelets in some chronic forms of DIC may actually cause shortening of the PT and aPTT or thrombocytosis (or both), even though elevated levels of D-dimers indicate secondary fibrinolysis in such cases. Elevated circulating D-dimers are nonspecific, but normal levels have a high negative predictive value for DIC.[8]

The most difficult differential diagnosis of DIC occurs in patients who have coexisting liver disease. The coagulopathy of liver failure (see the later section on liver failure) is often indistinguishable from that of DIC, partly because advanced hepatic dysfunction is in fact accompanied by a state of DIC. In liver failure, the combination of decreased synthesis of clotting factors, impaired clearance of activated clotting factors, secondary fibrinolysis, and thrombocytopenia from portal hypertension and hypersplenism may make the coagulopathy virtually impossible to differentiate from DIC. The coagulopathy associated with postpartum hemorrhage is rarely caused by DIC alone; there may also be varying proportions of dilutional coagulopathy, localized consumption, and increased fibrinolysis. Thrombotic microangiopathies including thrombotic thrombocytopenic purpura and hemolytic-uremic syndrome, the syndrome of "hemolysis, elevated liver enzymes, and low platelet count" (HELLP) in obstetric patients, and other forms of platelet consumption and thrombocytopenia (Chapter 158) are not accompanied by activation of clotting factors or secondary fibrinolysis; therefore, the PT, aPTT, thrombin time, and D-dimers are generally normal in these disorders. Schistocytes, often with frank hemolysis, are much more prominent in the peripheral smear in thrombotic thrombocytopenic purpura and hemolytic-uremic syndrome (Chapter 158) than in DIC. One situation where DIC and thrombotic microangiopathy can overlap and even coexist is in patients with cancer-associated thrombotic microangiopathy. These patients typically have bone marrow involvement and systemic microvascular metastases, either in the setting of known metastatic cancer or unexpectedly on presentation.

TREATMENT

Successful treatment of DIC (Table 161-2) requires that the underlying cause be identified and eliminated. All other therapies, including hemodynamic support, replacement of coagulation factors and platelets, and pharmacologic inhibitors of coagulation and fibrinolysis, are just temporizing measures. Because of the difficulty of testing this complex syndrome with multiple causes by controlled, randomized clinical trials, current guidelines for treatment are generally not based on high-grade evidence.[9]

In many patients with asymptomatic, self-limited DIC who have only laboratory manifestations of the coagulopathy, no treatment may be necessary. In patients with DIC who are actively bleeding or who are at high risk for bleeding, the blood component treatments of choice are transfusions of platelets to improve the thrombocytopenia and fresh-frozen plasma to replace all consumed coagulation factors and to correct the prolonged PT and aPTT. In the absence of robust evidence-based guidelines for the treatment of DIC, an

TABLE 161-2 TREATMENT OF DISSEMINATED INTRAVASCULAR COAGULATION

Identify and eliminate the underlying cause
No treatment if mild, asymptomatic, and self-limited
Hemodynamic support, as indicated, in severe cases
Blood component therapy
- *Indications:* active bleeding or high risk for bleeding
  - Fresh-frozen plasma
  - Platelets
  - In some cases, consider cryoprecipitate, antithrombin III

Drug therapy
- *Indications:* heparin for DIC manifested by thrombosis or acrocyanosis and without active bleeding; antifibrinolytic agents are generally contraindicated except with life-threatening bleeding and failure of blood component therapy

DIC = disseminated intravascular coagulation.

international consensus group recommended VTE prophylaxis in critically ill DIC patients, switching from pharmacologic to mechanical prophylaxis in the case of bleeding and maintaining platelets at greater than 20,000. For some patients who have particularly profound hypofibrinogenemia, the additional transfusion of cryoprecipitate, a plasma concentrate that is enriched in fibrinogen, may be useful. The theoretical concern that these blood products could "fuel the fire" and exacerbate the DIC has not been supported by clinical experience.

The use of pharmacologic inhibitors of coagulation and fibrinolysis in DIC is controversial. Heparin is of theoretical benefit because it blocks thrombin activity and quenches intravascular coagulation and the resultant secondary fibrinolysis. In practice, heparin might exacerbate the bleeding tendency in acute DIC. Heparin is usually reserved for special forms of DIC, including those manifested by thrombosis or acrocyanosis and forms that accompany cancer, vascular malformations, retained dead fetus, and possibly acute promyelocytic leukemia, in which active bleeding is not present. A meta-analysis of randomized controlled trials of anticoagulant therapy specifically in patients with sepsis and sepsis-induced DIC showed an increased risk of bleeding but significant reduction in mortality only in patients who had DIC.[A1] In cases of DIC in which thrombosis or acral ischemia predominates, unfractionated heparin should be used by continuous infusion because of its short half-life and reversibility in the event of increased bleeding. Monitoring the aPTT in the presence of DIC may be problematic, so heparin infusion in this setting should be followed mainly by clinical response and improvement in results of other tests of coagulation (e.g., thrombocytopenia). Antifibrinolytic agents, including ε-aminocaproic acid and tranexamic acid, are generally contraindicated in DIC. By blocking the secondary fibrinolytic response to DIC, these drugs cause unopposed fibrin deposition and may precipitate thrombosis. Antifibrinolytic agents may be effective in decreasing life-threatening bleeding in DIC, however, particularly in extreme cases in which aggressive blood component replacement fails to control the hemorrhage; in such situations, simultaneous infusion of low doses of heparin is needed to reduce the risk for thrombosis.

Antithrombin III and recombinant human soluble thrombomodulin[10] may have some efficacy in improving laboratory parameters of DIC, but neither reduces mortality significantly. Specific surgical treatments and pharmacotherapy may be required for treatment of DIC in patients with aortic aneurysm or vascular malformations.

LIVER FAILURE

Bleeding complications in patients with advanced liver disease (Chapters 139 and 140) can be severe and even fatal and directly account for about 20% of the deaths associated with hepatic failure. Procoagulant abnormalities often coexist. The extent of the bleeding tendency depends on the severity and type of liver disease involved. However, the hemostatic profile in liver failure is unrelated to the Model for End-stage Liver Disease (MELD) score (Table 139-2).[11] About one third of deaths in patients undergoing liver transplantation are attributable to perioperative hemorrhage.

PATHOBIOLOGY

The pathophysiologic mechanism of bleeding in liver failure is multifactorial. The complexity of the systemic coagulopathy of hepatic disease is not surprising inasmuch as the liver is the principal organ site for the synthesis of almost all the coagulation and fibrinolytic factors as well as their inhibitors. (Hepatocytes synthesize all the clotting factors except for von Willebrand factor [vWF], which serves as a physiologic "carrier" and stabilizer of factor VIII, so the elevated levels of vWF that are seen in liver disease can enable near-normal circulating levels of factor VIII despite diminished synthesis of the latter.) Thus, the abnormal hemostasis of liver failure is accompanied by opposing antithrombotic and prothrombotic alterations. Unfortunately, currently available laboratory tests of coagulation, with the possible future exception of thromboelastography (Chapter 157), cannot measure the net effect of the complex, incongruous hemostatic forces that are at work at any given time on clinical bleeding or thrombotic risk in a patient with liver disease. For example, the PT/international normalized ratio (INR) is still accepted as a valid prognostic marker of liver failure, but can no longer be considered a reliable indicator of bleeding tendency in these patients. Although the degree of prolongation of the PT/INR was commonly used in the past to guide treatment with fresh-frozen plasma (FFP) or prothrombin complex concentrate (PCC), it is now recognized that it is not a useful predictor of bleeding after surgery or an invasive procedure. This explains why having certain prolongations of the PT/INR and aPTT as a function of liver disease cannot be regarded as being functionally "auto-anticoagulated"; this notion is a seriously misleading fallacy.

The opposing hemostatic forces at work due to liver failure include (1) decreased *total* levels of circulating clotting factors (caused by consumption of the factors), (2) hypo- or dysfibrinogenemia, (3) enhanced fibrinolysis, and (4) increased levels of fibrin degradation products that act as circulating anticoagulants. All these forces promote bleeding, with simultaneously (1) increased levels of *activated* clotting factors (caused by impaired hepatic clearance), (2) decreased levels of the physiologic anticoagulant proteins antithrombin III (AT III), protein C and protein S (caused by consumption of those proteins), (3) elevated levels of von Willebrand factor and factor VIII, and (4) low plasminogen, all promoting thrombosis. Two factors that may tip the balance more toward a bleeding than a thrombotic phenotype in most of these patients are thrombocytopenia and anatomically vulnerable sites of bleeding in the GI tract, such as esophageal and gastric varices, gastritis (congestive gastropathy), and hemorrhoids.

There is an increased incidence of deep vein thrombosis and/or pulmonary embolism in patients with chronic liver disease (ranging from 0.5 to 6% in different studies). There is an even higher risk of portal vein thrombosis (ranging from 7 to 18% in different series; Chapter 129).[12]

Quantitative and qualitative abnormalities of platelets also contribute to the bleeding diathesis of liver failure. Congestive splenomegaly secondary to portal hypertension causes increased pooling of platelets in the spleen (hypersplenism). The resultant thrombocytopenia, the degree of which generally correlates with spleen size, rarely causes a reduction in the platelet count to less than 30,000/μL. In alcoholic patients, suppression of bone marrow thrombopoiesis by the acute toxic effects of alcohol or folate deficiency may contribute to the thrombocytopenia. Qualitative platelet abnormalities have also been described in patients with liver disease.

Liver transplantation (Chapter 140) poses special problems to the coagulation system. During the 2-hour or so anhepatic stage of surgery, defined as the time from physical removal of the liver from the recipient to recirculation of the graft, the complete cessation of synthesis of coagulation factors causes further prolongation of the PT and aPTT. Release of tissue plasminogen activator from the newly grafted liver leads to increased fibrinolysis and transient exacerbation of bleeding risk in the postoperative period.

CLINICAL MANIFESTATIONS

The most common hemorrhagic complication of liver disease is gastrointestinal bleeding, which is usually caused by anatomic abnormalities and exacerbated by the systemic coagulopathy of liver failure. Bleeding from other mucosal sites, extensive ecchymoses, or more serious hemorrhage into the retroperitoneum or central nervous system generally indicates more significant derangements of the coagulation system.

The severe coagulopathy in patients with liver disease makes liver biopsy a potentially hazardous procedure. The PT and platelet count may be the best guides to bleeding risk, but they lack reliability as predictors of risk of bleeding with liver biopsy. In general, liver biopsy can be performed safely if the platelet count is higher than 50,000/μL. The American Association for the Study of Liver Diseases has concluded that the bleeding risk-benefit ratio of liver biopsy must be carefully considered on a case-by-case basis.

DIAGNOSIS

Although the PT and aPTT are often prolonged in patients with advanced liver disease, the PT tends to be a more sensitive assay early in the course; a disproportionate prolongation of the aPTT should raise suspicion of a coexisting coagulation abnormality, such as a lupus anticoagulant or clotting factor inhibitor. A prolonged PT is also a useful prognostic indicator of poor outcome in patients with cirrhosis, acute acetaminophen hepatotoxicity, and acute viral hepatitis; in acute viral hepatitis, it is a better index of prognosis than are serum albumin and transaminases. A disproportionate prolongation of the thrombin time should suggest the presence of dysfibrinogenemia. Hypersplenism (Chapter 154), possibly associated with nutritional folate deficiency or the acute toxic effects of alcohol on bone marrow, often causes mild to moderate thrombocytopenia in patients with liver disease. Thrombocytopenia in liver disease can also be due to impaired synthesis of thrombopoietin, the primary megakaryocytopoietic growth factor (Chapter 142). However, consideration should be given to other coexisting causes of thrombocytopenia if the platelet count is significantly less than 30,000/μL.

The coagulopathy of liver failure is often indistinguishable from that of DIC, in part because some degree of DIC is in fact a necessary accompaniment of advanced liver disease. In general, patients with DIC have more marked decreases in levels of factor VIII and increases in D-dimer than do patients with liver failure.

A combination of conventional coagulation tests usually does not provide an accurate overall assessment of in vivo hemostasis in patients with advanced liver disease at any given time. Global coagulation tests, such as thrombelastography (ROTEM), thrombin generation assay, and clot waveform analysis (Chapter 157), would seem to lend themselves ideally to assessing bleeding or thrombotic risk and monitoring the overall hemostatic state of a complex coagulopathy like the one encountered in patients with liver disease. While ROTEM is increasingly used perioperatively in liver transplantation, the clinical utility of these global coagulation assays in chronic liver disease has not yet been well validated. In a randomized study of patients with advanced cirrhosis with active coagulopathy and bleeding, a thromboelastography-guided transfusion strategy led to a significantly lower use of blood components compared with standard of care, without failure to control bleeding, failure to prevent rebleeding, or mortality.[A2]

TREATMENT

Simple clinical coagulation tests such as the PT/INR are of little value in predicting bleeding problems in patients with liver disease,[13] and there is a dearth of evidence that blood component transfusions can predictably avert bleeding complications based on certain cut-off values of PT/INR or platelet count. These observations have driven a significant movement toward more restrictive transfusion strategies in patients with liver disease. Restrictive transfusion policies are now widely used in liver transplantation and have led to significant reductions in intraoperative blood loss and red cell transfusion requirements. By reducing central venous pressures, and consequently portal pressures, performing intraoperative phlebotomy has decreased blood loss with liver transplantation.

Routine transfusion of FFP for prophylaxis of bleeding in coagulopathic liver disease patients is not recommended because patients are unlikely to benefit.[14] Response to FFP is unpredictable and usually does not fully normalize the PT/INR even when multiple units are transfused, in part because FFP and especially stored thawed plasma itself often does not have an INR of less than 1.3. Some institutional guidelines have recommended empirically giving an intravenous dose of vitamin K, which may slightly reduce the PT/INR in liver failure, as well as transfusing cryoprecipitate if the plasma fibrinogen is less than 100 mg/dL (as a concentrated source of fibrinogen) in patients with or without active bleeding who are undergoing invasive procedures. There is little experience with the efficacy of four-factor prothrombin complex concentrate (PCC, Kcentra), which is currently approved for urgent reversal of vitamin K antagonists. Therapeutic plasma transfusion (10 mL/kg) is usually reserved for patients who are actively bleeding despite other treatments, including platelet transfusions if indicated.

In addition to the uncertainty regarding platelet count thresholds for platelet transfusion in patients with liver disease, there are other considerations in those who have portal hypertension with congestive splenomegaly and hypersplenism. Normally, about one third of the total peripheral platelet pool is sequestered in the spleen at any given time. In a patient with hypersplenism, platelet sequestration in the spleen can expand to as much as 90%, depending on the size of the spleen. Much of this splenic platelet pool can be mobilized into the circulation with catecholamines. It is unknown whether this phenomenon also occurs in response to endogenous catecholamines, but it is plausible that the stress of a hemostatic challenge could induce a transient increase in platelet counts, making the baseline level of thrombocytopenia in these patients a significant underestimation of what actually occurs in vivo. Related to the potentially marked expansion of the splenic platelet pool with hypersplenism, transfusion of a given amount of platelets often does not produce the expected "bump" in platelet count, and more units of platelets might be needed to achieve a calculated recovery in peripheral blood. The use of a thrombopoietin-receptor agonist to increase the platelet count is contraindicated based on a randomized trial using eltrombopag to increase the platelet count of thrombocytopenic patients (platelets <50,000 per μL) with chronic liver disease, which was prematurely terminated because of an excess of cases of portal vein thrombosis in the treatment group.

Because of the increased risk of thrombosis, as well as bleeding, in patients with chronic liver disease, prophylactic anticoagulation, especially when hospitalized or immobilized, should not be withheld. Prophylactic doses of low-molecular-weight heparin are safe to use. If there is coexisting kidney disease that precludes its use, prophylactic doses of unfractionated heparin or warfarin can be substituted, although monitoring of the latter may be complicated by a preexisting prolonged INR. In patients who are actively bleeding or have a very low platelet count, mechanical thromboprophylaxis can be substituted for pharmacologic thromboprophylaxis.

VITAMIN K DEFICIENCY

Vitamin K is required for γ-carboxylation of glutamic acid residues of the procoagulant factors II (prothrombin), VII, IX, and X and the anticoagulant factors protein C and protein S via the enzyme, γ-glutamyl carboxylase (GGCX). This post-translational modification normally renders these proteins functionally active in coagulation. The PT is more sensitive than the aPTT in detecting vitamin K deficiency states because factor VII, the only vitamin K–dependent factor that is in the extrinsic pathway of coagulation, is the most labile of these proteins.

The two major sources of vitamin K are dietary intake and synthesis by the bacterial flora of the intestine. In the absence of malabsorption, nutritional deficiency alone rarely causes clinically significant vitamin K deficiency. However, when eradication of gut flora is combined with inadequate dietary intake, as commonly occurs when critically ill patients in intensive care units have no oral intake and are receiving broad-spectrum antibiotics for prolonged periods, clinically significant vitamin K deficiency can be observed. Vitamin K deficiency can also develop in patients receiving total parenteral nutrition unless the infusions are supplemented with vitamin K. Certain mutations of the gene encoding GGCX can also cause a bleeding diathesis.

Vitamin K is absorbed predominantly in the ileum and requires the presence of bile salts. Clinically significant vitamin K deficiency occurs with malabsorption of fat-soluble vitamins secondary to obstructive jaundice (Chapter 141) or with malabsorption caused by intrinsic small bowel diseases, including celiac sprue, short bowel syndrome, and inflammatory bowel disease (Chapters 126 and 127).

Warfarin acts as an anticoagulant by competitive antagonism of vitamin K. Rare cases of hereditary deficiency of the vitamin K–dependent coagulation factors may cause a lifelong bleeding tendency.

Correction of vitamin K deficiency, when it is clinically significant, can be achieved with oral supplementation, unless malabsorption is present, in which case parenteral vitamin K (10 mg subcutaneously daily) should be administered. Patients on vitamin K antagonist therapy who have a supratherapeutic INR between 4.5 and 10.0 without bleeding are not likely to benefit from vitamin K administration in addition to stopping the anticoagulant.[A3] Emergency treatment of bleeding caused by vitamin K deficiency is transfusion of fresh-frozen plasma or four-factor prothrombin complex concentrate.

GENERAL REFERENCES

For the General References and other additional features, please visit Elsevier eBooks+ at https://ebooks.health.elsevier.com.

Grade A References

A1. Umemura Y, Yamakawa K, Ogura H, et al. Efficacy and safety of anticoagulant therapy in three specific populations with sepsis: a meta-analysis of randomized controlled trials. *J Thromb Haemost.* 2016;14:518-530.

A2. Kumar M, Ahmad J, Maiwall R, et al. Thromboelastography-guided blood component use in patients with cirrhosis with nonvariceal bleeding: a randomized controlled trial. *Hepatology.* 2020;71:235-246.

A3. Khatib R, Ludwikowska M, Witt DM, et al. Vitamin K reversal of excessive vitamin K antagonist anticoagulation: a systematic review and meta-analysis. *Blood Adv.* 2019;3:789-796.

162

TRANSFUSION MEDICINE

BETH H. SHAZ AND CHRISTOPHER D. HILLYER

Blood transfusion can be lifesaving and is currently the safest it has ever been. However, blood transfusion is associated with multiple adverse outcomes, including both noninfectious and infectious complications. The benefits and risks of transfusion can be considered for each patient using evidence-based, multidisciplinary approaches to reduce unnecessary transfusions and improve patients' outcomes. As a result, the number of units of blood transfused has declined substantially in the United States and worldwide. In the United States, for example, about 10.6 million units of red blood cells (RBCs) are now transfused annually, a decrease from the high of 14.8 million units in 2008.[1]

BLOOD COMPONENTS

The majority of blood collections are whole blood, which can then be separated into plasma, platelets, and red blood cell (RBC) components. In the United States, 85% of RBC units are manufactured from whole blood and more than 90% of platelet components are collected by apheresis.

The majority of blood is transfused as component therapy, tailored to the need of a specific patient. Blood components such as RBCs, plasma, platelets, or granulocytes are obtained either from donation of whole blood or via apheresis (Table 162-1). Each component is stored under their respective optimal conditions; RBCs are refrigerated with additive solutions to improve long-term storage, plasma is frozen to preserve clotting factors, and platelets are stored at room temperature to preserve function and post-transfusion survival. As needed, components can be modified (e.g., irradiated) or selected (e.g., hemoglobin S negative) to meet specific patient requirements.

WHOLE BLOOD

Whole blood contains RBCs, platelets, and plasma. It is stored refrigerated unless used shortly after collection. The shelf-life depends on the storage conditions and preservation solution used. Whole blood provides oxygen-carrying capacity (RBCs) and coagulation support (plasma and platelets). Whole blood has largely been replaced by individual blood components because most patients only require one component (RBCs, platelets, or plasma).

However, whole blood can be useful particularly for trauma patients. The military uses a walking donor program for fresh whole blood, which is stored at 22° C for less than 24 hours. This product has addressed blood component shortages, particularly for platelet products, in austere environments. For civilian trauma, some institutions use cold stored (2° to 6° C) whole blood, which may or may not be leukoreduced (i.e., depleted of leukocytes).

RED BLOOD CELL COMPONENTS

RBC components are usually prepared from whole blood by removing 200 to 250 mL of plasma after centrifugation. RBC components can also be manufactured by apheresis, which can collect two components from a single donor. RBC components are stored at 1° to 6° C, which allows for 42-day storage. General characteristics of RBC components include 130 to 240 mL of RBCs, 50 to 80 g of hemoglobin, and 150 to 250 mg of iron per unit. The total volume (250 to 350 mL), and hematocrit (55 to 80%), vary depending on the volume of blood collected (450 versus 500 mL) and the specific preservative and additive solution used, which also determine its shelf life. RBCs have a hematocrit of 65 to 80% and a shelf life of 21 days when stored in citrate-phosphate-dextrose (CPD), a hematocrit of 65 to 80% and a shelf life of 35 days when stored in CPDA-1, and a hematocrit of 55 to 65% and a shelf life of 42 days when stored in additive solutions. In the United States, most RBC components are stored in additive solutions and contain small amounts of plasma, platelets, and leukocytes, unless the latter have been removed by leukoreduction filtration (which also removes platelets). Canada and many countries in Europe have a universally leukoreduced blood supply.

RED BLOOD CELL COMPONENT MODIFICATION

RBCs and other blood components can be modified to mitigate the complications of transfusion, such as transmission of infectious agents, and to enhance the preservation of rare components. Modified blood components include leukoreduced, irradiated, pathogen reduced, frozen (also known as cryopreservation), and washed components.

TABLE 162-1 BLOOD PRODUCT CHARACTERISTICS

PRODUCT	VOLUME	COMPOSITION	STORAGE CONDITIONS	STORAGE LENGTH	COMMENTS
Red blood cells	300-350 mL	200 mL RBCs, 30-40 mL plasma, 100-110 mL anticoagulant and additive solution	1-6° C	CPD: 21 days CPDA-1: 35 days AS: 42 days	• Leukoreduced: <5 × 10^6 leukocytes • Red blood cells must be ABO compatible with patient plasma • D compatible for females with childbearing potential
Platelets	50 mL per whole blood derived platelet component; 200-400 mL/apheresis component	Platelets suspended in sufficient plasma or platelet additive solution	20-24° C with constant gentle agitation	5 days or 7 days with additional bacterial mitigation Pooled in an open system: 4 hrs	• Whole blood derived platelets: 5.5 × 10^{10} platelets/unit • Whole blood derived platelets into pools of 4-6 units • Apheresis platelets: 3 × 10^{11} platelets • Pool or apheresis, leukoreduced: <5 × 10^6 leukocytes • ABO or D compatible is not required
Plasma	200-250 mL	One mL of plasma contains one unit of coagulation factor activity	−18° C; 1-6° C after thawing	Frozen shelf life: 1 yr FFP/FP24/PF24RT24 after thaw: 24 hrs Thawed plasma: 5 days	• FFP: Plasma frozen within 8 hrs of phlebotomy • FP24: Plasma frozen within 24 hrs of phlebotomy • PF24RT24: Plasma frozen within 24 hrs after phlebotomy held at room temperature up to 24 hrs after phlebotomy • Thawed plasma: FFP/FP24/FP24RT24 stored for up to 4 days beyond outdate • Plasma must be ABO compatible with patient RBCs • D compatible is not required
Cryoprecipitate	10-15 mL/unit	80-120 units Factor VIII, >150 mg Fibrinogen, Factor XIII, vWF	−18° C; room temperature after thawing	Frozen shelf life: 1 yr Thawed/pooled in an open system: 4 hrs Thawed/pooled in a closed system: 6 hrs	• ABO and RhD compatible cryoprecipitate is not required

AS = additive solution; CPD = citrate-phosphate-dextrose (anticoagulant); CPDA = citrate-phosphate-dextrose-adenine (anticoagulant); FFP = fresh frozen plasma; RBCs = red blood cells; vWf = von Willebrand factor.

Leukoreduction

To remove 99.9% of the white blood cells (yielding $<5 \times 10^6$ white blood cells per component), most RBC and platelet components transfused in the United States are leukoreduced. This process decreases the risk of febrile nonhemolytic transfusion reactions, transfusion-transmitted cytomegalovirus (CMV) and other leukocyte-transmitted infections, HLA alloimmunization, and a transient depression of the immune system after transfusion.

Irradiation and Cryopreservation

Irradiation of cellular blood components prevents transfusion-associated graft-versus-host disease (GVHD). Irradiation of RBCs shortens their storage period.

Freezing of RBCs extends their storage capability to 10 or more years. RBCs with rare phenotypes can therefore be frozen and banked for prolonged periods and be more readily available for patients who have antibodies to high-frequency antigens or rare combinations of antigens. After thawing, frozen RBCs must be washed to remove the cryoprotectant (glycerol). Because washed cellular blood components are depleted of plasma proteins, they are the preferred products for patients with a history of allergic, anaphylactoid, or anaphylactic reactions. Washed RBCs expire 24 hours after washing.

Pathogen Reduction

Pathogen reduction inactivates nucleic acids in viruses and bacteria and thus reduces the risk of transfusion-transmitted pathogens, both known and unknown. It also inactivates residual white blood cells, thereby eliminating the need for irradiation. Pathogen-reduced platelets[2] and plasma are used preferentially in some European countries and are increasingly being used in the United States. Pathogen-reduced plasma, particularly plasma treated with a solvent detergent, has a very low adverse event rate. RBC components derived from pathogen-reduced whole blood are approved in Europe, the Middle East, and Africa and are undergoing clinical trials for approval in other countries. Pathogen-reduced RBCs have a shortened shelf-life. In the United States, pathogen-reduced cryoprecipitate is approved for use in acquired fibrinogen deficiency or for replacement of factor XIII or von Willebrand factor when specific factor concentrates are not available.

PLATELET COMPONENTS

Platelet components can be produced from whole blood or apheresis collections and generally have a volume of approximately 300 mL. Platelets derived from whole blood are commonly referred to as *random donor platelets, platelet concentrates*, or *buffy coat platelets*. Each unit derived from whole blood contains approximately 0.5×10^{11} platelets. Typically 5 units are pooled to provide a therapeutic dose of 3.0×10^{11} platelets. Platelets collected by apheresis (or plateletpheresis) are referred to as *single donor platelets* or *apheresis platelets*. The required minimum content for a platelet component collected by apheresis is 3.0×10^{11} platelets, but many apheresis-derived platelet collections contain two or three times the required minimum and are therefore split to make multiple platelet components from a single collection. Outside the United States, platelets are made from whole blood using the buffy coat method. These are then pooled and stored in either platelet additive solution or a single donor's plasma. Platelet components can be stored for up to 7 days.

Platelet components are screened for the presence of bacteria to prevent septic transfusion reactions. Also, platelet and plasma components are prepared to reduce the risk of transfusion-related acute lung injury by selecting male or never-pregnant female donors or testing previously pregnant donors for HLA antibodies. Finally, platelets stored in platelet additive solutions have less plasma and thus are less likely to result in allergic reactions and hemolytic reactions due to ABO incompatibility between the donor and recipient.

Another product modification, cold-stored platelets, is emerging for use in trauma or during major bleeding. In the United States, cold-stored (1° to 6° C) platelets are approved with a 14-day shelf life when standard room temperature platelets are not available. These platelets remain in circulation less than 24 hours compared to 5 to 7 days for platelets stored at room temperature.

PLASMA COMPONENTS

Plasma components can be produced from whole blood after centrifugation and removal of RBCs or by apheresis. Notably, the following information applies to the United States, but other countries have simpler terms for their plasma components. *Fresh frozen plasma* (FFP) is frozen at −18° C or colder within 8 hours of collection. Plasma frozen at −18° C or colder within 24 hours of collection is referred to as *plasma frozen within 24 hours after phlebotomy. Plasma frozen within 24 hours after phlebotomy held at room temperature up to 24 hours after phlebotomy* prepared from apheresis collections is also available. Once frozen, plasma has a frozen shelf life of 1 year. Prior to transfusion, plasma must be thawed to 30° to 37° C, a process that takes 20 to 30 minutes. Thawed plasma should be transfused immediately or stored at 1° to 6° C for up to 24 hours. Thawed plasma can be stored for up to 4 additional days at 1° to 6° C to prevent wastage. FFP contains approximately 1 IU/mL of each clotting factor. From a clinical perspective, all plasma products are essentially equivalent.

Other plasma components which are less commonly used include *cryoprecipitate-reduced plasma* and *liquid plasma*. Cryoprecipitate-reduced plasma, which is the plasma remaining after cryoprecipitate is removed, is mostly deficient in factor VIII, fibrinogen, von Willebrand factor, factor XIII, and fibronectin. The sole clinical indication for cryoprecipitate-reduced plasma is in the treatment of thrombocytopenic thrombotic purpura (Chapter 158). Liquid plasma, stored at 1° to 6° C, is separated from whole blood and transfused no later than 5 days after the expiration date of the whole blood. This product contains viable lymphocytes, so it requires irradiation to prevent transfusion-associated graft-versus-host disease in high-risk recipients, such as patients who are immunocompromised.

CRYOPRECIPITATE

Cryoprecipitate is manufactured by thawing FFP at 1° to 6° C. During this thawing process, a precipitate forms (the cryoprecipitate), is separated, and is refrozen. Cryoprecipitate is selectively enriched in fibrinogen, fibronectin, factor VIII, von Willebrand factor, and factor XIII. Cryoprecipitate and its supernatant (cryoprecipitate-poor plasma) are separately refrozen and stored for up to 1 year after collection.

Each unit of cryoprecipitate contains at least 150 mg fibrinogen and 80 IU of factor VIII. A single 10 to 15 mL unit of cryoprecipitate should increase the fibrinogen concentration by approximately 50 mg/dL per 10 kg of body weight. Most blood centers provide prepooled cryoprecipitate, which typically consists of 5 units of cryoprecipitate and which is easier for the hospital transfusion service to prepare. For adult patients, the typical order is a dose of 5 to 10 units of cryoprecipitate.

GRANULOCYTES

Granulocytes have a 24-hour shelf life and are stored at room temperature without agitation. Mostly they are collected by apheresis using hydroxyethyl starch to improve collection. In order to increase the number of granulocytes collected, the donor may be stimulated with steroids to yield components with approximately 1×10^{10} granulocytes and donors stimulated with steroids and granulocyte colony-stimulating factor (G-CSF; Chapter 142) to yield components with approximately 1×10^{11} granulocytes. Apheresis granulocytes have approximately 200 mL volume, 10 to 50 mL of RBCs, 3×10^{11} platelets (equivalent to a platelet component), and plasma. All granulocytes should be irradiated, cannot be leukoreduced, and should be transfused as soon as possible.

PRETRANSFUSION TESTING

Routine pretransfusion testing of blood components includes receipt of an appropriately labeled patient specimen by the transfusion service, testing of the patient's specimen for ABO group and D type and for the presence of unexpected antibodies, and crossmatching of RBC components with the patient's sample.

In emergency situations and before crossmatch compatible blood components are available, group O RBCs and group AB plasma (some institutions use group A plasma) may be appropriately transfused.

Critical to safe blood transfusion is a properly labeled pretransfusion blood specimen from the intended transfusion recipient. Most hemolytic transfusion reactions are caused by misidentification or labeling errors in pretransfusion blood specimens. Radio-frequency identification technology improves the safety and efficiency.

A "type and screen" involves typing the patient's RBCs for ABO and Rh (also known as RhD or D) type, as well as screening the patient's plasma for clinically significant RBC antibodies. A "type and crossmatch" also includes the selection, crossmatching, and reserving of appropriate RBC components for the transfusion recipient. Many institutions have a maximum surgical blood order schedule, which indicates when a type and screen is ordered and how many components should be reserved for each type of surgical procedure.

RBC antibodies of clinical significance are formed in response to pregnancy or transfusion; they may cause hemolysis or shortened survival of transfused RBCs carrying the reciprocal antigen (i.e., acute or delayed hemolytic transfusion reaction). For this reason, the intended recipient's plasma is screened for the presence of these unexpected antibodies prior to RBC transfusion. If a patient has a clinically significant antibody, the transfusion service will select and reserve the appropriate RBC components that do not carry the reciprocal antigen. The process of identifying a patient's RBC antibody and crossmatching the appropriate RBC components can take hours or even days, depending on the antibody or antibodies found. It can be particularly problematic when the intended recipient has autoantibodies (Chapter 146).

How far in advance a specimen can be drawn is determined by institutional policies. In patients with a negative antibody screen and no history of transfusion or pregnancy in the preceding 3 months, specimens may be drawn up to 1 month before surgery. However, if the patient has been transfused or has been pregnant in the preceding 3 months, a pretransfusion specimen is valid only for 3 days. Most hospitalized patients require a new specimen every 3 days.

ABO/D COMPATIBILITY

Individuals naturally have antibodies against the ABO groups they do not carry (i.e., group O individuals have anti-A and anti-B, group A individuals have anti-B, group B individuals have anti-A, and group AB individuals have none). RBC components must be major ABO compatible and usually D compatible. Group O is the universal RBC component because the RBCs carry no A or B group antigens, whereas group AB RBCs can only be transfused to group AB individuals, group A RBCs can only be transfused to group A or AB individuals, and group B RBCs can only be transfused to group B or AB individuals. Incompatible RBC transfusions may result in acute hemolytic transfusion reactions.

In contrast, D-negative individuals do not make anti-D unless exposed to D-positive RBCs through previous pregnancy or transfusion. D-negative females of childbearing potential must receive D-negative RBCs, unless unavailable in emergency situations, to prevent anti-D formation which may result in hemolytic disease of the fetus and newborn. If there is a shortage of D-negative RBCs, males and females not of childbearing potential (usually defined as age ≥50 years old) can receive D-positive components. The risk of anti-D formation from D-positive RBC unit is about 10 to 20%.

Plasma, which contains antibodies, should be minor ABO compatible such that group AB plasma is the universal product. Group A plasma can be transfused to group A or O individuals, group B to group B or group O individuals, and group O to group O individuals. Group A plasma is being used in massive transfusion settings due to the limited availability of group AB plasma (4% of the population is group AB). This practice appears safe, particularly given that these patients are receiving group O RBCs and are switched to type-specific components once the blood type is known. Plasma is not D-matched because no RBCs are in the product.

Platelets are typically transfused with ABO matching. ABO compatibility results in higher post-transfusion platelet count increment. To decrease the risk of hemolytic transfusion reactions from incompatible plasma, low titer (of anti-A) group O products are used. Risk of anti-D with D-positive to D-negative patients is less than 1%. Granulocytes should be major ABO compatible due to their contamination with RBC and subsequent risk of acute hemolytic transfusion reaction.

BLOOD SAFETY

Adverse events of blood transfusion occur in 0.2% of transfusions, and about 7% of these events are serious. Adverse events can be classified as acute (within hours) or delayed (days to years), and as noninfectious or infectious (Table 162-2 and Table 162-3).[3] Infectious risks include emerging infections, such as *Babesia*, and traditional infections, such as hepatitis B or C. With improvement in donor screening for transmissible diseases, more focus has been on reducing noninfectious transfusion reactions.[4,5]

NONINFECTIOUS ADVERSE EFFECTS OF BLOOD TRANSFUSION

ACUTE HEMOLYTIC TRANSFUSION REACTION

Acute hemolytic transfusion reactions occur when preformed recipient antibodies bind to transfused RBC antigens, thereby resulting in the formation of an antigen-antibody complex.[6] This complex activates the complement cascade and causes intravascular hemolysis. Most commonly, acute hemolytic transfusion reactions are severe reactions due to ABO incompatibility, usually because transfused RBC antigens are incompatible with the recipient's plasma (e.g., group A RBCs into group O recipient), and less commonly when transfused plasma contains antibodies against the recipient's RBC antigens (e.g., group O plasma into group A recipient). Acute hemolytic transfusion reactions can also be associated with antigen-antibody complexes outside of the ABO system. The destruction of RBCs also may result in mechanical hemolysis unrelated to the transfusion.

The incidence of acute hemolytic transfusion reactions is approximately 1 : 110,000 transfusions, and these rates have substantially decreased over time. About 70% of transfusion reactions are due to RBCs and 30% due to platelet transfusions. ABO-incompatible RBC transfusions most commonly occur with mistransfusion, when the patient receives an incorrect unit. Mistransfusion is usually caused by human error, including improper identification of the intended recipient during pretransfusion sample collection, improper ABO typing of the blood component or the intended recipient, or improper identification of the recipient or the blood component at the time of transfusion.

CLINICAL MANIFESTATIONS AND DIAGNOSIS

The signs and symptoms of acute hemolytic transfusion reactions are fever, chills/rigors, anxiety, chest and abdominal pain, flank and back pain, nausea, vomiting, dyspnea, hemoglobinuria, diffuse bleeding, and oliguria/anuria. If

TABLE 162-2 NONINFECTIOUS TRANSFUSION-ASSOCIATED EVENTS

TRANSFUSION-ASSOCIATED ADVERSE EVENT	RISK PER UNIT TRANSFUSED IN THE UNITED STATES
Acute hemolytic transfusion reaction	≈1 : 110,000 transfusions
Febrile nonhemolytic transfusion reaction	≈1 : 1100
Allergic transfusion reaction	≈1 : 1200 ≈1 : 15,500 severe
Transfusion-associated circulatory overload	≈1 : 9000
Transfusion-related acute lung injury	≈1 : 140,000
Hypotensive transfusion reactions	≈1 : 32,000
Transfusion-associated dyspnea	≈1 : 28,000
Delayed hemolytic transfusion reaction	≈1 : 32,000
Delayed serologic transfusion reaction	≈1 : 8000
Transfusion-associated graft-versus-host disease	<1 : 10,000,000
Post-transfusion purpura	≈1 : 10,000,000

TABLE 162-3 INFECTIOUS DISEASE WINDOW PERIOD AND RESIDUAL RISK

TEST	WINDOW PERIOD (DAYS)	RESIDUAL RISK OF TRANSFUSION
HIV MP-NAT	9	≈1 : 1,800,000
HIV EIA	21	
HCV MP-NAT	7	≈1 : 1,600,000
HCV EIA	51-58	
HBsAg	30-38	≈1 : 300,000
HBV NAT	40-50 (MP) and 15-34 (ID)	≈1 : 1,500,000
HTLV	80	≈1 : 3,300,000
Syphilis		1 reported case in the United States in the last 50 years
Chagas disease		7 reported cases in the U.S.; none since testing
WNV NAT		Last case in 2012
Bacterial contamination		1 : 200,000-1,000,000 with addition of multiple mitigation strategies

EIA = enzyme immunoassay; HBsAg = hepatitis B virus surface antigen; HBV NAT = hepatitis B virus nucleic acid test; HCV = hepatitis C virus; HIV = human immunodeficiency virus; HTLV = human T-cell leukemia-lymphoma virus; ID = individual donor nucleic acid testing; MP-NAT = mini-pool nucleic acid testing; WNV NAT = West Nile virus nucleic acid test.

an acute hemolytic transfusion reaction is suspected, the transfusion should be stopped immediately, the reaction should be reported to the transfusion service for investigation, and the unit should be returned to the blood bank. Diagnosis is based on laboratory evidence of hemolysis (e.g., decreased hemoglobin, decreased haptoglobin, hemoglobinuria, and elevated lactate dehydrogenase) and evidence of incompatible blood transfusion (e.g., positive direct antiglobulin test and incompatible crossmatch). Approximately 50% of ABO-incompatible RBC transfusions have no adverse effect, but 5% are fatal.

TREATMENT AND PREVENTION

Treatment includes saline infusion (and potentially the addition of low-dose dopamine) to maintain blood pressure and adequate urine output; a diuretic (e.g., furosemide) to increase renal blood flow; and plasma, cryoprecipitate, platelets, and heparin as needed for disseminated intravascular coagulopathy (Chapter 161).

Acute hemolytic transfusion reactions can be mitigated by decreasing the risk of ABO incompatible blood transfusion. Mislabeling of patient samples remains the major factor contributing to ABO incompatibility. Processes to address this problem include improved tracking and labeling of specimens, use of radiofrequency identification systems, and policies to require two separate blood draws for ABO typing prior to releasing type-specific RBC components.

Febrile Nonhemolytic Transfusion Reaction

Febrile nonhemolytic transfusion reaction, with an incidence of approximately 1 : 1100 transfusions, is defined as a temperature increase of 1° C or more or greater than 38° C and/or chills/rigors occurring within 4 hours of cessation of transfusion.[7] The incidence of febrile nonhemolytic transfusion reactions has significantly decreased with the widespread use of leukoreduction.

By definition, the temperature increase cannot be attributed to other etiologies. In platelet components, febrile nonhemolytic transfusion reactions are caused by leukocyte-derived cytokines that accumulate in the component during storage. With RBC components, these reactions are caused by donor leukocytes interacting with patient white blood cell antibodies.

If a febrile nonhemolytic transfusion reaction is suspected, the transfusion should be stopped and reported to the transfusion service to exclude a more serious transfusion-associated adverse event. Supportive care should be administered.

Allergic Transfusion Reaction

Allergic transfusion reactions have an overall incidence of approximately 1 : 1200 transfusions. Most allergic reactions are mild, but about 8% are severe. Platelet transfusions are the blood component most often associated with allergic reactions. Platelets stored in platelet additive solution have less plasma and thus a decreased allergic reaction rate of 0.3% compared with 0.8% for platelets stored in plasma. Solvent/detergent-treated plasma from pooled donors also has lower allergic reaction rates. Anaphylactic reactions (Chapter 233) may be secondary to anti-IgA, which can occur in patients with IgA deficiency.

Mild reactions consist of urticaria with or without generalized pruritus or flushing. More severe symptoms include hoarseness, stridor, wheezing, dyspnea, hypotension, gastrointestinal symptoms, and shock. Patients who have severe allergic reactions should be tested for IgA deficiency and the presence of anti-IgA.

TREATMENT AND PREVENTION

Mild reactions can be treated by temporarily stopping the transfusion and administering antihistamines, whereas severe reactions require discontinuation of the transfusion and treating with epinephrine, H1-receptor antagonists, and corticosteroids. (Chapter 233). Premedication with antihistamines decreases the incidence of allergic reactions, but is recommended only in patients who have a history of allergic reactions. If anti-IgA is identified, the patient should receive plasma components from IgA deficient donors or washed RBC and platelets components.

Transfusion-Associated Circulatory Overload

Transfusion-associated circulatory overload, with an incidence of approximately 1 : 9000 transfusions, results from circulatory overload following transfusion. Risk factors are age older than 70 years, a post-transfusion B-type natriuretic peptide (BNP) greater than 1000 pg/mL, a positive fluid balance of greater than 3 L, and more units transfused within 6 hours. Symptoms and signs include dyspnea, tachypnoea, decreased oxygen saturation, orthopnea, cough, chest tightness, cyanosis, hypertension, and headache. These signs and symptoms usually present at the end of transfusion but may occur up to 12 hours post-transfusion. Diagnosis is based on the presence of fluid overload and elevated levels of BNP or NT-pro BNP (Chapter 45). Management includes discontinuing the transfusion, diuretic therapy, oxygen supplementation, and sitting the patient upright (Chapter 46).

Transfusion-Related Acute Lung Injury

Transfusion-related acute lung injury (TRALI), with an incidence of approximately 1 : 140,000 transfusions, is noncardiogenic pulmonary edema that is associated with the transfusion and that occurs within 6 hours of cessation of transfusion.[8] The incidence of transfusion-related acute lung injury has substantially decreased[9] with the implementation of male-only, HLA antibody–negative, or nulliparous female plasma and platelet donors. Additionally, solvent/detergent-treated plasma has rarely been associated with cases of transfusion-related acute lung injury.

Transfusion-related acute lung injury is most commonly seen following platelet transfusions, and the majority of events are serious. Patient-related risk factors include higher IL-8 levels, liver surgery, chronic alcohol use disorder, shock, higher peak airway pressure while being mechanically ventilated, current smoking, positive fluid balance. Transfusion-related risk factors include the receipt of plasma from female donors and a higher volume of HLA class II human neutrophil antigen positive antibodies. Signs include hypoxemia with radiographic evidence of bilateral infiltrates. Transfusion-related acute lung injury is caused by neutrophil and pulmonary endothelial activation, usually a result of transfused donor white blood cell antibodies, including human leukocyte antigen (HLA) antibodies and human leukocyte antigen antibodies. These donor antibodies react with the recipient's white blood cells in the pulmonary vasculature, thereby causing leukoagglutination, activation of the complement cascade, cytokine release, and pulmonary edema. More rarely, transfusion-related acute lung injury is caused by the converse mechanism in which recipient white blood cell antibodies react against transfused donor white blood cells.

When hypoxemia occurs within 6 hours of transfusion in the absence of other risk factors for acute lung injury, the transfusion-related acute lung injury is called type 1, whereas it is called type 2 in patients who have such risk factors or already have at least mild preexisting acute respiratory distress syndrome or risk factors for it (e.g., pneumonia, inhalation injury, trauma, sepsis, drowning, pancreatitis, burn, shock, cardiopulmonary bypass, or drug overdose).

TREATMENT AND PROGNOSIS

In cases of suspected transfusion-related acute lung injury, the transfusion should be discontinued. Medical management is primarily supportive, commonly with supplemental oxygen and endotracheal intubation if needed. Diuresis is not indicated, and the role of corticosteroids is unclear. The majority of patients improve within 2 to 4 days, although transfusion-related acute lung injury has a 5 to 10% mortality rate.

Hypotensive Transfusion Reactions

Hypotensive transfusion reactions, with an incidence of approximately 1 : 32,000, are usually associated with transfusions of RBCs or platelets. These reactions appear to be related to the generation of bradykinin, thereby resulting in vasodilation and hypotension. Hypotensive reactions have most commonly been reported in association with the use of negatively charged bedside leukoreduction filters in patients being treated with angiotensin-converting enzyme inhibitors. The use of prestorage leukoreduction in lieu of bedside leukoreduction limits the incidence of these reactions. Hypotensive transfusion reactions typically resolve with cessation of transfusion.

Transfusion-Associated Dyspnea

Transfusion-associated dyspnea, with an incidence of approximately 1 : 28,000 transfusions, results in acute respiratory distress within 24 hours of transfusion cessation. It is a diagnosis of exclusion, when allergic reactions, transfusion-associated circulatory overload, and transfusion-related acute lung injury have been excluded.

Delayed Hemolytic and Serologic Transfusion Reaction

Delayed hemolytic transfusion reactions, with an incidence of approximately 1 : 32,000 transfusions, occur when RBC transfusion causes an alloantibody response, thereby resulting in decreased RBC survival. If an alloantibody response is noted in the absence of RBC destruction, it is termed a delayed *serologic* transfusion reaction, which has an incidence of approximately 1 : 8000 transfusions. If alloantibodies are formed within days of transfusion, it is presumed to be an anamnestic alloantibody response in an individual who had previously formed antibodies, usually from an earlier transfusion or pregnancy. If alloantibodies are formed within weeks of transfusion, it is presumed to be a primary alloantibody response.

Delayed hemolytic transfusion reactions are characterized by an unexpected decrease or less than expected increase in the recipient's hemoglobin post-transfusion. Other signs and symptoms, which are typically much less severe than those associated with acute hemolytic transfusion reactions, include fever, chills, jaundice, malaise, back pain, and rarely renal failure. To prevent future reactions, the patient should receive antigen-negative RBCs for future transfusions. The primary mitigation strategy is prophylactic RBC antigen matching.

A severe form of delayed hemolytic transfusion reaction is hyperhemolytic transfusion reaction. This rare reaction, which is most often reported in patients who have sickle cell disease (Chapter 149) or thalassemia (Chapter 148), results in destruction of both donor and recipient RBCs, thereby leading to more severe anemia. Additionally, the patients usually have reticulocytopenia. RBC alloantibodies or autoantibodies may or may not be present. The pathophysiology remains unclear. Treatment includes erythropoietin, intravenous immunoglobulin, corticosteroids, rituximab, tocilizumab, and eculizumab under expert supervision. Future RBC transfusions should be administered cautiously.

Transfusion-Associated Graft-versus-Host Disease

Transfusion-associated graft-versus-host disease (GVHD), with an incidence of less than 1 : 10,000,000 transfusions, results from the engraftment of transfused viable donor lymphocytes in an immunosuppressed recipient. The donor lymphocytes subsequently mount an immune response against the recipient, thereby resulting in pancytopenia, an erythematous rash or even generalized erythroderma, liver dysfunction, and gastrointestinal symptoms. Unlike GVHD associated with hematopoietic progenitor cell transplantation (Chapter 163), transfusion associated-GVHD has a nearly 100% fatality rate due to the profound pancytopenia.

Patients at increased risk for transfusion associated-GVHD include individuals with congenital immunodeficiencies, Hodgkin disease, acute leukemia, or other hematologic malignancies, as well as patients undergoing hematopoietic progenitor cell transplantation. Patients who receive HLA-matched blood components or blood components from close relatives, granulocyte transfusions, intrauterine transfusions, or neonatal red cell exchange are also at increased risk. At-risk patients should receive irradiated or pathogen-reduced cellular blood components, which prevent leukocytes from engrafting.

Post-Transfusion Purpura

Post-transfusion purpura, with an incidence of approximately 1 : 10,000,000 transfusions, is an immune thrombocytopenia caused by antiplatelet alloantibodies, most often anti-HPA-1a (Chapter 158). All types of blood components have been implicated, with transfusion triggering an antibody response to platelet antigens.

Post-transfusion purpura is characterized by acute, profound thrombocytopenia (platelet count <10,000/μL), unexplained purpuric rash, bruising, or mucosal bleeding 1 to 3 weeks post-transfusion. Thirty percent of affected patients have major hemorrhage, and 10% of patients have fatal hemorrhage. Diagnosis is based on the clinical presentation and the identification of platelet-specific alloantibodies. The primary treatment for post-transfusion purpura is intravenous immunoglobulin under expert supervision.

INFECTIOUS COMPLICATIONS OF TRANSFUSION

Criteria for transfusion-transmission of pathogens include: an asymptomatic infectious phase in the donor; an agent's viability during storage; a seronegative recipient population; and an agent capable of causing disease post-transfusion. The transfusion-transmitted infection rate is about 1 : 225,000, and this rate has substantially decreased over time worldwide. Higher rates occur with platelet transfusions, and the majority are severe reactions. About 50% of the reactions are bacterial and about 50% are parasitic, with rare viral transmission.

Blood safety relies upon several measures, including careful donor screening by questionnaire, the use of good manufacturing practices, and donor and component screening for infectious diseases. Currently, in the United States, blood donors are screened for infection with hepatitis B virus, hepatitis C virus, HIV-1 and HIV-2, human T-cell lymphotropic viruses (HTLV) types I and II, West Nile virus (WNV), syphilis, and *Trypanosoma cruzi*. Additionally, donors may be screened for cytomegalovirus and *Babesia* in high epidemic areas of the United States. Platelet components are also screened for bacterial contamination unless they have been pathogen-reduced.

Bacterial Contamination

The risk of a septic reaction is approximately 1 : 200,000 to 1,000,000 transfusions, with the risk decreasing as additional platelet bacterial contamination mitigation strategies are implemented.[10] Platelet components are primarily associated with bacterial contamination due to their storage at room temperature. The implementation of multiple steps for platelet units, including skin cleansing, diversion pouch, and bacterial screening, has resulted in approximately two-thirds decrease in septic reactions. Pathogen reduction decreases bacteria loads by more than four logs for most organisms, although several septic reactions have been reported from pathogen-reduced platelet transfusion in the United States[11] Additional mitigation strategies implemented in the United States and other countries reduce septic reactions to less than 1 : 500,000 transfusions include delayed or repeat bacterial culture and use of point-of-issue bacterial screening.[12]

Septic reactions should be suspected if the transfused patient has fever (≥38° C with rise ≥1° C) with rigors, hypotension, shock, tachycardia, dyspnea, or nausea/vomiting. The transfusion should be promptly stopped, supportive care should be instituted, and blood samples should be drawn for culture (aerobic and anaerobic times two) prior to initiating antibiotics. Thrombocytopenic neutropenic patients are most at risk for septic reactions, mostly due to *Staphylococcal aureus.*

Virus

Hepatitis B (Chapter 134) virus has an estimated transfusion transmission risk of approximately 1 : 1,500,000 transfusions. In the United States, blood components are screened by testing for Hepatitis B surface antigen (HBsAg), anti-HBc, and HBV nucleic acid testing (NAT).

Hepatitis C has an estimated transfusion transmission risk of approximately 1 : 1,600,000 transfusions. In the United States, blood components are screened by testing for anti-HCV and HCV NAT.

Human immunodeficiency virus (HIV) has an estimated transfusion transmission risk of approximately 1 : 1,800,000 transfusions. HIV-2 is found mainly in West Africa. In the United States, blood components are screened by testing for anti-HIV-1/HIV-2 and HIV-1/HIV-2 NAT.

Human T-cell lymphotropic virus (Chapter 360) has an estimated transfusion transmission risk of approximately 1 : 3,300,000 transfusions. In the United States, blood components are screened for HTLV-I and HTLV-II by testing for anti-HTLV-I/II.

Donor screening has substantially reduced the number of transfusion-transmitted cases of West Nile virus (Chapter 352), with the most recent U.S. case being reported in 2012. In the United States, blood components are screened by West Nile virus NAT. To improve testing logistics and cost, testing is initially performed on pooled samples, and then this process continues until increased regional disease activity is detected, at which time testing is on individual samples.

Four suspected cases of transfusion-transmitted Zika virus (Chapter 352) have been reported, all in Brazil, and none were associated with clinical sequelae in the recipients. Zika NAT testing was performed in the United States from 2016 to 2021, but then the FDA determined that Zika virus is no longer a relevant transfusion-transmitted infection. Now, neither testing nor pathogen reduction is required.

Other Infections

In the United States, blood components are screened for syphilis (Chapter 295) by nontreponemal or treponemal tests. No transfusion-transmitted syphilis infections have been reported in the last several decades due to the spirochete's poor viability during storage.

In the United States blood components are screened for *T. cruzi*, which is the causative agent of Chagas disease (Chapter 318), by testing for anti–*T. cruzi* antibody. In the United States, donors are tested only at their first donation. Since the advent of screening, no transfusion-related cases have been reported.

Screening of blood donors for *Babesia* (Chapter 324) is performed using either NAT or pathogen reduction in high epidemic states to prevent transfusion-transmitted babesiosis. The implementation of screening has decreased the incidence of transfusion-transmitted *Babesia,* which is dependent on the donor's residence and travel.

Many other pathogens have been reported to be transfusion transmitted, including *Anaplasma phagocytophilum* (Chapter 324), parvovirus B19 (Chapter 342), hepatitis A (Chapter 134), Dengue virus (Chapter 352), variant Creutzfeldt-Jakob disease (Chapter 371), and malaria (Chapter 316). Donors are screened by donor history questionnaire for malaria in the United States. Plasma for further manufacturing is tested for parvovirus B19 and hepatitis A.

INDICATIONS FOR BLOOD TRANSFUSION (TABLE 162-4)

RED BLOOD CELL TRANSFUSIONS

RBC transfusions are used to treat anemia when patients require increased oxygen carrying capacity, based on their individual clinical status and coexisting medical conditions. In an average adult, one RBC component (unit) should increase the hemoglobin by about 1 g/dL and the hematocrit by about 3%.

Almost 50 randomized controlled trials[A1,A2,13] have compared restrictive (hemoglobin between 7.0 g/dL and 8.0 g/dL) versus liberal (hemoglobin between 9.0 g/dL and 10.0 g/dL) transfusion thresholds in a variety of clinical contexts, including medical and surgical adult patients. Transfusing at lower versus higher hemoglobin levels results in equivalent rates of mortality, myocardial infarction, stroke, pneumonia, thrombosis, and infection. Clinical situations in which a higher transfusion threshold (e.g., >8.0g/dL) should be considered are patients who have symptomatic anemia, an acute coronary syndrome, an acute myocardial infarction,[A3] severe thrombocytopenia, or who require chronic transfusions. The COVID-19 pandemic resulted in sustained blood shortages worldwide, particularly for RBC products, thereby resulting in the adoption of blood conservation strategies, including splitting products and altering transfusion practices.[14]

PLATELET TRANSFUSIONS

Platelet transfusions are given to prevent or treat bleeding in thrombocytopenic patients (Chapter 158). Platelet transfusion may also be considered in patients with qualitative defects in platelet function. The threshold to transfuse platelets is determined by the patient's platelet count combined with underlying disease and the presence of clinical bleeding.

To prevent bleeding in patients with low platelet counts, patients can be transfused platelets prophylactically.[15] Platelets are indicated in patients with therapy-induced hypoproliferative thrombocytopenia at a platelet count of 10,000/μL or less. Platelet transfusions are also indicated in patients who are having an elective central venous catheter placement with a platelet count of less than 20,000/μL, patients having elective diagnostic lumbar puncture or non-neuraxial surgery with a platelet count of less than 50,000/μL, and in patients having major elective neurosurgery with a platelet count of less than 100,000/μL.

TABLE 162-4 EVIDENCE-BASED TRANSFUSION TRIGGERS

BLOOD COMPONENT	COMMONLY ACCEPTED INDICATIONS	TYPICAL INCREASE
RBC	Hb <7.0 g/dL Hb< 8.0 g/dL acute coronary syndrome/myocardial infarction	Hb: 1 g/dL or Hct: 3% after one unit of RBC
Platelets	<10,000/μL hospitalized adult patients with therapy-induced hypoproliferative thrombocytopenia <20,000/μL if febrile/septic, central venous catheter, or other minor procedures <50,000/μL if surgery, lumbar puncture, invasive procedure, or active bleeding <100,000/μL neurosurgery or central nervous system bleeding	30-60,000/μL after one platelet dose (a single apheresis component or 4-6 whole blood derived platelet concentrates [3 × 10^{11} platelets])
Plasma	Massive transfusion (plasma : RBC: 1 : 2) INR >2.0 prior to invasive procedure Replacement fluid for plasma exchange for thrombotic thrombocytopenic purpura	10-15 mL/kg increases factor levels by ≈20%
Cryoprecipitate	Fibrinogen <150 mg/dL with bleeding	≈7 mg/dL increase in fibrinogen per unit

Hb = hemoglobin; Hct = hematocrit; ICH = intracranial hemorrhage; INR = international normalized ratio; PCC = prothrombin complex concentrate; RBC = red blood cell.

Platelets also are administered therapeutically in patients who have low platelet counts, generally less than 50,000/μL, and if they are actively bleeding. Platelet transfusions are also indicated in patients who have undergone cardiac surgery with cardiopulmonary bypass, exhibit perioperative bleeding, and are either thrombocytopenic or have evidence of platelet dysfunction. In patients who have a massive hemorrhage, platelets should be administered at an appropriate ratio to RBC transfusions. Platelet transfusion is not recommended for patients who have an intracranial hemorrhage while receiving antiplatelet therapy.[A4]

In adults, a typical platelet dose is a single apheresis component or four to six whole blood-derived platelet concentrates pooled (3×10^{11} platelets). Lower dose platelet transfusions (e.g., $1.1 \times 10^{11}/m^2$ or $2.2 \times 10^{11}/m^2$) result in similar bleeding outcomes but require more platelet transfusions per patient.

The response to platelet transfusion can be assessed by a decrease in clinical bleeding and by measuring the post-transfusion increment in platelet count about 15 to 60 minutes after transfusion. A typical dose of platelets should increase the patient's platelet count by 30,000 to 60,000/μL.

A more formal evaluation of the platelet increment can be performed using the corrected count increment, which accounts for both the patient's size (via body surface area) and the number of platelets in the transfused component. The corrected count increment is calculated as:

$$\frac{\text{Body surface area}(m^2) \times \text{Platelet count increment} \times 10^{11}}{\text{Number of platelets transfused}}$$

A 1-hour corrected count increment greater than 7.5 is considered acceptable, whereas a corrected count increment value less than 7.5 is suggestive of platelet refractoriness.

Many clinical conditions can decrease the expected post-transfusion increment in the platelet count, including fever, sepsis, disseminated intravascular coagulation, splenomegaly with hypersplenism, active bleeding, and platelet or HLA alloantibodies or autoantibodies. ABO-compatible transfusions result in higher post-transfusion increment than ABO-incompatible transfusions. Patients who have multiple platelet transfusions may develop antibodies that blunt the response of the platelet count, and evaluation of platelet refractoriness usually includes screening for HLA compatibility and platelet antibodies. In this situation, HLA epitope-matched platelet transfusions provide a better response than standard HLA antigen-matched transfusions, with each epitope mismatch reducing the platelet count response by about 15%.[A5]

PLASMA TRANSFUSIONS

Plasma transfusions are generally used either to prevent or treat bleeding in patients with acquired coagulopathies. For the majority of patients with congenital coagulopathies, the specific and appropriate clotting factor concentrate should be administered (Chapter 160), such as von Willebrand factor, factor VIII, factor IX, fibrinogen, factor X, factor VIIa, factor XIII, prothrombin complex concentrate, and C1 inhibitor concentrate. These factors are either purified and virally inactivated human or recombinant proteins. If the specific factor is not available, plasma should be transfused.

Plasma should be administered to massively hemorrhaging patients at an appropriate ratio to red blood cell transfusions. Plasma can also be used to treat or prevent major bleeding in patients with multiple coagulation factor deficiencies, including disseminated intravascular coagulopathy (Chapter 161) and liver failure (Chapter 140).

Plasma is also indicated as replacement fluid for plasma exchange in patients with thrombotic thrombocytopenic purpura (Chapter 158) and other diseases.[16] Plasma may also be used as part of the replacement fluid for patients at risk of coagulation factor depletion, particularly patients who are on daily plasma exchange with albumin as replacement fluid.

The only clinical indication for plasma cryoprecipitate-reduced and thawed plasma cryoprecipitate reduced is thrombotic thrombocytopenic purpura (Chapter 158). The only indication for liquid plasma is for initial treatment of patients undergoing massive transfusion.

Plasma transfusion is not recommended for warfarin-related serious hemorrhage unless prothrombin complex concentrate is not available. Prothrombin complex concentrate, specifically 4-factor (factors II, VII, IX, and X), should be used instead of plasma for the rapid reversal of warfarin in patients who experience bleeding or require urgent surgery (Chapter 161). Plasma is not recommended for reversal of novel oral anticoagulants (e.g., direct thrombin inhibitors and direct factor Xa inhibitors).

The typical dose of plasma is 10 to 15 mL/kg. Because each plasma component is 200 to 300 mL, an average adult dose is 3 to 5 plasma components (units). Coagulation factors are expected to increase by approximately 20% immediately after plasma infusion.

CRYOPRECIPITATE TRANSFUSIONS

Cryoprecipitate is used for fibrinogen replacement when levels fall below 100 mg/dL in acquired hypofibrinogenemia with disseminated intravascular coagulopathy (Chapter 161), liver failure (Chapter 140), the anhepatic phase of liver transplantation (Chapter 161), and massive transfusion with dilution coagulopathy. Cryoprecipitate may also be used for management of intracranial bleeding related to thrombolytic therapy (tissue plasminogen activator). Pathogen-reduced cryoprecipitated fibrinogen concentrate, which is derived from pathogen-reduced plasma, is useful for the treatment and control of bleeding associated with fibrinogen deficiency.

GRANULOCYTE TRANSFUSIONS

Granulocytes are sometimes transfused in neutropenic patients with life-threatening infections (Chapters 153 and 260). However, their benefit in such patients is unproven.[A6]

INDICATIONS FOR COMPONENT MODIFICATION

LEUKOREDUCTION

The majority of RBC and platelet products are leukoreduced prior to storage. Leukoreduction removes white blood cells from the unit to mitigate febrile nonhemolytic transfusion reactions, HLA alloimmunization, CMV transmission, and transfusion-related immunomodulation. Thus, leukoreduction is indicated in patients at risk for these complications, such as potential transplant patients, patients with a history of febrile nonhemolytic transfusion reactions, pregnant patients, and immunocompromised patients.

CYTOMEGALOVIRUS SERONEGATIVE

For the mitigation of transfusion-transmitted cytomegalovirus, patients at risk for cytomegalovirus disease should receive leukoreduced, cytomegalovirus seronegative,[A7] or pathogen-reduced blood components. Such at-risk patients include transplant candidates, transplant recipients, patients undergoing chemotherapy, pregnant women, and immunocompromised patients.

IRRADIATION

Irradiation or pathogen reduction, which inactivates white blood cells so they cannot replicate, is used to prevent transfusion-associated graft-versus-host disease. Indications for irradiation include congenital immunodeficiency; stem cell transplantation; Hodgkin disease; use of purine analogue drugs, anti-CD32, or other drugs that alter T-lymphocyte function; intrauterine transfusion; neonatal exchange transfusion; leukemia; lymphoma; intense chemotherapy; congenital heart disease (DiGeorge syndrome); and aplastic anemia. Products from blood relatives, HLA match products, and granulocyte products should be irradiated.

PATHOGEN REDUCTION

Pathogen reduction mitigates the need for irradiation, cytomegalovirus seronegative blood products, testing for *Babesia*, and bacterial screening. Currently, this technology is mostly used in platelets and plasma. For plasma, solvent/detergent treated, pooled plasma product, or pathogen-reduced plasma product is available. The incidence of transfusion-related acute lung injury and allergic reactions with solvent detergent-treated pooled plasma is much lower than the risk with other plasma products.

For pathogen-reduced platelets data show: uncertainty as to whether pathogen-reduced platelets increase the risk of any bleeding, no evidence of difference in the incidence of clinically significant bleeding complications, probably no difference in all-cause mortality, probably no difference in serious adverse events, an increased risk of developing platelet refractoriness, an increased requirement for platelet transfusions, a shorter time interval between transfusions, and lower corrected platelet count increment compared with standard platelets.[A8]

SPECIFIC CLINICAL SETTINGS

Perioperative Alternatives to Allogeneic Transfusion

Autologous Donations

Patients may donate their own blood in the weeks prior to elective surgery. The advantages of such "preoperative autologous donation" include decreased risk of infectious disease transmission, decreased risk of alloimmunization to donor antigens, and the ready availability of compatible blood products if the patient requires rare RBC components. Its disadvantages include additional cost, potential adverse reactions associated with autologous blood donation, and the development of iatrogenic preoperative anemia associated with phlebotomy. These components are more expensive than allogeneic components because they are specially handled to ensure that they are transfused only to the intended recipient. Further concerns include bacterial contamination, transfusion-associated circulatory overload, and the potential for mislabeling. Additionally, the wastage rate for autologous components is about 60%, thereby suggesting that most autologous donations are unnecessary. As a result, routine use of autologous components is not recommended.

Directed Donors

Individuals who donate blood components for use by a specific patient, typically a family member or friend, are referred to as "directed donors." Although directed donors are typically motivated by compassion for the patient, components from directed donations are not safer than components from volunteer donations. Directed donors may intentionally or unintentionally omit information that might otherwise preclude them from donating, and this omission may compromise the safety of the resulting product. Nevertheless, directed donations from relatives may be medically desirable when a patient requires HLA-matched components or RBCs with a rare phenotype. All directed donations from blood relatives should be irradiated to prevent transfusion-associated-graft-versus-host disease.

Reinfusion of Recovered Blood

To salvage and reinfuse blood lost during a surgical procedure, intraoperative blood recovery is an option. The simplest approach is direct reinfusion of recovered blood without washing. In this method, recovered blood is collected, anticoagulant is added, and blood is reinfused. Recovered blood also can be washed with saline prior to reinfusion. Blood recovered by these methods must be reinfused within 4 hours or, if stored at 1° to 6° C, within 24 hours of the start of collection.

Cell salvage can be set up to meet the needs of patients who refuse blood transfusion, such as some Jehovah Witnesses. Potential contraindications to intraoperative blood recovery include a contaminated surgical site, blood collected from surgical procedures for cancer with the potential risk of tumor cell contamination, and blood collected in surgical sites that contain medications.

In the process of acute normovolemic hemodilution, intraoperative removal of whole blood into standard collection bags is replaced simultaneously with crystalloid or colloid of equal volume. Hemodilution reduces RBC loss because a bleeding patient with an iatrogenically lowered hematocrit loses fewer RBCs. The removed whole blood is stored in the operating room and reinfused in reverse order of collection. This approach allows for the components with the highest hematocrit to be transfused last, presumably when surgical bleeding has been controlled. The whole blood also has functioning platelets and coagulation factors. The iatrogenic anemia can compromise oxygen transport, but this problem is usually mitigated by the decrease in blood viscosity. If kept at room temperature, the collected components must be used within 8 hours of collection; if stored at 1° to 6° C, they must be used within 24 hours of collection.

Most patients tolerate the transfusion of autologous blood collected postoperatively from draining serosal cavities. Adverse effects can include respiratory distress, hypotension with anaphylaxis, and fever. Blood collected postoperatively must be used within 6 hours of collection.

MASSIVE TRANSFUSION

Massive transfusion is defined as transfusion of 10 or more RBC components (units) within 24 hours. Other definitions of massive transfusion include replacement of 50% of total blood volume within 3 hours or blood loss exceeding 150 mL per minute. Current practice is for a 1 : 1 : 1 or 1 : 1 : 2 ratio of plasma : platelets : RBCs during massive transfusion. In patients with severe trauma, a 1 : 1 : 1 ratio can reduce the rate of exsanguination within 24 hours and provide better hemostasis compared with a 1 : 1 : 2 ratio, but overall rates of complications and mortality are no different at 24 hours and 30 days.[A9] As a result, the 1 : 1 : 2 ratio remains the most commonly recommended transfusion ratio. Other options include the use of whole blood,[17] tranexamic acid, and the decision to transfuse guided by thromboelastography to assess clotting under expert supervision. Randomized trials have demonstrated improved survival with prehospital plasma transfusion when transport times are longer than 20 minutes.[A10]

HEMOGLOBINOPATHIES

Patients with hemoglobinopathies, such as thalassemia (Chapter 148) and sickle cell disease (Chapter 149), often require chronic transfusion. Patients who have sickle cell disease are at especially high risk of forming alloantibodies.

The use of prophylactic antigen matching has decreased alloimmunization rates from about 50% to 10% with limited matching (D, C, E, K antigens) and 5% with extended matching (D, C, E, K, Jk^b, Fy^a antigens). Additionally, individuals of African descent have variant Rh genes so may phenotype as positive but make alloantibodies to the antigen. As a result, genotyping for RBC antigens in this population is helpful to determine the appropriate antigen-negative component product. Providing units based on the patient's genotype has increased post-transfusion hemoglobin levels and transfusion intervals. Lastly, RBC units for sickle cell patients are hemoglobin S negative and labeled as such.

Patients with thalassemia (Chapter 148) may require chronic lifelong transfusion as frequently as every 2 to 5 weeks to maintain pretransfusion hemoglobin levels above 9 to 10.5 g/dL in order to promote normal growth and physical activity and suppress bone marrow activity. The predominant transfusion complication in these patients is iron overload.

PATIENT BLOOD MANAGEMENT

The goals of a patient blood management program include increasing awareness of evidence-based transfusion guidelines, reducing the likelihood of a transfusion, minimizing blood loss, improving blood utilization, continuously educating clinicians, and standardizing metrics. Implementation of patient blood management programs have decreased blood utilization, decreased cost, and improved patient care. Optimizing RBC mass includes the preoperative evaluation of anemia, the timing of surgery, and the optimization of postoperative erythropoiesis. Minimizing blood loss includes management of the risk of bleeding, meticulous surgical technique, blood sparing devices, blood conservation strategies, maintenance of normothermia, use of hemostatic agents, monitoring for postoperative bleeding, blood salvage, minimizing iatrogenic blood loss, managing anticoagulation, and prophylaxis for gastrointestinal hemorrhage. Optimizing physiologic anemia reserve includes estimating blood loss compared with the patient's tolerance, formulating a patient-specific blood management plan, optimizing cardiac output and oxygenation, optimizing anemia reserve, maximizing oxygen delivery, minimizing oxygen consumption, avoiding and treating infections, and using restrictive transfusion thresholds.

To decrease unnecessary use of blood products, general principles include:[18,19]

1. Do not transfuse more units than necessary. Transfuse using a restrictive threshold. Consider transfusing a single unit of RBCs in stable, nonbleeding hospitalized patients, and then checking the patient's hemoglobin and clinical status prior to further transfusions.
2. Do not proceed with elective surgery prior to evaluating and treating anemia.
3. Do not transfuse RBCs for iron deficiency if patients are hemodynamically stable. Iron-deficient patients should receive oral or intravenous iron.
4. Do not use blood products to reverse warfarin. Patients can generally be reversed with vitamin K alone. Prothrombin complex concentrates should be used in the setting of serious bleeding or the need for emergent surgery. Do not transfuse plasma to correct a mildly elevated INR (<1.8).
5. Do not perform serial blood counts on clinically stable patients. Repeat blood draws can result in iatrogenic anemia.
6. Do not transfuse O-negative blood except to O-negative patients and in emergencies for women of childbearing potential with unknown blood group. O-negative RBCs are in chronic short supply and should be restricted to patients who need them.
7. Do not transfuse AB plasma to non-AB patients except in emergency situations in which ABO blood type is unknown. Group A plasma can also be used for emergency transfusions.

GENERAL REFERENCES

For the General References and other additional features, please visit Elsevier eBooks+ at https://ebooks.health.elsevier.com.

Grade A References

A1. Carson JL, Stanworth SJ, Dennis JA, et al. Transfusion thresholds for guiding red blood cell transfusion. *Cochrane Database Syst Rev.* 2021;12:CD002042.

A2. Trentino KM, Farmer SL, Leahy MF, et al. Systematic reviews and meta-analyses comparing mortality in restrictive and liberal haemoglobin thresholds for red cell transfusion: an overview of systematic reviews. *BMC Med.* 2020;18:1-14.

A3. Ducrocq G, Gonzalez-Juanatey JR, Puymirat E, et al. Effect of a restrictive vs liberal blood transfusion strategy on major cardiovascular events among patients with acute myocardial infarction and anemia: the REALITY randomized clinical trial. *JAMA.* 2021;325:552-560.

A4. Baharoglu MI, Cordonnier C, Al-Shahi Salman R, et al. Platelet transfusion versus standard care after acute stroke due to spontaneous cerebral haemorrhage associated with antiplatelet therapy (PATCH): a randomised, open-label, phase 3 trial. *Lancet.* 2016;387:2605-2613.

A5. Marsh JC, Stanworth SJ, Pankhurst LA, et al. An epitope-based approach of HLA-matched platelets for transfusion: a noninferiority crossover randomized trial. *Blood.* 2021;137:310-322.

A6. Price TH, Boeckh M, Harrison RW, et al. Efficacy of transfusion with granulocytes from G-CSF/dexamethasone-treated donors in neutropenic patients with infection. *Blood.* 2015;126:2153-1561.

A7. Mainou M, Alahdab F, Tobian AA, et al. Reducing the risk of transfusion-transmitted cytomegalovirus infection: a systematic review and meta-analysis. *Transfusion.* 2016;56:1569-1580.

A8. Estcourt LJ, Malouf R, Hopewell S, et al. Pathogen-reduced platelets for the prevention of bleeding. *Cochrane Database Syst Rev.* 2017;7:CD009072.

A9. Holcomb JB, Tilley BC, Baraniuk S, et al. Transfusion of plasma, platelets, and red blood cells in a 1:1:1 vs a 1:1:2 ratio and mortality in patients with severe trauma: the PROPPR randomized clinical trial. *JAMA.* 2015;313:471-482.

A10. Pusateri AE, Morre EE, Moore HB, et al. Association of prehospital plasma transfusion with survival in trauma patients with hemorrhagic shock when transport times are longer than 20 minutes: a post hoc analysis of the PAMPer and COMBAT clinical trials. *JAMA Surg.* 2020;155:e195085.

163 HEMATOPOIETIC CELL TRANSPLANTATION

NELSON J. CHAO AND ARMAND KEATING

Hematopoietic cell transplantation is a procedure by which hematopoietic stem and progenitor cells are infused intravenously to restore hematopoiesis and immune function following a chemotherapy conditioning regimen, with or without radiation therapy, that ablates the endogenous hematopoietic and immune system.[1] Stem cells used for hematopoietic cell transplantation are of hematopoietic origin, in contrast to the more primitive pluripotent stem cells (i.e., embryonic stem cells) that are considered for regenerative therapy because of their ability to differentiate into virtually any somatic cell. Hematopoietic cell transplantation is now a standard treatment for many hematologic malignancies, immunodeficiency states, enzyme deficiencies (e.g., Hurler syndrome [Chapter 192]), and defective hematopoietic states (e.g., severe aplastic anemia [Chapter 151]).[2] In addition, hematopoietic cell transplantation can also treat hemoglobinopathies, immune deficiency states, and selected autoimmune diseases.[3] The infused hematopoietic stem/progenitor cells can give rise to all blood elements, including cells of the immune system, and they may be genetically modified to enhance their function. Furthermore, hematopoietic stem/progenitor cells may be manipulated ex vivo and used in the burgeoning field of regenerative medicine. Taken together, hematopoietic cell transplantation is a major component and foundation of the broader field of cellular therapy (Chapter 34).

The three cell sources for hematopoietic cell transplantation are syngeneic (i.e., cells from an identical twin), allogeneic (i.e., cells from a nonidentical donor), and autologous (i.e., reinfusion of one's own cells). The determination of the type of hematopoietic cell transplantation that a patient receives is based on the disease to be treated, the disease state (e.g., initial treatment vs. treatment of recurrent disease), the urgency with which the disease needs to be treated, the availability of a donor, and the time necessary to obtain hematopoietic stem/progenitor cells from a donor.

Hematopoietic stem/progenitor cells may be obtained from bone marrow (by serial aspirations from the posterior iliac crests while the donor is under general anesthesia), peripheral blood (after stimulation with hematopoietic growth factors such as granulocyte colony–stimulating factor [G-CSF] or plerixafor [a CXCR4 antagonist], followed by leukapheresis), or umbilical cord blood. In current practice, peripheral blood is the source for hematopoietic stem/progenitor cells in approximately 90% of autologous transplants and in approximately 70% of allogeneic transplants because of the relative ease of procurement and the donor's rate of hematopoietic recovery after infusion compared with cells derived from bone marrow.

Hematopoietic stem/progenitor cells may be infused fresh or after cryopreservation, which involves processing the cells in culture medium containing dimethyl sulfoxide (DMSO), placing them in specialized plastic bags, controlled freezing, and then storing in the vapor phase of liquid nitrogen until needed. Cord blood hematopoietic stem/progenitor cells are collected at the time of delivery, cryopreserved, and stored. For allogeneic donation, cells may also be infused on the day of collection. For autologous donation, cells are almost always cryopreserved.

ALLOGENEIC HEMATOPOIETIC CELL TRANSPLANTATION

The distinctive characteristics of allogeneic hematopoietic cell transplantation are that the stem cell graft allows for the establishment of a new immune system in addition to reconstitution of white blood cells, red blood cells, and platelets. The new immune system can be a major advantage if the immunologic response is directed against malignant cells, referred to as the graft-versus-leukemia or graft-versus-tumor effect, which potentially can eradicate disease and reduce the chance of disease relapse. However, if the immunologic response is directed against antigens present on normal tissues, the graft-versus-host response can result in the destruction of normal organs and is clinically described as graft-versus-host disease (GVHD). The risk for both graft rejection (host-versus-graft reaction) and GVHD rises with the degree of human leukocyte antigen (HLA) disparity between the donor and the recipient as well as the degree of immune suppression.

The clinical importance of the role that immunocompetent donor T cells play in mediating a graft-versus-tumor effect is exemplified by the increased rates of relapse in patients who receive allogeneic bone marrow grafts from which T cells had been removed (T-cell depletion), an inverse correlation between relapse and severity of GVHD, and increased rates of relapse after syngeneic or autologous hematopoietic cell transplantation in patients who have received similar conditioning regimens. However, the most compelling evidence for the importance of T cells mediating the graft-versus-tumor effect is the clinical observation that infusion of allogeneic T cells alone, termed a *donor lymphocyte infusion*, at a time remote from the transplant conditioning regimen can successfully eradicate leukemia that has persisted or recurred after allogeneic hematopoietic cell transplantation. Nevertheless, the clinical effectiveness of graft-versus-tumor can vary widely among different malignancies.

Because of the immunologic barriers that can result in graft rejection and GVHD, allogeneic hematopoietic cell transplantation requires that the donor and the recipient share as many key genes as possible. The most important of these are HLAs (Chapter 38), which are derived from the MHC located on chromosome 6. The HLA loci include HLA-A, HLA-B, HLA-C, DR, DP, and DQ. A single set of major histocompatibility complex (MHC) alleles, described as a haplotype, is inherited from each parent, thereby resulting in HLA pairs. A clinical "match" means that HLAs in the donor match the HLAs in the patient.

The choice of donor for an allogeneic hematopoietic cell transplantation takes into account several factors, including the patient's specific disease and disease state (i.e., remission vs. relapse) and the time that is required for obtaining hematopoietic stem/progenitor cells from a donor. A fully HLA-matched sibling is the preferred donor source because the risks for graft rejection and GVHD are lowest. The probability of having an HLA match with a single sibling is 25% and increases with the number of siblings within a specific family. This probability can be estimated using the following formula: chance of having an HLA-matched sibling $= 1 - (0.75)^n$, where n is the number of potential sibling donors. There is approximately a 1% chance of a crossover event (i.e., genetic material switched between chromosomes during meiosis), primarily between the HLA-A and the HLA-B loci. The clinical outcomes for allogeneic hematopoietic cell transplantation using a sibling with a single HLA mismatch are similar to those with a fully HLA-matched sibling.

For patients who lack an HLA-identical sibling donor, the alternative sources for allogeneic hematopoietic stem/progenitor cells include a fully HLA-matched volunteer unrelated donor, a fully or partially HLA-matched cord blood unit, or a partially HLA-matched first-degree family member. HLA genes are highly polymorphic, so the odds that any two unrelated individuals are HLA identical for main loci are less than 1 in 10,000. However, tens of millions of people worldwide are currently listed as potential volunteer donors, so a donor can be found for about 50% of all patients for whom a search is initiated. The probability of identifying a suitable volunteer donor is highly dependent on race because of varying degrees of HLA diversity. For example, for persons of northern European extraction, the probability of a match can be as high as 90%. In contrast, minority populations may have less than a 20% probability of a match because of fewer volunteer donors and a higher degree of genetic variation.

It usually takes about 2 to 4 months to locate and fully evaluate an unrelated donor, which may be too long for some patients with rapidly progressive malignancies. When a suitable volunteer is not available or a donor is needed more urgently, alternative sources can be considered, including partially HLA-matched ("haploidentical") relatives or umbilical cord blood. Haploidentical hematopoietic stem/progenitor cells are readily available but have increased risks for graft rejection and GVHD. These risks can be reduced by either ex vivo or in vivo T-cell depletion methods, but T-cell depletion may lead to delayed immune reconstitution and competency after transplantation, thereby increasing the risks for infection and recurrent disease. However, post-transplantation cyclophosphamide for GVHD prophylaxis has markedly increased the clinical use of haploidentical donors.

Umbilical cord blood hematopoietic stem/progenitor cells, which are taken at the time of delivery and stored in cord blood banks, are readily available within 2 to 4 weeks when needed. Because of the unique immature biology of lymphocytes in umbilical cord blood, these transplants are associated with less GVHD; consequently, the HLA-matching requirements are less strict, and two or three HLA mismatches may be acceptable. However, the small volume (50 to 150 mL) of cord blood that can be collected limits the number of hematopoietic stem/progenitor cells and often prohibits their use in adults because successful engraftment correlates with the number of cells per patient body weight. The limitation of cell dose can be overcome by the use of more than one cord blood unit and the ability to expand cord blood cells ex vivo, thereby resulting in engraftment rates similar to other cell sources. One significant disadvantage is that the use of a cord blood unit eliminates the probability of obtaining additional cells if the graft fails or if a donor lymphocyte infusion is required.

After a source of allogeneic stem cells has been identified, patients then receive a pretransplant regimen with the intent of "conditioning" or "preparing" them for the infusion (Fig. 163-1). These conditioning regimens are designed to be adequately immunosuppressive to overcome the host-versus-graft reaction and permit engraftment. They also are designed to eradicate the primary tumor in patients with an underlying malignancy. Most conditioning regimens use chemotherapy alone or a combination of total body irradiation or total nodal irradiation with chemotherapy. The doses of total body and total lymphoid irradiation vary between 200 and 1440 cGy. The most commonly used chemotherapy for conditioning regimens is an alkylating agent (e.g., cyclophosphamide, busulfan, thiotepa) combined with immunosuppressive drugs such as fludarabine. Conditioning regimens also may contain monoclonal antibodies that target T cells (e.g., antithymocyte globulin, alemtuzumab).

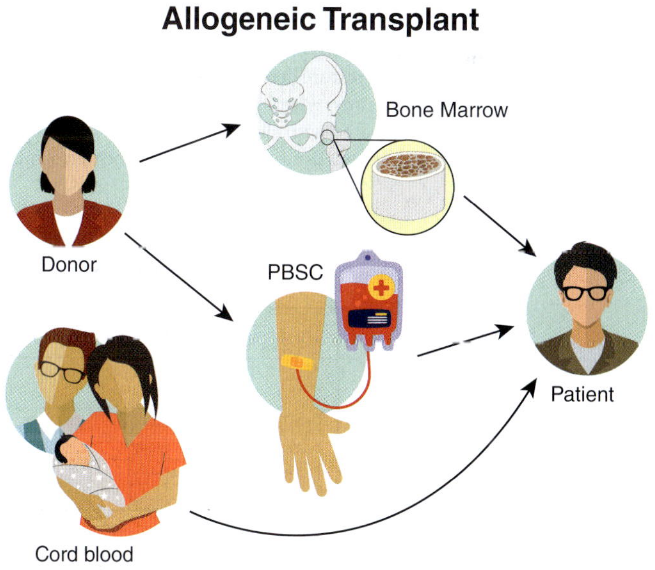

FIGURE 163-1. The process of allogeneic hematopoietic cell transplantation. (1) The patient receives a conditioning regimen of chemotherapy and/or radiation therapy that is used to both eliminate the underlying malignancy and suppress the immune system to prevent rejection of the allogeneic hematopoietic stem cells. (2) Allogeneic hematopoietic stem cells are then collected directly from the bone marrow or from the blood of a related or unrelated stem cell donor and infused intravenously into the donor. (3) After the infusion of the hematopoietic stem cells, the patient receives immunosuppressant drugs to help prevent the development of graft-versus-host disease (GVHD). PBSC = peripheral blood stem cells. (Image courtesy of the National Marrow Donor Program.)

The choice of a specific conditioning regimen depends on the disease being treated, and the doses of chemotherapy and radiation are highly variable. When the doses result in a degree of myelosuppression and immunosuppression that is nearly universally fatal without the infusion of hematopoietic stem/progenitor cells as a rescue product, they are referred to as myeloablative.

Allogeneic hematopoietic cell transplantation with myeloablative conditioning regimens has been performed successfully in patients older than age 60 years, but survival after transplantations declines with increasing age, thereby limiting the application of allogeneic transplantation to a minority of patients who potentially could benefit from this procedure. However, the demonstration that an immune-mediated graft-versus-tumor effect plays a central role in the therapeutic efficacy of allogeneic hematopoietic cell transplantation led to the development of less intensive conditioning regimens that are adequately immunosuppressive to permit the engraftment of donor cells but associated with decreased toxicities compared with myeloablative regimens. Another advantage of less intensive conditioning is that it can be delivered outside of the hospital setting, so that patients receive their care in the outpatient setting and are able to stay in a local apartment or their actual home if they live close to the center. Although the reduced doses of radiation and chemotherapy result in decreased antitumor activity and are associated with higher rates of recurrent disease after transplantation, these "nonmyeloablative" and "reduced-intensity" conditioning regimens have markedly increased the potential option of allogeneic hematopoietic cell transplantation for older patients and patients with preexisting comorbidities.

SYNGENEIC HEMATOPOIETIC CELL TRANSPLANTATION

The major advantage of a syngeneic hematopoietic cell transplantation from an identical twin is that it is not associated with GVHD or graft rejection, thereby resulting in a relatively low risk for treatment-related morbidity and mortality. Syngeneic hematopoietic cell transplantation, as with allogeneic transplantation, also avoids potential contamination with malignant cells. The major disadvantage of syngeneic transplantation is that it does not provide the graft-versus-leukemia effect associated with allogeneic transplantation. However, since far less than 1% of patients have an identical twin, syngeneic transplantation is rarely an option.

AUTOLOGOUS HEMATOPOIETIC CELL TRANSPLANTATION

The major rationale for autologous hematopoietic cell transplantation with the patient's own cells is that certain malignancies, such as leukemias and lymphomas, have a steep dose-response curve to chemotherapy and, to a relative degree, radiation. However, the associated limitation of higher doses of chemotherapy or radiation attenuates myelosuppressive effect. The infusion of autologous hematopoietic stem/progenitor cells (and for that matter, allogeneic and syngeneic cells) can restore hematopoiesis after the prior administration of high-dose chemotherapy, with or without radiation. The major advantages of autologous as compared with allogeneic transplantation are that the patient can serve as his or her own donor and that it may be performed in older patients with significantly lower morbidity and mortality because of the absence of GVHD. Although patients undergoing autologous hematopoietic cell transplantation have higher relapse rates than patients undergoing allogeneic transplantation, the lower rates of other complications seem to translate into similar long-term outcomes. Nevertheless, the higher conditioning doses of chemotherapy before autologous hematopoietic cell transplantation can be associated with more morbidity than conventional doses of chemotherapy.

INDICATIONS FOR TRANSPLANTATION

An estimated 90,000 hematopoietic cell transplantations are performed annually worldwide, primarily for the treatment of hematologic malignancies, bone marrow failure states, and immune and enzyme deficiencies (Fig. 163-2).

Acute Myeloid Leukemia

Allogeneic hematopoietic cell transplantation is capable of resulting in the long-term survival of 10% of patients with otherwise refractory acute myeloid leukemia (AML; Chapter 168).[4] By comparison, cure rates of 40 to 70% have been reported with hematopoietic cell transplantation performed during a first complete remission, and rates of 20 to 40% have been achieved in patients treated while in a second or subsequent complete remission. In randomized trials of patients with AML in first complete remission, both autologous and allogeneic hematopoietic cell transplantation provide improved leukemia-free survival compared with conventional chemotherapy. In terms of overall survival, however, meta-analyses demonstrate improvement with allogeneic hematopoietic cell transplantation compared with nonallogeneic treatments for AML in first complete remission in patients who have intermediate- and high-risk cytogenetics but not in patients who have good-risk AML.[A1] Data also indicate the importance of molecular mutations. For example, intermediate-risk AML with a normal karyotype represents a highly heterogeneous group with respect to prognosis based on molecular mutation status. Approximately one third of patients with normal-karyotype AML harbor the *FLT3*-internal tandem mutation, which carries a poor prognosis and may benefit from HLA-matched related hematopoietic cell transplantation, regardless of the presence of other mutations.

Acute Lymphoblastic Leukemia

Conventional chemotherapy provides excellent outcomes for childhood acute lymphoblastic leukemia (ALL), except for ALL associated with the Philadelphia chromosome (Chapter 168). In adults, however, remission, though frequently attained after intensive induction therapy, is commonly followed by relapse. Adverse prognostic factors include the presence of the Philadelphia chromosome, a high white blood cell count, advancing age, and the presence of minimal residual disease. Studies suggest that consolidation therapy including hematopoietic cell transplantation after initial chemotherapy improves overall survival compared with conventional chemotherapy alone, particularly for those who are Philadelphia chromosome–positive. For both pediatric and adult patients with relapsed ALL, the overall prognosis is relatively poor, and the general treatment strategy is to obtain a second complete remission and then proceed to an allogeneic hematopoietic cell transplantation.

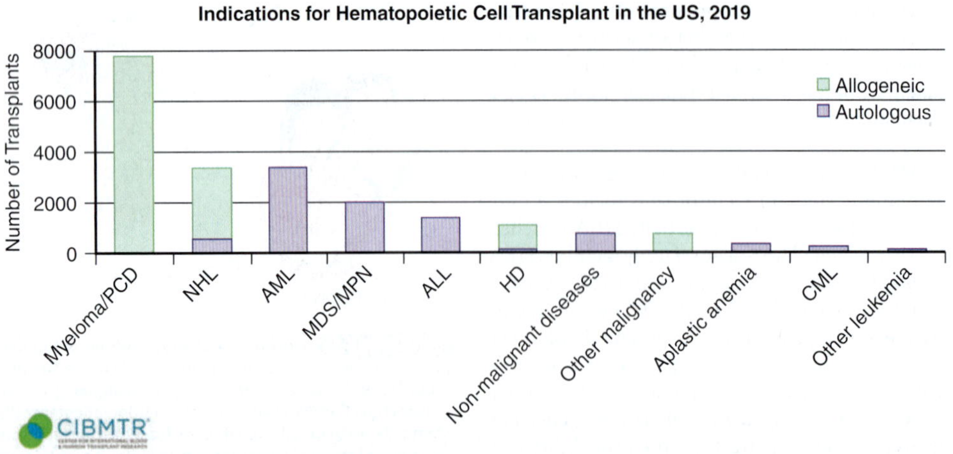

FIGURE 163-2. Indications for hematopoietic cell transplantation in the United States as reported to the Center for International Blood and Marrow Transplant Research. ALL = acute lymphocytic leukemia; AML = acute myeloid leukemia; CML = chronic myelogenous leukemia; HD = Hodgkin disease; MDS/MPN = myelodysplastic syndrome/myeloproliferative neoplasms; NHL = non-Hodgkin lymphoma. (Courtesy of the Center for International Blood and Marrow Transplant Research.)

Myelodysplastic Syndrome

The only known curative treatment for myelodysplastic syndrome (Chapter 167) is allogeneic hematopoietic cell transplantation. Unfortunately, the vast majority of patients are not considered candidates for this therapy for many reasons, including advanced age (the median age at diagnosis is in the seventh to eighth decade of life), comorbid diseases, the inability to identify a suitable donor, and the patient's preferences. The best results have been obtained in younger patients, who are earlier in their disease course and have not received any prior therapy. Increasing evidence suggests that reduced-intensity allogeneic hematopoietic cell transplantation may benefit even considerably older patients with myelodysplastic syndrome. A randomized trial of patients with myelodysplastic syndrome or secondary AML showed that a busulfan-based reduced-intensity conditioning regimen resulted in at least a 2-year relapse-free and overall survival, similar to that after a myeloablative conditioning regimen for allogeneic stem cell transplantation.[A2]

Chronic Myeloid Leukemia

In patients with chronic myeloid leukemia (CML; Chapter 170), hematopoietic cell transplantation is reserved for patients who are resistant to or intolerant of treatment with tyrosine kinase inhibitors, especially those who develop an accelerated phase or blast crisis CML. Although results of allogeneic hematopoietic cell transplantation are poor for accelerated-phase or blast-crisis disease, some patients may respond to tyrosine kinase inhibitors after transplantation.

Myeloproliferative Neoplasms

Myeloproliferative neoplasms, such as primary myelofibrosis, polycythemia vera, and essential thrombocythemia (Chapter 152), usually are chronic in nature but can progress to a "spent" phase and evolve into myeloid metaplasia, which is characterized by bone marrow fibrosis and a generally poor prognosis with transformation into acute leukemia and a median survival of less than 3 years. Conventional treatment options are limited at this stage, and the accepted standard of care for myeloid metaplasia/myelofibrosis is allogeneic hematopoietic cell transplantation, especially nonmyeloablative transplantation because of the older age of most patients with this condition.

Non-Hodgkin Lymphoma

Syngeneic, allogeneic, and autologous hematopoietic cell transplantation have all been reported to yield long-term, disease-free survival and an apparent cure for patients with advanced non-Hodgkin lymphoma (Chapter 171). Based on its risk-benefit ratio and availability, the standard of care for patients with primary refractory or chemotherapy-sensitive relapsed non-Hodgkin lymphoma of specific histologies (including diffuse large B-cell lymphoma) has been autologous hematopoietic cell transplantation. For mantle cell lymphoma, autologous hematopoietic cell transplantation appears to improve progression-free and possibly overall survival when used as part of frontline therapy, especially when combined with maintenance rituximab posttransplantation.[A3] The development of chimeric antigen receptor (CAR) T cells for lymphomas may challenge this sequence depending on the results of ongoing trials.

However, the graft-versus-tumor effect against various non-Hodgkin lymphoma histologies is very heterogeneous, and consensus is currently lacking regarding for which histology allogeneic hematopoietic cell transplantation is appropriate. For example, autologous transplantation can result in disease-free survival rates as high as 60% in patients with indolent follicular non-Hodgkin lymphoma,[A4] but late relapses after transplantation and the long overall survival observed with current medical therapy have reduced the role for hematopoietic cell transplantation despite its graft-versus-tumor effects.

Hodgkin Lymphoma

Based on a small prospective randomized trial conducted in the early 1990s, autologous hematopoietic cell transplantation has become the standard of care for patients with primary refractory and relapsed Hodgkin lymphoma (Chapter 172) whose disease nevertheless remains sensitive to chemotherapy. The usual approach is first to treat these patients with second-line chemotherapy and then with high-dose chemotherapy and autologous hematopoietic cell transplantation. Allogeneic transplantation has had a limited role because of the efficacy of autologous transplantation and the significant treatment-related toxicities associated with myeloablative allogeneic transplantation, but reduced-intensity allogeneic transplantation can be an option, especially in patients who relapse after autologous transplantation.

Multiple Myeloma

Although immunomodulatory derivatives and proteasome inhibitors are highly effective for the treatment of multiple myeloma (Chapter 173), early autologous hematopoietic cell transplantation, when feasible, remains the standard of care.[5] Prospective comparisons of single versus tandem autologous transplants give conflicting results, although overall survival rates appear similar. Single-arm and randomized trials support the use of a second autologous transplantation for patients who relapse after the first autologous transplantation, provided the duration of response was more than 1 year after the initial transplantation.

Solid Tumors

High-dose chemotherapy plus transplantation has had success in the treatment of some chemotherapy-sensitive solid tumors, including germ cell tumors and childhood cancers such as neuroblastoma and Wilms tumor. In patients who have germ cell tumors that are not cured by platinum-based chemotherapy regimens, high-dose chemotherapy and autologous hematopoietic cell transplantation has resulted in prolonged disease-free survival, even in patients with refractory disease.

Nonmalignant Conditions

Allogeneic hematopoietic cell transplantation can lead to long-term, disease-free survival in more than 50% of patients with severe aplastic anemia (Chapter 151). When compared with standard immunosuppressive therapy, allogeneic transplantation is more likely to produce a complete and durable reversal of the hematologic abnormalities. Patients with aplastic anemia who are less heavily transfused have better outcomes with allogeneic transplantation. For patients with less severe aplastic anemia, patients older than 40 years, and patients without a matched sibling donor, a trial of immunosuppression therapy is usually appropriate before consideration of allogeneic transplantation (Chapter 151).

Hematopoietic cell transplantation is also an effective treatment for other nonmalignant disorders, including thalassemia (Chapter 148), sickle cell disease (Chapter 149), immunodeficiency disorders, and enzyme deficiency states, primarily in children and young adults. Hemoglobinopathies can be cured by allogeneic hematopoietic cell transplantation, but new approaches such as gene therapy and the application of the clustered regularly interspaced short palindromic repeats (CRISPR) and CRISPR-associated protein 9 (CRISPR-Cas9) system may supplant hematopoietic cell transplantation (Chapter 34).[6] In thalassemia, the best transplant results have been obtained in pediatric patients with HLA-identical sibling donors. Adults tend to have more advanced disease with greater iron overload and more organ dysfunction; hence, they have high treatment-related mortality. Studies with nonmyeloablative regimens are ongoing. There is less experience with sickle cell disease (Chapter 149), partly because of reluctance to contemplate allogeneic hematopoietic cell transplantation in patients with an unpredictably variable clinical course.

For severe autoimmune disease, including systemic lupus erythematosus, rheumatoid arthritis, scleroderma, and multiple sclerosis, hematopoietic cell transplantation can reconstitute the immune system without the patient's native autoreactive T-cell clones. Trials have demonstrated clinically significant responses in patients with severe scleroderma (Chapter 246) and advanced multiple sclerosis (Chapter 380). In adults with severe scleroderma, for example, a randomized trial of myeloablative autologous hematopoietic cell transplantation showed long-term benefits, including improved event-free and overall survival, compared with 12 monthly infusions of cyclophosphamide.[A5]

COMPLICATIONS AFTER HEMATOPOIETIC STEM CELL TRANSPLANTATION

Improved supportive measures have led to a steady improvement in the outcomes of hematopoietic cell transplantation. Early complications, which are associated with all forms of hematopoietic cell transplantation, include direct organ toxicities from the conditioning regimen (e.g., mucositis) as well as prolonged cytopenias that can predispose to infections and bleeding.[7] Allogeneic hematopoietic cell transplantation also can be associated with acute and chronic GVHD. Long-term complications, particularly secondary malignancies, require that patients continue to be monitored for the remainder of their lives. A simple tally of the number of comorbid conditions can reliably predict nonrelapse mortality and survival and is useful for counseling patients before transplantation. Blood biomarkers may also become useful for predicting complications after transplantation, including the future occurrence of GVHD and its responsiveness to therapy, as well as nonrelapse mortality.

GRAFT-VERSUS-HOST DISEASE (GVHD)

Around the time of engraftment, patients are at risk for the development of GVHD, which represents the most important clinical challenge with allogeneic hematopoietic cell transplantation.[8] GVHD occurs when donor T cells recognize recipient antigens as foreign and attack these cells/organs. The pathophysiology involves many other cell types, cytokines, and even an important interaction with the host's microbiome, primarily the gut microbiome.[9]

GVHD can be either acute,[10] generally presenting within the first 100 days after transplantation, or chronic,[11] generally presenting after the first 100 days. However, clinical features of both acute and chronic GVHD may be observed at any time following allogeneic hematopoietic cell transplantation, and clinical manifestations rather than time after transplantation may best determine whether the GVHD syndrome is considered acute or chronic.

The incidence of clinically significant GVHD (grades II to IV) in recipients of HLA-matched sibling grafts (T-cell replete) using tacrolimus and methotrexate for GVHD prophylaxis is approximately 30 to 40%. The incidence of grades II to IV GVHD in recipients of HLA-matched unrelated donor grafts is approximately 50 to 80%.

ACUTE GRAFT-VERSUS-HOST DISEASE (GVHD)

The broad category of acute GVHD includes "classic" acute GVHD, occurring within 100 days after transplantation or donor lymphocyte infusion, as well as "persistent," "recurrent," or "late" acute GVHD, occurring beyond 100 days after transplantation or donor lymphocyte infusion. Risk factors for acute GVHD include HLA mismatch, a female donor (particularly a multiparous donor), more advanced age of the patient and the donor, cytomegalovirus seropositivity of the donor or patient, use of an unrelated donor, or use of a T-cell-replete versus T-cell-depleted graft.

CLINICAL MANIFESTATIONS

Acute GVHD primarily affects the skin, gastrointestinal tract, and liver. The skin manifestations range from a maculopapular rash to generalized erythroderma or desquamation. The severity of gastrointestinal GVHD is based on the amount of diarrhea per day and the presence of an ileus. The severity of liver GVHD is scored on the basis of the bilirubin level. Organs may be involved in isolation or simultaneously.

DIAGNOSIS

Histologic confirmation can be valuable to exclude other possibilities, such as infection. Mild GVHD of the skin may demonstrate vacuolar degeneration and infiltration of the basal layer by lymphocytes. With more advanced disease, histologic findings of necrotic dyskeratotic cells with acantholysis may progress to frank epidermolysis. In the liver, early GVHD may be difficult to distinguish from hepatitis of other causes. A clinical grading system (Table 163-1) correlates with clinical outcome.

TABLE 163-1 CLASSIFICATION OF PATIENTS WITH ACUTE GRAFT-VERSUS-HOST DISEASE

CLINICAL STAGING

STAGE	SKIN	LIVER	GUT
+	Rash <25% BSA	Total bilirubin 2-3 mg/dL	Diarrhea 500-1000 mL/day
++	Rash 25%-50% BSA	Total bilirubin 3-6 mg/dL	Diarrhea 1000-1500 mL/day
+++	Generalized erythroderma	Total bilirubin 6-15 mg/dL	Diarrhea >1500 mL/day
++++	Desquamation and bullae	Total bilirubin >15 mg/dL	Pain, with or without ileus

CLINICAL GRADING STAGE

GRADE	SKIN	LIVER	GUT	PS
0 (none)	0	0	0	0
I	+ to ++	0	0	0
II	+ to +++	+	+	+
III	++ to +++	++ to +++	++ to +++	++
IV	++ to ++++	++ to ++++	++ to ++++	+++

BSA = body surface area; PS = performance status.

PREVENTION

The best approach to GVHD is prevention.[12] The prophylactic use of cyclosporine plus methotrexate is equivalent to the combination of tacrolimus plus sirolimus in terms of reducing the incidence and severity of acute GVHD and improving survival after allogeneic cell transplantation.[A6] In a nonrandomized study, the addition of sitagliptin, which inhibits dipeptidyl peptidase 4, reduced acute GVHD from its usual 30 to 40% incidence rate to less than 10%.[13]

Cyclosporine has significant toxicities, including hypertension, nephrotoxicity, hypomagnesemia, risk for seizures, hypertrichosis, gingival hyperplasia, tremors, and anorexia. Tacrolimus closely resembles cyclosporine in mechanism of action, spectrum of toxicities, and pharmacologic interactions. For allogeneic hematopoietic cell transplantation, prophylactic immunosuppression is not lifelong; when immunologic tolerance is established, immunosuppressive agents can be slowly withdrawn and discontinued.

Another strategy to prevent GVHD is to deplete the donor's T cells from the graft. The disadvantage of this approach is its association with increased rates of relapsed disease and infection. Furthermore, overall survival does not seem to be improved.

TREATMENT

Moderate to severe GVHD (grades II to IV) requires treatment, and the mainstay of therapy is corticosteroids. Methylprednisolone (1 to 2 mg/kg/day) achieves responses in 40 to 60% of patients, and higher doses of steroids are beneficial. For steroid-refractory GVHD, oral ruxolitinib (10 mg twice daily) can provide a durable 6-month response in 90% of patients and nearly double median overall survival from 6.5 months to 11.1 months as compared with alternative therapies,[A7] such as antithymocyte globulin or various monoclonal antibodies (e.g., daclizumab, infliximab). In general, acute GVHD of the skin is most responsive to treatment, whereas GVHD of the liver is least responsive. Unfortunately, the fatality rate for steroid-refractory acute GVHD may still be as high as 50%.

CHRONIC GRAFT-VERSUS-HOST DISEASE (GVHD)

Chronic GVHD, which occurs in 20 to 50% of long-term survivors, occurs most commonly between 100 days and 2 years after transplantation and has polymorphic features similar to a number of autoimmune diseases. Chronic GVHD is classified as classic chronic GVHD, which consists only of manifestations that can be ascribed to chronic GVHD, or as acute and chronic GVDH overlap syndrome, in which features of both acute and chronic GVHD appear together. These distinctions are clinically relevant because "late-onset" acute GVHD and overlap syndrome subsets have been associated with poor survival.

Chronic GVHD is most likely to develop in older patients who also had acute GVHD or received peripheral blood rather than bone marrow grafts. In 20% of cases of chronic GVHD, however, there is no history of prior acute GVHD.

CLINICAL MANIFESTATIONS

Common manifestations include the sicca syndrome (Chapter 247); lichen planus–like skin rash; scleroderma-like skin changes (Chapter 246);[14] esophageal, intestinal, and vaginal fibrosis; obstructive lung disease with or without pneumonitis; and an elevated alkaline phosphatase level with or without hyperbilirubinemia. Underlying immunologic deficiencies, including hypogammaglobulinemia, are common and place patients at increased risk for infectious events. Adverse prognostic factors include thrombocytopenia, a progressive clinical presentation, extensive skin involvement, and an elevated bilirubin level.

DIAGNOSIS

Historically, chronic GVHD has been considered as limited, with localized skin involvement and minimal or no liver involvement, or extensive, with generalized skin involvement with or without other organ involvement. Chronic GVHD is usually a clinical diagnosis although biopsy is sometimes needed. The severity of GVHD can be graded in transplant centers based on the severity of disease for each affected organ/site at any given time.

TREATMENT

Treatment of chronic GVHD, which is guided by the extent of disease, should be initiated before patients develop functional impairment. Treatment usually begins with corticosteroids (e.g., prednisone 0.5 to 1 mg/kg/day). Ruxolitinib (10 mg twice daily) can prolong median failure-free survival from about 6 months to more than 18 months in glucocorticoid-refractory disease.[A8] Belumosudil (200 mg daily) is another potential option with an overall response rate of about 75%.[15] Ibrutinib (420 mg twice daily)[16] and pomalidomide (0.5 to 2 mg daily)[A9] are other alternatives.[17] Ibrutinib is also useful for glucocorticoid-refractory chronic GVHD. Other potential therapies include extracorporeal photopheresis, cyclosporine, ultraviolet light treatments, monoclonal antibodies, and methotrexate. Given that the most common cause of death in patients with chronic GVHD remains infection, all patients with GVHD should receive prophylactic antibiotics (penicillin 500 mg twice daily) for encapsulated bacteria, with or without intravenous immunoglobulin, depending on serum levels.

Graft Rejection

Graft rejection occurs when immunologically competent cells of host origin destroy the transplanted cells of donor origin. This complication occurs more commonly in patients who receive transplants from alternative source such as cord blood or HLA-mismatched donors, in T-cell-depleted transplants, and in patients with aplastic anemia. Graft rejection also occurs if the conditioning regimen is not sufficiently immunosuppressive to facilitate engraftment of donor cells.

Infections

Infections are a major cause of morbidity and mortality after all forms of hematopoietic cell transplantation but especially following allogeneic transplantation (Chapter 260) because of prolonged use of immunosuppression for the prevention or treatment of GVHD.[18] Bacterial infections are frequently related to central venous catheters.

Among fungal infections, candida (Chapter 310) and aspergillus (Chapter 311) infections typically occur in patients receiving prolonged high-dose corticosteroids for the treatment of GVHD. In such patients, prophylactic antifungal treatment (e.g., fluconazole 400 mg daily) and anti–*Pneumocystis jirovecii* (e.g., one double strength trimethoprim-sulfamethoxazole tablet daily) is necessary.[19]

Viral infections include reactivation of cytomegalovirus (Chapter 347), human herpesvirus 6, BK virus (Chapter 341), and Epstein-Barr virus (Chapter 348) infections. Letermovir prophylaxis (480 mg orally daily through day 100) can significantly reduce the risk of cytomegalovirus reactivation.[A10] Varicella zoster vaccination (Chapter 346) can significantly reduce zoster reactivation[A11] in post-transplantation patients, but the live vaccine should not be used. These patients are also susceptible to seasonal respiratory viruses. Influenza vaccination (Chapter 332) and revaccination for common childhood infections (Chapter 15) are required after transplantation.[20] Vaccines for COVID-19 are recommended once blood counts and CD4 counts have recovered.

Cardiac Toxicity

Most transplant centers screen potential patients for underlying cardiac abnormalities that would place them at a potentially increased risk during the procedure. Despite this screening, however, a small number of patients experience a cardiac arrhythmia (Chapters 51 to 53), heart failure (Chapters 45 and 46), or cardiac ischemia (Chapter 57), either acutely during the transplantation or at a later time, often due to the large volumes of fluids administered during the procedure or from the added physiologic stress. A pericardial effusion (Chapter 62) can develop during or after transplantation, especially in patients with initial disease or radiation therapy near that area. An idiosyncratic cardiomyopathy, associated with the administration of high doses of cyclophosphamide, has been documented in a small number of patients. Viral cardiomyopathies (Chapter 47) also can be seen.

Engraftment Syndrome

Engraftment syndrome occurs when the neutrophil count recovers after either autologous or allogeneic hematopoietic cell transplantation. Engraftment syndrome consists of a constellation of symptoms and signs that may include fever, erythrodermatous skin rash, and noncardiogenic pulmonary edema. In its most extreme forms, patients also develop acute renal failure and diffuse alveolar hemorrhage. These clinical findings reflect the manifestations of increased capillary permeability and extensive release of cytokines. Corticosteroid therapy (typically prednisone at 0.5 mg/kg) is often dramatically effective for engraftment syndrome, particularly for its pulmonary manifestations.

Pulmonary Toxicities

Pulmonary toxicities are common during and after transplantation. Patients who receive certain chemotherapeutic agents, such as 1,3-bis (2-chloroethyl)-1-nitrosourea (BCNU; carmustine) have an increased incidence of chemotherapy-induced lung tissue damage, which usually occurs several weeks after transplantation and can be treated successfully with the prompt initiation of corticosteroid therapy (e.g., prednisone 1 mg/kg, with tapering initiated after response is achieved, usually within 2 weeks). In addition to these complications, patients who are undergoing allogeneic hematopoietic cell transplantation are at increased risk for pneumonitis, caused by cytomegalovirus (Chapter 347) and fungal infections, because of the patient's increased immunosuppression, and idiopathic adult respiratory distress syndrome (Chapter 90) or interstitial pneumonia (Chapter 80). Chronic GVHD also can manifest as bronchiolitis obliterans in the lung.

Liver Toxicity

The most common liver complication associated with transplantation is veno-occlusive disease/sinusoidal obstruction syndrome of the liver (Chapter 136). Symptoms associated with these complications include jaundice, tender hepatomegaly, ascites, and weight gain. Progressive hepatic and multiorgan system failure can develop in the most severe cases. Predisposing factors appear to be previous hepatic injury, use of estrogens, and high-dose intensity conditioning. Defibrotide (6.25 mg/kg every 6 hours for a minimum of 21 days) is approved by the FDA to treat advanced veno-occlusive disease in the setting of hematopoietic stem cell transplantation.

Renal Toxicity

Acute renal failure requiring dialysis occurs infrequently during transplantation, although patients with underlying renal dysfunction are at risk for this complication. An idiopathic or cyclosporine-induced hemolytic-uremic syndrome (Chapter 158) can be seen after allogeneic transplantation, can result in end-stage renal disease, and poses a high risk of mortality. Thrombotic microangiopathy also can lead to acute renal injury. Nephrotic syndrome and membranous nephropathy (Chapter 107) have been described in long-term survivors; these complications seem to be associated more commonly with chronic GVHD and nonmyeloablative conditioning.

Secondary Malignancies

One complication of chemotherapy, radiation therapy (especially total body radiation), or both used to treat malignancy and condition patients for hematopoietic cell transplantation is the development of a secondary malignancy. Secondary AML or myelodysplastic syndrome can occur after autologous transplantation. After allogeneic transplantation, the overall incidences of secondary malignancies are 2.2% at 10 years and 6.7% at 15 years. Solid malignancies occur in up to 15% of patients 15 years after hematopoietic cell transplantation with myeloablative conditioning, with no plateau in the incidence rates.[21] Within the first 1 to 2 years, the most common malignancies are Epstein-Barr virus–related lymphoproliferative disorders (Chapter 348)[22]; solid tumors are more likely to occur more than 3 years after transplantation. Risk factors include the use of antithymocyte globulin to treat GVHD, the use of a T-cell-depleted allogeneic graft, HLA incompatibility, and perhaps total body radiation. This high incidence stresses the importance of careful long-term follow-up.

Infertility and Hypogonadism

Many of the preparative regimens used for transplantation are associated with a high incidence of permanent sterility, especially regimens containing total body radiation. However, successful pregnancies have occurred in some patients after other regimens, particularly in younger patients. A reproductive endocrinologist should be consulted before transplantation when future fertility is important. Gynecomastia occasionally occurs in males.

Endocrine Dysfunction

Iatrogenic Cushing syndrome (Chapters 204 and 208) and diabetes (Chapter 210) can occur and are commonly due to long-term corticosteroid therapy for chronic GVHD. Particularly disabling are steroid-induced myopathy (Chapter 28), avascular necrosis of the hip (Chapter 229), and osteoporosis (Chapter 225). Because many patients take corticosteroids for many months, tapering can be associated with malaise, nausea, hypotension, and musculoskeletal pains. In these situations, slower tapering over several months or reintroduction of physiologic replacement doses (e.g., 7.5 to 10 mg/day of prednisone) is appropriate. Hypothyroidism (Chapter 207) is typically related to the use of total body radiation or local radiation to the head and neck for lymphoma or other cancer.

Osteoporosis occurs in 50 to 60% of patients after hematopoietic cell transplantation. The major contributing causes include hypogonadism, secondary hyperparathyroidism caused by low serum calcium levels, and post-transplantation corticosteroid therapy. Bone mineral density should be evaluated before and after transplantation; osteopenia should be treated as appropriate with bisphosphonates, calcium, vitamin D, estrogen, and testosterone (Chapter 225).

FUTURE DIRECTIONS

There has been much progress in increasing the efficacy and safety of hematopoietic cell transplantation and in expanding the application of this treatment to more patients.[23] Areas currently under development that may further improve the use and efficacy of transplantation include continuous improvements in supportive care for transplant patients and the broadened use of alternative donors. Recurrence of disease remains the primary cause of treatment failure after both autologous and allogeneic hematopoietic cell transplantation in malignant diseases.[24] Better treatments are necessary for the treatment of GVHD and innovative studies are ongoing. Future progress depends on the ability to identify safer and better-targeted antitumor therapies that can be incorporated into transplantation regimens or given as maintenance therapy without increasing toxicity or attenuating graft-versus-tumor responses. Novel cellular therapies, including genetic modification of lymphocytes to enhance cancer-killing activity, such as chimeric antigen receptor (CAR) T cells (Chapter 34), hold considerable promise.

GENERAL REFERENCES

For the General References and other additional features, please visit Elsevier eBooks+ at https://ebooks.health.elsevier.com.

Grade A References

A1. Li D, Wang L, Zhu H, et al. Efficacy of allogeneic hematopoietic stem cell transplantation in intermediate-risk acute myeloid leukemia adult patients in first complete remission: a meta-analysis of prospective studies. *PLoS ONE*. 2015;10:1-16.

A2. Kröger N, Iacobelli S, Franke GN, et al. Dose-reduced versus standard conditioning followed by allogeneic stem-cell transplantation for patients with myelodysplastic syndrome: a prospective randomized phase III study of the EBMT (RICMAC Trial). *J Clin Oncol*. 2017;35:2157-2164.

A3. Le Gouill S, Thieblemont C, Oberic L, et al. Rituximab after autologous stem-cell transplantation in mantle-cell lymphoma. *N Engl J Med*. 2017;377:1250-1260.

A4. Berinstein NL, Bhella S, Pennell NM, et al. Prolonged clinical remissions in patients with relapsed or refractory follicular lymphoma treated with autologous stem cell transplantation incorporating rituximab. *Ann Hematol*. 2015;94:813-823.

A5. Sullivan KM, Goldmuntz EAS, Keyes-Elstein L, et al. SCOT Study Investigators. Myeloablative autologous stem-cell transplantation for severe scleroderma. *N Engl J Med*. 2018;378:35-47.

A6. Törlén J, Ringdén O, Garming-Legert K, et al. A prospective randomized trial comparing cyclosporine/methotrexate and tacrolimus/sirolimus as graft-versus-host disease prophylaxis after allogeneic hematopoietic stem cell transplantation. *Haematologica*. 2016;101:1417-1425.

A7. Zeiser R, von Bubnoff N, Butler J, et al. Ruxolitinib for glucocorticoid-refractory acute graft-versus-host disease. *N Engl J Med*. 2020;382:1800-1810.

A8. Zeiser R, Polverelli N, Ram R, et al. Ruxolitinib for glucocorticoid-refractory chronic graft-versus-host disease. *N Engl J Med*. 2021;385:228-238.

A9. Curtis LM, Ostojic A, Venzon DJ, et al. A randomized phase 2 trial of pomalidomide in subjects failing prior therapy for chronic graft-versus-host disease. *Blood*. 2021;137:896-907.

A10. Marty FM, Ljungman P, Chemaly RF, et al. Letermovir prophylaxis for cytomegalovirus in hematopoietic-cell transplantation. *N Engl J Med*. 2017;377:2433-2444.

A11. Winston DJ, Mullane KM, Cornely OA, et al. Inactivated varicella zoster vaccine in autologous haemopoietic stem-cell transplant recipients: an international, multicentre, randomised, double-blind, placebo-controlled trial. *Lancet*. 2018;391:2116-2127.

XVI

ONCOLOGY

164 APPROACH TO THE PATIENT WITH CANCER

JAMES H. DOROSHOW

INTRODUCTION TO THE CANCER PATIENT

Conveying or receiving an initial diagnosis of cancer, or the knowledge that cancer has recurred, is among the most difficult of human enterprises, and no amount of either specialized training or forewarning can adequately assuage the intensity of the emotions associated with these encounters. Patients often experience a storm of feelings that may limit useful discussion immediately following the receipt of a diagnosis of cancer. Even the most well-informed patient typically has difficulty processing the complexities of his or her individual situation, including the range of additional diagnostic tests that may be required and the potentially vast array of treatment options and outcomes that lie ahead. And yet, at some point prior to the initiation of treatment, the physician and the patient must discuss the diagnosis, its implications, and therapeutic alternatives. Because of the wide range of potential prognoses (from curable disseminated testicular cancer to the limited lifespan of patients with locally advanced gastric or pancreatic cancer), it is often useful for family members or close friends to be present in the consulting room when detailed discussions of the complexities of either disease or therapy are conducted, both to provide emotional support and to be another "set of ears" during the visit. It is helpful to ask patients directly: "What do you understand about your diagnosis and treatment?" Family members or close associates of the patient may also be especially helpful in developing a written or digital record of the questions posed to and answered by health care providers; many patients find such a record to be especially helpful for later reference.

If the physician is not familiar with the latest treatment options, prompt referral to a specialist, whether a surgical oncologist, radiation oncologist, or medical oncologist, is imperative. The generalist should not be a therapeutic nihilist unless she or he is intimately involved in the field and is well versed in the potential risks and benefits of currently available therapies and clinical trials.

DIAGNOSIS

Diagnostic possibilities are protean for the wide range of human malignancies that may be discovered either in the presence of nonspecific but foreboding symptoms or signs (severe weight loss [see Fig. 118-4], hematuria [see Fig. 100-3], jaundice [see Fig. 133-1]) or in asymptomatic individuals (e.g., during a routine physical examination).[1] The importance of the medical history and physical examination, however, must be emphasized *whether or not* a pathologic diagnosis of cancer has already been confirmed. One of the most important considerations that underlies the approach to both the diagnostic evaluation and choice of cancer treatment (surgical, radiation, and/or systemic therapy) is the patient's basic physiologic condition or "performance status" (Table 164-1). For example, a past medical history of prolonged tobacco smoking (Chapter 363) is not only relevant to a possible diagnosis of lung cancer but also to the ability of a patient to tolerate potentially curable multimodality treatment. Underlying evidence of excessive alcohol consumption (Chapter 364) may play a role in both the tolerance for and metabolism of systemic chemotherapeutic agents. Family histories of cancer can provide prognostic indicators as well as suggest molecularly guided treatment approaches in, for example, women with possible *BRCA1*-related breast or ovarian cancer. It is also critical to assess the environment of care, including the patient's support systems, which may be sorely tested by the experience of a cancer diagnosis and the interventions that ensue. Finally, the physical examination will define the extent of certain sites of measurable malignancy—for example, palpable lymph nodes or enlargement of the spleen or liver—as well as the patient's muscle strength, the presence of possible malignant effusions, and potential central or peripheral neuropathies reflective of metastatic disease or paraneoplastic syndromes. Most importantly, however, the evaluation provides the treating physician with an initial sense of the patient's well-being, or lack thereof, prior to the initiation of therapy.

TABLE 164-1 KARNOFSKY AND ZUBROD PERFORMANCE SCALES

KARNOFSKY PERFORMANCE STATUS SCALE	
VALUE	**LEVEL OF FUNCTIONAL CAPACITY**
100	Normal, no complaints, no evidence of disease
90	Able to carry on normal activity, minor signs or symptoms of disease
80	Normal activity with effort, some signs or symptoms of disease
70	Cares for self, unable to carry on normal activity or to do active work
60	Requires occasional assistance but is able to care for most needs
50	Requires considerable assistance and frequent medical care
40	Disabled, requires special care and assistance
30	Severely disabled; hospitalization is indicated, although death is not imminent
20	Hospitalization is necessary; very sick, active supportive treatment necessary
10	Moribund; fatal processes progressing rapidly
0	Dead
EASTERN COOPERATIVE ONCOLOGY GROUP (ZUBROD) PERFORMANCE SCALE	
PERFORMANCE STATUS	**DEFINITION**
0	Asymptomatic
1	Symptomatic; fully ambulatory
2	Symptomatic; in bed <50% of day
3	Symptomatic; in bed >50% of day
4	Bedridden

Diagnostic Procedures

After a lesion has been found, either on physical examination or following radiographic studies prompted by abnormal laboratory results, a percutaneous biopsy is often indicated for pathologic evaluation. The biopsy must be representative of the entire tumor and be robust enough in size that appropriate investigations (e.g., special immunohistologic stains, flow cytometry, cytogenetics, hormone assays, molecular testing) can be performed before treatment is initiated. If questions remain as to whether the lesion is benign or malignant or about its proper classification, consideration should be given to additional biopsies, and consultation with a reference pathologist may be indicated.

Molecular testing is increasingly useful for the early diagnosis of asymptomatic malignancy.[2] For example, a small number of cases of occult cancer may be subsequently diagnosed among pregnant women whose noninvasive prenatal testing results show discordance with the fetal karyotype.[3] Similarly, analysis of blood for circulating tumor cells (termed a liquid biopsy) can screen for some early cancers or a recurrence of tumor after treatment.

The wide range of molecularly targeted and immunotherapeutic agents active in solid tumors (see Table 164-2 for an abbreviated list of commonly used medications in cancer and https://www.cancer.gov/about-cancer/treatment/drugs/cancer-type for a full listing of all drugs approved by the U.S. Food and Drug Administration) has focused attention on obtaining sufficient tissue so that essential molecular studies (DNA sequencing, RNA expression analyses, FIH [fluorescence in situ hybridization], and immunologic profiling) are performed to guide choices among treatments. Although tumors removed by surgical resection are routinely of sufficient size to permit the full range of diagnostic examinations, active involvement of a skilled interventional radiologist or endoscopist is often required to produce both the size and number of tumor biopsies required for modern cancer therapeutic decision making. Emergent treatment is rarely required before appropriate pretreatment evaluations can be performed. For some tumor sites such as the colon (Chapter 179), one predominant histology is seen, but critical molecular features of the tumor (presence or absence of a mutant *Ras* oncogene) can define therapy. For other tumors, such as in the lung (Chapter 177), the distinction between

TABLE 164-2 U.S. FDA-APPROVED DRUGS COMMONLY USED FOR THE SYSTEMIC TREATMENT OF CANCER*

DRUG NAME	DRUG CLASS AND/OR MECHANISM	PHARMACOKINETICS/METABOLISM	TOXICITY	INDICATIONS†
Abiraterone acetate (Zytiga)	Inhibits androgen biosynthesis	Do not take with food; inhibits CYP2D6	Joint swelling or discomfort; edema; monitor liver enzymes	Metastatic prostate cancer
Acalabrutinib (Calquence)	Bruton kinase inhibitor	Avoid with proton pump inhibitors, strong CYP3A inhibitors or inducers, and patients with severe hepatic impairment	Opportunistic infection, cytopenias, atrial tachyarrhythmias, headache, diarrhea, musculoskeletal pain	CLL, small lymphocytic lymphoma, mantle cell lymphoma
Afatinib (Gilotrif)	Selective covalent inhibitor of EGFR, HER2, and HER4; inhibits wild-type and selected EGFR mutants	Interacts with P-gp inhibitors which may require dose reduction; dose reduction for moderate renal dysfunction	Acneiform eruption; hypokalemia; diarrhea, stomatitis, and nausea; altered liver function studies; decreased creatinine clearance	NSCLC first line with *EGFR* exon 19 deletions or exon 21 (L858R) mutation as detected by appropriate diagnostic test
Alectinib (Alecensa)	Tyrosine kinase inhibitor inhibiting *ALK* gene abnormalities and *RET* mutations; can inhibit certain *ALK* mutations that follow treatment with crizotinib	Hepatic metabolism by CYP3A4; excreted in the feces	Bradycardia; CK elevations; interstitial pneumonitis	ALK-positive metastatic NSCLC progressive on crizotinib
Amivantamab-vmjw (Rybrevant)	Human *EGFR* and *MET* bispecific antibody targeting *EGFR* exon 20 insertion mutations	Disrupts *EGFR* and *MET* signaling by blocking ligand binding and degrading *EGFR* and *MET*; terminal half-life of about 11 days	Rash; infusion reactions; paronychia; stomatitis; pruritus	NSCLC with *EGFR* exon 20 insertion mutations in patients who have progressed on platinum-based chemotherapy
Anastrozole (Arimidex)	Nonsteroidal aromatase inhibitor; blocks estrogen production selectively	Well absorbed from GI tract, maximum plasma levels within 2 hr; half-life is 50 hr; extensively metabolized in liver; despite hepatic and renal clearance being important, no adjustments needed for abnormal function of these organs because of the wide therapeutic index of this drug	Very well tolerated; asthenia, headache, and hot flashes occur in less than 15% of women; diarrhea, abdominal pain, anorexia, nausea, and vomiting occur in 10% or less; thrombophlebitis has been reported	As adjuvant therapy of breast cancer and for treatment of postmenopausal women with breast carcinoma who have progressed while being treated with tamoxifen
Apalutamide (Erleada)	Androgen receptor inhibitor	If no prior orchiectomy, prescribe a gonadotropin-releasing hormone analog concurrently	Ischemic cardiovascular events, fractures, fatigue, arthralgia, rash, decreased appetite, falls, weight decreased, hypertension, hot flush, diarrhea	Metastatic castration-sensitive prostate cancer or nonmetastatic castration-resistant prostate cancer
Arsenic trioxide (Trisenox)	Novel arsenical differentiating agent	Half-life of this compound is unknown; it is methylated in the liver and eliminated in the urine	The "differentiation syndrome" is dose limiting and includes leukocytosis, fever, dyspnea, chest pain, tachycardia, hypoxia, and sometimes death; corticosteroids seem to benefit this syndrome; QT prolongation is common; common adverse effects include rash, pruritus, headache, arthralgias, anxiety, bleeding, nausea, and vomiting; liver and renal toxicity are uncommon	Relapsed acute promyelocytic leukemia
L-Asparaginase (Elspar), colaspase	Naturally occurring enzyme derived from *Escherichia coli* or *Erwinia carotovora* that cleaves asparagine, an essential amino acid required by rapidly proliferating cells	After IV or IM injection, the drug is metabolized intravascularly by proteolysis; elimination half-life of 8-30 hr	Hypersensitivity can be life-threatening, requiring anaphylaxis precautions and a 2-unit test dose; coagulopathy is common and requires monitoring; nausea, vomiting, abdominal cramps, anorexia, elevated liver function tests, and transient renal insufficiency are common; lethargy, somnolence, fatigue, depression, and confusion are seen, as are pancreatitis and fever	ALL; also used in AML, late-stage CML, CLL, and non-Hodgkin lymphomas
Atezolizumab (Tecentriq)	Humanized monoclonal antibody that binds the programmed death ligand 1 (PD-L1) downregulating anti–T-cell function	No dosage adjustment for mild renal or hepatic insufficiency	Rash; endocrinopathies; immune hepatitis, pancreatitis, pneumonitis, colitis, adrenal insufficiency, diabetes; peripheral edema; fatigue; fever	NSCLC; small cell lung cancer; advanced urothelial cancer patients ineligible for or who have progressed after platinum-containing therapy; hepatocellular cancer; melanoma
Avelumab (Bavencio)	Programmed death ligand-1 (PD-L1) blocking antibody	Can cause fetal harm	Immune-mediated pneumonitis, hepatitis, colitis, endocrinopathies, nephritis; fatigue; musculoskeletal pain; rash; diarrhea	Adult and pediatric patients (12 yr of age and older) with metastatic Merkel cell carcinoma; renal cell carcinoma; urothelial carcinoma
Axitinib (Inlyta)	Avoid strong CYP3A inhibitors or reduce dose	Decrease dose 50% for CYP3A inhibitors, renal, hepatic impairment	Diarrhea, hypertension, fatigue, nausea	Advanced renal cell carcinoma after one treatment failure

TABLE 164-2 U.S. FDA-APPROVED DRUGS COMMONLY USED FOR THE SYSTEMIC TREATMENT OF CANCER*—cont'd

DRUG NAME	DRUG CLASS AND/OR MECHANISM	PHARMACOKINETICS/METABOLISM	TOXICITY	INDICATIONS†
Azacytidine (Vidaza)	Antimetabolite; induces hypomethylation of DNA, either inducing apoptosis or restoring normal function; at higher doses, acts as a cytidine analog	Not orally bioavailable; metabolized by the liver and excreted in urine; elimination half-life of 4 hr	Myelosuppression is dose limiting; leukopenia, thrombocytopenia, and transient elevation of liver function tests are common; nausea and vomiting and abdominal pain are common	Myelodysplastic syndromes
Bacillus Calmette-Guérin (TICE BCG, TheraCys), BCG	Immunostimulant/vaccine; induces a cellular immune response at the site of instillation	BCG is a live, attenuated bacteria culture; it does not enter the body in viable form; it has no detectable pharmacokinetic fate; in rare cases, a clinical infection can result from treatment, indicating invasion of the body at site of administration into systemic circulation	Urinary symptoms predominate, including dysuria, hematuria, hesitancy, urgency, frequency, and secondary infection; other toxicities include fever, chills, malaise, myalgias/arthralgias, anorexia, nausea, vomiting, and anemia; clinical mycobacterial infection is rare and generally seen only in immunocompromised patients	Intravesical instillation for noninvasive bladder cancer after removal of papillary tumors; also used for some experimental vaccine programs as an adjuvant to the vaccine
Belinostat (Beleodaq)	Histone deacetylase inhibitor; results in accumulation of acetyl groups on histone and nonhistone proteins causing cell cycle arrest and apoptosis	Hepatic metabolism via *UGT1A1* and CYP2A6; excreted in urine	Myelosuppression; peripheral edema and prolonged QT interval; rash; nausea and vomiting; fatigue	Relapsed peripheral T-cell lymphoma
Bendamustine (Treanda)	Alkylating agent	Reduce dose for hematologic toxicity	Nausea, pyrexia, vomiting, hematologic abnormalities	CLL and B-cell non-Hodgkin lymphoma
Bevacizumab (Avastin)	Recombinant humanized monoclonal antibody that binds to all forms of VEGF, preventing binding to its receptors	Administered by IV infusion; half-life is 20 days; the fate of parent drug and metabolites is unknown	Asthenia, pain, nausea/vomiting, diarrhea, anorexia, stomatitis, dermatitis, hypertension, proteinuria; infusion-related reactions rare; hemoptysis, hemorrhage, delayed wound healing, GI perforations; increased risk of thromboembolic events can be severe or fatal	Metastatic colorectal cancer and NSCLC; renal cell carcinoma
Bicalutamide (Casodex)	Nonsteroidal antiandrogen	Well absorbed orally; highly protein bound; converted to inactive metabolites in liver via oxidation and glucuronidation; half-life of several days	Constitutional symptoms predominate, including hot flashes, decreased libido, depression, weight gain, edema, gynecomastia, early disease-site pain (flare reaction), and constipation; nausea, vomiting, anorexia, diarrhea, and dizziness are uncommon; dyspnea, anemia, fever, and rashes are rare	Stage D2 prostate cancer, in combination with an LHRH agonist agent
Binimetinib (Mektovi)	Mitogen-activated protein kinase 1 and 2 inhibitor	Reduce dose if moderate or severe hepatic impairment	Cardiomyopathy, retinopathy, interstitial lung disease, hepatotoxicity, rhabdomyolysis	Unresectable or metastatic melanoma with a *BRAF* V600E or V600K mutation
Bortezomib (Velcade)	Proteasome inhibitor	Metabolized in the liver by CYP2C19 and 3A4; dose reduction for hepatic dysfunction	Cardiovascular; peripheral neuropathy; skin rash; nausea and diarrhea	Multiple myeloma; mantle cell lymphoma
Brentuximab vedotin (Adcetris)	CD30-directed antibody conjugate	Monitor patients taking CYP3A inducers or inhibitors	Progressive multifocal leukoencephalopathy; peripheral neuropathy; neutropenia	Hodgkin lymphoma and anaplastic large cell lymphoma
Brigatinib (Alunbrig)	Multikinase inhibitor	Interacts with strong CYP3A inhibitors; requires dose reduction; avoid grapefruit juice	Hypertension; skin rash; fatigue; increased liver function tests	ALK-positive NSCLC for patients who have progressed on crizotinib
Capecitabine (Xeloda)	Oral antimetabolite prodrug	Readily absorbed by the GI tract, metabolized in vivo to fluorouracil in the liver by carboxylesterase and cytidine deaminase, and then in turn in the peripheral tissues and tumor tissue by thymidine phosphorylase	Myelosuppression and palmar-plantar erythrodysesthesia are dose limiting; diarrhea, fatigue, stomatitis, and hyperbilirubinemia are uncommon; nausea, vomiting, and rash are rare	Metastatic breast cancer and metastatic colorectal cancer; used also in head and neck squamous cell cancer
Cabazitaxel (Jevtana)	Microtubule inhibitor	Caution for patients taking strong CYP3A inducers or inhibitors	Neutropenia and hypersensitivity	Metastatic hormone refractory prostate cancer when docetaxel fails
Cabozantinib	Inhibits many receptor tyrosine kinases; anti-angiogenic	55-hour half-life; take without food	Perforations, fistulas, and hemorrhage	Metastatic medullary thyroid cancer; advanced renal cell carcinoma; advanced hepatocellular cancer

Carboplatin (Paraplatin), Carbo, CBDCA	Atypical alkylator; produces intrastrand and interstrand cross-links in DNA via association bonds with the platinum molecule, leading to DNA strand breakage during replication	Rapidly cleared from the blood stream after IV infusion, with a terminal half-life of 2.5 hr; it is cleared largely as unchanged drug by the kidneys	Hemorrhage; thrombocytopenia	Ovarian cancer and used extensively in testicular cancer, squamous cell cancers of the head and neck and cervix, and lung cancer
Carfilzomib (Kyprolis)	Proteasome inhibitor	Drug-drug interactions unlikely; no adjustment for renal impairment; no experience with hepatic impairment	Fatigue, anemia, nausea, thrombocytopenia, dyspnea, diarrhea, and pyrexia; monitor for cardiac, pulmonary, tumor lysis, infusion reactions, thrombocytopenia	Multiple myeloma
Ceritinib (Zykadia)	Inhibitor of ALK tyrosine kinase as well as *ROS1*; also inhibits IGF-1R and the insulin receptor	Metabolized by CYP3A in the liver; dose reduction if concomitant strong CYP3A inhibitors are administered	Bradycardia; QTc prolongation; nausea, vomiting; hyperglycemia; interstitial pneumonitis	NSCLC that is *ALK* positive by an appropriate diagnostic test; demonstrated activity in crizotinib-resistant NSCLC xenograft models
Cetuximab (Erbitux)	Recombinant humanized monoclonal antibody, targeting *EGFR*; competitively inhibits growth factor binding, inhibits autophosphorylation and cell signaling	Metabolism poorly understood; half-life 5-7 days with minimal clearance by kidneys or liver	Infusion reaction, characterized by rapid-onset dyspnea, fever, chills, urticaria, flushing, angioedema, and hypotension, is seen in 40-50% of patients; acneiform rash is common; constitutional symptoms; hypomagnesemia; interstitial lung disease is rare	Metastatic colorectal cancer, head and neck cancer in combination with radiation
Cisplatin (Platinol)—cDDP, DDP, cisplatinum, cis-diamminedichloro-platinum (II)	Atypical alkylator; produces intrastrand and interstrand cross-links in DNA via association bonds with the platinum molecule, leading to DNA strand breakage during replication	After IV infusion, rapid distribution to tissues takes place, and the drug is over 90% protein bound	Nephrotoxicity is dose limiting for an individual dose, and neurotoxicity, especially painful peripheral neuropathy, is dose limiting for cumulative doses; myelosuppression is mild; nausea and vomiting are common but manageable, and anorexia and diarrhea are common; cumulative ototoxicity is also common; chronic renal magnesium and potassium wasting is common and sometimes not reversible; elevated liver transaminases can be seen, whereas alopecia and cardiac conduction abnormalities are rare; adequate renal perfusion and urine output are critical for minimizing renal toxicity; therefore prehydration and adequate posttreatment hydration are used, usually with normal saline solution with or without mannitol, potassium, and magnesium	Used for almost every class of solid tumor and lymphoma; FDA approved for testicular and ovarian cancer and transitional cell carcinoma
Cobimetinib (Cotellic)	Inhibitor of *MEK1* and *MEK2* in the MAPK cascade	Detoxified in the liver by CYP3A4 and UGT2B7; use of strong CYP3A4 inhibitors should be avoided; excreted in feces	Cardiotoxicity; rhabdomyolysis; rash; retinopathy; bleeding	Metastatic or unresectable melanoma for patients with *BRAF* V600E or V600K mutations in combination with vemurafenib
Copanlisib (Aliqopa)	PI-3 kinase inhibitor	Avoid concomitant strong CYP3A inducers and reduce dose of strong CYP3A inhibitors	Hyperglycemia, hypertension, neutropenia, thrombocytopenia, diarrhea, severe cutaneous reactions, nausea, lower respiratory tract infections	Relapsed follicular lymphoma after at least two prior systemic therapies
Crizotinib (Xalkori)	ALK kinase inhibitor; also inhibits *cMET*	Avoid strong CYP3A inhibitors, inducers, or substrates	Hepatotoxicity; pneumonitis; QT interval prolonged	*ALK*-positive NSCLC
Cyclophosphamide	Alkylating agent	Metabolized to its active alkylating species by mixed function oxidases in hepatic microsomes including CYP2A6 and 3A4; decreased activation to therapeutic species in the face of severe hepatic dysfunction	Myelosuppression; immunosuppression; hemorrhagic cystitis; myocarditis; pneumonitis; secondary malignancies; infertility; hyponatremia; veno-occlusive disease; nausea and vomiting; mucositis	Hodgkin and non-Hodgkin lymphoma; leukemias; ovarian cancer; breast cancer; retinoblastoma; neuroblastoma
Cytarabine	Antimetabolite that inhibits DNA polymerase after activation to its nucleotide triphosphate, is incorporated into DNA and RNA and blocks cell cycle progression from G1 to S phase	Metabolized in the liver and excreted by the kidney	Myelosuppression; immunosuppression; CNS, cardiac, and pulmonary toxicity; infection; fever, bone and chest pain and rash within hours of administration (Ara-C syndrome); nausea, diarrhea; mucositis; hepatic dysfunction	AML in adults and children

TABLE 164-2 U.S. FDA-APPROVED DRUGS COMMONLY USED FOR THE SYSTEMIC TREATMENT OF CANCER*—cont'd

DRUG NAME	DRUG CLASS AND/OR MECHANISM	PHARMACOKINETICS/METABOLISM	TOXICITY	INDICATIONS†
Dabrafenib (Tafinlar)	BRAF kinase inhibitor; selectively inhibits BRAF V600E mutated kinase	Metabolized to active form by CYP isoforms in the liver; absorption delayed by a high-fat meal	Decreased LVEF; skin rash, alopecia, keratoacanthoma and squamous cell carcinoma, palmar-plantar erythrodysesthesia; hyperglycemia; diarrhea; lymphopenia and anemia; abnormal liver function tests	Metastatic or unresectable melanoma with BRAF V600 E mutation or in combination with trametinib if either BRAF V600E or V600K mutations present; NSCLC if BRAF V600E mutation detected by an approved test
Dasatinib (Sprycel)	Multikinase inhibitor including Bcr-Abl and Src	Use with caution in patients with hepatic impairment; CYP3A4 inhibitors: may increase dasatinib drug levels; avoid or monitor closely and consider reducing dose; CYP3A4 inducers: may decrease dasatinib drug levels; avoid or consider increasing dose; antacids: may decrease dasatinib drug levels; avoid simultaneous administration; if needed, administer the antacid at least 2 hr prior to or 2 hr after the dose; H2 antagonists/proton pump inhibitors: may decrease dasatinib drug levels; consider antacids in place of H2 antagonists or proton pump inhibitors	Myelosuppression, bleeding events, fluid retention, diarrhea, headache, musculoskeletal pain, and rash	(Ph+) chronic myeloid leukemia (CML) in chronic phase, or chronic, accelerated, or myeloid or lymphoid blast phase Ph+ CML with resistance or intolerance to prior therapy including imatinib, or Philadelphia chromosome–positive acute lymphoblastic leukemia (Ph+ ALL) with resistance or intolerance to prior therapy
Daunorubicin	Anthracycline antitumor antibiotic; pleiotropic effects including free radical formation, topoisomerase II inhibition; altered mitochondrial function	After IV bolus, widely distributed and metabolized in liver to active and inactive metabolites; half-life of the parent drug is 18 hr, and 25 hr for active metabolite daunorubicinol	Daunorubicin is a vesicant; precautions are necessary; myelosuppression is dose limiting; alopecia, nausea, vomiting, and stomatitis are common; diarrhea, rash, elevated liver function tests, and transient arrhythmias are uncommon; dose-related cardiomyopathy is uncommon below cumulative doses of 400-500 mg/m^2	AML and ALL
Decitabine (Dacogen)	Antimetabolite; inhibits DNA methyltransferase, causing hypomethylation of DNA; this may induce apoptosis or restore normal function to genes that control cellular differentiation and proliferation	Deaminated by cytidine deaminase, found in liver, granulocytes, gut, and blood; elimination half-life is 30 min	Myelosuppression; nausea, vomiting, abdominal pain; constitutional symptoms; elevated liver functions, blood sugar, low serum magnesium, low serum potassium; respiratory toxicity	Myelodysplastic syndromes
Denosumab (Xgeva)	Monoclonal antibody; RANK ligand inhibitor	No drug interaction studies; more hypocalcemia for creatinine clearance <30 mL/min	Use calcium and vitamin D to treat or prevent hypocalcemia; fatigue/asthenia, hypophosphatemia, and nausea; osteonecrosis of jaw	Bone metastases from solid tumors; not in multiple myeloma; giant cell tumor of bone
Dexrazoxane (Zinecard)—ADR-529, ICRF-187	Iron-chelating agent that serves as a free-radical scavenger/cytoprotectant; widespread and rapid	Metabolism is mostly hepatic; half-life is 3-4 hr; parent drug and metabolites are excreted by the kidneys; hepatic impairment not studied; renal impairment suggests 50% dose reduction	Dexrazoxane appears to worsen slightly the leukopenia induced by doxorubicin; mild nausea and vomiting are common; fever, stomatitis, fatigue, anorexia, and hypotension are uncommon; seizure, respiratory arrest, deep venous thrombosis, and significant liver toxicity are rare	Prevent doxorubicin-induced cardiomyopathy
Docetaxel (Taxotere), RP-56976	Docetaxel is a semisynthetic taxane, a class of compounds that inhibit the mitotic spindle apparatus by stabilizing tubulin polymers, leading to death of mitotic cells	After a 1-hr infusion, docetaxel is widely distributed, with elimination half-life of 1 hr and a terminal half-life of 18 hr; extent and by-products of metabolism are not well known; the main excretion route is biliary	Myelosuppression is universal and dose limiting; alopecia is also universal; edema and fluid accumulation, including pleural effusions and ascites, are common and can be dose limiting; fluid accumulation is partially preventable with corticosteroid treatment before and after each cycle of docetaxel; mild sensory or sensorimotor neuropathy is common; mucositis and diarrhea are common and usually mild; hypersensitivity reactions are uncommon and can largely be prevented through premedication with corticosteroids and antihistamines; rash and elevated liver function tests are uncommon	Metastatic breast cancer and first- and second-line NSCLC

Doxorubicin (Adriamycin, Rubex), Adria, hydroxydaunorubicin	Anthracycline antitumor antibiotic; pleiotropic effects including free radical formation, topoisomerase II inhibition; altered mitochondrial function	After an IV dose, it is widely distributed in tissues and is 70% protein bound; it is metabolized in the liver to active and inactive forms; it has an elimination half-life of 18 hr or more; most of the drug and metabolites are excreted through the biliary route	Doxorubicin is a potent vesicant, and extravasation precautions are a must; myelosuppression is universal and usually dose limiting with each individual cycle; cardiotoxicity is common and can be dose limiting, although usually subclinical; chronic, cumulative cardiomyopathy is expected when the total dose exceeds 450 mg/m^2; this toxicity can be lessened by the addition of dexrazoxane or by longer infusions; acute cardiac effects, including arrhythmias, are less often seen and are unpredictable; nausea and vomiting are common but manageable; diarrhea and stomatitis are common but usually mild; alopecia, rash, and hyperpigmentation are common	Approved for a variety of cancers and used for many more; most commonly used for breast carcinoma, adult sarcomas, pediatric solid tumors, Hodgkin disease, non-Hodgkin lymphomas, and ovarian cancer
Doxorubicin, liposomal (Doxil)	Novel liposomal preparation of the anthracycline doxorubicin	Doxorubicin metabolized in the liver; significant plasma levels of the principal metabolite, doxorubicinol, not observed with the liposomal preparation, likely because of slow distribution of free doxorubicin to liver; half-life of liposomes in plasma is 55 hr	Myelosuppression is mild but dose limiting; palmar-plantar erythrodysesthesia is common and can occasionally be severe and dose limiting; stomatitis and nausea are common but usually mild; alopecia is uncommon; acute infusion reactions including chest pain, back pain, dyspnea, and wheezing can occur uncommonly	Recurrent metastatic ovarian cancer and AIDS-related Kaposi sarcoma; also used commonly in metastatic breast cancer and multiple myeloma
Durvalumab (Imfinzi)	Human monoclonal antibody that inhibits binding of PD-L1 to PD-1 and CD80, enhancing antitumor effects of T cells	May need to reduce dose or discontinue in the presence of treatment-related nephritis or hepatitis	Hepatotoxicity; renal toxicity; rash; endocrinopathies; colitis and diarrhea; infusion reactions; pneumonitis	Locally advanced or metastatic urothelial carcinoma following progression on platinum-based therapy; extensive stage small cell lung cancer; NSCLC
Enasidenib (IDHIFA)	Inhibitor of the enzyme isocitrate dehydrogenase (IDH2) targeting the R140Q, R172S, and R172K mutant variants of IDH2 to reduce 2-hydroxyglutarate levels and reestablish myeloid differentiation	Hepatic metabolism by way of multiple CYP isoforms and UGTs; primarily excreted in the feces; reduce dose for bilirubin >3 times ULN	Differentiation syndrome (black box warning): fever, respiratory distress, pleural and pericardial effusions, edema, multiorgan dysfunction—must be treated with corticosteroids; electrolyte imbalance; hepatotoxicity; nausea, vomiting, diarrhea; tumor lysis syndrome	AML patients with IDH2 mutations defined by an appropriate diagnostic test
Entrectinib (Rozlytrek)	Tropomyosin receptor kinase inhibitor	Avoid moderate and strong CYP3A inducers, reduce dose with moderate and strong CYP3A inhibitors	Heart failure, CNS side effects, skeletal fractures, hepatotoxicity, hyperuricemia, QT interval prolongation, vision disorders	Metastatic *ROS1*-positive NSCLC
Enzalutamide (Xtandi)	Androgen receptor signaling inhibitor	Take with or without food; 2C8 substrate; no other pathways need adjustments	Fatigue, musculoskeletal pain, dizziness, weakness	Metastatic castrate-resistant prostate carcinoma
Epirubicin (Ellence)	Anthracycline; pleiotropic effects including free radical formation, topoisomerase II inhibition; altered mitochondrial function	Metabolized primarily by liver; parent drug and metabolites glucuronidated and excreted in bile much more than via renal clearance; reduce doses for mild to moderate hepatic dysfunction; severe hepatic dysfunction is contraindicated; half-life is 30-35 hr	Myelosuppression is universal and dose limiting; alopecia is expected; this drug is a vesicant, and precautions must be taken to avoid extravasation into soft tissue around veins; nausea and vomiting are common but usually manageable; stomatitis is common; fatigue is common; detectable cardiac dysfunction at somewhat higher cumulative doses than doxorubicin; secondary leukemia is rare	Adjuvant therapy after optimal surgical treatment of localized breast cancer with involved axillary lymph nodes
Erdafitinib (Balversa)	FGFR kinase inhibitor	Avoid moderate CYP2C9 or strong CYP3A4 inhibitors, moderate or strong CYP2C9 or CYP3A4 inducers, CYP3A4 substrates, OCT2 substrates	Central serous retinopathy retinal pigment epithelial detachment, hyperphosphatemia, stomatitis, fatigue, increased creatinine level, diarrhea, dry mouth, palmar-plantar erythrodysesthesia syndrome	Locally advanced or metastatic urothelial carcinoma with FGFR3 or FGFR2 genetic alterations progressing despite chemotherapy
Eribulin mesylate (Halaven)	Microtubule inhibitor	Reduce dose in patients with hepatic impairment and moderate renal impairment	Neutropenia, peripheral neuropathy, monitor for QT prolongations, nausea, fatigue	Persons with metastatic breast cancer who have previously received at least two chemotherapeutic regimens for the treatment of metastatic disease; prior therapy should have included an anthracycline and a taxane in either the adjuvant or metastatic setting

TABLE 164-2 U.S. FDA-APPROVED DRUGS COMMONLY USED FOR THE SYSTEMIC TREATMENT OF CANCER*—cont'd

DRUG NAME	DRUG CLASS AND/OR MECHANISM	PHARMACOKINETICS/METABOLISM	TOXICITY	INDICATIONS[†]
Erlotinib (Tarceva)	Targeted agent	Inhibits the tyrosine kinase domain of the EGFR, leading to inhibition of EGFR autophosphorylation and signaling	Acneiform rash; diarrhea; interstitial lung disease	Second- or third-line therapy of NSCLC; pancreatic cancer, in combination with gemcitabine
Erythropoietin (Epogen, Procrit), EPO, epoetin alpha	Hematopoietic growth factor; stimulates erythrocytic precursors	Detectable in plasma for 24 hr after dosing; distributed to volume approximating total blood volume; degraded by proteolysis within blood compartment; half-life is 4-27 hr; onset of therapeutic effect takes at least 7 days; excretion of intact peptide is negligible	Hypertension is common but usually mild and not dose limiting; injection site pain is common but mild; flulike syndrome and diaphoresis are uncommon; nausea and vomiting are rare; seizures have been reported in patients undergoing dialysis who receive the drug; iron deficiency anemia can occur after prolonged therapy, and concomitant iron dosing may increase effectiveness of erythropoietin; hematocrit values should be monitored closely during therapy to prevent polycythemia and hyperviscosity	The oncology indication is chemotherapy-induced anemia that is symptomatic; also used for anemia of chronic renal failure and HIV-associated anemia
Etoposide (Vespid), VP-16, epipodophyllotoxin; also available as etoposide phosphate (Etopophos)	Plant alkaloid; topoisomerase II inhibitor; partially cell cycle dependent	Etoposide phosphate is rapidly converted to etoposide after IV infusion; etoposide itself is extensively protein bound, is metabolized in liver, and has a half-life of about 10 hr; 50% of oral etoposide is absorbed via GI tract, requiring oral doses to be twice as high as parenteral doses; excreted both unchanged in urine and as metabolites in bile	Myelosuppression, primarily leukopenia, is universal and dose limiting; nausea and vomiting are common with PO administration but rare when the drug is given by IV; stomatitis and diarrhea are rare with normal doses but common with high doses; alopecia is mild or absent; hepatic toxicity and neurologic effects (peripheral neuropathy and CNS changes) are rare; hypotension can occur with rapid administration of etoposide but does not occur commonly when etoposide phosphate is infused over 5 min; secondary AML has been reported after etoposide	Germ cell tumors and SCLC; also used for lymphomas, AML, brain tumors, non-SCLC, and as high-dose therapy in the transplant setting for breast cancer, ovarian cancer, and lymphomas
Everolimus (Afinitor)	m-TOR inhibitor	Hepatic impairment: for advanced HR+ BC, advanced PNET, advanced RCC, or renal angiomyolipoma with TSC patients with hepatic impairment, reduce the starting dose. Strong CYP 3A4 inhibitors: avoid concomitant use. Moderate CYP 3A4 and/or PgP inhibitors: if combination is required, use caution and reduce dose. Strong CYP 3A4 inducers: avoid concomitant use. If combination cannot be avoided, increase dose.	Noninfectious pneumonitis: monitor for clinical symptoms or radiologic changes; fatal cases have occurred. Infections: increased risk of infections, some fatal. Monitor for signs and symptoms, and treat promptly. Oral ulceration: mouth ulcers, stomatitis, and oral mucositis are common. Cases of renal failure (including acute renal failure), some with a fatal outcome, have been observed. Laboratory test alterations: elevations of serum creatinine, blood glucose, and lipids may occur. Decreases in hemoglobin, neutrophils, and platelets may also occur. Monitor renal function, blood glucose, lipids, and hematologic parameters prior to treatment and periodically thereafter. Avoid live vaccines and close contact with those who have received live vaccines. Advanced HR+ BC, advanced PNET, advanced RCC: most common adverse reactions include stomatitis, infections, rash, fatigue, diarrhea, edema, abdominal pain, nausea, fever, asthenia, cough, headache, and decreased appetite. Renal angiomyolipoma with TSC: most common adverse reaction is stomatitis. SEGA with TSC: most common adverse reaction (incidence ≥30%) are stomatitis and respiratory tract infection.	Postmenopausal women with advanced hormone receptor-positive, HER2 negative breast cancer (advanced HR+ BC) in combination with exemestane after failure of treatment with letrozole or anastrozole. Adults with progressive neuroendocrine tumors of creatic origin (PNET) that are unresectable, locally advanced, or metastatic. Adults with advanced RCC after failure of treatment with sunitinib or sorafenib. Adults with renal angiomyolipoma and TSC not requiring immediate surgery. Pediatric and adult patients with TSC who have SEGA that requires therapeutic intervention but cannot be curatively resected.
Exemestane (Aromasin)	Hormonal agent, steroidal aromatase inhibitor	40% of oral exemestane is absorbed from GI tract and increased by a fatty meal; it is highly protein bound in plasma; exemestane is metabolized in liver by cytochrome P450 3A4 and aldoketoreductases	Although generally well tolerated, exemestane is expected to cause or exacerbate hot flashes or intermittent flushing in some women; fatigue and mild nausea are common; vomiting, headache, and dyspnea are uncommon; it is teratogenic and should not be used in premenopausal women	Estrogen-responsive metastatic breast cancer in postmenopausal women whose disease has progressed while undergoing prior hormonal therapy

Filgrastim (Neupogen), G-CSF	Hematopoietic growth factor, relatively specific for the granulocyte lineage	After a bolus SQ injection, peak plasma levels of filgrastim occur in 2-6 hr, whereas the elimination half-life is generally 7 hr or less; metabolism is via proteolysis in the blood compartment; the intact molecule is largely absent from bile or urine	Mild bone pain is common; low-grade fever, myalgias, arthralgias, and transient hypotension are uncommon, as are hyperuricemia and elevations of lactate dehydrogenase and alkaline phosphatase; leukocytosis leading to hypoxia or capillary leak syndrome has been reported; anaphylaxis or allergic reaction is rare	Approved for minimization of granulocytopenia after myelosuppressive chemotherapy; also used to speed recovery of granulocytes in the setting of neutropenic fever after chemotherapy, for myelodysplastic syndromes, for congenital agranulocytosis, for cyclic neutropenia, and for mobilization of peripheral blood stem cells from patients or donors for transplant
Fludarabine (Fludara), FAMP	Purine nucleotide analog antimetabolite; only partially cell cycle–dependent	Fludarabine is available only by the parenteral route; after IV administration, the drug is metabolized to 2-fluoroara-A and widely distributed in tissues; it has an elimination half-life of 9-10 hr; the drug and metabolite are excreted primarily by the kidneys	Neurotoxicity, including cortical blindness, confusion, somnolence, coma, and demyelinating lesions, is dose limiting, but the lower doses that are conventionally used rarely produce these adverse effects; at these doses, mild myelosuppression is the most common toxicity, with cumulative lymphopenia being the most clinically important; nausea, vomiting, and other GI toxicities are rare; alopecia and rash are also rare	Approved for the treatment of CLL; also used for low-grade lymphomas and for AML
5-Fluorouracil (Adrucil, Efudex), 5-FU	Pyrimidine antimetabolite; inhibitor of thymidylate synthase; partially cell cycle dependent	80% of IV drug is metabolized to inactive dihydro-5-FU by dihydropyrimidine dehydrogenase in the liver; the rest of the drug is activated to fluorodeoxyuridine monophosphate in target cells; elimination half-life is 20 min; excretion is via the kidneys	GI toxicities, primarily mucositis for bolus injections and diarrhea for prolonged infusions, are dose limiting; rare patients with dihydropyrimidine dehydrogenase deficiency have excessive GI toxicity; myelosuppression is generally less with continuous infusion schedules; nausea and vomiting are uncommon and mild; dermatitis and other cutaneous toxicities, including hand-foot syndrome, are common; cerebellar ataxia and myocardial ischemia are rare	Approved for colon, rectum, gastric, pancreas, and breast carcinomas and used for a wide range of other neoplasms in combination regimens; used for intrahepatic arterial infusion for liver metastases from GI tumors; also used topically for various cutaneous neoplasms and disorders
Flutamide (Eulexin)	Nonsteroidal antiandrogen	Good oral bioavailability, with peak plasma levels after an oral dose at 1-2 hr; metabolized to active and inactive forms in the liver; half-life is 8-10 hr	Generally well tolerated; gynecomastia, galactorrhea, and impotence are common; nausea, vomiting, diarrhea, mild myelosuppression, myalgias, and elevated liver function tests are rare	Prostate carcinoma
Fulvestrant (Faslodex) estrogen receptor antagonist	Binds to the ER, leading to degradation and loss of ER from the cell	Peak plasma levels reached in 7 days, half-life is 40 days; metabolized by the liver microsomal P4503A4 systems	Constitutional symptoms, including hot flashes; peripheral edema; nausea, vomiting	ER+ metastatic breast cancer in postmenopausal women
Gemcitabine (Gemzar)	Antimetabolite; gemcitabine is a nucleoside analog that exhibits cell cycle–dependent and S-phase–specific cytotoxicity, likely because of inhibition of DNA synthesis	After IV infusion, the drug is rapidly distributed and has a half-life of less than 2 hr; it is metabolized throughout the body to inactive forms; parent drug and metabolite are excreted principally by the kidneys	Myelosuppression, including anemia, is mild but dose limiting; nausea and vomiting are mild but common; diarrhea and edema are sometimes seen; elevated transaminases are common, as is fever during drug administration; hematuria and proteinuria are uncommon; acute dyspnea and rash are uncommon; paresthesias and CNS depression are rare	Advanced pancreatic adenocarcinoma, NSCLC, and metastatic breast cancer; also extensively used in bladder cancer
Hydroxyurea (Hydrea)—hydroxycarbamide	Antimetabolite; inhibitor of ribonucleotide reductase, which converts nucleotides to the deoxyribose forms for DNA synthesis; cell cycle dependent	The drug is well absorbed; drug levels peak in the blood 2 hr after the dose is administered; half-life is 2-5 hr; metabolism to inactive forms in the liver; renal excretion is the route of elimination	Myelosuppression is common and dose limiting; other toxicities include rash, headache, fever, and hyperuricemia; nausea and vomiting are uncommon; liver toxicity and serious neurologic toxicity are rare	FDA approved for CML; commonly used for other myeloproliferative disorders; also used occasionally for metastatic melanoma, refractory ovarian carcinoma, and squamous cell carcinoma of the cervix and the head and neck
Ibrutinib (Imbruvica)	Irreversible inhibitor of Bruton tyrosine kinase altering B-cell receptor signaling	Hepatic metabolism by CYP3A and CYP2D6; dose reduction for hepatic dysfunction	Myelosuppression; cardiovascular; fatigue; skin rash; hyperuricemia; diarrhea, nausea; dry eyes; musculoskeletal pain	CLL and small lymphocytic lymphoma; mantle cell lymphoma; marginal zone lymphoma; Waldenström macroglobulinemia; chronic GVHD
Idelalisib (Zydelig)	Phosphatidylinositol 3-kinase delta inhibitor; results in apoptosis of malignant B cells	Metabolized in the liver by aldehyde oxidase and CYP3A	Hepatotoxicity; allergic reactions; myelosuppression; diarrhea; cutaneous reactions; infection; pneumonitis	Second-line therapy of CLL in combination with rituximab; follicular B-cell NHL; small lymphocytic lymphoma

TABLE 164-2 U.S. FDA-APPROVED DRUGS COMMONLY USED FOR THE SYSTEMIC TREATMENT OF CANCER*—cont'd

DRUG NAME	DRUG CLASS AND/OR MECHANISM	PHARMACOKINETICS/METABOLISM	TOXICITY	INDICATIONS[†]
Ifosfamide (Ifex)	Classic alkylating agent; not cell cycle dependent	After an intravenous dose, ifosfamide is activated by hepatic microsomal enzymes; it is then converted to inactive metabolites in the liver; the active form of the drug is the same as that for cyclophosphamide; the elimination half-life of the drug is 7-15 hr; the metabolites and some unchanged drug are excreted in the urine	Myelosuppression, hemorrhagic cystitis, and CNS toxicity are all fairly common and can be dose limiting; hemorrhagic cystitis can largely be prevented by co-administration of the uroprotective agent mesna, and nausea and vomiting are minimized with modern antiemetic regimens; the CNS toxicity, including lethargy, stupor, coma, myoclonus, and seizures, is usually mild and completely reversible; it is worse with impaired renal function; renal dysfunction, usually reversible, is also seen with ifosfamide; hepatic toxicity, diarrhea, and rash are rare	Approved for the treatment of recurrent germ cell tumors; used for many other tumor types, including adult sarcomas, lymphoma, Hodgkin disease, breast cancer, and ovarian cancer
Imatinib (Gleevec)	Bcr-Abl tyrosine kinase inhibitor; also inhibits platelet-derived growth factor (PDGF), c-Kit, and stem cell factor (SCF)	Rapid oral absorption; metabolized in the liver by CYP3A4; AUC increased by severe hepatic dysfunction; dose reduction for renal dysfunction	Edema, ascites, chest pain; fatigue; skin rash; increased LDH; nausea, diarrhea; muscle cramps; increased serum creatinine and liver function tests	CML; ALL that is Philadelphia chromosome positive; gastrointestinal stromal tumors; myelodysplastic syndrome associated with PDGF receptor gene rearrangements
Infigratinib (Truseltiq)	Receptor tyrosine kinase inhibitor that blocks fibroblast growth factor receptors FGFR1, FGFR2, FGFR3; blocks FGFR signaling from activating receptor mutations and gene fusions	Metabolized by CYP3A4; excreted in feces. Steady-state concentrations increased by 50-100% in patients who have mild to moderate liver dysfunction, so the dose must be reduced. Avoid coadministration of proton pump inhibitor.	Hyperphosphatemia requiring monitoring and dose adjustment	Unresectable or locally advanced/metastatic cholangiocarcinoma with *FGFR2* fusion or other rearrangement
Ipilimumab (Yervoy)	Human CTLA-4–blocking antibody	No formal pharmacokinetic drug interaction studies have been conducted; no clinically important differences in clearance of ipilimumab were found between patients with renal impairment and patients with normal renal function; no clinically important differences in clearance of ipilimumab were found between patients with mild hepatic impairment and normal hepatic function	Immune-mediated adverse reactions; fatigue, diarrhea, pruritus, rash, and colitis	Unresectable or metastatic melanoma; NSCLC; mesothelioma; renal cell cancer; hepatocellular cancer; colorectal cancer (MSI-high)
Irinotecan (Camptosar)—CP T-11	Semisynthetic camptothecin, which functions as a topoisomerase I inhibitor; partly cell cycle dependent	Converted partially from active lactone form to inactive carboxylate form; active metabolite of irinotecan, SN-38, also exists in lactone and inactive carboxylate form in equilibrium in plasma; SN-38 is inactivated by glucuronidation in the liver; SN-38 is responsible for the majority of antitumor activity attributed to parent drug; half-life of irinotecan is 8 hr, whereas half-life of SN-38 is 12 hr	Myelosuppression, primarily neutropenia, is common and dose limiting; diarrhea is also common and can be dose limiting; diarrhea can occur as part of a cholinergic syndrome, along with cramping, nausea, and vomiting, during or immediately after drug administration or for several days after drug administration; anticholinergic and antidiarrheal agents will curtail the immediate diarrhea and other GI symptoms partially but are less effective in treating the delayed diarrhea; flushing, rash, and alopecia are common; significant hepatic, renal, neurologic, or pulmonary toxicities are rare	Irinotecan is FDA approved for refractory or recurrent metastatic colon cancer, and it has now been used in other malignancies, including lung cancer, ovarian cancer, and lymphoma
Ixabepilone (Ixempra)	Microtubule inhibitor	In combination with capecitabine, must not be given to patients with AST or ALT >2.5 × ULN or bilirubin >1 × ULN; dose reduction is recommended when administering ixabepilone as monotherapy to patients with hepatic impairment; no formal renal impairment study; inhibitors of CYP3A4 may increase plasma concentrations of ixabepilone; dose of ixabepilone must be reduced with strong CYP3A4 inhibitors; inducers of CYP3A4 may decrease plasma concentrations of ixabepilone; alternative therapeutic agents with low enzyme induction potential should be considered	Peripheral neuropathy: monitor for symptoms of neuropathy, primarily sensory; neuropathy is cumulative, generally reversible, and should be managed by dose adjustment and delays; myelosuppression: primarily neutropenia; monitor with peripheral blood cell counts and adjust dose as appropriate; hypersensitivity reaction: must premedicate all patients with an H1 antagonist and an H2 antagonist before treatment; fatigue/asthenia, myalgia/arthralgia, alopecia, nausea, vomiting, stomatitis/mucositis, diarrhea, and musculoskeletal pain	Combination with capecitabine is indicated for the treatment of metastatic or locally advanced breast cancer in patients after failure of an anthracycline and a taxane; as monotherapy is indicated for the treatment of metastatic or locally advanced breast cancer in patients after failure of an anthracycline, a taxane, and capecitabine

Ixazomib (Ninlaro)	Inhibits 20 S proteasome	Absorption decreased by high-fat meals; hepatic metabolism; reduce dose for CrCl <30 mL/min and for total bilirubin >1.5 ULN	Myelosuppression; skin rash; peripheral neuropathy	Multiple myeloma in combination with lenalidomide and dexamethasone as second-line therapy
Lapatinib (Tykerb)	EGRF and HER2 tyrosine kinase inhibitor	Extensive metabolism spread over several enzymes	Hepatotoxicity; decreased left ventricular ejection fraction; diarrhea; some QT interval prolongation	HER2+ breast cancer, with capecitabine; treatment with anthracycline, taxane, trastuzumab failed
Larotrectinib (Vitrakvi)	Neurotrophic receptor tyrosine kinase inhibitor	Avoid strong CYP3A4 inhibitors, strong CYP3A4 inducers, and sensitive CYP3A4 substrates	Neurotoxicity, hepatotoxicity, nausea, vomiting, dizziness, cough, constipation, diarrhea	Metastatic or unresectable solid tumors with a neurotrophic receptor tyrosine kinase gene fusion
Lenalidomide (Revlimid)	Antiangiogenesis agent, immunomodulator	Mechanism of action not fully characterized; an immunomodulatory agent that inhibits angiogenesis in some cells; inhibits bone marrow secretion of IL-6, VEGF, and TNF-α	Myelosuppression; diarrhea, rash, fatigue; increased risk of DVT and PE	Transfusion-dependent anemia due to low- or intermediate-risk myelodysplasia with 5q deletion; multiple myeloma
Lenvatinib (Lenvima)	Multitargeted tyrosine kinase inhibitor *(VEGFR, FGFR, PDGFR, KIT, RET)*	Metabolized in the liver by CYP3A and aldehyde oxidase; dose reduction for hepatic insufficiency	Hypertension; alters thyroid suppression with TSH elevation and hypothyroidism; gastrointestinal toxicity and bowel fistula formation; hepatotoxicity; skin toxicity; hypocalcemia; renal toxicity	Renal cell carcinoma in combination with everolimus; differentiated thyroid cancer that is radioactive iodine refractory
Letrozole (Femara)	Nonsteroidal aromatase inhibitor	Letrozole has nearly 100% bioavailability, is metabolized in the liver, glucuronidated, and excreted by the kidneys; half-life is 2 days; with daily administration, steady-state plasma levels are reached in 2-6 wk	This drug is generally well tolerated; muscle aches and nausea are uncommon; hot flashes and fatigue are uncommon; weight change, urticaria, and dyspepsia are rare	Metastatic estrogen-responsive breast cancer in postmenopausal patients
Leucovorin calcium (Wellcovorin) citrovorum factor, folinic acid, FA, LV	Tetrahydrofolate derivative and enzyme cofactor for thymidylate synthase and other purine and pyrimidine synthesis steps; bypasses the dihydrofolate reductase step, which is inhibited by methotrexate and therefore can be used to "rescue" normal cells from the toxicity of methotrexate after high doses are administered; in addition, leucovorin potentiates the toxicity of fluoropyrimidines such as fluorouracil by strengthening the association of the drug	Leucovorin has excellent bioavailability by the oral or parenteral route; it is oxidized in cofactor reactions throughout the body and is also partly metabolized; it has an elimination half-life of 2-4 hr; excreted in the urine	Leucovorin is generally very well tolerated; it occasionally causes stomach upset or nausea, rash, diarrhea, and headache; allergic reactions have been reported	Used for rescue of high-dose methotrexate therapy for a variety of neoplasms and as a potentiator of fluoropyrimidines therapy in GI malignancies, particularly colorectal cancer
Leuprolide acetate (Lupron)—leuprorelin acetate	Gonadotropin-releasing hormone agonist, which serves to paradoxically shut down the pituitary release of gonadotropins with chronic exposure; this results in a dramatic decrease in gonadal estrogens and androgens and growth inhibition of hormone-dependent neoplasms	After an SQ injection, about 90% of the drug is eventually absorbed; the depot form of the drug is absorbed slowly over days, whereas the injectable solution is absorbed over several hours; the elimination half-life of the drug once in the serum is 3 hr; metabolism and excretion are not well delineated but are clinically unimportant	Usually well tolerated, but adverse effects can affect many systems, including endocrine (hot flashes, impotence, gynecomastia, breast tenderness, diminished libido, amenorrhea, atrophic vaginitis, increased cholesterol); GI (nausea, constipation, anorexia, diarrhea); hepatic (elevation of transaminases); dermatologic (rash, changes in body hair composition, pruritus); and neuropsychiatric (insomnia, depression, emotional lability, lethargy, memory loss); significant cardiac toxicity is rare	Approved for the treatment of hormone-dependent advanced prostate cancer; also used for breast cancer and endometriosis
Lurbinectedin (Zepzelca)	Alkylating agent	Avoid strong or moderate CYP3A inhibitors and strong or moderate CYP3A inducers	Myelosuppression, hepatotoxicity, increased creatinine level, hyperglycemia, nausea, musculoskeletal pain, constipation, dyspnea, decreased sodium level	Metastatic SCLC progressing despite platinum-based chemotherapy

TABLE 164-2 U.S. FDA-APPROVED DRUGS COMMONLY USED FOR THE SYSTEMIC TREATMENT OF CANCER*—cont'd

DRUG NAME	DRUG CLASS AND/OR MECHANISM	PHARMACOKINETICS/METABOLISM	TOXICITY	INDICATIONS[†]
Methotrexate (Mexate, Folex, others)—MTX, amethopterin	Antifolate antimetabolite; interferes with nucleotide synthesis by inhibiting dihydrofolate reductase; cell cycle dependent	Good oral bioavailability at low doses; after oral or IV dosing, it is distributed throughout the body water compartment; it will accumulate in "third-space" fluid compartments and exhibit prolonged toxicity and therefore should be used with caution, if at all, in patients with significant pleural or peritoneal fluid; minimally metabolized in the liver; half-life is 3 hr; even low concentrations of drug after most of the drug is eliminated can contribute to significant toxicity; therefore dosing based on renal function is critical; excretion of this drug is mostly renal	Myelosuppression is expected and is usually dose limiting; stomatitis and diarrhea are common; nausea and vomiting are uncommon; renal toxicity is uncommon and usually reversible but can be severe; many types of skin reactions can occur but are uncommon; pulmonary fibrosis and hepatic fibrosis are rare; encephalopathy is rare with moderate- to low-dose therapy but is more common with high doses, intrathecal administration, or concomitant CNS radiation; it can be severe and permanent	Approved for a wide spectrum of malignant and nonmalignant diseases; most often used for acute leukemias, lymphomas, breast cancer, bladder cancer, squamous cell cancers, and sarcomas
Midostaurin (Rydapt)	Tyrosine kinase inhibitor targeting *FLT3, FLT3 ITD, KIT, PDGFR, VEGFR2,* and *PKC* family	Metabolized by CYP3A4 in the liver	Cardiovascular (edema and QTc prolongation); headache and fatigue; electrolyte abnormalities and hyperglycemia; nausea and vomiting; myelosuppression; abnormal liver function tests; infection	FLT3 mutation-positive AML in combination with cytarabine and daunorubicin; mast cell leukemia; systemic mastocytosis
Neratinib (Nerlynx)	Irreversible inhibitor of EGFR and HER2 kinases	Hepatic metabolism by CYP3A4; dose reduction for severe hepatic dysfunction	Severe diarrhea with dehydration; hepatic toxicity requiring careful monitoring of liver function	Adjuvant therapy of HER2-positive breast cancer following adjuvant trastuzumab-associated therapy
Nilotinib (Tasigna)	Kinase inhibitor including Bcr-Abl	Dose adjustment may be required for hematologic and nonhematologic toxicities and drug interactions; lower starting dose is recommended in patients with impairment (at baseline); do not consume food for at least 2 hr before the dose is taken and for at least 1 hr after	Prolongs QT interval; rash, pruritus, headache, nausea, fatigue, myalgia, nasopharyngitis, constipation, diarrhea, abdominal pain, vomiting, arthralgia, pyrexia, upper respiratory tract infection, back pain, cough, and asthenia; hematologic adverse drug reactions include myelosuppression: thrombocytopenia, neutropenia, and anemia	Newly diagnosed adult patients with Philadelphia chromosome–positive chronic myeloid leukemia (Ph+ CML) in chronic phase; also, the treatment of chronic and accelerated phase Ph+ CML in adult patients resistant to or intolerant to prior therapy that included imatinib
Niraparib (Zejula)	Poly (ADP-ribose) polymerase enzyme inhibitor	Metabolized by carboxylesterases and then glucuronidated	Hypertension; skin rash; fatigue; nausea and constipation; myelosuppression; weakness and back pain; hepatic dysfunction	Ovarian and primary peritoneal cancers in complete or partial response following platinum-containing chemotherapy
Nivolumab (Opdivo)	Human anti-PD-1 monoclonal antibody; releases PD-1 pathway inhibition to improve immune response	Prolonged (>20 day) half-life	Endocrinopathies; colitis; encephalitis; pneumonitis; hypophysitis; rash; if severe may require systemic corticosteroids; infusion reactions	Colorectal cancer with microsatellite instability-high (MSI-H) or mismatch repair deficient (dMMR) that is metastatic and has progressed following fluoropyrimidine, oxaliplatin, and irinotecan; head and neck squamous cell cancer that is recurrent or progressed on platinum-containing chemotherapy; Hodgkin lymphoma; metastatic melanoma; NSCLC; advanced renal cancer; advanced urothelial cancer; esophageal cancer or gastroesophageal junction adenocarcinoma; hepatocellular cancer; mesothelioma; squamous cancer of the head and neck
Obinutuzumab (Gazyva)	Anti-CD20 monoclonal antibody; upon binding to CD20 on B cells, initiates ADCC	No dosage adjustments for renal or hepatic dysfunction	Hypophosphatemia; hypocalcemia; hyperkalemia; blood count suppression; altered liver and kidney function; infection; cough	CLL previously untreated in combination with chlorambucil; follicular lymphoma in combination with bendamustine in patients refractory to rituximab-containing regimens

Octreotide, octreotide long-acting (Sandostatin, Sandostatin LA), l-cysteinamide	Synthetic peptide analog of somatostatin; inhibits other GI peptide actions, such as serotonin, insulin, glucagon, and gastrin	Not orally bioavailable but rapidly absorbed after SQ administration; metabolized by hydrolysis throughout the body; no active metabolites; half-life of elimination is about 1.5 hr; intact drug is cleared via the kidneys	GI adverse effects are dose limiting and include abdominal pain, vomiting, loose stool, occasional fat malabsorption, bloating, and cholelithiasis; elevations of liver function tests can also occur, but frank hepatitis is rare; skin reactions, such as pain at the injection site or flushing, rash, or skin thinning, are sometimes seen; constitutional symptoms, including rhinorrhea, xerostomia, sweating, throat discomfort, and vertigo, can be bothersome; hyperglycemia or hypoglycemia can occur; cardiac side effects, including angina, congestive heart failure, and hypotension or hypertension, are uncommon; anxiety, depression, fatigue, and anorexia are uncommon, and seizures are rare	Approved for carcinoid tumors causing carcinoid syndrome and for vasoactive peptide–secreting tumors; also used for refractory diarrhea, either cancer related or treatment related, in patients with cancer
Olaparib (Lynparza)	Inhibitor of poly (ADP-ribose) polymerase enzyme; produces synthetic lethality in BRCA1/2-deficient tumor cells	Hepatic metabolism by CYP3A4; Cmax increased in patients with mild hepatic dysfunction; avoid concomitant use of CYP3A inhibitors	Peripheral edema; fatigue and headache; skin rash; nausea and abdominal pain; anemia and lymphopenia; myalgias; increased serum creatinine	*BRCA*-mutant ovarian cancer previously treated with three or more lines of therapy; maintenance therapy for ovarian cancer in complete or partial remission following platinum-based therapy
Osimertinib (Tagrisso)	Irreversible inhibitor of EGFR tyrosine kinase; binds to mutant forms of EGFR (*T970M*, *L858R*, exon 19 deletions); less active against wild-type EGFR	Metabolized by CYP3A and excreted in the feces; avoid concomitant use of strong CYP3A4 inducers	Bone marrow suppression; cardiotoxicity, decline in LVEF and prolongation of QTc; skin rash; impaired fertility; diarrhea; keratitis; pneumonitis	Metastatic NSCLC that is *T790M* mutation positive
Oxaliplatin (Eloxatin)	Platinating agent; DNA disrupted via intrastrand and interstrand cross-links with two strong platinum association bonds in the molecule, which induces apoptosis beyond a certain level of DNA damage in malignant cells	After IV administration, rapid distribution into tissues occurs, as well as rapid spontaneous conversion via hydrolysis into active drug and metabolites; the terminal half-life is long (>300 hr) but represents minimal plasma levels of the hydrolyzed drug; elimination of platinum metabolites is via the kidneys	Neurotoxicity, in the form of a transient neuropathy with each dose and a persistent, cumulative typical sensory polyneuropathy, is very common and dose limiting; myelosuppression is expected but mild and only sometimes dose limiting; fatigue and nausea are common but mild; diarrhea, stomatitis, edema, cough, hypersensitivity reactions, and extravasation injury are rare	Approved for metastatic colorectal cancer in combination with 5-FU/leucovorin
Paclitaxel (Taxol, Onxol)	Naturally occurring taxane molecule; inhibits depolymerization of tubulin in the spindle apparatus, thereby inducing apoptosis in dividing cells	After IV administration, the drug exhibits a large volume of distribution and undergoes metabolism in the liver; the elimination half-life is 15-50 hr; excretion of drug and metabolites is predominantly via the bile	Paclitaxel is an irritant or mild vesicant when extravasated into subcutaneous tissue; myelosuppression, predominantly neutropenia, is expected and is dose limiting; shorter infusions of the same dose produce less neutropenia; mucositis is also very common, particularly with longer infusions; peripheral neuropathy is common, usually mild, and increases with cumulative dose; acute neuromyopathy is also common and occurs for several days after each dose; this syndrome may require opiate analgesics to control pain; cardiovascular adverse effects, including hypertension, hypotension, premature contractions, and bradyarrhythmias, are common but rarely require intervention; hypersensitivity reactions to paclitaxel, including urticaria, wheezing, chest pain, dyspnea, and hypotension, are common but are reduced in frequency and severity by premedication with corticosteroids and histamine-1 and histamine-2 antihistamines (the recommended regimen is dexamethasone, 20 mg PO 12 and 6 hr prior to paclitaxel and diphenhydramine, 50 mg, and cimetidine)	Approved for salvage therapy in ovarian cancer and for breast cancer in both the metastatic and adjuvant settings; used also in persons with lung cancer, head and neck cancer, and bladder cancer
Paclitaxel, protein bound (Abraxane)	Taxane; an albumin-bound form of paclitaxel with a mean particle size of approximately 130 nanometers	No change in patients with mild to moderate hepatic dysfunction	Neutropenia, thrombocytopenia, anemia, hypersensitivity reactions, hypotension, cardiovascular events, dyspnea, cough, sensory neuropathy, arthralgias/myalgias, nausea/vomiting, asthenia	Metastatic breast cancer after failure of combination chemotherapy or relapse with 6 mo of adjuvant chemotherapy; also approved for NSCLC

TABLE 164-2 U.S. FDA-APPROVED DRUGS COMMONLY USED FOR THE SYSTEMIC TREATMENT OF CANCER*—cont'd

DRUG NAME	DRUG CLASS AND/OR MECHANISM	PHARMACOKINETICS/METABOLISM	TOXICITY	INDICATIONS†
Palbociclib (Ibrance)	Reversible small molecule inhibitor of cyclin-dependent kinases 4 and 6 affecting cell cycle progression through the G1/S phase	Metabolized by the liver by CY3A and sulfotransferase; avoid simultaneous use of strong CYP3A inhibitors	Fatigue; alopecia and skin rash; nausea, stomatitis, diarrhea, infection; blood count suppression, infection	Advanced breast cancer that is ER positive, HER2 negative in combination with an aromatase inhibitor as initial therapy for postmenopausal women
Pamidronate (Aredia), APD, aminohydroxypropylidene diphosphonate	Organic bisphosphonate; inhibitor of bone resorption by osteoclasts	After IV administration, the drug concentrates in the bone, spleen, and liver; its metabolism is not well characterized; it has a terminal half-life of about 27 hr; 50% of the parent drug is eliminated in the urine	Pamidronate is usually quite well tolerated; hypotension, syncope, tachycardia, and even atrial fibrillation have been reported uncommonly during the infusion; hypocalcemia, hypophosphatemia, hypokalemia, and hypomagnesemia occur commonly but only rarely require intervention; nausea, vomiting, and somnolence are rare	Approved for malignancy-induced hypercalcemia; may lead to pain relief and even tumor shrinkage of bone metastases in multiple myeloma, breast cancer, and prostate cancer
Panitumumab (Vectibix)	Recombinant, fully humanized IgG2 kappa monoclonal antibody that binds specifically to EGFR, competitively inhibiting ligand binding to the receptor	Steady-state levels are reached by the third infusion; elimination half-life is about 7.5 days	Rash, which may be severe; diarrhea; infusion reactions; hypomagnesemia; pulmonary fibrosis	Previously treated EGFR-expressing metastatic colorectal cancer
Panobinostat (Farydak)	Histone deacetylase inhibitor, affects chromatin remodeling	Hepatic metabolism in part through CYP3A; reduce dose for hepatic dysfunction	ECG abnormalities; fatigue; electrolyte abnormalities; diarrhea; blood count suppression; infection; hyperbilirubinemia	Multiple myeloma in combination with bortezomib and dexamethasone in patients who have received 2 prior regimens
Pazopanib (Votrient)	Inhibits large number of tyrosine kinases	Take without food; reduce dose for mild to moderate hepatic impairment; avoid severe hepatic impairment; interacts with many metabolizing enzymes	Diarrhea, hypertension, nausea, anorexia, vomiting, hair color depigmentation	Renal cell carcinoma; also approved for soft tissue sarcoma
Pembrolizumab (Keytruda)	Human monoclonal antibody against programmed cell death-1 (PD-1) activity that inhibits negative immune regulation to enhance antitumor effects	Long half-life (22 days)	Peripheral edema; rash; fatigue; endocrinopathies; electrolyte abnormalities; hyperglycemia; nausea, diarrhea, colitis; abnormal liver function tests	Squamous cell cancers of the head and neck; Hodgkin lymphoma, melanoma, microsatellite instable (MSI-H) or mismatch repair deficient solid tumors and colorectal cancers that have no alternative treatment options; NSCLC first-line metastatic in patients with high (50%) PD-L1 expression that are EGFR or ALK negative and first-line therapy for metastatic nonsquamous NSCLC in combination with pemetrexed and carboplatin; urothelial carcinoma that has progressed on platinum-containing therapy; triple-negative breast cancer; cervical cancer; cutaneous squamous cell cancer; endometrial cancer that is MSI-high; esophageal, gastric, and gastroesophageal junction adenocarcinoma; hepatocellular cancer; Merkel cell carcinoma; renal cell cancer; primary large B-cell lymphoma
Pemetrexed (Alimta)	Antimetabolite; inhibits folate-dependent enzymes thymidylate synthetase, dihydrofolate reductase, and glycinamide ribonucleotide formyltransferase, which are involved in the de novo synthesis of thymidine and purine nucleotides, leading to inhibition of DNA and RNA synthesis and function; metabolized intracellularly to its highly active polyglutamated form	Excreted in urine with 90% of drug unchanged	Myelosuppression; nausea, vomiting, diarrhea; rash; dyspnea and fatigue	Mesothelioma and NSCLC

Pertuzumab (Perjeta)	HER2/neu receptor antagonist antibody; HER2 testing: perform using FDA-approved tests by laboratories with demonstrated proficiency	Of 402 patients who received Perjeta in the randomized trial, 60 patients (15%) were 65 yr of age and 5 patients (1%) were 75 yr of age; no overall differences in efficacy and safety of Perjeta were observed between these patients and younger patients; based on a population pharmacokinetic analysis, no significant difference was observed in the pharmacokinetics of pertuzumab between patients <65 yr (n = 306) and patients ≥65 yr (n = 175)	Left ventricular dysfunction: monitor LVEF and withhold dosing as appropriate; reactions, hypersensitivity reactions/anaphylaxis: monitor for signs and symptoms; if a significant infusion-associated reaction occurs, slow or interrupt the infusion and administer appropriate medical therapies; in combination with trastuzumab and docetaxel: diarrhea, alopecia, neutropenia, nausea, fatigue, rash, and peripheral neuropathy	First-line HER2+ metastatic breast cancer
Pomalidomide (Pomalyst)	Immunomodulator, analog of thalidomide, decreases proliferation of myeloma cells, enhances T-cell–mediated immunity, and has antiangiogenic properties	Metabolized by CYP3A4 and CYP1A2; systemic exposure increased by hepatic dysfunction; avoid use with concomitant CYP1A2 inhibitors; reduce dose for renal or hepatic dysfunction	Thromboembolism; hematologic toxicity; hepatotoxicity; hypersensitivity; neurotoxicity; confusion; tumor lysis syndrome; fatigue; nausea; diarrhea; infection	Multiple myeloma in combination with dexamethasone as third-line therapy
Ponatinib (Iclusig)	Kinase inhibitor	For strong CYP3A inhibitors: reduce dose if co-administration cannot be avoided; renal or hepatic impairment not studied	Arterial thrombosis and hepatotoxicity have boxed warnings; nonhematologic adverse reactions (≥20%) were hypertension, rash, abdominal pain, fatigue, headache, dry skin, constipation, arthralgia, nausea, and pyrexia; hematologic adverse reactions included thrombocytopenia, anemia, neutropenia, lymphopenia, and leukopenia	CML and Philadelphia chromosome–positive acute ALL
Ramucirumab (Cyramza)	Monoclonal antibody targeting the vascular growth factor receptor 2, inhibiting endothelial cell proliferation and angiogenesis	Half-life 14 days	Infusion reaction; hypertension; proteinuria; arterial thrombosis; GI perforation; bleeding	Metastatic colorectal cancer in combination with FOLFIRI following progression on FOLFOX and bevacizumab; gastric cancer as a single agent or in combination with paclitaxel following progression on a fluoropyrimidine- or platinum-containing regimen; NSCLC in combination with paclitaxel for advanced disease after platinum-based treatment
Regorafenib (Stivarga)	Inhibits many membrane and intracellular kinases including *RET, VEGFR, KIT, PDGFR, FGF, TIE2, DDR2, TrkA, Eph2A, RAF-1, BRAF,* and *CSF1R*	Take with food; decreased exposure with strong inducers of CYP3A	Hepatotoxicity, fatigue, decreased appetite, hand-foot skin reaction	Previously treated metastatic colorectal cancer; gastrointestinal stromal tumor; hepatocellular carcinoma
Ribociclib (Kisqali)	Small molecule inhibitor of cyclin-dependent kinases 4 and 6; produces G1 cell cycle arrest; combined with aromatase inhibitors leads to enhanced tumor cell growth control	Metabolized in the liver by CYP3A4	Bone marrow suppression; hepatotoxicity with abnormal liver function; QT prolongation; peripheral edema; fatigue; alopecia; skin rash; hypokalemia; nausea and diarrhea; increased serum creatinine	Advanced breast cancer for patients with HR-positive, HER2-negative disease in combination with an aromatase inhibitor as initial endocrine therapy
Rituximab (Rituxan)	Monoclonal antibody directed against the B-cell surface antigen CD20	When given IV, it is taken up by B lymphocytes and then degraded throughout the body by proteolysis, with a wide-ranging serum half-life of 11-105 hr (mean 60 hr) with the first dose; there is no appreciable excretion of this polypeptide	Fever, chills, and malaise are common during administration, even with premedication with acetaminophen and diphenhydramine; other infusion-related symptoms include nausea, vomiting, flushing, urticaria, angioedema, hypotension, dyspnea, bronchospasm, fatigue, headache, rhinitis, and pain at disease sites; these symptoms are generally self-limited, improve with slowing of the infusion, and resolve after infusion; short-lived myelosuppression, abdominal pain, and myalgia are uncommon; arrhythmias and angina pectoris are rare	Relapsed or refractory low-grade or follicular, CD20-positive, B-cell lymphomas

TABLE 164-2 U.S. FDA-APPROVED DRUGS COMMONLY USED FOR THE SYSTEMIC TREATMENT OF CANCER*—cont'd

DRUG NAME	DRUG CLASS AND/OR MECHANISM	PHARMACOKINETICS/METABOLISM	TOXICITY	INDICATIONS†
Rucaparib (Rubraca)	Inhibits poly (ADP-ribose) polymerase enzyme isoforms essential for DNA repair; increased cell killing in tumors deficient in BRCA1/2 repair pathway	Metabolized by CYP2D6 in the liver	Fatigue and dizziness; skin rash; increased cholesterol; nausea, constipation; diarrhea; blood count suppression; increased liver function tests; increased serum creatinine; weakness; dyspnea; fever	Advanced ovarian cancer in the presence of *BRCA* mutations (germline or somatic) detected by an approved diagnostic test as third-line therapy
Ruxolitinib (Jakafi)	Janus kinase signaling inhibitor	With or without food; reduce dose 50% with strong CYP3A inhibitors, moderate renal or hepatic impairment	Thrombocytopenia, anemia, bruising, dizziness, headache	Intermediate- or high-risk myelofibrosis
Sacituzumab govitecan-hziy (Trodelvy)	Trop-2–directed antibody and topoisomerase inhibitor conjugate	Individuals who are homozygous for the uridine diphosphate-glucuronosyl transferase 1A1 (UGT1A1)*28 allele are at increased risk for neutropenia	Neutropenia, severe diarrhea, hypersensitivity reactions, nausea, vomiting, anemia, alopecia, constipation, rash, abdominal pain	Metastatic triple-negative breast cancer despite at least two prior therapies
Selinexor (Xpovio)	Nuclear export inhibitor	95% protein bound; metabolized by liver	Thrombocytopenia, neutropenia, gastrointestinal toxicity, hyponatremia, serious infection, neurologic toxicity	With dexamethasone for relapsed or refractory multiple myeloma despite at least four prior therapies; or refractory diffuse large B-cell lymphoma, including disease arising from follicular lymphoma, after at least two lines of systemic therapy
Sonidegib (Odomzo)	Hedgehog pathway inhibitor that binds and inhibits Smoothened, a transmembrane protein essential for hedgehog signaling	Metabolized in the liver by CYP3A	Fatigue; alopecia; hyperglycemia; abnormal liver function tests; anemia; increased CK, muscle pain; increased serum creatinine	Locally advanced basal cell carcinoma recurrent after surgery or radiation therapy
Sorafenib (Nexavar)	Oral multikinase inhibitor that interacts with multiple intracellular (CRAD, BRAF) and cell surface kinases (KIT, FLT-3, VEGFR-2, and PDGFR); may inhibit angiogenesis	Metabolized in the liver; drug and metabolites are excreted primarily in the feces	Skin toxicity with rash and hand-foot syndrome; nausea, vomiting, anorexia, diarrhea; asthenia, pain, arthralgias; hypertension; bleeding events, especially in anticoagulated patients; cardiac ischemia; myelosuppression	Advanced renal cell carcinoma
Sotorasib (Lumakras)	Selective, orally active inhibitor that covalently binds to Cys12 of KRAS; inhibits signaling only in tumors that exhibit the KRAS-G12C mutation	Avoid proton pump inhibitors and histamine-2 receptor antagonists	Drug-induced hepatitis with increased ALT/AST requires monitoring of liver function tests; interstitial lung disease; diarrhea; musculoskeletal pain; nausea; fatigue	Adults with *KRAS-G12C*-mutated locally advanced or metastatic NSCLC
Sunitinib maleate (Sutent)	Inhibits PDGFR-A, PDGFR-B, and VEGFR1-3, stem cell factor receptor, FLT-3, CSF-1R, and the neurotrophic factor receptor; this inhibition inhibits tumor growth and metastases	Metabolized in the liver with elimination primarily in the feces; half-life is 40-60 hr for the drug and 80-110 hr for its primary metabolite	Cardiotoxicity—usually reversible; bleeding event, epistaxis most common; hypertension; myelosuppression; nausea, vomiting; rash; liver function test alterations	Advanced renal cell carcinoma; second-line therapy for GIST cell tumors; also approved for pancreatic neuroendocrine tumors
Talazoparib (Talzenna)	PARP inhibitor	Reduce dose if moderate renal impairment (creatinine clearance 30-59 mL/min)	Myelodysplastic syndrome, AML, myelosuppression, nausea, headache, vomiting, alopecia, diarrhea	Germline *BRCA*-mutated HER2-negative locally advanced or metastatic breast cancer
Tamoxifen (Nolvadex)	Nonsteroidal antiestrogen; cytostatic effects on estrogen-dependent and nondependent malignant cells	Tamoxifen has good oral bioavailability, is metabolized in the liver, and has an elimination half-life of about 7 days; neither tamoxifen nor its major metabolite is found in the bile or urine	Tamoxifen is usually very well tolerated; constitutional symptoms are most prevalent and usually dose limiting; hot flashes, sweating, mood changes, weight gain or loss, and stomach upset are most common; nausea, vomiting, diarrhea, and constipation are less common; menstrual changes, including significant vaginal bleeding, are uncommon; venous thromboembolism, myelosuppression, and retinopathy are rare	Approved for the treatment of breast cancer, generally in postmenopausal patients or those with ER+ tumors; the same dose has been approved for chemoprevention of breast cancer in high-risk individuals; higher doses are used for melanoma and pancreatic cancer
Tazemetostat (Tazverik)	Methyltransferase inhibitor	Avoid strong and moderate CYP3A inhibitors and strong and moderate CYP3A inducers	Fatigue, nausea, vomiting, constipation, upper respiratory tract infection, musculoskeletal pain, abdominal pain	Metastatic or unresectable locally advanced epithelioid sarcoma, relapsed or refractory follicular lymphoma with an EZH2 mutation or no alternative treatment options

Temozolomide (Temodar)	Atypical alkylator (semiselective DNA methylator) drug sharing the same active metabolite as dacarbazine, MTIC but, unlike dacarbazine, is spontaneously converted to MTIC and also penetrates the blood-brain barrier effectively	Temozolomide had good bioavailability, enhanced by an empty stomach; after absorption into the blood stream, it is spontaneously converted to the active moiety MTIC; peak plasma concentrations occur in about 1 hr; the elimination half-life is about 1.8 hr; parent drug, MTIC, and other metabolites are eliminated in the urine	Myelosuppression is expected and dose-limiting; it may be cumulative; nausea is common but generally mild and treatable; headache and fatigue are common; rash or other cutaneous reactions are uncommon; infections are common in this population, and some are probably caused by immunosuppression that is known to occur with temozolomide	Approved for treatment of recurrent high-grade astrocytomas; used commonly for other gliomas and also for metastatic melanoma
Temsirolimus (Torisel)	Inhibitor of mTOR	Antihistamine pretreatment is recommended; dose reduction is required in patients with mild hepatic impairment; strong inducers of CYP3A4/5 and inhibitors of CYP3A4 may affect concentrations of the primary metabolite, sirolimus; if alternatives cannot be used, dose modifications are recommended	Hypersensitivity/infusion reactions (including some life-threatening and rare fatal reactions) can occur early in the first infusion; patients should be monitored throughout the infusion; monitor for symptoms or radiographic changes of ILD; if ILD is suspected, discontinue drug, and consider use of corticosteroids and/or antibiotics; bowel perforation may occur; evaluate fever, abdominal pain, bloody stools, and/or acute abdomen promptly; elderly patients may be more likely to experience certain adverse reactions, including diarrhea, edema, and pneumonia	Advanced renal cell carcinoma
Tepotinib (Tepmetko)	Tyrosine kinase inhibitor that blocks signaling through a *MET* exon 14 skipping mutation	Avoid use with strong CYP3A and P-gp inhibitors; metabolized in the liver and excreted in feces	Edema; fatigue; nausea; diarrhea; interstitial lung disease; hepatotoxicity	NSCLC with *MET* exon 14 skipping mutation
Tisagenlecleucel (Kymriah)	Anti-CD19 CAR–T-cell immunotherapy	No contraindications	Cytokine release syndrome; neurologic toxicity	ALL B-cell precursor type refractory to primary therapy
Topotecan (Hycamtin), hycamptamine	Semisynthetic camptothecin molecule; an inhibitor of topoisomerase I, which is required by cells for both transcription and replication	After IV administration, the drug is not extensively metabolized, and it has an elimination half-life of about 3 hr; a significant portion of the drug is excreted unchanged in the urine	Myelosuppression, especially leukopenia, is expected and dose limiting; thrombocytopenia and anemia are common but mild; nausea, vomiting, and diarrhea are common but usually not severe; headache, fever, fatigue, anorexia, malaise, and elevated liver function tests are also common; hypertension, tachycardia, urticaria, renal insufficiency, hematuria, neuropathy, and mucositis are uncommon	Approved for the treatment of refractory, relapsed ovarian carcinoma and for relapsed small cell lung cancer; also used in myeloid leukemias
Trabectedin (Yondelis)	Alkylating agent that binds the minor groove of DNA-producing adducts	Avoid strong CYP3A inhibitors or inducers	Neutropenic sepsis; rhabdomyolysis; hepatotoxicity; cardiotoxicity; fetal harm	Unresectable or metastatic liposarcoma or leiomyosarcoma after prior anthracycline therapy
Trametinib (Mekinist)	Selective inhibitor of mitogen-activated extracellular kinase (MEK) 1 and 2; decreases cellular proliferation; combination with BRAF inhibitors increases inhibition of MAPK pathway	Deacetylated and glucuronidated in liver; no dose adjustments for mild renal or hepatic dysfunction	Cardiovascular (hypertension, decreased LVEF); acneiform rash and palmar-plantar erythrodysesthesia; diarrhea; anemia; peripheral edema	Advanced melanoma in patients with *BRAF* V600E or V600K mutations alone or in combination with dabrafenib; metastatic NSCLC with *BRAF* V600E mutation in combination with dabrafenib
Aldo-trastuzumab emtansine (Kadcyla)	Antibody-drug conjugate targeting HER2; composed of trastuzumab covalently linked to a maytansine derivative (DM1) with microtubule inhibitory properties; after binding to HER2, it is internalized with release of DM1 and tubulin disruption	Metabolized in the liver by CYP3A4	Hepatotoxicity; left ventricular dysfunction; infusion reaction; pneumonitis; blood count suppression	HER2-positive metastatic breast cancer previously treated with trastuzumab and a taxane
Fam-trastuzumab deruxtecan-nxki (Enhertu)	HER2-directed antibody and topoisomerase inhibitor conjugate	Intravenous infusion only, but not with sodium chloride	Interstitial lung disease, neutropenia, left ventricular dysfunction, nausea, vomiting, fatigue, alopecia, constipation, anemia, diarrhea, thrombocytopenia	Unresectable or metastatic HER2-positive breast cancer despite two or more prior anti-HER2-based regimens

TABLE 164-2 U.S. FDA-APPROVED DRUGS COMMONLY USED FOR THE SYSTEMIC TREATMENT OF CANCER*—cont'd

DRUG NAME	DRUG CLASS AND/OR MECHANISM	PHARMACOKINETICS/METABOLISM	TOXICITY	INDICATIONS[†]
Trastuzumab (Herceptin)	Genetically engineered humanized mouse monoclonal antibody directed against HER2/neu growth factor receptor that is overexpressed in many invasive breast carcinomas; mechanism of action for clinical activity in breast cancer is unknown but may be complement-mediated cell lysis, antibody-dependent cellular cytotoxicity, or induction of apoptosis	Binding studies show strong binding to cells overexpressing HER2/neu molecules; very little else is known regarding the distribution and metabolic fates of this molecule; half-life should be very short with minimal distribution outside the vascular compartment and minimal clearance by kidneys or liver (similar to other monoclonal agents)	Common toxicities include acute fever, chills, nausea, vomiting, and headache; trastuzumab seems to worsen leukopenia, anemia, and diarrhea when given with chemotherapy compared with chemotherapy alone; also, trastuzumab may have uncommon acute cardiotoxicity, which may add to the more common anthracycline-induced cardiotoxicity; therefore, the use of trastuzumab with doxorubicin is not indicated by the FDA	Approved for HER2/neu overexpressing metastatic or locally advanced breast cancer; has shown clinical benefit as a single agent and in conjunction with paclitaxel-based chemotherapy; also approved for gastric cancer
Tucatinib (Tukysa)	HER2 tyrosine kinase inhibitor	Avoid strong CYP3A inducers, moderate CYP2C8 inducers, strong CYP2C8 inhibitors, CYP3A substrates, and P-gp substrates	Diarrhea, hepatotoxicity	In combination with trastuzumab and capecitabine for advanced unresectable or metastatic HER2-positive breast cancer despite other anti-HER2 regimens
Umbralisib (Ukoniq)	Oral kinase inhibitor active against PI3K-delta and casein kinase CK1-epsilon	No dosage reduction required for mild renal or hepatic dysfunction; rapidly absorbed and excreted predominantly in feces	Neutropenia; diarrhea; noninfectious colitis; hepatotoxicity; cutaneous reactions	Marginal zone lymphoma relapsed or refractory following at least one prior anti–CD20-based regimen; follicular lymphoma relapsed or refractory after at least three lines of systemic therapy
Vandetanib (Caprelsa)	Kinase inhibitor	The concomitant use of known strong CYP 3A4 inducers may reduce drug levels of vandetanib and should be avoided. No clinically significant drug interaction was shown with vandetanib and the potent CYP 3A4 inhibitor, itraconazole. The administration of vandetanib with agents that may prolong the QT interval should be avoided. In total, 18% of medullary thyroid cancer patients treated with vandetanib were age 65 yr or older, and 3% were 75 yr and older. No overall differences in safety and efficacy were observed between elderly and younger patients. No adjustment in starting dose is required for patients over 65 yr of age. There are limited data for patients over the age of 75 yr. Limited data for renal or hepatic impairment point toward dose reductions	QT prolongation: sudden death has been reported. Monitor electrocardiograms and levels of serum potassium, calcium, magnesium, and TSH at baseline, 2-4 wk and 8-12 wk after starting treatment, and every 3 mo thereafter and following dose adjustments. Dose reduction as appropriate. Stevens-Johnson syndrome resulting in death has been observed. Severe skin reactions may prompt permanent discontinuation of the drug. Interstitial lung disease resulting in death has been reported. Interrupt dosing and investigate unexplained dyspnea, cough, and fever. Appropriate measures should be taken for ILD. Ischemic cerebrovascular events, hemorrhage, heart failure, diarrhea, hypothyroidism, hypertension, and reversible posterior leukoencephalopathy syndrome have been observed. Other common adverse events: diarrhea, rash, acne, nausea, hypertension, headache, fatigue, upper respiratory tract infections, decreased appetite, and abdominal pain. The most common laboratory abnormalities were decreased calcium, increased ALT, and decreased glucose	Thyroid cancer unresectable locally advanced or metastatic
Vemurafenib (Zelboraf)	Inhibits V600E serine-threonine and other kinases	Take with or without food; inhibits CYP1A2, 2D6; enhances CYP3A	Produces cutaneous squamous cell carcinoma, hypersensitive and dermatologic reagins, QT prolonged, liver lab abnormalities	Metastatic *BRAF*+ melanoma
Venetoclax (Venclexta)	BCL-2 inhibitor	Take with meal and water; prophylaxis for tumor lysis syndrome with anti-hyperuricemic agents and adequate hydration; do not use strong inhibitors of CYP3A at initiation and during ramp-up phase	Tumor lysis syndrome; neutropenia; fetal harm; diarrhea, nausea; anemia; upper respiratory tract infection	CLL with 17p deletion, per FDA-approved test, after at least one prior therapy

Vinorelbine (Navelbine), 5′-noranhydrovinblastine, NVB	Semisynthetic vinca alkaloid; inhibitor of tubulin polymerization and thereby mitosis; G2-phase specific	Metabolized by the liver and has an elimination half-life of about 24 hr; excretion is predominantly in the bile	Vinorelbine is a mild vesicant, requiring extravasation precautions; myelosuppression, mostly leukopenia, is expected and dose limiting; significant nausea and vomiting are uncommon; neurotoxicity in the form of neuropathy is less common and milder than that seen with vincristine; tumor pain during administration has been reported; acute reaction such as dyspnea, chest pain, and wheezing have occurred during administration and may be prevented by premedication with corticosteroids	Approved for the treatment of relapsed metastatic breast cancer and for NSCLC as a single agent or combined with a platinating agent
Vismodegib (Erivedge)	Hedgehog pathway inhibitor	Safety and effectiveness have not been established for hepatic or renal impairment; absorption is saturable as evidenced by the lack of dose-proportional increase in exposure after a single dose of 270 mg or 540 mg vismodegib; may be taken without regard to meals because the systemic exposure of vismodegib at steady state is not affected by food	The most common adverse reactions (incidence of ≥10%) are muscle spasms, alopecia, dysgeusia, weight loss, fatigue, nausea, diarrhea, decreased appetite, constipation, arthralgias, vomiting, and ageusia. Advise patients not to donate blood or blood products while receiving vismodegib and for at least 7 mo after the last dose.	Metastatic basal cell carcinoma or locally advanced basal cell carcinoma that has recurred following surgery or patients who are not candidates for surgery and who are not candidates for radiation
Zoledronic acid (Zometa)	Bisphosphonate inhibitor of bone metastases	Zoledronic acid is poorly absorbed by the GI tract and is therefore given as an IV infusion; it is not metabolized and is excreted by the kidneys; it has a plasma terminal elimination half-life of about 150 hr	Zoledronic acid is generally well tolerated; the most common infusional adverse effect is fever, which is usually mild and treatable; nausea and constipation are also common; dyspnea, fatigue, diffuse pain, rash, and headache are uncommon; renal insufficiency is uncommon and generally reversible after discontinuation of the drug, but it is more likely with higher doses than with the approved and recommended 4-mg dose	Approved for treatment of hypercalcemia of malignancy and for prevention of pathologic fractures in multiple myeloma and solid tumors with known bone metastases

*Full listing of all FDA-approved agents appears online at https://www.cancer.gov/about-cancer/treatment/drugs/cancer-type.

†Note that indications may change based on the results of clinical trials and other data.

ABMT = autologous bone marrow transplantation; AC = accelerated phase; ADCC = antibody-dependent cell-mediated cytotoxicity; ADP = adenosine diphosphate; AIDS = acquired immunodeficiency syndrome; ALK = anaplastic lymphoma kinase; ALL = acute lymphoblastic lymphoma; ALT = alanine aminotransferase; AML = acute myelogenous leukemia; AST = aspartate aminotransferase; AUC = area under the curve; BC = breast cancer; BID = twice a day; CK = creatine kinase; CLL = chronic lymphocytic leukemia; CML = chronic myelogenous leukemia; CNS = central nervous system; CP = chronic phase; CTCL = cutaneous T-cell lymphoma; CTLA-4 = cytotoxic T-lymphocyte antigen 4; CYP = cytochrome; D5W = 5% dextrose in water; dATP = deoxyadenosine triphosphate; DMHHT = demethyl-homoharringtonine; DVT = deep vein thrombosis; ECG = electrocardiogram; EGFR = epidermal growth factor receptor; ER = estrogen receptor; FAMP = fludarabine monophosphate; FDA = Food and Drug Administration; 5-FU = 5-fluorouracil; FSH = follicle-stimulating hormone; G6PD = glucose-6-phosphate dehydrogenase; G-CSF = granulocyte-colony stimulating factor; GGT = gamma-glutamyltransferase; GI = gastrointestinal; GIST = gastrointestinal stromal tumor; GM-CSF = granulocyte-macrophage colony-stimulating factor; GnRH = gonadotropin-releasing hormone; GVHD = graft-versus-host disease; HDAC = histone deacetylase; HIV = human immunodeficiency virus; HMM = hexamethyl melamine; HR-positive = hormone receptor positive; HRT = hormone replacement therapy; HSC = hematopoietic stem cell; IFN = interferon; IGF = insulin-like growth factor; IgG2 = immunoglobulin G2; IL = interleukin; ILD = interstitial lung disease; IM = intramuscular; INR = International Normalized Ratio; IV = intravenous; LDH = lactate dehydrogenase; LH = luteinizing hormone; LHRH = luteinizing hormone–releasing hormone; LVEF = left ventricular ejection fraction; MAPK = mitogen-activated protein kinase; MDS = myelodysplastic syndrome; MET = mesenchymal epithelial transition factor receptor; MOPP = mechlorethamine, vincristine, procarbazine, and prednisone; MSI = microsatellite instability; MTIC = 5-(3-,ethyltriazen-1-yl)imidazole-4-carboxamide; mTOR = mammalian target of rapamycin; NHL = non-Hodgkin lymphoma; NSAIDs = nonsteroidal anti-inflammatory drugs; NSCLC = non–small cell lung cancer; PARP = poly (ADP-ribose) polymerase; PDGF = platelet-derived growth factor; PD-L1 = programmed death ligand 1; PE = pulmonary embolism; P-gp = P-glycoprotein; PI = phosphoinositide; PNET = progressive neuroendocrine tumor; PO = by mouth; PT = prothrombin time; RANK = receptor activator of nuclear factor–κB; RCC = renal cell carcinoma; SCLC = small cell lung cancer; SEGA = subependymal giant cell astrocytoma; SQ = subcutaneous; TID = three times a day; TNF = tumor necrosis factor; TSC = tuberous sclerosis; TSH = thyroid-stimulating hormone; UGTs = UDP-glucuronosyltransferases; ULN = upper limit of normal; VEGF = vascular endothelial growth factor.

As indicated throughout this chapter, the pace has accelerated for approvals of new drugs and new indications. Updated information should be checked on the FDA website (www.fda.gov/drugs) or other authoritative sources.

From Collins JM. Cancer pharmacology. In: Niederhuber JE, Armitage JO, Doroshow JH, Kastan MB, Tepper JE, eds. *Abeloff's Clinical Oncology*, 5th ed. Philadelphia: Churchill Livingston; 2014.

small cell lung cancer and non–small cell lung cancer is critical for treatment. For breast cancer (Chapter 183), the treating physician is interested in a variety of factors, such as histology, tumor grade, the presence (and its degree) or absence of estrogen and progesterone receptor proteins, the presence of HER2/neu overexpression, and other molecular characteristics. The rapidly increasing sophistication of molecular diagnostics has also greatly improved the potential to localize cancers of unknown primary origin (see the section Cancer of Unknown Origin later in this chapter).

Staging and Multidisciplinary Evaluation

After a tissue diagnosis has been established, careful staging is required to determine the extent of disease. The American Joint Committee on Cancer staging system, which is the standard in the United States, is based on the TNM (tumor, node, metastasis) system that is anatomically and pathologically based. The approach to staging from a clinical perspective depends on the type of cancer, but it commonly includes computed tomography (CT), magnetic resonance imaging (MRI), and, increasingly, positron emission tomography (PET) and PET-CT. These studies are supplemented by routine hematologic and chemistry profiles, tumor markers, and molecular characterization (when appropriate), as well as by bone marrow aspiration and biopsy in some cases.

The goal of tumor staging is to define the extent of a patient's disease. Tumor stage provides critical prognostic information that will inform the therapeutic approach that is most appropriate. Accurate staging involves delineating the magnitude of the tumor determined by imaging procedures, as well as confirming the pathologic limits of disease spread from tissues removed at surgery. In essence, for most solid tumor patients, the tumor stage will establish whether the treatment will focus on a local (usually confined to an organ), regional, or disseminated pattern of malignancy and can determine whether the expected outcome of therapy is curative or palliative. Conversely, hematopoietic malignancies are often disseminated at diagnosis and demand their own prognostic classifiers.

The focus of the staging evaluation is to identify potential sites of metastases and to establish indicator lesions with which to monitor therapy. For most solid tumors, CT scans can accomplish both goals; however, in some circumstances, other imaging modalities are more appropriate for therapeutic monitoring (e.g., MRI when central nervous system [CNS] metastases are likely [e.g., small cell lung cancer], or combined PET/CT imaging to establish that a given lesion is likely to be metabolically active and malignant, or in diseases in which early metabolic responses to treatment can be confirmed [such as for gastrointestinal stromal tumors]). In patients with established advanced disease, indicator lesions for therapeutic monitoring should be carefully chosen prior to the initiation of treatment, be well documented in the medical record, and be evaluated with the minimum frequency of imaging procedures required for accurate follow-up, consistent with evidence-based medical practice or the clinical protocol on which the patient is entered.

The consulting medical oncologist may often be advised by a local tumor board composed of other medical, surgical, and radiation oncologists, pathologists, radiologists, and members of the cancer care team (oncology nurses, social workers, and palliative care specialists). In such a multidisciplinary environment, the patient's overall prognosis can be reviewed and alternatives for care, including standard therapy, possible clinical trials, a second opinion, or no treatment, can be considered. The outcome of such an evaluation is usually viewed by patients and families as an important component in the coordinated development of an overall plan for either further diagnostic procedures or therapy. Finally, many oncologists actively participate in clinical trials that may make investigational drugs or other investigational procedures available for patients, or they may suggest referral to a tertiary cancer center where disease-specific or molecularly defined clinical trials are available.

TREATMENT

Therapeutic Plan

Intention of Treatment

Based on the multidisciplinary evaluation of an accurately staged patient, the chosen intent of treatment may be curative or palliative. Whether or not this choice is made during a formal tumor board or multidisciplinary case conference, clarity must be reached regarding the specific choice of therapeutic options (and their potential risks and benefits, overall goals, and alternatives) when considered in the context of the wishes of the patient and family. This issue is particularly relevant when the side effects of treatment are substantial (such as for the multidisciplinary management of non–small cell lung cancer or esophageal cancer). For cancers that are amenable to surgery, resection is often an initial alternative if the patient is a suitable candidate for anesthesia and is otherwise in acceptable condition in terms of comorbid illnesses (Chapter 399). Determination of the patient's performance score (see Table 164-1) is a simple means of assessing functional status. If life expectancy is limited or if the patient is not a good candidate for surgery, more limited approaches to palliative radiation or systemic therapy may be appropriate. Substantial data indicate that the extent of surgery required for an optimal long-term outcome may be reduced for certain solid tumors through the use of presurgical, so-called "neoadjuvant" chemotherapy, often as part of an "organ-sparing" approach. Concomitant or sequential multimodality treatments also have the potential to produce long-term disease-free remissions. When the best therapeutic outcomes require the combined skills of surgical, radiation, and medical oncologists, the need for coordination of care among a variety of specialists becomes paramount and the use of predefined treatment regimens critical.

Therapeutic Paradigm and Therapeutic Index

The therapeutic paradigm in oncology, although still directed at improving the multidisciplinary care model, has begun to change from one focused on delivering treatments at the "maximally tolerated dose" for normal tissues to therapy that is personalized based on both the molecular characteristics of the patient's tumor as well as any individual germline features that could modify treatment tolerance (Chapter 166). Based on the rapid expansion of information regarding somatic mutations in human malignancies and the ability to produce therapeutic molecules that can target specific defects in tumoral DNA repair, growth factor signaling, energy balance, or immunocompetence, for example, the current approach to cancer therapeutics involves the use of predictive molecular markers ("biomarkers") whenever possible to guide all modalities of cancer care for the benefit of unique cancer patients. Hence, the focus of oncologists is on the elaboration of treatments that can be administered with a high therapeutic index, defined as the comparison of the amount of treatment that is effective as compared with the amount that causes toxicity. The goal of precision cancer medicine therapy is to minimize toxicity to normal tissues and to preserve quality of life by advancing therapies or procedures that are targeted only to the specific molecular dependencies of the patient's tumor.

Surgical Therapy

Surgery is used to biopsy a suspected lesion, remove the primary tumor, bypass obstructions, provide palliation, and prevent cancers in patients at very high risk because of genetic predispositions or chronic inflammatory states. Surgical staging also establishes the extent of disease. For example, patients with ovarian cancer (Chapter 184) benefit from surgical "debulking" to remove all visible disease, leave minimal residual tumor, and thereby enhance the effectiveness of systemic treatment. Placement of a venous access device at the time of surgery, if considered proactively, may eliminate the need for a second procedure.

Risk-reducing bilateral mastectomy and risk-reducing salpingo-oophorectomy are options for the primary prevention of breast (Chapter 183) and ovarian cancers in individuals who are genetically predisposed to these malignancies. Although these operations provide considerable efficacy in terms of cancer prevention, they can be associated with profound adverse physical and psychosexual effects. Decisions to proceed with such risk-reducing surgery are complex and emotionally charged. Patients require clearly understandable information and counseling, as well as adequate time and support to think through their options.[4]

Surgery remains the most common method to cure localized cancers such as breast cancer (Chapter 183), colorectal cancer (Chapter 179), and lung cancer (Chapter 177), but it is limited by the location of the tumor, its extension, and distant metastases.[A1] Even if a tumor cannot be removed, surgical biopsy provides confirmation of the diagnosis and additional tissue for molecular analysis. Occasionally, an obstructing lesion can be bypassed to provide palliation.

In specific circumstances when the primary tumor has been controlled, removal of a single metastasis (metastasectomy) can result in long-term survival; an example is resection of a solitary liver metastasis found at the time of colectomy for colorectal cancer (Chapter 179). A variety of surgical techniques, such as radiofrequency ablation or cryoablation, can also be used to treat hepatic metastases in carefully selected patients. Adjuvant chemotherapy is often given after surgery in this situation to treat microscopic metastases.

The careful application of reconstructive surgery after a disfiguring procedure is critical to long-term physical and emotional well-being. Examples include postmastectomy breast reconstruction (Chapter 183) and plastic surgical procedures to correct deformities following head and neck surgery (Chapter 176).

Radiation Therapy

Ionizing radiation (Chapter 18) can be delivered using beams of high-energy rays, known as *teletherapy*, via a linear accelerator; by brachytherapy, through the application of sealed radioactive implants, seeds, wires, or plaques; and intravenously by using radioisotopes, either directly or attached to antibodies or other targeting molecules.[5] Radiation interacts with water molecules to induce free radical species, including hydroxyl radicals, which damage DNA, proteins, and lipid membranes, thereby leading to cell death. As with chemotherapy, radiation therapy is most effective against rapidly dividing cells that are well oxygenated. Radiation-induced DNA damage may also increase sensitivity to chemo- or immunotherapy.

The utility of radiation therapy is limited by the inapparent extension of disease outside a local treatment field, by the location of tumors next to normal structures that must be preserved, and by the presence of distant metastases. Normal tissue tolerance, which varies across different organs and tissues, often prevents the use of radiation doses that could uniformly eradicate cancers. Radiation therapy is also limited by tumor hypoxia: large, bulky tumors are frequently relatively radioresistant, whereas well-oxygenated tumors can be more effectively treated at lower doses. In addition to acute radiation-related toxicities (Chapter 18), late effects of radiation therapy include second malignancies, such as breast cancers that may occur decades after administering thoracic radiation fields during curative treatment for Hodgkin disease.

Radiation therapy can be used as primary treatment, as part of multimodality therapy, in the adjuvant setting, and for palliation. As a single modality, radiation therapy can be curative for early-stage malignancies such as laryngeal cancer (Chapter 176), cervical cancer (Chapter 184), and prostate cancer (Chapter 186). Breast-conserving surgery (Chapter 183) requires the use of radiation to treat the remaining breast. Partial irradiation techniques using three-dimensional planning with external beam radiation can be used in selected patients with appropriately placed and sized breast cancers. For certain patients who have localized prostate cancer (Chapter 186), implanted radioactive seeds of gold or palladium offer an alternative to surgery or external beam radiation therapy.

Intensity-modulated radiation therapy (IMRT) permits more exact tailoring of the dose to the target, thereby reducing damage to the surrounding normal tissues. Stereotactic radiation therapy or gamma knife techniques allow the treatment of primary or metastatic brain tumors (Chapter 175) measuring up to 3 cm with enhanced accuracy, thereby minimizing damage to normal brain. An analogous approach may help patients whose primary tumor has been controlled and who have a limited number of metastatic lesions. Particle-based treatment with protons can deliver higher radiation doses locally. However, no randomized studies demonstrate its superiority over other approaches that use computational techniques (e.g., IMRT) to improve the specificity of the delivery of radiation. However, proton therapy is generally recommended for some uveal melanomas, base-of-skull tumors, and a few pediatric malignancies.

Low- to moderate-dose palliative radiation is used to ameliorate symptomatic cancer when cure is no longer the goal. For instance, radiation therapy can improve symptoms from brain metastases (Chapter 175), relieve pain from bone lesions (Chapter 187), relieve some obstructing lesions, and sometimes improve hemoptysis caused by lung cancer (Chapter 177) or bleeding from a gynecologic malignancy (Chapter 184). Bone-seeking radioisotopes of samarium, strontium, or radium may relieve pain from bone metastases in prostate cancer (Chapter 186) or breast cancer (Chapter 183).

Systemic Therapy

Cancer Pharmacology

Principles

The fundamental goal of cancer pharmacology is the development of treatments that can be matched to the intrinsic sensitivity of specific tumors and that can be delivered in concentrations that affect the molecular target of interest with an acceptable therapeutic index. Three properties of all cancer therapeutic agents underlie their clinical utility: pharmacogenetics of the drug (how the germline or somatic expression of genes alters normal tissue toxicity or antitumor efficacy); action of the drug (pharmacodynamics, or what the drug does to the tumor/body); and delivery of the drug (pharmacokinetics, or what the body does to the drug).

Pharmacogenetics

Pharmacogenetics, which is the study of inherited interindividual differences in drug disposition and effects, is important in cancer therapy because genetic polymorphisms in drug-metabolizing enzymes may be responsible for the variations in efficacy and toxicity that are observed with many chemotherapeutic agents. Drugs potentially affected by polymorphisms include the thiopurines, 5-fluorouracil, irinotecan, taxanes, and platinum agents. In patients who are heterozygous or homozygous for deficiencies in metabolizing enzymes, toxicity can be dramatically enhanced. Testing for pharmacogenetic variations that predict for altered normal tissue tolerance is currently available for thiopurines and irinotecan.

Molecular Targeting and Pharmacodynamics

Molecular diagnostic testing, which began with testing to predict the antitumor activity of hormonal and anti-HER2 therapeutics, is now relevant to a wider range of tumors for which molecularly targeted and immunotherapeutic anticancer agents are useful only after demonstration of specific molecular abnormalities.[6] Examples of such diagnostic/drug pairs include the prototypical *BCR-ABL* mutation in chronic myelogenous leukemia and imatinib; *EGFR* mutations in lung adenocarcinomas and erlotinib; *ALK* tyrosine kinase translocations in lung adenocarcinomas and crizotinib; *BRAF*^{V600E} mutations in melanoma and vemurafenib, *NTRK* fusions and larotrectinib; and *KRAS* mutations in various solid tumors. Molecular targeting can also involve the expression of mismatch repair genes and immunologic checkpoint inhibitors.

Pharmacokinetics and Drug Delivery

Dose selection in oncology is a critical issue, primarily because anticancer agents have among the smallest therapeutic ratios in all of medicine. When tumors are responsive to treatment, higher doses may or may not be more effective but are likely to be more toxic to normal tissues. The clearance of a drug from both the systemic circulation and, potentially, from specific physiologic compartments (CNS, pleural, or peritoneal effusions), as evidenced by its systemic exposure, is the most important determinant of the recommended dose for a particular patient. Clearance, which is a composite of all the routes and mechanisms by which the drug can be eliminated from the body, determines dosing and dose adjustments in the face of changes in drug metabolism, transport, or altered organ function. Although a clear understanding of drug half-lives is important to establish initial dosing schedules, systemic exposure will be the actual determinant of the dose of drug that can be safely administered. Another aspect of drug delivery is the use of body surface area dosing versus flat dosing (using fixed amounts of a drug) in oncologic practice. Although dosing based on body surface area has a long history in oncology, very little data support this approach; for most agents in common use, empirically determined pharmacokinetic variability from patient to patient is far greater than what could reasonably be determined by dosing based on weight or surface area.

Routes of Drug Dosing

Although some agents require intravenous administration, oral agents that permit outpatient therapy are increasingly being used. The oral route of administration highlights drug delivery issues, such as adherence (does the patient take his/her medication), variability in absorption (due to food effects), emesis prior to drug absorption, first-pass metabolism in the liver or intestine, and difficulties in swallowing. For example, whether the orally administered anti-HER1/2 drug lapatinib is taken with food or on an empty stomach can alter its absorption by as much as 10-fold.

In addition to intravenous or oral dosing, anticancer drugs may be used for intrathecal delivery (to overcome the blood-brain barrier) in the treatment or prevention of meningeal spread of leukemia; for intravesicle therapy of early-stage bladder cancer; for intra-arterial delivery of fluoropyrimidines or other agents to treat hepatic metastases from colon cancer or hepatocellular carcinoma; and for intraperitoneal administration of drugs such as platinum agents for ovarian cancer therapy. In almost all cases, administration of anticancer agents by other than the oral or intravenous routes requires intimate involvement of an oncologic specialist.

Clinical Trials

Clinical trials in oncology are defined by the steps in which new diagnostic approaches, therapeutic agents, or procedures are tested to determine whether they will become part of the standard care for cancer patients. During interventional (rather than observational) clinical trials, specific treatments or procedures are assigned to participants, and the effects of the interventions are measured. For trials of new oncologic drugs, the U.S. Food and Drug Administration (FDA) recognizes several states in the drug development process. Exploratory studies of new drugs examined for the first time in humans (phase 0 trials) may be conducted in a limited number of patients to define a drug's mechanism of action or biodistribution and to guide subsequent dosing in larger studies. Phase I trials use a variety of dose-escalation strategies to define the maximum dose that can be safely administered to humans and the most appropriate schedule for drug administration, as well as the pharmacokinetic and pharmacodynamic profile of the drug. Phase II trials often enroll 50 to 150 subjects and focus on testing the drug to determine its effectiveness and side effect profile in a specific malignancy (or for a specific cancer-related molecular abnormality). If a drug demonstrates anticancer activity in a phase II study, phase III trials are performed to compare the usefulness of an investigational treatment to a control group of patients who receive the standard of care; patients in most phase III studies are randomly assigned to the new or standard treatment to avoid a biased assessment of the results of the study. Finally, after approval of a new drug by the FDA, usually based on the results of phase III studies, phase IV trials may be performed to collect safety information on larger patient populations to define the prevalence of side effects that may be rare but serious.

Traditionally designed phase II trials test one treatment at a time in heterogenous groups of patients and are therefore not an efficient use of clinical resources. Adaptive multigroup clinical trials have the potential to answer several questions simultaneously and more efficiently by matching targeted therapies to the cancer patients who are most likely to benefit from them. Some trials for breast cancer, for example, use a platform to compare up to 12 experimental therapies with a single, common control group in subgroups of breast cancer patients with 10 distinct biomarker signatures.[7] New drugs enter the platform as they emerge from phase I testing and exit the platform with an estimate of the chances of future success in a phase III trial of prespecified size. Despite some significant unresolved issues, the adaptive strategy is likely to become an important addition to the inventory of clinical trial designs. Another approach is so-called master protocols, which evaluate one or more agents against a specific molecular characteristic possessed by the tumor rather than its histology.[8]

Drug Interactions

Many drug interactions affect the toxicity profile of anticancer agents, usually because concomitant administration of a second drug changes the clearance of the cancer therapeutic, thereby potentially enhancing side effects if the clearance is decreased or diminishing efficacy because of reduced drug exposure.

Most often these interactions occur because one drug affects the metabolism of the other by inhibiting or enhancing the activity of cytochrome P-450 isoforms (such as CYP3A) in the liver. This interaction is particularly true for agents administered orally, such as imatinib, crizotinib, enzalutamide, pazopanib, and lapatinib. Concomitant drug-related as well as pharmacogenetic variations in proteins that affect the transport of anticancer agents across tumor and normal cell membranes, such as efflux pumps, also affect the sensitivity or resistance of many classes of cancer drugs. For example, certain drugs that are well-known inducers of hepatic metabolism (e.g., phenytoin and rifampin) also induce the expression of drug transport proteins.

Combination Therapy

Virtually all curative chemotherapy regimens developed for hematologic malignancies or solid tumors use combinations of active agents. Combination chemotherapy is usually superior to the use of single agents in adjuvant and neoadjuvant therapy as well. The improved results achieved by combination chemotherapy can be explained in several ways. Mechanisms of resistance to any particular single agent are almost always present in the tumor genome at diagnosis, even in clinically responsive tumors. Tumors that are initially "sensitive" to systemic therapy rapidly acquire resistance to single agents, either as a result of selection of a preexisting clone of resistant tumor cells or because of a variety of potential acquired molecular changes (e.g., increased drug efflux, enhanced DNA repair, insensitivity to apoptosis) that lead to clinical drug resistance. Combination therapy may address these phenomena by providing a broader range of mechanisms of drug action against initially resistant tumor cells, thereby preventing or slowing the selection of resistant clones.

The development of combination systemic therapy regimens follows a set of principles (Table 164-3). For standard cytotoxic agents, each drug in the combination must be active against the tumor, and all drugs must be given at an optimal dose and on an appropriate schedule. The drugs should have different mechanisms of antitumor activity as well as different toxicity profiles, and the drugs should be given at consistent intervals for the shortest possible treatment time. The use of molecularly targeted agents in combination requires that each agent engages its specific target and that the combination enhances the inhibition of the tumor's growth. Toxicities of targeted agents should be moderate to allow prolonged administration and maximum target inhibition.

Therapeutic Settings

Systemic therapy is used in a variety of settings with or without and before, during, or after surgery and radiation therapy (Table 164-4). Considerable experimental evidence suggests that cancers are most sensitive to chemotherapy during early stages of growth because of higher growth fractions and shorter cell cycle times. As a result, a given dose of a cytotoxic drug may exert a greater therapeutic effect against a rapidly growing tumor than against a larger quiescent tumor.

Neoadjuvant therapy, also called primary or induction systemic therapy, is used before surgery or radiation therapy to decrease the size of locally advanced cancers, thereby permitting a more complete surgical resection or eradication of undetectable metastases. Neoadjuvant therapy also affords an opportunity to evaluate the effectiveness of treatment by histologic and molecular analysis of resected tissue. This approach is most often used for locally advanced breast cancer (Chapter 183).

Organ-sparing therapy is another use of chemotherapy, radiation therapy, or both to salvage organs that would have been surgically removed if cure were the intended result. This technique is often effective in patients with cancers of the larynx (Chapter 176), esophagus (Chapter 178), and anus (Chapter 179).

Adjuvant chemotherapy is used in patients whose primary tumor and all visible evidence of cancer (e.g., regional lymph nodes) have been surgically removed or treated definitively with radiation, but in whom the risk of recurrence is high because of involved lymph nodes or certain morphologic or biologic characteristics of the cancer. Common examples include cancers of the breast (Chapter 183) and colon (Chapter 179). The typical end points of chemotherapy, such as shrinkage of measurable tumor on serial radiographic studies, are not available in this situation; instead, relapse-free survival and overall survival are the principal measures of a treatment's effect. The benefit of adjuvant therapy cannot be assessed in individual patients who receive it, so decisions about its use must be based on evidence from clinical trials.

Assessment of Response

Assessment of the response to therapy (usually performed using RECIST [Response Evaluation Criteria in Solid Tumors]) depends largely on the tumor's size, as determined by either direct measurement or diagnostic imaging studies, using predefined categories. The categories of response are "complete response," with total absence of tumor and correction of tumor-associated changes measured twice at least 4 weeks apart; "partial response," defined as 30% or greater reduction in the sum of the longest diameters of up to five target lesions per organ, confirmed by repeat measurement 4 weeks later; "progressive disease," characterized by either 20% or greater increase over the smallest sum of the longest diameters of target lesions or the development of new tumors; and "stable disease," defined as meeting criteria for neither partial response nor progressive disease. Leukemias are assessed by bone marrow biopsies and molecular diagnostic tests for residual disease, and multiple myeloma is typically assessed by the measurement of monoclonal proteins, peripheral blood counts, and percentages of malignant plasma cells in bone marrow samples, as well as imaging of bone lesions. Accurate assessment of response following systemic therapy is essential because of the tight relationship between the degree of response and the duration of disease control.

Classes of Therapeutic Agents

Cytotoxic Agents, Targeted Small Molecules, and Antibodies

An understanding of the pharmacologic properties and therapeutic indications of the most commonly used cytotoxic and molecularly targeted chemotherapeutic agents and antibodies approved by the FDA (see Table 164-2) is critical for prescribing physicians and is also important for physicians who participate in the patient's care. Current information should be sought from the manufacturer before therapy is initiated.

The administration of chemotherapy should be overseen by specifically trained individuals because of the dual acute risks of hypersensitivity reactions and extravasation. No doses or schedules are universally recommended because these agents are often used in combination, and the doses of each drug may need to be reduced when the compounds are combined, as well as when they are prescribed to patients who may have impaired liver or kidney function or a higher risk of adverse effects.

Unless otherwise specified, most cytotoxic chemotherapeutic agents may produce some degree of nausea and vomiting, myelosuppression, alopecia, mucositis, and/or diarrhea after treatment; many agents are also teratogenic, mutagenic, and carcinogenic. Specific drugs (see Table 164-2) often can be used to prevent agent-specific toxicities.

Small molecule anticancer agents with more precisely targeted mechanisms of action have become a standard part of oncologic practice (see Table 164-2). Although the molecular dependencies within the tumor cells against which these drugs are targeted are broad in scope, including tyrosine kinase growth factors or their receptors, they are functionally much more specific than prior generations of systemic cancer therapies. This specificity allows for a better appreciation of the clinical situations in which certain drugs might be beneficial, as well as the possibility of developing agents for use in specific tumors based on their genetic susceptibilities. The toxicity profiles of molecular targeted agents most often reflect alterations that are produced in biochemical pathways that control normal organ function, rather than a general pattern of toxicity consistent with injury to rapidly growing tissues, such as the bone marrow or gastrointestinal tract.

TABLE 164-3 PRINCIPLES OF COMBINATION THERAPY

CYTOTOXIC AGENTS	MOLECULARLY TARGETED DRUGS
Drugs are each active against the tumor	Agent has therapeutic effect on molecular pathway in vivo
Drugs have different mechanisms of action	Agents have complementary effects on the same target or other targets in the same pathway or pathways that cross-talk to control tumor growth
Drugs have different clinical toxicities to allow full doses of each to be administered	Toxicities do not overlap with cytotoxics and are moderate to low to allow prolonged administration. Consider physiologic consequences of target engagement in relation to toxicity profile
Intermittent intensive therapy is preferred to continuous treatment for cytoreduction and reducing immunosuppression	Schedule is chosen to maximize target inhibition

TABLE 164-4 COMMON EXAMPLES OF THERAPEUTIC SETTINGS

ADJUVANT THERAPY	NEOADJUVANT THERAPY	ORGAN-SPARING THERAPY	COMBINATION CHEMOTHERAPY
Stage I and II breast cancer Stage III colorectal cancer Stage II lung cancer	Stage III breast cancer	Anal cancer Laryngeal cancer Esophageal cancer	Metastatic solid tumors* Hematologic malignancies

*Usually palliative.

The development of monoclonal antibodies directed against proteins or other molecular determinants of cancer cells represents an additional approach to molecular targeting of systemic therapy. Examples include cetuximab (targeting the epidermal growth factor receptor), rituximab (targeting the B-cell CD20 surface antigen), and trastuzumab[A2] (which blocks HER2). These monoclonal antibodies can be used alone or in the form of recombinant bispecific or multispecific antibodies that provide multifunctional receptor targeting, they can be labeled with a radioactive molecule, or they can be conjugated to another cytotoxin to enhance cell killing. Radioimmunoconjugate approaches have been most effective in the treatment of non-Hodgkin lymphoma (Chapter 171) and chronic lymphocytic leukemia (Chapter 169). The effectiveness of monoclonal antibodies in specific tumor types is not identical to small molecules developed against the same target, in part because of the induction of immunologically mediated mechanisms of tumor cell killing that are unique to antibodies.

A major challenge with targeted therapy for malignancies is that drug resistance often develops. Cancers are characterized by extensive intratumor genetic heterogeneity, and resistance to molecularly targeted therapies can arise from the selected growth of preexisting subclones that are present within the bulk of the tumor and that carry drug-resistant mutations, which have a survival advantage for the tumor.[9]

Hormonal Therapies

Endocrine or hormonal therapy is almost entirely limited to breast cancer (Chapter 183) and prostate cancer (Chapter 186). Many premenopausal breast cancers are thought to be under the influence of ovarian estrogens, and hormonal deprivation (ablation) may produce long-term responses in properly selected patients (patients whose tumors express estrogen and/or progesterone receptors and who have predominantly soft tissue or bone disease). The antiestrogen tamoxifen is effective against breast cancer, and it may decrease the incidence of contralateral breast cancers in both premenopausal and postmenopausal women with breast cancer (Chapter 183). Tamoxifen also has an estrogen-like activity that is responsible for an increased rate of endometrial cancers. Postmenopausal women who are candidates for hormonal therapy may also respond to tamoxifen; however, aromatase inhibitors (e.g., anastrozole, letrozole, exemestane), which decrease the conversion of metabolites in fat and muscle into estrogen, are more effective than tamoxifen as first-line therapy in both the adjuvant and metastatic settings.

Prostate cancer (Chapter 186) is usually androgen-dependent, and androgen deprivation can produce meaningful responses. The recent introduction of more potent inhibitors of androgen biosynthesis (abiraterone) and androgen receptor-mediated signal transduction (enzalutamide) has further enhanced the range and effectiveness of androgen deprivation therapy for this disease.

The corticosteroids (Chapter 28), typically prednisone or dexamethasone, are widely used in the treatment of hematologic and oncologic cancers. In Hodgkin disease (Chapter 172), the non-Hodgkin lymphomas (Chapter 171), and multiple myeloma (Chapter 173), corticosteroids have antitumor activity. In solid tumor patients, they are used as antiemetics, for the symptomatic relief of cerebral edema in cases of CNS metastases (Chapter 175), or as an adjunct to radiation therapy for spinal cord metastases.

Epigenetic Therapies

Just as DNA mutations contribute to the progression of tumors, epigenetic alterations in the transcription of DNA also participate in the growth of tumors and their resistance to chemotherapy (Chapter 166). The two best characterized epigenetic mechanisms are DNA methylation and histone modification. DNA methylation is controlled by DNA methyltransferases, whereas histone modification (acetylation) is controlled by histone acetyltransferases. The DNA methyltransferase inhibitors (azacitidine and decitabine) produce durable responses and survival benefit in patients with myelodysplastic syndrome (Chapter 167) and acute myelogenous leukemia (Chapter 168). The histone deacetylase inhibitors (vorinostat and romidepsin) have clinical benefit for the treatment of cutaneous T-cell lymphoma (Chapter 171).

The DNA methyltransferase inhibitors also have an immune-based mechanism of action. Current clinical trials are testing the combination of epigenetic therapy plus immunotherapy in cancer treatment.[10]

Immunotherapy

Cancer immunotherapy blocks the processes by which tumors suppress the immune system. These agents have yielded dramatic clinical benefits for patients with a remarkably wide variety of advanced cancers, including melanoma, kidney, bladder, head and neck, esophageal, gastric, triple-negative breast, hepatocellular, and lung cancers, as well as Hodgkin and non-Hodgkin lymphoma. Immune checkpoint therapy targets regulatory pathways in T cells to enhance their antitumor immune responses. The goal of immune checkpoint blockade is not to activate the immune system to attack particular targets on tumor cells, but rather to remove inhibitory pathways that block effective antitumor T-cell responses. The survival of men and women with metastatic melanoma (Chapter 188) is significantly increased following treatment with antibodies (anti-CTLA-4 ipilimumab and anti-PD-1 nivolumab) that neutralize proteins that protect tumor cells against destruction by the immune system.[11] PD-1 antibodies also provide a survival benefit compared with platinum-based chemotherapy for patients with non–small cell lung cancer. Additional antibodies that target other immunologic checkpoint molecules (anti-PD-L1) provide substantive clinical benefits for patients with melanoma, renal cancer, non–small cell lung cancer, and a variety of other solid tumors and lymphomas. However, a broad range of toxicities can be associated with the use of checkpoint inhibitor therapy.[12]

Another approach to cancer immunotherapy is through adoptive cell transfer, which involves the engineering of the patient's own immune cells to recognize and attack their own tumors. In this form of treatment (CAR T-cell therapy),[13] T cells collected from a patient are genetically engineered to produce special receptors on their surface called "chimeric antigen receptors" (or "CARs"). Targeted CAR T cells have provided impressive responses in patients with B-cell malignancies and led to their FDA approval for an increasing number of indications despite a high risk of side effects, including cytokine release syndrome and acute neurologic complications.

Drugs for Prevention or Treatment of Toxicity

In addition to the hematopoietic growth factors used to reduce the adverse effects of systemic cancer therapies on the bone marrow (discussed later under Management of Complications), drugs have been developed to ameliorate important side effects of cytotoxic chemotherapy (see Table 164-2). These agents include dexrazoxane, which is an iron chelating agent that can prevent the cardiac toxicity of the anthracyclines (doxorubicin and daunorubicin); leucovorin, which can diminish the hematologic side effects of folic acid antagonists; and mesna, a thiol-containing compound that blocks damage to the bladder mucosa from metabolites of cyclophosphamide. Uridine triacetate is FDA-approved for the treatment of patients who receive an overdose of fluorouracil or capecitabine or who develop severe or life-threatening toxicities within 4 days of receiving them.

Bone Marrow or Hematopoietic Stem Cell Transplantation

Because the major dose-limiting toxicity of most chemotherapeutic agents is myelosuppression, pluripotent stem cells can be harvested from bone marrow, peripheral blood, or, less often, cord blood before marrow-damaging chemotherapy so that these stem cells can be reinfused later (Chapter 163). This technique is most effective for acute leukemias (Chapter 168), relapsed lymphomas (Chapter 171), and germ cell tumors (Chapter 185). The effectiveness of the approach is limited more by the inability to eradicate cancer cells than by the inability to achieve engraftment. Transplants may be syngeneic (from an identical twin), autologous (from oneself), allogeneic (from a matched donor such as a sibling or parent), or from a matched unrelated donor. Nonablative hematopoietic transplants that do not completely abolish myelopoiesis reduce toxicity and allow the treatment of older and medically infirm patients.

Special Treatment Populations

Obesity

Up to 40% of obese patients receive limited doses of chemotherapy that are not based on actual body weight. Concerns about toxicity or overdosing based on the use of actual body weight in obese patients with cancer are unfounded. Evidence-based practice guidelines recommend that full cytotoxic chemotherapy doses be used to treat obese patients with cancer, especially when the goal of treatment is cure.

Pregnancy

Cancer during pregnancy (Chapter 221) is not uncommon, with breast, cervical, ovarian, and thyroid cancers; melanoma; and hematologic malignancies being most frequent.[14] Cancer during pregnancy is an emotionally charged challenge, and clinical decision making is complicated by ethical, moral, cultural, and religious issues. If surgery can be safely accomplished, it may be the best course, even if it is only a temporizing measure. Radiation therapy carries the very real risk of radiation exposure to the fetus, and staging is almost always suboptimal and confined to ultrasound examinations. When the disease requires chemotherapy, both the mother and fetus must be taken into account. For example, drug clearance and gastrointestinal absorption are different during pregnancy, and placental transfer, fetal pharmacokinetics, and placental excretion can influence effective and safe drug dosing. Many commonly used chemotherapeutic drugs are classified by the FDA as category D (positive human fetal risk, but the benefits in pregnant women may be acceptable despite the risk) or category X (studies in humans and animals have shown fetal malformations or there is evidence of fetal risk based on human evidence). If the mother's condition permits, chemotherapy (including anthracyclines and taxanes) should be deferred during the first trimester and used to treat only life-threatening situations during the third trimester after extensive counseling with the parents.

The preservation of fertility is particularly challenging for women with newly diagnosed hematologic malignancies, breast cancer, sarcoma, and some pelvic cancers, for which combinations of alkylating agent chemotherapy, pelvic radiotherapy, and/or surgery are most likely to cause premature ovarian insufficiency. Options for the preservation of fertility include cryopreservation of embryos, mature oocytes, or ovarian tissue (Chapter 218).[15]

Geriatrics

An increasing proportion of cancers occur in an older population. The physiologic changes that develop with age (Chapter 23) include decreased excretion of drugs and metabolites from the kidneys, decreased volume of distribution of water-soluble drugs, and increased susceptibility to myelosuppression, cardiomyopathy, and neuropathy, related in part to comorbid conditions (Chapter 24). As a general rule, the suitability of an older patient for therapy can be determined by a comprehensive geriatric assessment (Chapter 23) that evaluates the patient's function, comorbidity, nutrition, medications, and resources. Age itself is not a barrier to surgery; rather, the patient's performance status and the comprehensive geriatric assessment should determine the likelihood of a good recovery. Tolerance of radiation therapy seems to remain largely intact with increasing age. Chemotherapy decisions are also based on performance status and the comprehensive geriatric assessment. Dosage adjustments are also made, when appropriate, for glomerular filtration rates for patients ages 65 years and older. The use of lower chemotherapy doses based on age alone is not advisable and may result in ineffective treatment.

Organ Dysfunction

Alterations in drug clearance (Chapter 25) play a critical role in the safe administration of anticancer agents. Alterations in pharmacokinetic parameters per se may occur with or without important changes in toxicity. Where evidence exists, chemotherapeutic drug doses must be modified in the setting of renal or hepatic dysfunction (see Table 164-2).

Immunocompromised Patients

The increasing proportion of patients who survive long-term after hematopoietic cell transplantation or with hematologic malignancies are at risk of complications related to their markedly compromised immune systems. Such patients are less likely to develop protective antibodies after vaccination, are more likely to have a variety of infections (Chapter 260), and tend to become sicker with their infections. For example, patients who have hematologic malignancies have significantly lower rates of seroconversion following vaccination against SARS-CoV-2 and have higher rates of hospital admission and mortality following SARS-CoV-2 infection than do patients who have solid tumors.[16]

Management of Complications

Supportive Care

Nutritional Support

Nutrition is always a concern for patients who are newly diagnosed with cancer, even if they have not experienced weight loss. Significant weight loss is an adverse prognostic factor for several cancers, especially lung cancer.

Malnourished patients should be evaluated by a dietitian to determine whether they are ingesting sufficient calories (Chapter 198) and whether dietary supplements might be needed. Some patients, such as patients with head and neck cancers (Chapter 176) or esophageal cancers (Chapter 178), may require parenteral nutrition through a percutaneous gastrostomy tube. Total parenteral nutrition (Chapter 198) is rarely indicated.

Patients are often concerned about whether their diet contributed to development of the cancer and whether diet can influence the results of therapy. In most settings, neither of these scenarios is the case. Larger-than-recommended doses of vitamins are also not helpful and may be toxic (Chapter 199). Current or contemplated use of over-the-counter and/or alternative medications (Chapter 30) must be determined because they can have potentially important interactions with chemotherapeutic agents.

Psychosocial Support

Patients with a recent cancer diagnosis have increased risks of death from cardiovascular causes, especially during the first week after diagnosis. The associated anxiety, depression, and fear experienced by many patients commonly require substantial ongoing psychosocial support, which may exceed what the immediate family can provide. In this setting, patients often benefit from participation in support groups or from direct one-on-one counseling, as well as from efforts to improve communication across all levels of care and support systems.

Hematopoietic Growth Factors

Growth factors, such as granulocyte colony-stimulating factor (G-CSF) and granulocyte-macrophage colony-stimulating factor (GM-CSF), speed the recovery of the white blood cell count, thereby often permitting chemotherapy to be given on schedule, without reducing the dosage (Chapter 142).[A3] However, such therapy does not decrease hospitalizations or improve survival. Consensus guidelines[17] can help determine which individuals are at greatest risk for febrile neutropenia (Chapter 153) and are more likely to benefit from pre-emptive treatment. Correction of anemia with erythropoiesis-stimulating agents (epoetin alfa and darbepoetin alfa) may be associated with complications of adverse cardiovascular events and even potentially tumor progression (Chapter 144).[18]

Prevention of Pathologic Bone Fractures

Bisphosphonates (e.g., pamidronate and zoledronate) are very effective not only for the treatment of tumor-induced hypercalcemia but also to reduce pathologic fractures in bones with metastatic lesions (Chapter 187), particularly from breast cancer (Chapter 183), prostate cancer (Chapter 186), and myeloma (Chapter 173). Bisphosphonates are also used to treat osteoporosis caused by chemotherapy-induced premature menopause in young women with breast cancer (Chapter 225). Denosumab (a human monoclonal antibody that binds to RANK ligand, which is a protein that is found on osteoclasts and is involved in bone breakdown) is superior to zoledronic acid for the prevention of skeletal-related events in cancer patients with bone metastases.[A4] Compared with placebo, adjuvant denosumab administered subcutaneously every 6 months reduces the risk of clinical fracture in postmenopausal women whose breast cancer is being treated with aromatase inhibitors, without any added toxicity.[A5]

Symptom Management

Effective management of symptoms is critical to successful delivery of either curative or palliative treatment and maintenance of a patient's quality of life.

Nausea and Vomiting

Patients continue to fear chemotherapy because of the risk of nausea and vomiting. Antiemetics (Table 118-5), typically used in combination,[19] have made this side effect much less debilitating. Chemotherapeutic drugs can be ranked according to their probability of causing nausea and vomiting, with prophylactic treatment given accordingly. The availability of the serotonin 5-hydroxytryptamine type 3 (5-HT_3) receptor antagonists (dolasetron, granisetron, ondansetron) has dramatically improved the ability to control nausea and vomiting completely. More emetogenic regimens require combination therapy with a corticosteroid (usually dexamethasone), a 5-HT_3 antagonist, and a benzodiazepine (e.g., lorazepam) or the neurokinin-1 receptor antagonist aprepitant. Aprepitant is particularly useful for the treatment/prevention of delayed nausea and vomiting. The combination of a neurokinin-1 receptor antagonist with dexamethasone and a 5-HT3 receptor antagonist is even better to control carboplatin-induced emesis.

Pain Control

Oncologists use a variety of scales to evaluate pain control (Chapter 26), which can be accomplished with a variety combination of analgesics, both non-narcotic and narcotic. Pharmacologic treatment should start with nonsteroidal anti-inflammatory drugs (NSAIDs) such as aspirin or acetaminophen, progress through ibuprofen and related drugs (see Table 26-4), and then through combinations of NSAIDs and narcotics (see Table 26-6) to stronger narcotics.[20] Newer narcotics are available in both short-duration and long-duration forms; some dermal patches provide benefit for 72 hours and are ideal for patients who have severe pain and who are unable to take oral medications. Oral transmucosal fentanyl is more effective than standard-release morphine in this setting. Painful oral mucositis, a common complication of intensive therapy for hematologic malignancies, can be treated with local measures or with recombinant human keratinocyte growth factor (Chapter 393). Oral anti-*Candida* drugs that are absorbed or partially absorbed from the gastrointestinal tract can help prevent pain from oral candidiasis (Chapter 310); both pharmacologic and psychosocial interventions (e.g., relaxation training, cognitive-behavioral therapy, and other education- and skills-based approaches) are complementary approaches that have real but relatively modest effects on both the severity of pain and its interference with daily activities.

Malignant Effusions

Accumulations of fluid and malignant cells in the pleural (Chapter 86), peritoneal, or pericardial spaces (Chapter 62) are common complications of epithelial and hematopoietic malignancies that frequently produce a significant array of symptoms, either at the time of diagnosis or accompanying tumor progression. Malignant pleural effusions (Chapter 86) are most commonly associated with cancers of the lung and breast or lymphomas, may be the result of lymphatic obstruction or direct invasion of pleural membranes, and can produce significant degrees of dyspnea, cough, or pain that require therapy. Diagnostic thoracentesis of sufficient volume (>60 mL), with cytologic analysis of the pleural effusion, has a reasonably high diagnostic yield for malignancy (60 to 90%). In patients with previously untreated lymphoma, breast cancer, or small cell lung cancer, objective response to the initiation of systemic chemotherapy may provide long-term symptomatic relief. However, in patients with recurrent lung or breast cancer, for example, pleural effusions that are confirmed to contain malignant cells may present difficult ongoing therapeutic challenges. For symptomatic patients, therapeutic thoracentesis, usually under ultrasound guidance, is required and may need to be repeated to reduce dyspnea. When frequent thoracenteses over short intervals are needed, drainage of the pleural space is combined with a chest thoracostomy and the instillation of a sclerosing compound (talc, doxycycline) that will initiate an inflammatory response of sufficient magnitude to obliterate the pleural space (Chapter 86). Such pleurodesis is usually at least temporarily successful in preventing fluid recurrence in most patients. When it is no longer successful, placement of an indwelling pleural catheter may provide long-term symptomatic relief of dyspnea.

Malignant ascites (peritoneal effusion) occurs most frequently in patients with intra-abdominal malignancies (gastric, ovarian, pancreatic, and primary peritoneal cancers) but also can be observed in patients with advanced breast and lung cancers or lymphoma. Malignant ascites may be caused in part by increased permeability of the tumor vasculature as a result of overexpression of vascular endothelial growth factor, by the overproduction of inflammatory cytokines in the peritoneal space, or by lymphatic blockade secondary to carcinomatosis. Ultrasound-guided paracentesis provides relief of bloating, dyspnea, and the pain of abdominal distension. However, paracentesis must be repeated, with an associated risk of dehydration, loss of protein, electrolyte imbalance, bleeding, infection, and kidney dysfunction. If paracentesis is required more often than once per week, prompt placement of a permanent catheter should be considered to allow self-drainage, even though these devices carry a significant risk of infection.

Malignant pericardial effusions (Chapter 62) are most commonly related to direct extension or metastatic spread from lung or breast cancers, melanomas, and hematologic malignancies. As is the case for other malignant effusions, image-guided pericardiocentesis with cytologic examination of the fluid that has been evacuated will frequently provide diagnostic confirmation of malignancy. Furthermore, the removal of even a relatively modest amount of fluid (<50 mL) may, at least partially, relieve the hemodynamic compromise produced by the effusion. The approach to a patient with malignant pericardial effusions is dictated by hemodynamic status (which can drive the choice between emergency pericardiocentesis or elective pericardiostomy) and by the predicted sensitivity of the inciting tumor to systemic therapy (e.g., untreated lymphoma versus chemotherapy-resistant lung cancer).

ENDOCRINE MANIFESTATIONS OF CANCER

Clinical syndromes associated with ectopic hormone production may pose special diagnostic dilemmas, can produce a significant degree of morbidity or even death in cancer patients, and may be difficult to treat (Table 164-5). Management of these syndromes involves the simultaneous treatment of both the cancer and the syndrome caused by excessive hormone production. Many of the endocrine manifestations of cancer[21] are caused by the production of small polypeptide hormones by tumors, some of which are derived from specific types of neuroendocrine cells. These cells are widely dispersed in a wide variety of organs, are often of neural crest origin, and can produce biogenic amines. The hormones produced from these tumors include adrenocorticotropic hormones (corticotropin, ACTH), calcitonin, vasoactive intestinal peptide, growth hormone–releasing hormone, corticotropin-releasing hormone (CRH), somatostatin, and other peptides. A second group of tumors, generally derived from squamous epithelium, produces parathyroid hormone–related proteins (PTHrP) and vasopressin.

TABLE 164-5 SOME CLINICAL SYNDROMES OF ECTOPIC HORMONE PRODUCTION

Humoral hypercalcemia
Parathyroid hormone–related protein
Squamous cell carcinoma
Breast cancer
Neuroendocrine tumors
Renal cell cancer
Melanoma
Prostate cancer
Increased calcitriol
Lymphoma
Benign conditions: sarcoid, berylliosis, tuberculosis, fungal infections
Corticotropin
Proopiomelanocortin
Small cell lung cancer
Pulmonary carcinoid
Medullary thyroid cancer
Islet cell tumor
Pheochromocytoma
Ganglioneuroma
Corticotropin-releasing hormone
Medullary thyroid cancer
Paraganglioma
Prostate cancer
Islet cell tumors
Human chorionic gonadotropin
Choriocarcinoma
Testicular embryonal cell carcinoma
Seminoma
Hypoglycemia
Insulinoma
Sarcomas or large retroperitoneal tumors
Inappropriate antidiuretic hormone secretion
Small cell lung cancer
Squamous cell head and neck cancer
Erythropoietin
Renal cell cancer
Hepatocellular carcinoma
Pheochromocytoma
Benign conditions: cerebellar hemangioblastoma, uterine fibroids

HYPERCALCEMIA OF MALIGNANCY

Humoral hypercalcemia (Chapter 227) is one of the most common endocrine syndromes related to an underlying malignancy. One of the most common causes of hypercalcemia of malignancy[22] is the ectopic production of parathyroid hormone–related protein, with resulting activation of the PTH receptor, an increase in the differentiation of osteoclasts, and increased bone resorption and consequent hypercalcemia. Ectopic parathyroid hormone–related protein (rather than PTH itself) can be produced by several different types of cancer, most characteristically squamous cell cancer, breast cancer, renal cell cancer, and prostate cancer, as well as by neuroendocrine tumors and melanoma (see Table 164-5). Increased production of calcitriol, which increases the absorption of calcium and suppresses levels of serum PTH, is another cause of malignant hypercalcemia, most commonly in patients with lymphoma. Bone metastases (Chapter 187), particularly in patients with breast cancer and myeloma, may produce hypercalcemia due to increased local production of PTHrP or other cytokines that increase bone resorption.

TREATMENT

The treatment of malignant hypercalcemia is similar to hypercalcemia that is caused by hyperparathyroidism (Chapter 227). The reversal of dehydration and the initiation of a saline diuresis should begin promptly; patients with a serum calcium in excess of 13 mg/dL should be treated with a bisphosphonate initially, with extended use of the bisphosphonate for the prevention of bone fractures and recurrence of hypercalcemia (Chapter 227).

OTHER ECTOPIC HORMONE SYNDROMES

Inappropriate secretion of ACTH is rare but resembles pituitary Cushing disease (Chapter 208). Tumors that produce corticotropin-releasing hormone include medullary thyroid cancer, prostate cancer, and islet cell neoplasms. Ectopic ACTH syndrome may manifest as classic Cushing syndrome, with easy bruisability, centripetal obesity, muscle wasting, hypertension, diabetes, and metabolic alkalosis. However, many patients with ectopic ACTH-producing cancers progress too quickly to develop prominent cushingoid manifestations clinically. Profound hypokalemia may predominate without the classic features of Cushing syndrome in patients with small cell lung cancer (Chapter 177).

Tumor-associated hypoglycemia (Chapter 211), although uncommon, may be the result of the overproduction of insulin by islet cell tumors; insufficient hepatic gluconeogenesis related to loss of functional hepatic mass by metastatic disease; or overexpression of insulin-like growth factor II, which can activate the insulin receptor in patients who have large retroperitoneal sarcomas or hepatocellular carcinomas. In each of these cases, treatment with frequent small feedings can be prescribed; however, successful symptomatic management of hypoglycemia may be difficult without control of the primary tumor mass or metastases.

The clinical syndrome of inappropriate secretion of antidiuretic hormone (Chapter 102) is caused by ectopic production of vasopressin, primarily in patients who have small cell lung cancer (Chapter 177) or squamous cancers of the head and neck (Chapter 176), and occasionally in patients with primary brain tumors (Chapter 175). This syndrome is characterized by hyponatremia, hypo-osmolality, excessive urine sodium excretion, and an inappropriately high urine osmolality for the low serum osmolality despite normal kidney, adrenal, and thyroid function. The hyponatremia in this condition is euvolemic. Fluid (free water) restriction can provide adequate short-term management of symptomatic hyponatremia, but treatment with demeclocycline, which blocks the effects of vasopressin on the kidney, provides more effective long-term therapy (Chapter 102).

PARANEOPLASTIC SYNDROMES

The term *paraneoplasia*, which means "alongside cancer," has been commonly used to denote a cancer's remote effects that cannot be attributed either to direct invasion or to distant metastases. These syndromes (Table 164-6)[23] affect up to 15% of patients with cancer; if patients with cachexia are excluded, however, the incidence probably drops to only a few percent.

Up to two thirds of paraneoplastic syndromes arise before an associated malignancy is diagnosed. In some cases, the paraneoplastic syndrome may be associated with relatively small tumors, and recognition of these associations may lead to earlier diagnosis and possibly more effective therapy. Furthermore, one of the hallmarks in defining a paraneoplastic syndrome is that the course of the syndrome generally parallels the course of the tumor. As a result, effective treatment of the underlying malignancy is often accompanied by improvement or resolution of the syndrome. Conversely, recurrence of the cancer may be heralded by the return of systemic symptoms.

TABLE 164-6 EVALUATION AND DIAGNOSIS OF PARANEOPLASTIC SYNDROMES

Characterize abnormality; obtain laboratory studies and biopsy as necessary
Carefully elicit any additional symptoms and signs
Eliminate common causes
If there is no obvious etiology, consider a paraneoplastic syndrome
If findings are consistent with a known syndrome, screen for underlying malignancy
If signs and symptoms are consistent with a known paraneoplastic syndrome, undertake a search for an unknown primary cancer or recurrence or progression of a known primary tumor
Screening should include a careful physical examination including breast, gynecologic, and prostate evaluations; basic hematology, chemistry, and urine studies; chest radiograph; and mammogram
Computed tomography (CT) of the abdomen and pelvis or positron emission tomography (PET) scan is indicated if there are any suspicious symptoms, signs, or laboratory abnormalities of cancer
Antibody testing for paraneoplastic neurologic syndromes and/or skin biopsy should be performed as indicated
Consider treatment of cancer and/or appropriate palliative treatment, including immunosuppressive therapy for paraneoplastic symptoms when possible

NEUROLOGIC PARANEOPLASTIC SYNDROMES

A variety of neurologic paraneoplastic syndromes[24] can complicate many different cancers, with small cell lung cancer (Chapter 177) being an especially common cause (Table 164-7). Lambert-Eaton myasthenic syndrome (Chapter 390) mimics myasthenia gravis clinically, with the exception that strength improves rather than deteriorates with sustained voluntary contraction. Paraneoplastic encephalitis, subacute sensory neuropathies (Chapter 388), and sensory ganglionopathies are also commonly associated with small cell lung cancer. Symptoms often include asymmetric numbness and paresthesias, as well as posterior column signs of loss of proprioception and vibratory sensation. Paraneoplastic cerebellar degeneration may be acute-onset and can mimic a cerebellar tumor (Chapter 175). Plasma cell dyscrasia and some lymphoproliferative neoplasms are associated with demyelinating peripheral neuropathies and with motor neuron symptoms that may mimic amyotrophic lateral sclerosis (Chapter 387). Polymyositis and dermatomyositis (Chapter 248) can be associated with a variety of tumors.

Paraneoplastic neurologic syndromes are more common with advanced tumors and are uncommonly the initial presenting manifestation, except perhaps with small cell cancers of the lung, plasma cell dyscrasias, and other

TABLE 164-7 PARANEOPLASTIC NEUROLOGIC SYNDROMES

NEUROLOGIC SYNDROME	CLINICAL MANIFESTATIONS	DIAGNOSIS	ANTIBODY AND ASSOCIATED MALIGNANCY
Lambert-Eaton myasthenic syndrome (Chapter 390)	Proximal lower limb weakness, with improvement in strength after several seconds of sustained voluntary contraction	Electromyogram showing *increased* muscle action potential with repeated nerve stimulation >10 Hz (opposite of myasthenia gravis)	Anti-VGCC or anti-SOX1 in small cell lung cancer (>80%)
Paraneoplastic encephalomyelitis/subacute sensory neuropathy (Chapter 383)	Subacute patchy or asymmetrical numbness, burning or aching paresthesias, and sensory ataxia with loss of proprioception and vibration sense	Clinical diagnosis supported by circulating antibodies and elevated cerebrospinal fluid protein levels with a lymphocytosis	Usually anti-Hu in small cell lung cancer; others include anti-SOX1 and anti-amphiphysin (small cell lung cancer, neuroblastoma), anti-Ma (small cell lung cancer, breast cancer), and anti-Trk (various carcinomas and lymphomas)
Paraneoplastic cerebellar degeneration	Often abrupt onset of dysarthria, ataxia, and oculomotor dysfunction	Clinical diagnosis supported by the presence of circulating antibodies, which also can be found in patients who have a variety of cerebellar disorders but no evidence of cancer; cerebrospinal fluid pleocytosis and elevated protein levels	Anti-Yo, anti-SOX1, or anti-Ri (breast, ovarian, and other gynecologic malignancies); anti-Hu (breast cancer); anti-Tr and anti-GluR (small cell lung cancer); and anti-Ma (Hodgkin lymphoma, various carcinomas)
Limbic encephalopathy (Chapter 383)	Subacute amnestic syndrome, affective disorder, seizures	Improvement common with treatment of underlying tumor	Anti-Hu, anti-amphiphysin, anti-SOX1, anti-VGKC, and anti-AMPA (small cell lung cancer); anti-Ta (testicular and breast cancers)
Stiff-person syndrome (Chapter 380)	Progressive muscle stiffness and rigidity, with intermittent and painful muscle spasms	Electromyogram showing continuous firing of motor unit potentials; may respond to muscle relaxants and improve with cancer therapy	Anti-amphiphysin (breast and small cell lung cancers) and anti-GAD (breast cancer)
Neuromyotonia (Chapter 390)	Diffuse muscle stiffness and cramps	Responds to treatment of tumor and immunosuppression	Anti-VGCC (thymoma)
Demyelinating neuropathies (including chronic demyelinating polyneuropathy, mononeuritis multiplex; Chapter 388)	Sensory more common than motor	IgM paraprotein may cross-react with myelin-associated glycoprotein, cryoglobulins	Plasma cell and lymphoproliferative neoplasms, osteosclerotic myeloma, POEMS, small cell lung cancer, other carcinomas
Necrotizing myelopathy	Symptoms associated with specific levels of spinal cord dysfunction; rapid deterioration and death		Variety of carcinomas and lymphomas
Motor neuron disease (Chapter 387)	Similar to amyotrophic lateral sclerosis with progressive weakness	Paraproteinemia	Plasma cell and lymphoproliferative neoplasms
Polymyositis/dermatomyositis (Chapter 248)	Proximal muscle weakness, skin lesions (Chapter 248)	May improve with treatment of cancer	Variety of carcinomas

AMPA = α-amino-3-hydroxy-5-methyl-4-isoxazolepropionic acid; GAD = glutamic acid decarboxylase; GluR = glutamate receptor; IgM = immunoglobulin M; POEMS = polyneuropathy, organomegaly, endocrinopathy, monoclonal protein, and skin changes associated with osteosclerotic myeloma; VGCC = voltage-gated calcium channel; VGKC = voltage-gated potassium channel.

lymphoproliferative diseases. Paraneoplastic neurologic syndromes may show some response to effective treatment of the tumor, but they can also progress despite such therapy.

DERMATOLOGIC PARANEOPLASTIC SYNDROMES

Associations between cutaneous syndromes and underlying malignancies may be difficult to confirm. Generally, the skin condition and cancer follow a parallel course, and the two diagnoses should be made at about the same time. Some skin lesions are almost always associated with malignancy. Others, however, are nonspecific and are most commonly seen with nonmalignant conditions, thereby making it difficult or impossible to connect the skin disease with the underlying malignancy. In addition, biopsies of the skin lesion are usually nonspecific and show features identical to what are seen when the same lesion occurs without a malignant condition. The formation of tumor-related autoantibodies has rarely been associated with dermatologic paraneoplastic syndromes, although inflammatory cell infiltration may be seen.

Recognition of cutaneous manifestations of malignancy can be critical for the early diagnosis and successful treatment of cancer,[25] but some syndromes are seen only with advanced, incurable disease. Cutaneous manifestations include direct involvement of the skin with tumor as well as the remote effects of cancer. Both specific and nonspecific dermatologic adverse effects are also seen with cytotoxic chemotherapeutic agents, including alkylating agents, antimetabolites, anthracyclines, tyrosine kinase inhibitors, and immunotherapies.

One of the best-known paraneoplastic syndromes is acanthosis nigricans (Chapter 408 and Fig. 408-14), the pathogenesis of which is unclear. The tumor may produce factors that activate insulin-like growth factors or the insulin receptor in skin. Many tumors are known to produce transforming growth factor-α (TGF-α), which might activate epidermal growth factor receptors in the skin, causing hyperpigmentation and thickening. The skin lesions arise as velvety, verrucous hyperpigmentation of the neck, axilla, groin, and mucosal membranes, including the lips, periocular area, and anus. Although acanthosis nigricans clearly occurs as a benign entity associated with obesity and endocrinopathy, its appearance in older adults, especially when it includes mucosal lesions, is highly associated with malignancies of the gastrointestinal tract as well as with other adenocarcinomas. The lesions often regress with successful treatment of the underlying tumor.

RHEUMATOLOGIC PARANEOPLASTIC SYNDROMES

The possibility of an underlying occult malignancy should be considered[26] in patients who have rheumatic disorders with an atypical clinical presentation, particularly older patients, patients who have coexisting systemic symptoms, and patients who respond unexpectedly poorly to usual antirheumatic treatments. Chemotherapeutic agents can also cause rheumatic adverse effects.

One of the more common and specific rheumatologic paraneoplastic syndromes is hypertrophic osteoarthropathy,[27] which arises as an oligoarthritis or polyarthritis of the distal joints, with clubbing (Fig. 39-9), tender periostitis of the distal long bones, and noninflammatory synovial effusions (also see Chapter 254). Hypertrophic osteoarthropathy may affect up to 10% of patients with adenocarcinoma of the lung and is also seen with a variety of other pulmonary malignancies, including lung metastases from other primary sites. The etiology is unknown. Laboratory studies often reveal an elevation in the erythrocyte sedimentation rate; bone radiographs show linear ossification of the distal long bones separated by a radiolucent zone from the underlying cortex (Fig. 164-1).

TREATMENT

Treatment is symptomatic with anti-inflammatory agents. Successful treatment of the underlying tumor may also improve the signs and symptoms of this syndrome.

RENAL AND HEPATIC PARANEOPLASTIC SYNDROMES

The most common renal paraneoplastic syndrome is membranous glomerulonephritis, which can include nephrotic-range proteinuria, edema, hypertension, hypoalbuminemia, and microscopic hematuria (Chapter 100). The most common associated cancers include adenocarcinoma of the lung (Chapter 177), breast cancers (Chapter 183), and gastric adenocarcinomas (Chapter 178). Lymphoproliferative disorders, especially Hodgkin disease (Chapter

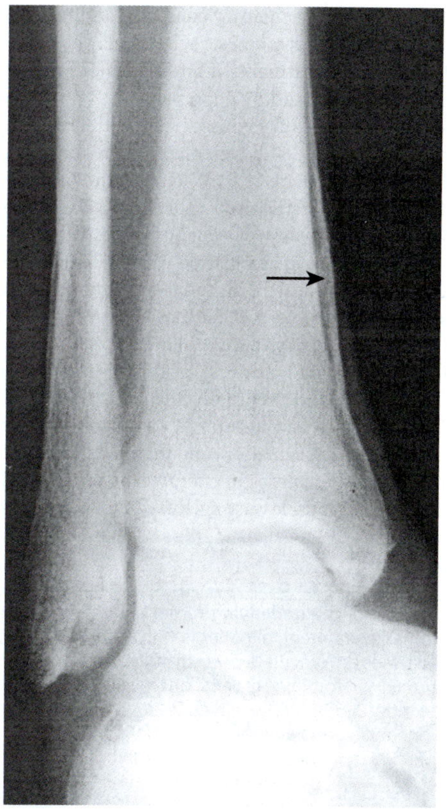

FIGURE 164-1. Hypertrophic pulmonary osteoarthropathy characterized by periosteal elevation of the tibia (*arrow*). (Courtesy Dr. Lynne S. Steinbach.)

172), can cause minimal-change nephropathy. Renal microangiopathy can be seen with cryoglobulinemia associated with hepatitis C–related hepatocellular carcinoma (Chapter 181). Paraneoplastic hepatopathy with elevated liver enzymes and abnormal synthetic function can be seen with renal cell cancer (Chapter 182) without evidence of direct hepatic involvement by the tumor.

HEMATOLOGIC PARANEOPLASTIC SYNDROMES

The most common immunologic paraneoplastic syndrome is thrombosis (Chapters 67 and 68). Some patients have hemorrhagic paraneoplastic syndromes, especially disseminated intravascular coagulation (Chapter 161), that can be seen in nearly all patients with acute promyelocytic leukemia (Chapter 168). Acquired von Willebrand disease (Chapter 159) may be seen in rare cases of lymphoproliferative and myeloproliferative disorders, and increased fibrinolysis can occur in patients with advanced prostate cancer (Chapter 186).

Anemia of chronic disease (Chapter 144) is a common finding in cancers of all types. Pure red cell aplasia (Chapter 151) is a rare condition associated with benign or malignant thymomas (Chapters 86 and 390).

Paraneoplastic hemolytic anemia (Chapter 147) can be seen with warm- or cold-reacting antibodies, especially in patients with chronic lymphocytic leukemia (Chapter 169). Microangiopathic hemolytic anemia (Chapter 147) with thrombocytopenia is a common complication of a variety of adenocarcinomas. Erythrocytosis is seen in tumors that produce erythropoietin, including renal cell cancers (Chapter 182), hepatocellular carcinomas (Chapter 181), and cerebellar hemangioblastomas (Chapter 175).

Patients with advanced cancer can develop leukocytosis caused by cytokines in the absence of infection. Eosinophilia (Chapter 156) can be seen with lymphoproliferative diseases, including Hodgkin disease. Paraneoplastic thrombocytosis (Chapter 152) is caused by tumors that produce interleukin-6 or thrombopoietin.

FEVER AND CACHEXIA

Fever (Chapter 260), night sweats, and cachexia are nonspecific symptoms that, when seen in the absence of infection or a known disorder, suggest the diagnosis of an underlying malignancy. Cytokines clearly play a pathogenetic role in inducing both fever and cachexia. TNF-α, interleukins (particularly IL-1 and IL-6), and interferon-γ, which result in a catabolic state, are produced directly by the tumor or by tumor-associated host inflammatory cells, such as macrophages. Cytokines may produce fever directly by acting at the level of the hypothalamic thermoregulatory center. In addition to the burden of tumor and the production of cytokines, cachexia may be caused or worsened by the side effects of cancer treatment, by intestinal blockage or malabsorption caused by tumor infiltration, and by depression.

Fever is generally cyclic and may be associated with drenching night sweats. Symptoms resolve with successful treatment of the underlying tumor, and return of fever usually heralds relapse. When treatment of the tumor is not possible or is ineffective, NSAIDs (see Table 26-4) or corticosteroids given around the clock significantly improve quality of life. Although cancer-related fever is most commonly seen in association with malignant lymphoproliferative disease (Chapters 171 and 172), renal cell carcinoma (Chapter 182), and leukemias (Chapters 168 to 170), it may also occur with other cancers, particularly in the face of extensive hepatic metastases.

Cachexia, or cancer wasting syndrome, is probably the single most common paraneoplastic syndrome and eventually affects up to 80% of patients with cancer. Cachexia appears to be caused by a combination of protein wasting, malabsorption, immune dysregulation, and increased glucose turnover in the setting of tumor-induced increases in energy expenditure. This syndrome is characterized by anorexia, muscle wasting, loss of subcutaneous fat, and fatigue.

TREATMENT

Successful treatment of the underlying tumor reverses the process. By comparison symptomatic treatment for patients with advanced disease is modestly successful at best. Megestrol acetate given in high concentrations in liquid form (400 to 800 mg/day) can improve appetite and result in weight gain, but at the cost of fluid retention. Anamorelin, which is an oral ghrelin-receptor agonist with appetite-enhancing and anabolic activity (100 mg orally once daily), provides a favorable clinical response, including a significant increase in lean body mass.[A6,A7]

TUMOR LYSIS SYNDROME

Tumor lysis syndrome can be a major complication of the rapid response of hematologic malignancies and occasionally solid tumors to successful chemotherapy.[28] The sudden release of cellular contents (especially potassium, phosphate, and nucleic acids) can lead to deposition of uric acid and calcium phosphate in renal tubules. Clinical manifestations can include renal failure, seizures, and cardiac arrhythmias. Laboratory findings include elevated serum levels of uric acid, potassium, and phosphorus, with a decreased calcium level.

TREATMENT AND PROGNOSIS

The risks of complications from tumor lysis syndrome can be reduced by vigorous hydration and the prophylactic administration of allopurinol (300 mg daily), started at least 24 hours before chemotherapy and continued until uric acid levels normalize (Chapter 252). Another option is the therapeutic use of rasburicase (0.15 mg/kg intravenously, usually once, but it can be given daily for up to 5 days if needed).[29]

CANCER OF UNKNOWN PRIMARY ORIGIN

Some cancers present with biopsy-confirmed visceral or nodal metastases in the absence of an obvious primary lesion. Subsequent clinical evaluation, with a comprehensive history, physical examination, complete blood cell count, screening chemistries, chest and abdominal CT scans, and other radiologic studies directed by specific symptoms or signs can often identify the primary tumor site and clarify the extent of metastatic disease. When a primary tumor cannot be located despite such a clinical evaluation, the patient is classified as having *cancer of unknown primary origin*. Additional clinical, pathologic, and genetic evaluation can sometimes identify the primary site, but in up to 90% of patients a primary site may never be identified throughout their subsequent clinical course.

In patients whose primary cancer site remains undetectable, the primary site has presumably remained small or, less likely, regressed spontaneously. Approximately 4% of all cancer patients have metastatic disease without a known primary site, and autopsies identify a primary site in only about 50% to 70% of these patients. Cancer of unknown primary site increases with advancing age, but it occurs with about equal frequency in men and women.

DIAGNOSIS

The initial clinical, radiographic, and pathologic evaluations should focus not only on identifying a primary site but also on trying to identify tumors for which specific treatments may be most beneficial.

Biopsy and Pathologic Evaluation

The diagnosis of metastatic cancer should first be confirmed by biopsy of the most easily accessible lesion. A fine-needle aspiration is often adequate to confirm the diagnosis of cancer, but it will not provide adequate material for optimum pathologic evaluation. A larger surgical or core needle biopsy should be performed if technically feasible.

In about 60% of patients with cancer of unknown primary site, the initial microscopy will identify an adenocarcinoma. Other common light microscopy findings include poorly differentiated carcinoma (25%), squamous cell carcinoma (10%), and poorly differentiated neoplasm (inability to distinguish among carcinoma, lymphoma, sarcoma, and melanoma; 5%).

For poorly differentiated tumors, additional pathologic evaluation is required. An immunohistochemical stain usually can determine the lineage (e.g., carcinoma vs. lymphoma vs. sarcoma) of a "poorly differentiated neoplasm," and it sometimes can identify germ cell tumors or neuroendocrine carcinoma. More than 50% of such patients will have a lymphoma, for which treatment can be highly effective.

In patients with adenocarcinoma, immunohistochemical stains can narrow the diagnostic spectrum, particularly when interpreted in conjunction with clinical features. In several situations, immunohistochemical stains are quite specific, including prostate-specific antigen (PSA) for prostate cancer (Chapter 186), estrogen and progesterone receptors for breast cancer (Chapter 183), and leukocyte common antigen for non-Hodgkin lymphoma (Chapter 171). Other diagnoses suggested by immunoperoxidase staining include melanomas (Chapter 188), sarcomas (Chapter 187), and neuroendocrine tumors. Occasionally, electron microscopy or analysis for tumor-specific chromosomal abnormalities (i12p in germ cell tumors, Chapter 185; t11 : 22 in Ewing tumor; immunoglobulin gene rearrangements in non-Hodgkin lymphoma, Chapter 171) are useful in the evaluation of poorly differentiated tumors if results of other pathologic studies are inconclusive.

Since cancers usually retain gene expression profiles that are similar or even identical to their tissue of origin, modern molecular profiling can correctly predict the origin of more than 90% of metastatic cancers by finding such tissue-specific gene expression patterns.[30] Although the accuracy of genetic profiling is uncertain in patients with cancer of unknown primary origin, in part because most primaries never become manifest, current data suggest a similarly high accuracy rate. As a result, molecular tumor profiling is now a routine complement to pathologic evaluation and is indicated whenever a tissue of origin is not definitive on histologic examination.

Search for the Primary Site

After completion of the brief and focused evaluation needed to make the initial diagnosis of cancer of unknown primary origin, any additional diagnostic studies should be carefully targeted (Table 164-8). The value of positron emission tomography (PET) in identifying a primary site is unclear because it has not been shown to provide increased information above and beyond CT scanning.[31] Other routine radiologic and endoscopic evaluations of asymptomatic areas are rarely helpful for identifying a primary site and, as a result, are not recommended. Levels of serum tumor markers, including carcinoembryonic antigen, CA-125, CA-19-9, and CA-15-3, are frequently elevated in patients with carcinoma of unknown primary site, but such elevations are nonspecific and are not useful for inferring a primary site. They can, however, be useful to monitor a patient's response to treatment.

Specific clinical findings warrant additional diagnostic evaluation. In all men with metastatic adenocarcinoma, a serum PSA level should be measured. Mammography and breast MRI are routine components of the evaluation of women with metastatic adenocarcinoma, particularly if clinical features are consistent with metastatic breast cancer (e.g., axillary node involvement, pleural effusion, lytic or blastic bone metastases). In patients who are younger than age 50 years and who have poorly differentiated carcinoma, serum human chorionic gonadotropin and α-fetoprotein (AFP) levels are indicated to screen for germ cell tumors. If metastatic squamous carcinoma involves cervical lymph nodes, a thorough endoscopic head and neck evaluation, from the nasopharynx to the larynx, and biopsy of any suspicious areas are indicated (Chapter 176). In patients who have low cervical adenopathy but no identifiable primary site in the head or neck on endoscopic examination, fiberoptic bronchoscopy should also be considered. In patients with metastatic squamous carcinoma involving inguinal lymph nodes, all perineal structures should be carefully inspected, including by anoscopy, a urologic evaluation, and a pelvic examination in women.

TABLE 164-8 CANCER OF UNKNOWN PRIMARY ORIGIN: RECOMMENDED EVALUATION AFTER INITIAL LIGHT MICROSCOPIC DIAGNOSIS

DIAGNOSIS	CLINICAL EVALUATION*	SPECIAL PATHOLOGIC STUDIES
Adenocarcinoma (or poorly differentiated adenocarcinoma)	PET CT of the chest and abdomen Men: serum PSA Women: mammography, breast MRI Colonoscopy (patients with colon cancer "profile") Additional directed radiologic or endoscopic studies to evaluate abnormal symptoms, signs, laboratory values	Men: PSA stain Women: estrogen and progesterone receptor stains (if clinical features suggest metastatic breast cancer) Molecular tumor profiling
Poorly differentiated carcinoma	PET CT of the chest and abdomen Serum hCG and AFP Additional directed radiologic or endoscopic studies to evaluate abnormal symptoms, signs, and laboratory values	Immunoperoxidase staining Molecular tumor profiling Electron microscopy (if other studies are indeterminate or conflicting)
SCC, cervical nodes	PET Direct laryngoscopy with visualization; biopsy of the nasopharynx, pharynx, hypopharynx, and larynx Fiberoptic bronchoscopy (if laryngoscopy results are negative)	—
SCC, inguinal nodes	PET Complete examination of perineal area (including pelvic examination) Anoscopy Cystoscopy	—

*In addition to a history, physical examination, complete blood cell counts, chemistry profile, and chest radiograph.

AFP = α-fetoprotein; CT = computed tomography; hCG = human chorionic gonadotropin; MRI = magnetic resonance imaging; PET = positron emission tomography; PSA = prostate-specific antigen; SCC = squamous cell carcinoma.

From Hainsworth J, Greco FA. Approach to the patient with cancer. In: Goldman L, Schafer AI, eds. *Cecil Medicine*, 25th ed. Philadelphia: Elsevier; 2015.

TREATMENT AND PROGNOSIS

Site-Specific Therapy Directed by Molecular Tumor Profiling

Site-specific treatment of metastatic tumors, as characterized by their molecular profiling,[32] is the standard treatment (Table 164-9), and empiric chemotherapy should be reserved for the minority of patients whose tumors cannot be classified by molecular profiling. In general, the response to treatment and subsequent survival are consistent with the predicted types of cancer, and median survival is at least twice as long for patients who have more responsive tumors. Targeted treatment results in a median survival of 12.5 months, but some patients remain progression-free for more than 5 years.[A8]

Adenocarcinoma

Women with Axillary Lymph Node Metastases

Metastatic breast cancer should be suspected in any woman who has axillary lymph node involvement with adenocarcinoma, particularly if an alternative metastatic site is not evident. In these patients, pathologic evaluation of the initial lymph node biopsy should include staining for estrogen and progesterone receptors and for *HER-2* expression; elevated levels strongly suggest the diagnosis of breast cancer.

When no other metastases are identified, these women should be treated as if they had stage II breast cancer, which is potentially curable with appropriate therapy (Chapter 183). Modified radical mastectomy identifies a breast primary site in about 45 to 80% of women, even when the breast examination and mammographic findings are normal. Axillary lymph node dissection followed by radiation therapy to the breast appears to give results similar to those of mastectomy, although these two options for primary therapy have not been compared directly. Adjuvant systemic therapy should follow standard guidelines for treating women with stage II breast cancer.

Women with Peritoneal Carcinomatosis

Adenocarcinoma involving the peritoneum in women usually originates from the ovary (Chapter 184), although carcinomas arising in the gastrointestinal tract or breast can occasionally produce this syndrome. Diffuse peritoneal carcinomatosis can occasionally occur in women who have histologically normal ovaries or who have had previous bilateral oophorectomy. The peritoneum is frequently the only site of tumor involvement, and serum CA-125 levels are usually elevated. When histologic features suggest ovarian cancer, this syndrome has been called *peritoneal papillary serous carcinoma* or *primary extraovarian serous carcinoma*.

Even when the histologic features are not typical, women with adenocarcinoma of unknown primary site involving the peritoneum often have cancers that are biologically similar to ovarian cancer (Chapter 184). In such patients, treatment should follow guidelines for stage III ovarian cancer. A full laparotomy with maximal surgical cytoreduction should be performed when feasible, and it should be followed by combination chemotherapy with a taxane/platinum-containing regimen. Serial measurement of serum CA-125 levels can accurately assess the efficacy of treatment. Some patients may have complete responses and long-term survival, particularly when initial surgical cytoreduction leaves minimal residual disease. A similar syndrome of peritoneal carcinomatosis that is responsive to chemotherapy for ovarian cancer has rarely been reported in men.

Men with Skeletal Metastases or Elevated Serum Prostate-Specific Antigen Levels

Metastatic prostate cancer (Chapter 186) should be suspected in men who have an adenocarcinoma that predominantly involves bone, particularly if the metastases are blastic. An elevated serum PSA level or PSA tumor immunostaining confirms the diagnosis of prostate cancer. Occasionally, men who have adenocarcinoma of unknown primary site and metastatic patterns that are unusual for prostate cancer (e.g., lung metastases, mediastinal lymph node metastases) nevertheless have elevated serum PSA levels. Such patients should be treated according to guidelines for advanced prostate cancer. Androgen ablation produces excellent responses and substantial palliation in most patients.

Single Metastatic Lesion

Occasionally, a single metastatic lesion containing adenocarcinoma or poorly differentiated carcinoma is identified, and a complete evaluation reveals absolutely no other evidence of disease. Such single lesions may be a single lymph node, a subcutaneous site, or visceral lesions in liver, lung, bone, brain, or adrenal gland. One possibility is that an unusual primary tumor is mimicking a metastatic lesion (e.g., a subcutaneous nodule from a primary apocrine or sebaceous carcinoma rather than a metastasis). This possibility can usually be excluded on clinical or pathologic grounds, and PET scanning is useful to exclude other metastatic lesions.

In patients who have only a single identifiable lesion, definitive local therapy is recommended. Based on the site of the tumor, such therapy may include surgical resection, radiation therapy, or both. Although most such patients eventually have other evidence of metastatic disease, local treatment can provide substantial palliation, and some patients experience a significant disease-free period. The role of adding systemic chemotherapy to definitive local therapy is uncertain, but younger patients who have poorly differentiated carcinoma or adenocarcinoma are often treated with a short course of a taxane/platinum-based regimen.

Colon Cancer Profile

In a patient who has cancer of unknown primary origin, a colon cancer profile includes metastases seen predominantly in the liver, peritoneum, or both; an adenocarcinoma that has histologic features typical of gastrointestinal origin; and typical immunohistochemical staining (CK20 positive, CK7 negative, and CDX-2 positive). Patients who have such a profile should be treated according to guidelines for metastatic colorectal cancer (Chapter 179).

TABLE 164-9 CANCER OF UNKNOWN PRIMARY ORIGIN: SPECIFIC PATIENT SUBSETS AND RECOMMENDED TREATMENT

SUBSET-IDENTIFYING FEATURES		
HISTOLOGIC	**CLINICAL**	**TREATMENT RECOMMENDATIONS**
Adenocarcinoma	Women, isolated axillary adenopathy	Treat as stage II breast cancer
Adenocarcinoma, poorly differentiated carcinoma	Women, peritoneal carcinomatosis (occasionally men?)	Treat as stage III ovarian cancer
Adenocarcinoma	Men, elevated PSA or blastic bone metastases	Treat as advanced prostate cancer
Adenocarcinoma, poorly differentiated carcinoma	Single metastatic lesion	Definitive local therapy (resection or radiation therapy [or both]) with or without chemotherapy
Adenocarcinoma	Colon cancer profile	Treat as metastatic colorectal cancer
Squamous cell carcinoma	Cervical adenopathy	Treat as locally advanced head or neck cancer
Squamous cell carcinoma	Inguinal adenopathy	Definitive local therapy (node dissection with or without radiation therapy) with or without chemotherapy
Poorly differentiated carcinoma	Young men with midline tumor or elevated hCG or AFP	Treat as extragonadal germ cell tumor
Neuroendocrine carcinoma, poorly differentiated	Diverse clinical presentations	Treat as advanced stage small cell lung cancer
Neuroendocrine carcinoma, well differentiated	Usually liver metastases	Treat as metastatic carcinoid tumor

AFP = α-fetoprotein; hCG = human chorionic gonadotropin; PSA = prostate-specific antigen.
From Hainsworth J, Greco FA. Approach to the patient with cancer. In: Goldman L, Schafer AI, eds. *Cecil Medicine*, 25th ed. Philadelphia: Elsevier; 2015.

Squamous Cell Carcinoma

Squamous cell carcinoma of unknown primary site is relatively uncommon. Most patients are middle aged or elderly with a long history of substantial use of alcohol or tobacco or both.

Cervical Adenopathy

When the cervical lymph nodes, especially in the upper or midcervical area, are involved with squamous cell carcinoma, a primary site should be suspected in the head and neck region (Chapter 176). Nevertheless, a complete endoscopic evaluation will not identify a primary tumor in about 15% of such patients. When the endoscopic evaluation is negative, PET scanning can identify a primary head and neck lesion in about 25% of such patients, so it should be part of the initial evaluation.

In patients with a squamous cell carcinoma of unknown primary site, concurrent chemotherapy and radiation therapy are recommended as for locally advanced squamous cell carcinoma arising in the head and neck.[33] Combined modality therapy results in 50 to 60% 5-year disease-free survival rates. A node larger than 2 cm and the presence of multiple involved lymph nodes are adverse prognostic features (Chapter 176).

Inguinal Adenopathy

Metastatic squamous cell cancer occasionally can be found in an inguinal lymph node. In most such cases the primary site can be identified in the perineal or anorectal area. For the occasional patient in whom no primary site is identified, local therapy with inguinal lymph node dissection, with or without radiation therapy, can result in long-term survival. Combined-modality treatment with concurrent chemotherapy and radiation therapy has improved survival and even led to cure in patients with several types of squamous cell carcinomas that originate in this region (e.g., cervix, anus, bladder). Although data are incomplete, a reasonable approach is the addition of chemotherapy with a platinum–5-fluorouracil regimen, as used for locally advanced carcinoma of the cervix (Chapter 184).

Poorly Differentiated Carcinoma

Extragonadal Germ Cell Cancer Syndrome

Young men who have clinical features suggestive of extragonadal germ cell tumors, such as tumors that are located in the mediastinum or retroperitoneum or tumors that are associated with elevated serum levels of human chorionic gonadotropin (hCG) or alpha fetoprotein, should be treated according to guidelines for extragonadal germ cell tumors (Chapter 185). Some of these patients can be proven to have germ cell tumors by identifying an i12p chromosomal abnormality even when the diagnosis is not possible with other standard pathologic techniques. Approximately 30 to 40% of such patients achieve complete responses and long-term survival after chemotherapy with cisplatin, etoposide, and bleomycin as used for advanced germ cell tumors.

Anaplastic Lymphoma

An appropriate initial pathologic evaluation should identify most histologically atypical lymphomas. Occasionally, immunohistochemical staining for leukocyte common antigen is negative or cannot be adequately performed in patients with anaplastic lymphoma. In some of these patients, the type of tumor can be identified using other immunohistochemical stains (e.g., Ki-1, CD-30), molecular genetic analysis (detection of immunoglobulin gene rearrangements), or molecular tumor profiling. All patients whose lymphomas are identified by special pathologic studies should be treated using standard guidelines for aggressive non-Hodgkin lymphoma (Chapter 171).

Neuroendocrine Carcinoma

In approximately 10% of poorly differentiated carcinomas, neuroendocrine features are identified by either immunohistochemical staining or electron microscopy. Treatment of these patients is as described for neuroendocrine carcinoma (see later).

Other Poorly Differentiated Carcinomas

Most patients with poorly differentiated carcinoma have no clinical or pathologic features that can be used to identify a specific treatment. Such patients have a poor prognosis, similar to that of patients who have adenocarcinoma of unknown primary site, and their treatment should follow similar guidelines.

Neuroendocrine Carcinoma

Poorly Differentiated Neuroendocrine Carcinoma or Small Cell Anaplastic Carcinoma

High-grade neuroendocrine tumors can be reliably identified using readily available immunohistochemistry stains. Although the origin of these tumors is unknown, they frequently are very sensitive to combination chemotherapy. For example, platinum–etoposide chemotherapy, as prescribed for small cell lung cancer (Chapter 177), can provide an overall response rate in approximately 60% of patients, including complete responses in 15 to 20% of patients. In patients who have locoregional disease, post-chemotherapy radiation therapy is also reasonable. Peptide receptor radionuclide therapy with ^{177}lutethium dotatate is also useful for the treatment of neuroendocrine tumors.

Low-Grade (Carcinoid-Type) Neuroendocrine Tumors

Some low-grade neuroendocrine tumors present at a metastatic site, usually in the liver and usually with histologic features that suggest a carcinoid tumor (Chapter 213) or an islet cell tumor of gastrointestinal origin (Chapter 211). The clinical syndromes may be dominated by the secretion and action of vasoactive peptides (e.g., serotonin, vasoactive intestinal peptide, gastrin). As with other carcinoid tumors, these tumors often are relatively indolent, so patients can often survive for several years despite multiple liver metastases. Unlike poorly differentiated neuroendocrine tumors, however, these tumors tend to be relatively resistant to chemotherapy, so intensive combination regimens should usually be avoided. Treatment, which should follow guidelines for metastatic carcinoid tumors (Chapter 213), may include somatostatin analogues, local ablative procedures (e.g., surgical resection, radiofrequency ablation, chemoembolization), targeted agents (e.g., sunitinib, everolimus), or fluorouracil-based chemotherapy regimens.

Empiric Chemotherapy

A substantial proportion of patients with adenocarcinoma or poorly differentiated carcinoma of unknown primary site do not fit into a defined clinical subset for which targeted treatment is available. In such patients, empiric chemotherapy (usually taxane–platinum or gemcitabine–platinum combinations) can provide modest benefit, with response rates of 30 to 45% and a median survival of 9 to 11 months. However, empiric chemotherapy regimens are best avoided, and patients are better served by the best possible site-specific treatment, guided by the tumor's likely site of origin based on molecular tumor profiling.

SURVIVORSHIP AND FOLLOW-UP

Approximately 4% of the U.S. population (≈14 million people) is living with a history of cancer, and about 60% of cancer survivors are age 65 years or older. As a result, a large number of individuals are living longer as cancer survivors from the conclusion of active treatment to the time of recurrence or death from another condition. These patients have specific needs, including a defined program of surveillance to detect recurrence or second cancers and the late effects of cancer treatment; intervention to treat the consequences of the cancer and its treatment (such as lymphedema, fatigue, and psychosocial distress); prevention of new cancers by changes in diet, behavior, and physical activity[34,A9] (Chapter 165); and the institution of a coordinated program of care that may require a variety of specialty services.[35] Long-term follow-up can be optimized by the provision of a survivorship care plan that provides a comprehensive summary of all diagnostic and therapeutic procedures undergone, toxicities experienced, and therapeutic outcomes, as well as a specific program for stress management[36] and for individualized follow-up care.[A10] Although definitive follow-up regimens do not exist for most cancers, evidence-based templates for common malignancies have been developed by the American Society of Clinical Oncology and the National Comprehensive Cancer Network. In addition, issues of survivorship also affect caregivers, who often experience a high degree of psychological distress during and after the period of active treatment.

GENERAL REFERENCES

For the General References and other additional features, please visit Elsevier eBooks+ at https://ebooks.health.elsevier.com.

Grade A References

A1. Altorki N, Wang X, Kozono D, et al. Lobar or sublobar resection for peripheral stage IA non-small-cell lung cancer. *N Engl J Med.* 2023;388:489-498.
A2. Early Breast Cancer Trialists' Collaborative group. Trastuzumab for early-stage, HER2-positive breast cancer: a meta-analysis of 13 864 women in seven randomised trials. *Lancet Oncol.* 2021;22:1139-1150.
A3. Wang Y, Chen L, Liu F, et al. Efficacy and tolerability of granulocyte colony-stimulating factors in cancer patients after chemotherapy: a systematic review and Bayesian network meta-analysis. *Sci Rep.* 2019;9:15374.
A4. Chen J, Zhou L, Liu X, et al. Meta-analysis of clinical trials to assess denosumab over zoledronic acid in bone metastases. *Int J Clin Pharm.* 2021;43:2-10.
A5. O'Carrigan B, Wong MH, Willson ML, et al. Bisphosphonates and other bone agents for breast cancer. *Cochrane Database Syst Rev.* 2017;10:CD003474.
A6. Garcia JM, Boccia RV, Graham CD, et al. Anamorelin for patients with cancer cachexia: an integrated analysis of two phase 2, randomized, placebo-controlled, double blind trials. *Lancet Oncol.* 2015;16:108-116.
A7. Katakami N, Uchino J, Yokoyama T, et al. Anamorelin (ONO-7643) for the treatment of patients with non-small cell lung cancer and cachexia: results from a randomized, double-blind, placebo-controlled, multicenter study of Japanese patients (ONO-7643-04). *Cancer.* 2018;124:606-616.
A8. Goyal L, Meric-Bernstam F, Hollebecque A, et al. Futibatinib for *FGFR2*-rearranged intrahepatic cholangiocarcinoma. *N Engl J Med.* 2023;388:228-239.
A9. Liu MG, Davis GM, Kilbreath SL, et al. Physical activity interventions using behaviour change theories for women with breast cancer: a systematic review and meta-analysis. *J Cancer Surviv.* 2022;16:1127-1148.
A10. Bower JE, Partridge AH, Wolff AC, et al. Improving biobehavioral health in younger breast cancer survivors: Pathways to Wellness trial secondary outcomes. *J Natl Cancer Inst.* 2023;115:83-92.

165

EPIDEMIOLOGY OF CANCER

RULLA M. TAMIMI

CANCER BURDEN AND TRENDS

GLOBAL STATISTICS

Cancer is a major public health concern worldwide. The World Health Organization (WHO) estimates that cancer is the first or second leading cause of death before age 70 years in the majority of countries.[1] In 2020, 19.3 million new cases of cancer were diagnosed globally, and almost 10 million deaths were attributable to cancer (Fig. 165-1). Among women, breast cancer (24.5%) is the leading cause of incident cancer followed by colorectal cancer (9.4%), and breast cancer (15.5%) is the leading cause of cancer mortality followed by lung cancer (13.7%). Among men, lung cancer (14.3%) is the leading cause of incident cancer followed by prostate cancer (14.1%), and lung cancer (21.5%) is the leading cause of cancer mortality followed by liver cancer (10.5%). The burden of cancer varies substantially by geographic region and is impacted by factors such as the age of the population, the prevalence of cancer risk factors, screening and treatment practices, and a country's social and economic development. For example, the incidence and mortality of cervical cancer (Chapter 184) is quite low in high-income countries compared with low-income countries because of cervical cancer screening and vaccination for human papillomavirus.

UNITED STATES STATISTICS

In the United States, cancer is the second leading cause of death after heart disease. In 2020, more than 1.8 million new cases of cancer were diagnosed, and over 600,000 deaths were attributed to cancer. Over the past 50 years, the United States has experienced substantial changes in the incidence of several types of cancer as a reflection of patterns of exposure to risk factors as well as access to and utilization of cancer screening (Fig. 165-2).[2,3] For example, the dramatic increase in the incidence of prostate cancer (Chapter 186) in the 1990s reflected widespread prostate-specific antigen (PSA) testing in men and the resulting detection of asymptomatic disease. This increase was then followed by a dramatic decline in the reported incidence of prostate cancer in 2007 to 2014, largely attributable to changes in the screening guidelines of the United States Preventive Task Force (USPTF), which recommended against routine PSA screening because of concerns regarding overdiagnosis and overtreatment. Similar to prostate cancer, the incidence of breast cancer (Chapter 183) increased in the late 1980s with widespread adoption of mammographic screening. However, incidence rates for breast cancer have remained relatively stable, with slight increases observed in the last 20 years, thought to be attributable to continued increases in body mass index and trends in reproductive patterns (e.g., later age at first birth and lower parity). The incidence rates for colorectal cancer (Chapter 179) have been declining for both men and women since the mid-1980s, likely reflecting colorectal cancer screening practices that can detect precancerous lesions and prevent cancers from occurring. Incidence rates for lung cancer (Chapter 177) closely mirror smoking patterns in the population, although the decline in incidence rates is more pronounced in men than in women. Some of this sex difference may be related to differences in the initiation and cessation of smoking, but a greater percentage of lung cancers in women occur in nonsmokers.

By 2040, estimates suggest that breast cancer will be the most common cancer in the United States, followed by melanoma, lung cancer, and colorectal cancer. In terms of cancer death, lung cancer is projected to remain first, followed by pancreatic cancer, liver and biliary cancer, colon cancer, and breast cancer.[4]

CANCER RISK FACTORS

DEMOGRAPHIC FACTORS

Increasing age is an important risk factor for most cancers, with more than one-third of new cancers in the United States occurring in people age 75 years or older. Age likely represents the accumulation of biologic changes that influence carcinogenesis (Chapter 166). However, these biologic changes occur at different rates in different people depending on their underlying genetics and exposures across the life course. Additionally, cancers at different sites have unique patterns of incidence across the age continuum.

For cancers that occur in both men and women, cancer incidence rates tend to be higher in men (Fig. 165-2). At least some of these sex differences may be attributable to differences in the prevalence of relevant risk factors. For example, the prevalence of smoking has changed over time, but current smoking and smoking-related cancers continue to be higher in men in most countries.

Cancer incidence and mortality rates vary by race and ethnicity.[5] These differences are multifactorial and reflect differences in risk factors and access to high-quality preventive care, screening, and cancer treatments. Across all cancer sites, Black men in the United States have about a 20% higher cancer death rate than do White men. Similarly, Black women in the United States have about a 12% higher death rate than do White women, despite having a lower incidence rate. Black and Hispanic patients are often diagnosed at later stages of cancer, in part reflecting lower rates of screening. Overall cancer mortality rates mask disparities for specific cancers. For example, although Hispanic and Asian individuals have lower overall cancer mortality, their incidence and mortality of liver cancer are higher than in the White population.

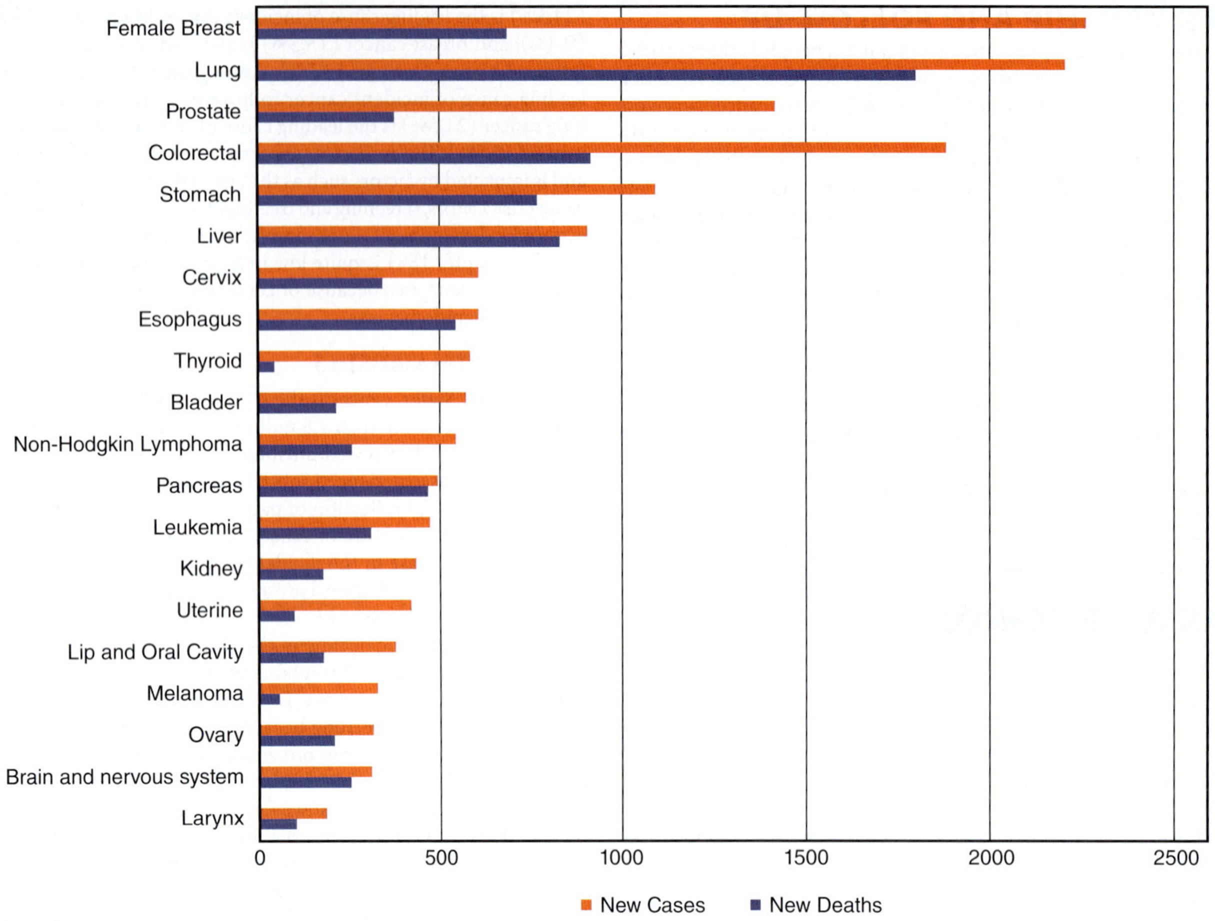

FIGURE 165-1. **Rank order of the top 20 cancers worldwide.** Worldwide cancer incidence and mortality in 2020. (Data from Sung H, Ferlay J, Siegel RL, et al. Global Cancer Statistics 2020: GLOBOCAN estimates of incidence and mortality worldwide for 36 cancers in 185 countries. *CA Cancer J Clin*. 2021;71:209-249.)

ENVIRONMENTAL AND LIFESTYLE FACTORS

Potentially modifiable environmental and lifestyle risk factors are major contributors to the development of cancer.[6,7]

Tobacco

Tobacco use (Chapter 363), and in particular cigarette smoking, is a leading cause of death from cancer. In the United States, almost 30% of cancer deaths are estimated to be attributable to tobacco smoking.[8] Strong evidence links tobacco smoking as a cause for a number of cancers, including lung, oral cavity, nasal cavity, nasopharynx, oropharynx, hypopharynx, larynx, esophagus, stomach, pancreas, liver, kidney, ureter, bladder, and cervix, as well as myeloid leukemia. Chewing tobacco also markedly increases the risk of oral and pharyngeal cancers. Significant advances in tobacco control have resulted in dramatic declines in the prevalence of smoking. Despite these successes, an estimated 22% of the global adult population smokes tobacco. Smoking rates vary widely by region and sex. China has the highest prevalence of adult male smoking (29%), whereas the United States has the highest prevalence of adult female smoking (10%).

Despite success in efforts to reduce cigarette smoking, the emergence of new tobacco products (e.g., vapes, sheesha, flavored tobacco products) has created new public health and equity issues. Additionally, tobacco control has been less successful in specific segments of the population, especially related to sexual orientation and gender identity (Chapter 215).

Obesity and Height

Consistent evidence links excess body weight (Chapter 201) with the risk of cancer at multiple sites. The risk is strongest (a three-fold increase in risk) for endometrial and esophageal cancers and more modest (relative risks of 1.5 to 3.0) for cancers of the kidney, liver, pancreas, and stomach, as well as for multiple myeloma and meningioma. The lowest relative risks (1.0 to 1.5) are for colorectal, postmenopausal breast, gallbladder, ovarian, and thyroid cancers.

The biologic mechanisms that have been proposed to underlie these associations include chronic inflammation, hyperinsulinemia/insulin resistance, insulin-like growth factor (IGF)-1 pathways, and the impact of obesity on circulating sex steroids. Given the strong association between adiposity and many cancers, maintaining a healthy body weight is an important recommendation for cancer prevention. For example, the marked weight loss after bariatric surgery is associated with a significant reduction in the incidence of cancer.[9]

Strong evidence links certain cancers with adult height independent of obesity. For example, adult height is positively associated with the risks of colorectal, ovarian, and breast cancer.[10] In a nationwide study in Sweden, every 10 cm increase in height was associated with about a 20% increased risk of cancer in women and about a 10% increased risk of cancer in men.[11] All cancer sites showed a positive association, with the strongest relative risk (35 to 40%) for malignant melanoma. Height may reflect a larger number of cells at risk of transformation, or adult height may reflect energy intake or exposures to growth factors early in life. For example, levels of IGF-1 in childhood are strongly correlated with height.

Diet and Alcohol

Although the association between adiposity and the risk of cancer is consistent across a number of cancer sites, the association between food groups and nutrients is not. Reasonable prevention recommendations specifically related to diet include: eat a diet rich in whole grains, vegetables, fruits, and beans; limit consumption of fast foods and/or other processed foods high in fat, starches, or sugars; limit consumption of red and processed meats;[12] and limit consumption of sugar-sweetened beverages (Chapter 13).

Alcohol (Chapter 364) is responsible for about 4% of cancers worldwide.[13] The magnitude of association is strongest for oral and pharyngeal cancers as well as esophageal squamous cell carcinoma, but alcohol is also associated with liver and colorectal cancer. For female breast cancer, the association is modest, with a relative risk of 1.6. No convincing evidence links alcohol to other common cancers such as prostate or lung cancers.

Most epidemiologic studies show a dose–response relationship, with increasing amounts of alcohol conveying higher risks regardless of the type of alcohol consumed. The primary hypothesized mechanism is via metabolites,

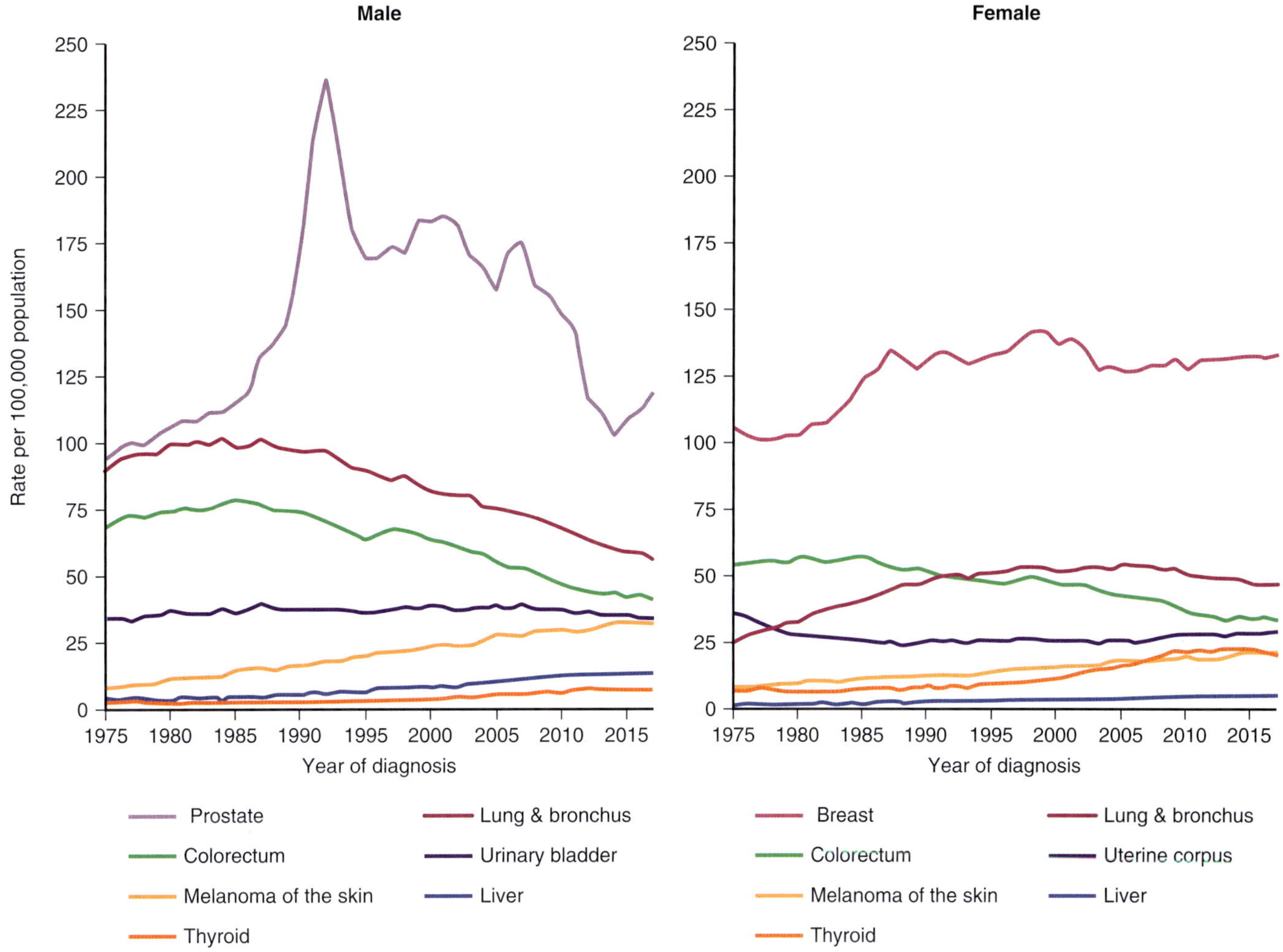

FIGURE 165-2. **Trends in incidence rates for selected cancers by sex, United States, 1975-2017.** (Reproduced from Siegel RL, Miller KD, Fuchs HE, et al. Cancer statistics, 2021. *CA Cancer J Clin.* 2021;71:7-33.)

such as acetaldehyde, which have carcinogenic and mutagenic properties. Alcohol's link to breast cancer probably is partly related to its association with increased levels of total and bioavailable estrogen in premenopausal women, as well as elevated plasma levels of estrogen and increased plasma estradiol levels in postmenopausal women. Additionally, alcohol consumption can indirectly impact the risk of cancer by its association with increases in body mass index.

Physical Activity

Physical activity (Chapter 14) has been hypothesized to reduce the risk of cancer, but the epidemiologic data are not entirely consistent, perhaps because of imperfect measurement of physical activity and the difficulty of separating the direct effects of physical activity from the effects of concomitant adiposity and obesity. The primary hypothesized mechanisms relate to the impact of physical activity on circulating hormones (e.g., sex steroids, insulin and insulin-like growth factors, adipokines), inflammation, immune function, and oxidative stress.

For example, pooled data suggest that higher levels of leisure time physical activity are associated with a reduced risk of 13 cancers,[14] with the strongest associations (>20% reduced risk when comparing the 90th percentile to the 10th percentile) for esophageal adenocarcinoma and cancers of the liver, lung, kidney, gastric cardia, and endometrium, as well as for myeloid leukemia. Moderate associations (10 to 20% reduced risk) are seen for colon, head and neck, rectal, bladder, and breast cancers, as well as for multiple myeloma. After adjusting for body mass index, endometrial, liver, and gastric cancer were no longer significantly associated with physical activity, whereas the relative risk for other cancer sites were only modestly reduced, thereby suggesting that physical activity is a risk factor independent of its relationship to body mass index. The relationship between increased physical activity and a reduced risk for breast cancer and colorectal cancer has also been confirmed using mendelian randomization analysis.[15]

Given the robust evidence and wide impact on reduced risk of several cancer sites, promoting physical activity should be a key component of cancer prevention efforts. For cancer prevention, adults should get at least 2.5 hours/week of moderate-intensity physical activity or 1.25 hours/week of vigorous-intensity physical activity.

Infectious Agents

Eleven infectious pathogens are classified as group 1 carcinogens (i.e., carcinogenic to humans), and an estimated 13% of all cancer cases worldwide are attributable to infections.[16]

The four agents with the greatest impact on cancer in rank order are *Helicobacter pylori* (non–cardia gastric adenocarcinoma; Chapter 178), high-risk human papillomavirus (Chapter 344; cervix, head and neck, and anal carcinoma), hepatitis B virus (Chapter 135), and hepatitis C virus. Almost all cervical cancers (Chapter 181) are attributable to high-risk subtypes of human papillomavirus. Hepatitis B virus is a DNA virus that can cause hepatocellular carcinoma; among carriers of hepatitis B virus, the lifetime risk of hepatocellular carcinoma (Chapter 181) is estimated to be 10 to 25%. Together, these four infectious agents explain >90% of all infection-related cancers globally. The age-standardized incidence rates for infection-attributable cancers vary considerably by geographic region. For example, although *H. pylori* is the most important infectious cause of cancer globally, the age-standardized incidence rates vary by more than five-fold from Eastern Asia, where they are highest, to North America, where they are lowest.

HORMONES

Endogenous Estrogens and Androgens

Several lines of evidence suggest that estrogens play a central role in the cause of female cancers. For example, the risk of breast cancer increases with increasing circulating levels of estrogen. Estrone, estrone sulfate, and free estradiol are similarly related to risk.

Androgens have been hypothesized to increase the risk of breast cancer either directly, by increasing the growth and proliferation of breast cancer cells, or indirectly, by their conversion to estrogen. In postmenopausal women, testosterone and other androgens have been positively associated with the risk of breast cancer. Among premenopausal women, data are much more limited, but statistically significant positive associations are also seen for testosterone, androstenedione, and dehydroepiandrosterone.[17]

Androgens are implicated in cancers of the prostate and breast. Total castration and androgen suppression are successful treatments for advanced prostate cancer,[18] but the association of circulating free testosterone with the risk of developing prostate cancer is more modest.[19]

Exogenous Hormones

Worldwide, the estimated 151 million women who use oral contraceptives represent 16% of women of reproductive age.[20] Most combined oral contraceptives contain ethinyl estradiol (or mestranol, which is metabolized to ethinyl estradiol; Chapter 220) plus a progestin. Patterns of use have changed considerably over time, with both increased duration of use and a trend toward younger age at first use.

The use of oral contraceptives is associated with a modest increased risk of breast cancer for current or recent users. Among women younger than age 50 years, the risk of breast cancer is about 20% higher in women who are current or recent users of hormonal contraceptives compared with nonusers, and a longer duration of use is associated with increased risk.[21] In contrast, the use of oral contraceptives has been associated with lower risks of colorectal, endometrial, and ovarian cancers.[22]

Some menopausal hormone therapies also increase the risk of breast cancer, but formulations and patterns of use have varied over time. The addition of a progestin to estrogen regimens has become increasingly common to minimize or eliminate the increased risk of endometrial hyperplasia and cancer associated with unopposed estrogens. Accumulating data suggest that the addition of a progestin increases the risk of breast cancer beyond that associated with estrogen alone, with stronger associations observed with longer durations of use. Furthermore, different formulations, routes of administration, and regimens may impact the association with breast cancer.[23] Postmenopausal hormonal therapy also appears to increase the risk of ovarian cancer.[24] By comparison, postmenopausal hormone therapies are associated with lower risks of colorectal, esophageal, and gastric cancers. Given the substantial evidence implicating postmenopausal hormone therapies in breast cancer, women and their physicians should carefully consider their risks and benefits (Chapter 222).

IONIZING RADIATION

Exposure to ionizing radiation (Chapter 18) causes somatic DNA mutations. The long-term effects of high levels of ionizing radiation on the risk of cancer is best estimated from people who were exposed to the atomic bombings in Japan in 1945 and to large nuclear disasters in Chernobyl and Fukushima. In atomic bomb survivors in Hiroshima and Nagasaki, excess cases of leukemia were observed by 3 years after exposure, and an excess risk of solid tumors was observed by 10 years after exposure. Sites of excess risk included bladder, breast (female), lung, brain, thyroid, colon, esophagus, ovary, stomach, and liver. For all of these types of cancer, the magnitude of risk increased as the radiation dose increased and as the age at exposure decreased.

MOLECULAR AND GENETIC EPIDEMIOLOGY

The integration of molecular tools in epidemiologic studies has allowed for robust insights into the causes of cancer. For example, aflatoxin is produced by a fungus, which can contaminate stored grain and nuts. Although animal studies demonstrated aflatoxin was carcinogenic, the association between the dietary intake of aflatoxin and liver cancer in humans was difficult to demonstrate until biomarkers of exposure (e.g., urinary metabolites of aflatoxin and DNA adducts reflecting exposure) were identified and showed strong evidence of a causal association.

The assessment of biomarkers for cancer epidemiologic research spans the continuum of disease from germline genetic susceptibility, markers of exposure (e.g., presence of cancer causing virus or cotinine), markers of internal dose (e.g., DNA adducts), markers of effective dose (e.g., somatic mutational patterns), or markers of tumor heterogeneity and prognosis (e.g., molecular subtypes). The landscape of molecular epidemiology has evolved over time as newer tools have demonstrated validity in stored biospecimens. Large-scale genome-wide association studies (GWAS) studies have led to the identification of single nucleotide polymorphisms (SNPs) that are associated with disease. Polygenic risk scores can incorporate multiple SNPs associated with a disease into a single score. Inclusion of a polygenic risk score to risk assessment models can significantly improve the ability to predict the development of breast and prostate cancer and may help develop more personalized cancer screening protocols.

CANCER CONTROL: PREVENTION AND TREATMENT

Cancer control refers to reducing the burden of cancer in the population, whether by reducing the incidence of and mortality from cancer or by improving the quality of life for patients who are being treated for and living with cancer (Fig. 165-3). Cancer prevention, screening, and early detection are critical for reducing the incidence and mortality from cancer.

PRIMARY PREVENTION

Primary prevention refers to strategies targeted at reducing exposure to established cancer risk factors. Cancer prevention efforts can be multifaceted by targeting individuals, medical recommendations, schools, neighborhood planning, and federal policies. Most notably, tobacco control efforts (Chapter 363) have had a substantial impact on the declining incidence and mortality rates attributable to lung cancer. Tobacco control efforts have included educational efforts to reduce the initiation of smoking and to increase the uptake of smoking cessation programs (Chapter 363). Policy changes have resulted in the implementation of tobacco-free public places, workplaces, and multiunit residential settings.

Vaccinations against carcinogenic infections are another successful approach for reducing the incidence of cancer. Vaccination programs for human papillomavirus (Chapter 344) and hepatitis B virus (Chapter 134) are two strategies to reduce the incidence rates of cervical and liver cancer,

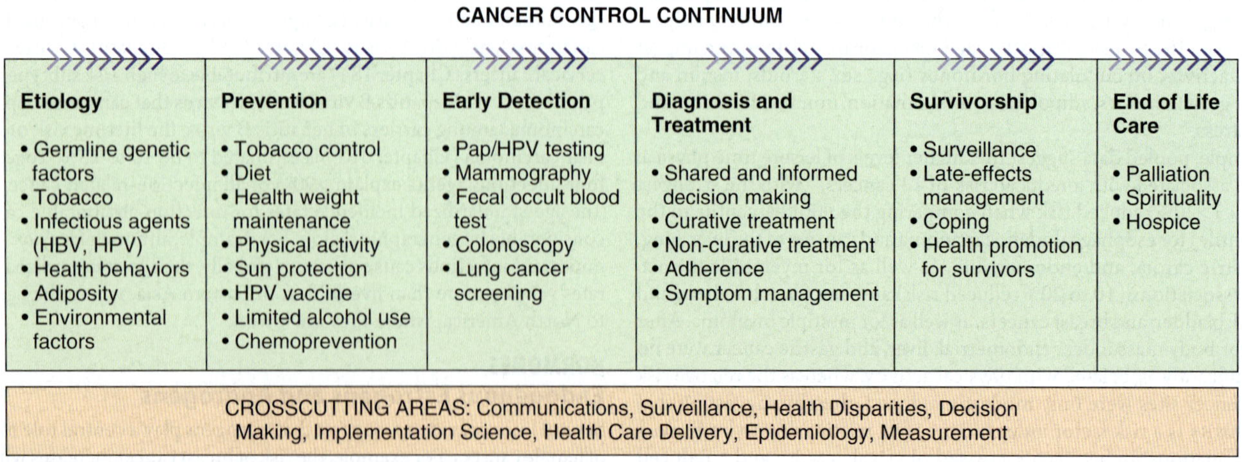

FIGURE 165-3. **The Cancer Control Continuum.** Examples and opportunities to impact cancer morbidity and mortality along the continuum. HBV = hepatitis B virus; HPV = human papillomavirus.

respectively. For example, a nationwide neonatal hepatitis B virus immunization program launched in Taiwan in 1984 reduced the incidence rate for hepatocellular carcinoma by 80%, and the mortality rate declined by over 90%.[25] Several clinical trials have demonstrated the efficacy and safety of vaccines for human papillomavirus,[A1] with data already showing reductions in cervical cancer[A2] and human papillomavirus–related oropharyngeal cancer.[A3] Because large-scale nationwide human papillomavirus vaccination programs were not initiated until 2007, it is too early to observe major declines in cancer incidence rates given the latency period, but widespread vaccination programs could lead to the elimination of cervical cancer. Major challenges that remain are related to the implementation of programs to improve both access and adherence.

Other established modifiable cancer risk factors include obesity (Chapter 201), physical inactivity (Chapter 14), poor diet (Chapter 13), and alcohol consumption (Chapter 364). Diets and behaviors aimed at maintaining healthy weights throughout life have the potential to reduce the risk of several cancers. Limiting alcohol consumption and being physically active also can reduce the risk of cancer.

SECONDARY PREVENTION

Secondary prevention refers to strategies aimed at reducing mortality from cancer. Screening is often a central part of secondary prevention because the goal of screening is to detect cancer in a presymptomatic state. Screening programs are well established for a number of cancers. For cervical cancer, initial success was observed with widespread screening using the Papanicolaou smear, and human papillomavirus–based screening strategies have demonstrated even greater efficacy when compared with cytology alone (Chapter 184).[A4] The incidence rates for colorectal cancer have been falling in the United States (see Fig. 165-2), largely due to the success of screening programs (with stool-based tests, sigmoidoscopy, and colonoscopy), which are now recommended to begin at ages 45 to 49 years (Chapters 12 and 179).[A5]

Widespread PSA testing for prostate cancer (Chapter 186) and mammography for breast cancer (Chapter 183) have resulted in dramatic increases in the reported incidence of these two cancers. Both approaches have also likely led to reductions in cancer-specific mortality, despite concerns about overdiagnosis and overtreatment of some of the lesions detected through these screening programs. Given concerns regarding harms related to PSA screening, the U.S. Preventive Services Task Force modified its recommendations in 2018 to advise that the decision to undergo PSA screening should be made at the individual level through shared decision making.[A6]

Lung cancer screening with low-dose computed tomographic scanning is beneficial for high-risk individuals, in whom it can reduce mortality by about 25 to 33% in the following 10 years.[A7,A8] The U.S. Preventive Services Task Force guidelines now recommend it for persons who are at high risk (e.g., adults ages 50 to 80 years with a >20 pack-year smoking history who either currently smoke or have quit within the past 15 years) of lung cancer (Chapters 12 and 177).[26] Unfortunately, the uptake of lung cancer screening has been slow, especially in diverse populations,[27] with <5% of eligible persons undergoing screening,[28] presumably reflecting a lack of awareness on the part of the physician and the patient, confusion regarding recommendations, limited access to screening, and the stigma associated with smoking and lung cancer.[29]

TREATMENT

The availability of cancer treatments, including surgery, radiation, and chemotherapy, varies significantly across the world, with fewer treatments in lower-income countries (Chapter 5) and by socioeconomic status and ethnicity even in higher-income countries (Chapter 4). Access to high-quality cancer care impacts patients' outcomes and survival. As treatment improves, the prevalence of cancer rises, thereby emphasizing the need to addresses cancer survivorship care (Chapter 164).

GENERAL REFERENCES

For the General References and other additional features, please visit Elsevier eBooks+ at https://ebooks.health.elsevier.com.

Grade A References

A1. Huh WK, Joura EA, Giuliano AR, et al. Final efficacy, immunogenicity, and safety analyses of a nine-valent human papillomavirus vaccine in women aged 16-26 years: a randomised, double-blind trial. *Lancet*. 2017;390:2143-2159.
A2. Arbyn M, Xu L, Simoens C, Martin-Hirsch PP. Prophylactic vaccination against human papillomaviruses to prevent cervical cancer and its precursors. *Cochrane Database Syst Rev*. 2018;5:CD009069.
A3. Tsentemeidou A, Fyrmpas G, Stavrakas M, et al. Human papillomavirus vaccine to end oropharyngeal cancer. A systematic review and meta-analysis. *Sex Transm Dis*. 2021;48:700-707.
A4. Ogilvie GS, van Niekerk D, Krajden M, et al. Effect of screening with primary cervical HPV testing vs cytology testing on high-grade cervical intraepithelial neoplasia at 48 months: the HPV FOCAL randomized clinical trial. *JAMA*. 2018;320:43-52.
A5. Lin JS, Perdue LA, Henrikson NB, et al. Screening for colorectal cancer: updated evidence report and systematic review for the US Preventive Services Task Force. *JAMA*. 2021;325:1978-1998.
A6. U.S. Preventative Services Task Force, Grossman DC, Curry SJ, Owens DK, et al. Screening for prostate cancer: US Preventative Services Task Force Recommendation Statement. *JAMA*. 2018;319:1901-1913.
A7. de Koning HJ, van der Aalst CM, de Jong PA, et al. Reduced lung-cancer mortality with volume CT screening in a randomized trial. *N Engl J Med*. 2020;382:503-513.
A8. Jonas DE, Reuland DS, Reddy SM, et al. Screening for lung cancer with low-dose computed tomography: updated evidence report and systematic review for the US Preventive Services Task Force. *JAMA*. 2021;325:971-987.

166 CANCER BIOLOGY AND GENETICS

BEN HO PARK

INTRODUCTION

Cancer is a collection of many different diseases and is often not uniformly categorized by even the tissue of origin. For example, hormone receptor–positive breast cancers are distinct in biology, prognosis, and treatment compared with hormone receptor–negative breast malignancies. A unifying feature shared by all human cancers is that they have a genetic basis, even though familial cancer syndromes are relatively uncommon compared with sporadic cancers. However, both heritable and sporadic cancers require the accumulation of DNA mistakes or alterations that lead to a step-wise progression of events, ultimately resulting in cancer. These DNA alterations are typically classified as mutations, copy number changes, and gene rearrangements. Cancer also results when DNA undergoes epigenetic changes that do not involve alterations to the DNA sequence but produce modifications that result in either the silencing or activation of genes in an aberrant fashion.

CANCER IS A DISEASE OF CUMULATIVE DNA ALTERATIONS

When the balance of cell proliferation as compared with cell death or quiescence is perturbed, either due to abnormally increased proliferation or to decreased cell death or stasis, the initial steps of carcinogenesis have begun. Genes that mediate cell proliferation and cell death are often the early drivers of cancer, and many of these genes are mutated or altered in diverse types of cancer.

Two broad categories of cancer genes are termed *oncogenes* and *tumor suppressor genes*. Oncogenes, which are the accelerators of cancer growth, drive abnormal cell proliferation through various mechanisms. Common oncogenes that are often mutated or altered in human cancers include *KRAS*, *BRAF*, *PIK3CA*, and *ERBB2* (HER2). The functions of oncogenes are diverse, but many mutations and alterations that occur in oncogenes constitutively activate critical growth promoting pathways that then drive cellular proliferation. Conversely, tumor suppressor genes act as the brakes of cell growth. Their normal function is to control cell cycling by monitoring and stopping proliferation when appropriate. Any disruption in the function of tumor suppressor genes would predictably lead to a net gain in cell numbers, possibly even without additional contributions of increased cell proliferation. Examples of tumor suppressor genes commonly mutated in human cancers include *TP53*, *CDKN2A*, *CDKN2B*, and others. Most cancers have genetic alterations involving both tumor suppressor genes and oncogenes, but the types of genetic alterations and consequences for therapies can vary dramatically between different malignancies.

DNA ALTERATIONS IN ONCOGENES AND TUMOR SUPPRESSOR GENES

Given the distinct yet complementary roles of oncogenes and tumor suppressor genes, it is perhaps not surprising that certain types of genetic alterations are associated more frequently with one or the other class of genes. Activating mutations within oncogenes, for example, tend to be heterozygous (i.e., only

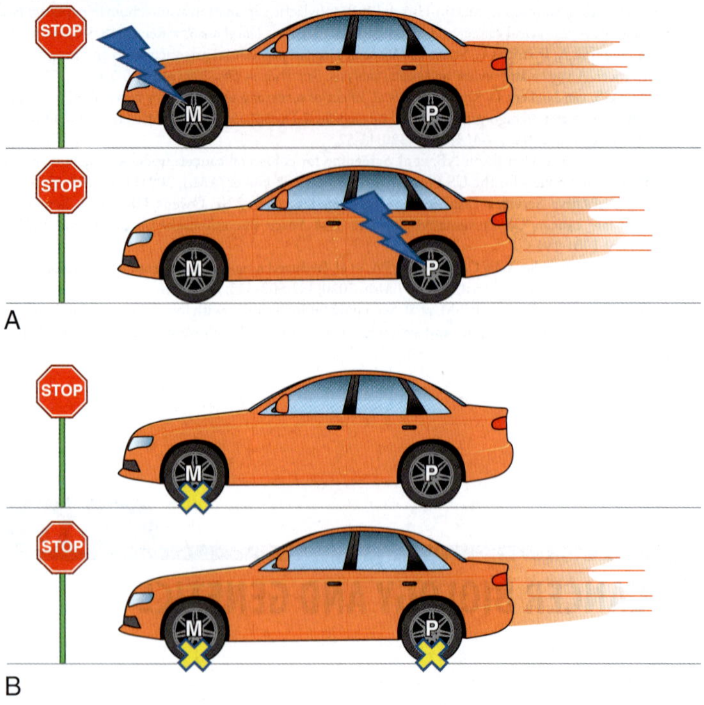

FIGURE 166-1. **Oncogenes and tumor suppressor genes: the accelerators and brakes of cancer. A,** Oncogenes act as the accelerators of cancer cells, driving forward even when the cell should stop (STOP sign). Oncogenic alterations such as mutations can occur in either the maternal allele (M front axle) or paternal allele (P rear axle) and will therefore cause the cell to continue to proliferate. In contrast (**B**), tumor suppressor genes are the brakes of the cell cycle. If a mutation or alteration disables only the front brakes or only the rear brakes (maternal allele; M front axle in figure), the cell can still obey stop signals. However, if both front (M axle) and rear (paternal allele; P rear axle) are disabled, the cell continues to go forward through normal stop signaling. Blue lightning bolts represent gain-of-function mutations in oncogenes; yellow X marks represent loss-of-function mutations in tumor suppressor genes.

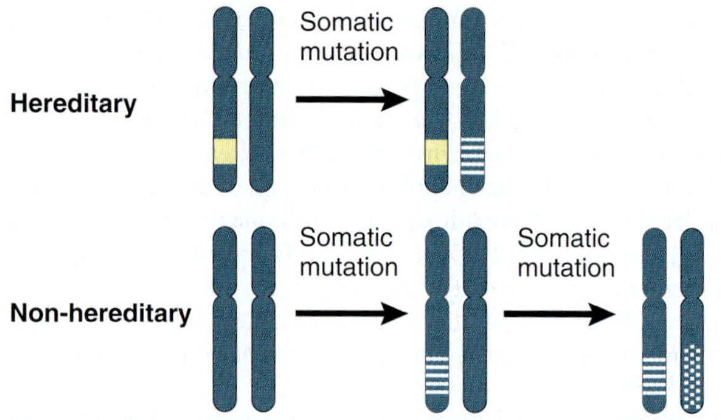

FIGURE 166-2. **Knudson's two-hit model of cancer development.** Biallelic inactivation (yellow band) is required for tumor initiation. In familial cancer syndromes, the first "hit" is inherited in the germline, requiring only a single somatic second "hit" (white stripes) to initiate carcinogenesis. In sporadic tumors, the first hit occurs in a single cell, and still requires the second somatic "hit" to occur in the same cell in order for tumor initiation to ensue. (Originally appearing in Jozwiak J, Jozwiak S, Wlodarski P. Possible mechanisms of disease development in tuberous sclerosis. *The Lancet Oncology*. 2008:Jan;9[1]:73-9.)

one allele is mutated) because a gain-of-function mutation would exert an effect even in the presence of the normal protein still being produced by the other wild-type allele (Fig. 166-1A). These mutations in oncogenes typically occur in regions that are known to regulate the corresponding protein's activity, such as kinase domain mutations that render the protein constitutively activated. An increased copy number of an oncogene can have a similar effect. Other examples are translocations and rearrangements, such as when the *BCR-ABL* translocation juxtaposes two genes so that the oncogene's normal function is in an "always on" state. In contrast, tumor suppressor genes generally require a loss-of-function genetic alteration, which by necessity usually requires alterations in both alleles of the cell (Fig. 166-1B). Accordingly, loss-of-function mutations observed in many tumor suppressor genes generally lead to premature truncation of the protein, such as nonsense mutations and insertion/deletion frameshift mutations. In addition, larger genomic alterations, such as deletions or loss of an entire gene or chromosome, are another mechanism for inactivating tumor suppression. Beyond these generalizations in the types of genetic alterations seen in oncogenes and tumor suppressor genes, exceptions also exist. For example, *TP53* is a tumor suppressor gene, yet the most frequent mutations found in human cancers are missense mutations, rather than frame shifts or deletions. These common missense mutations confer a dominant negative effect and prevent the p53 protein from forming tetramers, thereby usually resulting in a loss-of-function, although gain-of-function mutations in *TP53* have also been described. In contrast, certain deletions in the epidermal growth factor receptor (EGFR) gene (*ERBB1*) eliminate autoregulatory domains, thereby resulting in constitutive activation of this oncogene. Ultimately the nature and type of mutations in oncogenes and tumor suppressor genes are predicated on the domains of the protein that would readily lend themselves to activate or inactivate the gene, respectively.

GERMLINE VERSUS SOMATIC DNA ALTERATIONS IN CANCER

The human body is composed of trillions of cells, and each cell generally contains two copies (diploid) of the genome. Mature red blood cells and platelets are among the few cell types that are devoid of DNA, and gametes (i.e., ova and sperm) have only one copy of the genome (haploid), thereby allowing the zygote to inherit a haploid genome from each parent. DNA obtained from normal cells is often referred to as germline because it is derived from parental ova and sperm, which are also termed germ cells. By definition, germline DNA (sometimes also referred to as constitutional DNA) is heritable in that humans receive all their DNA from both parents. Any mutations that are present in a heterozygous fashion in germline DNA can be passed down to progeny, with a 50/50 chance of inheriting the mutant allele.

The majority of germline DNA alterations that lead to familial cancer syndromes are mutations in tumor suppressor genes.[1] In fact, the strictest genetic definition of a tumor suppressor is an alteration in a gene that predisposes to tumor formation. Indeed, pedigrees from families with hereditary predispositions to cancer have shed much light on the nature of tumor suppressor genes, including the "two-hit" hypothesis as well as the identification of key tumor suppressor genes such as *RB1, BRCA1, BRCA2* and *APC*. Since biallelic inactivation of a tumor suppressor is required to initiate cancer, familial cancer syndromes would be expected to follow an autosomal recessive pattern of inheritance. However, the majority of tumor suppressor genes are lethal to the embryo if two mutant copies are present in the zygote, so homozygosity is rarely seen in families with known mutations of a given tumor suppressor gene. Rather, a "second hit" (or inactivation of the second allele) occurs only in the cell or cells that are destined to become a tumor (Fig. 166-2). This second loss-of-function event can occur in a number of different ways, including loss of the gene, a new mutation, or epigenetic silencing. Regardless of the mechanism, because this second event occurs only in a single cell and therefore will not be present in gametes, these alterations are referred to as somatic changes. Because the human body has trillions of cells, the lifetime chance that any single cell in an individual who has inherited one mutant allele in a tumor suppressor gene will obtain a "second hit" is quite high; as a result, the pattern of inheritance for familial cancer syndromes is generally autosomal dominant. However, cancer is a result of the accumulation of many DNA alterations, so even the complete loss of function of a tumor suppressor gene is generally not sufficient to form a mass or tumor (Fig. 166-3). This requirement explains why, despite the autosomal pattern of inheritance, many familial cancer syndromes have incomplete penetrance (i.e., not all carriers will develop cancer).

Germline DNA alterations that predispose to tumor and cancer formation also explain the relatively earlier onset of diagnosis for familial cancers relative to sporadic counterparts. In the former, the initiation of cancer is accelerated because every diploid cell in the body has a lifelong functional loss of one of the two tumor suppressor genes. In the sporadic situation, by comparison, this "first hit" must occur somatically in any given cell.

With the advent of large cancer DNA sequencing, the complexity of human cancers has become apparent. Although these studies generally support the notion that most cancers arise from a stepwise accumulation of somatic genetic mutations and alterations that result in early proliferative changes, precancerous tumors, and then invasive disease, notable exceptions exist. For instance, pathogens such as viruses can initiate or predispose an individual to cancer. As an example, cells that are infected with human papillomaviruses (Chapter 344) can express proteins that inactivate key tumor suppressor genes such as p53 and RB. This suppression, which is to the advantage of the virus because cell proliferation is needed for viral replication, also establishes a situation akin

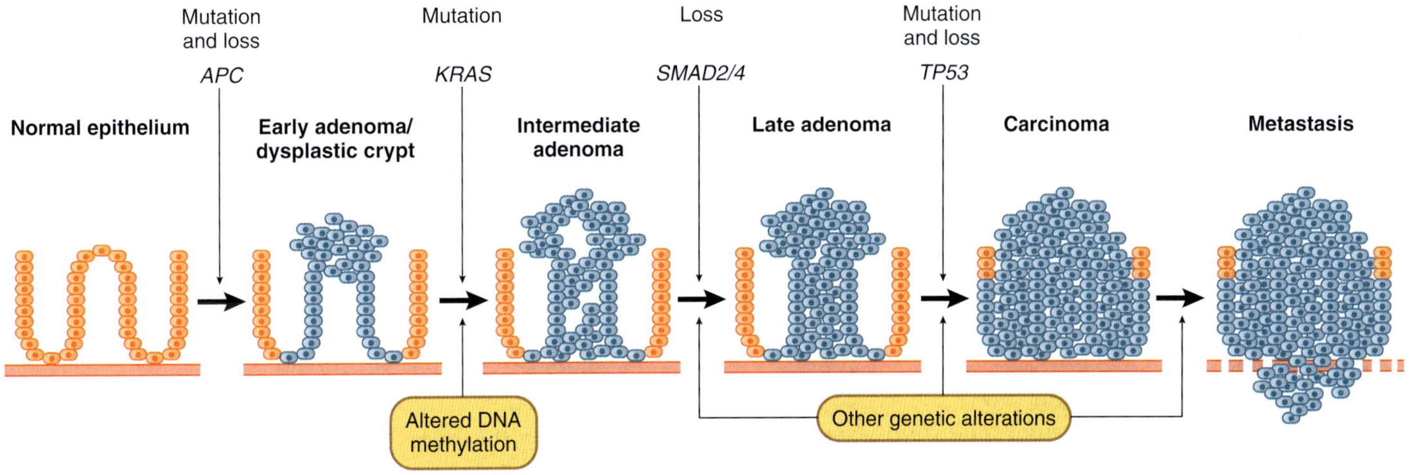

FIGURE 166-3. **The stepwise progression from normal colonic epithelium to invasive cancer.** Progression from normal epithelium through adenoma to colorectal carcinoma is characterized by accumulated genetic and epigenetic alterations of oncogenes and tumor suppressor genes, also known as "the Vogelgram" after Bert Vogelstein, MD. (From Davies RJ, Miller R, Coleman N. Colorectal cancer screening: prospects for molecular stool analysis. *Nature Reviews Cancer*. 2005;Mar;5[3]:199-209.)

to acquiring mutations within tumor suppressor genes. Similar to nonviral cancers, however, this suppression is an initiating event that is not sufficient to form a tumor because additional genetic events are required for a truly invasive cancer.

Sequencing studies have also shown that the number of mutations or genetic alterations required for carcinogenesis is highly variable, especially when considering the requirements for distant metastases. However, statistical analyses in pancreatic cancers suggest that two alterations may be sufficient.[2] Genomic and epidemiologic data suggest that increased cellular proliferation can be associated with an increased risk of cancer, but that the development of mutations, and therefore cancer, has a strong element of randomness or "bad luck."[3]

GENETIC INSTABILITY, CLONAL EVOLUTION, AND TUMOR HETEROGENEITY

When normal cells divide, surveillance and repair mechanisms within the cells ensure that any DNA errors are corrected prior to cytokinesis (i.e., cell division). This process ensures near-perfect fidelity and prevents the emergence of diseases, such as cancer, that are related to somatic alterations in DNA. In cancer cells, such fail-safe mechanisms are disabled, thereby allowing cells to accumulate DNA mutations, copy number changes, and genomic rearrangements. But even more daunting is that the lack of DNA repair mechanisms leads to a dynamic, ongoing process of Darwinian evolution. As cancer cells continue to divide, each resultant cell is slightly different from the next with regard to their genomes. Deleterious mutations or alterations will result in cell death, whereas advantageous changes will enable a clonal growth expansion, even as additional mutations and alterations are continually occurring within this clonal population. Although some rare cancers are exceptions to this model, modern sequencing studies of metastases support this notion, with many cancer cells within the same patient harboring so-called "private" mutations. Although some of these mutations may have no functional consequence and are therefore termed "passenger" mutations, these mutations along with other genomic alterations underscore the ongoing genetic instability of human cancers.

This continuing clonal evolution sets the stage for the development of cancer. Hallmarks (see Table 166-1) include angiogenesis, evasion of the immune system, escape from cell death and tumor suppressors, and a sustained proliferative capacity—all due to genetic alterations that directly or indirectly arise from genetic instability. Some of the mechanisms of genetic instability have been elucidated and can be classified into two broad categories. Chromosomal instability is a more common type of genetic instability in human cancers and is exemplified by copy number alterations and rearrangements. Cancers with chromosomal instability are therefore more likely to have amplifications, deletions, and aneuploidy. Conversely, genetic instability at the nucleotide level is also a much less common but well-described phenomenon, and sequencing has revealed that such cancers have thousands of mutations within their genomes and are often diploid or near diploid in contrast to tumors with chromosomal instability. This increase in mutations has been frequently referred to as high "tumor mutation burden." Several genes have been shown to mediate chromosomal instability, and many genes have also been shown to

TABLE 166-1 HALLMARKS OF CANCER

- Self-sufficiency in growth signals
- Insensitivity to anti-growth signals
- Evading apoptosis
- Limitless replicative potential
- Sustained angiogenesis
- Tissue invasion and metastasis

- Reprogramming energy metabolism
- Evading immune response
- Genome instability and mutation
- Tumor-promoting inflammation

Hanahan and Weinberg proposed in 2000 that there are six essential alterations in cell physiology ("hallmarks of cancer") that collectively dictate malignant growth, listed in the first six bullets. (Hanahan D, Weinberg RA. The hallmarks of cancer. *Cell*. 2000;100:57-70.) A decade later, they updated the list by adding four additional hallmarks, listed in the last four bullets. (Hanahan D, Weinberg RA. Hallmarks of cancer: the next generation. *Cell*. 2011;144:646-674.) There have been subsequent attempts to simplify the list by merging some of these core traits of most cancers. (Fouad YA, Aanel C. Revisiting the hallmarks of cancer. *Am J Cancer Res*. 2017;7:1016-1036.)

regulate an increase in tumor mutation burden. The most notable example of the latter is the mismatch repair genes and their regulation of a specific form of mutation burden termed microsatellite instability. Tumors with microsatellite instability generally have a high tumor mutation burden and a relatively diploid genome. The genetic defects that lead to microsatellite instability are the inactivation of DNA mismatch repair genes. In normal cells the presence of these mismatch repair proteins will ensure that any DNA mistakes occurring with cell replication will be corrected. The mismatch repair system is especially important for recognizing and correcting DNA mistakes that occur at base pair "repeat" sequences including mono-, di-, tri- and tetra-nucleotide sequences such as AAAAA, ATATAT, ATCATCATC, and ACGTACGTACGT, respectively. These areas of DNA repeats are scattered throughout the human genome and are termed microsatellite sequences. Tumors with microsatellite instability have difficulty repairing these microsatellite regions during DNA replication due to the lack of mismatch repair proteins. As a result, mismatch repair gene mutations, alterations, and epigenetic silencing occur in tumors with microsatellite instability. Most notably, right-sided colon cancers often have epigenetic silencing of mismatch repair proteins, with the two most frequently affected genes being *MLH1* and *MSH2*. Although not growth suppressors, *MLH1* and *MSH2* meet the definition of a tumor suppressor because germline mutations in either of these genes lead to hereditary nonpolyposis colorectal cancers and other malignancies, such as ovarian and endometrial cancers, also known as Lynch syndrome.[4] Examples of hereditary cancer risk syndromes are summarized in Table 166-2.

The genetic instability that drives tumor heterogeneity often makes cancers refractory to treatment and cure. Even though a therapeutic agent may be effective in the majority of cancer cells within a population, preexisting mutations and other alterations will then be selected as a new dominant population. In essence, the same Darwinian evolution that leads to cancer and metastases

TABLE 166-2 COMMON FAMILIAL CANCER SYNDROMES

SYNDROME	GENE	ASSOCIATED TUMORS
TUMOR SUPPRESSOR MUTATIONS		
Cowden	*PTEN*	Breast, thyroid, endometrial, colorectal, kidney, melanoma
Familial adenomatous polyposis	*APC*	Colorectal, stomach, intestinal, hepatoblastoma, thyroid, pancreatic, adrenal, bile duct, medulloblastoma
Familial gastric carcinoma	*CDH1* (E-Cadherin)	Stomach, breast
Familial malignant melanoma	*CDKN2* ($p16^{INK4A}$ and $p14^{ARF}$), *CDK4*	Melanoma, pancreatic
Familial Wilms tumor	*WT1*	Wilms (kidney)
Hereditary leiomyomatosis and renal cell carcinoma	*FH*	Cutaneous leiomyomas, uterine leiomyomas (fibroids), renal cell carcinoma
Hereditary retinoblastoma	*RB1* (pRB)	Retinoblastoma
Hereditary paraganglioma	*SDHA, SDHB, SDHC, SDHD*, or *SDHAF2*(succinate dehydrogenase)	Paraganglioma, pheochromocytoma
Li-Fraumeni	*TP53* (p53)	Osteosarcoma, soft tissue sarcoma, leukemia, breast, brain, adrenal, melanoma, Wilms, stomach, colorectal, pancreatic, esophageal, lung, gonadal germ cells
Multiple endocrine neoplasia type 1	*MEN1*	Parathyroid, pituitary, islet cell, adrenal, carcinoid
Neurofibromatosis type 1	*NF1*	Neurofibroma, glioma, leukemia, breast, rhabdomyosarcoma, gastrointestinal stromal
Neurofibromatosis type 2	*NF2*	Neuromas, schwannomas, meningiomas, astrocytomas, gliomas
Peutz-Jeghers syndrome	*LKB1*	Colon, intestine, stomach, pancreas, cervix, ovary, testis, breast, thyroid
Von Hippel-Lindau	*VHL*	Kidney, adrenal, pheochromocytoma
DNA REPAIR GENE MUTATIONS		
Ataxia telangiectasia	*ATM*	Leukemia, lymphoma
Bloom	*BLM*	Leukemia, multiple solid tumors
Fanconi anemia	*FANCA, FANCC, FANCD2, FANCE, FANCF*, or *FANCG*	Leukemia, multiple solid tumors
Hereditary breast and ovarian cancer	*BRCA1* or *BRCA2*	Breast, ovary, pancreatic, fallopian tube
Lynch (hereditary nonpolyposis colon cancer)	*MLH1, MSH2, MSH6*, or *PMS2*	Colorectal, endometrial, stomach, breast, ovarian, intestinal, pancreatic, prostate, urinary tract, liver, kidney
MYH-associated polyposis	*MUTYH*	Colorectal, intestinal
Xeroderma pigmentosum	*XPA, XPC, ERCC2, ERCC3, ERCC4, ERCC5*, or *DDB2*	Skin (basal cells, squamous), melanoma, tongue, eye
ONCOGENE MUTATIONS		
Costello	*HRAS*	Papilloma, rhabdomyosarcoma, neuroblastoma
Noonan	*PTPN11, SOS1, KRAS, NRAS, RAF1*, or *BRAF* (Ras-Erk pathway regulators)	Leukemia, rhabdomyosarcoma, neuroblastoma
Familial malignant melanoma	*CDK4*	Melanoma
Multiple endocrine neoplasia type 2	*RET*	Thyroid, parathyroid, pheochromocytoma
Hereditary papillary renal cell carcinoma	*MET*	Type 1 papillary renal cell carcinoma

continues when the cancer is subjected to various chemotherapies and targeted therapies.

CANCER GENETICS AND TARGETED THERAPIES

A fundamental goal of translating genetic information about cancers is to use this knowledge for risk assessment, diagnosis, screening, and therapy. Targeted therapies are based on an understanding of how oncogenes and tumor suppressor genes drive cancer growth and then developing strategies to disrupt these mechanisms. One of the earliest examples is the *ERBB2* (HER2) oncogene and breast cancer. HER2 amplification occurs in 15 to 20% of breast cancers (Chapter 183) and is associated with an aggressive behavior and worse prognosis. The humanized monoclonal antibody, trastuzumab, was one of the first examples of a drug against a therapeutic target, because only patients with HER2 amplification/overexpression in their tumors appeared to derive benefit from this therapy. The successes of trastuzumab and additional HER2 targeted therapies (e.g., pertuzumab, neratinib, tucatinib, ado-trastuzumab, and trastuzumab deruxtecan) have changed the natural history of HER2-positive breast cancers such that they are now a highly favorable group with good prognosis (Chapter 183). This success serves as a strong reminder that understanding the underlying biology of cancer can lead to therapies that can have a dramatic impact on the disease.

Many other effective targeted therapies have shown noteworthy success (Table 166-3). Examples include imatinib, which inhibits the BCR-ABL fusion protein in chronic myelogenous leukemia (CML) (Chapter 170), thereby converting a once-fatal disease into a manageable chronic condition in which the majority of patients can now live out their natural lives.[5] In certain forms of lung cancer (Chapter 177), genomic alterations that occur with 1 to 10% frequency can be targeted with relatively specific drugs that can have a profound effect.[6]

The study of mechanisms of drug resistance has also led to an improved understanding of predictors of resistance and the development of targeted therapies that can overcome this resistance. For example, gefitinib and erlotinib are two small molecule inhibitors against certain activating mutations found within the EGFR oncogene in non–small cell lung cancers (Chapter 177). Remarkably, sequencing of tumors that developed resistance to these drugs revealed that many cancers acquired a specific recurrent mutation (i.e., T790M). Further laboratory research and clinical development led to approval of next-generation receptor tyrosine kinase inhibitors capable of overcoming cancers that harbored these mutations. Similar findings have also emerged for other diseases. As an example, accumulating evidence suggests that the emergence of resistance mutations in the estrogen receptor alpha (*ESR1*) gene's

TABLE 166-3 EXAMPLES OF TARGETED CANCER THERAPIES

THERAPEUTIC AGENT	TYPE	TARGET	DISEASE	INDICATION	COMPANION TEST
Imatinib Dasatinib Nilotinib	Small molecule	BCR-ABL	CML, ALL	Philadelphia chromosome–positive	Cytogenetic analysis, FISH, PCR
Ponatinib Bosutinib	Small molecule		CML and AML resistant to prior tyrosine kinase inhibitor therapy	Philadelphia chromosome–positive	Cytogenetic analysis, FISH, RT-PCR
Imatinib	Small molecule	c-Kit	Gastrointestinal stromal tumors	CD117 (c-Kit) positive	Immunohistochemistry (c-Kit PharmDx)
Cetuximab Panitumumab	Monoclonal antibody	EGFR	Colorectal cancer, head and neck	*KRAS* wild-type in colon cancer	PCR (*therascreen* KRAS RGQ Kit)
Gefitinib Erlotinib Afatinib Osimertinib	Small molecule	EGFR	NSCLC	Mutant EGFR	PCR (*therascreen* EGFR RGQ PCR Kit, cobas EGFR Mutation Test)
Trametinib/ dabrafenib Cobimetinib/ vemurafenib	Small molecule	MEK/BRAF	Melanoma	V600 mutant BRAF	PCR (THxID, cobas 4800 BRAF V600 Mutation Test)
Sotorasib	Small molecule	KRAS	Lung	G12C mutant KRAS	PCR (*therascreen* KRAS RGQ Kit) next-generation sequencing,
Trastuzumab Pertuzumab Trastuzumab emtansine (antibody drug conjugate of trastuzumab) Trastuzumab deruxtecan (antibody drug conjugate of trastuzumab)	Monoclonal antibody	HER2	Breast, stomach, gastroesophageal	HER2 positive	Immunohistochemistry (PATHWAY, InSite, Bond Oracle, HercepTest), FISH (Inform, PathVysion, SPOT-Light, HER2 CISH PharmDx)
Lapatinib Neratinib	Small molecule	HER2, EGFR	Breast	HER2 positive	HER2 testing as above
Bevacizumab	Monoclonal antibody	VEGF	NSCLC, metastatic colorectal, metastatic kidney, glioblastoma		
Ipilimumab	Monoclonal antibody	CTLA-4	Melanoma		
Pembrolizumab Nivolumab	Monoclonal antibody	PD-1	Melanoma, NSCLC, microsatellite instability–positive cancers, cancers with a high tumor mutation burden		Immunohistochemistry for PDL1, microsatellite testing, next-generation sequencing for high tumor mutation burden
Olaparib, rucaparib, talazoparib, niraparib	Small molecule	PARP1 (due to inactivation of BRCA pathway)	Breast, ovarian, prostate, pancreas	Germline and somatic *BRCA1* or *BRCA2* pathogenic variants	Next-generation sequencing of germline and/or tumor DNA

Companion tests in parentheses are U.S. Food and Drug Administration–stipulated tests for certain uses of the corresponding drug.
ALL = acute lymphoblastic leukemia; AML = acute myeloid leukemia; *BRCA1* = breast cancer gene 1; *BRCA2*; breast cancer gene 2; CML = chronic myelogenous leukemia; FISH = fluorescence in situ hybridization; NSCLC = non–small cell lung cancer; PARP = poly adenosine diphosphate-ribose polymerase; PCR = polymerase chain reaction; PDL1 = programmed death-ligand 1; RT-PCR = reverse transcription polymerase chain reaction.

ligand binding domain occur with relatively high frequency in patients whose metastatic hormone receptor-positive breast cancer (Chapter 183) is treated with aromatase inhibitors.[7] Strategies to overcome these *ESR1* mutations with newer combination endocrine therapies are being tested in clinical trials.

Although other resistance mutations have emerged through further sequencing efforts, additional clarity has been brought about with the understanding of gene mutations and their impact on signaling pathways. For example, given the sequence of events required for activation of the MAP kinase pathway (E-Fig. 166-1), it would be predicted that antibody therapies against EGFR would be ineffective in tumors that harbor an activating mutation in *KRAS*, because the activating "lesion" in this particular case is distal to EGFR. Therefore, inhibition of EGFR using a therapeutic monoclonal antibody would not yield any effect. This indeed was shown to be true and has led to the requirement for patients' tumors to be sequenced for *KRAS* prior to receiving anti-EGFR antibody therapies to ensure that only wild-type *KRAS* is present in the cancer.[8] The success and approval of mutation-specific KRAS inhibitors[9] may allow for future combination therapies.

Additional opportunities for therapeutic targeting have arisen through a better understanding of cancer genetics. "Synthetic lethality" is an idea originally based on the realization that the absence of the BRCA proteins would lead to a therapeutic vulnerability, which could be exploited because the noncancerous cells in the affected individual would still harbor 50% of a given BRCA protein due to the intact wild-type allele (Fig. 166-4). Hence, original laboratory studies demonstrated that poly adenosine diphosphate-ribose polymerase (PARP) inhibitors could effectively kill *BRCA* null cells but spare their wild-type counterparts.[10] These findings were rapidly translated into clinical trials that have led to the approval of PARP inhibitors for some ovarian (Chapter 184), breast (Chapter 183), pancreas (Chapter 180), and prostate (Chapter 186) cancers.

Although targeted therapies are generally initially approved in a single cancer tissue type, it is the target, not the particular cell type, that determines susceptibility to a targeted therapy. For example, HER2 amplified/overexpressing gastric cancers (Chapter 178) can respond to trastuzumab. Similarly, BRAF V600 oncogenic mutations generally respond to targeted

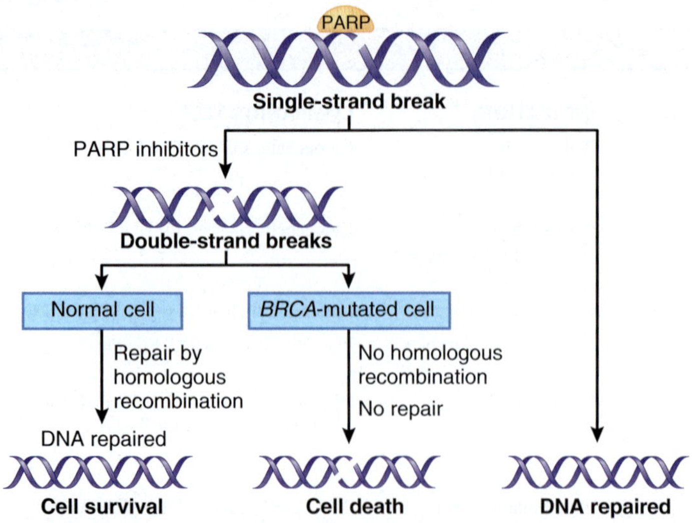

FIGURE 166-4. Poly(ADP-ribose) polymerase (PARP) inhibitors and synthetic lethality in BRCA null cells. PARP1 binds to DNA single-strand breaks that frequently occur during the cell cycle and recruits other enzymes to repair damaged DNA. Failure to repair DNA will eventually lead to further DNA damage and cell death. The BRCA pathway proteins can also repair this damaged DNA via homologous recombination. Because BRCA mediated cancers lack a BRCA protein, this ability to repair DNA via homologous recombination is lost. This is the basis for synthetic lethal and targeted therapy with PARP inhibitors in patients with BRCA-related cancers. DNA damage that occurs after inhibition of PARP activity cannot be repaired in BRCA null cancers, resulting in cell death. As BRCA proteins remain intact in noncancerous cells due to the retention of one functional copy of a *BRCA* gene, PARP inhibition selectively kills cancer cells. (From Sonnenblick A, de Azambuja E, Azim HA Jr, et al. An update on PARP inhibitors—moving to the adjuvant setting. *Nat Rev Clin Oncol.* 2015;12:27-41.)

therapies of V600 inhibitors, although colorectal cancers seem to be a notable exception.[11] Interestingly, suppression with BRAF V600 mutant inhibitors can lead to dysregulation of feedback networks in normal and cancerous cells. Combination therapies, including inhibitors of MEK, which is a molecule distal to BRAF in the MAP kinase pathway (E-Fig. 166-1), result in more efficacious therapy with fewer side effects. Another example of molecular targeted therapies is larotrectinib, which is an inhibitor of TRK proteins that have been made constitutively active via translocation of *TRK* genes with other genes, also known as fusion partners. This potent inhibitor has striking antineoplastic activity against a variety of tumor types, provided they have either a *TRK1*, *TRK2*, or *TRK3* translocation that leads to constitutive activation.[12] Both larotrectinib and entrectinib, which is another *TRK* inhibitor, are now FDA-approved for responsive cancer.

Research also led to the first approved antineoplastic therapy based upon the type of genetic instability. Melanomas and squamous cell lung cancers with high mutation burden are more likely to respond to immune check point inhibitors, in part because ultraviolet light and tobacco exposure, respectively, led to their high mutation burdens. Cancers with a high tumor mutation burden imparted by microsatellite instability have a significantly higher response rate to immune checkpoint inhibitor therapies, often even if such tumors have become refractory to all other therapies.[13]

CANCER GENETICS FOR DIAGNOSTICS

GENE EXPRESSION PROFILING FOR PROGNOSIS AND PREDICTION

The majority of RNA prognostic and predictive tests do not measure DNA alterations but instead assess relative levels of RNA within a tumor. These RNA levels are then used for various algorithms that have been validated for both prognostic information (i.e., the likelihood of recurrence and/or survival over a defined time frame) as well as predictive power (i.e., the likelihood of a patient benefitting from a given therapy). Several such tests have been validated in prospective trials[14] to help inform clinical decisions.

DIAGNOSTIC TESTS FOR TARGETED THERAPIES

Targeted therapies require genetic testing to select patients who will have the highest likelihood of responding to a given agent. For example, early studies of trastuzumab would likely have failed had patients not been preselected for HER2 amplification, given that the majority of breast cancers are HER2 negative. Next-generation sequencing (also see Chapter 33) involves generation of DNA "libraries" that are sequenced simultaneously (i.e., massively and in parallel), thereby generating terabytes or more of data. Redundant sequencing is needed to ensure that each nucleotide is sequenced enough times to differentiate true mutations from artifacts of the next-generation sequencing process. Each DNA molecule that is sequenced is then aligned against a reference genome to determine the presence or absence of mutations.

Because reference genomes are derived from a variety of sources, it is not always possible to distinguish a mutation from a normal variant that could exist within the population. As such, "germline sequencing and filtering" is becoming more commonplace for tumor sequencing. This technique entails obtaining a normal DNA sample from the patient whose tumor is being sequenced and subjecting the normal germline DNA to next-generation sequencing. After sequencing and alignment, the germline DNA is electronically subtracted from the tumor DNA to reveal only somatic mutations. Although this process can reduce the number of false-positive mutations, it also can potentially filter out important germline mutations that may have therapeutic relevance for a given cancer (e.g., *BRCA1*, *BRCA2*, *MLH1*, and *MSH2*). Newer bioinformatic methods may circumvent these issues by either not filtering germline mutations in key genes or identifying the likelihood of somatic versus germline mutations with the use of statistical algorithms.

Ongoing clinical trials are trying to exploit cancer DNA as a general diagnostic screening tool. For example, multitarget analysis of stool specimens using mutation testing, epigenetic markers, and a hemoglobin immunoassay has a relatively high sensitivity and specificity for detecting early-stage colorectal cancers,[15] and is now FDA-approved for colorectal cancer screening.

Next-generation sequencing has also brought to reality the concept of a "liquid biopsy," which is testing for circulating cell-free DNA for cancer diagnostics. All cells, cancerous and normal, shed DNA into the circulation.[16] This cell-free DNA can be isolated and analyzed by next-generation sequencing for a variety of purposes including identifying circulating tumor DNA using various substrates such as plasma, serum, urine, saliva, and others.[17,18] Next-generation sequencing, polymerase chain reaction testing, and other technologies have now become commonplace for detecting tumor mutations in the circulation.[19] Cell-free DNA is also being studied as a marker for residual cancer burden, response to therapies, and prognosis. In addition, asymptomatic clonal hematopoiesis, whereby precancerous stem cells accumulate genetic mutations that increase the risk of malignant transformation,[20] is another potential marker of prognosis. Interventions based on these new technologies have the potential to revolutionize how patients are treated for both early- and late-stage cancers, thereby allowing for precise knowledge of whether therapies are truly eradicating microscopic residual disease and effecting cures.

GENERAL REFERENCES

For the General References and other additional features, please visit Elsevier eBooks+ at https://ebooks.health.elsevier.com.

167

MYELODYSPLASTIC SYNDROMES

RICHARD M. STONE

DEFINITION

The myelodysplastic syndromes include a heterogeneous group of bone marrow failure syndromes collectively characterized by ineffective hematopoiesis that results in peripheral blood cytopenias, most commonly anemia.[1] In some patients, the distinction between myelodysplastic syndrome and acute myeloid leukemia (AML; Chapter 168) may be challenging.[2] Although the dominant clinical feature of myelodysplastic syndromes is bone marrow failure, myelodysplastic syndromes are clonal disorders and therefore classified as hematopoietic neoplasms by the World Health Organization (WHO) and other organizations.

EPIDEMIOLOGY

The incidence and prevalence of myelodysplastic syndromes have been difficult to estimate accurately, in part because of varying definitions and imprecise terminology historically, and also because myelodysplastic syndrome cases are incompletely captured by cancer registries. About 10,000 to 12,000 new cases are officially diagnosed each year, but analysis of Medicare claims suggests that the actual incidence of myelodysplastic syndromes is much higher, with at least 40,000 new U.S. cases per year—more than twice the incidence of AML. In addition, many geriatric patients have mild cytopenias and may have myelodysplastic syndromes that have been incompletely evaluated (e.g., they do not undergo bone marrow aspiration) and never are specifically diagnosed.

The primary risk factor for development of a myelodysplastic syndrome is aging, with disease resulting as a consequence of cumulative acquisition of somatic mutations in marrow stem cells. In Asia and Eastern Europe, a myelodysplastic syndrome is typically diagnosed at younger ages than in the West; in the United States, the median age at which myelodysplastic syndromes are diagnosed is about 71 years, whereas in China it is closer to 50 years. Overall, males are slightly more affected than females.

The rate at which myelodysplastic syndromes are diagnosed is slightly increased in workers in certain industries such as the petroleum industry and agricultural sector, probably because of exposure to agents that favor expansion of mutant clones. Individuals who have been exposed to ionizing radiation or to certain types of cytotoxic chemotherapy (i.e., alkylating agents such as chlorambucil or melphalan, or topoisomerase II inhibitors such as etoposide or doxorubicin) have an increased risk for developing myelodysplastic syndromes. The peak incidence at which a myelodysplastic syndrome is diagnosed after exposure to an alkylating agent or radiation is 5 to 10 years later, whereas it is 1 to 3 years after exposure to a topoisomerase inhibitor. This increased risk never completely disappears; even 50 years after the Hiroshima and Nagasaki atomic bomb events in Japan, radiation-exposed individuals continued to be diagnosed with myelodysplastic syndromes at a higher rate than the unexposed population. Patients with a chemotherapy or radiation exposure history are said to have therapy-related myelodysplastic syndromes.

PATHOBIOLOGY

Myelodysplastic syndromes are clonal disorders, by which it is meant that one or several stem or progenitor cells in the marrow that bear somatic gene mutations proliferate at the expense of healthy stem cells, and these mutation-bearing progeny eventually come to dominate the bone marrow. Clones can acquire additional mutations that give rise to subclones, which can contribute to progression of disease if they have a greater proliferation potential than the original mutant clone. The process of somatic mutation acquisition may be accelerated through exposure to radiation or DNA-damaging chemicals, but more important, such exposures can also select for small *TP53* or *PPM1D* mutant preexisting clones. The marrow microenvironment (i.e., nonhematopoietic stromal cells) appears to play an important role in supporting neoplastic clones.

Marrow cellularity is usually normal or increased in myelodysplastic syndromes, but excessive apoptosis (i.e., programmed cell death) of hematopoietic cells within the bone marrow accounts for the peripheral blood cytopenias. Although excessive apoptosis within the marrow characterizes earlier phases of myelodysplastic syndromes, as the disease progresses toward AML, intramedullary apoptosis may decrease. In addition, hematopoietic differentiation, which is disordered but still can proceed in earlier stages of the disease, may become completely impaired later in the disease course such that most developing hematopoietic cells are arrested at the myeloblast stage.

Large gains and losses of chromosomal material within the disease cells, detectable by routine metaphase karyotyping, are present in one half of patients with de novo myelodysplastic syndromes and in more than 80% of patients with therapy-related myelodysplastic syndromes. Genetic techniques such as array-based comparative genomic hybridization can uncover cryptic chromosomal deletions in some patients whose myelodysplastic syndromes are associated with normal karyotyping results.

More than 40 genes are now known to be recurrently mutated in myelodysplastic syndromes,[3] but most of these mutations are also commonly detected in AML and other myeloid neoplasms, albeit at different frequencies.[4] No single mutation dominates; myelodysplastic syndromes are associated with considerable genetic heterogeneity (Table 167-1). More than 90% of patients with myelodysplastic syndromes have at least one detectable clonal somatic mutation, which influences the clinical presentation and prognosis. Mutations affecting epigenetic patterning through DNA methylation and chromatin conformation (e.g., histone-DNA interactions) are common.[5] In addition, mutations affecting pre-mRNA splicing are frequent,[6] especially in patients with ring sideroblasts (i.e., erythroid precursors with abnormal perinuclear iron-containing mitochondria visible with Perls Prussian blue reaction) (see Fig. 167-1C); the specific genes that are mis-spliced and give rise to a myelodysplastic syndrome phenotype are as yet unclear.

Genetic bone marrow failure syndromes such as Schwachman-Diamond and Fanconi anemia (Chapter 151) are associated with myelodysplastic syndrome in children.[7] Up to 20% of adults with myelodysplastic syndrome may have a germline predisposition, and inherited forms of myelodysplastic syndrome, such as Schwachman-Diamond, may present in the sixth decade of life or later.

A subset of patients with pathologic findings that resemble a myelodysplastic syndrome will have autoimmune hematopoietic suppression, which may be driven by an expanded autoreactive T-lymphocyte population. Patients are more likely to have an immune component to their marrow failure if they are younger than 55 years and have a hypocellular marrow similar to what is seen in aplastic anemia, a normal chromosome pattern or trisomy 8 (rather than a more complex karyotype), a paroxysmal nocturnal hemoglobinuria cell population detectable by flow cytometry (Chapter 146), and HLA DR15 tissue type. Such patients may respond to immunosuppressive anti-T-cell therapies.

CLINICAL MANIFESTATIONS

Most patients with myelodysplastic syndromes come to medical attention because they have anemia. Anemia is present in 95% cases and is often macrocytic, but about 50% of patients also have neutropenia, thrombocytopenia, or both at the time of diagnosis.

The clinical course in myelodysplastic syndromes is dominated by complications of the cytopenias, including mucosal bleeding, recurrent infections, and exertional dyspnea and fatigue. Fatigue correlates poorly with the degree of anemia and may be in part due to cytokine release by the abnormal clonal cells. Paraneoplastic manifestations, including neutrophilic dermatosis (Sweet syndrome, Chapters 406 and 407), inflammatory arthritis, and other rheumatologic syndromes, occur in 10 to 15% of patients. Repeated transfusions of red cells can lead to transfusional hemosiderosis and organ dysfunction, including hepatic and cardiac disease. The frequency with which complications of iron overload occur, as well as the importance of chelation therapy in myelodysplastic syndromes, are controversial topics.[8]

DIAGNOSIS

Myelodysplastic syndromes are usually suspected when an older patient is discovered to have cytopenias, especially macrocytic anemia that is not due to B_{12} or folate deficiency, medication effect (e.g., methotrexate or azathioprine), or alcohol abuse. The blood count abnormality may be an incidental finding, but most patients with myelodysplastic syndromes are symptomatic with fatigue, dyspnea, and other cytopenia-associated symptoms.

The peripheral blood exhibits characteristic "dysplastic" cell morphologic abnormalities. In the peripheral blood, these abnormalities include hypogranular neutrophils, hypolobated neutrophils such as the two-lobed pseudo-Pelger-Hüet cell (Fig. 143-20), increased platelet size and platelet hypogranularity, poorly hemoglobinized red cells, and circulating early myeloid cells including a small number of myeloblasts (Chapter 143).

A bone marrow aspirate is required to make the diagnosis, and bone marrow core (trephine) biopsy is also useful and can provide information about the marrow architecture and overall marrow cellularity.[9] Maturation abnormalities in the bone marrow include megaloblastoid erythroid changes, multinucleated erythroid cells, ring sideroblasts, nuclear karyorrhexis, left-shifted myelopoiesis, hypogranular white cells, micromegakaryocytes, large hypernucleated megakaryocytes, or hypolobated megakaryocytes (Fig. 167-1). A mild increase in reticulin fibrosis is common in myelodysplastic syndromes, but severe reticulin fibrosis and collagen fibrosis are rare. Extramedullary hematopoiesis is uncommon in myelodysplastic syndromes, and the presence of splenomegaly or hepatomegaly should prompt consideration of another diagnosis. Metaphase cytogenetics is essential, whereas fluorescence in situ hybridization (FISH) is only necessary if karyotyping fails because of unsuccessful marrow aspiration. FISH abnormalities are rarely detected in patients for whom at least 20 metaphases can be counted during karyotyping. Flow cytometric immunophenotyping can provide useful diagnostic and prognostic information but should not be relied on to count blast proportion.

Although not technically required to make the diagnosis, a next generation sequencing panel can provide adjunctive diagnostic information. Genetic-clinical correlations including a thrombocytopenic prodrome in RUNX1 mutant patients and the association of GATA2 mutations with mycobacterial infections, warts, or monocytopenia. Patients with a *TP53* mutation may warrant identification because of their poorer prognosis.[10]

TABLE 167-1 GENE MUTATIONS ASSOCIATED WITH MYELODYSPLASTIC SYNDROMES AND FUNCTIONAL CLASS OF THE ASSOCIATED PROTEIN

RECURRENTLY MUTATED GENES	MUTATION FREQUENCY IN MDS	ADDITIONAL NOTES
SPLICEOSOME COMPONENTS (ALTER PRE-mRNA SPLICING)		
SF3B1	20-25%	Strongly associated with the presence of ring sideroblasts (60-80% of MDS-RS cases), often co-occurs with *DNMT3A* mutations; associated with more favorable outlook
U2AF1	5-10%	Often co-occurs with del(20q)
SRSF2	5-10%	More frequent in CMML (25-30%) than in MDS without proliferative features, often co-occurs with *RUNX1* or *ASXL1* mutations
ZRSR2	3-5%	
U2AF2, SFRA1, PRPF40B, SF1	<2% each	
EPIGENETIC PATTERN AND CHROMATIN CONFORMATION MODIFIERS		
TET2	20-25%	More frequent in CMML (~40%)
DNMT3A	10-15%	Low variant allele frequency mutations are also commonly found in the healthy elderly population
SETBP1	5-10%	More common in CMML; associated with adverse prognosis in that setting
ASXL1	10-20%	More frequent in CMML (~40%)
**EZH2*	6%	More frequent in CMML (~12%)
KDM6A	<2%	Rare in MDS, more frequent in CMML
IDH1, IDH2	<2%	More frequent in AML than MDS; amenable to targeted therapy with novel agents
PHF6	<1%	
ATRX	Rare	Associated with acquired α-thalassemia (hemoglobin H inclusions in red blood cells)
TRANSCRIPTION FACTORS/DNA REPAIR		
**RUNX1*	10-15%	Germline mutations cause Familial Platelet Disorder with propensity to AML (FPD-AML)
ETV6	<5%	Translocations common in AML; formerly known as *TEL*
MYBL2	<1%	
GATA2	Rare	Germline mutations cause familial MDS with monocytopenia
CEBPA	Rare	More frequently mutated in AML, germline mutations cause familial AML without preceding dysplasia
WT1	Rare	More frequently mutated in AML
**TP53*	5-10%	Associated with very poor prognosis; associated with t-MDS and with complex karyotype
TYROSINE KINASE SIGNALING		As a group, these genes are more often mutated in myeloid malignancies with a proliferative component
NRAS, KRAS, BRAF	5-10% collectively	*NRAS* mutations more common in CMML and AML; first mutations described in MDS (1987)
JAK2	<5%	More frequent in MDS/MPN with ring sideroblasts and thrombocytosis (MDS/MPN-RS-T) (50%)
CBL, CBLB	<5%	More frequently mutated in CMML than MDS
FLT3, MPL, KIT	<1%	*MPL* mutated in (5%) of MDS/MPN-RS-T; *FLT3* and *KIT* mutations are rare in MDS and much more common in AML
NF1	<1%	Germline mutations cause neurofibromatosis type 1
PTPN11	<1%	Rare in MDS, more frequent in JMML (30%)
OTHERS		
NPM1	<2%	Much more frequently mutated in AML
GNAS	<1%	
BCOR, BCORL1	<1%	More common in aplastic anemia
PIGA	<1%	Associated with a *PNH* clone; more common in paroxysmal nocturnal hemoglobinuria
UMODL1	<1%	
ZSWIM4	<1%	
PPM1D	1-3%	Associated with t-MDS
Cohesins (*RAD21, STAG1, STAG2, SMC3, SMC1A*)	5-10%	Despite role in chromatid segregation, not associated with numerical chromosome abnormalities

*Mutations that appear to be independently associated with poor outcomes in myelodysplastic syndromes (MDS).

AML = acute myeloid leukemia; CMML = chronic myelomonocytic leukemia; JMML = juvenile myelomonocytic leukemia; MDS = myelodysplastic syndromes; MDS-RS = MDS with ringed sideroblasts; MDS/MPN-RS-T = MDS/myeloproliferative neoplasm overlap syndrome with ring sideroblasts and thrombocytosis; pre-mRNA = precursor-messenger RNA; t-MDS = therapy-related myelodysplastic syndrome.

Data based on Bejar R, Levine R, Ebert BL. Unraveling the molecular pathophysiology of myelodysplastic syndromes. *J Clin Oncol.* 2011;29:504-515; Bejar R, Papaemmanuil E, Haferlach T, et al. Somatic mutations in MDS patients are associated with clinical features and predict prognosis independent of the IPSS-R: analysis of combined datasets from the International Working Group for Prognosis in MDS-Molecular Committee. *Blood.* 2015;126:907; and others.

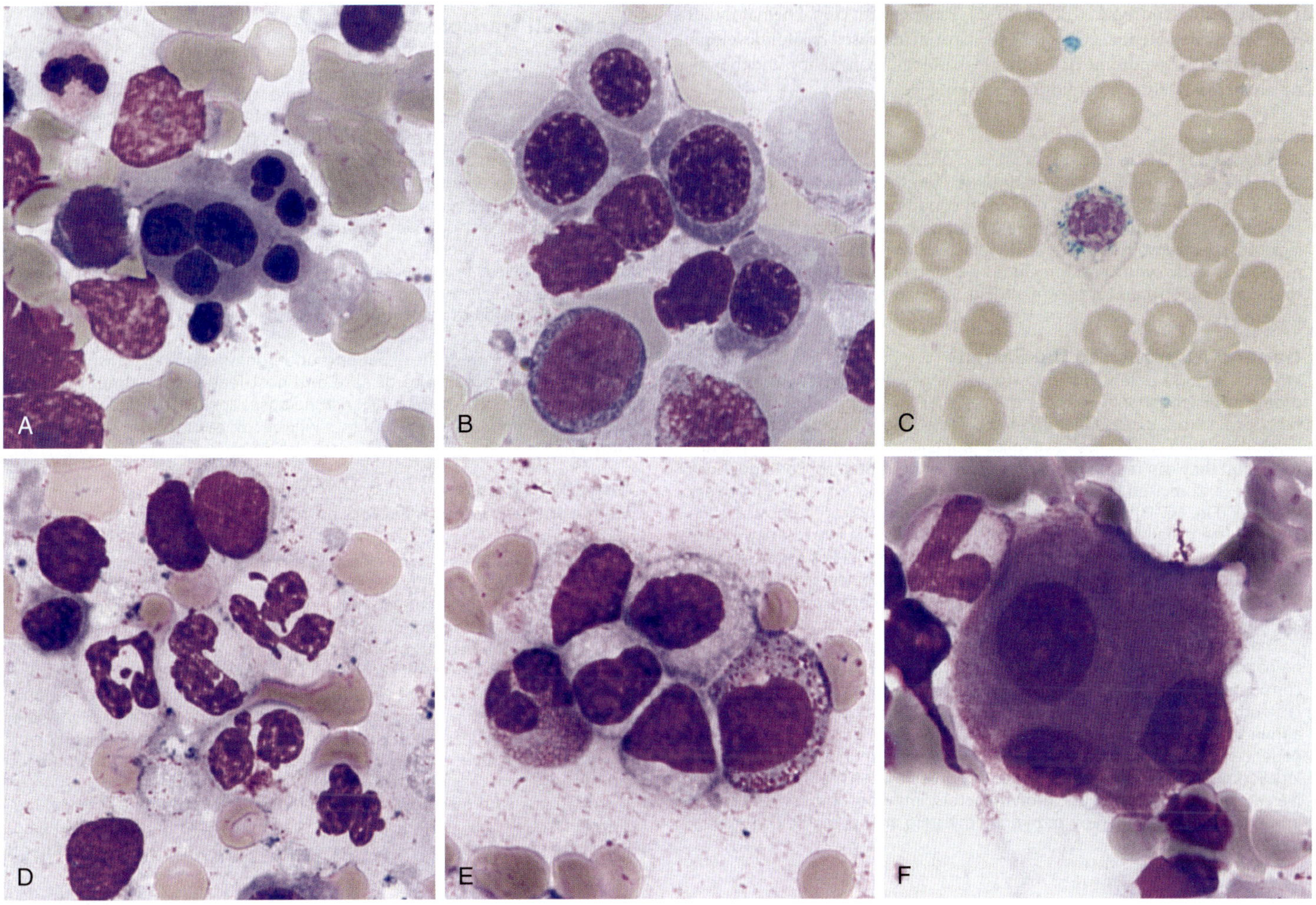

FIGURE 167-1. **"Dysplastic" cell morphologic abnormalities commonly observed in the peripheral blood or marrow patients with myelodysplastic syndromes. A, Multinucleated erythroid precursor. B, Megaloblastoid maturation of erythroid precursors with "open" nuclear chromatin. C, Ring sideroblast (pathologic erythroid precursor with iron granules surrounding at least one third of the nucleus). D, Hypogranular neutrophils. E, Pseudo-Pelger-Huët anomaly (hypolobated neutrophil). F, Abnormal nuclear lobation in a megakaryocyte—a "pawn ball" cell with three separated nuclei/nuclear lobes. *A, B, D,* and *F* are Wright-Giemsa stained marrow aspirate; *C* is Perls' Prussian blue reaction of marrow aspirate; *E* is Wright-Giemsa stained peripheral blood. (Courtesy Elizabeth A. Morgan, MD, PhD, Brigham & Women's Hospital, Boston, MA.)**

Diagnostic Criteria

Minimal diagnostic criteria for a myelodysplastic syndrome include the presence of one or more cytopenias, together with at least one additional feature. These features include: 5 to 19% marrow myeloblasts (although patients who have 10 to 19% marrow blasts may be classified as having myelodysplastic syndrome/acute myeloid leukemia);[11] an abnormal marrow karyotype with an acquired chromosome anomaly that is consistent with the diagnosis of a myelodysplastic syndrome;[12] or greater than 10% cells in any given hematopoietic linage that appears dysplastic (i.e., morphologically abnormal) in a patient in whom other causes of dysplastic cell morphology, such as nutritional deficiency or a drug effect, have been excluded.

Differential Diagnosis

Specific Other Diagnoses

Dysplastic hematopoiesis has a broad differential diagnosis, and other potential causes for cytopenias and morphologic abnormalities must be considered. This differential diagnosis includes nonclonal disorders such as B_{12} or folate deficiency (Chapter 150), copper deficiency (especially if ring sideroblasts are present), iron deficiency (Chapter 145), HIV infection, medication exposure (especially cytotoxic chemotherapy agents), or an immune disorder such as T-cell large granular lymphocyte (T-LGL) leukemia. In patients with isolated sideroblastic anemia (Chapter 145), it is important to exclude congenital sideroblastic anemias, including those due to germline mutations in *ALAS2*, which can present late in life.

Myelodysplastic syndromes must be distinguished from aplastic anemia (Chapter 151), which can be oligoclonal and associated with some of the same somatic mutations as myelodysplastic syndromes, but which is not typically associated with Pelger-Hüet cells or other morphologic abnormalities. The karyotype in aplastic anemia is usually (but not always) normal. Myelodysplastic syndromes can also be mistaken for a myeloproliferative neoplasm such as primary myelofibrosis (Chapter 152). Cases in which myelodysplastic syndrome features, such as cytopenias, overlap with myeloproliferative neoplasm features, such as leukocytosis and splenomegaly, include chronic myelomonocytic leukemia, which requires >1000 monocytes/μL in the blood to diagnose. The WHO categorizes myelodysplastic syndrome/myeloproliferative neoplasm overlap syndromes separately from myelodysplastic syndromes, and these cases have a distinct mutational spectrum.

Variants of Myelodysplastic Syndrome

Some patients with persistent cytopenias do not meet diagnostic criteria for a myelodysplastic syndrome, but no other diagnosis is apparent, even after detailed investigation.[13] This pattern has been termed *idiopathic cytopenias of undetermined significance* if a clonal somatic mutation is absent and *clonal cytopenias of undetermined significance* if a somatic myelodysplastic syndrome-associated mutation (e.g., *DNMT3A, TET2*) is present. Such patients should be followed over time because they have a risk for developing an overt myelodysplastic syndrome, especially if they have a clonal cytopenia of undetermined significance. More than 10% of the healthy population age 70 years or older have a somatic mutation in *DNMT3A, TET2*, or another myelodysplastic syndrome-associated gene; therefore, identification of a clonal mutation in the absence of any myelodysplastic syndrome feature (called *clonal hematopoiesis of indeterminate potential*) is not considered diagnostic of a myelodysplastic syndrome. If a patient has cytopenias even in the absence of characteristic myelodysplastic syndrome-associated morphologic abnormalities and a typical myelodysplastic syndrome-associated marrow cytogenetic abnormality (e.g., loss of chromosome 7 or deletion of the long arm of chromosome 5), the patient can be considered to have "unclassifiable myelodysplastic syndrome" (Table 167-2). Patients with clonal hematopoiesis of indeterminate potential (Chapter 142) have an increased risk for developing a myelodysplastic syndrome or another hematologic malignancy, and they also have an increased risk for cardiovascular mortality.[14]

TREATMENT

Given the heterogeneity of myelodysplastic syndromes and the wide spectrum of functional status and comorbid conditions among patients with myelodysplastic syndromes, treatment must be individualized.[15-17] Currently, lack of a specific well-characterized molecular target in most patients with myelodysplastic syndromes precludes a true biologically based approach to therapy. Algorithms for treatment (Fig. 167-2) are based primarily on the patient's prognosis.

General Approach to the Patient

When choosing a potential therapy for a patient with a myelodysplastic syndrome, clinicians should consider the patient's age,[18] comorbid conditions, functional status, disease biology, and disease kinetics. Some patients with myelodysplastic syndromes have mild cytopenias and minimal or no symptoms, and they can reasonably be observed without therapy. For higher-risk patients (e.g., revised International Prognostic Scoring System high or very high risk [Fig. 167-3]), immediate therapy is usually indicated because such patients are usually severely cytopenic and have a life expectancy of less than 2 years. For lower-risk patients (very low risk or low risk on the revised International Prognostic Scoring System or the Molecular International Prognostic Scoring System [https://mds-risk-model.com]), a more cautious approach is appropriate.

The only curative modality for a myelodysplastic syndrome is allogeneic hematopoietic stem cell transplantation (Chapter 163), so this option should be considered in developing a therapeutic plan if the patient is young enough and lacks other major medical problems. If transplantation is not the goal, prolonged administration of hypomethylating agents is generally indicated. In lower-risk patients who have a chromosome 5 abnormality, the immunomodulatory agent lenalidomide is the treatment of choice. For other lower-risk patients, supportive care alone, hematopoietic growth factors, immunosuppressive therapy, immunomodulatory therapy, or hypomethylating agents can be considered, depending on the clinical situation.

Stem Cell Transplantation

Allogeneic hematopoietic stem cell transplantation (Chapter 163) should be considered promptly and generally be performed if feasible in all patients who have higher-risk myelodysplastic syndromes, who are approximately age 75 years or younger, and who lack major comorbid conditions. Allogeneic transplantation also may lead to better outcomes than medical therapy alone in higher-risk patients age 55 years or older.[19-21] The optimal conditioning regimen is unclear.[A1] Reduced-intensity conditioning stem cell transplantation is feasible in adults up to age 75 years, whereas myelosuppressive stem cell transplantation is generally reserved for patients younger than age 55 years.

Because most patients with myelodysplastic syndromes are older and uncommonly have a younger sibling who is a suitable stem cell donor, azacitidine or decitabine (see DNA Hypomethylating Agents) may be useful to stabilize a patient before transplantation while the search for an unrelated donor is ongoing.

The long-term outcome of patients undergoing stem cell transplantation varies widely according to disease and host features. Treatment-related mortality is as high as a 15 to 20% risk. Relapses are unfortunately common, but approximately 40% of patients will become long-term disease-free survivors.

Supportive Care

Hematopoietic Growth Factors and Other Approaches to Cytopenias

Because most patients with myelodysplastic syndromes are anemic, the erythropoiesis-stimulating agents epoetin and darbepoetin[A2] are often used under expert supervision, even though these agents are not specifically approved by the U.S. Food and Drug Administration (FDA) for treatment of myelodysplastic syndromes. The benefits of erythropoiesis-stimulating agents are generally modest and of limited duration. Patients with lower baseline serum erythropoietin levels (<500 U/L, and especially <100 U/L) are more likely to respond to erythropoiesis-stimulating agents than are patients with higher baseline serum erythropoietin levels. For patients with ring sideroblasts, the addition of low-dose granulocyte colony-stimulating factor (G-CSF) to the erythropoiesis-stimulating agent may potentiate the erythropoietic response.

In patients who have lower-risk myelodysplastic syndromes (>15% ring sideroblasts, or >5% ringed sideroblasts and an SF3B1 mutation) and who have high erythropoietin levels or have become refractory to or intolerant of

TABLE 167-2 WORLD HEALTH ORGANIZATION SUBTYPES OF MYELODYSPLASTIC SYNDROME (MDS)

MDS SUBTYPE	DYSPLASIA	BLAST COUNT	OTHER FINDINGS
MDS with single-lineage dysplasia (MDS-SLD)	• Present in only 1 lineage (>10% of cells in that lineage)	• Peripheral blood: <1% • Bone marrow: <5%	• Cases with bilineage cytopenias may be included in this category, but marrow dysplasia must be limited to 1 lineage • Ring sideroblasts represent <15% of erythroid precursors
MDS with ring sideroblasts (MDS-RS)	• Present in the erythroid lineage (>10% of erythroid precursors); subtypes with single-lineage dysplasia (MDS-RS-SLD) and with multilineage dysplasia (MDS-RS-MLD)	• Peripheral blood: none • Bone marrow: <5%	• Anemia (normocytic/macrocytic) • Ring sideroblasts comprise ≥15% of erythroid precursors or if *SF3B1* mutation is present ≥5% of erythroid precursors
MDS with multilineage dysplasia (MDS-MLD)	• Present in 2 or more lineages (>10% of cells in each affected lineage)	• Peripheral blood: <1% • Bone marrow: <5%	• One or more cytopenias • No Auer rods • If ≥15% of erythroid precursors or if *SF3B1* mutation is present in ≥5% of erythroid precursors, represents MDS-RS-MLD
MDS with excess blasts-1 (MDS-EB-1)	• Present in 1 or more lineages (>10% of cells in each affected lineage)	• Peripheral blood: <5% • Bone marrow: 5-9%	• One or more cytopenias • No Auer rods • 2-4% blasts in the peripheral blood → MDS-EB-1
MDS with excess blasts-2 (MDS-EB-2)	• Present in 1 or more lineages (>10% of cells in each affected lineage)	• Peripheral blood: 5-19% • Bone marrow: 10-19%	• One or more cytopenias • The presence of Auer rods for any blast count <20% → MDS-EB-2
MDS with isolated deletion of chromosome 5q (5q− syndrome)	• Increased numbers of megakaryocytes, many small and with hypolobated/nonlobated nuclei • Minimal or no dysplasia in granulocytic lineage	• Peripheral blood: no or rare blasts (<1%) • Bone marrow: <5%	• Anemia (often macrocytic) with or without other cytopenias/thrombocytosis • No Auer rods • Interstitial or terminal deletion of the long arm of chromosome 5 with no or one other cytogenetic abnormality
MDS, unclassifiable	• Unequivocal, but present in <10% of cells of one or more lineages	• Peripheral blood: ≤1% • Bone marrow: <5%	• May progress to a specific MDS • Can also include cases otherwise classified as: MDS-SLD or MDS-MLD but with 1% blasts in peripheral blood; MDS-SLD but with pancytopenia • Cases with an MDS-associated chromosome abnormality (other than loss of the Y chromosome or trisomy 8 or deletion of chromosome 20) but without dysplasia can be included in this category

Data based on the 2016 WHO classification of hematopoietic and lymphoid neoplasms (Arber D, Orazi A, Hasserjian R, et al. The 2016 revision to the World Health Organization classification of myeloid neoplasms and acute leukemia. *Blood* 2016:127:2391-2405), which was a minor revision of the 2008 classification. Familial myeloid neoplasms are classified separately, as are therapy-related myeloid neoplasia and myelodysplastic syndromes with myeloproliferative neoplasm features.

- Consider clinical trial enrollment for all patients
- Supportive care (e.g., transfusions and antimicrobials as needed) for all patients; consider chelation
- Risk stratification using the Revised International Prognostic Scoring System (see Table 167-2) supplemented by molecular testing

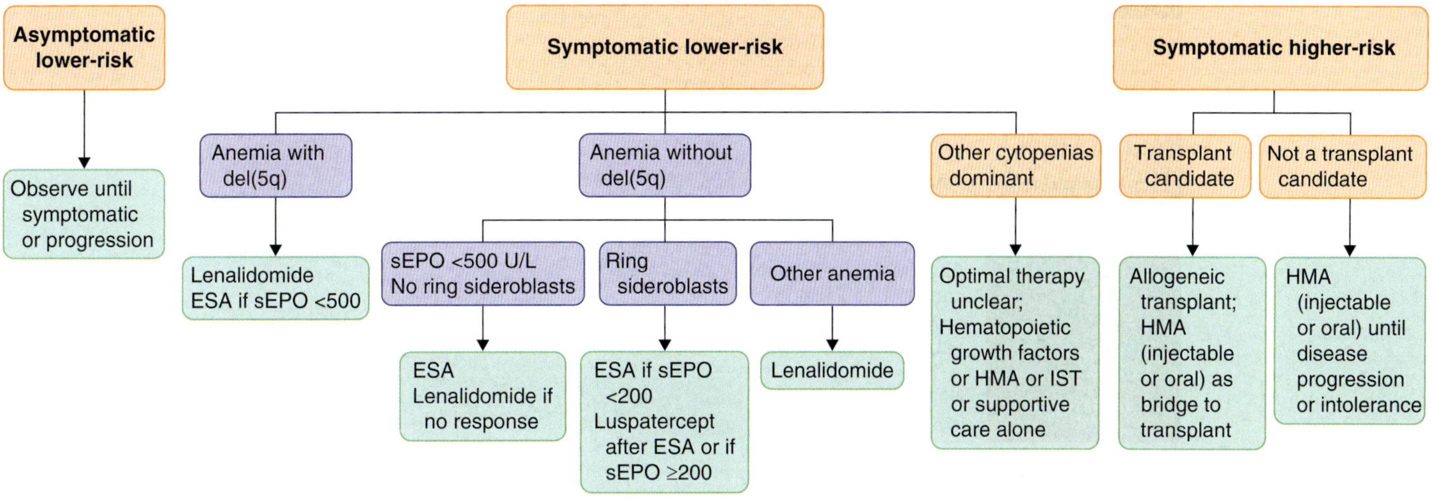

FIGURE 167-2. **Treatment algorithm in myelodysplastic syndromes.** EPO = erythropoietin; ESA = erythropoiesis-stimulating agent; HMA = DNA hypomethylating agent; IST = immunosuppressive therapy; sEPO = serum erythropoietin level. (Adapted from Steensma DP. Myelodysplastic syndromes current treatment algorithm 2018. *Blood Cancer J.* 2018;8:1-7.)

erythropoiesis-stimulating agents, luspatercept (1.0 to 1.75 mg/kg subcutaneously every 3 weeks) can reduce the severity of anemia by binding to cytokines that have a negative effect on erythropoiesis.[A3] A few patients will benefit from treatment with androgens, but the risk for prostate enlargement (in men) and other complications such as hepatotoxicity must be considered.

Myeloid growth factors such as G-CSF can ameliorate the neutropenia often seen in myelodysplastic syndrome patients but is not likely to reduce the risk for infections or provide other clinical benefits because of the frequency of neutrophil dysfunction in addition to neutropenia. Prophylactic antimicrobial agents have no clear role, but they can be considered in patients who have experienced recurrent infections or are at particularly high risk.

The thrombopoiesis-stimulating agents romiplostim and eltrombopag are not approved by the FDA for myelodysplastic syndromes and may induce progression to AML in some patients, but they may be useful in patients who have severe thrombocytopenia or clinically significant bleeding.[A4] Platelet transfusions should be used carefully in myelodysplastic syndrome patients because of the risk for alloimmunization. Prophylactic transfusion is appropriate only in patients with platelet counts less than 10,000/μL. Patients with mucosal bleeding and refractory thrombocytopenia may benefit from treatment with antifibrinolytic agents such as aminocaproic acid under expert supervision.

Iron Chelation Therapy

The multiple red blood cell (RBC) transfusions needed by some patients with myelodysplastic syndromes may cause iron overload and tissue injury, but the frequency with which this complication occurs is unclear. Furthermore, the toxicity and high cost of available chelators (e.g., deferasirox, deferiprone, or deferoxamine) makes their use controversial. A trial of iron chelation therapy is reasonable in patients with lower-risk disease and high transfusional burdens (e.g., more than 20 to 40 RBC units transfused).[A5]

Disease-Modifying Medical Therapy

DNA Hypomethylating Agents

Azacitidine and decitabine are two azanucleoside analogues that inhibit the enzyme DNA methyltransferase, thereby altering the cytosine methylation "epigenetic" status of DNA and changing gene expression. These agents have become the mainstay of therapy for most patients with higher-risk myelodysplastic syndromes, as well as for patients whose lower-risk myelodysplastic syndromes are refractory to other therapies.[22]

Azacitidine (75 mg/m^2 subcutaneously or intravenously daily for 7 days every month, given until disease progression or toxicity) can delay progression to AML, improve quality of life, and increase median survival from 15 to 24 months.[A6] Cytopenias and gastrointestinal symptoms are the most common adverse effects of this class of drugs.

Decitabine under expert supervision also can delay disease progression. Short courses of this agent may yield particular benefit in patients with lower-risk myelodysplastic syndrome.[A7] An oral formulation in combination with cedazuridine (i.e., a cytidine deaminase inhibitor that inhibits first-pass metabolism of the decitabine) provides responses similar to injectable decitabine.[23]

Although at least 50% of patients who receive a hypomethylating agent experience an improvement in at least one cytopenia, the risks of both neutropenia and thrombocytopenia are increased.[A8] These agents are not curative, and the median survival is less than 6 months when patients are unresponsive. No standard of care is available for patients whose disease worsens after treatment with hypomethylating agents. Options under study include[24] azacitidine with either magrolimab, venetoclax,[A9] or sabatolimab.

Immunomodulatory Agents

Patients with loss of chromosome 5q, either alone or in conjunction with other chromosomal abnormalities, have high response rates to lenalidomide, including a nearly 70% rate of transfusion independence and a greater than 30% rate of cytogenetic normalization persisting for a median of more than 2 years.[25] Lenalidomide (10 mg daily) is now the treatment of choice for lower-risk 5q– patients. In patients with lower-risk myelodysplastic syndromes without a chromosome 5 abnormality, the response rate to lenalidomide is approximately 35%; such responses persist for a median of 8 to 9 months.[26] In higher-risk myelodysplastic syndromes and AML with 5q–chromosomal abnormalities, however, it is less effective. Important adverse effects of lenalidomide include cytopenias, thrombosis, diarrhea, and rash.

Immunosuppressive Therapy

Patients who display a pathophysiology similar to aplastic anemia (e.g., T-lymphocyte-driven autoimmune attack against hematopoietic cells) may respond to anti-T-cell therapies, including antithymocyte globulin and calcineurin inhibitors under expert supervision. Younger patients with a normal karyotype, trisomy 8, paroxysmal nocturnal hemoglobinuria clones, or HLA DR15 status seem to have a higher likelihood of benefiting, but good predictive strategies for selecting patients for immunosuppressive therapy are lacking.

PREVENTION

At present there is no clear way by which myelodysplastic syndromes can be prevented, except avoiding known risk factors such as radiation exposure or alkylating agents. However, emerging clonal hematopoiesis following treatment for cancer or arising de novo can now be recognized at an early stage and may be amenable to intervention.[27]

PROGNOSIS

The natural history of myelodysplastic syndromes is highly variable. Approximately one half of patients will die of complications of the cytopenias, particularly infection due to neutropenia and functional neutrophil defects (i.e., impaired bactericidal activity due to hypogranularity). Among lethal infections in myelodysplastic syndromes, pneumonia and bacteremia are most common. Bleeding is the second most common disease-related cause of death. Anemia may exacerbate cardiovascular or cerebrovascular disease. Approximately 25% of patients will progress to AML, which is

Risk group	Included karyotypes	Median survival, years	25% of patients to AML, years	Proportion of patients in this group
Very good	del(11q), –Y	5.4	N/R	4%
Good	Normal, del(20q), del(5q) alone or with 1 other anomaly, del(12p)	4.8	9.4	72%
Intermediate	+8, del(7q), i(17q), +19, any other single or double abnormality not listed	2.7	2.5	13%
Poor	Abnormal 3q, –7, double abnormality include –7/del(7q), complex with 3 abnormalities	1.5	1.7	4%
Very poor	Complex with >3 abnormalities	0.7	0.7	7%

A

Parameter	Categories and associated scores				
Cytogenetic risk group	Very good	Good	Intermediate	Poor	Very poor
	0	1	2	3	4
Marrow blast proportion	≤2%	>2 – <5%	5 – 10%	>10%	
	0	1	2	3	
Hemoglobin	≥10 g/dL	8 – <10 g/dL	<8 g/dL		
	0	1	1.5		
Absolute neutrophil count	≥0.8 × 10^9/L	<0.8 × 10^9/L			
	0	0.5			
Platelet count	≥100 × 10^9/L	50 – 100 × 10^9/L	<50 × 10^9/L		
	0	0.5	1		

Possible range of summed scores: 0–10

B

Risk group	Points	% Patients (n = 7012; AML data on 6485)	Median survival, years	Median survival for patients <60 years	Time until 25% of patients develop AML, years
Very low	0–1.5	19%	8.8	Not reached	Not reached
Low	2.0–3.0	38%	5.3	8.8	10.8
Intermediate	3.5–4.5	20%	3.0	5.2	3.2
High	5.0–6.0	13%	1.5	2.1	1.4
Very high	>6.0	10%	0.8	0.9	0.7

C

FIGURE 167-3. **The 2012 Revised International Prognostic Scoring System (IPSS-R) for myelodysplastic syndromes. A, Cytogenetic abnormalities. B, Table for calculation of IPSS-R risk group. C, Outcomes by risk group. AML = acute myeloid leukemia. (Data from Greenberg PL, Tuechler H, Schanz J, et al. Revised international prognostic scoring system for myelodysplastic syndromes. *Blood* 2012;120:2454-2465.)**

usually a fatal complication.[28] Finally, because myelodysplastic syndromes are often diagnosed in elderly patients or people with a history of cancer, frailty and geriatric comorbid conditions contribute to death in at least one third of patients. The revised International Prognostic Scoring System (see Fig. 167-3) defines five different subgroups of myelodysplastic syndromes with varying risk for death and AML progression.

Molecular abnormalities (including mutations in *EZH2, TP53*, or *RUNX1*) are associated with poorer prognosis, and the Molecular International Prognostic Scoring System considers mutations in up to 17 genes to place patients into six prognostic categories.[29] Additionally, the presence of either a *TP53* or RAS pathway mutation predicts poor outcome after hematopoietic stem cell transplantation.

GENERAL REFERENCES

For the General References and other additional features, please visit Elsevier eBooks+ at https://ebooks.health.elsevier.com.

Grade A References

A1. Scott BL, Pasquini MC, Logan BR, et al. Myeloablative versus reduced-intensity hematopoietic cell transplantation for acute myeloid leukemia and myelodysplastic syndromes. *J Clin Oncol*. 2017;35:1154-1161.
A2. Platzbecker U, Symeonidis A, Oliva EN, et al. A phase 3 randomized placebo-controlled trial of darbepoetin alfa in patients with anemia and lower-risk myelodysplastic syndromes. *Leukemia*. 2017;31:1944-1950.
A3. Fenaux P, Platzbecker U, Mufti GJ, et al. Luspatercept in patients with lower-risk myelodysplastic syndromes. *N Engl J Med*. 2020;382:140-151.
A4. Dodillet H, Kreuzer KA, Monsef I, et al. Thrombopoietin mimetics for patients with myelodysplastic syndromes. *Cochrane Database Syst Rev*. 2017;9:CD009883.
A5. Angelucci E, Li J, Greenberg P, et al. Iron chelation in transfusion-dependent patients with low-to-intermediate-1 risk myelodysplastic syndrome: a randomized trial. *Ann Intern Med*. 2020;172:513-522.
A6. Almasri J, Alkhateeb HB, Firwana B, et al. A systematic review and network meta-analysis comparing azacitidine and decitabine for the treatment of myelodysplastic syndrome. *Syst Rev*. 2018;7:1-9.
A7. Sasaki K, Jabbour E, Montalban-Bravo G, et al. Low-dose decitabine versus low-dose azacitidine in lower-risk MDS. *NEJM Evid*. 2022;1:EVIDoa2200034.
A8. Gao C, Wang J, Li Y, et al. Incidence and risk of hematologic toxicities with hypomethylating agents in the treatment of myelodysplastic syndromes and acute myeloid leukopenia: a systematic review and meta-analysis. *Medicine (Baltimore)*. 2018;97:1-13.
A9. Dinardo CD, Jonas BA, Pullarkat V, et al. Azacitidine and venetoclax in previously untreated acute myeloid leukemia. *N Engl J Med*. 2020;383:617-629.

168 THE ACUTE LEUKEMIAS

ROLAND B. WALTER AND FREDERICK R. APPELBAUM

DEFINITION

Normal hematopoiesis (Chapter 142) requires tightly regulated proliferation and differentiation of pluripotent hematopoietic stem cells that become mature blood cells. Acute leukemia begins as a clonal disease that is the result of a malignant event in an early hematopoietic cell. Over time, subsequent mutational events give rise to full-blown leukemia that may be composed of multiple subclones. Instead of proliferating and differentiating normally, the affected cells give rise to progeny that fail to differentiate normally but continue to proliferate in an uncontrolled fashion. As a result, immature myeloid cells in acute myeloid leukemia (AML) or lymphoid cells in acute lymphoblastic leukemia (ALL)—typically called blasts—rapidly accumulate and progressively replace other cells in the bone marrow, thereby diminishing the production of normal red cells, white cells, and platelets. This loss of normal marrow function, in turn, gives rise to the common clinical complications of acute leukemia: anemia, infection, and bleeding. With time, the leukemic blasts pour out into the blood stream and eventually occupy the lymph nodes, spleen, and other organs. If untreated, acute leukemia is often rapidly fatal; most patients die within several weeks to months after diagnosis. With appropriate therapy, however, the natural history of acute leukemia can be markedly altered, and many patients can be cured.

EPIDEMIOLOGY

Incidence

An estimated 20,000 or so new cases of AML and 6600 or so new cases of ALL occur annually in the United States.[1] This incidence of acute leukemia has remained relatively stable in the United States over the past three decades, but there is substantial variation in incidence among and within world regions.[2]

In the United States, the annual deaths are about 11,500 from AML and about 1400 from ALL. Although acute leukemia accounts for only about 2% of cancer deaths, the impact of leukemia is heightened because of the young age of some patients. For example, ALL has a maximum incidence between ages 2 and 10 years, is the most common cancer in children younger than age 15 years, and accounts for one third of all childhood cancer deaths. The incidence of AML gradually increases with age, with a median age at diagnosis of about 67 years and without an early peak.

Determinants

In most cases, acute leukemia develops for no known reason, but sometimes a possible cause can be identified.

Genetic Predisposition

The concordance rate is virtually 100% in identical twins if one twin develops leukemia during the first year of life. An increasing number of germline mutations (e.g., in *RUNX1, CEBPA, GATA2, DDX41, ETV6, IKZF1, PAX5*, and *SAMD9*) are recognized to cause rare syndromes that can lead to acute leukemia without other manifestations.[3] The incidence of acute leukemia is markedly increased in syndromes involving defective DNA repair, such as Fanconi anemia and Bloom syndrome, and in bone marrow failure syndromes associated with ribosomal abnormalities (Chapter 151), including Diamond-Blackfan anemia, Shwachman-Diamond syndrome, and dyskeratosis congenita. Germline mutations in *TP53* (Li-Fraumeni syndrome) and abnormalities in chromosome number, as in Down and Klinefelter syndromes (Chapters 32 and 214), are also associated with an increased incidence of acute leukemia.

Radiation

Ionizing radiation (Chapter 18) is leukemogenic. The incidences of ALL, AML, and chronic myeloid leukemia (CML) are increased in patients given therapeutic radiation and among survivors of the atomic bomb blasts at Hiroshima and Nagasaki. The magnitude of the risk depends on the dose of radiation, its distribution in time, and the age of the individual. Greater risk results from higher doses of radiation delivered over shorter periods to younger patients. In areas of high natural background radiation (often from radon), chromosomal aberrations are reportedly more frequent, but an increase in acute leukemia has not been consistently found. Although some investigations have raised concern about the possible leukemogenic effects of extremely low-frequency nonionizing electromagnetic fields emitted by electrical installations, findings have been inconsistent across studies; if any such effect exists at all, its magnitude is very small.

Oncogenic Viruses

The search for a viral cause of leukemia has been pursued intensely, but only two clear associations have been found. Human T-cell lymphotropic virus type I (HTLV-I), an enveloped, single-stranded RNA virus, is a causative agent of adult T-cell leukemia (Chapter 360), spread either horizontally by sexual contact or blood products or vertically from mother to fetus. This distinct form of leukemia is found within geographic clusters in southwestern Japan, the Caribbean basin, and Africa. Because HTLV-I seropositivity was found with increasing frequency among heavily transfused patients and intravenous drug users, screening of blood products for antibodies to HTLV-I is now routine practice in blood banks in the United States. Epstein-Barr virus (Chapter 348), the DNA herpes family virus that causes infectious mononucleosis, is associated with the endemic African form of Burkitt lymphoma/leukemia (Chapter 171).

Chemicals and Drugs

Heavy occupational exposure to benzene and benzene-containing compounds, such as kerosene and carbon tetrachloride, may lead to marrow damage, which can take the form of aplastic anemia, myelodysplasia, or AML. A link between leukemia and tobacco use (Chapter 363) has been reported.

With the increasing use of chemotherapy and radiotherapy to treat other malignancies, as much as 10% of AMLs and a smaller percentage of ALLs are likely the consequence of prior cancer therapy. Exposure to alkylating agents such as melphalan and the nitrosoureas is associated with a risk for secondary AML, which often manifests initially as a myelodysplastic syndrome (Chapter 167), frequently with abnormalities of chromosomes 5, 7, and 8 but with no distinct morphologic features. These secondary AMLs typically develop 4 to 6 years after exposure to alkylating agents, and their incidence may be increased with greater intensity and duration of drug exposure. Secondary AML associated with exposure to topoisomerase II inhibitors, including the epipodophyllotoxins (teniposide or etoposide) and doxorubicin, tends to have a shorter latency period (1 to 2 years), lacks a myelodysplastic phase, has a monocytic morphology, and involves abnormalities of the long arm of chromosome 11 (band q23) or chromosome 21 (band q22). Because patients frequently receive combination chemotherapy, it is often difficult to identify a single causative agent. On average, secondary leukemia responds less well to treatment than does de novo disease.

PATHOBIOLOGY

Clonality and Cell of Origin

The acute leukemias are clonal disorders, and all leukemic cells in a given patient are descended from a common progenitor. The clonal nature of acute leukemia suggests that leukemic stem cells are capable of both self-renewal and proliferation. Leukemic stem cells in AML are rare among the leukemic mass, with a frequency of 0.2 to 10 per 10^6, and usually, but not invariably, are located within the primitive $CD34^{++}$ $CD38^{-}$ fraction. Less is known about the ALL stem cell.

Classification

The classification of acute leukemias is based on clinical, morphologic, immunophenotypic, cytogenetic, and molecular features (Table 168-1).

TABLE 168-1 WORLD HEALTH ORGANIZATION CLASSIFICATION OF ACUTE LEUKEMIAS (2016)

Acute Myeloid Leukemia (AML) and Related Neoplasms
AML with recurrent genetic abnormalities
AML with t(8;21)(q22;q22.1); *RUNX1-RUNX1T1*
AML with inv(16)(p13.1q22) or t(16;16)(p13.1;q22); *CBFB-MYH11*
APL with *PML-RARA*
AML with t(9;11)(p21.3;q23.3); *MLLT3-KMT2A*
AML with t(6;9)(p23;q34.1); *DEK-NUP214*
AML with inv(3)(q21.3q26.2) or t(3;3)(q21.3;q26.2); *GATA2, MECOM*
AML (megakaryoblastic) with t(1;22)(p13.3;q13.3); *RBM15-MKL1*
Provisional entity: AML with BCR-ABL1
AML with mutated NPM1
AML with biallelic mutations of *CEBPA*
Provisional entity: AML with mutated RUNX1
AML with myelodysplasia-related changes
Therapy-related myeloid neoplasms
AML, NOS
AML with minimal differentiation
AML without maturation
AML with maturation
Acute myelomonocytic leukemia
Acute monoblastic/monocytic leukemia
Pure erythroid leukemia
Acute megakaryoblastic leukemia
Acute basophilic leukemia
Acute panmyelosis with myelofibrosis
Myeloid sarcoma
Myeloid proliferations related to Down syndrome
Transient abnormal myelopoiesis (TAM)
Myeloid leukemia associated with Down syndrome
Blastic Plasmacytoid Dendritic Cell Neoplasm
Acute Leukemias of Ambiguous Lineage
Acute undifferentiated leukemia
Mixed phenotype acute leukemia (MPAL) with t(9;22)(q34.1;q11.2); *BCR-ABL1*
MPAL with t(v;11q23.3); *KMT2A* rearranged
MPAL, B/myeloid, NOS
MPAL, T/myeloid, NOS
B-Lymphoblastic Leukemia/Lymphoma
B-lymphoblastic leukemia/lymphoma, NOS
B-lymphoblastic leukemia/lymphoma with recurrent genetic abnormalities
B-lymphoblastic leukemia/lymphoma with t(9;22)(q34.1;q11.2); *BCR-ABL1*
B-lymphoblastic leukemia/lymphoma with t(v;11q23.3); *KMT2A* rearranged
B-lymphoblastic leukemia/lymphoma with t(12;21)(p13.2;q22.1); *ETV6-RUNX1*
B-lymphoblastic leukemia/lymphoma with hyperdiploidy
B-lymphoblastic leukemia/lymphoma with hypodiploidy
B-lymphoblastic leukemia/lymphoma with t(5;14)(q31.1;q32.3); *IL3-IGH*
B-lymphoblastic leukemia/lymphoma with t(1;19)(q23;p13.3); *TCF3-PBX1*
Provisional entity: B-lymphoblastic leukemia/lymphoma, BCR-ABL1–like
Provisional entity: B-lymphoblastic leukemia/lymphoma with iAMP21
T-Lymphoblastic Leukemia/Lymphoma
Provisional entity: Early T-cell precursor lymphoblastic leukemia
Provisional entity: Natural killer (NK) cell lymphoblastic leukemia/lymphoma

APL = acute promyelocytic leukemia; NOS = not otherwise specified.

Data from Arber DA, Orazi A, Hasserjian R, et al. The 2016 revision to the World Health Organization classification of myeloid neoplasms and acute leukemia. *Blood*. 2016;127:2391-2405.

Morphology

Leukemic blasts in AML are typically 12 to 20 µm in diameter, with discrete nuclear chromatin, multiple nucleoli, and cytoplasm that usually contains azurophilic granules (Fig. 168-1). Auer rods, which are slender, fusiform cytoplasmic inclusions that stain red with Wright-Giemsa stain, are virtually pathognomonic of AML (Fig. 168-2).

The leukemic cells in ALL tend to be smaller than AML blasts and relatively devoid of granules (see Fig. 168-1). ALL can be divided by French-American-British criteria based on size, nuclear chromatin appearance, nucleoli, and cytoplasm/granules. However, this morphologic classification scheme has been largely replaced by schemes that consider immunologic and cytogenetic characteristics.

Immunophenotyping

Immunophenotyping by multiparameter flow cytometry is used to determine lineage involvement of newly diagnosed acute leukemias and to detect aberrant immunophenotypes, thereby allowing quantification of measurable residual disease after therapy.

Acute Myeloid Leukemia

Most cases of AML express antigens seen on normal immature myeloid cells. The most immature forms of AML express CD34, CD117, and human leukocyte antigen (HLA)-DR, whereas more differentiated forms express CD13 and CD33. CD14, CD15, and CD11b are expressed by AMLs with monocytic features; erythroid leukemias express CD36, CD71, and CD235a (glycophorin A); and megakaryocytic AMLs express CD41 and CD61. In 10 to 20% of patients, otherwise typical AML blasts also express antigens usually restricted to B- or T-cell lineage (e.g., CD2, CD7, CD19, or CD56). Expression of a

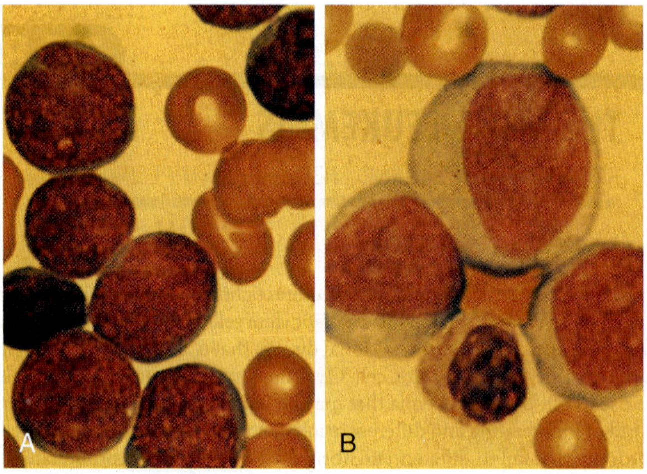

FIGURE 168-1. **Acute leukemia. A,** Acute lymphoblastic leukemia (ALL). **B,** Acute myeloid leukemia (AML). Lymphoblasts in ALL are smaller, with a higher ratio of nuclear to cytoplasmic material and less distinct nucleoli than in the myeloblasts in AML. The nucleoli in the myeloblasts are clear and "punched out."

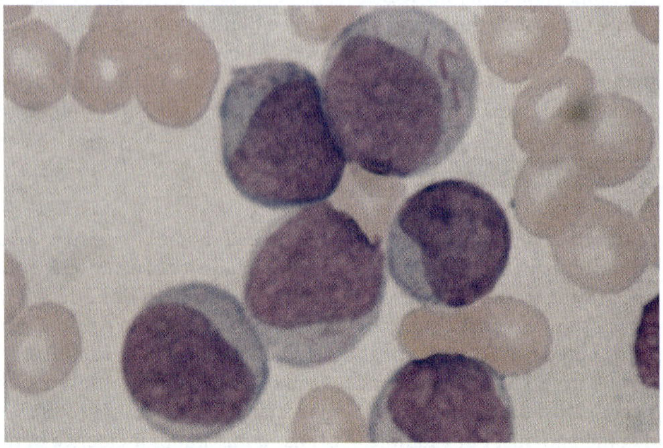

FIGURE 168-2. **Acute myeloid leukemia.** The myeloblasts in the smear show Auer rods as cytoplasmic inclusions.

single lymphoid antigen by AML cells does not change either the natural history or the therapeutic response of these leukemias.

Acute Lymphoblastic Leukemia

Approximately 75% of cases of ALL express B-lineage antigens and can be subdivided into four categories. The most immature group, previously called pro-B ALL, expresses the early B-cell antigens CD19 and/or CD22 but not CD10 and represents about 10% of cases of ALL. Approximately 50 to 60% of cases of ALL express CD19 and/or CD22 along with the common ALL antigen (CALLA, or CD10), a glycoprotein that is also found occasionally on normal early lymphocytes. CALLA-positive ALL is thought to represent an early pre–B-cell differentiation state. Approximately 10% of cases of ALL have intracytoplasmic immunoglobulin and were previously termed pre–B-cell ALL. The immunophenotypically most mature subset of B-cell ALL is signified by the presence of surface immunoglobulin and accounts for less than 5% of cases of ALL. In general, the best therapeutic outcomes among B-cell ALL types are with CALLA-positive ALL. The 25% of cases of ALL that express T-lineage antigens can be separated immunophenotypically into three groups: (1) those expressing CD7 but not CD1a or CD3 (currently recognized as early T-cell precursor lymphoblastic leukemia), (2) those expressing CD1a but not surface CD3 (previously termed thymic T-ALL), and (3) those expressing surface CD3 (previously termed mature T-ALL). In about 25% of patients with ALL, the leukemic cells may also express a myeloid antigen, but this antigen does not affect responses to current therapies. Although immunophenotyping remains important for ALL, the WHO currently classifies the ALLs largely based on cytogenetic and molecular features (see Table 168-1).

Acute Leukemia of Ambiguous Lineage

Acute leukemias of ambiguous lineage are rare cases with no evidence of lineage differentiation (i.e., acute undifferentiated leukemia) or with blasts that express definitive markers of more than one lineage (i.e., mixed phenotype acute leukemia). Mixed phenotype acute leukemia can contain either distinct blast populations of different lineages (bilineal) or a single population expressing features of both lineages (biphenotypic). In general, the prognosis of patients with acute undifferentiated leukemia or mixed phenotype acute leukemia is poor when treated with standard chemotherapy.

Cytogenetics and Molecular Biology

In most acute leukemias, an abnormality in chromosome number or structure is found. These abnormalities are (oligo)clonal, involving some or all of the malignant cells in a given patient; they are acquired and are not found in the patient's normal cells; and they are referred to as "nonrandom" because specific abnormalities are found in multiple cases and are associated with distinct morphologic or clinical subtypes of the disease. These abnormalities may simply entail the gain or loss of whole chromosomes, but more often they include chromosomal translocations, deletions, or inversions. When patients with acute leukemia and a chromosomal abnormality receive treatment and enter into complete remission, the chromosomal abnormality disappears; when relapse occurs, the abnormality often reappears. In many cases, these abnormalities have provided clues into the pathobiology of acute leukemia.

Acute Myeloid Leukemia

Translocations

The most common cytogenetic abnormalities seen in AML can be categorized according to their underlying biology and prognostic significance.[4,5] The translocation t(8;21) and the inversion inv(16) result in abnormalities of a transcription factor composed of core binding factor-α (CBF-α) and CBF-β. The translocation t(8;21) results in the fusion of CBF-α (*RUNX1*) on chromosome 21 with the *RUNXT1* gene on chromosome 8, whereas the inversion inv(16) results in the fusion of CBF-β (*CBFB*) on the q arm of chromosome 16 with the *MYH11* gene on the p arm. Both of these "core binding factor" AMLs (CBF-AMLs) are characterized by a high complete remission rate and relatively favorable long-term survival for the group as a whole. Comprehensive mutational profiling of CBF-AMLs does, however, reveal clinical prognostic as well as biologic heterogeneity within this pathogenetically unique category of patients.[6] An additional translocation with a favorable prognosis, t(15;17), involves two genes, *PML* and *RAR-α* (a gene encoding the α-retinoic acid receptor), and is invariably associated with acute promyelocytic leukemia. Other genetic alterations may cooperate with *PML-RARα* in the pathogenesis of acute promyelocytic leukemia. Translocations involving the *KMT2A* (previously: *MLL*) gene, located at chromosome band 11q23, are seen in 5 to 7% of AMLs. *KMT2A* is perhaps the most promiscuous oncogene partner in oncology, with more than 130 fusion partners identified. The prognosis of *KMT2A*-associated AML depends on the fusion partner, with t(9;11) predicting an intermediate prognosis but most others considered unfavorable. Trisomy 8 is among the most common nonrandom cytogenetic abnormalities seen in AML; it accounts for 9% of cases and carries an intermediate prognosis. Trisomies of chromosome 21, chromosome 11, and other chromosomes are sometimes seen as well. Deletions of part or all of chromosome 5 or 7 each account for 6 to 8% of cases of AML. These abnormalities are seen with greater frequency in older patients and in patients with AML secondary to myelodysplasia or prior exposure to alkylating agents, and they are associated with an unfavorable prognosis. The presence of multiple (three or more) cytogenetic abnormalities in individual cases of AML defines "complex cytogenetics" and also is associated with an unfavorable prognosis. Particularly unfavorable are cases with a monosomal karyotype (i.e., the presence of two or more distinct monosomies or one monosomy and another structural abnormality), at least partly because of their strong association with mutations in *TP53*.

TABLE 168-2 2017 EUROPEAN LEUKEMIANET CYTOGENETIC/MOLECULAR RISK STRATIFICATION OF AML

	SUBSET
Favorable	t(8;21)(q22;q22.1); *RUNX1-RUNX1T1* inv(16)(p13.1q22) or t(16;16)(p13.1;q22); *CBFB-MYH11* Mutated *NPM1* without *FLT3-ITD* or with *FLT3-ITD*$^{\text{low}*}$ Biallelic mutated *CEBPA*
Intermediate	Mutated *NPM1* and *FLT3-ITD*$^{\text{high}*}$ Wild-type *NPM1* without *FLT3-ITD* or with *FLT3-ITD*$^{\text{low}*}$ (without adverse-risk genetic lesions) t(9;11)(p21.3;q23.3); *MLLT3-KMT2A*[†] Cytogenetic abnormalities not classified as favorable or adverse
	t(6;9)(p23;q34.1); *DEK-NUP214* t(v;11)(v;q23.3); *KTM2A* rearranged T(9;22)(q34.1;q11.2); *BCR-ABL1*
Adverse	inv(3)(q21.3q26.2) or t(3;3)(q21.3;q26.2); GATA2, MECOM (EVI1) −5 or del(5q); −7; −17/abnl(17p) Complex karyotype,[‡] monosomal karyotype Wild-type *NPM1* and *FLT3-ITD*$^{\text{high}*}$
Adverse	Mutated *RUNX1*[§] Mutated *ASXL1*[§] Mutated TP53

*Low, low allelic ratio (<0.5); high, high allelic ratio (≥0.5).
†Takes precedence over rare, concurrent adverse-risk gene mutations.
‡Three or more unrelated chromosome abnormalities in the absence of one of the WHO-designated recurring translocations or inversions, that is, t(8;21), inv(16) or t(16;16), t(9;11), t(v;11)(v;q23.3), t(6;9), inv(3), or t(3;3).
§These markers should not be used as an adverse prognostic marker if they co-occur with favorable-risk AML subtypes.
AML = acute myeloid leukemia.

Mutations

Assaying for the status of genes that are frequently mutated in AML is slowly becoming standard, with increasing numbers of studies suggesting their utility both for prognosis (Table 168-2) and for the selection of treatment.[7] AML cells appear to carry, on average, about 10 to 15 mutations per cell, far less than found in epithelial cancers. Of these, on average five mutations are in genes recurrently mutated in AML (so-called driver mutations), with the remainder being considered as passenger mutations. Among the recurrently mutated driver mutations, several are of significant therapeutic and prognostic importance and thus are part of the standard evaluation of AML. *CEBPA*, a gene encoding a leucine zipper transcription factor involved in myeloid differentiation, is mutated in 4 to 15% of cases of AML. Biallelic mutations in *CEBPA* are associated with a more favorable prognosis. *NPM1* encodes a nucleolar phosphoprotein with multiple functions. Mutations in *NPM1* are found in approximately 30% of AML cases and are also associated with a more favorable prognosis. As for other genes, co-occurring mutations influence the prognostic significance of *NPM1* mutations. *FLT3* is a receptor tyrosine kinase and is mutated in 30 to 35% of AML patients, about one-fourth of the time as a point mutation and about three-fourths of the time as an internal tandem duplication. Mutations in *FLT3* are associated with a poorer clinical outcome, at least when found at a high allelic ratio. Other driver mutations recurrently mutated in AML include *DNMT3A*, *IDH1* and *2*, *NRAS* and *KRAS*, *RUNX1*, *TET2*, *ASXL1*, and *TP53*. Certain mutations (e.g., in *SRSF2*, *SF3B1*, *U2AF1*,

ZRSR2, ASXL1, EZH2, BCOR, or *STAG2*) are almost exclusively found in secondary AML and can be used to identify such cases molecularly.

Acute Lymphoblastic Leukemia

Translocations

The most common cytogenetic abnormality seen in adults with ALL is the Philadelphia chromosome, or t(9;22). This translocation results in fusion of the *BCR* gene on chromosome 22 to the *ABL1* tyrosine kinase gene on chromosome 9. The result is the constitutive activation of *ABL1*, but the precise mechanism by which this activity leads to leukemia is unclear. The *BCR-ABL1* fusion is associated with both ALL and CML (Chapter 170), with a difference in the breakpoint of *BCR* distinguishing the two. Specifically, a slightly smaller 190-kD fusion protein is usually found in ALL, whereas a larger 210-kD protein is characteristic of CML. The frequency of t(9;22) in ALL increases with age: it is found in approximately 5% of childhood cases and 25% of adults. Another translocation seen in adult B-cell ALL includes t(4;11), which is seen in 7% of cases, involves the *KMT2A* and *AF4* genes, and has a poor prognosis. t(8;14), which involves *MYC* and the immunoglobulin heavy chain gene, is the translocation associated with a leukemic variant of Burkitt lymphoma (Chapter 171). T-cell ALLs (Chapter 360) are frequently associated with translocations involving chromosomes 7 or 14 at the sites of T-cell receptor enhancer genes on these chromosomes. The other most common cytogenetic abnormalities seen in adult ALL include del(9p), seen in 5 to 9% of cases; del (6q), seen in 5 to 7%; and del(13q), seen in 3 to 5%.

Mutations

As in AML, directed and genome-wide evaluation of cases of ALL have revealed recurrent mutations in addition to those already identified through cytogenetics. Among the most common are mutations in *PAX5* and *IKZF1*, which are seen in 30 and 25% of cases of B-ALL, respectively, and mutations in *NOTCH1*, which are seen in 35% of cases of T-ALL. A poor-risk form of ALL termed Philadelphia chromosome–like ALL accounts for 20 to 25% of adult ALLs.[8] In this type of ALL, leukemia cells lack the classic *BCR-ABL1* translocation and, instead, have kinase-activating mutations in other genes in the same signaling pathway, including *CRLF2*, often in combination with mutations in *JAK2*.

CLINICAL MANIFESTATIONS

The signs and symptoms of acute leukemia, which result from decreased normal marrow function and invasion of normal organs by leukemic blasts, are usually rapid in onset, developing over a few weeks to a few months at most. Anemia, which is present at diagnosis in most patients, causes fatigue, pallor, headache, and, in predisposed patients, angina or heart failure. Thrombocytopenia is usually present, and approximately one third of patients have clinically evident bleeding at diagnosis, usually in the form of petechiae, ecchymoses, bleeding gums, epistaxis, or hemorrhage. Most patients with acute leukemia are significantly granulocytopenic at diagnosis. As a result, approximately one third of patients with AML and slightly fewer patients with ALL have significant or life-threatening infections, mostly of bacterial origin, when initially seen.

In addition to suppressing normal marrow function, leukemic cells can infiltrate other organs. In ALL, which tends to infiltrate normal organs more often than AML, enlargement of lymph nodes, liver, and spleen is common at diagnosis. Patients with T-ALL frequently have mediastinal masses. Bone pain, thought to result from leukemic infiltration of the periosteum or expansion of the medullary cavity, is a common complaint, particularly in children with ALL. Leukemic cells sometimes infiltrate the skin and result in a raised, nonpruritic rash—a condition termed *leukemia cutis*. Leukemic cells may infiltrate the leptomeninges and cause leukemic meningitis, typically manifested by headache and nausea. As the disease progresses, central nervous system (CNS) palsies and seizures may develop. Although less than 5% of patients with ALL have CNS involvement at diagnosis, the CNS is a frequent site of relapse, so CNS prophylaxis is an essential component of the treatment of ALL. Testicular involvement is seen in ALL, and the testicles are a frequent site of relapse.

In AML, collections of leukemic blast cells, often referred to as *chloromas* or *myeloblastomas* or *myeloid sarcomas*, can occur in virtually any soft tissue and appear as rubbery, fast-growing masses. Because the incidence of CNS disease is low in AML, there is no proven benefit of CNS surveillance or prophylaxis.

Certain clinical manifestations are unique to specific subtypes of leukemia. Patients with acute promyelocytic leukemia commonly have subclinical or clinically evident coagulation abnormalities, including disseminated intravascular coagulation (DIC; Chapter 161), caused by tissue thromboplastins released by the leukemic cells. AMLs with monocytic or myelomonocytic differentiation are most likely to have extramedullary involvement. Pure erythroid leukemia often has a long prodromal phase.

DIAGNOSIS

Abnormalities in peripheral blood counts are usually the initial laboratory evidence of acute leukemia, with anemia and thrombocytopenia being almost universal. Up to 25% of patients have severe thrombocytopenia (platelets <20,000/μL). Although most patients are granulocytopenic at diagnosis, the total peripheral white cell count is more variable; approximately 25% of patients have very high white cell counts (>50,000/μL), approximately 50% have white cell counts between 5000 and 50,000/μL, and about 25% have low white cell counts (<5000/μL). In most cases, blasts are present in the peripheral blood, although the percentage of blasts is quite low or absent in some patients.

The diagnosis of acute leukemia is typically established by marrow aspiration (or biopsy if an aspirate cannot be obtained), usually from the posterior iliac crest. Marrow aspirates and biopsy specimens are usually hypercellular and contain 20 to 100% blast cells, which largely replace the normal marrow (see Figs. 168-1 and 168-2). Occasionally, other abnormalities, such as marrow fibrosis (especially with acute megakaryoblastic leukemia) or bone marrow necrosis, are present in addition to the blast cell infiltrate. Marrow samples also should be evaluated for cytogenetic and molecular abnormalities, which are important for classification, prognostication, and guiding therapeutic decision making (see Table 168-2). A diagnostic lumbar puncture is generally recommended in all patients who have ALL but not in patients who have AML in the absence of CNS symptoms.

The prothrombin and partial thromboplastin times are sometimes elevated. In acute promyelocytic leukemia, reduced fibrinogen and evidence of DIC are often seen (Chapter 161). Other laboratory abnormalities frequently present include hyperuricemia, especially in ALL, and increased serum levels of lactate dehydrogenase. In cases of high cell turnover and cell death, evidence of *tumor lysis syndrome* (Chapter 164), including hypocalcemia, hyperkalemia, hyperphosphatemia, hyperuricemia, and renal insufficiency, may be noted at diagnosis. This syndrome, which is more commonly seen shortly after therapy is begun, can be rapidly fatal if untreated.

Differential Diagnosis

The diagnosis of acute leukemia is usually straightforward but can occasionally be difficult. Both leukemia and aplastic anemia (Chapter 151) can manifest with peripheral pancytopenia, but the finding of a hypoplastic marrow without blasts usually distinguishes aplastic anemia. An occasional patient has hypocellular marrow and a clonal cytogenetic abnormality, which establishes the diagnosis of myelodysplasia (Chapter 167) or hypocellular leukemia.

A number of processes other than leukemia can lead to the appearance of immature cells in the peripheral blood. Although other small round cell neoplasms can infiltrate the marrow and mimic leukemia, immunologic markers are effective in differentiating the two. *Leukemoid reactions* to infections such as tuberculosis can result in the outpouring of large numbers of young myeloid cells, but the proportion of blasts in marrow or peripheral blood almost never reaches 20% in a leukemoid reaction (Chapter 153). Infectious mononucleosis (Chapter 348) and other viral illnesses can sometimes mimic ALL, particularly if large numbers of atypical lymphocytes are present in the peripheral blood and the disease is accompanied by immune thrombocytopenia or hemolytic anemia.

TREATMENT AND PROGNOSIS

With the development of effective regimens of combination chemotherapy and advances in hematopoietic cell transplantation, many patients with acute leukemia can be cured. These therapeutic measures are complex and are best carried out at centers with appropriate support services and experience in treating leukemia. Because leukemia is often rapidly progressive, specific antileukemic therapy is typically started in a timely manner, usually within about 3 days of presentation. However, the time from diagnosis to treatment in AML is not related to survival, and it may be preferable to wait for a few extra days for genetic or other laboratory test results to become available in patients whose white blood cell counts are not rapidly increasing so that the best available treatment option can be determined. The goal of initial chemotherapy is to induce a complete remission with restoration of normal marrow function. In general, induction chemotherapy is intensive and is accompanied by significant toxicities. Therefore, patients should be stabilized to the extent possible before specific antileukemic therapy is begun.

Preparing the Patient for Therapy

The diagnosis of leukemia usually comes as a profound psychological shock to the patient and family. Therefore, in addition to stabilizing the patient hematologically and metabolically, it is worthwhile to have at least one formal conference in which the patient and family are advised about the meaning of the diagnosis and the consequences of therapy before treatment is initiated.

Severe bleeding usually results from thrombocytopenia, which can be reversed with platelet transfusions (Chapter 162). Once thrombocytopenic bleeding is stopped, continued prophylactic transfusions of platelets is warranted to maintain the platelet count higher than 10,000/μL. Occasionally, patients also have evidence of DIC (Chapter 161), usually associated with the diagnosis of acute promyelocytic leukemia. If acute promyelocytic leukemia is suspected as the cause, all-*trans*-retinoic acid should be started without waiting for molecular confirmation of the diagnosis (Table 168-3); the drug can be discontinued if the diagnosis is not confirmed. If active bleeding is due to DIC, low doses of heparin (50 U/kg) given intravenously every 6 hours can be of benefit. Platelets and fresh-frozen plasma (or cryoprecipitate) should be transfused to maintain the platelet count higher than 50,000/μL and the fibrinogen level greater than 100 mg/dL until the DIC abates. Whether heparin should be given prophylactically to patients with laboratory evidence of DIC but no active bleeding is an often debated but unsettled question.

In patients with fever and granulocytopenia, blood cultures should be obtained, and empiric broad-spectrum antibiotics should be started while awaiting guidance from the results of the blood cultures and sensitivities (Chapters 153 and 260). If the patient has an adequate granulocyte count, it is preferable to bring an infection under control before starting initial chemotherapy. However, patients often have infection but essentially no granulocytes; in this situation, delaying chemotherapy is unlikely to be beneficial.

Patients with very high blast counts may develop symptoms attributable to the effect of masses of these immature cells on blood flow (leukostasis). The role of leukapheresis and/or hydroxyurea in managing such patients is unclear. Randomized trials are lacking, but data in patients with AML and initial white cell counts greater than 100,000/μL show an early death rate of 20%, with neither leukapheresis nor hydroxyurea improving the outcome. Current guidelines thus suggest proceeding to cytoreductive treatment using planned induction therapy as soon as possible.

Before treatment, management in all patients should be aimed at preventing tumor lysis syndrome (Chapter 164). Patients should be hydrated and given allopurinol 100 to 600 mg orally or intravenously daily before chemotherapy is initiated. Allopurinol prevents the conversion of xanthine and hypoxanthine to uric acid but does not affect already formed uric acid. Patients who present with very high white cell counts may have uremia and anuria secondary to greatly increased serum uric acid levels and intratubular crystallization, even before starting therapy; these patients should be treated with intravenous rasburicase[9] under expert supervision to promote the catabolism of already-formed uric acid to allantoin. Urinary alkalinization is not recommended because it increases the possibility that xanthine and calcium phosphate will precipitate in the kidney.

Treatment of Acute Lymphoblastic Leukemia

After the patient's condition has been stabilized, antileukemic therapy should be started as soon as possible. Treatment of newly diagnosed ALL can be divided into three phases: induction of remission, postremission therapy, and CNS prophylaxis.[10]

Induction of Remission

The initial goal of treatment is to induce complete remission, defined as the reduction of leukemic blasts to undetectable levels and the restoration of normal marrow function. A number of different chemotherapeutic combinations can be used to induce remission; all include vincristine and prednisone, and most add L-asparaginase and daunorubicin, administered over a period of 3 to 4 weeks (Table 168-4). With such regimens, complete remission is achieved in 90% of children and 80 to 90% of adults. For adults age 18 to 59 years with CD20-positive, Philadelphia chromosome–negative ALL, the addition of rituximab (beginning with 375 mg/m^2 on days 1 and 7 and continuing for a total of 16 to 18 infusions) improves the outcome.[A1] Because vincristine, prednisone, and L-asparaginase are relatively nontoxic to normal marrow precursors, the disease often enters complete remission after a relatively brief period of myelosuppression. Failure to achieve complete remission is usually due to either the resistance of leukemic cells to the drugs or to progressive infection. These two complications occur with approximately equal frequency.

Postremission Chemotherapy

If no further therapy is given after induction of complete remission, relapse occurs in almost all cases, usually within several months. Chemotherapy after complete remission can be given in a variety of combinations, dosages, and schedules.

Consolidation chemotherapy refers to short courses of further chemotherapy, given in the hospital at doses similar to those used for initial induction. Consolidation chemotherapy usually involves different drugs than were successful for inducing the initial remission; alternatively, drug combinations can be rotated. Such drugs include high-dose methotrexate, cyclophosphamide, and cytarabine, among others. Most regimens include six to eight courses of intensive consolidation therapy. Maintenance involves the administration of low-dose chemotherapy on a daily or weekly outpatient basis for long periods. The most commonly used maintenance regimen in ALL combines daily 6-mercaptopurine and weekly or biweekly methotrexate. The optimal duration of maintenance chemotherapy is unknown, but it is usually given for 2 to 3 years. The use of more intensive regimens similar to those used in the treatment of pediatric ALL are tolerable in patients up to age 40 years and may improve outcomes compared with regimens initially developed for adults.

Central Nervous System Prophylaxis

Most chemotherapeutic agents that are given intravenously or orally do not penetrate the CNS well, and at least 35% of adults with ALL will develop CNS leukemia if no form of CNS prophylaxis is given. With prophylaxis, relapse in the CNS as an isolated event occurs in less than 10% of patients. Systemic chemotherapy with high-dose methotrexate (e.g., 200 mg/m^2 intravenously over 2 hours, followed by 800 mg/m^2 over 22 hours) and cytarabine (e.g., 3 g/m^2 over 2 hours every 12 hours for four doses) can achieve therapeutic drug levels within the CNS. Alternatives are intrathecal cytarabine, intrathecal methotrexate, intrathecal methotrexate combined with 2400 cGy radiation to the cranium, or 2400 cGy to the craniospinal axis.

Treatment of Burkitt-like ALL

Burkitt-like ALL (also called FAB L3 or mature B-cell ALL) is characterized by the presence of monoclonal surface immunoglobulin, cytogenetics showing t(8;14), and the constitutive expression of the *MYC* oncogene. Burkitt-like ALL, which accounts for 3 to 5% of adult cases of ALL, responds well to regimens that incorporate short, intensive courses of high-dose methotrexate (1.5 g/m^2 over 24 hours with leucovorin), cytarabine (3 g/m^2 over 2 hours every 12 hours for four doses), and cyclophosphamide (200 mg/m^2/day for 5 days); this regimen yields high rates of complete response and cures in about 50% of patients. The addition of rituximab may further improve outcomes.

Treatment of Philadelphia Chromosome–Positive ALL

Approximately 5% of pediatric cases and 25% of adult cases of ALL have cytogenetics showing t(9;22), the Philadelphia chromosome. The addition of a tyrosine kinase inhibitor such as imatinib, dasatinib, or ponatinib to conventional chemotherapeutic regimens can provide complete response rates equivalent to those seen in Philadelphia chromosome–negative ALL. Therapy with dasatinib (e.g., 70 mg twice daily for 84 days) and prednisone (e.g., 60 mg/m^2 per day for 24 days followed by a taper and discontinuing on day 32) alone without chemotherapy appears sufficient to allow the majority of older patients with Philadelphia chromosome–positive ALL to achieve an initial morphologic remission, but remissions typically are not durable.[11] However, subsequent treatment

TABLE 168-3 MANAGEMENT OF NEWLY DIAGNOSED ACUTE PROMYELOCYTIC LEUKEMIA

A. Induction—ATRA 45 mg/m^2 orally in divided doses daily plus arsenic trioxide 0.15 mg/kg daily until morphologic remission
B. Consolidation #1—oral arsenic trioxide 0.15 mg/kg/day 5 days/wk for 4 weeks every 8 weeks for total of 4 cycles, and ATRA 45 mg/m^2/day for 2 weeks every 4 weeks for total of 7 cycles

Or, if contraindications to arsenic:

A. Induction: Intravenous ATRA 45 mg/m^2 in divided doses daily plus idarubicin 12 mg/m^2 on days 2, 4, 6, 8
B. Consolidation: Intravenous ATRA 45 mg/m^2 × 15 days + idarubicin 5 mg/m^2 × 4 days × 1 cycle, then ATRA × 15 days plus mitoxantrone 10 mg/m^2 × 3 days × 1 cycle, then ATRA × 15 days + idarubicin 12 mg/m^2 × 1 day × 1 cycle

ATRA = all-*trans*-retinoic acid.

TABLE 168-4 MANAGEMENT OF NEWLY DIAGNOSED ADULT PHILADELPHIA CHROMOSOME–NEGATIVE ACUTE LYMPHOID LEUKEMIA UNDER EXPERT SUPERVISION

A. Induction (and courses 3, 5, 7)—cyclophosphamide 300 mg/m^2 over 3 hr q12h for 6 doses on days 1, 2, 3; doxorubicin 50 mg/m^2 on day 4; vincristine 2 mg/day on days 4 and 11; and dexamethasone 40 mg/day on days 1-4 and days 11-14
B. Consolidation (courses 2, 4, 6, 8)—MTX 200 mg/m^2 over 2 hr, followed by 800 mg/m^2 over 22 hr on day 1; high-dose cytarabine 3 g/m^2 over 2 hr q12h for 4 doses on days 2 and 3
C. Four intrathecal treatments of MTX 12 mg alternating with cytarabine 100 mg are given during the first four courses of systemic therapy

MTX = methotrexate.

with two cycles of blinatumomab (a bispecific antibody to CD19 on ALL cells and CD3 on T cells) can substantially increase the proportion of patients who achieve a molecular remission and is associated with survival expectations exceeding 90% at 18 months.[12]

Treatment of Relapsed ALL

Most relapses occur within 2 years after diagnosis, and most occur in the marrow. Occasionally, relapse is initially found in an extramedullary site such as the CNS or testes. Extramedullary relapse is usually followed shortly by systemic (marrow) relapse and should be considered part of a systemic recurrence. With the use of chemotherapeutic regimens similar to those used for initial induction, 50 to 70% of patients achieve at least a short-lived second remission. If the CNS or testes is the initial site of the relapse, specific therapy with chemotherapy and/or radiation to that site is also required along with systemic retreatment.

Because the prognosis of relapsed leukemia treated with standard chemotherapy alone is so poor, hematopoietic cell transplantation (Chapter 163) is usually recommended in this setting, especially if a morphologic remission is obtained with salvage therapy. Some alternatives to conventional multiagent salvage chemotherapy are available. For example, nelarabine when used as a single agent can induce complete remission in 30% of patients with recurrent T-ALL. The bispecific T-cell engager (BiTE) blinatumomab, which is composed of the single-chain variant fragments of anti-CD19 and anti-CD3 antibodies, improves disease-free and overall survival in patients with recurrent B-ALL[A2,A3] and in patients with B-ALL in first or second morphologic remission who have residual leukemia cells (i.e., measurable residual disease) quantified at more than 0.1%. Inotuzumab ozogamicin, which is a CD22 antibody conjugated to a highly toxic calicheamicin derivative, also can increase the complete remission rate, the duration of remission, and the progression-free survival in adults with relapsed or refractory B-ALL compared with standard intensive chemotherapy,[A4] but with an increased risk of sinusoidal obstruction syndrome (previously termed veno-occlusive disease; Chapter 129). Very high complete responses also have been reported in trials using chimeric antigen receptor T cells targeting CD19 or CD22[13,14] in B-ALL that is refractory or in second or later relapse. Cytokine release syndrome and neurologic toxicity are the most significant side effects.

Hematopoietic Cell Transplantation

The use of high-dose chemoradiotherapy followed by hematopoietic cell transplantation (Chapter 163) from a suitable donor can cure 20 to 40% of patients with ALL who fail to achieve an initial remission or who have a relapse after an initial complete remission; it can cure 50 to 60% of patients who undergo transplantation during a first remission. Despite considerable debate, several studies have reported improved survival when adults with high-risk or standard-risk ALL receive a hematopoietic stem cell transplant during a first remission rather than being treated with standard chemotherapy.[A5] The major limitations of transplantation are graft-versus-host disease, infections, and recurrent disease. If an HLA-identical sibling is not available, transplantation from a matched or partially matched unrelated donor or transplantation of cord blood from a partially matched unrelated donor can be conducted, with results that approach those seen with matched related donors.

Prognosis of ALL

A number of factors help predict the outcome in ALL, the most important of which are younger age, a lower white cell count at diagnosis, and favorable cytogenetics (Fig. 168-3). With currently available treatment regimens, 5-year survival has reached 90% for pediatric ALL. In adults, outcomes are less favorable, with 5-year survival rates of 65 to 75% in adolescents and young adults up to age 40 years, less than 20% in individuals older than age 60 years, and less than 45% overall.

Treatment of Acute Myeloid Leukemia

Remission Induction in Medically Fit Adults

Unless patients have contraindications to aggressive therapy, initial treatment generally includes a combination of an anthracycline and cytarabine (the latter at a dose of 100 to 200 mg/m^2/day for 7 days; Table 168-5) and leads to complete remission in 60 to 80% of patients.[15] Prospective randomized trials have demonstrated that for patients aged 65 years or less, idarubicin (10 to 12 mg/m^2/day for 3 days) or a higher dose of daunorubicin (60 to 90 mg/m^2/day for 3 days) is superior to the conventional daunorubicin dose of 45 mg/m^2/day for 3 days.[16] For acute myeloid leukemia with a mutation in isocitrate dehydrogenase 1, adding ivosidenib, which is an inhibitor of it, can prolong median overall survival from 8 months to 24 months.[A6] Profound myelosuppression always follows when these agents are used at doses capable of inducing complete remission. Approximately 50% of patients will have more than 5% blasts remaining in their marrow 1 week after completing the first cycle of induction. Many experts still recommend starting a second cycle in such circumstances, although the benefit of this approach has been questioned.

Persistence of blasts after the first cycle of induction appears to be associated with an increased risk of recurrent disease. In approximately 30% of cases, AML blasts will have mutations in *FLT3*. In such patients, the addition of the *FLT3* inhibitor midostaurin as part of induction (e.g., 50 mg twice daily on days 8 to 21), consolidation (e.g., 50 mg twice daily on days 8 to 21), and maintenance (e.g., 50 mg twice daily for 1 year) leads to improved disease-free and overall survival.[A7] The addition of the CD33 antibody-drug conjugate gemtuzumab ozogamicin to induction and, possibly, consolidation may reduce relapse and improve survival, particularly in patients with favorable-risk disease and, to a lesser extent, patients with intermediate-risk CD33-positive AML. Failure to achieve complete remission is usually due either to drug resistance or to fatal complications of myelosuppression. In older adults with therapy-related AML or AML with myelodysplasia-related changes, CPX-351, a liposomal formulation of cytarabine co-encapsulated with daunorubicin, leads to better survival than conventional chemotherapy.[A8] With the increasing availability of molecularly targeted agents and lower intensity regimens, a number of chemotherapeutic options are available for the initial therapy of AML in medically fit adults.[17]

Postremission Therapy

Intensive consolidation chemotherapy with repeated courses of daunorubicin and cytarabine at doses similar to those used for induction, high-dose cytarabine (1 to 3 g/m^2/day for 3 to 6 days), or other agents prolongs the average duration of remission and improves the chances for long-term, disease-free survival. The best results reported to date have generally been achieved with repeated cycles of high-dose cytarabine. Maintenance therapy with CC-486, an oral formulation of azacitidine, significantly improves median overall (from 15 to 25 months) and relapse-free (from 5 to 10 months) survival in older adults who are in remission after intensive induction/postremission therapy and cannot undergo allogeneic hematopoietic cell transplantation.[A9] In AML, recurrent leukemia occurs less often in the CNS (approximately 10% of cases) than in patients with ALL, most commonly in patients with monocytic or myelomonocytic differentiation of AML blasts. There is no evidence that CNS prophylaxis improves survival in AML.

Based on cytogenetics and molecular testing, the favorable outcomes after initial therapy are in patients who have t(8;21) or inv(16), patients who have

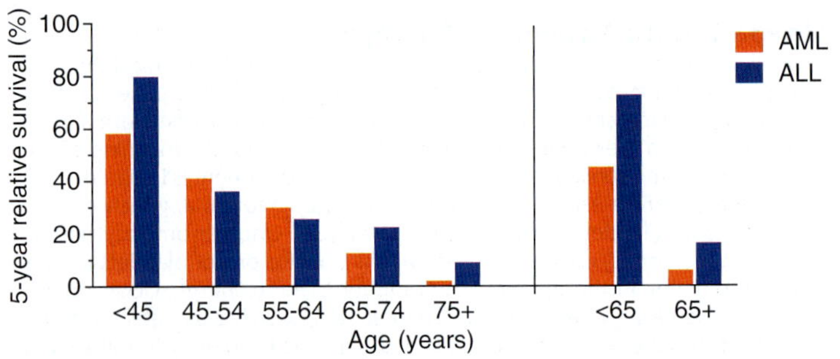

FIGURE 168-3. Shown are the 5-year survival rates (relative to age-matched controls) for adult patients with newly diagnosed acute myeloid leukemia (AML) on the left and acute lymphoblastic leukemia (ALL) on the right according to U.S. Surveillance, Epidemiology and End Results Program (SEER) data.

TABLE 168-5 MANAGEMENT OF NEWLY DIAGNOSED ACUTE MYELOID LEUKEMIA UNDER EXPERT SUPERVISION

A. Induction—daunorubicin 60-90 mg/m^2/day for 3 days (or idarubicin 10-12 mg/m^2/day for 3 days) and cytarabine 100-200 mg/m^2/day for 7 days
   1. At least for favorable-risk disease—add gemtuzumab ozogamicin 3 mg/m^2 (up to 4.5 mg) on days 1, 4, and 7
   2. For *FLT3*-mutated AML—add oral midostaurin 50 mg twice daily on days 8-21
   3. Older adults with therapy-related AML and AML with myelodysplasia-related changes—CPX-351 (100 mg/m^2 cytarabine, 44 mg/m^2 daunorubicin) on days 1, 3, and 5

B. Postremission
   1. Favorable risk—cytarabine 3 g/m^2 over 3 hr q12h on days 1, 2, and 3 every month for 4 months; may add gemtuzumab ozogamicin 3 mg/m^2 (up to 4.5 mg) on day 1 for first 2 cycles
   2. Intermediate risk—as for favorable risk; or, if HLA-matched related or unrelated donor exists, allogeneic hematopoietic cell transplantation
   3. Unfavorable risk—proceed to allogeneic transplantation if possible; if not, treat as for intermediate risk
   4. For *FLT3*-mutated AML—add oral midostaurin 50 mg twice daily on days 8-21
   5. Older adults with therapy-related AML and AML with myelodysplasia-related changes—CPX-351 (65 mg/m^2 cytarabine, 29 mg/m^2 daunorubicin) on days 1 and 3 for 1-2 cycles

AML = acute myeloid leukemia; CPX-351 = liposomal cytarabine-daunorubicin; *FLT3* = FMS-like tyrosine kinase 3; HLA = human leukocyte antigen.

normal cytogenetics but biallelic mutated *CEBPA*, and patients who have mutated *NPM1* and either wild-type *FLT3* or low-allelic-ratio *FLT3*-ITD (see Table 168-2). Intermediate-risk patients have normal cytogenetics without mutations in *NPM1*, *CEBPA*, and *FLT3* (or *FLT3*-ITD with a low allelic ratio) or with high-allelic-ratio *FLT3*-ITD in combination with a mutation in *NPM1*. Also at intermediate risk are patients with t(9;11) or those with cytogenetic abnormalities not classified as favorable or unfavorable. Patients with an unfavorable prognosis have high-allelic-ratio inv(3), t(6;9), −5 or del5, or −7 or del7; a high-allelic-ratio *FLT3*-ITD, and wild-type *NPM1*; mutations in *RUNX1*, *ASXL1*, or *TP53*; or complex cytogenetics (three or more independent chromosome abnormalities).

Treatment of Recurrent AML

Patients in complete remission by morphologic criteria (i.e., ≤5% blasts in the bone marrow) may still have some residual leukemic disease not identified by light microscopy. Both multiparameter flow cytometry-based methods, which rely on identification of abnormal immunophenotypes, and molecular-based methods detecting chimeric fusion proteins or somatic mutations can detect and quantify residual disease, which identifies patients with a high risk of subsequent recurrent disease and worse overall survival.

About 50% of patients whose AML recurs after initial chemotherapy can achieve a second remission after retreatment with daunorubicin-cytarabine or high-dose cytarabine. The likelihood of achieving a second remission is predicted by the duration of the first remission: 70% in patients whose first remission persisted beyond 2 years, compared with less than 15% in those whose first remission lasted less than 6 months. Enasidenib and ivosidenib, oral targeted inhibitors of mutant *IDH2* and *IDH1*, respectively, have been approved for the treatment of patients with recurrent *IDH*-mutated AML based on nonrandomized studies. For the treatment of patients with recurrent *FLT3*-mutated AML, the tyrosine kinase inhibitor gilteritinib (120 mg daily) improves median survival by about 3.5 months compared with standard salvage chemotherapy.[A10]

Second remissions tend to be short-lived, however, and few patients in whom relapse occurs after first-line chemotherapy are cured by salvage chemotherapy. Therefore, hematopoietic cell transplantation is generally indicated, especially if a morphologic remission is obtained with salvage therapy.

Hematopoietic Cell Transplantation

For patients with AML in whom an initial remission cannot be achieved or for those who relapse after chemotherapy, hematopoietic cell transplantation (Chapter 163) from an HLA-identical sibling offers the best chance for cure. Allogeneic transplant is most effective when performed in AML patients who are in complete remission both morphologically and by measurable residual disease testing. Patients with measurable residual disease at the time of transplant are at increased risk for post-transplant relapse.[18]

Meta-analyses confirm that allogeneic transplantation from an HLA-matched sibling improves survival compared with chemotherapy in patients who are in a first remission with unfavorable-risk disease. By comparison, the benefits of hematopoietic cell transplantation are less clear in patients with intermediate-risk disease and probably do not extend to patients with favorable-risk AML in remission, especially if the cytogenetics are favorable. The major limitations of allogeneic hematopoietic cell transplantation are lack of a matched sibling donor, graft-versus-host disease, infections related to immunosuppression, and recurrent disease. Because transplant-related toxicities increase with patient age, some centers limit hematopoietic cell transplantation to patients 65 years of age or younger. However, recent studies of reduced-intensity allogeneic transplantation have shown encouraging results in patients with AML in remission at ages up to 75 years. Allogeneic transplantation using HLA-matched unrelated donors results in survival essentially equivalent to that seen using matched siblings, although there is a higher incidence of complications. In experienced centers, survival outcomes with HLA-haploidentical donors have also approached those seen with HLA-matched patients. Similarly, cord blood transplantation results in cure rates similar to those seen with HLA-matched unrelated transplants and may result in reduced relapse rates in patients with measurable residual disease at the time of transplant. Autologous hematopoietic cell transplantation offers an alternative for patients without matched siblings to serve as donors. In randomized trials, autologous transplantation after consolidation chemotherapy has significantly prolonged the duration of disease-free survival for patients with AML in first remission, but it has not altered overall survival compared with chemotherapy alone.

Treatment of AML in Patients Not Candidates for Intensive Therapy

The benefits of intensive chemotherapy are reduced in older, medically less-fit patients. Traditional alternatives to intensive chemotherapy include supportive care alone, low-dose cytarabine, or use of a DNA methyltransferase inhibitor (e.g., azacitidine or decitabine). For example, in patients age 65 years or older with newly diagnosed AML, azacitidine can increase median overall survival from 6.5 months to 10.4 months compared with conventional care regimens (best supportive care or standard induction chemotherapy or low-dose cytarabine), and its safety was consistent with its known safety profile in other trials.[A11] The oral BCL2 inhibitor venetoclax combined with azacitidine can double the complete remission rate from 18% to 37% and increase median survival from 14.7 to 20.5 months compared with azacitidine alone.[A12] As a result, the combination of venetoclax and azacitidine has become a new standard of care for medically less-fit adults with newly diagnosed AML. Venetoclax also can be used with low-dose cytarabine. For the same target patient population, the hedgehog signaling pathway inhibitor glasdegib has been approved for use together with low-dose cytarabine based on data from a randomized trial showing an increase in median survival from 4.9 to 8.8 months.[A13] Uncontrolled studies suggest that a 10-day course of decitabine may be superior to shorter courses, especially in patients with adverse-risk AML, including those with *TP53* mutations.

In older patients with AML who are ineligible for intensive chemotherapy, single-agent gemtuzumab ozogamicin, as compared with best supportive care (including hydroxyurea), modestly improves overall survival without excess serious adverse events.[A14]

Prognosis of AML

Among patients in whom complete remission is achieved, 20 to 40% remain alive in continuous complete remission for more than 5 years, suggesting a probable cure. As with ALL, younger patients (see Fig. 168-3) and those with a low white cell count at diagnosis have a more favorable outcome.

Fifteen percent of patients with refractory disease can be saved by hematopoietic cell transplantation. If the transplant is performed earlier, the outcome is better: 50 to 60% of patients are cured if hematopoietic cell transplantation is performed during the first remission, but only approximately 30% of patients who are treated with hematopoietic cell transplantation at first relapse or during second remission are cured.

Patients who have a preleukemic phase before their disease evolves into acute leukemia and those whose leukemia is secondary to prior exposure to chemotherapy also have a poorer prognosis. Any measurable residual disease following induction and consolidation greatly increases the risk of subsequent relapse.

Treatment and Prognosis of Other Acute Leukemias

Treatment of Acute Promyelocytic Leukemia

The combination of all-*trans*-retinoic acid (45 mg/m²/day until complete remission is achieved) together with arsenic trioxide without any chemotherapy is superior to all-*trans*-retinoic acid plus an anthracycline for patients with low- to intermediate-risk acute promyelocytic leukemia (i.e., those who present with white blood cell counts <10,000/μL)[A15] and is preferred as first-line treatment.[19] For patients with high-risk disease, therapy with all-*trans*-retinoic acid/retinoic acid should be combined with either gemtuzumab ozogamicin or idarubicin, or all-*trans*-retinoic acid can be added to combination chemotherapy. Patients treated with all-*trans*-retinoic acid usually have their coagulation disorders corrected within several days. A unique toxicity of all-*trans*-retinoic acid in the treatment of acute promyelocytic leukemia is the development of hyperleukocytosis accompanied by respiratory distress and pulmonary infiltrates. This differentiation syndrome responds to temporary discontinuation of all-*trans*-retinoic acid and the addition of corticosteroids. In patients who have recurrent acute promyelocytic leukemia and who were not previously treated with all-*trans*-retinoic acid/arsenic trioxide or who have late relapse after all-*trans*-retinoic acid/arsenic trioxide therapy, arsenic trioxide (0.15 mg/kg/day until complete remission is achieved) ± all-*trans*-retinoic acid with or without an anthracycline or gemtuzumab ozogamicin is effective.

Treatment of Blastic Plasmacytoid Dendritic-Cell Neoplasm

Blastic plasmacytoid dendritic-cell neoplasm is a rare, aggressive malignancy with fewer than 1000 cases annually in the United States. With the newest WHO classification system, it is no longer considered a subtype of AML but, rather, considered a separate disease entity. In adults, it occurs primarily after age 60 years and in a 4:1 male:female ratio. The cause is the malignant proliferation of plasmacytoid dendritic cells that over-express CD123, the interleukin-3 receptor subunit alpha. In some patients, the disease can evolve from myelodysplastic syndrome (Chapter 167).

Bone marrow involvement typically presents as cytopenias. About 80% of patients have skin involvement, usually as brown to purple nodules, often accompanied by purpura. Lymphadenopathy, splenomegaly, and even central nervous system involvement can occur. Fatigue, fever, and night sweats are common. Skin or bone marrow biopsy shows immature plasmacytoid dendritic cells.

Tagraxofusp (SL-401) is an immunoconjugate consisting of IL-3 fused to a truncated diphtheria toxin (7 to 10 mg/kg on days 1 to 5 of each 21-day cycle)[20] that can result in remission in about 70% of cases. Hematopoietic cell transplantation is recommended during first remission. Chemotherapy regimens used for ALL and AML also can provide transient remission. In newly treated patients, about 50% survive for 2 or more years.

Management of Complications

Treatment of acute leukemia, especially AML, is accompanied by a number of complications, the two most serious and frequent being infection and bleeding. During the granulocytopenic period that follows induction and consolidation chemotherapy, the risk for bacterial infection is high. Antibiotic prophylaxis under expert supervision significantly decreases infection-related deaths in afebrile neutropenic patients, with the best results seen with quinolones. Despite prophylaxis, many patients become febrile while neutropenic, and patients can still develop important infections. The most common bacterial species vary somewhat from medical center to medical center, but *Staphylococcus* (primarily *S. epidermidis*; Chapter 267) and *Enterococcus* species (Chapter 270) are the most frequent gram-positive organisms, whereas *Pseudomonas aeruginosa* (Chapter 282) and enteric organisms such as *Escherichia coli* (Chapter 280) and *Klebsiella* species (Chapter 281) are the most common gram-negative organisms isolated.

Even if no cause for fever is found, bacterial infection should be assumed, and, in general, all patients with fever and neutropenia should receive broad-spectrum antibiotics (Chapters 153 and 260). Monotherapy with an intravenous antipseudomonal agent, such as a carbapenem (e.g., imipenem-cilastatin), a cephalosporin (e.g., cefepime), or an antipseudomonal penicillin (e.g., piperacillin-tazobactam), is recommended as empirical therapy. Vancomycin should not be part of standard coverage in most patients but may be used in those with suspected catheter infections or severe mucositis and in patients with hemodynamic instability or altered mental status. Combination therapy with other gram-negative agents (e.g., aminoglycosides) may be needed. Once begun, antibiotics should be continued until patients recover their granulocyte counts, even if they become afebrile first. If documented bacteremia persists despite appropriate antibiotics, the physician should consider removal of indwelling catheters.

Invasive fungal infections are also common following chemotherapy for acute leukemia and are associated with significant morbidity and mortality. Antifungal prophylaxis is associated with a significant reduction in death from fungal infection in patients with AML receiving induction chemotherapy. Posaconazoles is often considered to be more effective than fluconazole or itraconazole. In addition to being granulocytopenic, patients undergoing induction chemotherapy for leukemia have deficient cellular and humoral immunity, at least temporarily, and therefore are subject to infections common in other immunodeficiency states, including *Pneumocystis jirovecii* infection and a variety of viral infections. *P. jirovecii* infection can be prevented by the prophylactic use of trimethoprim-sulfamethoxazole. In cytomegalovirus (CMV)–seronegative patients, CMV-seronegative or leukocyte-reduced blood products should be used to prevent primary infection (Chapter 347). Herpes simplex (Chapter 345) can often complicate existing mucositis and can be prevented with prophylactic acyclovir. Acyclovir is also useful for the prevention and treatment of herpes zoster (Chapter 346).

Myeloid growth factors (granulocyte or granulocyte-macrophage colony-stimulating factor; Chapter 142), if given shortly after the completion of chemotherapy, shorten the period of severe myelosuppression by, on average, 4 days. In most studies, this accelerated recovery has resulted in fewer days with fever and less use of antibiotics, but it has not improved the complete response rate or altered survival and is currently not recommended after induction chemotherapy.

The platelet count that signals a need for platelet transfusion has been the subject of debate. Platelet transfusions from random donors are recommended at a threshold to 10,000/μL in patients without active bleeding. In contrast, a no-prophylaxis strategy results in more days with bleeding and a shorter time to first bleeding episode and therefore is not recommended.[21] In 30 to 50% of cases, patients eventually become alloimmunized and require the use of HLA-matched platelets (Chapter 162). Transfusion-induced graft-versus-host disease (Chapter 162), manifesting as a rash, low-grade fever, elevated values in liver function tests, and decreasing blood counts, can be prevented by irradiating all blood products before transfusion.

GENERAL REFERENCES

For the General References and other additional features, please visit Elsevier eBooks+ at https://ebooks.health.elsevier.com.

Grade A References

A1. Maury S, Chevret S, Thomas X, et al. Rituximab in B-lineage adult acute lymphoblastic leukemia. *N Engl J Med.* 2016;375:1044-1053.
A2. Kantarjian H, Stein A, Gokbuget N, et al. Blinatumomab versus chemotherapy for advanced acute lymphoblastic leukemia. *N Engl J Med.* 2017;376:836-847.
A3. Brown PA, Ji L, Xu X, et al. Effect of postreinduction therapy consolidation with blinatumomab vs chemotherapy on disease-free survival in children, adolescents, and young adults with first relapse of B-cell acute lymphoblastic leukemia: a randomized clinical trial. *JAMA.* 2021;325:833-842.
A4. Kantarjian HM, DeAngelo DJ, Stelljes M, et al. Inotuzumab ozogamicin versus standard therapy for acute lymphoblastic leukemia. *N Engl J Med.* 2016;375:740-753.
A5. Ribera JM, Morgades M, Ciudad J, et al. Chemotherapy or allogeneic transplantation in high-risk Philadelphia chromosome-negative adult lymphoblastic leukemia. *Blood.* 2021;137:1879-1894.
A6. Montesinos P, Recher C, Vives S, et al. Ivosidenib and azacitidine in *IDH1*-mutated acute myeloid leukemia. *N Engl J Med.* 2022;386:1519-1531.
A7. Stone RM, Mandrekar SJ, Sanford BL, et al. Midostaurin plus chemotherapy for acute myeloid leukemia with a FLT3 mutation. *N Engl J Med.* 2017;377:454-464.
A8. Lancet JE, Uy GL, Cortes JE, et al. CPX-351 (cytarabine and daunorubicin) liposome for injection versus conventional cytarabine plus daunorubicin in older patients with newly diagnosed secondary acute myeloid leukemia. *J Clin Oncol.* 2018;36:2684-2692.
A9. Wei AH, Döhner H, Pocock C, et al. Oral azacitidine maintenance therapy for acute myeloid leukemia in first remission. *N Engl J Med.* 2020;383:2526-2537.
A10. Perl AE, Martinelli G, Cortes JE, et al. Gilteritinib or chemotherapy for relapsed or refractory FLT3-mutated AML. *N Engl J Med.* 2019;381:1728-1740.
A11. Dombret H, Seymour JF, Butrym A, et al. International phase 3 study of azacitidine vs conventional care regimens in older patients with newly diagnosed AML with >30% blasts. *Blood.* 2015;126:291-299.
A12. DiNardo CD, Jonas BA, Pullarkat V, et al. Azacitidine and venetoclax in previously untreated acute myeloid leukemia. *N Engl J Med.* 2020;383:617-629.
A13. Cortes JE, Heidel FH, Hellmann A, et al. Randomized comparison of low dose cytarabine with or without glasdegib in patients with newly diagnosed acute myeloid leukemia or high-risk myelodysplastic syndrome. *Leukemia.* 2019;33:379-389.
A14. Amadori S, Suciu S, Selleslag D, et al. Gemtuzumab ozogamicin versus best supportive care in older patients with newly diagnosed acute myeloid leukemia unsuitable for intensive chemotherapy: results of the randomized phase III EORTC-GIMEMA AML-19 Trial. *J Clin Oncol.* 2016;34:972-979.
A15. Platzbecker U, Avvisati G, Cicconi L, et al. Improved outcomes with retinoic acid and arsenic trioxide compared with retinoic acid and chemotherapy in non-high-risk acute promyelocytic leukemia: final results of the randomized Italian-German APL0406 trial. *J Clin Oncol.* 2017;35:605-612.

169 CHRONIC LYMPHOCYTIC LEUKEMIA

JENNIFER R. BROWN

DEFINITION

Chronic lymphocytic leukemia is a mature B-cell malignancy in which the neoplastic cells share an immunoglobulin gene rearrangement. The disease involves the blood, bone marrow, lymph nodes, spleen, liver, and often other organs at the time of presentation, but clinical manifestations range from asymptomatic disease that may not require therapy for decades to rapidly progressive disease that soon can be life-threatening. Recent therapeutic advances using targeted therapies can provide prolonged progression-free survival.[1]

EPIDEMIOLOGY

Chronic lymphocytic leukemia (CLL) is the most common leukemia in the Western Hemisphere. In the United States, the annual incidence is over 20,000 cases, the prevalence is nearly 200,000, and approximately 4400 individuals die from the disease each year.[2] The lifetime risk of developing chronic lymphocytic leukemia is approximately 0.6%. From 2006 to 2021, both the incidence and death rates declined.

The median age at diagnosis is 70 years, with approximately one third of patients under age 65 years and 10% under age 55 years. Approximately twice as many men as women are diagnosed with chronic lymphocytic leukemia. The disease is more common among Whites than Blacks or Native Americans and is rare among Asians and Pacific Islanders, even when the latter have moved to the Western Hemisphere.

The risk factors for chronic lymphocytic leukemia are not well defined. Up to 10% of individuals with chronic lymphocytic leukemia have a first-degree relative with the disease. Epidemiologic studies suggest a five- to eight-fold increased risk for chronic lymphocytic leukemia among individuals with one affected first-degree relative, and a 27-fold increase in risk with two affected first-degree relatives. Although families have been reported with Mendelian inheritance over multiple generations, no highly penetrant risk mutations have been identified. However, genome-wide association studies have identified over 40 common alleles of low penetrance, and data suggest that rare variants in the *ATM* gene may also contribute.

Epidemiologic studies suggest a possible increase in risk with exposure to pesticides or living on a farm, but the data are not definitive. Chronic lymphocytic leukemia is recognized as a service-connected illness among Vietnam War veterans who were exposed to Agent Orange. Studies of exposure to radiation at the Chernobyl atomic plant are suggestive, but most studies have not shown a definite association between radiation exposure and the risk of chronic lymphocytic leukemia.

PATHOBIOLOGY

In many patients who have chronic lymphocytic leukemia, lymphoid-primed hematopoietic stem cells give rise to mature B-cells that expand and can become oligoclonal. The development and progression of one or more of these oligoclones is likely dependent on the acquisition of genetic events that lead to chronic lymphocytic leukemia. About 40% of patients with chronic lymphocytic leukemia carry what is called a stereotyped B-cell receptor, which has hundreds of types. These subgroups of B cell receptors are identical or almost identical to each other, a finding that strongly suggests a role for antigen stimulation in pathogenesis. Some stereotyped subsets of chronic lymphocytic leukemia lymphocytes with identical B cell receptors also carry the same genetic events.[3] Additionally, clones of chronic lymphocytic leukemia cells carry an epigenetic signature, which is similar to the developmental stage of the normal B-cell from which they arose. These genetic events, the B cell receptor structure, and the epigenetic signature all carry significant prognostic importance.

The B-Cell Receptor in Chronic Lymphocytic Leukemia

At the time when chronic lymphocytic leukemia is diagnosed, the population of B cells with a common immunophenotype by flow cytometry also carries and expresses a clonal, rearranged immunoglobulin heavy and light chain gene. Somatic hypermutation can be present, with up to 15% or more variations from germline.[4] Although the degree of somatic hypermutation is a continuum across chronic lymphocytic leukemia, the striking clinical observation is that the disease's behavior and outcome vary tremendously based on a dichotomous cutoff of 2% variation from germline. Patients whose chronic lymphocytic leukemia carries a mutated immunoglobulin heavy chain variable sequence that is more than 2% different from germline, called mutated IGHV, have an indolent course, sometimes not requiring therapy at all. By comparison, patients whose immunoglobulin heavy chain variable sequence is not mutated, defined as 2% or less different than germline and called unmutated IGHV, have higher risk disease. The biologic basis for this prognostic difference is unclear. The gene expression profile of both mutated and unmutated cells resembles a memory B cell and is more similar to each other than to any other normal or malignant B cell. Chronic lymphocytic leukemia with an unmutated immunoglobulin heavy chain variable sequence shows increased activation of the B-cell receptor, which drives survival and proliferation and is likely associated with increased clonal evolution over time. Most of the recurrently mutated cancer genes in chronic lymphocytic leukemia occur predominantly in cells with an unmutated immunoglobulin heavy chain variable sequence. In contrast, although chronic lymphocytic leukemias with mutated immunoglobulin heavy chain variable sequences have B cell receptors, activation is at a lower level, and these chronic lymphocytic leukemias are much less likely to have high risk cytogenetics and somatic mutations. Within a subset, chronic lymphocytic leukemia has similar clinical behavior, and some subsets have been associated with particular somatic mutations, thereby suggesting the possibility of codevelopment or crosstalk between B-cell receptor stimulation/selection and genetic abnormalities.[5]

Chromosomal Abnormalities

Chronic lymphocytic leukemia generally has a stable karyotype with few or no abnormalities, particularly at the time of diagnosis. In contrast to many other hematologic malignancies, balanced translocations are rare in chronic lymphocytic leukemia, which more commonly is associated with unbalanced deletions or amplifications but also usually has a quite stable karyotype. By fluorescence in situ hybridization (FISH) on interphase cells, the most common abnormalities in chronic lymphocytic leukemia are deletion 13q14, deletion 11q22, deletion 17p13, and trisomy 12.[6] Deletion 13q14, which is the most common abnormality in chronic lymphocytic leukemia, is seen in about 55% of patients and is the only abnormality that has been associated with favorable prognosis. In general, however, the prognosis of patients with deletion 13q14, trisomy 12, or normal cytogenetics follows what would be expected based on their *IGHV* mutation status. The highest risk abnormality is deletion 17p13, which deletes one copy of the *TP53* gene and is associated with the poorest prognosis. The second highest risk is deletion 11q22, which deletes one copy of the *ATM* gene. Both of these mutations are strongly associated with unmutated immunoglobulin heavy chain variable sequence, but mutated immunoglobulin heavy chain variable sequence mitigates the prognostic impact of the FISH abnormality. Other findings (e.g., deletion 6q22, trisomy 8, 8q gain, and 8p deletion) are relatively rare, especially at diagnosis, and have generally been associated with more aggressive disease. Cases with more than three to five abnormalities are associated with worse outcomes, but this information is not routinely used for determining prognosis.[7]

Recurrent Somatic Mutations

By next generation sequencing,[8] chronic lymphocytic leukemia has a relatively low mutation rate. Unlike Waldenstrom macroglobulinemia (*MYD88*; Chapter 173) and hairy cell leukemia (*BRAF*), chronic lymphocytic leukemia has no recurrent defining somatic mutation. The most common mutations in chronic lymphocytic leukemia occur in only 15 to 20% of patients and affect the *TP53* gene, *NOTCH1*, *SF3B1*, and *ATM*. Many other cancer genes are mutated in a few percent of cases, thereby making the disease genetically very heterogeneous. Some mutations can be clustered into affected pathways that are thought to be activated in most patients, either genetically or otherwise, and that may act cooperatively to induce disease.

Epigenetics

Methylation patterns in chronic lymphocytic leukemia correspond to the developmental pattern of the antecedent normal B cell and do not vary over the course of the disease.[9] The analysis of methylation patterns identifies three groups (low, intermediate, and high programmed chronic lymphocytic leukemia) that correspond to unmutated immunoglobulin heavy chain variable sequence, a mix of unmutated and mutated immunoglobulin heavy chain variable sequence, and mutated immunoglobulin heavy chain variable sequence.

Methylation can also silence genes that are sometimes deleted in chronic lymphocytic leukemia. For example, the most common recurrent genetic event in chronic lymphocytic leukemia is deletion 13q14, which removes the *miR-15* and *-16* genes that target *BCL-2*. When they are deleted, *BCL-2* is overexpressed. Interestingly, chronic lymphocytic leukemias that do not carry deletions of 13q14 typically have hypermethylation of that region, and the hypermethylation effectively silences *miR-15* and *-16*. This example of alternative mechanisms resulting in the same key pathogenetic event is believed to apply to other pathways in chronic lymphocytic leukemia (e.g., *NOTCH1* can be activated both mutationally or through stimulation by the microenvironment).

Immune Dysfunction

Patients with chronic lymphocytic leukemia display significant defects in immune function, including hypogammaglobulinemia and functional T-cell defects. Hypogammaglobulinemia can be present at diagnosis and progresses as the burden of disease increases. T cells show evidence of chronic stimulation, with exhaustion that also worsens with an increasing burden of disease. The number of T cells is often increased, but the cells are dysfunctional. Regulatory T cells are also increased. These defects do not always translate into infections in individual patients, but collectively patients with chronic lymphocytic leukemia have a substantially increased risk of infection.

CLINICAL MANIFESTATIONS

More than 75% of patients with chronic lymphocytic leukemia are asymptomatic at diagnosis. Diagnosis is most commonly made when a complete blood count obtained at the time of a routine physical examination or evaluation for an unrelated medical issue shows lymphocytosis. Alternatively, some patients may be identified when small lymph nodes (Chapter 154) are detected on a routine medical examination or sometimes on a mammogram.

Patients who present with symptomatic disease generally have larger lymph nodes, show signs or symptoms of splenomegaly (Chapter 154), have fatigue or dyspnea from anemia, or demonstrate petechiae or bruising from thrombocytopenia. Systemic (B) symptoms of fevers, chills, night sweats, or weight loss are very unusual except when chronic lymphocytic leukemia is very advanced.

Disease-Related Complications

Infectious Complications and Vaccination

Patients with chronic lymphocytic leukemia are immunosuppressed even at the time of diagnosis and are at increased risk of bacterial and viral infections, including reactivations of herpes virus and an increased mortality from coronavirus-2019 (COVID-19) infection. Sinus infections (Chapter 394) are particularly problematic.

Autoimmune Complications

Autoimmune complications, which can occur in up to 25% of patients with chronic lymphocytic leukemia, typically manifest as autoimmune hemolytic anemia (Chapter 146) or immune thrombocytopenia (Chapter 158), or very rarely autoimmune neutropenia (Chapter 153). Systemic autoimmune complications can occur but are also rare.

Autoimmune cytopenias can also arise as a complication of therapy, including purine analogues as well as newer targeted therapies, but they more commonly develop in the setting of progressive chronic lymphocytic leukemia. For many patients who develop an autoimmune complication, the problem is recurrent over the course of disease.

Secondary Malignancies

Additional cancers are common among people with chronic lymphocytic leukemia, probably related to immune suppression and perhaps genetic predisposition. Melanoma and non-melanoma skin cancers (Chapter 188) are especially increased, and non-melanoma skin cancers can be more invasive and more dangerous than in individuals without chronic lymphocytic leukemia. Common solid tumors including prostate (Chapter 186), breast (Chapter 183), colon (Chapter 179), and lung cancer (Chapter 177) are also increased.

Richter Transformation

Richter transformation, which is the development of an aggressive lymphoma in the context of underlying chronic lymphocytic leukemia, affects about 5% of patients,[10] especially heavily pretreated patients. The majority of lymphomas are diffuse large B-cell lymphomas (Chapter 171) that are clinically and genetically related to the underlying chronic lymphocytic leukemia. Patients commonly present with symptoms that include a rapidly enlarging lymph node, severe B symptoms, fatigue, and/or an elevated lactate dehydrogenase level. Biopsy is required to establish the diagnosis, and a positron emission tomographic (PET) scan is often helpful to target the area to biopsy. Diffuse large B-cell transformation that is clonally unrelated to the underlying chronic lymphocytic leukemia represents about 10 to 20% of cases and typically occurs in previously untreated patients.

DIAGNOSIS

The diagnosis of chronic lymphocytic leukemia should be suspected when an elevation of circulating lymphocytes leads to an elevated total white blood count, usually without any other associated abnormalities on the complete blood count. The peripheral blood smear typically shows an increase in mature appearing lymphocytes with smudge cells, which are an artifact when the fragile lymphocytes of chronic lymphocytic leukemia break open, thereby leaving the appearance of a smudge (Fig. 169-1 and E-Fig. 169-1). Higher numbers of smudge cells are associated with more indolent disease.

The most useful test for establishing a diagnosis of chronic lymphocytic leukemia is peripheral blood flow cytometry for lymphoid markers, which determine the immunophenotype of the circulating cells and often are definitive in establishing the diagnosis of chronic lymphocytic leukemia (Table 169-1). The classic immunophenotype in chronic lymphocytic leukemia includes expression of B-cell markers CD19 with dim CD20 and dim surface immunoglobulin; CD23; and the T-cell marker CD5.

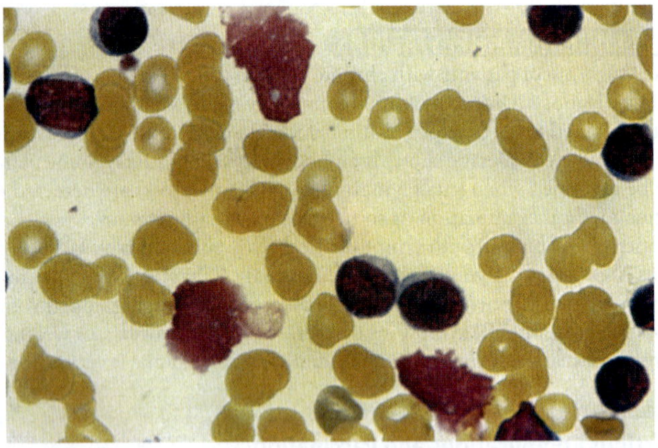

FIGURE 169-1. Chronic lymphocytic leukemia. Peripheral smear shows that the predominant leukocytes are "normal," mature-appearing lymphocytes, with occasional "smudge" cells. (Courtesy Andrew Schafer, MD.)

Differential Diagnosis

Infections such as Epstein-Barr virus (Chapter 348) and cytomegalovirus (Chapter 347) can present with marked lymphocytosis (Chapter 153). However, these and other reactive lymphocytoses are often more pleomorphic on the peripheral blood smear as compared with the lymphocytes of chronic lymphocytic leukemia. Furthermore, flow cytometry will be definitive in the occasional confusing case.

Small Lymphocytic Lymphoma

Small lymphocytic lymphoma (Chapter 171) also has the same immunophenotype as chronic lymphocytic leukemia and historically has been distinguished from chronic lymphocytic leukemia only because its initial presentation is with lymphadenopathy, with less than 5000/μL B lymphocytes in the blood. Currently, chronic lymphocytic leukemia and small lymphocytic lymphoma are considered the same disease and the choice of therapy is the same, so this distinction is of limited importance.

Monoclonal B-Cell Lymphocytosis

Essentially all patients diagnosed with chronic lymphocytic leukemia have had a preexisting subclinical phase called monoclonal B-cell lymphocytosis.[11] Monoclonal B-cell lymphocytosis is diagnosed when the circulating number of B lymphocytes is less than 5000/μL in the absence of cytopenias, lymphadenopathy, or splenomegaly. Many patients with this very low level of lymphocytosis have been told that they have chronic lymphocytic leukemia, when in fact they only meet criteria for monoclonal B-cell lymphocytosis. These monoclonal lymphocytic cells may be detected up to 77 months prior to the diagnosis of chronic lymphocytic leukemia. Although all patients with chronic lymphocytic leukemia have a pre-existing monoclonal B-cell lymphocytosis phase, most patients with monoclonal B-cell lymphocytosis will not progress to develop chronic lymphocytic leukemia.

Monoclonal B-cell lymphocytosis as detected by highly sensitive flow cytometry is very rare before age 40 years, but its prevalence increases to approximately 5% at age 60 years and as high as 45% at age 85 years. The incidence of monoclonal B-cell lymphocytosis is about twice as high among individuals in families with chronic lymphocytic leukemia compared with the general population of similar age.

Monoclonal B-cell lymphocytosis is divided into low-count (<500/μL monoclonal B-cells) disease, which is not detectable on a complete blood count and has a distinct pattern of B-cell receptor gene usage, and high-count (>500/μL but <5000μL monoclonal B-cell lymphocytosis) disease, which is usually identified on a complete blood count and has a B-cell receptor pattern gene usage that is similar to low-risk chronic lymphocytic leukemia.[12] High-count monoclonal B-cell lymphocytosis carries a 1 to 2% per year risk of progressing to chronic lymphocytic leukemia that requires therapy and about a 30% risk of becoming chronic lymphocytic leukemia over 7 years of follow-up, with the primary predictor of progression being a higher lymphocyte count at baseline. However, only 75% of high-count monoclonal B-cell lymphocytosis have a chronic lymphocytic leukemia phenotype, and careful clinical evaluation is warranted to exclude alternative diagnoses including non-Hodgkin lymphomas (Chapter 171).

Other Lymphoid Diseases

Other lymphoid diseases that can present with similar lymphocytosis on a blood smear include marginal zone lymphoma, lymphoplasmacytic lymphoma, mantle cell lymphoma, follicular lymphoma (Chapter 171), and hairy cell

TABLE 169-1 TYPICAL IMMUNOPHENOTYPE OF CHRONIC LYMPHOCYTIC LEUKEMIA COMPARED WITH OTHER B-CELL MALIGNANCIES

DISEASE	CD5	CD10	CD19	CD20	CD23	CYCLIN D1	SURFACE IMMUNOGLOBULIN
Chronic lymphocytic leukemia	+	–	+	+ (dim)	+	–	+ (dim)
Mantle cell lymphoma	+	–	+	+ (mod/bright)	–	+	+ (mod/bright)
Marginal zone lymphoma	–/+	–	+	+ (mod/bright)	–/+	–	+ (mod/bright)
B-prolymphocytic leukemia	–/+	–	+	+ (bright)	–	–	+ (bright)
Follicular lymphoma	–	+	+	+	+	–	

Adapted from Byrd J. Chronic lymphocytic leukemia. In: Goldman L, Schafer AI. *Goldman-Cecil Medicine*. 26th ed. Philadelphia: Elsevier; 2020.

leukemia. More aggressive B-cell lymphomas and mature T-cell leukemia/lymphoma (Chapter 171) can also circulate in the blood but are not difficult to distinguish morphologically from chronic lymphocytic leukemia.

Marginal zone lymphoma (Chapter 171) that is predominantly circulating or splenic is usually the most challenging disease to differentiate from chronic lymphocytic leukemia. Marginal zone lymphoma and lymphoplasmacytic lymphoma are typically negative for both CD5 and CD10, but they can sometimes express CD5 dimly. In these situations, clinical features and cytogenetic or mutational profiles (see Table 169-1) can help establish the most likely diagnosis, but some patients also exhibit features that span more than one diagnosis.

Among the low-grade B-cell diseases, CD5 positivity with CD10 negativity is a key differentiator that excludes follicular lymphoma, which is typically CD10 positive, and hairy cell leukemia, which is typically CD5 negative as well as positive for CD103, CD11c, and CD25. The other B-cell disease that expresses CD5 is mantle cell lymphoma, which can usually be distinguished from chronic lymphocytic leukemia because of the absence of CD23 and positivity for expression of cyclin D1 by immunohistochemistry and/or presence of t(11;14) juxtaposing the cyclin D1 gene with the immunoglobulin heavy chain gene.

Staging and Prognostic Factors

Chronic lymphocytic leukemia can be staged clinically using the Rai system (Table 169-2), which is based on the assessment of lymphadenopathy and organomegaly on physical examination as well as on the complete blood count. However, most patients are diagnosed with early-stage disease, and additional testing (Table 169-3) is useful to help inform prognosis. Among these risk factors, *TP53* aberration and immunoglobulin heavy chain variable mutational status are the most important.

TREATMENT

General Considerations

Very few patients with chronic lymphocytic leukemia require therapy at the time of diagnosis. Asymptomatic patients without cytopenias can be observed, sometimes for decades, and up to 30% of patients never require disease specific therapy. Nevertheless, referral to a specialist is important to confirm the diagnosis, to educate patients about complications, and to provide appropriate counseling and reassurance so patients can adjust to the diagnosis and to the possibility of not receiving therapy for a seemingly ominous condition.

Guidelines suggest the initiation of therapy when cytopenias reach a critical level (e.g., hemoglobin concentration <10 g/dL, platelet count <80-100,000/μL) or when patients develop bulky progressive or symptomatic lymphadenopathy (>10 cm), splenomegaly, significant disease-related symptoms, or difficult-to-control autoimmune hemolytic anemia or immune thrombocytopenic purpura.[13,14] The absolute lymphocyte count itself is not an indication for therapy, although its increase over time often correlates with slowly progressive anemia, thrombocytopenia, and increasing infections that can herald the need for therapy.

Before the initiation of therapy, a full-body computed tomographic scan should be considered in patients who have lymphadenopathy, and a bone marrow biopsy should be considered in patients who have cytopenias. Prognostic markers, such as del(17p), *TP53* mutation, and karyotype analysis, can evolve over time and should be reassessed before each new line of therapy (Table 169-3). Immunoglobulin heavy chain variable sequence mutation status remains stable and does not need to be repeated. If possible, any recommended vaccinations should be completed. Screening for prior hepatitis B infection is important because most therapies reactivate hepatitis B. Chronic active hepatitis B carriers should be on suppressive therapy (Chapter 135) with no detectable viral load before the initiation of any therapy.

Choosing among Medications

Classes of therapy in current use in chronic lymphocytic leukemia include Bruton tyrosine kinase inhibitors, venetoclax (a BCL-2 inhibitor), phosphatidylinositol 3-kinase inhibitors, chemotherapy, immunotherapy, chemoimmunotherapy, and cellular therapy (Table 169-4). Choices are generally determined by the patient's age and comorbid conditions, as well as their disease specific prognostic factors, particularly *TP53* alterations and immunoglobulin heavy chain variable mutation status (Fig. 169-2). Targeted therapies appear to be consistently superior to traditional chemotherapy for both initial treatment and treatment for relapsed or refractory disease (Table 169-5). Once therapy is required, most patients should receive targeted treatment with continuous Bruton tyrosine kinase inhibitor therapy with or without obinutuzumab, or time-limited therapy with venetoclax plus obinutuzumab. Young, fit patients who have favorable mutated immunoglobulin heavy chain gene (IgHV) mutation status and low-risk cytogenetics have the potential of cure with fludarabine/cyclophosphamide/rituximab chemoimmunotherapy.

Most patients are not diagnosed until after age 70 years and are even older by the time that treatment is initiated. Cardiac conditions and the possible need for anticoagulation should be considered prior to beginning treatment with Bruton tyrosine kinase inhibitors, whereas renal dysfunction is an important consideration before venetoclax therapy.[15]

Bruton Tyrosine Kinase Inhibitors

Chronic lymphocytic leukemia cells are dependent on signaling through the B-cell receptor for their growth and survival, and this signaling depends on Bruton tyrosine kinase. When Bruton tyrosine kinase is lost in the germline,

TABLE 169-2 THE RAI STAGING SYSTEM OF CHRONIC LYMPHOCYTIC LEUKEMIA

CLINICAL FEATURES	STAGE
Lymphocytosis only	0
Lymph node enlargement	1
Spleen or liver enlargement (by physical examination)	2
Anemia (hemoglobin <11 g/dL)	3
Thrombocytopenia (platelets <100,000/μL)	4

From Byrd J. Chronic lymphocytic leukemia. In: Goldman L, Schafer AI. *Goldman-Cecil Medicine*. 26th ed. Philadelphia: Elsevier; 2020.

TABLE 169-3 USEFUL TESTS IN THE EVALUATION OF PATIENTS WITH CHRONIC LYMPHOCYTIC LEUKEMIA

Immunophenotype (flow cytometry) – lymphoma markers
IGHV mutational status
Interphase FISH (deletion of 13q, 11q or 17p; trisomy 12)
Stimulated karyotype
TP53 mutation by next-generation sequencing
β_2-microglobulin level
Serum immunoglobulin levels

FISH = fluorescence in situ hybridization.

TABLE 169-4 THERAPIES USED IN CHRONIC LYMPHOCYTIC LEUKEMIA

THERAPY	MECHANISM OF ACTION
TARGETED THERAPIES	
Ibrutinib	Irreversible inhibition of BTK
Acalabrutinib	Second-generation irreversible inhibition of BTK
Zanubrutinib	Second-generation irreversible inhibition of BTK
Venetoclax	Inhibition of BCL-2 function
Idelalisib	Reversible inhibition of PI3Kδ
Duvelisib	Reversible inhibition of PI3Kδ,γ
BIOLOGIC THERAPIES	
Obinutuzumab	CD20-directed antibody with enhanced ADCC and direct killing
Rituximab	CD20-directed antibody with ADCC, CDC, and direct killing
Corticosteroids	Microenvironment effect and activation of the steroid receptor
CHEMOTHERAPY	
Chlorambucil	Alkylator/DNA damage
Cyclophosphamide	Alkylator/DNA damage
Bendamustine	DNA damage
Fludarabine	Purine analogue; inhibition of DNA and RNA synthesis and splicing

ADCC = antibody-dependent, cellular-mediated cytotoxicity; BTK = Bruton tyrosine kinase; CDC = complement-dependent cytotoxicity; PI3K = phosphoinositide 3-kinase.

patients lack mature B cells and have agammaglobulinemia as a result. The inhibitor of Bruton tyrosine kinase, ibrutinib (starting dose 420 mg orally daily), binds to Bruton tyrosine kinase covalently, thereby leading to its permanent inactivation.[16] Overall response rates are over 90%, most high-risk patients respond with at least somewhat durable responses, especially when the drug is continued as first-line therapy, and progression-free survival is improved compared with chemoimmunotherapy.[A1–A4]

Continuous therapy with ibrutinib is not possible in many patients because of significant side effects[17] related to the fact that it is not specific for Bruton tyrosine kinase but also potently inhibits 19 other kinases. Second-generation covalent Bruton tyrosine kinase inhibitors, which are more specific and better tolerated, include acalabrutinib (starting at 100 mg orally twice daily), which is FDA approved for the treatment of chronic lymphocytic leukemia at any stage of the disease based on randomized trials demonstrating over a 90% response rate[A5] and improved progression-free survival compared primarily to chemoimmunotherapy.[A6,A7] Zanubrutinib, which has a unique pharmacokinetic profile that maintains circulating drug levels throughout the dosing interval in addition to acting as a covalent inhibitor, is FDA approved for related B-cell malignancies and chronic lymphocytic leukemia. Both acalabrutinib and zanubrutinib[A8] are as efficacious and are substantially better tolerated than ibrutinib in relapsed chronic lymphocytic leukemia, with acalabrutinib showing significant reductions in the cumulative incidence of hypertension, arthralgia, bleeding, and diarrhea.[A9] Both acalabrutinib and zanubrutinib are tolerated by patients who have discontinued ibrutinib because of intolerance. Zanubrutinib also can improve progression-free survival compared with ibrutinib in relapsed CLL, with significantly fewer adverse events.[A10] In the United States, patients with chronic lymphocytic leukemia, particularly patients who are older or have comorbid conditions that put them at particular risk for complications of ibrutinib, should receive a second-generation Bruton tyrosine kinase inhibitor rather than ibrutinib.

With Bruton tyrosine kinase inhibitors, chronic lymphocytic leukemia cells are redistributed from lymph nodes, spleen, or bone marrow into peripheral blood, often resulting in an increase in the white count (called redistribution lymphocytosis) over the first few weeks of therapy, followed by stabilization and slow decline thereafter. Some patients will eventually achieve a normal white blood cell count, whereas other patients will have persistent stable elevation for years. Lymph nodes shrink rapidly and markedly, thereby allowing evaluation of response despite the increase in white count. Cytopenias also improve, sometimes rapidly but sometimes slowly over up to 6 months. Bruton tyrosine kinase inhibitors do not readily induce apoptosis in chronic lymphocytic leukemia cells, so they do not clear all disease. As a consequence, most patients have durable partial responses but the Bruton tyrosine kinase inhibitor must be continued indefinitely to sustain response.

Complications of Bruton tyrosine kinase inhibitors include a high incidence of cardiac side effects, particularly atrial fibrillation (in 10 to 20% of patients after 2 years on therapy) and hypertension (incidence ranging from 23 to 75% depending on the series), but ventricular arrhythmias, sudden death, conduction block, heart failure, and stroke can also occur. All of these side effects appear to be substantially less likely with acalabrutinib[A11] and zanubrutinib. All Bruton tyrosine kinase inhibitors can cause significant bruising and bleeding, so they must be discontinued for 7 days before and after any major surgical procedure and for 3 days before and after any minor procedure. The covalent Bruton tyrosine kinase inhibitors can be combined safely with single drug anti-platelet therapy (i.e., aspirin), but care must be taken if they are to be combined with anticoagulation, and dual anti-platelet therapy is usually best avoided. If anticoagulation is needed, warfarin is contraindicated and direct oral anticoagulants are preferred. Other side effects frequently leading to the discontinuation of ibrutinib include arthralgias, fatigue, infections, and cytopenias.

Venetoclax

Venetoclax inhibits BCL-2, which is universally overexpressed in chronic lymphocytic leukemia, and blocks apoptosis through direct binding and inhibition of pro-apoptotic proteins. Venetoclax, which is specific for BCL-2, is efficacious in patients with relapsed refractory chronic lymphocytic leukemia, in whom it can provide complete remissions. For example, 2 years of treatment with venetoclax plus rituximab is significantly better than bendamustine plus rituximab in terms of response rates, progression-free survival, and overall survival in heavily pretreated patients.[A12,A13] Even in previously untreated patients, 1 year of treatment with venetoclax plus obinutuzumab is superior to chlorambucil-obinutuzumab with

TABLE 169-5 REPORTED SUCCESS RATES FOR TREATMENT OF CHRONIC LYMPHOCYTIC LEUKEMIA

TREATMENT	PROGRESSION-FREE SURVIVAL	OVERALL SURVIVAL
PREVIOUSLY UNTREATED PATIENTS		
Fludarabine, cyclophosphamide, and rituximab	50% at 57 months	50% at 12.7 years
Bendamustine and rituximab	50% at 42 months	92% at 3 years
Chlorambucil and obinutuzumab	50% at 29 months	Not available
Acalabrutinib	78% at 48 months	88% at 48 months
Acalabrutinib and obinutuzumab	87% at 48 months	93% at 48 months
Venetoclax and obinutuzumab	74% at 48 months	85% at 48 months
Ibrutinib	70% at 5 years	83% at 5 years
RELAPSED OR REFRACTORY DISEASE		
Ibrutinib	50% at 52 months	55% at 7 years
Acalabrutinib	62% at 45 months	>90% at 16 months
Venetoclax	50% at 25 months	84% at 24 months
Venetoclax and rituximab	50% at 54 months	82% at 5 years

Adapted and updated from Burger JA. Treatment of chronic lymphocytic leukemia. *N Engl J Med.* 2020;383:460-473.

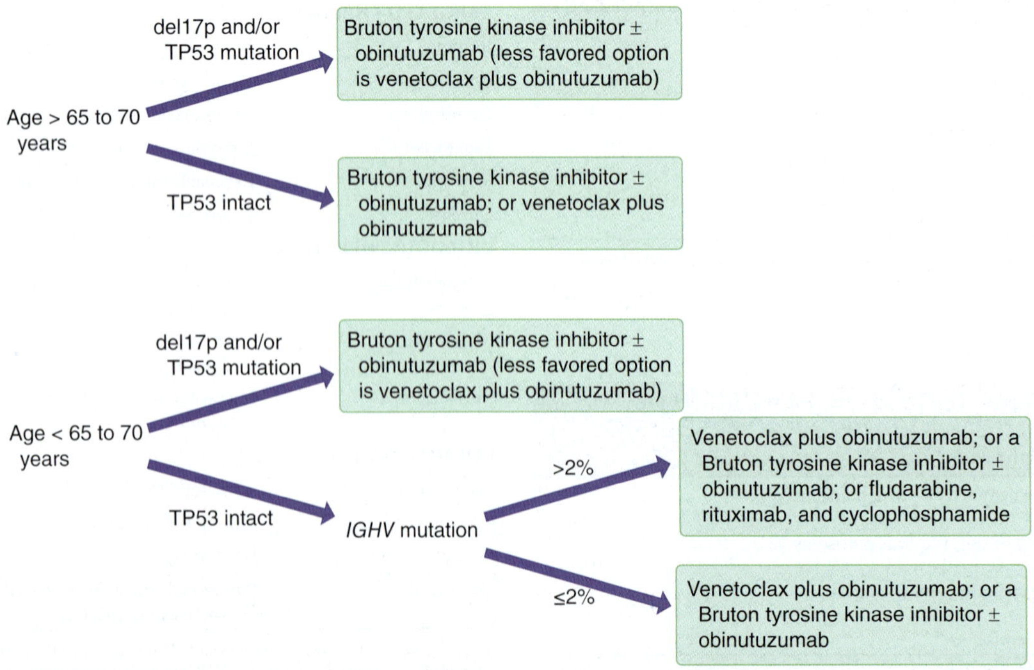

FIGURE 169-2. **Guide to the initial treatment of chronic lymphocytic leukemia.** *IGHV* = immunoglobulin heavy chain variable region.

marked improvement in progression-free survival and deep remissions without detectable residual disease in over 50% of patients,[A14] but all patients eventually relapse. Current investigations are focusing on combining venetoclax with Bruton tyrosine kinase inhibitors, also in time-limited regimens.[18,19] For example, 1 year of ibrutinib plus venetoclax is effective in older patients or patients with comorbid conditions.[A15] The goal of these time-limited regimens is to achieve deep remissions that allow patients substantial time without therapy, with the potential to resume therapy if and when relapse occurs. Venetoclax is also active in chronic lymphocytic leukemia patients whose disease has progressed on a prior Bruton tyrosine kinase inhibitor therapy, albeit with less durability than when it is used as frontline therapy or in patients at the time of first relapse.

The primary side effect of venetoclax is rapid induction of tumor cell death, thereby leading to potentially life-threatening tumor lysis syndrome (Chapter 164). As a result, approved administration starts at a low dose (20 mg orally daily) and is then increased weekly over 5 weeks to the full planned dose of 400 mg orally daily, with laboratory monitoring under expert supervision to avoid the tumor lysis syndrome. Venetoclax is very well tolerated, but other side effects include myelosuppression, nausea, vomiting, and diarrhea.

Immunotherapy

The most successful form of immunotherapy in chronic lymphocytic leukemia is monoclonal antibody therapy. CD20 is a B-cell specific antigen, so off-target effects are limited.

Obinutuzumab is a humanized, glycoengineered anti-CD20 antibody with antibody-dependent cellular cytotoxicity against tumor cells. Obinutuzumab provides better clinical responses and progression-free survival compared with rituximab, so it generally is the antibody of choice in chronic lymphocytic leukemia. For example, obinutuzumab is more potent than rituximab, however, and leads to a significant benefit in terms of progression-free survival when added to acalabrutinib.

The addition of rituximab to ibrutinib has no benefit for progression-free survival.[A16] Rituximab is now mostly used to treat autoimmune cytopenias or in combination with venetoclax.

Chemoimmunotherapy

The combination of CD20 antibodies with chemotherapy leads to synergistic benefit, with nearly universal overall response as well as a marked increase in rates of complete remission (30 to 70%) and durable remissions. For example, the addition of rituximab to chemotherapy with fludarabine plus cyclophosphamide increases overall response, complete response, progression-free survival, and overall survival. Patients with a mutated immunoglobulin heavy chain gene can achieve very prolonged progression-free survival with this regimen, with more than 50% still in remission at 12 years follow-up, thereby suggesting possible cure. Patients with unmutated immunoglobulin heavy chain genes generally experience relapse, but a subset with trisomy 12 can also have durable benefit. Fludarabine/cyclophosphamide/rituximab is preferred over bendamustine rituximab in terms of progression-free survival.[A17] The side effects of fludarabine/cyclophosphamide/rituximab include myelosuppression and a risk of secondary myeloid malignancy, both of which are worse with increasing age, thereby leading to the recommendation that fludarabine/cyclophosphamide/rituximab be considered only in young, fit patients with normal renal function.

Bendamustine plus rituximab can be used palliatively in older patients. Additionally, for older, less-fit patients, the combination of obinutuzumab plus chlorambucil is well tolerated and superior to chlorambucil alone. However, targeted therapy with a Bruton tyrosine kinase inhibitor or with venetoclax plus obinutuzumab provides better progression-free survival if it can be tolerated.[A18]

Phosphatidylinositol 3-kinase (PI3K) δ inhibitors

Like the Bruton tyrosine kinase inhibitors, the PI3Kδ inhibitors also inhibit B-cell receptor signaling downstream of the B-cell receptor. Options include idelalisib (150 mg orally twice daily) and duvelisib (25 mg orally twice daily). Because of substantial toxicity when used as front-line therapy (e.g., neutropenia, bacterial and opportunistic infections, severe colitis, pneumonitis, and elevated aminotransferase levels), these agents are limited to patients who have relapsed chronic lymphocytic leukemia after at least two prior regimens, both Bruton tyrosine kinase inhibitors and venetoclax, or who have comorbid conditions that preclude the use of these drugs.[20]

Refractory Disease

Patients with disease that has progressed despite continuous Bruton tyrosine kinase inhibitor therapy can respond to venetoclax, but durability is limited. Patients whose disease has progressed after both a Bruton tyrosine kinase inhibitor and venetoclax have limited treatment options, because neither PI3K inhibitors nor chemoimmunotherapy have established activity in this particular setting.

For refractory disease, allogeneic stem cell transplantation (Chapter 163) holds the promise of potential cure, but treatment-related mortality is 10 to 20%, and many patients have long-term chronic graft-versus-host disease. Furthermore, the efficacy of transplant is strongly dependent on the patient being in a deep remission, which is often not achievable.

Autologous chimeric antigen receptor (CAR) T-cell therapy is an emerging option for refractory disease. This treatment involves the engineering of the patient's own T cells with a chimeric T cell antigen receptor against a target on the B-cell malignancy, most commonly CD19. CAR T therapy has revolutionized the treatment of relapsed diffuse large B-cell lymphoma (Chapter 171), but results to date in chronic lymphocytic leukemia have been more modest. Possible explanations include the difficulty of collecting autologous T cells due to prior therapy, impaired function of collected T cells due to immune dysfunction, and impaired expansion of the CAR T cells either in vitro or in vivo after infusion, again due to the immune milieu related to chronic lymphocytic leukemia. The coadministration with Bruton tyrosine kinase inhibitors may mitigate some of these problems, but it is not known whether CAR T therapy has the same potential for cure that is offered by allogeneic stem cell transplantation.

Disease-Related Complications

Infections

Patients should be evaluated promptly for any fever, with a low threshold for antibiotic treatment with antimicrobial agents. Vaccination is strongly recommended, including yearly influenza vaccine, COVID-19 vaccine,[21] pneumococcal 20-valent conjugate vaccine followed at least 2 months later by pneumovax (which is then repeated every 5 years), and herpes zoster vaccination (Chapter 15). Studies generally demonstrate measurable but reduced response to these vaccines in patients with chronic lymphocytic leukemia, owing to their immune dysfunction. Patients with chronic lymphocytic leukemia should not receive live-attenuated vaccines because of the risk of disseminated disease arising from the vaccine. If patients have low IgG levels and develop recurrent bacterial infections, intravenous immune globulin replacement under expert supervision can substantially mitigate these infections. For sinus infections, regular sinus irrigation can help substantially.

Autoimmune Complications

When patients with chronic lymphocytic leukemia develop an autoimmune cytopenia, it can be treated with corticosteroids, the anti-CD20 antibody rituximab, or cyclosporine under expert supervision. When these complications develop in the setting of progressive disease, definitive therapy is required for the chronic lymphocytic leukemia.

Malignancy

Patients with chronic lymphocytic leukemia are advised to minimize exposure to ultraviolet light, use highly effective sunscreen, have regular dermatology examinations, and complete all other age-appropriate cancer screening. The treatment of any malignancies is generally the same as in other patients if it can be tolerated.

Richter Transformation

Diffuse large B-cell lymphoma (Chapter 171) can be cured with standard combination chemotherapy for lymphoma (Chapter 171) in previously untreated patients, but the median survival, even with aggressive therapy, is poor when the lymphoma occurs in previously heavily treated patients.

Hodgkin lymphoma (Chapter 172) is much less common. Hodgkin disease (Chapter 172) responds to standard combination chemotherapy for Hodgkin lymphoma and has a natural history like that of de novo disease.

PROGNOSIS

Deletion of 17p containing the *TP53* gene is associated with shorter time to needing treatment, poorer progression-free survival, and shorter overall survival. However, the era of targeted therapies has substantially improved outcome for these patients, with high response rates to targeted therapy albeit still generally shorter progression-free survivals.[22] Deletion 11q, which affects the *ATM* gene, is associated with a pattern of bulky lymphadenopathy, shorter time to treatment, and a shorter durability of remission; however, targeted therapies appear to mitigate this impact. *NOTCH1* mutation is another higher risk mutation that has been associated with an increased risk of Richter transformation. β_2 microglobulin is an extracellular protein component of the human leukocyte antigen (HLA) class 1 complex that associates with prognosis in many B-cell malignancies, most notably multiple myeloma but also chronic lymphocytic leukemia.

Immunoglobulin heavy chain variable sequence status similarly predicts shorter survival for early-stage patients, with older data from before the era of targeted therapy showing that unmutated *VH* genes predict an approximately 8-year survival compared with over 24 years for patients who have mutated *VH* genes. However, continuous Bruton tyrosine kinase inhibitor therapy can control disease for prolonged periods even in patients with unmutated immunoglobulin heavy chain variable sequence.

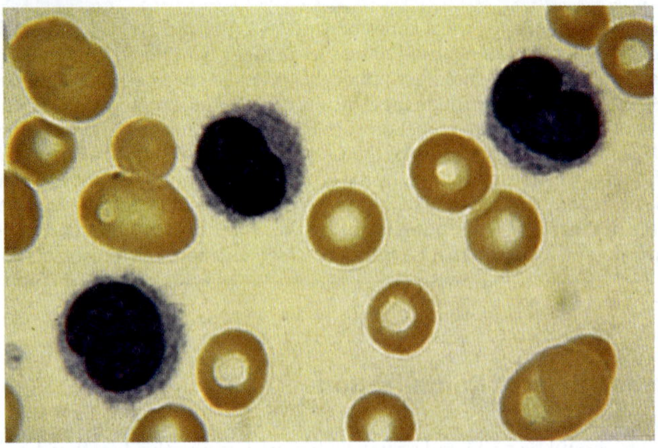

FIGURE 169-3. **Hairy cell leukemia.** Peripheral smear shows hairy cells with blue-gray cytoplasm; fine, hairlike projections (resembling ruffles); and oval or slightly indented nuclei with loose chromatin and indistinct nucleoli. (Courtesy Andrew Schafer, MD.)

OTHER CHRONIC LYMPHOCYTIC LEUKEMIAS

HAIRY CELL LEUKEMIA

Hairy cell leukemia, which is an indolent mature B-cell leukemia, is about five times more common in men than women and usually presents in patients aged 50 to 70 years. Most patients present with pancytopenia and marked splenomegaly without lymphadenopathy.[23] Typical mature hairy cells (which have thin cytoplasmic projections, a kidney-shaped nucleus, and one or two distinct nucleoli; Fig. 169-3) infiltrate the bone marrow, spleen, and liver. Because of a paucity of monocytes, tubercular and fungal infections are common. Diagnosis is based on finding the typical cells in the bone marrow. This leukemia is treated under expert supervision with purine analogues, which often lead to prolonged progression-free survival.[24] Vemurafenib, which is an oral BRAF inhibitor, combined with an anti-CD20 antibody also has substantial activity.[25]

PROLYMPHOCYTIC LEUKEMIA

In B-cell prolymphocytic leukemia, more than >55% of the circulating lymphocytes are prolymphocytes. These prolymphocytes are much larger than normal lymphocytes and have a typically round nucleus, with one clear punched-out nucleolus. Approximately 60% of patients have a translocation targeting *MYC*, and about 40% have a 17p deletion affecting *TP53*. B-cell prolymphocytic leukemia is quite rare as a presenting diagnosis, but some patients with chronic lymphocytic leukemia, typically patients with a 17p deletion, have a subset of cells that are similar to prolymphocytic leukemia cells. As the disease progresses, the distinction can pose a diagnostic dilemma, but the immunophenotype of B-cell prolymphocytic leukemia typically will differ from chronic lymphocytic leukemia by expressing surface immunoglobulin and CD20 brightly, not expressing CD23, and sometimes not expressing CD5. The targeted B-cell receptor pathway inhibitors that are effective in chronic lymphocytic leukemia also are effective for prolymphocytic leukemia, so the need to distinguish between these two diseases may be less important.

LARGE GRANULAR LYMPHOCYTIC LEUKEMIA

Large granular lymphocyte leukemia is discussed in Chapter 151.

GENERAL REFERENCES

For the General References and other additional features, please visit Elsevier eBooks+ at https://ebooks.health.elsevier.com.

Grade A References

A1. Shanafelt TD, Wang XV, Kay NE, et al. Ibrutinib-rituximab or chemoimmunotherapy for chronic lymphocytic leukemia. *N Engl J Med.* 2019;381:432-443.

A2. Woyach JA, Ruppert AS, Heerema NA, et al. Ibrutinib regimens versus chemoimmunotherapy in older patients with untreated CLL. *N Engl J Med.* 2018;379:2517-2528.

A3. Allan JN, Shanafelt T, Wiestner A, et al. Long-term efficacy of first-line ibrutinib treatment for chronic lymphocytic leukaemia in patients with TP53 aberrations: a pooled analysis from four clinical trials. *BR J Haematol.* 2022;19:947-953.

A4. Barr PM, Owen C, Robak T, et al. Up to 8-year follow-up from RESONATE-2: first-line ibrutinib treatment for patients with chronic lymphocytic leukemia. *Blood Adv.* 2022;6:3440-3450.

A5. Byrd JC, Woyach JA, Furman RR, et al. Acalabrutinib in treatment-naive chronic lymphocytic leukemia. *Blood.* 2021;137:3327-3338.

A6. Ghia P, Pluta A, Wach M, et al. ASCEND: phase III, randomized trial of acalabrutinib versus idelalisib plus rituximab or bendamustine plus rituximab in relapsed or refractory chronic lymphocytic leukemia. *J Clin Oncol.* 2020;38:2849-2861.

A7. Sharman JP, Egyed M, Jurczak W, et al. Acalabrutinib with or without obinutuzumab versus chlorambucil and obinutuzmab for treatment-naive chronic lymphocytic leukaemia (ELEVATE TN): a randomised, controlled, phase 3 trial. *Lancet.* 2020;395:1278-1291.

A8. Tam CS, Brown JR, Kahl BS, et al. Zanubrutinib versus bendamustine and rituximab in untreated chronic lymphocytic leukaemia and small lymphocytic lymphoma (SEQUOIA): a randomised, controlled, phase 3 trial. *Lancet Oncol.* 2022;23:1031-1043.

A9. Byrd JC, Hillmen P, Ghia P, et al. Acalabrutinib versus ibrutinib in previously treated chronic lymphocytic leukemia: results of the first randomized phase III trial. *J Clin Oncol.* 2021;39:3441-3452.

A10. Brown JR, Eichhorst B, Hillmen P, et al. Zanubrutinib or ibrutinib in relapsed or refractory chronic lymphocytic leukemia. *N Engl J Med.* 2023;388:319-332.

A11. Htut TW, Han MM, Thein KZ. Acalabrutinib-related cardiac toxicities in patients with chronic lymphocytic leukemia: a meta-analysis of randomized controlled trials. *J Immunother Precis Oncol.* 2021;5:43-47.

A12. Kater AP, Wu JQ, Kipps T, et al. Venetoclax plus rituximab in relapsed chronic lymphocytic leukemia: 4-year results and evaluation of impact of genomic complexity and gene mutations from the MURANO phase III study. *J Clin Oncol.* 2020;38:4042-4054.

A13. Seymour JF, Kipps TJ, Eichhorst B, et al. Venetoclax-rituximab in relapsed or refractory chronic lymphocytic leukemia. *N Engl J Med.* 2018;378:1107-1120.

A14. Fischer K, Al-Sawaf O, Bahlo J, et al. Venetoclax and obinutuzumab in patients with CLL and coexisting conditions. *N Engl J Med.* 2019;380:2225-2236.

A15. Kater AP, Owen C, Moreno C, et al. Fixed-duration ibrutinib-venetoclax in patients with chronic lymphocytic leukemia and comorbidities. *NEJM Evid.* 2022;1:1-13.

A16. Burger JA, Sivina M, Jain N, et al. Randomized trial of ibrutinib vs ibrutinib plus rituximab in patients with chronic lymphocytic leukemia. *Blood.* 2019;133:1011-1019.

A17. Eichhorst B, Fink AM, Bahlo J, et al. First-line chemoimmunotherapy with bendamustine and rituximab versus fludarabine, cyclophosphamide, and rituximab in patients with advanced chronic lymphocytic leukaemia (CLL10): an international, open-label, randomised, phase 3, non-inferiority trial. *Lancet Oncol.* 2016;17:928-942.

A18. Moreno C, Greil R, Demirkan F, et al. First-line treatment of chronic lymphocytic leukemia with ibrutinib plus obinutuzumab versus chlorambucil plus obinutuzumab: final analysis of the randomized, phase III iLLUMINATE trial. *Haematologica.* 2022;107:2108-2120.

170

CHRONIC MYELOID LEUKEMIA

JERALD RADICH

DEFINITION

Chronic myeloid leukemia (CML) is a hematopoietic stem cell disease caused by the reciprocal translocation of gene sequences from the breakpoint cluster region (*BCR*) gene on chromosome 22 with the tyrosine kinase sequences of the Abelson (*ABL*) gene on chromosome 9. On a cytogenetic level, this results in an elongated chromosome 9 and a shortened chromosome 22, the latter known as the Philadelphia (Ph) chromosome. The unique chimeric fusion protein, *BCR-ABL*, is a constitutively active tyrosine kinase that drives the pathogenesis of the disease. Thus, *BCR-ABL* represents the target for tyrosine kinase inhibitor therapy as well as a direct measure of disease burden. As described further below, there can be cases of "Ph-" CML, where the Ph chromosome is not detected, but other methods (fluorescence in situ hybridization [FISH], polymerase chain reaction [PCR]) can detect the chimeric *BCR-ABL*. There is no *BCR-ABL*-negative CML, and such diseases as "atypical" CML and chronic neutrophilic leukemia have distinct genetic features that identify them as unique disease entities (discussed briefly later).

CML is categorized in different phases (chronic, accelerated, and blast phases) based on bone marrow and peripheral blood blast counts, additional cytogenetic abnormalities besides the Ph chromosome, and clinical features such as fever. There are several classification schemes, including those proposed by the European Leukemia Network and the World Health Organization (WHO). The main difference between the European Leukemia Network and WHO classifications is the definition of accelerated phase and blast phase: the European Leukemia Network defines accelerated phase as peripheral or bone marrow blast counts of at least 15% to less than 30%, and blast phase as blasts counts greater than or equal to 30%, whereas in the WHO classification, these values are at least 10 to 20% and greater or equal to 20%, respectively. Of note, the WHO criteria are rarely used in clinical practice or clinical trials. More than 75% of CML cases in the developed world are diagnosed in the chronic phase, whereas the proportion of cases of advanced (accelerated and blast) phase disease is higher in the developing world. Untreated chronic phase CML will eventually progress to advanced phase within a mean period of approximately 3 to 5 years, and when disease reaches blast crisis, the natural history is survival of less than 1 year.

EPIDEMIOLOGY

The incidence of CML is fairly uniform throughout the world, affecting about 1 to 1.5 per 100,000 of the adult population each year.[1] In the Western industrialized world, CML represents approximately 15% of all adult and less than 5% of all childhood leukemias, with a median age of onset of about 65 years. The median age appears to be earlier in the developing world. As a result of the spectacular success of tyrosine kinase inhibitor therapy (see later), the prevalence of CML is increasing steadily because the average duration of the disease has lengthened appreciably.

There are no described "CML families." The greatest risk factor for CML is radiation exposure, particularly in Japanese atomic bomb blast survivors. Although *ABL* sequences are found in the Abelson murine leukemia retrovirus, no infectious agent for human CML has been described.

PATHOBIOLOGY

The Ph chromosome is an acquired cytogenetic abnormality present in all leukemic cells of the myeloid lineage and in some B cells and T cells in CML patients. It is formed as a result of a reciprocal translocation of genetic material of chromosomes 9 and 22 expressed as t(9;22)(q34;q11) (Fig. 170-1). The Ph chromosome is found in more than 90% of CML patients, whereas approximately 5% of cases have translocations that involve chromosomes 9, 22, and others as well. The remaining 5% of patients with clinical and hematologic features consistent with CML have undetectable Ph chromosome, but *BCR-ABL* can be detected by FISH (which detects the DNA fusion) or reverse transcription–polymerase chain reaction (RT-PCR), which detects the chimeric mRNA.

Three possible breakpoints in the *BCR* gene exist, including breaks in the *major* breakpoint cluster region (M-BCR) in the intron between exons e13 and e14 or in the intron between exons e14 and e15.[2] These breakpoints account for more than 95% of CML cases. The breakpoint in the *ABL* gene is varied and can occur broadly upstream of exon a2. Thus, the two possible common *BCR* breakpoints, merging with the *ABL* breakpoint, can yield two slightly different chimeric *BCR-ABL* genes, which yields a longer e13a2 or slightly smaller e14a2 transcript. Both transcripts are translated into a 210-kD BCR-ABL tyrosine kinase ($p210^{BCR\text{-}ABL}$) that has greatly enhanced tyrosine kinase activity compared with the normal ABL protein. Rarely in CML, the breakpoint *BCR* occurs 5′ to the common breakpoint between exons e1 and e2 in an area designated the *minor* breakpoint cluster region (m-bcr). This produces the e1a2 mRNA, yielding a smaller *BCR-ABL* fusion gene ($p190^{BCR\text{-}ABL}$). Curiously, although this genetic alteration is uncommon in CML, it accounts for roughly half of the cases of Ph chromosome–positive acute lymphoblastic leukemia (ALL).

Very rarely, a breakpoint in the so-called *micro* breakpoint cluster region (μ-bcr) results in e19a2 chimeric mRNA and a larger 230-kD BCR-ABL protein ($p230^{BCR\text{-}ABL}$). This molecular lesion appears to be associated with the rare Ph chromosome–positive chronic neutrophilic leukemia.

The normal ABL protein is a nonreceptor tyrosine kinase with important roles in signal transduction and the regulation of cell growth. Normal ABL protein migrates between the cytoplasm and nucleus. The chimeric BCR-ABL protein, however, associates with the cytoplasmic membrane and is constitutively active with increased kinase activity, causing activation of numerous signal transduction pathways, including MYC, RAS, STAT, JUN, and phosphatidylinositol-3 kinase. Unlike many multihit models of carcinogenesis, the single *BCR-ABL* lesion thus appears to influence cell cycling, differentiation, and apoptosis, causing DNA genetic instability and attenuation of the DNA damage response. In murine models, *BCR-ABL* can cause myeloproliferative diseases similar to human CML, although chronic phase has been difficult to simulate until recent sophisticated genetically engineered murine models coupled inducible *BCR-ABL* with the genetic scrambling of the Sleeping Beauty transposon. In vitro studies suggest that *BCR-ABL* expression allows cells to become cytokine independent, protects cells from apoptotic responses to DNA damage, and increases adhesion of hematopoietic cells to extracellular matrix proteins.

The progression to advanced phase disease will eventually occur in all cases not treated with a tyrosine kinase inhibitor or allogeneic transplantation, and advanced phase disease is not curable without transplant (even in the age of tyrosine kinase inhibitors). Progression is associated with a further block in differentiation, with death coming from the eventual absence of normal platelets (bleeding) or white blood cells (infection). Blast counts increase and new cytogenetic abnormalities accumulate. The most common cytogenetic changes in progression are an additional Ph chromosome, trisomy 8, isochrome i(17q), and trisomy 19. Gene expression profiling suggests that the bulk of the

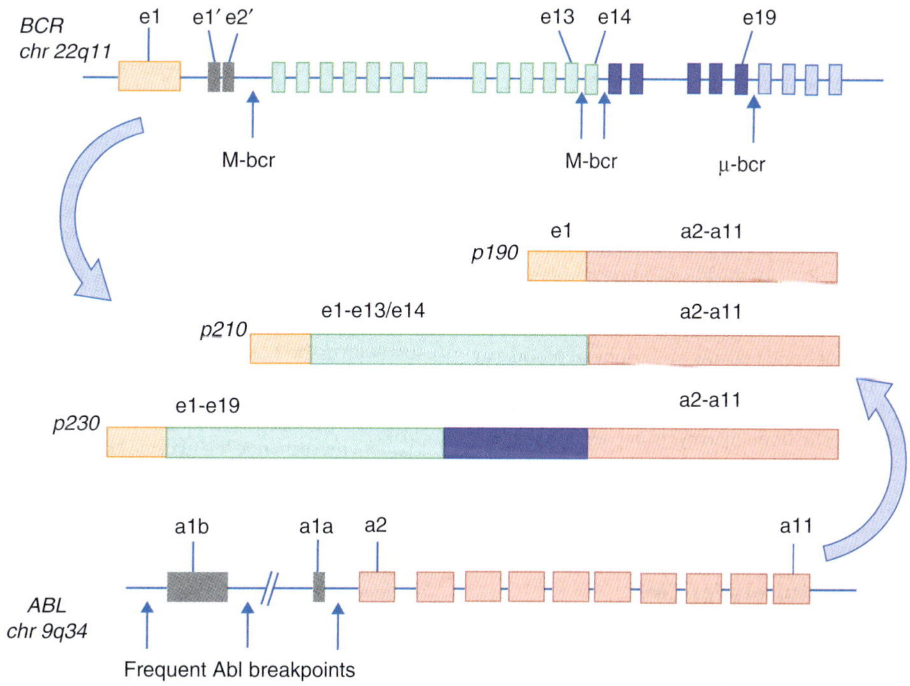

FIGURE 170-1. *BCR* and *ABL* gene breakpoints. The *BCR* gene (from chromosome 22) contains three primary breakpoint regions (denoted the "major breakpoint cluster" [M-bcr]; "minor breakpoint cluster" [*m-bcr*]; and "micro breakpoint cluster" [*μ-bcr*]). Gene rearrangement at the *M-bcr* site results in either of two p210 fusion proteins, composed of *BCR* exons 1-13 or exons 1-14 (*orange* and *green*) fused to *ABL* exons 2-11 (*pink*). Gene rearrangement at *m-bcr* site results in the p190 fusion protein, composed of *BCR* exon 1 (e1) (*orange*) fused to *ABL* exons 2-11 (a2-a11) (*pink*). Gene rearrangement at the *μ-bcr* site results in the p230 fusion protein, composed of *BCR* exons 1-19 (*orange, green*, and *purple*) fused to *ABL* exons 2-11 (*pink*). The *BCR* e1′ and e2′ are included in the fusion gene, but splicing events result in loss of RNA from the *BCR-ABL* transcript. Fusion transcripts may additionally include *ABL* exons 1a or 1a/1b with exons 2-11, depending on the *ABL* breakpoint region. Not to scale.

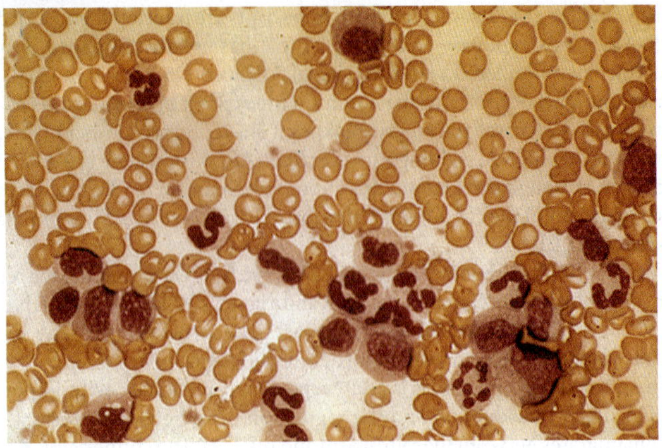

FIGURE 170-2. Chronic myeloid leukemia, chronic phase. Peripheral smear shows leukocytosis, with representation by the entire spectrum of leukocyte differentiation, ranging from myeloblasts to mature neutrophils. (Courtesy Andrew Schafer, MD.)

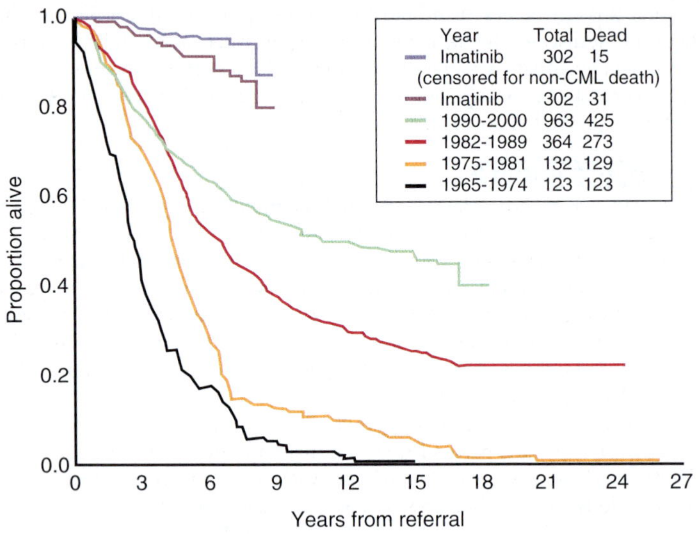

FIGURE 170-3. Survival of patients with Ph chromosome–positive chronic myeloid leukemia (CML) in chronic phase CML. In single-institutional studies, industry-sponsored trials, and national reports where tyrosine kinase inhibitor therapy has full penetration, the estimated 8- to 10-year survival rates are high. The survival rates are lower where tyrosine kinase inhibitor treatment penetration is not optimal. (From Bjorkholm M, Ohm L, Eloranta S, et al. Success story of targeted therapy in chronic myeloid leukemia: a population-based study of patients diagnosed in Sweden from 1973-2008. *J Clin Oncol.* 2011;29:2514-2520, and Chen Y, Wang H, Kantarjian H, et al. Trends in chronic myeloid leukemia incidence and survival in the United States from 1975-2009. *Leuk Lymphoma.* 2013;54:1411-1417.)

genetic changes triggering progression occur from the transition of chronic to accelerated phase, with relatively minor genetic changes occurring from accelerated to blast phase. In keeping with the stem cell origin nature of CML, in about 25% of blast phase cases, the predominant blast expansion is in the lymphoid, not myeloid, lineage.

CLINICAL MANIFESTATIONS

Most CML patients (>90%) present in chronic phase, often diagnosed incidentally during routine examination and blood cell counts. Symptoms, when present, usually include fatigue and abdominal discomfort from splenomegaly. More extreme constitutional symptoms of weight loss, bone pain, fever, and night sweats are more commonly associated with advancing disease. This has practical clinical relevance because although the tyrosine kinase inhibitors used to treat CML (discussed later) are generally well tolerated, compliance early in the treatment course can be challenging because the medications can make patients feel worse than they felt before they were diagnosed.

DIAGNOSIS

Patients generally present with leukocytosis, often accompanied by thrombocytosis and anemia (Fig. 170-2). Basophilia and eosinophilia are common. Without any other obvious explanation for a high white blood cell (WBC) count, the diagnosis of CML can be entertained.[3]

In CML, the diagnostic and monitoring target is the chimeric *BCR-ABL* gene, whether this is at the chromosome level (metaphase cytogenetics), at the DNA level (FISH), or by chimeric mRNA transcript (RT-PCR).

Diagnostic Work-Up

The diagnostic work-up for the suspected CML patient is fairly straightforward, and the goal is to establish both the diagnosis and the phase of disease. A bone marrow aspirate should be evaluated for, at minimum, morphology (to determine blast count) and cytogenetics (to look for the Ph chromosome and other cytogenetic abnormalities that would classify the patient as advanced phase). FISH can be used if the cytogenetic test fails and can be done on peripheral blood if need be. The RT-PCR assay of bone marrow or peripheral blood can be useful to define a "baseline" for later disease monitoring during therapy but is not required. Using peripheral blood RT-PCR testing for *BCR-ABL* can establish diagnosis, but initial diagnostic bone marrow is needed for staging.

TREATMENT

Tyrosine kinase inhibitors are the cornerstone of treatment for CML (Fig. 170-3).[4,5]

Frontline Tyrosine Kinase Inhibitors for CML

There are four FDA-approved tyrosine kinase inhibitors for newly diagnosed chronic phase CML, the "first-generation" tyrosine kinase inhibitor imatinib and three "second-generation" agents, dasatinib, nilotinib, and bosutinib (Table 170-1).[6–8] All work by competitively binding to the adenosine triphosphate (ATP)-binding pocket of BCR-ABL, thus blocking phosphate passage to other downstream signaling effector proteins. In addition, each tyrosine kinase inhibitor has a unique pattern of "off-target" kinase inhibition, which likely explains how the different toxicities of the agents can provide a 67% complete cytogenetic response compared with 7% in the control arm. After more than a decade of follow-up, the cumulative rate of complete cytogenetic response with imatinib is 80 to 85%, with an estimated freedom from progression to progressive disease and overall survival of 92% and 83%, respectively.[A1] Moreover, roughly half all patients with a complete cytogenetic response obtain a major molecular response.

However, the long-term follow-up studies showed that more than 40% of patients discontinue imatinib therapy. These failures of imatinib are roughly divided into thirds: primary resistance to tyrosine kinase inhibitors, intolerance, and resistance/progression after an initial response. Second-generation TKIs (nilotinib, dasatinib, and bosutinib; Table 170-2)[A2–A4] produce superior short-term responses, as measured by rate of complete cytogenetic response and major molecular response by 12 months of therapy. In addition, the second-generation tyrosine kinase inhibitors produce a higher proportion of "deep" molecular responses (which may influence the potential for tyrosine kinase inhibitor discontinuation, discussed later). Transformation to advanced phase disease is less frequent. However, long-term survival has not been significantly different between imatinib and the second-generation tyrosine kinase inhibitors.

Several trials have also compared standard (400 mg/day) to high-dose (600 to 800 mg/day) imatinib. These studies consistently show that high-dose imatinib can yield similar short- and long-term outcomes as the second-generation tyrosine kinase inhibitors. However, these higher doses are less well tolerated and are discouraged as initial therapy in newly diagnosed chronic phase cases.

Toxicities of Tyrosine Kinase Inhibitors

The common side effect of tyrosine kinase inhibitors is myelosuppression, which is less problematic in imatinib than the second-generation tyrosine kinase inhibitors (with grade 3 or 4 cytopenias occurring in roughly 10% vs. more than 20% for imatinib and the second-generation tyrosine kinase inhibitors, respectively). In addition, each tyrosine kinase inhibitor has a unique side-effect profile (see Table 170-1). The tyrosine kinase inhibitors tend to be "cross-tolerant" in that if a patient must change the tyrosine kinase inhibitor because of a particular side effect, it is unlikely that the same complication would be found with another tyrosine kinase inhibitor. Chronic fatigue (mostly correlated with musculoskeletal pain and muscular cramps) is especially problematic for imatinib users and is the side effect that most affects quality of life, although fluid retention is also a problem. Pleural effusion is an adverse event for dasatinib and can be found in about 20% of patients (as opposed to 1% with imatinib). In addition, reversible pulmonary arterial hypertension is a rare (about 5%) but serious side effect with dasatinib. Nilotinib can cause a prolongation of the QT interval and is associated with an increased risk for peripheral arterial occlusive disease. Bosutinib's primary toxicity is diarrhea, which can occur in up to 70% of patients. Ponatinib has a strong association with hypertension and carries a black box warning regarding hepatotoxicity and vascular occlusion. Indeed, arterial and venous thrombosis and occlusions occurred in approximately 30% of CML patients receiving the drug who had highly resistant disease, and these events happened in cases with and without cardiovascular risk factors. Peripheral and

TABLE 170-1 THERAPY OF CHRONIC MYELOID LEUKEMIA WITH OUTCOMES AND MOST FREQUENT SIDE EFFECTS

SETTING	DRUGS	CCyR (%)	SURVIVAL (%)	NOTABLE SIDE EFFECTS (TOP THREE)
Frontline	Imatinib	65% at 5 years	83% at 11 years	Muscle spasms (41%), edema (37%), hypophosphatemia (28%)
	Dasatinib	86% at 2 years	91% at 5 years	Neutropenia (29%), pleural effusion (28%), diarrhea (21%)
	Nilotinib	85% at 4 years	94% at 54 months	Rash (38%), headache (32%), fatigue (23%)
	Bosutinib	77% at 1 year	N/A	Diarrhea (70%), increased ALT (23%), thrombocytopenia (14%)
Second/third line	Dasatinib	50% at 5 years	71% at 6 years	
	Nilotinib		85% at 3 years	*For all TKIs given as third-line agents, same side effects occur with higher frequency*
	Bosutinib	40% at 2 years	92% at 2 years	
	Ponatinib	45% at 2 years	90% at 2 years	
	Omacetaxine	10% at 2 years	85% at 2 years	Cytopenias

ALT = alanine aminotransferase; TKI = tyrosine kinase inhibitor.

TABLE 170-2 TWELVE-MONTH RESPONSES IN THE ENESTND, DASISION, AND BOSUTINIB TRIALS

	ENESTND TRIAL			*DASISION TRIAL*		*BFORE TRIAL*	
RESPONSE	NIL300 BID	NIL400 BID	IM 400	DAS 100	IM 400	BOS 400	IM 400
CCyR	80%	78%	65%	83%	72%	77%	66%
MMR	44%	43%	22%	46%	28%	47%	37%
AP/BC	0.7%	0.4%	4.2%	1.9%	3.5%	2%	3%

AP/BC = patients progressing to accelerated phase and blast crisis; bid = twice daily; CCyR = complete cytogenetic remission; DAS = dasatinib; IM = imatinib; MMR = major molecular response; NIL = nilotinib.

coronary occlusion are seen to a lesser degree with bosutinib and are least likely in patients treated with imatinib.

Monitoring Tyrosine Kinase Inhibitor Therapy

The day-to-day management of tyrosine kinase inhibitor side effects is detailed extensively in the National Comprehensive Cancer Network guidelines.[9] The response to therapy must be carefully monitored and assessed. Many studies have shown that peripheral blood quantitative monitoring of mutant *BCR-ABL* transcript by RT-PCR is a sensitive and reliable measure of disease burden and correlates with short-term and long-term outcomes. Because of the exquisite sensitivity of the *BCR-ABL* assay (with an estimated detection limit of 1 CML cell in 10^5 normal cells), peripheral blood testing is the foundation of *monitoring* treatment (www.NCCN.org and www.leukemia-net.org). Indeed, quantitative PCR testing of *BCR-ABL* transcript is recommended as the only monitoring test needed during therapy. Follow-up bone marrow aspirates and cytogenetics are reserved for patients who fail to meet treatment milestones or relapse while on therapy (see later).

A complete hematologic response is the normalization of peripheral blood counts, and it occurs in more than 90% of patients within 3 months of starting tyrosine kinase inhibitor therapy. A cytogenetic response is based on the number of Ph chromosomes found on a metaphase preparation of at least 20 cells. A major cytogenetic response occurs when 0 to 35% of metaphases are positive for Ph chromosomes. A complete cytogenetic response is when no Ph chromosomes are found. Complete cytogenetic response correlates strongly with a high overall survival, and a peripheral blood value *BCR-ABL* allele burden of 1% correlates with a complete cytogenetic response.

A molecular response measures peripheral blood *BCR-ABL* as a ratio to a control (wild-type) gene (*BCR, ABL*, or *GUSB*, depending on the reference laboratory), set to an international scale (IS). A three-log reduction (0.1% IS) is termed a major molecular response and correlates with a superior progression-free survival and overall survival compared with patients with a lesser response. Deeper responses are based on the log reduction in the BCR-ABL load (e.g., MR4 represents a four-log reduction from baseline). The use of the terms "undetectable" and "negative" BCR-ABL is discouraged because the absence of BCR-ABL can be from either low actual disease burden or poor laboratory performance.

Discontinuation of Tyrosine Kinase Inhibitor Therapy

In in vitro studies, the "CML stem cell" appears impervious to tyrosine kinase inhibitor therapy, and therefore it was assumed that patients would have to remain on a tyrosine kinase inhibitor for life because discontinuation would simply allow the stem cell reservoir to proliferate, assuring certain relapse. However, about 40 to 50% of patients who have been without detectable *BCR-ABL* for several years remain in molecular remission for more than 2 years after tyrosine kinase inhibitor therapy is discontinued.[10,11] The minimum pre-discontinuation time appears to be at least 2 years of a deep response. Since about a year is required to obtain a deep response, most patients will have had at least 3 years of therapy. The rapidity of the BCR-ABL decline after initiating therapy ("halving time") and the detection of BCR-ABL by ultrasensitive techniques prior to discontinuation are associated with an increased or decreased chance of treatment-free remission, respectively.[12,13] Most (>90%) relapsing patients respond well and quickly to the reintroduction of therapy, although not all achieve similarly deep responses. Progression to advanced phase disease after discontinuation is exceedingly rare. However, the long-term consequences of discontinuation are unknown, and patients and physicians who wish to try discontinuation are advised to enroll in a clinical trial.

Which Tyrosine Kinase Inhibitor for Frontline Therapy?

Both the National Comprehensive Cancer Network and the European Leukemia Network are agnostic in regard to which tyrosine kinase inhibitor should be used as frontline therapy. Some practical considerations include:

1. *What are the treatment goals?* For an older patient, controlling the disease and extending survival without undue toxicity are primary goals, and these can be accomplished with imatinib. On the other hand, a younger patient may be interested in childbearing and/or discontinuation of tyrosine kinase inhibitor therapy. In this setting, starting with a second-generation tyrosine kinase inhibitor may be the best choice because the likelihood of a deep response is greater.
2. *What is the status of the disease?* Patients who present in chronic phase by morphologic and cytogenetic criteria may be in a high-risk group given a high WBC count and spleen size. In cases in which advancing phase disease is suspected, the use of the more potent second-generation tyrosine kinase inhibitor may have merit.
3. *What is the status of the patient?* Many patients may have comorbidities that can affect drug choice. Of the three agents available, imatinib has the longest track record and seems to be relatively free of long-term side effects. Nilotinib is associated with troublesome side effects in patients with the metabolic syndrome and has a higher incidence of vascular occlusive events compared with imatinib. Dasatinib has the highest risk for producing pleural effusions and is associated with pulmonary artery hypertension in a small subset of patients. Lastly, bosutinib can cause considerable diarrhea.

Resistance to Tyrosine Kinase Inhibition

Primary resistance to imatinib is defined as the failure to normalize peripheral blood counts (which typically occurs 1 to 3 months after initiating therapy). In clinical trials this occurs in less than 10% of cases. This can be confused with poor compliance for reasons noted previously because studies have shown that poor adherence significantly affects the likelihood of patients ever achieving a major molecular response or deeper response, or losing cytogenetic response; they have a nearly 30% chance of losing complete cytogenetic response compared with only about 2% in highly adherent patients. Beyond the strict definition of primary resistance, a failure to reach molecular response milestones at 3 and 6 months bodes poorly (see later), and the fact that patients with a poor early response have a higher likelihood of early progression to advanced phase disease suggests a biologic relationship between primary resistance and progression.

Acquired or "secondary" resistance describes the phenomenon of an early response to therapy, with subsequent resistance and a rise in *BCR-ABL* transcript levels. In roughly 25 to 50% of cases, this is caused by a single base pair mutation in the *ABL* kinase domain, resulting in a change in protein conformation, with an alteration of the binding of tyrosine kinase inhibitors and the resulting inhibition of *BCR-ABL*. Thus far, more than 100 such mutations have been discovered. It is not clear whether these mutations are present at a very low level even at diagnosis and emerge under the selective pressure of the tyrosine kinase inhibitor, or whether they arise during therapy. In vitro methods have been used to describe the relative inhibitory effects of different tyrosine kinase inhibitors with different mutations, and this can be useful in selecting which tyrosine kinase inhibitor one should use as second-line therapy in cases of resistance. The detection of the T315I mutation is of special note because only one tyrosine kinase inhibitor (ponatinib) is effective with this particular mutation. The T315I mutation becomes more prevalent with increasing patterns of resistance and tyrosine kinase inhibitor substitution, so although unusual at the first signs of resistance, it is quite common in the setting of multiple tyrosine kinase inhibitor failure.

Treatment Milestones for Frontline Therapy in Chronic Phase CML

The National Comprehensive Cancer Network and the European Leukemia Network recommend a set of treatment milestones associated with survival outcomes (Table 170-3). The major prognostic milestones are (1) the achievement of a complete cytogenetic response (or its near equivalent, a *BCR-ABL* of ≤1% IS) should occur by 12 months of therapy; (2) thereafter, achievement of a major molecular response (*BCR-ABL* ≤0.1% IS) is desirable because this level of disease burden is associated with a very low rate of resistance and progression; and (3) deeper responses (MR4.0 and lower) that are sustained may allow for tyrosine kinase inhibitor discontinuation. The failure to reach milestones, or the loss of milestones, should prompt consideration of change to another tyrosine kinase inhibitor and mutation testing to inform the decision of which tyrosine kinase inhibitor to use as second-line therapy.

The treatment response of a complete cytogenetic response at 12 months of tyrosine kinase inhibitor therapy is a prognostic indicator of long-term survival with imatinib or second-generation tyrosine kinase inhibitors. For example, for chronic phase patients receiving either imatinib or second-generation tyrosine kinase inhibitors, the 3-year progression-free survival and overall survival rates for patients with and without a 12-month complete cytogenetic response were 98%/99% and 67%/94%, respectively. Achievement of a major molecular response is associated with continued complete cytogenetic response, less disease progression to advanced phases, and a better overall survival compared with patients without a major molecular response. For example, in the IRIS study, the 10-year overall survival rate was 91% for patients with a major molecular response at 12 months versus 85% in those without a major molecular response. Similar benefits of achieving a major molecular response are seen in patients receiving second-generation tyrosine kinase inhibitors.

Recent attention has shifted to even earlier assessment of disease burden as measured by peripheral blood *BCR-ABL* allele burden at 3 and 6 months of therapy (early molecular response, or EMR). The *BCR-ABL* cutoff of 10% IS or less (good prognosis) versus more than 10% IS (bad prognosis) has been evaluated after frontline therapy with imatinib, dasatinib, and nilotinib, and the early molecular response is consistently associated with short- and long-term outcomes across all tyrosine kinase inhibitors. A retrospective study of chronic phase CML patients treated with imatinib first-line therapy found that patients with 3-month BCR-ABL levels of 10% IS or less had overall survival and progression-free survival rates of 93% (both), whereas patients with more than 10% IS had inferior rates of 57% (both). This trend has been shown in several other retrospective and randomized trials. In addition, cytogenetic and molecular responses also differ based on early molecular response. For example, dasatinib-treated patients with good EMR had a 5-year complete cytogenetic response, a major molecular response, and MR4.5 rates of 94%, 87%, and 54%, whereas patients with poor early molecular response had rates of 41%, 38%, and 5%, respectively.

Second-Line Therapy—Tyrosine Kinase Inhibitors and Other Approaches

For second-line therapy, the second-generation tyrosine kinase inhibitors have quite similar efficacy.[A5,14,15] Single-arm studies suggest that these agents will yield a complete cytogenetic response in 30 to 50% of relapsed cases (much higher in cases in which a tyrosine kinase inhibitor switch was precipitated by a lack of tolerance to the first-line agent). The progression-free survival rate for second-line tyrosine kinase inhibitor therapy is more than 70% (see Table 170-1). At 5-year follow-up, however, only one third of patients remain on treatment. If or when subsequent relapse occurs, a third-line agent can be used, but in this setting, responses are unusual. The possible exception is ponatinib, which in the setting of multiple-resistant or T315I mutations, achieved a complete cytogenetic response of more than 70%, with 2-year progression-free survival rates of about 70%. The more frequent use of ponatinib for resistance has been constrained by its significant vascular side effects, however.

TABLE 170-3 DRUG FAILURE MILESTONES THAT SUGGEST NEED FOR A CHANGE IN TYROSINE KINASE INHIBITOR

TIME POINT AFTER INITIATION OF TKI THERAPY	RESPONSE MILESTONE
3 months	No CHR* Ph+ >95% *BCR-ABL* >10% IS†
6 months	*BCR-ABL* >10% IS Ph+ >35%
12 months	*BCR-ABL* >1% Ph+ >0%
Any time after 12 months	Loss of CHR Loss of CCyR Loss of MMR (*BCR-ABL* >0.1% IS) *ABL* kinase domain mutations New clonal cytogenetic abnormality

*Recommendations for milestones by the National Comprehensive Cancer Network and the European Leukemia Network.

†The National Comprehensive Cancer Network considers change for these patients if the patient has not had treatment interruptions from toxicity or adherence. The European Leukemia Network assesses early molecular response at 6 months.

CCyR = complete cytogenetic response; CHR = complete hematologic response; IS = international scale; MMR = major molecular response; Ph = Philadelphia chromosome; TKI = tyrosine kinase inhibitor.

In heavily pretreated CML patients with resistance to or unacceptable side effects from tyrosine kinase inhibitors, asciminib (10 to 200 mg once or twice daily), an allosteric inhibitor that binds a myristoyl site of the BCR-ABL1 protein, thereby locking BCR-ABL1 into an inactive conformation through a mechanism distinct from all other ABL kinase inhibitors, can provide a major molecular response in about 25 to 50% of patients.[16,A6]

A key question for patients with resistant disease who are placed on a salvage tyrosine kinase inhibitor regimen is when to judge efficacy because allogeneic stem cell transplantation would be the next strategy. Two different studies support an evaluation of response after 3 months of therapy. If a major cytogenetic response is not achieved, the progression-free survival is dramatically different compared with patients achieving a major cytogenetic response. If a patient is a transplantation candidate, a formal search can be initiated at the same time as the initiation of a second-line tyrosine kinase inhibitor because it usually requires 3 months to identify an unrelated donor. Thus, an assessment can be made as to adequacy of tyrosine kinase inhibitor response and availability of a donor at 3 months. If the patient has a good response, tyrosine kinase inhibitor therapy is continued; if the response is poor, the patient can move to transplantation.

Allogeneic Hematopoietic Stem Cell Transplantation

Before the advent of tyrosine kinase inhibitor therapy, allogeneic transplantation was the treatment of choice for newly diagnosed CML. Most centers reported survival rates of 75 to 85%, 25 to 40%, and 10 to 20% for chronic, accelerated, and blast phase disease, respectively. The results are similar for those with related and unrelated matched donors. Currently, transplantation is reserved for salvage therapy for those few patients who cannot tolerate tyrosine kinase inhibitors, patients with highly resistant disease, and those with advanced phase disease.[17,18] Several studies have shown that prior tyrosine kinase inhibitor therapy does not have an adverse effect on transplant-related mortality and that patients who undergo transplantation because of intolerance to tyrosine kinase inhibitors have survival rates similar to untreated historical controls. In additions, studies have shown that patients with T315I mutations have similar outcomes as historical controls.

Who Should Undergo Allogeneic Transplantation in the Era of Tyrosine Kinase Inhibitors?

Reasonable indications might include the following:

1. *Intolerance of tyrosine kinase inhibitors*. Tyrosine kinase inhibitors tend to be cross-tolerant, meaning that if a particular toxicity occurs with tyrosine kinase inhibitor "A," it is unlikely to occur with agent "B." However, rare patients cannot tolerate any tyrosine kinase inhibitors. For these patients, bone marrow transplantation is encouraged.
2. *Primary tyrosine kinase inhibitor failure* (e.g., failure to reach the National Comprehensive Cancer Network or European Leukemia Network guidelines, such as lack of a cytogenetic response by 3 to 6 months, less than major cytogenetic response by 12 months, or complete cytogenetic response by 18 months). These patients should receive a trial of a different tyrosine

kinase inhibitor, but it is prudent to make sure these patients are evaluated for transplantation and undergo HLA typing. Failure of the second agent in this setting would be a reasonable indication at least prompting evaluation for bone marrow transplantation.

3. *Secondary resistance.* When patients become resistant to a frontline agent, the probability of achieving a complete cytogenetic response with a second-line agent is 50% or less. In addition, the probability of such patients failing second-line therapy and developing progression or a T315I mutation is greatly increased compared with tyrosine kinase inhibitor-naïve patients.
4. *Patients with T315I mutation.* Ponatinib is highly effective in chronic phase patients with the T315I mutation, and most patients should initially be started on this agent. However, there is considerable risk for venous and arterial occlusive disease, so patients with a high risk for vascular events or who are young and might need to be on ponatinib for many years should consider the transplantation option. The protein synthesis inhibitor omacetaxine is also approved in this setting, although responses are few and short lived.
5. *Accelerated or blast phase disease.* The rare patients who present with accelerated phase respond well to tyrosine kinase inhibitor therapy and might not need transplantation (although it is worthwhile to begin looking for a donor early in these cases). Patients who present in blast crisis should get intensive therapy (often chemotherapy combined with a tyrosine kinase inhibitor) and move to transplantation when a donor is identified. Patients who progress to advanced phase disease while on a tyrosine kinase inhibitor have a median survival of less than 1 year and need transplantation in short order.
6. *Clonal abnormalities with myelodysplasia.* Clonal changes in Ph chromosome–negative cells occur in about 5% of patients in complete cytogenetic response. In most cases, these do not seem to affect the natural history. However, rare patients have a −5 or −7 abnormality associated with features of myelodysplastic syndrome and should consider bone marrow transplantation.

Treatment of Patients with Advanced Phase CML

It is rare for CML to present in advanced phase disease. Indeed, a patient who presents in lymphoid or myeloid blast crisis is difficult to distinguish from de novo ALL or acute myeloid leukemia (AML; Chapter 163).

Rarely, patients present with advanced phase disease defined by a modest increase in blast counts or the Ph chromosome with other clonal cytogenetic abnormalities. In this case, upfront treatment with a single-agent tyrosine kinase inhibitor regimen is often quite effective, yielding results similar to chronic phase disease. Results are different, however, in chronic phase CML, in which patients who progress to advanced phase disease while on tyrosine kinase inhibitors have a median survival of less than 1 year. Both dasatinib and bosutinib (but not nilotinib) are approved for the treatment of blast phase CML. In general, the blast phase of CML is treated with ALL- or AML-like chemotherapy (Chapter 163), with the addition of a tyrosine kinase inhibitor. Another potentially useful drug approved for chronic and accelerated phase disease is omacetaxine (also known as homoharringtonine), an inhibitor of protein synthesis. The major side effect is myelosuppression, and its role is generally as a bridge to allogeneic transplantation, which is the only potential curative therapy in patients with advanced phase disease in the face of tyrosine kinase inhibitor treatment. The survival rates after allogeneic transplantation are, roughly, for chronic phase more than 80%, accelerated phase 40 to 50%, and blast phase 10 to 20%.

PROGNOSIS

Several clinical and pathologic features at diagnosis or shortly thereafter are associated with long-term response. The strongest prognostic feature is the phase of disease.

Numerous risk scores have been used to predict long-term outcomes. Each combines clinical factors (e.g., age, spleen size) with laboratory values, and all work with a high degree of intrascore system correlation (Table 170-4). The scores typically divide patients into low-, intermediate-, and high risk categories, with survival and progression correlating with risk group. The Sokal Index, developed in 1984 for chronic phase patients, is the most commonly used and places patients into risk categories based on age, blast count, spleen size, and platelet count. The Hasford score was developed from patients on interferon and adds peripheral blood counts to the Sokal measures. The more recently developed European Treatment and Outcome Study requires only an assessment of the spleen size and percent basophils in blood. All of these scores have online calculators for easy determination of score. At diagnosis, they prove a reasonable guide to predict outcome. These scores work similarly in cases treated with first- and second-generation tyrosine kinase inhibitors alike.

TABLE 170-4 CLINICAL SCORING SYSTEMS USED IN RISK-STRATIFYING CML PATIENTS

	SOKAL	HASFORD	EUTOS
Age	x	x	
Spleen size	x	x	x
Blast (peripheral)	x	x	
Basophilia		x	x
Eosinophilia		x	
Thrombocytosis	x	x	

EUTOS = European Treatment and Outcome Study for CML; Hasford = Hasford score for CML; Sokal = Sokal Index for CML (https://www.mdcalc.com/sokal-index-chronic-myelogenous-leukemia-cml).

Additional Cytogenetic Abnormalities

The presence of major additional chromosomal abnormalities (trisomy 8, isochromosome 17q, second Ph chromosome, and trisomy 19) at diagnosis is generally associated with negative prognostic impact on survival and disease progression to accelerated or blast phase. Patients with major route additional chromosomal abnormalities at the time of diagnosis have longer times to cytogenetic and molecular responses and shorter progression-free survival and overall survival than patients with t(9;22), t(v;22), loss of Y chromosome, or other minor additional chromosomal abnormalities. For example, 5-year survival rates are about 91%, 87%, 89%, 92%, and 52%, respectively, for patients with t(9;22), t(v; 22), loss of Y chromosome, minor route additional chromosomal abnormalities, and major route additional chromosomal abnormalities. Other studies have reported that some of the minor route additional chromosomal abnormalities, such as 11q23 and 3q26 rearrangements, are also associated with poor prognosis. Another study found that the presence of trisomy 8, loss of Y chromosome, or second Ph chromosome had no adverse impact on treatment response and survival, whereas the presence of isochromosome 17q, del7q, or 3q26.2 rearrangements was associated with lower response rates and inferior survival. The concurrent presence of two or more additional chromosomal abnormalities is associated with a poor prognosis.

Next-generation sequencing has shown that chronic phase patients who respond poorly to treatment and who progress to advanced phase disease have a higher prevalence of mutations in genes commonly associated with acute leukemia (e.g., *ASXL1, RUNX1, IZF1*). However, these markers are not currently used in routine clinical treatment algorithms.

Molecular Response

The peripheral blood monitoring of *BCR-ABL* transcripts has a very important role in CML management for the following reasons: (1) the depth of molecular responses is associated with outcomes (the achievement of a major molecular response is a "safe harbor" because disease resistance or progression is extremely rare after this low level of disease burden is achieved); (2) the kinetics of response appears to predict outcome because the rate of achieving the 3-month response is important and patients with a *BCR-ABL* of more than 10% IS at the 3-month mark do poorly compared with patients whose disease recedes more rapidly; and (3) deeper responses, beyond a major molecular response, are becoming increasingly more important as experience, trials, and treatment strategies move toward treatment discontinuation for those patients with a prolonged deep molecular response. Several studies have shown that a proportion of selected patients with persistently undetectable *BCR-ABL*, as defined by at least a 4- or 4.5-log read depth (the so-called "deep molecular response"), may discontinue tyrosine kinase inhibitor therapy without molecular relapse of their disease.

CHRONIC MYELOMONOCYTIC LEUKEMIA AND ATYPICAL CHRONIC MYELOPROLIFERATIVE DISEASES

DEFINITION AND EPIDEMIOLOGY

The chronic non-*BCR-ABL* leukemias are diseases that feature components of both myeloid dysplasia and proliferation. The WHO classifies chronic myelomonocytic leukemia (CMML), juvenile CMML, chronic neutrophilic leukemia (CNL), and atypical CML (aCML) among the myelodysplastic/myeloproliferative disorders (Chapters 152 and 167). Chronic neutrophilic leukemia and atypical CML are poorly named because they do not involve the *BCR-ABL* rearrangement. In CMML, there is an expansion of the monocytic population in the peripheral blood and bone marrow, whereas in CNL, the neutrophil population is increased.

These diseases are quite rare, and indeed, their incidence is difficult to accurately estimate. CMML is estimated to have an incidence of less than 0.5/100,000, and aCML and CNL are even rarer. The median age at diagnoses for these diseases is approximately 65 to 75 years.

PATHOBIOLOGY

There is no singular distinguishing genetic feature of CMML. Clonal cytogenetic abnormalities are seen in about 30% of cases, and mutations in greater than 90%. The most common mutations are in genes associated with mRNA splicing (e.g., *SF3B1*), cytokine signaling (e.g., *NRAS*), and epigenetic modification (e.g., *TET2*). On the other hand, mutations in *CSF3R* are present in more than 60% of aCML and CNL patients, and this mutation is unusual in other myeloid leukemias and myelodysplastic syndrome. In addition, one fourth of cases of aCML will have a point mutation in the *SETBP1* gene.

CLINICAL MANIFESTATIONS AND DIAGNOSIS

Like CML, the signs and symptoms are often nonspecific. The first clue to the diagnosis is usually abnormal peripheral blood WBC counts, which in CMML would demonstrate monocytosis, and may include neutropenia, anemia, and thrombocytopenia. Splenomegaly is quite common in these diseases. The work-up will be negative for the Ph chromosome or molecular evidence of *BCR-ABL*. The bone marrow typically shows myeloid hyperplasia and dysplasia of the myeloid lineage (and sometimes other lineages).[19]

The WHO definition of CMML requires a persistent (at least 3 months) peripheral blood monocytosis of more than 1000/μL and more than 10% of the entire WBC differential. In addition, the peripheral blood and bone marrow myeloblasts plus monoblasts plus promyelocytes must be less than 20% of the total WBC differential; if it is higher, it is classified as AML. Chronic neutrophilic leukemia and atypical CML are not so strictly defined.

TREATMENT AND PROGNOSIS

The median survival for these diseases is less than 3 years, with death arising from either transition to acute leukemia or from complications of cytopenias. There is no curative therapy outside of allogeneic stem cell transplantation.[20] Patients with CMML may benefit from a trial of hypomethylating agents (with an overall response rate of ~30 to 40%) or opt for disease control (if they have a highly proliferative disease) with hydroxyurea under expert supervision.[21] For CMML there is a roughly 20% risk of transformation to acute myeloid leukemia (AML) after 3 years from diagnosis. If transition to AML occurs, induction therapy is often attempted, especially as a bridge to rapid transplantation. In atypical CML and chronic neutrophilic leukemia, mutations in *CSF3R* appear to cause aberrant signaling through SRC or JAK2, depending on where the mutation occurs. Thus, clinical trials are exploring targeted therapy inhibiting SRC and JAK in these rare patients.

GENERAL REFERENCES

For the General References and other additional features, please visit Elsevier eBooks+ at https://ebooks.health.elsevier.com.

Grade A References

A1. Hochhaus A, Larson RA, Guilhot F, et al. Long-term outcomes of imatinib treatment for chronic myeloid leukemia. *N Engl J Med*. 2017;376:917-927.

A2. Kantarjian HM, Hughes TP, Larson RA, et al. Long-term outcomes with frontline nilotinib versus imatinib in newly diagnosed chronic myeloid leukemia in chronic phase: ENESTnd 10-year analysis. *Leukemia*. 2021;35:440-453.

A3. Cortes JE, Saglio G, Kantarjian HM, et al. Final 5-year study results of DASISION: the dasatinib versus imatinib study in treatment-naive chronic myeloid leukemia patients trial. *J Clin Oncol*. 2016;34:2333-2340.

A4. Brümmendorf TH, Cortes JE, Milojkovic D, et al. Bosutinib versus imatinib for newly diagnosed chronic phase chronic myeloid leukemia: final results from the BFORE trial. *Leukemia*. 2022;36:1825-1833.

A5. Cortes JE, Khoury HJ, Kantarjian HM, et al. Long-term bosutinib for chronic phase chronic myeloid leukemia after failure of imatinib plus dasatinib and/or nilotinib. *Am J Hematol*. 2016;91:1206-1214.

A6. Rea D, Mauro MJ, Boquimpani C, et al. A phase 3, open-label, randomized study of asciminib, a STAMP inhibitor, vs bosutinib in CML after 2 or more prior TKIs. *Blood*. 2021;138:2031-2041.

171

NON-HODGKIN LYMPHOMAS

JULIE M. VOSE AND JAMES O. ARMITAGE

DEFINITION

Lymphomas are solid tumors of the immune system. Increasing knowledge of the biology of the immune system has led to a corresponding increase in the understanding of these malignancies. In addition to better systems of classification and clinical evaluation, this new knowledge has led to the development of new therapies. Beneficial treatment is available for essentially every patient with non-Hodgkin lymphoma. The overall survival of lymphoma patients has increased steadily over the past 40 years, and many patients can be cured.

EPIDEMIOLOGY

In the United States, an estimated 80,000 or so new cases of non-Hodgkin lymphoma are diagnosed in annually, and about 20,000 patients to die of this disease each year. Non-Hodgkin lymphomas account for about 5% of new cancers in the United States and result in about 3% of cancer deaths. The U.S. lifetime risk for developing non-Hodgkin lymphoma is estimated to be 2.4% (1 in 42) for men and 1.9% (1 in 52) for women.[1] The incidence rate increases dramatically with age and is higher in Whites than in other ethnic groups.

Geographic differences in the incidence of non-Hodgkin lymphomas vary as much as five-fold. The highest rates are seen in the United States, Europe, and Australia, whereas lower rates are seen in Asia. Even more striking are geographic differences in the incidence of certain types of non-Hodgkin lymphoma, such as Burkitt lymphoma, follicular lymphoma, extranodal natural killer (NK)/T-cell nasal lymphoma, and adult T-cell leukemia/lymphoma.

In the United States the incidence rate for non-Hodgkin lymphomas increased by about 3 to 4% yearly from 1950 and the beginning of the 21st century, likely related to increased longevity, to the acquired immunodeficiency syndrome (HIV/AIDS) epidemic (Chapter 353), to occupational and environmental exposures (e.g., agricultural chemicals), to improvements in imaging techniques, and to improvements in the ability of pathologists to diagnose lymphoma. Since then, the incidence rate for non-Hodgkin lymphoma has reached a plateau, and the death rate from the disease has been declining.

PATHOBIOLOGY

For most cases of non-Hodgkin lymphoma, the cause is unknown, although genetic, environmental, and infectious agents have been implicated (Table 171-1).

Genetic Factors

Familial non-Hodgkin lymphoma clusters have been described, with a slightly higher risk for non-Hodgkin lymphoma among siblings and first-degree relatives of patients with lymphoma or other hematologic malignancies. The incidence of non-Hodgkin lymphoma has been associated with polymorphisms in a variety of genes related to immunity, including chemokines, tumor necrosis factor, interleukin-10 (IL-10), and lymphotoxin-α. Polymorphisms in other genes related to the cell cycle and apoptosis have also been associated with an increased risk for developing lymphoma.

Immune System Abnormalities

Several inherited disorders increase the risk for developing non-Hodgkin lymphoma as much as 250-fold (see Table 171-1). In some of these conditions, the lymphoma may be related to Epstein-Barr virus (Chapter 348). For example, patients with X-linked lymphoproliferative disorder have mutations in the *SH2D1A* gene, which encodes proteins that regulate the host immune response against Epstein-Barr virus–infected cells; individuals with this disorder may develop fatal infectious mononucleosis or non-Hodgkin lymphoma after primary exposure to Epstein-Barr virus. Acquired immunodeficiency states are also associated with an increased risk for non-Hodgkin lymphoma. For example, post-transplantation lymphoproliferative disorders (Chapter 348) occur in as many as 20% of solid organ transplant recipients, related to the proliferation of B lymphocytes that have been transformed during immunosuppressive therapy. The risk for non-Hodgkin lymphoma is also increased more than 100-fold in patients infected with the human immunodeficiency virus (HIV, Chapter 355). Almost all central nervous system (CNS) lymphomas

TABLE 171-1 FACTORS ASSOCIATED WITH THE DEVELOPMENT OF NON-HODGKIN LYMPHOMA

Inherited immune disorders
Severe combined immunodeficiency disease
Common variable immunodeficiency disease
Wiskott-Aldrich syndrome
Ataxia-telangiectasia
X-linked lymphoproliferative disorder
Autoimmune lymphoproliferative syndrome
Acquired immune disorders
Solid organ transplantation
Acquired immunodeficiency syndrome (AIDS)
Rheumatoid arthritis and systemic lupus erythematosus
Sjögren syndrome
Hashimoto thyroiditis
Celiac disease
Drug related
Methotrexate for autoimmune disorders
JAK1/2 inhibitor for myelofibrosis
Azathioprine for autoimmune disorders
Anti–tumor necrosis factor agents (e.g., infliximab, adalimumab)
Infectious agents
Epstein-Barr virus
Human T-lymphotropic virus type 1
Human herpesvirus type 8
Hepatitis C virus
Helicobacter pylori
Borrelia burgdorferi
Chlamydia psittaci
Campylobacter jejuni
Coxiella burnetii
Occupational and environmental exposure
Herbicides
Organic solvents
Ultraviolet light
Diet
Smoking

and approximately 50% of other lymphomas in patients with the acquired immunodeficiency syndrome (AIDS) are related to Epstein-Barr virus. Some studies have shown a two-fold increase in the incidence of non-Hodgkin lymphomas among patients with rheumatoid arthritis (Chapter 243), and the risk for marginal zone lymphomas is increased approximately 30- to 40-fold in patients with Sjögren syndrome (Chapter 247). Increases in the incidence of thyroid lymphoma are seen in patients with Hashimoto thyroiditis (Chapter 207). Enteropathy-type T-cell lymphomas are associated with celiac disease (Chapter 126). Patients with the autoimmune lymphoproliferative syndrome, associated with mutations in the *FAS* gene, also appear to be at higher risk for developing lymphoma.

Infectious Agents

Epstein-Barr virus (Chapter 348) is associated with the majority of post-transplantation lymphoproliferative disorders and many HIV/AIDS-associated lymphomas. This viral genome is detectable in more than 95% of cases of endemic Burkitt lymphoma and in approximately 15 to 35% of cases of sporadic Burkitt lymphoma and AIDS-associated lymphomas. This virus is also associated with Epstein-Barr virus-positive diffuse large B-cell lymphoma of elderly people, plasmablastic lymphoma, and extranodal NK/T-cell lymphoma.

The human T-lymphotropic virus type 1 (HTLV-1; Chapter 360) is detectable in virtually all cases of adult T-cell leukemia/lymphoma. The risk for lymphoma is approximately 3% in patients infected with HTLV-1. In endemic areas, up to 50% of all non-Hodgkin lymphomas may be related to HTLV-1.

Human herpesvirus-8 (HHV-8, Kaposi sarcoma–associated herpesvirus; Chapter 359), which is associated with expansion of the B-cell population, is also associated with primary effusion lymphoma (see later) in immunocompromised patients and with multicentric Castleman disease. Patients with primary effusion lymphoma are often coinfected with Epstein-Barr virus.

Epidemiologic evidence has linked hepatitis C virus (Chapter 135) to lymphoplasmacytic lymphoma associated with type II cryoglobulinemia, nodal marginal zone lymphoma, and splenic marginal zone lymphoma. Chronic antigenic stimulation from this virus may lead to the emergence of malignant B-cell clones.

Helicobacter pylori is associated with gastric lymphoma (Chapter 178) of extranodal marginal zone/mucosa-associated lymphoid tissue (MALT). Colonized patients develop gastritis from chronic antigenic stimulation mediated by T cells, which respond to *H. pylori*–specific antigens and emergence of malignant B-cell clones. *Borrelia burgdorferi* (associated with Lyme disease, Chapter 296) has been associated with marginal zone B-cell lymphoma of the skin. Evidence also links *Chlamydia psittaci* (Chapter 294) with ocular adnexal lymphomas, *Campylobacter jejuni* with immunoproliferative small intestinal disease (Chapter 279), and *Coxiella burnetii* with diffuse large B-cell and follicular lymphoma.

Environmental and Occupational Exposure

Agricultural chemicals have been associated with an increased risk for developing non-Hodgkin lymphomas, and the strongest associations involve phenoxy herbicides such as 2,4-dichlorophenoxyacetic acid (2,4-D), which was also a component of Agent Orange. An increased risk has also been associated with ionizing radiation (Chapter 18), organic solvents, and nitrates in drinking water, although contradictory results have been reported. Some studies have also linked non-Hodgkin lymphomas to high-fat diets and ultraviolet radiation (Chapter 18). The risk for non-Hodgkin lymphoma is increased approximately 20-fold after treatment for Hodgkin lymphoma (Chapter 172). Heavy smokers (Chapter 363) have an increased risk for developing follicular lymphoma. Low levels of vitamin D have been associated with increased risk for recurrent lymphoma, as well as poor outcome. Anti–tumor necrosis factor (anti-TNF) agents might be associated with an increased risk for developing lymphoma, particularly hepatosplenic T-cell lymphoma. Breast implants also are associated with the development of anaplastic large cell lymphoma.

Pathology

Non-Hodgkin lymphomas are derived from cells of the immune system at varying stages of differentiation. In some cases, the cell of origin is directly linked to the morphology, immunophenotype, and clinical behavior of the lymphoma (E-Fig. 171-1 and Table 171-2).

The transformation of cells from the normal immune system into malignant lymphoma reflects the acquisition of specific genetic abnormalities. In many cases, cytogenetic studies can identify chromosomal translocations that underlie the development or progression of the lymphoma. In most cases of non-Hodgkin lymphoma, the activation of proto-oncogenes is the major abnormality, but occasionally chromosomal translocations can lead to fusion genes that code for chimeric proteins. In addition, some cases are associated with deletion of tumor suppressor genes. Specific genetic abnormalities are associated with some specific subtypes of non-Hodgkin lymphoma (Table 171-3). It is becoming clear that the tumor microenvironment from cells of the host immune system is important in tumor cell survival and response to therapy.

Classification

The updated 2016 World Health Organization (WHO) classification integrates genetic data into the clinicopathologic classification (Table 171-4). This classification divides lymphomas on the basis of B-cell or T/NK-cell origin and whether they are derived from primitive precursor cells or from more mature "peripheral" cells. Specific clinical and pathologic entities are recognized within each of these groupings. In the United States and Europe, 85 to 90% of non-Hodgkin lymphomas are B cell in origin.

The most frequent type is diffuse large B-cell lymphoma, which represents about 30% of all non-Hodgkin lymphomas worldwide. The next most frequent type is follicular lymphoma, which represents about 20% of cases. Follicular lymphoma is relatively more frequent in North America and Western Europe and less frequent in Asia. Less common types, each representing between 5 and 10% of all non-Hodgkin lymphomas, are extranodal marginal zone/MALT lymphomas, peripheral T-cell lymphomas, small lymphocytic lymphoma, and mantle cell lymphoma. Other types each represent less than 2% of non-Hodgkin lymphomas seen in the United States.

The non-Hodgkin lymphomas recognized in the WHO classification have clinically distinctive characteristics (Table 171-5), such that an experienced hematopathologist can accurately classify 85% or more of patients by WHO criteria when adequate material is available. Some diagnoses, such as follicular lymphoma, can be made with a high degree of accuracy without immunologic or genetic studies. The diagnosis of T-cell lymphomas cannot be made accurately without immunophenotyping. Cytogenetic studies and molecular genetic studies (fluorescence in situ hybridization, or FISH) can help resolve difficult differential diagnoses. For example, the presence of a t(8;14) translocation supports the diagnosis of Burkitt lymphoma, whereas a t(11;14) with cyclin D1 overexpression can confirm the diagnosis of mantle cell lymphoma (see Tables 171-2 and 171-3).

TABLE 171-2 TYPICAL IMMUNOPHENOTYPES OF COMMON NON-HODGKIN LYMPHOMAS

LYMPHOMA	CD20	CD3	CD10	CD5	CD23	OTHER
Small lymphocytic	+	−	−	+	+	
Lymphoplasmacytic	+	−	−	−	−	Cytoplasmic immunoglobulin^{+}
Extranodal marginal zone MALT	+	−	−	−	−	
Nodal marginal zone	+	−	−	−	−	
Follicular	+	−	+	−		
Mantle cell	+	−	+	+		Cyclin D1^{+}
Diffuse large B cell	+	−				
Mediastinal large B cell	+	−				
Burkitt	+	−	+	−		TdT^{-}
Precursor T lymphoblastic	−	+/−				TdT^{+}, CD1a$^{+/-}$, CD7^{+}
Anaplastic large T cell	−	+/−				CD30^{+}, CD15^{-}, EMA^{+}, ALK$^{+/-}$
Peripheral T cell	−	+/−				Other pan-T variable

ALK = anaplastic lymphoma kinase; EMA = epithelial membrane antigen; MALT = mucosa-associated lymphoid tissue; TdT = terminal deoxynucleotidyl transferase.

Gene expression profiling has allowed the identification of distinct subsets of patients with diffuse large B-cell lymphoma (DLBCL). Patients with histologically identical lymphomas can be divided into those with gene expression patterns resembling normal germinal center B cells (GCBs), those whose tumors resemble activated post–germinal center B cells (ABCs), or those with patterns resembling that seen in Hodgkin lymphoma. The last pattern is most frequently found in young women who present with large mediastinal masses. Use of immunohistochemistry to subdivide diffuse large B-cell lymphoma into germinal center B cell subtype and activated post–germinal center B cell subtype is widely used but does not correlate perfectly with DNA microarray results. Using a combination of exome and transcriptome sequencing, array-based DNA copy-number analysis, and targeted amplicon resequencing of selected genes, diffuse large B-cell lymphoma can be further subtyped based on shared genomic abnormalities.

TABLE 171-3 CHROMOSOMAL TRANSLOCATIONS CHARACTERISTIC OF NON-HODGKIN LYMPHOMA

LYMPHOMA SUBTYPE	TRANSLOCATION	GENES INVOLVED	FREQUENCY (%)
Diffuse large B cell	t(3q27) t(14;18)(q32;q21) t(18;14)(q24;q32)	*BCL6* *IgH, BCL2* *MYC (c-Myc), IgH*	35 15-20 <5
Burkitt	t(8;14)(q24;q32) t(8;22)(q24;q11) t(2;8)(p12;q24)	*MYC, IgH* *MYC, IgL* *IgK, MYC*	100% have one of these, most commonly t(8;14)
Follicular	t(14;18)(q32;q21)	*IgH, BCL2*	~90
Mantle cell	t(11;14)(q13;q32)	*BCL1, IgH*	>90
ALCL	t(2;5)(p23;q35)	*ALK, NPM*	>80 of ALK+ ALCLs
MALT	t(11;18)(q21;q21) t(14;18)(q21;q32) t(1;14)(p22;q32)	*API2, MALT1* *IgH, MALT1* *BCL10, IgH*	35 20 10

ALCL = anaplastic large cell lymphoma; ALK = anaplastic lymphoma kinase; MALT = mucosa-associated lymphoid tissue.

CLINICAL MANIFESTATIONS

The most common presentation of non-Hodgkin lymphoma is lymphadenopathy (Fig. 171-1; Chapter 154). In many cases, patients notice cervical, axillary, or inguinal adenopathy and seek a physician's advice. In general, lymph nodes containing lymphomas are firm, nontender, and not associated with a regional infection. In other patients, lymphadenopathy occurring in sites such as the mediastinum or retroperitoneum causes symptoms such as chest pain, cough, abdominal pain, and back pain. More extensive disease can also cause symptoms related to the superior vena cava syndrome, spinal cord compression, and renal insufficiency (associated with ureteral compression).

Non-Hodgkin lymphomas are often associated with systemic symptoms that may lead to the diagnosis. The most obvious symptoms, termed B symptoms, are fever, night sweats, and unexplained weight loss. Any of these symptoms without an obvious cause should lead a physician to consider the diagnosis of lymphoma. Other, less characteristic symptoms include fatigue, which is frequently present at the time of diagnosis if the patient is questioned carefully, and pruritus.

Non-Hodgkin lymphomas can involve essentially any organ in the body, and malfunction of that organ can cause symptoms that lead to the diagnosis. Examples include neurologic symptoms with primary brain lymphoma (Chapter 175), shortness of breath with MALT lymphomas in the lung, epigastric pain and vomiting with gastric MALT lymphomas or diffuse large B-cell lymphomas (Chapter 178), bowel obstruction with small bowel lymphomas (Chapter 179), testicular masses with diffuse large B-cell lymphoma (Chapter 185), and skin lesions with cutaneous lymphomas (Chapter 407). Many lymphomas involve the bone marrow and occasionally cause extensive myelophthisis (Chapter 151) and bone marrow failure. These patients may present with infections, bleeding, and anemia.

Non-Hodgkin lymphomas can also manifest with a variety of immunologic abnormalities. For example, autoimmune hemolytic anemia (Chapter 146) and immune thrombocytopenia (Chapter 158) can be the presenting manifestations of non-Hodgkin lymphoma, especially small lymphocytic lymphoma/chronic lymphocytic leukemia as well as other subtypes, including diffuse large B-cell lymphoma. Peripheral neuropathies (Chapter 388), often associated with overproduction of a monoclonal protein, can be seen in a variety of subtypes but are most characteristic of lymphoplasmacytic lymphoma; sometimes they are also seen with POEMS syndrome (polyneuropathy, organomegaly, endocrinopathy, M protein, skin changes; Chapter 173). Paraneoplastic neurologic complications of non-Hodgkin lymphoma include demyelinating polyneuropathy, Guillain-Barré syndrome, autonomic dysfunction, and peripheral neuropathy. Paraneoplastic syndromes (Chapter 164) associated with non-Hodgkin lymphoma can affect the skin (e.g., pemphigus), kidney (e.g., glomerulonephritis), and miscellaneous organ systems (e.g., vasculitis, dermatomyositis, cholestatic jaundice).

DIAGNOSIS

Each new patient with a non-Hodgkin lymphoma should be thoroughly evaluated in a systematic manner (Table 171-6). The diagnosis of non-Hodgkin lymphoma must be considered in patients with compatible clinical presentations and then confirmed by an adequate biopsy read by an experienced hematopathologist. The diagnosis should never be inferred, and patients should not be treated until the diagnosis is confirmed by biopsy. Similarly, patients who achieve a complete remission with initial therapy should not be treated for presumed relapse on the basis of symptoms or abnormal images without a biopsy. Because subtle pathologic distinctions may alter therapy, the most important issue in managing non-Hodgkin lymphoma is to establish an accurate diagnosis.

The differential diagnosis in patients with non-Hodgkin lymphoma is broad. Any cause of lymphadenopathy or splenomegaly can potentially be confused with non-Hodgkin lymphoma (Chapter 154).[2] However, this confusion is resolved by an appropriate biopsy. Core needle biopsies can occasionally be used for a primary diagnosis if the specimen is handled properly. Fine-needle aspirates should not be used to diagnose lymphoma, because they preclude an accurate diagnosis of the specific subtype of non-Hodgkin lymphoma. In most cases, an excisional biopsy is necessary (and is always preferred) for the

TABLE 171-4 2016 REVISION OF THE WHO CLASSIFICATION OF NON-HODGKIN LYMPHOMA

MATURE B-CELL NEOPLASMS
Chronic lymphocytic leukemia/small lymphocytic lymphoma
Splenic marginal zone lymphoma
Hairy cell leukemia/lymphoma
Splenic B-cell lymphoma/leukemia, unclassifiable
Splenic diffuse red pulp B-cell lymphoma
Hairy cell leukemia-variant
Lymphoplasmacytic lymphoma
Waldenström macroglobulinemia
Extranodal marginal zone lymphoma of mucosa-associated lymphoid tissue (MALT)
Nodal marginal zone lymphoma
Follicular lymphoma
In situ follicular neoplasia*
Duodenal-type follicular lymphoma*
*Large B-cell lymphoma with IRF4 rearrangement**
Primary cutaneous follicle center lymphoma
Mantle cell lymphoma
In situ mantle cell neoplasia*
Diffuse large B-cell lymphoma (DLBCL), NOS
Germinal center B-cell type*
Activated B-cell type*
T-cell/histiocyte-rich large B-cell lymphoma
Primary DLBCL of the central nervous system (CNS)
Primary cutaneous DLBCL, leg type
EBV^+ DLBCL, NOS*
*EBV^+ mucocutaneous ulcer**
DLBCL associated with chronic inflammation
Lymphomatoid granulomatosis
Primary mediastinal (thymic) large B-cell lymphoma
Intravascular large B-cell lymphoma
ALK^+ large B-cell lymphoma
Plasmablastic lymphoma
Primary effusion lymphoma
$HHV8^+$ DLBCL, NOS*
Burkitt lymphoma
High-grade B-cell lymphoma with *MYC* and *BCL2* and/or *BCL6* rearrangements
High-grade B-cell lymphoma, NOS*
B-cell lymphoma, unclassifiable, with features intermediate between DLBCL and HL
MATURE T AND NK NEOPLASIA
Chronic lymphoproliferative disorder of NK cells
Hydroa vacciniforme-like lymphoproliferative disorder*
Adult T-cell leukemia/lymphoma
Extranodal NK-/T-cell lymphoma, nasal type
Enteropathy-associated T-cell lymphoma
Monomorphic epitheliotropic intestinal T-cell lymphoma*
*Indolent T-cell lymphoprolifeative disorder of the GI tract**
Hepatosplenic T-cell lymphoma
Subcutaneous panniculitis-like T-cell lymphoma
Mycosis fungoides
Sézary syndrome
Primary cutaneous $CD30^+$ T-cell lymphoproliferative disorders
Lymphomatoid papulosis
Primary cutaneous anaplastic large cell lymphoma
Primary $\gamma\delta$ T-cell lymphoma
Primary cutaneous $CD8^+$ aggressive epidermotropic cytotoxic T-cell lymphoma
*Primary cutaneous acral CD8+ T-cell lymphoma**
Primary cutaneous $CD4^+$ small/medium T-cell lymphoproliferative disorder*
Peripheral T-cell lymphoma, NOS
Angioimmunoblastic T-cell lymphoma
*Follicular T-cell lymphoma**
*Nodal peripheral T-cell lymphoma with TFH phenotype**
Anaplastic large-cell lymphoma, ALK+
Anaplastic large-cell lymphoma, ALK^-
*Breast implant-associated anaplastic large-cell lymphoma**
POST-TRANSPLANT LYMPHOPROLIFERATIVE DISORDERS (PTLD)
Plasmacytic hyperplasia PTLD
Infectious mononucleosis PTLD
Florid follicular hyperplasia PTLD*
Polymorphic PTLD
Monomorphic PTLD (B- and T-/NK-cell types)

Provisional entities are listed in italics; *denotes changes from the 2008 classification (shown in Volume 25); ALK = anaplastic lymphoma kinase; EBV^+ = Epstein-Barr virus-positive; GI = gastrointestinal; HL = Hodgkin lymphoma; NK = natural killer; NOS = not otherwise specified; TFH = T follicular helper. This table does not include the lymphoid leukemias, plasma cell dyscrasia, and Hodgkin lymphoma (see Chapter 172).
Modified from Swerdlow SH, Campo E, Pileri SA, et al. The 2016 revision of the World Health Organization classification of lymphoid neoplasms. *Blood* 2016;127:2375-2390.

initial diagnosis. A second biopsy should be performed if sufficient material is not obtained with the first attempt.

Staging and Prognostic Systems

After diagnosis, a meticulous staging evaluation is necessary to estimate prognosis and determine therapy. Staging requires a careful history and physical examination; complete blood count; renal and hepatic function tests; serum lactate dehydrogenase (LDH) level; either computed tomography (CT) of the chest, abdomen, and pelvis or positron emission tomography (PET), which can often replace CT scanning when done on a combined PET/CT machine; and bone marrow biopsy (might not be necessary in patients with diffuse large B-cell lymphoma if the PET/CT scan showed bone marrow involvement). PET can identify initial sites of involvement and, after treatment, can distinguish persisting lymphoma from residual fibrosis in masses seen on CT. The most common staging system is the Ann Arbor classification, which separates patients into four stages based on anatomic sites of disease (Table 171-7). In addition, each stage is subdivided into A (no defined general symptoms) and B (unexplained weight loss >10% of body weight in the previous 6 months, unexplained temperature >38° C, or night sweats) categories. Known sites of disease can be re-evaluated after treatment to evaluate the response to therapy.

Although a wide variety of patient factors (e.g., age, symptoms, LDH level) and tumor factors (e.g., bulk, gene expression pattern, proliferation rate) can affect treatment outcomes, two prognostic systems can help in choosing therapy and determining an accurate prognosis. The International Prognostic Index (Table 171-8) is the most widely used method to predict treatment outcome and survival. This index is based on five adverse factors (age >60 years, performance status ≤2, elevated serum LDH level, two or more extranodal sites of disease, Ann Arbor stage III or IV), which are summed to give the score. This index was developed for patients with diffuse aggressive lymphoma (predominantly diffuse large B-cell lymphoma), but it can be used to predict treatment outcome with any subtype. For patients younger than 60 years, an abbreviated index that uses only reduced performance status, elevated serum LDH level, and high stage can be applied. Because patients with follicular lymphoma rarely have a reduced performance status or a large number of extranodal sites, an alternative index termed the Follicular Lymphoma International Prognostic Index was developed. It substitutes more than four nodal areas of involvement and a hemoglobin value less than 12 g/dL as staging criteria and is better for predicting the outcome of treatment for follicular lymphoma.

At the end of therapy, patients should undergo restaging, which involves repeating previously abnormal tests to prove the patient has achieved a complete remission. For most subtypes of lymphoma, the best definition of a complete remission is a PET/CT scan that has a score of Deauville 1, 2, or 3. The Deauville score uses the intensity of uptake in the mediastinum and liver as an internal control and is the most widely used system for documenting remission (Table 171-9).

TREATMENT

Lymphomas may behave in an indolent or an aggressive manner. The behavior of many of these neoplasms is distinctive, but within each category, behavior is frequently influenced by disease site, tumor bulk, and performance status of the patient. Some lymphomas can be managed, at least initially, with observation, whereas other situations are medical emergencies, such as spinal cord compression. Three questions should be considered before starting therapy: (1) Does treatment have curative potential? (2) Can treatment prolong survival? (3) Will treatment alleviate symptoms? When treatment is appropriate, genomic profiling is typically recommended to guide therapy and inform prognosis.[3]

SPECIFIC TYPES OF NON-HODGKIN LYMPHOMAS

PRECURSOR T-CELL AND B-CELL LYMPHOMAS

Precursor T-cell and B-cell lymphomas are nodal or other solid tissue infiltrates of cells that are morphologically and immunophenotypically identical to the immature cells seen in B-cell or T-cell acute lymphoblastic leukemia (Chapter 168). Patients who have predominantly nodal disease with minimal or no involvement of the bone marrow are frequently classified as having *lymphoblastic lymphoma,* whereas those with more than 25% neoplastic cells in the marrow are classified as having *lymphoblastic leukemia.* These distinctions are arbitrary and reflect the stage of disease rather than different diagnoses. These neoplasms are more common in children than in adults.

TABLE 171-5 PRESENTING CLINICAL CHARACTERISTICS OF COMMON NON-HODGKIN LYMPHOMA SUBTYPES

TYPE OF LYMPHOMA	MEDIAN AGE (yr)	MALE (%)	STAGE (%) I	STAGE (%) IV	B SYMPTOMS (%)	BONE MARROW INVOLVED (%)
B-CELL LYMPHOMAS						
Small lymphocytic	65	53	4	83	33	72
Lymphoplasmacytic	63	53	7	73	13	73
Extranodal marginal zone MALT	60	48	39	31	19	14
Nodal marginal zone	58	42	13	40	37	32
Follicular	59	42	18	51	28	42
Mantle cell	63	74	13	71	28	64
Diffuse large B cell	64	55	25	33	33	16
Mediastinal large B cell	37	34	10	31	38	3
Burkitt	31	89	37	38	22	33
PRECURSOR B/T-CELL LYMPHOMAS						
Precursor T lymphoblastic	28	64	0	75	21	50
T-CELL LYMPHOMAS						
Anaplastic large T cell	34	69	19	39	53	13
Peripheral T cell, NOS	61	55	8	65	50	36

B symptoms = fevers, night sweats, and weight loss; MALT = mucosa-associated lymphoid tissue; NOS = not otherwise specified.
Adapted from Armitage JO, Weisenburger DD, for the Non-Hodgkin Lymphoma Classification Project. New approach to classifying non-Hodgkin lymphomas: clinical features of the major histologic subtypes. *J Clin Oncol*. 1998;16:2780-2795.

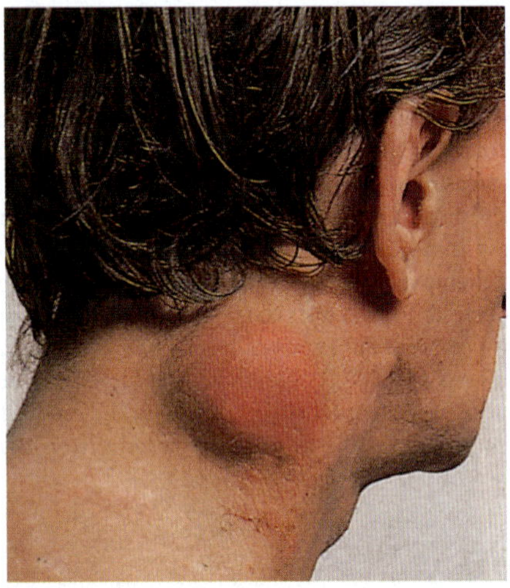

FIGURE 171-1. Non-Hodgkin lymphoma. Despite the redness of the skin over the enlarged lymph node in this patient, the lesion was completely painless. (From Forbes CD, Jackson WF. *Color Atlas and Text of Clinical Medicine*, 3rd ed. London: Mosby; 2003.)

TABLE 171-7 STAGING OF NON-HODGKIN LYMPHOMA

STAGE	DESCRIPTION
I	Involvement of a single lymph node region (I) or a single extralymphatic organ or site (I_E)
II	Involvement of two or more lymph node regions on the same side of the diaphragm (II) or localized involvement of an extralymphatic organ or site and one or more lymph node regions on the same side of the diaphragm (II_E)
III	Involvement of lymph node regions on both sides of the diaphragm (III), which may also be accompanied by localized involvement of an extralymphatic organ or site (III_E) or by involvement of the spleen (III_S) or both (III_{SE})
IV	Diffuse or disseminated involvement of one or more extralymphatic organs or tissues with or without associated lymph node enlargement
Subtypes	
A	No B symptoms
B	B symptoms: unexplained weight loss ≥10% of body weight in prior 6 months, unexplained fever with temperature >38° C, or night sweats

Adapted from Carbone PP, Kaplan HS, Musshoff K, et al. Report of the Committee on Hodgkin Disease Staging Classification. *Cancer Res*. 1971;31:1860-1861.

TABLE 171-6 TYPICAL EVALUATION OF A PATIENT NEWLY DIAGNOSED WITH NON-HODGKIN LYMPHOMA

1. Biopsy to establish diagnosis
2. Careful history and physical examination
3. Laboratory evaluation
   A. Complete blood count
   B. Chemistry screen, including lactate dehydrogenase
4. Imaging studies
   A. Computed tomography (CT) of chest, abdomen, and pelvis
   B. Positron emission tomography (can often replace the CT scan)
5. Additional biopsies
   A. Bone marrow
   B. Any other suspicious site if results would change therapy (i.e., lumbar puncture)

B-cell precursor lymphomas frequently manifest as solid tumors with involvement of the skin and bones, whereas T-cell neoplasms typically manifest as a mediastinal mass in young males. Involvement of the CNS is common in T-cell lymphomas. Approximately 90% of patients who present with lymphoblastic lymphoma have a T-cell phenotype, whereas about 85% of patients who present with acute lymphoblastic leukemia have a B-cell phenotype.

TREATMENT AND PROGNOSIS

Patients with either T-cell lymphoblastic lymphoma or precursor B-cell lymphoblastic lymphoma are typically treated with regimens modeled after those used for acute lymphoblastic leukemia (Chapter 168). These regimens frequently contain cytarabine and high-dose methotrexate, and they often include maintenance therapy. CNS prophylaxis with intrathecal chemotherapy, high-dose methotrexate, or cranial irradiation is often a component of these regimens. Adverse prognostic characteristics include CNS involvement, stage IV disease, and an elevated LDH level.

TABLE 171-8 INTERNATIONAL PROGNOSTIC INDEX

CATEGORY	SCORE (NO. OF RISK FACTORS)
ALL PATIENTS*	
Low	0 or 1
Low intermediate	2
High intermediate	3
High	4 or 5
AGE-ADJUSTED INDEX, PATIENTS ≤60 YEARS†	
Low	0
Low intermediate	1
High intermediate	2
High	3

*Adverse factors for all patients: age >60 yr, ↑LDH, performance status 2-4, >1 extranodal site, Ann Arbor stage III or IV.

†Adverse factors for patients ≤60 yr: ↑LDH, performance status 2-4, Ann Arbor stage III or IV.

LDH = lactate dehydrogenase.

Adapted from Shipp M, Harrington D, Anderson J, et al. A predictive model for aggressive non-Hodgkin lymphoma. *N Engl J Med.* 1993;329:987-994.

TABLE 171-9 THE DEAUVILLE SCORE FOR ASSESSING POSITRON EMISSION TOMOGRAPHY/COMPUTED TOMOGRAPHIC SCANS TO MEASURE PATIENT RESPONSES TO THERAPY

CRITERIA

1. No uptake related to lymphoma
2. The highest uptake in any site of lymphoma is less than or equal to to the uptake by the mediastinum
3. The highest uptake by any site of lymphoma is greater than the uptake by the mediastinum, but less than or equal to the uptake by the liver
4. The uptake by any site of lymphoma is greater than the uptake by the liver
5. The presence of new sites of uptake or substantial increases in the standardized uptake value in previous sites of lymphoma, or both

MATURE B-CELL LYMPHOMAS

SMALL LYMPHOCYTIC LYMPHOMA AND CHRONIC LYMPHOCYTIC LEUKEMIA

Small lymphocytic lymphoma is defined as a lymph node or other tissue infiltrate that is morphologically and immunophenotypically identical to chronic lymphocytic leukemia (Chapter 169). Patients frequently are symptom free, and the diagnosis is often made when blood counts are performed for other reasons. Patients frequently have lymphadenopathy or splenomegaly. Fatigue is common. Hypogammaglobulinemia can occur and may lead to an increased susceptibility to infection.

TREATMENT AND PROGNOSIS

The median survival time is more than 10 years for patients without adverse characteristics, and these patients often can be managed initially with observation. Therapy is necessary for patients who develop extreme fatigue or have systemic symptoms, for those with rapidly progressive or symptomatic lymphadenopathy or splenomegaly, and for those who develop cytopenias. Management (Chapter 169) must be individualized because therapy is unlikely to be curative, and patients are often elderly.[4] Allogeneic hematopoietic stem cell transplantation may be curative, but few patients are candidates for this approach. Patients may develop autoimmune thrombocytopenia (Chapter 158), autoimmune neutropenia (Chapter 153), and red blood cell aplasia (Chapter 151). These disorders may respond to treatment with corticosteroids, intravenous immune globulin, anti-CD20 monoclonal antibodies such as rituximab or obinutuzumab, cyclosporine, or splenectomy, as used in patients without underlying lymphoma.

A poor prognosis is associated with advanced stage and systemic symptoms, unmutated immunoglobulin heavy chain genes, and genetic abnormalities such as del(17p) or *TP53* mutation. As many as 10% of patients exhibit transformation to diffuse large B-cell lymphoma (Richter syndrome), which is associated with a poor prognosis.

EXTRANODAL MARGINAL ZONE LYMPHOMA OF MUCOSA-ASSOCIATED LYMPHOID TISSUE (MALT LYMPHOMA)

The WHO classification of lymphomas recognizes three groups of marginal zone lymphomas (MZL): (1) splenic MZL, (2) nodal MZL, and (3) extranodal MZL of the MALT type (MALT lymphoma).[5] The marginal zone B cells in general are continuously exposed to exogenous antigens and have a physiologically reduced threshold for triggering proliferation, which may predispose them to malignant transformation. The first two types of marginal zone lymphomas are discussed later (section on "Rare Types of B-Cell Lymphoma"). They have different diagnostic criteria, behavior, and therapeutic implications.

MALT lymphomas are indolent lymphomas that originate in association with epithelial cells and are seen most commonly in the gastrointestinal tract, salivary glands, breast, thyroid, orbit, conjunctiva, skin, and lung. Gastric MALT lymphomas are frequently associated with infection by *H. pylori* (Chapter 125). The majority of cases are stage I or II at diagnosis, although in some series as many as 30% disseminate to bone marrow or other sites. These lymphomas tend to remain localized for extended periods.

TREATMENT AND PROGNOSIS

Local treatment with surgery or radiation therapy cures a high proportion of localized neoplasms. Even in patients who have more than one extranodal site, locations can sometimes be successfully treated with local therapy. Patients without symptoms can be monitored closely without therapy until symptoms progress. Patients with symptoms can be treated with rituximab, single-agent chemotherapy, or combinations similar to the treatment of follicular lymphoma (see later).[6]

About 75% of patients with gastric MALT lymphomas achieve remission after eradication of *H. pylori* (see Chapter 125), and more than 90% remain in remission for prolonged periods of time. Nonresponders are more likely to have submucosal invasion by endoscopic ultrasonography, lymph node metastases, or the t(11;18) chromosomal translocation. Approximately 25% of patients progress, of whom about 25% develop diffuse large B-cell lymphoma. Gastric MALT lymphoma that does not respond to antibiotics can be treated with radiation, rituximab as a single agent (similar to its use in follicular lymphoma), or several traditional combination chemotherapy regimens (see Table 171-10).

FOLLICULAR LYMPHOMA

Follicular lymphoma is derived from germinal center B cells. The hallmark t(14;18)(q32;q21) translocation of follicular lymphomas occurs early in B-cell development, caused by an error in VDJ ("variable," "diversity," and "joining" gene segments) recombination.[7] Follicular lymphoma is the most frequent of indolent or low-grade lymphomas in the United States. Follicular lymphoma is divided into three grades based on the proportion of large, transformed cells (centroblasts).

Patients with follicular lymphoma are frequently asymptomatic. The most common presenting complaint is painless lymphadenopathy. Some patients have cough or dyspnea related to pulmonary or mediastinal involvement or pleural effusions. Other patients have symptoms of abdominal pain or fullness related to subdiaphragmatic or splenic disease. A minority of patients have systemic symptoms of fevers, night sweats, or weight loss.

The clinical behavior and treatment of follicular lymphoma grades 1 and 2 are the same. Some grade 3 follicular lymphomas have a more aggressive clinical course and are treated similarly to diffuse large B-cell lymphoma (see later). This distinction between grade 3a (indolent behavior) and 3b (aggressive behavior) is based on the presence or absence of sheets of centroblasts, although this separation may not be reproducible among pathologists.

TREATMENT AND PROGNOSIS

Watch and Wait

A "watch and wait" approach is reasonable in asymptomatic elderly patients, patients with other medical illnesses, and in other selected patients who have low-grade follicular lymphoma and who are asymptomatic, have no disease involvement in sites that might be dangerous, and desire to avoid therapy as long as possible.[8] Such patients can sometimes be observed for long periods before treatment is required. However, modern treatment options may improve the survival of a large proportion of patients with follicular lymphoma.

TABLE 171-10 COMBINATION CHEMOTHERAPY REGIMENS FOR NON-HODGKIN LYMPHOMA

REGIMEN	DOSE	DAYS OF ADMINISTRATION	FREQUENCY
R-CHOP			**EVERY 21 DAYS**
Cyclophosphamide	750 mg/m² IV	1	
Doxorubicin	50 mg/m² IV	1	
Vincristine	1.4 mg/m² IV*	1	
Prednisone, fixed dose	100 mg daily PO	1-5	
Rituximab	375 mg/m² IV	1	
R-EPOCH†			**EVERY 21 DAYS**
Etoposide	50 mg/m²/day IV‡	1-4	
Doxorubicin	10 mg/m²/day IV‡	1-4	
Vincristine	0.4 mg/m²/day IV‡	1-4	
Cyclophosphamide	750 mg/m² IV	5	
Prednisone	60 mg/m² bid PO	1-5	
Rituximab	375 mg/m² IV	1	
R-CVP			**EVERY 21 DAYS**
Cyclophosphamide	1000 mg/m² IV	1	
Vincristine	1.4 mg/m² IV*	1	
Prednisone, fixed dose	100 mg daily PO	1-5	
Rituximab	375 mg/m² IV	1	
B-R			**EVERY 28 DAYS**
Bendamustine	90 mg/m²/day IV	1-2	
Rituximab	375 mg/m² IV	1	

*Vincristine dose is often capped at 2 mg total.
†Doses are adjusted based on myelosuppression with previous cycle.
‡Continuous infusion.
bid = twice daily; IV = intravenous; PO = oral.

Localized Disease

Approximately 5 to 15% of patients have localized disease (stage I or minimal stage II disease) at diagnosis. These lymphomas are typically treated with involved-field radiation, preferably with 24 Gy in 12 equal fractions,[A1] and most series report 10-year disease-free survival rates of approximately 50% and overall survival rates of about 50% at 20 years.[9]

Advanced Disease

Most patients with follicular lymphoma have extensive disease at diagnosis. The median survival time of these patients has improved after the addition of rituximab and is now 10 to 20 years. Spontaneous regression also has been described. However, as many as 30 to 50% of patients experience transformation to a more aggressive histology—usually diffuse large B-cell lymphoma. Transformation is frequently associated with new systemic symptoms, rapidly progressive lymphadenopathy, an aggressive clinical course, and a poor prognosis.

Most patients with follicular lymphoma eventually require treatment because of systemic symptoms, symptomatic or progressive lymphadenopathy, splenomegaly, effusions, or cytopenias. In elderly patients, patients who are poor candidates for intensive chemotherapy regimens, and patients who want to avoid the side effects of chemotherapy, single-agent rituximab (375 mg/m² intravenously, given weekly for 4 consecutive weeks) yields an objective response rate of well over 50%. The median duration of response is approximately 1 to 2 years for patients who receive no additional therapy, but the response can be extended with ongoing administration of rituximab once every 2 or 3 months or by repeating the initial four doses every 6 months.[10] When rituximab is combined with standard chemotherapy regimens (see Table 171-10) or with lenalidomide, the response rate, duration of response, and survival are increased compared with the chemotherapy regimen alone.[A2,A3] Maintenance rituximab extends the duration of remission but not overall survival.[A4] An alternative is obinutuzumab, which can provide longer progression-free survival but at the expense of more side effects, without improving overall survival.[A5]

Salvage Therapy

Most patients respond to initial chemotherapy. However, follicular lymphoma recurs in the majority of patients with advanced-stage disease. Patients who relapse usually respond to additional therapy, sometimes with the same agents, although the duration of response becomes progressively shorter with repeated courses of therapy.[11] For patients with disease that is refractory to rituximab, the combination of obinutuzumab plus bendamustine is preferable to bendamustine alone.[A6] Copanlisib, which is a pan-class PI3K inhibitor has also shown promising results when added to rituximab.[A7] Alternative therapies include lenalidomide with rituximab, or standard chemotherapies. Radiation therapy also may be useful for patients with a localized site of symptomatic disease.

Prolonged remissions have been observed after autologous hematopoietic stem cell transplantation. Allogeneic hematopoietic stem cell transplantation may cure some patients with relapsed follicular lymphoma but has more toxicity than autologous transplants. Chimeric antigen receptor (CAR) T-cell therapy (Chapter 164) has shown promise as salvage therapy in patients with relapsed or refractory B-cell lymphomas and is now FDA approved for patients whose follicular lymphoma has failed two prior therapies.[12]

MANTLE CELL LYMPHOMA

Mantle cell lymphoma is a B-cell neoplasm composed of small lymphoid cells that may resemble small lymphocytic lymphoma or follicular lymphoma. It is most common in elderly patients and is usually at an advanced stage at the time of diagnosis. Males are more frequently affected, and extranodal disease, especially involvement of the bone marrow, Waldeyer ring, and the gastrointestinal tract, is common. Mantle cell lymphoma is the most common cause of multiple lymphomatous polyposis, and many oncologists recommend that the gastrointestinal tract be evaluated with endoscopy during the initial evaluation.

Some patients present with involvement of the peripheral blood as well as the bone marrow, a clinical picture that resembles chronic lymphocytic leukemia (Chapter 169). The lymphocytes in both disorders are $CD5^+$, but the t(11;14) translocation[13] and overexpression of cyclin D1 seen in mantle cell lymphoma usually allow an accurate diagnosis.

TREATMENT AND PROGNOSIS

Occasional patients, particularly patients with a leukemic presentation, may have an indolent course without initial therapy. However, the median survival of mantle cell lymphoma has significantly improved with new therapies.[14] The combination of bendamustine plus rituximab and regimens that incorporate high-dose cytarabine are efficacious, as is the combination of lenalidomide plus rituximab. Ibrutinib added to rituximab plus bendamustine can significantly prolong remission-free survival[A8] and is commonly part of standard therapy. Substituting bortezomib (1.3 mg/m² on days 1, 4, 8, and 11) for vincristine (VR-CAP rather than R-CHOP) can improve the median progression-free survival seen with R-CHOP alone by about 40% (from 14 to about 25 months) in newly diagnosed patients.[A9] Maintenance rituximab seems to prolong the duration of remission.

Autologous hematopoietic stem cell transplantation is widely used for patients in their first remission. The Bruton tyrosine kinase inhibitors such as ibrutinib or acalabrutinib are very active and are part of standard therapy for relapsed disease.[15] If such therapy is not successful, anti-CD19 CAR T-cell therapy may provide a complete response in about 60% of patients.[16] Allogeneic transplantation can be curative but is associated with considerable morbidity and mortality.

The elderly comprise the majority of the patients with mantle cell lymphoma. For patients who are not too frail, 4-year overall survival of greater than 80% can be achieved with rituximab and moderate intensive chemotherapy such as R-CHOP followed by rituximab maintenance or R-bendamustine.

DIFFUSE LARGE B-CELL LYMPHOMA

Diffuse large B-cell lymphomas are the most common type of non-Hodgkin lymphoma, but their morphology and genetic features are heterogeneous. Signs and symptoms are similar to those of other subtypes, although patients are more likely to have B symptoms.[17]

The 2016 WHO classification of non-Hodgkin lymphomas has identified several variants and subtypes of diffuse large B-cell lymphoma (see Table 171-4). Many of these histologic or genetic subtypes or variants share the same standard treatment approach as used for diffuse large B-cell lymphoma. Other subtypes present unusual clinical syndromes or specific therapeutic problems.

TREATMENT

Localized Disease

As many as 30% of patients with diffuse large B-cell lymphoma have stage I or minimal stage II disease. These patients are occasionally cured with radiation therapy alone, but initial treatment with chemotherapy alone or combined with radiation therapy is more effective.[18] In the United States, most patients are treated with R-CHOP (see Table 171-10). Some patients can be treated with fewer courses of chemotherapy if radiotherapy is included. For patients with bulky disease, a complete course of chemotherapy is usually used with or without radiotherapy. Some physicians advocate the use of PET scans to shorten the duration of therapy or eliminate the need for radiotherapy in complete responders.

Advanced Disease

R-CHOP is still the most widely used regimen for adults of all ages with advanced-stage diffuse large B-cell lymphoma. Among patients older than age 60 years, 75% achieve a complete response, with a 10-year progression-free survival rate of about 35% and a 10-year overall survival rate of about 45%. In younger patients, the outcome is better. No advantage has been found for R-EPOCH over R-CHOP (see Table 171-10).[A10] Autologous stem cell transplantation in first remission may benefit very high-risk patients. Although not yet FDA approved for this purpose, the antibody-drug conjugate polatuzumab vedotin combined with R-CHP (rituximab-cyclophosphamide-doxorubicin-prednisone) can improve progression-free survival of diffuse large B-cell lymphoma patients compared with R-CHOP.[A11]

Salvage Therapy

A variety of chemotherapy regimens for patients who relapse after attaining a remission with initial chemotherapy commonly contain agents such as cisplatin, cytarabine, etoposide, carboplatin, and ifosfamide. Response rates exceeding 50% can be observed with these combinations, although no more than 10% of patients achieve long-term disease-free survival. High-dose therapy followed by autologous hematopoietic stem cell transplantation has become accepted therapy for patients with relapsed diffuse large B-cell lymphoma. Approximately 20 to 50% of these patients attain long-term disease-free survival, depending on their response to conventional salvage chemotherapy. Lenalidomide and ibrutinib seem to particularly benefit patients with activated B-cell (ABC) subtype. Other agents used as second- or third-line treatments include polatuzumab-vedotin plus bendamustine or rituximab or tafasitamab plus lenalidomide.[19,20] Autologous CD-19–directed, CAR T-cell therapy is now FDA approved for relapsed or refractory disease, especially with high-risk features.[21,A12]

Subtypes of Diffuse Large B-Cell Lymphoma

Approximately 30% of diffuse large B-cell lymphomas originate in extranodal sites. Presentation in certain extranodal sites is associated with unique clinical behaviors that may necessitate diagnostic studies or additional therapy beyond what is used for patients with nodal presentations.

Primary Mediastinal Large B-cell Lymphomas

Primary mediastinal large B-cell lymphomas originate in the thymus and are most common in young women. This subtype shares genetic features with classic Hodgkin lymphoma. This entity is distinguished by the presence of a mediastinal mass, which usually causes symptoms of cough, chest pain, or superior vena cava syndrome. A very large mass (>10 cm) or the existence of a malignant pleural effusion is associated with a worse prognosis.

TREATMENT AND PROGNOSIS

Mediastinal large B-cell lymphoma is treated with the same chemotherapy regimens used for diffuse large B-cell lymphoma, followed, in some cases, by consolidative radiation therapy.[22] R-EPOCH is more likely than R-CHOP (see Table 171-10) to achieve a durable remission without the need for radiotherapy. Relapses often occur in extranodal sites such as the CNS, lungs, gastrointestinal tract, liver, ovaries, and kidneys.

Intravascular Large B-cell Lymphoma

Intravascular large B-cell lymphoma is an aggressive lymphoma caused by cells that infiltrate the lumens of small blood vessels. Widespread extranodal involvement is common. Focal neurologic deficits and mental status changes are frequent. Cases are often diagnosed at autopsy, although durable responses to combination chemotherapy have been described.

Primary Effusion Lymphoma

Primary effusion lymphoma is associated with HHV-8 (Chapter 359) and is seen in HIV-infected and other immunosuppressed patients.[23] Effusions occur in serous body cavities. Peripheral lymphadenopathy is not seen. Prognosis is poor despite chemotherapy.

Primary CNS Lymphoma

Primary CNS lymphoma (Chapter 175) is increasing in incidence. Patients with primary CNS lymphoma (Chapter 175) commonly have ocular involvement, and all patients with this diagnosis should have a slit lamp examination.

TREATMENT AND PROGNOSIS

Surgical resection usually is not performed for primary CNS lymphoma, and the primary role of surgery is for diagnosis. Primary lymphomas of the CNS are very sensitive to corticosteroids, but some patients can be cured with chemotherapy regimens incorporating high-dose methotrexate (alone or in combination with other agents such as cytarabine, temozolomide, and rituximab) with or without autologous bone marrow transplant.[24] For primary CNS lymphoma, whole-brain radiotherapy is not as good as chemotherapy,[A13] does not add to the benefit achieved by chemotherapy alone, and is associated with increased neurologic toxicity.

Plasmablastic Lymphoma

Plasmablastic lymphoma is most often seen in patients with HIV infection and frequently presents with involvement of the head and neck. This tumor does not express CD20 and thus does not benefit from treatment with rituximab.

Primary Cutaneous Diffuse Large B-cell Lymphoma

Primary cutaneous diffuse large B-cell lymphoma of the leg (leg type) is one of two presentations of B-cell lymphoma in the skin.[25] This tumor occurs mostly in older patients and follows an aggressive course. This neoplasm must be distinguished from primary cutaneous follicle center lymphoma, which might also be diagnosed as a cutaneous diffuse large B-cell lymphoma but follows an indolent course and requires only local therapy.

Double-Hit, Triple-Hit, and Gray-Zone Lymphomas

Double-hit, triple-hit, and gray-zone lymphomas have rearrangements of *MYC* in combination with *BCL2* and/or *BCL6*. These tumors are now incorporated into an entity called high-grade B-cell lymphoma with rearrangements of *MYC* and *BCL2* and/or *BCL6*. Gray-zone lymphomas may have features intermediate between diffuse large B-cell lymphoma and Burkitt lymphoma or features intermediate between mediastinal diffuse large B-cell lymphoma and classic Hodgkin lymphoma.

TREATMENT AND PROGNOSIS

These lymphomas have a poor outcome when treated with standard chemotherapy regimens. More aggressive regimens such as DA-R-EPOCH (dose-adjusted etoposide, prednisone, vincristine, cyclophosphamide, and doxorubicin) may improve the outcome of the double- or triple-hit lymphomas.

Testicular, Gastric, and Intestinal Large B-Cell Lymphomas

Large B-cell lymphoma occasionally originates in the testis or gastrointestinal tract.

TREATMENT AND PROGNOSIS

Treatment of primary testicular lymphoma, the most common testicular cancer in men older than age 60 years (Chapter 185), usually consists of orchiectomy followed by combination chemotherapy. Relapse in the contralateral testicle is common, and radiation is usually given to the entire scrotal bed. CNS involvement is common, and prophylactic intrathecal chemotherapy is usually recommended. Late relapses occur frequently.

Diffuse large B-cell lymphoma of the stomach and gastrointestinal tract is treated differently from gastric MALT lymphoma, even if patients have is a history of prior MALT lymphoma. Patients can be cured with surgery and adjunctive radiation or chemotherapy, although surgery is rarely performed for gastric lymphomas because of the morbidity associated with gastric resection. Patients should be treated with chemotherapy regimens used for other diffuse large B-cell lymphomas. Radiation therapy is sometimes used after chemotherapy, although the role of combined-modality treatment is not defined.

BURKITT LYMPHOMA

Burkitt lymphoma is a highly aggressive B-cell lymphoma that is more common in children and immunosuppressed individuals than in healthy adults (see later).[26] Widespread extranodal involvement is common. The endemic form of Burkitt lymphoma is seen most frequently in children who reside in equatorial Africa. Involvement of bones of the jaw is common in this form. The sporadic form of Burkitt lymphoma is seen most commonly in children in the United States. Males are more frequently affected. Both children and adults frequently have bulky abdominal disease, sometimes with involvement of the kidneys, ovaries, and breasts. Bone marrow involvement is seen in about one third of cases.

TREATMENT

Tumors may progress extremely rapidly, so therapy should be started as soon as possible. Tumor lysis syndrome (Chapter 164) may occur because of the frequent presence of bulky disease, the high rate of tumor proliferation, and the extreme sensitivity of the tumor to chemotherapy. Patients are usually treated with specialized high-intensity regimens, including rituximab, of relatively short duration.[A14] Treatment with the R-CHOP regimen used for diffuse large B-cell lymphoma has a poor outcome, but excellent results have been described with R-EPOCH. CNS prophylaxis with intrathecal chemotherapy or high-dose methotrexate is required. Cure rates well in excess of 50% are typical with appropriate therapy.[27]

RARE TYPES OF B-CELL LYMPHOMA

Several rare types of lymphoma have distinct clinical features.

Lymphoplasmacytic Lymphoma

Lymphoplasmacytic lymphoma is an indolent lymphoma that frequently involves the bone marrow, peripheral blood, and spleen. Patients frequently have an immunoglobulin M (IgM) paraprotein that may lead to symptoms of hyperviscosity, autoimmune phenomena, or neuropathies. Plasmapheresis can reduce symptoms of hyperviscosity.

TREATMENT AND PROGNOSIS

Chemotherapy with alkylating agents, combination chemotherapy, or fludarabine all in combination with rituximab may be used. Ibrutinib and other Bruton tyrosine kinase (BTK) inhibitors have shown significant activity in lymphoplasmacytic lymphoma, and the combination of ibrutinib plus rituximab has resulted in significantly higher rates of progression-free survival than rituximab alone.[A15]

Splenic Marginal Zone Lymphoma

Splenic marginal zone lymphoma is an indolent lymphoma that usually manifests with splenomegaly and lymphocytosis. A monoclonal gammopathy is frequently seen. Peripheral lymphadenopathy is unusual. Anemia and thrombocytopenia may respond to splenectomy.

TREATMENT AND PROGNOSIS

Chemotherapy with single agents or anthracycline-based combinations may be useful, and when the lymphoma is associated with hepatitis C, antiviral therapy may be effective (Chapter 134 and 135). This lymphoma appears to be particularly responsive to rituximab with or without bendamustine. Bruton kinase inhibitors are also very useful for marginal zone lymphoma treatment.[28]

Nodal Marginal Zone B-cell Lymphoma

Nodal marginal zone B-cell lymphoma is an indolent disorder that is usually associated with generalized lymphadenopathy. The clinical course and prognosis are similar to those of follicular lymphoma, and it is usually treated in a similar manner.

Small Intestinal Immunoproliferative Disease

Small intestinal immunoproliferative disease, which is a disorder seen most frequently in the Middle East, begins as a polyclonal process and can progress to a large B-cell lymphoma. The process is often associated with *C. jejuni* infection (Chapter 279). Early in the disease, patients may respond to antibiotics, and frank lymphoma may respond to combination chemotherapy regimens.

MATURE T-CELL LYMPHOMAS (PERIPHERAL T-CELL LYMPHOMAS)

Peripheral (or mature) T-cell lymphomas are neoplasms of post-thymic T cells. These include relatively indolent disorders such as mycosis fungoides and $CD30^+$ cutaneous lymphoproliferative disorders, but most patients diagnosed with peripheral T-cell lymphoma have an aggressive neoplasm.[29] Peripheral T-cell lymphomas represent only 10% of the non-Hodgkin lymphomas occurring in the United States. Unfortunately, the treatment for these lymphomas has not progressed as rapidly as the treatments for B-cell lymphomas.

MYCOSIS FUNGOIDES

Mycosis fungoides (often referred to as *cutaneous T-cell lymphoma*) is an indolent malignancy that is most common in middle-aged and older adults.[30] The clinical course is usually a slow progression from isolated patches or plaques to thickened, more widespread plaques and then to multiple cutaneous tumors that may ulcerate (Chapter 407). A subset of patients presents with generalized erythroderma and circulating tumor cells, called *Sézary syndrome*. Lymph node and visceral involvement may occur late in the course of the disease.

TREATMENT

Cutaneous radiation therapy may be curative for patients with limited patch or plaque disease. Patients with early-stage disease (<10% body surface area) are frequently treated with skin-directed therapy that may include ultraviolet radiation, topical steroids, or topical nitrogen mustard.

Patients with more advanced disease frequently benefit from total skin electron beam therapy or extracorporeal photopheresis. Medical treatments include brentuximab vedotin, with[A16] or without[A17] standard chemotherapy, bexarotene (a selective retinoid X receptor agonist), interferon-α, retinoids, monoclonal antibodies, histone deacetylase inhibitors (vorinostat, romidepsin), and mogamulizumab (a monoclonal antibody directed against C-C chemokine receptor 4).[A18]

Unfortunately, treatments are usually only palliative.[31] Results with autologous hematopoietic stem cell transplantation are usually poor, although allogeneic stem cell transplantation has yielded promising results in some selected young patients.

ADULT T-CELL LYMPHOMA/LEUKEMIA

Adult T-cell lymphoma/leukemia, which is associated with HTLV-1 infection (Chapter 360), is most commonly seen in southern Japan and the Caribbean. Most infected patients are asymptomatic, and the lifetime risk for developing adult T-cell lymphoma/leukemia is approximately 3%.

Patients may have acute leukemia, aggressive lymphoma, or an indolent lymphoproliferative disease. Patients with aggressive disease present with generalized lymphadenopathy, hepatosplenomegaly, cutaneous infiltration, and hypercalcemia. Many patients have characteristic circulating tumor cells with a "flower" or "cloverleaf" nucleus.

TREATMENT

Patients with indolent disease can sometimes be monitored without therapy. Aggressive disease is usually treated with combination chemotherapy, but there is no consensus on the best regimen. Historically, the 5-year survival rate has been less than 10%, although recent trials have reported better outcomes.

$CD30^+$ CUTANEOUS LYMPHOPROLIFERATIVE DISORDERS

These disorders represent a spectrum of diseases that may have an identical histologic appearance and overlapping clinical manifestations. Treatment decisions are often based on the clinical behavior of the lesions. These lymphomas express CD30 but do not express the anaplastic lymphoma kinase (ALK) protein (see later).

Lymphomatoid Papulosis

Lymphomatoid papulosis is a "histologically malignant" clonal disorder consisting of erythematous or skin-colored papules that frequently undergo spontaneous ulceration and necrosis over a period of weeks. The prognosis is excellent, although patients may eventually develop lymphoma.

Primary Cutaneous Anaplastic Large Cell Lymphoma

Primary cutaneous anaplastic large cell lymphoma occurs most commonly in men and undergoes frequent spontaneous regression. The 5-year survival rate is greater than 90%. Treatment usually consists of local measures (surgery or radiation), although chemotherapy may be required.

PRIMARY SYSTEMIC ANAPLASTIC LARGE CELL LYMPHOMA

Anaplastic large cell lymphoma is an aggressive CD30$^+$ T-cell non-Hodgkin lymphoma that is seen most frequently in young males.[32] B-cell lymphomas with similar morphology can occur, but they have clinical features identical to other diffuse large B-cell lymphomas and are not considered part of this disease. A morphologically similar but biologically unrelated and clinically distinct neoplasm, primary cutaneous anaplastic large cell lymphoma, occurs predominantly in older adults and represents part of the spectrum of cutaneous CD30$^+$ lymphoproliferative disorders (see earlier). Primary systemic anaplastic large cell lymphoma frequently has a t(2;5) chromosomal translocation that leads to overexpression of ALK, a protein not normally detectable in lymphoid cells.

Patients usually have lymphadenopathy, and involvement of the skin, bone, and gastrointestinal tract may be observed.

A newly described entity of anaplastic large cell lymphoma of the breast is associated with breast implants. When localized, patients may be cured with surgery, including removal of the implant.

TREATMENT

Patients are usually treated with chemotherapy regimens such as CHOP with or without the addition of etoposide. Patients whose tumors express ALK have an excellent outcome, and 5-year survival rates of 70 to 90% have been observed. ALK-negative anaplastic large cell lymphoma is more common in older patients and is associated with an inferior response rate and shorter survival time. Autologous hematopoietic stem cell transplantation may be curative for patients who relapse. The anti-CD30 antibody-drug conjugate brentuximab vedotin is highly active for patients with relapsed disease and may be incorporated into primary therapy.[A19] Patients whose lymphomas express ALK usually respond to the ALK inhibitor crizotinib.

Anaplastic large cell lymphoma of the breast extends beyond the breast capsule. It is treated similarly to advanced-stage anaplastic large cell lymphoma.

PERIPHERAL T-CELL LYMPHOMAS, UNSPECIFIED

The largest group of patients with peripheral T-cell lymphomas is defined in the WHO classification as having "peripheral T-cell lymphoma, unspecified." These patients' signs and symptoms are similar to those of patients with aggressive B-cell lymphomas, although systemic symptoms (fevers, night sweats, and weight loss) and extranodal involvement are frequent. The diagnosis of peripheral T-cell lymphoma requires immunophenotyping to demonstrate the T-cell origin.

TREATMENT

Patients are generally treated with the same regimens used for diffuse large B-cell lymphomas (e.g., CHOP with or without etoposide), often in combination with upfront autologous hematopoietic stem cell transplantation, although the outcome is substantially worse. Belinostat is a histone deacetylase inhibitor that has some activity in peripheral T-cell lymphoma.[33] Patients who relapse after complete remission can sometimes be cured with hematopoietic stem cell transplantation.

UNUSUAL SUBTYPES OF T-CELL LYMPHOMA

Angioimmunoblastic T-cell Lymphoma

Angioimmunoblastic T-cell lymphoma is associated with generalized lymphadenopathy, fever, weight loss, skin rash, and polyclonal hypergammaglobulinemia. Results of therapy are similar to those for peripheral T-cell lymphoma, unspecified.

Extranodal NK/T-cell Lymphoma

Extranodal NK/T-cell lymphoma usually occurs in extranodal sites, especially the nose, palate, and nasopharynx. Involvement of the nose and face leads to the syndrome that was previously called lethal midline granuloma. This disorder is unusual in the United States, but it is frequent in Southeast Asia and Latin America. Patients with localized disease often can be cured with aggressive combination radiation therapy and chemotherapy.[34] Patients with widespread disease have a poor prognosis. These patients frequently respond to L-asparaginase.

Hepatosplenic T-cell Lymphoma

Hepatosplenic T-cell lymphoma is characterized by sinusoidal infiltration of the spleen, liver, and bone marrow, which leads to hepatosplenomegaly, systemic symptoms, and cytopenias. Lymphadenopathy is unusual. Hepatosplenic T-cell lymphoma is more commonly occurs in young men, and this disease can occur in the setting of immune dysfunction. The prognosis is poor.

Enteropathy-type T-cell Lymphoma

Enteropathy-type T-cell lymphoma is usually seen in patients with gluten-sensitive enteropathy (Chapter 126). Patients typically present with abdominal pain and diarrhea and sometimes with bowel perforation. Treatment of celiac disease with a gluten-free diet may reduce the risk for lymphoma. The prognosis in undernourished patients is poor, but more fit patients can sometimes be cured with intensive chemotherapy and autologous bone marrow transplant.

Subcutaneous Panniculitis-like T-cell Lymphoma

Subcutaneous panniculitis-like T-cell lymphoma manifests with multiple subcutaneous nodules and is often misdiagnosed as panniculitis. Patients with disseminated disease can have a syndrome consisting of fevers, weight loss, hepatosplenomegaly, pancytopenia, and phagocytosis of blood cells (hemophagocytic syndrome). Patients sometimes respond to combination chemotherapy regimens used for diffuse large B-cell lymphoma, interferon, and radiation therapy, but long-term disease-free survival is unusual.

SPECIAL CLINICAL SITUATIONS

The diagnosis and management of patients with the various types of non-Hodgkin lymphoma can be profoundly influenced by the site of origin of the lymphoma and by certain clinical characteristics of the individuals affected with the disease. Examples of the latter include lymphoma in patients who are severely immunosuppressed because of HIV infection or a prior transplant, elderly patients with lymphoma, and pregnant patients with lymphoma.

LYMPHOMA IN AIDS

Non-Hodgkin lymphoma is an AIDS-defining illness in HIV-infected individuals (Chapters 355 and 359), and the risk for developing a non-Hodgkin lymphoma is increased more than 150-fold after the diagnosis of another AIDS-defining illness.[35] Most cases are diffuse large B-cell lymphomas or Burkitt lymphomas. AIDS-associated lymphomas behave aggressively and frequently involve the CNS and other unusual sites, such as the gastrointestinal tract, anus, rectum, skin, and soft tissue. Factors associated with poor survival include low CD4 counts, poor performance status, older age, and advanced stage. The incidence of AIDS-associated non-Hodgkin lymphoma has declined, and the prognosis has improved considerably.

TREATMENT

Patients are generally treated in the same manner as nonimmunocompromised patients, and the prognoses are similar. Intrathecal prophylaxis is generally recommended because of a higher risk for CNS involvement.

POST-TRANSPLANT LYMPHOPROLIFERATIVE DISEASE

The risk for developing a non-Hodgkin lymphoma is also markedly increased in patients who have received a solid organ transplant. The histologic appearance of these lymphomas is variable, but they frequently resemble aggressive lymphomas in nonimmunocompromised patients. Epstein-Barr virus (Chapter 348) is almost always the causative agent. Similar disorders can be seen in patients who are treated with methotrexate and other drugs for autoimmune disorders and in recipients of allogeneic hematopoietic stem cell transplants, especially if the transplants are T-cell depleted. These post-transplantation lymphoproliferative disorders, which may develop within weeks after surgery, are more common in patients who receive aggressive immunosuppression after transplantation. Involvement of extranodal sites is common, and lymphoma frequently involves the transplanted organ.

TREATMENT

Post-transplantation lymphoproliferative disorders may respond to reduction or withdrawal of immunosuppression.[36] Acyclovir or ganciclovir can be considered, because these lymphomas are usually related to Epstein-Barr virus, but this practice is controversial. High response rates are also seen with rituximab. Other patients require treatment with combination chemotherapy regimens including rituximab.

NON-HODGKIN LYMPHOMA IN ELDERLY PATIENTS

More than 50% of patients who develop non-Hodgkin lymphomas are older than age 60 years, and the prognosis is generally worse for elderly patients. These poorer outcomes are related to increased toxicity of drug therapy, lower remission rates, increased rates of relapse, and higher death rates from cardiovascular disease and causes other than the lymphoma itself. Older patients are more likely to have other adverse prognostic characteristics (see Table 171-8), which also contribute to poorer outcomes. The practice of arbitrary dose reductions based solely on age should be discouraged if patients have a good performance status and no comorbid illnesses.

NON-HODGKIN LYMPHOMA AND PREGNANCY

Non-Hodgkin lymphoma in pregnancy involves major clinical and ethical issues, and a multidisciplinary approach is needed. Although chest radiographs are generally considered safe, ultrasound examination is usually used instead of CT for staging in the abdomen and pelvis.

TREATMENT

Treatment occasionally can be delayed until after delivery. However, most women have a lymphoma that is potentially curable, and delays in treatment may decrease the chance for cure. Other patients have conditions such as superior vena cava syndrome that require immediate treatment. After the first trimester, full-dose standard therapy such as R-CHOP may be used. Several studies indicate high probabilities of cure without significantly increased adverse long-term physical or intellectual deficits for the child. Although it is reasonable to offer therapeutic abortion for women in the first trimester, chemotherapy also may be successful in this situation. Regimens using methotrexate or abdominal radiation must be avoided.

DISEASES SOMETIMES CONFUSED WITH LYMPHOMA

A variety of conditions are associated with lymphadenopathy that can be confused with lymphoma. The most common atypical lymphoid proliferations that can be confused with lymphoma are florid reactions to immune stimulation. Follicular hyperplasia with diffuse proliferation of B cells and T cells can be seen in a variety of autoimmune diseases (e.g., Sjögren syndrome [Chapter 247], systemic lupus erythematosus [Chapter 245], rheumatoid arthritis [Chapter 243]) and infectious processes (e.g., Epstein-Barr virus [Chapter 348], cytomegalovirus [Chapter 247], cat-scratch disease [Chapter 291]). If the definitive diagnosis of lymphoma cannot be made even after immunologic and molecular studies, the patient should be closely observed. The clinical course or subsequent biopsies can usually resolve the confusion.

Castleman Disease

Castleman disease, or angiofollicular lymph node hyperplasia, usually appears with a hyaline vascular pattern of lymphoid proliferation, but a subset of patients has hyperplastic lymphoid follicles and sheets of plasma cells.[37] Patients with Castleman disease often present with a localized lymphoid mass, but some patients have a systemic illness with fevers, night sweats, weight loss, and fatigue. Frequently, the systemic symptoms of Castleman disease are related to excessive production of IL-6. Castleman disease in HIV-infected patients is frequently associated with HHV-8 (Chapter 358).

TREATMENT

Patients with disseminated and plasma cell–rich forms of Castleman disease may occasionally progress to lymphoma. Patients with localized Castleman disease can be treated with surgical removal, radiation therapy, or occasionally observation if asymptomatic.[38] Patients with systemic disease may respond to treatment with high-dose corticosteroids and/or rituximab. Patients with overexpression of IL-6 frequently benefit from treatment with an anti–IL-6 antibody. For example, siltuximab (a chimeric monoclonal antibody against interleukin 6 at 11 mg/kg intravenous infusion every 3 weeks) can provide durable responses in about one third of HIV-negative patients.[39] If other treatments fail, patients sometimes benefit from combination chemotherapy regimens, autologous or allogeneic hematopoietic stem cell transplantation, or both.[40] The mammalian target of rapamycin (mTOR) inhibitor sirolimus also is a potentially promising agent.

Sinus Histiocytosis with Massive Lymphadenopathy

Sinus histiocytosis with massive lymphadenopathy, also known as Rosai-Dorfman disease (Chapter 154), manifests as bulky lymphadenopathy in children and young adults. Extranodal sites such as the skin, upper airways, gastrointestinal tract, and CNS can be involved. The disease is usually self-limited, but it has been associated with autoimmune hemolytic anemia.

Kikuchi Disease (Histiocytic Necrotizing Lymphadenitis)

Kikuchi disease (histiocytic necrotizing lymphadenitis) is a disease of unknown origin that most commonly affects young women. Symptoms most commonly consist of painless cervical lymphadenopathy that is often accompanied by fever, flulike symptoms, and rash. Treatment is symptomatic, and manifestations usually resolve within weeks or months.

IgG4-related Disease

IgG4-related disease is a systemic immune-mediated fibrosing inflammatory disease in which various organs are infiltrated by IgG4-positive plasma cells (Chapter 254). Patients often have accompanying asymptomatic lymphadenopathy that usually responds to corticosteroids.

GENERAL REFERENCES

For the General References and other additional features, please visit Elsevier eBooks+ at https://ebooks.health.elsevier.com.

Grade A References

A1. Hoskin P, Popova B, Schofield O, et al. 4 Gy versus 24 Gy radiotherapy for follicular and marginal zone lymphoma (FoRT): long-term follow-up of a multicentre, randomised, phase 3, non-inferiority trial. *Lancet Oncol.* 2021;22:332-340.

A2. Leonard JP, Trneny M, Izutsu D, et al. AUGMENT: a phase III study of lenalidomide plus rituximab versus placebo plus rituximab in relapsed or refractory indolent lymphoma. *J Clin Oncol.* 2019;37:1188-1199.

A3. Morschhauser F, Nastoupil L, Feugier P, et al. Six-year results from RELEVANCE: lenalidomide plus rituximab (R^2) versus rituximab-chemotherapy followed by rituximab maintenance in untreated advanced follicular lymphoma. *J Clin Oncol.* 2022;40:3239-3245.

A4. Bachy E, Seymour JF, Feugier P, et al. Sustained progression-free survival benefit of rituximab maintenance in patients with follicular lymphoma: long-term results of the PRIMA study. *J Clin Oncol.* 2019;37:2815-2824.

A5. Marcus R, Davies A, Ando K, et al. Obinutuzumab for the first-line treatment of follicular lymphoma. *N Engl J Med.* 2017;377:1331-1344.

A6. Cheson BD, Chua N, Mayer J, et al. Overall survival benefit in patients with rituximab-refractory indolent non-Hodgkin lymphoma who received obinutuzumab plus bendamustine induction and obinutuzumab maintenance in the GADOLIN study. *J Clin Oncol.* 2018;36:2259-2266.

A7. Matasar MJ, Capra M, Özcan M, et al. Copanlisib plus rituximab versus placebo plus rituximab in patients with relapsed indolent non-Hodgkin lymphoma (CHRONOS-3): a double-blind, randomised, placebo-controlled, phase 3 trial. *Lancet Oncol.* 2021;22:678-689.

A8. Wang ML, Jurczak W, Jerkeman M, et al. Ibrutinib plus bendamustine and rituximab in untreated mantle-cell lymphoma. *N Engl J Med.* 2022;386:2482-2494.

A9. Robak T, Jin J, Pylypenko H, et al. Frontline bortezomib, rituximab, cyclophosphamide, doxorubicin, and prednisone (VR-CAP) versus rituximab, cyclophosphamide, doxorubicin, vincristine, and prednisone (R-CHOP) in transplantation-ineligible patients with newly diagnosed mantle cell lymphoma: final overall survival results of a randomised, open-label, phase 3 study. *Lancet Oncol.* 2018;19:1449-1458.

A10. Bartlett NL, Wilson WH, Jung SH, et al. Dose-adjusted EPOCH-R compared with R-CHOP as frontline therapy for diffuse large B-cell lymphoma: clinical outcomes of the Phase III Intergroup Trial Alliance/CALGB 50303. *J Clin Oncol.* 2019;37:1790-1799.

A11. Tilly H, Morschhauser F, Sehn L, et al. Polatuzumab vedotin in previously untreated diffuse large B-cell lymphoma. *N Engl J Med.* 2022;386:351-363.

A12. Locke FL, Miklos DB, Jacobson CA, et al. Axicabtagene ciloleucel as a second-line therapy for large B-cell lymphoma. *N Engl J Med.* 2022;386:640-654.

A13. Houillier C, Taillandier L, Dureau S, et al. Radiotherapy or autologous stem-cell transplantation for primary CNS lymphoma in patients 60 years of age and younger: results of the intergroup ANOCEF-GOELAMS randomized phase II PRECIS study. *J Clin Oncol.* 2019;37:823-833.

A14. Ribrag V, Koscielny S, Bosq J, et al. Rituximab and dose-dense chemotherapy for adults with Burkitt's lymphoma: a randomised, controlled, open-label, phase 3 trial. *Lancet.* 2016;387:2402-2411.

A15. Dimopoulos MA, Tedeschi A, Trotman J, et al. Phase 3 trial of ibrutinib plus rituximab in Waldenström's macroglobulinemia. *N Engl J Med.* 2018;378:2399-2410.

A16. Horwitz S, O'Connor OA, Pro B, et al. Brentuximab vedotin with chemotherapy for CD30-positive peripheral T-cell lymphoma (ECHELON-2): a global, double-blind, randomised, phase 3 trial. *Lancet.* 2019;393:229-240.

A17. Prince HM, Kim YH, Horwitz SM, et al. Brentuximab vedotin or physician's choice in CD30-positive cutaneous T-cell lymphoma (ALCANZA): an international, open-label, randomised, phase 3, multicentre trial. *Lancet.* 2017;390:555-566.

A18. Kim YH, Bagot M, Pinter-Brown L, et al. Mogamulizumab versus vorinostat in previously treated cutaneous T-cell lymphoma (MAVORIC): an international, open-label, randomised, controlled phase 3 trial. *Lancet Oncol.* 2018;19:1192-1204.

A19. Horwitz S, O'Connor OA, Pro B, et al. The ECHELON-2 trial: 5-year results of a randomized, phase III study of brentuximab vedotin with chemotherapy for CD30-positive peripheral T-cell lymphoma. *Ann Oncol.* 2022;33:288-298.

172

HODGKIN LYMPHOMA

JOSEPH M. CONNORS AND KERRY J. SAVAGE

DEFINITION

Hodgkin lymphoma, one of the B-cell lymphomas, consists of two major types: classic Hodgkin lymphoma, with a characteristic neoplastic cell, the Hodgkin-Reed-Sternberg cell; and the much less common (~10% of cases) nodular lymphocyte-predominant Hodgkin lymphoma, with a characteristic predominance of small lymphocytes. Both types have a distinct natural history, and most important, an excellent response to treatment, with the large majority of patients being cured. Highly effective multiagent chemotherapy is the cornerstone of treatment. Carefully selected patients may require the addition of radiation or, if the lymphoma recurs after primary treatment, high-dose chemoradiation therapy and autologous hematopoietic cell transplantation. The major challenge to clinicians managing this neoplasm is to cure the disease while minimizing long-term toxicity.

EPIDEMIOLOGY

The incidence of Hodgkin lymphoma varies substantially around the world. The highest rates occur in the United States, Canada, Switzerland, and northern Europe. Intermediate rates are seen in southern and eastern Europe and low rates in eastern Asia. No clear explanation for this variation has been found. Postulated reasons include differences in the age at onset or genotype of an associated Epstein-Barr virus infection; crowding during childhood as a result of lower socioeconomic status, predisposing to passage of an as-yet-undiscovered infectious vector; and intrinsic genetic differences in susceptibility.

Approximately 30,000 new cases are diagnosed annually in North America and Europe. The age-adjusted incidence of Hodgkin lymphoma declined modestly over the 20 years before 1990 but has leveled off since then at approximately 2.7 per 100,000. Age-adjusted annual mortality is 0.5 per 100,000. Hodgkin lymphoma occurs slightly more often in men and is seen more frequently in Whites than Blacks and much less frequently in Asian populations. Much of the difference in incidence between Whites and Blacks in North America can be attributed to the higher incidence seen in higher socioeconomic classes. The cumulative lifetime risk for Hodgkin lymphoma is approximately 1 in 250 to 1 in 300 in North America.

The incidence of Hodgkin lymphoma is bimodal in age distribution, rising from very low in childhood to an early peak in young adulthood (25 to 30 years) and a later peak in late adulthood (>50 years). In the Western world, only about 5% of cases occur in persons younger than 15 years of age and 5% in individuals older than 70 years of age. In contrast, the age distribution in the Indian subcontinent is strongly shifted into childhood.

PATHOBIOLOGY

The cause of Hodgkin lymphoma remains unclear. It is not associated with exposure to radiation, chemicals, biocidal agents, working in health care–related professions, or previous tonsillectomy. The leading suspect remains Epstein-Barr virus, based on much suggestive evidence but no definitive proof.[1]

Epstein-Barr Virus

Epstein-Barr virus is a large B-lymphocyte tropic herpesvirus (Chapter 348). Approximately 90% of the general population acquires infection by early adulthood. In the developing world, this infection usually occurs in childhood, but in developed countries, infection is often delayed into the teens, when it is associated with the syndrome of infectious mononucleosis in up to 30% of new cases. A history of infectious mononucleosis increases the likelihood for subsequent Hodgkin lymphoma three-fold. Antibodies to the viral capsid antigen reach higher levels in patients with Hodgkin lymphoma than in controls, and these higher levels appear several years before the neoplasm. In situ hybridization studies have demonstrated that the Hodgkin-Reed-Sternberg cells in approximately 50% of cases of Hodgkin lymphoma contain Epstein-Barr virus-encoded small RNA. In these cases, virtually all the Hodgkin-Reed-Sternberg cells are positive for the virus; the Epstein-Barr virus genome is amplified 50-fold or more in Hodgkin-Reed-Sternberg cells; and is monoclonal in an individual patient's Hodgkin-Reed-Sternberg cells. In some populations, virtually all cases of Hodgkin lymphoma occur in Epstein-Barr virus–positive individuals (<15 or >65 years of age; non-European ancestry; low socioeconomic status), but up to 50% of patients in developed countries do not have Epstein-Barr virus in their Hodgkin-Reed-Sternberg cells. Thus, although Epstein-Barr virus may play an important role in the development of Hodgkin lymphoma, that role is neither straightforward nor universal.

Genetic Factors

Circumstantial evidence for a genetic contribution to the etiology of Hodgkin lymphoma comes from studies showing that Hodgkin lymphoma is almost 100-fold more likely to develop in the monozygotic twin of an affected individual than in a dizygotic twin. First-degree relatives of individuals with the disease have up to a five-fold increased risk for development of the lymphoma. Genome-wide association studies have identified multiple genetic risk variants, which have been detected primarily in immune-related genes. For example, variants in *GATA3*, *IL13*, and genes controlling the expression of HLA class II molecules have been associated with the Epstein-Barr virus–negative nodular sclerosing subtype of classic Hodgkin lymphoma, which is seen predominantly in adolescents and young adults.

Polymerase chain reaction–based genotypic analysis has demonstrated the clonal derivation of Hodgkin-Reed-Sternberg cells, including identical *p53* mutations from multiple Hodgkin-Reed-Sternberg cells extracted from a single biopsy specimen, thereby unequivocally establishing clonality. The presence of clonal immunoglobulin gene rearrangements from multiple cells in the same biopsy specimen also confirms a B-cell origin.[2] Only a few rare cases with a T-cell genotype have been reported. Finally, identification of cells with identical immunoglobulin gene rearrangements, both at diagnosis and at relapse, verify that the B-cell clonality of the disease is preserved over time.

Aneuploidy and hyperploidy consistent with the multinucleated nature of Hodgkin-Reed-Sternberg cells are frequent, but no consistent chromosomal translocations have been detected. Several susceptibility loci for Hodgkin lymphoma have been localized to active chromatin with an overrepresentation of determinants of B-cell development and immune response.

Despite their B-cell origin, the neoplastic cells of Hodgkin lymphoma are incapable of making intact antibodies, perhaps because they lack the ability to make the transcription factors necessary to activate the immunoglobulin promoter. B cells that are incapable of manufacturing antibody should undergo apoptosis and immune destruction, but the Hodgkin-Reed-Sternberg cells avoid cell death by activating NFκB and thereby impeding apoptosis and inducing immune blockade by overexpressing checkpoint inhibitors such as programmed cell death ligands 1 and 2.

CLINICAL MANIFESTATIONS

Hodgkin lymphoma is usually manifested as lymphadenopathy (Chapter 154), typically in the cervical, axillary, or mediastinal areas for the predominant classic Hodgkin lymphoma, and only about 10% of patients present with nodal disease below the diaphragm. Although peripherally located nodes seldom reach large size, very large mediastinal masses or, less often, retroperitoneal masses can develop with only modest symptoms. Lymph node involvement in Hodgkin lymphoma is usually painless, but an occasional patient notes discomfort in involved nodal sites immediately after drinking alcohol.

Approximately 25% of patients with Hodgkin lymphoma have constitutional symptoms. The classic B symptoms—significant weight loss (>10% of baseline), night sweats, and persistent fever—usually signal widespread or locally extensive disease and imply a need for systemic treatment. Generalized pruritus, occasionally severe, can antedate the diagnosis of Hodgkin lymphoma by up to several years. Some patients have symptoms suggestive of a growing mass lesion, such as cough or stridor as a result of tracheobronchial compression from mediastinal disease or bone pain secondary to metastatic involvement. Because Hodgkin lymphoma can rarely involve the bone marrow extensively, an occasional patient presents with symptomatic anemia or incidentally noted pancytopenia. Paraneoplastic neurologic or endocrine syndromes (Chapter 164) have been reported with Hodgkin lymphoma but are rare.

DIAGNOSIS

The diagnosis of classic Hodgkin lymphoma is based on recognition of Hodgkin-Reed-Sternberg cells (Fig. 172-1) or Hodgkin cells (or both) in an appropriate cellular background in tissue sections from a lymph node or extralymphatic organ, such as bone marrow, lung, or bone. Fine-needle aspiration biopsy is not adequate for the diagnosis of Hodgkin lymphoma. Open biopsy and standard histochemical staining are required to establish the diagnosis unequivocally and to determine the histologic subtype.[3]

Hodgkin lymphoma can typically be classified into well-described subtypes (Table 172-1), including a relatively new category of lymphocyte-rich classic Hodgkin lymphoma, which must be distinguished from nodular lymphocyte-predominant Hodgkin lymphoma. The most common subtype is nodular sclerosing, which has characteristic coarse bands of sclerosis surrounding nodules composed of typical Hodgkin-Reed-Sternberg cells in the usual background mixture of reactive and inflammatory cells.

In classic Hodgkin lymphoma, scattered large Hodgkin-Reed-Sternberg cells either are multinucleated or have large polyploid nuclei. Variations include mononuclear cells that are similar to the usual polylobated or multinuclear cells but have only one large nucleus with a prominent nucleolus, as well as lacunar cells, which are Hodgkin-Reed-Sternberg variants with abundant cytoplasm that has retracted as an artifact of formalin fixation. The infrequent Hodgkin-Reed-Sternberg cells are usually present in a background mixture of polyclonal lymphocytes, eosinophils, neutrophils, plasma cells, fibroblasts, and histiocytes. A high number of associated macrophages has been demonstrated to be a strong predictor of treatment resistance. Occasionally, granulomas form with a prominent histiocytic component. In contrast, in nodular lymphocyte-predominant Hodgkin lymphoma the cellular pattern predominantly consists of small lymphocytes and scattered histiocytes, epithelioid histiocytes, and characteristic large neoplastic lymphocytic cells ringed by non-neoplastic T lymphocytes.

The immunophenotype of the neoplastic cells in Hodgkin lymphoma can help identify the specific subtype. Typically, the Hodgkin-Reed-Sternberg cells stain positively for CD30 (90 to 100% of cases), CD15 (75 to 85% of cases), and B-cell-specific activating protein (BSAP), which is the product of the *PAX5* gene (>90% of cases). CD20, a generally reliable marker of B-cell lineage, is positive in about 40% of cases of classic Hodgkin lymphoma, but usually only in a minority of cells, and the staining can be weak. In contrast, nodular lymphocyte-predominant Hodgkin lymphoma almost always stains strongly positive for CD20 and for the specialized B-cell markers CD79a and CD45 but is negative for CD30 and CD15. Anaplastic large cell lymphoma (Chapter 171) is positive for CD30 but reliably negative for CD15, CD20, and CD79a.

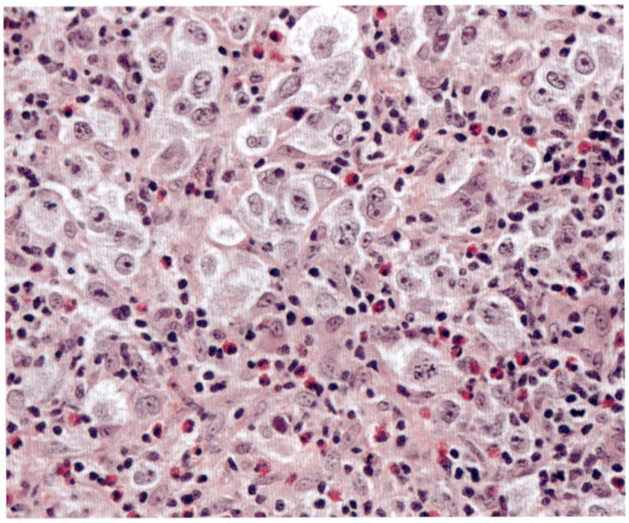

FIGURE 172-1. **Nodular sclerosing Hodgkin lymphoma.** This figure shows a typical case of classic nodular sclerosing Hodgkin lymphoma with many lacunar cells, occasional diagnostic Hodgkin-Reed-Sternberg cells, and the characteristic background of lymphocytes and eosinophils. (Photomicrograph courtesy of Randy D. Gascoyne, MD, British Columbia Cancer Agency.)

TABLE 172-1 WORLD HEALTH ORGANIZATION CLASSIFICATION OF HODGKIN LYMPHOMA SUBTYPES

SUBTYPE NAME	FREQUENCY (%)*
Classic Hodgkin lymphoma	
Nodular sclerosing	60
Lymphocyte rich	3
Mixed cellularity	9
Lymphocyte depleted	1
Nodular lymphocyte-predominant Hodgkin lymphoma	8
Hodgkin lymphoma, not otherwise classifiable	19

*Frequency based on all new cases (N = 2488) seen in British Columbia from January 1998, when the category of lymphocyte-rich classic Hodgkin lymphoma became well established, to December 2020.

Differential Diagnosis

Depending on the site of occurrence and associated symptoms, the differential diagnosis of Hodgkin lymphoma includes non-Hodgkin lymphoma (Chapter 171), primary mediastinal B cell lymphoma, mediastinal gray zone lymphoma, germ cell tumors (Chapters 184 and 185), thymoma (Chapter 390), sarcoidosis (Chapter 83), histiocytosis (Chapter 155), and tuberculosis (Chapter 299). However, the specific diagnosis is readily determined by obtaining an adequate biopsy specimen for review by an experienced hematopathologist. T-cell/histiocyte–rich B-cell lymphoma (Chapter 171) is distinguished from nodular lymphocyte-predominant Hodgkin lymphoma, which it otherwise closely resembles, by being CD30 negative but positive for IgD mantle cells and follicular dendritic cell networks. Proceeding to a biopsy early in the assessment of patients with lymphadenopathy (Chapter 154), especially of the mediastinum, often saves time and avoids delay in diagnosis. With appropriate biopsy procedures to investigate enlarged central thoracic or intra-abdominal lymph nodes, the diagnosis of Hodgkin lymphoma seldom presents difficulty. The immunophenotype helps distinguish Hodgkin lymphoma from other diseases. The combination of appropriate immunohistopathologic evaluation by an expert hematopathologist and clinical assessment has virtually eliminated difficulties with the differential diagnosis. Problems mostly arise when inadequate or improperly processed material is all that is available for diagnosis.

Staging

Physical Examination

The stage of Hodgkin lymphoma can be established by using readily available imaging and laboratory tests (Fig. 172-2 and Table 172-2). The evaluation should start with a careful history to search for the presence of localizing signs, such as bone pain, or the constitutional symptoms of fever, weight loss, or night sweats or comorbid conditions that may affect the safe delivery of planned treatment. The physical examination may identify lymphadenopathy or organomegaly.

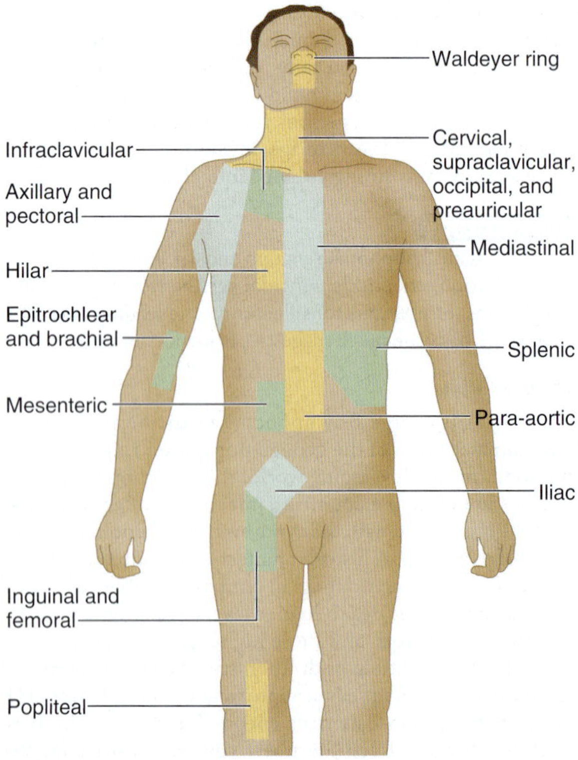

FIGURE 172-2. **Anatomic definition of lymph node regions for staging of Hodgkin disease.** (From Kaplan HS, Rosenberg SA. The treatment of Hodgkin disease. *Med Clin North Am.* 1966;50:1591-1610.)

TABLE 172-2 TESTS REQUIRED FOR STAGING OF HODGKIN LYMPHOMA

Complete history to search for B symptoms (fever, weight loss, night sweats) or other symptomatic problems suggesting more advanced disease
Physical examination for lymphadenopathy or organomegaly
Complete blood count
Serum creatinine, alkaline phosphatase, lactate dehydrogenase, bilirubin, and protein electrophoresis (including serum albumin level)
Chest radiograph, posteroanterior and lateral views
Computed tomography scan of the neck, thorax, abdomen, and pelvis
Fluorodeoxyglucose positron emission tomography with computed tomography (PET/CT)

TABLE 172-3 MODIFIED ANN ARBOR STAGING SYSTEM FOR HODGKIN LYMPHOMA

STAGE	INVOLVEMENT
I	Single lymph node region (I) or one extralymphatic site (I_E)
II	Two or more lymph node regions, same side of the diaphragm (II), or local extralymphatic extension plus one or more lymph node regions, same side of the diaphragm (II_E)
III	Lymph node regions on both sides of the diaphragm (III); may be accompanied by local extralymphatic extension (III_E)
IV	Diffuse involvement of one or more extralymphatic organs or sites
A	No "B" symptoms
B	Presence of at least one of the following: Unexplained weight loss >10% of baseline during 6 months before staging Recurrent unexplained fever >38° C Recurrent night sweats

Laboratory Testing

Laboratory testing should include blood cell counts and the erythrocyte sedimentation rate, assessment of liver and renal function, serum albumin level, serum protein electrophoresis, and serologic testing for human immunodeficiency virus (HIV) as well as hepatitis B and C. Bone marrow aspiration and biopsy have been rendered unnecessary by fluorodeoxyglucose positron emission tomography (PET).

Imaging

Imaging techniques to evaluate Hodgkin lymphoma continue to evolve (Fig. 172-3). All patients should undergo contrast-enhanced computed tomography (CT) scanning of the neck, thorax, abdomen, and pelvis with slices at intervals of 1 cm or less. Magnetic resonance imaging is occasionally useful when the extent of bone or soft tissue involvement must be determined precisely or for a patient with an absolute contraindication to the use of intravenous contrast agents.

Positron Emission Tomography

Fluorodeoxyglucose PET is more sensitive and specific than CT or gallium scanning both for staging and for assessment of residual masses after treatment, and it is now considered mandatory for staging and following patients with Hodgkin lymphoma.[4-6] For staging, PET imaging reliably detects Hodgkin lymphoma and therefore precludes the need for a bone marrow aspirate or biopsy and is very useful for the assessment of residual masses during or after planned treatment, thereby allowing better selection of patients who should receive altered or additional therapy, especially radiotherapy.

Staging System

The Ann Arbor staging system with the Cotswold modification (Table 172-3) categorizes patients into four stages. The spleen and the lymphoid tissue of the Waldeyer ring each count as nodal sites in this system. Stage IV is reserved for diffuse extranodal disease, which for all practical purposes is disease in the bone marrow, lung, bone, or liver. Hodgkin lymphoma at any other extranodal site should prompt questioning of the diagnosis or a search for HIV infection.

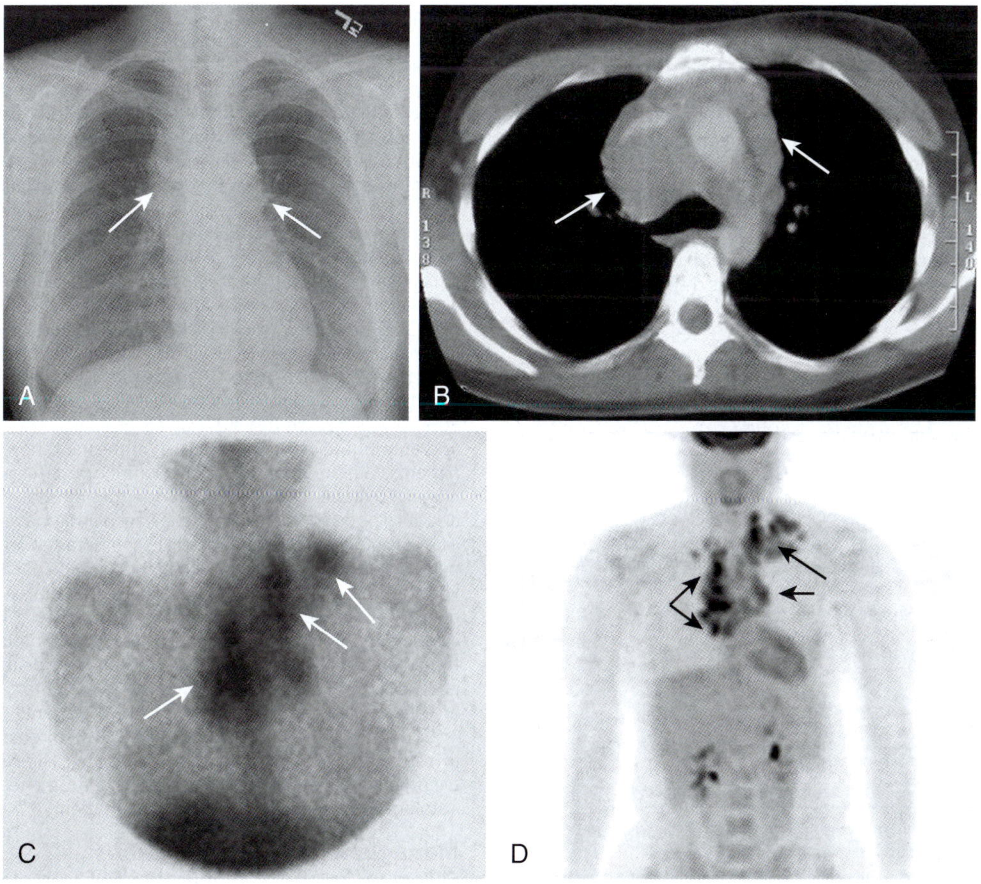

FIGURE 172-3. **Imaging of Hodgkin lymphoma.** Bulky Hodgkin disease as seen on chest radiograph (**A**), computed tomography (CT) of the chest (**B**), gallium scan (**C**), and positron emission tomography (PET) (**D**). The *arrows* indicate sites of disease. Note that the PET and CT scans provide more detailed information than the chest radiograph and gallium scan.

Bulky disease is defined as the presence of any tumor mass with the largest diameter of 10 cm or more. The E lesion designation identifies patients whose limited extranodal extension of Hodgkin lymphoma could be included in a reasonable involved field of irradiation. As part of staging, patients are further subdivided into those with or without fever, night sweats, or weight loss (B symptoms).

TREATMENT

Hodgkin lymphoma is usually cured.[7] Patients who are event-free at 2 years have an excellent outcome regardless of baseline prognostic factors, although they have an enduring increased risk of death from all causes compared with the general population.[8] Accurate diagnosis, staging, and delivery of appropriate combined-modality treatment and multiagent chemotherapy require a multidisciplinary team, including pathologists, experts in diagnostic imaging, medical and radiation oncologists, nurses, and support staff. The necessity to balance greater efficacy of initial treatment, which often requires an increase in intensity and therefore toxicity, against troublesome and occasionally fatal late complications has encouraged a long-term perspective and careful monitoring for late treatment-related side effects.

Patients with stage III or IV disease or bulky disease are defined as having advanced disease, whereas patients without these characteristics have limited-stage disease. In Europe, patients with limited disease are further subdivided into those with favorable and unfavorable outcomes. Cure rates exceed 90 to 95% for patients with nonbulky stage IA or IIA (limited) disease. However, for patients with advanced-stage disease, independent predictors of progression include sex, age, stage, hemoglobin level, white blood cell count, lymphocyte count, and serum albumin level. Current treatment results indicate a spread from 60 to 80% from the worst to best prognosis groups.[9] A straightforward plan of treatment for the 90% of patients in whom Hodgkin lymphoma is diagnosed between the ages of 16 and 70 years can be based on clinical stage, the presence of B symptoms, and bulk of the largest tumor mass (Table 172-4).

Treatment of Limited-Stage Hodgkin Lymphoma

More than 95% of the one third of patients with Hodgkin lymphoma initially found to have limited-stage disease can be cured regardless of the site of occurrence, the presence of disease above or below the diaphragm, or the histologic subtype. The challenge is to achieve this goal with the least toxicity and cost.[10]

Treatment with two cycles of ABVD (Adriamycin [doxorubicin], bleomycin, vinblastine, and dacarbazine under expert supervision) chemotherapy followed by involved-field or involved site irradiation cures nearly 95% of patients with limited-stage disease; nearly completely eliminates the risk for infertility, premature menopause, and leukemia; and minimizes cardiopulmonary toxicity.[11] However, three cycles of chemotherapy alone is a viable alternative for patients who have limited-stage Hodgkin lymphoma and who have a complete metabolic response, as documented by PET scan, because the reduction in the risks of exposure to radiation offset a slightly higher risk of progressive disease.[A1] For the minority whose lymphoma does not completely regress after three cycles as assessed by PET scanning, the addition of radiation is indicated.

In some European centers, limited-stage Hodgkin lymphoma is divided into favorable (lacking adverse prognostic factors) and unfavorable (bulky mediastinal mass, extranodal extension, elevated erythrocyte sedimentation rate, or involvement of three or more lymph node areas). Patients with limited-stage, favorable Hodgkin lymphoma are treated as described above, but more-intensive approaches have been tested for limited-stage but unfavorable Hodgkin lymphoma with these adverse prognostic factors. In such patients, two cycles of BEACOPP (bleomycin, etoposide, doxorubicin, cyclophosphamide, vincristine, procarbazine, and prednisone) followed by two cycles of ABVD under expert supervision plus involved-field radiotherapy significantly improves tumor control compared with four cycles of ABVD before involved-field radiotherapy, but long-term overall survival is not better.[A2] The addition of a checkpoint inhibitor (e.g., nivolumab or pembrolizumab) either before or concomitantly with four cycles of AVD under expert supervision appears to improve outcome for patients with limited stage, unfavorable Hodgkin lymphoma, in whom it can induce a progression-free survival of >98%,[12,13] but the role for checkpoint inhibitors awaits the results of ongoing clinical trials.

Treatment of Advanced-Stage Hodgkin Lymphoma

Formerly, in advanced-stage Hodgkin lymphoma (stages IIIA, IIIB, IVA, IVB, and in some cases bulky stage II), ABVD for six cycles under expert supervision had been the most widely used regimen.[14] If the PET scan had become negative after two cycles of ABVD, bleomycin could be safely omitted from the remaining four cycles.[A3] More recently, however, the addition of brentuximab vedotin, an anti-CD30 antibody-drug conjugate to doxorubicin, vinblastine, and dacarbazine (A+AVD), has been shown to improve both 5-year progression-free and overall survival compared with ABVD in previously untreated stage III or IV Hodgkin lymphoma and has become standard.[A4,A5] A negative PET scan at the end of chemotherapy distinguishes between residual fibrosis and persistent lymphoma and identifies the 75% of patients with a residual mass who do not require radiation therapy.[A6,A7]

An alternative to ABVD chemotherapy for advanced-stage Hodgkin lymphoma in patients less than 60 years of age is escalated BEACOPP (bleomycin, etoposide, doxorubicin, cyclophosphamide, vincristine, procarbazine, and prednisone under expert supervision; see Table 172-4), either by itself[15] or used only for patients with a positive interim PET scan after two cycles of ABVD. PET scan results also can guide the intensity of BEACOPP therapy and allow reductions in future doses in patients without detectable residual disease.[A8] Alternatively, BEACOPP may be switched to ABVD if the PET scan is negative after two cycles.[A9,A10] Assessing the appropriateness of escalated BEACOPP for advanced-stage Hodgkin lymphoma requires consideration of potential secondary treatments for those not cured by primary therapy. About 50% of such patients can be effectively treated with high-dose chemoradiation therapy and autologous hematopoietic cell transplantation (Chapter 163). Thus, although escalated BEACOPP offers better initial disease control, randomized trials have failed to demonstrate its superior overall survival compared with ABVD.[A11,A12]

Management of Refractory or Relapsed Hodgkin Lymphoma

For most patients whose Hodgkin lymphoma persists or recurs despite primary chemotherapy, high-dose chemoradiation therapy (e.g., BEAM [carmustine, etoposide, cytarabine, and melphalan] under expert supervision) and autologous hematopoietic cell transplantation is the recommended treatment, if feasible. Approximately one third of patients whose disease progresses during or within 3 months of initial multiagent chemotherapy (refractory Hodgkin lymphoma) and about two thirds of patients who relapse more than 3 months after multiagent chemotherapy (relapsed Hodgkin lymphoma) can be cured using high-dose chemoradiation therapy and autologous hematopoietic cell transplantation.[16] Two special subgroups may be exceptions. Patients who are initially stage I to III but who relapse solely in originally involved but unirradiated lymph nodes and without B symptoms or extranodal disease may obtain up to a 40 to 50% cure rate with wide-field irradiation, and patients who relapse without B symptoms more than 1 year after completion of primary chemotherapy also may achieve up to a 30 to 40% cure rate with additional chemotherapy with or without irradiation. However, these two subgroups may achieve up to an 80% 10-year disease-free survival rate after high-dose chemoradiation therapy and autologous hematopoietic cell transplantation. Thus, data suggest that patients with progressive Hodgkin lymphoma after primary chemotherapy for advanced-stage disease should undergo high-dose chemoradiation therapy and autologous hematopoietic cell transplantation regardless of the characteristics of the relapse. After high-dose chemoradiation therapy and autologous hematopoietic cell transplantation, the addition of consolidative brentuximab vedotin improves outcomes by eliminating approximately one third of the relapses that would have otherwise occurred.[A13,A14] For patients who relapse despite high-dose chemoradiation therapy and autologous hematopoietic cell transplantation, blockade of the programmed death 1 (PD-1) pathway with checkpoint inhibitors (e.g., nivolumab[A15] or pembrolizumab[A16,17]) can induce an objective response in more than 70% of patients.

Chimeric antigen receptor T-cells (CAR-T) directed against CD30 is being investigated for relapsed Hodgkin lymphoma. If efficacious, this approach may eventually become an alternative to high-dose chemoradiation therapy and autologous hematopoietic cell transplantation.[18]

Management of Complications

Follow-up and Late Complications of Treatment

Most adult patients with Hodgkin lymphoma are cured and experience minimal long-term toxicity from their treatment. However, the risk for certain late effects

TABLE 172-4 TREATMENT PLAN FOR HODGKIN LYMPHOMA BASED ON STAGE

GROUP	STAGE	TREATMENT
Limited	IA or IIA, no bulky disease*	ABVD† × 2 + IRRT or ABVD × 3 If complete remission, no further treatment If partial remission, add IRRT or a checkpoint inhibitor × 8 doses + AVD × 4
Advanced	IB, IIB, or any stage III or IV or bulky disease, any stage	ABVD† × 6 or A+AVD × 6 or escalated BEACOPP† × 4-6
Refractory/ Relapsed	All stages	Second line chemotherapy followed by high-dose chemoradiation therapy and autologous hematopoietic cell transplantation

*Bulky refers to disease with the largest diameter of any single mass equal to or greater than 10 cm.
†See text for drugs in each regimen. Optimal dosing must be individualized.
A+AVD = brentuximab vedotin, doxorubicin, vinblastine, and dacarbazine; ABVD = Adriamycin [doxorubicin], bleomycin, vinblastine, and dacarbazine; BEACOPP = bleomycin, etoposide, doxorubicin, cyclophosphamide, vincristine, procarbazine, and prednisone; IRRT = involved region radiotherapy.

TABLE 172-5 MONITORING AFTER SUCCESSFUL PRIMARY TREATMENT OF HODGKIN LYMPHOMA

RISK/PROBLEM	INCIDENCE/RESPONSE
Relapse	Ten to 30% of patients experience relapse. Careful attention should be directed to lymph node sites, especially if previously involved with disease and not treated with radiation. New persistent focal symptoms such as bone pain should be investigated with appropriate laboratory and imaging studies.
Dental caries	Neck or oropharyngeal irradiation may cause decreased salivation. Patients should have regular dental care and should make their dentist aware of the previous irradiation.
Hypothyroidism	After thyroid irradiation at doses sufficient to cure Hodgkin lymphoma, at least 50% of patients eventually become hypothyroid. All patients who have been exposed to neck irradiation should have an annual TSH level determined. Patients whose TSH level becomes elevated should be treated with lifelong thyroxine replacement in doses sufficient to suppress TSH levels to low normal (Chapter 207).
Cardiac complications	Coronary heart disease, especially in patients exposed to mediastinal radiation, anthracyclines, or both.
Infertility	ABVD is not known to cause permanent gonadal toxicity, although temporary oligospermia or irregular menses may persist for 1 to 2 years after treatment. Direct or scatter radiation to gonadal tissue may cause infertility, amenorrhea, or premature menopause, but this adverse event seldom occurs with the current fields used for the treatment of Hodgkin lymphoma. In general, women who continue menstruating are fertile, but men require semen analysis to provide a specific answer.
Secondary neoplasms	Although uncommon, certain secondary neoplasms occur with increased frequency in patients who have been treated for Hodgkin lymphoma: acute myelogenous leukemia; thyroid, breast, lung, gastric, pancreatic, colorectal, and cervical cancers; non-Hodgkin lymphoma; and melanoma. It is appropriate to "be vigilant" for these neoplasms for the remainder of the patient's life because they may have a lengthy induction period.

ABVD = doxorubicin (Adriamycin), bleomycin, vinblastine, and dacarbazine; TSH = thyroid-stimulating hormone.

warrants careful but not intrusive follow-up and selective intervention (Table 172-5). At the conclusion of treatment, a thorough reassessment of the initial sites of lymphoma should be completed to provide post-treatment baseline measurements. Patients should be seen by a specialist knowledgeable in the management of lymphoma, preferably about every 3 months for 2 years, after which follow-up can be switched to the patient's family physician every 6 months for 3 years, then annually. Patients should be strongly encouraged to refrain from smoking, to perform careful breast and skin examinations on a regular basis, and to undergo annual immunization for influenza, immunization for pneumococcus at diagnosis and 5 years after treatment, and immunization for diphtheria and tetanus every 10 years (Chapter 15). Patients who have received radiation to the head or neck area should follow a vigorous program of dental prophylaxis in anticipation of the deleterious effect of reduced saliva production and should have their thyroid-stimulating hormone (TSH) level checked annually in recognition of the 50% risk for eventual hypothyroidism.

Other potential long-term sequelae of the treatment of Hodgkin lymphoma include second malignancies. Radiation therapy–related solid tumors—most commonly nonmelanoma skin cancers, lung, breast, and colorectal malignancies—have a median latency period of more than 14 years after treatment. Chemotherapy-related myelodysplasia (Chapter 167) and acute myeloid leukemia (Chapter 168) are more likely to be caused by alkylating agents that are included in regimens like MOPP (mechlorethamine, vincristine, procarbazine, and prednisone) and BEACOPP, a risk minimized with ABVD, and have shorter latency periods (median of 3 years) after treatment. Despite the trend toward smaller radiation target volumes, lower radiation doses, and less toxic chemotherapy regimens, the risk of solid cancers has not appreciably changed among patients who were treated during the 1990s as compared with patients who were treated during earlier decades.[19] However, more recently treated female survivors of Hodgkin lymphoma appear to have a reduced risk of breast cancer, and the risk of hematologic malignancies has clearly decreased among 5-year survivors who were treated in the most recent study period, probably reflecting the declining use of alkylating agent–based chemotherapy.

Long-term (usually >10 years after treatment) cardiovascular complications include coronary artery disease (related to mediastinal irradiation) and cardiomyopathy (caused by the cardiotoxicity of anthracycline chemotherapy). The median interval between the initial treatment of Hodgkin lymphoma and the development of coronary artery disease is approximately 19 years. There is a linear, no-threshold relationship between mean heart dose of radiation therapy and development of coronary artery disease in survivors of Hodgkin lymphoma, so the reduced radiation exposure to the heart in current radiation therapy protocols should reduce cardiovascular risk in the future. Chemotherapy, particularly alkylating agents in MOPP and BEACOPP but not ABVD regimens, can cause permanent infertility. Long-term survivors of childhood Hodgkin lymphoma (median age at diagnosis of 15 years) are at increased risk for neurocognitive impairment.

Special Problems in the Management of Hodgkin Lymphoma

Hodgkin Lymphoma During Pregnancy

Between 0.5 and 1.0% of cases of Hodgkin lymphoma occur coincident with pregnancy (Chapter 221). When the lymphoma is discovered during pregnancy, it is almost always possible to keep it under control and allow the pregnancy to go to full term.

Standard staging tests (see Table 172-2) should be completed, except that imaging requiring radiation must be minimized. For example, abdominal ultrasonography can identify bulky retroperitoneal disease, and a single posteroanterior radiograph of the chest, with proper shielding, can identify bulky mediastinal disease.

Patients can often continue the pregnancy to term without any treatment of the lymphoma. If symptomatic or progressive disease develops, ABVD chemotherapy can be given in the second and third trimester with very low risk for injuring the fetus. An attractive alternative to multiagent chemotherapy is intermittent single-agent vinblastine, given in the lowest dose that can control symptoms until delivery, followed by a full course of six to eight cycles of multiagent chemotherapy after delivery.

Hodgkin Lymphoma and Acquired Immunodeficiency Syndrome

In patients with HIV infection, the incidence of Hodgkin lymphoma is increased as much as 5- to 10-fold, and the lymphoma manifests differently and pursues a more aggressive natural history (Chapter 359). Hodgkin lymphoma in HIV-positive individuals is almost always associated with Epstein-Barr virus within Hodgkin-Reed-Sternberg cells. The histology is much more likely to be mixed cellularity or lymphocyte depleted. The disease commonly involves extranodal sites, especially the bone marrow. More than 80% of patients have advanced-stage disease, and most patients have B symptoms.

Patients are prone to opportunistic infections, and the interaction of chemotherapeutic agents with other medications may compromise the patient's ability to tolerate treatment. Meticulous attention to drug-drug interactions is required to avoid drug toxicity and adverse pharmacokinetic effects that might compromise the potential for cure.[20] The best approach is a combination of highly active antiretroviral agents (Chapter 357); vigorous supportive care with antiherpetic agents (Chapter 345), antifungal agents (Chapter 307), and neutrophil-stimulating growth factors (Chapter 142); and standard multiagent chemotherapy. With appropriate supportive care, regimens such as ABVD can be delivered. However, more-severe-than-normal toxicity must be anticipated. With appropriate supportive care and careful choice of highly active antiretroviral therapy to avoid drug interactions that compromise delivery of full chemotherapy doses, cure rates and long term survival rates for Hodgkin lymphoma have become comparable to those seen in HIV-negative individuals.[21]

Hodgkin Lymphoma in the Elderly Population

Elderly patients with Hodgkin lymphoma have a worse outcome. For example, the 5-year overall survival rate falls from an average of about 80% in patients younger than age 65 years to less than 50% in patients older than age 65 years as a reflection of the impact of comorbid conditions that may lead to incomplete staging and inadequate adherence to standard treatment protocols. By comparison, elderly patients achieve outcomes equivalent to those of younger patients when they undergo complete staging and receive full doses of planned chemotherapy. The best approach for elderly patients is to attempt to treat them in a manner similar to younger patients, with vigorous supportive care and the addition of neutrophil growth factors such as filgrastim or pegfilgrastim under expert supervision if necessary to enable safe delivery of full doses. In patients over age 70 years or with preexisting pulmonary or cardiac disease, it might be necessary to reduce the dose of bleomycin or omit doxorubicin.

FUTURE DIRECTIONS

The ability to profile multigene expression patterns and identify genetic polymorphisms associated with specific malignancies may provide better insight into the molecular genesis of Hodgkin and other lymphomas. Molecular methods to monitor minimal residual disease, in addition to the current practice of following only imaging and clinical evaluations, may transform treatment paradigms. Determining levels of circulating tumor DNA holds particular promise for such monitoring. The role of checkpoint inhibitors is likely to evolve as more trials are reported.[22] Therapeutic agents more specifically targeted at the malignant Hodgkin-Reed-Sternberg cells, such as those coupling an antibody to the CD30 antigen with a cellular toxin, hold substantial promise to improve treatment outcomes.

GENERAL REFERENCES

For the General References and other additional features, please visit Elsevier eBooks+ at https://ebooks.health.elsevier.com.

Grade A References

A1. Radford J, Illidge T, Counsell N, et al. Results of a trial of PET-directed therapy for early-stage Hodgkin's lymphoma. *N Engl J Med.* 2015;372:1598-1607.
A2. Gillessen S, Plütschow A, Fuchs M, et al. Intensified treatment of patients with early stage, unfavourable Hodgkin lymphoma: long-term follow-up of a randomised, international phase 3 trial of the German Hodgkin Study Group (GHSG HD14). *Lancet Haematol.* 2021;8:e278-e288.
A3. Johnson P, Federico M, Kirkwood A, et al. Adapted treatment guided by interim PET-CT scan in advanced Hodgkin's lymphoma. *N Engl J Med.* 2016;374:2419-2429.
A4. Connors JM, Jurczak W, Straus DJ, et al. Brentuximab vedotin with chemotherapy for stage III or IV Hodgkin's lymphoma. *N Engl J Med.* 2018;378:331-344.
A5. Ansell S, Radford J, Connors JM, et al. Overall survival with brentuximab vedotin in stage III or IV Hodgkin's lymphoma. *N Engl J Med.* 2022;387:310-320.
A6. Gallamini A, Rossi A, Patti C, et al. Consolidation radiotherapy could be safely omitted in advanced Hodgkin lymphoma with large nodal mass in complete metabolic response after ABVD: final analysis of the randomized GITIL/FIL HD0607 trial. *J Clin Oncol.* 2020;38:3905-3913.
A7. Borchmann P, Plütschow A, Kobe C, et al. PET-guided omission of radiotherapy in early-stage unfavourable Hodgkin lymphoma (GHSG HD17): a multicentre, open-label, randomised, phase 3 trial. *Lancet Oncol.* 2021;22:223-234.
A8. Kreissl S, Goergen H, Buehnen I, et al. PET-guided eBEACOPP treatment of advanced-stage Hodgkin lymphoma (HD18): follow-up analysis of an international, open-label, randomised, phase 3 trial. *Lancet Haematol.* 2021;8:e398-e409.
A9. Casasnovas RO, Bouabdallah R, Brice P, et al. Positron emission tomography-driven strategy in advanced Hodgkin lymphoma: prolonged follow-up of the AHL2011 phase III Lymphoma Study Association study. *J Clin Oncol.* 2022;40:1091-1101.
A10. Stephens DM, Li H, Schöder H, et al. Five-year follow-up of SWOG S0816: limitations and values of a PET-adapted approach with stage III/IV Hodgkin lymphoma. *Blood.* 2019;134:1238-1246.
A11. Carde P, Karrasch M, Fortpied C, et al. Eight cycles of ABVD versus four cycles of $BEACOPP_{escalated}$ plus four cycles of $BEACOPP_{baseline}$ in stage III to IV, International Prognostic Score ≥ 3, high-risk Hodgkin lymphoma: first results of the phase III EORTC 20012 Intergroup Trial. *J Clin Oncol.* 2016;34:2028-2036.
A12. Merli F, Luminari S, Gobbi PG, et al. Long-term results of the HD2000 trial comparing ABVD versus BEACOPP versus COPP-EBV-CAD in untreated patients with advanced Hodgkin lymphoma: a study by Fondazione Italiana Linfomi. *J Clin Oncol.* 2016;34:1175-1181.
A13. Moskowitz CH, Walewski J, Nademanee A, et al. Five-year PFS from the AETHERA trial of brentuximab vedotin for Hodgkin lymphoma at high risk of progression or relapse. *Blood.* 2018;132:2639-2642.
A14. Ansell SM, Radford J, Connors JM, et al. Overall survival with brentuximab vedotin in stage III or IV Hodgkin's lymphoma. *N Engl J Med.* 2022;387:310-320.
A15. Ansell SM, Lesokhin AM, Borrello I, et al. PD-1 blockade with nivolumab in relapsed or refractory Hodgkin's lymphoma. *N Engl J Med.* 2015;372:311-319.
A16. Kuruvilla J, Ramchandren R, Santoro A, et al. Pembrolizumab versus brentuximab vedotin in relapsed or refractory classical Hodgkin lymphoma (KEYNOTE-204): an interim analysis of a multicentre, randomised, open-label, phase 3 study. *Lancet Oncol.* 2021;22:512-524.

173

PLASMA CELL DISORDERS

S. VINCENT RAJKUMAR

DEFINITION

Plasma cell disorders are neoplastic or potentially neoplastic diseases associated with the clonal proliferation of immunoglobulin-secreting plasma cells (Table 173-1). These disorders are characterized by the secretion of electrophoretically and immunologically homogeneous (monoclonal) proteins that represent intact or incomplete immunoglobulin molecules. Monoclonal proteins are commonly referred to as M proteins, myeloma proteins, or paraproteins.

Syndromes associated with plasma cell disorders and monoclonal proteins include premalignant disorders (monoclonal gammopathy of undetermined significance; MGUS), smoldering multiple myeloma, malignant neoplasms (multiple myeloma, Waldenström macroglobulinemia), as well as disorders primarily related to the unique properties of the secreted monoclonal protein (cryoglobulinemia, immunoglobulin light chain [AL] amyloidosis, light chain deposition disease; see Table 173-1).[1]

Serum Immunoglobulins

Intact immunoglobulins consist of two heavy (H) polypeptide chains of the same class and subclass and two light (L) polypeptide chains of the same type (Chapter 35). The heavy polypeptide chains are designated by Greek letters: γ in immunoglobulin G (IgG), α in immunoglobulin A (IgA), μ in immunoglobulin M (IgM), δ in immunoglobulin D (IgD), and ε in immunoglobulin E (IgE). The light chain types are kappa (κ) and lambda (λ). Both heavy chains and light chains have "constant" and "variable" regions with respect to the amino acid sequence. The class specificity of each immunoglobulin is defined by a series of antigenic determinants on the constant regions of the heavy chains (γ, α, μ, δ, and ε) and the two major classes of light chains (κ and λ). The amino acid sequence in the variable regions of the immunoglobulin molecule corresponds to the active antigen-combining site of the antibody.

In the majority of clonal plasma cell disorders, *intact* immunoglobulin molecules are secreted as monoclonal (M) proteins. In addition, there can also be abnormal secretion of excess monoclonal *free* light chains (FLCs) that are released without being bound to immunoglobulin heavy chains. In some patients, heavy chain expression is completely lost, and only monoclonal free light chains (commonly referred to as Bence Jones proteins) are secreted. Even less frequently, only heavy chains are secreted, resulting in heavy chain diseases (HCDs). Rare patients with multiple myeloma secrete no identifiable immunoglobulin ("nonsecretory myeloma").

Identification of Monoclonal Proteins

Protein electrophoresis of the serum and urine detects M protein as a narrow peak (like a church spire) on the densitometer tracing or as a dense, discrete band on agarose gel (Fig. 173-1). Electrophoresis also permits quantitation of M proteins. Monoclonal light chains (Bence Jones proteins) are rarely seen on serum electrophoresis but are easily detected on urine electrophoresis. Urine electrophoresis requires a 24-hour urine collection.

When a peak or band is first seen on protein electrophoresis, immunofixation of the serum and urine should be performed to identify the heavy and light chain type of the M protein. Immunofixation is also a more sensitive test than protein electrophoresis, and it should always be performed in conjunction with electrophoresis when multiple myeloma or related disorders are first suspected so as to detect small, unmeasurable M proteins that may be missed on electrophoresis. Immunofixation is particularly important in oligosecretory myeloma, primary amyloidosis, and solitary plasmacytoma, as well as after successful treatment of multiple myeloma or macroglobulinemia. In these instances, a small M protein can be concealed within the normal β or γ areas of the electrophoresis gel and may be overlooked. Mass spectrometry can be

TABLE 173-1 PLASMA CELL PROLIFERATIVE DISORDERS

I. Premalignant monoclonal gammopathies
  A. Monoclonal gammopathy of undetermined significance (MGUS)
    1. IgM MGUS
    2. Non-IgM MGUS
    3. Light chain MGUS
  B. Biclonal and triclonal gammopathies of undetermined significance
  C. Smoldering multiple myeloma
II. Malignant monoclonal gammopathies
  A. Multiple myeloma (IgG, IgA, IgD, IgE, and light chain only)
  B. Plasma cell leukemia
  C. POEMS syndrome
  D. Solitary plasmacytoma
  E. Solitary plasmacytoma with minimal marrow involvement
  F. Waldenström macroglobulinemia (IgM)
III. Heavy chain diseases (HCDs)
  A. γ-HCD
  B. α-HCD
  C. μ-HCD
IV. Cryoglobulinemia (types I, II, and III)
V. Immunoglobulin light chain amyloidosis

Ig = immunoglobulin; POEMS = polyneuropathy, organomegaly, endocrinopathy, monoclonal plasma cell disorder, and skin changes.

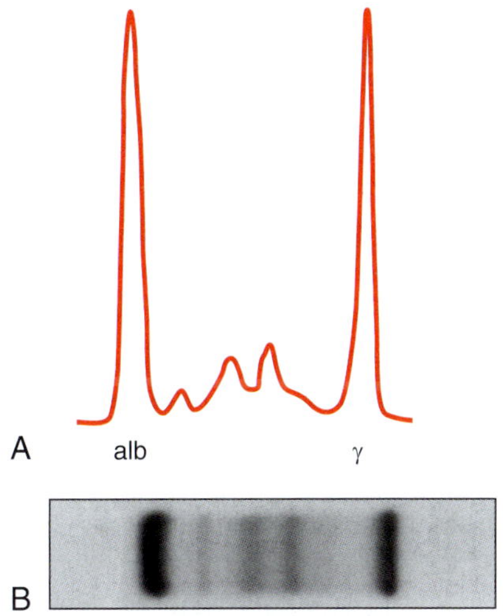

FIGURE 173-1. **Serum protein electrophoresis showing a monoclonal (M) protein. A,** Monoclonal pattern of serum protein as traced by a densitometer after electrophoresis on agarose gel: tall, narrow-based peak of γ mobility. alb = albumin. **B,** Monoclonal pattern from electrophoresis of serum on agarose gel (anode on the left): dense, localized band representing monoclonal protein of γ mobility. (From Kyle RA, Katzmann JA. Immunochemical characterization of immunoglobulins. In: Rose NR, Conway de Macario E, Folds JD, et al., eds. *Manual of Clinical Laboratory Immunology*, 5th ed. Washington, DC: ASM Press; 1997:156, with permission of the American Society for Microbiology.)

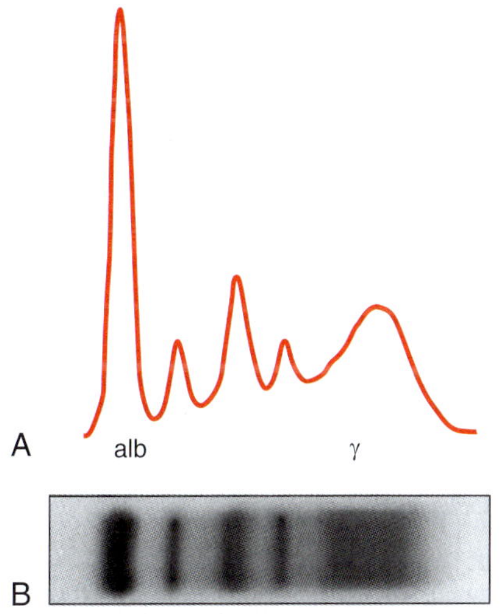

FIGURE 173-2. **Serum protein electrophoresis showing increased polyclonal immunoglobulins. A,** Polyclonal pattern from a densitometer tracing of agarose gel: broad-based peak of γ mobility. alb = albumin. **B,** Polyclonal pattern from electrophoresis of agarose gel (anode on the left). The band at the right is broad and extends throughout the γ area. (From Kyle RA, Katzmann JA. Immunochemical characterization of immunoglobulins. In: Rose NR, Conway de Macario E, Folds JD, et al., eds. *Manual of Clinical Laboratory Immunology*, 5th ed. Washington, DC: ASM Press; 1997:156, with permission of the American Society for Microbiology.)

used instead of immunofixation to identify the M protein more accurately (E-Figs. 173-1 and 173-2).

Monoclonal proteins must be distinguished from an excess of polyclonal immunoglobulins (one or more heavy chain types and both κ and λ light chains, usually limited to the γ region), which produce a broad-based peak or broad band (Fig. 173-2). This finding is associated with chronic infectious or inflammatory states.

Detection of Serum Free Light Chains

The serum free light chain assay measures the level of free κ and λ immunoglobulin light chains (i.e., light chains that are not bound to intact immunoglobulin). An abnormal κ/λ free light chain ratio (normal range, 0.26 to 1.65) indicates a significant excess of one light chain type versus the other and is interpreted as representing a monoclonal elevation of the corresponding light chain type. The serum free light chain assay is more sensitive than electrophoresis or immunofixation in detecting free monoclonal light chains and is useful in the diagnostic evaluation of plasma cell disorders and in risk stratification.

MONOCLONAL GAMMOPATHY OF UNDETERMINED SIGNIFICANCE

DEFINITION

Monoclonal gammopathy of undetermined significance (MGUS; formerly called *benign monoclonal gammopathy*) is a premalignant clonal plasma cell disorder characterized by the presence of a serum M protein in persons who lack evidence of multiple myeloma, macroglobulinemia, amyloidosis, or other related diseases. MGUS is defined by a serum M protein concentration lower than 3 g/dL, less than 10% clonal plasma cells in the bone marrow, and absence of myeloma-defining events. The main clinical significance of MGUS is its lifelong risk of transformation to myeloma or related malignancy at a fixed but unrelenting rate of 1% per year.[2] There are three major types of MGUS: IgM MGUS, non-IgM MGUS, and light chain MGUS (Table 173-2).

EPIDEMIOLOGY

Most patients in whom a serum M protein is detected have MGUS (E-Fig. 173-3). The prevalence of MGUS in the general population increases with age, from approximately 1% in persons 50 to 60 years old to greater than 5% in those older than 70 years. The age-adjusted prevalence is higher in males than in females and is twice as high in Blacks compared with Whites (E-Table 173-1). The prevalence of MGUS and of multiple myeloma is increased among blood relatives of individuals with monoclonal gammopathies.

PATHOBIOLOGY

The etiology of MGUS is unknown, but age, male gender, family history, immunosuppression, and exposure to certain pesticides are known risk factors. It is hypothesized that infection, inflammation, or other antigenic stimuli, acting in concert with the development of cytogenetic abnormalities in the plasma cells, are the initiating pathogenetic events in most patients. Approximately 40% of MGUS is associated with plasma cell translocations involving the immunoglobulin heavy chain (IgH) locus on chromosome 14q32 (IgH translocated MGUS), 40% with trisomies involving odd-numbered chromosomes (hyperdiploid MGUS), 15% with both trisomies and IgH translocations, and the remaining with other cytogenetic abnormalities. The primary IgH translocations seen in MGUS commonly involve one of five recurrent partner chromosome loci: 11q13 (*CCND1* [cyclin D1 gene]), 4p16.3 (*FGFR-3* and *MMSET*), 6p21 (*CCND3* [cyclin D3 gene]), 16q23 (*c-maf*), and 20q11 (*mafB*). On flow cytometry, normal plasma cells are preserved and reside alongside the clonal cells.

CLINICAL MANIFESTATIONS

MGUS is asymptomatic and is usually diagnosed incidentally on laboratory testing. Patients with MGUS progress to multiple myeloma or related malignancy at a rate of approximately 1% per year. Patients with IgM MGUS are at risk of progression to Waldenström macroglobulinemia, while patients with non-IgM MGUS and light chain MGUS are at risk of progression to multiple myeloma. All forms of MGUS carry a risk of progression to AL amyloidosis.

DIAGNOSIS

MGUS represents a limited, nonmalignant expansion of monoclonal plasma cells. MGUS is differentiated from multiple myeloma and smoldering multiple myeloma by the level of the M protein, the percentage of plasma cells in the bone marrow, and the presence or absence of anemia, renal failure, hypercalcemia, or lytic bone lesions (Table 173-2).[3] Because anemia and renal insufficiency are relatively common in the elderly population with MGUS, the causes of these conditions should be carefully investigated with adequate laboratory studies. Only patients with strong evidence of end-organ damage thought to be directly related to a plasma cell disorder can be considered to have myeloma or a related malignancy.

Although a reduction in the levels of the immunoglobulin classes other than M protein (i.e., the normal polyclonal or background immunoglobulins) is more frequently seen in multiple myeloma or Waldenström macroglobulinemia, such reductions also occur in almost 40% of patients with MGUS.

TABLE 173-2 CRITERIA FOR THE DIAGNOSIS OF PLASMA CELL DISORDERS

DISORDER	DISEASE DEFINITION
IgM monoclonal gammopathy of undetermined significance (IgM MGUS)	All three criteria must be met: 1. Serum IgM monoclonal protein <3 g/dL 2. Bone marrow lymphoplasmacytic infiltration <10% 3. No evidence of anemia, constitutional symptoms, hyperviscosity, lymphadenopathy, or hepatosplenomegaly that can be attributed to the underlying lymphoproliferative disorder
Non-IgM monoclonal gammopathy of undetermined significance (MGUS)	All three criteria must be met: 1. Serum monoclonal protein (non-IgM type) <3 g/dL 2. Clonal bone marrow plasma cells <10%* 3. Absence of end-organ damage such as hypercalcemia, renal insufficiency, anemia, and bone lesions (CRAB) that can be attributed to the plasma cell proliferative disorder
Light chain MGUS	All criteria must be met: 1. Abnormal FLC ratio (<0.26 or >1.65) 2. Increased level of the appropriate involved light chain (increased κ FLC in patients with ratio >1.65 and increased λ FLC in patients with ratio <0.26) 3. No immunoglobulin heavy chain expression on immunofixation 4. Absence of end-organ damage that can be attributed to the plasma cell proliferative disorder 5. Clonal bone marrow plasma cells <10% 6. Urinary monoclonal protein <500 mg/24 h
Smoldering multiple myeloma	Both criteria must be met: 1. Serum monoclonal protein (IgG or IgA) ≥3 g/dL, or urinary monoclonal protein ≥500 mg per 24 h and/or clonal bone marrow plasma cells 10-60% 2. Absence of myeloma-defining events or amyloidosis

Multiple myeloma	Both criteria must be met:
	1. Clonal bone marrow plasma cells ≥10% or biopsy-proven bony or extramedullary plasmacytoma
	2. Any one or more of the following myeloma-defining events:
	• Evidence of end-organ damage that can be attributed to the underlying plasma cell proliferative disorder, specifically:
	  • Hypercalcemia: serum calcium >0.25 mmol/L (>1 mg/dL) higher than the upper limit of normal or >2.75 mmol/L (>11 mg/dL)
	  • Renal insufficiency: creatinine clearance <40 mL per minute or serum creatinine >177 μmol/L (>2 mg/dL)
	  • Anemia: hemoglobin value of >2 g/dL below the lower limit of normal or a hemoglobin value <10 g/dL
	  • Bone lesions: one or more osteolytic lesions on skeletal radiography, computed tomography (CT), or positron emission tomography-CT (PET-CT)
	• Clonal bone marrow plasma cell percentage ≥60%
	• Involved: uninvolved serum free light chain (FLC) ratio ≥100 (involved free light chain level must be ≥100 mg/L)
	• >1 focal lesions on magnetic resonance imaging (MRI) studies (at least 5 mm in size)

Solitary plasmacytoma	All four criteria must be met: 1. Biopsy-proven solitary lesion of bone or soft tissue with evidence of clonal plasma cells 2. Normal bone marrow with no evidence of clonal plasma cells 3. Normal skeletal survey and MRI (or CT) of spine and pelvis (except for the primary solitary lesion) 4. Absence of end-organ damage such as hypercalcemia, renal insufficiency, anemia, or bone lesions (CRAB) that can be attributed to a lymphoplasma cell proliferative disorder
Solitary plasmacytoma with minimal marrow involvement†	All four criteria must be met: 1. Biopsy-proven solitary lesion of bone or soft tissue with evidence of clonal plasma cells 2. Clonal bone marrow plasma cells <10% 3. Normal skeletal survey and MRI (or CT) of spine and pelvis (except for the primary solitary lesion) 4. Absence of end-organ damage such as hypercalcemia, renal insufficiency, anemia, or bone lesions (CRAB) that can be attributed to a lymphoplasma cell proliferative disorder

*A bone marrow can be deferred in patients with low-risk MGUS (IgG type, M protein <1.5 g/dL, normal free light chain ratio) in whom there are no clinical features concerning for myeloma.
†Solitary plasmacytoma with 10% or more clonal plasma cells is considered multiple myeloma.
FLC = free light chain; Ig = immunoglobulin; MRI = magnetic resonance imaging.
Reproduced from Rajkumar SV, Dimopoulos MA, Palumbo A, et al. International Myeloma Working Group updated criteria for the diagnosis of multiple myeloma. *Lancet Oncol* 2014;15:e538-e548.

Association of MGUS with Other Diseases

MGUS is associated with numerous diseases. However, because 3% of the general population older than 50 years has MGUS, it is often difficult to determine whether these reported associations are causal or coincidental. Associations that have been verified based on epidemiologic studies include peripheral neuropathy (Chapter 388), proliferative glomerulonephritis, deep vein thrombosis (Chapter 68), osteoporosis (Chapter 225), and lymphoproliferative disorders (Chapter 171). A secondary form of MGUS also occurs with immunosuppression after organ transplantation (Chapter 38) and autologous or allogeneic stem cell transplantation (Chapter 163). M proteins also occur in the sera of some patients with CLL (Chapter 169) but have no recognizable effect on the clinical course.

Approximately 5% of patients with sensorimotor peripheral neuropathy of unknown cause (Chapter 388) have an associated monoclonal gammopathy (monoclonal gammopathy–associated peripheral neuropathy).[4] Patients with IgM MGUS–associated peripheral neuropathy have a slowly progressive distal acquired demyelinating symmetric (DADS) presentation, with predominantly sensory symptoms beginning in the distal ends of the extremities and extending proximally. In contrast, non-IgM MGUS neuropathy may present similar to chronic inflammatory demyelinating polyneuropathy (CIDP) with both proximal and distal involvement and with more motor symptoms. A causal relationship between MGUS and peripheral neuropathy is usually assumed in younger patients and those without other conditions known to cause neuropathy in whom the neuropathy is severe and progressive. Therapeutic approaches include intravenous immunoglobulin or rituximab for IgM monoclonal proteins and plasmapheresis or prednisone for non-IgM monoclonal proteins.

Monoclonal gammopathy is also felt to be the underlying cause of approximately 50% of idiopathic proliferative glomerulonephritis (Chapter 107), including membranoproliferative glomerulonephritis and C3 glomerulopathy. Certain skin disorders are also known to be associated with MGUS. Lichen myxedematosus (papular mucinosis, scleromyxedema) (Chapter 407) is associated with an IgG γ protein. Pyoderma gangrenosum and necrobiotic xanthogranuloma are other associated skin disorders.

TREATMENT

No treatment is necessary for MGUS (Fig. 173-3).[5] A baseline bone marrow biopsy and bone imaging can be omitted in patients who appear clinically to have low-risk, uncomplicated MGUS, small IgM MGUS, or light chain MGUS with a free light chain ratio less than 8. Bone imaging can also be omitted in patients who have IgM MGUS and in whom bone disease is not suspected. Low-risk patients (Table 173-3) should be evaluated in 6 months and, if stable, require no further follow-up until symptoms suggestive of myeloma or related disorders occur. In all other patients with MGUS, electrophoresis, serum free light chains, complete blood count, and creatinine and calcium levels should be repeated at 6 months and, if stable, yearly thereafter.

PROGNOSIS

Differentiating a patient with MGUS in whom the disorder will remain stable for life from one in whom multiple myeloma, macroglobulinemia, or a related disorder will eventually develop is difficult when the M protein is first recognized. The size and type of the M protein at diagnosis of MGUS and an abnormal serum free light chain ratio are prognostic factors for progression (see Table 173-3).[6] Overall, about one third of patients progress to a symptomatic monoclonal gammopathy over 10 or more years.[7]

BICLONAL GAMMOPATHIES

Biclonal gammopathies occur in at least 5% of patients with clonal plasma cell disorders. A biclonal gammopathy of undetermined significance (analogous to MGUS) accounts for about two thirds of such patients. The remainder have multiple myeloma, macroglobulinemia, or other lymphoproliferative diseases. Rarely, triclonal gammopathies may occur.

MULTIPLE MYELOMA

DEFINITION

Multiple myeloma is a malignancy of plasma cells characterized by bone marrow infiltration and extensive skeletal destruction resulting in anemia, bone pain, and fractures. Multiple myeloma (commonly referred to as *myeloma*) is defined by the presence of 10% or more clonal plasma cells on bone marrow examination, M protein in serum or urine (except in the case of nonsecretory myeloma), and evidence of one or more myeloma-defining events (see Table 173-2). Patients with multiple myeloma must be differentiated from those with MGUS and smoldering multiple myeloma.[8]

EPIDEMIOLOGY

Multiple myeloma accounts for 1% of all malignant disease and slightly more than 10% of hematologic malignancies in the United States. The annual

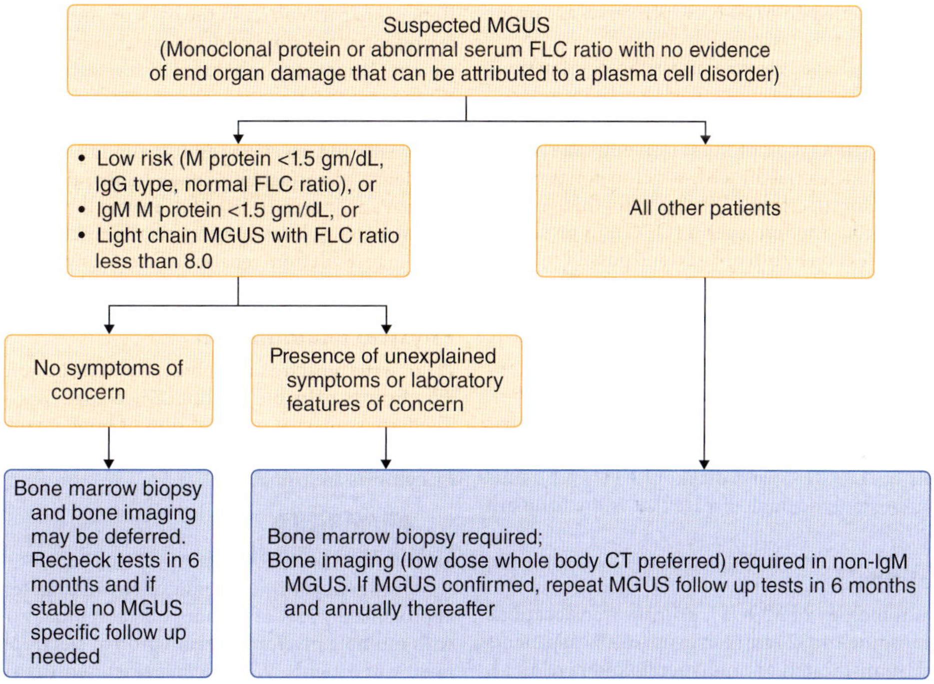

FIGURE 173-3. **Approach to diagnosis and management of monoclonal gammopathy of undetermined significance.** CT = computed tomography; FLC = free light chain ration; MGUS = monoclonal gammopathy of undermined significance.

TABLE 173-3 RISK OF PROGRESSION OF MONOCLONAL GAMMOPATHY OF UNDETERMINED SIGNIFICANCE TO MYELOMA OR RELATED DISORDERS

RISK GROUP	RELATIVE RISK	CUMULATIVE ABSOLUTE RISK OF PROGRESSION AT 20 YR (%)*	CUMULATIVE ABSOLUTE RISK OF PROGRESSION AT 20 YR ACCOUNTING FOR DEATH AS A COMPETING RISK (%)†
Low risk: serum M protein <1.5 g/dL, IgG subtype, normal free light chain ratio (0.26-1.65)	1	5	2
Low-intermediate risk: any one factor abnormal	5.4	21	10
High-intermediate risk: any two factors abnormal	10.1	37	18
High risk: all three factors abnormal	20.8	58	27

*Estimates in this column represent the risk of progression, assuming that patients do not die of other causes during this period.
†Estimates in this column represent the risk of progression calculated by using a model that accounts for the fact that patients can die of unrelated causes during this time.
Ig = immunoglobulin.
Adapted from Rajkumar SV, Kyle RA, Therneau TM, et al. Serum free light chain ratio is an independent risk factor for progression in monoclonal gammopathy of undetermined significance (MGUS). *Blood*. 2005;106:812-817.

incidence of multiple myeloma is approximately 4 per 100,000. The incidence of multiple myeloma in Blacks is almost twice that in Whites. Multiple myeloma is slightly more common in men than in women. The median age of patients at the time of diagnosis is about 65 years; only 2% of patients are younger than 40.

PATHOBIOLOGY

The cause of multiple myeloma is unclear. Exposure to radiation, benzene, and other organic solvents, herbicides, and insecticides may play a role. Multiple myeloma has been reported in familial clusters of two or more first-degree relatives and in identical twins.

Almost all cases of myeloma evolve from a premalignant MGUS phase, although the MGUS is clinically recognized before the diagnosis of myeloma in only a small minority of patients. The progression of MGUS to myeloma suggests a simple, random, two-hit genetic model of malignancy in which the risk of progression is fixed (approximately 1% per year) regardless of the duration of MGUS. Unfortunately, the precise mechanisms of progression are unknown, although several potentially pathogenetic abnormalities have been described in the clonal plasma cells. The two main events associated with progression of MGUS to multiple myeloma appear to be *RAS* mutations and *MYC* abnormalities. Deletions involving 17p and 1p and amplification of 1q occur with disease progression in multiple myeloma and are associated with adverse prognosis. These changes cause dysregulation of the NF-κB and other signaling pathways. Normal plasma cell differentiation is also affected. Changes in the bone marrow microenvironment likely play a major role in the pathogenesis, including induction of angiogenesis and abnormal paracrine loops involving cytokines such as interleukin-6 (IL-6), which serves as a major growth factor for plasma cells.

The lytic bone lesions, osteopenia, hypercalcemia, and pathologic fractures in patients with myeloma are a result of abnormal osteoclast activity induced by the neoplastic plasma cells, as well as inhibition of osteoblast differentiation. Osteoclasts are activated by stimulation of the transmembrane receptor RANK (receptor activator of nuclear factor κB), which belongs to the tumor necrosis factor (TNF) receptor superfamily. The ligand for this receptor (RANKL) also has a decoy receptor, osteoprotegerin (OPG). In myeloma, there is an increase in RANKL expression by osteoblasts (and possibly plasma cells), accompanied by a reduction in the level of OPG. The resultant increase in the RANKL/OPG ratio causes osteoclast activation and increased bone resorption and turnover (Chapter 225). Other factors that may play a role in osteoclast activation include increased levels of macrophage inflammatory protein–1-alpha (MIP-1-alpha), stromal derived factor alpha (SDF-alpha), IL (interleukin)-3, IL-1 beta, and IL-6. In addition to these changes that promote osteoclast activation, simultaneous suppression of osteoblasts is mediated by increased levels of IL-3, IL-7, and dickkopf 1 (DKK1). This combination leads to the pure osteolytic bone disease that is the hallmark of multiple myeloma.

Cytogenetic Abnormalities

As discussed earlier (see Pathobiology of MGUS), primary translocations involving the IgH loci (chromosome 14q32) are seen in up to 40% of patients with multiple myeloma (IgH-translocated or nonhyperdiploid myeloma). Approximately 40% of patients do not have IgH translocations but have evidence of trisomies (hyperdiploid myeloma), 15% have both IgH translocations and trisomies, and 5% have other abnormalities. Although IgH translocations and trisomies originate at the MGUS stage, the response to therapy and prognosis of myeloma are affected by the specific underlying abnormality (Table 173-4). Besides these primary cytogenetic abnormalities, other abnormalities (termed secondary cytogenetic abnormalities) occur as late events during the course of symptomatic myeloma; these include deletion of 17p, deletion of 1p, and amplification of 1q.

CLINICAL MANIFESTATIONS

Many patients are asymptomatic because they are detected early based on incidental laboratory testing. Smoldering (asymptomatic) multiple myeloma is defined by the presence of an M protein level greater than 3 g/dL in serum or 10 to 60% clonal plasma cells in bone marrow in the absence of anemia, renal insufficiency, hypercalcemia, or skeletal lesions. Clinically, patients with smoldering multiple myeloma are similar to patients who have MGUS but carry a much higher risk for progression to myeloma or a related malignancy: 10% per year for the first 5 years, 5% per year for the next 5 years, and 1 to 2% per year thereafter. Even patients who meet the full criteria for multiple myeloma may be asymptomatic and be detected only by an evaluation of laboratory abnormalities.

TABLE 173-4 STAGING AND PROGNOSTIC FACTORS IN MULTIPLE MYELOMA

STAGE/RISK FACTOR
Stage I (serum albumin >3.5, serum beta-2-microglobulin <3.5, no high-risk cytogenetics, and normal serum lactate dehydrogenase level)
Stage II (neither stage I nor stage III)
Stage III (serum beta-2-microglobulin >5.5 and either high-risk cytogenetics [t(4;14), t(14;16), or del(17p)] or elevated serum lactate dehydrogenase level)
High-risk myeloma (any one of the following): Translocations of t(14;16), t(14;20), t(4;14) Deletion of 17p Amplification of 1q p53 mutation
Standard-risk myeloma Translocations of t(11;14), t(6;14) Trisomies
Poor performance status
Increased circulating plasma cells
Plasmablastic morphology

History

Bone pain, particularly in the back or chest and less often in the extremities, is present at the time of diagnosis in more than two thirds of patients. The patient's height may be reduced by several inches because of vertebral collapse. Weakness and fatigue are common and are often associated with anemia. The incidence of infections is increased in patients with multiple myeloma. The propensity for infection results from impairment of the antibody response, deficiency of normal immunoglobulins, and neutropenia. Myeloma patients also have an increased risk of deep vein thrombosis, although some myeloma treatments (e.g., lenalidomide) may themselves cause thrombosis. Other symptoms may result from renal insufficiency, hypercalcemia, nephrotic syndrome, radiculopathy, or AL amyloidosis (Chapter 174).

Physical Examination

Pallor is the most frequent physical finding in patients with multiple myeloma. The liver is palpable in about 5% of patients and the spleen in only 1%. Tenderness may be noted at sites of bone involvement. Radiculopathy may be caused by spinal compression fractures. Occasionally, extramedullary plasmacytomas are palpable.

DIAGNOSIS

Laboratory Findings

A normocytic, normochromic anemia (Chapter 144) is present initially in approximately 75% of patients, but it eventually occurs in nearly every patient with multiple myeloma. Serum protein electrophoresis shows an M protein in 80% of patients. With the increased sensitivity of serum immunofixation, an M protein can be detected in 93% of patients. When these serum studies are combined with urine electrophoresis plus immunofixation, an M protein can be detected in 97% of patients with myeloma.[9] The serum free light chain assay is more convenient and can be used in place of urine studies in the diagnostic evaluation. The type of M protein is IgG in 52%, IgA in 21%, light chain only in 16%, IgD in 2%, and biclonal gammopathy in 2%; the light chain type is κ in 65% of cases and λ in 35%. In 3% of patients, no secreted M protein can be identified; these patients are considered to have nonsecretory myeloma.

In the bone marrow, clonal plasma cells account for greater than 10% of all nucleated cells in 96% of patients (Fig. 173-4 and E-Figs.173-4 and 173-5). In 4% of patients, bone marrow examination shows less than 10% plasma cells, even though the patient otherwise meets the criteria for myeloma; because bone marrow involvement in myeloma may be focal rather than diffuse, repeated bone marrow examinations or biopsy of a discrete bone or extramedullary lesion may be required. In most cases, the plasma cells in myeloma are cytoplasmic Ig^+, $CD38^+$, $CD45^-$, $CD138^+$, and CD 56^+. Only 20% express CD20. The clonality of the plasma cells is established using the κ/λ ratio by immunohistochemistry or flow cytometry (E-Fig. 173-6). The κ/λ ratio is abnormal in myeloma (either >4 : 1, indicating a clonal κ population, or <1 : 2, indicating a clonal λ population). This is helpful for differentiating monoclonal plasma cell proliferation in multiple myeloma from reactive plasmacytosis.

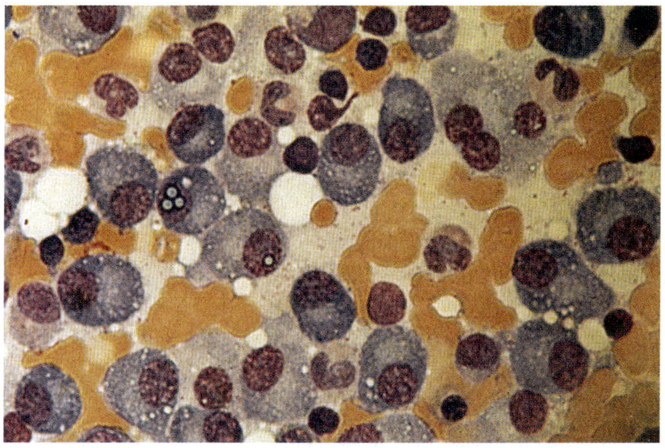

FIGURE 173-4. **Multiple myeloma.** A bone marrow aspirate shows a predominance of plasma cells.

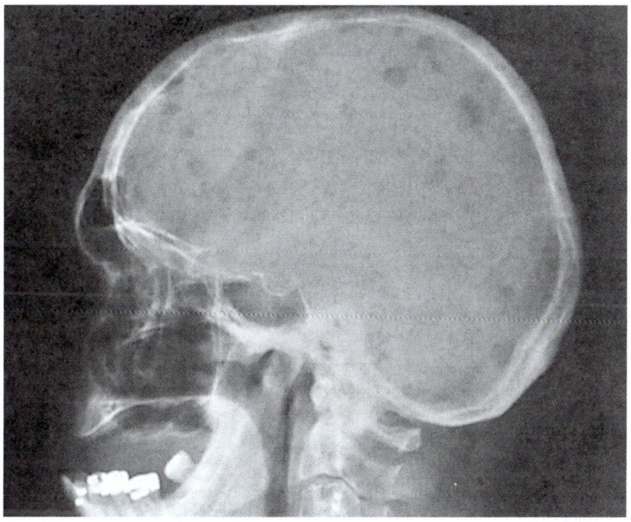

FIGURE 173-5. **Skull radiograph showing multiple lytic lesions.**

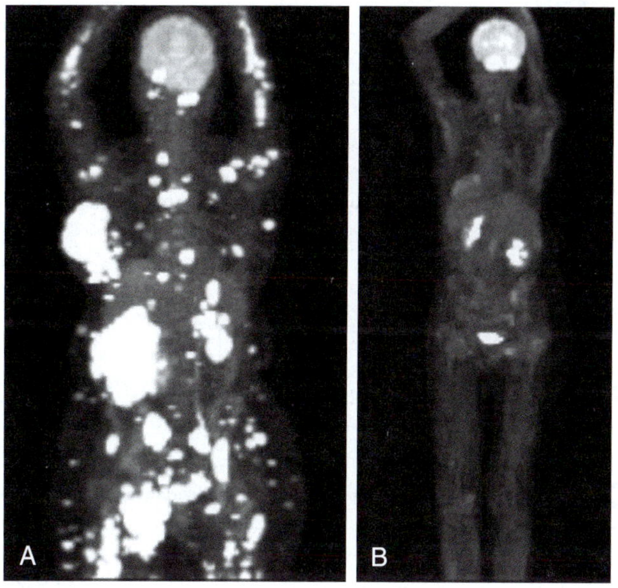

FIGURE 173-6. **Positron emission tomography in multiple myeloma. A,** Extensive bony and extramedullary disease. **B,** Significant improvement after systemic chemotherapy for myeloma.

Radiologic Findings

Conventional radiographic studies reveal abnormalities consisting of punched-out lytic lesions (Fig. 173-5), osteoporosis, or fractures in nearly 80% of patients. The vertebrae, skull, thoracic cage, pelvis, and proximal ends of the humerus and femur are the most frequent sites of involvement. Conventional radiographs are not sensitive, and low-dose whole body computed tomography and positron emission tomography (PET) are now the preferred imaging modalities to assess bone disease in multiple myeloma (Fig. 173-6).[10] Magnetic resonance imaging (MRI) is useful in patients in whom there is doubt about the magnitude of the disease burden and in those who have spinal involvement.

Organ Involvement

Renal

Renal insufficiency, defined as a creatinine level greater than 2 mg/dL, is observed in 20% of patients with multiple myeloma at diagnosis. The two major causes of renal insufficiency are light chain cast nephropathy *(myeloma kidney)* and hypercalcemia. Light chain cast nephropathy is characterized by the presence of large, waxy, laminated casts in the distal and collecting tubules. The casts are composed mainly of precipitated monoclonal light chains. The extent of cast formation correlates directly with the amount of free urinary light chain and with the severity of renal insufficiency. Hypercalcemia, which is present in 15 to 20% of patients initially, is a major and treatable cause of renal insufficiency. It results from destruction of bone. Other contributing factors include dehydration and hyperuricemia.

Besides light chain cast nephropathy and hypercalcemia, there are other mechanisms by which renal dysfunction can occur in myeloma and related plasma cell disorders. For example, light chain amyloidosis (Chapter 174) occurs in nearly 10% of patients with myeloma and may produce nephrotic syndrome, renal insufficiency, or both. Acquired Fanconi syndrome (Chapter 108), characterized by proximal tubular dysfunction, results in glycosuria, phosphaturia, and aminoaciduria. Deposition of monoclonal light chains in the renal glomerulus (light chain deposition disease) may also produce renal insufficiency and nephrotic syndrome. Monoclonal gammopathy–associated proliferative glomerulonephritis presents with hematuria and renal insufficiency.

Neurologic

Radiculopathy (Chapter 369), which is the single most frequent neurologic complication of multiple myeloma, usually occurs in the thoracic or lumbosacral area and results from compression of the nerve by the vertebral lesion or by the collapsed bone itself. Compression of the spinal cord occurs in up to 10% of patients. Peripheral neuropathy (Chapter 388) is uncommon in multiple myeloma and, when present, is generally caused by amyloidosis. Rarely, myeloma cells diffusely infiltrate the meninges. Intracranial plasmacytomas almost always represent extensions of myelomatous lesions of the skull. True involvement of the central nervous system is rare and is associated with poor prognosis.

Other Systemic Involvement

Hepatic infiltration, pleural effusions, or ascites suggests progression to plasma cell leukemia. Similarly the development of multiple extramedullary plasmacytomas is also a sign of more aggressive disease biology.

TREATMENT

Smoldering Multiple Myeloma

Treatment for patients with smoldering multiple myeloma depends on the risk of progression. Risk factors for progression include serum monoclonal protein greater than 2 gm/dL, serum free light chain ratio greater than 20, and bone marrow plasma cells greater than 20%. Patients with zero or one risk factor are considered to have low- or intermediate-risk smoldering multiple myeloma, respectively. Patients with two or three risk factors are considered to have high-risk smoldering multiple myeloma.[11]

Patients with low- or intermediate-risk smoldering multiple myeloma should not be treated until evidence of multiple myeloma develops (Fig. 173-7).[12,13] The standard of care for low- and intermediate-risk smoldering multiple myeloma is observation every 3 to 4 months. In patients with high-risk smoldering multiple myeloma, therapy for approximately 2 years with lenalidomide (25 mg on days 1 to 21 of a 28-day cycle) or with lenalidomide plus low-dose dexamethasone (40 mg once per week) can significantly reduce the risk of progression to symptomatic multiple myeloma, the development of end-organ damage,[A1] and overall mortality.[A2]

Multiple Myeloma

The approach to the treatment of multiple myeloma (Fig. 173-8) is increasingly targeted and personalized under expert supervision.[14] Response to therapy and minimal residual disease assessment is assessed using standard International

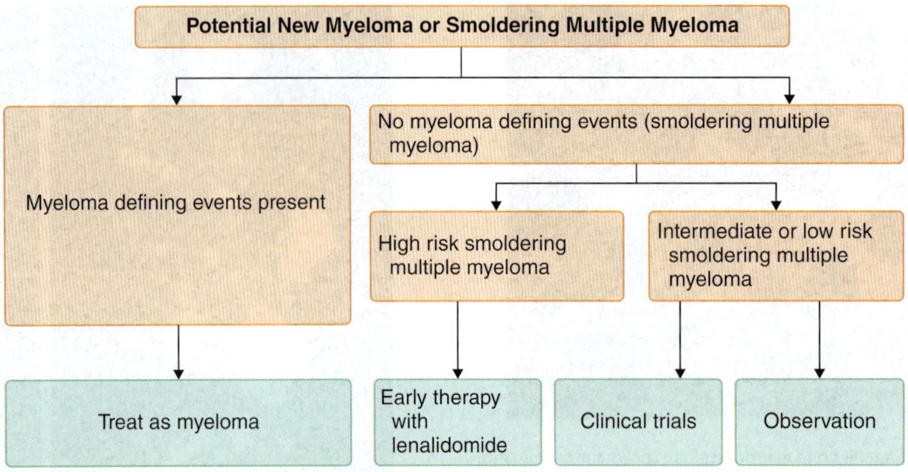

FIGURE 173-7. **Approach to the management of smoldering multiple myeloma.**

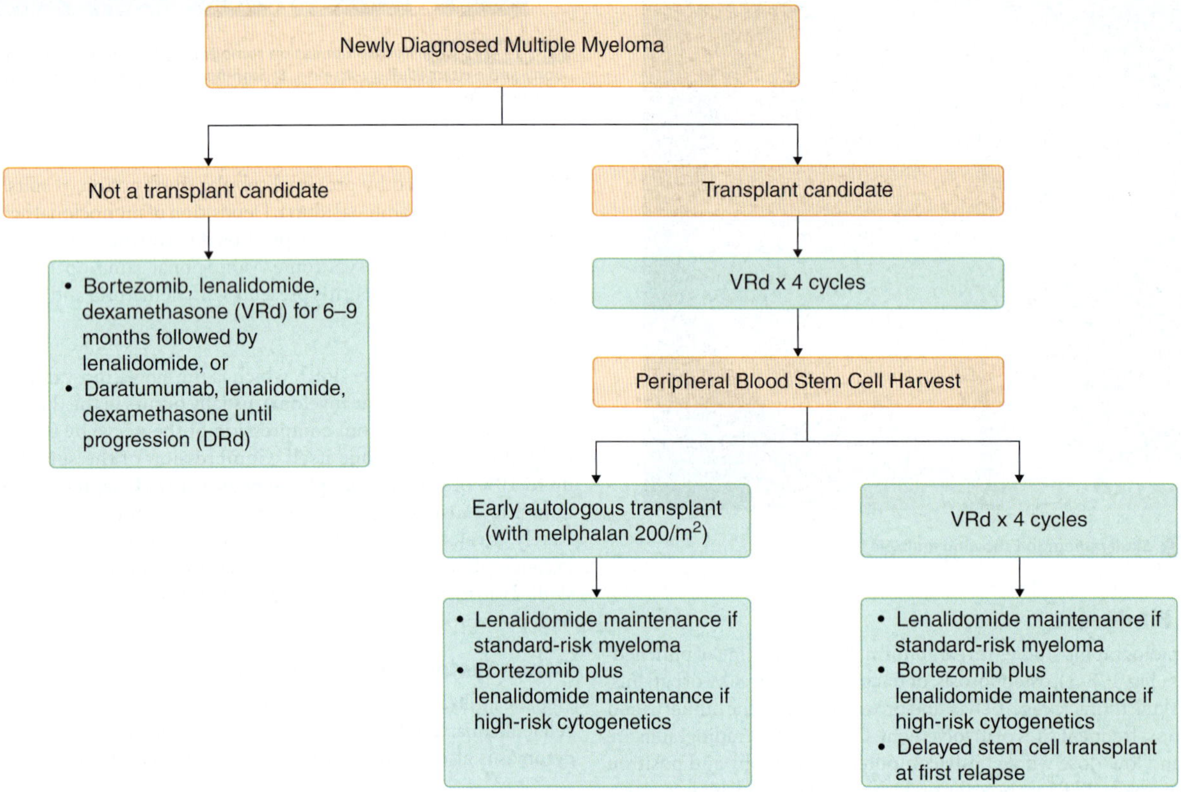

FIGURE 173-8. **Approach to newly diagnosed multiple myeloma.** DRd = daratumumab, lenalidomide, and dexamethasone; VRd = bortezomib-lenalidomide-dexamethasone.

Myeloma Working Group criteria.[15] Although achieving a minimal residual disease-negative state is associated with better survival, therapy usually is not changed based on the presence of minimal residual disease.

Initial Therapy of Patients Who Are Candidates for Autologous Stem Cell Transplantation

In the approximately 50% of patients with newly diagnosed multiple myeloma who are considered candidates for autologous stem cell transplantation based on good performance status, no or limited comorbid conditions, and younger physiologic age (<65 to 70 years), autologous peripheral blood stem cell transplantation (Chapter 163) with high-dose chemotherapy improves overall survival in comparison to conventional chemotherapy. Autologous transplantation is not curative, but it prolongs event-free and overall survival.[16]

Initial therapy typically consists of bortezomib, lenalidomide, and dexamethasone (VRd) for approximately 3 to 4 months followed by stem cell collection,[A3] but adding daratumumab may provide even better results[A4,A5] and can be considered in patients with high-risk myeloma. Alternative induction regimens include the combination of daratumumab, lenalidomide, and dexamethasone (DRd)[A6] or the combination of bortezomib, cyclophosphamide, and dexamethasone (VCD) (Table 173-5). Lenalidomide plus low-dose dexamethasone (40 mg once a week) is associated with superior overall survival compared with lenalidomide and high-dose dexamethasone (40 mg on days 1 to 4, 9 to 12, and 17 to 20). Toxicities of lenalidomide include deep vein thrombosis, and all patients must be treated with prophylactic aspirin or an anticoagulant.

After induction therapy, peripheral blood stem cells adequate for one to two stem cell transplants are collected with the use of granulocyte colony-stimulating factor with or without plerixafor or cyclophosphamide to aid in mobilization. Autologous stem cell transplantation (Chapter 163) is performed with melphalan 200 mg/m^2 as the conditioning regimen, followed by infusion of peripheral blood stem cells.

Early stem cell transplantation is often preferred[A7] because its mortality is low (<1%), and it avoids the inconvenience, cost, and potential side effects of prolonged chemotherapy. However, an equally good alternative approach in patients with standard-risk newly diagnosed myeloma is to delay transplantation until the first relapse.[A8] With this latter strategy, stem cells are collected and cryopreserved for future use after initial therapy. Patients then continue

TABLE 173-5 SELECTED REGIMENS FOR THE TREATMENT OF MULTIPLE MYELOMA

REGIMEN	USUAL DOSING SCHEDULE*
Bortezomib-cyclophosphamide-dexamethasone (VCd or CyBord)	Cyclophosphamide 300 mg/m² orally on days 1, 8, 15 and 22 Bortezomib 1.3 mg/m² intravenously on days 1, 8, 15, 22 Dexamethasone 40 mg orally on days on days 1, 8, 15, 22 Repeated every 4 wk
Bortezomib-lenalidomide-dexamethasone (VRd)	Bortezomib 1.3 mg/m² intravenous days 1, 8, 15 Lenalidomide 25 mg oral days 1-14 Dexamethasone 20 mg on day of and day after bortezomib (or 40 mg days 1, 8, 15, 22) Repeated every 3 wk
Carfilzomib-lenalidomide-dexamethasone (KRd)	Carfilzomib 20 mg/m² on cycle 1 and 27 mg/m² on subsequent cycles, intravenously on days 1, 2, 8, 9, 15, 16 Lenalidomide 25 mg oral days 1-21 Dexamethasone 20 mg on day of and day after bortezomib (or 40 mg days 1, 8, 15, 22) Repeated every 4 wk
Daratumumab-lenalidomide-dexamethasone (DRd)	Daratumumab 16 mg/kg intravenously weekly for 8 wk, and then every 2 wk for 4 mo, and then once monthly Lenalidomide 25 mg oral days 1-21 Dexamethasone 40 mg days 1, 8, 15, 22 Lenalidomide-dexamethasone repeated in usual schedule every 4 wk
Daratumumab-bortezomib-lenalidomide-dexamethasone (DVRd)	Daratumumab 16 mg/kg intravenously weekly × 8 wk, and then every 2 wk for 4 mo, and then once monthly Bortezomib 1.3 mg/m² intravenous days 1, 8, 15 Lenalidomide 25 mg oral days 1-14 Dexamethasone 40 mg days 1, 8, 15, 22 Bortezomib, lenalidomide, dexamethasone repeated every 3 wk
Elotuzumab-lenalidomide-dexamethasone (ERd)	Elotuzumab 10 mg/kg intravenously weekly × 8 wk, and then every 2 wk Lenalidomide 25 mg oral days 1-21 Dexamethasone 40 mg days 1, 8, 15, 22 Lenalidomide-dexamethasone repeated in usual schedule every 4 wk
Ixazomib-lenalidomide-dexamethasone (IRd)	Ixazomib 4 mg oral days 1, 8, 15 Lenalidomide 25 mg oral days 1-21 Dexamethasone 40 mg days 1, 8, 15, 22 Repeated every 4 wk
Daratumumab-bortezomib-dexamethasone (DVd)	Daratumumab 16 mg/kg intravenously weekly × 8 wk, and then every 2 wk for 4 mo, and then once monthly Bortezomib 1.3 mg/m² subcutaneously on days 1, 8, 15, 22 Dexamethasone 20 mg on day of and day after bortezomib or 40 mg days 1, 8, 15, 22 Bortezomib-dexamethasone repeated in usual schedule every 4 wk

*All doses need to be adjusted for performance status, renal function, blood counts, and other toxicities; doses of dexamethasone and/or bortezomib recommended have been reduced based on subsequent data showing lower toxicity and similar efficacy with reduced doses. Daratumumab can be given using a subcutaneous formulation instead of the intravenous route. Duration of therapy for all regimens varies under expert supervision depending on the disease phase.

Modified from Rajkumar SV. Multiple myeloma: 2020 update on diagnosis, risk-stratification, and management. *Am J Hematol.* 2020;95:548-567.

initial therapy for a few more months, followed by maintenance. Delayed stem cell transplantation is performed at the time of first relapse. The choice of early versus delayed transplantation is usually based on the patient's preferences and other clinical conditions, but early transplantation is often recommended.

Following stem cell transplantation, the long-term outcome is improved by lenalidomide maintenance (10 mg per day). In high-risk multiple myeloma, bortezomib maintenance is administered every 2 weeks in combination with lenalidomide (see Table 173-4 for definitions of standard and high-risk myeloma).

Allogeneic Bone Marrow Transplantation

Allogeneic transplantation for myeloma is best performed in the context of clinical trials or as second-line salvage therapy in selected high-risk patients who are willing to accept the high treatment-related mortality rate associated with the procedure.[17]

Initial Therapy of Patients Who Are Not Candidates for Transplantation

Approximately 50% of newly diagnosed patients are not considered candidates for stem cell transplantation either due to advanced age, poor performance status, or associated comorbidities. Initial therapy consists of either bortezomib/lenalidomide/dexamethasone (VRd) for approximately 9 months followed by lenalidomide maintenance, or daratumumab/lenalidomide/dexamethasone (DRd) given until disease progression. Ixazomib/lenalidomide/dexamethasone is used occasionally for high-risk patients who are unable to access parenteral therapy.[A9] Bortezomib/cyclophosphamide/dexamethasone (VCd) can be used as an alternative if lenalidomide is not available or in the setting of severe renal failure.

Treatment of Relapsed Refractory Myeloma

Almost all patients with multiple myeloma eventually relapse. The general goal is to select a regimen that contains more than two drugs that the patient has not received or to which the disease is or has become refractory. The duration of remission in relapsed multiple myeloma decreases with each regimen. All of the active agents discussed here can be used alone and in combination under expert supervision for the treatment of relapsed multiple myeloma.

The approach to therapy at relapse is complex, and a number of factors must be considered, including response to prior therapy, duration of prior remission, aggressiveness of the relapse, and eligibility for stem cell transplantation.[18] In general, if relapse occurs more than 6 months after stopping therapy, reinstitution of the initial chemotherapy regimen is reasonable. If patients have elected to undergo delayed transplant, then autologous transplantation should be considered. Similarly, eligible patients who have had a reasonable response to a prior autologous transplantation (>18 months without maintenance therapy or >36 months with maintenance therapy) may be considered for a second transplantation. In most patients, one of the triplet regimens (see Table 173-5) is used for the treatment of relapse, with each subsequent relapse treated with sequential regimens that contain drugs that are different than the ones used before. Patients with relapsed refractory myeloma should also be considered for clinical trials.

Specific Options for Relapsed Multiple Myeloma

Thalidomide, lenalidomide, and pomalidomide are closely related immunomodulatory drugs that form the backbone of numerous myeloma treatment regimens. Lenalidomide is better tolerated than thalidomide and has proven efficacy in relapsed myeloma. The starting dose of lenalidomide is 25 mg orally on days 1 to 21, every 28 days. Pomalidomide is a newer, more potent analogue of lenalidomide. All three drugs are associated with a risk of deep vein thrombosis, and therefore routine antithrombotic prophylaxis is needed.

Bortezomib, which is a selective proteasome inhibitor, is useful in relapsed multiple myeloma. The usual dose is 1.3 mg/m² administered subcutaneously on days 1, 8, 15, and 22 every 28 days. The once-weekly subcutaneous dosing is associated with significantly lower neuropathy than the twice-weekly intravenous schedule. The most common adverse events are gastrointestinal side effects, fatigue, and neuropathy. Newer proteasome inhibitors that have since been found to be effective in myeloma include carfilzomib and ixazomib.[A10,A11]

Both daratumumab and isatuximab (both of which target CD38) as well as elotuzumab (targeting SLAMF7) are monoclonal antibodies that are effective in the treatment of relapsed multiple myeloma.[A12–A14] Daratumumab can be administered subcutaneously instead of intravenously without loss of efficacy and is better tolerated.[A15] Several triplet regimens using these agents have been developed for use in relapsed multiple myeloma.

Newer options for the treatment of relapsed refractory myeloma are teclistamab (bispecific antibody),[19] idecabtagene vicleucel (ide-cel; chimeric antigen receptor T [CAR-T] cell therapy),[20] and ciltacabtagene autoleucel (cilta-cel, which is another CAR-T product).[A16] These approaches target the B-cell maturation antigen that is almost universally expressed on the surface of plasma cells. The major toxicity with bispecific antibody and CAR-T therapies are cytokine release syndromes and neurologic complications. Venetoclax (a bcl-2 inhibitor) has significant activity against the t(11;14) subtype of myeloma but is not recommended in other cytogenetic types due to an adverse effect on overall survival.[A17] Other less commonly used options for relapsed myeloma include bendamustine and selinexor (exportin-1 inhibitor).[A18] In addition, traditional chemotherapeutic agents such as doxorubicin are also of benefit in selected patients. Promising investigational agents include newer bispecific antibodies (such as elranatamab, cevostamab, and talquetamab)[21] that target specific antigens expressed on myeloma cells.[22]

Role of Radiation Therapy

Palliative radiation in a dose of 20 to 30 Gy should be limited to patients who have multiple myeloma with disabling pain and a well-defined focal process that has not responded to chemotherapy and to patients with spinal cord compression from a plasmacytoma. Analgesics in combination with chemotherapy can usually control the pain (Chapter 26).

Management of Complications

Hypercalcemia

Hypercalcemia, which is present in 15 to 20% of patients at diagnosis, should be suspected in patients who have anorexia, nausea, vomiting, polyuria, polydipsia, constipation, weakness, confusion, or stupor. If hypercalcemia is untreated, renal insufficiency may develop. Hydration, steroids, and bisphosphonates (zoledronic acid or pamidronate) are recommended and will correct hypercalcemia in almost all patients (Chapter 227).

Renal Insufficiency

The most common cause of acute renal failure is light chain cast nephropathy in patients who have excess excretion of monoclonal protein in urine (myeloma kidney). Aggressive treatment of acute renal failure due to light chain cast nephropathy is critical for long-term overall survival. If the patient is not oliguric, intravenous fluids and furosemide are needed to maintain a high urine flow rate (100 mL/hour). Allopurinol (300 mg daily) is necessary if hyperuricemia is present. If the underlying cause is thought to be light chain cast nephropathy based on clinical findings (e.g., serum free light chains >150 mg/dL) or renal biopsy, plasmapheresis is recommended daily for 5 days to reduce the levels of circulating light chains.[23] Hemodialysis is necessary for symptomatic azotemia. The mainstay of therapy is aggressive treatment of myeloma with a combination regimen such as bortezomib/cyclophosphamide/dexamethasone or daratumumab/bortezomib/cyclophosphamide/dexamethasone or bortezomib/thalidomide/dexamethasone under expert oversight.

Infection

Prompt, appropriate therapy for bacterial infections is necessary. Prophylactic antibiotics such as trimethoprim-sulfamethoxazole should be considered in patients taking high-dose corticosteroids.[24] Acyclovir should be given as prophylaxis against herpes zoster in patients receiving bortezomib. Intravenously administered immunoglobulin is reserved for patients with hypogammaglobulinemia and recurrent severe infections. Pneumococcal and influenza immunizations (Chapter 15) should be given to all patients. COVID vaccination (Chapter 337) is recommended for all patients, and booster doses should also be given as needed.

Skeletal Lesions

Patients should be encouraged to be as active as possible but to avoid trauma. Zoledronic acid (4 mg intravenously over at least 15 minutes every 4 weeks) or pamidronate (90 mg infused intravenously over a 4-hour period every 4 weeks) is recommended for all patients with myeloma bone disease. These agents reduce the incidence of bone pain, pathologic fractures, and spinal cord compression and may improve overall survival. After 1 to 2 years the dosing can be reduced to once every 3 months in patients who are stable to minimize the risk of osteonecrosis of the jaw, which is a complication of long-term bisphosphonate therapy. Denosumab is an alternative agent that can be used in patients who are unable to tolerate zoledronic acid or pamidronate. Kyphoplasty is useful in selected patients with vertebral fractures.

Spinal cord compression from an extramedullary plasmacytoma (Chapter 369) should be suspected in patients who have severe back pain, weakness or paresthesia of the lower extremities, or bladder or bowel dysfunction. Initial treatment is with dexamethasone-based therapy and/or radiation therapy. If the neurologic deficit increases, surgical decompression is necessary.

Miscellaneous Complications

Symptomatic hyperviscosity (see later) is less common than in Waldenström macroglobulinemia. Anemia that persists despite adequate treatment of underlying myeloma often responds to erythropoietin (Chapter 144).

PROGNOSIS

Multiple myeloma is considered incurable at present, but survival has improved significantly in recent years. The median survival is approximately 6 to 7 years in patients who are older than age 65 years, and approximately 12 years in patients who are less than age 65 years and who are eligible for stem cell transplantation, but it varies widely according to clinical stage and risk stratification factors (Table 173-4). In some patients, an acute or aggressive terminal phase is characterized by rapid tumor growth, pancytopenia, soft tissue subcutaneous masses, decreased M protein levels, and fever; survival in this subset is generally limited to a few months.

VARIANT FORMS OF MULTIPLE MYELOMA

PLASMA CELL LEUKEMIA

Patients who have multiple myeloma with more than 5% plasma cells in the peripheral blood differential count and/or an absolute plasma cell count of 500/μL or greater are considered to have plasma cell leukemia.[25] Plasma cell leukemia is classified as primary when it is diagnosed in the leukemic phase (60%) or as secondary when there is leukemic transformation of a previously recognized multiple myeloma (40%). Patients with primary plasma cell leukemia are younger and have a greater incidence of hepatosplenomegaly and lymphadenopathy, a higher platelet count, fewer bone lesions, a smaller serum M protein component, and better survival than do patients with secondary plasma cell leukemia.

TREATMENT AND PROGNOSIS

Current treatments are generally unsatisfactory. An aggressive initial treatment regimen under expert supervision is a reasonable strategy. Options include bortezomib/dexamethasone/thalidomide/cisplatin/doxorubicin/cyclophosphamide/etoposide (VDT-PACE) or daratumumab plus bortezomib/lenalidomide/dexamethasone, followed by autologous stem cell transplantation and subsequent maintenance therapy with bortezomib plus lenalidomide. Nonetheless, the prognosis of primary plasma cell leukemia is significantly worse than high-risk multiple myeloma.

NONSECRETORY MYELOMA

Patients with nonsecretory myeloma have no M protein in either serum or urine and account for only 3% of cases of myeloma. To establish the diagnosis, the clonal nature of bone marrow plasma cells should be confirmed by immunoperoxidase, immunofluorescence, or flow cytometric methods. Treatment and survival are similar to those in patients with typical myeloma. The serum free light chain assay is abnormal in more than 60% of patients and can be used to monitor the response to therapy.

OSTEOSCLEROTIC MYELOMA (POEMS SYNDROME)

Osteosclerotic myeloma is characterized by polyneuropathy, organomegaly, endocrinopathy, M protein, and skin changes (POEMS).[26] Almost all patients have a λ-type M protein. The major clinical features are a chronic inflammatory-demyelinating polyneuropathy with predominantly motor disability and sclerotic skeletal lesions. The bone marrow usually contains less than 5% plasma cells, and hypercalcemia and renal insufficiency rarely occur. The diagnosis is confirmed by identification of monoclonal plasma cells obtained at biopsy of an osteosclerotic lesion.

If the lesions are in a limited area, radiation therapy substantially improves the neuropathy in more than 50% of patients. If the patient has widespread osteosclerotic lesions, treatment is with autologous stem cell transplantation or other systemic therapy similar to that used for myeloma.[27]

SOLITARY PLASMACYTOMA (SOLITARY MYELOMA) OF BONE

The diagnosis of solitary bone plasmacytoma is based on histologic evidence of a solitary tumor consisting of monoclonal plasma cells identical to those in multiple myeloma. In addition, PET-CT (or whole body CT) or MRI of the spine and pelvis must show no other lesions of myeloma, and the bone marrow aspirate must contain no evidence of clonal plasma cells. An M protein may be present in serum or urine at diagnosis, but persistence of the M protein after radiation therapy is associated with an increased risk for progression to multiple myeloma. Treatment consists of radiation in the range of 40 to 50 Gy. Patients with an apparent solitary plasmacytoma who have limited (<10%) clonal marrow involvement are considered to have solitary plasmacytoma with minimal marrow involvement (Table 173-2). The risk of recurrence or progression to multiple myeloma within 3 years is approximately 10% in patients with solitary plasmacytoma versus 60% in patients with solitary plasmacytoma and minimal marrow involvement.

EXTRAMEDULLARY PLASMACYTOMA

Extramedullary plasmacytomas outside the bone marrow are most commonly found in the upper respiratory tract (80% of cases), especially in the nasal cavity and sinuses, nasopharynx, and larynx. Extramedullary plasmacytomas may also occur in the gastrointestinal tract, central nervous system, urinary bladder, thyroid, breast, testes, parotid gland, or lymph nodes. Extramedullary plasmacytomas may be solitary,[28] or they may occur in the context of existing myeloma. The diagnosis of solitary extramedullary plasmacytoma is based on detection of a plasma cell tumor in an extramedullary site, absence of clonal plasma cells on bone marrow examination, and absence of other bony or extramedullary lesions on radiographic studies. Treatment of solitary extramedullary plasmacytoma consists of either complete surgical resection or tumoricidal irradiation. The plasmacytoma may recur locally, metastasize to regional nodes, or, rarely, develop into multiple myeloma. Prognosis is generally better in patients with solitary extramedullary plasmacytoma, compared with solitary bony plasmacytoma.

WALDENSTRÖM MACROGLOBULINEMIA (PRIMARY MACROGLOBULINEMIA)

Waldenström macroglobulinemia is the result of the uncontrolled proliferation of lymphocytes and plasma cells in which an IgM M protein is produced. The median age of patients at the time of diagnosis is about 65 years, and approximately 60% are male. The cause is unknown, but familial clusters have been reported. A recurrent mutation of the *MYD88* gene (*MYD88 L265P*) is present in most patients with Waldenström macroglobulinemia and is thought to be relatively specific for this disease.

CLINICAL MANIFESTATIONS

Weakness, fatigue, and bleeding (especially oozing from the oronasal area) are common initial symptoms. Blurred or impaired vision, dyspnea, weight loss, neurologic symptoms, recurrent infections, and heart failure may occur. In contrast to multiple myeloma, lytic bone lesions, renal insufficiency, and amyloidosis are rare. Physical findings include pallor, hepatosplenomegaly, and lymphadenopathy. Retinal hemorrhages, exudates, and venous congestion with vascular segmentation ("sausage" formation) may occur. Sensorimotor peripheral neuropathy is common. Pulmonary involvement is manifested by diffuse pulmonary infiltrates and isolated masses.

Laboratory Evaluation

Almost all patients have moderate to severe normocytic, normochromic anemia. The serum electrophoretic pattern is characterized by a tall, narrow peak or dense band that is of the IgM type on immunofixation. Quantitative IgM levels are high. A monoclonal light chain is detected in the urine of 80% of patients, but the amount of urinary protein is generally modest.

The bone marrow aspirate is often hypocellular, but the biopsy is hypercellular and extensively infiltrated with lymphoid cells and plasma cells or lymphoplasmacytic cells. The number of mast cells is frequently increased. Rouleaux formation is prominent (Chapter 143), and the sedimentation rate is markedly increased. About 10% of cases may have an associated type I cryoglobulinemia (see later).

DIAGNOSIS

Diagnosis requires the combination of typical symptoms and physical findings, the presence of an IgM M protein, and 10% or greater lymphoplasmacytic infiltration of the bone marrow.[29]

Diagnostic Criteria and Differential Diagnosis

The diagnostic criteria are IgM monoclonal gammopathy (regardless of the size of the M protein), 10% or greater bone marrow infiltration (usually intertrabecular) by clonal lymphocytes that exhibit plasmacytoid or plasma cell differentiation, and a typical immunophenotype (e.g., surface IgM^+, $CD5^{+/-}$, $CD10^-$, $CD19^+$, $CD20^+$, $CD23^-$) that would satisfactorily exclude other lymphoproliferative disorders, including CLL (Chapter 169) and mantle cell lymphoma (Chapter 171).

Patients who meet the diagnostic criteria for Waldenström macroglobulinemia but who have less than 3 g/dL IgM protein at diagnosis have sometimes been classified as having "lymphoplasmacytic lymphoma with an IgM M protein" (Chapter 171). However, except for hyperviscosity, the clinical picture, therapy, and prognosis for these patients do not differ from those of patients with an IgM level of 3 g/dL or greater; thus, these patients are also considered to have Waldenström macroglobulinemia by the current definition.

Asymptomatic patients with 10% or greater lymphoplasmacytic infiltration of the bone marrow are considered to have smoldering Waldenström macroglobulinemia. Multiple myeloma, CLL, and MGUS of the IgM type must be excluded.

TREATMENT AND PROGNOSIS

Patients should not be treated unless they have anemia; constitutional symptoms such as weakness, fatigue, night sweats, or weight loss; hyperviscosity; or significant hepatosplenomegaly or lymphadenopathy. The most common regimens used as front-line therapy are the combination of ibrutinib plus rituximab,[A19] bendamustine plus rituximab, or dexamethasone/rituximab/cyclophosphamide.[30]

For relapse, the agents used as initial therapy can be given alone or in combination. Zanubrutinib, which is a more selective Bruton tyrosine kinase inhibitor, has comparable activity to ibrutinib and may be better tolerated.[A20] Autologous stem cell transplantation can be considered for eligible patients with relapsed disease. Other options under expert supervision include venetoclax, cladribine, or fludarabine (with or without rituximab); lenalidomide-based or bortezomib-based regimens; and other regimens used in the treatment of non-Hodgkin lymphoma (Chapter 171).

Spuriously low hemoglobin and hematocrit levels may occur because of the increased plasma volume from the large amount of intravascular M protein. Symptomatic hyperviscosity should be treated by plasmapheresis. The median survival of patients with macroglobulinemia is in excess of 5 to 7 years.

HYPERVISCOSITY SYNDROME

Hyperviscosity syndrome occurs when patients with Waldenström macroglobulinemia have high levels of serum IgM M protein (>5 g/dL) and occasionally in those with myeloma, especially of the IgA type. For any given level of paraprotein, IgM or IgA is more likely than IgG to cause hyperviscosity because the former circulate as pentamers or dimers, respectively, in contrast to monomeric IgG. Chronic nasal bleeding and oozing from the gums are the most frequent symptoms of hyperviscosity, but postsurgical or gastrointestinal bleeding may also occur. Retinal hemorrhages are common, and venous congestion with sausage-like segmentation and papilledema may be seen (Fig. 173-9). The patient occasionally complains of blurring or loss of vision. Dizziness, headache, vertigo, nystagmus, decreased hearing, ataxia, paresthesias, diplopia, somnolence, and coma may occur. Hyperviscosity can precipitate or exacerbate heart failure. Most patients have symptoms when the relative viscosity is greater than 4 cP, but the relationship between serum viscosity and clinical manifestations is not precise.

TREATMENT

Patients with symptomatic hyperviscosity should be treated with plasmapheresis and with chemotherapy to treat the underlying malignancy. Plasma exchange of 3 to 4 L with albumin should be performed daily until the patient is asymptomatic. Plasma exchange is rapidly effective (two to three exchanges) for IgM M proteins, which are primarily intravascular. For IgG M proteins, however, multiple attempts may be needed because a significant amount of IgG can exist in the extravascular space.

HEAVY CHAIN DISEASES

The heavy chain diseases are characterized by the presence of an M protein consisting of a portion of the immunoglobulin heavy chain in serum, urine, or both. These heavy chains are devoid of light chains and represent a lymphoplasma cell proliferative process. The three major types are γ-heavy chain disease, α-heavy chain disease, and μ-heavy chain disease.

γ-HEAVY CHAIN DISEASE

Patients with γ-heavy chain disease often initially have a lymphoma-like illness, but the clinical findings are diverse and range from an aggressive

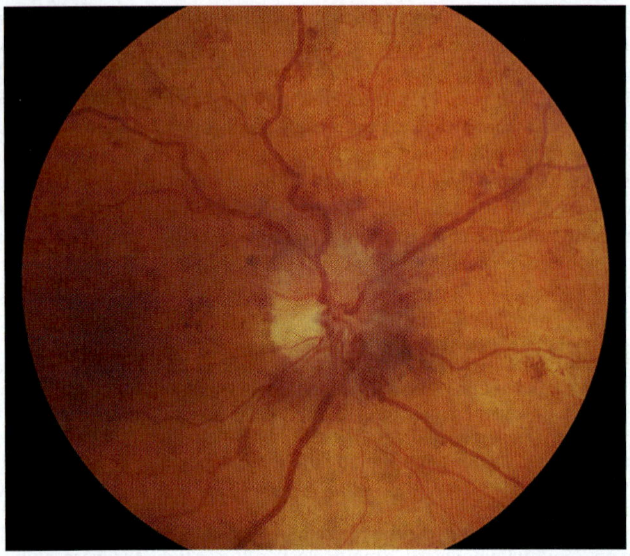

FIGURE 173-9. Hyperviscosity syndrome. Right eye retinal image in a patient with Waldenström macroglobulinemia and hyperviscosity syndrome showing sausaging (focal venular dilations), intraretinal hemorrhages, microaneurysms, and peripapillary cotton-wool spots and disc swelling (papilledema).

lymphoproliferative process to an asymptomatic state. Hepatosplenomegaly and lymphadenopathy occur in about 60% of patients. Anemia is found in approximately 80% initially and in nearly all eventually. The electrophoretic pattern often shows a broad-based band more suggestive of a polyclonal increase than an M protein. The diagnosis depends on the identification of an isolated monoclonal γ-heavy chain on serum immunofixation, without evidence of either monoclonal κ or λ light chain expression.

TREATMENT AND PROGNOSIS

Treatment is indicated only for symptomatic patients and consists of chemotherapy with regimens used to treat non-Hodgkin lymphoma (Chapter 171), such as cyclophosphamide, vincristine, and prednisone. The prognosis of γ-heavy chain disease is variable and ranges from a rapidly progressive downhill course of a few weeks' duration to the asymptomatic presence of a stable monoclonal heavy chain in serum or urine.

α-HEAVY CHAIN DISEASE

α-Heavy chain disease, which is the most common form of heavy chain disease, occurs in patients from the Mediterranean region or the Middle East, generally in the second or third decade of life. About 60% of patients with α-heavy chain disease are men. Most commonly the gastrointestinal tract is involved, and severe malabsorption with diarrhea, steatorrhea, and weight loss is noted (Chapter 126). Plasma cell infiltration of the jejunal mucosa is the most frequent pathologic feature. Immunoproliferative small intestinal disease is restricted to patients with small intestinal lesions who have the pathologic features of α-heavy chain disease but do not synthesize α-heavy chains.

The serum protein electrophoretic pattern is normal in about 50% of cases. In the remainder, an unimpressive broad band may appear in the α_2 or β region. The diagnosis depends on identification of an isolated monoclonal α-heavy chain on serum immunofixation, without evidence of either monoclonal κ or λ light chain expression. The amount of α-heavy chain in urine is small.

TREATMENT AND PROGNOSIS

In the absence of therapy, α-heavy chain disease is typically progressive and fatal. The usual treatment consists of antibiotics, such as tetracyclines, and the eradication of any concurrent parasitic infection. Patients who do not respond adequately to antibiotics are given chemotherapy similar to that used to treat non-Hodgkin lymphoma, for example, the cyclophosphamide, hydroxydaunomycin, vincristine (Oncovin), and prednisone (CHOP) regimen (Chapter 171).

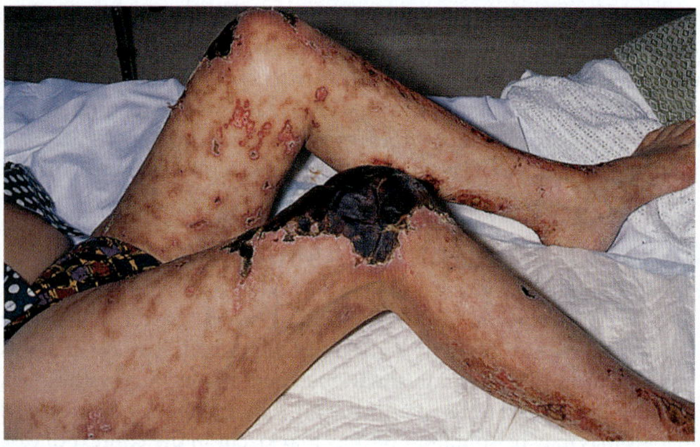

FIGURE 173-10. Skin infarction in cryoglobulinemia. The skin has a reticulated pattern as a result of leakage of red blood cells from damaged skin capillaries. Necrosis and ulceration have occurred in peripheral sites because of vessel blockage. This patient eventually required plastic surgery. (From Forbes CD, Jackson WF. *Color Atlas and Text of Clinical Medicine*, 3rd ed. London: Mosby; 2003.)

μ-HEAVY CHAIN DISEASE

μ-Heavy chain disease disease is characterized by the demonstration of an isolated monoclonal μ-chain fragment on serum immunofixation, without evidence of either monoclonal κ or λ light chain expression. The serum protein electrophoretic pattern is usually normal, except for hypogammaglobulinemia. Bence Jones proteinuria is found in two thirds of cases. Lymphocytes, plasma cells, and lymphoplasmacytoid cells are increased in the bone marrow. Vacuolization of the plasma cells is common and should suggest the possibility of heavy chain disease.

TREATMENT AND PROGNOSIS

Treatment is with corticosteroids and alkylating agents. The course of μ-heavy chain disease is variable, and survival ranges from a few months to many years.

CRYOGLOBULINEMIA

Cryoglobulins are plasma proteins that precipitate when cooled and dissolve when heated. They are designated as idiopathic or essential when they are not associated with any recognizable disease. Cryoglobulins are classified into three types: type I (monoclonal), type II (mixed monoclonal plus polyclonal), and type III (polyclonal).[31]

TYPE I CRYOGLOBULINEMIA

Type I (monoclonal) cryoglobulinemia is most commonly of the IgM or IgG class, but IgA and Bence Jones cryoglobulins have been reported. Most patients, even with large amounts of type I cryoglobulin, are completely asymptomatic from this source. Others with monoclonal cryoglobulins in the range of 1 to 2 g/dL may have evidence of vasculitis with pain, purpura, Raynaud phenomenon, cyanosis, and even ulceration and sloughing of skin and subcutaneous tissue (Fig. 173-10) on exposure to cold because their cryoglobulins precipitate at relatively high temperatures. Type I cryoglobulins are associated with macroglobulinemia, multiple myeloma, or MGUS.

TREATMENT

Therapy for patients with symptomatic type I cryoglobulinemia and significant symptoms is similar to that for Waldenström macroglobulinemia for the IgM type and multiple myeloma for the non-IgM type.

TYPE II CRYOGLOBULINEMIA

Type II (mixed) cryoglobulinemia typically consists of an immune complex of IgM M protein and polyclonal IgG, although monoclonal IgG or monoclonal IgA may also be seen with polyclonal IgM. Serum protein electrophoresis generally shows a normal pattern or a diffuse, polyclonal hypergammaglobulinemic pattern. The quantity of mixed cryoglobulin is usually less than 0.2 g/dL. Despite the monoclonal component, most patients do not have a clonal plasma cell disorder; rather, they have serologic evidence of infection with hepatitis C virus (Chapter 135). At present, hepatitis C is thought to be the cause of most cases of type II cryoglobulinemia.

Most clinical manifestations are related to the development of vasculitis and include palpable purpura, livedo reticularis, polyarthralgias, and neuropathy. Involvement of the joints is symmetrical, but joint deformities rarely develop. Raynaud phenomenon, necrosis of the skin, and neurologic involvement may be present. In almost 80% of renal biopsy specimens, glomerular damage can be identified. Nephrotic syndrome may result, but severe renal insufficiency is uncommon.

TREATMENT

Treatment should target the underlying hepatitis C infection (Chapter 135). Administration of corticosteroids is often needed to control vasculitis. Agents to treat the monoclonal component, such as cyclophosphamide or rituximab, are used if there is no response. Plasmapheresis (with a warmed circuit) is helpful in the acute management of symptoms by removing circulating immune complexes.

TYPE III CRYOGLOBULINEMIA

Type III (polyclonal) cryoglobulinemia does not have a monoclonal component and is not associated with a clonal plasma cell proliferative disorder. Type III cryoglobulins are found in many patients with chronic infections or inflammatory diseases and are usually of no clinical significance unless associated with hepatitis C infection.

GENERAL REFERENCES

For the General References and other additional features, please visit Elsevier eBooks+ at https://ebooks.health.elsevier.com.

Grade A References

A1. Lonial S, Jacobus S, Fonseca R, et al. Randomized trial of lenalidomide versus observation in smoldering multiple myeloma. *J Clin Oncol.* 2020;38:1126-1137.
A2. Mateos MV, Hernández MT, Giraldo P, et al. Lenalidomide plus dexamethasone versus observation in patients with high-risk smouldering multiple myeloma (QuiRedex): long-term follow-up of a randomised, controlled, phase 3 trial. *Lancet Oncol.* 2016;17:1127-1136.
A3. Durie BGM, Hoering A, Abidi MH, et al. Bortezomib, lenalidomide and dexamethasone vs. lenalidomide and dexamethasone induction followed by lenalidomide and dexamethasone maintenance in patients with newly diagnosed myeloma without intent for immediate autologous stem cell transplant: results of the randomised phase III SWOG trial S0777. *Lancet.* 2017;389:519-527.
A4. Moreau P, Attal M, Hulin C, et al. Bortezomib, thalidomide, and dexamethasone with or without daratumumab before and after autologous stem-cell transplantation for newly diagnosed multiple myeloma (CASSIOPEIA): a randomised, open-label, phase 3 study. *Lancet.* 2019;394:29-38.
A5. Voorhees PM, Kaufman JL, Laubach J, et al. Daratumumab, lenalidomide, bortezomib, and dexamethasone for transplant-eligible newly diagnosed multiple myeloma: the GRIFFIN trial. *Blood.* 2020;136:936-945.
A6. Facon T, Kumar SK, Plesner T, et al. Daratumumab, lenalidomide, and dexamethasone versus lenalidomide and dexamethasone alone in newly diagnosed multiple myeloma (MAIA): overall survival results from a randomised, open-label, phase 3 trial. *Lancet Oncol.* 2021;22:1582-1596.
A7. Richardson PG, Jacobus SJ, Weller EA, et al. Triplet therapy, transplantation, and maintenance until progression in myeloma. *N Engl J Med.* 2022;387:132-147.
A8. Attal M, Lauwers-Cances V, Hulin C, et al. Lenalidomide, bortezomib, and dexamethasone with transplantation for myeloma. *N Engl J Med.* 2017;376:1311-1320.
A9. Facon T, Venner CP, Bahlis NJ, et al. Oral ixazomib, lenalidomide, and dexamethasone for transplant-ineligible patients with newly diagnosed multiple myeloma. *Blood.* 2021;137:3616-3628.
A10. Dimopoulos M, Quach H, Mateos MV, et al. Carfilzomib, dexamethasone, and daratumumab versus carfilzomib and dexamethasone for patients with relapsed or refractory multiple myeloma (CANDOR): results from a randomised, multicentre, open-label, phase 3 study. *Lancet.* 2020;396:186-197.
A11. Moreau P, Masszi T, Grzasko N, et al. Oral ixazomib, lenalidomide, and dexamethasone for multiple myeloma. *N Engl J Med.* 2016;374:1621-1634.
A12. Dimopoulos MA, Oriol A, Nahi H, et al. Daratumumab, lenalidomide, and dexamethasone for multiple myeloma. *N Engl J Med.* 2016;375:1319-1331.
A13. Moreau P, Dimopoulos MA, Mikhael J, et al. Isatuximab, carfilzomib, and dexamethasone in relapsed multiple myeloma (IKEMA): a multicentre, open-label, randomised phase 3 trial. *Lancet.* 2021;397:2361-2371.
A14. Dimopoulos MA, Dytfeld D, Grosicki S, et al. Elotuzumab plus pomalidomide and dexamethasone for multiple myeloma. *N Engl J Med.* 2018;379:1811-1822.
A15. Mateos MV, Nahi H, Legiec W, et al. Subcutaneous versus intravenous daratumumab in patients with relapsed or refractory multiple myeloma (COLUMBA): a multicentre, open-label, non-inferiority, randomised, phase 3 trial. *Lancet Haematol.* 2020;7:e370-e380.
A16. Rodriguez-Otero P, Ailawadhi S, Arnulf B, et al. Ide-cel or standard regimens in relapsed and refractory multiple myeloma. *N Engl J Med.* 2023;388:1002-1014.
A17. Kumar SK, Harrison SJ, Cavo M, et al. Venetoclax or placebo in combination with bortezomib and dexamethasone in patients with relapsed or refractory multiple myeloma (BELLINI): a randomised, double-blind, multicentre, phase 3 trial. *Lancet Oncol.* 2020;21:1630-1642.
A18. Grosicki S, Simonova M, Spicka I, et al. Once-per-week selinexor, bortezomib, and dexamethasone versus twice-per-week bortezomib and dexamethasone in patients with multiple myeloma (BOSTON): a randomised, open-label, phase 3 trial. *Lancet.* 2020;396:1563-1573.
A19. Dimopoulos MA, Tedeschi A, Trotman J, et al. Phase 3 trial of ibrutinib plus rituximab in Waldenström's macroglobulinemia. *N Engl J Med.* 2018;378:2399-2410.
A20. Tam CS, Opat S, D'Sa S, et al. A randomized phase 3 trial of zanubrutinib vs ibrutinib in symptomatic Waldenstrom macroglobulinemia: the ASPEN study. *Blood.* 2020;136:2038-2050.

174

AMYLOIDOSIS

MORIE A. GERTZ AND ANGELA DISPENZIERI

The amyloidoses are protein-misfolding diseases caused by a precursor protein that undergoes a conformational change, which in turn triggers the formation of amyloid fibrils that damage different organs. Amyloidosis can be either localized or systemic. In systemic amyloidosis (Table 174-1), amyloid deposition occurs at sites distant from where the precursor protein is formed.[1] In localized amyloidosis, the deposits form exclusively where the precursor protein is synthesized. Despite differences in structure and function, amyloid fibrils formed by all these various precursor proteins share a cross-β structure and form 2- to 5-nm-diameter filaments that either coil together or form laterally adherent fibrils with distinct intensities at 4.7 and 10 angstroms.

SYSTEMIC AMYLOIDOSIS

EPIDEMIOLOGY

The incidence of AL (formerly called primary) amyloidosis is about 12 per million persons per year. In one large series confirmed by mass spectroscopy, about 60% of cases were immunoglobulin amyloidosis, about 30% were transthyretin or TTR amyloidosis, and only about 3% were secondary amyloidosis. Familial amyloidosis mostly involves mutated transthyretin but also includes other rare mutations (Table 174-1). Wild-type TTR amyloidosis is often clinically unrecognized and is much more common than originally believed.

SYSTEMIC LIGHT CHAIN AMYLOIDOSIS

PATHOBIOLOGY

In rare cases, light chain amyloidosis can be familial, owing to a mutation in the light chain gene, rather than caused by a monoclonal plasma cell dyscrasia. Immunoglobulin light chain amyloidosis is characterized by a clonal population of bone marrow plasma cells that produces a monoclonal light chain of the κ or λ type, as either an intact molecule or a fragment. The light chain protein, instead of conforming to the α-helical configuration of most proteins, misfolds and forms a β-pleated sheet.[2] This insoluble protein is deposited in tissues and interferes with organ function. The β-pleated sheet configuration is responsible for the tinctorial properties; when the protein is stained with Congo red and viewed under polarized light, apple-green birefringence is demonstrated and is required for the diagnosis.

CLINICAL MANIFESTATIONS

The presenting symptoms can be diverse and are mimicked by far more common disorders (Table 174-2). The signs include tongue enlargement with dental indentations (Fig. 174-1) and "pinch" or periorbital purpura (Fig. 174-2), which is a result of vascular fragility. The signs are specific but lack sensitivity in that they are present in no more than 15% of patients.

Renal Involvement

The kidney is commonly involved in AL amyloidosis (58% of cases). The diagnosis should be suspected in any patient who presents with nondiabetic nephrotic-range proteinuria (Chapter 100).[3] One third of patients with AL amyloidosis have nephrotic syndrome that is manifested with dramatic increases in the blood cholesterol level (median, 270 mg/dL), and urinalysis for proteinuria should be done in patients with a sudden increase in the serum cholesterol

TABLE 174-1 SYSTEMIC AMYLOIDOSES

DISEASE	CAUSE	AFFECTED ORGANS
AL (Light chain) amyloidosis (formerly primary amyloidosis)	Immunoglobulin light chain	Heart, kidney, liver, nerve
AL (Heavy chain) amyloidosis	Immunoglobulin heavy chain	Kidney, liver, heart
TTRwt (formerly senile cardiac) amyloidosis	Accumulation of wild-type transthyretin	Heart, vessels, soft tissues (especially ligaments)
TTRm (formerly familial) amyloidosis	Hereditary mutation of transthyretin	Heart, kidney, peripheral nervous system
ALECT2	No mutation etiology not known	Kidney, liver
AA (Secondary) amyloidosis	Overproduction of serum amyloid A protein because of chronic inflammation	Kidney, liver, spleen
AB2 M wild-type (dialysis-related) amyloidosis	Acquired copper-triggered oligomerization of β_2-microglobulin	Musculoskeletal system
AB2 M variant amyloidosis	Hereditary variant of β_2-microglobulin	Autonomic nervous system
ALYS	Hereditary mutation of lysozyme	Kidney, liver, spleen
ApoAI amyloidosis	Hereditary mutation of apolipoprotein AI	Kidney, heart, liver
ApoAII amyloidosis	Hereditary mutation of apolipoprotein AII	Kidney
ApoAIV amyloidosis	Hereditary mutation of apolipoprotein AIV	Kidney
ApoCII amyloidosis	Hereditary mutation of apolipoprotein C II	Kidney
ApoCIII amyloidosis	Hereditary mutation of apolipoprotein C III	Kidney
AFib amyloidosis	Hereditary mutation of fibrinogen α chain	Kidney
AGel (Finnish hereditary) amyloidosis	Hereditary mutation of gelsolin	Cornea, facial and peripheral nerves, skin
ACys amyloidosis	Hereditary mutation of cystatin C	Peripheral nervous system, skin
ABri amyloidosis	Hereditary mutation of BriPP	Microvasculature of the brain

Apo = apolipoprotein; BriPP = Bri precursor protein; wtTTR = wild-type transthyretin.
Adapted from Blancas-Mejia LM, Ramirez-Alvarado M. Systemic amyloidoses. *Annu Rev Biochem*. 2013;82:745-774.

TABLE 174-2 SYMPTOMS, SIGNS, AND SYNDROMES OF SYSTEMIC AMYLOIDOSIS

SYMPTOMS AND SIGNS
Common symptoms: fatigue, edema, dyspnea, anorexia, paresthesias
Rare symptoms: claudication, joint pain and stiffness, sicca syndrome
Common signs: periorbital purpura, glossomegaly, hepatomegaly
Rare signs: waxy infiltration of eyelids, shoulder pad sign
SYNDROMES
Nondiabetic nephrotic syndrome
Nonischemic cardiomyopathy with an echocardiogram showing "hypertrophy"
Hepatomegaly or increased alkaline phosphatase with no imaging abnormality
Peripheral neuropathy with monoclonal gammopathy of undetermined significance or chronic inflammatory demyelinating polyneuropathy with autonomic features
Atypical monoclonal gammopathy of undetermined significance or myeloma with monoclonal light chains and modest marrow plasmacytosis

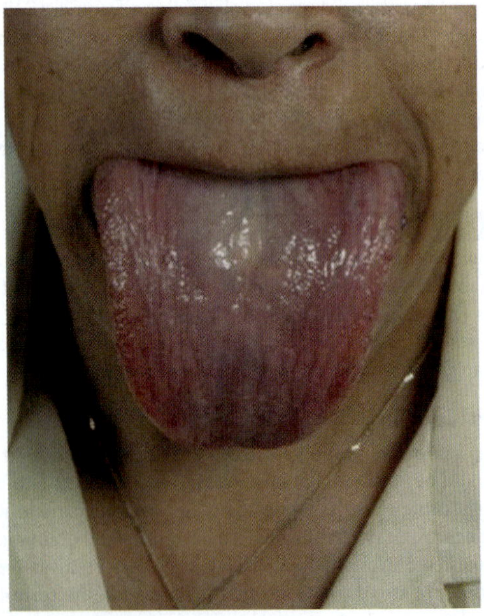

FIGURE 174-1. **Macroglossia (or glossomegaly) in a patient with amyloidosis.** (From Esplin BL, Gertz MA. Current trends in diagnosis and management of cardiac amyloidosis. *Curr Probl Cardiol*. 2013;38:53-96.)

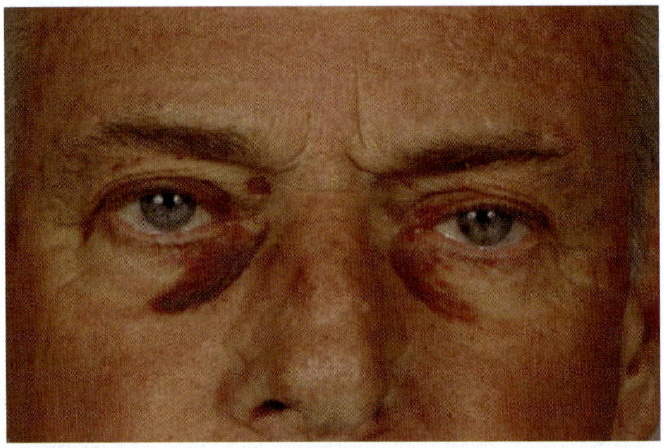

FIGURE 174-2. **Periorbital purpura in amyloidosis.** (From Kitchens CS. Purpura and other hematovascular disorders. In: Kitchens CS, Konkle BA, Kessler CM, eds. *Consultative Hemostasis and Thrombosis*. 3rd ed. Philadelphia: Elsevier; 2012.)

level. Ten percent of renal biopsy specimens from patients with nondiabetic nephrotic syndrome are subsequently shown to be involved by amyloidosis. The incidence of bleeding after percutaneous renal biopsy is not increased in patients with AL amyloidosis.

Cardiac Involvement

The heart is involved in approximately 70% of patients with AL amyloidosis, and the presentation of disease is subtle because fatigue is often the only manifestation.[4] Because amyloid heart disease (Chapter 47) is a disorder of diastolic failure, the typical findings of cardiomyopathy (enlarged cardiac silhouette, depressed ejection fraction, and pulmonary vascular redistribution) are absent. The effect of amyloidosis on the heart is poor filling during diastole. Patients have low end-diastolic volume and, as a consequence, poor stroke volume, despite a completely normal ejection fraction.[5] Cardiac conduction abnormalities (Chapter 51) are common and can be a presenting clinical manifestation. Patients with amyloidosis rarely have symptoms of ischemic heart disease. Imaging is typically not helpful, and liver uptake is homogeneous. Liver biopsy is not associated with an increased rate of bleeding.

Neuropathy

The peripheral neuropathy (Chapter 388) associated with AL amyloidosis (seen in approximately 15% of patients) begins in the lower extremities, is symmetrical, and is generally sensory or mixed sensorimotor. When a monoclonal protein is recognized, frequent diagnoses are chronic inflammatory demyelinating polyneuropathy and neuropathy associated with monoclonal gammopathy of undetermined significance. Associated autonomic neuropathy occurs in approximately 4% of patients and can be characterized by orthostatic hypotension, which may be misattributed to cardiac failure.

Carpal tunnel syndrome (Chapter 384) occurs in approximately 10 to 15% of patients. It is not clinically distinguishable from the syndrome associated with repetitive stress injury but may fail to improve after surgical release.

Gastrointestinal/Liver

Autonomic dysmotility of the bowel is a common associated finding (Chapter 122). It can be upper intestinal, leading to pseudo-obstruction and recurrent emesis, or lower intestinal, characterized by alternating obstipation and fecal incontinence. Diarrhea caused by autonomic failure can be misdiagnosed as collagenous colitis when eosinophilic deposits are found in the bowel mucosa on hematoxylin-eosin staining in the absence of Congo red staining.

The liver is involved in 10 to 20% of patients with AL amyloidosis, and the typical presentation is hepatomegaly with an increased serum alkaline phosphatase value. Increased aminotransferase levels and hyperbilirubinemia are generally late signs. Many patients undergo evaluation for suspected malignant disease due to liver enlargement.

Other Symptoms

Rarely, patients present with spontaneous splenic rupture. Acquired deficiency of coagulation factor X (Chapter 160) is specific to AL amyloidosis and can be associated with severe hemorrhage. Interstitial lung disease, pseudoclaudication, periarticular deposits, and unexplained weight loss rarely are presenting symptoms.

DIAGNOSIS

AL amyloidosis is particularly difficult to diagnose. No single imaging procedure or laboratory study is diagnostic for AL amyloidosis. The clinician must therefore be aware of the possibility of amyloidosis, or it may be overlooked.[6]

In a patient with nondiabetic proteinuria, cardiomyopathy without ischemic risk factors, unexplained hepatomegaly, peripheral or autonomic neuropathy, or carpal tunnel syndrome, amyloidosis is not the most likely cause. The classic physical finding of periorbital purpura occurs in only 10% of patients, is often limited to petechial eruptions over the eyelids, and is easily overlooked. Enlargement of the tongue occurs in 10 to 15% of patients; therefore, although it is specific, it is not sensitive for the diagnosis. AL amyloidosis in patients with an enlarged tongue may be unrecognized, or these patients may be evaluated for acromegaly or undergo unnecessary tongue biopsies because of the suspicion of squamous cell cancer.

Initial Testing

When a patient presents with a compatible clinical syndrome, immunofixation of serum and a urine-free light chain assay should be completed before invasive diagnostic studies are performed (Fig. 174-3). Simple electrophoresis without immunofixation is inadequate because the monoclonal proteins are quantitatively very small in most patients and will not cause a detectable peak on serum protein electrophoresis. When these three diagnostic studies are used in combination, the sensitivity is 100%. The existence of a monoclonal protein, however, is not sufficiently specific to establish the diagnosis of AL amyloidosis.

With modern testing, a monoclonal component can be found in approximately 25% of patients with ATTRwt amyloidosis, so typing of the amyloid tissue is critical. If a monoclonal protein is not found, three possibilities exist: (1) the patient does not have amyloidosis; (2) if the patient is known to have amyloidosis, it may be localized rather than systemic; or (3) if the patient is known to have systemic amyloidosis, it may be ATTRwt (senile systemic) or ATTRm (familial type) rather than the light chain type (see later section on other forms of amyloidosis).

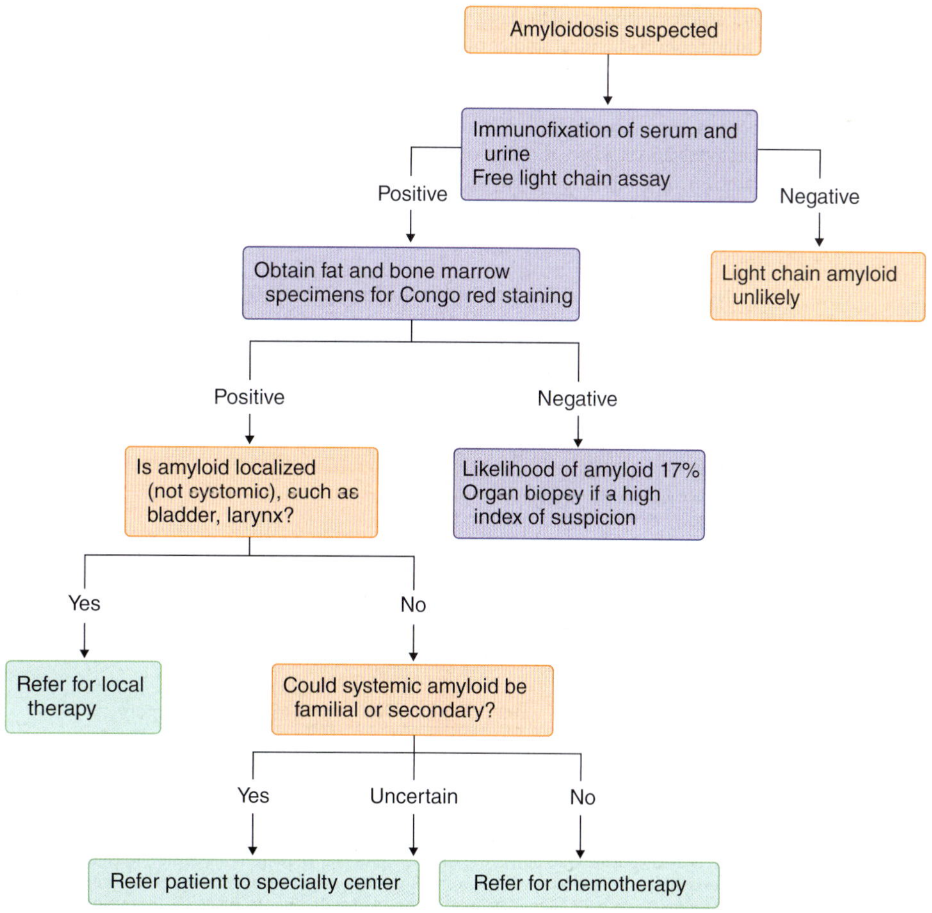

FIGURE 174-3. Algorithm for the cost-effective pursuit of a diagnosis of systemic light chain amyloidosis.

Differential Diagnosis

Systemic AL amyloidosis can be confused with early multiple myeloma (Chapter 174). Patients who present with vague symptoms of fatigue and edema are found to have a monoclonal protein in the urine, and a bone marrow biopsy specimen shows a clonal plasmacytosis with a median of 10% plasma cells in the bone marrow. These patients are often considered to have atypical multiple myeloma when the underlying amyloid syndrome is unrecognized. Taken together, a misdiagnosis of myeloma kidney or demyelinating neuropathy is made when an adequate diagnostic evaluation to exclude amyloidosis has not been performed.

Systemic AL amyloidosis also must be distinguished from systemic amyloidosis associated with inherited amyloid cardiomyopathies and neuropathies (familial amyloidoses) or cardiac amyloidosis caused by deposition of aberrant transthyretin. By definition, AL amyloidosis is a plasma cell dyscrasia (Chapter 174); therefore, virtually all patients have a detectable immunoglobulin abnormality by immunofixation of the serum or urine, or they have abnormal results on a serum immunoglobulin free light chain assay.

Definitive Testing

In view of the grave prognosis associated with AL amyloidosis, the diagnosis must be confirmed by biopsy (with Congo red staining) in all cases.[7] Subcutaneous fat aspiration is an outpatient procedure that has a 24-hour turnaround time, recognizes amyloid deposits in 70% of patients, and is the initial diagnostic test that should be performed to confirm AL amyloidosis. Bone marrow is a second convenient biopsy site, and this test is often required to exclude the possibility of associated multiple myeloma. Bone marrow biopsy is positive in 50% of patients. When both subcutaneous fat aspiration and bone marrow biopsy are combined, amyloid is detected in approximately 80% of patients. The remaining patients should have biopsy of the appropriate involved organ: the kidney when proteinuria is the presenting symptom, the heart when cardiomyopathy is recognized, the liver in patients who have hepatomegaly and an increased alkaline phosphatase value, or the nerve if sensorimotor functional loss is present. These latter procedures are quite invasive and often are not required for definitive diagnosis of AL amyloidosis.

Once amyloid deposits are detected in tissues, further diagnostic evaluation is required (Fig. 174-3). The presence of a monoclonal protein in the serum or urine and the presence of congophilic deposits in tissue do not verify that amyloidosis is light chain in origin. Further diagnostic studies are essential to classify the type of amyloid before therapy is initiated. Immunohistochemical studies on the tissue may be useful, but misfolding of the amyloid light chain often prevents epitopes from being recognized by commercial antisera; as a result, false-negative and false-positive results are common. Mass spectrometric analysis of the amyloid deposit can be performed on paraffin-embedded tissue and validates the type of amyloid by direct amino acid sequencing, thereby leaving no question about the origin of the amyloid protein as an immunoglobulin light chain. Alternatively, immunoelectron microscopy can be used to type the amyloid. Each of these tests have a specificity of nearly 100% for light chain amyloidosis.

When the heart is involved, electrocardiography frequently shows a pseudoinfarct pattern, which can be interpreted as demonstrating silent ischemic infarction; this finding can lead to coronary angiography, which is invariably negative (unless the patient has coincidental coronary artery disease). Echocardiography shows thickening of the heart walls and a hyperreflective granular texture (see Fig. 47-8) due to amyloid infiltration but can be misinterpreted as showing left ventricular hypertrophy. Enhancement on magnetic resonance imaging with gadolinium is delayed in approximately 70% of patients with cardiac amyloidosis. Myocardial enhancement is associated with increased ventricular mass and impaired left ventricular systolic function. Technetium pyrophosphate (Tc^{99} PYP) imaging of the heart can be supportive of a diagnosis of ATTR amyloidosis (see E-Fig. 44-4).

TREATMENT

AL amyloidosis was previously thought to be untreatable and invariably fatal. With current therapy,[8] complete response rates of over 50% are reported, and the median duration of survival is upward of 5 years.[9] Agents to reverse the misfolding of the protein and render it soluble would be ideal, but they are currently investigational. The source of the immunoglobulin light chain is the clonal plasma cell population in the bone marrow. All known therapies are directed at destruction of the plasma cell clone.

The two treatment choices are traditional-dose chemoimmunotherapy with or without high-dose chemotherapy with autologous stem cell transplantation. Most patients are not candidates for high-dose therapy because of age, advanced cardiac dysfunction, or renal insufficiency. High-dose melphalan is a feasible approach in selected patients with light chain amyloidosis and is associated with a high rate of hematologic and organ responses that lead to prolonged survival (Fig. 174-4). Current therapies include combinations of melphalan, cyclophosphamide, dexamethasone, bortezomib,[10] and lenalidomide. Treatment under expert oversight with a combination of daratumumab, which is a human monoclonal antibody against CD38 (1800 mg subcutaneously),[11] bortezomib (1.3 mg/m^2 weekly), cyclophosphamide (300 mg/m^2 orally weekly), and dexamethasone (40 mg weekly) can produce rapid and complete hematologic responses in the majority of patients with light chain amyloidosis with few side effects.[A1] Even without the daratumumab, the triplet of bortezomib, cyclophosphamide, and dexamethasone can result in slightly more than 50% of patients not requiring additional treatment for at least 7 years.[12] Effective plasma cell directed therapy has been associated with resolution of nephrotic syndrome, cardiac failure, and hepatomegaly.

For rescue therapy (Fig. 174-5), expert oversight is required. One option is pomalidomide plus dexamethasone.[13] Another option is to add daratumumab, which can provide a rapid hematologic response and a 2-year survival of about 75% as a single agent.[14,A2] Investigational venetoclax appears to have high activity in patients whose plasma cells express t(11;14).

For patients with chronic renal failure, kidney transplantation (Chapter 117) is an option.[15] Antibodies to amyloid fibrils are being tested.

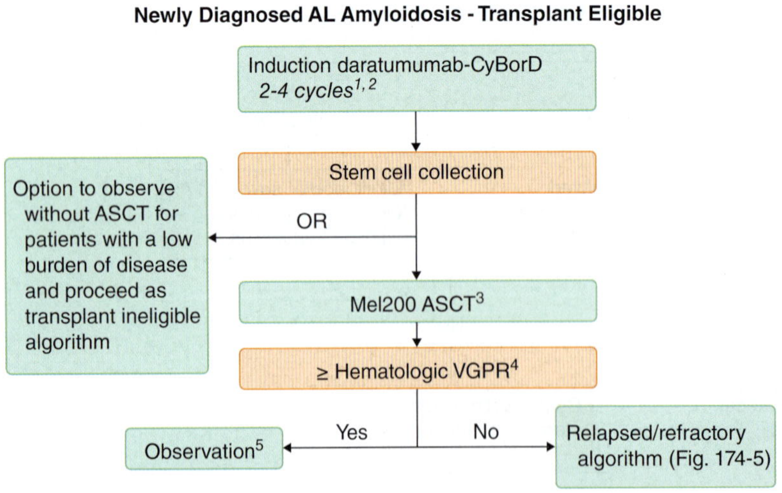

FIGURE 174-4. Treatment for newly diagnosed AL amyloidosis patients who are transplant-eligible. [1]Consider adding doxycycline for at least a year. [2]If daratumumab is not accessible, CyBorD is an acceptable alternative regimen (weekly bortezomib only). [3]For CrCl <30, use Mel 140 mg/m^2. [4]Decision to change therapy if in VGPR but < CR is based on a number of clinical factors, re-refer to amyloid center of excellence. [5]For patients with overt multiple myeloma, use myeloma-type maintenance; consider for BMPCs ≥20% and high-risk FISH (del 17p, t(4;14), t(14;16) and t(14;20)). Please refer for myeloma mSMART guidelines for choice of maintenance. https://www.mayoclinic.org/medical-professionals/cancer/news/msmart-a-clear-and-simple-guide-for-treating-patients-with-multiple-myeloma/mqc-20506750. ASCT = autologous stem cell transplant; BMPC = bone marrow plasma cells; CyBorD = cyclophosphamide, bortezomib, dexamethasone; Mel = melphalan; VGPR = very good partial remission.

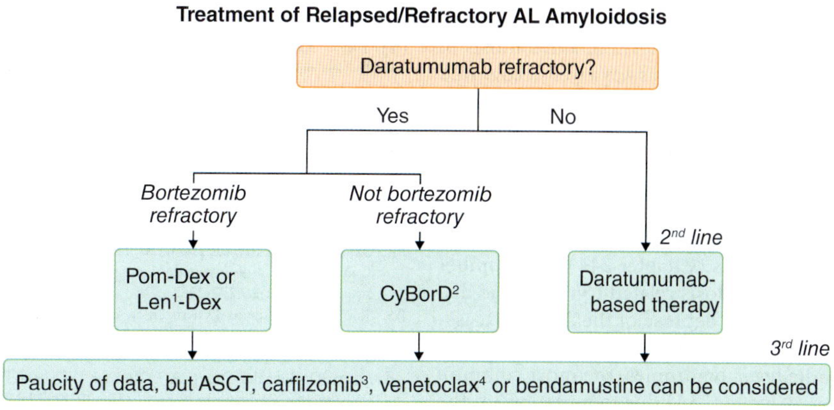

FIGURE 174-5. **Treatment of relapsed/refractory AL amyloidosis.** [1]Starting dose of lenalidomide should be no higher than 15 mg/d. [2]Melphalan-dexamethasone and ixazomib-dexamethasone are appropriate if patient has significant neuropathy. [3]Not recommended in patients with cardiac involvement. [4]For patients with t(11;14). Be cautious of infection risk. ASCT = autologous stem cell transplant; CyBorD = cyclophosphamide, bortezomib, dexamethasone; Dex = dexamethasone; Len = lenalidomide; Pom = pomalidomide.

PROGNOSIS

Patients who have AL amyloidosis and a baseline difference of less than 50 mg/L between circulating involved and uninvolved free light chain (i.e., low free light chain burden) have a better outcome.[16] This assay also can measure the therapeutic effect of interventions because the light chain level is quantifiable and reproducible.[17] Successful therapy is characterized by a 50% reduction in the abnormal free light chain level, but it is uncertain whether patients who do not achieve this level of response should be subjected to more intensive treatment in an effort to remove this pathogenic amyloid serum precursor.

The outcome of patients with light chain amyloidosis is highly dependent on the extent of cardiac involvement (Chapter 47), including myocardial dysfunction and arrhythmias. Doppler echocardiography allows quantitative measurements of diastolic function and reflects the slowing of blood flow into the ventricular chamber as the noncompliant left ventricle fills. This "stiffness," measured by the deceleration time, provides useful information and correlates well with survival.

Cardiac biomarkers are extremely sensitive measures of myocardial function, are reproducible, and can be used not only for prognosis but also to follow cardiac response after effective therapy.[18] The serum troponin value is a powerful predictor of survival in patients with amyloidosis, and the N-terminal pro–brain natriuretic peptide value also predicts survival. With the advent of routine hemodialysis, death due to renal failure is uncommon.

OTHER SYSTEMIC AMYLOIDOSES

ATTRwt AMYLOIDOSIS

ATTRwt amyloidosis (formerly known as senile systemic amyloidosis) results from the deposition of a normal serum protein, transthyretin, in the myocardium. Most patients are older than age 70 years.

The clinical presentation of ATTRwt is not distinguishable from that of cardiac light chain amyloidosis. The diagnosis of ATTRwt is supported when a cardiac technetium pyrophosphate scan is positive (see E-Fig. 44-4) in the absence of a monoclonal protein. ATTRwt is the only type of amyloid that can be made without a tissue diagnosis. When a monoclonal protein is present, however, confirmation of the type of amyloid requires analysis of the Congo red–positive tissues by mass spectrometry or immunoelectron microscopy.

TREATMENT AND PROGNOSIS

Tafamidis (61 mg once daily), an oral agent that prevents misfolding of TTR into amyloid configuration, is the only approved therapy for ATTRwt. Elevated levels of NT-pro-brain natriuretic peptide and/or troponin, a reduced eGFR, and a decreased left ventricular ejection fraction are adverse risk factors. The median survival is 3.6 years.

FAMILIAL AMYLOIDOSIS

Familial (or hereditary) amyloidosis is uncommon in the United States and represents only 3% of cases of systemic amyloidosis. The precursor protein of the amyloid determines the clinical phenotype (Table 174-1).

Among the 100 or more transthyretin point mutations, one important form of familial amyloidosis in the United States is a *TTR* allele in which isoleucine is substituted for valine at gene position 152 resulting in the TTR protein V122I. Approximately 4% of Black Americans are heterozygotes for *ATTRV122I*, which increases the risk of incident heart failure by 50% but not the risk of mortality.[19] The gene mutation *ATTRV50M* causes a late-onset transthyretin familial amyloid polyneuropathy. Less common causes of hereditary systemic amyloidoses include destabilizing mutations or deletions of lysozyme, apolipoprotein AI,[20] apolipoprotein AII, apolipoprotein AIV, fibrinogen α chain, gelsolin, and cystatin C.

CLINICAL MANIFESTATIONS AND DIAGNOSIS

Patients may present with the full clinical spectrum associated with amyloidosis, including cardiomyopathy, peripheral neuropathy, autonomic neuropathy, and/or proteinuria, depending on the precursor protein.[21] Diagnosis, typically by biopsy in the early stages, is essential to allow for timely treatment to prevent or delay disease progression. Myocardial radiotracer uptake on bone scintigraphy using technetium (Tc^{99}) pyrophosphate (PYP; see E-Fig. 44-4) or 3,3-diphosphono-1,2-propanodicarboxylic acid (DPD) is greater than 99% sensitive and 86% specific for cardiac mutant and wild-type ATTR cardiac amyloidosis, with false-positive results almost exclusively from uptake in patients with cardiac light chain amyloidosis.[22] Guidelines encourage genetic counseling and routine presymptomatic genetic testing.[23]

TREATMENT AND PROGNOSIS

Transthyretin amyloid cardiomyopathy is now a treatable condition.[24,25] Tafamidis (20 to 80 mg daily), which binds noncooperatively to the two thyroxine sites on the tetrameric form of transthyretin and thereby prevents its dissociation into monomers, can slow progression of transthyretin amyloid cardiomyopathy and reduce all-cause mortality.[A3] At 30 months, the 80-mg dose appears to be more efficacious, in terms of cardiac function as well as mortality.[A4] Patisiran (generally 0.3 mg/kg with a capped dose of 30 mg intravenously every 3 weeks) is a small interfering RNA drug that blocks the production of transthyretin; it can decrease ventricular wall thickness, reduce adverse cardiac outcomes,[A5] and slow the progression of the polyneuropathy.[A6] Similarly, inotersen (284 mg subcutaneously weekly) also can slow the progression of polyneuropathy and improve quality of life.[A7] Diflunisal (an FDA–approved generic nonsteroidal anti-inflammatory drug at 250 mg twice daily) can slow the rate of progression of the familial TTR amyloidosis–associated polyneuropathy.[26] Diflunisal complexes to the thyroxine binding sites on the tetrameric form of transthyretin, stabilizes it, and thus inhibits the release of the transthyretin monomer required for amyloidogenesis.

Because this disease is characterized by systemic accumulation of polymerized transthyretin in the peripheral nerves and systemic organs, liver transplantation stops the major production of amyloidogenic transthyretin. Selected patients with familial amyloidosis and polyneuropathy have benefited from liver transplantation. In the future, the availability of gene silencing therapy[27] may reduce the need for liver transplantation.

For transthyretin-related amyloidosis, the median historical survival was 5 to 15 years depending on the organs involved. The effect of newer medications on life expectancy is encouraging but uncertain. The estimated probability of 10-year survival in patients with familial amyloid polyneuropathy can be as high as 90 to 100%.

SECONDARY SYSTEMIC AMYLOIDOSIS

Systemic secondary amyloidosis is now the rarest form of amyloidosis in Western countries.[28] Previously, secondary amyloidosis was a well-recognized consequence of uncontrolled sustained inflammation, usually infectious, and causes included tuberculosis and osteomyelitis. Cystic fibrosis (Chapter 77), bronchiectasis (Chapter 78), decubitus ulcers, and skin abscesses related to subcutaneous injection of illicit drugs remain modern-day infectious causes. Secondary amyloidosis can also occur in patients with difficult-to-control inflammatory syndromes, including Crohn disease (Chapter 127), juvenile arthritis, and ankylosing spondylitis (Chapter 244). The number of patients who develop secondary amyloidosis related to rheumatic diseases has declined markedly, at least in part because of the use of disease-modifying antirheumatic therapy.[29] Familial forms of secondary amyloidosis are associated with familial periodic fever syndromes, the most common being familial Mediterranean fever (Chapter 254) due to mutations in the tumor necrosis factor receptor.

Organ damage results from the extracellular deposition of proteolytic fragments of the acute phase reactant serum amyloid A as amyloid fibrils. The distribution of deposits is mostly in the kidney, spleen, liver, and intestines.

Secondary amyloidosis patients typically present with proteinuria, nephrotic syndrome, or renal dysfunction. Diarrhea related to intestinal involvement (22%) and thyromegaly (9%) also occur.

TREATMENT

Suppression of the inflammatory process results in regression of tissue amyloid deposits. Therefore, monitoring of patients with chronic, active inflammatory disease by serial testing of serum amyloid A, C-reactive protein, microalbuminemia, proteinuria, and other indicators of amyloid development, as well as possibly determination of the *SAA1* genotype, can guide management. Anti–tumor necrosis factor-α agents have markedly reduced the incidence of secondary amyloidosis from inflammatory arthritis. Interleukin-1 inhibitors (e.g., anakinra) have been used successfully under expert oversight for patients who have inherited periodic fever syndromes (Chapter 254).

LOCALIZED AMYLOIDOSIS

Localized amyloidosis can be confused with systemic amyloidosis. However, patients with localized amyloidosis do not have a demonstrable monoclonal protein in the serum or urine and have a normal free light chain ratio. The location of the amyloid deposits also can be a clue to the localized nature.

Typical sites for localized amyloid deposition include the ureter, bladder, urethra, and prostate. Most forms of cutaneous amyloidosis are localized, although nodular cutaneous amyloidosis can occur in systemic light chain amyloidosis. Tracheobronchial and laryngeal amyloidosis and nodular pulmonary amyloidosis are localized and are not associated with a plasma cell dyscrasia. Nodular pulmonary amyloidosis is often diagnosed after thoracotomy or transcutaneous biopsy. Most cases of laryngeal amyloidosis are found when the patient presents to an otorhinolaryngologist with hoarseness and amyloid deposits are found on endoscopic biopsy. The localized amyloidosis found in Alzheimer disease (Chapter 371) is chemically unrelated to light chain amyloidosis, and patients with light chain amyloidosis do not have an increased risk of dementia.

TREATMENT AND PROGNOSIS

Management can be supportive or localized to the deposition, and patients generally do not require systemic therapy. For genitourinary amyloidosis, therapy entails cystoscopic resection or intravesical instillation of dimethyl sulfoxide. Laryngeal, tracheobronchial, and cutaneous amyloidosis can be treated with a variety of local agents under expert supervision with varying degrees of success. Overall, however, localized amyloidosis has a much better prognosis than does systemic amyloidosis.

GENERAL REFERENCES

For the General References and other additional features, please visit Elsevier eBooks+ at https://ebooks.health.elsevier.com.

Grade A References

A1. Kastritis E, Palladini G, Minnema MC, et al. Daratumumab-based treatment for immunoglobulin light-chain amyloidosis. *N Engl J Med.* 2021;385:46-58.

A2. Dimopoulos MA, Terpos E, Boccadoro M, et al. Daratumumab plus pomalidomide and dexamethasone versus pomalidomide and dexamethasone alone in previously treated multiple myeloma (APOLLO): an open-label, randomised, phase 3 trial. *Lancet Oncol.* 2021;22:801-812.

A3. Maurer MS, Schwartz JH, Gundapaneni B, et al. Tafamidis treatment for patients with transthyretin amyloid cardiomyopathy. *N Engl J Med.* 2018;379:1007-1016.

A4. Damy T, Garcia-Pavia P, Hanna M, et al. Efficacy and safety of tafamidis doses in the Tafamidis in Transthyretin Cardiomyopathy Clinical Trial (ATTR-ACT) and long-term extension study. *Eur J Heart Fail.* 2021;23:277-285.

A5. Solomon SD, Adams D, Kristen A, et al. Effects of patisiran, an RNA interference therapeutic, on cardiac parameters in patients with hereditary transthyretin-mediated amyloidosis. *Circulation.* 2019;139:431-443.

A6. Adams D, Gonzalez-Duarte A, O'Riordan WD, et al. Patisiran, an RNAi therapeutic, for hereditary transthyretin amyloidosis. *N Engl J Med.* 2018;379:11-21.

A7. Benson MD, Waddington-Cruz M, Berk JL, et al. Inotersen treatment for patients with hereditary transthyretin amyloidosis. *N Engl J Med.* 2018;379:22-31.

175 TUMORS OF THE CENTRAL NERVOUS SYSTEM

INGO K. MELLINGHOFF AND LISA M. DEANGELIS

Central nervous system (CNS) tumors can involve the brain or the spinal cord, may be benign or malignant, and may be primary or metastatic. In the United States, about 80,000 new primary brain tumors and other nervous system tumors are diagnosed annually, and about one-third of primary CNS tumors are malignant. In contrast, intracranial metastases are five times more common than primary brain tumors.

Over 100 different types and subtypes of brain and spinal cord tumors arise from cells that make up the CNS (Table 175-1). Because CNS tumors grow within the CNS and rarely if ever metastasize to other organs, conventional tumor staging approaches are not applicable, so histopathologic and molecular features are used to categorize CNS tumors. Histopathologic features that suggest more aggressive growth include cytologic atypia, increased mitotic rate, microvascular proliferation, and regional necrosis. Tumors lacking these features are still able to grow within the CNS and to cause progressive neurologic disability, and they may acquire a more malignant phenotype over time. Tumor grading includes histologic features[1,2] as well as molecular information. In difficult cases, DNA methylation patterns can help assign a tumor subtype.

BRAIN TUMORS

Extra-axial primary brain tumors arise within the intracranial cavity but are not tumors of brain tissue. Although they produce neurologic symptoms and signs by compressing the underlying brain, almost all extra-axial tumors are benign. Since the brain is rarely invaded, complete surgical excision is often feasible.

In contrast, intra-axial primary brain tumors tend to invade brain tissue diffusely, and none can be completely excised surgically. Most primary intra-axial brain tumors are gliomas, including the astrocytomas, oligodendrogliomas, and ependymomas.

CLINICAL MANIFESTATIONS

A patient with a brain tumor can present with generalized and/or lateralizing symptoms and signs. Generalized symptoms, which include headache, lethargy, personality change, nausea, and vomiting, typically reflect the increased intracranial pressure that often accompanies cerebral tumors. Lateralizing symptoms, which reflect the specific location of the tumor, include hemiparesis, hemisensory deficits, aphasia, visual field impairment, and seizures (Table 175-2).

TABLE 175-1 WORLD HEALTH ORGANIZATION CLASSIFICATION (WHO) OF BRAIN TUMORS

GLIOMAS, GLIONEURONAL TUMORS, AND NEURONAL TUMORS
Adult-type Diffuse Gliomas
Astrocytoma, IDH-mutant
Oligodendroglioma, IDH-mutant, and 1p/19q-codeleted
Glioblastoma, IDH-wildtype
Pediatric-type Diffuse Low-grade Gliomas
Pediatric-type Diffuse High-grade Gliomas
Diffuse midline glioma, H3 K27-altered
Diffuse hemispheric glioma, H3 G34-mutant
Diffuse pediatric-type high-grade glioma, H3-wildtype and IDH-wildtype
Infant-type hemispheric glioma
Circumscribed Astrocytic Gliomas
Pilocytic astrocytoma
Pleomorphic xanthoastrocytoma
Subependymal giant cell astrocytoma
Glioneuronal and Neuronal Tumors
Ependymal Tumors
CHOROID PLEXUS TUMORS
EMBRYONAL TUMORS
Medulloblastoma
Other CNS embryonal tumors
PINEAL TUMORS (INCLUDING PINEOBLASTOMA, OTHERS)
CRANIAL AND PARASPINAL NERVE TUMORS (INCLUDING NEUROFIBROMA, SCHWANNOMA, OTHERS)
MENINGIOMAS
MESENCHYMAL, NON-MENINGOTHELIAL TUMORS
MELANOCYTIC TUMORS
HEMATOLYMPHOID TUMORS
Lymphomas, including Primary CNS Lymphoma
Histiocytic tumors
GERM CELL TUMORS
TUMORS OF THE SELLAR REGION
Craniopharyngioma
Pituitary adenoma/PitNET

CNS = central nervous system; IDH = isocitrate dehydrogenase; PitNET = pituitary neuroendocrine tumor.
Abridged and modified from Louis DN, Perry A, Wesseling P, et al. The 2021 WHO classification of the tumors of the central nervous system: a summary. *Neuro Oncol.* 2021;23:1231-1251.

Symptoms of brain tumors can be produced by tumor that directly invades the brain parenchyma, when tumor and edema compress brain tissue, when obstruction to cerebrospinal fluid (CSF) is directly caused by the tumor or by a shift of brain tissue, and when herniation occurs. Invasion and compression typically produce lateralizing symptoms, whereas obstruction of the flow of cerebrospinal fluid and herniation typically produce generalized symptoms but can also cause false localizing signs, such as an abducens nerve palsy as a result of diffuse increased intracranial pressure.

Headache (Chapter 367) is a presenting symptom of approximately 35% of brain tumors. It is more common in younger than in older patients and more common in patients who have rapidly growing tumors than in patients whose tumors have evolved slowly. Local growth of the tumor may cause mental and cognitive abnormalities (e.g., aphasia, alexia, agnosia) or general impairment (e.g., lethargy, confusion, word finding difficulty, apathy).

Most patients have symptoms that progress during a week to a few months. A sudden intensification of symptoms may precipitate the patient's initial visit to the physician, but a careful history usually reveals symptoms that predated the acute deterioration and slowly worsened over time. Two exceptions are the new appearance of a seizure in a previously asymptomatic individual (Chapter 372) and sudden hemorrhage into a tumor.

Seizures (Chapter 372) affect approximately one-third of patients with brain tumors, and they are especially common as the presenting and only symptom of a low-grade tumor. The seizures, which are focal because they originate at the site of the tumor, may remain restricted (e.g., focal motor seizures), or they may generalize secondarily to produce loss of consciousness, sometimes so quickly that the focal signature is missed by the patient or even an observant witness.

TABLE 175-2 FOCAL CLINICAL MANIFESTATIONS OF BRAIN TUMORS

FRONTAL LOBE
Generalized seizures; focal motor seizures (contralateral); expressive aphasia (dominant side); behavioral changes; dementia; gait disorders; incontinence; hemiparesis (contralateral)
BASAL GANGLIA
Hemiparesis (contralateral); movement disorders (rare)
PARIETAL LOBE
Receptive aphasia (dominant side); spatial disorientation (nondominant side); cortical sensory dysfunction (contralateral); hemianopia (contralateral); agnosias
OCCIPITAL LOBE
Hemianopia (contralateral); visual disturbances (unformed)
TEMPORAL LOBE
Complex partial (psychomotor) seizures; generalized seizures; olfactory and complex visual auras; behavioral changes; visual field defect; language disorder (dominant side)
CORPUS CALLOSUM
Dementia (anterior); memory loss (posterior); asymptomatic (middle); behavioral changes
THALAMUS
Sensory loss (contralateral); language disorder (dominant side); behavioral changes
MIDBRAIN/PINEAL
Paresis of vertical eye; pupillary abnormalities; precocious puberty (boys)
SELLA/OPTIC NERVE/PITUITARY
Endocrinopathy; bitemporal hemianopia; monocular visual defects; ophthalmoplegia (cavernous sinus)
PONS/MEDULLA
Cranial nerve dysfunction; ataxia; nystagmus; spasticity; weakness; sensory loss
CEREBELLOPONTINE ANGLE
Deafness (ipsilateral); loss of facial sensation (ipsilateral); facial weakness (ipsilateral); ataxia
CEREBELLUM
Ataxia (ipsilateral or gait); nystagmus

DIAGNOSIS

A careful history and physical examination (Chapter 366) should assess cognitive function (Chapter 361) and search for any lateralizing signs. Routine hematologic and blood chemistry tests should be obtained to exclude a metabolic cause of mental status changes (Chapter 361). However, urgent brain imaging is required when the diagnosis of a brain tumor is suspected.

Brain Imaging

Magnetic resonance imaging (MRI) should be performed both without and with intravenous administration of gadolinium, preferably using a standardized brain tumor imaging protocol. A well-performed MRI identifies any intracranial tumor, and a normal MRI effectively excludes a neoplasm.

The MRI of some extra-axial tumors (e.g., acoustic neuromas, meningiomas) is so characteristic that histologic confirmation is not required. A non–contrast-enhancing infiltrative lesion that is visible primarily on T2-weighted or fluid-attenuated inversion recovery images is most consistent with a low-grade glioma (Fig. 175-1). A contrast-enhancing lesion with an area of central necrosis and surrounding edema is most likely to be a glioblastoma or possibly a brain metastasis.

MRI is far superior to computed tomography (CT) for the diagnosis of brain tumors and should be obtained in all patients with a suspected intracranial tumor. A CT scan, even with the administration of contrast material, may miss low-grade tumors and tumors in the posterior fossa, so a CT scan should be obtained only in patients who cannot undergo MRI.

In less clear cases, functional imaging techniques can be helpful to distinguish a brain tumor from other CNS lesions. Examples include cerebral blood volume (perfusion MRI), loss of tumor cellularity (diffusion-weighted MRI), the flow of contrast agent across a damaged blood-brain barrier (dynamic contrast-enhanced MRI), or the abundance of certain metabolites (MR spectroscopy).

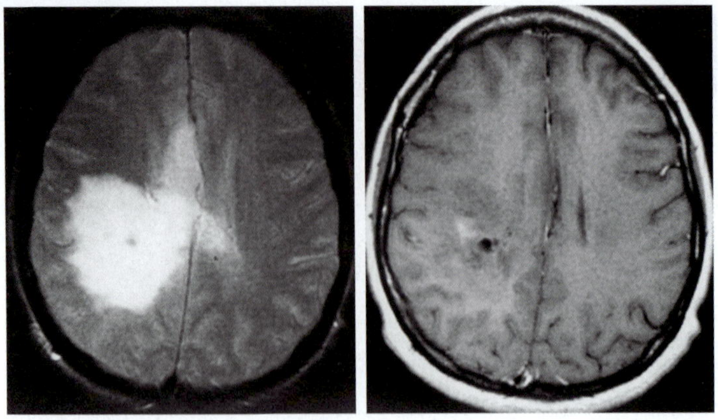

FIGURE 175-1. Glioma. Magnetic resonance imaging of a low-grade glioma. *Left*, T2-weighted image. *Right*, T1-weighted image, gadolinium contrast with minimum enhancement.

Malignant tumors, for example, are associated with an increased choline : *N*-acetylaspartate ratio and may contain areas with elevated levels of lactate and lipid. Functional MRI, which measures cerebral blood flow when areas of cortex are activated, may guide a safer and more complete surgical resection by localizing critical neurologic functions and their relationship to the tumor. Angiography no longer has a diagnostic role, but angiographic embolization is occasionally useful preoperatively to reduce the vascularity of some meningiomas, thereby making a complete resection safer.

Biopsy

Biopsy is typically part of a surgical procedure to remove the tumor to the greatest degree that is safe. However, most lesions that cannot be resected are still amenable to biopsy for diagnostic purposes. Stereotactic biopsy can reach lesions in almost any area of the brain with minimal morbidity. The risks of stereotactic biopsy include an inadequate tissue sample to make a diagnosis, a tissue sample that does not accurately reflect the most malignant grade of the tumor, and a procedure-related complication. Hemorrhage that causes neurologic impairment occurs in only 2% of stereotactic biopsies, typically in patients with glioblastomas. Unfortunately, some tumors, such as brain stem gliomas, are in such critical locations that biopsy should not be attempted.

Other Diagnostic Approaches

Electroencephalography (EEG) can be useful when a patient with a brain tumor has prolonged or unexplained confusion or stupor and for whom nonconvulsive status epilepticus is a consideration. Intraoperative monitoring is used frequently to help guide resection of epileptogenic cortex adjacent to or within the brain tumor tissue or to perform intraoperative mapping of critical functions to facilitate a safe, complete resection.

Cerebrospinal fluid analysis has a limited role in the diagnosis of most intracranial neoplasms. In primary CNS lymphoma (Chapter 171), however, the diagnosis may be established on cerebrospinal fluid cytologic examination in about 15% of patients. The sensitivity of cerebrospinal fluid cytology in the diagnosis of CNS lymphoma increases when it is combined with flow cytometry and is further enhanced by immunophenotypic and molecular genetic analyses of the cerebrospinal fluid. Rarely, a lumbar puncture is required to exclude inflammatory conditions or other processes that may be confused with a primary brain tumor. Lumbar puncture must be avoided in patients with cerebellar tumors because the release of pressure through the spinal needle may result in herniation of the cerebellar tonsils through the foramen magnum. The ability to detect tumor-derived DNA and circulating tumor cells in cerebrospinal fluid from some patients with CNS tumors may be helpful to monitor the tumor's evolution and response to therapy without the need for neurosurgical procedures.

Differential Diagnosis of Brain Tumors

Patients who present with symptoms of raised intracranial pressure or the new onset of central neurologic symptoms, such as hemiparesis or seizure, must be evaluated urgently. Prompt neuroimaging discloses a mass, and the radiographic features narrow the differential diagnosis (Table 175-3). Extra-axial tumors, such as a meningioma or acoustic neuroma, can be confused with a dural metastasis. Low-grade intra-axial tumors, which are nonenhancing on MRI, have been confused with infections such as herpes encephalitis (Chapter 383) when they involve the temporal lobe. Contrast-enhancing intra-axial tumors can be confused with a stroke (Chapter 376), brain abscess (Chapter 382), or focal plaque of demyelination (Chapter 380). Subacute infarction can show brisk contrast enhancement, usually in a gyral pattern, unlike brain tumors in which enhancement is primarily in the white matter; however, the two are occasionally indistinguishable radiographically. Brain abscesses (Fig. 382-1) typically have a thinner enhancing wall than a malignant tumor and have restricted diffusion. Despite careful evaluation, patients thought to have a malignant glioma occasionally are found at surgery to have a brain abscess. A single large plaque of demyelination can also be confused radiographically with a brain tumor and sometimes the diagnosis can be established only by biopsy.

When MRI suggests a primary brain tumor, an extensive systemic search for a possible source of metastasis is rarely required. Brain metastases are more common than primary brain tumors, but most occur in patients with known cancer, typically with active systemic disease. If an obvious systemic cancer is not revealed by a thorough physical examination, chest radiograph, routine blood tests, and urinalysis, the patient should proceed to craniotomy. Even if a brain metastasis is found at surgery, resection of a single brain metastasis is the appropriate treatment, and the pathologic examination of the lesion guides the subsequent search for the primary tumor.

TABLE 175-3 DIFFERENTIAL DIAGNOSIS OF INTRACRANIAL TUMORS

INFECTION
Brain abscess (Chapter 382)
Bacterial
Fungal
Parasitic (e.g., cysticercosis; Chapter 325)
Herpes encephalitis (Chapter 383)
VASCULAR DISEASE
Stroke (Chapter 376)
Intracranial hemorrhage (Chapter 377)
INFLAMMATORY CONDITIONS
Granuloma (sarcoid; Chapter 83)
Multiple sclerosis (Chapter 380): tumefactive single large lesion
VASCULAR MALFORMATIONS
Cavernous angiomas (Chapter 377)
Venous angiomas (Chapter 377)
CONGENITAL ABNORMALITIES
Cortical dysplasia (Chapter 385)
Heterotopia (Chapter 385)

TREATMENT

The treatment for all brain tumors can be divided into two main categories: symptomatic therapy and tumor-directed therapy (Table 175-4). Symptomatic treatment addresses cerebral edema, thromboembolic disease, and seizures, all of which can contribute substantially to clinical symptoms caused by the tumor.

Management of Symptoms

Corticosteroids (typically dexamethasone starting at 8 to 12 mg/day) decrease the vasogenic edema that often surrounds primary and metastatic brain tumors. Clinical improvement may begin within minutes, and patients frequently improve dramatically within 24 to 48 hours. This dose is then adjusted to find the lowest dose that alleviates neurologic symptoms. Once- or twice-daily dosing is preferred for maintenance therapy over more frequent dosing. After definitive treatment is instituted, many patients can be tapered off their corticosteroid completely. Chronic high-dose corticosteroid therapy is associated with substantial side effects (Chapter 28) and should be avoided if possible. Common side effects include insomnia, steroid myopathy, gastrointestinal complications, and opportunistic infections. Patients who will be taking corticosteroids for 6 weeks or longer should receive prophylaxis against *Pneumocystis jirovecii* (Chapter 313). Antibodies that block the effects of vascular endothelial growth factor (VEGF), such as bevacizumab, can be very effective in the management of symptomatic cerebral edema and can reduce corticosteroid requirements.

Venous thromboembolism affects about 25% of patients who have brain tumors. All patients undergoing neurosurgery should have pneumatic compression boots in the postoperative period to reduce the incidence of venous thromboembolism. Prophylactic anticoagulants (Chapter 68) also have been used successfully in the immediate postoperative period without increasing postoperative hemorrhage. Appropriately regulated anticoagulation (Chapter 70) is the optimal therapy for deep vein thrombosis and is not associated with an increased risk for intracerebral hemorrhage. Inferior vena cava filters can be used for patients who have deep vein thrombi or pulmonary emboli and who cannot be fully anticoagulated.

TABLE 175-4 TREATMENT OF BRAIN TUMORS

SYMPTOMATIC TREATMENT
Glucocorticoids
Antiepileptics
Venous thromboembolism prophylaxis and treatment
TUMOR-DIRECTED THERAPY
Surgery
Radiation therapy
Chemotherapy or other systemic therapy

Anticonvulsant medications (Chapter 372) are administered to any patient who has had a seizure, but prophylactic anticonvulsants should not be prescribed for patients who have never had a seizure, except in the immediate perioperative period. When used, the dose of antiepileptic agents generally should be tapered beginning 2 to 3 weeks after craniotomy.

Tumor-Directed Therapies

Surgery

Complete excision is the goal for a primary brain tumor. Surgical excision can often be accomplished for primary extra-axial tumors, such as meningiomas and acoustic neuromas, unless their intracranial location makes resection impossible. Tumors of the skull base are particularly difficult to remove, and partial resection for decompression is often performed to preserve neurologic function. The safe boundaries for resecting cortical lesions while preserving function often can be elucidated by preoperative functional MRI and intraoperative cortical mapping. However, lesions involving critical structures, such as the brain stem or thalamus, cannot be excised safely.

Complete excision can cure an extra-axial primary brain tumor and is associated with prolonged survival and better neurologic outcome, even in patients with primary intra-axial tumors. In patients with malignant and lower grade gliomas, gross total excision, as measured by postoperative neuroimaging, is associated with prolonged survival. However, most low-grade gliomas are not amenable to gross total excision, and only partial excision is usually feasible. In patients with high-grade gliomas, macroscopic tumor frequently can be removed completely, but microscopic disease that infiltrates surrounding brain tissue always remains.

Radiation Therapy

A course of external beam radiation therapy is delivered in small daily fractions to a total cumulative dose usually between 45 and 60 Gy. Dividing the treatment into small daily fractions permits sublethal repair in normal tissues and markedly reduces the neurologic toxicity that is associated with cerebral irradiation. External beam radiation, which is the most effective nonsurgical treatment of brain tumors, doubles median survival time of patients with malignant primary brain tumors or metastatic lesions. Radiation therapy can also be useful for recurrent meningiomas and acoustic neuromas. However, it only rarely cures any of these lesions, and most patients develop recurrent disease despite maximal radiation therapy.

Stereotactic radiosurgery delivers high fractions of focused radiation therapy that spare normal surrounding tissue. The technique is generally limited to tumors that are 3 cm in diameter or smaller and is less useful for malignant gliomas because of their infiltrative nature.

The neurologic complications of radiation therapy, which are usually observed months to years after completion of treatment, include radionecrosis, dementia, and leukoencephalopathy. The incidence is reported as less than 5%, and most patients die of their brain tumor before the delayed consequences of treatment can be observed. However, in long-term survivors (e.g., patients with lower grade glioma or children with medulloblastoma), the late consequences of radiation therapy are important. Dementia accompanying radiation-induced leukoencephalopathy can progress and result in severe neurologic impairment. Radionecrosis can mimic recurrent tumor with a large contrast-enhancing lesion on MRI. Corticosteroids under expert supervision can reduce the edema and sometimes are sufficient to treat small areas of radionecrosis. However, if the lesion is sufficiently large, resection may be required to decompress the mass and reduce the corticosteroid requirement. Laser interstitial thermal therapy is also a possible therapeutic approach for intractable radionecrosis.

Systemic Therapy

Systemic medical therapies vary depending on the type and grade of the tumor. Currently, all such regimens are palliative rather than curative, except for some patients who have CNS lymphomas.

SPECIFIC TYPES OF PRIMARY BRAIN TUMORS

MENINGIOMAS

EPIDEMIOLOGY AND PATHOBIOLOGY

Meningiomas are the most common primary CNS tumors and are usually benign. Between 10 and 15% of meningiomas are atypical or malignant variants with a more aggressive course.[3] Meningiomas are more common in women and may be multiple in about 10% of patients with sporadic meningioma.

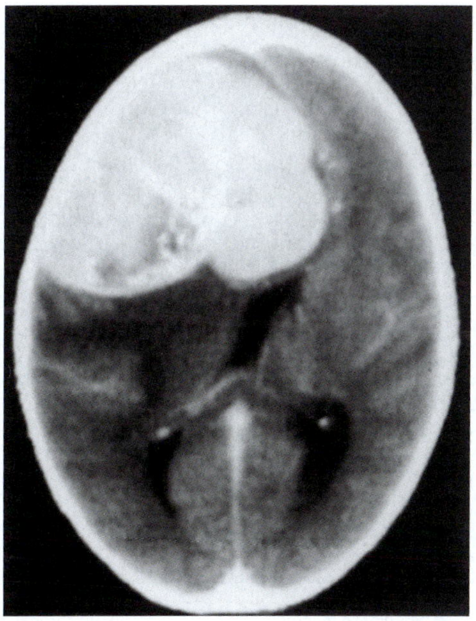

FIGURE 175-2. **Meningioma.** Computed tomography scan with contrast enhancement of a meningioma in a patient who presented with mild cognitive deficits, illustrative of the size that a slow-growing tumor can attain in the brain. The tumor was completely resected.

Exposure to ionizing radiation elevates the risk for meningioma. Meningiomas are occasionally part of a familial syndrome and occur with increased frequency in patients with neurofibromatosis type 2 (NF2; Chapter 385). Inactivation of *NF2* is seen in approximately 50% of sporadic tumors. Other genes are also mutated frequently in meningioma (e.g., *SMO*, *AKT1*, *KLF4*, *TRAF7*), but the role of these alterations in the development or growth of meningioma remains to be defined.

CLINICAL MANIFESTATIONS AND DIAGNOSIS

Meningiomas grow slowly and produce symptoms that are insidious in onset and typically slowly progressive. Frequently, meningiomas are completely asymptomatic and are identified on neuroimaging done for another purpose, such as head trauma.

Tumors can reach a considerable size (Fig. 175-2), but they grow so slowly that the brain accommodates to the progressive compression. Meningiomas typically occur in specific locations: over the convexity, along the falx and parasagittal area, in the olfactory groove, at the base of the skull near the sphenoid bone, in the cavernous sinus (Fig. 175-3), in the cerebellopontine angle, and in the foramen magnum. Cortical and parasagittal tumors typically are manifested with seizures or progressive hemiparesis. Tumors in the anterior cranial fossa can cause slowly progressive cognitive and personality changes. Meningiomas at the base of the skull are manifested with cranial neuropathies and gait difficulties when the brain stem is compressed.

On MRI, meningiomas have a characteristic appearance consisting of a diffusely enhancing, dural-based lesion that is associated with a thin enhancing dural tail that extends from the tumor. The radiographic features are often so characteristic that biopsy is not required and surgery is performed for therapeutic purposes only. The radiographic differential diagnosis includes the less common hemangiopericytoma and dural metastasis. Most meningiomas are not accompanied by significant edema, but marked edema is seen with high-grade malignant lesions or the secretory variant.

TREATMENT AND PROGNOSIS

If small meningiomas are discovered in the absence of clinical symptoms or the symptoms are minor, lesions may be monitored with serial images because growth can be so slow. If treatment is indicated, complete resection is often curative, but even completely resected benign tumors may recur in as many as 20% of cases, so radiologic follow-up is essential. Tumors at the base of the skull often cannot be resected completely and tend to recur despite successive attempts at surgical resection. Stereotactic radiosurgery may be an alternative to surgery if the lesion is small or if patients have progressive or residual tumor.[4] External beam radiation therapy may slow progression of recurrent lesions and is essential for the treatment of malignant meningiomas.

DNA methylation profiling and determination of *CDKN2A/B* gene copy loss can provide prognostic information. No effective systemic therapy has been identified for recurrent meningioma.[5]

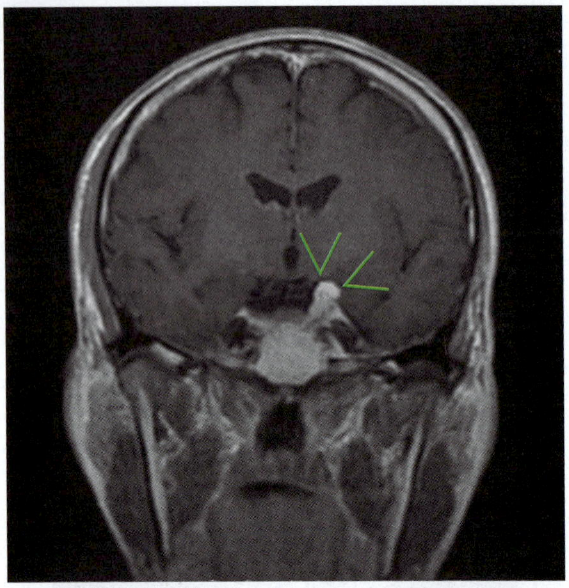

FIGURE 175-3. Skull base meningioma. A post-gadolinium coronal magnetic resonance image demonstrating a small left meningioma arising from the clinoid.

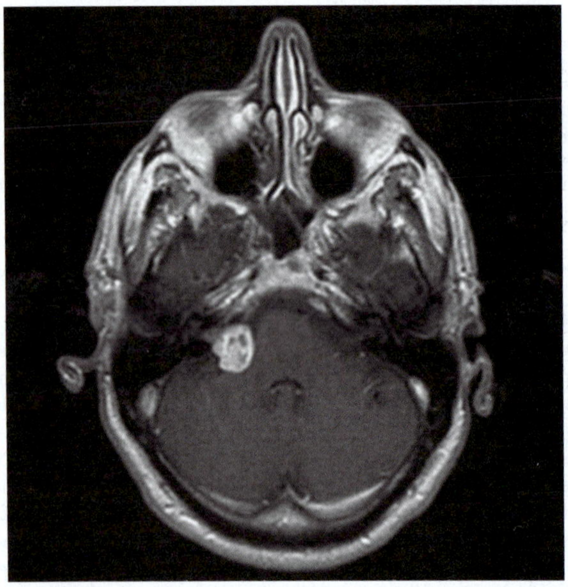

FIGURE 175-4. Vestibular schwannoma. A post-gadolinium magnetic resonance image demonstrating a large right vestibular schwannoma. The origin can be seen in the acoustic canal, but the tumor has grown into the cerebellopontine angle, where it is compressing the brainstem.

VESTIBULAR SCHWANNOMAS

Vestibular schwannomas, also called acoustic neuromas (Chapter 396), are benign tumors that arise from the eighth cranial nerve. Vestibular schwannomas are twice as common in women as in men, with a peak incidence between ages 40 and 60 years. Sporadic vestibular schwannomas are unilateral, whereas bilateral vestibular schwannomas are pathognomonic of neurofibromatosis type 2 (Chapter 385).

CLINICAL MANIFESTATIONS AND DIAGNOSIS

Vestibular schwannomas usually arise from the vestibular portion of the nerve and typically are manifest by unilateral hearing loss, sometimes preceded or accompanied by tinnitus and a sensation of dizziness or unsteadiness but not true vertigo (Chapter 396). The slow, progressive enlargement of the tumor produces ipsilateral facial numbness or weakness by compressing the fifth or seventh cranial nerve, respectively. Tumors originate within the internal auditory meatus but grow out of the acoustic canal and into the cerebellopontine angle, where they can compress the brain stem and cause ataxia and ipsilateral cerebellar signs.[6] Cranial MRI with gadolinium delineates even small acoustic neuromas with ease (Fig. 175-4).[7]

TREATMENT

Treatment is often surgical, but stereotactic radiosurgery is an effective alternative, especially for lesions smaller than 3 cm.[8] Tumors should be treated when they are small to preserve facial nerve function and hearing.

PITUITARY ADENOMAS

Pituitary adenomas are discussed in Chapter 205.

OTHER EXTRA-AXIAL PRIMARY BRAIN TUMORS

Pineal Tumors

Pineal region tumors include pineal parenchymal tumors, such as pineocytomas and the more aggressive pineoblastomas, and germ cell tumors, including germinomas and non-germinomatous germ cell tumors. Pineal region tumors all have a characteristic clinical presentation that includes Parinaud syndrome, which consists of paresis of upward gaze, poor pupillary reaction to light with brisk reaction on accommodation, impairment of convergence, and convergence-retraction nystagmus. Some of these lesions may also cause hydrocephalus and symptoms of increased intracranial pressure. Germinomas can be completely cured with focal radiation therapy, whereas non-germinomatous germ cell tumors are more aggressive and frequently relapse despite chemotherapy plus cranial irradiation.

Chordomas and Lipomas

Chordomas are rare tumors of residual notochordal tissue. They usually occur at the base of the skull, are locally invasive, and are characterized by multiple recurrences despite surgery and radiation therapy. Proton radiotherapy may be recommended for skull-based lesions that are adjacent to critical structures. Small molecule inhibitors of oncogenic signaling pathways (e.g., imatinib, sorafenib) have been reported to produce responses and clinical benefit in some patients with recurrent disease.

Lipomas are benign tumors that can occur in midline structures, particularly near the corpus callosum. They can be cured by complete removal.

Arachnoid Cysts

Arachnoid cysts are not tumors but can manifest with headache, seizures, or focal neurologic symptoms if they become large enough to compress underlying brain tissue. Many are completely asymptomatic and are found incidentally on neuroimaging. Only symptomatic cysts require removal.

GLIOMAS

DEFINITION

Gliomas comprise a heterogenous group of tumors.[9] Diffuse gliomas include types that primarily occur in adults and types that primarily occur in children. All diffuse astrocytic tumors with mutations in isocitrate dehydrogenase (IDH) 1 or 2 are considered a single type (*astrocytoma, IDH-mutant*) and then graded as grade 2 (previously called *diffuse astrocytoma, IDH-mutant*), grade 3 (previously called *anaplastic astrocytoma, IDH mutant*), or grade 4 (previously called *glioblastoma, IDH-mutant*). For IDH-wildtype diffuse astrocytic tumors, the diagnosis of glioblastoma, IDH-wildtype should be made if the tumor shows microvascular proliferation or necrosis or 1 or more of 3 genetic parameters: a *TERT* promoter mutation, *EGFR* gene amplification, or combined gain of chromosome 7 and loss of chromosome 10. All grade 2 to 4 gliomas are diffuse and infiltrate widely into the brain, and the lower grade lesions may progress to higher grade tumors over time. Grade 1 lesions such as the pilocytic astrocytoma are extremely low-grade focal tumors that have a separate designation; they are more common in children, may be associated with neurofibromatosis type 1, and are often cured by complete surgical excision.

EPIDEMIOLOGY

Gliomas occur at any age, but the peak is ages 20 to 30 years for grade 2 lesions, age 40 years for grade 3 tumors, and age 55 to 60 years for glioblastoma. For all grades of glioma, men are more frequently affected than women, and White persons are significantly more frequently affected than Black persons. Gliomas are typically single lesions, but multifocal disease is seen in approximately 5% of patients with high-grade tumors.

PATHOBIOLOGY

At least 95% of gliomas are sporadic, and only 5% occur in patients with a family history of brain tumor. Furthermore, patients with a familial history of glioma usually do not fall into a well-recognized hereditary syndrome.

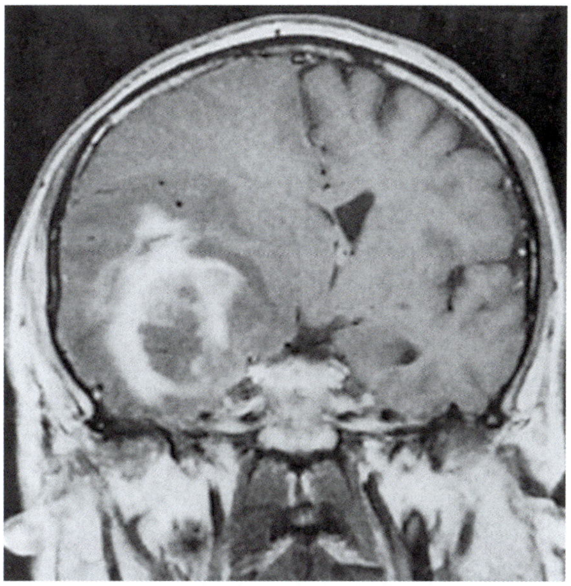

FIGURE 175-5. **Temporal lobe glioblastoma.** This T1-weighted gadolinium-enhanced magnetic resonance image shows a typical ring configuration of contrast material with central necrosis and marked mass effect.

Neurofibromatosis 1 (von Recklinghausen disease; Chapter 385) is associated with an increased incidence of gliomas, particularly in the optic pathway, hypothalamus, and brain stem. Gliomas also occur with increased frequency in Turcot and Lynch syndromes (Chapter 179), in which colorectal neoplasms are seen in association with a variety of CNS tumors. Somatic mutations of IDH1 and IDH2 have been identified in most lower grade gliomas.

CLINICAL MANIFESTATIONS AND DIAGNOSIS

Patients with gliomas often present with seizures, headache, and lateralizing signs such as hemiparesis, aphasia, or a visual field deficit. IDH-mutant astrocytomas and oligodendroglial tumors have a variable course, with the oligodendrogliomas being more indolent. These young adults often present with isolated seizures that can be controlled easily with antiepileptic agents.

On MRI, low-grade gliomas typically appear as diffuse, non-enhancing lesions with a propensity to occur in the frontal lobe and insular cortex (see Fig. 175-1). High-grade gliomas, which typically enhance with contrast material, occur in the cortical white matter and are accompanied by significant surrounding edema. Glioblastomas frequently have regions of central necrosis (Fig. 175-5), and hemorrhage can occur in 5 to 8% of patients.

TREATMENT AND PROGNOSIS

For all gliomas, treatment frequently involves surgery, radiation therapy, and chemotherapy.[10] The surgical goal of complete removal of all visible disease is often impossible; even when possible, residual tumor remains. The extent of resection can be optimized using intraoperative MRI guidance and fluorescence-guided resection using 5-aminolevulinic acid. The adequacy of resection is best assessed on a postoperative MRI, without and with gadolinium, performed within 24 to 96 hours after surgery. Glioma resections with intraoperative stimulation and cortical mapping are associated with fewer severe neurologic deficits and more extensive resection. Surgical removal usually improves neurologic function and reduces dependency on corticosteroids.

Age is the single most important clinical prognostic factor; younger patients live substantially longer than older patients. Tumors of any histology or grade with an IDH mutation have a significantly better prognosis than the identical tumor that is IDH-wildtype. Performance status, duration of symptoms, and whether a complete resection has been achieved are also strong predictors of improved outcome and prolonged survival.

Glioblastoma, IDH-Wildtype, Grade 4

All glioblastomas should be treated with postoperative radiation therapy to a dose of approximately 60 Gy. Hypofractionated radiotherapy is superior to standard radiation therapy in elderly patients with glioblastomas, especially in patients older than age 70 years.

The alkylating agent temozolomide (75 mg/m^2 daily orally), administered concurrently with radiation therapy and followed by adjuvant temozolomide (150 to 200 mg/m^2 for 5 consecutive days every 4 weeks for six cycles), can significantly improve median survival from 12.1 months to 14.6 months and more than double the 2-year survival rate to 26% compared with radiation therapy alone. Patients whose tumors contain a methylated promoter of the O6-methylguanine-DNA methyltransferase (MGMT) DNA repair gene benefit most from the addition of temozolomide.[11] In glioblastoma patients who have received standard radio-chemotherapy, the combination of maintenance temozolomide plus low-intensity alternating electric fields, which are delivered to the tumor through a portable medical device that is applied to the scalp, can improve progression-free survival and overall survival compared with maintenance temozolomide alone.[A1] The addition of bevacizumab, a monoclonal antibody that blocks vascular endothelial growth factor (VEGF), can be helpful to control cerebral edema, but it does not prolong survival and is not recommended for routine use in patients with newly diagnosed glioblastoma.

In almost all patients, the glioblastoma recurs following initial therapy. Recurrences can be treated with reoperation, stereotactic radiosurgery, tumor-treating fields, systemic agents, or a combination of approaches.[A2] Commonly used systemic therapies include temozolomide rechallenge, bevacizumab, and lomustine (alone or in combination with procarbazine and vincristine) under expert supervision.[12] A second course of radiation with concurrent bevacizumab is generally well tolerated and can prolong disease control.[A3] Chemotherapy is generally well tolerated and associated with minimal toxicity. Elderly patients, however, often do poorly, so alternative treatment approaches may be preferable. Since none of the currently available treatment approaches have been proven to prolong survival in recurrent glioblastoma, patients with recurrent glioblastoma should be encouraged to participate in a clinical trial whenever possible.

The median overall survival time for patients with glioblastoma is about 15 months. Key prognostic factors include patient age and performance status, as well as the presence or absence of *IDH* gene mutation and O6-methylguanine-DNA methyltransferase promoter methylation.

Astrocytomas, IDH Wildtype, Grade 2/3

No large randomized data exist to guide treatment decisions for patients with IDH-wildtype astrocytomas. Immediate postoperative radiation and chemotherapy, as described for the treatment of glioblastoma, are often used. However, close observation may be appropriate for young patients whose grade 2 tumors have undergone gross total resection.

Astrocytomas, IDH-Mutant, and All Oligodendrogliomas

For IDH-mutant astrocytomas and oligodendroglial tumors, resection should be performed at diagnosis. If a complete resection is achieved and the patient is younger than age 40 years, these patients have an excellent prognosis and may be followed with serial imaging alone to avoid long-term neurotoxicity from cranial irradiation.

For incompletely resected grade 2 tumors and for all grade 3 tumors, regardless of the degree of resection, however, immediate postoperative radiation plus adjuvant chemotherapy is recommended.[13] Postoperative radiation with adjuvant temozolomide is recommended for IDH-mutant astrocytomas.[A4] The combination of radiotherapy and chemotherapy with procarbazine, lomustine, and vincristine is superior to radiotherapy alone for patients with anaplastic oligodendroglial tumors.[A5]

Treatment is also instituted immediately after initial surgery in patients who have progressive neurologic symptoms or intractable seizures. It is also given at recurrence, sometimes following re-resection. Grade 2 tumors can transform to a higher-grade malignant neoplasm, a change that typically is associated with the appearance of contrast enhancement on MRI. Resection or a biopsy may be necessary in these patients to establish a change in grade, which often determines the appropriate dose of radiotherapy (60 Gy for high-grade lesions and about 54 Gy for low-grade tumors). Re-resection is followed by radiation therapy plus chemotherapy if patients have not received it previously. Salvage regimens include lomustine alone, bevacizumab, temozolomide (150 to 200 mg/m^2 for 5 days every 4 weeks for anywhere from 6 to 24 cycles), and carboplatin under expert supervision.

Optic and Brain Stem Glioma

Optic gliomas, which can involve the optic nerve or optic chiasm, are usually associated with neurofibromatosis type 1 (Chapter 385). Optic gliomas are typically pilocytic tumors that can have an indolent course, including rare spontaneous regression. Optic gliomas often are not amenable to surgical resection, and they can have a stuttering clinical course, with periods of visual loss punctuated by prolonged periods of visual stability. When necessary, radiation therapy or even chemotherapy may be useful under expert supervision, but often no treatment is required.

Brain stem gliomas usually involve the pons and less often the medulla or midbrain. Brain stem gliomas are most commonly seen in children in the first decade of life but can be found even in elderly people. Brain stem gliomas can have a low-grade or high-grade histology, but outcome is primarily determined by the location of the tumor. In general, most brain stem gliomas have a dismal outcome, with survival of 1 year or less, but relatively benign variants occasionally occur, especially in adults with tumors in the medulla or midbrain.

Medulloblastoma

Medulloblastomas usually occur in the vermis of the cerebellum and principally affect children and young adults. Boys outnumber girls by about 2 : 1, and peak onset is age 7 years. Medulloblastoma in postpubertal patients and adults is rare and usually affects the cerebellar hemisphere.

Transcription profiles have identified four distinct subclasses that include the Wnt subtype (10% of tumors) driven by a stabilizing mutation in *CTNNB1* (β-catenin), which has an excellent prognosis; the SHH subtype (30% of tumors) with mutations in *PTCH1, SMO, GLI2,* or *SUFU,* which has an intermediate prognosis; group 3 (25% of tumors), which has an increased expression of *MYC* and has the worst prognosis; and group 4 (35% of tumors), which is characterized by isochromosome 17q and marked male predominance.[14] Medulloblastomas have a characteristic clinical presentation, with ataxia (due to cerebellar and brain stem involvement), headache, nausea, and vomiting (due to increased intracranial pressure from obstructive hydrocephalus).

TREATMENT AND PROGNOSIS

Aggressive surgery with complete excision is strongly associated with improved outcome. Surgery is always followed by craniospinal radiation therapy.

Adults with medulloblastoma should receive adjuvant multiagent chemoradiotherapy (e.g., vincristine, lomustine or cyclophosphamide, and cisplatin) under expert supervision. This treatment is associated with 5-year overall survival rates of up to 70% in adults with medulloblastoma despite its considerable toxicity.

Whether molecular subclasses should supersede clinical stratification or dictate the selection of treatment is unknown. The SHH-driven tumors may respond to Smo inhibitors.

Therapy of medulloblastoma often results in delayed complications in survivors, including intellectual deficits, growth impairment, and endocrinologic dysfunction. Late relapses and secondary neoplasms compromise long-term outcome.

Ganglioglioma

Gangliogliomas possess both a glial component and a neoplastic neural component (ganglion cell). Some low-grade gangliogliomas are indolent and do not require additional treatment after surgical extirpation. Patients with anaplastic tumors may fare better than patients with malignant gliomas, but recurrence is the rule despite surgery and radiation therapy. Gangliogliomas and other circumscribed astrocytic gliomas, glioneuronal, and neuronal tumors frequently harbor somatic mutations in the *BRAF* gene and respond to inhibitors of the RAF-MEK signaling axis.[15]

PRIMARY CENTRAL NERVOUS SYSTEM LYMPHOMA

Primary CNS lymphomas are associated with immunodeficiency states, particularly acquired immunodeficiency syndrome and organ transplantation, and are seen with increased frequency among the apparently immunocompetent population, in whom the median age at diagnosis is about 60 years. These tumors are usually diffuse large B-cell non-Hodgkin lymphomas identical to systemic diffuse large B-cell lymphoma (Chapter 171).

CLINICAL MANIFESTATIONS AND DIAGNOSIS

The tumor can involve the cerebrospinal fluid, eye, and brain, where it is multifocal in about 40% of patients at presentation (Fig. 175-6). Biopsy is usually the preferred surgical approach.

TREATMENT

In contrast to all other brain tumors, surgical resection may not be associated with improved survival and can cause significant neurologic morbidity. Chemotherapy is the primary treatment, and high-dose methotrexate (3 to 8 g/m^2 on alternate weeks for 3 to 12 months) is the most important chemotherapeutic agent.[16] In most patients, radiation therapy is avoided because the necessary whole brain irradiation causes significant cognitive impairment when it is combined with chemotherapy and does not prolong survival. Corticosteroids (e.g., dexamethasone 8 to 16 mg/day), which are frequently used as part of the chemotherapeutic regimen, not only help manage the associated cerebral edema but also can cause tumor regression. Ibrutinib, which is an inhibitor of Bruton tyrosine kinase, has antitumor activity in recurrent or refractory primary CNS lymphoma.

With the use of multiagent chemotherapy, with or without cranial irradiation, median survival is 3 to 5 years. Younger patients who receive high-dose chemotherapy and autologous stem cell transplantation may have a 60 to 70% chance of cure.[A6]

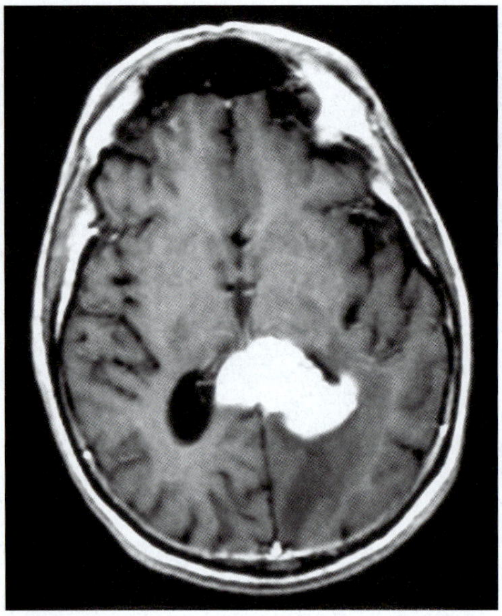

FIGURE 175-6. Primary central nervous system (CNS) lymphoma. A post-gadolinium magnetic resonance image demonstrating a diffusely enhancing splenial lesion. The periventricular location and absence of central necrosis are characteristic of primary CNS lymphoma.

OTHER INTRA-AXIAL PRIMARY BRAIN TUMORS

Rare, intra-axial cerebral tumors include ependymomas, which are optimally treated with surgical excision followed by radiation therapy.[17] Choroid plexus papillomas and carcinomas may be manifested with hydrocephalus or lateralizing signs. Resection may be sufficient for benign papillomas, but carcinomas rapidly recur even when postoperative radiation therapy is also used. Colloid cysts of the third ventricle are benign tumors that can cause obstructive hydrocephalus; they may be treated with a third ventriculostomy or with resection by use of an intraventricular endoscope.

Hemangioblastomas occur primarily in the cerebellum but can also occur in the spinal cord and the hemispheres. About 15% of patients with a hemangioblastoma have the autosomal dominant disorder von Hippel-Lindau disease (Chapter 385), which is characterized by hemangioblastomas in the CNS and retina, renal cell carcinoma, pheochromocytoma, endolymphatic sac tumors, and cysts in a variety of visceral organs. Hemangioblastomas are treated by surgical excision and require radiation therapy only for recurrence. Complete removal usually results in cure. The HIF-2α inhibitor belzutifan has shown promising antitumor activity against CNS hemangioblastomas in patients with von Hippel-Lindau disease.[18]

BRAIN METASTASIS

EPIDEMIOLOGY

Metastases are the most common intracranial tumors in adults. Every systemic cancer is capable of metastasizing to the brain. Melanoma (Chapter 188) has the greatest propensity to spread to the CNS, but the most common causes of CNS metastases are cancers of the lung (Chapter 177) and breast (Chapter 183). CNS metastases are being seen with greater frequency because patients with systemic cancers have prolonged survival with better treatments. In most patients with brain metastases, CNS disease develops late in the course of their illness, but a brain metastasis may be the initial presentation of a systemic cancer. In most of these patients, lung cancer is the primary site; in some, however, a primary site is never identified (Chapter 164).

CLINICAL MANIFESTATIONS AND DIAGNOSIS

Patients with brain metastases present with progressive neurologic symptoms and signs that typically include headache, seizures, and lateralizing signs. Metastases are best diagnosed by cranial MRI with gadolinium (Fig. 175-7). All lesions can be clearly seen by MRI, which is better than CT for visualizing the posterior fossa. Metastases, which are usually well-circumscribed lesions at the gray matter–white matter junction, are often associated with extensive edema. Hemorrhage into a metastasis occurs most frequently with metastases from melanoma, renal cancer, or thyroid cancer. Because brain metastases from lung cancer are so common, however, they are the most common hemorrhagic type. Sometimes, hemorrhage into a brain metastasis is best visualized by noncontrast head CT.

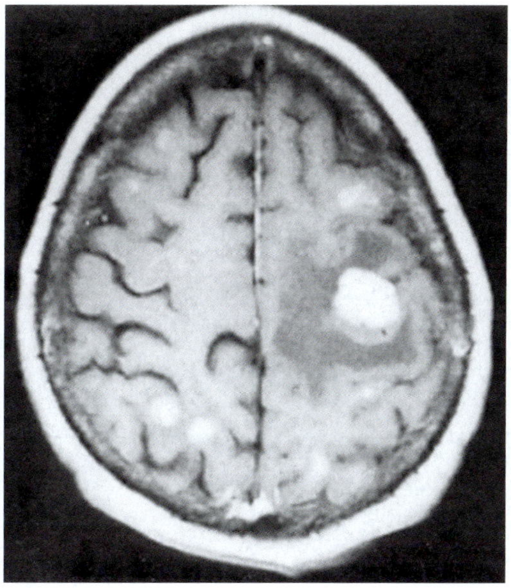

FIGURE 175-7. **Brain metastasis. Multiple metastases from breast carcinoma are seen on this T1-weighted gadolinium-enhanced magnetic resonance image. The multiple smaller tumors were not visible on computed tomography, even after a contrast agent was given.**

TREATMENT

The survival of patients with brain metastasis has been improved in recent decades by the increasingly individualized refinement of radiosurgical techniques and the development of more effective systemic therapies. Corticosteroids, especially dexamethasone (8 to 12 mg daily), are useful for symptomatic brain metastases. Anticonvulsant medications (Table 372-6) are required in patients who have seizures but are not recommended prophylactically in patients without seizures.[19]

Surgery

Because brain metastases do not widely infiltrate into brain tissue and tend to have a pseudo-capsule around them, they can be completely excised surgically. Complete removal of a single brain metastasis can substantially prolong life and maintain neurologic function. If multiple lesions can be completely resected, these patients do as well as patients in whom a single lesion has been removed.

Radiation Therapy

Postoperative whole brain radiation therapy significantly improves control of CNS disease after resection of a single brain metastasis, but it does not prolong survival because patients die of progressive systemic tumor.[20] The use of postoperative whole brain radiation therapy is frequently decided on an individual basis, but increasingly partial brain radiotherapy or stereotactic radiosurgery to the postoperative bed are used instead to avoid irradiating the entire brain. Nonetheless, many patients with multiple brain metastases are best treated with a course of whole brain radiation therapy, most commonly 3 Gy in 10 fractions for a total of 30 Gy. Stereotactic radiosurgery, with either a gamma knife that delivers gamma radiation from multiple cobalt sources or a linear accelerator that delivers x-rays to a highly focused area involving the tumor, has been effective for the treatment of patients with one to three brain metastases, resulting in less cognitive deterioration at 3 months, with no difference in overall survival compared with whole brain radiotherapy.[A7,A8] Growing evidence suggests the use of stereotactic radiosurgery for as many as 10 brain metastases.

Most patients tolerate radiosurgery without difficulty, but the procedure is occasionally complicated by seizures or acute swelling that causes more neurologic dysfunction. Approximately 20 to 30% of patients develop radiation necrosis, which may be indistinguishable clinically and on MRI from recurrent tumor. One advantage of stereotactic radiosurgery is that most of the normal brain is not exposed to the radiation.

Systemic Therapy

Chemotherapy is used to treat brain metastases from highly chemosensitive primary cancers, such as testicular cancer (Chapter 185), small cell lung cancer (Chapter 177), and, to a lesser extent, breast cancer (Chapter 183). Bevacizumab under expert supervision can be effective in progressive brain metastases or radionecrosis after stereotactic radiosurgery. Chemotherapy also has increasingly been used in asymptomatic patients in whom brain metastases are identified at diagnosis on a screening MRI examination and who require chemotherapy for their systemic disease. Brain metastases will frequently respond in a fashion comparable to other systemic sites of disease.

The choice of agents is based on the primary type of cancer and the patient's prior drug exposures under expert supervision. For patients with *BRAF*-mutant melanoma (Chapter 188), for example, the combination of BRAF plus MEK inhibition (dabrafenib plus trametinib) can achieve intracranial responses.[21] Similarly, systemic immunotherapy with nivolumab plus ipilimumab can provide clinically meaningful intracranial activity against asymptomatic melanoma brain metastases.[A9] Upfront systemic therapy with the combination of the HER2 kinase inhibitor tucatinib, capecitabine, and trastuzumab can be considered for the treatment of asymptomatic brain metastases in HER2-positive metastatic brain cancer patients (Chapter 183) who were previously treated with trastuzumab, pertuzumab, and trastuzumab-emtansine (T-DM1).[A10] Systemic therapy with newer-generation CNS-penetrant tyrosine kinase inhibitors, rather than radiation or surgery, is increasingly used for the initial treatment of lung cancer patients (Chapter 177) whose tumors harbor EGFR mutations, anaplastic lymphoma kinase (ALK) translocations, c-ROS oncogene 1 (ROS1)-rearrangements, RET fusions, or MET exon-14-skipping mutations.

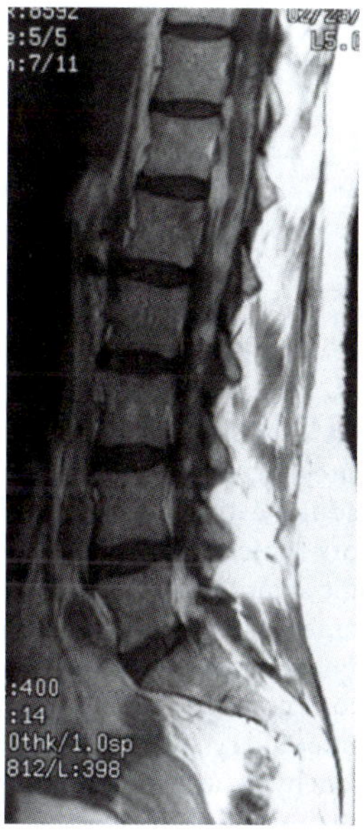

FIGURE 175-8. **Leptomeningeal metastases. Gadolinium-enhanced magnetic resonance imaging of the lumbosacral spine in a patient with leptomeningeal metastases from melanoma. Multiple enhancing nodules are seen on the cauda equina, and the conus medullaris and lower spinal cord are encased by tumor.**

INTRACRANIAL LEPTOMENINGEAL METASTASIS

The brain is the most common intracranial site of metastases, but systemic cancer can spread to the dura and the leptomeninges as well. Dural metastases most commonly arise from breast (Chapter 183) or prostate (Chapter 186) cancer, frequently from a metastasis in the overlying calvaria.

CLINICAL MANIFESTATIONS AND DIAGNOSIS

Metastasis to the leptomeninges is often manifested as multifocal neurologic symptoms and signs. These metastases involve the cranial nerves to cause diplopia or bulbar palsy (E-Fig. 175-1); the cervical and lumbar roots to cause limb pain or weakness; and the intracranial space to cause headache, nausea, vomiting, and elevated intracranial pressure. The diagnosis is established by the presence of tumor cells in the cerebrospinal fluid, by cytologic examination or novel techniques to identify isolated cancer cells, or by neuroimaging that definitively outlines tumor in the subarachnoid space (Fig. 175-8).

TREATMENT

Treatment frequently involves radiation therapy to symptomatic sites. Intrathecal chemotherapy, usually through an intraventricular cannula (Ommaya reservoir), or systemic chemotherapy with agents or doses that penetrate into the cerebrospinal fluid are also used under expert supervision.

TABLE 175-5 SPINAL TUMORS

EXTRADURAL	
Metastasis	
Primary bone tumors arising in the spine	
	Chordoma
	Osteogenic sarcoma
	Chondrosarcoma
	Plasmacytoma
INTRADURAL EXTRAMEDULLARY	
Meningiomas	
Neurofibromas	
Schwannomas	
Lipomas	
Arachnoid cysts	
Epidermoid cysts	
Metastasis	
INTRAMEDULLARY	
Ependymoma	
Glioma	
Hemangioblastoma	
Lipoma	
Metastasis	

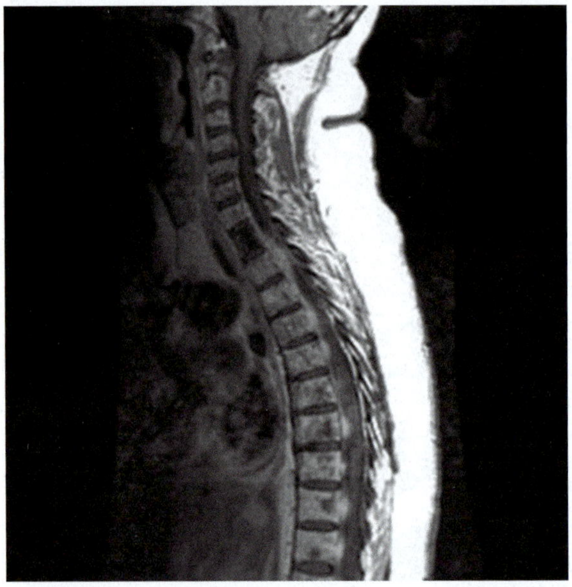

FIGURE 175-9. Multilevel epidural spinal cord compression. This patient with metastatic breast cancer has multiple areas of ventral epidural tumor seen throughout the thoracic spine on this post-gadolinium sagittal magnetic resonance image.

SPINAL TUMORS

Spinal tumors can be categorized according to the anatomic area they involve: extradural, intradural extramedullary, and intramedullary (Table 175-5). Extradural tumors typically arise from the bone elements of the spine and cause neurologic symptoms and signs by compressing the spinal cord. Intradural but extramedullary tumors arise from the pachy-meninges or nerve roots (meningiomas or schwannomas) and can cause either radicular symptoms or spinal cord compression. Most intradural extramedullary tumors are benign. Intramedullary spinal cord tumors are rare; they arise from the spinal cord parenchyma and have a biology that is similar to the biology of brain tumors.

EXTRADURAL TUMORS

Most extradural tumors originate from a metastasis to the bone elements of the spine, typically the vertebral body and occasionally the vertebral lamina or spinous process. Expansile growth of the bone tumor impinges on the spinal canal and, if untreated, compresses the spinal cord or the nerve roots as they exit the intervertebral foramina. Whereas most of these lesions arise from bone metastases, extradural tumors can also arise from paravertebral metastases that can grow through the intervertebral foramina and into the epidural space without affecting surrounding bone structures. Very rarely, a direct metastasis to the epidural space is also seen. The most common primary cancers that cause extradural metastases are prostate cancer (Chapter 186), breast cancer (Chapter 183), lung cancer (Chapter 177), and the lymphomas (Chapters 171 and 172). Hematologic malignant neoplasms may be associated with paravertebral disease that grows through the intervertebral foramina. Less common are primary tumors of the spine, including chordomas, osteogenic sarcomas, plasmacytomas, and chondrosarcomas.

CLINICAL MANIFESTATIONS

Extradural tumors cause neurologic symptoms and signs by compressing the spinal cord. Although the mass is a primary bone tumor or a metastasis from a distant source, 98% of patients present with pain that is usually localized to the site of the tumor. Because the spine has more thoracic than cervical or lumbar vertebrae, the tumor and pain are likely to be in the middle or high back, a site that is a less common site for benign pain (Chapter 369). Back pain often precedes the development of any other neurologic symptom or sign, frequently by weeks and occasionally by months. Motor impairment and sensory symptoms are present in about 50% of patients, whereas sphincter disturbances are found in only about 25% of patients.

DIAGNOSIS

Severe back pain in a patient with cancer should be evaluated by MRI, which does not require intravenous administration of contrast material. Plain films of the spine, bone scans, or even CT scans may show bone disease, but epidural tumor can only be seen only on MRI (Fig. 175-9). Furthermore, MRI is the only technique that can reveal paravertebral or direct epidural metastasis. Patients who cannot have an MRI study should be imaged by CT with sagittal reconstruction images.

The differential diagnosis of extradural tumors includes epidural abscess (Chapter 382), acute or subacute epidural hematomas (Chapter 369), herniated intervertebral discs (Chapter 369), spondylosis (Chapter 369), epidural lipomatosis, and, rarely, extramedullary hematopoiesis. On occasion, a percutaneous needle biopsy or decompressive laminectomy is required to make a definitive diagnosis.

TREATMENT

Epidural metastases require immediate treatment because patients can develop acute and unpredictable neurologic deterioration resulting in paraplegia.[22] Patients should be started on high-dose corticosteroids (usually >20 mg of intravenous dexamethasone), which rapidly relieve pain and may contribute to neurologic recovery.

Surgery followed by postoperative radiation therapy is superior to radiation therapy alone for preserving the ability to walk and may prolong survival in a wide population of patients with metastatic spinal cord compression. However, it may not benefit patients who are age 65 years and older.

Stereotactic radiosurgery is also an effective option to treat epidural metastases, either initially or at the time of relapse.[A11] It is much easier to preserve neurologic function than to reverse impairment, so clinically silent areas of extradural tumor that are detected on MRI should be treated before neurologic compromise develops. Patients with epidural metastasis can have a good neurologic outcome if they are treated before the onset of severe neurologic compromise, but their overall survival is usually short because of the presence of widespread metastatic disease.

Patients whose primary tumor arises in the spine, such as an osteogenic sarcoma (Chapter 187), should undergo definitive surgery. The need for postoperative radiation therapy is based on the tumor's histology.

INTRADURAL EXTRAMEDULLARY TUMORS

MENINGIOMAS

Spinal meningiomas are benign, slow-growing tumors that occur primarily in middle-aged women and are predominantly located in the thoracic region.

Back pain is a common symptom, but about 25% of patients have no pain and present with slowly progressive neurologic dysfunction, typically a gait disorder that has been progressing, frequently for years. Spinal MRI with gadolinium clearly delineates the lesion. Surgical resection is curative, and a complete resection can usually be accomplished easily.

NERVE SHEATH TUMORS

Nerve sheath tumors include schwannomas and neurofibromas. Both typically arise from the dorsal root, and the first symptom is often radicular pain that precedes symptoms of spinal cord compression by months or even years. Some patients with spinal neurofibroma or schwannoma have neurofibromatosis type 1 (Chapter 385), but most do not. The diagnosis is clearly established by gadolinium-enhanced MRI of the spine. The treatment is surgical, and complete removal results in cure.

METASTASES

Metastasis to the spinal leptomeninges can be manifested as an intradural extramedullary lesion. A single large tumor nodule can cause focal symptoms and signs referable to that spinal level. In most patients, however, multiple levels of the neuraxis are involved, and patients have multifocal neurologic symptoms and signs. Cervical and lumbosacral radicular pain, as well as sensory and motor loss, are seen in more than half of patients. The diagnosis is established by gadolinium-enhanced MRI showing multifocal nodules or sometimes a layer of cells coating the spinal cord or nerve roots (see Fig. 175-9). If imaging is negative, the diagnosis can be established by demonstrating tumor cells in the cerebrospinal fluid.

TREATMENT

Because of the diffuse nature of the disease, surgery is not an option. Treatment is complicated and frequently requires radiation therapy to symptomatic sites of disease, intrathecal chemotherapy best administered through an intraventricular cannula (Ommaya device) and occasionally systemic chemotherapy under expert guidance. Radiation therapy can ameliorate neurologic symptoms, particularly pain, but the disease often has a relentless progressive course, and results in death in 3 to 6 months despite aggressive therapy.

INTRAMEDULLARY TUMORS

Intramedullary spinal cord tumors are similar to neoplasms that arise in brain parenchyma. The most common spinal cord tumors are ependymomas and astrocytomas. Hemangioblastomas (particularly in association with von Hippel-Lindau disease), lipomas, and, rarely, intramedullary metastases are also seen.

CLINICAL MANIFESTATIONS AND DIAGNOSIS

All intramedullary tumors have a similar clinical presentation, and pain is a common initial symptom. Signs of spinal cord dysfunction subsequently ensue and reflect the location of the lesion. In addition, some intramedullary tumors are accompanied by a syrinx (Chapter 389), which can contribute to symptoms. The classic signs of intramedullary spinal cord lesions, such as dissociated sensory loss, sacral sparing, and early sphincter problems, are not sufficiently reliable to distinguish intramedullary from extramedullary lesions. The diagnosis is established by gadolinium-enhanced and T2-weighted MRI (Fig. 175-10).

TREATMENT

Surgery is the first therapeutic intervention, both to obtain a definitive diagnosis and to resect the lesion. Complete resection of spinal cord tumors is possible, particularly in the case of ependymomas and hemangioblastomas. However, spinal cord tumors are rare, and only neurosurgeons experienced in removal of this type of lesion should perform the procedure. High-grade gliomas and residual ependymomas should be treated with postoperative radiation therapy. Low-grade astrocytomas of the spinal cord can be treated with radiation therapy when the patient develops symptomatic neurologic impairment. Presymptomatic treatment does not prevent the development of impairment nor necessarily delay it. Intramedullary metastases do not require surgery because the diagnosis is usually straightforward. Radiation therapy provides limited benefit because these patients typically have other CNS metastases.

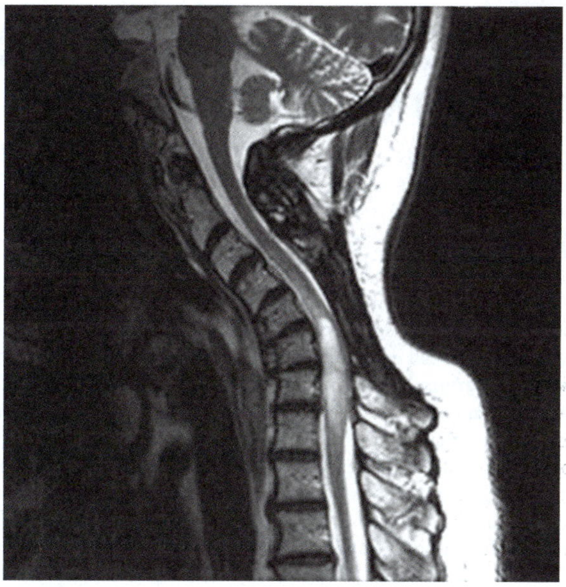

FIGURE 175-10. Spinal cord astrocytoma. T2-weighted sagittal magnetic resonance image demonstrating a lower cervical intramedullary low-grade astrocytoma; no enhancement was evident.

GENERAL REFERENCES

For the General References and other additional features, please visit Elsevier eBooks+ at https://ebooks.health.elsevier.com.

Grade A References

A1. Stupp R, Taillibert S, Kanner A, et al. Effect of tumor-treating fields plus maintenance temozolomide vs maintenance temozolomide alone on survival in patients with glioblastoma: a randomized clinical trial. *JAMA.* 2017;318:2306-2316.

A2. McBain C, Lawrie TA, Rogozinska E, et al. Treatment options for recurrent glioblastoma: a network meta-analysis. *Cochrane Database Syst Rev.* 2021;5:CD013579.

A3. Tsien CI, Pugh SL, Dicker AP, et al. NRG Oncology/RTOG1205: a randomized phase II trial of concurrent bevacizumab and reirradiation versus bevacizumab alone as treatment for recurrent glioblastoma. *J Clin Oncol.* 2023;41:1285-1295.

A4. van den Bent MJ, Tesileanu CMS, Wick W, et al. Adjuvant and concurrent temozolomide for 1p/19q non-co-deleted anaplastic glioma (CATNON; EORTC study 26053-22054): second interim analysis of a randomised, open-label, phase 3 study. *Lancet Oncol.* 2021;22:813-823.

A5. Lassman AB, Hoang-Xuan K, Polley MC, et al. Joint final report of EORTC 26951 and RTOG 9402: phase III trials with procarbazine, lomustine, and vincristine chemotherapy for anaplastic oligodendroglial tumors. *J Clin Oncol.* 2022;40:2539-2545.

A6. Houillier C, Dureau S, Taillandier L, et al. Radiotherapy or autologous stem-cell transplantation for primary CNS lymphoma in patients age 60 years and younger: long-term results of the randomized phase II PRECIS study. *J Clin Oncol.* 2022;40:3692-3698.

A7. Gaebe K, Li AY, Park A, et al. Stereotactic radiosurgery versus whole brain radiotherapy in patients with intracranial metastatic disease and small-cell lung cancer: a systematic review and meta-analysis. *Lancet Oncol.* 2022;23:931-939.

A8. Hartgerink D, Bruynzeel A, Eekers D, et al. Quality of life among patients with 4 to 10 brain metastases after treatment with whole-brain radiotherapy vs. stereotactic radiotherapy: a phase III, randomized, Dutch multicenter trial. *Ann Palliat Med.* 2022;11:1197-1209.

A9. Long GV, Atkinson V, Lo S, et al. Combination nivolumab and ipilimumab or nivolumab alone in melanoma brain metastases: a multicentre randomised phase 2 study. *Lancet Oncol.* 2018;19:672-681.

A10. Lin NU, Borges V, Anders C, et al. Intracranial efficacy and survival with tucatinib plus trastuzumab and capecitabine for previously treated HER2-positive breast cancer with brain metastases in the HER2CLIMB trial. *J Clin Oncol.* 2020;38:2610-2619.

A11. Sahgal A, Myrehaug SD, Siva S, et al. Stereotactic body radiotherapy versus conventional external beam radiotherapy in patients with painful spinal metastases: an open-label, multicentre, randomised, controlled, phase 2/3 trial. *Lancet Oncol.* 2021;22:1023-1033.

176

HEAD AND NECK CANCER

JULIE E. BAUMAN

DEFINITION

Head and neck cancer arises from the mucosal linings of the upper aerodigestive tract, sinonasal cavities of the face, major or minor salivary glands, or the structures of the base of skull including cranial nerves. The dominant histology, squamous cell carcinoma, comprises more than 95% of cancers of the oral cavity, pharynx, larynx, and paranasal sinuses (Fig. 176-1). Due to the sun-exposed cutaneous surface area of the scalp and face, nonmelanomatous skin cancers, in particular basal cell carcinoma and squamous cell carcinoma, are also frequent within the head and neck. Other less common neoplasms occurring within the anatomic structures of the head and neck include sarcoma as well as cutaneous or mucosal melanoma, which are treated according to the principles for these mesodermal malignancies (Chapters 187 and 188, respectively).

Oral Cavity

The margins of the oral cavity extend superiorly from the skin-vermillion border of the upper lip to the junction of the soft and hard palates, inferiorly from the skin-vermillion border of the lower lip to the circumvallate papillae, and laterally to the anterior tonsillar pillars. The structures of the oral cavity include the mucosal lip, buccal mucosa, upper and lower alveolar ridges, retromolar trigone, floor of the mouth, hard palate, and oral or mobile tongue.

Nasopharynx

The margins of the nasopharynx start anteriorly at the posterior choana and extend along the superior, posterior, and lateral walls to a theoretical plane between the free edge of the soft palate and the posterior pharyngeal wall. The structures of the nasopharynx include the fossae of Rosenmüller, the superior surface of the soft palate, and the mucosal linings of the eustachian tube and choanal orifices.

Oropharynx

The margins of the oropharynx extend from the plane of the superior surface of the soft palate to the superior surface of the vallecula, or hyoid bone. The structures of the oropharynx include the base of the tongue (the lingular tonsil), the palatine tonsils, the glossotonsillar sulcus, the inferior surface of the soft palate and uvula, the anterior and posterior tonsillar pillars, and the continuity of the lateral and posterior pharyngeal walls. Oropharyngeal squamous cell carcinoma largely arises from the rich lymphoreticular tissue of the lingular and palatine tonsils.

Hypopharynx

The margins of the hypopharynx extend from the plane of the superior border of the vallecula to the plane of the lower border of the cricoid cartilage. The structures of the hypopharynx include the pyriform sinuses, the lateral and posterior hypopharyngeal walls, and the postcricoid region.

Larynx

The margins of the larynx include anteriorly the anterior surface of the epiglottis, the thyroid cartilage, and the anterior arch of the cricoid cartilage; posterolaterally the aryepiglottic folds and arytenoids; superolaterally the tip and lateral borders of the epiglottis; and inferiorly the plane of the inferior border of the cricoid cartilage. The structures of the larynx include the epiglottis and false cords (supraglottic larynx), the true vocal cords (glottis), and the subglottis.

Salivary Glands

The salivary glands of the head and neck comprise the major salivary glands, which include the parotid, submandibular, and sublingual glands, as well as the minor salivary glands, which are scattered throughout the lining of paranasal sinuses, oral cavity, pharynx, and larynx. Approximately 6 to 8% of head and neck cancers arise from the salivary glands. Although the unified biologic function of salivary glands is the production and secretion of saliva, salivary gland tumors are histologically, genetically, and prognostically diverse. The three most common histologies are mucoepidermoid carcinoma, adenoid cystic carcinoma, and salivary duct carcinoma, which presents de novo or arises from a preexisting pleomorphic adenoma.

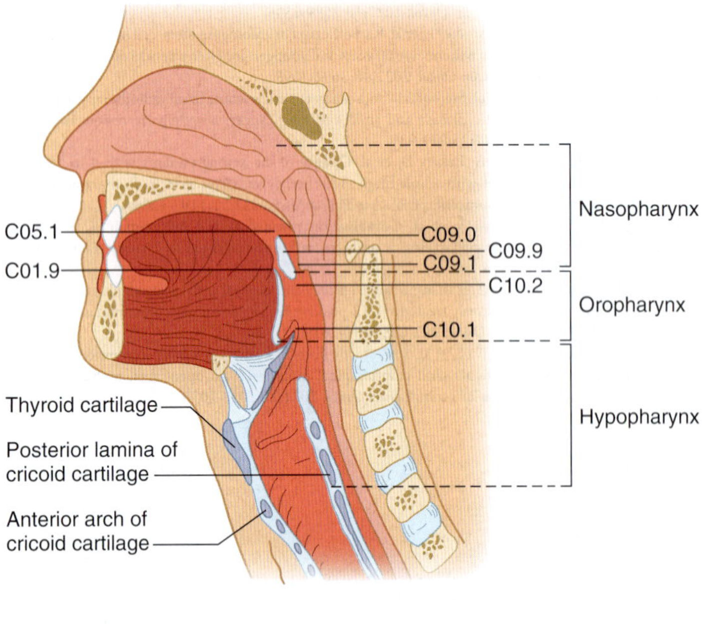

FIGURE 176-1. **More than 95% of head and neck cancers arise from the mucosal surfaces of the upper aerodigestive tract.** Specific anatomic sites are associated with unique etiologies, including environmental and viral risk factors, and underpin modern staging systems and treatment paradigms.

EPIDEMIOLOGY

Head and neck cancer is the seventh most common incident cancer worldwide. Among the more than 900,000 index cases of head and neck squamous cell carcinoma estimated in 2020, the substantial majority was caused by environmental carcinogenesis.[1]

Viruses

Human Papillomavirus

Oropharyngeal squamous cell carcinomas also can be caused by oncogenic human papillomaviruses (HPVs). Oral HPV 16 infection (Chapter 344) is responsible for about 80% of oropharyngeal cancers in the United States and is the cause of the ongoing epidemic of oropharyngeal squamous cell carcinoma predominantly occurring in males across all inhabited continents. Patients who are diagnosed with HPV-associated oropharyngeal squamous cell carcinoma have a lower median age at diagnosis, 58 years, than patients with environmental head and neck squamous cell carcinoma. The male:female incidence ratio is approximately 5 : 1.

Oral HPV infection is sexually transmitted and consistently associated with oral sexual behavior, including oral-oral, oral-genital, and oral-anal exposures. The prevalence of oral oncogenic HPV infection has two distinct peaks among males: between ages 25 and 30 years and 55 and 60 years, whereas the median age at diagnosis of HPV-associated oropharyngeal squamous cell carcinoma is 58 years. Thus, the estimated latency period between initial oral HPV infection and the development of oropharyngeal squamous cell carcinoma is approximately 10 to 30 years.

In the United States, the proportion of oropharyngeal squamous cell carcinoma cases infected with HPV has increased substantially. Furthermore, the incidence of human papillomavirus–associated oropharyngeal squamous cell carcinoma in the United States surpassed the incidence of cervical cancer in 2016. Incidence rates of HPV-associated oropharyngeal squamous cell carcinoma also have been rising in Europe, Australia, Asia, Brazil, and Peru, although large regional, racial, and ethnic variations exist as demonstrated by lower rates in Central Europe, some regions of Latin America, and among Blacks and Hispanics in the United States.

Epstein-Barr Virus

The dominant risk factor for nasopharyngeal carcinoma is infection with the Epstein-Barr virus (Chapter 348), which is an endemic cause of nasopharyngeal carcinoma in Southeast Asia, North Africa, and circumpolar indigenous populations, where the median age of diagnosis is age 50 years.[2] Head and neck cancer related to the oncogenic Epstein-Barr virus is also predominantly observed in males, with a male:female incidence ratio of approximately 3 : 1.

Human Immunodeficiency Virus (HIV)

The age-standardized incidence of HPV-associated and HPV-negative head and neck squamous cell carcinoma is three-fold higher in HIV-infected individuals than in the general U.S. population. Although the excess in tobacco-related cancers is decreasing in this population, likely due to declining tobacco use, the excess of HPV-associated head and neck squamous cell carcinoma is increasing. Unlike cervical cancer, HPV-associated oropharyngeal squamous cell carcinoma is not considered an AIDS-defining cancer. Nonetheless, the prevalence of oral HPV infection in HIV-infected people is inversely related to the $CD4^+$ T-cell count, thereby indicating that HIV-induced immunosuppression and the associated failure to control oncogenic HPV are major contributors to rising incidence rates.

Environmental Carcinogens

The risk of environmental head and neck squamous cell carcinoma increases with age, with diagnosis at a median age of 66 years. Environmental risk factors can be proximal, when modifiable individual behavior causes direct carcinogen exposure from tobacco, alcohol,[3] or the areca nut (Chapter 165). Depending upon the world region, approximately half of attributable risk for head and neck cancer is explained by such proximal environmental risk factors. Distal environmental risk factors also pose a substantial burden in developing countries when unavoidable exposures to secondhand smoke, industrial pollution, pestilence, or war are especially associated with low socioeconomic status. Incidence patterns for head and neck cancer caused by environmental carcinogenesis vary in relationship to exposure patterns. In the populations of the United States, Hong Kong, and the Republic of Korea, for example, the incidence of environmental head and neck squamous cell carcinoma is declining in parallel to decreased overall use of tobacco, whereas the incidence is rising in Taiwan, England, and Peru.[4]

Occupational exposures associated with head and neck cancer include the group 1 human carcinogen solvents, polycyclic aromatic hydrocarbons, and heavy metals. For head and neck cancer, the strongest data point to formaldehyde for nasopharynx cancer, polycyclic aromatic hydrocarbons for larynx cancer, chlorinated solvents for all head and neck squamous cell carcinoma anatomic sites, and wood dust for sinonasal cancer.

Leukoplakia

The minority of oral squamous cell cancers are preceded by precancerous lesions, termed *oral potentially malignant disorders*. Acquired potentially malignant disorders, including *leukoplakia* (mucosal white patches or plaques that cannot be rubbed off) and *erythroplakia* (a fiery red patch that cannot be characterized clinically or pathologically as any other diagnosis; Chapter 393), are associated with the consumption of tobacco and alcohol.[5] The presence of loss of heterozygosity within an oral potentially malignant lesion is associated with higher risk of progression to oral cancer within the lesion itself or at another site within the carcinogen-exposed epithelium and is useful for risk stratification.[6]

Sex and Genetic Risk Factors

Males demonstrate a significantly higher risk than females for head and neck squamous cell carcinoma, whether caused by environmental carcinogens or oncogenic viruses. The male:female ratio for HPV-unrelated head and neck squamous cell carcinoma parallels the sex-specific prevalence of tobacco, alcohol, or areca nut use in any geographic area. For instance, the age-adjusted incidence rate of oral cavity cancer among men ranges from 1 to 16 per 100,000 population as compared with 0 to 10 per 100,000 among women. Despite a similar prevalence of anogenital HPV infection between adult males and females, males have significantly higher rates of oral HPV infection. In a population-based, cross-sectional study in the United States, 1.6% of men versus 0.3% of women harbored oral HPV 16. The disparity in HPV oral infection is reflected in the incidence rate of HPV-associated oropharyngeal squamous cell carcinoma, in which the male:female ratio ranges from 2.7 to 5.7. Plausible biologic explanations for this disparity are two-fold: oral HPV infections are cleared more slowly by males, and the linear dose-response relationship between lifetime number of sexual partners and the prevalence of oral HPV infection exists uniquely among males, thereby suggesting that males less frequently develop protective anti-HPV antibodies when exposed to anogenital HPV than do females.[7]

Genetically inherited disorders associated with oral leukoplakia and high risk of progression to head and neck squamous cell carcinoma include the rare bone marrow failure syndromes dyskeratosis congenita, which is caused by aberrant telomere biology, and Fanconi anemia, which is caused by inherited mutations in DNA repair genes (Chapter 151).

Dietary Factors

A reduced risk for head and neck squamous cell carcinoma has been associated with diets rich in fruits and vegetables, in particular the *Brassica* genus of cruciferous vegetables. Crucifers are rich in isothiocyanates, which are phytochemicals that potently induce cytoprotective enzymes that could mitigate the impact of environmental carcinogens including benzene, polycyclic aromatic hydrocarbons, and mutagenic aldehydes found in tobacco smoke and air pollution. People with incident environmental head and neck squamous cell carcinoma have lower serum levels of several micronutrients, including vitamin A and beta carotene, which may be surrogates for lower intake of fruits and vegetables.

Ionizing Radiation

Ionizing radiation was first recognized as a risk factor for both benign and malignant salivary gland tumors among long-term survivors of the Hiroshima and Nagasaki, Japan, atomic bombs. Increased odds of salivary gland tumors are also observed in people treated with therapeutic radiation during childhood, with evidence of a dose-response relationship. Unlike head and neck squamous cell carcinoma, salivary gland tumors are not associated with tobacco exposure, with the single exception of the benign Warthin tumor.

PATHOBIOLOGY

Environmental Carcinogenesis

The transformation of oral epithelial cells by environmental carcinogens is based on the principle of multistep carcinogenesis, in which the accumulation of structural and functional DNA damage drives stepwise clonal evolution. Loss of heterozygosity, also known as allelic imbalance, has been quantified across the histopathologic spectrum of hyperplasia, dysplasia, and carcinoma in situ to model malignant transformation. In essence, environmentally induced head and neck squamous cell carcinoma is characterized by loss of function of tumor suppressor genes and genes that influence NOTCH signaling.[8] A central, early molecular event is loss of heterozygosity at 9p21, which is the locus of the *CDKN2A* gene. *CDKN2A* encodes p16, which is a tumor suppressor that regulates cell cycle traversal from the G1 to S-phase. Mutation of *TP53* is a later molecular event. Mutations of *CDKN2A* and *TP53* are the most common genetic alterations in HPV-negative head and neck squamous cell carcinoma and are observed in 57% and 84% of cases, respectively. Moreover, expression of p16 is lost due to epigenetic silencing in an additional 30% of tumors, thereby leading to the histopathologic classification of HPV-negative head and neck squamous cell carcinoma as "p16-negative." *PIK3CA*, which encodes the alpha subunit of phosphoinositide-3-kinase (PI3K), is the most commonly mutated oncogene in HPV-negative head and neck squamous cell carcinoma.[9] Nongenomic activation of the oncogenes epidermal growth factor receptor (EGFR) and cyclooxygenase-2 (COX2) is induced by tobacco smoke and also increases during oral epithelial transformation. Aberrant activation of PI3K, EGFR, and COX2 contributes to uncontrolled cellular proliferation while subverting an appropriate apoptotic response to DNA damage.

Viral Carcinogenesis

HPV, which is a member of the *Papillomaviridae* family, is an epitheliotropic, double-stranded, circular DNA virus with more than 170 distinct genotypes (Chapter 344). The viral life cycle is strictly dependent upon the cellular differentiation program of the keratinocyte, and viral oncogene expression is coordinated with cellular division and stratification. Members of the alpha genus infect mucosa, and high-risk anogenital genotypes, including HPV 16 and 18, are the established cause of cervical cancer. HPV genotype 16 also has a predilection for the lymphoid-rich mucosa of the oropharynx, and it comprises more than 95% of DNA isolated from oropharyngeal squamous cell carcinoma specimens. In particular, the early genes, E6 and E7, are transcribed in the basal and parabasal cell layers. The E6 and E7 oncoproteins degrade two critical tumor suppressors, p53 and retinoblastoma, respectively. Retinoblastoma is a nuclear protein that serves as the major G1 checkpoint in cell cycle regulation. The functional loss of retinoblastoma and p53 permit unbridled cellular proliferation. As the keratinocyte stratifies into the spinous epithelium, late viral genes are expressed, including the L1 and L2 capsid proteins. Ultimately, progenitor virions are encapsidated and released from the anuclear, cornified keratinocytes. In an HPV-transformed malignancy, late viral gene expression is lost, and the virus fails to complete its life cycle. However, the E6 and E7 oncoproteins are preserved and necessary for maintenance of the transformed phenotype.

The mutational spectrum of HPV-associated oropharyngeal squamous cell carcinoma is distinct from that of HPV-negative disease. Although p53 dysfunction appears to be a universal requirement for squamous epithelial transformation, in HPV-associated oropharyngeal squamous cell carcinoma, this dysfunction is accomplished by the degradation of p53 protein by the E6 oncoprotein. Thus, in HPV-infected cells there is little selective advantage for *TP53* mutations, which are rarely identified in this setting. Likewise, genomic alterations in *CDKN2A* are not observed. In fact, as a consequence of negative feedback inhibition, p16 is upregulated as E7 degrades retinoblastoma, resulting in the histopathologic classification of HPV-positive oropharyngeal squamous cell carcinoma as "p16-positive." Diffuse nuclear and cytoplasmic immunohistochemical (IHC) staining for p16 is an accepted surrogate for HPV in oropharyngeal squamous cell carcinoma. The most common genomic alteration in HPV-associated oropharyngeal squamous cell carcinoma, found in approximately 50% of cases, is mutation or amplification of the oncogene *PIK3CA*. The selection for gain-of-function alterations in *PIK3CA* results in hyperactive PI3K pathway signaling, and the associated pro-proliferative, antiapoptotic phenotype may initially enhance the viral life cycle.

Immunology

Whether caused by environmental carcinogens or HPV oncogenes, head and neck squamous cell carcinoma demonstrates a markedly suppressive immune profile. Although immunogenic tumor antigens exist in head and neck squamous cell carcinoma, as confirmed by circulating T lymphocytes specific for p53 and the E6/E7 oncoproteins, head and neck squamous cell carcinoma evades recognition by selective loss of human leukocyte antigen I as well as antigen processing machinery. Head and neck squamous cell carcinoma also induces a tumor-permissive cytokine profile, in which immunosuppressive cytokines such as TGF-β, interleukin-6, and vascular endothelial growth factor predominate over immune-stimulatory cytokines such as IFN-γ or interleukin-12. Head and neck squamous cell carcinoma also demonstrates critical defects in immune effector cells. Tumor-infiltrating lymphocytes demonstrate low expression of costimulatory T-cell receptors, such as OX40 and CD137, and high expression of coinhibitory receptors, including the immune checkpoints cytotoxic T-lymphocyte–associated antigen 4 (CTLA-4) and programmed death 1 (PD-1).

Molecular Landscape of Salivary Gland Cancers

Approximately 90% of cases of mucoepidermoid carcinoma, which is the most common malignant salivary gland tumor, have the *MECT1-MAML2* gene fusion, which is now considered a genomic hallmark and used to establish pathologic diagnosis. Most adenoid cystic carcinomas harbor a gene rearrangement with the transcription factor *NFIB*, including *MYB-NFIB*, which is regulated by IGF1R in an AKT-dependent manner by overexpression of insulin growth factor receptor 1 (IGFR1). Secretory carcinoma, previously known as mammary analogue secretory carcinoma, is associated with *NTRK* gene fusions. Salivary duct carcinoma almost uniformly expresses the androgen receptor. Otherwise, salivary duct carcinoma demonstrates different genetic fingerprints depending upon whether it arises de novo or from a preexisting pleomorphic adenoma. De novo salivary ductal carcinoma frequently harbors somatic mutations in *HRAS*, *PIK3CA*, or both, whereas salivary ductal carcinoma from a preexisting pleomorphic adenoma is commonly enriched for HER2neu amplification.

CLINICAL MANIFESTATIONS

Oral Cavity Cancer

Proximal risk factors for oral cavity cancer include oral tobacco, tobacco smoke, areca nut (betel quid), alcohol, and poor dentition. Oral cavity cancers typically present at an early stage with the chief complaint of a persistent mouth sore, ulcer, or mass lesion.[10] Due to rich innervation, cancers of the mobile tongue are often painful and functionally interfere with the oral phase of eating. Dysarthria, but not hoarseness, can also be associated with larger lesions of the oral cavity.

HPV-Associated Oropharyngeal Squamous Cell Carcinoma

Risk factors for HPV-associated oropharyngeal squamous cell carcinoma include lifetime number of sexual partners and male sex. Although not pathognomonic, HPV-associated oropharyngeal squamous cell carcinoma typically presents with a small, asymptomatic T1-2 primary tumor and a persistent neck mass. Among squamous cell carcinomas of unknown primary metastatic to the cervical neck, the majority are p16-positive, and the primary is usually localized within the tonsil or base of the tongue. If an oropharynx tumor is more advanced, patients can present with globus sensation, throat pain, otalgia, dysphagia, odynophagia, or hemoptysis.

HPV-Unrelated Oropharyngeal Squamous Cell Carcinoma and Hypopharynx Cancer

Behavioral risk factors for HPV-unrelated oropharyngeal squamous cell carcinoma and hypopharynx cancer include tobacco smoke and alcohol. Due to occult anatomy, HPV-negative oropharynx and hypopharynx cancers often present with locally advanced T3-4 tumors that cause throat pain, dysphagia, or weight loss.

Larynx Cancer

Proximal risk factors for larynx cancer include tobacco smoking and alcohol use. Laryngeal cancers frequently present with hoarseness as early-stage T1-2 disease (Chapter 397). More advanced tumors can present with airway obstruction that requires emergent tracheostomy.

Nasopharyngeal Carcinoma

More than 70% of cases of nasopharyngeal carcinoma occur in Southeast Asia, although its incidence is declining worldwide. A painless cervical mass is the most common mode of presentation. Other associated symptoms include epistaxis, unilateral nasal obstruction, conductive hearing loss, and cranial nerve involvement.

Salivary Gland Tumors

Salivary gland tumors have a varied presentation depending upon the site of origin, with chief complaints including an uncomplicated parotid or submandibular mass, a new or growing oral or oropharyngeal lesion, dysphagia, cough, hoarseness, and even airway obstruction. A rare presentation is Bell palsy (Chapter 388) of cranial nerve VII, which courses through the deep parotid gland where occult tumors can be missed by routine inspection and palpation. The typical presentation of Bell palsy is acute, flaccid facial paralysis without an obvious parotid mass. If no mass is evident, cranial nerve VII palsy may initially be treated with steroids and antiviral therapy (Chapter 388), but follow-up for resolution is critical. An atypical presentation, such as a prodrome of unilateral facial twitching or spasm, slow progression over 1 month or more, or nonresolution after 4 months should trigger magnetic resonance imaging and referral to an otolaryngologist.

Other Head and Neck Tumors

Lymphomas frequently manifest either as neck nodes or in the lymphoid tissues of the ring of Waldeyer (Chapters 171 and 172). The tonsil is a preferred site for mantle cell and undifferentiated lymphomas. Solitary, extramedullary plasmacytoma (Chapter 173) can also occur in the nasopharynx or paranasal sinuses. Sarcomas (Chapter 187) in the head and neck include osteogenic sarcomas and nerve sheath tumors. Paragangliomas can be extensive, multicentric, and vascular. Rhabdomyosarcomas have a predilection for the orbit and sinuses. Melanomas and squamous cell cancers can be accompanied by neck adenopathy or parotid lesions.

DIAGNOSIS

Evaluation of a Neck Mass

In adults, particularly adults over age 40 years, a new neck mass requires a disciplined diagnostic approach with high suspicion for malignancy (Fig. 176-2). The mass, which can be a cystic mass, an enlarged lymph node, or a collection of lymph nodes (Chapter 154), should be considered cancer unless proved otherwise. In an adult male, HPV-associated oropharyngeal squamous cell carcinoma most commonly presents as a new painless neck mass. In endemic regions, Epstein-Barr virus–related nasopharyngeal carcinoma most commonly presents with a painless cervical neck mass, often in association with unilateral nasal obstruction and/or epistaxis. Supraclavicular masses usually are related to primary tumors below the clavicles, whereas submental, upper cervical, and midcervical neck masses almost always derive from head and neck tumors.

The differential diagnosis is framed by a detailed medical and social history, including assessment for time course; antecedent or current upper respiratory, dental, or sinus infection; epistaxis; dysphagia or odynophagia; otalgia; hoarseness; hemoptysis; B symptoms (fever, drenching night sweats, or weight loss); tobacco and alcohol habits; prior tobacco-related malignancy; prior

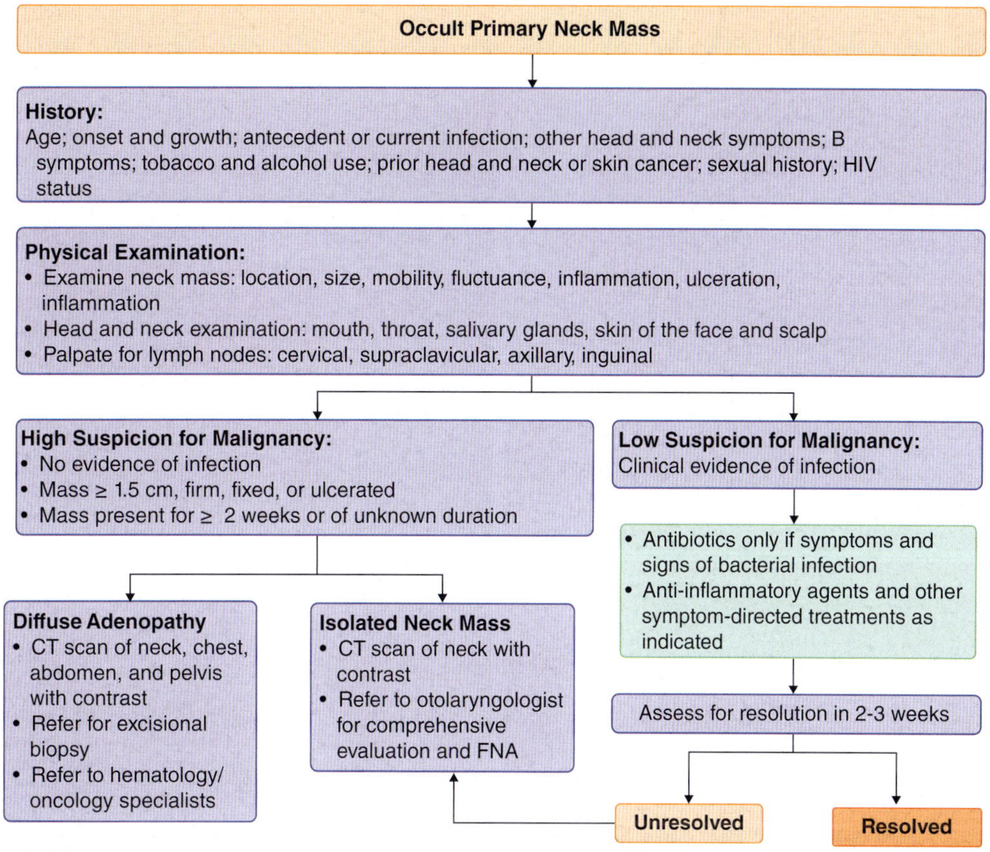

FIGURE 176-2. **Evaluation of an occult neck mass. B symptoms = fever, drenching night sweats, weight loss (>10% over 6 months); CT = computed tomography; FNA = fine needle aspiration; HIV = human immunodeficiency virus. (Adapted from Pynnonen MA, Gillespie MB, Roman B, et al. Clinical practice guideline: evaluation of the neck mass in adults. *Otolaryngol Head Neck Surg*. 2017;157[2 Suppl]:S1-S30.)**

skin cancer; sexual history; and HIV status. The physical examination should encompass the head and neck, including inspection and palpation of the oral cavity, oropharynx, and major salivary glands; inspection of the skin of the face and scalp; and a thorough examination of lymph nodes, including sites outside the neck.

The primary tumor site for an isolated upper cervical neck mass is most commonly found in the oropharynx (base of the tongue and tonsil), but salivary gland cancers, lymphomas, melanomas, and nonmelanoma skin cancers can also present in this manner. In East and Southeast Asia, a new neck mass also requires close examination of the nasopharynx.

Systemic symptoms or enlarged lymph nodes at other sites suggest lymphoma, whereas tenderness, warmth, and erythema suggest an infectious cause. Intraparotid nodes most commonly are metastases from skin malignancies. If the history and physical examination suggest reactive lymphadenopathy based on evidence of current or antecedent infection (Chapter 154), a brief course of observation or treatment with antimicrobial or anti-inflammatory medications is appropriate, but re-evaluation for resolution is critical. In all cases, a neck mass that persists for more than 3 weeks in an adult should prompt referral to an otolaryngologist to evaluate the patient for a potential malignancy.

Pathology

In the evaluation of a persistent neck mass, the initial test should be a fine needle aspiration (FNA) of the mass. Excisional biopsy is reserved for cases in which initial or repeat FNA is nondiagnostic and panendoscopy has identified no primary or when the baseline suspicion for lymphoma is very high due to extensive adenopathy outside of the neck (Chapter 154).

Ultimately, cytology or histology must confirm the diagnosis of head and neck squamous cell carcinoma. Environmental head and neck squamous cell carcinoma is associated with well to poorly differentiated cells, whereas well-differentiated tumors demonstrate unique features of keratinization including the presence of "keratin pearls" (Fig. 176-3 A and B). HPV-associated oropharyngeal squamous cell carcinoma is commonly associated with poorly differentiated or basaloid histology and lacks keratin pearls (Fig. 176-3 C and D). For oropharyngeal or unknown primary tumors, HPV status must be determined because it influences both staging and prognosis. The most widely used and accepted standard is immunohistochemistry for the cell cycle protein p16; diffuse nuclear and cytoplasmic staining in more than 70% of tumor cells signifies an HPV-positive tumor (Fig. 176-3E). Of note, p16 immunohistochemistry is not a direct measurement of the HPV 16 virus or its oncoproteins; rather, p16 overexpression confirms the presence of functionally relevant E7 oncoprotein. As such, p16 immunohistochemistry is not considered a surrogate for HPV infection outside of the oropharynx. Alternative methods for establishing the HPV status of oropharyngeal squamous cell carcinoma include in situ hybridization for HPV 16 DNA, multiplex polymerase chain reaction (PCR) for high-risk HPV genotypes, and detection of E6 and E7 mRNA by reverse transcription PCR.

Staging

Once a pathologic diagnosis of head and neck squamous cell carcinoma is established, the staging evaluation includes the following procedures:

- Complete head and neck examination with mirror or fiberoptic examination of the oropharynx, hypopharynx, larynx, and nasopharynx as indicated.
- Head and neck imaging. Locoregional staging is accomplished by a computed tomography (CT) or magnetic resonance imaging (MRI) scan of the primary and neck.
- Chest imaging. Less than 10% of patients with head and neck squamous cell carcinoma present with distant metastatic disease at diagnosis; however, distant metastases, when present, typically occur in the lungs. As a result, a diagnostic chest CT scan is a recommended component of staging; combined positron emission tomography (PET)/CT may also be considered, particularly in patients who have locally advanced tumors or nodal disease. Since patients with tobacco-related head and neck squamous cell carcinoma have a high risk for a second primary upper aerodigestive malignancy, including a head and neck, esophageal, or lung primary, a chest CT or PET/CT is also routinely indicated in such patients.
- The utility of panendoscopy under anesthesia with direct laryngoscopy, esophagoscopy, and bronchoscopy depends on expert consultation.

Each head and neck squamous cell carcinoma primary site has a staging system (Table 176-1). Staging for oral cavity tumors incorporates depth of invasion, tumor size, and invasion of adjacent structures. p16-positive (HPV-associated) oropharyngeal squamous cell carcinoma is distinguished from p16-negative oropharyngeal squamous cell carcinoma by a separate TNM staging system. p16-negative oropharyngeal squamous cell carcinoma is

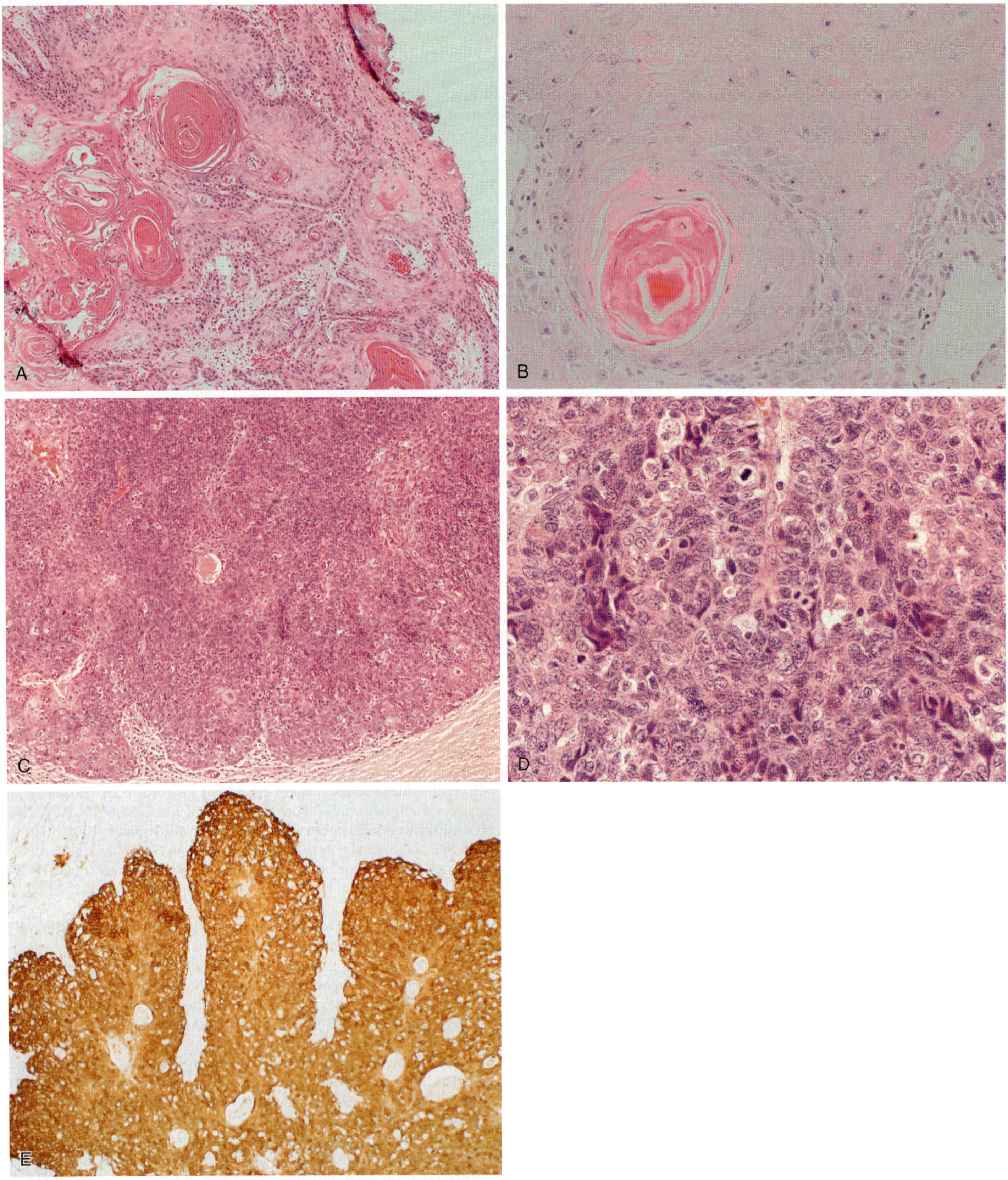

FIGURE 176-3. **Head and neck squamous cell carcinoma histology and immunohistochemistry. A,** The jagged outlines of well-differentiated squamous cell carcinoma tongues are associated with stromal desmoplastic reaction (low power). **B,** Keratin pearls, abnormal squamous cells forming concentric layers, are associated with well-differentiated squamous cell carcinoma (high power). **C,** Basaloid squamous cell carcinoma is frequently associated with human papillomavirus (HPV) infection, here demonstrating a highly infiltrative pattern of nests composed of poorly differentiated cells with pushing borders (low power). **D,** The basaloid squamous cell carcinoma cells demonstrate high nuclear to cytoplasmic ratios and numerous mitotic figures (high power). **E,** HPV-associated oropharyngeal squamous cell carcinoma shows poorly differentiated histology and diffuse nuclear and cytoplasmic staining for the p16 protein (high power).

grouped with hypopharynx cancers owing to the common etiology of environmental carcinogenesis, contiguous anatomy, and similarly poor prognosis. For hypopharynx and p16-negative oropharyngeal squamous cell carcinoma, tumor staging incorporates both size and invasion of adjacent structures. Staging of larynx cancer uniquely includes vocal cord mobility, where vocal cord fixation constitutes a T3 tumor irrespective of size. Due to distinct biology, patterns of spread, and natural history, nasopharyngeal carcinoma has its own staging system.

TABLE 176-1 CLINICAL PRIMARY TUMOR STAGING SYSTEM FOR HEAD AND NECK SQUAMOUS CELL CARCINOMA

TUMOR	LARYNX	LIP & ORAL CAVITY	HYPOPHARYNX	OROPHARYNX (p16-NEGATIVE)	OROPHARYNX (p16-POSITIVE)
T0	NA	NA	NA	NA	No primary identified
TX	Primary tumor cannot be assessed	Primary tumor cannot be assessed	Primary tumor cannot be assessed	Primary tumor cannot be assessed	NA
Tis	Carcinoma in situ	Carcinoma in situ	Carcinoma in situ	Carcinoma in situ	NA
T1	*Supraglottis*: Tumor limited to one subsite of supraglottis with normal vocal cord mobility *Subglottis*: Tumor limited to the subglottis *Glottis*: Tumor limited to the vocal cord(s) (may involve anterior or posterior commissure) with normal mobility	Tumor ≤2 cm, ≤5 mm depth of invasion (DOI) Note: DOI is depth of invasion and not tumor thickness	Tumor limited to one subsite of hypopharynx and/or ≤2 cm	Tumor ≤2 cm	Tumor ≤2 cm
T1a	*Glottis*: Tumor limited to one vocal cord				
T1b	*Glottis*: Tumor involves both vocal cords				
T2	*Supraglottis*: Tumor invades mucosa of more than one adjacent subsite of supraglottis or glottis or region outside the supraglottis (e.g., mucosa of base of tongue, vallecula, medial wall of pyriform sinus) without fixation of the larynx *Subglottis*: Tumor extends to vocal cord(s) with normal or impaired mobility *Glottis*: Tumor extends to supraglottis and/or subglottis, and/or with impaired vocal cord mobility	Tumor ≤2 cm, DOI >5 mm and ≤10 mm *or* tumor >2 cm but ≤4 cm, and ≤10 mm DOI	Tumor invades more than one subsite of hypopharynx or an adjacent site, or >2 cm but ≤4 cm without fixation of hemilarynx	Tumor >2 cm but ≤4 cm	Tumor >2 cm but ≤4 cm
T3	*Supraglottis*: Tumor limited to larynx with vocal cord fixation and/or invades any of the following: postcricoid area, preepiglottic space, paraglottic space, and/or inner cortex of thyroid cartilage *Subglottis*: Tumor limited to larynx with vocal cord fixation and/or invasion of paraglottic space and/or inner cortex of the thyroid cartilage *Glottis*: Tumor limited to the larynx with vocal cord fixation and/or invasion of paraglottic space and/or inner cortex of the thyroid cartilage	Tumor >4 cm *or* any tumor >10 mm DOI	Tumor >4 cm in greatest dimension or with fixation of hemilarynx or extension to esophagus	Tumor >4 cm or extension to lingual surface of epiglottis	Tumor >4 cm or extension to lingual surface of epiglottis
T4	Moderately advanced or very advanced	Moderately advanced or very advanced local disease	Moderately advanced or very advanced local disease	Moderately advanced or very advanced local disease	Moderately advanced local disease Tumor invades the larynx, extrinsic muscle of tongue, medial pterygoid, hard palate, or mandible or beyond Note: Mucosal extension to lingual surface of epiglottis from primary tumors of the base of the tongue and vallecula does not constitute invasion of the larynx
T4a	*Supraglottis*: Moderately advanced local disease. Tumor invades through the outer cortex of the thyroid cartilage and/or invades tissues beyond the larynx (e.g., trachea, soft tissues of neck including deep extrinsic muscle of the tongue, strap muscles, thyroid, or esophagus) *Subglottis*: Moderately advanced local disease. Tumor invades cricoid or thyroid cartilage and/or invades tissues beyond the larynx (e.g., trachea, soft tissues of neck including deep extrinsic muscles of the tongue, straps muscle, thyroid, or esophagus) *Glottis*: Moderately advanced local disease. Tumor invades through the outer cortex of the thyroid cartilage and/or invades tissues beyond the larynx (e.g., trachea, cricoid cartilage, soft tissues of neck including deep extrinsic muscle of the tongue, strap muscles, thyroid, or esophagus)	*Lip*: Tumor invades through cortical bone or involves the inferior alveolar nerve, floor of mouth, or skin of face (i.e., chin or nose) *Oral cavity*: Tumor invades adjacent structures only (e.g., through cortical bone of the mandible or maxilla, or involves the maxillary sinus or skin of the face) Note: Superficial erosion of bone/tooth socket (alone) by a gingival primary is not sufficient to classify a tumor as T4	Tumor invades thyroid/cricoid cartilage, hyoid bone, thyroid gland, or central compartment soft tissue Note: Central compartment soft tissue includes prelaryngeal strap muscles and subcutaneous fat	Tumor invades the larynx, extrinsic muscle of tongue, medial pterygoid, hard palate, or mandible Note: Mucosal extension to lingual surface of epiglottis from primary tumors of the base of the tongue and vallecula does not constitute invasion of the larynx	

TABLE 176-1 CLINICAL PRIMARY TUMOR STAGING SYSTEM FOR HEAD AND NECK SQUAMOUS CELL CARCINOMA—cont'd

TUMOR	LARYNX	LIP & ORAL CAVITY	HYPOPHARYNX	OROPHARYNX (p16-NEGATIVE)	OROPHARYNX (p16-POSITIVE)
T4b	Tumor invades prevertebral space, encases carotid artery, or invades mediastinal structures	Tumor invades masticator space, pterygoid plates, or skull base and/or encases the internal carotid artery	Tumor invades prevertebral fascia, encases carotid artery, or involves mediastinal structures	Tumor invades lateral pterygoid muscle, pterygoid plates, lateral nasopharynx, or skull base or encases carotid artery	
CLINICAL REGIONAL LYMPH NODE STAGING					
NX	Regional lymph nodes cannot be assessed				Regional lymph nodes cannot be assessed
N0	No regional lymph node metastases				No regional lymph node metastases
N1	Metastasis in a single ipsilateral lymph node, ≤3 cm and ENE(-)				≥1 ipsilateral lymph node, none >6 cm
N2	Assigned an N2 subcategory as identified below				Contralateral or bilateral lymph nodes, none >6 cm
N2a	Metastasis in a single ipsilateral lymph node >3 cm but <6 cm and ENE(-)				NA
N2b	Metastases in multiple ipsilateral lymph nodes, non >6 cm and ENE(-)				NA
N2c	Metastases in bilateral or contralateral lymph nodes, non >6 cm and ENE(-)				NA
N3	Assigned an N3 subcategory as identified later				Lymph node(s) >6 cm
N3a	Metastasis in a lymph node >6 cm and ENE(-)				NA
N3b	Metastasis in any node(s) and clinically overt ENE(+)				NA
OROPHARYNX (p16+) PROGNOSTIC STAGE GROUPS					
M0*	T0	T1	T2	T3	T4
N0	I	I	I	II	III
N1	I	I	I	II	III
N2	II	II	II	II	III
N3	III	III	III	III	III
*When M1, the stage group is IV for any N and T.					
LARYNX, LIP, AND ORAL CAVITY, HYPOPHARYNX, OROPHARYNX (p16–) PROGNOSTIC STAGE GROUPS					
M0*	T1	T2	T3	T4a	T4b
N0	I	II	III	IVA	IVB
N1	III	III	III	IVA	IVB
N2	IVA	IVA	IVA	IVA	IVB
N3	IVB	IVB	IVB	IVB	IVB
*When M1, the stage group is IVC for any N and T.					

ENE = extranodal extension; NA = not applicable.

AJCC Cancer Staging Manual, 8th ed. Chicago: American Joint Committee on Cancer and Springer; 2017.

TREATMENT

Multidisciplinary Team

In head and neck squamous cell carcinoma, both the cancer itself and its treatment place patients at risk for acute and long-term compromise of critical human functions, including speaking, eating, and breathing. Treatment by a multidisciplinary team composed of a surgical, medical, and radiation oncologist with specific expertise in head and neck cancer optimizes both oncologic and functional outcomes. Early consultation with specialists in dental sciences, nutrition, and speech and language pathology is also optimal. Given the social and behavioral risk factors associated with HPV-negative head and neck squamous cell carcinoma, the integration of patient navigators, social workers, and behavioral medicine specialists into the clinical management team can be particularly beneficial for addressing social isolation, transportation barriers, housing and food security, treatment compliance, and addiction.

Because more than 90% of index head and neck squamous cell carcinoma diagnoses are stage I to IVb, initial treatment in the vast majority is curative in intent (see https://www.nccn.org/professionals/physician). The multidisciplinary team must optimally deploy and sequence three key modalities: surgery, radiation therapy, and systemic therapy.

Treatment Modalities

The primary curative modality for head and neck squamous cell carcinoma is either surgery or radiation therapy, whereas systemic therapy serves as an adjunct to radiation therapy.[11] The selection of a specific multimodality treatment plan is tailored to anatomic site, stage, organ preservation, and goals of care.[12,13]

Surgery

In head and neck surgery, the advent of minimally invasive endoscopic procedures incorporating transoral CO_2 laser microsurgery or robotic surgery has markedly limited the morbidity of surgical exposure to the oropharynx. Avoiding violation of the soft tissue framework of the head and neck, including muscles, ligaments, and bones, decreases hospital stay and enhances function and cosmesis compared to historical open procedures.[14]

Radiation Therapy

The dissemination of intensity-modulated radiation therapy techniques,[15] including image-guided radiation therapy, improves the precision and accuracy of delivery of radiation therapy to the tumor and regional nodes while sparing intricate and vulnerable head and neck structures. Intensity-modulated radiation therapy reduces the important long-term morbidity of xerostomia (dry mouth). Although hyperfractionated radiation therapy is superior to conventional fractionation and is an appropriate standard of care when concomitant chemotherapy is not indicated, the value of altered fractionation regimens is uncertain when concomitant chemotherapy is used.[A1]

Systemic Therapies

Systemic therapies used in head and neck cancer include cytotoxic chemotherapy, molecular targeted therapy, and immunotherapy under expert supervision. The core cytotoxic chemotherapies are cisplatin, 5-fluorouracil, and docetaxel. Cisplatin is used in both the primary setting, concurrent with radiation therapy, or as first-line treatment for recurrent/metastatic disease. 5-Fluorouracil and docetaxel are predominantly used in the recurrent/metastatic setting. Cetuximab, which is a murine-human chimeric IgG1 monoclonal antibody against EGFR, is used during definitive radiation therapy for patients who are not candidates for cisplatin and may be used in the recurrent/metastatic setting. Nivolumab and pembrolizumab, which are IgG4 monoclonal antibodies against PD-1, are indicated in the recurrent/metastatic setting and are under investigation for curative intent.

Oral Cavity Cancer

Cancers of the oral cavity are resistant to radiation and are preferably managed with primary surgery, which generally should include lymph node dissection at the time of the primary surgery.[16] The advancement of modern reconstruction techniques, including free tissue transfer with microvascular reconstruction, has enhanced functional and cosmetic outcomes. In the clinically negative (N0) neck, sentinel node biopsy provides equivalent survival and lower morbidity compared with modified radical neck dissection.[A2]

The recommendation for adjuvant radiation therapy is based on the presence of adverse pathologic features, including extension to extracapsular lymph nodes, positive surgical margins, a pT3-4 primary tumor, N2-3 nodal disease, and perineural or lymphovascular invasion. The addition of concurrent cisplatin chemotherapy to adjuvant radiation therapy under expert guidance improves locoregional control and survival in patients with pathologic high-risk head and neck squamous cell carcinoma, defined as the presence of extracapsular nodal extension or a positive surgical margin.

HPV-Unrelated Oropharyngeal Squamous Cell Carcinoma and Hypopharynx Cancer

The majority of patients with hypopharyngeal and p16-negative oropharyngeal squamous cell carcinoma present with locally advanced disease and are treated with an organ preservation approach (i.e., primary radiation therapy). In stage III or higher disease, concurrent systemic therapy with cisplatin or cetuximab under expert supervision increases locoregional control and survival compared with radiation therapy alone, with cisplatin generally being preferable to cetuximab. The decision to offer concurrent systemic therapy also depends upon physiologic fitness, because both acute and late toxicities are magnified in patients who are frail or have a low performance status. Although concurrent cisplatin improves locoregional control in people over age 70 years, it does not improve survival, probably because of competing comorbid conditions or late toxic effects such as aspiration pneumonia. Cetuximab has a more favorable systemic toxicity profile than cisplatin, with fewer renal, bone marrow, and otologic adverse events, so concurrent cetuximab-radiation therapy is an appropriate standard of care for locally advanced head and neck squamous cell carcinoma in patients who are unfit for cisplatin.[17]

HPV-Associated Oropharyngeal Squamous Cell Carcinoma

Patients with HPV-associated oropharyngeal squamous cell carcinoma have a markedly better prognosis than their HPV-negative counterparts, whether treated with primary surgery or radiation therapy. Treatment standards under expert supervision include definitive (chemo)radiation therapy or minimally invasive, transoral surgery followed by adjuvant (chemo)radiation therapy. When a definitive radiation approach is selected, cisplatin-radiation therapy is superior to cetuximab-radiation therapy and remains the standard of care.[A3,A4] Deintensification strategies under investigation include induction chemotherapy followed by lower-dose radiation therapy, minimally invasive surgery followed by lower-dose versus standard adjuvant radiation therapy,[A5] and lower-dose radiation therapy with either concurrent cisplatin or nivolumab.[A6]

Larynx Cancer

An important general principle for the treatment of larynx cancer is preservation of a functional larynx.[18] Maintaining the larynx without adequacy of its three key functions, airway patency, pharyngeal swallowing, and voice, is not an appropriate goal. For patients with early-stage T1-2 larynx cancer, single-modality treatment with either radiation therapy or larynx preservation surgery results in 90% long-term laryngectomy-free survival.

For patients with locally advanced larynx cancer, the combination of radiation therapy and chemotherapy under expert supervision is the preferred approach for organ preservation. The two evidence-based standards include cisplatin-based induction chemotherapy followed by definitive radiation therapy or concurrent cisplatin-radiation therapy.

Evidence also supports the feasibility of larynx preservation in appropriately selected patients with limited T4 disease. Patients who are likely to be more appropriate for up-front total laryngectomy include patients who have destructive tumors affecting both vocal cords, patients who are frail or have a poor performance status, and patients who are unlikely to adhere to a 7-week radiation therapy program that requires daily attendance.

Nasopharyngeal Carcinoma

Radiation therapy is the cornerstone of curative treatment for localized nasopharyngeal carcinoma. Radiation therapy alone is noninferior to chemoradiotherapy for low-risk localized disease,[A7] but induction chemotherapy with cisplatin and gemcitabine prior to concurrent cisplatin-radiation therapy significantly improves recurrence-free and overall survival compared with chemoradiotherapy alone in patients with locoregionally advanced disease.[A8] Neck dissection is recommended if locoregional treatment fails or disease recurs. For recurrent/metastatic disease, the addition of camrelizumab (an anti-PD-1 antibody) to gemcitabine plus cisplatin increases progression-free survival and is now a first-line standard.[19,A9]

Salivary Gland Malignancies

The primary curative-intent treatment for salivary gland malignancies is surgery, followed by reconstruction. Adjuvant radiation therapy is frequently offered for stage III-IVb disease. In recurrent or metastatic disease, platinum-based chemotherapy remains a palliative option, but its clinical activity is limited, and targeted molecular approaches are an increasingly utilized option under expert oversight. The TRK inhibitor larotrectinib can yield a response rate of 75% for tumors that harbor an *NTRK* gene fusion, including salivary gland cancers,[A10] and this agent compares favorably with cytotoxic chemotherapy. Combined androgen blockade can provide about a 40% overall response rate with excellent tolerability in patients who have advanced salivary duct carcinoma. HER2neu-enriched tumors may respond to ado-trastuzumab emtansine or other clinically available HER2 inhibitors.[20] The existence of multiple unique gene fusions within salivary gland cancers also raises the promise of immunotherapy against the peptide neoantigens translated from these fusion sites.

Recurrent/Metastatic Head and Neck Squamous Cell Carcinoma

For patients with locally advanced head and neck squamous cell carcinoma, the major cause of mortality is failure of locoregional control. In a minority of patients with isolated locoregional relapse, salvage surgery or re-irradiation can lead to durable long-term disease control but at the expense of substantial morbidity.[21] For oligometastatic pulmonary disease, metastasectomy may occasionally be curative, particularly in patients who have HPV-associated cancer.

The majority of patients with locoregional recurrence and/or distant metastatic disease are candidates for palliative systemic therapy, depending upon performance status, comorbidities, and goals of care. The standard palliative systemic management of recurrent/metastatic head and neck squamous cell carcinoma is pembrolizumab (an anti-PD-1 monoclonal antibody), either as monotherapy or in combination with platinum and 5-fluorouracil[A11,A12] under expert supervision unless contraindicated by an autoimmune disorder. For the platinum-refractory disease, either nivolumab or pembrolizumab improves survival relative to single-agent chemotherapy or cetuximab.[A13] Treatment with PD-1 checkpoint blockade can provide long-term disease control in 10 to 20% of patients with recurrent/metastatic head and neck squamous cell carcinoma. HPV-specific immunotherapies under development include T cells engineered with a T-cell receptor targeting HPV-16 E7[22] and therapeutic HPV vaccines.[23]

Supportive and Palliative Care

Due to its anatomic location, head and neck squamous cell carcinoma and its treatment impact fundamental human functions, including voice, facial expression, eating, and breathing.[24] The care team must address both physical and psychological distress, often stemming from pain, nausea, malnutrition, fatigue, impaired communication, and social isolation. Even when cured from head and neck cancer, survivors experience a high burden of symptoms, including psychological distress and poor quality of life. Survivors have a high rate of suicide, almost twice that of survivors of cancers at other sites. In patients with recurrent/metastatic head and neck cancer, the burden of symptoms is particularly profound at the end of life, especially when locoregional disease is uncontrolled. The unique palliative challenges in this setting include the management of foul-smelling, ulcerative masses; decisions regarding the palliative role of enteral feeding tubes or tracheostomy; and preparation of the patient and caregivers for acute terminal events resulting from loss of airway or carotid exsanguination. Due to the unique burden of symptoms across the natural history of head and neck squamous cell carcinoma, early and continuous involvement of palliative care specialists is ideal.

PREVENTION

Environmental Head and Neck Squamous Cell Carcinoma

Patients with an index HPV-negative head and neck squamous cell carcinoma develop a second primary tumor of the upper aerodigestive tract at the alarming rate of 3 to 6% per year. The most important strategy for decreasing primary or secondary risk for head and neck squamous cell carcinoma is withdrawal of the offending carcinogen.[25] Although tobacco cessation reduces the incidence of second primary tumors, the risk is not reduced in the first 5 years and never returns to baseline. Although high-dose isotretinoin, a synthetic vitamin A analog, can reverse oral premalignant lesions and prevent second primary tumors following an index head and neck squamous cell carcinoma, isotretinoin is too toxic for chronic administration, and the risk returns to baseline upon its discontinuation. Ongoing investigations focus on whole plant-based interventions and on therapies aimed to reprogram the permissive immune microenvironment that tolerates oral epithelial transformation.

HPV-Associated Head and Neck Squamous Cell Carcinoma

HPV vaccination (Chapters 15 and 344) has an estimated 93% efficacy for preventing oral HPV[A14] and likely will prevent HPV-associated oropharyngeal cancer, although randomized clinical trials designed to demonstrate a reduction in HPV-associated oropharyngeal carcinoma are impractical because of the long latency period. HPV vaccination is recommended for all males and females ages 9 to 26 years and can be administered from ages 27 to 45 years after shared decision making.[26] The high risk of subsequent oropharyngeal cancers among persons who harbor oral HPV[27] raises the possibility of future minimally invasive screening protocols.

PROGNOSIS

Environmental Head and Neck Squamous Cell Carcinoma

The prognosis of HPV-negative head and neck squamous cell carcinoma is dependent upon stage and performance status. Although patients with stage I to II disease have an overall 5-year survival of 60 to 90%, the corresponding survival rate for patients who present with locally advanced stage III to IVb disease is only 30 to 50%. At the time of locoregional or distant metastatic relapse, median survival with modern palliative systemic therapy is 1 year.

HPV-Associated Head and Neck Squamous Cell Carcinoma

Patients with HPV-associated oropharyngeal squamous cell carcinoma have a more favorable prognosis than patients with HPV-negative cancer. Patients with stage I to II disease experience a 5-year overall survival of 72 to 89%. In nonsmokers with stage I to II disease, the 5-year overall survival rates approach 95%. Patients with stage III HPV-associated oropharyngeal squamous cell carcinoma have an intermediate prognosis, with a 5-year overall survival of 46 to 72%. When patients with HPV-associated oropharyngeal squamous cell carcinoma develop recurrent/metastatic disease, median survival is approximately 2 years, twice the survival rate for HPV-negative head and neck squamous cell carcinoma. This survival disparity in the recurrent/metastatic setting may be explained by better prognostic characteristics, including younger age and lower comorbidity scores, as well as the enhanced sensitivity of HPV-transformed cancers to chemotherapy.

Nasopharyngeal Cancer

Intensity-modulated radiation therapy can achieve locoregional control in >90% of stage I to II nasopharyngeal carcinomas. For locoregionally advanced disease, 5-year survival is about 85% with induction plus concurrent chemotherapy. Current median survival rates are about 29 months for metastatic disease.[28]

Salivary Gland Cancers

Prognosis is favorable in the setting of stage I to II disease, intermediate in the setting of stage III to IVb disease, and poor in the setting of stage IVc disease. For adenoid cystic carcinomas, the primary tumor is often well controlled following surgery and/or radiation, but the disease may relapse years later with involvement of cranial nerves and the base of the skull. Delayed lung metastases are also a common feature, so these patients are frequently followed for a decade or more by their treating oncologists.

GENERAL REFERENCES

For the General References and other additional features, please visit Elsevier eBooks+ at https://ebooks.health.elsevier.com.

Grade A References

A1. Lacas B, Bourhis J, Overgaard J, et al. Role of radiotherapy fractionation in head and neck cancers (MARCH): an updated meta-analysis. *Lancet Oncol.* 2017;18:1221-1237.

A2. Garrel R, Poissonnet G, Moyà Plana A, et al. Equivalence randomized trial to compare treatment on the basis of sentinel node biopsy versus neck node dissection in operable T1-T2N0 oral and oropharyngeal cancer. *J Clin Oncol.* 2020;38:4010-4018.

A3. Gillison ML, Trotti AM, Harris J, et al. Radiotherapy plus cetuximab or cisplatin in human papillomavirus-positive oropharyngeal cancer (NRG Oncology RTOG 1016): a randomised, multicentre, non-inferiority trial. *Lancet.* 2019;393:40-50.

A4. Mehanna H, Robinson M, Hartley A, et al. Radiotherapy plus cisplatin or cetuximab in low-risk human papillomavirus-positive oropharyngeal cancer (De-ESCALaTE HPV): an open-label randomised controlled phase 3 trial. *Lancet.* 2019;393:51-60.

A5. Ferris RL, Flamand Y, Weinstein GS, et al. Phase II randomized trial of transoral surgery and low-dose intensity modulated radiation therapy in resectable p16+ locally advanced oropharynx cancer: an ECOG-ACRIN cancer research group trial. *J Clin Oncol.* 2022;40:138-149.

A6. Yom SS, Torres-Saavedra P, Caudell JJ, et al. Reduced-dose radiation therapy for HPV-associated oropharyngeal carcinoma (NRG Oncology HN002). *J Clin Oncol.* 2021;39:956-965.

A7. Tang LL, Guo R, Zhang N, et al. Effect of radiotherapy alone vs radiotherapy with concurrent chemoradiotherapy on survival without disease relapse in patients with low-risk nasopharyngeal carcinoma: a randomized clinical trial. *JAMA.* 2022;328:728-736.

A8. Zhang Y, Chen L, Hu GQ, et al. Final overall survival analysis of gemcitabine and cisplatin induction chemotherapy in nasopharyngeal carcinoma: a multicenter, randomized phase III trial. *J Clin Oncol.* 2022;40:2420-2425.

A9. Yang Y, Qu S, Li J, et al. Camrelizumab versus placebo in combination with gemcitabine and cisplatin as first-line treatment for recurrent or metastatic nasopharyngeal carcinoma (CAPTAIN-1st): a multicentre, randomised, double-blind, phase 3 trial. *Lancet Oncol.* 2021;22:1162-1174.

A10. Drilon A, Laetsch TW, Kummar S, et al. Efficacy of larotrectinib in TRK fusion-positive cancers in adults and children. *N Engl J Med.* 2018;378:731-739.

A11. Harrington KJ, Burtness B, Greil R, et al. Pembrolizumab with or without chemotherapy in recurrent or metastatic head and neck squamous cell carcinoma: updated results of the phase III KEYNOTE-048 study. *J Clin Oncol.* 2023;41:790-802.

A12. Cohen EEW, Souliéres D, Le Tourneau C, et al. Pembrolizumab versus methotrexate, docetaxel, or cetuximab for recurrent or metastatic head-and-neck squamous cell carcinoma (KEYNOTE-040): a randomised, open-label, phase 3 study. *Lancet.* 2019;393:156-167.

A13. Ferris RL, Blumenschein G Jr, Fayette J, et al. Nivolumab for recurrent squamous-cell carcinoma of the head and neck. *N Engl J Med.* 2016;375:1856-1867.

A14. Tsentemeidou A, Fyrmpas G, Stavrakas M, et al. Human papillomavirus vaccine to end oropharyngeal cancer. A systematic review and meta-analysis. *Sex Transm Dis.* 2021;48:700-707.

177

LUNG CANCER AND OTHER PULMONARY NEOPLASMS

FADLO R. KHURI

Lung cancers grow from a single abnormal cell or small group of abnormal cells to develop into large macroscopic masses that may be several centimeters in diameter. Most lung cancers originate from the bronchial epithelium and are termed carcinomas. Primary noncarcinoma lung cancers are less common and include carcinoid, pulmonary blastomas (more common in younger patients), and sarcomas. Abnormal lung tissues range in histologic grade from mildly atypical cells to aggressive cancers. Lesions such as atypical adenomatous hyperplasia are considered preinvasive lesions, with a continuum of cellular atypia through adenocarcinoma.

BRONCHOGENIC LUNG CANCER

DEFINITION

Lung cancer, or bronchogenic carcinoma, is a proliferative malignant neoplasm arising from the primary respiratory epithelium. Lung cancer is generally divided into two major histologic groups: *non–small cell lung cancer* (NSCLC), which accounts for approximately 85% of all lung cancers, and *small cell lung cancer* (SCLC).

EPIDEMIOLOGY

Lung cancer is by far the leading cause of cancer-related mortality globally. An estimated 2.2 million new cases diagnosed worldwide each year account for nearly 11% of all cancers and cause an estimated 1.8 million annual deaths. Among men, lung cancer is the most common malignant neoplasm (worldwide incidence rate of 31.5 per 100,000), whereas in women, lung cancer incidence (14.6 per 100,000) trails breast, cervix, and colon cancers. The incidence and mortality related to lung cancer in men have declined during the last two decades in Western countries but continue to increase in the developing world.[1] In women, lung cancer deaths are increasing in most regions of the world. The most dramatic increases in lung cancer incidence and death globally are in China, which has experienced over a 4.5-fold increase in lung cancer–related deaths during the past 3 to 4 decades.

Risk Factors

Cigarette smoking is the most common risk factor for lung cancer, with roughly 85% of lung cancer patients having a tobacco-smoking history and approximately 50% being former smokers (defined as free from smoking for at least 12 months before diagnosis). The risk for developing lung cancer correlates with the number of cigarettes smoked per day and the cumulative duration of smoking time.[2] Patients with a smoking history of at least 20 to 30 pack-years (defined as one pack per day of cigarettes for 20 to 30 years) are at substantially increased risk for lung cancer.

Since the release of the first U.S. Surgeon General's Report on the Hazards of Smoking in 1964, the prevalence of cigarette smoking has declined considerably in the United States but continues to increase at an alarming rate in developing and third world countries. As a result, the number of cases of lung cancer diagnosed annually is likely to rise during the next few decades, and it is estimated that the majority of lung cancer cases will occur outside the United States and Europe by the year 2030. Smoking cessation is associated with a gradual reduction in risk of developing lung cancer, although it does not reach that of a never-smoker. Second-hand exposure to smoke is another risk factor that contributes to nearly 1% of all cases of lung cancer.

Because only about 11% of heavy smokers develop lung cancer, genetic susceptibility to lung cancer also appears to play a role. Patients with a family history of early lung cancer (before 60 years of age) have a two-fold higher risk for developing lung cancer. Women appear to be at a higher risk for lung cancer at the same smoking exposure level as that of men.

Occupational exposure to asbestos leads to an estimated four-fold higher risk of lung cancer, with cigarette smoking having an additive effect on risk. The latency between asbestos exposure and the development of lung cancer is several decades, and risk is related to the duration of exposure as well as to the quantity and the type of asbestos fiber. However, all forms of asbestos are carcinogenic.

Radon exposure has also been implicated in the development of 5 to 8% of lung cancer cases. Household exposure to radon, which results from the radioactive decay of uranium, is high in certain geographic regions. Exposure to ionizing radiation in the form of therapeutic radiation or frequent diagnostic radiographic tests is also associated with a higher risk for developing lung cancer. Similarly, exposures to metals (including arsenic, nickel, and chromium), silica, and general air pollution (including biomass fuels such as coal and wood smoke) are also associated with the risk of lung cancer but to a lesser degree compared with ionizing radiation. The human immunodeficiency virus is associated with a 3.6-fold increased risk of developing lung cancer.

PATHOBIOLOGY

Pathology

Lung cancer is broadly subdivided into NSCLC and SCLC on the basis of their distinct histopathology, biologic behavior, and response to therapies. NSCLC comprises *adenocarcinoma*, *squamous cell carcinoma*, and *large cell carcinoma* subtypes. In addition to morphologic features, immunohistochemical studies are important in establishing the histologic subtype of NSCLC.

Adenocarcinomas

Adenocarcinoma has increased in incidence over the past several decades and now represents over 50% of all lung cancers. Never-smokers who develop lung cancer most frequently have adenocarcinoma. Adenocarcinoma has a higher predilection for developing distant metastases compared with squamous cell lung cancers. Adenocarcinoma specimens usually stain positive for cytokeratin 7, thyroid transcription factor-1 (TTF-1), and Napsin-A, but they stain negative for cytokeratin 20.

Lung adenocarcinoma can be divided into preinvasive, minimally invasive, and invasive types. *Atypical adenomatous hyperplasia* refers to a localized proliferative lesion consisting of atypical type II pneumocytes or Clara cells and measuring less than 5 mm. *Adenocarcinoma in situ*, which refers to lesions that are smaller than 3 cm and that lack any invasive characteristics, was previously referred to as bronchioloalveolar carcinoma or noninvasive adenocarcinoma. Lesions 3 cm or smaller with a predominantly lepidic pattern and with invasion of less than 5 mm in greatest dimension are referred to as *minimally invasive adenocarcinoma*. Invasive adenocarcinoma represents nearly 90% of all cases of adenocarcinoma. Based on the predominant characteristic features, it is categorized as lepidic, acinar, papillary, micropapillary, or solid predominant with mucin production.

Squamous Cell Carcinoma

Squamous cell lung cancer is decreasing in incidence in the United States, most likely because of the changing smoking habits of the population. Squamous tumors of the lung are generally centrally located and are almost always seen in patients with a significant smoking history. Squamous dysplasia and squamous cell carcinoma in situ are preinvasive lesions that can develop into invasive cancers.

The majority of squamous cell tumors stain positive for p40 and p63, which are members of the p53 family of proteins, whereas adenocarcinomas occasionally stain positive for p63. On the basis of these findings, a panel of markers including TTF-1, p63, and p40 is frequently evaluated in diagnostic specimens of patients with lung cancer to identify the histologic subtype accurately (E-Table 177-1).

Large Cell Carcinoma

Large cell carcinoma represents 3 to 4% of NSCLC and is characterized by a high mitotic rate, necrosis, and morphologic features of NSCLC. Large cell tumors stain positively for neuroendocrine markers such as chromogranin A and synaptophysin. Large cell carcinoma is often difficult to diagnose accurately owing to an abundance of necrotic tissue and a poor degree of differentiation, so diagnosis requires an adequate tissue specimen. Large cell carcinoma is strongly associated with a history of prior smoking.

Small Cell Lung Cancer

SCLC is diagnosed in approximately 13% of lung cancer cases in the United States, and its incidence has gradually declined during the past several decades. SCLC is strongly associated with smoking and is rare in never-smokers. Pathologic diagnosis can be challenging because of an abundance of necrotic tissue but is established by characteristic features, such as a high degree of mitosis and necrosis. The diagnostic evaluation of SCLC includes immunostaining for TTF-1, chromogranin, synaptophysin, and CD56. Approximately 15% of SCLC specimens have mixed morphology with components of NSCLC.

Molecular Pathology

Whole-genomic sequencing has revealed that the mutational burden in specimens of adenocarcinomas from the lungs of persons who have never smoked is a log order of magnitude lower than the mutational burden in the lungs of persons who have ever smoked. Characteristic cytosine-adenine (C→A) nucleotide transversions are associated with tobacco exposure and are seen predominantly in lung adenocarcinomas from smokers rather than from those who have never smoked. The cause of the increasing number of lung cancers among never-smokers is unclear, but affected individuals are more likely to harbor certain genetic alterations in the tumor, such as mutations in the gene encoding epidermal growth factor receptor (EGFR) and rearrangement in the gene encoding anaplastic lymphoma kinase (ALK).[3]

Oncogenes

In lung adenocarcinoma, nearly two thirds of patients harbor an oncogenic mutation that can potentially be targeted with specific agents (E-Fig. 177-1A).[4] The most common are mutations involving *KRAS, EGFR, BRAF, HER2, MET*, and *PIK3CA* and gene rearrangements involving *ALK, RET*, and *ROS1*. *KRAS* mutations are present in approximately 25% of lung adenocarcinomas and are usually associated with cigarette smoking. The most common sites of mutation in *KRAS* include codons 12, 13, and 61, where the resulting amino acid substitutions cause impaired GTPase activity and constitutive activation of RAS signaling.

Mutations in *EGFR* are observed in nearly 15% of White and almost 40% of Asian patients with lung adenocarcinomas. Deletion mutations in exon 19 and a point mutation in exon 21 are located in the tyrosine kinase–binding domain of the receptor and result in constitutive activation of the signaling pathway, thereby leading to proliferation, evasion of apoptosis, and enhanced angiogenesis. Patients with *EGFR*-activating mutations can derive robust and durable clinical benefit from treatment with EGFR tyrosine kinase inhibitors; however, most of the benefit is limited in duration and within 12 to 24 months, and nearly 60% of patients treated with first- or second-generation inhibitors will develop a secondary mutation in exon 20(T790M) that confers resistance to this therapy. In some patients with lung adenocarcinomas, this exon 20(T790M) mutation can also be found de novo along with an exon 19 or 21 mutation before exposure to EGFR tyrosine kinase inhibitor therapy. Another common mechanism of acquired resistance to EGFR tyrosine kinase inhibitor therapy is amplification of the growth factor receptor c-Met.

In approximately 5% of patients with lung adenocarcinomas, gene rearrangement involving *ALK* is observed. Clinical features associated with the *ALK* gene rearrangement include never-smokers, signet ring features on histopathologic evaluation, and younger age. The fusion gene results from inversion or translocation of portions of the *echinoderm microtubule-associated protein-like 4 (EML4)* with the *ALK* gene and leads to activation of downstream signals that can be inhibited by specific ALK kinase inhibitors such as crizotinib. The *ALK* gene rearrangement can be detected by fluorescence in situ hybridization or by immunohistochemistry. Other fusion abnormalities involving the *RET* and *ROS1* genes are each observed in 1% of lung adenocarcinoma specimens. It is noteworthy that *EGFR* and *KRAS* mutations and *ALK* gene rearrangements are usually mutually exclusive.

Squamous cell carcinoma has an entirely different spectrum of molecular abnormalities (E-Fig. 177-1B), including common mutations in *p53, PTEN, PIK3CA, KEAP1, DDR2*, and *RB1*. Amplification of the gene for *fibroblast growth factor receptor* (FGFR) is also noted in 10 to 20% of squamous cell lung cancers.

Tumor Suppressor Genes

The function of multiple tumor suppressor genes (e.g., *p53, Rb, LKB1*, and a number of genes found on the short arm of chromosome 3 [*3p*]) is frequently lost in lung cancer. Mutation or loss of *p53* correlates with cigarette smoking and is detected in some preneoplastic lesions of the lung. Mutations of *p53* are common in both NSCLC (≈50%) and SCLC (≈80%). Mutations in *LKB1* are also common in NSCLC. The *STK11/LKB1* gene, which encodes a *serine/threonine kinase*, regulates cell polarity and functions as a tumor suppressor. One of the earliest genetic abnormalities in lung cancer occurs during the deletion of genetic material on chromosome 3p (p14 to p23). The deletion occurs in approximately 50% of NSCLC and 90% of SCLC patients. The *FHIT* (fragile histidine triad) gene (3p14.2), which is abnormal in many lung cancers, may function as a tumor suppressor gene by limiting tumor growth and enhancing apoptosis. The Rb protein is not expressed in 90% of SCLC because of mutation or deletion. In NSCLC, Rb is normally expressed, but when Rb is phosphorylated, uncontrolled cell division can occur.

Epigenetics

Epigenetic modifications involving changes in DNA methylation are common in lung cancer and include hypomethylation, dysregulation of DNA methyltransferase I, and hypermethylation. Genes that are methylated in NSCLC include *p16, RARB, RASSFIA, MGMT* (methylguanine-methyltransferase), and death-associated protein kinase (DAP-kinase). Hypermethylation in lung cancer can often silence tumor suppressor genes, thereby promoting dysregulated cell growth. Silencing of tumor suppressor genes in histologically normal lymph nodes in patients with resectable NSCLC is associated with higher likelihood of disease relapse.

CLINICAL MANIFESTATIONS

Currently, only 15% of patients with lung cancer are asymptomatic when they are initially diagnosed. These early lung cancers often are manifested as a pulmonary nodule (defined as a rounded opacity, well or poorly defined, measuring up to 3 cm in diameter), first seen incidentally on a chest radiograph obtained for other reasons (e.g., a preoperative study) or on a screening computed tomographic (CT) scan.

Most patients have symptoms and signs that are caused by the pulmonary lesion itself: local tumor growth, invasion, obstruction, intrathoracic-regional tumor spread to lymph nodes and adjacent structures, distant extrathoracic spread of disease, or a paraneoplastic syndrome. Common presenting symptoms of lung cancer include cough, dyspnea, pain, hemoptysis, and weight loss. Anorexia occurs in about 30% of patients, fatigue in one third of patients, and anemia and fever in 10 to 20% of patients. More than 80% of patients initially have three or more symptoms or signs as a result of the lung cancer. Because the majority of patients with lung cancer have other tobacco-related cardiopulmonary diseases, such as chronic obstructive pulmonary disease (Chapter 76) and ischemic heart disease (Chapters 56 to 58), these overlapping symptoms often result in a delay in diagnosis of the underlying malignant disease. Symptoms that can result from local invasion or metastasis of the tumor include headache, bone pain, airway obstruction, cough, and hemoptysis. Paraneoplastic syndromes (Chapter 164) associated with lung cancer include the syndrome of inappropriate antidiuretic hormone (Chapter 102), hypercalcemia (Chapter 227), pulmonary hypertrophic osteoarthropathy (Chapter 254 and Fig. 254-1), Eaton-Lambert myasthenic syndrome (Chapter 390), and Cushing syndrome (Chapters 164 and 208). Hypercalcemia is common in squamous cell histology, whereas the syndrome of inappropriate antidiuretic hormone, Eaton-Lambert myasthenic syndrome, and Cushing syndrome are most commonly associated with SCLC.

DIAGNOSIS

Solitary Pulmonary Nodule

Asymptomatic solitary pulmonary nodules less than 3 cm in diameter with normal surrounding lung architecture are found incidentally in up to 0.2% of chest radiographs.[5] A solitary pulmonary nodule can be the first sign of early lung cancer, but about 95% of such lesions are noncancerous and most often are granulomas or intrapulmonary lymph nodes. Smaller nodules are likely to be benign. The potential for these lesions to be malignant increases with the patient's age, the size of the nodule, the nodule's rate of growth, a history of smoking, and any changes compared with prior imaging studies.

The evaluation (Fig. 177-1) begins with computed tomographic (CT) scanning. Nodules are categorized as small solid (<8 mm), large solid (≥8 mm), or subsolid. Subsolid nodules are divided into ground-glass nodules (no solid component) and part-solid nodules (both ground-glass and solid components). The likelihood of malignancy is <1% for nodules that are less than 6 mm and 1 to 2% for solid nodules that are 6 mm to 8 mm. These low-risk nodules can be monitored with serial CT scans. A pulmonary nodule that has not changed in size for more than 2 years is probably benign.

For larger nodules, which have a higher likelihood of malignancy, CT characteristics suggestive of malignancy include irregular margins, spiculation, invasion of adjacent structures, lymphadenopathy, and distant metastases.[6] Further imaging is warranted (e.g., positron emission tomography [PET]), and suspicious nodules should undergo definitive biopsy. For nodules that are partly solid, diagnostic strategies are typically guided by the size of the solid component.

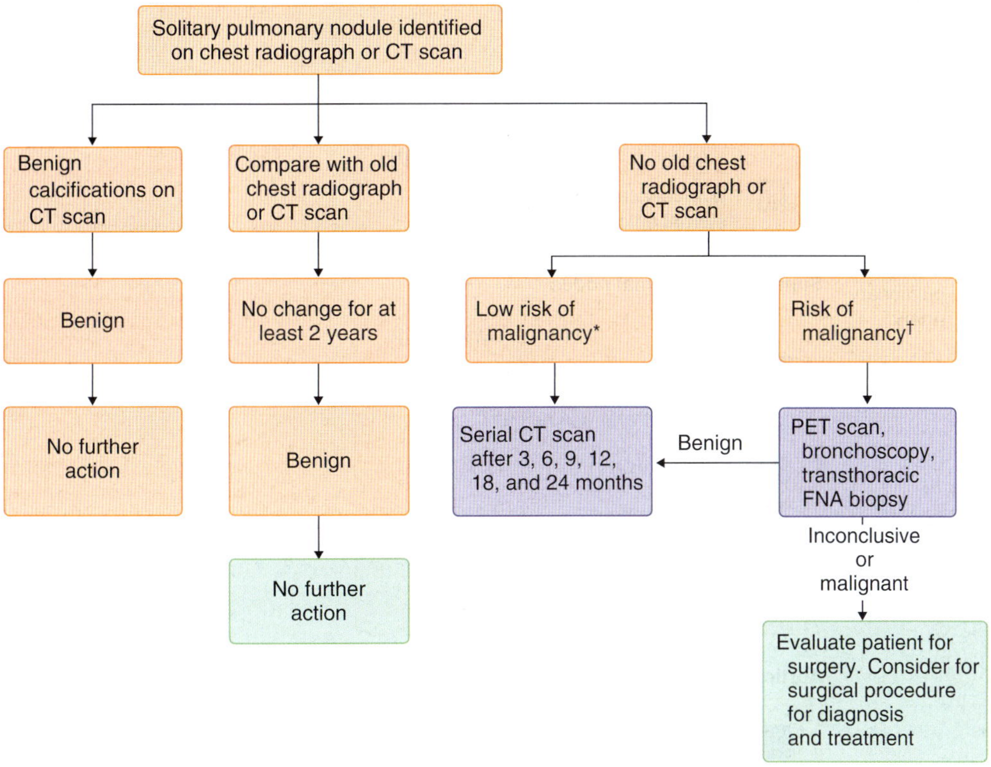

FIGURE 177-1. Evaluation of a patient with a solitary pulmonary nodule. *Patient with a minimal or absent history of smoking and other known risk factors for the development of lung cancer and a nodule 8 mm or smaller. †Patient with a history of smoking and other risk factors for the development of lung cancer and a nodule 8 mm or larger. CT = computed tomography; FNA = fine-needle aspiration; PET = positron emission tomography.

Noncancerous causes of a solitary pulmonary nodule include granulomatous diseases (e.g., sarcoidosis [Chapter 83] and histoplasmosis [Chapter 308], coccidiomycosis [Chapter 308], rheumatoid arthritis [Chapter 243]) and benign hematomas, as well as scars from prior pulmonary infections.

In screening studies, new solid nodules are detected at each round of screening in 5 to 7% of individuals. New nodules have a high probability of malignancy even when small, thereby suggesting more aggressive follow-up of new nodules that appear upon serial screening CT than for nodules that are detected at baseline imaging.

Initial Evaluation

With the advent of CT screening, a greater percentage of patients with lung cancer are being diagnosed before the onset of symptoms. In patients with clinical or radiographic findings suggestive of lung cancer, CT scans of the chest and abdomen are indicated to determine the location of the primary tumor, involvement of mediastinal lymph nodes (Fig. 177-2), and spread to other anatomic sites.

Invasive Diagnostic Procedures

Establishing the Diagnosis

Accurate diagnostic characterization of lung cancers is essential because the presence or absence of mediastinal nodal metastases is crucial in determining prognosis, assessing resectability, and selecting the appropriate treatment strategy for primary lung cancer.[7] For patients with localized lung tumors that are suggestive of cancer, it is reasonable to proceed with surgical resection without a diagnostic biopsy if all other potential causes are excluded. Commonly, however, a biopsy is necessary to establish the diagnosis of lung cancer and to define its histology before proceeding with surgery. The most accessible site with the least invasive method is the preferred approach to obtaining diagnostic tissue. Although a fine-needle aspiration procedure is often adequate to establish diagnosis and can be accomplished by a transthoracic approach or by bronchoscopy, the yield is often inadequate to conduct molecular studies. Therefore, a core needle biopsy to obtain sufficient tissue is recommended for patients with suspected lung cancer.[8]

For patients who present with pleural or pericardial effusions, transthoracic aspiration of fluid is typically sufficient for diagnosis and staging. Cell blocks prepared from the fluid can be used to conduct molecular studies, although the success rate depends on the number of viable cancer cells in the specimen. The diagnostic yield of pleural fluid in patients with malignant effusion is approximately 50 to 70%. In instances in which repeated aspiration of pleural fluid is nondiagnostic, a video-assisted thoracoscopy procedure might be necessary to establish diagnosis.

Staging Thoracic Disease

Enlarged lymph nodes identified by CT or positron emission tomography (PET) require histologic confirmation. Whether all patients require invasive mediastinal staging before surgical resection or other local treatment is uncertain because only 5 to 15% of patients who have peripheral T1 tumors and a negative mediastinum by CT or PET scanning have mediastinal nodal metastases.

Transbronchial needle aspiration allows staging of the mediastinum during diagnostic bronchoscopy. The sensitivity of transbronchial needle aspiration is dependent on the size and location of the lymph nodes (see Fig. 177-2) as well as on the size of the needle and is best suited for large, clinically positive lymph nodes. Endobronchial ultrasound can guide transbronchial fine-needle aspiration and provide an overall sensitivity approaching 90%. When combined with esophogeal ultrasound-guided fine-needle aspiration (which provides access to lymph node stations 7, 8, and 9), the sensitivity can exceed 90%. Other diseases that are also associated with enlarged and metabolically active mediastinal lymph nodes include sarcoidosis, tuberculosis, and multiple infectious causes, generally of a fungal (e.g., histoplasmosis, coccidioidomycosis), atypical bacterial, or viral nature, so nodal tissue must be obtained.

Mediastinoscopy involves surgical assessment of mediastinal lymph nodes to determine tumor involvement. Cervical mediastinoscopy (which provides access to lymph nodes at stations 2, 4, 7, and often 10) has a complication rate of 2% but with few life-threatening complications. With video mediastinoscopy, sensitivity and specificity exceed 97%. Anterior mediastinotomy provides access to lymph node stations 5 and 6 (aortic and aortopulmonary window), which are generally not accessible with cervical mediastinoscopy.

Diagnostic Imaging

In conjunction with standard thoracic imaging procedures, additional sites of disease may require evaluation based on presenting complaints. The most common sites of lung cancer metastases include the contralateral lung, liver, adrenal gland, bones, and brain. Imaging of the brain is recommended to evaluate for metastasis in patients with suggestive symptoms and signs as well as in

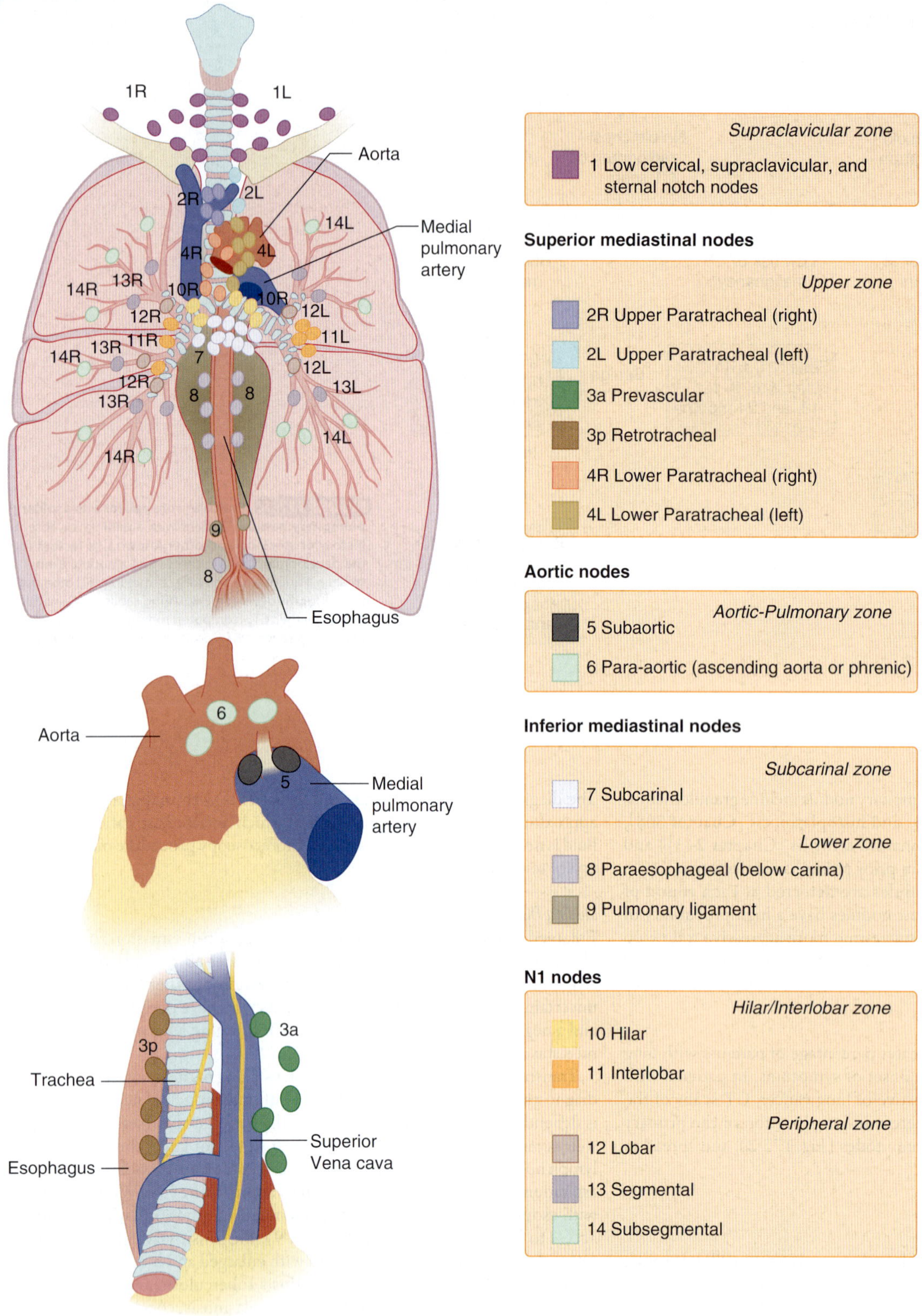

FIGURE 177-2. **The International Association for the Study of Lung Cancer (IASLC) lymph node map.** Included is the proposed grouping of lymph node stations into "zones" for the purposes of prognostic analyses. (From Rusch VW, Asamura H, Watanabe H. The IASCL lung cancer staging project. A proposal for a new international lymph node map in the forthcoming seventh edition of the TNM classification for lung cancer. *J Thorac Oncol*. 2009;4:568-577.)

patients who have a lung adenocarcinoma larger than 3 cm and evidence of mediastinal nodal involvement. Magnetic resonance imaging (MRI) and CT scan with contrast enhancement are both acceptable modalities to evaluate for brain metastases, but MRI is preferred for its superior sensitivity. Radionuclide study of the bones is indicated in patients with bone pain or an unexplained elevation in serum alkaline phosphatase level.

PET scanning is part of staging in patients with localized lung cancer. MRI scan of the chest may be useful in determination of invasion of surrounding structures, such as the brachial plexus, in patients with tumors involving the superior sulcus of the lung, but its use in staging is generally restricted to preoperative settings.

Staging

Staging (Table 177-1) based on the size of the tumor, the presence of involved lymph nodes, and the presence of metastases guides therapeutic choices and is the most important determinant of prognosis in patients with lung cancer. The tumor size is categorized as less than 2, 2 to 3, 3 to 4, 4 to 5, 5 to 6, and then 7 cm. Currently, satellite nodules in the same lobe as the primary tumor

TABLE 177-1 TREATMENT BY AMERICAN JOINT COMMITTEE ON CANCER (AJCC) STAGE

	T	N	M	MEDICALLY FIT	MEDICALLY UNFIT
Stage IA and IB	1a, 1b, 1c, 2a	0	0	Surgery	SBRT
Stage IIA/B	T1-3	0/1	0	Surgery plus adjuvant chemotherapy	Thoracic radiation
Stage IIIA	X-3	1/2	0	Multimodality therapy	
	4	X	0		
Stage IIIB	X-4	2/3	0	Concurrent chemoradiation and immunotherapy	
Stage IIIC	1-4	3		Concurrent chemoradiation and immunotherapy	Sequential chemoradiotherapy
Stage IVA	X	X	1a/b	Systemic therapy	
Stage IVB	X	X	1c	Systemic therapy; radiation for palliation	

M = metastasis; N = node; SBRT = stereotactic body radiation therapy; T = tumor.
From *AJCC Cancer Staging Manual*, 8th ed. New York: Springer-Verlag; 2018.

are categorized as T3, and nodules in another lobe of the ipsilateral lung are characterized as T4. Malignant pleural or pericardial effusion constitutes M1 disease. Presence of metastases within the thorax constitutes M1a, and extrathoracic disease is classified as M1b because patients with M1a disease have a slightly better prognosis than those with M1b.

Molecular Testing

A full gene expression profile can improve the diagnostic accuracy of the biopsy for detecting lung cancer and is often helpful for therapeutic decisions. Guidelines recommend routine molecular testing for *EGFR* mutation and *ALK* translocation in all newly diagnosed patients with advanced-stage lung adenocarcinoma. For patients with tumors of squamous cell histology, routine molecular testing is not yet recommended, but randomized clinical trials using this approach are in progress.

TREATMENT

Non–Small Cell Lung Cancer

Treatment for non–small cell lung cancer includes surgery, radiation, and medications, depending on the stage of the tumor and the fitness of the patient.[9,10]

Surgery

Surgical management plays the major role in the treatment of patients with stage I, stage II, and selected stage III NSCLC. However, nearly 40% of patients with early-stage lung cancer are not candidates for surgery because of limiting comorbid conditions. The commonly used parameters for inoperability include pulmonary functions with baseline forced expiratory volume in the first second of expiration (FEV_1) of less than 40%, predicted postoperative FEV_1 of less than 30%, and severely limited diffusion capacity. Such patients are referred to as medically inoperable despite the presence of localized disease and may be candidates for stereotactic body radiation therapy.

Lobectomy is the standard surgical procedure for patients who have localized lung cancer and who are medically fit. If anatomic resection cannot be achieved with lobectomy, bilobectomy or pneumonectomy might be necessary. Sleeve resection refers to removal of the tumor along with the bronchus and anastomosis of the remaining ends of the bronchial tree. Surgical resection can be achieved by performing an open thoracotomy or by video-assisted thoracoscopic surgery (VATS; Chapter 87), which is associated with lower morbidity, faster recovery from surgery, and better ability to administer postoperative systemic therapy.[A1] The ability to achieve an R0 resection (defined as no gross or microscopic tumor at the resection margins) is critical, and surgery should not be attempted if this outcome is not deemed feasible based on the preoperative evaluation. For patients with positive surgical margins, re-resection should be attempted whenever it is feasible. If not, postoperative radiation therapy should be administered. Robotic resection of lung cancers, including robotic lobectomy and pneumonectomy, has increased in use but is not as widely used as are VATS approaches.

Sublobar resections are not recommended because of the higher risk of local recurrence. An exception to this rule is for patients with peripheral tumors smaller than 2 cm, for which studies have demonstrated excellent outcomes.[A2]

Tumors involving the superior sulcus are managed with preoperative chemoradiotherapy to enhance tumor resectability and to gain local and distant tumor control. The decision to perform surgery for these anatomically challenging tumors depends on the extent of local invasion, involvement of the brachial plexus, and mediastinal lymph node involvement.

For stage III NSCLC with mediastinal nodal involvement, surgery alone is associated with a poor outcome, and chemoradiotherapy followed by surgery does not improve survival compared with chemoradiotherapy alone. For patients with multistation N2 disease or bulky nodal disease, surgical resection is not recommended. Clearance of mediastinal nodes after induction therapy might be the most important predictor of benefit from surgical resection, which calls for restaging of the mediastinum after induction therapy if surgery is contemplated.

Surgery can be considered under certain situations in patients with oligometastatic disease.[11] Surgical resection of both the primary and a solitary brain metastasis can result in 5-year survival rates of approximately 20%. Limited data also suggest resection of oligometastatic disease to the adrenal glands, but similar approaches with solitary metastasis at other distant sites are not recommended. This approach cannot be recommended for patients with mediastinal nodal involvement. Spinal cord compression (Chapter 164) is often a surgical emergency.

Radiation Therapy

Radiation therapy is an important part of multimodality therapy for NSCLC. It plays a major role in curative therapy for stage I to III disease and palliation of stage IV disease.

Stage I and Stage II NSCLC

Stereotactic body radiation therapy, which involves the delivery of high-dose radiation to a limited tumor volume after stereotactic localization, is an effective treatment option for patients who have T1 and node-negative T2 tumors but who are medically inoperable because of comorbid illness.[A3] In such patients, radiation therapy over three to five fractions can provide local control in almost 90% of cases. Stereotactic body radiation therapy also has considerable efficacy for peripheral tumors. Radiation therapy is also indicated for patients with positive surgical margins after surgery for early-stage NSCLC but not for patients with negative surgical margins or with involved mediastinal nodes.

Stage III NSCLC

Whereas surgery is appropriate for patients with T3N1 disease, radiation therapy results in improved outcomes for patients who have involvement of mediastinal lymph nodes.[12] A subset of N2-positive patients might benefit from multimodality therapy involving neoadjuvant chemoradiation followed by surgical resection, including stage IIIA patients with single-station or microscopic lymph node involvement and disease amenable to resection with lobectomy or bilobectomy. Preoperative radiation generally consists of 45 Gy once daily, but a dose of 60 Gy also is associated with acceptable safety results.

For patients with unresectable stage III disease, thoracic radiation therapy to a dose of 60 to 66 Gy in once-daily fractions with concurrent (rather than sequential) chemotherapy is the recommended treatment and is associated with a 5-year survival rate of 20 to 25%. The main adverse events include esophagitis and pneumonitis (depending on the extent of normal lung tissue and the dose of radiation received by normal lung tissue) that can occur immediately after radiation therapy or 6 to 9 months later.

Hyperfractionated radiation administered as two or three fractions per day is preferable to once-daily fractionation, particularly in squamous cell carcinoma, but logistical constraints have limited the adoption of this approach. In stage III patients, prophylactic cranial radiation can significantly decrease the risk of developing symptomatic brain metastases but does not improve survival.[A4]

Stage IV NSCLC

In patients with advanced-stage NSCLC, radiation therapy can be effective for palliation of spinal cord compression, brain metastasis, airway obstruction, hemoptysis, and pain. Spinal cord compression is usually managed with 30 Gy of external beam radiation therapy plus high-dose corticosteroids, but surgical decompression should precede radiation therapy when neurologic compromise is early and the patient has well-controlled systemic disease (Chapter 164).

For multiple brain metastases or oligometastatic disease not amenable to surgical resection, whole-brain radiation therapy (30 to 37.5 Gy given in 10 to 15 fractions) can be administered. Stereotactic radiosurgery can be used instead of whole-brain radiation therapy when low-volume brain metastases are limited to one to three lesions and when-brain lesions progress after whole-brain radiation therapy.

A short course of radiation therapy can provide pain control at sites of bone metastases or chest wall involvement. Palliative radiation therapy is also administered at 30 to 45 Gy during 2 to 3 weeks before the initiation of systemic therapy in patients who have systemic disease and who present with hemoptysis or postobstructive pneumonia.

Systemic Therapy

Systemic therapy refers to the use of cytotoxic agents, molecularly targeted therapy, or immunotherapy. Although it was initially developed for patients with advanced-stage lung cancer, the high propensity for metastasis of lung cancer

TABLE 177-2 TARGETED AGENTS IN LUNG CANCER THERAPY

MOLECULAR TARGET	FDA-APPROVED AGENTS
EGFR	Erlotinib Gefitinib Afatinib Osimertinib Necitumumab Dacomitinib
ALK translocation	Crizotinib Ceritinib Alectinib Brigatinib Lorlatinib
ROS1 rearrangement	Crizotinib Entrectinib
VEGF	Bevacizumab Ramucirumab
B-Raf V600E	Dabrafenib/trametinib
NTRK gene fusion	Larotrectinib Entrectinib
MET exon 14 skip mutation	Capmatinib
RET gene fusion	Selpercatinib Pralsetinib

ALK = anaplastic lymphoma kinase; EGFR = epidermal growth factor receptor; MET = metastatic; NTRK = neurotrophic tyrosine kinase; RET = rearranged during transfection; ROS1 = c-ros oncogene 1; VEGF = vascular endothelial growth factor.

cells has extended the use of systemic therapy to patients with earlier stages of the disease. A number of effective and well-tolerated cytotoxic agents are now used for the routine care of patients with lung cancer. In addition, many targeted agents (Table 177-2) have replaced standard chemotherapy as first-line agents for patients with specific mutations, and others are under clinical investigation.

Systemic Therapy in Early-Stage NSCLC

Even in the setting of optimal surgery, patients with early-stage NSCLC remain at high risk for disease recurrence or metastases due to the presence of micrometastasis, which can increasingly be quantified by the evaluation of circulating tumor cells or circulating tumor DNA. In stage IA disease, the potential benefits of chemotherapy are largely outweighed by the risks, and the overall effect is detrimental. For stage IB disease, adjuvant therapy may improve survival in patients whose tumors are larger than 4 cm, but this observation has yet to be validated in prospective trials. Drug options include cisplatin/vinorelbine or newer and better tolerated agents such as taxanes, gemcitabine, and pemetrexed under expert supervision. For stage II and stage IIIA NSCLC, four cycles of adjuvant cisplatin-based two-drug combination regimens under expert supervision provide a 5 to 15% absolute improvement in 5-year survival rates and are the standard of care.

Consistent with the success of molecularly targeted therapies in advanced-stage NSCLC, osimertinib can prolong disease-free survival in patients whose EGFR-mutated tumors have been treated with surgery and adjuvant chemotherapy.[A5] Efforts are underway to evaluate ALK inhibitors and immune checkpoint inhibitors in the adjuvant and neoadjuvant settings.

Locally Advanced NSCLC

For patients whose stage III disease is not amenable to surgical resection, concomitant administration of cisplatin or carboplatin-based chemotherapy plus radiation therapy under expert supervision is superior to sequential therapy. With modern combined chemoradiotherapy regimens, cure rates of nearly 20 to 25% are achieved in locally advanced NSCLC, with esophagitis and pneumonitis being the main toxicities. The addition of 12 months of consolidation therapy with durvalumab (a PD-L1 inhibitor) can improve survival to 43% at 5 years[A6] in patients with nonprogressive disease following chemoradiotherapy, and this approach is now the standard of care.

Advanced-Stage NSCLC

In patients with advanced-stage NSCLC, platinum-based systemic therapy under expert supervision improves overall survival and quality of life compared with supportive care alone. Carboplatin is a better tolerated outpatient option, and its dose-limiting toxicity is thrombocytopenia. Cisplatin treatment may be slightly more efficacious but is associated with nausea, emesis, nephrotoxicity, and neurotoxicity, although the availability of highly effective antiemetic agents has greatly improved its tolerability. Two-drug combination regimens are superior to monotherapy, with survivals in the 10- to 11-month range, and are recommended. Options to add to platinum-based therapy under expert supervision include etoposide, vinblastine, vindesine, vinorelbine, taxanes, gemcitabine, irinotecan, and pemetrexed (Table 177-3), with the choices among them based on consideration of toxicity, the preference of the patient, schedule, and cost. Combinations of three cytotoxic agents are not recommended because of their higher toxicity without a meaningful incremental benefit.

TABLE 177-3 CHEMOTHERAPY REGIMENS IN ADVANCED NON-SMALL CELL LUNG CANCER

FIRST-LINE THERAPY	SECOND-LINE THERAPY
Cisplatin/docetaxel	Docetaxel +/− ramucirumab
Cisplatin/gemcitabine	Pemetrexed (non-squamous tumors)
Cisplatin/pemetrexed (non-squamous tumors)	Gemcitabine
Cisplatin/vinorlebine	Vinorelbine
Cisplatin/paclitaxel	
Carboplatin/paclitaxel +/−bevacizumab	
Carboplatin/docetaxel	
Carboplatin/pemetrexed (non-squamous tumors)	
Carboplatin/vinorelbine	
Carboplatin/gemcitabine	

Targeted Systemic Therapies

Although targeted agents have shown great efficacy against lung cancer, they are unfortunately not curative. Resistance is universal to these agents, and therapy is usually continued until the disease progresses or unacceptable toxicity develops.

In patients with an activating *EGFR* mutation, treatment with gefitinib or erlotinib is associated with improvements in progression-free survival and quality of life compared with platinum-based chemotherapy, and adding gefitinib to platinum-based therapy prolongs survival compared with gefitinib alone.[A7] Afatinib, which is an irreversible EGFR tyrosine kinase inhibitor, is superior to chemotherapy[A8] in patients who have an activating *EGFR* mutation. Dacomitinib and osimertinib, which are second- and third-generation agents, respectively, appear to be more efficacious than earlier agents.[A9,A10] Osimertinib is also associated with favorable effects against brain metastases, which are a common clinical problem in patients with EGFR-mutated NSCLC.

The VEGF antibody bevacizumab is useful for advanced NSCLC with non-squamous histology, in which it significantly improves overall survival and progression-free survival when added to carboplatin and paclitaxel chemotherapy. Notable adverse events include bleeding, hypertension, proteinuria, and neutropenia.

In *ALK*-positive advanced-stage NSCLC, second-generation ALK inhibitors (ceritinib,[A11] alectinib,[A12] brigatinib,[A13] and lorlatinib[A14]) are now preferred over crizotinib as first-line therapeutic options. Lorlatinib is also used for patients who develop acquired resistance to prior ALK inhibitors.

BRAF-V600E mutations are observed in 1 to 2% of NSCLC. The combination of dabrafenib plus trametinib can result in response rates of 60% or more.[13] *RET* fusions are also oncogenic drivers in 1 to 2% of patients with NSCLC, and a durable response with acceptable toxicity is seen with selpercatinib[14] in untreated and platinum-treated patients with *RET* fusion-positive NSCLC.

KRAS G12C mutations account for approximately 40% of all KRAS mutations in NSCLC. Sotorasib and adagrasib, which are inhibitors of the KRAS G12C mutation, can provide a 35% response rate and median progression-free survival of about 7 months in advanced-stage NSCLC.[15,16] In patients whose tumors express human epidermal growth factor receptor 2 (HER2), transtuzumab deruxtecan can provide durable benefit.[17]

Immunotherapy

Inhibition of the programmed death (PD-1) ligand pathway with monoclonal antibodies reverses T-cell exhaustion and results in activation of host antitumor immune responses. Nivolumab, pembrolizumab, and cemiplimab are monoclonal antibodies against the PD-1 receptor, whereas atezolizumab and durvalumab are monoclonal antibodies against its ligand (PD-L1). Pembrolizumab can provide superior overall survival when added to or used instead of platinum-based chemotherapy for first-line therapy.[A15] For patients with PD-L1 expression level >50%, pembrolizumab monotherapy is associated with a 5-year survival rate of 32%. Atezolizumab[A16] and cemiplimab[A17] are also effective as monotherapy for first-line treatment for patients with PD-L1 expression ≥50%. Toripalimab and atezolizumab are also incrementally beneficial in combination with standard chemotherapy.[A18,A19] Nivolumab is effective as neoadjuvant therapy for resectable NSCL[A20] and also improves survival when combined with ipilimumab as a first-line therapy, with improvement in overall survival compared with chemotherapy.[A21] Another approach involving two cycles of platinum-based chemotherapy in combination with nivolumab and ipilimumab has also shown superiority over chemotherapy alone regardless of PD-L1 expression level or histology. Sugemalimab has also shown benefit with or after chemotherapy as first-line[A22] or secondary[A23] treatment of NSCLC.

Based on these results, these agents are now front-line therapy of advanced NSCLC, thereby representing a major shift in the treatment paradigm for advanced NSCLC. Specifically, for patients with PD-L1 >50%, which represents approximately 25 to 30% of NSCLC, immune checkpoint inhibitor monotherapy is the present standard of care; for PD-L1 <50% or negative disease, either the combination of chemotherapy with immunotherapy or the combination of ipilimumab and nivolumab is considered an acceptable first-line therapy option. In these patients, immunotherapy is used for a maximum duration of 2 years in patients who demonstrate clinical benefit. The main toxicity associated with these agents is autoimmune events, with pulmonary toxicity being the most serious; fortunately, the majority of these events are treatable with appropriate supportive and immunosuppressive therapy.

Role of Histology in Choice of Chemotherapy

Preferred chemotherapy regimens can vary for different histologic subtypes of NSCLC. For example, cisplatin-pemetrexed is preferred for nonsquamous advanced-stage NSCLC, whereas cisplatin-gemcitabine is preferred for squamous cell tumors. Nanoparticle albumin-bound paclitaxel (nab-paclitaxel) is associated with a favorable response rate in patients with advanced squamous NSCLC. Furthermore, the monoclonal antibody necitumumab added to gemcitabine and cisplatin is better than gemcitabine and cisplatin alone for patients with advanced squamous NSCLC.[A24]

Maintenance Therapy

Immunotherapy is now the major maintenance therapy, with the optional application of chemotherapy. Pemetrexed is the only cytotoxic agent that has specifically shown benefit as maintenance therapy. Single-agent maintenance therapy also is useful in patients who have a demonstrated clinical benefit from four cycles of platinum-based combination chemotherapy. Current therapeutic strategies employ either a "switch maintenance" approach, which uses an alternative cytotoxic or targeted agent that has not been previously administered, or "continuation maintenance," which involves continuing only the nonplatinum agent beyond four cycles.

Salvage Therapy

Virtually all patients with advanced NSCLC will eventually experience progressive disease regardless of the extent of benefit from first-line chemotherapy. Salvage therapy for these patients under expert supervision provides a modest but real improvement in survival. For patients who did not receive immune checkpoint inhibitors as part of first-line therapy, immune checkpoint inhibitors are the preferred salvage therapy, with a response rate of approximately 20%, an overall survival of 12 to 13 months, and a favorable toxicity profile. In patients who have received prior checkpoint inhibitor therapy, docetaxel (75 mg/m^2 every 3 weeks) improves survival compared with best supportive care or first-generation cytotoxic agents. Ramucirumab, a monoclonal antibody against VEGFR2 receptor, in combination with docetaxel provides a modest improvement in overall survival. Compared with docetaxel, pemetrexed has similar efficacy as salvage therapy and a more favorable toxicity profile, but its use is restricted to patients with nonsquamous histology. Overall, current salvage therapy options are associated with response rates of less than 10%, with a median progression-free survival of 3 months and overall survival of 8 months. Combinations of cytotoxic or targeted agents have not resulted in improved survival and are not recommended for salvage therapy.

Management of Special Populations of Patients

In the United States, the median age at diagnosis of lung cancer is 70 years, and elderly patients represent a growing subset of lung cancer patients. Aging is associated with a lower tolerance for systemic therapy, thereby making current physical function and prospective quality-of-life considerations important factors in the choice of systemic treatment.

For patients with a targetable mutation, appropriate targeted therapy can be administered regardless of the performance status in view of the greater potential for benefit. The use of immune checkpoint inhibitors, guided by PD-L1 expression level, is also appropriate for this patient population. However, bevacizumab is associated with a narrow therapeutic index in nonsquamous cancers in older patients, and it is recommended only with great caution.

Platinum-based combinations are superior to single-agent therapy for patients with a good performance status. Nevertheless, single-agent chemotherapy has a survival benefit compared with supportive care in elderly patients and is often more appropriate for selected patients with a poor performance status.

Small Cell Lung Cancer

For small cell lung cancer, the role of surgery is limited to the less than 5% of patients who present with peripheral lung lesions without mediastinal nodal involvement. Surgery may also be useful in the 10 to 15% of patients whose SCLC has a mixed histology with features of NSCLC.

For patients with limited-stage SCLC, radiation therapy (70 Gy on a once-daily fractioned schedule or 45 Gy on a twice-daily schedule) in combination with chemotherapy can achieve cure for approximately 20 to 30% of patients.[18] Earlier initiation of radiation therapy appears superior to a delayed approach, and twice-daily radiation therapy fractions are better than once-daily. Prophylactic cranial irradiation is associated with a modest improvement in 5-year survival for patients who have limited-stage SCLC and who achieve complete remission after combined modality therapy.

TABLE 177-4 SYSTEMIC THERAPY REGIMENS IN ADVANCED SMALL CELL LUNG CANCER

FIRST-LINE THERAPY	SECOND-LINE THERAPY
Cis- or carboplatin/etoposide	Platinum rechallenge
Cis- or carboplatin/irinotecan	Topotecan
Cis- or carboplatin/etoposide/durvalumab	Irinotecan
Carboplatin/etoposide/atezolizumab	Lurbinoctedin
	Nivolumab
	Pembrolizumab

However, approximately two thirds of patients present with extensive-stage SCLC, defined as having metastatic disease outside of the chest or having large-volume intrathoracic disease that cannot be cured with surgery or treated with radiation therapy.[19] SCLC is characterized by excellent initial sensitivity to systemic chemotherapy, although the disease commonly recurs regardless of the extent of the initial response.

Four to six cycles of cisplatin and etoposide under expert supervision is the standard chemotherapy. Carboplatin is an acceptable alternative in the treatment of extensive-stage disease. The addition of four to six cycles of immune checkpoint inhibitors (e.g., durvalumab, atezolizumab, and serplulimab) results in modest improvement in overall survival,[A25,A26] but disease recurs at a median of 4 to 6 months (Table 177-4).

Disease that progresses during or within 90 days of administration of cisplatin-based chemotherapy is referred to as refractory relapse. Topotecan can provide a response rate of 20% and improve the symptom profile but not overall survival in randomized studies. The combination of cisplatin, etoposide, and irinotecan can significantly improve overall survival compared with topotecan alone but with a higher incidence of febrile neutropenia.[A27] Other agents under study include lurbinectedin, which demonstrated a response rate of 35% in a phase 2 study of patients with relapsed/refractory SCLC.[20]

Surveillance and Follow-Up

The importance of smoking cessation cannot be overemphasized, given the high risk of enhanced complications of chemotherapy and the higher incidence of second primary tumors in lung cancer survivors. Patients should be provided with counseling and behavioral therapy and other treatment modalities to assist their efforts to discontinue smoking (Chapter 363).

CT scans are commonly used to follow patients who undergo surgical resection or chemoradiotherapy, but the relative merits of CT scan versus chest radiography, the frequency of evaluation, and the role of PET scans are unclear. For patients with advanced-stage disease, CT scans are used to assess response to therapy after every two or three cycles of treatment. In view of the proven role for salvage therapy, patients who are in follow-up after combination chemotherapy should be closely observed for development of new symptoms or clinical deterioration in addition to periodic radiographic studies.

Supportive Care

Respiratory therapy should be offered and strongly recommended to patients with dyspnea after surgery or chemoradiotherapy. Because a high proportion of these patients also have smoking-related pulmonary diseases, referral to a pulmonologist should be considered in symptomatic patients. Overall, a team approach that includes supportive care personnel, oncologic psychiatrists, nutritionists, oncologists, and appropriate additional specialists should be used to ensure the return of lung cancer survivors to normalcy to the fullest extent possible.

Because the cure rate for lung cancers is only 16%, even in the most advanced health care systems, early discussion and institution of palliative and supportive care (Chapter 3) are therefore critical to maximize quality of life. The early integration of supportive care not only helps maintain and improve quality of life but also may produce a meaningful impact on overall survival. Among family members of elderly patients who died with advanced-stage lung cancer, perceptions of better end-of-life care were associated with earlier enrollment in hospice care, avoidance of ICU admissions, death outside the hospital, and advanced care planning consistent with patients' preferences.

PREVENTION

Primary Prevention

Primary prevention of lung cancer focuses on ways to prevent individuals from smoking and promotion of smoking cessation (Chapter 363), which remain the most effective means to prevent lung cancer. The Environmental Protection Agency recommends that the household radon level be less than 4 picocuries/liter of air, and simple remedial methods are available to reduce radon exposures above this threshold. Trials of supplemental β-carotene, vitamin E, and selenium have been unsuccessful.

Secondary Prevention

Screening with annual low-dose CT scans in high-risk individuals is associated with a 20% reduction in lung cancer mortality and a 6.7% reduction in all-cause mortality. Nearly 80% of patients diagnosed with lung cancer with low-dose CT have stage I, II, or IIIA disease amenable to curative therapy. Among patients with a positive CT scan, 96.4% are deemed false positive after additional evaluation.[A28] Screening with low-dose CT is most beneficial among patients who are at highest risk and prevents very few deaths among those at lowest risk. These results have led to the adoption of low-dose CT for early detection of lung cancer by major health organizations, including the U.S. Preventive Services Task Force.[21] Because overly frequent screening has associated harms, increasing the interval between screens in persons with a negative low-dose CT result might be warranted.

PROGNOSIS

The use of targeted therapies has resulted in a substantial 50% decline in the annual mortality rate among patients diagnosed with NSCLC, and such patients now have a 35% chance of dying from a cause other than lung cancer.[22] Adenocarcinoma in situ and minimally invasive adenocarcinoma have a more than 95% 5-year survival rate when they are treated with surgical resection, thereby making the establishment of a precise pathologic diagnosis of great significance. Large cell carcinoma is often associated with an aggressive clinical course and poor survival rates, even when it is found in the setting of early-stage disease.

For SCLC, the median survival of untreated extensive-stage disease is less than 2 months, but platinum-based chemotherapy results in response rates of 50 to 70% and a median survival of 9 to 11 months. Survival for SCLC has not changed considerably over the past two decades.

OTHER PULMONARY NEOPLASMS

MALIGNANT MESOTHELIOMA

Malignant pleural mesotheliomas are generally related to asbestos exposure, with a peak risk for developing the disease 30 to 35 years after the initial exposure. Additional possible risk factors include radiation and the SV40 virus.

Mesothelioma is generally diagnosed in the fifth to seventh decade of life (median age 60 years), with a male-to-female preponderance of 5 : 1. Common symptoms include dyspnea (60%) and chest wall pain or discomfort (60%).

Chest radiographs and CT scan usually reveal pleural thickening (Fig. 86-6). Tumor progression and symptoms are generally the result of local progression, and symptomatic distant metastases are a late occurrence. Cytologic evaluation of pleural fluid to establish diagnosis is difficult and often inaccurate. The diagnosis is generally made by a biopsy procedure under CT guidance or thoracoscopically, including VATS if necessary. Several staging systems have been proposed, but none has achieved complete acceptance.

TREATMENT AND PROGNOSIS

Treatment, depending on the extent of disease, commonly includes surgery (thoracoscopy with sclerosis, pleurectomy, extrapleural pneumonectomy), radiation therapy, and, often, chemotherapy.[23] With rare exceptions, no single modality has significantly improved survival rates, and neither chemotherapy nor radiation therapy provides long-term palliation or relief of symptoms. Combination chemotherapy with pemetrexed and cisplatin can provide symptomatic relief in patients with advanced, unresectable malignant mesothelioma.

Immunotherapy with nivolumab[A29] or with nivolumab plus ipilimumab[A30] can improve overall survival, and the combination of chemotherapy with immune checkpoint inhibition has yielded promising results. The addition of bevacizumab to pemetrexed plus cisplatin can improve overall survival but just from 16.1 to 18.8 months and at the cost of manageable toxic effects.[A31]

NEUROENDOCRINE AND OTHER LUNG TUMORS

Carcinoid Tumors

Carcinoid tumors (Chapter 213) of the lung account for 1 to 2% of all lung neoplasms. These neuroendocrine tumors trace their origin to the Kulchitsky cell present in bronchial epithelium. Typical and atypical carcinoids differ in the number of mitoses (<2 per 10 high-power fields vs. 2 to 10 per 10 high-power fields, respectively), nuclear pleomorphism (absent vs. present), and regional lymph node metastases (5 to 15% vs. 20 to 28%). Distant metastases at initial evaluation are unusual (<20%). Carcinoid tumors are not associated with cigarette smoking, are twice as common in women as in men, usually occur in patients younger than age 40 years, and arise in the perihilar area of the lung. Treatment of bronchial carcinoid tumors is based on the stage of the disease. Mediastinal staging is usually followed by surgical resection. With mediastinal lymph node involvement, radiation therapy is recommended for typical carcinoid tumors if surgery cannot be performed. For atypical carcinoid or metastatic disease, chemotherapy (etoposide plus cisplatin every 3 weeks for four cycles) plus radiation therapy is commonly used, but there is no evidence for the benefit of one therapy over another. Patients with typical or low-grade carcinoid tumors usually live for many years, with a 10-year survival of >90%, whereas patients with atypical carcinoid tumors have a 5-year survival rate of about 60 to 90%.

Large Cell Neuroendocrine Carcinoma

Large cell neuroendocrine carcinoma is an aggressive neuroendocrine tumor that does not meet the criteria for carcinoid, atypical carcinoid, or SCLC. Treatment is usually with platinum agents and etoposide under expert supervision.

Salivary Gland Carcinomas

Salivary gland carcinomas (Chapter 176) include mucoepidermoid carcinoma and adenoid cystic carcinoma, which represent approximately 0.2% of lung cancers. These slow-growing neoplasms arise from the bronchial glands and are usually treated with surgery.

Primary Lung Sarcoma and Lymphoma

Primary sarcomas of the lung are very rare and include malignant fibrous histiocytoma, fibrosarcoma, leiomyosarcoma, rhabdomyosarcoma, epithelioid hemangioendothelioma, angiosarcoma, and liposarcoma (Chapter 187). The primary treatment is surgery. Depending on the size and grade of the tumor and whether the margins are clear, radiation therapy or chemotherapy may also be given. A subset of sarcomatoid carcinoma of the lung is likely to harbor MET 14 exon skipping mutations that could be amenable to targeted therapy.

Primary lymphomas of the lung are also very rare, accounting for approximately 0.3% of all primary lung cancers. The most common type is a low-grade small lymphocytic lymphoma, for which surgery and chemotherapy are the usual treatments (Chapter 171).

GENERAL REFERENCES

For the General References and other additional features, please visit Elsevier eBooks+ at https://ebooks.health.elsevier.com.

Grade A References

A1. Bendixen M, Jorgensen OD, Kronborg C, et al. Postoperative pain and quality of life after lobectomy via video-assisted thoracoscopic surgery or anterolateral thoracotomy for early stage lung cancer: a randomised controlled trial. *Lancet Oncol.* 2016;17:836-844.

A2. Saji H, Okada M, Tsuboi M, et al. Segmentectomy versus lobectomy in small-sized peripheral non-small-cell lung cancer (JCOG0802/WJOG4607L): a multicentre, open-label, phase 3, randomised, controlled, non-inferiority trial. *Lancet.* 2022;399:1607-1617.

A3. Ball D, Mai GT, Vinod S, et al. Stereotactic ablative radiotherapy versus standard radiotherapy in stage 1 non-small-cell lung cancer (TROG 09.02 CHISEL): a phase 3, open-label, randomised controlled trial. *Lancet Oncol.* 2019;20:494-503.

A4. De Ruysscher D, Dingemans AC, Praag J, et al. Prophylactic cranial irradiation versus observation in radically treated stage III non-small-cell lung cancer: a randomized phase III NVALT-11/DLCRG-02 study. *J Clin Oncol.* 2018;36:2366-2377.

A5. Wu YL, Tsuboi M, He J, et al. Osimertinib in resected EGFR-mutated non-small-cell lung cancer. *N Engl J Med.* 2020;383:1711-1723.

A6. Antonia SJ, Villegas A, Daniel D, et al. Overall survival with durvalumab after chemoradiotherapy in stage III NSCLC. *N Engl J Med.* 2018;379:2342-2350.

A7. Hosomi Y, Morita S, Sugawara S, et al. Gefitinib alone versus gefitinib plus chemotherapy for non-small-cell lung cancer with mutated epidermal growth factor receptor: NEJ009 study. *J Clin Oncol.* 2020;38:115-123.

A8. Soria JC, Felip E, Cobo M, et al. Afatinib versus erlotinib as second-line treatment of patients with advanced squamous cell carcinoma of the lung (LUX-Lung 8): an open-label randomised controlled phase 3 trial. *Lancet Oncol.* 2015;16:897-907.

A9. Mok TS, Cheng Y, Zhou X, et al. Improvement in overall survival in a randomized study that compared dacomitinib with gefitinib in patients with advanced non-small-cell lung cancer and EGFR-activating mutations. *J Clin Oncol.* 2018;36:2244-2250.

A10. Ramalingam SS, Vansteenkiste J, Planchard D, et al. Overall survival with osimertinib in untreated, EGFR-mutated advanced NSCLC. *N Engl J Med.* 2020;382:41-50.

A11. Shaw AT, Kim TM, Crinò L, et al. Ceritinib versus chemotherapy in patients with ALK-rearranged non-small-cell lung cancer previously given chemotherapy and crizotinib (ASCEND-5): a randomised, controlled, open-label, phase 3 trial. *Lancet Oncol.* 2017;18:874-886.

A12. Peters S, Camidge DR, Shaw AT, et al. Alectinib versus crizotinib in untreated ALK-positive non-small-cell lung cancer. *N Engl J Med.* 2017;377:829-838.

A13. Camidge DR, Kim HR, Ahn MJ, et al. Brigatinib versus crizotinib in ALK-positive non-small-cell lung cancer. *N Engl J Med.* 2018;379:2027-2039.

A14. Shaw AT, Bauer TM, de Marinis F, et al. First-line lorlatinib or crizotinib in advanced ALK-positive lung cancer. *N Engl J Med.* 2020;383:2018-2029.

A15. O'Brien M, Paz-Ares L, Marreaud S, et al. Pembrolizumab versus placebo as adjuvant therapy for completely resected stage IB–IIIA non-small-cell lung cancer (PEARLS/KEYNOTE-091): an interim analysis of a randomised, triple-blind, phase 3 trial. *Lancet Oncol.* 2022;23:1274-1286.

A16. Herbst RS, Giaccone G, de Marinis F, et al. Atezolizumab for first-line treatment of PD-L1-selected patients with NSCLC. *N Engl J Med.* 2020;383:1328-1339.
A17. Gogishvili M, Melkadze T, Makharadze M, et al. Cemiplimab plus chemotherapy versus chemotherapy alone in non-small cell lung cancer: a randomized, controlled, double-blind phase 3 trial. *Nat Med.* 2022;28:2374-2380.
A18. Felip E, Altorki N, Zhou C, et al. Adjuvant atezolizumab after adjuvant chemotherapy in resected stage IB-IIIA non-small-cell lung cancer (IMpower010): a randomised, multicentre, open-label, phase 3 trial. *Lancet.* 2021;398:1344-1357.
A19. Wang Z, Wu L, Cheng Y, et al. Toripalimab plus chemotherapy for patients with treatment-naive advanced non–small-cell lung cancer: a multicenter randomized phase III trial (CHOICE-01). *J Clin Oncol.* 2023;41:651-663.
A20. Forde PM, Spicer S, Lu M, et al. Neoadjucant nivolumab plus chemotherapy in resectable lung cancer. *N Engl J Med.* 2022;386:1973-1985.
A21. Paz-Ares L, Ciuleanu TE, Cobo M, et al. First-line nivolumab plus ipilimumab combined with two cycles of chemotherapy in patients with non-small-cell lung cancer (CheckMate 9LA): an international, randomised, open-label, phase 3 trial. *Lancet Oncol.* 2021;22:198-211.
A22. Zhou Q, Chen M, Jiang O, et al. Sugemalimab versus placebo after concurrent or sequential chemoradiotherapy in patients with locally advanced, unresectable, stage III non-small-cell lung cancer in China (GEMSTONE-301): interim results of a randomised, double-blind, multicentre, phase 3 trial. *Lancet Oncol.* 2022;23:209-219.
A23. Zhou Q, Chen M, Jiang O, et al. Sugemalimab versus placebo after concurrent or sequential chemoradiotherapy in patients with locally advanced, unresectable, stage III non-small-cell lung cancer in China (GEMSTONE-301): interim results of a randomised, double-blind, multicentre, phase 3 trial. *Lancet Oncol.* 2022;23:209-219.
A24. Thatcher N, Hirsch FR, Luft AV, et al. Necitumumab plus gemcitabine and cisplatin versus gemcitabine and cisplatin alone as first-line therapy in patients with stage IV squamous non-small-cell lung cancer (SQUIRE): an open-label, randomised, controlled phase 3 trial. *Lancet Oncol.* 2015;16:763-774.
A25. Goldman JW, Dvorkin M, Chen Y, et al. Durvalumab, with or without tremelimumab, plus platinum-etoposide alone in first-line treatment of extensive-stage small-cell lung cancer (CASPIAN): updated results from a randomized, controlled, open-label phase 3 trial. *Lancet Oncol.* 2021;22:51-65.
A26. Cheng Y, Han L, Wu L, et al. Effect of first-line serplulimab vs placebo added to chemotherapy on survival in patients with extensive-stage small cell lung cancer: the ASTRUM-005 randomized clinical trial. *JAMA.* 2022;328:1223-1232.
A27. Goto K, Ohe Y, Shibata T, et al. Combined chemotherapy with cisplatin, etoposide, and irinotecan versus topotecan alone as second-line treatment for patients with sensitive relapsed small-cell lung cancer (JCOG0605): a multicentre, open-label, randomised phase 3 trial. *Lancet Oncol.* 2016;17:1147-1157.
A28. Jonas DE, Reuland DS, Reddy SM, et al. Screening for lung cancer with low-dose computed tomography: updated evidence report and systematic review for the US Preventive Services Task Force. *JAMA.* 2021;325:971-987.
A29. Fennell DA, Ewings S, Ottensmeier C, et al. Nivolumab versus placebo in patients with relapsed malignant mesothelioma (CONFIRM): a multicentre, double-blind, randomised, phase 3 trial. *Lancet Oncol.* 2021;22:1530-1540.
A30. Baas P, Scherpereel A, Nowak AK, et al. First-line nivolumab plus ipilimumab in unresectable malignant pleural mesothelioma (CheckMate 743): a multicentre, randomised, open-label, phase 3 trial. *Lancet.* 2021;397:375-386.
A31. Zalcman G, Mazieres J, Margery J, et al. Bevacizumab for newly diagnosed pleural mesothelioma in the Mesothelioma Avastin Cisplatin Pemetrexed Study (MAPS): a randomised, controlled, open-label, phase 3 trial. *Lancet.* 2016;387:1405-1414.

178 NEOPLASMS OF THE ESOPHAGUS AND STOMACH

ADAM J. BASS AND ANIL K. RUSTGI

NEOPLASMS OF THE ESOPHAGUS

DEFINITION

The esophagus (Chapter 124) is a hollow tubular organ with primary physiologic functions related to contraction to permit propulsion of solid and liquid food contents into the stomach. The mucosa is a stratified squamous epithelium that covers the submucosa and muscle; the latter is skeletal muscle in the proximal esophagus and smooth muscle in the mid-distal esophagus. Cancers of the esophagus may be classified broadly into epithelial versus nonepithelial cancers. Benign epithelial tumors are referred to as squamous cell papillomas. Malignant epithelial tumors are classified into two main subtypes: esophageal squamous cell carcinoma and esophageal adenocarcinoma. Other, less common, esophageal epithelium-derived cancers include verrucous squamous cell carcinoma, adenosquamous carcinoma, adenoid cystic carcinoma, and mucoepidermoid carcinoma. Benign nonepithelial tumors include leiomyoma, granular cell tumors, fibrovascular polyp, hemangioma, lymphangioma, lipoma, and fibroma. Malignant nonepithelial tumors include leiomyosarcoma and other sarcomas, metastatic carcinoma (e.g., originating from breast or lung), and lymphoma.

ESOPHAGEAL SQUAMOUS CELL CARCINOMA

EPIDEMIOLOGY

Esophageal squamous cell carcinoma is the more common type of esophageal cancer worldwide and is a major cause of cancer-related mortality.[1] Esophageal squamous cell carcinoma may have rates of up to 100 per 100,000 population in what is often termed the *Central Asian belt*, including regions around the Caspian Sea, Iran, India, and China; other areas of high incidence include some Mediterranean countries and Eastern Africa. In the United States, esophageal squamous cell carcinoma is more common among Black males than White males, with risks of 15.1 per 100,000 compared with 2.9 per 100,000, respectively. Rates are 2 to 3 times higher in men than in women. Although the U.S. incidence of esophageal squamous cell carcinoma is low in both men and women younger than age 50 years, the incidence increases with advancing age.

Risk Factors

Hereditary esophageal squamous cell carcinoma is exceedingly rare, and is associated with a desquamating condition termed *tylosis palmaris et plantaris*. This desquamation most dramatically affects the hands and feet but extends to the esophagus as well. Another uncommon condition, Plummer-Vinson syndrome or Paterson-Brown Kelly syndrome, entails glossitis, cervical esophageal webs, and iron deficiency anemia. In both conditions, it is likely that chronic inflammation triggers the cascade of events that culminate in esophageal squamous dysplasia and esophageal squamous cell carcinoma.

Most esophageal squamous cell carcinoma cases are related to cigarette smoking or alcohol consumption, especially in combination, because their deleterious effects appear to be synergistic. Chemical carcinogens that are present in both include *N*-nitroso compounds, polycyclic aromatic hydrocarbons, and aromatic amines. The relative risk for esophageal squamous cell carcinoma is 6.2-fold higher in persons who smoke more than 25 cigarettes daily. Cessation of cigarette smoking is helpful in attenuating risk after 10 years of abstinence. Cigarette smokers who drink beer and whiskey have a 10- to 25-fold enhanced risk of developing esophageal squamous cell carcinoma. Vitamins A, B_{12}, C, and E; folic acid; and certain minerals (zinc, selenium, molybdenum) exert direct or indirect antioxidant effects, and their deficiencies impair epithelial and tissue homeostasis and regeneration.

Other risk factors for esophageal squamous cell carcinoma (Table 178-1) include achalasia (Chapter 124), which is a disorder that involves agangliosis of the Auerbach plexus, thereby resulting in dysphagia, chest pain, and weight loss, among other symptoms. The emergence of esophageal squamous cell carcinoma may be observed 10 to 20 years after the identification of achalasia. Because head and neck squamous cell carcinoma (Chapter 176) shares many of the same environmental and lifestyle risk factors with esophageal squamous cell carcinoma, particularly alcohol use and tobacco smoking, head and neck squamous cell carcinoma and esophageal squamous cell carcinoma may occur synchronously or metachronously. In different parts of the world, esophageal

TABLE 178-1 RISK FACTORS FOR ESOPHAGEAL CANCER

Esophageal squamous cell cancer
Tylosis palmaris et plantaris
Achalasia
Plummer-Vinson syndrome
Cigarette smoking
Alcohol
Chronic lye ingestion
Dietary deficiencies (minerals, vitamins)
Human papillomavirus (HPV) infection
Radiation injury
Celiac sprue
Esophageal adenocarcinoma
Gastroesophageal acid reflux
Bile reflux
Obesity
Barrett esophagus

squamous cell carcinoma is also associated with chronic esophageal stricture due to lye ingestion, consumption of maté (a hot herb-based beverage), celiac sprue, infection with human papillomavirus (HPV) (especially genotypes HPV-16, HPV-18, and HPV-33), and radiation injury.

PATHOBIOLOGY

Esophageal squamous cell carcinoma involves the transition from normal squamous epithelium to squamous dysplasia to cancer. The initiation, progression, and metastatic potential of esophageal squamous cell carcinoma are associated with a number of genetic alterations, including overexpression of epidermal growth factor receptor (*EGFR*) and cyclin D1 oncogenes, as well as inactivation of *TP53*, *p16INK4A*, and p120-catenin (*p120ctn*) tumor suppressor genes. The frequency of these changes varies greatly based upon various studies, but the oncogenic alterations generally appear early in dysplasia and early esophageal squamous cell carcinoma, whereas the inactivation of tumor suppressor genes appears as later events in established primary and metastatic esophageal squamous cell carcinoma. From a genomic viewpoint, the SOX-2 transcription factor, which is important in the pluripotent capacity of somatic cells, is an important gene involved in the pathogenesis of esophageal squamous cell carcinoma. Conditional knockout of the *p120ctn* tumor suppressor gene in the esophagus of mice results in invasive esophageal squamous cell carcinoma. Deep DNA sequencing has confirmed these genetic alterations and revealed a lower frequency of other alterations, such as inactivation of chromatin-modifying enzymes.

CLINICAL MANIFESTATIONS

Symptoms and Signs

Although esophageal squamous dysplasia is typically not associated with symptoms, esophageal squamous cell carcinoma, which has a predilection for the proximal to mid-esophagus, may be associated with dysphagia, odynophagia, atypical or typical chest pain, gastrointestinal bleeding, nausea, vomiting, weight loss, and malnutrition. Esophageal squamous cell carcinoma may metastasize to local lymph nodes, lung, liver, and bone. Symptoms attributable to metastatic esophageal squamous cell carcinoma may include bone-related pain, dyspnea, and evidence of jaundice and liver failure, depending upon the extent of metastatic disease.

Physical Examination

Weight loss may result in general cachexia and muscle wasting. The patient should be evaluated for changes in hair, skin integrity, and nail beds as a reflection of malnutrition. Lymphadenopathy may be detected in the anterior cervical and supraclavicular regions. Hepatomegaly and complications of liver disease may herald metastatic disease to the liver.

Laboratory Studies

A progressive iron deficiency anemia may be due to chronic indolent upper gastrointestinal bleeding. Additional abnormalities may be reflected in metabolic disturbances, such as metabolic alkalosis due to vomiting and hypernatremia due to dehydration. Liver enzyme abnormalities, both hepatocellular and cholestatic, may reflect metastasis to the liver. Paraneoplastic hypercalcemia is uncommon. Esophageal squamous cell carcinoma has no specific markers, but an elevated carcinoembryonic antigen (CEA) level and levels of cell-free DNA from tumor cells may be used to aid in monitoring for recurrent disease after therapy.

DIAGNOSIS

An upper gastrointestinal contrast radiographic study can show a filling defect due to the mucosal lesion or impaired transit of contrast due to luminal growth (Chapter 119). However, definitive diagnosis involves direct visualization with upper endoscopy (Chapter 120). Once the mass is visualized, biopsies are necessary to confirm the diagnosis and to enable genomic studies. Fine-needle aspiration can provide a rapid diagnostic assessment in the procedure room. Esophageal squamous cell carcinoma may involve local lymph nodes, which are best detected by endoscopic ultrasound; as needed, samples can then be analyzed by cytopathology following fine-needle aspiration. Endoscopic ultrasound is routinely used also to gauge depth of invasion, which guides the use of neoadjuvant therapy in node-negative localized cases.

Evaluation of metastatic disease involves chest and abdominal computed tomography (CT) scans. Bone scan might be useful in patients who are symptomatic with bone-related pain. Positron emission tomography (PET) is increasingly used to assess metastatic disease. In totality, these diagnostic modalities also allow for staging of esophageal squamous cell carcinoma, which is important in guiding therapeutic options.

TREATMENT

Surgical Therapy

Surgery is the cornerstone of therapy for curative intent, but adjuvant chemotherapy or chemoradiation markedly improves outcomes.[2] Depending upon the location of the esophageal squamous cell carcinoma, either total esophagectomy or subtotal esophagectomy is pursued.[3] For the latter, jejunal or colonic interposition can be done.

Surgical techniques include transthoracic, transhiatal, and radical en bloc resections. Increasing surgical proficiency in performing esophagectomy improves short-term as well as long-term mortality results in esophageal cancer. In selected patients, minimally invasive esophagectomy[4] can provide equivalent or better perioperative mortality, morbidity, and oncologic outcomes compared with open surgery.[A1–A3]

In patients who are medically unfit for surgery or in whom surgery is likely to result in high morbidity (e.g., tumors in the cervical esophagus), definitive chemoradiation is often pursued as an alternative to surgical therapy. Salvage esophagectomy after definitive chemoradiotherapy can offer acceptable short- and long-term outcomes in selected patients whose esophageal cancers are treated at experienced centers.

Medical Therapy

Neoadjuvant or adjuvant combination chemoradiotherapy under expert supervision is more effective than surgery alone for improving the survival of patients with resectable esophageal cancer.[A4] For patients who have localized node-positive or more advanced esophageal cancer, outcomes are improved by neoadjuvant chemoradiation with about 40 Gy of radiation plus either carboplatin with paclitaxel[A5] or cisplatin with vinorelbine.[A6] Adjuvant nivolumab can enhance survival in patients who have residual disease despite chemoradiation and surgery.

In patients who have metastatic esophageal squamous cell carcinoma, first-line platinum-containing cytotoxic chemotherapy should be combined with immune checkpoint inhibition using nivolumab,[A7,A8] camrelizumab,[A9] toripalimab,[A10] or pembrolizumab.[A11] For patients who have unresectable or metastatic disease, palliative therapy includes endoscopically placed expandable prosthetic stents (to open the nearly obstructed lumen and to allow passage of food contents), percutaneous endoscopic gastrotomy tubes (to deliver nutrition to the stomach distal to the mass lesion), total parenteral nutrition, pain control, and systemic chemotherapy.[5]

PROGNOSIS

The 5-year survival for treated esophageal squamous cell carcinoma is dependent upon stage and types of therapies used. For stages T1 and T2 without lymph node involvement, surgery alone may be curative in more than 60% of cases. Major postoperative complications, which occur in about one third of patients, exert a long-lasting negative effect on health-related quality of life in patients who survive for 5 years after esophagectomy for cancer. Dyspnea, fatigue, eating restrictions, sleep difficulty, and gastroesophageal reflux progressively worsen more during follow-up in patients who suffer such major postoperative complications compared with patients without major surgical complications.

ESOPHAGEAL ADENOCARCINOMA

EPIDEMIOLOGY

Esophageal adenocarcinoma has an age-adjusted annual incidence of 1.3 per 100,000. It affects Whites more than Blacks, males much more than females (3:1 to 5.5:1), and increases in incidence after age 40 years. The incidence of esophageal adenocarcinoma is increasing dramatically in developed countries, especially in the United States (by 4 to 10% annually) and Western/Northern Europe.[6]

Risk Factors

Obesity (central) is an important risk factor for esophageal adenocarcinoma (see Table 178-1), perhaps because it is related to either mechanical factors that foster greater gastroesophageal reflux disease (GERD) or, more likely, the release of proinflammatory adipokines, cytokines, and chemokines that track to the esophagus. The major recognized precursor of esophageal adenocarcinoma is Barrett esophagus (Chapter 124), which is the replacement of the normal stratified squamous epithelium by an incomplete small intestinal epithelium (metaplasia) that projects from the gastroesophageal junction into the distal esophagus in a distal-proximal gradient (Chapter 124). In turn, Barrett esophagus is fostered by GERD as well as by an admixture of bile acids in the acid refluxate. A small subset of patients with Barrett esophagus may progress to esophageal adenocarcinoma through intermediate stages of low-grade and high-grade dysplasia. In Barrett esophagus, one case of esophageal adenocarcinoma is estimated to arise in every 55 to 441 patient-years, a rate that corresponds to an approximately 125-fold increased risk for esophageal adenocarcinoma compared with the risk in the general population.

PATHOBIOLOGY

In Barrett esophagus, metaplasia in the distal esophagus results in a small intestinal epithelium with columnar enterocytes and secretory goblet cells, but without Paneth cells or enteroendocrine cells—hence the designation of incomplete intestinal metaplasia.[7] By itself, the metaplasia of Barrett esophagus cannot become esophageal adenocarcinoma. However, if and when Barrett esophagus transitions to low-grade and high-grade dysplasia, risk for esophageal adenocarcinoma increases dramatically. Barrett esophagus is associated with abnormal DNA ploidy as well as genetic alterations in epidermal growth factor receptor signalling, *TP53*, and *p16INK4A*. Emerging data demonstrate that markers, including mutation of TP53 and detection of aneuploidy, can identify patients whose Barrett esophagus has the greatest risk of progressing to cancer.

Esophageal adenocarcinoma can be distinguished from gastroesophageal adenocarcinomas (so-called gastroesophageal junctional cancer) and gastric cardia adenocarcinomas based on its location, although genomic data demonstrate remarkable similarity between esophageal and gastric adenocarcinomas. Whole-genome approaches show gains and losses of chromosomal regions that might lead to identification of known and previously unknown genes critical in the pathogenesis of esophageal adenocarcinoma.

CLINICAL MANIFESTATIONS

Symptoms and Signs

A small subset (about 5 to 15%) of patients who have gastroesophageal reflux disease may develop Barrett esophagus. However, millions of people are affected with gastroesophageal reflux disease, and most patients who have gastroesophageal reflux disease do not undergo upper endoscopy. Patients with Barrett esophagus may or may not have symptoms related to gastroesophageal reflux disease. Chronic gastroesophageal reflux disease with Barrett esophagus may be associated with distal esophageal strictures. Patients with esophageal adenocarcinoma may suffer from dysphagia, odynophagia, upper gastrointestinal bleeding, chest pain, nausea, vomiting, early satiety, weight loss, and malnutrition.

Physical Examination

Examination of the patient may reveal signs consistent with malnutrition and weight loss. Hepatomegaly may be present, and lymphadenopathy may be a sign of metastasis. Paraneoplastic syndromes are unusual with esophageal adenocarcinoma.

Laboratory Studies

Patients with esophageal adenocarcinoma may have iron deficiency anemia (from occult upper GI bleeding), metabolic derangements, and abnormal liver enzyme tests owing to metastatic disease. The CEA level may be elevated as a tumor serologic marker, although it is not a diagnostic test.

DIAGNOSIS

It is important to ensure that esophageal adenocarcinoma is not mistaken for a benign entity such as a primary esophageal motility disorder. Barium swallow radiography may lead to the suspicion of Barrett esophagus and can diagnose luminal mass lesions consistent with esophageal adenocarcinoma in the distal esophagus. However, the mainstay of diagnosis is upper endoscopy. If the extent of Barrett esophagus is 3 cm or less, it is termed *short-segment Barrett esophagus*; if it is more than 3 cm, it is referred to as *long-segment Barrett esophagus*. This distinction is important because the risk for esophageal adenocarcinoma in long-segment Barrett esophagus is greater than in short-segment Barrett esophagus. Unlike the pinkish-white hue of the normal esophageal mucosa, esophageal adenocarcinoma has a characteristic salmon-colored mucosa that can be visualized at the gastroesophageal junction, with frondlike projections in a proximal direction. Endoscopic mucosal biopsies from the Barrett esophagus region (with control biopsies from the normal esophagus and gastric cardia) are required for histopathologic diagnosis. Features of dysplasia are best appreciated in the absence of reflux-related esophagitis, which can lead to nuclear architectural distortion. Hence, gastric acid production should be suppressed with proton pump inhibitor therapy (Table 124-1) for 6 to 8 weeks prior to biopsy.

TREATMENT

The principles for surgical resection and neoadjuvant therapy after chemoradiation and surgical resection are similar to what is recommended for squamous cell esophageal carcinoma. However, the impact of neoadjuvant chemoradiation is more modest in esophageal adenocarcinoma. In the setting of residual disease despite chemoradiation and surgery, adjuvant nivolumab can improve survival.[A12]

Systemic therapies for advanced and metastatic esophageal adenocarcinomas are analogous to what are recommended for adenocarcinomas of the stomach, including immune checkpoint therapies in concert with chemotherapy for first-line treatment under expert supervision. For tumors that overexpress the HER2 protein, targeted therapies are recommended under expert oversight. Patients with esophageal cancers often have serious comorbid conditions (e.g., obesity, heart disease, emphysema, and malnutrition) that limit treatment options after first-line therapy. For advanced, unresectable tumors, self-expanding stents, often with localized brachytherapy, can provide palliation.[8]

PREVENTION

If the patient has Barrett esophagus metaplasia, upper endoscopy should be repeated every 3 years. However, low-grade dysplasia (with confirmation by an expert pathologist) requires surveillance endoscopy every 6 to 12 months. High-grade dysplasia, if properly evaluated by the pathologist, may require reconfirmation, but then leads to either medical (radiofrequency ablation or endoscopic mucosal resection) or surgical intervention because of the possibility of missed contiguous esophageal adenocarcinoma (Chapter 124). Radiofrequency ablation reduces the progression of low-grade dysplasia or possibly high-grade Barrett esophageal dysplasia to cancer. Endoscopic mucosal resection is used for Barrett esophagus–related high-grade dysplasia or Barrett esophagus associated with intramucosal (tumor stage T1a) esophageal adenocarcinoma.[9] Endoscopic ultrasound may be helpful in discriminating between high-grade dysplasia and esophageal intramucosal adenocarcinoma.

PROGNOSIS

Localized disease detected by careful follow-up of patients with residual Barrett esophagus can be cured. With localized disease, long-term survival can exceed 50%, with higher rates among patients with complete responses to neoadjuvant therapy. However, esophageal adenocarcinoma carries among the most dismal survival rates within oncology. The overall 5-year survival is about 20%, because the disease is diagnosed at an advanced stage, it has a propensity to relapse after surgical therapy, and the efficacy of chemoradiation is modest. Whether adjuvant immune checkpoint therapy and the introduction of new agents will substantially improve survival remains to be proven.

NEOPLASMS OF THE STOMACH

DEFINITION

Gastric neoplasms are predominantly malignant, and nearly 90 to 95% of these tumors are adenocarcinomas. Less frequently observed malignant diseases include lymphomas, especially non-Hodgkin lymphoma, and sarcomas such as leiomyosarcoma. Benign gastric neoplasms include leiomyomas, carcinoid tumors, and lipomas.

ADENOCARCINOMA OF THE STOMACH

EPIDEMIOLOGY

The great geographic variation in the incidence of gastric cancer worldwide indicates that environmental factors influence the pathogenesis of gastric carcinogenesis. Further support for this notion comes from observations that groups emigrating from high-risk to low-risk areas, such as Japanese individuals moving to Hawaii and Brazil, acquire the low risk of the area into which they emigrate, presumably because of adoption of the endogenous lifestyle and exposure to different environmental factors.[10]

TABLE 178-2 CONDITIONS PREDISPOSING TO OR ASSOCIATED WITH GASTRIC CANCER

ENVIRONMENTAL
Helicobacter pylori infection
Dietary: excess of salt (salted pickled foods), nitrates/nitrites, carbohydrates; deficiency of fresh fruit, vegetables, vitamins A and C, refrigeration
Low socioeconomic status
Cigarette smoking
GENETIC
Familial gastric cancer (rare)
Associated with hereditary nonpolyposis colorectal cancer
Blood group A
PREDISPOSING CONDITIONS
Chronic gastritis, especially atrophic gastritis with or without intestinal metaplasia
Pernicious anemia
Intestinal metaplasia
Gastric adenomatous polyps (>2 cm)
Postgastrectomy stumps
Gastric epithelial dysplasia
Ménétrier disease (hypertrophic gastropathy)
Chronic peptic ulcer

Gastric adenocarcinoma was the most frequently observed malignant disease in the world until the mid-1980s, and it remains extremely common among men in certain regions such as tropical South America, some parts of the Caribbean, and Eastern Europe. Regardless of gender, it remains one of the most common malignancies in Japan and China. Nevertheless, incidence is decreasing worldwide.[11,12]

Whereas gastric cancer was the most common cancer in the United States in the 1930s, its annual incidence has steadily decreased to fewer than 10,000 new cases per year. The U.S. incidence is about 1.8-fold higher in non-Whites and is highest among Korean Americans.[13] However, although the incidence of gastric adenocarcinoma localized to the distal stomach has declined, the incidence of proximal gastric and gastroesophageal junctional adenocarcinomas has been steadily increasing in the United States, a finding that perhaps reflects differences in pathogenic factors.

Typically, gastric cancer occurs between ages 50 and 70 years and is uncommon before age 30. The rates are higher in men than in women by 2:1. However, rates of the diffuse histologic form of gastric cancer are rising in younger women for reasons that are not understood. In the United States, gastric cancer is more common in Black men and women compared with White men and women.

Risk Factors

Risk factors for the development of gastric adenocarcinoma can be divided into environmental and genetic factors as well as precursor conditions (Table 178-2). For example, *Helicobacter pylori* infection is significantly more common in patients with noncardia gastric cancer than in matched control groups. Unlike distal gastric cancer emerging in the setting of intestinal metaplasia, where metaplasia is typically precipitated by *H. pylori*, adenocarcinomas near the gastroesophageal junction appear to be inversely associated with *H. pylori*. Epidemiologic studies of high-risk populations have also suggested that genotoxic agents such as *N*-nitroso compounds may play a role in gastric tumorigenesis. *N*-nitroso compounds can be formed in the human stomach by nitrosation of ingested nitrates, which are common constituents of the diet. High nitrate concentrations in soil and drinking water have been observed in areas with high death rates from gastric cancer. Atrophic gastritis (Chapter 125), with or without intestinal metaplasia, is observed in association with gastric cancer, especially in endemic areas. Pernicious anemia (Chapter 150) is associated with a several-fold increase in gastric cancer. Atrophic gastritis and intestinal metaplasia likely represent intermediary steps to gastric cancer. The achlorhydria associated with gastritis related to *H. pylori* infection, pernicious anemia, or other causes favors the growth of bacteria that are capable of converting nitrates to nitrites. At the same time, most patients with atrophic gastritis do not develop gastric cancer, a finding suggesting that neither atrophic gastritis nor achlorhydria alone is responsible.

Benign gastric ulcers do not appear to predispose patients to gastric cancer. However, patients who have a gastric remnant after subtotal gastrectomy for benign disorders have an increased relative risk for gastric cancer of 1.5 to 3.0 by 15 to 20 years after surgery.

PATHOBIOLOGY

Gastric adenocarcinomas can be divided into two types based on the Lauren classification[14]: intestinal and diffuse. The intestinal type (typically in the distal stomach with ulcerations and often preceded by premalignant lesions) is declining in incidence in the United States, but adenocarcinomas in the area of the cardia/gastroesophageal junction have increased. By contrast, the diffuse type involves widespread thickening of the stomach, especially in the cardia, and it often affects younger patients; this form may present as linitis plastica, which is a nondistensible stomach with the absence of folds and a narrowed lumen caused by infiltration of the stomach wall with tumor. Diffuse-type gastric cancers harbor mucin-producing cells. Other conditions that may result in linitis plastica include lymphoma (Chapter 171), tuberculosis (Chapter 299), syphilis (Chapter 295), and amyloidosis (Chapter 174).

Key histopathologic features of gastric cancer include the degree of differentiation, invasion through the gastric wall, lymph node involvement, and the presence or absence of signet ring cells within the tumor itself. Other pathologic manifestations include a polypoid mass, which may be difficult to distinguish from a benign polyp. Early gastric cancer, a condition that is common in Japan and has a relatively favorable prognosis, consists of superficial lesions with or without lymph node involvement. These lesions can be classified as group I, polypoid; group II, fungating ulcer with sharp raised margins; group III, ulcer with poorly defined infiltrative margins; and group IV, infiltrative, mostly intramural lesion, not well demarcated.

The leading hypothesis explaining the way in which *H. pylori* predisposes to gastric cancer risk is the induction of an inflammatory response, in which IL-1β may be pivotal. Chronic *H. pylori* infection also leads to chronic atrophic gastritis with resulting achlorhydria, which in turn favors bacterial growth that can convert dietary nitrates to nitrites. These nitrites, in combination with genetic factors, promote abnormal cellular proliferation, genetic mutations, and eventually cancer.

Genetics

Gastric cancer patients have a two- to three-fold higher family history of the disease, thereby suggesting a genetic contribution. Furthermore, germline or inherited mutations in the genes for E-cadherin and α-catenin, albeit rare, have been described in diffuse hereditary gastric cancer, which is seen in young patients. In addition, in Lynch syndrome (Chapter 179), patients have associated extracolonic cancers, including gastric cancer. Patients with familial adenomatous polyposis also have an increased risk of distal (antral) gastric adenocarcinoma. Blood group A is also associated with a higher incidence of gastric cancer, even in nonendemic areas.

Gene expression data have identified molecular subtypes linked to distinct patterns of molecular alterations that are associated with differences in disease progression and prognosis. Examples include Epstein-Barr virus–related tumors, tumors with microsatellite or chromosomal instability, and a diffuse histologic subtype that often has decreased genomic instability.[15] Gastric tumors with chromosomal instability bear striking similarity to esophageal adenocarcinomas. Both the activation of oncogenes and the inactivation of tumor suppressor genes can be promoted by processes including chromosomal instability, aberrant DNA methylation, and microsatellite instability. Loss of *p53* is common, especially in the chromosomal instability class of gastric cancers. The inactivation of *p53* in precancerous gastric lesions suggests that mutation of *p53* is an early event in gastric carcinogenesis.

CLINICAL MANIFESTATIONS

Symptoms and Signs

In its early stages, gastric cancer may be asymptomatic or produce only nonspecific symptoms that make early diagnosis difficult. Later symptoms include bloating, dysphagia, and epigastric pain. Early satiety or vomiting may suggest partial gastric outlet obstruction, although gastric dysmotility can contribute to the vomiting with nonobstructive tumors. Epigastric pain reminiscent of that associated with peptic ulcer occurs in about one fourth of patients, but the pain is not relieved by food or antacids in most patients with gastric cancer. Pain that radiates to the back may indicate that the tumor has penetrated the pancreas. When dysphagia is associated with gastric cancer, this symptom suggests a more proximal gastric tumor at the gastroesophageal junction or in the fundus.

Signs of gastric cancer include bleeding, which can result in iron deficiency anemia (Chapter 145) that produces weakness, fatigue, and malaise, as well as rare, more serious cardiovascular and cerebrovascular consequences. Perforation related to gastric cancer is unusual. Gastric cancer metastatic to the liver can lead to right upper quadrant pain, jaundice, and fever. Lung metastases can cause cough, hiccups, and hemoptysis. Peritoneal carcinomatosis can lead to malignant ascites unresponsive to diuretics. Gastric cancer can also metastasize to bone.

Physical Examination

In the earliest stages of gastric cancer, the physical examination may be unremarkable. At later stages, patients become cachectic, and an epigastric mass may be palpated. If the tumor has metastasized to the liver, hepatomegaly with jaundice and ascites may be present. Portal or splenic vein invasion and thrombosis can cause splenomegaly. Lymph node involvement in the left supraclavicular area is termed a Virchow node, and periumbilical nodal involvement is called a Sister Mary Joseph node. The fecal occult blood test may be positive. Metastasis to the ovary is termed Krukenberg tumor.

Paraneoplastic syndromes (Chapter 164) may precede or occur concurrently with gastric cancer. Examples include Trousseau syndrome (Chapter 67), which is recurrent migratory superficial thrombophlebitis indicative of a possible hypercoagulable state; acanthosis nigricans, which arises as raised and hyperpigmented skin lesions of the flexor areas, neck, axilla, groin, and mucosal membranes; neuromyopathy with involvement of the sensory and motor pathways; and central nervous system syndromes with altered mental status and ataxia.

Laboratory Studies

Laboratory studies may reveal iron deficiency anemia. Microangiopathic hemolytic anemia has also been reported. Abnormalities in liver tests generally indicate metastatic disease. Hypoalbuminemia is a marker of malnutrition. Protein-losing enteropathy is rare but can be seen in Ménétrier disease (Chapter 125), which is another predisposing condition. Serologic test results, such as CEA and CA72.4 (typically not used), may be abnormal. Although these tests are not recommended for initial diagnosis, they may be useful for monitoring disease after surgical resection.

DIAGNOSIS

The diagnostic accuracy of upper endoscopy with biopsy and cytologic examination approaches 95 to 99% for both types of gastric cancer. Cancer may arise as a small mucosal ulceration, a polyp, or a mass (Fig. 178-1). In some patients, gastric ulceration may first be noted in an upper gastrointestinal barium contrast study. A benign gastric ulcer is associated with a smooth, regular base, whereas a malignant ulcer is associated with a surrounding mass, irregular folds, and an irregular base. Although these and other radiographic characteristics historically helped to predict benign versus malignant disease, upper gastrointestinal endoscopy with biopsy and cytologic examination is mandatory whenever a gastric ulcer is found on a radiologic study, even if the ulcer has benign characteristics.

Endoscopic ultrasonography is very helpful in both the diagnosis and staging of gastric cancer. The extent of tumor, including gastric wall invasion and local lymph node involvement, can be assessed by endoscopic ultrasound (Fig. 178-2), which provides information complementary to that obtained from CT scans. Endoscopic ultrasound can help guide aspiration biopsies of lymph nodes to determine malignant involvement. CT of the chest, abdomen, and pelvis should be performed to document lymphadenopathy and extragastric organ (especially lung and liver) involvement. In some centers, staging of gastric cancer entails bone scans because of the proclivity of gastric cancer to metastasize to bone.

TREATMENT

Surgical Therapy

The primary chance for cure of gastric cancer is surgical resection, which is possible in 25 to 30% of cases.[16] If the tumor is confined to the distal stomach, subtotal gastrectomy is performed, with resection of lymph nodes in the porta hepatis and the pancreatic head. When early gastric cancer is confined to the mucosa, endoscopic mucosal resection may be an alternative. By contrast, tumors of the proximal stomach require total gastrectomy to obtain an adequate margin and to remove lymph nodes; distal pancreatectomy and splenectomy are usually also performed as part of this procedure, which carries higher mortality and morbidity rates. The addition of para-aorta nodal dissection does not improve survival. Even if a curative procedure is not possible because of metastasis, limited gastric resection may be necessary for patients with excessive bleeding or obstruction. However, gastrectomy followed by chemotherapy is no better than chemotherapy alone for advanced gastric cancer that is not surgically curable.[A13] If cancer recurs in the gastric remnant, limited resection may again be necessary for palliation. Most recurrences of either type of gastric cancer are in the local or regional area of the original tumor.

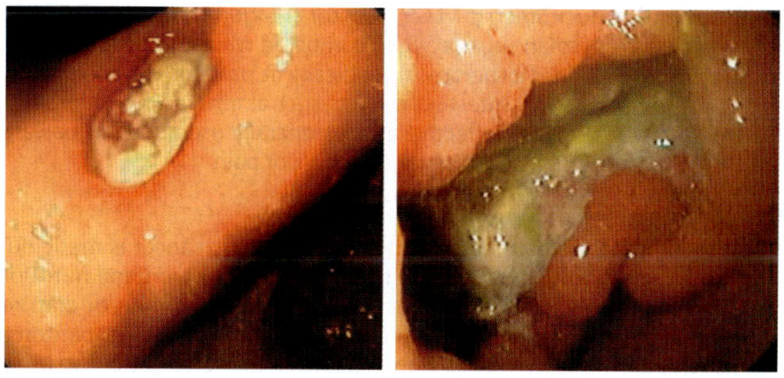

FIGURE 178-1. Benign (*left*) and malignant (*right*) gastric ulcer. Note the shaggy, thickened, and overhanging edges of the cancer. (Courtesy Pankaj Jay Pasricha, MD.)

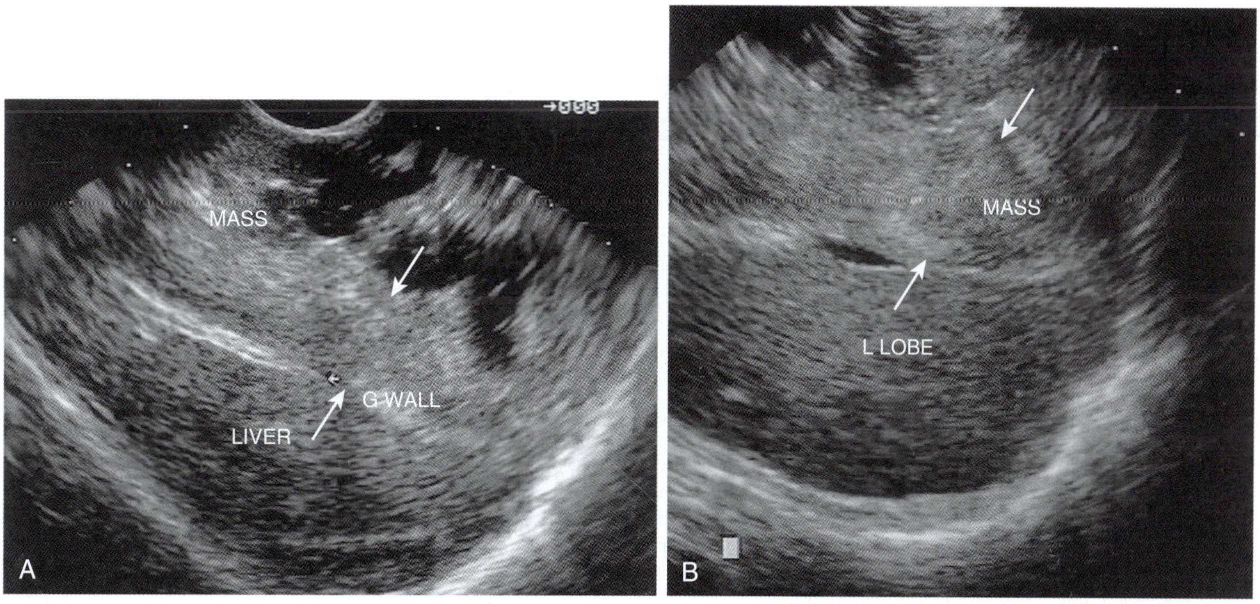

FIGURE 178-2. Gastric mass. Endoscopic ultrasonography depicting a large gastric mass that is compressing the liver and gallbladder wall (A) and, on a different view, the left lobe of the liver (B).

Medical Therapy

Gastric cancer is often responsive to chemotherapy.[17,18] Single-agent chemotherapy, which provides partial response rates of 20 to 30%, is reserved for patients with a poor performance status. Otherwise, combination chemotherapy increases overall survival compared with single-agent chemotherapy in metastatic disease as well as in the neoadjuvant and adjuvant treatment of nonmetastatic disease.[A14]

In patients who have gastric cancer and who undergo surgery with curative intent, the addition of perioperative chemotherapy can improve survival. For example, the combination of epirubicin, cisplatin, and fluorouracil, given both preoperatively and postoperatively, improves 5-year survival from 23 to 36% in patients with resectable gastroesophageal cancer. Perioperative therapy with a combination of fluorouracil, leucovorin, oxaliplatin, and docetaxel (Table 178-3) can extend median survival to 50 months and is increasingly used in medically fit patients.[A15] However, postoperative chemoradiotherapy does not improve overall survival compared with postoperative chemotherapy in patients whose resectable gastric cancers are treated with adequate preoperative chemotherapy and surgery.[A16]

For advanced or metastatic disease, combination regimens emphasize two-drug therapies, typically 5-fluorouracil or capecitabine with platinum. First-line therapy is now being increasingly supplemented with immune checkpoint inhibitors; their benefit is most notable in patients whose tumors express PD-L1,[A17] but patients whose tumors demonstrate microsatellite instability or are positive for Epstein–Barr virus may also be especially sensitive to PD-1 therapy.

Some gastric cancers have overexpression of the human epidermal growth factor receptor 2 (HER2, also called ERBB2). In patients with advanced gastric or gastroesophageal junction cancers showing overexpression of HER2, the addition of trastuzumab (a humanized monoclonal anti-HER2 antibody) to chemotherapy increases survival from 11.1 months to 13.8 months. The addition of the immune checkpoint inhibitor pembrolizumab is now approved in combination with trastuzumab and chemotherapy for first-line therapy in all ERBB2+ patients with metastatic disease.

Following resistance to first-line therapy, trastuzumab deruxtecan (which is an antibody-drug conjugate consisting of trastuzumab, a cleavable tetra-peptide-based linker, and a cytotoxic topoisomerase I inhibitor) can increase median survival by about 4 months and is now approved for second-line usage.[A18] The combination of ramucirumab (a VEGF receptor antagonist) plus paclitaxel can modestly increase median survival when compared with supportive care.

Empiric third-line chemotherapy in medically fit patients can include regimens utilized in other gastrointestinal cancers, such as irinotecan/5-fluorouracil. Radiation therapy alone is ineffective and is generally used only for palliative purposes in the setting of bleeding, obstruction, or pain.

Other Management

Critical in the management of the patient with gastric cancer is meticulous attention to nutrition (jejunal enteral feedings or total parenteral nutrition), correction of metabolic abnormalities that arise from vomiting or diarrhea, and treatment of infection from aspiration or spontaneous bacterial peritonitis. Patients with early gastric cancer who receive *H. pylori* eradication treatment have a reduced risk for metachronous gastric carcinoma.[A19] To maintain lumen patency, endoscopic laser treatment or prosthesis placement can be used in a palliative fashion.

TABLE 178-3 COMMON CHEMOTHERAPY REGIMENS FOR GASTRIC CANCER

NEOADJUVANT/PERIOPERATIVE THERAPY
For Medically Fit Patients: FLOT (5-fluorouracil, leucovorin, oxaliplatin, docetaxel) given as 4 preoperative and 4 postoperative 2-week cycles
METASTATIC CANCER FIRST LINE
5-fluorouracil and platinum chemotherapy backbone with immune checkpoint inhibitor (PD-1) for PD-L1+ (or can be used more broadly in PD-L1-); for ERBB2/HER2+ patients, add trastuzumab and pembrolizumab and consider addition of an anti-EGFR antibody

PREVENTION

In patients who have a family history of gastric cancer in a first-degree relative and who are infected with *H. pylori*, *H. pylori* eradication therapy reduces the risk of gastric cancer by about 75%.[A20] Such treatment also has reduced the incidence of gastric cancer by 40 to 50% in high-risk patients in Southern China[A21] and in patients who have precancerous lesions.[A22] Whether such treatment is equally effective in lower-risk populations is not known.[19]

PROGNOSIS

In aggregate, the overall 5-year survival rate of patients with gastric cancer is less than 10%. Approximately one third of patients who undergo a curative resection are alive after 5 years. In patients with early gastric cancer that is confined to the mucosa and submucosa, surgical resection can be curative and improves the 5-year survival rate to more than 50%.

Prognostic factors include anatomic location and nodal status. Distal gastric cancers without lymph node involvement have a better prognosis than proximal gastric cancers with or without lymph node involvement. Other prognostic factors include depth of penetration and tumor cell DNA aneuploidy. Linitis plastica and infiltrating lesions have a much worse prognosis than polypoid disease or exophytic masses.

LYMPHOMA OF THE STOMACH

EPIDEMIOLOGY

Gastric lymphoma represents about 5% of all malignant gastric tumors and is increasing in incidence. Most gastric lymphomas are non-Hodgkin lymphomas (Chapter 171), and the stomach is the most common extranodal site for non-Hodgkin lymphomas. Patients with gastric lymphoma are generally younger than patients with gastric adenocarcinoma, but the male predominance remains.

CLINICAL MANIFESTATIONS

Patients commonly present with symptoms and signs similar to those of gastric adenocarcinoma. Lymphoma in the stomach can be a primary tumor, or it can be secondary to disseminated lymphoma.

B-cell lymphomas (Chapter 171) of the stomach are most commonly large cell with a high-grade type. Low-grade variants in the setting of chronic gastritis and are termed mucosa-associated lymphoid tissue (MALT) lymphomas. MALT lesions are strongly associated with *H. pylori* infection.

DIAGNOSIS

Radiographically, primary gastric lymphomas usually arise as ulcers or exophytic masses; diffusely infiltrating lymphoma is more suggestive of secondary lymphoma. As a result, upper gastrointestinal contrast imaging usually shows multiple nodules and ulcers for a primary gastric lymphoma and typically has the appearance of linitis plastica (see earlier) with secondary lymphoma. As with gastric adenocarcinoma, however, upper endoscopy with biopsy and cytologic examination are required for diagnosis and have an accuracy of nearly 90%. Apart from conventional histopathologic analysis, immunoperoxidase staining for lymphocyte markers is helpful in diagnosis. As with gastric adenocarcinoma, proper staging of gastric lymphoma involves endoscopic ultrasound, chest and abdominal/pelvic CT scans, and bone marrow biopsy as needed.

TREATMENT

Treatment of gastric diffuse large B-cell lymphoma is best pursued with combination chemotherapy with or without radiation therapy (Chapter 171). For MALT lesions, eradication of *H. pylori* infection with antibiotics should be attempted[20] (Chapter 125), but patients with refractory lesions that are confined to the stomach can sometimes be cured with chemoradiotherapy (Chapter 171).

OTHER MALIGNANT TUMORS OF THE STOMACH

Leiomyosarcoma (Chapter 187), which constitutes approximately 1% of all gastric cancers, usually occurs as an intramural mass with central ulceration. Symptoms may include bleeding accompanied by a palpable mass. Leiomyosarcomas are often relatively indolent; surgical resection yields a 5-year survival rate of about 50%. Metastasis can occur to lymph nodes and the liver. Other gastric sarcomas include liposarcomas, fibrosarcomas, myosarcomas, and neurogenic sarcomas.

Most gastrointestinal stromal tumors (GISTs; Chapter 187) have been associated with activating mutations in the C-*kit* gene; a subset of such tumors is associated with mutations in the platelet-derived growth factor receptor (*PDGFR*) gene.[21] C-*kit* mutations are also found in chronic and acute myelogenous leukemia (Chapters 168 and 170), and approximately 50% of GISTs respond to imatinib mesylate (400 mg daily or 400 mg twice daily for *KIT* exon 9 mutant; Chapter 170), which is typically continued for at least 3 years.[A23] If imatinib is not successful, sunitinib increases survival. If both fail, regorafenib[A24] or ripretinib[A25] under expert supervision can prolong survival.[22] Pimitespib, which is a heat shock protein 90 inhibitor, may be useful when tyrosine kinase inhibitors are no longer successful.[A26] Carcinoid tumors (Chapter 213) may begin in the stomach and are curable by removal if they have not yet spread to the liver.

Other primary tumors can spread to the stomach. In addition to lymphomas, primary lung (Chapter 177) and breast (Chapter 183) cancers as well as malignant melanoma (Chapter 188) can metastasize to the stomach.

LEIOMYOMAS AND BENIGN TUMORS

Leiomyomas (Chapter 187), which are smooth muscle tumors of benign origin, occur with equal frequency in men and women and are typically located in the middle and distal stomach. Leiomyomas can grow into the lumen, with secondary ulceration and consequent bleeding. Alternatively, they can expand to the serosa with extrinsic compression. Endoscopy may reveal a mass that has overlying mucosa or mucosa replaced by ulceration. On upper gastrointestinal imaging, leiomyomas are usually smooth with an intramural filling defect, with or without central ulceration. However, benign leiomyomas can be difficult to distinguish from their malignant counterparts radiographically or endoscopically, so tissue diagnosis is imperative. Symptomatic leiomyomas should be removed, but those without associated symptoms do not require therapy.

Other benign gastric tumors include lipomas, neurofibromas, lymphangiomas, ganglioneuromas, and hamartomas, the last associated with Peutz-Jeghers syndrome (Chapter 179) or juvenile polyposis (when restricted to the stomach).

ADENOMAS

Gastric adenomas and hyperplastic polyps are unusual but may be found in middle-aged and elderly patients. Polyps may be sessile or pedunculated. Although isolated gastric adenomatous polyps are generally asymptomatic, some patients may have dyspepsia, nausea, or bleeding. Gastric adenomas and hyperplastic polyps are smooth and regular on upper gastrointestinal series, but the diagnosis must be confirmed by upper endoscopy with biopsy. Pedunculated polyps that are larger than 2 cm or that have associated symptoms should be removed by endoscopic snare cautery polypectomy, whereas large sessile gastric adenomatous polyps may require segmental surgical resection. If polyps progress to an intermediary stage of severe dysplasia or culminate in cancer, treatment is the same as for gastric adenocarcinoma.

GENERAL REFERENCES

For the General References and other additional features, please visit Elsevier eBooks+ at https://ebooks.health.elsevier.com.

Grade A References

A1. Mariette C, Markar SR, Dabakuyo-Yonli TS, et al. Hybrid minimally invasive esophagectomy for esophageal cancer. *N Engl J Med.* 2019;380:152-162.

A2. van der Sluis PC, van der Horst S, May AM, et al. Robot-assisted minimally invasive thoracolaparoscopic esophagectomy versus open transthoracic esophagectomy for resectable esophageal cancer: a randomized controlled trial. *Ann Surg.* 2019;269:621-630.

A3. Nuytens F, Dabakuyo-Yonli TS, Meunier B, et al. Five-year survival outcomes of hybrid minimally invasive esophagectomy in esophageal cancer: results of the miro randomized clinical trial. *JAMA Surg.* 2021;156:323-332.

A4. Pasquali S, Yim G, Vohra RS, et al. Survival after neoadjuvant and adjuvant treatments compared to surgery alone for resectable esophageal carcinoma: a network meta-analysis. *Ann Surg.* 2017;265:481-491.

A5. Shapiro J, van Lanschot JJB, Hulshof M, et al. Neoadjuvant chemoradiotherapy plus surgery versus surgery alone for oesophageal or junctional cancer (CROSS): long-term results of a randomised controlled trial. *Lancet Oncol.* 2015;16:1090-1098.

A6. Yang H, Liu H, Chen Y, et al. Long-term efficacy of neoadjuvant chemoradiotherapy plus surgery for the treatment of locally advanced esophageal squamous cell carcinoma: the NEOCRTEC5010 randomized clinical trial. *JAMA Surg.* 2021;156:721-729.

A7. Doki Y, Ajani JA, Kato K, et al. Nivolumab combination therapy in advanced esophageal squamous-cell carcinoma. *N Engl J Med.* 2022;386:449-462.

A8. Janjigian YY, Shitara K, Moehler M, et al. First-line nivolumab plus chemotherapy versus chemotherapy alone for advanced gastric, gastroesophageal junction, and oesophageal adenocarcinoma (CheckMat 649): a randomised open-label, phase 3 trial. *Lancet.* 2021;398:27-40.

A9. Luo H, Lu J, Bai Y, et al. Effect of camrelizumab vs placebo added to chemotherapy on survival and progression-free survival in patients with advanced or metastatic esophageal squamous cell carcinoma: the ESCORT-1st randomized clinical trial. *JAMA.* 2021;326:916-925.

A10. Wang ZX, Cui C, Yao J, et al. Toripalimab plus chemotherapy in treatment-naïve, advanced esophageal squamous cell carcinoma (JUPITER-06): a multi-center phase 3 trial. *Cancer Cell.* 2022;40:277-288.e3.

A11. Sun JM, Shen L, Shah MA, et al. Pembrolizumab plus chemotherapy versus chemotherapy alone for first-line treatment of advanced oesophageal cancer (KEYNOTE-590): a randomised, placebo-controlled, phase 3 study. *Lancet.* 2021;398:759-771.

A12. Kelly RJ, Ajani JA, Kuzdzal J, et al. Adjuvant nivolumab in resected esophageal or gastroesophageal junction cancer. *N Engl J Med.* 2021;384:1191-1203.

A13. Fujitani K, Yang HK, Mizusawa J, et al. Gastrectomy plus chemotherapy versus chemotherapy alone for advanced gastric cancer with a single non-curable factor (REGATTA): a phase 3, randomised controlled trial. *Lancet Oncol.* 2016;17:309-318.

A14. Iacovelli R, Pietrantonio F, Maggi C, et al. Combination or single-agent chemotherapy as adjuvant treatment of gastric cancer: a systematic review and meta-analysis of published trials. *Crit Rev Oncol Hematol.* 2016;98:24-28.

A15. Al-Batran S-E, Homann N, Pauligk C, et al. Perioperative chemotherapy with fluorouracil plus leucovorin, oxaliplatin, and docetaxel versus fluorouracil or capecitabine plus cisplatin and epirubicin for locally advanced, resectable gastric or gastro-oesophageal junction adenocarcinoma (FLOT4): a randomised, phase 2/3 trial. *Lancet.* 2019;393:1948-1957.

A16. Cats A, Jansen EPM, van Grieken NCT, et al. Chemotherapy versus chemoradiotherapy after surgery and preoperative chemotherapy for resectable gastric cancer (CRITICS): an international, open-label, randomised phase 3 trial. *Lancet Oncol.* 2018;19:616-628.

A17. Shitara K, Özgüroğlu M, Bang YJ, et al. Pembrolizumab versus paclitaxel for previously treated, advanced gastric or gastro-oesophageal junction cancer (KEYNOTE-061): a randomised, open-label, controlled, phase 3 trial. *Lancet.* 2018;392:123-133.

A18. Shitara K, Bang YJ, Iwasa S, et al. Trastuzumab deruxtecan in previously treated HER2-positive gastric cancer. *N Engl J Med.* 2020;382:2419-2430.

A19. Choi IJ, Kook MC, Kim YI, et al. Helicobacter pylori therapy for the prevention of metachronous gastric cancer. *N Engl J Med.* 2018;378:1085-1095.

A20. Choi IJ, Kim CG, Lee JY, et al. Family history of gastric cancer and *Helicobacter pylori* treatment. *N Engl J Med.* 2020;382:427-436.

A21. Yan L, Chen Y, Chen F, et al. Effect of Helicobacter pylori eradication on gastric cancer prevention: updated report from a randomized controlled trial with 26.5 years of follow-up. *Gastroenterology.* 2022;163:154-162.e3.

A22. Ford AC, Yuan Y, Moayyedi P. *Helicobacter pylori* eradication therapy to prevent gastric cancer: systematic review and meta-analysis. *Gut.* 2020;69:2113-2121.

A23. Joensuu H, Eriksson M, Sundby Hall K, et al. Survival outcomes associated with 3 years vs 1 year of adjuvant imatinib for patients with high-risk gastrointestinal stromal tumors: an analysis of a randomized clinical trial after 10-year follow-up. *JAMA Oncol.* 2020;6:1241-1246.

A24. Kang YK, George S, Jones RL, et al. Avapritinib versus regorafenib in locally advanced unresectable or metastatic GI stromal tumor: a randomized, open-label phase III study. *J Clin Oncol.* 2021;39:3128-3139.

A25. Blay JY, Serrano C, Heinrich MC, et al. Ripretinib in patients with advanced gastrointestinal stromal tumours (INVICTUS): a double-blind, randomised, placebo-controlled, phase 3 trial. *Lancet Oncol.* 2020;21:923-934.

A26. Kurokawa Y, Honma Y, Sawaki A, et al. Pimitespib in patients with advanced gastrointestinal stromal tumor (CHAPTER-GIST-301): a randomized, double-blind, placebo-controlled phase III trial. *Ann Oncol.* 2022;33:959-967.

179 NEOPLASMS OF THE SMALL AND LARGE INTESTINE

EDWARD CHU

NEOPLASMS OF THE SMALL INTESTINE

EPIDEMIOLOGY

Small bowel malignancies are relatively rare and account for only approximately 3% of all cancers involving the gastrointestinal (GI) tract and less than 0.5% of all cancers in the United States. In 2022, an estimated 11,790 new cases of small bowel cancers will be diagnosed, and this disease accounts for nearly 1960 deaths annually.[1] The four major histologic subtypes, which make up over 90% of small bowel cancers, include carcinoid, adenocarcinoma, lymphoma, and gastrointestinal stromal tumors (GISTs). Over the past several decades, the incidence of small bowel tumors, and in particular carcinoid tumors, has increased significantly, in part because of improved diagnostic techniques.

For small bowel tumors, the mean age at diagnosis is 65 years. Sarcomas and lymphomas present at a slightly younger age, in the range of ages 60 to 62 years, whereas adenocarcinomas and carcinoid tumors present at a mean age of 68 years. These cancers are slightly more common in men compared with women and in Blacks compared with Whites.

PATHOBIOLOGY

Adenocarcinomas typically arise from adenomas, and the adenoma-carcinoma process is driven by specific genetic alterations.[2] Large-scale genomic analysis has identified distinct genomic differences between small bowel adenocarcinomas and colorectal cancers. *HER2* point mutations, microsatellite instability, and high tumor mutational load are more common in small bowel adenocarcinomas, and potentially targetable mutations in *PIK3CA* and *MEK1* also are seen. Small bowel adenocarcinomas comprise approximately 35 to 40% of all malignant small bowel tumors, and the duodenum is the most common site of presentation in the small bowel. The majority of these adenocarcinomas are moderately or well differentiated.

Small bowel carcinoids (Chapter 213) are derived from enterochromaffin cells in the crypts of Lieberkühn, and they account for up to 40 to 45% of cancers that arise in the small bowel. Carcinoids are typically well-differentiated cancers and, in contrast to adenocarcinomas, they tend to occur in the distal ileum. Up to 30% of cases are multifocal. Other less common small bowel neuroendocrine tumors include gastrinomas and somatostatinomas (Chapter 213). Small cell cancers occur rarely in the small bowel.

About 15% of small bowel cancers are malignant connective tissue tumors. GISTs, which are derived from the interstitial cells of Cajal, account for approximately 85% of the connective tissue tumors in the small bowel (Fig. 179-1). GISTs most commonly present in the duodenum, and they often resemble soft tissue sarcomas morphologically (Fig. 179-2). However, in contrast to classic sarcomas, GISTs express the c-Kit protein (CD117). Soft tissue sarcomas, such as leiomyosarcomas, present more commonly in the stomach and rarely in the small bowel (Chapter 187).

Primary GI lymphomas represent the most common location for extranodal lymphomas, and the second most common site in the GI tract is the small intestine. The non-Hodgkin histopathologic subtype is most commonly observed, and they account for nearly 10% of all small bowel cancers. The ileum is the most common region for these extranodal GI lymphomas, presumably because this region of the small intestine is rich in submucosal lymphoid follicles. These cancers may be low- or high-grade in nature. Although they are most commonly of B-cell origin (Chapter 171), they can also arise from precursor T lymphocytes.

The small intestine is also a site for metastatic spread of advanced solid cancers. Metastatic spread can occur via direct invasion, hematogenous spread, or extension of peritoneal metastases. For example, the small bowel is the most common GI site for metastatic malignant melanoma (Chapter 188). Ovarian (Chapter 184), breast (Chapter 183), lung (Chapter 177), and other GI cancers (Chapter 178) can also spread to the small bowel.

Benign tumors originating in the small bowel include adenomas, lipomas, and leiomyomas. Desmoids, hamartomas, and hemangiomas are other benign tumors but are relatively rare. These benign tumors usually present in the distal small bowel.

Predisposing Conditions

Age is an important risk factor for small bowel cancers as it is for colorectal cancer. These cancers occur in the older age population, with a mean age of 66 years. Chronic mucosal inflammatory conditions are linked to the development of small bowel adenocarcinomas and lymphoma. Inflammatory bowel disease (Chapter 127), in particular Crohn disease, is associated with an increased risk of adenocarcinoma within the involved region of the small intestine, and the risk of small bowel adenocarcinoma increases with extent and duration of small bowel involvement. Patients with chronic immunodeficiency states and autoimmune disorders, such as celiac disease (Chapter 126), are at increased risk for developing small bowel adenocarcinomas and small bowel lymphoma.

A number of dietary factors, including red meat, salt-cured and smoked food, refined sugar, and alcohol, are associated with an increased risk of small bowel adenocarcinomas. Although tobacco exposure and obesity may increase the risk of small bowel cancers, the data on the potential role of these two factors are conflicting.

Several familial polyposis syndromes are associated with small bowel neoplasms. Familial adenomatous polyposis syndrome is associated with a 100% risk of developing colorectal cancer, and patients with this familial colorectal cancer syndrome have a 4 to 12% lifetime risk of developing cancers in the duodenum or periampullary region. The risk of cancer is related to the number of polyps and to their size, histologic type, and degree of dysplasia. Hereditary nonpolyposis colon cancer is associated with an 80% lifetime risk of colorectal cancer and a 1 to 4% lifetime risk of small bowel cancer, which represents a 100-fold increased risk when compared with the general population. Hereditary nonpolyposis colorectal cancer–associated small bowel cancers tend to present 10 to 20 years earlier than the usual age of onset for small bowel cancer. Peutz-Jeghers syndrome is associated with a 57% lifetime risk of GI cancers, with colorectal cancer the most common tumor followed by small bowel adenocarcinoma.

CLINICAL MANIFESTATIONS

Small bowel malignant tumors are usually associated with symptoms, whereas benign tumors are asymptomatic in up to 50% of patients. The most common symptom is abdominal pain. Other symptoms include weight loss, nausea and vomiting, reduced appetite, fatigue, GI bleeding, and symptoms related to GI obstruction. Duodenal primary tumors, and especially tumors in the periampullary region, can be associated with obstructive jaundice.

Small bowel carcinoid tumors are usually asymptomatic. With advanced disease and especially in the presence of hepatic metastasis, they secrete bioactive amines that can lead to symptoms typically associated with the carcinoid syndrome: flushing, wheezing, diarrhea, and right-sided heart failure (related to valvular fibrosis) (Chapter 213). Systemic symptoms are more frequent with tumors that originate in the jejunum or ileum.

Patients with lymphoma may present with evidence of lymphadenopathy, hepatomegaly, and intestinal obstruction (e.g., abdominal distention and hyperperistalsis). GI lymphomas also may present with constitutional symptoms, such as fever, night sweats, and weight loss. Benign tumors usually are incidental findings, although larger tumors may eventually cause obstruction or bleeding.

DIAGNOSIS

The diagnosis of small bowel cancer is often delayed due to its rare and nonspecific presentation. The mean duration of symptoms prior to making a definitive diagnosis of small bowel cancer ranges from 8 to 10 months. In patients with small bowel tumors, the physical examination is typically unremarkable, although some patients develop a palpable mass, distended abdomen, or ascites. Patients with a primary duodenal tumor may present with scleral icterus and jaundice resulting from biliary obstruction.

The common laboratory findings may include iron deficiency anemia (Chapter 145) or elevations in hepatic enzymes (aspartate aminotransferase [AST], alanine aminotransferase [ALT], alkaline phosphatase). The serum bilirubin level can be elevated in patients who have liver metastases or biliary obstruction. In small bowel adenocarcinoma, serum levels of the carcinoembryonic antigen (CEA) may be elevated, especially in advanced cases, but this

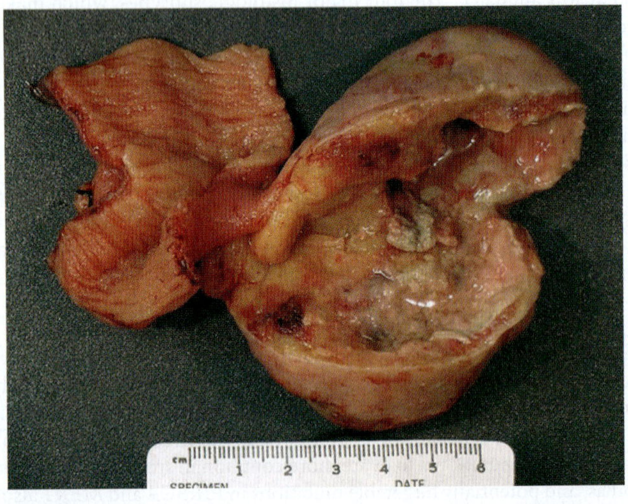

FIGURE 179-1. Small bowel gastrointestinal stromal tumor with ulceration.

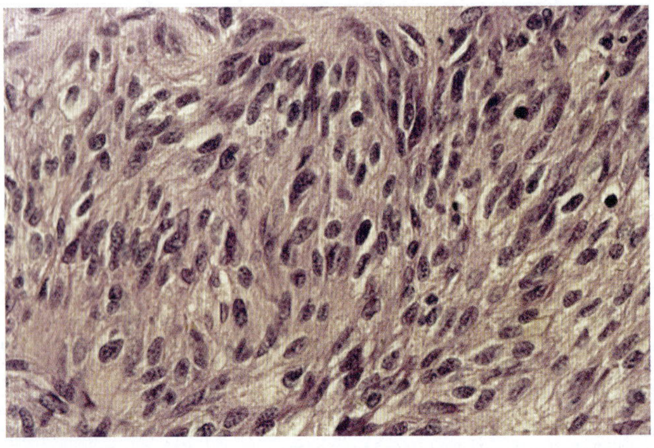

FIGURE 179-2. Histopathology of gastrointestinal stromal tumor (GIST).

marker is neither sensitive nor specific for routine diagnosis because several tumor types may present with elevated levels. In patients with neuroendocrine tumors, elevated levels of serotonin, chromogranin A, tumor-specific bioactive amines (e.g., gastrin), or urinary 5-hydroxyindoleacetic acid (5-HIAA) are commonly observed.

Imaging is required to diagnose and stage small bowel tumors, but no imaging modality is optimal.[3] Standard imaging techniques include upper GI series with small bowel follow-through, enteroclysis, transabdominal ultrasound, computed tomography (CT) scan, or magnetic resonance imaging (MRI). Enteroclysis is a double-contrast imaging study that is superior to an upper GI series with small bowel follow-through, and it has greater sensitivity to detect malignant small bowel tumors. A major limitation of enteroclysis is the inability to detect flat lesions. CT scanning of the abdomen is the most common imaging modality used in daily clinical practice, and this imaging modality is good for diagnosing primary tumors as well as metastatic disease. MRI appears to be superior to CT, especially as it relates to the detection of liver metastases as well as characterizing soft tissue sarcomas.

Carcinoids and primary neuroendocrine tumors are best imaged with nuclear medicine scans with indium-111 octreotide and/or meta-iodobenzylguanidine (MIBG). Over 90% of carcinoid tumors express somatostatin receptors, and the octreotide scan using the indium-111 tracer has high sensitivity (80 to 100%). A wide variety of small bowel cancers, including adenocarcinomas, lymphomas, and GISTs, may display uptake on positron emission tomograph (PET) scanning. However, PET is not useful for diagnosing carcinoid tumors because they are not typically FDG-avid.

Video capsule endoscopy (Chapter 120) uses a wireless endoscopic device to visualize the entire small bowel. The primary indication for video capsule endoscopy is to evaluate GI bleeding of an unknown source. In about 2 to 3% of patients who undergo capsule endoscopy for GI bleeding, a tumor is found. Capsule endoscopy can also assess the small intestine in patients who have familial adenomatous polyposis and Peutz-Jeghers syndrome, but its clinical utility as a routine screening test in such patients is unknown.

Deep enteroscopy techniques (Chapter 120) facilitate the intubation of the small bowel using long endoscopes. The small bowel may be examined antegrade (from the mouth) or retrograde (from the colon), thereby permitting direct examination of most of the small bowel. These methods are more invasive than capsule endoscopy but have the potential advantages for tissue biopsy, immediate polypectomy, and direct control of bleeding.

Staging

Staging for small bowel tumors varies by histology. Adenocarcinomas, GISTs, and neuroendocrine cancers are typically staged using specific classifications within the American Joint Committee on Cancer's (AJCC) TNM system. In contrast, non-Hodgkin lymphomas (Chapter 171) are staged in accordance with a modified Ann Arbor system originally used for the staging of Hodgkin disease (Chapter 172).

TREATMENT

Surgery

Surgical removal is the treatment of choice for localized small bowel tumors, with the extent of the surgical resection dependent on the tumor's histology and location. For adenocarcinomas in the first two portions of the duodenum, extensive pancreaticoduodenectomy is usually required, whereas small bowel carcinomas of the distal small intestine may require segmental or wide local resection of the tumor and the regional lymph nodes. En bloc resection is recommended for low-grade endocrine tumors, including regional lymph nodes. In contrast, GISTs do not require lymphadenectomy, unless the lymph nodes are grossly abnormal at the time of surgery. Surgery is not usually a primary treatment approach for lymphomas but can be considered for low-stage lymphomas. Surgery may also be required to treat complications such as bowel obstruction or perforation. Benign small bowel tumors, such as incidental lipomas, may simply be observed. Small adenomas can be removed by endoscopic polypectomy, but periampullary villous adenomas may require pancreaticoduodenectomy (Video 179-1).

Adjuvant Therapy

The role of adjuvant therapy depends on the specific type of small bowel cancer. Small bowel adenocarcinomas are generally treated similarly to colorectal cancer, with 6 months of fluoropyrimidine-based systemic chemotherapy under expert guidance for patients with lymph node involvement. Completely resected, moderately differentiated neuroendocrine cancers do not require adjuvant therapy.

For high-risk GISTs, postoperative imatinib reduces recurrence, and 3 years of treatment improves survival compared with 1 year of treatment, especially in patients with certain *Kit* exon 11 deletions as well as deletions that involve exon 11 codons 557 or 558. Emerging clinical data suggest that 5 years of adjuvant imatinib therapy may confer additional clinical benefit to patients with high-risk GISTs.[4] For other soft tissue sarcomas, adjuvant therapy has no definitive role following surgical resection. Postoperative systemic chemotherapy is recommended for both low- and high-grade lymphomas (Chapter 171).

Metastatic Disease

Metastatic small bowel carcinomas are generally treated with systemic chemotherapy regimens known to be effective against colorectal cancer, but no treatment regimen is standard.[5,6] For patients with metastatic GISTs, imatinib therapy yields median survival rates of nearly 4 years, with an estimated 10-year survival rate of about 20%.[A1] When resistance to imatinib develops, sunitinib and/or regorafenib are effective second-line treatments under expert guidance. For metastatic carcinoids that are surgically unresectable, somatostatin analogues, such as octreotide and lanreotide, are the main treatment options (Chapter 213), but agents such as 5-fluorouracil, streptozocin, and doxorubicin have been used with modest clinical activity (see Table 164-2).

PREVENTION

In patients with any of the various familial colon cancer syndromes (including familial adenomatous polyposis, hereditary nonpolyposis colorectal cancer, and Peutz-Jeghers syndrome), regular surveillance of the small intestine is required. Patients with familial adenomatous polyposis also should undergo regular screening esophagogastroduodenoscopy as part of their initial diagnostic evaluation and again at intervals of 1 to 5 years, depending on the presence and degree of duodenal polyposis. Patients with hereditary nonpolyposis colorectal cancer are also at increased risk for small bowel carcinomas, which may, in fact, be the first manifestation of their disease. Hereditary nonpolyposis colorectal cancer–associated small bowel cancer typically presents at a younger age (median, 39 years), and the duodenum is the most common site of disease (about 50% of cases). Screening should be started at age 30 years. Patients with sporadic small intestine adenomas and patients with carcinoid tumors should undergo colonoscopy given their higher risk of colonic neoplasia. Currently, no specific guidelines are available for the routine surveillance of patients with resected small bowel carcinomas.

PROGNOSIS

The overall prognosis for small bowel cancers depends on the specific pathologic subtype. For small bowel carcinomas, the 5-year survival is 50 to 85% for stage I to III patients but only 5% for stage IV. Tumor site is an important determinant of prognosis, with survival rates being worse for primary duodenal tumors compared with ileal or jejunal primary tumors. Other factors associated with poor prognosis include poor differentiation, lymph node involvement, distant metastases, and lymphovascular invasion. The tumor mutational burden and SMAD4 mutations may potentially be useful biomarkers for predicting the prognosis in small bowel cancers.[7]

Carcinoids (Chapter 213) are typically indolent, and 5-year survival rates range between 50 and 95% depending on the stage of disease. The prognosis of small intestine GISTs depends on the primary site (distal tumors have a worse prognosis), size, and mitotic activity, as well as the adequacy of surgical resection. However, 5-year survival rates approach 80% with imatinib therapy, even when complete surgical resection is not possible. For small intestinal lymphomas, the 5-year survival rate is over 60% but varies by histologic subtype.

NEOPLASMS OF THE LARGE INTESTINE

EPIDEMIOLOGY

In the United States, colorectal cancer is the third most common cancer, with an annual incidence of approximately 150,000. It is also the second-leading cause of cancer death, with approximately 53,000 deaths each year. Worldwide, an estimated 1.2 million new cases of colorectal cancer are diagnosed each year, and about 600,000 patients die from it. In the average individual, the lifetime risk of developing colorectal cancer is high, about 1 in 20.

About 75% of large bowel cancers arise in the proximal colon. Colorectal cancer is more common in the elderly, with a median age of approximately 73 years, but about 10% of cases are in patients younger than age 50 years. The overall incidence and mortality of colorectal cancer have declined significantly over the past 2 decades, especially for patients older than 50 years of age. However, this decline has not occurred equally in all populations and varies according to age. For example, the incidence of colorectal cancer in adults younger than age 50 years has increased by more than 20% since 2000, and this rise has been driven by tumors in the distal colon and rectum.[8] The incidence in individuals between ages 20 and 49 years has also been increasing, with the largest increase, approaching 90%, in Hispanics ages 20 to 29 years.[9] The overall incidence of left-sided or distal colon cancer has decreased, likely because of effective distal large bowel screening, but the incidence of right-sided or proximal colon cancer has been steadily increasing in the United States.

Colorectal cancer is slightly more common in men than in women, and men, on average, develop the disease 5 to 10 years younger than women. The mortality associated with colorectal cancer is also 25% higher in men. Of all the ethnic groups in the United States, Blacks have the highest rates of colorectal cancer, and they are diagnosed an average of 5 to 10 years earlier than White patients, with an especially increased frequency under age 50 years. The mortality associated with this disease is 20% higher in Blacks than in Whites.

Risk Factors

Sporadic colorectal cancer accounts for 80 to 85% of cases, and the main risk factors include older age, male sex, African ancestry, family history, inflammatory bowel disease, obesity, diabetes mellitus and insulin resistance, tobacco use, and alcohol use. The consumption of red meat or processed foods and reduced intake of fiber, green leafy vegetables, and fruits also contributes to the risk of colorectal cancer. The presence of certain intestinal microbiota, including bacteria (*Streptococcus bovis*, *Fusobacterium*, and various *E. coli* strains) and viruses (human papillomavirus), may be risk factors. Factors associated with a reduced risk of colorectal cancer include greater physical activity and exercise; higher dietary intake of fiber, fruit, and vegetables; regular use of aspirin and nonsteroidal anti-inflammatory agents; and supplementation with folic acid, calcium, and vitamin D.

Age is the strongest risk factor for sporadic colorectal cancer, with risk increasing substantially starting at age 50 years. Nevertheless, 10 to 12% of colorectal cancers are diagnosed before age 50 years.[10] Family history is important, even in the absence of defined familial colon cancer syndromes. If a first-degree relative has colorectal cancer, a person's risk for developing colorectal cancer is two- to three-fold higher, with the risk rising to five- to six-fold when two first-degree relatives have colorectal cancer. Even if a first-degree relative has an adenoma, the risk of colorectal cancer is increased two-fold. Patients with a history of ulcerative colitis or Crohn disease (Chapter 127) have a 60% higher risk of colorectal cancer[11] compared with the general population, and the risk is related to the extent and duration of large bowel involvement.

PATHOBIOLOGY

Adenocarcinomas comprise more than 90% of colorectal cancers. Other relatively rare histologic subtypes include neuroendocrine cancers, epidermoid carcinomas, hamartomas, lymphomas, and sarcomas (including GISTs). Composite tumors are also observed, most commonly adenocarcinomas with neuroendocrine features.

Adenocarcinomas

Colorectal adenocarcinomas arise from the columnar glandular epithelium of the mucosa. Mucinous cancers make up the large majority of colorectal cancer, whereas only about 20% do not produce mucin. Mucinous cancers tend to develop in the right side of the colon. The medullary carcinoma subtype is characterized by large, eosinophilic cells and has a heavy infiltration of tumor-infiltrating lymphocytes. These tumors exhibit a high degree of microsatellite instability because they are deficient in one or more of the mismatch repair proteins. Medullary carcinomas arise more commonly on the right side of the colon, are seen in older women, and are less likely to spread to lymph nodes. Signet ring cancer is characterized by large numbers of single tumor cells with nuclear displacement by intracytoplasmic mucin.

Carcinogenesis for colorectal adenocarcinomas is caused by a multistep process when multiple genetic alterations occur over time (Fig. 179-3) in one or more of three pathways: chromosomal instability, microsatellite instability, and CpG island methylator phenotype. The chromosomal instability pathway, which accounts for up to 70% of cases of sporadic colorectal cancer, is most commonly related to mutations in the *APC* (tumor suppressor gene) and in the *KRAS* gene (proto-oncogene that regulates transduction of mitogenic signals across cell membranes). In familial adenomatous polyposis, germline mutations in *APC* are the result of chromosomal instability that leads to aneuploidy (imbalance in chromosome number), genomic amplifications, and loss of heterozygosity (cells have only one gene allele because of the loss of individual chromosomes during mitosis). Several other gene mutations lead to colorectal cancer, including the colon cancer (*MCC*) gene (a tumor suppressor gene), p53 (a key regulator of the cell cycle), *VEGF*, *MYC*, *MET*, *LYN*, and *PTEN*. Many of the mutational events have downstream effects on the Wnt signaling pathway.

The microsatellite instability pathway is a result of defects in DNA mismatch repair. Microsatellites are short repeating nucleotide sequences that are prone to errors because of their repetitive nature. Microsatellite instability–high tumors are caused by defects in the function of mismatch repair genes, especially *MLH1*, *MSH2*, *MSH6*, and *PMS2*. Germline mutations in these genes cause HNPCC (Lynch syndrome), but silencing of *MLH1* by hypermethylation is the most common molecular mechanism underlying mismatch repair defects in sporadic colorectal cancer. Microsatellite instability–high tumors are more

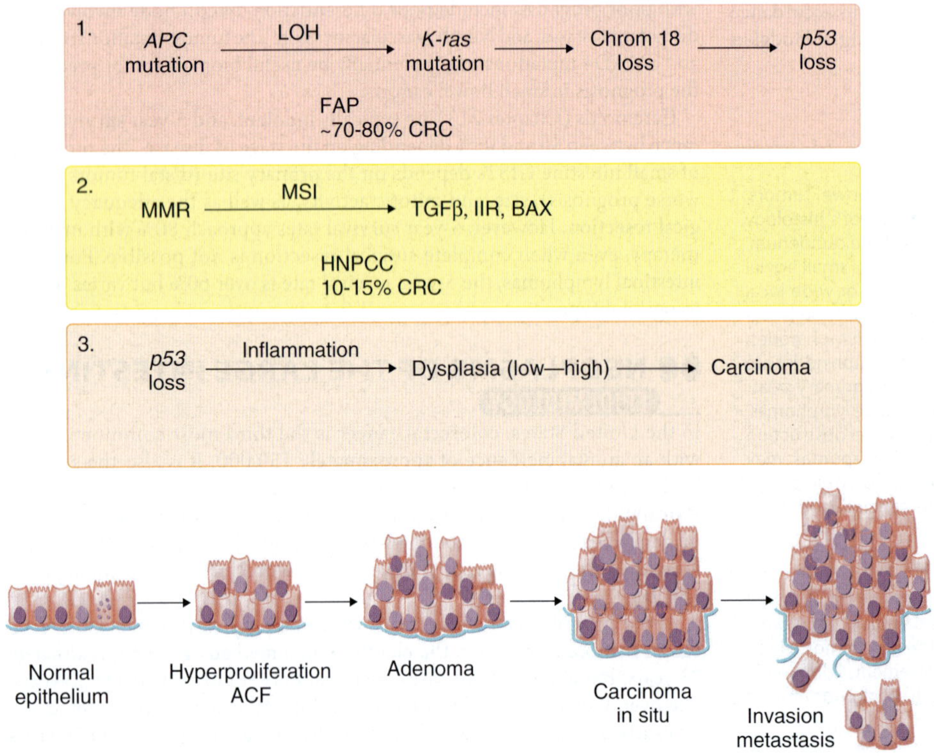

FIGURE 179-3. **The molecular basis of colorectal cancer.** Sequence-specific genetic alterations result in the transition from normal large bowel epithelium to invasive cancer. *Panel 1* demonstrates chromosomal instability, *Panel 2* illustrates microsatellite instability, and *Panel 3* shows the CpG island methylator phenotype. ACF = aberrant crypt foci; *APC* = adenomatous polyposis coli; BAX = apoptosis-related proteins; CRC = colorectal cancer; FAP = familial adenomatous polyposis; HNPCC = hereditary nonpolyposis colorectal cancer; IIR = type II receptor; LOH = loss of heterozygosity; MMR = mutation mismatch repair; MSI = microsatellite instability; TGF-β = transforming growth factor-β.

common in women and in the right colon, and they are often poorly differentiated and associated with a lymphocytic infiltration.

In the CpG island methylator phenotype pathway, hypermethylation of DNA promoter regions silences tumor suppressor genes, thereby leading to carcinogenesis. In colorectal cancer, hypermethylated genes include *APC*, *MCC*, *MLH1*, and *MGMT*. CpG island methylator phenotype-high tumors often have *BRAF* mutations, are poorly differentiated, have mucinous or signet ring morphology, and are microsatellite instability high. The precursor is likely to be a sessile serrated adenoma.

Neuroendocrine Cancers

Neuroendocrine cancers include carcinoid tumors (Chapter 213) and small cell carcinomas. Carcinoid tumors are the second most common colorectal neoplasms after adenocarcinomas, and are more common in non-Whites. In the distal bowel, carcinoids rarely are hormonally inactive.

Epidermoid Carcinomas

Epidermoid carcinomas are usually of the squamous cell subtype. They tend to be more common in women and Hispanic patients. More than 90% of epidermoid carcinomas are located in the rectum, and they tend to be moderately or poorly differentiated.

Lymphomas

Primary large intestinal lymphomas (Chapter 171) make up about 10 to 20% of all GI lymphomas but less than 1% of all colorectal cancers. The cecum is the most common site, and they are more common in males and in the elderly. The large majority of these large bowel lymphomas are of B-cell origin.

Sarcomas

Large bowel sarcomas are relatively rare, and a majority are leiomyosarcomas (Chapter 187). These tumors commonly present in the rectum, where they are usually localized at the time of diagnosis, regardless of their grade. GISTs and Kaposi sarcomas (Chapter 359) occur in the large bowel.

POLYPS OF THE COLON

A polyp is a grossly visible epithelial-cell mass that protrudes out from the intestinal mucosal surface into its lumen. A polyp may be flat, sessile, or pedunculated (attached by a stalk). Polyps can be non-neoplastic or neoplastic (adenomatous). Polyps usually are asymptomatic but can occasionally cause bleeding, prolapse, or obstruction. Non-neoplastic polyps are not premalignant, but neoplastic polyps can become a true cancer.

FAMILIAL COLORECTAL CANCER SYNDROMES

Several well-defined familial syndromes are associated with an increased risk for colorectal cancer. These syndromes include hereditary nonpolyposis colorectal cancer (HNPCC), Muir-Tore syndrome, familial adenomatous polyposis, Gardner syndrome, Turcot syndrome, *MUTYH*-associated polyposis, Peutz-Jeghers syndrome, and juvenile polyposis (Table 179-1).

Hereditary Nonpolyposis Colorectal Cancer

Hereditary nonpolyposis colorectal cancer (HNPCC), also known as Lynch syndrome, is the most common hereditary colorectal cancer syndrome and accounts for approximately 2% of all cases of colorectal cancers. The cause is a highly penetrant, autosomal dominant, loss-of-function germline mutation in genes (*MLH1, MSH2, MSH6*, and *PMS2*) that repair DNA base pair mismatches occurring during DNA replication.[12]

CLINICAL MANIFESTATIONS AND DIAGNOSIS

Although patients may have several adenomas, the diffuse polyposis characteristic of familial adenomatous polyposis is not typically observed. Synchronous and metachronous tumors are common. Colon cancers associated with HNPCC have a right-sided predominance (before the splenic flexure). These cancers are often poorly differentiated but generally have a better prognosis than typical sporadic colorectal cancers. Patients with HNPCC also have a higher risk for other solid tumors, especially endometrial cancer, as well as cancers of the ovary (Chapter 184), stomach (Chapter 178), small bowel, pancreas (Chapter 180), hepatobiliary tract (Chapter 181), and ureter (Chapter 182).

The median age for diagnosis of HNPCC is the mid-40s, which is 25 to 30 years younger than the age of presentation for sporadic colorectal cancer. Testing of patients for HNPCC includes testing the tumor for microsatellite instability and staining for the protein products of mismatch repair genes (*MLH1, MSH2, MSH6*, and *PSM2*).[13] A positive screen does not definitively diagnose HNPCC, because up to 15% of sporadic colorectal cancers may have these features. Germline testing of peripheral blood is generally preferred, but saliva or a buccal swab also can be tested to confirm the presence of mutations in one of the mismatch repair genes and to make the definitive diagnosis of HNPCC.

The Amsterdam criteria define HNPCC: (1) an HNPCC-associated cancer (colorectal cancer or cancers of the stomach, small bowel, renal pelvis, ureter, or endometrium) has been diagnosed in three or more relatives, one of whom is a first-degree relative of the other two, in the absence of familial adenomatous polyposis; (2) colorectal cancer has developed in at least two successive generations; and (3) one or more family members was diagnosed before age 50 years, with one being a first-degree relative of the other two. The revised Bethesda criteria define HNPCC when: (1) colorectal cancer is diagnosed in a patient younger than 50 years of age; (2) synchronous or metachronous colorectal cancer or other Lynch syndrome–associated tumors are diagnosed, regardless of age; (3) colorectal cancer has a high degree of microsatellite instability in a patient younger than 60 years of age; (4) colorectal cancer is diagnosed in one or more first-degree relatives with a Lynch syndrome cancer, with one of the cancers diagnosed at younger than 50 years of age; (5) colorectal cancer is diagnosed in two or more first-degree or second-degree relatives with a Lynch syndrome cancer, regardless of age.

Muir-Torre Syndrome

The Muir-Torre syndrome is a rare autosomal dominant syndrome that is an HNPCC subtype. Muir-Torre syndrome also arises from mutations in DNA mismatch repair genes (*hMLH1, hMSH2*, and *MSH6*), and patients present with colorectal cancer, genitourinary tract cancers, and skin lesions, including keratoacanthomas and sebaceous tumors.

TABLE 179-1 GENERAL FEATURES OF INHERITED COLORECTAL CANCER SYNDROMES

SYNDROME	POLYP HISTOLOGY	POLYP DISTRIBUTION	AGE OF ONSET	RISK OF COLON CANCER	GENETIC LESION	CLINICAL MANIFESTATIONS	ASSOCIATED LESIONS
Familial adenomatous polyposis	Adenoma	Large intestine, duodenum	16 yr (range, 8-34 yr)	100%	5q (*APC* gene)	Rectal bleeding, abdominal pain, bowel obstruction	Desmoids, CHRPE
Peutz-Jeghers syndrome	Hamartoma	Large and small intestine	First decade	Slightly above average	19p (*STK11*)	Possible rectal bleeding, abdominal pain, intussusception	Orocutaneous melanin pigment spots, other tumors
MUTYH-associated polyposis	Adenoma	Large intestine, duodenum	45-50 yr (range, 13-60 yr)	75% (range, 50-100%)	1p (*MUTYH* gene)	Rectal bleeding, abdominal pain, bowel obstruction	CHRPE, osteomas
Juvenile polyposis	Hamartoma (rarely adenoma)	Large and small intestine	First decade	≈9%	*PTEN, SMAD4, BMPR1*	Possible rectal bleeding, abdominal pain, intussusception	Pulmonary AVMs
Hereditary nonpolyposis colon cancer	Adenoma	Large intestine	40 yr (range, 18-65 yr)	30%	Mismatch repair genes*	Rectal bleeding, abdominal pain, bowel obstruction	Other tumors (e.g., ovary, uterus, pancreas, stomach)

*Including hMSH2, hMSH3, hMSH6, hMLH1, hPMS1, and hPMS2.
AVM = arteriovenous malformation; CHRPE = congenital hypertrophy of the retinal pigment epithelium.

Familial Adenomatous Polyposis

Familial adenomatous polyposis is an autosomal dominant condition with incomplete penetrance and is the result of a mutation in the adenomatous polyposis coli *(APC)* gene.[14] Patients have hundreds to thousands of adenomatous polyps (Fig. 179-4) that occur relatively evenly throughout the colon and that usually appear by early in the second decade of life. GI symptoms usually develop in the third or fourth decade, and nearly every untreated patient develops colorectal cancer by age 40 years. Small bowel adenomas, usually in the duodenum, are seen in 45 to 90% of cases, and periampullary duodenal cancer develops in about 10% of patients. Patients with an attenuated form of familial adenomatous polyposis have fewer than 100 colonic adenomas with a right colon predominance and develop colorectal cancer about 10 years later.

Gardner Syndrome

Gardner syndrome is a subtype of familial adenomatous polyposis and is also the result of mutations in the *APC* gene. It is characterized by extra-intestinal clinical features, including soft tissue tumors (e.g., lipomas, sebaceous cysts, and fibrosarcomas), supernumerary teeth, desmoid tumors, osteomas (particularly mandibular), mesenteric fibromatosis, and congenital hypertrophy of the retinal pigment epithelium. Gardner syndrome and familial adenomatous polyposis differ because of variations in the location of the *APC* mutation, modifying genes, and environmental factors. However, the adenomatous polyps in Gardner syndrome and in familial adenomatous polyposis have similar malignant potential, so screening and treatment recommendations also are similar.

Turcot Syndrome

Turcot syndrome is the combination of colorectal polyposis, colorectal cancer, and central nervous system malignancy. *APC* gene mutations cause two-thirds of cases, whereas the other one-third result from the same DNA mismatch repair gene mutations that are seen in HNPCC. The central nervous system malignancies include medulloblastomas, glioblastomas, and ependymomas.

MUTYH-Associated Polyposis

MUTYH-associated polyposis is an autosomal recessive syndrome caused by mutations in the *MUTYH* gene (also called MYH [mutY homologue]). Underlying defects in base excision repair as well as acquired mutations in the *APC* gene and other genes (e.g., *KRAS*) lead to colonic polyposis and an increased risk of developing colorectal cancer. About 0.4 to 0.7% of patients who develop colorectal cancer have a homozygous *MUTYH* mutation. The phenotype is similar to attenuated familial adenomatous polyposis. Patients have up to hundreds of adenomas throughout the colon and may also have multiple hyperplastic polyps as well as serrated adenomas. Compared with familial adenomatous polyposis, the colorectal cancers of *MUTYH*-associated polyposis are more likely to be right-sided, with an average age of onset at 45 to 50 years. Extra-colonic features include gastroduodenal polyps, duodenal carcinoma, breast cancer, ovarian cancer, bladder cancer, skin cancer, osteomas, and congenital hypertrophy of the retinal pigment epithelium.

Peutz-Jeghers Syndrome

Peutz-Jeghers syndrome is a rare but highly penetrant autosomal dominant syndrome caused by a mutation in the serine-threonine kinase *(STK11)* gene located on chromosome 19p. Nearly all patients have characteristic melanin spots on their lips, buccal mucosa, and skin. The average age at diagnosis is the third decade. The syndrome is characterized by benign hamartomatous polyps predominantly in the small intestine, stomach, and colon, occasionally accompanied by adenomatous and hyperplastic polyps. The most common symptoms are small bowel intussusception, obstruction, and GI bleeding. Nearly 50% of patients develop a malignancy by age 65 years, most commonly in the small intestine, stomach, colon, pancreas, testes, breast, ovary, cervix, or uterus. Because genetic testing is not widely available, first-degree relatives should be screened annually from birth, looking especially for melanotic spots, precocious puberty, and testicular tumors.

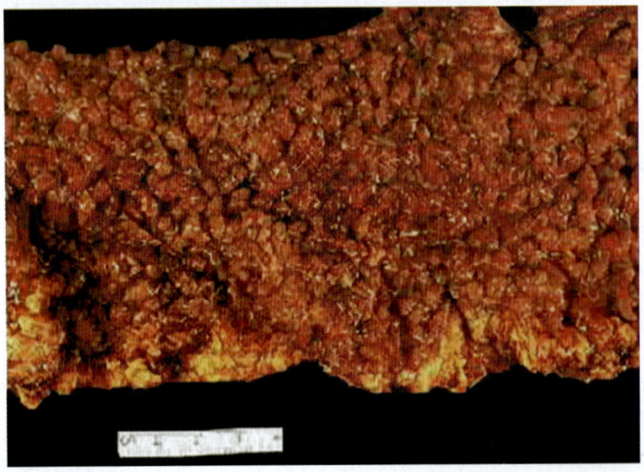

FIGURE 179-4. Resected colon of a patient with familial adenomatous polyposis.

Juvenile Polyposis

Familial juvenile (non-neoplastic, hamartomatous) polyposis is a rare (<1 in 100,000 births) syndrome in which patients develop 10 or more hamartomatous, non-neoplastic polyps (histologically distinct from those seen in Peutz-Jeghers syndrome) throughout their GI tract. This syndrome results from a highly penetrant autosomal dominant mutation in the *SMAD4*, *PTEN*, or *BMPR1A* gene. Symptoms and signs include abdominal pain, rectal bleeding, intestinal obstruction, and anemia by early adolescence. Pulmonary arteriovenous malformations are also seen. The risk of malignancy can be as high as 20%, with a median age of 37 years.[15]

NON-NEOPLASTIC POLYPS

About 50% of all large bowel polyps in average-risk individuals older than age 50 years are non-neoplastic (nonadenomatous) polyps. Nonadenomatous polyps can be hyperplastic, inflammatory, lymphoid, or juvenile. Hyperplastic polyps usually are caused by abnormal maturation of the mucosal epithelial cells. Hyperplastic polyps usually are small and seen mostly in the distal sigmoid colon and rectum. Hyperplastic polyps are not premalignant.

Patients with inflammatory bowel disease (Chapter 127) often have inflammatory pseudopolyps that are distinguished from neoplastic polyps only by biopsy. Lymphoid polyps contain exaggerated intramucosal lymphoid tissue. Juvenile polyps are focal hamartomatous malformations that are caused by abnormal development of the lamina propria and that are usually seen in the rectum of young children.

SERRATED POLYPS

Sessile serrated adenomas are neoplastic lesions with a right colon predominance and a high malignant potential.[16] Serrated polyps present with a disorganized and distorted crypt growth pattern. Because they are sessile or flat, they can be difficult to visualize on endoscopy. Their pathogenesis is via hypermethylation of CpG islands ("CIMP-high") and the *MLH1* mismatch repair gene, in the presence of *BRAF* mutations. As a result, serrated polyps exhibit a high degree of microsatellite instability.

Traditional serrated adenomas are rare and histologically distinct from sessile serrated adenomas. They commonly exhibit high-grade dysplasia and oftentimes carcinoma in situ.

ADENOMATOUS POLYPS

Adenomatous chronic polyps (adenomas) are benign glandular tumors with malignant potential. On pathologic examination, they can have evidence for low- or high-grade dysplasia. Adenomatous polyps have an anatomic distribution similar to colorectal adenocarcinoma, can vary in size, and may be sessile, flat, or pedunculated. Adenomatous polyps are the precursor lesions for colorectal adenocarcinoma. Furthermore, screening, early detection, and removal of adenomatous polyps substantially reduce the risk of subsequent colorectal cancer.

EPIDEMIOLOGY

Adenomatous polyps are relatively common and become more common with age: more than 15% of healthy women and more than 25% of healthy men over age 50 years have adenomas. The prevalence of adenomas tends to be higher in Western countries and wherever colorectal cancer is more common. In addition to defined genetic risks seen in familial colorectal cancer syndromes, sporadic adenomas have a familial component. For example, if a first-degree relative has an adenomatous polyp, an individual's risk is increased. In the United States, Blacks have a higher risk relative to Whites of European descent, whose risks, in turn, are similar to those of Asian and Hispanic individuals.

PATHOBIOLOGY

The epithelial cells in the large bowel undergo continuous self-renewal, with complete turnover every 3 to 8 days. Adenomatous polyps are caused by the sequence-specific acquisition of mutations that favor cell proliferation over cell death. Undifferentiated cells accumulate at the luminal surface, continue to divide, and eventually form an adenomatous tissue mass.

Adenomas can be tubular, villous, or tubulovillous. Most adenomas (70 to 85%) removed at colonoscopy are tubular; they typically are small, pedunculated, and composed of dysplastic glands that divide and branch out from the mucosal surface. Tubular adenomas rarely have high-grade dysplasia or carcinoma in situ. By comparison, villous adenomas (<5% of all adenomas) are usually large, sessile, and composed of dysplastic epithelium that projects into the intestinal lumen. Villous adenomas often have high-grade dysplasia or even carcinoma in situ. Tubulovillous adenomas (10 to 25% of all adenomas) include both tubular and villous components. An adenoma is considered "advanced" if it is at least 1 cm in size or has villous histology or high-grade dysplasia. Patients with advanced adenomas or three or more adenomas have a much higher risk of developing synchronous or metachronous colorectal cancer. In a patient who has a first documented adenoma, the risk of an additional adenoma is 30 to 50%.

CLINICAL MANIFESTATIONS

Most adenomatous polyps are asymptomatic and discovered only at the time of colorectal screening. Some patients, however, may present with an asymptomatic positive stool occult blood test or overt evidence of a lower GI bleed. Less than 5% of all adenomas will eventually develop into carcinomas: 1 to 3% of polyps smaller than 1 cm, 10% of polyps between 1 and 2 cm, and 40% of polyps larger than 2 cm. All adenomas contain some level of dysplasia, and higher-grade dysplasia carries a 30% risk of undergoing malignant transformation.

DIAGNOSIS

Colonic and rectal polyps and cancer can be diagnosed by several methods, including endoscopy, barium radiography, or CT colography (virtual colonoscopy). Colonoscopy is the preferred method because of its high accuracy and ability to perform a biopsy of and remove most polyps immediately. Nevertheless, colonoscopy may miss 6 to 12% of large (≥1 cm) polyps and 5% of cancers. By comparison, barium enemas miss about 50% of polyps that are larger than 1 cm. CT colography is sensitive for detecting large (>1 cm) polyps (>85%) and for detecting cancers (96%) but much less sensitive and specific for polyps smaller than 1 cm. Although CT colography is noninvasive and relatively quick, it still requires bowel preparation and exposes the patient to ionizing radiation. Nonpolypoid (flat and depressed) colorectal neoplasms, which are more likely to be carcinomatous than are polypoid lesions, are found on colonoscopy in almost 10% of asymptomatic and symptomatic adults but are much less likely to be diagnosed by barium radiography or CT colography.

Flexible sigmoidoscopy can be used to screen average risk asymptomatic individuals, but it detects only 50 to 60% of all polyps and cancers. Patients with polyps detected by barium radiography, CT colography, or flexible sigmoidoscopy should undergo colonoscopy to remove the lesion and to search for additional polyps or mass lesions. This need for subsequent colonoscopy underscores the attractiveness of using it as the initial screening modality.

TREATMENT

Neoplastic polyps should be removed endoscopically to reduce the risk of subsequent colorectal cancer. A pedunculated adenoma usually can be removed intact by snare polypectomy (Video 179-2), whereas sessile polyps may require piecemeal snare resection. Pathologic evaluation should assess the presence or absence of cancer; if malignant tissue is identified, it should be evaluated for its histologic grade, vascular and lymphatic spread, and adenoma-free margin. Unfavorable histopathologic factors that require prompt surgical resection after endoscopic polypectomy include poorly differentiated histology, vascular invasion, lymphatic invasion, and incomplete resection. Malignant pedunculated polyps can be treated with endoscopic resection alone if the cancer is confined to the submucosa and no unfavorable histologic features are present. When a malignant sessile polyp is removed endoscopically, the potential risk of recurrence or lymph node involvement must be weighed against the risks of definitive surgery in each individual patient.

PROGNOSIS

Patients who have undergone endoscopic removal of a previously diagnosed adenomatous or sessile serrated polyp are at increased risk for the subsequent development of adenomas and colorectal cancer. The recommended surveillance post-resection depends on the primary lesions, size, and histology, as well as the number of adenomas (Table 179-2).[17] If a low-risk patient has just 1 or 2 small tubular adenomas, surveillance colonoscopy can be delayed for 5 to 10 years. By comparison, patients who have multiple (>2) adenomas, large (≥1 cm) adenomas, adenomas with villous or high-grade histology, or numerous (>10) adenomas, should undergo repeat colonoscopy within 3 years. After removal of a large (≥2 cm) adenoma or the piecemeal resection of any adenoma, colonoscopy should be repeated within 6 months to determine whether the original resection was complete. For sessile serrated polyps smaller than 10 mm without dysplasia, surveillance colonoscopy is recommended at 5 years, but the recommended interval is 3 years if the serrated polyp showed high-grade dysplasia or was a traditional serrated adenoma (Video 179-3).

ADENOCARCINOMA OF THE COLON AND RECTUM

CLINICAL MANIFESTATIONS

Patients with early-stage colon cancer are typically asymptomatic, and the cancer is usually discovered upon routine screening. Symptoms usually arise when the tumor grows into the bowel lumen or when the tumor invades adjacent anatomic structures. Common symptoms related to colorectal cancer include lower abdominal pain, change in bowel function, GI bleeding (Chapter 121), anemia, and alterations in stool caliber. Anorexia, weight loss, and fatigue may develop, and liver metastases can be manifested by hepatomegaly, jaundice, abdominal fullness, or ascites.

Symptoms also depend on the primary site (Fig. 179-5). Proximal lesions more frequently present with iron deficiency anemia (Chapter 145) resulting from occult blood loss. For lesions that occur in the distal colon, the usual presenting symptoms include a change in bowel habits, such as constipation or diarrhea, and hematochezia. Tumors arising in the rectum usually present with changes in stool caliber, rectal bleeding, and rectal pain. In some cases when the rectal tumor involves sacral nerve plexi, significant neuropathic pain may be present.

TABLE 179-2 COLONOSCOPY SURVEILLANCE INTERVALS

MOST ADVANCED FINDING	INTERVAL
No polyps or small (<10 mm) hyperplastic polyps	10 yr
1-2 adenomas, <1 cm	5-10 yr
3-10 adenomas or adenoma with villous features, ≥1 cm, or with high-grade dysplasia	3 yr
>10 adenomas	<3 yr
Sessile adenoma ≥ 2 cm, piecemeal excision	2-6 mo
Serrated lesions:	
• <10 mm, no dysplasia	5 yr
• ≥10 mm or dysplasia	3 yr

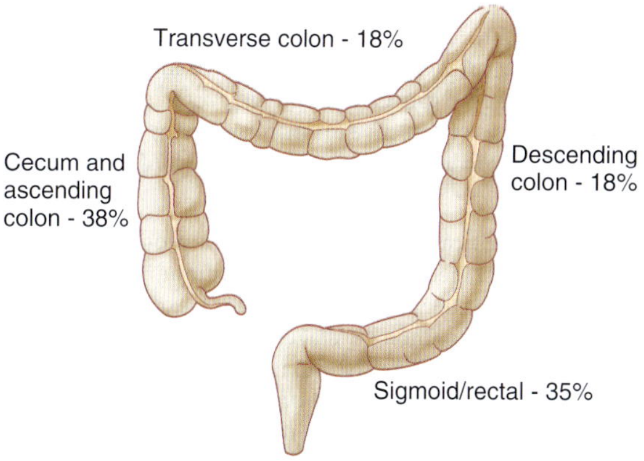

FIGURE 179-5. Sites of development of large bowel adenocarcinoma.

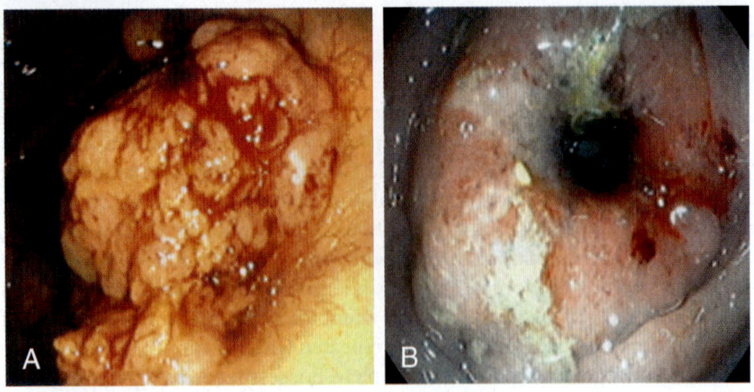

FIGURE 179-6. Colonoscopy appearance of large bowel adenocarcinomas. A, Exophytic growth within the bowel lumen. B, "Apple core" stricturing lesion.

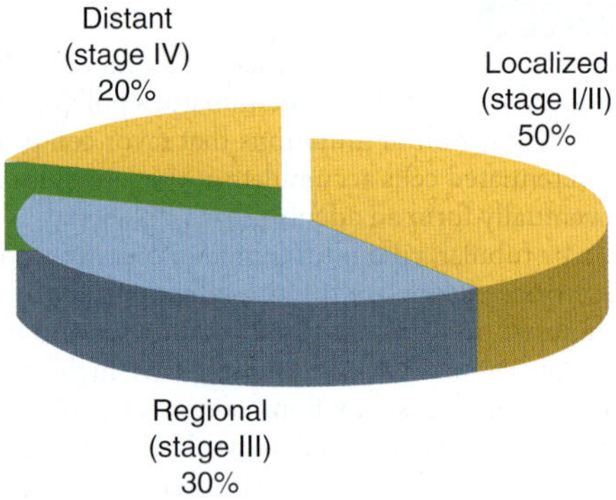

FIGURE 179-7. Stage of disease at time of initial presentation.

DIAGNOSIS

A careful history, physical examination, and radiologic evaluation are important in making the diagnosis. The patient should be questioned about a history of adenomatous polyps or colorectal cancer, a history of inflammatory bowel disease, and any family history of colorectal cancer or other solid tumors. On physical examination, extra-intestinal lesions characteristic of Peutz-Jeghers syndrome or Gardner syndrome may be noticed. Metastatic disease to the liver or lymph nodes may present with hepatosplenomegaly or lymphadenopathy, and abdominal fullness or ascites may reflect peritoneal involvement. Digital rectal examination may reveal a mass in the distal rectal region or spread of the tumor to the rectal shelf or pelvis. Examination of the stool may show frank or occult blood in up to 80% of advanced cases. Iron deficiency anemia and elevated liver enzymes (AST, ALT, and alkaline phosphatase) and serum bilirubin may aid in the diagnosis. The peripheral blood levels of the tumor markers (CEA and CA19-9) may be elevated, but these serum markers are relatively insensitive and can be elevated in other solid tumors.

The approaches for making the definitive diagnosis of colorectal cancer are similar to those used to detect adenomatous polyps. Colonoscopy is considered the standard for all patients with occult blood in their stools, unexplained iron deficiency anemia, or symptoms and signs suggestive of colorectal cancer (Fig. 179-6).

For rectal cancer, endoscopic ultrasound combines high-frequency ultrasonography with video endoscopy. This procedure is superior to CT to stage the tumor by accurately determining the degree of invasion as well as detecting and sampling any enlarged lymph nodes. Endoscopic ultrasound also is highly sensitive for detecting recurrent rectal cancer after a low anterior resection. MRI also can accurately stage rectal cancer and may be preferable to endoscopic ultrasound.

Consensus guidelines recommend CT scans of the chest, abdomen, and pelvis because advanced liver metastases or involvement of other sites often preclude immediate surgical resection of the primary tumor. PET scans can confirm systemic disease and are useful before resection of a solitary metastatic site and in patients who have a rising CEA or new symptoms suggestive of progressive disease, despite no change in their CT scans. PET scans also may be used to evaluate abnormal lesions seen on CT. However, PET has no specific role in the routine evaluation of patients with colorectal cancer. Plain chest radiographs are not sufficiently sensitive to detect the presence of metastatic lesions in the lungs, and plain abdominal films are useful only to aid in the diagnosis of bowel obstruction.

Histopathologic analysis is critical for making the diagnosis of colorectal cancer. Additional studies to evaluate immunohistochemical expression of certain key cellular proteins may be helpful in identifying adenocarcinomas of colorectal cancer origin. For example, cytokeratin 20 (CK20) and caudal-type homeobox 2 (CDX2) are two of the most sensitive and specific markers used to help diagnose colorectal cancer. Immunohistochemistry also can be helpful in making the diagnosis of defective mismatch repair by testing for the protein expression of the four main MMR genes: *MLH1, MSH2, PMS2,* and *MSH6.*

Staging

Accurate staging is critical for determining both prognosis and treatment. Colorectal cancer is staged according to the tumor, node, and metastasis (TNM) classification system based on the physical examination, radiography, endoscopy, surgery, and pathologic stage: stage I cancers penetrate into but not through the bowel wall (T1–2N0M0); stage II cancers penetrate through the bowel wall and can involve nearby organs but do not spread to regional lymph nodes; stage III cancers involve regional lymph nodes (Fig. 179-7); and stage IV disease spreads to the liver, lung, lymph nodes, and peritoneum. In the United States, about 50% of patients present with stage I or II disease, 30% with stage III disease, and 20% with advanced, metastatic disease. In general, primary tumors that arise in the colon follow an orderly spread to the regional lymph nodes, then to the liver, and then to the lungs and other distant sites. In contrast, because of the dual venous drainage of the rectum to the portal vein and inferior vena cava, primary rectal tumors may spread via hematogenous dissemination to the lungs before any liver involvement.

TREATMENT

Surgery

Surgical resection is the primary treatment for early-stage, locally confined colon cancer (stage 0 and stage I). Highly selected patients with site-limited metastatic disease (stage IV) also may undergo surgery with curative intent. Curative surgery aims to remove the primary tumor with tumor-free margins, as well as to remove the primary feeding arterial vessel and corresponding lymphatics en bloc. A minimum of 12 lymph nodes should be removed and examined microscopically for accurate staging. Synchronous colon cancers can be removed individually by subtotal colectomy. Any adjacent adherent structures should be resected en bloc. Prophylactic oophorectomy is not recommended, but if one ovary is grossly involved, the other should be removed as well given the risk of contralateral involvement. Laparoscopic resection is as safe and effective as open resection and requires a modestly shorter recovery time.[18]

For rectal cancer, the main goal of surgery is to preserve the function of the anal sphincter. For cancers involving the distal rectum, the recommendation is total mesorectal excision with en bloc removal of the lymphovascular and fatty envelope surrounding the rectum. For upper rectal tumors, by comparison, tumor-specific mesorectal excision (en bloc removal of the mesorectum 5 cm distal to the tumor) is sufficient. For minimal-risk (T1 disease, size <3 cm, well differentiated, within 8 cm of the anal verge, no lymphovascular invasion, and less than one third circumferential) low rectal cancers, local transanal excision is acceptable. Postoperatively, increased bowel frequency is common, and some patients develop fecal incontinence or evacuation dysfunction (Chapter 131). As such, the main focus in patients with rectal cancer is to preserve the function of the anal sphincter.

Obstructing tumors should be immediately resected with bowel re-anastomosis. Proximal diversion may be the only initial option for an advanced unresectable cancer, with future resection followed by ostomy closure if the primary tumor responds to the point where it can later be removed. Endoscopic stenting may sometimes relieve acute obstruction. Perforated bowel must be resected, with or without diversion, prior to re-anastomosis. In patients who present with synchronous colorectal cancer and unresectable metastases, an asymptomatic primary tumor can be treated safely with systemic medical therapy without surgery, with a low probability that serious complications will require immediate surgical intervention.

Post-Surgical Surveillance

Active surveillance is recommended after surgical resection of early-stage colon and rectal cancer because the risk for recurrent disease is highest within the first 2 to 3 years after surgery and adjuvant chemotherapy for patients with stage II or III cancer. The American Society of Clinical Oncology recommends a history and physical examination every 3 to 6 months for 5 years, annual chest and abdominal CT scans for 3 years after resection of high-risk primary tumors, and the addition of pelvic CT scanning for primary rectal cancer. However, CT plus CEA screening at 12 and 36 months appears to be as good as more frequent screening for stage II and III disease.[A2] Colonoscopy should be performed 1 year after the completion of adjuvant chemotherapy, and, if completely negative, every 5 years thereafter. Serum CEA levels should be measured every 3 to 6 months for 5 years.

Radiation Therapy

Radiation therapy is usually not considered as a treatment option for surgically resected early-stage colon cancer nor for the treatment of a primary colon cancer when metastatic disease is present. The major role for radiation therapy is in the combined modality treatment of locally advanced rectal cancer. Certain colorectal cancers are at high risk for locally recurrent disease, such as T4 tumors with penetration to a fixed structure especially within the pelvic region, may be considered for postoperative radiation therapy. However, no randomized clinical trials have documented benefit of radiation therapy in this setting. Palliative radiation therapy also may be considered to control tumor-related symptoms when metastatic colon cancer spreads to bone, brain, liver, and lung.

Stereotactic radiation therapy can be useful for metastatic colorectal cancer patients with liver metastases. The 1- and 2-year local control rates are about 90%, with few reports of major toxicity. This approach is a reasonable and safe alternative for patients who have fewer than four liver metastatic lesions and who are unable to undergo surgery or any other treatment options.

Systemic and Combination Therapies

The backbone of the treatment of colorectal cancer, in both the adjuvant and metastatic disease settings, is 5-fluorouracil. Although 5-fluorouracil has modest activity as a single agent, its clinical efficacy is enhanced by prolonged infusion and by coadministration with the reduced folate leucovorin. Two other cytotoxic agents commonly used to treat metastatic colorectal cancer are irinotecan (a topoisomerase I inhibitor) and oxaliplatin (a third-generation platinum analogue; see Table 164-2). Biologic agents are available to target the vascular endothelial growth factor (VEGF) signaling pathway (bevacizumab, aflibercept, and ramucirumab), the epidermal growth factor receptor (EGFR) pathway (cetuximab and panitumumab), and tyrosine kinases that are involved in cell growth, proliferation, angiogenesis, invasion, and metastasis (regorafenib).

Patients with resected stage I colon cancer have an extremely high cure rate, approaching 95%, with surgery alone, and do not need adjuvant systemic therapy (Table 179-3).[A3] For stage II patients, the risk of relapse is higher (about 25% at 3 years), and combined treatment with 5-fluorouracil and leucovorin provides modest clinical benefit.[18] However, stage II tumors that express high levels of microsatellite instability have a better prognosis than tumors with microsatellite stable disease, and survival in such patients is worse when they are treated with 5-fluorouracil. Adjuvant chemotherapy is not recommended for stage II, microsatellite instability–high disease. For high-risk stage II disease (defined by obstruction, perforation, lymphovascular invasion, perineural invasion, and fewer than 12 lymph nodes in the surgical resection specimen), the benefit from adjuvant chemotherapy is similar to that seen for stage III colon cancer. Patients with high-risk stage II disease and good performance status should receive 6 months of adjuvant therapy with combination chemotherapy that includes 5-fluorouracil, leucovorin, and oxaliplatin (FOLFOX) or an alternative combination regimen of capecitabine and oxaliplatin (XELOX/CAPOX; Table 179-3) under expert supervision, with the decision potentially guided by the presence or absence of the circulating tumor DNA.[A4] Both FOLFOX and XELOX/CAPOX significantly prolong disease-free survival and overall survival compared with fluoropyrimidine monotherapy. For patients who have comorbid illnesses and who are unable to tolerate aggressive combination chemotherapy, fluoropyrimidine monotherapy with infusional 5-fluorouracil or oral capecitabine under expert supervision is a reasonable alternative.

In patients with stage III colon cancer, 5-year disease survival rates range from 25 to 85%, depending on the number of lymph nodes that are positive in the surgical resection specimen. The usual recommendation for patients with node-positive stage III disease is to receive adjuvant systemic therapy (E-Fig. 179-1). For patients with good performance status and no comorbid illnesses, aggressive treatment with the FOLFOX regimen significantly improves long-term survival rates and represents current standard care. XELOX/CAPOX appears to be as good as FOLFOX in patients of all ages. For patients who are not candidates for aggressive cytotoxic chemotherapy, fluoropyrimidine monotherapy with either infusional 5-fluorouracil or oral capecitabine is an appropriate option. Several randomized trials show that 3 months of adjuvant therapy is as good as 6 months of therapy in lower risk patients with T1 to T3 disease and only 1 to 3 positive lymph nodes. In contrast, for stage III patients with more than 4 lymph nodes, standard 6 months of adjuvant therapy provides greater clinical benefit than 3 months of therapy, albeit at a higher cost of adverse events. CAPOX rather than FOLFOX is now viewed as a preferred option for adjuvant therapy.

TABLE 179-3 TREATMENT OF EARLY-STAGE COLON CANCER ACCORDING TO DISEASE STAGE

STAGE	SURGICAL TREATMENT	ADJUVANT CHEMOTHERAPY
I	Colectomy with en bloc removal of regional lymph nodes	Observation
II (MSI-H/dMMR)	Colectomy with en bloc removal of regional lymph nodes	Observation
II (MSS/pMMR and no high-risk features)	Colectomy with en bloc removal of regional lymph nodes	Observation *OR* Consider capecitabine (6 months) or 5-FU/leucovorin (6 months)
II (MSS/pMMR and high-risk features)	Colectomy with en bloc removal of regional lymph nodes	FOLFOX (6 months) or CAPOX (3 months) *OR* Capecitabine (6 months) or 5-FU/leucovorin (6 months) for patients who cannot tolerate aggressive chemotherapy
III (low-risk)	Colectomy with en bloc removal of regional lymph nodes	CAPOX (3 months) or FOLFOX (3-6 months) *OR* Consider capecitabine (6 months) or 5-FU/leucovorin (6 months) for patients who cannot tolerate aggressive chemotherapy
III (high-risk)	Colectomy with en bloc removal of regional lymph nodes	CAPOX (3-6 months) or FOLFOX (6 months) *OR* Consider capecitabine (6 months) or 5-FU/leucovorin (6 months) for patients who cannot tolerate aggressive chemotherapy

MSI-H/dMMR = microsatellite instability-high/defective mismatch repair; MSS-H/pMMR = microsatellite stable/proficient mismatch repair.

Rectal Adenocarcinoma

The risk of local recurrence is much greater for rectal cancer, so the therapeutic approach for patients with primary rectal adenocarcinoma is distinct from that for primary colon cancer. Rectal cancer patients require accurate preoperative staging with endoscopic rectal ultrasound or rectal MRI for precise definition of the size, extent, and depth of invasion of the rectal tumor as well as lymph node involvement. For patients with stage I rectal cancer, surgical resection is sufficient with no need for additional adjuvant treatment with either radiation or chemotherapy. However, higher-risk patients (T2 disease, T1 with poorly differentiated histology, perineural or lymphovascular invasion, or close margins) should receive postoperative pelvic irradiation with or without 5-fluorouracil chemotherapy.

Radiation therapy is considered standard therapy for patients with locally advanced stage II and III rectal adenocarcinomas to decrease local relapse rates, improve the chance of sphincter preservation, and possibly improve survival. The major issues to consider relate to timing (preoperative or postoperative) and duration (short or long), as well as whether to combine it with fluoropyrimidine-based chemotherapy. Short-course 5-day preoperative irradiation without chemotherapy, as is practiced in certain countries in Europe, may be considered when tumor downsizing is not necessary. When short-course radiation is used, postoperative systemic adjuvant therapy is recommended with either a fluoropyrimidine alone (stage II) or a fluoropyrimidine-oxaliplatin combination regimen (node-positive disease).

For locally advanced rectal cancer, which includes lymph node involvement or large bulky tumors, a 5-day course of radiotherapy followed by either 6 cycles of CAPOX or 9 cycles of FOLFOX chemotherapy, can significantly reduce 3-year disease-related treatment failure[A5] and is now considered a standard treatment. With this neoadjuvant approach, induction systemic chemotherapy is administered first and followed by chemoradiation, with the goal of downstaging the primary tumor as well as reducing the risk of distant metastatic spread. Adjuvant chemotherapy is usually administered after surgical resection.

For stage II/III disease, however, the optimal chemotherapy regimen has yet to be determined. Fluoropyrimidine monotherapy with either infusional 5-fluorouracil or oral capecitabine is usually recommended if patients have no evidence of lymph node involvement in the surgical resection specimen and if the primary tumor has been significantly downstaged. If not, however, oxaliplatin-based chemotherapy regimens with either FOLFOX or XELOX/CAPOX are usually recommended.

Metastatic Colorectal Cancer

Metastatic colorectal cancer is treated with the same approach, regardless of the primary site of origin (colon versus rectum).[19,20] Metastatic colorectal cancer is becoming a chronic disease, and the key issue is to ensure that patients are treated in a continuum of care approach with exposure to all of the active agents within the therapeutic armamentarium. Current systemic cytotoxic chemotherapies in combination with various biologic agents (Chapter 29) have improved median overall survival to nearly three years (E-Fig. 179-1).[21]

First-Line Chemotherapy

For first-line treatment, the cytotoxic chemotherapy FOLFOX and FOLFIRI regimens provide virtually identical progression-free survival and overall survival,[A6] with a median overall survival of nearly 23 months. Interestingly, long-term results seem to be similar regardless of which drug (oxaliplatin or irinotecan) is combined first with 5-fluorouracil. However, the toxicity pattern varies, depending on which drug is given; irinotecan is commonly associated with GI side effects, whereas oxaliplatin treatment can lead to peripheral sensory neuropathy.

Biologic Therapy

ANTI–VASCULAR ENDOTHELIAL GROWTH FACTOR ANTIBODIES. In metastatic colorectal cancer patients with wild-type RAS, the addition of the anti-VEGF antibody bevacizumab or the anti-EGFR antibody cetuximab to cytotoxic chemotherapy (either FOLFOX or FOLFIRI) provides equivalent clinical benefit, with a median progression-free survival of 10.6 months and a median overall survival of 30 months. If disease progresses, bevacizumab can be continued in combination with second-line cytotoxic chemotherapy. Aflibercept plus FOLFIRI improves survival compared with FOLFIRI alone in patients who progress despite oxaliplatin treatment. Ramucirumab is approved for use in combination with FOLFIRI in the second-line treatment of metastatic colorectal cancer. Cross-trial comparisons suggest equivalent clinical efficacy among bevacizumab, aflibercept, and ramucirumab, but aflibercept is significantly more toxic and ramucirumab is much more expensive than bevacizumab.

ANTI–EPIDERMAL GROWTH FACTOR ANTIBODIES. For epidermal growth factor receptor (EGFR) positive chemorefractory disease, two monoclonal antibodies (cetuximab and panitumumab) have nearly identical single-agent activity, and both agents can be effectively combined with FOLFIRI or FOLFOX chemotherapy in the first-line treatment setting to improve overall response rates and progression-free survival. However, these anti-EGFR antibodies should be used only in patients whose tumors express wild-type *RAS* and *BRAF*. Unfortunately, even in the setting of wild-type *RAS*, only about 30% of patients will respond to anti-EGFR therapy. Right-sided tumors derive little benefit from cetuximab, whereas left-sided tumors derive significantly greater clinical benefit from cetuximab compared with bevacizumab. Although bevacizumab is effective in both left- and right-sided tumors, its clinical efficacy is also much greater in left-sided tumors.[22]

Programmed Death 1 Blockade

Immunotherapy with an anti–programmed death 1 (PD-1) immune checkpoint inhibitor (pembrolizumab or nivolumab) is useful in patients who have metastatic disease that has progressed despite treatment with a fluoropyrimidine, oxaliplatin, and irinotecan.[23] These antibodies stimulate the T-cell immune response, thereby leading to T-cell activation and proliferation. For microsatellite instability–high or mismatch repair defective metastatic colorectal cancer,[A7] pembrolizumab is superior to 5-fluorouracil-based chemotherapy, regardless of whether patients are also receiving bevacizumab or cetuximab, with median progression-free survival doubled from 8.2 months to 16.5 months. Furthermore, patients who are treated with pembrolizumab immunotherapy have fewer treatment-related adverse events and a significantly improved health-related quality of life.[A8] The combination of nivolumab plus ipilimumab, an antibody that targets cytotoxic T-lymphocyte–associated protein 4 (CTLA4), is also associated with encouraging progression-free survival and overall survival at 12 months in patients with microsatellite instability–high or mismatch repair defective metastatic colorectal cancer, and this combination immunotherapy regimen appears to provide enhanced clinical efficacy when compared with anti-PD-1 monotherapy.[24]

BRAF *V600E* Inhibition

The 8% of patients whose metastatic cancer expresses the *BRAF* V600E mutation have an overall poor prognosis,[25] but a triplet combination of encorafenib (a *BRAF* inhibitor), cetuximab (an anti-EGFR antibody), and binimetinib (a MEK inhibitor) can improve survival compared with standard irinotecan-based chemotherapy plus cetuximab.[A9] This regimen is now considered standard of care for metastatic disease with this specific mutation.

Other Agents

Regorafenib (a multikinase inhibitor) and TAS-102 (a combination of trifluridine and tipiracil) are agents that have nearly identical clinical activity and improve median progression-free survival and overall survival in patients with progressive disease. In general, TAS-102 has a more manageable safety profile and does not require as many dose reductions or treatment delays. Sotorasib and adagrasib under expert supervision are options for solid tumors with the *KRAS*-G12C mutation.[26,27]

Locally Directed Treatment of Metastatic Disease

For select patients with metastatic colorectal cancer, complete resection of isolated hepatic or pulmonary metastases may provide long-term survival.[28] For hepatic metastasectomy, 5-year survival rates are in the 30 to 50% range. In patients initially deemed to have surgically unresectable metastatic disease, preoperative systemic therapy improves response rates. For patients with wild-type *RAS* disease, cytotoxic chemotherapy with FOLFOX or FOLFIRI in combination with cetuximab or panitumumab appears to offer the best chance for cytoreduction of the metastatic liver disease and successful surgical resection. In the setting of mutant *RAS* metastatic colorectal cancer, the anti-VEGF antibody bevacizumab combined with chemotherapy provides an objective response rate approaching 70% with successful surgical resection approaching 30%. In patients with initially unresectable *RAS* mutant colorectal liver metastases, bevacizumab combined with mFOLFOX6 can increase the resectability of liver metastases and improve survival compared with mFOLFOX6 alone.[A10] After patients have recovered from their surgical procedure, which usually requires 4 to 5 weeks, 6 months of adjuvant chemotherapy with FOLFOX is usually recommended.

Radio frequency ablation can be used for patients whose liver metastases are deemed to be surgically unresectable because of their anatomic location or because the patient is too debilitated to undergo hepatic resection. An alternative strategy is to administer fluoropyrimidine chemotherapy via the hepatic artery through an intraarterial catheter. Selective internal radiation therapy embolizes radiolabeled spheres into the hepatic artery for the treatment of liver metastases.[A11] Stereotactic body radiation therapy is also a reasonable and safe alternative for patients who have liver-limited metastatic colorectal cancer and who are unable to undergo surgery.

PREVENTION

Screening

The role of screening is to reduce colorectal cancer-related mortality by removing any precursor adenomas and by detecting true cancers at an earlier, more curable stage. For average-risk individuals, the relatively long latency between adenoma development and the development of cancer is of the order of 8 to 12 years, thereby making colorectal cancer a highly preventable disease using colonoscopy with polypectomy.[A12] For sporadic colorectal cancer, age is the major risk factor; for this reason, most patients should begin screening at age 45 years. The wide range of options for average-risk individuals (Table 179-4) can be divided into two distinct categories: stool tests for occult blood or abnormal DNA; and structural tests, which include colonoscopy, flexible sigmoidoscopy, CT colography, and double-contrast barium enema, used alone or in combination.[29] In asymptomatic adults age 50 to 69 years, one-time colonoscopy and fecal immunochemical testing are equally effective at identifying the presence of colorectal cancer, although a greater number of adenomas are identified by colonoscopy (Chapter 120). Current professional society guidelines recognize multiple screening options but recommend structural tests that can both detect and prevent colorectal cancer. For example, the American Cancer Society now recommends screening average-risk adults for colorectal cancer starting at age 45 years and high-risk individuals starting before age 40 years (or 10 years before the age when the youngest relative was diagnosed with colorectal cancer). Colonoscopy, flexible sigmoidoscopy, or a stool-based test are recommended for average-risk patients, but flexible sigmoidoscopy or colonoscopy is recommended for high-risk patients. For individuals in good health and expected to live at least more than 10 years, routine screening should continue up through age 75 years. Individuals between ages 76 to 85 years should consult with their primary health care provider as to whether screening should be continued.[30] The general recommendation is to discontinue colorectal cancer screening in individuals who are older than 85 years of age.

Patients with ulcerative colitis (Chapter 127) are 10 to 20 times more likely to develop colorectal cancer than the general population, with a 25-year cumulative incidence of about 12%. The risk is even higher in patients who have both primary sclerosing cholangitis (Chapter 141) and ulcerative colitis. If Crohn disease (Chapter 127) involves more than one-third of the colon, the risk of colorectal cancer risk is increased 6- to 8-fold. Patients with ulcerative colitis or extensive Crohn disease should have screening colonoscopy every 1 to 2 years, starting 8 to 10 years after the disease is first diagnosed. The main goal is to identify the presence of dysplasia. Multifocal low-grade dysplasia or any dysplasia that cannot be excised endoscopically is an indication for colectomy. In familial adenomatous polyposis, the *APC* gene mutation can be identified in up to 85% of affected individuals and is useful for screening.

Fecal occult blood testing detects the presence of hemoglobin from bleeding tumors. Guaiac-based testing decreases colorectal cancer mortality by 15 to 33%, with the mortality benefit persisting for 30 years. However, immunochemical-based tests have higher sensitivities and specificities than guaiac tests, and they identify 2.5-fold more advanced adenomas and colorectal cancers than do guaiac-based tests. Furthermore, they do not require any dietary restrictions and require only one stool specimen. As a result, immunochemical-based tests are now the preferred fecal occult blood test.[31] Fecal occult blood tests should be repeated on an annual basis, and any positive test should prompt colonoscopy.

TABLE 179-4 SCREENING METHODS FOR COLORECTAL CANCER*

TEST	INTERVAL
TESTS THAT DETECT ADENOMATOUS POLYPS OR CANCER	
Colonoscopy	Every 10 yr
Flexible sigmoidoscopy†	Every 5 yr
CT colography†	Every 5 yr
Double-contrast barium enema†	Every 5 yr
TESTS THAT DETECT PRIMARILY CANCER†	
Fecal occult blood tests	
• High-sensitivity guaiac-based fecal occult blood test	Annually
• Fecal immunochemical test	Annually
Stool DNA	Interval uncertain

*Beginning at age 45 for average-risk individuals.
†Positive test should prompt full colonoscopy.
CT = computed tomography.

The rationale for stool DNA tests is that both adenomas and carcinomas contain altered DNA, which is shed continuously in the stool. These stool DNA tests contain a panel designed to detect exfoliated DNA markers, including *KRAS* mutation, aberrant *NDRG4* and *BMP3* methylation, and beta-actin. Stool DNA testing identifies up to about 90% of patients with colorectal cancer and 40% of patients with advanced adenomas.[32] In a large colorectal cancer screening trial, the sensitivity of the multitarget stool DNA test for detecting colorectal cancer was 92% with stool DNA testing compared with 74% with fecal immunochemical testing, and the sensitivity for detecting advanced precancerous lesions and polyps with high-grade dysplasia was also significantly higher with stool DNA testing. However, stool DNA testing is more costly and associated with a higher false-positive rate. The optimal screening interval for stool DNA testing has not been clearly defined.

Flexible sigmoidoscopy (Chapter 120) is an endoscopic procedure that examines the rectum and distal colon up to the splenic flexure. It is performed with minimal bowel preparation, does not require sedation, and can be performed in the office by primary care doctors, nurses, or physician's assistants. This procedure detects distal cancers or polyps with the same accuracy as colonoscopy. If an adenoma is found on sigmoidoscopy, colonoscopy is required because of the high risk of synchronous polyps or cancer in the more proximal colon. Screening with flexible sigmoidoscopy (with subsequent colonoscopy as indicated) can reduce the incidence of both distal and proximal colorectal cancer by about 30%, with a significant 50% decrease in mortality from distal colorectal only. A single flexible sigmoidoscopy continues to provide significant protection against both incidental and fatal colorectal cancer for at least 15 to 17 years.[A13]

Colonoscopy (Chapter 120) allows complete visualization of the colon and removal of any visualized polyps. As such, colonoscopy is both diagnostic and preventive.[A14] Screening colonoscopy detects cancer in about 1% of patients, advanced adenoma (size >10mm, villous histology, or high-grade dysplasia) in 5 to 10% of patients, and 1 or more adenomas in at least 20% of patients. The major complication rate of screening colonoscopy is less than 3 per 1000, with more than half of such complications related to a polypectomy. After colonoscopic polypectomy, the incidence of colorectal cancer is reduced by 75 to 90%. In patients whose adenomas are detected and removed by colonoscopy, the subsequent risk of death from colorectal cancer is 50% lower than otherwise expected, with most of the benefit attributable to the removal of low-risk adenomas. The highest risk of subsequent colorectal cancer is in patients whose removed adenomas were 20 mm or greater in diameter or had high-grade dysplasia.[33] The benefit of colonoscopy is higher if it is performed by an experienced gastroenterologist. If the initial screening colonoscopy is completely normal, future screening can be deferred for 10 years. Re-screening is recommended more frequently in patients with positive findings (see Table 179-2).[34]

CT colography (virtual colonoscopy) obtains two- and three-dimensional images of the entire colon via multidetector CT scanning (Chapter 119). A rectal tube is used to infuse gas to distend the bowel for better imaging. The sensitivity is 85 to 92% for large polyps (≥10 mm), with a specificity of 83 to 89%, and about 65% for polyps 5 mm or larger. Its 96% sensitivity for detecting colorectal cancer is similar to colonoscopy. Because CT colography is less sensitive than colonoscopy for detecting lesions smaller than 10 mm and substantially less sensitive for detecting high-risk sessile serrated polyps, colonoscopy is the preferred screening procedure. Colon capsule endoscopy appears to be better than CT colography, but neither is as accurate as colonoscopy.[A15] If used, CT colography screening should begin at age 45 years and be repeated every 5 years. Discovery of a polyp larger than 5 mm requires colonoscopy.

Double-contrast barium enema (Chapter 119) can evaluate the mucosal surface of the entire colon. This test has a sensitivity of 85 to 97% for detecting colorectal cancers but only 48 to 73% for detecting large adenomas. Given this low sensitivity and the small but real risk of ionizing radiation, this imaging procedure is not recommended for routine screening.

Chemoprevention

NSAIDs[A16] and aspirin[A17,A18] reduce the formation of adenomas and inhibit the development of colon cancer by inhibiting cyclooxygenase and the subsequent generation of prostaglandin. In patients with familial adenomatous polyposis, sulindac (150 mg daily) and celecoxib can cause existing adenomas to regress and inhibit the formation of new adenomas. Aspirin also reduces the recurrence of adenomas by up to 20 to 40%, with pooled data suggesting up to a 70% reduction in the incidence of colorectal cancer when at least 75 mg of aspirin daily is taken for 5 or more years. Epidemiologic studies also show that regular users of NSAIDs have a lower risk of developing colorectal cancer. Calcium supplementation decreases the rate of metachronous adenomas by 20%, and total calcium intake greater than 1400 mg per day is associated with a significantly lower risk of colon cancer than an intake of less than 600 mg per day. Observational studies suggest that higher levels of 25-hydroxyvitamin D3 (25[OH]D) are associated with a reduced risk of colorectal cancer and also improved survival after its diagnosis. In patients with stage III colon cancer, adjuvant vitamin D supplementation is associated with a significant improvement in recurrence-free survival and overall survival. However, aspirin, NSAIDS, and calcium are not routinely recommended to prevent colorectal cancer, although they may be considered on an individual basis.

Dietary Prevention

Epidemiologic studies have identified a correlation of colorectal cancer with diets high in fat and low in fiber, green leafy vegetables, and fruits; physical inactivity; smoking; and excessive alcohol use. Increased fish consumption is associated with a lower incidence of colorectal cancer, and supplementation with the omega-3 fatty acid eicosapentaenoic acid can decrease the burden of polyps in familial adenomatous polyposis. However, randomized trials of modest dietary changes (10% less fat, 25 to 75% more fiber, 50% more fruits and vegetables) have not reduced the incidence of adenomas or colorectal cancers over 3 to 8 years of follow-up. It is possible that more prolonged dietary modification may be required to effect significant changes in the molecular events that mediate the development of adenomas and/or colorectal cancer.

PROGNOSIS

The overall prognosis for patients with colorectal cancer is mainly dependent on stage (Fig. 179-8), but up to 50% of patients who initially present with early-stage disease will recur with metastatic involvement. Five-year survival is approximately 90 to 95% for stage I disease and declines considerably to less than 10% for stage IV metastatic disease. The prognosis for stage III colorectal cancer can range from 65 to 70% for patients with only one or two lymph nodes and down to less than 25% for those with high-risk disease and more than four positive lymph nodes. Corresponding rates for rectal cancer are slightly inferior to those for colon cancer. In addition to stage, other factors that are associated with poorer outcomes in patients with early-stage colon cancer who undergo potentially curative resection include signet ring histology, high tumor grade, lymphovascular and perineural invasion, absence of host lymphoid response, evidence for obstruction or perforation preoperatively, high preoperative serum CEA levels, positive surgical margins, and microsatellite-stable disease.

Mucinous adenocarcinomas are associated with a worse overall prognosis than nonmucinous subtypes. By comparison, the medullary subtype has a relatively favorable prognosis.

Interestingly, the prognosis of colorectal cancers is not dependent on the size of the primary tumor. However, the location of the primary tumor is an important prognostic factor, with left-sided primary tumors associated with a significantly better prognosis compared with right-sided tumors. Moreover, the effect of tumor location is independent of other important clinical factors, including stage, race, and use of adjuvant chemotherapy.

Molecular biomarkers also correlate with the prognosis of all stages of colorectal cancer. *KRAS* mutations are present in 30 to 40% of colorectal cancer, and are associated with a worse prognosis. These mutations lead to constitutive

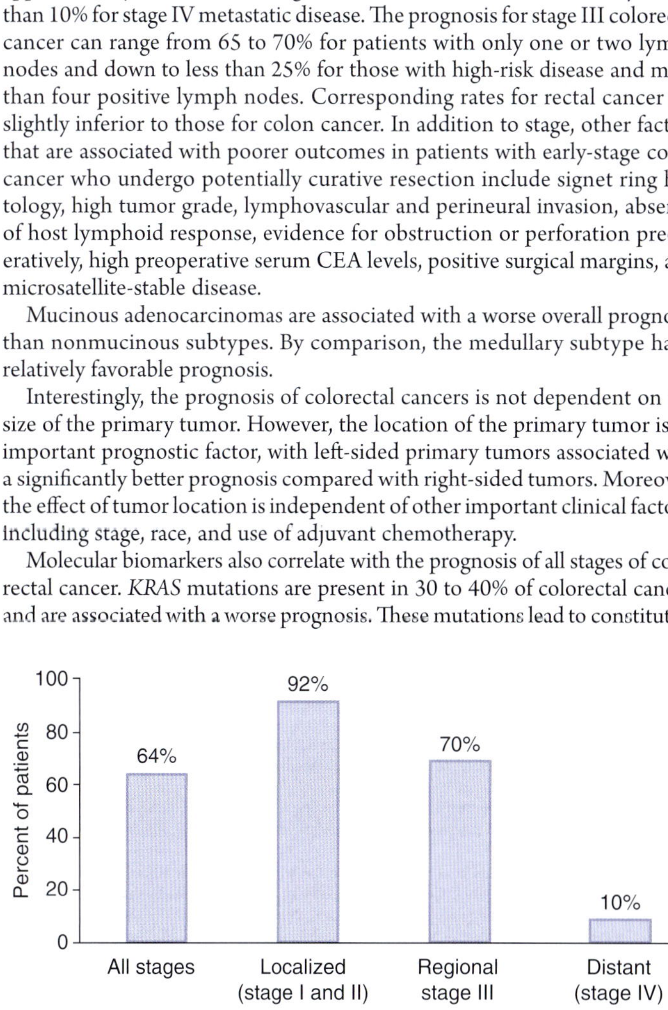

FIGURE 179-8. Five-year survival of colon cancer by disease stage.

activation of the RAS-RAF-MAPK signaling pathway downstream of EGFR, which render tumors resistant to anti-EGFR antibody therapy with cetuximab or panitumumab. *NRAS* mutations occur in only about 5% of colorectal cancer patients, and these mutations also confer resistance to anti-EGFR therapy. *BRAF* mutations, which are seen in 5 to 10% of colorectal cancer patients, are associated with poor prognosis and also predict resistance to anti-EGFR therapy.

More detailed molecular subtyping may be even more predictive. One approach groups colorectal cancers into four types—microsatellite instability immune, canonical, metabolic and mesenchymal—based on such profiling.

The poorly differentiated neuroendocrine cancers, such as true small cell carcinoma, are the most aggressive, commonly present with hepatic and other distant metastases, and have a poor overall prognosis. In contrast to carcinoids, however, poorly differentiated neuroendocrine cancers are more responsive, at least initially, to systemic chemotherapy.

GENERAL REFERENCES

For the General References and other additional features, please visit Elsevier eBooks+ at https://ebooks.health.elsevier.com.

Grade A References

A1. Casali PG, Zalcberg J, Le Cesne A, et al. Ten-year progression-free and overall survival in patients with unresectable or metastatic GI stromal tumors: long-term analysis of the European Organisation for Research and Treatment of Cancer, Italian Sarcoma Group, and Australasian Gastrointestinal Trials Group Intergroup phase III randomized trial on imatinib at two dose levels. *J Clin Oncol.* 2017;35:1713-1720.

A2. Wille-Jørgensen P, Syk I, Smedh K, et al. Effect of more vs less frequent follow-up testing on overall and colorectal cancer-specific mortality in patients with stage II or III colorectal cancer: the COLOFOL randomized clinical trial. *JAMA.* 2018;319:2095-2103.

A3. Kemeny MM, Zhao F, Forastiere AA, et al. Phase III prospectively randomized trial of perioperative 5-FU after curative resection for colon cancer: an intergroup trial of the ECOG-ACRIN Cancer Research Group (E1292). *Ann Surg Oncol.* 2022;30:1099-1109.

A4. Tie J, Cohen JD, Lahouel K, et al. Circulating tumor DNA analysis guiding adjuvant therapy in stage II colon cancer. *N Engl J Med.* 2022;386:2261-2272.

A5. Bahadoer RR, Dijkstra EA, van Etten B, et al. Short-course radiotherapy followed by chemotherapy before total mesorectal excision (TME) versus preoperative chemoradiotherapy, TME, and optional adjuvant chemotherapy in locally advanced rectal cancer (RAPIDO): a randomised, open-label phase 3 trial. *Lancet Oncol.* 2021;22:29-42.

A6. Venook AP, Niedzwiecki D, Lenz HJ, et al. Effect of first-line chemotherapy combined with cetuximab or bevacizumab on overall survival in patients with KRAS wild-type advanced or metastatic colorectal cancer: a randomized clinical trial. *JAMA.* 2017;317:2392-2401.

A7. André T, Shiu K-K, Kim TW, et al. Pembrolizumab in microsatellite-instability-high advanced colorectal cancer. *N Engl J Med.* 2020;383:2207-2218.

A8. Andre T, Amonkar M, Norquist JM, et al. Health-related quality of life in patients with microsatellite instability-high or mismatch repair deficient metastatic colorectal cancer treated with first-line pembrolizumab versus chemotherapy (KEYNOTE-0177): an open-label, randomised, phase 3 trial. *Lancet Oncol.* 2021;22:665-677.

A9. Kopetz S, Grothey A, Yaeger R, et al. Encorafenib, binimetinib, and cetuximab in BRAF V600E-mutated colorectal cancer. *N Engl J Med.* 2019;381:1632-1643.

A10. Tang W, Ren L, Liu T, et al. Bevacizumab plus mFOLFOX6 versus mFOLFOX6 alone as first-line treatment for RAS mutant unresectable colorectal liver-limited metastases: the BECOME randomized controlled trial. *J Clin Oncol.* 2020;38:3175-3184.

A11. Wasan HS, Gibbs P, Sharma NK, et al. First-line selective internal radiotherapy plus chemotherapy versus chemotherapy alone in patients with liver metastases from colorectal cancer (FOXFIRE, SIRFLOX, and FOXFIRE-Global): a combined analysis of three multicentre, randomised, phase 3 trials. *Lancet Oncol.* 2017;18:1159-1171.

A12. Lin JS, Perdue LA, Henrikson NB, et al. Screening for colorectal cancer: updated evidence report and systematic review for the US Preventive Services Task Force. *JAMA.* 2021;325:1978-1997.

A13. Juul FE, Cross AJ, Schoen RE, et al. 15-Year benefits of sigmoidoscopy screening on colorectal cancer incidence and mortality: a pooled analysis of randomized trials. *Ann Intern Med.* 2022;175:1525-1533.

A14. Bretthauer M, Løberg M, Wieszczy P, et al. Effect of colonoscopy screening on risks of colorectal cancer and related death. *N Engl J Med.* 2022;387:1547-1556.

A15. Cash BD, Fleisher MR, Fern S, et al. Multicentre, prospective, randomised study comparing the diagnostic yield of colon capsule endoscopy versus CT colonography in a screening population (the TOPAZ study). *Gut.* 2021;70:2115-2122.

A16. Tomić T, Domínguez-López S, Barrios-Rodríguez R. Non-aspirin non-steroidal anti-inflammatory drugs in prevention of colorectal cancer in people aged 40 or older: a systematic review and meta-analysis. *Cancer Epidemiol.* 2019;58:52-62.

A17. Emilsson L, Holme Ø, Bretthauer M, et al. Systematic review with meta-analysis: the comparative effectiveness of aspirin vs. screening for colorectal cancer prevention. *Aliment Pharmacol Ther.* 2017;45:193-204.

A18. Burn J, Sheth H, Elliott F, et al. Cancer prevention with aspirin in hereditary colorectal cancer (Lynch syndrome), 10-year follow-up and registry-based 20-year data in the CAPP2 study: a double-blind, randomised, placebo-controlled trial. *Lancet.* 2020;395:1855-1863.

180 PANCREATIC CANCER

DANIEL LAHERU

DEFINITION

More than 90% of pancreatic tumors are adenocarcinomas that arise from the ductal epithelium. Other major tumors of the pancreas include acinar cell, intraductal papillary mucinous neoplasm, mucinous cystic neoplasm, mixed histology, endocrine malignancies, carcinoid tumors, lymphomas, and a variety of rare sarcomas.

EPIDEMIOLOGY

Pancreatic ductal adenocarcinoma has one of the highest mortality-to-incidence ratios of any disease. Although it represents the tenth leading cause of cancer in the United States, it is the fourth leading cause of cancer-related deaths because most patients will die from their disease. By the year 2030, pancreatic cancer is expected to be the second leading cause of cancer-related death behind only lung cancer. Each year in the United States, approximately 50,000 individuals die from pancreatic adenocarcinoma or its complications.[1] The incidence of pancreatic cancer is slowly increasing based on the changing demographics of the U.S. population. In the United States, Blacks have a higher incidence and mortality from pancreatic cancer compared with Whites, although the incidence rate is not increasing as fast in Blacks as in Whites.[2] The risk of developing pancreatic adenocarcinoma increases with age, with a mean onset at age 71 years. The risk is equivalent in men and women, with an average lifetime risk for developing pancreatic adenocarcinoma of about 1 in 78. Globally, 70% of all pancreatic cancer cases occur in people living in advanced economies, with about 470,000 worldwide deaths in 2020.[3]

Smoking tobacco, as well as passive exposure to tobacco smoke in the environment, contributes significantly to the development of pancreatic adenocarcinoma and is also associated with a reduction in survival among patients with pancreatic cancer.[4] Occupational hazards that have been associated with an enhanced risk of developing pancreatic adenocarcinoma include exposure to chlorinated hydrocarbon solvents and heavy metals.

Most pancreatic adenocarcinoma cases are sporadic and occur without a history of the disease in first-degree relatives. Germline mutations in cancer susceptibility genes are commonly identified, even in patients without a significant family history of cancer.[5] Some pancreatic adenocarcinomas occur in association with other cancers or diseases, but most do not occur in association with a defined syndrome.

However, approximately 10% of pancreatic adenocarcinomas occur in families with a history of pancreatic adenocarcinoma.[6] In such families, the risk of developing pancreatic adenocarcinoma is increased seven-fold compared with the general population.[7] Premalignant cystic lesions of the pancreas also occur in families with pancreatic cancer. In addition to mutations of the *PALB2* gene in 3% of these families, mutations have also been identified in *ATM* or *BRCA2*, which are critical partners in the DNA damage repair pathway, as well as in *p16*.

Chronic pancreatic inflammation from alcohol misuse or genetic anomalies significantly increases the risk of being diagnosed with pancreatic adenocarcinoma. Pro-inflammatory cytokines contribute to the progression from premalignant lesion to advanced tumor.

New-onset insulin-dependent diabetes after age 50 years can be an indicator of pancreatic cancer.[8] Long-standing type 1 and type 2 diabetes mellitus may increase the risk of pancreatic adenocarcinoma. For example, the increase in obesity in the U.S. population and the concomitant increase in associated diabetes mellitus are strongly associated with an enhanced lifetime risk of developing pancreatic adenocarcinoma. Epidemiologic studies also note a relationship between type 3c diabetes (diabetes related to pancreatic disease and characterized by a severe deficiency of all glucoregulatory hormones) and the development of pancreatic adenocarcinoma. Patients with type 3c diabetes appear to have the highest associated risk of developing pancreatic adenocarcinoma, especially in the setting of coexisting chronic pancreatitis. Type 3c diabetes is also a consequence of pancreatic adenocarcinoma in approximately 30% of patients.

PATHOBIOLOGY

Pancreatic cancer is caused by inherited (germline) and acquired (somatic) mutations in cancer-causing genes. Oncogenes and tumor suppressor genes contribute to the growth of the tumor itself as well as to the surrounding microenvironment. A major advance in understanding the development of pancreatic cancer has been the appreciation that the majority of pancreatic adenocarcinomas progress sequentially from histologically normal ductal epithelium to low-grade pancreatic intraepithelial neoplasia, to high-grade pancreatic intraepithelial neoplasia, to invasive carcinoma. This process is associated with the accumulation of specific gene alterations (Fig. 180-1).

The *KRAS* oncogene, located on chromosome 12, is the most frequently mutated oncogene in pancreatic cancer in (>90% of tumors). It encodes a membrane-bound protein that has GTP-ase activity and is involved in signal transduction. When activated by mutation, typically a point mutation in codon 12, the functions of *KRAS* are independent of growth factor control, thereby leading to chronic activation of its downstream signaling partners (*PI3K*, *MAPK*, and *RAF*), the inhibition of apoptosis, the activation of the cell cycle, migration, angiogenesis, cytoskeletal remodeling, and unchecked proliferation. *KRAS* oncogenic dose variation plays an important role in pancreatic cancer tumorigenesis, progression, and metastasis.[9]

The tumor suppressor *CDKN2A/TP16*, which is a cell cycle control gene, is commonly inactivated in pancreatic cancer, with 80 to 95% loss of activity leading to increased cell cycle progression. *TP53* is activated by DNA damage to stop cell cycle progression and repair damaged DNA or initiate apoptosis. Mutations in this tumor suppressor gene are commonly found in 50 to 75% of pancreatic tumors. Inactivation of *SMAD4* (DPC4), which is involved in regulating cell cycle progression through the transforming growth factor (TGF)-β pathway, is observed in over 50% of pancreatic cancers and is associated with worse prognosis and the development of metastases. Inactivation of *RB1* (in <10% of pancreatic cancers) and *STK11* (responsible for Peutz-Jeghers syndrome) is also observed.

Several major signaling pathways are involved in pancreatic tumorigenesis. Hedgehog (Hh) signaling, critical in embryogenesis, regulates the cell cycle and apoptosis, aids in the formation of tumor stroma, and is often upregulated and abnormal in pancreatic cancers. The NOTCH pathway, which is also important in normal embryogenesis to prevent terminal differentiation of cells until appropriate, can be abnormally activated in pancreatic cancer, thereby allowing cells to remain in an undifferentiated state that contributes to tumor growth. When the Wnt pathway is activated, β-catenin is stabilized and migrates into the nucleus, where it activates its target genes. The epidermal growth factor receptor (EGFR), TGF-β, and JAK/STAT pathways are also abnormal in pancreatic cancer cells and lead to the promotion of cell growth, proliferation, differentiation, and survival. Epigenetic modification, the process by which gene expression is altered by mechanisms other than changes in the actual DNA sequence, also has a role in pancreatic cancer tumorigenesis.[10]

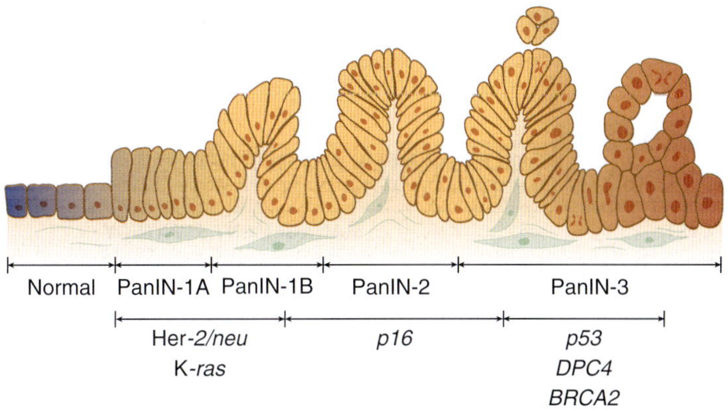

FIGURE 180-1. **Genetic progression model of pancreatic adenocarcinoma. Molecular changes in the development of pancreatic ductal adenocarcinoma begin with early changes that include telomere shortening and development of mutations in *KRAS*; these are followed by loss of p16 function and expression of cyclin D1. Late changes include expression of p53 and loss of SMAD4/DPC4. PanIN = pancreatic intraepithelial neoplasia.**

Shortening of telomeres and overexpression of microRNAs lead to chromosomal instability and dysregulation of gene expression, respectively.

In addition to cancer cells themselves, the tumor microenvironment is composed of stromal cells, inflammatory cells, and endothelial cells that all play a particularly important role in the growth of pancreatic cancer. Cancer cells secrete growth factors, including insulin-like growth factor (IGF)-1, fibroblast growth factor (FGF), TGF-β, vascular endothelial growth factor (VEGF), and platelet-derived growth factor (PDGF), that stimulate pancreatic stellate cells (also called myofibroblasts) to secrete excess amounts of extracellular matrix. In turn, the matrix and its stromal cells secrete cytokines and growth factors that promote the growth, invasion, and dissemination of cancer cells. This matrix also protects pancreatic cancer cells from apoptosis and generates a desmoplastic reaction that interferes with the delivery of chemotherapy to the tumor site. The local presence of TGF-β also leads to decreased activity of helper T-cells and thereby suppresses the body's immune reaction against pancreatic cancer cells.

CLINICAL MANIFESTATIONS

Many pancreatic tumors are asymptomatic when they are diagnosed by an imaging study obtained for an unrelated reason. The symptoms of early pancreatic adenocarcinoma are often subtle and include nonspecific gastrointestinal complaints (nausea, vague abdominal pain), fatigue, and weight loss of undetermined etiology. Epigastric pain and obstructive jaundice often prompt the initial diagnostic work-up of the biliary tree but are frequently late symptoms that are associated with advanced local or regionally disseminated disease. Because approximately 75% of pancreatic carcinomas are located in the head of the pancreas, clinical presentations are often related to compression or invasion of the biliary tree or pancreatic ducts. Deep or superficial venous thrombosis (Trousseau syndrome) is not infrequent, either early or late in the presentation of pancreatic adenocarcinoma. Observation of a palpably distended gallbladder (from obstruction of the distal common bile duct), or Courvoisier sign, is uncommon.

The laboratory abnormalities that accompany pancreatic adenocarcinoma at presentation include anemia and elevations of serum levels of bilirubin, alkaline phosphatase, and aminotransferases. A majority of patients eventually develop signs of obstructive jaundice as well as hyperglycemia, which reflects associated diabetes mellitus.

Early pancreatic intraepithelial neoplasia lesions are asymptomatic, and cystic lesions of the pancreas often remain asymptomatic. Some are discovered on abdominal imaging performed for other purposes, with some estimates that 2 to 15% of patients undergoing abdominal magnetic resonance imaging (MRI) may have unsuspected pancreatic cysts. Most small lesions do not cause symptoms and otherwise would remain undetected unless they later caused acute symptoms that would precipitate an abdominal computed tomographic (CT) scan. Large cysts may cause vague symptoms, but obstructive jaundice is uncommon. Most intraductal papillary mucinous neoplasms are asymptomatic, but some patients present with obstructive jaundice or with pancreatitis.

DIAGNOSIS

Differential Diagnosis

The differential diagnosis of pancreatic adenocarcinoma includes conditions that can present as a solid pancreatic mass, including acute (or an exacerbation of chronic) pancreatitis (Chapter 130), ampullary or distal cholangiocarcinomas (Chapter 181) with associated biliary obstruction and jaundice, and nonadenocarcinomatous cystic pancreatic neoplasms.

A high proportion of incidental cysts among patients without a history of pancreatitis are neoplastic. High-resolution CT may provide a presumptive diagnosis when characteristic features are present. MRI can identify any communication between the cyst and the pancreatic duct. Endoscopic ultrasonography can differentiate benign from malignant lesions if it finds a solid mass or invasive tumor.

Cystic Neoplasms

Cystic lesions of the pancreas can be categorized into non-neoplastic (e.g., pseudocysts; see Chapter 130) and neoplastic cystic lesions.[11] Cystic neoplasms can be subcategorized into mucin-producing and non-mucin-producing cystic neoplasms.[12] Cystic neoplasms that do not produce mucin include serous cystadenomas, which do not have increased risk of cancer, papillary cystic neoplasms, and cystic pancreatic neuroendocrine tumors.

Serous cystadenomas occur more commonly in women and are nearly always benign. Though usually asymptomatic, they can be symptomatic as they enlarge. The pathology shows a well-circumscribed fibrous capsule containing numerous small fluid-filled cysts.

Mucinous cystic neoplasms, which nearly always occur in the pancreatic body or tail in women, comprise about 50% of pancreatic tumors removed in contemporary surgical series. About one third are discovered incidentally on radiographic imaging for other purposes, but patients also may present with pain, an abdominal mass, or weight loss. A thick fibrous capsule contains cysts lined by mucin-producing duct-like cells. About 30% of mucinous cystic neoplasms have evidence of invasive adenocarcinoma with a variable prognosis.

Intraductal papillary mucinous neoplasms are mucin-producing lesions that, unlike mucinous cystic neoplasms, communicate with the main pancreatic duct. Their intraductal dysplastic epithelium resembles colorectal villous adenomas, with papillae covered by columnar epithelium and the occasional goblet cell with extensive mucin production. These neoplasms often contain at least low-grade dysplasia and are always premalignant and require follow-up.

Imaging

A computed tomographic (CT) scan with oral and intravenous contrast and thin cuts through the pancreas is the imaging procedure of choice when pancreatic adenocarcinoma is suspected. CT scans can provide information regarding the presence of metastatic disease, vascular invasion, and potential for resection. Malignancy is more common when the cyst is greater than 3 cm, has a solid component, or is associated with a dilated pancreatic duct greater than 1 cm, but malignancy is less clearly associated with the rate of growth on serial imaging studies. Consensus recommendations[13] include MRI of pancreatic cysts identified on CT imaging; endoscopic ultrasonography and fine-needle aspiration for pancreatic cysts with concerning features on MRI; and cytologic and biomarker evaluation of aspirated fluid.[14]

Endoscopic ultrasound may provide additional information for preoperative assessment, including by guiding fine-needle aspiration biopsy. However, the typical desmoplastic reaction that can encase pancreatic adenocarcinomas increases the possibility of false-negative biopsy findings. Patients with locally advanced or metastatic disease should have their diagnosis confirmed pathologically by fine-needle biopsy of the primary site or of a metastasis.

Biomarkers and Screening

Analysis of cyst fluid can correctly identify up to 90% of pancreatic cysts that would not require surgery.[15] No serum- or tumor-based biomarkers or biomarker panels are both sensitive and specific enough for accurate early detection in clinical practice, but multianalyte blood tests that can detect and localize surgically resectable cancers, including pancreatic cancers, are promising.[16] CA19.9 is the most commonly used tumor biomarker for monitoring therapeutic progress in pancreatic adenocarcinoma, but the assay lacks specificity and cannot be used for early detection. Endoscopic ultrasound is useful for the evaluation of cystic lesions and permits sampling of cystic fluid for genetic markers associated with the development of pancreatic adenocarcinoma in cancer-prone families, as well as for cytologic studies. Some data suggest a potential benefit from annual screening using MRI, magnetic resonance cholangiopancreatography, or endoscopic ultrasound in asymptomatic adults who are carriers of the high-risk *CDNK2A* mutation.

TREATMENT

Pancreatic Cysts

Patients with pancreatic cysts that have concerning features (cyst ≥ 3 cm, a dilated main pancreatic duct > 1 cm, presence of an associated solid component or clinical symptoms such as jaundice) should be referred for fine-needle aspiration guided by endoscopic ultrasound. If the cytology is consistent with either high-grade dysplasia or invasive pancreatic cancer, these patients are commonly offered surgical resection (Table 180-1).[17] In contrast, patients whose features do not warrant resection should undergo MRI surveillance every 1 to 2 years for up to 5 years.[18]

Serous cystadenomas are benign abnormalities that do not connect to pancreatic ducts and warrant surgery only if symptomatic. Mucinous cystadenomas, which are precursors of pancreatic adenocarcinoma, are overtly malignant in 15% of patients and require surgical resection. Intraductal papillary mucinous neoplasms of the pancreas may contain malignant elements in about 40% of patients particularly in patients with concerning features, and should be removed surgically.

Pancreatic Cancer

Surgical Candidates

Surgery offers the only chance to cure pancreatic cancer.[19] Tumors are considered resectable if a clear fat plane is present around the celiac and superior mesenteric arteries and if the superior mesenteric and portal veins are patent. If the superior mesenteric vein and/or the portal vein is involved, that portion of the vein must be judged to be reconstructible. After surgery, the somatostatin analogue pasireotide (900 mg subcutaneously twice daily for 7 days beginning in the morning of surgery) may reduce the risk of a fistula leak with abscess. Unfortunately, tumor will recur in the majority of patients who undergo resection, including local recurrence in approximately 40% of patients.

Adjuvant and Neoadjuvant Therapy

Decisions regarding chemotherapy should be made in a multidisciplinary manner to achieve the most timely and coordinated therapy.[20] Participation in clinical research protocols should be encouraged.

Adjuvant therapy, typically started 1 to 2 months after surgery to allow the patient to recover from the complications associated with the underlying cancer as well as from the surgery itself, is indicated under expert oversight to decrease the risk and delay the onset of locoregional and metastatic recurrence. FOLFIRINOX (oxaliplatin, irinotecan, fluorouracil, and leucovorin) is the standard of care for patients who have a good performance status,[A1] but the rate of serious side-effects (including peripheral neuropathy) is higher compared with gemcitabine. If gemcitabine is chosen, adding capecitabine can increase survival by about 10 weeks.[A2] Another option for patients with resectable pancreatic cancers is neoadjuvant FOLFIRINOX or neoadjuvant nab-paclitaxel plus gemcitabine for 3 months preoperatively followed by 3 months postoperatively.[A3,A4]

Borderline Surgical Candidates

Neoadjuvant (presurgical) therapy can downstage 15 to 40% of borderline[A5] tumors, thereby allowing patients to undergo surgery with a higher likelihood of complete resection.[21] Neoadjuvant therapy also spares some patients the risks and stress of a complex surgical procedure, because rapidly developing metastatic disease may be detected by routine restaging following the completion of neoadjuvant treatment. Unfortunately, chemotherapy-resistant cancer can be demonstrated in 15 to 35% of patients initially considered for surgery in this setting.

The use of neoadjuvant treatment also guarantees that almost all patients will receive some form of chemotherapy or chemoradiation because they do not have any postoperative complications from which to recover. The chemoradiation component of neoadjuvant therapy also decreases local recurrence rates in patients who undergo surgery.

Local Recurrence

The complications associated with local recurrence include abdominal pain, risk for bowel obstruction, gastrointestinal bleeding, and recurrent biliary obstructions. Chemoradiation versus chemotherapy alone for locally advanced pancreatic cancer can decrease the risk for local recurrence but has not improved median survival compared with chemotherapy alone.[A6]

Unresectable or Metastatic Disease

First-line therapy for unresectable or metastatic pancreatic cancer is FOLFIRINOX or gemcitabine plus nab-paclitaxel (Table 180-2).[22] Nanoliposomal irinotecan in combination with fluorouracil and folinic acid extends survival with a manageable safety profile in patients with metastatic pancreatic adenocarcinoma who previously received gemcitabine-based therapy.[A7] Gemcitabine has also been combined with targeted therapies, such as the EGFR inhibitor erlotinib, but with a very modest improvement on overall survival.[23]

In the small percentage of patients with germline mutations in *BRCA1* or *BRCA2*, olaparib (300 mg twice daily) can prolong progression-free survival by about 3.5 months in patients who have been received a platinum-containing regimen for a minimum of 4 months and have been at least stable radigraphically.[A8] In patients with KRAS G12C mutations, sotorasib is a promising experimental therapy.[24]

Thromboembolism

Advanced pancreatic cancer is associated with a high risk of venous thromboembolic complications. Current guidelines do not recommend routine thromboprophylaxis for all patients with active pancreatic cancer, but this prophylaxis

TABLE 180-1 GUIDELINES FOR ASYMPTOMATIC INCIDENTAL PANCREATIC CYSTS

CYST	MANAGEMENT STRATEGY
Either (a) a solid component and dilation of the main pancreatic duct of >5 mm or (b) suspicious EUS-guided FNA	EUS-guided FNA. Surgery if high-grade dysplasia or cancer, with follow-up MRI every 2 years after surgery; if benign, no follow-up required.
Size <3 cm, no solid component, no dilation of main pancreatic duct	MRI at 1, 3, and 5 years: if changes, EUS-guided FNA; if stable at 5 years, discontinue screening.

EUS = endoscopic ultrasound; FNA = fine needle aspiration; MRI = magnetic resonance imaging.
Vege SS, Ziring B, Jain R, et al. American Gastroenterological Association Institute guideline on the diagnosis and management of asymptomatic neoplastic pancreatic cysts. *Gastroenterology*. 2015;148:819-822.

TABLE 180-2 SELECTED METASTATIC PANCREATIC CANCER STUDIES

STUDY	CHEMOTHERAPY	MEDIAN SURVIVAL (MO)	1-YEAR SURVIVAL (%)
Burris (1997)* N = 126	5-FU vs. gem	4.4 vs. 5.6 (P = .0025)	2 vs. 18
Cunningham (2009)† N = 533	Gem ± capecitabine	7.4 vs. 6 (P < .05)	26 vs. 19
Conroy (2011)‡ N = 343	Gem v. FOLFIRINOX	6.8 vs. 11.1 (P < .0001)	17 vs. 36
Van Hoff (2013)§ N = 861	Gem ± nab-paclitaxel	8.5 vs. 6.7 (P < .001)	35 vs. 22 (P < .001)

*Burris H, Storniolo AM. Assessing clinical benefit in the treatment of pancreas cancer: gemcitabine compared to 5-fluorouracil. *Eur J Cancer*. 1997;33 Suppl 1:S18-S22.
†Cunningham D, Chau I, Stocken DD, et al. Phase III randomized comparison of gemcitabine versus gemcitabine plus capecitabine in patients with advanced pancreatic cancer. *J Clin Oncol*. 2009;27:5513-5518.
‡Conroy T, Desseigne F, Ychou M, et al. FOLFIRINOX versus gemcitabine for metastatic pancreatic cancer. *N Engl J Med*. 2011;364:1817-1825.
§Von Hoff DD, Ervin T, Arena FP, et al. Increased survival in pancreatic cancer with nab-paclitaxel plus gemcitabine. *N Engl J Med*. 2013;369:1691-1703.
5-FU = 5-fluorocil; FOLFIRINOX = combination chemotherapy with oxaliplatin, irinotecan, fluorouracil, and leucovorin; gem = gemcitabine; NR = not reported.

can be considered for patients who are at high risk.[25] Thromboprophylaxis with enoxaparin (Chapter 70) is feasible and effective.[A9] Another options is rivaroxaban (see Table 70-6).[A10]

Palliative Care

Because many patients suffer from biliary obstruction, diarrhea, pain, and malnutrition, palliative care (Chapter 3) can provide great benefit. Surgery can also play an important palliative role; patients whose tumors are unresectable may experience symptomatic improvement after a biliary or gastric bypass procedure, depending on the site of obstruction. Endoscopic placement of both biliary and duodenal stents may also improve pruritus, pain, or other complications of biliary tract obstruction. Palliative care for patients with pancreatic adenocarcinoma necessitates scrupulous attention to pain management (Chapter 26), often with a multidisciplinary approach, as well as maintenance of hydration and adequate nutrition.

Prevention

Even though premalignant intraductal papillary mucinous neoplasms or pancreatic mucinous neoplasms can be detected by imaging, screening is not currently recommended in asymptomatic adults.[26] However, consensus guidelines recommend that pancreatic cancer surveillance be considered for select high-risk individuals (based on family risk or germline mutation status) and that any evaluations should be conducted in a research protocol by experienced multidisciplinary teams.[27,28]

Prognosis

Among patients with a serous cystic neoplasm followed beyond 1 year, the size increases in about 40%, is stable in about 55%, and decreases in about 5%. Serous cystadenocarcinomas develop in only about 0.1% of patients at an average follow-up of 3 years.[29]

The overall 5-year survival for all patients with pancreatic cancer is less than 5%, because the cancer is advanced when clinically detected. Once patients are diagnosed, only 15 to 20% initially have resectable and potentially curable disease. In patients with early-stage disease, median survival has improved from 20 to 24 months to 54 months with adjuvant FOLFIRINOX. Patients with locally advanced (about 25 to 30% of patients at presentation) and metastatic (about 50 to 60% of patients at presentation) disease have median survivals of 8 to 14 months and 4 to 6 months, respectively. T-cell immunity has been linked to the exceptional outcome of the few long-term survivors, and neoantigen quality has been identified as a biomarker for immunogenic tumors.

GENERAL REFERENCES

For the General References and other additional features, please visit Elsevier eBooks+ at https://ebooks.health.elsevier.com.

Grade A References

A1. Conroy T, Hammel P, Hebbar M, et al. FOLFIRINOX or gemcitabine as adjuvant therapy for pancreatic cancer. *N Engl J Med*. 2018;379:2395-2406.

A2. Neoptolemos JP, Palmer DH, Ghaneh P, et al. Comparison of adjuvant gemcitabine and capecitabine with gemcitabine monotherapy in patients with resected pancreatic cancer (ESPAC-4): a multicentre, open-label, randomised, phase 3 trial. *Lancet*. 2017;389:1011-1024.

A3. Birrer DL, Golcher H, Casadei R, et al. Neoadjuvant therapy for resectable pancreatic cancer: a new standard of care. Pooled data from 3 randomized controlled trials. *Ann Surg*. 2021;274:713-720.

A4. Sohal DPS, Duong M, Ahmad SA, et al. Efficacy of perioperative chemotherapy for resectable pancreatic adenocarcinoma: a phase 2 randomized clinical trial. *JAMA Oncol*. 2021;7:421-427.

A5. Versteijne E, van Dam JL, Suker M, et al. Neoadjuvant chemoradiotherapy versus upfront surgery for resectable and borderline resectable pancreatic cancer: long-term results of the Dutch randomized PREOPANC trial. *J Clin Oncol*. 2022;40:1220-1230.

A6. Hammel P, Huguet F, van Laethem JL, et al. Effect of chemoradiotherapy vs chemotherapy on survival in patients with locally advanced pancreatic cancer controlled after 4 months of gemcitabine with or without erlotinib: the LAP07 randomized clinical trial. *JAMA*. 2016;315:1844-1853.

A7. Wang-Gillam A, Li CP, Bodoky G, et al. Nanoliposomal irinotecan with fluorouracil and folinic acid in metastatic pancreatic cancer after previous gemcitabine-based therapy (NAPOLI-1): a global, randomised, open-label, phase 3 trial. *Lancet*. 2016;387:545-557.

A8. Golan T, Hammel P, Reni M, et al. Maintenance olaparib for germline BRCA-mutated metastatic pancreatic cancer. *N Engl J Med*. 2019;381:317-327.

A9. Pelzer U, Opitz B, Deutschinoff G, et al. Efficacy of prophylactic low-molecular weight heparin for ambulatory patients with advanced pancreatic cancer: outcomes from the CONKO-004 trial. *J Clin Oncol*. 2015;33:2028-2034.

A10. Vadhad-Raj S, McNamara M, Venerito M, et al. Rivaroxaban thromboprophylaxis in ambulatory patients with pancreatic cancer: results from a pre-specified subgroup analysis of the randomized CASSINI study. *Cancer Med*. 2020;9:6196-6204.

181 LIVER AND BILIARY TRACT TUMORS

ROBIN K. KELLEY AND ALAN P. VENOOK

DEFINITION

Cancers arising from the liver and biliary tract include hepatocellular carcinoma, cholangiocarcinoma, and gallbladder adenocarcinoma, as well as other less common malignant histologies (E-Table 181-1, Fig. 181-1). Cholangiocarcinomas are further subclassified by their anatomic location along the biliary tract: intrahepatic (also known as peripheral) or extrahepatic, which includes hilar (also known as Klatskin tumors) and distal locations. These cancers collectively represent the third leading cause of cancer death worldwide and are rising in incidence.

The liver is also a frequent site of metastasis from other primary cancers. The diagnosis of liver tumors must distinguish metastatic disease from primary liver tumors.

EPIDEMIOLOGY

Hepatocellular Carcinoma

Hepatocellular carcinoma is the most common primary tumor of the liver and the third leading cause of cancer death worldwide.[1] It accounts for approximately 900,000 new cases and 830,000 deaths each year. More than 80% of hepatocellular carcinomas occur in developing countries (Fig. 181-2), owing to an increased prevalence of risk factors, particularly hepatitis B virus and hepatitis C virus (Chapter 134), but rates are also increasing in developed nations (E-Table 181-2).[2] Hepatitis B and hepatitis C viruses together account for more than 80% of all hepatocellular carcinomas worldwide. Alcoholic cirrhosis is another classic predisposing factor.[3] However, nonalcoholic fatty liver disease has surpassed both viral hepatitis and alcoholic cirrhosis as the leading cause of hepatocellular carcinomas in the United States.[4]

Nonalcoholic fatty liver disease can lead to steatohepatitis, cirrhosis, and hepatocellular carcinoma.[5] When hepatocellular carcinoma develops in patients with nonalcoholic liver disease without preceding cirrhosis, it is more likely to present at an older age, with a larger tumor burden, and with higher rates of recurrent tumor compared with tumors that develop after patients already have cirrhosis.[6]

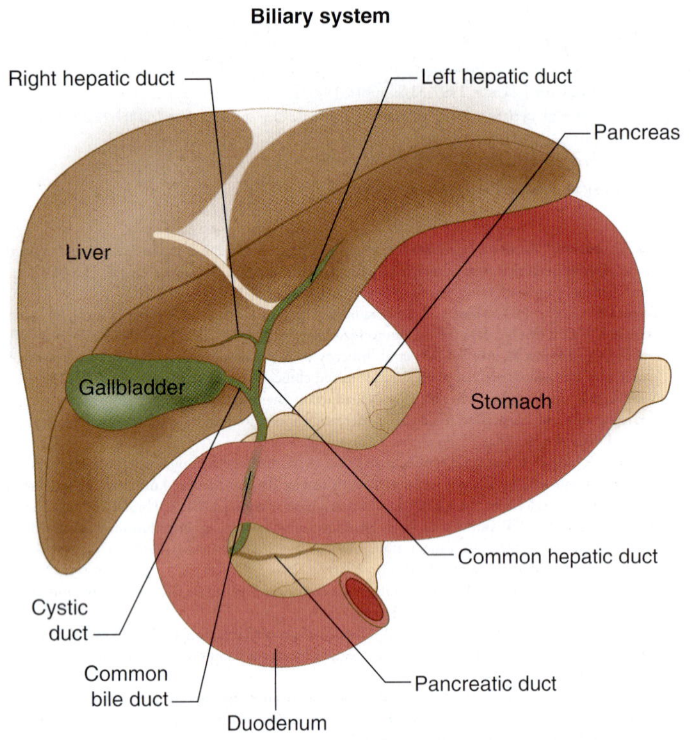

FIGURE 181-1. **Anatomy of the liver and biliary tract.** Hepatocellular carcinoma arises from liver parenchyma, and cholangiocarcinomas arise from the biliary ductal epithelium within (intrahepatic or peripheral) or outside of (extrahepatic) the liver. Tumors arising from the confluence of the right and left bile duct at the hepatic hilum are called hilar cholangiocarcinoma or Klatskin tumors.

Hepatitis B virus is endemic in regions such as Asia and sub-Saharan Africa, and it can be vertically transmitted from mother to fetus in utero. Hepatitis C virus, which may be acquired by intravenous drug use or from blood transfusion (Chapter 134), is another important risk factor for hepatocellular carcinoma. In patients who have cirrhosis caused by hepatitis C virus, the estimated annual risk for developing hepatocellular carcinoma is 3 to 5% per year. Other risk factors for hepatocellular carcinoma include hepatitis D virus (which requires coinfection with hepatitis B virus to be pathogenic), hereditary hemochromatosis (Chapter 196), α_1-antitrypsin deficiency (Chapter 132), primary biliary cirrhosis (Chapter 141), autoimmune hepatitis (Chapter 135), male gender, and dietary exposure to fungal aflatoxins.

Biliary Tract Cancers

Cholangiocarcinoma is the most common primary biliary tract malignancy and the second most common primary cancer of the liver after hepatocellular carcinoma. The incidence of intrahepatic cholangiocarcinoma appears to be increasing. Although most cases are sporadic, the risk for cholangiocarcinoma is increased in patients who have primary sclerosing cholangitis (Chapter 141), inflammatory bowel disease (Chapter 127), viral hepatitis (Chapter 135), congenital choledochal cysts or other structural abnormalities of the biliary tract, chronic pancreatitis (Chapter 130), obesity (Chapter 201), fluke infections (Chapter 326) and other causes of chronic cholangitis, bile duct adenomas, Caroli disease, and diabetes mellitus (Chapter 210).

Gallbladder adenocarcinomas are rare in the United States[7] but account for about 220,000 cases per year worldwide. The incidence varies geographically, with higher incidence rates reported in India and areas of South America and Asia. Risk factors for gallbladder adenocarcinoma include female gender, chronic cholelithiasis, chronic cholecystitis, history of gallbladder polyps, and abnormalities of the common bile duct (Chapter 141). Calcification of the gallbladder ("porcelain gallbladder") is often considered a risk factor, but it is only weakly associated with the development of cancer.

Other Primary Liver Cancers

Other primary tumors of the liver are much less common, with poorly understood risk factors. Chronic inflammatory conditions, including viral hepatitis, may be associated with the development of combined-histology liver tumors. Exposure to polyvinyl chloride has been implicated in the development of hepatic angiosarcomas. The fibrolamellar variant of hepatocellular carcinoma

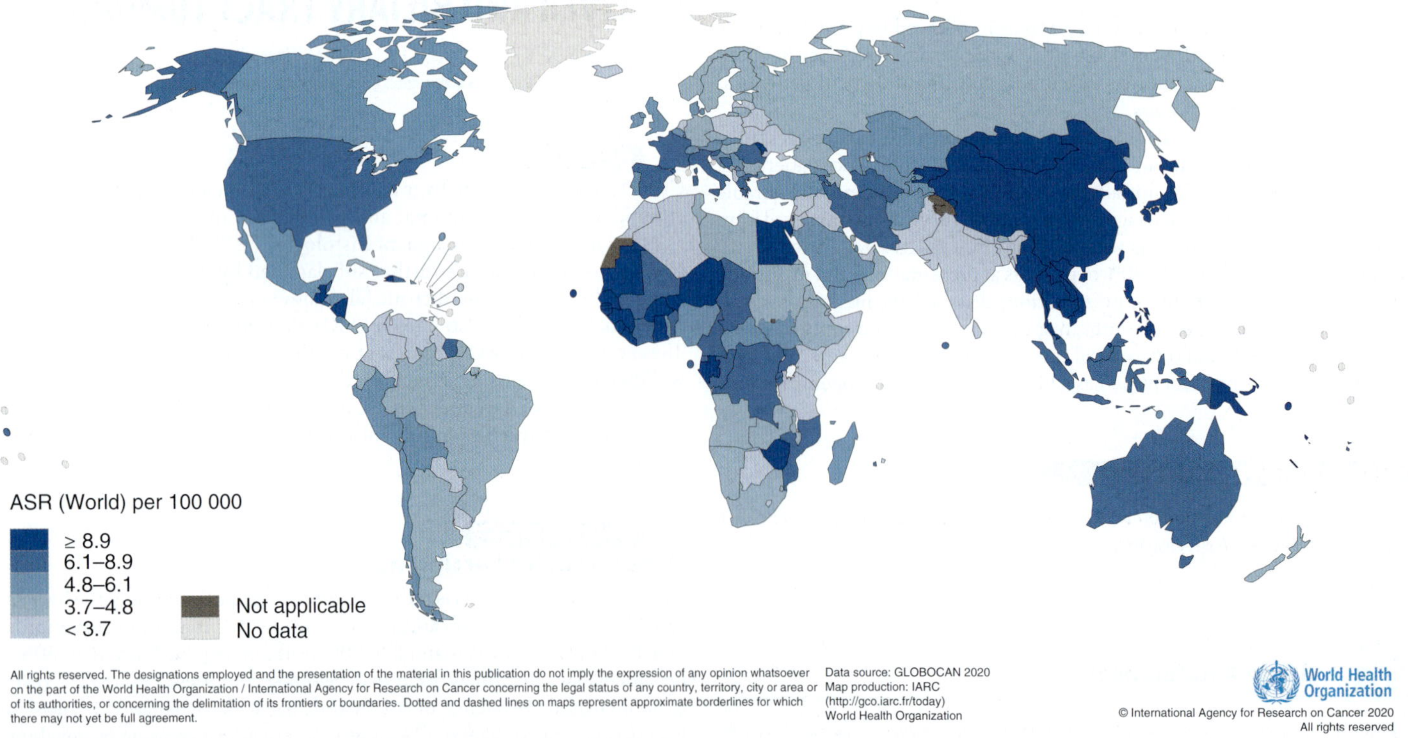

FIGURE 181-2. **Estimated worldwide age-standardized incidence rates of liver cancer.** The incidence rates are highest in Asia and parts of Africa.

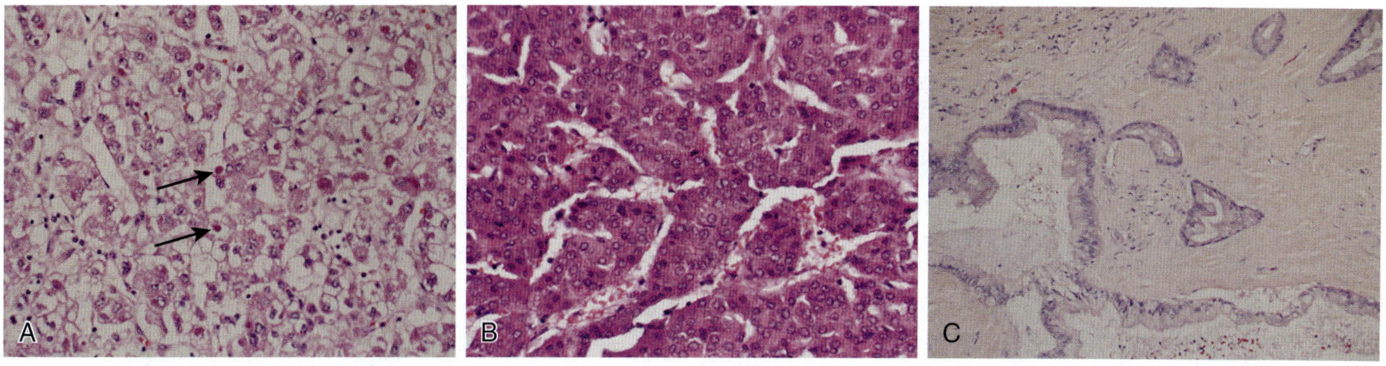

FIGURE 181-3. Histology of hepatocellular carcinoma and cholangiocarcinoma. A, Hepatocellular carcinoma (40×) with clear cell features and Mallory hyaline inclusions (*arrows*). B, Hepatocellular carcinoma (40×) with trabecular pattern and small cell change. C, Hilar cholangiocarcinoma (20×) with dense fibrous stromal reaction. (Courtesy Dr. Linda Ferrell, Department of Pathology, University of California, San Francisco.)

may occur more commonly in females. Hepatoblastoma tumors occur in infants and children, but almost never in adults.

PATHOBIOLOGY

Hepatocellular Carcinoma

Hepatocellular carcinoma is an epithelial neoplasm that arises from malignant transformation of liver hepatocytes (Fig. 181-3A and B). In the majority of cases, the pathogenesis of hepatocellular carcinoma is thought to be a multistep process triggered by underlying liver injury (such as from viral hepatitis, steatohepatitis, alcohol, iron overload, or exposure to aflatoxin). Subsequent inflammation, necrosis, regeneration, cell turnover, and proliferation[8] result in the progressive accumulation of genetic damage and somatic (acquired) mutations. Activation of oncogenes or inactivation of tumor suppressor genes, dysplasia, and subsequently carcinoma can arise. Promoter mutations that result in activation of the *TERT* gene, which encodes telomerase reverse transcriptase, are seen in approximately 45% of cases, inactivation of the tumor suppressor *TP53* is seen in about 30% of cases, and activation of the oncogene β-catenin (*CTNNB1*) gene is seen in about 25% of cases. Alterations in *Wnt*, cell cycle, and chromatin-remodeling pathways also have been described.

In hepatitis B-associated hepatocellular carcinoma, a unique mechanism of malignant transformation is direct integration of viral DNA into the host genome. This integration appears to favor specific loci, including activation of the *TERT* gene promoter.

Biliary Tract Cancers

Cholangiocarcinomas are a histologically diverse group of epithelial cancers that may arise from multiple different liver cell types, including biliary epithelial cells or hepatic progenitor cells, and are often surrounded by a dense stroma with cancer-associated fibroblasts (see Fig. 181-3C). Cholangiocarcinomas are associated with underlying inflammation and cholestasis, which activate growth factors and a proliferative response. Overexpression of *Notch1* and *AKT* has been implicated in a process by which hepatocytes are converted into the cholangiocytic precursors of intrahepatic cholangiocarcinoma. Molecular and genomic subtypes of biliary tract cancers can also be defined by mutational status and gene expression profiles.[9] For example, isocitrate dehydrogenase-1 (*IDH1*) gene mutations and fibroblast growth factor receptor-2 (*FGFR2*) gene fusions each occur in approximately 15% of intrahepatic cholangiocarcinomas.

CLINICAL MANIFESTATIONS

General Considerations

Liver masses, regardless of their cause, can be asymptomatic and may be detected during evaluation of abnormal liver chemistry tests (Chapter 133) or an imaging procedure obtained for an unrelated issue. In patients with known cirrhosis or other risk factors for hepatocellular carcinoma (see E-Table 181-2), an asymptomatic liver tumor also may be identified by surveillance imaging and/or monitoring of the serum alpha-fetoprotein (AFP) level.

Regardless of their histologic subtype, primary tumors of the liver can manifest with right upper quadrant pain, mass effect causing early satiety or obstructive symptoms, nausea, bleeding, and biliary obstruction. All of these tumors have metastatic potential, so they also can less commonly present with constitutional symptoms (e.g., weight loss, fevers, or night sweats) or signs or symptoms of metastatic disease (e.g., bone pain or a pathologic fracture). Paraneoplastic syndromes are rare in hepatobiliary cancers but can include the hypercalcemia of malignancy as well as erythrocytosis from the production of erythropoietin by tumor (Chapter 164).[10]

Hepatocellular Carcinoma

The clinical presentation of hepatocellular carcinoma can vary according to the extent of tumor and the degree of underlying liver dysfunction. Some patients may be asymptomatic, particularly when diagnosed by surveillance imaging and/or by an elevation in the AFP level. In cases with hepatic decompensation triggered by a growing tumor, patients present with symptoms of worsening liver function and portal hypertension (Chapter 139), including new ascites, encephalopathy, gastrointestinal bleeding, or jaundice, especially in the presence of associated portal vein thrombosis. In other cases, tumor involvement of the sensitive liver capsule can cause chronic progressive upper abdominal pain. The sudden onset acute pain suggests bleeding into the tumor or rupture. Constitutional symptoms such as cachexia, fatigue, and weight loss may be present with advanced stages.

On physical examination, patients with hepatocellular carcinoma may have an enlarged liver with tenderness, and a palpable mass lead to the diagnosis of hepatocellular carcinoma. A bruit may be auscultated over the liver surface, particularly with large and rapidly growing tumors. Ascites, jaundice, signs of portal hypertension (e.g., caput medusae and splenomegaly), and asterixis may be variably present if hepatic function has decompensated. The AFP level is elevated in approximately 70% of cases but is not diagnostic.

Biliary Tract Cancers

Extrahepatic cholangiocarcinomas most often manifest with signs and symptoms of biliary obstruction, such as jaundice, pruritus, pale stools, dark urine, anorexia, nausea, and weight loss. Intrahepatic cholangiocarcinomas can also cause obstruction, but generally only when extensive disease is present. Less commonly, complications such as biliary fistulas and hemobilia can occur.

Gallbladder cancers are often diagnosed incidentally during cholecystectomy, but some cases can be associated with right upper quadrant pain, biliary colic, or a tender and palpable mass. Biliary obstruction can lead to infections of the biliary tract (cholangitis), with symptoms including right upper quadrant pain, fever, chills, nausea, vomiting, and jaundice (Chapter 141). Cholangitis can lead to complications such bacteremia (most commonly with gram-negative enteric pathogens), sepsis, and abscess formation.

DIAGNOSIS

General Considerations

The approach to patients with a liver mass requires assessment of risk factors and extent of any underlying liver disease. The diagnostic evaluation, staging, and treatment options are guided by whether underlying liver disease is present as well as by its extent. The differential diagnosis for hepatocellular carcinoma and biliary tract cancers includes benign liver lesions (such as hemangiomas, adenomas, abscesses, and regenerative nodules), malignant tumors of other primary liver histologies, mixed-histology tumors, and metastatic disease.

Hepatocellular Carcinoma

Whether the patient has an asymptomatic liver mass or has a mass discovered because of symptoms, it must be evaluated promptly (see Fig. 132-6). Hepatocellular carcinoma is unique in oncology in that a diagnosis can be made radiographically without tumor tissue sampling in the appropriate clinical

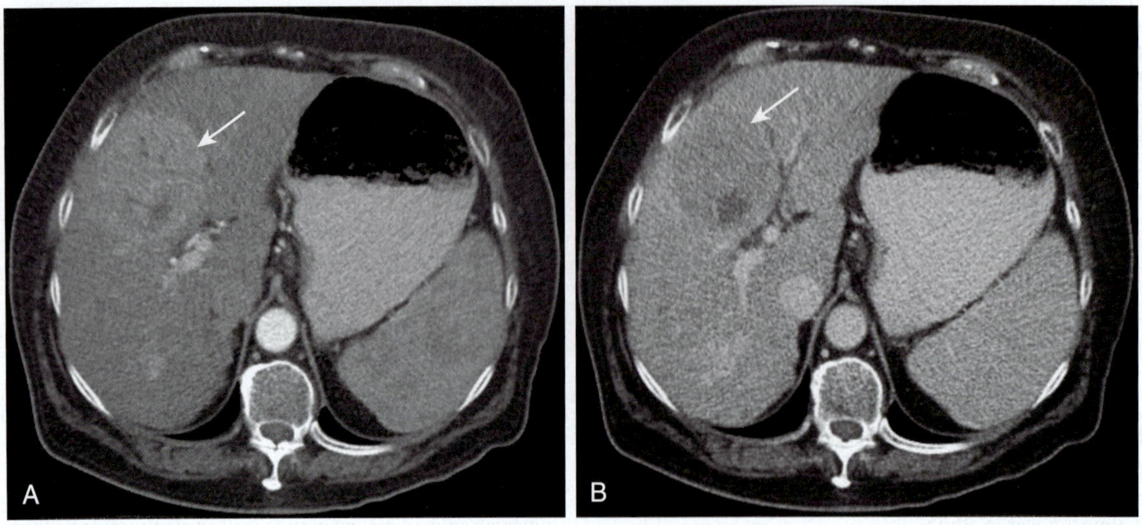

FIGURE 181-4. **Imaging of hepatocellular carcinoma.** In this contrast-enhanced computed tomography scan of the liver of a patient with hepatocellular carcinoma, a tumor in the right hepatic lobe demonstrates arterial phase enhancement (*arrow*, **A**) followed by "wash-out" in the portal venous phase (*arrow*, **B**). The bright arterial enhancement of hepatocellular carcinoma lesions on contrast-enhanced imaging studies is due to the propensity of this tumor to parasitize blood supply from the hepatic artery, whereas the normal hepatic parenchyma derives the majority of its blood supply from the portal vein.

context.[11] For the diagnostic evaluation of liver tumors, either magnetic resonance imaging (MRI) or computed tomography (CT) with multiple phases of contrast administration (including arterial, portal venous, and delayed phases) is recommended. In patients with risk factors for hepatocellular carcinoma (see E-Table 181-2), a nodule of at least 1 cm featuring arterial phase enhancement with decreased enhancement during the portal venous phase of contrast (known as "washout") is sufficient for a radiographic diagnosis (Fig. 181-4A and B).

A biopsy is warranted to confirm the diagnosis of hepatocellular carcinoma if diagnostic imaging criteria are not met. Because of the rare risk of seeding tumor along the needle track, biopsy should be performed at an expert center. When the first biopsy is inconclusive in patients whose liver nodules were found during the follow-up for chronic liver disease (e.g., fibrosis or no definitive focal lesion), a second biopsy of a suspicious lesion is indicated because its yield is as high as for the first biopsy.[12] An elevated AFP level is not sufficiently sensitive or specific for the diagnosis of hepatocellular carcinoma in cirrhotic patients with a liver mass.

Once a patient has been radiographically and/or pathologically diagnosed with hepatocellular carcinoma, the staging for extent of disease requires cross-sectional imaging of the chest, abdomen, and pelvis; an AFP measurement; and a bone scan if symptoms or signs of bone metastases (such as bone pain or markedly elevated alkaline phosphatase value) are present. Staging of hepatocellular carcinoma also requires a thorough assessment of underlying liver function, which affects prognosis and treatment options independent of the extent of the tumor.

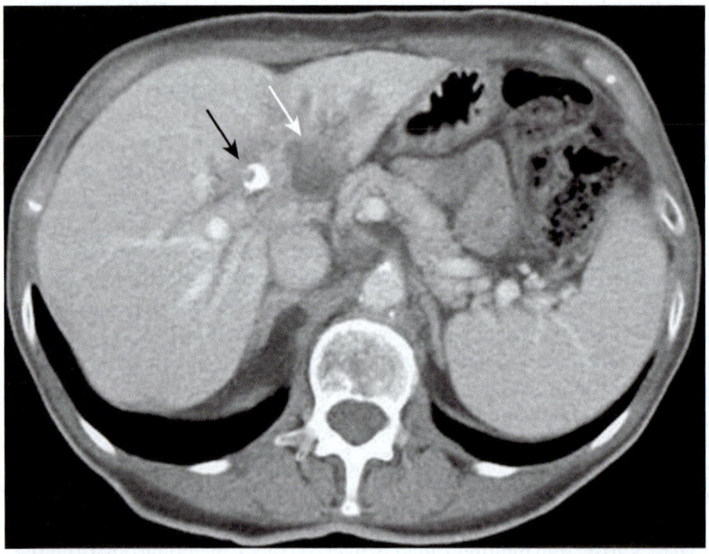

FIGURE 181-5. **Imaging of cholangiocarcinoma.** This computerized tomography image with contrast in portal venous phase depicts an infiltrative hilar cholangiocarcinoma (Klatskin tumor) extending into the left hepatic lobe (*white arrow*) with an endobiliary stent in place (*black arrow*).

Biliary Tract Cancers

For the diagnosis of biliary tract cancers, endoluminal approaches, such as by endoscopic retrograde cholangiopancreatography (ERCP) cytologic brushing or endoscopic ultrasound fine-needle aspiration, are preferred in patients whose early-stage disease may be amenable to curative surgery or transplantation. Cholangiography (by ERCP or magnetic resonance cholangiogram) may be indicated for both diagnostic and therapeutic purposes (such as stent placement), particularly if biliary obstruction is present. Staging of biliary tract and other rarer types of liver cancer generally includes cross-sectional imaging of the chest, abdomen, and pelvis. A mass in the gallbladder fossa suggests primary gallbladder cancer. Unlike hepatocellular carcinoma, cholangiocarcinomas characteristically display progressive enhancement during the portal venous phase of contrast imaging (Fig. 181-5). Biliary obstruction and ipsilateral hepatic lobe atrophy and contralateral hypertrophy may be present and can sometimes obscure identification of the actual tumor mass.

For biliary tract cancers, CA-19-9 and carcinoembryonic antigen (CEA) tumor markers may be elevated and can help to monitor response to treatment, although levels can be confounded if biliary obstruction and hyperbilirubinemia are present. Upper and lower endoscopy are indicated to exclude metastatic disease in patients who are diagnosed with likely intrahepatic cholangiocarcinoma, which otherwise can be difficult to discriminate from metastatic disease radiographically and histologically. Diagnostic laparoscopy should be considered to exclude peritoneal disease before undertaking a laparotomy for curative resection in patients with newly diagnosed gallbladder adenocarcinoma and cholangiocarcinoma because imaging may not detect peritoneal metastases, which would affect surgical decision making.

TREATMENT

General Considerations

The treatment of patients with hepatobiliary cancers requires management of underlying liver disease or obstruction as well as the tumor itself. In patients with active hepatitis B virus infection or prior exposure, close monitoring of liver function and viral load is advisable; antiviral therapy (Chapter 135) may be required to prevent reactivation, which can occur with immunosuppressive therapy (Chapter 29). Management of liver tumors in patients with cirrhosis may necessitate treatment for complications of portal hypertension or liver dysfunction (Chapter 139). In patients with biliary tract cancers, biliary obstruction (Chapter 141) is a common complication that often requires endoscopic stent placement, percutaneous drainage, or antibiotic therapy if cholangitis develops. The doses of chemotherapy agents and of medications used for supportive care may require adjustment depending on the degree of liver dysfunction.

Hepatocellular Carcinoma

Surgery and Ablation

The treatment of early stages of hepatocellular carcinoma depends on the degree of liver dysfunction.[13] In patients who have localized hepatocellular carcinoma and preserved liver function without significant portal hypertension, surgical resection can be curative, with 5-year survival rates of approximately 60 to 80% in carefully selected patients. Among patients who have increasing degrees of portal hypertension, however, surgical outcomes are significantly poorer. For individuals with contraindications to surgery or inadequate projected future function of the liver remnant, ablation of small tumors (by radiofrequency, microwaves, or ethanol injection) can provide long-term control and is sometimes curative. Adjuvant systemic therapy does not improve outcomes after surgery or ablation for hepatocellular carcinoma.

If patients have one lesion 5 cm or smaller or up to three lesions 3 cm or smaller each without any evidence of vascular involvement or extrahepatic spread, and are not candidates for resection because of the tumor's location or inadequate hepatic reserve, orthotopic liver transplantation (Chapter 140) can provide long-term survival similar to that of patients undergoing transplantation for cirrhosis without cancer. Patients who have larger tumors may be accepted for transplantation at selected centers, often accompanied by liver-directed treatments such as embolization or ablation to control the tumor burden while awaiting transplant.

Embolization

When the hepatocellular carcinoma tumor burden exceeds criteria for transplantation or surgery but remains limited to the liver, liver-directed therapies can delay progression and prolong survival but are not likely to be curative. Transarterial chemoembolization, which delivers embolic material usually mixed with chemotherapeutic agents[A1] via arterial catheters directly to vascular tumors within the liver (Fig. 181-6), can prolong survival in patients who have intermediate-stage hepatocellular carcinoma. Radioembolization using yttrium-90 bound to glass or resin microspheres is another option.

Systemic Therapy for Advanced Disease

For patients with more advanced stage hepatocellular carcinoma, conventional cytotoxic chemotherapy agents do not improve survival. The combination of atezolizumab (a programmed death [PD]-L1 immune checkpoint inhibitor) and bevacizumab (a VEGF inhibitor) under expert supervision significantly improves progression-free survival, overall survival, and quality of life compared with sorafenib,[A2] which was the prior standard of care. As a result, it has become the standard of care for advanced hepatocellular carcinoma in patients with Child-Turcotte-Pugh A liver function (see Table 139-2).[14] Sorafenib also can significantly prolong survival, but tumors shrink in fewer than 5% of patients. Lenvatinib (a multikinase inhibitor that targets VEGFR and fibroblast growth factor receptors) is not inferior to sorafenib.[A3] The addition of other targeted therapies or chemotherapy to sorafenib has not improved outcomes over sorafenib monotherapy.

After progression on first-line therapy, the multikinase inhibitors regorafenib and cabozantinib improve survival compared with placebo.[A4,A5] The vascular endothelial growth factor receptor 2 inhibitor, ramucirumab, alco can improve survival in patients who have an elevated alpha-fetoprotein tumor marker greater than 400 ng/mL.[A6]

Monotherapy with either pembrolizumab and nivolumab can provide a durable objective tumor response in 15 to 20% of patients but has not improved overall survival.[15] The combination of nivolumab plus the ipilimumab can achieve objective responses in over 30% of patients,[16] but its impact on survival has not been established.

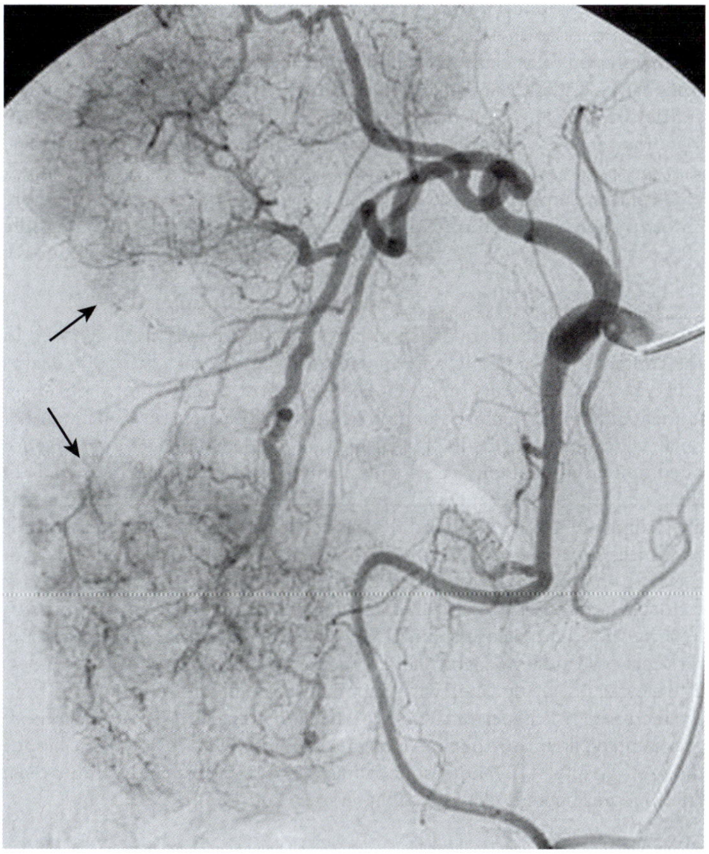

FIGURE 181-6. Transarterial chemoembolization of hepatocellular carcinoma. This common hepatic artery angiogram from a 42-year-old woman with hepatitis B shows two distinct areas of "tumor blush" corresponding to underlying hepatocellular carcinoma lesions (*arrows*) that were treated by transarterial chemoembolization. (Courtesy Dr. Nicholas Fidelman, Department of Interventional Radiology, University of California, San Francisco.)

Biliary Tract Cancers

Surgery

Surgical resection is the definitive therapy for patients with localized biliary tract cancers,[17,18] including gallbladder cancer.[19] For patients with distal cholangiocarcinoma, a Whipple pancreaticoduodenectomy may be required. Liver transplantation for early-stage hilar cholangiocarcinoma after neoadjuvant chemotherapy and/or chemoradiation may be an option at certain centers in highly selected patients.

For gallbladder cancer, cholecystectomy with en bloc hepatic resection and porta hepatis lymphadenectomy is recommended for patients with a gallbladder mass identified preoperatively on imaging or intraoperatively. A staging laparoscopy may be performed in advance to exclude occult peritoneal carcinomatosis. For patients with early-stage gallbladder cancer diagnosed incidentally on review of surgical pathologic findings after a cholecystectomy performed for benign causes, patients with tumors invading no deeper than the lamina propria (T1a) and negative surgical margins may be treated with observation only. If tumor invasion extends to the muscular layer (T1b) or beyond, patients should be referred to a specialized center for consideration of additional hepatic resection and lymphadenectomy.

Other Therapies

For patients with cholangiocarcinoma and gallbladder cancers, adjuvant chemotherapy, radiation, or chemoradiation can improve survival rates after surgical resection.[20] For example, the addition of adjuvant capecitabine for 6 months significantly prolongs overall survival and recurrence-free survival following resection of cholangiocarcinoma or gallbladder cancer and has become a standard adjuvant option.[A7]

In patients with advanced biliary tract cancers not amenable to resection, the addition of the immune checkpoint inhibitor durvalumab to combination chemotherapy (gemcitabine plus cisplatin) improves survival compared with chemotherapy alone.[A8] After progression on gemcitabine plus cisplatin chemotherapy, the combination of 5-fluorouracil plus oxaliplatin (FOLFOX) can improve survival compared with supportive care.[A9] Genomically targeted therapies, including *IDH1* and *FGFR2* inhibitors, have shown benefit for mutation-defined subsets. For example, the IDH1 inhibitor ivosidenib improves progression-free survival in patients whose cholangiocarcinomas harbor *IDH1* mutations.[A10] The FGFR inhibitors pemigatinib and infigratinib can provide durable responses in patients whose cholangiocarcinomas are positive for *FGRF2* fusion.[21] For the rare subset of patients whose cholangiocarcinomas are mismatch repair (MMR) pathway–deficient, pembrolizumab can provide durable responses and prolongs survival.[22]

End-of-Life Care

Palliative care and end-of-life care (Chapter 3) play an integral role in management of patients who have primary hepatobiliary cancers because most patients progress and succumb to their cancer or to complications within a relatively short period of time. Palliative care specialists and social workers provide important ancillary services in the end-of-life care for patients with hepatobiliary cancers. Referral to hospice care (Chapter 3) may be appropriate when patients have progressed on standard anticancer therapies and/or are ineligible for further anticancer therapy because of extent of disease, liver dysfunction, poor performance status, or patient preferences.

As with most advanced cancers, pain control (Chapter 26), treatment of nausea (see Table 118-5) and constipation (see Table 122-3), and family and social support are essential. Pain management in patients with prior or active substance abuse disorder (Chapter 365) may be complicated by tolerance and/or dependency. In some cases, patients and caregivers may require providers' reassurance before using opiates or other analgesics for pain control because of concerns about addiction. Bone metastases may require palliative radiation or stabilization procedures. Patients with advanced stages of hepatobiliary cancers, particularly hepatocellular carcinoma, are also at risk for developing complications of end-stage liver disease, such as intractable ascites, jaundice, pruritus, encephalopathy, infections, and gastrointestinal bleeding (Chapter 121). Diuretic therapy, therapeutic paracentesis, and endoscopic management of gastrointestinal bleeding may be required. In biliary tract cancers, biliary obstruction and recurrent cholangitis also may require endoscopic or percutaneous biliary drainage (Chapter 141)[23] and antibiotic therapy for palliation.

In the United States, hepatocellular carcinoma is associated with a high incidence of health disparities (Chapter 4) related to immigrant status, being a member of racial or ethnic minority, and lower socioeconomic status. Clinicians must have an awareness of cross-cultural issues surrounding disclosure of diagnosis, pain control, use of alternative therapies, and end-of-life care.

PREVENTION

Screening and surveillance for hepatocellular carcinoma is associated with improved outcomes in selected populations with cirrhosis,[24] but routine screening and surveillance remains controversial even for high-risk populations. Hepatitis B virus vaccination and treatment programs (Chapters 134 and 135) can reduce the incidence of hepatocellular carcinoma. Treatment of chronic hepatitis C infection my reduce the risk of hepatocellular cancer by about one-third, but the risk still appears to be perhaps 20-fold higher than in the general population. Prevention and treatment of alcohol-related disorders, obesity, and other conditions associated with nonalcoholic fatty liver disease are appropriate measures to mitigate risk factors and to minimize ongoing liver injury, but prospective evidence regarding any reduction in the risk of cancer is limited. Some data suggest that low-dose aspirin can significantly lower the risk of hepatocellular carcinoma and liver-related mortality in patients with chronic viral hepatitis.[25]

Limited evidence to support preventive measures or screening for biliary tract cancers. Patients who have primary sclerosing cholangitis (Chapter 141) are at increased risk for cholangiocarcinoma. Periodic screening by noninvasive imaging and serum CA-19-9 marker measurements may be considered, but supporting data are limited.

PROGNOSIS

The prognosis of patients with hepatocellular carcinoma and biliary tract cancers is generally poor. For patients with hepatocellular carcinoma or intrahepatic cholangiocarcinoma, the overall 5-year survival rate across stages is approximately 20%. Hepatocellular carcinomas associated with steatohepatitis and alcoholic liver disease have a similar clinical course, even though the characteristic features underlying these two diseases are different.

For the minority of patients whose hepatocellular carcinomas or intrahepatic cholangiocarcinomas are diagnosed at a localized stage of disease, the 5-year relative survival rate approaches 30%, but 5-year cause-specific survival rates generally approximate or exceed 60% when patients with early stages of disease undergo curative ablation, surgery, or transplantation. For patients who are diagnosed with metastatic hepatocellular carcinoma or cholangiocarcinoma, the 5-year survival rate is less than 5%, and the median overall survival is less than 1 year.

For patients with gallbladder adenocarcinoma, the overall 5-year survival rate ranges from approximately 50% for patients who have stage I tumors to less than 5% for patients who have metastatic disease. The rate of metastatic recurrence is high even among patients who have resectable gallbladder carcinoma. The prognosis of patients with rarer types of primary liver cancers such as fibrolamellar hepatocellular carcinoma, hepatic endothelioid hemangioendothelioma, or hepatic angiosarcoma is highly variable.

GENERAL REFERENCES

For the General References and other additional features, please visit Elsevier eBooks+ at https://ebooks.health.elsevier.com.

Grade A References

A1. Yang B, Liang J, Qu Z, et al. Transarterial strategies for the treatment of unresectable hepatocellular carcinoma: a systematic review. *PloS One.* 2020;15:e0227475.

A2. Finn RS, Qin S, Ikeda M, et al. Atezolizumab plus bevacizumab in unresectable hepatocellular carcinoma. *N Engl J Med.* 2020;382:1894-1905.

A3. Kudo M, Finn RS, Qin S, et al. Lenvatinib versus sorafenib in first-line treatment of patients with unresectable hepatocellular carcinoma: a randomised phase 3 non-inferiority trial. *Lancet.* 2018;391:1163-1173.

A4. Bruix J, Qin S, Merle P, et al. Regorafenib for patients with hepatocellular carcinoma who progressed on sorafenib treatment (RESORCE): a randomised, double-blind, placebo-controlled, phase 3 trial. *Lancet.* 2017;389:56-66.

A5. Abou-Alfa GK, Meyer T, Cheng AL, et al. Cabozantinib in patients with advanced and progressing hepatocellular carcinoma. *N Engl J Med.* 2018;379:54-63.

A6. Zhu AX, Finn RS, Galle PR, et al. Ramucirumab in advanced hepatocellular carcinoma in REACH-2: the true value of α-fetoprotein. *Lancet Oncol.* 2019;20:e191.

A7. Primrose JN, Fox RP, Palmer DH, et al. Capecitabine compared with observation in resected biliary tract cancer (BILCAP): a randomised, controlled, multicentre, phase 3 study. *Lancet Oncol.* 2019;20:663-673.

A8. Oh D-Y, Ruth He A, Qin S, et al. Durvalumab plus gemcitabine and cisplatin in advanced biliary tract cancer. *NEJM Evidence.* 2022;1:EVIDoa2200015.

A9. Lamarca A, Palmer DH, Wasan HS, et al. Second-line FOLFOX chemotherapy versus active symptom control for advanced biliary tract cancer (ABC-06): a phase 3, open-label, randomised, controlled trial. *Lancet Oncol.* 2021;22:690-701.

A10. Zhu AX, Macarulla T, Javle MM, et al. Final overall survival efficacy results of ivosidenib for patients with advanced cholangiocarcinoma with IDH1 mutation: the phase 3 randomized clinical ClarIDHy trial. *JAMA Oncol.* 2021;7:1669-1677.

182

TUMORS OF THE KIDNEY, BLADDER, URETERS, AND RENAL PELVIS

DEAN F. BAJORIN

RENAL CELL CARCINOMA

DEFINITION

Cancers of the kidney are a heterogeneous group of neoplasms, the majority of which are of epithelial origin and malignant. Renal cell carcinoma, classically referred to as clear cell carcinoma or hypernephroma, is not a single malignancy. Rather, renal cell carcinoma comprises a group of distinguishable entities (Table 182-1), each with a strong relationship between its morphologic and genetic features.[1] The metastatic potential depends on the histologic subtype and ranges from the most virulent conventional clear cell carcinomas (65% of total tumors but accounting for 90% of the metastases), to the more indolent papillary and chromophobe carcinomas (25% of the total but only 10% of the metastases), and to the benign oncocytomas (10% of all tumors).

EPIDEMIOLOGY

Over 75,000 new tumors of the kidney and renal pelvis are diagnosed in the United States annually, and they result in approximately 14,000 deaths each year. These cancers represent the sixth most common form of cancer in men and the ninth most common in women. The increase in incidence of renal cell cancers may be in part related to early detection as a consequence of computed tomography (CT) and magnetic resonance imaging (MRI) of the abdomen for other medical conditions. The ratio of males to females is approximately 2 : 1 to 3 : 1, and the incidence is highest in Black Americans and lowest in Asians and Pacific Islanders. The mean age at diagnosis is in the sixth to seventh decade of life. Aside from genetic predisposition, risk factors associated with renal cell carcinoma include cigarette smoking, obesity, hypertension, and the use of diuretics.[2] Obese persons have an increased risk for renal cell carcinoma, and the risk rises with increasing body mass index. The elevated risk associated with diuretic use is difficult to distinguish from the increased risk associated with hypertension. Renal cell carcinoma is more prevalent in patients with pre-existing renal injury,[3] such as polycystic kidney disease (Chapter 112), horseshoe kidney (Chapter 113), and chronic renal failure requiring hemodialysis (Chapters 116 and 117).

PATHOBIOLOGY

Renal Cell Carcinoma

Clear cell renal cell carcinoma constitutes approximately 65% of renal tumors (Table 182-2) and is believed to be derived from the proximal convoluted tubule. It is generally solitary and well circumscribed, with a golden yellow color that results from the abundant cytoplasmic lipid. Higher-grade tumors

TABLE 182-1 CLASSIFICATION OF RENAL CELL TUMORS ACCORDING TO THE 2016 WHO CLASSIFICATION

CURRENT RENAL CELL TUMOR SUBTYPES
Clear cell (conventional) renal cell carcinoma* (65-70%)
Papillary (chromophil) renal cell carcinoma* (15-20%)
Chromophobe renal cell carcinoma* (5-7%)
Collecting duct carcinoma*
Renal medullary carcinoma*
Mucinous tubular and spindle cell carcinoma*
RCC, unclassified*
Oncocytoma
Papillary (chromophil) adenoma
NEW RENAL CELL TUMOR SUBTYPES
Multilocular cystic renal neoplasm of low malignant potential
Mi T family translocation renal cell carcinoma*
Tubulocystic renal cell carcinoma*
Acquired cystic disease–associated renal cell carcinoma*
Clear cell papillary renal cell carcinoma*
Succinate dehydrogenase–deficient renal cell carcinoma*
Hereditary leiomyomatosis and associated renal cell carcinoma*

*Malignant.

Tumor subtypes comprising the percentages of all renal cell carcinomas (in parentheses), respectively.

Mi T = microphthalmia transcription factor; WHO = World Health Organization.

Adapted from Inamura K. Renal cell tumors: understanding their molecular pathological epidemiology and the 2016 WHO classification. *Int J Mol Sci.* 2017;18:2195. The revised 2016 WHO classification added the new tumor subtypes to the 2013 International Society of Urological Pathology (ISUP) Vancouver Classification of Renal Neoplasia (Srigley JR, Delahunt B, Eble JN, et al. *Am J Surg Pathol.* 2013;37:1469-1489).

TABLE 182-2 HISTOLOGIC SUBTYPES, GENETICS, AND SYNDROMES

HISTOLOGIC SUBTYPE	PERCENT	MAJOR GENETIC/ MOLECULAR DEFECTS	ASSOCIATED SYNDROMES
Conventional clear cell	75	LOH 3p mutation of 3p26 (*VHL*)	Von Hippel-Lindau hereditary renal cell carcinoma (RCC)
Papillary 1	5	*MET* gene mutation 7q34	Hereditary papillary renal cell carcinoma (HPRCC)
Papillary 2	10	Fumarate hydratase (*FH*)1q42.1	Hereditary leiomyomatosis renal cell carcinoma (HLRCC)
Chromophobe	5	Birt-Hogg Dubé 17p11.2 (*FLCN*)	Birt-Hogg Dubé
Oncocytoma	9.7	Birt-Hogg Dubé 17p11.2 (*FLCN*)	Familial oncocytoma Birt-Hogg Dubé
Collecting duct	0.4	−18, −Y	Renal medullary carcinoma

Modified from Zambrano N. Histopathology and molecular genetics of renal tumors. *J Urol.* 1999;162:1246-1258.

contain less lipid and glycogen. Approximately 50% of the tumors exhibit either a solid or acinar growth pattern that is characterized by solid sheets of tumor cells accompanied by a rich capillary vascular network.

Clear cell renal cell carcinoma is characterized by the loss of genetic material from the short arm of chromosome 3 (3p) and mutations in the von Hippel-Lindau (*VHL*) gene.[4] In patients with von Hippel-Lindau disease (Chapter 385), these losses and mutations occur in virtually all cases. The more common sporadic tumors also have somatic mutations and hypermethylation in the same region in approximately 75 to 80% of cases. Conventional clear cell tumors have a mutation in the *VHL* gene, which is inactivated by a point mutation or by epigenetic gene silencing by promoter methylation. The loss of *VHL*, which is responsible for ubiquination and degradation of the hypoxia-inducible factor (HIF), leads to upregulation of HIF-responsive genes responsible for angiogenesis and cell growth. Two of these upregulated genes are platelet-derived growth factor (PDGF) and vascular endothelial growth factor (VEGF), which are pro-angiogenic proteins that are thought to induce the neovascularity in both primary and metastatic clear cell cancers. Patients with von Hippel-Lindau disease more commonly develop tumors at an earlier age and frequently have multiple tumors. Other tumors associated with the syndrome include central nervous system hemangioblastomas, pancreatic neuroendocrine tumors, pheochromocytomas, retinal angiomas, and epididymal cystadenomas (Chapter 385). Molecular characterization of renal cell carcinoma shows alterations in genes responsible for maintenance of chromatin states such as *PBRM1*, the SWI/SNF chromatin remodeling complex including *ARID1A* and *SMARCA4*, and members of the P13K/AKT pathway.

Papillary Renal Cell Carcinomas

Papillary renal cell carcinomas comprise from 7 to 14% of primary epithelial renal neoplasms. The majority of patients present with unilateral tumors. Multifocality, either bilateral or multifocal lesions in the same kidney, is present in approximately 45% of cases. The majority of these tumors exhibit a broad morphologic spectrum, including papillary, papillary-trabecular, and papillary-solid areas; associated necrosis is a common finding. The classic papillary pattern is characterized by discrete papillary fronds lined by neoplastic epithelial cells and containing a central fibrovascular core, easily recognized on low magnification.

The majority of sporadic papillary renal cell carcinomas are characterized by trisomy of chromosomes 7 and 17 and loss of chromosome Y. Chromophobe renal cell cancers have genetic loss on chromosomes 1 and Y, as well as combined chromosomal losses affecting chromosomes 1, 6, 10, 13, 17, and 21. Hereditary papillary renal cell cancer is a result of germline mutations and activation of the *MET* proto-oncogene, which is located on chromosome 7q. These cells have aberrant hepatocyte growth factor receptors that are unable to deactivate after binding by the growth factor. Somatic *MET* gene amplifications also are observed in approximately 10% of cases of sporadic papillary renal cancer.[5]

These tumors are divided into type 1 and type 2 lesions, based on cytologic features and genetic differences. Comprehensive molecular characterization shows that type 1 and type 2 papillary renal cell carcinomas are clinically and biologically distinct.

Chromophobe Renal Cell Cancer

Chromophobe renal cancers account for 6 to 11% of renal epithelial tumors. Characteristically, these tumors are solitary and discrete but not encapsulated. The typical histologic findings consist of large round-to-polygonal cells with well-defined cell borders and pale basophilic cytoplasm admixed with a smaller population of polygonal cells with eosinophilic cytoplasm. These tumors may be quite large at diagnosis, with resectable tumors reported as big as 23 cm.

Other Renal Tumors

Hereditary leiomyomatosis renal cell carcinoma, which is characterized by alteration of the gene fumarate hydratase, is associated with uterine leiomyomas (more common) or leiomyosarcoma (rare), cutaneous nodules (leiomyomas), and type 2 papillary renal cell carcinoma, which is often solitary and frequently develops metastases. Birt-Hogg-Dubé syndrome is a rare disorder predominantly associated with chromophobe renal cancers but in which clear cell and chromophobe/oncocytic tumors can develop. Birt-Hogg-Dubé syndrome is characterized by fibrofolliculomas, pulmonary cysts, pneumothorax, and bilateral renal tumors. The gene associated with Birt-Hogg-Dubé syndrome has been mapped to 17p and expresses a novel protein, folliculin, whose function is not yet fully characterized.

CLINICAL MANIFESTATIONS

The majority of patients are asymptomatic at presentation, with about 50% of tumors detected by an abdominal ultrasound, a CT scan, or an MRI obtained for unrelated medical reasons. The next most common presentation is with asymptomatic hematuria, often microscopic. The classic presenting triad of hematuria, a palpable mass, and pain is now unusual, and less than 5% of patients have a palpable mass at presentation. The more common manifesting symptoms are anemia, weight loss, malaise, and anorexia (Table 182-3). Patients who present with renal cell carcinoma frequently have associated paraneoplastic syndromes (Chapter 164).[6] Hypercalcemia (Chapter 227) is observed in approximately 20% of patients and can be due to the secretion of parathyroid hormone, parathyroid hormone–like peptide, and interleukin-6 (IL-6), which stimulate osteoclastic bone resorption. Other associated syndromes include hypertension, erythrocytosis (from ectopic erythropoietin production), and the rare Stauffer syndrome, which is liver dysfunction without hepatic metastases and which resolves after surgical resection of the tumor.

TABLE 182-3 PRESENTING SYMPTOMS AND SIGNS OF RENAL CELL CARCINOMA (BOTH LOCALIZED AND METASTATIC DISEASE)

SYMPTOMS AND SIGNS	PERCENT
Anemia	52
Hepatic dysfunction	32
Weight loss	23
Hypoalbuminemia	20
Malaise	19
Hypercalcemia	13
Anorexia	11
Thrombocytosis	9
Night sweats	8
Fever	8
Hypertension	3
Erythrocytosis	4
Chills	3

Modified from Kim HI, Belldegrun AS, Freitas DG, et al. Paraneoplastic signs and symptoms of renal cell carcinoma: implications for prognosis. *J Urol*. 2003;170:1742-1746.

TABLE 182-4 TNM STAGING OF RENAL CELL CARCINOMA

TUMOR, NODE, AND METASTASIS CLINICAL CLASSIFICATION	
T—Primary Tumor	
TX	Primary tumor cannot be assessed
T0	No evidence of primary tumor
T1	Tumor 7 cm or less in greatest dimension, limited to the kidney
T1a	Tumor 4.0 cm or less in greatest dimension, limited to the kidney
T1b	Tumor more than 4 cm but not more than 7 cm in greatest dimension, limited to the kidney
T2	Tumor more than 7 cm in greatest dimension, limited to the kidney
T2a	Tumor more than 7 cm but less than or equal to 10 cm in greatest dimension, limited to the kidney
T2b	Tumor more than 10 cm, limited to the kidney
T3	Tumor extends into major veins or the perinephric tissues or into the ipsilateral adrenal gland and but not beyond the Gerota fascia
T3a	Tumor extends into renal vein or its segmental branches or pelvicalyceal system, or invades perirenal and/or renal sinus fat but not beyond the Gerota fascia
T3b	Tumor extends into the vena cava below the diaphragm
T3c	Tumor extends into the vena cava above the diaphragm or invades the wall of the vena cava
T4	Tumor invades beyond the Gerota fascia (including contiguous extension into the ipsilateral adrenal gland)
N—Regional Lymph Nodes	
NX	Regional lymph nodes cannot be assessed
N0	No regional lymph node metastasis
N1	Metastasis in regional lymph node(s)
M—Distant Metastasis	
Mx	Distant metastasis cannot be assessed
M0	No distant metastasis
M1	Distant metastasis
STAGE GROUPING	
Stage I	T1 N0 M0
Stage II	T2 N0 M0
Stage III	T1 N1 M0
	T2 N1 M0
	T3a N0 or N1 M0
	T3b N0 or N1 M0
	T3c N0 or N1 M0
Stage IV	T4 N0 M0
	T4 N1 M0
	Any T Any N M1

AJCC = American Joint Committee on Cancer.
Adapted from *AJCC Staging Manual*, 8th ed. New York: Springer International Publishing; 2017.

DIAGNOSIS

Ultrasonography, CT, and MRI can help distinguish benign from malignant lesions. Ultrasound can distinguish small simple cysts from solid lesions. For other renal cystic lesions, CT or MRI can define three categories: likely benign lesions that require no follow-up; lesions that are usually benign (generally smooth wall of no more than 3 mm with enhancing septa) but require repeat imaging at 6 months, 12 months, and then annually for 5 years; or thicker-walled or irregularly enhancing lesions that require biopsy.

CT is the most reliable method for evaluating solid lesions.[7] The preferred CT scan for renal masses can be divided into four phases, including the precontrast images, the arterial phase (~25 seconds after injection), the nephrographic phase (~90 seconds into the injection), and the excretory phase. The most important phases for imaging renal tumors are the precontrast and nephrographic images because renal lesions appear low in density in contrast to the uniformly enhanced renal parenchyma. The arterial phase is helpful for identifying renal arteries and small hypervascular masses. The excretory phase aids in assessing the collecting system and the renal pelvis. Lack of enhancement is consistent with a hemorrhagic or inflammatory cyst that can mimic a solid lesion. Macroscopic fat in a solid renal mass suggests an angiomyolipoma.

The complete evaluation for patients with suspected renal cell carcinoma should include a complete blood count, a chemistry profile, and a CT scan of the chest, abdomen, and pelvis. CT scan is also helpful for detecting regional metastases and for indicating when partial nephrectomy is feasible. MRI is useful for imaging tumors in patients who have poor renal function and in whom intravenous contrast may be contraindicated. MRI is also helpful for delineating any thrombi that may be extending into the renal vein or inferior vena cava, and magnetic resonance angiography can determine the number and location of renal arteries in patients who are candidates for partial nephrectomy. Once the evaluation is complete, the clinical stage is assessed using the Tumor, Node, Metastasis (TNM) system (Table 182-4). A bone scan is indicated for patients with clinically advanced disease, hypercalcemia, bone pain, and/or an elevated alkaline phosphatase level.

TREATMENT

Renal Cell Carcinoma

Localized Disease

The increasing prevalence of small tumors discovered incidentally on imaging has resulted in a marked increase in the use of partial nephrectomy rather than complete nephrectomy. For tumors of 7 cm or less, partial nephrectomy by the open or minimally invasive laparoscopic technique provides local tumor control and survival similar to radical nephrectomy. Partial nephrectomy preserves some renal function and reduces the risk for renal insufficiency over time. Partial nephrectomy is further supported by the fact that approximately 35% of renal cortical tumors are indolent papillary or chromophobe carcinomas.

Radical nephrectomy is generally preferred for large and centrally localized tumors that have effectively replaced the majority of the normal renal parenchyma, tumors associated with regional adenopathy (of benign or malignant etiology), tumors that extend into the inferior vena cava or right atrial vein, and even when metastatic disease is evident.[8] Radical nephrectomy can be performed laparoscopically or by an open technique through a flank, transperitoneal, or transthoracic approach. The ipsilateral adrenal gland is also removed, but a regional lymph node dissection is optional and controversial.

Renal cell carcinomas are resistant to both radiation therapy and cytotoxic chemotherapy, so neither modality is useful for adjuvant therapy after nephrectomy. However, sunitinib (a tyrosine kinase inhibitor that targets vascular endothelial growth factor [VEGF])[A1] and pembrolizumab (an antibody that inhibits programmed death-1 [PD-1] receptors)[A2] under expert oversight are effective as adjunctive treatment in patients at high risk for recurrence after nephrectomy.

Metastatic Disease

Surgery

Approximately 30% of patients with renal cell carcinoma present with metastatic disease, usually with pain from either an unresectable primary tumor or skeletal metastases, and an additional 20 to 30% of patients with surgically resected primary tumors will relapse with metastases.[9] Radiation therapy is frequently used for palliation of bone metastases and for patients with multiple brain metastases. Palliative nephrectomy is sometimes used to provide symptomatic relief of pain. In other patients, surgical resection of the primary tumor can be considered, even in the presence of metastatic disease,[A3] but this approach is now less common with the advent of more effective systemic therapies. However, resection of metastatic sites of disease (metastasectomy) may extend survival in selected patients and may even cure a subset of patients.[10] The patients most likely to benefit from surgical resection of metastatic disease have a disease-free interval of greater than 1 year after nephrectomy, a solitary site of metastasis, and lung metastases.

Medications

Current consensus recommendations[11] are to use anti–PD-1 antibodies (nivolumab, pembrolizumab, or avelumab) in combination with either tyrosine kinase inhibitor therapy (e.g., axitinib, cabozantinib, lenvatinib, and sorafenib) or anti-CTLA antibodies (e.g., ipilumimab) under expert supervision for first-line treatment of metastatic clear cell carcinoma. Nivolumab in combination with either cabozantinib[A4] or ipilumimab[A5] provides significantly better progression-free and overall survival compared with sunitinib monotherapy, except perhaps for patients who have favorable risk factors. Pembrolizumab in combination with a tyrosine kinase inhibitor, either lenvatinib[A6] or axitinib,[A7,A8] is also superior to sunitinib monotherapy in terms of both progression-free and overall survival. Pembrolizumab plus either axitinib or lenvatinib is recommended in all patients irrespective of risk, whereas nivolumab plus ipilumimb is recommended in patients with intermediate and poor risk features. Common side effects with tyrosine kinase inhibitors include fatigue, diarrhea, hypertension, and hand-foot syndrome (a condition in which blisters appear at sites of physical contact).

Two drugs targeting the mammalian target of rapamycin (mTOR) pathway, everolimus and temsirolimus, are effective for the treatment of renal cell carcinoma. Everolimus, an oral mTOR inhibitor, is used most frequently based on clinical benefit in patients who have been previously treated with sunitinib or sorafenib. Belzutifan (a small molecule inhibitor of hypoxia-inducible factor-2) is useful for patients who have cancers associated with *VHL* mutations. Side effects include anemia, hypoxia, fatigue, increased glucose, headache, and nausea; both the anemia and the hypoxia can be severe.

Non–Clear Cell Cancer

For non–clear cell renal carcinoma, evidence supports sunitinib under expert supervision as the recommended treatment.[A9] Cabozantinib, as a single agent or in combination with immune therapy, is another potential agent.

PREVENTION

No interventions are proven to prevent renal cancers. However, the risk may decrease by 20 or so years after smoking cessation. Avoiding obesity also may decrease the risk. Whether controlling hypertension will reduce the risk is uncertain.

PROGNOSIS

Progression-free survival and overall survival rates for resected nonmetastatic renal cortical tumors substantially differ according to multiple factors, including age, size, grade, and pathologic state. Overall, 5-year survival rates are 90 to 95% for localized disease, 70% for disease with regional spread, and only 15% for disease with distant spread. Of the more common histologic subtypes of renal cell carcinoma, the prognosis of clear cell renal cell carcinoma is less favorable than that of papillary renal cell carcinoma; chromophobe renal cell carcinoma is the most favorable.

In patients with metastatic disease, clinical features associated with poorer natural history include low performance status, a hemoglobin concentration below 12 g/dL, an albumin-corrected calcium level above 10.2 mg/dL, an absolute neutrophil count above 7000/µL, a platelet count above 400,000/µL, and absence of prior nephrectomy. Survival directly correlates with the number of these pretreatment risk factors. For example, in patients who are treated with modern combination therapy, 85% of patients with zero risk factors survive for 30 months compared with about 70% for one risk factor, 60% for two risk factors, 40% for three risk factors, and 30% for four to six factors.[12] In patients who have solitary metastases after otherwise successful surgical therapy, long-term survival is seen after metastasectomy in the lung (up to 45%) and even in the brain (up to 20%) lesion.

BLADDER CANCER

DEFINITION

A spectrum of tumors arises from the urothelial lining of the bladder, renal pelvis, ureters, and urethra. The vast majority of tumors originate in the bladder, with a minority originating in the upper tracts (renal pelvis and ureters) and even fewer from the proximal urethra. Transitional cell carcinoma is the most common histologic type. Although transitional cell cancers possess a variable natural history, they have a proclivity for multifocality, high recurrence rates, and progression to higher pathologic stages. These tumors are generally grouped into the three broad categories of non–muscle-invasive, muscle-invasive, and metastatic disease, each of which differs in clinical behavior, prognosis, and primary management. For non–muscle-invasive tumors, the aim is to prevent recurrences and progression to a more advanced stage. In muscle-invasive disease, the medical challenge is to integrate the modalities of surgery, chemotherapy, and/or radiation to optimize cure and minimize morbidity. For metastatic disease, chemotherapy is used to palliate the symptoms of most patients, but there is a subset of patients for whom combination chemotherapy may result in long-term cure. Long-term cure is directly related to stage and grade, ranging from 99% for low-grade Ta tumors to up to 15% for metastatic disease.

EPIDEMIOLOGY

An estimated 80,000 or so new cases of bladder cancer are diagnosed in the United States annually, and approximately 17,000 patients die from this disease each year. The overall 77% 5-year survival rate for all stages results in a prevalence of more than 500,000 people living with bladder cancer in the United States. The ratio of males to females is 3:1, and bladder cancer is the fourth most common cancer in men. It is estimated that men have a 1 in 27 chance of developing this cancer in their lifetimes, whereas the risk is 1 in 89 for women. Bladder cancer is twice as prevalent in Whites as in Black Americans and is less frequently observed in Asians. The vast majority of patients (90%) are over age 50 years at diagnosis, with a median age of 73 years.

Carcinogens or their metabolites implicated in the carcinogenesis of bladder cancer are believed to be excreted in the urine, where they can act directly on the urothelial lining. The latency period from initial exposure to the development of cancer is almost 20 years, so it can be difficult to establish a definitive cause-and-effect relationship between a putative carcinogen and the development of disease. Cigarette smoking is the leading risk factor for bladder cancer and is believed to contribute to 50% of the cancers in men and 25% of the cancers in women.[13] A longer duration of exposure is associated with a higher risk than a more intense exposure (in cigarettes/day) over a shorter time period. Overall, smokers have a two-fold to four-fold higher relative risk for bladder cancer than nonsmokers. Smoking is associated with cellular atypia of the urothelium. Individuals who never smoke have atypia in only 4% of cases, whereas atypia is seen in 50% of smokers.

Polycyclic aromatic hydrocarbons such as 2-naphthylamine, 4-aminobiphenyl and benzidine, and benzene or exhausts from combustion gases are associated with an increased risk for bladder cancer. Occupations reported to be at higher risk include aluminum workers, dry cleaners, manufacturers of preservatives and polychlorinated biphenyls, and pesticide applicators. Arylamines, also implicated in carcinogenesis, are metabolically activated to electrophilic compounds by N-hydroxylation in the liver by cytochrome P-450 IA2 and detoxified by N-acetylation; studies suggest that individuals with a fast oxidizer and slow acetylator phenotype are at highest risk. Occupations associated with a higher exposure to arylamines, such as workers in the dye, rubber, or leather manufacturing industries, are believed to be at higher risk for developing bladder cancer. *Schistosoma haematobium* infection (Chapter 326) enhances formation of carcinogenic N-nitroso compounds and results in an increased risk for both squamous and transitional cell carcinomas of the bladder. An association has been observed between squamous cell carcinoma (but not transitional cell tumors) and the presence of chronic urinary tract infections seen in paraplegics and patients with chronic bladder stones and indwelling Foley catheters. The chemotherapy agent cyclophosphamide can increase the risk for bladder cancer nine-fold when used chronically, and phenacetin-containing compounds have been implicated in the development of tumors of the renal pelvis and ureters.

PATHOBIOLOGY

Urothelial tumors occur anywhere along the urinary tract, including the renal pelvis, ureters, bladder, and the urethra. Over 90% of tumors originate in the bladder, 8% in the renal pelvis, and the remaining 2% in the ureter and urethra. Transitional cell carcinomas comprise 90 to 95% of urothelial tumors; squamous cell (keratinizing) tumors (3%), adenocarcinomas (2%), and small cell tumors (1%) are the remainder. Mixed-histology tumors, consisting of predominantly transitional cell carcinoma with areas of squamous, adenocarcinomatous, or neuroendocrine elements, are frequently observed.[14] Squamous cell tumors are more frequent in the distal urethra, and adenocarcinomas occur in the embryonal remnant of the urachus on the dome of the bladder and in periurethral tissues. In endemic areas of *S. haematobium* infections (such as Egypt; Chapter 326), 40% of tumors are squamous cell carcinomas. Rare tumors of the bladder include lymphoma (Chapter 171), sarcoma (Chapter 187), and melanoma (Chapter 188).

The majority (70 to 80%) of newly detected bladder cancers are classified as non–muscle-invasive tumors and include exophytic papillary tumors confined to the mucosa (Ta), tumors invading the lamina propria (T1), and carcinoma in situ (CIS). Non–muscle-invasive bladder tumors are typically graded according to the World Health Organization/International Society of Urologic Pathology (WHO/ISUP) grading system as low grade and high grade. If the grading system is not specified, a numeric system can be used: well differentiated (G1), moderately differentiated (G2), poorly differentiated (G3), and undifferentiated (G4). Grading is more important for noninvasive Ta tumors because almost all invasive bladder tumors (T1 or greater) are high grade. Primary carcinoma in situ without a concurrent Ta or T1 tumor constitutes 1 to 2% of new bladder cancer cases. More frequently, tumor in situ is found in the presence of multiple papillary tumors, either immediately adjacent to another lesion or involving remote mucosa in the bladder. Tumor in situ is, by definition, high-grade disease. T1 tumors are an aggressive, invasive malignancy. Virtually all T1 tumors are high grade, and 50% have associated tumors in situ. Disease recurs in 50% of patients by 1 year and in 90% within 5 years. At the time of diagnosis, a minority of primary tumors invade the muscularis propria (T2), extend to perivesicular fat (T3), or extend into immediately adjacent organs (T4); all primary tumors stage T2 or higher are high grade.

Genetic predisposition may also play a role in the development of urothelial cancer. About 15% of patients have germline variants in DNA-damage repair genes (e.g., *BRCA2, BRCA1, MSH2, CHEK2, ERCC3, NBN*, and *RAD50*), and about 40% of affected patients have biallelic inactivation.[15]

Recurrences may be clonal in origin. The epidermal growth factor receptor (EGFR) is highly expressed (~80%) in bladder cancers, whereas the HER2/Neu growth factor receptor is less frequently expressed (~50 to 70%). Studies suggest that higher expression of these receptors is associated with a more advanced and/or more aggressive phenotype of disease. Bladder cancer has a very high somatic mutation rate (7.7 per megabase) compared with that of other cancers, exceeded only by lung cancer and melanoma. Epigenetic modifying genes *MLL2, ARID1A, KDM6A*, and *EP300* are significantly mutated in bladder cancer; approximately 75% have at least one inactivating mutation. Genes that regulate the cell cycle are also frequently mutated, including *TP53* in 49% and *RB1* in 13% of tumors. Mutations and/or amplifications of *FGFR, ERBB2, MDM2*, and *EGFR* occur in a minority of tumors and represent potential therapeutic targets.

CLINICAL MANIFESTATIONS

Hematuria is the manifesting symptom in 80 to 90% of bladder cancers, but patients also may present with a urinary tract infection. Urinary frequency and nocturia may be present as a consequence of either irritative symptoms or a reduced bladder capacity. Pain, when present, typically reflects the location of the bladder tumor. Lower abdominal pain may occur as a result of a bladder mass, and rectal discomfort and perineal pain can result from tumors that invade the prostate or pelvis. Tumors of the renal pelvis, ureter, or bladder in which the ureteral orifice is obstructed can cause hydronephrosis, reduced renal function, and flank pain. Patients with more advanced disease can present with anorexia, fatigue, weight loss, or pain from a metastatic bone lesion. The physical examination is frequently unremarkable in patients who present with bladder tumors because the vast majority of patients have organ-confined tumors.

DIAGNOSIS

Individuals over age 40 years who develop hematuria should have an evaluation for the presence of urothelial cancer (Fig. 100-3), including urinary cytology, cystoscopy, and imaging of the urinary tract by either an ultrasound or CT scan. Urinary biomarkers currently are neither sufficiently sensitive nor specific for the diagnosis of bladder cancer,[16] and a small proportion of cases can be missed even if biomarkers are combined with urinary cytology.

The mainstay of diagnosis and staging is the cystoscopic evaluation under anesthesia to determine if a palpable mass (either mobile or not) is present. A nonmobile tumor mass is indicative of disease that invades the pelvic sidewall and that is unlikely to be resectable. Urine is obtained to evaluate for the presence of malignant cells. A cystoscope is inserted to inspect the bladder and detail the size, number, location, and growth pattern (papillary or solid) of all lesions.

All visible disease undergoes transurethral resection to determine the histologic subtype and depth of invasion. Adequate evaluation, particularly in large tumors that may be invasive, requires that muscle be identified in the pathologic specimen. Repeat biopsy of the resected area is occasionally required to ensure that no muscle invasion is present, because invasion into muscle requires consideration of surgical removal of the bladder rather than endoscopic resection of the tumor. Biopsies from any areas of erythema are performed to assess for carcinoma in situ. The urethra is inspected during withdrawal of the cystoscope, and biopsies are taken if clinically indicated. Patients with positive cytologic findings but no apparent tumor within the bladder undergo selective retrograde catheterization of the ureters up to the renal pelvices to determine whether upper tract disease is present.

The decision whether to obtain images of the abdomen and pelvis is based on the results of cystoscopy and the pathology of the tumor. Either CT or magnetic resonance urogram can evaluate the upper urinary tracts, and CT or MRI may distinguish whether a tumor extends to the perivesical fat (T3), prostate, or vagina (T4) and whether regional lymph nodes are involved (N+). For larger, invasive tumors, the presence or absence of distal metastases can be documented by physical examination, CT of the abdomen and pelvis, a chest radiograph, and radionuclide bone scan.

All patients with carcinoma of the bladder or related sites are staged using the TNM system (E-Table 182-1). The TNM system categorizes the depth of invasion of the primary tumor, nodal metastases in the pelvis (or retroperitoneum for upper tract disease) on the basis of the number and size of regional nodal involvement, other nonregional lymph node sites, and any visceral sites of disease.

TREATMENT

Non–Muscle-Invasive Disease

The standard treatment for non–muscle-invasive tumors is a complete endoscopic resection. Additional treatment in the form of adjuvant intravesical therapy depends on the number of lesions, the size, the depth of invasion, and the number of prior tumors in that individual. Immediate postresection intravesicular gemcitabine significantly reduces the risk of recurrence in patients who are at high risk of recurrence and progression because of multifocal or large lesions, high-grade papillary lesions, T1 tumors, carcinomas in situ, or a combination of these factors.[A10] Intravesical therapy is not warranted for Ta tumors that are low grade, and it is never advised for muscle-invasive tumors because agents instilled in the bladder do not penetrate beyond a few layers of cells. After allowing sufficient time for healing after the endoscopic resection, intravesical therapy is most frequently initiated with the immunologic agent bacillus Calmette-Guérin (BCG) weekly for 6 weeks, followed by a prolonged maintenance schedule.[17] BCG is highly effective for eradicating tumors in situ, with 70% of patients disease-free at 1 year and 40% at 10 years. Occasionally, other chemotherapeutic agents or cytokines are used under expert oversight when BCG is contraindicated. Bladder toxicity caused by urothelial irritation from BCG includes bladder irritability or spasms, hematuria, and pain on urination. A rare complication of BCG is development of a systemic tuberculosis infection requiring treatment with systemic antituberculosis agents (Chapter 299).

The majority of patients develop new tumors, 30% of which progress to a higher stage, so vigilant surveillance at 3-month intervals for the first year should include cystoscopy, urine cytology, and repeat transurethral resection when indicated. If disease persists, either a repeat course of BCG treatment or even an immediate cystectomy may be recommended. Pembrolizumab is useful for high grade, non–muscle-invasive bladder cancer that either does not respond to BCG or relapses within 12 months after BCG therapy.[18]

Selected tumors in the ureter or renal pelvis can be managed by ureteroscopic resection, sometimes accompanied by the instillation of BCG through the renal pelvis, or by nephroureterectomy. Tumors of the prostatic urethra are frequently managed by cystoprostatectomy, particularly if a complete resection cannot be accomplished.

Muscle-Invasive Tumors

For patients whose tumors are infiltrating the muscularis propria, the standard of care in the United States and Europe is a radical cystectomy and pelvic lymphadenectomy because of the high incidence of cancer extending into the perivesicular fat or into regional lymph nodes.[19,20] A prostatectomy is also performed in men; in women, the urethra, uterus, fallopian tubes, ovaries, and anterior vaginal wall are removed. Urinary flow can be directed through either a conduit diversion or a continent reservoir. With a conduit diversion, urine is drained directly from the ureters to a loop of small bowel that is anastomosed to the skin surface with no internal reservoir. Urine is collected in an external appliance. Alternatively, a low-pressure continent reservoir can be created from a detubularized segment of bowel attached to the abdominal wall with a continent stoma that can be self-catheterized at regular intervals. Low-pressure reservoirs also can be anastomosed to the urethra, thereby creating an internal orthotopic neobladder that permits the patient to void via the normal urethra.[21] The standard pelvic lymphadenectomy includes the distal common iliac, external iliac, obturator, presacral, and hypogastric nodes; improved survival and decreased local recurrence are associated with removal of an increased number of lymph nodes. Radical cystectomy is effective at providing long-term disease control in 75 to 80% of patients with organ-confined disease, in approximately 50% of patients whose tumors extend into the perivesical tissues, and in up to one third of patients with regional lymph node involvement. Complications of cystectomy include recurrent urinary infections, hyperchloremic acidosis, oxalate stones, incontinence, and impotence.

For muscle-invasive bladder cancer, neoadjuvant chemotherapy with cisplatin-based combinations before cystectomy increases survival.[22] To be eligible, patients must have normal renal and cardiac function, as well as a good performance status. Immediate cystectomy followed by standard adjuvant chemotherapy is no better than neoadjuvant chemotherapy.[A11] However, nivolumab is recommended for 1 year after surgery for patients with pathologic features that carry a high risk of recurrence, even if they were treated with neoadjuvant chemotherapy.[A12]

Some patients prefer a nonsurgical, bladder-sparing approach using radiation treatment rather than a cystectomy. Radiation with chemotherapy sensitization (e.g., with cisplatin, gemcitabine, and mitomycin plus 5-fluorouracil) under expert supervision is preferred over radiation alone because of better tumor control. The best candidates for this approach are patients who have a solitary early-stage lesion and no evidence of hydronephrosis. This tri-modality treatment for bladder preservation first requires a successful, near-complete transurethral resection of tumor followed by concurrent chemotherapy and radiation. External beam treatments are typically delivered in five daily fractions per week, at conventional fractions of about 1.8 Gy to a total treatment dose of approximately 65 Gy. Toxicities include inflammation of the skin, impotence, fatigue, and irritative symptoms from the bladder and bowel, but persistent proctitis is rare. In this approach, cystectomy is reserved for patients whose disease failed to achieve complete response.

Metastatic Disease

Metastatic disease in the pelvic lymph nodes is very frequent despite a normal preoperative CT scan. Bilateral pelvic lymph node dissection in addition to cystectomy improves survival.

Patients with metastatic disease are treated with either platinum-based chemotherapy or immunotherapy with checkpoint blockade inhibitors targeting either PD-1 or PD-L1 under expert supervision.[23] Cisplatin-based chemotherapy is the standard first-line treatment based on the potential for cure. The two most commonly used regimens are either gemcitabine plus cisplatin or the four-drug regimen of methotrexate, vinblastine, doxorubicin, and cisplatin. The most frequently observed toxicities include anemia, thrombocytopenia, neutropenic fever, mucositis, and fatigue. The median survival of patients treated with either regimen is approximately 14 months, and the 5-year survival is 15% or less. Favorable prognostic factors include a good performance status and metastatic disease limited to the lymph nodes. When medical comorbid conditions preclude the use of cisplatin, immunotherapy with pembrolizumab can be considered instead of carboplatin-based chemotherapy if the tumor is positive for PD-L1.[24] After first-line chemotherapy, avelumab maintenance therapy can significantly prolong survival in patients whose disease did not progress during chemotherapy.[A13] Durable responses can also be obtained in patients with progressive disease by using pembrolizumab or nivolumab.[A14] The antibody-drug conjugate enfortumab vedotin can be considered for patients with progressive cancer despite chemotherapy and/or immunotherapy.[A15] Sacituzimab govitecan, another antibody-drug conjugate, is also useful for patients who were previously treated with chemotherapy and immunotherapy; myelosuppression is the most common toxicity.[25] For patients whose previously treated tumors harbor mutations or fusions in the fibroblast growth factor receptor (FGFR) 2 or 3 genes, the oral pan-FGFR inhibitor erdafitinib can be beneficial.[26] Common side effects include hyponatremia, stomatitis, and asthenia.

PREVENTION

Screening of asymptomatic individuals for hematuria increases the probability of diagnosing bladder cancer at an earlier stage but does not improve survival and is not routinely recommended.

PROGNOSIS

Cancer of the urinary bladder is a common but heterogeneous disease. The natural history of a urothelial tumor is to recur either at the same location or at a separate site in the urothelial tract and at the same or a more advanced stage. Non–muscle-invasive TaG1 lesions are easily treated with endoscopic resection alone and almost never progress.

Without treatment, about 60% of tumors in situ progress to more invasive disease within 5 years. Endoscopic resection plus intravesicular BCG immunotherapy can substantially reduce recurrence and progression, with 5-year disease-free survival rates of 60%.

Muscle-invasive disease is most frequently cured with an integrated approach of systemic chemotherapy for micrometastases followed by cystectomy and pelvic lymphadenectomy; cure rates for T2 tumors can be as high as 80% with this multimodality approach. Bladder-sparing approaches associated with an improved quality of life are possible using external beam radiation. The 5-year disease-free survival with this approach is approximately 50%, with the majority of surviving patients retaining a normally functioning bladder.

Metastatic urinary bladder cancer is a fast-growing and often lethal malignancy; despite aggressive chemotherapy, only about 15% of patients are disease-free at 5 years. Even in this chemotherapy-refractory setting, modern immunotherapy can potentially cure a subset of patients.

CANCERS OF THE RENAL PELVIS AND URETERS

Approximately 10% of transitional cell carcinomas are upper tract tumors that occur in the ureters and the renal pelvis. These tumors can arise either de novo or in the setting of prior tumors. The risk for developing an upper tract tumor approaches 25% by 10 years in patients who have multifocal carcinoma in situ of the bladder.

These tumors are morphologically similar to the tumors in the bladder and behave in a similar manner. Hematuria is the most common manifesting symptom, although patients with large tumors and/or ureteral obstruction can present with flank pain. A CT scan or MRI is used to stage the extent of primary disease and to detect regional metastases. Upper tract transitional cell carcinomas are staged according to the TNM system (see E-Table 182-1).

Low-grade tumors can be treated endoscopically, but high-grade tumors are most commonly treated with a nephroureterectomy. In contrast to bladder cancer, regional lymphadenectomy is not routinely performed. In renal pelvic tumors, the ureter is also removed because of the high risk for multifocal tumors along the entire upper tract and the inability to monitor the ureteral stump accurately postoperatively.

Adjuvant systemic chemotherapy under expert oversight with either cisplatin plus gemcitabine or carboplatin plus gemcitabine confers a survival advantage for patients whose tumors have pathologic features deemed at high risk for relapse.[A16] For advanced nonsurgical disease, treatment options include chemotherapy, immunotherapy, antibody drug conjugates, and targeted therapies similar to the approach used for primary bladder cancer. These upper tract urothelial tumors generally have the same responses to treatment and clinical outcomes as does bladder cancer.

GENERAL REFERENCES

For the General References and other additional features, please visit Elsevier eBooks+ at https://ebooks.health.elsevier.com.

Grade A References

A1. Ravaud A, Motzer RJ, Pandha HS, et al. Adjuvant sunitinib in high-risk renal-cell carcinoma after nephrectomy. *N Engl J Med.* 2016;375:2246-2254.

A2. Powles T, Tomczak P, Park SH, et al. Pembrolizumab versus placebo as post-nephrectomy adjuvant therapy for clear cell renal cell carcinoma (KEYNOTE-564): 30-month follow-up analysis of a multicentre, randomised, double-blind, placebo-controlled, phase 3 trial. *Lancet Oncol.* 2022;23:1133-1144.

A3. Méjean A, Ravaud A, Thezenas S, et al. Sunitinib alone or after nephrectomy in metastatic renal-cell carcinoma. *N Engl J Med.* 2018;379:417-427.

A4. Choueiri TK, Powles T, Burotto M, et al. Nivolumab plus cabozantinib versus sunitinib for advanced renal cell carcinoma. *N Engl J Med.* 2021;384:829-841.

A5. Motzer RJ, Tannir NM, McDermott DF, et al. Nivolumab plus ipilimumab versus sunitinib in advanced renal-cell carcinoma. *N Engl J Med.* 2018;378:1277-1290.

A6. Motzer R, Alekseev B, Rha SY, et al. Lenvatinib plus pembrolizumab or everolimus for advanced renal cell carcinoma. *N Engl J Med.* 2021;384:1289-1300.

A7. Powles T, Plimack ER, Soulières D, et al. Pembrolizumab plus axitinib versus sunitinib monotherapy as first-line treatment of advanced renal cell carcinoma (KEYNOTE-426): extended follow-up from a randomised, open-lavel, phase 3 trial. *Lancet Oncol.* 2020;21:1563-1573.

A8. Rini BI, Plimack ER, Stus V, et al. Pembrolizumab plus axitinib versus sunitinib for advanced renal-cell carcinoma. *N Engl J Med.* 2019;380:1116-1127.

A9. Fernández-Pello S, Hofmann F, Tahbaz R, et al. A systematic review and meta-analysis comparing the effectiveness and adverse effects of different systemic treatments for non-clear cell renal cell carcinoma. *Eur Urol.* 2017;71:426-436.

A10. Messing EM, Tangen CM, Lerner SP, et al. Effect of intravesical instillation of gemcitabine vs saline immediately following resection of suspected low-grade non-muscle-invasive bladder cancer on tumor recurrence: SWOG S0337 randomized clinical trial. *JAMA.* 2018;319:1880-1888.

A11. Sternberg CN, Skoneczna I, Kerst JM, et al. Immediate versus deferred chemotherapy after radical cystectomy in patients with pT3-pT4 or N+ M0 urothelial carcinoma of the bladder (EORTC 30994): an intergroup, open-label, randomised phase 3 trial. *Lancet Oncol.* 2015;16:76-86.
A12. Bajorin DF, Witjes JA, Gschwend JE, et al. Adjuvant nivolumab versus placebo in muscle-invasive urothelial carcinoma. *N Engl J Med.* 2021;384:2102-2114.
A13. Powles T, Park SH, Voog E, et al. Avelumab maintenance therapy for advanced or metastatic urothelial carcinoma. *N Engl J Med.* 2020;383:1218-1230.
A14. Bellmunt J, de Wit R, Vaughn DJ, et al. Pembrolizumab as second-line therapy for advanced urothelial carcinoma. *N Engl J Med.* 2017;376:1015-1026.
A15. Powles T, Rosenberg JE, Sonpavde GP, et al. Enfortumab vedotin in previously treated advanced urothelial carcinoma. *N Engl J Med.* 2021;384:1125-1135.
A16. Birtle A, Johnson M, Chester J, et al. Adjuvant chemotherapy in upper tract urothelial carcinoma (the POUT trial): a phase 3, open-label, randomised controlled trial. *Lancet.* 2020;395:1268-1277.

183 BREAST CANCER AND BENIGN BREAST DISORDERS

NANCY E. DAVIDSON

BREAST CANCER

EPIDEMIOLOGY AND PATHOBIOLOGY

Invasive breast cancer, which is the most common nonskin cancer in women in the United States, is diagnosed in approximately 290,000 women annually and results in approximately 43,000 deaths each year.[1] Worldwide, about 2.25 million cases are diagnosed annually.[2] The incidence and mortality from breast cancer appear to be declining in the United States and parts of Western Europe, likely because of a decreased use of postmenopausal hormone replacement therapy (Chapter 222), early detection by screening mammography, and widespread use of adjuvant systemic therapy.

Breast cancer is largely a disease of women, but it occurs in men at an incidence of approximately 1% of the incidence seen in women. A second critical risk factor is age. Approximately 75% of breast cancer cases in the United States are diagnosed in women older than age 50 years.

Family history is a third critical risk factor (Table 183-1). Approximately 20% of breast cancers occur in women with a family history of breast cancer, and a diagnosis of breast cancer in first-degree relatives before age 50 years especially increases the risk. Of breast cancer cases, 5 to 8% occur in high-risk families. Familial breast cancer syndromes that are associated with known molecular abnormalities include the breast-ovarian cancer syndrome, which is linked to germline mutations in the breast cancer susceptibility genes, *BRCA1* and *BRCA2*. These mutations, which include specific breast cancer cluster regions within these genes, are inherited in an autosomal dominant fashion. Germline mutation in either of these *BRCA* genes is associated with a 50 to 85% lifetime risk for developing breast cancer.

Other hereditary cancer syndromes (Chapter 166) include the Li-Fraumeni syndrome (which is linked with germline mutations in the *p53* tumor suppressor gene), Cowden syndrome (which is associated with inherited mutations in the *PTEN* gene), and germline loss-of-function mutations in *PALB2*, *CHEK2*, and other DNA repair genes. In addition to these high-penetrance genetic susceptibility syndromes, low-penetrance genetic associations include single nucleotide polymorphisms in a variety of genes.

Reproductive risk factors that result in prolonged exposure of the breast to estrogen include early menarche, late menopause, nulliparity, and late first pregnancy. The association between postmenopausal obesity and breast cancer likely reflects estrogen exposure as well.

Certain types of preexisting breast pathology, including atypical hyperplasia and lobular carcinoma in situ, are also associated with increased risk of breast cancer. Breast density as assessed by mammography may also be a risk factor.

Exogenous environmental factors that may predispose to breast cancer include ionizing radiation during adolescence, prolonged use of combined estrogen plus progesterone hormone replacement therapy (but not estrogen therapy alone),[A1] ongoing use of oral contraceptives, and alcohol consumption. Large studies have failed to show any convincing association between breast cancer and exposure to estrogenic pesticides or to a high-fat diet.

CLINICAL MANIFESTATIONS

Breast cancer usually manifests as an asymptomatic abnormality on a screening mammogram. However, patients sometimes have a physical change in the breast, including a mass[3] or asymmetrical thickening, nipple discharge, or skin or nipple changes. These abnormalities are commonly first detected by the patient but also may first be noted on a routine physical examination by a clinician.[4]

A milky discharge is seldom associated with a malignant diagnosis, but a clear or bloody nipple discharge is of great concern, and a bloody discharge is frequently caused by an intraductal papilloma. Breast pain is common, especially as a premenstrual symptom in premenopausal women, but it may also be associated with an underlying malignancy.

Paget disease of the nipple is a form of adenocarcinoma that involves the skin and ducts and is manifested as nipple excoriation. Inflammatory breast cancer is characterized by a constellation of redness, warmth, and edema that often reflects infiltration of tumor cells into the dermal lymphatics of the breast, and can mimic simple mastitis.[5]

Although most breast cancers are localized or relatively localized at the time of diagnosis, metastatic disease can be seen at the time of presentation or up to decades later. Common metastatic sites include bone, with pain and pathologic fractures (Chapter 187); liver metastases, with elevations of liver enzymes and sometimes jaundice; pleura, with malignant effusions (Chapter 86); central nervous system, with space occupying lesions and spinal cord compression (Chapter 175); and pericardium, with effusions (Chapter 62). Breast cancer is also a common cause of a hypercoagulable state (Chapter 67) manifested by deep vein thrombosis of the legs and even thromboses of the upper extremity (Chapter 68).

DIAGNOSIS

Patients who have an asymptomatic mammographic abnormality or any of the clinical manifestations associated with breast cancer, whether initially noted by the patient or by an examining clinician, require a careful history and breast examination, including palpation for potentially suspicious axillary lymph nodes. A careful history should focus on family history and exposure to estrogens and hormone replacement therapy. The physical examination should

TABLE 183-1 RISK FACTORS FOR BREAST CANCER IN WOMEN

RELATIVE RISK >4.0
Age (65+ vs. <65 yr, although risk increases across all ages until age 80 yr)
Biopsy-confirmed atypical hyperplasia
Certain inherited genetic mutations for breast cancer, including *BRCA1, BRCA2, p53, CHEK2, PALB2, PTEN*
Ductal carcinoma in situ
Lobular carcinoma in situ
Mammographically dense breasts (compared with least dense)
Personal history of early-onset (<40 yr) breast cancer
Two or more first-degree relatives with breast cancer diagnosed at an early age
RELATIVE RISK 2.1-4.0
Personal history of breast cancer (40+ yr)
High endogenous estrogen or testosterone levels (postmenopausal)
High-dose radiation to chest
One first-degree relative with breast cancer
RELATIVE RISK 1.1-2.0
Alcohol consumption
Ashkenazi Jewish heritage
Diethylstilbestrol exposure
Early menarche (<12 yr)
Height (tall)
High socioeconomic status
Late age at first full-term pregnancy (>30 yr)
Late menopause (>55 yr)
Never breastfed a child
No full-term pregnancies
Obesity (postmenopausal)/adult weight gain
Personal history of endometrial or ovarian cancer
Proliferative breast disease without atypia (usual ductal hyperplasia and fibroadenoma)
Recent and long-term use of menopausal hormone therapy containing estrogen and progestin
Recent oral contraceptive use

Modified from American Cancer Society. *Breast Cancer Facts & Figures 2017-2018.* ACS; Atlanta, GA: 2017; Hu C, Hart SN, Gnanaolivu R, et al. A population-based study of genes previously implicated in breast cancer. *N Engl J Med.* 2021;384:440-451.

include inspection of the breasts for changes in shape, skin color, or dimpling with the patient's hands above their head and on the hips; palpation of the breasts in the upright and reclining positions using a standard approach of circles, wedges, or lines to cover the entire breast; and examination of the axillary, supraclavicular, and infraclavicular lymph nodes. If the abnormality was not detected by a screening mammogram, a mammogram should be obtained promptly.

If the breast examination and bilateral mammography are normal in patients who have localized noncyclic breast pain, ultrasound or magnetic resonance imaging (MRI) may be used to exclude the small possibility of a malignancy. Bilateral breast imaging is always recommended to identify any unsuspected lesions in the contralateral breast that may also require evaluation.

For both clinically occult and clinically apparent lesions, pathologic evaluation is mandatory to establish a diagnosis. An outpatient core needle biopsy should be guided by mammography, ultrasonography, or MRI if the lesion is not palpable. In patients who have clear or bloody nipple discharge, ductography and ductoscopy may help to identify the inciting lesion, but excisional biopsy may be required.

These technologies generally permit an accurate diagnosis that can be followed by definitive treatment, but the concordance among pathologists is only about 96% for the diagnosis of invasive carcinoma, about 85% for ductal carcinoma in situ or fully benign biopsies, and as low as 50% for atypia. Further expert evaluation is required when biopsy of a suspicious lesion yields equivocal diagnosis after needle aspiration or core biopsy.

Staging and Prognostic and Predictive Markers

Breast cancers are staged from I to IV, with stages I and II representing early-stage disease, stage III signaling more locally advanced disease, and stage IV denoting metastatic disease. Outcomes are highly correlated with stage of disease.

Anatomic staging (Table 183-2) considers just the tumor's size (T), nodal involvement (N), and metastases (M) and should only be used in global regions where biomarker tests are not routinely available. Most patients with breast cancer present with anatomic stage I or II disease in the absence of symptoms. In such patients, basic laboratory studies can be limited to blood counts, chemistry panel, and a chest radiograph, because more extensive radiologic evaluation is not warranted because of low yield. In contrast, women with clinical evidence of stage III or IV disease should undergo more intensive evaluation of common sites for metastases, including lung, liver, and bone, using computed tomography (CT) and positron emission tomographic (PET) radionuclide scanning.

However, all patients with invasive cancers (anatomic stage 1 A or higher) also should undergo pathological prognostic staging, which incorporates a number of biomarkers (including histologic grade, expression of estrogen and progesterone receptors and HER2 proteins, and sometimes multigene panels).[6] By integrating data derived from analysis by genomic DNA copy number arrays, DNA methylation, exome sequencing, messenger RNA arrays, microRNA sequencing, and reverse-phase protein arrays, breast cancers can be divided into at least four molecular subsets: luminal A and B, HER2, and basal. The luminal subtypes frequently express the estrogen receptor-α, but luminal A appears to be associated with a better prognosis and higher likelihood of response to endocrine therapy than luminal B. The basal subtype is dominated by tumors that lack expression of the estrogen receptor-α, the progesterone receptor, or HER2—the so-called triple-negative breast cancer that lacks a readily identified molecular target. Multigene assays can identify early-stage steroid receptor–positive breast cancers that will benefit from the addition of chemotherapy to endocrine therapy and may identify women with a poor prognosis.[A2] Whole-genome sequencing of the breast cancer also may help to pinpoint avenues for precise diagnostics and targeted therapy.

Germline testing for *BRCA1* and *BRCA2* mutations through a multigene panel should be part of the evaluation of women with clinical features suggestive of a hereditary breast cancer syndrome (e.g., a personal diagnosis of breast cancer at age 45 years or younger or of ovarian cancer at any age, a personal diagnosis of triple-negative breast cancer at age 60 years or younger, multiple family members with early-onset breast or ovarian cancer, bilateral breast cancer, or Ashkenazi Jewish heritage). Careful counseling about the implications of positive or negative results and about the limitations of testing is a prerequisite for testing.[7]

Less than 10% of women present initially with metastatic disease. Advanced disease is more commonly diagnosed in women who have a previous diagnosis of early breast cancer for which they have received treatment. Common sites for metastases include bone, soft tissues, lung, liver, and brain. If metastatic disease is suspected, relevant hematologic, biochemical, and radiographic evaluation is indicated to assess the location and severity of involvement. Because of the importance of the diagnosis, pathologic confirmation is preferred to verify recurrent disease, exclude other diagnoses, and reassess of biologic features such as the expression of estrogen receptors, progesterone receptors, and HER2. Elevation of tumor markers (e.g., CA-27-29, carcinoembryonic antigen) or the presence of circulating tumor cells or circulating free tumor DNA is not diagnostic of recurrent disease, although these markers may be useful adjuncts in the assessment of the effects of therapy.

TABLE 183-2 ANATOMIC STAGING OF BREAST CANCER

STAGE	DESCRIPTION
NONINVASIVE	
0	• Ductal carcinoma in situ; no invasion of the duct's basement membrane or adjacent normal tissue
INVASIVE	
1A	• Breast tumor ≤ 2 cm, no spread beyond the breast and no involved lymph nodes
1B	• No breast tumor, but microscopic (>0.2 mm to ≤2 mm) metastases in axillary lymph nodes OR • Tumor ≤ 2 cm in the breast plus involved lymph nodes
IIA	• No tumor in the breast, but macroscopic (>2 mm) tumor in one to three axillary lymph nodes OR • Tumor ≤ 2 cm in breast, with spread to axillary lymph nodes OR • Tumor > 2 cm to ≤5 cm in the breast, no spread to axillary lymph nodes
IIB	• Tumor > 2 cm but ≤5 cm in the breast, spread to one to three axillary lymph nodes OR • Tumor > 5 cm in the breast, no spread to axillary lymph nodes
IIIA	• Tumor > 5 cm in the breast, spread to axillary and/or internal mammary nodes • Metastases in four to nine axillary lymph nodes or in internal mammary nodes regardless of presence or size of tumor in the breast
IIIB	• Tumor spread to chest wall and/or skin of the breast regardless of size of tumor in the breast; may also be seen to axillary or internal mammary tumor nodes
IIIC	• Tumor of any size with spread to ≥10 axillary lymph nodes OR • Tumor spread to infraclavicular or supraclavicular lymph nodes OR • Tumor spread to both axillary lymph nodes and internal mammary nodes
METASTATIC	
IV	• Spread of tumor to other parts of the body such as liver, lung, or bone

TREATMENT

The treatment of breast cancer should be tailored to its stage and biology.[8] For example, tumors that express the estrogen receptor-α, the progesterone receptor, or both, are responsive to endocrine therapy, whereas tumors that lack both seldom respond to such therapy. Overexpression of the HER2 protein is associated with response to the HER2-targeted therapies.[9] Evidence that links expression of the estrogen receptor, the progesterone receptor, or HER2 to the efficacy of chemotherapy is equivocal.

In Situ Carcinoma

In countries where screening mammography is widely used, in situ carcinomas account for 20 to 25% of newly diagnosed cases of breast cancer (see Table 183-3).

Ductal Carcinoma In-Situ

Most in situ breast tumors are ductal carcinoma in situ (DCIS) lesions, which are associated with approximately a 30% risk for the development of subsequent invasive breast cancer in the same breast. The risk for metastatic breast cancer with a diagnosis of DCIS is extremely small. As a consequence, management decisions are centered on the involved breast, and axillary lymph node evaluation is not routinely performed. Total mastectomy has a high likelihood of cure, but lumpectomy with conservation of the breast is appropriate for many women with DCIS. Sufficient excision to obtain tumor-free margins is critical. Careful examination of the specimen and postexcision mammography are crucial to confirm that the DCIS has been adequately excised. The size and grade of the lesion are other important determinants of local outcome.

Radiotherapy plus lumpectomy decreases the likelihood of in situ or invasive recurrence compared with lumpectomy alone, but women who have favorable histologic findings and who are willing to undergo close surveillance are candidates for local excision alone. In addition, the use of oral tamoxifen (20 mg daily) or an aromatase inhibitor (e.g., oral anastrozole 1 mg daily) for 5 years can reduce the likelihood of recurrent ipsilateral breast cancer or a new contralateral breast cancer by approximately 50%.

Lobular Carcinoma In Situ

Controversy continues over whether lobular carcinoma in situ (LCIS) is truly a malignant lesion. LCIS is usually an incidental finding on a breast biopsy that

TABLE 183-3 CARCINOMA IN SITU: DUCTAL VERSUS LOBULAR

FEATURE	LOBULAR CARCINOMA IN SITU	DUCTAL CARCINOMA IN SITU
Age	Younger	Older
Palpable mass	No	Uncommon
Mammographic appearance	Not detected on mammography	Microcalcifications, mass
Immunophenotype	E-cadherin negative	E-cadherin positive
Usual manifestation	Incidental finding on breast biopsy	Microcalcifications on mammography or breast mass
Bilateral involvement	Common	Uncertain
Risk and site of subsequent breast cancer	25% risk for invasive breast cancer in either breast over remaining lifespan	At site of initial lesion; 0.5% risk/yr of invasive breast cancer in opposite breast
Prevention	Consider tamoxifen or raloxifene or aromatase inhibitor	Consider tamoxifen or aromatase inhibitor if estrogen receptor positive
Treatment	Yearly mammography and breast examination	Lumpectomy ± radiation; mastectomy for large or multifocal lesions

was performed for other indications, and it appears to be associated with a 25% risk for the development of invasive breast cancer in either breast. Women with LCIS are generally managed expectantly with regular breast examination and imaging. Bilateral total mastectomy is sometimes considered for women whose LCIS is associated with other risk factors for breast cancer or with extreme anxiety. Women with LCIS are candidates for tamoxifen (20 mg daily), raloxifene (60 mg daily), or an aromatase inhibitor (e.g., anastrozole 1 mg daily) as a risk-reduction strategy.

Early Stage Invasive Breast Cancer

Surgery

Breast conservation surgery with lumpectomy plus radiotherapy provides identical survival rates to modified radical mastectomy (removal of the breast and lymph nodes) for women with stages I and II breast cancer. Medical contraindications to breast conservation therapy include multifocal disease, previous radiotherapy, ongoing pregnancy that precludes the timely use of radiotherapy, poor cosmesis, and patient preference. Patients who undergo mastectomy should be counseled about the availability of autologous tissue and implant options for reconstruction, either at the time of surgery or any time thereafter.[10]

For women who have small tumors and a clinically negative axilla, no further local evaluation is needed. For adequate staging of larger tumors, however, the involvement of axillary lymph nodes must be determined. To minimize the incidence of postoperative lymphedema associated with lymph node dissection,[11] a radioactive tracer, blue dye, or both are injected into the area around the primary breast tumor and tracked to the dominant axillary lymph node (the sentinel node), which can be located and removed by the surgeon. If the sentinel node is tumor free or if the burden of disease in sentinel nodes is low, no further axillary surgery is required. Women who have palpable axillary nodes or who have extensively involved sentinel nodes should be counseled to undergo axillary dissection.

Adjuvant Radiotherapy

Women who have undergone lumpectomy alone have a breast cancer recurrence rate of up to 40%, whereas the rate of recurrence is less than 10% with whole-breast radiotherapy, often administered on an accelerated schedule.[12] Women who are older than age 65 years and who receive tamoxifen for low-risk estrogen receptor–positive tumors will have a lower rate of local recurrence but no benefit in terms of distant recurrence or survival.[A3] In women who have positive axillary nodes or high-risk characteristics despite negative nodes, radiation therapy appears to reduce recurrence rates but provides little if any overall survival benefit.

Women who have undergone mastectomy also likely gain a survival advantage from postoperative radiation therapy if they have more than three involved lymph nodes. For women who have involvement of one to three nodes, the potential benefit is smaller, and expert consultation is helpful.

Adjuvant Systemic Therapy

Neoadjuvant Chemotherapy

Women frequently receive several adjuvant interventions, including chemotherapy, radiotherapy, endocrine therapy, and/or anti-HER2 therapy. For clinically

TABLE 183-4 (NEO)ADJUVANT TREATMENT GUIDELINES FOR PATIENTS WITH EARLY-STAGE INVASIVE BREAST CANCER

PATIENT GROUP	TREATMENT
HORMONE RECEPTOR–POSITIVE (ER- AND/OR PR-POSITIVE) BREAST CANCER	
Low tumor burden	
≤0.5 cm pN0	Consider adjuvant hormonal therapy
0.6-1.0 cm well differentiated and no unfavorable features pN0	Consider adjuvant hormonal therapy
>1 cm	Adjuvant hormonal therapy ± adjuvant chemotherapy (may use genomic testing)
Intermediate or high tumor burden and unfavorable biology	
	Adjuvant hormonal therapy + adjuvant chemotherapy; may consider abemaciclib
HORMONE RECEPTOR–NEGATIVE (ER- AND PR-NEGATIVE) BREAST CANCER	
≤0.5 cm and pN0	No adjuvant therapy
All other tumors	(Neo)adjuvant chemotherapy; consider pembrolizumab
HER2 POSITIVE	
	Anti-HER2 therapy should be added to the suggested treatment above for all node-positive patients and considered for pN0 tumors that are >5 mm

Modified from National Comprehensive Cancer Network Guidelines and 2021 St. Gallen Conference. Available at http://www.nccn.org. and Ann Oncol 32:1216-1235, 2021.

node-positive tumors or tumors larger than 2 cm, neoadjuvant preoperative checkpoint inhibitor therapy with pembrolizumab plus chemotherapy is standard treatment for triple-negative breast cancer, and neoadjuvant anti-HER2 therapy plus chemotherapy should be considered for HER2-positive breast cancer.[13] Otherwise, neoadjuvant chemotherapy improves the rate of breast conservation but does not enhance disease-free or overall survival.[A4]

Adjuvant Chemotherapy

After definitive local therapy for early breast cancer, adjuvant chemotherapy, endocrine therapy, biologic therapy, or a combination of these approaches aims to suppress or eradicate clinically occult micrometastases. Recommendations for adjuvant systemic therapy are based on menopausal status, lymph node status, tumor size, the extent of expression of the estrogen receptor, progesterone receptor, HER2 proteins in breast cancer cells, and certain multigene tests (Table 183-4).[14]

Adjuvant therapy results in a proportional reduction in risk for recurrence across all patients regardless of risk for recurrence, so the absolute benefit of adjuvant systemic therapy is greatest for patients who have the greatest risk for recurrence. However, women who have a high clinical risk but a low genomic risk for recurrence based on a 70-gene signature gain little benefit from adjuvant chemotherapy.

Adjuvant chemotherapy may be administered before or after radiotherapy. Adjuvant endocrine therapy should be delayed until after completion of chemotherapy. The benefit of trastuzumab for HER2-positive cancers appears to be optimized when it is coadministered with taxane chemotherapy rather than following completion of the taxane.

ADJUVANT ENDOCRINE THERAPY. Tamoxifen (20 mg/day for 5 to 10 years) improves outcomes in women of all ages with estrogen receptor– or progesterone receptor–positive breast cancer.[A5] Its side-effect profile includes an increased risk for thromboembolic events and uterine cancer, especially in postmenopausal women, because of its estrogen agonist properties. Potential benefits include promotion of bone density and lowering of cholesterol. Tamoxifen is the preferred adjuvant endocrine therapy for premenopausal women and for men.

Luteinizing hormone–releasing hormone (LHRH) agonists (e.g., leuprolide 3.75 mg intramuscularly monthly) can temporarily and reversibly suppress ovarian function when used in combination with an aromatase inhibitor (e.g., exemestane 25 mg daily) or tamoxifen (20 mg daily) and can improve disease-free survival in women who are premenopausal and are at sufficient risk for recurrence to warrant adjuvant chemotherapy.[A6] Administration of goserelin (a gonadotropin-releasing hormone agonist to protect ovarian function at 3.6 mg subcutaneously monthly) with chemotherapy may protect against permanent ovarian failure, thereby reducing the risk for early menopause and improving prospects for subsequent fertility.[A7]

In postmenopausal women, the primary source of estrogen is the conversion of androgens synthesized by the adrenal glands to estrogen through the activity of CYP19 or aromatase in peripheral tissues such as mammary and adipose tissues. The aromatase inhibitors (anastrozole 1 mg daily; letrozole 2.5 mg daily; and exemestane 25 mg daily) specifically inhibit this conversion, thereby leading to further estrogen deprivation in older women. Multiple trials suggest that an aromatase inhibitor is preferred over tamoxifen in postmenopausal women and in premenopausal women who are receiving an LHRH agonist for estrogen receptor–positive breast cancer because these inhibitors reduce recurrence rates by about 30% (proportionately) compared with tamoxifen.[A8,A9] Side effects include postmenopausal symptoms, osteoporosis, fractures, and arthralgias. Aromatase inhibitors are not useful for receptor-negative breast cancer, and they should not be used as monotherapy in premenopausal women or men with breast cancer. The simultaneous administration of aromatase inhibitor plus tamoxifen does not improve outcome over aromatase inhibitor alone, but the addition of abemaciclib (a CDK4/6 inhibitor) to an aromatase inhibitor can provide additional benefit for women who have high-risk early breast cancer.[A10]

The duration of endocrine therapy appears to be quite important. Five years of adjuvant endocrine therapy is associated with better outcomes than shorter periods, and 10 years of tamoxifen appears to be better than 5 years. However, the benefit of extending aromatase inhibitor therapy beyond 5 years is unproven.[A11] The greatest benefit of longer term therapy is probably prevention of contralateral breast cancer.

ADJUVANT ANTI-HER2 THERAPY. The transmembrane HER2/neu protein is overexpressed in approximately 15 to 20% of breast cancers, generally because of gene amplification. Adding 1 year of therapy with trastuzumab (a monoclonal antibody to HER2) to chemotherapy reduces the risk for recurrence by approximately 50% in women with high-risk or residual invasive HER2-positive early breast cancer.[A12] Questions remain regarding long-term risks and benefits, the use of trastuzumab in the absence of chemotherapy, and the role of other anti-HER2 agents such as lapatinib, pertuzumab, neratinib, and trastuzumab emtansine in addition to or in place of trastuzumab. Neratinib is beneficial when used as adjuvant therapy for 1 year after a year of trastuzumab-containing therapy, and emtansine is beneficial for women who have residual breast cancer after neoadjuvant chemotherapy.[A13]

ADJUVANT CHEMOTHERAPY. The benefit of conventional adjuvant chemotherapy varies by age and nodal status, with its greatest absolute benefit in women who are younger than age 50 years, in whom it decreases the 15-year risk of breast cancer mortality from 42 to 32%. Effective combination regimens may include anthracyclines, taxanes, antimetabolites, and cyclophosphamide, preferably for 3 to 6 months at standard doses under expert oversight. Careful use of colony-stimulating agents can minimize neutropenia, accelerate administration of chemotherapy, and improve responses,[A14] but current evidence argues against the use of erythroid-stimulating agents for chemotherapy-induced anemia. Acute side effects of therapy are nausea and vomiting, bone marrow suppression, and hair loss; all are reversible, and the first may be mitigated by the use of modern antiemetics. Induction of menopause is related to the type and duration of chemotherapy and the age of the patient; most women older than 40 years will suffer drug-induced menopause. Doxorubicin-related cardiomyopathy is noted in approximately 1% of women who receive doxorubicin-containing adjuvant chemotherapy. Use of standard adjuvant chemotherapy regimens results in a very small increase in the incidence of acute leukemia but not of other second tumors.

OTHER ADJUVANT APPROACHES. One year of the oral poly (ADP ribose) polymerase (PARP) inhibitor, olaparib, is indicated for adjuvant treatment of patients who have BRCA-mutated, HER2 negative, high-risk early breast cancer and who have been treated with neoadjuvant or adjuvant chemotherapy.[A15] The combination of pembrolizumab with chemotherapy in the neoadjuvant and adjuvant setting improves outcomes for early triple-negative breast cancer.[A16]

Follow-Up of Early-Stage Breast Cancer Survivors

Substantial evidence can guide follow-up of asymptomatic survivors of early-stage breast cancer (Table 183-5). More aggressive testing does not provide incremental value.

Stage III Breast Cancer

Approximately 10% of breast cancers present as locally advanced or inoperable stage III tumors that are characterized by large primary tumor, fixed tumor or lymph nodes, or neoplastic invasion of the skin or chest wall. Inflammatory breast cancers also are categorized as stage III. Because as many as one third of women with locally advanced breast cancer also have distant metastases at the time of diagnosis, an evaluation for metastatic disease is often indicated even in asymptomatic patients.

Combined-modality therapy is used under expert supervision to maximize control of local disease and distant micrometastases. Several months of preoperative endocrine therapy or chemotherapy can result in tumor regression in most patients, thereby allowing definitive breast surgery of some type to be performed. Postoperative radiotherapy is generally used to enhance local control, and some studies suggest that administration of further chemotherapy, hormone therapy, anti-HER2 therapy, or a combination thereof (depending on the features of the cancer) is then desirable.

TABLE 183-5 FOLLOW-UP GUIDELINES FOR PATIENTS WITH EARLY-STAGE BREAST CANCER: AMERICAN SOCIETY OF CLINICAL ONCOLOGY GUIDELINES

PROCEDURE OR TEST	FREQUENCY
History and physical examination* (eliciting of symptoms of breast cancer)	Every 3-6 mo for first 3 yr, every 6-12 mo for next yr, then yearly
MAMMOGRAPHY	
Mastectomy patients	Yearly
Lumpectomy patients	Yearly
Pelvic examination	Age appropriate
Breast self-examination	Monthly
Complete blood cell counts and chemistry studies	The literature does not support the use of these tests
Chest radiography, bone scans, PET scans, breast MRI, liver imaging, and tumor marker studies	Not recommended for routine follow-up in asymptomatic patients
Patient education regarding signs and symptoms of recurrence	Each visit

*Limited evaluation: assess for pain, dyspnea, weight loss, and other major changes in function. The limited examination should include an assessment of nodes, axillae, lumpectomy or mastectomy site, contralateral breast, chest, and abdomen. Patients should be instructed regarding symptoms of recurrence.

MRI = magnetic resonance imaging; PET = positron emission tomography.

Modified from Khatcheressian JL, Hurley P, Bantug E, et al. Breast cancer follow-up and management after primary treatment: American Society of Clinical Oncology clinical practice guideline update. *J Clin Oncol.* 2013;31:961-965.

Stage IV or Metastatic Breast Cancer

Whenever possible, biopsy of a putative metastatic lesion should be performed to confirm the diagnosis of metastatic breast cancer and assess biological markers to guide systemic therapy.[15] Although seldom curable, advanced breast cancer is a highly treatable illness. Palliation or prevention of symptoms without excess toxicity is the primary goal of treatment.

General Approach

The role of surgery in metastatic breast cancer is limited. However, surgery is useful in certain circumstances, such as resection of a chest wall nodule or solitary brain metastasis, or orthopedic stabilization to treat or prevent a long-bone fracture. Pleural (Chapter 86) and pericardial (Chapter 62) effusions should be drained percutaneously but often require more definitive local therapy.

Radiotherapy is a mainstay in the management of advanced disease. It may be used at any time during the patient's course to treat localized disease such as chest wall recurrence, brain metastases, or painful bony metastases.

Systemic treatment is the primary mode to manage disseminated disease. Key principles for the selection of therapy include maximal palliation of symptoms, minimization of treatment-related toxicity, and prevention of disease complications (Fig. 183-1).

Endocrine Therapy

Endocrine therapy under expert supervision is preferred as the first intervention for metastatic breast cancer whenever feasible because of its favorable therapeutic index. Factors that support the use of endocrine therapy include the expression of hormone receptors, a long disease-free interval, and absence of symptoms or visceral disease. More than 50% of women who meet these criteria respond to an initial course of hormone therapy, with a median response duration of 9 to 12 months. Length of response is a good predictor for the likelihood of response to a second course of endocrine therapy when the first agent fails. A second course of endocrine therapy is less likely to be successful, and the duration of response is shorter; again, duration of response predicts for likelihood of success with third-line therapy. In some women, this approach can result in good disease control with little toxicity for several years.

Several months of therapy are needed before the efficacy of a newly introduced endocrine therapy can be assessed. Patients and clinicians should be aware of the possibility of treatment-related tumor flare with worsening symptoms and increased circulating tumor markers within the first few weeks of treatment. This response is usually of short duration and should not be confused with progressive disease.

Available hormone therapies include the selective estrogen receptor modulator (SERM) tamoxifen, the selective estrogen receptor–degrading agent fulvestrant, the aromatase inhibitors, and ovarian suppression by oophorectomy or LHRH agonists. Selection under expert oversight is usually made on the basis of efficacy, toxicity, and menopausal status. Serial administration of agents is the norm, but the combination of the aromatase inhibitor anastrozole with fulvestrant is superior to anastrozole alone or to sequential anastrozole and

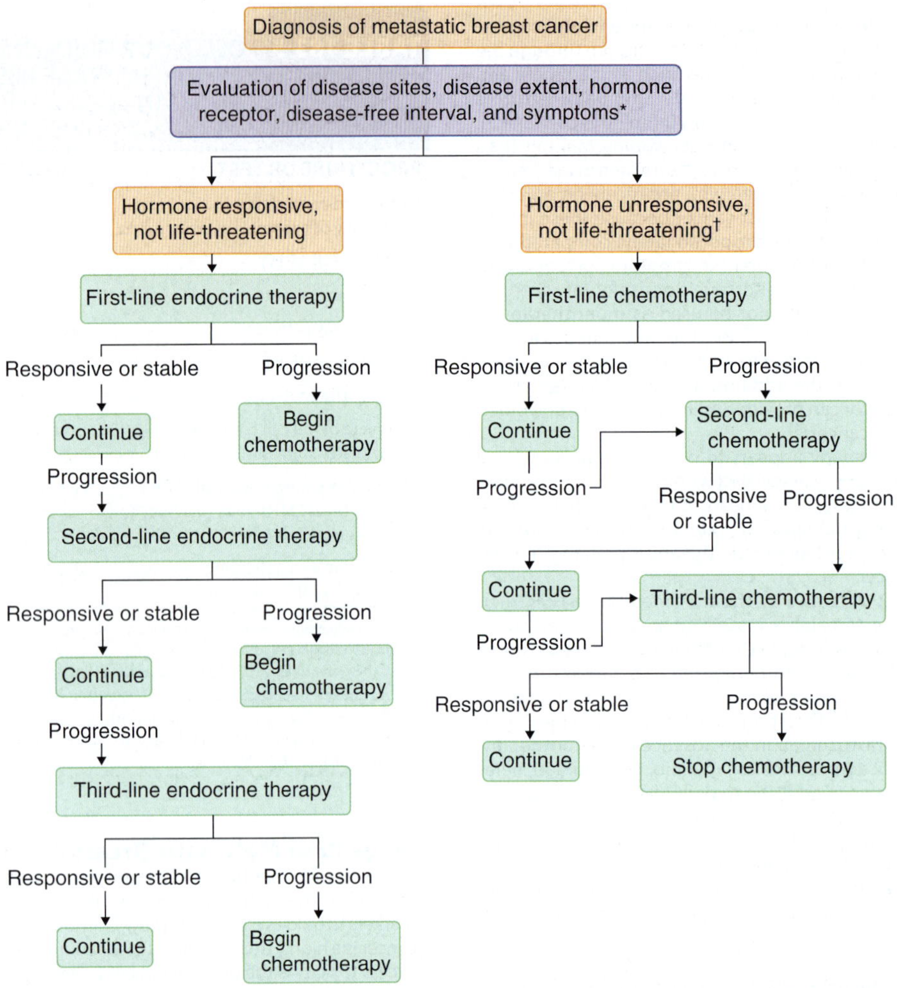

FIGURE 183-1. **An algorithm used for the systemic treatment of stage IV breast cancer.** *Consider use of bisphosphonate or denosumab if bone involvement and use of a CDK4/6 inhibitor with first-line endocrine therapy. †Consider integration of anti-HER2 therapy if the tumor overexpresses HER2 or pembrolizumab for triple-negative metastatic breast cancer.

fulvestrant.[A17] Other combination therapies (with the possible exception of ovarian suppression plus tamoxifen) do not improve outcomes.

Inhibitors of cyclin-dependent kinases 4 and 6 (e.g., palbociclib, ribociclib, and abemaciclib), which promote progression from the G1 phase to the S phase of the cell cycle, are now commonly used with endocrine therapy to improve outcomes. For example the combination of ribociclib plus letrozole increases survival[A18] in postmenopausal women with hormone-receptor-positive metastatic disease.

In patients who have PIK3CA-mutated hormone receptor–positive HER2-negative advanced breast cancer and who have previously received combination endocrine plus CDK4/6 inhibitor therapy, the addition of alpelisib (a PI3Kα-specific inhibitor) improves progression-free survival.[A19] Everolimus (but not temsirolimus) combined with an aromatase inhibitor can also improve progression-free survival compared with an aromatase inhibitor alone in patients with hormone receptor–positive advanced breast cancer previously treated with nonsteroidal aromatase inhibitors.

HER2-Expressing Tumors

Trastuzumab monotherapy under expert supervision can provide partial or complete tumor regression in about 30% of women who have metastatic HER2-overexpressing breast cancer. Concurrent trastuzumab with paclitaxel also increases the rate and duration of response as well as survival compared with paclitaxel alone for women with newly diagnosed HER2-overexpressing metastatic breast cancer. Seven other anti-HER2 agents now available for treatment of advanced breast cancer in the United States include the oral small molecule inhibitors (e.g., neratinib, tucatinib, and lapatinib), monoclonal antibodies (pertuzumab, which inhibits HER dimerization, as well as margetuximab-cmkb), and conjugates of a cytotoxic agent to trastuzumab (trastuzumab emtansine or trastuzumab deruxtecan).[16] The addition of pertuzumab to trastuzumab and docetaxel significantly improves outcomes in first-line treatment of metastatic HER2-positive breast cancer, whereas trastuzumab deruxtecan is preferred over trastuzumab emtansine in the second-line setting.[A20] Adding tucatinib to trastuzumab and capecitabine also can prolong survival in heavily pretreated patients.[A21]

Other Biologic Agents

The poly-ADP-ribose polymerase (PARP) inhibitors of DNA repair show activity in women with *BRCA* mutant breast cancer. Two inhibitors, olaparib[A22] and talzoparib,[A23] are now approved for use in women with germline *BRCA1*- or *BRCA2*-mutant advanced breast cancer.

Bevacizumab, which is a monoclonal antibody that targets the vascular endothelial growth factor, has only modest activity in metastatic breast cancer, whether used as monotherapy or in addition to taxane-based chemotherapy.

Chemotherapy

Most women with advanced breast cancer eventually become unresponsive to endocrine and other targeted therapies, at which time they become candidates for palliative chemotherapy. Serial chemotherapy under expert oversight is the norm. Patients receive two to four cycles of therapy and then are re-evaluated for stabilization or improvement. The duration of therapy varies depending on response, but quality of life is often better with continued therapy until the disease progresses, provided that side effects are tolerable.

Active agents include cyclophosphamide, doxorubicin, methotrexate, paclitaxel, docetaxel, vinorelbine, capecitabine, gemcitabine, carboplatin, ixabepilone, pegylated doxorubicin, eribulin, nano-albumin–bound paclitaxel, and sacituzumab govitecan-hziy. However, pembrolizumab may be combined with chemotherapy in patients who have advanced triple-negative breast cancer that expresses PD-L1.[A24]

As with endocrine therapy, response rates and duration diminish with each successive change in therapy. High-dose chemotherapy combined with autologous stem cell or bone marrow support is not of incremental benefit. A difficult question for patient and doctor is when to stop chemotherapy. No consensus guidelines indicate when to discontinue chemotherapy, but many patients and physicians move to a program of supportive care if two successive chemotherapy regimens fail to produce a tumor response or to stabilize the disease.

Supportive Care

Bone Health

Because palliation of symptoms and prevention of complications of metastatic disease are the primary goals of treatment for advanced breast cancer, careful attention to supportive care is vital. Bone is the most common site of metastasis in breast cancer, and bone disease can be a source of significant morbidity. The regular administration of a bisphosphonate such as zoledronate or pamidronate or the anti-RANKL monoclonal antibody denosumab (Chapter 225), in addition to endocrine therapy or chemotherapy, can reduce pain and the incidence of skeletal complications in metastatic disease. Bisphosphonates are sometimes used as adjuvant therapy to try to reduce the rate of recurrent breast cancer in the bone and to improve breast cancer survival in early-stage postmenopausal patients, and denosumab (60 mg subcutaneously every 6 months) is another alternative in this setting.[A25]

Postmenopausal Symptoms

Postmenopausal symptoms (Chapter 222) are common in breast cancer survivors as a consequence of therapy or of natural aging. In general, hormone replacement therapy should be avoided in women with a history of breast cancer. A short course of treatment can be considered in patients who have early-stage breast cancer who have truly disabling symptoms. Topical estrogens are considered for women with vaginal dryness that does not respond to lubricants. Otherwise, vasomotor symptoms may be reduced by nonhormonal therapies (Chapter 222).

Lymphedema

Lymphedema develops in the ipsilateral arm in up to 15% of women after treatment for early breast cancer. Its incidence is lower with sentinel lymph node procedures and meticulous radiotherapy. Prevention includes avoidance of trauma and possibly exercises. Early recognition of symptoms is key. Affected patients should be referred to specialists for consideration of treatments such as manual drainage or the use of compression stockings or pumps.

Breast Cancer During Pregnancy

The risk for breast cancer is slightly increased during and just after pregnancy (Chapter 221). Suspicious breast findings during pregnancy should be investigated vigorously. Surgical therapy can be safely performed for breast cancer after the first trimester of pregnancy, but radiotherapy should be delayed until after delivery. Certain adjuvant chemotherapy regimens can be safely administered in the second and third trimesters of pregnancy under expert oversight. Administration of antimetabolites should be avoided because of the potential for damage to the placenta. Initiation of endocrine therapy is generally delayed until after delivery. Pregnancy after a diagnosis of early breast cancer does not appear to increase the risk for metastatic disease. The major considerations for women contemplating pregnancy should be its timing with regard to endocrine therapy, which may require 5 or more years to complete, as well as the underlying risk for recurrent breast cancer.

Breast Cancer in Men

Men account for not more than 1% of breast cancer cases.[17] Failure of the patient or health care provider to diagnose the disease means that it may be diagnosed at a later stage. Germline DNA repair gene mutations (especially *BRCA2*) are associated with breast cancer in men, and men with breast cancer should be offered genetic counseling and testing of relevant genes.[18] Most breast cancers in men express the estrogen receptor, and treatment recommendations for these men are generally similar to those for postmenopausal women.[19]

PREVENTION

Current strategies to prevent breast cancer include surgical, chemopreventive, and lifestyle modification approaches.

Prophylactic Mastectomy and Oophorectomy

Prophylactic mastectomy appears to reduce the risk for developing breast cancer by approximately 90% in individuals who are at high risk because of a strong family history or carriage of a germline *BRCA1* or *BRCA2* or related mutation. However, women who opt for prophylactic mastectomy must be counseled about the possibility that cancer may develop in remnants of breast tissue that persist after prophylactic mastectomy. In carriers of *BRCA* mutations, prophylactic oophorectomy can decrease the incidence of breast cancer by approximately 50%, presumably because of a reduction in ovarian steroids.

Chemoprevention

Tamoxifen (20 mg daily) reduces the risk of invasive breast cancer by about 40% in high-risk women (i.e., women who are age 60 years or older, have a diagnosis of lobular carcinoma in situ, or are ages 35 to 59 years with a constellation of risk factors that, when combined, result in a 1.67% or greater risk for breast cancer within 5 years).[20] Side effects include an increased risk for endometrial cancer and thromboembolic events in women over age 50 years. Raloxifene (60 mg daily) reduces the incidence of breast cancer in postmenopausal women who are at average risk of breast cancer but at elevated risk for cardiovascular disease, but it is less effective than tamoxifen for preventing invasive breast cancer in high-risk postmenopausal women. Raloxifene is associated with fewer uterine cancers but the same risk for thromboembolic events compared with tamoxifen. Other aromatase inhibitors (exemestane or anastrozole) also lower the incidence of breast cancer by approximately 50% in moderate- to high-risk postmenopausal women.[A26] Based on these data, the U.S. Preventative Services Task Force recommends tamoxifen, raloxifene, or aromatase inhibitors for women who have an increased risk of breast cancer and a low risk of adverse effects from these medications.[21,22]

TABLE 183-6 BREAST CANCER SCREENING IN WOMEN WITHOUT KNOWN GENETIC MUTATIONS (E.G., *BRCA1* OR *BRCA2*) OR FAMILIAL BREAST CANCER SYNDROME

TEST	ACS	USPSTF
Mammography	For average risk: Annual aged 45-54 yr Biennial (or annual) aged 55 yr and older if healthy and life expectancy ≥10 yr Option if 40-44 yr	Individual decision before age 50 Every 2 yr, aged 50-74 yr; insufficient evidence aged ≥75 yr
Clinical breast examination	Not recommended	Insufficient evidence to support
Breast self-examination	Not recommended	Not recommended

ACS = American Cancer Society; USPSTF = U.S. Preventive Services Task Force.

A vitamin A derivative, fenretinide, showed some impact as a chemopreventive agent for secondary prevention in premenopausal breast cancer survivors but has not found a place in routine practice. Finally, large epidemiologic studies have raised the possibility that aspirin or certain statins might also decrease breast cancer risk, but these agents have not yet been prospectively tested.

Lifestyle Modification

Regular exercise, especially during adolescence, may be associated with reduced risk of breast cancer. By extrapolation from the epidemiologic studies, abstinence from alcohol might slightly reduce the risk for breast cancer. A low-fat diet has not been shown to prevent breast cancer.

Screening

Conventional breast self-examination is not an effective screening tool, so many experts now promote breast awareness rather than regular breast self-examination. Breast examinations by a clinician have not been rigorously assessed, but the combination of examination plus mammography appears to decrease mortality from breast cancer by approximately 20% for average-risk women of all ages and by 25 to 30% in women over age 50 years. Considerable controversy continues over the value of screening mammography in women ages 40 to 50 years and women over age 70 years, as well as the optimal interval between mammograms for women ages 50 to 70 years. For example, a large randomized trial of annual mammography screening in women ages 40 to 49 years showed a 25% reduction in mortality from breast cancer at 10 years but no further reduction over the next 12 years.[A27] Currently, the American Cancer Society does not recommend clinical breast examination for cancer screening among average-risk women at any age, but it recommends annual screening mammography for women at standard risk for breast cancer starting at age 45 years (with opportunity to begin at age 40 years) and biennial screening (with opportunity to continue annual screening) beginning at age 55 years. In contrast, the U.S. Preventive Services Task Force and the American College of Physicians recommend that women between ages 40 and 50 years of age be counseled about the risks and benefits of screening mammography and that screening mammography can be used at 2-year intervals for women ages 50 to 74 years (Table 183-6). However, women ages 40 to 49 years with a two-fold increased risk for breast cancer have benefit-to-harm ratios for biennial screening mammography similar to average-risk women ages 50 to 74 years. In general, screening is unlikely to be worthwhile for women with a life expectancy of less than 10 years.

The survival benefits of mammography come at the cost of false-positive results that lead to anxiety and further evaluation.[23] By various estimates, more than 50% of women who are screened by mammography have false-positive results over 10 years of screening, and 7 to 9% are recommended for breast biopsy. Other studies have estimated an overdiagnosis rate of 3.3% for invasive cancer and from 18 to 32% for carcinoma in situ. The radiation exposure from mammography is estimated to cause 2 to 11 deaths per 100,000 screened women. Furthermore, some analysts suggest that the reduction in breast cancer mortality after the introduction of screening mammography is mostly a result of improved therapy rather than earlier diagnosis.

Screening mammography fails to diagnose approximately 10 to 15% of breast cancers, and screening MRI should be considered for women whose predicted risk for breast cancer exceeds 20%. MRI also can detect breast cancer in the contralateral breast in 3% of women with a newly diagnosed breast cancer whose contralateral mammogram showed no abnormality.

For women with dense breasts, digital mammography may be more useful than conventional mammography. Another alternative is adjunctive ultrasonography, which similarly increases sensitivity and the detection rate of cancers but also has significantly more false positive results.

Supplemental MRI also increases the sensitivity for diagnosing cancer in women with extremely dense breasts.[A28,A29] However, the use of MRI in the general population is limited by the fact that it is highly sensitive but lacks specificity. As a result, MRI has not translated into improved selection of surgical treatments or a reduction in the number of operations.

PROGNOSIS

Five-year life expectancy is 99% for localized disease and over 85% for regional disease. For stage III disease, multimodality therapy results in a 5-year disease-free survival rate of approximately 50%. The median survival after diagnosis of metastatic breast cancer is 2 to 3 years, although the range is great, and a small cadre of long-term survivors has been described. Poor prognosis is associated with high lymph node burden, poor histologic grade, large tumor size, absence of expression of estrogen receptors or progesterone receptors, and overexpression of HER2. Recent clinical trials document small improvements in survival with newer therapies.

BENIGN BREAST LESIONS

Benign breast disease includes mastalgia (pain and tenderness), mastitis (including infectious and noninfectious inflammatory conditions), trauma, and benign tumors.[24]

MASTALGIA

Mastalgia can be caused by trauma or by extramammary conditions, such as myocardial ischemia, pneumonia, pleural irritation, esophageal spasm, costochondritis, rib fracture, and varicella-zoster virus (preceding the skin eruption). After these conditions have been excluded, mastalgia is considered to be a benign condition that is self-limited. It can be cyclical or noncyclical in timing (where it is thought to be related to hormonal activity), and it may occur in postmenopausal women, even in the absence of hormone replacement therapy.

MASTITIS

Mastitis, which is caused by breast inflammation or infection, can occur in either nonlactating or lactating women. The typical presentation in nonlactating women is occurrence in their 40s with the acute onset of severe breast pain and tenderness followed by erythema and swelling that tends to be localized in the nipple-areolar area. In most cases, the cause is rupture of dilated subareolar ducts, followed by an inflammatory response to leakage of intraductal contents into periductal tissue. Infection is difficult to exclude, and patients are often treated with empirical antibiotics (e.g., oral cephalexin 250 mg every 6 hours or dicloxacillin 250 mg every 6 hours). If symptoms do not resolve within 7 to 10 days on antibiotics, ultrasound is required to exclude abscess.[25] If an abscess is found, incision and drainage are required. The most important differential diagnosis with mastitis is inflammatory carcinoma, and failure to improve with antibiotics or to find an abscess should lead to evaluation by a breast surgeon.

Mastitis in lactating women is often due to infection caused by a break in the skin of the nipple or milk stasis. *Staphylococcus aureus, Staphylococcus albus*, and sometimes *Escherichia coli, Corynebacteria*, or streptococci are the most common pathogens. Treatment requires antibiotics and removal of milk.

NONPROLIFERATIVE AND PROLIFERATIVE BENIGN BREAST LESIONS

The most common nonproliferative breast condition is fibrocystic breast disease, which is now more appropriately called *fibrocystic changes*. Fibrocystic changes are observed clinically in up to 50% of women and histologically in 90% of women. Lesions are composed of varying amounts of fibrosis and cysts, sometimes associated with calcifications and inflammation. Simple or complex cysts should be aspirated with ultrasound guidance and, when the fluid is not clear, sent for cytologic analysis.

Other nonproliferative benign breast lesions that can initially present as tumor-like processes include fibroadenomas (which are seen in about 25% of women and are usually solitary, sharply demarcated, smooth lesions in younger patients); phyllodes tumor (previously known as cystosarcoma phyllodes); and intraductal papillomas, which are solitary lesions that may be accompanied by bloody nipple discharge. Less-common nonproliferative benign breast lesions include inflammatory fat necrosis, which follows surgical or blunt trauma and generally resolves spontaneously; lymphocytic mastitis, which may be seen in diabetic patients; and granulomatous mastitis, which is associated with foreign body reactions (e.g., silicone and paraffin for breast augmentation and reconstruction after cancer surgery), sarcoid (Chapter 83), or certain infections.

Proliferative benign breast lesions include ductal or lobular hyperplasia. Atypical hyperplasias are associated with increased risk for breast cancer.

Overall, the relative risk for breast cancer for women with biopsy-proved benign breast disease is 1.5 to 1.6 compared with women in the general population, with this increased risk persisting for at least 25 years after the original biopsy. The relative risk for developing cancer is 4.24 with atypia, 1.9 with proliferative changes without atypia, and 1.3 with nonproliferative lesions. However, about 50% of the later cancers arise in the contralateral breast, thereby suggesting that these findings are more a marker than a cause of subsequent breast cancers.

GENERAL REFERENCES

For the General References and other additional features, please visit Elsevier eBooks+ at https://ebooks.health.elsevier.com.

Grade A References

A1. Chlebowski RT, Anderson GL, Aragaki AK, et al. Association of menopausal hormone therapy with breast cancer incidence and mortality during long-term follow-up of the Women's Health Initiative randomized clinical trials. *JAMA*. 2020;324:369-380.

A2. Piccart M, van't Veer LJ, Poncet C, et al. 70 gene signature as an aid for treatment decision in early breast cancer: updated results of the phase 3 randomized MINDACT trial with an exploratory analysis by age. *Lancet Oncol*. 2021;22:476-488.

A3. Kunkler IH, Williams LJ, Jack WJL, et al. Breast-conserving surgery with or without irradiation in early breast cancer. *N Engl J Med*. 2023;388:585-594.

A4. Early Breast Cancer Trialists' Collaborative Group (EBCTCG). Long-term outcomes for neoadjuvant versus adjuvant chemotherapy in early breast cancer: meta-analysis of individual patient data from ten randomised trials. *Lancet Oncol*. 2018;19:27-39.

A5. Pan H, Gray R, Braybrooke J, et al. 20-year risks of breast-cancer recurrence after stopping endocrine therapy at 5 years. *N Engl J Med*. 2017;377:1836-1846.

A6. Francis PA, Pagani O, Fleming GF, et al. Tailoring adjuvant endocrine therapy for premenopausal breast cancer. *N Engl J Med*. 2018;379:122-137.

A7. Lambertini M, Moore HCF, Leonard RCF, et al. Gonadotropin-releasing hormone agonists during chemotherapy for preservation of ovarian function and fertility in premenopausal patients with early breast cancer: a systematic review and meta-analysis of individual patient-level date. *J Clin Oncol*. 2018;36:1981-1990.

A8. Early Breast Cancer Trialists' Collaborative Group (EBCTCG). Aromatase inhibitors versus tamoxifen in early breast cancer: patient-level meta-analysis of the randomized trials. *Lancet*. 2015;386:1341-1352.

A9. Early Breast Cancer Trialists' Collaborative Group (EBCTCG). Aromatase inhibitors versus tamoxifen in premenopausal women with oestrogen receptor-positive early-stage breast cancer treated with ovarian suppression: a patient-level meta-analysis of 7030 women from four randomised trials. *Lancet Oncol*. 2022;23:382-392.

A10. Harbeck N, Rastogi P, Martin M, et al. Adjuvant abemaciclib combined with endocrine therapy for high-risk early breast cancer: updated efficacy and Ki-67 analysis from the monarchE study. *Ann Oncol*. 2021;32:1571-1581.

A11. Gnant M, Fitzal F, Rinnerthaler G, et al. Duration of adjuvant aromatase-inhibitor therapy in postmenopausal breast cancer. *N Engl J Med*. 2021;385:395-405.

A12. Early Breast Cancer Trialists" Collaborative Group (EBCTCG). Trastuzumab for early-stage HER-2 positive breast cancer: a meta-analysis of 13,864 women in seven randomized trials. *Lancet Oncol*. 2021;22:1139-1150.

A13. von Minckwitz G, Huang CS, Mano MS, et al. Trastuzumab emtansine for residual invasive HER2-positive breast cancer. *N Engl J Med*. 2019;380:617-628.

A14. Early Breast Cancer Trialists' Collaborative Group (EBCTCG). Increasing the dose intensity of chemotherapy by more frequent administration or sequential scheduling: a patient-level meta-analysis of 37, 298 women with early breast cancer in 26 randomised trials. *Lancet*. 2019;393:1440-1452.

A15. Tutt ANJ, Garber JE, Kaufman B, et al. Adjuvant olaparib for patients with BRCA1 or BRCA2-mutated breast cancer. *N Engl J Med*. 2021;384:2394-2405.

A16. Schmid P, Cortes J, Dent R, et al. Event-free survival with pembrolizumab in early triple-negative breast cancer. *N Engl J Med*. 2022;386:556-567.

A17. Mehta RS, Barlow WE, Albain KS, et al. Overall survival with fulvestrant plus anastrozole in metastatic breast cancer. *N Engl J Med*. 2019;380:1226-1234.

A18. Hortobagyi GH, Stemmer SM, Burris HA, et al. Overall survival with ribociclib plus letrozole in advanced breast cancer. *N Engl J Med*. 2022;386:942-950.

A19. André F, Ciruelos E, Rubovszky G, et al. Alpelisib for PIK3CA-mutated, hormone receptor-positive advanced breast cancer. *N Engl J Med*. 2019;380:1929-1940.

A20. Cortes J, Kim SB, Chung WP, et al. Trastuzumab deruxtecan versus trastuzumab emtansine for breast cancer. *N Engl J Med*. 2022;386:1143-1154.

A21. Murthy RK, Loi S, Okines A, et al. Tucatinib, trastuzumab, and capecitabine for HER2-positive metastatic breast cancer. *N Engl J Med*. 2020;382:597-609.

A22. Robson M, Im SA, Senkus E, et al. Olaparib for metastatic breast cancer in patients with a germline BRCA mutation. *N Engl J Med*. 2017;377:523-533.

A23. Litton JK, Rugo HS, Ettl J, et al. Talazoparib in patients with advanced breast cancer and a germline BRCA mutation. *N Engl J Med*. 2018;379:753-763.

A24. Cortes J, Rugo HS, Cescon SA, et al. Pembrolizumab plus chemotherapy in advanced triple-negative breast cancer. *N Engl J Med*. 2022;387:217-226.

A25. Gnant M, Frantal S, Pfeiler G, et al. Long-term outcomes of adjuvant denosumab in breast cancer. *NEJM Evid*. 2022;1.

A26. Cuzick J, Sestak I, Forbes JF, et al. Use of anastrozole for breast cancer prevention (IBIS-II): long-term results of a randomised controlled trial. *Lancet*. 2020;395:117-122.

A27. Duffy SW, Vulkan D, Cuckle H, et al. Effect of mammographic screening for age 40 years on breast cancer mortality (UK Age trial): final results of a randomized, controlled trial. *Lancet Oncol*. 2020;21:1165-1172.

A28. Comstock CE, Gatsonis C, Newstead GM, et al. Comparison of abbreviated breast MRI vs digital breast tomosynthesis for breast cancer detection among women with dense breasts undergoing screening. *JAMA*. 2020;323:746-756.
A29. Bakker MF, de Lange SV, Pijnappel RM, et al. Supplemental MRI screening for women with extremely dense breast tissue. *N Engl J Med*. 2019;381:2091-2102.

184 GYNECOLOGIC CANCERS

DEBORAH K. ARMSTRONG

Gynecologic cancers are not common, but earlier diagnosis is always associated with improved survival and a greater chance for cure. Although most care is provided by gynecologic surgeons and oncologists, patients may first present to other physicians with signs or symptoms that require evaluation. Furthermore, all physicians share responsibility for encouraging recommended cancer screening.

CERVICAL CANCER

EPIDEMIOLOGY

Cancer of the uterine cervix is the third most common gynecologic cancer in the United States. A more than 80% decrease in the incidence of cervical cancer since the 1950s is related to screening, initially for abnormal cervical cytology with the Papanicolaou (Pap) test and now for high-risk human papillomavirus (HPV) infection. These demographic trends are seen throughout the developed world, yet cervical cancer remains a major cause of cancer-related deaths in women worldwide, particularly in Central and South America and in Africa, owing to lack of access to screening and treatment. In the United States, over 14,000 new cases of cervical cancer and over 4000 cancer-related deaths occur annually.[1]

HPV infection is central to the development of preinvasive and invasive disease and is detected in more than 99% of cervical cancers.[2] Risk factors for cervical cancer (Table 184-1) are mostly related to increased risk of acquiring HPV or increased virulence of HPV infection.

Of the more than 200 strains of HPV (Chapter 344), about 40 infect the genital tract. Low-risk HPV causes genital warts, whereas high-risk HPV causes cancers of the anogenital tract, including cervical, vaginal, vulvar, anal, and penile cancers, as well as oral and throat cancers. Among the approximately one dozen high-risk HPVs, two types, HPV 16 and HPV 18, cause 70% of cervical cancers, and HPV types 31, 33, 45, 52, and 58 cause an additional 20% of cases. HPV is transmitted sexually through genital-genital or genital-oral contact, and the majority of sexually active individuals will be infected with HPV at some time, usually near the beginning of sexual activity, even though its transmission is significantly diminished with the use of condoms.

PATHOBIOLOGY

HPVs are small, nonenveloped, double-stranded DNA viruses protected by a capsid formed by late proteins, L1 and L2 (Chapter 344). The regulation of viral gene expression is complex and controlled by host cellular and viral transcription factors. HPV infection occurs at the basal cell layer of stratified squamous epithelial cells, thereby resulting in cellular proliferation, with pathologic findings from benign hyperplasia to dysplasia to invasive carcinoma. The E6 and E7 proteins of the high-risk HPV types act as viral oncoproteins that suppress normal, negative growth regulation. E6 binds to and degrades the tumor suppressor protein p53, thereby inhibiting normal apoptotic cell death, contributing to immortalization of HPV-infected cells. Similarly, E7 binds to and degrades the pRB tumor suppressor protein and targets cellular cyclins and cyclin-dependent kinases that are critical for cell cycle regulation. Both E6 and E7 have immunosuppressive effects that contribute to immune evasion and induction of peripheral tolerance in cytotoxic T lymphocytes.

HPV infects cutaneous and mucosal epithelial tissues with tropism for the anogenital tract. Most HPV infections are transient, asymptomatic, and without clinical consequences. They clear within 1 to 2 years. In about 10% of infected women, HPV DNA will continue to produce viral proteins, thereby resulting in persistent infection. In some cases, the HPV DNA is silenced, thereby resulting in latency of variable duration, but can be reactivated later. The persistence of HPV in a latent state requires maintenance of the viral genome in the infected cell, either as an episome or integrated into the host cell DNA. Persistent HPV infection is necessary for the development of precancerous cervical changes and, subsequently, cervical cancer.

TABLE 184-1 RISK FACTORS FOR CERVICAL CANCER

- Human papillomavirus
- Early onset of sexual activity
- Multiple sexual partners
- History of genital warts
- Multiparity
- Lower socioeconomic status
- Cigarette smoking
- Long-term use of oral contraceptive agents
- Human immunodeficiency virus infection
- Immunodeficiency state
- In utero diethylstilbestrol (DES) exposure
- Hispanic and Black American women

The cervical cells targeted by HPV are in the squamocolumnar junction, where the squamous cells of the ectocervix meet the columnar cells of the endocervix. The position of the squamocolumnar junction migrates with age and is altered by hormonal and reproductive factors. The susceptibility of the squamocolumnar junction to the carcinogenic effects of HPV is higher in adolescents and younger women and declines with hormonal maturation of the cervix. The carcinogenic effects of HPV take approximately a decade to develop into malignancy. Cervical cancer presents at a median age of 48 years.

CLINICAL MANIFESTATIONS AND DIAGNOSIS

Early-stage cervical cancer is largely asymptomatic, and detection is generally made by colposcopy and biopsy for abnormalities that are detected by screening. Cervical cancer frequently spreads by local extension to the uterine corpus, vagina, bladder, and parametria. In advanced stages, patients may present with pain with intercourse, vaginal discharge or bleeding, pelvic pain, or abnormalities of bowel, bladder, or sexual function.

In advanced cases, direct visualization of the cervix may reveal an obvious lesion for biopsy. In these cases, Pap smear is not adequate for diagnostic purposes, and the patient should be referred for biopsy.

Careful and thorough clinical evaluation by a gynecologic oncologist is required. In addition to pelvic and rectovaginal examination, staging may include examination under anesthesia, cystoscopy, proctoscopy, and imaging such as magnetic resonance imaging (MRI), computed tomography (CT), or positron emission tomography (PET).

TREATMENT AND PROGNOSIS

The treatment of cervical cancer is guided predominantly by the stage of the disease (Table 184-2). Survival from cervical cancer is higher when women are managed by a gynecologic oncologist, and prompt referral is important. In addition to clinical stage, treatment decisions must consider the patient's age, desire for fertility, and comorbid conditions, as well as the size of the tumor.

In some cases, a cervical cone biopsy (excision of a cone-shaped circumferential wedge from the cervix, the transformation zone, and at least a portion of the endocervical canal, called conization) or loop electrosurgical excision procedure (LEEP) may be sufficient for women with microscopic disease.[A1]

However, treatment of low-volume disease limited to the cervix is generally radical hysterectomy, although simple hysterectomy is an alternative in very-low-risk disease. In women undergoing radical hysterectomy, open surgery is indicated because it provides better disease-free survival compared with minimally invasive approaches (e.g., laparoscopic or robot-assisted laparoscopic).[A2] In limited situations in which the preservation of fertility is desired, a radical trachelectomy (removal of the cervix only) can be performed.

When hysterectomy reveals invasion of the lymphovascular space, deep cervical stromal involvement, larger-than-expected tumor size, positive surgical margins, parametrial involvement, or nodal involvement, adjuvant postoperative radiation therapy[A3] is typically recommended under expert supervision (see Table 184-2). Patients with stages IIB to IVA cancers should be treated with definitive chemoradiation therapy using radiation-sensitizing weekly cisplatin in combination with radiation therapy. Patients with persistent recurrent or metastatic cervical cancer are generally treated with systemic therapy containing a platinum taxane doublet. Bevacizumab, which is an antibody to vascular endothelial growth factor (VEGF), provides an incremental survival benefit when combined with initial chemotherapy for advanced cervical cancer.[A4] The immune checkpoint inhibitor pembrolizumab can be combined with chemotherapy, with or without bevacizumab, for patients whose tumors express PD-L1.[A5]

Highly selected patients with a central recurrence of cervical cancer may be candidates for pelvic exenteration, which is a very morbid procedure that cures 25 to 50% of patients. Otherwise, recurrent cervical cancer, though treatable, is usually not curable. Systemic chemotherapy under expert supervision is the usual approach. Palliative localized radiation may be used to manage symptoms.

TABLE 184-2 APPROACH TO CERVIX CANCER BY STAGE*

STAGE	BRIEF DEFINITION	USUAL TREATMENT
0	Carcinoma in situ	Conization, hysterectomy†
I	Cervical cancer confined to the uterus	
IA1	Microscopic stromal invasion <3 mm plus invasion of the lymphovascular space‡	Conization, hysterectomy† Radical hysterectomy or CRT
IA2	Microscopic stromal invasion 3 to 5 mm	Radical hysterectomy or CRT
IB1	Visible lesion ≤4 cm in greatest dimension§	Radical hysterectomy or CRT
IB2	Visible lesion >4 cm in greatest dimension	Radical hysterectomy or CRT
II	Limited cervical cancer spread beyond the uterus	
IIA	Tumor beyond the uterus, no parametrial involvement	
IIA1	Visible lesion ≤4 cm in greatest dimension	Radical hysterectomy or CRT
IIA2	Visible lesion >4 cm in greatest dimension	Radical hysterectomy or CRT
IIB	Parametrial extension	CRT
III	Pelvic extension of cervical cancer	
IIIA	Tumor involves lower third of the vagina but no pelvic wall extension	CRT
IIIB	Tumor extends to pelvic wall, hydronephrosis, or regional nodes	CRT
IVA	Involvement of mucosa of bowel or bladder	CRT
IVB	Distant metastatic disease	Chemotherapy¶

*Cervical cancer is staged clinically, radiographically, and pathologically. Staging may include findings at examination under anesthesia, imaging, and pathology, where available, to supplement clinical findings with respect to tumor size and extent, in all stages. Gynecologic cancers are most commonly staged using the FIGO (Fédération Internationale de Gynécologie et d'Obstétrique) staging system.
†If positive margins after cone, repeat cone or perform hysterectomy.
‡Hysterectomy recommended for lymphovascular space invasion.
§Chemoradiation therapy (CRT) includes weekly cisplatin treatment with definitive radiation therapy.
¶Initial chemotherapy for metastatic disease is generally a platinum taxane doublet with bevacizumab. Pembrolizumab can be added to chemotherapy for patients whose tumors express PD-L1.

PREVENTION

Human Papillomavirus Vaccine

Routine HPV vaccination should be given at ages 11 to 12 years, regardless of gender or gender identity, but can be given as early as age 9 years (Chapters 15 and 344). A two-dose series given 6 to 12 months apart is now recommended for any child who initiates vaccination before age 15 years. The vaccination is also indicated for previously unvaccinated adults up to age 45 years (see Table 344-2). Vaccination of males is critical not only to prevent the spread of HPV to female partners but also to prevent HPV-associated head and neck cancers (Chapter 176).

Pregnancy testing is not required before HPV vaccination, but vaccination should be delayed in pregnant women. Vaccination after treatment for cervical intraepithelial neoplasia types 2 and 3 may decrease the incidence of recurrence.

Three different HPV vaccines are approved by the FDA, but only the nine-valent vaccine is currently available in the United States. Trials of all three vaccines document a high level of safety.[A6] More than 97% of healthy vaccine recipients develop antibodies to HPV vaccine types after vaccination. All of the vaccines are highly effective in preventing sequelae of high-risk HPV in males and females, with 97% or greater efficacy.[A7] HPV vaccination also decreases invasive and pre-invasive cervical cancers in an age-dependent manner. The reduction in the incidence of cervical cancer and stage 3 cervical intraepithelial neoplasm is 87% for vaccination at ages 12 to 13 years, 62% for vaccination at age 14 to 16 years, and 34% for vaccination at ages 16 to 18 years compared with an unvaccinated cohort.[3]

A clinician's recommendation is one of the strongest drivers of adherence to vaccine recommendations. In the United States, about 75% of teens have received at least one dose of HPV vaccine, and nearly 60% are fully vaccinated, with rates slightly higher for females and in metropolitan areas. Lack of parental understanding about the necessity and safety of HPV vaccination appears to be the main reason why these rates are not higher. The U.S. Centers for Disease Control and Prevention (CDC) provides tools for clinicians to guide their recommendations, with an emphasis on cancer prevention.[4]

TABLE 184-3 CERVICAL CYTOLOGY AND HISTOPATHOLOGY

Dysplasia	Very mild	CIN1	LSIL
	Mild	CIN1	LSIL
	Moderate	CIN2	HSIL
	Severe	CIN3	HSIL
Carcinoma	In situ	CIN3	HSIL
	Invasive		

CIN = cervical intraepithelial neoplasia; HSIL = high-grade squamous intraepithelial lesion; LSIL = low-grade squamous intraepithelial lesion.

Screening Recommendations

The three options for cervical cancer screening are cervical cytology (Papanicolaou [Pap] test) alone, high-risk HPV testing, or cervical cytology and high-risk HPV testing together ("co-testing"). The U.S. Preventive Services Task Force and the American College of Obstetrics and Gynecology recommend cervical cytology every 3 years from ages 21 to 29 years, then cervical cytology every 3 years; high-risk HPV testing every 5 years from ages 30 to 65 years; or co-testing every 5 years from ages 30 to 65 years. The American Cancer Society recommends starting cervical cancer screening at age 25 years, with a high-risk HPV test alone every 5 years until age 65 years.

Adenocarcinoma may be better detected by HPV testing.[5,6] Screening is not recommended in women whose cervix has been removed, women younger than age 21 years, or women older than age 65 years who have previously been adequately screened. HPV vaccination status does not affect screening recommendations, so women who have been vaccinated against HPV should still follow these guidelines. Longer and more frequent screening are recommended for women who have had a positive Pap or HPV test, women who are at high risk for cervical cancer because of immunosuppression (e.g., HIV infection, organ transplantation, or long-term use of corticosteroids), or women who have had in utero exposure to diethylstilbestrol (DES).[7]

Interpretation of Screening Tests

Pap smear results are typically reported as normal, atypical squamous cells of undetermined significance (ASC-US), low-grade squamous intraepithelial lesion (LSIL), high-grade squamous intraepithelial lesion (HSIL), or atypical glandular cells. These cytologic findings generally correlate with subsequent histologic findings of varying degrees of dysplasia, cervical intraepithelial neoplasia (CIN), and carcinoma in situ or invasive carcinoma (Table 184-3). However, cytologic results may be associated with a subsequent histologic finding that is either more or less severe, so the results of cervical cytology are generally not used alone to make a definitive diagnosis or initiate treatment.

The recommended follow-up of an abnormal screening test follows an algorithm that incorporates current and prior test results, screening history, and age to estimate the risk of precancer. The finding of atypical squamous cells of undetermined significance conveys a low risk for progression to carcinoma. A low-grade squamous intraepithelial lesion, particularly in young women, is generally caused by a transient HPV infection. A high-grade squamous intraepithelial lesion is more likely to be associated with persistent HPV infection and a higher rate of progression to invasive cervical cancer. Colposcopy is recommended for most patients with positive HPV tests and abnormal Pap tests. The presence of atypical glandular cells on cervical cytology is a significant marker for premalignant disease of the cervix or endometrium, and evaluation should include testing of both these sites.

The colposcope is a lighted binocular microscope that magnifies the tissue of interest. Cervical colposcopy is used to examine the entire surface of the cervix, with emphasis on the squamocolumnar junction and transformation zones. Abnormal colposcopic findings are used to choose the sites to biopsy. In addition to cervical biopsy, repeat cervical cytology (with HPV testing, if indicated) and endocervical curettage may be obtained. The pathologic findings will guide follow-up and therapy, if necessary. Women with high-risk cytologic findings during pregnancy can still undergo colposcopy, although the endocervical curettage is omitted.

PROGNOSIS

Five-year survival rates are 92% for localized disease, about 60% for disease that has spread regionally, and about 20% for disease with distant spread. Cervical cancer survivors are also at risk for HPV-associated oropharyngeal (Chapter 176) and anal (Chapter 131) cancer.

The predominant site of recurrence for cervical cancer is locoregional at the vaginal apex or pelvic sidewall. Distant metastatic spread to lymph nodes, peritoneum, liver, lung, or bone can also be seen.

Median overall survival for individuals with advanced disease is less than 18 months. Death is usually associated with local recurrence and may also be associated with organ dysfunction such as hydronephrosis, bowel obstruction, and the formation of fistulas.

ENDOMETRIAL CANCER

Endometrial cancer arises from the inner epithelial lining of the uterus and is the most common gynecologic cancer in women in the United States. Most cancers are adenocarcinomas, but other rare histologic types include squamous cell, small cell, and transitional cell carcinomas.

EPIDEMIOLOGY

Endometrial cancer rates are rising in parallel with increasing obesity rates, with an estimated 67,000 new cases of endometrial cancer and 13,000 cancer-related deaths in the United States annually. Endometrial cancer is the fourth most common cancer in women after breast, lung, and colorectal cancers. Nearly 3% of women in the United States are expected to develop the disease. The average age of endometrial cancer diagnosis is 60 years, and it is rare in women before age 45 years. Endometrial cancer is more common in White women but has a higher mortality rate in Black women. A major factor for the development of endometrial cancer is estrogen exposure. Trends in the incidence of endometrial cancer may be largely explained by trends in exposure to endogenous estrogens and the use of exogenous estrogen in perimenopausal and postmenopausal women. Obesity is related to increased circulating estrogens due to increased aromatase activity in adipose tissue, thereby contributing to the conversion of adrenal androgens to estrogen (Table 184-4).

Women with a history of complex atypical hyperplasia have a nearly 30-fold risk for subsequently developing endometrial cancer. As the population ages, the incidence of endometrial cancer increases. The combination of improved life expectancy, decreasing parity, and rising rates of diabetes and obesity make endometrial cancer an increasing challenge in many developing and middle-income countries.

Most endometrial cancers are sporadic, but a small percentage (3 to 5%) of endometrial cancers are attributed to a genetic predisposition. Women with a family history of endometrial cancer are at a 1.5- to 2-fold increased risk for the disease. Lynch syndrome (also called *hereditary nonpolyposis colorectal cancer* [HNPCC; Chapter 179]) is the most common genetic syndrome associated with endometrial cancer and is caused by germline mutations in one of the DNA mismatch repair genes, *MLH1, MSH2, MSH6, PMS2*, or *EPCAM* (Chapter 166). Women with Lynch syndrome have up to a 80% lifetime risk for colorectal cancer and up to a 60% risk for developing endometrial cancer.

Cowden syndrome is a rare condition resulting from a mutation in the *PTEN* tumor suppressor gene. The lifetime risk for endometrial cancer is 13 to 20% in women with Cowden syndrome, a five-fold elevation compared with the general population.

PATHOBIOLOGY

More than 80% of endometrial cancers (type 1 endometrial cancers) are related to estrogen. The remaining 10 to 20% (type 2 endometrial cancers) are estrogen independent but share some risk factors with type 1 endometrial cancers, such as low parity, early age at menarche, and diabetes. The distinction between types 1 and 2 endometrial cancer is based on differences in histology and clinical outcomes, with type 2 having a poorer prognosis (Table 184-5). Type 1 malignancies tend to present with uterine-confined disease, generally have a better overall prognosis than the type 2 cancers, and often retain expression of hormone receptors. On a molecular level, type 1 tumors are more likely to be diploid, have loss of *PTEN*, retain wild-type *p53*, and be associated with microsatellite instability. Conversely, type 2 endometrial cancers are poorly differentiated; have serous, clear cell, or carcinosarcoma histology; often first present at advanced stages; and are at higher risk for disseminating. At the molecular level, type 2 endometrial cancers are higher grade, more frequently have aneuploidy, harbor mutations or loss of *p53*, and rarely express estrogen and progesterone receptors.

Endometrioid cancers include four subtypes (Fig. 184-1): *POLE* ultramutated, microsatellite instability hypermutated, copy number low (*TP53* wild-type), and copy number high (*TP53* mutated). In addition, about 25% of endometrioid tumors share characteristics with serous tumors, including extensive copy number alterations, few DNA methylation changes, low estrogen receptor and progesterone receptor expression, and frequent *TP53* mutations.

TABLE 184-4 RISK FACTORS FOR ENDOMETRIAL CANCER

- Complex atypical hyperplasia
- Unopposed estrogen exposure
- Obesity
- Increasing age
- Nulliparity
- Diabetes mellitus
- Early menarche, late menopause
- Tamoxifen use
- Family history of endometrial cancer
- Lynch syndrome (hereditary nonpolyposis colorectal cancer [HNPCC])
- Cowden syndrome

TABLE 184-5 TYPE 1 VERSUS TYPE 2 ENDOMETRIAL CANCERS

	TYPE 1 ENDOMETRIAL CANCERS	TYPE 2 ENDOMETRIAL CANCERS
Hormonal impact	Estrogen dependent	Estrogen independent
Histology	Endometrial adenocarcinoma	Clear cell or serous carcinosarcoma
Patient population	Younger, obese, perimenopausal	Older, thin, postmenopausal
Frequency	80-85%	15-20%
Prognosis	Lower grade; earlier stage; lower mortality rate	More aggressive; higher mortality rate
Molecular and genomic characteristics	ER/PR-positive; MSI	*P53* mutations; *ERBB2* overexpression

ER = estrogen receptor; MSI = microsatellite instability; PR = progesterone receptor.

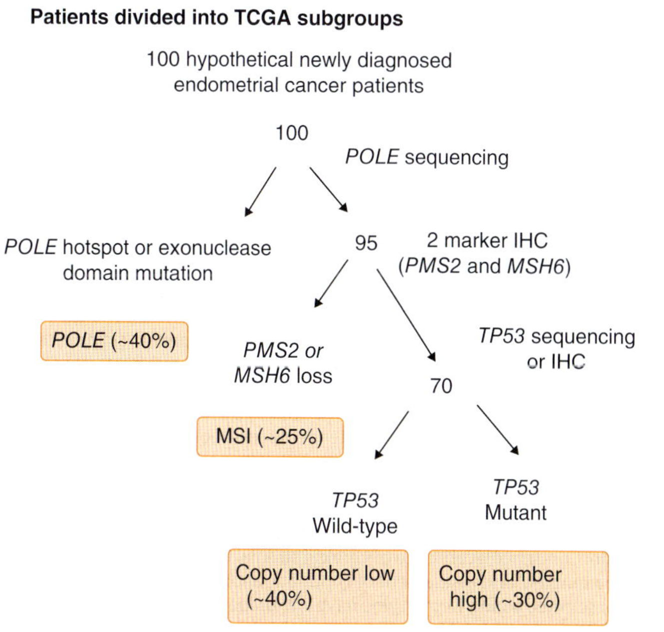

FIGURE 184-1. Suggested potential schema for molecular classification of endometrial cancer using sequencing and immunohistochemistry results to segregate patients into the molecular subtypes previously defined by The Cancer Genome Atlas (TCGA). IHC = immunohistochemistry; MSI = microsatellite instability; POLE = polymerase ε; TCGA = The Cancer Genome Atlas. (From MacKay HJ, Levine DA, Bae-Jump VL, et al. Moving forward with actionable therapeutic targets and opportunities in endometrial cancer: NCI clinical trials planning meeting report on identifying key genes and molecular pathways for targeted endometrial cancer trials. *Oncotarget*. 2017;8:84579-84594.)

About 30 to 40% of women with endometrioid endometrial cancer will have evidence of microsatellite instability, sometimes as a result of germline mutations in DNA mismatch repair genes (e.g., in Lynch syndrome), but more commonly from noninherited alterations, such as hypermethylation of the *MLH1* promoter or somatic mutations in the DNA mismatch repair genes that result in loss of protein expression. The proteins involved in mismatch repair correct errors that spontaneously occur during DNA replication, such as base mismatches or short insertions and deletions. Cells with deficient mismatch repair accumulate errors, creating novel microsatellite fragments. Mismatch repair–deficient cells have a marked increase in mutations: 1700 on average, compared with just 70 in a typical cancer cell. These mutations result in production of abnormal proteins that are recognized by the immune system as foreign.

CLINICAL MANIFESTATIONS AND DIAGNOSIS

The primary manifestation of endometrial cancer is postmenopausal vaginal bleeding (Chapter 218). Pap test results sometimes show signs of an abnormal endometrium. Any report of postmenopausal bleeding or of a suspicious finding on a Pap smear requires a thorough evaluation to exclude endometrial cancer. The initial approach to suspicious bleeding is pelvic examination, ultrasound imaging, and endometrial biopsy.

Special Considerations for Testing in Endometrial Cancer

Tumor tissue can be used to identify patients with abnormal DNA mismatch repair expression using immunohistochemistry for the four mismatch repair proteins. PCR to test for microsatellite instability requires tumor and normal tissue. Immunohistochemistry is frequently used because of the lower cost of this testing. In some cases, the etiology of loss of DNA mismatch repair protein expression can be identified by tumor tissue methylation testing. Tumors with deficient mismatch repair, regardless of site of origin, have a high response rate to immunotherapy with the PD-1 inhibitors pembrolizumab and dostarlimab, and an additional substantial fraction will have prolonged stable disease. All women who are diagnosed with endometrial cancer should undergo systematic clinical screening for Lynch syndrome (review of personal and family history) and/or molecular screening.

High-Risk Subtypes

Three high-risk histologic subtypes of endometrial cancer warrant special consideration: carcinosarcoma, serous carcinoma, and clear cell carcinoma. Uterine carcinosarcomas are rare, aggressive, biphasic neoplasms that contain high-grade malignant epithelial and mesenchymal elements. The mesenchymal component may resemble any one of a number of high-grade sarcomas. At the time of diagnosis, approximately one third of patients will have disease spread beyond the uterus. Uterine carcinosarcomas have frequent *TP53* mutations and are thus considered type 2 tumors. Uterine serous carcinomas are very aggressive neoplasms with a very high propensity for spread, including to distant sites in the upper abdomen, even when confined to the endometrium. Clear cell carcinomas are characterized by clear and often eosinophilic cells, and they are often aggressive.

TABLE 184-6 APPROACH TO ENDOMETRIAL CANCER BY STAGE*

STAGE	BRIEF DEFINITION	TREATMENT
I	Tumor confined to the uterine corpus	
IA	<50% myometrial invasion	TH, BSO, ± vag brachy†
IB	≥50% myometrial invasion	TH, BSO, ± vag brachy†
II	Cervical stromal involvement	TH, BSO, EBRT ± vag brachy‡
IIIA	Tumor involving uterine serosa and/or adnexa	TH, BSO, systemic therapy ± EBRT ± vag brachy
IIIB	Vaginal or parametrial involvement	TH, BSO, systemic therapy ± EBRT ± vag brachy§
IIIC1	Pelvic lymph node involvement	TH, BSO, systemic therapy ± EBRT ± vag brachy
IIIC2	Para-aortic lymph node involvement	TH, BSO, systemic therapy ± EBRT ± vag brachy
IVA	Tumor invades bladder or bowel	TH, BSO, systemic therapy ± EBRT ± vag brachy
IVB	Distant metastases, inguinal node involvement	TH, BSO, systemic therapy ± EBRT ± vag brachy

*Endometrioid histology.
†EBRT and systemic therapy can be considered for those with high-grade disease or adverse risk factors.
‡Systemic therapy can be considered for those with high-grade disease.
§Vaginal brachytherapy is recommended for stage IIIB.
BSO = bilateral salpingo-oophorectomy; EBRT= external beam radiation therapy; TH = total hysterectomy; vag brachy = vaginal brachytherapy.

TREATMENT

Fortunately, most women will have localized disease that is amenable to surgery. In almost all cases of pathologically confirmed endometrial cancer, hysterectomy with surgical staging is recommended. Minimally invasive surgery with a laparoscopic or robotic approach has largely replaced open surgical procedures for apparent uterine-confined disease. Total hysterectomy, bilateral salpingo-oophorectomy, peritoneal cytology (washings), and lymph node assessment are recommended. Visual inspection of the upper abdomen and pelvic surfaces is important to exclude extrauterine disease. Common sites of spread for endometrial cancer include the ovaries, pelvic or periaortic lymph nodes, and peritoneum. Sentinel node biopsy is an alternative at centers with expertise in these surgical methods. Comprehensive pathologic evaluation should include histologic subtype and grade, size and location of tumor, depth of myometrial invasion, presence or absence of cervical stromal involvement, involvement of the parametria, and assessment of lymphatic and vascular invasion.

For selected young women who have low-grade endometrial cancer and who desire to preserve fertility, or in women who are not medically fit for surgery, continuous progestin-based therapy with repeat endometrial sampling every 3 to 6 months can be considered. Radiation is another option for women with an absolute contraindication to surgical management.

Adjuvant Therapy

Surgical staging (Table 184-6) and identified risk factors guide recommendations for adjuvant, postoperative therapy. Risk factors include increasing age, invasion of the lymphovascular space, histology, tumor size, tumor grade, involvement of the lower uterine segment, or cervical stromal (glandular) involvement.[8,9]

For select women with uterine-confined disease, adjuvant, post-hysterectomy radiation with vaginal brachytherapy and/or external beam whole pelvic radiation therapy is sometimes considered.[A8] Systemic therapy has typically been with paclitaxel and carboplatin under expert supervision. Adjuvant treatment can reduce the risk for recurrence but may not have a significant impact on survival because of its toxicities. Numerous ongoing studies are evaluating the value of adding immunotherapy to initial chemotherapy.[10]

Advanced and Recurrent Disease

For women with adnexal, parametrial, or nodal involvement (stage III disease) or disseminated (stage IV) disease, systemic chemotherapy is as good as chemotherapy plus radiation.[A9] For women with distant metastases at the time of diagnosis, surgical debulking along with radiation for palliation is sometimes considered, but systemic chemotherapy is the standard of care.

For women with recurrent disease, systemic therapy is standard treatment. For low-grade tumors that are hormone receptor–positive, hormonal therapy under expert supervision can sometimes provide long-term treatment benefits. Progestational agents have traditionally been the backbone of hormonal treatment and can be used alone or with tamoxifen, but aromatase inhibitor therapy with everolimus or with palbociclib also has shown benefit.[A10]

Expert recommendations for systemic chemotherapy depend on prior treatment and time to recurrence. Bevacizumab alone or in combination with chemotherapy may be considered. In patients who have previously had chemotherapy, pembrolizumab or dostarlimab can be used for women who have a high tumor mutation burden or those whose tumor is deficient in the expression of DNA mismatch repair or has high microsatellite instability. Pembrolizumab in combination with lenvatinib can be used regardless of microsatellite status and is superior to second-line chemotherapy.[A11]

High-Risk Subtypes

High-risk subtypes (carcinosarcomas, serous carcinomas, and clear cell carcinomas) are more aggressive, have a higher propensity for advanced disease at diagnosis, and have a poorer overall prognosis. Systemic chemotherapy with or without radiation under expert supervision is recommended for almost all stages of these high-risk histologies. Uterine serous carcinomas and carcinosarcomas frequently overexpress ErbB2 (HER2), and HER2-directed therapy with trastuzumab should be added to chemotherapy when they do. For endometrial clear cell carcinomas, paclitaxel and carboplatin are considered standard therapy.

PREVENTION

On reaching menopause, all women should be informed about the risks and symptoms of endometrial cancer and strongly encouraged to report any unexpected vaginal bleeding or spotting to their physicians. No standard endometrial cancer screening is recommended for the general population.

The identification of Lynch syndrome in women with endometrial cancer can lead to the prevention of a second cancer in the patient and prevention of new, incident cancers in family members by using risk-reducing strategies and heightened surveillance.[11] Women with Lynch syndrome should be offered endometrial cancer screening with transvaginal ultrasound and endometrial biopsy annually starting at age 35 years. Hysterectomy with bilateral salpingo-oophorectomy is recommended for women with Lynch syndrome after the completion of childbearing.

PROGNOSIS

Five-year survival rates are about 92% for tumors that are confined to the corpus of the uterus but fall to about 75% if the tumor invades the cervical stroma, 50% with local or regional spread, and only 15% if the tumor invades either the bladder or bowel. Typical sites of recurrent endometrial cancer include local pelvic disease and distant metastases to the upper abdomen or lung. The risk for local pelvic recurrence is lower in patients who have received radiation therapy.

Uterine serous carcinomas represent less than 10% of endometrial cancers but are responsible for more than 30% of endometrial cancer mortality. Uterine carcinosarcomas account for less than 5% of uterine malignancies but have a poor overall prognosis. Endometrial clear cell carcinomas are rare tumors that have an aggressive clinical behavior and a poor outcome.

Survivors of endometrial cancer are at higher risk for a number of long-term cardiovascular problems compared with their cancer-free counterparts, including thrombophlebitis, pulmonary heart disease, and atrial fibrillation. In survivors of endometrial cancer, obesity is associated with lower health-related quality of life.

OVARIAN AND FALLOPIAN TUBE CANCER

DEFINITION

The ovary has three types of cells, all of which can become malignant: the ovarian epithelial cells that form the surface of the ovary; the supporting stromal cells that provide structural support to the follicles, maintain cellular organization within the ovary, and differentiate into steroid-secreting cells necessary to promote oocyte development and ovulation; and the ova that are the female germ cells necessary for reproduction. *Ovarian cancers* refer to epithelial ovarian cancers, cancers of the fallopian tube, and primary peritoneal cancers. Tumors of the ovarian epithelium, along with the cells of the fallopian tube and cells that line the peritoneal cavity give rise to what is commonly referred to as *ovarian epithelial malignancies.*

EPIDEMIOLOGY

Approximately 20,000 new cases of ovarian cancer are diagnosed annually in the United States Unfortunately, most women have advanced disease at diagnosis, and 13,000 women die annually of their disease. As a result, ovarian cancer has the highest mortality rate of all gynecologic malignancies. Because the incidence of ovarian cancer is highest in developed countries where parity is lower, diets are higher in fat, and women have longer life expectancies, its incidence is highest in North America and Europe but lower in much of Asia and sub-Saharan Africa. The lifetime risk for ovarian cancer in women in the United States is 1:70, or 1 to 2%. The median age of onset for ovarian cancer is 60 to 65 years, although women with a genetic predisposition to ovarian cancer may develop the disease in their 40s or 50s.

Although risk factors for ovarian cancer have been identified (Table 184-7), the cause of most ovarian cancers is not known. More frequent lifetime ovulation is associated with increased risk, and factors that suppress ovulation (e.g., pregnancy, use of oral contraceptives, and prolonged lactation) are associated with a decreased risk. Most of these risk factors are modest, with the exception of genetic predisposition related to inherited germline mutations in cancer-predisposing genes.

The risk of ovarian cancer is lower in women who have had a tubal ligation, which may result in necrosis of the fallopian tube and death of tubal epithelial cells. A weak association with the use of powder in the genital area has been suggested by case-control studies but is controversial and not substantiated by cohort studies.[12,13]

Approximately 80% of ovarian cancers are sporadic, but about 15 to 20% can be linked to autosomal dominant germline mutations.[14] *BRCA1* and *BRCA2* are the most common mutations, identified in about 15% of patients with advanced ovarian cancer (Chapter 166). Inherited mutations in these genes are associated with a 5- to 30-fold increase in the lifetime risk of ovarian cancer and with a significantly increased risk for breast and other cancers (Table 184-8). In addition to *BRCA1* and *BRCA2*, other genes associated with an increased ovarian cancer risk include *ATM, BRIP1, PALB2, BARD1, RAD51C, RAD51D*, and the Lynch syndrome genes (*MSH2, MLH1, PMS2*, and *MSH6*).[15] These genes combined are responsible for the remaining 5% of advanced ovarian cancers with an identified germline mutation. Most of these genes have a lower penetrance and may increase the lifetime risk of ovarian cancer to 5 to 15% or less.

TABLE 184-7 RISK FACTORS FOR OVARIAN CANCER

Increasing age
Factors associated with increased lifetime ovulation
- Early menarche
- Late menopause
- Nulliparity
- Infertility
- Use of ovulatory stimulating drugs
- Family history of ovarian cancer

Genetic predisposition
- *BRCA1* and *BRCA2*
- Lynch syndrome
- Other genes
- Decreased ovarian cancer risk
- Use of oral contraceptives
- Prolonged lactation
- Increased parity
- Tubal ligation

TABLE 184-8 *BRCA1* AND *BRCA2* PENETRANCE: CUMULATIVE LIFETIME CANCER RISK

	GENERAL POPULATION	*BRCA1*	*BRCA2*
Breast cancer	13%	50-72%	40-69%
Ovarian cancer	1-2%	35-60%	10-27%
Prostate cancer	11%	15-25%	15-25%
Pancreatic cancer	1-2%	Two-fold increase	Two- to five-fold increase

PATHOBIOLOGY

Histopathologic evaluation can identify several subtypes of epithelial ovarian cancer, the most common being serous, mucinous, clear cell, and endometrioid cancers. Endometrioid and clear cell carcinomas are much more common in early-stage ovarian cancer. By comparison, more than 80% of patients with advanced disease have high-grade, serous ovarian cancer, which is the best-understood ovarian cancer.

It is now clear that a significant portion, perhaps the majority, of serous ovarian cancers arise from the fallopian tube. The process of malignant transformation of the fallopian tube's epithelium is characterized by *p53* mutation, increased proliferation, cytologic atypia, detachment and exfoliation, metastasis, and implantation on peritoneal surfaces, including the ovary.[16]

CLINICAL MANIFESTATIONS AND DIAGNOSIS

Small adnexal masses are usually silent,[17] and most symptoms are related to disseminated disease within the abdomen and pelvis. The symptoms of dissemination include bloating, increased abdominal girth, early satiety, pelvic or abdominal pain, dyspareunia, and bowel or bladder complaints.

Ultrasonography or CT of the abdomen and pelvis will usually identify adnexal abnormalities and may also demonstrate ascites, lymphadenopathy, and omental or peritoneal involvement. Peritoneal fluid cytology can sometimes be diagnostic, but percutaneous biopsy of an apparently isolated adnexal mass is not recommended because of the potential for tumor spillage and spread of an otherwise localized tumor into the peritoneal cavity.

CA-125 is a glycoprotein encoded by the *MUC16* gene that is often significantly elevated in the serum of patients with ovarian cancer and can support the diagnosis of ovarian cancer. An elevated CA-125 alone is not diagnostic of ovarian cancer, because it can be elevated with other malignancies and with benign processes, especially conditions that affect the abdominal and peritoneal surfaces. It is also frequently normal when tumors are confined to the fallopian tube and/or ovary.

Ovarian cancer is often associated with inherited cancer-predisposing genes (Chapter 166). All women with ovarian cancer should undergo genetic counseling and consider genetic testing.

TREATMENT AND PROGNOSIS

Surgery and Neoadjuvant Therapy

In patients who are eligible, treatment of ovarian cancer starts with surgery, which should be performed by a gynecologic oncologist, preferably in a hospital with a high volume of ovarian cancer cases. Surgery makes the pathologic diagnosis and stages the patient's disease. Initial surgery should include an exploratory laparotomy, a total abdominal hysterectomy, bilateral salpingo-oophorectomy, omentectomy, removal of ascites or peritoneal washings, and, in certain circumstances, lymph node dissection. The diaphragm and upper abdomen should be inspected, and biopsies should be obtained. The goal of initial surgery, which may include peritonectomy and/or bowel resection, is to remove all visible disease. The improved outcome with resection of disseminated disease is somewhat unique to ovarian cancer and may reflect the propensity for peritoneal spread rather than lymphatic or hematogenous dissemination. If complete resection is not achievable, a maximal cytoreduction effort is still useful because of the direct correlation between volume of residual tumor and survival. Patients are characterized after initial surgery as R0 (zero visible residual disease) if no visible disease remains, optimally debulked when all visible disease is smaller than 1 cm, and suboptimally debulked if disease of 1 cm or greater remains at completion of surgery.

Primary cytoreductive surgery is recommended over neoadjuvant chemotherapy for women with a high likelihood of achieving optimal cytoreduction with acceptable morbidity.

However, if optimal debulking is not considered feasible because of the volume and location of disease, four or fewer cycles of neoadjuvant chemotherapy should precede debulking surgery.[A12] Outcomes for patients who are treated with neoadjuvant chemotherapy are not as good as for patients who can have all visible tumor removed or who can have optimal debulking before chemotherapy, their outcomes are similar to patients who have suboptimal initial debulking.

At the completion of primary surgery, the tumor's histology is identified, and the tumor is staged based on surgical and pathologic findings (Table 184-9). Up to 85% of patients have disease beyond the ovary at the time of diagnosis, and 75 to 80% will have stage III or IV disease. More than 85% of patients with advanced stages III and IV disease have serous histology, whereas clear cell and endometrioid histologies comprise approximately 50% of stages I and II disease.

For stage IA or IB, grade 1 tumors, disease recurs in less than 5% of patients, so postoperative observation without adjuvant chemotherapy is recommended. Grade 2 tumors are rare, and treatment recommendations for nonserous stage I, grade 2 tumors are individualized. Three to six cycles of chemotherapy (typically a platinum-taxane combination, but pegylated liposomal doxorubicin and carboplatin can also be considered) under expert oversight are recommended for stage I, grade 3 and stage IC disease. Six cycles are preferred for serous tumors, whereas three cycles may be sufficient for endometrioid, clear cell, and mucinous tumors.

For patients who have stage II disease or who have stage III disease with no residual tumor or with optimally debulked tumor after surgery, six cycles of platinum-based combined intravenous and intraperitoneal treatment can be considered. Patients who have suboptimal stage III or stage IV disease should receive intravenous platinum-based therapy with or without bevacizumab.

Advanced Disease

Most patients with advanced disease respond to initial therapy and enter a clinical remission, but the vast majority will eventually relapse. As a result, additional maintenance therapy should be considered under expert oversight after completion of initial chemotherapy. The most commonly used maintenance treatments are bevacizumab, which is used with and after initial chemotherapy, and poly-ADP-ribose polymerase (PARP) inhibitors.[18,19] PARP inhibitors (rucaparib, olaparib, or niraparib) for 2 to 3 years after platinum-based therapy can help maintain remission, with the greatest benefits seen in *BRCA*-associated homologous recombinant deficiency (HRD)–positive ovarian cancers.[A13,A14]

Patients who experience a recurrence more than 6 to 12 months after completion of initial platinum-based therapy are considered platinum-sensitive and are usually retreated with another platinum-containing doublet. Patients whose disease recurs less than 6 months after completion of prior platinum-based therapy are considered platinum-resistant and are typically treated with non-platinum single-agent therapy. Bevacizumab added to treatment of platinum-sensitive or platinum-resistant disease can improve response to therapy and delay recurrence.[A15] In select patients with a late, platinum-sensitive recurrence, cytoreductive surgery followed by chemotherapy[20] is better than chemotherapy alone.[A16]

A much smaller fraction of familial ovarian cancers are linked to Lynch syndrome (HNPCC) or have microsatellite instability or somatic loss of DNA mismatch repair function. As in endometrial cancer, ovarian cancers that are deficient in mismatch repair will have a high rate of response to immune checkpoint inhibitor therapy with pembrolizumab.

TABLE 184-9 APPROACH TO OVARIAN CANCER BY STAGE

STAGE	BRIEF DEFINITION	TREATMENT
I	Tumor confined to the ovary or fallopian tube	
IA	No surface involvement	
	Grade 1/2	Staging laparotomy, observation*
	Grade 3	Staging laparotomy, 3-6 cycles IV chemotherapy
IB	Tumor confined to both ovaries or fallopian tubes	
	Grade 1/2	Staging laparotomy, observation
	Grade 3	Staging laparotomy, 3-6 cycles IV chemotherapy
IC	Surface involvement, positive ascites or washings	
	Capsule rupture or surgical spill	Staging laparotomy, 3-6 cycles IV chemotherapy
II	Disease spread limited to the pelvis	
IIA	Extension/Implants on the uterus, ovaries or fallopian tubes	Staging laparotomy, 3-6 cycles chemotherapy[†,§]
IIB	Extension to other pelvic tissues	Staging laparotomy, 3-6 cycles chemotherapy[†,§]
III	Tumor involving upper abdomen or regional nodes	
IIIA	Microscopic disease beyond the pelvis ± RP nodes	Staging laparotomy, 6 cycles IV or IVIP chemotherapy[†,§]
IIIB	≤2 cm disease beyond the pelvis ± RP nodes	Staging laparotomy, 6 cycles IV or IVIP chemotherapy[†,§]
IIIC	>2 cm disease beyond the pelvis ± RP nodes	Staging laparotomy, 6 cycles IV chemotherapy[‡,§]
IVA	Pleural effusion, positive cytology	Staging laparotomy, 6 cycles IV chemotherapy[‡,§]
IVB	Liver/spleen parenchyma, inguinal node involvement	
	Extraabdominal metastases	Staging laparotomy, 6 cycles IV chemotherapy[‡,§]

*Staging laparotomy includes exploratory laparotomy, a total abdominal hysterectomy with bilateral salpingo-oophorectomy, omentectomy, removal of ascites or peritoneal washings, and lymph node dissection.

†Combined intravenous and intraperitoneal chemotherapy can be considered for stage II patients and for R0 or optimally debulked stage III patients with less than 1 cm residual disease.

‡For patients unlikely to be successfully debulked with initial surgery, neoadjuvant chemotherapy with interval debulking can be considered.

§Maintenance PARP inhibitor therapy can be considered for responding patients with stage II-IV disease.

IV = intravenous; IVIP = intravenous/intraperitoneal; RP = retroperitoneal.

Less Common Histologies

A number of less common ovarian histologies have been identified (Table 184-10). Borderline tumors, also known as *low malignant potential tumors*, are a distinct group that is characterized by a lack of invasion (although it may spread within the peritoneal cavity), slow growth, and overall indolent behavior. These tumors tend to occur in younger women and are managed primarily with surgical resection as necessary. Low-grade ovarian cancers also have a lower growth fraction but have characteristics of invasion. These tumors have lower responses to chemotherapy and are more responsive to hormonal therapies. Mucinous cancers involving the ovary are commonly metastatic from a gastrointestinal primary that may be occult. Mucinous ovarian cancers are less responsive to standard ovarian chemotherapy regimens, and many require the use of agents used in treatment of gastrointestinal cancers (Chapter 179) under expert supervision.[21] As with endometrial carcinosarcomas, ovarian carcinosarcomas are biphasic neoplasms with malignant epithelial and mesenchymal elements. Carcinosarcomas are also less responsive to typical ovarian cancer treatments and may be more responsive to ifosfamide-based therapies under expert supervision. Clear cell carcinomas are frequently associated with endometriosis involving the ovary and are characterized by *ARID1A* driver mutations. These tumors are also less responsive to standard ovarian cancer therapies.

PREVENTION

Screening for ovarian cancer is not recommended in women who do not have symptoms. Neither serum CA-125 levels, alone or in combination with other markers, nor transvaginal ultrasound benefits the general population, and these tests are of limited value even in high-risk women.[A17]

TABLE 184-10 LESS COMMON OVARIAN HISTOLOGIES AND TREATMENT RECOMMENDATIONS

- **Borderline** (also known as low malignant potential [LMP]):
  - Observation
  - Complete surgical staging without invasive implants
- **Low-grade serous/endometrioid**
  - Hormonal therapy or
  - Chemotherapy ± hormonal therapy
- **Mucinous:**
  - Poor response to standard ovarian cancer chemotherapy, consider gastrointestinal-targeted therapies or regimens (5-fluorouracil, capecitabine, oxaliplatin)
- **Carcinosarcoma:**
  - Treated with standard ovarian cancer chemotherapy or an ifosfamide-containing regimen
- **Clear cell carcinoma:**
  - Associated with endometriosis, *ARID1A* driver mutations; less responsive to standard ovarian cancer chemotherapy

TABLE 184-11 OVARIAN CANCER: STAGE AND SURVIVAL

STAGE	PROPORTION OF PATIENTS		5-YR SURVIVAL
I	15%		90%
II	<5%		70%
III	70%	85% (II–IV)	25-50%
IV	10%		10-15%

Few strategies are available to prevent ovarian cancer. The use of oral contraceptive agents (Chapter 220) for 5 years or longer reduces the incidence of ovarian cancer by about 50%. For high-risk women, such as women with *BRCA1* or *BRCA2* mutations, prophylactic removal of the fallopian tubes and ovaries is recommended beginning at age 35 years and when childbearing is complete. Such surgery is the most effective approach to reduce the risk of ovarian cancer but is associated with complications of early menopause (Chapter 222). Given the role of the fallopian tube in ovarian carcinogenesis, the opportunistic removal of the fallopian tubes is increasingly recommended for primary prevention of epithelial ovarian malignancies.[22] This approach entails removal of the fallopian tubes in average-risk women undergoing pelvic surgery for another indication and allows preservation of the ovary without interruption of ovarian hormonal function. Common procedures that could potentially include opportunistic salpingectomy include hysterectomy for benign indications and in place of tubal ligation for women who desire sterilization.

PROGNOSIS

Recurrence and overall survival are related to stage of disease (Table 184-11). Ovarian cancer most commonly recurs at the prior sites of disease, typically in the abdominal or pelvic peritoneum or the pelvic and para-aortic nodes. Many patients with recurrent ovarian cancer will have significant bowel problems, including obstipation, constipation, and intermittent bowel obstruction.

Five-year survival rates for epithelial ovarian cancer are about 93% for localized disease, 75% for disease that has spread regionally, and 30% for disease with distant spread. Survival rates are reasonably similar for primary fallopian tube cancers and somewhat better for germ cell and stromal cell tumors. Women with *BRCA1/2*-mutated ovarian cancer survive longer than do women with sporadic ovarian cancer.

OTHER GYNECOLOGIC CANCERS

Malignant transformation can occur in every part of the müllerian tract. Other much less common types of gynecologic cancers include gestational trophoblastic disease, stromal and germ cell ovarian tumors, uterine sarcomas, and cancers of the vagina and vulva. Patients with these tumors should be referred to experts in the care and treatment of gynecologic cancer patients. Gestational trophoblastic disease is a group of pregnancy-related disorders resulting from a pathologic conceptus. The cells that form such tumors arise from trophoblastic tissue that will form the placenta. Gestational trophoblastic diseases range from benign hydatidiform moles to malignant choriocarcinoma. Ovarian germ cell tumors have strong homology with testicular cancer, including early age of onset, and a high cure rate with current therapies. Ovarian stromal tumors are typically early stage and usually cured with surgery alone but may require systemic therapy if advanced or recurrent.

The most common uterine sarcomas are leiomyosarcoma and endometrial stromal sarcoma. Leiomyosarcoma, which is a malignant tumor of smooth muscle, develops in the myometrium. Surgical resection is the treatment of choice. Neither adjuvant chemotherapy nor radiotherapy is useful for stage I disease, but recurrent leiomyosarcoma is most commonly treated with chemotherapy. Endometrial stromal sarcomas are commonly low grade and responsive to hormonal therapy, but when high grade, they are treated similarly to leiomyosarcomas. Cancers of the vagina and vulva are typically HPV-related cancers and are treated similarly to cervical cancer. Topical imiquimod is as effective as surgery for vulvar intraepithelial neoplasia.[A18]

Survivors of all forms of gynecologic cancers—whether of the cervix, endometrium, or ovary—are at risk for future sexual dysfunction as well as alterations of bowel and bladder function. They also must be counseled and often treated regarding the consequences of early menopause.

APPROACH TO SURVIVORS OF GYNECOLOGIC CANCERS

Survivors of gynecologic cancers are at continuous risk for both local and distant recurrences. Most gynecologic cancers that recur will do so within the first 5 years, but later recurrences can occur, particularly with low-grade disease. The treating oncology team will have primary responsibility for surveillance, but internists and primary care physicians may be called on to evaluate new symptoms, laboratory abnormalities, or physical examination findings.

Radical hysterectomy may disrupt the autonomic nervous system in the pelvis, thereby leading to bowel and/or bladder dysfunction. Pelvic lymphadenectomy, performed as part of many gynecologic cancer surgeries, can lead to lymphedema. Women treated with whole pelvic radiation therapy can suffer from bowel and bladder dysfunction and sexual dysfunction. Bladder problems may include urgency, incontinence, and chronic cystitis with loss of bladder elasticity and distensibility. Rectal problems include pain, diarrhea or constipation, rectal urgency, and incomplete stool evacuation or fecal incontinence. Radiation can also lead to pelvic insufficiency fractures with associated pain in up to 10% of patients.

Gynecologic cancer surgery and treatment are commonly associated with sexual dysfunction, which is multifactorial and related to fatigue from treatment, emotional and physical stresses of disease, surgery, and sequelae of systemic therapy. Vaginal stenosis, dryness, and dyspareunia are common. Resection of the upper vagina included in cervical cancer surgery may lead to a shortened vagina. Sexual dysfunction is increased after pelvic radiation but is also documented in women who have had surgery alone.

Most gynecologic cancer surgery will include removal of the ovaries. In premenopausal women, the result is abrupt menopause with its attendant short- and long-term sequelae (Chapter 222). In addition, even when the ovaries are preserved, as in younger cervical cancer patients, the ovarian blood supply may be compromised, thereby resulting in premature ovarian failure. For many gynecologic cancers, the use of hormone replacement therapy is contraindicated and should be used only after consultation with the oncology care team.

Cisplatin and paclitaxel, which are commonly used in all gynecologic cancers, can result in peripheral neuropathy, which can be permanent in many women. Cisplatin can also result in renal injury and renal electrolyte wasting, including loss of potassium, magnesium, and calcium. Bevacizumab is used in most gynecologic cancers, sometimes as prolonged maintenance in patients who are in remission. Bevacizumab toxicities, many of which are cumulative, include hypertension, proteinuria, bleeding or clotting, interference with wound healing, bowel perforation or fistula formation, and reversible posterior leukoencephalopathy syndrome. Patients whose ovarian cancer, especially BRCA-associated ovarian cancer, is treated with poly-ADP ribose polymerase (PARP) inhibitors are at increased risk for secondary hematologic malignancies, specifically myelodysplastic syndrome (Chapter 167) and acute myelogenous leukemia (Chapter 168). Persistent cytopenias or other unexplained abnormalities in blood counts in patients treated with this class of agents should prompt a thorough hematologic evaluation.

All gynecologic cancer survivors should be encouraged to adopt a healthy lifestyle, including increased physical activity (Chapter 14) and dietary modifications (Chapter 13). Fatigue, depression, and mood disorders are common in cancer survivors. These factors have a significant impact on quality of life and may persist many years, even decades, after treatment. Gynecologic cancer survivors may benefit from seeing a counselor or therapist to help with emotional issues associated with cancer treatment and recovery.

UTERINE FIBROIDS

The most common pelvic tumors in women are uterine fibroids, which are present in up to 40% of women during their reproductive years and up to 70 to 80% by 50 years of age.[23] Germline mutations in the *FH* (fumarate hydratase) gene are associated with early onset of uterine and cutaneous leiomyomas and renal cell cancer. Other implicated somatic mutations include the *MED12* gene on the X chromosome. Since fibroids require estrogen and progesterone, they can grow rapidly in early pregnancy but typically shrink after menopause.

Fibroids are usually asymptomatic. However, fibroids can cause pelvic discomfort and substantial uterine bleeding. Fibroids often can be detected by careful physical examination, but ultrasonography is confirmatory.

Fibroids themselves are benign and not premalignant. However, about 1 per 1100 to 1 per 1500 women under age 45 years may also have uterine cancer.

TREATMENT

The definitive treatment for fibroids is hysterectomy, but less invasive options are often preferable.[24] An anti-progesterone agent (e.g., oral mifepristone, 5 mg daily for 6 months or 10 mg daily for 3 months) or ulipristal acetate 5 or 10 mg per day for 13 weeks can effectively reduce fibroid size and symptoms.[A19] However, their benefits usually are transient. Oral gonadotropin-releasing hormone antagonists (e.g., elagolix at 300 mg twice daily[A20] or relugolix 40 mg once daily[A21]) combined with daily estradiol (1 mg) and norethindrone acetate (0.5 mg) can reduce fibroid-associated heavy menstrual bleeding and preserve bone density. Nonsteroidal anti-inflammatory drugs (e.g., naproxen or mefenamic acid) also are useful for discomfort. Hysteroscopic myomectomy can remove submucosal fibroids and preserve childbearing capacity, and myomectomy (open, laparoscopic, or hysteroscopic) provides better outcomes than uterine-artery embolization.[A22] For other symptoms, options include focused ultrasound surgery, radiofrequency ablation, and surgical myomectomy. Power morcellation has fallen out of favor because of the low but real chance of spreading malignant tissue that can appear as fibroids on imaging.

GENERAL REFERENCES

For the General References and other additional features, please visit Elsevier eBooks+ at https://ebooks.health.elsevier.com.

Grade A References

A1. Greene SA, De Vuyst H, John-Stewart GC, et al. Effect of cryotherapy vs loop electrosurgical excision procedure on cervical disease recurrence among women with HIV and high-grade cervical lesions in Kenya: a randomized clinical trial. *JAMA.* 2019;322:1570-1579.
A2. Ramirez PT, Frumovitz M, Pareja R, et al. Minimally invasive versus abdominal hysterectomy for cervical cancer. *N Engl J Med.* 2018;379:1895-1904.
A3. Gupta S, Maheshwari A, Parab P, et al. Neoadjuvant chemotherapy followed by radical surgery versus concomitant chemotherapy and radiotherapy in patients with stage IB2, IIA, or IIB squamous cervical cancer: a randomized controlled trial. *J Clin Oncol.* 2018;36:1548-1555.
A4. Tewari KS, Sill MW, Penson RT, et al. Bevacizumab for advanced cervical cancer: final overall survival and adverse event analysis of a randomised, controlled, open-label, phase 3 trial (Gynecologic Oncology Group 240). *Lancet.* 2017;390:1654-1663.
A5. Colombo N, Dubot C, Lorusso D, et al. Pembrolizumab for persistent, recurrent or metastatic cervical cancer. *N Engl J Med.* 2021;385:1856-1867.
A6. Huh WK, Joura EA, Giuliano AR, et al. Final efficacy, immunogenicity, and safety analyses of a nine-valent human papillomavirus vaccine in women aged 16-26 years: a randomised, double-blind trial. *Lancet.* 2017;390:2143-2159.
A7. Arbyn M, Xu L, Simoens C, et al. Prophylactic vaccination against human papillomaviruses to prevent cervical cancer and its precursors. *Cochrane Database Syst Rev.* 2018;5:CD009069.
A8. Yi L, Zhang H, Zou J, et al. Adjuvant chemoradiotherapy versus radiotherapy alone in high-risk endometrial cancer: a systematic review and meta-analysis. *Gynecol Oncol.* 2018;149:612-619.
A9. Matei D, Filiaci V, Randall ME, et al. Adjuvant chemotherapy plus radiation for locally advanced endometrial cancer. *N Engl J Med.* 2019;380:2317-2326.
A10. Slomovitz BM, Filiaci VL, Walker JL, et al. A randomized phase II trial of everolimus and letrozole or hormonal therapy in women with advanced, persistent or recurrent endometrial carcinoma: a GOG Foundation study. *Gynecol Oncol.* 2022;164:481-491 .
A11. Makker V, Colombo N, Casado Herráez A, et al. Lenvatinib plus pembrolizumab for advanced endometrial cancer. *N Engl J Med.* 2022;386:437-448.
A12. Wright AA, Bohlke K, Armstrong DK, et al. Neoadjuvant chemotherapy for newly diagnosed, advanced ovarian cancer: Society of Gynecologic Oncology and American Society of Clinical Oncology clinical practice guideline. *Gynecol Oncol.* 2016;143:3-15.
A13. Monk BJ, Parkinson C, Lim MC, et al. A randomized, phase III trial to evaluate Rucaparib monotherapy as maintenance treatment in patients with newly diagnosed ovarian cancer (ATHENA-MONO/GOG-3020/ENGOT-ov45). *J Clin Oncol.* 2022;40:3952-3964.
A14. Tattersall A, Ryan N, Wiggans AJ, et al. Poly(ADP-ribose) polymerase (PARP) inhibitors for the treatment of ovarian cancer. *Cochrane Database Syst Rev.* 2022;2:CD007929.
A15. Coleman RL, Brady MF, Herzog TJ, et al. Bevacizumab and paclitaxel-carboplatin chemotherapy and secondary cytoreduction in recurrent, platinum-sensitive ovarian cancer (NRG Oncology/Gynecologic Oncology Group study GOG-0213): a multicentre, open-label, randomised, phase 3 trial. *Lancet Oncol.* 2017;18:779-791.
A16. Harter P, Sehouli J, Vergote I, et al. Randomized trial of cytoreductive surgery for relapsed ovarian cancer. *N Engl J Med.* 2021;385:2123-2131.
A17. Menon U, Gentry-Maharaj A, Burnell M, et al. Ovarian cancer population screening and mortality after long-term follow-up in the UK Collaborative Trial of Ovarian Cancer Screening (UKCTOCS): a randomised controlled trial. *Lancet.* 2021;397:2182-9322.
A18. Trutnovsky G, Reich O, Joura EA, et al. Topical imiquimod versus surgery for vulvar intraepithelial neoplasia: a multicentre, randomised, phase 3, non-inferiority trial. *Lancet.* 2022;399:1790-1798.
A19. Murji A, Whitaker L, Chow TL, et al. Selective progesterone receptor modulators (SPRMs) for uterine fibroids. *Cochrane Database Syst Rev.* 2017;4:CD010770.
A20. Schlaff WD, Ackerman RT, Al-Hendy A, et al. Elagolix for heavy menstrual bleeding in women with uterine fibroids. *N Engl J Med.* 2020;382:328-340.
A21. Al-Hendy A, Lukes AS, Poindexter AN 3rd, et al. Treatment of uterine fibroid symptoms with relugolix combination therapy. *N Engl J Med.* 2021;384:630-642.
A22. Manyonda I, Belli AM, Lumsden MA, et al. Uterine-artery embolization or myomectomy for uterine fibroids. *N Engl J Med.* 2020;383:440-451.

185 TESTICULAR CANCER

LAWRENCE H. EINHORN

EPIDEMIOLOGY

Testicular cancer has an annual incidence of about 8700 cases per year in the United States and accounts for only 1% of all male malignancies.[1] Nevertheless, it is the most common carcinoma in men ages 15 to 35 years.[2] In the United States, testicular cancer is four to five times more common in White men compared with men of other ethnicities,[3] but incidence rates are rising in Asian/Pacific Islander and Hispanic men.[4] Men who have cryptorchidism have a 10- to 40-fold increased risk for the development of testicular cancer in the undescended testis, but even the normally descended testis in these men has a higher risk for malignancy. Testicular cancer is associated with drinking alcohol, overweight and obesity, and elevated blood lipid levels.[5]

PATHOBIOLOGY

More than 95% of testicular tumors are germ cell cancers.[6] Rare tumor types include lymphoma (especially in older men and often bilateral), Leydig cell, and Sertoli cell tumors. Non–germ cell tumors do not secrete serum α-fetoprotein or human chorionic gonadotropin and do not respond to platinum-based chemotherapy.

Of germ cell tumors, about half are seminomas and half are nonseminomas. Nonseminomas include embryonal cell carcinomas, yolk sac tumors, choriocarcinomas, and teratomas (with/without seminoma). Both seminomas and nonseminomas typically have amplification or aneuploidy with a gain of genetic information at the 12p position on the short arm of chromosome 12.[7]

CLINICAL MANIFESTATIONS

A testicular cancer may be first detected by the patient or a physician as a painless lump, often about the size of a pea. However, most patients present with unilateral pain or swelling of the testis or scrotum. Enlarging metastatic retroperitoneal nodes may cause flank pain as a presenting symptom. Less commonly, testicular cancer may be first suspected during a couple's evaluation for infertility when the male partner is found to have oligospermia. Pulmonary symptoms of chest pain, cough, or dyspnea are seen only with extensive hematogenous spread to the lungs. Significant elevation of the serum human chorionic gonadotropin level may produce gynecomastia.

Compared with nonseminomas, seminomas occur in men one to two decades older, never secrete α-fetoprotein,[8] have normal or modest elevation of human chorionic gonadotropin, and usually present with disease localized in the testis (stage I). Initial spread is lymphatic to ipsilateral retroperitoneal nodes, and hematogenous spread to lungs is rare.

DIAGNOSIS

Careful testicular examination is mandatory. With the patient standing or lying supine, the testes are gently palpated with the thumb and second or third fingers. Patients with a palpable mass or persistent orchialgia should be suspected of having testicular cancer. History of cryptorchidism or flank pain further raises the possibility of cancer. The differential diagnosis includes epididymitis, hydrocele (which may be secondary to cancer), torsion, or a varicocele.

Testicular ultrasound is the diagnostic modality of choice in all suspicious cases.[9] A hypoechogenic intratesticular mass is almost always malignant and requires referral to a urologist (Fig. 185-1). Orchiectomy will diagnose the type of tumor. Embryonal cell carcinoma is positive for CD30, and seminoma is positive for CD117 and placental alkaline phosphatase. Most germ cell tumors are positive for OCT 3/4 and micro-RNA371.[10]

The evaluation for metastatic disease is dependent on signs, symptoms, and histology. In all cases, serum levels of human chorionic gonadotropin and α-fetoprotein should be obtained, and an abdominal computed tomographic (CT) scan should be performed.

Patients with testicular cancer are staged according to the anatomic extent of disease and presence or absence of detectable levels of serum human chorionic gonadotropin and α-fetoprotein post-orchiectomy. Lymphatic spread of a testicular germ cell cancer is detected on abdominal CT scanning with nodes more than 1 cm in the interaortocaval area for a right-sided primary tumor and left periaortic area for left-sided primary tumor. Nodal disease below the diaphragm constitutes stage II, and nodal spread above the diaphragm to posterior mediastinal or supraclavicular nodes is stage III. Hematogenous dissemination to lungs, or liver, bone, or brain is also classified as stage III. A chest radiograph or CT scan is routine for nonseminoma or for stage II seminoma. If a patient has cryptorchidism, scrotal violation, vasectomy, or prior inguinal hernia surgery, a pelvic CT scan also should be obtained. Head CT or magnetic resonance imaging is indicated only if the patient has signs or symptoms of central nervous system disease. Positron emission tomography is not indicated.

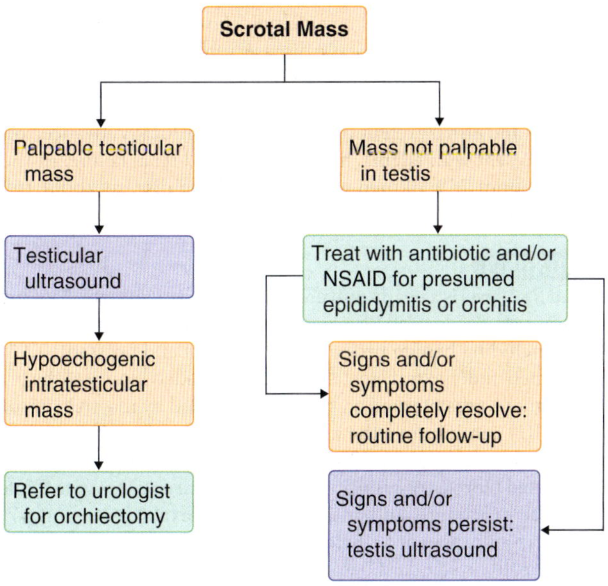

FIGURE 185-1. **Management of a scrotal mass or orchialgia.** NSAID = nonsteroidal anti-inflammatory drug.

TREATMENT

Initial treatment primarily depends on the stage of disease at presentation.[11,12]

Local and Regional Disease

Seminomas

Approximately 70% of seminomas are initially diagnosed with clinical stage I disease. Risk factors for micro-metastases include a primary tumor larger than 4 cm or involvement of the rete testis. Absence of either feature results in a 95% cure rate with orchiectomy alone. Presence of either adverse pathologic finding translates to an 80% cure rate with orchiectomy alone. A persistent or rising level of human chorionic gonadotropin indicates metastatic spread that requires chemotherapy, even in the absence of metastases on CT scans or physical examination. The half-life is 18 to 24 hours for human chorionic gonadotropin and 5 days for α-fetoprotein. As a result, the α-fetoprotein might require 6 weeks to normalize in a patient who had a preorchiectomy α-fetoprotein level of 1000 ng/mL even if stage I disease was cured with orchiectomy alone.

Although a single course of carboplatin or radiotherapy is an option,[13] the preferred recommendation for all clinical stage I seminomas is surveillance, with history and physical examination, serum levels of human chorionic gonadotropin and α-fetoprotein, and abdominal CT (with pelvic CT if indicated) every 4 months in year 1, every 6 months in year 2, and annually in years 3 to 5. Patients who relapse on surveillance still have a nearly 100% cure rate with either abdominal irradiation or cisplatin-based combination chemotherapy. Selected patients with early stage II disease can undergo retroperitoneal lymph node dissection to avoid late complications from chemotherapy or radiotherapy.

TABLE 185-1 DEFINITIONS OF POOR-RISK AND INTERMEDIATE-RISK DISEASE

POOR-RISK (ALL NONSEMINOMA)
hCG > 50,000 mIU/mL*
AFP > 10,000 ng/mL*
Nonpulmonary visceral metastases (e.g., bone, liver, or brain)
Primary mediastinal nonseminomatous germ cell tumor
INTERMEDIATE-RISK
Nonpulmonary visceral metastases in seminoma
hCG 5000-50,000 mIU/mL*
AFP 1000-10,000 ng/mL*

*Measured post-orchiectomy at start of chemotherapy.
AFP = α-fetoprotein; hCG = human chorionic gonadotropin.

Nonseminomatous Germ Cell Tumors

Patients who present with clinical stage I disease can be managed initially with orchiectomy alone and observation (surveillance), retroperitoneal lymph node dissection, or a single course of bleomycin/etoposide/cisplatin combination chemotherapy. All three options lead to an eventual 98 to 100% cure rate. Most relapses occur the first year and are detected by screening with a history, physical examination, and serum levels of human chorionic gonadotropin and α-fetoprotein every 2 months, as well as chest radiography plus an abdominal CT scan every 4 months. All studies should be repeated every 6 months during year 2 and annually in years 3 to 5. Risk factors for relapse on surveillance are vascular invasion in the orchiectomy specimen or embryonal carcinoma as the predominant cell type. Clinical small-volume stage II disease (1- to 3-cm nodes) is often managed by retroperitoneal lymph node dissection, which is best performed at a tertiary center with a nerve-sparing procedure to prevent retrograde ejaculation. Patients with bulky stage II or stage III disease are treated with cisplatin combination chemotherapy.

Chemotherapy for Disseminated Disease

Cisplatin combination chemotherapy under expert oversight can cure 70% of cases. Bleomycin/etoposide/cisplatin combination chemotherapy for three or four courses is the standard chemotherapy for disseminated testis cancer. About 60% of patients who require chemotherapy have good-risk metastatic disease.[14] Risk stratification, based on the amplitude of the serum human chorionic gonadotropin and α-fetoprotein levels and the presence of nonpulmonary visceral metastases, separates patients into good-risk (90% cure rate with three courses of chemotherapy), intermediate-risk (75% cure rate with three to four courses of chemotherapy), and poor-risk (50 to 60% cure rate with four courses of chemotherapy) (Table 185-1).

Second- or third-line therapy still has curative potential, either with standard-dose salvage chemotherapy (with ifosfamide/cisplatin plus either paclitaxel or vinblastine) or high-dose carboplatin/etoposide followed by peripheral blood stem cell transplantation under expert oversight.[15] Cure rates range from 25 to 85%, depending on second- versus third-line chemotherapy, the patient's characteristics, and the type of tumor. Selected patients with localized relapse are appropriate for salvage surgical procedures such as retroperitoneal lymph node dissection.

Late relapse beyond 2 years is uncommon but can occur in 2 to 3% of patients who have achieved a complete remission. Late relapse usually manifests by a rise in the serum α-fetoprotein level. The optimal approach is to identify the site of metastases and to perform surgical resection if feasible. Platinum-based chemotherapy without post-chemotherapy surgery can produce temporary remissions but few cures.

PREVENTION

Surgical correction of cryptorchidism before puberty reduces the risk of testicular cancer, but abnormalities in the testicle itself may explain both the cryptorchidism and the risk of cancer. Physicians should examine the testes carefully in men, especially men ages 15 to 40 years. Although self-examination has been associated with an earlier stage of diagnosis of testicular cancer,[16] the U.S. Preventive Services Task Force does not recommend it because of its limited accuracy for this rare condition and its tendency to generate needless testing.[17] However, patients who have been cured of their testis cancer have a 2% probability of a second unrelated germ cell cancer in the contralateral testis. These high-risk individuals should be instructed in self-examination. Physician examination of the remaining testis should be a routine component of follow-up examinations.

PROGNOSIS

Testicular cancer is the most curable solid tumor, with 10-year survival rates of 95% for stages I to III and 80% for disseminated disease that requires chemotherapy. The amplitudes of serum levels of human chorionic gonadotropin and α-fetoprotein are independent prognostic variables for cure with cisplatin combination chemotherapy. However, potential sequelae in long-term survivors include a 2.5- to 3-fold increased risk of a second malignancy,[18] especially acute myeloid leukemia[19] and prostate cancer,[20] from chemotherapy or irradiation, cardiovascular disease, ototoxicity with tinnitus and high-frequency hearing loss, infertility, and psychosocial issues.[21] The great majority of survivors work full-time and lead healthy and productive lives. Patients with metastatic disease should not be denied curative platinum combination chemotherapy because of these late complications. Health maintenance, including exercise, abstinence from tobacco, avoidance of obesity, and management of the blood pressure and lipid profile, is crucial. Hypogonadism with low testosterone levels can increase the risk for the metabolic syndrome.

GENERAL REFERENCES

For the General References and other additional features, please visit Elsevier eBooks+ at https://ebooks.health.elsevier.com.

186

PROSTATE CANCER

KATHLEEN A. COONEY AND ELISABETH I. HEATH

EPIDEMIOLOGY

Prostate cancer is the most common nonskin cancer that affects U.S. men, with approximately 270,000 new cases diagnosed annually and approximately 35,000 deaths each year. Worldwide, approximately 1.4 million cases of prostate cancer are diagnosed annually and lead to approximately 375,000 deaths each year. The disease is the most common cancer among men in much of Europe, North America, and Australia, but lower rates are observed in Asia. Higher mortality rates are observed in sub-Saharan Africa and the Caribbean, likely because of much lower rates of early detection.

In developed countries, the widespread use of screening with prostate-specific antigen (PSA) testing, beginning in the early 1990s, led to a rapid increase in the reported annual incidence of prostate cancer, mostly attributable to the identification of asymptomatic cases. Since 1992, however, the reported incidence rate of prostate cancer has fallen by 50%,[1] first because of an acceleration of diagnosis for early prevalent cases and subsequently because of more conservative recommendations regarding PSA screening.

The three well-recognized risk factors for prostate cancer are advanced age, ethnicity, and family history.[2] Prostate cancer is rarely diagnosed before age 40 years, and the average age of onset is approximately age 68 years. In the United States, non-Hispanic Black men have the highest incidence of prostate cancer (171.6 cases/100,000 population age adjusted) and the highest mortality (38.3/100,000) from the disease. In contrast, Asian/Pacific Islander men have the lowest incidence and mortality (53.8/100,000 and 8.8/100,000, respectively). About 10% of all prostate cancers in the United States are early onset, diagnosed at or before age 56 years; such men are more likely have a genetic component to their disease. The risk of prostate cancer is related to the number of affected family members, regardless of whether the first-degree relatives are affected, and the presence of early-onset disease in the pedigree. Familial clustering of prostate cancer appears to be related to genetic factors, with no evidence that shared environment contributes to familial clustering.[3] Other possible risk factors include high consumption of dietary fats, high intake of calcium, exposure to dioxin, and prior prostatitis.

PATHOBIOLOGY

Most prostate cancers are adenocarcinomas and arise from the epithelial cells that line the prostate gland. Prostate-specific antigen (PSA) is an androgen-regulated serine protease that is produced by epithelial cells in the prostate gland as well as by cancers that arise from these cells. High grade prostatic intraepithelial neoplasia and atypical small acinar proliferation are precursor lesions.

The PTEN protein is commonly lost in aggressive prostate cancers, generally through genomic deletion. Transposition of the transmembrane protease gene *TMPRSS2* to the ETS family member *ERG* gene, thereby creating the *TMPRSS2-ERG* fusion, is seen in 40 to 50% of prostate cancers, especially in White men. Other molecular abnormalities that are seen in cases without an ETS gene fusion include: overexpression of the serine peptidase gene *SPINK1*; recurrent point mutations in the transcriptional repressor gene *SPOP*; loss and/or mutations in the *CHD1* gene; and alterations in members of the RAS/RAF gene family. Metastatic and/or castrate-resistant prostate cancers often have aberrations in the androgen receptor, *TP53*, and *RB1* genes in addition to loss of PTEN.

Rare nonsynonymous mutations in the transcription factor *HOXB13* are associated with a three- to four-fold increased risk of prostate cancer.[4] Prostate cancer is also increased in carriers of *BRCA1* and *BRCA2* mutations. About 12% of men with metastatic prostate cancer have a germline mutation in a DNA repair gene.[5]

Histologies other than adenocarcinomas are reported in less than 5% of cases. Ductal and intraductal cancers may be related to germline DNA repair gene mutations.

CLINICAL MANIFESTATIONS

In the United States and most developed countries, the majority of men who are diagnosed with prostate cancer are asymptomatic and have tumors that are discovered by PSA screening. Men who have localized disease may complain of a variety of lower urinary tract symptoms, including urinary retention, frequency, and nocturia. Other symptoms may include hematuria and hematospermia. For men who present with metastatic disease, symptoms may include fatigue, weight loss, and bone pain. Spinal cord compression (Chapters 164 and 175) can be heralded by increasing and well-localized back pain that is associated with weakness and urinary retention. Some men with locally advanced prostate cancer may present with edema, hypertension, and renal failure. At the time of diagnosis, about 75% of men will have localized disease, about 15% will have regional disease, and about 10% will have distant disease.

DIAGNOSIS

An elevated PSA level is a nearly universal finding in patients who have prostate cancer.[6] However, an elevated PSA level can be caused by many noncancerous conditions including benign prostatic hypertrophy and prostatitis (Chapter 114). Most men undergo transrectal ultrasound-guided biopsy of the prostate gland to diagnose prostate cancer, but biopsy guided by magnetic resonance imaging (MRI) can improve the accuracy of the biopsy.[A1,A2] Since prostate cancer is often multifocal, usually 10 to 12 cores are obtained , but MRI-directed targeted biopsies of suspicious areas alone are an alternative.[A3] Infection is a risk of the procedure, and antibiotic prophylaxis (e.g., a single 750mg oral dose of ciprofloxacin or a single 160/800 mg oral dose of trimethoprim/sulfamethoxazole) is standard before the procedure. A routine urine culture can be obtained before the procedure to guide prophylactic prebiopsy and postbiopsy treatment if bacteria are detected (Chapter 263). Since bleeding is another procedural risk, anticoagulant and/or antiplatelet medications are ideally discontinued for the procedure and restarted afterwards.

Prostate cancers are graded by their Gleason score (Table 186-1), which grades the histology of the most frequent patterns on biopsy and then sums the two scores.

TABLE 186-1 GLEASON SCORING SYSTEM

PATTERN	CRITERIA
1	Prostate cancer is well differentiated, with small and well-formed glands that closely resemble normal prostate tissue
2	A moderately differentiated carcinoma in which glands are well-formed but larger and with more tissue between them
3	A moderately differentiated carcinoma in which glands are recognizable but the cells are darker, have an infiltrative pattern, and are beginning to invade the surrounding tissue
4	A poorly differentiated carcinoma with few recognizable glands and cells that are invading the surrounding tissue in neoplastic clumps
5	Anaplastic carcinoma with few recognizable glands and with sheets of cells throughout the surrounding tissue

TABLE 186-2 STAGING OF PROSTATE CANCER

TUMOR (T)	NODES (N)	METASTASIS (M)	PSA (ng/mL)	GLEASON SCORE	STAGE
T1-T2	N0	M0	<10	6	I
T1-T2	N0	M0	≥10 to <20	6	IIA
T1-T2	N0	M0	<20	3+4=7	IIB
T1-T2	N0	M0	<20	4+3=7	IIC
T1-T2	N0	M0	<20	8	IIC
T1-T2	N0	M0	≥20	≤8	IIIA
T3-T4	N0	M0	Any	≤8	IIIB
Any T	N0	M0	Any	9-10	IIIC
Any T	N1	M0	Any	Any	IVA
Any T	Any	M1	Any	Any	IVB

M0 = no tumor spread to distant sites; M1 = tumor spread to distant sites; N0 = no tumor spread to regional lymph nodes; N1 = tumor spread to regional lymph nodes; PSA = prostate-specific antigen; T1 = tumor too small to be seen or felt on physical examination; T2 = tumor confined to the prostate gland; T3 = tumor invades the seminal vesicles or extends beyond the prostate gland; T4 = tumor extends to adjacent structures.

For Gleason score, see Table 186-1.

Atypical small acinar proliferation is observed in approximately 5% of prostate biopsies, and between 30 to 50% of individuals with this finding will have invasive cancer on repeat biopsy. Men whose biopsies show high-grade prostatic intraepithelial neoplasia or atypical small acinar proliferation are generally reevaluated at 6- to 24-month intervals and should be considered for biomarker tests or imaging to aid in cancer diagnosis if appropriate. Benign findings on a prostate biopsy include atrophy, adenosis, atypical adenomatous hyperplasia, and acute or chronic inflammation.

Staging

The initial risk stratification and staging of prostate cancer combines clinical and pathologic features as well as imaging results to establish the extent of cancer. Prostate cancer is staged based on the degree of elevation of the PSA level, the primary tumor's Gleason score and local extent, whether the tumor has spread to regional or distant lymph nodes or nearby structures, and whether it has spread to bone or distant organs (Table 186-2). Imaging studies are key to determine the extent of local disease as well as the presence of any metastatic disease. For local disease, transrectal ultrasound and magnetic resonance imaging (MRI) scans are preferred to determine the size of the prostate gland, to localize nodules, and to detect invasion into adjacent structures.[7] A bone scan and computed tomographic (CT) scan are preferred to assess metastatic disease. Positron emission tomography (PET)/CT scan can also assist not only in initial staging but also in assessing biochemically recurrent disease. The most common imaging tracers to detect small-volume disease in soft tissue and/or in bone are C-11 choline or F-18 fluciclovine rather than F-18 fluorodeoxyglucose (FDG), which is routinely used in other common cancers. Prostate-specific membrane antigen can be targeted using Ga-68 PSMA-11 and 18F-DCFPyl as tracers.[8]

Germline genetic testing is recommended for men who have prostate cancer and who have one or more of the following: high-risk, very-high-risk, regional, or metastatic prostate cancer; Ashkenazi Jewish ancestry; or a strong family history of prostate cancer or other epithelial cancers such as breast, ovarian, colorectal, or endometrial cancers.

TABLE 186-3 TREATMENT OF PROSTATE CANCER

EXTENT OF CANCER	THERAPEUTIC OPTIONS
Stage I	Observation Active surveillance External-beam radiation therapy or brachytherapy Radical prostatectomy with or without pelvic lymph node dissection
Stage II	Active surveillance External-beam radiation therapy or brachytherapy Radical prostatectomy with or without pelvic lymph node dissection
Stage IIIA	Androgen-deprivation therapy plus either external-beam radiation therapy or brachytherapy Radical prostatectomy with pelvic lymph node dissection
Stage IIIB, IIIC, IVA, or IVB	External-beam radiation therapy, and/or brachytherapy plus androgen-deprivation therapy, and/or docetaxel Radical prostatectomy with pelvic lymph node dissection
Biochemical PSA relapse	Observation Salvage external-beam radiation therapy Salvage radical prostatectomy Androgen-deprivation therapy
Metastatic hormone-sensitive prostate cancer	Androgen-deprivation therapy, docetaxel, abiraterone, enzalutamide, apalutamide, darolutamide
Metastatic castration-resistant prostate cancer	Androgen-deprivation therapy, docetaxel, cabazitaxel, abiraterone, enzalutamide, darolutamide, sipuleucel-T, olaparib, rucaparib, radium 223, pembrolizumab, lutetium 177 vipivotide tetraxetan

TREATMENT

Prostate cancer exhibits extensive clinical heterogeneity, and some men may be treated aggressively for cancers that will never cause clinical symptoms. Treatment decisions are based not only on risk stratification and the stage of disease but also on the side effects of treatment (Table 186-3).[9,10]

Localized Disease

A number of treatment options are available for patients who have localized prostate cancer (Table 186-3).

Watchful Waiting and Active Surveillance

Observation (watchful waiting) is an option for men who have competing causes of death that are likely to shorten life-expectancy to less than 10 years.[A4] Another strategy is active surveillance, which includes PSA testing every 6 months, a digital rectal examination once a year, repeat prostate biopsies potentially every 12 months, and consideration of MRI spectroscopy.[11,A5] Ki-67 is a marker of proliferation, and high staining for Ki-67 and/or loss of PTEN may identify patients who may require more aggressive treatment.[12]

Curative Therapy

Both radical prostatectomy and radiation therapy can achieve a high cure rate for early disease. The preferred option should consider the patient's wishes, experience, and expectations. Referral to the appropriate specialist or team is highly encouraged to provide a balanced explanation of the impacts of each option on bowel, bladder, and sexual function, as well as other systemic side effects.

Radical prostatectomy is an option for patients who have clinically localized disease and a life expectancy of more than 10 years.[A6] Laparoscopic and robot-assisted radical prostatectomy are commonly performed rather than open radical prostatectomy to reduce the length of hospital stay as well as blood loss, surgical complications, urinary incontinence, and erectile dysfunction.[A7] In patients in whom the probability of nodal involvement is high, a pelvic lymph node dissection should be performed, typically at the time of prostatectomy. An extended pelvic lymph node dissection removes all nodes in the external iliac vein, pelvic side wall, bladder wall, floor of the pelvis, and internal iliac artery.

Another curative treatment option for patients with clinically localized disease is radiation therapy,[A8] delivered either as external beam radiation therapy with photons or protons or by brachytherapy.[13] Intensity-modulated external beam radiation therapy (19 treatments of 3.4 Gy each rather than 39 treatments of 2.0 Gy each) or ultrafractionated therapy (7 treatments of 4.1 Gy each) provide equivalent outcomes.[A9,A10] Three-dimensional image-guided radiation therapy localizes the tumor daily to ensure proper positioning, so as to localize therapy to the prostate and minimize the dose to the surrounding normal organs, such as the bladder and rectum. Proton therapy delivers highly conformal doses to the prostate with less radiation to the surrounding normal tissue, but it does not improve clinical outcomes despite its substantially higher costs.[14] Brachytherapy (seed implantation or interstitial radiation therapy), which delivers radioactivity directly to the prostate, can be used alone for patients who have early-stage, low-risk prostate cancer or in combination with external beam radiation therapy for patients who have higher-risk disease.[15]

High-Risk Disease

For patients who have high-risk stage II disease or have stage III disease, the higher risk of nodal and micrometastatic disease warrants radical prostatectomy, commonly followed by radiation therapy. For these high-risk patients, neoadjuvant androgen deprivation therapy[16] should precede surgery and radiation to increase the likelihood of achieving cure.[A11] High-intensity focal ultrasound, focal cryotherapy, and focal laser ablation are experimental approaches for localized disease, but they are associated with high recurrence rates and currently cannot be recommended for routine use.

Biochemical Recurrent Disease

Patients who undergo initial definitive therapy should undergo follow-up PSA testing every 6 to 12 months for the first 5 years and then annually thereafter. For patients who have lymph node–positive disease, PSA testing and a physical examination every 3 to 6 months are warranted. Imaging studies are not indicated as part of routine monitoring.

About 40% of men treated with definitive local therapy may experience biochemical recurrence within 10 years owing to residual or recurrent disease. After radical prostatectomy, the PSA level should be undetectable, and a biochemical recurrence is defined as a PSA level of 0.2 ng/mL or higher, confirmed at two different time points. In contrast to the immediate effect of surgery, the maximal effect of radiation therapy can occur up to 2 years later, and even then the PSA remains detectable because normal prostate cells continue to make PSA. After radiation therapy, recurrence is defined as a rising PSA level more than 2 ng/mL above its post-treatment nadir or a doubling of the PSA level within a 3-month period.

Salvage therapy should be initiated promptly for recurrent or residual disease after prostatectomy or radiation therapy. Depending on the degree of rise of the PSA level, on imaging results to search for local recurrence or distant disease, and on the type of prior definitive local therapy, options to treat recurrence vary but include PET/CT imaging guided radiation therapy[A12] and androgen deprivation therapy[A13] under expert supervision.

Androgen Deprivation Therapy

For patients with recurrent or advanced disease, the goal of systemic therapy is to reduce the testosterone level either surgically by bilateral orchiectomy or medically by androgen deprivation therapy (i.e., medical castration). Medical options under expert supervision include gonadotropin-releasing hormone (GnRH) agonists and antagonists. In the majority of patients treated with either class of agent, levels of serum testosterone decline to castration levels within 30 days of initial treatment.

GnRH agonists, which are synthetic analogs of GnRH, bind to the GnRH receptor in the anterior pituitary and can lead to a temporary surge of luteinizing hormone and hence in testosterone. As a result, patients who have significant metastatic disease can acutely deteriorate unless the amount of circulating testosterone is reduced by pretreatment with an antiandrogen or androgen receptor antagonist, such as oral flutamide, bicalutamide, or nilutamide. GnRH agonists, which are available either as injectables or implants, include leuprolide, goserelin, triptorelin, and histrelin.

GnRH antagonists, which are synthetic analogs of the gonadotropin-releasing hormone that is produced by the hypothalamus, prevent GnRH from binding to its receptors in the anterior pituitary. As a result, levels of luteinizing hormone are reduced, and then testosterone levels are reduced. Because GnRH antagonists have a direct mechanism of action, a flare response does not occur. Available GnRH antagonists under expert oversight, either as injectables or oral agents, are degarelix or relugolix.

Side effects with both GnRH agonists and antagonists reflect low testosterone levels. Common symptoms and signs for which patients should be monitored include hot flashes, weight gain, fatigue, osteoporosis, increased levels of serum cholesterol, loss of muscle mass, loss of libido, and increased blood pressure. The cumulative incidence of major adverse cardiovascular events (e.g., nonfatal myocardial infarction, nonfatal stroke, and all-cause death) is about 50% less with relugolix than with leuprolide.[A14]

Metastatic Prostate Cancer

Most metastatic prostate cancers are initially hormone-sensitive and respond to androgen deprivation, but nearly all tumors eventually become nonsensitive.[17]

Metastatic, Hormone-Sensitive Prostate Cancer

In patients who have metastatic disease, another systemic agent typically is added to androgen deprivation therapy because intensification of treatment with either docetaxel or a newer generation hormonal agent can significantly improve survival. For example, the addition of docetaxel to androgen-deprivation therapy in patients with hormone-sensitive disease extends median overall survival by 17 months compared with androgen therapy alone[A15] in patients who have high-volume disease, defined by presence of visceral metastasis or four or more bone lesions, including at least one beyond vertebral bodies and pelvis. In such patients, attaining a PSA level ≤ 0.2 ng/mL at 7 months is prognostic for longer overall survival.

Newer generation hormonal agents used under expert oversight include abiraterone, enzalutamide, apalutamide, and darolutamide, each of which blocks the androgen receptor and improves overall survival in both low- and high-volume disease when added to androgen deprivation therapy compared to androgen deprivation therapy alone.[A16-A19] Unlike abiraterone, treatment with enzalutamide and apalutamide does not require replacement glucocorticoid treatment.

Metastatic, Castration-Resistant Prostate Cancer

General Approach

Despite the success achieved by androgen deprivation and hormonal therapy, castration-resistant disease ultimately emerges, as evidenced by rising PSA levels despite testosterone levels that confirm castration. Under expert supervision, the treatment plan for patients with metastatic, castration-resistant prostate cancer should be guided by the location and burden of metastasis, the prior treatment that was received when disease was hormone-sensitive, symptoms, and molecular status. Single-agent treatment is usually preferred.

When PSA levels rise during treatment with androgen deprivation therapy and first-generation antiandrogens, androgen deprivation therapy (a GnRH agonist or antagonist) is generally continued indefinitely, but withdrawal of the antiandrogen may temporarily reverse the rise in PSA. If patients were treated with docetaxel, retreatment with docetaxel may be reasonable if the progression occurred more than 12 months after it was last used. If progression occurs quickly after docetaxel treatment in hormone-sensitive disease, cabazitaxel can be utilized. If patients received a newer-generation hormonal therapy, another similar agent should not be used. Instead, another agent with a different mechanism of action, such as docetaxel, should be considered. Abiraterone, enzalutamide, and darolutamide are FDA-approved agents in metastatic, castration-resistant prostate cancer, but apalutamide is not FDA-approved in this setting. The emergence of lethal and aggressive prostate cancer with neuroendocrine/small cell features requires treatment with combination chemotherapy (cisplatin/carboplatin and etoposide).

In addition to chemotherapy and novel hormonal therapy, other FDA-approved agents include immunotherapy, poly (ADP-ribose) polymerase (PARP) inhibitors, and bone-targeting agents such as radium-223. For patients whose tumors are microsatellite instability-high (MSI-H), mismatch repair deficient (dMMR), or tumor mutational burden-high (≥10 mutations/megabase cancer), pembrolizumab, a programmed death receptor-1 (PD-1) blocking antibody, is effective. Sipuleucel-T is an autologous cellular immunotherapy that is designed to induce an immune response targeted against prostatic acid phosphatase, which is an antigen that is expressed in prostate cancer. This agent is indicated for treatment of asymptomatic or minimally symptomatic metastatic, castration-resistant prostate cancer regardless of the type of prior therapy.[18] The toxicities related to sipuleucel-T are related to acute infusion reactions and include fatigue, fever, chills, and nausea.

Men with prostate cancer due to DNA repair gene mutations respond well to poly (ADP-ribose) polymerase (PARP) inhibitors. Men with prostate cancer in the setting of mutations in one of the mismatch repair genes associated with Lynch syndrome may benefit from immunotherapy. If the molecular profiling reveals a deleterious or suspected deleterious germline or somatic homologous recombination repair gene in patients who have progressed following prior treatment with chemotherapy and/or abiraterone or enzalutamide, treatment with PARP inhibitors (including olaparib and rucaparib) is useful.[A20,A21] The toxicities include anemia, pneumonitis, and diarrhea.

Radium 223, an α-particle-emitting radioactive therapeutic agent, is indicated for the treatment of patients with symptomatic bone metastasis and no known visceral metastatic disease. Similar to the other agents, the overall survival with this agent is nearly 4 months better compared with placebo. The toxicities from radium-223 include bone marrow suppression and an increased risk of fractures, but adding bone-strengthening agents may reduce the risk of fractures. Combination of radium-223 with other agents is not currently recommended.

Theranostics represent another therapeutic class of drugs. A targeted radioligand therapy, ^{177}Lu-PSMA-617, targets prostate specific membrane antigen, which is highly expressed in prostate cancer, as demonstrated by a positive prostate specific membrane antigen PET/CT scan.[A22]

Supportive Care

Optimization of quality of life requires careful management of the symptoms as well as the side effects of treatment. Goals of care in the management of patients with advanced or metastatic prostate cancer should be established early and revisited frequently by a multidisciplinary team of experts. For example, androgen deprivation therapy, whether given short or long term, has side effects that require collaboration with primary care physicians and appropriate subspecialists, including cardiology, endocrinology, and/or orthopedics. Bone health also requires supplemental vitamin D and calcium as well as bisphosphonates, depending on bone density and the risk of fractures (Chapter 225). Fortunately, many therapeutic options and clinical trials are available.

PREVENTION

Screening

Randomized trials show that PSA screening can somewhat reduce prostate-cancer-specific mortality but probably not overall mortality despite the potential side-effects of biopsies and procedures.[A23,A24] Based on these data, the U.S. Preventive Services Task Force recommended against routine PSA screening in 2012 and now recommends that men ages 55 to 69 years be informed about the potential benefits and harms of PSA-based screening, so that they can make individualized decisions. For higher-risk men, such as men with a positive family history, screening probably should be encouraged. By comparison, routine screening is not recommended in men ages 70 years and older.[19]

PSA testing has a high sensitivity but low specificity because conditions such as benign prostatic hypertrophy and prostatitis (Chapter 114) can cause false-positive elevations. A PSA level above 4 ng/mL will detect 70 to 80% of tumors, but age-specific thresholds are 2.5 ng/mL for men ages 40 to 49 years, 3.5 ng/mL for men ages 50 to 59 years, 4.5 ng/mL for men ages 60 to 69 years, and 6.5 ng/mL for men ages 70 to 79 years. When the PSA is 4 to 10 ng/mL, a free PSA percentage below 25% can detect 95% of cancers while avoiding 20% of unnecessary biopsies. Another approach, especially for older men with concomitant benign prostatic hypertrophy, is to divide the PSA level in ng/mL by the size of the prostate in mL on ultrasonography; a value less than 0.09 ng/mL/cc is strongly suggestive of benign disease. When biopsy is being considered, magnetic resonance imaging guidance[A25] is generally preferred over ultrasonography-guided biopsy, and both are preferred over unguided biopsy.

Chemoprevention

Finasteride and dutasteride, which are 5α-reductase inhibitors that are commonly prescribed for benign prostatic hypertrophy (Chapter 114), reduce the risk of developing of prostate cancer.[A26] However, neither medication is FDA-approved to prevent prostate cancer because initial studies raised concerns that 5α-reductase inhibitors increased the risk of higher-grade prostate cancer. Interestingly, recent evidence from long-term follow-up studies of men with access to modern screening options questions this concern.[20]

PROGNOSIS

At the time of diagnosis, 5-year survival rates are 100% for localized disease, 100% for regional disease, and 30% for disseminated disease. However, 10-year PSA progression-free survival rates are lower: about 70 to 80% for well-differentiated tumors treated with either surgery or radiation therapy; 50 to 70% for intermediate-risk tumors; and 30% for high-risk tumors. The decrease in screening since the more conservative U.S. guidelines were promulgated has resulted in a small but real increase in the incidence of metastatic prostate cancer[21] and in prostate-cancer–specific mortality rates.[22]

Adverse prognostic markers include Gleason score at the time of prostatectomy, reappearance of PSA after complete prostatectomy, and the PSA doubling time. Bone metastases may be seen. For androgen-responsive metastatic disease, median survival generally ranges from 2 to 6 years depending on the tumor's characteristics. The median survival period for men with metastatic castration-resistant prostate cancer is about 3 years.

Rare ductal and intraductal tumors have a poorer prognosis. Small-cell or neuroendocrine carcinomas are characterized by lack of responsiveness to androgen deprivation as well as rapid progression, with lytic bone lesions and visceral disease.

GENERAL REFERENCES

For the General References and other additional features, please visit Elsevier eBooks+ at https://ebooks.health.elsevier.com.

Grade A References

A1. Ahdoot M, Wilbur AR, Reese SE, et al. MRI-targeted, systematic, and combined biopsy for prostate cancer diagnosis. *N Engl J Med.* 2020;382:917-928.

A2. Nordström T, Discacciati A, Bergman M, et al. Prostate cancer screening using a combination of risk-prediction, MRI, and targeted prostate biopsies (STHLM3-MRI): a prospective, population-based, randomised, open-label, non-inferiority trial. *Lancet Oncol.* 2021;22:1240-1249.

A3. Hugosson J, Månsson M, Wallström J, et al. Prostate cancer screening with PSA and MRI followed by targeted biopsy only. *N Engl J Med.* 2022;387:2126-2137.

A4. Wilt TJ, Jones KM, Barry MJ, et al. Follow-up of prostatectomy versus observation for early prostate cancer. *N Engl J Med.* 2017;377:132-142.

A5. Hoffman KE, Penson DF, Zhao Z, et al. Patient-reported outcomes through 5 years for active surveillance, surgery, brachytherapy, or external beam radiation with or without androgen deprivation therapy for localized prostate cancer. *JAMA.* 2020;323:149-163.

A6. Bill-Axelson A, Holmberg L, Garmo H, et al. Radical prostatectomy or watchful waiting in prostate cancer—29-year follow-up. *N Engl J Med.* 2018;379:2319-2329.

A7. Yaxley JW, Coughlin GD, Chambers SK, et al. Robot-assisted laparoscopic prostatectomy versus open radical retropubic prostatectomy: early outcomes from a randomised controlled phase 3 study. *Lancet.* 2016;388:1057-1066.

A8. Hamdy FC, Donovan JL, Lane JA, et al. 10-year outcomes after monitoring, surgery, or radiotherapy for localized prostate cancer. *N Engl J Med.* 2016;375:1415-1424.

A9. Dearnaley D, Syndikus I, Mossop H, et al. Conventional versus hypofractionated high-dose intensity-modulated radiotherapy for prostate cancer: 5-year outcomes of the randomised, noninferiority, phase 3 CHHiP trial. *Lancet Oncol.* 2016;17:1047-1060.

A10. Fransson P, Nilsson P, Gunnlaugsson A, et al. Ultra-hypofractionated versus conventionally fractionated radiotherapy for prostate cancer (HYPO-RT-PC): patient-reported quality-of-life outcomes of a randomised, controlled, non-inferiority, phase 3 trial. *Lancet Oncol.* 2021;22:235-245.

A11. Attard G, Murphy L, Clarke NW, et al. Abiraterone acetate and prednisolone with or without enzalutamide for high-risk non-metastatic prostate cancer: a meta-analysis of primary results from two randomised controlled phase 3 trials of the STAMPEDE platform protocol. *Lancet.* 2022;399:447-460.

A12. Jani AB, Schreibmann E, Goyal S, et al. ^{18}F-fluciclovine-PET/CT imaging versus conventional imaging alone to guide postprostatectomy salvage radiotherapy for prostate cancer (EMPIRE-1): a single centre, open-label, phase 2/3 randomised controlled trial. *Lancet.* 2021;397:1895-1904.

A13. Pollack A, Karrison TG, Balogh AG, et al. The addition of androgen deprivation therapy and pelvic lymph node treatment to prostate bed salvage radiotherapy (NRG Oncology/RTOG 0534 SPPORT): an international, multicentre, randomised phase 3 trial. *Lancet.* 2022;399:1886-1901.

A14. Shore ND, Saad F, Cookson MS, et al. Oral relugolix for androgen-deprivation therapy in advanced prostate cancer. *N Engl J Med.* 2020;382:2187-2196.

A15. Kyriakopoulos CE, Chen YH, Carducci MA, et al. Chemohormonal therapy in metastatic hormone-sensitive prostate cancer: long-term survival analysis of the randomized phase III E3805 CHAARTED trial. *J Clin Oncol.* 2018;36:1080-1087.

A16. Fizazi K, Foulon S, Carles J, et al. Abiraterone plus prednisone added to androgen deprivation therapy and docetaxel in de novo metastatic castration-sensitive prostate cancer (PEACE-1): a multicentre, open-label, randomised, phase 3 study with a 2 × 2 factorial design. *Lancet.* 2022;399:1695-1707.

A17. Armstrong AJ, Azad AA, Iguchi T, et al. Improved survival with enzalutamide in patients with metastatic hormone-sensitive prostate cancer. *J Clin Oncol.* 2022;40:1616-1622.

A18. Chi KN, Agarwal N, Bjartell A, et al. Apalutamide for metastatic, castration-sensitive prostate cancer. *N Engl J Med.* 2019;381:13-24.

A19. Smith MR, Hussain M, Saad F, et al. Darolutamide and survival in metastatic, hormone-sensitive prostate cancer. *N Engl J Med.* 2022;386:1132-1142.

A20. de Bono J, Mateo J, Fizazi K, et al. Olaparib for metastatic castration-resistant prostate cancer. *N Engl J Med.* 2020;382:2091-2102.

A21. Fizazi K, Piulats JM, Reaume MN, et al. Rucaparib or physician's choice in metastatic prostate cancer. *N Engl J Med.* 2023;388:719-732.

A22. Sartor O, de Bono J, Chi KN, et al. Lutetium-177-PSMA-617 for metastatic castration-resistant prostate cancer. *N Engl J Med.* 2021;385:1091-1103.

A23. Ilic D, Djulbegovic M, Jung JH, et al. Prostate cancer screening with prostate-specific antigen (PSA) test: a systematic review and meta-analysis. *BMJ.* 2018;362:k3519.

A24. Fenton JJ, Weyrich MS, Durbin S, et al. Prostate-specific antigen-based screening for prostate cancer: evidence report and systematic review of the US Preventive Services Task Force. *JAMA.* 2018;319:1914-1931.

A25. Eklund M, Jäderling F, Discacciati A, et al. MRI-targeted or standard biopsy in prostate cancer screening. *N Engl J Med.* 2021;385:908-920.

A26. Goodman PJ, Tangen CM, Darke AK, et al. Long-term effects of finasteride on prostate cancer mortality. *N Engl J Med.* 2019;380:393-394.

187 MALIGNANT BONE TUMORS, SARCOMAS, AND OTHER SOFT TISSUE NEOPLASMS

ROBIN L. JONES

BONE TUMORS

Primary bone tumors include osteosarcomas, chondrosarcomas, and Ewing sarcoma. These rare tumors, which arise from the normal cellular components of bone and can potentially metastasize, have an incidence of 1.8 new cases per 100,000 population per year and account for only 0.2% of all cancers. Tumors that originate in other organs can metastasize to bone and represent the vast majority of bone cancers in adults.

CLINICAL MANIFESTATIONS AND DIAGNOSIS

Patients who have either primary malignant or benign bone tumors can present with pain, swelling, and sometimes pathologic fracture of the involved bone.

Metastatic tumors to bone also can be similarly symptomatic but are often first suspected based on imaging tests that are obtained to stage the tumor. Imaging of a primary bone tumor includes plain radiographs, magnetic resonance imaging (MRI), and computed tomography (CT). On imaging, malignant tumors generally have irregular, poorly defined borders, a wide area of transition, evidence of cortical bone destruction, periosteal reaction, and soft tissue extension.

When imaging suggests a malignant primary bone tumor, the patient should be referred to an orthopedic oncologist to perform a diagnostic biopsy. An improperly performed biopsy can potentially change a tumor that is resectable by limb salvage to a tumor that requires amputation. Staging evaluation should include both a CT scan and a bone scan.

MAJOR PRIMARY MALIGNANT BONE TUMORS

OSTEOSARCOMA

Osteosarcoma, which is the most common bone sarcoma, accounts for approximately 35% of all primary bone tumors. Osteosarcomas have a bimodal age distribution, with the highest incidence before age 20 years and a second peak after age 60 years.[1] About 60% of cases occur in males. The most common primary sites in the younger age group are the metaphyses of long bones and the extremities, especially the distal femur, proximal tibia, and proximal humerus. In older adults, the primary anatomic sites are more varied.

Most osteosarcomas are sporadic, but the incidence is higher among families with germline gene mutations or deletions, such as retinoblastoma (about 60% of familial cases), *TP53* (Li-Fraumeni syndrome, about 40% of familial cases), or rarely the *RecQ DNA helicase* genes (Rothman-Thompson, Werner, or Bloom syndrome). Prior radiation and Paget disease (Chapter 228) are also risk factors, particularly for older individuals.

On histologic examination, osteosarcomas contain varying amounts of osteoid as well as cartilage and fibrous tissue. The typical radiologic appearance consists of a mixture of osteoblastic and osteolytic features with periosteal elevation.

TREATMENT

Management generally consists of neoadjuvant chemotherapy followed by surgical resection and then adjuvant chemotherapy.[2] Most patients can undergo limb salvage surgery rather than amputation. For patients under age 40 years, the most widely used chemotherapy schedule consists of methotrexate, doxorubicin, and cisplatin under expert supervision. Some patients with solitary or oligometastatic disease can undergo surgery with curative intent, but the evidence base is limited. A number of salvage chemotherapy schedules can be considered, including gemcitabine/docetaxel and ifosfamide/etoposide.

PROGNOSIS

With current multidisciplinary management, including complete surgical resection and multiagent chemotherapy, the overall survival of patients with osteosarcoma is on the order of 65%.[3] A higher percentage of tumor necrosis (>90%) following neoadjuvant chemotherapy portends a better prognosis. However, the outcome for patients with metastatic osteosarcoma is poor.

CHONDROSARCOMA

Chondrosarcomas, which are the second most common bone sarcoma (25% of cases), are characterized by malignant differentiation of hyaline cartilage.[4] The peak incidence is in the fifth to seventh decades. The pelvis, proximal femur, and proximal humerus are the most common primary sites, and patients can present with long-standing swelling and/or pain. Approximately 15% of chondrosarcomas arise from preexisting peripheral osteochondromas and harbor mutations in the exostosis (*EXT1 or EXT2*) gene. The other 85% arise in a central location, some in preexisting enchondromas. The majority of chondrosarcomas (90%) are low or intermediate grade, but the 10% of chondrosarcomas that are high-grade exhibit much more metastatic potential.

The pathologic distinction between low-grade chondrosarcoma and benign central enchondromas can be challenging, but size greater than 5 cm and axial location are very suggestive of malignancy. On imaging, chondrosarcomas often have a mixed sclerotic and lytic appearance.

TREATMENT AND PROGNOSIS

Complete surgical resection with clear margins is the mainstay of management for all grades of chondrosarcoma. The overall 5-year survival rate is about 75%, and most patients who survive for 4 years also survive for 10 years or longer.[5] Unfortunately, these tumors are relatively insensitive to radiation and chemotherapy, although these modalities may be considered in the palliative setting.

EWING SARCOMA

Ewing sarcoma, which accounts for approximately 15% of bone sarcomas, commonly has a characteristic translocation between *EWS* and *ETS* family transcription factors. The most common translocation [t(11;22)(q24;q12)] between *EWSR1* and *FLI1* occurs in approximately 85% of cases, but other fusion genes are also found. Although Ewing sarcoma most commonly presents in bone, it can also arise in soft tissue, in which case it is called extraosseous Ewing sarcoma.

The peak incidence for Ewing sarcoma is in the second decade, but about 20% of cases occur in older patients. This disease mainly occurs in Whites of European origin. Patients can present with a systemic illness, characterized by intermittent low-grade fever, leukocytosis, and anemia. Ewing sarcoma has a predilection for the diaphyseal region of long bones, pelvis, and ribs.

On imaging, these tumors frequently have associated soft tissue involvement and can also have a permeative or "moth-eaten" appearance and a multilayered "onion-skin" periosteal reaction. Special pathologic input is critical in establishing the diagnosis, particularly in distinguishing Ewing sarcoma from other small, round, blue cell tumors.

TREATMENT AND PROGNOSIS

Patients are generally treated with neoadjuvant chemotherapy followed by surgery/radiation and then adjuvant chemotherapy.[6] A commonly used combination under expert guidance is dose-intensive vincristine, doxorubicin, and cyclophosphamide alternating with ifosfamide and etoposide.[A1]

With multiagent chemotherapy, the 5-year event-free survival rate is about 70%. The outcome for patients with clinically detectable metastatic disease is poor. A number of salvage therapies can be used, including cyclophosphamide/topotecan, irinotecan/temozolomide, and gemcitabine/docetaxel.

METASTATIC TUMORS TO BONE

Metastatic bone disease from hematogenous spread[7] is an important cause of cancer-related morbidity. Breast cancer (Chapter 183) in women and prostate cancer (Chapter 186) in men are the most common tumors that metastasize to bone. Other tumors that often develop bone metastases include lung (Chapter 177), thyroid (Chapter 207), gastrointestinal tract (Chapter 179), and kidney (Chapter 182) cancers.[8]

A plain radiograph can show blastic (typical of prostate cancer) or lytic (e.g., myeloma; Chapter 173) lesions. However, most bone metastases have a mixed appearance. A radiologic survey should be performed in a patient who has known bony metastatic disease or who presents with bone pain to identify other possible metastatic lesions. CT scanning or MRI can help determine the risk of fracture. Radionuclide bone scans can also identify the extent of metastatic bone disease and evaluate response to treatment, but the bone scan may be negative in tumors such as myeloma that cause purely lytic lesions. If patients have no symptoms and a low risk of developing bone metastases, routine screening is not recommended.

TREATMENT

Pathologic fractures or lesions at imminent risk of fracture are generally treated with surgical fixation. Painful lesions with no risk of fracture are treated with external-beam radiation. Dexamethasone (two 4-mg dexamethasone tablets at least 1 hour before the start of radiation treatment and then every day for 4 days after radiotherapy) can reduce the risk of a radiation-associated flare of pain. Systemic palliative therapy for bone metastases[9] should follow standard guidelines for the specific tumor type, and treatment can include bisphosphonates (Chapter 225), denosumab, and endocrine and/or chemotherapy.

PREVENTION

Treatment with bisphosphonates under expert supervision can prolong the time to a first skeletal event in patients with breast cancer (Chapter 183), prostate cancer (Chapter 186), and myeloma (Chapter 173).[A2] The optimal schedule and duration of therapy remain to be defined.

PROGNOSIS

The prognosis of patients with metastatic cancer to bone depends on the specific type of tumor but typically is poor because it represents late-stage disease.

SOFT TISSUE SARCOMAS

DEFINITION

Sarcomas, which are malignant tumors of mesodermal origin, account for approximately 1% of all adult cancers. These tumors of connective tissue can occur in almost any anatomic location. In addition, they are very heterogeneous, with more than 100 different histologic subtypes, each with unique underlying biology and clinical behavior.[10]

EPIDEMIOLOGY

The incidence of soft tissue sarcomas in the United States is about 13,000 cases per year. Individuals who are at high risk for developing sarcomas include patients with Li-Fraumeni syndrome (Chapter 166), retinoblastoma (Chapter 391), neurofibromatosis (Chapter 385), malignant peripheral nerve sheath tumor, gastrointestinal stromal tumors (GISTs; Chapter 179), and familial polyposis (Chapter 179). Prior radiation treatment (e.g., for breast cancer, cervical cancer, or lymphoma) also increases the risk of developing a sarcoma in the radiation field. Occupational exposure to polyvinyl chlorides is associated with increased risk of hepatic angiosarcomas. Chronic lymphedema is also a risk factor for the development of angiosarcoma (Stewart-Treves syndrome). However, the vast majority of soft tissue sarcomas are sporadic with no known risk factor.

PATHOBIOLOGY

Soft tissue sarcomas can be divided into tumors with a complex karyotype (e.g., leiomyosarcoma, undifferentiated pleomorphic sarcoma, and angiosarcoma) and tumors with a simple karyotype. Tumors with simpler karyotypes include translocation-associated sarcomas (e.g., myxoid liposarcoma and synovial sarcoma), sarcomas with specific kinase mutations (notably gastrointestinal stromal tumors), tumors with simple genetic alterations (amplifications of *CDK4* and *MDM2* in dedifferentiated liposarcoma), and tumors with gene activation (e.g., *INI1* loss in rhabdoid tumors, *NF1* in malignant peripheral nerve sheath tumor, and *NTRK* fusions in soft tissue sarcomas).

CLINICAL MANIFESTATIONS AND DIAGNOSIS

The diversity of primary anatomic sites and the rarity as well as the heterogeneity of histologic subtypes can make the diagnosis and management of sarcomas challenging. Even within a particular subtype of sarcoma (e.g., leiomyosarcoma), clinical manifestations can be remarkably heterogeneous. Clinical behavior can range from an indolent tumor that can grow over decades (e.g., well-differentiated liposarcoma) to highly aggressive, life-threatening diseases (e.g., angiosarcoma). Sarcomas on the extremities often present with a slowly growing, nontender mass, but over 99% of such masses are benign soft tissue tumors of fat, muscle, fibrous or vascular tissue, or peripheral nerves rather than malignant sarcomas.[11]

The primary anatomic distribution of soft tissue sarcomas is approximately 40% on the lower extremities, 20% on an upper extremity, 20% in the abdomen or pelvis, 10% on the trunk, and 10% in the head and neck. The blood stream is the primary means of dissemination, and sarcomas very rarely spread to lymph nodes. Notable subtypes that can spread to lymph nodes include epithelioid, clear cell, and certain vascular sarcomas.

Initial investigation of a suspected sarcoma should include imaging of the primary site. MRI is preferred for sarcomas on the extremities, chest wall, head, or neck. CT scans are preferred to evaluate sarcomas of the abdomen and pelvis, as well as to define the possible presence of metastatic disease in the lungs and bone.

A core biopsy of the mass should be performed to make the histologic diagnosis. The biopsy tract should be in the direction of the future incision. Because of the challenges of histopathologic diagnosis, fine-needle aspiration is not performed except occasionally in gastrointestinal stromal tumors.

Because of their heterogeneous pathobiology, specialized pathologic review is needed to confirm the diagnosis of sarcoma. The most common histologic subtypes are gastrointestinal stromal tumor, undifferentiated pleomorphic sarcoma, leiomyosarcoma, and liposarcoma.

TREATMENT

Improperly performed surgical procedures can have a negative impact on outcome, so patients with a suspected sarcoma should be evaluated and treated by an experienced multidisciplinary team.[12]

Localized Sarcomas

The mainstay of management of localized sarcomas is limb-preserving complete surgical resection with clear margins plus radiation therapy. For large, high-grade soft tissue sarcomas of the extremities or trunk, preoperative neoadjuvant radiation is generally recommended over postoperative adjuvant radiation[13] because of its lower dose, smaller field size, and consequently reduced fibrosis and edema despite a higher wound complication rate than with adjuvant radiation.

For retroperitoneal sarcomas, an aggressive surgical approach, including resection of adjacent structures even in the absence of clear invasion, may improve local control. The role of neoadjuvant radiation in potentially operable retroperitoneal sarcomas is uncertain.

The role of neoadjuvant/adjuvant chemotherapy for soft tissue sarcomas other than large, high-grade tumors of the extremity and trunk remains controversial. Neoadjuvant/adjuvant chemotherapy provides a survival advantage in embryonal rhabdomyosarcoma and soft tissue Ewing sarcoma. If given under expert oversight, standard neoadjuvant chemotherapy (epirubicin/ifosfamide) is as good as histology-tailored chemotherapy.

Progressive or Metastatic Disease

Despite optimal management, about 50% of patients with high-grade localized soft tissue sarcomas progress to locally recurrent or metastatic disease. Such progression is usually within the first 3 years, but late spread can be seen with more indolent tumors. Some patients with low-volume, asymptomatic, and indolent disease may initially undergo active surveillance. For patients with solitary or oligometastatic disease, local therapy, including surgery, radiation, ablation, and embolization techniques, can be effective.[14]

However, the mainstay of management of metastatic disease is palliative chemotherapy. First-line palliative therapy generally consists of an anthracycline-based regimen, and the combination of doxorubicin plus trabectedin under expert supervision provides longer progression-free survival compared with doxorubicin alone.[A3] The combination of doxorubicin and ifosfamide is usually reserved for patients with symptomatic and rapidly progressive disease. Adding olaratumab (a monoclonal antibody that blocks subunit alpha of the platelet-derived growth factor receptor) to doxorubicin is of no incremental value.[A4] Pazopanib (a multitarget tyrosine kinase inhibitor) may be as effective and safe as doxorubicin for the initial treatment of patients over age 60 years.[A5]

For certain histologic subtypes, specific therapies can be considered under expert oversight. Examples include paclitaxel for angiosarcoma; aromatase inhibitors for endometrial stromal sarcoma and low-grade leiomyosarcoma; antiangiogenic agents (pazopanib/sunitinib) in alveolar soft part sarcoma and solitary fibrous tumor; tropomyosin receptor kinase inhibitors (e.g., larotrectinib or entrectinib) for sarcomas with *NTRK* fusions;[15] tazemetostat (a selective EZH2 inhibitor) for epithelioid tumors with a loss of INI1/*SMARCB1* expression;[16] and ALK inhibitors in *ALK*-mutated inflammatory myofibroblastic tumors.

For second-line systemic therapy, the combination of gemcitabine plus docetaxel or gemcitabine plus dacarbazine is preferred over single-agent therapy. Among patients with advanced pretreated liposarcoma and leiomyosarcoma, trabectedin can significantly prolong progression-free survival (median 4.2 vs. 1.5 months, respectively) but not overall survival compared with dacarbazine,[A6] whereas eribulin may prolong overall survival but not progression-free survival.[A7] In patients with pretreated advanced sarcomas, pazopanib can prolong median progression-free survival but not overall survival.

PROGNOSIS

Approximately 50 to 60% of patients with localized sarcoma are cured with optimal management. However, sarcomas encompass a range of different diseases with variable prognoses. The risk of recurrence varies depending on the tumor's grade, size, anatomic location, depth, and histologic subtype. Furthermore, the primary anatomic site can also be important; for example, the outcome following resection of a cutaneous sarcoma is excellent, whereas the prognosis of a cardiac sarcoma is poor.

The prognosis for patients with metastatic disease is limited, with a median overall survival between 12 and 18 months. However, prognosis varies depending on the volume of metastatic disease, histologic subtype, and location. For most sarcomas, however, current chemotherapeutic regimens have improved median survival from 12 months to approximately 18 to 20 months.

GASTROINTESTINAL STROMAL TUMORS

Gastrointestinal stromal tumors are the most common mesenchymal tumor of the gastrointestinal tract. About 85% of cases have activating mutations in *KIT* or *PDGFRA*.[17] Gain-in-function mutations in KIT and PDGFRA receptors lead to constitutive, ligand-independent activation of downstream signaling pathways. Most gastrointestinal stromal tumors express CD117 and DOG1, and CD34 is also expressed in about 70% of cases.[18]

Gastrointestinal stromal tumors occur throughout the gastrointestinal tract, most commonly in the stomach or small intestine. They typically are vascular tumors, frequently presenting with bleeding into the bowel or the abdominal cavity. Mass effects of gastrointestinal stromal tumors may cause abdominal pain or bowel obstruction, and they sometimes are palpable on physical examination. However, most gastrointestinal stromal tumors are detected by imaging, endoscopic screening for colon cancer, or surgical exploration.

TREATMENT

Surgery is the mainstay of management for localized disease,[19] but patients at high risk for progression should be treated with at least 3 years of adjuvant imatinib,[A8] which provides durable benefit in a high proportion of patients. For patients whose gastrointestinal stromal tumors recur or do not respond to imatinib, treatment with sunitinib, regorafenib, or ripretinib can provide sustained benefit (Chapter 178).[A9,A10]

DESMOID TUMORS/AGGRESSIVE FIBROMATOSIS

Desmoid fibromatosis is a very rare, monoclonal, fibroblastic proliferation. Between 80 and 95% of desmoid tumors harbor mutations in the *β-catenin* gene (*CTNNB1*), which leads to nuclear accumulation of β-catenin protein. This tumor lacks metastatic potential but is locally invasive, has a high local recurrence rate, and is characterized by an unpredictable clinical course.

TREATMENT

The general consensus is that a period of initial active surveillance is appropriate for most asymptomatic patients because spontaneous regressions can occur. Local treatment options include surgery, radiation, isolated limb perfusion, and ablation techniques under the expert oversight of an experienced multidisciplinary team. Sorafenib is of proven value for prolonging progression-free survival for advanced and refractory tumors.[A11] Other systemic therapies include tamoxifen/nonsteroidal anti-inflammatory drugs, liposomal doxorubicin, imatinib, navelbine, and methotrexate/vinorelbine.

GENERAL REFERENCES

For the General References and other additional features, please visit Elsevier eBooks+ at https://ebooks.health.elsevier.com.

Grade A References

A1. Brennan B, Kirton L, Marec-Bérard P, et al. Comparison of two chemotherapy regimens in patients with newly diagnosed Ewing sarcoma (EE2012): an open-label, randomised, phase 3 trial. *Lancet.* 2022;400:1513-1521.

A2. Hortobagyi GN, Van Poznak C, Harker WG, et al. Continued treatment effect of zoledronic acid dosing every 12 vs 4 weeks in women with breast cancer metastatic to bone: the OPTIMIZE-3 randomized clinical trial. *JAMA Oncol.* 2017;3:906-912.

A3. Pautier P, Italiano A, Piperno-Neumann S, et al. Doxorubicin alone versus doxorubicin with trabectedin followed by trabectedin alone as first-line therapy for metastatic or unresectable leiomyosarcoma (LMS-04): a randomised, multicentre, open-label phase 3 trial. *Lancet Oncol.* 2022;23:1044-1054.

A4. Tap WD, Wagner AJ, Schöffski P, et al. Effect of doxorubicin plus olaratumab vs doxorubicin plus placebo on survival in patients with advanced soft tissue sarcomas: the ANNOUNCE randomized clinical trial. *JAMA.* 2020;323:1266-1276.

A5. Grünwald V, Karch A, Schuler M, et al. Randomized comparison of pazopanib and doxorubicin as first-line treatment in patients with metastatic soft tissue sarcoma age 60 years or older: results of a German intergroup study. *J Clin Oncol.* 2020;38:3555-3564.

A6. Demetri GD, von Mehren M, Jones RL, et al. Efficacy and safety of trabectedin or dacarbazine for metastatic liposarcoma or leiomyosarcoma after failure of conventional chemotherapy: results of a phase III randomized multicenter clinical trial. *J Clin Oncol.* 2016;34:786-793.

A7. Schöffski P, Chawla S, Maki RG, et al. Eribulin versus dacarbazine in previously treated patients with advanced liposarcoma or leiomyosarcoma: a randomised, open-label, multicentre, phase 3 trial. *Lancet.* 2016;387:1629-1637.

A8. Joensuu H, Eriksson M, Sundby Hall K, et al. Survival outcomes associated with 3 years vs 1 year of adjuvant imatinib for patients with high-risk gastrointestinal stromal tumors: an analysis of a randomized clinical trial after 10-year follow-up. *JAMA Oncol.* 2020;6:1241-1246.

A9. Kang YK, George S, Jones RL, et al. Avapritinib versus regorafenib in locally advanced unresectable or metastatic GI stromal tumor: a randomized, open-label phase III study. *J Clin Onol.* 2021;39:3128-3139.

A10. Blay J-Y, Serrano C, Heinrich MC, et al. Ripretinib in patients with advanced gastrointestinal stromal tumours (INVICTUS): a double-blind, randomised, placebo-controlled, phase 3 trial. *Lancet Oncol.* 2020;21:923-934.

A11. Gounder MM, Mahoney MR, Van Tine BA, et al. Sorafenib for advanced and refractory desmoid tumors. *N Engl J Med.* 2018;379:2417-2428.

188 MELANOMA AND NONMELANOMA SKIN CANCERS

LYNN M. SCHUCHTER

MELANOMA

EPIDEMIOLOGY

The incidence of melanoma continues to rise rapidly worldwide, but mortality rates are declining. Each year in the United States, nearly 100,000 new cases of invasive melanoma are detected, and approximately 7000 patients die from melanoma.[1] Melanoma is the leading cause of death from cutaneous malignant disease, and it accounts for 1 to 2% of all cancer deaths in the United States.

The rising incidence is attributed to increasing sun exposure, especially early in life, as well as to more aggressive diagnosis[2] and even over-diagnosis.[3] Melanoma affects all age groups, with a median age at diagnosis of 63 years. Melanoma is largely a disease of Whites, with a very low incidence in Black Americans, Asians, and Hispanics.

Risk Factors

Risk factors for melanoma include family history of melanoma, prior melanoma or nonmelanoma skin cancer, inherited genetic susceptibility, and sun exposure. Artificial exposure to UV radiation by indoor tanning beds is likewise a risk factor for melanoma.[4] Individuals who have blond or red hair, blue eye color, and freckles have a tendency to burn rather than to tan and have higher rates of melanoma. The pattern of sun exposure may also be important; intermittent intense exposure, rather than chronic sun exposure, may carry a higher risk for melanoma.

Individuals with an increased number of typical or benign moles, atypical moles, or dysplastic nevi (Figs. 188-1 and 188-2) also have an increased risk for melanoma. Atypical moles or dysplastic nevi are important precursor lesions of melanoma and serve as markers for increasing risk. For example, individuals with dysplastic nevi have a 6% lifetime chance of developing melanoma, and this risk increases to as high as 80% in individuals who have dysplastic nevi and a strong family history of melanoma.

PATHOBIOLOGY

Exposure to sunlight, especially ultraviolet (UV) radiation (Chapter 18), is the major causative factor for the development of melanoma. Melanomas originate from melanocytes, which are located predominantly in the basal cell layer of the epidermis and use the enzyme tyrosinase to synthesize melanin pigment, which serves to protect against UV damage (Chapter 403). In persons of color, however, exposure to UV light may not be an important risk factor.[5]

Somatic mutations in primary and metastatic melanoma primarily involve the mitogen activated protein kinase pathway (MAPK). The point-mutation burden increases from benign through intermediate precursor lesions to melanoma, with strong genetic evidence of the effects of UV radiation detectable at all evolutionary stages. Activating mutations in the *BRAF* gene can be found in approximately 50% of melanomas, and 20% of melanomas are associated with a mutation in the *NRAS* gene. Distinct patterns of genetic alterations are found in primary melanomas based on anatomic location and extent of sun exposure.[6] For example, melanomas that originate on mucous membranes, acral skin (soles, palms), and skin with chronic sun damage (i.e., lentigo maligna melanoma) have frequent mutations in *KIT*. Uveal melanoma is associated with mutations in *GNAQ/GNA11*. Monosomy of chromosome 3 and somatic mutations in the gene encoding BRCA1-associated

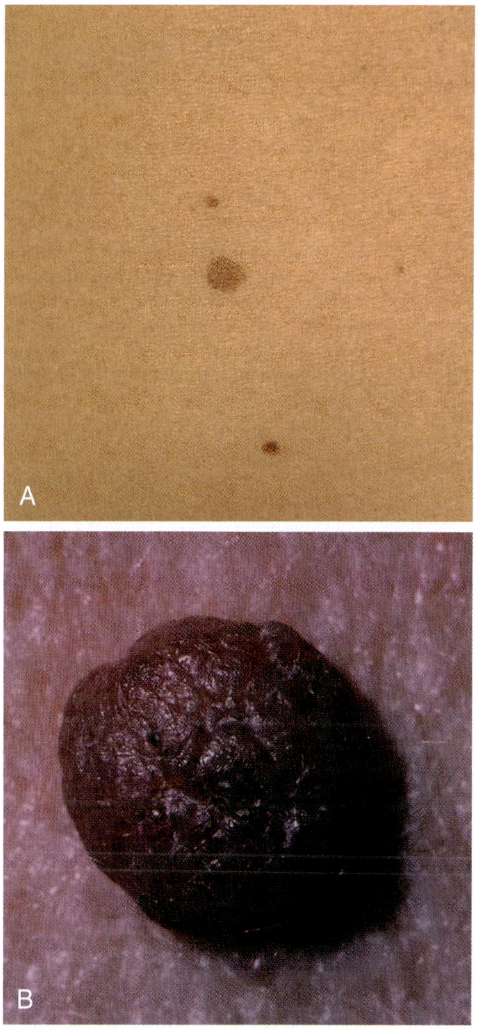

FIGURE 188-1. Nevi. A, Common benign nevus. B, Dermal nevus.

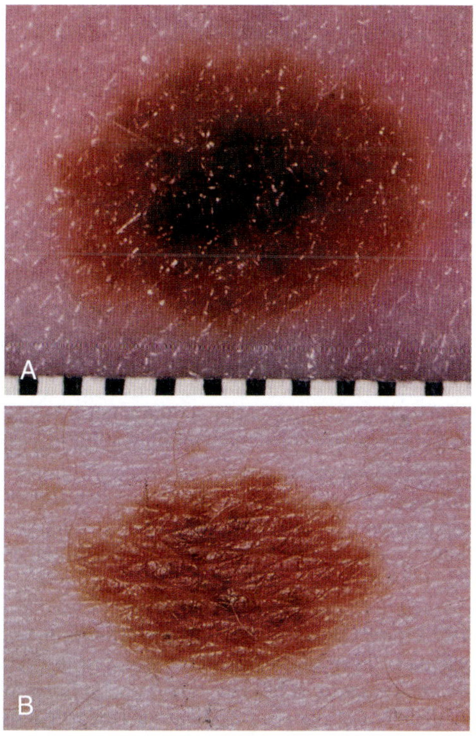

FIGURE 188-2. Dysplastic nevi. A and B, Examples of dysplastic nevi.

protein (BAP1) on chromosome 3 are associated with worse outcome and the development of metastatic melanoma. The discovery of somatic mutations in melanoma and associated aberrant signal transduction pathways has provided the basis for the development of molecularly targeted therapy for patients with advanced melanoma.[7]

Inherited Genetics

Approximately 10% of patients with melanoma have a family history of melanoma. Several chromosomal loci determine susceptibility to melanoma. The most important locus is *p16/CDKN2A*, which is on chromosome 9p21. This gene is a member of a class of molecules that play a central role in cell cycle regulation. Of the members of melanoma-prone families, 25 to 40% have mutations in this gene. The risk for developing cutaneous melanoma in an individual who is a *CDKN2A* carrier is between 30 and 90% by age 80 years and varies by geographic location.

Genetic variability in the melanocortin-1 receptor (MC1R) plays a key role in pigmentation of skin and hair, and this variability has been implicated in a predisposition to melanoma. Carriers of a pathogenic mutation in the *BRCA2* familial breast cancer gene have an increased risk of developing cutaneous melanoma. Germline mutations in *BAP1* gene are linked to the BAP1 tumor predisposition syndrome. Both uveal and cutaneous melanoma have been described in this syndrome, which is also associated with mesothelioma and renal cell cancer.

CLINICAL MANIFESTATIONS

Early detection and recognition of melanoma are key to improving survival. The signs of early melanoma are based on the clinical appearance of the pigmented lesion and a change in the shape, color, or surface of an existing mole. Most patients report a preexisting mole at the site of the melanoma. Itching, burning, or pain in a pigmented lesion should increase suspicion, although melanomas often are not associated with local discomfort. Bleeding and ulceration are signs of a more advanced melanoma. Most melanomas are varying shades of brown, but they may be black, blue, or pink. The ABCDEs for the recognition of melanoma are asymmetry, border irregularity, color variation, diameter greater than 6 mm, and evolution or a change in a skin lesion. The "ugly duckling" sign is recognizing a skin lesion that looks different from other skin lesions and is therefore suspicious.

Cutaneous melanoma has been divided into four subtypes. Superficial spreading melanoma, which accounts for 70% of all melanomas, can be located on any anatomic site (Fig. 188-3). Lentigo maligna melanoma, which represents 4 to 10% of all melanomas, tends to occur more commonly in chronically sun-exposed skin in older patients, frequently on the head and neck (Fig. 188-4); clinically, it appears as a macular (flat) lesion, with varying degrees of color, usually brown. Nodular melanoma (Fig. 188-5) accounts for 15 to 30% of melanomas and manifests as a rapidly enlarging, elevated, or polypoid lesion, often blue or black. These lesions can also be amelanotic and lack pigment and have more of a pink color. The ABCDE rule does not always apply as well to nodular melanomas. Acral lentiginous melanoma manifests as a darkly pigmented, flat to nodular lesion on the palm, on the sole, or subungually; sunlight is not thought to play a causative role in this form of melanoma. Histologic subtype does not directly correlate with clinical behavior. However, recent data suggest that histologic subtype may correlate with specific genetic abnormalities. For example, superficial spreading melanoma may be associated with *BRAF* mutation, and lentigo maligna melanoma may be associated with *KIT* mutation.[8]

Ocular melanomas arise from the pigmented layer of the eye. Uveal melanoma is the most common intraocular malignancy of adults. Melanomas can also arise from noncutaneous sites, including mucosal epithelium in the gastrointestinal tract, anorectal area, genitourinary tract, and nasal and nasopharyngeal mucosa. Melanomas of the vulva and vagina are relatively rare. In general, mucosal melanomas are diagnosed at a more advanced stage of disease. The mainstay of treatment is surgical.

DIAGNOSIS

Biopsy of the Primary Lesion

Any skin lesion suggestive of melanoma should be sampled by biopsy with complete excision, including a 1- to 2-mm margin of normal skin and some subcutaneous fat. Lesions that can be confused with melanoma include blue nevi, pigmented basal cell carcinoma, seborrheic keratosis, and hemangiomas (Table 188-1). Both molecular and cellular criteria can distinguish common nevi from dysplastic nevi.

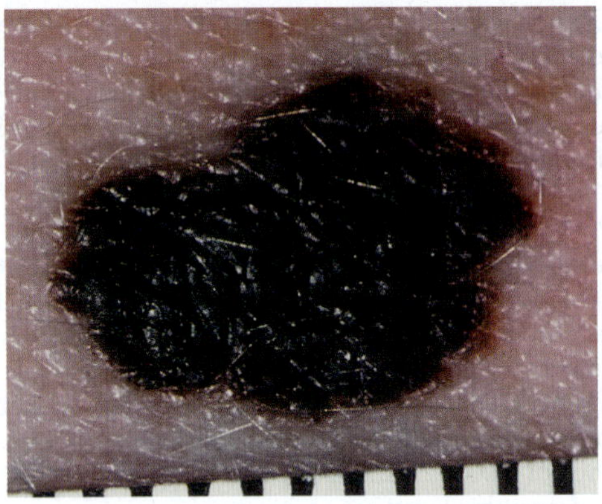

FIGURE 188-3. Superficial spreading melanoma.

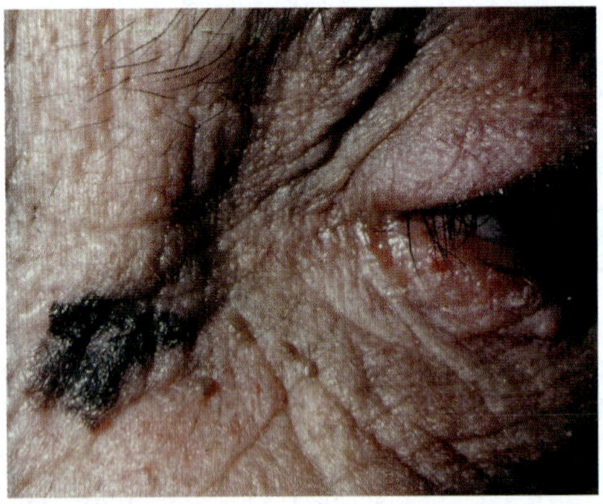

FIGURE 188-4. Lentigo maligna melanoma.

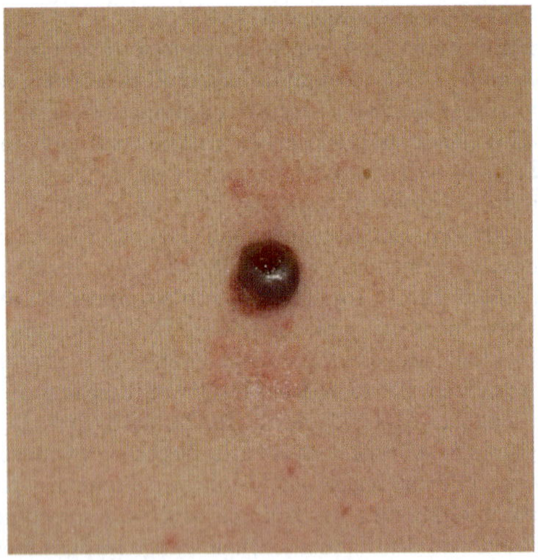

FIGURE 188-5. Nodular melanoma.

An incisional biopsy may be necessary for lesions that are too large for complete excision. Shallow shave biopsies, curettage, cryosurgery, laser, and electrodessication are contraindicated in lesions suggestive of melanoma.

Activating mutations in the *BRAF* gene are present in approximately 50% of melanomas, and all patients with advanced cutaneous melanoma should have their tumors assessed for the presence or absence of a *BRAF* mutation. Almost 80% of *BRAF* mutations are V600E, with most of the remainder consisting of V600K.

Sentinel Lymph Node Biopsy

Sentinel lymph node mapping is considered a critically important surgical staging tool[9] and should be performed whenever the melanoma is ulcerated or when the original biopsy reveals a melanoma with a depth of more than 1 mm or an increased mitotic rate (Fig. 188-6). For melanomas that are less than 1 mm thick, the likelihood of regional lymph node involvement is approximately 5%, so sentinel lymph node mapping is not routinely recommended for thin melanomas unless patients have adverse prognostic features such as ulceration and/or high mitotic count.

TABLE 188-1 CLINICAL FEATURES OF COMMON NEVI, DYSPLASTIC NEVI, AND MELANOMAS

DISEASE	CHARACTERISTICS
Common acquired nevi (moles)	These tend to be small, flat, and round; the border is regular, smooth, and well defined; the color is homogeneous, usually no more than two shades of brown; any site is affected; lesions are usually <6 mm (see Fig. 188-1).
Dysplastic nevi (atypical moles)	These occur predominantly on the trunk; they tend to be large, usually >5 mm, with a flat component; the border is characteristically fuzzy and ill defined. The shape can be round, oval, or misshapen. The color is usually brown but can be mottled with dark brown, pink, and tan. Some individuals have only one to five moles; others have more than 100 (see Fig. 188-2).
Melanoma	The border is more irregular; lesions tend to be larger, often >6 mm; substantial heterogeneity of color is noted, which can be tan-brown, dark brown, black, pink, red, gray, blue, or white.

The sentinel lymph node biopsy is generally performed at the same time as the wide excision of the primary tumor and must be performed prior to the wide excision.[A1] The morbidity of sentinel lymph node biopsy is relatively low, and the staging information is critically valuable.

Sentinel lymph node biopsy accurately evaluates whether microscopic melanoma cells involve regional lymph nodes. The technique relies on the concept that specific regions of the skin drain specifically to an initial lymph node within the regional nodal basin through an organized pathway of afferent lymphatic channels. Sentinel lymph node biopsy is performed by injecting the primary melanoma site with blue dye (isosulfan blue), radiolabeled colloid, or both. When both modalities are used in combination, a sentinel node can be identified in 98% of patients; biopsy of the node accurately determines whether melanoma cells have metastasized to that specific lymph node basin.

Staging

Staging and prognosis for melanoma are based on the TNM system, in which T refers to tumor, N to nodes, and M to metastasis.[10] Stages I (limited to the epidermis) and II (extending into the dermis) indicate clinically localized primary melanoma, stage III indicates regional involvement (lymph nodes or in-transit metastases), and stage IV is metastatic disease beyond the regional lymph nodes (i.e., lung, liver, brain).

Comprehensive Clinical Evaluation

The initial evaluation of a patient with melanoma should include a personal history, a family history, a total skin examination, and palpation of regional (draining) lymph nodes. The focus is to identify risk factors, signs, or symptoms of metastases, dysplastic nevi, and additional melanomas. A chest radiograph and liver enzyme tests may be performed at the discretion of the physician. Most patients who present with melanoma do not have distant metastatic disease at presentation, so extensive evaluations with computed tomography (CT) to search for distant metastases have an extremely low yield and are not indicated in asymptomatic patients. More extensive staging evaluation with CT or positron emission tomography (PET) can be considered in patients who have high-risk disease (primary melanoma >4 mm thick or node-positive disease), in whom the risk for distant metastatic disease is higher, or for mutations in *BRAC2*.

In patients who have a family history of melanoma, testing for mutations in the *p16/CDKN2A* locus can be informative. For patients or family members who are thought to be at risk for a hereditary cancer melanoma syndrome, referral to a genetic counselor should be considered to learn about the risks and benefits of genetic testing, the role of surveillance strategies, and their potential impact on medical management.

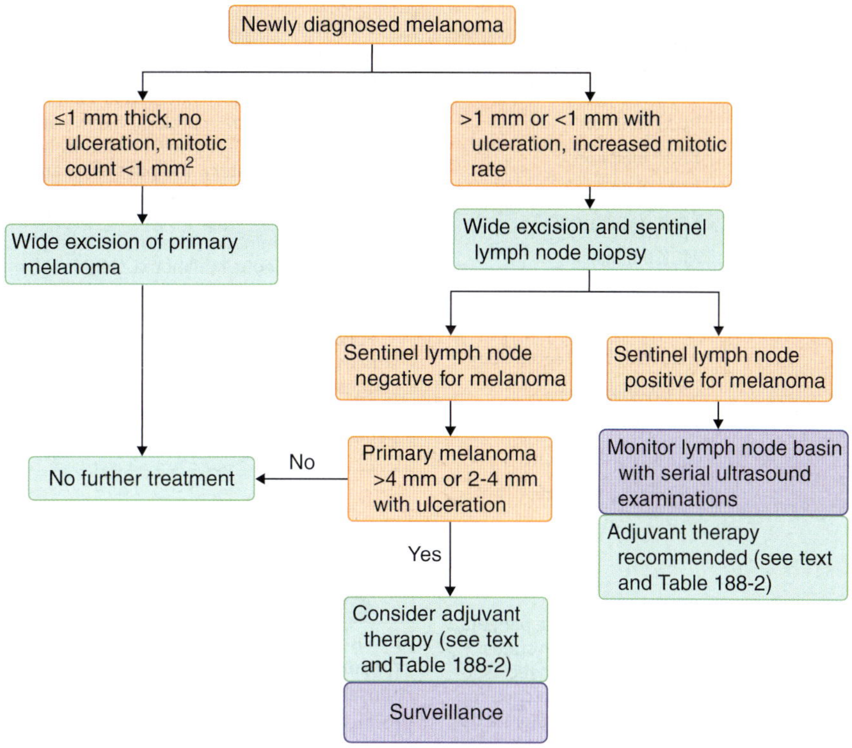

FIGURE 188-6. Treatment algorithm for newly diagnosed melanoma.

TREATMENT

Staging guides treatment decisions, including primary treatment, surveillance strategies, adjuvant therapy, and optimal management of patients with advanced melanoma.[11]

Primary Melanoma

After melanoma is diagnosed, the standard treatment is surgical excision of the primary lesion with consideration of an assessment of the regional nodal basin using sentinel lymph node mapping and biopsy (see Fig. 188-6). The extent of the surgery depends on the thickness of the primary melanoma, and most wide excisions can be performed with primary closure without skin grafting. For melanoma in situ, excision with a 0.5-cm border of clinically normal skin is sufficient. For melanomas less than 1 mm thick, a 1-cm margin is recommended. If the thickness is between 1 and 4 mm, a 1- to 2-cm margin is recommended. For melanomas thicker than 2 mm, a 2-cm resection margin also is sufficient and safe.[A2] In cosmetically sensitive areas (face) or anatomically difficult areas (ear, hands), the desired margin may be difficult to achieve, but at least a 1-cm margin should be obtained whenever possible.

Normal Regional Lymph Nodes

If the patient does not require a sentinel lymph node biopsy (see Fig. 188-6) or if the sentinel lymph node biopsy is negative for melanoma, no further lymph node surgery is required. For patients who have stage IIB (>2 to <4 mm thick with ulceration or >4 mm thick without ulceration) and stage IIC (>4 mm thick with ulceration) node-negative melanoma, pembrolizumab under expert supervision can increase recurrence-free survival from 77 to 88% compared with placebo.[A3] The decision to offer adjuvant therapy to stage II melanoma patients requires expert consultation regarding its overall benefits and risks.

Stage III Disease

If the sentinel lymph node biopsy is positive for melanoma in a patient who does not otherwise have clinically apparent lymph node involvement, a completion lymph node dissection does not improve survival, and patients can be observed with ultrasonography monitoring.[A4] For patients with clinically enlarged regional lymph nodes, however, surgical (therapeutic) lymphadenectomy is the preferred treatment following pathologic confirmation of melanoma. The goal is to provide long-term, disease-free survival and reduce local morbidity of enlarged lymph nodes. In this patient population, neoadjuvant therapy or systemic therapy administered before surgery may be an appropriate option to consider, especially as part of a clinical trial.

Adjuvant Therapy for Stage III Melanoma

For patients who have completed surgical resection of the melanoma, the decision of whether to recommend adjuvant therapy is based upon characteristics of the primary tumor (thickness, mitotic count, ulceration status) and the involvement of regional lymph nodes. All patients with stage III melanoma should have their tumor assessed for the *BRAF* mutation. For patients with resected stage III (node positive) melanoma, adjuvant therapy with immunotherapy or targeted therapy under expert supervision is recommended to improve recurrence-free survival.[12] Options include adjuvant anti-PD-1 therapies (e.g., pembrolizumab or nivolumab), targeted therapy with dabrafenib and trametinib in *BRAF* mutant melanoma, or participation in a clinical trial. For example, anti-PD-1 antibody with nivolumab provides a higher rate of recurrence-free survival compared with ipilimumab (a CTLA4 inhibitor) and with much fewer adverse immune side effects.[A5,A6] Pembrolizumab can increase the 3-year rate of relapse-free survival from 44 to 64% compared with placebo.[A7]

For patients with BRAF V600 mutant melanoma, anti-PD-1 therapy is the preferred option, but another option under expert supervision is adjuvant targeted therapy with dabrafenib (BRAF inhibitor) plus trametinib (MEK inhibitor), which can increase the 5-year relapse-free survival from 36 to 52%.[A8]

Advanced Melanoma (Stage IV)

Melanoma can metastasize to virtually any organ, especially the lung, skin, liver, and brain. Treatment must be individualized under expert supervision based on the overall condition of the patient, the burden of disease, symptoms, prior treatment, a molecular analysis for the presence of a mutated *BRAF* gene, and eligibility for immunotherapy.[13] The initial focus of treatment is immunotherapy: either anti-PD-1 antibody monotherapy (nivolumab or pembrolizumab) or in combination with ipilimumab, even in patients with *BRAF* mutations. For patients with a *BRAF* mutation, another option is combination targeted therapy with *BRAF* and MEK inhibitors (vemurafenib and cobimetinib, dabrafenib and trametinib, or encorafenib and binimetinib) or immunotherapy (Table 188-2).[A9]

Immunotherapy

The overall response rate of metastatic melanoma to monotherapy with an anti-PD-1 antibody is about 25 to 35%. Responses are sometimes delayed, and disease may progress before it stabilizes or regresses. Nivolumab as first-line treatment is superior to dacarbazine[A10] or ipilimumab.[A11] Pembrolizumab also is superior to ipilimumab.[A12]

Treatment with PD-1 inhibitors is associated with immune-related adverse events including enterocolitis, hepatitis, dermatitis, and endocrinopathies such as hypopituitarism, hypothyroidism, and type 1 diabetes mellitus. Rare but serious immune-mediated pneumonitis or myocarditis can occur and requires careful monitoring. Tumor expression of PD-L1 may correlate with higher

TABLE 188-2 TREATMENTS FOR MELANOMA

AGENT	MECHANISM OF ACTION
Dabrafenib	BRAF inhibitor
Vemurafenib	BRAF inhibitor
Encorafenib	BRAF inhibitor
Binimetinib	MEK inhibitor
Trametinib	MEK inhibitor
Cobimetinib	MEK inhibitor
Pembrolizumab	Anti-PD-1 blocking antibody
Nivolumab	Anti-PD-1 blocking antibody
Ipilimumab	CTLA-4 inhibitor
Atezolizumab	Anti PD-L1 antibody
Nivolumab + relatlimab	Anti-PD-1 + Anti LAG 3
Talimogene laherparepvec	Oncolytic viral therapy

response rates but is not an adequate biomarker of response because patients may or may not have a response regardless of their PD-L1 expression status.[14]

The combination of anti-CTLA-4 and anti-PD-1 immunotherapy (dual-checkpoint blockade) under expert supervision is now the preferred approach for treatment of patients with stage IV melanoma when patients can tolerate its toxicity. In large trials of patients with either resected stage IV or metastatic melanoma, the combination of ipilimumab (which blocks CTLA-4) plus nivolumab is superior to either agent alone, with a median survival exceeding 5 years.[A13] Grades 3 to 4 treatment-related adverse events occur in about 50% of patients, including elevations of alanine aminotransferase levels, diarrhea, and colitis. Dose interruption of immunotherapy and corticosteroids are the mainstays of treatment for this side effect mediated by T-cell activation and proliferation.

Two immune checkpoint inhibitors, relatlimab (which targets LAG-3) and nivolumab, can be combined; compared with nivolumab alone, this combination can provide longer progression-free survival for patients who have advanced melanoma.[A14] Tumor-infiltrating lymphocyte therapy is another newer option for advanced melanoma.[A15]

BRAF Inhibitors and MEK Inhibitors

BRAF inhibitors can provide dramatic antitumor activity with an approximately 50% response rate. BRAF inhibitors (vemurafenib, dabrafenib, and encorafenib) and MEK inhibitors (trametinib, cobimetinib, and binimetinib) are indicated for *BRAF*-mutated melanoma but should not be used in *BRAF* wild-type tumors. Combination therapy with BRAF and MEK inhibition results in increased response rates, with improvement in progression-free and overall survival over monotherapy, and it is considered a standard treatment option (dabrafenib plus trametinib, vemurafenib plus cobimetinib, and encorafenib plus binimetinib).[A16] Although clinical activity of the selective BRAF inhibitors is impressive, complete responses are uncommon, and most patients develop progressive disease owing to acquired drug resistance.

The most common toxicities from *BRAF*-targeted therapy include fever, dermatologic complications (e.g., rash, photosensitivity, squamous cell carcinoma, keratoacanthoma, hyperkeratoses), arthralgia, fatigue, nausea, and diarrhea. The combination of encorafenib plus binimetinib is less likely to cause fever.[A17] Secondary tumors, including second primary melanomas, rapid expansion of chronic myelomonocytic leukemia, and mucosal cancers, have been reported.

Brain Metastases

Brain metastases occur in 10 to 50% of patients with advanced melanoma. Common symptoms include headache, seizures, or focal neurological symptoms. Nivolumab and ipilimumab[A18] have activity in the central nervous system and have improved prognosis for some of these patients. As a result, patients who have brain metastases should be considered for systemic therapy in addition to local measures, such as stereotactic radiotherapy or surgery. After such local measures, whole brain radiation does not add incremental benefit.[A19]

Surveillance and Follow-Up

Patients should be educated on the clinical characteristics of melanoma, the importance of safe sun exposure strategies, and the performance of monthly self-examinations of the skin. Patients should be followed regularly for evidence of local or regional recurrence, distant metastatic disease, and a second primary melanoma. The intensity of the surveillance and the extent of the investigation are influenced by risk for recurrence, with more frequent follow-up visits in patients who have thicker tumors or node-positive disease because these patients are at greater risk for recurrence.

For patients with low-risk melanoma (≤1 mm), visits are recommended every 6 months for 2 years and then annually. The surveillance guidelines for patients with high-risk melanoma include evaluation every 6 months for 5 years. After 5 years, patients are seen once a year. Patients are generally followed for 10 years. However, lifelong dermatologic examination is recommended, particularly for patients with dysplastic nevi or a family history of melanoma.

In general, a history and physical examination are performed at each visit. Periodic laboratory studies and other imaging studies are performed at the discretion of the treating physician. The physical examination should include a thorough skin examination because at least 3% of patients develop an additional primary cutaneous melanoma. Regional lymph nodes should be thoroughly examined, especially in patients without prior nodal surgery. The examination should also consider the frequency of metastases to lung, liver, and brain.

Follow-up studies may include a complete blood cell count and chemistry studies, including liver enzyme tests. An elevated lactate dehydrogenase level suggests metastatic melanoma. CT scans of chest/abdomen and pelvis or PET/CT scans are often performed every 6 months for 5 years after diagnosis in patients who have stage III melanoma.

PREVENTION

The most important measures to prevent melanoma are to reduce excessive sun exposure, particularly to the midday sun, and to avoid sunburns. Behavioral counseling should be encouraged[15] but is not of proven benefit.[A20] Sunscreen products with a sun protection factor (SPF) of 15 or greater and protective clothing are recommended. Data from some population studies support the use of sunscreen to prevent melanomas.[16] Sunscreens block primarily UVB rays, which are considered to be the major causative agent of cutaneous cancers. Newer sunscreen products also block UVA rays, which may contribute to the risk for melanoma. Use of these sunscreens has not been associated with reduction in bone mineral density or an increase in fractures in adults.[17]

Screening for skin cancer, whether by self-examination or by a health care provider, is controversial (Chapter 12)[18] and may lead to over-diagnosis and over-treatment.[19] Many public health experts do not recommend screening for adults in the general population, but some organizations do. On the basis of the type and number of nevi, family history of melanoma, prior melanoma, and history of severe sunburns, clinicians can identify patients who are at high risk for melanoma and who may benefit from screening programs. In several population studies, screening has detected melanomas at an earlier, curable stage. Physicians, other health care providers, and the public should be educated regarding the early signs of melanoma and the need for prompt biopsy of a suspicious pigmented lesion.

Patients with clinically atypical nevi (see Fig. 188-2), particularly patients who have a family history of melanoma, require a regular dermatologic surveillance program. Regular skin examinations should be performed every 6 to 12 months, preferably with the use of serial photography.

Numerous chemoprevention studies have been conducted aimed at reducing the development of melanoma, and none have proved effective.

PROGNOSIS

As with most malignancies, the outcome of melanoma depends on the stage and extent of disease at presentation. For localized melanoma, the most important prognostic factor is involvement of regional lymph nodes. The most important prognostic factor related to the primary tumor is the depth of invasion of the melanoma in millimeters. Increasing thickness is associated with an increased risk for recurrence, regional lymph node involvement, and death from melanoma. Patients whose melanomas are thinner than 1 mm have about a 99% 5-year survival and an 80 to 90% 10-year survival. For patients whose melanomas are thicker than 4 mm, the 10-year survival rate was 40 to 50% in the preimmunotherapy era but is improving. Other poor prognostic factors related to the primary melanoma include the presence of ulceration, an increasing level of invasion, a high mitotic rate, and the presence of microscopic satellites.

Regional lymph node involvement (stage III) has a major impact on survival, with 5-year survival rates of about 70%, depending on the number of involved lymph nodes. With modern treatment approaches, some patients with metastatic melanoma have a prolonged disease-free survival and a small subset of patients may be cured. Many have remarkable improvements in symptoms and quality and duration of life. The median overall survival of patients with disseminated melanoma has increased from 9 months before 2011 to almost 5 years now.

Patients with multiple primary melanomas may have a similar survival time as patients with single primary melanomas.[20] Melanomas that arise on the extremity tend to have a better prognosis, and women tend to do better than men.

BASAL AND SQUAMOUS CELL SKIN CANCER

Nonmelanoma skin cancer (basal and squamous cell carcinoma) is the most common malignant disease in the United States. Although national statistics are imprecise, an estimated 3.3 million Americans are diagnosed each year with basal cell or squamous cell skin cancer. Squamous cell carcinoma accounts for 20%, and most of the remainder are basal cell carcinoma.

EPIDEMIOLOGY

Overall, skin cancer incidence rates are rising[21] because of increased recreational sun exposure, longer life expectancy, and depletion of the ozone layer.[22] More than 99% of nonmelanoma skin cancers occur in Whites. These skin cancers are most often seen in elderly persons, especially individuals with fair skin and long-standing sun exposure. However, nonmelanoma skin cancers are increasingly being seen in people in their 30s and 40s. The lifetime risk for developing basal cell carcinoma is 30%.

PATHOBIOLOGY

Basal cell carcinoma arises from a pluripotential stem cell within the skin. Acquired mutations in the patched gene 1 (*PTCH1*), a tumor suppressor gene in the hedgehog signaling pathway, have been identified in cases of sporadic basal cell carcinoma. Sporadic basal cell carcinoma is also associated with mutations in the genes encoding p53 and RAS.

Squamous cell carcinoma of the skin is a malignant disease of epidermal keratinocytes. Many such carcinomas are derived from actinic keratosis, a precursor that appears as a rough, scaly, often erythematous papule, which often is more apparent on palpation than on visual examination. Estimates of the likelihood of progression of actinic keratosis to squamous cell carcinoma range from 0.025% to as high as 20%. Mutations in the gene encoding the p53 protein and in the RAS oncogene have been found in both actinic keratosis and squamous cell carcinomas. Mutations in *p16* have also been reported in squamous cell carcinomas.

Risk Factors

The most important risk factor is exposure to UV radiation from sunlight. The most clearly established association is with UVB radiation, but increasing evidence suggests that UVA is probably carcinogenic as well (Chapter 18). The timing and pattern of sun exposure are associated with different types of skin cancer. In general, squamous cell carcinoma is associated with cumulative sun exposure and occurs most frequently in areas maximally exposed to the sun (e.g., the face, back of hands, and forearms). Intermittent, intense exposure to the sun, particularly in childhood, is associated with an increased risk for basal cell carcinoma. Evidence suggests a dose-response relationship between artificial UV radiation exposure by use of tanning beds and the risk for skin cancers, especially basal cell carcinoma, and the association is stronger for individuals with a younger age at exposure. Individuals who have fair skin, light-colored eyes, red hair, a tendency to burn rather than tan, and a history of severe sunburns are at increased risk for nonmelanoma skin cancers. Other risk factors, primarily for squamous cell carcinoma, include chronic arsenic exposure, therapeutic radiation, chronic inflammatory skin conditions, psoralen plus UVA (PUVA) treatment for psoriasis and other diseases, as well as exogenous (e.g., after organ transplantation) or endogenous (e.g., chronic lymphocytic leukemia) immunosuppression. Long-term use of certain drugs with photosensitizing properties, including some antihypertensive agents (e.g., calcium-channel blockers, β-blockers), can also increase the risk for skin cancer. Most cases in Black American patients are associated with scarring or burns rather than UV exposure. Human papillomavirus infection (Chapter 344) has also been implicated in some squamous cell carcinomas, particularly in autosomal dominant epidermodysplasia verruciformis.

Basal cell carcinoma can be seen in association with several conditions, including the basal cell nevus syndrome (also called nevoid basal cell carcinoma syndrome or Gorlin syndrome), albinism, and xeroderma pigmentosum. The basal cell nevus syndrome is a rare autosomal dominant disorder caused by germline mutations in the patched gene (*PTCH*).

CLINICAL MANIFESTATIONS

Basal Cell Carcinoma

Approximately 90% of basal cell carcinomas occur on sun-exposed areas such as the face, neck, ears, scalp, and arms. The nose is the most common site. Typical basal cell carcinoma appears as slowly growing, shiny, skin-colored to pink translucent papules with telangiectasia and a "pearly," rolled border (Fig. 188-7). As the tumor grows, the center may become ulcerated and bleed, although usually without associated pain or tenderness.

Squamous Cell Carcinoma

Squamous cell skin cancer usually appears on areas of skin that are heavily damaged by sun exposure. The most common sites include the head, neck, back, forearms, and dorsum of the hand. Clinically, squamous cell carcinoma occurs as a discrete scaly erythematous papule on an indurated base that can develop on normal-appearing skin or on an actinic keratosis (Fig. 188-8). The lesion may grow over time and may become ulcerated, itchy, or painful and may bleed. Keratoacanthoma is a variant that is characterized by rapid growth and a crateriform appearance with a central plug. Bowen disease, or squamous cell carcinoma in situ, manifests as an erythematous, scaly, sharply defined plaque.

Untreated squamous cell carcinoma may cause significant local destruction. Most metastases develop in regional lymph nodes, although metastases may also occur in lung, liver, brain, skin, or bone. For patients with lymph node metastases, the 5-year survival rate is less than 50%.

DIAGNOSIS

The diagnosis of basal and squamous cell carcinoma is frequently suspected by inspection alone, but histologic confirmation is usually indicated. Either a shave or a punch biopsy technique is acceptable. Care should be taken to include the base of the lesion if a shave biopsy technique is used.

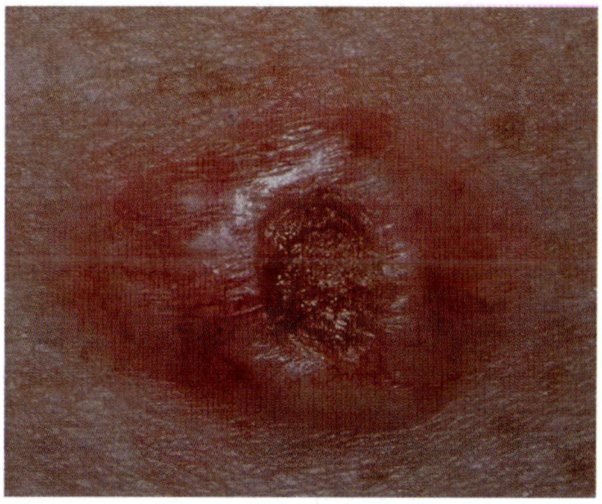

FIGURE 188-7. Basal cell carcinoma.

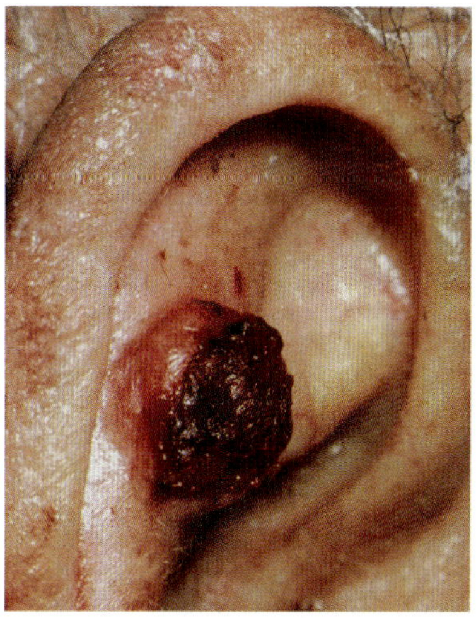

FIGURE 188-8. Squamous cell carcinoma of the skin.

TREATMENT

Basal Cell Carcinoma

Basal cell carcinomas are classified as low or high risk based on their clinical features, location, and histology.[23] Treatment options include cryotherapy (liquid nitrogen), electrosurgery (i.e., curettage and electrodessication), topical treatment (i.e., 5-fluorouracil, photodynamic therapy, or imiquimod),[A21] surgical excision, Mohs surgery, or radiation therapy. Mohs microsurgery involves serial excisions of a skin cancer with subsequent microscopic examinations for residual tumor, providing histologic control of the surgical margins to achieve the lowest recurrence rate while maximally preserving uninvolved tissue.[24] The procedure should be considered when treating recurrent cases; microscopically aggressive forms, such as the morpheaform subtype; lesions more than 2 cm in greatest diameter; and tumors of the ears, eyelids, nose, nasolabial folds, and lips.

For advanced and metastatic basal cell carcinomas, targeted therapy with vismodegib and sonidegib (which are inhibitors of the hedgehog signaling pathway) under expert supervision can provide objective tumor responses in 30 to 43% of patients and a complete response in 20% of patients. Side effects associated with therapy include muscle spasms, taste abnormalities, diarrhea, and fatigue. Patients often have an excellent long-term response after the drug is discontinued; if not, most patients respond when it is restarted. Immunotherapy with cemiplimab, which is an anti-PD-1 antibody, is also effective for patients who have locally advanced or metastatic basal cell carcinomas.[25]

Squamous Cell Carcinoma

As with basal cell carcinoma, squamous cell carcinoma can also be cured by traditional surgical excision or Mohs surgery, cryotherapy, topical therapies, and radiation therapy.[26] Topical 5-fluorouracil, photodynamic therapy, and imiquimod can also be useful for in situ squamous cell carcinoma. The optimal approach for a specific patient requires consideration of likelihood of the lesion recurring or metastatic potential, cosmetic factors, and the expertise of the treating physicians.

Mohs micrographic surgery provides the lowest recurrence rate, with cure rates greater than 90%. Mohs microsurgery is especially useful for recurrent tumors or lesions that have an increased risk for metastasis. Cemiplimab under expert supervision also can provide high response rates in patients with locally advanced or metastatic squamous cell carcinoma.[27] The PD-1 antibody pembrolizumab is also useful for patients with advanced squamous cell carcinoma,[28] provided that the squamous cell carcinoma was not a consequence of immunosuppression from organ transplantation. Cetuximab, a monoclonal antibody that targets epidermal growth factor receptor (EGFR), has some antitumor activity in patients with advanced squamous cell carcinoma of the skin.

PREVENTION

Primary prevention strategies are aimed at reducing long-term sun exposure. Public education and patient education should encourage the regular use of sunscreens with an SPF of 15 or greater, especially in childhood, and sun-protective clothing (e.g., a broad-brimmed hat). Avoidance of tanning salons and minimizing of total sun exposure, especially to the midday sun, is recommended. The thinning of the ozone layer has been linked to increased UV radiation and increases in the incidence of nonmelanoma skin cancers. Currently, no evidence indicates that total body skin examination is effective at reducing mortality or morbidity from nonmelanoma skin cancer. In one randomized trial of patients who had two or more nonmelanoma skin cancers in the prior 5 years, oral nicotinamide (vitamin B_3, 500 mg twice daily) safely reduced new nonmelanoma skin cancers and actinic keratosis by 20 to 30%.[A22]

PROGNOSIS

Basal cell carcinoma rarely metastasizes, and cure rates range from 90 to 99% with a variety of treatments. Although the mortality rate is low, these cancers may result in significant morbidity owing to invasive local growth with potential disfigurement and destruction of skin, bone, and cartilage.

Unlike basal cell carcinoma, squamous cell carcinoma carries a 0.5 to 5% risk for metastasis. Higher risk lesions are larger than 2 cm, are moderately or poorly differentiated, have perineural involvement, are located on the ear or the lip, arise in scars, or occur in immunosuppressed patients.

GENERAL REFERENCES

For the General References and other additional features, please visit Elsevier eBooks+ at https://ebooks.health.elsevier.com.

Grade A References

A1. Crystal JS, Thompson JF, Hyngstrom J, et al. Therapeutic value of sentinel lymph node biopsy in patients with melanoma: a randomized clinical trial. *JAMA Surg*. 2022;157:835-842.

A2. Utjés D, Malmstedt J, Teras J, et al. 2-cm versus 4-cm surgical excision margins for primary cutaneous melanoma thicker than 2 mm: long-term follow-up of a multicentre, randomised trial. *Lancet*. 2019;394:471-477.

A3. Luke JJ, Rutkowski P, Queirolo P, et al. Pembrolizumab versus placebo as adjuvant therapy in completely resected stage IIB or IIC melanoma (KEYNOTE-716): a randomised, double-blind, phase 3 trial. *Lancet*. 2022;399:1718-1729.

A4. Faries MB, Thompson JF, Cochran AJ, et al. Completion dissection or observation for sentinel lymph node metastasis in melanoma. *N Engl J Med*. 2017;376:2211-2222.

A5. Weber J, Mandala M, Del Vecchio M, et al. Adjuvant nivolumab in resected stage III or IV melanoma. *N Engl J Med*. 2017;377:1824-1835.

A6. Wolchok JD, Chiarion-Sileni V, Gonzales R, et al. Long-term outcomes with nivolumab alone versus ipilimumab in patients with advanced melanoma. *J Clin Oncol*. 2022;40:127-137.

A7. Eggermont AMM, Blank CU, Mandalà M, et al. Adjuvant pembrolizumab versus placebo in resected stage III melanoma (EORTC 1325-MG/KEYNOTE-054): distant metastasis-free survival results from a double-blind, randomised, controlled, phase 3 trial. *Lancet Oncol*. 2021;22:643-654.

A8. Dummer R, Hauschild A, Santinami M, et al. Five-year analysis of adjuvant dabrafenib plus trametinib in stage III melanoma. *N Engl J Med*. 2020;383:1139-1148.

A9. Atkins MB, Lee SJ, Chmielowski B, et al. Combination dabrafenib and trametinib versus combination nivolumab and ipilimumab for patients with advanced *BRAF*-mutant melanoma: the DREAMseq trial—ECOG-ACRIN EA6134. *J Clin Oncol*. 2023;41:186-197.

A10. Ascierto PA, Long GV, Robert C, et al. Survival outcomes in patients previously untreated BRAF wild type advanced melanoma treated with nivolumab: three-year follow-up of a randomized phase 3 trial. *JAMA Oncol*. 2019;5:187-194.

A11. Larkin J, Chiarion-Sileni V, Gonzalez R, et al. Combined nivolumab and ipilimumab or monotherapy in untreated melanoma. *N Engl J Med*. 2015;373:23-34.

A12. Schachter J, Ribas A, Long GV, et al. Pembrolizumab versus ipilimumab for advanced melanoma: final overall survival results of a multicentre, randomised, open-label phase 3 study (KEYNOTE-006). *Lancet*. 2017;390:1853-1862.

A13. Livingstone E, Zimmer L, Hassel JC, et al. Adjuvant nivolumab plus ipilimumab or nivolumab alone versus placebo in patients with resected stage IV melanoma with no evidence of disease (IMMUNED): final results of a randomised, double-blind, phase 2 trial. *Lancet*. 2022;400:1117-1129.

A14. Tawbi HA, Schadendorf D, Lipson EJ, et al. Relatlimab and nivolumab versus nivolumab in untreated advanced melanoma. *N Engl J Med*. 2022;386:24-34.

A15. Rohaan MW, Borch TH, van den Berg JH, et al. Tumor-infiltrating lymphocyte therapy or ipilimumab in advanced melanoma. *N Engl J Med*. 2022;387:2113-2125.

A16. Robert C, Grob JJ, Stroyakovskiy D, et al. Five-year outcomes with dabrafenib plus trametinib in metastatic melanoma. *N Engl J Med*. 2019;381:626-636.

A17. Dummer R, Ascierto PA, Gogas HJ, et al. Overall survival in patients with BRAF-mutant melanoma receiving encorafenib plus binimetinib versus vemurafenib or encorafenib (COLUMBUS): a multicentre, open-label, randomised, phase 3 trial. *Lancet Oncol*. 2018;19:1315-1327.

A18. Tawbi HA, Forsyth PA, Algazi A, et al. Combined nivolumab and ipilimumab in melanoma metastatic to the brain. *N Engl J Med*. 2018;379:722-730.

A19. Hong AM, Fogarty GB, Dolven-Jacobsen K, et al. Adjuvant whole-brain radiation therapy compared with observation after local treatment of melanoma brain metastases: a multicenter, randomized phase III trial. *J Clin Oncol*. 2019;37:3132-3141.

A20. Henrikson NB, Morrison CC, Blasi PR, et al. Behavioral counseling for skin cancer prevention: evidence report and systematic review for the US Preventive Services Task Force. *JAMA*. 2018;319:1143-1157.

A21. Jansen MHE, Mosterd K, Arits A, et al. Five-year results of a randomized controlled trial comparing effectiveness of photodynamic therapy, topical imiquimod, and topical 5-fluorouracil in patients with superficial basal cell carcinoma. *J Invest Dermatol*. 2018;138:527-533.

A22. Chen AC, Martin AJ, Choy B, et al. A phase 3 randomized trial of nicotinamide for skin-cancer chemoprevention. *N Engl J Med*. 2015;373:1618-1626.

INDEX

Page numbers followed by "*f*" indicate figures, "*t*" indicate tables, and "*b*" indicate boxes.

A

B

F

J

K

S

V

GUIDE TO THE APPROACH TO COMMON SYMPTOMS, SIGNS, LABORATORY ABNORMALITIES, SCREENING, AND TREATMENTS

	CHAPTER	SPECIFIC TABLES OR FIGURES
SYMPTOMS		
Constitutional		
Poor appetite	118	Table 118-1
Fever	259, 260	Figures 260-1, 260-2, 260-3, 260-4; Tables 259-1, 259-2, 259-3, 259-4, 259-5, 259-6, 259-7
Obesity	201	Figure 201-1; Table 201-4
Snoring, sleep disturbances	374	Figures 374-5, 374-6
Weight loss	118, 200	Figure 118-4; Table 118-4
Head, Eyes, Ears, Nose, Throat		
Headache	367	Tables 367-1, 367-2, 367-3
Visual loss, transient	391, 392	Tables 391-2, 392-1
Ear pain	394	Table 394-8
Hearing loss	396	Figure 396-1
Ringing in ears (tinnitus)	396	Figure 396-2
Vertigo	396	Figure 396-3
Loss of smell or taste	395	Table 395-1
Nasal congestion, rhinitis, or sneezing	394	Figure 394-5; Tables 394-3, 394-5, 394-7
Dry mouth	393	Table 393-7
Hoarseness	397	
Sore throat	397	Tables 397-1, 397-2
Cardiopulmonary		
Cardiac arrest	50	Figures 50-2, 50-3; Table 50-1
Chest pain	39, 123	Tables 39-2, 123-8, 123-9
Cough	71	Figure 71-1; Tables 71-2, 71-3
Dizziness	39, 49, 396	Figure 49-1; Table 396-1
Hemoptysis	71	Figure 71-3; Tables 71-6, 71-7
Palpitations	39, 49	Figure 49-1; Tables 39-4, 49-8
Shortness of breath	39, 71	Figure 71-2; Table 71-5
Syncope	49	Figure 49-1; Tables 49-1, 49-2, 49-3, 49-4, 49-6, 49-7, 49-8
Gastrointestinal		
Abdominal pain		
Acute	118, 128	Figures 118-1, 118-2; Tables 118-2, 118-3, 128-1
Chronic	118, 123	Figure 118-3; Table 118-2
Anal pain	131	
Constipation	122, 123	Figures 122-3, 123-1; Table 122-2
Diarrhea	123, 126	Figures 123-1, 126-1, 126-2, 126-3, 126-4
Dysphagia, odynophagia	118, 124	Table 118-1
Fecal incontinence	131	Figure 131-5
Heartburn/dyspepsia	118, 123, 124, 125	Figures 118-6, 124-2; Tables 123-3, 123-4, 125-1
Hematemesis	121, 139	Figure 121-3; Table 121-1
Melena, blood in stool	121	Figures 121-3, 121-4, 121-6; Table 121-4
Nausea and vomiting	118	Figure 118-5; Table 118-5
Genitourinary		
Dysuria	263, 264	Tables 263-3, 263-5, 264-2
Erectile dysfunction	216	Figure 216-4; Table 216-9
Frequency	263	Table 263-3
Genital ulcers or warts	264	Table 264-1
Hematuria	100	Figure 100-3
Hot flashes	222	Tables 222-3, 222-4
Incontinence	115	Tables 115-1, 115-2, 115-3
Infertility, female	218, 222	Table 218-5
Infertility, male	216	Figures 216-2, 216-3; Table 216-7
Menstrual irregularities	218	Figure 218-3; Tables 218-4, 218-5, 218-6

	CHAPTER	SPECIFIC TABLES OR FIGURES
Polyuria	102	Figure 102-5; Table 102-10
Renal colic	111	Figure 111-1
Scrotal mass	185	Figure 185-1
Vaginal discharge	264	
Musculoskeletal		
Neck pain	369	Figures 369-4, 369-7; Tables 369-3, 369-4
Back pain	369	Figures 369-4, 369-5, 369-6; Tables 369-3, 369-5
Joint pain	236	Figures 236-1, 236-3; Tables 236-1, 236-3
Extremities		
Edema		
Bilateral	39	Figure 39-7
Unilateral	68	Figure 68-2; Table 68-2
Claudication	65	Tables 65-3, 65-4
Limb ischemia (acute)	65	Figure 65-4; Table 65-2
Neurologic		
Gait abnormalities	366	Table 366-2
Memory loss	371	Figures 371-1, 371-2; Tables 371-1, 371-2, 371-3, 371-4, 371-5, 371-6, 371-7, 371-8
Seizures	372	Tables 372-1, 372-2, 372-3, 372-4, 372-5, 372-6
Sensory loss	366, 388	Figure 388-1; Tables 388-1, 388-3
Weakness	366, 388, 389, 390	Tables 366-1, 388-2, 389-1, 389-2, 389-4
Integumentary		
Alopecia	409	Tables 409-1, 409-3
Bleeding abnormalities	157	Tables 157-1, 157-2, 157-3
Hirsutism	409	
Hives	232, 407	Figure 232-2; Tables 232-1, 407-1, 407-2
Nail disorders	409	Table 409-4
Pigmentation abnormalities	408	Table 408-2
Rash	259, 403, 408	Figure 403-1; Tables 259-2, 403-1, 403-2, 403-3, 403-4, 403-5, 403-6, 403-8, 408-5
SIGNS		
Vital Signs		
Abnormal vital signs	7	Tables 7-1, 7-2, 7-3
Fever	259, 260	Figures 260-1, 260-2, 260-3, 260-4; Tables 259-1, 259-2, 259-3, 259-4, 259-5, 259-6, 259-7, 260-2
Heat illness/hyperthermia	95	Tables 95-1, 95-2, 95-3
Hypothermia	7, 95	Tables 95-4, 95-5, 95-6
Bradycardia	7, 49, 51	Figures 49-2, 49-3; Tables 51-1, 51-2, 51-3
Tachycardia	7, 49, 52, 53	Figures 49-2, 49-3; Tables 52-1, 52-2, 52-3, 53-2
Hypertension	64	Tables 64-4, 64-5, 64-6, 64-7, 64-8, 64-9, 64-10, 64-11, 64-12
Hypotension/shock	7, 92	Figures 92-1, 92-2, 92-3, 93-2, 94-1; Tables 92-1, 93-1, 93-2, 93-3
Respiration alteration	7, 74, 90	Tables 74-1, 74-2, 90-2
Head, Eyes, Ears, Nose, Throat		
Eye pain	391	Table 391-3
Jaundice	133	Figure 133-1; Tables 133-1, 133-2, 133-3
Nystagmus	392	Table 392-4
Papilledema	391, 392	Figure 391-25; Table 392-2
Pupillary dilatation	392	Figure 392-4
Red eye	391	Tables 391-4, 391-6
Strabismus	392	Figure 392-6
Rhinitis	394	Tables 394-1, 394-3
Sinusitis	394	Tables 394-2, 394-4, 394-5
Oral ulcers and discolorations	393	Tables 393-1, 393-2, 393-3, 393-4
Salivary gland enlargement	393	Table 393-6

GUIDE TO THE APPROACH TO COMMON SYMPTOMS, SIGNS, LABORATORY ABNORMALITIES, SCREENING, AND TREATMENTS—cont'd

	CHAPTER	SPECIFIC TABLES OR FIGURES
Neck		
Lymphadenopathy	154	Tables 154-1, 154-2, 154-3, 154-4
Neck mass	176	Figure 176-2
Thyroid nodule	207	Figure 207-5
Thyromegaly/goiter	207	Figures 207-1, 207-3
Breast		
Breast mass	183	
Lungs		
Wheezes	71	Table 71-4
Cardiac		
Carotid pulse abnormalities	39	Figure 39-4
Heart murmur or extra sounds	39	Figure 39-5; Tables 39-7, 39-8
Jugular venous distention	39	Table 39-6
Abdomen		
Abdominal swelling/ascites	128, 139	Table 139-3
Acute abdomen	118, 128	Figure 118-2; Table 128-1
Hemorrhoids	131	Figures 131-1, 131-2; Table 131-1
Hepatomegaly	132	Figure 132-5
Rectal bleeding/positive stool	121, 179	Figures 121-3, 121-4, 121-6; Table 121-4
Splenomegaly	154	Table 154-5
Musculoskeletal/Extremities		
Arthritis	236	Figures 236-1, 236-2; Table 236-3
Clubbing	39, 254	Figures 39-9, 254-1
Cyanosis	39, 66	Figures 39-8, 66-12
Edema	39	Figure 39-7
Raynaud phenomenon	66	Figure 66-9
Neurologic		
Autism spectrum	385	Table 385-1
Coma	373	Tables 373-1, 373-2, 373-3, 373-4, 373-5, 373-6
Delirium	361	Figure 361-1; Tables 361-1, 361-2, 361-3
Movement disorders	378, 379	Tables 378-1, 378-2, 378-3, 378-4, 379-1, 379-2, 379-3, 379-4, 379-5, 379-6, 379-7, 379-8
Neuropathy	388	Figure 388-1; Tables 388-1, 388-2, 388-3, 388-4
Psychiatric disturbances	362	Tables 362-1, 362-2, 362-3, 362-4, 362-5, 362-6, 362-7, 362-8, 362-9, 362-10, 362-11, 362-12, 362-13, 362-14
Stroke	376, 377	Figure 376-1; Tables 376-2, 376-5, 376-6, 377-5, 377-6
Skin and Nails		
Mole	188	Table 188-1
Nail diseases	409	Table 409-4
COMMON LABORATORY ABNORMALITIES		
Hematology/Urinalysis		
Anemia	144	Figure 144-3; Tables 144-2, 144-3, 144-4, 144-5, 144-6, 144-7, 144-8, 144-9
Eosinophilia	156	Figure 156-1; Tables 156-1, 156-2
Leukocytosis	153	Figure 153-4; Table 153-1
Lymphocytosis	153	Table 153-3
Monocytosis	153	Table 153-2
Neutropenia	153	Figure 153-7; Tables 153-4 and 153-5
Neutropenia with fever	260	Figures 260-1, 260-2, 260-3, 260-4
Polycythemia	152	Table 152-4
PT or PTT prolongation	157	Figure 157-4
Thrombocytopenia	158	Figure 158-1; Tables 158-1, 158-3
Thrombocytosis	152	Table 152-5
Urinalysis	100, 106	Figure 100-3; Tables 100-2, 106-5